Sixth Edition

Forfar & Arneil's

Textbook of Pediatrics

Forfar & Arneil's Textbook of Pediatrics, Sixth edition
Multimedia CD-ROM

ELSEVIER CD-ROM LICENCE AGREEMENT

PLEASE READ THE FOLLOWING AGREEMENT CAREFULLY BEFORE USING THIS PRODUCT. THIS PRODUCT IS LICENSED UNDER THE TERMS CONTAINED IN THIS LICENCE AGREEMENT ("Agreement"). BY USING THIS PRODUCT, YOU, AN INDIVIDUAL OR ENTITY INCLUDING EMPLOYEES, AGENTS AND REPRESENTATIVES ("You" or "Your"), ACKNOWLEDGE THAT YOU HAVE READ THIS AGREEMENT, THAT YOU UNDERSTAND IT, AND THAT YOU AGREE TO BE BOUND BY THE TERMS AND CONDITIONS OF THIS AGREEMENT. ELSEVIER LIMITED ("Elsevier") EXPRESSLY DOES NOT AGREE TO LICENSE THIS PRODUCT TO YOU UNLESS YOU ASSENT TO THIS AGREEMENT. IF YOU DO NOT AGREE WITH ANY OF THE FOLLOWING TERMS, YOU MAY, WITHIN THIRTY (30) DAYS AFTER YOUR RECEIPT OF THIS PRODUCT RETURN THE UNUSED PRODUCT AND ALL ACCOMPANYING DOCUMENTATION TO ELSEVIER FOR A FULL REFUND.

DEFINITIONS As used in this Agreement, these terms shall have the following meanings:

"Proprietary Material" means the valuable and proprietary information content of this Product including without limitation all indexes and graphic materials and software used to access, index, search and retrieve the information content from this Product developed or licensed by Elsevier and/or its affiliates, suppliers and licensors.

"Product" means the copy of the Proprietary Material and any other material delivered on CD-ROM and any other human-readable or machine-readable materials enclosed with this Agreement, including without limitation documentation relating to the same.

OWNERSHIP This Product has been supplied by and is proprietary to Elsevier and/or its affiliates, suppliers and licensors. The copyright in the Product belongs to Elsevier and/or its affiliates, suppliers and licensors and is protected by the copyright, trademark, trade secret and other intellectual property laws of the United Kingdom and international treaty provisions, including without limitation the Universal Copyright Convention and the Berne Copyright Convention. You have no ownership rights in this Product. Except as expressly set forth herein, no part of this Product, including without limitation the Proprietary Material, may be modified, copied or distributed in hardcopy or machine-readable form without prior written consent from Elsevier. All rights not expressly granted to You herein are expressly reserved. Any other use of this Product by any person or entity is strictly prohibited and a violation of this Agreement.

SCOPE OF RIGHTS LICENSED (PERMITTED USES) Elsevier is granting to You a limited, non-exclusive, non-transferable licence to use this Product in accordance with the terms of this Agreement. You may use or provide access to this Product on a single computer or terminal physically located at Your premises and in a secure network or move this Product to and use it on another single computer or terminal at the same location for personal use only, but under no circumstances may You use or provide access to any part or parts of this Product on more than one computer or terminal simultaneously.

You shall not (a) copy, download, or otherwise reproduce the Product or any part(s) thereof in any medium, including, without limitation, online transmissions, local area networks, wide area networks, intranets, extranets and the Internet, or in any way, in whole or in part, except for printing out or downloading nonsubstantial portions of the text and images in the Product for Your own personal use; (b) alter, modify, or adapt the Product or any part(s) thereof, including but not limited to decompiling, disassembling, reverse engineering, or creating derivative works, without the prior written approval of Elsevier; (c) sell, license or otherwise distribute to third parties the Product or any part(s) thereof; or (d) alter, remove, obscure or obstruct the display of any copyright, trademark or other proprietary notice on or in the Product or on any printout or download of portions of the Proprietary Materials.

RESTRICTIONS ON TRANSFER This Licence is personal to You, and neither Your rights hereunder nor the tangible embodiments of this Product, including without limitation the Proprietary Material, may be sold, assigned, transferred or sublicensed to any other person, including without limitation by operation of law, without the prior written consent of Elsevier. Any purported sale, assignment, transfer or sublicense without the prior written consent of Elsevier will be void and will automatically terminate the Licence granted hereunder.

TERM This Agreement will remain in effect until terminated pursuant to the terms of this Agreement. You may terminate this Agreement at any time by removing from Your system and destroying the Product and any copies of the Proprietary Material. Unauthorized copying of the Product, including without limitation, the Proprietary Material and documentation, or otherwise failing to comply with the terms and conditions of this Agreement shall result in automatic termination of this licence and will make available to Elsevier legal remedies. Upon termination of this Agreement, the licence granted herein will terminate and You must immediately destroy the Product and all copies of the Product and of the Proprietary Material, together with any and all accompanying documentation. All provisions relating to proprietary rights shall survive termination of this Agreement.

LIMITED WARRANTY AND LIMITATION OF LIABILITY Elsevier warrants that the software embodied in this Product will perform in substantial compliance with the documentation supplied in this Product, unless the performance problems are the result of hardware failure or improper use. If You report a significant defect in performance in writing to Elsevier within ninety (90) calendar days of your having purchased the Product, and Elsevier is not able to correct same within sixty (60) days after its receipt of Your notification, You may return this Product, including all copies and documentation, to Elsevier and Elsevier will refund Your money. In order to apply for a refund on your purchased Product, please contact the return address on the invoice to obtain the refund request form ("Refund Request Form"), and either fax or mail your signed request and your proof of purchase to the address indicated on the Refund Request Form. Incomplete forms will not be processed. Defined terms in the Refund Request Form shall have the same meaning as in this Agreement.

YOU UNDERSTAND THAT, EXCEPT FOR THE LIMITED WARRANTY RECITED ABOVE, ELSEVIER, ITS AFFILIATES, LICENSORS, THIRD PARTY SUPPLIERS AND AGENTS (TOGETHER "THE SUPPLIERS") MAKE NO REPRESENTATIONS OR WARRANTIES, WITH RESPECT TO THE PRODUCT, INCLUDING, WITHOUT LIMITATION THE PROPRIETARY MATERIAL. ALL OTHER REPRESENTATIONS, WARRANTIES, CONDITIONS OR OTHER TERMS, WHETHER EXPRESS OR IMPLIED BY STATUTE OR COMMON LAW, ARE HEREBY EXCLUDED TO THE FULLEST EXTENT PERMITTED BY LAW. IN PARTICULAR BUT WITHOUT LIMITATION TO THE FOREGOING NONE OF THE SUPPLIERS MAKE ANY REPRESENTIONS OR WARRANTIES (WHETHER EXPRESS OR IMPLIED) REGARDING THE PERFORMANCE OF YOUR PAD, NETWORK OR COMPUTER SYSTEM WHEN USED IN CONJUNCTION WITH THE PRODUCT, NOR THAT THE PRODUCT WILL MEET YOUR REQUIREMENTS OR THAT ITS OPERATION WILL BE UNINTERRUPTED OR ERROR-FREE. EXCEPT IN RESPECT OF DEATH OR PERSONAL INJURY CAUSED BY THE SUPPLIERS' NEGLIGENCE AND TO THE FULLEST EXTENT PERMITTED BY LAW, IN NO EVENT (AND REGARDLESS OF WHETHER SUCH DAMAGES ARE FORESEEABLE AND OF WHETHER SUCH LIABILITY IS BASED IN TORT, CONTRACT OR OTHERWISE) WILL ANY OF THE SUPPLIERS BE LIABLE TO YOU FOR ANY DAMAGES (INCLUDING, WITHOUT LIMITATION, ANY LOST PROFITS, LOST SAVINGS OR OTHER SPECIAL, INDIRECT, INCIDENTAL OR CONSEQUENTIAL DAMAGES ARISING OUT OF OR RESULTING FROM: (I) YOUR USE OF, OR INABILITY TO USE, THE PRODUCT; (II) DATA LOSS OR CORRUPTION; AND/OR (III) ERRORS OR OMISSIONS IN THE PROPRIETARY MATERIAL.

IF THE FOREGOING LIMITATION IS HELD TO BE UNENFORCEABLE, OUR MAXIMUM LIABILITY TO YOU IN RESPECT THEREOF SHALL NOT EXCEED THE AMOUNT OF THE LICENCE FEE PAID BY YOU FOR THE PRODUCT. THE REMEDIES AVAILABLE TO YOU AGAINST ELSEVIER AND THE LICENSORS OF MATERIALS INCLUDED IN THE PRODUCT ARE EXCLUSIVE.

If the information provided in the Product contains medical or health sciences information, it is intended for professional use within the medical field. Information about medical treatment or drug dosages is intended strictly for professional use, and because of rapid advances in the medical sciences, independent verification of diagnosis and drug dosages should be made.

The provisions of this Agreement shall be severable, and in the event that any provision of this Agreement is found to be legally unenforceable, such unenforceability shall not prevent the enforcement or any other provision of this Agreement.

GOVERNING LAW This Agreement shall be governed by the laws of England and Wales. In any dispute arising out of this Agreement, you and Elsevier each consent to the exclusive personal jurisdiction and venue in the courts of England and Wales.

Sixth Edition

Forfar & Arneil's

Textbook of Pediatrics

Edited by

Neil McIntosh DSc(Med) FRCP(Edin) FRCP(Lond) FRCPCH
Professor of Child Life and Health, University of Edinburgh, Edinburgh, UK

Peter J Helms MBBS PhD FRCP(Edin) FRCPCH
Professor of Child Health, University of Aberdeen, Aberdeen, UK

Rosalind L Smyth MA MBBS MD FRCPCH
Brough Professor of Paediatric Medicine, University of Liverpool, Liverpool, UK

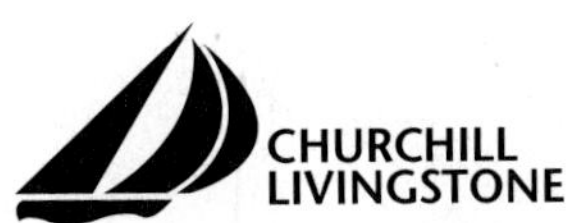

Edinburgh London New York Oxford Philadelphia St Louis Sydney Toronto 2003

CHURCHILL LIVINGSTONE
An imprint of Elsevier Limited

First edition 1973
Second edition 1978
Third edition 1984
Fourth edition 1992
Fifth edition 1998

ISBN 0 443 07192 6

British Library Cataloguing in Publication Data
A catalogue record for this book is available from the British Library

Library of Congress Cataloging in Publication Data
A catalog record for this book is available from the Library of Congress

Note
Medical knowledge is constantly changing. Standard safety precautions must be followed, but as new research and clinical experience broaden our knowledge, changes in treatment and drug therapy may become necessary or appropriate. Readers are advised to check the most current product information provided by the manufacturer of each drug to be administered to verify the recommended dose, the method and duration of administration, and contraindications. It is the responsibility of the practitioner, relying on experience and knowledge of the patient, to determine dosages and the best treatment for each individual patient. Neither the Publisher nor the editors assume any liability for any injury and/or damage to persons or property arising from this publication.

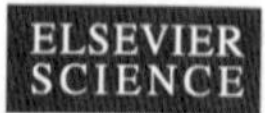

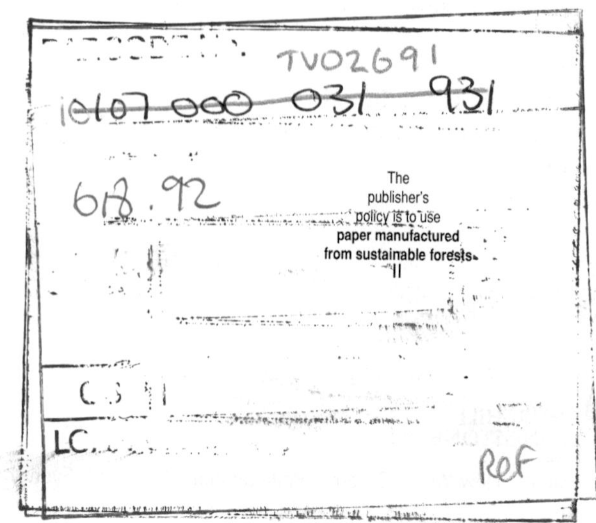

Printed in Spain

Commissioning Editor: Judith Fletcher
Project Development Manager: Sheila Black
Project Manager: Rory MacDonald
Illustration Manager: Mick Ruddy
Design Manager: Jayne Jones
Illustrator: Tim Loughhead

Contents

Section 2
PERINATAL/NEONATAL MEDICINE

Section 3
THE SPECIALITIES

Section 4
INVESTIGATIONS AND THERAPY

Contributors

Ishaq Abu-Arafeh MBBS MD MRCP FRCPCH
Consultant Paediatrician
Department of Paediatrics
Stirling Royal Infirmary
Stirling, UK

Nicholas Archer MA FRCP FRCPCH
Consultant Paediatric Cardiologist
Honorary Clinical Senior Lecturer
John Radcliffe Hospital
Oxford, UK

Peter D Arkwright MRCPCH, DPhil
Lecturer in Child Health
University Department of Child Health
Booth Hall Children's Hospital
Manchester, UK

Gillian Baird FRCPCH
Consultant Paediatrician
Newcomen Centre
Guy's Hospital
London, UK

Alastair J Baker MB BChir MA MD FRCP FRCPCH
Consultant Paediatric Hepatologist
King's College Hospital
London, UK

Susan Beath BSc MB BS MRCP
Consultant Paediatric Hepatologist
The Liver Unit
Birmingham Children's Hospital
Birmingham, UK

Thomas F Beattie MB FRCS(Ed) FFAEM DCH MSc
Consultant in Paediatric Accident and Emergency Medicine
Accident and Emergency Department
Royal Hospital for Sick Children
Edinburgh, UK

Neville Richard Belton BSc PhD CChem MRSC FRCPCM
Honorary Fellow
Department of Child Life and Health
University of Edinburgh
Edinburgh, UK

W Michael Bisset BSc MBchB DCH MSc MD FRCP FRCPCH
Consultant Paediatric Gastroenterologist
Department of Medical Paediatrics
Royal Aberdeen Children's Hospital
Aberdeen, UK

Paula Bolton-Maggs FRCP FRCPCH FRCPath MA
Consultant Paediatric Haematologist and Haemophilia
Centre Director
Department of Haematology
Royal Liverpool Children's Hospital NHS Trust,
Alder Hey
Liverpool, UK

Bernard J Brabin MB ChB MSc PhD FRCPC FRCPCH
Professor of Tropical Paediatrics, University of Liverpool
Liverpool, UK
Professor of Tropical Child Health, University of Amsterdam
Amsterdam, Netherlands
Honorary Consultant, Community Child Health
Royal Liverpool Children's NHS Trust, Alder Hey
Liverpool, UK

Colin Bruce MBChB FRCS FRCS (Orth)
Consultant Paediatric Orthopaedic Surgeon
Department of Orthopaedics
Alder Hey Hospital
Liverpool, UK

Neil Buist MB ChB FRCPE DCH
Professor of Pediatrics
Pediatrics Department
Doerubecher Children's Hospital
Portland, OR, USA

Frances Bu'Lock MD MRCP
Consultant Paediatric Cardiologist
Glenfield Hospital
Leicester, UK

Nigel Peter Burrows MD FRCP
Consultant Dermatologist and Associate Lecturer
Department of Dermatology
Addenbrooke's Hospital
Cambridge, UK

Andrew Bush MD FRCP FRCPCH
Reader in Paediatric Respirology
Department of Paediatrics
Royal Brompton Hospital
London, UK

Gary E Butler MD FRCP FRCPCH
Consultant Paediatric & Adolescent Endocrinologist
Senior Clinical Lecturer in Paediatrics
Paediatric Endocrine Department
Leeds General Infirmary
Leeds, UK

Catherine Cale MB ChB PhD MRCP MRCPath
Consultant Paediatric Immunologist
Department of Immunology
Great Ormond Street Hospital
London, UK

Harry Campbell MD FRCP Edin FFPHM
Reader in Epidemiology
Public Health Sciences
University of Edinburgh
Edinburgh, UK

Andrew Cant BSc MD FRCP FRCPCH
Consultant in Paediatric Immunology & Infectious Diseases
Paediatric Immunology and Infectious Disease Unit
Newcastle General Hospital
Newcastle upon Tyne, UK

Michael Clarke MB ChB BSc DCH FRCP FRCPCH
Consultant Paediatric Neurologist
Department of Neurology
Stepping Hill Hospital
Stockport, UK

Andrew Gavin Cleary BSc (Hons) MBChB MRCPCH
Specialist Registrar in Paediatric Rheumatology
Department of Paediatric Rheumatology
Alder Hey Hospital
Liverpool, UK

J Brian S Coulter MD FRCPI FRCPCH DCH
Senior Lecturer in Tropical Child Health
Honorary Consultant Paediatrician
Royal Liverpool Children's NHS Trust
Liverpool School of Tropical Medicine
Liverpool, UK

David Lockhart Cowan MBChB FRCSE
Consultant Otolaryngologist RHSC Edinburgh
Honorary Senior Lecturer
University of Edinburgh Medical School
Ear, Nose & Throat Department
Royal Hospital For Sick Children
Edinburgh, UK

Steve Cunningham MBChB PhD MRCP
Consultant Respiratory Paediatrician
Department of Respiratory and Sleep Medicine
Royal Hospital for Sick Children
Edinburgh, UK

Timothy J David MB ChB MD PhD FRCP FRCPCH DCH
Professor of Child Health and Paediatrics
Honorary Consultant Paediatrician
The University of Manchester
Manchester, UK

Joyce E Davidson BSc (Hons) MBChB MRCP FRCPCH
Consultant in Paediatric Rheumatology
Department of Paediatric Rheumatology
Alder Hey Hospital
Liverpool, UK

E Graham Davies MA FRCPCH
Consultant Paediatrician/Immunologist
Great Ormond Street Hospital for Sick Children
London, UK

Ruth E Day MBChB FRCP
Consultant Paediatrician
Department of Neurology and Child Development
Royal Hospital for Sick Children
Glasgow, UK

P Barton Duell MD
Associate Professor of Medicine
Division of Endocrinology, Diabetes and Clinical Nutrition
Oregon Health & Science University
Portland, OR, USA

Tim Eden MB BS MRCP(UK) FRCP(E) FRCP FRCPath FRCPCH
Professor of Paediatric Oncology
Academic Unit of Paediatric Oncology
Christie Hospital NHS Trust & Royal Manchester Children's Hospitals
Manchester, UK

Christine Edwards BSc PhD RNutr
Senior Lecturer in Human Nutrition
Department of Human Nutrition
Glasgow University
Glasgow, UK

Heather Elphick MBChB MRCP MRCPCH MD
Lecturer in Child Health
Institute of Child Health
Alder Hey Children's Hospital
Liverpool, UK

Greg Enns MB ChB
Assistant Professor of Pediatrics
Director, Biochemical Genetics Program
Stanford University School of Medicine
Stanford CA, USA

Jeremy Farrar MBBS MRCP BSc DPhil
Senior Lecturer
University of Oxford Research Unit
The Centre for Tropical Diseases
Ho Chi Minh City, Vietnam

Colin D Ferrie BSc(Hons) MBChB MD MRCP FRCPCH
Consultant Paediatric Neurologist
Department of Paediatric Neurology
The General Infirmary at Leeds
Leeds, UK

Alistair Fielder FRCP FRCS FRCOphth
Professor of Ophthalmology
Department of Ophthalmology
The Western Eye Hospital
London, UK

Brian W Fleck BSc(Hons) MBChB MD FRCS(Ed) FRCOph
Consultant Ophthalmic Surgeon
Honorary Clinical Senior Lecturer
Princess Alexandra Eye Pavilion
Edinburgh, UK

Peter Fleming MB ChB PhD FRCP(C) FRCP FRCPCH
Professor of Infant Health and Developmental Physiology
Institute of Child Health
Royal Hospital for Children
Bristol, UK

Yvonne Freer RGN RM RSCN BSc Mid PhD
Research & Practice Development
Neonatal Intensive Care Unit
Simpson Memorial Maternity Pavilion
Edinburgh, UK

Anne S Garden FRCOG ILTM
Director of Medical Studies
Faculty of Medicine
University of Liverpool
Liverpool, UK

Andrew R Gennery MD MRCP MRCPCH DCH Dip Med Sci
Senior Lecturer
Honorary Consultant in Paediatric Immunology
Paediatric Immunology & Infectious Diseases Unit
Newcastle General Hospital
Newcastle upon Tyne, UK

Diana Gibb MD FRCPCH MSc
Senior Lecturer in Paediatric Epidemiology
MRC Clinical Trials Unit
University College London Medical School
London, UK

K Michael Gibson PhD FACMG
Director, Biochemical Genetics Laboratory
Department of Pediatrics and Molecular & Medical Genetics
Oregon Health & Science University
Portland, OR, USA

Barbara Elaine Golden BSc MBBCh BAD MD FRCPI FRCPCH DCH RNutr
Clinical Senior Lecturer & Honorary Consultant in International Child Health
Department of Child Health
University of Aberdeen Medical School
Aberdeen, UK

Ann Goldman MB FRCP FRCPCH
Consultant in Paediatric Palliative Care
Symptom Care Team
Great Ormond Street Children's Hospital
London, UK

John M Goldsmid MSc PhD FRCPath FACTM FIBiol FASM FRCPA (Hon)
Professor of Medical Microbiology
Discipline of Pathology
University of Tasmania
Hobart, Australia

Isky Gordon FRCR FRCP FRCPCH
Consultant in Paediatric Radiology
Great Ormond Street Children's Hospital
London, UK

John R W Govan BSc PhD DSc
Professor of Microbial Pathogenicity
Department of Medical Microbiology
University of Edinburgh Medical School
Edinburgh, UK

Stephen M Graham MB BS FRACP DTCH
Clinical Research Fellow
Wellcome Trust Research Laboratories
Blantyre, Malawi

Markus Grompe MD
Professor
Department of Pediatrics and Molecular & Medical Genetics
Oregon Health & Science University
Portland, OR, USA

Henry Halliday MD FRCPS FRCP FRCPCH
Honorary Professor of Child Health and Consultant Neonatologist
Department of Child Health
The Queen's University of Belfast
Belfast, UK

Helga Hanks BSc MSc DipPsych
Consultant Clinical Psychologist
St James University Hospital
Leeds, UK

Khalid N Haque FRCP FRCPCH FPAMS FICP FAAP MBA DCH DTMRH
Senior Lecturer / Consultant Neonatalogist
Department of Neonatology
St Helier Hospital
Carshalton, UK

Cary Harding MD
Assistant Professor
Department of Pediatrics and Molecular & Medical Genetics
Oregon Health & Science University
Portland, OR, USA

C Anthony Hart MBBS BSc PhD FRCPCH FRCPath
Professor of Medical Microbiology
Department of Medical Microbiology
University of Liverpool Medical School
Liverpool, UK

Paul T Heath FRACP FRCPCH
Senior Lecturer, Honorary Consultant
Paediatric Infectious Diseases Unit
St George's Hospital
London, UK

Peter J Helms MBBS PhD FRCP(Edin) FRCPCH
Professor of Child Health
University of Aberdeen
Aberdeen, UK

John Henderson MD FRCP FRCPCH
Consultant Paediatrician
Department of Respiratory Medicine
Bristol Royal Hospital for Children
Bristol, UK

George M A Hendry MB BS DMRD FRCR
Consultant Paediatric Radiologist
Radiology Department
Royal Hospital for Sick Children
Edinburgh, UK

Tom Hilliard BM BCh MA MRCPCH
Special Registrar in Respiratory Paediatrics
Department of Respiratory Medicine
Bristol Royal Hospital for Children
Bristol, UK

Peter Hoare DM FRCPsych
Senior Lecturer, University of Edinburgh
Honorary Consultant Psychiatrst
Child & Family Mental Health Service
Royal Hospital for Sick Children
Edinburgh, UK

Christopher James Hobbs BSc FRCP FRCPCH
Consultant Paediatrician
Department of Community Paediatrics
St James University Hospital
Leeds, UK

Richard Howard MB FRCA
Consultant Anaesthetist
Great Ormond Street Children's Hospital
London, UK

Mary Imelda Hughes MB BCh FRCPCH
Consultant Paediatric Neurologist
Department of Paediatric Neurology
Royal Manchester Children's Hospital
Manchester, UK

Robert Hume BSc (Hons) MBChB PhD FRCPEdin, FRCPH
Professor of Developmental Medicine
Tayside Institute of Child Health
University of Dundee
Dundee, UK

David Isaacs MBBChir MD FCRPCH FRACP
Clinical Professor
Department of Immunology & Infectious Diseases
The Children's Hospital at Westmead
Westmead, Australia

Omar Ismayl MD MSc MRCPCH
Consultant Neurologist
Department of Paediatric Neurology
Royal Manchester Children's Hospital
Manchester, UK

Huw Jenkins MB BChir MA MD FRCP FRCPCH
Consultant Paediatric Gastroenterologist
Department of Child Health
University Hospital of Wales
Cardiff, UK

Cheryl A Jones MBBS(Hons) PhD FRACP
Head, Herpesvirus Research Unit
Honorary Consultant in Infectious Diseases
Department of Immunology and Infectious Diseases
The Children's Hospital at Westmead
Sydney, Australia

Christopher J H Kelnar MA MD FRCPCH FRCP
Consultant Paediatric Endocrinologist
Reader in Child Health
Section of Child Life and Health
Department of Reproductive & Developmental Sciences
University of Edinburgh
Edinburgh, UK

Alastair I G Kerr MB ChB FRCS(Edin & Glas)
Consultant Otolaryngologist
Ear, Nose and Throat Department
Royal Hospital for Sick Children
Edinburgh, UK

Denise J Kitchiner MD FRCP FRCPCH
Consultant Paediatric Cardiologist
Cardiac & ITU Directorate
Royal Liverpool Children's Hospital
Liverpool, UK

Nigel J Klein BSc MBBS MRCP PhD
Senior Lecturer and Consultant in Infection and Immunity
Institute of Child Health
London, UK

David Koeller MD
Associate Professor of Pediatrics and Molecular & Medical Genetics
Oregon Health & Science University
Portland, OR, USA

Sailesh Kotecha MA FRCPCH PhD
Senior Lecturer
Consultant in Child Health
Department of Child Health
University of Leicester
Leicester, UK

Ian A Laing MA MD FRCPE FRCPCH
Clinical Director of Neonatology
Neonatal Unit
Royal Infirmary of Edinburgh
Edinburgh, UK

David Lalloo MB BS MD FRCP
Senior Lecturer in Tropical Medicine
Liverpool School of Tropical Medicine
Liverpool, UK

Malcolm Levene MB BS MRCP MD FRCP FRCPCH FMedSc
Professor of Paediatrics and Child Health
Department of Paediatrics
Leeds General Infirmary
Leeds, UK

Leesa Linck MD
Adjunct Assistant Professor of Pediatrics and Molecular & Medical Genetics
Oregon Health & Science University
Portland, OR, USA

Diana N J Lockwood BSc MD FRCP
Consultant Physician & Leprologist
Hospital for Tropical Diseases
London, UK

Stuart Logan MB ChB MSc(FPID) MSc (Politics) MRCP FRCPCH
Senior Lecturer in Paediatric Epidemiology
Honorary Consultant in Child Health
Department of Paediatric Epidemiology
Institute of Child Health
London, UK

Gordon Alexander MacKinlay MB BS CRCP FRCSEd FRCS
Senior Lecturer
Department of Clinical Surgery
University of Edinburgh
Consultant Paediatric Surgeon
Department of Paediatric Surgery
Royal Hospital for Sick Children
Edinburgh, UK

Janice Main FRCP (Edin and Lond)
Senior Lecturer in Infectious Diseases and Medicine
Imperial College School of Medicine
St Mary's Hospital
London, UK

Guy Makin BA BMBCh PhD MRCP
Lecturer in Paediatric Oncology
Academic Unit of Paediatric Oncology
Christie Hospital
Manchester, UK

Timothy R Martland MB ChB MRCP MRCPCH
Consultant Paediatric Neurologist
Department of Paediatric Neurology
Royal Manchester Children's Hospital
Manchester, UK

Alexander McCall-Smith LLB PhD FRSE
Professor of Medical Law
School of Law
University of Edinburgh
Edinburgh, UK

Mary McGraw MB ChB DCH FRCP FRCPCH
Consultant Paediatric Nephrologist
Bristol Royal Hospital for Children
Bristol, UK

Kieran McHugh FRCR FRCPI DCH, LMCC
Consultant Paediatric Radiologist
Radiology Department
Great Ormond Street Hospital for Children
London, UK

Neil McIntosh DSc(Med) FRCP(Edin) FRCP(Lond) FRCPCH
Professor of Child Life and Health
University of Edinburgh
Edinburgh, UK

Sheila McKenzie MD FRCPCH
Consultant in Paediatrics
Department of Paediatrics
Queen Elizabeth Children's Services
London, UK

Ian McKinlay BSc(Hon) MBChB DCH FRCP FRCPCH
Senior Lecturer in Child Health
McKay Gordon Centre
Manchester, UK

Craig M Mellis MBBS MD MPH FRACP
Professor of Paediatrics & Child Health, University of Sydney
Department of Paediatrics and Child Health
The Children's Hospital at Westmead
Westmead, Australia

Malcolm E Molyneux MD FRCP FMedSci
Professor of Medicine
(Malawi-Liverpool-Wellcome Trust Research Programme, College of Medicine, University of Malawi, and School of Tropical Medicine, University of Liverpool, UK)
Blantyre, Malawi

E Richard Moxon MA FRCPCH FMEDSci
Head, Department of Paediatrics
Head, Molecular Infectious Diseases Group
University of Oxford
Oxford, UK

Simon Newell MD FRCPCH FRCP
Consultant in Neonatal Medicine and Paediatric Gastroenterology
Regional NICU
Leeds Teaching Hospitals
Leeds, UK

Richard Newton MD FRCP FRCPCH
Consultant Paediatric Neurologist
Department of Paediatric Neurology
Royal Manchester Children's Hospital
Manchester, UK

Angus Nicoll FFPHM FRCP FRCPCH
Director
PHLS Communicable Disease Surveillance Centre
London, UK

Caroline Pao MBBS MRCP
Research Fellow
Royal London Hospital
London, UK

James Paton HD FRCPCH FRCPS (Glasgow)
Reader in Paediatric Respiratory Disease
Department of Child Health
Royal Hospital for Sick Children
Glasgow, UK

Michael Patton MA MSc MB ChB FRCP FRCPCH
Professor of Medical Genetics
SW Thames Regional Genetic Service
St George's Hospital
London, UK

Gale A Pearson MB BS MRCP FRCPCH
Consultant in Paediatric Intensive Care
Intensive Care Unit
The Birmingham Children's Hospital
Birmingham, UK

Stavros Petrou BSc MPhil PhD
Health Economist
National Perinatal Epidemiology Unit
Institute of Health Sciences
Oxford, UK

John Reilly BSc PhD
Senior Lecturer
Department of Human Nutrition
University of Glasgow
Glasgow, UK

Janet M Rennie MA MD FRCP DCH
Consultant & Senior Lecturer in Neonatal Medicine
Department of Child Health
King's College Hospital
London, UK

Sam Richmond MBBS FRCP FRCPCH
Consultant Neonatologist
Neonatal Unit
Sunderland Royal Hospital
Sunderland, UK

Irene A G Roberts MD FRCP FRCPath DRCOG
Professor of Paediatric Haematology
Department of Haematology
Hammersmith Hospital
London, UK

Stephen C Robson MD MRCOG MBBS
Professor of Fetal Medicine
Department of Obstetrics & Gynaecology
Royal Victoria Infirmary
Newcastle upon Tyne, UK

Mary Rose MBBS FRCA
Consultant Paediatric Anaesthetist
Department of Anaesthetics
Royal Hospital for Sick Children
Edinburgh, UK

Peter T Rudd MD FRCPCH
Consultant Paediatrician
Royal United Hospital
Bath, UK

Martin Runciman MBBS MRCP MRCPCH
Pediatric Cardiologist
Pediatric Cardiology Associates
Colorado Springs, CO, USA

Nick Rutter MD FRCP FRCPCH
Professor of Paediatric Medicine
Queen's Medical Centre
Nottingham, UK

George Rylance MB FRCPCH
Consultant in Paediatrics
Department of Child Health
Royal Victoria Infirmary
Newcastle-upon-Tyne, UK

Alison Salt MBBS MSc DCH FRCPCH FRACP
Consultant Development Paediatrician
Neurodisability Service
Great Ormond Street Hospital for Sick Children
London, UK

Jo Sibert MA MD FRCP FRCPCh DCH D.OHRCOG
Professor of Community Child Health
Department of Child Health
University of Wales College of Medicine
Vale of Glamorgan, UK

Jonathan Skinner MBChB MD FRCPCH FRACP
Paediatric Cardiologist
Department of Pediatric Cardiology
Greenlane Hospital
Auckland, New Zealand

Rosalind L Smyth MA MBBS MD FRCPCH
Brough Professor of Paediatric Medicine
University of Liverpool
Institute of Child Health
Alder Hey Children's Hospital
Liverpool, UK

Robert D Steiner MD
Associate Professor and Head of Division of Metabolism
Department of Pediatrics and Molecular & Medical Genetics
Oregon Health & Science University
Portland, OR, USA

Ben James Stenson MBChB MD FRCP FRCPCH
Consultant Neonatologist
Neonatal Unit
Simpson Memorial Maternity Pavilion
Edinburgh, UK

Terence Stephenson BSc BM BCh DM FRCP FRCPCH
Professor of Child Health
Academic Division of Child Health
School of Human Development
Nottingham, UK

Steven Sturgiss MBChB MD MRCOG
Consultant in Fetal Medicine
Fetal Medicine Unit
Royal Victoria Infirmary
Newcastle upon Tyne, UK

William Tarnow-Mordi BA(Cantab) MBChB MRCP (UK) DCH
Professor of Neonatal Medicine
Neonatal Intensive Care Unit
Westmead Hospital
Sydney, Australia

C Mark Taylor FRCP FRCPCH DCH
Consultant Paediatric Nephrologist
Department of Nephrology
Birmingham Children's Hospital
Birmingham, UK

Angela Thomas MBBS PhD FRCPEd FRCPCH FRCPath
Consultant Paediatric Haematologist
Department of Haematology
Royal Hospital for Sick Children
Edinburgh, UK

Pamela Tomlin MA FRCP FRCPCH DCH
Consultant Paediatric Neurologist
Paediatric Neurology
Royal Preston Hospital
Preston, UK

Russell Viner MBBS FRCPCH FRACP FRCP PhD
Consultant in Adolescent Medicine & Endocrinology
Department of Paediatrics
Middlesex Hospital
London, UK

Alan R Watson MBChB FRCP(Ed) FRCPCH
Consultant Paediatric Nephrologist
Special Senior Lecturer, University of Nottingham
Children & Young People's Kidney Unit
City Hospital
Nottingham, UK

Michael Watson MBBS FRACP FRCPA DTMorh MPM & TM
Staff Specialist Paediatric Infectious Diseases & Clinical Microbiology
Department of Immunology & Infectious Diseases
The Children's Hospital at Westmead
Sydney, Australia

Lawrence T Weaver MA MD FRCP FRCPCH DCH
Samson Gemmell Professor of Child Health
Department of Child Health
University of Glasgow
Glasgow, UK

Philip D Welsby FRCP(Ed)
Consultant in Infectious Diseases
Infectious Disease Unit
Western General Hospital
Edinburgh, UK

Alastair Graham Wilkinson MBBS MA MRCP FRCR
Consultant Paediatric Radiologist, X-Ray Department
Royal Hospital for Sick Children
Edinburgh, UK

Anthony F Williams BSc MBBS DPhil FRCP FRCPCH
Senior Lecturer
Department of Child Health
St George's Medical School
London, UK

Bridget A Wills BMedSci BMBS MRCP DTM&H
Clinical Senior Lecturer in Paediatrics
University of Oxford - Wellcome Trust Clinical Research Unit
Ho Chi Minh City, Vietnam

David Wilson MD FRCP FRCPCH
Senior Lecturer in Paediatric Gastroenterology and Nutrition
Department of Child Life and Health
University of Edinburgh
Edinburgh, UK

Dieter Wolke PhD
Professor in Lifespan Psychology and Deputy Director of Avon Longitudinal Study of Parents and Children (ALSPAC)
University of Bristol
Bristol, UK

C Mae Wong BMedSci(Hons) MRCP MRCPCH
Rivendell Research Fellow in Neonatology
Department of Child Life and Health
University of Edinburgh
Edinburgh, UK

Siobhan M E Wren MBBS MRCOphth
Registrar in Ophthalmology
Department of Ophthalmology
Imperial College
London, UK

Christopher Wren MB ChB
Consultant Paediatric Cardiologist
Department of Paediatric Cardiology
Freeman Hospital
Newcastle upon Tyne, UK

Jane Wynne D (of Univ) MB ChB FRCP FRCP Ch
Consultant Community Paediatrician
Honorary Senior Lecturer-Leeds University
Leeds Community & Mental Health Unit
Leeds, UK

Preface

One of the most important developments in the 21st century has been the acknowledgment that clinical practice should be embedded, where possible, in a sound evidence base. The editors of this new edition of *Forfar & Arneil's Textbook of Pediatrics* recognised this development and set contributors the challenging task of ensuring that the statements and recommendations made were based on the most robust clinical research available. The objective assessment of evidence and the formulation of secure recommendations from that evidence are gathering pace. However, in child health, the evidence base, with the possible exception of disciplines such as oncology and neonatology, is not as comprehensive or as well defined as we would wish. This edition of Forfar and Arneil is different from those before. The whole book has been revised and updated and the chapter authors and editors have been asked to incorporate where possible, secure evidence for therapy, diagnosis, aetiology and prognosis. This evidence is incorporated into the individual chapters, and in chapter reference lists it is starred for easy reference. We believe that the result is the most comprehensive, evidence-based, general textbook of pediatrics available to date. Our ability to access best evidence has been greatly enhanced by the rapid advances in information technology and electronic publishing, and consequently another important new feature for this edition is a CD ROM of the text in which references listed in Pubmed can be accessed via the internet. We would like to acknowledge the outstanding contributions of the many individual authors and our chapter editors, without whom this ambitious project would not have been possible. It has been a great privilege to work with them. We would also like to thank our own secretaries for their unstinting help (Elaine Forbes, Mary Dow and Moira Saphier) over the weeks they have dealt with the many questions from authors and have kept us on schedule.

This enterprise began with Churchill Livingstone as the publishers and progressed through Ballière Tindall to Harcourt, but we are now part of the Elsevier organisation. There have been many highly professional people involved in all of these organisations as the editions have developed. We hope that this new 6th edition, as a first of its type and ready for the evidence-based world, will be well received by you, the reader, and become as trusted a friend and guide as have preceding editions.

Neil McIntosh
Peter J Helms
Rosalind L Smyth
2003

Section 1

Foundations for health and practice

1

Evidence-based child health

Rosalind L Smyth

INTRODUCTION

Evidence-based pediatrics and child health has been defined as 'the integration of clinical information obtained from a patient, with the best evidence available from clinical research and experience and the application of this knowledge to the prevention, diagnosis or management of disease in that child'.[1] This definition has been adapted from an earlier one by Sackett and colleagues[2] who have consistently argued that there is an art to medicine, as well as objective scientific knowledge, and that both are essential to the clinical encounter. Within the classical clinical method, as taught in medical schools and beyond, the diagnostic approach starts with a history, leads on to a clinical examination and utilizes, if required, special investigations. In the process of history taking, the clinician integrates the case specific features of the patient's own story with their accumulated case expertise. For example, the differential diagnosis and mode of history taking in two children presenting with cough will be very different, if in one, it is elicited that she has experienced fever and night sweats and is recently returned from India, and in the other, recurrent wheeze and hay fever are accompanying symptoms. In taking a history, one constantly updates the differential diagnoses and redirects one's questioning as each new item of information is elicited. Indeed, it is this ability to take a history in a directive and efficient manner that distinguishes the experienced clinician from the new clinical student.

Sackett and colleagues have long argued that the clinical examination should be studied rigorously to establish which features are predictive of specific diagnoses. For example, they have reviewed studies that evaluated the accuracy of signs recommended for use in the diagnosis of chronic obstructive pulmonary disease.[3] They found, that for all the signs reviewed, the sensitivity, specificity and likelihood ratios varied considerably between studies, and were far short of what would be required for an ideal diagnostic test.[3]

It is only the final part of the diagnostic process, the use of special investigations, for which there are clear criteria for assessment of the validity of clinical evidence.[2] Conventionally, diagnostic tests are judged by their sensitivity (proportion of patients with the target disorder who have positive tests) and specificity (proportion of patients without the target disorder who have negative tests). However a concept which gives more useful information than sensitivity or specificity about the performance of a test, is known as the likelihood ratio. For example, suppose you are assessing a child with failure to thrive and malabsorption. You estimate that the probability of the child having celiac disease is around 10%. Before suggesting to the parents that the child should undergo a small intestinal biopsy, you want evidence that the probability of the child having celiac disease is greater than 1 in 10. You wish to know whether a test which detects antiendomysial antibodies in the serum, will, if positive, increase the probability of the child having celiac disease.

A publication from South America has evaluated both serum immunoglobulin A (IgA) antigliadin antibodies and serum IgA-class antiendomysial antibodies and compared them with findings of subtotal, or total villous atrophy on small intestinal biopsy (the reference standard).[4] The blood samples were taken at the same time as the small intestinal biopsy, so it appeared that the reference standard was applied independently of the diagnostic tests being evaluated and the reference standard was applied objectively to all patients. The sensitivity of antiendomysial antibodies in the detection of celiac disease was 97%, with a specificity of 84.6%. This study, therefore, provides at least level 2 evidence concerning the validity of this diagnostic test (Table 1.1).

The likelihood ratio is the ratio of the probability of the test result in patients with the disease to the probability of the test result in patients without the disease. It enables an updated 'post-test' probability to be calculated from the pretest probability, using the results of appropriate studies. The likelihood ratio of a positive test result is calculated from the sensitivity and specificity as follows:

$$LR+ = \text{sensitivity}/(1 - \text{specificity})$$

From the example of antiendomysial antibodies provided above, the study we have found would suggest the following:

$$LR+ = 97\%/15\%, \text{ or approximately } 6.$$

If this is applied to the estimated pretest probability, provided in the example above, of 10%, or odds of 1:9, a positive test result will convert these pretest odds to a post-test odds of 6:9, or a post-test probability of 40%. Most clinicians would consider that a small intestinal biopsy should be performed in a child who has a probability of 40% of having celiac disease.

Table 1.1 Oxford Centre for Evidence-Based Medicine levels of evidence (May 2001)

Level	Therapy/prevention, etiology/harm	Prognosis	Diagnosis	Differential diagnosis/symptom prevalence study	Economic and decision analyses
1a	SR (with homogeneity*) of RCTs	SR (with homogeneity*) of inception cohort studies; CDR† validated in different populations	SR (with homogeneity*) of Level 1 diagnostic studies; CDR† with 1b studies from different clinical centers	SR (with homogeneity*) of prospective cohort studies	SR (with homogeneity*) of Level 1 economic studies
1b	Individual RCT (with narrow confidence interval‡)	Individual inception cohort study with ≥ 80% follow-up; CDR† validated in a single population	Validating** cohort study with good††† reference standards; or CDR† tested within one clinical center	Prospective cohort study with good follow-up****	Analysis based on clinically sensible costs or alternatives; systematic review(s) of the evidence; and including multiway sensitivity analyses
1c	All or none§	All or none case-series	Absolute SpPins and SnNouts††	All or none case-series	Absolute better-value or worse-value analyses††††
2a	SR (with homogeneity*) of cohort studies	SR (with homogeneity*) of either retrospective cohort studies or untreated control groups in RCTs	SR (with homogeneity*) of Level >2 diagnostic studies	SR (with homogeneity*) of 2b and better studies	SR (with homogeneity*) of Level >2 economic studies
2b	Individual cohort study (including low quality RCT; e.g. < 80% follow-up)	Retrospective cohort study or follow-up of untreated control patients in an RCT; Derivation of CDR† or validated on split-sample§§§ only	Exploratory** cohort study with good†††reference standards; CDR† after derivation, or validated only on split-sample§§§ or databases	Retrospective cohort study, or poor follow-up	Analysis based on clinically sensible costs or alternatives; limited review(s) of the evidence, or single studies; and including multiway sensitivity analyses
2c	'Outcomes' research; ecological studies	'Outcomes' research		Ecological studies	Audit or outcomes research
3a	SR (with homogeneity*) of case-control studies		SR (with homogeneity*) of 3b and better studies	SR (with homogeneity*) of 3b and better studies	SR (with homogeneity*) of 3b and better studies
3b	Individual case-control study		Non-consecutive study; or without consistently applied reference standards	Non-consecutive cohort study, or very limited population	Analysis based on limited alternatives or costs, poor quality estimates of data, but including sensitivity analyses incorporating clinically sensible variations
4	Case-series (and poor quality cohort and case-control studies§§)	Case-series (and poor quality prognostic cohort studies***)	Case-control study, poor or non-independent reference standard	Case-series or superseded reference standards	Analysis with no sensitivity analysis
5	Expert opinion without explicit critical appraisal, or based on physiology, bench research or 'first principles'	Expert opinion without explicit critical appraisal, or based on physiology, bench research or 'first principles'	Expert opinion without explicit critical appraisal, or based on physiology, bench research or 'first principles'	Expert opinion without explicit critical appraisal, or based on physiology, bench research or 'first principles'	Expert opinion without explicit critical appraisal, or based on physiology, bench research or 'first principles'

Produced by Bob Phillips, Chris Ball, Dave Sackett, Doug Badenoch, Sharon Straus, Brian Haynes, Martin Dawes since November 1998.

Notes—Users can add a minus-sign '-' to denote the level that fails to provide a conclusive answer because of:

- EITHER a single result with a wide confidence interval (such that, for example, an ARR in an RCT is not statistically significant but whose confidence intervals fail to exclude clinically important benefit or harm)
- OR a systematic review with troublesome (and statistically significant) heterogeneity.
- Such evidence is inconclusive, and therefore can only generate Grade D recommendations.

Table 1.1 Cont'd

* By homogeneity we mean a systematic review that is free of worrisome variations (heterogeneity) in the directions and degrees of results between individual studies. Not all systematic reviews with statistically significant heterogeneity need be worrisome, and not all worrisome heterogeneity need be statistically significant. As noted above, studies displaying worrisome heterogeneity should be tagged with a '-' at the end of their designated level.

† Clinical Decision Rule (these are algorithms or scoring systems which lead to a prognostic estimation or a diagnostic category).

‡ See note #2 for advice on how to understand, rate and use trials or other studies with wide confidence intervals.

§ Met when *all* patients died before the treatment became available, but some now survive on it; or when some patients died before the treatment became available, but *none* now die on it.

§§ By poor quality *cohort* study we mean one that failed to clearly define comparison groups and/or failed to measure exposures and outcomes in the same (preferably blinded), objective way in both exposed and non-exposed individuals and/or failed to identify or appropriately control known confounders and/or failed to carry out a sufficiently long and complete follow-up of patients. By poor quality *case-control* study we mean one that failed to clearly define comparison groups and/or failed to measure exposures and outcomes in the same (preferably blinded), objective way in both cases and controls and/or failed to identify or appropriately control known confounders.

§§§ Split-sample validation is achieved by collecting all the information in a single tranche, then artificially dividing this into 'derivation' and 'validation' samples.

†† An 'Absolute SpPin' is a diagnostic finding whose *S*pecificity is so high that a *P*ositive result rules-*in* the diagnosis. An "Absolute SnNout" is a diagnostic finding whose *S*ensitivity is so high that a *N*egative result rules-*out* the diagnosis.

‡‡ Good, better, bad and worse refer to the comparisons between treatments in terms of their clinical risks and benefits.

††† *Good* reference standards are independent of the test, and applied blindly or objectively to applied to all patients. *Poor* reference standards are haphazardly applied, but still independent of the test. Use of a non-independent reference standard (where the 'test' is included in the 'reference', or where the 'testing' affects the 'reference') implies a level 4 study.

†††† Better-value treatments are clearly as good but cheaper, or better at the same or reduced cost. Worse-value treatments are as good and more expensive, or worse and equally or more expensive.

** Validating studies test the quality of a specific diagnostic test, based on prior evidence. An exploratory study collects information and trawls the data (e.g. using a regression analysis) to find which factors are 'significant'.

*** By poor quality prognostic cohort study we mean one in which sampling was biased in favor of patients who already had the target outcome, or the measurement of outcomes was accomplished in < 80% of study patients, or outcomes were determined in an unblinded, non-objective way, or there was no correction for confounding factors.

**** Good follow-up in a differential diagnosis study is > 80%, with adequate time for alternative diagnoses to emerge (e.g. 1–6 months acute, 1–5 years chronic).

RCT, randomized controlled trial; SR, systematic review.

Grades of recommendation:

A. Consistent Level 1 studies
B. Consistent Level 2 or 3 studies *or* extrapolations from Level 1 studies
C. Level 4 studies *or* extrapolations from Level 2 or 3 studies
D. Level 5 evidence *or* troublingly inconsistent or inconclusive studies of any level

'Extrapolations' are where data are used in a situation which has potentially clinically important differences from the original study situation.

What should the clinician do, though, if the test is negative? The likelihood ratio of a negative test result is calculated as follows:

$$LR- = (1 - \text{sensitivity})/\text{specificity}$$

For our example, this is:

$$LR- = 3\%/85\% \text{ or } 0.04.$$

So a negative test result will convert our pretest odds of 1:9 or 10% to around 0.4%. It will be up to the clinician to judge whether a small intestinal biopsy is necessary in a child with an estimated 0.4% probability of having celiac disease.

For those familiar with statistical methods, it will be evident that the concept of likelihood ratios has been adopted from the Bayesian approach to statistical inference. The first step in any Bayesian analysis is to establish a prior probability distribution for the value of interest (e.g. probability of a child having a diagnosis of gluten sensitive enteropathy). The clinical evidence is then used to update the prior distribution to a posterior distribution using Bayes theorem. This is analogous to the intuitive process in clinical history taking, where the probabilities of having one of a number of different diagnoses are updated as each new piece of information is elicited. In an evidence-based medicine approach, we start with a prior view about whether, for example, a drug treatment will improve clinical outcomes for an individual patient. This view may be informed by knowledge of the patient's preferences, cost of therapy and so on. This prior view is then updated by the results of a randomized controlled trial of the drug treatment, in a group of patients similar to our patient, which shows clear improvement in the outcomes we consider important. This evidence is integrated with our prior beliefs, to enable a clinical decision to be made. Many have argued that the natural statistical framework for evidence-based medicine is a Bayesian approach to decision making,[5] both for the individual patient and for health policy.[6]

In an article entitled 'Narrative-based medicine in an evidence-based world',[7] Greenhalgh quotes a scenario, referred to as 'Dr Jenkins's hunch', which goes as follows: 'I got a call from a mother who said that her little girl had had diarrhea and was behaving strangely. I knew the family well and was sufficiently concerned to break off my Monday morning surgery and visit immediately.' Dr Jenkins' subsequent actions resulted in the child recovering from meningococcal septicemia. To many this may seem like a fortunate fluke, and indeed meningococcal septicemia presents rarely in primary care. No guideline could have reliably prompted Dr Jenkins' action. However the doctor was integrating his clinical intuition (mothers rarely use the word 'strangely' to describe their children's behavior), his acquaintance with the family (known to be sensible and uncomplaining), with current best evidence (prognosis of meningococcal septicemia, with and without early administration of parenteral penicillin) to take a course of action which saved a child's life. Greenhalgh rejects the notion that the 'narrative of illness experience' and the 'intuitive and subjective' aspects of clinical method run counter to evidence-based medicine.[7] In making clinical decisions, either informally, by integrating new evidence with our prior views, or formally, by using Bayesian analysis, the framework exists to ensure that clinical evidence can play an explicit part in the process.

THE PRACTICE OF EVIDENCE-BASED MEDICINE

Traditionally there are four basic steps described in this approach. The first is to frame a clinically relevant question and to focus it in a way which can be answered. This is not as trivial a step as it may at first appear. The key elements of a well framed question include a description of:

1. the patient or population;
2. the intervention or exposure;
3. the comparison intervention or exposure (if relevant); and
4. the clinical outcome(s) of interest.

Such an approach can be applied whether the issue is one of diagnosis, prognosis or therapy.

For example, let us consider the following scenario. You are the clinical director of an accident and emergency department in a children's hospital. You have noted that in children who attend the department with a diagnosis of asthma, there appears to be a very high rate of subsequent reattendance. You are interested in interventions which may prevent reattendance and improve the care of children with frequent acute asthma exacerbations. It has been suggested that a strategy of review of such children in a clinic, within a week of their original attendance, by an experienced asthma nurse practitioner, with careful attention to education of the child and family about asthma, may be useful in reducing such reattendances. To investigate this further you may, therefore, formulate the following question 'in children with asthma who attend a hospital accident and emergency department (population), does early review at an asthma nurse led clinic (intervention), compared with no such review (comparison intervention), reduce the risk of reattendances with acute asthma at the accident and emergency department (outcome)?'

Having defined the question, the second step is to undertake a comprehensive review of the best available clinical evidence. This is likely to involve searching electronic databases (e.g. Medline, EMBASE, CINAHL and *The Cochrane Library*). The development of search strategies for these databases often involves expertise of information scientists who can adjust the search strategy to maximize finding all relevant studies (which increases sensitivity), but at the expense of identifying many irrelevant articles (decrease specificity).

Having retrieved all potentially relevant articles which address the question, the third step is to critically appraise them. Tools have been developed to appraise studies evaluating diagnostic tests, prognostic markers, treatments, adverse effects and systematic overviews.[2] In the example provided above, you will have been searching for studies which are used to evaluate the effectiveness of treatments. There are many different study designs which may address this type of question. A hierarchy of such study designs has been developed with the most rigorous at the top and the least rigorous at the bottom (Fig. 1.1). The primary research study, which is considered to be the gold standard in assessing treatments, is the randomized controlled trial. The key element in this design is that the allocation of patients to the treatment group or to the comparison group is done randomly, and thus the observed differences between the treatment and the comparison group(s) will be due to the experimental treatment alone rather than to biases which may be introduced by patient characteristics, physician preferences, etc. However, even given this robust study design, the methodological quality of randomized controlled trials may be subject to biases in other ways and these can be evaluated appropriately by checklists.[2]

The fourth step, which is to apply the evidence in clinical practice, is the point at which clinical expertise and patient values are integrated with the best available external evidence. To do this, the clinician needs to ask two questions concerning the evidence that s/he has appraised. The first is 'is this evidence sufficiently robust for me to be confident in its application?' and the second is 'is

Systematic Review of Randomized Controlled Trials
Confirmed Randomized Controlled Clinical Trials
Single Randomized Controlled Clinical Trial
Non-Randomized Controlled Clinical Trial
Case Controlled Observational Studies
Analysis of Large Computer Databases
Case Series with Historical Controls
Case series, Literature Control
Uncontrolled Case Series
Anecdotal Case

Fig. 1.1 Research pyramid of study designs used to assess the efficacy of treatments.

this study applicable to the patient (or population) about whose care I am deciding?'.

Practitioners of evidence-based medicine have long argued that it should not be conducted from ivory towers, by individuals who have little patient contact. If it is to be applicable it needs to be practiced by all clinicians, not least because the questions or question posed need to be relevant to routine practice. However, as will be apparent from the brief description above, the second and third steps of this approach can be very laborious. This has led to the development of a number of shortcuts which will enable the clinician to move easily from step one to step four. To be reliable, such shortcuts must use rigorous methods. One of the most attractive and reliable of these tools is the development systematic reviews. As will be seen from Table 1.2, the systematic review is now regarded by many as the most rigorous study design for providing information about treatments. The term *systematic* or *scientific* review is used to distinguish them from more *traditional* or *narrative* type reviews of topic areas conducted by experts in the field.

SYSTEMATIC REVIEWS

Narrative reviews have become a regular feature of many medical journals. Such reviews may be very informative, lively and interesting and are usually well illustrated. They are popular because clinicians are busy and have limited time to try and assimilate all primary research which is relevant in a particular area. However, if judged as scientific work which provides summaries of the evidence, which can be used to guide diagnosis or treatment, they are very subject to bias and are therefore unreliable. A study by Antman et al[8] examined the temporal relationship between the appearance of results in the literature for randomized controlled trials of treatments of myocardial infarction and the recommendations of clinical experts from textbook chapters and review articles. They found that review articles continued to recommend treatments that have been shown to be ineffective, or even harmful, and on occasions failed to mention important advances in treatment.

These deficiencies led to the concept of systematic reviews, which should adopt a rigorous scientific methodology to eliminate systematic bias or random error, as would be expected of investigators undertaking primary clinical research. The methodology for systematic reviews is outlined in Table 1.2. First the reviewer needs to state the hypothesis that they wish to investigate and then prospectively define a comprehensive search strategy to identify all potentially relevant studies. This strategy will almost certainly include searching electronic databases but may involve other methods such as those designed to access unpublished studies, to ensure that the studies accessed are representative of all the research conducted in a particular area. The protocol for the review should state prospectively what studies will be considered eligible for inclusion, defined according to study design, type of participant, intervention, (or exposure) and comparison intervention or exposure. The outcomes of interest are stated prospectively. The protocol should also state how the quality of the included studies will be assessed.

Having determined which studies are to be included and assessed them for methodological quality, the reviewer then extracts the relevant data and analyzes it. This may involve statistical methods such as meta-analysis. This enables the data from a number of different studies to be aggregated so that a pooled effect size can be estimated. There are many examples where individual studies, usually because they are too small, fail to show that an intervention is either beneficial or harmful. By combining the results from all potentially relevant studies, such benefit or harm has been clearly demonstrated. This enables questions to be answered such as 'does this treatment have a beneficial effect?' and also 'what is the size of the effect?'.

There now exists a database of systematic reviews of randomized controlled trials of interventions across the whole range of health care. This is *The Cochrane Library*,[9] which, at the time of writing, contains over 1000 such systematic reviews. These reviews have been prepared by the Cochrane Collaboration, an international body dedicated to producing systematic reviews of the effects of health care using randomized controlled trials as the primary study design. *The Cochrane Library* is produced as a CD-ROM, is updated quarterly and is accessible on the Internet (http://hiru.mcmaster.ca/cochrane/centres/canadian/). This means that systematic reviews can also be updated to take account of new knowledge.

Although well conducted systematic reviews are regarded as being at the top of the hierarchy of study designs to evaluate the effectiveness of treatments, they can be misused or be badly conducted. Therefore systematic reviews need also to be appraised and there are checklists available for doing this. Jadad et al,[10] for example, have published an evaluation of reviews and meta-analyses of treatments used in asthma. Of the 50 reviews that they considered, 40 were found to have serious methodological flaws. Included within these 40 were six reviews funded by the pharmaceutical industry. All but one of these six reviews had

Table 1.2 How to conduct a systematic review

1. State objectives and hypotheses
2. Outline eligibility criteria, stating types of study, types of participant, types of intervention and outcomes to be examined
3. Perform a comprehensive search of all relevant sources for potentially eligible studies
4. Examine the studies to decide eligibility (if possible with two independent reviewers)
5. Construct a table describing the characteristics of the included studies
6. Assess methodological quality of included studies (if possible with two independent reviewers)
7. Extract data (with a second investigator if possible), with involvement of investigators if necessary
8. Analyze results of included studies, using statistical synthesis of data (meta-analysis), if appropriate
9. Prepare a report of review, stating aims, materials and methods and describing results and conclusions

Courtesy of Craig JV, Smyth RL. Evidence based practice manual for nurses. Edinburgh: Churchill Livingstone, 2002.

results and conclusions that favored the intervention related to the company which sponsored the review. Reassuringly they found that Cochrane Reviews had higher overall quality scores than reviews published in other scientific journals. The Cochrane Collaboration has made strenuous efforts to ensure that its methodology reduces bias to a minimum and has also guarded against biases which may be introduced by authors with conflicts of interest, e.g. significant support from the pharmaceutical industry. This methodology and the external appraisal by individuals such as Jadad provide reassurance that systematic reviews produced by the Cochrane Collaboration are reliable sources of information for the clinician.

EVIDENCE-BASED CHILD HEALTH

The evidence-based medicine movement was initially advanced by practitioners of internal medicine, but, more recently, pediatricians have become leading proponents. The scope of a number of Cochrane Collaborative Reviews Groups (such as the Cystic Fibrosis and Genetic Disorders Group) covers areas that deal mainly with illnesses of childhood. In addition, the Cochrane Child Health Field has recently become registered with the Cochrane Collaboration. One of its main aims will be, within Cochrane Reviews, to increase the focus on health needs of children. However, one feature that this discipline of evidence-based health care has highlighted is that when children's health is compared to adult health care, research questions in children may have been addressed either not at all or by small, poorly designed studies.[11] This was the case when all randomized trials published during a 15-year period in a specialist pediatric journal were examined. In this review sample sizes were found to be generally small and only a small proportion of studies were multicenter.[12] Subspecialty areas within pediatrics have also been reviewed, such as cystic fibrosis,[13] pediatric rheumatology[14] and community pediatrics[15] and the conclusions about the volume and quality of the research contained therein have been similar. Indeed this edition of Forfar & Arneil, which has asked contributors to be more explicit about the evidence that they cite, has led to contributors expressing frustration at the lack of level 1 evidence available for them to access in many different disease areas.

There are a number of different reasons why it is more difficult to undertake clinical trials and other rigorous studies in children than in adults. There are obvious ethical dilemmas. For example, research on a new therapy must first be conducted in adults before studies are undertaken in children. However, if data from a study of a therapy in adults show a clear advantage for a drug over placebo, does equipoise still exist and is it ethical to repeat such a study in children? Such ethical dilemmas need to be considered clearly and dispassionately by individuals who are advocates for the interests of children. However, there are many examples of therapies which have different effects depending on the stage of the disease process or the age of the patient, including, for example, the sedative effects of phenobarbital in adults, but its frequent association with hyperactivity in children.

There are other practical problems. Generally the proportions of children affected by chronic diseases are smaller than in adults and even for common childhood diseases such as asthma, the condition may be more heterogeneous than in adults and diagnostic criteria less precise. Outcome measures which have been developed and validated in adults, such as quality of life measures are unlikely to be appropriate or feasible for young children and infants.

All of these difficulties have led to a dearth of clinical evidence by which practitioners wishing to practice evidence-based child health. However, there are encouraging signs that as well as identifying the deficiencies in the evidence, initiatives are being made to promote research that will meet these needs. For example, the Food and Drug Administration in the USA mandated in 1997 that new drugs brought to the market should be tested in children unless there were compelling reasons not to do so and within the UK, the Cystic Fibrosis Trust has established a clinical trials group to facilitate the conduct of high quality multicenter trials.

HOW TEXTBOOKS ENSURE THAT THEY ARE EVIDENCE BASED

Most manuals written for evidence-based practitioners do not consider textbooks to be a valuable source of information. Sackett et al[2] in the relevant section in their textbook *Evidence-based Medicine* state 'we begin with textbooks only to dismiss them' later stating 'while we may find some useful information in text books about the pathophysiology of clinical problems it is best not use them for establishing the cause, diagnosis, prognosis, prevention or treatment of a disorder'. Part of the problem is that the material published in textbooks is written some time (often some years) before the book is published. Thus textbooks rapidly become out of date. Publishers have realized this and are trying to address this with strategies such as providing regular electronic updates more frequently than the published paper editions.

However, some textbooks have been found not to include information which is current at the time they are written. *The Oxford Textbook of Medicine* has been criticized for including a statement in its second edition concerning the clinical benefits of thrombolysis for patients who had had a myocardial infarction, which stated that these benefits had not been established. This statement was made some years after this therapy had been shown, in a systematic review of randomized controlled trials to reduce the risk of premature death after myocardial infarction.[16] By way of further illustration Jefferson[17] described his experience in conducting a Cochrane Review of the effects of cholera vaccine. Although much of the data available for this review concerned older, killed whole cell cholera vaccine, the reviewers were aware that the killed whole cell vaccine had been discouraged as it had become widely accepted that it had a low efficacy and short duration of effect, required multiple doses and was less effective in children under 5 than in adults. However, the systematic review found that the efficacy of the vaccine compared with placebo was over 50% in both the first 7 months and in the first year and just under 50% in the second year and that most of the trials achieved this efficacy using a single dose. Vaccine efficacy in the first year was also as great in children under 5 as in older people. The reviewers concluded that the level and duration of efficacy of the killed whole cell cholera vaccine had been underestimated in the literature and that the incidence of adverse effects had been overestimated. A further survey of journal editors and authors of reviews of cholera vaccines concluded that many narrative reviews had been written using the so called 'desk drawer method'. This involved including the evidence that was known to reviewers, but not assembling it or evaluating it systematically. Now that over 1000 Cochrane Reviews and over 300 000 randomized controlled trials of interventions are available on *The Cochrane Library*, there can be no excuse for the reviewer, or indeed textbook writer, not to consult *The Cochrane Library* when considering treatments for the condition or conditions they are writing about.

Many textbooks now contain the term 'evidence-based' within their title. These fall into two groups. Firstly the manuals that aim to instruct the clinician on how to practice evidence-based medicine and secondly textbooks which purport to present evidence-based information which has been synthesized in a rigorous manner and presented in an easily accessible format. Such textbooks include *Evidence-based Pediatrics and Child Health*[18] and *Clinical Evidence.*[19] *Clinical Evidence,* which states at the outset that it is 'not a textbook of medicine' is rather a handbook, or a reference guide, of topics of wide general interest in health care. In the 'Compendium of evidence', at the start of the book, the methods used are clearly presented. However, its question and answer presentation, limitation to interventions and incomplete coverage of all subjects within its scope make it a rather different from a textbook such as this one. *Evidence-based Pediatrics and Child Health* describes itself as a 'melding of a textbook of evidence-based medicine and a clinical pediatric text addressing common conditions'. The first section of this book provides readers with the skills needed to practice evidence-based child health, while the second and third sections address common pediatric conditions. Again the format is in a question and answer framework, with illustration by scenarios. Within the second and third sections, only those specific questions for which evidence is available are considered and as a consequence much of clinical pediatrics is not discussed.

A large and complete textbook of pediatrics such as this one needs to provide a detailed consideration of all aspects of a condition, not just diagnosis, prognosis, prevention and treatment (which are more amenable to evidence-based approaches). Moyer and Elliott[1] refer to two sorts of questions which may be used by the reader in trying to elicit information about a topic, including background information such as: what is Cornelia de Lange syndrome, what is the incidence of tracheoesophageal fistula with esophageal atresia and what is meant by the term apoptosis? These are distinguished from 'foreground' questions relating to, for example, benefits or adverse effects of therapy. Textbooks therefore need to consider the definition, pathophysiology and clinical presentation of conditions as well as diagnosis, prognosis, prevention or treatment of the disorder.

In considering how textbook writers put this information together in a readable format it is helpful to consider how this process has evolved over decades or even centuries. Bristowe in the preface to the 1876 first edition of his *Theory and Practice of Medicine*[20] states his primary aim as 'to give in a readable form as much information as I could within a limited space'. He describes his practice of 'in every case to read the subject up carefully; to compare the knowledge thus acquired or renewed with the results of my own experience, in those cases in which I had any experience; and then, having taken a more or less definite view of the whole subject and while my mind was still full of it, and its details, to write as clear and as comprehensive an account as I was capable of'. He states that this method of procedure will partly explain 'the prevailing absence of notes, quotations and references to authorities'. This textbook, which ran to over 1000 pages, was written entirely by Bristowe and contained no references. Indeed it was unusual for textbooks to contain more than a few references per chapter until the middle of the twentieth century. The method used by Bristowe is similar to that used by many authors today, and the depth of the individual's experience contributes to the richness of the narrative and thus its readability.

So whilst retaining these traditional methods for the provision of background information we have, however, asked all authors to search for and use the best available evidence when presenting 'foreground' information. The methods that we have used to do this will be discussed in the next section.

CLINICAL EVIDENCE WITHIN THE 6TH EDITION OF FORFAR & ARNEIL

For this edition of Forfar & Arneil the editors gave specific instructions to contributors to ensure that their contributions were as evidence-based as possible. The contributors were asked to identify, where possible, 'level 1 evidence'. This system of grading evidence and recommendations was chosen because it is widely used and has been developed over the last 20 years. The table which contributors were asked to use (Table 1.1) is available on the Website of the Oxford Centre for Evidence-based Medicine (http://cebm.jr2.ox.ac.uk).[21] This type of approach has been used in other evidence-based textbooks.[22] The editors appreciated that in a number of areas there may not be level 1 evidence available, but to distinguish this category of evidence from the remainder, authors were asked to identify references to level 1 evidence with an asterisk (*). This approach may be considered inadequate by some evidence-based proponents but was felt to be an important step in ensuring that the standard of information available from this textbook was as high as possible. The grading system used has some problems and a number of these are acknowledged (http://cebm.jr2.ox.ac.uk). For example, definitions of homogeneity (with respect to systematic reviews) and narrow confidence intervals (with respect to randomized controlled trials) are open to considerable interpretation and may not adequately distinguish high quality studies from those of poor quality.

SUMMARY

Clinical decision making is a complex process. Evidence-based medicine proponents endorse the importance of clinical expertise, which uses narrative skills to integrate the information provided by the clinical method. In practicing evidence-based medicine, clinicians integrate this information with that provided by sound clinical research. When tensions arise in this approach, it is usually because the narrative/intuitive paradigm has been discarded and decision making is predicated on the 'evidence' alone. Systematic reviews are the result of rigorous research, using methodology which is designed to reduce bias. As such they can provide reliable summaries of evidence. This methodology has been most comprehensively developed for systematic reviews of randomized controlled trials, but is being developed for other study designs. By searching databases of systematic reviews, such as those contained within *The Cochrane Library*, the clinician can obtain high quality evidence rapidly and reliably and enhance his/her clinical practice.

REFERENCES (* Level 1 evidence)

1 Moyer V, Elliott E. Preface. In: Moyer V, Elliott E, Davis R, et al, eds. Evidence based pediatrics and child health. London: BMJ Books; 2000.

2 Sackett DL, Richardson WS, Rosenberg W, et al. Evidence-based medicine: how to practice and teach EBM. London: Churchill Livingstone; 2000.

3 McAlister F, Straus S, Sackett DL. Why we need large, simple studies of the clinical examination: the problem and a proposed solution. Lancet 1999; 354:1721–1724.

4 de Rosa S, Litwin N, de Davila M, et al. The correlation of IgA-class antigliadin and antiendomysial antibodies (AGA-IgA–EmA-IgA) with the intestinal histology in celiac disease

(CD). Acta Gastroenterol Latinoam 1992; 22:161–167.

5 Ashby D, Smith AFM. Evidence-based medicine as Bayesian decision-making. Stat Med 2000; 19:3291–3305.

6 Lilford R, Braunholtz D. The statistical basis of public policy: a paradigm shift is overdue. BMJ 1996; 313:603–607.

7 Greenhalgh T. Narrative based medicine in an evidence based world. BMJ 1999; 318:323–325.

8 Antman EM, Lau J, Kupelnick B, et al. A comparison of results of meta-analyses of randomized control trials and recommendations of clinical experts. JAMA 1992; 268:240–248.

9 Cochrane Library. The Cochrane Library, Issue 3, 2001. Oxford: Update Software.

10 Jadad AR, Moher M, Browman G, et al. Systematic reviews and meta-analyses on treatment of asthma: critical evaluation. BMJ 2000; 320:537–540.

11 Smyth RL, Weindling AM. Research in children: ethical and scientific aspects. Lancet 1999; 354 (suppl 2):SII21–SII24.

12 Campbell H, Surry S, Royle E. A review of randomised controlled trials published in *Archives of Disease in Childhood* from 1982–1996. Arch Dis Child 1997; 79:192–197.

13 Cheng K, Smyth RL, Motley J, et al. Randomized controlled trials in cystic fibrosis (1966–1997) categorized by time, design, and intervention. Pediatr Pulmonol 2000; 29:1–7.

14 Feldman B, Giannini E. Where's the evidence? Putting the clinical science into pediatric rheumatology. J Rheumatol 1996; 23:1502–1504.

15 Polnay L. Research in community child health. Arch Dis Child 1989; 64:981–983.

16 Chalmers I, Haynes B. Systematic reviews: reporting, updating, and correcting systematic reviews of the effects of health care. BMJ 1994; 309:862–865.

17 Jefferson T. What are the benefits of editorials and non-systematic reviews? BMJ 1999; 318:135.

18 Moyer VA, Elliott EJ, Davis RL, et al, eds. Evidence-based pediatrics and child health. London: BMJ Books; 2000.

19 Barton S. Clinical evidence. London: BMJ Publishing; 2001.

20 Bristowe J. Theory and practice of medicine. London: Smith, Elder & Co; 1882.

21 Website of Oxford Centre for EBM. http://cebm.jr2.ox.ac.uk Oxford Centre for Evidence-based Medicine; 2001.

22 Feldman W. Evidence-based pediatrics. Ontario: BC Decker, 2000.

23 Canadian Task Force on the Periodic Health Examination. The periodic health examination. Can Med Assoc J 1979; 121:1193–1254.

24 Sackett DL. Rules of evidence and clinical recommendations on use of antithrombotic agents. Chest 1986; 89(2 suppl):2S–3S.

25 Cook DJ, Guyatt GH, Laupacis A, et al. Clinical recommendations using levels of evidence for antithrombotic agents. Chest 1995; 108(4 suppl):227S–230S.

26 Yusuf S, Cairns JA, Camm AJ, et al. Evidence-based cardiology. London: BMJ Publishing; 1998.

2

Epidemiology of child health

Stuart Logan

INTRODUCTION

Children under 15 comprise about one-third of the world population, with three-quarters living in less developed countries. Children's health varies enormously across the world. In 1999 the under-5 mortality was 6 per 1000 in industrialized countries but 173 per 1000 in sub-Saharan Africa. There has been a decline in mortality rates at all ages in childhood throughout the world in the last 50 years, but the rate of decline has been much slower in poorer countries and has recently stopped or even reversed in some of the poorest.

Understanding the patterns of health and disease is important in planning health and social policies and in monitoring change over time. It is important to recognize the limitations of the data that are available. If the statistics are to be useful for comparing between areas and over time, effective systems must be in place to collect the data and there must be consistency of definitions. In many parts of the world, such systems are rudimentary, although considerable progress has been made in ensuring agreed definitions at least for the principal measures of birth and mortality.

This chapter will review the patterns of mortality and morbidity amongst children in industrialized countries and examine the major determinants of health at a population level. The situation in less developed parts of the world is discussed further in Chapter 8.

In describing the health of children at a population level we are usually forced to rely on measures of mortality or morbidity. Measures of health rather than disease are philosophically attractive but have proved problematic in practice. Although a number of tools have been developed to measure quality of life in childhood their application at a population level has been limited and they have mainly proved useful in clinical trials or in the investigation of the effects of specific conditions.

MORTALITY RATES

DEFINITIONS

Any infant who breathes, has a heart beat or pulsation of the umbilical cord is defined as a 'live birth', irrespective of gestation or the duration of the signs of life. It seems likely that at least some very premature infants who fulfil this definition are not in fact registered as live births and that, as the frontiers of neonatal intensive care have been pushed back over time, this proportion has changed. A stillbirth is defined now as being a child born at 24 or more weeks postconception who shows no signs of life, although, up until 1992, the definition required that they were born at least 28 weeks postconception.

The definitions of the various perinatal, neonatal and infant moratality rates (IMRs) are shown graphically in Figure 2.1. The denominator for the stillbirth and perinatal mortality rates is the number of still and live births while that for the other rates is the number of live births.

The under-5 mortality rate, widely used, particularly in poorer countries, is defined as the annual number of deaths in children under 5 years of age per 1000 live births. Age-specific death rates are the number of deaths in an age group per 1000 individuals in that age group.

PATTERNS OF MORTALITY

There have been dramatic changes in life expectancy in developed countries over the last century. In 1901, average life expectancy for women in the UK was 48 years, but by 1997 was 79.6 years. Life expectancy for men in the UK, although lower than for women, at 74.4 years, has also risen greatly. Although death rates at all ages have declined, much of this change has been due to the rapid decrease in deaths in childhood, particularly in the first half of the century. Changes in death rates during childhood over time for England and Wales are shown in Figure 2.2.[1]

Deaths in the first year of life

Of all deaths in childhood (age 0–14), 70% occur within the first year of life, 46% within the first month and 35% within the first week (Fig. 2.3).[1] The decline in the rate of stillbirths and infant mortality in England and Wales is shown in Figure 2.4.[1] The figure does not show stillbirths for the last two data points, as the change in definition mentioned above means that the rates are no longer

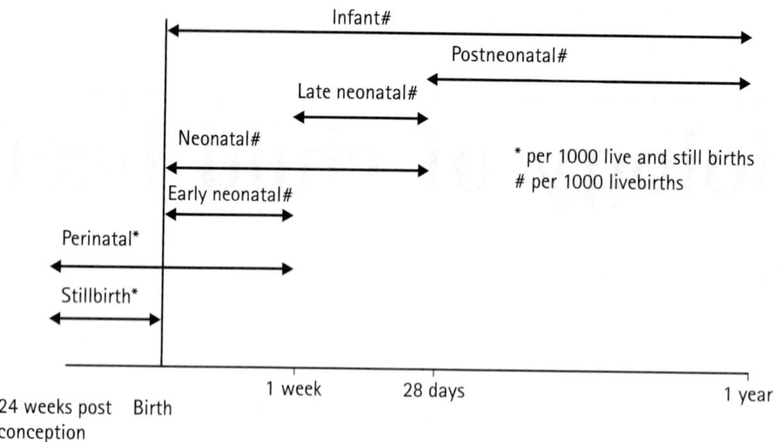

Fig. 2.1 Definitions of some mortality rates in the neonatal period and infancy.

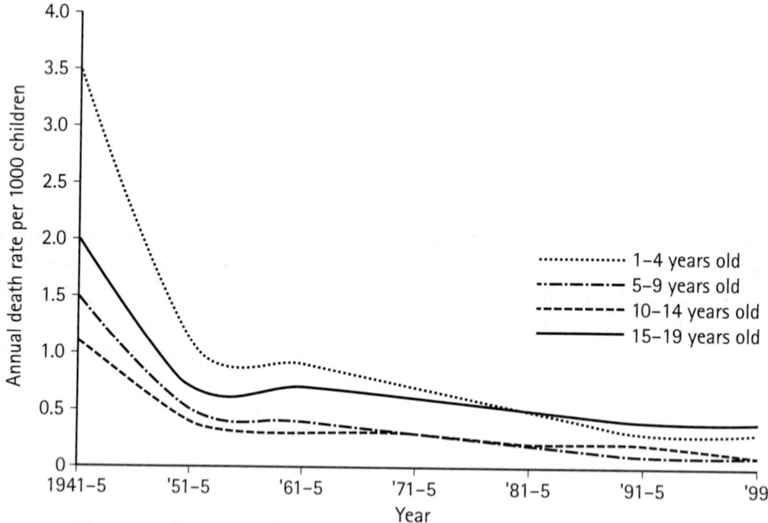

Fig. 2.2 Death rates in children in England and Wales over time.[1]

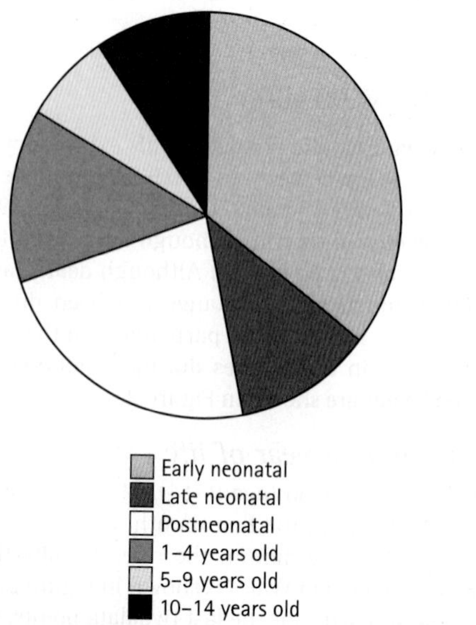

Fig. 2.3 Proportion of deaths in childhood by age of occurrence.[1]

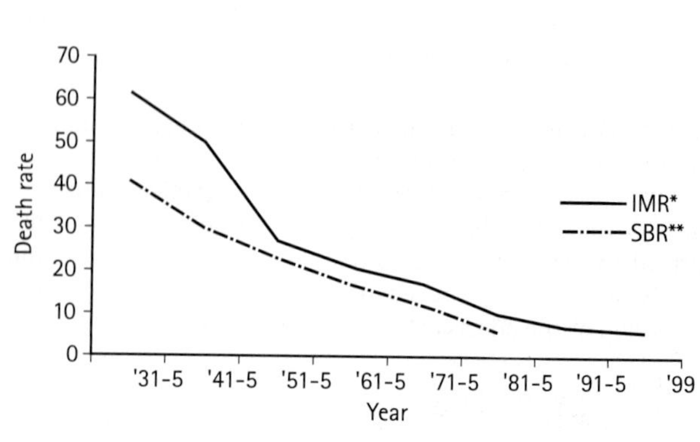

Fig. 2.4 Changes in stillbirth (SBR) and infant (IMR) mortality rates over time (England and Wales).[1]

comparable. The decline in infant mortality reflects declines in both neonatal and postneonatal mortality rates.

In the neonatal period, a substantial proportion of deaths are related to congenital anomalies and prematurity. The main causes of death in this age group for 1979 and 1999 are listed in Table 2.1. Congenital anomalies are an important cause of death in the neonatal period although the birth prevalence of many anomalies appears to have declined, particularly that of anomalies of the central nervous system (Fig. 2.5).[2] While part of this decline appears to relate to the widespread introduction of screening for neural tube defects in pregnancy there has also been a substantial decline in incidence, possibly related to changes in diet or the use of periconceptual folate supplements.

Congenital anomalies remain an important cause of death after the neonatal period, accounting for 24% of all deaths between 1 month and 1 year of age in England and Wales in 1999. In spite of a substantial fall in the risk of sudden infant death syndrome in the 1990s, this condition still accounted for around 20% of postneonatal deaths in the UK in 1999, a similar proportion to that related to infections. As with older children, injuries and poisoning are responsible for a significant number of deaths in the first year of life, but in this age group, the much higher rates of death from other conditions mean that they are responsible for a relatively small proportion of all deaths.

Even within the industrialized world there are substantial variations in IMRs (Table 2.2).[3] While there is an obvious relationship between mortality rates and wealth there are some surprising anomalies. For example, the USA has an IMR twice that of Sweden. To some extent, this appears to be related to differences in IMRs in different population groups within the same country. In the USA, in 1998, the IMR for infants born to white mothers was 6.0 per 1000 compared to 14.1 per 1000 for infants with black mothers, and different states reported IMRs ranging from 4.3 in New Hampshire to 13.2 in the District of Columbia.[3]

Birth weight, reflecting both gestation and intrauterine growth, is the strongest predictor of the risk of death in the first year of life (Fig. 2.6).[4] In large part, differences in mortality between, for instance, Sweden and the UK and between different ethnic groups in the USA are accounted for by differences in the birth weight distribution. The proportion of babies by birth weight group in England and Wales in 1999 is shown in Figure 2.7 In recent decades there has been a small overall increase in mean birth weight in many industrialized countries, largely accounted for by an increase in the proportion of babies born weighing > 3500 g. There has also, however, been an increase in the proportion of babies born weighing less than 2500 g, in the USA from 6.7% of live-born infants in 1984 to 7.5% in 1997. This partly reflects increasing numbers of twins and higher order births, which in the USA now comprise almost 3% of all births.[3]

Table 2.1 Categories of 'main cause of deaths' for neonatal deaths in 1999 (England and Wales)*

Condition	Percentage of deaths
Congenital anomalies	17.1
Prematurity	32.7
Respiratory distress syndrome	5.5
'Other respiratory conditions'	10.4
Infections	5.8
Intrauterine anoxia and birth asphyxia	3.6
Birth trauma	5.6

*Since 1986 changes in classification mean that it is not possible to ascribe deaths to a single cause but only to record the proportion which mention a condition as a 'main cause' on the death certificate.

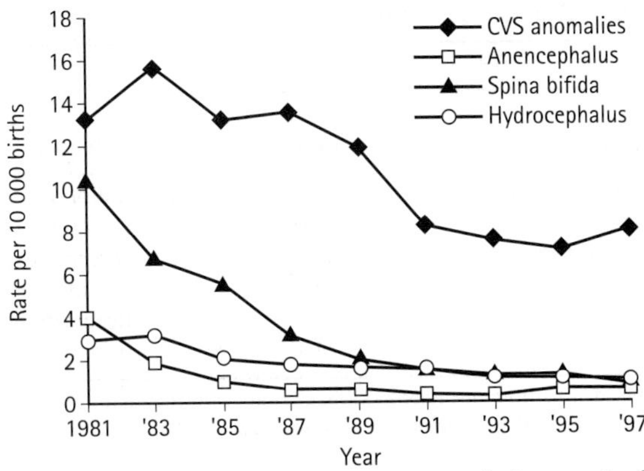

Fig. 2.5 Notifications of some important congenital anomalies.[2]

Deaths in older children

The risk of death drops rapidly after the first year of life; in the UK to around 27 per 100 000 children aged 1–4 and to 12 per 100 000 aged 5–14 compared to a risk of death in the first year of life of 580 per 100 000 live births. Death rates then begin to rise again after the age of 15, particularly in boys and largely as a result of the increasing risk of injuries.[1]

As shown in Figure 2.2, the risk of death from all causes in childhood has been falling throughout the last 50 years. Rates of death from unintentional injury in children have also fallen, but injury and poisoning remain responsible for the greatest proportion of deaths in older children. Table 2.3 compares the most common attributable causes of death in children aged 1–14 in 1955, 1985 and 1999, in England and Wales. Very similar patterns are seen in the USA[3] although unintentional injury rates are higher than in England and Wales and homicide is a far more important cause of death in children. In 1998 in the USA, homicide accounted for some 6.1 % of deaths in children aged 1–14 compared to 1.8% in England and Wales. Amongst adolescents aged 15–19 in the USA in 1998, accidents were responsible for 46.4% of deaths and homicide for 16.3%. In both the UK and USA the risks of non-intentional and intentional injuries are substantially higher in boys than in girls.

MORBIDITY IN CHILDHOOD

Morbidity data are more difficult to obtain and to interpret than mortality data, which are generally easily available and reasonably

Table 2.2 Infant mortality rates (IMRs) for some selected industrialized countries (1997)[3]

Country	IMR (per 1000 live births)
Sweden	3.6
Norway	4.1
Switzerland	4.5
Austria	4.7
Germany	4.9
The Netherlands	5.0
France	5.1
Italy	5.5
United Kingdom	5.9
Belgium	6.1
Ireland	6.2
New Zealand	6.6
United States	7.2
Portugal	8.4

Table 2.3 Deaths (age 1–14) for some important main categories in 1955, 1985 and 1999 in order of frequency (England and Wales)

1955		1985		1999	
Category	Percentage of deaths	Category	Percentage of deaths	Category	Percentage of deaths
Injury and poisoning	25.0	Injury and poisoning	33.6	Injury and poisoning	23.1
Respiratory disease*	13.0	Congenital anomalies	15.3	Malignant disease	18.4
Malignant disease	11.7	Malignant disease	14.0	Diseases of the CNS	13.0
Infectious disease	9.4	Diseases of the CNS	9.4	Respiratory disease*	9.6
Congenital anomalies	8.7	Respiratory disease*	6.2	Congenital anomalies	8.2
Diseases of the GIT	4.1	Infectious disease	4.0	Infectious disease	6.3

*Includes deaths from pneumonia. CNS, central nervous system; GIT, gastrointestinal tract.
Note: changes in the classification of disease over time mean that the categories may not be strictly comparable.

reliable. However such data are essential if one is to build up a picture of the health of the population.

HEALTH SERVICE USE

Children are heavy users of health services and routine service data can provide useful information about patterns of morbidity. A number of different sources of health service data are available in the UK, some derived directly from the use of services and some from special surveys such as the annual 'General Household Survey' which includes self-reported health and use of services.[5] Somewhat confusingly, these often cover different components or combinations of components of the UK. All these routine data have to be interpreted with some caution. Changes in admission rates over time for instance may reflect changes in classification either by health professionals or those who code the data, changes in thresholds for admission or real changes in incidence.

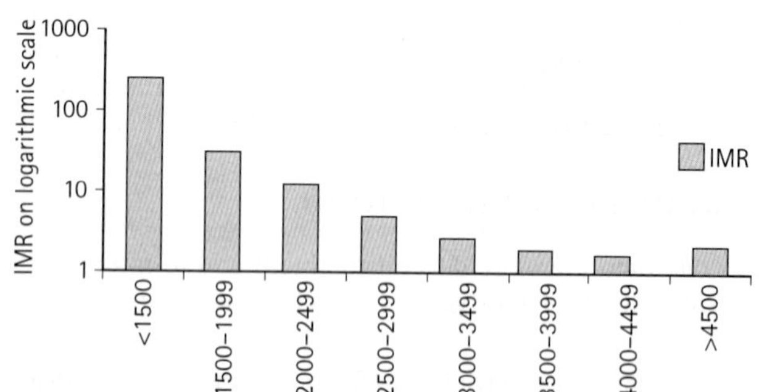

Fig. 2.6 Infant mortality rate (IMR) by birth weight in grams.[4]

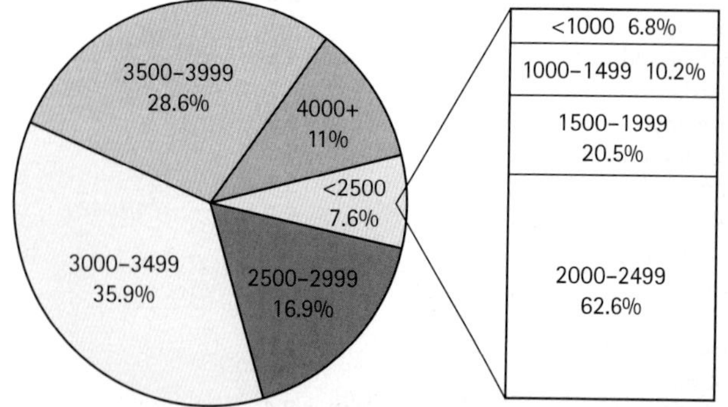

Fig. 2.7 Proportion of live births by birth weight in grams.[6]

Admission of children to hospital is relatively common. In the UK, in 1995, around 8% of 0–4-year-olds and 4% of 5–15-year-olds reported being admitted to hospital at least once in the previous year. There has been a steady decline in both the proportion and the average length of stay in hospital over time. The two most important reasons for admission in 5–14-year-olds are respiratory conditions, (including asthma), and injuries, each accounting for about 16% of admissions. A further 10% are admitted with non-specific 'signs and symptoms', while in 1995, otitis media accounted for an astonishing 6.6% of all admissions in this age group.

Children are also frequent visitors to accident and emergency departments and to general practitioners (GPs). More than 10% of British children report going to an accident and emergency department over a 3 month period. Those under 5 visit a GP on average seven times per year and those between 5 and 15, three times per year. Data collected in Scotland suggest that the commonest reasons for these GP visits are upper respiratory tract infections, otitis media, coughs, sore throats and other minor conditions.

CHRONIC DISEASE AND DISABILITY

Data on chronic disease and disability are relatively poor, even in countries with highly developed health systems. In the UK, one generally has to rely on special studies for this information. Unfortunately there are often problems with the representativeness of the samples and with the quality of the definitions used.

The General Household Survey, mentioned earlier, asks a representative group of people in the UK to report on their own and their children's health. One of the questions asks whether they have a longstanding illness and whether it limits their activities. In 1995, the parents of 13% of 0–4 and 19% of 5–15-year-olds said that their child had a longstanding illness and 4% and 8%, respectively, said that this limited their child's activities.

Reliable information on the prevalence of disability in childhood, except for the prevalence of a few well-defined conditions such as Down syndrome, is particularly difficult to find. Such information may also be difficult to interpret, as children's functional abilities form a continuum, and the point at which one labels the child as 'disabled' is arbitrary. A national survey in the UK, published in 1989, reported on parents' perceptions of whether their children were disabled.[6] Overall 3% of 0–15-year-olds were reported to have a disability. The rates by functional category and age group are shown in Figures 2.8–2.10.[6]

Estimates of the prevalence of cerebral palsy, the most common form of serious physical disability in childhood, are available from a number of countries. Most recent studies in industrialized countries report rates of cerebral palsy between 2 and 3 per 1000 infants surviving the neonatal period. In the UK,

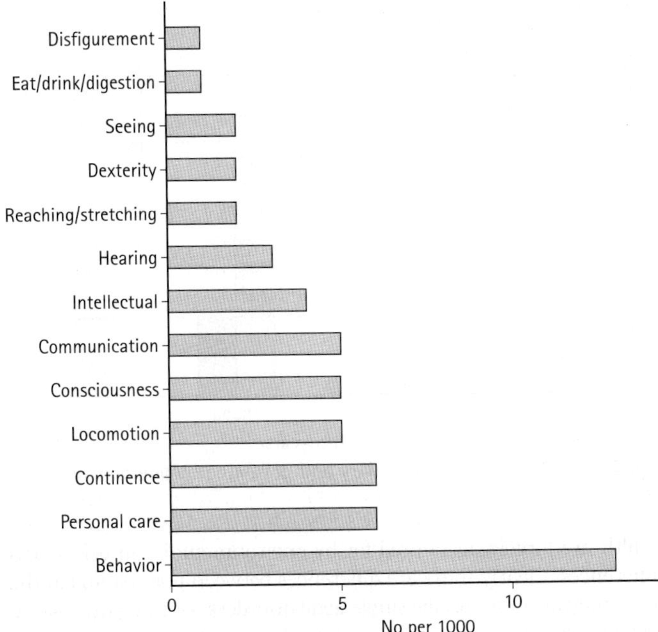

Fig. 2.8 Rates of disability per 1000 children aged 0–4 by functional category (Great Britain, 1985–1989).[6]

rates appear to have risen, with one study reporting a change between 1964 and 1968 and 1989 and 1993 from 1.68 to 2.45/1000 neonatal survivors.[7] The rate in babies born weighing > 2500 g has remained virtually constant over this period while at least some studies suggest that the rate in smaller babies has risen. As this is happening against a background of falling neonatal mortality in small infants, it may suggest that some infants, who would in earlier times have died in the neonatal period, are now surviving with cerebral palsy. There have also been increases in the life span of children with cerebral palsy, which will further increase the overall prevalence of cerebral palsy in the population.

It is generally believed that the life expectancy of children with a number of other chronic conditions has also increased, which is again likely to raise the prevalence of such conditions in the population. A survey carried out in one health district attempted to ascertain what proportion of children suffer from non-malignant 'life-threatening' conditions.[8] These were defined as conditions as a result of which the child had at least a 50% likelihood of dying before the age of 40 and included conditions such as cystic fibrosis, chronic renal failure and conditions causing central nervous system degeneration. The overall prevalence among children aged 0–19 was 1.2/1000, suggesting a large burden on families and services.

Mental health problems are extremely common in children and adolescents. Recent studies indicate that approximately one in five children and adolescents suffers from some type of mental health problem, although the prevalence is highly dependent on the definitions used.[9] Mental health problems include both profoundly disabling conditions such as autism and childhood psychoses and milder conditions such as attention deficit hyperactivity disorder and conduct disorder. One recent study in the UK has suggested that the prevalence of all autistic spectrum disorders is 62.6/10 000, although the prevalence of classical autism is much lower.[10] While it has been suggested that there has been a rise in the prevalence of these conditions, it is more likely that this represents changes in case definition and in professional awareness over time. Most of these children will continue to have significant problems throughout childhood and adulthood. Even apparently milder psychological problems such as behavioral difficulties in young children can have profound effects on the quality of families' lives. Garalda & Bailey[11] reported recently that, in one urban area in the UK, almost a quarter of 7–12-year-olds visiting a GP had a psychiatric disorder.

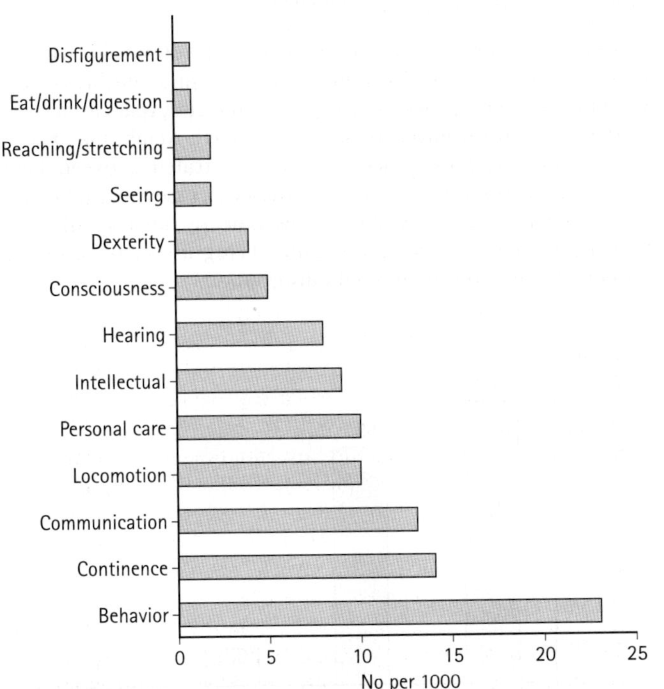

Fig. 2.9 Rates of disability per 1000 children aged 5–9 by functional category (Great Britain, 1985–1989).[6]

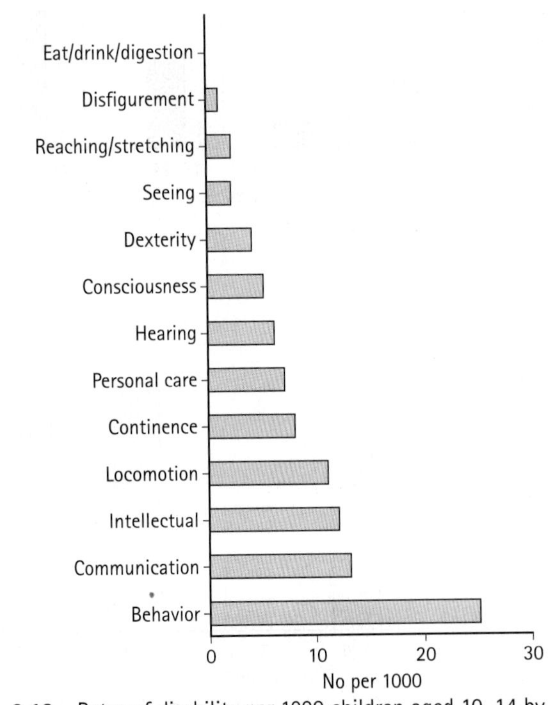

Fig. 2.10 Rates of disability per 1000 children aged 10–14 by functional category (Great Britain, 1985–1989).[6]

POPULATION DETERMINANTS OF CHILD HEALTH

The health of an individual is determined by a complex interaction between genetic factors, health behaviors and environmental influences.

AGE AND SEX STRUCTURE OF THE POPULATION

Between the ages of 5 and 15 the risk of death and severe illness is at its lowest, before rising again. Death rates are higher in boys than girls at all ages (Fig. 2.11).[1] The magnitude of the difference varies with age, rising from around 25% higher in boys from birth until 15 and then becoming more than twice as great in adolescence and early adulthood (Fig. 2.12).[1] Much of this increasing discrepancy between the sexes is due to the much higher rates of unintentional injuries in males, particularly later in childhood and adolescence. The death rates from all injuries and poisoning (which includes the small numbers of deaths due to intentional injuries) in the UK are shown in Figure 2.13,[1] broken down by age and sex.

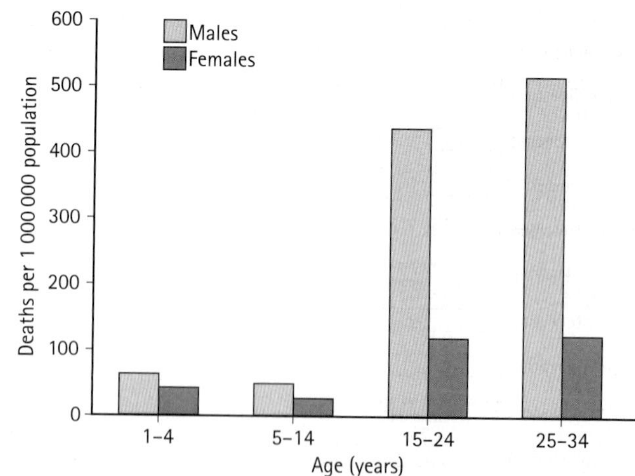

Fig. 2.13 Death rates from injury and poisoning by age and sex.[1]

GENETIC FACTORS

At an individual level there is no doubt that genetic factors play an important role in determining health status. At a population level however, there is little evidence that they have a significant effect on overall health. The genetic differences between human sub-populations are in fact very small and it appears that differences in health are largely accounted for by environmental and behavioral differences. Clearly there are differences between populations in the frequency of some specific single gene disorders – for instance, sickle cell disease is uncommon in northern Europeans and cystic fibrosis is uncommon in Africans – but these contribute relatively little to the health experience on a population level. In other words, an individual's genetic makeup is important in determining their risk of ill health within a particular subpopulation who share common experiences, but not in explaining the differences between these subpopulations. This is borne out by numerous studies of immigrant populations which suggest that, the longer they spend in a new country and the more they adopt the lifestyle of that country, the more nearly their health experience comes to resemble that of the native population. Most differences that continue to exist between immigrant groups and the native population can be explained on the basis of either behavioral or socioeconomic factors.

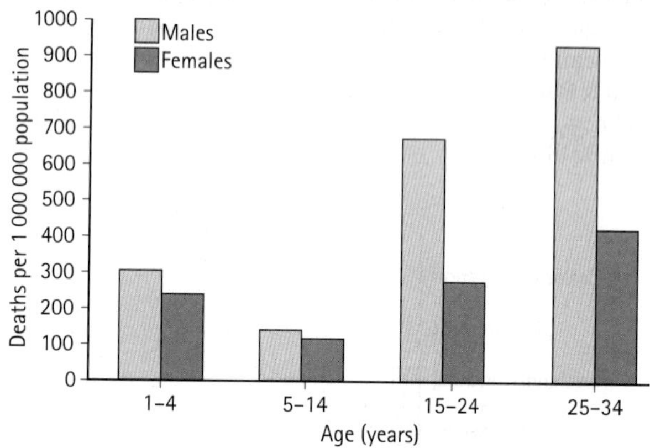

Fig. 2.11 Death rates by age and sex.[1]

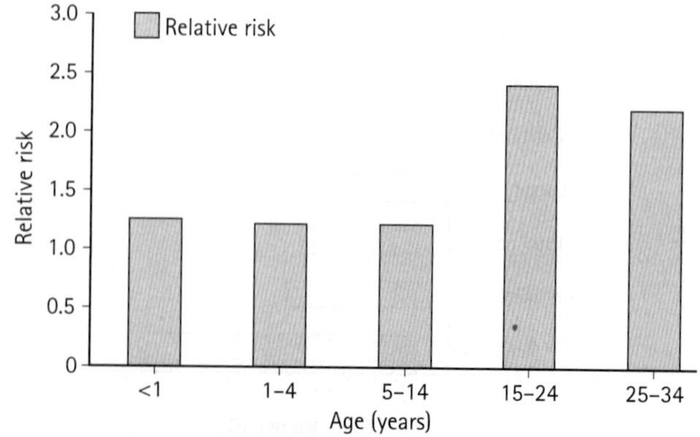

Fig. 2.12 Relative risk of death in males compared to females by age group.[1]

BIRTH WEIGHT AND GESTATION

Birth weight, reflecting both gestation and intrauterine growth, is a powerful predictor of mortality (Fig. 2.6) and morbidity (e.g. cerebral palsy, Fig. 2.14)[12] in childhood. In recent years it has been recognized that the effects of suboptimal birth weight may persist throughout life, with links being demonstrated between birth weight and cardiovascular and respiratory disease in adulthood. It appears that these adverse effects have a nearly linear relationship with birth weight rather than simply being associated with the lower extreme of the birth weight distribution.

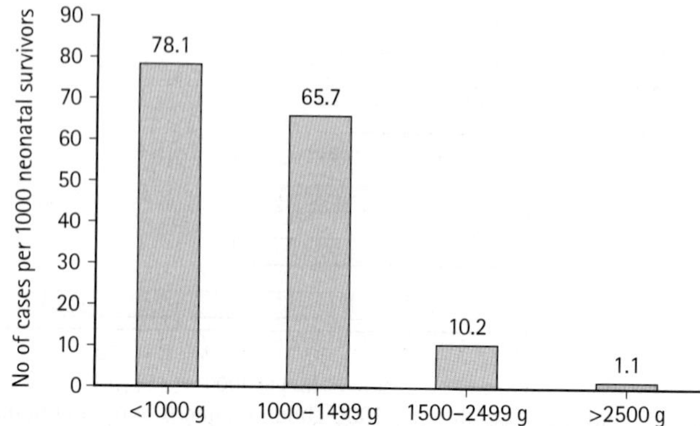

Fig. 2.14 Prevalence of cerebral palsy by birth weight.[12]

Many of the determinants of both prematurity and poor intrauterine growth remain to be elucidated, although some specific conditions such as pre-eclamptic toxemia are important in individuals. Poor intrauterine growth is associated with smoking during pregnancy and with socioeconomic deprivation. Diet has often been suggested as a possible cause of intrauterine growth retardation but good evidence for this is lacking, except for the effects of extreme malnutrition.

PHYSICAL ENVIRONMENT

While some specific environmental hazards have been clearly identified, the links between others such as damp, overcrowded housing or atmospheric pollution and ill health have been difficult to determine. Many of these, possibly disadvantageous, conditions tend to occur in combination with each other and with socioeconomic disadvantage, making it difficult to disentangle their effects. Many pollutants in the environment or in food are so widespread that investigation is difficult. It is also possible that it is the interactions between such pollutants that are important, which further complicates attempts to quantify their effects. It could be argued that, in these circumstances, it may be appropriate to accept lower levels of evidence before proceeding to action, sometimes referred to as the precautionary principle, than would generally be required for reaching conclusions about causal links.

SOCIAL FACTORS

Socioeconomic status (SES) is a powerful predictor of health outcome within all societies. Within poor countries, this is unsurprising, given that SES is linked to the availability of basic necessities including food and shelter. What is perhaps remarkable is that the link remains strong even in rich industrialized countries. What may seem equally surprising is that the differences exist, not simply between the poorest members of society and the rest of the population, but, for many important health outcomes, there is something approaching a linear relationship between SES and adverse outcome.

How best to measure SES in childhood remains a source of debate. It is clearly a complicated concept and it seems likely that different aspects of disadvantage will be important for different health outcomes. In the UK, SES has traditionally been measured using an occupational classification, the Registrar General's classification of social class. This scheme, first employed around the beginning of the twentieth century, assigns all occupations to six (originally five) groups based on a notion of a hierarchy of status (Table 2.4). Children are assigned to a social class based on the occupation of the 'head of the household', usually the father, or the mother if no father is present. It has been suggested that this may be a relatively poor measure of SES, especially for children, but it does have the advantage of having been used over a long period so that changes over time can be documented. Other classifications have been developed based on factors such as maternal education, income, access to material goods such as motor cars or telephones, type of housing and the nature of the area in which the family lives. Although the strength of the association between SES and a particular outcome may vary according to the measure used, the direction of effect is virtually always the same.

The effects of SES are observable from the beginnings of life, with a strong relationship between birth weight and SES. Figure 2.15[13] shows the proportion of infants born below 2500 g in SES deciles in one region of the UK (based on the characteristics of the small area in which they live).[13] Perhaps even more striking is the proportion of infants born weighing above 3500 g (regarded as being an optimum birth weight) in different SES deciles (Fig. 2.16).[13] In both figures there is a clear gradient across the different social groups. The magnitude of this effect is illustrated by the fact that this study reported that, if the whole population had the risk seen in the richest 10%, this would avoid 30% of all births below 2500 g and 32% of births below 1500 g.

In the UK in 1987–1991 the difference in life expectancy between children in social classes I and II and those in social class V was 5.2 years for boys and 3.4 years for girls.[14] The differences in mortality across social classes are present within each age group in childhood (Figs 2.17 and 2.18).[4,14] Particularly marked differences are seen in mortality from injuries and poisoning between the social classes; in 1989–1992 the risk of death from this cause in children in social class V was five times as high as that in social class I (Fig. 2 19).[15]

Table 2.4 The Registrar General's classification of social class

Social class	Description
I	Professional occupations (e.g. lawyer, doctor)
II	Intermediate occupations (including most managerial groups e.g. teacher, nurse)
IIINM	Non-manual skilled occupations (e.g. shop assistant, clerk)
IIIM	Manual skilled occupations (e.g. plumber)
IV	Partly skilled occupations (e.g. bus conducter, postman)
V	Unskilled occupations (e.g. laborer)

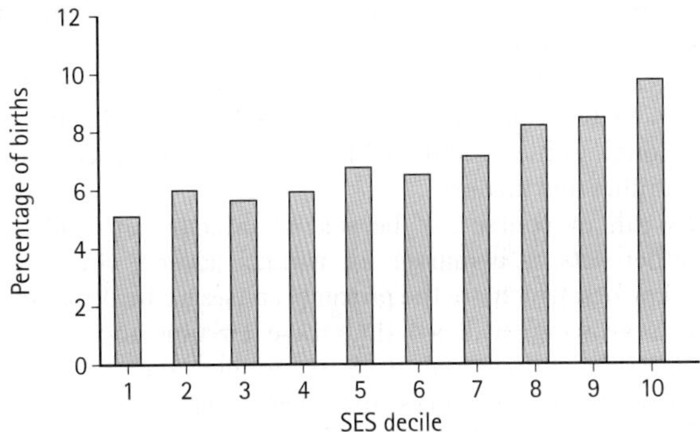

Fig. 2.15 Percentage of births <2500 g by SES decile in the West Midlands, UK.[13]

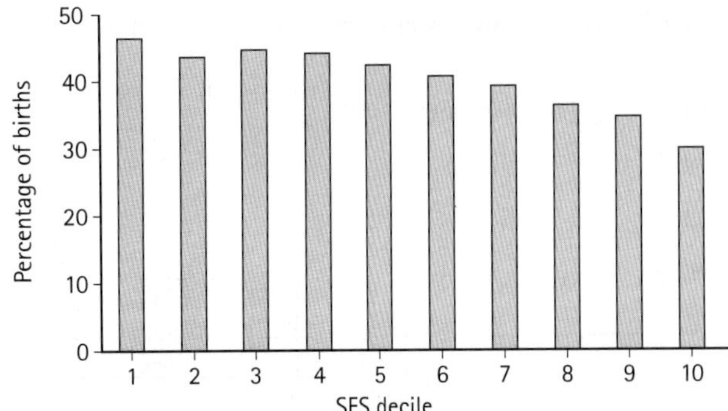

Fig. 2.16 Percentage of births >3500 g by SES decile in the West Midlands, UK.[13]

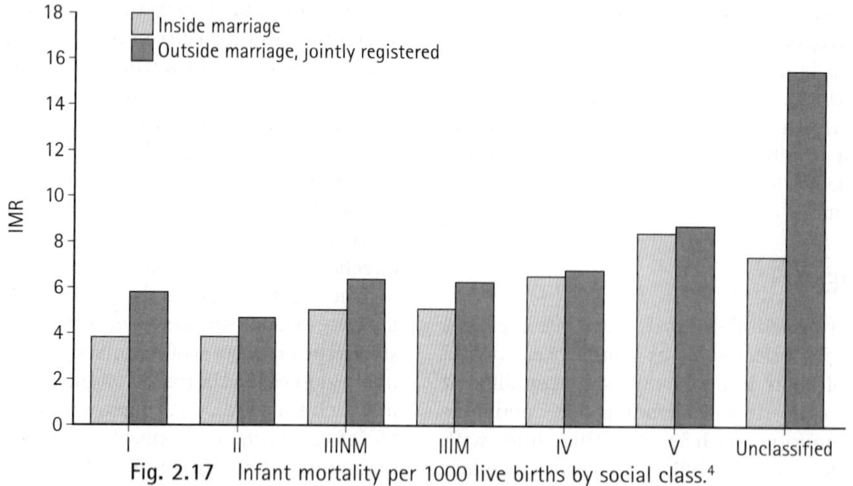

Fig. 2.17 Infant mortality per 1000 live births by social class.[4]

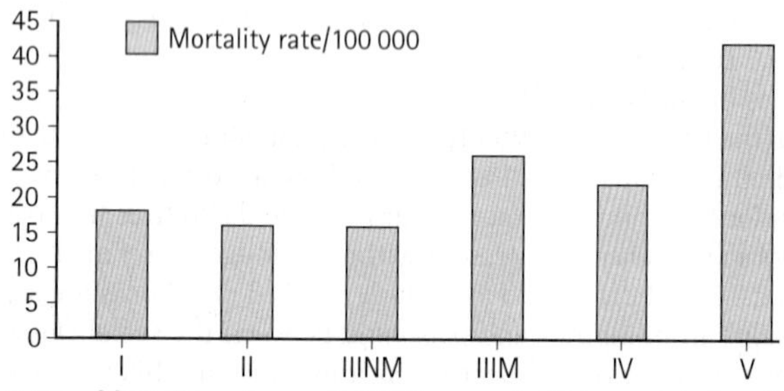

Fig. 2.18 Mortality rate per 100 000, ages 1–15 by social class.[14]

Similar differences are seen for most measures of morbidity, where figures are available, with large differences being shown between social groups for the risk of admission to hospital, for severe respiratory infections and for behavioral problems. Finally, SES in early childhood strongly predicts the likelihood of educational achievement, which in turn predicts later job opportunities and income.

SES can of course not be said to directly cause ill health, but rather acts as a marker for various adverse circumstances and behaviors, which are the proximal causes for health outcomes. There is growing evidence that these circumstances cumulate over the life course and that the longer a child spends in adverse social circumstances, the greater the risk of poor health outcome.

HEALTH BEHAVIORS

There is considerable evidence of the deleterious effects of a number of health behaviors by parents and children on the health of children. Smoking by parents, and by children, in particular, is a major cause of many adverse outcomes including intrauterine growth retardation, sudden infant death syndrome and respiratory disease. At least in the UK and the USA, smoking is much more common amongst people in poorer social circumstances and is likely to be one of the mechanisms through which SES has its effects on children's health. This close relationship between SES and smoking does, however, hamper efforts to estimate the magnitude of the effect of smoking per se as its effects may be confounded by other adverse circumstances.

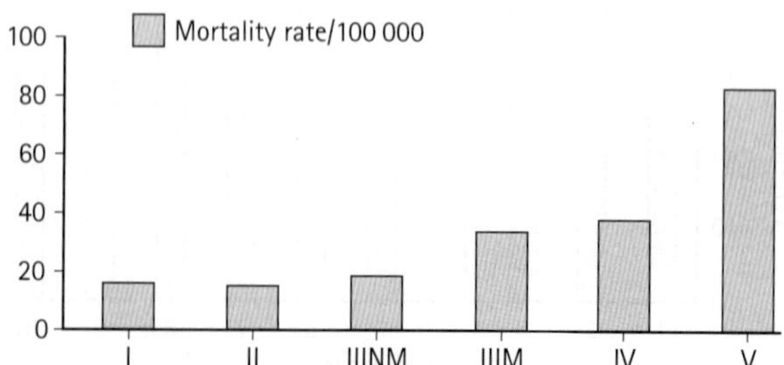

Fig. 2.19 Mortality rate per 100 000, from injuries and poisoning, ages 1–15 by social class.[15]

Harmful effects of poor diet and lack of exercise in childhood have also been suggested. Increases in the proportion of children who are overweight or obese have been reported in the UK and USA: one recent UK study reported that 22% of children aged 7–11 were overweight and 11.3% obese.[16] As there is substantial tracking between fatness in childhood and adulthood, this may have important implications for the risk of cardiovascular disease and type 2 diabetes in later life. It has been suggested that these increases are likely to reflect declining levels of physical activity and the increasing consumption of convenience foods, although clear evidence is lacking.

HEALTH SERVICES

Until recent years there has been surprisingly little evidence that health services are an important determinant of children's health. The obvious exceptions are immunization and public health measures such as the provision of safe water supplies. Even for those diseases preventable by immunization, much of the decline in mortality preceded the introduction of immunization. It is nonetheless true that immunization has been associated with dramatic declines in deaths from measles, polio, meningococcal disease and other conditions which were major causes of deaths into recent times.

It is clear that the major determinants of child health lie outside the realm of curative services and are related to social and environmental factors. However, in rich societies, the rates of mortality have fallen to very low levels and the importance of the effective management of relatively uncommon conditions has become proportionately more important in determining mortality rates. For instance, the widespread use of antenatal steroids in women in preterm labor and of surfactant in premature infants has led to substantial declines in mortality from idiopathic respiratory distress syndrome in neonates. Similarly, as malignant disease accounts for an increasing proportion of childhood deaths, improvements in cure rates due to medical management can have significant effects on childhood mortality rates.

While health services can significantly ameliorate the consequences of many diseases they can also result in an increased prevalence of children with significant morbidity. Some of the children who are saved from death may survive with significant morbidity and may be kept alive for long periods in spite of their disabilities. It is important that clinicians recognize both the importance of factors outside their control in determining children's health and the potential societal consequences of advances in technology.

REFERENCES (* Level 1 evidence)

1 Mortality data for England and Wales is summarised in publications from the Office for National Statistics. Available: http://www.statistics.gov.uk/

2 Office for National Statistics. Congenital anomaly statistics: notifications. Series MB3 no. 15. London: The Stationery Office; 2001.

3 Guyer B, Hoyert DL, Martin JA, et al. Annual summary of vital statistics – 1998. Pediatrics 1999; 104:1229–1246.

4 Office of National Statistics. Mortality statistics: childhood, infant and perinatal. Series DH3 no. 32. London: The Stationery Office; 2001.

5 Office for National Statistics. Living in Britain: results from the 2000/1 General Household Survey. London: The Stationery Office; 2001.

6 Bone M, Meltzer H. The prevalence of disability among children. OPCS Surveys of Disability in Great Britain, report 3. London: HMSO; 1989.

7 Colver A, Gibson M, Hey EN, et al. Increasing rates of cerebral palsy across the severity spectrum in north-east England 1964–1993. Arch Dis Child 2000; 83:F7–F12.

8 Lenton S, Stallard P, Lewis M, et al. Prevalence and morbidity associated with non-malignant, life-threatening conditions in childhood. Child Care Health Dev 2001; 27(5):389–398.

9 Target M, Fonagy P. The psychological treatment of child and adolescent psychiatric disorder. In: Royh A, Fonagy P, eds. What works for whom? A critical review of pschotherapy research. New York: The Guilford Press; 1996:263–320.

10 Chakrabati S, Fombonne E. Pervasive developmental disorders in pre-school children. JAMA 2001; 285:3093–3099.

11 Garalda ME, Bailey D. Children with psychiatric disorder in primary care. J Child Psychol Psychiatry 1986; 27:612–624.

12 Pharoah POD, Cooke T, Johnson MA, et al. Epidemiology of cerebral palsy in England and Scotland, 1984–9. Arch Dis Child Fetal Neonatal Ed 1998; 79:F21–F25.

13 Bambang S, Spencer NJ, Gill L, et al. Socioeconomic status and birthweight: comparison of an area-based measure with the Registrar General's social class. J Epidemiol Community Health 1999; 53:495–498.

14 Office for National Statistics. Health inequalities. Series DS no. 15. London: The Stationery Office; 1997.

15 Roberts I, Power C. Does the decline in child injury mortality vary by social class? A comparison of class specific mortality in 1981 and 1991. BMJ 1996; 313:784–786.

16 Rudolf MCJ, Sahota P, Barth JH. Increasing prevalence of obesity in primary school children: a cohort study. BMJ 2001; 322:1094–1095.

3

History taking and physical examination

C Mae Wong, Ian A Laing

INTRODUCTION

Successful interpretation of a pediatric patient's problems is dependent upon a thorough history and physical examination. In an era of increased availability of near-patient testing and sophisticated laboratory and imaging investigations, it remains important that sound basic clinical skills are preserved.[1] History taking and physical examination should be goal oriented, targeted to confirm or refute a likely diagnosis or list of differential diagnoses, rather than being too broad ranging and non-specific. However, goal-oriented methods are best learnt through practice. For the purposes of this chapter, a wider scope will be discussed.

AGE-APPROPRIATE CONSULTATION AND COMMUNICATION SKILLS

A medical consultation is frequently a source of anxiety for children and their parents. Sitting or kneeling to be at eye level with a child is reassuring and a white laboratory coat is unnecessary. Introduce yourself, shake hands, and ask what the child likes to be called. Never use 'it' in reference to a child at any age and do not get the gender wrong. Maintain good eye contact throughout and smile if appropriate. Toys and quiet music can be useful adjuncts, and complimentary remarks or social conversation usually win cooperation.

The history of the presenting complaint should be directed to the child whenever possible. Open questioning is recommended. Older children can provide much detail, and even a younger child can give useful information with age-appropriate questioning. If possible, ascertain what descriptive words each child commonly uses for various symptoms. The parents should then be asked for information that the child cannot give, as well as their personal observations. It is also essential to find out what their main concerns are and to address these. Mothers and parents of younger children generally give more accurate histories, regardless of education or occupation.[2] Whenever a history is obtained from a third party, although astute parental observation can be of benefit, limitations such as misinterpretation and bias must also be bornein mind.

The physical examination can be used to obtain important clinical information, assist development, and teach children and parents about health and lifestyle choices. Adapting examination techniques to the child's developmental level improves these results.[3] Children can be divided by age groups into:

Neonates	First 28 days of life
Infants	First year
Preschool children	1 to 4 years
School children	5 to 15 years
Adolescents	13 to 19 years

INTERDISCIPLINARY ASSESSMENTS

Whether dealing with routine child health surveillance or with behavioral difficulties, school problems or allegations of abuse, interdisciplinary assessments are valuable. Parent and teacher interviews may assist in implementing changes towards a child's continuing care.[4]

CONFIDENTIALITY WITH ADOLESCENTS

The teenage years can be a difficult time of transition. Effective care at this age can help preserve good health, development, and future opportunities, yet adolescents tend to underutilize health care resources due to concerns about confidentiality. Substance abuse, sexually transmitted diseases and unplanned pregnancy are examples of health issues that are more readily discussed in confidence with parents absent. Children with chronic illnesses who have attended outpatient clinics with parents for years, may, as adolescents, benefit from a confidential consultation to discuss sensitive issues. Good communication is vital to enable the parents to understand and allow their adolescent's move towards self-responsibility for health care. The adolescents must also be aware of circumstances that may require disclosure of confidential information, such as a life-threatening emergency. The General Medical Council has produced Standards of Practice on Patient Confidentiality, and the American Academy of Pediatrics has a policy statement on Confidentiality in Adolescent Health Care, both available on respective web sites (www.gmc-uk.org and www.aap.org).

CULTURAL AWARENESS

With increased ethnic diversity in the UK, it is important for health service providers to be both culturally aware and culturally sensitive.[5] There are ethnic differences in indicators of child health status, such as birth weight and infant mortality. Some pathological conditions are also more common in particular racial groups (Table 3.1). There are variations in rate of growth and development,[6] and screening and immunization requirements and uptake may also differ.

When there are ethnic differences between the caregiver and child, special attention must be paid to language, socioeconomic status, religious beliefs and cultural traditions. The caregiver must be aware that cultural differences can influence perceptions of health, illness and treatments. Verbal and non-verbal communication, as well as expression of symptoms, can be different. There may also be heightened anxiety for the child and parents.

Table 3.1 Diseases commoner to particular ethnic groups

Ethnic groups	Diseases
African	Sickle cell disease, glucose-6-phosphate dehydrogenase deficiency, tuberculosis, HIV
Amish	Ellis–van Creveld syndrome
Ashkenazi Jews	Gaucher disease, Tay–Sachs disease, breast and ovarian cancers, other autosomal recessive diseases
Asian Indians	Tuberculosis, autosomal recessive diseases
Chinese	Nasopharyngeal carcinoma, glucose-6-phosphate dehydrogenase deficiency
Hopi Indians	Oculocutaneous albinism
Mediterranean	Thalassemia, glucose-6-phosphate dehydrogenase deficiency
Yupik Eskimos	Congenital adrenal hyperplasia

POVERTY

Unfortunately, poverty can be linked to racial and cultural background. There are inevitable inequalities in the global village, and health service providers should therefore also be aware of those children at greater risk of malnutrition, health difficulties and delayed development.

TELEPHONE CONSULTATIONS

In rural areas, telephone consultations can form a substantial part of basic health care. Common complaints include cough, diarrhea and rashes. Certain vital questions, such as breathing difficulty with cough, abdominal pain and state of hydration with diarrhea, and the characteristics of rashes, give clues to illness severity in place of examining the child. These should form a fundamental part of the telephone history taking and yet the majority tend to be overlooked.[7]

CLINICAL HISTORY

In addition to the standard information on name, age, sex and race of the child, the accompanying adult and their relationship to the child should also be recorded.

PRESENTING COMPLAINT

Open questioning should lead to a chronological description of events that should initially be obtained uninterrupted. Different presenting complaints will then require different lines of specific questioning (Table 3.2). In addition, information should be acquired on any previous treatment sought or obtained for the current illness, whether the illness is affecting school attendance, and possible infectious contacts if relevant. If the problem is behavioral or emotional, it may be prudent to discuss sensitive issues in the child's absence.

PAST MEDICAL HISTORY

Previous illnesses

Infant records, health visitor records and baby books may help. Previous illnesses should be listed in chronological order and hospital admissions recorded. Ask specifically about childhood infections, such as measles, mumps, rubella and chickenpox.

Table 3.2 Clinical history points and relevant amplification

System	Symptom	Amplification
General	Pyrexia and night sweats	Duration, method of ascertaining temperature, rigors, sheet changing
	Weight loss	Amount, method of weighing, duration, other symptoms
	Rashes	Site, size, number of lesions, color, nature (petechiae, purpura, macules, papules, pustules, vesicles, bullae, ulcers), associated pain or pruritus
	Cyanosis	Peripheral or central, intermittent or persistent, association with environmental temperature
	Pain	Onset, nature, duration, severity, precipitating factors, relieving factors, associated symptoms, treatment sought
Respiratory	Discharge from nose, eyes or ears	Nature and duration
	Sore throat or earache	Localization, associated pyrexia or other respiratory symptoms
	Cough	Character, duration, exacerbating factors, sleep disturbance, association with pain, whoop, vomiting, other respiratory symptoms, nature of sputum
	Stridor	Associated color change or apnea
	Wheeze	Precipitating or exacerbating factors, diurnal variation, home peak flow testing
	Snoring	Change in cry or voice, mouth breathing
	Dyspnea	At rest or with exercise, intermittent or persistent, nocturnal or diurnal, association with cough, cyanosis or breath-holding
	Apnea	Duration, association with infection or airway obstruction
Cardiovascular	Breathlessness	At rest, or exertion or with feeding
	Tiredness and lethargy	Exercise tolerance, interest in play
	Slow feeding	Associated breathlessness
	Poor weight gain	Dietary intake
	Pallor or cyanosis	Intermittent or persistent, associated with crying or straining
Gastrointestinal	Appetite and feed tolerance need for special diet	Temporary or persistent impairment, food faddism, parental attitudes towards diet, vitamin or other supplementation
	Dysphagia	Often functional food refusal rather than organic, in organic dysphagia food is swallowed but soon regurgitated
	Thirst	Assess total daily intake of fluid and output of urine
	Vomiting	Amount, frequency, association with feeds, effortless or projectile, bilious or bloodstained, association with pain or impairment of consciousness
	Constipation	Consistency, frequency, pain on defecation
	Diarrhea	Nature of stool, consistency, frequency, presence of blood
	Abdominal pain	Site, nature, timing, duration, intermittent or constant, aggravation by breathing or movement, relationship of feeds, bowel movements or micturition, association with other gastrointestinal symptoms, sore throat, cough or purpura
	Jaundice	Onset, duration, nature of stool and urine, associated vomiting
Genitourinary	Incontinence or bed-wetting	Day or night, deterioration from before or regression in development, associated urinary symptoms, parental reaction, stress or bullying, treatment sought or tried
	Increased urinary frequency	Recent change in pattern, urine volume
	Dysuria	Pain, burning or cry related to micturition
	Change in odor or appearance of urine	Associated urinary symptoms, hematuria
Neurodevelopmental	Headaches	Site, manner of onset, severity, associated symptoms, aura
	Visual disturbances	Fixation and following, myopia or hypermetropia, color blindness, colliding with objects, associated symptoms
	Speech	Delay in onset or regression, nature, difficult comprehension or expression
	Hearing	Unresponsiveness or inattentiveness, functional or organic, family history
	Fits, Faints, Floppiness	Time, duration, frequency, tonic and clonic components, state of consciousness, known triggers, associated color change, oculogyrus, choking or incontinence, injury sustained
	Abnormalities in posture, gait or coordination	Deterioration from before or regression in development, falling and injury
	Involuntary movement	Nature, aggravating factors, injury suffered as a result
	Changes in mood, activity or behavior	Performance in normal play and household activities, interest in surroundings and excursions, tiring easily
	School performance	Normal or special school, extra support, bullying

Birth history

This is especially relevant with infants and younger children. Details should be elucidated regarding:

- mother's health during pregnancy and exposure to any drugs or radiation;
- place of child's birth;
- gestational age at birth;
- mode of delivery and presentation;
- birth weight and Apgar score;
- problems around birth or need for admission to a special care baby unit;
- method of feeding;
- vitamin K prophylaxis.

Growth and development

These are detailed in Chapters 7 and 13. The following questions about achievement of major milestones usually suffice:

- smiling, head control, fixing and following;
- sitting independently, crawling or bottom shuffling, walking;
- age at first spoken word;
- result of the 8-month hearing test or neonatal audiological screening;
- ability to use a cup and spoon;
- ability to understand and obey simple commands;
- ability to identify different parts of the body;
- age at successful toilet training.

However, further details are appropriate if chronic illness, growth or neurological problems are the presenting complaint. Particular attention should then be paid to dissociated development. For example, specific delay in language acquisition may indicate hearing impairment or speech disorder, and standing with assistance before sitting could signal spastic diplegia. Approximately 15% of children with cognitive impairment achieve normal motor milestones in infancy.

SCHOOL PERFORMANCE

Besides being a helpful 'ice-breaker', this is a useful question to identify developmental problems or the impact of a chronic illness on older children. The name and type of school also give useful information on social background.

FEEDING AND DIET

Illness can temporarily impair feeding, but more persistent disturbance of feeding could signal chronic organic disease, food faddism, or an emerging eating disorder. There may also be unusual parental ideas regarding diet.

DRUG HISTORY AND ALLERGIES

List all medications taken including dosage, frequency and duration. Establish what drugs have already been prescribed for the current illness. Remember to ask also about non-drug allergies.

IMMUNIZATIONS

It is important to ask about immunizations in more detail than whether they are 'up-to-date'. For example, bacillus Calmette–Guérin (BCG) vaccination status in an Asian child with respiratory symptoms is relevant. Measles, mumps and rubella (MMR) vaccination uptake has been less than optimal due to adverse media reporting and there will be children with an incomplete immunization schedule for this triad of infections. Check for booster updates. The current UK immunization program is detailed in Chapter 8.

FAMILY HISTORY

A complicated family history may be better illustrated with a coded family tree (genogram) than in words (Fig. 3.1). Genograms have been shown to enable more thorough history taking, especially regarding family structure, major life events, repetitive illnesses, and family relationship.[8,9] They are also easily interpreted accurately when a standardized version is used.[9] Ask tactfully about consanguinity if an autosomal recessive condition is suspected, especially in certain ethnic and religious groups.

SOCIAL HISTORY

With sensitive questioning, information should be obtained about the parents' occupations, smoking status, type and nature of home. If relevant, further details should be sought on whether there is travel or residence abroad, single parenthood, financial problems, drug abuse (including alcohol) or difficulties with the law. Psychosocial and basic demographic history documentation tends to be poor,[10] yet can be an important indicator to causes for recurrent visits to pediatric emergency departments.

PHYSICAL EXAMINATION

The child's dignity should always be preserved. Children should not be separated from their parents unnecessarily and it is often much easier auscultating a quiet child on a parent's knee than an upset one on the bed. Establish a rapport with the parents as children quickly sense a lack of compassion. Minimize the number of people in the room. Let the parents do the undressing of the child. It may be considerate to use blankets or maintain partial clothing for older children. Ask permission before examining an older child or adolescent.

Engaging the cooperation of the child allows for much easier and efficient physical examination. Play or turning the

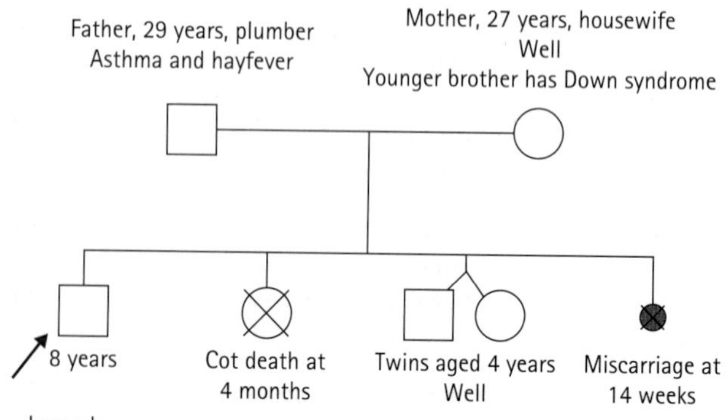
Father, 29 years, plumber
Asthma and hayfever
Mother, 27 years, housewife
Well
Younger brother has Down syndrome
8 years
Cot death at
4 months
Twins aged 4 years
Well
Miscarriage at
14 weeks
Legend:
• Squares indicate males and circles female
• The index case is marked with an arrow
• The birth order should be set out from left to right
• A crossed out symbol indicates a death
• Spouses are connected with lines, separations and divorces indicated by slash lines running through the lines
• Birth, marriage, divorce, or death dates may be indicated by the initial and date (e.g. b.89)

Fig. 3.1 Example of a genogram.

examination into a little game can calm a frightened child. Speak to the child in reassuring tones and draw conversations into topical books, cartoons or toys. Let the child handle the stethoscope or otoscope. The physical examination should commence only when the child's confidence has been gained. Be opportunistic: auscultate sleeping children with a warm stethoscope before waking them up for the rest of the examination. Unpleasant procedures should be left until the end, for example otoscopy, pharyngeal inspection, hip or rectal examinations. Be aware of the child's response throughout.

GENERAL ASSESSMENT

This should have begun to take place even during history taking. Document any dysmorphic features. The child's activity and behavior, as well as interaction with others, can be observed during conversation. The facies may reveal whether the child is well or ill or in pain. Such an initial overall assessment has been found to be a key skill in evaluating febrile children, but has limited sensitivity and its accuracy varies with experience.[11,12] Observe the child's standard of hygiene.

Activity, behavior and parent–child interaction

The level of activity and type of behavior can be a good clue to illness severity. Watching the parent–child interaction can provide subtle clues to psychosocial disruptions within the family. Some parents overdominate their children while others make no attempt to control them.

State of nutrition

The axillae, abdomen, buttocks and thighs give indications of loose skin and creasing with weight loss and malnutrition.

GROWTH PARAMETERS

Weight, height and head circumference should be plotted on appropriate centile charts. Accurate measurements are vital. Parent-held records might be more useful for identifying trends in growth if it is the first consultation. Use the most up-to-date charts available, which will be more representative of the current population, and remember that there are special charts for different age groups and children with Down syndrome.

A neonate normally loses up to 12% of body weight in the first few days of life, but should regain birth weight by 10 days of age, and subsequently gain approximately 30 g per day. Birth weight is doubled by 5 months and tripled at about 1 year. A young child's expected weight in kilograms can then be estimated from the formula: age in years plus 4, multiplied by 2.

Standing height, or crown–heel length in infants, usually correlates with weight. At birth, length is approximately 50 cm, increasing to 75 cm at 1 year and 100 cm at 4 years. Subsequently there should be an annual gain of approximately 5 cm. Remember that body proportions change with age (Fig. 3.2).

Head circumference is routinely measured as the maximal occipitofrontal circumference. At birth, the average is 35 cm, increasing to 40 cm at 3 months and 47 cm at 1 year. The subsequent annual increase is 0.5 cm from 2 to 7 years, and 0.3 cm from 8 to 12 years.

The trend in weight, length or head circumference gain is more significant than any absolute value. Dissociation between any of the anthropometric parameters may indicate underlying disease, such as hypothyroidism, malnutrition, obesity, or Marfan syndrome (for growth charts, see Ch. 13).

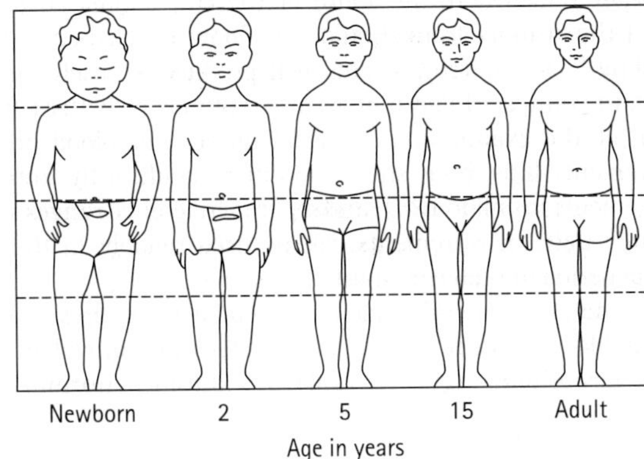

Fig. 3.2 Body proportions at different ages.

TEMPERATURE

This should be recorded in degrees Celsius. Normal core temperature should be 36.5–37.5°C. Temperature can be measured at various sites (sublingual, rectal, tympanic or axilla) as well as using different devices (mercury thermometer, digital thermometer, tympanic infrared thermometer, or color-change chemical thermometer). Rectal, sublingual and tympanic temperatures correspond to core temperature better than axillary temperature.[13–15] Axillary temperatures are accurate in neonates, being representative of sublingual or rectal temperatures and detecting pyrexia with a sensitivity of 98%.[16,17] However, in older infants and children, axillary temperatures perform less well and detect pyrexia with a sensitivity of only 47%.[16] One degree Celsius should be added to the axillary temperature for any child older than a month of age.[17] Temperature readings also take longer to stabilize using the axillary route: the thermometer should be left in place for 4 min as opposed to 2 min for the oral or rectal routes.[16] Forehead liquid crystal strips are even less accurate than axillary temperature.[17]

Age, presence of fever,[18] and environment[19,20] can affect device accuracy. Digital and color-change chemical thermometers correlate well with glass/mercury thermometers in infants.[19] Infrared tympanic membrane thermometry is a newer development. Tympanic membrane temperature recordings have also been evaluated for use in infants, and have been validated for well preterm infants down to 27 weeks gestation,[20,21] although some earlier studies reported poor detection of pyrexia.[22,23]

BLOOD PRESSURE

Practice in pediatric blood pressure measurement has been found to vary widely in the UK, with further variation in what are deemed to be acceptable limits for normal blood pressure.[24,25] Pediatric normograms are available as blood pressure changes with age.[26,27]

The gold standard for blood pressure measurement is invasive continuous intra-arterial waveform readings. Apart from allowing trend monitoring to look for gradual changes in status, the pattern of the waveform may indicate pathology, such as a bisferiens peak in persistent ductus arteriosus.[28] Non-invasive methods include the manual auscultatory method, and also automatic oscillometric and Doppler methods. Non-invasive oscillometric measurements have been found to be reliable in healthy settled neonates.[29] Pulse oximetry waveform systolic blood pressure measurements are a newer development that may be useful in patients on transport, but require further validation for regular use.[30]

Non-invasive blood pressure should be measured with an appropriate cuff, where the width of the cuff should cover two-thirds of the distance from shoulder to elbow. Labeled cuffs can be misleading.[31] Too narrow a cuff will produce a falsely elevated reading. In younger children, measurement may be better left until the end of the examination to avoid upset. Calf blood pressure measurements have been shown to differ significantly from arm measurements in children[32,33] and separate reference ranges should be used.[33] Calf measurements can be used reliably in the early neonatal period in preterm infants.[34]

In neonates, a general guide to acceptable blood pressure is for the mean blood pressure to be at least numerically equivalent to the infant's gestational age.[35,36] Table 3.3 outlines normal blood pressure ranges for older children.

EXAMINATION OF INDIVIDUAL SYSTEMS

In clinical pediatric practice, examination should ideally be by region rather than by individual systems, so that the child is minimally disturbed or handled. However, for the purposes of this chapter, individual systems will be detailed. Tables 3.4 and 3.5 provide possible interpretations for some common physical signs. Landmarks for a child's chest are shown in Figure 3.3.

MORPHOLOGY

The head, face, neck, eyes, ears, mouth, hands and feet can all give clues to normal or abnormal morphology (Table 3.4). Different head shapes are shown in Figure 3.4. The anterior fontanelle is diamond-shaped and measures approximately 2.5 cm across at birth, although this can vary widely due to different degrees of molding. It closes at about 18 months. The posterior fontanelle measures 0.5 cm and closes soon after birth. Tension should be assessed. The cranial sutures tend to be heaped up from molding, but may occasionally be prematurely fused due to craniosynostosis. Widely separated sutures may indicate hydrocephalus or raised intracranial pressure. If suspected, auscultation over various cranial regions may yield cranial bruits of an arteriovenous malformation.

Ear position, size and shape should be noted. A normally positioned ear should have its upper third set above a horizontal line at eye level. For eyes, distance apart may be determined in terms of inner-canthal, midpupillary or outer-canthal measurements. Normograms for these and ear length are available in textbooks of morphology.[37]

SKIN AND MUCOUS MEMBRANES

Overall inspection of the skin for cyanosis, jaundice or rashes is made. Causes of common rashes are listed in Table 3.4. The mucous membranes are a poor guide to anemia, but may be useful for estimating state of hydration.

RESPIRATORY

Inspection for cyanosis and finger clubbing should be performed. If respiratory tract infection is the presenting complaint, note conjunctival suffusion, nasal congestion and discharge, ear-pulling, or excessive salivation.

Record respiratory rate. Chest infection is unlikely in the absence of tachypnea.[38] Periodic breathing, where respirations are irregular with intermittent apneic pauses up to 10 s, is a common occurrence in infants and neonates. Describe the chest shape, including hyperinflation, Harrison's sulci, scoliosis, pectus excavatum or pectus carinatum. The chest is almost circular in transverse section in neonates, with the ratio of anteroposterior to transverse diameter falling to the adult value of 0.75 by 3 years of age. Chest expansion from full expiration to full inspiration can be measured at the nipple line in cooperative older children, and should be 4 cm or more. Look for asymmetry during chest movement. Infants tend to have prominent abdominal breathing movements.

Signs of respiratory distress in children include recession or indrawing (sternal, subcostal, intercostal, supraclavicular or tracheal tug), nasal flaring, grunting, and use of accessory muscles of respiration. Characteristic coughs may give the diagnosis, such as the seal-barking cough of croup or the moist, rattly cough of bronchiolitis. Even before formal auscultation, an inspiratory stridor or expiratory wheeze may be audible. However, remember that a critically ill asthmatic may not wheeze but have a 'silent chest' due to a severely diminished tidal volume. This is an emergency.

Palpation for tracheal deviation is unpleasant and probably unhelpful in younger children. Percussion comparing both sides of the chest may occasionally identify extensive consolidation or effusion, or a pneumothorax. However, if this procedure is likely to upset a sensitive child, it should be omitted or left until after auscultation, as it seldom yields additional information. Chest transillumination for a pneumothorax may be used in neonates.[39]

Auscultation for breath sounds and added sounds should be performed. Vocal resonance and whispering pectoriloquy may be used in cooperative older children as in adults. Transmitted sounds from the upper respiratory tract and contralateral chest are common in younger children, and normal breath sounds tend to sound more intense than in adults. In infants and neonates, extensive lung disease may be present with minimal signs on auscultation.[38] Finally, palpate the neck for lymphadenopathy or other masses. Otoscopy and pharyngeal examination are left until the end. Remember that the external auricular canals are highly sensitive.

CARDIOVASCULAR

Significant cardiac disease is usually associated with poor growth. Other general signs to look for include cyanosis, pallor, tachypnea, dyspnea, and sweating. Finger clubbing may not be obvious before

Table 3.3 Normal ranges or values for physiological variables across different ages

Sign	Preterm neonate	Term neonate	Up to 1 year	1–5 years	10 years
Heart rate (beats per min)	120–160	100–140	80–120	70–100	60–80
Blood pressure (mm/Hg)					
Systolic	*Mean* BP at least numerically equivalent to gestational age		80	85	95
Diastolic			50	55	60
Respiratory rate (breaths per min)	40–60	30–50	20–40	20–30	15–20

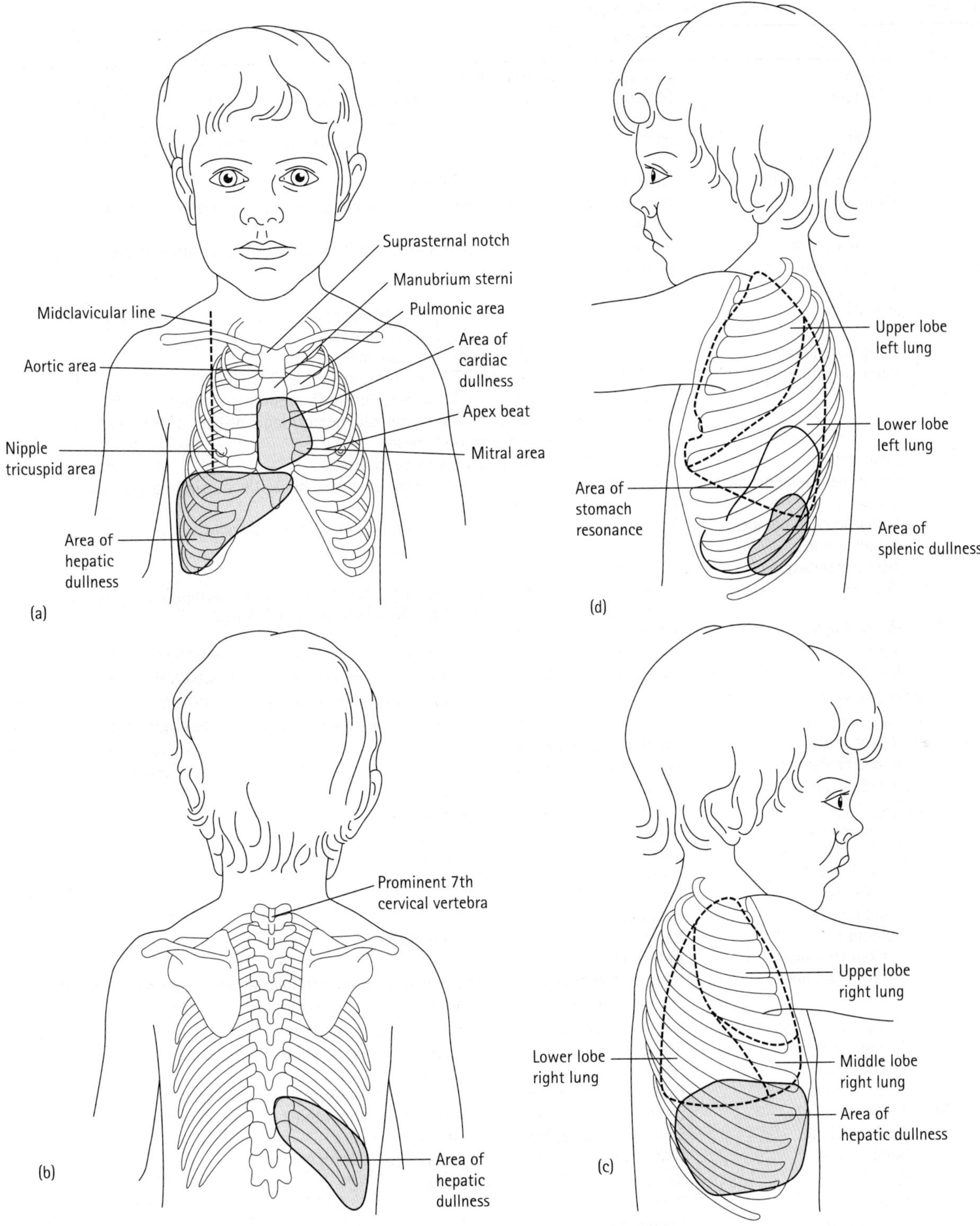

Fig. 3.3 Landmarks in a child's chest: (a) anterior, (b) posterior, (c) right lateral, (d) left lateral.

6 months of age, even in cyanotic congenital heart disease. Assess pulse characteristics as you would for an adult. The resting pulse rate is quicker in neonates and infants than in older children (Table 3.3). Palpate the brachial rather than radial pulse in infants. The femoral pulses are best felt with the hips extended and abducted. Weak femoral pulses may be a better indicator of coarctation of the aorta in tachycardic infants than assessing radiofemoral or brachiofemoral delay. The jugular venous pressure is often difficult to assess in younger children but prominent pulsation may be seen in tricuspid regurgitation and cannon waves in congenital heart block.

Look for the scars of previous cardiothoracic surgery. Be aware that modern advances in laparoscopic surgery may result in lack of the traditionally recognized scars.

Table 3.4 Common physical signs and their possible causes

System	Sign	Possible causes
Skin	Albinism	Inherited, Chediak–Higashi syndrome
	Alopecia	Stress, protein deficiency, iron or zinc deficiency, hypopituitarism, rapid weight loss, SLE, hypothyroidism, thyrotoxicosis, diabetes mellitus, renal failure, drugs
	Bruising	Hemophilia, non-accidental injury, leukemia, ITP, liver failure, scurvy, Cushing's syndrome, drugs
	Butterfly rash	SLE, photodermatitis
	Café-au-lait spots	Neurofibromatosis, tuberous sclerosis
	Cyanosis	Congenital cyanotic heart disease, persistent pulmonary hypertension, cardiovascular collapse, respiratory failure
	Depigmentation	Pityriasis versicolor or alba, vitiligo, postinflammatory, hypopituitarism, leprosy
	Dermographism	Allergy or hypersensitivity
	Herald patch	Pityriasis rosea, drugs
	Hirsutism	Congenital adrenal hyperplasia, pituitary–gonadal tumors, hypothyroidism, steroid therapy, Albright syndrome, mucopolysaccharidoses
	Lymphadenopathy	Infection, chronic inflammation, lymphoma, metastases
	Petechiae/purpura	Meningococcal septicemia, ITP, vasculitis, leukemia, DIC, Henoch–Schönlein purpura, Waterhouse–Friderichsen syndrome, Cushing's syndrome, congenital infection, neonatal alloimmune thrombocytopenia, hemorrhagic disease of the newborn, infective endocarditis, trauma, drugs
	Scaly rash	Seborrheic dermatitis, pityriasis rosea, psoriasis
	Spider nevi/telangiectasia	Liver cirrhosis, thyrotoxicosis, systemic sclerosis, hepatitis, ataxia telangiectasia
	Striae	Cushing's syndrome or disease
	Subcutaneous nodules	Neurofibromatosis, tuberous sclerosis, rheumatic fever, sarcoid
	Target lesions	Erythema multiforme, Stevens–Johnson syndrome
	Tissue crepitations	Subcutaneous emphysema
	Vesicles	Herpes zoster, herpes simplex, impetigo, contact dermatitis, pemphigus, pemphigoid, incontinentia pigmenti, epidermolysis bullosa, burns, drugs
	White forelock	Waardenburg syndrome
	Xanthoma	Hyperlipidemia, diabetes, cholestasis
	Xeroderma	Ichthyosis, hypothyroidism, seborrheic dermatitis, eczema, psoriasis
Head	Microcephaly	Congenital infection, chromosomal abnormality, perinatal asphyxia
	Macrocephaly	Hydrocephalus, achondroplasia, gigantism, mucopolysaccharidoses, familial megalencephaly
	Acrocephaly	Apert and Crouzon syndromes
	Brachycephaly	Positional, Down syndrome
	Dolichocephaly	Ex-preterm infant
	Plagiocephaly	Positional, coronal suture craniosynostosis
	Scaphocephaly	Sagittal suture craniosynostosis
	Prominent occiput	Edward syndrome, Beckwith–Wiedemann syndrome
	Frontal bossing	Rickets, chondrodysplasia, storage diseases
	Craniotabes	Rickets, prematurity
	Scalp defects	Patau syndrome
	Bulging fontanelle	Raised intracranial pressure, meningitis
	Sunken fontanelle	Dehydration
	Delayed fontanelle closure	Rickets, hypothyroidism, hydrocephalus, chondrodysplasias and chondrodysgeneses, other chromosomal abnormality
Face and neck	Moon face	Cushing's syndrome or disease, Prader–Willi syndrome
	Triangular face	Russell–Silver syndrome, osteogenesis imperfecta, Turner syndrome
	Coarse face	Hypothyroidism, mucopolysaccharidoses
	Micrognathia	Familial, Pierre–Robin sequence, other chromosomal abnormalities
	Torticollis	Sternomastoid tumor, corpus striatum or labyrinthine disease, 11th cranial nerve palsy
	Neck webbing	Turner syndrome, Noonan syndrome
	Saddle nose	Down syndrome, chondrodysplasias, fetal teratogenicity
Eyes	Aniridia	Aniridia–Wilm's tumor association
	Blue sclera	Osteogenesis imperfecta
	Buphthalmos	Congenital glaucoma
	Cataract	Congenital infection, Down syndrome, galactosemia, Alport syndrome, diabetes mellitus, malnutrition, trauma, ocular tumors, retrolental fibroplasia
	Chorioretinitis	Congenital cytomegalovirus infection
	Choroidal tubercles	Tuberous sclerosis
	Coloboma of eyelid	Treacher–Collins and Goldenhar syndromes
	Coloboma of iris	Idiopathic, CHARGE syndrome, Patau syndrome
	Corneal clouding	Hurler syndrome, other mucopolysaccharidoses
	Enophthalmos	Dehydration, malnutrition, Horner syndrome
	Exophthalmos	Thyrotoxicosis, cerebral, optic or orbital tumor, neurofibromatosis, malignant hypertension, Apert and Crouzon syndromes, Cushing's disease

(Continued)

Table 3.4 *(Continued)*

System	Sign	Possible causes
	Epicanthic folds	Down syndrome, other chromosomal abnormalities
	Hypertelorism	Various chromosomal abnormalities
	Hypotelorism	Holoprosencephaly syndrome, Patau syndrome
	Lens dislocation	Marfan syndrome, homocystinuria
	Lid retraction	Thyrotoxicosis
	Miosis	Bright light, convergence, narcotics, sympathetic nerve paralysis, Horner syndrome, drugs
	Mydriasis	Darkness, thyrotoxicosis, anxiety, iritis, inflammatory adhesions, coma, drugs
	Nystagmus	Normal in some infants and with watching moving object, labyrinthine and vestibular disease, brainstem lesions, central vision loss, septo-optic dysplasia, Friedreich's ataxia
	Optic atrophy	Glaucoma, retinal ischemia, optic neuritis, retinitis pigmentosa
	Papilledema	Raised intracranial pressure, optic neuritis, hypertension
	Periorbital edema	Nephrotic syndrome
	Ptosis	Bell's palsy, Horner syndrome, myasthenia gravis, 3rd cranial nerve palsy, congenital
	Racoon sign	Basal skull fracture
	Retinal hemorrhages	Non-accidental injury, trauma, leukemia, hypertension, bacterial endocarditis, bleeding diathesis
	Retinal pigmentation	Congenital infection, mucopolysaccharidoses, Laurence-Moon-Biedl syndrome
	Strabismus	Intermittent normal in neonates, fixed due to birth trauma, raised intracranial pressure, 3rd, 4th or 6th cranial nerve palsy, severe miosis, chromosomal abnormality
	Sunsetting	Hydrocephalus
	Xanthelasma	Hyperlipidemia, cholestasis
Ears	Low-set ears	Branchial developmental abnormalities, various chromosomal abnormalities
	Malformed auricles	Various chromosomal abnormalities
	Deafness	Familial, congenital infection, postmeningitis, branchial developmental abnormalities, other metabolic and chromosomal abnormalities
	Pre-auricular tags or pits	Beckwith–Wiedemann syndrome, Treacher-Collins syndrome, may be associated with deafness
	Earlobe crease	Beckwith–Wiedemann syndrome
Mouth	Xerostomia	Anxiety, pyrexia, dehydration, diabetes mellitus and insipidus, cystic fibrosis, drugs
	Risus sardonicus	Tetanus
	Stomatitis	Iron deficiency, herpes simplex, Stevens–Johnson syndrome, Kawasaki disease
	Cleft lip/palate	Idiopathic, Pierre-Robin syndrome, Patau syndrome, fetal teratogenicity
	Smooth philtrum	Fetal alcohol syndrome
	Blue gums	Lead poisoning
	Gum hypertrophy	Chronic phenytoin administration
	Glossoptosis	Down syndrome
	Macroglossia	Hypothyroidism, Beckwith–Wiedemann syndrome, mucopolysaccharidoses, other storage diseases
	Strawberry tongue	Scarlet fever, vitamin B deficiency
	White tongue	Milk, thrush, leukoplakia
	Anodontia/hypodontia	Osteochondrodysplasias, ectodermal dysplasia, Down syndrome
	Enamel hypoplasia	Tuberous sclerosis, Williams syndrome, Prader–Willi syndrome
Cardiovascular	Tachycardia	Exercise, pain, hypovolemia, infection, thyrotoxicosis, cardiac failure, anaphylaxis, pheochromocytoma, drugs
	Bradycardia	Hypothyroidism, heart block, raised intracranial pressure, hypothermia, cardiac failure, drugs
	Hypertension	Anxiety, renal disease, pheochromocytoma, aortic coarctation, raised intracranial pressure, Conn's and Cushing's syndromes, SLE, drugs
	Hypotension	Cardiac failure, hypovolemia, cardiogenic or septic shock, anaphylaxis, Addison's disease, electrolyte imbalance, hypothyroidism, drugs
	Atrial fibrillation	Wolff–Parkinson–White syndrome, thyrotoxicosis, rheumatic valve disease, carditis
	Bounding pulse	Pyrexia, thyrotoxicosis, anemia, hypercarbia
	Collapsing pulse	Aortic regurgitation, PDA, VSD, heart block, thyrotoxicosis, hyperdynamic circulation
	Plateau pulse	Aortic stenosis, aortic coarctation
	Pulsus paradoxus	Severe asthma, pericardial effusion or tamponade, constrictive pericarditis
	Gallop rhythm	Left ventricular failure, cardiac dilatation, constrictive pericarditis
	Systolic murmur	Physiological, VSD, PDA, ASD, pulmonary stenosis, aortic coarctation, aortic stenosis, hyperdynamic circulation, mitral regurgitation, tricuspid regurgitation, cardiomyopathy
	Diastolic murmur	Venous hum, PDA, large VSD, mitral stenosis, aortic regurgitation, pulmonary regurgitation, tricuspid stenosis
	Thrill	Palpable murmur
	Pericardial rub	Pericarditis, rheumatic fever, pleurisy, pneumonia
	Bruits	Artery stenosis, arteriovenous malformation
	Thrust/heave	Apical – left ventricular hypertrophy, lower left sternal edge – right ventricular hypertrophy
Respiratory	Barrel chest	Emphysema, asthma
	Pectus carinatum	Asthma, rickets, chromosomal or metabolic abnormalities
	Pectus excavatum	Asthma, rickets, chromosomal or metabolic abnormalities
	Thoracic rosary	Rickets

(Continued)

Table 3.4 *(Continued)*

System	Sign	Possible causes
	Barking cough	Croup
	Hemoptysis	Airway trauma, foreign body inhalation, infection, malignancy, arteriovenous malformation, bleeding diathesis
	Stridor	Croup, epiglottitis, laryngitis, laryngomalacia, infectious mononucleosis, diphtheria, subglottic hemangioma or cyst
	Wheeze	Asthma, bronchitis
	Bronchial breathing	Normal in young children, pneumonia
	Coarse crepitations	Bronchiolitis, bronchiectasis
	Fine crepitations	Pulmonary edema, atelectasis, pneumonia
	Pleural rub	Pleurisy, pneumonia, pulmonary thrombosis
	Hyperventilation	Anxiety, pain, pyrexia, metabolic acidosis, infection, hypoxia, drugs, Rett syndrome
	Hypoventilation	Raised intracranial pressure, drugs, lung disease
Gastrointestinal	Abdominal distension	Intestinal obstruction, ileus, peritonitis, ascites, masses, pregnancy, organomegaly
	Scaphoid abdomen	Congenital diaphragmatic hernia
	Abdominal mass	Organomegaly, tumor, fluid, hernia, cyst, abscess, pregnancy
	Hernias	Ex-preterm infant, hypothyroidism, Beckwith–Wiedemann syndrome, mucopolysaccharidoses
	Omphalocele	Idiopathic, Beckwith–Wiedemann syndrome, Patau syndrome, Edward syndrome
	Hepatomegaly	Congestive cardiac failure, any cause of infectious hepatitis, metabolic or liver storage disease, malignancy
	Splenomegaly	Infectious mononucleosis, infective endocarditis, portal hypertension, leukemia, lymphoma, hemolytic anemia, malaria
	Abdominal rigidity	Peritonitis
	Rebound tenderness	Peritonitis
	Visible peristalsis	Pyloric stenosis, acute intestinal obstruction
	Shifting dullness	Ascites
	Fluid thrill	Ascites
	Borborygmi	Intestinal obstruction, toxic enteritis
	Pale stool	Pancreatic insufficiency, bile duct obstruction
	Melena	Upper intestinal bleeding, iron therapy
	Green stool	Intestinal hurry, starvation
	Anal defects	VATER association, caudal regression sequence
Nervous	Hypertonia	Upper motor neurone lesions, extrapyramidal lesions, asphyxia, kernicterus, raised intracranial pressure, meningitis, cerebral palsy
	Hypotonia	Lower motor neurone lesions, prematurity, cerebellar lesions, myopathies, metabolic and chromosomal abnormalities
	Clasp-knife rigidity	Upper motor neurone lesion
	Cog-wheel rigidity	Extrapyramidal lesions, cerebral palsy
	Neck stiffness	Meningeal irritation
	Opisthotonus	Meningitis, cerebellar lesions, tetanus
	Myoclonus	Upper motor neurone lesions
	Brisk tendon reflexes	Upper motor neurone lesions, thyrotoxicosis, anxiety, tetanus
	Diminished tendon reflexes	Peripheral neuropathies, hypothyroidism, syringomyelia, lower motor neurone lesions
	Muscle fasciculation	Lower motor neurone lesions, muscular dystrophies, hypocalcemia, thyrotoxicosis, depolarizing drugs
	Athetosis	Kernicterus, juvenile Huntington's chorea, Wilson's disease, Lesch–Nyhan syndrome, basal ganglia or extrapyramidal lesions, drugs
	Chorea	Rheumatic fever, Huntington's chorea, Sydenham's chorea, Wilson's disease, kernicterus, thyrotoxicosis, SLE, Lesch–Nyhan syndrome, drugs
	Ataxia	Ataxia–telangiectasia, Angelman syndrome, Cockayne syndrome, cerebellar or brainstem lesions, drugs (including alcohol and antiepileptics), vestibular neuronitis
	Intention tremor	Cerebellar or brainstem lesions, Friedreich's ataxia, mercury poisoning
	Postural tremor	Anxiety, thyrotoxicosis, alcohol, Wilson's disease, cerebellar lesions, drugs
	Dysdiadochokinesia	Cerebellar lesions
	Asterixis	Encephalopathy, liver failure, metabolic disease
	Meningomyelocele	Maternal folate deficiency, fetal teratogenicity, chromosomal abnormality
	Encephalocele	Meckel–Gruber syndrome
Locomotor	Scoliosis	Congenital vertebral anomaly, developmental abnormality, disc prolapse, Marfan syndrome, Coffin–Lowry syndrome
	Buffalo hump	Cushing's disease, steroid therapy
	Short limbs	Chondrodysplasias, osteogenesis imperfecta, fetal varicella syndrome
	Cubitus valgus	Turner syndrome
	Fixed flexion deformities	Arthrogryposis multiplex congenita usually due to oligohydramnios sequence
	Joint erythema	Septic arthritis, inflammatory arthropathy, rheumatic fever
	Joint hypermobility	Familial, enthesopathy, Marfan syndrome, Ehlers–Danlos syndrome, acromegaly

(Continued)

Table 3.4 *(Continued)*

System	Sign	Possible causes
	Myotonia	Myotonic dystrophy, hyperkalemia
	Muscular atrophy	Lower motor neurone lesions, muscular dystrophies, prolonged immobilization
	Muscular hypertrophy	Duchenne's muscular dystrophy
Hands and feet	Finger or toe clubbing	Chronic cardiac, respiratory or gastrointestinal disease, congenital cyanotic heart disease, tumors, suppurative disease
	Koilonychia	Iron deficiency anemia
	Nail pitting	Eczema, psoriasis, chronic paronychia, alopecia areata
	Thickened nail	Psoriasis, chronic paronychia or fungal infection, lichen planus
	Onycholysis	Trauma, fungal infections, eczema, psoriasis, diabetes, drugs
	Splinter hemorrhages	Infective endocarditis, blood dyscrasias, eczema, psoriasis, trauma
	Arachnodactyly	Marfan syndrome
	Brachydactyly	Down syndrome, Ellis van Creveld syndrome
	Camptodactyly	Edward syndrome
	Clinodactyly	Down syndrome, other chromosomal abnormalities
	Polydactyly	Familial, Patau syndrome, other chromosomal abnormalities
	Syndactyly	Acrocephaly–syndactyly syndrome, various chromosomal abnormalities
	Thumb hypoplasia	Thrombocytopenia–absent radius syndrome, Fanconi anemia, Holt–Oram syndrome
	Single transverse palmar crease	Normal, chromosomal abnormality
	Wrist drop	Radial nerve lesion, peripheral neuropathy, muscular dystrophy
	Talipes equinovarus	Positional, oligohydramnios sequence, muscular dystrophy, chromosomal abnormality
	Pes cavus	Familial, Friedreich's ataxia, spina bifida, sacral dermoid
	Pes planus	Physiological lax ligaments, tarsal coalition, cerebral palsy, polio
	Peripheral edema	Cardiac failure, venous thrombosis, hypoproteinemia, nephrotic syndrome, renal failure, prolonged immobilization
	Carpopedal spasm	Hypocalcemia
Reproductive	Gynecomastia	Puberty, obesity, thyrotoxicosis, pituitary–adrenal–gonadal disease, liver disease, drugs
	Galactorrhea	Normal in some newborns, pituitary–adrenal tumors, hormonal therapy, thyroid disease, pregnancy and nursing
	Ambiguous genitalia	Congenital adrenal hyperplasia, hermaphroditism, Prader–Willi syndrome, other chromosomal abnormality
	Cryptorchidism	Delayed testicular descent, causes of ambiguous genitalia
	Testicular mass	Hydrocele, hernia, tumor, orchitis

ASD, atrial septal defect; CHARGE (syndrome), ocular coloboma, heart defects, atretic choanae, retarded growth or development, genital hypoplasia, and ear anomalies; DIC, disseminated intravscular coagulopathy; ITP, idiopathic thrombocytopenic purpura; PDA, patent ductus arteriosus; SLE, systemic lupus erythematosus; VATER, vertebral defects, imperforate anus, tracheoesophageal fistula, and radial and renal dyspalasia; VSD, ventricular septal defect

Table 3.5 Eponymous signs

Eponymous sign	Sign description	Possible causes
Austin Flint murmur	Murmur at apex, onset with third heart sound and loudest at mid diastole	Aortic regurgitation
Argyll Robertson pupil	Small unequal pupils that react to convergence but not to light	Neurosyphilis, diabetes
Battle's sign	Retromastoid bruising behind ears	Petrous bone fracture
Beau's ridges	Transverse ridging of nail plate	Hypoalbuminemia, steroid therapy, cytotoxics, severe illness
Brushfield spots	Focal areas of iris stromal hyperplasia giving appearance of white spots	Down syndrome
Charcot joint	Severely disorganized, arthritic joint which is pain-free	Tabes dorsalis, diabetic neuropathy, leprosy, myelomeningocele
Cheyne–Stokes respiration	Respirations that decrease in frequency, then stop temporarily before restarting and building up again	Damage to cerebral respiratory center terminal stage
Corrigan's sign	Vigorous pulsation of major head and neck arteries causing head or ears to move	Aortic regurgitation, PDA, VSD
Cullen's sign	Spontaneous umbilical bruising	Hemoperitoneum
Dance's sign	Right iliac fossa depression in distressed infant	Intussusception
Epstein's pearls	Epithelial inclusions along midline of hard palate	Normal in neonates
Erb's palsy	Arm held adducted and internally rotated, extended at elbow, with forearm and palm pronated	C5/6/7 damage
Gottron's sign	Scaly patches over dorsal finger joints, with subungual erythema and cuticular telangiectasia	Polymyositis, dermatomyositis

(Continued)

Table 3.5 *(Continued)*

Eponymous sign	Sign description	Possible causes
Graham Steel murmur	Soft, high pitched murmur in second left intercostal space in early diastole	Pulmonary regurgitation from pulmonary hypertension
Harrison's sulcus	Chest deformity with subcostal groove along attachment of diaphragm	Chronic asthma, rickets
Henoch–Schönlein purpura	Extensive purpuric and ecchymotic lesions on extensor surfaces of limbs	Idiopathic, post-streptococcal, drug-induced
Hoffmann's reflex	Foot dorsiflexion causes calf muscle pain	Calf thrombophlebitis or cellulitis
Jacobsen–Holdsnedt phenomenon	Mediastinum displaced away from affected side during expiration on X-ray	Unilateral obstructive emphysema, e.g., foreign body inhalation
Janeway lesion	Small purplish nodules on palms or soles	Infective endocarditis
Kayser–Fleischer ring	Green–brown ring at outer edge of cornea	Wilson's disease
Kehr's sign	Left shoulder tip pain with acute abdomen	Splenic rupture
Koplik spots	Gray spots in the mucous membranes of the mouth	Measles
Kussmaul breathing	Deep sighing respirations	Diabetic ketoacidosis, uremia, other metabolic acidosis, neurogenic hyperpnea
Murphy's sign	Pain and interruption of inhalation during palpation of right upper abdominal quadrant	Cholecystitis

PDA, patent ductus arteriosus; VSD; ventricular septal defect.

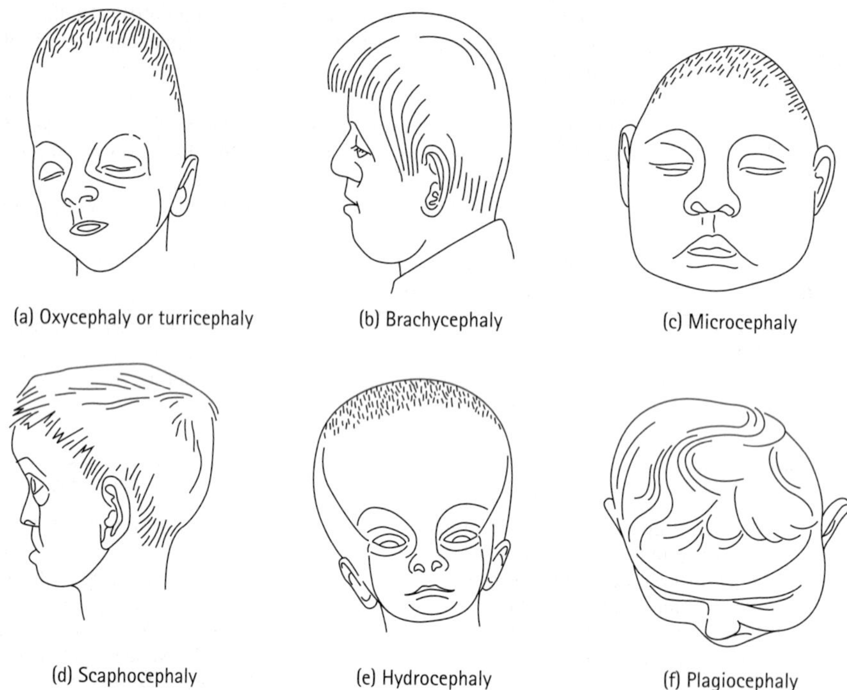

Fig. 3.4 Head shapes.

Also note any chest deformity and look for the apex position. The apex beat is normally in the fourth or fifth intercostal space in the midaxillary line, but may be more lateral in neonates and infants. Prominence of the left anterior chest wall may indicate cardiac enlargement. Use the palm of the hand to locate a precordial heave or thrill. An apical thrust indicates left ventricular hypertrophy while a heave at the lower left sternal edge suggests right ventricular hypertrophy.

Auscultate at the apex to identify the heart sounds. These should be assessed carefully even if the instantly obvious finding is a loud murmur. The first heart sound tends to be single, and the second split with splitting varying during respiration. A third heart sound at the apex is common in infants and younger children. Proceed to other auscultation positions (Fig. 3.5).[40] Heart murmurs should be described in detail, including site, timing, propagation and variation with position. They are graded as follows:

Grade 1 – barely audible;
Grade 2 – quiet;
Grade 3 – easily audible;
Grade 4 – easily audible with a thrill;
Grade 5 – loud and with a thrill, audible with stethoscope held off the chest wall;
Grade 6 – audible without a stethoscope.

Examples of commonly heard murmurs are:

- benign flow murmur – musical vibratory low-pitched systolic murmur, best heard at apex or lower left sternal edge;

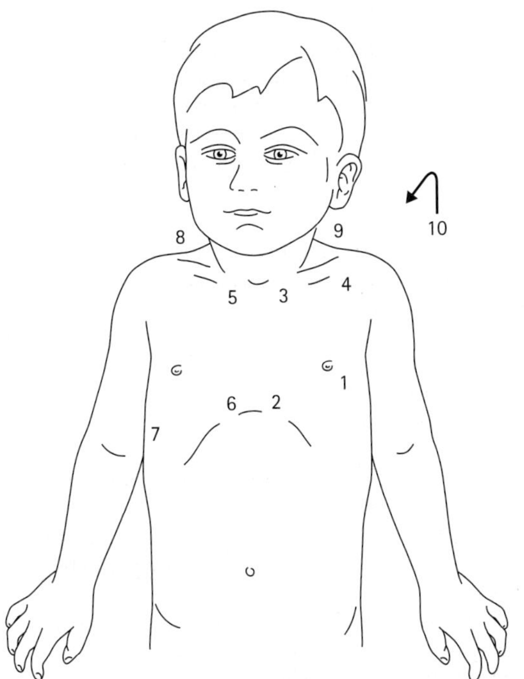

Fig. 3.5 Auscultation positions. Recommended order of auscultation: 1, apex 2, left lower sternal edge; 3 left upper sternal edge; 4 left infraclavicular; 5, right upper sternal edge; 6, right lower sternal edge; 7 right midaxillary line; 8, right side of neck; 9 left side of neck; 10, posteriorly. (From Laing & McIntosh[40] with permission of Baillière Tindall)

- venous hum – low-pitched humming systolic/diastolic murmur at neck and infraclavicular area; absent when supine and eliminated by compressing neck veins;
- peripheral pulmonary artery branch stenosis – blowing high-pitched systolic murmur at left infraclavicular area with radiation to the back;
- ventricular septal defect – louder, harsher systolic murmur at lower left sternal edge or apex, heard throughout systole (pansystolic);
- persistent ductus arteriosus – often musical, commonly purely systolic in the infant but being a continuous murmur at left infraclavicular area, with radiation to the back in the older child, full pulses;
- aortic stenosis – systolic murmur at right infraclavicular area, perhaps with an ejection click, radiating to neck;
- atrial septal defect – blowing systolic murmur at left infraclavicular area with widely split and fixed second heart sound.

As a general guide, a murmur is likely to be innocent if it is soft, systolic, with normal heart sounds, and no other abnormal cardiovascular findings. The diagnosis of murmurs is notoriously difficult and inaccurate.[41,42] However, non-specialized pediatricians should still be able to differentiate those children with true innocent murmurs from those who would benefit from further investigation.[43]

Signs of cardiac failure include tachypnea, dyspnea with feeding, short feeds, sweating, tachycardia, gallop rhythm, crepitations of pulmonary edema, and poor weight gain or unexpected sudden weight gain. Hepatosplenomegaly, limb edema and cyanosis are late signs. Other longer-term indicators of cardiac well-being include growth rate, general demeanour and exercise tolerance.

ABDOMINAL

In children, the classical position for abdominal examination may not always be obtainable. Fractious young children may have to be examined when prone or sitting hugging a parent. Examination may frequently have to be performed with the child on a parent's lap.

Inspect the abdomen for distension, discoloration, visible peristalsis and superficial abnormalities, such as hernias and prominent veins. A child with peritonitis is unlikely to be active or move around, but will probably be lying still.

Palpation should be performed with warm hands, using the flat of the hand (Fig. 3.6). Start away from the site of any pain. Watch the child's face for apprehension or reaction to pain. In a crying child, the abdomen is relaxed briefly during inspiration, allowing palpation. The liver may be felt normally up to 1 cm below the right inferior costal margin in the midclavicular line, and the spleen tip below the left. Splenic enlargement is towards the right iliac fossa in older children, but towards the left iliac fossa in infants. Kidneys may be easily felt in neonates and slim children. Record positions of masses or tenderness with a diagram. Masses in the groin may be lymph nodes, hernias or gonads. Note guarding, rebound tenderness and quality of bowel sounds. Abdominal percussion should be performed if relevant. Examination of stools is important.

Examination for a pyloric tumor should be performed when the infant is feeding. Sitting on the infant's left, the left hand should be placed flat on the abdomen with fingers directed towards the right hypochondrium, below the liver edge and lateral to the rectus muscle. Gentle depression of the fingers allows palpation of the tumor, most easily after vomiting.

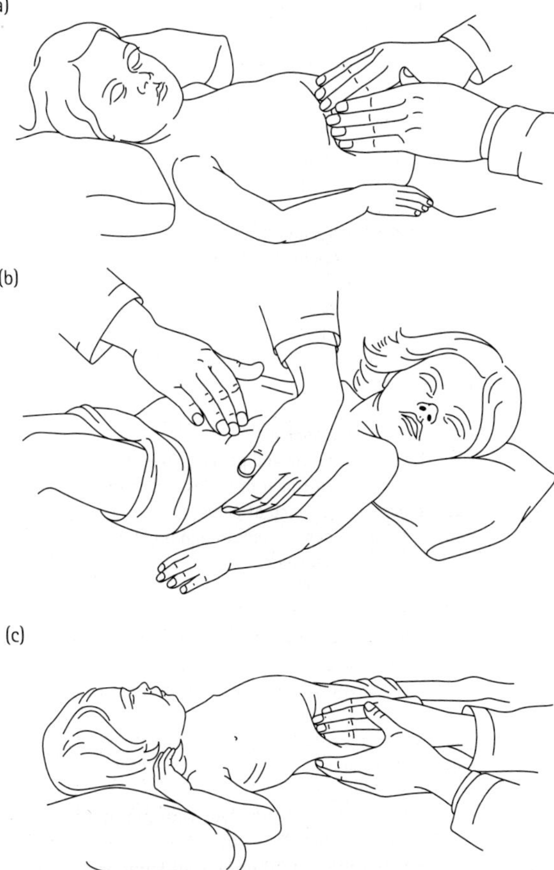

Fig. 3.6 Palpation: (a) liver, (b) spleen, (c) kidney.

SEXUAL MATURATION

Genitalia should be examined for ambiguity, congenital abnormalities and excoriation or abnormal discharge if relevant. In girls, look for labial adhesions and clitoral enlargement. In boys, testicular descent should be checked. Cold examining fingers and a brisk cremasteric reflex may cause testicular retraction that mimics maldescent. To differentiate the two, start palpation from the inguinal area and move distally. The scrotal quality also gives a clue to the diagnosis. Check for other scrotal masses, hypospadias and note the size and shape of the penis. The foreskin should not be forcibly retracted in infants and young boys.

Pubertal grading is illustrated in Figure 3.7.[40] For easier recall, stages 1 and 5 are fully infantile and fully adult respectively, and hence only 2, 3 and 4 need to be remembered.

In sexual abuse, the presence of a normal history with an abnormal examination has been shown to decrease diagnostic accuracy,[44] highlighting the importance of accurate sensitive history taking when sexual abuse has been suspected.

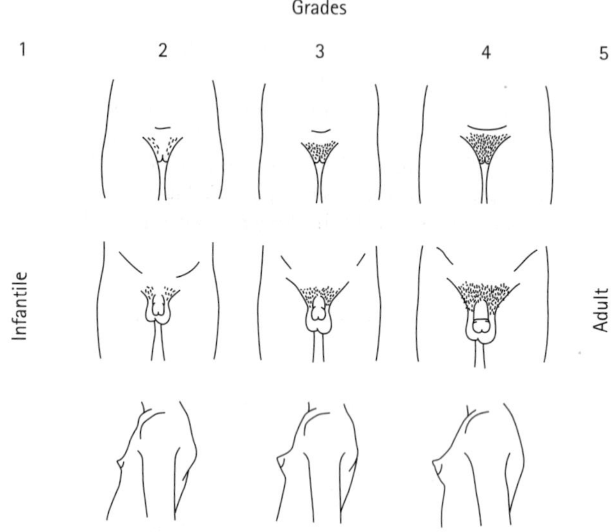

Girls – breast development:
Stage 1: as in early childhood
Stage 2: breast bud
Stage 3: breast and areola enlarging
Stage 4: areola and papilla form a secondary mound distinct from enlarging breast
Stage 5: mature

Boys – genital development:
Stage 1: testes, scrotum and penis as in early childhood
Stage 2: some enlargement of testes and scrotum
Stage 3: early lengthening of penis
Stage 4: enlarged penis in length and breadth, with glans development
Stage 5: adult genitalia

Girls and boys – pubic hair:
Stage 1: no pubic hair
Stage 2: sparse growth of pubic hair on each side of penile root or on labia
Stage 3: darker coarse hair meeting on symphysis
Stage 4: adult hair, no spread to medial surface of thighs
Stage 5: adult in quantity and type with spread to medial surface of thighs

Fig. 3.7 Pubertal development grading. (From Laing & McIntosh[40] with permission of Baillière Tindall)

NERVOUS SYSTEM

The classical full examination of the nervous system may be possible in older children, but flexibility, patience and skill are needed to assess younger ones. The first clues to the well-being of the central nervous system come from the child's level of alertness, behavior and willingness to play, observed during history taking. Grade a decreased level of consciousness using the Glasgow Coma Scale (see Ch. 20).

Note abnormal tone, posture or movements. Look for muscle fasciculation or wasting and myoclonus. Note incoordination and gait abnormalities. Tone, power and coordination can be tested in cooperative older children as in adults. For younger children, power and coordination are better assessed during observation of normal play or other activity rather than by formal examination. Sensation is also often difficult to test reliably in younger children. Cutaneous nerve segments are shown in Figure 3.8.[45] Most reflexes can be elicited as in adults. Neonatal reflexes are outlined in Table 3.9. Some useful neurological signs are given in Table 3.6.

Cerebral palsy can be defined in terms of type of movement abnormality, or affected area. Types of movement abnormality are as follows:

1. spasticity and rigidity – damage to pyramidal tracts;
2. dyskinesia – damage to extrapyramidal tracts;
3. ataxia – damage to cerebellum;
4. mixed picture of the above;
5. persistent hypotonia – rare.

Affected areas are:

1. quadriplegia – all four limbs;
2. diplegia – either upper or lower limbs, usually lower;
3. hemiplegia – one half of the body.

Cranial nerve testing can be performed on most children as a game, using methods similar to those for adults (Table 3.7). Improvisation will be required in younger children. Hearing can be tested crudely by distraction testing, or more formally by otoacoustic emissions, auditory brainstem evoked responses, and multifrequency audiometry. Vision can be crudely tested in neonates by moving an object held less than 30 cm from their eyes and watching for fixation and following. Infants are more likely to fix and follow on a human face than other shapes.

LOCOMOTOR

The locomotor examination is intertwined with examination of the nervous system and development. Mild versions of genu varum, genu valgum, tibial torsion, and positional talipes equinovarus are not uncommon in infants and young children. It is therefore important to be aware of the variations in normal that may apply. However, some specific disorders of the skeletal system are associated with certain syndromes (Table 3.4).

Inspect the child's overall morphological appearance and head shape. Test the neck for full range of movement to exclude torticollis. Examination for scoliosis, kyphosis and lordosis should be made with the child first standing erect. True scoliosis can be demonstrated if an apparent hemithoracic convexity persists on bending down forwards. Look in the lumbosacral area for a tuft of hair marking spina bifida occulta.

Examine the upper and lower limbs for any deformities and check for symmetry of both sides. Measurements of limb lengths may be relevant and normograms are available in textbooks of morphology.[37] Note the number of digits. Ask about pain before proceeding to move any limbs. Remember that pain may be referred, such as hip pathology presenting as pain in the knee. Crepitus, deformity, pain on movement, and local tenderness will indicate

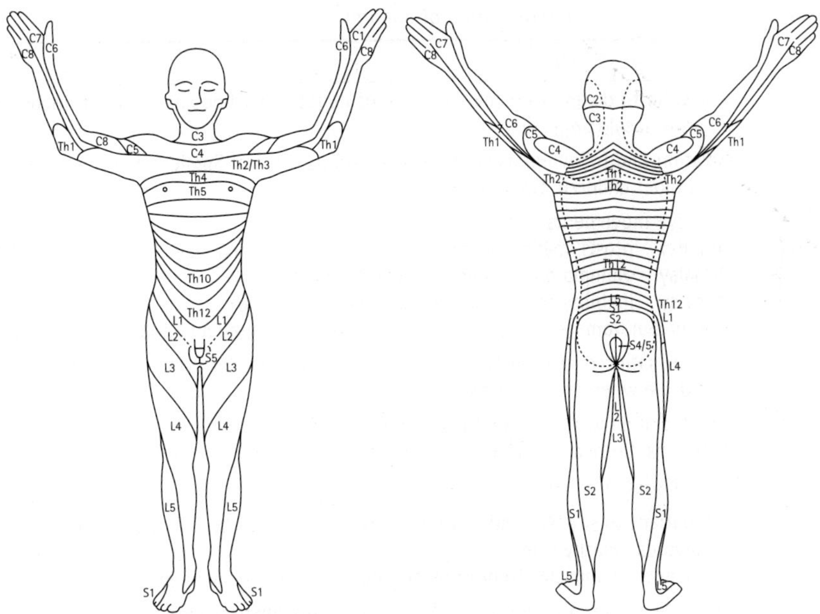

Fig. 3.8 Cutaneous nerve segments. From Geigy[45] with permission.

Table 3.6 Neurological and locomotor tests

Test name	Test description	Possible causes
Babinski's sign	Stroking lateral plantar surface from heel to toes causes extension of great toe	Normal in infants, upper motor neurone lesions
Barlow's test	With one hand stabilizing pelvis, the other hand abducts infant's hip. Pressure is then applied backwards and outwards with the thumb on the inner upper thigh while abducting same hip in an attempt to dislocate an unstable hip	Unstable hip
Bragaard test	Dorsiflexion of foot following straight leg raising causes pain in leg and lumbar region	Sciatic nerve root impingement
Brudzinski's sign	Flexing head causes legs to be drawn up	Meningeal irritation
Chvostek's sign	Tapping facial nerve lightly causes contraction of ipsilateral facial muscles	Hypocalcemia
Gower's maneuver	Child getting up from floor by walking hands up legs	Duchenne muscular dystrophy
Kernig's sign	With hip flexed, any attempt to straighten knee results in hamstring or lumbar spasm	Meningeal irritation
Lachman's test	With knee almost fully extended, tibia can be moved forward on femoral condyle	Anterior cruciate ligament laxity or rupture
McMurray test	Flex hip and knee to 90 degrees. Grasp heel with one hand and steady knee with other. Slowly extend knee using heel movement, while palpating joint line. Do with tibia in external and internal rotation. A clunk indicates displaced cartilage	Cartilage displacement in knee
Moro reflex	See Table 3.9	
Ortolani's test	With one hand stabilizing pelvis, abduct hip and press forward with middle finger on greater trochanter. A dislocated hip can be felt to slip forward into joint again with a 'clunk'	Congenital dislocation of the hip
Romberg's sign	Closing eyes while standing with feet together causes severe swaying or falling over	Proprioceptive or vestibular deficit, posterior column lesion, intoxication
Simmond's test	With patient lying prone, squeezing calf results in absence of plantarflexion of foot	Ruptured Achilles tendon
Thomas test	With patient supine, place one hand between lumbar spine and couch. Flex normal hip to limit to straighten lumbar spine. Opposite leg with rise off couch if fixed flexion deformity present	Flexion deformity of hip
Trendelenburg's test	While standing, pelvis tilts down towards side on which leg is lifted. Opposite side is impaired	Congenital dislocation of the hip, muscular dystrophy
Trousseau's sign	Circumferential pressure of limb causes carpopedal spasm	Hypocalcemia, alkalosis, Bartter syndrome

Table 3.7 Testing of cranial nerves and possible interpretation of abnormalities

Cranial nerve	Methods of testing
I (Olfactory)	Ask child to distinguish smell. Beware of negative findings in young or uncooperative child, or in nasal congestion
II (Optic)	Fixation and following as crude test in infants. Formal Snellen charts and visual field testing in older children. Ophthalmoscopy
III (Oculomotor) IV (Trochlear) VI (Abducens)	Test eye movements in all directions III palsy – ptosis, mydriasis, lateral deviation of affected side IV palsy – diplopia on looking downwards and medially VI palsy – inability to look laterally with affected side Horner syndrome – ptosis, miosis, anhidrosis of affected side (paralysis of sympathetic branch)
V (Trigeminal)	Test sensation over forehead, cheeks and jaw. Test motor function by palpating masseter muscle when teeth clenched
VII (Facial)	Test facial movements. Forehead wrinkling differentiates upper from lower motor neurone lesions. Corneal sensation is supplied by the facial nerve but testing it is unpleasant
VIII (Auditory)	Test hearing and balance
IX (Glossopharyngeal) X (Vagus)	Ask patient to say 'Ah' and examine movement of palate. Palate is drawn towards healthy side
XI (Spinal accessory)	Test trapezius muscle strength by shrugging against resistance
XII (Hypoglossal)	Ask patient to protrude tongue. Tongue deviates towards paralyzed side

an underlying fracture. Bony injuries may be secondary to non-accidental injury.

Joints should also be examined after asking about pain. Assess range of movement, temperature, swelling and associated pain. Deformity may indicate dislocation or severe joint destruction. A patellar tap indicates synovial effusion.

Further useful tests of the neurological and locomotor systems are given in Table 3.6.

INVASIVE EXAMINATIONS

These should be left until the end of the physical examination as they are likely to distress the child.

Otoscopy

Make sure the speculum is of an appropriate size. An erythematous, bulging, acutely inflamed tympanic membrane may be seen, or a duller, retracted membrane of chronic otitis media. Perforations tend to occur in the upper part of the membrane. The child should be held as in Figure 3.9.[40]

Pharyngeal inspection

This may occasionally be performed successfully without the use of a spatula. Inspect the shape of the palate and uvula. Ask the child to say 'Ah' to check for symmetrical movement of the soft palate and examine the tonsils and fauces. If not visualized, then a spatula should be used to induce the gag reflex by touching the posterior pharyngeal wall. Note any inflammation, exudate, or membrane formation on the tonsils or posterior pharyngeal wall. With an uncooperative child, hold as demonstrated in Figure 3.10.

Rectal examination

Rectal examination is usually unnecessary in children unless bowel obstruction or sexual abuse is suspected. There may be anal fissuring, trauma, or prolapse. Rectal examination should be performed with the lexaminer's well-lubricated fifth finger in infants and younger children. Note material on the withdrawn finger.

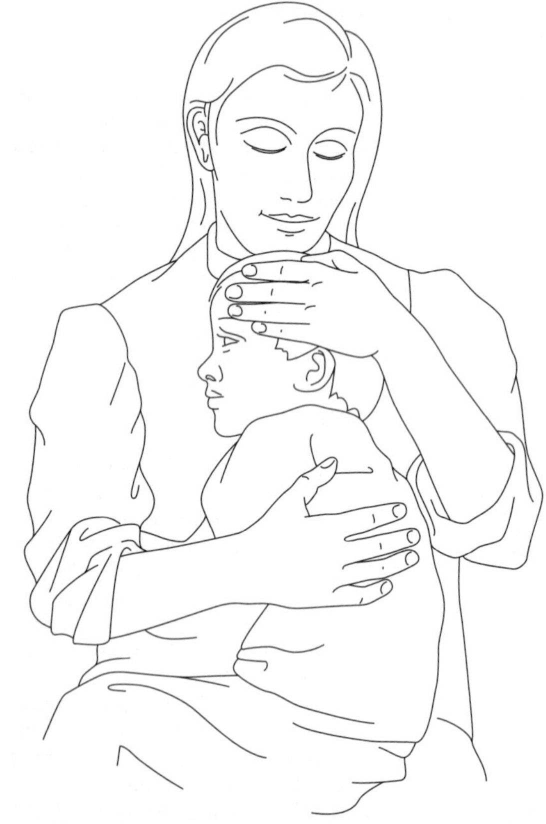

Fig. 3.9 Method of holding a child for otoscopy. (From Laing & McIntosh[40] with permission of Baillière Tindall)

THE NEWBORN

NEONATAL HISTORY

Many of the same principles described in general pediatric history taking (see above) apply to the neonate. Most information is obtained from the mother, the father and the obstetric and

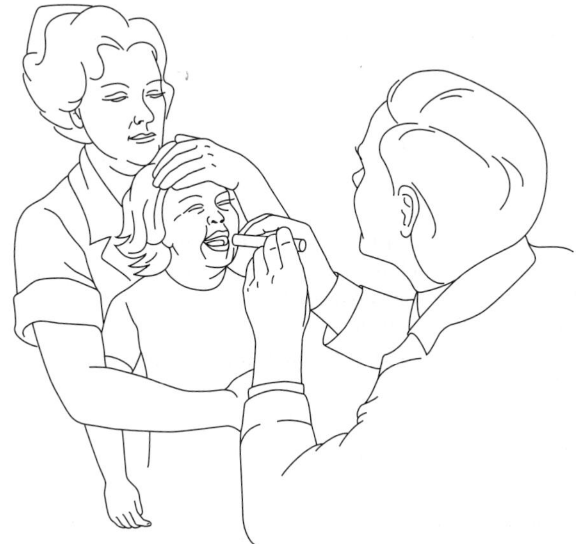

Fig. 3.10 Examining the mouth – uncooperative child.

midwifery case records. Usually babies are born without complications and prove to be entirely well on clinical examination. Neonates may however present with complications which can include premature or postmature delivery, congenital abnormalities and infections. The parents may or may not have had previous warning of such complications. Father and mother may both be overwrought, their hopes and expectations shattered. They may be consumed with guilt, however unjustified this may seem. What may seem a simple problem to the clinician takes on enormous proportions to the infant's parents at this emotional time. History receiving must therefore be sensitive, gentle and with understanding and empathy towards the inevitable parental anxiety.

The following should be recorded.

Date of examination:
Name of infant:
Date of infant's birth:
Race/ethnicity/native language:
Place of birth:
Presenting history (see general history taking above):

Maternal history

Important details of the maternal history include:

- maternal age;
- parity and outcome of previous pregnancies, including fetal or neonatal deaths and their causes;
- previous infertility;
- rubella status;
- chronic maternal illness;
- sexually transmitted diseases including herpes and human immunodeficiency virus (HIV)/acquired immune deficiency syndrome (AIDS);
- uterine anomaly.

Current pregnancy

Important details of the current pregnancy include:

- current gestation;
- previous suspicion of large for dates or small for dates fetus;
- results of fetal testing, e.g. ultrasonography, amniocentesis or biophysical profile;
- drug history including recent glucocorticoids, labor suppressants or antibiotics;
- drug abuse including tobacco, alcohol and other drugs (whether prescribed or not);
- recent infections and exposures;
- health during this pregnancy, including diabetes (type A?, gestational?, insulin dependent?), urinary tract infections, hypertension and any proteinuria;
- complications of pregnancy, including vaginal bleeding, infections, hydramnios, oligohydramnios.

Labor and delivery

The following should be accurately recorded from the obstetric/ midwifery case record:

- time of onset of labor;
- whether labor spontaneous or induced;
- timing and therefore duration of rupture of membranes;
- abnormalities of liquor including volume and staining, e.g. with meconium;
- presenting part;
- duration of first stage (min);
- duration of second stage (min);
- mode of delivery, e.g. Cesarean section or assisted delivery, and include the indication for the procedure;
- problems encountered during labor including details of cardiotocographic tracings, observation of presence of meconium, cord noted to be round the neck or any fever or vaginal discharge noted.

Infant at birth

The following details of the child's early minutes of life should be documented:

- gender;
- birth weight;
- condition and appearance at birth, e.g. pallor, grunting, irritability, coma;
- Apgar scores (see below);
- resuscitation required and its timing;
- drugs given, including vitamin K, and by what route.

Observations of placenta and umbilical cord

The weight of the placenta is normally one-fifth to one-sixth of that of the infant. It may demonstrate calcification, infarcts, a retroplacental clot, or indeed a hitherto unsuspected remnant of a twin (fetus papyraceous). If there is a known multiple pregnancy, it is important to document carefully the number of chorions and amnions. This information may contribute strongly to the establishment of zygosity. Monochorionic twins are monozygotic, whereas dichorionic twins may be either monozygotic or dizygotic.

The cord vessels usually consist of two arteries and one vein. The cord may contain a true knot.

Dr Virginia Apgar designed the Apgar score as a system of evaluating an infant in the delivery room at 1 and 5 min of age.[46] Nowadays it is common also to quote Apgar scores at 10 min and occasionally beyond. The Apgar score is often filled in retrospectively by clinicians present at the resuscitation and its main use now may be the documentation of the newborn infant's progress as the minutes pass rather than a primary guide to interventions (Table 3.8).

NEONATAL EXAMINATION

Examination of the newborn is part of child health surveillance.[47] The purpose of carrying out a newborn examination is fourfold: to provide parental reassurance that the child appears to be normal, to identify any congenital abnormalities, to detect illnesses such as

Table 3.8 Apgar scoring system

Features evaluated	0 points	1 point	2 points
Heart rate	0	< 100	> 100
Respiratory effort	Apnea	Irregular/shallow/ gasping	Vigorous/crying
Color	Pale/blue	Pale or blue extremities	Pink
Muscle tone	Absent	Weak	Normal/flexed
Response to stimuli	Absent	Grimace	Active/sneeze/cry

infection, and to gather statistical data such as weight and head circumference for monitoring the population's health.

Abnormalities, mainly orthopedic problems, are found in almost 9% of infants during the examination.[48] Nevertheless it is important to emphasize the limitations of the newborn examination. The examiner is trying to identify any abnormalities that may be present at the time. Often however congenital abnormalities cannot be identified during this first examination. Hypoplastic left heart syndrome may show no symptoms or signs in the first days of life. Some congenital metabolic conditions become evident only after a significant intake of milk over a period of days. Most cases of cerebral palsy are caused in utero and yet clinical evidence of muscle stiffness or neurodevelopmental delay may be absent for several months. Parents should be informed, preferably in writing, about the purpose of newborn examination and they should be told that not all problems are evident at birth.

Routine examination of the neonate should be carried out ideally in front of both parents: if mother is well enough she should always be present. This is an ideal opportunity for the clinician to reassure parents about any uncertainties they may have. The pediatrician should never be patronizing or judgmental. Some parents may never have handled an infant before, while some may be highly experienced. Questions must always meet with a full and sympathetic response.

Examination of the neonate must be carried out in a well-lit warm room that is free of draughts. The clinician should avoid handling an infant immediately after or immediately before a feed. Talking to the infant will soothe both infant and parent and will contribute greatly to the success of the consultation. It is a council of perfection to state that one should always be systematic in the examination of a newborn baby. The truth is one must frequently be opportunist. Some aspects of the examination may need to be deferred, e.g. when attempting direct ophthalmoscopy it may not be possible, on day 1, to see a satisfactory red reflex because puffiness of the infant's eyes may prevent adequate visualization. Equally, the yelling baby may require to be fed before adequate auscultation can exclude the presence of a heart murmur. In general it is advisable to keep uncomfortable procedures to the end, e.g. examination of the hips for dislocation or dislocatability.

Each pediatrician may wish to adopt and practice an individual system of examination. Provided it is complete and accurate then that is satisfactory. One possible scheme is as follows:

GENERAL INSPECTION
INSPECTION OF SKIN AND RELATED TISSUES
EXAMINATION OF HEAD, NECK, EARS, NOSE AND MOUTH
CARDIOVASCULAR EXAMINATION
RESPIRATORY EXAMINATION
ABDOMINAL EXAMINATION
NEUROLOGICAL EXAMINATION
FINAL INSPECTION

General inspection

Before touching or undressing the newborn infant, look carefully. A neurologically normal term infant will be flexed and fairly symmetrical, whereas a preterm infant, or one who is profoundly hypotonic, may adopt a more extended position. The following questions may be readily answered.

- Does the child look well?
- Is the appearance that of an appropriately grown infant?
- Is the respiration rate normal? (see Table 3.3)
- Are there any congenital abnormalities visible? (e.g. a rash or skin tags)
- Is the child at rest or is there evidence of irritability?
- If crying, is this of normal pitch and volume?

The observer should record the weight, crown–heel length and occipitofrontal circumference on a centile chart appropriate to that population. Note that infants in Scandinavian countries are larger than those from the Far East. There are specialized centile charts for products of multiple pregnancies and for infants with Down syndrome. The clinician may then undress the child, speaking soothingly all the while. The following should then be examined and documented.

Skin and related tissues

- Abnormality of color, e.g. jaundice, pallor, plethoric appearance, rash. Jaundice is always an abnormal finding in the first 24 h of life and always needs investigation. Pallor may be due to anemia or peripheral vasoconstriction. Plethora may be caused by peripheral vasodilatation or by polycythemia. If a rash is present, describe its distribution, size, color, presence of discrete macules or papules, and any areas of pus, bleeding or exudation. Occasionally a 'harlequin' appearance is seen where the infant is lying on one side and the dependent side is red and the non-dependent side is pale. The appearance is often episodic and usually resolves spontaneously. The 'stork's beak mark' occurs in 30–50% of newborns and is commonest as a pink discoloration at the nape of the neck, the eyelids and on the glabella. The port wine stain or nevus flammeus is a red or purple macule which is permanent and most common on the face (see association with Sturge–Weber syndrome). The strawberry nevus is a raised red tumor on the dermis, and, although most appear postnatally, 20% of them are present at birth. Central cyanosis is the blue color identified in the child who is hypoxic or polycythemic. Acrocyanosis is a very common feature in the early minutes and hours of life and describes the blue periphery of a neonate which contrasts with the pinkness observed centrally in the well-oxygenated infant. Pallor is caused by anemia or vasoconstriction, but occasionally a fair-skinned baby may seem to be pale. The word plethora implies an overload, but in practice it is used to describe the marked redness seen in vasodilatation, polycythemia or volume overload. Icterus refers to the yellow color seen on the skin of a jaundiced infant.
- Texture, e.g. dry, wrinkled or vernix-covered. Ichthyosis refers to a scaly, fish-like texture of the skin. Describe any blisters or bullae seen. The term 'collodion baby' refers to a varnished appearance of the skin seen in postmaturity, lamellar ichthyosis and congenital ichthyosiform erythroderma.

- Look for specific characteristic findings, e.g. Mongolian blue spot (bluish, often large and over buttocks, back and thighs, often fading towards the end of the first year of life). Count and measure any pigmented nevi. Other common appearances on the newborn skin include milia, sebaceous gland hyperplasia, acne neonatorum, erythema toxicum, nappy dermatitis and monilial dermatitis: see detailed descriptions of these appearances in Chapter 28.
- Trauma. Subcutaneous fat necrosis may occur as hard plaques under the skin where there has been local trauma, e.g. as a result of compression by forceps. Document any scalp cuts and bruises, e.g. from forceps or cardiotocography leads.
- Palpable lymph nodes are present in one-third of normal newborn infants, especially in the inguinal cervical and axillary areas.[49]

Head and neck

Describe the shape of the baby's head according to Figure 3.4. Molding of the head is especially common in the first 24 h of life. Caput succedaneum refers to the soft boggy feeling overlying the cranium where molding has occurred: it is most commonly felt at the vertex. It represents subdermal edema. Rarely the edema may be associated with significant bleeding under the skin tissues which may extend under the aponeurosis causing a subgaleal hemorrhage.

A cephalhematoma is a subperiosteal hemorrhage which is usually benign. It is most commonly felt as a swelling over one of the parietal bones, and its borders are restricted to the periosteal margins. In 15% of cases the cephalhematoma is bilateral.

Note whether the anterior fontanelle is open, and if so does the skin feel sunken, flat or bulging? There is a wide range of size of the anterior fontanelle in newborns and this is usually of little significance in the absence of craniosynostosis or rasied intracranial pressure.[50] Feel all the sutures and comment on whether they are over-riding (feels like a shallow step), split apart (e.g. by raised intracranial pressure) or fused together (synostosis). Rarely the skull bones are thin and fragile (craniotabes): the sensation is said to be like pressing on a table-tennis ball, but this procedure is contraindicated. Aplasia cutis most commonly shows as a small area of alopecia and absence of skin in the midline of the vertex such that the periosteum of the underlying parietal bones is visible.

An encephalocele is a congenital swelling, most commonly seen as a herniation through cranium bifidum, particularly seen in the midline occipitally. It may consist of meninges alone, or else meninges plus brain tissue.

Eyes

The eyes may be puffy in the first 2 days of life and inspection of the eyeballs and visualization of the retinas may be very difficult. If so, make arrangements for the eyeballs to be examined later in the first week of life. Examination of the eyes should include the eyebrows and eyelashes, eyelids and lacrimal system. Look for any congenital abnormality, and for symmetry of the eyes. Icterus may be seen and, particularly in pigmented races, may be the best sign of neonatal jaundice. Also ensure that there is no clouding of the optical media (cornea, lens and vitreous). Subconjunctival hemorrhages show as localized bleeding into the tissues anterior to the choroid. Look for a discharge of pus and surrounding erythema. Microphthalmia may be a significant finding in infants with multiple congenital abnormalities, including chromosomal anomalies and intrauterine infections such as toxoplasmosis.

A hyphema will show as a red fluid level over the iris which varies with the child's position. The eye may show a coloboma which presents as a sector-shaped defect in the iris. Inspect with an ophthalmoscope to ensure that the red reflex is seen. Failure to see the red reflex may indicate that a cataract is present. One recent study showed that only 35% of infant cataracts were detected at birth.[51] Increased size of the eyeball, firmness to palpation and haziness of the iris may indicate glaucoma (buphthalmos).

Nose

Check that the nares are both patent. This is most easily done by occluding each nostril in turn and observing that the infant continues to breathe through the other nostril.

Mouth

Inspect the overall shape of the mouth. Note any smallness of the jaw (hypomandibularism or micrognathia).

Tongue. True macroglossia occurs as a large tongue protruding from the mouth. In Down syndrome there is protrusion of a normal or even small tongue through the rather neat mouth (glossoptosis, not macroglossia).

Often a lingual frenulum is identified in the midline, joining the tongue to the floor of the mouth. True tongue tie is uncommon.

Pale colored inclusion cysts may be seen on the tongue.

Palate. Describe any cleft lip or palate. Is the cleft lip midline, unilateral or bilateral? Does it involve the alveolus? Is it associated with cleft of the hard palate? Discrete white Epstein's pearls are small inclusion cysts and are most commonly found on the hard palate close to the midline.

Gum. A congenital epulis may occur as a firm mass, usually fixed to the maxillary mucosa and occasionally protruding from the mouth. On the gum, eruption cysts may be observed prior to the eruption of neonatal teeth. These early teeth are part of the normal deciduous complement. Poorly developing neonatal teeth may be loose and should be extracted.

Mucosa. The buccal mucosa and the mucous membrane of the tongue may show white discoloration. This may be due to curdled milk from the last feed, or from thrush. Scraping the discoloration gently will easily remove the milk, but thrush tends to be very adherent and produces a little local bleeding when removed. A mucous cyst on the floor of the mouth is known as a ranula: it is related to the sublingual or submandibular salivary ducts.

Ear

The normal ear shows a great deal of variation in shape of the pinna. The helix may be temporarily folded due to local pressure in utero. Low-set ears are often defined as those where the helix joins to the cranium at a level below a plane including the corners of the inner canthi.

Auricular skin tags are seen as excrescences, often anterior to the pinna. Occasionally they occur on the cheek in a line joining the pinna to the lateral corner of the mouth.

Transverse earlobe creases may be seen in Beckwith–Wiedemann syndrome.

Neck

Asymmetry of the neck is often due to fetal posture and usually resolves over days or weeks. Torticollis is usually caused by shortening of the sternocleidomastoid muscle, often from a fibrosed hematoma (tumor only in the Greek sense of a swelling). Torticollis can be associated with cervical spine abnormalities. Look also for a branchial sinus or cyst, which is most commonly seen anterior to the sternomastoid muscle. A cystic hygroma is a large soft swelling in the neck, often unilateral. It consists of local proliferation of lymph vessels. A goitre may be identified at birth as a trilobed enlargement of the thyroid isthmus and its lateral lobes.

Cardiovascular examination

The following comments supplement the detailed description of pediatric cardiological examination (see above). It is important to note that, while congenital heart disease occurs in approximately 6 per 1000 live-born infants, routine examination of the newborn will detect only 45% of these.[52]

Inspection may show central cyanosis only in good lighting conditions but pulse oximetry will help to confirm suspicions that the newborn child may be blue. The infant with congenital heart disease may or may not be tachypneic.

With the child undressed in a warm room, time the respiratory rate and note any respiratory distress including indrawing or use of accessory muscles of respiration. Is the apex beat visible and prominent? Record the heart rate. The heart rate of the normal newborn may be as slow as 80 beats per min when the child is asleep and as high as 160 beats per min when roused and upset.

The femoral pulses may be most easily felt by the examiner's thumbs placed gently at either femoral triangle with the hips moderately abducted. Radiofemoral delay can be a difficult sign in the newborn, and any child with low volume femoral pulses needs coarctation of the aorta excluded. Four-limb blood pressures are mandatory in this situation: normally the lower limbs have higher blood pressure than upper limbs, and any reversal of this in the face of low volume or absent femoral pulses requires immediate referral to a pediatric cardiologist. Note that in the neonatal period, while the ductus arteriosus is open, femoral pulses may be readily palpable even in the face of coarctation of the aorta.

Palpate the abdomen and measure the size of the liver in the midclavicular line. The apex of the heart may be best palpated by the palm of the examiner's hand. Record the position of the apex and document any heave or thrill.

Systematic auscultation is important if all abnormalities are to be identified. The bell of the stethoscope is best for low-pitched sounds and should be used initially to auscultate at the apex. The diaphragm of the stethoscope is better at high-pitched sounds and murmurs and should be used in all positions. One suggested scheme of examination is shown in Figure 3.5.[40]

Because the heart rate of the newborn is faster than that of an older child or adult, the examiner may be limited in being certain of some signs, e.g. fixed splitting of the second heart sound in atrial septal defect. Nevertheless it is usually straightforward to describe the rate, the quality of the first and second heart sounds, whether splitting of the second heart sound is detected, any additional heart sounds and the presence or absence of murmurs.

In the early days of life it is common to hear only a systolic murmur in patency of the ductus arteriosus. This is because the pulmonary and systemic blood pressures are initially similar and left-to-right shunting of blood through the ductus is limited. The typical ductal murmur with the diastolic component is not heard in the early days of life. Although large volume pulses may be a useful sign of the significance of the ductus arteriosus in older children, in the neonatal period this is largely subjective. If a patent ductus is causing the child to be dyspneic or the apex beat to be prominent, then the ductus is significant irrespective of the pulse findings.

Respiratory examination

Inspection of the respiratory system is again essential prior to handling the infant. The normal sleeping respiratory rate may vary from 20 to 40 breaths per min, but the hungry or crying or cold neonate may have a respiration rate above 60 breaths per min. Accurately count the rate over 15 s and record the estimate per min. Extra breathing sounds, e.g. stridor, should also be recorded prior to handling the infant. Describe also any abnormality of the shape of the chest wall.

Suprasternal, intercostal or subcostal indrawing may be due to upper or lower respiratory tract disease. In the newborn period stridor and indrawing which begin on the second or third day of life and appear to get worse in an otherwise well child may be due to laryngomalacia. Any sign of respiratory distress must alert the examiner to the possibility of infection. Percussion of the newborn's chest is rarely helpful. It will make the infant cry, so that further respiratory examination is very difficult and is therefore not recommended.

Auscultation for respiratory purposes should be carried out anteriorly, laterally and posteriorly and always symmetrically. Crepitations and rhonchi should be documented.

Abdominal examination

Inspect the abdomen and perineum prior to handling the infant. Mild abdominal distension is common in the neonate and may reflect gastric distension after a recent feed or swallowed air during crying. Because the anterior abdominal wall has poorly developed musculature in the newborn, the intestines may be seen. Clearly defined laddering of the intestines may reflect intestinal obstruction. Divarication of the recti is common and is readily palpable as separation of the musculature of the anterior abdominal wall in a line running vertically upwards from the umbilicus to the xiphisternum.

Inspect the umbilicus for an omphalocele, gastroschisis or umbilical hernia. An umbilical hernia is covered with skin and subcutaneous tissue, an omphalocele (or exomphalos) shows protruding intestines covered by a thin layer of peritoneum, and a gastroschisis emerges from a defect in the anterior abdominal wall above the umbilicus and is not covered with any membrane. A small amount of bleeding from the umbilicus is not uncommon in the early days of life, but this should lead the examiner to check that the infant has received vitamin K supplementation. A halo of erythema round the umbilicus should alert the examiner to a possible omphalitis which may require urgent treatment. A granuloma of the umbilicus is usually diagnosed later when there has been delayed separation of the cord remnant and granulation tissue shows as a local swelling in the umbilical stump. It must be differentiated from omphalocele: the granuloma feels 'velvety' and does not contain intestines. Indirect inguinal hernias are not infrequent in the newborn, especially in boys, and particularly in preterm infants with chronic lung disease. Check that any hernia can be readily reduced. This is best done by sustained gentle upward pressure on the bowel from the direction of the scrotum towards the inguinal canal. Such infants should be placed on a pediatric surgeon's urgent outpatient list.

Examination of the abdomen is otherwise very similar to that of the older child. Gentle, warm hands placed flat on the abdomen will obtain more information than uncomfortable fingertips. Superficial palpation should always precede deeper exploration of the abdomen. In the neonate the kidneys may often be palpable especially if ballotted. Remember that the neonate's spleen tends to enlarge down the left flank rather than towards the right iliac fossa (Fig. 3.12).[40]

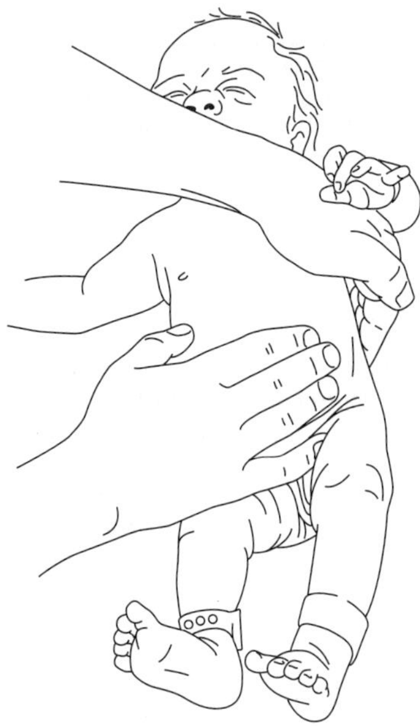

Fig. 3.11 Palpating spleen/kidey. (From Laing & McIntosh[40] with permission of Baillière Tindall)

The neonatal perineum

Examination of female genitalia should be done gently. A milky substance is seen quite commonly in the vagina: this is a normal phenomenon and is not to be confused with an infected discharge. Later in the first week of life it is also quite common to see a little vaginal bleeding ('pseudomenses') as the child withdraws from maternal hormonal influence. Gentle retraction of the labia majora may reveal a mucosal tag attached to the wall of the vagina: this needs no treatment. In preterm infants the labia majora are often retracted laterally and cause the labia minora to appear more prominent, and even sometimes give a masculinized appearance. This will resolve over the subsequent weeks.

Male genitalia should be inspected for any abnormality of the shape or size of penis or scrotum. The position of the outlet of the urethra should be at the tip of the penis and if there is any doubt the mother should be asked to witness the urinary stream. Males usually have the appearance of phimosis at birth, and no attempt should be made to retract the child's foreskin. Hypospadias may be glandular or at any position along the ventral shaft of the penis. Epispadias is less common but occasionally the urethral outlet can be seen on the dorsal aspect of the penis. Chordee is a tethering of the foreskin and often causes the glans to be curved ventrally. A hydrocele is a common swelling of the scrotum, diagnosed because it readily transilluminates, and normally resolves spontaneously over a few weeks. Cryptorchidism is an important diagnosis to make in the newborn period. Maldescent of one or both testes should be carefully excluded. Usually the right testis descends from the abdomen into the scrotum later than the left testis, and the latter usually takes up a lower position in the scrotum. Hands should always be warm for this inspection. It may be difficult reliably to palpate the testes in infants with a large pad of suprapubic fat. A retractile testis may be felt just below the inguinal canal. Occasionally it is necessary to re-examine the child in an outpatient clinic several weeks later.

Neurological examination

The newborn infant is relatively unsophisticated and therefore neurological examination (Table 3.9) is more limited than in older children.

Inspection is crucial. The neonate should be fairly symmetrical in posture and movement. Any asymmetry should be recorded. The child with postdelivery Erb's palsy may show poverty of movement and medial rotation of the forearm along with inability to extend the ipsilateral wrist. The child with a facial nerve palsy may show poor movement of the cheek muscles and poor downturning of the mouth on the ipsilateral side during crying. Inspection of the newborn infant may reveal muscle wasting, e.g. in an infant with talipes equinovarus. Fasciculation is rare in the newborn infant.

Sensory examination is largely limited to withdrawal from stimuli, e.g. stroking of the child's feet. Painful stimuli should never be inflicted on the infant. The eyesight of a newborn infant can be checked crudely, in the alert state, by carrying the child to a dark corner where he may open his eyes wide and then to a brightly lit area such as a window in daylight, whereupon the infant will screw up his eyes in response to the bright light. Formal referral to an expert ophthalomolgist should be carried out where the infant's visual capabilities are in doubt. Hearing can be tested by a startle response to loud sounds, but it is hoped that in the near future universal neonatal audiological screening will be available in the UK.

Tone is defined as the resistance to passive movement across a joint. Decreased tone in the newborn is a rather subjective judgment but becomes more reliable with experience. Normal infants may feel 'floppy' after a large feed. Infants with Down syndrome are undoubtedly hypotonic. It is possible on careful examination to demonstrate central (largely truncal) and peripheral (largely limb) hypotonia. Hypotonic infants may adopt a rather frog-like posture with abducted hips and extended elbows. Back arching, neck arching, limb extension and stiffness may be indicative of meningitis, asphyxia or an intracranial hemorrhage. Tremulousness of the newborn is relatively common, but occasionally may reflect a subarachnoid hemorrhage or drug withdrawal. Infrequent jerks in light sleep are common and normal. Regular clonic or tonic jerks must always be considered abnormal.

Establishing that the infant has normal power is also somewhat subjective at birth. The examiner is looking for strong symmetrical limb and truncal movements. The assessment of overall power is very dependent on the state of arousal of the infant.

Demonstration of primitive reflexes may seem at first blush to be pointless, except perhaps as the display of a candidate's prowess in examinations. This is not completely true. The infant with an asymmetrical Moro response may be shown to have a previously unsuspected fracture of the clavicle. Persistence of the primitive reflexes into later infancy may be the first signs of neuro-developmental abnormality. Demonstration of primitive reflexes is often done clumsily and inefficiently. The following schema is one way of ensuring that most reflexes are inspected in a logical flow which ensures that the infant is minimally disturbed.

Carry out the reflexes in the following order: grasp response of feet, grasp response of hands, pull to sit, ventral suspension, pelvic response to back stimulation, vestibular responses, place and step reflexes, Moro reflex, root and suck responses, and finally the tonic neck reflex. All of these reflexes require practice and some of them are very arousal–dependent.

During stimulation of the plantar aspect of the feet and palmar aspect of the hand be sure that the response is not inhibited by inadvertent stimulation of the dorsal aspects of feet and hands. While gently pulling the child towards a sitting position, note that the sternocleidomastoid muscles bilaterally anticipate the pull to sit, providing momentary flexion at the neck before head lag occurs (Fig. 3.13).[40] During ventral suspension, the examiner should witness good neck extension which is relatively mature in the newborn infant. Pelvic response to stimulation of the back and

Table 3.9 Neonatal reflexes

	How elicited	Time of appearance	Usual time of disappearance of those reflexes which are time limited	Possible significance if abnormal
Primitive reflexes				
Cranial nerve reflexes (relevant cranial nerves)				
Sucking (IX, X, XII)	On feeding	Birth	When voluntary control of feeding achieved at 6–9 months	General neurological depression, hypotonia, immaturity or bulbar palsy
Swallowing (IX, X, XII)	On feeding	Birth	When voluntary control of feeding achieved at 6–9 months	General neurological depression, hypotonia, immaturity or bulbar palsy
Rooting (V)	On light contact with infant's cheek the infant turns towards the point of contact	Birth	9 months	General neurological depression, hypotonia, immaturity or bulbar palsy
Glabella (V, VII)	A sharp tap on the glabella produces momentary tight closure of the eyes	Birth	Variable persistence	Apathy or facial palsy if absent; accentuated in hyperexcitability
Head turn to light (II)	With infant supine light from a diffuse source is allowed to fall on one side and then on the other side of the infant's face and he turns his head to the light (the infant must be in a quiet relaxed state)	Several weeks	–	General neurological depression, hypotonia, ?impaired vision
Pupillary (II, also III and V)	Shade one eye with the hand for a moment or two and then withdraw it	Birth	–	General neurological depression, ?impaired vision
Optic blink (II)	Shine a bright light suddenly at the eyes	Birth	–	General neurological depression, ?impaired vision
Doll's eye (III, IV, VI)	Turn head slowly to right or left watching position of eyes (normally eyes do not move with head)	Birth	2 weeks	Ophthalmic muscle palsies (ophthalmoplegia)
Acoustic blink (VIII)	Clap the hands about 30 cm from the infant's head. Avoid producing an air stream across the face. Rapid habituation – no response to test – normally achieved	After a few days	–	?Impaired hearing
Labyrinthine (rotation) (VIII, also III, IV, VII)	(a) Hold baby upright with examiner's hands under infant's arms. Spin round so that baby turns with examiner, first one direction then other (the head should turn towards direction in which baby is being turned)	Birth	–	Disturbed vestibular function or ophthalmoplegia
	(b) Baby similarly held but head held firmly by examiner's forefinger and middle finger which, on each side, are extended upwards against the side of the baby's head. Similar rotation (the baby's eyes should turn towards the turning direction)			Disturbed vestibular function or ophthalmoplegia
Gag (IX, X, XII)	Touch posterior pharynx, e.g. with spatula	Birth	–	General neurological depression or bulbar palsy

(Continued)

Table 3.9 *(Continued)*

	How elicited	Time of appearance	Usual time of disappearance of those reflexes which are time limited	Possible significance if abnormal
Cough (IX, X, XII)	Generated spontaneously on irritation of the respiratory passages	Weak for several weeks after birth	–	General neurological depression
Cutaneous reflexes				
Palmar/foot grasp	Place the examiner's forefinger in the palm/sole of the infant's hand/foot which then closes round the examiner's finger maintaining a grip	Birth	2–3 months (palmar), 7–8 months (foot)	General neurological depression, hypotonia: hemisyndromes, Erb palsy or clavicular fracture. May persist beyond normal time in spastic cerebral palsy
Abdominal	Stroke a pin or thumbnail from the side to the center of the abdomen (a response is only possible if muscles are fully relaxed)	7 days	–	Absence does not necessarily imply abnormality
Anal	Contraction of the external anal sphincter when the skin round it is stroked with a pin	Birth	–	Damage to sacral cord (e.g. spina bifida)
Cremaster	Stroking the medial side of the thigh with a pin or thumbnail results in pulling up of the testes	10 days	–	Absent in spinal cord lesion
Withdrawal	On pricking the sole of the foot with a pin there is rapid flexion of the hip, knee and foot	Birth	–	Hemisyndromes; absent or weak in spina bifida and after breech delivery with extended legs
Plantar (Babinski)	Stroking the foot along the lateral side with pin or thumbnail produces dorsal flexion of the big toe and spreading of the other toes in infancy (and plantar flexion of the other toes in older children who are walking). Do not mistake a grasp reflex of the foot for a flexor plantar response	Birth	–	Defects of lower spinal cord, hemisyndromes
Extensor reflexes				
Asymmetrical tonic neck	With baby in supine position rotate the head to one side. This produces increased tone in, and partial extension of, the arm and leg on the side to which the head is rotated, and there may be flexion of the arm and leg on the contralateral side	1 month	3–5 months	Medullary or spinal cord damage. Readily elicited in immature infant. May persist beyond normal time in cerebral palsy
Crossed extensor reflex	Passively extend one lower limb pressing the knee down, and with a pin stimulate the sole of the foot of this fixated leg. Flexion and slight abduction of the unstimulated lower limb normally occurs	A few days after birth	1 month	Absent in lesions of spinal cord and weak in peripheral nerve damage
Trunk incurvation (Galant)	Stroke a pin or thumbnail along the paravertebral line about 3 cm from the midline from the shoulder to the buttock (the back should curve with the concavity to the stimulated side)	5–6 days	7–8 days	Hemisyndromes; spinal cord damage – with indication of segmental level

(Continued)

Table 3.9 *(Continued)*

	How elicited	Time of appearance appearance	Usual time of disappearance of those reflexes which are time limited	Possible significance if abnormal
Perez	Elicited as for Galant but by stroking over central vertebral spines (the infant arches backwards, the buttocks rise and the anus dilates)	5–6 days	–	As for trunk incurvation reflex
Moro	Hold baby in supine position with shoulders and back supported on left hand and arm of the examiner and head (occiput) on the right hand. Allow the head to fall back suddenly (catching it again with the right hand after it has fallen a short distance) while the rest of the body remains supported. The arms rapidly abduct and come together again with an embracing movement and the legs flex	Birth	2–3 months	General neurological depression, hypotonia. Prolongation of tonic phase of response in immaturity. Hemisyndromes, fractured clavicle or humerus. May persist beyond normal time in cerebral palsy
Hand opening	Stroke the dorsum of the hand	Birth	2–3 months	General neurological depression; hemisyndrome
Progression				
Walking/stepping	Hold infant in standing position and place foot on a flat surface. The leg extends to take the infant's weight (supporting reaction), the opposite leg flexes then extends, and as it takes weight the original leg flexes	4 days	2 months	General neurological depression, hypotonia: paresis of lower limbs
Placing	With the baby held upright between the hands of the examiner the dorsal part of the foot is brought lightly in contact with the edge of the table. Normally the baby flexes knee and hip and places foot on the table	4 days	5–9 months	General neurological depression, hypotonia: paresis of lower limbs
Crawling	Infant prone. Crawling movements may occur spontaneously but can be reinforced by the examiner pressing his thumb gently into the sole of the infant's foot (the crawling reflex is more easily elicited in the immature infant than the walking reflex)	4 days	4 months	General neurological depression, hypotonia; paresis of lower limbs
Tendon reflexes				
Jaw jerk	Sharp tap on the examiner's index finger placed on patient's chin below the lip	2 days	–	Absent in brainstem lesions or 5th cranial nerve damage; exaggerated in hyperexcitability, e.g. hypocalcemia
Biceps	A tap on the examiner's finger placed on the biceps muscle causes contraction of the muscle	2 days	–	Absent in general neurological depression and hypotonia; exaggerated in hyperexcitability
Knee jerk	A tap on the patellar tendon with the knee in the flexed position produces quadriceps contraction	2 days	–	Absent in general neurological depression and hypotonia; exaggerated in hyperexcitability
Ankle	With infant prone, knee slightly flexed and the fore part of the foot held lightly in the examiner's hand a tap over the tendo Achillis produces plantar flexion of the foot (response better felt than seen)	Birth	–	Absent in general neurological depression and hypotonia; exaggerated in hyperexcitability
Ankle clonus	Rapid dorsiflexion of the foot with the examiner's hand on the distal part of the sole produces a succession of rapid contractions of the calf muscle (only briefly sustained in normal infant)	Birth	–	Absent in general neurological depression and hypotonia; exaggerated in hyperexcitability

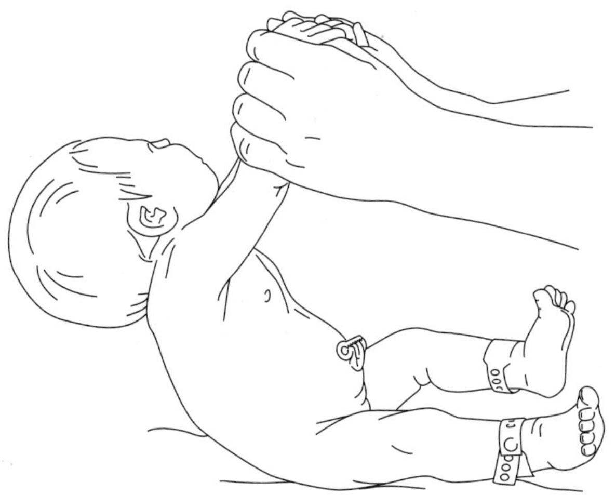

Fig. 3.12 Pull to sit. (From Laing & McIntosh[40] with permission of Baillière Tindall)

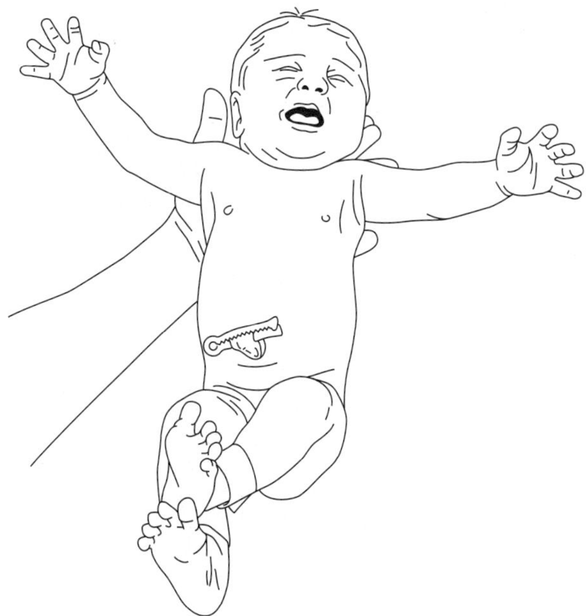

Fig. 3.13 Moro reflex. (From Laing & Mcintosh[40] with permission of Baillière Tindall)

flanks should be symmetrical. Vestibular responses are best demonstrated by holding the child upright, and then rotating in an arc. The eyes are seen to gaze in the direction of travel. After a few days it is normal to observe optokinetic nystagmus during this movement. The place and step reflexes are often very arousal dependent: the place response is elicited by stimulating the dorsum of the infant's foot on the edge of the examination table. The step response occurs as a walking movement when the ventral surfaces of the child's feet are placed on the table.

The Moro response should always be carried out with the infant's pelvis safely on the examining couch. The trunk is supported at an acute angle to the couch. The examiner's hand supports the head, and then allows the baby's trunk and head to drop by an inch or so. The normal response involves symmetrical abduction of both arms, spreading of the fingers and is often followed by a rather jerky adduction of the arms as though the hands were reaching for an unseen security (Fig. 3.14).[40]

Efficient infant feeding depends on rooting, sucking, swallowing and defending the airway. The first two can be tested by gentle stimulation of the baby's cheek. The hungry child will immediately root as though for a nipple. Sucking is often very vigorous.

The tonic neck reflex is the most unreliable and difficult to achieve of all the primitive reflexes. In theory, if the recumbent infant's head is turned to the left, then the left arm and leg will extend and the right arm and leg will flex (Fig. 3.15).[40] In theory the tonic neck reflex appears at 37 weeks' gestation but is most prominent at 1 month of age.

Final inspection

After the examination of systems, it is appropriate to carry out a final inspection of the infant. One recommended practice is to begin at the top and progress carefully to the feet. The scalp should again be inspected and palpated for any abnormalities. All aspects of the head and neck should be reinspected as above. The upper limbs and hands should be examined, the fingers and thumbs counted and the palmar creases visualized. Any oligodactyly, polydactyly or syndactyly are noted. The palmar creases of both hands are inspected: remember that a small percentage of the normal population may have single palmar creases. The chest and abdomen should be reinspected and the whole of the vertebral column palpated. Breast engorgement of the child may cause understandable parental anxiety, and yet is benign and resolves spontaneously. The presence of the sacrum and coccyx should be recorded particularly for the infant of a diabetic mother, in whom sacral agenesis is an associated finding. A hairy or pigmented patch over the lower spine may reflect spina bifida occulta. A sacrococcygeal pit is a very common phenomenon and is usually benign, but it is important to visualize the bottom of the blind-ending of the pit to ensure that it is not in communication with the spinal cord: the pit is particularly significant if above S2. The anus should be examined to ensure firstly that it is present and secondly to record any anal fissure. The anus may occasionally be malpositioned either anteriorly or posteriorly, and its patency should be checked by inspection and with evidence of the passage of meconium. If there is any pouting of the anal fissure then the sphincter should be gently stimulated to inspect muscle reactivity. Rectal examination is not a routine part of clinical examination of the newborn: it can cause trauma including the creation of an anal fissure. If it is clinically indicated it should be carried out by the examiner's well-lubricated fifth finger.

The legs are then examined and any deformations or malformations are recorded. The toes are counted and any over-riding is noted. Talipes equinovarus is not uncommon in the newborn period, but it is always essential to check that the foot and ankle can easily achieve the correct position with gentle manipulation. Because of the fetal position in utero, the neonate may have forefoot adduction and tibial bowing, both of which are normal phenomena.

Finally an examination for dislocation of the hip is carried out (Fig. 3.15).[40] Nowadays we should refer to 'developmental dysplasia of the hip' (DDH) because it is believed that some of the dysplasias identified at 1 year of life may not have been evident as dislocation or dislocatability at the time of birth. The incidence of DDH can only be presumed and depends on the care and experience of the examiner, and the population of infants being examined. It may be around 1 in 1000 in the UK.[53] The subject is complex and has been reviewed in detail on behalf of the American Academy of Pediatrics.[54] This part of the examination should be carried out on a firm but comfortable surface. The thighs are inspected for symmetry of the thigh creases.

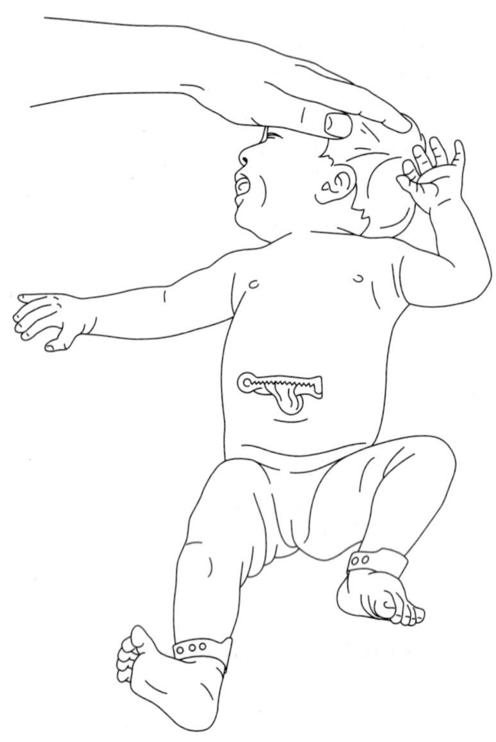

Fig. 3.14 Tonic neck reflex. (From Laing & McIntosh[40] with permission of Baillière Tindall)

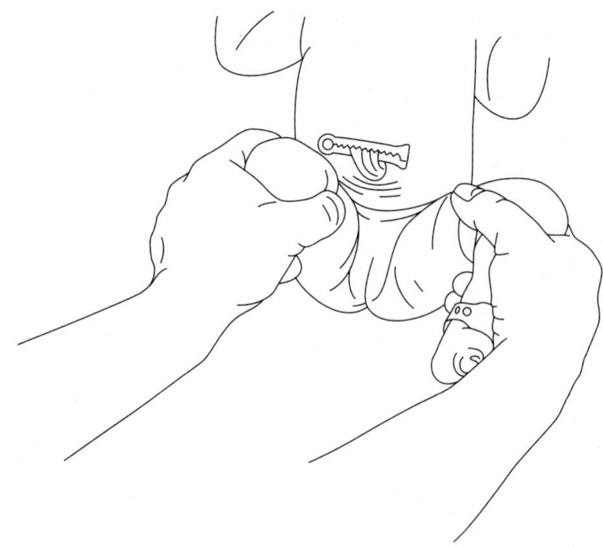

Fig. 3.15 Hip examination. (From Laing & McIntosh[40] with permission of Baillière Tindall)

The Ortolani procedure is then carried out as shown in Figure 3.15. Each hip should be examined separately. The thighs are held with the knees flexed and the examiner's thumb on the medial aspect of the thigh. The upper end of the thigh is moved laterally and then downwards on to the examining table. The thigh is then abducted. Any clunk felt indicates dislocatability of the hip. Dislocated hips are diagnosed when the femoral head is felt to be very lax and a clunk is produced without the above lateral and downward movement being required. Minor clicks are frequently felt during the examination of normal hips and are often generated at the hip or knee by tendon movements. Whenever there is doubt the examiner should refer the infant for a senior opinion, including if available an orthopedic surgeon with expertise in pediatrics. An ultrasound screening program is available in some centers to aid in the diagnosis of hip dislocation.

CONCLUDING REMARKS

High quality examination of the newborn can be achieved only with experience, and all professionals must seek advice when in doubt. At the end of the examination of the newborn, the clinician should allow time for the parents to ask any questions they may have. A few reassuring replies at this stage may prevent hours of parental anxiety. The clinician should appear enthusiastic about the child and congratulate the parents on their baby. Where abnormalities have been identified, there should be a clear written plan of treatment and follow-up. Parents should also be informed about the most appropriate sources of advice for their infant's care in the coming days and weeks.

REFERENCES (* Level 1 evidence)

1 Miall LS, Davies H. An analysis of paediatric diagnostic decision-making: how should students be taught? Med Educ 1992; 26:317–320.

*2 Pless CE, Pless IB. How well they remember. The accuracy of parent reports. Arch Pediatr Adolesc Med 1995; 149:553–558.

3 Vessey JA. Developmental approaches to examining young children. Pediatr Nurs 1995; 21:53–56.

4 Dworkin PH, Woodrum DT, Brooks KS, et al. Pediatric-based assessment: children with school problems. J School Health 1981; 51:325–329.

5 Kune-Karrer BM, Taylor EH. Toward multiculturality. Implications for the pediatrician. [Review] [17 refs]. Pediatr Clin North Am 1995; 42:21–30.

6 Danker-Hopfe H, Delibalta K. Menarcheal age of Turkish girls in Bremen. Anthropol Anz 1990; 48:1–14.

7 Greitzer L, Stapleton FB, Wright L, et al. Telephone assessment of illness by practicing pediatricians. J Pediatr 1976; 88:880–882.

*8 Rogers JC, Cohn P. Impact of a screening family genogram on first encounters in primary care. Fam Pract 1987; 4:291–301.

9 Jolly W, Froom J, Rosen MG. The genogram. J Fam Pract 1980; 10:251–255.

10 Green J, Sullivan AL, Jureidini J. Shortcomings in psychosocial history taking in a paediatric emergency department. J Paediatr Child Health 1998; 34:188–191.

11 McCarthy PL, Jekel JF, Stashwick CA, et al. History and observation variables in assessing febrile children. Pediatrics 1980; 65:1090–1095.

12 McCarthy PL, Jekel JF, Stashwick CA, et al. Further definition of history and observation variables in assessing febrile children. Pediatrics 1981; 67:687–693.

*13 Schmitz T, Bair N, Falk M, et al. A comparison of five methods of temperature measurement in febrile intensive care patients. Am J Crit Care 1995; 4:286–292.

*14 Robinson JL, Seal RF, Spady DW, et al. Comparison of esophageal, rectal, axillary, bladder, tympanic, and pulmonary artery temperatures in children. J Pediatr 1998; 133:553–556.

*15 Erickson RS, Woo TM. Accuracy of infrared ear thermometry and traditional temperature methods in young children. Heart Lung 1994; 23:181–195.

16 Osinusi K, Njinyam MN. Comparison of body temperatures taken at different sites and the reliability of axillary temperature in screening for fever. Afr J Med Med Sci 1997; 26:163–166.

17 Shann F, Mackenzie A. Comparison of rectal, axillary, and forehead temperatures. Arch Pediatr Adolesc Med 1996; 150:74–78.

18 Wilshaw R, Beckstrand R, Waid D, et al. A comparison of the use of tympanic, axillary, and rectal thermometers in infants. J Pediatr Nurs 1999; 14:88–93.

19 Leick-Rude MK, Bloom LF. A comparison of temperature-taking methods in neonates. Neonatal Network 1998; 17:21–37.

20 Hicks MA. A comparison of the tympanic and axillary temperatures of the preterm and term infant. J Perinatol 1996; 16:261–267.

21 Bailey J, Rose P. Axillary and tympanic membrane temperature recording in the preterm neonate: a comparative study. J Adv Nurs 2001; 34:465–474.

*22 Yetman RJ, Coody DK, West MS, et al. Comparison of temperature measurements by an aural infrared thermometer with measurements by traditional rectal and axillary techniques. J Pediatr 1993; 122:769–773.

23 Muma BK, Treloar DJ, Wurmlinger K, et al. Comparison of rectal, axillary, and tympanic membrane temperatures in infants and young children. Ann Emerg Med 1991; 20:41–44.

24 Lip GY, Beevers M, Beevers DG, et al. The measurement of blood pressure and the detection of hypertension in children and adolescents. J Hum Hypertens 2001; 15:419–423.

25 Goonasekera CD, Dillon MJ. Measurement and interpretation of blood pressure. Arch Dis Child 2000; 82:261–265.

*26 de Swiet M, Fayers P, Shinebourne EA. Blood pressure in first 10 years of life: the Brompton study. BMJ 1992 ;304:23–26.

*27 de Man SA, Andre JL, Bachmann H, et al. Blood pressure in childhood: pooled findings of six European studies. J Hypertens 1991; 9:109–114.

28 Gevers M, Van Genderingen HR, Van der Mooren K. Bisferiens peaks in the radial artery pressure wave in newborn infants: a sign of patent ductus arteriosus. Pediatr Res 1995; 37:800–805.

29 Sarici SU, Alpay F, Okutan V, et al. Is a standard protocol necessary for oscillometric blood pressure measurement in term newborns? Biol Neonate 2000; 77:212–216.

30 Gilmore B, Hardwick W, Noland J, et al. Determination of systolic blood pressure via pulse oximeter in transported pediatric patients. Pediatr Emerg Care 1999; 15:183–186.

31 Arafat M, Mattoo TK. Measurement of blood pressure in children: recommendations and perceptions on cuff selection. Pediatrics 1999; 104:e30.

*32 Short JA. Noninvasive blood pressure measurement in the upper and lower limbs of anaesthetized children. Paediatr Anaesth 2000; 10:591–593.

33 Crapanzano MS, Strong WB, Newman IR, et al. Calf blood pressure: clinical implications and correlations with arm blood pressure in infants and young children. Pediatrics 1996; 97:220–224.

34 Kunk R, McCain GC. Comparison of upper arm and calf oscillometric blood pressure measurement in preterm infants. J Perinatol 1996; 16:89–92.

*35 Cunningham S, Symon AG, Elton RA, et al. Intra-arterial blood pressure reference ranges, death and morbidity in very low birthweight infants during the first seven days of life. Early Hum Dev 1999; 56:151–165.

36 Engle WD. Blood pressure in the very low birth weight neonate. Early Hum Dev 2001; 62:97–130.

37 Jones KL. Smith's recognizable patterns of human malformation 5th edn. Philadelphia International: WB Saunders; 1997.

38 Margolis P, Gadomski A. Does this infant have pneumonia? JAMA 1998; 279:308–313.

39 Kuhns LR, Bednarek FJ, Wyman ML, et al. Diagnosis of pneumothorax or pneumomediastinum in the neonate by transillumination. Pediatrics 1975; 56:355–360.

40 Laing I, McIntosh N. Paediatric history and examination. London: Baillière Tindall; 1994.

41 Pelech AN. Evaluation of the pediatric patient with a cardiac murmur. [Review] [44 refs]. Pediatr Clin North Am 1999; 46:167–188.

42 Haney I, Ipp M, Feldman W, et al. Accuracy of clinical assessment of heart murmurs by office based (general practice) paediatricians. Arch Dis Child 1999; 81:409–412.

43 Hansen LK, Birkebaek NH, Oxhoj H. Initial evaluation of children with heart murmurs by the non-specialized paediatrician. Eur J Pediatr 1995; 154:15–17.

44 Ashworth CS, Fargason CA Jr, Fountain K, et al. Impact of patient history on residents' evaluation on child sexual abuse. Child Abuse Negl 1995; 19:943–951.

45 Geigy JR. Folia Medica scientific table. Basle, S.A., Switzerland.

46 Apgar V. A proposal for new method of evaluation of the newborn infant. Anesth Analg 1953; 32:260.

47 Hall DMB, ed. Health for all children. A programme of child health surveillance. Oxford: Oxford University Press; 1989.

48 Moss GD, Cartlidge PHT, Speidel BD, et al. Routine examination in the newborn period. BMJ 1991; 302:878–879.

49 Banji M, Stone RK, Kaul A, et al. Palpable lymph nodes in healthy newborns and infants. Pediatrics 1986; 8:573.

50 Faix RG. Fontanelle size in black and white term newborn infants. J Pediatr 1982; 100:304.

51 Rahi JS, Dezateus C. National cross sectional study of detection of congenital and infantile cataract in the United Kingdom: role of childhood screening and surveillance. BMJ 1999; 318:362–365.

52 Wren C, Richmond S, Donaldson L. Presentation of congenital heart disease in infancy: implications for routine examination. Arch Dis Child 1999; 80:F49–F53.

53 Leck I. An epidemiological assessment of neonatal screening for dislocation of the hip. J Roy Coll Physicians Lond 1986; 20:56–62.

*54 American Academy of Pediatrics. Clinical practice guideline: early detection of developmental dysplasia of the hip. Pediatrics 2000; 105(4):896–905.

4

Ethical and legal aspects of pediatrics (incl. consent)

Ben Stenson, Alexander McCall-Smith

INTRODUCTION

Everyone involved in the care of children has a duty of care which compels them to promote the best interests of the child and by doing so to maximize the child's potential to achieve optimal physical, mental and social health. Decisions or recommendations made on behalf of children, as well as being medically appropriate, must be consistent with contemporary ethical reasoning and be legal. To the fullest extent permissible they should be joint decisions involving all those with a legitimate role in the partnership of care and they must respect the human rights of everyone whose life may be affected by them. It is essential to take into account the views of the child if these are ascertainable. In most everyday clinical situations the options available are relatively straightforward, the communication is harmonious and everyone involved agrees on the appropriate course of action. However, when situations are more complex, placing ethical or legal principles in conflict with one another and requiring decisions to be weighed and balanced, major difficulties can arise. Many clinicians are ill equipped to deal with these situations.[1] Until recently, little emphasis has been placed in medical curricula on ethical and legal issues.

The actions of health professionals are subject to external scrutiny more than ever before. Highly publicized enquiries into standards of practice in relation to postmortem examinations, organ retention, research conduct and children's cardiac surgery (see appendix) have tested the trust of the public in the medical profession. Doctors need to become comfortable with the fact that their recommendations may be questioned rather than accepted uncritically, both at the time they are made and later in retrospect once the outcome of a clinical situation is known. Practicing medicine under these circumstances requires familiarity with ethical reasoning, legal issues and the professional standards of behavior expected by regulatory bodies as well as with technical medical information. The aim of this chapter is to provide basic guidance in these matters. The same broad principles governing conduct apply wherever medicine is practiced but legal matters vary significantly by jurisdiction. The legal issues discussed here represent the position in UK jurisdictions. Guidance on professional matters can be found on the General Medical Council web site (see appendix).

CHILDREN'S RIGHTS

The United Nations Convention on the Rights of the Child[2] was endorsed by the UK Government in 1991 and deals specifically with children's rights. In October 2000, as a result of the Human Rights Act 1998,[3] rights contained in the European Convention on Human Rights[4] also became incorporated into UK law. These rights apply to minors as well as to adults. The rights under the European Convention have not yet been extensively legally tested in the UK, so it is presently unclear how this legislation will impact on pediatric practice. In simple terms, clinicians should examine whether their decisions or actions interfere with any person's human rights and if so, whether that interference is justifiable. Up-to-date information about developments in the application of this new legislation can be obtained from the British Medical Association web site (see appendix). The rights of one individual can often conflict with the rights of another and determining which right carries most importance in a given situation can be difficult. Clinicians are encouraged to seek legal advice if they are in doubt in these matters. As far as health issues are concerned, the main rights which are likely to affect practice are the right to life (article 2 of the Convention), the right not to be subjected to inhuman or degrading treatment (article 3), and the right to private and family life (article 8). Some other rights may be relevant, including the right to marry and found a family (article 12, which may affect fertility questions), and the right not to be subjected to discrimination (article 14). The precise effect of these rights in the health context is not yet settled, but Human Rights Act-based arguments have already been taken into account in a number of important cases involving treatment decisions. Article 2 issues have arisen in relation to right to treatment and cessation of treatment cases, as have issues raised under article 3. At this stage, however, it might be pointed out that human rights are not given absolute protection under the Convention: the interests of others, and of the State, have to be taken into account in assessing how a right will be interpreted in a particular case. This allows for the balancing of parental rights with the rights of children and the rights of the State. It is also open to individual jurisdictions to approach these rights in their characteristic way: there is no single philosophy which will be enforced on all signatories to the Convention. Thus, in the UK the existing body of case law and principle based on the concept of the best interests of the child remains an important building block of the law and must be taken into account alongside human rights claims.

THE BEST INTERESTS OF CHILDREN

At the center of issues relating to the care of children is the requirement to safeguard the best interests of the child. A person's best interests are not definable in simple terms of physical health. A complex interaction of physical, emotional and social factors is involved. Personal beliefs and values give each individual a unique perspective of their best interests. The health gains of a procedure alone may not therefore be sufficient to determine a clear best interest. If the child does not wish to be treated or investigated it may not be justifiable to do so. The negative impact on the child and on relationships with the child of performing a procedure against their wishes may outweigh the health benefit obtainable. Adults are free to make choices that to others might seem unwise and to take actions that place themselves at risk of harm. Children who are in the process of developing competency as decision makers do not enjoy the same degree of autonomy. Until they become competent, others have rights and responsibilities to decide on their best interests for them. When a child's best interests are being judged by a proxy decision maker it is important to attempt to separate the interests of the child from those of the decision maker to determine whose interests are being met. At the same time the interests of an individual are dependent on their relationships with others so this may not be straightforward.

There are many reasons why caregivers and parents or young people may evaluate best interests differently. Health care professionals tend to be enthusiasts for positive action in response to health problems. They are strongly motivated to improve outcomes and tend to believe that scientific advances will help them to do so. If treatments are not working there is a natural urge to look for new alternatives and a reluctance to accept failure. This so-called technological imperative[5] could affect a clinician's balance in favor of using treatments to which a patient or a different clinician might not wish to agree. The converse is also true. Experienced clinicians can sometimes be more pessimistic than parents or young people about what the future might hold.[6] Assessments made by able-bodied people of the quality of life of disabled people are often more negative than the assessments made by the disabled themselves.

The views of clinicians about the same clinical situation often differ[7] and they evolve over time in the light of changing experience.[8,9] Inevitably, some clinicians would recommend treatment when others might believe it inappropriate. Clinicians have their own values and their recommendations are significantly related to their age, religious affiliation, religious activity, gender and specialization.[10] This suggests that treatment recommendations may be prone to arbitrariness unless they are openly shared with others. It is important for clinicians to analyze whether their personal beliefs may affect the advice or treatment that they offer patients and to be open about this in order that patients can see another professional if they wish. The values and experiences of parents and young people are likely to be equally variable. They may not yet have had cause in life to address seriously what their own values are and there may be differences between children and parents or between parents in this respect. Absolute religious beliefs may dictate that people wish to decide in a particular way whatever the consequences.

Whilst there is a commanding presumption in favor of life, it is generally agreed that in certain circumstances a person's best interests may not be served by medical efforts to prolong their life. There is not complete consensus in these matters and in individual cases it is important to make every effort to ensure that adequate communication has taken place to establish the views of all of the parties to a decision.

COMMUNICATION

Honest, open communication is an essential foundation of ethical practice. Many differences of opinion originate from misunderstandings or inadequate information. The input of time required for optimal communication is substantial but the investment is usually repaid in the form of greater trust and confidence on the part of patients and parents. Communication is a two-way process and should involve substantial listening as well as talking. When information has been shared and decisions or recommendations have been made openly there are greater grounds for confidence in their validity.

There are many barriers to communication. Children begin life completely dependent on others with little or no communication skills or decision-making capacity and require proxy decision makers. As they develop greater reasoning powers and understanding it becomes increasingly important to recognize their evolving capacities and include them in decision making and communication according to their wishes. Whether they are fully competent to decide issues for themselves or not, children generally have viewpoints and questions which should be listened to and responded to. Information should not generally be withheld from children who want it, nor given to those who do not. Providing the required information in an appropriately comprehensible form may be difficult and time consuming.

Sometimes distress about an illness or pain resulting from it may make it difficult for people to take in new information. Cultural or language barriers can add to the problem. Differences of opinion amongst the wider family can arise. Differences in communication style or language may mean that quite different messages are received when people communicate similar information. Some issues are just too complex. Clinicians, parents and young people may differ in the degrees of importance that they attach to individual components of the information communicated, so feedback should be sought to ensure that information needs are being met. Parents interviewed after difficult experiences have expressed a lack of involvement in decision making.[11]

If there is a clear medical recommendation, it should be made. Giving expert guidance about health matters is a fundamental duty and patients expect it. Few people want to be presented with statistical facts and risks and be left to make a decision alone. Good factual information is essential. Medical uncertainty should be acknowledged. It should be clearly established what is known, what can still be discovered and what is currently unknowable.[12]

In difficult circumstances, the child or the parents may have trusted friends or advisers who they feel will provide helpful support to them if they are involved.

An offer to organize a second opinion may be appropriate. Interpreters can help to overcome language barriers. Discussion with the family's religious adviser may give an insight into the background to specific moral standpoints. There is a need to revisit information and decisions with families to maintain ongoing confidence in them.

Communication should always be truthful and realistic. Information about risks and benefits should reflect local experience as well as the outcomes described in the medical literature. In cases of possible medical error patients and parents should be informed and this should be documented. It may occasionally be justifiable to withhold information but only if disclosing it would cause serious harm to the patient or another person. The General Medical Council publication Good Medical Practice outlines professional standards on which continuing medical registration is dependent.

> *'If a patient under your care has suffered harm, through misadventure or for any other reason, you should act immediately to put matters right, if that is possible. You must explain fully and promptly to the patient what has happened and the likely long and short term effects. When appropriate you should offer an apology. ... In the case of children the situation should be explained honestly to those with parental responsibility and to the child, if the child has sufficient maturity to understand the issues.'*[13]

Sometimes parents and professionals may feel that giving a child full details is not in their best interests although this should be the exception, rather than the rule.

CONSENT AND THE COMPETENCY OF CHILDREN

Rights to autonomy mean that every individual can determine what happens to his or her body. In the absence of consent, any act of touching by another person, including medical treatment, may form the basis of a legal claim for damages.[14] Consent, implied or expressed, makes such acts of touching lawful and, in normal circumstances, medical treatment should only proceed in the presence of a valid consent. There are exceptions to this: an unconscious patient may be treated without consent if it is unreasonable to delay treatment until consent can be obtained; non-consensual treatment for a mental disorder may also be authorized by mental health legislation.

Consent requires competence, and children are one group where this competence may not be present. In such cases, consent is obtained on the child's behalf from a parent, guardian, or other person exercising parental powers. In certain cases, the power to authorize treatment in the face of parental objection may be exercised by the State. Both under English[15] and Scots law,[16] a person aged 16 or over has the capacity to consent to medical treatment. A valid consent may still be given, though, by a child under the age of 16, provided that the nature and implications of the treatment can be understood. Whether or not a child has the capacity to consent depends, then, on the maturity of the individual and on the complexity of the issues that have to be decided. A comparatively young child may be able to give consent to an uncomplicated procedure with no long term implications for health (minor surgery, for example, or the administration of an antibiotic to combat an infection) whereas it will clearly require considerably greater understanding to consent to procedures involving greater risk. The law does not, and cannot set out precise criteria for determining capacity: this will entail an assessment of the facts of each case.

Once a child is deemed competent to consent to treatment it is not necessary to have parental consent as well. Only a single valid consent is required to enable treatment to proceed legally. The child should be encouraged to involve the parents but this choice belongs to the competent child. A parental refusal of consent cannot over-ride the consent of a competent child as once the child is seen to be capable of acting in his/her own best interests there is no need for a proxy decision maker. Although it may seem logical from this position that a child who is competent to consent to medical treatment should also be competent to refuse it, the courts have deemed children who refused medical treatment where a parent had consented not to be competent and have allowed treatment to proceed against the wishes of the child. In the case of *Re W*,[17] a 16-year-old girl refused treatment for anorexia nervosa in spite of the grave threat which the illness posed to her health. Although she was legally entitled to consent to treatment, the court ruled that the power to consent to treatment did not imply a power to refuse treatment and that parental consent in such circumstances would over-ride the child's opposition until such time as the child reaches the age of majority (18 years). This means that provided that parental consent is obtained, treatment in the best interests of the child may be imposed even if the child satisfies legal criteria of competence. This is justified on the grounds that there is a difference between consent to treatment and its refusal; the latter requires greater maturity and understanding than the former. Ultimately, the need to preserve life may over-ride other considerations. In *Re M*[18] the court authorized a heart transplant operation in the case of a 15-year-old girl who expressed strong objections to further treatment. This was done on the explicit grounds that the need to preserve her life outweighed the risks entailed and her possible future feelings of resentment over her wishes being ignored.

A Human Rights Act challenge to this position is conceivable. Both article 3 and article 8 of the Convention provide some protection for the realm of private decision making. It could be argued that subjecting a competent child to a strongly resisted procedure constitutes inhumane treatment, although this would have to be balanced against parental rights under article 8 to make decisions relating to family life. It is unlikely, though, that a court would allow a child to embark on a life-threatening course of action (even with parental approval). The law is prepared to be paternalistic in relation to the decisions which children make. Certainly autonomy may be encouraged, but it would be a negation of the principle of respect for autonomy to allow choices which would prevent the development of the full autonomy which comes with adulthood.

CONFIDENTIALITY

Adults should be able to assume that health care professionals dealing with personal information about them will maintain confidentiality. Confidentiality may be broken but only when consent (expressed or implicit) is given for disclosure or where it becomes necessary to breach confidence to protect others from a risk of serious harm. When children have been deemed competent their right to confidentiality must be respected, as long as this is judged to be in their best interests. (This was established legally in the case of *Gillick v. West Norfolk and Wisbech Area Health Authority*).[19] When serious issues are being considered the competent child should be encouraged to involve their parents but the choice belongs to the competent child. Less mature children may also wish for matters to remain confidential. They too should be encouraged to share information with their parents voluntarily and their confidence should not be broken lightly. If the information involves serious matters relating to the health or well-being of the incompetent child, the health care professional will have to disclose the information but they should not do so without informing the child of their intention and explaining their reasons for disclosing the information. In cases of abuse or neglect there is a responsibility to disclose information to the social services to protect the child from possible harm. It may be justifiable not to inform the child of your intention to disclose information but only if doing so would introduce a serious risk to their health and well-being.

Medical records are confidential, which means that parents may not see the medical records of their competent child without their permission. Children have a right of access to their own records under the Access to Health Records Act 1990,[20] provided that the child is capable of understanding the nature of its application for access (section 4 of the Act). This right of access to the record may be exercised by the parent or guardian on behalf of the child. As in the case of an application by an adult to see medical records, information can be withheld when the person holding the record believes that disclosing it will cause serious harm to the patient or another person.

Where personal health information potentially attributable to an individual is published or presented, consent should be sought for the disclosure, although under section 60 of the Health and Social Care Act 2001[21] the non-consensual use of identifiable patient information for the purposes of research and the improvement of treatment services may be authorized in certain circumstances. In the normal case, the consent to the use of identifiable patient information should specify the ways in which the information will be disclosed. When such information is disclosed for research purposes to others who are not directly involved in the care of the patient, consent should also be sought. Anonymized information is not protected in the same way, and considerable benefit is obtained from clinical improvement activity and research work in which clinicians analyze their patient information databases and the anonymized databases of others. Such work would become impracticable if individual patient consent was required and there would be a potential for considerable loss of health benefit to patients.

PARENTAL RESPONSIBILITY

Very young children cannot participate in decision making and for this reason parents are accorded the power to make decisions on their behalf. This right resides morally with parents because they can generally be expected to safeguard the interests of their child to a greater degree than anyone else.[22] But parental rights do not amount to ownership, and it is implicit in parental rights that they be exercised for the benefit of the child and not for the benefit of the parents. Parents must therefore always act in the best interest of the child. Of course, biological parenthood does not guarantee that this duty will be fulfilled. Some parents neglect their children or deliberately harm them. Even if they are acting in good faith and on the basis of strongly held religious beliefs, parents are not permitted to endanger their children by their decisions. The Children Act 1989,[23] which applies in England and Wales, and the Children (Scotland) Act 1995,[24] which is the equivalent Scottish legislation, state that the duty to care for the child and to raise him/her, to moral, physical and emotional health is the fundamental task of parenthood and the only justification for the authority that it confers.

In the case of young children who are not competent to decide for themselves, consent for medical treatment should be obtained from someone with parental responsibility under the Act. The biological parents are the legal parents unless a child has been adopted but biological parenthood does not necessarily confer parental responsibility under the Act. The mother has parental responsibility, and so does the father, provided that he was married to the mother at the time of the conception or the birth or if he marries her after the birth. Once a parent has obtained parental responsibility, it is not lost in the event of divorce. It is possible that the Human Rights Act could be used by unmarried fathers to establish their parental responsibility through their right to enjoy family life if the mother of the child is not permitting them involvement.

A parent is not always available. The person who has care of the child under these circumstances (e.g. a grandparent or carer) has a responsibility under the Children Act to do

> *'what is reasonable in all the circumstances of the case for the purposes of safeguarding or promoting the child's welfare'.*

This could in theory include giving consent to medical treatment but in an emergency, where serious harm might result from delay, treatment can proceed without consent in any case. Carers should not give consent if they know that the parent is likely to object.

In England, Wales and Northern Ireland, if the parents are not married, the father can gain parental responsibility by entering into a parental responsibility agreement with the mother and registering it in the Principal Registry of the Family Division of the High Court. There is an intention on the part of the Government to change the legislation to give parental responsibility to fathers who sign a child's birth certificate along with the mother, but this has not yet happened. A father can also be granted parental responsibility by a court. Adoptive parents have parental responsibility. The courts can grant parental responsibility to others such as a guardian or a local authority where the child is made the subject of a care order or a residence order. The parental responsibility that accompanies these orders lasts for the duration of the order. The court itself can also give consent to treatment on behalf of a child and can make specific issue orders or prohibited steps orders limiting parental responsibility in specified circumstances. The High Court can make the child a ward of court, which requires all important decisions about the welfare of the child to be referred to the court. In an emergency the High Court is available at all hours and if appropriate, a duty judge can be obtained through the security officer at the Royal Courts of Justice. The judge may deal with the issue by telephone or in person. A medical adviser should be available to speak to the judge in such circumstances.

In Scotland, unmarried fathers can gain parental responsibility through a voluntary parental responsibility agreement with the mother, registered in the Books of Council and Session. Fathers can also apply to the Sheriff Court or the Court of Session for an order granting them parental responsibilities and rights. Adults can gain parental responsibility by being appointed as guardians or on the order of a court. The Court of Session can give consent on behalf of a child who is not competent but probably cannot over-ride the refusal of a competent young person, although this has not been tested. As in the rest of the UK, the courts are available at all hours if necessary and can respond promptly. Both the Sheriff Court and the Court of Session can make decisions about medical issues. Contact should be made with the local Sheriff Court or with the Keepers office and if appropriate a Sheriff or Judge Depute will be contacted. As before, a medical adviser should be available via telephone or in person to answer any questions. The court can make specific issue orders or prohibited steps orders.

In Scotland the Children's Hearing System is another means for resolving issues relating to the care of children. If someone believes that a child requires compulsory measures of supervision, a reporter investigates and decides whether a ground for referral to a Children's Hearing is established, for example that the child is likely to suffer serious impairment in health or development due to a lack of parental care. If such a ground is established a hearing is arranged. If the young person and the parents accept the ground for referral, the hearing can then decide on the case and issue an appropriate order. If the ground is not accepted then the case must be determined by a Sheriff Court. If the Sheriff decides that the ground is valid the case is returned to the Children's Hearing, otherwise it is dismissed. The Children's Hearing can decide on supervision orders.

Because the courts can respond within hours to difficult situations involving consent it is the responsibility of the practitioner who embarks on treatment without a valid consent to be sure that there was a risk of serious harm had they not done so. It may be that the practitioner has later to defend their action.

DUTY OF CARE OF THE HEALTH PROFESSIONAL

The clinician has an ethical and legal duty of care to protect the life and health of his or her patients. Treatment decisions should be consistent with the basic ethical principles of beneficence and non-maleficence, which require that the benefits must outweigh the burdens. In the UK, doctors alone have the right to decide whether a treatment is medically appropriate and patients have no right to insist on treatment from a doctor if that doctor does not consider it to be in their best interests. Similarly, parents have no right to obtain such treatments for their children. The courts cannot oblige doctors to undertake any specific medical intervention, even if parents wish to insist on it.

Several UK cases have turned upon this issue. In *Re C (a minor)*,[25] a decision of the Family Division of the High Court of England and Wales, there was a difference of opinion between the parents and the doctors of a 16-month-old child suffering from spinal muscular atrophy. The medical view was that further ventilation in the event of a collapse was futile, a view which was not shared by the parents, who for religious reasons believed that everything possible should be done to save human life. The court declined to endorse the parental view. In *R v. Cambridge District Health Authority, ex parte B*,[26] the parents of a child requiring a treatment with a limited chance of success challenged the decision of the area health authority that this treatment was not justified. This was unsuccessful, the Court of Appeal accepting that decisions have to be made about the allocation of resources and that parents could not upset such hard decisions, provided that they were reasonably reached by those making them.

Parental wishes were at the center of two life-or-death cases, *Re T (a minor) (wardship: medical treatment)*[27] and, more recently, *Re A (children)*.[28] In *Re T* a parental decision to refuse a liver transplant for a child suffering from biliary atresia was upheld, even although medical opinion was that this could add several years to the child's life. This was an exceptional case and in *Re A (children)*, the highly publicized conjoined twins, parental opposition to surgery to separate the child was over-ruled.

If the clinician is being pressed to administer a treatment deemed inappropriate, then all efforts should be made to resolve the situation through further communication. If these efforts do not succeed then the clinician should go to reasonable lengths to find an alternative clinician for the family, although if good decision-making practices have been followed there may not be one easily identifiable. If these measures do not succeed and the clinician has the support of his colleagues then he should not treat. The parents should be informed of their right to obtain judicial review if they wish. If the medical reasoning has been sound and the clinician's colleagues support him then there is a strong prospect that the decision not to treat will be upheld. If a doctor refuses to give a treatment then this decision may later be legally challenged on the grounds that it amounts to a failure to discharge the duty of care owed to the patient. If there has been such a failure, then this may amount to negligence, the presence of which is determined by applying the test of whether the doctor has acted in accordance with the practice accepted by a responsible body of medical practitioners skilled in that particular art (the *Bolam* test).[29] In other words, a specialist must practice with the ordinary skill of his/her speciality.

Doctors have no legal authority to institute treatments in the absence of consent but they have a duty of care and a moral responsibility to institute emergency treatment deemed to be in the child's best interests. If there is doubt as to the best interests in an emergency, then this same duty should compel them to act on the presumption that the child would want to be saved, at least until there has been time for further consideration. Under these circumstances, if the action satisfied the *Bolam* test it is highly likely (even if not absolutely certain) that the courts would support it. This residual uncertainty provides some safeguard to ensure that doctors use their capacity to trump the parental proxy rights in an emergency responsibly. In the absence of any urgency doctors have neither moral nor legal justification to proceed without consent.

If the patient or parents refuse consent to important but non-urgent treatment, attempts should again be made to resolve the dispute through further communication. A second opinion, particularly from an acknowledged expert, may help. If these measures do not succeed and the clinician has the support of his colleagues in the view that the treatment is strongly in the best interests of the child, then judicial resolution should be sought. Again the sharing of the information with colleagues and presence of their support will increase the chances that the court will endorse the doctor, but if the decision-making process has lacked balance then the court will rightly support the alternative position. One viewpoint is that an approach for judicial resolution might relocate the conflict concerning the child's best interests to be between the State and the family and take the pressure off the relationship between the family and the clinician. In reality it probably just relocates the conflict from the consulting room to the courtroom without substantially changing the individuals involved, the balance of power or the nature of the conflict.[30]

WITHHOLDING OR WITHDRAWING LIFE-PROLONGING TREATMENT IN CHILDREN

Difficult ethical decisions in medical practice may result from our increased ability to sustain life in patients who, in years past, would not have survived. When little or nothing could be done, death was accepted as inevitable and perhaps 'for the best'. As medical advances have enhanced our ability to prolong life, increasingly penetrating questions have been asked about the wisdom of using modern medical technology to save or sustain life in all circumstances; about what some view as the unnecessary and cruel prolongation of dying; and about the medical, moral and legal justification of continuing 'futile' treatment in patients who are not dying. Arguments about the relative roles and responsibilities for making such decisions continue to occupy not only those directly involved, but have also engaged the attentions of lawyers, philosophers, theologians and others. All those involved in the care of the child have a duty to act in the child's best interests. Yet the defining of those best interests is problematic when it includes opening up to the possibility that they may be best served by withholding or withdrawing life-prolonging treatment.

Although there is a strong presumption in favor of life it has to be recognized that life cannot always be sustained and that sometimes, even with optimal treatment, death is inevitable. Treatment can also be burdensome and futile and if it serves no useful purpose it is unethical to continue it. A competent adult can decide for him or herself whether or not treatment is in their best interests. Young people can participate in these matters too, even if not fully competent, and it is important to involve them if they wish. Some people, however, through immaturity or disability are not able to share in decision making and parents and professionals are left with the awesome responsibility of making decisions on their behalf.

It may become clear that the quality of life experienced by a person if given treatment, will be likely to be so afflicted as to be intolerable. This is a contentious issue on which there will never be complete consensus. Those involved in decision making must recognize that many people with severe handicap enjoy a life of high quality and do not view disability as negatively as some able-bodied people do. A quality of life that would seem intolerable to an able-bodied person would not necessarily be unacceptable to someone who has only known that experience. It is important, then, not to devalue disabled people and to respect their contribution to society. They have the same human rights as others and should not be discriminated against. Quality of life is determined externally by the inputs of others as well as by internal factors and there are ways of improving the lives of disabled people. At the same time, most people recognize that there is a degree of severe handicap, which includes a loss of awareness and an inability to interact with others or the environment, that no reasonable person would want to endure. Medical treatment that prolonged survival of this nature without prospect of recovery would not be seen by most to be in an individual's best interests.

It is clear from the medical literature that it is common practice for life-prolonging treatment to be withdrawn. Around 30% of deaths in neonatal units[31] and up to 65% of deaths in pediatric intensive care units[32] follow a decision to withdraw treatment. Since many of the issues raised by life and death dilemmas are moral and not medical, some commentators, notably philosophers and lawyers, believe that doctors and parents are not competent to make such decisions on their own and that the law should dictate this process. This view should be treated with caution. These decisions are very delicate and complex ones, and the very particular moral claims of the parents must be recognized. Not every decision needs to be made by a court, and indeed it would be impossible for medicine to function if doctors were constantly looking over their shoulders at the law. At the same time, the protection of human life is a matter of central concern for the law, and therefore any medical and parental decisions must be made against a background of certain legal limits to what may be done. Within these limits there remains considerable room for nuanced and sensitive decisions to be made by those most intimately involved in the life of the child and its medical care.

The starting point of any discussion of this issue is the stark proposition that any deliberate act intended to bring life to an end is normally the crime of murder. This is the case even if the person carrying out the act acted with the motive of ending the victim's suffering (euthanasia). Although there have not been many prosecutions of doctors in the UK for killing their patients with this motive in mind, this is more because of the difficulty of getting juries to convict in such cases than in any ambiguity in the law. Nor is there any indication that the law will be changed in this country; only a handful of jurisdictions have legislated to allow euthanasia (The Netherlands, Belgium and the Northern Territory of Australia, where the State law was over-ruled by Federal legislation). This legal prohibition of euthanasia does not, however, prevent the appropriate and medically-indicated use of pain-killing drugs which will have the incidental effect of shortening the life of the patient. This is justified by the doctrine of double effect, which holds that pursuing a legitimate goal (in this case, pain relief) is justified even if this will have the inevitable effect of causing an undesirable event (the death of the patient). It is important, though, that drugs of this nature are not administered in such a way as to cause death virtually immediately: this might be taken as an indication that the death of the patient is the principal goal.

Euthanasia is one thing, but the withdrawal or denial of treatment is quite another matter. It has long been accepted that it is lawful to withdraw life-prolonging treatment if it is no longer in a person's best interests and that it is lawful to withhold treatment for the same reason. This has been established in a series of cases in which the courts have considered the circumstances in which it is proper to withdraw support for infants and young children for whom the prognosis is bleak. In most of these cases the courts have readily recognized that where a child's suffering would be intense and where no reasonable quality of life could be achieved, then it is futile to continue with treatment. An example of such a decision is *A National Health Service Trust v. D*,[33] in which the child in question had been born with chronic and worsening lung disease and suffered in addition from heart failure, hepatic and renal dysfunction as well as severe developmental delay. There was a difference of opinion in this case between the parental and medical views as to whether resuscitation should be attempted in future; the court endorsed the medical conclusion of futility. In reaching its conclusion, the court also addressed arguments based on European Convention rights. In particular, the court said that the decision not to resuscitate was compatible with article 2 of the Convention (the right to life). It also expressed the view that such a course of action was in accordance with article 3, which requires that a person should not be subjected to inhumane or degrading treatment; undue prolongation of life through excessively zealous treatment could infringe the right to die with dignity. This decision is significant, in that it demonstrates that human rights provisions will not be interpreted in such a way as to oblige doctors to provide treatment in those circumstances where their clinical and indeed human judgment suggests otherwise.

The practice of withholding or withdrawing life-prolonging treatment is acknowledged and endorsed by the British Medical Association[34] and by the Royal College of Paediatrics and Child Health.[35] There is presently no legal requirement for the involvement of the courts in medical decisions of this nature, nor a general belief that their involvement would be helpful. It is clearly desirable, though, that decisions of such gravity, made on behalf of dependent individuals, are not made by a single person but reflect the views of a body of people with an intimate involvement in the situation. This is required as a safeguard against the possibility that a decision could be overly influenced by the polarized views or values of one person. Openness should promote better decision making. Clear documentation of the issues being addressed, the individuals involved and their viewpoints is an important part of this. Nor should decisions of this nature be rushed. In emergencies where the appropriate course of action is unclear and a plan has not been documented, trainee doctors should administer life-sustaining treatment until a senior and more experienced doctor arrives.

With these safeguards in place it is reassuringly uncommon for parents to think later that the wrong decision was made.[36] It is not essential for there to be unanimity of views on the part of the medical team. There should be substantial consensus and the weight attributed to individual dissent will depend on the experience and knowledge of the person expressing it.

Withdrawal of life-prolonging treatment does not imply withdrawal of care. Care which is directed at maintaining the comfort and dignity of the patient (palliative care) is always required. The clinical team should continue to consider the child's physical, emotional and spiritual needs. Food and fluid should usually be offered (but not forced) on a regular basis. The role of assisted feeding by nasogastric tube or gastrostomy can be a source of difficulty. There is a spread of opinion as to what circumstances determine whether this is a life-prolonging medical treatment, a comfort measure or a basic necessity. In some circumstances such as the persistent vegetative state it may be seen to be in a person's best interests for feeding or intravenous fluids to be withdrawn. It is important to consider whether these measures are benefitting the patient. These issues must be handled sensitively, taking into account the views of the family and the staff.

Where consideration is being given to withdrawal of treatment, there may be a number of treatments in use, such as mechanical ventilation, antibiotics, analgesics or sedatives and paralyzing agents. It is not appropriate to wait for the effect of the medications to wear off before withdrawing the ventilation. This would effectively be giving one futile treatment because you were already giving another. Analgesics should be continued after the withdrawal of ventilation. The primary intention of administering analgesics is to control pain and distress and this has a clear benefit to the patient. A side-effect of opioids may be that they suppress breathing and could shorten life; however this is not the purpose for which they are being administered. As discussed above, this situation of double effect is recognized and accepted in law. The situation is a little more finely balanced in the case of paralyzing agents. If ventilation is withdrawn in a paralyzed patient, death will certainly follow shortly afterwards. These agents are generally being given to facilitate ventilation in a critically ill patient with severe cardiopulmonary failure. Under these circumstances death is inevitable after withdrawal of ventilation whether paralyzing agents are being used or not. Paralyzing agents may therefore reasonably be continued up to the point that ventilation is withdrawn but should not be administered after extubation. In the absence of cardiopulmonary failure, paralyzing agents are unlikely to be in clinical use and should not be given to patients who are not going to be ventilated.

In 1997 the Ethics Advisory Committee of the Royal College of Paediatrics and Child Health published a guidance document for professionals about withdrawing or withholding life-prolonging treatment from children.[35] The document is available from the College and remains current. The document highlights a number of axioms on which ethical decision making about the withholding or withdrawal of life-prolonging treatment may be based.

1. There is no significant ethical difference between withdrawing (stopping) and withholding treatments, given the same ethical objective.
2. Optimal ethical decision making concerning children requires open and timely communication between members of the health care team and the child and family, respecting their values and beliefs and the fundamental principles of ethics and human rights.
3. Parents decide on behalf of children who are unable, for whatever reason, to express preferences, unless they are clearly acting against the child's best interests or are unable, unwilling or persistently unavailable to make such decisions on behalf of their child.
4. The wishes of a child who has obtained sufficient understanding and experience in the evaluation of treatment options should be given substantial consideration in the decision-making process.
5. The antecedent wishes and preferences of the child, if known, should also carry considerable weight given that conditions at the time for action match those envisaged in advance.
6. In general, resolution of disagreement should be by discussion, consultation and consensus.
7. The duty of care is not an absolute duty to preserve life by all means. There is no obligation to provide life-sustaining treatment if its use is inconsistent with the aims and objectives of an appropriate treatment plan or if the benefits of that treatment no longer outweigh the burden to the patient.
8. It is ethical to withdraw life-sustaining treatment if refused by a competent child; or from children who are unable to express wishes and preferences when the health care team and parent/carers agree that such treatment is not in the child's best interests.
9. A redirection of management from life-sustaining treatment to palliation represents a change in beneficial aims and objectives and does not constitute a withdrawal of care.
10. The range of life-sustaining treatments is wide and will vary with the individual circumstances of the patient. It is never permissible to withdraw procedures designed to alleviate pain or promote comfort.
11. There is a distinction to be drawn between treatment of the dying patient and euthanasia. When a dying patient is receiving palliative care, the underlying cause of death is the disease process. In euthanasia, the cause of death is the intended lethal action.
12. It follows that use of medication and other treatments which may incidentally hasten death may be justified if their primary aim is to relieve suffering. The Ethics Advisory Committee of the Royal College of Paediatrics and Child Health does not support the concept of active euthanasia.
13. Legal intervention should be considered when disputes between the health care team, the child, the parents and carers cannot be resolved by attempts to achieve consensus.

The guidance document outlines five situations where it is reasonable to consider the withdrawal or withholding of life-prolonging treatment from children.

1. **The Brain Dead Child.** When brainstem death is confirmed by two medical practitioners, the patient is by definition dead, even if their organs continue to function with medical assistance (note, however, that this is not necessarily the legal definition of death). The criteria for establishing brain death are not fully applicable to neonates because of issues related to brain maturity so this situation only applies to older children.
2. **The Permanent Vegetative State.** This is defined as a state of unawareness of self and environment in which the patient breathes spontaneously, has a stable circulation and shows cycles of eye closure and eye opening which simulate sleep and waking, for a period of 12 months following a head injury or 6 months following other causes of brain damage. In such circumstances treatment, including tube feeding, may be withdrawn whilst making the patient comfortable by nursing care.
3. **The No Hope/Chance Situation.** The child has such severe disease that life-sustaining treatment simply delays death without significant alleviation of suffering.
4. **The 'No Purpose' Situation.** This is the most difficult and contentious category. The patient may be able to survive with

treatment, but the degree of physical or mental impairment will be so great that it is unreasonable to expect them to bear it. The child in this situation will never be capable of taking part in decisions regarding treatment or its withdrawal. The Ethics Advisory Committee of the Royal College of Paediatrics and Child Health envisage an 'impossibly poor life' either now or in the future.

5. **'The Unbearable Situation'.** The child and/or family feel that in the face of progressive and irreversible illness further treatment is more than can be borne. They wish to have a particular treatment withdrawn or to refuse further treatment irrespective of the medical opinion on its potential benefit. Oncology patients who are offered further aggressive treatment might be included in this category.

'In situations that do not fit with these five categories, or where there is dissent or uncertainty about the degree of future impairment, the child's life should always be safeguarded by all in the health care team in the best way possible.'

Decisions about withdrawing or withholding life-prolonging treatment are likely to be based on probabilities rather than on certainties. Parents need to be prepared for what might follow. Death may take minutes or hours or may not occur. Protracted deaths are particularly stressful for parents and may cause them to doubt the wisdom of the decision. There is a danger that withdrawing or withholding treatment in a child who goes on to survive may mean that the eventual outcome is worse than would otherwise have been the case. Unexpected survivors need ongoing support, evaluation and respect.

GENETIC TESTING (see also Ch.12)

Recent progress in elucidating the genetic basis of disease has been beyond all expectation and continued progress is likely. This carries great potential to improve health through new approaches to the diagnosis, treatment and prevention of illness. Further progress must be made before gene therapy becomes widespread but diagnosis and screening are already widely established. This gives rise to a number of ethical issues.[37] Rare and serious diseases which affect the health of children can be detected and this has obvious potential benefit to children. The new science also offers increasing capacity to detect predisposition to illnesses or even behavioral traits that may affect individuals only in adulthood. The results of such tests may have marked adverse effects on a child and on their future potential. As well as the person being tested, genetic tests also affect many others who are related to them. They may influence parental reproductive decisions. They may cast doubt on parenthood. They may raise similar issues for siblings. False positive and false negative results can cause considerable anxiety. Genetic tests should therefore only be used with caution, informed consent and adequate counseling. In general, tests on children should only be performed when a direct benefit to the child is anticipated during childhood. If the test will give information that will not have great relevance to the child until adulthood, then it should be deferred until the child is competent to decide for him or herself whether or not to agree to testing. This cautious approach to the genetic testing of children has been endorsed in the UK by the Government's Advisory Committee on Genetic Testing and by its successor body, the Human Genetics Commission (see appendix).

Consent to genetic testing raises questions which have yet to be firmly settled. In the case of routine non-genetic tests carried out in a clinical context, all that is required is that there should be consent to the necessary medical procedures (by the competent child or by the parent or guardian). It is not necessary, then, to explain the implications of every biochemical test, for example, which will be carried out on a sample. Where, however, the test has particular significance [such as an human immunodeficiency virus (HIV) test], then the person giving consent should know the nature of the test being proposed. Genetic tests have special features, which should be explained in general terms to the patient. In particular, genetic tests may have implications for other family members, and if this is the case then this should be discussed with the parent (and with the child, if the child is sufficiently mature to understand what is entailed by the information). Further questions are raised by multiplex testing, which may involve testing for a number of different genetic characteristics through devices capable of detecting numerous DNA sequences. It may be unrealistic to expect a full explanation to be given of everything that such a test may do, and for this reason consent should be valid if it is explained to the patient that a number of genetic characteristics may be revealed by the test and that this information may be retained on the record. Obviously this must be done sensitively, as nothing will be gained by giving complicated explanations which may serve only to alarm the patient unnecessarily. In respect of consent to testing, all that the law requires is that the doctor should give the patient that amount of information which is reasonable in the circumstances. A sound sense of current professional consensus on these issues is probably as good a guide as any as to how the matter should be approached.

Paternity testing may be requested by parents. This should not be performed without the involvement of both parents unless authorized by a court. Courts usually determine that testing is in the interests of the child. The child and family may need a lot of support and counseling. Guidelines on this subject are now available (see appendix).

RESEARCH

There is no doubt that medical research is in the best interests of children. Without it medicine would be unable to progress, ineffective treatments would not be discarded, effective new treatments not introduced, and dangerous ones not identified. Carrying on in ignorance where properly conducted research could determine the optimal path is unethical. However, whilst research may benefit society it can sometimes be of little benefit to the individual under study. This may be irrelevant in the case of competent adults, who can consent to participate in ethical research even if it is of no therapeutic benefit to them. The involvement of children in research is more problematic. Research which is of potential therapeutic benefit to the child is acceptable, and can be consented to by the parent on behalf of the child. Non-therapeutic research, however, is of no benefit to the child, unless, possibly, the child has a sibling or other close relative who suffers from the condition which is the subject of research. In such a case, it is possible to argue that the child benefits from helping to advance knowledge of a condition which affects him or her through the family link. There are other ways in which participation might be in the best interests of the child. Patients enrolled in studies tend to experience some improvement in their clinical outcomes when compared with similar patients who are not being studied.[38] This inclusion benefit may relate to the closer supervision necessary to perform successful research. Where there is no such justification, then it must be asked whether it is either ethical or legal to involve children in non-therapeutic research.

There is widespread agreement that it is ethical to use children in medical research provided that the research in question involves a negligible risk of harm to the child. There is a range of views as to how this risk is to be assessed. The legal position on this issue is more complex. It has been suggested in the past that the law prevented participation by children even in non-risky research on the grounds that parental consent, which would be needed, cannot be given in respect of anything which is not in the best interests of the child. In this view it would be impossible, then, for a parent ever to agree to something from which the child would not benefit. However, the more reasonable view has emerged that a parent may consent to that which does not actually threaten the child's interests. This would mean that non-therapeutic research on children is permissible, with parental consent, as long as the risk is negligible. This issue remains to be pronounced upon by the courts, but it is likely that the view expressed immediately above would prevail.

It should be stressed that if the child is old enough to have views on involvement, these views should be taken into account (even if the child does not have the capacity to consent in general). If a research procedure involves discomfort, and the child objects, then it would be unethical to continue with the procedure. From the legal point of view it would clearly not be in the child's best interests to proceed with unwelcome procedures.

In 2000, The Ethics Advisory Committee of the Royal College of Paediatrics and Child Health published guidelines for the ethical conduct of medical research involving children.[39] Six principles were outlined.

1. Research involving children is important for the benefit of all children and should be supported, encouraged and conducted in an ethical manner.
2. Children are not small adults; they have an additional, unique set of interests.
3. Research should only be done on children if comparable research on adults could not answer the same question.
4. A research procedure which is not intended directly to benefit the child subject is not necessarily either unethical or illegal.
5. All proposals involving medical research on children should be submitted to a research ethics committee.
6. Legally valid consent should be obtained from the child, parent or guardian as appropriate. When parental consent is obtained, the agreement of school-age children who take part in research should also be requested by researchers.

Consent is required for research studies which involve touching people in some way or using their blood or tissues. The same basic principles apply as when consent is obtained for treatment or examination. The person must be given adequate information to enable them to understand the nature and purpose of the research and weigh up its risks and benefits. The consent will otherwise be invalid. This so-called informed consent can be difficult to achieve when the individual may already be heavily burdened with complex information.[40] People who have given written consent do not always remember that they did so. Recollection of the information that they were given is often poor and their understanding of what they consented to may be incorrect.[41] For these reasons researchers should regard the consent process as being ongoing throughout the duration of their involvement with any patient from whom they obtain consent. They should maintain awareness on the part of the child and the parents that they are enrolled in a study, explaining any procedures, tests or treatments that are being used, making clear whether they are part of standard care or are being performed specifically for the purposes of the study. Wherever possible, a reasonable amount of time should be allowed between informing a family about a research study and obtaining consent. This can be impracticable in some studies where interventions are performed under pressure of time, e.g. in the immediate newborn period. The child and family should be aware that they are free to withdraw from a study at any time without penalty. Important details about the study should be given in the form of a printed information sheet which the patient can keep, as well as communicated verbally. Financial rewards should not be offered to families other than reasonable expenses. Pressure should not be exerted. If the child and family wish to know the final results of the research then these should be made available to them as soon as is practicable. There may be considerable delay in this if long term follow-up requires blinding to be maintained.

Agreeing to participate in a research project is an altruistic act, which may involve the patient experiencing increased uncertainty, anxiety or discomfort. It may also involve taking significant risks where treatments for serious conditions are being compared. Study design should seek to minimize this and should involve peer review and where appropriate, lay advice. The ethics committee and the process of peer review are important to ensure that the balance of risk and benefit of a study is appropriate. The peer review may be very important because the local ethics committee alone may not be fully equipped to evaluate the research question. If the research will take place in five or more centers it must be reviewed by a multicenter research ethics committee.

Statistical advice should be sought, to determine that the study has adequate power to answer the question it sets out to address. Poorly designed research is unethical research. Often the results of studies can be disappointing, with no positive finding. It is still important to attempt to get such studies published to avoid other workers repeating the study and burdening future participants unnecessarily. Failure to publish negative results is an important source of bias in the published literature. Traditionally this has been made difficult by the competition for publication in a limited amount of journal space. With advances in technology this problem should lessen as electronic publishing will provide the space for studies that cannot compete successfully for mainstream scientific journal exposure.

A great deal of research is commercially sponsored.[42] As well as potentially affecting the outcomes of future patients, the results of such studies may be of considerable economic importance to individuals or companies. Clinicians entering into agreements to organize such studies should not do so if they are not given a say in the study design, access to the full data and freedom to publish the data, even if the results are not flattering to the product in question. At the time of submission for publication, authors should disclose all financial interests between themselves and others that might influence their work.

Sometimes circumstances can arise that justify the use of new medical treatments or procedures that have not yet been evaluated by research. This activity is a form of research and should only be undertaken with the informed consent of those involved after open honest communication of the limitations of knowledge about the treatment in question and with close monitoring.

MENTAL HEALTH CARE

When treating people for mental illness the same ethical principles apply as when treating others. The Mental Health Acts[43,44] describe statutory powers which allow patients to be detained in hospital and treated for mental illness in the interests of their own health. There is no specific statutory authority to treat physical disorders of those receiving treatment under the Mental Health Acts. Psychiatric treatment can proceed without consent where a patient has been compulsorily admitted under the relevant Act. Children or young people who have been detained under the Mental

Health Acts have the right to a hearing either before a tribunal or, in Scotland, the Sheriff Court. The tribunal, or court, may order the discharge of a detained patient if the patient is found not to have a mental disorder of a nature or degree justifying detention in hospital. Alternatively, even if there is a disorder present, discharge may be ordered if the detention is not justified in the interests of the patient's health or safety, or in order to protect others.

ROLE FOR ETHICS COMMITTEES

Given the difficulty faced by many caregivers in unravelling the complexities of ethical and legal situations, there may be a role for institutional ethics committees to provide advice, education and support.[45] In the USA their development has been encouraged by professional bodies.[46] In the UK, any medical decision made would remain the legal and professional responsibility of the doctor concerned. Doctors and nurses do not express widespread support for a decision-making role for such committees[1] and neither do parents.[47] However, sometimes conflicts between parents and clinicians can become personalized and it is possible that under these circumstances recommendations made by an ethics committee may be more palatable to the parents than those made by the clinician. A clear need for education of health care staff in the ethical and legal background to these situations has been identified.[1]

APPENDIX - INFORMATION RESOURCES

ETHICAL AND LEGAL ISSUES

Consent, Rights and Choices in Health Care for Children and Young People. BMJ Books, London 2001. This book gives an excellent detailed overview of many of the issues discussed in this chapter.

ROYAL LIVERPOOL CHILDREN'S ENQUIRY

The Royal Liverpool Children's Inquiry Report (The Redfern Report). London: The Stationery Office, 2001. http://www.rlcinquiry.org.uk/

NORTH STAFFS ENQUIRY

NHS Executive West Midlands Regional Office. Report of a review of the research framework in North Staffordshire Hospital NHS Trust (Griffiths report). Leeds: NHS Executive, 2000 http://www.doh.gov.uk/wmro/northstaffs.htm. See also: Hey E, Fleming P, Sibert B, Markovitch H. Learning from the sad, sorry saga at Stoke. Archives of Disease in Childhood 2002; 861:1–3.

BRISTOL ENQUIRY

Public Inquiry into Children's Heart Surgery at the Bristol Royal Infirmary 1984–1995. In: Learning from Bristol. London: Stationery Office, 2001 (Cmnd 5207). http://www.bristol-inquiry.org.uk/

GENERAL MEDICAL COUNCIL

Standards of practice on which ongoing professional registration within the UK depend are outlined on the General Medical Council web site at http://www.gmc-uk.org/. This site covers a broad range of issues including duties of a doctor, good medical practice, medical research guidance, withholding and withdrawing treatment, confidentiality, consent, and guidance for doctors asked to circumcize male infants.

BRITISH MEDICAL ASSOCIATION

Up-to-date information about the impact of the European Convention on Human Rights on medical practice within the UK can be obtained from the BMA web site at http://www.bma.org.uk/

HUMAN GENETICS COMMISSION

http://www.hgc.gov.uk/business_publications.htm. Includes: 'Whose hands on your genes?' (November 2000) – A consultation document on the uses of human genetic information, followed by a report on this subject (May 2002). The Human Genetics Commission has endorsed the report of the Advisory Committee on Genetic Testing for late-onset disorders (1998), which includes advice on the genetic testing of children (http://www.doh.gov.uk/genetics/lodrep.htm).

PATERNITY TESTING

Code of Practice and Guidance on Genetic Paternity Testing Services (Department of Health Guidance Document). http://www.doh.gov.uk/genetics/paternity.htm.

PUBLICATION ETHICS

Guidelines on good publication practice have been published by the Committee on Publication Ethics. http://www.publicationethics.org.uk/

REFERENCES (* Level 1 evidence)

1 McHaffie HE, Fowlie PW. Life and death decisions. Doctors and nurses reflect on neonatal practice. Hale: Hochland and Hochland; 2000.
2 UN Convention on the Rights of the Child.
3 Human Rights Act 1998.
4 European Convention on Human Rights.
5 Guillemin JH, Holmstrom LL. Mixed blessings: intensive care for newborns. New York: Oxford University Press; 1986.
6 Streiner DL, Saigal S, Burrows E, et al. Attitudes of parents and health care professionals toward active treatment of extremely premature infants. Pediatrics 2001; 108:152–157.
7 Lantos JD, Singer PA, Walker RM, et al. The illusion of futility in clinical practice. Am J Med 1989; 87:81–84.
8 Lorber J. Ethical problems in the management of myelomeningocoele. J Roy Coll Surg 1975; 10:47.
9 Lorber J, Salfield SA. Result of selective treatment of spina bifida cystica. Arch Dis Child 1981; 56:822–830.
10 Todres ID, Krane D, Howell MC, et al. Pediatricians' attitudes affecting decision making in defective newborns. Pediatrics 1977; 60: 197–201.
11 Pinch WJ, Spielman ML. Parental voices in the sea of neonatal ethical dilemmas. Issues Comp Pediatr Nurs 1989; 12:423–425.
12 Laing IA, Halley GC. Enough is enough – when to stop neonatal care. Curr Pediatr 1995; 5:53–58.
13 General Medical Council. Good medical practice. London: GMC; 1998.
14 Mason JK, McCall Smith RA. Law and medical ethics. London: Butterworths; 1999: 244–288.

15 Family Law Reform Act 1969.
16 Age of Legal Capacity (Scotland) Act 1991.
17 Re W (a minor) (medical treatment) [1992] 4 All England Law Reports 627.
18 Re M [1999] 2 FLR 1097.
19 Gillick v. West Norfolk and Wisbech Area Health Authority [1985] 1 All England Law Reports 402 (HL).
20 Access to Health Records Act 1990.
21 Health and Social Care Act 2001.
22 Archard D. Children rights and childhood. London: Routledge; 1993.
23 Children Act 1989.
24 Children (Scotland) Act 1995.
25 Re C (a minor) [1998] 1 FLR 384.
26 R v. Cambridge District Health Authority, ex parte B [1995] 2 All England Law Reports 129.
27 Re T (a minor)(wardship: medical treatment) [1997] 1 All England Law Reports 906.
28 Re A (children) (conjoined twins: surgical separation) [2000] 4 All ER 961.
29 Bolam vs Friern Hospital Management Committee [1957] 2 All England Law Reports 118.
30 Stenson B, McIntosh N. The rights and duties of parents in the neonatal unit: the limits of informed consent. Semin Neonatol 1998; 3:291–296.
31 Report of the House of Commons Select Committee on Medical Ethics 1994; 1:47.
32 Balfour-Lynn IM, Tasker RC. At the coalface – medical ethics in practice. Futility and death in paediatric medical intensive care. J Med Ethics 1996; 22:279–281.
33 A National Health Service Trust v. D. [2000] 2 FLR.
34 British Medical Association. Withholding and withdrawing life prolonging medical treatment. Guidance for decision making. BMJ Books; 2000 (see www.bmjpg.com/withwith/ww.htm for full text)
35 Royal College of Paediatrics and Child Health, Ethics Advisory Committee. Withholding or withdrawing life saving treatment in children. A framework for practice. London: Royal College of Paediatrics and Child Health, 1997.
36 McHaffie HE, Lyon AJ, Hume R. Deciding on treatment limitation for neonates: the parents' perspective. Eur J Pediatr 2001; 160:339–344.
37 American Academy of Pediatrics, Committee on Bioethics. Ethical issues with genetic testing in pediatrics. Pediatrics 2001; 107:1451–1455.
38 Lantos JD. The 'Inclusion benefit' in clinical trials. J Pediatr 1999; 134:130–131.
39 McIntosh N, Bates P, Brykczynska G, et al. Guidelines for the ethical conduct of medical research involving children. Royal College of Pediatrics and Child Health: Ethics Advisory Committee. Arch Dis Child 2000; 82:177–182.
40 Anonymous. Your baby is in a trial. (Editorial). Lancet 1995; 345:805–806.
41 Snowdon C, Garcia J, Elbourne D. Making sense of randomisation: responses of parents of critically ill babies to random allocation of treatment in a clinical trial. Soc Sci Med 1997; 45:1337–1355.
42 Davidoff F, DeAngelis CD, Drazen JM, et al. Sponsorship, authorship and accountability. Lancet 2001; 358:854–856.
43 Mental Health Act 1983.
44 Mental Health (Scotland) Act 1984.
45 Larcher VF, Lak B, McCarthy J. Paediatrics at the cutting edge; do we need clinical ethics committees? J Med Ethics 1997; 23:245–249.
46 American Academy of Pediatrics, Committee on Bioethics. Guidelines on forgoing life-sustaining medical treatment. Pediatrics 1994; 93:532–536.
47 Lee SK, Penner PL, Cox M. Comparison of the attitudes of health care professionals and parents toward active treatment of very low birth weight infants. Pediatrics 1991; 88:110–114.

5

Child abuse and social aspects of pediatrics

Christopher J Hobbs, Jane M Wynne, Helga G I Hanks

INTRODUCTION

The recognition of the importance of social relationships in the child's growth and development has paralleled the explosion of interest in the psychosocial aspects of health and disease. Fundamental changes in practice have followed the wider appreciation of the psychological and social needs of children. This chapter will focus on child abuse and neglect in all its forms and with the social aspects of child health. The latter will include groups of children designated as being in need.

Child abuse and neglect represents a legally defined concept where significant harm results from acts of commission or omission on the part of others, usually someone with responsibility of care for the child.

A child is defined as being in need if their health or development is likely to be significantly impaired, or further impaired, without the provision of services, or if they are disabled (section 17 Children Act 1989). Considerable change in practice has taken place in the decade since the implementation of the Children Act. The emphasis has been on closer working with families who are seen as 'in partnership' with professionals. There has also been emphasis on less intrusion into family life. Pediatricians have needed to acquire new skills and knowledge and to adapt to the needs of multidisciplinary working. Services must be designed to meet the needs of children and their families. This chapter will look towards the information needs of pediatricians in this difficult and sometimes stressful part of pediatric practice.

The evidence base for many major social decisions taken in children's lives is far from robust. However social work based research in the early 1990s[1] has provided new information on which current services are being refocused. Child abuse is an area of active research, from a pediatric point of view, reflecting its inclusion as a subject heading in Index Medicus in 1965. The pediatrician must be conversant with the complex and sometimes controversial literature on the diagnosis and management of abuse and neglect. Expertise will be needed to advise families, professionals and statutory agencies (local authorities, police, courts) of any pediatric aspects. Decisions are based on a mixture of experience, evidence and opinion. There is room for both medical and social science in the pursuit of good outcomes for children. However services must be judged by how far aims are being realized. It should not be sufficient to believe that something works, it needs to have been shown to work.

CHILDREN IN THE UK IN THE TWENTY-FIRST CENTURY

Child rearing is complex and ever more so as society changes and the demands on children and parents differ from previous generations. The changes have occurred more quickly in the last century as traditions are lost. The support of nuclear families may be inadequate, whilst the extended family is far away and scattered and may be able to offer little practical help. Needs and expectations of children are high. Children cannot wait for their needs to be met. What is not learned as an infant, particularly in terms of emotional and social development, may have serious long term consequences. There is also increasing concern about 'The fetal origins of adult disease'.[2] Deaths from ischemic heart disease are more common in men who were small at birth (LBW) and at 1 year. Later work showed an association with LBW and an increase in blood pressure and impaired glucose tolerance. Improved nutrition of the mother and avoidance of cigarette smoking would be the most effective ways to reduce fetal growth retardation. Good parenting appears to be a buffer against later adversity, be it poverty, bereavement, or war. Loved children have greater resilience. Whilst the responsibility for child rearing is primarily with the parents, the State also has a role in providing services to support families.

The Children Act 1989 concentrated on legal intervention and the balance of needs of children, their long term welfare and need for protection. The philosophy of the Children Act is to view the child as a person in their own right and, in general, children are better brought up within their family. Parents are expected to take responsibility for their children and local authorities have statutory responsibility to provide support through services for families, where the child is defined as being in need. The local authority also has statutory responsibility to protect children who are suffering, or at risk of suffering, significant harm. There are some groups of children who do not benefit fully from the Act. These include families living in poverty, children aged 0–17 years who are regularly physically punished (parents have a right to hit), children in the care of the local authority, children in secure units, and refugee children. The implementation of the Act is slow, unwieldy and expensive. The concept of 'a child in need', whilst a positive notion, requires financing if needs are to be met. Working Together to Safeguard Children (1999)[3] gave guidance to professionals, which must now give reference to the Human Rights Act (1998):

1. There are certain fundamental rights for all citizens.
2. Article 2 gives the right to life.
3. Article 3 outlaws torture, inhuman or degrading treatment or punishment.
4. Article 6 gives the right to a fair trial.

CHILDREN AND THE FAMILY

Children in the UK are usually brought up in families with two parents. There are changes in the composition of families moving towards fewer children in nuclear families and geographically distant from the extended family. Families are smaller, with 25% of women choosing to have no children. The birth rate overall is 1.7 infants per woman, except for families who have settled recently in the UK. In families from Bangladesh and Pakistan, where 37% of the community are under 16 years, divorce and separation of the parents is low but unemployment and poverty are high.

In the UK, overall in the 1970s, there were 8% of lone parents – usually a mother. By 1999, 25% of children were brought up by a lone mother, and 2% by a lone father. Of lone mothers 14% were aged 16–24 years. Although 30% of infants are born outside marriage, 70% live with both parents. During childhood, 30% of children will experience divorce. Divorce troubles children and 28% of calls to the confidential children's helpline 'Childline', are about worries concerning divorce. In 1998, 55% of divorcing couples in England and Wales had one or more children aged less than 16 years. Of these children 45% were between 5 and 10 years of age and 26% of children less than 5 years of age. Lone parents occur most frequently in black families and least often in Asian families.

TEENAGED PARENTS

In the UK in 1999, 90 000 conceptions were to a mother less than 20 years of age. In 8000 conceptions the mother was less than 16 years. Half of the conceptions by mothers under the age of 16 years were aborted but fewer in social class IV and V. The pregnancies are notable for poor antenatal health, LBW babies, and increased infant mortality rate (Table 5.1). Infant and mother have more ill health than expected. The rate of conception is 10 times greater in social class V than social class I. One in eight teenaged mothers has a second infant in 2 years. Girls in local authority care are especially at risk; 25% are pregnant by 16 years and 50% by 18 years. These mothers have little or no educational achievement; they have emotional problems and a poor home background. The relationship between the parents is often short lived and 50% break down in the first year. The father is more likely to have been excluded from school, be unskilled or unemployed or have been in custody. Like the mother they have also had a socially deprived childhood, are more likely to smoke cigarettes and drink alcohol to excess. Violence to partner and child is common.

THE SOCIALLY DEPRIVED CHILD

One-third of children in the UK live in households with an income of less than half the national average. 2001 has seen the beginning of

Table 5.1 The effect of poverty on mortality

Mortality rate	IMR	PNM	NM	PMR	SBR
Social class I	7	3	3.0	6.6	3.4
Social class V	11.8	6	5.9	9.6	6.8
Lone parent	14.5	9	6.1	9.1	4.9
NCWP	14.2	6.5	6.8	18	n/a

IMR, infant mortality rate; NM, neonatal mortality rate; PNM, postnatal mortality rate; PMR, perinatal mortality rate; SBR, stillbirth rate; NCWP, new Commonwealth and Pakistan (all rates/100 000 live births)

a reversal, with a modest increase in income in the poorest households. The socially deprived child is more likely to be from an ethnic minority, have a poor diet, be disabled, live in a cold house in poor repair, be at greater risk of house fires and have poor play and child care facilities. The leading cause of death age 0–19 years in the UK is injury and poisoning (47%) strongly linked to social deprivation (Table 5.2). Clean drinking water, better nutrition, and to a lesser extent, immunization, antibiotics and universal health care, have improved child survival, but the most important determinant of well-being is social advantage (Office of Population Census and Surveys 1841–1983). Social disadvantage is associated with an increase in child morbidity from chest infection, ear infection, eczema, mental health illness, accidents and poisoning, LBW, and neglect. Maternal factors linked to social disadvantage include cigarette, alcohol and substance abuse, poor antenatal care and inadequate diet, neglect and family violence. Exacerbating the above are homelessness, substandard housing and inadequate play areas.

POVERTY IN THE UK

The number of children living in poverty is one of the highest in Europe.[4] One in eight children live in profound poverty. Black and ethnic minorities are over-represented in low income groups and many households with a disabled child are 'the poorest of the poor'. Low income is associated with fuel and food poverty. This leads to failure to thrive in some cases. Poor families are unable to afford child care and adults remain unemployed, caught in the poverty trap. Unemployment and low income is associated with child maltreatment especially physical abuse and neglect. Marital stress is increased by the stress of relentless poverty. Poverty is associated with neglect, behavior and conduct disorder, truanting, school failure and crime.[5] The intergenerational cycle of poverty leads to malnourished mothers who have LBW infants perpetuating the risk of illness through adult life. Different strategies are needed to provide good health and limit the consequences of social deprivation and isolation. It is known that the inverse care law[6] or social exclusion is associated with poor health and very poor access to health services (one in seven children in the inner city have no GP). Families need adequate income, housing which is dry, warm and safe, education, which is tailored to the needs of the children and services which target the children at most disadvantage. Target groups are the homeless, children in care, traveling families (30 000 in the UK), children from ethnic minorities, runaways, refugees and children in custody.

CHILD ABUSE AND NEGLECT

DEFINITION

Child abuse and neglect is defined as 'Acts of omission or commission by a parent or guardian that are judged by a mixture of community values and professional expertise to be inappropriate or damaging'.[7] Harm, as defined in the Children Act 1989, means ill treatment or the impairment of health (physical or mental) or development (physical, intellectual, emotional or behavioral). Significant harm means noteworthy or important and the context is 'when compared with that which would reasonably be expected of a similar child'. Ill treatment includes physical abuse, sexual abuse, emotional abuse and all forms of ill treatment.

Child abuse includes various terms – battered baby syndrome, non-accidental injury, child sexual abuse, and child cruelty. From the wider and global perspective, the term child maltreatment is favored. The National Commission of Inquiry into the Prevention of Child Abuse[8] adopted an all-inclusive definition: 'Child abuse consists of anything which individuals, institutions, or processes do, or fail to do, which directly or indirectly harms children or damages their prospects of safe and healthy development into adulthood'. For clinicians this definition is too all-inclusive and the definition given above is preferable. Child maltreatment encompasses physical abuse, sexual abuse, emotional abuse and neglect including failure to thrive. Other forms of abuse are recognized, e.g. Munchausen syndrome by proxy abuse (also known as factitious illness, fabricated illness or pediatric condition falsification) but usually registered under one of the above categories.

INCIDENCE AND PREVALENCE OF ABUSE AND NEGLECT IN UK

Incidence is the number of new cases occurring in a given time period. *Prevalence* refers to the proportion of the population that has been abused at some time during the course of childhood. The number of officially reported cases grossly underestimates the scale of the problem. On 31st March 2000 there were 30 300 children on child protection registers in England. The registered categories (by percentage of total) are shown in Table 5.3.[9] Mixed categories are incorporated into main categories in this table. Children may therefore appear in more than one category, which explains why the sum exceeds 100%.

Prevalence figures are based on samples of adults or parents describing their own or their children's experiences. These reveal far higher numbers than appear in statistics of reported cases. Based on recent research, The National Commission of Inquiry into the Prevention of Child Abuse and Neglect[8] estimated that at least 150 000 children annually suffer severe physical punishment, up to 100 000 each year have potentially harmful sexual experience and 350 000–400 000 live in environments consistently low in warmth and high in criticism (emotional neglect). A recent study of 18–24-year-olds[10] found that many problems were located in the family: 10% said their families were not loving and relationships not close; 33% experienced a lot of stress at home including divorce or separation of parents, illness, bereavement, unemployment and homelessness; and 14% had to regularly assume parental responsibilities because of parental illness, disability, or personal problems including substance abuse. Violence was a common experience for many children: 26% had witnessed violence between parents at least once and for 5% this was a constant or frequent occurrence; 7% suffered serious physical abuse in their family.

Table 5.2 The effect of poverty on accidents and accident mortality

	All accidents	Road traffic accident	Mortality – all causes Age 1–4	Mortality – all causes Age 5–9	Mortality – all causes Age 10–15
Social class 1	23/100 000	1.5/100 000	1/100 000	1/100 000	1/100 000
Social class 5	50/100 000	7/100 000	2/100 000	1.7/100 000	1.4/100 000
Lone parent			2.2/100 000	2.56/100 000	4.1/100 000

Table 5.3 Child protection registered categories (From DOH 2000[9])

Category	Percentage
Neglect	46
Physical abuse	29
Emotional abuse	18
Sexual abuse	8
Categories not recommended	1

In addition 6% suffered serious absence of physical care, 6% serious emotional maltreatment and 5% serious absence of supervision. Sexual abuse was reported more often in situations outside the home. Of the sample 1% were abused by parents or carers, 3% by other relatives, 11% by known but unrelated people, and 4% by strangers or someone just met.

FAMILY VIOLENCE

People are more likely to be killed or physically assaulted in their own homes by other family members than anywhere else or by anyone else. Family violence occurs in all social strata and is exacerbated by stress – financial, mental health problems and pregnancy. There were 41 527 rapes, stabbings and beatings in England and Wales in 2000, perpetrated on partners. Only an estimated 10% are reported to the police. There appeared to be a gradual but real rise of 7% during 2001. Family violence involves fetal abuse, child abuse, spouse abuse, courtship abuse, elder abuse, sibling abuse and parent abuse. It accounts for 25% of all violent crimes and 25% of all women will be abused at some time in the context of the home. Two women are killed each week. Evidence also links animal abuse with child abuse. Spouse abuse usually involves abuse of women by men but the reverse is encountered. Marital violence is estimated to affect 11–28% of all marriages.[11] It includes emotional, physical and sexual abuse. In the UK, 47% of female murders are the result of women being killed by their partners.[12]

DOMESTIC VIOLENCE

Domestic violence (DV) affects children in many ways. Around 90% of children are in the same or next room when incidents occur so stories of parents protecting children from the consequences are to be treated with caution. One-third of children present try to protect their mother. Therefore emotional abuse occurs in 75–100% of children in the household. Children may show a range of emotional responses, e.g. nightmares, disrupted sleep, bed wetting, depression, running away, and 13% are hurt by accident when caught in the crossfire.[13] The child may also be abused: 27–59% of child protection cases in two studies included a history of domestic violence.[14,15] DV is associated with child sexual abuse (CSA) in as many as one in three of children in the household. The child may end up living in a refuge.[16] DV affects women in many ways. Physically abused women are more likely to hit their own children. A mother's ability to parent may be impaired. Women who suffer DV are 15 times more likely to abuse alcohol, nine times more likely to abuse drugs, three times more likely to suffer depression and five times more likely to attempt suicide than non-abused mothers.[17] DV may begin or escalate during pregnancy causing direct harm to the fetus.

PHYSICAL ABUSE

A physically abused child is defined as 'any child who receives physical injury (or injuries) as a result of acts (or omissions) usually on the part of his parents or guardians'. The definition includes actual or likely physical injury to a child, or failure to prevent physical injury (or suffering) to a child. Deliberate poisoning, suffocation and Munchausen syndrome by proxy are usually included in this category. Physical abuse (non-accidental injury) is usually perpetrated by the child's carers. It has been recognized as an assault, i.e. abuse, from when 'battered babies' were first described.

Common pattern of injuries in infancy includes skull, rib and long bone fractures, bruising anywhere (but note that the head, neck and chest are more common), retinal hemorrhages and subdural hematomas. It is now recognized that any inflicted injury, which results in bruising, even if the intention was 'discipline or chastisement' has resulted from too hard a blow. The cause of injuries varies; in infancy they are more likely to be inflicted, whereas older children are more likely to have accidents. Death due to abuse is most common in infancy. Of severe head injuries in infancy 95% are due to abuse.[18]

Over the last 20–30 years attitudes are slowly changing and hitting children is less acceptable, although the percentage of 4–7 year olds who are hit remains high in the UK. Smith et al[19] found that in 'ordinary' families 90% of children are hit at sometime. In 14% the punishment was severe. Mothers hit more than fathers. Children who were severely punished were more likely to be aggressive including to their siblings. Physical punishment has been outlawed by several European countries. In the UK 'reasonable chastisement' remains the legal description of an adult inflicting pain on a child. In the UK there is a long tradition of hitting and beating. Although the punishment is legitimate at the beginning of the hitting, the force used may increase and become clearly abusive. The abuser may admit that he had used too much force and the punishment was now abusive. In the UK pressure groups initially campaigned against corporal punishment in schools (STOPP), and now against any physical punishment (EPOCH, children and violence). The physical abuse of children is increasingly seen as part of family violence and violence in society as a whole.

Other important aspects of violence have been demonstrated in research studies. Drugs and alcohol play an important part in violence. Alcohol abuse has been recorded in more than 25% of child protection conferences. Injury may begin when the child is still in utero and be severe. Women and mothers in particular are involved in more violence than is generally recognized. Perpetrators of physical abuse to the child are more often female (mothers in particular). Bullying affects most school children at sometime during their education and may escalate to cause serious injury or death, possibly suicidal. Incidence, management and prevention of bullying has been described.[20,21]

INCIDENCE AND PREVALENCE OF PHYSICAL ABUSE

Incidence

There are no reliable incidence figures currently available. In the past NSPCC annual statistics[22] revealed that 1.5–2% of all children were physically abused by the age of 17 years with 55% boys and 45% girls.

Half were aged 0–4 years, a quarter each were 5–9 and 10–14 years. One in eight were aged less than 1 year. Of the cases, 0.6% were classified as fatal, 9% serious and 90% moderate. There were an estimated 200–230 non-accidental deaths each year but only around a third of these appeared in official figures. Of serious head injuries 70% occurred in children less than 1 year old.

Prevalence

The UK study[10] of 2869 young people aged18–24 years, found that 25% (27% male, 23% female) had experienced violent treatment as a child (21% by parents – mother 49%, father 40%). Lower socioeconomic groups experience higher levels of family violence but the connection is less clear with sexual abuse.[22a] Fourteen per cent suffered intermediate abuse (irregular violence); 12% reported injuries including bruises, head injuries, fractures and burns; 7% had an injury of sufficient severity to cause pain lasting at least 24 h; 6% hit on bottom with a hard implement; 4% grabbed round the neck and choked and 1% burned or scalded intentionally. Of those who had experienced physical discipline or violence, 17% on reflection thought their treatment too harsh, 7% thought it was 'child abuse'. Smith et al[19] reported on 403 ordinary families. Mothers, some fathers and children provided information about routine parental control strategies. Common strategies were spanking or slaps 58%, pushing/shoving 41%, kicked, beaten or punched 8%, threatened with knife or gun 3%. Most children were affected. Of infants < 12 months 75% had been hit and by age 4 years, 97% children had been smacked and 14% of children suffered severe physical punishment (defined as likely to lead to physical or psychological harm). This was linked to poor marital relationship, family violence and aggression between siblings but not to marital status, social class or poor housing. Mothers hit more often than fathers even when child care equally shared.

Presentation

Physical abuse presents less often by direct report from child, parent or other third party. Whilst occasionally malicious, many reports are true and need investigation. More often the abuse presents with an injury. Parents or relatives take the child for help, e.g. to hospital, GP. There may be repeated presentation for injury or minor complaints sometimes to different hospitals. The injuries are typically not consistent with the history – i.e. too many, too severe, wrong kind, wrong distribution, wrong age. There are some typical injuries, which strongly suggest abuse, e.g. bruising or fractures to an immobile infant; multiple injuries following a moderate fall; severe head injury in infant or toddler; subdural hematoma and retinal hemorrhage, cigarette or immersion burns. The jigsaw picture is built up (Fig. 5.1) with other signs of abuse, which include neglect, failure to thrive, and sexual abuse. Unusual behavior in the parents including delay in seeking medical advice, lack of cooperation with treatment or admission, aggression toward staff add important information to the picture. The injury may be discovered incidentally, in school, nursery or through contact with another relative. Parents may deny knowledge of the injury and provide no explanation.

Other features include a discrepant history, which changes with repeated telling, with who tells (father, mother, child), and to whom

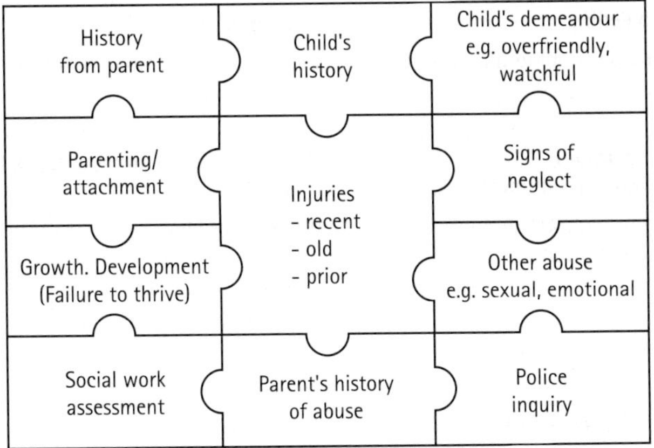

Fig. 5.1 Jigsaw of physical abuse. Key elements in the diagnosis of physical abuse assembled into a jigsaw picture.

told (doctor, social worker, police). The story is often vague, unclear, speculative, and the incident unwitnessed. Unreasonable delay in seeking help or care for the child, e.g. following a fracture or serious burn or scald, may be linked to denial, e.g. child not in pain or didn't cry. Minimization of symptoms is common.

There may be a crisis of care, violence between parents, breakup of a partnership or marriage and psychiatric illness in a parent. Trigger factors may precipitate a parent's violence, e.g. inconsolable crying, feeding difficulty, wetting or soiling, stealing or lying. The parent may have a history of abuse or local authority care. Alcohol or substance abuse is common. Unrealistic expectations of the child coupled to poor understanding of child development are described. The child is expected to love and accept his parents (and be put in the position of role reversal, or parenting the parents). Obsessional and rigid patterns of child rearing may be expressed in other ways (for example a meticulously clean and tidy home) and can create stresses and tensions. Social isolation from friends, extended family and professionals reflects poor social support and increased stress. The child may exhibit anxious or insecure attachment, frequent admissions to hospital, frequent 'accidents' or a 'tendency to bruise easily'. He may be seen as different, e.g. handicapped. The family may be characterized by unstable parental relationships, violence, separation and divorce with little extended family support. Other parental factors include lack of education, low intelligence, poor parenting skills, youth and especially immaturity, and criminality. A tendency to repeat the cycle of abuse from generation to generation is common. Environmental: effects of cold, damp, overcrowded housing, nowhere for the children to play, and enforced proximity all add to the picture.

PATTERNS OF INJURY IN PHYSICAL ABUSE

Superficial injury

Bruises

Present in 90% of physically abused children, these are the commonest injury. Blood escapes from the intravascular space into the tissues as a result of trauma, resulting in visible discoloration if superficial in site. The site, pattern and number are relevant to the diagnosis of non-accidental injury. Accidental bruises are found over bony prominences in about 30–40% of normal children after 9 months to 1 year of age and result from painful injury. Up to 12 bruises may be found in a normal active mobile child with appropriate protection.[23]

Abusive bruises may be present in larger numbers in unusual sites, and there may be characteristic patterns. Bruises in premobile infants are particularly worrying. Important sites for non-accidental bruises are buttocks, lower back and outer thighs. Inner thigh and genital area suggest either sexual abuse or punishment for perceived toileting misdemeanors. The penis may be pinched or pulled and sometimes tied with string, hairs or rubber bands. Injury to the head and neck include slap marks on the sides of the face and ears, extending onto the scalp, and strangulation marks around the neck. Bruising to the external ear is unusual following accidents because of the protective effect of the triangle created by the shoulder, skull and base of neck. Other common sites strongly associated with abuse are lower jaw, mastoid, eyes and mouth. Black eyes can occur in normal school children from direct injury but from a penetrating orbital injury or a very hard blow to the forehead for blood to track down around one or both eyes. Mouth injury includes upper lip and frenulum bruising/tearing which may follow forced feeding or a punch. An old tear of the frenulum will persist. On the limbs proximal sites are more typical of abuse than the distal (accidental sites). Also uncommonly injured accidentally is the trunk (chest and abdomen). Lower abdominal bruises suggest sexual abuse. Characteristic patterns of bruises include hand marks (pinch, grasp, slap, punch), marks left by implements (belt, looped flex, stick, shoe, ligature), bites – adult, child (size) and animal (shape, presence of puncture marks in dog bites), kicks (large irregular shaped bruises), petechiae over head, neck and upper chest from chest pressure/crushing, localized petechiae from skin traction or stretching.

Aging bruise. The unpredictable nature and time scale of the appearance, change in color and disappearance of bruises make reliable aging impossible. Studies agree that a yellow color indicates that a bruise is older than 18 h.[24,25] The differential diagnosis of bruising is discussed in Table 5.4.[26]

Bone injuries

Skeletal injury is associated with severe force. 85% of fractures occur before the age of 5 years . Leventhal et al[27] studied 215 consecutive children under 3 years of age with 253 fractures: 24.2% were categorized as abuse, 8.4% unknown and 67.4% unintentional. Under 1 year of age 39% were abusive whereas from 2 to 3 years only 8%. Radiological features assist with ageing (Table 5.5).[28]

Accidental fractures in young children

Falls of up to 1 m carry a low risk of fracture. Fractures of the clavicle or a hairline linear parietal skull fracture occasionally follow. Serious head injury is extremely rare. Genuine falls from outside buildings of three stories usually result in survival but significant injury is quite likely. From five stories mortality increases to 50%. Of 338 falls in day care, only one child sustained a serious head injury.[29] Falls downstairs[30] result in occasional fractures of skull or distal limb bone, unless in a baby walker when more serious injury may follow. Usually a single site abrasion or bruise results. Head injury is unusual, but possibly more common, if the child is dropped over stairs from a carer's arms.

The history is important in diagnosis. In accidental injury there is prompt presentation, a clear history of an accident, development of immediate pain, loss of function and swelling. In abuse, the history of injury is vague, inconsistent (e.g rolled off settee sustaining a skull fracture) or absent. Medical attention may be later sought for swelling or loss of function. Sometimes a fracture may present coincidentally, e.g. rib fracture on chest X-ray for bronchiolitis. Fractures, whether caused accidentally or as a result of abuse, are variably associated with bruising. The absence of bruising does not assist in establishing the cause. The specificity of abuse with different types of fractures is seen in Table 5.6.[28]

Mechanisms of injury

Metaphyseal lesions are caused by indirect forces of pulling or twisting.

Posterior rib fractures, often multiple and bilateral result from compression when the infant is grasped around the chest by both hands when shaken or thrown. Skull fractures result from impact with a hard object. Long bone fractures are either transverse, spiral, oblique transverse or oblique. Simple mechanical theory dictates that transverse fractures are the result of angulation, as can occur following a direct blow. Oblique transverse fractures result from angulation (or bending) with axial loading (or compression). Spiral fractures result from axial twists with or without axial loading. Oblique fractures are the result of angulation and axial twisting in the presence of axial loading. Axial loading applies to bones, e.g. tibia, which are weight bearing at the time of injury.[31]

Fractures of specific bones

Femur. It is reported that 60–83% of femoral fractures, under 12 months of age, are due to abuse.[27,32–34] Trivial injury or minor fall is unlikely to cause this fracture in a healthy child. In abuse, the fracture follows violent twisting or swinging of the child by the leg. A major fall (e.g. from a first floor window) could generate sufficient force. The fracture type carries no specificity for abuse except metaphyseal, which occurs more often at the distal end.

Tibia. This bone is commonly fractured in abuse. Toddler fracture can arise with relatively minor trauma. Toddler fracture is an undisplaced oblique fracture of the distal tibial shaft in children from 9 months to 3 years, from when weight bearing is just

Table 5.4 Differential diagnosis of bruising (From Hobbs et al 1999[26])

Presentation	Differential diagnoses	Features	Investigations
?Bruise	Blue spots, hemangioma, café-au-lait spots, prominent veins	Static lesions, no evolution with time	Follow-up, re-examine
?Bruise	Bleeding disorder, e.g. ITP, hemophilia, hemorrhagic disease of newborn, platelet disorder	Bruising with minimal trauma – usual accidental ones. Family history, prolonged bleeding	Hematological investigations (Tables 5.2 and 5.3) Chapter 21
?Bruise	Infection, vasculitis: meningococcal septicemia, disseminated intravascular coagulation	Ill child, rapidly developing purpuric rash	Blood culture, lumbar puncture, hematology
	Henoch–Schönlein disease	Distribution of purpura joint, abdominal, renal involvement	Urine microscopy, urine dipstick for protein
?Bruise	Allergy – periorbital swelling	History of allergy, contact dermatitis, appearance, evolution	IgE, eosinophilia
?Bruise	Skin disease:		
	Ehlers–Danlos syndrome	Low elasticity, poor wound healing, easy bruisability, muscular hypotonia	Seek dermatology opinion
	Erythema nodosum, other skin disease	painful, warm, erythematous swellings, usally pretibial and joint pain	Biopsy
?Bruise	Ink, paint, dye, dirt	Removable	Soap and water

ITP, idiopathic thrombocytopenic purpura

Table 5.5 Dating fractures (From Kleinman 1987[28])

Resolution of soft tissue change	4–10 days
Periosteal new bone formation	10–14 days
Loss of fracture line definition	14–21 days
Soft callus	14–21 days
Hard callus	21–42 days
Remodelling	1 year

beginning.[35] The child is unable to weight bear. Radiological findings may be subtle and easily missed. Relatively less force is required and there is usually an absence of local swelling and bruising. More severe forces, such as those leading to a displaced spiral or oblique fracture, are unlikely to be accidental.

Humerus. This is frequently injured in abuse (Fig. 5.2). Thomas et al[34] found 14 humeral fractures in all children up to the age of 3, of which 11 were judged to have been abusive. All the abusive fractures were diaphyseal or distal metaphyseal, and the accidental ones supracondylar. In abuse, the infant is violently grasped by the arm, pulled, swung or jerked, resulting in a range of fractures to the shaft and to both ends of the bone.

Hands and feet. Injuries to the digits, metatarsals or metacarpals are occasionally found in abuse. There may be little indication of injury clinically, and direct impact is thought to account for some of these. Fusiform swelling of the digits may mimic juvenile arthritis.

Other long bones. The clavicle is commonly fractured in childhood. A lateral fracture, less common than midshaft fracture, is more suggestive of abuse. Scapular and sternal fractures, which usually result from direct impact (blows), are highly suggestive of abuse although uncommon.

Rib fractures. Rib fractures comprise 5–27% of fractures in abuse. Cardiopulmonary resuscitation rarely, if ever, causes rib fractures and can be safely disregarded as a factor.[36,37] Rib fractures less commonly occur in motor vehicle accidents, rickets, osteoporosis, surgery and osteogenesis imperfecta. Rib fractures are frequently multiple and bilateral and most often situated posteriorly near the costotransverse process articulation. Fractures can also occur further anteriorly and are sometimes multiple in the same rib. A physical sign of rib fracture, which has been ignored, is clicking or a grating feeling in the rib cage.[38]

SKULL FRACTURES AND HEAD INJURY

Indicators of skull fracture include: localized boggy swelling (hematoma) of scalp, bleeding or cerebrospinal fluid (CSF) from nose or ear, or rarely a palpable defect.

Skull fractures cannot be readily aged. Swelling persists around 1 week.

Confusion with aberrant sutures can occur but the presence of swelling is confirmatory of fracture. Patterns of skull fractures[39] can assist in assessing likely cause. Fractures should be accurately described and measured on the radiograph or at postmortem. Single linear fracture consists of an unbranched line in straight, zig-zagged or angled configuration. The fracture margins are closely opposed with the maximum width between them usually no more than 1–2 mm and often less than 1 mm. Multiple or complex described fractures where there is more than one fracture or a single fracture has multiple components including a branching pattern. There may be a stellate configuration with several branching lines converging on a central point. Depressed fracture is where the normal curvature of the skull is interrupted by the inward displacement of bone. Growing fractures are widened linear fractures, usually > 3 mm at maximum width. They may continue to enlarge over time, sometimes with the formation of a leptomeningeal cyst. The most commonly fractured bone, in accident or abuse, is the large and prominent parietal bone.[27,40] Frontal fractures are uncommon, either in abuse or accident, whilst occipital fractures have a special predominance in abuse. A depressed occipital fracture is virtually pathognomonic of abuse. Fractures of the temporal bone, anterior and middle fossae are uncommon and usually follow severe trauma.

Significance of skull fractures

Skull fracture is common in the severely battered child. Violent shaking may result in serious intracranial injury without skull fracture but if impact against a blunt object has occurred skull fracture may also be present. Accidental fracture in young children usually follows falls of greater than 3 feet. The impact surface is also relevant. Diagnosis depends on inconsistency of injury with history, presence of other injuries and other features in the 'jigsaw'. Differentiation simply on the basis of fracture characteristics is not possible. Findings associated with greater severity of impact (complex, multiple, larger depressed areas, wide or growing, involving more than one bone, basal, occipital, associated with intracranial injury) should be accompanied by a history of appropriate severity. Uncomplicated linear parietal fractures are the most frequently encountered fractures following both abuse and accident.[40]

A complete skeletal survey is required in the investigation of suspected child abuse. The presence of a fracture, or other suspicious injury or unexplained death in an infant or toddler should prompt consideration of the need for this. Where positive, repeat survey may reveal additional information.[41] The differential diagnosis of fractures includes birth trauma, intrinsic bone disease (osteogenesis imperfecta, metabolic bone disease, copper deficiency) and rarely osteomyelitis or disuse osteoporosis.

INTRACRANIAL INJURY

This is the major cause of death from physical abuse, which is the leading cause of head injury in the first year of life. The prevalence of subdural hemorrhage from abuse is 14.5 to 24.6/100 000 births aged 0–1 and 7.28 to 12.8 aged 0–2 years.[42,43] Intracranial

Table 5.6 Specificity of radiological findings (From Kleinman 1987[28])

High specificity	Moderate specificity*	Common but low specificity*
Metaphyseal lesions	Multiple fractures especially bilateral	Linear parietal skull
Posterior rib fractures	Fractures of different ages	Shafts of long bones
Scapular and sternal fractures	Epiphyseal separations	Clavicle
Spinous process fractures	Vertebral body fractures and subluxations	
	Digital fractures	
	Complex skull fracture	

* Lesions of moderate and low specificity become high when history of trauma is absent or inconsistent with injuries.

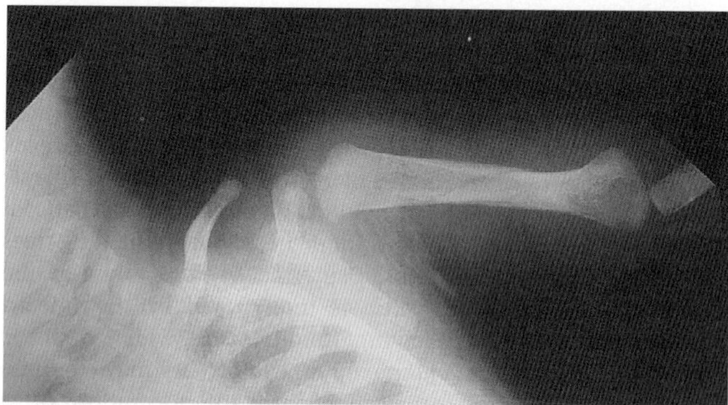

Fig. 5.2 A 4 month female infant taken to the hospital emergency department because of distress when arm was moved. History that the previous day she had slipped when her father had been bathing her and he had grabbed her arm. Spiral fracture of right humerus is seen on radiograph. There are also healing fractures of the R 5th and 6th ribs. The child was originally sent away from hospital until the radiologist noted the rib fractures. The combination of spiral fracture and rib fracture is physical abuse.

injury arises from combinations of violent shaking, impact and hypoxia. The peak age is 0–6 months. The pathology of abusive head injury includes scalp injury (bruises, traumatic subgaleal hematoma), skull fracture, subdural, extradural, subarachnoid and intraventricular hemorrhage, cerebral injury including diffuse axonal injury, tears, contusion, hemorrhage and edema. Eye injury is frequently associated.

Presentation and diagnosis

Reece & Sege et al[44] compared head injury in relation to etiology. Table 5.7[44] summarizes the main differences between accidents and abuse.

Shaken baby syndrome (whiplash shaken, shaken-impact)

This term is applied to a clinical picture in which the causative mechanism of injury is thought to be severe repeated shaking probably with impact in most cases.[45] Affected infants show evidence of acute or chronic symptoms and signs, which may be subtle and non-specific. There is a spectrum of severity at presentation from a well child with enlarging head, to a severely ill one requiring resuscitation. Important symptoms include drowsiness, unconsciousness, poor feeding, irritability, fits, pallor, floppiness, vomiting, sudden collapse, breathing difficulties, signs of other injury, large head, apnea and delayed development. Infants may present as 'cot death'. Diagnosis is commonly missed or delayed.[46]

Table 5.7 Head injury in childhood (From Reece & Sege 2000[44])

	Accident	Abuse
287 children (1 week to 6.5 years)	81%	19%
Mean age (years)	2.5	0.7
Subdural hemorrhage	10%	46%
Subarachnoid hemorrhage	8%	31%
Retinal hemorrhages	2%	33%
Associated cutaneous injury	16%	50%
Mortality	2%	13%

Clinical findings include full to normal fontanelle, low hemoglobin, and bilateral or unilateral retinal hemorrhages (50–75% of infants). Computed tomography (CT) shows intracranial hemorrhage, characteristically convex subdural hematomas of varying and sometimes different ages. In the acute stage these are small (10–15 ml is a typical volume), but may enlarge with time and repeated injury. Injury to the brain is important in predicting outcome and may include cerebral contusion, laceration, diffuse traumatic axonal injury, intracerebral hemorrhage and edema, which may be a terminal event. Magnetic resonance imaging (MRI) permits more accurate dating of injury. Other injuries include bruises from grasping or head impact and rib, skull and long bone fractures. Cervical cord injury is also encountered. Differential diagnosis of subdural hemorrhage includes clotting disorder (hemophilia, vitamin K deficiency), severe accidental trauma, birth injury, and rare causes including alpha-1 glutaric aciduria in which frontal atrophy is accompanied by widened CSF space around the frontal lobes. Investigations for unexplained intracranial hemorrhage include CT and MRI, clotting studies, skeletal survey, examination by an ophthalmologist, and a mutiagency child protection investigation.

ABDOMINAL INJURY[26]

Abusive abdominal injury, although less common than head injury, is a significant cause of death. Delayed presentation and absence of a history of injury or localized bruising can delay diagnosis and treatment. Kicks, punches, stamping or standing on the child results in injury to solid or hollow viscera. Stomach, duodenum, duodenojejunal flexure, jejunum ileum may be perforated. Hemorrhage results from rupture of a major vessel or laceration, contusion, hematoma of liver, spleen, duodenum, pancreas, mesentery or kidney.

MUNCHAUSEN SYNDROME BY PROXY (FABRICATED, FICTITIOUS, FALSIFIED ILLNESS)[47]

The term Munchausen syndrome by proxy is being slowly replaced by fabricated, fictitious or falsified illness. This form of abuse results from the production or presentation of false illness in the child by an adult, usually a parent. Related behaviors include mothering to death, doctor shopping, overanxious parents. Munchausen syndrome describes behavior in adults who fabricate symptoms and signs of illness in themselves. The syndrome requires a parent who exhibits the behavior ('the perpetrator') and assumes the sick role by proxy, a child who is dependent and unable to prevent the deception and a doctor who is deceived into accepting the child as ill. The parent positively gains attention and care for themselves as the 'good' parent of a sick child, as well as status with friends and family, and continual social, professional and most of all personal gratification. Other rewards may be financial, through disability allowance, social, through relationships with health care staff, but these are not essential parts of the syndrome. Addiction to hospitals has been described. Additional gains may be acquired, e.g. through the media, active participation in parent support groups and from the legal process if cases go to court. Harm results from the betrayal of trust by the adult of the child. Some see this as emotional abuse, which is pervasive and may include lack of empathy, cruelty, dishonesty, deception and disregard of the child's needs and rearing the child into an illness dependent person. Harm also results from the effects of unnecessary, often invasive, investigation, admission, treatment and restriction of the child's life. Prevalence is unknown. Incidence in one study was 0.5/100 000 under 16 years, 2.8/100 000 under 1 year.[48]

CLINICAL PRESENTATION

Excessively heavy case notes are a characteristic feature. Frequent admission to hospital and attendance at several clinics for a variety of complaints soon lead to case notes which run into more than one volume. Attendance at other hospitals in the area, as well as at the GP's surgery, is common. Symptoms and signs are produced which don't resolve, and there is constant production of new, varied symptoms and signs. The child's clinical appearance is not consistent with the description of his symptoms. The parents' response to the serious clinical picture, which they communicate, of their child is inappropriate. There is ever-increasing pressure by the parents to discover what is wrong – a plea for investigations, enthusiasm for admission. Progress of the clinical condition is not as expected or diagnosis does not fit a typical pattern. The parent may use medical terms, e.g. describes 'black tarry stools', and has unusual medical knowledge. There may be a medical or nursing background. Efforts to achieve diagnosis and treatment are unsuccessful and frustrated. The doctor may become involved and driven to further investigate (in order to fulfill the parents' demands to show what a good and thorough doctor they are) and treat despite seeing a 'well child'.[49]

SPECIFIC PRESENTATIONS

Non-accidental poisoning was one of the first forms of factitious illness to be described.[50] The drugs used may be prescribed for child or for mother or purchased separately. A wide range of substances has been described including salt poisoning. Toxicology screening, when there is no specific suspected substance, can be hit or miss. Induction of acute asphyxia, apnea and collapse by suffocation is a potentially fatal form of illness induction. Suffocation is also responsible for some cases of apparent sudden infant death syndrome.[51] The perpetrator is with the infant when he collapses and calls for help. Covert video surveillance has confirmed this form of abuse.[52] There are few physical findings in the suffocated child. Occasional periorbital petechiae or bleeding from the nose or mouth are described. Other commonly encountered symptoms include fits, apnea and 'funny turns', diarrhea, passage of blood either in urine or stool. Some of these accounts may be difficult to verify or disprove as factitious.

Failure to thrive can be induced by deliberately not feeding the child (the milk was poured down the sink). The mother insists on feeding her own child, is reluctant to leave the ward and may say the child feeds well but is observed not to gain weight. This encourages the doctor to believe that 'there must be something medically the matter with the child' although further investigations fail to reveal it. Rubbing or otherwise injuring the skin, including the application of caustic substances can induce skin rashes. The fabricated and bizarre nature of these can be recognized by an experienced clinician. For an up to date analysis of this form of abuse see Eminson & Postlethwaite.[53]

EMOTIONAL ABUSE

> *'Rather than casting psychological maltreatment as an ancillary issue, subordinate to other forms of abuse and neglect, we should place it as the centerpiece of efforts to understand family functioning and to protect children' Garbarino et al (1988).*[7]

Emotional maltreatment and its consequences have been difficult to tease out and quantify. Garbarino et al[7] clarified the clinical response and showed that emotionally abused children suffered both short and long term sequelae following emotional abuse. If the carers continue to abuse the child emotionally there follows more psychological damage with the inevitable consequences for adult life. This has also been the experience in the UK[1] with graphic description of the 'corrosiveness' of long term abuse causing psychological impairment or even significant harm.

The carers abuse the child by constant criticism, undermining, calling names, threatening with abandonment, or demanding behavior which involves having to behave in an unreasonable way in order to appease the aggressive parent. Psychological consequences in the child will be inevitable. When a child is used for adults' sexual exploits, for begging, stealing, or separated from their peers and other social contacts it is damaging to them.[26] Garbarino et al[7] and others recognized these consequences and also that both short and long term effects were difficult to reverse and treat. Egeland et al[54] concluded, from a follow-up study, that emotional abuse has serious long term consequences for children's social and intellectual development.[55] Rohner & Rohner[56] identified two patterns of rejection by parents of their children. In the first, the mental attitude of hostility is converted into behavioral aggression towards the child. In the second, the mental attitude of indifference is manifested in the neglect of the child's physical and emotional needs. In either case the child's perception is that they are neither valued nor loved. This is experienced as mental cruelty by the child and undermines their self-esteem, ability to make relationships and trust others. Further they are unable to distinguish between those people who mean well by them and those who do not. Emotional abuse almost always occurs in conjunction with physical abuse, sexual abuse and neglect. It can take place in an environment of good physical care in a materially advantaged family whilst inflicting as much damage as experienced by the emotionally abused, socially deprived child.

The case of Victoria Climbié highlights the most cruel aspects of this abuse. She was left in a cold bathroom stripped of clothes, hungry, with no physical or human warmth and protection. Children in affluent homes may be emotionally maltreated in more subtle ways. These include continual rejection, criticism, demands made upon them that are socially and age inappropriate, made to feel frightened, and deprived of love and affection.

DEFINITIONS

Iwaniec[57] defines emotional neglect as

> *'...the passive ignoring of a child's emotional needs, lack of attention and stimulation, and parental unavailability to care, to supervise, to guide, to teach, and to protect'.*

Whiting[58] said that

> *'emotional neglect occurs when meaningful adults are unable to provide necessary nurturance, stimulation, encouragement, and protection for the child at various stages of development'.*

Iwaniec also includes crippling overprotection of a child. Whiting[58] wrote of the consequences of this type of abuse, which inhibits a child's optimal functioning, and

> *'this is a result of subtle or blatant omission or commission experienced by the child, which causes handicapping stress on the child'*

Garbarino et al[7] quoted a 1976 manual which describes a psychological condition as determined by a psychiatrist, psychologist or pediatrician apparently caused by acts or omissions of a parent or person responsible for a child (including the refusal of appropriate treatment) which:

1. renders the child chronically and severely anxious, agitated, depressed, socially withdrawn, psychotic, or in reasonable fear that life and/or safety is threatened;
2. makes it extremely likely that the child will become chronically and severely anxious, agitated, depressed, socially withdrawn, psychotic or in reasonable fear that life and/or safety is threatened; or
3. seriously interferes with the child's ability to accomplish age-appropriate developmental milestones, or school, peer and community tasks.

Glaser[59] quoted a definition used in a conference on psychological abuse of children and youth (1983):

> *'Psychological maltreatment of children and youth consists of acts of omission and commission, which are judged by community standards and professional expertise to be psychologically damaging. Such acts are committed by individuals, singly or collectively, who, by their characteristics (e.g. age, status, knowledge, organisational form) are in a position of differential power that renders a child vulnerable. Such acts damage immediately, or ultimately, the behavioral, cognitive, affective or physical functioning of the child.'*

This definition has been widely accepted and used by many who work in this field.

The Department of Health definition in 'Working Together to Safeguard Children'[3] states that

> *'Emotional abuse is the persistent emotional ill-treatment of a child such as to cause severe and persistent adverse effects on the child's behavior and emotional development.'*
>
> *The child feels worthless or unloved, inadequate, or valued only insofar as they meet the needs of another person. It may feature age or developmentally inappropriate expectations being imposed on children. It may involve causing children frequently to feel frightened or in danger, or the exploitation or corruption of children. Some level of emotional abuse is involved in all types of ill treatment of a child, though it may occur alone.'*

INCIDENCE OF EMOTIONAL ABUSE

During the year ending 31st March 2000, 4800 (17%) children were registered as solely emotionally abused.

PRESENTATION

Some of the clinical features of emotional abuse and neglect are very obvious, particularly when children and others around them can describe how they have been treated. Emotional abuse is one form of abuse which may be seen in the consulting room in front of the pediatrician. Observation of the parents' behavior and of the child is essential. Quiet and demure behavior should not be taken as a sign that all is well when the history would suggest that the child has experienced emotional maltreatment. Equally, some children who present being very angry and aggressive may show these behaviors because they are acting out some of their feelings. Working with other professionals, including psychologists, social workers, therapists and psychiatrists is essential.

PARENT–CHILD RELATIONSHIPS

The relationship between parents/carers and their children is pivotal. A number of dimensions of emotionally abusive or inappropriate relationships have been described.[59] Some children are persistently negatively treated by carers, always called names, never their real name, told they are bad, mad, stupid, are always blamed, belittled on a consistent basis, or are told that they have inherited negative characteristics from which they cannot escape. Also included are those behaviors of adults towards children, which are harsh and overcontrolling.

Another dimension is seen in parents who make their love and care dependent on the condition that the children do exactly as they are told. This does include inappropriate behavior for the children but approved of by the adults. A third dimension is when parents have inappropriate expectations of their children which can include blaming them inappropriately, leaving children alone or separating from them frequently without explanation. Children are asked to deceive on their behalf, are overprotected and do not have the opportunity to explore, They may be inappropriately involved in sexual and/or criminal behaviors, for instance the effects of witnessing spousal violence or rape. A final dimension is the situation when carers are emotionally unavailable. Whatever the reason for such lack of caretaking it is damaging to children over time.

Important features of emotional abuse and neglect are shown in Table 5.8.[60]

NEGLECT

Neglect is widespread. Recognition of this insidious, pervasive and damaging form of abuse has been gradually increasing. Neglect is less well understood in terms of theory. This is reflected in the shortage of literature about neglect, the small number of research studies, and the absence of professional training for practitioners in neglect. There is much truth in the term 'Neglect of Neglect'.[61] The child has a right to expect, and the adult caretaker has a duty to provide: food, clothing, shelter, safekeeping, nurturance and teaching. Failure to provide these constitutes neglect.[62] Working Together[63] limited the definition to severe cases:

> *'The persistent or severe neglect of a child, or the failure to protect a child from exposure to any kind of danger, including cold or starvation or extreme failure to carry out important aspects of care, resulting in the significant impairment of the child's health or development, including non-organic failure to thrive.'*

Neglect therefore is most commonly thought of as the absence of adequate parental care and supervision.

PREVALENCE

Cawson et al[10] reported that serious absence of care was experienced by 6% of children. This included frequently going hungry; frequently having to go to school in dirty clothes; not being taken to the doctor when ill (under age of 12 years) and regularly having to look after themselves because parents went away, or had problems such as drugs or alcohol; being abandoned or deserted; or living in a home with dangerous physical conditions. The study also found that one or more of these criteria, and an additional criterion of often expected to do own laundry before the age of 12, were experienced with less frequency by a further 9% of the sample.

Table 5.8 Key features of emotional abuse and neglect at different developmental ages (From Skuse 1997[60])

Key features in:	Infants	Preschool children	School children
Physical	Failure to thrive Recurrent and persistent minor infections Frequent attendance at casualty departments Unexplained bruising Severe nappy rash	Short stature Microcephaly Unkempt and dirty	Short stature Poor hygiene Unkempt apearance
Development	General delay	Language delayed Attention span limited Socioemotional immaturity	Learning difficulties Lack of self-esteem Poor coping skills Socioemotional immaturity
Behavior	Attachment disorders: anxious, avoidant Lack of social responsiveness	Overactive Aggressive and impulsive Lack of social responsiveness Indiscriminate friendliness Seeks physical contact from strangers	Disordered or few relationships Self-stimulating or self-injurious Lack of social behavior Unusual patterns of defecation or urination or both

Generally there were few distinctions by socioeconomic grade, although poorer grades more often experienced serious absence of care. Fewer subjects self-assessed as not having been well cared for (4%) and 2% felt they had been neglected.

More children are placed on child protection registers in England and Wales under the category of neglect than any other. Neglect may also include neglect of basic emotional needs. In practice physical neglect is usually associated with emotional deprivation, whereas emotional abuse may occur in the absence of physical neglect. It is estimated that 3% of children live in a home that is consistently 'low in warmth and high in criticism'.[1] This constitutes emotional neglect.

CLINICAL FEATURES

It is important to build a jigsaw picture, carefully collecting information together from a number of different sources (Table 5.9). There are a number of conditions, which in the absence of a fully explanatory medical cause indicate neglect. A lack of attachment to the parent or, conversely, anxious or avoidant attachment to the parent, is an important finding. The parents fail to provide emotional nurturance for emotional growth. The children are left unattended and in unsafe situations or in unnecessary risk for emotional or physical harm by the caretaker's omission or commission. Failing to send a child to school also results in the child not being stimulated. Developmental delay, especially in language and social development, is a constant finding. Social development may be aberrant, with lack of age appropriate and consistent limit setting. Finally, the child is not given needed preventive or curative medical care.

The child exhibits signs of delayed development, lack of stimulation and behavioral problems including aggression. He may experience physical injury, sexual abuse, disinhibited sexuality, poor hygiene, be hungry, have feeding problems and an inadequate diet. Failure to thrive frequently follows and a range of untreated health problems and inappropriate medical requests. The parents or caregivers will often have experienced poor parenting, and have a history of neglect or abuse themselves. They may have experienced the care system or prison. There is often a history of substance abuse, mental illness or learning disability. They have an inability to nurture and a lack of bonding to the child. Their parenting skills are poor and the home is frequently disorganized and mismanaged.

The family is characterized by high stress levels, violence, and unrealistic expectations of the child. The parents' needs are put first and patterns of scapegoating and lack of boundaries are common. There is a general lack of supervision of the child, who is left with frequent inappropriate carers in an open house situation. Many families are known to social services, but resistance and non-cooperation with statutory agencies are common. Failure to keep appointments and poor school attendance are characteristic. A background of poverty and social deprivation is linked to debts, financial problems, unemployment and reliance on benefits.

Table 5.9 The 'jigsaw' in the diagnosis of neglect

Denial of problems by parents (may have learning problems)	History from child – bullied, no friends, aggressive	'Attention seeking'. Concern by nursery school of standard of care
Physical symptoms, e.g. pain from dental caries	Poor physical condition – dirty, thin hair, nappy rash Deprivation hands and feet	Growth – stunted/fails to reach potential height
Development delayed, e.g. language, social skills	Poor compliance with treatment, e.g. asthma	Increased risk of accidents: road traffic accident fire, drowning
Supportive network, i.e. with family and friends – little effect as share similar problems	Poverty with poor housing, diet, parents with poor health (physical and mental), little education	Large number of involved professionals – health visitor, school nurse, social worker, home care, housing, GP, pediatrician, etc.

The family frequently live in poor housing and suffer social isolation or exclusion.

Clinical examination findings are of a cold, dirty child, inappropriately dressed, with infestation, inattention to grooming, chronic nappy and other rashes and excessive decayed, unfilled or missing teeth. Deprivation hands and feet (red or blue and swollen) may be present and reflect cold injury. There will be failure to thrive, stunted height, anemia (usually from dietary iron deficiency), and, sometimes, other nutritional deficiencies including vitamin D deficient rickets. Delay in development affects especially language and social development but less often motor. A history of excessive accidents including ingestions and scars from old injury signals a lack of protection. Signs of abuse, physical or sexual are often present. Untreated conditions (e.g. squints), disfiguring minor untreated conditions, untreated infection (e.g. otitis media with discharge), unusual severe presentation of illness, repeated infection (e.g. gastroenteritis), are typical. Behavior patterns may include attention seeking, indiscriminate seeking of contact, angry or aggressive, isolation – child living in own world and appearing cut off, chaotic and showing a lack of understanding of others.

Neglect is a major factor in child death linked to malnutrition and poor care, which lowers resistance to infection. Injury, the leading cause of death in childhood, and lack of supervision are linked. Parents may fail to respond to illness leading to sudden and unexpected death. Failure to use preventive health care, for example immunization, is an additional factor contributing to excessive mortality. Parental drug abuse may result in an intoxicated adult, or accidental ingestion by the child. Under-reporting and recognition of neglect and child death are both common.

MANAGING NEGLECT

A balance has to be struck between informal and formal interventions and treatment. Failure to thrive (FTT) and neglect are clearly child protection issues. Neglected children receive help under both child protection and child in need procedures.

Whichever system is used, careful assessment is needed to establish why parents are failing and whether the parents are motivated to change. How can parents and child be supported? Is the extended family able to support?

Intervention must be planned, focused and systematic. Separate interventions may be required for parents and for child. There are many approaches. Coordinated team-working provides for effective use of resources, prevents duplication of effort and supports professionals in not feeling defeated. The pediatrician's role includes careful and objective monitoring of the child and family for progress toward acceptable levels of growth and development. The time scale may be longer than with other forms of maltreatment. A realistic framework is required for when to call it a day and seek other approaches for the child. Prevention programs, some of which have been positively evaluated, include health visiting, sure start, parenting programs, adult literacy. Professionals must be well supported. They may offer the best prospect of limiting the effects of multiple deprivation and neglect.

OUTCOMES FOR NEGLECTED CHILDREN

Neglect is insidious, chronic and affects children in many ways. Signs of cognitive and socioemotional delays appear early in the child's life. Left unattended, poor outcomes are more likely. Failure is in all walks of life including education, job prospects, social and intellectual functioning. Links between neglect and mental illness, substance abuse, offending behavior and general adjustment have been established. The outlook is not uniformly gloomy and much can be done to improve it. The presence of an attentive person taking genuine interest in the child at some time is important. This person needs to be identified and supported. It is vital therefore to recognize neglectful patterns of parenting and to seek with the help of others to provide appropriate resources for the child and family.

FAILURE TO THRIVE

Non-organic failure to thrive (NOFTT) is appropriately considered along with child abuse and neglect. FTT occurs when an infant or child fails to achieve the expected growth, as assessed by measurements of weight and height. NOFTT refers to children who are growth retarded secondary to malnutrition. NOFTT is a form of nutritional neglect where the infant or child is fed inadequate calories for normal growth. Children who fail to thrive show long term deficits in physical growth, cognitive functioning and emotional and social development. The child may also fail to achieve full potential in other parameters of development. An important aspect of NOFTT is the part parental relationships play in a child's growth and development; hence its inclusion in this chapter. NOFTT is an outcome of inadequate nutrition and nurturing which expresses itself in the child's poor weight and growth. FTT is commonly encountered in pediatric practice. In community surveys 5% of inner city children failed to thrive of which 94% of cases were of non-organic origin.[64]

Presentation and diagnosis is frequently delayed. Identification of cases is often the result of professional surveillance activity. Cases from more affluent families, without overt signs of neglect or expressed feeding difficulty, are more likely to remain undiagnosed.[65] The emotional impact of NOFTT on families and professionals can be considerable and denial of the problem is frequent. Whole population screening, using growth data, has been used effectively to identify cases.[66] Case finding relies upon identification of the slowest growing infants in the population. This will include infants who show temporary faltering of growth, which corrects spontaneously or with minimum intervention. By the time the condition has fully developed, it is best to use the terminology of 'growth failure' or 'failure to thrive' to indicate the severity of the condition. There are currently discussions around these issues as some professionals wish to reduce what they feel is the stigmatizing effect on parents of the term 'failure to thrive'. However caution is required in the use of any euphemism, which could distract attention from the serious consequences of NOFTT for the child.

Whilst NOFTT typically develops in the early months of postnatal life, the condition may develop in the second and subsequent years, including adolescence. The syndrome is distinct from the spectrum of eating disorders, which have a different causation, and require a different treatment approach.

Definitions based on anthropometric data or formulae alone are likely to miss cases. The addition of clinical examination improves diagnostic accuracy. Serial growth measurements are essential for accurate diagnosis. There are various abnormal growth patterns in FTT. They include falling centiles, parallel poor centiles, markedly discrepant height and weight centiles, growth discrepancy from the family pattern, retrospective improvement of growth with changes in life situation, and dipping or saw tooth patterns.[26] The clinical picture is of a small, chronically underweight child with poor skinfold thickness, mid upper arm circumference and head growth and variable stunting. Developmental delays are most marked in the areas of speech and language and social function, including social responsiveness, affect and activity level.[67] Behavioral and emotional signs are frequent and variable and many parents express difficulty in the care of these children. Feeding and sleeping patterns are commonly disturbed. Contrary to traditional views, many of these children are overactive, restless and show poor quality of concentration and play skills. Inactivity and social withdrawal are seen as poor prognostic signs.

NOFTT is associated with various risk factors common for maltreatment generally. Poor quality of maternal attachment may be associated with a range of stresses. A difficult pregnancy or one where the child was unwanted or the result of rape or abuse, including incest, increases the risk. Maternal postnatal depression, drug or alcohol abuse, and domestic violence may increase the risks of the infant not thriving. A parent's own preoccupation with food and body weight may affect feeding patterns and may lead to withholding of food from the infant. Lack of parenting skills, emotional hostility, parental indifference, withdrawal and rejection are common features of NOFTT, emotional abuse and neglect. Many neglected children also fail to thrive and there are clearly links with physical and sexual abuse, although the majority of children attending pediatric clinics show no signs of these abuses. There are also factors which can be located in the child. The child may be the opposite sex from the one which the mother desired, or may have been born at the end of a woman's reproductive life, after she thought her family was complete. Congenital malformation and disability of any kind may be factors. The child's temperament, significance or meaning to the parents may also be relevant.[68,69] Some of these reasons help to explain why NOFTT may affect only one child in a family with other children. The importance of nutrition in the genesis of NOFTT cannot be overstated. Feeding the child inadequate calories can result from an inappropriate diet, restricting foods rich in calories, prolonged milk (including breastfeeding) to the exclusion of other foods, infrequent feeding, or feeding under hostile, restrictive, tense or forced conditions. A preoccupation with adult style 'healthy eating', a 'meals with no snacks regime', aversion to the mess involved with feeding young children and rigid child care practices, may contribute to mealtime misery and food refusal.

Mothers of children failing to thrive show less frequent verbal and physical contact, less positive reinforcement and warmth. They talk to, play with and cuddle these children less often than mothers of children who are thriving. Where mothers have both children who were growing normally and those who were failing to thrive they say that they get on better with the thriving ones. Some mothers describe feelings of helplessness and despair when attempting to feed their children. Others reported little or no pleasure from their baby or a disturbance in their sense of the child belonging to them.

MANAGEMENT

The clinician's role is to provide a clinical environment which is warm, supportive, nurturing, and free as far as possible from the negative feelings which may be engendered by parents who fail to feed and nurture their offspring. A multidisciplinary approach is favored[70] and has been shown to be effective in inducing catch up growth by encouraging extra and frequent feeding of calorie rich foods. Enhancing parenting in all areas as well as in feeding practice can be offered by involvement with family centers, and through the application of targeted programs. Home-based programs of care by skilled professional helpers have been shown to be effective.[71] Regular, but not obsessive, monitoring of growth, target setting and an outpatient program of support are essential features of the treatment regime. In the author's practice the use of nasogastric tube feeding and proprietary dietary supplements have not contributed positively to the management of NOFTT.

Medical diagnosis relies on history and examination. Dietary assessment is notoriously difficult and there are various approaches.[72] Observation of feeding at home or in the clinic or hospital ward is essential to a fuller understanding of the issues around food for the family and child. Screening for iron deficiency and urinary tract infection are recommended, but more complex laboratory investigation should be restricted to that clinically indicated on the basis of the clinical history and examination. There is ample evidence from various studies that routine investigation is unlikely to be helpful.

CONSEQUENCES OF NOFTT

There is both morbidity and mortality associated with NOFTT. Death is linked to abuse and neglect as well as to infectious diseases which arise from it. The symptoms and signs of infection may be modified by serious undernutrition. Failure to thrive is associated with sudden and unexpected death in infancy.[73,74] The major area of concern remains the substantial morbidity that arises from undernutrition at important and critical times in the development of the individual. Effects have been clearly demonstrated in clinical samples, but in community surveys the effects have been more difficult to demonstrate. Follow-up of clinical series suggests that for many children some improvement in growth can be expected with or without intervention over time. Neurodevelopmental attainment is frequently delayed with children who have failed to thrive showing reduced scores on tests of language development, reading age, social maturity and verbal intelligence on follow-up in school.[75]

SEXUAL ABUSE

DEFINITION

> *'The sexual exploitation of children is referred to as the involvement of dependent, developmentally immature children and adolescents in sexual activities that they do not fully comprehend, are unable to give informed consent to and that violate the social taboos of family roles'.*[76]

Child sexual abuse (CSA) entered into society's consciousness in England at Cleveland in 1987. The Report of the Inquiry into Child Abuse in Cleveland[77] noted that,

> *'We have learned during the Inquiry that sexual abuse occurs in children of all ages, including the very young, to boys as well as girls, in all classes of society and frequently within the privacy of the family'.*

However the professionals who were involved in the Cleveland crisis wrote:

> *'Child sexual abuse is a problem which depends on silence and secrecy. We have experienced something of what happens to abused children when they attempt to speak: we have been disbelieved, rejected and silenced'.*[78]

The current debate struggles to acknowledge the importance of sexual abuse in child and adult mental health and the difficulties of recognition, diagnosis, protection and treatment of children.

EPIDEMIOLOGY

CSA has been encountered in all human societies. The prevalence in various countries[79] range in women from 7% in Finland, to 36% in Austria, and for men, from 3% in Sweden and Switzerland to 29% in Austria. In the UK, CSA occurs more often outside the family[80] and involves perpetrators of both sexes, with a heavy male predominance. In a UK student sample, one in two young women and one in four young men had experienced sexual abuse before age 18 years. Sexual abuse was broadly defined to included exposure or 'flashing'. What is included within a definition of CSA has a major effect on the prevalence figure. Also, 95% of children failed to report to a person in authority, although half told a friend or other close person.[80] The National Commission of Inquiry into the Prevention of Child Abuse (1996) estimated that 100 000 children are 'exposed to potentially harmful sexual experiences' every year.[8] These figures are different from those derived from the single UK incidence study.[81] The figure was 0.9 per 1000 for established cases (0.34 for boys, 1.49 for girls).

A recent prevalence study[10] of 2869 young adults age 16–24 years (1235 men and 1634 women) defined sexual abuse as no consent, or consent when the age difference between victim and perpetrator was 5 years or more and the individual aged 12 years or less. They found that the prevalence of CSA was 1% by parents/carers (mostly physical contact); 3% by other relatives (2% contact, 1% non-contact); and 11% by other known people (8% physical contact, 3% non-contact); 4% by strangers or person just met (2% of each type); 7% suffered indecent exposure with more than a third by a stranger. Most abuse, except indecent exposure, involved repeated incidents. A significant number experienced sexual acts by non-relatives or by age peers, including boy or girlfriends, friends of brothers or sisters and fellow pupils or students.

It is not known how often predatory pedophiles are responsible for the abuse revealed in these studies. Certain high profile individuals receive disproportionately greater publicity in professional and public circles. Experience has determined that in schools and residential children's homes, the activities of pedophile staff has gone unchecked for many years. Clinical experience (a more accurate measure than retrospective prevalence data) indicates that the abuse involves children of all ages but with many under the age of 5 years.[82] Clinical samples are heavily weighted toward the poorer end of the social spectrum, but sexual abuse is probably encountered equally in all social classes. A quarter to a third of all reported abuse is committed by perpetrators under 18 years. The majority of reported perpetrators are male. Women abuse more often than is generally believed. In clinical practice generational patterns of CSA are commonly encountered.

PATTERNS OF ABUSE

CSA occurs in varied social settings. Intrafamilial abuse includes within the nuclear and extended family, adoptive and foster families. Family friends, lodgers or close acquaintances may be involved. Extrafamilial abuse is by adults frequently known to the child, including neighbors, family friends, schoolfriends, parents, and abuse within 'sex rings'. Institutional abuse occurs within schools, residential children's establishments, day nurseries, holiday camps, cubs, brownies, boy scouts and other organizations both secular and religious. Street or stranger abuse includes assaults on children in public places including child abduction. Sexual abuse may exist with other forms of abuse, e.g. physical, emotional. Organized and ritual abuse is described. There are overlaps between these different settings. For example, many of the children in sex rings were found to have been abused at home. Often ringleaders had been victims of parental abuse and had recruited other children into the ring. Other children were deprived of attention at home and vulnerable to the rewards of 'prostitution', but had not been sexually abused within their homes. Multiple abuse, episodes occur in half the cases from community research samples and over 75% of clinical cases. Children who have once been sexually abused appear to be at greater risk of further abuse by the same or different perpetrator.

Acts involved in sexual abuse

Such acts can be classified as contact or non-contact. Contact involves touching, fondling or oral contact of breast or genitals. There may be insertion of fingers or objects into vulva or anus. Masturbation may be by adult of him/herself in the presence of the child, including ejaculation onto the child, by adult of child or by child of adult. Intercourse is vaginal, anal or oral, whether actual or attempted in any degree. This is usually with adult as the active party but in some cases a child may be encouraged to penetrate the adult. Rape is attempted or achieved penile penetration of the vagina. Other genital contact includes intercrural intercourse where the penis is laid between the legs or genital contact with any part or the child's body, e.g. a penis rubbed on child's thigh.

Prostitution involves any of the above abuse, which includes the exchange of money, gifts or favors and applies to both boys ('rent boys') and girls. Cases have been encountered where parents have prostituted their children aged as young as 3 years. Non-contact abuse involves exhibitionism (flashing), pornography (photographing sexual acts or anatomy), showing pornographic images (photographs, films, videos) and erotic talk (telling children titillating or sexually explicit stories). Other sexual exploitations include sadistic activities, e.g. burning a child's buttocks or genital area.

EFFECTS OF SEXUAL ABUSE

Childhood sexual abuse is undoubtedly harmful. At best it is unpleasant, at worst extremely frightening and painful, physically and psychologically, for the child. Even older children, sufficiently physically mature to experience pleasurable sexual sensations, are hurt and suffer from its effects. Children say that they do not like it, wish it to stop and convey pain and discomfort when attempting to talk about it.

The accommodation syndrome[83] describes the situation when a child is caught up in a sexually abusive relationship and develops an adjustment pattern to the abuse. An understanding of this usual behavior pattern is vital in assisting children, including explaining in court why a child relates in a particular way. The five stages of the CSA accommodation syndrome are secrecy, helplessness, accommodation, delayed disclosure and retraction. This pattern is most clearly seen when the abuser is a trusted caregiver, for example a parent or parent figure. Children are told not to tell. Threats of physical violence, but often promises of withdrawal of love and affection, are all that are needed to secure silence. The child fears disapproval or punishment, and attempts to tell confirm these worst fears. Retaliation certainly occurs. Older children understand the implications for the family of a police investigation: possible imprisonment of father, loss of income, stigmatization, shame and the possibility that they may be held responsible. Children choose to maintain the conspiracy of secrecy and silence. Helplessness reflects the fact that children are unable to stop the abuse. Although they may resist at least initially, they find that it is less trouble to lie still, pretend to be asleep and switch off. In this way they attempt to protect themselves. This behavior is often reflected in the ease with which children are medically examined (some children go to sleep).

Children will not cry out or struggle to protect themselves and this is often misinterpreted as willing compliance, both by the abuser and society at large.

The cost that the child pays for the abandonment of active resistance is insecurity, victimization and a loss of psychological well-being and self-esteem. The child is helpless, powerless and has no-one to whom she can turn. Entrapment and accommodation follow. The child feels that there is no way out of the situation. The only active role the child can play is to hold herself responsible. In sensing that what is happening is both wrong and bad, she attempts to make amends. The victim therefore scapegoats herself, leaving the abuser free of experiencing the child's hostility. Self-blame and guilt are almost universal feelings shared by sexually abused children. In addition the child faces other pressures. There is the need to protect other children. The abuser may tell the child that if he stops abusing her he may have to turn to other, possibly younger children. Secondly there is a need to protect the other parent, the family home and integrity of the family. Seemingly the child has the power to destroy the family, but the responsibility to keep it together. Parent and child roles have been subtly reversed. The child has accommodated to the situation at the expense of herself and her needs. The loss of childhood describes how the child is forced into a pseudoadult role. Once in this position, other adults easily view the child as a consenting and willing participant in the situation and come to doubt the child's statements if later the truth is revealed. The child who is able to accommodate effectively to the abuse will cover up the reality in order to protect the parent, but also to allow herself space for survival. It is not unusual for children, for example, to flourish at school where they feel protected and safe, effectively splitting off that part of their life from the threats and insecurity of home. Children's capacity to develop different personalities to cope with their complex feelings leads to psychological disintegration and the multiple personality states seen in some adult survivors. Finally disclosure is very often delayed and followed by retraction. It is likely that many children never disclose their sexual abuse. They may attempt to within the family, but less often outside. Many adult victims disclosing in later life indicate that they never told.

Long term effects

There are few studies of medically diagnosed groups, with a predominance of intrafamilial cases. A case controlled study of children aged 7 years or less at diagnosis[84] found high levels of morbidity 8 years after diagnosis. Social, educational and health morbidity disadvantaged many children. Educational problems, adverse behaviors (aggressive and sexualized behavior) and chronic health problems (soiling, wetting, abnormal growth, and mental health problems) were common. A third experienced further abuse, and a quarter spent time in care or were adopted. Almost a third had a surname change, and cases experienced significantly more moves of home and school than controls.

Long term effects in adults include mental health problems, sexual adjustment difficulties, social dysfunction and child rearing difficulties. Depression, suicide, self-injury, poor self-esteem, alcohol and/or drug abuse, prostitution, marital difficulties, aversion to sexual contact and fertility control problems are linked. Some children repeat the cycle of abuse as adults, others may be over-protective, or have a fear of closeness. Delinquency, criminal behavior/offending, acts of violence and adoption of the victim role are other effects.

Women are more likely to internalize their distress whereas men may cope by exhibiting more aggressive and angry behavior. High rates of CSA history were found in various diagnostic groups of women. These included patients with multiple personality disorder, eating disorders, chronic pelvic pain, psychosexual disorders, and depression. The risk for depression is up to four times greater in those abused sexually as children than those not.

THE DIAGNOSTIC PROCESS IN CSA

The process of diagnosis is often complex and involves information gathering by other agencies including social services and the police.[3,63] The diagnosis, considered a jigsaw (Fig. 5.3), is assembled from the history, physical examination and laboratory investigation. Physical, emotional and sexual abuse may coexist. Growth, development and behavior should be considered.

Clinical presentation and diagnosis

Disclosure by the child may be the central piece of the 'diagnostic jigsaw'. Disclosure is a clinically useful concept to describe the process by which a child, who has been sexually abused, gradually comes to inform the outside world of her plight.[85] Deliberate fabrication is unusual and largely restricted to older children. Young children cannot fantasize specific sexual acts not experienced. The incidence of false allegations ranges from 2–8% in samples, which including a variety of situations. Higher figures are reported from allegations made during the course of custody and access disputes. However, these allegations must also be taken seriously. False allegations arise in different ways. They may arise in an adult's mind, either a carer or professional, be erroneous but sincere or false. A parent may misinterpret a child's statement, behavior, or a physical condition. A parent might indoctrinate a child into believing that someone had abused them, an interview may be frankly suggestive, or a parent may suffer from a delusion. Group contagion has been suggested as another mechanism, but sexual abuse may occur to groups of children. Finally a child who makes a false allegation may do so at the request of a parent, or for revenge – the 'true' false allegation.

Disclosure is favored in various situations. These include an overwhelmingly impossible situation at home and the presence of a sensitive friend or helper, e.g. school teacher. If the abuser loses contact (e.g. divorce) this may encourage disclosure. Educational strategies, telephone lines and good luck (right opportunity at the right time) also influence the process. Children usually disclose to a chosen, trusted person, for example a friend, family member or professional (teacher, school nurse, doctor). After initial 'disclosure' and a strategy discussion between professionals, a formal interview will take place. In the UK this is performed jointly by a social worker and police officer.

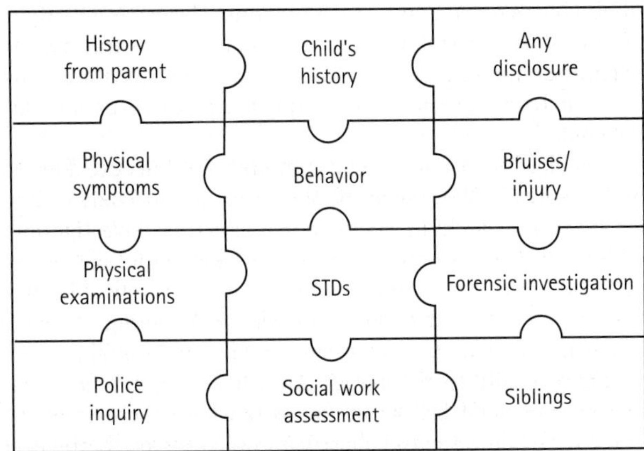

Fig. 5.3 Jigsaw of sexual abuse. Key elements in the diagnosis of sexual abuse assembled into a jigsaw picture.

Interviews of children, in child abuse investigations, are undertaken by appropriately trained staff, working to prescribed standards, acceptable to the legal process. Memorandum of Good Practice[86] provides guidance on the process of interviewing and video recording. The number of investigative interviews should be kept to a minimum. Most children, who are ready to talk, are able to disclose the details of their abuse in 1–2 interviews. Other frightened children may disclose after months to years. Children with communication difficulties, or who have English as a second language, need interviewers with particular skills.

Current research in the UK shows that children who do give evidence have more anxiety symptoms up until the trial than those who do not give evidence. This anxiety persists for the following 12 months, before falling to the levels of those who don't give evidence. The sexually abused child's predicament is that most do not tell anyone who can act to protect them. The child has been exploited and misused by an abuser who is more powerful than the child. The disclosure is frequently delayed, the child is often disbelieved, subtly or openly admonished or silenced.

The abuser's use of grooming and manipulation encourages the child to feel responsible for the abuse and sequelae, e.g. family breakup. Disclosure occurs in situations of relative safety, for example bedtime, to trusted adult or in foster care. Play materials, including anatomically complete dolls, drawing, and plasticine may help the child explain their experiences were the child has delayed expressive language, or has difficulty in using appropriate language.

Types of interview include 'screening' usually with a parent present. Questions must be open and not leading. 'Investigative' interviews can be used as evidence in civil or criminal proceedings. 'Facilitative' interviews are held when there are high levels of suspicion, children with learning difficulties, communication difficulties, psychiatric disorder associated with the abuse, or where there have been considerable delays since allegations were first made. These require special knowledge and skill.

PHYSICAL INDICATORS OF CSA

Sexual abuse may present with a physical symptom or indicator. This may be the only sign in infants, young children or children with communication difficulty. Caution is needed in the interpretation of signs and symptoms and time needed to build up the diagnostic jigsaw. Physical complaints include vaginal or anal pain, soreness, bleeding or discharge. Important presentations include sexually transmitted disease, pregnancy, vaginal foreign body, genital or anal injury, and recurrent urinary symptoms most notably dysuria. Genital bleeding must always be investigated. If the girl is prepubertal, the most common cause is trauma either accidental or non-accidental injury (sexual abuse). Rare causes, e.g. vulval hemangioma, tumor and lichen sclerosus should be considered.

Rectal bleeding occurs most commonly after infective diarrhoea or with fissures.[87] Bleeding in the absence of fissures may be due to other disorders such as rectal polyp. Further investigation is required. Anal fissures may be caused by the painful passage of a large hard stool, and fecal masses are usually palpable in the abdomen. A fissure is defined as 'a break in the lining of the anal canal, usually extending from inside the canal to the anal verge, and traveling vertically to the verge'. Anal fissures are differentiated from the superficial breaks in the skin where there is perianal soreness for whatever cause; diarrhea, threadworms, streptococcal infection, or seborrheic dermatitis. Here the break in the skin does not cross the anal verge into the anal canal. Anal fissures are caused by stretching of the anal margin to a point where splitting occurs, giving a triangular tear with the apex within the anal canal. The etiology of the fissure, whether organic or caused by an object inserted forcibly cannot easily be deduced from its appearance. However, substantial fissures are more likely to follow abuse. Fissures are also seen in inflammatory bowel disease, for example Crohn's disease, but other signs and symptoms will be apparent in the presence of systemic illness. Anal fissures cause pain on defecation and are associated with anal spasm. They bleed initially, but usually heal over 1–3 weeks. Healing is impaired if the fissures are deep or persistently stretched, as in untreated constipation or continuing abuse. These fissures are seen as a deep, wide cleft, usually anteriorly or posteriorly. Healing may take months and result in scarring, including a skin tag as a marker of previous trauma. Anal fissures are seen most commonly in infancy, associated with significant constipation and are usually superficial and may be multiple. They are uncommon in the school-aged child. Some abused children become constipated.

Vulvitis and vaginitis in prepubertal girls is common. Maternal estrogen thickens the vaginal mucosa at birth and causes slightly acidic secretions. These effects cease after 4–6 weeks and the mucosa becomes thin with pH neutral until puberty. Prepubertal girls are prone to vulvitis, possibly relating to relative estrogen deficiency. Specific infections are influenced by estrogen status. *Trichomonas* grows poorly in the absence of estrogen, but the reverse is the case for gonococcus (*Neisseria gonorrhoeae*) and *Chlamydia*. Causes of vulvitis include poor hygiene, sensitivity, e.g. to bubblebath, soaps, threadworms (possibly causing irritation but rarely observed in the vulva), atopic eczema, seborrheic dermatitis, sexual abuse (causing local trauma and secondary infection), excessive and inappropriate washing, sexually transmitted disease (STD) and other infections, e.g. *Streptococcus*, *Candida*. Masturbation is not a cause of vulvitis, unless self-mutilation, as occurs in some sexually abused children, is seen. Symptoms caused by vulvitis include soreness, itchiness and burning on micturition.

Symptoms of vulvovaginitis are the same as for vulvitis with the addition of vaginal discharge. A high proportion of prepubertal girls who have been sexually abused complain of 'soreness' and have a vulvitis or vulvovaginitis on examination. This is probably due to rough handling leading to mucosal abrasions with secondary infection. Genitourinary symptoms, including vulvovaginitis, associated with soreness, discharge, or recurrent sterile dysuria, should encourage CSA to be considered. Causes of vaginal discharge include non-specific, group A beta-hemolytic *Streptococcus*, *Staphylococcus aureus*, *Haemophilus influenzae*, *Gardnerella vaginalis*, STD, and vaginal foreign body.

Dysuria

Following CSA, pain or frequency on micturition or even traumatic hematuria may be seen in boys and girls resulting from urethral trauma. Bruising, swelling, inflammation or dilatation may be seen. Urine microscopy and culture differentiate urinary tract infection from local inflammation. A history of recurrent dysuria is common in girls who have been sexually abused. Of girls under 6 years, 20% have genitourinary symptoms. Difficulty in passing urine and occasionally retention is seen with more serious trauma. Urethral pathology is uncommon and includes urethral caruncle, hemangioma, prolapse and polyp.

Masturbation

Masturbation does not ordinarily cause any abnormal physical signs. Excessive masturbation is described in some abused children. It describes the behavior of children who are continually rubbing their genitalia in public, both digitally and also rubbing against furniture, knees or any firm surface. This may be the child's response to the need for sexual arousal, or comfort, or due to vulval irritation secondary to trauma or infection. If masturbation alone causes a vulvitis this is abnormal and indicates self-mutilation and is highly correlated with CSA.

Genital and other self-mutilation

Self-mutilation is recognized in abused adolescents and is increasingly being appreciated, in young children (Fig. 5.4), where excessive scratching may cause deep lacerations, which bleed or become secondarily infected. Children burn, pinch and cut themselves. The mutilation may affect face, neck, arms, abdomen and arms, less commonly the genitalia or anus.

Foreign bodies

Vaginal or anal insertion of foreign bodies is unusual. Younger prepubertal girls are unaware they have a vagina. Presentation is with bleeding, purulent discharge and odor. Insertion, causing stretching of the hymen, results in pain and often bleeding. CSA must be considered if a child is seen with a vaginal foreign body. Episodes may be repeated.[88] Herman-Giddens[89] found that 11 of 12 prepubertal girls with foreign bodies were either confirmed or suspected victims of sexual abuse. Rectal foreign bodies are more rarely seen and associated with sadistic rape in older children.

STD (Table 5.10)[90]

STD is diagnosed in 3–13% of sexually abused children, with higher rates in older children. The presence of an STD in a child usually leads to suspicion of CSA. Various modes of transmission of STD to a child exist. The presence of a STD provides corroborative evidence of CSA and Table 5.11 gives a guide to the probability of abuse.[90]

Full penetrative intercourse (vaginal or anal) is not necessary for infection. Orogenital sex and intercrural contact may transmit pathogens. Infections can occur asymptomatically so there is a case for routine screening where sexual abuse is being considered. Infections encountered include gonorrhea, which with the exception of neonatal ophthalmia or vaginitis, is strong evidence of sexual abuse. Genital/anal warts have an incubation which may be several months and up to 2 years. Infection represents possible

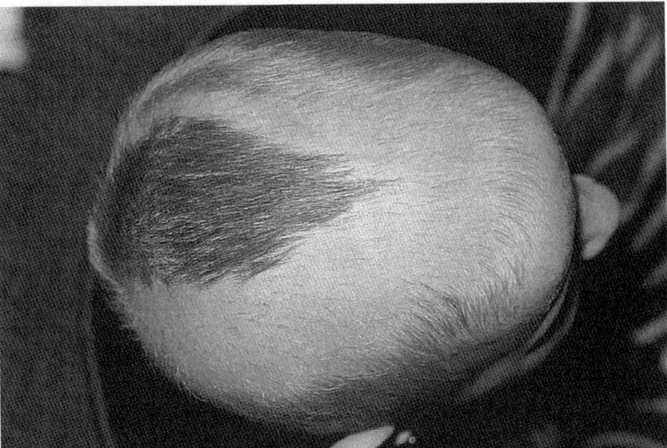

Fig. 5.4 Traumatic hair loss in a 4-year-old girl which was self-inflicted. Genital examination revealed an unusual shaped hymen with a posterior tear. During the investigation it became apparent that she was being sexually abused by her parents and grandparents. Her hair regrew in foster care.

Table 5.10 Transmission of STDs in children (From Royal College of Physicians 1997[90])

In utero	HIV, syphilis, HPV
Perinatal	Trachomatis, gonorrhea, HSV, HPV, HIV, TV
Direct contact	
Non-sexual/auto inoculation	HPV, HSV
Fomite transmission	? TV
Consensual sexual contact	All STD
Sexual abuse	All STD

HIV, human immunodeficiency virus; HPV, human papillomavirus; HSV, herpes simplex virus; TV, *Trichomonas vaginalis*.

sexual abuse. Sexual contact is the most usual mode of transmission. *Chlamydia* has an incubation of 7–14 days. Neonates may develop conjunctivitis, but in a child over 3 years sexual transmission is likely. The incubation period for *Trichomonas* is 1–4 weeks and if the child is over 6 weeks then sexual transmission is virtually certain. Herpes simplex, either type I or II is likely to be sexually transmitted. Bacterial vaginosis suggests the possibility of sexual abuse. Other infections rarely encountered in the UK in children are hepatitis B, syphilis and HIV. These are likely to have been transmitted sexually if other routes of transmission can be excluded.

Links with other forms of abuse

Physical abuse and CSA are closely related.[91] Approximately one in six physically abused children was sexually abused and one in seven of sexually abused children was physically abused, including fatal cases. All physically abused children must be assessed, for sexual abuse. Patterns of injury may be suggestive, but in many cases there is nothing to suggest sexual abuse. Common patterns include sadistic injury (burns are a good example), injuries around genital area and lower abdomen or breasts and restraint type injuries (grips marks to buttocks, thighs, knees or arms). Severe and fatal physical abuse may occur when the abuser acts to terrorize or silence them. Neglected children suffer higher levels of sexual abuse.

Psychological and behavioral signs

Complaints, which are of psychological origin, are important because they draw attention to the child's distress. Common, but non-specific, symptoms include recurrent abdominal pains especially between 5 and 10 years of age and headaches, including migraine, are more common as children grow into adolescence. Anorexia and eating disorders are relatively common in adolescence and have significant morbidity and mortality. CSA is an important antecedent. Although girls predominate, both sexes may be affected. Constipation, soiling and encopresis are associated with CSA. Constipation involves difficulty or delay in the passage of feces. Soiling is the frequent passage of liquid or semi-solid feces into clothing. Encopresis is the passage of feces of normal or near normal consistency into socially inappropriate places (including clothing). Constipation and soiling are occasionally linked to CSA. Encopresis is usually associated with considerable emotional trauma and therefore with emotional abuse and CSA. Factors contributing to constipation include training too young, punitive parenting and disorganized household. Delayed development, anxiety, and fear also contribute. In CSA retention of feces is seen as a response to stress, especially in anal abuse. Abused children may experience extreme anger. Encopresis may be an expression of this anger and be associated with smearing of feces and other

Table 5.11 Incubation period for sexually transmitted infections and probability of sexual abuse, (From Royal College of Physicians 1997[90])

Incubation period	Probability of abuse
Gonorrhea: 3–4 days	*** (** if child <1 year)
Chlamydia trachomatis: 7–14 days	** (*** if child > 3 years)
†HSV: 2–14 days	**
Trichomonas vaginalis: 1–4 weeks	*** (if child > 6 weeks)
HPV: 1 months–several months or longer	* (** if not perinatally acquired AAP)‡
Bacterial vaginosis	*
Syphilis: up to 90 days	*** (having excluded congenital infection)
HIV: majority seroconvert within 3 months	* (exclude material infection)
Hepatitis B: up to 3 months	*(exclude material infection)

* Possible ; ** probable; *** strong probability.
† HSV (herpes simplex virus) incubation period possibly longer.
‡ AAP (American Academy of Pediatrics) suggests ** probability of abuse if human papillomavirus (HPV) not perinatally acquired.

destructive behavior. Other children, who may be depressed and fearful, express their distress through soiling. Encopresis may act as a protection for the child. 'If I'm smelly and dirty he'll leave me alone'. Stopping the abuse may lead to dramatic cure of an intractable problem.

One cause of secondary daytime or nocturnal enuresis is abuse including CSA. Some abused children only become dry when they feel safe and protected. Amongst persistent day-wetters there are increasing numbers of recognized victims of CSA. Behavioral disturbance is a common manifestation of CSA. The range of behavior is wide. Rare presentation with psychotic symptoms may be precipitated by the stress of coping with sexual abuse in a vulnerable personality. Sexually explicit behavior and play is relatively specific for CSA. Others are non-specific, for example conduct disorder or deterioration in school performance. Mental deterioration, with loss of skills in language and play, and general social withdrawal[92] have been described. The differential diagnosis in these children includes autism, attention deficit hyperactivity disorder, schizophrenia and neurodegenerative conditions such as lipidosis. Sexualized behavior includes excessive or indiscriminate masturbation, preoccupation with genitals, or seeking to engage others in differentiated sexual behavior, sexual aggression, prostitution and extreme sexual inhibition in teenagers. All are closely linked to CSA. Aggressive behavior is another commonly associated behavior.

PEDIATRIC ASSESSMENT IN CSA[26]

The pediatric assessment of the sexually abused child should be undertaken by appropriately trained pediatricians. There are both pediatric and forensic aspects to the assessment and in some cases a joint examination with a forensic physician may assist in the collection of forensic evidence. The assessment should take place in an appropriate and safe environment, with such equipment that is required readily available. The doctor must be chaperoned at least for the physical examination. The doctor must have a knowledge of the signs and symptoms which sexually abused children show as well as a knowledge of sexually transmitted diseases. He must be aware of and sensitive to the complex psychological issues in CSA. Increasingly the doctor is expected to have experience in the use of the colposcope, in obtaining good quality images and in interpreting the findings.

Emphasis is on a whole child assessment rather than examination of his or her genitalia/anus. The aims are to assess any injury and determine if abuse has occurred and its nature. It may be necessary to collect forensic evidence and document physical signs associated with abuse. The assessment should start and assist the process of psychological healing. Additional referral or treatment may be required for any consequences of the abuse including STD, pregnancy and psychological trauma. Both the child's and parent's histories, including details of any disclosure of abuse, are recorded. Other significant history includes previous medical contacts, the child's general health and any specific complaints. An examination where no abnormality is found cannot exclude CSA. In a study to evaluate the physical signs associated with CSA, of 382 sexually abused girls, mean age 5.8 years, 71% had normal findings on examination including 48% who had a history of penetration which included interlabial rather than vaginal.[93] Other authors agree.[88,94] Healing occurs rapidly and scarring is uncommon.[82] Changing physical signs suggest healing, reabuse, or that a disease process is evolving.

GENITAL EXAMINATION IN PREPUBERTAL GIRLS

The colposcope is increasingly used in clinical practice.[95] It provides a good light source, magnification and a facility for photography or videophotography. The colposcope may help in subtle cases to confirm normality or abnormality. The advantages and disadvantages are shown in Table 5.12. Photographs are used to discuss findings with colleagues, peer review, teaching, and second opinions, thereby avoiding the need for re-examination and medicolegal work. Children handle the examination well and are not 'retraumatized'.[96]

Normal anatomy

The hymen is the membrane across the opening of the vagina. The newborn and infant has a hymen both thick and redundant under the effects of maternal estrogen. As estrogen effect wanes the hymen changes, becoming thinner, flatter and with a sharp edge. This change has taken place in 75% of girls by 3 years of age[97] (Table 5.13).[98] The hymen continues in this form, thin, with a sharp edge and clearly visible vessels during childhood until puberty, when it once again becomes estrogenized. The pubertal hymen is thick, paler, redundant, sleeve-like or fimbriated. There is often a white physiological vaginal discharge. Hymenal elasticity increases with pubertal development and the capillary network is obscured. Congenital absence of hymen is probably rare[99] but 3–4% have hymenal variants such as tags and transverse bands.

Variations in central hymenal opening before puberty include: thin and crescentic, annular, frilly, septate, cuff-like and punctate. A vertical hymenal septum may be associated with a septate vagina

Table 5.12 The advantages and disadvantages of using a colposcope

Advantages in use of colposcope	Disadvantages in use of colposcope
Non-invasive technique	Expensive (but robust)
Good light and magnification	Relatively non-portable
Facilities for non-intrusive photography	May discourage unaided examination
Acceptable to child, parents, doctor	Danger of overinterpretation of minor signs

Table 5.13 Changes in hymenal configuration in early life (From Herman-Giddens & Frothingham 1987[98])

Configuration of hymen	Newborn	At 3 years
Annular	72%	38%
Crescentic	1%	55%
Fimbriated	19%	2%
Sleeve	6%	5%

and bicornuate uterus. Ultrasound examination in older children will delineate the extent of the problem. Hymenal tags are relatively common in the newborn and are occasionally seen in older children too as a redundant tag of tissue usually attached inferiorly. Imperforate hymen or microperforate hymen is very uncommon. Primary or congenital imperforate hymen is smooth, distinguishing it from a secondarily imperforate hymen, which has been traumatized and has a thickened, disorganized appearance.[100]

Physical signs[101]

Signs depend on the type of abuse, time interval from the last assault (healing may be very rapid), chronicity of abuse and presence of infection. The following are thought to be significant signs:[90,102] diagnostic signs of abuse include a fresh laceration of hymen (digital, penile, other penetration), or an old laceration of hymen with or without healing, with scarring and interruption of hymenal margin (hymenal penetration); attenuation of the hymen, often posteriorly or laterally and narrow hymenal rim refer to reduction in hymen substance. Pregnancy and positive 'forensic tests' provide other firm diagnostic signs. Supportive signs are more commonly encountered. These include a notch in posterior hymenal edge with or without scarring (penetration). A notch is usually normal in the ventral 180 degrees of hymen,[90] but opinion is divided and asymmetrical notches anteriorly may also be considered traumatic. Acute injuries to genitalia, such as localized erythema, edema, minor abrasions (seen in all types of contact abuse) are also considered supportive. A scar at the posterior fourchette may follow a shearing or splitting injury and is supportive evidence. A hymenal orifice with a transverse diameter of 1.5 cm is considered supportive, although such wide diameters are occasionally seen in children who have not been abused. Foreign body in vagina, STD, physical injury to external genitalia, grip marks, 'love-bites', and other non-accidental injury are all seen as supporting a diagnosis of sexual abuse. Some examiners place emphasis on unusual behavior during examination and other signs of emotional abuse and neglect. Other signs which are less clear in terms of significance include a pouting or dilated urethral orifice (on labial traction it may be normal to see dilatation) thought to follow vigorous rubbing or insertion of objects into the urethra.

Visualization of the hymenal opening is achieved by labial separation, involving gentle pressure downwards and laterally, and supplemented with labial traction, where the labia are lifted forwards and outwards. Hymenal opening dimensions vary according to the method used. A gaping hymenal orifice is one, which is clearly open with abduction of the legs but with no manipulation of the labia, and is suggestive of abuse. If the posterior part of the hymen is not clearly visualized on traction and appears rolled, examination of the child in the knee–chest position permits better visualization as the hymen unfolds.

Hymenal opening diameter depends on both techniques of examination and measurement.[103] Measurement may be by tape, photograph, or glass rod. Hymenal orifice diameter increases a little with age, up to 4 mm at 4 years, 7 mm at onset of puberty and 10 mm at completion of puberty. For various reasons, less significance is now placed on this sign. The range of normality is wide, the measurement influenced by the state of relaxation of the child and method of examination used, and the measurement is difficult to make accurately. The hymenal opening is usually symmetrical in mid-childhood. Marked asymmetry, for example a small notch at 11 o'clock and a marked notch at 1 o'clock or other sharp angles, square angles or distortions of the hymenal margin should be noted as signs of possible previous trauma. Minor bumps in the margin are probably normal variants but bumps in association with a distorted hymenal margin and a disrupted vascular pattern seen especially posteriorly and laterally are seen in association with abuse.

Vaginal ridges running vertically down the vagina are normal and may cause a smooth bump at the hymenal margin. Scars are very unusual. They may be visible at the posterior fourchette after a 'splitting or shearing injury'.[90] The scar is seen as a thickened, white irregular area, which disrupts the usual lacy vascular pattern. Labial fusion is the partial or complete adherence of the labia minora and is commonly seen in infancy and early childhood, often in association with nappy rash. It occurs secondary to denudation of the upper squamous epithelial layer of the labial mucosa with the formation of a thin connective tissue bridge and is caused by inflammatory disorders, including vulvitis and nappy rash, or trauma as in CSA.

THE PHYSICAL EXAMINATION OF PUBERTAL AND POSTPUBERTAL GIRLS

Older children understand the significance of what has happened as well as the consequences. Examination therefore may be more difficult. Consent, which will be better informed and understood, may be refused. A teenager may permit only limited examination for example of the 'love bites' on her neck. The girl may accept an appointment for a further examination in 2–3 weeks, a period of time the social worker may use to help the girl prepare herself.

This age group is at particular risk of STD, especially if sexually promiscuous. Long term effects include infertility and risk of cancer. Pregnancy becomes a possibility and teenage pregnancy and CSA are related. Simple inspection of the estrogenized hymen is an unreliable way to assess abnormal physical signs associated with sexual abuse. Use of cotton-tipped swab, Glaister rods and other such devices assist in assessment of recent or old hymenal injury. Digital examination if tolerated provides additional information. At puberty the 'usual' hymenal opening is about 1.0 cm and even the examiner's smallest finger is likely to cause discomfort. With this diameter it may be inferred that penile penetration is unlikely and digital penetration infrequent, if at all. The smallest tampon is less than 1 cm and may cause a little stretching.[104,105] An index finger, which measures 1.5 cm, inserted without discomfort would clearly be consistent with digital penetration. Two-finger examination, with ease, would correspond to a diameter of 3.5–4.5 cm and be consistent with penile penetration. If penetration has been infrequent the girl may complain of discomfort. Repeated vaginal intercourse leads to a widened, lengthened vagina eventually with loss of vaginal rugae. In practice a history of tampon/pad usage is not of great significance. More important is a history of consensual sexual activity in assessing the significance of genital findings. Speculum examination is used in postpubertal girls, for example to swab the cervix for gonorrhea. If a child is badly traumatized and there is marked vaginal bleeding it is likely that a speculum examination will be needed to identify the source of the bleeding. In this situation a general anesthetic is necessary. Rape, in this context, is defined as penile penetration of a female child's genitalia no matter to what degree. Investigations and management for rape victims include complete forensic swabs, a STD screen and HIV testing as indicated. Postcoital contraception is offered. Prophylactic antibiotics are not usually indicated unless it is known that the assailant is infected. The child and other family members are usually referred for counseling.

DIFFERENTIAL DIAGNOSIS OF GENITAL FINDINGS

Accidental genital injury may be suggested as the cause of a genital injury, which is really the result of an assault. Whatever the cause, any injury will be painful, with immediate bleeding and a dramatic history. Straddle injuries occur when the child falls astride a climbing frame, crossbar of a bicycle, or furniture. Forced compression of soft tissues between the object straddled and underlying bony pubic symphysis and rami cause anterior injury, i.e. to the mons, clitoris, urethra and anterior labia majora and minora. The injury may be linear, asymmetrical, and coincide with the bone, with marked swelling, and bruising in the traumatized tissue, and on occasion laceration. The hymenal opening is not dilated. Accidental penetration of the labia is less common[106] and seen typically between 18 months and 3 years after a history of falling astride toys or steps. Minor bruising and small, 0.5–1.0 cm, lacerations of the labia minora, which may bleed profusely, may result. The laceration, which is indistinguishable from those caused by fingernails in CSA, heals rapidly without scarring. Tearing due to forced abduction of the legs is rare. Splitting of the midline structures has been described when the girl's legs were forcibly parted during abuse. Laceration of the posterior fourchette may follow clumsy attempts at penetration. Masturbation does not cause damage unless it is part of self-mutilation, usually following CSA.

Female genital mutilation involves partial or total removal of the external genitalia. The practice, which is cultural, seeks to reduce sexual responsiveness. Elderly women perform it in unsanitary and hazardous situations resulting in complications of pain, shock, hemorrhage, urinary retention and sepsis. Longer term problems include abscesses, fistulae, scarring, dyspareunia, incontinence and problems in childbirth. It is illegal and therefore a form of child abuse in the UK under the Prohibition of Female Circumcision Act (1985). The practice originates from parts of Africa including Eritrea, Ethiopia and Somalia. It is estimated that in the UK 10 000 girls and young women who have come from these countries are at risk.

Harmful genital care practices in children are also considered a form of abuse.[107] The practice involves painful washing of the genitalia, frequent and ritualistic inspections, applications of creams, and various medications for 'genital soreness', discharge and perceived infection.

Skin disorders include nappy rash (ammoniacal dermatitis) atopic or seborrheic eczema and lichen sclerosus. The latter condition is increasingly recognized and may give an initial impression of trauma. There may be bleeding from hemorrhagic blisters and purpura may look like bruises. The girl may complain of 'burning' or an intense itch. Ivory or white shiny macules and papules form homogenous hypopigmented atrophic areas on the vulva and often perianal skin in a 'figure of eight pattern'. Areas of vasculitis or purpura with ecchymoses may be seen. Fissures are common perianally. There may be a superadded infection and vulvovaginitis. Confusion with sexual abuse is described. Trauma including CSA has been suggested as a possible etiological factor,[108] but this has not been firmly established. Treatment is with corticosteroid cream of moderate to high potency until the child is asymptomatic. The condition waxes and wanes and the girl should take responsibility for applying the creams herself, as she grows older, to avoid application becoming abusive. Boys do not appear to have the perianal disorder,[90] but a disorder which is said to be equivalent to lichen sclerosus, xeroderma obliterans, involves the penis. Congenital vascular lesions are small vascular lesions on the labia minora or the perineum and look like a bruise. Follow-up will clarify the situation. Fungal nappy rash may be seen in association with oral candidiasis. This is uncommon in older girls.

GENITAL EXAMINATION OF BOYS

Sexual abuse of boys is readily overlooked. Whilst male genital injury may be less commonly encountered, diagnosis of its cause may be more difficult. In many instances, the abuse will leave no signs, but there may be abrasions, bite marks, bruises, lacerations, edema and inflammation or burns of the penile shaft, glans or foreskin. Burns and bruising to the scrotum also occur, although an accidental cause of scrotal bruising is a straddle injury. Injuries may sometimes represent a non-sexualized punishment, e.g. for bedwetting.[90]

ANAL EXAMINATION

Anal abuse occurs to children of both sexes and at any age.[109] It is more difficult for victims and professionals to discuss and is often denied. Penile penetration is possible in preschool children and although there is a small risk of rectal perforation, this is usually encountered only in the very young child or infant. In the UK, the act of penile anal penetration is termed buggery, in the USA, sodomy. Physical signs may or may not be present and vary with factors such as degree of force, use of lubricant, method of abuse, frequency and duration of the abuse and time interval between last act and examination. Signs vary in significance and specificity for abuse. Most signs heal completely, although a major laceration can result in scarring. The child may be examined in left lateral or knee–chest position and findings vary with both position used and length of time of observation (Table 5.14 and Fig. 5.5).

The differential diagnosis of anal signs includes perianal streptococcal infection, skin disease (lichen sclerosus, eczema, nappy rash), inflammatory bowel disease (Crohn's disease), and hemolytic uremic syndrome (megacolon and rectum with anal dilatation). Bleeding may be caused by a rectal polyp. Other causes include *Shigella* or *Salmonella*, or a fissure from constipation. Congenital abnormality and some normal appearances need to be distinguished, for example the midline raphe and shiny depressed areas, which look like scars, directly anterior or posterior. Neurological disorders which lead to a lax anal sphincter are occasionally encountered. Rare causes include rectal or sacral tumor. Accidental injury is uncommon.

FORENSIC SAMPLING IN SEXUAL ABUSE

Forensic samples are those examined in forensic science laboratories. They comprise evidential samples and controls.[110] Materials, which may be sampled in CSA, include stains for blood, semen, saliva, vaginal fluid, lubricants and feces. Debris includes pubic hair, other materials (e.g. hairs, fibers), which are of limited importance where the child and perpetrator share the same domestic environment. Clothing, bedding, furniture and carpets may be richer sources of forensically important materials as they are less likely to be washed than the child. Time limits have been established for the detection of spermatozoa and seminal fluid. These vary according to body site (Table 5.15).[110]

Table 5.14 Physical signs in the anal and perianal region

Site	Lesion	Description	Cause
Skin	Erythema	Reddening	Non-specific infection (NB streptococcal cellulitis), poor hygiene, trauma
	Thickening, lichenification	Swelling with reddening, cracks, pigmentation	Skin disorder, e.g. eczema, lichen sclerosus
	Loss of anal folds	Loss of fold pattern, smooth pink shiny skin	Chronic abuse
	Scars	Fan-shaped linear, heaped up skin, distorted fold pattern	Secondary to fissures from any etiology if severe enough
	Perianal warts, vesicles	Often multiple raised lesions scattered on and around anus	Human papillomavirus infection (various types)
	Threadworm infection	Small white cotton-like worms at margin – reddening and excoriation from scratching	*Enterobius vermicularis*
Anal margin	Edema	Tyre sign – swelling of margin	Recent trauma from stretching and shearing as in penetration
	Bruising	Non-draining discolored patches	Severe trauma
	Hematoma of anal verge	Discrete swelling on margin	Severe trauma
	Skin tag	Mound or flap of skin at any point around circumference	Secondary to fissure Unknown how often congenital
	Fissure	Break in lining of canal which usually extends onto anal verge. Variable depth, length and width. Single or multiple, acute or chronic	Stretching of anal margin – severe constipation or anal penetration Crohn's disease Very uncommon in normal children
	Anal verge defect or deficit	Skin covered indentation in anal margin	Uncertain – possible site of old healed fissure
Perianal area	Venous congestion	Purple or blue/black discoloration, flat or raised around a portion or whole circumference	May be normal in infancy Seen after anal penetration Avoid prolonged examination
	Funneled perianal area	Deep set fixed funnel appearance	Infrequent in older children/adolescents. Reflects chronic penetrative abuse
External sphincter	Shortening or eversion of the anal canal	Anorectal junction is approximated to anal orifice (turned inside out)	Associated with repeated anal abuse in first 2–3 years Sphincter is lax
	Laxity	On gentle traction or parting the buttocks anus appears open or gapes	Neurological disorder (patulous anus), severe chronic constipation with relaxed sphincter Anal penetrative abuse
	Gaping (open anal canal)	Widely gaping anus which does not contract or relax – 'visible hole'	Recent acute penetration – transient phenomenon
External and internal sphincter	Reflex anal dilatation	On separation of buttocks, both sphincters relax allowing observation through anus into rectum Orifice is circular, 5–20 mm diameter with dynamic opening and closing Some children able to perform at will	Anus dilates when contents (feces, wind) evacuated but otherwise closed Possible link to surgical manipulation/ use of suppositories, hemolytic uremic syndrome, inflammatory bowel disorder Associated with chronic anal abuse

It is important that there are agreed procedures to maintain the chain of evidence including the use of correct sampling methods, labeling, storage and transport of specimens.

DEATHS FROM CHILD ABUSE

Infanticide is legally defined as 'the killing of a child under the age of 12 months by the child's mother when the balance of her mind is disturbed because she had not fully recovered from the effect of childbirth or lactation' (Infanticide Act 1938). Filicide refers to killing of a child by either parent. Homicide is usually the result of a single fatal assault whereas death from child abuse occurs in association with assault and neglect over a much longer period.[111] Child homicide and fatal abuse have differences and may be distinct.[112–114] In England and Wales, children account for between 11 and 25% of homicide victims. The majority of perpetrators are parents. Child abduction and murder by a stranger is relatively rare. Between the years 1984 and 1993, 57 children were murdered by

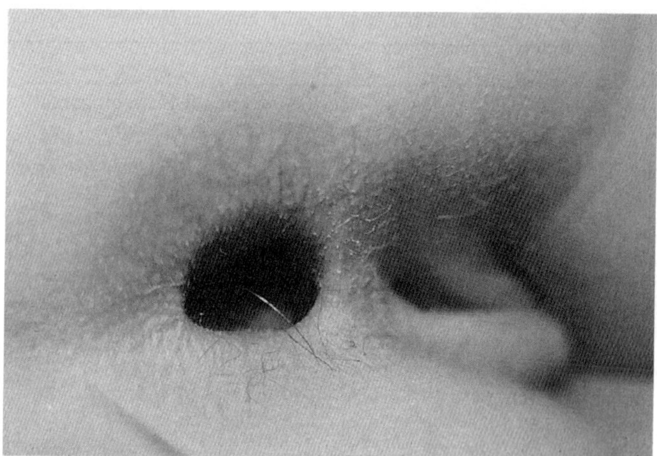

Fig. 5.5 Girl aged 12 years who shows thickened perianal skin with reddening and reflex anal dilatation with stool visible in the rectum. These signs slowly resolved over 12 months after she was taken into protective care. She disclosed anal abuse by her father repeated three times weekly over the preceding 6 years.

strangers, i.e. between five and six per year.[114] Child abuse deaths are considerably more common. In the USA, five children per day, and in the UK, one to two children per week, are killed by caretakers. In the UK, these figures have remained stable over the last 20 years with minor fluctuations in rate from year to year although a 40% increase has been reported for 2001. Official figures are likely to underestimate the true scale of fatal child abuse because where findings are in any way doubtful, parents are given the benefit of the doubt, because of the tragic circumstances accompanying the death of a child. In the USA the introduction of child death review teams has highlighted this problem further.[115] The risk of death decreases with increasing age (Table 5.16).

Factors responsible for parents killing their children are complex. Wilczynski[116] classified deaths into a number of different categories. Retaliation occurred when anger meant for the person's partner was displaced onto the child. There is usually a background of severe marital conflict and domestic violence. Jealousy of, or rejection by, the child may also trigger fatal abuse. Usually a male partner felt resentful because it was not his child, or the child received too much attention from the mother, or the child appeared rejecting of him. Many deaths are linked to the child being unwanted, frequently involving the mother. The child is unplanned or unwanted from conception. Newborn killings are included. Handicapped children may represent older unwanted children with feelings of rejection for the child developing after birth. Discipline killings follow attempts to discipline the child for behavior which the parent finds irritating. Altruistic killings apply to children who are suffering or severely handicapped. It is important to recognize the importance of parental mental health problems in child killings.

Table 5.15 Time limits for detection of spermatozoa and seminal fluid (From Jenkins & Lewington 1997[110])

Site	Spermatozoa	Seminal fluid
Vagina	6 days	12–18 h
Anus	3 days	3 h
Mouth	12–14 h	–
Clothing/bedding	Until washed	Until washed

Times limits shorter in prepubertal girls.

Table 5.16 UK child homicides in 1992

	Number	Offences per million children
Infants (under 1 year)	38	48
Toddlers (1 to 4)	25	89
Children (5 to 15)	40	5
Total children (< 16)	103	

Psychotic parents or those who have distorted perceptions of themselves, may be at risk. Links between child death and Munchausen syndrome by proxy (falsified illness) are well established. Only very rarely is self-defence an explanation. Parental psychiatric morbidity is common in fatal or near fatal child abuse. Falkov[111] identified around a third of cases with a history of psychiatric morbidity most often in the mother: psychosis (40%), depression (20%), personality disorder (20%), and Munchausen syndrome by proxy (8%). Few cases of puerperal psychosis and alcohol related problems were found, but drug dependence occurred with an increased frequency.

Clinical presentation of fatal child abuse varies. The severely battered infant or child is usually accurately diagnosed, but more difficult is the case where unexpected death occurs where occult injury is found. Cot death may mimic death due to suffocation and Munchausen by proxy. Neglect can be overlooked. A child may be deliberately or passively left in dangerous situations for example near water or alone in a house with fire hazards. Deliberate poisoning requires awareness and toxicology. Recurrent unexplained deaths have been shown to be the result of abuse in certain well-publicized cases. Child death has long been associated with sexual assault where stranger abduction is involved, but parallel domestic situations, of CSA also occur.

MANAGEMENT OF CHILD ABUSE

(See Working Together[3] for details of current national guidelines for the interagency protection of children from abuse and neglect. Each area should have locally established procedures.)

The concept of children's rights is a recent one. In the twentieth century, for the first time in England and Wales, Parliament placed the responsibility and duty onto local authorities to protect children at risk of harm and provide support for families. The need for a child centered legal system is increasingly accepted. The Children Act (1989), whilst progressive, has experienced difficulties with family (domestic) violence, violence and contact arrangements and delay in court proceedings, which are usually detrimental to the child. Adversarial hearings continue to dominate court practice. Gradually the needs of children have been accepted as being different from those of adults and children's welfare is the main interest of the Family Court. Criminal courts in England and Wales have a low age of criminal responsibility, at 10 years, and in Scotland it is 8 years. 'Doli incapax' which allowed some discretion between 10 and 13 years has been erased. Young offenders are frequently victims of abuse and neglect. Many have drifted into the care system ill-educated and 30% on leaving care have a reading age of less than 7 years. Family support is lacking due to geographically distant units.

During the 1970s Maria Colwell, aged 7 years, was killed by her stepfather, after being returned from the care of her aunt and uncle, who had looked after her for most of her life. Over the last 15 months of her life she was severely maltreated: neglected, physically and emotionally abused and failed to thrive.[117] Not only were children not protected by local authorities, but decisions were not always geared to the needs of children. Assessments are increasingly thorough and there is a growing evidence base for care planning. If children have been in care for 6 months or longer they are likely to remain in care for the rest of their childhood. There is increasing evidence of the irreversible nature of the damage done by abuse and 'It is clear that early deleterious experiences can have significant negative effect on the developing brain that may be long term'.[118] Flexible and individual child care plans are encouraged in the High Court. Children's rights are now incorporated in the proceedings and the child's view sought and discussed. The welfare checklist gives structure to this. Table 5.17[119] illustrates the factors involved, which influence the likelihood of success or failure of rehabilitation after abuse has occurred.

THE RESPONSIBILITIES OF HEALTH PROFESSIONALS IN CHILD PROTECTION

All health professionals in the NHS, private sector and other agencies play an essential part in ensuring that children and families receive the care, support and services they need in order to promote children's health and development.[3] In the context of child protection, it is the child whose interests are paramount. The welfare of children must always be regarded as of primary importance, as their age and vulnerability renders them powerless to protect their own interests. All those working in the field of health have a professional responsibility to protect children, and their participation in interagency support to social service departments is essential, if the interests of children are to be safeguarded. Comprehensive service specifications for services for children, of which child protection is a key component, should be drawn up by purchasers in conjunction with providers and other relevant agencies such as social services and education.

CONSENT FOR EXAMINATION

This is sought from the person with parental responsibility. This may be both parents, if married, single mother or unmarried father and others by application to court. Older 'Gillick competent' children may give their own consent. In an emergency, consent may be unavailable. Legal advice may need to be sought if there is sufficient time. The General Medical Council provides guidance to doctors on the issue of consent. The most recent position is that disclosure of information is allowable to

> *'...an appropriate responsible person or statutory agency, in order to prevent further harm to the patient'.*

Disclosure may require justification, as may non-disclosure.

CHILD IN NEED (Fig. 5.6)

A 'Child in Need' is the description of a large number of children who have extra needs as described by the Children Act (1989) and who, unless given support, as children are unlikely to achieve or maintain, or have the opportunity of achieving or maintaining, a reasonable standard of health or development, without the provision of services from a Local Authority. The child's health or development is likely to be significantly impaired, or further impaired, without the provision of such services. This of course also includes the disabled child. Development includes physical, intellectual, emotional, social and behavioral development. Health is defined as physical or mental health. Over half the children who have been sexually abused have mental health problems, such as depression, post-traumatic stress disorder or behavioral problems. Abused children living away from home have even higher levels of distress.[120] Reabuse rates are high wherever the placement. The Needs Assessment was introduced in 2000 by the Government to provide a framework shared by social services, education, youth justice and health to assess and begin to understand the child and family and their particular needs. The assessments from different professional points of view will overlap as '...they are rooted in child development'. This is part of a multidisciplinary philosophy where it is imperative to integrate various aspects of the work. The aims firstly are to identify the

Table 5.17 Factors involved in success or failure following abuse (After Jones 1998)[119]

Factors	Rehabilitation poor prognosis	Rehabilitation better prognosis
Abuse	Severe injury, CSA sadistic, neglect, MSBP	Less severe abuse Severe but no denial & compliant
Child	Very young Disability	Behaves well, later onset, One caring adult
Parent	Antisocial, aggressive, denial, learning problem, substance abuse Abuse in childhood	Non-abusing parent Compliant, no denial Responsibility taken Responsive to therapy
Parenting and parent/child	Poorly attached, lack empathy, own needs first Abuse in childhood	Normal attachment with empathy, some competence
Family	Pervasive family Violence Poor negotiating skills	No other violence Non-abusive partner Can change Supportive family
Professional	Lack of resources Ineptitude	Family work well with child and professionals
Social	Isolated Violent unsupportive neighborhood	Good child care Volunteer networks Social support

MSBP, Munchausen syndrome by proxy

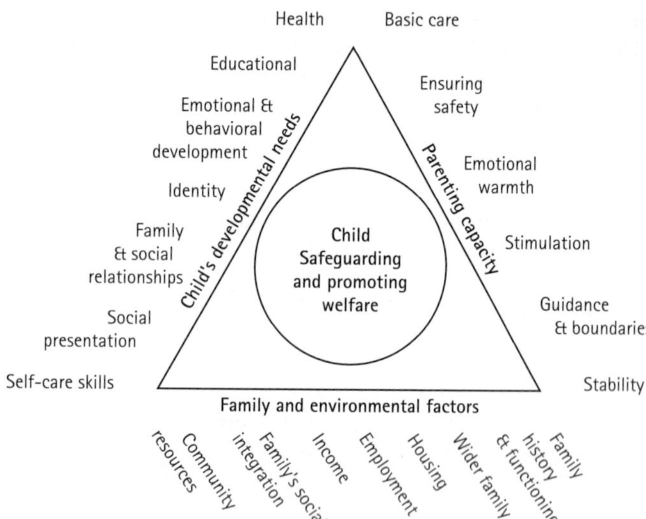

Fig. 5.6 The assessment framework.

developmental needs of the child, and how far they are being met. Secondly it is vital to assess the parent's capacity to meet their child's needs. Thirdly the assessment will examine what intervention is needed. In some cases it is necessary to determine how to prevent further offending. Treatment and support services should be available. There has to be an ongoing appraisal of the intervention, for example by asking such questions as 'is the child safe?', 'is the parenting improving?', 'are behaviors such as childhood violence receiving appropriate attention?'.

Pediatricians with an interest in development may be of considerable assistance in assessing the child in need and offering follow-up in terms of monitoring and intervening as appropriate in growth and development. They should be able to provide an objective opinion of progress or the reverse. The needs of the child and carer change over time and continuous assessment should be sensitive to this, and also the reaction of the carers, who may find the intervention increasingly stressful. Detailed proforma are available.[121]

CHILDREN LIVING AWAY FROM HOME

Current practice is to support children, when at all possible, in their own home. The difficulty of providing good alternative care and the poor outcome for many children who have been through the 'care system' have hastened the debate. The level of abuse in all residential institutions[122] and also foster homes, children's homes[123] and adoptive homes have added to this major shift from 'protection' to family support. The research base, on which to make such far-reaching decisions, is limited. In any event these decisions, which often concern a child and family with special needs and a past history of abuse, are complex. The levels of reabuse remain high and outcome uncertain, with considerable morbidity and mortality.

The current view is that an infant who has been severely abused should be assessed and plans made, without undue delay, for the long term. From all the referrals to social services, because of concerns of possible abuse, less than 1% are in public care after 6 months.[1] There is real concern that children will drift into care, as they grow older, and become further damaged and increasingly difficult to manage. The number of children in public care is 0.05–0.1%, with two-thirds in foster care. The remainder are with their own family on a court order, with the extended family, in children's schools or homes and a few are in secure units. The children's background shows substantial vulnerability. They come from families with five to six times the expected number of single parents and five times as many have experienced poverty. At entry into public care, around 40% are the subject of a statutory order, with the remainder accommodated. Many children are small and malnourished. Teenage girls may be obese and pregnancy is common when the young woman leaves care. Immunization is frequently incomplete and dental, vision and hearing checks missed. Many children are developmentally delayed, have poor social skills. Wetting, soiling, sleep problems, and feeding difficulties are common (Table 5.18).[124,125] Poor attachment is frequent. Mental health problems have often existed from an early age and many children have behavior disturbance. Early abuse of alcohol, glue, and drugs is common. A quarter of children in care are on the Child Protection Register when they enter. Private fostering has been increasing and 10 000 vulnerable children are involved (Table 5.19). However only 10% of local authorities have a social worker dedicated to these children who are often non-English speaking.[126] The care of children away from home can be thought of as a continuum from day care, respite care, short and long term fostering (including children with disability and children on remand), residential (homes, schools, secure units) to adoption.[127] Of children that are fostered, 38% have been in care more than 3 years and 22% more than 5 years.[121]

For any child in alternative care the concept of a triangle with the child at one corner and the alternative carer and birth parents at the others emphasizes the complex influences on the child. Ideally the placement of a child into foster care is planned to be able to meet the child's needs and provide a stable and safe home.[122] Despite an excess number of places to foster children, 70% are admitted to care as an emergency. It is not surprising that the child is usually moved between three and four times by 6 months.

PEDIATRIC ASSESSMENT OF THE CHILD IN CARE

This is a legal requirement to be performed 6 monthly for children under 2 years and 12 monthly thereafter, to assess the child. It should involve a full pediatric assessment. The emphasis is on mental health, developmental, educational progress and family history. Medical reports are written for the adoption panel. The 'Quality Protects' and 'Children First' (1995) are two initiatives in England and Wales to improve health for children in care. Adoption assessment requires a detailed medical history for the child and family, to include illnesses such as schizophrenia, which may have genetic implications. Post adoption emotional and behavioral problems are common, especially in older children, and are

Table 5.18 The health of looked after children

Kahn (1989)[124]	An excess of intercurrent infections Bedwetting & emotional problems
McCann et al (1996)[125]	Study of mental disorder in care/adolescence: 20% anxiety; 22% conduct disorder; 23% depressed 1/10 ill health 1/5 hearing/visual problem >1/2 educational problem >1/2 behavioral problems <1/5 fully immunized 1/4 pregnant on leaving care

Table 5.19 Pattern of care in the UK

1970s	22 000 children/year available to adopt (9000 infants)
1990s	150 infants available for adoption 55 000 children in care 14 000 in residential care – 85% > 11 years Behavior problems, sibling groups difficult to place 6000 adoptions each year (4000 adopted by step-parents, other relatives) 10 000 children awaiting adoption 2162 children adopted from care/year
Private fostering	More stringent regulations expected as a recommendation of Victoria Climbie enquiry No. of private foster homes: 19 in 1994 to 120 in 2001
Breakdown of adoption	20% of children > 3 years 50% > 10–11 years
Contact	30–40% adoptions include on going contact with birth family
Foster care	27 000 /33 000 fostered in England and Wales – unplanned in more than 75% – 40% moved two to five times in next 6/12 months
Statutory outcome	< 60% court order, 10% 'looked after', 20% with relatlives

particularly difficult for parents who were previously childless. Post adoption counseling services may be required.

ADOPTION

An Adoption Bill is to be re-presented in 2001/2002 in England and Wales to improve efficiency and decrease delay. In 'Adoption Proceedings-a new approach',[128] there are designated adoption centers, staffed by adoption staff and an adoption judge, who will offer continuity and ultimately make the adoption order.

The principal features of the law are that the child's welfare is paramount. Children will be placed for adoption rather than freed for adoption. Various placement orders will be made including contact orders, which may be made in the adoption proceedings. Restrictions are made on the removal of an adopted child, avoidance of delay is sought and there will be a National Adoption Register. An amendment also made to the Children Act (1989) is that an unmarried father may take on parental responsibility upon registering as 'father' and a step-parent may acquire parental responsibility.

CHILD PROTECTION AND PARENTAL SUBSTANCE AND ALCOHOL ABUSE

There is an increase in parental substance and alcohol abuse in the UK year upon year with consequent increase in child rearing problems. A lifestyle of alcohol, drugs, cigarettes may leave the child at serious risk.[129] The Department of Health[122] has given guidance as to ongoing assessment and support of children and their parents. In pregnancy the fetus may be damaged, stillborn, born prematurely, suffer intrauterine growth retardation, be infected with hepatitis B or HIV. It is considered that a woman who drinks over 21 units of alcohol per week puts her fetus at risk of fetal alcohol syndrome. During the neonatal period, the infant may be ill from the consequences of substance abuse. In infancy, there is an increased risk of sudden infant death syndrome (SIDS), neglect and abuse. In childhood, there may be developmental delay, learning difficulty and behavioral problems. At all ages, the child is at risk of all types of maltreatment. Of children on the Child Protection Register parental substance abuse, including alcohol, is a common cause for concern in up to about half the cases in some areas. The outcome for the child born addicted to heroin is variable. Increased mortality and breakdown of parental care are more serious outcomes. In addition to the biological factors which affect the outcome, the lifestyle of the parents puts the child at risk. The parent may not always be available to care. Drugs, especially methadone, may be left out and ingested by young children and in some cases the carer may use drugs to pacify the baby.

THE HEALTH CARE FOR REFUGEE CHILDREN[130]

Recent figures from the Association of Directors of Social Services indicate that there are approximately 23 000 accompanied children in the UK, and approximately 6000 unaccompanied minors. The refugees live in temporary accommodation, with many in bed and breakfast hotels. Referrals because of abuse and neglect are not uncommon. Living in poor, crowded housing on low income has a negative effect on physical and mental health. The children may have difficulty in gaining places in school and their education and development suffer. Children usually have English as a second language. Refugee children have an entitlement to health care (16 years and younger) but not to Welfare foods (note the mother may be HIV positive and so unable to breastfeed). Mobility may lead to difficulties for the child and family who are unable to register with a GP and so do not receive appointments for immunization, for example. Health visitors and school nurses are helpful in 'tracking' children. Children who are 16–18 years and unaccompanied may be treated as adults. All refugees are likely to be emotionally upset, having lost family members, friends, a homeland, and may have been tortured.

REFERENCES (* Level 1 evidence)

1 Messages from Research. Child protection. Studies in child protection. Department of Health. London: HMSO; 1995.

2 Robinson R. The fetal of origins adult disease. BMJ 2001; 322:375–376.

3 Working Together to Safeguard Children. A guide to inter-agency working to safeguard children. London: The Stationery Office; 1999.

4 Department of Social Security. Households below the average income (children living in poverty). London: The Stationery Office; 2000.

5 Schorr LB. Within our reach – breaking the cycle of deprivation. New York: Doubleday; 1988.

6 Webb E. Children and the inverse care law. BMJ 1998; 316:1588–1591.

7 Garbarino J, Guttman E, Seeley JA. The psychologically battered child. San Francisco: Jossey-Bass; 1988.

8 Childhood Matters. Report of the National Commission of Inquiry into the prevention of child abuse. Chairman Lord Williams of Mostyn. 2 vols. London: The Stationery Office; 1996.

9 Department of Health. Children and young people on Child Protection Register in England. London: Governmental Statistical Service; 2000.

*10 Cawson P, Wattam C, Brooker S, et al. Child maltreatment in the United Kingdom. A study of the prevalence of child abuse and neglect. London: NSPCC; 2000.

11 Dobash RE, Dobash RF, Kavanagh K, et al. Wifebeating: the victims speak. Victimology 1987; 2(3/4):608–622.

12 Home Office. Criminal statistics: England and Wales. London: HMSO; 1993.

13 NCH. The hidden victims. Children and domestic violence. London: NCH Action for Children; 1994.

14 Gibbons J, Conroy S, Bell C. Operating the child protection system: a study of child protection practices in English local authorities. London: HMSO; 1995.

15 Farmer E, Owen Child protection practice: private risks and public remedies. London: HMSO; 1995.

16 Mullins A. Making a difference: practice guidelines for professionals working with women and children experiencing domestic violence. London: NCH Action for Children; 1997.

17 Stark E, Flitcraft A. Women at risk: domestic violence and women's health. London: Sage; 1996.

*18 Billimire ME, Myers PA. Serious head injury in infants: accident or abuse? Pediatrics 1985; 75:340–342.

*19 Smith M, Bee P, Heverin A, et al. Parental control within the family: the nature and extent of parental violence to children. In: Messages from Research. Child protection. London: HMSO; 1995.

20 Elliott M. Stop bullying. Booklet for parents and children. London: Kidscape; 1991.

21 Dawkins JL, Hill P. Bullying: another form of abuse? In: David TJ, ed. Recent advances in paediatrics. Vol. 13. Edinburgh: Churchill Livingstone; 1995.

22 Creighton SJ, Noyes P. Child abuse trends in England and Wales 1983–87. London: NSPCC; 1989.

22a Corby B. Child abuse: toward a knowledge base. Bukingham: Open University Press; 2000.

*23 Roberton DM, Barbor P, Hull D. Unusual injury? Recent injury in normal children and children with suspected non-accidental injury. BMJ 1982; 285:1399–1401.

*24 Stephenson T, Bialas Y. Estimation of the age of bruising. Arch Dis Child 1996; 74:53–55.

*25 Langlois NEI, Gresham GA. The ageing of bruises: a review and study of the colour changes with time. Forensic Sci Int 1991; 50:227–238.

26 Hobbs CJ, Hanks HGI, Wynne JM. Child abuse and neglect. A clinician's handbook. London: Churchill Livingstone; 1999.

*27 Leventhal JM, Thomas SA, Rosenfield NS, et al. Fractures in young children – distinguishing child abuse from unintentional injuries. Am J Dis Child 1993; 147:87–92.

28 Kleinman PK. Diagnostic imaging of child abuse. Baltimore: Williams & Wilkins; 1987.

*29 Chadwick DL, Salerno C. The rarity of serious head injury in day care centers. Letter to Editor. J Trauma 1993; 35:968.

30 Joffe M, Ludwig S. Stairway injuries in children. Pediatrics 1988; 82:457–461.

31 Alms M. Fracture mechanics. J Bone Joint Surg 1961; 43:162–166.

32 Anderson WA. Significance of femoral fractures in children. Ann Emerg Med 1982; 11:174–177.

33 Gross RH, Stranger M. Causative factors responsible for femoral fractures in infants and young children. J Pediatr Orthopaed 1983; 3:341–343.

*34 Thomas SA, Rosenfield NS, Leventhal JM, et al. Long bone fractures in young children: distinguishing accidental injuries from child abuse. Pediatrics 1991; 88:471–476.

*35 Schravat BP, Harrop SN, Kane TP. Toddler's fracture. J Accid Emerg Med 1996; 13:59–61.

36 Feldman KW, Brewer DK. Child abuse, cardiopulmonary resuscutation and rib fractures. Paediatrics 1984; 73:339–342.

*37 Spevak MR, Kleinman PK, Belanger PL, et al. Cardiopulmonary resuscitation and rib fractures in infants. JAMA 1994; 272:617–618.

38 Carty H. Clicking ribs – a clinical sign of rib fractures. Arch Dis Child 2002; 86(1):67.

39 Hobbs CJ. Skull fracture and the diagnosis of abuse. Arch Dis Child 1984; 59:246–252.

40 Meservy CJ, Towbin R, McLaurin RL, et al. Radiographic characteristics of skull fractures resulting from child abuse. Am J Roentgenol 1987; 149:173–175.

*41 Kleinman PK, Nimkin K, Spevak M, et al. Follow-up skeletal survey in suspected child abuse. Am J Roentgenol 1996; 167:893–896.

42 Jayawant S, Rawlinson A. Gibbon J, et al. Subdural haemorrhages in infants: population based study. BMJ 1998; 317:1558–1561.

43 Hobbs CJ, Childs AM, Wynne JM, et al. Subdural haematoma and effusion (hygroma) in infancy. An epidemiological study. Part 1 Presentation, aetiology and diagnosis. Submitted for publication 2002.

*44 Reece RM, Sege R. Childhood head injury – accidental or inflicted. Arch Pediatr Adolesc Med 2000; 154:11–15.

*45 Duhaime AC, Alario AJ, Lewander WJ, et al. Head injury in very young children: mechanisms, injury types, and ophthalmologic findings in 100 hospitalized patients younger than 2 years of age. Pediatrics1992; 90:179–185.

*46 Jenny C, Hymel K, Ritzen P, et al. Analysis of missed cases of abusive head trauma. JAMA 1999; 281:621–626.

47 Meadow R. Munchausen syndrome by proxy – the hinterland of child abuse. Lancet 1977; 2(8033):343–345.

48 McClure RJ, Davis PM, Meadow SR, et al. Epidemiology of Munchausen syndrome by proxy, non-accidental poisoning, and non-accidental suffocation. Arch Dis Child 1996; 75:57–61.

49 Schreier HA, Libow JA. Hurting for love – Munchausen by proxy syndrome. New York: The Guildford Press; 1993.

50 Rogers D, Tripp J, Bentovim A, et al. Non-accidental poisoning: an extended syndrome of child abuse. BMJ 1976; 1:793–796.

51 Meadow R. Suffocation, recurrent apnoea and sudden infant death. J Pediatr 1990; 117:351–357.

*52 Southall DP, Plunkett MCB, Banks MW, et al. Covert video recording of life threatening abuse: lessons for child protection. Pediatrics 1997; 100:735–760.

53 Eminson M, Postlethwaite RJ, eds. Munchausen syndrome by proxy abuse: a practical approach. Oxford: Butterworth-Heinemann; 2000.

54 Egeland B, Sroufe A, Erickson M. The developmental consequence of different patterns of maltreatment. Child Abuse Negl 1983; 7:459–469.

55 Hanks HGI, Stratton P. Consequences and indicators of child abuse. In: Wilson K, James A, eds. The child protection, 2nd edn. Edinburgh: Baillière Tindall; 2002.

56 Rohner R, Rohner E. Antecedents and consequences of parental rejection: a theory of emotional abuse. Child Abuse Negl 1980; 4(3):189–198.

57 Iwaniec D. The emotionally abused and neglected child. Chichester: John Wiley; 1995.

58 Whiting L. 'Defining emotional neglect'. Child Today 1976; 5:2–5.

59 Glaser D. Emotional abuse. In: Hobbs C, Wynne J, eds. Baillière's clinical paediatrics – child abuse. Vol. 1, No. 1. London: Baillière Tindall; 1993.

60 Skuse DH. Emotional abuse and neglect. In: Meadow R, ed. ABC of child abuse, 3rd edn. London: BMJ Publishing Group; 1997.

61 Stone B. Child neglect: practitioner's perspectives. Child Abuse Rev 1998; 7:87–96.

62 Rosenberg D, Cantwell H. The consequences of neglect – individual and societal. In: Hobbs CJ, Wynne JM, eds. Baillière's clinical paediatrics. International practice and research in child abuse. London: Bailliere Tindall; 1993.

63 Working Together under the Children Act 1989. A guide to arrangements for inter-agency co-operation for the protection of children from abuse. London: HMSO; 1991.

64 Skuse DH, Wolke D, Reilly S. Failure to thrive: clinical and developmental aspects. In: Remschmidt H, Schmidt MH, eds. Developmental psychopathology. New York: Hogrefe & Huber; 1992.

*65 Batchelor JA, Kerslake A. Failure to find failure to thrive. London: Whiting & Birch; 1990.

66 Wright CM. A population approach to weight monitoring and failure to thrive. In: David

TJ, ed. Recent advances in paediatrics. Vol. 13. Edinburgh: Churchill Livingstone; 1995:73–87.
67 Frank DA, Drotar D. Failure to thrive. In: Reece RM, ed. Child abuse. Medical diagnosis and management. Philadelphia: Lea & Febiger; 1994.
68 Thomas A, Chess S, Birch, H, et al. Behavioural individuality in early childhood. New York: New York University Press; 1963.
69 Stratton PM. Biological pre-programming of infant behaviour. J Child Psychol Psychiatry 1983; 24:301–309.
70 Hobbs CJ, Hanks HGI. A multidisciplinary approach for the treatment of children with failure to thrive. Child Care Health Dev 1996; 22:273–284.
*71 Rayner P, Rudolf MC, Cooper K, et al. A randomised control trial of specialist health visitor intervention for failure to thrive. Arch Dis Child 1999; 80(6):500–506.
72 Moores J. Non-organic failure to thrive – dietetic practice in a community setting. Child Care Health Dev 1996; 22:251–259.
73 Hobbs CJ, Wynne JM, Gelletlie R. Leeds inquiry into infant deaths: the importance of abuse and neglect in sudden infant death. Child Abuse Rev 1995; 4:329–339.
74 Knowleden J, Keeling J, Nicholl JP. Postneonatal mortality. Report of a multicentre study. London: DHSS; 1985.
75 Hufton IW, Oates RK. Non organic failure to thrive. A long term follow up. Paediatrics 1977; 59:73–77.
76 Schechter M, Roberge L. Child sexual abuse. In: Helfer R, Kempe C, eds. Child abuse and neglect: the family and the community. Cambridge, Mass: Ballinger; 1976.
77 Butler-Sloss E. Report of the inquiry into child abuse in Cleveland 1987. London: HMSO; 1988.
78 Richardson S, Bacon H. Child sexual abuse: whose problem? Reflections from Cleveland. Birmingham: Venture Press; 1991.
79 Finkelhor D. The international epidemiology of child sexual abuse. Child Abuse Negl 1994; 18(5):409–417.
*80 Kelly L, Regan L, Burton S. An exploratory study of the prevalence of sexual abuse in a sample of 16–21 year olds. London: University of North London; 1991.
81 Northern Ireland Research Team. Child sexual abuse in Northern Ireland. Belfast: Greystone; 1991.
*82 Hobbs CJ, Wynne JM. Child sexual abuse – an increasing rate of diagnosis. Lancet 1987; ii:837–841.
83 Summit R. The child sexual abuse accommodation syndrome. Child Abuse Negl 1983; 1:177–193.
*84 Frothingham TE, Hobbs CJ, Wynne JM, et al. Follow up study eight years after diagnosis of sexual abuse. Arch Dis Child 2000; 83:132–134.
85 Jones DPH. Interviewing the sexually abused child. London: Royal College of Psychiatrists; 1992.
86 Memorandum of good practice on video recorded interviews with child witnesses for criminal proceedings. London: HMSO; 1992.
87 Raine PAM. Investigation of rectal bleeding. Arch Dis Child 1991; 66:279–280.
88 Royal College of Physicians. Physical signs of sexual abuse in children (report of working party of RCP). 1st edn. London: Royal College of Physicians; 1991.
89 Herman-Giddens ME. Vaginal foreign bodies and child sexual abuse. Arch Pediatr Adolesc Med 1994; 148:195–200.
90 Royal College of Physicians. Physical signs of sexual abuse in children (report of working party of RCP). 2nd edn. London: Royal College of Physicians; 1997.
91 Hobbs CJ, Wynne JM. The sexually abused battered child. Arch Dis Child 1990; 65:423–427.
92 Corbett J, Harris R. Progressive disintegrative psychosis in childhood. J Child Psychol Psychiatry 1977; 18:211–219.
93 Marshall WN, Puls T, Davidson C. New child abuse operation in an era of increased awareness. Am J Dis Child 1988; 142:664–667.
94 Muram D. Child sexual abuse: relationship between sexual acts and genital findings. Child Abuse Negl 1989; 13:211–216.
95 Woodling BA, Heger A. The use of the colposcope in the diagnosis of sexual abuse in the pediatric age group. Child Abuse Negl 1986; 10:111–114.
96 Steward MS, Schmitz M, Steward DS, et al. Children's anticipation of and response to colposcopic examination. Child Abuse Negl 1995; 19(8):997–1005.
*97 Berenson AB. A longitudinal study of hymenal morphology in the first 3 years of life. Pediatrics 1995; 95:628–631.
98 Herman-Giddens ME, Frothingham T. Prepubertal female genitalia: examination for evidence of abuse. Pediatrics 1987; 80(2):203–208.
*99 Jenny C, Kuhns MLD, Arakawa F. Hymens in newborn female infants. Pediatrics 1987; 80(3):399–400.
100 Berkowitz CD, Elvik SL, Logan MA. Labial fusion in pre-pubertal girls: a marker for sexual abuse? Am J Obstet Gynecol 1987; 156:16–20.
101 Hobbs CJ, Wynne JM. Physical signs of child abuse, 2nd edn. London: WB Saunders; 2001.
102 American Academy of Pediatrics. Guidelines for the evaluation of sexual abuse of children. Pediatrics 1999; 103(1):186–191.
*103 McCann J, Wells R, Voris J, et al. Comparison of genital examination techniques in prepubertal girls. Pediatr Clin North Am 1990; 85:182–187.
*104 Emans J, Wood E, Allred E, et al. Hymenal findings in adolescent women: impact of tampon use and consensual sexual activity. J Paediatr 1994; 125:153.
105 Woodling BA, Kossoris PD. Sexual misuse, rape, molestation and incest. Pediatr Clin North Am 1981; 28:481–499.
106 West R, Davies D, Fenton T. Accidental vulval injuries in children. BMJ 1989; 298:1002–1003.
107 Herman-Giddens ME. Harmful genital care practices in children. JAMA 1989; 261(4):577–579.
108 Warrington SA, de San Lazaro C. Lichen sclerosus et atrophicus and sexual abuse. Arch Dis Child 1996; 75:512–516.
109 Hobbs CJ, Wynne JM. Buggery in childhood – a common syndrome of child abuse. Lancet 1986; iii:793–796.
110 Jenkins D, Lewington F. The significance of forensic medical samples which may be taken in suspected child sexual abuse. In: Physical signs of sexual abuse in children, 2nd edn. London: Royal College of Physicians of London; 1997.
111 Falkov A. Fatal child abuse and parental psychiatric disorder. DOH – ACPC series report no 1. London: Department of Health; 1996.
112 Greenland C. Preventing CAN deaths: an international study of deaths due to child abuse and neglect. London: Tavistock; 1987.
113 Gelles RJ. Physical violence, child abuse and child homicide: a continuum of violence or distinct behaviours? Human Nature 1991; 2(1):59–72.
114 Browne KD, Lynch MA. The nature and extent of child homicide and fatal abuse [editorial]. Child Abuse Rev 1995; 4:309–316.
115 McClain PW, Sacks JJ, Froelke RG, et al. Estimates of fatal child abuse and neglect, United States, 1979 through 1988. Pediatrics 1993; 91(2):338–343.
116 Wilczynski A. Child killing by parents: a motivational model. Child Abuse Rev 1995; 4:365–370.
117 DHSS. The report of the Committee of Inquiry into the care and supervision provided in relation to Maria Colwell. London: HMSO; 1974.
118 Glaser D. Child abuse and neglect and the brain: a review. J Child Psychol Psychiatry 2000; 41(1):97–117.
119 Jones DPH. The effectiveness of intervention. In: Adcock M, White R, eds. Significant harm: its management and outcome, 2nd edn. Croydon: Significant Publications; 1998.
120 Farmer E, Pollock S. Sexually abused and abusing children in substitute. Chichester: John Wiley; 1998.
121 Department of Health. Assessing children in need and their families – practice guidelines and assessment recording forms. London: The Stationery Office; 2000.
122 Utting W. People like us. The report of the review of the safeguards for children living away from home. The Department of Health. The Welsh Office. London: The Stationery Office; 1997.
123 Hobbs GF, Hobbs CJ, Wynne JM. Abuse of children in foster and residential care. Child Abuse Negl 1999; 23:1239–1252.
124 Kahn B. The physical and mental health of children in care. In: Kahn B, ed. Child care and research policy and practice. London: Hodder & Stoughton; 1989.
125 McCann JB, James A, Wilson S, et al. Mental disorder in adolescents. BMJ 1996; 313:1529.
126 ADSS. Children looked after by local authorities in England year ending 31.03.02. Available: http://www.doh.gov.uk/public/state3.htm
127 Payne H. Fostering and adoption – the paediatrician's role. Curr Paediatr 2001; 11(1):40–45.
128 PIU Report. Prime minister's review of adoption. London: The Cabinet Office; 2000.
129 Forrester D. Parent substance misuse and child protection in a British sample. Child Abuse Rev 2000; 9:235–246.
130 Lynch MA. Providing health care for refugee children and unaccompanied minors. Med Confl Surv 2001; 17(2): 25–130.

6

Preventive pediatrics

Harry Campbell

Any child's health, development, and welfare reflect the interaction of genetic endowment (see Ch. 12), family and social circumstances, and environment from conception, through pregnancy, childbirth and beyond. The provision of adequate, appropriate and hygienic food, water, housing, clothing and a healthy temperature are widely recognized as the basic rights of every child because they promote health and prevent disease.[1] Security, stability, a loving family and appropriate stimulation provide the necessary social environment for normal emotional and intellectual development.[2] Social and economic policy can have an important impact on child health.[3] In contrast, medical science and health services have made, and can make, only a limited contribution to prevention of ill health. The greater impact of political action, economic progress, improved education and social change is shown by falling morbidity and mortality long before antibiotics, vaccines and high-technology medicine became available (Fig. 6.1). Thus child health action has been considered to involve 'placing the health of children and their families in their full social, political and economic context' and to be 'the responsibility of decision makers in all organizations in all sectors of the economy'.[4] The health of the child's mother is also an important factor in determining the health of the child, whether this be, for example, in ensuring proper antenatal care of mothers with diabetes or treating and supporting mothers with psychiatric problems or alcohol addiction. It is in this context that this chapter presents the actions that can be taken principally by health services to promote child health and development and prevent childhood illness and handicap. The UN Convention on the Rights of the Child places a clear responsibility on the State to provide access to preventive care (article 24). Preventive medicine usually requires skilled teamwork to work with children and their families, often with colleagues outside the health services such as teachers and social workers.

There is increasing attention given to the *equitable* delivery of these services so that vulnerable groups of children (such as those in families of displaced peoples or asylum seekers or travellers or those from economically deprived areas) receive the recommended preventive care. Additional special services may be required to reach these children. It may be important to monitor access to services across these groups to ensure that due attention is given to inequity of access.

Renewed interest in the 'life course approach to health' has highlighted the long term health implications of the fetal and early childhood environment.[5,6] Thus preventive action in childhood can not only lead to improvement in child health but may also be an effective intervention against some of the common diseases of public health importance in the adult population.

Preventive actions relevant to promoting child health in developing countries are presented in Chapter 8.

PRINCIPLES OF PREVENTION

Primary prevention implies specific measures which reduce the incidence of bodily impairment or disease by controlling causes or risk factors (e.g. vaccination against poliomyelitis to prevent poliovirus infection and its attendant risks of paralysis, the use of condoms to prevent human immunodeficiency virus (HIV) infection, antenatal folate supplementation, fluoridation of drinking water or road safety legislation).

Secondary prevention aims to treat patients either in order to cure them or to reduce the more serious consequences of disease through early diagnosis and treatment. It thus aims to detect disease at an early preclinical or clinical stage in order to reverse the disease process or to result in a less severe disease outcome. This reduces the prevalence of the disease (e.g. screening for

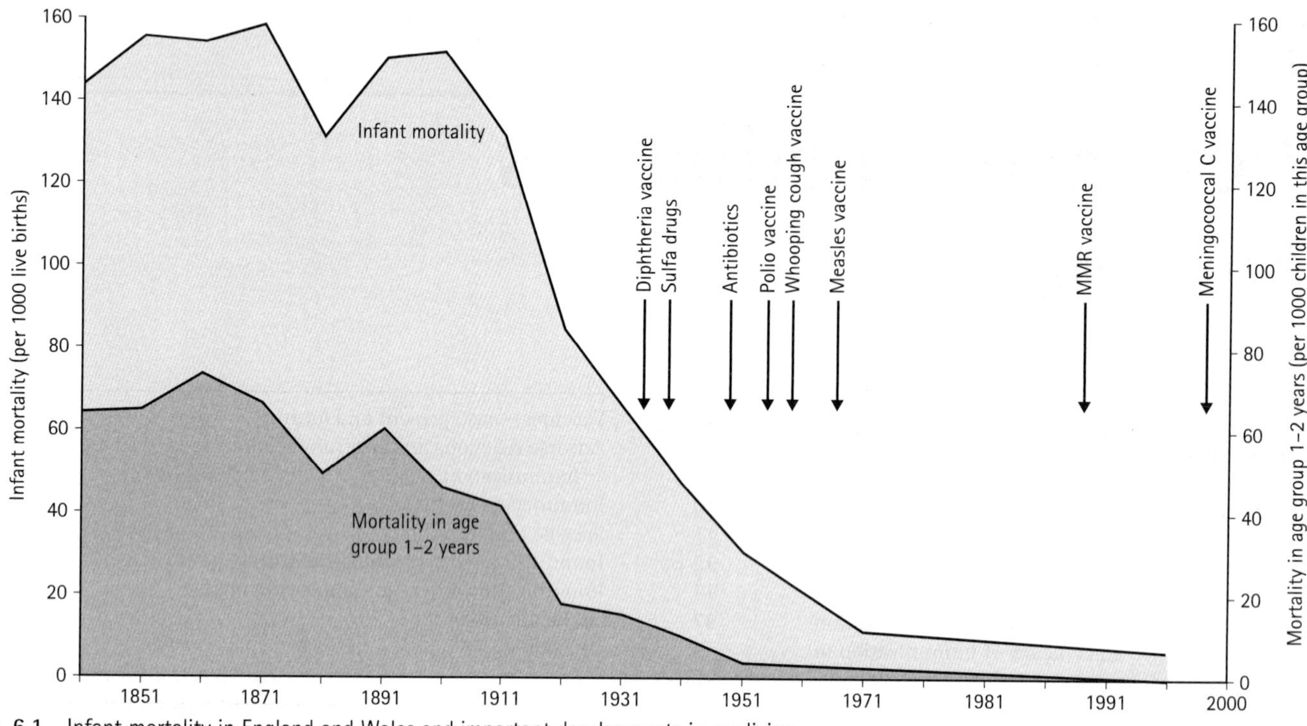

Fig. 6.1 Infant mortality in England and Wales and important developments in medicine.

hypothyroidism in neonates permits early replacement of deficient thyroxine and prevents the disabilities of cretinism or otoacoustic emission screening for hearing loss). The term secondary prevention can also be applied to the termination of pregnancy to avoid the birth of a fetus with a recognized severe impairment.

Tertiary prevention aims to reduce the progress or complications of established disease, thus limiting its impact. It consists of measures to reduce impairments and disabilities from the disease or injury and so minimize any handicap which may result. Thus after developmental screening (secondary prevention) has revealed motor, visual or hearing impairments before disabilities have become apparent, consequent early application of remedial measures (tertiary prevention) may limit the adverse effects of such impairments. For example, tertiary prevention through the rehabilitation of children with polio can enable them to take part in daily social life and bring about a great improvement in the well-being of these children.

PREVENTIVE MEASURES

PRECONCEPTUAL PREVENTION

Genetic factors in either parent, the present and past health of the mother, her age, her diet, her habits (e.g. smoking, alcohol), the frequency of her pregnancies, her previous immunizations (e.g. rubella and tetanus) and her social class are all factors which can potentially influence the health of her infant before it is conceived. Control or elimination of adverse factors will play an important part in prevention, e.g. the introduction of anti-D immunoglobulin for rhesus (Rh) negative mothers has significantly reduced the incidence of Rh incompatibility (see Ch 10, Gastrointestinal problems and jaundice of the neonate) and adequate consumption of folic acid before conception and during the first 2–3 months of pregnancy significantly reduces the risk of neural tube defects.[7,8]

PREVENTIVE MEASURES DURING PREGNANCY

Early pregnancy

In early pregnancy preventive measures include the avoidance of teratogenic drugs and the prevention and cure of infections which might damage the fetus (Ch. 9). The following drugs and chemicals have been found to be associated with fetal defects: diphenylhydantoin (phenytoin), trimethadione, paramethadione, valproic acid, carbamazepine, thioureas, carbimazole, methimazole, isotretinoin, vitamin A, etretinate, thalidomide, warfarin, methotrexate, corticosteroids, androgens, progestins, diethylstilbestrol, iodine, lithium, mercury and chlorobiphenyls. A number of other drugs and chemicals have featured in retrospective studies or case reports but associations with fetal defects have not been confirmed by subsequent investigations (see Stevenson[9] for a further discussion). Exposure to abdominal X-rays should be avoided, but there is no evidence that ultrasound examinations are harmful to the fetus. The effects of a pregnant woman's smoking or alcohol (Ch. 9) consumption on her fetus are now well recognized and demand preventive action. Smoking can lead to intrauterine growth retardation, certain congenital anomalies and fetal loss. In addition, smoking during pregnancy has emerged as a major risk factor for sudden infant death syndrome in studies carried out after the widespread recommendations on infant sleeping position led to a reduction in the number of infants found dead in the prone position.[10,11] Excessive alcohol ingestion (above 1 oz absolute alcohol daily in early pregnancy) can lead to the fetal alcohol syndrome.[12] Routine screening for a number of conditions such as neural tube defects, rhesus hemolytic disease and maternal diabetes should be carried out (see Table 6.1).[13] The 77% reduction in the birth

Table 6.1 Current genetic screening programs in the UK (modified from Nuffield 1993[13])

Age group	Disease	Population screened	Type of screening test	Comments
Neonatal	Phenylketonuria	All newborn infants	Indirect	
	Hypothyroidism	All newborn infants	Indirect	
	Sickle cell disease	All newborn in some areas; confined to certain ethnic groups in others	Indirect	Also detects carriers
	Cystic fibrosis	Some areas only (still at pilot stage)	Indirect	
	Duchenne muscular dystrophy	Pilot studies	Indirect	
	Other rare metabolic disorders	Family testing	Usually indirect	
Later childhood		NONE IN THE UK		
Premarital and prepregnancy	Cystic fibrosis	Pilot projects in general practice	Direct	Detects 85–90% of carriers
During pregnancy	Rhesus hemolytic disease	All mothers	Indirect	
	Diabetes mellitus	All mothers	Indirect	Fetuses have expert fetal anomaly scanning
	Congenital malformations	Most fetuses	Routine ultrasound	Confirm with fetal anomaly ultrasound
	Down syndrome	1. All mothers in some areas	Serum screening tests	Amniocentesis with chromosome tests on fetus required for confirmation
		2. All mothers over 35–37	Chromosome tests on fetus	
	Neural tube defects (spina bifida and anencephaly)	All mothers in many areas	Indirect	Confirm with fetal anomaly ultrasound
	Hemoglobin disorders	All mothers not of North European origin	Indirect	Detects carriers
	Cystic fibrosis	Pilot studies	Direct	Detects 85–90% of carriers

prevalence of neural tube defects in the last 25 years is in part due to improved prenatal detection and selective termination of pregnancy. A link between low folate intake and neural tube defects has led to a national recommendation for all women to take oral folate supplements during pregnancy.[7,14–16] The risk of hyaline membrane disease can be reduced in preterm babies by the administration of steroids to the mother before or during preterm labor.[17]

Individuals with a family history of a genetic disorder may undergo genetic testing. In the last 10 years there have been major advances in the understanding of the molecular basis of medical disorders and in the development of new techniques to identify genes associated with disease. Most of the genes for the more common inherited disorders have now been identified (see Ch. 12). This in turn often makes prenatal detection and genetic counseling possible.[18,19] In conjunction with this there have been advances in prenatal diagnosis, e.g. by amniocentesis (Ch. 9), ultrasound techniques and biopsy of chorionic villus (Ch. 9). Secondary prevention by termination of pregnancy has therefore become more widely practiced.

Late pregnancy

In late pregnancy the welfare of the fetus and ultimate health of the child can be influenced significantly by competent obstetric management including the various techniques for fetal monitoring (see Ch. 9). There is a growing body of evidence that prenatal factors may contribute to important chronic diseases in adulthood such as hypertension and coronary heart disease.[5,20–22]

PREVENTION IN THE NEONATAL PERIOD

Good intrapartum obstetric care and subsequent effective monitoring, investigation and treatment of the many disorders from which the newborn infant may suffer are important preventive measures. Such disorders include asphyxia, birth injury, low birth weight and hyperbilirubinemia (see Ch. 10). Vitamin K should be given to all babies at birth. The British Paediatric Association (now the Royal College of Paediatrics and Child Health) recommended oral vitamin K 500 μg at birth with a repeated dose at 4–6 weeks for breast-fed babies only (See Ch. 10, Hematological problems of the newborn). However, there has been concern that although oral vitamin K is effective in preventing early hemorrhagic disease of the newborn, it is ineffective in preventing late disease in settings in which compliance in taking repeated oral doses is low.[23] Concerns about the possible increased incidence of childhood leukemia and cancer have been substantially allayed by the results of recent large case control studies which have shown no increased risk.[23–25]

The promotion of breast-feeding is an important preventive measure. Breast-feeding reduces the risk of diarrheal disease, lower respiratory infections, otitis media, necrotizing enterocolitis, and other serious neonatal infections.[26] Recent evidence has linked lack of breast-feeding with poorer intellectual development, possibly due to the lack of certain long chain fatty acids, essential for normal brain development, in most breast milk substitutes.[27,28] Frequent breast-feeds given over a prolonged period also significantly reduce fertility and the birth interval, with indirect benefits to both mother and infant.[29]

WHO and UNICEF are coordinating a global initiative (the Baby Friendly Hospital Initiative) to promote breast-feeding and to improve health service support for breast-feeding mothers. Many hospital routines and practices discourage women from breast-feeding or make it difficult for them to do so successfully.[30–32] Good practice guidelines have been developed for maternity hospitals. Improving hospital practices and staff skills in line with these guidelines has been shown to improve breast-feeding rates across all ethnic and socioeconomic groups.[26,33,34] Policy statements on breast-feeding by pediatric associations have been used to raise awareness amongst pediatric staff of the need to promote breast-feeding, to promote good practice and to advocate for inclusion of breast-feeding topics in the undergraduate medical and nursing curricula and in postgraduate courses for pediatricians, obstetricians, general practitioners, midwives and maternal and child health nurses.[35] The risks of (HIV) viral transmission are now better understood, leading to guidelines for the management of HIV-positive mothers to reduce the vertical transmission. The additional risk of mother to child HIV infection conferred by breast-feeding has been estimated (by meta-analysis of published studies) to be 14% (95% confidence interval 7–22%). This is increased in the presence of clinical mastitis and breast abscess[36] (See also Ch. 25).

Screening procedures

A number of preventive screening procedures are used in the neonatal period (see Table 6.1). These include: examination for congenital dislocation of the hips (see Ch. 10), Examination of the neonate); the careful routine examination of all newborn infants,[37] and a number of specific biochemical screening tests [e.g. for metabolic disorders such as phenylketonuria and galactosemia, and for congenital hypothyroidism (Table 6.1)]. In some regions routine genetic screening for Duchenne muscular dystrophy (Wales) and cystic fibrosis (Victoria State, Australia; Wisconsin, USA) has been carried out for a number of years.[38]

PREVENTION IN INFANCY AND CHILDHOOD

Breast-feeding should be maintained for at least 3 months. Its protective action against diarrheal and respiratory disease persists throughout the first year of life.[39] In infancy and childhood curative medicine can have an important preventive role. Early diagnosis and effective treatment of diseases such as meningitis, pneumonia, otitis media, osteomyelitis and patent ductus arteriosus can prevent chronic illness or permanent handicap in some children following these conditions.

Accidents cause nearly half of all deaths at ages 1–19 years in the UK.[40] The cause of the accidents, and therefore the preventive action, varies with the age of the child. Important preventive measures include: using appropriate child car restraints; road safety education; child-proof containers for drugs; home safety devices such as stair gates and fire alarms; the design and installation of safe playground apparatus and surfaces; and the proper supervision of children near water (see Ch. 32).

Sudden infant death syndrome. Infants should be put to sleep on their backs and should not be overwrapped nor exposed to cigarette smoke in the home. These measures have been shown to substantially reduce the incidence of sudden infant death syndrome.[41] Recent studies, carried out in several countries after reductions in sudden infant death rates which followed health education campaigns promoting these messages, have highlighted the fact that further declines could be achieved by reducing maternal smoking.[42,43]

Immunization against polio, pertussis, tetanus, diphtheria, measles, mumps, *Haemophilus influenzae* type b, tuberculosis and, in some settings, hepatitis B continue to be important routine preventive measures for all children (see below). Newer vaccines against pneumococcal disease and chickenpox have been introduced in some populations and are likely become more widely employed in the coming years.

A healthy *diet* should be promoted. Dietary guidelines have been published by many authorities.[44–47] These combine concerns about achieving recommended daily intakes of selected essential nutrients with the need to reduce risks of chronic diseases of adulthood which are partly attributed to diet. In addition, in certain circumstances supplements may be necessary, e.g. iron for premature babies, iodine where specific deficiency is endemic, vitamins A, C and D for breast-fed babies after 6 months of age.[48] The diet should contain adequate sources of available iron. Recent studies in the UK have shown a prevalence of iron deficiency anemia of up to 25% in young children, particularly in some ethnic minority communities. Effects on mental and motor development can be reversed if treatment is prompt. Much dental caries can be prevented by fluoride supplements where local water supplies are deficient. There is evidence that diet and other factors in childhood can contribute directly to health problems in adult life.[49]

Exposure to *harmful chemicals* in the diet, water or environment should be prevented or reduced, e.g. lead and passive smoking.

The prevention of *carcinogenesis* by chemicals or ionizing radiation has aroused scientific and political interest in recent years. The relative risks and potential for prevention require further study. Pediatricians should be aware of the relative amount of radiation involved in various diagnostic imaging techniques (Ch. 39).

Preventive drug prophylaxis still has a place in the secondary prevention of meningococcal disease,[50,51] in the primary and secondary prevention of rheumatic fever[51,52] (Ch. 40), protecting the heart from bacterial endocarditis (Table 19.4), preventing tuberculosis in susceptible contacts (Ch. 26, Tuberculosis), malaria prophylaxis (Ch. 26, Malaria) and perhaps most commonly of all, in anticonvulsive therapy.

A structured program of child health promotion should be carried out to prevent disease and to detect problems affecting growth and development at an early stage. This should comprise both primary prevention through health promotion activities and secondary prevention through child health surveillance (Table 6.2).[53] Health promotion should incorporate a coordinated and determined effort to address issues such as accident prevention, good nutrition and dental care, and full immunization coverage. There should be sufficient flexibility in any program to allow health staff to give more attention and time to families with complex needs and to decide the specific input which is most appropriate to the needs of individual children. Child health surveillance should include only those activities which have been shown to be safe and effective, and which meet the well-established criteria for screening tests.[54] Child health surveillance programs have been recommended in a number of countries. The UK Royal College of Paediatrics and Child Health has laid out a recommended program encompassing components of screening, immunization, monitoring and oversight, individual health education/promotion and population-based health promotion (summarized in Table 6.3)[53] based on a critical consideration of the published data on effectiveness of these approaches.[53] Details of these recommendations are published intermittently.[53] It is important that there are good referral arrangements to specialist services when abnormalitiesare detected. At a district or regional level existing national child health surveillance policies should be adopted[37] and local health promotion policies on the issues noted above should be developed. Personal child health records should be made available to all families and their use by both families and health staff encouraged.

All health professionals in contact with children should be alert to the possibility of *child abuse*, particularly in cases of repeated multiple or unusual trauma or burns, or in children with developmental delay.[55] Prompt recognition can prevent future abuse and can identify the need for counseling or specific treatment.[56,57]

The UK Education Act 1981 required that health authorities inform education departments of children who may have *special educational needs*. A full assessment of the child is then made and a statement of special educational needs produced. This system involves the parents of the child in the assessment and focuses on the needs of the child rather than on categorization of the child by diagnostic labeling. These children often require medical support also and this is usually best provided by a multidisciplinary team such as those found in child development centers or 'district handicap teams'. The aim of these procedures is tertiary prevention – to limit the handicap which can result from specific impairments by early recognition of the child's medical and educational needs and then appropriate intervention.

PREVENTION IN LATER CHILDHOOD AND ADOLESCENCE

The prevention of smoking, alcohol addiction, abuse of drugs and related substances, unplanned and unwanted teenage pregnancy, sexually transmitted diseases including HIV and acquired immune

Table 6.2 Suggested model for quality standards and outcome measures for child health surveillance (From Blair 2001[53] with permission of BMJ Publishing)

Structure

Waiting room/clinic area
Suitable temperature of the room (comfortable for child in vest)
Adequate seating
Generally clean room
Someone to welcome parents
Toys in waiting area
Notice board on child health issues
Pram park (lockable) or space for prams in waiting room
Appropriate child health records available
Full set of standard growth charts available
(boys/girls/weight/height/head circumference)
Relevant child health leaflets freely available
Baby weighing scales (electronic)
Scales suitable for weighing a child
Provision for private discussion with a parent
Provision for breast-feeding in private
Child toilet seat/potty in toilets

Examination room
Toys available
Suitable temperature for child in vest
Measuring mat (standard)
Appropriate height measure
Tape measure
Equipment for development assessment, e.g. crayons/paper/cubes

Safety
Electrical, e.g. plug covers, wires
Furniture, e.g. no sharp corners at head height, radiators, stacked chairs
Fire exits/stair safety, e.g. open stairs, low windows
Toys/play material, e.g. broken toys
Clinical equipment, e.g. sharps bins, scissors out of reach of children

(Continued)

Table 6.2 *(Continued)*

Other comments
Staff should be suitably trained
If vaccines kept for immunizations:
fridge thermometers (max/min) present
fridge temperature checked daily
Provision of interpreters where necessary

Process
When a parent and child attend a baby clinic:
They should be made welcome
There should be opportunity for the parent to ask questions
Weights should be recorded in the appropriate records and explained
Time should be spent with the parent, questions answered/ explanations/reassurance given
Possibility of discussion in a private room should be offered
Appropriate follow-up arrangements should be made

Baby clinics should have:
An appointment system allowing parents to attend with and without an appointment
A doctor and health visitor available to be seen by parents

At each child health surveillance review:
Parental concerns should be discussed
Physical assessment of the child should be made
Assessment of developmental progress should be made
Weight and, if appropriate, height and head circumference should be measured accurately and compared with standard centile charts
Health education issues should be discussed
Immunizations should be reviewed
Results should be recorded in the personal child health record
Appropriate follow-up arrangements should be made
There should be a call up system
There should be a recall system for non-attenders

Other comments
There should be liaison between doctors and health visitors
Child health surveillance should be seen as a continuous process and not a system of checks at specific ages
In this health authority (HA), the program of child health surveillance reviews that is followed should be consistent with the HA preschool child health surveillance policy and the HA personal child health record

Outcome
Parent satisfaction
Parents will feel able to discuss their concerns:
with their health visitor
with their doctor
Parents will feel welcome at the baby clinic
Parents should have the results of any assessment explained to them so that they can understand

Uptake and timeliness of child health surveillance reviews (preschool targets)
All babies should have neonatal examination during first 48 h of life
90% of 10–14 day reviews should be done by 4 weeks
90% of 6–8 week reviews should be done by 12 weeks
90% of 6–9 month reviews should be done by 10 months
90% of 18–24 month reviews should be done by 28 months
90% of 3 year reviews should be done by 3 years 9 months

Immunization rates
95% of children should be fully immunized by 2 years

Table 6.3 Summary of recommended UK child health program (From Blair 2001[53] with permission of BMJ Publishing)

Age	Review and screening procedures	Immunization	Health promotion
Newborn	*Review:* Family history Pregnancy Birth *Full physical examination including:* Weight Heart and pulses Hips Birth marks Testes Head circumference plotted Eyes (exclude cataracts and squint) Guthrie test after 6 days (phenylketonuria, hypothyroidism) Sickle cell (if indicated) *Consider:* Risk factors for hearing loss If high risk then refer for otoacoustic emission, brainstem auditory evoked response	BCG (high risk) Hep B (if mother is a carrier)	Cot death prevention Feeding technique Nutrition Baby care Crying Sleep Car safety Family planning Passive smoking Dangers of shaking baby Sibling management
10–14 days	Guided by results and review of neonatal check Assess and establish levels of support and assistance required Review sickle cell and thalassemia test (if appropriate)	Review BCG and Hep B status Introduce to immunization program and obtain informed consent	Nutrition Breast-feeding Passive smoking Accident prevention: bathing, scalding and fires Explanation of tests and results Encouraging parents to request results of all tests Significance of prolonged jaundice Depression, coping and help (parents/carers)
6–8 weeks	*Review*: Parental concerns, e.g. vision, hearing, activity Risk factors including significant family history *Full examination including:* Weight Head circumference Length Centile plotting Hip check Testes Eyes: red reflex, squint, movement, tone and general development Heart and pulses Report Guthrie results back to parents	1st DT Pert Hib/Pol Meningococcal C	Immunization Nutrition and dangers of early weaning Accidents: fires, falls, overheating, scalds Recognition of illness in babies and what to do Fever management Crying Sleeping position Passive smoking Review of car safety Depression (parents/carers)
2–4 months	Parental concerns	2nd and 3rd DT Pert Hib/Pol Meningococcal C	Weighing as appropriate Maintain previous health promotion Promotion of language and social development Deter future use of baby walkers
6–9 months	Hip check Distraction hearing test (catch up for missed neonatal screen, infants moving in) Discussion of developmental progress, asking specifically about vision, hearing and language development		Parental concerns Nutrition Accident prevention: fires, choking, scalding, burns, gate guard, etc. Review of transport in cars

(Continued)

Table 6.3 *(Continued)*

Age	Review and screening procedures	Immunization	Health promotion
	Check weight and head circumference as required or if parental concern Observe behavior and look for squints		Dental care Play and development needs
13 months		MMR	
18–24 months	Parental concerns, behavior, vision and hearing Observe gait Emphasize value of comprehension and social communication in relation to speech development (speech and language screening tests) Measure height and plot	Review immunization status	*Safety*: Accident prevention: falls from heights, drowning, poisoning, road safety *Development:* Language and play Management and behavioral issues Promote positive parenting Toilet training Diet, nutrition, prevention of iron deficiency
39–42 months	Enquiry and discussion of vision, squint, hearing, behavior, language acquisition, development – referral as necessary Education needs and choices Notification of any special educational needs and choices Measure height and plot Check testicular descent has been recorded, if not examine Where concerns are: hearing impairment, perform test (e.g. McCormick toy discrimination test)	Check immunization status DT/polio (preschool booster) 2nd MMR	*Safety*: Accident prevention: burns, road safety, drowing, poisoning, falls from heights *Development:* Language and play socialization Management of behavior issues School readiness Nutrition/diet Dental care Toilet training
5 years school entrant	Review preschool record including a check for record of testicular and heart examination School entrant review – parent and school nurse Establish teachers/parental concerns Height (plot and compare with previous measurements), weight and hearing sweep Visual acuity (Snellen) Observation of gait and fine motor skills	Review of immunization status	Obtain consent for planned program and health checks Access to school health School health surveillance program Sleep Friendships/settling at school Accident prevention, road safety, stranger danger Dentist, dietician Management of medicines at school Care in the sun
Year 3 (school) 7–8 years	Teacher concerns Review of records Height, weight, vision General health check Issues raised by child		Accident prevention, road safety, safety at play, stranger danger Friendships Exercise, nutrition and dental care Care in the sun
Year 7 (school) 11–12 years	Visual acuity Color vision General health check Issues raised by young person Support for individual programs of care		Accident prevention Relationships Exercise/nutrition Smoking Dental care Management of medication in school Puberty/sexual health Care in the sun
Year 8 (School) 12–13 years		Heaf test BCG	
Year 10 (School) 14–15 years	General health check including height, weight, vision where concerns Issues raised by young person	Td/polio booster	Substance abuse: alcohol, smoking, drugs, solvents Diet/exercise Testicular self-examination, promotion of cervical cytology Sexual health

(Continued)

Table 6.3 *(Continued)*

Age	Review and screening procedures	Immunization	Health promotion
			Promotion of general practitioner well woman/man check Information about health services, e.g. teenage clinics health shop dental health Careers Stress management
Year 11 (School) 15–16 years	Self-referral – issues raised by students	Information to school leavers on need for immunizations as adult catch up immunization	Self-referral – issues raised by students

BCG, bacillus Calmette-Guérin; DT, diphtheria, teanus; Hep B, hepatitis B; Hib, *Haemophilus influenzae* b; MMR, measles, mumps, rubella; Pert, pertussis; Pol, polio; Td, tetanus, adult-type vaccine with low potency diphtheria vaccine.

deficiency syndrome (AIDS), family breakdown, and child abuse and neglect is particularly challenging. Considerable medical, social, economic and, in the view of some, spiritual or moral resources are required to meet these challenges. In addition health professionals need to collaborate in school health promotion programs to promote healthy lifestyles in young people, including adequate regular exercise and a healthy diet.

The health risks of smoking are well recognized. In a national survey carried out in 1990 a quarter of 15-year-olds were found to be regular smokers. In recent years research has shown that more boys than girls smoke in mid-teen years.[58,59] It has been estimated that there are over 500 000 smokers aged 11–15 years in the UK, with about 100 000 of them likely to die as a result of their tobacco consumption.[60] Health professionals should routinely ask about smoking in older children and their parents, and provide advice and help where necessary on stopping smoking. Parents who cannot stop smoking should be encouraged not to smoke in the house or in front of their children. Health services should actively support any effective and appropriate action against the promotion of cigarettes and tobacco.[61]

A national study in 1989 showed that 26% of 16–17-year-olds in the UK drank more than 8 units of alcohol on at least one occasion during a 1-week period.[62] Concern over alcohol use in adolescents is based not only on related health problems (e.g. one-third of all accidental deaths in 16–19-year-olds are associated with alcohol) but also on drunkenness and its related social problems.

In addition:

1. The abuse of volatile substances and drugs such as marijuana, heroin and cocaine has increased among adolescents in recent years.
2. Approximately 1% of girls aged 14–15 years in the UK conceive each year and over half of these result in abortion.
3. Levels of physical activity decline in teenage years so that over one-third of young men aged 16–24 years and over half of young women do not take regular exercise.
4. National dietary surveys have shown that nutrient and energy intakes are generally adequate but that iron intake in teenage girls is low and the contribution of fat to energy intake is higher than currently recommended.[61]

Responses to these problems require action in the early teenage years before the problem is fully manifest. A combination of interventions to reinforce negative views of the unhealthy behavior must be mixed with the promotion of a positive view of health and of healthy behaviors such as non-smoking as the norm. Action needs to involve not only a wide range of health, education and social work professionals but also relevant voluntary agencies and young people themselves through peer projects and requires to be part of an overall strategy involving both national and local action. Action can be taken in a stepped fashion with:

- *broad* messages or action aimed at the general population at low risk (e.g. warnings about binge drinking or the use of recreational drugs at parties); and
- *more focused* messages or action for subgroups at higher risk and finally leading to;
- *individual action* and support for young people who are, for example, dependent on substances and at greatest risk to themselves and their community.[63]

Health professionals who care for children should maintain a high level of awareness and know where and how to seek assistance when faced with these problems.

Schools represent an opportunity to develop 'health action sites' for students to receive health education/promotion messages and improved access to care. An integrated child health service could include screening, diagnostic, treatment and health counseling services covering management of medical emergencies, medication delivery, services for children with special health care needs and health screening.[64] These services operate most successfully when they are fully integrated with other community and hospital health and related social services. An international network of 'health promoting schools' has developed this model further by harnessing a wide variety of schools policies to promote child health within schools, e.g. by providing affordable and tasty healthy food options and promoting a healthy diet, by ensuring there are sufficient opportunities for physical activity such as through organized sports, adopting and enforcing no-smoking policies and making the school environment safer and more attractive.

In all these areas there is an increasing recognition of the need to adopt evidence-based action based on systematic reviews of randomized controlled trials or other evidence of effectiveness of interventions. In recent years randomized controlled trials have been carried out across a wide range of child health interventions including: counseling and community schemes to improve smoke alarm usage,[65] home visiting by nurses to improve parenting and quality of home environment[66] and prevent childhood injury[67] and interventions to reduce passive smoke exposure in homes.[68]

PREVENTION AND PROTECTION THROUGH IMMUNIZATION

THE IMPORTANCE AND EFFICACY OF IMMUNIZATION IN PREVENTION OF DISEASE

Immunization is the deliberate stimulation of an immune response in a person by giving a specific 'vaccine' to protect against an infectious disease.[69,70] The vaccine is usually a protein similar to part of a virulent infectious organism that can be recognized by the individual's immune system which then produces antibodies and cell-mediated immunity against the antigen in the vaccine.

Active immunity is the protection produced by the individual and the effects are usually long lasting. *Passive immunity* protects by injected antibodies, either in the form of human immunoglobulin or produced by some other biological process. This produces immediate protection which only lasts for some weeks or months, until the donated antibodies are broken down or used up by the individual.

The immediate goal of immunization is to prevent disease in individuals, but the ultimate goal is to eliminate or even eradicate a communicable disease. *Herd immunity* exists if the number of people in a community who have active immunity against an infection exceeds a critical level. Above this, susceptible individuals are unlikely to contact someone with the infection. In this way transmission falls or stops without universal immunity.[71]

Immunization is a simple, economic and effective form of control for some infectious diseases. The efficacy of immunization depends on the vaccines available, the biological and social response of individuals, the epidemiology, modes of transmission and reservoirs of pathogens, and the health service infrastructure for delivering the immunization.

VACCINES – PAST, PRESENT AND FUTURE

A vaccine is a protein antigen, originally derived from or similar to a bacterium, virus or protozoon, used for active immunization. The term was previously used exclusively for smallpox vaccine derived from cowpox lymph (from Latin *vacca*, a cow). It is now used for all forms of vaccines.

Vaccines may be live, killed, toxoids or genetically engineered.

A *live attenuated vaccine* is one which produces active immunity by causing a mild 'infection'. A virulent organism is weakened, usually by multiple subcultures in unfavorable conditions, so that it produces an antigenic response without the serious consequences of a wild organism infection. Crossreacting organisms are another type of live vaccine which causes the body to produce a defense against the virulent strain. The bacillus Calmette–Guérin (BCG) vaccine is an example of this. The BCG is a strain of *Myobacterium bovis* which was isolated and attenuated by Calmette and Guérin in 1906 at the Pasteur Institute and is now used widely for vaccination against tuberculosis (TB).[72] There are new candidate organisms being tested to replace BCG against TB.[73]

Killed, or *inactivated vaccine* is prepared from virulent organisms or preformed antigen inactivated by heat, phenol, formaldehyde or some other means. Classical pertussis vaccine is an example of a whole-cell killed and inactivated vaccine. Such vaccines usually require a series of spaced injections to produce an immune response.

Component vaccines use parts of pathogens as antigens and the newer pertussis vaccines are examples of this.[74,75] Polysaccharide meningococcal and pneumococcal vaccines are derived from the mucopolysaccharide coat of specific bacteria.[76] The response to polysaccharide vaccines is incomplete and unreliable and consequently these have sometimes been conjugated with other antigens in an attempt to improve the immunological response. An example is the linkage of *Haemophilus. influenzae* or pneumococcal polysaccharide with the pertussis antigen of diphtheria–pertussis–tetanus (DPT) vaccine[77] and diphtheria toxoid[78] to produce a vaccine conjugate capable of stimulating T cells and thus eliciting immunological memory. An adjuvant is another product, for example an aluminum compound, combined with a vaccine to increase antigenicity and prolong the effect as in diphtheria and tetanus toxoids.

Toxoids also induce active immunity. A toxoid is an inactivated toxin preparation. The serious consequences of some diseases are due to toxins released by the organisms when they infect the patient. Diphtheria and tetanus toxins are examples of this. Toxoids from these produce antibodies which inactivate the toxins but do not kill the bacteria.

Vaccinology is the application of molecular biology to produce the vaccines of the future.[79] Conventional vaccine development depended upon the identification and isolation of an infectious agent, the production of that organism in a culture system, killing or attenuation of the organism and then the testing of the resulting antigen for potency and safety. Molecular biology has opened the way to the identification of key antigenic sites in organisms, an epitope or short sequence of amino acids which is responsible for the specific interaction between antibody and antigen.[80] It is possible to develop vaccines of small specific proteins, synthetic polypeptides or even 'naked' DNA, which can act as immunogens.[81] There are also methods of synthesizing such specifically sequenced proteins and polypeptides by recombinant DNA techniques. These may be enhanced by using new adjuvants like viral liposomes, i.e. viral antigens attached to lipid spheres and immune stimulated complexes ('iscoms') which induce aggregates of viral protein.

Combination vaccines are being increasingly developed.[82] The internationally sponsored Children's Vaccine Initiative announced the goal of developing a vaccine that could immunize the newborn with one orally administered dose against the major vaccine-preventable diseases.[83] More modest goals are the combination of six antigens in a single shot: diphtheria, tetanus, pertussis, *H. influenzae* b, hepatitis B and inactivated polio vaccine. Components must be very concentrated and compatible with each other and with preservatives and adjuvants.[84]

ADVERSE REACTIONS AND CONTRAINDICATIONS TO IMMUNIZATION

No child should be denied immunization without serious thought about the consequences, both for the individual child and the community. There are many false contraindications to immunization (see Table 6.4), as opposed to the true contraindications (Table 6.5) discussed below.

Adverse reactions may be due to faulty administration, for example abscesses due to unsterile needles or syringes, or to inherent properties of the vaccines.

Both minor and major side-effects of vaccination cause parental anxiety and undermine professional confidence in the benefits of immunization. The situation has been confused by anecdotal information, inadequate epidemiological studies and mass media speculation. Much debate has concerned the pertussis component of the DPT vaccine in the UK.[85] Evidence indicates that the serious side-effects of both pertussis and measles vaccines are much less than the risks and morbidity of the clinical diseases in the first few

Table 6.4 FALSE contraindications to immunization

Illnesses or treatments
- Minor illnesses, e.g. mild upper respiratory infection
- Chronic diseases of heart, lung and kidneys
- Treatment with antibiotics or locally acting corticosteroids, i.e. by topical application or inhalation
- Stable neurological condition such as Down syndrome, cerebral palsy, spina bifida
- Malnutrition or under a particular weight
- Dermatoses, eczema or localized skin infection
- Recent or imminent surgery

Personal or family medical history
- Personal or family history of allergy, asthma, eczema, hay fever, etc.
- Previous history of measles, pertussis, rubella, mumps, *Haemophilus influenzae*, polio or other specific infection
- Family history of adverse reaction to immunization
- Family history of convulsions
- Jaundice at birth or prematurity: do not postpone immunization
- Contact with an infectious disease
- Older than the usual age for immunization

Note: some of these conditions constitute priority or high risk groups for immunization, for example low birth weight infants, those with Down syndrome, asthma, congenital heart disease, chronic lung disease and infants with HIV-1 antibody positive mothers.

years of life (Table 6.6[86,87]). No case of subacute sclerosing panencephalitis (SSPE) has ever been attributed to measles vaccine. After 3 years of intensive case finding the British National Childhood Encephalopathy Study found so few cases that it

> *'could not say conclusively whether or not pertussis can cause permanent brain damage if such damage occurs at all'.*[88]

When the risk from a disease becomes very small, as with paralytic poliomyelitis in Europe, the small risk of vaccine associated paralytic poliomyelitis (VAPP) from live oral polio vaccine (OPV) becomes relatively more important and may warrant a reconsideration of vaccination policy.[89,90] A more recent example in the UK involved public concern about a link between measles, mumps and rubella (MMR) vaccination and inflammatory bowel disease and autism. Despite the absence of any good scientific evidence to support these links a loss of public confidence led to declining uptake of MMR vaccine and fears of impending outbreaks. Recent reviews of the evidence by various independent expert groups have helped inform health professionals and encourage them to continue to promote MMR vaccination.[91]

Side-effects of DPT vaccination

Minor reactions

There are significantly different rates of these reactions between various vaccine lots and endotoxin content from reputable commercial manufacturers.[92] Minor reactions are quite frequent in 20–50% of vaccines. Local reactions include inflammation, induration or a painless nodule at the site of injection. These are progressively more common after the first injection. Constitutional upsets include fever, screaming, crying more than usual or persistently (more than 5 h in the first 12).

Serious reactions

In normal infants a neurological reaction such as a prolonged convulsion occurs after about 1 in 100 000 injections. Most result in no permanent damage. Encephalopathy and brain damage can

Table 6.5 TRUE contraindications to immunization

Summary of contraindications
1. Acute illness
2. Previous severe reaction to immunization
3. Immune deficiency or suppression, acquired or induced
4. Progressive or uncontrolled CNS disease
5. Specific situations with whole cell pertussis or some live vaccines

Definite contraindications – general
- Severe febrile illness. Immunization might superimpose adverse effects on the illness, or manifestations of the disease may wrongly be attributed to immunization. Postpone immunization

Definite contraindications – pertussis
- Definite history of severe adverse reactions from previous dose of the vaccine, usually DPT
- General reactions include fever above 39.5°C, anaphylaxis, bronchospasm, laryngeal edema, collapse, prolonged unresponsiveness or inconsolable screaming within 72 h
- Severe local reaction, implies extensive induration or inflammation around the injection site
- Definite convulsion within 72 h of administration of a previous dose of DPT
- Progressive neurological disease, e.g. uncontrolled epilepsy or tuberous sclerosis

Definite contraindications – live vaccines
- Patients with immune deficiency or those with impaired response due to leukemia, malignant disease and those with AIDS. Those who are HIV Ab positive with symptoms may be given killed vaccines
- Those being treated with large doses of corticosteroids or other immunosuppressive treatments, e.g. following organ transplantation
- Within 3 weeks of another live vaccine [but oral polio vaccine (OPV), measles, rubella or BCG vaccine may be given simultaneously with another live viral vaccine]
- Within 3 weeks before or 3 months after a dose of normal immunoglobulin
- Allergy to hens' eggs if severe, e.g. anaphylaxis or generalized urticaria (these are relatively rare)
- BCG vaccine should not be given to those with:
  - generalized specific skin conditions; if eczema exists, vaccination should be in an area of healthy skin
  - positive skin sensitivity test to tuberculin protein; an interval of at least 3 weeks should be allowed between BCG and any live vaccine
- Patients with tuberculosis should not receive measles vaccine unless on full treatment for TB

Circumstances requiring individual consideration
- Children with a personal history of convulsions or 'febrile convulsions' (they can usually be immunized)
- Children with first degree relatives with epilepsy may have a fit after measles or MMR vaccine. However, the possibility of a fit is 10 times as great with an infection of measles. In these circumstances the matter should be discussed with parents, the vaccine should be given and they should be supplied with a pediatric dose of rectal diazepam and instructions about what to do if a convulsion occurs
- Documented evidence of cerebral damage in neonatal period including twitching and clonic episodes
- Stable abnormality of the CNS, including spina bifida and cerebral palsy

Note: previously these last two conditions were, but are no longer, accepted contraindications to DPT and measles immunization. Children in these categories do require special, individual consideration, a weighing of risk and benefit in each case
- In chronic heart, kidney and lung disease, including cystic fibrosis, failure to thrive and treated TB, MMR immunizations are recommended in the UK
- Diarrhea or vomiting is considered a reason to postpone OPV in the UK, but in many countries it is given, and an extra dose is recommended after recovery

Table 6.6 Estimated rates of adverse events following DPT and measles immunizations per 100 000 injections compared to complication rates of natural pertussis and measles per 100 000 cases (Modified from Galazka et al 1984[86] and WHO 1996[87])

	Pertussis		Measles	
Condition	Pertussis disease per 1000 000 cases	DPT immunization per 100 000 injections	Measles disease per 100 000 cases	Measles immunization per 100 000 injections
Encephalopathy or encephalitis	90–4000	0.2	50–400	0.1
Convulsions	600–8000	0.3–90	500–1000	0.02–190
Death	100–4000	0.2	10–10 000	0.02–0.3

occur in the first year of life in immunized and non-immunized children. No completely reliable estimate can be made of the risk. Whole-cell pertussis vaccination has been associated very rarely with seizures and hypotensive–hyporesponsive episodes which seem to be reduced by approximately two-thirds when acellular pertussis vaccine is used.

Contraindications to pertussis and other vaccines

There is limited factual information about major side-effects and specific contraindications due to their relative rarity and under-reporting. Moreover, confusion occurs because of background disease, emotion because of ignorance, guilt and fear of litigation. Doctors and health visitors are unsure about contraindications and in about 40% of the cases advised against pertussis and measles vaccinations, the reasons for withholding were invalid.[93] Table 6.6 gives the estimated rates of adverse reactions set out by the WHO EPI unit, compared with the risks from the relevant diseases.

There is general agreement about certain definite contraindications, but continuing uncertainty about other factors (Table 6.5). Even when a specific list of contraindications is given, there can be significant problems of interpretation of these. In the UK less than 5% of children have contraindications to DPT and less than 1% to measles vaccine with current guidelines.[94]

IMMUNIZATION SCHEDULES

Immunization schedules are the basic framework for the delivery of immunizations to individuals and the community. No one schedule is applicable to all countries and communities of the world and several national programs are changing in response to local factors. The timing of the first immunizations is a compromise between the developing maturity of the infant's immune system and the risk of infection from virulent organisms.[95] Maternal transplacental immunoglobulin G (IgG) protects infants against many infections for the first few months of life. It is an incomplete protection, particularly against pertussis, but is satisfactory against measles and rubella. Consequently pertussis immunization should be provided early in situations where this disease is prevalent. The production of a satisfactory primary antigen response is vital. Unless this is achieved, subsequent immunizations or infections will not produce an adequate recall response to effect protection. This is particularly relevant for inactivated vaccines.

Basic principles

The aim is to reach the majority of children before the age when exposure to natural infection occurs. Which vaccines are included and the ages at which they are delivered depends on the age-specific risks of disease, response to vaccines, risks of complications, potential interference from maternal antibody, cost of vaccine and health service infrastructure. No child should be denied immunization without serious thought about the consequences, both for the individual child and for the community. The schedule should also be simple so that it can be remembered by staff and parents and should fit in with other aspects of health care such as developmental screening. The optimal age for starting immunization depends on both host immunological maturity and local disease epidemiology. In developing countries where TB and poliomyelitis may infect young children, immunization can be started soon after birth.[73,96] In communities where pertussis is still a problem, this vaccine should be given early in the first year since cases before 6 months of age have a higher morbidity and mortality. Where measles is a major threat in the first year of life, vaccine should be given early despite the fact that the response will be less than optimal. The most appropriate age for measles immunization depends on the age-specific attack rate in a particular community. In industrialized countries measles immunization may be deferred until 12–15 months of age since early risk of infection is not great and the vaccine works optimally only after 12 months. In countries where measles may occur much earlier the WHO recommends immunization at 9–12 months, preceded by an extra dose at 6 months of age in high risk situations.

The correct timing of immunizations of different vaccines is of great importance if an adequate primary immune response is to be obtained. Three current immunization schedules (for the UK, the USA and that recommended by the WHO) are set out in Table 6.7.[88] The UK schedule completes primary immunization by 6 months of age, minimizing the number of drop-outs. The introduction of a *H. influenzae* b (Hib) immunization program in the UK in 1992 has led to the rapid reduction of invasive cases of *H. influenzae* infection.[97] Recent changes to the US schedule[98,99] include:

- the withdrawal of the previously recommended rotavirus vaccine administered at 2, 4 and 6 months of age in 2000 due to a possible causal relation to this vaccine with intussusception;
- the adoption of a heptavalent protein polysaccharide conjugate pneumococcal vaccine;
- the change from OPV to inactivated poliovirus vaccine (IPV) to eliminate the risk of vaccine-associated paralytic polio;
- the change from DPT to diphtheria-tetanus–acellular pertussis (DtaP) to reduce the incidence of adverse effects associated with pertussis immunization;
- the use of separate DtaP and Hib conjugate vaccines for primary immunization due to concern about reduced immune response to Hib with DtaP/Hib combination products.

In all countries, if an immunization schedule has been interrupted or has not been completed it is not necessary to start the schedule afresh. The course should be completed with the remaining doses administered at the recommended intervals.

Table 6.7 A comparison of three selected immunization schedules, recommended for use in the UK and USA and by the World Health Organization

Recommended age	UK[88] main schedule	USA†	WHO (1996) expanded program on immunization
Birth–neonatal period	BCG and Hep B-1 for special at risk groups	Hep B-1	OPV-1 BCG Hep B-1a
2 months	DPT-1, OPV-1 Hib-1, Men C-1 Hep B-2 for special at risk groups	DTaP-1, IPV-1 Hep B-2 Hib-1, PCV-1	OPV-2, DT-1 Hep B-1b
3 months	DPT-2, OPV-2 Hib-2, Men C-2		OPV-3, DPT-2 Hep B-2
4 months	DPT-3, OPV-3 Hib-3, Men C-3	DTaP-2, IPV-2 Hib-2, PCV-2	OPV-4, DPT-3 Hep B-3
6 months	Hep B-3 for special at risk groups	DTaP-3, IPV-3 Hep B-3 Hib-3, PCV-3	(Measles MV‡)
7 months			
8 months			
9 months			Measles (MV) Yellow fever (YF)
10 months			
11 months			
12 months	MMR-1 at 12–15 months or at any age after 12 months	MMR-1	
15 months		Hib-4, PCV-4 Var	
18 months		DTaP-4	(DPT-4 in countries with good pertussis control)
2 years	Hep A (given in selected high risk groups between 2 and 16 years of age)		
4–5 years	DT, OPV-4 MMR-2	DTaP-5 IPV-4 MMR-2	
10–14 years	BCG	Hep B (catch up) Var (catch up)	
14–16 years	Td OPV or IPV	Td	
Adult	RV OPV (IPV in special circumstances)		

†, Advisory Committee on Immunization Practices of the American Academy of Pediatrics 1996; BCG, bacillus Calmette–Guérin; DPT, diphtheria, pertussis, tetanus; DT, diphtheria, tetanus; DTaP, diphtheria, tetanus and acellular pertissis (may replace DPT); Hep A, hepatitis A vaccine; Hep B, hepatitis B-1a (where perinatal risk is hogh), B-1b (standard regimen); Hib, *Haemophilus influenzae* b polysaccharide conjugate vaccine; IPV, inactivated polio vaccine; MMR, measles. mumps, rubella; MV‡, measles vaccine (give early extra dose in situations of high risk); OPV, oral polio vaccine; PCV, 7-valent pneumonoccal polysaccharide conjugate vaccine; RV, rubella vaccine; Td, tetanus, adult-type vaccine with low potency diphtheria vaccine; Var, live attenuated vaccine, varicella-zoster; YF, yellow fever vaccine in all countries at risk.

Developing country schedules

In developing countries booster immunization schedules present financial and logistic problems so the main emphasis is on primary immunization as part of basic health care. The priority for the WHO is to deliver the primary immunization series to over 90% of infants and thus reduce the burden of these diseases. Low birth weight infants, whether due to premature birth or intrauterine growth retardation, or both, should generally be immunized with the same schedule as for normal weight, full-term infants.[95] In addition to the standard WHO schedule, other vaccines are available and recommended for use in specific geographic areas, for example Japanese encephalitis and pigbel vaccines. Others like Hib may not yet be affordable in some developing countries. This is a striking example of global inequity in child health care – the children at lowest risk of Hib disease receive immunization whilst the children at highest risk have no access to immunization, resulting in hundreds of thousands of child deaths each year.

Mass immunization campaigns are an integral part of the global polio eradication strategy; they are now also recommended by WHO for use in measles elimination programs. They can have a dramatic impact as the first phase of an elimination strategy, especially where health infrastructure is limited. Such campaigns should not be isolated events, but part of the long term strategy.[87]

In conclusion, a schedule should be epidemiologically relevant, immunologically effective, operationally feasible and socially acceptable. At a global level child health advocacy (see below) is required to promote equitable access to essential vaccines for all children in the world since immunization (with WHO Expanded Programme of Immunization vaccines) represents a highly cost effective child health promotion strategy in all world populations.

SPECIFIC IMMUNIZATIONS

Measles and rubella in the UK

The earlier UK schedule for rubella immunization, targeting only schoolgirls, and the relatively poor uptake of measles vaccine in the 1980s left cohorts of older children susceptible to these diseases and outbreaks were predicted. In November 1994 there was a major campaign to immunize all children aged 5–16 years old with measles and rubella vaccine (MR). In England 92% of the target 7.1 million children received MR vaccine. Susceptible individuals were reduced to less than a third, and measles cases fell to a fifth of the number reported the previous year.[100] Adverse reactions were reported as 1 in 2600, but serious neurological reactions were only 1 in 78 000 doses, and anaphylaxis or allergy within 24 h only in 1 in 65 000 doses. This may overestimate attributable risk. The serious reactions were significantly less than would have been expected with the diseases. There is need for better awareness of the benefits as well as the adverse reactions to sustain public confidence in immunizations.

Poliomyelitis (live oral, killed injectable or both) vaccines

WHO, in partnership with various groups, has set the objective of the global eradication of polio. Eradication from the Americas was achieved in 1991, using OPV. However, the Advisory Committee on Immunization Practices (ACIP) of the USA recommended that the country adopt a sequential poliomyelitis immunization schedule – two doses of IPV followed by two doses of OPV.[90,101] The USA schedule now recommends IPV alone for primary immunization in order to eliminate the risk of 1 case per 2.5 million doses of OPV (vaccine associated paralytic polio). OPV is only to be used for unvaccinated children traveling to polio endemic areas, children of carers who do not accept the recommended number of IPV vaccine injections, and for any mass vaccination campaigns should this ever be necessary to respond to an outbreak. The WHO does not support this policy: it believes that global eradication is possible with OPV, and the US change in policy promotes a misconception that OPV is inadequate.[102] Recent epidemics indicate that the problem was a failure to vaccinate rather than OPV vaccine failure.[103] Moreover, IPV would be too expensive for many developing countries. Global eradication might cost $500 million, but thereafter there will be no risk of VAPP and an annual saving of $1500 million.[102]

Pertussis acellular vaccines

Whole-cell vaccines, suspensions of killed *Bordetella pertussis* organisms, have been both effective in reducing the disease and unsatisfactory because of adverse reactions. The organisms contain a number of antigens; pertussis toxin, pertactin, filamentous hemagglutinin and several fimbrial antigens. These have been separated and used in combinations in acellular vaccines. Even whole-cell vaccines have differences in composition due to different strains and manufacture. Many trials of acellular vaccines have been conducted.[75,104] Although there are disputes about which combinations of antigens are best,[105] the acellular vaccines had efficacies which approached and sometimes exceeded the comparison whole-cell vaccines, and all had fewer and milder adverse reactions. The common (e.g. fever, pain, redness) and uncommon (i.e. seizures and hypotensive–hyporesponsive episodes) adverse events are reduced by about two-thirds compared with whole-cell vaccines. Seven effective acellular pertussis vaccines are licensed in one or more countries, four have been licensed in the USA. Acellular pertussis vaccines are now recommended in routine childhood immunization schedules in the USA.

In the UK acceptance of whole-cell vaccine is currently high and switching to acellular products will increase cost with little improvement in uptake. Other considerations may be more important; the purified acellular vaccines may be easier to mix with other antigens in the combined vaccines that seem likely in the future.[106] There is evidence of pertussis outbreaks in older children and adults in the USA, and acellular vaccines with lower reactogenicity will be more acceptable as boosters. Clinical trials in the UK are in progress to evaluate reactogenicity and immunogenicity of acellular pertussis and combined vaccines. It is probably only a matter of time before they are incorporated in the routine schedule.

Varicella vaccine

Despite a relatively low complication rate, varicella is an important cause of child morbidity and mortality since infection is almost universal. Varicella vaccine, from an attenuated varicella-zoster virus, has been licensed for use in healthy children in the USA since 1995. Controlled trials demonstrated the vaccine to be 70–90% effective at preventing varicella and more than 95% effective at preventing severe varicella. Protection appears to last for at least 20 years in line with experience with other live vaccines (e.g. measles, rubella) which induce long term immunity. Because of the exacting storage requirements for varicella vaccine, postlicensure studies have been important to determine vaccine performance. Between 1995 and 1999 varicella incidence and hospitalizations declined by 80% in all age groups (90% among 1 to 4-year-old children). There are arguments about the costs and benefits, the immunization schedule and who it should be given to. In the UK it is likely to be restricted initially to those at greatest risk, especially immunocompromised children.[107,108] Cost–benefit studies in the USA concluded that when both direct medical and indirect societal costs were considered, a routine varicella immunization program for healthy children was cost beneficial.[109] Studies do not support the theoretical concerns that immunization may lead to an increased incidence of herpes zoster or an unacceptable rate of infection among vaccinees. Immunization may increase the mean age of varicella infection but the overall reduction in the numbers of cases of adult varicella should offset this problem but will require close surveillance after introduction of the vaccine.[110]

Pneumococcal conjugate vaccine

Streptococcus pneumoniae remains a major cause of childhood morbidity and mortality. At least 1 million children die from pneumococcal disease each year, making it the largest bacterial cause of death globally.[111] In addition antimicrobial resistance to pneumococcus is increasing.[112,113] A new 7-valent protein polysaccharide conjugate vaccine has recently been licensed in the USA and is expected to obtain a European license by 2005. The conjugate vaccine has the effect of changing the antigen to T cell dependent leading to an anamnestic response to future infection. Although the threshold antibody level which confers protection is unknown at present, pneumococcal conjugate vaccines elicit higher antibody responses than pneumococcal polysaccharide vaccines, induce mucosal antibody and immunological memory and are likely to have a higher efficacy in preventing both invasive and non-invasive disease. The conjugate pneumococcal vaccines contain 7–11 serotypes that cause the majority of pneumococcal disease in young children. The 7-valent conjugate vaccine includes serotypes 4, 6B, 9V, 14, 18C, 19F and 23F. In the 9-valent and 11-valent vaccines, serotypes 1 and 5 and serotypes 1, 3, 5, and 7F are added respectively. In the USA, the 7-valent vaccine would cover above 80% of invasive and 65% of non-invasive pneumococcal disease in children under 6 years of age.

Antibody responses to pneumococcal conjugate vaccines vary with serotypes and vaccine formulations. Studies in developed and developing countries have reported that the pneumococcal conjugate vaccines are immunogenic in infants aged 6–8 weeks. Antibody levels at 7 months of age after a series of three doses, range from 0.5 to 4.29 μg/ml for the poor immunogenic serotypes to 1.13 to 14.09 μg/ml for the most immunogenic serotypes. It has been suggested that antibody levels of 0.3 μg/ml may afford protection against invasive disease caused by serotypes 3, 4, 6A, 8, 14, 19F and 23F in children. Studies in patients with immunocompromised disorders (HIV, Hodgkin's and sickle cell diseases) and recurrent respiratory infections have shown that pneumococcal conjugate vaccines are capable of inducing higher antibody responses than the polysaccharide vaccine.

A large scale double blind randomized controlled clinical trial from the 3-year Northern California Kaiser Permanente study among 37 000 children using Wyeth–Lederle's 7-valent pneumococcal CRM_{197} conjugate vaccine[114] has shown the vaccine to be highly effective in preventing invasive disease in children under the age of 2 years, among whom it also reduces the incidence and severity of otitis media. The vaccine also appears to be safe and immunogenic. The adverse reactions to conjugate pneumococcal vaccines are minimal and comparable to 23-valent polysaccharide vaccine and other routine pediatric vaccines.

The vaccine currently licensed in the USA contains serotypes which are associated with multidrug resistant invasive strains. Studies in other countries have shown a significant reduction in nasopharyngeal carriage in vaccinated infants and children. Data from South Africa showed a reduction of over 50% in nasopharyngeal carriage in vaccine serotypes in infants immunized at 6, 10 and 14 weeks. This suggests that universal childhood vaccination with pneumococcal conjugate vaccine has the potential to produce herd immunity and decrease the spread of antibiotic resistant pneumococcal disease in children. Nevertheless, studies in South Africa and Gambia found that colonization with non-vaccine serotypes was increased in vaccinees compared to controls. Therefore, continued surveillance data are essential to monitor the long term colonization effects of widespread use of conjugate vaccines in future. Health economic studies in the USA have concluded that infant immunization with pneumococcal conjugate vaccine has the potential to be cost effective. If the vaccine costs were less than the manufacturer's list price of $58 for each dose, vaccination could even be cost saving.[115]

Group c meningococcal conjugate vaccine

Meningococcal infection is the most common infectious cause of death in children and young people up to the age of 20 years in the UK. The age groups at highest risk of meningococcal disease are children under 1 year of age, followed by those 1–5 years of age and then adolescents 15–19 years of age. A new conjugated vaccine containing group C meningococcal polysaccharide conjugated to a non-toxic derivative of diphtheria toxoid (CRM 197) or tetatnus toxoid was introduced into the UK immunization schedule in 1999 (Table 6.7). Group C accounts for about 30% of cases of meningococcal disease in the UK, but the majority of cases under 2 years of age. Similr to the Hib conjugate vaccine, the MenC conjugate vaccine produces a T cell dependent antibody response which is immunogenic in infants and young children and induces immunological memory. It does not provide protection against group A or C meningococcal disease. The MenC vaccine has not been found to be associated with serious adverse effects and does not appear to afect seroconversion of other vaccines. Contraindications include previous hypersensitivity reaction to MenC vaccine or to the vaccine carrier proteins.

Hepatitis B vaccine

Hepatitis B vaccination aims to prevent symptomatic hepatitis in adolescents and adults, chronic carriage of hepatitis B and primary hepatic cancer in adults. Hepatitis B vaccine is effective and safe and is recommended in many countries in a four-dose childhood schedule (see Table 6.7). Universal immunization is cost effective in countries with high endemicity. In these settings it is important to commence immunization in neonates since this has the greatest impact on carriage, the main reservoir of infection (due to the inverse relationship between age and risk of chronic carriage). Universal immunization is less cost effective in countries with low endemicity. In these settings selective immunization targeted at high risk groups is common. However these programs are often poorly implemented and do not protect against horizontal transmission in early childhood.[116] Concerns about thiomersal (an organic compound containing mercury) has led to the development of thiomersal-free hepatitis B vaccines.

IMMUNIZATION FOR INTERNATIONAL TRAVEL

Small children now travel with their parents to every corner of the globe. Such visits may expose children to infectious diseases no longer endemic in Europe and North America and to conditions which, although preventable, are not normally covered in a routine immunization program. As the disease incidence and health regulations are constantly changing, up to date advice should be sought from appropriate authorities. Basic preventive measures should always be observed: careful food hygiene, breast-feeding, protection from insects which transmit infections, etc.

Barnett & Chen [117] reviewed recommendations for immunization of children involved in international travel. A list of immunizations to be considered for children traveling outside Europe and North America is shown in Table 6.8. Young children should have their full course of routine immunization appropriate to their home country. It may be advisable to give some immunizations at a rather earlier age than in the UK schedule. For example, BCG vaccine should be given in the first few months of life if the child is traveling to an area of high TB infectivity. If the risk from measles is high, this immunization may be given at 6–11 months of age and repeated between 12 and 15 months of age.

IMMUNIZATION COVERAGE – IMPROVING UPTAKE

Causes of poor uptake

In some communities immunization appears to have a low priority and false beliefs sometimes obstruct immunization. In parts of Southeast Asia measles used to be considered a disease which children had to have and overcome in order to grow up strong and healthy. In Europe there are many public fears about the dangers of adverse reactions from vaccines. Many of these are false and even what is true is sometimes exaggerated by the media. Professional fear of litigation in some countries encourages health workers to advise against vaccination in all cases where there is any doubt at all. Health workers in a number of countries, including the UK, are not entirely clear about the contraindications for immunization.[118] They then tend to extend contraindications to groups who really require immunization, such as children who fail to thrive or have recurrent infections (see Table 6.4). Conflicting advice undermines the confidence of both the public and the profession.

Table 6.8 Vaccines and pretravel preparation for children

1. Make sure that routine immunizations are up to date
2. If going to a high risk area consider
   - BCG for neonates and children
   - Hepatitis B
   - Hepatitis A
   - Yellow fever
   - Typhoid
   - Cholera
   - Japanese encephalitis
   - Rabies
   - Meningococcal meningitis
   - Influenza

Improving knowledge, information and training

1. Use a simple schedule which is not changed more often than necessary.
2. Written guidelines should be available for staff and a simplified version for parents.
3. There should be a referral system for cases in which there is uncertainty about immunization.
4. Training specific to immunization counseling should be given to all those involved.
5. Clear instructions are required for dealing with anaphylaxis or other emergencies which are occasionally associated with immunization.[119]

Operational measures

In any country an immunization policy with definite targets and clear allocation of responsibility is essential. The person in overall charge should be specified and also which members of the team are responsible for vaccines, supplies, recall of the children and the practicalities of immunization. Immunization should be clearly recognized as an activity of nurses and auxiliaries who are appropriately supported by a doctor trained and interested in the topic.

The immunization schedule should be coordinated with other activities of the health service. Times of developmental assessment and school entry examination are appropriate for reviewing the immunization status and 'sweeping up' any missed immunizations. Opportunistic immunization should also be available at outpatient and hospital services, accident and emergency departments and at school entry examinations.

Immunization clinics should be near to the community and held at hours which are convenient for the parents. In some services domiciliary and home visit immunizations may need to be available. A local back-up team is required for training, inquiries and emergencies. Those responsible for the service should respond quickly and with sensitivity to special needs and emergencies, such as alarm caused by severe side-effects. The public should be informed about the purpose and plan of immunization campaigns through local channels of communication. Conflict about immunizations in the media seriously damages confidence. Immunization records should be appropriate to the health service. Sometimes these are parent-retained, computerized or held by the doctors and clinics. Often a combination of record systems is required. It is essential that immunization uptake is recognized as a key indicator of health care. All those involved in the immunization service should receive regular feedback so they can understand how their particular part of the service is working in relation to the targets of child immunization.

Practical issues

Many practicalities are involved in running an effective immunization program. These include appropriate training, care of vaccines, maintenance of equipment and correct administration of the vaccines, when and how they should be given. Personnel need to know how to prepare for and conduct an immunization session. The health education opportunity of an immunization program needs to be utilized by appropriate preparation and materials. Finally, evaluating an immunization program both at a local and regional level is important. Many of these issues have been clearly and systematically set out in *Immunization in Practice – A Guide for Health Workers who Give Vaccines*, by the World Health Organization,[120] in which guidelines to improve vaccine coverage are set out (see Table 6.9).

Table 6.9 World Health Organization guidelines about immunization

Unnecessary restrictions on immunizations limit the coverage and effectiveness of a program. The WHO Global Program of Immunization urges health workers to consider the following points:

1. Health workers should use every opportunity to immunize eligible children
2. No vaccine is entirely without side-effects, but the risk of disease far outweighs the risks of vaccines, especially in developing countries
3. BCG and OPV can be safely and effectively given to newborns
4. DPT can be given from the second month of life
5. Measles vaccine, in countries where the disease affects many before 1 year, should be given at 9 months, possibly earlier for high risk
6. Do not give DPT to a child who had a severe reaction to a previous dose (see above). Complete the schedule with DT vaccine
7. Do not withhold OPV during diarrhea, but give an extra dose as soon as possible after recovery
8. Malnourished children particularly need protection
9. Low fever, mild respiratory infections, diarrhea and minor illnesses are *not* contraindications to immunization
10. Every hospitalized child should be individually considered for immunization. Some benefit from admission immunization, e.g. measles, if there are cases in the ward. Review the immunization status of all children at discharge, and give appropriate vaccines
11. The decision to withhold immunizations has potentially serious consequences. It should only be advised after careful consideration and usually a second opinion

CHILD HEALTH ADVOCACY

In order to achieve improvements in child health in any population wider action needs to accompany the specific measures noted above. There is a need to advocate for promoting action within society (e.g. on socioeconomic circumstances and inequalities, quality of the environment, housing, nutrition and education) that will lead to improvements in child health or reductions in inequalities in child health. Child health advocacy often begins with an individual child or family and then may extend into local, regional or even national public health action. It involves taking action to promote health beyond treatment of a medical condition. This action can be taken as an individual or collectively. Specific steps in individual pediatrician advocacy have been described by Waterston & Tonniges:[121]

- identifying a preventable problem in one child;
- helping that child overcome the problem;
- drawing conclusions in relation to the factors that led to the problem in the first place;
- identifying the means to tackle these factors;
- influencing government or policy makers to change or reform the system that fostered these factors or introduce appropriate legislation.

Waterston gives as an example of such individual advocacy the work of Hugh Jackson who cared for a child who died of an accidental drug overdose and whose later action led to the development of legislation requiring the use of childproof medication.[121]

Collaborative action of pediatricians and other professionals involved in child health can advocate effectively against the tobacco industry or the motor industry or baby milk manufacturers.

REFERENCES (* Level 1 evidence)

1 UNICEF. Facts for life. New York: United Nations Children's (Emergency) Fund; 1989.

2 Inequalities in health. The Black report and the health divide. London: Penguin Books; 1988.

3 Spencer NJ. Child poverty and deprivation in the UK. Arch Dis Child 1991; 66:1255–1257.

4 Kohler L. Child public health: a new basis for child health workers. Eur J Pub Health 1998; 8:253–255.

5 Marmot ME, Wadsworth MEJ, eds. Fetal and early childhood environment and long-term health implications. Br Med Bull 1997; 53:81–96.

6 Kuh D, Ben-Shlomo YA. A life course approach to chronic disease epidemiology. Oxford: Oxford University Press; 1997.

*7 MRC Vitamin Study Research Group. Prevention of neural tube defects: results of the MRC vitamin study. Lancet 1991; 338:131–137.

*8 Czeizel AE, Dudas L. Prevention of the first occurrence of neural-tube defects by periconceptional vitamin supplementation. N Engl J Med 1992; 327:1832–1835.

9 Stevenson RE. The environmental basis of human anomalies. In: Stevenson RE, Hall JG, Goodman RM, eds. Human malformations and related anomalies. Vol 1. Oxford Monographs on Medical Genetics, number 27. Oxford: Oxford University Press; 1993.

10 Daltveit AK, Oyen N, Skjaereven R, et al. The epidemic of SIDS in Norway 1967–93: changing effects of risk factors. Arch Dis Child 1997; 77:23–27.

11 Arnestead M, Anderson M, Vege A, et al. Changes in the epidemiological pattern of sudden infant death syndrome in southeast Norway, 1984–1998: implications for future prevention and research. Arch Dis Child 2001; 85:108–115.

12 Golding J. The environment and child health. In: Harvey D, Miles M, Smyth D, eds. Community child health and paediatrics. Oxford: Butterworth-Heinemann; 1995.

13 Nuffield Council on Bioethics. Genetic screening: ethical issues. London: Nuffield Council; 1993.

14 Smithells RW, Shephard S, Schorah CJ, et al. Possible prevention of neural tube defects by periconceptional vitamin supplementation. Lancet 1980; i:339–340.

15 Smithells D. Vitamins in early pregnancy. BMJ 1996; 313:128–129.

*16 Laurence KM, James N, Miller MH, et al. Double blind randomised controlled trial of folate treatment before conception to prevent recurrence of neural tube defects. BMJ 1981; 282:1509–1511.

*17 Crowley P. Antenatal steroids for the prevention of respiratory distress syndrome in preterm babies. In: Enkin MW, Keirse MJNC, Renfrew MJ, Neilson JP, eds. The Cochrane pregnancy and childbirth database. Cochrane updates. Oxford: Update Software; 1993

18 House of Commons Science and Technology Committee. Human genetics: the science and its consequences. London: HMSO; 1995.

19 Motulsky AG. Predictive genetic testing. Am J Hum Genet 1994; 55:603–605.

20 Barker DJ. The fetal and infant origins of disease. Eur J Clin Invest 1995; 25:457–463.

21 Barker DJ. Fetal origins of coronary heart disease. BMJ 1995; 311:171–174.

22 Law CM, Barker DJ. Fetal influences on blood pressure. J Hypertens 1994; 12:1329–1332.

23 Zipursky A. Vitamin K at birth. BMJ 1996; 313:179–180.

24 Ansell P, Bull D, Roman E. Childhood leukaemia and intramuscular vitamin K: findings from a case-control study. BMJ 1996; 313:204–205.

25 Von Kries R, Gobel U, Hachmeister A, et al. Vitamin K and childhood cancer: a population based case-control study in Lower Saxony, Germany. BMJ 1996; 313:199–202.

26 Campbell H, Jones IJ. Breastfeeding in Scotland. Scottish Needs Assessment Programme. Glasgow: Scottish Forum for Public Health Medicine; 1994.

27 Lucas A, Morley R, Cole TJ, et al. Breast milk and subsequent intelligence quotient in children born preterm. Lancet 1992; 339:261–264.

28 Florey CV, Leech AM, Blackhall A. Infant feeding and mental and motor development at 18 months of age in first born singletons. Int J Epidemiol 1995; 24:S21–S26.

29 McNeilly AS. Effects of lactation on fertility. Br Med Bull 1979; 35:151–154.

30 Anonymous. A warm chain for breastfeeding. Lancet 1994; 344:1239–1241.

31 Campbell H, Gorman D, Wigglesworth A. Audit of the support for breastfeeding mothers in Fife maternity hospitals using adapted Baby Friendly Hospital materials. J Public Health Med 1995; 17:450–454.

32 Beeken S, Waterston T. Health service support of breastfeeding – are we practising what we preach? BMJ 1992; 305:285–287.

*33 Perez-Escamilla R, Pollitt E, Lohnerdal B, et al. Infant feeding policies in maternity wards and their effect on breastfeeding success: an analytical overview. Am J Public Health 1994; 84:89–97.

34 Phillip BL, Merewood A, Miller LW, et al. Baby-friendly hospital initiative improves breastfeeding initiation rates in a US hospital setting. Pediatrics 2001; 108:677–681.

35 Australian College of Paediatrics. Policy statement on breastfeeding. J Paediatr Child Health 1998; 34:412–413.

36 Michie CA, Gilmour J. Breastfeeding and the risks of viral transmission. Arch Dis Child 2001; 84:381–382.

37 Hall DMB. Health for all children: a programme of child health surveillance. Oxford: Oxford Medical Publications; 1996.

38 Fenton-May J, Bradley DM, Sibert JR, et al. Screening for Duchenne muscular dystrophy. Arch Dis Child 1994; 70:551–552.

39 Howie PW, Forsyth S, Ogston SA, et al. Protective effect of breastfeeding against infection. BMJ 1990; 300:11–16.

40 Jarvis S, Towner E, Walsh S. Accidents. In: Department of Health: The health of our children. London: HMSO; 1996.

41 Department of Health. The sleeping position of infants and cot death: report of the Chief Medical Officer's Expert Group. London: HMSO; 1993.

42 Dwyer T, Ponsonby AL. Sudden infant death syndrome. BMJ 1996; 313:180–181.

43 Blair PS, Fleming PJ, Bensley D, et al. Smoking and the sudden infant death syndrome: results from 1993–95 case-control study for confidential inquiry into stillbirths and deaths in infancy. Confidential enquiry into stillbirths and deaths regional coordinators and researchers. BMJ 1996; 313:195–198.

44 American Academy of Pediatrics. Committee on nutrition recommendations. Nutr Rev 1976; 34:248.

45 Department of Health and Social Security. Diet and cardiovascular disease (COMA report). Reports on health and social subjects: number 28. London: HMSO; 1984.

46 British Medical Association. Diet, nutrition and health. Report of the Board of Science and Education. London: Camelon Press; 1986.

47 Scottish Home and Health Department. Working party for the Chief Medical Officer of Scotland 1993. The Scottish diet. Edinburgh: SOHHD; 1993.

48 Clark B, Wharton B. Food and nutrition. In: Harvey D, Miles M, Smyth D, eds. Community child health and paediatrics. Oxford: Butterworth-Heinemann; 1995.

49 Falkner F. The prevention in childhood of health problems in adult life. Geneva: WHO; 1980.

50 Kristiansen B. Secondary prevention of meningococcal disease. BMJ 1996; 312:591–592.

51 Massell BF, Chute CG, Walker AM, et al. Penicillin and the marked decrease in morbidity and mortality from rheumatic fever in the United States. N Engl J Med 1988; 318:280–286.

52 Dajani AS, Bisno AL, Chung KJ, et al. Prevention of rheumatic fever. Circulation 1988; 78:1082–1086.

53 Blair M. The need for and the role of a coordinator in child health surveillance/promotion. Arch Dis Child 2001; 84:1–5.

54 Wilson JMG, Jungner G. Principals and practice of screening for disease. Geneva: WHO; 1968.

55 HMSO. Effective intervention: child abuse. Guidelines on co-operation in Scotland. Edinburgh: HMSO; 1990.

56 Green AH. Child sexual abuse: immediate and long term effects and intervention. J Acad Child Adolesc Psychiatry 1993; 32:890–902.

57 Glaser D. Treatment issues in child sexual abuse. Br J Psychiatry 1991; 159:769–782.

58 Charlton A. Smoking. In: Harvey D, Miles M, Smyth D, eds. Community child health and paediatrics. Oxford: Butterworth-Heinemann; 1995.

59 Holland WW, Fitzsimons B. Smoking in children. Arch Dis Child 1991; 66:1269–1274.

60 Amos A. Young people, tobacco and 1992. Health Educ J 1991; 50:26–30.

61 Power C. Health related behaviour. In: Department of Health: The health of our children. London: HMSO; 1996.

62 Goddard E. Drinking in England and Wales in the late 1980s. OPCS. London: HMSO; 1991.

63 Bonomo Y, Bowes G. Putting harm reduction into an adolescent context. J Paediatr Child Health 2001; 37:5–8.
64 American Academy of Pediatrics. School health centers and other integrated school health services. Pediatrics 2001; 107:198–201.
*65 DiGuiseppi C, Higgins JPT. Systematic review of controlled trials of interventions to promote smoke alarms. Arch Dis Child 2000; 82:341–348.
*66 Kendrick D, Elkan R, Hewitt M, et al. Does home visiting improve parenting and the quality of the home environment? A systematic review and meta-analysis. Arch Dis Child 2000; 82:443–451.
67 King WJ, Klassen TP, LeBlanc J, et al. The effectiveness of a home visit to prevent childhood injury. Pediatrics 2001; 108:382–388.
68 Emmons KM, Hammond K, Fava JL, et al. A randomised trial to reduce passive smoke exposure in low-income households with young children. Pediatrics 2001; 108:18–24.
69 Ada AL. Modern vaccines. The immunological principles of vaccination. Lancet 1990; 335:523–526.
70 Moxon ER. Modern vaccines. The scope of immunisation. Lancet 1990; 335:448–451.
71 Anderson RM, May RM. Modern vaccines. Immunization and herd immunity. Lancet 1990; 335:641–645.
72 Fine PEM, Rodrigues LC. Modern vaccines. Mycobacterial diseases. Lancet 1990; 335:1016–1020.
73 WHO. (WHO/GPV/95.05) Report of the Scientific Advisory Group of Experts. Geneva: WHO; 1995.
74 Moxon ER, Rappuoli R. Modern vaccines. *Haemophilus influenzae* infections and whooping cough. Lancet 1990; 335:1324–1329.
75 Edwards KM, Decker MD. Acellular pertussis vaccines for infants. N Engl J Med 1996; 334:391–392.
76 Shann F. Modern vaccines. *Pneumococcus* and *influenzae*. Lancet 1990; 335:898–901.
77 Lepow ML, Peter G, Glode MP, et al. The response of infants to *Haemophilus influenzae* type b polysaccharide vaccine conjugate with diphtheria–tetanus–pertussis antigen. J Infect Dis 1984; 149:950–955.
78 Lepow ML, Samuelson JS, Gordon LK. Safety and immunogenicity of *H. influenzae* type b polysaccharide-diphtheria toxoid conjugate vaccine (PPP-D) in infants. J Infect Dis 1987; 156:591–596.
79 Plotkin SA. Vaccination in the 21st century. J Infect Dis 1993; 168:29–37.
80 Brown F. Modern vaccines. From Jenner to genes – the new vaccines. Lancet 1990; 335:587–590.
81 Donnely JJ, Ulmer JB, Liu MS. Immunisation with DNA. J Immunol Methods 1994; 176:145–152.
82 Plotkin SA, Fletcher MA. Combination vaccines and immunization visits. Pediatr Infect Dis J 1996; 15:103–105.
83 Robbins A. The children's vaccine initiative. Am J Dis Child 1993; 147:152–153.
84 Insel RA. Potential alterations in immunogenicity by combining or simultaneously administering vaccine components. Ann N Y Acad Sci 1995; 754:35–47.
85 Hinman AR, Orenstein WA. Modern vaccines. Immunisation practice in developed countries. Lancet 1990; 335:707–710.
86 Galazka AM, Lauer BA, Henderson RH, et al. Indications and contraindications for vaccines used in the Expanded Programme on Immunization. Bull World Health Organ 1984; 62:357–366.
87 WHO. (WHO/EPI/GEN/95.03 Rev.1) Global programme for vaccines and immunization. Immunization policy. Geneva: WHO; 1996.
88 Immunization against infectious disease. London: HMSO; 1996.
89 Beale AJ. Modern vaccines. Polio vaccines: time for a change in immunisation policy? Lancet 1990; 335:839–842.
90 Plotkin SA. Inactivated polio vaccine for the United States: a missed vaccination opportunity. Pediatr Infect Dis J 1995; 14:835–839.
91 Elliman DAC, Bedford HE. MMR vaccine – worries are not justified. Arch Dis Child 2001; 85:271–274.
92 Baraff LJ, Manclark CR, Cherry JD, et al. Analysis of adverse reactions to diphtheria and tetanus toxoids and pertussis vaccine potency and percentage of mouse weight gain. Pediatr Infect Dis J 1989; 8:502–507.
93 National Immunisation Study. Factors influencing immunisation uptake in childhood. Horsham: Action Research for the Crippled Child; 1989.
94 Nicoll A, Jenkinson D. Decision making for routine measles/MMR and whooping cough immunisation. BMJ 1988; 297:405–407.
95 Anonymous. (Editorial). Routine immunisation of preterm infants. Lancet 1990; 335:23–24.
96 Hall AJ, Greenwood BM, Whittle H. Modern vaccines. Practice in developing countries. Lancet 1990; 335:774–777.
97 Hargreaves RM, Slack MP, Howard AJ, et al. Changing patterns of invasive *Haemophilus influenzae* disease in England and Wales after introduction of the Hib vaccination programme. BMJ 1996; 312:160–161.
98 American Academy of Pediatrics. Recommended childhood immunisation schedule – US January–December 2000. Pediatrics 2000; 105:148.
99 American Academy of Pediatrics. Recommended childhood immunisation schedule – US January–December 2001. Pediatrics 2001; 107:202.
100 Cutts FT. Revaccination against measles and rubella. BMJ 1996; 312:589–590.
101 Frankel D. US group urges immunisation change. Lancet 1995; 346:1151.
102 Hull HF, Lee JW. Sabin, Salk or sequential? Lancet 1996; 347:630.
103 Ward NA, Hull HF. Polio eradication. Lancet 1995; 345:318.
104 Edwards KM, Meade BD, Decker MD. Comparison of 13 acellular pertussis vaccines: overview and serologic response. Pediatrics 1995; 96:548–557.
105 Preston NW, Matthews RC. Components of acellular pertussis vaccines. Lancet 1996; 347:764.
106 Miller E. Acellular pertussis vaccines. Arch Dis Child 1995; 73:390–391.
107 Gershon AA. Varicella vaccine: its past, present and future. Pediatr Infect Dis J 1995; 12:742–752.
108 Ross LF, Lantos JD. Immunisation against chickenpox. BMJ 1995; 310:2–3.
109 American Academy of Pediatrics. Varicella vaccine update. Pediatrics 2000; 105:136–141.
110 Skull SA, Wang EEL. Varicella vaccination – a critical review of the evidence. Arch Dis Child 2001; 85:83–90.
111 WHO. Pneumococcal vaccines – WHO position paper. Wkly Epidemiol Rec 1999; 74:177–184.
112 Dagan R, Yagupsky P, Goldbart A, et al. Increasing prevalence of penicillin resistant pneumococcal infections in children in southern Israel: implications for future immunization policies. Pediatr Infect Dis J 1994; 13:782–786.
113 Klugman K. Pneumococcal resistance to antibiotics. Clin Microbiol Rev 1990; 3:171–196.
*114 Black S, Shinefield H, Fireman B, et al. Efficacy, safety and immunogenecity of heptavalent pneumococcal conjugate vaccine in children. Pediatr Infect Dis J 2000; 19:187–195.
115 Choo S, Finn A. New pneumococcal vaccines for children. Arch Dis Child 2001; 84:289–294.
116 MacIntyre CR. Hepatitis B vaccine: risks and benefits of universal neonatal vaccination. J Paediatr Child Health 2001; 37:215–217.
117 Barnett E, Chen R. Children and international travel: immunizations. Pediatr Infect Dis J 1995; 14:982–992.
118 Wood D, Halfon N, Pereya M, et al. Knowledge of the childhood immunization schedule and of contraindications to vaccinate by private and public providers in Los Angeles. Pediatr Infect Dis J 996; 15:40–45.
119 Nicoll A, Elliman D, Begg NT. Immunisation – causes of failure and strategies and tactics for success. BMJ 1989; 299:808–812.
120 WHO. Immunization in practice. A guide for health workers who give vaccines. Oxford: Oxford University Press; 1989
121 Waterston T, Tonniges T. Advocating for children's health: a US and UK perspective. Arch Dis Child 2001; 85:180–182.

7

Developmental pediatrics

Ruth E Day revised by Gillian Baird (with assessment of vision by Alison Salt)

INTRODUCTION

Developmental pediatrics is concerned with the processes of children's learning and competent adaptation to the environment from birth to adulthood. There are three purposes:

1. to promote optimal physical and mental health and development for all children, applying principles of prevention of impairment, wherever possible, and to reduce, where possible, disability and handicap (Table 7.1);
2. to ensure early diagnosis and effective treatment of impairments of body, mind and personality;
3. to discover the cause and means of preventing such impairments.

Increasingly pediatricians and all others concerned with the professional care of children will find their time spent with chronic illness, chronic physical or mental disability, learning or behavioral problems. Acute illnesses are likely to be shorter, self-limiting or more rapidly responsive to treatment. This chapter looks at the process of development, how it can be observed and how abnormalities can be identified and interpreted. The context for observing a child's development is the family, school and community. Family, educational, social, cultural, spiritual, economic, environmental and political forces act favorably or unfavorably, but always significantly, on the health and functioning of children.[1]

THEORIES OF CHILD DEVELOPMENT

There is a particularly long developmental period in humans, which must be adaptive for social and cognitive competence. Childhood marks the change from the entirely dependent baby into the mature independent adult. During this period the child:

1. builds up a store of knowledge about the environment;
2. learns motor skills to survive;
3. learns a language with which to communicate and think;
4. develops a sense of self, self-regulation of emotions and behavior and the coping strategies for successful interpersonal relationships.

Philosophical views of child development (e.g. Rousseau) were replaced last century by the more scientific approaches of direct observation of children's behavior and the work of experimental researchers. Theories have included:

1. the 'maturational' view exemplified by Gesell (i.e. developmental progression depends upon neurological maturation);
2. 'behavioral' (i.e. changes in the environment are the most important influence in shaping the child);
3. 'psychoanalytic/psychosocial' theories of Freud and Erikson (unconscious motivations);
4. 'cognitive' theories developed by Piaget, which emphasize stages of development and the mental process of constructing knowledge from interaction with the environment that builds the next stage upon the previous one.

All these theories continue to influence the ways in which we think about a child's development. Mental growth and development are dependent both on maturation of the nervous system and on experience. At 5 months the fetus has the full adult complement of 12 billion or more nerve cells. As the fetus and infant grow, the developing interconnections between these cells result in patterns of behavior that are generally similar, but the acquisition of knowledge and the refinement of skills depend on the child's

Table 7.1 Definitions of impairment and disability. There are many definitions and the term is used differently in different legislation

The Children Act 1989

'A child in need' is unlikely to achieve or maintain or to have the opportunity of achieving or maintaining, a reasonable standard of health or development without the provision for the child of services by a local authority.

The health or development of 'a child in need' is likely to be significantly impaired or further impaired, without the provision for the child of such services.

A disabled child is 'a child in need'.

The Disability Discrimination Act 1995

This Act defines a disable person as someone who has: 'a physical or mental impairement which has a substantial and long-term adverse effect on his/her ability to carry out normal day to day activities'.

The World Health Organization International Classification (ICDH)

Impairment is 'a loss or abnormality of body structure or of a physiological or psychological function'.

Disability is 'the functional effect of any impairment'.

Handicap is 'the limitation or prevention of fulfilment in life normal for that individual because of impairment or disability'.

The new ICDH-2

The concept of disability is replaced by the 'activity' of an individual and the extent of their functioning.

The concept of handicap is replaced by measure of participation.

opportunity to observe, copy and experiment. Neuronal maturation of the brain continues into postnatal life and myelination is completed in sensory and motor areas first and association areas last. Neural systems stabilize to optimal patterns of functioning via a process of reorganization and subtraction within neonatal architectural constraints and biases, which lead to recruitment of specific pathways. There is a capacity for plasticity, which becomes less flexible with age. At an anatomical level, the resultant brain–behavior relationships show domain specificity (e.g. specific areas devoted to language processing and learning).

1. Nativist or innate theories continue to be influential, for example in language learning[2] and motor development – theories of self-organization.[3]
2. 'Modern social learning constructivist' theories emphasize cognitive processes as mediators of environmental/behavioral influences.
3. Bronfenbrenner's 'ecological theories' emphasize the importance of the context in which children grow up, the goodness of fit and other features of the environment (i.e. the family situation, parents working, early child care and the wider cultural influences).
4. Vygotsky emphasized the immediate context for social learning, described as the 'zone of proximal development', as that area where the child cannot manage a task independently but can do more with supportive assistance. This is particularly relevant to his views of the development of language and thinking where social meaning is conferred on language and actions by the social sharing of ideas with others.
5. More mechanistic learning models and 'connectionist' theories are based on information processing and the perception, conception, storage, manipulation, transformation and retrieval of information. They are also based on the limitations that these processes place on functioning through memory capacity and attentional skills such as selection, shifting, inhibition, multi- and crossmodal functions, speed of processing, the development of automaticity and metacognitive skills, such as knowing about things and making comparisons and judgments. These are universal learning mechanisms incorporating theories of efficiency such that the mental resource and effort that is devoted to interaction with the environment and problem solving for the individual is minimized while retaining flexibility and increasing hierarchy and coherence.

'Dynamic systems' theory integrates all the above elements. Children actively construct their understanding of the world by interacting with it, thus developing schemes and strategies that can be applied to a wide variety of situations. Intelligence reflects the child's capacity to initiate and assimilate new experiences and to profit by past experience.

FACTORS THAT AFFECT DEVELOPMENT

NATURE VS NURTURE

Although there is now little disagreement that there are both genetic and environmental contributions to development of intelligence and personality, the nature/nurture debate continues. The contribution of each is complex because both the individual and the environment are continuously changing over time and the interaction between them, which molds psychological growth, is fluid and dynamic.[4] The genetic influences on a child's development extend to the environment also, through the parental phenotype.

ENVIRONMENTAL RISK FACTORS

Environmental factors may act in two ways:

1. by affecting the perceptual or effector organs and brain biologically at any stage from prenatally onwards;
2. by altering the child's opportunity to learn by limiting or expanding his experience – psychosocial factors.

PSYCHOSOCIAL FACTORS

In general, people rather than physical elements are the most important factors in the environment of the young child. The parents are responsible for giving the child the opportunities to enable learning, form relationships and develop social understanding. Most crucially, if the infant does not develop a sense of trust in people and attachment from that first relationship with a parent then he or she is more likely to have lifelong difficulties with relationships. Various factors affect the parents' capacity to cope well with the task of child rearing and provision of an optimal learning environment. Resilience to life events is related to temperament as well as to family factors of warmth, cohesion and support and other sources of external support.

Temperament

Temperament is a major influence on all aspects of adaptive development as well as social–emotional development, both through the effect on the child's adaptation to the environment and their personal regulation, but also through the effect on the caregivers/parents and broader social context. Temperament can be seen from the earliest weeks as a mix of activity, adaptability, attention and emotional responses. Continuities of temperament over time have been well documented. For example, high reactors as infants are more inhibited in new situations at age 4 years.[5] Particular patterns are:

1. the easy child;
2. the slow-to-warm up child;
3. the difficult child.

Current research emphasizes both 'emotionality' and 'self-regulation' as important. Differences within children may mean that some are more sensitive than others to maternal 'sensitivity', which is thought to be an important influence on attachment in infancy.

Parenting style and parental mental illness

Depression in mothers in the postnatal period is associated with effects on children's social–emotional development and their later academic achievements. Parental inconsistency in methods of behavioral control is linked to children's behaviour problems. However, a diversity of methods of parental control of children's behavior is normal and a balance of approaches – e.g. praise and punishment – is important, providing a 'good enough' environment for most children. The emotional context is particularly important. Parental conflict is adverse in affect. The social learning environment that promotes moral development is warm not punitive, emphasizes others' feelings and perspectives and models appropriate behavior. Children continue to practice skills if they are rewarded or the behavior is reinforced. A young baby hits an object during an involuntary action. If it makes a noise or looks attractive he or she is likely to try again and thus the process of exploring the environment starts. If when babies wave their arms around and make a noise there is no feedback or response from their environment or they are shouted at, they are likely to stop exploring and keep quiet. It has been suggested that in this way severe deprivation in the first year of life can affect children's ability to learn for the rest of their lives. The more infants see and hear the more they want to see and hear later.

Deprivation

Children from deprived environments (especially where neglect is prominent) tend to show developmental delay, particularly of language.[6,7] Children best learn the meaning of words when the word and the object are closely and frequently associated. The child deprived of simple play with adults does not have the opportunity to hear language related to the immediate environment. He or she may be surrounded by more complex visual and auditory stimuli from the television or older siblings, but will be unable to interpret and learn from these stimuli because of their complexity or because of interference from background noises.

Recent studies of children who have been adopted from Romanian orphanages attest both to the resilience and the vulnerability of developmental processes. When reassessed at the age of 4 years, those children adopted within the UK by the age of 6 months had shown cognitive catch up, despite having shown severe physical and developmental retardation. Those adopted after 6 months of age showed catch up, but not to the same extent.[8,9] Social, cognitive and interactive development are particularly, but not exclusively, at risk. Age of adoption was a greater predictor of outcome than nutritional state, but multiple factors make the precise separation of effects difficult.

BIOLOGICAL FACTORS

A child's development may be affected by abnormalities of brain function, of special senses or of effector organs such as the limbs and muscles, either as part of innate development or acquired through some damaging event such as illness or accident.

Brain damage or dysfunction

Brain damage or dysfunction may affect all areas of function or only specific areas of function. Diffuse insults may produce specific dysfunction because of the vulnerability of a particular area of the brain at the time of insult (e.g. periventricular leukomalacia preterm and basal ganglia damage due to hypoxia at term).

Influences may be:

1. prenatal – through genetics, or maternal disease (e.g. placental insufficiency causing nutritional deficiencies, toxins and infections, in the perinatal period);
2. postnatal – for example illness, non-accidental injury, accidents and deficiencies.

Deficiencies are likely to be rare in developed countries, but iron deficiency anemia has effects on development, and a number of studies show that the milk given to premature newborns affects cognitive development.[10]

The effects of certain types of brain damage (e.g. cranial irradiation) may not be immediately apparent, but only materialize when new learning is attempted. Concepts of neural plasticity are invoked in the context of damage, although some areas of differentiated function appear to show less of this (e.g. the primary motor cortex) than others.

Effects of early occurring brain injury are often attenuated relative to later injury, for example the effects of stroke on language development in children with dominant hemisphere, but unilateral, cerebral damage. In this situation language learning is relatively unimpaired if they are under 6 or 7 years of age. In many children who have so-called 'developmental disorders', for example dyslexia and language disorder, there is no evidence of brain damage, but newer imaging techniques identify specific areas and/or processes of dysfunction, often in the context of a strong family history.[11]

Chromosome abnormalities

Chromosome abnormalities (see Ch. 12) may influence development through effects on general learning processes, as well as specific effects, and can result in the development of specific and recognizable behavioral phenotypes, for example:

1. Prader–Willi (early feeding difficulties and hypotonia, learning problems and later eating/hunger control disorder, see Chapter 13);
2. Smith–Magenis (severe mental retardation with severe sleep disturbance, behavior problems of aggression and self-mutilation and the stereotyped behavior of upper body hugging).

Single and multiple gene disorders

Many developmental disorders are increasingly being recognized as having substantial genetic predisposition, but are referred to as complex conditions with multigene effects likely to be caused by normal variations within genes rather than mutations as in single gene defects. Thus the genes which cause a developmental problem may vary between individuals, which may account for the variations in phenotypic manifestations of disorders such as autism.

Defects of special senses

Defects of special senses most commonly affect vision and hearing (rarely smell) and can result in a severe restriction of the information a child receives, which is essential to normal development. When impairments are severe it is obvious that development will be affected. When impairments are less severe, or intermittent, as in the case of secretory otitis media, it is more difficult to assess the effect on development; however, where other impairments exist, the effect is likely to be cumulative.

Defects of effector organs – structural and movement disorders

Disorders of movement may be due to abnormality of the brain (cerebral palsy), spinal cord (paraplegia), nerves (spinal muscular atrophy) or muscles (dystrophy). These disorders have a direct effect on movement and also limit the child's experience. The child who cannot move independently does not experience space and distance and cannot reach things to manipulate them. It is important for parents and therapists to recognize this and to provide the child with compensatory experience. Limb deficiencies have similar effects.

Those disorders where there is no central brain involvement are less complex from the learning point of view, but some disorders that predominantly affect muscles (e.g. muscular dystrophy) have a significant effect on learning through a direct brain effect.

Other structural problems, such as facial disorders and cleft palate, influence development through direct effects (e.g. speech articulation), indirect effects (e.g. conductive hearing loss) or associated learning problems (as in chromosome 22 abnormalities: the velocardiofacial syndrome).

Sex and development

Although the mediation is unknown and texts of milestones of development do not necessarily differentiate, there are some differences between boys and girls in development. For example, in the MacArthur study of language acquisition boys were on average 1 month behind girls, but the difference accounted for less than 2% of the variation within and across ages.[12] Nearly all the developmental disorders are more common in boys than girls. One theory – that of Geschwind & Galaburda[13] – suggest that the influence of testosterone is to delay maturation of specific processes within the brain.

Gestational age

Gestational age is a relevant consideration for children under 24 months of age. Convention and arithmetic suggest that full correction for gestation should be made up to this time, but clinically there should be caution and this author's rule-of-thumb is to use less than the whole correction from 12 months onwards, especially in cognitive skills.

Compounding effects of impairments

Biological and social factors may interact. When there is a biological abnormality, psychosocial factors become even more important determinants of the child's future, but it is precisely in this situation that parental resources are stretched. The child with a disability may have particular characteristics that are likely to make it harder for the parents to react to him or her, for example the child may not smile or may go rigid when picked up and thereby not elicit the normal mothering response. This can result in a vicious cycle, with the child becoming more disabled than originally expected. The severely visually impaired child may withdraw into self-stimulation, the rarely handled child with cerebral palsy becomes more rigid. The child with a communication disorder such as autism may not respond as expected, so caregiver behavior changes.

The more competent, less stressed parents may well have resources to consciously modify their reaction and provide for the child's special needs. The less competent or more stressed parents are less likely to be able to do this.

NORMAL DEVELOPMENT

Previous texts by Sheridan[14] and Illingworth[15] are classic texts in developmental pediatrics.

A developmental framework is essential for understanding a child's functioning and behavior and should be conceived over a life time course. It is traditional to describe child development as steps or stages of ages and in various fields of behavior, for example prenatal, infancy (from birth to 24 months), childhood (2–5/6 years), in areas such as physical, motor, adaptive, cognitive and language, personal, social and emotional. This should not detract from the fact that a child's development at any specific age is an integrated whole and over time is a continuous process. The integration of all aspects of development through to adolescence is shown in Table 7.2.

Descriptions of development tend to focus on universals rather than individual differences. They also tend to focus on skills acquired rather than processes of learning. Age is an ambiguous variable and is often a proxy for other processes (e.g. brain maturation). Change and continuity both need to be emphasized for individuals. At a number of time points critical periods occur with consequent disturbances to development. For example the presence of a cataract in a child's eye that prevents visual information reaching the visual cortex may result in failure to develop vision unless the cataract is removed within the first weeks of life. Whether there is firm evidence for other critical periods for learning social or cognitive skills remains contentious.

The following section looks at the sequence and process of development in different areas.

PHYSICAL GROWTH

Physical growth is discussed in Chapter 13. Hormones affect development and behavior, but physical and mental growth may be dissociated.

MOTOR SKILLS

Figure 7.1 gives a description of motor development at different ages.

The acquisition of motor skills depends on:

1. the loss of primitive reflexes (the fetus moves in utero and the newborn infant shows movements, some of which are reflexly determined – after birth, reflex movements that initially may be useful have to disappear before purposeful controlled movements can develop – the asymmetric tonic neck reflex, most evident at 2–3 months, may contribute to the development of visually directed grasping but its persistence, as in some children with cerebral palsy, interferes with bimanual manipulative skills);
2. the development of a body schema or image through interpretation of proprioceptive, vestibular, tactile and visual information;
3. the development of postural control, which depends on reflex adjustment of tone in a large number of muscles in response to visual and proprioceptive feedback;
4. an increasing ability to interpret the visual information in the environment in order to judge, for example, distance, depth, rajectory and weight correctly;
5. the development of movement patterns which are rapidly adjustable in response to environmental circumstances so that actions are smooth, refined and economical, and where movements are increasingly separable from each other (e.g. arm and hand reach without whole body movement – as happens in cerebral palsy).

Postural control develops in a cephalocaudal direction starting with head control, then progressing with sitting,

Table 7.2 Integration of all aspects of development through to adolescence.

Ages (years)	0–1	1–2	3–5	6–12	12+
Stages	Infant	Toddler	Preschool	School	Adolescent
Motor	Sitting → Stand → Walk →Run				
	Grasp →Finger/thumb grip →Handedness →Bimanual coordination for complex tasks				
Cognitive and play	Sensorimotor →	Representational (defining by use) →	Imaginative and pretence		
	manipulative →	Matching → Categorization (perceptually obvious) →	(conceptual)		
	Object permanence →	Concrete thinking (increasingly symbolic) →		Abstract thinking	
	Means–end →	Increasing linking of events →		Dual representation of ideas and theory of mind	
	Observation → Imitation				
Communication	Joint action →	Increasing sharing			
	Joint attention (both initiated and receptive) →	Reciprocity and conversation			
Language	Recognizes familiar setting and shows understanding in context →	Increasing understanding of meaning of words outside familiar context →		Increasing understanding of abstract concepts (e.g. time, distance, motions)	
Speech	Babble → Gesture → Point → Words →Sentences →Understands and uses range of facial communicative and emotional expressions				
Social/emotional	Smiles in response				
		Egocentric →Increasing awareness of other needs			
	Dependent caregiver/attachment →	Explores from secure base →		Peer group play Individual friends →	Extended peer group
	Friendly to all →	Stranger awareness			
	Fed → Feeds self →	Increasing independence dressing, feeding, continence			
Moral	Aware of action/reaction →	Self/other action on others →	Rules →		Ideals
Attention	Distractible/ single channel →	Own control			
Psychosexual		Gender identity → Gender-typed behavior		→ Single sex play	→ Sexual object choice

standing, walking and running. The child cannot develop sophisticated movements without first achieving postural control. All forms of movement are sequential postural adjustments, so that without resting tone or balance, movement is uncontrolled. Primitive neonatal reflexic behavior declines as both gross and fine controlled movements increase. Preferred head turning, which is seen maximally at 2–3 months, should disappear thereafter. Like the other primitive reflexes, persistence may be a sign of abnormality. The secondary protective reflexes of propping and saving, which develop from 20 weeks onwards, are developmental and can be absent or abnormal in motor disorders.[16] Mirror movements may be a feature of normal motor development.

SENSORY AND PERCEPTUAL DEVELOPMENT

Specific domains process the perceptions of vision, hearing, smell and touch and their components (e.g. movement, form, color and dimension for vision). There may be critical periods for speech sound processing recognition as well as visual information. The principles of information processing apply: for example speed, intermodal and crossmodal integration, such as the coordination of vision and hearing perception at 3 months. The meaning (conceptual understanding) of what is seen builds probably on innate recognition patterns (e.g. of the face).

Vision

At birth the newborn eyeball is short and the ciliary muscles immature. The focal length for clearest vision is thus near to the baby and helped by high contrast. Movement, form and color are all perceived early. The infant scans the edges of shapes first and then internal features, showing pattern preferences (e.g. of faces rather than jumbled features). By 6–7 months the baby not only recognizes faces but discriminates between facial expressions (e.g. happy or fearful). Various ingenious experiments show that by 6–7 months, depth perception, as well as an understanding that shapes stay the same whether you are close or far away, is present (what is called size and shape constancy). The visual cortex appears to be highly specific and to show critical periods for its development – brain plasticity does not extend to other areas taking over its function. A significant visual impairment will affect all areas of development because the child's awareness of, and ability to interact with, the environment is different.

Sound perception

The ear is fully developed at birth and sound perception is possible in utero. Speech perception and recognition of voices of different

Position	Newborn	4 weeks	6 weeks	8 weeks	12 weeks	16 weeks	20 weeks	24 weeks
Supine	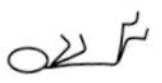	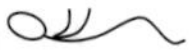			Head midline, finger play 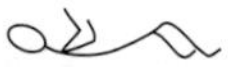		Head lifted more 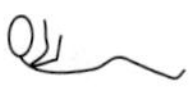	Rolls from prone to supine. Head lifed spontaneously, legs lifted, foot play 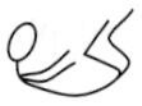
Pull to sit	No head control 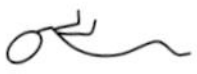	Almost complete head lag	Head lag not quite complete 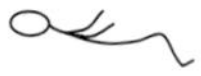		Good head control - only moderate head lag 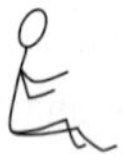		Head lifted in anticipation of being picked up 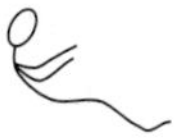	Pull to sit - head lifted off couch when about to be pulled up - hands are held up to be lifted
Sitting	Curved back 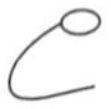	Held in sitting position may hold head up momentarily 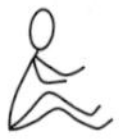		Head is held up but recurrently bobs forwards	Holds head steady and erect for several seconds, lumbar curve 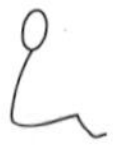	Held in sitting position - holds head well up constantly - looks actively around but head still wobbles if examiner causes sudden movement of trunk	Partial response to sideways tilt of trunk, righting but not propping with arm 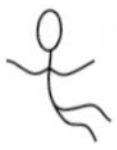	Sits in high chair for few moments (supported); sits propped forwards 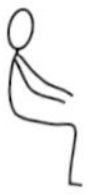
Prone	Legs tucked under 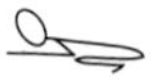	Momentarily holds chin off couch	Lifts chin off couch. Legs extended 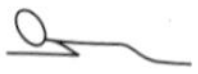		Prone - lifts head and upper chest off couch - bearing weight on forearms 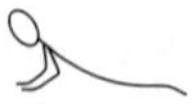 Good head control	Curvature of back - now only in lumbar region compared with rounded back of earlier weeks		Prone - weight borne on hands with extended arms - chest and upper part of abdomen being off the couch 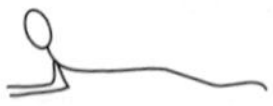
Ventral suspension in prone position with hand under abdomen	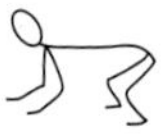		Momentary tensing of neck muscles should be noted	Ventral suspension holds head up so that its plane is in line with that of the body 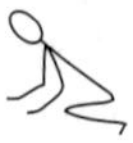				Partial forward parachute 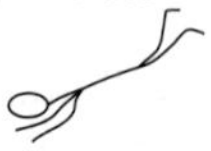
Standing	Automatic stepping 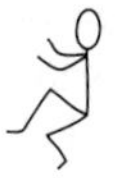				Off feet 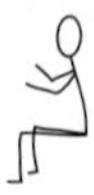			Held in standing position - bears large fraction of weight Downward parachute response, feet meet ground plantigrade when baby held and rapidly lowered (not shufflers) 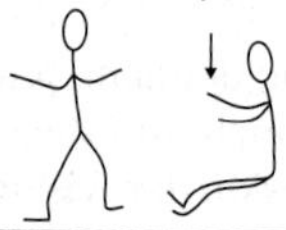

Fig. 7.1 Summary of development of spontaneous movement and posture control.

Continued

Position	28 weeks	32 weeks	36 weeks	40 weeks	44 weeks	48 weeks	1 year	15 months	18 months
Supine	Supine - spontaneously lifts head off couch, rolls from supine to prone								
Sitting	Sits with hands forward for support	Sits for a few moments when unsupported. 90% at 8 months 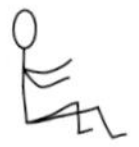	Sits steadily for 10 minutes, leans forward and recovers balance (cannot lean sideways)	Sits steadily without risk of falling over except for occasional accident Pulls self to sitting position, goes forward from sitting to prone and from prone to sitting	Sitting - can lean over sideways	Sitting - can pivot, can turn round and pick up objects 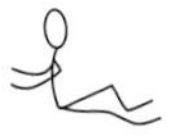			Seats itself in chair often by a process of climbing up, standing, turning round and sitting down
Prone	Prone - bears weight on one hand		Prone - in trying to crawl may progress backwards - may progress by rolling	Creeps pulling self forward with hands, abdomen on couch	Prone - crawls (abdomen off couch) 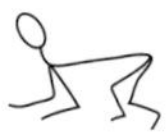		Prone - walks on hands and feet like a bear - may shuffle on buttocks and hands 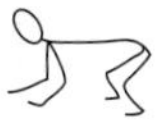	Creeps upstairs	
Evoked responses	Puts arm out to save if tilted off balance - sideways prop 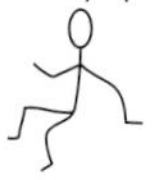	Full propping response both sides And tilt response 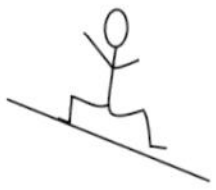		Forward parachute response, forward descent to ground, arms and hands extended 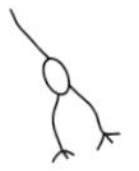	Oblique suspension. Baby held under pelvis sideways arm and leg extended 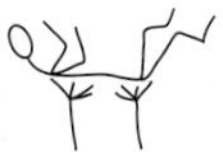				

Fig. 7.1 *(Continued)*

speakers are present shortly after birth. The capacity for smell and touch as well as the other senses are similarly developed at birth and play an important part in the perceptual learning about the environment.

Crossmodal perception

Crossmodal perception (i.e. the integration of information from different senses) is demonstrable within the first months and contributes to the conceptual development of the meaning of experiences stored in memory and the expectation of constancy of experience – shown experimentally as confusion. The 'meaning' that the child is able to attach to sensations and perceptions is the cognitive end point and this depends not only on the process of perception and conception, but the social and cultural context, which attaches meaning as well.

Fine motor skills

Figure 7.2 shows normal manipulative, visual and hearing development.

Once a child achieves reliable postural control, increasingly accurate manipulative skills can be developed – integration of visual input and motor output is essential for normal acquisition of these skills. Grasping is shown in Figure 7.3.[17] Voluntary and accurate release are as essential as grasping for later manipulative skills. Handedness (which hand is dominant) is clear in many children by 24 months and is expected in the majority by 42 months. Delayed development of which hand is dominant is frequently associated with specific as well as general learning difficulties.

From the age of 3 years manual competence can be assessed in component skills:

1. use of tools (e.g. putting a bead in a screw top jar, putting a pen together);
2. imitation of gestures (these can be miming, how to brush hair after being shown a hairbrush or a picture of one, or copying hand postures that are increasingly complex and may or may not be symbolic) – miming the use of a familiar object is a skill shown by 5 years; all others show a steady progression to the age of 12 years;[18]
3. learning a sequence of motor actions and writing/drawing.

Perceiving shapes correctly and being able to reproduce them are essential for reading and writing (the orientations of p, q, b and d are particularly delayed in dyslexia). The ability to match shapes

Position	28 weeks	32 weeks	36 weeks	40 weeks	44 weeks	48 weeks	1 year	15 months	18 months
Standing	Standing position - can maintain extension of hips and knees for short period when supported. Bounces with pleasure having previously sagged at hips and knees	Readily bears whole weight on legs when supported	Stands holding on to furniture 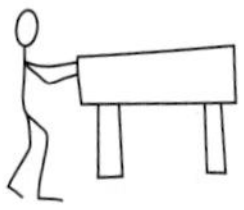	Pulls to standing position	When standing holds on - lifts and replaces one foot	Walks sideways holding on to furniture. Walks with two hands held	Walks with one hand held May stand unsupported for a moment 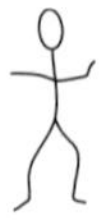 Walking alone	Can get into standing position without support, walks without help with broad base - high stepping gait and steps of unequal length and direction. (The maturity of the gait must be noted from now onward.) The wide base decreases as balance improves and arms are released for carrying 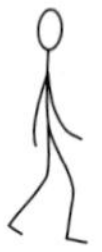 Lower guard	Walks well with feet only slightly apart - pulls toys as he walks - climbs stairs holding rail or helping hands. Runs rather stiffly - seldom falls. Throws ball without falling 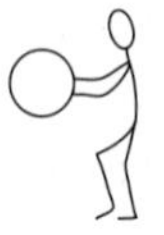 Squat and rise

Position	21 months	2 years	2.5 years	3 years	4 years	5 years	By 10 years
Walking skills	Walks backwards in imitation - picks up object from floor without falling, walks upstairs two feet per step	Goes upstairs alone, and down holding on, two feet per step	Jumps on both feet - walks on tiptoe when asked - kicks a large ball	Goes upstairs one foot per step - downstairs two feet per step Jumps off bottom step - stands on one foot for a few seconds	Runs, avoiding objects easily Goes up and downstairs one foot per step	Skips, hops, dances	Walks heel to toe backwards Can do 'fog' tests - walk on outer borders of feet with arms loose at sides
Other skills				Rides tricycle, catches well-directed ball with arms outstretched		Throws and catches a ball well enough to join in group games, but catching with one hand is not reliable until 9–10 years	

Fig. 7.1 (*Continued*)

can be demonstrated by the use of form boards with different shapes (e.g. circles, squares and triangles), which have to be fitted into the appropriate space on the board. The ability to copy shapes is shown by asking the child to copy a three-brick bridge (3 years) and five-brick bridge (5 years). The ability to copy shapes with a pencil starts with a vertical line (second year) and a horizontal line and circle (third year). This progresses to letters and more complex shapes requiring juxtaposition of vertical, horizontal and oblique lines (Bender Gestalt test, see p. 131).

Harris[19] devised a scoring system giving age norms for the ability to draw a man. Such ability is related to control of pencil movement, ability to reproduce shapes and concept of body image. By 3 years the

Age	Manipulation	Vision	Hearing
4 weeks		Watches mother when she talks to him. Looks at a dangling toy in line of vision and follows briefly	Quiets to familiar voice
8 weeks	Hands more frequently open	Follows dangling toy from side to side past midline, eyes show fixation and convergence in focusing	
12 weeks	Watches movement of own hands, pulls at clothes, shows a desire to grasp objects and holds rattle briefly when placed in hands	Follows dangling toy from one side to the other through 180° and vertically	Turns to familiar sounds in supine
16 weeks	Hands come together, approaches objects with hands – often fails to reach. Plays for longer periods with object placed in hand	Recognizes objects, for example familiar toy	Turns head towards a sound
20 weeks	Two-handed scoop for object Arm movements increasingly better controlled to reach directly for objects	Smiles at self in mirror	Recognizes individual voices, listens to conversation
24 weeks	Manipulation – reaches and grasps objects on table surface with raking palmar grasp. Puts hands up to hold bottle, drops one object if holding when another offered	Sees ands recognizes at adult distance Looks at falling objects	Turns to sounds when sitting if sounds on ear level Distraction tests used to test functional hearing
36 weeks	Has learned to transfer objects from one hand to another and can hold an object in each hand. Uses index finger approach to touch objects, can pick up small object between finger and thumb. Enjoys releasing objects over the side of cot or chair	Sees crumbs on floor Looks for fallen objects out of sight	Locates sounds made above and below ear level and at greater distance
1 year	Has mature prehension and can release object precisely. Can now hold two cubes in one hand, brings one cube in each hand together in the midline and imitates clicking and tries to build two cubes	Recognizes pictures of objects	Recognizes tunes and tries to join in Locates sounds above ear level
15 months	Can takes objects out of container and replace more precisely (e.g. pegmen in wooden boat)	100s and 1000s used for near vision	Distraction test to specific frequencies used
18–24 months	Refinement of release enables the child to build cubes to an increasing height and post objects accurately through holes. Increasing control of finger movements can be used by the child to manipulate tools (e.g. spoon, crayon) and pages of a book. Initially pencils are held with a fisted cylindrical palmar grip then a high shaft pronated grip		

Fig. 7.2 Development of manipulation, vision and hearing.

(*Continued*)

Age	Manipulation	Vision	Hearing
24–36 months	Learns to use a more adult grip, turn single page carefully, stack eight bricks (90% by 30 m) and take off socks 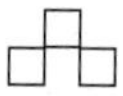 33–36 m 80% at 39 m Copies ○ from model 36–39 m □ ○ △ Shapes inserted 24 m Insert puzzle-pieces recognized at 30 m and orientated 33 m Draws man	Tested with matching letters from 2+ years. Can use the Kay pictures from 24 months (naming pictures) but monocular testing difficult before 42 months Sonksen-Silver linear chart from 30 m	Hearing tested by pointing at toys/pictures from 24 months chosen for their range of component sounds (e.g. McCormick toys) and by conditioning to sounds from 30 months (to put an object in a box when a sound is heard). This leads on to pure tone audiometry; individual ears may be tested in some children at 3 years
4 years	Holds a pencil in the adult way, a dynamic tripod, is able to cut with scissors and thread beads Copies from model 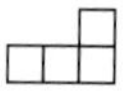 39–42 m 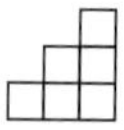 48 m 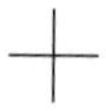 Man 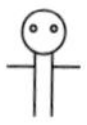	Monocular testing possible in majority	Speech/word tests and pure tone audiometry in each ear
5 years	Shows great precision in hand movements and in the use of tools. Can cut a strip of paper neatly, and when building bricks holds the cubes with the ulnar fingers tucked in and hand diagonal to get a better view. Can feed tidily with a spoon and fork, dress and brush teeth. Refinement of finger movements can be demonstrated by increasing speed at inserting pegs in a board and threading beads Copies 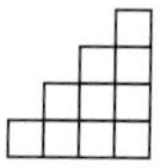 □ 60 m △ 66 m 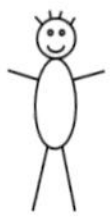 50 m+	Screening recommended by orthoptists in school	Audiometric screening recommended in school

Fig. 7.2 (*Continued*)

child has just learned to draw a circle and during the next year will add to this – vertical lines to represent legs, horizontal lines as arms and one or two features such as eyes and mouth (Fig. 7.4). It is not until 5 years that arms and legs are appropriately placed on a trunk (Fig. 7.5) At this age children can also draw a square and therefore a house with windows (some can do this at a younger age; Fig. 7.6).

LANGUAGE, SPEECH AND COMMUNICATIVE DEVELOPMENT

An essential feature of human life is the use of a system of symbols for communication and thought. The attachment of names to objects and actions is an essential prerequisite not only for language but also for thinking. If we had no such system we would need to produce the object itself each time we wished to discuss it. This is just what an infant or a child with a learning disability does. It is conventional to consider 'speech' separately from 'language' and both as having 'receptive' and 'expressive', or 'input' and 'output' components. The component structures of language are:

1. the phonological (the perception and production of sounds to words and sentences);
2. the semantics and syntax (words, their meaning, the small grammatical features – morphemes and rules combining words in sentences).

Pragmatics refers to the understanding and use of language in context.

Overview of theories applied to speech, language and communicative development

Theories of language development range from the structural linguistic to the functional social and from language as a

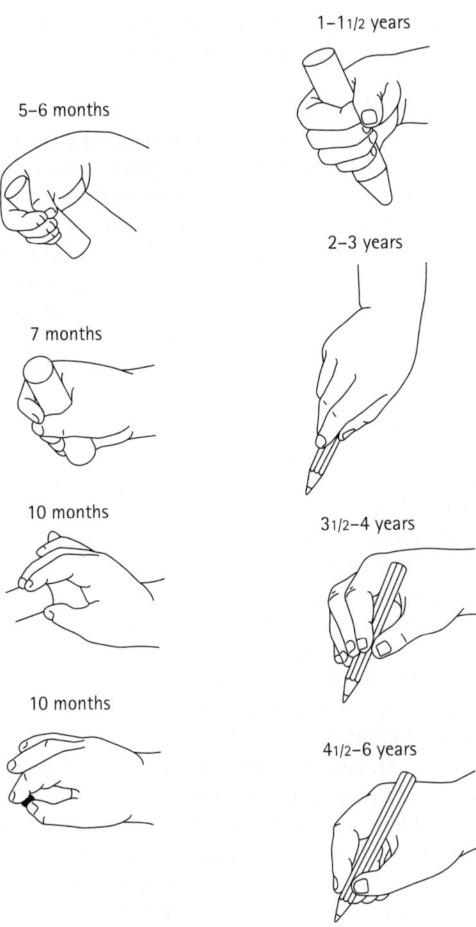

Fig. 7.3 Grasping. (Illustrations from The Erhardt Development Prehension Assessment, from Developmental Hand Dysfunction, 2nd edn.[17] Copyright © 1994 by Rohda P Erhardt. Published by Erhardt Developmental Products, Maplewood MN 55119, USA. Reprinted by permission.)

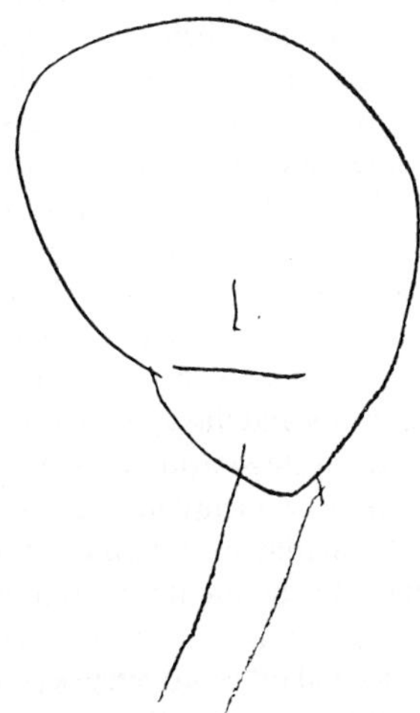

Fig. 7.4 By 3 years the child has learned to draw a circle and during the next year will add to this – vertical lines to represent legs, horizontal lines as arms and one or two features such as eyes and mouth.

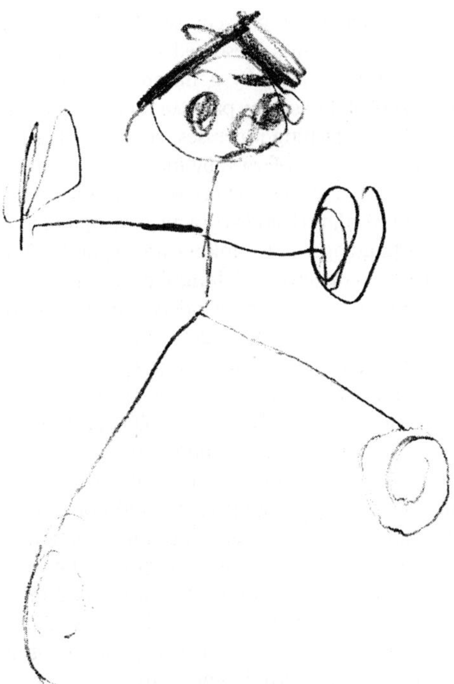

Fig. 7.5 It is not until 5 years that arms and legs are appropriately placed on a trunk.

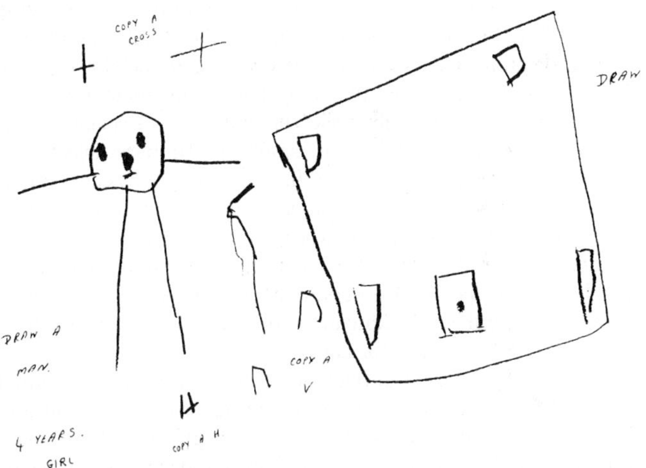

Fig. 7.6 At 5 years, children can draw a square and therefore a house with windows.

domain-specific skill to a continuity of general cognitive processes applied to linguistic symbols.

Chomsky[2] proposed that the brain must be preprogrammed to extract and master the specific grammatical structures of spoken language. He introduced the concept of the 'language acquisition device', suggesting the nativist view that language is a robust and preprogrammed biological function, separate, to some extent, from other intellectual functions and dependent only to a limited extent on environmental input. Some children with specific language impairments have a particular problem with acquisition of grammatical morphemes, leading to the search for particular grammatical markers of language impairment.

The 'decoding–encoding' motor programming – execution aspects of structural linguistic speech and language learning – have led to theories of abnormalities of auditory processing and auditory short term memory and a psycholinguistic model of assessment and remediation.

'Connectionist theories' of computer simulated parallel processing combine sensitivity to language input with dependence on a learning architecture in the brain. Models have been described for the learning of past tenses of verbs, vocabulary, concept words and syntax. Learning takes place as the system is presented with regular and then irregular verbs and is modulated by a number of weighted activations assessing the probability of any particular ending for any particular verb stem. General learning processes, such as imitation and context bound chunk learning, followed by increasing symbolic representational development and abstraction with creativity, are thought to be important in word, verb and syntactic development.

The degree to which language and thinking are separable has taxed theorists. Vygotsky[20] conceives of language as a speech processing/word formation system developing independently and, for technical perfection and intelligibility, dependent upon a domain-specific learning system. However, the meaning of the speech processed and used depends on the social context in which it is learned, and this has its basis in the social cognitive ability of the child as well as the environment and responsiveness of the parent/caregiver. Thus language acquisition is inseparable from the development of social communication, both verbal and non-verbal, and the social relationship. The meaning of communication is learned in a social cultural context and requires broader social–cognitive skills to interpret the meaning of all the coordinated forms of communication, such as body posture, facial expression, eye gaze, tone of voice, speech and gestures, which are all smoothly combined in the adult – the pragmatics of language use.

The child is an active partner in language acquisition. Babies have an innate social interest in other humans, displaying an early ability to perceive aspects of the face and the meaning of facial expressions and posture, actions and sounds in varying combinations, and are therefore programmed to develop an interest in human communication. The baby responds to facial expression and tone of voice (6 months) long before he understands the meaning of words. The baby seeks the 'meaning' of social actions from a number of cues, especially emotions. Mothers reflect back certain things babies do and give them meaning. Physical actions are usually easy to interpret. The understanding that the focus of an adult's visual attention is likely to be what they are talking about, is an important cognitive step. The child's understanding that objects have labels is helped by the spontaneous behavior of adults who when they see children looking at or pointing to an object, will tend to name it (e.g. 'yes, that's the cat').

The child and parent develop 'joint' attention through shared actions.[21] The child learns to coordinate his or her attention and interest between an object and person, seen in gaze switching, facial expressions and vocalizing. The baby uses sounds in a reciprocal or turn-taking manner before they are intelligible as words. Early conversations have all the important elements of social discourse, initiating, responding and repair (i.e. making some effort if the exchange breaks down). Towards the end of the first year, the baby shows increasing awareness of self and others and becomes an intentional communicator, also showing anticipation of the parents' actions, intentions and feelings, and checking the parents' response to new situations by observing their facial expression ('social referencing').

The initiation of shared interest with an adult by the child is a very good marker of normally developing social communication skills in a child of 12–18 months. Gaze switching and the frequency of this behavior in a play situation is easily observed. Communication accompanied by eye gaze has greater social meaning. The child learns to form predictions of complexes of behaviors. Early joint attention skills are deficient in children with autism[22] and representational forms of communication may not be understood as having relevant meaning. In blind children, establishing meaning can be particularly difficult. For the deaf child in a speaking household this can also be a problem. For the learning disabled child (e.g. Down syndrome) it is a slow process needing more time for both assimilation and response.

Vocalization and speech

The development of vocalization and speech depends upon an intact motor learning system as well as hearing speech, and evolves rapidly from a limited repertoire of sounds during the first few months. From about 6 months onwards, the sound patterns take on the qualities of adult speech. By the end of the first year, the sound patterns of the child's 'native' language are established and the ability to discriminate the sounds of other languages diminishes (e.g. 9-month-olds prefer to listen to native words rather than non-native). They learn to reproduce pairs of syllables by integrating the sequences in which they are presented as well as the rhythm (at 6 months babies are sensitive to the rhythm, but not the sequences of syllables). Strings of babble become more connected, intonation takes on the pattern of adult speech and the child begins to imitate phrases and words. At this stage, the words and sentences may not be analyzed into their component parts. The child may copy a whole word or phrase by the rhythm it makes.

Children vary in their rote memory capacity for memorizing chunks of speech. Constant practice in making sounds reinforces motor patterns, which become increasingly automatic. The amount of babble is correlated with early vocabulary. Abnormal or infrequent speech sounds in the first year can be a marker of later speech and language problems or deafness. The alert parent will note such signs, but often only in the second child.

At the early stages of communicative development some children may tend to use gestures without also using spoken words, while other children use both gestures and words. Bates et al[23] suggested that this reflected individual variation in communicative style or preference. The developmental sequelae of these different early communicative styles are not known. Fenson et al[24] suggested that symbolic and communicative gestures may act as a 'bridge'[25] from word comprehension to word production.

Pointing behavior is particularly important because it indicates a precise referent on the part of the child rather than undifferentiated need and is a precursor of symbolic development.

Two reasons for pointing behaviors can be observed.

1. Proto-imperative 'indicating' behaviors represent the child's demand for needs to be met. This may be done by pointing or vocalization. Such behaviors do not necessarily involve any shared interest or attention (or mental idea of other people).
2. In contrast, proto-declarative communicative behaviors are a preverbal effort to direct the adult's attention to an event or object. This purpose of pointing is to 'share' interest with another person. Proto-declarative behaviors correlate highly with the emergence of first words, and predict in normal development the vocabulary at 20 months and the sentence length at 28 months.

During the first 10-word stage words may be largely imitative or bound to context, they may be formulaic and learned in association with a particular event and may be presymbolic. The words are not necessarily securely fixed in the mental representational linguistic system.

The first words that a child utters are very dependent upon shared referents with parents, for example in the Korean culture, verbs are commoner than nouns; the opposite is true in English speakers. The proportion of early vocabulary that consists of context-bound phrases (names of people and objects) or communicative social words (such as 'look' or 'here y'are', or words such as 'more' and 'gone') in a way that was thought to describe two extremes of language learning, referential or expressive, varies. Most children use both styles.

Language and thinking are intimately related as the child learns to map words onto existing thoughts or concepts and the learning of a word can stimulate new concepts. While acquiring early vocabulary the child's next cognitive stage is the move from the primary and simple associative use of the sounds of language to a more symbolic, representational and decontextualized use. Overextensions are common at this stage (e.g. 'daddy' for all men).

Comprehension of language is in advance of expression in normal development. Nouns are the largest class of words in early vocabularies. When new words are used, a child tries to find a meaning for them. The development of grammar does not seem to depend on repeating adult structures; rather children seem to extract the rules of grammar and experiment for themselves, sometimes to comical effect – for example:

Lucy: 'Squeak, squeak – that's what mouses does.'
Mother: 'That's what mice do.'
Lucy: 'What do mices does?'[26]

Wide normal range

As with many skills of development there is a wide normal variation in the acquisition of speech and language (e.g. in the MacArthur scales[23]). At 16 months children in the top 10% produce 154words, those in the lowest 10% produce none; 80% of children at 16 months understand between 78 and 303 words (–1.28 SD to +1.28 SD). Severe delays have predictive significance, but there is no best age for determining milder speech and language delays. Also a child who is delayed at 18 months will not necessarily be delayed at 3 years.

SOCIAL LEARNING, SELF AND OTHERS, PLAY AND ADAPTIVE SKILLS

Social learning, self and others, play and adaptive skills include:

1. the child's social reactions to other persons and to peers through the development of attachments and social understanding;
2. development of self-awareness and self-regulation;
3. mastery of skills such as feeding, elimination and dressing.

The normal development of cognitive and adaptive skills, play, language comprehension and speech, communication and social interaction is outlined in Table 7.3.

Table 7.3 Normal development of cognitive and adaptive skills, play, language comprehension and speech, communication and social interaction

Age	Play	Personal skills	Communication/ social interaction	Comprehension	Speech
6–8 weeks			Smiles responsively when mother talks to/smiles at. Opens and closes mouth imitatively		
3 months	Interested in everything seen/ increasing intention to touch objects		Vocal turntaking, gurgles/coos with pleasure. Generally social to friendly adult but knows caregiver	Regularly localizes speaker with eyes	Often vocalizes with two or more different syllables
6 months	Reaches for and grasps toys, usually both hands- takes to mouth. Watches objects disappear – no sustained searching. Excited by familiar toy	Tries to hold cup/bottle, poor tipping	Shares interest by gaze and gesture in peek-a-boo game. Makes noise to get attention. Tries to imitate (e.g. tongue protrusion). Smiles at image of self in mirror	Situational understanding of familiar phrase and angry/ friendly voices. Localizes and recognizes different speakers	Occasionally vocalizes with four or more different syllables at one time. Non-specific indication of emotion/ need etc. but tries to attract attention vocally
9 months	Persistent in getting toys. Transfers toys hand-to-hand, bangs toys (7 m). Looks for objects that disappear. Stage of 'sensorimotor' play and early 'cause and effect'. Pulls string to get toy	Interested in mirror play. Aware of different types of clothing. Finger feeds and early chewing. Some anticipation of familiar events	Responds to parental 'indicating' gesture. Beginnings of imitation of gesture (e.g. waves-bye-bye, claps hands 10 months) and shows joint attention – ability to switch gaze between object and person to share interest. Understands and takes part in lap games with anticipation, demanding of repeated 'games' (e.g. peek-a-boo). Now more wary of strangers	Regularly stops activity in response to 'no'. Responds to own name and names of familiar people (e.g. 'daddy'). Understands gestures (e.g. gives toys or other objects to a parent on verbal request) but may not yet have skills of release	Intonated babble with sequences of sounds. Babble more complete with different vowels and consonants. Imitates sounds. Attracts attention to self frequently
Around 12 months	'Container' play putting objects in and out. Interested in picture book. Finds hidden objects. Shows recognition of familiar objects (e.g. brush, telephone, cup and spoon and car). Less mouthing, may 'cast' – throw objects on floor. Imitates actions with objects (e.g. clicks bricks, rings bell, tries to build bricks)	Cooperates with dressing by putting arms up. Drinks from beaker held by self	Points to indicate need. Separation anxiety on leaving parent common. Quite distractible and switches to new dominant stimulus easily. Repeats performance to be laughed at	Generally shows intense attention and response to speech over prolonged periods of time – understands people's names and familiar words (e.g. 'shoes'/responds to familiar requests)	'Talks' to toys and people throughout the day using long verbal patterns – protowords, or words accompanying communicative gesture. Shakes head for 'no'

(Continued)

Table 7.3 (Continued)

Age	Play	Personal skills	Communication/ social interaction	Comprehension	Speech
Around 15 months	Early definition by use of play on self (e.g. brushes hair or mother's hair). Builds two-cube tower. Uses pencil to mark paper. Plays to and fro game with ball or truck	Increasing awareness of self/others shown in shift of object play from self to doll, use of me/ mine pronouns and awareness of aspects of self in mirror Increasingly persistent in attaining goals May indicate when wet	Frequent communication initiated by child accompanied by showing and bringing of toys and pointing for interest and need. Follows adult point at object	Simple requests in context. Recognizes and identifies many named in familiar surroundings. Points to pictures in book	More frequent use of words with meaning, final or beginning consonant often missing. Asks for objects by vocalizing and pointing
Around 18 months	Uses real and toy objects appropriately. Briefly imitates everyday domestic and personal activities. Shows preference in play. May use dolly/teddy to feed/put to bed. Builds a tower of three bricks. Can match circular shapes in insert puzzle	Feeds self with spoon without rotating it at mouth Takes off hat/shoes Bowel control often attained Alternates between clinging and resistance	Attends to own choice of activity, but attention can be caught by calling name and producing new toy. Verbally requests and comments Watches others play and plays near them	Listens to adult and identifies two or more familiar objects on request from a group of four or more familiar objects. Generally understands more than 100 words in familiar setting	Begins repeating words overheard in conversation – uses minimum of 10–20 words spontaneously – range of vowels and m, p, b, t, d, n (mean 50–100)
Around 24 months	Play now more toy based linking actions (e.g. feed doll and then put to bed). Builds tower of six/seven bricks. Turns pages of book singly. Copies line with pencil. Able to play for more lengthy periods of time Turns door knob and unscrews lids	Dry by day, pulls pants up and down Helps with simple putting away when asked Understands spills and tries to rectify Behavior can be active and oppositional	Mainly with adult still – watches other children. Simple chase games develop Wants to please adult/shows off	Recognizes new words daily at an ever-increasing rate. Listens to conversations and responds. Carries out simple instructions. Understands objects by function (e.g. which one do we sit on). Points to several body parts	Speaks more and more new words each week, gesture used less often. Echoes some of the adult's speech. Puts words together in phrases 'me go'. Verbally very demanding
Around 36 months	Builds tower of eight cubes. Vivid make believe. Understands stories, can make plans. Beginning to draw recognizable man with head, eyes, legs. Copies circle and can do simple inset puzzle (orientate and insert all pieces) and match colors. Can unbutton buttons. Tries to cut with scissors. Able to show sustained concentration	Feeds with spoon and fork Shows a sense of danger Understands rules, right and wrong behavior related to self – more amenable. Can remove front opening garment and many other clothes Attends to toilet needs without help	Can share, comfort others distressed. Plays with other children. Affectionate and confiding Shows understanding that others can 'know' things. Shows sense of humor Understands polite behavior	Understands on/in/under/ big/little. Can give full name, age and sex. Beginning to count. Understands why, who, how many and questions such as 'what should you do when you're hungry?'	Uses sentences of three-four word phrases, personal pronouns, plurals and prepositions. Asks 'what', 'where' and beginning to ask 'why'? Relates own experiences. Able to have simple conversations. Immaturities of articulation still common but mostly intelligible
Around 48 months	Able to show sustained concentration More extended make-believe Draws man with body Copies cross and six brick steps	Aware of being in a group and expected behaviors		Understands concepts of number up to 3, colors, listens to a short story and can answer simple questions about it. Can listen to and answer two-part question and understand some words relating to feelings. Likes rhymes	Sentences of four-eight words, mostly grammatically correct. Counts to 10. Talks about experiences and can retell a simple story. Uses approximately 1500 words
Around 5–6 years	Copies square (5) and triangle (6) and ten-brick step from a model. Draws a man with head, body and features and a house with windows	Can care for most toilet needs independently. Can dress self except for shoe laces	Can have conversations, tell jokes and discuss emotions. Able to retell in a different way to assist others' understanding. Most children show 'first order theory of mind' (i.e. that someone else can 'know' something that is different and may be incorrect) Makes friends and has a preferred friend	Knows simple time concepts, can follow three commands together. Can define common objects in terms of use and answer 'what if' questions. Understands common opposite (e.g. hot/cold). Follows instructions given in a group. Can tell an unfamiliar story from pictures	Speech completely intelligible including consonant blends (e.g. Sh, th), rate, pitch and volume

Social learning, becoming aware of self and others, and the development of other play and adaptive skills marks the change from a dim awareness of self and mother to an understanding of the complex rules of social behavior and interaction. Even neonates are socially competent, in that they are able to elicit the attention of their parents. It has been shown that mothers respond to their babies' behavior more often than the other way round. Thus features of infant temperament and his or her potential for social communicative drive and competence will be relevant to how the parent behaves. Studies of blind babies and their mothers show how easy it is for parents to miss cues for communication when they are not conventional. The non-initiating, non-responding, autistic child soon trains a parent not to initiate interaction. The parent of the baby with Down syndrome needs to wait for the often rather slower initiating and responding behavior so that the rhythmic turn taking of communication is not lost.

Babies respond to the human face and to objects quite differently. In response to a face their eyes widen, posture is relaxed and by 6 weeks a smile arises. This simple milestone is a very reliable indicator of abnormality if delayed beyond 8 weeks. During the latter half of the first year babies lose their indiscriminate warm response to all people and begin to recognize familiar adults and to become wary of strangers. They develop a strong attachment to their caretakers and separation at this time and during the second year of life is particularly distressing to a child. Securely attached children who are confident of their mother's warm presence are able during the second year to begin to explore and to achieve mastery of feeding and elimination.

An important stage of social cognitive development is that of joint attention (described in the language section above) shown in the transition from dyadic to triadic attention (from focus on object or focus on person to focus on object then switching focus to person and back again to object). The latter involves the sharing of focus, which is the indication of interest by the child and recognition that there is mutuality of meaning with the parent and the sharing of an idea. Such behavior appears to be the precursor of social understanding of others' feelings and perspectives, the knowing that other people have minds. Understanding other people's emotions is an important part of learning about them and sharing those feelings may lead to the development of empathy. Emotional 'knowing' and 'display' may not be the same as understanding the thinking of other minds (a connected but possibly separable skill).[27] Understanding and using the knowledge of how someone else might feel is also an important component of moral development.

In normal development, children initiate joint attention. They direct their parents to something they are interested in and respond to parental behavior that does the same, shown by gaze shifts to share looking at things and following index finger pointing. The social referencing behavior of children, in new situations, when they scan the faces of people, but especially parents, to give them cues about how they should then respond, is seen in the last trimester of the first year.

The child shows increasing independence from adults and awareness of self in relation to others during the second and third year, and this is observable both in play and language use.

During the nursery years (3–5 years) children's horizons widen as they are faced with a new social world of adults and other children. The child becomes less egocentric and learns how to play with other children, taking into account their wishes and needs, although the cognitive capacity to consider two perspectives simultaneously and reflect upon them in a judgmental way does not mature until nearer 8 or more years.

Behavior should get easier as reasoning becomes more possible and the child learns about 'deferment'. Instead of just reacting, children cognitively appraise and interpret events. The personal memories that form the basis of reflection are constructed from the experiences of the child woven into a mental schema or narrative of representations and feelings. Ideas of truth and moral rightness develop. For example, young school-age children (but not preschoolers) can accept an action by someone who is mistaken in their belief, but not where they are morally wrong. Thus it is alright to give more food to boys than girls if you believe they need more but not if it is done because it is OK to be nicer to boys![28] Moral development, the rules and conventions of interpersonal behavior, require both the behavioral opportunities for learning (i.e. example, reinforcement, rules/punishment) and the cognitive skills to be able to take perspectives and self-reflect. The environment needs to be:

1. warm;
2. not punitive;
3. model what is appropriate;
4. emphasize other people's feelings and perspectives.

The child obtains final mastery of dressing and toileting self-help skills, and by 5 years of age is ready for school. The child is, however, still essentially home based in outlook and influences. During the primary school years, the rules of the group become increasingly important, so that by 10 years of age they are often quoted to parents in a rather rebellious way. At this age boys and girls tend to form separate groups or gangs and the peer group social perspective becomes more important. The teenager is able to think in the abstract, work out the principles behind actions and is therefore able to become more independent. Freeing from parental authority is associated with a desire for acceptance and popularity in the peer group. However, developing sexual maturity is associated with many other concerns, which are dealt with in the chapter on adolescence (see Ch. 34).

COGNITIVE AND LEARNING DEVELOPMENT

Children learn about their world by listening, observing, copying and experimenting. The world of infants is very small and their repertoire of skills limited. They learn about their world through observation, by reaching and grasping objects and by copying sounds and actions. In contrast, toddlers are mobile and their worlds are large. Their motor skills are greater and they begin to attempt constructional tasks, thereby learning about aspects such as size, shape, the properties of objects and space.

The child is an active participant in the learning process. Progress depends upon not only the learning opportunities, but the learning strategies and processes within the child. Information processing in infants is related to later cognitive abilities in memory and speed of processing, thus in visual recognition tasks, habituation, learning, object permanence and attention, including crossmodality.

In older children, the features of new problem solving that are linked to learning are variability, ability to shift focus, frequency of self-correction and diversity of strategies.

Problems with the learning process

In some infants, perceptual processing that depends upon innate recognition may be damaged and perceptual attributes that lead to salience may not be perceived. Perception that depends upon temporal processing may be slowed and crossmodality may be impaired. Meaning may be more easily accessed visually (i.e. what is seen may make more sense than what is heard). Infants learn from the repeated familiar and respond to difference – a learning style used in the 'habituation to repeat stimulus' in developmental experiment.

Learning from the familiar needs repeated stimulus and is enhanced if as many features as possible are fixed and what is remembered depends upon the match between context and item. This is a stage of normal development referred to as 'context bound' learning, when children recognize their own cups or shoes, for example, but not 'cupness' or a sentence said by one person in one place, but not another. Some children get stuck in this stage and require a sustained high degree of contextual or environmental sameness to show a skill. This is particularly shown in autism.[29]

Children learn from 'contingency' – the event that follows within 3–5 s of their action. This may be disrupted by a number of mechanisms, such as:

1. failure of the adult to make the response (depressed/mentally ill caregiver);
2. the child not giving a clear enough signal (as for those who are blind or who have cerebral palsy).

Aspects of maternal or caregiver behavior that promote learning need to be sensitively adjusted to developmental level. Thus at 2 years of age, language input needs to be explicitly directive and adult actions tied to the focus of child interests. By 3 years less parental directive is needed because the child has more language and is learning to manage own goal setting and problem solving skills.

Play complexity is enhanced by caregiver behaviors that maintain a child's focus of attention rather than redirect it. Children also learn more through the process of learning itself. For example, learning particular names of shapes accelerates shape learning generally, as though attention to the 'shape concept' allows noticing of 'shapeness'. The child's ability to inhibit and select responses and to try alternatives is crucial to all cognitive learning. This is seen in the progression from the 'trial and error' approach, where repeatedly forcing the square into the round hole is a less useful strategy than trying alternative placements with inset puzzles, which shows more flexibility of mental skills.

The progress from sensorimotor play, from mouthing to manipulation at 6–10 months, then to imitation and definition by use play by 12 months is followed by increasing creativity in play. Make-believe play with dolls, in which the child is reconstructing events observed, is an important element of this period. It indicates early symbolic representation and concept formation. The child begins to use language to direct or describe the action of his play, and as command of language improves the need to act out the events decreases. Lack of ideas, failure of pretence and inability to play constructively are indications of a developmental problem.

The cognitive stage of mental symbolic development allows more complex thinking, including reflection and planning. Symbols (words) facilitate thinking about, and reference to, situations that are not in the 'here and now'. The answering of simple questions dealing with non-present situations presents difficulty as late as 3 years. Even primary and junior school children still tend to be concrete in their way of thinking (i.e. real objects, here and now). Early in school life, judgments are made intuitively on superficial appearances. With increasing experience and language at their disposal, children can imagine complex situations, think out the most appropriate solution and anticipate the outcome. This requires the ability to think abstractly and imaginatively. Thus, children develop logical thinking from assimilating experience into schemes or general laws that they can apply to a range of situations. The use of symbols also helps to inhibit prepotent responses of behaviors and allows increasing distancing from the 'here and now' (rather like the red card in football games). Children are developing skills of representation and object substitution in the second year, but the skill of mentally comparing reality with representation (dual reality) is not clearly seen in research studies until aged 3 years. For example, children shown where an object is hidden in a scale model of a room can find it in the real room at 3 years, but not at 30 months. At 3–6 years, children get increasingly skilled at knowing that others can hold particular views, even false views, and thus have what has been called a 'theory of mind'. In the classic Wimmer and Perner task, roughly half the 4–5-year-olds could correctly show 'knowing', whereas over 90% of 6–9-year-old children were correct.[30] This understanding of children's thinking is highly relevant when considering children's perceptions of events and their reporting of them.

DETECTING AND ASSESSING DEVELOPMENTAL PROBLEMS

Developmental impairments, learning and behavior problems are common. One of the aims of a child health service is to detect any impairment early enough to ameliorate or even prevent secondary disability and handicap. The debate is concerned with 'how' and 'which problems' at 'what ages' are significant.

SCREENING

Screening is the presumptive identification of unrecognized disease or defect by the application of tests, examinations or other procedures that can be applied to a whole population. The criteria of Wilson & Jungner[31] Cochrane & Holland[32] need to be applied to any condition and to any screening test (Table 7.4).

Table 7.4 The criteria of Wilson & Jungner[31] and Cochrane & Holland[32]

1. The condition being sought for should be an important health problem for both the individual and the community
2. There should be an acceptable form of treatment for those with recognized disease or some other form of useful intervention should be available (e.g. genetic advice)
3. The natural history of the condition should be adequately understood
4. There should be a recognizable latent or early symptomatic stage
5. Equity of access across a geographic area must be ensured
6. There should be a suitable test for detecting the early or latent stage that is acceptable to the population. The distribution of test value should be known with an agreed cutoff, high sensitivity, specificity and high positive predictive value
7. There must be an agreed method of diagnosis in the screen positive and there must be systems in place for adequate diagnosis and counseling. It is important to note that there are dangers to overinclusiveness in the 'at risk' group. Research has shown that the worry of a false positive screen does not disappear easily
8. There should be an agreed policy on who should be treated
9. The treatment in the presymptomatic stage should be able to favorably influence the course and prognosis of the disease
10. It is important to ensure that all the above criteria for a screening program are met before primary care groups and districts embark upon it. Experience has shown that it is much more difficult to stop than to start a widespread program
11. The cost of case finding which should include the cost of diagnosis and treatment should be economically balanced in relation to the possible expenditure on medical care as a whole and the constant treatment of the patient does not present until the disease reaches the symptomatic stage
12. Case finding should be a continuing process

Any test has to be simple, quick, easy to interpret, acceptable to parents, accurate and repeatable. It should be:

1. Sensitive – that is it should have the ability to give a positive finding if the person has the impairment.
2. Specific– that is, it should have an ability to give a negative result in a person with no impairment.

In considering sensitivity and specificity the prevalence of the disease is very important. The ideal is high sensitivity and high specificity, but in practice one is usually at the expense of the other.

Screening for developmental impairments

Enthusiasm for early detection of impairments by professionals led to a program of universal developmental checks added to visits to 'well baby' clinics at several time points in the preschool years in the UK and the use of specific screening tests. Of the impairments that potentially affect development, hearing impairment is one of those that would meet the criteria listed in Table 7.4. The 'health visitor distraction test' although reliable in skilled hands, did not show adequate sensitivity when applied across the population, but the cochlear echo test should meet all criteria.

Inspection of the eyes looking for obvious ocular pathology is recommended as part of the neonatal examination, but thereafter screening for impairment of vision and for refractive errors or amblyopia, using visual acuity measures, is not recommended until 4 years of age. Then screening should be carried out by orthoptists because of the difficulty of training and achieving good enough results using behavioral tests carried out by a variety of people on small children.

Screening for developmental impairment presents particular problems. Not only is development a continuous process, but the range of normal in almost all areas is wide, so that the cut-off for definite abnormality is not always clear. Neither is the best time point for judging this clear. Continuity of developmental problems is concerned with the predictive outcome of a particular delay at any moment in time.

The continuity from very early developmental assessment depends upon the number of skill areas that show impairment and their degree. Thus, for example, a delay in one area of development alone is much less predictive than delays in all. Also, as a generalization, the younger the child, the less easy it is to be predictive about the outcome and hence the necessity of intervention. What is a 'case' is not always clear. This is especially true in child development, when there is frequently considerable overlap in the developmental item between those who have a problem and those who do not. It is a particular problem in the consideration of screening for language delays because separation from disorders is not clear cut.[33,34]

Comparisons are usually made with norm-based measures, but as the example of walking delay at 18 months shows, clear cut-offs at any particular age are bound to include a mix of biologically based abnormality, general learning problems and normal variants.[35] Another problem with developmental assessment is that what is most important in the long term for any particular child is the integration of their skills and functions with the emotional and behavioral regulation necessary for adapting to their environment, for example, being able to problem solve. Thus developmental tasks that do not assess integrated functions or fail to take into account how the child functions 'on line' in real life may miss very significant impairments. The concept of using very specific screening tests for general development, including language, has not been found to fulfil the Cochrane & Holland criteria as outlined in Table 7.4, and has led to review of the recommendations and the conclusion that current screening for many developmental problems is untenable. The reader is referred to *Health for all Children*[36] and the American Academy of Pediatrics statement.[37] This has to be balanced against the findings that parents want to know about developmental problems early and that early intervention shows positive effects. For example, there is increasing evidence that appropriately targeted intervention improves outcomes in children with autistic spectrum disorders (reviewed by the National Research Council[38]), but a screening study of the general population showed at best moderate sensitivity only.[39,40]

Such a professionally initiated activity as developmental screening, using tests, also negates the immensely important role that parents have in detecting developmental impairments. Most very severe impairments of motor or visual or general learning skills, not detected at birth, are detected by parents. Two-thirds of children with cerebral palsy had this diagnosis confirmed by 24 months, in a recent population-based study, and 89 out of 145 were detected by the parent or other family member (Baird & Scrutton, unpublished data).

This leaves the much more difficult minor disabilities and developmental problems in the preschool years to be detected by other means. What families require is a rapid response to their concerns by way of a full assessment, which should lead to effective planning of management. Access to health service resources is an issue and many districts have had to develop imaginative schemes to ensure that particular ethnic groups, travelers and asylum populations receive both health and developmental care. There are particular challenges attached to 'looked after' children who may change geographic location frequently yet have mixed complex problems.

Using parental knowledge

Glascoe[41,42] has developed and evaluated an interesting model of seeking developmental concerns and evaluating the response needed using a simple series of questions, which has the advantage of being able to be used at any age in the preschool years, the PEDS – Parents' Evaluation of Developmental Status (1997). She has found that parental concerns, carefully elicited, have a 75–80% sensitivity to childhood disability and 70–80% specificity for normal development. These questions are intended to be asked of parents.

1. Do you have any concerns about your child's learning, development or behavior?
2. Do you have any concerns about how your child talks and makes speech sounds?
3. Do you have any concerns about how your child understands what you say?
4. Do you have any concerns about how your child uses his or her hands or feet to do things?
5. Do you have any concerns about how your child uses his or her arms or legs?
6. Do you have any concerns about how your child behaves?
7. Do you have any concerns about how your child gets along with others?
8. Do you have any concerns about how your child is learning to do things for him or herself?
9. Do you have any concerns about how your child is learning preschool or school skills?
10. Do you have any other concerns?

Glascoe[42] has shown that parents who have no concerns (and where there is no literacy/language barrier) tend to have children without disabilities. Decisions about who to assess further can be based on the results of the PEDS. For example, a parent who has two or more significant concerns about the child should be referred for appropriate assessment without more screening. One significant concern should elicit a further screen in the appropriate skill and this improves specificity.

Surveillance

In the UK, current recommendations are that, rather than a professional model of testing all children by regular developmental checks, using something like the Denver Developmental Screening Test (which has limited sensitivity and specificity), there should be 'a parent partnership model'. In this model, emerging skills in development are discussed with parents on a regular basis in the preschool years. Parental concern can be responded to rapidly and an area of specific concern can be further evaluated by the use of a test.

It is thought that leaving the onus of initiation of concern entirely to parents would lead to inequity of health care, with the likelihood that those members of society most in need would find themselves least able to access care (the so-called 'inverse care' law). The job of the professional is to respond to parental concerns to help a parent see that there is a concern, to bring the parents to the point of seeking advice, and to provide assistance and a pathway to do so.

The concept of parent/professional partnership in which either can initiate contact is called 'surveillance'. This is not necessarily a particularly good or popular term as it has connotations of 'big brother'. As part of this process, a number of other health related activities may be encompassed in the primary care aim of ensuring a good enough environment for all aspects of physical and mental health development. For example, accident prevention, positive health promotion including eating advice and the prevention of further diseases through the immunization program.[36]

Responding to parental concern

Any parental concern should be taken extremely seriously. It must be the experience of all pediatricians that parental concern is ignored at one's peril. Fictitious illness is less common than the parent being right and the professional failing to recognize it.

One of the goals of a District Health Service is rapid response to developmental concern by referral to a profession or group of professionals with the training and competence to adequately assess the presence or absence of impairment by means of a 'developmental assessment and examination' in a way that meets the wide cultural needs of a population and differences in parent style and needs.

Such an examination will usually take place away from the child's normal environment and will follow the pattern of history, observation of the child's specific engagement on tasks and then a physical examination.

A major change in the examination of young children with possible developmental problems is the number of norm-based psychometrically constructed tests with standard methods of administration available that examine or test behavior in a number of areas and provide a profile of development.

PROBLEMS WITH DEVELOPMENT

For the infant and very young child

For the infant and very young child (i.e. under 18 months), most major defects will present neonatally, at the at-risk follow-up clinic or to the family. The presenting developmental concerns are those of disorders of motor development, vision and hearing, and general development, static and progressive. Many children with visual and motor impairments also have other learning problems.

After 18 months of age

After 18 months of age, problems with speech and language, global delays, motor competence and behavior problems typically present.

It is conventional to describe 'delays' of development (meaning normal but slow patterns of skill acquisition) and 'disorders' (where the pattern is abnormal). In practice the two coincide frequently and distinction may not be possible or even logical.

Estimates of prevalence of neurodevelopmental problems are shown in Table 7.5.[43]

Developmental assessment

Developmental assessment starts with 'information gathering' from all who know the child either informally or more formally using checklists. It then encompasses the 'interview' with parents/caregivers and the 'examination' of the child. The process results in a conclusion, if possible a diagnosis with an etiological explanation, but always a plan of action to meet needs.

Knowledge of the normal patterns of child development enables us to assess the developmental level of a particular child. Comprehensive professional assessment is or should be multidisciplinary. Families need to understand the process of

Table 7.5 Neurodevelopmental problems and estimates of their prevalence in parentheses[43]

Learning impairments
1. Severe learning disability (3.5/1000)
2. Moderate learning difficulties IQ 50–70 (1.8%)
3. Specific learning difficulty including dyslexia (underestimated at 2%)
4. Down syndrome (1/1000)

Motor impairments
1. Cerebral palsy (2.5/1000) – hemiplegia (30%); diplegia (20%); other types (50%)
2. Clumsy child syndrome – developmental coordination disorder (5%); deficits in attention, motor control and perception (1–3%) (overlaps with attention deficit disorder and with hyperactivity)
3. Neural tube defects (1/1000)
4. Hydrocephalus (0.1/1000)

Neuromuscular disorders
1. Duchenne muscular dystrophy (3/100 000)
2. Other neuromuscular disorders

Other chronic neurological disorders
1. Neurodegenerative disorders
2. Other chronic neurological disorders – survivors of brain infections, such as meningitis or encephalitis; damaged survivors of head injury; brain malformations
3. Epilepsy (0.8%) – usually associated with other disorders to require child development service

Speech, language and communication disorders
1. Severe speech language disorder (5/1000)
2. Autistic spectrum disorders (including Asperger's syndrome) (6/1000)

Visual impairment
1. Partially sighted (0.4/1000)
2. Blind (0.3/1000)

Hearing impairment
Significant impairment (> 50 dB loss in better ear) (1.5/1000)

Many children have two or more coexisting disorders

Associated problems
1. Behavior (up to 30%)
2. Nutrition/gastroesophageal reflux/constipation
3. Recurrent respiratory infection
4. Orthopedic deformities
5. Other medical problems (e.g. asthma)
6. Social and family problems

assessment to be able to share in it. The process needs to be sensitive to, and assess, the family's needs, awareness, concerns and broader cultural issues. It should occur as locally to the child's home as possible. This requires flexibility and an emphasis on needs and family centered services rather than being professionally driven.

All services should aim to:

1. enhance the parents' understanding of their child;
2. promote the relationship between parent and child;
3. support families as the most significant caregivers;
4. identify services to meet needs, provide practical help and emotional support;
5. use language that is understood by all;
6. evaluate barriers to service use by families.

The history

The general aspects of taking a history described in Chapter 3 apply to the child who presents with developmental problems. Here we comment on particular aspects of importance (Table 7.6).

History taking should cover family history, social and family environment and the pre-, peri- and postnatal history, looking particularly for the risk factors as outlined above. It is then followed by more detailed questions both about particular concerns of the parent and what would be expected in other skilled areas.

Certain risk factors increase the likelihood of a developmental impairment. These could be medical disorders of known etiology, such as Down syndrome. Biological risks may be:

1. prenatal, for example use of drugs or alcohol, severe toxemia and viral infections;
2. perinatal factors, such as prematurity, low birth weight, obstetric complications;
3. neonatal factors, such as neonatal encephalopathy, infections (e.g. sepsis or meningitis) and severe hyperbilirubinemia;
4. postnatal factors, such as injury or non-accidental injury, meningitis, encephalitis, exposure to toxins, severe continuous failure to thrive and severe epilepsy;
5. certain factors, in the family history, visual and hearing as well as specific learning.

Environmental risks, such as a parent with mental retardation or significant mental health problems, history of abuse or neglect and concerns about parent/child interaction would increase the likelihood of a developmental impairment.

Developmental history. It used to be implied that parents were not particularly good informants about their children's development, but this was partly a function of asking detailed questions about age of acquisition of particular skills, which might have passed some time before. Asking open-ended questions and then asking for examples elicits the most reliable history.

What all parents are very good at remembering is whether or not they had concerns and if so what the concerns were about. They are particularly good at observing current behavior if the right questions are asked. Parents' interpretation of what their child does may be incorrect (e.g. he understands everything), but their observations are usually accurate (e.g. he will fetch his shoes only if they are visible). Parents find accurate estimates of comprehension difficult, as do professionals, unless a specific test is carried out. Examples of questions to ask at specific ages are given in Table 7.7. Between 18 and 24 months is a particularly good time to note any delays of communication, for example not pointing or not using gaze to regulate communication. Between 24 and 30 months is a particularly good time to note delays in language development, because the child should move quickly from single words to putting words into simple sentences.

Some semistructured interviews of history taking have been developed for certain situations, for example the Diagnostic Interview Schedule for Communication Disorder (DISCO 2000) developed for detailed history of both normal and abnormal patterns of development where a child might be suspected of having an autistic spectrum disorder, and the Autism Diagnostic Interview.[44] Parents are unreliable in their recall of when milestones were passed, but it is important to determine the rate of development of skills in order to establish whether the child has always had a problem or whether there is any possibility of regression (deterioration or loss of skills). If the latter is suspected then the exploration of etiology follows a different path from that of a static non-progressive disorder. If there is a suggestion of regression, it is useful to inquire at what age the child was at his best and to jog memories with questions such as 'What sort of things was he doing last Christmas that he cannot do now?.

Past history is directed at elucidating any cause for the problems, either real or wrongly attributed by the parents. Ruling out the latter (e.g. mother working or being depressed as a cause of autism) can reduce or remove parents' guilt and help them in accepting the child's difficulties.

It is particularly important that problems are not wrongly attributed (e.g. to obstetric intervention or pertussis immunization), which might result in missing a genetic problem.

Events such as 'cord around the neck' rarely if ever cause problems or forceps delivery if carried out to protect the infant. What is important is the reason for intervention (e.g. fetal distress), which may have resulted in brain damage, and the condition of the baby at birth, for example low Apgar core (< 5 at 5 and 10 min), poor feeder, fits.

General health. The child's general health and any illnesses can be very relevant and must be inquired about and explored.

Family history. Family history is extremely important and inquiries must be made about first and second degree relatives: parents, siblings, aunts, uncles and cousins. A diagnosis, even if very definite, must not be taken at face value and must be pursued if it might be relevant (e.g. a reported diagnosis of spina bifida in a male cousin turned out to be muscular dystrophy).

In boys with learning disability a history of affected males on the mother's side must be very carefully pursued. The parents may need to be examined (e.g. child with hypotonia whose mother has myotonic dystrophy).

Social history. Social history is important not only because of its role in etiology, but also because social factors may affect the family's capacity to cope with a child with a disability.

Table 7.6 Topics to be asked about in the history

Growth and any medical problems
Feeding
Behavior
Vision
Hearing
Motor skills, including manipulation
Communication, speech and language
Play and social relationships
Self-help and personal skills
Drive and motivation for learning

Examination: observations and interactive assessment

Gesell[45] stated that psychological/developmental examination should be regarded 'not as a series of achievement tests but as a means of eliciting significant behavior, which calls for diversified

Table 7.7 Examples of specific questions to ask about children at different ages

Age	Questions
8 months	Does your child take solids from a spoon?, ...hold the bottle?. Does your child have any problems sleeping? ... see you across a room and follow movement?, ... see crumbs on the floor?, ...turn round and locate a speaker? ...seem to be aware of quiet sounds in a room that cannot be seen? ... show an awareness of strangers? ... understand 'no' in a tone of voice? ... like playing social games such as 'beep-bo' and making babble sounds Does your child sit alone and get into the crawl position? ... pass objects from hand to hand? ... show some use of index finger?
15 months	Does your child help with feeding by holding a loaded spoon? ...help with dressing by putting arms up appropriately? Is your child easy to manage? How does your child sleep? Does your child have tantrums? Are there any concerns about your child's vision? Are there any signs of a squint? Does your child respond to being talked to even in a quiet voice? Is your child walking? If not walking, pulling to standing and walking round the furniture? Does your child seem unsteady? How does your child communicate (pointing is usual at this age plus some vocalization)? Does your child understand the names of people? Could your child show you a part of his body by pointing? Does your child like to copy you and do things with you showing domestic imitation? Does your child play with toys knowing what they are for and show an ability to put for example peg men in and out of boats, bricks in and out of a box?
24 months	Can your child feed himself with a spoon? ...drink from an open cup? Do you have any worries about your child's behavior, for example temper tantrums, sleeping? Can your child see in the distance and nearby? Does your child hear and respond both to voice and other sounds? Can your child run? ...climb the stairs? Is your child unsteady? Can your child build bricks and play a simple posting box game? Does your child show pretend play and imagination with a dolly or a teddy? Can your child play for several minutes with toys on his own? Does your child understand the names of objects? Can your child point to several parts of his body or go and get something from another room for you? Does your child use at least 20 words to communicate? Is your child beginning to put words together? Does your child bring things to show you? ...point at things to engage your interest? ...show a drive and curiosity about the environment?
30 months	Can your child feed himself? Is your child starting to be toilet trained? Are there worries about your child's behavior, compliance and listening? At this age the child should be able to sit with an adult looking at a book for several minutes Are their any concerns about your child's vision and hearing? Can your child run? ...jump? ...kick a ball? ...scribble with a pencil? Does your child understand questions such as 'put it in something' or 'which one is for drinking'? Does your child show imaginative play sequences with toys and talk during the play? Does your child ask questions and use sentences of two to four words? Is your child beginning to be interested in what other children are doing and start to chase them?
36 months	Can your child use a spoon, fork and a knife? Are there any particular problems with eating? This is a common time for food fads Is your child toilet trained by day? Can your child put on some clothes? Are there any management problems with your child? Can your child listen to a short story with pictures? Can your child run, catch a ball, kick it and climb stairs? ...hold a pencil and copy a circle? Can your child match colors and replace shapes in a board? Does your child understand and ask questions, for example 'where?', 'what?' and 'why?'? ...use sentences of four to five words and have conversations? Can your child be understood by strangers? Is your child able to describe in a picture what is happening and what people are doing, not just point out single items? Can your child now play interactively with other children of the same age?
48-60 months	Can your child use a knife and fork neatly? Can your child go to the toilet alone? Can your child undress and put on most clothes? Are there any problems at home? ... difficulties with playing with peers? Can your child see and hear? Can your child go up and down stairs without difficulty quite steadily? Can your child understand concepts of shape, color, time and sentences containing negatives? Could your child describe the picture sequence story understanding that the events on one page may be reflected in subsequent events on the following page? Can your child use a pencil to copy a circle and a cross and draw a man?

analysis rather than a meager recording of success and failure'. The examiner needs to set the context that will most easily show the spontaneous and elicited behaviors that he or she wishes to observe. Tables 7.8 and 7.9 and Figure 7.7 set the framework for observation.

The developmental examination should take place in a room with toys appropriate for the child and with one or both parents present. There should be a chair and table suitable for the child to sit at. A history is then taken, all the time observing the child's behavior and interaction with parents. This period of talking to the parents enables the child to get used to the environment and to see that the parents accept strange people. Toys and other play materials, appropriate for the age of the child, should be available (e.g. cause and effect toys, a bell, bricks, truck, doll or teddy, tea-set or other dolls' house toys for the 18-month-old and for the older child, crayons and pencil and paper and books with single pictures and stories). These are separate from those required for tests.

It is particularly valuable to allow time with a suitable selection of toys available for the child for observation before immediately setting a structure and interacting with the child. This is because, in certain developmental problems, children are able to function very well when a helpful adult interacts with them, makes particular demands and sets the structure for how they should organize their responses. However, when left to his or her own devices the child is unable to organize his or her environment and may not be able to generate any ideas, and this will be shown in limited and somewhat repetitive play. The child may not be able to organize his or her attention in which case he or she will flit going from one object to another. Such difficulties will not be apparent from the more structured interview.

One of the cardinal rules of developmental assessment is not only to look at what the child does but 'look at how they do it'; thus all the time the quality of response is to be evaluated as well as the actual achievement. Unstructured time allows the examiner to see what ideas a child has and capacity for organizing his or her own play. However, it is equally important to set a context for structured social observations in response to specific cues or 'presses' from the examiner. This has been formalized in a play-based observation for possible autism, the Autism Diagnostic Observation Schedule.[46]. Following the history and informal observations, more structured and standardized tests for general and specific areas of development may be used (Table 7.10).[19,46–48]

Normal range

The range of normal for attaining some skills is so wide that children with impairments may well fall within it. Conversely many children whose milestones fall outside the normal range (i.e. 97th centile) are normal. It may not be possible to diagnose mild learning difficulties or language disorder or clumsiness before a child is 18 months to 2 years of age because the more complex skills involved are not exhibited earlier.

Some children may initially show abnormalities that disappear, only for the child to have other associated difficulties later (e.g. language delay resolving, but later reading and spelling problems; minor motor signs in the first year resolving, but with clumsiness appearing later).

Look for patterns of development suggestive of normal variation

Some developmental patterns cause delay in the acquisition of other milestones (e.g. shuffling is associated with late walking). The mean age of walking in children who 'bottom shuffle' is 16–17 months and the 90th centile is 23 months.[49,50]

Look for patterns of development that suggest abnormal development

Besides looking for the acquisition of normal developmental skills, it is also important to look for skills that are present at an earlier stage which should have disappeared and are abnormal beyond a certain age. For example, mouthing is a normal pattern of investigation of the environment at 7–8 months, but after that hand and vision examination increasingly take the place of mouthing.

Persistent mouthing of objects beyond 18 months is indicative of a general learning problem. Persistent casting (throwing forwards or to the side) is a normal behavior at 12 months, but not at 24 months or beyond, and hand regard is a normal behavior at 3–4 months.

Some behaviors are abnormal at any age, for example the persistent visual inspection of objects out the corner of the eye seen in young children with autism. However, some of the excited arm/body actions seen persistently in older children with autism are also seen in normal development at the age of 6–9 months.

Importance of skill delays

Delays in some areas of development are more important for long term learning than others, for example:

1. Developmental delay in motor skills only is of much less long term significance than persistent significant delays in language and cognitive skills.
2. Self-help competence, for example toilet training, feeding and dressing, can also be dissociated from the level of general learning.
3. Some skills (e.g. symbolic play and language) reflect understanding of the environment and are therefore better indicators of intellectual ability than are purely motor skills for example.

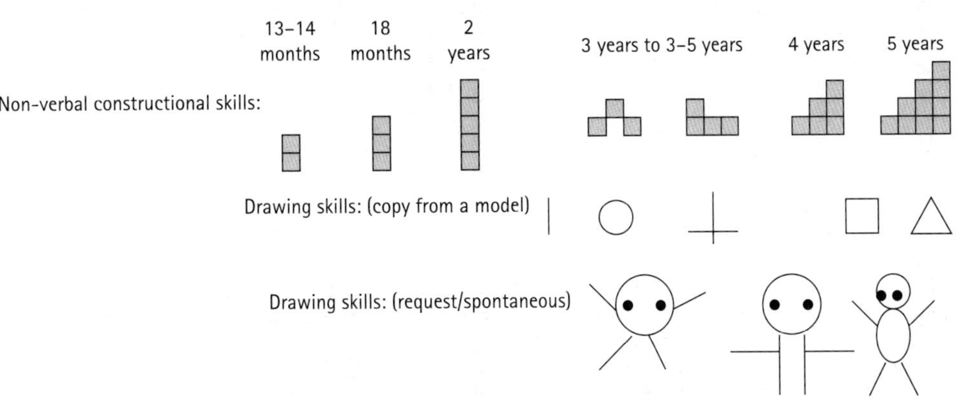

Fig. 7.7 Constructional and drawing skills.

Table 7.8 Framework for making developmental observations – birth to 13 months (Courtsey of AJ Sharma)

	Newborn	3 months	4 months	6 months	8 months	9 months	12 months	13 months
POSTURE/GROSS MOTOR MOVEMENTS AND REFLEXES								
Supine	Head to side	Head in midline Hands open Finger play		Lifts head spontaneously				
Pull to sit	No head control		Good head control	Lifts head in anticipation				
Sitting	Flopping forward	Head held up Back curved	Straight back	Sits with hands for support	Sits with no support			
Ventral suspension		Good head control	Most primary reflexes (e.g. Moro's) markedly lessen by this age and are not present by 6 months		Forward parachute			
Prone		Shoulders up on forearms		Chest off on hands				
Supported standing				Weight bears Downward parachute		Stands holding on	Walks hands held	Walks alone (18 months age limit)
HAND FUNCTION/FINE MOTOR: *Look for the way of approaching with one or both hands, grasping and releasing spontaneously and on request*								
	Persisting fisting beyond 2 months is abnormal		Reaches with one hand-5–6 months, mouths 6 months Transfers from hand to hand 7 months		Index finger approach	Pincer grasp 9–10 months Releases brick in a container	Mature grasp of 1 inch brick	Can give a toy on request
VISUAL BEHAVIOR								
Visual fixation and following	Looks towards bright light	Follows face beyond midline	Follows objects 180°		Fixes on 1 mm sweets			
HEARING BEHAVIOR								
Response to sound	Startle	Searches for sound		Turns head towards sound				
LANGUAGE AND COMMUNICATION: *Observe vocalization and gestures to attract other's attention, to indicate needs, in response to others' vocalization and to share emotions*								
		Cooing		Babbling	Responds to own name	Understands words in context	First word with meaning	
PERSONAL–SOCIAL: *Note awareness of parents/carers and strangers, initiation of interactions and response to others' approaches*								
	Smiles responsively 6 weeks			Stranger awareness 6–7 months	Waves bye-bye		Points to request and show	
PLAY: *Observe exploration and free play, use of real size and small toys on self and others and initiation and response to social games (e.g. peek-a-boo, pat-a-cake)*								
				Bangs and mouths	Looks for fallen toy, pulls string to get toy	Plays pat-a-cake, explores with finger	Holds phone to ear	Uses cup/ spoon/brush on self

Table 7.9 Framework for making developmental observations – 15 months to 5 years

	15 months	18 months	2 years	2.5 years	3 years	3.5 years	4 years	5 years
FINE-MOTOR/PERCEPTUAL COORDINATION: *Note spontaneous effort, attention to directions, ability to copy from a model, response to help and praise, attention to task and quality of movements*								
Constructional skills with 1 inch cubes	Two cubes 14 months	Three cubes	Six cubes	Puts three cubes in a row for a train	Makes a train with a chimney 39 months	Three-brick bridge from a model	Steps of six cubes from a model	Steps of 10 cubes from a model
Pencil grasp and drawing			In prone at distal end	Middle of pencil	Mature grasp (tripod grasp)			
	Makes a mark on paper	Straight scribble	Circular scribble	Line in imitation	Copies: O	Copies: +	Copies square 4–4.5 years	Copies triangle
Shape sorting (visuospatial skills)		Simple shapes circles and squares	Circles, squares and triangles	Six-shape sorter	Good scanning of shape sorter before putting shape in and rotating shapes to align – little or no pushing of shapes			
LANGUAGE, COMMUNICATION AND SOCIAL INTERACTION: *Note speech quality, use of language: to express need, comment, describe, share interest and initiating and responding for conversation*								
Understanding	Simple requests in context: give me...	Knows two to three body parts	Gives two or more objects on requests	Prepositions: in, on. Gives objects by function	Preposition under/size big/little	Size, color		
Communication and social interaction	Initiates communication, shows, points	Many spontaneous words, repeats words	Puts two words together in phrases		Sentences of three or more words, personal pronouns. Can give full name and sex. Asks what/where questions.		Joined sentences, speech mainly clear	
PLAY AND SOCIAL INTERACTION: *Note initiating interactions and responding to parent/examiner/other children and use of eye contact and gestures*								
	Brushes own/ mother's hair	Brushes doll's hair, may feed/put to bed doll/teddy	Plays with small toys, relates two toys. Watches other children		Develops sequence with small toys. Plays with other children. Can share. Offers comfort			

Table 7.10 Psychometric tests in common use

Test	Age range tested	Training required to carry out test	Areas tested[a]
Complete profile			
Bayley scales of infant development	2 months to 3 years	Professionals including pediatricians	Mental, motor and behavior
Griffiths scales	0–8 years	Clinicians trained to administer it	Locomotor, personal social, hearing and speech, eye–hand and performance
British Ability Scales BAS 11	2–17 years	Psychologists	Verbal and non-verbal reasoning/attainments and diagnostic scales
WPPSI-R – Wechsler Preschool and Primary Scale of Intelligence	3–7 years	Psychologists	Two scales, verbal and performance, with five subtests in each, VIQ and PIQ and IQ derived
WISC – Wechsler Intelligence Scales for Children WISC111 UK-R	6–16 years	Psychologists	Two scales, verbal and performance, with five subtests in each
Stanford–Binet intelligence scale	2 years to adult	Psychologist	Recent revision
Schedule of growing skills	0–5 years	Any professional	Profile of development in nine areas – based on Sheridan. Gives a general developmental overview
Miller assessment for preschoolers	2.9–5.8 years	Any professional	Identifies developmental delays in sensori-motor and cognitive abilities in verbal and non-verbal areas
Kaufman assessment battery for children	2–12 years	Psychologist	3 scales, sequential, simultaneous processing and attainments. Mental processing composite derived. There is an adolescent extension scale
Developmental neuropsychological assessment NEPSY	3–12 years	Psychologist	Attention/executive function; language; sensorimotor functions; visuospatial processing; memory and learning
Language			
Reynell DLS – Developmental Language Scale Now RDLS111 (1997)	1–7 years	Speech therapists, psychologists, some teachers	Verbal comprehension and verbal expression; (NFER)
TOWK - Test of Word Knowledge	5–17 years	Any professional, usually SLT	Detailed evaluation of semantic development and lexical knowledge. 7 subtests
Picture vocabulary test (Peabody or British)	2–8 years	Any professional,	Tests single word vocabulary. The child selects picture most appropriate for the given word (NFER)
CELF – Clinical Evaluation of Language Function	6–18 years	Any professional, usually speech therapist	Eleven subtests that probe different aspects of complex language functioning
Speech/articulation tests EAT – Edinburgh Articulation Test	3–8 years	Speech therapist	Picture naming task to assess English sound system
Preschool CELF	3–6.11 years	Any professional, usually SLT	Three receptive and three expressive subtests probing different aspects of language function
Renfrew Action Picture test RAPT	3–8 years	SLT	Picture description task designed to elicit specific information and grammar
Renfrew Bus Story	3–8 yrs	SLT	Story retelling task with pictures. Scored for information, grammar and sentence length
Preschool language scales	2 weeks–6 years	Any professional usually SLT	A developmentally based assessment combining parental report and direct test – best aged 1–4 years
Non-verbal intelligence tests – suitable for those with impaired hearing			
Ravens progressive matrices	5 years to adult	Any professional	A series of pictures or designs with one part missing (NFER)
Snijders–Ooman non-verbal psychometric test	Aged 2 years +		Reasoning and spatial abilities subtests
Leiter International performance test-R	Age 2–20		Visualization and reasoning battery, also attention and memory

(*Continued*)

Table 7.10 (continued)

Test	Age range tested	Training required To carry out test	Areas tested[a]
Visuomotor and motor tests			
Goodenough–Harris drawing test (Harris[19])	3–15 years	Any professional	The child is asked to draw a man and a score is derived from the content and converted to a mental age
Bender Gestalt test	4 years to adult	Test of perceptuomotor function	Nine designs for the child to copy
Movement Assessment Battery for Children (see review by Wiart & Darrah[47], for comparison with other gross motor tests)	4–12 years	Any professional, usually physio-therapist or occupational therapist	Eight items divided into three subsections; manual dexterity, ball skills, and static and dynamic balance
Frostig – DTVP – Developmental Test of Visual Perception	4–8 years		Five areas are tested: eye motor coordination, figure ground, constancy of shape, position in space and spatial relationships (NFER)
Developmental test of visuomotor integration (Beery)	3–17 years		Developmental sequence of geometric forms to be copied with paper and pencil
Test of visual perceptual skills (Gardner) or the motor-free test of visual perceptual skills (revised)	4–12 years with upper age band available		Non-verbal assessment by matching figures
Matrix analogy test	5–17 years		A series of designs with one part missing divided into four sections: pattern completion, reasoning, sequencing and spatial visualization
Memory and attention tests			
Children's memory scale	5–16 years	Psychologists	Verbal and visual immediate and delayed memory
Rivermead behavioural memory test	5–10 years	Psychologists	Everyday memory problems, episodic and prospective
Test of everyday attention for children	6–16 years	Psychologists	Sustained and selective attention and impulsivity
Play test			
Symbolic play test of Lowe & Costello	1–3 years	Any professional	Four groups of toys presented without verbal instructions. Results in an age equivalent score
Observational scale for autism ADOS (Lord et al)[46]			Social interaction, communication and imaginative play observed
Tests for those with visual impairment			
Reynell Zinkin scales	Birth to 5 years	Any professional	Five subscales: social adaptation, sensorimotor understanding, exploration of environment, response to sound and verbal comprehension, expressive language. Also a communication subscale for children with additional problems
Behavior scales			
Vineland adaptive behavior scales	0–adult	Any professional	Survey or interview form – semistructured carer interview for assessment of communication, daily living skills, socialization and motor skills plus a maladaptive section
Strengths and difficulties questionnaire (Goodman)			Teacher and parent version summarizes behavior problems in prosocial, hyperactivity, conduct, emotional and peer group areas
Other behavior schedules (see O'Brien et al[48])			

[a]Most of these tests are available from NFER – Nelson, Danville House, Windsor 1DF, or The Psychological Corporation SLT, speech and language therapist.

Prematurity

Make allowance for prematurity under 12 months.

Child's performance

The child may not perform at his or her best, and if this is suspected will need to be seen again. It is always helpful to ask parents if the child that you have seen and the competencies or difficulties that you have encountered are typical. Parents are more likely to accept an opinion if they think the child has behaved typically and it is based on two periods of observation. Children may be able to perform a very successful examination in a structured environment with a helpful skilled adult giving full attention. Drive, motivation and the emotional regulation that is related to temperament will all influence the learning style of the child.

Observe over time

It is not always possible to be certain about a child's development on a single assessment. Skills need to be developed in sharing uncertainty with parents and a need to be observed over time.

Motor skills, vision and hearing

Make sure that the motor, vision and hearing systems are functioning normally before making judgments about the rest of the child's development.

Assessment of motor development

To assess motor development in the child under 2 years:

1. watch first;
2. then place in prone, supine, pull to sit, stand, ventral suspension and look for the secondary protective responses as illustrated (Fig. 7.8).[51] Assess tone, symmetry and spontaneous movements and then compare the motor development with other maturity milestones.

Differential diagnosis. Problems with motor development are most likely to present concerns in the first 2 years of life, although 'clumsiness' is a common associated problem in many other developmental delays. Note, however, that early walking does not exclude other developmental problems.

The differential diagnosis of delay in motor milestones is:

1. a normal variant – for example shuffler, roller, asymmetric head turner, toe walker – ask about family history; shuffling and other patterns may have a genetic predisposition;
2. global delay/general learning difficulties/mental retardation;
3. cerebral palsy/other neurological disorder;
4. early presentation of developmental coordination problems – hypotonia and delay;
5. connective tissue disorder.

Clues on examination are scissoring on downward parachute in diplegia (Fig. 7.9);[51] adopting a sitting posture on downward parachute, as in bottom shufflers (Fig. 7.10).

Definite persistent handedness at 6–9 months may indicate pathology.

Headlag on 'pull to sit' after 8 months is abnormal.

Not walking by 18 months is delayed in a prone developing crawler.

An example of an evidenced-based approach to assessing motor delay is given in Case study 1 on page 138.

Four common tests used to assess motor skills are reviewed in Wiart & Darrah.[47] As with all tests the emphasis is on knowing the tests and whether each test measures what it purports to measure and whether that is what is needed for that particular child.

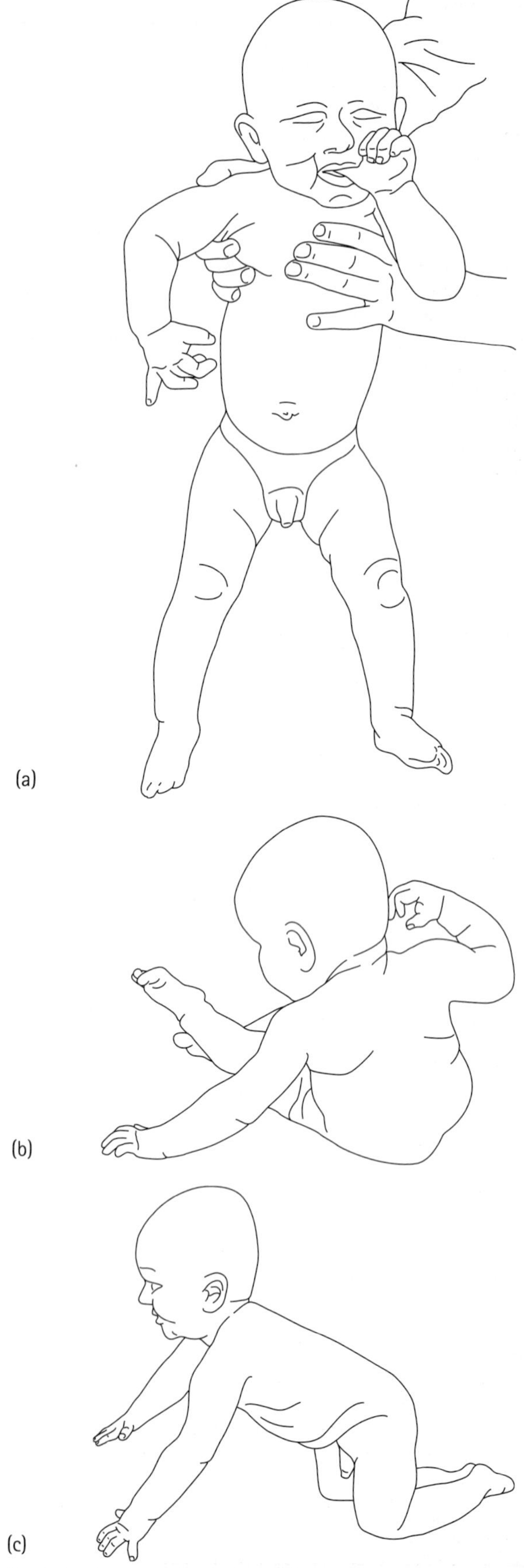

Fig. 7.8 Downward parachute (a), sideways parachute (b), and forward parachute (c). (After Milani-Comparetti & Gidoni 1967[51])

Oromotor skills

A significant impairment of central origin affecting motor development will affect oral skills, as demonstrated in delayed sucking (and with a severe cerebral palsy in abnormal swallowing and breathing). Less severe difficulties may not be so obvious until solids are introduced when textures, lumps, chewing and drooling problems may present.

Assessment of vision

Significant visual impairment has a potentially serious and complex impact on all areas of development, including cognition, language, social, gross and fine motor abilities. Early recognition and specialist rehabilitative support are essential.

Assessment of vision in children should include history and examination. The history should cover:

1. any parental concern about the child's vision;
2. visual behavior relevant to the child's age (see Fig. 7.2);
3. suspected squint.

Examination of the eyes includes assessment of:

1. any gross ocular pathology (including ophthalmoscopy);
2. the pupillary response to light;
3. eye movements (smooth pursuit and saccades);
4. squint – checking that the corneal reflection of a light is in the same position in the two eyes and by doing the cover test (in the cover test each eye is covered in turn while the child visually fixates on an object and a note is made of whether the uncovered eye moves to take up fixation).

Visual assessment includes:

1. measurement of visual acuity – ability to distinguish separation of two visual targets and therefore to distinguish detail;
2. detection vision – ability to recognize/detect individual targets.

The Snellen letter chart was the accepted standard for measurement of acuity until recent years. The acuity is expressed as the distance at which a particular letter size is seen by a person with normal vision. The result is given as a pseudofraction – on top the distance tested at (the standard distance being 6 m or 20 feet), and below the size of the letter seen, thus 6/6 is normal vision and 6/60 very poor vision.

The LogMAR (log of the minimal angle of resolution) is now the increasingly accepted standard. In this test the letter sizes change by more even steps. The results are expressed as a decimal, thus the line of letters equivalent to 6/6 is 0 and 6/60 is 0.1 and each letter recognized contributes to the acuity result, as a proportion of the number of letters on each line. Letter charts with reduced type are used for near vision in both tests. Measurement of acuity by standard adult methods is reliably possible from the age of about 5 to 6 years.

In younger children tests need some adaptation to allow for several developmental issues, but this does not require compromise of the adult standard after 2.5–3 years.[52]

Although young children cannot name letters, by the age of 2.5–3 years over 85% of children are able to match letters and by 3 years most children can do so.[53] Difficulties with attention control arise at a test distance of 6 m and children also have difficulty understanding the task when several lines of letters are presented simultaneously. Visual acuity should be measured if possible in each eye separately; however, a significant proportion of children under 3.5 years of age are unable to accept occlusion of one eye (46% of 2.5–3-year-olds and 73% of 3–4 year-olds will accept occlusion). In this age group it is therefore advisable to obtain a measure with both eyes open before attempting to cover one eye.

To address all these issues Sonksen and Silver devised a test of visual acuity, the Sonksen–Silver Acuity System[52] based on the

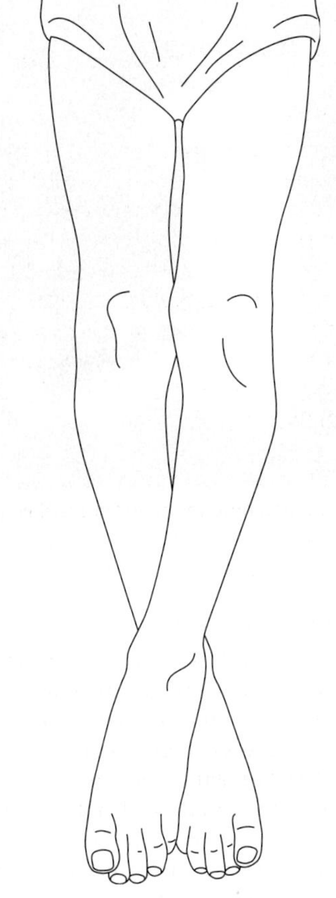

(a)

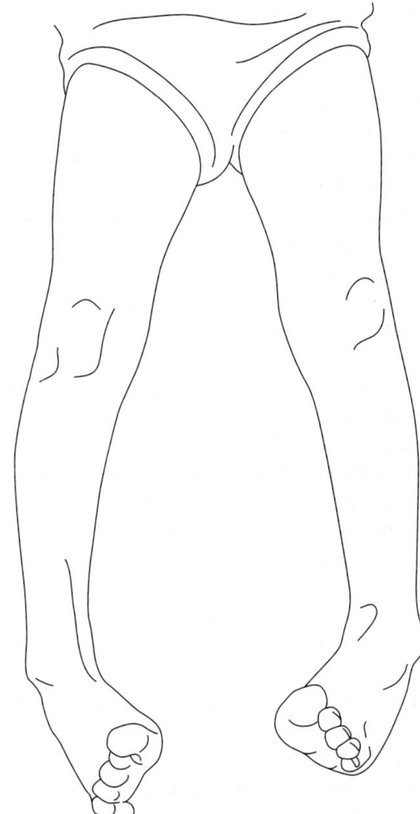

(b)

Fig. 7.9 Downward parachute in (a) spastic cerebral palsy, (b) dystonic cerebral palsy. (After Milani-Comparetti, Gidoni 1967[51])

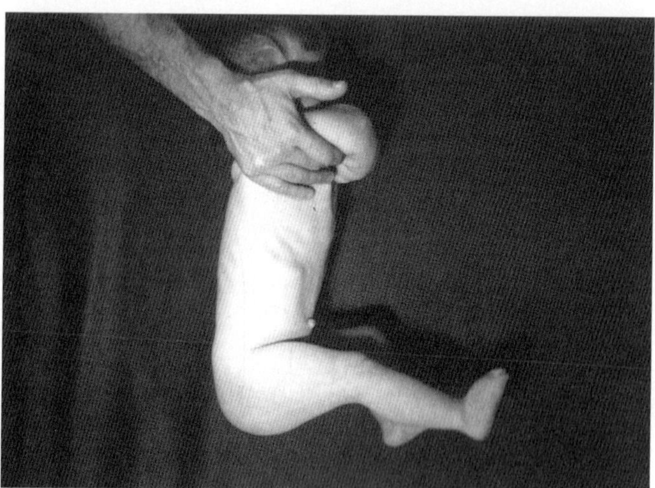

Fig. 7.10 Downward parachute in a bottom shuffler. (Courtesy of D Scrutton.)

Snellen standard. Cards, each with a single row of letters of each size, using the six letters known to be least confusing for young children,[14] with a key card for letter matching and a training booklet are used. Seating the child at a small table and using a test distance of 3 m also improves concentration and cooperation with the test. Using this test, an acuity measure for both eyes can be obtained in 78% of 2.5–3-year-olds, and in the majority of children after 3 years. Similar adaptations have been made to a logMAR based test, which is currently under development. Other tests designed for younger children include the Cambridge crowding test and Keeler logMAR test.

Sheridan[54] devised a test (STYCAR letter test) that involved the presentation of single letters of decreasing size at 3 m. This is still widely used for young children, but these tests have been shown to significantly overestimate acuity, especially in children with amblyopia, by as much as three lines and therefore linear acuity (as above) should be measured wherever possible.

The Kay Picture Test[55] is similar to the STYCAR letter test, but uses pictograms designed to be of equivalent proportions to Snellen letters and can provide an estimate of acuity in children from 18 months to 2–2.5 years, when children are unable to match letters. They do then require the vocabulary to name the pictures. This test is said to be accurate to within one line of Snellen acuity, and tests near and distance vision.

Visual acuity can be measured from 2 months using forced choice preferential looking as on Keeler or Cardiff Acuity Cards.[56] In this test the infant is shown two targets on a card. One is uniformly gray and the other has either black and white stripes (Keeler) or a pictogram similar to the Kay pictures (Cardiff). The stripes or pictograms become sequentially narrower or smaller on each card according to a standard scale. An infant will automatically look toward the more interesting visual target until they reach the limit of their acuity.

Opticokinetic nystagmus may be demonstrated in the clinic setting using an opticokinetic drum with black and white stripes of varying diameter. Nystagmus will not be elicited at the limits of the child's acuity (i.e. the stripe width is too small for the child to discriminate).

Visual acuity gradually improves with age. This has been demonstrated using grating acuity in infancy and using the Sonksen–Silver Acuity System. A vision of 6/6 is only achieved in 90% of children by 5.7 years with both eyes and 6.4 years with each eye separately.[53] In the infant, evaluation of vision should begin with observation of detection vision. Near detection will include observing the child fix and follow a silent object presented at about 30 cm from the face. In the first weeks of life the infant will be most likely to follow the examiner's face and may ignore other objects. Infants show little interest in small objects on a table top until 9 months. By 9–12 months, near detection vision may be tested by observing visual fixation on one small sweet (a one hundred and thousand measuring 1.2 mm), placed on a dark contrasting background. In children with normal vision, immediate and sharp fixation is expected. Children with significant visual impairment (equivalent of 6/60 or greater measured with Keeler cards) may show visual awareness of this small sweet, but they show slower fixation, inexact location and peering. Inability to locate this target therefore suggests a child has very severe visual impairment and could be registered blind.

Distance detection can be measured by establishing the size of the smallest object the child can see at a particular distance. Sheridan designed a test using ten white balls of standardized diameter, which are either rolled on a dark strip horizontal to the line of the infant's gaze at 3 m from the child, or mounted on sticks for presentation from behind a dark screen (STYCAR graded balls test). This test is most appropriate in children from the age of 9 months to around 15 months because it relies on a young child's attention being drawn to the major stimulus in the environment (as in the distraction hearing test); after this age it is less reliable. It is important to note that visualization of even the smallest ball does not denote perfect vision, and rolling the ball considerably enhances its visibility. These tests can be helpful in assessing children with severe visual impairment and for some children with learning disabilities who are not able to do the letter tests.

Assessment of vision in the child with a visual impairment. In the child with visual impairment, the largest sized letters may not be recognized at 3 m and so the distance of testing is reduced until the letters are identified. In children with the most severe visual impairment, measurement of acuity at a distance may be more difficult or impossible. A methodical approach to the observation of functional (near and distance detection) vision should therefore be made. Care needs to be taken in interpretation, because the detection of small objects at near distance may lead to an overestimation of vision (see above).

A description of the size of object, the visual complexity and the distance recognized, can be used to provide advice to parents and the professionals working with them about toys and educational material that will be appropriate for learning.

A useful visual scale for near detection vision in the most visually impaired has been developed by Sonksen (personal communication) using visual targets of standardized size, ranging from a light source in a darkened room, a large, light-reflecting dangling ball through to smaller non-light reflecting targets. The distance from the target and the child's ability to fixate and/or follow can then be recorded. The Stycar fixed or rolling balls, everyday objects and pictures may be shown, initially at 3 m and then moving in methodically to 2, 1, 0.5 and less than 0.5 m. The distance at which the target is recognized is then recorded. The test material should only be presented once because a child may be able to make an intelligent guess when it is re-presented.

The ability to identify pictures both near and at a distance by a child with visual impairment will vary with the level of background contrast and the level of detail required for recognition within the picture. A child may recognize a clear picture of a dog on a white background, but fail to pick out the same picture on less well contrasted background or when part of a more complex picture.

Sonksen & Macrae[57] devised a picture recognition test using a selection of Ladybird pictures graded according to visual complexity. Advice to teachers about this is essential, because much educational material is presented in a visually complex way and at a distance.

Objective measurement of vision may also be obtained by measuring the electrical response from the retina (the electroretinogram) and the visual cortex to a given visual stimulus (the visual evoked potential). The response to a simple flash and to graded check patterns can be recorded.[58] A variety of ocular and visual problems occur in children:

1. Some children have no ocular problems but appear to have visual impairment. They are likely to have cortical impairment where the problem lies in the interpretation of what is processed visually.
2. Sometimes there is a delay – so called delayed visual maturation – in which the visual behaviors outlined in Figure 7.2 are all slower, often by months. Such children usually have other developmental impairments, which become clearer with time.
3. Some children, often with more profound neurological damage, have more permanent cortical visual problems. In these children vision may show apparent variability. Movements may be seen, but not the level of discriminating detail that allows recognition of objects.
4. Visuoperceptual skills, which are particularly at risk in premature babies under 32 weeks' gestation and affect pattern recognition and topographical skills can be assessed with specific tests.
5. Specific area or domain (brain anatomical site) defects may cause very specific defects (e.g. proposognosia – a difficulty of face recognition, which is usually, but not invariably, an acquired brain damage deficit).
6. Eye movement disorders, such as ocular motor apraxia may present with signs of early visual impairment, but by deploying motor control skills, with maturity the visual acuity is shown to be unimpaired.

The awareness of the impact of visual impairment on development and techniques to ameliorate this have been shown to be successful in promoting visual development.[59]

Testing hearing

Persistent hearing loss can significantly impair speech and language development. Treatment is either by removal of the cause (in the case of middle ear effusion, or 'glue', causing conductive loss) or by aiding, either with conventional hearing aids or with a cochlear implant (in the case of sensorineural loss) and special teaching. Such interventions can change the outcome for young children and early detection is therefore a high child health priority, with 1–2 per 1000 children having sensorineural hearing loss. Even if a child 'passes' his neonatal screening he may develop a hearing loss later due for example to secretory otitis media or later onset of sensorineural loss; therefore passing the neonatal screening test should not be seen as a final statement of normality.[60] Parental concerns should always be noted and hearing tests should be arranged after an illness such as meningitis and should form part of the evaluation of speech delay. Tests of hearing and competence in applying them need to be part of the skills of early child care and surveillance. A history suggestive of 'risk' for hearing impairment should be elicited but reliance on this alone for screening will miss significant numbers of children (family history, ototoxic drugs, meningitis, NICU/SCBU experiences, structural palatal abnormality). Children with other developmental disorders need particular attention to hearing tests as the effects of impairment tend to be cumulative on function.

Tests of hearing are divided into those reliant on child cooperation and are subjective and those that do not and are objective.

Objective tests.

1. *Otoacoustic emissions.* This technique is applicable to the infant of any age, can be carried out in the neonatal period and has a sensitivity and specificity that makes it suitable for universal screening. However, it is only a screen of cochlear function and definitive threshold estimation requires brainstem evoked response testing.
2. *Brainstem evoked response audiometry [or auditory brainstem response (ABR) assessment].* This technique requires a still or sleeping subject, and may therefore require sedation. The stimulus sound is delivered by headphones or insert earphones. The most common stimulus is a broad-band 'click' which facilitates neural synchronicity but contains most energy in the mid- to high-frequency range, limiting threshold estimation to these frequencies. In threshold ABR assessment, responses are recorded at different stimulus intensities, allowing threshold estimation. Diagnostic ABR involves the examination of the morphology and latencies of waves recorded at higher intensities, allowing assessment of the site of lesion in cases of known impairment.

Subjective (behavioural) tests. These rely on cooperation and developmental level. They are thus also a guide to the developmental level of function of the child (Fig. 7.2). The tests can be used at any age, depending on the functional level, i.e. a child or young person with learning difficulties may still be best tested using distraction or visual reinforcement audiometry techniques (perhaps with modifications) at any age. Care needs to be taken to distinguish between hearing acuity, auditory attention and speech processing and comprehension. For example, children with autism may hear normally or even show apparent hypersensitivity to specific sounds, but may not show any attention to adult speech. Children with disorders of attention may also be able to hear normally but not show sustained attention to listening tasks (or any other tasks). Children with speech delay may be slower processors of speech and language, present as poor listeners and later be shown to have poor auditory short term memories. However, they can usually hear normally, but may show apparent impairment in subjective tests.

1. *Distraction test and visual reinforcement audiometry.* The ability to locate sounds at ear level is mature by 7–8 months and prior to otoacoustic emissions was used for universal screening. The technique requires a well and alert baby, not in an overactive or distressed state, a quiet room, two people who are trained and skilled in the technique and an adult to hold the child who is instructed to remain neutral and non-responsive. The adult in front (the distractor) gains and controls the child's attention with a toy, which is then removed or covered. Within one second of the removal of the distracting object, out of sight, the other adult (or, rarely, a mechanical device) introduces a sound stimulus. The test stimuli should be frequency specific, and include voice (both low frequency and high – e.g. a sibilant 'ss'), a specially designed rattle (high frequency) and electronically generated 'warble' tones. The usual response is a full head turn to locate the stimuli. Minimal sound levels eliciting a reliable response can be measured using a sound level meter and the stimuli are designed to test the range of frequencies needed for speech development. The location ability on ear level at 6–7 months, above and below ear level at 8 months and above the head at 12 months are markers of perceptual/cognitive maturation. However, babies of 9 and more months also learn to play games and check who is

behind them! Other common invalidators of this test are visual cues (including shadows and/or reflections visible to the baby), auditory cues (e.g. creaking shoes, floors) and even olfactory cues.

2. For this, and other, reasons *visual reinforcement audiometry (VRA)* is an important technique. In VRA the child is generally seated, again on an adult's lap, between loudspeakers. Warble tone stimuli are presented, initially at suprathreshold level, and the child's attention drawn (by a tester seated in front of the child) to a visual reward (often a bright or animated toy hidden behind smoked glass) which is illuminated briefly. Once the child has associated the auditory stimulus with the reward the stimulus level is reduced and the reward delayed until the child has begun to search for it (a positive response). In this way assessment of threshold can be performed for stimuli at different frequencies. The visual reward has been shown to elicit more responses than the social reward used in distraction testing, and the electronic stimuli used in VRA can be more accurately calibrated in terms of level and frequency. There are many reasons why these tests may not work well, but a failure to respond on the baby's part should be taken seriously as a developmental as well as a hearing concern.
3. *Behavioural tests:*
   a) Speech discrimination tests. The principle is choosing toys or pictures of objects that are paired and demand careful listening and hearing to discriminate, for example cup/duck, plate/plane. Children can start to cooperate with such speech tests from 24 months although many cannot manage the full 14 toys of the McCormick test (a popular example) at that age, as there are too many. Speech tests in the form of word lists can be used for all ages. The child sits at the table with the examiner checking that all toys can be identified at normal speaking voice and then with the voice lowered and the mouth covered, the child is asked to show each in turn. For younger children the 'cooperative test' can be performed in which the child is asked to 'give' toys to 'mummy' (or 'daddy'), 'teddy' or 'dolly', allowing assessment of speech discrimination.
   b) Conditioning/performance tests. From 30 months and by 36 months children can carry out an action in response to a stimulus and have sufficient control to wait for the stimulus. The stimulus used is a machine emitting tones of a range of frequency and decibel level. The technique is a conditioning one. The child, sitting at the table, puts a brick in a box or a pegman in a boat every time the adult says 'go'. After managing this, the child listens for a tone and puts the brick in, or similar action. Once the child can do this action reliably, the child usually quickly learns to wear headphones and each ear can then be tested individually using pure tones (i.e. tones containing only one frequency), producing a pure tone audiogram – the gold standard hearing test. The ability to manage such tests can be a guide to developmental maturity.

Testing children with developmental disorders. The above tests can all be adapted for use with children with disabilities. Those with visual impairment do not show the same turning to locate sounds in the distraction tests. Those with motor impairments may also have difficulty with location and/or hand actions. Non-cooperative tests are increasingly frequently employed to confirm normal hearing.

Problems with speech, language and communication

Speech and language delays. Speech and language delays are among the commonest developmental problems in children, and parental concern should always be taken seriously. A problem with speech and language may be an indicator of a broader developmental problem and all children must have their hearing tested.

Comorbidities are common and together with severity are important in prognosis.

In general, children have significant problems if they do not babble in the first year, have less than 10 words at 2 years and are not speaking in sentences by 3 years. Most children have adult syntax and grammar by 4 years and are intelligible to most people.[61] These milestone absolutes, however, ignore the qualitative impairments in the use of speech and language for social communication, which are such a key part of social skills.

A problem affecting speech or expressive language only is generally regarded as being less severe in terms of long term significance compared with comprehension problems. However, the view that expressive disorders all have normal receptive skills is less tenable, as increasing research has shown subtle problems not previously found on cruder tests. Many children have problems in all areas of speech, language and communication.

Various attempts have been made to devise classification systems, based on linguistic criteria, regardless of causation. It is helpful to think of speech and language as means for getting needs met, sharing interests and for mental representation for thinking abstractly – an inner language.

Getting needs met can be non-verbal or verbal. Examples of the former are not using another person at all but going to get something, either directly, or by pulling a chair over and climbing up! Alternatively the child may bring an object (e.g. a bottle because a drink is wanted), or take the parent by the hand or pull/push towards the object. Such forms of communication are neither social nor symbolic in that there is no representation of the object (or idea).

Language and communication have forms and functions. The forms (i.e. speech, gestures, facial expressions), their maturity and complexity and how well they are coordinated together, need to be assessed as well as the functions of the forms – needs met, comments, requests, frequency (both initiation and response).

Verbal communication for 'needs met' can be words/sounds or gestures or the written symbol/word may substitute for spoken words. Concerns about reciprocity in communication are often not noted in young children, even when quite extreme under the age of 18 months, and especially in a first child. By this age, children should show not only an increasing understanding of phrase and interest in people talking to them, but a desire to share, show and take turns with pointing use both for needs and interests. Persistent failure to do this may indicate a social communicative problem. Indeed, a lack of gaze monitoring, in combination with a lack of pointing for interest and simple pretend play, by 18 months of age was highly predictive of autism in the CHAT screening study.[40] The same study showed that over 97% of 16 000 children were able to follow an adult pointing at a distant object, were using pointing themselves to get their needs met and show things, and 93% were said by their parents to show pretend play by 21 months age.

Some children with speech and language delays will be slow in all aspects of these skills. Those with speech/articulation problems will have better comprehension and communication, but poor unintelligible speech and may have oromotor delay.

A common clinical presentation is seen in young children with language learning disability in the transition from associatively learned words to symbolic language. Parents report that the child reaches the stage of imitating word forms, but then stops progressing and may indeed lose those first words. One explanation may be that these children have not truly mastered the connection between words spoken and representational meaning and have failed to progress to the higher levels of language learning. Another common experience is for parents to say that children produce words only in situations of extreme emotional provocation or only once and never again; the explanation is likely to be that the language is attached to very particular contexts. Rapid word learning, 'fast mapping', is a skill of normal language acquisition that is significantly poorer in language impairments. A prolonged period before the child moves from single words to sentences is also more common in delayed and disordered development.

Even experts can overestimate the child's comprehension of language. Where there are any concerns, specific tests should be carried out.

Behavior

Food fads, sleep problems, night waking, problems of compliance and temper tantrums are part of normal development between 2 and 5 years of age, and show some continuity through those years. When the behaviors of normal development are functionally impairing for parent and child then they may or may not be called a disorder, but they certainly warrant assessment and intervention. Any developmental impairment puts a child at risk of psychiatric disorder, particularly severe learning and communication difficulties. Extremes of temperament also contribute to risk, as do family factors such as maternal mental ill health, family conflict, school-based difficulties and any other problem with parent–child interaction.

LEARNING IMPAIRMENTS

The terminology of neurodevelopmental impairments leading to functional disability continues to be problematic and different in the USA, the UK and Europe. For example, learning disability is the preferred term in the UK for what would be referred to as mental retardation in the USA. This is defined as an impairment in intellectual learning and adaptive skills to a degree that significantly impairs normal function and on standardized tests falls outside two standard deviations below the mean. Although the implication is that all aspects of development will be affected, in practice this is variable. In severe to profound learning difficulties motor development is usually slower. This may be evident in delayed achievement of milestones, but with a normal pattern of motor development with or without floppiness (hypotonia). However, it is quite possible for a child to show normal acquisition of motor milestones and still have a very significant mental and adaptive impairment. Even within mental and adaptive skills certain strengths and weaknesses are common rather than uncommon. A distinction is made between:

1. general learning difficulties;
2. specific learning difficulties.

It is common, however, for these distinctions to be blurred and overlap in practice.

SPECIFIC NEURODEVELOPMENTAL IMPAIRMENTS

The term 'specific' is used to mean that the skill in question is more delayed than would be expected from the overall level of cognitive ability. Although it is convenient to classify these as covering different functional domains, in practice overlaps of impairment are common. This reflects the more common problem, seen in children, of integration of information processing in a developing brain, rather than the 'damage model' which comes from the study of adults, where brain behavior relationships may be much more specifically anatomically located. Both delay and disorder (differences in developmental pattern) occur in the problem area and often it is difficult to separate these elements. Specific neurodevelopmental impairments include:

1. specific developmental disorders of speech and language;
2. specific developmental disorders of acquired academic skills, for example reading, spelling and mathematics;
3. specific developmental disorders of motor function (clumsy child);
4. autistic spectrum disorders (also called the pervasive developmental disorders) – these disorders are usually classified in the international classification systems under the psychiatric disorders section, but can properly be considered as neurodevelopment impairments;
5. specific developmental impairments of attention (usually with impulsivity and distractability plus or minus hyperactivity and with failure of inhibition control as the likely underlying difficulty);
6. specific impairments of memory (short or long term episodic or declarative) and learning;
7. specific developmental impairment of executive function.

Developmental impairments of attention, with or without hyperactivity, are usually classified under the psychiatric disorders, but the range of functional impairments is due not only to a failure of inhibition. Often there are additional problems with other processes of executive function (i.e. the planning, organizing and carrying through of ideas and actions) and hence are included here as a neurodevelopmental impairment.

All neurodevelopmental impairments place the child at increased risk of additional developmental impairments and behavior problems, which may be of sufficient severity for a psychiatric disorder diagnosis. All these neurodevelopmental impairments have their origin in brain function, either at a neuroanatomical or neurochemical level and can present as behavioral or emotional problems as well as deficits in input (perception) or output functions (e.g. in speaking or recording). They are probably underdiagnosed.

Combinations of developmental impairments that are particularly common are those of attention and motor perception with or without language and learning delay. These are referred to as Delayed Attention and Motor Perception (DAMP) by Scandanavian clinicians. The autistic spectrum disorders are frequently associated with language learning difficulties and problems with motor coordination. These neurodevelopmental impairments are all described in Chapter 20.

The developmental assessment of these varying problems requires analysis and description using appropriate tools for the child's age often by a multidisciplinary team.

PHYSICAL EXAMINATION

A full examination should be carried out as described in Chapter 3. Some aspects are particularly important if the child has a developmental or neurological problem and these will be commented on. The physical examination is generally left to the end because the child may become upset and this would interfere with the developmental examination.

Motor examination

Motor examination is best carried out by observing the child's movement patterns and posture. This can be done during the developmental examination, when the child is walking, speaking and handling material (e.g. tendency to keep the forearm pronated and rather deliberate finger movements in mild spasticity). Indeed after observing the child, one should have a good idea of the nature and extent of any motor problem and examination of tone, reflexes and power is largely confirmatory.

Compare both sides of the body

It is useful to compare the two sides of the body and to determine the child's hand preference. The motor skill, tone, reflexes or the size of the limbs may be significantly asymmetrical suggesting hemisphere dysfunction and therefore focal pathology (mild hemiparesis and visuospatial difficulties).

Head circumference

Head circumference must always be measured and plotted on a centile chart and compared with the child's height and, if there is any discrepancy, with the parents' head circumference (as this is the usual reason for a large head).

Optic discs

Examination of the optic discs and fundi is difficult, but can be very valuable in diagnosing particular disorders (septo-optic dysplasia) as well as raised intracranial pressure.

Appearance

Dysmorphic features and congenital malformations must be looked for because they may suggest a particular syndrome or etiology (e.g. fetal alcohol syndrome).

Skin

The skin should be carefully examined for pigmented and depigmented spots.

Growth

Height, weight and growth rate should be determined as these may indicate a condition such as hypothyroidism.

Mental state

The child's mental state should be observed, for example is the child hyperactive, impulsive? Does the child concentrate well? Is the child having absence or other seizures?

Is there more than one problem?

It is important to remember that the child with one problem may have others and is more likely to do so.

EVALUATION AND INTERPRETATION

The purpose of assessment is to come to a conclusion about whether there is an impairment in development, make a diagnosis and seek to intervene positively to improve outcome and function for the child and family. Evaluation and interpretation of the historical, observational and test data should lead to:

1. a profile of the child – both assets and difficulties (Table 7.11);
2. a management plan to be agreed with parents and to include ways of implementing it (Table 7.12);
3. appropriate onward referrals for intervention, specific therapy, genetic advice;
4. ensuring voluntary services and social services benefits are discussed and arranged [if the child is likely to have special educational needs then there is a duty to inform, with parental permission, the education department so that they can make their own assessment – using the legal framework (Code of Practice Guidelines in the UK[62])], additional resource may be allocated based on a level of need;
5. family support through social services, including respite as needed;
6. written record of findings and discussion to be given to parents;

Table 7.11 Child profile

Diagnosis of the presenting condition
Any other specific neurodevelopmental impairments
Level of intellectual function
Medical condition, either associative or causative, to include a hypothesis about etiology that might need tests for confirmation or refuting
Associated psychosocial situations that may or may not be thought to be causative or contributory
Style of learning/motivation and needs

Table 7.12 Aims of appropriate onward referrals for intervention, specific therapy, genetic advice

Reinforcing acquired skills
Teach developmentally appropriate skills
Provide missed experience
Make use of other skills to overcome difficulties
Use learning style to promote learning

7. further appointment to discuss report and plan, key worker as an ideal, further information and counseling as needed and date for further appointment.

Disclosure discussion

Most importantly it is necessary to develop skills of talking with parents, understanding their reaction to any possible problem in their child. The sharing of information about possible impairment and disability (disclosure discussion) has been the subject of audit and research, which show how important the occasion is in its impact and how training can affect satisfaction.[63]

Important principles are:

1. valuing the child;
2. respecting parents and families;
3. how to tell;
4. who should be there;
5. tuning in to parents: effective communication;
6. next steps: practical help and information.

INTERPRETATION OF ABNORMAL DEVELOPMENT USING AN EVIDENCE-BASED APPROACH AND DEVELOPMENTAL ASSESSMENT FINDINGS

Case study 1: The child of 18 months who is not yet walking64

A boy is referred because of failure to walk independently at 18 months. Does this matter?

Not walking by 18 months places the child outside the 90th centile for British children. A literature search shows one relevant study of such children, an epidemiological survey[35] and that less than 10% of such children had a neurological impairment, 11% had delays in other developmental areas. Bottom shuffling and a family history of late walking were common.[50] Although there is no clear evidence base to assess the yield of further physical examination or exclusion by family history of motor variants, there are two questions that are discriminatory:

1. Is the motor pattern deviant (e.g. toe walking or a pronated position of forearms suggesting spasticity) or does it look normal for a younger child? Observe the nature of the child's movement pattern and examine tone and reflexes, and look for any persistent primitive reflexes and fasciculation.

2. Is development in other areas normal or abnormal? At this age language and symbolic play should be looked at as well as adaptive competencies (e.g. shape sorting). If the child has a significant motor disorder affecting hand function the methods used to determine intellectual ability will need to be modified (e.g. eye pointing to named objects).

How likely is this to be a presentation of muscular dystrophy?

The incidence of muscular dystrophy in male births is 1 in 3802. Of children with muscular dystrophy 50% walk by 18 months of age (although later walking than the family pattern suggests is common). Muscular dystrophy is noted because the child's motor competence falls away from the normal trajectory, even though progress continues to be made for the first few years of life (e.g. running is invariably impaired or the child presents with more general delays such as speech). The risk of muscular dystrophy because of late walking is 1 in 228 for a boy not walking at 18 months; however, if other causes of late walking can be excluded and there is any suggestion of developmental delay generally, a creatine phosphokinase (CPK) estimation is advised.

Most likely etiology in this child

1. History suggests global developmental delay and a maternal male cousin with learning disability. Investigations would be fragile X chromosome and a CPK.
2. History is of preterm delivery, 2 days' ventilation and no family history. Examination shows that the child tends to sit with a curved back and stands propped on toes with legs crossed. The diagnosis is spastic diplegia.

It is always extremely important to ascertain whether or not there is any question of regression because this would lead to another chain of inquiry and investigation.

Case study 2: The child who is saying only a few single words by 30 months

At 30 months many children will be putting two or even three words together and most will have quite large vocabularies. The possible causes of language delay are part of normal variation, specific language delay or disorder, general learning disability (mental retardation), deafness, autism, severe environmental deprivation.

A difficulty with speech (output unclear) may be due to specific motor disorders or other neurological disorders.

In order to discriminate between these it is necessary to determine the child's:

1. understanding of language;
2. ability in non-language areas – drawing, brick building, shapes, symbolic play;
3. understanding and use of non-verbal communication and social interactive and sharing behavior (e.g. gesture, facial expression, response to and initiation of communication) – this can be observed in a play-based assessment and the peer social play assessed at nursery;
4. quality of speech – are the few words clear? – does the child speak jargon using normal speech sounds and intonation?;
5. pattern of speech development: is it following the normal lines or is it deviant in any way (e.g. use of the word rhinoceros before mum and dad)?

A persistent receptive language problem is of more global significance than an expressive problem only. From the Whitehurst and Fischel study[65] most 2-year-old children with 10 words only had caught up by 5 years of age. In another study, however, children with delays in speech and language at 4–5 years still showed impairments in language-based literacy skills in their teens.[66] A family history of language delay might support a genetic predisposition, which is common in developmental language disorder.

Hearing should be checked in all children – even if it is not the main cause. A mild loss may be making a child with a potentially mild developmental language disorder worse.

John's language problem

John's profile on the Griffiths test shows that his ability in non-language areas is normal, so he does not have a global learning disability. His symbolic play is also normal. He is a social child who understands and uses pointing and some simple gestures. His social skills with peers, play and imaginative skills show that he is not therefore autistic. His understanding of language is a little delayed, but not as much as his expressive skills. The words he has are clear and he uses normal sounding jargon. There is nothing deviant about his language development; it is simply delayed. There is a history that his father had been slow to talk and later on had reading and spelling problems. The home environment is satisfactory. Hearing is tested and found to be normal.

John therefore has a developmental language delay for which there is probably a genetic predisposition. As his language comprehension is reasonable and he is beginning to use words he is likely to make steady progress. It is possible he will also have reading and spelling problems at school. He should be reviewed by a speech and language therapist to make sure his progress is satisfactory, and to offer parents advice on how to encourage language development and anticipate any problems with phonological awareness predictive of reading delay.

CHILD DEVELOPMENT TEAMS AND CENTERS IN THE UK

A child development service includes the specialist services for assessment and management of children with disabilities including physical and learning disabilities, hearing, vision, speech and language problems. These children require a different kind of service from that required by most children attending hospital or other pediatric clinics.

At one end of the spectrum there is the child with multiple disabilities, complex neurological problems or physical problems compounded by psychological and behavioral difficulties. Most pediatricians would agree that such children need a dedicated multidisciplinary service that differs from that of an ordinary pediatric consultation.

At the other end of the spectrum is a group of children who sometimes require reviews by a team of professionals with complementary skills and experience, while at other times the child and his or her family might best be dealt with by just one member of the group. In the UK these services are provided on a district basis serving a population of about 250 000–300 000 people. Legislation and guidelines provide the framework for service provision.[67]

1. The multidisciplinary team works directly with the child and family in special and mainstream schools and nurseries, in community clinics and in the child's home, provides advice to the local education authority, and contributes towards statements and reviews under the 1993 Education Act and Code of Practice (2001), together with responsibilities relating to social services under the Children Act.
2. Core team members are usually a pediatrician, speech therapist, physiotherapist, occupational therapist, psychologist, nurse/health visitor, teacher, social worker and administrator.
3. It is important that child development services have comprehensive local knowledge in order to provide the best possible packages of

care. This means that good collaborative working relationships must be built up with primary care, education, social services, parent groups and voluntary groups. Government directives that emphasize the importance of 'joined up care' and local planning for provision and purchasing of services should be joint between health, education and social services.

4. Access to services via 'a single front door' is important. A single organizational and information base for all children with special needs is preferable to provide an integrated service.
5. Parental representatives should be involved in planning and in the running of child development services.
6. The majority of children are seen by the child development center between 0 and 5 years of age. However, there is an important ongoing commitment for review and treatment of a number of children with special educational needs in mainstream or special schools in collaboration with the education department. Continuity of care from preschool to school age is important. The client group includes children and young people with developmental disability up to the age of 19 years.
7. Handover arrangements should be made for transfer to adult services (where available) during the teenage years. A transitional care plan should be drawn up in collaboration between health, social services and education, including the resource team for adults with learning difficulties.
8. Primary health care (including general practitioners and health visitors) has a particular role to play in the detection and ascertainment of children with disability. Liaison should be close, with provision of support, training, clear referral criteria and lines of communication with regular audit to ensure best practice.
9. Supporting hospital pediatric services should be available at a convenient location, with established lines of communication and referral criteria. Inpatient admissions to acute services should use a system to inform the ward staff on how to care for and communicate with the disabled child. 'Seamless' models of service provision are to be encouraged. Combined protocols for management could be devised. The needs of adolescents and young adults for appropriate inpatient accommodation should be considered both for medical needs and acute mental health issues.
10. Tertiary specialist services for childhood disability may be provided within larger teaching districts. In smaller health districts, children needing these services should be able to easily access them in the nearest center. Combined outreach clinics may also be set up.
11. It is desirable for one professional to take on the role of key worker in order to provide a single point of contact and coordination for the family's care package. Initially this is likely to be the team health visitor; however, the family will often make this selection for themselves. Specialist health visitors working in the field of childhood disability have a vital role in service delivery. They are in a particularly good position to form supportive relationships with families, to help them use services appropriately and to act as advocates and intermediaries for the family. The role may pass to different professionals either inside or outside the child development team as the child grows.
12. Ideally, child psychiatry should be part of the child development service rather than being supplied from a different unit since a number of conditions benefit from combined input.
13. Other professionals who are not core members of the child development team provide important additional services and combined clinics can work well for a number of these services. These include a pediatric ophthalmologist, orthoptist and peripatetic teacher for the visually impaired; audiology, hearing aid service, peripatetic teacher for the hearing impaired; dietitian; a clinic for severe neurological feeding impairment; specialist dentistry; orthopedic surgery, with access to gait analysis and to a spinal unit, good orthotic support; specialist radiology (X-ray, computed tomography, magnetic resonance imaging, videofluoroscopy); specialist neurophysiology (electroencephalography, auditory and visual evoked responses); podiatry; a neuropathic bladder
14. Respite care is an essential requirement of families whose children have severe disability.
15. Written information for the family is essential. A special health record for disabled children enables parents to know exactly what services and which health professionals are involved, where they can be reached and to give them information about their child's special needs. Advice about benefits should be readily available.
16. Services should be sensitive to the particular needs of ethnic and cultural minorities.
17. Clear guidelines should exist for the management of child protection issues.

Milner et al[68] provide a checklist suitable for monitoring services for children and families with special needs.

REFERENCES (*Level 1 evidence)

1 American Academy of Pediatrics. Committee on Community Health Services. The pediatrician's role in community pediatrics. Pediatrics 1999; 103:1304–1307.

2 Chomsky N. Language and mind. New York: Harcourt Brace Jovanovitch; 1972.

3 Thalen E, Smith L. A dynamic systems approach to the development of cognition and action. Cambridge, MA: Bradford MIT; 1994.

4 Plomin R. Genetics of childhood disorders III. Genetics and intelligence. J Am Acad Child Adolesc Psychiatry 1999; 38:786–788.

5 Kagan J, Snidman N, Arcus D. Childhood derivatives of high and low reactivity in infancy. Child Dev 1998; 69:1483–1493.

6 Culp R, Watkins RV, Lawrence H, et al. Maltreated children's language and speech development: abused, neglected, and abused and neglected. First Language 1991; 11:377–391.

7 Croft C, Andersen-Wood L, and the English and Romanian Study Team, Institute of Psychiatry. Language development following severe early deprivation. Conference presentation at Afasic Third International Symposium; 1999.

*8 Rutter M, and the English and Roumanian Adoptees (ERA) Study Team. Developmental catch-up and deficit following adoption after severs global early deprivation. J Child Psychol Psychiatry 1998; 39:465–476.

*9 O'Connor T, Rutter M, Beckett C, and the English and Roumanian Adoptees Study Team. The effect of global severe deprivation on cognitive competence: extension and follow-up. Child Dev 2000; 71:376–390.

*10 Lucas A, Morley R, Cole TJ, et al. Breast milk and subsequent intelligence quotient in children born preterm. Lancet 1992; 339:261–264.

11 Brunswick N, McCrory E, Price CJ, et al. Explicit and implicit processing of words and pseudowords by adult developmental dyslexics: a search for Wernicke's Wortschatz? Brain 1999; 122:1901–1917.

12 Fensom L, Bates E, Dale P, et al. Measuring variability in early child language: don't shoot the messenger. Child Dev 2000; 71:323–328.

13 Geschwind N, Galaburda A. Cerebral lateralization: biological mechanisms, associations

and pathology: I. A hypothesis and a program for research. Arch Neurol 1985; 42:428–429.
14 Sheridan MD. The developmental progress of infants and young children, 3rd edn. London: HMSO; 1975.
15 Illingworth R. Development of the infant and young child, 9th edn. Edinburgh: Churchill Livingstone; 1987.
16 Milani-Comparetti A, Gidoni EA. Routine developmental examination in normal and retarded children. Dev Med Child Neurol 1967; 9:631–638.
17 Erhardt R. Developmental hand dysfunction: theory, assessment and treatment. San Antonio: The Psychological Corporation; 1994.
18 O'Hare A, Gorzkowska J, Elton R. Development of an instrument to measure manual praxis. Dev Med Child Neurol 1999; 41:597–607.
19 Harris DB. Children's drawings as measures of intellectual maturity. New York: Harcourt, Brace & World; 1963.
20 Vygotsky LS. Thought and language. Cambridge, MA: Harvard University Press; 1986.
21 Bruner J. Child's talk: learning to use language. New York: WW Norton; 1983.
22 Mundy P. Joint attention and social–emotional approach behavior in children with autism. Dev Psychopathol 1995; 7:63–82.
23 Bates E, Dale P, Thal D. Individual differences and their implications for theories of language development. In: Fletcher P, MacWhinney B, eds. The handbook of child language. Oxford: Blackwell; 1995.
24 Fenson L, Dale PS, Resnick JS, et al. MacArthur's communicative development inventories. San Diego: Singular Publishing; 1993.
25 Volterra V, Erting CJ, eds. From gesture to language in hearing and deaf children. Berlin: Springer; 1990.
26 Crystal D. Listen to your child. Middlesex: Penguin Books; 1986.
27 Astington JW, Jenkins JM. Theory of mind development and social understanding. In: Dunn J, ed. Connections between emotions and understanding in development. Special Issue of J Cognit Emot 1995:151–167.
28 Wainryb C, Shaw L, Maianu C. Tolerance and intolerance: children's and adolescents' judgments of dissenting beliefs, speech, persons and conduct. Child Dev 1998; 69:1541–1555.
29 Stanley O, Dolby S. Learning in pre-school children with neurological disability. Arch Dis Child 1999; 80:481–484.
30 Wimmer H, Perner J. Beliefs about beliefs: representation and constraining function of wrong beliefs in young children's understanding of deception. Cognition 1983; 13:103–128.
31 Wilson J, Jungner G. Principles and practice of screening for disease. Public Health Papers No. 34. Geneva: WHO; 1968.
32 Cochrane A, Holland W. Validation of screening procedures. Br Med Bull 1969; 27:3–8.
33 Law J, Boyle J, Harris F, et al. The feasibility of universal screening for primary language delay: findings from a systematic review. Dev Med Child Neurol 2000; 42:190–200.
34 Law J, Boyle J, Harris F, et al. Screening for primary language delay: a systematic review of the literature. Health Technol Assess 1998; 2:1–184.
*35 Chaplais JD, Macfarlane A. A review of 404 late walkers. Arch Dis Child 1984; 59:512–516.
36 Hall DMB. Health for all children. The Report of the Joint Working Party on Child Health Surveillance. 3rd ed. Oxford: Oxford University Press; 1996.
37 American Academy of Pediatrics. Committee on Children with Disabilities. Screening infants and young children for developmental disabilities. Pediatrics 1994; 93:863–865.
38 National Research Council. Educating children with autism. Committee on Educational Interventions for Children with Autism. Division of Behavioral and Social Sciences and Education. Washington: National Academy Press; 2001.
*39 Baird G, Charman T, Baron-Cohen S, et al. A screening instrument for autism at 18 months of age: a six-year follow-up study. J Am Acad Child Adolesc Psychiatry 2000; 39:694–702.
40 Baird G, Charman T, Cox A, et al. Screening and surveillance for autism and pervasive developmental disorders. Arch Dis Child 2001; 84:468–475.
41 Glascoe F. A method for deciding how to respond to parents' concerns about development and behavior. Ambul Child Health 1999; 5:197–208.
42 Glascoe FP. The value of parents' concerns to detect and address developmental and behavioural problems. J Paediatr Child Health 1999; 35:1–8.
43 British Association for Community Child Health. Child Development and Disability Group of the RCPCH. Standards for child development services. A guide for commissioners and providers. London: Royal College of Paediatrics and Child Health; 2001.
44 Lord C, Rutter M, Le Couteur A. Autism diagnostic interview – revised. J Autism Dev Disord 1994; 24:659–686.
45 Gesell A. The first five years of life. London: Methuen; 1950.
46 Lord C, Risi A, DiLavore P, et al. The autism diagnostic observation schedule – generic. Los Angeles: The Western Psychological Corporation; 1999.
47 Wiart L, Darrah J. Review of four tests of gross motor development. Dev Med Child Neurol 2001; 43:279–285.
48 O'Brien G, Pearson J, Berney T, et al. Measuring behaviour in developmental disability: review of existing schedules. Dev Med Child Neurol 2001: 43(suppl).
49 Robson P. Shuffling, hitching, scooting or sliding: some observations in 30 otherwise normal children. Dev Med Child Neurol 1970; 12:608–617.
50 Robson P. Prewalking locomotor movements and their use in predicting standing and walking. Child Care Health Dev 1984; 10:317–330.
51 Milani-Comparetti A, Gidoni EA. Pattern analysis of motor development and its disorders. Dev Med Child Neurol 1967; 9:625–630.
52 Sonksen PM. The assessment of vision in the preschool child. Arch Dis Child 1993; 68:513–516.
53 Salt A, Sonksen P, Wade A, et al. The maturation of linear acuity and compliance with the Sonksen–Silver acuity system in young children. Dev Med Child Neurol 1995; 3:505–514.
54 Sheridan MD. The clinical assessment of visual competence in babies and young children. In: Smith V, Kean J, eds. Visual handicap in children. London: Heinemann; 1979.
55 Kay Picture Test. PO Box 156, Coventry CV8 3LJ. 1983.
56 Teller DY, McDonald MA, Preston K, et al. Assessment of visual acuity in children: the acuity card procedure. Dev Med Child Neurol 1986; 28:779–789.
57 Sonksen PM, Macrae AJ. Vision for coloured pictures at different acuities. Dev Med Child Neurol 1987; 29:337–347.
58 Mackie RT, McCulloch DL. Assessment of visual acuity in multiply handicapped children. Br J Ophthalmol 1995; 79:290–296.
59 Sonksen P, Petrie A, Drew K. Promotion of visual development of severely visually impaired babies: evaluation of a developmentally based program. Dev Med Child Neurol 1991; 33:320–335.
60 Fortnum HM, Summerfield AQ, Marshall DH, et al. Prevalence of permanent childhood hearing impairment in the United Kingdom and implications for universal neonatal screening: questionnaire based ascertainment study. Br Med J 2001;323:536–539.
61 Wells G. Language development in the pre-school years. Cambridge: Cambridge University Press; 1985.
62 Code of Practice Guidelines in the UK. Special educational needs, code of practice. Department of Education and Skills 581/2001; http://www.dfes.gov.uk
63 Baird G, McConachie H, Scrutton D. Parents' perceptions of disclosure of the diagnosis of cerebral palsy. Arch Dis Child 2000; 83:475–480.
64 Dorling J, Salt A. Assessing developmental delay; evidenced based case report. Br Med J 2001; 323:148–150.
65 Whitehurst GJ, Fischel JE. Early developmental language delay: what, if anything, should the clinician do about it? J Child Psychol Psychiatry 1994; 35:613–648.
*66 Stothard S, Snowling M, Bishop D, et al. Language impaired preschoolers: a follow-up to adolescence. J Speech Lang Hear Res 1998; 41:407–418.
67 Lloyd-Evans A. Standards for child Development services. Produced for the British Association of Community Child Health. London: Royal College of Paediatrics and Child Health; 2001.
68 Milner J, Bungay C, Jellinek D, et al. Needs of disabled children and their families. Arch Dis Child 1996; 75:399–404. service.

8

International child health

Bernard J Brabin

INTRODUCTION

This chapter sets out some dimensions and trends in child health affecting children in an international context. It also reviews the services attempting to tackle these problems at the start of the third millennium.

Child health worldwide is profoundly affected by economic, social, behavioral, political, scientific and technological factors, many of which are changing at an unprecedented rate in both the industrialized and developing worlds. Millions of children live in circumstances which place their survival, protection and development at significant risk.[1] One in four live in unsuitable conditions. 250 million work in hazardous and exploiting labor, many of whom have no access to education. In sub-Saharan Africa there are 10 million acquired immune deficiency syndrome (AIDS) orphans. Each year about 11 million children die before reaching their fifth birthday. More than 98% of these deaths occur in less developed countries and in Africa most occur before a child reaches a health facility.

In the developing world, there are differences of environment, inequalities of natural assets and maldistribution of resources. The result is many impoverished families and a large burden of morbidity and mortality on their children. There are an increasing number of factors contributing to disease re-emergence, especially malaria, tuberculosis and sexually transmitted diseases. Poverty and population growth mean that many families and countries have little to spend on health care which leads to a cycle of poverty, violence and disease.

When planning to improve standards of health, essentials must come first. An adequate water supply in each community, satisfactory housing, agricultural aids, productive employment, stable markets, appropriate energy sources and improved female literacy and adolescent health. For the health of children the essentials also include sufficient and appropriate food, and a safe, stable and stimulating environment. A capable mother can compensate for many other deficiencies. Doctors and pediatricians should be aware that they can do little to influence many factors that limit the health of the world's children. Diagnosing and treating the sick child are important tasks, but the role of pediatricians includes informed advocacy, speaking out for children and supporting parents. Although the health of a child is dependent on many groups and individuals in general, ultimately it depends on one in particular – his or her mother.

THE STATE OF THE WORLD'S CHILDREN 2001 (UNICEF)

Children of the world live in very varied environments and circumstances. The social, economic, demographic and environmental factors which affect their health and well-being are set out in a detailed set of tables at the end of each year's UNICEF report, *The State of the World's Children*. A few of the many facts from the 2001 report have been summarized in Table 8.1. Countries are grouped together by region and developmental status. The three types under consideration are industrialized countries, developing countries and the least developed countries (columns 6–8 in Table 8.1). There are about 10 times as many children in developing and least developed countries compared with industrial countries. Also in the developing and least developed countries children make up 37–50% of the total population. In contrast, in industrialized countries children constitute only about 20% of the population, but there is a higher proportion of people in the older age groups.

Table 8.1 International comparisons: children's health, mortality and associated factors

	Sub-Saharan Africa (1)	Middle East & North Africa (2)	South Asia (3)	East Asia & Pacific (4)	Latin America & Caribbean (5)	Industrialized countries (6)	Developing countries (7)	Least developed countries (8)
Population under 18 years (millions)	306	149	557	599	193	189	1858	310
Population under 5 years (millions)	101	42	163	160	54	50	538	100
Under-5 mortality rates*								
1960	258	247	244	212	153	37	222	283
1999	173	63	104	45	39	6	90	164
Annual urban population growth % (1990–1995)	4.7	3.3	3.2	2.9	2.3	0.8	3.0	4.8
Nutrition: percentage of children (1999–2000)								
moderate to severe wasting**	10	8	17	6	2	–	10	12
moderate to severe stunting	37	24	48	24	17	–	33	45
Adult literacy rate 1995–1999								
Male (%)	64	74	69	91	89	–	81	63
Female (%)	46	53	43	79	87	–	66	44
Education: percentage reaching grade 5 primary (1995–1999)	66	88	54	87	76	99	73	61
Percentage births attended by trained health personnel (1995–2000)	37	69	29	66	83	99	52	28
GNP† per capita ($US), 1999	503	2106	443	1057	3806	26157	1222	261
GNP† per capita: annual growth rate 1990–1999 (%)	0.1	0.3	3.8	6.6	1.8	1.7	3.3	2.2
Total fertility rate‡ 1999	5.4	3.7	3.3	2.0	2.6	1.6	2.9	4.9

Source: The State of the World's Children (UNICEF 2001[3])

*The number of deaths of children under 5 years of age per 1000 live births. More specifically this is the probability of dying between birth and exactly 5 years of age.

**Moderate to severe wasting and stunting means those that are below –2 standard deviations from the median weight for height or height for age of a reference population

†Gross national product, expressed in current US dollars. GNP per capita growth rates are average annual growth rates that have been computed by fitting trend lines to the logarithmic values of GNP per capita at constant market prices for each year of the time period

‡The number of children that would be born per woman according to the prevailing age-specific fertility rates.

The under-5 mortality rate (U5MR) is an important measure of the development of countries and the well-being of their children. The U5MR is the number of children who die before completing 5 years of age per 1000 live-born children in a country or community. In industrialized countries the U5MR has decreased from 37 in 1960 to 6 in 1999. The decrease in the least developed countries is from 283 to 164. Thus in 1960 a child born into the least developed countries had 7.7 times the chance of dying before age 5, compared with a child born in an industrialized country. By the mid-1990s a child from the least developed countries had 27 times the chance of dying before its fifth birthday compared with one in an industrialized country. Many factors influence the U5MR, for example food availability, educational opportunity, human immunodeficiency virus (HIV) prevalence, immunization coverage, etc., but the most striking differences are in the per capita income. In industrialized countries this is virtually 100 times that of the least developed countries.

The large number of developing countries in the world have been divided by UNICEF into five groups (columns 1–5 in Table 8.1). These countries are characterized by having a high proportion of the population in the pediatric age group (31–48%) and a relatively low but variable gross national product (GNP) per capita, often with great contrasts of wealth and poverty within individual countries. In general these countries all had a high U5MR (153–258) 40 years ago, and have been able to cut this figure by more than half by the late 1990s, except for sub-Saharan Africa. Some regions have seen a remarkable decrease in mortality among infants and children, for example the Middle East and North Africa and East Asia and the Pacific. In these regions the U5MR is approximately a quarter of what it was 40 years ago. The sub-Saharan Africa region has had a poor improvement of the U5MR. It has been hit by a series of catastrophies: droughts; political instability and coups; drops in world prices of its raw materials; and the epidemic of HIV infection, associated with other diseases and particularly tuberculosis. The emergence of drug resistant malaria has also contributed.

Table 8.2 summarizes the mean levels and variation of infant and child mortality rates for the Demographic and Health Surveys in developing countries, 1986–1998.[2] Of the component mortality rates which together make up the U5MR, the rate under 1 year of age makes up 62% of the U5MR. The rate of child mortality at 2–4 years has the greatest variation.

TRENDS IN CHILD MORTALITY IN DEVELOPING COUNTRIES

The U5MR is used as a principal indicator in the UNICEF tabulations (Table 8.1). Using this measurement has several advantages. First it relates to an end result of the development process rather than an 'input' such as school enrollment level, per capita calorie availability, or the number of doctors per 1000 population – all of which are means to an end. Second, the U5MR is the result of a wide variety of inputs: the nutritional health and the health knowledge of mothers; the level of immunization and use of oral rehydration; the availability of maternal and child health services including prenatal care; income and food accessibility in the family; clean water and sanitation; and the overall safety of the child's environment. Third, the U5MR is less susceptible than some measures, for example per capita GNP, to 'distortions of the average'. This is because the natural scale does not allow the children of the rich to be 1000 times as likely to survive, even if the man-made scale does permit them to have 1000 times as much money. In other words it is much more difficult for a wealthy minority to affect a nation's U5MR. It therefore presents a more accurate, if far from perfect, picture of the health status of the majority of children and the society in which they live.

The speed of progress in reducing U5MR can be measured by calculating its average annual reduction rate (AARR). Unlike the comparison of absolute changes, the AARR reflects the fact that the lower limits to the U5MR are approached only with increasing difficulty. This is because when the U5MR is low, a higher proportion of the deaths is due to the rarer and less easily preventable diseases like congenital malformations and malignancy. As the lower levels of under-5 mortality are reached, the same absolute reduction obviously represents a greater percentage of reduction. The AARR therefore shows a higher rate of progress for say a 10-point reduction if that reduction happens at the lower level of under-5 mortality. The GNP per person, expressed in US dollars, is an index of wealth or poverty of a country. When the AARR is used in conjunction with GNP growth rates, the U5MR and its reduction rate gives a picture of the progress being made by any country or region, and over any period of time, towards achieving some of the most essential human needs.

Mortality among infants and children has been declining in most developing countries from the mid-1980s and throughout the 1990s. However this decline has recently slowed, stopped, or reversed itself in some countries of sub-Saharan Africa. It is likely that there have been improvements in a wide range of factors which explain the mortality decline. The two most important groups of factors associated with the decline in mortality have been reported as the proportion of malnourished children and of those living in poor environmental conditions (poor water supply, sanitation and housing). Pregnancy and perinatal medical care were also important factors.[2]

Figure 8.1 shows the U5MR change in three African countries relative to the rate in 1981 and the corresponding HIV prevalence among adults at the end of 1999.[3] Today 1.3 million children under 15 years of age live with HIV/AIDS, and with 5.4 million new HIV infections in 1999 alone, the worst is yet to come. HIV infection and the resurgence of malaria are important factors related to the

Table 8.2 Mean level and variation of infant and child mortality rates for the Demographic and Health Surveys in developing countries, 1986–1998

	Mortality rate*				
Value	Neonatal	Post-neonatal	Infant (<1 year)	Age 2–4 years	Under 5 years
Minimum	16.3	5.1	24.7	29.1	31.6
Maximum	67.9	93.4	144.3	218.7	273.8
Mean†	33.4 (11.4)	36.3 (19.9)	69.7 (19.1)	95.0 (48.9)	112.4 (60.6)

*Mortality rates for neonates, infants and children under the age of 5 years are expressed as the number of deaths per 1000 births in a given period. Other mortality rates (postneonatal, child at age 2–4 years) are expressed as the number of deaths per 1000 survivors at the younger age.
†Values in parentheses are standard deviations
Source: Modified from Rutstein 20002

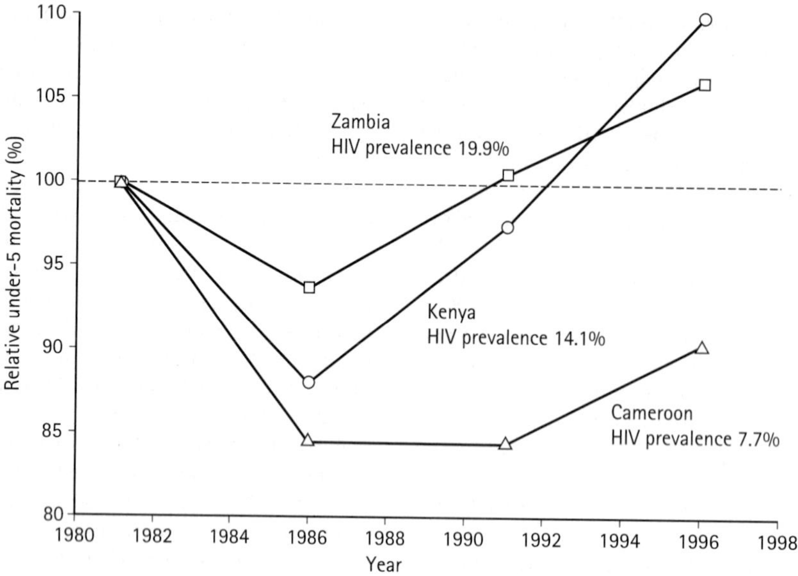

Fig. 8.1 HIV and mortality among children under 5 years old in selected African countries.[3] HIV prevalence rate is among adults at the end of 1999. (From UNICEF 2001[3] with permission)

reversal of mortality trends in some African countries. There is a continuing need to reduce deaths amongst children with greater efforts to control these infectious diseases. Population pressure at the national or household level is also relevant as this affects child care. The data shown in Table 8.1 give the total fertility rate for each country and it can be seen that regions which have achieved substantial reductions in their U5MR have also achieved significant reductions in fertility.

Reduction of maternal mortality is also a major goal because of its implications for the health and development of millions of children and families around the world. The estimated number of maternal deaths in 1995 for the world was 515 000. Of these over half (273 000) occurred in Africa, about 42% occurred in Asia, about 4% in Latin America and the Caribbean, and less than 1% in the more developed regions of the world.[4] The low percentage of births attended by trained health personnel (Table 8.1) is linked to high maternal mortality in large parts of sub-Saharan Africa. This is a particular cause for concern in settings with a high prevalence of HIV/AIDS where the need for skilled care during labor and childbirth is critical.

GLOBAL CONSTRAINTS ON CHILD HEALTH

ECONOMIC FACTORS

The Declaration and Plan of Action of the 1990 World Summit for Children set out future international goals – at the highest political level – to reduce rates of mortality and disease, malnutrition and illiteracy, and to reach specific targets by the year 2000. These goals included one-third reduction in the 1990 U5MR, halving of maternal mortality rates and rates of malnutrition among the world's under 5's, a reduction in the incidence of low birth weight to less than 10%, high immunization coverage (>90%) and completion of primary education (>80%), safe water supplies, acceptance of the rights of the child and family planning initiatives. In the 10 years since the summit, the situation for children has improved, but these goals have not been reached in many poor countries. The attainment of such goals depends on political factors and economic constraints affecting sustainable development. Many of the poorest countries rely on concessional lending and as a group they contain 80% of the world's population categorized as living in poverty. In this situation debt overshadows basic social services.

The term 'adjustment' refers to a range of economic policies which have mostly been supported by loans from the World Bank and International Monetary Fund. These new loans broadly represent an attempt to strengthen the balance of payments by shifting towards a market-orientated system. The debt crisis and falling export prices reduced foreign exchange for most developing countries and the substantial loans available allowed countries to reduce these burdens and support the commodity process. This may be viewed as an unavoidable response to the debt crisis. Adjustment has potentially important effects on health and education, through its effects on market prices and employment. Households may have lower incomes which affect health-related activities, and reduced government spending may reduce health provision and educational opportunities. User-fees reduce access to clinic facilities and schools.

There has been little systematic evaluation of how structural adjustment policies and the terms of trade relate to child health and welfare. However, an analysis by the Save the Children Fund[5] strongly questions whether this approach is wise. Using examples such as the cost of immunization and the new tuberculosis epidemic it illustrates that outside agencies may be getting it wrong – mainly by failing to support national structures in sustaining health care over the long term. Key aspects for the future may be based on adapting economic and health strategies to local circumstances and devolving decision making to communities.

GENDER RELATED FACTORS

The concept of childhood as a time free from gender is only true of children from wealthier families in the world. Gender has two components – biological and cultural. For girls, in many less developed countries the emphasis is on their reproductive role and this becomes established in childhood. The focus on the vulnerability of girls arises partly because of this, but also because of discrimination against them in many societies due to male attitudes and a preference for sons over daughters. Parents favor sons because of the labor and old age security they provide and because they carry the family line. This discrimination limits access to food and medical facilities for girls which can have serious consequences for their health. Death rates for girls, after the neonatal period, are consistently higher than for boys of the same age in many less developed countries, particularly in the Indian subcontinent.

One measure of a child's position is the parental willingness to send him or her to school. In less developed countries deeply rooted traditional and religious attitudes often limit girls' educational and employment opportunities. For example in Pakistan, literacy rates are about 21% for women and 47% for men and only 35% of girls are enrolled in primary school, which is half the enrollment rate for boys. It is important that girls are enabled to reach their full intellectual and social potential in their own right. The aim should not be solely to produce reproductively efficient mothers.

In many countries programs that empower women lead to improvements in children's lives. Women's relative powerlessness in society can make them more likely to be infected with HIV,[6] more vulnerable to violence and abuse and easier targets in armed conflicts. It also plays a major role in how children are cared for within their homes, in who makes the decisions about them and how they are provided for. Gender discrimination is a frequent occurrence and it should be replaced by an environment in which boys and girls are equally valued.

MATERNAL EDUCATION AND CHILD SURVIVAL

The quality of family child health care is more often associated with maternal than paternal schooling and there is a close relationship between child mortality and the length of formal schooling of the mother. Even after adjustment for economic factors, 1–3 year maternal education is associated with a fall of 20% in childhood mortality. This relationship exists in all major regions of the developing world and in countries with either well developed or poorly developed health care systems.[7] Literacy programs for adults who received no childhood education also show these benefits.[8]

When girls can assume some independence even when unmarried, they are more likely to remain in school. When older women are allowed to appear in public on their own initiative, then mothers are more likely to take action for a sick child and not wait to consult husbands or brothers. With more autonomy, women will be more likely to treat their daughters like their sons, providing better nutrition and health care. For these reasons a marked degree of female autonomy is probably essential for significant child mortality reduction in less developed countries.[9] Several studies have demonstrated a close association between maternal education and infant and child mortality. The key analysis was by Caldwell[10] who surveyed data from Ibadan, Nigeria, and demonstrated that the mother's education was a more decisive determinant of child survival than economic well-being. Although other studies have confirmed these initial findings the various mechanisms, or intervening factors, which lead to the lower mortality are not well understood. More equitable treatment of daughters, and sons plays some role, but factors, affecting water use, housing quality, and use of preventive and curative services are also important. Little is known about the intervening role of health beliefs and domestic practices, although these are probably very important.

The education advantage in survival is less pronounced during the neonatal period and higher male mortality rates during the first 4 weeks of life are reported. This is consistent with the overwhelming evidence that in childhood, male biological risk, as opposed to cultural risk, of death is higher than that for females.

CHILD EXPLOITATION

Child labor

Children are exploited because they are vulnerable. Families in least favored circumstances will be those who are most likely to send their children out to work. Children from lower socioeconomic groups are those most likely to be sent to work and to be malnourished. Evidence for this comes from a study of childhood malnutrition and child labor in rural India.[11] Conversely, children kept at home to help with household duties and child care may not be able to attend school. Many children must combine domestic tasks in the home with waged labor outside; others are required to stay at home in order to free adults for labor outside the home.

In view of the lack of reliable statistical data at national level, it is not possible to assess the trend of child labor over time. There are indications that the number has increased since 1980 in some developing countries. According to a recent International Labor Organization estimate, the number of working children between the ages of 5 and 14 years in developing countries is 250 million, of whom 120 million work full-time.[12] Approximately 61% of child workers are in Asia, 32% in Africa and 7% in Latin America. Child labor also exists in industrialized cities in South Europe.

The employment of young children is a serious problem, particularly in rural areas where it is not unusual for children to start work at the age of 5 or 6 years.

Culturally related exploitation

Behaviors and attitudes acceptable in some areas and eras may be viewed as detrimental in others. Cross-cultural perspectives in child maltreatment depend on circumstances and should be considered in the context of:

1. Cultural differences in child-rearing practices
2. Departure from culturally acceptable behavior
3. Societal harm of children which is beyond control of parents or care-takers.[13]

Parents who exploit and abuse their children are themselves often under stress and a high proportion have a poor education. Premature, mentally retarded and physically disabled children may be at particular risk.

In some societies girls are considered an important asset to families (e.g. Cambodia) as, according to tradition, husbands come to live with their wives' family, becoming an asset for income generation. For this reason girls are less likely to be abandoned.

Child prostitution, pornography and trafficking

The commercial sexual exploitation of children has in recent years become a matter of international concern. About 1 million children in Asia are victims of the sex trade and the number is increasing in Africa and Latin America. The situation is becoming even more serious, because children are being sold and taken secretly across national borders. Girls may have a high economic value fetching hundreds of dollars when sold into the sex grade as virgins. The consequences for children are far reaching and can be fatal.

Case studies reveal the depth of the trauma and many such children are unable to return to normal activities.

Slavery and similar practices

The most vulnerable children are those in forced labor systems, the most common of these being debt bondage. In South Asia the number of children employed in this way is estimated at several tens of millions. The lenders manipulate the system making it impossible for the family to repay the debt. A family can remain bonded for generations. In West Africa, trafficked children who sell water in African markets is commonplace.[14]

Child soldiers

One of the most deplorable developments in recent years has been the increasing use of children as soldiers. Recently in many countries, thousands of children under the age of 16 have fought in wars. Such children have experienced the psychological trauma of violence, captivity, sexual abuse, undernutrition and torture and the effects of this on their psychological development is difficult to determine. In Uganda, trauma rehabilitation centers have been established to help abducted children rescued from areas of conflict.[15] These provide counseling and nursing services and are facilitated by social workers to enable resettlement of children to their parents or next of kin. Similar initiatives have been developed in other war torn zones.

Street children

Most of the literature on street children concerns boys. There is no adequate information on the numbers of children who live on the streets or the comparative proportion of boys and girls who engage in specific street trade. It is estimated there are 50 000–100 000 street children who manage to survive in Calcutta, India; and in Phnom Penh estimates vary between 5000 and 10 000. Such estimates do not account for the fluctuations of the street population, who may not live solely on the street but maintain links with the family. These numbers do not account for some of the most exploited children – girls sold into prostitution and hired labor – and they do not account for the full number of orphaned and abandoned children. In 1991 it was estimated that in Cambodia 1 in every 13 children had lost at least one parent and 45% of these have lost both parents. Traditionally, such children are cared for by the extended family, but as this support is reduced by the effects of war or the HIV epidemic, then many children cater for their own needs. Not all these children are orphaned and many may be runaways who are escaping violence in the home. Common factors cited by children themselves as reasons they were on the street include poverty, hunger, family disharmony and violence.

The problems and dangers faced by street children relate to their hazardous occupations, for example sifting rubbish with bare hands and feet. Some are sexually abused and become infected with sexually transmitted diseases. In Honduras 44% of street children were sexually active and almost all had been treated for sexually transmitted diseases.[16] They live in fear of bullying and losing their earnings as they have no safe place to keep them or their meager belongings. In a study of 30 child street hawkers in Port Harcourt, Nigeria, the children complained of adult abuse (13%), sexual harassment (42%, both boys and girls), education deprivation (17%), and disliking their work (27%). In traffic-polluted city centers such as Lagos, where a high number of street hawkers are children, air pollution resulting in respiratory morbidity is likely to be a significant hazard. A particular cause for concern are the Indian temple prostitutes, termed devadasis, who are low-caste girls estimated to be over 100 000 in number and who are given to temples of the goddess Yellema by their parents. These girls are sexually exploited from early puberty by devotees and have almost no option but to become prostitutes.[17]

Seeking solutions to these problems involves a range of measures from immediate service provision to tackling the root causes. Many non-government agencies are involved in this work. Fyfe[18] presents five stages to assist working children which extend into tackling the 'root causes':

1. education and training (providing access to schooling);
2. welfare services (to disadvantaged children in the community as a whole, and not only to those in residential centers; rehabilitation of children leaving the sex industry);
3. protected work (placement schemes and sheltered workshops, community-based care at specific sites);
4. advocacy (emphasis on child rights, youth networks and local support groups);
5. regulation and enforcement (support for the training of police; child-specific provision within the court and prison systems).

PROBLEMS FACING HEALTH SERVICES

Competition between various health initiatives is dependent on internal resource allocation and severe problems in financing health initiatives, particularly in sub-Saharan Africa, emerged in the 1980s. The demand for health services has also increased due to population growth, successful social mobilization and the AIDS pandemic with tuberculosis and other associated infections. In some countries this has led to an inadequate availability of medicines, equipment and a failure to pay health worker salaries.

Although communities can provide to some extent for themselves they still require access to health services and these services should provide what people want. People do not accept poor quality services just because they are there and this leads to underutilization. Health Sector Reform has emerged as a priority for refining policies and reforming structures through which health improvements are implemented in developing countries. The main components emphasize decentralization in order to promote efficiency and public accountability. Governments of developing countries have to ensure that the appropriate share of public resources is allocated to health in a way that satisfies users who should also exercise some control over them. These initiatives have to be achieved in countries where per capita expenditure on health is about 2% of that in established market economies. Can this be achieved in a health sector where staff are unmotivated and sometimes poorly trained, where patients face long clinic times at inconvenient hours and there are frequently inadequate supplies and drugs? In the private sector financial exploitation may occur with no safeguards against unnecessary or even dangerous treatments. Hospital management in most less developed countries is a relatively neglected area, partly as a consequence of the international focus on primary health care.

When mothers arrive at a clinic, giving priority to very sick children is also essential. Introducing 'triage' (French: to sort) into first level health facilities is necessary for efficient screening for very sick children. Assigning children on simple clinical signs and symptoms into urgent or less urgent cases is required and the selection for earlier treatment needs to be explained to the parents.

A recent assessment of hospital facilities in seven less developed countries showed that the quality of hospital care for seriously ill children is greatly affected by the following:[19]

1. poorly organized and delayed triage;
2. inappropriate inpatient or emergency treatment;
3. poor monitoring of patients;
4. inadequate training of physicians and nurses;
5. lack of guidelines for standard case management;
6. sporadic lack of essential drugs;
7. understaffing, particularly at night.

It is hard not to conclude that the majority of children in many developing countries, despite international initiatives of larger institutions, do not have access to simple and affordable health care and yet this is an essential part of their fundamental human right.

INTERNATIONAL RESPONSES TO IMPROVE CHILD HEALTH

THE RIGHTS OF THE CHILD

Children's rights is a concept which is clearly related to the law. A child's rights approach to improving the situation for children in less developed countries establishes through recognition, but not necessarily legislation, the needs of children in health, education and security. The United Nations Convention on the Rights of the Child received universal ratification in 1993 from its member states. The Convention with its 52 articles provides a set of principles and standards for the planning and practice of pediatrics and child health for all children and young people up to the age of 18 years. The main article recognizes that every child has an inherent right to life and states that parties shall ensure to the maximum extent possible the survival and development of the child.[20] The main article concerned with the provision of health services is Article 24 which says that *all* children and young people under 18 years old have the right to 'the enjoyment of the highest attainable standard of health'. This includes such principles as:

- steps to reduce infant and child mortality;
- providing primary health care;
- providing pre- and postnatal care;
- providing basic health promotion information;
- developing preventive health care services.

Those providing services should also allow children to have their own views about their health and treatment and the services which affect them. This includes children with disabilities who have a right to appropriate services and support. Those from indigenous populations and ethnic, linguistic and religious minorities have the right to enjoy and practice their own cultures. Equal opportunities in education should be provided to children who are unable to attend school regularly.

Implementing the Convention in developing countries is restricted because of these realities. Nevertheless in daily work those responsible for child care may look to the Convention as a source of authority in advocating children's rights. This is especially important for the most deprived and vulnerable children and those who are chronically sick, as it counterbalances complacent or defeatist views concerning the prospects for improving child life and health in poor countries.[21]

INTERNATIONAL PARADIGMS IN CHILD HEALTH

Against the background of global constraints on child health there have been significant achievements and sustained international efforts (Fig. 8.2). The World Health Organization (WHO) has established targets related to Health for All, including one which may realistically be achieved – the elimination of paralytic polio within the next few years. A number of international development targets have been agreed by the United Nations (UN). Two of the most important are the reduction by two-thirds in the mortality rates for infants and children under the age of 5 years by 2015 and the reduction by half of people living in extreme poverty by 2020. Paradigms for improving child health in the 1970s and 1980s concentrated on specific themes: growth monitoring, oral rehydration for diarrheal disease, breast-feeding promotion, immunization and family planning strategies. These were part of a global strategy. Much of this effort has had a community basis, linked to the implementation of primary health care. In a wide variety of ways, grass-roots, services which used local personnel and simple methods had shown that it was possible, without great expense and advanced technology, to reduce mortality and morbidity rates.[22]

During the 1990s UN agencies have increased their efforts in the areas of Safe Motherhood, the management of acute respiratory

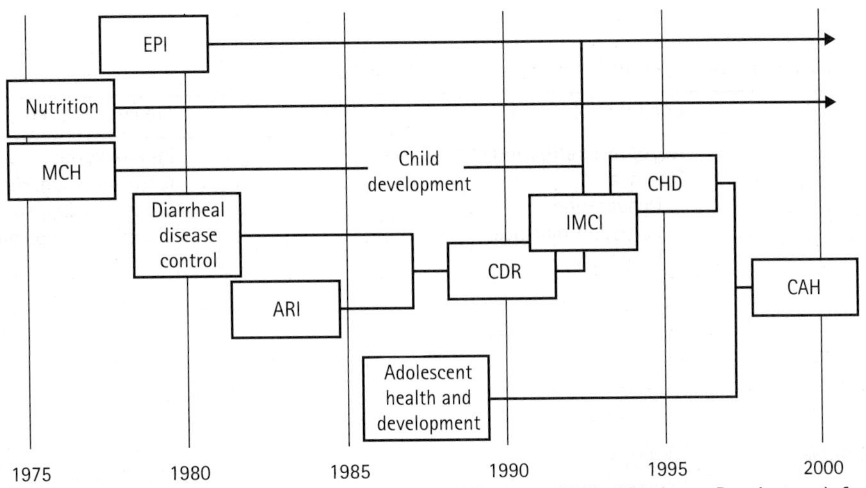

Fig. 8.2 The evolution of child and adolescent health and development programs in WHO; ARI, Acute Respiratory Infection Control; CAH, Child and Adolescent Health; CHD: Child Health and Development; CDR Communicable Disease Research; EPI, Expanded Program on Immunization; IMCI, Integrated Management of Childhood Illness, MCH, Material and Child Health.

infections, adolescent health and poliomyelitis eradication. WHO and UNICEF are now developing a program termed 'Integrated Management of the Sick Child' (IMCI).[23] The core IMCI intervention is integrated case management of the five most important causes of childhood deaths in developing countries – acute respiratory infections (ARI) (19%), diarrhea (19%), measles (7%), malaria (5%) and perinatal complications (18%). Half of all of these are complicated by malnutrition. The strategy includes a range of other preventive and curative interventions which aim to improve practices in the health facilities and at home. In addition to the leading causes of childhood mortality, the IMCI guidelines also address other common associated conditions (Table 8.3). The IMCI strategy also promotes a number of interventions such as immunization, vitamin A supplementation and drug supply management.[24]

A minimum level of knowledge, skill and supplies is required to ensure health care of a reasonable quality. This includes availability of a short list of essential drugs for outpatient use. Health workers require a simple timing device for counting the respiratory rate, a liter measure for preparation of oral rehydration salts (ORS), a weight scale and a thermometer. A list of essential drugs for integrated outpatient management of the sick child proposed by WHO/UNICEF is shown in Table 8.4.[25]

Integrated management of the sick child by health workers who are not doctors, although not a new concept,[26] is attractive because it addresses major health needs and could be cost effective. The algorithms developed for this program have not yet been fully evaluated in areas with varying endemicity of common childhood diseases. The approach addresses the sick child as a whole and not single diseases. Disease-specific control programs for diarrhea and pneumonia have been comprehensively evaluated and show good efficacy in reducing child mortality, particularly in research settings (Table 8.5). Their implementation on a program basis requires good and regular health staff supervision and active health promotion. The supervisory aspects of these activities are easily neglected, greatly reducing their impact and cost effectiveness.

The above concept acknowledges the coexistence of several illnesses in many children; for example those children living in malaria endemic areas may have clinical malaria together with diarrhea and/or pneumonia. Therefore the presence of respiratory or gastrointestinal symptoms does not exclude malaria. The prompt diagnosis and treatment of malaria, without microscopy, is a priority but is difficult because fever alone cannot be presumed to indicate malaria and presenting symptoms and signs vary according to the level of malaria transmission and hence acquired immunity.[27] Therefore 'observation areas' for regular checking of diagnosis are necessary in health facilities in order to review management before outpatient discharge. Malaria microscopy remains the key element in malaria diagnosis.

Following the adoption of a global malaria control strategy, emphasizing improved case management as the main priority, the WHO made an effort to estimate the number of actual clinical malaria attacks per year, arriving at an estimate of 300–500 million clinical cases each year for 1991 and 1993. Estimates of malaria mortality were quoted as varying from 1.5 to 3 million.[28–30] New strategies to combat malaria have also focused on the use of impregnated bed nets, which have been shown to reduce child mortality significantly in research settings, and the use of combination antimalarial therapy to prevent the emergence of drug resistant strains of *Plasmodium falciparum* parasites.

IMPROVING PERINATAL HEALTH

Most mortality and morbidity in the perinatal and neonatal periods is preventable. The causes are often classified as maternal, obstetric and fetal. They include factors such as poor maternal health and poor care during pregnancy, inappropriate management of maternal complications and delivery and lack of appropriate care for the newborn, especially the resuscitation of mildly asphyxiated babies. The significance of these factors will vary from place to place.[31] A valuable summary of available information on perinatal mortality has been compiled by the Maternal Health and Safe Motherhood Programme of WHO.[32] Improved malaria control in pregnancy is essential as *P. falciparum* infection during pregnancy is the most important cause of low birth weight in first pregnancies in women living in highly malarious areas.

Lower perinatal mortality will result from interventions addressing the needs of the newborn – resuscitation when necessary (adequate provision of bag and masks), immediate breast-feeding (for example ensuring implementation of the baby-friendly initiative of UNICEF) (Table 8.6), warm, clean and hygienic delivery conditions and cord care, and early detection (or prevention) of perinatal infections or neonatal diseases. The prevention and management of anemia and control of malaria in pregnancy will reduce the low birth weight risk and improve survival.[33] The mother–baby package[34] introduced by WHO's Maternal Health and Safe Motherhood Programme in 1995

Table 8.3 Interventions included in the IMCI guidelines for first-level health workers

	Conditions covered by case management	Preventive interventions
Generic version	Acute respiratory infections Diarrhea Dehydration Persistent diarrhea Dysentery Meningitis, sepsis Malaria Measles Malnutrition Anemia Ear infection	Immunization Nutrition counseling Breast-feeding support Vitamin A supplementation
Using the *IMCI Adaptation Guide*	HIV/AIDS Dengue hemorrhagic fever Wheeze Sore throat	Periodic deworming

Table 8.4 Essential drugs for outpatient management of the sick child

- Oral rehydration salts
- Oral first and second line antibiotics
- Oral first and second line antimalarials
- Iron tablets
- Vitamin A capsules
- Paracetamol
- Mebendazole
- Tetracycline eye ointment
- Gentian violet for application to skin and mouth
- Quinine for intramuscular use
- Chloramphenicol for intramuscular use

Table 8.5 Intervention studies: impact of ARI programs on mortality in children under 5 years

Place	Reduction in ARI mortality (%)	Reduction in overall mortality (%)
Matlab, Bangladesh	51	30
Gadchiroli, India	54	30
Haryana, India	42	24
Kediri, Indonesia	67	41
Jumla, Nepal	–	28
Kathmandu Valley, Nepal	62	40
Abbotabad, Pakistan	56	55
Bohol, Philippines	25	13
Bagamayo, Tanzania	30	27

Source: WHO program for acute respiratory infections

Table 8.6 Ten steps for successful breast-feeding

1. Have a written breast-feeding policy that is routinely communicated to all health care staff
2. Train all health care staff in skills necessary to implement this policy
3. Inform all pregnant women about the benefits and management of breast-feeding
4. Help mothers initiate breast-feeding within an hour of birth
5. Show mothers how to breast-feed, and how to maintain lactation even if they are separated from their infants
6. Give newborn infants no food or drink other than breast-milk, unless medically indicated
7. Practice rooming-in – allow mothers and infants to remain together 24 h a day
8. Encourage breast-feeding on demand
9. Give no artificial teats or pacifiers (also called dummies or soothers) to breast-feeding infants
10. Foster the establishment of breast-feeding support groups and refer mothers to them on discharge from the hospital or clinic

comprises a cluster of cost-effective interventions. The emphasis is on the birth attendant who can ensure carefully monitored deliveries and life-saving interventions, should complications occur. The mother–baby package offers a minimum list of essential interventions (Table 8.7). Low cost technologies for the newborn are especially important in developing countries. In community settings simple delivery kits enabling hygienic cutting and tying of the umbilical cord are essential for use by traditional birth attendants in order to reduce the risk of hemorrhage and neonatal tetanus.

One of the cheapest appropriate technologies for low birth weight newborn babies is close skin-to-skin contact with the mother. This is one of the ideas behind the kangaroo method which has been shown to be effective in reducing neonatal mortality. Late clamping of the umbilical cord can also increase red cell mass in the newborn baby, reducing the risk for subsequent development of infant anemia.[35]

Table 8.7 Mother–baby package: essential interventions

- Family planning to reduce incidence of unwanted and mistimed pregnancies
- Basic maternal care to all women
- Protection and support for early and exclusive breast-feeding
- Reduce anemia in pregnant women
- Reduce sexually transmitted diseases in pregnant women
- Reduce maternal deaths due to complications of abortions
- Reduce maternal deaths due to hemorrhage
- Reduce maternal deaths due to prolonged/obstructed labor
- Reduce maternal deaths due to puerperal sepsis
- Eliminate neonatal tetanus
- Reduce neonatal deaths due to birth asphyxia
- Reduce neonatal deaths associated with neonatal hypothermia
- Reduce ophthalmia neonatorum

IMMUNIZATION STRATEGIES

Neonatal tetanus (NT) is the second leading cause of death from vaccine-preventable diseases among children worldwide.[36] The number of NT cases globally decreased from 31 849 in 1988 to 15 716 in 1997 and 60% of cases were from China, India and Pakistan. The goal of NT elimination was adopted by the World Summit for Children in 1990. Elimination was defined as less than 1 case per 1000 live births. The primary strategies for achieving the goal include:

1. vaccination of pregnant women with at least two doses of tetanus toxoid; and
2. provision of clean delivery services to all pregnant women.

Additional strategies of supplemental vaccination in targeted 'high risk' areas has been implemented during the 1990s. There is also a need to improve immunization of adolescents in view of the sustained low vaccination coverage in pregnant women.[37,38] Missed opportunities for immunization can reach 30–40% in some under-5s clinics.

Polio transmission has been interrupted in the Region of the Americas, the Western Pacific and the European Regions. The eradication of polio in more than 100 countries including many with extremes of climate, access, poor health systems and internal conflicts have demonstrated the effectiveness of polio eradication strategies. Progress has been achieved through effective National Immunization Days and surveillance for acute onset flaccid paralysis. There has been a decrease in the number of virus strains in many endemic countries and polio virus type 2 is on the verge of extinction.

Based upon efforts to control measles in the Western Hemisphere and the UK, global measles eradication is technically feasible with available vaccines. A goal of global measles eradication should be established with a target date during 2005–2010. The effort should build on the success of poliomyelitis eradication.

NUTRITIONAL STRATEGIES

Local, national, international and non-governmental organizations have been working on the problem of malnutrition in many different ways for decades. A key focus of nutritional assessment has centered on growth monitoring using a Road to Health chart. Numerous forms of this chart are used by different countries but the simplest version uses an upper line which is usually the 50th percentile for boys and a lower line which is the third percentile for girls. The reference values are often the National Centre for Health Statistics (NCHS) standards (Fig. 8.3). The successful use of this chart depends on supervision of attendants and the availability of a suitable community nutrition program and referral facilities for malnourished children.

There have been changes in the profile of nutrition-related diseases during the last 20 years in several developing countries. In sub-Saharan Africa severe food shortages and, in places, near famine exists, while in Southeast Asia severe protein–energy malnutrition (PEM) has declined. Florid acute micronutrient deficiencies such as pellagra and keratomalacia have also declined, whereas chronic micronutrient deficiencies have become the major nutritional problems. These are iron and folate deficiency, goiter and other iodine deficiency disorders and the less severe forms of vitamin A deficiency. The possibility that zinc deficiency could have a bearing on PEM, vitamin A deficiency and anemia should be seriously considered. Zinc is a component of key enzymes and is involved in protein synthesis; its deficiency could therefore aggravate PEM. Micronutrients play a life-saving role in developing countries. Three of them – vitamin A, iron and iodine – have been shown to profoundly affect child survival, women's health, educational achievement, adult productivity and overall resistance to illness. Vitamin D and calcium deficiency leading to rickets is a significant problem in groups with limited sun exposure. Rickets also occurs in immigrant populations who maintain cultural and dietary practices predisposing to vitamin D deficiency. Cereal-based diets rich in phytate and common in most developing countries will predispose to insufficient absorption of calcium, iron and zinc.

Nutritional interventions to address these problems have been grouped into the following categories: household food security, nutrition and infectious disease control; caring capacity; controlling micronutrient deficiencies; and therapeutic nutrition through rehabilitation. Most interventions in the field of micronutrient nutrition have concentrated on deficiencies of vitamin A, iron and iodine, in concordance with the priorities set by the World Summit for Children in 1990.[39] Significant mortality reduction has been reported in several community vitamin A supplementation trials (Table 8.8)[40] primarily due to reduced severity and complications from measles and severe diarrhea. In the longer term more attention must be given to improving vitamin A and iron intake in the diet.[41]

Other micronutrients such as zinc, copper and riboflavin warrant attention, not least because of nutrient interactions and multiple deficiencies. This has drawn attention to multimicronutrient supplementation strategies, although these will be costly.

Control of infectious disease as well as dietary/nutritional interventions are essential to break the infection–malnutrition cycle. Iron-infection interventions have recently been reviewed.[42]

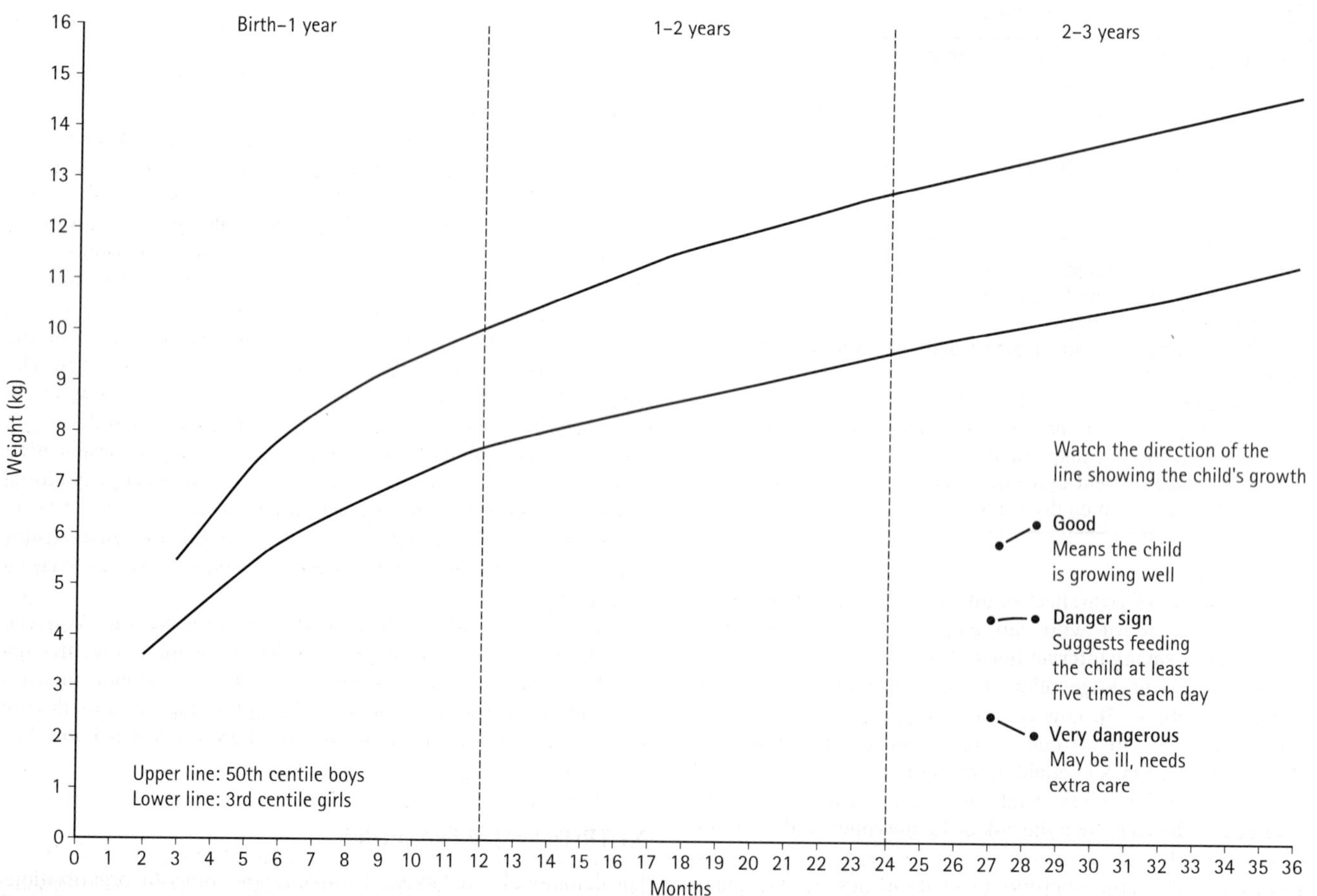

Fig. 8.3 An example of a Road to Health Chart for Growth Monitoring using the NCHS standards.

Table 8.8 Major community mortality prevention trials using vitamin A supplementation

Study	Year	Country	Vitamin A supplement	Reported mortality reduction
Aceh	1986	Indonesia	Large dose every 6 months	34%
Bogor	1988	Indonesia	Vitamin A-fortified monosodium glutamate	45%
NNIPS	1991	Nepal	Large dose every 4 months	30%
Jumla	1992	Nepal	One large dose with follow-up at 5 months	29%
Tamil Nadu	1990	India	Weekly RDA*	54%
Hyderabad	1990	India	Large dose every 6 months	6% (ns**)
Khartoum	1992	Sudan	Large dose every 6 months	+6% (ns)
VAST	1993	Ghana	Large dose every 4 months	19%

* A weekly dose was given, providing the recommended dietary allowance (RDA).
** Not statistically significant.
Source: McLaren & Frigg 1997[40]

Improved dietary management of infection is important. This includes:

- continuation of breast-feeding (Table 8.6);
- maintenance of diet during infection, especially in persistent diarrhea;
- administration of vitamin A in the management of measles and severe diarrhea;
- the use of ORS in diarrhea;
- dietary support in chronic infections;
- use of low dose oral iron in anemia even if associated with malaria parasitemia;[43]
- treatment of intestinal parasites.

The dietary prevention of infection includes promoting exclusive breast-feeding for 4–6 months, and continued breast-feeding into the second year of life. The debate continues over breast-feeding versus formula feeding as a strategy for the interruption of breast milk transmission of HIV in resource poor settings. Exclusive breast-feeding for the first three months of life may be as safe as formula feeding and much safer than mixed feeding in preventing viral transmission. This issue has recently been reviewed.[44] Satisfactory weaning foods are essential. Prevention of low birth weight by improving both nutritional status during pregnancy and lactation and malaria control in pregnancy are priorities.

Therapeutic nutrition

Nutritional rehabilitation of individual undernourished children has a conventional sequence consisting of the resuscitation phase, first refeeding phase, rehabilitation itself and then preparation for returning home. The interventions in these phases are well described.[45,46] Nutritional rehabilitation is considered satisfactory when the child reaches 100% of reference weight for height. The child must be closely monitored throughout this 6- to 8-week period. This may not imply a lengthy stay in hospital as rehabilitation may continue in an appropriate center or preferably at home.

In summary, malnutrition is an extremely complex condition. A comprehensive understanding of its ecology is necessary to plan long term solutions. The central role of women in interventions has been well demonstrated. There is no single way to eradicate malnutrition, but there are workable, sustainable strategies in which health workers and communities can cooperate.

SCHOOL HEALTH

The success of child-survival programs has created new challenges for the third millennium: to improve the quality of life of the survivors and to help children to realize their full potential through a reduction in their burden of disease. For school-age children this implies the prevention of morbidity to promote not only physical but also intellectual development.[47] The aim of improving health may be sufficient cause for health interventions in school children, but this need is greatly enhanced because good health is important for education.[48] The fact that children assemble daily in one place – their school – provides an opportunity to deliver mass treatments through an existing infrastructure to a group in the community that bears a high burden of disease. The promotion of child health through helminth control has received a high priority since school-age children are prime targets for treatment in areas where prevalence of infection with intestinal worms or schistosomes is greater than 50%. The WHO now recommends the mass treatment of school-age children although a lower threshold may be applied if undernutrition is widespread.

ADOLESCENT HEALTH (see also Ch. 34)

Adolescents are defined by WHO as young people between the ages of 10 and 19 years. Out of 1.2 billion adolescents worldwide, about 85% live in developing countries. Adolescence is a period of change – at the younger end are girls and boys, most of whom are not yet sexually active. At the older end are physically mature young men and women, many of whom are sexually active and in many cases, have children of their own.

In younger adolescents undernutrition and stunting are prevalent in both girls and boys. Some may require tetanus vaccination if they were not fully immunized as babies. As girls enter puberty they may know little about menstruation and how pregnancy occurs. The majority of first sexual contacts among adolescents are unprotected leading to high rates of pregnancy, sexually transmitted and HIV infections. At all ages interpersonal violence and sexual abuse is increasing, with girls especially victimized.

The lives of adolescents are at risk because society does not provide them with the skills, the health services and the support they need as they physically and socially mature. WHO, UNICEF and the United Nations Population Fund (UNFPA) are advocating a common agenda to address adolescents' needs and advocate[49] creating safe and supportive environments through:

- promoting delayed marriage and child-bearing;
- expanding access to education and training;
- providing income-earning opportunities;
- providing information and skills;
- expanding access to health services.

In 2001 the WHO presented the findings of a Global Consultation on Adolescent Friendly Health Services. Its aims were to develop a common understanding of the health and development related needs of adolescents, to define best practices and to develop a consensus on global research and an action agenda to make it easier for adolescents to access the health services they need. The meeting supported implementation of a package of health services for adolescents, and this should provide a good basis for action in future. Promoting the healthy development of young people in the second decade of life is one of the most important long term investments that any society can make.[50]

THE DISABLED CHILD

Children in developing countries are more likely to suffer from one of the preventable causes of disability, such as paralytic poliomyelitis, and are least likely to receive help and understanding. Disability is closely associated with poverty. Estimates of prevalence vary greatly because of varying definitions. WHO and UNICEF estimates are between 5 and 10%. The organization of services for these children depends on both community-based and institutional approaches to rehabilitation. Institutional approaches have the disadvantage that they are expensive, 'patient orientated', urban, can be difficult to integrate into other activities and are usually run by well-trained professionals. Community-based rehabilitation (CBR) refers more to therapeutic measures applied by families to the disabled in their own homes. The focus is on the child in the community and the role of the professional is supportive. Local technologies and self-help become more important. Through this approach help can be given to many more children of all ages. The movement towards CBR has increased throughout the 1980s and important lessons have been learnt. These are reviewed in a report from The Netherlands.[51] Regular newsletters (*CBR News*) are also published by the Appropriate Health Resource and Technologies Action Group (AHRTAG).

REFUGEE HEALTH

The United Nations has defined a refugee as a person who:

> *'owing to a well founded fear of being persecuted for reasons of race, religion, nationality, membership of a particular social group or political opinion is outside the country of his nationality and is unable, or owing to such fear, is unwilling to avail himself of the protection of that country; or who is unable to, or owing to such fear, is unwilling to return to it'.* [52]

Guidelines have been produced for pediatricians concerning the health of refugee children.[52] Refugee children in developing countries are often vulnerable to disease and malnutrition because their situation has arisen in an emergency context. A practical approach to children's health in emergencies has been reviewed by Health Link Worldwide.[53]

The annual average of refugees has been growing steadily throughout the 1990s. Exile usually destabilizes children who find themselves in a new culture and often exposed to new infectious agents. Epidemic disease is a particular risk amongst refugees and includes measles, malaria, scabies, dysentery and cholera. Evidence of previous hepatitis B virus (HBV) infection may be common amongst refugees and immigrants originating from areas of high HBV prevalence. This has implications for close contacts of carriers who may benefit from immunization.[54]

REFERENCES (* Level 1 evidence)

1 Costello A, White H. Reducing global inequalities in child health. Arch Dis Child 2001; 84:98–102.

2 Rutstein SO. Factors associated with trends in infant and child mortality in developing countries during the 1990s. Bull World Health Organ 2000; 78(10):1256–1270.

3 United Nations Children's Fund. The state of the world's children. New York: UNICEF; 2001.

4 World Health Organization. Maternal mortality in 1995: estimates developed by WHO, UNICEF, UNFPA. Geneva: WHO; 2001.

5 Save the Children Fund. Poor in health. London: Save the Children Fund; 1996.

6 Brabin L. Clinical management and prevention of sexually transmitted diseases: a review focusing on women. Acta Trop 2000; 75:53–70.

7 Cleland J, Van Ginneken JK Maternal education and child survival in developing countries: the search for pathways of influence Soc Sci Med 1988; 27:1357–1368.

8 Sandiford P, Cassel J, Montengro M, et al. Impact of women's literacy on child health and its interaction with access to health services. Popul Studies 1995; 49:5–17.

9 Caldwell JC. Routes to low mortality in poor countries. Popul Dev Rev 1986; 12(2):171–220.

10 Caldwell JC. Education as a factor in mortality decline: an examination of Nigerian data. Popul Studies 1979; 33:395–413.

11 Satyanarayan K, Prasanna KT, Rao NBS. Effect of early childhood undernutrition and child labour on growth and adult nutritional status of rural Indian boys around Hyderabad. Hum Nutr Clin Nutr 1986; 400:131–139.

12 Amsterdam Child Labour Conference. Combating the most intolerable forms of child labour: a global challenge. The Netherlands: Ministry of Social Affairs and Employment; 1997.

13 Tsitoura S. Child abuse and neglect. In: Lindstrom B, Spencer N, eds. Social paediatrics. Oxford: Oxford University Press; 1995:310–330.

14 Dottridge M. Child slavery in West Africa and beyond. Ending violence against children. Global Future: World Vision J Hum Dev 2001; Third Quarter:1–25.

15 Omona G, Matheson KE. Uganda: stolen children, stolen lives. Lancet 1998; 351:442.

16 Wright JD, Kaminsky D, Wittig M. Health and social conditions of street children in Honduras. Am J Dis Child 1993;147:279–283.

17 Ennew J. Defining the girl child: sexuality, control and development. VENA J 1994; 6:51–56.

18 Fyfe A. Child labour. Cambridge: Polity Press; 1989.

19 Nolan T, Angos P, Cunha AJLA, et al. Quality of hospital care for seriously ill children in less developed countries. Lancet 2001; 357:106–110.

20 Her Majesty's Stationery Office (HMSO). The UN Convention on the Rights of the Child. London: HMSO; 1991.

21 Southall DP, Burr S, Smith RD, et al. The child-friendly healthcare initiative (CFHI): healthcare provision in accordance with the UN convention on the Rights of the Child. Pediatrics 2000; 106:1054–1064.

22 Newell KW. Health by the people. Geneva: WHO; 1975.

23 Nicoll A. Integrated management of childhood illness in resource-poor countries: an initiative from the World Health Organization. Trans Roy Soc Trop Med Hyg 2000; 94:9–11.

24 World Health Organization. Management of childhood illness in developing countries: Rationale for an integrated strategy. WHO/ CHS/CAH/98.1A: Rev 1. Geneva: WHO; 1998.

25 Pécoul B. Access to essential drugs in poor countries: a lost battle? J Am Med Assoc 1999; 281(4):361–367.

26 Morley DC. Paediatric priorities in the developing world. London: Butterworths; 1973.

27 Pagnoni F, Convello N, Tiendrebeogo J, et al. A community-based program to provide prompt and adequate treatment of presumptive malaria in children. Trans Roy Soc Trop Med Hyg 1997; 91:512–517.

28 World Health Organization. Weekly Epidemiol Rec 1993; 34:245–258.

29 World Health Organization. Weekly Epidemiol Rec 1994; 42:309–314, 43:317–321.

30 World Health Organization. Weekly Epidemiol Rec 1996; 71:17–32.

31 Scrimshaw NS, Schunch B. Causes and consequences of intrauterine growth retardation. Eur J Clin Nutr 1998; 52(Suppl):S1–S103.

32 World Health Organization. Perinatal mortality, a listing of available information.

Maternal Health and Safe Motherhood Programme. Family and reproductive health. Geneva: WHO; 1996.

33 Brabin BJ, Hakimi M, Pelletier D. An analysis of anemia and pregnancy-related maternal mortality. J Nutr 2001; 131:604S–615S.

34 World Health Organization. Mother–baby package. Implementing safe motherhood in developing countries. (WHO/FHE/MSM/94.11.) Geneva: WHO; 1994.

*35 Grajeda R, Perez-Escamilla R, Dewey KG. Delayed clamping of the umbilical cord improves hematologic status of Guatemalan infants at 2 months of age. Am J Clin Nutr 1997; 65:425–431.

36 World Health Organization. Progress towards the global elimination of neonatal tetanus, 1990–1998. Weekly Epidemiol Rec 1999; 10:73–80.

37 Brabin L, Fazio-Tirrozzo G, Shaid S, et al. Tetanus antibody levels among adolescent girls in developing countries. Trans Roy Soc Trop Med Hyg 2000; 94:455–459.

38 World Health Organization. Global strategies, policies and practices for immunisation of adolescents: a review. Geneva: WHO; 1999.

39 Stoltzfus RJ, Dreyfuss ML. Guidelines for the use of iron supplements to prevent and treat iron deficiency anaemia. International Nutritional Anemia Consultative Group (INACG), World Health Organization (WHO) and United Nations Children's Fund (UNICEF). Washington: ILSI Press; 1998.

40 McLaren DS, Frigg M. Sight and life manual on vitamin A deficiency disorders (VADD) 1st edn. Basel: Task Force Sight and Life; 1997.

41 Brabin BJ, Premji Z, Verhoeff F. An analysis of anaemia and child-related mortality. J Nutr 2001; 131:636S–648S.

42 Oppenheimer S. Iron and its relation to immunity and infectious disease. J Nutr 2001; 131:616S–636S.

43 NACG Consensus Statement. Safety of iron supplementation programs in malaria endemic areas. Washington DC: International Life Science Institute; 1999.

44 Saloojee H, Violari A. HIV infection in children. BMJ 2001; 323:670–674.

45 World Health Organization. Management of severe malnutrition. A manual for physicians and other senior health workers, Geneva: WHO; 1998.

46 World Health Organization. Management of the child with a serious infection or severe malnutrition. Guidelines for care at the first-referral level in developing countries. Geneva: WHO; 2000.

*47 World Health Organization. A critical link. Interventions for physical growth and psychological development. A review. Department of Child and Adolescent Health and Development. Geneva: WHO; 1999.

48 Partnership for Child Development. Better health nutrition and education for the school age child. Trans Roy Soc Trop Med Hyg 1997; 91:1–2.

49 World Health Organization. Programming for adolescent health and development. WHO Technical Report Series 886. Geneva: WHO; 1999.

50 World Health Organization. Department of Child and Adolescent Health and Development. Global consultation on adolescent friendly health services. Geneva: WHO; 2001.

51 Schulpen TWJ, de Waal FC. Crippling disorders in children, a global problem. Trop Geograph Med 1993; 45:196–268.

52 Royal College of Paediatrics and Child Health. The health of refugee children. Guidelines for paediatricians. London: RCPCH; 1999.

53 Child Health Dialogue. Children's health in emergencies: a practical approach. London: Health Link Worldwide; Oct–Dec 1999.

54 Aweis D, Brabin BJ, Beeching NJ, et al. Hepatitis B prevelence and risk factors for HBsAg carriage amongst Somali households in Liverpool. Comm Dis Public Health 2001; 4:357–252.

Section 2

Perinatal/Neonatal medicine

9

Fetal medicine

Stephen C Robson, Steven Sturgiss

PRENATAL SCREENING AND DIAGNOSIS OF CONGENITAL ABNORMALITIES

Congenital abnormalities occur in 3–4% of newborn infants and are responsible for between 10 and 15% of perinatal deaths and 30–40% of postneonatal deaths.[1] Even if not lethal, many congenital abnormalities cause long term morbidity. The benefits of prenatal diagnosis include enhanced parental and neonatal preparedness and optimization of delivery. For those anomalies likely to be associated with death and/or significant disability, parents can be offered pregnancy termination. Antenatal screening for trisomy 21 receives much attention, but structural malformations account for 63% of therapeutic pregnancy terminations for fetal abnormalities.[2]

MATERNAL SERUM SCREENING

Maternal serum screening (MSS) for trisomy 21 is carried out with a combination of maternal age and biochemical analytes. Measurements of alpha-fetoprotein (AFP) and human chorionic gonadotrophin (hCG) in the second trimester constitute the double test; the addition of unconjugated estriol (μE3), or μE3 and inhibin A make the triple and quadruple tests, respectively. The detection rates for trisomy 21 with the double (60%), triple (68%) and quadruple tests (79%) are all substantially greater than using maternal age alone. These test characteristics are based on a false positive rate (FPR) of 5% and a threshold for offering invasive testing of 1 in 200-250. More recently, pregnancy associated plasma protein-A (PAPP-A) and hCG have been used as first trimester serum markers, with a detection rate of 63%.

ULTRASOUND

FIRST TRIMESTER

Structural anomalies

First trimester anatomy screening identifies 32–65% of major structural abnormalities in low risk populations, and 57–74% in high risk cases. The anomalies that have been detected in the first trimester include anencephaly, holoprosencephaly, cystic hygroma, multicystic kidneys, megacystis and anterior abdominal wall defects.

Nuchal translucency

Screening with nuchal translucency (NT), measured as the maximum thickness of the subcutaneous tissue overlying the cervical spine at 11–14 weeks, identifies 74–82% of fetuses with trisomy 21 for a FPR of 5%. NT also acts as a marker for other trisomies (18, 13), sex chromosome abnormalities, syndromic disorders and structural abnormalities including cardiac defects (Table 9.1); in one large study 56% of the major cardiac anomalies

Table 9.1 Anomalies associated with nuchal translucency in euploid fetuses

Cardiac	Other structural
Tetralogy of Fallot	Diaphragmatic hernia
Hypoplastic left heart	Pentalogy of Cantrell
Transposition of the great arteries	Exomphalos
Coarctation of the aorta	Body stalk anomaly
Aortic stenosis or atresia	Caudal regression
Ventricular and atrioventricular septal defects	Achondrogenesis
Other complex cardiac defects	
Genetic syndrome	**Other conditions**
Mucopolysaccharidosis type VII	Homozygous alpha-thalassemia
Zellweger	Twin–twin transfusion syndrome
Spinal muscular atrophy	Parvovirus infection
Noonan	
Robinow	
Cleidocranial dysplasia	
Jarcho–Levin syndrome	

Table 9.2 Sensitivities of routine ultrasonography for the detection of anomalies in organ systems

	Total n	(%)
Central nervous system		
Anencephaly	29/29	(100)
Spina bifida	18/22	(82)
Hydrocephaly	8/20	(40)
Holoprosencephaly	3/5	(60)
Other	9/13	(69)
Total	*67/89*	*(75)*
Cardiovascular system		
Septal defects	4/54	(7)
Transposition	0/9	(0)
Other complex heart	18/78	(23)
Total	*22/41*	*(16)*
Urinary tract		
Obstructive uropathy	164/171	(96)
Renal agenesis	10/11	(91)
Renal dysplasia	13/24	(54)
Other	7/9	(78)
Total	*194/215*	*(90)*
Thoracic abnormalities		
CCAM	6/6	(100)
Diaphragmatic hernia	8/13	(62)
Pleural effusion	1/3	(33)
Other	2/5	(40)
Total	*17/27*	*(63)*
Abdominal/gastrointestinal		
Exomphalos	9/9	(100)
Gastroschisis	6/6	(100)
Small bowel obstruction	2/5	(40)
Esophageal atresia	2/11	(18)
Other	2/25	(8)
Total	*21/56*	*(38)*

Summary data from five studies of routine ultrasonography in low risk populations.[6–10]
CCAM, congenital cystic adenomatoid malformations.

occurred in fetuses with a NT above the 95th centile at 10–14 weeks' gestation.[3] Others have demonstrated that the prevalence of major cardiac defects in euploid fetuses with NT > 3.5 mm is 5–6%. However, the sensitivity of NT screening for cardiac abnormalities is low (15%). The overall chance of delivering a healthy infant declines with increasing NT; 86% at 3.5–4.4 mm, 77% at 4.5–5.4 mm, 67% at 5.5-6.4 mm, and less than 31% for an NT > 6.5 mm.[4]

Combining NT measurements and maternal serum PAPP-A and hCG in the first trimester increases the detection rate for trisomy 21 to 86% for the same FPR of 5%. Integrating first trimester NT and serum screening with second trimester MSS increases the detection rate for trisomy 21 to 95%. Alternatively, FPRs can be reduced to < 1% while maintaining sensitivity at ~80%.

Strategies incorporating first trimester ultrasonography have the additional benefits of providing parents with early reassurance and the early detection of non-viable and multiple pregnancies. It is perceived that termination of pregnancy in the first, as compared to the second trimester, is safer and less likely to result in psychological sequelae. Termination prior to 15 weeks of pregnancy can be carried out by suction aspiration, obviating the need for a medical procedure involving vaginal expulsion of the conceptus. However, recent evidence suggests that the emotional responses to termination for an abnormal fetus are independent of the gestational age and method of termination.[5] Other potential problems with early pregnancy screening include the narrow time interval for screening and diagnosis, the higher loss rate of chorionic villus sampling compared with amniocentesis, lack of pathological confirmation of diagnosis, and the high spontaneous loss rate in abnormal pregnancies (particularly trisomies and cystic hygroma).

SECOND TRIMESTER

Structural anomalies

Ultrasound screening between 18 and 20 weeks of pregnancy identifies 61–85% of fetal anomalies in low risk populations.[6–10] The sensitivities for individual anomalies are shown in Table 9.2. Although one large trial[11] reported very poor detection rates (17%), subsequent analysis indicated that the low sensitivities were due in part to poor sonographer training. A recent meta-analysis of eight studies showed that, when compared with selective examination, routine second trimester screening is associated with earlier diagnosis of twin pregnancy and a reduced incidence of induction of labor for post-term pregnancy,[12] but no apparent benefit in terms of perinatal mortality. It is likely that this result is explained by the rarity of perinatal deaths (~10 per 1000), variable detection rates, and some parents opting to continue their pregnancy even when a lethal anomaly is diagnosed.

Markers of chromosomal anomalies

Many aneuploid fetuses exhibit major structural anomalies and/or minor findings of little or no functional significance (soft markers). For each soft marker, a likelihood ratio for aneuploidy is calculated from the ratio of the frequencies in affected and normal fetuses. Likelihood ratios (LRs) for potential ultrasound markers associated with trisomy 21 are shown in Table 9.3. Maternal age is used for the prior risk, and the risk factors applied sequentially when more than one is present. A normal scan without anomalies or soft markers reduces the risk for trisomy 21 by about 40–45% (i.e. LR 0.6).

Table 9.3 Ultrasound markers for trisomy 21

Songraphic feature	Likelihood ratio for trisomy 21
Nuchal fold 6+mm	10.0
Echogenic bowel	5.5
Short femur	2.5
Mild pyelectasis	1.5
Choroid plexus cyst	1.5
Sandal gap	1.5

SAFETY OF ULTRASOUND

Ultrasound induces thermal effects and gas bubble formation (cavitation). There is no evidence of teratogenesis in humans despite the widespread use of prenatal ultrasound for more than 20 years. Newnham et al[13] reported that mothers exposed to five or more third trimester ultrasound examinations delivered babies weighing about 25 g less than controls. These results have not been confirmed in other studies. Case control or randomized controlled studies have shown small but significant increases in speech problems, dyslexia, abnormal grasp, and non-right handedness.[12] However, there is little consistency between these studies, which are all prone to methodological problems including errors due to chance in multiple hypothesis testing.

MANAGEMENT OF PRENATALLY DETECTED STRUCTURAL ANOMALIES

PRINCIPLES OF MANAGEMENT

The prenatal diagnosis of a fetal malformation should prompt referral to a clinician with expertise in the antenatal management of such conditions. Regional fetal medicine centers have been established with core teams of experts specialized in ultrasonography, invasive assessment and intrauterine therapy. The initial management includes a detailed characterization of the malformation, as well as a thorough search for associated anomalies. Many structural anomalies are associated with an increased risk of chromosome abnormalities, and the management will usually include the offer of prenatal karyotyping. Parents are provided with considerate, empathetic and knowledgeable counseling based, wherever possible, on relevant prenatal literature. The prognosis for lesions diagnosed during pregnancy is often very different from those diagnosed after delivery. A single clinician leads and coordinates this process, which often includes colleagues in genetics, neonatology and neonatal surgery. Decisions regarding further testing, surveillance during pregnancy, and the time and place of delivery are individualized according to the underlying problem.

Termination of pregnancy (TOP) in the UK is allowable at any gestation if there is a substantial risk of serious handicap. The interpretation of risk and handicap, and by implication the decision to offer termination of pregnancy, is presently at the discretion of the clinician(s) involved with the case. The Royal College of Obstetricians and Gynaecologists has issued guidelines recommending fetocide for TOPs after 22 weeks' gestation.[14]

CENTRAL NERVOUS SYSTEM (CNS)

Ventriculomegaly

Ventriculomegly (ventricular width ≥ 10 mm) describes dilatation of the lateral ventricles whereas hydrocephalus refers to a pathological increase in intracranial cerebrospinal fluid which is usually associated with increased intracranial pressure and enlargement of the fetal head. Ventriculomegaly occurs in 0.05 to 0.3% of all pregnancies.

The causes of ventriculomegaly include constitutional increase in size, obstruction to the flow of fluid through the ventricular system, other CNS anomalies (e.g. neural tube defects, hemorrhage, or migration defects), infection (cytomegalovirus, toxoplasmosis, adenovirus), genetic disorders and karyotype abnormalities (trisomies 21, 18 and 13, as well as triploidy and translocations). Associated anomalies are found in 70% of cases. Additional investigations should include fetal echocardiography, and an infection screen. Consideration should be given to magnetic resonance imaging for the detection of agenesis of the corpus callosum which increases the likelihood of underlying CNS pathology.

In general, the prognosis for fetuses with ventriculomegaly and other abnormalities is very poor. However, quantification of individual risk for adverse outcome when the underlying diagnosis is unclear can be difficult. The management and prognosis for fetuses with isolated ventriculomegaly are influenced by the severity of the ventricular dilatation.

Mild ventriculomegaly

In mild ventriculomegaly (ventricular width 10–14 mm), 2–3% of fetuses with apparently isolated mild ventriculomegaly will have a karyotype anomaly. If all investigations are normal, about 90% of fetuses will have a normal outcome. There is preliminary evidence that fetuses with ventricular widths between 10 and 12 mm have normal outcomes as has been reported in 97% of cases.[15] Serial scans are undertaken throughout pregnancy to monitor the ventricular size. Resolution of the ventriculomegaly occurs in about one-third of cases and increases the chance of a normal outcome.

Severe ventriculomegaly

For severe ventriculomegaly (ventricular width ≥15 mm), the incidence of chromosome abnormalities is ~10%. With apparently isolated severe ventriculomegaly the neonatal/infant mortality rate is ~50%, with about 50% of surviving infants exhibiting abnormal neurodevelopment.[16] Where severity has been reported, about 20% were mildly affected and 80% moderate to severe. Postnatal ventriculoperitoneal shunting is required in 60% of cases. For parents continuing their pregnancy, serial scans should be undertaken to monitor ventricular size. In cases with rapidly progressive disease and/or hydrocephalus, delivery should be considered as soon as fetal maturity can reasonably be assumed. There is no benefit from routine cesarean section, but the macrocephaly can be severe enough to preclude vaginal delivery. In-utero ventriculoperitoneal shunting does not improve outcome, and frequently results in intracranial hemorrhage with in-utero demise. Cephalocentesis may be justified to avoid traumatic delivery but also has a very high mortality.

Spina bifida

The incidence of neural tube defects in the UK has declined from 5.5 to 1.0 in 1000 over the last 20 years. Part of this reduction might be due to periconceptual folate supplementation which reduces the incidence of neural tube defects by 75%.[17] The ultrasound features include widening of the spinal posterior ossification centers (dysraphism), a sacular protrusion and/or a defect in the overlying skin. Virtually all cases of myelomeningocele manifest cranial features including microcephaly, scalloping of the frontal bones (lemon sign), ventriculomegaly, obliteration of the cisterna magna and/or an absent or abnormally shaped cerebellum (banana sign) as a consequence of the Arnold–Chiari malformation. Associated anomalies occur in most other systems, but the commonest are urogenital anomalies (9%) including renal agenesis, horseshoe kidneys and ureteral duplications. Karyotype abnormalities, mainly trisomy 18, occur in 2% of apparently isolated cases.

In general, higher, more extensive and open lesions are associated with a worse outcome, but the correlations between ultrasound findings and outcomes are imprecise. Infant mortality rates are about 35%. It has been reported that between 68 and 73% of patients will have normal intelligence, 61–77% will be mobile, and that 19–25% will void urine normally. In general, about 10% of infants manifest minimal or no symptoms, whereas another 10% have very severe disability encompassing immobility, marked intellectual dysfunction and severe incontinence.

Agenesis of the corpus callosum

Agenesis of the corpus callosum (ACC) is found in 1 in 19 000 unselected autopsies and 2.3% of children with mental retardation. The corpus callosum can be identified with coronal ultrasound views after 20 weeks' gestation. However, these views are not part of the standard ultrasound scan, and it is likely that many cases are unrecognized. In low-risk cases, the diagnosis will only be made through identification of associated anatomic alterations including mild ventriculomegaly, absence of the cavum septum pellucidum, and enlargement or upward displacement of the third ventricle.

In total, 80% of cases are associated with other anomalies including hydrocephalus, Dandy–Walker syndrome, neuronal migration disorders and aneuploidy (trisomies 13 and 18). Normal outcome occurs in 85% of cases with apparently isolated ACC and in 13% of cases with additional scan abnormalities.[18]

Holoprosencephaly

Holoprosencephaly is characterized by failed septation of the midline forebrain structures, and is frequently accompanied by midfacial abnormalities. The forebrain abnormalities are subdivided into lobar, semilobar, and alobar types according to increasing degree of failed septation. Population-based studies suggest a prevalence of 1.1 to 1.2 cases/10 000 pregnancies.[19] Associated syndromic (including Smith–Lemli–Opitz, Hall–Pallister, pseudotrisomy 13, and Meckel) and structural anomalies are common. Trisomy 13, the most commonly identified cause, and other chromosomal abnormalities (trisomy 18 and rearrangements or deletions) account for nearly 50% of cases.

The prognosis is very poor; overall, about 70% of affected infants die within 1 year, and all diagnosed infants exhibit developmental delay, which is often severe. It is possible that individuals with subtle forms of undiagnosed lobar holoprosencephaly exist with little or no neurological abnormality. Even when a case of holoprosencephaly appears to be sporadic, the recurrence risk (13–14%) remains higher than with other major malformations. The high incidence of syndromic and subtle familial cases and the high recurrence rates emphasize the importance of full investigation and detailed postnatal counseling.

Dandy–Walker malformation

Dandy–Walker malformation (DWM) describes agenesis or hypoplasia of the cerebellar vermis with communication between the fourth ventricle and the cisterna magna. Chromosome abnormalities are present in 15–45% of cases and around 45% have other CNS anomalies, including holoprosencephaly, ventriculomegaly and neuronal migration defects. Non-CNS structural and syndromic anomalies are present in two-thirds of cases. Prenatal series report a 40% risk of fetal or neonatal death and almost all reported survivors are symptomatic with developmental/motor delay, seizures and spasticity. It is possible that isolated DWM is associated with a lower risk of neurodevelopmental problems, but very few genuinely isolated cases have been reported.

URINARY TRACT

Hydronephrosis

Renal pelvic dilatation (RPD) is diagnosed in up to 1% of pregnancies. The diagnosis, as well as the grading of severity, is based on the anteroposterior diameter of the renal pelvis; measurements of ≥ 5.0 mm at 20 weeks' gestation and ≥ 7.0 mm at 36 weeks are more than 2 standard deviations (SDs) above the mean.[20] Other workers[21] have claimed that using a threshold of 4 mm at 20 weeks of pregnancy increases the sensitivity for detecting significant pathology from 53 to 76%. Antenatal RPD can be a variant of normal or can be secondary to urinary tract pathology [pelviureteric junction obstruction, vesicoureteric reflux (VUR), vesicoureteric junction obstruction, posterior urethral valves and obstruction in a duplex system]. Bladder and/or ureteric dilatation suggest the presence of lower urinary tract uropathy, but their absence does not exclude this possibility. The presence of caliectasis is associated with an increased likelihood of significant disease.

Mild RPD

Many kidneys with apparently isolated mild RPD (pelvis 5–10 mm) will be normal postnatally; FPRs have varied between 45 and 90%. Mild RPD progresses in-utero to moderate or severe dilatation in 4% of cases and therefore a follow-up scan should be performed at 30–32 weeks' gestation. Even when the dilatation remains mild, VUR occurs in up to 15% of cases. An ultrasound scan should be performed 3–4 days after delivery. Many units recommend antibiotic prophylaxis, as well as investigation for VUR for those babies with postnatal hydronephrosis. Relatively few (3–7%) fetuses with mild renal pelvic dilatation will ultimately require surgery.

Moderate or severe RDP

Between 42 and 64% of fetuses with apparently isolated moderate (pelvis 11–15 mm) RPD will have significant renal pathology, as will almost all with severe (pelvis > 15 mm) dilatation. The overall prognosis for fetuses with isolated unilateral dilatation is usually excellent. A more cautious approach needs to be taken with bilateral disease. The long term outcome is usually good but is dependent on the degree of antenatal dilatation. Reduction or absence of amniotic fluid suggests severe renal dysfunction and a very poor prognosis, especially if diagnosed in the second trimester before lung development is complete. Serial scans should be undertaken to assess the degree of dilatation and amniotic fluid volume. Progressive dilatation and/or diminution of amniotic fluid volume near term (37 weeks) are indications for delivery. Surgical intervention is required in about 50% of cases with moderate renal pelvic dilatation, and 76–100% with severe dilatation.

Renal agenesis

Unilateral renal agenesis occurs in 1 in 1000 pregnancies, and bilateral renal agenesis 1 in 4000. Bilateral renal agenesis is always associated with severe oligohydramnios from about 15 weeks' gestation. Earlier in pregnancy, a large proportion of the amniotic fluid originates from the fetal membranes. The differential diagnosis of severe oligohydramnios includes other causes of impaired urine production (bilateral multicystic kidney disease, urinary tract obstruction), fetal growth restriction and amniorrhexis. The sonographic demonstration of kidneys and bladder is very difficult in the absence of amniotic fluid. Transvaginal and color Doppler sonography may help but a definitive diagnosis often requires amnioinfusion and occasionally infusion of fluid into the fetal abdomen.

Low urinary tract obstruction

Posterior urethral valves (PUV) are the most common cause of severe lower urinary tract obstructive uropathy, occurring in 1 in 5000–8000 male fetuses. Ultrasonographic appearances include a dilated thick-walled bladder, a dilated posterior urethra, and oligohydramnios. The obstruction is classified as complete when there is anhydramnios, or incomplete when the amniotic fluid volume is normal or slightly reduced. The most important differential diagnosis is severe bilateral VUR producing the megacystis–megaureter association. However, with reflux, the bladder is often thin-walled and the liquor volume is normal. Urethral atresia can also lead to severe bladder dilatation and has a worse prognosis because of the associated cloacal anomalies. Associated abnormalities are seen in 43% of fetuses and include cardiac anomalies, bowel rotation, imperforate anus and vesicorectal fistula. Karyotype abnormalities occur in up to 8% of cases.

The prognosis for PUV is dependent on the degree of obstruction and the extent of renal dysplasia.

Complete obstruction

Complete obstruction is associated with anhydramnios and a very poor prognosis as a consequence of renal dysplasia and pulmonary hypoplasia. Decompression of the dilated bladder with a vesicoamniotic shunt can increase amniotic fluid volume and protect the fetus from pulmonary hypoplasia. Shunt placement is only worthwhile in fetuses with satisfactory residual renal function, as assessed with ultrasonography and measurement of urinary electrolytes after vesicocentesis. Kidneys with bilateral cystic change will always be severely dysplastic. Normal ranges have been established for fetal urinary sodium, calcium, phosphate, osmolality and beta 2-microglobulin. In borderline cases, analysis of fresh urine from a repeat vesicocentesis after 2–3 days can provide more definitive results. The complications of shunt placement include chorioamnionitis, anterior abdominal wall defects, and fetal demise; the overall procedure-related fetal loss rate is about 5%. With appropriate case selection, survival rates of 67% have been reported after vesicoamniotic shunt procedures.[22] However, even when the shunt works satisfactorily, many fetuses develop renal dysplasia requiring renal support within the first year of life.

Incomplete obstruction

Fetuses with no or mild oligohydramnios throughout pregnancy are protected from pulmonary hypoplasia and are very likely to survive. Some degree of renal dysplasia is common, but the severity is highly variable and difficult to predict. Vesicocentesis might be indicated in those fetuses with borderline amniotic fluid volume. Management during pregnancy should include serial scans to monitor amniotic fluid volume and renal appearances.

Cystic kidney disease

Multicystic renal dysplasia is the commonest form of cystic kidney disease diagnosed in-utero. Bilateral disease occurs in 23% of cases, and is characterized by paraspinal cystic masses, a non-visible bladder, and severe oligohydramnios. Pulmonary hypoplasia is invariable resulting in neonatal death. The prognosis for unilateral disease is dependent on the presence of contralateral renal anomalies, which occur in up to 39% of cases and include renal agenesis, renal hypoplasia, pelviureteric junction obstruction and VUR. Reflux occurs in 15% of cases, but is not always apparent prenatally. If the contralateral kidney appears normal, and there are no apparent systemic anomalies, the prognosis is excellent. A further ultrasound scan should be carried out in the third trimester of pregnancy to monitor the size of the diseased kidney. Postnatal investigations should include a renal scan and a micturating cystourethrogram with antibiotic cover.

Autosomal recessive and dominant renal cystic disease are usually only diagnosed in cases with a family history. The management is individualized according to the underlying pathology and degree of in-utero renal dysfunction as assessed from amniotic fluid volume. Specialist neonatal nephrologic advice is required.

ABDOMINAL WALL

Exomphalos

Exomphalos is an incomplete return of the abdominal contents into the abdominal cavity, which is complete by 11–12 weeks' gestation. The incidence is 1–3 per 1000 pregnancies. The lesion is highly variable in size and appears as an anterior extrusion of abdominal contents contained within a sac which occasionally ruptures. The umbilical vein will be seen coursing through the sac, in contrast to a gastroschisis where the cord insertion is intact. Other abnormalities are common. Cardiac malformations are seen in up to 50%, limb abnormalities in 30%, and karyotype abnormalities in 28–36%, mainly trisomy 18. The smaller umbilical hernias, and lesions diagnosed early in pregnancy (< 15 weeks) are associated with even higher rates of aneuploidy. Associated genetic anomalies include the Beckwith–Wiedemann and de Lange syndromes.

Survival rates for isolated lesions are in excess of 90%, but some babies will require staged repairs and need to be in hospital for many weeks. Larger lesions are associated with reduced survival rates (33–80%), as is the presence of additional abnormalities. Periodic ultrasound surveillance should be undertaken, but the incidence of complications such as bowel constriction is low. There is no merit in routine cesarean section, but this might be justified for the very extensive lesions where the fetal liver is completely extruded.

Gastroschisis

A gastroschisis is a herniation of the intra-abdominal contents through a defect in the abdominal wall, usually just to the right of the cord insertion. The ultrasonographic features include free loops of bowel floating in the amniotic fluid, associated with an intact cord insertion. Gastroschisis is not usually associated with other anomalies, but some studies have reported cardiac anomalies in up to 5% of cases. About 50% of fetuses will be small for gestational age (SGA), and there is an increased risk of hypoxic intrauterine death. Intestinal atresias or stenosis secondary to intestinal ischemia are reported in up to 30% of cases. Survival rates for isolated cases without liver herniation approach 95%. Management should include periodic surveillance during pregnancy to establish fetal size, growth, placental function and bowel status. Bowel luminal diameters of 11–17 mm have been associated with an increased incidence of bowel complications at surgery. Delivery should be in a unit with neonatal surgical facilities. There is no merit in routine cesarean section.

THORAX

Diaphragmatic hernia

Left sided congenital diaphragmatic hernia (CDH) is usually suspected when the fetal heart is displaced to the right side of the chest, and/or the stomach is seen in the thoracic cavity. If neither of these signs is evident, the diagnosis is often missed. The prenatal diagnosis of a right sided CDH is especially difficult; the echogenicity patterns of the fetal lung, liver and small intestine are very similar. About 60% of CDHs evade prenatal diagnosis. Associated anomalies occur in 30% of cases, and include abnormalities of the cardiovascular, genitourinary, musculo-skeletal, and central nervous systems, as well as aneuploidy (mainly trisomy 18) in 10–15% of cases. Reported survival rates for isolated lesions diagnosed in-utero are 50–60% but this falls to 10% when there are coexistent anomalies. The prognosis is dependent on contralateral lung development, but ultrasound assessment of lung size and growth is imprecise. Early diagnosis, the presence of liver in the chest, hydramnios and hydrops are associated with a worse outcome, but the relationship between these factors and prognosis is poor. The lung area:head circumference ratio measured with ultrasonography, or lung volume assessed with magnetic resonance imaging might be more predictive of outcome.

Management should include fetal echocardiogropahy and ultrasound scans every 2 weeks during the third trimester to look for hydramnios and hydrops. Delivery should be in a unit with specialist neonatal and pediatric surgical facilities. There is no contraindication to vaginal delivery.

Cystic adenomatoid malformation

Congenital cystic adenomatoid malformations (CCAM) are classified on the basis of ultrasound appearances as macrocystic (type 1), mixed (type 2) or microcystic (type 3). Microcystic lesions appear predominantly echogenic, whereas macrocystic lesions contain one or more unilocular cysts. The differential diagnosis includes CDH, pulmonary sequestration, and bronchial atresia. In difficult cases, intrathoracic instillation of fluid helps differentiate a CDH. Doppler color flow imaging may visualize a direct vascular connection to the aorta in sequestration. Associated anomalies are rare but hydrops can occur as a result of distortion of the thoracic great arteries/veins, or myocardial dysfunction.

The prognosis for a CCAM in the absence of hydrops is very favorable. In about 20–30% of cases, there is partial or apparently complete resolution of the lesion in-utero. Ultrasound scans should be performed every 4 weeks to exclude hydrops, but this rarely develops if it is not present at diagnosis. The place of delivery can be decided according to the size of the lesion. The prognosis for fetuses with hydrops is much less favorable. However, even when hydrops is present in early pregnancy, serial scans have documented apparent shrinkage and resolution of the lesion with disappearance of the hydrops.

GASTROINTESTINAL ABNORMALITIES

Duodenal atresia

Duodenal atresia affects 1 in 5000 pregnancies. The typical ultrasonographic appearances include a 'double-bubble', with the stomach and dilated duodenum forming similarly sized and connected fluid-filled structures, and hydramnios which can predispose to premature labor. The diagnosis is not usually evident before the end of the second trimester. Associated anomalies include vertebral defects, imperforate anus, tracheoesophageal fistula with esophageal atresia, and radial and renal dysplasia (complex) (VATER) association and trisomy 21, which is present in 30% of cases. The prognosis for fetuses with isolated duodenal atresia is very good. Regular ultrasound surveillance should be carried out to monitor amniotic fluid volume. Hydramnios can be severe and warrant amnioreduction.

Other bowel obstruction

The appearance of multiple fluid-filled bowel loops suggests small bowel obstruction. Precise localization of the obstruction is not possible, but the greater the number of dilated bowel loops and the greater the dilatation, the more distal the atresia. Conversely the greater the volume of amniotic fluid, the more proximal the obstruction. Associated anomalies external to the gut are uncommon. The prognosis is usually excellent, but the outlook needs to be more guarded when multiple atresias are suspected. Serial ultrasound scans are performed to monitor amniotic fluid volume. Amnioreduction is occasionally required.

Meconium ileus

Meconium ileus should be suspected when the bowel is dilated and hyperechogenic. Virtually all cases are due to cystic fibrosis, which can usually be confirmed with parental and fetal genotyping. About 96% of the cystic fibrosis gene mutations have been characterized and can be identified with DNA studies. The immediate prognosis for meconium ileus is good, but the longer term prognosis is determined by the underlying condition.

CARDIAC ABNORMALITIES

Congenital heart disease occurs in 0.4–1.0% of live births and accounts for 35% of infant deaths secondary to congenital disease. Screening using the four-chamber view of the fetal heart will detect about 20% of cardiac abnormalities. Sensitivity is increased by incorporating views of the arterial connections. Chromosomal anomalies have been reported in up to 30% of fetuses with prenatally detected heart disease; trisomy 18 is detected as frequently as trisomy 21, with Turner's syndrome the next most common. Karyotype analysis should include a search for microdeletions localized to the long arm of chromosome 22 (22q11) which result in DiGeorge syndrome.

A detailed discussion about the diagnosis and management of the individual cardiac abnormalities amenable to prenatal diagnosis is outwith the scope of this chapter. Interested readers are referred to Allan et al.[23] The prognosis for malformations detected with prenatal ultrasonography is usually worse than for those first seen after delivery. Counseling should be undertaken by clinicians specializing in the field of prenatal echocardiography.

SKELETAL DYSPLASIAS

The commonest lethal skeletal dysplasia seen prenatally is thanatophoric dysplasia with an incidence of 1 in 10 000 births. Other lethal dysplasias include achondrogenesis (1 in 40 000 births) and osteogenesis imperfecta (1 in 55 000). The prenatal diagnosis of skeletal dysplasias is complex and beyond the scope of this chapter. Interested readers are referred to Griffin.[24] Frequently, the precise diagnosis is not made until after delivery or autopsy. The lethal anomalies can usually be identified by either severe micromelia (long bone lengths >4 SDs below the mean for gestation), narrow chest dimensions, or associated anomalies.

INVASIVE PROCEDURES AND FETAL SURGERY

The commonest indication for invasive testing is to establish the fetal karyotype in situations of high risk such as advanced maternal age, abnormal MSS or the ultrasonographic visualization of anomalies or soft markers. The number of monogenic disorders amenable to prenatal diagnosis by polymerase chain reaction (PCR) analysis of DNA is increasing rapidly, but there are a few metabolic disorders that can only be diagnosed by enzyme assay. Other indications include suspected fetal infection and alloimmunization.

All invasive procedures should be performed with real-time ultrasound guidance by appropriately trained and experienced operators. The Royal College of Obstetricians and Gynaecologists has recently issued guidelines suggesting that operators should undertake a minimum of 30 amniocenteses a year in order to maintain skills.[25]

AMNIOCENTESIS

Amniocentesis can be carried out from 15 weeks' gestation onwards. Early (11–14 weeks) amniocentesis is more hazardous than either chorionic villus sampling (CVS) or second trimester amniocentesis.[26] The cells in the amniotic fluid are mostly in interphase, and are prepared for metaphase analysis by culture in flasks for 2–3 weeks. More rapid culture on cover slips reduces reporting time to 7–10 days, but is more costly. Rapid detection of trisomy 21 and other trisomies is possible with fluorescent in situ hybridization (FISH) and quantitative PCR, but the information provided is probe specific.

The only randomized controlled study of pregnancy outcomes following amniocentesis reported a procedure-related loss rate before viability of 1%.[27] Procedure-related losses occur up to 6 weeks after the test, but the maximal risk appears to be within 1–2 weeks. Experienced operators have lower complication rates; those undertaking < 50 procedures in 3 years had a single pass success rate of 82% compared with 93% for those carrying out > 50 procedures.[28] It is likely that the majority of losses occur as a result of infection.

CHORIONIC VILLUS SAMPLING

CVS in the first trimester of pregnancy can be performed transabdominally or transcervically using biopsy forceps or aspiration. Direct chromosome preparations from the cytotrophoblast provide provisional information about the fetal karyotype within 48 h. Rapid culture of the mesenchymal core allows full cytogenetic analysis using G-banding and also obviates diagnostic errors due to mosaicism in the fetus and/or placenta (see below). Chorionic villi are also an excellent source of DNA, supplying sufficient amounts for most molecular genetic techniques without prior culture. It is recommended that CVS is performed after 10 weeks of pregnancy when there is no increased risk of severe limb deficiencies and the hypoglossia/hypodactyly syndrome. Transabdominal placental sampling can also be performed in the second and third trimesters, but is more prone to failure as a result of reduced mitotic activity of the cytotrophoblast.

Meta-analysis of three randomized trials[29] showed pregnancy loss rates before viability to be significantly greater following first trimester CVS compared to midtrimester amniocentesis (odds ratio, OR 1.37, 95% confidence interval, CI 1.18–1.60.) However, a large number of the CVS procedures were carried out using a transcervical approach, which is associated with a higher incidence of procedure-related miscarriage.

Diagnostic errors can occur due to confined placental mosaicism (CPM), where aneuploid cells (mosaic and rarely non-mosaic) occur in the placenta but not in the fetus. In one large series, mosaicism was present in 30 (1.2%) of 2483 CVS cases.[30] Confined placental mosaicism within the cytotrophoblast will be apparent in the direct preparation, but not the longer term mesoderm culture. For those cases where the long term culture confirms the mosaicism, or shows mosaicism not found on direct analysis, further investigation is warranted with either an amniocentesis, fetal blood sample or skin biopsy.

FETAL BLOOD SAMPLING BEFORE LABOR

Fetal blood can be obtained from the umbilical vein, the intrahepatic vein, or the heart from about 18 weeks' gestation onwards. The main indications for fetal blood sampling are urgent fetal karyotyping after 18 weeks and measurement of hematologic parameters in fetuses at risk of alloimmune anemia or thrombocytopenia. Other indications include suspected fetal infection, later pregnancy DNA analysis, assessment of fetal acid–base status, and investigation of mosaic results from either amniocentesis or CVS.

The post-procedure pregnancy loss rate following fetal blood sampling is about 1%. Loss rates are related to the indication for sampling; in one study loss rate was 1.5% for prenatal diagnostic procedures, 14% for fetuses with suspected placental dysfunction and 25% for fetuses with fetal hydrops.[31]

OTHER TISSUE BIOPSIES

Fetal skin biopsies are performed for suspected dermatological disorders such as harlequin ichthyosis or congenital bullous epidermolysis. Skin biopsies are also potentially useful in the investigation of fetuses with a suspected mosaic karyotype. Fetal liver and muscle biopsies have also been reported, but there are few indications.

FETAL SURGERY

Despite many advances in prenatal diagnosis, the fetus remains inaccessible. Established in-utero therapeutic procedures include transabdominal intravascular transfusion of red cells or platelets, as well as placement of pleuroamniotic and vesicoamniotic shunts. The transplacental route is used for the delivery of antiarrhythmic agents for the treatment of complex cardiac arrhythmias.

The desire to perform more complex surgical treatments led to the development of open fetal surgery for conditions such as CDH, sacrococcygeal teratoma, CCAM of the lungs and obstructive uropathies. In severe form these conditions have a very poor prognosis due in part to progressive organ damage throughout the second trimester. In open surgery, the fetus is partially extracted, undergoes surgery, and is then returned to the amniotic cavity. Success rates have been severely limited by the high incidence of preterm labor, premature rupture of membranes and placental abruption. The median interval between surgery and delivery is 4 weeks with a median gestational age at delivery of only 25 weeks.

Endoscopic fetal surgery is less traumatic to the uterus and membranes, and is associated with fewer complications. In a recent series of 15 endoscopic fetal tracheal occlusion procedures for severe CDH, two mothers (13%) delivered within 2 weeks of surgery.[32] The mean duration of pregnancy after surgery was 38 days, and there were five (33%) survivors. Prenatal tracheal occlusion obstructs the normal egress of lung fluid, increases transpulmonary pressure, leading to enhanced lung growth. Other possible indications for endoscopic fetal surgery include amniotic bands and obstructive uropathies. Fetal surgery is an intriguing future development, but rigorous assessment is required before these techniques become more widely available.

ASSESSMENT OF FETAL SIZE AND WELL-BEING

DEFINITIONS

Perinatal mortality and morbidity are linked not only to gestational age but also to fetal growth. Antenatal detection of fetal growth restriction (FGR) is therefore one of the primary aims of antenatal care. Screening has focused on the detection of the small fetus but it is only recently that obstetricians have appreciated the differences between size and growth. Size is an endpoint, typically weight at birth, whereas growth is the process by which this endpoint is reached. Size is determined by a combination of local factors in tissues and organs, together with systemic nutritional and endocrine factors. Genetic influences, which are the primary determinant of fetal size, probably act primarily at the local level.

Small for gestational age refers to a fetus that is below a specific weight or anthropometric threshold. The commonly used thresholds for clinical and ultrasonic measurements are the 10th and 5th centiles. Approximately 40% of SGA infants are growth restricted as assessed by morphometric measures of wasting [ponderal index, midarm to head circumference (MAC:HC) ratio, skinfold thickness]. These fetuses have failed to achieve their genetically programmed growth potential usually because of placental dysfunction and/or maternal disease. The remainder of SGA infants are thought to be constitutionally small.

SGA fetuses are at greater risk of stillbirth, acidemia at birth, low Apgar scores, neonatal complications, neurodevelopmental impairment and non-insulin dependent diabetes and hypertension in later life. They are therefore the single largest group of fetuses tested for well-being. The reason that studies of SGA infants have shown poor perinatal outcome is likely to be due to the high incidence of true FGR in this group. Morbidity is much commoner in SGA infants with evidence of wasting and there is little evidence that small infants who reach term without evidence of growth restriction are at increased perinatal risk.[33]

ETIOLOGY OF FGR

The etiology of FGR is diverse but can be broadly classified according to the site of the primary pathology (Fig. 9.1). Some factors (e.g. maternal smoking) may affect fetal growth through several mechanisms. Genetic alterations associated with FGR can be divided into chromosomal anomalies, CPM and syndromes. Overall 4–7% of SGA fetuses will be aneuploid, the commonest abnormalities being triploidy and trisomies 13, 18 and 21. In CPM two or more cell lines with different karyotypes are present, both being derived from the same zygote. Cytogenetic abnormalities restricted to the placenta that have been associated with FGR include trisomy 16, trisomy 22 and trisomy 9. Growth restriction is also part of the phenotype of a large number of syndromes, some of which involve a primary disturbance of bone growth (e.g. osteogenesis imperfecta) and others associated with generalized (proportionate) reduction in body growth (e.g. Silver–Russell syndrome).

Congenital viral infection probably accounts for up to 5% of FGR. A causal relationship is clear for cytomegalovirus and rubella virus but probably also exists for varicella-zoster and human immunodeficiency viruses.

Abnormalities of uteroplacental perfusion and stem artery structure underlie a significant proportion of preterm FGR. Failure of extravillous trophoblast invasion and spiral artery transformation, leading to placental ischemia, is generally associated with maternal pre-eclampsia. However identical changes can be seen in the

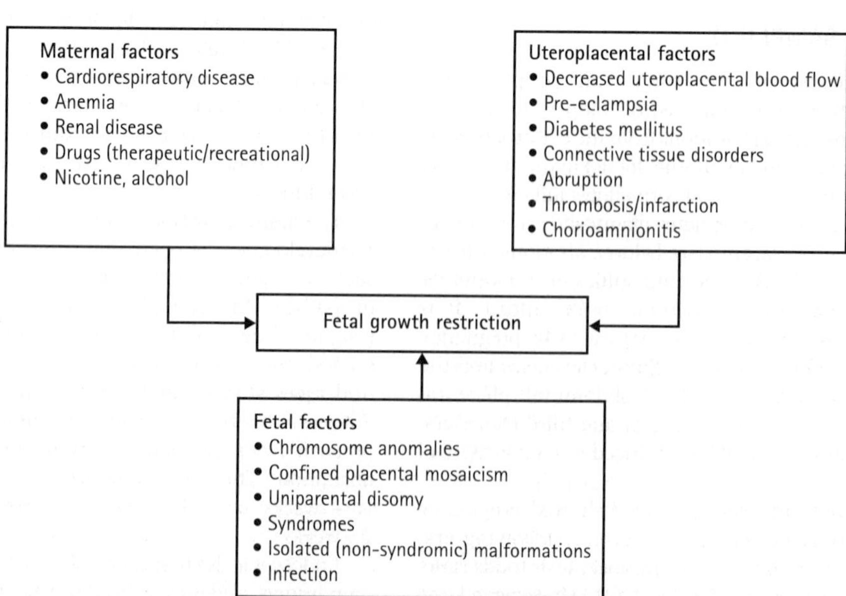

Fig. 9.1 Etiology of fetal growth restriction according to site of primary pathology.

myometrial spiral arteries of 60–80% of growth restricted fetuses born to women without hypertension.

SCREENING AND DIAGNOSIS OF SGA/FGR

Clinical assessment

Methods of detecting SGA fetuses include antenatal clinical examination, measurement of symphysis–fundal height (SFH), fetal anthropometry and ultrasound estimated fetal weight (EFW). All measurements require an accurate estimation of gestational age for correct interpretation. There is clear evidence that all women should have their date of delivery calculated from ultrasound measurements rather than menstrual dates. Fetal crown–rump length prior to 13 weeks' gestation and biparietal diameter (BPD) between 16 and 24 weeks' gestation are equally accurate (95% prediction interval ± 5 days).

Abdominal palpation remains a routine part of obstetric examination, despite the fact that the sensitivity for detection of a SGA infant is only 20–30% and the positive predictive value (PPV) no greater than 40%. Measurement of SFH is an alternative and although early studies reported sensitivities of 56–86% and specificities of 80–93%, more recent studies have suggested the technique is no better than palpation at detecting SGA. A systematic review identified one controlled trial which showed that SFH measurement did not improve perinatal outcome.[34]

Serial SFH measurements may improve sensitivity and specificity as may the use of customized SFH charts. The customized antenatal growth chart displays computer generated curves for fetal weight and SFH, adjusted for physiological variables (maternal height, weight at booking, parity and ethnic group). One controlled trial has shown that use of customized charts improved detection rate of SGA infants [48% vs 29%, OR 2.2 (95% CI 1.1–4.5)] and reduced the number of women admitted (OR 0.6, 95% CI 0.4–0.7).[35] SFH should be measured at each antenatal assessment after 24 weeks of pregnancy. Ultrasound assessment is indicated if the SFH falls below the 10th centile.

Ultrasound anthropometry

A large number of ultrasonic anthropometric measurements have been used to predict fetal size but abdominal circumference (AC) and EFW are the most accurate.[36] Fetal AC is measured at the level of the hepatic vein. Fetal weight can be calculated from a variety of formulae incorporating routine ultrasonic anthropometric measurements [AC, BPD, HC and femur length (FL)]. Systematic review suggests that an AC < 10th centile has the highest sensitivity, predicting 84% of SGA infants in high risk women with an overall OR of 18 (95% CI 10–34).[36] Reported sensitivities for EFW < 10th centile are lower and more variable (33–89%) although the overall OR is higher [39 (95% CI 29–52)]. FPRs are comparable (20–25%) but can be reduced by the use of customized ultrasound charts which adjust for physiological variables; in one study 27.5% of cases classified as SGA using an unadjusted EFW < 10th centile were reclassified as appropriate-for-gestational age (AGA) using the customized cut-off.[37] Fetuses identified as small by customized charts are more likely to suffer adverse perinatal outcome; the OR for stillbirth was 6.1 (95% CI 5.0–7.5) for fetuses classified as SGA by customized charts but AGA by population charts compared with 1.2 (CI 0.8, 1.9) for those classified as SGA by population charts but normal by customized charts.[38] Fetal anthropometric ratios (e.g. HC:AC and FL:AC) have been used to assess body proportionality but they are less predictive of SGA than AC or EFW and there is no evidence that disproportion adds to the prognostic significance over and above the severity of growth restriction. None of the biophysical tests used to assess fetal well-being (see below) is good at diagnosing a small or growth restricted fetus.

Despite the evidence that ultrasound anthropometry is effective at detecting small fetuses, there is no evidence that routine late pregnancy ultrasound in low risk or unselected women confers benefit to mother or baby; systematic review of seven randomized trials (25 000 women) suggests that, while screened women are less likely to deliver post-term [OR 0.69 (95% CI 0.58–0.81)], perinatal mortality is no different [OR 1.12 (95% CI 0.75–1.68)].[39] Most of these studies investigated the value of a one-off measurement of size rather than the trend (reflecting growth).

Reference charts of AC and EFW, derived from longitudinally collected measurements, can be used to assess fetal growth although the optimal method of quantifying changes remains to be determined. Fetal weight increases by approximately 1% per day [mean 25 (SD 5) g/day] after 32 weeks' gestation. Several studies have confirmed that serial measurements of AC and EFW are superior to single estimates in the prediction of wasting at birth and perinatal morbidity; a change in EFW SD (z) score of ≥ −1.5 [the optimal cut-off determined from receiver operating characteristic (ROC) curve analysis] detects 80% of babies with an abnormal MAC:HC ratio (OR 14.6 [95% CI 2.8–76.5]) and 54% of babies with suboptimal neonatal outcome (OR 3.6 [95% CI 1.3–9.5]).[40] Where growth restriction is suspected, measurements of size should be performed every 2 weeks as shorter intervals increase the FPR.

Uterine artery Doppler

Because of the association between abnormal placentation and FGR, there has been considerable interest in the ability of uterine artery Doppler to predict pre-eclampsia and FGR. Uterine arteries can be readily identified transabdominally with color flow Doppler and reproducible waveforms obtained by pulsed Doppler. A positive test (defined as an abnormal waveform ratio and/or a diastolic notch) between 20 and 24 weeks predicts pre-eclampsia, FGR and perinatal death in low and high risk populations. In women at high risk the pooled LR for a SGA infant is 2.7 (95% CI 2.1–3.4) for a positive result and 0.7 (95% CI 0.6–0.9) for a negative result.[41] Comparable figures for perinatal death are 4.0 (95% CI 2.4–6.6) and 0.6 (95% CI 0.4–0.9). These results suggest that the clinical usefulness of the test is limited; in the quoted overview an abnormal result increased the pretest probability of SGA from 18% to only 37%.[41] However the test is more predictive of FGR necessitating delivery before 34 weeks' gestation (LRs > 5). There is also accumulating evidence that several of the analytes used in maternal serum screening for Down syndrome (e.g. hCG and alpha-fetoprotein) can also be used to screen for pre-eclampsia and FGR. Thus in the future we may be able to offer multiparameter screening for 'poor placentation' between 16 and 24 weeks.

ASSESSMENT OF FETAL WELL-BEING

Principles

Fetal death from hypoxic ischemia may occur acutely, as a result of a sudden insult (e.g. cord accident or placental abruption), or may be the result of chronic placental dysfunction. In the latter case, FGR (but not necessarily SGA) is invariably present. Our understanding of the adaptive responses and consequences of progressive fetal hypoxemia is primarily derived from animal studies but antenatal fetal blood sampling has provided important insights into human FGR. In the face of progressive hypoxemia (fetal pO_2 > 2 SDs below mean for gestation) the fetus makes a number of circulatory and metabolic adaptations to optimize the available oxygen and nutrient supply. With progressive placental insufficiency the fetus becomes academic (pH > 2 SDs below mean for gestation) and ultimately suffers end-organ damage prior to death. Up to 40% of severely growth restricted fetuses (AC > 2 SDs below the mean for gestation) are academic. This is an important outcome as there is evidence that chronic fetal acidemia is associated with reduced neurodevelopmental outcome as assessed by Griffiths neurodevelopmental quotient at a mean age of 29 [range 12–52] months.[42]

A number of biophysical tests are available to assess fetal well-being. These include Doppler ultrasound, cardiotocography (CTG), amniotic fluid volume (AFV) and the biophysical profile score (BPS). For many of these tests the relationship between test result and antenatal hypoxemia/acidemia has been defined, thereby obviating the need for fetal blood sampling which carries a significant risk in FGR. In this context a normal test result implies the absence of acidemia and therefore fetal well-being. As the only effective intervention available to the obstetrician is delivery, the presence of fetal well-being justifies expectant management, at least prior to term, unless there is coexistent maternal disease necessitating delivery. When the test is abnormal, the likelihood of acidemia and the risk of end-organ damage/death with further expectant management have to be balanced against the risks of premature delivery.

Umbilical artery Doppler

Reproducible Doppler velocity waveforms can be obtained from the umbilical artery (UA) using pulsed Doppler. A variety of descriptive indices have been used to characterize the waveform including pulsatility index (PI), resistance index and systolic:diastolic ratio. Mean PI declines during pregnancy with the 95th centile value falling from around 2.0 at 20 weeks to 1.4 at term. Waveform indices are independent of the angle of ultrasound insonation and reflect downstream blood flow resistance. With progressive placental damage and vascular occlusion, PI increases and in some cases this may progress to absent or even reversed end-diastolic velocities (A/R EDV). Between 40 and 45% of fetuses with an elevated PI (but EDV present) are hypoxemic and 20–30% are acidemic. In contrast 80–90% of fetuses with AEDV are hypoxemic and 45–80% are acidemic. Loss of EDV is a key finding which has a profound impact on outcome and management. Overall perinatal mortality in this group is around 40%,[43] justifying delivery on this finding alone after 33 weeks' gestation and possibly earlier.

Systematic review of randomized trials in high risk pregnancies (mainly in association with hypertensive disorders and FGR) has indicated that management based on UA Doppler significantly improves important obstetric outcomes, including fewer admissions [OR 0.56 (95% CI 0.42–0.72)] and fewer labor inductions [OR 0.83 (95% CI 0.74–0.93)].[44] There was also a trend to reducing perinatal mortality [OR 0.71 (95% CI 0.50–1.01)]. There is also evidence that UA Doppler is superior to CTG and the BPS in predicting outcome in SGA fetuses and that it reduces use of resources.[45] Thus UA Doppler should be the primary mode of fetal monitoring in the high risk fetus. Screening low risk fetuses by UA Doppler however does not reduce perinatal mortality or morbidity and is not recommended.

Fetuses with a normal UA Doppler and normal anatomy can be managed as a 'normal small fetus'; in this group twice weekly monitoring results in earlier deliveries and more inductions of labor than fortnightly monitoring without any difference in neonatal morbidity.[46] Thus provided UA Doppler and fetal growth remain normal, fortnightly surveillance can be maintained until delivery. Fetuses with abnormal UA Doppler, especially those with A/R EDV, require more intensive surveillance, usually under the supervision of a specialist obstetrician. The average interval between loss of EDV in the UA and the development of a terminal CTG is 7 days although the range is wide (1 day to more than 4 weeks). Gestational age > 30 weeks, the presence of maternal hypertension and Doppler venous abnormalities are associated with a reduced interval. The optimal monitoring strategy in this group is unclear and may involve targeted fetal Doppler (arterial and venous), BPS or both. Quality randomized trials are urgently needed in this area.

Fetal arterial and venous Doppler

Redistribution of cardiac output to the cerebral circulation is one of the earliest signs of hypoxemia. This is reflected by an increase in the umbilical artery:middle cerebral artery (MCA) PI ratio to greater than 1 (~95th centile) or a decrease in the middle cerebral artery PI. Despite being a sensitive indicator of hypoxemia, there is no evidence that MCA Doppler is a better predictor of adverse outcome than UA Doppler. However the absence of cranial redistribution may provide better negative prediction in the preterm fetus; when gestational age at first Doppler was less than 32 weeks, the MCA PI had a sensitivity of 95.5% and a negative predictive value of 97.7% (negative LR 0.10) for major adverse outcome (death, neurological complications and necrotizing enterocolitis).[47] Compared to fetuses without cranial redistribution, those with cerebral sparing appear to have no long term adverse neurodevelopmental effects although larger follow-up studies are needed.

Fetal venous Doppler abnormalities generally follow loss of EDV in the UA and are thought to reflect ventricular function and, to a lesser extent, cardiac afterload. Waveforms from the ductus venosus (DV) show a systolic and a diastolic peak followed by a trough ('a' wave) related to atrial contraction. With increasing hypoxemia, the 'a' wave decreases and then reverses and pulsations may be evident in the umbilical vein (UV); 90% of fetuses with these findings are acidemic and they have the highest sensitivity for perinatal death and serious morbidity.[48] Many regard reversal of the DV 'a' wave and/or UV pulsations as indications for delivery irrespective of biophysical parameters. As myocardial function worsens, tricuspid valve regurgitation may appear and there may be a loss of brain sparing with normalization of the MCA PI. These are pre-terminal events and fetal death is likely within 48 h.

Biophysical profile scoring (BPS)

The BPS incorporates CTG, AFV and three dynamic ultrasound variables (fetal movement, fetal breathing and fetal tone). Each component is scored 0 (abnormal) or 2 (normal). A total score of 8 or 10 is normal and excludes acidemia.[49] Perinatal mortality within 7 days of a normal BPS is ≤ 1 per 1000 and no test has a lower false negative rate. Scores of 4 or less are regarded as abnormal; > 90% of fetuses will be acidemic and 50% will have an umbilical vein pH < 7.25. Adverse outcome increases with declining score: perinatal mortality increases from 12.5% with a score of 4 to 100% with a score of 0 without intervention (and 43% despite intervention), while the rate of cerebral palsy increases from ~2 to 25% respectively.[49] A score of 6 is equivocal necessitating repeat testing, usually within 12–24 h. Systematic review of four poor quality studies (fewer than 3000 subjects) indicates that BPS does not improve perinatal outcome but insufficient data are available to assess the true value of the test.[50] Given the absence of benefit from randomized trials and that the BPS is a time consuming test, it is not recommended for primary surveillance in high risk fetuses. However, based on the results of observational studies, BPS may have a role in monitoring preterm fetuses with A/R EDF in the UA when a normal score allows continued expectant management.

CTG and AFV have been used in isolation as tests of fetal well-being although there is little evidence to support this. The CTG records autonomic reflexes superimposed on intrinsic cardiac activity. In addition to the baseline fetal heart rate (FHR) and variability, the CTG records periodic changes (accelerations and decelerations). Two 15 beats/min accelerations lasting ≥ 15 s in a 20 min period are regarded as reassuring. Preterm accelerations are less marked. Unlike the BPS where only 0.7% of tests are abnormal (score ≤ 4) and 1.7% are equivocal, up to 15% of CTGs will be non-reassuring. This proportion increases as gestation declines. A non-reassuring CTG is a poor predictor of perinatal death within 7 days (< 10%). The features most predictive of acidemia are reduced FHR variability (< 5 beats/min) and decelerations (positive predictive value 65 and 75% respectively). When both are present (so-called 'terminal' CTG), the overall mortality rate is around 45%. Use of CTG in high risk pregnancies is not associated with better perinatal outcome; in fact systematic review of four randomized trials showed a trend towards increasing perinatal mortality in the CTG group (OR 2.85, 95% CI 0.99–7.12).[51] Computerized analysis of the CTG provides a more objective measure of FHR variability; several parameters have been studied but the short term variability (STV) appears to be the most useful; around 60% of fetuses with a STV < 3.5 ms (the optimal cut-off from ROC curve analysis) are acidemic. Computer systems have been shown to be more accurate predictors of umbilical acidemia than clinical experts but it is unclear whether use of this technology (as opposed to visual analysis) improves perinatal outcome.

There are many definitions for reduced AFV but the two most widely accepted are a maximum vertical pocket < 2 cm or a four quadrant amniotic fluid index (AFI) < 5 cm. Both correlate very poorly with actual AFV and neither accurately predicts perinatal outcome. Systematic review of 18 studies indicated that an AFI < 5 cm was associated with an increased risk of cesarean section for fetal distress (relative risk, RR 2.2, 95% CI 1.5–3.4) and Apgar score < 7 at 5 min (RR 5.2, 95% CI 2.4–11.3),[52] but not with neonatal acidosis. Large observational studies have shown an association between reduced AFV and perinatal mortality but the predictive value is poor (< 10%). There is little evidence to support intervention with isolated oligohydramnios (with a normal UA Doppler).

The sequence and timing of circulatory changes in FGR with progressive hypoxemia/acidemia have been determined and are summarized in Figure 9.2. In a serial study of preterm growth restricted fetuses, 73% showed this pattern of Doppler deterioration prior to emergency delivery (median gestation of 30 weeks) for a BPS of ≤6.[52] In the majority, Doppler deterioration was confined to the week prior to delivery, was most marked for the UA and DV and was complete 24 h before BPS decline. The decline in BPS typically involved cessation of breathing movements 2–3 days before delivery, followed by a decline in AFV and then a loss of fetal movement and tone on the day of delivery.

Organization of screening

Women with risk factors for FGR and fetal acidemia/perinatal mortality (Table 9.4) should have ultrasound screening for fetal size and well-being by AC/EFW and UA Doppler. The timing and frequency of assessment will be determined by the degree of risk. A single screen at 32–34 weeks may be appropriate but where risk is high (e.g. previous stillbirth associated with FGR), 2 weekly surveillance from 26 weeks is justified. We use uterine artery Doppler to guide management; women with normal uterine waveforms at 23 weeks are not followed up until 34 weeks while those with positive waveforms have serial ultrasound assessment from 26 to 28 weeks.

Our management guidelines following the initial AC/EFW and umbilical artery Doppler are shown in Figure 9.3. We regard the presence of A/R EDF in the UA as an indication for daily BPS and venous Doppler studies. Deterioration of the DV Doppler, with reversal of the 'a' wave, usually heralds a decline in the BPS. Unless parents have made an informed decision not to intervene due to the expected poor prognosis (< 500 g and < 27 weeks' gestation) we would deliver when the BPS became abnormal or when a gestational age of 34 weeks was attained. However the benefit of using the BPS rather than abnormalities

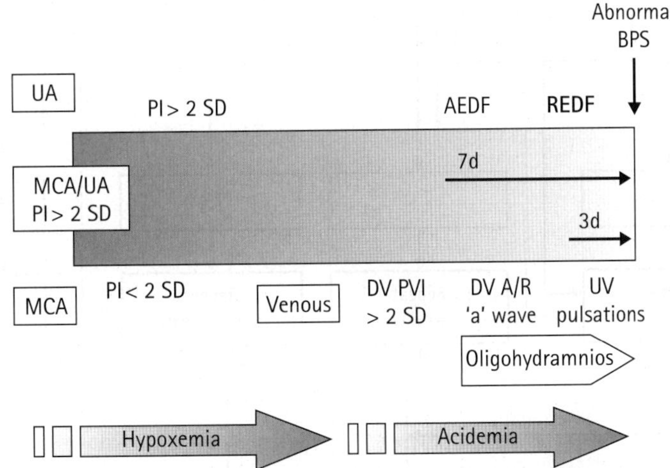

Fig. 9.2 The sequence and timing of Doppler changes in FGR with progressive hypoxemia/acidemia. Doppler changes are usually (but not invariably) preceded by a decline in fetal growth (as assessed by serial changes in abdominal circumference or weight). AEDF, absent end diastolic frequencies; BPS biophysical profile score; d, days; DV A/R, ductus venosus absent/reversed; MCA, middle cerebral artery; PI, pulsatility index; PVI, peak velocity index; REDF, reversed end diastolic frequencies; SD, standard deviation; UA, umbilical artery; UV, umbilical vein.

Table 9.4 Indications for ultrasound assessment to assess fetal size and well-being

Maternal medical history	Current pregnancy history
Hypertension	SFH < 10th centile
Antiphospholipid syndrome	Pregnancy-induced hypertension
Sickle cell disease	Antepartum hemorrhage
Renal disease	Oligohydramnios
Cardiopulmonary disease	Post-term
Insulin dependent diabetes mellitus	Abnormal uterine artery Doppler waveforms
	Elevated maternal AFP
Previous obstetric history	
Stillbirth	
Pre-eclampsia	
SGA infant	
Cesarean section for fetal distress	
Placental abruption	

AFP, alpha-fetoprotein; SFH, symphysis–fundus height; SGA, small for gestational age.

in the DV (or other venous Doppler) waveform to time delivery have not been studied. In this group, we routinely offer cesarean section as in excess of 75% will develop fetal distress if exposed to labor.

MULTIPLE PREGNANCIES

TWINS

Perinatal complications

Perinatal mortality in twins is about five times greater than in singletons. The majority of adverse outcomes occur as a result of either preterm delivery, which occurs in 30–50% of twin pregnancies, or FGR. The predominant prenatal prognostic factor for twins is chorionicity. Relative to dichorionic twins, monochorionic twins are at greater risk of fetal loss at 10–24 weeks' gestation (12.2% vs 18.0%), perinatal mortality (2.8% vs 1.6%), preterm delivery < 32 weeks (9.2% vs 5.5%) and birth weight < 5th centile in both twins (7.5% vs 1.7%).[53] The marked increase in the number of second trimester losses is a consequence of the fetoplacental vascular anastamoses that are present in more than 98% of monochorionic pregnancies. Hemodynamic imbalance between the two circulations is responsible for acute and chronic transfusion syndromes.

Prenatal ultrasonography in twins

Prenatal ultrasonographic assessment of fetal sex and placental/membrane morphology is highly accurate in predicting chorionicity. The lambda sign, an echogenic chorionic tissue projection into the base of the intertwin membrane, is evident in all dichorionic pregnancies at 10–14 weeks' gestation but disappears by the 20th week in about 7% of dichorionic pregnancies with fused

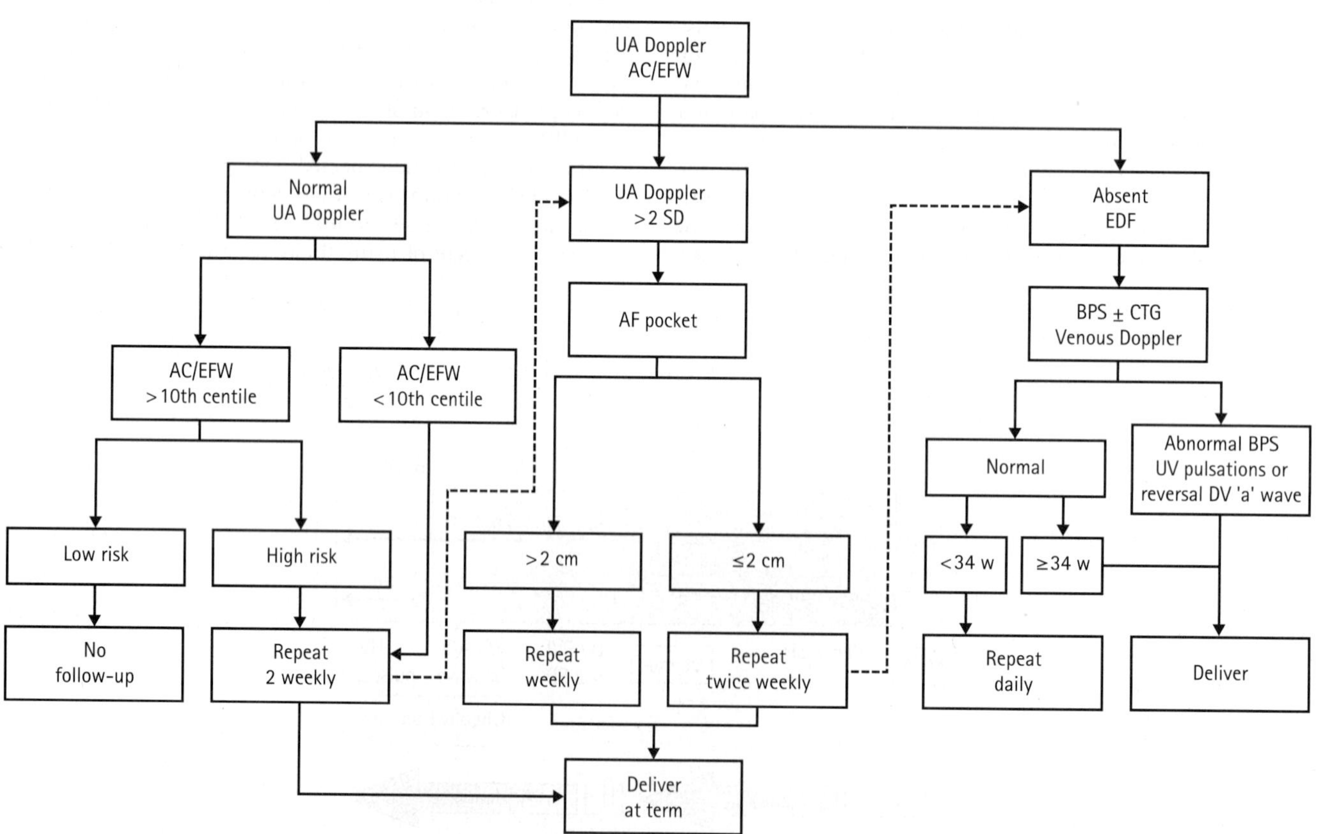

Fig. 9.3 Guidelines for management of high risk fetuses based on ultrasound morphometry and umbilical artery (UA) Doppler. We base the decision to deliver fetuses with absent or reversed end diastolic frequencies (A/R EDF) prior to 34 weeks on the biophysical profile scoring (BPS). Randomized trials are needed to determine if this is a better strategy than using Doppler alone. AC/EFW, abdominal circumference/estimated fetal weight; AF, amniotic fluid; CTG, cardiotocography; DV, ducts venosus; EDF, end diastolic frequencis; SD standard deviation; UV, umbilical vein.

placenta. Monochorionic twins should be scanned every 2–3 weeks in the second trimester to look for evidence of transfusion pathology. All twins should be scanned every 3–4 weeks from 24 weeks onwards to monitor growth and well-being.

Discordant size and growth

A 20–25% discordance in size between twins is associated with an increased incidence of adverse pregnancy outcomes. The differential diagnosis includes constitutional size difference, uteroplacental dysfunction, and fetal abnormalities as well as twin–twin transfusion syndrome (TTTS) in monochorionic twins. Detailed ultrasonography including Doppler analysis of the umbilical, fetal and uteroplacental circulations will usually determine the etiology. A meta-analysis of three studies has shown that fetal surveillance with biometric measurements and UA Doppler ultrasound was more effective than biometric assessment alone at preventing unexplained fetal deaths (OR 0.15, 95% CI 0.03–0.67).[54] The assessment of fetal well-being is based on the same principles as for singletons, but decisions regarding premature delivery need to consider the outcome of the healthy twin.

Twin-twin transfusion syndrome

The TTTS occurs in about 10–15% of monochorionic twins and accounts for 17% of perinatal deaths. The syndrome develops when there is unbalanced shunting of blood from one twin (the donor) to the other (the recipient) through arteriovenous anastomoses in the placenta. The donor twin progressively becomes anemic, growth restricted, and oliguric. The resulting oligohydramnios can be so severe that the donor becomes shrouded in the amniotic membrane ('stuck twin'). The recipient becomes plethoric, polyuric, and develops cardiomegaly and cardiac failure manifest as hydrops. The polyuria leads to hydramnios which predisposes to miscarriage and/or extreme prematurity.

Mortality rates for the severe form of TTTS approach 95%. Several treatment options are available:

Serial amnioreduction

Therapeutic amniocentesis reduces the amniotic fluid volume and/or pressure, thereby reducing the risk of preterm birth and amniorrhexis. The procedure sometimes results in reappearance of fluid in the donor sac. This might reflect alterations in the hemodynamic characteristics of the shunt caused by a reduction in hydrostatic pressure. Serial amnioreduction improves survival rates to between 33 and 83%, but neurological disability in survivors occurs in 5–32% of cases as a result of either ongoing chronic transfusion, or acute shunts associated with fetal cardiovascular instability and/or single fetal demise.[55]

Endoscopic laser coagulation of placental vascular anastamoses

Endoscopic laser coagulation obliterates the communicating placental vessels between the twins. A combination of ultrasonography and direct vision are used to examine systematically the chorionic plate along the whole length of the intertwin membrane and identify the crossing vessels. Initial reports suggest a fetal survival rate of 55%, with at least one survivor in 73% of cases. An advantage of this treatment is that the potential for further intertwin vascular shunting is much reduced, possibly explaining the apparent low incidence (4–5%) of neurological disability in survivors.[56]

Selective feticide

The spontaneous death of one twin is often associated with either loss of the sib, or resolution of the hydramnios. Selective feticide of one twin with a mechanical procedure, such as umbilical cord ligation, has been reported with good short term results. However, there is concern regarding the potential for acute transfer of blood into the placenta of the demised twin.

Single fetal demise

Single fetal death occurs in 0.5–6.8% of twin pregnancies. The earlier twins are diagnosed, the more likely one twin is to demise. The three major factors affecting outcome are the gestational age at death, the cause of death and the chorionicity of the twins. With dichorionic twins, provided the cause of death is intrinsic to the dead twin, complications are unusual. However, the death of a monochorionic twin may be followed by cerebral infarction in the survivor, as well as renal, hepatic and cutaneous damage. In 13 studies, single fetal death was associated with serious morbidity in 24% of 119 surviving monochorionic children.[57] It is likely that the cause of the neurological damage is acute exsanguination of the surviving twin into the circulation of the dead twin through placental vascular anastomoses.

The optimal management of single fetal death ≥ 36 weeks' gestation is elective delivery. For dichorionic twins remote from term, an expectant approach leads to enhanced maturity and an increased chance of survival. For the survivors of monochorionic single fetal deaths, there is debate as to whether the optimal management is delivery or expectant. However, delivery is unlikely to improve outcome if the reason for neurological injury is acute hypoperfusion immediately after the demise of the sib. Thus a conservative approach is usually adopted with serial ultrasound follow-up to look for ventriculomegaly, porencephaly, and microcephaly.

Fetal anomalies

Fetal anomalies are more common in twin pregnancies, particularly monozygous twins, compared to singletons (OR 1.25, 95% CI 1.21–1.28).[58] Even in monozygous twins it is more common for twins to be discordant for anomalies. When ultrasound or genetic studies demonstrate that twins are discordant for a major anomaly, parents are faced with a choice between continuation, TOP, or selective feticide. The risks of selective feticide are dependent on gestation and chorionicity. In dichorionic twins, selective feticide with intracardiac injection of potassium chloride is associated with miscarriage rates varying between 5% at 11–12 weeks and 15% at 16–20 weeks' gestation. The chance of co-twin demise is much reduced if the procedure is carried out during the third trimester after fetal maturity is established, but parents find this option emotionally more difficult.

Selective feticide in monochorionic twins is problematic. Potassium chloride injected into the heart of the abnormal twin might enter the circulation of the normal twin through placental vascular connections. Umbilical cord ligation or diathermy is less likely to cause immediate co-twin demise, but there is concern regarding the potential for acute exsanguination into the placenta of the dead twin.

Monoamniotic twins

About 1% of twins are monoamniotic. Mortality rates (10–40%) are greater than for all other forms of twins due to the increased incidence of fetal anomalies, cord entanglement, prematurity and trauma during labor. Fetal deaths from cord entanglement usually occur before 24 weeks and are very unusual after 30 weeks of pregnancy. Prophylactic early delivery at ≤ 32 weeks' gestation by cesarean section is no longer recommended, but there is ongoing debate about the optimal timing and mode of delivery. Serial scans with color flow Doppler are carried out from 24 weeks' gestation to look for cord entanglement which prompts daily biophysical testing and consideration of delivery if there is evidence of fetal compromise.

HIGHER ORDER MULTIPLES

The natural incidence of triplets is ~1 in 8000 pregnancies. With assisted reproductive techniques, the incidence has increased to between 1 in 850–2000. The mean gestation at delivery is 33 weeks with a mean birth weight of 1800 g. Preterm delivery at less than 28 weeks' gestation occurs in 7% of cases, and at less than 32 weeks in 28%. Perinatal mortality rates vary from 41 to 66 per 1000 pregnancies. Cerebral palsy occurs in about 3% of long term survivors. For quadruplets, perinatal mortality rates are between 67 and 104 per 1000, with cerebral palsy occurring in 10% of survivors. The outcomes for higher order multiple pregnancies are even worse.

Multifetal pregnancy reduction (MFPR)

Although advances in prenatal and neonatal care have resulted in significant improvement in perinatal mortality for higher order multiple pregnancies, there remains concern about long term morbidity for both the offspring and the family. One option is MFPR which is usually performed by intrathoracic injection of potassium chloride. Success rates of 100% are typical.

The majority of pregnancies are reduced to twins. This leaves 'margin for error' if there is a problem with a remaining fetus. The frequency of complications, mainly miscarriage or preterm delivery, is a function of the starting number of fetuses (Table 9.5).[59] The outcome for pregnancies reduced to twins is comparable to non-reduced twins. There is some debate as to whether MFPR is justified for triplets, but there are no doubts that outcomes are improved for quadruplets and higher order multiple pregnancies.

ALLOIMMUNIZATION

RED CELL ANTIBODIES

When maternal antibodies to antigens on fetal red cells cross the placenta they can result in hemolysis. The risk of hemolytic disease of the newborn (HDN) requiring treatment is dependent on the red cell antigen (Table 9.6). Transplacental fetomaternal hemorrhage (FMH) is the most common cause of alloimmunization. Heterologous blood transfusion is the second, but is the most common cause of sensitization to the uncommon antigens. Of the five major antigenic loci determining rhesus (Rh) status (C, D, E, c, e), D is the most immunogenic, followed by c. Approximately 85% of the Caucasian population are RhD positive, 45% being homozygous for the D antigen. Routine screening for red cell antibodies is undertaken at booking and around 30 weeks of pregnancy. Alloimmunization is now sufficiently uncommon that all cases at risk of significant hemolysis should be managed by, or in collaboration with, a regional center.

Anti-D prophylaxis

Anti-D immunoglobulin (Ig) should be given to all non-sensitized RhD negative women within 72 h of the delivery of a RhD positive infant. A dose of 100 µg (500 iu) is capable of suppressing immunization by 4–5 ml RhD positive cells. A Kleihauer test is routinely undertaken to detect larger FMH requiring additional anti-D Ig. Prophylaxis is also given after potentially sensitizing events during pregnancy (e.g. antepartum hemorrhage, invasive prenatal diagnosis) and after therapeutic TOP, ectopic pregnancy, and uterine evacuation of a spontaneous or incomplete abortion. Between 1 and 1.5% RhD negative women develop anti-D antibodies during a first or subsequent pregnancy due to 'silent' FMH. Evidence from several studies indicates 100 µg of anti-D Ig at 28 and 34 weeks can reduce this to 0.2% or less and antenatal prophylaxis is now recommended.

Management of women with anti-D

Once anti-D antibodies are detected the father's RhD type should be determined. Significant hemolysis does not occur with anti-D concentrations ≤ 4 iu/ml and there is no need for intervention. Antibody testing should be repeated monthly to 28 weeks and fortnightly thereafter. Above 4 iu/ml there is a risk of anemia but this is not accurately predicted by anti-D concentration; between 4 and 15 iu/ml mild to moderate anemia, requiring postnatal transfusion, may occur but severe anemia (hemoglobin < 7 g/dl) is uncommon. Above 15 iu/ml, and particularly in the presence of rapidly rising levels, the risk of severe anemia has been reported to be as high as 50%. Where there is a risk of significant hemolysis and the partner is heterozygous for the RhD antigen, fetal RhD genotyping using PCR on amniotic fluid is reliable. This can now be performed on fetal cells sorted from the maternal circulation.

Traditionally the risk of anemia has been assessed by spectrophotometric determination of amniotic fluid bilirubin in women with anti-D > 4 iu/ml. The shift in optical density (OD) is measured at a wavelength of 450 nm (ΔOD 450) and the result plotted on a graph according to gestational age. The original charts published by Liley have three ascending zones indicating the risk of severe anemia between 28 and 40 weeks. Amniocentesis is usually repeated every 2 weeks and management is dictated by the trend; a progressive rise in ΔOD 450 towards or into the upper zone indicates the need for further action (delivery or fetal blood sampling). The timing of the first amniocentesis is dependent on the anti-D level, the rate of rise and the previous rhesus history. It is assumed the

Table 9.5 Multifetal pregancy reduction: pregnancy losses or deliveries as a function of starting number (S) before reduction

		Losses	Deliveries				
	N	< 24 wks n (%)	25–28 wks n (%)	29–32 wks n (%)	33–36 wks n (%)	37+ wks n (%)	Mean GA
S 6+	96	22 (22.9)	11 (11.5)	11 (11.5)	33 (34.4)	19 (19.8)	33.6
S 5	170	29 (17.1)	9 (5.3)	21 (12.4)	55 (32.4)	56 (32.9)	34.5
S 4	653	90 (13.0)	32 (4.9)	68 (10.4)	221 (33.8)	242 (37.1)	35.0
S 3	759	58 (7.6)	25 (3.3)	57 (7.5)	263 (34.7)	356 (46.9)	35.5
S 2	111	10 (9.0)	4 (3.6)	4 (3.6)	12 (10.8)	81 (73.0)	35.6

Collaborative data from 1789 patients having multifetal pregnancy reduction to twins, or singletons when reducing from twins.[59] GA, gestational age.

Table 9.6 Red cell antigens causing hemolytic disease of the newborn (HDN)

Can cause severe HDN and intrauterine death	Severe HDN uncommon
Rhesus – D, c, e, C, E	Kidd – JK^a
Kell	Duffy – Fy^a
	Kp $^{a\ or\ b}$
	k
	S
Severe HDN rare	**Never cause HDN**
Fy^b	Le $^{a\ or\ b}$
Jk^b	p
Lu^a	
Hutch	
M,	
N,	
s,	
U	

disease will become worse with each RhD positive pregnancy. Assessment of risk based on amniotic fluid bilirubin has several disadvantages, apart from the cumulative risk of increased sensitization and amnionitis with repeated procedures; reliable data are not available before 28 weeks and even in the third trimester 10% of predictions are erroneous.

Several ultrasonic parameters have been evaluated as non-invasive predictors of anemia. Hydrops is a reliable but late sign of severe anemia. Weekly ultrasound surveillance to detect early signs of ascites will miss many fetuses with significant anemia. Furthermore once hydrops has developed, transfusion is more hazardous and less effective. Measurements of liver size, spleen size and umbilical vein diameter are unreliable predictors of anemia. In contrast, there is accumulating evidence that fetal middle cerebral artery Doppler is a reliable non-invasive test; in the most comprehensive study to date, the sensitivity of an increased peak velocity of systolic blood flow was 100% with a FPR of 12% (positive LR 8.5, 95% CI 4.7–15.6, negative LR 0.02, 95% CI 0.00–0.25).[60] Whether cerebral Doppler can replace amniocentesis is currently the focus of randomized trials.

The extent of anemia is assessed by measurement of fetal hematocrit (or hemoglobin). The risk of increased sensitization, especially with transplacental passage of the needle, and fetal death suggests that fetal blood sampling should be reserved for fetuses perceived to be at highest risk. Intravascular transfusions are begun when the fetal hematocrit declines below 30% (less than the 2.5th centile after 20 weeks). The timing of subsequent blood sampling in fetuses with a hematocrit > 30% is determined by the strength of the positive direct antiglobulin test and the fetal reticulocyte count. Compatible (RhD negative), fresh, leukocyte depleted blood, resuspended in saline to a hematocrit of ~70–75%, is transfused into either the umbilical vein (at the placental cord insertion) or the intrahepatic vein. The volume of blood required to attain the desired hematocrit (typically 40–50%) can be estimated from the initial fetal and donor hematocrits together with the estimated fetoplacental blood volume. The second transfusion is arbitrarily undertaken 2 weeks after the first. The timing of subsequent transfusions is then determined from the fall in hematocrit which becomes more consistent over time (typically ~1%/day) as fetal erythropoiesis is suppressed and only donor blood is circulating. Intraperitoneal transfusion is less effective and associated with a greater risk of fetal death compared with intravascular transfusion. Furthermore combining intraperitoneal and intravascular transfusion confers no advantage. The aim with fetal transfusion is to reach a gestational age of at least 36 weeks before delivery.

Mortality rate per intravascular transfusion is ~3%, with higher rates reported when transfusion is required prior to 20 weeks' gestation and in hydropic fetuses. Overall 84% of fetuses (94% without hydrops and 74% with hydrops) requiring in-utero transfusion will survive[61] with < 10% suffering developmental problems.[62] Postnatal exchange transfusion is rarely necessary when there have been at least two antenatal transfusions. Top-up transfusions are frequently necessary because of late anemia prior to resumption of normal erythropoiesis.

Management of women with other alloantibodies

Anti-c antibodies can be quantitated accurately and management of women with anti-c levels > 4 iu/ml follows similar guidelines to anti-D. Antibody levels for other red cell antibodies are measured by indirect antiglobulin test. The reciprocal of the highest dilution of serum that causes agglutination is the titer. Severe hemolysis rarely, if ever, occurs with titers ≤ 1 in 32 with the exception of anti-Kell where severe anemia has been reported with titers as low as 1:2. In Kell disease the main cause of fetal anemia is erythroid suppression rather than hemolysis. Determination of the partner's Kell status is vital as only 9% will be Kell positive, with virtually all being heterozygous. Thus very few fetuses of women with anti-Kell are actually at risk. The role of amniocentesis in monitoring women with alloantibodies other than anti-D is controversial. Certainly for anti-Kell and anti-E there is evidence that ΔOD 450 measurements may be falsely reassuring and where the risk of severe anemia is high, fetal blood sampling is necessary.

PLATELET ANTIBODIES

In alloimmune thrombocytopenia (AIT), maternal antiplatelet antibodies to a paternally derived platelet antigen, usually PLA1, cross the placenta and destroy fetal platelets. Neonatal AIT occurs in 1 in 2000–5000 births with intracranial hemorrhage (ICH) in 15–20% of cases. Between 30 and 50% of ICH occurs in-utero, usually after 30 weeks' gestation. The mother is healthy and her first child is affected in 50% of cases. Recurrence rates are very high (> 85%).

Management is controversial but fetal blood sampling at 22–24 weeks allows determination of fetal platelet count in at risk cases. If severe thrombocytopenia (platelet count < 50×10^9/L) is confirmed intravenous immunoglobulin (1 g/kg/week) has been shown to raise platelet count in some cases. Because the response is not consistent repeat fetal blood sampling 2–4 weeks later is necessary. A falling platelet count, particularly to < 20×10^9/L , is an indication for platelet transfusion. Transfusion raises the platelet count for only a few days and therefore needs to be repeated weekly. Platelet transfusions are more likely to be complicated by fetal bradycardia and death than red cell transfusions and therefore delivery around 34 weeks, usually by cesarean section, is appropriate. Where the initial platelet count is > 50×10^9/L it is reasonable to repeat blood sampling 4–6 weeks later.

REFERENCES (* Level 1 evidence)

1 Northern Regional Maternity Survey Office Annual Report 1995. Newcastle-upon-Tyne: Survey Office; 1997.

2 Boyd PA, Chamberlain P, Hicks NR. 6-year experience of prenatal diagnosis in an unselected population in Oxford, UK. Lancet 1998; 352:1567–1569.

3 Hyett JA, Moscoso G, Nicolaides KH. First trimester nuchal translucency and cardiac septal defects in fetuses with trisomy 21. Am J Obstet Gynecol 1995; 172:1411–1413.

4 Souka AP, Krampl E, Bakalis S, et al. Outcome of pregnancy in chromosomally normal fetuses with increased nuchal translucency in the first trimester. Ultrasound Obstet Gynecol 2001; 18:9–17.

5 Statham H, Solomou W, Chitty L. Prenatal diagnosis of fetal abnormality: psychological effects on women in low-risk pregnancies. Best Practice Res Clin Obstet Gynaecol 2000; 14:731–747.

6 Chitty LS, Hunt GH, Moore J, et al. Effectiveness of routine ultrasonography in detecting fetal abnormalities in a low risk population. BMJ 1991; 303:165–169.

7 Shirley IM, Bottomley F, Robinson VP. Routine radiographer screening for fetal abnormalities in an unselected low risk population. Br J Radiol 1992; 65:564–569.

8 Luck CA. Value of routine ultrasound scanning at 19 weeks: a four year study of 8849 deliveries. BMJ 1992; 304:1474–1478.

9 Bernaschek G, Stuempflen I, Deutinger J. The value of sonographic diagnosis of fetal malformations: different results between indication-based and screening-based investigations. Prenat Diagn 1994; 14:807–812.

*10 Crane JP, LeFevre ML, Winborn RC, et al. A randomized trial of prenatal ultrasonographic screening: Impact on the detection, management and outcome of anomalous fetuses. Am J Obstet Gynecol 1994; 171:392–399.

*11 Ewigman BG, Crane JP, Frigoletto FD, et al. Effect of prenatal ultrasound screening on perinatal outcome. New Engl J Med 1993; 329:821–827.

*12 Neilson JP. Ultrasound for fetal assessment in early pregnancy (Cochrane Review). In: The Cochrane Library, Issue 4. Oxford: Update Software; 2001.

*13 Newnham JP, Evans SF, Michael CA, et al. Effects of frequent ultrasound during pregnancy: a randomised controlled trial. Lancet 1993; 342:887–891.

14 Royal College of Obstetricians and Gynaecologists. Termination of pregnancy for fetal abnormality. London: RCOG; 1996.

15 Vergani P, Locatelli A, Strobelt N, et al. Clinical outcome of mild fetal ventriculomegaly. Am J Obstet Gynecol 1998; 178:218–222.

16 Sparey C, Robson S. Fetal cerebral ventriculomegaly. Fetal Mat Med Rev 1998; 10:163–179.

*17 Lumley J, Watson L, Watson M, et al. Periconceptional supplementation with folate and/or multivitamins for preventing neural tube defects. [Systematic Review] Cochrane Pregnancy and Childbirth Group Cochrane Database of Systematic Reviews. Issue 4, 2001.

18 Gupta JK, Lilford RJ. Assessment and management of fetal agenesis of the corpus callosum. Prenat Diagn 1995; 15:301–312.

19 Bullen PJ, Rankin JM, Robson SC. Investigation of the epidemiology and prenatal diagnosis of holoprosencephaly in the North of England. Am J Obstet Gynecol 2001; 184:1256–1262.

20 Scott JE, Wright B, Wilson G, et al. Measuring the fetal kidney with ultrasonography. Br J Urology 1995; 76:769–774.

21 Anderson N, Clautice-Engle T, Allan R, et al. Detection of obstructive uropathy in the fetus: predictive value of sonographic measurements of renal pelvic diameter at various gestational ages. Am J Radiol 1995; 164:719–723.

22 Johnson M, Bukowski TP, Reitleman C, et al. In utero surgical treatment of fetal obstructive uropathy: a new comprehensive approach to identify appropriate candidates for vesico-amniotic shunt therapy. Am J Obstet Gynecol 1994; 170:1770–1779.

23 Allan L, Hornberger L, Sharland G. Textbook of fetal cardiology. London: Greenwich Medical Media; 2000.

24 Griffin DR. Skeletal abnormalities. In: James DK, Steer PJ, Weiner CP, et al., eds. High risk pregnancy. London: WB Saunders; 1999:465–488.

25 Royal College of Obstetricians and Gynaecologists. Amniocentesis. Clinical Guideline No. 8. London: RCOG; 2001.

*26 Canadian Early and Mid Trimester Amniocentesis Trial Group. Randomized trial to assess safety and fetal outcome of early and midtrimester amniocentesis. Lancet 1998; 351:243–249.

*27 Tabor A, Philip J, Madsen M, et al. Randomised controlled trial of genetic amniocentesis in 4606 low-risk women. Lancet 1986; i:1287–1293.

28 Silver RK, Russell TK, Kambich MP, et al. Midtrimester amniocentesis. Influence of operator caseload on sampling efficiency. J Reprod Med 1998; 43:191–195.

*29 Alfirevic Z, Gosden CM, Neilson JP. Chorion villus sampling versus amniocentesis for prenatal diagnosis. [Systematic Review] Cochrane Pregnancy and Childbirth Group Cochrane Database of Systematic Reviews. Issue 4, 2001.

30 Kalousek DK, Vekemans M. Confined placental mosaicism. J Med Genet 1996; 33:529–533.

31 Maxwell D, Johnson P, Hurley P, et al. Fetal blood sampling and pregnancy loss in relation to indication. Br J Obstet Gynaecol 1991; 98:892–897.

32 Flake AW, Crombleholme TM, Johnson MP, et al. Treatment of severe congenital diaphragmatic hernia by fetal tracheal occlusion: clinical experience with 15 cases. Am J Obstet Gynecol 2000; 183:1059–1066.

33 Soothill PW, Bobrow CS, Holmes R. Small for gestational age is not a diagnosis. Ultrasound Obstet Gynecol 1999; 13:225–228.

*34 Neilson JP. Symphysis–fundal height measurement in pregnancy. Cochrane Database Syst Rev 2000; CD000944.

*35 Gardosi J, Francis A. Controlled trial of fundal height measurement plotted on customised growth charts. Br J Obstet Gynaecol 1999; 106:309–317.

36 Chang TC, Robson SC, Boys RJ, et al. Prediction of the small for gestational age infant; which ultrasonic measurement is best? Obstet Gynecol 1992; 80:1030–1038.

37 Mongelli M, Gardosi J. Reduction of false-positive diagnosis of fetal growth restriction by application of customized fetal growth standards. Obstet Gynecol 1996; 88:844–848.

38 Clausson B, Gardosi J, Francis A, et al. Perinatal outcome in SGA births defined by customised versus population-based birthweight standards. Br J Obstet Gynaecol 2001; 108:830–834.

*39 Bricker L, Neilson JP. Routine ultrasound in late pregnancy (after 24 weeks gestation). Cochrane Database of Systematic Reviews. Issue 3, 2001.

40 Robson SC, Chang TC. Measurement of human fetal growth. In: Hanson MA, Spencer JAD, Rodeck CH, eds. Fetus and neonate physiology and clinical applications. Vol 3 (Growth). Cambridge: Cambridge University Press; 1995:297–325.

41 Chien PFW, Arnott N, Gordon A, et al. How useful is uterine artery Doppler flow velocimetry in the prediction of pre-eclampsia, intrauterine growth retardation and perinatal death? An overview. Br J Obstet Gynaecol 2000; 107:196–208.

42 Soothill PW, Ajayi RA, Campbell S, et al. Relationship between fetal acidemia at cordocentesis and subsequent neurodevelopment. Ultrasound Obstet Gynecol 1992; 2:80–83.

43 Karsdorp VHM, van Vugt JM, van Geijn HP, et al. Clinical significance of absent or reversed end-diastolic velocity waveforms in umbilical artery. Lancet 1994; 344:1664–1668.

*44 Neilson JP, Alfirevic Z. Doppler ultrasound for fetal assessment in high risk pregnancies. [Systematic Review] Cochrane Pregnancy and Childbirth Group Cochrane Database of Systematic Reviews. Issue 3, 2001.

45 Soothill PW, Ajayi RA, Campbell S, et al. Prediction of morbidity in small and normally grown fetuses by fetal heart rate variability, biophysical profile and umbilical artery Doppler studies. Br J Obstet Gynaecol 1993; 100:742–745.

*46 McCowan LM, Harding JE, Roberts AB, et al. A pilot randomized trial of two regimes of fetal surveillance for small-for-gestational age fetuses with normal results of umbilical artery Doppler velocimetry. Am J Obstet Gynecol 2000; 182:81–86.

47 Fong KW, Ohlsson A, Hannah ME, et al. Prediction of perinatal outcome in fetuses suspected to have intrauterine growth restriction: Doppler US study of fetal, cerebral, renal and umbilical arteries. Radiology 1999; 213:681–689.

48 Baschat AA, Gembruch U, Reiss I, et al. Relationship between arterial and venous Doppler and perinatal outcome in fetal growth restriction. Ultrasound Obstet Gynecol 2000; 16:407–413.

49 Manning FA. Fetal biophysical profile: a critical appraisal. Fetal Mat Med Rev 1997; 9:103–123.

*50 Alfirevic Z, Neilson JP. Biophysical profile for fetal assessment in high risk pregnancies. [Systematic Review] Cochrane Pregnancy and Childbirth Group Cochrane Database of Systematic Reviews. Issue 3, 2001.

*51 Pattison N, McCowan L. Cardiotocography for antepartum fetal assessment. [Systematic Review] Cochrane Pregnancy and Childbirth Group Cochrane Database of Systematic Reviews. Issue 3, 2001.

*52 Chauhan SP, Sanderson M, Hendrix NW, et al. Perinatal outcome and amniotic fluid index in the antepartum and intrapartum periods: a meta-analysis. Am J Obstet Gynecol 1999; 181:1473–1478.

53 Sebire NJ, Snijders RJ, Hughes K, et al. The hidden mortality of monochorionic twin pregnancies. Br J Obstet Gynaecol 1997; 104:1203–1207.

*54 Giles W. Doppler ultrasound in twin pregnancies. Fetal Mat Med Rev 2001; 12.

55 Mari G, Roberts A, Detti L, et al. Perinatal morbidity and mortality rates in severe twin–twin transfusion syndrome: results of the International Amnioreduction Registry. Am J Obstet Gynecol 2001; 185:708–715.

56 Ville Y, Hecher K, Gagnon A, et al. Endoscopic laser coagulation in the management of severe twin-to-twin transfusion syndrome. Br J Obstet Gynaecol 1998; 105:446–453.

57 Van Heteren CF, Nijhuis JG, Semmekrot BA, et al. Risk for surviving twin after fetal death of co-twin in twin–twin transfusion syndrome. Obstet Gynecol 1998; 92:215–219.

58 Mastroiacovo P, Castilla EE, Arpino C, et al. Congenital malformations in twins: an international study. Am J Med Genet 1999; 83:117–124.

59 Evans MI, Dommergues M, Wapner RJ. International collaborative experience of 1789 patients having multifetal pregnancy reduction: a plateauing of risks and outcomes. J Soc Gynecol Invest 1996; 3:23–26.

60 Mari G, Deter RL, Carpenter RL, et al. Noninvasive diagnosis by Doppler ultrasonography of fetal anaemia due to maternal red-cell alloimmunization. New Engl J Med 2000; 342:9–14.

61 Schumacher B, Moise KJ. Fetal transfusion for red blood cell alloimmunization in pregnancy. Obstet Gynecol 1996; 88:137–150.

62 Doyle LW, Kelly EA, Rickards AL, et al. Sensorineural outcome at 2 years for survivors of erythroblastosis treated with fetal intravascular transfusion. Obstet Gynecol 1993; 81:931–935.

10

The newborn

Edited by Neil McIntosh, Ben Stenson

INTRODUCTION

DEFINITIONS – WORLD HEALTH ORGANIZATION (WHO)

GESTATION (INDEPENDENT OF BIRTH WEIGHT)

1. Preterm = less than 36 completed weeks of gestation (258 days).
2. Full term = between 37 weeks and 41 completed weeks of gestation (259–293 days).
3. Post-term or postmature = more than 42 weeks (294 days).

Dates are taken from the first day of the last menstrual period. Conception is presumed to be approximately 2 weeks after this date. Ultrasound dates are based on conception and have to be altered to fit with the dates estimated from the last menstrual period.

BIRTH WEIGHT (INDEPENDENT OF GESTATION)

1. Low birth weight (LBW) = less than 2500 g.
2. Very low birth weight (VLBW) = less than 1500 g (accepted by convention).
3. Extremely low birth weight (ELBW) (USA – very, very low birth weight) = less than 1000 g (accepted by convention).

SIZE FOR GESTATION (Fig. 10.1)

1. Small for gestation (SGA) = less than 10th centile in weight expected for gestation (small for dates).
2. Appropriate for gestation (AGA) = between 10th and 90th centiles of weight expected for gestation.
3. Large for gestation (LGA) = more than 90th centile in weight expected for gestation.

NB: The expected weight centiles will vary with the population. The terms immature, premature and dysmature should no longer be used.

AGE

In utero

1. Less than 1 week = fertilized egg to the formation of the blastocyst.
2. 1–12 weeks = embryo.
3. 12 weeks–delivery = fetus.
4. 24 weeks or more = current period of 'legal' viability in the UK.

In the UK it is uncommon to terminate a pregnancy after 20 weeks of gestation, though it is legal through to term for major fetal anomaly or maternal life-threatening problem.[1]

Abortion is the expulsion of the dead fetus prior to 24 weeks' gestation (168 days). A dead fetus expelled after this time is a *stillbirth*. Note that a live-born baby is a baby of *any gestation* that has signs of life (e.g. only a heart beat) at delivery. Many miscarriages before 20 weeks' gestation will show signs of life.

The neonate

1. Perinatal period = the period from 24 weeks' gestation or the time of the live-birth if less than 24 weeks' gestation, to 7 days of postnatal age.
2. Early neonatal period = the first 7 days of life of a live-born infant of *any* gestation.
3. Late neonatal period = 8–28 days after birth.
4. Neonatal period = the first 28 days of life of a live-born infant of *any* gestation.
5. Infancy = the first year of life.

MORTALITY RATES

1. Stillbirth rate = number of stillbirths per 1000 total births.
2. Perinatal mortality rate (PMR) = number of stillbirths + early (up to 7 completed days) neonatal deaths per 1000 total births.
3. Neonatal mortality rate (NNMR) = number of deaths in the first 28 days per 1000 live births.
4. Infant mortality rate (IMR) = number of deaths in the first 365 days per 1000 live births.

Maternity units should collect the figures for PMR, NNMR and also neonatal deaths before discharge from hospital. Reduction of NNMR simply by postponing the deaths out of the neonatal period is not the aim of neonatal care. Bronchopulmonary dysplasia, infection and necrotizing enterocolitis (NEC) are the current problems that lead to late deaths after 28 days. The 'corrected' WHO neonatal mortality rate is the number of deaths in the first 28 days of life (birth weight greater than 1000 g) per 1000 live births.

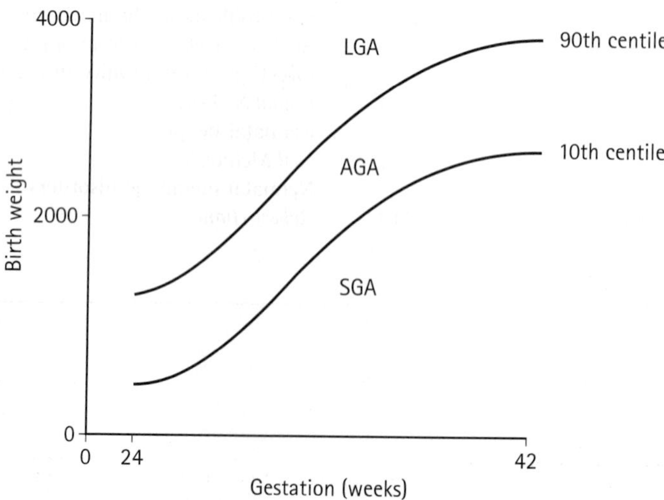

Fig. 10.1 Size for gestation based on population centiles for birthweight with gestation: LGA, large for gestational age; AGA, appropriate for gestational age; SGA, small for gestational age (less than the 10th centile expected weight for gestation).

EPIDEMIOLOGY AND EVIDENCE BASED NEONATAL CARE

Most clinical decisions must be based on incomplete evidence. However, a sound understanding of epidemiology allows us to select the best available evidence for clinical policy.

COMPARISONS OF THE PREVALENCE OF NEONATAL MORTALITY AND MORBIDITY

Accurate estimates of the burden of disease are important for planning services and for first generating and then testing hypotheses about the underlying causes of disease and the appropriate interventions. Hospital based estimates of the prevalence of disease are open to substantial selection bias. Prospective, population based estimates of the prevalence of neonatal mortality and morbidity are more reliable, but still require considerable caution in their interpretation. Apparent differences in prevalence between different populations may reflect variations in many factors, such as definitions, accuracy and completeness of ascertainment, genetic and biological causes, socioeconomic factors and the provision and quality of services.

Table 10.1[2–10] illustrates recent population based estimates of neonatal mortality and morbidity among survivors in a range of settings. Compared with England and Wales neonatal mortality in China was 70% greater for all infants and nearly 10-fold greater for infants of very low birth weight (under 1500 g). This is more likely to reflect differences in socioeconomic development and in the provision and organization of perinatal care than differences in the definition or ascertainment of neonatal mortality. The approximately 60% increase in neonatal mortality for very low birth weight infants in England and Wales versus Australia is more difficult to explain. Variations in ascertainment might be important. Marginally viable infants of extremely low birth weight who are born alive and then die without being resuscitated or weighed may not always be registered as live births and the registration of live-born infants of less than 1000 g can vary considerably between regions and countries. However, neonatal mortality was over 50% greater in England and Wales than in Australia for infants between 1000 and 1499 g, a group in which variation in registration of live births is less likely. This difference in birth weight specific mortality may be consistent, at least in part, with differences in the organization of perinatal care.[11]

Definitions and degrees of ascertainment of cerebral palsy can also vary. The risk increases with decreasing gestation or birth weight. In England and Scotland in 1984–1989 the birth weight specific prevalence of cerebral palsy ranged from 1.1 per 1000 neonatal survivors in infants weighing 2500 g or more to 78.1 in infants weighing less than 1000 g.[4] Despite this, Table 10.1 shows relatively consistent estimates of the prevalence of cerebral palsy of between 2.1 and 3.3 per 1000 live births in various European population based studies of infants born between 1981 and 1996. Within the same geographical populations, the prevalence fell from 3.3 to 2.3 per 1000 between 1981 and 1990 in Slovenia but remained relatively constant at between 2.0 and 2.5 per 1000 live births between 1967 and 1985 in Western Australia.[8] In China, the prevalence of cerebral palsy has recently been estimated as 1.6 per 1000 live births, with evidence of a rise between 1990 and 1997.[3] Compared with developed countries, substantially fewer infants of low birth weight in China survive to be old enough to be diagnosed as having cerebral palsy. When adjusted for birth weight, using the distribution of birth weights in Australia as a standard, the prevalence of cerebral palsy in China was 2.8 per 1000 live births.

Table 10.1 Prevalence of neonatal mortality and early and late morbidity in various population-based studies

Outcome	Rate	Source
Neonatal mortality for all infants	4.0 per 1000 live births	England and Wales, 1996[2]
	6.8 per 1000 live births	China, 1993–1996[3]
Neonatal mortality for infants of less than 1500 g birth weight	129 per 1000 live births	Australia, 1996[3]
	197 per 1000 live births	England and Wales, 1996[2]
Neonatal mortality for infants of 1000–1499 g birth weight	39.7 per 1000 live births	Australia, 1996[3]
	59.1 per 1000 live births	England and Wales, 1996[2]
	581 per 1000 live births	China, 1993–1996[3]
Cerebral palsy* in surviving children for infants of all birth weights	1.6 per 1000 live births	China, 1993–1996[3]
	2.1 per 1000 live births	England and Scotland 1998[4]
	2.12 per 1000 live births	Sweden, 1991–1994[5]
	2.3 per 1000 livebirths	Slovenia, 1990[6]
	2.57 per 1000 live births	Alberta, 1985–1996[7]
	2.0–2.5 per 1000 live births	Western Australia, 1967–1985[8]
	3.3 per 1000 live births	Slovenia, 1981[6]
Chronic lung disease** in infants of less than 28 weeks' gestation: number (%)	22.9% (752/3285)	Australia and New Zealand, 2000[9]
Chronic lung disease** in infants of 28–31 weeks' gestation: number (%)	12.3% (261/2188)	Australia and New Zealand, 2000[9]
Retinopathy of prematurity, treated with cryotherapy or laser therapy, in babies born at less than 28 weeks' gestation: number (%)	7% (59/845)	Australia and New Zealand, 2000[9]
	15.9% (47/295)	Northern Region, UK, 1990-1994[10]

* Cerebral palsy: a chronic disability of central nervous system origin characterized by aberrant control of movement or posture, appearing early in life and not as a result of a progressive disease.

** Chronic lung disease: requiring supplementary oxygen, mechanical ventilation or continuous positive airway pressure at 36 weeks' postmenstrual age, among infants admitted to neonatal units.

Table 10.1 shows that the rate of chronic lung disease can also vary considerably in infants of different gestational age. As with cerebral palsy, appropriate comparisons of chronic lung disease between populations can only be made after standardizing for differences in the distribution of gestational age (or its proxy, birth weight).

Severe retinopathy of prematurity requires treatment with cryotherapy or laser therapy. Using similar criteria, the prevalence of treatment for severe retinopathy in infants of less than 28 weeks' gestation appeared to be less than half in Australia in 2000 than in the Northern Region of England between 1990 and 1994, despite greater rates of survival for these infants in Australia. Furthermore, the risk of severe retinopathy among survivors between neonatal units within the Northern Region varied by more than fourfold, from 6.2% to 27.7%. These differences are consistent with the hypothesis that contrasts in clinical practice, such as target ranges of oxygen saturation, may contribute to variations in the rate of severe retinopathy.[10] This hypothesis merits rigorous examination in a randomized controlled trial.

HOW CAN WE ESTABLISH CAUSE AND EFFECT?

Deciding which risk factors cause or contribute to illness, or which treatments are effective, is a fundamental problem that requires careful judgment. Sir Austin Bradford Hill developed a number of guidelines that are helpful. The most important are that there should be evidence:

1. of a strong association (strength);
2. that exposure to the risk factor occurred before onset of disease (temporality);
3. of a plausible biological explanation (plausibility);
4. that the association is supported by other investigations in different settings (consistency and coherence);
5. of reversibility of the effect – if the causal factor is removed the effect should also disappear;
6. of a dose–response effect, so that the greater the exposure to the risk factor, the greater the chance of disease (biological gradient);
7. no convincing alternative explanation, for example a strong confounding variable (specificity).

Not all the criteria are necessary to decide about causation in any particular setting.

IMPORTANCE OF RANDOMIZED CONTROLLED TRIALS IN MINIMIZING SYSTEMATIC BIAS

In general, the best evidence about whether treatments are effective comes from randomized controlled trials. Random allocation of treatments is the most reliable way of minimizing bias, because it ensures that the innumerable variables that would otherwise confound comparisons tend to be evenly balanced between the treated and control groups. In fact, *random allocation balances all confounding variables, regardless of whether or not they are known or measured.* This is a major advantage over non-randomized comparative studies, in which we must attempt to identify and account for every potentially important confounding variable to protect against bias, which may well be an impossible task. Table 10.2 shows how randomization achieved a close balance in the mean maternal age and in the distribution of gestational ages of their babies among 4809 mothers with preterm prelabor rupture of the membranes. The mothers were randomized to four combinations of antibiotics in the ORACLE 1 trial in the treatment of preterm prelabor rupture of membranes.[12]

IMPORTANCE OF ADEQUATE SAMPLE SIZE IN MINIMIZING RANDOM ERROR

Despite its importance in reducing systematic bias, randomization is not enough to ensure reliable evidence. Another essential feature of any comparison is achieving a sample size that is large enough to minimize random error. Figure 10.2 shows that surprisingly large sample sizes would be necessary to demonstrate that a particular surfactant therapy reduced the risk of mortality in hyaline membrane disease by one-third, from 15% to 10%. A trial with 600 or more per group would be needed to demonstrate this with reasonable certainty, while trials with less than 300 per group are likely to be inconclusive. To detect even more moderate treatment differences than this, trials would need to be even larger. In the OSIRIS surfactant trial,[13] 2690 babies were judged to be at high risk of respiratory distress syndrome (RDS) when less than 2 h of age. These were randomly allocated to either early administration or delayed selective administration and 96% versus 73% received surfactant, at median ages of 118 and 182 min. The risk of death or dependence on extra oxygen at the expected date of delivery was significantly reduced by one-sixth, or 16% [95% confidence interval (CI) 25% to 7%], among infants allocated early administration.

ABSENCE OF EVIDENCE OF EFFECT IS NOT THE SAME AS EVIDENCE OF NO EFFECT

The problem of inadequate sample size is a major barrier to evidence based neonatal care. Most perinatal and neonatal randomized controlled trials, and most systematic reviews of randomized controlled trials, are inconclusive (i.e. $P \geq 0.05$ and the CI for the treatment effect is wide and includes 1.0) because they

Table 10.2 Balancing effect of randomization on descriptive variables in the ORACLE 1 trial

	Erythromycin (N = 1190)	Co-amoxiclav N = 1205	Both N = 1189	Neither N = 1225
Maternal age (years) Mean (SD)	27.5 (6.1)	28.0 (6.0)	27.8 (6.1)	27.9 (6.1)
Gestation at entry (days) (median, range)	223 (109–258)	223 (136–258)	224 (119–258)	222 (128–258)
< 26 weeks	121 (10·2%)	127 (10·5%)	139 (11·7%)	136 (11·1%)
26–28 weeks	186 (15·6%)	173 (14·4%)	162 (13·6%)	195 (15·9%)
29–31 weeks	303 (25·5%)	317 (26·3%)	290 (24·4%)	302 (24·7%)
32–36 weeks	580 (48·7%)	588 (48·8%)	598 (50·3%)	592 (48·3%)

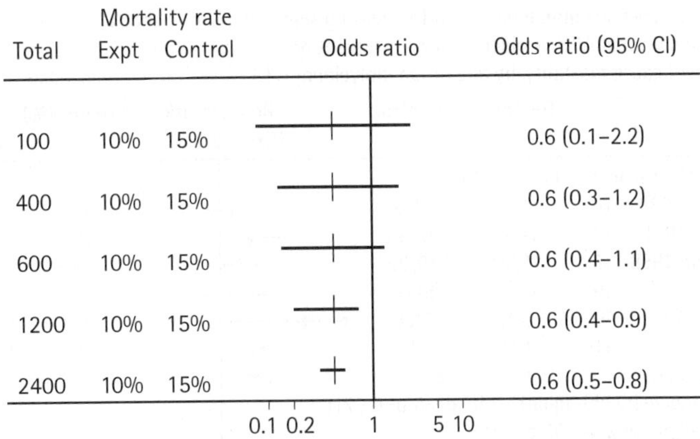

Mortality rate
Total
Expt
Control
Odds ratio
Odds ratio (95% CI)
100
10%
15%
0.6 (0.1–2.2)
400
10%
15%
0.6 (0.3–1.2)
600
10%
15%
0.6 (0.4–1.1)
1200
10%
15%
0.6 (0.4–0.9)
2400
10%
15%
0.6 (0.5–0.8)
0.1 0.2
1
5 10

Fig. 10.2 Effect of sample size on results of randomized controlled trials of a surfactant therapy that reduces mortality from respiratory distress syndrome from 15% to 10%. Even with 600 (300 per group) the result is likely to be inconclusive, with the 95% confidence interval overlapping 1.0. Surprisingly large sample sizes are needed to demonstrate moderate treatment benefits conclusively. If this surfactant therapy only reduced mortality from 15% to 12%, even larger sample sizes would be needed to reliably demonstrate this.

are based on insufficient numbers. This point is illustrated in Figure 10.2. If the surfactant therapy had only been studied in a trial with 300 per group that yielded an inconclusive result, it would have been a mistake to conclude that this treatment did not work. This kind of mistake is known as a type II error. Inconclusive results do not always prove that the treatments are ineffective, and often larger numbers are needed before reliable conclusions can be drawn. On this basis, most perinatal and neonatal treatments remain inadequately evaluated. For many important clinical questions, multicenter national and international collaboration would be needed to achieve sufficiently large samples to overcome these limitations.[14]

SYSTEMATIC REVIEWS AND META-ANALYSES OF RANDOMIZED CONTROLLED TRIALS

Another strategy for minimizing the constraints of inadequate sample size is to pool the results of several smaller trials, after first performing a systematic review by searching for all relevant trials and impartially assessing each for validity according to predefined criteria. Those trials which satisfy the criteria for validity are pooled together in a meta-analysis, to provide a larger randomized sample with which to test the study hypotheses. This process is routinely employed in the Cochrane Library's database of systematic reviews of controlled trials.[15] Figure 10.3[16–27] shows a meta-analysis from a systematic review of randomized controlled trials of polyclonal intravenous immunoglobulin (IVIG) in the treatment of sepsis and septic shock, in 11 trials with a total of 492 adults and neonates. There was a 36% reduction in relative risk of death in those who received IVIG among all 492 patients (relative risk 0.64, 95% CI 0.51–0.80). However, all the trials were small and the reviewers cautiously concluded that the totality of the evidence was not yet sufficient to support a robust conclusion of benefit.

There was a 30% reduction in relative risk of mortality in neonates, which was not statistically significant. To conclude from this that polyclonal IVIG is not effective in neonates could well be a mistake (a type II error). A more appropriate conclusion is that a further, definitive neonatal trial is needed. The reviewers concluded that polyclonal IVIG significantly reduced mortality and is a promising adjuvant in the treatment of sepsis and septic shock. They recommended further studies before the intervention is introduced into routine practice.

Relative risk and odds ratio

- The relative risk of death is the rate in the treated group divided by the rate in controls.
- If treatment is ineffective, death rates must be about equal between treatment and controls, and the true relative risk will be 1.0. This is shown in the Cochrane Library diagram as the vertical line, which indicates no treatment difference.
- In the trial by Schedel[20] the death rate was 2/27(=7.4%) in the treated group and 9/28 (=32.1%) in controls. The estimated relative risk of death was 7.4/32.1=0.23. This number is also known as the 'point estimate' of the relative risk.
- In the same trial, the odds of death in the treated group was 2/25 (0.04) and 9/19 (0.47) in the controls. The odds ratio for death in treated versus controls was 0.08/0.47=0.17. This is larger than the relative risk of death. When sample sizes are large, the relative risk and odds ratio tend to be similar.

Confidence intervals and statistical significance

- The horizontal line around the point estimate is the 95% CI, which represents the play of chance.
- For the trial by Schedel,[20] the 95% confidence interval was 0.05–0.97. As this does not include 1.0 (the horizontal line finishes to the left of the vertical line) it indicates a statistically significant difference, or a treatment benefit.
- If the 95% confidence interval had included 1.0 (i.e. overlapped the vertical line) the trial result would not have been statistically significant.
- The larger the trial sample size, the narrower the CI (and the larger the solid square around the point estimate).
- In the meta-analysis of the subgroup of six trials in adults with sepsis, all six point estimates are less than 1.0 (to the left of the vertical line), indicating a consistent trend. Note that four of the CIs included 1.0 (overlapping the vertical line) indicating that these four trials were not statistically significant.
- However, when the results of all six trials in adults were pooled, the overall point estimate of the relative risk of death was 0.62, with a narrow CI of 0.49–0.79. This indicates a highly statistically significant treatment benefit in adults, with a 38% reduction in relative risk of death.

Review: Intravenous immunoglobulin for treating sepsis and septic shock
Comparison: Polyclonal IVIG vs placebo or no intervention
Outcome: All cause mortality, by age group, polyclonal IVIG

Study		Treatment	Control	Relative risk (fixed) 95% CI	Weight (%)	Relative risk (fixed) 95% CI
Polyclonal IVIG vs placebo, adults, ACM						
De Simone 1988	16	7/12	9/12		8.5	0.78 (0.44, 1.39)
Dominioni 1991	17	11/29	22/33		19.3	0.57 (0.34, 0.96)
Grundmann 1988	18	15/24	19/22		18.6	0.72 (0.51, 1.03)
Just 1986	19	6/13	9/16		7.6	0.82 (0.40, 1.70)
Schedel 1991	20	2/27	9/28		8.3	0.23 (0.05, 0.97)
Wesoly 1990	21	8/18	13/17		12.6	0.58 (0.33, 1.04)
Subtotal (95% CI)		49/123	81/128		74.9	0.62 (0.49, 0.79)
Test for heterogeneity chi-square=3.85 df=5 p=0.5711						
Test for overall effect Z=-3.93 p=0.00						
Polyclonal IVIG vs placebo, neonates, ACM						
Chen 1996	22	2/28	1/28		0.9	2.00 (0.19, 20.82)
Erdem 1993	23	6/20	9/24		7.7	0.80 (0.34, 1.86)
Haque 1988	24	1/30	6/30		5.6	0.17 (0.02, 1.30)
Shenoi 1999	25	7/25	7/25		6.6	1.00 (0.41, 2.43)
Weisman 1992	26	2/14	5/17		4.2	0.49 (0.11, 2.13)
Subtotal (95% CI)		18/117	28/124		25.1	0.70 (0.42, 1.18)
Test for heterogeneity chi-square=3.59 df=4 p=0.4650						
Test for overall effect Z=-1.34 p=0.18						
Total (95% CI)		67/240	109/252		100.0	0.64 (0.51, 0.80)
Test for heterogeneity chi-square=7.49 df=10 p=0.6786						
Test for overall effect Z=-3.92 p=0.00						

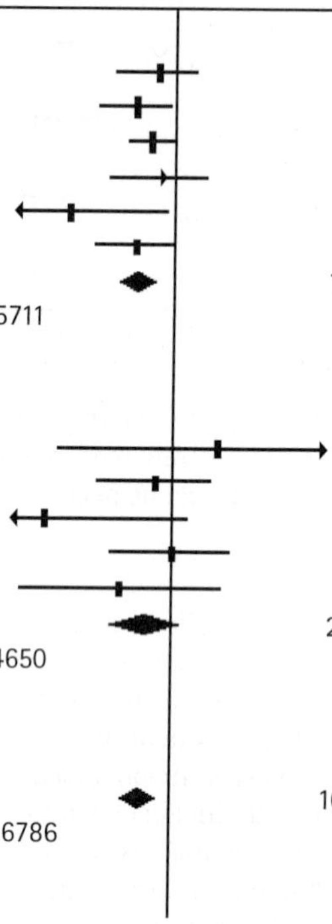

Fig. 10.3 How to read a meta-analysis. (From Alejandria et al 2002[27])

- In the meta-analysis of the subgroup of five trials in neonates with sepsis, all five CIs included 1.0 (overlapping the vertical line), indicating that none of the trials was statistically significant.
- After pooling the results of these five trials in neonates, the point estimate for the relative risk of death was 0.70 and the 95% CI was 0.42–1.18. As this includes 1.0 it is not a statistically significant result. There is thus insufficient evidence currently to conclude benefit in neonates.
- When all 11 trials in adults and neonates were pooled, the net relative risk of death was 0.64, with a 95% CI of 0.51–0.80. This indicates a highly statistically significant result in patients overall, with a 36% reduction in relative risk of death (95% CI 20–49%).

Heterogeneity between trials

- In the six trials in adults, the test for heterogeneity yielded a non-significant result (P = 0.5711) confirming no heterogeneity. The CIs of all six trials overlapped with each other, which also suggests no heterogeneity between them. If there had been heterogeneity between trials, many authors would not have performed a meta-analysis.
- In the five trials in neonates, there was also no heterogeneity. Similarly there was no heterogeneity when all 11 trials were pooled.

WHY RISK ADJUSTMENT IS IMPORTANT IN NON-RANDOMIZED COMPARISONS

Many clinical questions cannot be answered by randomized controlled trials. For example, whether some neonatal intensive care units (NICUs) are more effective than others cannot be investigated by randomly allocating babies to be transferred to some units versus others. Non-randomized comparative studies are essential. However, it is important to adjust for variations in risk in any research that does not equalize risks through randomization. Risk adjustment first requires strict definition of each specific outcome. Then each risk factor is measured and weighted accordingly. Severity of illness scores are a special form of risk adjustment. The leading newborn illness severity scores, such as score for neonatal acute physiology (SNAP), clinical risk index for babies (CRIB) and the Berlin score[28–30] rely on physiology based items from bedside vital signs and laboratory tests. The process of weighting risk factors usually involves building multivariate models and then establishing their validity, discriminatory power, calibration and reliability.[31] It is imperative that risk adjustment takes account of more than just one factor, such as birth weight. NICUs that treat patients with greater severity of illness may have greater birth weight adjusted mortality than others, despite providing an excellent standard of care.

USE OF RISK ADJUSTMENT FOR QUALITY IMPROVEMENT OR BENCHMARKING

The simplest form of benchmarking is a time trend in one institution. However, a NICU with poor performance, such as high rates of nosocomial infection, can improve each year without recognizing how serious the problem is. The most informative comparisons are against several similar NICUs. Although using the network average is politically neutral and mathematically sound, it does not identify NICUs with the best performance, for example the lowest risk adjusted rates of bacteremia. These NICUs both illustrate achievable goals and may represent 'best practices'. Benchmarking refers to both the best performing sites and the process of comparing outcomes. Some NICUs may be top performers in some outcomes, but not in others.

THE EFFECTS OF SAMPLE SIZE IN BENCHMARKING

In a multicenter cross sectional comparison of birth weight adjusted mortality rates between 13 NICUs in the UK, CIs remained wide and overlapping even after adjusting for illness severity using CRIB.[32] A longitudinal comparison of hospital mortality among nine NICUs over 6 years showed that the annual rankings and apparent performance of individual NICUs fluctuated substantially from year to year and were therefore too unstable to justify any intervention. The authors concluded that annual comparisons of risk adjusted mortality rates may not be reliable indicators of performance and that any action prompted by these underpowered comparisons would have been equally likely to have been beneficial, detrimental or irrelevant.

A more reliable approach to monitoring performance is to undertake prospective studies of outcomes in large groups of hospitals and test whether variations in outcome are associated with differences in prespecified organizational characteristics. The UK Neonatal Staffing Study[33] was a prospective cohort study of risk adjusted outcomes in relation to unit size, nursing and consultant provision and daily workload. It demonstrated that although larger units dealt with sicker patients and had higher crude mortality, there was no difference in adjusted mortality among units in relation to size, or nursing or consultant provision after accounting for differences in patient risk and illness severity. However, there was a linear increase in risk adjusted mortality in relation to total unit workload, measured as percentage of maximum occupancy. Infants were 80% more likely to die if admitted to a UK unit at full versus lowest occupancy and 50% more likely to die if admitted at full versus half occupancy. This relationship was not explained by selection bias of sicker infants at high occupancy (Fig. 10.4).[33] This type of evidence, of the effects of excessive workload on risk adjusted outcome, could not have been obtained in a randomized controlled trial, but only in an observational study.

BENCHMARKING BY COMPARING PROCESS RATHER THAN OUTCOME

It may frequently be more useful to compare the implementation of evidence based measures of the process of care, particularly those

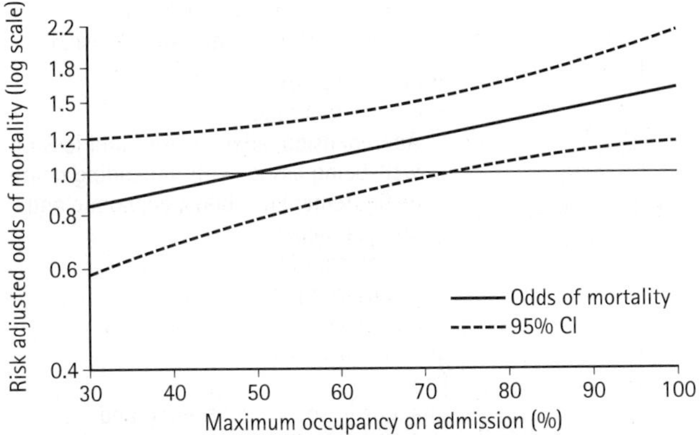

Fig. 10.4 Percentage maximum occupancy on admission by risk-adjusted odds of mortality. (From UK Neonatal Staffing Study Collaborative Group 2002[33])

proven effective in randomized controlled trials, rather than measures of risk adjusted outcome. Mant & Hicks[34] showed that comparing the appropriate use of proven treatments for myocardial infarction between hospitals would substantially reduce the number of patients needed and speed up the identification of significant differences in hospital performance. However, to be valid, comparisons require that all patients eligible to receive the treatments are included in all hospitals. Given the current evidence supporting a policy of prophylactic surfactant use, an audit of performance, measured as the proportions of eligible infants receiving prophylactic surfactant, could detect differences in process between hospitals long before finding differences in mortality rates. Richardson et al[31] showed that differences in performance between hospitals A and B could be detected more rapidly and reliably by comparing the proportion of eligible infants receiving prophylactic surfactant (process) than by comparing mortality rates (outcomes). Similar benchmarking of the process of care can be applied to the use of antenatal corticosteroid administration.[35]

THE ECONOMICS OF NEWBORN CARE

INTRODUCTION

The improved survival chances of immature infants and the diffusion of new technologies for mature infants, have increased the demand for neonatal care.[36] This has generated considerable debate about the correct level of funding for neonatal care. Economic evaluation provides a framework for assessing the costs and benefits of care, and for identifying the combination of human and material inputs that maximize health benefits or other measures of social welfare. This section outlines the methods of economic evaluation of health care and describes the key economic issues raised by studies of neonatal care.

Perspective and coverage of economic study

The first stage of any economic evaluation requires specification of the study objective. The study objective determines the perspective that should be adopted and the time period or coverage that should be considered. The perspective of an economic evaluation usually falls into one of three categories: health service, public sector or societal. Conditions requiring neonatal care are likely to have resource consequences for sectors of the economy other than the health service, as well as for individuals. Low birth weight babies may require support from social service departments after discharge from hospital. The parents of sick neonates may have to forego other productive activities (paid or unpaid work) to spend time with them; their transport costs to and from the neonatal unit may be considerable, and care for other children may be required.[37] As a result, economic evaluations of neonatal care should be conducted from a broad perspective.

The time period or coverage of the evaluation should depend upon the extent to which the resource consequences of health care activities accrue into the future. Neonates requiring intensive care may have additional health care needs (hospital readmissions or increased contacts with other health professionals), educational needs, and care requirements for everyday living. There may be broader resource consequences. Many mothers of low birth weight infants who intend to return to work after the birth either postpone doing so, reduce their hours or leave the workforce altogether. This is usually associated with a reduction in family income; a 20% reduction is cited in one paper,[38] a 32% reduction in another.[37] Table 10.3 lists the potential resource requirements that should be considered by economic studies of neonatal care.

Measurement of quantities of resource use

Once the perspective and coverage of the economic evaluation have been specified, the quantities of resources attributable to the health care program must be estimated. Resource quantities can be estimated within randomized clinical trials or by comparison of data from routine health service information sources, primary surveys, reviews of published studies or from expert opinion (Delphi panels). It is unlikely that a complete profile of resource use can be obtained from a single source. Less well controlled sources are usually needed, especially in the extrapolation from intermediate to long term outcomes. Whatever source of data is used, the validity of the method adopted depends upon the degree to which the resource quantities are representative of the forms of care and contexts defined for the evaluation. Although randomized controlled trials confer the advantage of minimizing bias in comparisons between forms of care, the clinical trial protocol may induce additional resource use. Furthermore, the patients recruited into randomized controlled trials are often atypical of the context relevant to the subject for the economic evaluation.[39]

Measurement of unit costs of elements of resource use

In economic evaluations of health care interventions, unit costs have to be estimated for each element of resource use. In the USA, where there is a comprehensive system of billing and fee-for-service payment, unit costs can be relatively easily identified for each item of resource use, such as neonatal intensive bed days, outpatient visits, diagnostic tests and investigative procedures. However, unit costs often reflect provider charges, which have been shown to include elements arising from corporate financial decisions.[40]

It is difficult to establish the unit costs of care outside the USA because of the absence of itemized billing. In European countries, unit costs tend to come from a variety of sources because of the lack

Table 10.3 Examples of costs attributable to conditions requiring neonatal care

Direct costs *Hospital service costs* Equipment: Cots and bassinets Overhead heaters Resuscitaires Incubators Transport incubators Ventilators Humidifiers Cardiorespiratory monitors Apnea monitors Blood pressure monitors Pulse oximeters Oxygen monitors Transcutaneous gas monitors Temperature monitors Cassette infusion pumps Syringe pumps Phototherapy units ECG machines Defibrillators Fiberoptic light sources Blood gas analysers Other side ward analysers Ultrasound Head boxes Air/O_2 blenders Flow meters Breast pumps Electronic scales Portable suction pumps Medical and surgical services: Pediatric surgery Ophthalmology Cardiology Cardiac surgery ENT Neurosurgery Plastic surgery Orthopedic surgery	Medical and surgical supplies: Dressings Linen Clothing Direct patient support: Drugs Parenteral nutrition Milk, feeds and catering Medical gases Imaging Physiotherapy Total pathology Staff costs: Medical staff Nursing staff Support staff Support services: Electricity Coal/oil/gas Water/sewerage Local government taxes Portering Cleaning Laundry Hospital administration Postage and telephone Medical records Ambulance services *Community service costs* Day care services Prescribed medications General practitioners Practice nurses Physiotherapists Speech therapists Hearing therapists Nutritionists Counselors Psychologists Psychiatrists	Community pediatricians Social workers Volunteers *Direct non-medical costs* Additional educational support Respite care Hospital visiting costs Additional child care costs Additional help with housework Adaptations to home Dietary requirements Additional bedding Additional clothing Repairs to home Additional heating requirements *Indirect costs* Changes in productivity resulting from: Changes in health status Morbidity Mortality Income lost by family members Foregone leisure time Time spent by patient seeking medical services Time spent by family and friends attending patients (e.g. hospital visits) *Intangible costs* Psychosocial costs: Apprehension, anxiety, grief and loss of well-being assoc. with impending death, disfigurement,disability, economic and physical dependence Social isolation Family conflict Valuations others put on patients' health and well-being Pain Changes in social functioning and activities of daily living

of readily available cost data. The data may come from nationally available published studies, salary review boards for health service personnel, locally held data sources or ad hoc studies reported in the literature. Additionally, the unit cost data may be generated from first principles at the study sites themselves using small accounting studies. These accounting studies may use a number of methods including time and motion studies, diary methods, work sampling, interviews with key caregivers, case note analysis and patient activity databases.[41]

Estimating total costs of care

The total costs of health care programs can be estimated by applying unit costs to each component of resource use (the *bottom-up* costing approach). Once total costs are expressed in monetary terms, adjustments must be made to account for costs external to the institutional accounting system, those *opportunity costs* (or foregone benefits) which are not reflected in the estimated total costs. For example, unpaid volunteers in a hospital may not add to the hospital's wage bill, but their labor still represents a true cost of the running of the hospital. They contribute to the hospital's output, and their labor is a cost to society in the sense that it could have been more productively used in another sector during that time or spent on leisure activities. Similarly, a policy of increased staff levels in the neonatal unit may reduce the number of staff available for routine postnatal support in the maternity unit. This could affect outcomes such as breast-feeding success or postnatal infection rates, and it is incumbent on economic analysts to incorporate the resource consequences of such adverse outcomes into their evaluations.

It is possible that other adjustments have to be made to the estimated costs of a health care program. Most unit costs reflect the *average costs* of production. Under certain circumstances, it may be more appropriate for unit costs to reflect the *marginal costs* of production, that is, the additional costs of changes in the production of a program.[42] Unit cost estimates from previous years should be adjusted using a health care specific price index, such as the National Health Service Hospital and Community Health Services Index, to reflect a more recent price level. Finally, costs accruing into the future should be *discounted* or reduced to present levels to take account of differences in potential productivity of resources over time.

COMBINATION OF DATA ABOUT CHANGES IN COSTS AND OUTCOMES

Once the resource implications of the health care program have been measured and valued, economic evaluation requires an assessment of the program's impact on health outcomes or other measures of social welfare. The incremental cost of achieving a unit of health gain (or other measure of social welfare) is calculated and expressed as a ratio. Although the various forms of economic evaluation consider the same categories of costs, they differ in their approach to measuring and valuing the consequences of health care programs. *Cost effectiveness analysis* is the commonest approach. It compares the costs of a health care program to its consequences, measured in natural or physical units such as lives saved or episodes of RDS avoided. Assessments of clinical effectiveness for incorporation within the cost effectiveness ratio can come from a single clinical study, a systematic overview of several studies, or an ad hoc synthesis of several sources. However, the gold standard remains the randomized, double blind controlled trial.[43]

Cost utility analysis is a refinement of cost effectiveness analysis in that it constructs a single index of outcomes that reflects preferences for each possible outcome. Preferences for different outcomes depend on prevailing ethical and moral standards about life, death and disability, and tend to vary between population groups.[44] Potential instruments for measuring health outcomes within a cost utility framework include the quality-adjusted life year (QALY),[45] the healthy years equivalent (HYE)[46] and the saved young life equivalent (SAVE).[47] A number of cost utility analyses of neonatal interventions have attempted to value the long term disability of surviving low birth weight infants in terms of QALYs and explored the impact on the cost effectiveness of the interventions. A study from Canada by Boyle et al[48] and a study from Australia by Kitchen et al[49] were based on outcomes for population based cohorts before and after access to neonatal intensive care was expanded. For babies born at less than 1000 g, the studies estimated a cost per additional survivor of between £84 490 and £174 040 (1998 prices). The cost-effectiveness ratio fell to between £4440 and £15 790 when the outcome of neonatal intensive care was measured in terms of an additional life year gained, and fell to between £4190 and £38 030 when the outcome was measured in terms of an additional QALY gained.

The final form of economic evaluation is *cost benefit analysis* which measures the costs and consequences of health care programs in the same monetary units and attempts to ascertain whether the programs can be justified per se, that is, whether the benefits of the program exceed its cost. Studies that have attempted to weigh up the overall life time social costs and benefits of neonatal intensive care in monetary units[48,50,51] have concluded that there would be a net economic loss for babies born at less than 1000 g, but that neonatal intensive care could provide a net gain for bigger babies. The results of these studies have been contentious, partly because of the methods for valuing survival. This was done by estimating the long term care costs and subtracting them from potential earnings of survivors. Even if one accepts this as a good measure of social costs and benefits, the studies were based on limited information about the life expectancy and long term disability for low birth weight survivors, and about likely life time care needs and earning patterns. These comparisons of costs and effects of increased access to neonatal intensive care were based on historical comparisons. It is therefore likely that the estimated change in effects may be biased.

EXPRESSING UNCERTAINTY ABOUT ECONOMIC ESTIMATES

The final stage of economic evaluation is to express uncertainty around the calculated cost effectiveness, cost utility or cost benefit estimates. In the absence of stochastic data for all variables, health economists commonly use sensitivity analysis to explore the implications of uncertainty surrounding the values of key economic parameters.[52] This may take many forms, including simple one-way sensitivity analysis (variation of values of single component variables); multiway sensitivity analysis (simultaneous variation of multiple variables); and scenario analysis (multiple variables are set at their 'best' and worst' values). Sensitivity analysis has rarely been used in economic studies of neonatal care which makes it difficult to judge whether the conclusions of many economic studies are meaningful and robust.[53] In recent years, the methods for calculating CIs for incremental cost effectiveness ratios have also developed considerably. These methods include confidence boxes, confidence ellipses, the Taylor series expansion, Fieller's theorem and non-parametric bootstrapping.[54] However, no published economic studies of neonatal care have applied these methods to calculate CIs for cost effectiveness ratios.[53] It is imperative that these approaches are applied if decision-makers are to assess the uncertainty surrounding cost effectiveness estimates of neonatal care.

RESULTS OF ECONOMIC RESEARCH

There are an increasing number of economic studies of neonatal care.[53] In general these show that:

1. the *per diem* hospital cost (i.e. the average cost per patient day) tends to be inversely related to the duration of hospital stay;
2. staff costs form the largest category of costs;
3. key cost generating activities, such as transportation of the neonate to and from the neonatal unit, are commonly overlooked;
4. the per-patient cost of neonatal intensive care tends to be inversely related to birth weight;
5. the per-patient cost of neonatal intensive care is also related to mortality with survivors incurring higher initial costs than infants who die;
6. the per-patient cost of neonatal intensive care increases with intensity of care; and
7. the per-patient cost of neonatal intensive care is related to the degree of surgical intervention undergone and the level of assisted ventilation received by the infant.

Methodological differences between studies make comparisons of data about the cost effectiveness or cost utility of different neonatal interventions difficult. The early economic evaluations of neonatal intensive care estimated the net economic benefits of introducing a new form of health care. Once neonatal intensive care had become widely established economic analysts focused on the economic impact of the introduction of exogenous surfactant and increased use of antenatal corticosteroids. Over the coming years, it is likely that economic analysts will evaluate the impact of recent developments in care such as head cooling, whole body cooling, liquid ventilation, IVIG therapy and high frequency oscillation ventilation.

THE NORMAL FETAL–NEONATAL TRANSITION

The most vital change immediately after birth is for the lungs to expand to take in air. If lung expansion fails, death will occur quite rapidly and shortly after the umbilical cord is clamped. Almost as important as lung expansion is the change from the fetal type circulation, where the cardiac output bypasses the lungs, to the postnatal pattern where the cardiac output from the right side of the heart will perfuse the lungs and be oxygenated (Fig. 10.5). Less urgent changes in the other organ systems must take place over the next days and weeks in order to ensure a viable postnatal existence.

THE LUNGS (Fig. 10.6)

The lungs of the fetus in utero are filled with a unique fluid which near term is being produced at a rate of about 3 ml/kg/h. Clearance

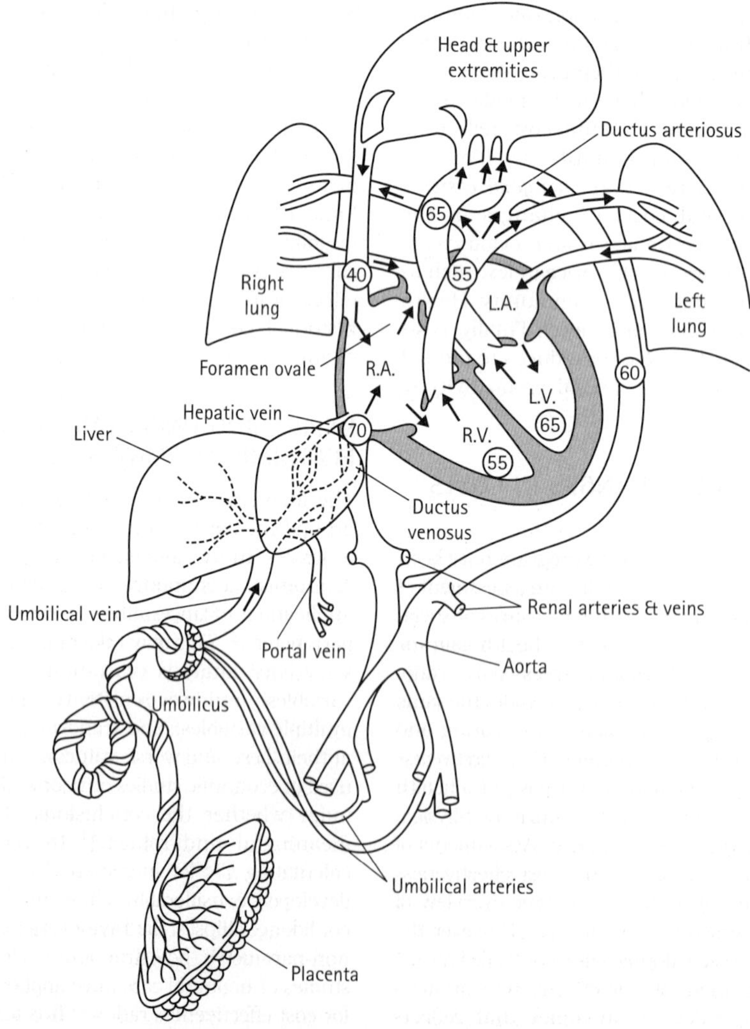

Fig. 10.5 Fetal circulation. The circled figures indicate oxygen saturation at various points, e.g. blood 70% saturated at point where inferior vena cava enters right atrium. L. A., left atrium; L. V., left ventricle; R. A., right atrium; R. V., right ventricle.

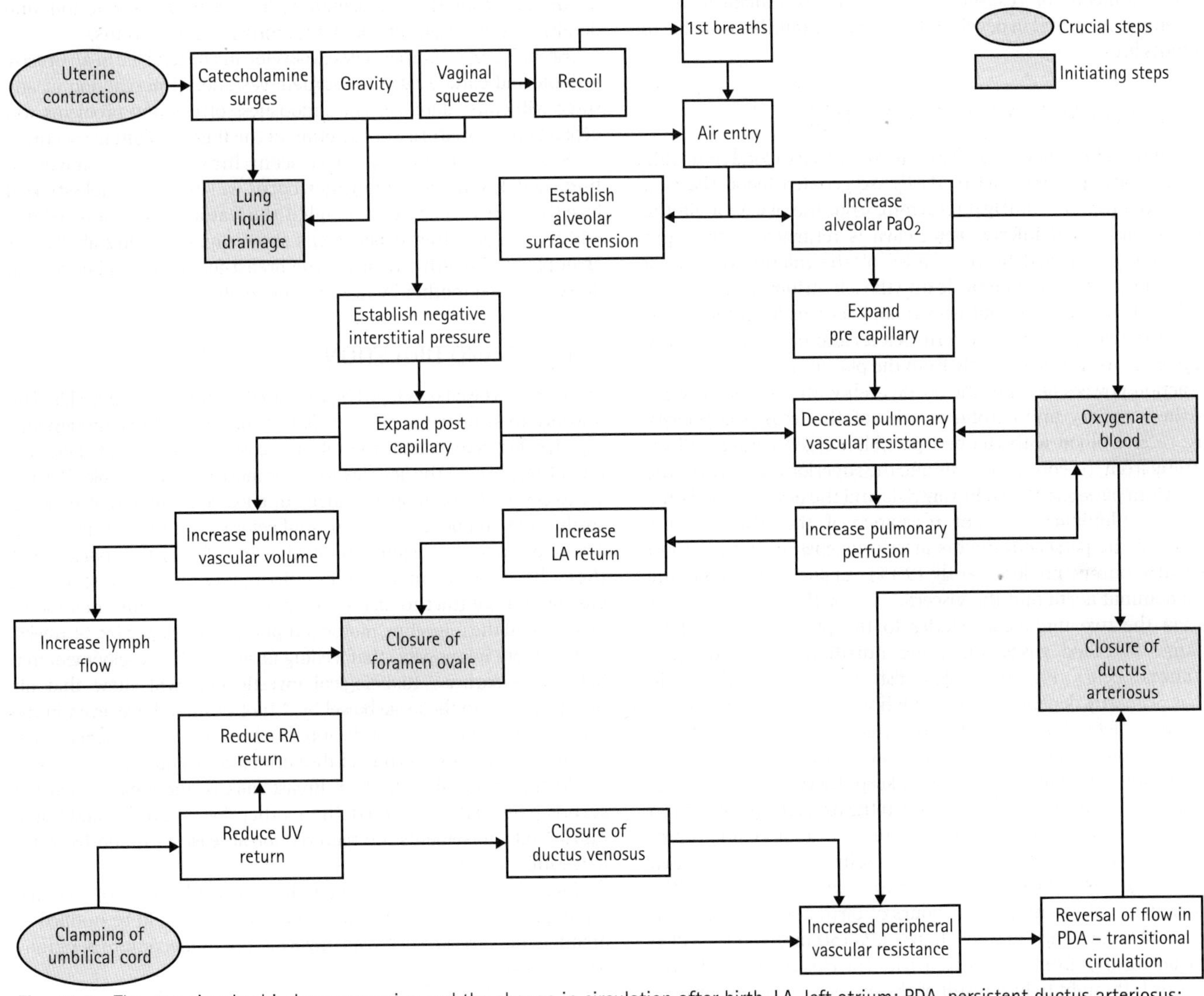

Fig. 10.6 The steps involved in lung expansion and the change in circulation after birth. LA, left atrium; PDA, persistent ductus arteriosus; RA, right atrium; UV, umbilical vein.

of this fluid is crucial for successful air breathing and begins during labor. Each uterine contraction has been shown to generate surges of fetal catecholamines which reduce the rate of lung liquid secretion and, as labor progresses, lead to active resorption. Elective delivery of the baby before labor will lead to babies being born with wet lungs which result in transient tachypnea of the newborn (p. 256, TTN). Additional lung fluid is dispersed during the second stage of labor by a compression force of up to 160 cm of water and the elastic recoil from this vaginal squeeze may draw up to 50 ml of air into the chest. Where a mother delivers her infant from a squatting position, further fluid drains by gravity in the vertex delivery. Cesarean section can reduce the effectiveness of all these mechanisms to give an increased incidence of respiratory problems from wet lungs, but even the normal vaginally delivered infant will have a quantity of fluid in his lungs at the moment of birth.

The first gasps or cries of the baby achieve a transthoracic pressure of 70–90 cm of water and a tidal wave of air passes into the upper respiratory passages and larynx. This air initiates Head's paradoxical reflex which potentiates the first gasp. The Valsalva maneuver achieved by the infant crying against a partially closed glottis pushes further fluid from the airway through to the lymphatics. The first breath may generate a pressure as high as 70–120 cm water and may achieve a volume of 80 ml of air in the lungs. The gasps occurring immediately after birth are crucial for the success of air breathing. It is not clear which of the many stimuli that occur after birth are most important in initiating breathing. It may be the deluge of sensory information as the baby delivers – tactile (midwife's hands), thermal (air temperature in the delivery room and evaporation of liquor from the skin), noise, position, light, gravity, pain, etc. It is likely that chemoreceptor input caused by hypoxia and hypercarbia in the last moments before delivery (physiological asphyxia) are also important; however, severe hypoxia and acidemia may depress the respiratory center.

There are two major reasons for the failure of the lungs to expand at birth:

1. the lungs may be unable, physically, to expand either because they have failed to develop properly in utero (e.g. Potter's syndrome, prolonged liquor leakage, diaphragmatic hernia) or because the airway is obstructed (congenital laryngeal web, acquired meconium aspiration);
2. the brain may fail to initiate the expansion of the lungs (e.g. extreme immaturity, oversedation with obstetric prescribed narcotics or brain damage occurring during either the pregnancy or the delivery).

Effective means of resuscitation at birth are crucial in these situations (p. 204) and in developed countries should be available to all infants born.

HEART AND CARDIOVASCULAR SYSTEM

The left and right ventricles of the fetus both receive blood returning from the body (cf. after birth). Partly oxygenated blood (PaO_2 = 3.7–4.7 kPa (25–35 mmHg)) returning from the placenta via the ductus venosus and inferior vena cava is returned to the right atrium but is deflected by the 'valve' of the inferior vena cava through the patent foramen ovale into the left atrium. In utero only 5–10% of the cardiac output goes to and returns from the lungs; therefore the blood passing from the left atrium to the left ventricle is largely the oxygenated supply from the placenta. Left ventricular contraction powers blood to the aortic arch with its major vessels; thus the coronary and carotid arteries of the fetus, the priority areas, receive blood with the best possible oxygen content. Blood returning from the coronary sinus and the superior vena cava to the right atrium passes to the right ventricle and the pulmonary trunk. The high pulmonary vascular resistance of the fetus and the presence of the persistent ductus arteriosus ensure that the right ventricular output predominantly (90%) supplies the descending and abdominal aorta and the viscera. 50% of the abdominal flow goes via the two umbilical arteries to the placental bed where exchange of blood gases and other nutritional and excretory substances occurs (Fig. 10.6). The distribution of blood flow in utero is primarily dependent on the high vascular resistance of the unexpanded fetal lung and the low vascular resistance of the placenta. Fetal pulmonary arterioles have a thick medial muscle layer. The low fetal PaO_2 is thought to keep the vessels constricted. With the first gasps there is a rapid rise in the oxygen tension within the alveoli, and the arteriolar musculature relaxes and pulmonary perfusion occurs. The sudden increase in pulmonary venous return of well-oxygenated blood to the left atrium functionally closes the foramen ovale within minutes or hours of birth and this now well-oxygenated blood (PaO_2 greater than 7 kPa (50 mmHg)) is ejected up the aortic arch from the left ventricle. The closure of the ductus arteriosus is thought to be a result of the increased oxygen content. The ductal muscle in utero is maintained in a relaxed state by the combination of the relative hypoxia and the presence of high circulating levels of prostaglandins produced by the placenta.

The clamping of the umbilical cord raises the systemic vascular resistance and, as a consequence, blood may pass in the reverse direction through the persistent ductus. This 'transitional circulation' may revert back to the fetal situation (right to left) if satisfactory oxygenation is not achieved (persistent pulmonary hypertension in the newborn, p. 277). Functional closure of the ductus usually takes place within the first 24 h (and usually much earlier) after birth but before this, a systolic murmur may be present at the base of the heart from transient left to right ductal flow. After birth the pulmonary artery pressure falls from about 25–40 mmHg on the first day to 15 mmHg after 6 weeks. During this time there is a rise in the systemic blood pressure from 45–55 mmHg to approximately 70 mmHg.

BRAIN AND CENTRAL NERVOUS SYSTEM

The brain and central nervous system develop steadily through fetal life, infancy and childhood. There are no dramatic changes that occur with or because of birth itself although sensory experience following birth is obviously different. At birth the cerebellum is more maturely developed than the cerebrum. Neuronal development and dendritic connections are more evident and myelination is already occurring from the oligodendroglia. Cerebral myelination and dendritic connections are predominantly postnatal events.

Brainstem and higher reflexes develop in late fetal life in an orderly fashion and can be used to estimate gestation. Interruption at any stage will cause damage. The seriousness of ensuing problems will depend on the maturity of the brain at the time the damage occurs.

Some recognition patterns seem innate in the newborn. Immediately after birth many newborns will follow a simple stylized face through 180 degrees though if the features are scrambled this will not occur. Other experiments show rapid learning ability; for example by the fifth day of life the breast-fed infant will be able to detect his own mother by his sense of smell.

THE GUT AND DIGESTION

Swallowing is well developed by the fourth month of in utero life. The inability to swallow in utero leads to hydramnios. Sucking develops rapidly after birth; usually the baby increases the number of sucks in a burst from 5–6 on the first day to 30 or more by day 3. Babies born at 28 weeks' gestation may also suck but good coordination of sucking, swallowing and breathing is unusual before 34–35 weeks' gestation. The importance of sucking and swallowing after birth is obvious but these have to be matched by the ability of the rest of the gastrointestinal tract to digest and absorb the food. Intestinal motor activity and the migrating motor complex are developed by 34 weeks' gestation but it is possible that feeding facilitates this development in a baby born earlier.[55] Radiological investigation will show that air usually passes to the large bowel by 2 h of postnatal age, even in the very preterm infant. Most of the intestinal enzymes are present at birth but their full activity and that of the various gastrointestinal hormones are further induced by feeding. Breast milk is undoubtedly and not surprisingly better tolerated than other food and no additional nutritional supplements are required for at least 4–5 months of life in the full-term infant.

Meconium should be passed within 24 h of birth (95%). Should the baby fail to pass meconium, medical staff should be notified as an intestinal atresia, Hirschsprung's disease or meconium ileus may be the cause.

THE KIDNEYS AND RENAL FUNCTION

Dynamic measurements of bladder volume by ultrasound show that the fetus at full term will be producing 7 ml of urine/kg/h; thus glomerular filtration from the full complement of nephrons (present by 35 weeks' gestation) is considerable. Fine control of water balance in utero has been the concern of the placenta and after birth both glomerular and tubular immaturity mean that fluid and electrolyte insults on the newborn are poorly tolerated. The glomerular filtration rate (GFR) of the term infant is only 10 ml/min/m^2, increasing to 15 ml/min/m^2 by the end of the first week. Renal blood flow is low at birth and the juxtaglomerular nephrons are preferentially perfused. Sodium resorption is well developed in the full-term infant (though not in the preterm) as the tubules are comparatively mature and the circulating aldosterone levels are high. The maximum urine osmolality is relatively low, not because of the baby's inability to secrete the antidiuretic hormone, arginine vasopressin (AVP), from the posterior pituitary but because the low solute and nitrogen content of breast milk result in a low solute concentration of the interstitial compartment of the medulla. Increasing the protein intake of the infant increases the maximum urine osmolality that is possible.

The renal bicarbonate threshold is low and there may be limited hydrogen ion excretion due to reduced phosphate availability. Both of these may lead to acidosis. The tubular cells are also less able to produce ammonia. This is more marked in preterm infants particularly with high protein and acid loads and leads to the late metabolic acidosis of prematurity.

The breast-fed infant receives low solute food with adequate nitrogen and calories: there is little stress on the kidneys. Unmodified cows' milk or solids contain too much solute and nitrogen and can rapidly lead to metabolic difficulties such as cows' milk tetany (p. 362) and hypernatremia (p. 220).

Congenital abnormalities of the kidney and renal excretory systems lead to metabolic upset developing over the first days or weeks of life depending on their severity. The common coexistence of pulmonary hypoplasia with complete renal agenesis (Potter's syndrome) ensures this abnormality presents as an acute respiratory difficulty, usually with rapid death.

LIVER FUNCTION

Immaturity of liver function leads to jaundice (p. 278) and also to the newborn's inability to tolerate drugs which are usually excreted via the biliary tree. The 'gray baby' syndrome is due to increased free and conjugated chloramphenicol levels in the serum leading to vomiting, poor sucking, respiratory distress, abdominal distention, diarrhea and eventually collapse. Liver immaturity may be a factor in the development of hemorrhagic disease of the newborn (p. 307) though damage to the liver from hypoxia and an inadequate supply of vitamin K are likely to be more important components.

BLOOD

The fetal hemoglobin (Hb) predominant in the full-term newborn (80%) is ideal for oxygen uptake across the placenta at the low oxygen tensions that are present in utero. After birth this fetal Hb is less able to unload oxygen at the tissues. Red cell 2,3-diphosphoglycerate levels increase rapidly in the newborn period to improve oxygen delivery and release, and the oxygen dissociation curve shows a shift to the right.

The blood volume of the newborn depends on the age at which the umbilical cord is clamped. Clamping within the first 15 s after delivery leads to a blood volume of around 75 ml/kg but delayed clamping increases this, the contracting uterus expelling blood from the sinuses of the placenta to the baby (Fig. 10.7).[56] If the cord is not clamped for 3 min after delivery, the blood volume may be 95–100 ml/kg. In the term baby this is associated with a higher incidence of respiratory problems and jaundice but in the preterm infant, where the Hb and red cell volume at birth tend to be lower, a 30 s delay in cord clamping with the newborn infant lower than the placenta may reduce the respiratory problems and the subsequent requirement for top-up blood transfusions.

ENDOCRINE SYSTEM

Numerous hormonal changes take place during labor and immediately after birth which allow the infant to adjust to the change in the environment and the loss of the placental supply of nutrients and minerals. There is a rapid surge in thyroid hormones, thought to be a response to cold exposure. Cortisol and adrenocorticotropic hormone (ACTH) rise with labor and peak a few hours after delivery in response to stress. Intact pituitary, thyroid, parathyroid, adrenal and pancreatic function are required to maintain glucose, calcium and electrolyte homeostasis. Babies with disorders of pituitary function may present with hypoglycemia or prolonged jaundice, and this may be associated with midline structural abnormalities of the brain (septo-optic dysplasia). Inborn errors of adrenocortical steroid synthesis (congenital adrenal hyperplasia) can present with ambiguous genitalia and/or salt loss.

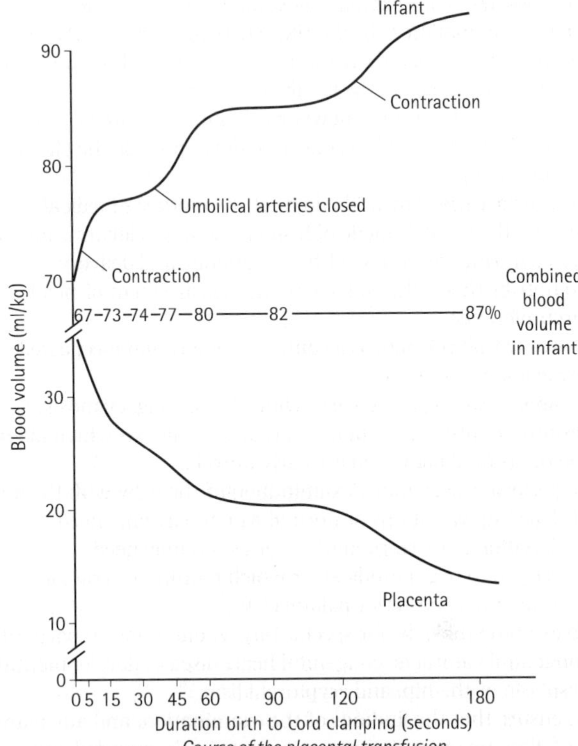

Fig. 10.7 Variation in infants' blood volume with time of clamping of the umbilical cord. (From Smith & Nelson 1976[56] with permission)

THE IMMUNE RESPONSE AND INFECTION

Once delivered from the protected environment of the uterus, the baby is subjected to many potentially infectious agents. Immunoglobulin G (IgG) transferred actively across the placenta in the last trimester of pregnancy will last for only a short time (up to 6 months). During this time the infant must develop his own antibodies. Although both B and T cells are potentially functional in utero the virginal experience (in relation to foreign antigen) in the uterus leads to a gap of cell mediated immunity in the neonatal period. It is sensible for people overtly suffering with viral or bacterial infections not to be intimately involved with the management of newborn infants. Exposure to a pathogen leads to a response at a rate similar in the baby to that seen in older age groups. Absence of either B or T cell functions after birth leads to severe infections and if the diagnosis is not considered, the infant may die (Ch. 25).

ROUTINE CARE OF THE FULL-TERM INFANT

EXAMINATION OF THE NEONATE

It is standard practice in the UK and many other countries for all newborn babies to have a formal clinical examination in the first few days of life. This is often referred to as the routine newborn examination and it can be defined as the detailed professional examination in the first few days of life of a baby who, at the start of the examination, is thought to be well and without significant problems. Examination of a baby to whom attention has been drawn, for example because of cyanosis, feeding problems, apneic episodes or an obvious congenital anomaly, is not a routine newborn examination.[57] In the UK, where most births take place in maternity units rather than the mother's home, this examination usually takes place before the family returns home.

The aims of the routine newborn examination are as follows:

- To ascertain the family's concerns and to provide the chance to discuss them.
- To consider the baby in the light of the mother's medical history, the family's medical history and any relevant concerns raised during the course of the pregnancy and delivery.
- To note birth weight and a baseline measurement of head circumference.
- To verify that the baby is feeding acceptably and has passed urine and meconium.
- To appreciate the presence of clinical signs (e.g. cyanosis, respiratory distress, or inappropriate drowsiness) which identify the occasional baby who is clearly unwell.
- To perform a systematic examination of the baby with the aim of detecting variations of normal which may only need explanation (e.g. 'stork marks'); or which may need investigation (e.g. jaundice); or which require referral for treatment (e.g. posterior palatal cleft).[58]
- To examine the baby for specific target conditions, in particular congenital cataracts, congenital heart disease, developmental dysplasia of the hip, and cryptorchidism.[59]
- To ensure that the findings of the examination, and any plans for follow-up or treatment, are appropriately recorded and effectively communicated to the parents and to those involved in providing future health care to the family.

The mother's handling of her baby while the history is taken and her behavior during the examination will usually alert the doctor to any problem in the developing relationship between mother and baby. The doctor should also consider the following points: Is the baby satisfactorily nourished? Has the weight gain been satisfactory since birth? If not, is the artificial feed being taken well, or is the mother persevering with breast-feeding when she is not actually producing any milk?

EFFECTIVENESS OF THE ROUTINE NEWBORN EXAMINATION

Many of the aims of the routine newborn examination, particularly the identification of babies with specific target conditions, fit well with the UK National Screening Committee definition of screening. This body defines screening as 'the systematic application of a test or inquiry, to identify individuals at sufficient risk of a specific disorder to warrant further investigation or direct preventive action, amongst persons who have not sought medical attention on account of symptoms of that disorder'.[60] The effectiveness of such programs should be the subject of regular scrutiny.

The criteria for appraising the viability, effectiveness and appropriateness of screening programs were set out by Wilson & Jungner[61] and enlarged upon by Cochrane & Holland.[62] If applied to the routine newborn examination these would essentially demand that the examination can detect significant malformations reliably and accurately; that the conditions so detected would, if left undetected, result in a worse outcome for the baby; that the conditions are treatable; and that the mode of examination is acceptable to the parents. These criteria have recently been further developed in the UK by the National Screening Committee.[60]

In these days of increasing patient expectations it is important not to exaggerate the effectiveness of the routine newborn examination. When evaluated as a screening test for the four target conditions mentioned below, the routine newborn examination does not perform particularly well. Some justification for including these target conditions in the newborn examination and some idea of the performance of the examination in the detection of affected children can be found in the next few paragraphs.

CONGENITAL CATARACT

Congenital cataract occurs in about 2–3 per 10 000 births in the UK and is well recognized as a preventable cause of blindness.[63] All babies should have their eyes examined and the presence of a red reflex confirmed as part of the routine newborn examination. If a red reflex is not clearly seen then urgent referral for ophthalmological examination is justified. The early surgical removal of dense opacities together with early postoperative refractive correction produces the best results in terms of visual acuity.[64] Delaying surgical correction of congenital cataracts beyond the age of 8 weeks results in a measurable reduction in the quality of vision when compared with correction before this age.[65] Most ophthalmologists would wish to remove cataracts well before this age. A recent study in the UK has shown that only 35% of infant cataracts were detected at routine newborn examination.[66]

CONGENITAL HEART DISEASE

Unrecognized heart disease carries a serious risk of avoidable mortality, morbidity and handicap.[67] However, detecting congenital cardiac malformations in the newborn period is difficult for a number of reasons.[68] The prevalence of congenital cardiac malformation is low at about 6 per 1000 births and most babies with congenital cardiac malformation show no signs or symptoms of heart disease in the newborn period.[69] Murmurs can be heard in about 1–2% of babies undergoing routine newborn examination but less than half of these murmurs indicate congenital cardiac malformation.[70] Conversely, of babies with congenital cardiac malformation, less than half have a murmur in the newborn period.[57] Finally the most dangerous diagnoses (left ventricular outflow tract obstructions) have a combined prevalence of only 1:1500[69] and usually only become symptomatic once they are already established on a rapidly deteriorating course which can lead to death in a matter of hours.[71] It is thus perhaps not surprising that the routine newborn examination only detects about 45% of congenital cardiac malformations and that serious conditions are no more likely to be detected than less serious ones.[57]

DEVELOPMENTAL DYSPLASIA OF THE HIP

Developmental dysplasia of the hip (DDH) resulting in dislocation at about 1 year of age could be expected to occur in about 1 per 1000 live births in the UK in the absence of screening.[72] Even though universal screening was introduced in this country in 1969,[73] a national review 30 years later suggests that the number of children receiving surgery for this condition has not been reduced.[74] Results from South Australia appear more successful, though this is exaggerated by their presumption that all positive neonatal findings represented true cases.[75]

However, screening for this condition aims to achieve good hip structure and function, not merely to avoid surgery. No study has yet looked at the quality of hips in surgically treated screened and unscreened cases. In the past places with a special interest in this condition screening program have been estimated to detect a little over 60% of cases at a 'cost' of splinting 10 or more false positives for every true case.[72] The number of cases unnecessarily treated may be able to be safely reduced if ultrasound examination is included in the assessment of possible cases. Primary screening with ultrasound is unlikely to be helpful.[76] Complications can result from non-surgical treatment.[77] An extensive review of the literature and various detection strategies are outlined in a clinical practice guideline recently issued by the American Academy of Pediatrics and its technical report.[78,79]

CRYPTORCHIDISM

About 2% of term male babies have one or both testes undescended but most of these will descend in the first few months of life, probably as a result of the postnatal testosterone surge.[80] Many of those that have not descended by the age of 4 months will probably not descend until puberty when human chorionic gonadotrophin and testosterone levels increase once again. Most surgeons regard boys as cryptorchid if one or both testes are not descended at 1 year of age. In the cohort studied by Scorer and Farrington in the 1950s this definition applied to 0.8%.[80]

While it is reasonably clear that cryptorchidism is associated with both reduced fertility[81] and an increased risk of testicular malignancy[82] it is less clear that either of these risks are reduced by orchidopexy.[83] However, histological changes occur in testes not brought down in the first 2 years of life which are not apparent in those brought down earlier.[84]

WHO PERFORMS THE ROUTINE NEWBORN EXAMINATION

In the UK at the present time most routine newborn examinations are performed by junior medical staff attached to a pediatric department for a period lasting perhaps 6 months. Training to perform such examinations is not standardized and supervision is variable. Recent data have shown that when neonatal nurse practitioners are responsible for performing these examinations the results are significantly improved.[85] This is probably due to two factors, firstly nurse practitioners receive specific training before taking on this responsibility and secondly nurse practitioners are likely to remain in post for considerably longer, and thus are likely to gather considerably more experience of the examination than the average pediatric senior house officer.

A detailed description of a suitable approach to neonatal history taking and examination is given in Chapter 3.

LABOR WARD ROUTINES

AIRWAY

Around 95% of term infants establish spontaneous respiration by 1 min of age and rapidly become vigorous and pink. Suctioning these infants after delivery is unnecessary and may provoke bradycardia and apnea. Even if there was meconium staining of the liquor, airway suctioning after delivery of vigorous infants carries no advantage.[86] A significant proportion of the infants who end up needing extensive resuscitation after birth cannot be predicted in advance of delivery. This is one of the reasons that justify a recommendation that all infants should be delivered in hospital. Although they are clinically pink, healthy term infants without breathing difficulties still have oxygen saturations in the low 80s at the time of the 5 min Apgar score.[87] There is no evidence that they benefit from oxygen supplementation.

THERMAL STABILITY

Newborn infants lose heat rapidly, particularly if they have low birth weight. They should be dried with a warm towel as soon as possible after birth. This only takes seconds and should not prevent close contact between the baby and the mother from being established promptly. The delivery room should be kept warm and draught free. Routinely bathing infants in the delivery room is not beneficial and places them at risk of hypothermia.

CORD CARE

The cord should be clamped with a disposable clamp or tied twice with a cord ligature to prevent accidental hemorrhage. The optimal timing of cord clamping and the preferred position of the infant in relation to the mother prior to cord clamping remain uncertain.[88] Delayed clamping of the cord in preterm infants increases blood volume and may be advantageous. In term infants the increased blood volume may decrease the risk of later anemia but this must be balanced against the risk of occasional polycythemia and volume overload.

SUCKLING

With a minimum of delay, the infant should be given to the mother. Skin to skin contact between the baby and mother will help keep the baby warm and encourage early suckling, which promotes successful breast-feeding.

APGAR SCORES

The condition of the infant should be continually assessed during the first minutes of life. A policy of assigning Apgar scores at 1 and 5 min of age helps to ensure that assessment takes place (p. 203).

OTHER ISSUES

Mistaken identity must be prevented strenuously. Someone who was present at the birth should stay with the baby at all times until two identity labels have been securely fastened to the baby, particularly if the baby is removed from the birthing room for resuscitation. At some point, the baby should be weighed. Vitamin K should be given (p. 307) and the baby should be inspected for congenital malformations, dysmorphic features and signs of illness.

POSTNATAL WARD ROUTINES

Unless they are unwell, babies should generally remain with their mother rather than be admitted to a separate nursery. A further assessment of the general well-being and temperature of the infant should be made at the time of admission to the postnatal ward.

Long postnatal ward stays in healthy mothers and infants used to be the norm but discharge home soon after birth is now increasingly common. This means that an increasing proportion of the problems which occur during neonatal adaptation now develop after discharge and require readmission to hospital.[89] High levels of support for mothers and infants in the community are required to prevent occasional serious morbidity. Hypernatremic dehydration due to inadequate milk intake in breast-fed infants is increasingly recognized[90] and kernicterus has begun to reappear after a long absence.[91]

At some point in the newborn period the infant should be thoroughly examined by someone competent in neonatal hip examination, auscultation and ophthalmoscopy (Ch. 3) for newborn examination). Once milk feeds are established, a capillary blood sample is collected onto filter paper (the Guthrie test). This is used for screening for hypothyroidism, phenylketonuria and galactosemia and is also archived. A formidable array of tests is now possible on these samples and many new screening tests are proposed but not yet routine. Archived blood spots have also been used for population-based research and anonymous screening.

VITAL FUNCTIONS

Most infants (95%) are observed to pass urine during the first 24 h after birth. Those who do not probably micturated at the time of delivery. By 48 h 99% of infants have micturated and failure to do so should prompt further assessment. Meconium is also passed soon after birth by most infants. Failure to do so by 24 h may indicate an underlying cause such as Hirschsprung's disease or meconium ileus and further investigation may be required if there is clinical suspicion. Infants should be kept under review until normal meconium passage has been documented.

After 2–3 days of milk feeding the dark green meconium (bile stained intestinal secretions, intestinal debris and cells) becomes mixed with milk stool and after a further 2–3 days yellow milk stools are present. Delay in the development of changed stools in a breast-fed infant should prompt assessment of the adequacy of the milk intake. There is wide variation between healthy infants in the frequency of passage of stool in the first weeks. Breast-fed infants tend to pass loose yellow stools that may be mistaken for diarrhea, many times per day. The stool frequency of formula fed infants tends to be lower and the consistency more solid.

Most babies lose weight in the days after birth. A 10% weight loss in the first 4 days is common as excess extracellular fluid is excreted. Thereafter, provided that the milk intake is adequate a steady pattern of weight gain of approximately 25 g/day is observed. The weight gain may be established more slowly in breast-fed infants and this can undermine maternal confidence in breast-feeding. A very small number of breast-fed infants do not establish an adequate milk intake, continue to lose weight and develop hypernatremic dehydration which can be life threatening.[90] They are often felt to have been feeding satisfactorily although clues to an inadequate intake may have been present such as delay in developing changed stool. One approach to preventing this problem is to weigh all breast-fed infants at the time of the Guthrie test with the aim of identifying excess weight loss before illness develops.

Vomiting is common in the healthy newborn but may be a sign of abnormality. Occasional mucus or milk vomits are acceptable. Bilious or blood-stained vomits require prompt investigation (p. 281). The commonest explanation for blood-stained vomits in the newborn period is maternal blood swallowed, either during delivery or when feeding from a cracked nipple.

The umbilical stump remains a potential portal for infection until it has healed. It is important to keep the area clean as the stump necroses and separates. Some advocate the regular application of surgical spirit, chorhexidine powder, or antispectic dyes to the umbilical stump. Trials of these practices in the developed world do not demonstrate them to be advantageous.[92] Periumbilical erythema indicates infection and requires prompt medical review.

Mothers may require support and education in the basics of baby care, including feeding, feed preparation, bathing and temperature control. If the environmental temperature is warm enough for the mother to be clothed only in a nightdress then the baby should be warm enough in a babygrow under two blankets. Overheating is probably as common as hypothermia in term infants. Both may be dangerous. Epidemiological data demonstrate that the incidence of sudden infant death syndrome is lower when infants sleep supine rather than prone.

GENITALIA

Routine circumcision is a non-medical ritual that should not be imposed on infants of either sex.

FEEDING THE FULL-TERM NEWBORN

Immediately after the umbilical cord is cut, the newborn infant must change from total parenteral nutrition, obtained by the transplacental route, to enteral nutrition. The gut has been prepared by fetal enteral nutrition, and trophic gut hormone levels rise rapidly after birth. Some babies will not tolerate enteral feeding, due either to anomalies of the gastrointestinal tract or concomitant disease. In this case, parenteral nutrition is used, although often and preferably, combined with some enteral feeding. Most clinical trials in infant nutrition have had serious methodological flaws, and many nutrition policies are decided by tradition or anecdote.

BREAST MILK

The milk of the mother has been uniquely developed to be appropriate in composition for the human newborn infant (Table 10.4). The rise in prolactin from the anterior pituitary during pregnancy is inhibited from producing milk by the high pregnancy levels of progesterone

Table 10.4 Composition of milks

Per 100 ml	Colostrum	Mature breast milk	Drip breast milk (foremilk)	Unmodified cows' milk	*Whey based	Casein based
Energy (kcal)	67	70	45	65	67	67
Protein (g)	2.3	1.34	1.0	3.2	1.5	1.6
Fat (g)	2.95	4.2	2.2	3.8	3.6	3.6
Carbohydrate (g)	5.7	7.1	6.5	4.7	7.2	7.0
Sodium (mg)	50	19		77	23	22
Calcium (mg)	48	27		137	66	56
Phosphorus (mg)	16	14		91	42	44
Iron (μg)	100	50		45	700	800
Vitamin A (μg)	161	60		23	60	75
Vitamin C (μg)	7.2	5.2		1.1	8.0	9.0
Vitamin D (μg)	0.04	0.1		0.02	1.0	1.1
Vitamin E (mg)	1.5	0.24		0.06	0.6	0.74
Vitamin B_6 (mg)	–	0.018		0.05	0.04	0.06

* Aptamil First and SMA White are two commercial full-term baby formulae respectively, available in Europe from Milupa Ltd (Nutricia NV, Netherlands) and from SMA Nutrition (Wyeth, UK).

but with the delivery of the baby, further prolactin secretion and the withdrawal of other circulating hormones (progesterone, estrogens and placental lactogen) leads to lactogenesis. Nipple stimulation (suckling) exaggerates prolactin production; thus after birth the baby is literally switching on the mother's milk production. Nipple stimulation also causes secretion of oxytocin from the posterior pituitary which leads to contraction of the myoepithelial cells surrounding the milk-filled lactiferous sinuses to cause milk ejection (the let-down reflex). Oxytocin release (and let-down) may also come from visual, auditory and other stimuli.

Over the first 48–72 h the secretions from the breast (colostrum) are high in protein, hormones, immunoglobulins and white cells but are low in volume. After this time the milk 'comes in' sometimes causing extreme tenseness and tenderness of the breasts. Continued suckling by the infant empties the breast and stimulates further milk production. Once the baby is feeding well the breast will be emptied in about 5 min and further time is for emotional and physical satisfaction of mother and baby as much as for nutrition. Breast milk is variable in composition both with the stage of lactation and as the feed progresses (towards the end of the feed, it is high in fat and calories).

Breast-feeding has multiple advantages for the full-term newborn infant, although few have been proven in studies providing level 1 evidence – it is unlikely that a randomized controlled trial of breast-feeding would ever be considered ethically permissible. Breast milk contains multiple anti-infective substances, including immunoglobulins, and well-designed cohort studies have shown that breast-feeding in the first 3 months of life, even in developed countries, confers protection against gastrointestinal and respiratory infection throughout infancy.[93] Breast-feeding also protects against the development of obesity, the commonest nutritional problem in children in the developed world.[94] Breast-feeding may prevent later common chronic diseases in childhood and adult life, such as type 1 diabetes, celiac disease, and inflammatory bowel disease, but many of the case-control studies performed to date lack methodological rigor.[95–99] Epidemiological evidence suggests that breast-feeding is protective against sudden infant death syndrome.[100,101] No studies have conclusively demonstrated improved neurodevelopmental outcome in full-term infants fed with breast milk, rather than infant formula, in the developed world. In the UK, local and national policies have resulted in an increase in the rate of breast-feeding. The prevalence of breast-feeding as the initial feed in the UK has increased from 66% in 1995 to 69% in 2000.[102] The UNICEF UK Baby Friendly Initiative aims to promote and support breast-feeding,[103] and is now endorsed in many maternity units in the UK. Breast-feeding is of even more importance in the developing world. There are few absolute contraindications to breast-feeding. These would include rare metabolic problems in the infant, such as galactosemia; some maternal drug therapy, such as cytotoxic agents; and an HIV-positive mother. In the developing world, the risk of HIV transmission may be outweighed by the anti-infective properties of breast milk, and this is at present an active focus of research.

BREAST MILK SUBSTITUTES (Table 10.4)

Formula feeds are derived from cows' milk. Although the overall calorie density of unmodified cows' milk (65 cal/100 ml) is similar to human breast milk, the composition is very different. Modification involves reducing the high protein and particularly casein concentration and substituting lactalbumin (whey protein). The high sodium and phosphate concentrations are reduced, iron and vitamin D are added and the fatty acid composition is made more like breast milk. New additions to term formulas continue to appear. A recent Cochrane review[104] concludes that there is currently little evidence from random controlled trials (RCTs) of long chain polyunsaturated fatty acid supplemented term formula to show improvement in visual or general development. Despite accepting that modified formulae are generally safe when made up as recommended with a sterile water supply, breast milk is the gold standard nutrient for newborn infants. In the developed world, where water supplies are well prepared, there is usually no problem using a powdered milk formula, but in the developing world where water supplies are frequently contaminated their use may lead to disastrous gastroenteritis, other infections and death.

Milk derived from soya or other sources (rice, goats) are not indicated for the feeding of normal newborn infants and may be very dangerous.

PRACTICAL BREAST-FEEDING

Successful breast-feeding depends on both the mother and infant being relaxed. It is more difficult for the mother to relax in a hospital environment; and hospital, medical and midwifery routines may further compromise breast-feeding. For these reasons, UNICEF developed 'The 10 steps to successful breast-feeding', a set of evidence based standards to measure the quality of breast-feeding support in the maternity services.[103] These state that all providers of maternity services should: have a written breast-feeding policy that is routinely communicated to all health care staff; train all health care staff in the skills necessary to implement the breast-feeding policy; inform all pregnant women about the benefits and management of breast-feeding; help mothers initiate breast-feeding soon after birth; show mothers how to breast-feed and how to maintain lactation even if they are separated from their babies; give newborn infants no food or drink other than breast milk, unless medically indicated; practice rooming-in, allowing mothers and infants to remain together 24 h a day; encourage breast-feeding on demand; give no artificial teats or dummies to breast-feeding infants; and foster the establishment of breast-feeding support groups and refer mothers to them on discharge from the hospital or clinic. Units which implement them can be accredited as Baby Friendly, and currently more than 13 000 hospitals worldwide have this award. Of note, almost all maternity units in the UK are working to implement these steps; by February 2002, nine Scottish maternity units had obtained the Baby Friendly Initiative Award.

Over the first 24 h the baby may only wish to feed three to four times and may be quite sleepy between feeds. Soon, the baby at the breast will be demanding feeds nearly 2-hourly; the baby is switching on mother's supply at this stage. After the milk has come in the baby will settle down by 10–12 days to 3- to 4-hourly feeds in most instances. Failure of breast-feeding may occur, especially if inadequate support is given to the mother, and this is most commonly associated with early (< 48 h) hospital discharge. It is associated with both hypernatremic dehydration and early malnutrition. Prevention lies in prenatal and perinatal education and support, and early follow-up after discharge. Breast and formula-fed infants should have similar growth patterns to 3 months of age; after this, breast-fed infants tend to gain less weight and have a lower fat mass than formula fed infants, probably due to infant self-regulation of energy mass. New growth charts based on breast-fed infants during the first year of life are currently being developed. The prevalence of breast-feeding in the UK once the baby is aged 4 weeks has remained at 42% in the two most recent national infant feeding surveys, performed in 1995 and 2000.[102]

PRACTICAL BOTTLE-FEEDING

The practice of using ready-to-feed milk in hospitals is convenient, but means that the mother who has chosen to bottle-feed may not have seen or made up a bottle of milk when she returns home. Midwives should ensure that the mother who is choosing to bottle-feed sees how to prepare such a bottle. Powdered milk must be reconstituted in the way stated on the packet, with water that has boiled and cooled a few minutes previously. The practice of adding extra scoops is still not uncommon in Western cultures and may be dangerous if the baby has a free water loss from any cause, though hypernatremia is uncommon with modern commercial milks. Bottles and teats should be carefully cleaned soon after use, and if not steam sterilized should be kept in a 1% hypochlorite solution to ensure sterility.

After the first few days of life the bottle-fed baby usually demands food about 4-hourly. If the baby is demanding food more often and is irritable it may be that thirst rather than hunger is the problem and clear fluid (boiled and cooled water is best) may be needed.

THE HIGH RISK NEWBORN

BIRTH TRAUMA

A birth injury is a potentially avoidable mechanical injury occurring during labor or delivery (thus excluding damage from amniocentesis or intrauterine transfusion). Asphyxia and injury may occur together as the identification of a fetus in suboptimal condition inevitably leads to a rushed delivery. Even competent obstetric intervention in this situation may lead to injury but it is often possible that more serious damage such as severe asphyxia or death may have been prevented. Improvements in antenatal care and obstetric practice have reduced the incidence of birth trauma but where obstetric provision is poor, injuries are both common and severe. In the Western world, possibly because of the low incidence, obstetric anxiety and guilt may be an inevitable sequel to each case. It is important that information is given to the parents immediately problems are identified in order to avoid misunderstandings and recrimination. Sensitive counseling is a most important aspect of management. Estimates of incidence are meaningless as the frequency varies with the quality of obstetric practice but the more difficult or prolonged the labor and delivery, the more likely it is that trauma will occur. Conditions predisposing to injury are listed in Table 10.5.

SOFT TISSUE INJURIES

Abrasions and blisters from forceps or vacuum deliveries, punctures from scalp electrodes or blood samples and incisions from hurried cesarean sections lead to potential infection sites. Bruises from trauma may be severe in preterm deliveries and extensive into the buttocks following breech deliveries leading later to jaundice and anemia and occasionally disseminated intravascular coagulation. Vitamin K should be given and phototherapy considered early. The sternomastoid tumor is originally a hemorrhage. Do not call it a tumor in front of parents. It may require passive physiotherapy. Petechiae are common over the head and neck following shoulder dystocia, face presentation or a nuchal cord. Subconjunctival hemorrhages are common in spontaneous deliveries (the mother may be worried about the baby's vision – reassure). Subcutaneous fat necrosis may be from obvious pressure from forceps or mother's pelvis, the thickened rubbery skin sometimes softening with resolution. This necrosis may occur over the back of head, cheek, outside of upper arm or greater trochanter of the femur. No treatment is required. Fractures (Table 10.6), deformity or pseudoparalysis may be observed and crepitations or later callus may be palpable. Pain relief is important.

Table 10.5 Conditions predisposing to birth injury

Poor maternal health	Cephalopelvic disproportion
Maternal age (very young and old)	Hydrocephalus
Grand multiparity	Macrosomia
Twins (particularly the second)	Dystocia
Prematurity/low birth weight	Contracted pelvis
Malpresentation	Instrumental delivery

INTRA-ABDOMINAL INJURIES

Hepatosplenomegaly (e.g. rhesus hemolytic disease), coagulation disorders and hypoxia, breech deliveries and cardiac massage all predispose to *subcapsular hematomas of the liver and spleen*. Anemia, pallor, tachycardia and tachypnea may be the presenting features or rupture may occur (immediately or days later) to give hypovolemic shock and death. *Adrenal hemorrhages* may follow severe infection, severe asphyxia or coagulation disorder. Hypovolemic shock with a flank mass and overlying skin discoloration may be evident. Adrenal failure may require treatment and later calcification may occur. All hemorrhages predispose to jaundice. Ultrasound assists in diagnosis.

EXTRACRANIAL INJURIES

The *caput succedaneum* (present at birth) is a serosanguineous subcutaneous effusion over the presenting part in a vaginal delivery. It crosses the suture lines and disappears rapidly. *Subaponeurotic hemorrhages* are rare. They may follow vacuum deliveries or less commonly other instrumental deliveries. The hemorrhage is between the scalp aponeurosis and the periosteum and if it is massive it may present with hypovolemic shock and be fatal. Vitamin K (1 mg i.m.) should be given to all vacuum deliveries. Once diagnosed full clotting tests should be performed and 10 ml/kg of fresh frozen plasma should be given followed by crossmatched blood. Later there may be jaundice and anemia. The *chignon* is usual from a vacuum delivery and requires no treatment. A *cephalhematoma* may follow an instrumental or less commonly a spontaneous delivery. This subperiosteal hematoma is limited by each cranial bone and is probably always associated with a hairline fracture. There is no scalp discoloration and it appears *after* birth. Jaundice may develop and phototherapy may be required. The hematoma usually resolves over 2–8 weeks with hardening of the edge and at this stage may mimic a depressed fracture. Thickening of the diploë on skull X-ray may be apparent for years. The commonest site is parietal (sometimes bilateral) followed by frontal and then occipital. No treatment is required. Do *not* drain as this allows infection into the hematoma.

INTRACRANIAL INJURIES

Asphyxia and intracranial birth injury show similar clinical features and frequently coexist. Prenatal asphyxia or congenital abnormality may have initiated an instrumental delivery so it may

Table 10.6 Fractures

	Specific cause	Potential problem	Treatment	Comment
Skull				
Linear	1. Forceps pressure 2. Pubic pressure 3. Sacral pressure 4. Ischial spine pressure	Usually none, rarely subdural or extradural hemorrhage		
Depressed	Forceps	Underlying brain injury	1. If asymptomatic, none 2. If symptomatic, elevate	Prevent sustained cortical pressure
Occipital subluxation	Traction on spine in breech deliveries with head fixed in the pelvis	Rupture of underlying venous sinus		Usually fatal from subdural hemorrhage or tentorial tear
Clavicle (common)	1. Breech – extended arms 2. Difficult shoulder in vertex delivery	Associated brachial plexus injury	1. None – or if pain: treat pain 2. Bandage arm to chest with pad in axilla for 10 days	Prognosis excellent
Humerus	Breech – bringing down a displaced arm	Nerve damage	As for clavicle	Prognosis excellent
Femur	Extended breech	Sciatic nerve damage	1. Immobilize leg onto abdomen for 2–4 weeks (the in utero position) 2. Gallows traction	Position unimportant, molding will repair
Epiphyseal separation		Callus interferes with joint mobility and bone growth		1. On the upper femur, pain on external rotation 2. Outlook good
Nose	Dislocation of nasal cartilage	Difficulty feeding	1. Insert oral airway 2. Straighten surgically	Nares asymmetrical and nose flat

be impossible to attribute abnormal features neonatally or later neurodevelopmental problems to one cause rather than the other. It is also possible that prenatal asphyxia may make a baby more vulnerable to birth injury by causing a high venous pressure, acidosis or disordered coagulation.

Intraventricular hemorrhage (p. 321)

This hemorrhage usually found in preterm infants is not now thought to be related to birth injury. In the asphyxiated full-term infant the choroid plexus may bleed into the ventricle.

COMPRESSION HEAD INJURIES

Cephalopelvic disproportion and instrumental delivery will predispose to intracranial injury. In many cases there will be obvious extracranial injury. Hypoxic–ischemic encephalopathy and cerebral edema (p. 199) may contribute to the clinical signs. If intracranial hemorrhage is massive, resuscitation may prove impossible or when initially successful the infant may survive only a few hours with generalized hypotonia progressing later to rigidity with convulsions and deep gasping respirations. Supratentorial bleeds lead to a tense fontanel but posterior fossa bleeds do not. Head retraction may be marked, retinal hemorrhages may occur rapidly and the infant may have a high-pitched cry or may moan continuously. If unconscious the infant may make no sound.

Less severe hemorrhage leads to apathetic periods interspersed with periods of extreme irritability. The hemisyndrome may be evident with eyes and head turned to one side and paucity of movement on the other. Up to 50% of such infants convulse and tonic fits have a worse prognosis.

Subarachnoid hemorrhage

This may occur in preterm and term infants following perinatal hypoxia. The baby may be pale and irritable with a high-pitched cry, neck retraction and sometimes a full fontanel. Diagnosis is difficult by ultrasound but the presumptive diagnosis by lumbar puncture may be confirmed by computerized tomography (CT) scan.

Subdural hemorrhage (hematoma)

Tears of the tentorium cerebelli or less often the falx cerebri are rare nowadays. If the hemorrhage is not rapidly fatal and if it is supratentorial, localization leads to hematoma. Signs of cerebral irritation settle after 48–72 h but later in the first week the head circumference begins to increase fast and there is clinical deterioration. Vomiting is common. Diagnosis is by CT scan and treatment by subdural taps at the lateral edge of the anterior fontanel. Ultrasound may show midline shift but it is frequently difficult to see the subdural region to visualize the hemorrhage itself.

Management of intracranial injury

Any baby suspected of having an intracranial injury should be closely observed in an incubator with monitoring of PaO_2 and $PaCO_2$. Temperature, blood pressure, fluid balance, and metabolic problems of blood sugar, calcium and coagulation should be corrected.

Phenobarbital 4 mg/kg/12 h may help prevent convulsions but if these occur a loading dose of 20 mg/kg intravenously followed by the sedative dose should be used. Breakthrough convulsions may require diazepam, paraldehyde or phenytoin or other anticonvulsant (p. 202). Careful fluid balance is needed and it is wise to restrict intake initially to intravenous 10% dextrose at 50 ml/kg/24 h (to reduce edema secondary to inappropriate vasopressin secretion). Manual expression of the bladder may be needed.

The sedation is reduced from 48–72 h of age but is reintroduced if convulsions recur. Treatment may be required for cerebral edema (p. 199).

Prognosis

Prediction of late effects from brain damage is notoriously difficult. A recent Edinburgh study showed 9% died, 29% were handicapped (12% severely) and 62% were normal. The bad outcome is usually due to dyskinetic or hemiplegic cerebral palsy with some degree of mental retardation and sometimes epilepsy.

PERIPHERAL NERVE INJURIES

Sixth nerve palsy seen for a few days after birth is probably associated with cerebral edema and trapping of the nerve on the tentorium. *Facial nerve damage* (VII) is usually peripheral from forceps pressure or from pressure on the maternal pelvis (spontaneous deliveries). No facial movement or forehead movement is seen when the infant cries. The corner of the mouth droops with dribbling at feeds and the eye fails to close (this requires protection). Recovery usually occurs over weeks but if after months there has been no recovery surgical neuroplasty should be considered. Rarely a central nuclear agenesis leads, if one sided, to paralysis of the lower half of the face.

Brachial plexus injury occurs in about 4–5/1000 deliveries in Europe.[105] Neck retraction in breech deliveries or shoulder dystocia damages the upper brachial plexus roots to give *Erb palsy* (C5, C6) or *phrenic palsy* (C3, C4, C5). The arm is limp with forearm pronated and wrist flexed (waiter's tip position) from paralysis of deltoid, biceps, brachioradialis and long wrist extensors. Finger movements and therefore grasp reflex are normal. The biceps and Moro reflexes are absent on the affected side. Initial splinting of the arm to the side of the head probably makes little difference to the rate of recovery which is usually within 3 weeks (if severe it may take up to 2 years). In over 70% complete recovery is achieved. Shoulder contracture is frequent in those with delayed or incomplete recovery.[105] Phrenic involvement presents as acute cyanosis and irregular labored breathing. There are reduced breath sounds and an absent abdominal bulge on inspiration because of paradoxical diaphragmatic movement. Diagnosis is by ultrasound or fluoroscopy. Treatment is with oxygen and intravenous fluids and then the gradual introduction of enteral feeds. If there is no improvement in 2 months (on ultrasound), diaphragmatic plication is indicated to prevent recurrent infection and bronchiectasis. *Klumpke palsy* (C8, T1) may occur with a breech delivery when the arms are extended up beside the head and the lower roots are stretched. The hand and forearm are paralyzed and there may be an ipsilateral Horner's syndrome. Edema and hemorrhage cause temporary problems but avulsion leads to permanent disability. Traditional treatment strapping the upper limb to the trunk probably makes little difference to the rate of recovery. *Radial nerve* damage is temporary and leads to wrist drop. It may be due to fat necrosis involving the nerve but frequently no predisposing factor can be found. Treat with a cock up splint.

In general peripheral nerve injuries need gentle passive exercise of the limb several times a day with splinting to avoid contractures. If paralysis continues for more than 3 months, recovery is unlikely. Neuroplasty and tendon transplant have usually been considered at 3–4 years of age but there has been a recent move in brachial plexus injuries to explore and attempt repair at 3–6 months if there has been no improvement since birth.

SPINAL CORD INJURIES

Upper cervical cord injury may rarely be associated with rotational forceps deliveries and presents with quadriparesis and diaphragmatic paralysis.[106] The lower cervical or upper thoracic cord may be bruised or rarely transected by forceful longitudinal or lateral traction on the spine. Subluxation or fractures of the vertebrae may occur with breech deliveries where the head is hyperextended or in a vertex delivery with shoulder dystocia. Coincident brachial plexus injury is common. The infant may be normal at birth or shocked but paralysis with flaccidity below the lesion quickly occurs with accompanying constipation and urinary retention. Intercostal paralysis leads to respiratory recession (Fig. 10.8). Spinal reflex activity returns after a short time. The initial flaccidity and immobility are replaced after several weeks by rigid flexion at hip, knee and ankle with increased tone and spasms. Absent sensation

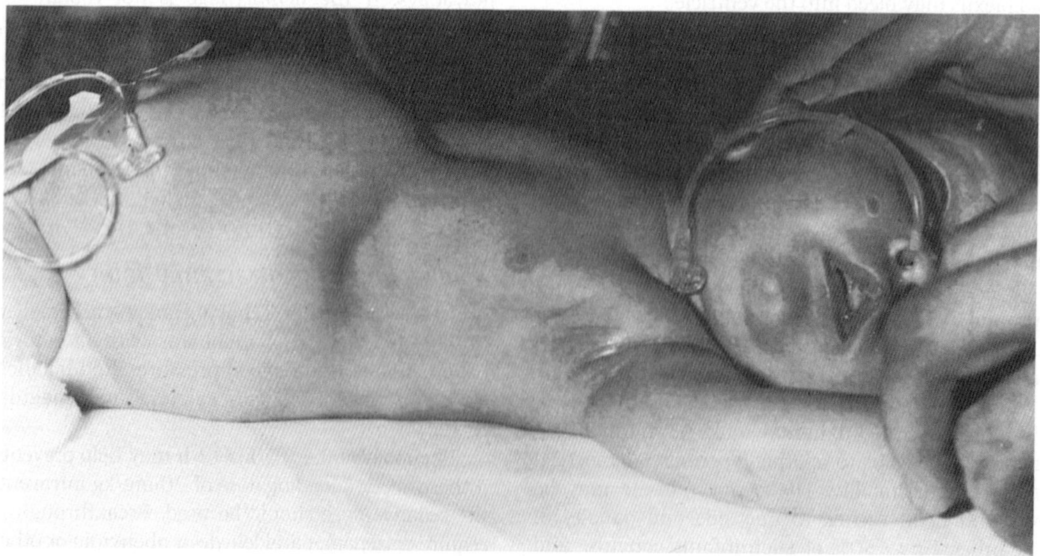

Fig. 10.8 Thoracic indrawing in newborn infant with broken neck.

and automatic bladder function necessitate treatment similar to that of the baby with a meningomyelocele (Ch. 20). Diagnosis may be confirmed by magnetic resonance imaging (MRI). There is no reparative treatment but multidisciplinary involvement inclusive of physiotherapy may prevent or reduce contractural difficulties in the future.

BIRTH ASPHYXIA

Birth asphyxia is the most common and important cause of preventable cerebral injury occurring in the neonatal period, but although asphyxia at birth is a commonly made diagnosis, there is no generally accepted definition for it. The term is used to imply an abnormal process and one that, if untreated, may cause permanent injury. Asphyxia, at a pathophysiological level, is the simultaneous combination of both hypoxia and hypoperfusion which impairs tissue gas exchange leading to tissue acidosis. Almost any organ can be affected, but the brain, myocardium, kidneys and bowel appear to be most sensitive to severe damage. Cerebral complications are the most devastating as full recovery may not occur and the child may be left with life-long neurological impairment and in some cases devastating disability.

THE FETAL RESPONSE TO HYPOXIC STRESS

Hypoxia, and to a lesser extent placental underperfusion, both hallmarks of asphyxia, are relatively common events during labor and ones to which the fetus is well adapted. These adaptations are summarized in Table 10.7, and each is discussed briefly below. It is most important to realize that these are physiological responses to perturbations in the fetal environment which are common enough during labor to be considered 'normal'.

Reflex activity

Certain diving marine mammals have the ability to redistribute their cardiac output to vital organs and to slow their heart rate to extraordinarily low levels in order to remain under water for up to an hour in some cases. The fetus has been shown to have adaptive mechanisms during periods of normal hypoxic stress of labor in some ways similar to those of the diving seal. There is a reduction of blood flow through the descending aorta, together with reflex bradycardia. This reflex is mediated through a number of mechanisms discussed below.

Table 10.7 Important physiological adaptations to short episodes of fetal hypoxic stress

Cardiovascular responses
'Diving seal' reflex
Redistribution of blood flow
towards brain, myocardium and adrenals
away from gut, lungs and carcass
Bradycardia
Increase in blood pressure
Regional cerebral blood flow changes
relative increase to brainstem
relative decrease to cerebral cortex
Autonomic responses
In premature animals:
net parasympathetic response
In full-term animals:
net sympathetic response
Catecholamine surge
Biochemical response
Glycolysis
switch from aerobic to anaerobic metabolism

Redistribution of blood flow

Episodes of hypoxemia cause a reduction in the fetal heart rate and an increase in blood pressure. This results in a net fall in cardiac output during the hypoxemic event. The overall reduction in cardiac output is more than compensated by a simultaneous redistribution of blood flow to vital organs with marked increase to the fetal brain, heart and adrenals. These increases occur at the expense of a redistribution of flow away from the placental circulation, lungs, gut and carcass. Although there is an increase of up to 100% in the total cerebral blood flow (CBF) during episodes of fetal hypoxia, regional CBF also shows consistent adaptive changes. Blood flow to the brain is distributed towards the phylogenetically more primitive regions, particularly the brainstem, at the expense of the cerebral cortices, thus protecting function in the most basic and 'vital' centers. During fetal stress, high levels of circulating cortisol are produced, which may mediate some of the vascular effects seen in the normal fetus during periods of hypoxia. The autonomic nervous system is also closely involved with the fetal responses to stress.

Glycolytic activity

Glucose and oxygen are the metabolic fuels of the developing brain. Metabolism can switch to anaerobic glycolysis during periods of hypoxia with the production of lactic acid. This is a normal metabolic adaptation. It has been known for three centuries that the immature animal is more resistant to asphyxia than more mature animals of the same species. This resistance is in part due to the increased resilience of the mature cardiovascular system, but the brain also appears to have greater resistance and this may be due to either augmented glycolytic ability (production of more fuel) or lower utilization of glucose by the brain.

Stress vs distress

It is clear from the above that the fetus is a beautifully adapted organism with a number of interrelated mechanisms to protect it from the rigors of labor, both hypoxic and ischemic. Stress is an invariable accompaniment of the birth process and one which the fetus is well able to withstand under most circumstances. Distress may result from a prolonged stress response and the two may merge as an imperceptible continuum. It may be extremely difficult to separate fetal stress from distress using currently available clinical methods. Fetal distress may occur as the result of a single period of hypoxia which is too long, or periods which occur too frequently. Currently, methods used to detect 'fetal distress' such as cardiotocography and fetal scalp pH assessments are really detecting degrees of fetal stress. These tests may be misinterpreted by the obstetrician as fetal distress, but an understanding of the fetal responses to the stress of uncompromised labor might encourage the fetus' medical attendants that s/he requires no assistance.

What is asphyxia?

There is no clinically accepted definition for asphyxia, although many suggested definitions have been put forward. The suggestion that asphyxia occurs when there is hypoxia together with accumulation of carbon dioxide and if prolonged this leads to an eventual state of respiratory and then metabolic acidosis ignores the fact that this may be an entirely normal sequence of physiological events. The clinical detection of acidosis as an indicator of asphyxia is discussed in more detail below. There is no single or widely accepted definition of 'birth asphyxia'. Some have recommended that the term 'birth asphyxia' should not be used,[107] but the concept that 'birth asphyxia' is a syndrome, or collection of features, with the exclusion of alternative conditions[108] is becoming more widely accepted.

Meconium staining of the amniotic fluid

Heavy or thick meconium staining is considered to be a marker of more prolonged or severe asphyxial episodes. Meconium staining is seen in approximately 15% of all labors and is present during labor in 11% of full-term pregnancies where there is no evidence, other than the meconium, of asphyxia.[109] This sign is poorly predictive of adverse outcome and, in one study, more than half of infants who had early neonatal seizures (a possible indicator of intrapartum asphyxia) showed no evidence of meconium staining. Furthermore, if cerebral palsy is taken as the endpoint of a major asphyxial event in the perinatal period, then 99.6% of normal birth weight infants with meconium staining had no evidence of this condition.[110]

Electronic fetal monitoring (EFM)

A normal fetal heart rate trace in labor appears to be a good indicator that metabolic acidosis is not developing, but a severely abnormal trace with late decelerations in the fetal heart rate is associated with significant fetal acidosis in only about 50% of cases. A recent Cochrane review[111] showed that there was a statistically significant reduction in neonatal seizures (RR 0.51, 95% CI 0.32–0.82) when EFM had been used, but no protective effect for 1 min Apgar scores, rates of admission to neonatal units, perinatal death or cerebral palsy. There was a statistically significant increased risk of delivery by cesarean section following use of EFM (RR 1.41, 95% CI 1.23–1.61). The increase in operative delivery appears to be reduced by analyzing electrocardiographic waveforms in addition to EFM when compared with EFM alone (OR 1.05, 95% CI 0.87–1.27).[112]

Acidosis

Acidosis is a marker of CO_2 accumulation (respiratory acidosis) and/or metabolic acidosis as the result of anaerobic metabolism. Severe fetal or cord blood acidosis is a marker of impaired tissue gas exchange, but there is no evidence that acidosis per se is a cause of further tissue damage. There is poor correlation between cord blood acidosis and depression of Apgar scores. Severe fetal acidosis (pH $\leq$ 7.00) occurs in 2.5 per 1000 term infants and is often taken as representing intrapartum compromise possibly severe enough to be associated with organ dysfunction, but a minority of these infants will show neurological complications.

Maladaptation at birth

The baby who is born in less than optimal condition may reflect a transient failure to adapt physiologically to the changes that occur at birth or may reflect ongoing fetal asphyxia. The most widely used descriptor of condition at and after birth is the Apgar score. It assesses five variables easily elicitable at birth (Table 10.8) and is a useful method for describing the condition of any infant at varying times from birth. Depression of the score may be due to factors such as gestational age, maternal medication, cardiovascular disease of the infant and a variety of congenital neuromuscular problems quite apart from asphyxia. The more immature the infant, the more the respiratory effort, muscle tone and reflex irritability will be reduced, irrespective of any degree of depression due to other causes. Premature infants born in optimal condition normally have a lower Apgar score than full-term infants also born in good condition.

In both preterm and full-term infants there is a direct relationship between severe depression of the Apgar score (0–3) at 5 min and risk of death,[113] but there is a poor predictive value of depressed Apgar score and neurological deficit. As well as being an insensitive predictive method, it is also poorly specific: 50% of children with cerebral palsy evident at 7 years of age had an optimal Apgar score of 7–10 at 1 min.[114]

Table 10.8 The Apgar score

Sign	0	1	2
Heart rate	Absent	< 100/min	> 100/min
Respiratory effort	Absent	Weak cry	Strong cry
Muscle tone	Limp	Some flexion	Good flexion
Reflex irritability on suctioning pharynx	No response	Some motion	Cry
Color	Pale	Centrally pink, peripherally blue	Pink all over

Attempts have been made to identify babies at high risk of neonatal seizures on the basis of very early neonatal markers. Poor condition, as measured by the combination of three factors at birth (Apgar score of $\leq$ 5 at 5 min, the need for intubation and a cord blood pH of $\leq$ 7.00), has been reported to increase the risk of neonatal seizures 340-fold.[115]

Hypoxic–ischemic encephalopathy (HIE)

This refers to a consistent pattern of abnormal neurological signs occurring in sequence over a period of the first days of life in response to a hypoxic–ischemic insult affecting the brain. This is discussed in detail below and is an important feature to be considered in the clinical diagnosis of 'birth asphyxia'.

Multiorgan involvement

A significant asphyxial insult to the fetus is likely to compromise a number of different organ systems of which the brain, kidneys and myocardium are particularly vulnerable, but bowel, endocrine and pulmonary complications may also occur. The presence of transient compromise to more than one organ is therefore a feature of a global asphyxial insult. Recently, reports have been published of babies with HIE who later developed cerebral palsy, but who have not shown multiorgan dysfunction.[116,117] In many of these cases, intrapartum asphyxia was documented to be of short duration (mean 32 min) and was severe and unexpected such as occurs with uterine rupture.[117]

HYPOXIC–ISCHEMIC ENCEPHALOPATHY

If the full-term brain has been compromised by an hypoxic–ischemic event (asphyxia) during delivery, it is likely that the infant will show a disturbance in neurological behavior, a state referred to as HIE. HIE cannot be reliably diagnosed in premature babies. Infants show a sequence of often transient encephalopathic behavior lasting often for days which is dependent on the severity and duration of the asphyxial event. Grading systems have been published to define the degree of encephalopathy[118,119] and Table 10.9 describes the major clinical features. Mild HIE recovers completely within 48–72 h and moderate HIE continues to show significant neurological signs for 7–10 days. Babies with severe HIE may remain persistently neurologically abnormal although the signs often improve prior to discharge home. Asphyxia is not the only cause of neonatal encephalopathy,[120] and alternative causes such as hypoglycemia and meningitis must be considered and excluded before HIE can be reliably used as a feature of

Table 10.9 The major clinical features for grading the severity of postasphyxial encephalopathy

Mild	Moderate	Severe
Irritability	Lethargy	Coma
Hyperalert	Seizures	Prolonged seizures
Normal tone	Differential tone (legs > arms) (neck extensors > flexors)	Severe hypotonia
Weak suck	Poor suck, requires tube feeds	No sucking reflex
Sympathetic dominance	Parasympathetic dominance	Coma, requires respiratory support

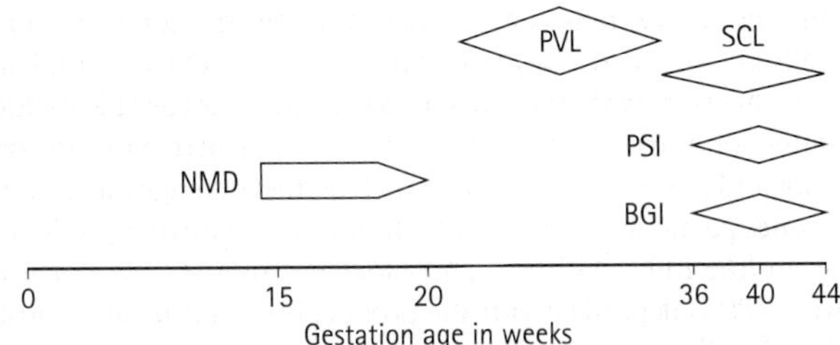

Fig. 10.9 Vulnerable periods for the development of different forms of pathology as the result of an hypoxic ischemic insult: NMD, neuronal migration disorder; PVL, periventricular leukomalacia; SCL, subcortical leukomalacia; PSI, parasagittal injury; BGI, basal ganglia injury.

postasphyxial insult. In particular, neonatal convulsions alone with clinical interseizure normality are not a feature of HIE, nor is the baby who shows an unchanging pattern of neurological abnormalities in the neonatal period. It has been suggested that in the majority of cases, 'neonatal encephalopathy' in full-term babies may not be due to intrapartum events, but may originate in the antepartum period.[121]

The severity of HIE is the best clinical method currently available to predict subsequent outcome following asphyxia (see section on outcome), but it has a number of disadvantages. Firstly, the severity of HIE can only be determined retrospectively as the clinical neurological features of asphyxia take some time to evolve. Secondly, other organs such as the kidneys and heart may be compromised due to asphyxia, but the fetus preserves blood flow to his brain thereby sparing cerebral function. The lack of encephalopathy does not necessarily indicate that the infant has not suffered from significant intrapartum asphyxia.

INCIDENCE

The incidence of HIE is reported to be 1.8–6.0 per 1000 full-term infants. It is estimated that approximately 2 per 1000 will show moderate to severe HIE which is a marker of the infant who has sustained potentially irreversible brain injury. The reported incidence of HIE has been shown to have fallen in more recent years although this may reflect a reduction in the least severe form of this condition.[122] A cohort of full-term infants born 1984–1988 had an incidence of 4.6 per 1000 compared with 7.7 per 1000 for a similar group born 1976–1980.[123]

PATHOLOGY

The type of brain pathology seen in infants depends on the duration and intensity of the asphyxial event and the gestational age of the baby at the time the insult occurred. The type of pathology expected with insults at different stages of development is summarized in Figure 10.9. An asphyxial insult occurring very early in development (< 20 weeks) may cause a disorder in neuronal migration, but by 20 weeks an asphyxial insult cannot damage the brain in the same way since all the neurones have completed their migration by then. A severe insult at 24–34 weeks of gestation is likely to cause periventricular leukomalacia (p. 321), but by 35 weeks of gestation brain maturation no longer predisposes to this type of pathology. By 35 weeks onwards a new watershed vulnerability is exposed and subcortical leukomalacia (p. 322) may occur. In the term brain and for a number of weeks after term an asphyxial insult may lead to damage primarily in the watershed distribution or in the basal ganglia.

As mentioned above the brain has the ability to redistribute regional cerebral blood flow away from the cortical areas to the more primitive brainstem, basal ganglia and cerebellum. The classical studies of Windle[124] and Myers[125] distinguished two forms of neuropathology dependent on the pattern of asphyxiating insult; the partial or intermittent model and the sudden and complete form. In partial fetal asphyxia (the clinically more common form) the cortical mantle is more likely to be affected in the parasagittal distribution whereas in the acute and total form of asphyxia, the lesions affect mainly the basal nuclei and brainstem. These patterns of damage are only seen in the term baby's brain as described above and can be recognized on brain imaging (see below).

Hemorrhage

Although intracranial hemorrhage is a common condition in premature infants, its incidence in more mature asphyxiated babies is much less. Subdural hemorrhage is the best described hemorrhagic lesion associated with birth asphyxia in full-term infants, but it probably occurs in only 5% of such infants. Some subarachnoid hemorrhage is commonly found at autopsy examination, but this is not usually severe and its frequency is not known in surviving infants. Hemorrhage may occur into the choroid plexus, cerebellum and thalamus in asphyxiated infants, but these are all relatively uncommon.

Cerebral edema

Two forms of cerebral edema have been described: cytotoxic and vasogenic edema, and both occur in the neonatal brain following asphyxia. Injury to the cellular pump mechanism causes sodium and water to enter the cell causing it to swell (cytotoxic edema). Injury to the blood–brain barrier causes it to become leaky and fluid enters the cerebral interstitial space with consequent swelling. This is known as vasogenic edema. Cerebral edema does not become apparent clinically until 24–48 h after the asphyxial event, by which time progressive swelling is obvious on macroscopic examination with flattening of the gyri and obliteration of sulci. Rarely, herniation of the uncus through the tentorium or cerebellar displacement through the foramen magnum is found. Cerebral edema may be detected either clinically or by imaging.

The causes of neuronal death

In recent years advances in neurobiology have advanced our understanding of how neuronal death ensues from an hypoxic–ischemic insult. The key to this process is excitotoxic activation of neuroreceptors which is particularly enhanced in the immature brain. A severe asphyxial event causes excessive accumulation of excitatory amino acid neurotransmitters such as glutamate which accumulates in the synaptic space. This results from increased release and reduced reuptake of glutamate and causes excessive stimulation of calcium channels. There are at least three glutamate-like receptor ligands, which are named from the agents that individually excite them and can be divided into either N-methyl-D-aspartate (NMDA) receptors or non-NMDA receptors. As a result of opening these channels, Ca^{2+} floods into the neurone disrupting intracellular processes and activating a cascade of abnormal biochemical events which results in cell death. This cascade includes generation of nitric oxide (a free radical) and peroxynitrate with activation of lipases and proteases which in turn damage intracellular membranes particularly of the mitochondria with further production of oxygen free radicals thus further fuelling the toxic cycle. During hypoxia, ATP is degraded with the production of adenosine, inosine and hypoxanthine. At resuscitation and reperfusion the enzyme xanthine oxidase uses any available oxygen to convert hypoxanthine or xanthine to uric acid with the production of large quantities of free radicals. This may cause progressive mitochondrial compromise.

It is now recognized that cell death occurs in one of two ways; necrosis and apoptosis which can be distinguished on histological examination. The former is an explosive process due to energy (adenosine triphosphate; ATP) depletion with disruption of nuclear and cytoplasmic membranes. Apoptosis refers to a genetically programmed energy requiring cell suicide reaction to an hypoxic–ischemic event leading to cell shrinkage. This appears to be much more prevalent in the immature than the mature brain subjected to an asphyxial insult and probably occurs significantly later than necrosis. Apoptosis is mediated by casapase activity (particularly caspase-3) derived from the mitochondrion and is probably stimulated by mitochondrial damage.

Selective brain injury evident on MRI occurs in regions of the immature brain which are particularly susceptible to excitotoxic activation including the basal ganglia, brainstem and perirolandic cortical region. Strategies to limit this brain damage in animal and human studies (see later) have exploited interruption of the biochemical cascade described here.

CLINICAL FEATURES

There is a characteristic sequence of abnormal clinical neurological signs associated with birth asphyxia. These have been well described and Table 10.9 lists the major clinical features. In the majority of cases the clinical pattern of HIE is only consistent for relatively mature newborn infants with a gestational age of 35 weeks or above. The very premature infant has a less well-developed nervous system and similar clinical signs may not be evident. In addition, other neuropathological conditions such as hemorrhage or periventricular leukomalacia are much more common in these infants, and any clinical signs are more likely to be related to these conditions. Nevertheless, very immature infants have been reported to develop the typical features of severe HIE, but this is rare. The description that follows is most relevant to the more mature infant.

Mild encephalopathy

Babies with mild encephalopathy exhibit relatively subtle abnormalities which last no longer than 3 days. They show no depression in conscious level, but are described as being 'hyperalert'. This refers to the appearance of hunger, yet not feeding well together with a wide-eyed gaze, but failure to fixate. They are overly responsive to external stimuli and show exaggerated and excessive numbers of spontaneous Moro reflexes. These babies often do not feed well and may need occasional gavage feeding. There is a net sympathetic effect with mydriasis and tachycardia. Clinically evident seizures are not a feature of mild encephalopathy.

Moderate encephalopathy

These children are more severely neurologically abnormal and show evidence of seizures. These may be relatively subtle including lip smacking, excessive sucking type movements as well as the more typical tonic or clonic convulsive activity. The infants also show differential tone. This refers to increased lower limb tone compared with that in the upper limbs as well as increased neck extensor tone compared with that of the neck flexors. This is best elicited by placing the baby in a sitting position with the head first extended and then flexed on the trunk. The baby's spontaneous movements are observed and if the infant holds his head in the extended position with little effort to flex it, then this confirms neck extensor muscle hypertonus. Lethargy is the other constant feature of moderate encephalopathy with reduction in spontaneous movements. The baby requires a higher sensory input to elicit a response. The Moro and other primitive reflexes are usually lost in the early stages, but the tendon jerks are often exaggerated. The infants show predominantly parasympathetic activity with relative bradycardia and constricted pupils. Recovery begins within the first week after birth and full recovery (if it occurs) may be delayed for a number of weeks.

Severe encephalopathy

These infants develop coma, although it may take several hours before the infants show severe respiratory depression and require mechanical ventilation. Seizures are also a prominent feature and these may be prolonged and very frequent. In the most severely asphyxiated infants, there may be no seizure activity either clinically or evident on electroencephalogram (EEG) monitoring as the brain's energy supply has been completely exhausted. Babies with severe encephalopathy are markedly hypotonic and show little spontaneous movement other than that due to seizures. Reflex activity is usually lost. These infants may die in the acute phase of their illness, but if they recover, their abnormal neurological signs may progress from hypotonia through to excessive hypertonia. Apparent neurological recovery may occur, but may take up to 6 weeks. Persistently abnormal neurological signs beyond this time are ominous predictors of subsequent cerebral palsy.

INVESTIGATION AND MONITORING TECHNIQUES

In clinical practice the main indications for investigation of cerebral function in babies with actual or suspected asphyxia is threefold; establishing a diagnosis, investigation where therapeutic intervention may be required or for prediction of outcome so that parents may be given the most accurate prognostic information.

Establishing a diagnosis

The diagnosis of 'birth asphyxia' is most commonly made on the basis of the clinical history and obstetric monitoring. It is always important to consider alternative causes for a baby's poor condition at birth or encephalopathy or an underlying cause for the asphyxial insult. Table 10.10 lists the main differential diagnosis for birth asphyxia and/or HIE. Meningitis must always be considered and a lumbar

Table 10.10 Differential diagnosis for HIE

Differential diagnosis for HIE
Meningitis (bacterial or viral)
Encephalitis (herpes simplex)
Inborn error of metabolism
Traumatic brain lesion (e.g. subdural hemorrhage)
Shock secondary to severe, acute antepartum or intrapartum hemorrhage
Congenital lung abnormality (e.g. diaphragmatic hernia)
Neuromuscular disorder (e.g. spinal muscular atrophy)
Maternal drug exposure (acute or chronic)
Congenital brain malformation (e.g. neuronal migration disorder)

puncture performed if there is any risk factor including prolonged rupture of the membranes, neonatal fever or systemic signs of infection. Neonatal herpes is another diagnosis which should be considered early and may mimic HIE. Metabolic disorders may produce an HIE-like syndrome, but lactic acidosis and hyperammonemia may also occur as a result of a severe asphyxial insult.

Investigation for therapeutic intervention

The two main treatable conditions which may require investigation are large subdural hemorrhage and subclinical convulsions. Ultrasound imaging is of particular value in the immature infant as hemorrhagic and ischemic lesions can be readily identified. Ultrasound imaging is of less value in the full-term infant as these lesions occur less frequently. The main role of ultrasound in the term baby who has suffered severe birth asphyxia is as a screening test to identify shift of the midline structures associated with large subdural hemorrhage. This is an uncommon lesion (see above) and, if suspected, a CT or MRI scan should be performed as the hemorrhage may require surgical evacuation.

Convulsions may be subtle and difficult to diagnose clinically or the baby may be paralyzed in order to facilitate mechanical ventilation and seizures will not be clinically evident. Electrical monitoring of cortical function is necessary to diagnose this condition in such infants. This may be performed by continuous amplitude integrated EEG (aEEG) also referred to as cerebral function monitoring (CFM). The signal is obtained by a pair of parietal electrodes and displayed in real-time by the baby's cot. Seizure activity lasting 20 s or more is easily recognized. Intermittent polygraphic EEG recordings can also be used to assess seizure activity. This will require more expertise in analyzing the traces and interpretation may be difficult outside of specialized centers. Electrocortical monitoring is most valuable for prognostic purposes (see below).

Intracranial hypertension due to cerebral edema is a commonly anticipated complication in asphyxiated infants, but in fact probably occurs in less than 50% of such infants and a sustained rise in pressure exceeding 15 mmHg is rare.[126] Measurement of raised intracranial pressure is unreliable by transfontanel devices and direct measurement by intracranial transducer is highly invasive and not indicated. There is no evidence that the medical treatment of raised intracranial pressure alters outcome.[127]

Prediction of outcome

The three main monitoring techniques which have been shown to predict outcome are brain imaging, electroencephalography and Doppler assessment of a major cerebral artery. These are discussed further in the section on prognosis (p. 204).

COMPLICATIONS

The fetus copes with an asphyxial event by a number of protective reflexes to preserve function to vital organs. Less well-perfused tissues may be particularly vulnerable to hypoxic–ischemic injury. Up to a third of full-term asphyxiated infants developed asphyxia-related complications in two different organ systems. The kidney appears to be most vulnerable, followed by the brain and then the heart. Gastrointestinal complications of asphyxia are uncommon. This section reviews organ damage at sites other than the brain.

Lungs

During intrapartum asphyxia, the fetus commonly passes meconium and gasping may occur due to brainstem compromise. The gasp causes meconium to be aspirated deep into the bronchial tree and this may cause a chemical pneumonitis with severe pulmonary hypertension and a high risk of air leak. The management of meconium aspiration is discussed on page 290. Those infants who are pharmacologically paralyzed in order to facilitate mechanical ventilation for this condition will not show clinical signs of encephalopathy and coincidental cerebral injury may not be recognized. These infants should have continuous EEG monitoring to assess cerebral function.

Cardiovascular system

Blood flow to the myocardium is preserved during asphyxial episodes, but cardiac compromise is a relatively common complication of hypoxic–ischemic injury. Myocardial dysfunction detected by Doppler ultrasound studies has been reported in 28–40% of asphyxiated infants.[128,129] Recognized complications include cardiogenic shock and hypotension, functional tricuspid incompetence secondary to acute cardiac dilation, arrhythmias and myocardial ischemia which may be diagnosed from the electrocardiogram.

Renal impairment

Acute tubular necrosis and oliguria occurs commonly following episodes of asphyxia. This usually recovers with supportive treatment alone. The incidence of renal impairment (oliguria) after birth asphyxia occurs in 23–55% of babies[130,131] and acute renal failure was reported in 19% of asphyxiated infants.[132] Acute retention of urine is also a relatively common complication following birth asphyxia and usually indicates very severe compromise, often associated with severe cerebral injury. Renal failure following asphyxia has also been reported to be due to myoglobinuria.

Gastrointestinal tract

NEC (see p. 285) is associated with hypoxic–ischemic events, but in mature infants this is rarely seen in conjunction with hypoxic–ischemic encephalopathy.

Metabolic disorders

One of the commonest metabolic complications of birth asphyxia is inappropriate antidiuretic hormone (ADH) secretion with concentrated urine, dilute plasma and hyponatremia. Transient hyperammonemia has been reported with asphyxia but the precise cause of this metabolic compromise is not known.

Hematological disorders

Disseminated intravascular coagulation (DIC) is a well-recognized complication of birth asphyxia and usually presents with excessive bleeding from puncture sites together with petechial hemorrhages. Secondary complications such as intracranial hemorrhages may occur as the result of the DIC.

MANAGEMENT

The management of birth asphyxia can be considered under a number of headings including diagnosis during the intrapartum period with rescue by expeditious delivery, effective resuscitation, general support of the infant, management of complications, brain-orientated intensive care and more speculative and novel treatments directed towards the early pathophysiology which leads to neuronal injury.

Intrapartum care

Modern obstetrics is directed towards the recognition of the high-risk fetus together with careful monitoring and early delivery if fetal distress is suspected. As discussed above, although there has been a marked increase in the proportion of pregnancies terminated by operative delivery, there is no evidence that electronic fetal monitoring reduces subsequent handicap.

Resuscitation

It is vital to ensure that the newborn infant is effectively resuscitated following intrapartum compromise and this may reduce the risk of subsequent complications. Neonatal resuscitation is discussed in detail on page 204.

General support

The asphyxiated infant may develop complications in almost any organ system and the infant who is recognized to have suffered from hypoxic–ischemic injury should be carefully monitored. Table 10.11 lists the categories of general support which should be considered. Any infant with major complications involving any organ system should be given the benefit of modern intensive care with very careful monitoring undertaken by experienced nursing and medical staff. The specific management of non-cerebral asphyxial injury is discussed elsewhere in this book. A particularly important and common complication of birth asphyxia is systemic hypotension and this should be detected by careful blood pressure monitoring. Undetected or inadequately treated hypotension will cause the already compromised brain to be further underperfused.

Brain-orientated care

Unfortunately there has been no advance in recent years in brain orientated management which has shown by randomized controlled trials to improve outcome. The practical management of moderate and severe HIE is listed in Table 10.12. More detailed discussion of some of these points is warranted.

Table 10.11 General methods for managing the asphyxiated infant and organ-related complications

General support	
Nurse in thermoneutral environment	
Avoid hypo- and hyperglycemia	
Measure blood gases:	
treat hypoxia with oxygen	
treat hypercarbia with IPPV	
Review infection risk and treat with antibiotics if appropriate	
Adequate hydration, do not dehydrate	
Treat hyperbilirubinemia	
Cardiovascular	
Hypotension	Plasma, inotrope support
Myocardial failure	Digoxin, inotrope support
Renal	
Oliguria	Careful assessment of fluid status
Acute tubular necrosis	Renal failure regimen Peritoneal dialysis if necessary
Pulmonary	
Meconium aspiration	Respiratory support
Metabolic	
Inappropriate ADHS	Restrict fluids
Hypoglycemia	Give glucose, but avoid inducing hyperglycemia
Hematological	
DIC	No specific therapy
Gastrointestinal	
NEC	Antibiotics, avoid enteral feeds

ADHS, antidiuretic hormone secretion; DIC, disseminated intravascular coagulation; IPPV, intermittent positive pressure ventilation; NEC, necrotizing enterocolitis.

Seizures

These are very common following intrapartum asphyxia and may be clinically evident or only detected on EEG monitoring. Treatment is often relatively unsuccessful and not infrequently multiple anticonvulsant medication may be necessary. It is likely that prolonged or frequent convulsions in neonates with already compromised cerebral function causes further neuronal injury,[133] but there is no evidence that abolition of all convulsions improves outcome. Exposing the infant to the minimum number of anticonvulsants is obviously important. It is not necessary to abolish all convulsions, but treatment should be started for frequent (> 2/h) or prolonged (≥ 1 min) convulsions. The following drugs are used to treat postasphyxial convulsions.

Phenobarbital. This is the first-line anticonvulsant for neonatal seizures. The loading dose is 20 mg/kg followed 12 h later by 6 mg/kg/24 h given twice daily. High-dose phenobarbital monotherapy has been suggested to be a useful method for treating seizures resistant to standard phenobarbital treatment.[134] They suggest that if seizures continue, a further infusion of 5–10 mg/kg of phenobarbital is given over a 10–15 min period and repeated every 20–30 min until seizures stop or the serum level of drug exceeds 40 µg/ml. Two-thirds of convulsing neonates responded to this form of management. More recently, a randomized (non-blinded) controlled study of phenobarbital (40 mg/kg over 1 h) prior to the onset of seizures in 20 severely asphyxiated babies showed that the outcome at 3 years was significantly better than in a similar group of babies where phenobarbital was only given after onset of seizures.[135] A meta-analysis of barbiturate treatment in asphyxia did not, however, show an overall beneficial effect when all such studies were considered together.[136]

Other anticonvulsants. Clonazepam can be used as a second-line anticonvulsant (100 µg/kg loading dose) followed by an intermittent dosage regimen every 24 h. Phenytoin is also widely used to treat ongoing convulsions but is contraindicated with lidocaine (lignocaine) (see below). The loading dose is 20 mg/kg intravenously, but maintenance therapy is very unpredictable in its effect and is not recommended in the neonatal period.

More recently, two other anticonvulsants have been used to treat asphyxiated infants; midazolam (0.05 mg/kg as a loading dose followed by 0.15 mg/kg/h) and lidocaine (lignocaine) 2 mg/kg loading dose followed by 6 mg/kg/h. There may be synergism between these drugs, and they may be a useful combination in

Table 10.12 Brain-orientated management. The dosages of the anticonvulsants are discussed in the text

Cerebral perfusion
- Carefully monitor blood pressure and maintain a mean arterial blood pressure > 40 mmHg in full-term infants

Seizures
- Treat initial seizures with phenobarbital
- If intermittent seizures, give paraldehyde
- If persistent seizures, consider:
  - phenytoin (avoid maintenance therapy)
  - clonazepam
  - midazolam
  - lidocaine (lignocaine)

Intracranial hypertension
- Give 20% less than daily fluid requirements
- If full fontanel and seizures, give mannitol 20% (1 g/kg), avoid if the baby is oliguric

babies with refractory seizures. The potentially cardiotoxic effects of lidocaine (lignocaine) are rarely seen except if phenytoin has been used prior to its administration.

Brain swelling

Treatment is commonly directed towards the prevention and reduction of raised intracranial pressure. It is traditional to keep asphyxiated infants relatively dehydrated by carefully monitoring serum electrolytes and urinary specific gravity to give just enough fluid to keep the infant on the dry side of normal hydration. Fluid restriction (20% less than daily requirements) is only necessary for the first 48 h of life.

There is no evidence that the treatment of cerebral edema or raised intracranial pressure improves outcome (see above). Mannitol has been shown to significantly reduce brain water in an animal model when given immediately after an asphyxial event[137] but it did not reduce the severity or distribution of brain damage. Although 20% mannitol infusion reduced intracranial pressure, we found no improvement in outcome in babies given intravenous mannitol.[138] The routine measurement of intracranial pressure is not indicated, but if the infant is neurologically abnormal and has a bulging fontanel, 20% mannitol may reduce intracranial hypertension and should be given as a 20% solution, 1 g/kg by continuous infusion over 20 min. Mannitol is contraindicated in the presence of oliguria or severe renal compromise as this may cause a rebound effect with increased swelling of the brain and an increase in pressure due to failure of the infant to excrete the drug.

In older children and adults with presumed or actual cerebral edema the $PaCO_2$ is usually adjusted to between 3.5 and 4 kPa. This reduces intracranial pressure by reducing intracranial blood volume but there is no evidence that this actually improves outcome. It is now apparent that hyperventilation with reduction in $PaCO_2$ increases neuropathology in immature experimental animals[139] and human premature infants.[140] Limited data in mature newborn animals do not suggest a similar adverse effect.[141] In the human infant there is no evidence that maintaining a $PaCO_2$ lower than the normal range is of any benefit and it is potentially dangerous in immature babies as cerebral ischemia may be induced.

Steroids have no effect on experimental global cerebral edema when given following birth asphyxia. Corticosteroid treatment may be associated with adverse outcome and should not be used.

Early prevention of neuronal injury

Intervention strategies to prevent or modify secondary neuronal death following an hypoxic–ischemic insult is the subject of much basic scientific research and has recently been well reviewed by Hagberg et al.[142] This is an exciting area for the future and randomized clinical trials are currently underway in severely asphyxiated human newborn infants to evaluate potential benefit of some of these forms of therapy. To date these new therapies are experimental and cannot be recommended.

Hypothermia

This therapy may have effects in many parts of the abnormal biochemical cascade leading to neuronal death including reduction of free radical production, excitotoxic amino acids and proinflammatory cytokines. There is evidence that hypothermia may have an important role in the reduction of apoptotic neuronal death. Studies of mild hypothermia (34–35°C) in various neonatal animal species[142] immediately after experimental hypoxic–ischemic insult suggests that there is protection against neuronal compromise. Human studies are underway using regional head cooling as well as total body cooling and reports suggest that this can be done safely,[143–145] but these studies are unfinished and there are no data on medium to long term outcome of survivors.

Allopurinol

The majority of free radicals are produced during resuscitation following an asphyxial insult. Xanthine oxidase inhibition with either allopurinol or oxypurinol reduces free radical production[146] and allopurinol given after an hypoxic–ischemic insult results in a significant reduction in cerebral edema and neuronal destruction.[147] A pilot study of allopurinol given after asphyxia in full-term infants has shown benefit in cerebral function although no follow-up data are yet available.[148] There is currently a randomized control trial in human babies of this form of treatment in The Netherlands.

PROGNOSIS

The outcome for birth asphyxia depends upon the criteria used to make the diagnosis. As discussed above, the diagnosis of birth asphyxia in premature infants is more difficult than in the full-term infant and obvious neuropathology evident on imaging is much more commonly detected in the premature group. The prognosis in premature infants is usually more accurately made on the basis of whether the infant has parenchymal hemorrhage or periventricular leukomalacia than how low the Apgar score was or the need for intubation or resuscitation. The prognosis related to these specific neuropathological events is discussed below.

Apgar scores

There is a close relationship between severe (Apgar 0–3) and moderate (Apgar 4–6) depression of Apgar score and mortality.[149] In preterm babies (26–36 weeks' gestation) with Apgar 0–3 at 5 min the neonatal mortality rate was 315 per 1000 infants compared to 5 per 1000 for similar infants with 5 min scores of 7–10. In term infants the neonatal death rate was 244 per 1000 in those born with Apgar scores 0–3 at 5 min.

Depression of Apgar scores is an insensitive method for predicting handicap in newborn infants. The risk of death or disability (cerebral palsy) in infants with severely depressed Apgar scores is shown in Table 10.13.[150] It is not until the Apgar score remains at 0–3 by 20 min that there is a relatively high risk of cerebral palsy. Such a small proportion of newborn infants have depression of the Apgar score to this degree as to make its predictive ability of little relevance. Thomson et al[151] reported that 93% of infants with an Apgar score of 0 at 1 min and/or 0–3 at 5 min were entirely normal at follow-up. Levene et al[152] graded the severity of Apgar score depression according to different criteria in an effort to

Table 10.13 Risk of death or cerebral palsy (CP) in infants with Apgar scores of 0–3 at varying times from birth (data from Nelson & Ellenberg 1981[150])

Age (min)	Death in first year <2500 g (%)	CP <2500 g (%)	Death in first year >2500 g (%)	CP >2500 g (%)
1	26	2	3	0.7
5	55	7	8	0.7
10	67	7	18	5
15	84	0	48	9
20	96	0	59	57

establish how predictive these scores were for serious impairment at a median age of 2.5 years. They found that an Apgar score of 5 or less at 10 min was the most sensitive for adverse outcome, but that this was far less good than a prediction based on encephalopathy.

HIE

Peliowski & Finer[153] have reported an overall outcome related to the severity of HIE. There was a remarkable consensus in prediction, although many of the grading systems had slight variations in detail. All referred to three grades of encephalopathy considered to be mild, moderate or severe. No infant with mild encephalopathy alone developed significant impairment. The median risk of impairment from five follow-up studies in full-term infants with moderate encephalopathy (seizures, but not coma) was 25% (range 17–27%) and for severe encephalopathy (seizures and coma) 92% died or were severely handicapped (range 75–100%).[154] Mortality in the group of infants with moderate HIE is 4.5%, compared with 62% mortality in those with severe HIE.[153] Of the surviving infants with moderate HIE, 20% were severely disabled and 71% in the severe HIE group. The accuracy of prognosis based on HIE is far better than Apgar scores or delay in establishing respiration. Follow-up at 8 years in survivors of HIE confirmed that the longer term prognosis was very poor for infants who had sustained severe HIE.[155] Those children who had sustained moderate HIE and who had no evidence of neurological impairment at 8 years nevertheless had a significant reduction in IQ (102) compared with those who had mild HIE (IQ 106) and a control group (IQ 112) ($p < 0.001$).

Brain imaging

CT appears to be a good predictor of subsequent outcome in asphyxiated full-term babies, but only if the scan is performed after the first week of life (see Levene[154] for review). This limits the value of the technique in the acute management of the severely asphyxiated infant in whom withdrawal of care is considered.

More recently MRI has been widely evaluated for its prognostic role in asphyxiated babies. The feature which is the best predictor in the first 10 days of life is abnormal signal in the posterior limb of the internal capsule (PLIC), best seen on IR sequences.[156] Abnormal or equivocal PLIC signal has a sensitivity of 90%, specificity of 100% and positive predictive value of 100% for abnormal outcome. More general abnormalities within the basal ganglia (usually including abnormal PLIC) are generally predictive of poor outcome and abnormalities with cortical highlighting in the perirolandic area often accompanies these abnormalities.[157,158]

Doppler

Doppler assessment is also an accurate predictor of adverse outcome in asphyxiated full-term infants.[159–162] A low Pourcelot Resistance Index (PRI) or a high mean flow velocity above 3 SD from the mean has a positive predictive value for adverse outcome of 94%.[159] These Doppler abnormalities appear within 12–60 h after birth.[159,162]

Electrocortical activity

Assessment of cerebral function by EEG is a very useful prognostic tool. An overview of four studies[153] found that a normal or mildly abnormal EEG had an excellent prognosis (likelihood ratio of adverse outcome 0.03, 95% CI 0.01–0.11) compared with a likelihood ratio of 1.56 (95% CI 0.82–2.96) for moderate EEG abnormality (slow wave activity). A severely abnormal EEG (burst suppression, low voltage or isoelectric EEG) gave a very poor prognosis with a likelihood ratio for adverse outcome of 18.60 (95% CI 6.88–50.00). Further studies published since this meta-analysis have confirmed these findings.[163,164]

Studies using aEEG assessment (CFM) have also shown that this technique gives accurate prognostic information following birth asphyxia.[160,165–167] Specific abnormalities predictive of poor outcome include an isoelectric or very low voltage (< 5 uV) trace or a discontinuous burst-suppression pattern.[168] Major abnormalities at 6 h or later were associated with a poor prognosis.[160] At 6 h of age the CFM was the best predictor of any test of outcome in asphyxiated full-term infants with a positive and negative predictive value of 84.2% and 91.7% respectively.

Practical approach to prognosis

At the present time there is no proven effective treatment in asphyxiated infants. It may be appropriate to recognize a group of infants with very poor prognosis so that an informed discussion about withdrawal of intensive care can be conducted with the parents. The author suggests that two separate assessments with both EEG (or CFM) and Doppler should be carried out at 6 h and 24 h. If the EEG (CFM) is severely abnormal at 6 and 24 h and the Doppler is abnormal at 24 h then the prognosis is extremely poor and the parents should be made aware of this.

RESUSCITATION IN THE NEWBORN

In Western countries relatively few mature newborn infants require active resuscitation at birth. In Sweden, just 1% of babies weighing over 2.5 kg required artificial ventilation, but significantly 20% of these were unexpected in babies with no obvious risk factors.[169] In the UK, a comparison between two large obstetric units found that there was a fivefold variation in the proportion of newborn infants who required intubation; 2% vs 10%. In the developing world it is estimated that 1 million babies a year die of asphyxia and that lack of simple airway interventions is a significant factor in many of these deaths. The more preterm the delivery, the more likely it will be that the baby needs active resuscitation.

The physiology of fetal hypoxia leading to the need for resuscitation at birth is well understood and has been known for many years. In recent years, a number of national and multidisciplinary groups have described optimal practice for neonatal resuscitation based on the best available scientific evidence.[170–172] Although there are some differences in detail between these recommendations these are relatively minor. Current recommendations are outlined in this section.

THE PHYSIOLOGICAL RESPONSE TO HYPOXIA

Our understanding of the newborn's response to hypoxia is based on neonatal animal experiments published in the 1960s[173,174] and is summarized in Figure 10.10.[174] At the onset of hypoxia there is a period of small-volume but rapid breaths lasting for several minutes followed by a period of primary apnea. Prior to primary apnea the heart rate and blood pressure are maintained. Once apnea occurs the heart rate falls, but with increasing stroke volume a good cardiac output is maintained with continued perfusion of the vital organs. At this stage the baby looks cyanosed.

If hypoxia continues then after a period of primary apnea lasting up to 5 min, spontaneous gasping occurs (10–15 per min) and this lasts for a further period of 5–6 min before a second period of apnea develops. This is referred to as terminal apnea and if nothing is done to resuscitate the animal at this time death will occur within another 10 min. During the period of primary apnea and subsequent gasping, blood pressure and heart rate are maintained, but with increasing metabolic acidemia. Cardiovascular deterioration commences with the onset of terminal apnea.

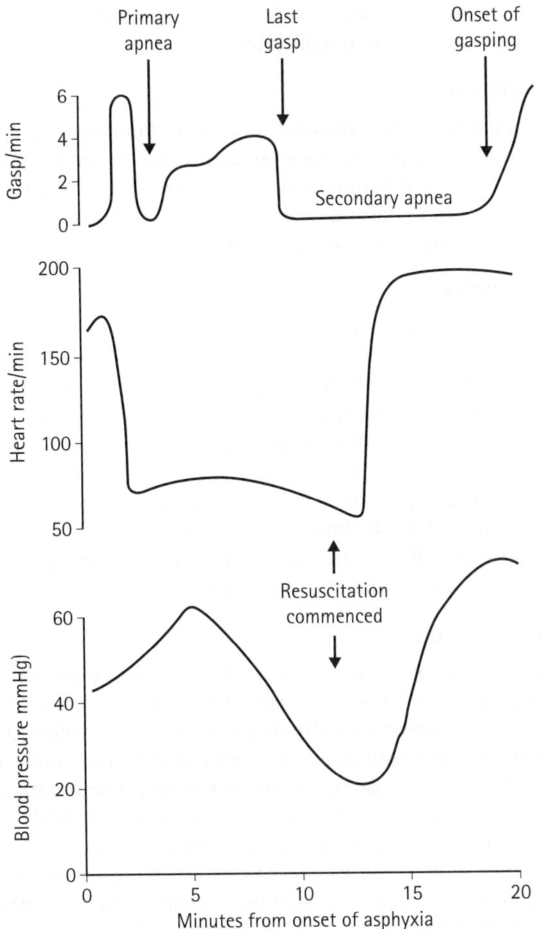

Fig. 10.10 The effects of asphyxia on a newborn animal showing primary and secondary apnea. (Redrawn from Dawes 1968[174] with permission of Blackwell Scientific Publications.)

These timings are based on rhesus monkey studies, but are likely to reflect the human situation although the timing of the sequence of events may be a little shorter than in monkeys.

THE PRINCIPLES OF NEONATAL RESUSCITATION

All babies must be born in an environment where they have rapid access to expert resuscitation skills. In home births there must be two attendants, one responsible for resuscitating the baby should this be necessary who has appropriate training and equipment in full working order. Most babies will require no active resuscitation other than gentle stimulation, but others are slow to adapt to their extrauterine environment and some active steps will need to be taken by caregivers. The vigor of the response will depend on the stage of the baby's reaction to the hypoxic event. The baby who is not breathing may start to breathe spontaneously if in the stage of primary apnea but will not if in secondary apnea. Whether the baby is in primary or secondary apnea may be difficult to determine clinically. Consequently, the attendant must undertake a measured response and be prepared to escalate resuscitative measures if the initial response is inadequate.

Many, but by no means all, infants who are born in a depressed state can be anticipated and Table 10.14 lists the indications for calling a pediatrician or other person competent to resuscitate the newborn infant.

Table 10.14 Indications for calling a pediatrician to be present at a delivery

Prematurity
Gestation < 36 weeks
Fetal distress
Thick meconium staining
Severely abnormal CTG
Fetal scalp acidosis (pH < 7.2)
Operative delivery
Any delivery under general anesthesia
Mid-cavity or rotational forceps
Multiple pregnancy
Significant antepartum hemorrhage
Fetal disease
Known major congenital abnormality
Rhesus disease

CTG, cardiotocograph

PREPARATION PRIOR TO DELIVERY

The pediatrician called for a high-risk delivery should spend some time prior to delivery acquainting himself with the mother's medical and antenatal history. It is important that he checks all the equipment that may be required prior to delivery and not rely on the fact that this should have been done by others.

Resuscitation trolley

A stop clock permanently fixed to the trolley is started at delivery, giving the operator a reference point for the duration of resuscitation. An integral overhead heater should be of fixed height above the infant with a dial to give variable temperature settings.

Medical gases

It is most important that both air and oxygen are readily available, together with appropriate reduction valves so that a variable and measurable flow of gas can be given to the infant. One gas line must be available for face mask oxygen and another that can be attached to an endotracheal tube (ET) via a Y-piece connector. The arm of the Y-piece not connected to the ET tube can be occluded by the pediatrician's thumb which will direct the gas mixture into the baby's lungs at regular intervals for predetermined periods of time. As well as controlling the flow of gas a blow-off valve must be fitted so that the baby's lungs are not overdistended by unacceptably high pressures. On many resuscitation trolleys a water manometer valve is used, set to blow off at a maximum of 30 cm of water.

Suction

The presence of suction apparatus on the resuscitation trolley is essential. This must also be fitted with an accurate valve device with a display of negative pressure as too high a suction pressure may damage the infant's respiratory tract. A variety of electric suction devices are manufactured for use in neonatal resuscitation and are perfectly acceptable. Mouth suction must not be used. A number of suction catheters of different sizes (FG 4, 6 and 8) must also be at hand with appropriate connectors to attach to the suction device.

Bag and mask

Bag and mask resuscitation equipment is essential in every hospital where babies are delivered or cared for and all staff must be familiar with their effective use. The method for appropriate bag and mask ventilation is described below. A number of different bags exist, the best being the Laerdal type. These are fitted with blow-off valves which can be adjusted to give a maximum inflation pressure. Tubing can be fitted to these devices so that the baby can be ventilated with additional oxygen. As well as the bag, a tight-fitting deformable Laerdal face mask is essential. These should be of variable sizes to fit the faces of the smallest and the biggest babies likely to be encountered. The technique is shown in Figure 10.11.[175] The baby's head is slightly extended and one hand elevates the mandible. The tightly fitting Silastic face mask covers the mouth and nose and is pressed down to form an airtight seal. The bag is then squeezed using two or three fingers just hard enough to produce good symmetrical chest expansion. More forceful inflation is unnecessary and dangerous.

Intubation equipment

Two laryngoscopes should be available with fresh batteries and these should be checked prior to delivery of the baby. A selection of endotracheal tubes should be present varying in size from 2.5 to 4.0 mm. The correct connector must also be available together with a malleable metal introducer. Reliable means of securing the tube to the baby's face should also be available and the assisting nurse must be skilled in the fixation of the tube. A stethoscope should be worn by the resuscitator prior to delivery of the baby.

A SCHEME FOR RESUSCITATION

A resuscitation must match the clinical condition of the baby. Most babies require nothing more than tactile stimulation, but babies born in a very poor condition (Apgar score ≤ 3 at 1 min) should if possible be intubated immediately by someone with advanced resuscitation skills. If such a person is not available, oxygen must be given by bag and mask until a more skilled person arrives. The techniques below should be practiced by all involved with the delivery of newborn infants. Each section follows if the previous one fails to achieve the desired result of a pink oxygenated baby in good condition.

Tactile stimulation

This is all that is necessary for the vast majority of babies. Dry the baby with a towel and clear the airway by gentle suction of mouth and nose. Blind pharyngeal suction may cause vagal stimulation with apnea and bradycardia and should be avoided. Flicking the toes or rubbing the baby's back may be effective if drying and clearing the airways are not effective.

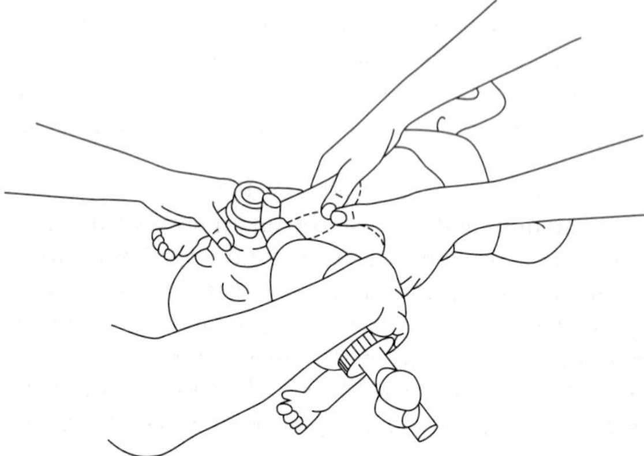

Fig. 10.11 Cardiorespiratory resuscitation. One operator inflates the baby's lungs with the bag and mask. The head is slightly extended and the chin pulled forward. The other operator gives external cardiac massage with hands encircling the chest. (From Levene et al 1987 with permission of Blackwell Scientific Publications.)

Open airway

If spontaneous breathing does not occur with stimulation, lie the baby on its back with the head looking up. Ensure that the neck is extended but not too far or this may obstruct the airway. Give chin support (Fig. 10.12). An oropharyngeal airway (Guedel) should be used if there is an orofacial abnormality such as cleft palate or hypoplastic chin.

Inflate lungs

This should initially be performed by a self-inflating bag and mask if the baby has not started breathing spontaneously by 30–60 s.[176] A soft round face mask of the appropriate size for the baby should be selected. The bag should have a blow-off valve of 30 cm of water and be connected to 100% oxygen flow at 5 L/min. Apply the mask to the baby's face ensuring a tight fit so that gas does not leak out. Inflate the lungs with pressures of 30 cm of water for 2–3 s each (five in all) to replace the lung fluid with oxygen. Premature babies (<30 weeks) usually require lower inflation pressures. Satisfactory oxygenation leads to an increase in the heart rate.

Ventilate lungs

If the baby does not breathe spontaneously after these five inflations give intermittent positive pressure ventilation (IPPV) at 30 breaths/min. Observe good movement of the chest wall with each breath. If the chest wall does not move consider the reason. Is the head in the correct position? Could there be a pneumothorax or pulmonary hypoplasia? Satisfactory oxygenation leads to an increase in heart rate. If spontaneous respiration has not occurred by a further 2 min consider the need for naloxone (see below). Intubation with continued ventilation is recommended if the baby is not breathing spontaneously by 2 min. Is there chest wall movement with each breath now? If not, consider why not. Is the endotracheal tube misplaced? Is there a pneumothorax? Could there be pulmonary hypoplasia? Call for help! Earlier intubation may be performed in babies born in poor condition (Apgar score ≤ 3 at 1 min) or those very preterm if personnel with advanced resuscitation skills are present. There is however, no evidence that outcome is improved by routinely intubating all very immature babies although this may be necessary prior to transportation to a neonatal unit.

Chest compression

If the heart rate has not improved despite adequate artificial ventilation chest compression is indicated. Use the two handed method shown in Figure 10.11. The thumbs should meet on the sternum in the line of the nipples with the fingers over the spine.

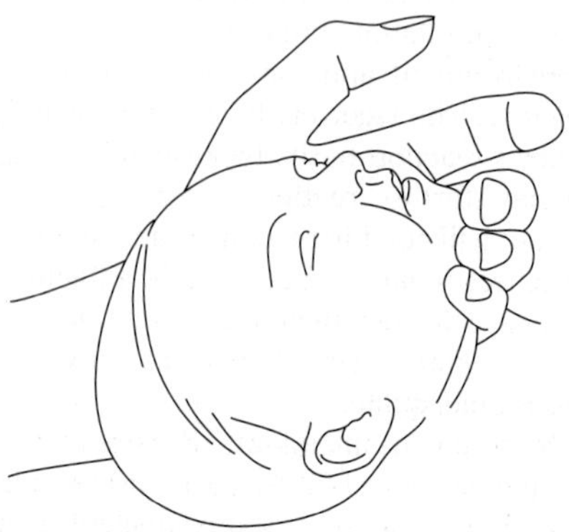

Fig. 10.12 Slight head extension with chin support to open airway.

Use enough force to compress the chest wall by one-third of its anteroposterior (AP) diameter. Coordinate compressions and ventilation in a ratio of 3:1 at a rate of 120 events/min to achieve 90 compressions and 30 breaths/min.

Drugs

Epinephrine (adrenaline) is the key drug to use when the heart rate remains < 60 beats/min (bpm) despite 30 s of adequate ventilation and chest compression. Give 10 μg/kg (0.1 ml/kg) of 1:10 000 solution down the ET tube. This can be repeated up to three times. Alternatively, if vascular access is available this can be given intravenously through an umbilical catheter.

If there is no improvement, re-evaluate the adequacy of ventilation. Consider hypovolemia – give 10 ml/kg of normal saline or dextrose saline. If still no improvement and significant time has passed and a senior experienced person is present, consider withdrawal of active treatment.

Naloxone is a specific opiate antagonist and is indicated if the baby is slow in establishing spontaneous respiration and the mother had received an opiate for pain relief with 4 h prior to delivery. The dose is 200 μg i.m. or 0.5 ml of 'adult' narcan. Smaller doses will have a short acting effect which may be significantly less than the duration of opiate toxicity in the newborn thereby requiring multiple doses. When given intravenously to term babies the plasma level peaks at 5–40 min and 30–120 min when given i.m.[177] The latter is the most appropriate route of administration. Do not give naloxone to the baby of an opiate dependent mother as this may cause acute and severe withdrawal symptoms in the baby.

Vascular access

Only epinephrine (adrenaline) can be given through the ET tube although the US recommendations include the option of giving naloxone down the tube. It is probably best given i.m. if there is reasonable tissue blood flow. If other drugs or fluid need to be given then the most rapid access is by cannulation of the umbilical vein. As a rough guide the radio-opaque cannula should not be inserted further than the distance from the umbilicus to the internipple line for it to lie in the inferior vena cava.

CONTROVERSIES IN NEONATAL RESUSCITATION

Sodium bicarbonate

The use of this substance routinely in neonatal resuscitation is not recommended as there are no neonatal studies showing a benefit. It should not be used during periods of brief cardiopulmonary resuscitation (CPR) and avoided unless there is adequate ventilation as expiration of CO_2 is necessary for it to have a buffer effect. The appropriate dose is 1–2 mmol/kg (2–4 ml/kg) of 4.2% solution given through the umbilical venous catheter.

Volume expansion

This should only be given when a baby is thought to be hypovolemic. This may occur as a result of prenatal bleeding, premature clamping of the cord, when the baby is held above the mother prior to cord clamping or with a nuchal cord and failure of adequate blood flow to the fetus from the placenta. If the baby is shocked at birth and is thought to have bled acutely then he should be given an infusion of O-negative blood immediately.

There remains considerable controversy about the role of albumin in treating hypovolemia. There is evidence from a Cochrane overview that mortality is higher when albumin is used compared with a crystalloid solution although there was only one neonatal study included in this review.[178] An isotonic crystalloid solution such as normal saline is recommended in both the British and American Neonatal Resuscitation guidelines. Give 10 ml/kg over 5–10 min initially and this can be repeated if necessary.

Resuscitation in air or 100% oxygen

There has been considerable debate about the benefit of initial resuscitation in air compared with 100% oxygen. Data from animal and human studies have been well reviewed by Saugstad[179] and show that oxidative stress was higher when 100% oxygen was used for early resuscitation. Three randomized control studies with allocation to one or other of these gas regimens at birth showed no major differences in outcome between the two groups except those given air had significantly better Apgar scores[180,181] and time to first breath was longer in the 100% oxygen group.[181,182] It is suggested that the effects of 100% oxygen may be more adverse in preterm infants than at term.[179] Despite these studies the consensus guideline on resuscitation from the UK and US recommend using 100% oxygen if assisted ventilation is required. Where an oxygen blender is available 40% oxygen may be an alternative.

Meconium stained liquor

Approximately 15% of babies are born with meconium staining of the liquor and in approximately 5% meconium aspiration syndrome (MAS) occurs. In the presence of severe prenatal hypoxia, gasping causes aspiration of meconium deep into the bronchial tree. In the USA 25–60% of infants with MAS require mechanical ventilation.[183,184] Strategies to reduce the risk of MAS include amnioinfusion to dilute the meconium prior to delivery and suctioning the oro- and nasopharynx after birth of the head and before delivery of the baby's trunk[185] although others have not shown a similar beneficial effect (see Wiswell[186] for review) and this technique remains of unproven benefit. In a large randomized control study of apparently vigorous babies born through meconium stained liquor, intubation and suctioning did not reduce the incidence of MAS compared with conservative management (seven in five). Chest compression immediately after birth to avoid aspiration of meconium is dangerous and should not be performed.

The US recommendations for resuscitation of a baby born through meconium stained liquor is initially thorough suctioning of the mouth, nose and pharynx with either a bulb syringe or 12F to 14F suction catheter as soon as the head is delivered and before the body emerges. After delivery, if the baby is in a *depressed* state (slow to establish regular breathing, reduced tone, or heart rate < 100 bpm) then immediate direct laryngoscopy should be performed with intubation/suctioning of any residual meconium from the trachea under direct vision. Saline lavage is not recommended. Delay gastric suctioning of meconium until initial resuscitation is complete. If the baby is vigorous intratracheal suctioning is not recommended.

Hypothermia

Controlled hypothermia to 35°C is currently being evaluated as a therapeutic modality in severe birth asphyxia (p. 197), but it is not appropriate to allow a baby to become cold during resuscitation. Hypothermia is particularly disadvantageous in preterm infants in whom it has been shown to increase mortality. Conversely, inadvertent hyperthermia must be avoided during resuscitation and this may occur as a result of an overhead warmer. This may cause an exacerbation of cerebral injury.

WHEN TO STOP RESUSCITATION

All babies should be considered for active resuscitation, unless they are macerated or show an obvious lethal congenital malformation.

In very immature babies of 23 weeks' gestation and below it is most appropriate to discuss with the parents prior to the delivery what the treatment options are. The parents should be encouraged to consider whether they wish their baby to receive resuscitation at birth and their views should be respected. If the baby is vigorous at birth it may be appropriate to resuscitate fully and transfer the baby to the neonatal unit where with time a more considered decision can be made about the continuation of intensive care. This option should be put to the parents prior to delivery of the infant.

In mature infants failure to achieve a spontaneous cardiac output after 10 min of vigorous resuscitation indicates a very poor prognosis and resuscitation should be abandoned. A more difficult situation is when the baby has a reasonable cardiac output but fails to breathe. Other causes of respiratory failure must first be considered such as maternal drug effect and neuromuscular disorders. If the baby is not breathing by 40 min and particularly if he remains extremely depressed with severe hypotonia, then further active resuscitation should be considered to be inappropriate. The most senior doctor available should make this decision. If there is any doubt it is best to take the baby to the NICU until such time as a full assessment can be made. It is much easier for the parents to mourn the loss of their baby if they are convinced that full resuscitation was attempted and they will come to terms with it better if they have time to understand the severe problems that are present. Parents should be encouraged to hold their baby when resuscitative efforts are abandoned.

THE SMALL FOR GESTATIONAL AGE INFANT (Fig. 10.13)

The WHO in 1950 defined a baby as small for gestational age (SGA) when it was below the 10th weight centile for gestation. At that time perinatal mortality of this group even in the Western world was very high. Obstetric deaths due to placental failure in utero and acute intrapartum asphyxia were relatively common. Neonatal problems such as pulmonary hemorrhage and hypoglycemia were inadequately treated and the mortality and morbidity from congenital rubella was commoner (immunization schedules were not introduced until 1966 in the UK). Times have now changed but the definition has not. With modern antenatal and intrapartum care it is unusual for the pediatrician to be confronted by an unexpectedly small baby. Intrauterine and peripartum asphyxia and death are rarities. Rubella embryopathy is much less common and ultrasound policies for infants early diagnosed as small may allow termination of pregnancy for a lethal congenital abnormality. Better feeding policies postnatally have made all but the smallest of light for dates babies (SGA) manageable with care on the postnatal wards. It is unlikely that the baby more than 1800 g birth weight will need to be transferred to the neonatal unit if delivery care and care on the postnatal wards are appropriate.[187]

ETIOLOGY

Maternal causes

Maternal causes are: in utero starvation and placental insufficiency [essential hypertension, pregnancy associated hypertension (PET), chronic renal disease, longstanding diabetes, heart disease in pregnancy, multiple pregnancy, poor socioeconomic circumstances with severe malnutrition, excess smoking, excess alcohol, living at high altitude]. Classically, placental insufficiency leads to asymmetric growth retardation, the weight being more affected than the length or particularly the head circumference. The obstetrician may identify this problem in utero, ultrasound showing a small abdominal and thoracic circumference and a relatively spared head circumference. Small mothers and elderly primigravidae tend to have smaller than average babies.

Fetal causes

Fetal causes are: congenital abnormality (chromosomal and many syndromes, e.g. Potter's) and congenital infection [rubella,

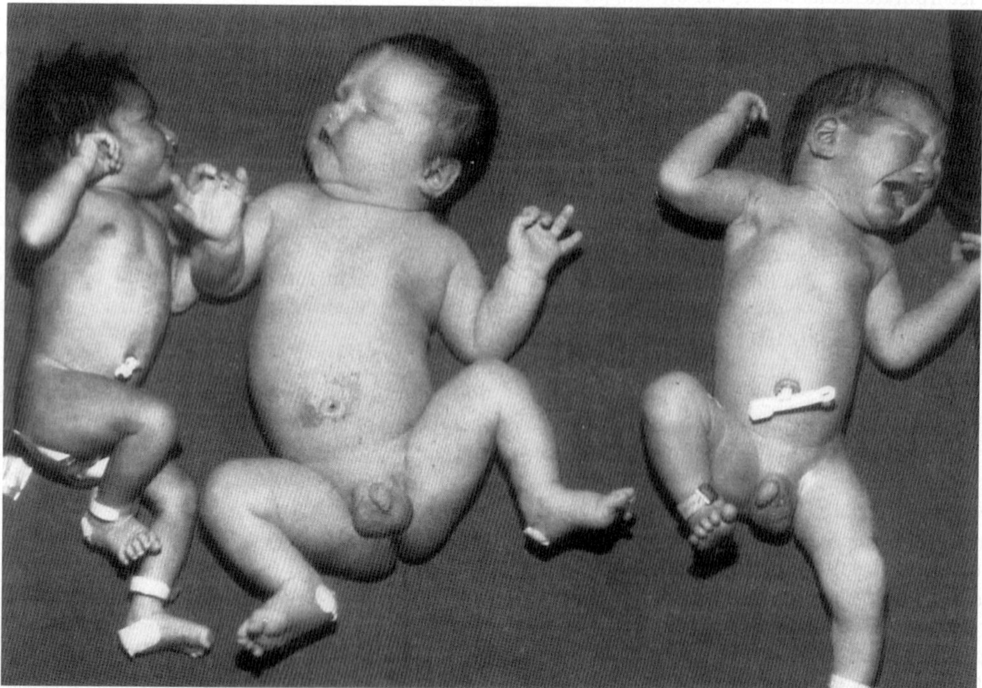

Fig. 10.13 Size with gestation. The baby on the left at 1.7 kg and 39 weeks is small for gestational age. The baby on the right is 1.9 kg and 34 weeks' gestation and is both appropriate for gestation and preterm. The center baby at 4.4 kg and 39 weeks' gestation is large for gestational age.

toxoplasmosis, cytomegalovirus (CMV), herpes simplex and syphilis] and early fetal toxins such as alcohol, phenytoin and warfarin. Such infants usually display symmetrical growth retardation, the head size being as retarded as the weight and length.

PROBLEMS OF THE SGA BABY

Hypoglycemia

Before modern neonatal treatment developed, 60% of preterm babies who were also SGA and 30% of full-term SGA babies developed hypoglycemia. Hypoglycemia may be present before birth. The etiology after birth is complex.

1. Reduced glycogen deposits (in liver, muscle and heart).
2. The brain and heart (but not the liver, spleen, thymus and adrenals) are large in proportion to the rest of the body and have high energy substrate demands.
3. A reduced catecholamine response to a falling blood sugar suggests that the adrenal medulla is failing with consequent reduced glycogenolysis.
4. Rapid glucose disappearance may in some cases be due to high insulin levels. However many infants show a reduced insulin response to a glucose load which suggests either a defect in peripheral glucose utilization or reduced insulin sensitivity.
5. Defective lipolysis is suggested by reduced levels of beta-hydroxybutyrate and lack of the normal inverse relationship between free fatty acids and blood sugar.
6. Hepatic gluconeogenesis is reduced. Frequently there are elevated levels of alanine, lactate and pyruvate and an alanine load does not provoke an appropriate increase in blood sugar. There may be a delay in the postnatal development of hepatic gluconeogenic enzymes.

Hypoglycemia may lead to neuroglycopenia. Clinical signs of apnea and convulsions do not occur until a blood sugar of less than 1 mmol/L has been present for several hours, probably because alternative substrates are available (glycerol, lactate, beta-hydroxybutyrate, acetoacetate). Nevertheless, Koh et al[188] have shown that auditory evoked potentials are compromised at much higher blood sugar levels so it is important to be obsessional in blood sugar management in these small infants.

Practically, in all except the very small for gestational age (less than 3rd centile), management can and should be on the postnatal ward where a specific management guideline should exist.

Breast-feeding mothers are encouraged to breast-feed 3-hourly, and prefeed dextrostix or BM stix are done after 6 h for 48 h. If hypoglycemia less than 2.6 mmol/L is detected, 8 ml/kg of formula are given after each breast-feed on day 1 and 12 ml/kg after each feed on day 2, if necessary by nasogastric tube. After 48 h, if there has been no hypoglycemia the bottle feeds after the breast can be withdrawn gradually as the mother's milk comes in.

Bottle-fed babies should be given 90, 120, 150 ml/kg/day respectively on each of the first 3 days of life. Prefeed dextrostix or BM stix should be done at 6, 9, 12, 18, 24, 30, 36 and 48 h. If the blood sugar is low, < 2.6 mmol/L, or the baby is asymptomatic add 2 ml/kg/feed of 50% dextrose. If the dextrostix is still low or the baby is vomiting or the hypoglycemia is symptomatic a drip of at least 90 ml/kg/24 h of 10% dextrose is required.

Hypoglycemia is unlikely to be problematic after 48 h of age if it has not been so beforehand.

A baby both small for gestational age and less than 1800 g should probably be admitted to the neonatal unit for observation and treatment.

Infants with transient diabetes mellitus are usually small for gestational age.

Hypothermia

SGA infants may be born with a temperature above mother's as the inefficient placenta will not exchange heat. The scraggy baby with large surface area:body weight ratio may cool fast after delivery if appropriate steps are not taken to prevent this (p. 224).

Polycythemia

The high altitude effect associated with poor placental oxygen transfer leads to increased packed cell volume, red cell mass and high erythropoietin levels. This may lead to viscosity problems after birth. Sheer stresses may reduce the platelet count and on rare occasions liberated platelet thromboplastins may set off disseminated intravascular coagulation (DIC). It is appropriate if the baby looks plethoric to do a venous packed cell volume (PCV) and also platelet count and clotting tests. Treatment with partial exchange transfusion may be required on occasions and vitamin K should be given (p. 303).

Neutropenia and thrombocytopenia

Severely SGA infants particularly those less than 1000 g birth weight may show neutropenia and thrombocytopenia.[189] Platelets may be reduced in number partly by the mechanisms mentioned above but it may be that the marrow in utero is more committed to manufacture of red cell series (high normoblasts) because of hypoxia and there is a temporary reduction in the ability to produce other cells after birth (red cell steal).

Hypocalcemia

This is less commonly seen now that babies are delivered in good condition by the obstetric team. It was probably related to perinatal asphyxia but the pathophysiology is not clear.

Infection

With modern management it is rare for SGA infants to develop a postnatal infection unless they are in addition very preterm.

Congenital abnormality

Of SGA babies, 3–6% have congenital abnormalities; these are usually obvious and lethal such as the chromosome abnormalities, Potter's syndrome and the baby with disseminated congenital infection.

Meconium aspiration

Rare with modern obstetric management.

Pulmonary hemorrhage

This was probably related to intrapartum asphyxia and polycythemia. Modern obstetric and pediatric practice should identify and rectify these problems before hemorrhage results.

Other humoral and metabolic abnormalities

High ammonia, urea and uric acid levels after birth may reflect the reduced calorie reserve of these infants or a protein catabolic state. High circulating cortisol, corticosterone and growth hormone levels have also been demonstrated at birth.

CLINICAL FEATURES OF SGA BABIES

A minority of infants will have obvious congenital abnormalities, chromosome defects or intrauterine infection. Most infants will be scraggy individuals with wasting, particularly of the thighs. The fingernails are mature and long and cracks and desquamation of the skin begin rapidly after birth. The infant is usually active and vigorous and apparently anxious lest his starved state in utero may continue after birth. Sucking is usually strong and the weight loss after birth is less than for an appropriately sized baby.

MANAGEMENT

Early obstetric diagnosis should be followed by a planned delivery in the presence of pediatric staff capable of skilled resuscitation. Labor and birth are asphyxial stresses so labor should be carefully monitored. The baby may be hypoglycemic at birth so a dextrostix should be performed immediately. If there are no signs of anomaly or infection the major pediatric concerns are to prevent hypothermia and hypoglycemia hopefully on the normal postnatal ward.

OUTCOME

Babies with asymmetric growth retardation usually catch up to within the normal centiles after birth whereas many symmetrically growth retarded infants do not. Unless they suffer symptomatic hypoglycemia, they will in all probability develop with a normal DQ and later IQ. Babies SGA because of syndromes, chromosome abnormalities and intrauterine infections will have a high neonatal mortality and later morbidity.

THE LARGE FOR GESTATIONAL AGE INFANT (Fig. 10.13)

By definition heavier than the 90th weight centile for gestation.

ETIOLOGY

1. Constitutionally large baby from heavy large mother.
2. Maternal diabetes or prediabetes – the infant of the diabetic mother (IDM) or the infant of the gestational diabetic mother (IGDM).
3. Severe erythroblastosis.
4. Other causes of hydrops fetalis and ascites.
5. Transposition of the great arteries (sometimes).
6. Syndromes:
   a. Beckwith–Wiedemann (BW) syndrome
   b. Sotos' syndrome
   c. Marshall syndrome
   d. Weaver syndrome.

PROBLEMS OF LARGE FOR GESTATIONAL AGE (LGA) BABIES

Birth asphyxia and trauma

Shoulder dystocia may delay delivery leading to low Apgars, acidosis, meconium aspiration and HIE, and the consequent interventions may lead to fractured clavicle or long bones, brachical plexus injury (Erb or phrenic palsy), subdural or cephalhematoma and skin bruising (later resulting in jaundice).

Hypoglycemia

The IDM, IGDM, baby with erythroblastosis and BW syndrome baby all have hyperinsulinism leading to reactive hypoglycemia after birth.

Polycythemia

Unusual.

Apparent large postnatal weight loss

A 5 kg baby may naturally lose more than 0.5 kg in weight over a few days (10% body weight being 500 g) even if supplied with adequate milk.

CARE OF THE PRETERM INFANT

DEVELOPMENTAL CARE

INTRODUCTION

Advances in medical technology have had a dramatic effect on the progress of neonatal care over the last century; not least in the way it is provided. Prematurely born infants were described as 'weaklings' or 'congenitally debilitated' and it was only with the turn of the last century that these infants were considered worthy of care and protection. Pierre Budin introduced the first premature baby unit and considered, as essential elements of treatment, the infant's temperature, feeding, disease process and the prevention of cross infection. Although he encouraged visiting by parents, when neonatal intensive care became more widespread after the Second World War they were discouraged and actively prohibited from sharing in their infant's care. This practice often led to poor parenting and neglect. Thus from the 1970s parent inclusion in care provision became the predominant theme of change in the social environment of the preterm infant: the physical environment and care giving practices evolved in parallel to advances in medical knowledge and technology.

Although these changes contributed to a reduction in neonatal mortality, prematurely born infants are liable to experience, in the absence of an apparent medical insult, medical complications, neurological impairments and a range of subtle cognitive and behavioral difficulties. It has been postulated that the sensory impact of the environment may partly contribute to these adverse neurodevelopmental outcomes.

THEORIES OF DEVELOPMENTAL CARE

For the fetus carried to term, the environment of the uterus provides a sensitive sensory experience appropriate to the needs of the developing brain. If prematurely born, the infant's rapidly developing brain becomes vulnerable to the unexpected and stressful environment of the NICU.[190] With the realization of this, the theoretical models underpinning the concept of developmental care consider the sensory and social impact of the environment.

There are two ways by which the 'environment' can exert effects on the newborn. *Direct* influences are those characteristics of the physical and care environment which affect sensory perception and lead to immediate responses detectable in the physiological, motor and state organization of the infant. Alternatively, if parents and staff are better informed and supported then they are able to provide better care for the infant. This is an *indirect* effect promoting the infant's development.[191] It is from these two premises that a broad category of interventions which support stabilization of infants as they receive neonatal intensive and special care and which promote optimal outcome by facilitating recovery and development in the infant and family is derived.

In a review of the ecology of the neonatal intensive care environment, Wolke[192] found a lack of recognition by the professional caregivers (nurses or doctors) of the effect of stimulation on the infant. He concluded that there was mismatch between the type, intensity and patterning of stimuli and the infant's developmental status. 'Developmental care' aims to provide an environment with care contingent upon an infant's ability to manage the experience and minimize unfavorable effects. In order to elucidate the value of a particular intervention, the caregiver must have knowledge of the infant's physiological stability, behavior and family relationships and an ability to interpret the findings in the context of the situation and furthermore be able to deliver appropriate care. The dimensions which have created the most interest are environmental influences (noise and light) and caregiving interventions (frequency of handling, positioning, comfort measures). Research has focused on the effects of one or more interventions, clustering of care and the provision of an individualized program of assessment and care on physiological parameters, sleep disturbance and long term neurobehavior of infants.[193]

ENVIRONMENTAL INFLUENCES

Noise/sound

Sound is measured as frequency (cycles/s) and intensity or pressure (decibels). By 26 weeks' postmenstrual age the anatomical and functional components of hearing are in place and for the fetus, both frequency and intensity of sound are attenuated by maternal tissue and fluid. Once born immature infants are exposed to moderate noise levels for weeks and months without having any control over the noise exposure. The mean noise levels outside the incubator are in the range 55–75 dB(A). This resembles the noise pollution found in a busy office environment. Incubators of the 1990s comply with UK safety standards which require that the mean noise level inside an incubator should not exceed 60 dB(A).

The frequency of hearing related disorders is greater in premature infants than term infants (approximately 13% of premature infants experience significant hearing loss compared to 2% of term infants) but there is little to suggest a cause and effect response between the NICU sound environment and the impairment. However data from animal studies suggest that the use of aminoglycoside antibiotics in combination with high intensity sound may, during critical periods of growth, cause cochlea hair cell damage.[194] Furthermore other conditions observed in premature infants have also been associated with hearing loss; for example hyperbilirubinemia, hyponatremia and asphyxia.

Concern has also been raised as to whether, in the absence of impairment of functional hearing, there is some alteration in the recognition and integration of sound. The high levels of continuous sound or 'white noise' and lack of rhythm mask the infant's ability to make associations between source and sound; it has been postulated that this may account for the difficulties which preterm infants experience with concept learning and recognition.

Despite the lack of confirmatory evidence of long term effects of noise on the LBW infant, there are some data suggesting that noise can have a disorganizing effect. Adverse physiological outcomes, for example bradycardia, apnea, hypoxemia and raised intracranial pressure, sleep disturbance and motor instability are associated with sudden loud noises.[192] Again the long term effects of these events are unknown but they are concerns which justify a need to modify sound levels within the NICU.

Reduction of noise pollution can be achieved by changing staff behavior. Radio playing should be eliminated in the unit, talking should be at a considerate low level and loud laughter should be discouraged. Cot-side ward rounds should be abandoned if no patient contact is necessary and no equipment should be placed on the incubator; incubator portholes should be opened and shut gently. With particularly sensitive infants, e.g. those withdrawing from maternal substance abuse, the application of earmuffs may be helpful in reducing the sensory overload. The telephone should not be placed in or immediately adjacent to the unit. Sounds from monitoring equipment should be muffled or be replaced by light signal systems. Opportunities to participate in function and design development of new equipment should be encouraged – staff should have the opportunity to comment on the effects of noise that is generated by equipment and/or alarms. Ideally, new nursery design should include soundproofing for ceilings, walls and floors, and manufacturers of medical equipment and incubators should be encouraged to reduce noise levels in their products. A no-noise policy should be applied at night-time. Indistinct background noise should be replaced by meaningful sounds such as gentle music or recordings of one of the parents reading stories. These should be played at a low sound level from a tape recorder from within the incubator and only when the infant is awake.

Light

Light is a form of energy which is measured as illuminance or intensity in lux (lumens/m^2) or foot-candles (lux/10 = 1 foot-candle) and irradiance (watts/cm^2) which is the amount of energy that is emitted over wavelength bands. The ambient levels described within NICUs vary from 24 to 150 foot-candles, but these increase with the use of supplementary light sources such as phototherapy lamps (300–400 foot-candles) and direct sunlight (1000 + foot-candles).

The levels experienced by infants depend upon postmenstrual age (reflecting anatomical and functional maturity), illness acuity, number and location of exposed windows, incubator/cot position within the unit and seasonal changes. In practice, the most fragile and immature of infants seem to receive the highest exposure of both natural and artificial light. For the recovering infant, the nature of exposure varies from continuous high or dim lighting to random cycling of varying illumination levels. These factors raise questions as to the effect of lighting on the developing retina and the behavioral and physiological responses of the infant to the varying conditions.

In response to the first concern, although preterm infants are at an increased risk for developing a variety of visual problems, the evidence examining the association between lighting levels and retinal damage is inconclusive.[194,195] Likewise, inconsistent findings are reported on the effect of varying lighting levels and patterns on physiological circadian rhythm development.[194] However one study has reported that infants exposed to cycled lighting spent more time in sleep than wakeful states, were able to enterally feed sooner and had greater weight gain than controls in an uncycled light environment.[196] The explanations considered for the positive effects of cycled lighting included a more rapid development of an endogenous circadian rhythm, influences of the hypothalamus and the anabolic effects of sleep. Slevin et al[197] showed that by introducing a quiet period where stimulation from light and noise were considerably reduced, staff activity and infant handling were also significantly less. It may be that this facilitated rest and reduced energy expenditure in the infants.

The literature has not demonstrated any benefit to the infant from being exposed to high intensity lighting; on the other hand it may promote physiological and motor arousal thereby restricting the infant from achieving meaningful rest or sleep or quiet alertness for social interaction. When considering modification to lighting there needs to be a balance between the desired infant response and close observation. Practical strategies should include use of incubator/cot covers, reducing en face stimulation from light and closure of window blinds; structural modifications might include use of uplighters and/or dimmer switches and individual space spotlights. Some consideration should be given to infants adjacent to those receiving phototherapy.

CAREGIVING

All care activity involves some form of handling. The literature will be discussed looking at the effects of frequency of handling, positioning of infants, and the use of comfort measures, for example non-nutritive sucking and containment.

Frequency of handling

Periods of undisturbed sleep (the normal sleep cycle being approximately 60 min long) are essential for optimal growth and development and should be a feature provided in the neonatal intensive care unit. In a recent review of infant handling in the NICU, Peters[198] demonstrated that this was unlikely to happen – infants were noted to be disturbed/handled between 2 and 10 times/h both day and night. Most handling was associated with routine care procedures, investigations/therapeutic interventions and monitoring equipment very little being concerned with parent interaction or comfort measures such as gentle touching or quiet talking. Handling by nursing and medical staff disrupts the young infant's sleep pattern and is associated with a significantly higher incidence of hypoxemia, bradycardia, apnea and behavioral distress.[199] These disruptions can lead to serious complications, which may endure into adulthood.[200]

It should be noted that infant responses to disturbance are variable and dependent upon central nervous system integrity, behavioral state and biorhythm cycle. Biorhythms are characteristic of all physiological functioning; they are repetitive, forming regular and predicable patterns with maturation of the cycle being affected by genetic potential, brain maturation and the environment.[201] Whilst heart rate, respiratory rate, blood pressure, temperature, secretion of several hormones, sleep and waking and feeding all have pronounced patterns, the effects of the provision of intensive care on these functions are unknown.

Not only is the frequency of handling important but also the number of activities involved with each handling episode. In the 1980s the concept and practice of clustering care was introduced – the purpose was to allow infants long periods of undisturbed rest. However recent data suggest this may be more harmful than beneficial. Anand[202] describes the evidence as indicating that prematurely born infants have a lower pain threshold than previously thought and that repeated stimuli further decreases the threshold. These cumulative events cause a phenomenon known as 'windup'. With this there is a prolonged increase in excitability of nociceptive pathways leading to chronic heightened sensitivity of infants to non-noxious stimuli, e.g. bathing and handling.[203] The effects of chronic hypersensitivity are unknown but Peters[198] reports on two studies where cardiovascular indices (heart rate and blood pressure) significantly alter according to the number the interventions per caregiving epoch rather than the duration of the episode.

In view of the literature presented it would be prudent to reduce the frequency of handling episodes and perhaps more importantly to reconsider the number of interventions clustered together at any one time.

Positioning

Positional disorders, which are frequently observed in prematurely born infants, include:

1. the 'frog-like' position – this disadvantages the infant in later months when attempting weight bearing activities;
2. the 'W' shoulder position – this reduces the infant's ability to bring his/her hands to midline and may restrict 'hand regard' and 'reaching to grasp' movements, and
3. craniofacial deformation – this may give rise to difficulty in head rotation and possible visual impairment.[204]

These disorders are attributed to the manner in which intensive care is provided, e.g. equipment fixation techniques, use of flat unyielding surfaces and inappropriately sized nappies, prolonged lying in either supine or prone position and the infant's inability to spontaneously counteract the effects of gravity. 'Supportive positioning' attempts to override these limitations by incorporating techniques and aids which promote physiological stability whilst encouraging a balance between flexion and extension and facilitating self-regulatory behavior. (Self-regulatory behavior includes facial exploration, hand to mouth activity, spontaneous and/or assisted seeking and holding on to equipment, soft rolls or toys and boundary searching and bracing.)

There is evidence that placing infants in particular positions with supportive bedding enhances physiological and behavioral outcomes.[205,206] The practice of placing infants prone is frequently observed when there is evidence of respiratory illness as there is improved oxygenation and ventilation in this position and less gastroesophageal reflux; to counteract resulting hip abduction and rotation, pelvic elevation has been advocated. This may be achieved by using small rolls placed under the infant's pelvis and trunk but it is important to ensure that the weight is not transferred to the femur. Utilization of the supine position requires a degree of 'nesting' to maintain a supported midline position of head, shoulders, trunk and hips. The desired hip and shoulder flexion can be achieved by lifting the infant's knees and arms away from the mattress surface and by supporting the elevation with soft bedding and the use of flexible boundaries; the containment should promote flexion but not restrict or prevent extension. Side lying minimizes the postural disorders associated with prone and supine positions. Limbs should be adducted and flexed towards the midline. Supporting boundaries must be flexible but firm enough to support the infant's back in achieving a rounded posture. This position enables the infant to engage in self-regulatory behavior.

Comfort measures

Interest in infant discomfort and pain has increased due to the understanding and knowledge of preterm infant perception of pain and the immediate and long term consequences to noxious experiences. Pain management is discussed elsewhere but there are a number of strategies that can be considered as developmental interventions for the purpose of reducing stress and discomfort and promoting comfort in the infant.

The concept of non-nutritive sucking stimulates much discussion and controversy. From a breast-feeding perspective there is concern that the early introduction of dummy/pacifier sucking will interfere with the successful establishment of breast-feeding. In full-term infants there is an association between the early introduction of dummies and restrictive breast-feeding practices. It has been postulated that dummy sucking may lead to ineffective suckling or alternatively as a 'calming' intervention where an underlying feeding problem has led to a reduction in milk production and hence a fretful and demanding infant. Conversely dummy sucking could be implemented because mothers are unable to spend quality time in breast-feeding or have a desire to wean the infant from the breast. However, in respect to prematurely born infants, no studies conducted using therapeutic non-nutritive sucking as an intervention could be found to support the association between the activity and restrictive breast-feeding. On the other hand, a systematic review of 20 studies found better bottle-feeding performance and behavior and a faster transition from tube to bottle-feeds.[207] The evidence on reducing heart rate and increasing oxygenation, greater nutrient absorption, faster intestinal transit times and better weight gain remain inconclusive. Furthermore it is found to be effective in decreasing the effect (as assessed using the Premature Infant Pain Profile) of a painful intervention (heelstick). The magnitude of the effect was greater when non-nutritive sucking was combined with the administration of 24% sucrose.[208]

Sucrose has been repeatedly found to lead to a calming response during painful interventions such as immunization.[209]

Containment and facilitative tucking

Containment is the term given for using bedding or 'nests' to provide boundaries for infants; facilitative tucking is a similar action but the caregiver's hands provide the boundaries. Not only do containment and facilitative tucking support postural development but these strategies also result in significantly less stress responses as denoted by a lower heart rate, improved oxygenation, less crying and fewer sleep state changes.[210,211]

SUPPORTIVE PARENTING

The philosophy of developmental care not only promotes the understanding of the infant's strengths and stresses and the techniques for promoting stability and growth, it also advocates parental competence and family/professional partnerships. Underpinning this belief is a vast literature base highlighting the immediate and long term consequences of premature birth and parent–infant separation. The resolution of the emotional crisis surrounding the birth of a premature infant and the development/acquisition of the knowledge and skills needed to be competent in understanding and interacting with an infant is clearly pivotal to successful parenting.[191]

The most important issue raised by parents is that they often feel that *open and honest communication* between themselves and professionals on medical and ethical issues is lacking. It is suggested that opportunistic conversations at the cot-side, with the many disruptions and lack of privacy that this entails inhibit meaningful discussion.[212] Parents wish a more sober and realistic appraisal of what neonatal medicine can and cannot do. They wish for honest communication, to be informed about treatment choices and to be involved in making decisions in medical situations involving high mortality and morbidity and regarding further highly invasive treatments for their infant.[213] The situation should be explained in language adapted for the parents. Instead of assuming that parents do not want to be involved, neonatal carers should consider parents as often wanting but not always able to be involved. Parents have little experience of premature birth and carers underestimate the difficulties parents experience in juggling these new emotional experiences and practical constraints with resuming daily responsibilities.

Simple changes can help to make parents more welcome:

- Encouragement by neonatal unit staff should not begin and end with providing parents with a booklet about the unit and explaining the equipment and medical condition of the infant. Nursing and medical staff should work with the parents to explore areas where the parents themselves can provide an important part of the care within a warm and trusting atmosphere. The lack of space and privacy are frequently cited as obstacles to positive parent interaction. Privacy is often considered as a strategy to promote breast-feeding but seldom offered to the parent who wishes to bottle feed or simply cuddle their infant. Parents can be encouraged to keep records of their infant's behavior, which are valuable for the medical and nursing team in designing an individual care plan for the patient. Parents can carry out tube feeding and hygiene care and in the transitional and special care nurseries, if given the information, can stimulate their infant at appropriate times and learn how to read the infant cues for sensitive interaction and care. Breast-feeding should be encouraged and facilities for rooming in should be available.
- The small infant and his environment (incubator or cot) can be made attractive by clothing and toys.
- The surroundings of the unit should be attractive and comfortable (i.e. wallpaper, pictures, etc.) and ideally should also allow for some privacy for the parents. The setting should be baby centered (e.g. mobiles, toys, etc.). Parents should have comfortable seating such as rocking chairs which also facilitate nursing in the post-intensive care nursery.
- There should be unrestricted access to neonatal units by parents, grandparents, siblings and close friends. Late night visits however should not interfere with the practice of reduced noise, light and handling for other infants in the nursery.
- Practical help in the form of financial support for traveling and caretaking arrangements (e.g. play areas for siblings) are important to enable parents to visit the unit. A direct telephone line should be available for parents.
- Self-help groups and educational classes for parents have been shown to be beneficial. Psychological support has been shown to reduce anxiety and depression.[214]
- Medical and nursing staff can only provide emotional support to parents if they themselves are emotionally available and coping. Support for the staff can be by various means including team work, staff support groups, and regular formal and informal meetings between the different professions to enhance the work ethos and atmosphere. Occasionally individual counseling may be warranted.

Parents are individuals with their own characteristics and needs. There is no easy recipe or approach which is right to help all parents cope. An individual care approach should be adopted for each member of each family to promote the contact necessary to encourage the development of the infant in the best way possible.

SPECIFIC PROGRAMS

Neonatal individualized care and assessment program – NIDCAP[215]

Over the last 15 years a number of studies have been carried out to determine the effectiveness of the neonatal individualized developmental care and assessment program. NIDCAP is based on close observation of an infant pre-, during and post-intervention. The infant's responses as observed through physiological alterations, facial expressions, general body movements, sleep/wake state and behavioral interaction are considered a measure of tolerance to the activity and form the basis for individual intervention recommendations.

Utilization of this program over the years has consistently shown that it decreases the need for ventilatory support or persistent oxygen supplementation and results in infants being discharged sooner than infants receiving conventional care.[215–219] Other studies have shown that infants receiving NIDCAP appear to have improved patterns of growth and advanced feeding ability as well as less severe intraventricular hemorrhage and chronic lung disease.[215,216,218]

In contrast to these studies Stevens[220] found no particular benefits from the intervention. However it was noted that when infants were reclassified in terms of physiological stability, the intervention group was found to be more stable than the control group. As the outcomes of the developmentally cared for infants were no worse than the control infants, it was considered that the interventions were effective in improving physiological stability and therefore were of benefit to the infant.

Criticisms of developmentally supportive care

Before implementing any change, the clinician must consider the validity of the evidence and any associated risks and benefits (including costs) of the proposed change. In respect to the current studies, there are acknowledged limitations. First design issues – the randomized control trial, the phase-lag design and retrospective data analysis are all flawed. Where randomization has taken place within a single unit the effects of contamination between the groups are impossible to control for; where phase-lag design is used there can be little control for clinical improvement initiatives or operational constraints; retrospective data seldom have accurate documentation reflecting either actual interventions or outcome measures. From a sampling perspective, the numbers of subjects recruited to each study are relatively small and often decided upon by using non-probability techniques. Poor control for severity of infant illness and lack of clarity in measurement descriptions and/or blinding in outcome evaluation make generalization of the results difficult. However these limitations are reflective of the knowledge and practices of the time as well as the constraints in conducting clinical research.

In terms of neurodevelopmental outcome, no published studies have identified adverse effects of the interventions or shown an increase in long term morbidity in infants receiving single interventions or the neonatal individualized developmental care and assessment program. Indeed some studies have shown neurodevelopmental improvements at 2 weeks post-term and at 6 and 9 months and 3 years of age.[215,216,221–223] NICU professionals need to acknowledge that critically ill newborns can be harmed not only by undertreatment but also by overtreatment, a feature now reflected in some legal proceedings.[224] The improvements demonstrated in these studies are persuasive for early implementation of treatment policies for the infant and family to be based on comfort and compassion as well as hard science.

SPECIAL CARE – FLUID BALANCE

Even the anephric fetus enjoys biochemical homeostasis but immediately following birth, the kidney becomes essential for chemical and fluid balance. The preterm infant is particularly vulnerable and dehydration and hyponatremia are the commonest problems.[225]

BODY WATER CONTENT AND DISTRIBUTION

Changes in body fluid related to delivery

At the time of delivery, stress hormones, including glucocorticoids, aldosterone, antidiuretic hormone and angiotensin[226] are all elevated in the newborn and may contribute to salt and/or water retention. Moreover, crystalloid fluids administered to laboring mothers equilibrate across the placenta and increase fetal extracellular fluid (ECF) volume. As a result, plasma sodium concentration in the newborn correlates closely with maternal plasma sodium concentration at delivery.[227]

Postnatal changes

The ratio of ECF to intracellular fluid (ICF) decreases in the immediate postnatal period owing to water loss from the ECF space. A postnatal weight loss of 5–8% is common in term infants, the nadir occurring around the fifth day with birth weight usually regained by the 10th day. An even greater percentage loss of 12–21% may occur in premature infants.[228]

Some of this weight loss is meconium, vernix and umbilical stump but most is water derived from the ECF space. The ECF is comprised of interstitial fluid and circulating blood and most of the early postnatal weight loss is due to a reduction in interstitial fluid volume since plasma volume is well maintained over the first week of postnatal life. The interstitial fluid is lost from the body as urine which is virtually isotonic[229] and the negative sodium and water balance and weight loss which result from this appear to be obligatory as these are not prevented by administration of water, sodium or both.[230]

WATER BALANCE

To maintain a stable water balance:
Water intake = water for growth
+ respiratory losses } insensible losses
+ transepidermal losses
+ sweat
+ urine } sensible losses
+ fecal losses

In addition, to achieve a 'normal' water balance, rather than maintaining the status quo, pre-existing deficits or overload must also be corrected.

Water for growth

Approximately 75% of increase in weight in utero is water. If the intra-uterine growth velocity of approximately 16 g/kg/24 h[231] is to be sustained in infants born preterm, 12 ml/kg/24 h of water intake will be diverted towards growth, mostly into the ICF space. This is equivalent to the water of oxidation generated from infant feeds (13.5 ml/kg/24 h for an infant fed on a regime of 120 kcal/kg/24 h).[232] If the infant is not being fed enterally or parenterally, this consideration of water for growth is irrelevant as intravenous crystalloid solutions contain no nitrogen for anabolism.

Respiratory water losses

Inspired air is humidified and warmed by the respiratory tract so that expired air leaves the nose and mouth almost fully saturated at a temperature of 35–36°C. The amount of water lost from the respiratory tract is inversely proportional to the humidity of the inspired air, highest when the inspired air is dry and non-existent when it is fully saturated. It will also depend on the minute volume, the product of tidal volume and respiratory rate. The amount is 7 ml/kg/24 h at an ambient humidity of 50% in term infants[233] and will be similar in preterm infants in the absence of respiratory disease. The management of the fluid balance of a tiny, very immature infant is therefore simplified if a high humidity (> 90%) is provided within the ventilator circuit.

Transepidermal water loss

Transepidermal water loss (TEWL) is the passive diffusion of water through the epidermis and is dependent on the ambient humidity and temperature. TEWL is low in the full-term newborn (6–10 ml/kg/24 h), lower than the child or adult. Values are higher in preterm infants and very high before 30 weeks' gestation in the early newborn period as a result of a poorly developed keratinized layer of the epidermis. As the stratum corneum rapidly matures in the first 2 weeks of life, TEWL falls towards term values.[234] There is an inverse correlation between TEWL and ambient relative humidity, so that TEWL is much higher if the surrounding air is dry and is abolished when it is fully saturated. The management of the fluid balance of a tiny, very immature infant is therefore simplified if a high ambient humidity is provided within the incubator, and this should be provided routinely for infants less than 30 weeks' gestation and less than 1000 g in the first week (Grade D, Level 5).[235] Humidification close to 100% is possible if the incubator ports are kept closed and will reduce TEWL by 50% in infants 24–27 weeks' gestation. TEWL is also increased by phototherapy and radiant heat. Infants nursed naked on radiant heaters can lose 200–300 ml/kg/day as TEWL.

Respiratory and transepidermal water loss together make up insensible water loss. This has been measured as insensible weight loss and is about 15 ml/kg/24 h for a term infant. Values in preterm infants are higher (especially in the very immature infant in the early neonatal period, because TEWL is so high), ranging from 15 to 120 ml/kg/24 h depending on the gestational age, postnatal age and the ambient conditions.[236] Insensible water loss is best derived by adding 7 ml/kg/24 h (respiratory water loss) to the values of TEWL shown in Table 10.15.[234]

Sweating

The ability to sweat is impaired in the term newborn compared with children or adults. If the heat stress is sufficient to raise the body temperature above 37.5°C, evaporative water loss increases by a factor of two to four. This means an increase from 15 to 30–60 ml/kg/24 h. Below 36 weeks' gestation sweating does not appear until a few days after birth and is limited compared with a term infant. Before 30 weeks' gestation, sweating is absent in the first 2 weeks and can be ignored in fluid balance consideration.

Fecal water loss

Allow 5–10 ml/kg/24 h unless the infant has diarrhea or an enterostomy.

Urinary losses

In the immediate period after birth, urine production falls and the urine becomes more concentrated. Failure to pass urine postnatally is not clinically significant until 24 h have elapsed (7% of neonates do not void in the first 24 h),[237] unless there are other pointers to a urogenital abnormality.

This oliguric period may be due to the high levels of antidiuretic hormone in the newborn following birth as there is no evidence of a fall in glomerular filtration rate (GFR). Indeed, over the first week of postnatal life, both GFR[238] and blood pressure increase in term and premature infants (see Tables 5.67 and 5.68, p. 199; Table 5.107, p. 257) and the initial period of oliguria and relatively concentrated urine is followed by a diuresis of isotonic or even hypotonic urine[239] and contraction of the ECF volume.

During early postnatal life, the kidney of even a full-term infant has a limited capacity to produce concentrated urine and fractional sodium excretion is high. In the VLBW infant, GFR varies from 0.4 to 1.0 ml/min/kg with a mean of 0.7 ml/min/kg at 26 weeks' gestation and 0.84 ml/min/kg at 33 weeks.[238] Given the reported maximum concentrating capacity of 800 mOsm/kg of urine (Table 10.16), compared to 1200 mOsm/kg of urine for an adult, and average renal solute load, fluid intake should be such as to maintain a minimum urine output of 1 ml/kg/h.

Table 10.15 Average values of transepidermal water loss (in ml/kg/24 h) at an ambient relative humidity of 50%. There is wide individual variation in the higher values. Data from Hammarlund et al[234]

	Postnatal age (days)						
Gestation (weeks)	1	3	5	7	14	21	28
25–27	110	71	51	43	32	28	24
28–30	39	32	27	24	18	15	15
31–36	11	12	12	12	9	8	7
37–41	6	6	6	6	6	6	7

WATER REQUIREMENTS

The aims of fluid management are to maintain satisfactory volumes of total body water (TBW), ICF and ECF, normal tissue perfusion, a normal blood pressure and a normal plasma sodium concentration. Changes in plasma sodium during the first week of life are usually due to changes in water balance rather than sodium balance.[230] For junior staff, a helpful maxim is that in the first week of preterm life, hyponatremia is usually due to excessive intravenous fluids and hypernatremia is usually secondary to inadequate fluid replacement in the face of excessive insensible losses.

COCHRANE REVIEW OF RESTRICTED VERSUS LIBERAL WATER INTAKE FOR PREVENTING MORBIDITY AND MORTALITY IN PRETERM INFANTS (THE COCHRANE DATABASE OF SYSTEMATIC REVIEWS 2000;[239] GRADE A, LEVEL 1A)

Four randomized controlled trials were included. Each study compared two groups, one of whom received more liberal water intake (the standard or control group) and the other restricted water intake. In the von Stockhausen study[240] (n = 56, 'most of whom were premature' – published in German), the prescribed water intake was given only during the first 3 days of life; in the Lorenz study[241] (n = 88, 750–1500 g), only during the first 5 days; in the Tammela study[242] (n = 100, < 1751 g), the prescribed water intake was begun within 24 h and continued up to 28 days; in the Bell study[243] (n = 170, 751–2000 g), the prescribed water intake was begun before 72 h and continued up to 30 days (Table 10.17).[240–243]

Outcomes

The planned interventions indeed occurred as judged by significantly greater postnatal weight loss in the restricted water intake groups. There was a trend towards less bronchopulmonary dysplasia in the restricted water intake groups but this was not statistically significant. There was no difference in intracranial hemorrhage. The risks of persistent ductus arteriosus, NEC and death (Table 10.18) were statistically significantly lower with restricted water intake in the overall analysis.

However, the mortality analysis included five infants in the Tammela study who died on the first day of life. It could be argued these were too early to be influenced by the fluid regime. If these five, who were all in the liberal fluid group, were excluded from analysis, restriction of water intake would no longer significantly affect the risk of death.

Interpretation

The results of the overall analysis were heavily influenced by the Bell study since this contained most participants. This study also continued the restriction for the longest duration. Moreover, all the infants were enrolled at least a decade ago and there would be few units in the UK now using fluid regimes in early postnatal life as liberal as those in these trials. These studies did not control for sodium intake and it is not clear how many infants were exposed to

Table 10.16 Normal renal function in newborn infants in the first week of life

Glomerular filtration rate	0.35–0.85 ml/kg/min
Urine flow rate	1.0–3.0 ml/kg/h
Urine osmolality	45–800 mOsm/kg

Table 10.17 Fluid regimes

	Restricted water intake (ml/kg/day)	Liberal water intake (ml/kg/day)
Von Stockhausen[240]	60	150
Lorenz[241]		
Day 1	65–70	80
Increasing gradually to day 5	80	140
Tammela[242]		
Day 1	50	80
Day 2	60	100
Day 3	70	120
Day 4	80	150
Day 5	90	150
Day 6	100	150
Day 7	120	150
Thereafter	150	200
Bell[243]	Mean 122 ml/kg/day throughout study period	Mean 169 ml/kg/day throughout study period

antenatal steroids or postnatal surfactant. There were only limited numbers of ELBW infants in these trial. As of October 2001, the most recent update of this Cochrane review (17.11.2000)[239] did not include the study by Kavvadia et al[237] referred to below and involving 168 infants, which may ultimately influence the overall analysis of the systematic review. Future work required in this regard is outlined in Table 10.19.

GESTATIONAL AGE AND POSTNATAL AGE

Fluid requirements depend on gestational age. The premature infant has a greater surface area to volume ratio, a thinner epidermis and more limited renal water conservation than a term infant. The premature infant is also more likely to require ventilation and phototherapy, and be nursed under a radiant heater.

Fluid requirements also vary with postnatal age, increasing during the first week of life to cope with the transition from oliguria to diuresis and reaching a plateau as water balance is restored and birth weight is regained. Fluid requirements do not fall again until after the first 6 months of life.

If the infant is fed enterally, all or part of the water requirement is delivered in breast or formula milk. If the infant is not fed, all the water must be administered intravenously, as 10% dextrose solution on the first day and 10% dextrose/0.18% saline thereafter (see section on sodium balance). Alternatively, the water requirement can be incorporated into a total parenteral nutrition regime.

In our unit, water requirements are given according to Table 10.20, and provided there is no water retention due to inappropriate secretion of ADH or excessive water loss due to transepidermal evaporation, plasma sodium concentration generally remains within the normal range as urinary losses are initially isotonic.

The fluid regime recommended in Table 10.20 may need to be modified in the light of continuing assessment of fluid balance or the presence of the conditions in Table 10.21.

CRYSTALLOID VERSUS COLLOID?

All of the above trials used crystalloid regimes. There has been recent controversy as to whether colloid administration may actually increase mortality in resuscitation and intensive care settings.[244] Colloid is not given to neonates routinely as part of their fluid balance management but is frequently used to attempt to treat metabolic acidosis and hypotension, although there are randomized trials which show sodium bicarbonate (Grade A, Level 1b)[245] and dopamine (Grade A, Level 1a)[246] are superior, respectively. These trials used surrogate outcomes and did not address improved morbidity or mortality. The possible role of colloid in the genesis of chronic lung disease (CLD) is discussed below.

ASSESSMENT OF WATER BALANCE

Water balance cannot be assessed independently of sodium balance. Together, they constitute the major solute and solvent of the ECF. Most clinical and laboratory observations give information about the ECF volume rather than ICF volume.

Clinical examination

Heart rate, systemic arterial blood pressure, central venous pressure and skin–core temperature gradient are all variables which are related to intravascular volume and cardiac output. However, these signs are crude monitors of fluid balance and tachycardia, hypotension and poor perfusion are features of decompensation

Table 10.18 Risks of persistent ductus arteriosus, necrotizing enterocolitis (NEC) and death

	Typical RR (95% CI)	Typical RD (95% CI)	Number needed to treat to prevent one case (95% CI)
Persistent ductus arteriosus	0.40 (0.26, 0.63)	−0.19 (−0.27, −0.11)	5.3 (3.7, 9.1)
NEC	0.30 (0.13, 0.71)	−0.08 (−0.14, −0.03)	11.9 (7.2, 33.3)
Death	0.52 (0.28, 0.96)	−0.06 (−0.12, −0.01)	15.9 (8.4, 167)

Table 10.19 Future work required

- ELBW infants
- Critical period over which water intake must be controlled
- A larger study to determine whether mortality really is reduced
- New trials with the previous 'restricted' regimes as the control arm and even greater restriction during the early postnatal period as the intervention arm, provided infants are nursed in incubators rather than under radiant warmers

ELBW, extremely low birth weight.

Table 10.20 Recommended daily fluid requirements (ml/kg/24 h)

	Day 1	Day 2	Day 3	Day 4	Day 5
Premature infants	60	90	120	120–150	120–150
Term infants	40	60	80	110	120–150

following significant hypovolemia. Moreover, many factors other than fluid balance modulate cardiovascular responses.

Classical signs of decreased interstitial fluid volume are sunken eyes, a depressed fontanel and reduced skin turgor but only semiquantitative interpretation is possible and this is much more difficult in premature infants in whom these skin changes may be less apparent. Nor is edema a reliable sign of fluid overload in the premature infant.[247]

Fluid balance charts

If obsessionally maintained, these are a helpful guide to monitoring fluid balance. Obviously they give no information about insensible losses and the cumulative arithmetic balance may become very misleading if these are overlooked. Sources of error in recording fluids administered are the omission of drug vehicle volumes and omission of the volumes of heparinized saline used to flush vascular cannulae. A common error in the 'out' column of the chart is the omission of blood sample volumes which may cause significant cumulative losses leading to anemia[248] and even hypovolemia.

Body weight

This is the best cot-side guide to TBW. Where fluid balance is important, the infant should be weighed daily, on the same scales and at the same time, particularly in relation to feeds. Serial body weights are of great help in distinguishing hyponatremia due to water overload from that due to sodium depletion.

Table 10.21 Fluid intake alterations

Conditions in which fluid restriction should be considered
- Persistent ductus arteriosus, especially if indometacin given
- Hypoxic–ischemic encephalopathy
- Severe respiratory distress
- Oliguric renal failure
- Inappropriate release of ADH

Conditions in which fluid requirements are increased
- VLBW infant with excessive insensible water loss
- Use of a radiant warmer
- Phototherapy
- Vomiting
- Diarrhea
- Polyuria (e.g. due to glycosuria or following relief of obstructive uropathy)

ADH, antidiuretic hormone; VLBW, very low birth weight.

A stable or increasing body weight may be falsely reassuring under circumstances in which TBW and intravascular volume do not move in parallel, e.g. concealed losses from the intravascular compartment into the so-called 'third space' in peritonitis, ileus, hydrops and congestive cardiac failure.

Urine flow rates

The normal range is given in Table 10.16. Catheterization should be avoided wherever possible but urine output must be assessed in all infants when fluid balance is considered critical, particularly if there is evidence of renal disease. Bag collections are more reliable in male infants but the adhesive used may damage the skin of a very immature infant. Alternatively, the infant may be nursed on a dimple plastic sheet and the urine collected with a syringe, or nursed on cotton wool which is weighed before and after micturition. All three methods also allow the collection of samples for urine chemistry (see below), urine pH, glucose testing, specific gravity and osmolality (Fig. 10.14).[249] A urine specific gravity of between 1.005 and 1.012 is desirable as the newborn kidney is not then at the limits of its concentrating or diluting capacity. Specific gravity and osmolality are unreliable in the presence of glycosuria or significant proteinuria.

Urine and plasma biochemistry

Plasma creatinine concentration is of limited value as an index of glomerular filtration in the newborn because:

1. initially the neonatal concentration mirrors the maternal concentration before birth;
2. non-creatinine cromogens interfere with measurement;
3. the normal range is wide.[238,250]

The interpretation of urinary electrolytes is difficult as the ranges encountered are so wide (Table 10.22).[251–253] Interpretation should always be made in the light of simultaneous plasma electrolytes and a clinical assessment. Moreover, fractional sodium excretion declines with increasing gestation and increasing postnatal age so that fluid intake is best adjusted to maintain a normal plasma sodium concentration rather than relying on urinary measurements.

Nevertheless, urinary chemistry is obviously of value in distinguishing oliguria due to hypovolemia when fluid intake should be increased from established renal failure when fluid intake should be restricted. Another cause of oliguria is inappropriate ADH secretion, and urinary electrolytes and osmolality are necessary for the definitive diagnosis before initiating fluid restriction. In VLBW infants, random urine creatinine concentration is related to instantaneous urine flow rate by the formula: urine flow rate (ml/kg/24 h) = 90/urine creatinine concentration (μmol/L). However, the 95% confidence limits are wide.[250]

Plasma albumin and colloid osmotic pressure

Albumin concentration accounts for 70% of colloid osmotic pressures (COP). The two measurements are closely correlated in the premature newborn and both increase postnatally, in a similar fashion to the increase in fetal albumin concentration in utero. However, low albumin concentrations correlate poorly with clinical edema[247] and although high albumin concentrations may reflect reduction in plasma volume ('hemoconcentration'), this relationship has not been demonstrated directly.

Packed cell volume

Packed cell volume (PCV) falls with decreasing gestation and increasing postnatal age, but with great variability between individuals, so that single measurements are a poor guide to fluid balance. However, if serial measurements of PCV (a simple and

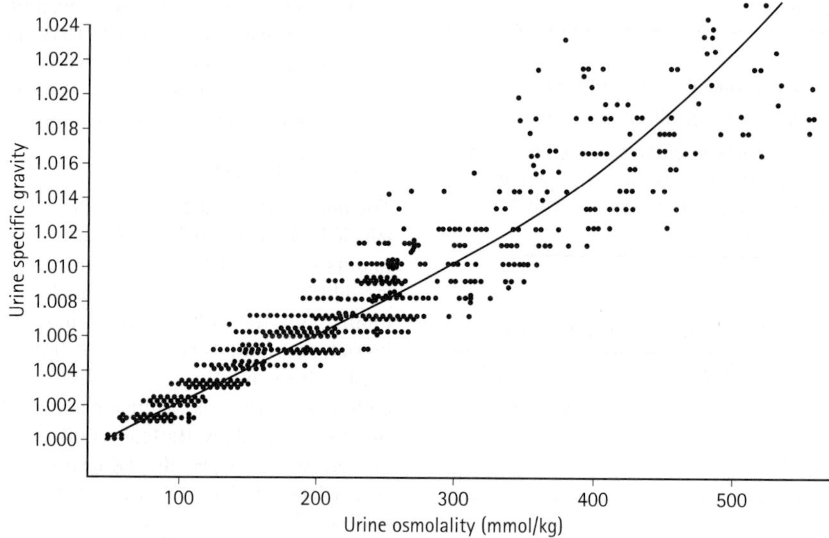

Fig. 10.14 Comparison of urinary specific gravity and urinary osmolality in 1000 urine samples. Third order regression line is shown: $r = 0.97$. (From Jones et al 1976[249] with permission)

reproducible task using a microhematocrit meter) show a rising trend in a sick infant, in whom erythropoiesis is usually depressed, then fluid intake is probably insufficient. Falling levels of PCV may be due to blood loss or hemodilution and are therefore difficult to interpret.

POSSIBLE CLINICAL CONSEQUENCES OF WATER OVERLOAD AND DEFICIENCY

Poor control of water balance leads to both volume and osmolar changes within body fluid compartments. The consequences of pure water overload and deficiency are discussed in the section on sodium under the headings hyponatremia and hypernatremia. Perhaps more common in the neonatal period is overload of water and sodium, which if it is isotonic expands only the ECF, and this has been implicated in the pathogenesis of a number of neonatal disorders.

Respiratory distress syndrome (RDS) and chronic lung disease (CLD)

In infants with RDS, the oliguric phase following birth persists for longer and there is correlation between the degree of oliguria and the minimum PaO_2.[254] There is also correlation between the duration of oliguria, the duration of oxygen therapy and the risk of bronchopulmonary dysplasia (BPD). The use of paralysis in RDS exacerbates this fluid retention as pancuronium is associated with passage of concentrated urine, peripheral edema and weight gain.[255] Colloid administration appears to adversely affect short term measures of lung function in the perinatal period.[256]

The orthodox view is that the onset of the diuretic phase precedes improvement in respiratory function but this has been questioned.[257,258] High levels of ADH[259] and angiotensin II have been reported in RDS, which would contribute to salt and water retention, and increased levels of atrial natriuretic peptide (ANP)[260] which would antagonize these hormones, have been reported during the diuretic phase of RDS.[261] The use of diuretics in the treatment of acute RDS and CLD has given differing results (see also Energy, fluid and electrolyte requirements, Chronic lung disease.

The role of fluid intake in CLD has been addressed in a recent randomized trial in 168 VLBW ventilated infants at high risk of CLD and routinely exposed to antenatal steroids and postnatal surfactant (Grade A, Level 1b).[237] The prescribed water intake was begun on the first day and continued up to 7 days (Table 10.23).

The importance of documenting actual intakes is emphasized by the fact that input actually exceeded the recommended regime by up to 26 ml/kg/day although variances from the trial protocol became smaller after the first 48 h of life.

Table 10.22 Normal reference values for urinary excretion

Term infants	Mean	SD
Sodium*	1.63	(0.78) mmol/kg/24 h
Potassium*	0.68	(0.31) mmol/kg/24 h
Creatinine†	0.45	(0.23) mmol/24 h
Urea‡	3.34	mmol/24 h
Preterm infants	**Median**	**Range**
Sodium§	2.23	(0.18–4.12) mmol/kg/24 h
Potassium§	0.75	(0.06–3.50) mmol/kg/24 h
Creatinine	0.06	(0.03–0.36) mmol/kg/24 h
Urea§	2.44	(0.67–7.04) mmol/kg/24 h

* Full-term, appropriate weight, breast-fed babies during the first and second weeks of life.[251]
† Normal full-term infants during the first month of life.[252]
‡ Normal full-term infants during the first week of life.[253]
§ Male infants, 24–36 weeks' gestation, during the first week of life (Stephenson & Broughton Pipkin, unpublished observations).

Outcomes

Significantly lower urine output in the restricted group indicated that the planned interventions indeed occurred. There were no significant differences in the two primary outcome measures, the proportions developing chronic lung disease or surviving without chronic lung disease. There were no differences in the secondary outcomes of persistent ductus arteriosus, intracranial hemorrhage, NEC and death. Significantly fewer infants who received the restricted regime required postnatal steroids after the first week (19% versus 43%). Postnatal steroids were prescribed for infants fully ventilator dependent beyond 7 days or in 40% O_2 after 3 weeks but it is unclear whether this was enforced by trial protocol or left to the clinicians' discretion. Since the duration of ventilation (median 7 days in both) and O_2 dependency (median 40 days in the restricted group and 38 in the standard group) was similar, it is difficult to explain the difference in steroid therapy except to note that the trial was not blinded.

Table 10.23 Prescribed fluid regimes

	Documented mean restricted fluid intake (crystalloid + colloid) (ml/kg/day)	Documented mean standard fluid intake (crystalloid + colloid) (ml/kg/day)
Day 1	66	86
Day 2	79	93
Day 3	84	114
Day 4	103	124
Day 5	121	142
Day 6	136	148
Day 7	146	159

In a post hoc analysis, volume of colloid infused was associated with duration of oxygen dependency. However, this was not a randomized intervention and results could be biased since colloid was probably prescribed to sicker infants.

Persistent ductus arteriosus (PDA)

PDA is extremely common in premature infants and this has been associated with high fluid intake.[243] The persistence of the duct may be partly due to failure of the usual postnatal contraction in ECF and this in turn may be responsible for the elevated levels of ANP found with persistent ductus arteriosus.[262,263] Moreover, prostaglandin E_2, which is the most potent dilator of the duct[264] is also involved in regulation of sodium balance, causing natriuresis. Elevated levels of PGE_2 may therefore be provoked by salt and water retention.

There has been no systematic trial of the place of fluid restriction in the treatment (as opposed to prevention) of PDA and, as in cardiac failure, it may be more rational to restrict sodium intake and maintain fluid and hence calorie intake, using diuretics to reduce fluid overload. Diuretics can also be used with indometacin in the treatment of PDA since PG E_2 synthesis is inhibited by indometacin and fluid retention may result (see p. 276).

In a number of other conditions, such as cardiac failure, renal failure or ascites, salt and water overload occurs as a *consequence* of organ dysfunction rather than as an etiological factor.

SPECIAL CARE – SODIUM AND POTASSIUM

BODY SODIUM CONTENT AND DISTRIBUTION

Sodium is the major extracellular cation. As the percentage of body weight which is ECF falls during fetal life, so the sodium content in the fetus falls from 94 mmol/kg at 25 weeks' gestation to 74 mmol/kg at term. However, with the continued increase in absolute fetal weight, there is a daily accretion of sodium in utero of about 1 mmol/kg/24 h.

Because of the isotonic contraction of the ECF following birth, there is an inevitable loss of sodium during the first week which averages 14 (range 6–22) mmol/kg. This loss cannot be prevented but may be excessive if sodium intake is inadequate.[265] Negative sodium balance is maximal on day 4 and becomes positive by day 6 or 7[266] provided sodium intake is maintained at 6–8 mmol/kg/24 h.

REGULATION OF SODIUM HOMEOSTASIS

The control of sodium and water balance is regulated by a number of homeostatic mechanisms to maintain a normal plasma sodium concentration (132–142 mmol/L) and normal circulating volume. Moreover, there must be a net stimulus to conserve sodium throughout childhood as this is essential for growth. The regulating mechanisms are:

1. sodium and water intake under the influence of thirst;
2. glomerular filtration rate which determines the amount of sodium and water delivered to the renal tubules;
3. reabsorption of sodium and water by the renal tubules and collecting ducts.

The healthy term infant can respond to thirst by demand feeding but an infant of less than 34 weeks' gestation has no control over intake. Moreover, as the rise in GFR over the first week outstrips the more gradual improvement in renal tubular sodium reabsorption, transient glomerulotubular imbalance develops and a high fractional sodium excretion results. Sodium sensors in the macula densa are stimulated by this high delivery of sodium to the distal tubule, as shown by correlation between urinary sodium and plasma renin even in very premature infants.[267] However, the immature nephron appears to be unresponsive to the high circulating concentrations of angiotensin II and aldosterone generated by this system. ANP levels are high in the immediate newborn period[268] and ANP inhibits the sodium-retaining actions of both angiotensin and aldosterone.[269]

This initial sodium-losing state continues until the end of the first week following which positive sodium balance ensues to ensure growth. Maturation of the aldosterone-dependent distal tubular reabsorption, which is gestation dependent but accelerated by birth, appears to be responsible for the transition to net sodium gain, since proximal tubular reabsorption is unchanged.

During the initial period of glomerulotubular imbalance, urine flow rates do not increase significantly[270] although GFR is increasing. This suggests that the collecting ducts are sensitive to ADH, the levels of which are high in the immediate newborn period.[266] The feedback control of ADH secretion is operative from 26 weeks' gestation (although inappropriate secretion of ADH also occurs commonly in this group[266]) and as a result plasma osmolality is normally maintained within a narrow range of 282–298 mOsm/kg despite variable water intake.

SODIUM BALANCE

To maintain a stable plasma sodium concentration and allow growth:

Sodium intake = sodium for growth (mostly increase in ECF)
+ sodium lost in urine
+ sodium lost in sweat (only after 36 weeks' gestation)
+ sodium lost in feces.

In a healthy term infant, urinary sodium losses (1–2 mmol/kg/24 h) far exceed the other terms in this equation. In VLBW infants, urinary sodium losses up to 20 mmol/kg/24 h are seen.[271] Sodium for growth is roughly 1–2 mmol per week over the first year of life and fecal sodium losses are trivial (0.23 mmol/kg/24 h) in the absence of diarrhea.

Therefore, for the first 24 h of life no sodium is required as there is oliguria. During the succeeding week, 4–8 mmol/kg/24 h should be adequate. Thereafter, term infants require as little as 1 mmol/kg/24 h whereas immature infants may require 8–12 mmol/kg/24 h if 'late' hyponatremia is to be avoided (see below). The needs of a term infant are ideally supplied by human breast milk which, with a nominal intake of 150 ml/kg/24 h, provides 4 mmol/kg/24 h on day 3 but only 1.2 mmol/kg/24 h after a month, the sodium concentration of breast milk naturally falling with time. Preterm human milk alone can rarely keep pace with the obligate renal losses in preterm infants of < 2 kg. Either preterm formulae should be used (sodium content 14–26 mmol/L) or fortified expressed breast milk. Sodium supplements may be required in addition, depending on plasma sodium concentration.

If parenteral fluids are given, the same sodium intakes as above can be achieved by giving 10% dextrose on day 1 and 10% dextrose and 0.18% saline (30 mmol/L NaCl) thereafter at the rates recommended in Table 10.20, thus delivering 4.5 mmol/kg/24 h of sodium by day 5 if 150 ml/kg/24 h 10% dextrose/0.18% saline is administered. Changes in plasma sodium concentration during the first week of life are more often due to changes in water balance than sodium balance[266] so the volumes of water suggested in Table 10.20 may need to be adjusted on the basis of frequent plasma sodium estimations.

In premature infants, a high incidence of 'late' hyponatremia is well recognized and, in contrast to the first postnatal week, this is due to total body sodium depletion (accompanied to a lesser extent by water depletion) and there is poor weight gain or even weight loss. The sodium depletion is due to prolongation of the period of obligate renal sodium loss, possibly due to a delay in endocrine maturation, so that plasma sodium concentration is dependent on sodium intake which must be increased accordingly, usually by oral supplements of 30% NaCl (5 mmol/ml).

HYPONATREMIA

The causes of hyponatremia (plasma sodium <130 mmol/L) are listed in Table 10.24. Water overload is the major cause during the first week of life but thereafter sodium depletion becomes more important. Under conditions of sodium depletion, initially the kidney loses water to maintain a normal plasma osmolality but eventually the need to conserve plasma volume becomes the overriding stimulus, there is *appropriate* release of ADH and hyponatremia occurs.

The clinical features of hyponatremia have three origins:

1. Hypotonia, lethargy and convulsions due to the hyponatremia, irrespective of the cause. These symptoms are not usually seen until plasma sodium falls below 125 mmol/L and are partly related to the acuteness of the fall.
2. Inappropriate weight gain with iatrogenic water overload in early postnatal life or weight loss with sodium depletion in later postnatal life.
3. Features associated with the underlying disease. The underlying cause should be treated but in the interim symptomatic treatment may be necessary to achieve a safe plasma sodium concentration. It is critical that a definitive diagnosis is made as the appropriate treatment may be either fluid restriction or sodium supplementation.

If there is water overload, renal failure or hyponatremia following indometacin treatment, restrict fluids rather than give more sodium.

If there is a sodium deficit, the number of millimoles required is given by the formula:

$$(135 - \text{plasma sodium concentration}) \times \text{body weight (kg)} \times 2/3$$

- Replace slowly over 24 h giving sodium intravenously by adding appropriate amounts of 30% NaCl (5 mmol/ml) to intravenous fluids.
- If plasma sodium < 120 mmol/L or infant irritable, apneic or convulsing, start resuscitation with a slow bolus of 15 ml/kg 0.9% saline (150 mmol/L).

Table 10.24 Causes of hyponatremia in the newborn

A. Water overload
  1. Maternal water overload prior to birth
  2. Iatrogenic water overload following birth
  3. Decreased free water clearance in a sick preterm infant
  4. Inappropriate release of antidiuretic hormone
     Cerebral disease (birth asphyxia, meningitis)
     Respiratory disease (pneumonia, pneumothorax)

B. Sodium depletion
  This is usually accompanied by a lesser degree of water depletion
  1. Excessive gastrointestinal losses (vomiting, diarrhea, nasogastric aspirate, enterostomy loss)
  2. Excessive removal (repeated drainage of ascites, pleural fluid or CSF)
  3. Excessive renal losses
     a. Primary renal tubular problems
        (i) 'late' hyponatremia of prematurity
        (ii) following relief of obstructive uropathy
        (iii) Fanconi's syndrome
        (iv) Bartter's syndrome
     b. Hypoadrenalism
        (i) congenital adrenal hyperplasia
        (ii) congenital adrenal hypoplasia
        (iii) hypoaldosteronism
        (iv) pseudohypoaldosteronism

HYPERNATREMIA

This is almost invariably the result of water depletion (Table 10.25). There is usually failure to thrive or weight loss and irritability, hypertonicity and convulsions may occur when plasma sodium exceeds 150 mmol/L. A 'doughy' quality of the skin and a paradoxically full fontanel may also suggest hypernatremic dehydration. The osmotic gradient favors maintenance of the ECF at the expense of the ICF and the diagnosis may be delayed as signs of hypovolemia and decreased skin turgor occur late.

Treatment is difficult as persistence of hypernatremia is associated with cerebral hemorrhage and renal vein thrombosis in the newborn but overaggressive correction may cause cerebral edema as water enters cells down the osmotic gradient. A solution of 0.9% saline should be used initially and the deficit should be corrected slowly over 48 h.

BODY POTASSIUM CONTENT AND DISTRIBUTION

Potassium is the major intracellular cation, 'of the soil and not the sea, of the cell and not the sap'. It is not surprising then that whilst fetal growth must be accompanied by a more than commensurate

Table 10.25 Causes of hypernatremia in the newborn

A. Water depletion
  1. Inadequate intake
  2. Excessive transepidermal water loss
  3. Excessive renal losses
     a. Glycosuria
     b. Diabetes insipidus

B. Sodium overload
  Isolated sodium overload is rare as water is usually retained with sodium. It is caused by the administration of hypertonic solutions, such as sodium bicarbonate

increase in total body potassium (as the ICF fraction of TBW increases), the potassium concentration in blood throughout life is virtually unchanged from 15 weeks' gestation.[272] Likewise, as only 2% of total body potassium is found in ECF, large changes may occur in total body potassium without significantly altering plasma potassium concentration. For example, in ventilated premature infants a negative potassium balance of 10% of total body potassium occurs over the first 4 postnatal days, but hypokalemia is a rare problem. Subsequently, positive potassium balance is restored and net potassium accumulation then continues at an average of 1 mmol/24 h over the first year of life (approximately 0.3 mmol/kg/24 h initially and 0.05 mmol/kg/24 h at 1 year). Nevertheless, plasma potassium concentration is a major determinant of the cell membrane potential and if significant changes do occur, they must be corrected quickly.

POTASSIUM BALANCE

Intake = potassium for growth
+ potassium lost in urine
+ potassium losses from the gastrointestinal tract

As with sodium balance, urinary losses far exceed the other terms, particularly during early newborn life when prostaglandin E_2 levels are high. As these levels decline, the distal tubule becomes more aldosterone responsive (leading to reabsorption of sodium from the tubular lumen in exchange for excretion of potassium) so that urinary potassium to sodium ratio continues to increase with postconceptional age. Urinary potassium excretion in VLBW infants is 1–5 mmol/kg/24 h.[271,273] Gastrointestinal losses are normally less than 0.5 mmol/kg/24 h but very significant cumulative losses of potassium can occur if there is prolonged nasogastric suction, ileostomy losses, diarrhea or ileus.

A daily potassium intake of 3 mmol/kg/24 h should be more than adequate. Human breast milk provides 2.25 mmol/kg/24 h (assuming 150 ml/kg/24 h intake). The sodium : potassium ratio in mature human breast milk is about one, the same as the ratio in the urine of healthy term infants.[271]

HYPOKALEMIA

Symptoms rarely occur until the plasma potassium concentration is more than 0.5 mmol/L below the lower limit of the normal range (3.0–6.6 mmol/L up to 1 month of age). A concomitant increase in plasma bicarbonate is common. The clinical features (weakness, hypotonia, hyporeflexia, lethargy) are extremely difficult to recognize in the newborn and therefore plasma potassium should be measured frequently in sick infants. Such infants should receive continuous cardiac monitoring (ECG features of hypokalemia are small T waves, depression of the ST sequence, and the appearance of U waves) because cardiac arrhythmias may occur. Loop diuretics and aminophylline[274] predispose to hypokalemia in the newborn and hypokalemia sensitizes the heart to digoxin.

Causes of hypokalemia are listed in Table 10.26. Treatment is by oral or intravenous (5 ml of 20% solution contains 1 g or 13 mmol) potassium chloride administration, depending on the infant's condition and the severity of the hypokalemia, and by reversal of the underlying cause if possible. Intravenous potassium supplements should not exceed a concentration of 40 mmol/L. ECG monitoring is mandatory, infusion through a central venous catheter is preferable (provided the tip is not in the right atrium), and potassium added to fluid in plastic containers must be well mixed to prevent adherence. Potassium should not be added to blood products as it may cause red cell lysis. Oral potassium supplements should be avoided in gastrointestinal disorders because they may cause vomiting, ulceration and stricture. Diuretics should be stopped if possible or the potassium-sparing aldosterone antagonist spironolactone added.

Table 10.26 Causes of hypokalemia in the newborn

Gastrointestinal losses
Vomiting or excessive nasogastric aspirate
Diarrhea
Enterostomy losses
Ileus
Renal losses
Bartter's syndrome
Fanconi's syndrome
Following relief of obstructive uropathy
Diuretic therapy
Alkalosis from any cause
Inadequate intake
Inadequate enteral or intravenous supplements

HYPERKALEMIA

The causes of hyperkalemia are listed in Table 10.27. Plasma potassium concentrations above the 'normal' range occur in 3.5% of infants under 1500 g, particularly sicker infants less than 28 weeks.[271,275] Acute rises in plasma potassium can occur with intravenous administration but apart from this, hyperkalemia due to excessive intake is rare because the kidney has a large reserve for potassium excretion. Hyperkalemia is more commonly due to a failure of excretion by the distal tubule, and this is supported by the finding of impaired renal function in 50% of cases of hyperkalemia in VLBW infants.[275] Altered Na^+, K^+ - ATPase cation pump function may contribute to this non-oliguric hyperkalemia of the preterm neonate.[276] Preterm infants have lower erythrocyte intracellular sodium concentrations and higher intracellular potassium concentrations suggesting Na^+, K^+-ATPase enzyme activity is increased.[277]

As with hypokalemia there may be apathy, weakness, hypotonia and hyporeflexia and also ileus. The ECG shows tall peaked T waves and arrhythmias occur in 60% of premature infants with serum potassium above 7.5 mmol/L, the commonest being supraventricular tachycardia.[275]

Hyperkalemia > 7.5 mmol/L requires urgent treatment (or 6.5–7.5 mmol/L if associated ECG abnormalities) to redistribute potassium into cells as measures to improve renal excretion are too slow. The myocardium is stabilized by intravenous calcium whilst the other measures in Table 10.28 take effect. Exchange transfusion with washed red cells has also been used effectively but needs further evaluation.

Table 10.27 Causes of hyperkalemia in the newborn

Excessive intake
Iatrogenic supplementation of i.v. fluids or parenteral nutrition
Inadequate excretion
Acute renal failure
Hypoadrenalism (especially congenital adrenal hyperplasia and hypoplasia)
Hypoaldosteronism

SPECIAL CARE – THERMOREGULATION

Children and adults maintain a constant deep body temperature over a wide range of ambient thermal conditions. This is achieved by physiological and behavioral responses that control the rate at which heat is produced or lost. The newborn infant is also homeothermic but control of body temperature can only be achieved over a narrower range of ambient conditions. The preterm infant has even greater difficulty in body temperature control, and the most immature infants behave at times as if they are poikilothermic – their body temperature tending to drift up and down with the ambient temperature. The aim in neonatal care is to provide a thermal environment which keeps body temperature in the normal range, and which does not stress the infant to produce or lose large amounts of heat. This is not just instinctive common sense. Several randomized controlled trials have shown that if sick or preterm infants are allowed to become cold their chances of becoming ill are higher, they do not grow as well and they are more likely to die (see Rutter[278] for references).

HEAT BALANCE

By the law of conservation of energy:

$$\text{heat production} = \text{heat lost by convection} + \text{radiation} + \text{evaporation} + \text{conduction}$$

Heat production

Heat is produced as a by product of cell metabolism. The lowest obligatory rate of heat production occurs when an individual is starved, quiet and resting (basal metabolic rate) but a newborn infant is rarely in this state. It is usual therefore to measure resting metabolic rate as the minimal rate of oxygen consumption in an infant who is lying still and asleep at least 1 h after a feed in a neutral thermal environment. Values depend on gestation and postnatal age. Heat production per unit area is lower in preterm infants, particularly below 28 weeks' gestation. In all infants there is a progressive rise over the first weeks of life so that by about 6 months of age adult values are reached.

Table 10.28 Management of hyperkalemia in the newborn

1. Intravenous 10% calcium gluconate 0.5 ml/kg over 5 min
2. Intravenous 4.2% sodium bicarbonate 4 ml/kg over 5 min. This should be given via a different vein or after flush to prevent precipitation
3. Intravenous salbutamol 4 µg/kg over 5 min – can repeat if necessary
4. A glucose + insulin infusion is less safe than salbutamol. Give 4 ml/kg 25% glucose + insulin 0.1 unit/kg infusion over 2 h. These should be mixed in the same syringe. The venous blood sugar and plasma potassium concentrations should be measured hourly and dialysis considered
5. Calcium resonium enema 0.5 g/kg, retained for at least 30 min. This can be repeated 8-hourly

All potassium administration, potassium-conserving diuretics and potentially nephrotoxic drugs should be stopped. Any prerenal failure due to hypovolemia should be corrected, sepsis should be treated (avoiding potassium-containing penicillin salts), and nutrition should be provided to minimize catabolism. The ECG should be monitored continuously

Heat loss

Convection

Heat is lost from the skin surface to the surrounding air by convection. Loss is high if the air is cold, the skin surface is exposed and there is rapid movement of air over the skin. A naked baby in a cold drafty room has a high convective heat loss.

Radiation

Heat is lost from the skin surface to the nearest surface that faces the skin by means of radiation. It varies with the temperature of that surface and its distance from the skin but is independent of the temperature of the intervening air. A naked infant can radiate large amounts of heat to the cool inner walls of an incubator even if the air is warm. An overhead warmer provides heat by radiation.

Evaporation

Heat is lost as water evaporates from the surface of the skin (560 cal/ml of water). Evaporative heat loss is low in mature infants unless they are sweating in response to heat stress. Losses are high in preterm infants who have a high TEWL due to passive diffusion of water vapor through the thin, poorly keratinized immature epidermis. A newly born infant wet with amniotic fluid loses heat as the skin dries.

Conduction

Newborn infants are not usually in direct contact with a structure of high thermal capacity, so conductive losses are small.

RESPONSE TO THERMAL STRESS

There is a range of environmental temperature over which an infant has a minimum rate of heat production and is not sweating. Small adjustments to thermal control can be made by alterations in posture, activity and skin blood flow, and deep body temperature remains constant within the normal range defined for children and adults. This is the thermoneutral range. The range widens and falls if the infant is well insulated by clothes and bedding but is narrow and high if the infant is small and naked. As environmental temperature falls below the lower end of the thermoneutral range, metabolic heat production increases (Fig. 10.15).[278] This may be partly due to increased activity but is mainly the result of oxidation of brown adipose tissue. This is distributed in the neck, between the scapulae and along the aorta. As the environmental temperature falls, nerve endings in the skin are stimulated, catecholamines are released and the brown adipose tissue is metabolized to produce heat. This is non-shivering thermogenesis. A term newborn infant can double his resting heat production in this way without any increase in activity. As environmental temperature continues to fall, heat production reaches a maximum (summit metabolism) and below this point the body temperature starts to fall. As environmental temperature rises above the upper end of the thermoneutral range, sweating occurs until a point is reached when the heat lost by sweating is not enough and body temperature starts to rise.

Non-shivering thermogenesis is impaired in preterm infants and there is doubt that it occurs at all in very immature infants. It is impaired in all newborn infants in the first 12 h after delivery, especially if there is asphyxia, hypoxia or maternal sedative administration. Sweating in response to heat stress occurs from birth in most infants beyond 36 weeks' gestation but takes 2 or 3 weeks to appear in the most immature infants. This is a result of

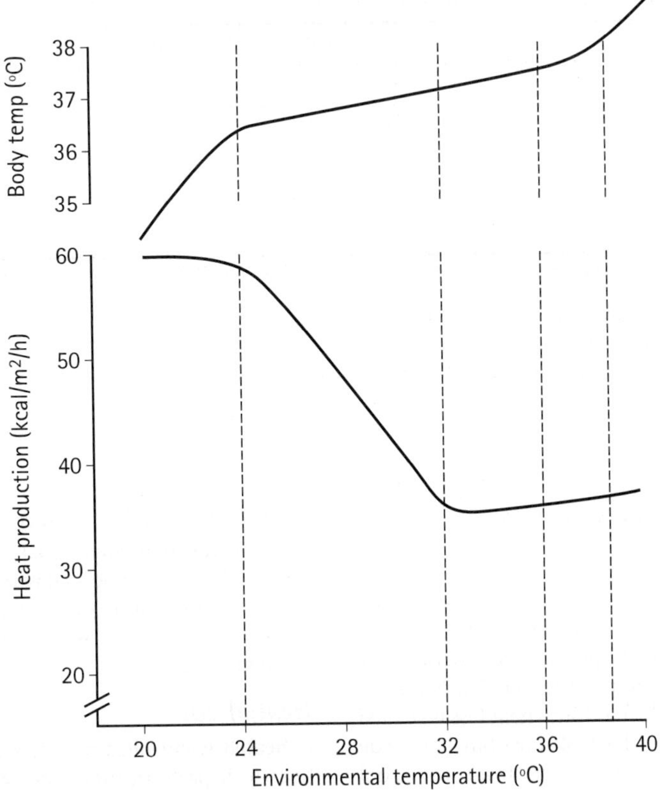

Fig. 10.15 The effects of environmental temperature on heat production and body temperature of a 1.9 kg infant of 34 weeks' gestation, nursed naked in surroundings of uniform temperature and moderate humidity. Between 32 and 36°C, heat production is minimal, there is no sweating, and the body temperature is normal (neutral thermal range). When the environmental temperature exceeds 36°C the infant sweats and above 38°C the body temperature rises rapidly. Below 32°C heat production increases by non-shivering thermogenesis, but below 24°C heat production has reached its maximum and body temperature rapidly falls. (From Rutter 1999[278])

neurological rather than glandular immaturity. Sweating is a relatively poor defense against overheating in the newborn because the production of sweat per unit area of skin is low compared with a child or adult. Alteration of skin blood flow by vasoconstriction and vasodilation results in an increase or decrease in the amount of heat lost by convection and radiation, particularly if the infant is unclothed. The term newborn can alter skin blood flow effectively but this is impaired in the very immature infant. Alteration of posture to increase or decrease the surface area available for heat loss by convection and radiation is important in thermoregulation. It occurs in the healthy term infant and to some extent in the preterm infant but not in the presence of illness.

BODY TEMPERATURE AND ITS MEASUREMENT

Measurement of body temperature in the newborn is a crude way of assuring the effectiveness of the thermal environment. It is clear from the heat production diagram that an infant has to be considerably heat or cold stressed for the body temperature to rise or fall outside the normal range. An infant can have a normal body temperature but still be too hot or too cold. The most immature and smallest infants who are nursed naked for observation have a very narrow neutral thermal range and a limited ability to respond to heat or cold. Their body temperature tends to rise and fall according to environmental conditions and therefore a normal temperature suggests a suitable environment. It is essential to record body temperature in infants nursed under radiant warmers as a check against overheating. Instability of body temperature, particularly a mild pyrexia, may be an early sign of infection.

Deep body temperature is usually measured as rectal temperature. Colonic temperature can be recorded with a soft flexible probe inserted several centimeters past the anal margin but such probes are easily extruded. Esophageal and tympanic membrane temperatures are only useful in research. Rectal temperature under-records deep body temperature especially if the bulb of the mercury in a glass thermometer is only just inserted into the anal canal – 3 cm in term and 2 cm in the preterm are recommended depths of insertion and at least half a minute is required to obtain a stable reading. The normal range is 36.6–37.1°C. Hemorrhage or bowel perforation are rare but well-described complications, and rectal temperature should not be measured in infants with colitis.

Axillary temperature is a reasonable guide to deep body temperature and is less invasive. The bulb of the thermometer should be held in the roof of the axilla with the infant's arm pressed against the side of the chest until a stable reading is obtained, usually by 3 min. The normal range is 36.3–37.0°C. Skin temperature reflects tissue insulation and environmental conditions as well as deep body temperature and is therefore less useful. However, if an infant lies on a skin temperature probe which is insulated on the outside, the recorded temperature is close to rectal temperature.

Table 10.29 Average incubator air temperatures needed to provide a suitable thermal environment for naked, healthy infants

	Environmental temperature					
Birth weight (kg)	37°C	36°C	35°C	34°C	33°C	32°C
Less than 1.0	For 1 day	After 1 day	After 2 weeks	After 3 weeks	After 4 weeks	After 6 weeks
1.0–1.5			For 10 days	After 10 days	After 3 weeks	After 5 weeks
1.5–2.0				For 10 days	After 10 days	After 4 weeks
2.0–2.5				For 2 days	After 2 days	After 3 weeks
More than 2.5					For 2 days	After 2 days

Note: 1. In a single-walled incubator the environmental temperature needs to be increased by 1°C for every 7°C difference between room and incubator temperature.
2. Infants below 1.0 kg and below 30 weeks' gestation need a humidified incubator in the first week of life.
3. Clothed infants need lower incubator temperatures.
4. Values are average ones but there is considerable variation in individual requirements.

From Hey 1975[281] and Sauer et al 1984[282]

PROBLEMS OF TEMPERATURE CONTROL IN THE PRETERM INFANT

The smaller and more immature the infant, the greater the difficulties in temperature control. The major problem is hypothermia and there are physical and physiological reasons for this. Size alone places the small infant at a thermal disadvantage. Heat production is related to mass which is low – heat loss is related to surface area which is relatively high. Lack of subcutaneous tissue means poor insulation of the heated core from the cool surroundings. A poorly developed stratum corneum results in a very high evaporative water and therefore heat loss. The ability to conserve heat by vasoconstriction and increase heat production by metabolism is reduced. Overheating is rarely a problem unless the infant is warmed by a very powerful heating device where output is uncontrolled.

MANAGEMENT OF THE THERMAL ENVIRONMENT

At delivery

The delivery room and operating theater are usually kept at a temperature considered suitable for adults but which is cold for the newborn. The naked infant loses heat by convection and radiation, and by evaporation of amniotic fluid from the wet skin. The body temperature of a small preterm infant can easily fall by 1°C every 5 min and this is particularly likely to occur if delivery takes place unexpectedly at home. The healthy term infant does not appear to suffer from this transient cold exposure at birth but in the preterm infant a fall in body temperature is associated with an increased risk of acidosis, hypoxia and respiratory distress. The newborn infant should be dried at delivery, wrapped in a warm dry blanket and given to the mother – skin to skin contact with the mother is an effective way of maintaining body warmth. Exposure for weighing, cord care and fixing of namebands should be minimized and bathing avoided. The small preterm infant should be dried, wrapped and removed to a warm environment as soon as possible. If an infant requires resuscitation, a supplementary heat source such as a radiant warmer is necessary.

Nursing

Most healthy term and preterm infants can be nursed clothed and wrapped in a blanket in a cot in a warm room. This is both comfortable and thermally safe. Very small infants may need to be nursed clothed in an incubator to provide a sufficiently warm ambient temperature.

Over 2 kg: nurse clothed, with bedding in a cot, in a room temperature of about 24°C.
1.5–2 kg: nurse clothed with a bonnet and bedding in a cot, in a room temperature of about 26°C.
Below 1.5 kg: nurse clothed with a bonnet, in an incubator temperature of 30–32°C.

Heated cot

A heated water-filled mattress can be used to provide conductive heat to a preterm infant nursed in a cot in the usual way. The mattress is a polyvinyl chloride bag, filled with 10 L of water and heated electrically by a foil pad, controlled to provide a set temperature between 35 and 38°C. It has been shown that it is just as effective as the incubator for keeping small babies warm. It results in similar rates of resting metabolism and growth.[279] Its advantages are that it is cheap, simple and does not depend on a constant unbroken supply of electricity (because of its stored heat), so that it is particularly useful in developing countries. It is also more comfortable for the infants and appealing to their mothers, but is only of use if the infants are healthy and do not need to be nursed naked for observation and access. It has been effectively used as a method of rewarming cold preterm infants.[280]

Incubator

The incubator provides a warm environment suitable for nursing small or sick infants, particularly if they need to be naked for observation and access. Air within the Perspex canopy is warmed by a heater and circulated by a fan. The heater output can be controlled in two ways. In air mode the incubator air temperature is set to a point between 30 and 37°C and the heater is thermostatically controlled to reach and maintain this temperature. In servo mode a thermister probe is taped to the infant's abdominal skin and the desired skin temperature is set – the heater output varies to provide an air temperature which maintains the set skin temperature. In practice, air mode control is simpler to use, safer and results in a very constant ambient air temperature regardless of the condition of the infant and the amount of care he is receiving. Servo control results in wide fluctuations in air temperature during periods of handling, the probe can become detached or wet, and the infant's own attempts at thermoregulation are overridden so that a fever is disguised.

Suggested air temperature (Table 10.29)[281,282] and skin temperature settings (Table 10.30)[278] for the two modes of control are shown. In a single-walled incubator the inner wall is cooler than the air in the canopy and the naked infant therefore loses heat by radiation as well as convection. This can be reduced by raising the

Table 10.30 Suggested abdominal skin temperature settings for infants nursed in servo mode incubators or under radiant warmers (From Rutter 1999[278])

Weight (kg)	Abdominal skin temperature (°C)
Less than 1.0	36.9
1.0–1.5	36.7
1.5–2.0	36.5
2.0–2.5	36.3
More than 2.5	36.0

temperature of the nursery, raising the incubator air temperature, using a radiant heat shield within the incubator which warms to the air temperature and shields the infant from the inner wall of the canopy, or by using a double-walled incubator.

In most infants it is not necessary to humidify the incubator air. In infants below 30 weeks' gestation, weighing less than 1 kg, evaporative water loss and therefore heat loss is high during the first few days of life and may exceed the infant's own heat production. Thus a very immature infant may have a subnormal deep body temperature although the incubator air temperature is on the maximum setting. Raising the humidity of the air around the body will reduce evaporative losses so that a normal body temperature can be achieved. Some (but not all) incubators have humidifiers which will produce an ambient relative humidity within the canopy of 90% or more (compared with 30–40% relative humidity without use of the humidifier). At such high humidity the infant's evaporative water and heat losses are very low, it is easy to control body temperature and fluid balance is simplified. Beyond 1 week of age the immature infant's skin has matured to such an extent that evaporative water and heat losses are less important and added humidity is no longer required. There is always the concern that use of humidity predisposes the infant to bacterial infection, particularly by *Pseudomonas* or *Klebsiella* species, although in practice this does not seem to be a major problem. The humidifier water should be drained and replaced with sterile water each day, with a brief period in between where the incubator is run dry. An alternative to humidifying the incubator air is the use of a waterproof covering over the infant. This raises the humidity close to the skin surface and therefore reduces evaporation – it reduces visibility though and when the covering is removed the evaporative losses are high.

The incubator provides a constant, bland thermal environment which keeps the infant's heat losses by radiation and convection to levels which are balanced by his own heat production. It is difficult to get at the infant for examination and practical procedures (not always a disadvantage) and parents sometimes find the physical barrier distressing.

Radiant warmer

The infant lies naked on a platform exposed to a radiant heat source suspended horizontally above him. The output of the heater is controlled by a temperature sensor in contact with the infant's skin, set to the desired temperature. The sensor should be taped to the abdomen or chest rather than a limb and should be shielded from the heat source. The normal range of abdominal skin temperature under neutral thermal conditions for infants of different size is shown in Table 10.30 – this is a good guide to the set temperature that should be chosen.

Since the infant is exposed to the cool drafty nursery air and walls, heat losses by convection and radiation are high when radiant warmers are used. Evaporative water loss is also increased as a result of the drafts and a direct effect of radiant heat on the infant's skin. These losses are all balanced by a large radiant heat gain from the powerful heater. Wide fluctuations in heater output occur, producing a very uneven, asymmetrical thermal environment compared with an incubator. In the more immature infants, evaporative water loss may lead to hypernatremia and dehydration. The wide fluctuations in thermal environment and high evaporative water losses can be conveniently reduced by placing a small clear plastic canopy over the infant – radiant heat can still reach the infant but heat losses by convection, radiation and evaporation are greatly reduced.

Radiant warmers are powerful devices and therefore inherently more hazardous than incubators. Overheating can occur and regular measurement of the infant's body temperature by an independent method is essential. If the heater is switched off, moved to one side or if something is interposed between the infant and the heat source, the infant's heat losses are very great and rapid cooling occurs. Their advantage is that they allow access to the infant for practical procedures whilst keeping the infant warm. They are ideally suited to the care of a small or large sick infant in the early neonatal period when the illness is evolving, but less suitable for the care of the stable or improving infant.

Both devices have been in use in neonatal intensive care for over 25 years and there is no evidence that either is superior. Several studies have shown that infants nursed under radiant warmers have higher rates of insensible water loss compared to infants nursed in incubators. A systematic review demonstrated a mean increase of about 23 ml/kg/day.[283] This increase in water loss results in a higher heat loss and therefore a slightly higher metabolic rate.

Transport

A small sick infant who is transferred from one hospital to another for intensive care is thermally vulnerable. The body temperature is often low before the journey, the ability to produce and conserve heat is limited, the outside temperature may be very low indeed and the transport incubator is less sophisticated than the usual nursing incubator. It is important to cover the infant to reduce radiant heat losses, which may be very high. A waterproof covering is useful if evaporative water loss is likely to be high. The infant therefore has to be monitored indirectly rather than by direct observation. In spite of the risk of cold stress during transport, studies have shown that body temperature does not usually fall during the journey but may actually increase.

Surgery

A newborn infant who needs surgery is at risk of cold stress. He is usually starved and drugged, thus reducing the normal metabolic response to cold. The operating theater may be a journey away, it is drafty and has cool walls and often cool air. The infant needs to be exposed for the operation and exposed moist organs lose heat by evaporation. To minimize cold stress and hypothermia, the infant should be well insulated before the journey to theater and the minimum area exposed for surgery in theater. The theater air temperature should be raised to 28–30°C and a supplementary source of heat such as an electric warming pad or radiant warmer should be provided.

DISORDERS OF BODY TEMPERATURE IN THE NEWBORN

A low body temperature (below 36°C)

Acute hypothermia in the newborn is not uncommon – it is usually mild (rectal temperature 34–36°C) but may be moderate (30–34°C) or severe (below 30°C). Of the several causes, accidental hypothermia due to cold exposure is the commonest, particularly in the moderate or severe cases. Accidental hypothermia is likely to occur in hospital when LBW infants require resuscitation or when infants are exposed to a cool delivery room or operating theater. If careful attention is paid to keeping infants warm after delivery it should happen infrequently. It commonly occurs when infants are born outside hospital, either unexpectedly or after a concealed delivery – if the infant is small, born into a toilet, abandoned, or inadvertently exposed to cold, severe hypothermia may result. Accidental hypothermia also occurs later on in the newborn period or early infancy because of inadvertent cold exposure due to inadequate clothing or cold thermal environments – it may occur chronically. Infants with bacterial sepsis or with respiratory syncytial virus (RSV) infection are prone to mild hypothermia – so too are infants in severe heart failure or with marked cyanosis. Malnutrition predisposes to hypothermia because of poor tissue insulation and an impaired metabolic response to cold. Hypothyroidism also results in an impaired metabolic response to cold. Drugs given to the mother which cross the placenta have a similar effect on the newborn infant, particularly the long-acting sedatives such as diazepam. Finally intentional hypothermia is used as an adjunct to cardiopulmonary bypass when newborn infants have major heart surgery – body temperature is lowered to about 28°C by surface cooling with ice to reduce the metabolic demands of the brain. The infants tolerate this brief, acute severe hypothermia well. Similar hypothermia appears to be an effective method for preventing brain damage in asphyxiated animals. It is currently undergoing trials as rescue therapy for newborn infants with severe birth asphyxia, both in the form of whole body and local head cooling.

Hypothermic infants develop symptoms when their deep body temperature falls below 34°C. They become lethargic, feed poorly, have a weak cry and reduced movements. If exposure to cold has been persistent there may be peripheral edema, sclerema and marked facial erythema in the presence of a strikingly cold skin – these are the features of neonatal cold injury. In very severe hypothermia there is profound bradycardia with slow, shallow respiration and the infant may appear to be dead. There are anecdotal reports of such infants being left for dead yet eventually making a full recovery. The diagnosis of hypothermia is made by recording a low rectal temperature – it is important that a low reading thermometer is used, not the standard clinical thermometer with a minimum reading of 35°C.

The treatment of accidental hypothermia is rewarming – if there is an underlying cause, this obviously needs to be treated too. There is limited information about the correct rate for rewarming cold infants. In cases of mild hypothermia rewarming can take place rapidly. In moderate or severe cases there is concern that rapid rewarming of the infant's surface causes peripheral vasodilation, diversion of blood from the core and therefore hypotension. Use of a plasma expander during rewarming has been advocated. Very slow rewarming over a period of several days has been used in infants with cold injury but after acute accidental hypothermia it appears to be safe to restore deep body temperature to normal over a few hours. This can be achieved using a radiant warmer, an incubator or a heated cot.[280]

Hypoglycemia may occur during rewarming – it should be anticipated and treated or better still prevented by a slow intravenous infusion of 10% dextrose. Care should be taken in interpreting blood gas results – a metabolic acidosis at 37°C is less severe at 30°C and should not be overenthusiastically treated. Abdominal distention is common as a result of ileus and feeding should not be started until a normal body temperature is achieved. NEC and hemorrhagic pulmonary edema have been described and are sinister complications. The reported mortality rate in severe hypothermia is 25–50% but this includes infants with overwhelming sepsis or congenital abnormalities that predisposed them to cold. Most survivors develop normally.

Table 10.31 Differences between a healthy infant who is overheated and a febrile infant with a raised set point (From Rutter 1999[278])

Overheated infant	Febrile infant
High rectal temperature	High rectal temperature
Warm hands and feet	Cool hands and feet
Abdominal exceeds hand skin temperature by less than 2°C	Abdominal exceeds hand skin temperature by more than 3°C
Pink skin	Pale skin
Extended posture	Lethargic
Healthy appearance	Looks unwell

A high body temperature (above 38°C)

An infant with a high body temperature may be febrile or overheated. A febrile infant has a high set point temperature and behaves as if cold. He makes physiological and behavioral responses which reduce heat loss, increase heat production and therefore raise body temperature. An overheated infant makes physiological and behavioral responses in an effort to increase heat loss and therefore lower body temperature. The distinction is an important one which can be made clinically (Table 10.31).[278] Overheated infants simply need a cooler environment, not a series of painful investigations to find an infective cause for the 'fever'. In a large study of term infants with a high body temperature, 90% were found to be overheated and only 10% had infection.

The newborn infant may develop a raised body temperature in the presence of infection but this is usually not marked. It may be masked if the infant is being nursed in a servo control incubator or radiant warmer. It is not known why serious infection in a newborn seems to elicit such a mild febrile response when mild infection in a toddler is often associated with a very high body temperature. Infection is not the only cause of a raised set point temperature in the newborn; it is also caused by a severe cerebral abnormality, either congenital (holoprosencephaly, hydranencephaly, encephalocele) or acquired (birth asphyxia). Such infants have hypothalamic dysfunction leading to poor temperature control.

Overheating is less common than accidental hypothermia in the newborn. It is invariably the cause of hyperpyrexia (rectal temperature above 41°C). Mild degrees occur when active, large infants are overwrapped and left in a warm room, or when small infants are overheated by an incubator or radiant warmer. Severe overheating occurs when there is electrical or mechanical failure of a warming device, or when an incubator is exposed to direct sunlight (this turns it into a greenhouse). It can also occur if infants are left in closed cars exposed to direct sunlight.

Mild overheating has been suggested as a predisposing factor in apnea of prematurity but is otherwise not dangerous. Severe overheating leading to hyperpyrexia has caused sudden death in the newborn without prior symptoms. In this context it is interesting that sudden death in infancy has been linked to overheating, and is described in families with a history of malignant hyperpyrexia and anhidrotic ectodermal dysplasia.

SPECIAL CARE – ENTERAL NUTRITION

The preterm baby has very little stored energy and urgently needs an adequate supply of food in order to survive beyond a few days. Subsequently, good nutrition is essential to promote the rapid growth which characterizes this period of life, and is important for long term outcome.[284] Nutrients can be provided either parenterally or enterally but the aim in all infants is to use full enteral feeding as soon as it is safe to do so. The section that follows reviews the balance of benefits and risks of enteral feeding and recommends suitable intakes, aimed at promoting growth and avoiding deficiencies.

DEVELOPMENT OF GUT FUNCTION

The motility, digestive and absorptive functions of the gut, and hence its ability to deal with food, develop in utero. Gut development continues postnatally and enteral feeding has an important influence on this. An understanding of gut development is essential to the discussion of benefits and risks of enteral feeding.

Sucking, swallowing, gastric emptying and small gut peristalsis are inefficient in the preterm baby.[285] The fetus begins to swallow at 16 weeks but in babies born before 34 weeks' gestation feeding behavior is characterized by short bursts of sucking, a small intake of milk, uncoordinated swallowing, and non-propagative, disorganized esophageal motor activity.[286] Lower esophageal sphincter pressure is low,[287] predisposing to gastroesophageal reflux. Gastric emptying time is prolonged to about twice that of the term infant, and is even longer in the presence of illness or when feeds are of high energy density, fat or carbohydrate content.[285] In the fetus small intestinal transit is seen from 30 weeks, but the normal pattern of migrating motor complexes and peristalsis is not observed until a few weeks later. The coincidence of nutritive sucking, swallowing and gut motor activity at about 34 weeks is a good example of developmental coordination.

Gastric acid production is present by 24 weeks' gestation. Pepsin production is low, but this does not appear to inhibit utilization of dietary protein and may enhance the passage of intact IgG and IgA into the small bowel. Pancreatic enzyme secretion is reduced in the term infant, and in the preterm infant levels of trypsin, lipase, amylase and bicarbonate secretion are further reduced.[288] In the preterm baby, studies using test meals have demonstrated inadequate intraluminal digestion of fat, protein and carbohydrate, but clinical malabsorption is rare. Fat absorption, for example, limited by low pancreatic lipase and low intraluminal bile salt concentration, may be improved by the high contribution of lingual and gastric lipase and bile salt dependant lipase in breast milk. Alpha-glucosidase (sucrase, maltase and isomaltase) activities are about 70–80% of normal at 32 weeks' gestation.[289] Lactase is at 25% of adult levels at 26 weeks and increases markedly towards term.[290]

Intestinal permeability is increased in the preterm baby and results in increased macromolecular transport across the epithelium.[291] This may be relevant to the development of NEC by allowing bacteria and their antigens to penetrate the gut wall.

INTRODUCTION OF ENTERAL FEEDS

The healthy preterm baby should be fed within 1 or 2 h of birth, in order to prevent hypoglycemia and to maintain hydration. Deciding when to feed enterally in intensive care is a contentious matter and practice varies widely.[292] Most would not attempt enteral feeding in the ill preterm infant, unstable in intensive care. In the preterm infant, stable on intensive care and receiving ventilatory assistance, should milk feeds be given? The main arguments for not feeding are the fear of milk aspiration into the lungs, respiratory embarrassment through gastric distention, and NEC (see Complications of feeding). With a cautious approach, however, many neonatal units successfully milk feed babies on ventilators. Milk feeds should be stopped for a period following extubation, to allow recovery of laryngeal protective reflexes.

The SGA infant also merits particular care. In intrauterine growth restriction (IUGR) with abnormal fetal Doppler studies, fetal gut perfusion is reduced, predisposing the infant to NEC.[293] A large European study showed no increase in NEC in infants with a history of abnormal fetal Doppler studies.[294] In infants with IUGR, notably those with the triad of IUGR, abnormal fetal Doppler studies and fetal echogenic gut, difficulty with enteral feeds is common.[295] It is now widespread practice to delay introduction of milk feeds in the infant who is SGA.[296] Our policy in the VLBW infant who has IUGR is to delay feeds for 24–48 h after birth then giving 0.5–1.0 ml/h for the first 24 h period, before increasing slowly. If such infants require intensive care, parenteral nutrition is given accompanied by trophic feeding (see below).

TROPHIC FEEDING (TF)

TF is also known as minimal enteral feeding, hypocaloric feeding and gut priming. It is an important advance in the use of enteral feeding, entailing the administration of small, nutritionally inconsequential amounts of milk in order to confer the benefit of milk feeds on the infant receiving parenteral nutrition.[297]

Physiology

Absence of enteral feeding is associated with reduced gastrointestinal growth and maturation. Gastric, intestinal and pancreatic weight and DNA content is reduced if milk is withheld, changes that occur in the first days of enteral starvation.[298,299] Bile flow is reduced and this may underly the high incidence of conjugated hyperbilirubinemia in infants on parenteral nutrition.

The administration of TF has major advantages in inducing maturation of gastrointestinal motor function,[300] an effect which is not seen if water is given. This translates to more rapid whole gut transit time in infants receiving TF.[301,302] Milk tolerance is improved with a reduction of 4 days in time to reach full feeds.[297,303] Gastric emptying is not altered in infants who have received TF (Fig. 10.16).[301]

TF induces surges in gut hormones[304] including motilin and enteroglucagon which are known to be trophic and promote normal motility. In animals, enteral feeds enhance digestive capacity, with increase in gastric lipase, intestinal lactase activity, and pancreatic responsiveness to glucose. In our trials, TF induced lactase activity measured in duodenal aspirate,[305] while the second RCT to examine this found increased lactase activity and parallel improvement in milk tolerance.[306] Chymotrypsin activity is not altered by TF.[305]

Clinical trials

The Cochrane review of TF concludes that there is no proven benefit, but does not analyse the two large, well-conducted and more recent RCTs.[302,303,307] It is clear when all available evidence from RCTs is considered that TF confers a reduction in time to full enteral feeds, improved milk tolerance, shorter hospital stay, more rapid full nipple feeding and accelerated growth in the first 6 weeks.[297] Avoidance of cholestatic jaundice has not been explored by studies with sufficient power. The most surprising result in our trial was a large reduction in culture positive sepsis with parallel

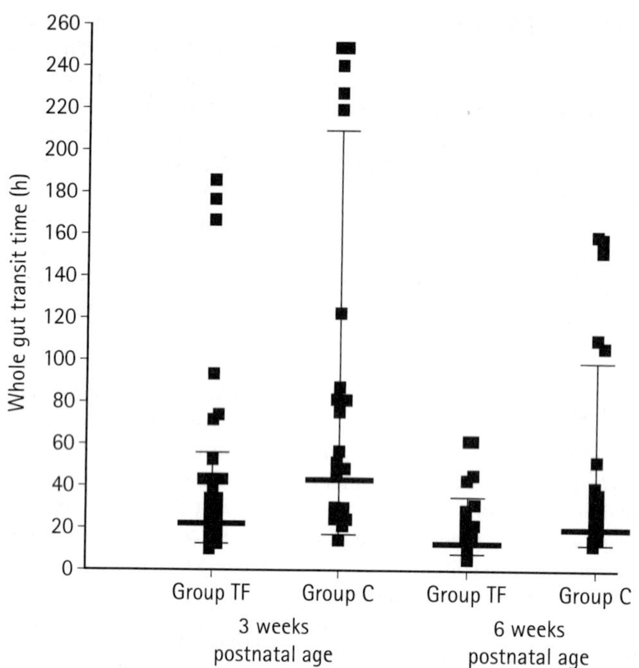

Fig. 10.16 Individual whole gut transit time at 3 and 6 weeks of postnatal age. Broad horizontal bars represent median; narrow horizontal bars interquartile ranges: $p < 0.05$ at 3 and 6 weeks. (Reproduced with permission, McClure & Newell 1999, Arch Dis Child Neonatal Ed, BMJ Publishing Group.[301])

decrease in days with elevated C-reactive protein in the infants who received TF.[303] An associated reduction in upper gut colonization with coagulase negative staphylococci may, in part, explain this observation.

None of the 10 RCTs examining TF has demonstrated any adverse effects.[297] There is no evidence to suggest an increase in respiratory problems. NEC was not increased by TF in over 600 infants randomized in trials. There has been no study comparing TF with faster feed introduction.

We introduce TF once infants have cardiovascular stability on intensive care provided there is no contraindication to milk feeds. Infants receiving TF should be monitored closely, and TF discontinued if the infant becomes unstable on intensive care, or shows problems with TF tolerance. It is our practice to discontinue TF for a period of 12 h after extubation.

NUTRITIONAL REQUIREMENTS OF THE PRETERM INFANT

Table 10.32 compares body composition of infants of 26 weeks' gestation and term. Fetal and infant metabolic demands differ, and nutrient requirements based on prenatal growth may not be appropriate for the preterm baby. Current consensus, however, is that the fetal growth curve seems a reasonable 'gold standard', and a growth rate falling far below it should be regarded as a risk factor for poor long-term outcome.[308] Composition of growth varies during late fetal life. For example, in the term infant, during the first weeks after birth over 40% of weight gain is fat and about 12% protein, whereas in late fetal life only 15–20% of the weight gain is fat, and protein accretion rates are higher. It is also extremely hard in the preterm infant to achieve fetal accretion rates of calcium (3 mmol/kg/day) and phosphate (2 mmol/kg/day).

The nutritional requirements of the preterm baby for the major nutrients, electrolytes, minerals, vitamins and trace elements remain a subject of debate. European consensus was reached by ESPGAN[309] and a trans-Atlantic agreement is now widely used.[308] Differences between the two recommendations are small in relation to the major nutrients. Aiming for a growth rate of 15–18 g/kg/day, the requirements of the preterm baby for the major nutrients (Table 10.33) and electrolytes, minerals, vitamins and trace elements (Table 10.34) are shown.

Table 10.32 Some aspects of body size and composition at 26 weeks' gestation and at term

	26 weeks	40 weeks
Weight	850 g	3500 g
Length	34 cm	51 cm
Brain weight	260 g	490 g
Body water	730 ml	2400 ml
Body sodium	70 mmol	280 mmol
Total nitrogen	10 g	60 g
Fat	6 g	540 g
Calcium	6 g	35 g
Phosphate	3 g	18 g

THE CHOICE OF MILK FOR THE PRETERM INFANT

The choice of milk has effects upon neurodevelopmental outcome and intelligence. All mothers of preterm infants should be encouraged to express their milk, which is the feed of choice.[310] Long term results with preterm formula are almost as good.[284] In intensive care, the chosen milk should meet nutritional requirements, be well tolerated, digested and absorbed and minimize risk of adverse effects, notably NEC.

Human milk

When the preterm mother's own milk is available, it is the feed of choice. In the preterm infant, human milk is better tolerated and full

Table 10.33 Requirements of the preterm baby for the major nutrients

Calories	130 kcal/kg/day
Water	150–180 ml/kg/day
Carbohydrate	16 g/kg/day
Fat	7 g/kg/day
Protein	3.5 g/kg/day

Table 10.34 Requirements of the preterm baby for electrolytes, minerals, trace elements and major vitamins

Sodium	2.5–5 mmol/kg/day
Potassium	2.5–3.5 mmol/kg/day
Chloride	2.5–3.5 mmol/kg/day
Calcium	2–3 mmol/kg/day
Phosphate	2–3 mmol/kg/day
Magnesium	0.5 mmol/kg/day
Iron	2 mg/kg/day
Copper	120 µg/kg/day
Zinc	1000 µg/kg/day
Vitamin A	1000 IU/day
Vitamin D	400 IU/day
Vitamin C	30 mg/day
Vitamin E	8 mg/day
Vitamin B_{12}	0.3 µg/day
Folic acid	50 µg/day

enteral feeding is achieved more rapidly than with formula,[311] gastric emptying is quicker[312] and stool frequency greater.

The advantages of human milk are now well established: considerable reduction in risk of NEC;[313] protection against gastrointestinal and respiratory tract infection in the first years of life;[314] reduction in atopic symptoms in infants with a family history of atopy;[315] and, most importantly, its association with optimal neurodevelopmental and intellectual outcome.[284,310] The semi-essential long chain polyunsaturated fatty acids contained in breast milk are structurally important in the central nervous system and may underlie this advantage of breast milk.[316] Breast milk may also protect against adult disease, like diabetes mellitus and Crohn's disease and confer protection against cardiovascular disease through nutritional programming, whereby early nutritional experience exerts a later effect upon health, independent of other influential factors during life.[317–319] Human milk also contains growth factors, IgA, and immunoprotective factors.

There are two main problems with human milk: it is not always available, and its energy, protein, calcium, phosphate and sodium content do not meet theoretical nutrient requirements despite optimal absorption of breast milk.

Breast milk varies in composition, and is particularly affected by gestation, postnatal age and method of collection. The mothers of term and preterm infants produce milk which is different in important respects during the first 2–3 weeks after birth. Preterm milk has about a three times higher concentration of sodium, protein and IgA, and a lower water content producing a general increase in the concentration of most constituents, but not calcium or phosphate. Method of collection is important, and drip milk is of lower energy content than expressed milk (Table 10.4). Banked donor milk from term mothers produces less good weight gain than either expressed preterm milk or preterm formula. Breast milk can be given in larger volumes than formula milk at around 180 ml/kg/day.

If donated milk is used, great care must be taken to prevent transmission of HIV[320] and hepatitis B and C, through screening of donors and pasteurization. Records are kept on all donors and recipients. This disincentive to the use of donor milk, has led to a reduction of milk banking.

Breast milk fortification

Fortification of breast milk is now used in most neonatal units in the UK.[292] Breast milk fortifiers are powders added to breast milk and increase energy, protein, carbohydrate, sodium, calcium and phosphate contents of the milk (Table 10.35). We have not found altered tolerance of feeds and gastric emptying during introduction of milk feeds is unchanged,[321] although with larger volume feeds it is less rapid.[322] Two studies have shown less good feed tolerance and one a trend towards increased risk of NEC, a feature which is not borne out in other studies.[323]

Growth and mineral accretion is improved with fortification[324] although the impact on long term outcome is not clear. At 18 months, infants given fortifier show no neurodevelopmental advantage over those whose milk was not fortified.[323] A recent trial exploring protein content of fortifier has shown improved growth and increase in head cirfumference with a higher protein content.[325]

The optimal use of breast milk fortifier and its ideal compostion is not established. In some centers fortifier is only used after growth failure is observed. Our practice is routinely to add it, once maternal breast milk is being produced and given in a volume exceeding 90 ml/kg/day. This strategy avoids fortification during the introduction of feeds when the infant's mother is producing milk with a naturally high nutrient content.

Preterm formula milks

The preterm formulae are based upon human milk. The principal differences are: more protein (approx. 1.8–2.5 g/100 ml); more energy (approx. 75–90 kcal/100 ml); higher sodium, calcium and phosphorus content; and the addition of iron and vitamins, especially D, E and the B complex. Some lactose is replaced with glucose or its polymers, and a small proportion of fat may be given as medium chain triglyceride to improve fat absorption. The addition of long chain polyunsaturates (see above), similar to those found in breast milk, has been shown to produce more rapid maturation of the visual pathway, and may confer neurodevelopmental advantage.[316] Purified sources of these fats are now added to formula milk. Preterm formulae work well, growth rates are good, nutritional deficiencies are rare, and long term outcome almost matches that seen with breast milk.[284]

Other milks

Term formula is not adequate for the preterm infant.[326] Preterm formula is given until an infant weighs 2.0– 2.5 kg. Most, who are

Table 10.35 Nutrient change in 100 ml breast milk after fortification

Nutrient	Energy (kcal)	Protein (g)	Carbohydrate (g)	Fat (g)	Sodium (mmol)	Calcium (mmol)	Phosphorus (mmol)
Increase	10–14	0.6–1.0	2.0–2.4	small	0.3–0.9	1.0–2.2	0.7–1.2

not breast-fed, then go on to a whey-dominant term formula. Many preterm infants remain underweight at term, and better weight gain may be seen after discharge home if a formula of composition between preterm and term formula is given.[327] Infants may compensate by taking a larger volume of formula, but male infants have increased linear growth and head circumference if fed a nutrient enriched formula for 6 months post-term.[328] A number of preterm post-discharge formulae are now available. Our policy is routinely to advise such a formula until 3 months post-term and to continue until 6 months depending upon observed growth. At no time during the first year of life is unprocessed cows' milk a suitable food for the preterm baby.

Special milks are occasionally required to treat cows' milk protein or lactose intolerance and inborn errors of metabolism. This should be done in collaboration with a pediatric dietitian. Soya milks have not been properly evaluated in the preterm baby and should probably be avoided. Goat's milk is suitable for goats.

FEEDING IN PRACTICE

No-one is in a better position to make individual decisions about feeding than the experienced neonatal nurse caring for an infant. Feeding policy and each infant's nutrition should be managed jointly by nursing and medical staff, while empowering the neonatal nurse to make feeding management decisions when necessary.

Enteral feeding should be introduced gradually and increased with care. Tolerance should be assessed and, whenever possible, infants should be weighed and measured regularly. It is reasonable to begin with 0.5–1 ml/h in a baby of less than 30 weeks' gestation, increasing by 0.5–1 ml every 6 h. In more mature babies, larger starting volumes and a faster rate of progress may be indicated. In a healthy baby, enteral feeds may be given at 75 ml/kg on day 1, 90 ml/kg on day 2, 120 ml/kg on day 3, 135 ml/kg on day 4 and 150 ml/kg on day 5, with subsequent increases up to a maximum of 180 ml/kg/day according to tolerance and growth rate. We routinely increase fortified breast milk or preterm formula feeds to 165 ml/kg/day, and breast milk or other formulae to 165–180 ml/kg/day. If enteral feeding is intended during intensive care but not achieved, parenteral feeding is mandated.

Full nipple feeding from breast or bottle depends upon maturity and health. In most it is achieved at a postmenstrual age of 34–37 weeks.

Avoidance of NEC

Trials of strategies aimed at preventing NEC are inherently difficult. The condition is unpredictable with variation in incidence that demands very large studies to obtain adequate power. There is some evidence for the following in order to avoid NEC during enteral feeding:

- use of breast milk;[313]
- avoidance of hyperosmolar feeds (addition of electrolyte supplements to milk);[329]
- rapid, incautious increase in feed volume;[330]
- careful introduction of milk in infants with IUGR;[293]
- control of infection in epidemic NEC (enteral aminoglycosides or immunoglobulins).[331]

Continuous or intermittent feeds?

Randomized studies of these two techniques show little difference, although bolus feeding improves milk tolerance.[332] If feeds are not tolerated, the alternative technique is worth trying!

Feeding tube placement

Meta-analyses of trials of tube placement have shown a 15% (95% CI 5–23%) increase in mortality in association with transpyloric feeding compared with gastric feeding.[333] Transpyloric feeding can no longer be recommended.

The choice between nasal and oral tube passage is more a matter of esthetics than of clinical importance. Nasal tubes are easier to fix but may increase resistance to air flow through the nose and increase the work of breathing. Most commonly fine bore nasogastric tubes are used.

Non-nutritive sucking (use of a dummy during gastric tube feeds) has no effect upon gastric emptying or nutrient absorption, but meta-analysis shows a mean reduction of hospital stay of 6 days (95% CI 2–10).[333]

Weaning from tube to breast or bottle feeds is usually a gradual process and most experienced neonatal nurses say that if rushed, it will take longer. There may be parental pressure to accomplish the task as soon as possible as the time for discharge approaches. Special soft teats are available for preterm babies and do seem to have some advantages over conventional teats.

NUTRITIONAL SUPPLEMENTS

Protein and energy

There is no need to routinely supplement fortified breast milk or preterm formula. Occasionally an energy supplement (glucose polymers or a mixture of glucose polymers and fat) is needed when larger feed volumes are not possible (e.g. heart failure). These supplements are usually well tolerated when added to milk at a rate up to 5 g/100 ml. Energy:protein ratio should not exceed 100 kcal/2 g of protein.

Vitamins

Vitamin deficiency states are rare, but in most centers vitamin supplements are given routinely to all VLBW infants. Breast milk will provide adequate amounts of most vitamins, but contains little vitamin D or vitamin K. Preterm formulae and breast milk fortifiers contain additional vitamins. All preterm infants should receive vitamin K (phytomenadione 0.25 mg) at birth for prevention of hemorrhagic disease of the newborn and in most this is given parenterally (p. 307). Extra vitamin K should be given i.m. if the preterm baby needs to undergo surgery, has clinical liver disease, or severe diarrheal illness during the first 4 months of life. A daily intake of vitamin D of 400 IU (10 μg) will prevent deficiency.

Routine use of a multivitamin preparation is common practice in breast- and formula-fed infants. The widely used Abidec (Warner Lambert), 0.6 ml/day, will provide enough vitamins A, B_6, C, and D. In most neonatal units, a multivitamin is given after discharge until full mixed feeds are established.

Sodium

The preterm infant requires 2.5–4 mmol/kg/day of sodium, usually as chloride. When intake is poor, urinary excretion may well exceed the intake, leading to poor growth and hyponatremia. Routine supplementation of fortified breast milk or preterm formula is not necessary. Initially after birth, preterm milk may contain 20 mmol/L of sodium but this falls over 2–3 weeks to levels seen in mature human milk, at about 7 mmol/L. This is one reason, as suggested above, to fortify breast milk only when lactation is established. If feeding with unfortified breast milk, a sodium supplement should be considered. Certainly, if a preterm baby is not growing well, it is always worth checking the serum and urinary sodium concentrations, as the response to an additional 2–4 mmol/kg/day of sodium (as chloride) can be dramatic. Serum concentrations should be monitored during therapy.

Calcium and phosphorus

Metabolic bone disease of prematurity (previously, osteopenia of prematurity or neonatal rickets) is largely due to substrate deficiency which is the almost inevitable consequence of preterm delivery. In fetal life, active transport across the placenta, during the final trimester, results in fetal accretion rates which cannot be matched by enteral or parenteral supplementation after birth because when sufficient calcium and phosphate is added to feeds, precipitation of insoluble salts occurs. It is, however, known that addition of calcium and phosphate to enteral feeds will result in improved bone mineral density and lower levels of alkaline phosphatase.[333,334]

Addition of calcium and phosphate to preterm formulae or fortified breast milk is usually unnecessary. If unsupplemented breast milk is used, a supplement of phosphorus (as buffered sodium phosphate: 1 mmol/kg/day) is recommended. Serum chemistry and alkaline phosphatase should be monitored. Adequate provision of substrate should prevent fractures although special care should be taken in infants exposed to sytemic steroids or long term diuretics.

Iron

Iron absorption from human milk is very efficient, but its iron content is low. The iron accretion rates of the third trimester cannot be achieved in the human milk fed preterm infant. Fortification and preterm formulae provide additional iron. The need to give a further supplement is contentious, but in many centers 2 mg/kg/day of iron is given from 6–8 weeks of age until about 12 months.

COMPLICATIONS OF FEEDING

Milk aspiration

Regurgitation of milk into the esophagus, as shown by esophageal pH monitoring, is common among preterm babies[335] but significant aspiration is uncommon in infants receiving milk feeds during intensive care. The extent to which milk aspiration contributes to chronic lung disease or recurrent apneic attacks remains uncertain, but in the infant who has atypical disease, with unexplained deterioration, or failure to respond to standard therapy, gastroesophageal reflux and aspiration should be considered. Prone positioning, thickening agents and smaller, more frequent, feeds may help. Xanthines may be withdrawn. A prokinetic, low dose of erythromycin may be used. There are few good trial data in this area.

Respiratory embarrassment resulting from gastric distention

When the lungs are normal, tube feeding has little or no effect on lung function, but when the lungs are abnormal a tube feed of only 5 ml of milk has been shown to produce a small reduction in arterial PO_2 for about 30 min. During suckling, a fall in arterial PO_2 and a small rise in arterial PCO_2 has been shown in preterm infants. It is important to be aware of this effect in babies recovering from RDS and those with bronchopulmonary dysplasia.

Food intolerance

Intolerance of cows' milk protein seems uncommon among preterm babies, perhaps reflecting the relative unresponsiveness of their immune system. It may present as colitis with fresh bleeding per rectum. Lactose intolerance is commoner, especially after NEC or gut surgery. Treatment by exclusion diet is appropriate as long as the substitute food is carefully chosen with the nutritional needs of the preterm baby in mind. The advice of the pediatric dietitian is most helpful.

NUTRITIONAL ASSESSMENT

The final validation of any nutritional regime is satisfactory growth, and prevention of deficiency states. Careful and frequent assessments of the growth of the preterm baby should be made. Weight, length and occipitofrontal circumference are measured at least weekly, and related to centile charts. In addition to the routine measurements, reference data are now available for skinfold thickness, mid-upper arm circumference (MUAC) and MUAC:head circumference ratio which can be used as indicators of fat deposition and lean body mass.

Hematological and biochemical assessments should be undertaken regularly to look for signs of nutritional deficiency such as: anemia due to iron deficiency; raised alkaline phosphatase and low serum phosphate related to metabolic bone disease; hypoalbuminemia suggesting absolute or relative protein deficiency; hyponatremia; hypocalcemia; metabolic acidosis due to excessive protein intake, etc.

Finally, growth monitoring and dietary advice are an important part of follow-up for the VLBW infant after discharge, and throughout the first year.

INTENSIVE CARE OF THE NEWBORN

ORGANIZATION OF NEONATAL INTENSIVE CARE SERVICES

It is now accepted that 1.0–1.9 intensive care cots are required per 1000 deliveries.[336] Each unit providing for anything other than anticipated normal deliveries should have special care back-up facilities. The belief by many obstetricians and pediatricians in the UK that a normal delivery is only diagnosable in retrospect has encouraged moves to ensure that all deliveries occur in hospital.

Although intensive care equipment can be bought for even small district units, nursing and medical staff have to be properly trained to use such 'high-tech' machinery or the baby may be at risk from the equipment itself. Continuous back-up maintenance and service support is needed for machines that are themselves in use all day every day. Without a certain critical level of expertise neonatal care becomes a very dangerous provision. It should only be carried out in recognized centers.[336]

HIERARCHY OF CARE

Every hospital concerned with the delivery of babies should *at all times* provide expertise for the resuscitation of the newborn – this can be by trained medical or nursing staff and it is the training of these staff that is critical. In addition, all district hospital maternity services should have a neonatal unit that can provide special care. This care can be given by midwives under the supervision of staff trained in neonatal care but the skill mix must be adequate. There should be medical personnel with pediatric experience on site at all times. The special care unit (level 1 care – USA) must be capable of providing safe temperature control, oxygen therapy, intravenous access and therapy, and treatment for hypoglycemia, hypocalcemia, hyperbilirubinemia and infection. Though not intended to carry out sophisticated intensive care, the special care unit must still provide expertise for the safe resuscitation and stabilization of the unexpected critically ill child with respiratory failure while help arrives.

The subregional center (level 2 – USA) will usually be sited in a larger hospital and will be able to offer short term neonatal intensive care to their own deliveries. Infants likely to require long periods of intensive care (e.g. the ELBW infant or infant requiring surgical treatment) would reasonably be diverted to the perinatal intensive care unit (ICU) which when busy could itself refer shorter term problems and high-dependency cases back. The subregional center should be capable of intensive care with the exception of surgery; its specialist staffing will be less broad.

Each region should have one or more perinatal ICUs (level 3 – USA) (Table 10.36) dealing with the very high-risk mother and infant. These centers not only provide care for all the most difficult medical and surgical problems of the region but also are intimately concerned with the improvements of standards in the region by specialist education and research. In the UK, extracorporeal membrane oxygenation (ECMO) is provided supraregionally at only three centers.

CATEGORIES OF NEONATAL CARE

In 1984 the categories of care required for babies were more clearly defined (see Definitions, p. 178). Despite these and other sensible recommendations made by multiple reports, few recommendations have been implemented. Although it is true that such organization is expensive, there is little doubt that it is extremely cost effective (see Economics of newborn care, p. 183). Most expensive is the trained neonatal nurse staffing – the intensive care bay should at all times have 1:1 trained nurse care – indeed a baby with severe pulmonary hypertension may require two nurses. In special care a nurse should never have care of more than four babies. Medical, laboratory and paramedical back-up services add in lesser costs.

Table 10.36 The perinatal intensive care unit (ICU) (at least one in every health region)

Facilities
1. Obstetric ICU facilities
2. Neonatal ICU facilities
   a. Minimum medical provision
      Senior House Officer (experienced in pediatrics) always on duty
      Specialist Registrar (experienced in neonates) always on duty
      Consultant (experienced in neonatal intensive care) always on call
   b. Nursing provision
      One neonatal intensive care nurse per intensive care baby per shift*
   c. 24-h back-up provisions
      Radiology service to the unit
      Biochemistry with blood gases and electrolytes
      Hematology service for diagnosis and transfusion
      Microbiological service
      Medical physics and electronics
   d. Specialist facilities – Surgery, cardiology, audiology, ophthalmology, pharmacy and physiotherapy

Responsibilities
1. Provision of medical neonatal intensive care
2. Provision of surgical neonatal intensive care
   THE BUCK STOPS HERE!
3. Administrative liaison within the region
4. Neonatal education for the region
   a. Ward rounds and seminars for nursing and medical visitors to the ICU
   b. Medical and nursing outreach by staff to the district and subregional centers
5. Regional audit
6. Training base for medical and neonatal nursing staff
7. Research
   Epidemiological, applied, basic

*Although recommended and ideal, the provision of one neonatal intensive care trained nurse per intensive care baby per shift is not available anywhere in the UK at this stage. One is forced back to stipulating that there be adequate overall numbers of trained nurses and a reasonable skill mix of trainers to trainees. This in fact means that most units are unable to take all the sick infants that they are asked to because of insufficient nursing staff.

TRANSPORT OF SICK OR HIGH-RISK NEONATES

Introduction

Except in the remoter areas of Scotland or under extreme weather conditions, road transfer is the usual means of transporting babies from one center to another in the UK. It is also the rule to use ambulances provided by the health service as these are available at all times. They have the added advantage that the crew have expert knowledge of the hospitals and the major and minor routes between them, thus enabling the use of alternative routes if traffic conditions are problematic and there is no police escort. It is usual for the ICU to provide the transport team to pick up the sick infant: the ambulance traveling with the emergency siren will get the expert team to the baby with the greatest possible speed. Returning the sick infant to the ICU should be done at a steady pace rather than a rush and, if there is a problem in transit, it is wise to stop and sort it out, not run for the home base. A police escort in the city can be a big advantage on the return journey. When the infant no longer requires intensive care, the local hospital sends a team to collect the infant, again using the local ambulance service.

Equipment

The equipment needed for transferring sick newborn infants is almost identical to that required in the ICU. The infant is stabilized in a portable transport incubator which enables management of the infant in the optimal thermal environment with good visibility and access. Full respiratory support must be possible using ventilator or continuous positive airway pressure (CPAP) and adjustable oxygen concentration. Ideally the inspired cases should be both warmed and humidified, but many older transport incubators do not allow this. All the supporting equipment such as laryngoscope, endotracheal tubes, chest drains, etc. and drugs must be available in a compact and portable travel case. Monitoring of respiratory and cardiovasular function should be possible. Except for diagnostic services (e.g. radiology and blood gases) the transport team should be fully equipped such that they are independent of the district hospital.

Indications

The indication for postnatal transfer is the perceived inability by the district hospital to provide a satisfactory level of diagnosis or care on that site, either at that moment or in the immediate future. This may be a result of lack of equipment or adequately trained staff. One important job of the ICU is to ensure that staff at district hospitals are given training, both in-service by outreach and by clinical meetings. A level of expertise is then always available for the management of stable but high-dependency problems on site. In this way the district hospital can take infants back before they are 'low risk' thus allowing a greater turnover of patients at the center.

Antenatal (in utero) transfer (Table 10.37)

With few exceptions the best portable incubator for the high-risk problem is the uterus, with delivery of the infant where support and

Table 10.37 Indicators for antenatal (in utero) transfer

1. Obstetric assessment of the high-risk fetus where urgent delivery is likely (e.g. IUGR, fetal cardiac rhythm disorder)
2. The severely ill mother (e.g. with pregnancy-associated hypertension) at an early stage of pregnancy with a potentially viable fetus
3. Early preterm labor where the referring hospital has inadequate facilities
4. Hemolytic disease with a severely affected fetus
5. Fetal malformation needing postnatal surgery
6. Prolonged and preterm rupture of the fetal membranes with resulting oligohydramnios
7. Any other situation where advanced neonatal resuscitation is anticipated

expertise are readily available. Such transfers should be with agreement between district and central obstetric consultants and should also involve the neonatal staff of the ICU. Mothers in advanced stages of preterm labor may need delivery peripherally to avoid the danger of a delivery in the ambulance. The mother with severe pregnancy-associated hypertension or antepartum hemorrhage should be stable before transfer and an obstetric doctor should accompany her.

PRACTICAL PARENTERAL NUTRITION

All units providing neonatal intensive and high dependency care must be able to provide optimal parenteral nutrition for sick, full-term and preterm infants; if not, the baby must be transferred to an appropriate center. All regimens should provide complete nutrition in terms of macronutrients (protein, carbohydrate and fat) and micronutrients, with minimal adverse nutritional or other consequences. The vast majority of energy and nutrient stores are laid down in the third trimester of pregnancy, so parenteral nutrition of the preterm infant must supply energy and nutrients not only to meet basic needs, but also to promote growth, which occurs at a rate of 15 g/kg/day or 1.5% of body weight at this stage.[337] About 10 years ago, it was stated that there was a dearth of well-designed studies of parenteral nutrition use in the newborn,[338] and despite the advent of evidence-based medicine and the Cochrane collaboration, there remain few high quality systematic reviews with homogeneous studies, and few randomized controlled trials of parenteral nutrition of the newborn without major methodological flaws.

INDICATIONS IN THE NEONATAL UNIT

Parenteral nutrition may provide all the nutritional requirements of the infant (total parenteral nutrition, TPN) or may more usually be supplemented by some enteral nutrition (partial parenteral nutrition, PPN). Trophic nutrition or 'minimal' enteral feeding should be started in all sick newborn infants,[339] except those at the highest risk of NEC.[337]

There are three major indications for parenteral nutrition in the neonatal unit:

1. surgical lesions such as omphalocele or gastroschisis, or following extensive bowel resection (PPN if possible, or TPN);
2. the medical (and surgical) treatment of NEC (usually TPN);
3. in immature and usually very premature infants where enteral feeds cannot be fully established, due to gastrointestinal immaturity (PPN preferably, unless high risk of NEC).

NUTRITIONAL REQUIREMENTS DURING PARENTERAL NUTRITION

Fluid and sodium

After birth, loss of interstitial fluid causes contraction of the extracellular compartment, and the resulting loss of sodium and water accounts in part for the early postnatal weight loss seen in all babies.[336] After this, growth can only be supported by a positive sodium balance. Some preterm babies have renal salt wasting, and thus very high sodium needs. Fluid needs vary depending upon maturity, postnatal age and environment, and may be huge in very immature infants; cohort and case control studies have suggested that excessive fluid intake in early life is associated with worse outcome in preterm infants in terms of chronic lung disease and NEC.

Energy

It has been suggested that a parenteral energy intake of 90 kcal/kg/day with adequate nitrogen intake will support weight gain in preterm infants at equivalent to the intrauterine rate.[338] The energy needs of the very preterm or ventilator dependent baby are likely to be higher.[340] Chronic energy imbalance is common in very preterm babies, particularly those with chronic lung disease, and a major problem is the shortfall between prescribed and actual energy intakes.[341] Multiple reasons will contribute to this shortfall, such as the need for fluid restriction, intolerance of standard dextrose infusions, witholding parenteral lipid due to concerns about clinical status, delay in commencing and advancing enteral feeds, and technical problems such as delay in re-establishing venous access. Only determined efforts to monitor and negate this shortfall in energy intake will help prevent the growth problems that are very common at hospital discharge of very preterm infants.[342]

Protein

Although milks provide between 2 and 4 g/kg/day of protein, most preterm infants receive only 2.5 g/kg/day of parenteral amino acids, and few randomized controlled studies have assessed higher intakes.[342] During evolution, the animal kingdom lost the enzyme capacity to synthesize nine amino acids. The infant is dependent upon supply from exogenous sources for these *essential* amino acids; the remainder are termed *non-essential*. A more accurate terminology has been created[343] which now divides amino acids into *indispensable* (equivalent to essential), *conditionally indispensable* (whose rates of biosynthesis may be inadequate, particularly during certain pathophysiological or metabolic states), and *dispensable* (no dietary need for preformed amino acids, but do contribute to non-specific nitrogen pool). The original parenteral amino acid solutions were protein hydrolysates, and were replaced by crystalline amino acid solutions, which were then specifically refined for use in children; problems such as hyperammonemia, metabolic acidosis and hyperphenylalaninemia were associated with the use of these in newborn infants. The latest amino acid preparations for neonatal TPN contain amino acids felt to be conditionally indispensable for the newborn. They have low phenylalanine contents, and are carbohydrate and electrolyte-free and are based upon the amino acid profile of either human breast milk or cord blood.[344] Table 10.38 shows the amino acid solution profile of two such preparations. For optimal nitrogen utilization adequate calories

Table 10.38 Amino acid profile of two solutions available in UK (each amino acid expressed as g/1000 ml)

	Vaminolact*	Primene 10%†
Indispensable		
Isoleucine	3.1	6.7
Leucine	7.0	10.0
Valine	3.6	7.6
Lysine	5.6	11.0
Methionine	1.3	2.4
Phenylalanine	2.7	4.2
Threonine	3.6	3.7
Tryptophan	1.4	2.0
Histidine	2.1	3.8
Conditionally indispensable		
Arginine	4.1	8.4
Cysteine	1.0	2.5
Glutamine	–	–
Glycine	2.1	4.0
Proline	5.6	3.0
Taurine‡	0.3	0.6
Tyrosine	0.5	0.45
Dispensable		
Alanine	6.3	8.0
Serine	3.8	4.0
Aspartic acid	4.1	6.0
Glutamic acid	7.1	10.0
Ornithine	–	2.49

* Fresenius Kabi, UK.
† Baxter, UK.
‡ Taurine is not synthesized into protein.

must also be provided, the ideal calorie to nitrogen ratio being between 150 and 250.

Fat

The absence of an intravenous lipid emulsion in early parenteral nutrition regimens led to a syndrome of essential fatty acid deficiency with inadequate growth and a scaly dermatitis. In the UK and Europe lipid solutions can be obtained as 10% or 20% concentrations; randomized controlled trials have demonstrated the superiority of the use of 20% emulsions.[345] These solutions are usually based on soya oil, although olive oil based solutions and solutions containing medium chain triglycerides are available; few studies have compared different types of solutions. Preterm infants can tolerate incremental increases up to 3.5–4.0 g/kg/day of parenteral lipid without side-effects.[342] Heparin increases the clearance of lipid from the circulation; there is a belief, not backed up by any evidence, that addition of 1 IU/ml to parenteral nutrition solutions preserves intravenous line patency and promotes lipolysis. Preterm infants have low concentrations of carnitine, required for oxidation of long chain fatty acids; a recent Cochrane review evaluated the many studies of supplemental carnitine in parenterally fed newborns, and concluded that there was no evidence to support its use.[346]

Carbohydrate

Term newborn have a significantly higher glucose requirement than older children, and preterm infants have the highest needs of all. It is usual to start with a 10% dextrose solution at approximately 6 g/kg/day (4 mg/kg/min), and to increase this incrementally if there is no hyperglycemia. Continuous insulin infusions have been used as an effective treatment of hyperglycemia in preterm infants.[342]

Vitamins and minerals

The vitamin and mineral requirements of preterm infants have often been poorly met in the past with parenteral feeding; a typical parenteral prescription that meets these is shown in Table 10.39.

TECHNIQUE OF PREPARATION, ADMINISTRATION AND MONITORING

As for all nutritional support, involvement of a multidisciplinary nutrition support team will optimize parenteral feeding. Prescription of TPN is often aided by the use of a computer program, although nutritional regimens should be individualized depending on the degree of prematurity, postnatal age, concurrent illness, enteral feed tolerance and presence of undernutrition requiring catch-up growth.[337] Whether the final solution is infused by central or by peripheral vein, it should be made up by pharmacy under laminar flow conditions to prevent contamination. It should be run through from the bag to the giving set delivery point so that all that is required on the neonatal unit is the linking of the sterile connection of the set to the intravenous line on the baby. The lipid should join the main set by a Y-connector just prior to this connection. The use of millipore filters is not backed up by reliable evidence. Covering the bags with colored polyethylene will reduce the photodegradation of vitamins.

Since Wilmore & Dudrick's original description in 1968,[347] central lines have frequently been used to give parenteral nutrition. This is because access to the circulation can be very difficult in infants, particularly if prolonged parenteral nutrition is required. Peripheral venous infusions have a limited life span and are associated with infiltration of the infusate and skin sloughs.[338] Frequent occlusion will result in increased handling of the baby and interruption of nutrient supply. Central access is usually provided by non-cuffed silicone catheters that are inserted percutaneously and threaded to a central position. Due to concerns about pericardial effusions, these are now usually placed close to, but not in, the right atrium. Monitoring of growth and biochemical and metabolic tolerance is mandatory with parenteral nutrition. A few infants, for example those with short gut syndrome, will require prolonged parenteral feeding in hospital or at home, and early liasion with pediatric gastroenterologists is advised.

COMPLICATIONS

1. Catheter related:
   a. Sepsis – bacterial or fungal.
   b. Thrombosis/obstruction.
   c. Hemorrhage.
   d. Extravasation of fluid from peripheral lines.
   e. Catheter displacement, breakage or removal.
2. Metabolic related:
   a. Cholestasis – often reversible, and reduced by minimal enteral feeding.
   b. Fat embolism, lipid overload – rare.
   c. Hyperglycemia and glycosuria.
   d. Hyperammonemia and acidosis – rare.

BLOOD GASES AND RESPIRATORY SUPPORT

Optimal respiratory support requires meticulous attention to blood gases, ventilator settings, blood pressure and infant behavior. To achieve appropriate gas exchange with minimal complications

Table 10.39 A typical parenteral nutrition prescription (150 ml/kg/day) for a 10-day-old infant of 1500 g with necrotizing enterocolitis (NEC)

Aqueous bag			Lipid bag	
Primene 10%*		40 ml	Intralipid 20%†	26 ml (3.5 g/kg/day)
Glucose 50% w/v		48 ml	Vitlipid Infant†	6 ml (4 ml/kg/day)
Solvito†		1.5 ml (1 ml/kg/day)		
Sodium chloride 30% w/v		0.7 ml		
Potassium acetate 2 mmol/ml		1.4 ml		
Addiphos†		0.6 ml		
Magnesium chloride 2 mmol/ml		0.15 ml		
Peditrace†		1.5 ml (1 ml/kg/day)		
Calcium gluconate 10% w/v		5.3 ml		
Water for injections		94 ml		
	Total:	*193 ml*		*32 ml*
Amino acids	3.75 g	(2.5 g/kg/day)		
Retinol	414 μg	(276 μg/kg/day)		
Nitrogen	0.6 g	(0.4 g/kg/day)		
Ergocalciferol	6 μg	(4 μg/kg/day)		
Carbohydrate	24 g	(16 g/kg/day)		
Tocopherol	3.84 mg	(2.56 mg/kg/day)		
Sodium	4.5 mmol	(3 mmol/kg/day)		
Phytomenadione	120 μg	(80 μg/kg/day)		
Potassium	3.7 mmol	(2.5 mmol/kg/day)		
Lipid	5.2 g	(3.5 g/kg/day)		
Calcium	1.2 mmol	(0.8 mmol/kg/day)		
Phosphate	1.2 mmol	(0.8 mmol/kg/day)		
Magnesium	0.3 mmol	(0.2 mmol/kg/day)		
Vitamin B_1	0.38 mg	(0.25 mg/kg/day)		
Vitamin B_2	0.54 mg	(0.36 mg/kg/day)		
Nicotinamide	6.0 mg	(4.0 mg/kg/day)		
Pantothenic acid	2.25 mg	(1.5 mg/kg/day)		
Biotin	9.0 μg	(6.0 μg/kg/day)		
Folic acid	60 μg	(40 μg/kg/day)		
Vitamin B_6	0.6 mg	(0.4 mg/kg/day)		
Vitamin B_{12}	0.75 μg	(0.5 μg/kg/day)		
Vitamin C	15 mg	(10 mg/kg/day)		
Copper	0.47 μmol	(0.31 μmol/kg/day)		
Zinc	5.7 μmol	(3.8 μmol/kg/day)		
Manganese	0.027 μmol	(0.018 μmol/kg/day)		
Selenium	0.038 μmol	(0.025 μmol/kg/day)		
Fluoride	4.5 μmol	(3.0 μmol/kg/day)		
Iodide	0.012 μmol	(0.008 μmol/kg/day)		

* Baxter, UK.
† Fresenius Kabi, UK.

requires knowledge of:
1. lung mechanics;
2. mechanisms of lung injury from ventilation;
3. the principles of gas exchange;
4. appropriate blood gas values;
5. measurement of blood gases.

LUNG MECHANICS

To inflate the lungs, work must be done against their elastic recoil and resistance. Even with adequate surfactant most of this recoil is attributable to surface tension. Lung compliance is the change in lung volume per unit change in pressure. This is proportional to the number of recruited alveoli and is therefore determined by the size of the lungs but is reduced by atelectasis or consolidation and improves as these improve. Resistance reflects airway caliber and increases with airway narrowing.

THE PRESSURE–VOLUME CURVE OF THE LUNGS

When lungs are inflated from complete atelectasis, large pressure changes are required to begin opening the alveoli. Once opened, they inflate easily and smaller changes in pressure achieve large changes in volume. As the alveoli become overdistended, further pressure changes add little volume. During deflation the alveoli do not collapse completely. Surfactant enables lung volume to remain higher per unit pressure than during inflation. Around 30 ml/kg body weight of gas remains in the lungs at end-expiration. This functional residual capacity (FRC) enables gas exchange to continue during expiration. Surfactant deficiency impairs deflation stability causing alveolar collapse, reduced FRC and impaired gas exchange. Once the alveoli collapse, high pressures are required to re-recruit them.

The time required to inflate or deflate the lungs depends on the tidal volume, the pressure applied and the resistance to flow. If resistance is high, as in chronic lung disease or endotracheal tube obstruction, the same volume takes longer to exchange. Where compliance is low, as in RDS, the recoil pressure is high and the lungs empty rapidly.

MECHANISMS OF VENTILATION – INDUCED LUNG INJURY

The same mechanisms of lung injury from ventilation operate in all age groups.[348,349] High volume injury (volutrauma) occurs when the airspaces are inflated to excess end-inspiratory volume. Low volume injury (atelectrauma) occurs when the lungs are allowed recurrently to collapse at end-expiration and are re-inflated with each breath. Both mechanisms cause epithelial disruption and alveolar capillary leak. This causes accumulation within the airspaces of proteinaceous material which inhibits surfactant function and adds further to the cycle. Injury may begin within minutes and is accompanied by inflammation, the persistence of which has been implicated in the pathogenesis of chronic lung disease.[350]

Respiratory support techniques should aim to maintain optimal alveolar recruitment and limit excess tidal volume. This is associated with lower mortality and more rapid resolution of pulmonary inflammation in adults.[351,352] There are no published trials examining this approach in neonates. A healthy, term infant breathes with a tidal volume of around 7–9 ml/kg.[353] In the presence of lung disease there may be less fully functional alveoli than normal. Ventilator tidal volumes of around 4–7 ml/kg may be more appropriate if focal overinflation is to be minimized.

Oxygen in high concentration generates free radicals. The preterm infant has poorly developed antioxidant lung defences and may be at greater risk of oxygen toxicity.

PRINCIPLES OF GAS EXCHANGE

If ventilation and perfusion are well matched, gas tensions in the blood equilibrate with those in the air spaces. Mechanisms of ventilation/perfusion mismatching and impaired gas exchange are illustrated in Figure 10.17.

Oxygenation

When alveoli collapse or are filled with blood, edema or exudate, blood perfusing them traverses the lungs without exchanging gas (right-to-left shunt). If the pulmonary vascular resistance is elevated, extrapulmonary right-to-left shunt can take place through the foramen ovale and ductus arteriosus. This occurs in association with acidosis, hypoxia, hypercarbia, lung disease or persistent pulmonary hypertension of the newborn and is worsened by low systemic blood pressure. High ventilator pressures may also compromise pulmonary blood flow. If cardiac output is low, the blood perfusing the alveoli has lower oxygen tension and higher carbon dioxide tension than normal and equilibration with alveolar gas may be incomplete. If blood volume is low the increased rate of recirculation may reduce the time available for equilibration. Inadequate alveolar ventilation results in lower alveolar oxygen tension and hypoxia.

Mild degrees of shunt can be corrected by increasing the inspired oxygen concentration. If the shunt is more substantial, increased inspired oxygen is ineffective. The vast majority of the oxygen carried in blood is bound to Hb. Relatively little can dissolve in the plasma. Once Hb is fully saturated, further large increases in oxygen tension (PO_2) generate small increases in total blood oxygen content as they only reflect increased dissolved oxygen in plasma. When fully saturated blood from alveoli with good ventilation/perfusion matching is mixed with large amounts of desaturated shunt blood, the mixture cannot be fully saturated. Severely compromised oxygenation can only be improved by decreasing the degree of shunt. This requires recruitment of unventilated alveoli or improvement of pulmonary perfusion. By improving pulmonary perfusion, correction of hypotension may improve gas exchange without alteration of the ventilator settings.

Carbon dioxide elimination

Carbon dioxide is more soluble in plasma than oxygen and its pulmonary diffusion capacity is greater. The relationship between blood carbon dioxide content and arterial carbon dioxide tension ($PaCO_2$) is linear. In respiratory failure or where there is right-to-left shunting, the carbon dioxide tension of blood returning from alveoli with good ventilation/perfusion matching can be lowered by increased alveolar ventilation. This can compensate for the elevated carbon dioxide of shunt blood and normalize $PaCO_2$. Alveolar ventilation or perfusion must be severely impaired before carbon dioxide elimination becomes problematic. Alveolar ventilation is proportional to minute ventilation, which is tidal volume multiplied by the number of breaths/min. Minute ventilation may be inadequate with poor respiratory drive, airway obstruction, widespread atelectasis or increased respiratory dead space.

MEASUREMENT OF BLOOD GASES

All neonatal units should have immediate 24 h access to a blood gas analyzer. Blood samples are usually obtained from an umbilical arterial catheter, or by indwelling catheter or needle puncture from the radial or posterior tibial arteries after assessing the collateral circulation. Use of end arteries (temporal, brachial or femoral) is less desirable because of the risk of irreversible ischemia.

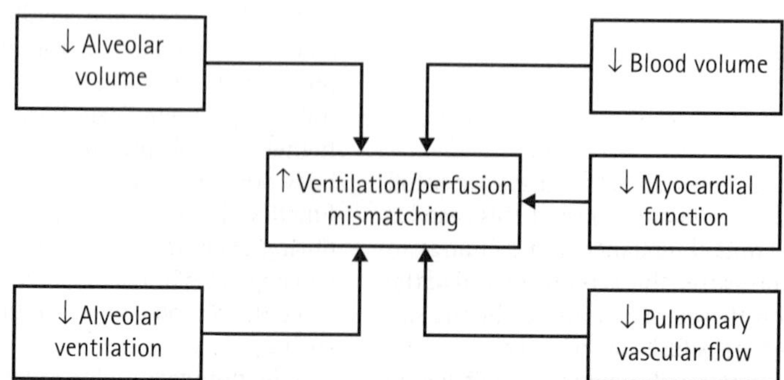

Fig. 10.17 Mechanisms leading to ventilation/perfusion mismatching.

Measurements of PO_2 in capillary or venous blood underestimate arterial oxygen tension (PaO_2) and cannot be relied on, even if the skin is warmed to 40°C. Capillary blood obtained by heel prick provides an acceptable estimate of arterial PCO_2, pH and base excess, but warming the heel to 40°C does not significantly improve accuracy of PO_2.[354]

Continuous monitoring of blood gas tensions or oxygen saturation is an important supplement to, but not a substitute for, intermittent sampling. Continuous measurements can be made by an indwelling device in the umbilical artery.[355] Transcutaneous monitors generate local hyperemia by gently heating the skin. Diffusion of gases through the skin then permits measurement of gas tensions. This technique is unreliable when the skin is poorly perfused or compressed and becomes less reliable as the skin thickens with age. In very immature infants, repeated reattachment of the transcutaneous (tc)PO_2 electrode can damage the skin. Pulse oximetry is easier and less invasive but gives less information. A probe transilluminates a body part and measures the light absorption characteristics of oxygenated Hb. Pulse oximeters can be used at all gestations, require no calibration and are not affected by changes in skin thickness or perfusion. The technique is very prone to movement artefact, although new signal processing techniques can reduce this problem.[356] In the steep portion of the oxygen–Hb dissociation curve, small changes in PO_2 cause large changes in O_2 saturation, so in this range the pulse oximeter reflects hypoxia and oxygen availability to tissues better than $tcPO_2$ measurements. In the flat portion of the oxygen–Hb dissociation curve large changes in PO_2 cause small changes in O_2 saturation, so hyperoxia cannot safely be excluded when transcutaneous Hb saturation ($tcSaO_2$) is 95–100% and $tcPO_2$ monitoring is more reliable.

RECOMMENDED BLOOD GAS VALUES

Present recommendations are based on physiological reasoning and clinical observations. There is a need for prospective trials which compare the outcomes of infants with different target blood gas values as the interventions introduced to normalize blood gases may be harmful.

Oxygenation (PaO_2, $tcPO_2$ and $tcSaO_2$)

Values for $tcPO_2$ and $tcSaO_2$ in the first weeks of life from healthy term and preterm infants[357,358] are shown in Table 10.40.[357,358] In preterm infants hyperoxia is associated with increased risk of chronic lung disease and retinopathy of prematurity.[359] Even modest variations in oxygen administration policy may be associated with significant changes in risk of adverse outcome.[360] There is considerable variation in policy between units.[361] At all gestations prolonged severe hypoxia causes organ damage. Until new data become available, a reasonable policy for preterm infants receiving respiratory support is to aim for PaO_2 or $tcPO_2$ between 6.7 and 10.7 kPa (50–80 mmHg) or $tcSaO_2$ between 86 and 94%.

Carbon dioxide tension

Hypercapnia produces pulmonary vasoconstriction, but cerebral vasodilatation. In a prospective study of 200 VLBW infants, $PaCO_2$ > 7 kPa (52.5 mmHg) was associated with both periventricular hemorrhage and periventricular leukomalacia.[362] Severe hypocapnia causes a profound reduction in cerebral blood flow, and has been associated with periventricular leukomalacia, intracerebral hemorrhage and cerebral palsy.[363–366]

Broad consensus in current practice is to keep $PaCO_2$ between 4.7 and 8 kPa (35–60 mmHg).[367] However in severe respiratory failure some authors *routinely* keep $PaCO_2$ between 6.7 and 8 kPa (50–60 mmHg) or higher, provided arterial pH remains above 7.25. By allowing lower ventilator pressures to be used this, it is suggested, may increase the number of infants surviving without chronic lung disease.[368–371] Whether allowing higher values of $PaCO_2$ may also increase the risk of cerebral insult and handicap in preterm infants is uncertain. Data from prospective trials in newborn infants are limited and inconclusive at present.[372] In the meantime a reasonable compromise is to aim for $PaCO_2$ between 5.3 and 7.0 kPa (40-52.5 mmHg) in preterm infants below 33 weeks' gestation during the first 3 days of life. In term infants or older preterm infants, higher levels of $PaCO_2$ are probably acceptable in order to limit ventilator pressures, provided acidosis is avoided. Iatrogenic hypocapnia should be avoided.

pH

Acidosis causes cerebral vasodilatation and alkalosis cerebral vasoconstriction. Acidosis may also promote pulmonary vasoconstriction and right-to-left shunting. In preterm infants, pH < 7.20 has been associated with periventricular hemorrhage[373] and pH < 7.1 with periventricular leukomalacia.[362] In VLBW infants pH < 7.20 has been associated with retinopathy of prematurity.[359] Acidosis may be due to tissue hypoxia, respiratory failure, excess acid load, renal dysfunction or inborn error of metabolism. It is unlikely that a pH value will have the same implications whatever its origins. Simultaneous measurements of plasma lactate may give additional information. Interventions aimed at altering pH should reflect the likely underlying explanation. On present information, a reasonable policy for infants receiving respiratory support is to keep pH between 7.25 and 7.45.

RESPIRATORY SUPPORT

Reducing the need for respiratory support by antenatal steroids

Treating mothers at risk of preterm delivery with antenatal steroids reduces infants' risks of RDS, death and brain damage by around 50%[374] and should be a standard of care subjected to routine

Table 10.40 Normal range of $tcPO_2$ and $tcSaO_2$ in healthy infants in air* (adapted from Mok et al 1986,[357] 1988[358])

	Awake	Quiet sleep	Active sleep
Term infants (*n* = 55)			
$TcPO_2$ (kPa†)			
Postnatal age			
<1 week	8.5–13.0	7.8–12.1	6.7–12.8
6 weeks	9.1–12.2	7.1–12.3	7.1–12.4
$TcSaO_2$ (%)			
Postnatal age			
<1 week	91.8–100	87.4–98.3	86.1–98.4
6 weeks	95.0–99.0	89.4–98.1	87.5–98.5
Preterm infants (*n* = 28)			
$TcPO_2$ (kPa†)			
Postconceptional age			
29–34 weeks	4.7–11.0	6.4–11.7	4.7–11.1
36–38 weeks	6.8–12.5	7.0–12.9	6.7–12.0
$TcSaO_2$ (%)			
Postconceptional age			
29–34 weeks	86.6–96.3	86.0–96.1	86.6–96.5
35–38 weeks	86.8–96.8	87.6–97.9	88.6–96.8

*No infant appeared cyanosed or had signs of respiratory distress during any of the studies.

† To convert oxygen tension in kPa to mmHg, multiply by 7.5.

audit.[375] There is presently no evidence that repeat courses are beneficial.

Continuous positive airway pressure

CPAP helps to establish and maintain alveolar recruitment. This protects against low-volume lung injury, improves gas exchange and reduces work of breathing. CPAP may also maintain the patency of the upper airways and reduce the frequency of apnea. Use of nasal CPAP in preterm infants after extubation is associated with a lower risk of extubation failure.[376] CPAP can be generated by placing the outlet tubing of a gas source under water (bubble CPAP), by a mechanical ventilator, or by a flow generated method (infant flow driver or Benveniste valve). None is proven to be clearly superior in clinical trials. Epidemiological data suggest that chronic lung disease may be observed less frequently when CPAP is preferred to mechanical ventilation.[377] Two current prospective randomized controlled trials (the IFDAS study and the COIN trial) may help to answer this question.

Nasal CPAP can be combined with surfactant administration to treat RDS.[378,379] Infants with worsening respiratory failure are sedated, intubated, surfactant is administered and the infants are extubated and returned to CPAP. This may reduce the number of infants that require ventilation but it has not been demonstrated to be superior to elective intubation soon after birth for prophylactic surfactant treatment. Further trials are required.

Indications for respiratory support by endotracheal tube

No consensus exists as to when to start intermittent positive pressure ventilation by endotracheal tube. Some start it electively at birth in the smallest infants, others use it as rescue therapy in infants failing on CPAP. Prolonged apnea, or progressive respiratory failure are the principal indications. Intubation can be hazardous. An endotracheal tube prevents laryngeal closure which removes the infant's capacity to maintain lung volume by grunting. Adequate positive end-expiratory pressure (PEEP) is required to prevent atelectasis. By narrowing the airway the resistive work of breathing is increased. The extra work is done by the ventilator except at low ventilator settings. Other complications include blockage or malplacement of the tube, airway injury, impaired mucociliary clearance, infection and aspiration, which all may contribute to chronic lung disease.

CONTROLLING GAS EXCHANGE BY MECHANICAL VENTILATION

Despite variations in the type and severity of neonatal respiratory disorders, alterations in ventilator settings often have predictable effects on oxygenation and $PaCO_2$. These are summarized in Tables 10.42 and 10.43.

Mean airway pressure and oxygenation

Herman & Reynolds[380] showed in infants with severe hyaline membrane disease a linear relationship between mean airway pressure and oxygenation, expressed as $A\text{-}aDO_2$ (Fig. 10.18).[380] Improved oxygenation was mainly attributed to improved alveolar inflation with reduced intrapulmonary right-to-left shunt. Increases in (1) peak pressure, (2) inspiratory:expiratory ratio and (3) positive end expiratory pressure were thought to (a) expand collapsed lung units, (b) hold them open longer and (c) prevent their collapse during expiration. With stiff lungs in severe disease, high mean airway pressures had no effect on cardiac output or arterial blood pressure. Stewart et al[381] achieved greater increases in oxygenation per unit

Table 10.41 Ventilator settings and gas exchange: methods of increasing oxygenation

Maneuver	Probable underlying mechanisms
1. ↑ FiO_2	a. ↑Saturation of alveolar capillary blood b. Relieving hypoxia can decrease pulmonary vascular resistance, reducing extrapulmonary right-to-left shunt through fetal channels
2. Adding CPAP	Maintains lung volume in spontaneously breathing infants with reduced lung compliance
3. ↑ PIP 4. ↑ PEEP 5. ↑ I:E ratio	These three maneuvers increase mean airway pressure (MAP), hence lung volume and oxygenation The stiffer the lungs, the greater the MAP needed for optimum lung expansion NB: In mild or improving disease, excessive MAP may cause hypoxia by obstructing the pulmonary circulation (causing right-to-left shunt) and it may also decrease cardiac output
6. Achieving synchronous ventilation	a. Maximizes efficiency of baby's contribution to gas exchange b. ?Minimizes compression of pulmonary circulation during ventilator inflation and consequently reduces right-to-left shunting
7. Correcting hypotension	If there is evidence of hypovolemia (systemic hypotension ± peripheral vasoconstriction), correcting it with an infusion of blood, plasma or an inotrope may reduce extrapulmonary right-to-left shunt, improving pulmonary perfusion and oxygenation without a change in ventilator settings
8. Exogenous surfactant	Increases alveolar recruitment and improves deflation stability by decreasing surface tension
9. Percutaneous oxygenation	Direct absorption of ambient oxygen by the immature skin (infants < 30 weeks' gestation)

CPAP, continuous positive airway pressure; I:E ratio, inspiratory:expiratory ratio; PEEP, positive end-expiratory pressure; PIP, Peak inspiratory pressure.

increase in mean airway pressure by raising PEEP than by adjusting inspiratory:expiratory ratio or peak inspiratory pressure (PIP). With earlier intervention and less severe lung disease shorter inspiratory times and faster rates were associated with improved outcomes.[382,383] High airway pressures are now seldom required. In mild disease, excess airway pressures may cause lung injury and impair gas exchange by compromising the pulmonary and systemic circulation. If oxygenation is good with low FiO_2 (fraction of inspired oxygen), high PEEP and long inspiratory times are inappropriate. However, extremely short inspiratory times may compromise lung inflation. Field et al[384] found a significant fall in tidal volume at inspiration times under 0.3 s.

Minute ventilation, carbon dioxide exchange and inadvertent PEEP

Herman & Reynolds[380] showed that $PaCO_2$ (a) falls with increasing ventilator rate (increased minute volume), and (b) rises with increases in PEEP (i.e. decreased minute volume). Bartholomew et al[385] showed that the average effect on tidal volume of a 1 cm H_2O change in PEEP was comparable that of a 2 cm H_2O change in PIP in infants with hyaline membrane disease. This probably reflects the sigmoid shape of the pressure–volume curve.

Inadvertent PEEP occurs when the expiration time is too short to allow adequate deflation before the next inflation is imposed.[386]

Table 10.42 Ventilator settings and gas exchange: methods of decreasing $PaCO_2$

Maneuver	Probable underlying mechanisms
1. Reduce excess CPAP	In a spontaneously breathing baby, excess CPAP a. Decreases compliance and tidal volume b. Obstructs the pulmonary circulation c. Increases the work of breathing
2. ↑ Ventilator rate	Increases minute volume
3. ↑ PIP 4. ↓ PEEP	Increases tidal volume and therefore minute volume
In severe disease, with stiff lungs:	
5. ↑ Inspiratory time	If expansion of the chest wall is poor and $PaCO_2$ is elevated, increasing the inspiratory time may improve alveolar ventilation and decrease $PaCO_2$. *Increasing the expiratory time may have the opposite effect*
In mild or improving disease, with compliant lungs:	
6. ↑ Expiratory time	Compliant lungs need longer to deflate. If expiratory time is too short, inadvertent PEEP is produced and alveolar ventilation is decreased. Inadvertent PEEP can be reduced by increasing expiratory time

CPAP, continuous positive airway pressure; PEEP, positive end-expiratory pressure; PIP, peak inspiratory pressure.

The gas trapped in the lungs increases the respiratory dead space and may compress the pulmonary circulation, impairing gas exchange. The intrapulmonary pressure does not fall as far as the PEEP set on the ventilator. Inadvertent PEEP may be dangerous[387] and is most likely when compliance is improving and airway resistance is elevated, as in chronic lung disease. Reducing the ventilator rate by lengthening expiration time may improve gas exchange under these circumstances by allowing more complete expiration.

HUMIDIFICATION

Bypassing the upper airway with an endotracheal tube makes the baby dependent on external humidification. Inadequate humidity slows mucociliary clearance causing viscid secretions and may predispose to pneumothorax and chronic lung disease.[388] The presence of condensate in the ventilator tubing indicates that relative humidity is close to 100% but unless the gas temperature is above 30.5°C the absolute humidity will be inadequate. Inspired gas temperature or humidity may vary considerably[389,390] and should be measured continuously, close to the patient's airway. Excess humidification may cause fluid overload, increased respiratory system resistance and surfactant dysfunction.

Table 10.43 WHO definitions

Impairment Any loss or abnormality of psychological, physiological or anatomical structure or function: in principle impairments represent disturbances at organ level.
Disability Any restriction or lack (resulting from an impairment) of ability to perform an activity in the manner or within the range considered normal for a human being. A disability thus reflects the consequences of an impairment in terms of functional performance and activity by an individual.
Handicap A disadvantage for a given individual resulting from an impairment or disability that limits or prevents the fulfillment of a role that is normal (depending on age, sex and social and cultural factors). Handicap thus reflects interaction with the surroundings and is a difficult outcome to use for comparison as it depends on attitudes within the family and society to disability.

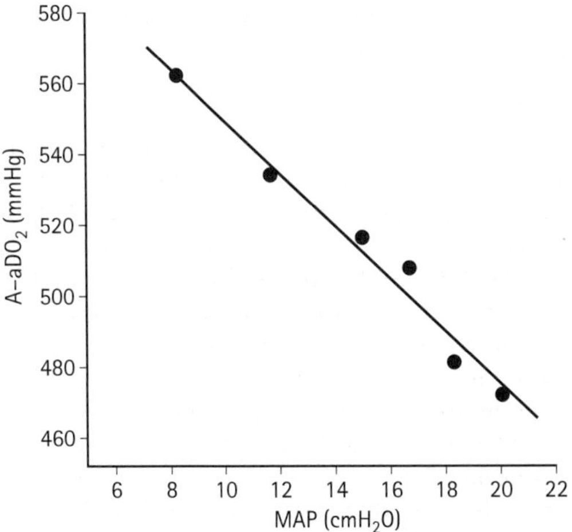

Fig. 10.18 Inverse relationship between mean airway pressure (MAP) and $A\text{-}aDO_2$ in severe hyaline membrane disease, indicating that MAP is directly proportional to oxygenation. (From Herman & Reynolds 1973[380] with permission)

ENDOTRACHEAL LAVAGE, SUCTION AND PHYSIOTHERAPY

Clearance of secretions by intermittent endotracheal tube lavage and suction reduces respiratory system resistance[391] and may prevent tube blockage. However, endotracheal suction is associated with hypoxia, bradycardia, increased blood pressure[392] and altered cerebral hemodynamics[393] and should be used in a measured way, particularly in the first 48 h of life when secretions are scant.

ADDITIONAL TECHNIQUES

The latest neonatal ventilators offer a wide range of new ventilation modes. These utilize the capacity to monitor the interaction between the baby and the ventilator and to measure flow and volume at the airway. The situation is made confusing by the lack of a standard terminology.

Synchronous ventilation modes

If the ventilator rate is set slightly faster than the spontaneous respiratory rate, many babies begin to breathe synchronously with the ventilator and show improved gas exchange.[394] Breath-sensing technology now eliminates the need for this entrainment. Modern ventilators can detect the onset of spontaneous inspiration quickly enough for a ventilator breath to be delivered in synchrony. To prevent the inflation continuing after the onset of spontaneous expiration, short inspiratory times are required. Inspiratory efforts can be measured directly at the patient airway or sensed by changes in the ventilator circuit pressure or flow, thoracic impedance, or pressure changes in a Grazeby capsule attached to the abdomen. Increased trigger sensitivity allows smaller respiratory efforts to be sensed but also promotes accidental triggering (autocycling) by other signals such as air leak around the endotracheal tube or water in the ventilator circuit. Autocycling is common[395] and may cause hypocapnia in triggered modes where the ventilator rate is unrestricted.

Synchronized intermittent mandatory ventilation mode (SIMV) leaves the clinician in control of ventilator rate, inspiratory time and pressures. The ventilator divides the minute into equal blocks of time determined by the set rate. In the first part of each time block (trigger window) the ventilator can sense an inspiratory effort and deliver a triggered breath. If no breath is sensed, a mandatory breath is delivered. There is then a brief refractory phase. Weaning is accomplished as the clinician chooses. The need for a preset inspiratory time and a refractory period in each time block limits effective SIMV to slower respiratory rates because the trigger window is narrow at higher rates.

In patient triggered ventilation mode (PTV), all inspiratory efforts made by the infant of greater than trigger threshold are rewarded by a ventilator breath. The infant determines the ventilator rate and the clinician the inspiratory time and pressures. A mandatory back-up rate is delivered in the event of apnea or failure to trigger. Weaning is accomplished by decreasing the pressures. Assist control is another term for PTV.

Neither SIMV nor PTV is superior to the other for weaning infants from the ventilator.[396] In comparison to conventional intermittent mandatory ventilation (IMV), tidal volume and gas exchange were superior to SIMV.[397,398] SIMV has also been associated with reduced variability in cerebral blood flow velocity.[399] In a multicenter randomized study enrolling 306 infants there was no clear advantage to SIMV over conventional IMV in terms of mortality or frequency of intraventricular hemorrhage.[400] Two randomized trials of PTV versus conventional IMV demonstrate no significant difference in clinical outcome between the two techniques.[401,402] A meta-analysis pooling the results of trials of both PTV and SIMV in comparison to conventional IMV suggests that synchronized modes may be associated with more rapid weaning from ventilation but not with altered clinical outcomes.[403]

Pressure support ventilation is a further adaptation of PTV where changes in flow at the airway are used to initiate and terminate inspiration, leaving the infant in control of everything except pressure. Volume guarantee allows the ventilator to adjust inspiratory pressure within preset limits according to the tidal volume measured on the preceeding breaths. Volume guarantee can be used in association with the other modes of ventilation. The value of these newer modes is presently unclear.

Paralysis

Greenough et al[403] demonstrated in randomized trials that ventilated infants breathing asynchronously sustain fewer pneumothoraces if paralysed with pancuronium. Shaw et al[404] found that routine paralysis of all ventilated infants was not more effective than selective treatment of those breathing asynchronously. Prolonged neuromuscular blockade is associated with decreased lung compliance[405] and edema. When pancuronium is administered rapid hypoxia can develop if ventilation is inadequate. With milder lung disease and gentle ventilation, paralysis is seldom required.

High frequency ventilation

High frequency ventilation describes any technique using ventilator rates of 60/min or more. It can be divided into three major types: high frequency positive pressure ventilation (HFPPV 60–150/min – see OCTAVE study group[382] and previous discussion on synchronous ventilation); high frequency oscillatory ventilation (HFOV 180–3000/ min); and high frequency jet ventilation (HFJV 200–600/min).

High frequency oscillatory ventilation

HFOV eliminates the large changes in lung volume generated with conventional ventilation. A continuous distending pressure is applied to establish and maintain alveolar recruitment. As with conventional ventilation, oxygenation is determined by the mean airway pressure. The FiO_2 becomes low once alveolar recruitment is established.[406] In addition, the ventilator produces oscillations in pressure, above and below the mean airway pressure, at around 10 Hz (3–50 Hz). These oscillations have little effect on the mean airway pressure but cause small volumes of gas to move in and out of the lungs. The tidal volume (typically around 2 ml/kg) is determined by the amplitude of the oscillations and is much lower than with conventional ventilation. Carbon dioxide elimination on HFOV is proportional to tidal volume squared.[407] Because of the high frequency employed, there is only time for around 10% of the pressure oscillation in the ventilator circuit to reach the airspaces. Increasing the frequency reduces the tidal volume.[408] Carbon dioxide elimination is optimal at around 10 Hz.[409] By maintaining alveolar recruitment and avoiding overinflation, both low-volume (atelectrauma) and high volume (volutrauma) lung injury may be avoided.

The indications for HFOV are unclear. Some infants with severe lung disease appear to be easier to stabilize on HFOV than conventional ventilation. A meta-analysis of trials of elective early HFOV versus conventional ventilation shows no advantage to routine early HFOV.[410,598] The UKOS trial which was completed in 2001 randomized 799 infants to elective early HFOV or conventional ventilation and showed no significant advantage to either technique (Calvert S, personal communication). In an uncontrolled prospective study, 21 out of 46 term or near-term infants with severe respiratory failure who were referred for extra-corporeal membrane oxygenation (ECMO) were successfully managed with HFOV without an increase in mortality or morbidity.[411] No clear advantage was demonstrated in a small randomized controlled trial[412] although some infants failing on conventional ventilation could be successfully managed with HFOV. In a randomized controlled trial of rescue HFOV in preterm infants with severe RDS, HFOV was associated with reduced risk of new air leak but increased risk of intraventricular hemorrhage and no effect on mortality or chronic lung disease.[413]

High frequency jet ventilation

The principles of ventilation strategy with HFJV are similar to those with HFOV.[414] With this technique high frequency positive pressure pulses of gas are introduced into the endotracheal tube through a cannula within its lumen. These pulses entrain additional gas through the endotracheal tube. Expiration is passive and is promoted by the use of low inspiratory to expiratory time (I:E) ratios. Rate, peak pressure and inspiratory time are controlled and tidal volume and mean airway pressure are dependent on them. The optimum frequency for carbon dioxide elimination tends to be lower than with HFOV. HFJV has been associated with improved gas exchange in RDS.[415] A meta-analysis of three small trials of elective high frequency jet ventilation for RDS suggests that HFJV may be associated with a decreased risk of chronic lung disease at 36 weeks' gestation.[416]

Extracorporeal membranous oxygenation

This technique uses an artificial membrane oxygenator to achieve gas exchange outside the body. It is used where there is severe reversible respiratory failure such as in persistent pulmonary hypertension of the newborn, severe lung disease, or diaphragmatic hernia. The rarity of such sick infants and the complexity of the treatment mean that it is only available in a few centers and infants must be transferred for treatment. Among 190 infants in severe respiratory failure, the risk of death or disability at 1 year was reduced by 50% among those randomly allocated to be transferred to an ECMO facility versus those who remained in their local center.[417] Exactly which infants should be referred for ECMO is unclear because nitric oxide, HFOV and surfactant treatment for term respiratory failure[599] reduce the need for ECMO but were not in widespread use when the UK ECMO study began. It is essential not to allow infants to die of potentially reversible respiratory failure without reaching an ECMO center. Sick infants should be discussed with an ECMO specialist early in their illness.

Pulmonary vasodilators

Pulmonary vasodilators may improve oxygenation where there is right-to-left shunt secondary to increased pulmonary vascular resistance. They have not been shown to reduce mortality. The most promising agent is nitric oxide. Others include prostacycline (PGI2), glyceryl trinitrate, nitroprusside, magnesium and tolazoline. Systemically administered vasodilators may cause hypotension.

Nitric oxide

Vascular smooth muscle relaxation is induced by an endogenous vasodilator previously known as endothelium derived relaxing factor, now known to be nitric oxide.[418] Inhaled nitric oxide is inactivated by combining with Hb to form metHb, which confines its effects to the lungs. Nitric oxide reacts with oxygen to form nitrogen dioxide, nitric and nitrous acid, raising issues of toxicity. US safety regulations recommend that nitrogen dioxide exposure should not exceed 5 parts per million (p.p.m.) in an 8 h period. Miller et al[419] found that in an infant ventilator circuit, nitric oxide concentrations greater than 80 p.p.m. resulted in nitrogen dioxide levels greater than 5 p.p.m. in the presence of 90% oxygen. Nitric oxide concentrations of less than 70 p.p.m. did not result in excess nitrogen dioxide. A meta-analysis of randomized trials of nitric oxide in term or near term infants with respiratory failure suggests that around 50% of infants show improved oxygenation and this is associated with a significant reduction in the number of infants who require ECMO.[420] A reasonable starting dose is 20 p.p.m. It is less clear whether preterm infants benefit from treatment.[421] When nitric oxide is discontinued, a rebound worsening of oxygenation is frequently observed whether or not the infant responded to treatment.[422] This is minimized if the nitric oxide is weaned down to 1 p.p.m. before it is discontinued. Methemoglobin levels, and NO_2 levels should be monitored. Because nitric oxide may inhibit platelet adhesion, caution is warranted in the presence of hemorrhage or thrombocytopenia.

Hyperventilation

Hyperventilation to unphysiological levels of pH > 7.6 can reverse extrapulmonary right-to-left shunt in severe pulmonary hypertension but its clinical value is questionable.[369,423] A similar effect is achieved through infusion of alkali to high pH.[424] Both maneuvers may cause cerebral ischemia and should not be preferred to nitric oxide treatment or transfer to an ECMO center.

Liquid ventilation

High surface tension at the air–water interface in immature lungs is virtually eliminated if they are filled with liquid. This has stimulated interest in using liquids as respiratory media. Perfluorocarbon liquids are biologically inert, will not mix with water, have low surface tension and high solubility for oxygen and carbon dioxide. Numerous animal studies of lung injury demonstrate improved gas exchange and lung mechanics during liquid ventilation or partial liquid ventilation. The techniques have shown promise in small, uncontrolled series of human infants,[425,426] but there are no published neonatal trials. In a randomized controlled trial in adults with acute respiratory distress syndrome (ARDS) partial liquid ventilation did not reduce duration of ventilation or 28 day mortality (Alliance Pharmaceutical Corp. Press Release, 21 May 2001). The results of a randomized trial in human infants which stopped recruiting in 1998 are not yet published.

NEURODEVELOPMENTAL OUTCOME

Survival with good health into childhood and beyond is the true measure of success of perinatal care. Severe neurodevelopmental disability remains the worst adverse long term outcome associated with prematurity. The types of neurological disability seen amongst preterm survivors include spastic diplegia, spastic hemiplegia and quadriplegia with and without intellectual impairment. Other problems include blindness, deafness and severe epilepsy. Minor motor problems, specific learning disorders and attention deficits are commonly recognized amongst school-age survivors.

The median prevalence of cerebral palsy in a meta-analysis of 111 studies reporting outcome of VLBW survivors was 7.7%.[427] The median prevalence of any disability in VLBW survivors was high at 25% with a positive correlation between the reported incidence of disability and length of follow-up. Follow-up studies from the USA report better survival and worse neurodevelopmental outcome than current European studies; the lower incidence of disability and higher mortality in Dutch preterm survivors when compared to those in Oxford, England was thought to reflect the more aggressive Dutch approach to the withdrawal of intensive care.[428] Time trends show that the prevalence of cerebral palsy is increasing, particularly amongst the VLBW population. The prevalence of cerebral palsy amongst babies born in the Mersey region between 1966 and 1977 was 1.5 per 1000 live births overall but 15.5 per 1000 live births amongst those born weighing less than 1500 g.[429] Subsequently the same group have shown a threefold increase in all types of cerebral palsy for infants of birth weight below 1500 g with a rate of 50:1000.[430] This figure is in remarkable agreement with those from the Western Australia register of cerebral palsy, the Scottish LBW study and a large geographical study in California.[431,432] Whilst increasing survival means that there has been a net gain of normal survivors amongst the VLBW group over time, these trends and the fact that disabilities are more often multiple in preterm infants can leave no room for complacency.

EVALUATING THE OUTCOME STUDIES

The vast literature reporting the outcome of preterm babies can be a minefield for the unwary reader. The results of outcome studies show a huge variation and there has been little improvement in methodology over time. A recent evaluation confirmed that there can be considerable selection bias.[433]

Population

Most reports of preterm morbidity are hospital based making it difficult to compare results as referral practices vary widely between units. Birth weight cut-offs are extensively used, perhaps the most frequent being the reporting of the outcome for babies less than 1500 g. Small for dates infants of around 30 weeks' gestation are over-represented in these reports. The ideal study would report results from an entire geographical region and contain information about the outcome of all pregnancies ending between 22 and 32 weeks' gestation. The recent EPICURE study comes closest to this, providing data on the outcome of all pregnancies ending between 20 and 25 weeks of gestation in the UK in 1995.[434] Recent reports remind us that babies of 32–36 weeks' gestation are also at increased risk of death and disability, and the population is larger than that of babies born at 23–25 weeks.[435,436]

Treatment of multiples

As many as a quarter of most preterm cohorts are one of a multiple delivery, and this trend seems set to continue. Some outcome studies exclude multiples, and many do not differentiate between singleton and multiple deliveries making specific counseling difficult. Although some researchers say that the outlook is not different for preterm twins compared to singletons there is increasing evidence that twinning is associated with an increased risk of cerebral palsy. This is particularly important when there is intrauterine death of a co-twin, where the risk of significant handicap may be as great as 1 in 10.[437]

Reason for prematurity

As more data accrue, it becomes possible to analyze outcome by etiology of prematurity. There are differences between the outcomes of babies born because of maternal pre-eclampsia (about 12% of preterm deliveries), prolonged rupture of membranes (22%), placental abruption (4%), IUGR (4%), idiopathic preterm labor (40%) or multiple pregnancy (20%). Chorioamnionitis carries a particularly high risk of subsequent periventricular leukomalacia and spastic diplegia.[438] The obstetric team's perception of the chance of survival has been shown to influence outcome.

Missing cases

Tracing the movements of babies is never easy. Frequent changes of surname and address are common and some leave the country of their birth altogether. Work from the Northern region of the UK continues to show that the last few babies remaining to be found in a follow-up study contain a disproportionate number of handicapped infants.[439] The reasons for the discrepancy include the fact that the parents of the handicapped infants are already busy with hospital attendances or that they do not wish to confront the adverse outcome. Studies reporting less than 95% follow-up are likely to be underestimating handicap and an ideal study would have 100% ascertainment.

Duration and timing of follow-up

The diagnosis of cerebral palsy cannot be made with any degree of confidence before 2 years, and may not be stable until 5 years or more. Late deaths will alter the denominator if the handicap rates are to be reported for survivors rather than for live births, another potential source of difficulty when trying to compare studies. Some report neonatal survival, some survival to discharge, and some survival to the time of late follow-up. There is a tendency to use cranial ultrasound results as a proxy for the more expensive and time-consuming neurodevelopmental assessments; this will underestimate the number of cases and is becoming less accurate as the incidence of large hemorrhages and 'periventricular leukomalacia' continues to reduce because periventricular leukomalacia is not reliably detected with ultrasound.

Definition of disability

This is perhaps the most variable of the many problems with the outcome studies. The WHO international classification of impairment, disabilities and handicap contains useful definitions which are listed in Table 10.43. Usually major handicap includes cerebral palsy, severe developmental delay (more than two or three standard deviations below the mean on the particular test used), blindness and deafness. There are differences of opinion regarding inclusion of conditions such as epilepsy and shunted hydrocephalus. The latter can cause impairment without disability, as can a mild hemiplegia. Types of cerebral palsy include spastic, ataxic, dyskinetic (athetoid and dystonic) and hypotonic and can involve a single limb through to quadriplegia. Few groups have enough subjects to allow analysis of outcome according to type of cerebral palsy: there are probably different associated antecedent variables for spastic diplegia, hemiplegia, athetosis and quadriplegia. Important associations may be missed by 'lumping' adverse outcome in small studies.

Minor disability, clumsiness, language disorder, school failure and behavior disorder are even more difficult to define and the wide range in the reported incidence between studies reflects this.

Diagnosis of disability

The tests used to diagnose disability should be reproducible and have been previously evaluated in an appropriate population in order to minimize problems such as intraobserver variability. At present there are a large number of tests applied at different ages by people of varying levels of experience and this can severely bias results. Well validated in this respect are the Bayley and Griffiths scales of infant development, and the Amiel-Tison method of neurological examination.

Control groups

In a cohort descriptive follow-up study of all children below a certain weight there can be no control group. Consideration needs to be given to the inclusion of control subjects such as term infants, however, particularly in view of the known effects of socioeconomic deprivation on the incidence of prematurity. As studies of preterm outcome begin to report school performance, variables such as birth order and social class will become relatively more important factors than they are in the current descriptions of the prevalence of major handicap.

OUTCOME RELATED TO BIRTH WEIGHT, RACE, SEX AND GESTATIONAL AGE

That the incidence of handicap increases with decreasing birth weight and gestational age was shown as early as 1956. Most large regional studies reporting the outcome of VLBW babies born during the last 50 years record serious disability in less than 10% of the survivors, increasing to 13–25% of affected children when moderate disability is included. The interaction of birth weight and gestational age on survival and disability can be studied by those who have access to large datasets. One approach is to calculate the birth weight ratio, which is the actual birth weight divided by the mean birth weight for the same gestational age.[440] A birth weight ratio of 0.8 corresponds to the 10th centile. This is a statistically useful tool because the number generated is a normally distributed continuous variable. In a cohort of 429 VLBW infants Morley and her colleagues[440] were unable to show any association between birth weight ratio and neurodevelopmental outcome at 18 months, but Cooke[441] reported that his population was skewed to the right, suggesting a higher mortality for very preterm growth retarded infants. Synnes et al[442] showed either a U-shaped curve or a negative correlation between mortality and weight at each gestational age between 23 and 26 weeks. A collaborative network in the USA has presented very valuable information based on a large recent cohort (1991–1992) which allow the calculation of mortality risk by sex, birth weight and gestational age.[443] Male sex has been associated with a doubling of the risk of death and/or handicap in almost every study which has included sex as a factor in logistic regression analysis. Some studies suggest an increased chance of survival amongst black preterm babies,[444] whereas others show the opposite.

In the longer term, most follow-up studies describe worse cognitive outcome for preterm SGA infants when compared with appropriate for gestational age controls.[445]

Outcome related to gestational age

22–23 weeks

Survival at 22 weeks' gestation has been described, but remains very rare. At 23 weeks the chance of a handicapped survivor outweighs that of a normal survivor, and many would argue that this means the parents should be fully informed of the experimental nature of intensive care at these low gestations.[446] The survival rate is now about 15% at 23 weeks, although the rate is much lower when it is recorded for all live-born babies, rather than amongst all those admitted to a neonatal unit[447] (Table 10.44, Fig. 10.19).[447–450]

24 weeks

Since the fourth edition of this book the survival rate for 24 week gestation infants has improved from virtually zero to about 30% (Fig. 10.19, Table 10.44). All the infants born at 24 weeks' gestation in The Netherlands during 1983 died and only one baby survived in the same year in the northern region of England. The Epicure study reported on all babies born between 22 and 25 weeks' gestation in the UK in 1995, of whom almost a third survived.[447] Similar results are now reported from Australia and Canada.[448,451] At least 30% of the survivors have a significant disability (Table 10.45,[434,448,451,452] Fig. 10.20), and in addition many more children have school failure.

25 weeks

Now 25 weeks marks the point at which 50% survival is reached. This is a dramatic change since the 1980s, and many obstetric units now adopt an aggressive approach to monitoring and delivery of babies at this gestation as a result. About 20% of the survivors have a major disability, with a similar proportion performing poorly at school, as at 24 weeks. Figure 10.19 bears a remarkable similarity to previous versions of this graph, with a consistent 10–12% of the whole cohort developing a major disability at follow-up. This observation has remained remarkably constant since the early 1980s, the only change being the proportion who die and who survive.[453] In some follow-up studies there has been an increase in disability in recent cohorts, largely due to retinopathy of prematurity rather than cerebral palsy.[454]

26–28 weeks

For the baby born between 26 and 28 weeks' gestation the risk of severe disability in survivors falls from about 20% to about 15% (Table 10.45). Perhaps surprisingly the risk of disability does not decrease markedly with increasing gestational age. The risk of dying correlates better with the degree of immaturity. Figure 10.20 expresses the information from the studies which report outcome related to gestational age. From this it can be seen that the chance of taking home a normal survivor (providing the baby survives long enough to be admitted to an ICU) increases from 8% at 23 weeks through 55% at 26 weeks to 75% at 28 weeks. This chance increases to about 85% at 30 weeks and above.

Very few studies have addressed the problem of predicting outcome prior to delivery. This is important as a significant number of very preterm babies will die during delivery or cannot be resuscitated. More information about the mother's chance of taking home a normal baby, which can be used to counsel her and to advise her obstetrician so that he or she can make an informed choice about the timing and mode of delivery is essential. Unfortunately at present such decisions have to be taken using very little information as there was no legal requirement to register stillborn deliveries below 28 weeks' gestation until 1992. The Northern Region team[455] have shown that neonatal death represents only a small proportion of fetal loss at low gestational ages, and that overall between 24 and 31 weeks' gestation 25% of deaths occurred antepartum or intrapartum. Intrapartum deaths accounted for only 5% of loss, meaning that the risks presented above can be helpful once the mother is established in labor with a live fetus.

SUMMARY

In summary, whilst it is generally true that survival increases and the percentage risk of handicap remains the same as pregnancy advances the accruing data show some gradation of risk. There are still insufficient good quality national studies on which to base important decisions. These data provide no justification for failure to offer intensive care at 25 or 26 weeks, whereas at 23 and 24 weeks the poor outcomes confirm that intensive care remains a risky option which should be fully discussed with parents.[446]

Outcome related to birth weight

Some studies continue to use birth weight as a criterion for enrolment, but these are less valuable now that there are good regional/population based data on outcome related to gestational age. The small for dates, growth retarded baby is at increased risk of mortality at low gestational ages. The degree of increase in risk is shown in the outcome data from Trent and in the USA.[443,449]

SENSORY HANDICAP

In addition to the cerebral palsy rate of about 7% in VLBW infant survivors there are a significant number of visually impaired children, often as a consequence of retinopathy of prematurity. About 3% are blind, and in addition many more have severe myopia: a quarter of the children followed by Saigal et al[456] were wearing prescription glasses. Deafness afflicts slightly fewer children but is still a problem in about 1–2%. Early diagnosis by screening can help limit the handicap resulting from this latter disability.

MINOR HANDICAPS AND SCHOOL FAILURE

Follow-up to school age and beyond has been reported for several cohorts of ex-preterm children. More of the children are left-handed, which has been suggested as a possible risk factor for a later risk of schizophrenia. More are hyperactive with a short attention span and thus require special help at school. The meta-analysis of Aylward[457] showed a mean reduction of six points in IQ when disabled survivors were excluded. There is a considerable overlap between behavioral disorders, neurodevelopmental abnormalities and school problems – 'clumsiness' may be a marker for this type of dysfunction. More (14%) Finnish LBW children born in 1966 than controls (6%) were educationally subnormal at the age of 14, but when the disabled survivors were excluded similar numbers succeeded in higher education.[458] The Bavarian follow-up study showed that ex-preterm children had significant problems with sequential and simultaneous information processing and language.[459]

OUTCOME RELATED TO CRANIAL ULTRASOUND APPEARANCE

Cohort screening of asymptomatic VLBW infants with cranial ultrasound has uncovered a high incidence of lesions involving

Table 10.44 Survival by gestational age from national and regional studies of babies born in the 1990s

Place	Year of birth	23 wks	24 wks	25 wks	26 wks	27 wks	28 wks	29 wks	30 wks	Reference
UK survival amongst live-born	1995	26/241 10.7%	100/382 26%	186/424 43%						Costeloe et al 2000[447]
UK survival after admission to NNU	1995	26/131 19.8%	100/298 33.5%	186/357 52%						Costeloe et al 2000[447]
Victoria, Australia	1991–92	5/52 9.6%	21/63 33%	51/88 57.9%	71/98 72.4%	77/100 77%				Doyle 2001[448]
Trent, UK	1994–97	8%	20%	40%	61%	78%	88%	93%	96%	Draper et al 1999[449]
East Anglia, UK	1995–97	1/38 2.6%	12/57 21%	34/68 50%	65/104 62%	96/129 74%	115/147 81%	134/153 87%	142/149 95%	Jag Ahluwalia, personal communication
South East Thames, UK	1998–2001	12/48 24%	65/132 49%	104/163 64%	175/206 85%	218/253 86%	329/362 91%	356/367 97%	443/457 97%	Tony Ducker, personal communication
Wales, UK	1993–94	1/22 4.5%	6/31 19.3%	19/41 46.3%	40/59 67.7%	39/57 68.4%	80/105 76%	124/130 95%		Cartlidge & Stewart 1997[450]
England, Wales and Northern Ireland, UK	1998–2000					86%	89%			CESDI project 8th annual report
		15%	30%	50%	70%	80%	90%	93%	95%	

NNU, neonatal unit

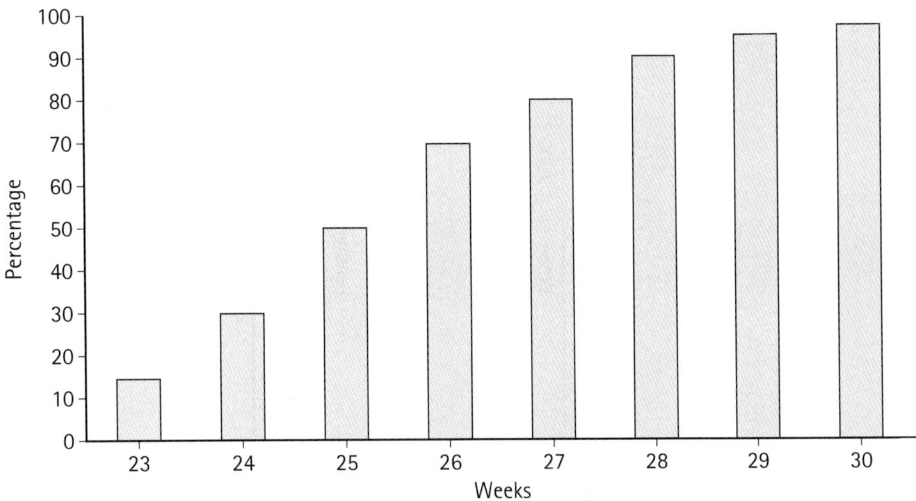

Fig. 10.19 Survival by gestational age at birth.

the periventricular zone. Although damage to premyelin cells abundant in this region provides a convenient explanation for the high prevalence of cerebral palsy, a causal relationship remains to be proven. Cysts in the parenchyma and cerebral atrophy indicate loss of white matter and are the strongest predictors yet found for cerebral palsy. Delayed myelination has been confirmed with later MRI studies, suggesting that the cysts are markers of even more diffuse injury to oligodendroglia. Ultrasound is a poor predictor of later periventricular leukomalacia diagnosed with MRI, detecting only about 30% of cases. Most studies are in remarkable agreement about the outcome of cystic change, showing a fivefold increase in the risk of cerebral palsy following ultrasound diagnosis of any parenchymal lesion, and a 15-fold increase in the presence of bilateral occipital periventricular leukomalacia. Accumulated experience is still relatively meager, however, and the predictions have wide confidence intervals due to the small numbers of cases. Visual handicap can be accurately predicted from ultrasound abnormalities. A normal scan is not therefore a guarantee of a normal outcome, although the chances are about 90%.[460]

Normal ultrasound scan

The outcome of over 3500 preterm infants enrolled in 18 studies has now been reported: over 2000 of these infants had a normal scan and of these 89% were normal at follow-up.[461] The risk of a significant disability is very small for a preterm infant who has a normal cranial ultrasound scan in the neonatal period, particularly if this is repeated before discharge. Only 128 of these children had a major handicap (6%: 95% CIs from 5 to 7).

Germinal matrix hemorrhage, subependymal hemorrhage

There is consistent agreement that the appearance of increased echodensity in the region of the germinal matrix capillary bed carries no increased risk of adverse outcome. This is also true for intraventricular hemorrhage which is not associated with ventricular enlargement.

Ventricular dilation and progressive hydrocephalus

The natural history of ventriculomegaly secondary to the presence of blood in the ventricular cavity in VLBW infants is that about 50% will progress to require a ventriculoperitoneal (VP) shunt insertion and the remainder will arrest or regress. Attempts at preventing the progression by early cerebrospinal fluid (CSF) drainage have proved unsuccessful. Many of these infants have associated parenchymal lesions of the brain making the assessment of risk due to persistent dilation alone very difficult. Most of the 127 infants with ventriculomegaly followed in the aforementioned large collaborative study had a poor outcome: only 11 of 112 were normal at 30 months.[462]

Non-cavitating transient parenchymal echodensity

This is perhaps the most variable of the ultrasound diagnoses discussed. The incidence with which a 'flare' or 'blush' is seen in the parenchyma surrounding the ventricle varies widely with the observer and the frequency of scanning. Graham et al[463] described a slightly increased risk related to a flare which persisted for 2 weeks compared to a normal ultrasound scan (8%). Appleton et al[464] found handicap in 4 of 15 (26%) survivors who had 'isolated and transient' intracerebral flares seen with ultrasound during the neonatal period. This lesion may not be completely benign but at the time of writing too few studies have accurately recorded this appearance to enable assessment of risk.

Persistent parenchymal echodensities and porencephalic cysts

A single large echodense area in the parenchyma of the brain may be the end result of one or several pathological events including venous infarction, secondary hemorrhage into an ischemic area or a primary hemorrhagic event due to transmission of a hypertensive peak or release of vasoactive substances. Large hemorrhages into the brain often cause death in VLBW infants so the number of survivors with this diagnosis is small. However, the overall risk of major neurodevelopmental handicap of 75% is the best estimate that can be given until more consensus regarding definition of diagnosis is reached.

Large parenchymal lesions often cavitate to form parenchymal cysts: these are associated with a similar risk of handicap of about 83%. As expected this abnormality is usually correlated with a hemiplegia rather than spastic diplegia. Parenchymal lesions predict motor outcome better than cognitive outcome and from the studies completed so far periventricular leukomalacia is more likely

Table 10.45 Summary of published literature reporting major disability in survivors (denominator is survival after admission) of babies born in 1990s

Place	Year of birth	23 wks	24 wks	25 wks	26 wks	27 wks	28 wks	29 wks	30 wks	Reference
UK survival after admission to NNU	1995	8/26 30%	24/100 24%	40/186 21%						Wood et al 2000[434]
Victoria, Australia	1991–92	2/5 40%	7/21 33%	13/51 25%	17/71 24%	5/77 6%				Doyle 2001[448]
North of England, UK	1991–94	0/1 0%	5/13 38%	8/36 22%	2/15 13%	10/28 35%				Tin et al 1997[452]
Montreal, Canada	1987–92		4/9 44%	5/24 21%	9/40 22%	9/72 12%	11/72 15%			Lefebvre et al 1996[451]
		40%	35%	20%	20%	15%	15%			

NNU, neonatal unit

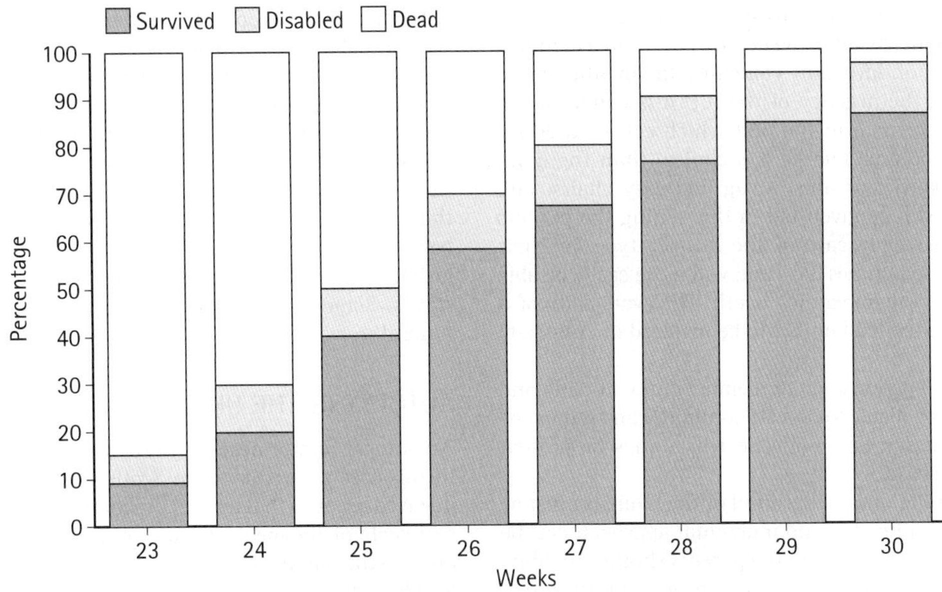

Fig. 10.20 Outcome by gestational age.

to be associated with a cognitive and motor defect than a parenchymal hemorrhagic lesion or porencephalic cyst.

Periventricular leukomalacia

There is no doubt that cystic periventricular leukomalacia is the most powerful predictor of cerebral palsy amongst the neonatal cranial ultrasound lesions so far described. In many cohort follow-up studies almost all the cases of cerebral palsy had bilateral occipital leukomalacia in the neonatal period. Cysts involving more than one zone have a particularly poor prognosis. Earlier studies, reporting an association between ventricular dilation and adverse outcome probably included some undiagnosed cases of periventricular leukomalacia owing to poor resolution of the older, 5 MHz skinheads. Single cysts and cysts confined to the frontal region have a better outcome than multiple bilateral occipital cysts, where the outlook is universally dismal. Too few studies have reported the outcome of anterior or central cysts to make it possible to give a confident prediction of a good outcome, although most of the reported survivors with single unilateral cysts or cysts confined to the frontal zone are normal at follow-up.

NEONATAL DEATH

Although neonatal deaths have become steadily less common, they are still frequent enough both on the labor ward and on the neonatal unit for consideration of best management to be important. NICUs have developed to rescue preterm and sick infants but there is still a steady trickle of deaths in a neonatal unit from congenital abnormality and the problems occurring in the very immature baby. With all formal nursing and medical training geared to rescue, the death of the patient is often regarded as failure. If it is an occasional event, a neonatal death may be rapidly 'set aside', but in a referral unit the frequency and regularity means that such events cannot be easily avoided. The emotional load of guilt and depression occurring with frequent deaths on a unit almost certainly plays a part in the high turnover of nursing staff and the incidence of 'burn out' in physicians. In the arena of neonatal intensive care, perinatal mortality meetings and more universally perinatal mortality statistics, highlight the unsatisfactory nature of death, yet many will be inevitable.

PARENTAL GRIEF

The grief of the parents after a neonatal death seems independent of the size of the offspring. Such grief is present even when the infant is non-viable or lives for only a very short time. It has also been shown that parents go through an identical reaction after a stillbirth. The failure of a mother to come to terms with a perinatal death can lead to emotional problems. Overt psychiatric problems are common in the 2 years after such an event but parents touching their infants before and after death can considerably reduce such sequelae. We now acknowledge that for the parents, the sensitive management of the death by the staff is as important as the rescue of life.

THE DEATH

The death of a baby in the neonatal unit is a very undignified event for the baby and the family, especially when 'rescue therapy' is applied until the last moment. It is difficult for the parents to express their true emotions in the ICU where staff are busy with other critically ill patients. It is difficult for staff to cope on the one hand with the rescue care for some patients and still provide sensitivity for grieving parents in the same nursery, and it is particularly difficult for parents of other babies in a unit with an open visiting policy.

The emphasis in neonatal death must be changed from a medical failure which must be rapidly forgotten to an event, tragic indeed, but in which the parents are if at all possible closely involved. Deaths in a neonatal unit should occur, if possible, with the parents present and life support can often be withdrawn with the baby in the mother's or father's arms. Thus in many instances the time of death is itself organized for the benefit of the parents. Death then becomes a reality and with this involvement parents may feel, in retrospect, that they have done their best for their infants by allowing death to occur in a dignified way in the presence of love and company. In an attempt to dissociate death from the urgency of the ICU it is helpful to set aside for the parents a room in the unit which can be used for terminal care. This room should be less clinical than the main nurseries with wallpaper, curtains, a rug and easy chairs. Full supportive care may still be given but in this setting the parents will be more able to supply care of the hospice type for their infant's last hours or sometimes days and will more easily be able to come to terms with the impending death. The availability of a special room allows extended families to be involved in culturally important ritual.

During the terminal period a senior member of the nursing and medical staff must be available to provide continuity and it must be made clear to the parents that someone will always be present unless they wish otherwise.

The cultural and religious background of the families must be acknowledged so that a flexible and individual approach can be developed. Discussions early on with the parents should elucidate their religious beliefs and standpoints and outside support from a priest, mullah, rabbi, etc. should be encouraged if indicated. The introduction of this support at an early stage in a critically ill infant is important as it allows more constructive relationships to develop than when the meeting is for the baptism of a terminally ill infant. Hospital chaplains and social workers are increasingly involved providing spiritual support with people representing the whole spectrum of faith communities as well as those of no faith background (i.e. not just Christian). The presence of young siblings can enrich the feeling of family togetherness at this time of grief and is unlikely to damage the siblings.[465] Ritual is important. If an emergency baptism is required this should be memorable with a proper silver christening bowl to facilitate baptism with meaning and dignity. I believe it is important to *suggest* to parents that they might like to hold or groom their dead infant. This is usually met with agitation and a certain degree of horror, particularly by European parents, but after a short time many mothers will request such involvement. In some instances parents have left the hospital to obtain their own baby clothes in which to dress their infant in the laying out process. Photographs of the infant will usually have been taken during life but if the life span has been short it is suggested that pictures of the dead infant are taken, often in the parents' arms (we have also in recent years seen the increasing use of video). Frequently the baby can be specially clothed to enable a better photograph for remembrance to be taken than the ones in life, which have had evidence of intensive care support. The neonatal unit can provide the parents with a bereavement folder which combines advice and information (to help them at this time) with mementos of their baby (lock of hair, name band, hand and foot prints, etc.).

THE IMMEDIATE AFTERMATH OF DEATH[466]

Their baby's death is an intensely private and personal experience for all parents. Many will wish to follow the customs of their own culture or the rights of their own particular religion and these wishes should be respected. It is important that no assumptions are made. It may be helpful to ask parents as sensitively and gently as possible to explain their needs. If language problems make this or any other discussion with parents difficult every effort should be made to find an appropriate and skilled interpreter. Parents who have a specific religious commitment may want to make contact with their minister, priest or other religious leader and he or she will probably advise them about their baby's funeral as well as provide support and help. Some parents who do not hold any particular religious belief will still find comfort with a simple ceremony in the hospital, perhaps in the hospital chapel with their families and the nursing and medical staff involved in the care of their infant taking part. This may be suggested bearing in mind that it is not appropriate for all parents. Parents will inevitably be bewildered by a neonatal death. It may be their first experience of losing a close relative and sensitivity is required by staff at all stages. Some parents wish to take their infant home before the funeral.

AUTOPSY IN THE UK

An autopsy may be necessary because the cause of death is unclear. In this case a coroner (or in Scotland, a procurator fiscal) will be involved because the medical practitioner is unable to issue a death certificate of the medical cause of death. In this situation it is not open to the parents to withhold their consent. If an autopsy is not legally required, a high quality hospital autopsy should be offered as a right to every parent who has lost a baby. This hospital autopsy may only be performed with full parental consent. I believe they should be asked because:

1. In 25% of autopsies further information is discovered which has a direct bearing on the counseling of the parents for the future.[467]
2. It is important for the medical staff to know that their diagnosis has been accurate. It is only in this way that medical science can progress.
3. At some stage in the future it is not uncommon that parents will have anxieties that something went undiscovered in their baby and that this led to the death.
4. Retained tissue as organ blocks may be helpful at a future date to make a specific genetic diagnosis.

Where the parents' consent is necessary, it is highly desirable that they can give their consent freely. An honest and unhurried approach to parents by a consultant or senior resident (not a junior staff member), explaining the reasons for an autopsy and what it involves, will help them to reach a decision. Parents will also feel more comfortable if the request is made as a normal rather than an exceptional procedure. Although the consent of only one parent is required by law, it is advisable that whenever possible parents should be asked to sign the consent form together. A duplicate copy of the consent form should be given to the parents to keep. It will help parents to make their decision if they are given clear information about the following:

1. Why it is thought an autopsy is necessary and why therefore their consent is being sought. Although many parents wish to be given the reason for their baby's death, many also find the thought of an autopsy very distressing. It is important that they can feel their baby is still theirs and not becoming a hospital specimen.
2. The possible outcome of the examination. While it should be explained that an autopsy can provide a definite cause of death, parents should also be warned that an indecisive result is possible.
3. Where, when and by whom the autopsy will be performed. Parents are also likely to want information and reassurance about the whereabouts of and their access to their baby and, if the autopsy is to be performed at another hospital, the body should not be removed to that hospital until the day of the

autopsy and should be returned as quickly as possible after the examination.

4. When, to whom and how the results of the autopsy will be made available. If you are not prepared to transmit the full information to the parents you should not be doing an autopsy.

Most parents feel anxious about giving their consent to an autopsy and need reassurance. A particular fear is the damage which will be done to their baby. With good practice by the pathologist (who can be introduced to the parents), it is possible for the baby to be restored and carefully dressed so as to be acceptable for the parents to see again before the funeral. If the parents are to hold their infant following the autopsy, they should be warned that he or she may be lightweight as in many cases the brain will be removed for later processing (this can only be done with parental consent). It may also be suggested that the parents might like to provide clothes including a bonnet for the baby to be dressed in after the autopsy or the parents may prefer a funeral director to prepare the baby for them.

The results of an autopsy are anxiously awaited by most parents and there should be a minimum of delay in providing parents not only with the results but also with the opportunity to discuss them fully. I believe that the full autopsy report should be sent to the parents with an appointment shortly after so that they can bring it and discuss it fully with the pediatrician involved. In this way they have both written information and the access to a pediatrician to discuss all the implications. If necessary the results can be discussed also with an obstetrician. If an autopsy shows the baby's death to be the result of a genetic disorder, parents should be offered the opportunity for later genetic counseling.

CERTIFICATION AND REGISTRATION PROCEDURES IN THE UK

When a baby is born alive and subsequently dies, irrespective of the gestation or the duration of life, the medical practitioner who attended the baby is required by law to issue a medical certificate giving the cause of death. This certificate is required to enable the death to be registered. If the cause of death is not immediately apparent the medical practitioner may have to report the death to the coroner (or in Scotland, a procurator fiscal). The law requires that all births and deaths be notified to the registrar of births and deaths. It is best if parents can deal with registration themselves and both together and this is necessary where the couple are unmarried and wish both parents' names entered on the certificate. The medical practitioner who attended the baby during his or her last illness will issue a medical certificate giving the cause of death. This certificate must be produced to the registrar of births and deaths within 5 days of the baby's death (8 days in Scotland). The registrar will issue a green certificate after registration (the certificate for disposal) to permit burial or cremation. This certificate is required before the funeral can take place. It is free of charge. The registrar will also issue, on request, a copy of a certified entry (a death certificate) for a small fee. It is helpful if parents are told in advance that this certificate is available since to many parents it is a valuable memento of their baby. Parents should be told in advance when registering a baby's death that the registrar can enter the baby's forename as well as the surname if they so wish. This may be particularly important for those parents where the baby died soon after birth, as they can then give some thought to the naming of the child, before registering the death.

Parents can apply to the Department of Social Security for a grant or loan to cover the funeral expenses. In Scotland, the health board will meet the funeral costs for stillborn babies and terminations.

THE FUNERAL IN THE UK

It is the parents' choice whether they wish to arrange a funeral privately or to accept a health authority's offer to arrange a funeral on their behalf, though the latter will only happen if the infant is stillborn or lives for only a very short time after birth. Ceremonies can take many different forms and may be religious or non-religious. The certificate of disposal (Form 14) issued after registration is needed by the undertaker before a cremation can take place but is not needed for a burial. It should be handed to the funeral director or if the parents have asked the hospital to take responsibility for the funeral, to the hospital. The funeral director involved will complete all necessary documentation according to the kind of funeral requested. It is also the parents' choice whether their baby is buried or cremated. The cremation of a baby leaves no remains whatsoever (ashes) and the parents should be aware of this. A baby cannot be cremated without the parents' formal consent. If the funeral is privately arranged the funeral director will organize all steps in conjunction with the parents. If on the other hand the parents wish for a hospital contract funeral, they must be aware that there may be some emotional risks in accepting this option. If there is any anxiety about this the parents can always contact the British Institute of Funeral Directors or the Stillbirth and Neonatal Death Society (SANDS).

GRAVES, MEMORIALS AND REMEMBRANCE

Depending on the funeral that the parents opt for, the baby may be buried with other babies in a common grave though this practice is becoming increasingly rare. Many parents find it comforting to know that their baby is buried with other babies but for others this is distressing and sometimes it takes a while before the grave is full (usually no more than 10 babies should be buried in one grave). Local authorities have often identified areas in cemeteries specifically for baby burials. Parents should be warned that unless they purchase exclusive right to burial, they do not have the right to erect any kind of memorial of their own. If the parents buy exclusive right of burial they can mark their baby's grave with a memorial provided that it complies with local regulations. All crematoria and some cemeteries have a book of remembrance for individual entries. Many specialist neonatal units also have a book of remembrance for infants dying in their units. This book may be located on the neonatal unit or in the hospital chapel. A full page can be allocated to each baby with a personal inscription designed by the parents. This can be made in copperplate writing. The parents can then see the book at any time by arrangement with the hospital chaplain or neonatal unit staff.

LATE BEREAVEMENT COUNSELING AND SUPPORT

It is now accepted that the aftercare of the parents and siblings is important for subsequent emotional well-being. The parents should be seen several times after the death of their infant. On the first occasion, usually on the day of death, sympathy is shown for the parents' situation. Explanation, I believe, is inappropriate at this stage and intrudes into the grief.

Over the next few days necessary formalities have to be completed and this can be a bewildering time. The parents need to be seen on the day after the death to explain what has to be done. If the mother is mobile (that is, not just postoperative after a cesarean section) it is appropriate to encourage both parents to complete the formalities together rather than the man take on an organizational role. A social worker or member of the clergy if indicated can frequently be involved in shepherding through these routines. It is also at this second interview that permission is asked for the autopsy (by a senior pediatrician). We do not pressurize parents for this permission but find it is exceptional for them to be unwilling when the reasons are explained unless there are cultural or religious differences and these can usually be resolved by contact with the local mosque or temple. The final task on this second visit is to guide the parents through a few of the reactions and emotions that they will suffer in the ensuing period.

At between 1 and 2 weeks after the death the parents are seen a third time. They will have received a copy of the autopsy report and this interview will explain the findings of the autopsy. If possible, the senior nurse who has been involved in the terminal events will also be present. The interview will last between 30 min and 1 h. It is important not to see the parents in the neonatal unit or in the middle of the busy outpatient session where other babies and infants intrude too easily into their consciousness. The distress and anxieties of the ensuing weeks are again raised and suggestions are made as to how best to deal with them. Finally at this time an appointment is given for an optional visit at about 3 months at which outstanding questions may be clarified and at which pathological grief, if present, should be evident (in which case professional counseling may be required). At all stages hospital social workers and chaplains should be informed (not necessarily to be active) of what is proceeding. The GP should have a full letter with regard to each interview. Genetic counseling should be arranged for the future if this is appropriate from the results of the autopsy.

VOLUNTARY SUPPORT ORGANIZATIONS

The Stillbirth and Neonatal Death Society (SANDS), 28 Portland Place, London W1B ILY (Tel. 0207 436 5881).

The British Institute of Funeral Directors, 140 Leamington Road, Coventry CV3 6JY (Tel. 024 7669 7160).

BOOKLETS

The Loss of Your Baby produced by the Health Education Council in conjunction with the Stillbirth and Neonatal Death Society and the National Association for Mental Health.

Saying Goodbye to Your Baby by Priscilla Alderson. Available from SANDS and the National Childbirth Trust, 9 Queensborough Terrace, London W2 3TB.

Miscarriage, Stillbirth and Neonatal Death: Guidelines for Professionals. Available from SANDS.

STAFF SUPPORT

With the realization that the support and understanding of health professionals can play a vital role in the eventual recovery of the parents, there has also come the realization that this involvement can itself cause depression and emotional stress in the staff. After a death I believe that it is important not only to analyze in detail traditional physiological and pathological events but also the stress aspects for the parents and the nursing and medical staff. Some units may feel it is important to involve formal psychiatric help in this process but regular discussion on a less formal basis (and at particular times of need) are as important (our regular involvement of chaplaincy staff with parents in a neonatal unit pays dividends for the staff themselves at 'crisis times'). In this way we hope that the people involved in a neonatal death and who will inevitably be under considerable stress will not reach the point of physical and emotional exhaustion.

PROBLEMS OF THE NEWBORN

PULMONARY DISORDERS AND APNEA

DEVELOPMENT OF THE LUNG

The viability of the preterm baby is limited by lung development. The airways begin as an outpouching from the primitive gut at 24 days. By 26 days two primary branches, which will form the major bronchi, can be discerned. This is called the *embryonic phase* and it ends about the 6th week. The *pseudoglandular phase*, from the 7th to 16th week, consists of branching of the endodermal tube into the surrounding mesenchyme. By 10 weeks cartilage is deposited in the bronchi and by 16 weeks formation of new bronchi is almost complete. The *canalicular phase*, from 16 to 26 weeks, comprises canalization of the airways, increased capillary growth and differentiation of type I pneumocytes (needed for gas exchange) from type II pneumocytes which produce surfactant. The terminal *saccular phase* begins from 24 to 26 weeks and continues until term. The terminal air sacs or alveoli appear as outpouchings of the bronchioles after 26 weeks and increase in number to form multiple pouches of a common chamber called the alveolar duct. From 26 weeks the capillary network, which arises at about 20 weeks from vascular structures in the mesenchyme, proliferates close to the developing airway to constitute the *alveolar phase* which continues postnatally until the age of 2 years. There is a continuum between antenatal and postnatal lung development. Normal alveolarization proceeds rapidly to achieve alveolar numbers that are between 20 and 50% of the adult number of 300×10^6 by 40 weeks' gestation. Normal lung development can be disrupted by antenatal events which lead to preterm birth. Before 24–26 weeks gas exchange must take place across terminal bronchioles into the developing capillary network.

Growth of the lung

Growth factors have a major role in lung growth and development. Over- or underexpression of these growth factors may lead to abnormal development such as cystic adenomatoid malformation (CAM) and tracheoesophageal fistula. Mechanical and humoral factors also influence growth of the fetal lung. Distention in the fluid-filled lung, with tracheal fluid acting as an internal template or splint, regulates lung growth. There are also external forces, which include the phasic negative pressure of fetal breathing and the tonic negative pressure of diaphragmatic tone. Normal lung growth is dependent upon fetal breathing movements but the mechanism is unclear. It is unlikely to be due to increased lung distention as only 1 ml of tracheal fluid is displaced during fetal breathing movements. Lung hypoplasia may be caused by oligohydramnios from renal agenesis, bladder neck obstruction or rupture of the membranes before 20 weeks. These lungs, although structurally immature with persistent cuboidal epithelium and lack of elastic tissue, are also biochemically immature containing low levels of phospholipids. Hypoplastic lungs may also result from absence of fetal breathing movements in babies with central nervous system anomalies, congenital muscle disorders or absent diaphragm. These lungs, although small, appear to be appropriately developed and have normal content of phospholipids. Pulmonary hypoplasia may also be caused by thoracic space-occupying lesions such as diaphragmatic hernia, lung cysts, or pleural effusions which may be associated with severe erythroblastosis.

Maturation of the lung

After birth alveolar stability is dependent upon the release of pulmonary surfactant into the lumen. Synthesis and release of surfactant rely more on humoral control mechanisms than mechanical factors. Alveolar type II cells, which synthesize surfactant, have microvilli on the luminal surface and contain lamellar bodies. They constitute 16% of alveolar cells but only 7% of the alveolar surface area and can differentiate to form the larger, thinner type I cell which covers the remaining 93% of the alveolar surface. The lamellar bodies (storage sites for surfactant) are first recognized at about 22 weeks. They contain about 80% phosphatidylcholine, mostly dipalmitoylphosphatidylcholine (DPPC) but also unsaturated phosphatidylglycerol (PG). PG is used as a marker of lung maturity and levels rise as phosphatidylinositol levels decrease towards term. Lamellar bodies also contain many enzymes and two protein groups, a glycoprotein of 28–36 kDa (SP-A) and two very hydrophobic low molecular weight proteins (SP-B and SP-C). A fourth surfactant apoprotein, SP-D, is not stored in the lamellar bodies and is secreted separately. SP-A and SP-D appear to have major roles in host defense of the lung whereas SP-B and SP-C have surface active properties. mRNA for SP-C appears before 20 weeks' gestation but mature SP-C does not appear in the airspaces until much later. Mature SP-B increases in amniotic fluid in late gestation and SP-A is the last surfactant protein to appear in amniotic fluid. The major pathway for surfactant synthesis uses choline incorporation (Fig. 10.21). The mechanisms controlling surfactant synthesis and secretion are not fully understood but humoral factors are important.

Humoral factors

Glucocorticoids

These induce both structural and biochemical changes in alveolar type II and type I cells. Glucocorticoids act on lung fibroblasts to produce fibroblast pneumocyte factor which in turn stimulates surfactant synthesis by alveolar type II cells. They also increase the numbers of lamellar bodies, the rate of choline incorporation into phosphatidylcholine, the amount of DPPC in tracheal fluid and the lung content of SP-A. The induction of fibroblast pneumocyte factor is relatively slow, which may account for the delayed clinical effect of maternal corticosteroid treatment.

Thyroid hormones

Thyroid hormones increase the synthesis of surfactant lipids in type II cells, probably by making the cells more responsive to fibroblast pneumocyte factor. They act earlier in the phospholipid biosynthetic pathway and are synergistic when used with glucocorticoids. Synthetic analogs of T_3 and thyrotropin releasing hormone (TRH) cross the placenta.

Insulin

Hyperinsulinemia is associated with reduced surfactant production. Insulin does not cross the placenta but in pregnancies complicated by maternal diabetes which is inadequately controlled fetal hyperinsulinemia is associated with an increased risk of neonatal RDS.

Catecholamines

Epinephrine but not norepinephrine decreases tracheal fluid secretion and increases surfactant release. The concentration of beta-adrenergic receptors in the lung increases at term and in response to glucocorticoids. Beta-adrenergic agents delay preterm labor; if used in association with betamethasone, they have a synergistic effect in preventing RDS.

Other hormones and agents

Prolactin levels are lower in babies with RDS. Estrogen, testosterone, epidermal growth factor, prostaglandins, cholinergic agonists and leukotrienes have all been postulated as having roles in fetal lung development. These roles remain to be defined but it is possible that many aspects of lung development are regulated by various hormones acting in concert.

$$\text{Choline} \xrightarrow[\text{Mg ATP}]{\text{Choline kinase}} \text{P-choline} \xrightarrow[\text{Mg ATP}]{\text{Cytidyl transferase}} \text{CDP-cholin}$$

$$\text{CDP-choline} \xrightarrow[\text{1,2-diglyceride}]{\text{cholinephosphotransferase}} \text{Phosphatidylcholin}$$

Fig. 10.21 Synthesis of phosphatidylcholine by choline incorporation.

Role of surfactant and fetal lung fluid

The fetal lung is filled with liquid secreted by the epithelium of potential air spaces. Absorption across the epithelium is initiated by increased circulating catecholamines associated with the contractions of labor. The air-filled lung after birth retains a thin fluid layer in the alveolus. Surface tension at this air–fluid interface tends to decrease its area and this must be overcome by the transpulmonary pressure, if alveolar collapse is to be avoided. Pulmonary surfactant forms an insoluble film at the alveolar air–liquid interface replacing water molecules in the surface layer and lowering surface tension. Alveolar stability during expiration is due to low surface tension from surfactant during surface compression. At functional residual capacity surface tension is close to zero, but without surfactant it would be 70 mN/m at 37°C.

Surfactant allows very low transpulmonary pressures to be used during normal respiration and also has a role in the host defense mechanisms of the lung mainly through the actions of the large hydrophilic proteins, SP-A and SP-D. The mechanisms controlling surfactant metabolism and secretion are still unclear. SP-B regulates surfactant protein metabolism and enhances the uptake of phospholipids by type II cells in vitro. Although beta-adrenergic agents have been shown to initially increase secretion, prolonged use could deplete surfactant stores if rate of synthesis is low. Lung inflation also stimulates surfactant secretion but this may be mediated by humoral mechanisms. SP-A and SP-D have a role in the feedback control of surfactant secretion. When surfactant is released the contents of the lamellar bodies are extruded into the alveoli. After secretion the tightly packed lamellae of the lamellar bodies are left as tubular myelin which does not appear to have an active role in lowering surface tension.

The surface film needs to be constantly replenished from freshly secreted surfactant and recycling occurs within the type II cells. As much as 85–90% of surfactant is recycled. The clearance of surfactant is rapid and may be increased in the newborn period or after hyperventilation. Specific proteins may regulate the clearance of surfactant back to type II cells and small amounts are also phagocytosed by alveolar macrophages and cleared up the airways.

Further reading

Warburton D, Schwarz M, Tefft D, et al. The molecular basis of lung morphogenesis. Mech Dev 2000; 92:55–81. (Review article with 258 references)

Cardoso WV. Transcription factors and pattern formation in the developing lung. Am J Physiol 1995; 269:L429–442. (Review article with 185 references)

Bolt RJ, van Weissenbruch MM, Lafebre HN, et al. Glucocorticoids and lung development in the fetus and preterm infant. Pediatr Pulmonol 2001; 32:76–91. (Review article with 256 references)
Jobe AH, Ikegami M. Lung development and function in preterm infants in the surfactant era. Annu Rev Physiol 2000; 62:825–846. (Review article with 98 references)
Curley AE, Halliday HL. The present status of exogenous surfactant for the newborn. Early Hum Dev 2001; 61:67–83. (Review article with 86 references)

RESPIRATORY DISTRESS SYNDROME (HYALINE MEMBRANE DISEASE)

RDS, also known as hyaline membrane disease because of the histological features at autopsy, is caused by surfactant deficiency and affects mainly preterm infants. The incidence is 2–3% of all births but it is important as it is responsible for the deaths of many preterm infants throughout the world each year. The incidence of RDS is inversely proportional to gestational age.[468] There is evidence that increased use of prenatal corticosteroid treatment and perhaps prophylactic surfactant therapy have led to a reduction in both the incidence and severity of RDS (Table 10.46).[469] Apart from prematurity certain other factors are known to affect the incidence of RDS (Table 10.47).

Pathogenesis

Deficiency of surfactant leads to alveolar collapse, reduced lung volume, decreased lung compliance and ventilation–perfusion abnormalities. Right-to-left shunting of up to 70% or more occurs through collapsed lung (intrapulmonary) or across the ductus arteriosus and the foramen ovale (extrapulmonary) if pulmonary hypertension is severe. Persistent hypoxemia (< 4 kPa) causes metabolic acidosis and respiratory acidosis will also be present because of alveolar hypoventilation. This further reduces surfactant production and affects pulmonary vascular resistance, myocardial contractility, cardiac output and arterial blood pressure. Perfusion of the kidneys, gastrointestinal tract, muscles and skin is reduced leading to edema and electrolyte disorders.

Surfactant deficiency in RDS is primary and due to immaturity, the normal pool size of 100 mg of phospholipids/kg at term is reduced to < 5 mg/kg in babies with severe RDS. In some babies there is sufficient surfactant at birth to sustain normal respiration but this is gradually used up so that a generally mild form of RDS presents some hours after birth. Surfactant may also be inactivated by plasma proteins leaking into the alveoli and this form of ARDS may be seen in infants born to mothers with severe pregnancy-induced hypertension. Usually after 2–3 days endogenous surfactant production begins and this is followed by clinical recovery. Surfactant replacement will hasten recovery and it does not delay the onset of endogenous surfactant production.

Table 10.46 Risk of RDS by gestational age groups

Gestation (weeks)	Risk of RDS (%)
< 27	41.5
27–28	54.0
29–30	44.6
31–32	37.2
33–34	12.0
35–36	2.0
37–42	0.1

After Rubaltelli et al[469]

Table 10.47 Factors affecting the incidence of RDS

Decrease	Increase
Intrauterine growth retardation	Asphyxia
Prolonged rupture of membranes	Erythroblastosis
Maternal steroid therapy	Maternal diabetes
? Maternal smoking	Maternal hypertension
Sickle cell disease	Antepartum hemorrhage
Heroin	Elective cesarean section
Alcohol	Second twin
Black infants	Family history
Girls	Boys

Pathology

Macroscopically the lungs appear collapsed and liver-like and sink in water. Microscopic examination shows generalized collapse of alveoli with eosinophilic membranes in infants surviving more than a few hours. The membranes begin to break up by the third day and are removed by macrophages. Sometimes there is frank pulmonary hemorrhage and interstitial emphysema. The muscle layer of the walls of the pulmonary arterioles is thickened and pulmonary lymphatics are dilated. Surfactant treatment may modify the pathological features of RDS reducing the incidence of epithelial necrosis, interstitial emphysema and pulmonary interstitial hemorrhage but increasing the incidence of intra-alveolar hemorrhage.

Clinical features

The disease has a wide spectrum of severity from mild respiratory distress lasting 2 or 3 days to a rapidly fatal illness causing death within a few hours. The early clinical signs are shown in Table 10.48. When at least two of these signs are present after the first hour of life and the chest radiograph is typical (see below) diagnostic criteria are fulfilled. Each of these clinical signs may be explained by disturbed lung function. Increased respiratory rate is caused by the demand of increased alveolar ventilation and is related to blood gas changes of hypercarbia and hypoxemia. Later slow or decreasing respiratory rate which may progress to apnea may be related to diaphragmatic muscle fatigue.

The sternal and intercostal recession or retractions are due to reduced lung compliance as a result of surfactant deficiency. Expiratory grunting results from expiration against a partially closed glottis in an attempt to prevent alveolar collapse. It may be absent in the very immature or seriously ill baby. Cyanosis is due to decreased arterial oxygen tension caused by right-to-left interatrial and ductus shunts and to increasing intrapulmonary shunting after the first 12 h of life due to perfusion of collapsed or poorly ventilated parts of the lungs. These right-to-left shunts contribute to total venous admixtures of up to 75% of the cardiac output.

In severe disease, immature babies or those with asphyxia may need positive pressure ventilation from birth. In more mature babies grunting and retractions are prominent and cyanosis may be

Table 10.48 Early clinical signs of RDS

Tachypnea (> 60/min)
Expiratory grunting
Sternal and intercostal recession
Cyanosis in room air
Delayed onset of respiration in very immature babies

Table 10.49 Non-respiratory clinical signs in severe RDS

Hypotonia	Jaundice
Decreased movements	Hypothermia
Edema	Abdominal distention
Loss of heart rate variability	Decreased urinary output

apparent from soon after birth. Oxygen concentrations of greater than 60% are often needed to abolish cyanosis, and respiratory failure with hypercarbia and acidosis frequently supervenes, so that mechanical ventilation becomes necessary. Clinical signs outside the respiratory system also occur (Table 10.49).

The classical signs of RDS have become outdated for two reasons. First, most of the babies cared for in neonatal units are very immature and they often present with apnea at birth and second, prophylactic surfactant treatment is widely practiced for these babies and this significantly modifies the clinical course and the chest radiographic appearances.

Investigations

The aims of these are to confirm the diagnosis and exclude disorders in the list of differential diagnoses (Table 10.50). The chest radiograph is the best way to confirm the diagnosis but there are two caveats; first, congenital pneumonia can have a similar picture often coexisting with RDS and second, surfactant treatment will rapidly improve the chest radiographic appearances.

The classical radiographic signs are a diffuse reticulogranular pattern of mottling of the lung fields and an 'air bronchogram' appearance due to air in the major bronchi being highlighted against the white opacified lung (Fig. 10.22). With increasing severity the granular areas increase and become confluent so that the lung has a homogeneous ground glass appearance and the heart borders are obscured. Grading of the severity of RDS using radiological criteria (Table 10.51) is useful although the use of CPAP or surfactant replacement may improve the radiographic appearances considerably. The radiological appearances may be atypical with asymmetry when the changes are more pronounced on the right side or are confined to the lower lobes. When the chest radiograph shows uneven distribution of reticulogranularity this may be due to underlying pneumonia or follow surfactant treatment.

Other investigations may be biochemical, hematological or microbiological. Serial analyses of pH and arterial blood gases are essential for clinical evaluation. Continuous measurements of oxygen and carbon dioxide tensions may be made transcutaneously, and oxygen saturation can be assessed non-invasively by pulse oximetry but this has a major disadvantage of failing to exclude hyperoxia. These measurements are necessary to follow the clinical course of a baby with RDS and to detect early signs of deteriorating respiratory function allowing effective interventions such as surfactant therapy, CPAP or assisted ventilation. Hematological and microbiological investigations are needed to exclude underlying infection especially that due to group B streptococcus (GBS).

Table 10.50 Differential diagnosis of RDS

Congenital pneumonia
Aspiration pneumonia
Meconium aspiration syndrome
Air leak – pneumothorax, pulmonary interstitial emphysema and pneumomediastinum
Transient tachypnea of the newborn
Lobar emphysema
Pulmonary hypoplasia
Diaphragmatic hernia
Heart failure
Persistent pulmonary hypertension
Asphyxia and raised intracranial pressure
Metabolic acidosis/inborn errors of metabolism
Congenital neuromuscular disorders
Anemia, hypovolemia and polycythemia

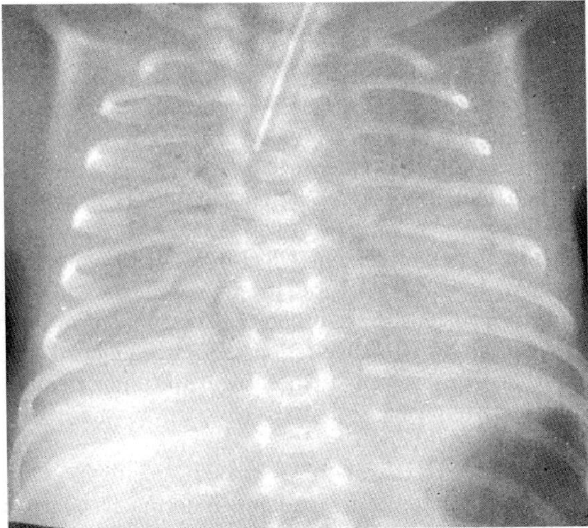

Fig. 10.22 Radiograph of severe RDS with widespread reticulogranular mottling and air bronchograms amounting to grade IV disease (see Table 10.51).

Natural history

The clinical course of classical RDS is that of increasing severity during the first 24–48 h of life, followed by a period of stability lasting another 48 h before improvement occurs. The severity of the disease may be expressed in terms of oxygen requirements and need for assisted ventilation. In the 24 h prior to recovery a diuresis usually occurs but diuretic therapy does not alter the course of RDS. The widespread introduction of surfactant therapy has meant that this natural history is unfamiliar to today's resident pediatricians although the occasional more mature infant with RDS is encountered who is not treated with surfactant.

Prevention

Antenatal glucocorticoid administration reduces the incidence and the severity of RDS provided 48 h of treatment is possible. Improved survival and reduced risk of complications such as pneumothorax, intraventricular hemorrhage and persistent ductus arteriosus but not bronchopulmonary dysplasia have also been demonstrated.[470] Combination treatment with glucocorticoids and thyrotropin releasing hormone has been abandoned following the publication of a study showing poorer outcomes.[471,472] Ambroxol if given intravenously for 5 days to women in preterm labor, appears to reduce the incidence of RDS. This drug is popular in some European

Table 10.51 Radiological grading of severity of RDS

Grade I	Fine reticulogranular mottling, good lung expansion
Grade II	Mottling with air bronchograms
Grade III	Diffuse mottling, heart borders just discernible, prominent air bronchograms
Grade IV	Bilateral confluent opacification of lungs ('whiteout')

countries but, because of the long treatment period and conflicting results from other studies[473] it is not used widely in the UK.

RDS may also be prevented or at least ameliorated if care is taken to prevent hypoxemia, acidosis and hypothermia in preterm babies. Gentle resuscitation at birth with early expansion of the alveoli or terminal airways in the preterm baby is very important and for babies of less than 30 weeks' gestation. This may be done by giving prophylactic surfactant or early use of CPAP.

Later surfactant replacement will also modify the course of RDS and in general the earlier it is given the greater the benefit.[474] Babies that might benefit most from prophylactic treatment at birth are those of less than 30 weeks' gestation, those needing endotracheal intubation for resuscitation or those who were not treated with prenatal corticosteroids.

Treatment

The objectives of treatment are to maintain normal blood gases, pH, biochemistry and physiology (blood pressure, temperature and renal function) and in addition to prevent complications of both the disease and the treatments. Surfactant replacement therapy is an effective way of accomplishing these objectives.[475] There are two basic types of surfactant, synthetic and natural and both have been shown to improve survival by about 40% and reduce the risk of pneumothorax by 30–70% in babies with RDS.[476–478] Recent studies and systematic reviews have shown that natural surfactants containing the proteins SP-B and SP-C are more effective than the protein-free synthetic surfactants[479–481] with improved survival and a reduced risk of pneumothorax compared to synthetic surfactants. One synthetic surfactant, Exosurf©, containing DPPC, tyloxapol and hexadecanol is still available for use.[482] There are many natural surfactant preparations, prepared from animal lungs: Survanta© (bovine), Alveofact© and Infasurf© (calf) and Curosurf© (porcine). The optimal dose of surfactant is about 100 mg/kg and repeated doses may be needed for babies who show relapse.[475] Synthetic surfactants may still have a role in the prevention of RDS whilst natural surfactants may be given to babies with moderate to severe RDS as soon after birth as possible or used prophylactically for very immature infants.[473]

Maintenance of temperature

Preterm infants should be nursed in an incubator or under a radiant warmer. In order to maintain adequate temperature in very preterm infants incubators need high humidity and double walls.

Maintenance of normoxemia

The aim is to achieve satisfactory oxygenation. For more mature babies (> 30 weeks) with spontaneous respiration, humidified oxygen may be given into a Perspex headbox. For very immature infants (< 30 weeks) or when respiratory failure supervenes, some form of assisted ventilation may be necessary (see below). Excessive handling should be avoided as this causes hypoxemia and leads to deterioration. Monitoring of oxygenation is essential as too little oxygen will cause hypoxemia, metabolic acidosis and tissue damage and too much oxygen has been associated with the development of retinopathy of prematurity. An initial right radial artery blood sample is helpful. An arterial catheter should be inserted in babies needing greater than 40% oxygen after the first hour (or greater than 30% oxygen in babies of less than 1200 g birth weight). Continuous methods of assessing oxygenation such as intravascular electrodes, transcutaneous monitors and pulse oximeters do not remove the need for intermittent arterial blood sampling to check calibration and measure pH, arterial carbon dioxide tension and base deficit. Oxygen delivery is affected by arterial oxygen tension, oxygen-carrying capacity, oxygen affinity, peripheral blood flow, temperature and pH. Fetal Hb allows more oxygen to be carried in the blood at any oxygen tension (greater affinity) but less oxygen will be released to the tissues. The newborn and especially the preterm infant also has a reduced level of 2,3-diphosphoglycerate (2,3-DPG) and oxygen delivery may be improved by giving transfusions of adult blood or exchange transfusion.

Correction of acid–base abnormalities

Respiratory acidosis due to raised arterial carbon dioxide tension is common in severe RDS. Hypercarbia can only be treated adequately by improving ventilation. Metabolic acidosis may arise from hypoxemia, hypotension, infection, renal failure, persistent ductus arteriosus or intraventricular hemorrhage. Treatment of the underlying cause, for example by increasing oxygen concentrations or giving blood or plasma transfusions, may be more appropriate than infusion of sodium bicarbonate. The aim should be to keep the pH above 7.25. If the base deficit becomes greater than 10 mmol/L then sodium bicarbonate should be considered. The dose may be calculated as follows:

$$\text{dose (mmol)} = \text{base deficit (mmol/L)} \times \text{weight (kg)} \times 0.3$$

Molar sodium bicarbonate 8.4% (1 mmol/ml) is the most frequently used alkali in clinical practice but it is hyperosmolar and rapid infusions have been associated with the development of intraventricular hemorrhages. Severe tissue injury may occur in the event of extravasation. It also has a high sodium content and will raise $PaCO_2$ unless ventilation is adequate.

In practice molar sodium bicarbonate should be diluted and given slowly (not faster than 1 mmol/min) by peripheral venous infusion. The total amount of bicarbonate should be restricted to 10 mmol/kg/day to lessen risks of hypernatremia and intraventricular hemorrhage.

Energy, fluid and electrolyte requirements

The preterm baby with RDS has reduced stores of carbohydrate (as glycogen), fat and protein (as skeletal muscle), and at the same time has increased metabolic requirements as a result of the extra work of breathing. Providing adequate exogenous sources of energy as parenteral nutrition for these sick babies is technically difficult, if not impossible. For the first 24–48 h protein and fat requirements are not met and in practice only an infusion of 10% dextrose in water at 60–90 ml/kg is given on the first day. Fluid requirements may be monitored by looking at *plasma sodium*, urine output and specific gravity, osmolality and by regular weighing. Excessive fluid intake is associated with increased risk of persistent ductus arteriosus, NEC and bronchopulmonary dysplasia.

Oliguria in severe RDS is not unusual for the first 48 h due to the effects of asphyxia, hypotension and possibly inappropriate ADH secretion. Care must be taken to avoid fluid and electrolyte overload. Subsequently, when the diuretic phase occurs, the large urinary losses mean that extra fluid, sodium and potassium intake will be necessary to prevent hyponatremia or hypokalemia (see pp. 220–221).

Parenteral nutrition in the form of amino acids and fat solutions can usually be started on the second or third day of life. Once the baby shows signs of recovery, extra energy should be provided in the form of enteral milk feeds.

Assisted ventilation

CPAP is a distending pressure which prevents alveolar collapse during expiration and thus improves oxygenation. Studies in infants of >1500 g show that it reduces mortality and the need for IPPV but increases the risk of pneumothorax.[483] The indications for using CPAP in RDS are not absolute and may depend upon the maturity of the baby (Table 10.52). CPAP should be considered for all spontaneously breathing infants of < 30 weeks and it can be used in infants who have been treated with surfactant.[484,485] Use of CPAP soon after birth may obviate the need for IPPV.

Methods of applying CPAP include facemask, face chamber, nasal prongs, nasopharyngeal tube and Gregory box but today nasal prongs using a ventilator circuit or a flow driver are generally used.[486] Variable flow nasal CPAP leads to greater lung recruitment than continuous flow nasal CPAP administered via prongs.[487] Underwater bubble CPAP was associated with a reduction of minute volume compared with ventilator-derived CPAP in preterm neonates ready for extubation.[488]

Mechanical ventilation is used to treat respiratory failure or intractable apnea (Table 10.53). For babies less than 30 weeks' gestation, $PaCO_2$ of > 8 kPa (60 torr) is usually accepted as an indication for IPPV. Use of mechanical ventilation requires considerable expertise and meticulous attention to detail by both medical and nursing staff. The quality of the intensive care team may determine outcome to a greater degree than the type of ventilator used. Suitable ventilators are pressure limited and time cycled, and allow variation of inspired oxygen concentration, flow rate, peak airway pressure, PEEP, ventilation rate and inspiratory and expiratory times. IPPV is performed through an endotracheal tube inserted through either the nose or mouth into the trachea. The initial ventilator settings employed will depend upon the maturity of the baby and the severity of the lung disease. For the baby less than 30 weeks' gestation with severe lung disease, the aim of IPPV should be to expand the lungs as early as possible with the lowest peak airway pressure possible. Peak airway pressures of 15–25 cmH_2O are often needed initially, with PEEP of 3–5 cmH_2O and ventilator rate of 60–120/min. These faster rates are preferred by smaller babies who may often be induced to breathe synchronously with the ventilator without resort to muscle relaxants.[489,490] Sedation with morphine or fentanyl should be considered for these babies. Inspiratory times of 0.3–0.5 s are used so that the I:E ratio is about 1:1. Mechanical ventilation of the more mature baby with severe RDS may need higher peak airway pressures and lower rates. Sometimes muscle relaxants and sedation with morphine or fentanyl are needed to prevent these babies 'fighting' the ventilator which will increase the risk of pneumothorax.

If gas exchange remains impaired in a ventilated infant after surfactant treatment, oxygenation may be improved by increased mean airway pressure (MAP) or use of high frequency oscillation (HFOV). Muscle relaxation with pancuronium (0.03 mg/kg) or vecuronium (0.05 mg/kg/h by infusion after a loading dose of 0.1 mg/kg) may be required. A further dose of surfactant should be given but the use of vasodilating drugs is controversial. Inhaled nitric oxide is an experimental therapy for preterm infants with RDS although it effectively lowers pulmonary hypertension in term babies.[491]

As the baby's condition improves the ventilator settings can be reduced. Peak airway pressure should be lowered first, along with inspired oxygen concentration. Later, ventilator rates can be lowered keeping inspiratory time constant at about 0.4–0.5 s to prevent air trapping. Following surfactant treatment ventilator settings can usually be reduced quite rapidly and an inspiratory time of 0.3 s is desirable. Intermittent mandatory ventilation (IMV) is possible with all of the newer pressure-limited ventilators and this allows ventilator rates to be lowered with the baby breathing as he or she wishes between each ventilator breath. A period of CPAP is sometimes tried before extubation but in the immature baby, longer periods of IMV (rates 10/min) may be necessary. Theophylline or caffeine has been used to successfully wean VLBW infants from mechanical ventilation.[492] Patient triggered ventilation may also have a role to play in weaning although it appears to be less effective in infants of < 28 weeks.[493] After extubation nasal CPAP probably reduces the need for re-intubation.[494,495]

Table 10.52 Indications for CPAP in RDS

1. Early treatment of infants < 30 weeks if good spontaneous respiratory effort
2. After surfactant treatment in infants > 27 weeks
3. For infants > 30 weeks and oxygen need > 30% to keep PaO_2 > 8 kPa (60 mmHg)
4. Recurrent apneic attacks
5. Weaning from IPPV and after extubation

Table 10.53 Indications for IPPV in RDS

1. Failure to establish respiration at birth
2. To administer surfactant at birth in infants < 27 weeks
3. To administer surfactant in infants > 27 weeks and < 32 weeks when they need > 30% oxygen
4. In infants > 32 weeks when respiratory failure develops
   pH < 7.20
   $PaCO_2$ > 9 kPa (68 mmHg)
   PaO_2 < 7 kPa (53 mmHg) in > 60% oxygen
5. Intractable apneic attacks not responding to other measures

Complications of RDS (Table 10.54)

Persistent ductus arteriosus (PDA)

The ductus arteriosus is likely to remain open in babies with severe RDS for a number of reasons: prematurity with poorly developed ductus musculature, reduced arterial oxygen tensions and inadequate metabolism of prostaglandins in the lungs.[496] Fluid overload and surfactant replacement may also increase the risk of PDA. The management is discussed on page 276.

Table 10.54 Complications of RDS

1. Persistent ductus arteriosus
2. Intraventricular hemorrhage
3. Pulmonary
   a. Air leaks
      Pneumothorax
      Pneumomediastinum
      Pulmonary interstitial emphysema
      Pneumopericardium
      Pneumoperitoneum
      Air embolism
      Subcutaneous emphysema
   b. Chronic lung disease
   c. Pneumonia
      Aspiration
      Bacterial
4. Complications of mechanical ventilation (see above)
5. Long term neurological sequelae

Intraventricular hemorrhage (IVH) (p. 321)

IVH can cause acute deterioration in infants with RDS and may be predisposed to by other causes of collapse such as pneumothorax.[497] Maintenance of physiological stability and prevention of air leak by manipulation of ventilator settings or surfactant replacement[498] has reduced the incidence of IVH in recent years.

Pulmonary air leaks (p. 260)

The incidence of these depends upon the severity of the RDS and the need for assisted ventilation. For babies with RDS not needing assisted ventilation the incidence is 5–10%. In the decades of the 1970s and 1980s, if CPAP was needed the incidence was about 10–15% and with IPPV 10–30%.[499] Since that time high rate ventilation, muscle relaxation and surfactant replacement,[476–478,498] together with better ventilators, have reduced the incidence of pneumothorax to less than 5%,[500] which means that many residents have not had much experience in insertion of chest drains.

Bronchopulmonary dysplasia or chronic lung disease (p. 267)

This condition was not described until after the introduction of mechanical ventilation to treat RDS.[501] Positive pressure ventilation with an endotracheal tube is necessary for its development, but other factors such as oxygen toxicity, infection and fluid overload probably have a significant role in pathogenesis. This form of 'ventilator lung' is rarely seen today but CLD is relatively common in very preterm infants and it is probably a form of chronic pulmonary inflammation associated with chorioamnionitis.[502,503] About 20% of babies needing mechanical ventilation for RDS will develop this complication[504] but infants with mild or no RDS can also develop CLD associated with infection and PDA.[505]

Pneumonia (p. 257)

Pneumonia may coexist with RDS or be secondary associated with the presence of an endotracheal tube. Cultures of tracheal aspirates are of limited use in diagnosis of secondary infection but may guide the choice of antibiotics should the infant deteriorate. The presence of both pus cells and organisms in tracheal aspirates, development of patchy opacity on chest radiograph and general deterioration often with positive blood cultures help to make the diagnosis.[506] Appropriate antibiotic treatment is then necessary. The role of chest physiotherapy is probably limited. Aspiration pneumonia may also be common and may cause acute deterioration. In one study it occurred in up to 80% of mechanically ventilated neonates.[507] Chest radiograph may show areas of collapse and consolidation especially in the right upper or right lower lobes. Antibiotic therapy and possibly gentle chest physiotherapy may be helpful.

Long term neurological sequelae (p. 243)

There is recent evidence that modern neonatal intensive care has not only reduced neonatal mortality very considerably, but has also improved the quality of survival. A major contributing factor is the improved understanding of the pathogenesis of RDS as well as improved methods of prevention and treatment. For babies of > 30 weeks' gestation, ventilatory techniques are now well standardized and technical difficulties are minimal. Babies in whom RDS is the primary indication for mechanical ventilation are unlikely to develop permanent brain injury unless there is severe asphyxia or extensive intraventricular hemorrhage. The role of fetal infection in causing white matter damage is under intensive study.[508,509] The introduction of surfactant therapy after 1988 was largely responsible for the sharp reduction in the RDS-specific infant mortality rate from 2 per 1000 births in 1970 to 0.4 per 1000 in 1995.[510]

TRANSIENT TACHYPNEA OF THE NEWBORN

This occurs in both term and preterm babies. First described in 1966[511] it has also been called type II RDS and wet lung disease.

Incidence

Transient tachypnea of the newborn (TTN) occurs in about 1% of births.[469] The risk is increased after cesarean section to about 4% but the timing of elective cesarean section is important with the risk decreasing from about 10% to 2% from 37 to 40 weeks' gestation.[512]

Etiology and pathogenesis

TTN has been attributed to delayed resorption of fetal lung fluid and predisposing factors include elective cesarean section, perinatal asphyxia, excessive maternal analgesia or hypothermia, maternal diabetes and male gender. Many of these factors are associated with increased production or decreased resorption of lung fluid. Catecholamine levels after elective cesarean section are lower than those following vaginal delivery with the result that fetal lung fluid production continues after birth.[513] The time of cord clamping is related to tachypnea after birth with delayed clamping being associated with an increased incidence of respiratory distress in both term and preterm babies. Late cord clamping leads to increased placental transfusion to the baby and may cause left ventricular dysfunction which has been found in echocardiographic studies of babies with transient tachypnea of the newborn.[514] Asphyxia exacerbates this left ventricular failure in some babies who resemble those with persistent fetal circulation.

Clinical presentation

Most affected babies are either large preterm or term infants with a male preponderance of three to one. Tachypnea is apparent from about 1 h after birth, with respiratory rates of up to 120/min. Subcostal recession, grunting and cyanosis may be present but are not prominent features. Affected babies have barrel chests with increase in anteroposterior diameter. Babies with a picture of persistent fetal circulation are uncommon, but present with marked cyanosis and often need mechanical ventilation.[515] A recent study has shown that infants born by elective delivery at 37–38 weeks are 120 times more likely to need ventilatory support than those born at 39–41 weeks.[516]

Diagnosis

The chest radiograph shows hyperinflated lung fields, perihilar opacities, increased vascular markings, fluid in the transverse fissure and small pleural effusions (Fig. 10.23). Two important differential diagnoses should be considered in atypical infants. Early onset GBS sepsis can mimic TTN initially but if unrecognized and untreated will be fatal. Blood culture, examination of gastric aspirate and full blood picture will help to make this diagnosis. Some forms of congenital heart disease, for example anomalous pulmonary venous drainage, can also mimic TTN. Chest radiograph and echocardiography are helpful if a cardiac anomaly is suspected.

Management

Oxygen is often needed for 2 or 3 days but respiratory failure is uncommon unless a pulmonary air leak or pulmonary hypertension occurs. Pulse oximetry may be useful in monitoring the oxygen needs of affected term babies. Only rarely are oxygen concentrations above 40% necessary. Penicillin should be given until GBS sepsis has been excluded. There is no evidence that furosemide (frusemide) treatment hastens recovery.[517]

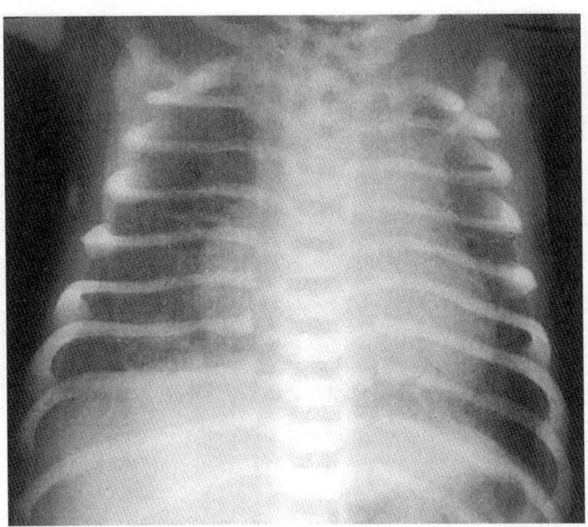

Fig. 10.23 Radiograph of TTN with overinflated lungs, fluid in the right costophrenic angle and horizontal fissure. The skinfold line seen at the right base may be mistaken for a pneumothorax.

Outcome

Most infants recover within 2–3 days and there are no long term sequelae. Up to 10% of babies develop pneumothoraces and a few may need mechanical ventilation. The mortality rate should approach zero and survivors should have normal neurodevelopment.[518] A multicenter study from Italy that included term and preterm infants reported a case fatality rate of 2%.[469]

PNEUMONIA

Pneumonia is probably the most common serious infection of the newborn baby. It may be either congenital or acquired, although intrapartum infection can occur and may not fit easily into either category (Table 10.55).

Incidence

Preterm babies are more commonly infected for at least three reasons. Firstly congenital infection may stimulate preterm labor, secondly preterm babies have problems with host defense mechanisms and thirdly they are more likely to need intensive care and thus be exposed to the risks of acquired infections. Early-onset pneumonia has been estimated to occur in 1.79 per 1000 live births.[519] Nosocomial infection causing pneumonia was found in about 8% of babies in a NICU.[520] Pneumonia as a complication of endotracheal intubation for mechanical ventilation has an incidence of about 30%.[506]

Pathogenesis

Pneumonia that is acquired congenitally or intrapartum (Table 10.56) usually presents within the first 4–6 h and may then be described as early onset. Nosocomial infections are usually late onset although colonization with organisms acquired intrapartum can lead to subsequent infection occurring after 7 days. This may occur in late onset GBS infections.

Table 10.55 Pathogenesis of neonatal pneumonia

Congenital (transplacental acquisition)
Intrapartum a. Ascending infection and chorioamnionitis b. Aspiration of infected secretions at delivery
Acquired Nosocomial – often during mechanical ventilation or late infection after colonization at birth

Transplacentally acquired pneumonia may be due to viruses (CMV, Coxsackie, herpes simplex and rubella), bacteria (*Listeria monocytogenes*, coliforms, pneumococci and streptococci) or toxoplasmosis.[518] The ascending route of infection is the most important in early-onset infection and the organisms found in the maternal genital tract and in the baby's lungs are very similar. Prolonged rupture of the membranes is commonly found in cases of ascending infection and as the duration of membrane rupture increases up to 3 days the incidence of chorioamnionitis increases to about 50% and neonatal infection to about 8%. Ascending infection can occur through intact membranes and cause illness or perinatal death,[521] although this is less common. Organisms involved in ascending infection are coliforms, streptococci, *Haemophilus influenzae*, pneumococci, staphylococci and herpes simplex virus.

Intrapartum aspiration of infected secretions can cause infection with *L. monocytogenes*, streptococci, herpes simplex and varicella. Nosocomial or environmentally acquired infection can be transmitted by hospital staff usually from poor handwashing. The organisms involved are staphylococci, streptococci and RSV. Sometimes infection is acquired from nursery equipment and the organisms involved are pseudomonas, serratia, klebsiella and listeria. Late-onset infection may also be due to delayed invasion of organisms acquired at birth. This typically occurs with certain serotypes of streptococci and listeria and is probably not preventable by prophylactic antibiotic use.

Early onset pneumonia

Clinical features

Intrapartum stillbirth may occur, but often the baby is born alive with signs of asphyxia and needs resuscitation. The onset of respiratory symptoms may be more gradual with a clinical picture very similar to that of RDS (Table 10.48). Helpful distinguishing features include temperature instability, hypotension, apneic spells and acidosis. Sometimes a skin rash or hepatosplenomegaly (listeriosis) will be present or the baby may be foul smelling (coliforms or bacteroides). The severity of respiratory distress is variable and some babies may have profound shock and metabolic upsets with right-to-left shunting and a clinical course resembling severe persistent fetal circulation whereas others have respiratory signs such as tachypnea.

A chest radiograph is necessary to exclude other causes of respiratory distress. With transplacentally acquired infection there are diffuse, interstitial opacities giving a ground glass, reticular pattern which may be indistinguishable from RDS or there may be extensive consolidation (Fig. 10.24). With ascending infection there may be alveolar involvement which produces bilateral coarse opacities which are much less uniform (Fig. 10.25). Air bronchograms may also be seen especially if the opacities become confluent.

Pneumonia acquired following aspiration is usually less evenly distributed on chest radiograph and may show as segmental or lobar collapse (Fig. 10.26).

Diagnosis

The clinical diagnosis is confirmed by culturing organisms from tracheal fluid, blood or gastric aspirate, although the last is less reliable. There is not time to wait for culture results before starting treatment and hematological (white cell and platelet counts) and biochemical (C-reactive protein) tests are not sensitive enough to be relied upon if negative. If in doubt, it is best to start antibiotics after cultures have been taken. Direct examination of gastric aspirate has been used to guide antibiotic therapy but any polymorphonuclear leukocytes present are probably of maternal origin and any

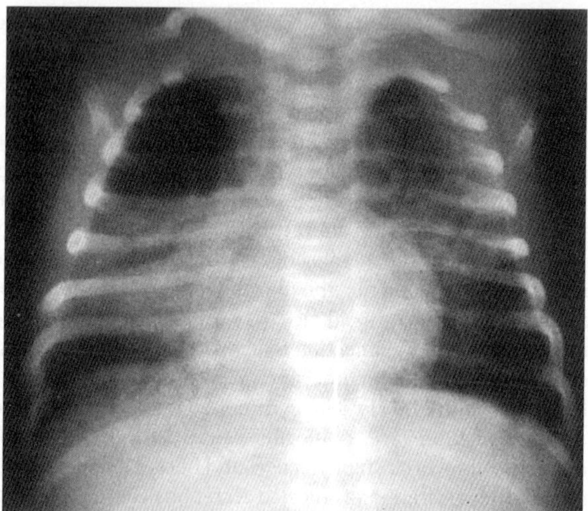

Fig. 10.24 Radiograph of congenital listeriosis showing extensive consolidation in both midzones but more marked on the right. An arterial catheter is seen with its tip at T7 and T8.

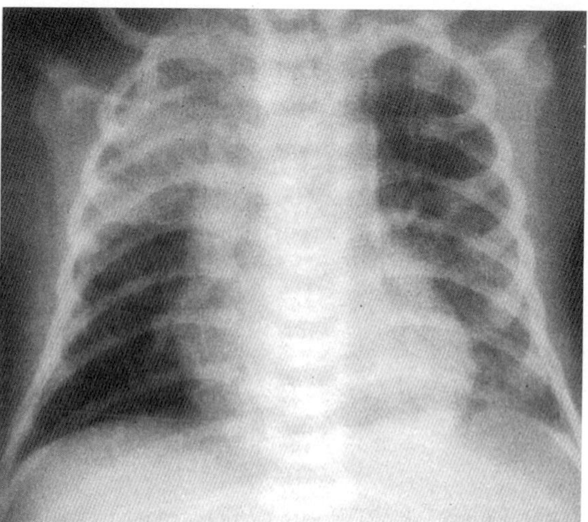

Fig. 10.26 Chest radiograph showing aspiration pneumonia with collapse and consolidation in right upper lobe.

organisms seen on Gram stain may be contaminants rather than the pathogens causing the pneumonia. If tracheal aspirate can be obtained and examined within 8 h of birth there is a good correlation between organisms seen and those subsequently cultured.

Differential diagnosis

This includes RDS, transient tachypnea of the newborn and meconium aspiration syndrome in addition to causes of severe asphyxia at birth including pulmonary hypoplasia. Sometimes these conditions can coexist so that if any doubt exists antibiotic cover especially for GBS infection should be given. Severe pneumonia may also be difficult to distinguish from cyanotic heart disease and persistent fetal circulation.

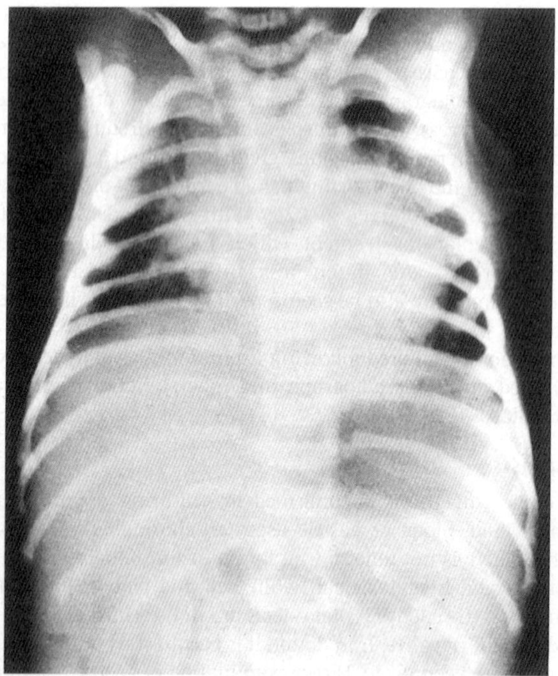

Fig. 10.25 Radiograph of intrauterine pneumonia from ascending infection showing patchy bronchopneumonic consolidation.

Management

Prevention. Early-onset GBS infection can be predicted from maternal risk factors such as prolonged rupture of the membranes, colonization of the genital tract, spontaneous preterm labor and maternal pyrexia in labor. When women with these risk factors who are known to be colonized with GBS are treated with intravenous penicillin in large doses during labor there is a significant reduction in neonatal infection.[522] Penicillin may also be effective in pregnancies complicated by infection with listeria, haemophilus and pneumococci but other Gram negative organisms and anaerobes will not usually be sensitive. A combination of ampicillin and metronidazole would improve the spectrum of cover in these high-risk cases. Recently the ORACLE study has demonstrated that maternal erythromycin improves neonatal outcome when there is preterm prelabor rupture of the membranes.[523]

Treatment. Babies born to mothers with the risk factors mentioned above should have cultures taken and be given antibiotic prophylaxis. There is no evidence that routine penicillin prophylaxis for all preterm babies is effective and this approach might increase the risk of Gram negative infections. Routine monitoring of the respiratory rate for 24 h on the postnatal ward has been shown to be effective in shortening the time to diagnosis and treatment of the occasional late-presenting case.[524]

For symptomatic infants with respiratory distress, penicillin therapy should be started after appropriate cultures have been taken; the antibiotic can be stopped after 48 h if the cultures are negative and the baby's condition improved or a clear diagnosis of non-infective illness has been made. If infection is strongly suspected, cultures become positive or the infant deteriorates, an aminoglycoside such as gentamicin should be added to the antibiotic regimen.

Treatment of the ill baby requires good resuscitation, stabilization and respiratory support, in addition to antibiotics given after cultures have been taken. Blood or plasma transfusion, inotropic drugs and correction of acidosis are all important. Penicillin or ampicillin and gentamicin or netilmicin in combination provide the best cover for early-onset pneumonia. Recently, cefotaxime has been advocated because of increased penetration into lung tissue.

Surfactant treatment may be helpful to treat respiratory failure due to surfactant inactivation in streptococcal pneumonia but the effect is less than in infants with RDS.[525]

Late-onset pneumonia

This may be associated with mechanical ventilation, aspiration, bacteremia or occur secondary to late invasion with an organism acquired during birth, e.g. GBS or *L. monocytogenes*. Occasionally unusual organisms such as chlamydia, candida, CMV, herpes simplex, RSV or mycoplasma are implicated although staphylococci and coliforms are much more commonly found.

Clinical features

Late-onset pneumonia occurs after 24 h and presents with signs of respiratory distress although preterm babies may develop apnea. There may be systemic signs with pyrexia in term babies and hypothermia in preterm ones. Bacteremia and meningitis can be present at the same time.

A chest radiograph is necessary for diagnosis, and culture of blood, tracheal aspirate and CSF should also be performed. The differential diagnosis includes persistent ductus arteriosus and heart failure, aspiration pneumonia, early chronic lung disease or an inborn error of metabolism.

Management

General supportive measures, antibiotics and perhaps gentle chest physiotherapy form the basis of management. Antibiotic selection must cover staphylococci and Gram negative organisms and if meningitis is suspected be capable of penetrating the CSF. A combination of flucloxacillin and netilmicin or one of the third generation cephalosporins, e.g. cefotaxime, is usually satisfactory. For pseudomonas infections ceftazidime is used and some staphylococcal infections respond only to vancomycin.

Outcome

Early-onset pneumonia has a high mortality of about 50% especially when due to GBS which often affects very immature babies who have septicemia with pneumonia. Late-onset pneumonia has a mortality rate of less than 15% despite its association with bacteremia and meningitis.

MECONIUM ASPIRATION SYNDROME

This is a serious and potentially preventable condition occurring usually in term and post-term babies.

Incidence

Meconium staining of the amniotic fluid is found in about 9% of deliveries at term, and at birth 56% of these babies have meconium in their trachea. However, only 20% of babies born through meconium-stained liquor develop pulmonary disease requiring oxygen supplementation or have a pulmonary air leak.[526] The incidence may be lower in the UK where obstetricians manage prolonged pregnancy more aggressively.[527,528]

Etiology and pathogenesis

In the term or post-term infant asphyxia prior to birth stimulates intestinal peristalsis and relaxation of the anal sphincter. Meconium passage is most likely to occur in the post-term baby, the term baby after asphyxia or the baby with IUGR. It rarely happens in the preterm baby of < 34 weeks' gestation as even with severe asphyxia the anal sphincter does not usually relax.

If meconium staining does occur in preterm labor one should consider an alternative cause such as congenital infection, especially that due to listeriosis[529] or GBS. Once meconium reaches the major airways, respiration after birth ensures distal migration into the smaller airways. This may lead to obstruction with air trapping and atelectasis and pneumothorax is a common complication.

Other factors producing lung disease are chemical pneumonitis and secondary bacterial infection. There may be abnormal pulmonary vascular spasm with arteriolar thickening causing pulmonary hypertension. Most babies with meconium aspiration syndrome have suffered from some degree of pre- or perinatal asphyxia and this by itself can cause pulmonary disease.

Clinical features

Affected babies are usually post-term or growth retarded. There may be meconium staining of the skin, umbilical cord and nails. The baby may present with respiratory distress from birth but the respiratory signs may gradually develop over 12 h with tachypnea, cyanosis, indrawing and a hyperinflated chest. There may be profound hypoxemia although hypercarbia is less common. Metabolic acidosis and hypoglycemia are common and postasphyxial signs may be found in the central nervous system, kidneys and heart. Pneumothorax complicates about 30% of cases of severe meconium aspiration syndrome.

Diagnosis

The diagnosis is made on the basis of meconium-stained amniotic fluid, presence of meconium in the trachea and radiological changes. On chest radiograph there is overinflation of the lungs with widespread coarse, fluffy opacities (Fig. 10.27). Sometimes the appearances are confined to the right lung or right upper lobe. Pneumothorax, pneumomediastinum and cardiomegaly may be present. There is usually slow radiological clearing over 10 days but in some babies the meconium disappears within 2–3 days possibly by ciliary action, phagocytosis or enzymatic lysis.[518]

Management

This comprises prevention by intervention in pregnancy, labor or at birth and the treatment of established aspiration.

Prevention

Meconium aspiration syndrome should be largely preventable by careful antenatal monitoring, rapid delivery for fetal distress and rapid resuscitation with tracheal suctioning at birth if indicated. A pediatrician skilled at neonatal resuscitation should

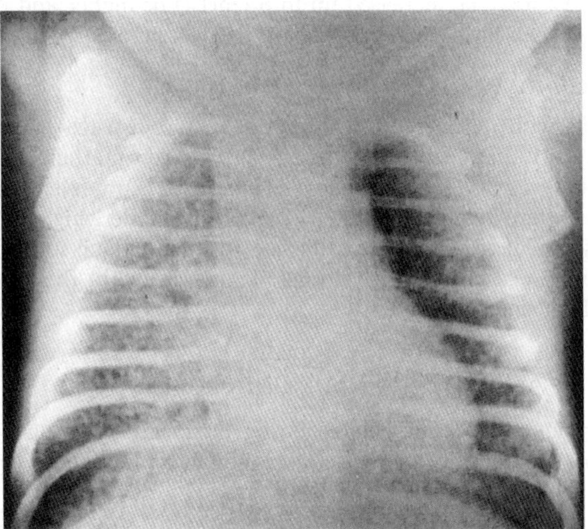

Fig. 10.27 Radiograph of meconium aspiration syndrome with overinflated lungs, depressed diaphragm and coarse modular opacities alternating with areas of focal overinflation.

attend all deliveries complicated by meconium staining of the amniotic fluid. If the meconium staining is thick and particulate ('pea soup'), an attempt to clear the mouth and pharynx should be made as soon as the head has been delivered. After birth the larynx should be inspected directly and, if meconium is found and especially if the baby is depressed, the trachea should be carefully intubated and any meconium aspirated from the airway.

Intubation of all meconium-stained babies and careful tracheal toilet had been advocated as a method of reducing mortality and severity of subsequent respiratory distress. Large randomized studies[530,531] and a subsequent systematic review[532] however, showed no benefit of routine endotracheal intubation in babies who were vigorous at birth. Intubation should be reserved for babies with signs of respiratory depression and asphyxia or those born through thick, particulate meconium-stained liquor. Tracheal aspiration using an endotracheal tube adaptor should be repeated until the trachea is cleared and saline lavage should be avoided as this may help to liquefy the meconium allowing it to pass distally.[518] Positive pressure ventilation should be postponed until tracheal aspiration has been completed.

Treatment

All babies with meconium below the vocal cords should be admitted to the neonatal unit for observation and further management. All symptomatic babies should have a chest radiograph performed and oxygen supplements as indicated by blood gas analyses. Babies with mild disease may need only humidified oxygen in a headbox. Gentle chest physiotherapy and postural drainage may be helpful but lung lavage should be avoided. Broad spectrum antibiotics should be given to treat any coexistent pneumonia or congenital sepsis. There is no benefit from the use of hydrocortisone and it may even delay recovery. Recently, surfactant treatment has been shown to hasten recovery but larger (150 mg/kg) and more frequent (6-hourly) doses are required[533] presumably to overcome inactivation of surfactant by meconium.

Severely asphyxiated babies with meconium aspiration often have multisystem involvement and require careful management. Mechanical ventilation may be indicated to treat respiratory failure and severe hypoxemia. Rapid ventilator rates with low PEEP are advised because of the risk of pneumothorax and cardiovascular side-effects. Muscle relaxation or sedation with morphine or fentanyl is often necessary. If hypoxemia due to right-to-left shunting persists the PEEP may be increased up to 6 cmH_2O or higher and use of inhaled nitric oxide might obviate the need for ECMO.

Outcome

Infants with mild disease who do not require assisted ventilation recover within a few days. Recent reports suggest mortality rates of about 10%.[518,534] Both mortality and long-term neurodevelopmental sequelae are related to the severity of the underlying perinatal asphyxia. There is an increased risk of asthma among survivors of meconium aspiration syndrome compared with the general childhood population.[535]

OTHER ASPIRATION PNEUMONIAS

Aspiration may occur before, during or after birth. Apart from meconium the substances aspirated may be amniotic fluid, blood, secretions or milk.

Incidence

This is unknown but early contrast radiography studies showed that 10–15% of newborn babies aspirate fluid into their lungs during the first few days after birth. It is likely that the incidence of milk aspiration in preterm babies has substantially decreased as a result of more widespread use of intravenous fluids which allows the volume of feeds to be gradually increased. Preterm babies with endotracheal tubes for mechanical ventilation probably aspirate secretions frequently; one study suggested that this occurred in 80% of such babies.[507]

Etiology

Aspiration can occur before birth and amniotic debris including squamous cells have been found in the lungs of stillborn babies. Aspiration of small amounts of fetal and maternal blood do not appear to cause major problems and are rapidly removed from the lungs. If purulent secretions are aspirated during birth there is an increased risk of subsequent bacterial pneumonia. Aspiration of milk may occur in the very preterm infant, those with swallowing disorders, and those with esophageal atresia and tracheoesophageal fistula. Before 34 weeks, sucking and swallowing are uncoordinated and most babies need gastric tube feeds. Aspiration of liquids may cause apnea as part of a protective laryngeal reflex.

Clinical features

Aspiration before or during birth may cause signs of asphyxia and immediate respiratory distress in the same way as meconium aspiration syndrome. Aspiration after birth presents with apneic or cyanotic attacks and there may be choking or signs of airway obstruction. After such an episode there may be tachypnea and indrawing.

Apart from immaturity, babies at risk of aspiration are those who have suffered asphyxia or those with neuromuscular disorders who may also have drooling, poor suck and myopathic facies. If there are recurrent episodes of aspiration, an underlying disorder such as H-type tracheoesophageal fistula or posterior laryngeal cleft should be excluded. In supine infants aspiration is most likely to occur into the right upper lobe and crepitations may be heard there. Occasionally there may be complete collapse of a lobe with shift of the mediastinum towards the affected side.

Diagnosis

The chest radiograph may be clear or show localized or diffuse opacities and areas of atelectasis. These changes are most frequently seen in the right upper lobe (Fig. 10.26). Aspirate from the lung may show fat-laden macrophages in babies who have aspirated milk or medium chain triglycerides. If gastroesophageal reflux is suspected, barium swallow, esophageal manometry or pH studies and endoscopy may be necessary.

Management

Direct laryngoscopy and careful suction of the airways should be performed to resuscitate babies who have aspirated. Supportive care includes oxygen to correct hypoxemia, intravenous fluids and the treatment of acidosis. Broad spectrum antibiotics should be given if the extent of the aspiration is large or the secretions aspirated appear to be infected. Careful nursing is important, gastric emptying is most rapid with the baby lying either prone or on the right side.

PULMONARY AIR LEAKS

These comprise pneumothorax, pulmonary interstitial emphysema, pneumomediastinum, pneumopericardium, pneumoperitoneum, subcutaneous emphysema and air embolism. They are related conditions of varying severity which have a common etiology and pathogenesis.[518]

Etiology and pathogenesis

Alveolar rupture occurs more commonly in the neonate than any other time of life. It is more likely to occur in states of hyperinflation of the chest and the risk is increased because of lack of pores of Kohn which are communications between alveoli.

Air leak occurs at the base of a group of alveoli and tracks into the perivascular sheath at the center of the pulmonary lobule. Air later tracks along the bronchovascular spaces to the hilum where it dissects into the mediastinum and pleural space. Air may also form subpleural blebs which can later rupture to cause a pneumothorax. Extension of air into the subcutaneous tissues of the neck will cause surgical emphysema, and down along perivascular or periesophageal tissue sheaths to form a pneumoperitoneum. A pneumothorax may result from high transpulmonary pressures generated by the first breath but it more usually arises later because of some underlying lung pathology such as RDS, aspiration syndromes, pulmonary hypoplasia and the need for positive pressure ventilation. Traumatic pneumothorax may occur from perforation of the lung by a suction catheter or a chest drain. Although the more mature lung ruptures at lower transpulmonary pressures than the immature lung, pneumothorax is commoner in the preterm baby who is more likely to have respiratory distress.

Pneumothorax

This is accumulation of air within the pleural cavity and usually occurs following a pneumomediastinum, although the latter may not be obvious clinically or radiologically.

Incidence

About 1% of term babies have an asymptomatic pneumothorax. Symptomatic pneumothorax is less common occurring in about 1 in 1000 live births. Prior to surfactant therapy mild RDS had an incidence of pneumothorax of about 5% increasing to 10–20% with continuous positive airway pressure and to 20–40% with positive pressure ventilation. However, since the introduction of surfactant therapy the incidence of pneumothorax has fallen to about 5% and many pediatric residents have no or little experience of chest drain insertion. Up to 10% of babies with transient tachypnea of the newborn and 40% of those with meconium aspiration syndrome develop pneumothoraces.[500]

Clinical presentation

Most babies with spontaneously occurring pneumothoraces who have no underlying lung pathology have minimal signs of respiratory distress and the pneumothorax is seen as an incidental finding on a chest radiograph taken for another reason. However, most significant pneumothoraces occur in babies with underlying pulmonary disease and the diagnosis should be suspected in any such baby whose condition suddenly deteriorates. If the baby is breathing spontaneously, tachypnea, grunting and cyanosis are often the presenting signs. In a unilateral pneumothorax there may be shift of the mediastinum (apex beat) away from the side of the pneumothorax and breath sounds may be reduced on the affected side. The affected hemithorax or the abdomen may appear distended because of increased tension within the pleural space. There may be hyper-resonance to percussion on the affected side and hypotension may occur because of venous compression and reduced cardiac output. With a small pneumothorax there may be an increase in cardiac output, heart rate and blood pressure so that continuous monitoring of blood pressure can help to make the diagnosis.[536]

In about 10% of babies pneumothoraces will be bilateral and this causes a major hemodynamic upset which for the very preterm baby may prove fatal.[537] In survivors there is an increased likelihood of intraventricular hemorrhage.[497]

Diagnosis

The chest radiograph confirms the diagnosis. Anteroposterior (AP) (Fig. 10.28) and lateral views should be taken.[538] The lateral will show air in the anterior mediastinum and the thymus may be lifted up, which may also be evident on the AP film (Fig. 10.29). If the pneumothorax is extensive there will be collapse of the lung and mediastinal shift away from the affected side (Fig. 10.28). Sometimes a pneumothorax may only be seen medially and may be mistaken for a pneumomediastinum. Ultrasound scanning may be helpful in distinguishing these.[539] For the baby who deteriorates suddenly, there may not be time to wait for a chest radiograph, and two alternative methods of confirming the diagnosis of pneumothorax have been used. For the baby in extremis diagnostic pleural aspiration using a needle, syringe and three-way tap can be performed without delay. The second or third intercostal space in the mid-clavicular line should be used for this procedure which is both diagnostic and therapeutic. Transillumination of the chest with a fiberoptic bright light can be used to rapidly diagnose large pneumothoraces in less severely ill babies. This technique is less useful for diagnosing small pneumothoraces or those occurring in term babies.

Treatment

No treatment is necessary if the infant is asymptomatic. For term babies with mild symptoms, breathing high oxygen concentrations to wash out nitrogen may accelerate resorption of gas loculated within the pneumothorax. The only satisfactory treatment of a tension pneumothorax is drainage, usually by insertion of a pleural catheter connected to a non-return valve such as an underwater seal drain. The catheter should be large bore and placed in the anterior mediastinal space with care to avoid perforation of the lung. Local anesthetic should be used before making a small skin incision and careful dissection of the intercostal muscle. Use of an artery forceps will prevent overpenetration of the trocar into the chest. Continuous suction of 10–20 cmH_2O may occasionally be needed to prevent reaccumulation of the pneumothorax. Simple needle aspiration may be successful and avoid the need for insertion of a chest drain especially when the pneumothorax is not under great tension.

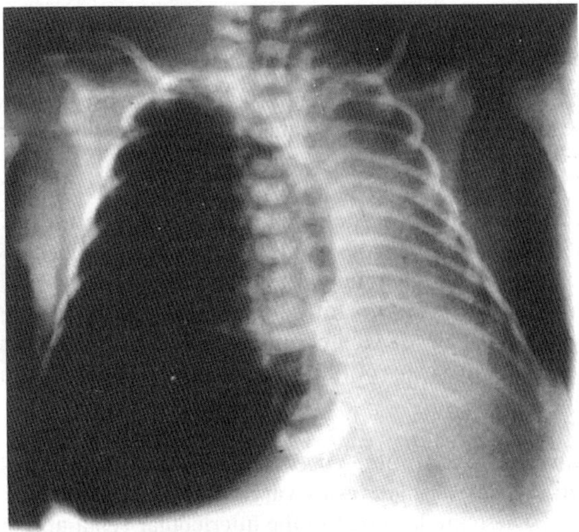

Fig. 10.28 Radiograph of a right tension pneumothorax with depression of the diaphragm and shift of the mediastinum to the left. There is also mediastinal herniation.

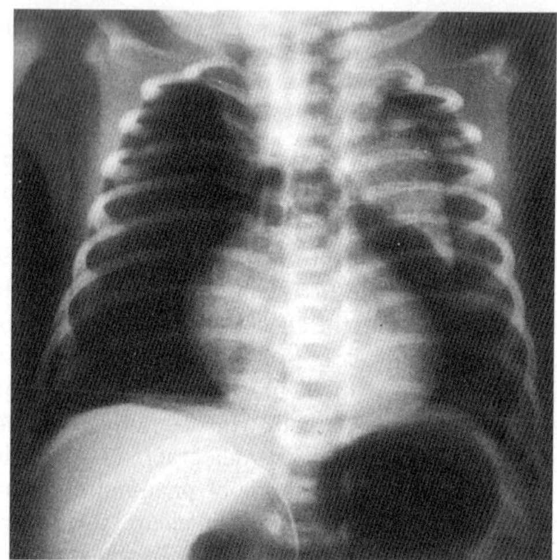

Fig. 10.29 Radiograph showing bilateral pneumothoraces and a large pneumomediastinum with elevation of the lobes of the thymus clear of the cardiac shadow (the sail sign). The endotracheal tube is shown with its tip in the right mainstem bronchus.

Careful fluid balance should be observed as increased vasopressin secretion, leading to fluid retention, may occur after a pneumothorax although this is not common.[540] Fibrin glue pleurodesis has been used to treat persistent pneumothorax with bronchopleural fistula.[541]

Prevention

The incidence of pneumothorax may be reduced by muscle relaxation for babies with severe RDS who need mechanical ventilation,[542] rapid rate conventional ventilators with reduced inspiratory time[543] and natural surfactant replacement used either prophylactically at birth in babies of < 30 weeks' gestation or to treat babies with severe RDS.[476]

Prognosis

Pneumothorax is associated with increased morbidity and mortality depending upon the nature of the underlying lung disease and the gestational age of the baby. Both mortality rate and intraventricular hemorrhage rate are approximately doubled following pneumothorax.

Pulmonary interstitial emphysema (PIE)

This is the presence of air in the interstitium or perivascular tissues of the lung and it is probably a prerequisite of all other forms of air leak.

Incidence

The true incidence is uncertain but interstitial emphysema has been described in about 10% of neonatal autopsies. The incidence in control groups of the randomized surfactant trials varies from 25 to 50%.[500] With the introduction of surfactant therapy, widespread use of CPAP and more gentle forms of assisted ventilation the incidence of PIE is likely to be much lower than this.

Pathogenesis

After alveolar rupture, air escapes into the pulmonary interstitium to form regular air-filled cysts varying from 0.1 to 1.0 cm in diameter. These are localized to the interlobular septa and extend radially from the hila of each lung to form a diffuse or a localized pattern. Lung function is impaired by compression of normal lung tissue, decreased compliance and obstruction of pulmonary blood flow. Interstitial emphysema is associated with raised leukocyte elastase levels in tracheal aspirates suggesting that intrauterine infection or prior lung injury may predispose.[544,545]

Clinical presentation

When interstitial emphysema is localized there may be no symptoms or the baby may gradually deteriorate. If the condition becomes diffuse there is progressive hypoxemia and ventilation–perfusion imbalance necessitating an increase in ventilator settings. There is usually decreased chest wall movement with hyperinflation of the chest and muffling of the heart sounds.

Diagnosis

The chest radiograph may show areas of translucency and collapse scattered throughout the lung fields rather like a snowstorm (Fig. 10.30). If the changes are localized to one lung there may be marked overinflation and shift of the mediastinum as in a tension pneumothorax. Pseudocysts may form within the pulmonary parenchyma beneath the visceral pleura or along fissure lines.

Treatment

For diffuse interstitial emphysema, fast rate mechanical ventilation using low pressures has been advocated and periods of fast rate hand bagging up to 140 breaths/min may also be of benefit. A more conservative approach has been suggested with postural drainage and chest physiotherapy especially in cases of unilateral interstitial emphysema under tension. More aggressive treatment has also been used to manage the severe unilateral form of interstitial emphysema and includes selective intubation of the normal lung to allow the emphysematous lung to collapse,[546] selective bronchial obstruction of the affected side, artificial creation of a pneumothorax by probing[547] or some form of surgical procedure. HFOV has been advocated as a method of treating PIE[548] but there have been no randomized trials.

Prognosis

Severe diffuse interstitial emphysema occurring soon after birth has a very high mortality rate. For babies weighing less than 1000 g, mortality at 67% is more than twice that of babies without interstitial emphysema.[549] Complications such as pneumothorax

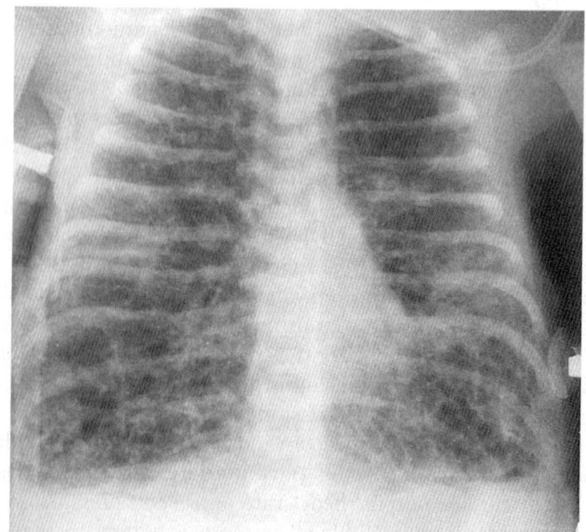

Fig. 10.30 Radiograph showing bilateral diffuse pulmonary interstitial emphysema with marked overinflation of the chest, lowered diaphragm and narrowed heart shadow.

and intraventricular hemorrhage are common and affected babies need prolonged ventilator support. Surviving infants have an increased risk of developing bronchopulmonary dysplasia.

Pneumomediastinum

Incidence

Pneumomediastinum probably occurs prior to all cases of pneumothorax but it often goes unrecognized.

Clinical presentation

Pneumomediastinum may occur with other air leaks or in isolation, when it is asymptomatic in over 90% of cases, being noticed incidentally on a routine chest radiograph. If there are symptoms the baby may have tachypnea, cyanosis and an overinflated chest which is hyper-resonant to percussion. Occasionally a large pneumomediastinum causes severe symptoms by compressing the heart and lungs.

Diagnosis

Confirmed by chest radiograph. The lateral view is most helpful to demonstrate air lying anteriorly. The thymus may be lifted off the mediastinum in the anteroposterior view giving rise to the 'sail sign' or 'spinnaker sign' (Fig. 10.29).

Treatment

In pneumomediastinum the air is loculated so that drainage is impracticable. The rate of absorption can be accelerated by breathing high oxygen concentrations provided that the infant is full term and there are no concerns about the effects of hyperoxia.

Pneumopericardium

This occurs in about 1.6% of babies with RDS.[537]

Clinical presentation

Occasionally asymptomatic but more usually presents with pallor, shock and hypotension due to cardiac tamponade. In most cases it is associated with other forms of air leak.

Diagnosis

Chest radiograph shows a complete ring of air around the heart. The transverse diameter of the heart is reduced if tamponade is present and substernal transillumination may be used to make a rapid diagnosis in the baby who suddenly deteriorates during mechanical ventilation.

Treatment

The only effective treatment for pneumopericardium with tamponade is immediate drainage of air from the pericardial sac using a needle and syringe directed anteriorly and superiorly from below the xiphisternum. Recurrence of tamponade is common and permanent drainage is often needed.

Prognosis

The mortality is high despite early drainage with more than half of affected babies dying.

Pneumoperitoneum

Air in the peritoneal cavity may be the result of a pulmonary air leak or a ruptured abdominal viscus.

Incidence

The incidence of pneumoperitoneum as a complication of mechanical ventilation is about 2%.[537]

Clinical presentation

This may be asymptomatic or present as abdominal distention. There are usually other signs of air leak (Fig. 10.31).

Treatment

Aspiration is only necessary if abdominal distention is severe enough to compromise ventilation.

Subcutaneous emphysema

This is rare in the neonate and when it does occur it is usually associated with pneumomediastinum. Air from the superior mediastinum passes along the perivascular fascia to the subclavicular area before spreading subcutaneously. Apart from swelling and a typically crackling feel to the affected skin there are few other signs and the air usually absorbs in a few days.

Air embolism (pneumatosis arterialis)

This is an uncommon and almost universally fatal condition which may present as air being withdrawn from an umbilical arterial catheter in an infant who has collapsed.[550] Air embolism results from rupture of pulmonary veins associated with raised intra-alveolar pressure during mechanical ventilation of very preterm babies. Affected babies have other forms of air leak and deteriorate acutely with pallor, bradycardia and hypotension. Chest and abdominal radiographs show gas shadows in the heart chambers and major arteries. Massive air embolism is usually fatal but one surviving baby has been reported where the embolism was minor.[551] There is no effective treatment and prevention involves avoidance of unnecessary barotraumas.[500] The introduction of surfactant therapy and gentler forms of assisted ventilation have greatly reduced the risk of this serious condition.

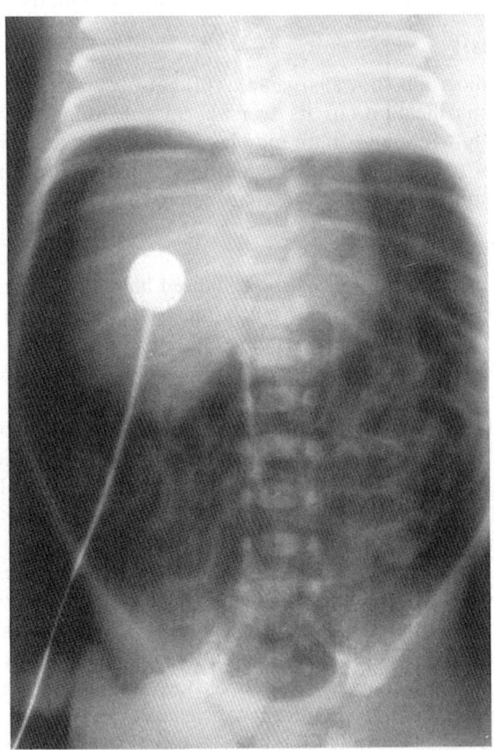

Fig. 10.31 Radiograph showing a large pneumoperitoneum with the liver clearly outlined by the air in the peritoneal cavity. The lungs appear collapsed and airless.

PULMONARY HEMORRHAGE

Sometimes called massive pulmonary hemorrhage, this poorly understood condition has a sudden onset and a high mortality.

Incidence

Isolated pulmonary hemorrhage is a rare condition occurring in approximately 1/1000 live births. Between 2 and 5% of babies with RDS develop pulmonary hemorrhage.[552]

Etiology and pathogenesis

Pulmonary hemorrhage can occur in SGA babies with no underlying lung disease but more usually there has been a history of severe perinatal asphyxia, hypothermia, rhesus isoimmunization, pneumonia, hypoglycemia, coagulation disorder or fluid overload, particularly when a persistent ductus arteriosus is present.[553] It is likely that pulmonary hemorrhage is a form of hemorrhagic pulmonary edema which occurs secondary to left ventricular failure and damage to pulmonary capillaries. The edema fluid usually has an hematocrit of less than 10% and is probably a filtrate from pulmonary capillaries. Pulmonary hemorrhage may sometimes be secondary to aspiration, hypoproteinemia and lung tissue damage from pneumonia, RDS, oxygen toxicity or mechanical ventilation. There is an association with surfactant treatment especially in the very immature infant treated with synthetic surfactant.[552,554]

Clinical presentation

The onset is frequently between the second and fourth day after birth when an infant with respiratory distress shows sudden deterioration with shock, cyanosis, bradycardia and apnea. Pink or red frothy fluid is aspirated from the mouth and lungs and the baby needs urgent resuscitation to prevent death. In ventilated babies, bloodstained fluid appears in the endotracheal tube during suctioning. Auscultation of the chest reveals widespread crepitations.

Diagnosis

Chest radiograph shows large areas of consolidation with areas of diffuse opacification. In its worst form the lungs may appear completely white and there may be cardiomegaly. Sometimes the diagnosis is only confirmed at autopsy when widespread intra-alveolar and interstitial hemorrhage is found.[555]

Treatment

Immediate resuscitation of the collapsed baby is important with endotracheal intubation for mechanical ventilation and volume expansion with blood or plasma. High PEEP may help to reduce bleeding by tamponade, and a diuretic such as furosemide (frusemide) may reduce pulmonary edema. If the ductus arteriosus is widely patent indometacin or ibuprofen should be administered intravenously. Correction of acidosis and underlying coagulation disorder is beneficial and antibiotics should be given if infection is suspected. Repeated doses of surfactant may be beneficial.[556]

Prognosis

Until recently massive pulmonary hemorrhage was invariably fatal but prompt use of mechanical ventilation and transfusions of fresh whole blood have improved the outlook.[518] A recent study has shown that severe pulmonary hemorrhage was associated with a fourfold increased risk of chronic lung disease, sevenfold risk of death and threefold risk of major intraventricular hemorrhage.[557] However, rather surprisingly there was no increase in long term morbidity at 2 year follow-up.

Prevention

Prevention is most important because of the poor outlook once major pulmonary hemorrhage has occurred. SGA babies should not be allowed to develop asphyxia, hypothermia, hypoglycemia or acidosis. Coagulation defects in these babies should be corrected early. In babies with RDS especially after surfactant treatment care should be taken to ensure that the ductus arteriosus is closed. There should be a low threshold for treatment with indometacin or ibuprofen.

DEVELOPMENTAL ANOMALIES OF THE LUNG

Pulmonary hypoplasia

In this condition, which is frequently bilateral, the lungs are smaller than normal. Unilateral hypoplasia may be primary but is more often associated with other congenital malformations such as diaphragmatic hernia.

Incidence

Pulmonary hypoplasia is present in 15–20% of early neonatal deaths and is now the commonest single abnormality at autopsy.[558] Milder cases survive and the condition is probably underdiagnosed.

Etiology and pathogenesis

Pulmonary hypoplasia occurs as a primary lesion in about 10% of cases but is most often associated with other malformations that restrict lung growth (Table 10.56). Pulmonary hypoplasia, as a result of oligohydramnios, is caused by the combined effects of reduced lung volume and impaired fetal breathing.

Clinical presentation

The diagnosis may be suspected prenatally if there has been prolonged rupture of the membranes especially if this occurs before 20 weeks or an ultrasound scan has demonstrated congenital diaphragmatic hernia or a chondrodystrophy. Babies with pulmonary hypoplasia may present at birth with signs of asphyxia and difficulties in resuscitation. Some of these babies have Potter's syndrome and do not survive; pneumothoraces readily develop during resuscitation. With less severe degrees of hypoplasia the presentation is less acute with mild but prolonged respiratory distress and oxygen dependency. Congenital diaphragmatic hernia must be excluded by chest radiograph (Fig. 10.32). Such a hernia is usually left sided, in 80% of cases occurring through the foramen of Bochdalek and there is displacement of the mediastinum to the right by stomach and bowel. About 25% of cases have associated congenital heart lesions which increase mortality.

Diagnosis

In life it is difficult to confirm the diagnosis unless an associated abnormality such as Potter's syndrome, diaphragmatic hernia, Jeune's syndrome or prolonged oligohydramnios is present. Sometimes chest radiograph shows small lungs with a bell-shaped

Table 10.56 Pathogenesis of pulmonary hypoplasia

1. Oligohydramnios: renal agenesis, urinary tract obstruction, prolonged rupture of the membranes
2. Lung compression: diaphragmatic hernia, lung cysts, pleural effusions, erythroblastosis, chondrodystrophies
3. Absent fetal breathing movements: anencephaly, neuromuscular disorders

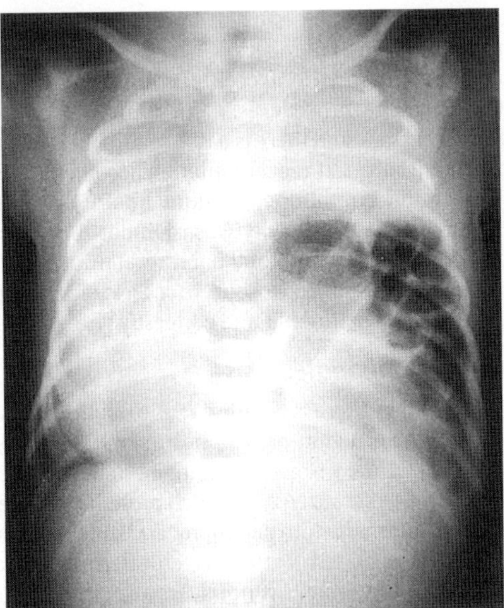

Fig. 10.32 Radiograph of a large left-sided diaphragmatic hernia with mediastinal shift to the right. Air in the stomach and intestine is due to resuscitation with bag and mask.

thorax. At autopsy lung:body weight ratio may be helpful in making the diagnosis provided that there is no postnatal complication such as pneumonia or pulmonary hemorrhage. A lung:body weight ratio of < 0.012 for babies over 28 weeks' gestation and < 0.015 for lower gestations is used to define pulmonary hypoplasia.[559] Strict confirmation of the diagnosis requires more sophisticated autopsy analysis such as radial alveolar counts or DNA estimation.

Management

The outlook depends upon the severity of the respiratory signs and the associated congenital anomalies. Severe pulmonary hypoplasia occurring with oligohydramnios is usually fatal but on occasions mechanical ventilation with high pressures has been successful in 'opening up' the lungs.[560] Although surfactant deficiency is present in some cases surfactant replacement therapy is usually not successful.[561] Babies with diaphragmatic hernia need surgical correction, but even with this, severe unilateral pulmonary hypoplasia can be associated with marked pulmonary hypertension which does not respond to mechanical ventilation or vasodilators such as inhaled nitric oxide. ECMO is less effective in treating congenital diaphragmatic hernia than other causes of respiratory failure in term infants.[562] For babies who survive the neonatal period, lung growth occurs and their prognosis improves.

Congenital lobar emphysema

This is an uncommon condition where overinflation of one or more lobes occurs secondary to bronchial obstruction or deficiency of bronchial cartilage. The left upper lobe and the right middle lobe are most commonly affected and the babies present with signs of respiratory distress and occasionally wheezing. Boys are affected twice as commonly as girls.[563] The chest radiograph may initially show lobar opacification due to fluid trapped beyond the obstruction but later the affected lobe becomes overdistended and there may be shift of the mediastinum (Fig. 10.33).

Bronchoscopy is often needed to make the diagnosis and to remove any cause of bronchial obstruction. If symptoms are slight, conservative management is preferred and continuous positive airway pressure may be beneficial. For babies with persistent respiratory failure, surgical excision of the affected lobe is necessary. In about 30% of affected babies there is an associated congenital heart defect.

(a)

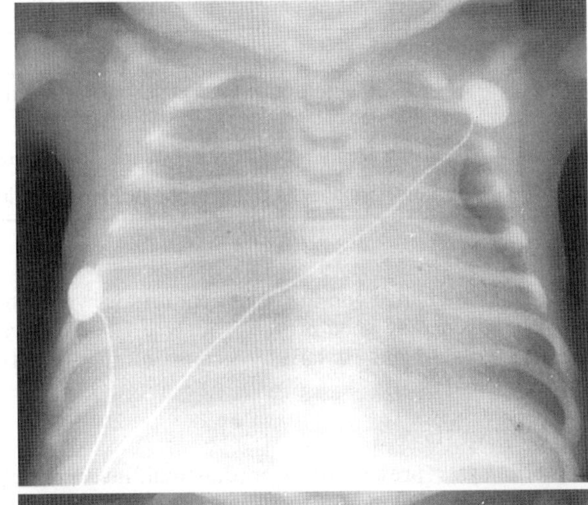

(b)

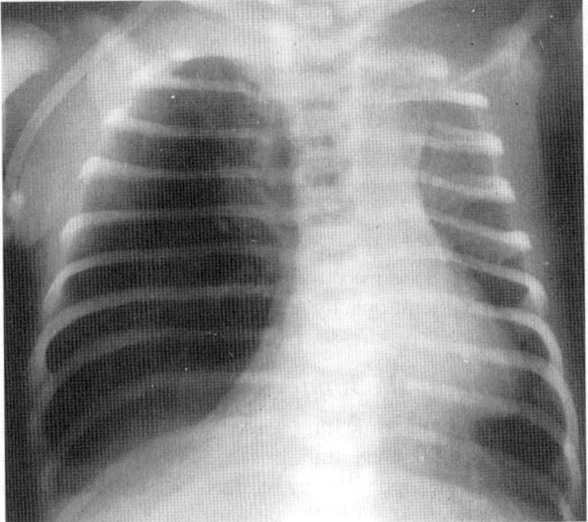

Fig. 10.33 (a) Congenital lobar emphysema showing retained lung fluid on the right as a result of bronchial obstruction, and displacement of the heart shadow to the left. (b) After 24 h with clearance of the lung fluid the right lung shows gross overinflation and the mediastinal displacement is more clearly demonstrated.

Cystic adenomatoid malformation

This is a rare form of congenital cystic disease of the lung which has three pathological types[564] (Table 10.57). Antenatal diagnosis by ultrasound is possible and in some cases the lesion seems to regress before birth. However, when ultrasound findings return to normal and neonatal chest radiograph is normal many congenital pulmonary lesions are still demonstrable on CT scanning so careful follow-up is still indicated.[565] Half of the affected babies are preterm and about one-quarter are stillborn with boys affected twice as commonly as girls. Polyhydramnios and hydrops occur in about one-third of cases. Associated anomalies include hydranencephaly and prune-belly syndrome. The middle or upper lobes are usually affected and the condition is unilateral. Affected babies present with respiratory distress soon after birth, and there may be mediastinal shift. Chest radiograph shows the cystic overdistention of the affected lung and the differential diagnosis includes lobar emphysema and diaphragmatic hernia. There may be an increased

Table 10.57 Types of cystic adenomatoid malformation (CAM)

Type	Frequency (%)	Features
I	70	Multiple large cysts which mimic type III lobar emphysema
II	20	Medium sized cysts (< 12 mm in diameter)
III	10	Small cysts evenly distributed in a bulky lung

risk of malignant change and therefore treatment is by lobectomy which gives a generally good prognosis in type I but survival is reduced in types II and III largely because of the severity of associated anomalies.

Other lung cysts

Neurenteric cysts present as a mediastinal mass on chest radiograph in association with vertebral anomalies. Gastrogenic cysts, containing gastric mucosa, may ulcerate and cause hemoptysis. Duplication cysts of the duodenum may extend through the diaphragm and, if associated with a vertebral anomaly, can cause meningitis.

Bronchogenic cysts

These may present as episodes of wheezing or stridor. They are found near the carina but may be radiolucent on chest radiograph. If bronchial obstruction occurs there may be retained lung fluid giving rise to confluent opacity of one lung or lobe on radiography. Antenatal diagnosis by ultrasound scan is possible.

Sequestration of the lung

This is a mass of embryonic lung tissue that does not communicate with the bronchial tree, and has a systemic rather than a pulmonary arterial supply. It may be intra- or extralobar and in the latter communication with the foregut, and other congenital anomalies including congenital heart disease are common. Males are more commonly affected and in about three-quarters of cases the sequestration is on the left side. Ultrasound can be used to make the diagnosis prenatally and hydrops fetalis may occasionally occur. Extralobar lesions are more likely to be symptomatic but abnormality on chest radiograph is the most usual presentation. A triangular density at the left lung base extending to the mediastinum gives rise to the 'scimitar sign'. Bronchoscopy, radionuclide scanning or aortography may be needed to confirm the diagnosis. In 65% of cases there are associated anomalies.[566] Surgery for intralobar sequestrations prevents repeated respiratory infections and may also be needed for extralobar lesions that are symptomatic.

Chylothorax

This is a form of pleural effusion in which chyle or lymphatic fluid appears in the pleural cavity. The condition is typically unilateral with 60% occurring on the right side and may be congenital or acquired, both being more common in males. In congenital or spontaneous chylothorax there is usually an anomaly of lymphatic drainage and chylous ascites and lymphedema may be associated. Acquired chylothorax may follow birth trauma or thoracotomy. About half of affected babies present with respiratory distress soon after birth and a further one-quarter have symptoms by the end of the first week. Breath sounds are reduced on the affected side and there is mediastinal shift away from this side. Chest radiography shows diffuse opacity with depressed diaphragm and mediastinal shift. A pleural tap will show clear yellow fluid soon after birth and only after feeding does the effusion appear chylous. The fluid is sterile and contains large numbers of lymphocytes and fat globules. Treatment is initially by thoracocentesis and most babies recover after a few drainage procedures. Occasionally several drainage attempts are necessary and there is a risk of protein and lymphocyte depletion in these babies. If reaccumulation becomes a problem, use of a milk formula containing medium chain triglycerides will reduce the production of chyle. Occasionally it is necessary to discontinue oral feeds and use total parenteral nutrition.

Pleural effusion can also occur in cases of hydrops fetalis, Turner's syndrome, pneumonia and congestive heart failure.

Pulmonary lymphangiectasis

In this rare condition there is bilateral cystic dilation of pulmonary lymphatics with obstruction of lymph drainage. Three types have been described: a primary isolated developmental defect accounting for 70% of cases; a generalized type which presents with generalized edema, malabsorption, hemihypertrophy and other anomalies; and thirdly a type associated with congenital heart disease and obstruction of pulmonary venous return (total anomalous pulmonary venous drainage, closure of atrial septum in hypoplastic left heart syndrome or pulmonary vein atresia).

There may be polyhydramnios and antenatal diagnosis by ultrasound scan is possible. Babies with primary lymphangiectasis are often born at term and have progressive respiratory distress which is usually fatal. Clinical and radiological features mimic RDS so that there is underdiagnosis of this condition. Chest radiograph may show reticulogranular mottling with hyperaeration, and dilated lymphatics may sometimes be seen. Confirmation of the diagnosis is by lung biopsy or at autopsy.

Choanal atresia

This obstruction to the nasal airway may be unilateral or bilateral, membranous or bony. The incidence is about 0.3 per 1000 births with girls affected twice as commonly as boys. About two-thirds of cases are unilateral and in about half there are associated anomalies such as coloboma, heart defects, micrognathia and tracheoesophageal fistula. If the obstruction is bilateral, babies often present with great distress at birth, although when crying they may remain pink. Babies with unilateral choanal atresia may be asymptomatic or present later with a purulent nasal discharge. The diagnosis may be confirmed by attempting to pass a fine feeding tube or suction catheter, although use of a radiopaque dye and radiograph is sometimes necessary. The infant with bilateral choanal atresia needs an oral airway or oral endotracheal intubation followed by a surgical procedure. A transnasal or transpalatal approach may be used to open the posterior choanae and patency is maintained by inserting silastic tubes for up to 2 months. Operative correction of unilateral choanal atresia may be postponed until the child is several years old.

Laryngomalacia

This is a condition where the larynx appears soft and flexible, associated with an elongated, floppy epiglottis and loose aryepiglottic folds which tend to be drawn over the glottis during inspiration. Also known as congenital laryngeal stridor, it needs to be distinguished from other causes of stridor such as vocal cord paralysis, vascular rings, laryngeal webs and cysts, and papillomata. The onset of stridor is usually on the second day of life but delay of up to 4 months is possible. Usually the stridor persists for less than 1 year. The diagnosis is confirmed by direct laryngoscopy which will help to exclude other causes of stridor. No specific treatment is required apart from reassurance of the parents although occasionally long term feeding problems and speech difficulties occur.

CHRONIC LUNG DISEASE

The prevalence of chronic pulmonary disorders has increased because of more intensive respiratory support and improved survival of small preterm babies. The term bronchopulmonary dysplasia (BPD) was coined over 30 years ago to describe damage to the lung from high volume mechanical ventilation.[501] It has largely been replaced by the term chronic lung disease (CLD) to describe a condition where a preterm infant requires oxygen supplementation beyond 28 days' or beyond 36 weeks' corrected age. The latter definition is preferable as many very immature infants may need oxygen at 28 days without having significant lung disease.[567] Wilson–Mikity syndrome was a term used to describe very preterm infants who developed CLD without having been treated with mechanical ventilation.[568] It is no longer recognized as an entity and has become subsumed within the heading of CLD. Rather than CLD being caused by 'ventilator-induced injury' it is now believed that chronic inflammation is important in its pathogenesis – 'from barotrauma to biotrauma'.[569] Chronic lung disease is common in small preterm babies who, although ventilator dependent for long periods, have not needed high pressures or oxygen concentrations[504] and may occur in infants who did not need assisted ventilation.[570]

Incidence

The incidence of CLD varies according to the definition with rates between 5 and 40% of VLBW infants being reported. To simplify the definition of CLD, it has recently been suggested that oxygen dependency and other signs of respiratory distress at a postconceptional age of 36 weeks be used.[567] With this definition the incidence of BPD in VLBW infants is about 10–20%.

Etiology and pathogenesis

Factors associated with the development of CLD are listed in Table 10.58. RDS is not an absolute prerequisite for CLD as babies treated with mechanical ventilation for apnea or meconium aspiration syndrome and babies without any initial respiratory disorder may subsequently develop CLD. Oxygen concentrations in excess of 60% are toxic to the lungs of newborn mice causing proliferative changes in the alveoli rather than the smaller airways. Perhaps the combination of 'oxygen plus pressure plus time' is important.[571] The role of pulmonary infection, frequently starting in utero has recently been shown to be a very important etiological factor.[503] Other factors important in the pathogenesis of CLD include pulmonary interstitial emphysema, persistent ductus arteriosus and fluid overload, and deficiency of vitamins A and E.[572]

Pathology

CLD or BPD is a disease of scarring and repair which affects lung growth. Histological abnormalities may be found in babies dying before the development of the clinical disease.[573] Babies dying of severe BPD have hyperinflated lungs with extensive destruction of alveoli causing widespread emphysema and fibrosis. There is also bronchial necrosis, peribronchial fibrosis and squamous metaplasia giving an obliterative bronchiolitis. Active epithelial regeneration is not uniform and there may be marked thickening of the intima of pulmonary arterioles causing progressive pulmonary hypertension.

Table 10.58 Factors associated with CLD

Chorioamnionitis
Respiratory distress syndrome
Congenital pneumonia
Mechanical ventilation
Oxygen therapy
Acquired pulmonary infection
Pulmonary interstitial emphysema
Persistent ductus arteriosus
Fluid overload
Vitamin A or E deficiency

Clinical presentation

The usual history is of a preterm baby treated with mechanical ventilation and surfactant for RDS whose condition improves and then deteriorates between 7 and 10 days with increasing oxygen requirements. Mild cases need increased inspired oxygen concentrations for a few weeks but in severe cases there may be progressive respiratory failure with ventilator dependence and later tachypnea, indrawing, wheezing and recurrent apnea with cyanotic spells. Cor pulmonale may develop secondary to pulmonary hypertension, and these babies show hepatomegaly, increased weight gain and edema which is often found in the face and neck region.[518]

Chest radiographs initially show generalized hazinesss which later can progress to hyperinflation, coarse streaking and cystic changes most marked at the lung bases (Fig. 10.34).

Management

One aspect of prevention is to limit ventilation and oxygen therapy to the shortest possible time. Management of infection, PDA and fluid balance are also important in trying to prevent CLD. Once established, CLD needs to be treated with adequate oxygen to maintain the arterial oxygen tension above 7 kPa as below this level there is an increase in pulmonary vascular resistance and a risk of cor pulmonale. Transcutaneous oxygen monitoring may underestimate PaO_2 beyond the age of 10 weeks so that pulse oximetry may be preferable.

Weaning from the ventilator may be helped by allowing $PaCO_2$ levels to rise to 7–9 kPa so that peak inspiratory pressures can be lowered. Reduced fluid intake, diuretic therapy and closure of the ductus arteriosus may all assist in weaning. Theophylline or caffeine has also been shown to improve lung function and shorten the duration of ventilation. Dexamethasone improves CLD in the short term allowing rapid weaning from the ventilator[574–576] but there are concerns about both short term complications (hyperglycemia, hypertension and gastrointestinal bleeding and perforation) and long term adverse effects on the central nervous system.[577] These concerns mean that their use should be limited to babies who are

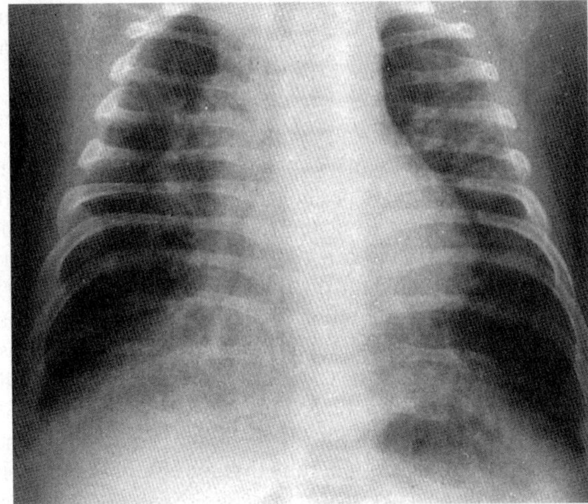

Fig. 10.34 Radiograph of severe CLD (formerly called BPD) with basilar emphysema, coarse stranding and cystic changes.

ventilator dependent and whose condition is deteriorating. The role of steroids in the prevention of CLD should be limited to study within a randomized trial where long term outcome is the primary endpoint (e.g. the DART study). Inhaled steroids might have a role to play as they appear to be as effective as dexamethasone but without the major short term adverse effects.[578] Adequate nutrition is important and supplemental calories may be given in the form of long chain glucose polymers so that fluid restriction is possible without reducing energy intake. Vitamin supplementation especially with vitamin A[579] may have a role to play. For a discussion on the risk–benefit of drugs for CLD see Sweet & Halliday.[580] Blood transfusions should be given to maintain adequate hematocrit. Chest infections should be promptly treated with antibiotics. In later infancy RSV infections may cause acute deterioration and immunization with a protective monoclonal antibody has been advocated in these babies. Experimental treatments include inhaled nitric oxide and surfactant replacement.[581]

Prognosis

Many babies with CLD require prolonged oxygen therapy which may conveniently be given via a nasal catheter. For babies needing low flow rates home oxygen therapy significantly shortens the period in hospital. Mortality in babies with severe CLD is about 25–30%. Surviving babies have frequent lower respiratory tract infections and often require hospital admission with persistent tachypnea, intermittent wheezing and subcostal retractions. Growth and development depend upon the severity of the lung disease and adverse perinatal events. Growth retardation is present in about one-third of survivors and major developmental defects in about 25%.

Chronic pulmonary infection

This may account for a small proportion of cases of CLD in the newborn. Infection with CMV may be congenital or acquired although pneumonitis is uncommon in congenitally infected babies.[582] Interstitial pneumonitis can also occur with congenital toxoplasmosis, rubella, varicella and herpes simplex virus. Acquired infections with enteroviruses, adenovirus, RSV and rhinovirus can cause acute pneumonitis.

Chlamydia may cause a late pneumonitis with tachypnea, cough and a chest radiograph showing disproportionately severe infiltrates and hyperinflation. Erythromycin treatment for 14 days is effective. Pneumocystis pneumonia has also been reported in preterm infants and should be treated with co-trimoxazole. One prospective study found chlamydia in 25%, ureaplasma in 21%, CMV in 20% and pneumocystis in 18% of preterm babies with pneumonitis.[583] How relevant this study of infants from the southern states of the USA is to a UK population of babies is unknown.

Subglottic stenosis

Subglottic stenosis may be congenital or acquired. Acquired subglottic stenosis is due to prolonged endotracheal intubation and occurs in a severe form in about 1% of ventilated babies. Use of endotracheal tubes that are too big, oral rather than nasal intubation and repeated intubations may increase the risk of subglottic stenosis. Presentation is with stridor and respiratory distress after extubation although there may be a delayed onset of symptoms for several months with difficulty apparently precipitated by an upper respiratory tract infection.

In mild cases treatment with high humidity and supplemental oxygen is sufficient, but use of dexamethasone or inhaled epinephrine (adrenaline) has been advocated in more severe cases prior to a trial of extubation. Sometimes tracheostomy is needed but cryosurgery[584] or minor surgery to split the cricoid cartilage anteriorly[585] have been successful as an alternative to tracheostomy which often proves difficult to close. Dilation of the narrowed segment at intervals by an experienced ENT surgeon may be necessary.

CONTROL OF BREATHING

Postnatal control of breathing is complex and involves chemical and non-chemical stimuli and respiratory reflexes. The inspiratory and expiratory centers in the brainstem are influenced by sensors (central and peripheral chemoreceptors) monitoring arterial blood and they maintain normal oxygen tensions and pH despite wide variations in oxygen demand and carbon dioxide production.

Chemical stimuli

Hypoxemia and hypercapnia are the most important chemical stimuli to respiration. For the first week after birth there are three phases of the respiratory response to hypoxemia:

1. stimulation of peripheral chemoreceptors causing transient hyperventilation in a warm environment;
2. central depression;
3. central stimulation by severe hypoxemia causing gasps.

Hypoxemia depresses ventilation and blunts the ventilatory response to hypercapnia. In the preterm baby these responses may persist for up to 6 weeks after birth. Breathing oxygen reduces ventilation by an effect on carotid body chemoreceptors but after several minutes hyperventilation occurs secondary to carbon dioxide retention.

The response to hypercapnia, mediated by hydrogen ion receptors in the medulla, increases with gestational and also with postnatal age.

Sleep state

In rapid eye movement (REM) sleep respiration is intrinsically driven with little chemical control. There is inhibition of intercostal muscles which results in distortion of the rib cage and this can lead to diaphragmatic fatigue with apnea. In non-rapid eye movement (NREM) sleep control of respiration is chemical rather than intrinsic and apnea is less common.

Respiratory reflexes

The Head and Hering–Breuer reflexes, arising from lung stretch receptors and mediated through the vagus nerve, are important in the modulation of respiratory center output in the newborn. Head's paradoxical reflex, which is present for the first few days after birth, causes an extra inspiratory effort when the upper airways are distended. Its importance is in aeration of lungs soon after birth. In the Hering–Breuer reflex sustained lung inflation inhibits respiration causing apnea in inspiration. This inflation reflex is stronger in preterm infants than term babies. The Hering–Breuer deflation reflex consists of an increase in respiratory rate in response to reduced lung volume and may also be important in the preterm baby. There are irritant receptors in the hypopharynx and larynx which, if stimulated by vigorous suctioning or cows' milk, cause apnea.

Apneic attacks

Apnea in the newborn is cessation of breathing for more than 20 s and this is significant if it is associated with bradycardia and/or cyanosis. Periodic breathing is a series of respiratory pauses of about 10 s duration alternating with periods of hyperventilation of up to 15 s and occurring at least three times per min. It is not associated with cyanosis and bradycardia and may be a physiological response in the preterm baby.[586]

Incidence

Apneic attacks occur in most infants of less than 30 weeks' gestation and in about half of babies of 30–32 weeks decreasing to less than 10% of babies at 34 weeks' gestation. Periodic breathing is also common, occurring in nearly all LBW babies and about one-third of term babies.

Etiology and pathogenesis

There are many clinical conditions that are associated with apnea (Table 10.59). Only after exclusion of the disorders listed from one to six can a confident diagnosis of apnea of prematurity be made. Immaturity of the brainstem respiratory neurones is probably a major underlying factor and apnea may also occur if the medullary centers are immature or depressed by hypoxia. There is some debate about the relationship between gastroesophageal reflux (GER) and apnea in infants. Episodes of apnea are seldom associated with GER and when they are associated obstructive apnea or to a lesser extent mixed apnea is followed by reflux.[587]

Pathophysiology

During a significant apneic attack the preterm baby has bradycardia, peripheral vasoconstriction and a variable alteration of blood pressure which may increase or decrease slightly. The interval between the onset of apnea and bradycardia varies between 2 and 30 s. There are three types of apnea based upon polygraphic recordings (Table 10.60). In preterm babies central apnea and mixed apnea occur with about equal frequencies.[586] The use of apnea monitors which detect chest wall movement and bradycardia will underestimate the incidence of apnea and suggest that isolated bradycardia is occurring.

Table 10.60 Polygraphic classification of type of apnea

1. Central apnea: simultaneous cessation of respiratory effort and air flow at the end of expiration. Probably due to cessation of motor output from the respiratory center in the brainstem
2. Obstructive apnea: cessation of airflow while respiratory effort continues. Seen in babies with the Pierre Robin syndrome for example
3. Mixed apnea: cessation of airflow with continued respiratory effort on some occasions and not on others. Both central and obstructive apneas occur during the same episode[588]

Diagnosis

The infant should be examined carefully to look for signs of infection, airway obstruction, seizures or persistent ductus arteriosus. Laboratory investigations might include full blood picture, blood culture, C-reactive protein (CRP), blood glucose, electrolytes and calcium.

Chest radiography, blood gas analysis and pH and examination of cerebrospinal fluid might also be indicated. Only after exclusion of infection, biochemical or drug causes of apnea can an infant be confidently labeled as having apnea of prematurity.

Treatment (Table 10.61)

All preterm babies < 34 weeks' gestation should have continuous monitoring of heart and respiratory rate until 5 days have elapsed without apnea. Pulse oximetry or transcutaneous oxygen monitoring is also desirable in less mature babies. Monitors which respond to chest wall movement (the apnea mattress, pressure sensor pad or pressure-sensitive capsule) will fail to detect obstructive apnea as long as respiratory movement continues. In order to detect obstructive or mixed types of apnea, the heart rate must also be monitored. Sometimes a simple adjustment of environmental temperature or feed frequency will prevent apneic attacks. During resuscitation, overzealous suctioning must be avoided as this stimulates irritant receptors in the pharynx and perpetuates the apnea and bradycardia. Many apneic attacks are self-resolving and provided bradycardia and hypoxemia do not occur these are probably not harmful to the baby.

Table 10.59 Clinical conditions associated with apnea

1. Hypoxemia: respiratory distress syndrome, pneumonia, chronic lung disease, recurrent aspiration, airway obstruction
2. Infection: septicemia or bacteremia, meningitis, necrotizing enterocolitis
3. Metabolic disorder: hypoglycemia, hypocalcemia, hypomagnesemia, hypernatremia, hyponatremia, acidosis
4. Central nervous system disorder: seizures, intracranial hemorrhage, drugs and drug withdrawal, kernicterus, cerebral malformation
5. Circulatory disorder: hypotension, congestive heart failure, persistent ductus arteriosus, anemia, polycythemia
6. Temperature instability: hyperthermia, hypothermia
7. Apnea of prematurity: diagnosis by exclusion

Repeated stimulation

Stimulation by stroking, gentle rubbing or rocking, e.g. rocking water beds, often prevents or shortens apneic attacks by increasing the input to the immature respiratory center by cutaneous, vestibular or proprioceptive pathways.

Intermittent bag and mask ventilation

When peripheral stimulation fails, bag and mask ventilation, using the same oxygen concentration as the baby is breathing, will stimulate spontaneous respiration without increasing the risk of retinopathy of prematurity.

Continuous positive airway pressure (CPAP)

CPAP reduces apnea by improving oxygenation and increasing functional residual capacity. It may also stabilize the chest wall and eliminate the Hering–Breuer deflation reflex. CPAP decreases the incidence of both mixed and obstructive apneas but does not affect central apneas so that it might work by helping to relieve upper airway obstruction. A nasopharyngeal tube or nasal prongs may be used to deliver the CPAP at 3–4 cmH_2O.

Drug therapy

Theophylline is useful in central as well as obstructive apnea and works by increasing the sensitivity of the respiratory center to hypercapnia, increasing minute ventilation and oxygen consumption. Other effects are stimulation of the diaphragm, positive

Table 10.61 Management of apnea

1. Immediate resuscitation
2. Exclude underlying cause (Table 10.59)
3. Lower environmental temperature 0.5°C
4. Correct mild hypoxemia and anemia
5. Repeated stimulation
6. Intermittent bag and mask ventilation
7. Continuous positive airway pressure
8. Drug therapy – caffeine, aminophylline, theophylline, doxapram
9. Mechanical ventilation

inotropic and chronotropic effects, mild diuresis and increased heat production through utilization of brown fat. Unwelcome effects include decreased cerebral blood flow and some uncertainty about long term outcome.[589] Dosage schedule and therapeutic range are shown in Table 10.62. Caffeine is also effective in treating apnea, and has a wider margin of safety than theophylline.[590,591] As there are concerns about potential long term adverse effects there is now a randomized trial of caffeine against placebo (CAP study) which should resolve the question of cost:benefit ratio. Doxapram is a direct respiratory stimulant which has undergone limited study in the treatment of neonatal apnea and has the side-effect of jitteriness and raised blood pressure.[592,593] It appears to have similar efficacy to the methylxanthines[594] but recent concerns about adverse long term neurological sequelae should severely limit the use of doxapram.

Antireflux medications do not reduce the frequency of apnea in preterm infants.[595]

Mechanical ventilation

This is reserved for babies whose apnea is resistant to other measures. Very immature infants and those with bacteremia often need mechanical ventilation and low inflating pressures should be used as lung compliance is usually normal.

Prognosis

Recurrent apnea has been associated with spastic diplegia and delayed development, especially if associated with an underlying cause but more recently uncomplicated recurrent apnea has been associated with a poor neurological outcome.[596] Overall mortality of babies with apnea < 33 weeks' gestation is one-third though this reflects the illness of the baby rather than the apnea per se. There appears to be no relationship between apneic spells in the neonatal period and subsequent sudden infant death syndrome (SIDS). Apnea can recur within 2 months of discharge from hospital if there is a respiratory infection or if general anesthesia is needed for surgery.[597]

NEONATAL CARDIOVASCULAR DISEASE

This section first considers normal perinatal cardiovascular changes (Fig. 10.6). Certain situations characteristically associated with the newborn period are then covered in detail. Congenital and acquired cardiac diseases are considered in Chapter 19.

PERINATAL CARDIOVASCULAR PHYSIOLOGY

Figure 10.5 illustrates fetal circulatory pathways. Labor and delivery trigger a number of cardiovascular events (Fig. 10.6), the occurrence of or failure of which have implications for the presentation and management of neonatal cardiovascular diseases.

Pulmonary vascular resistance

In healthy term babies the postnatal fall in pulmonary vascular resistance results in a rapid fall in right heart pressures over a few days with adult pulmonary to systemic pressure ratios being established by 2–3 weeks of age. Many factors can inhibit, delay or reverse pulmonary vasodilation in the newborn and these are listed with clinical examples in Table 10.63. The fall in resistance may occur more slowly in certain congenital cardiac abnormalities, such as atrioventricular septal defect (AVSD) and large ventricular septal defect (VSD). This delayed fall has implications for the time at which heart murmurs, clinical left-to-right shunting and heart failure develop. Thus, a very small VSD is more likely to produce a murmur in the first few days after birth than a large one, and a large VSD rarely causes heart failure in the first few weeks of life. In some congenital heart lesions, pulmonary vascular resistance never falls to normal and pulmonary vascular disease develops without clinical evidence of a large shunt ever having been present. This happens not infrequently in complete AVSD but can also happen with a large VSD, in both cases particularly if the child has Down syndrome.

Ductus arteriosus

As gestation progresses, ductal smooth muscle becomes less sensitive to dilating circulating prostaglandins and more sensitive to oxygen, a potent constrictor of the ductus. At term, increasing arterial oxygen tension causes functional closure of a normal ductus within the first 2–3 days in virtually all babies. In preterm babies without respiratory distress the time of ductal closure is similar.[600] Babies with structural abnormalities of the cardiovascular system may maintain ductal patency longer than normal before spontaneous closure occurs. There are two groups of congenital heart lesions which are critically dependent on ductal patency for the baby to remain alive (Table 10.64). The first group, those with duct-dependent pulmonary circulation, show appearance of or worsening in cyanosis on ductal closure. The second group are those conditions in which the systemic circulation is dependent on the ductus and collapse with gross heart failure occurs when the ductus closes. An important part of resuscitation in both these groups of infants is the use of prostaglandin E_1 or E_2 to reopen and maintain ductal patency. In addition babies with transposition without a large VSD will show a marked deterioration in oxygenation when the ductus closes. Persistent ductus arteriosus, either isolated or in association with other cardiac abnormalities, may also be a structural abnormality which will never close. If a normal ductus arteriosus is subject to abnormal conditions, its closure may be delayed. This situation is frequently seen in preterm babies with lung disease and may respond to prostaglandin synthetase inhibitor administration.

Foramen ovale

Increased pulmonary venous return after birth results in closure of the flap-like structure of the foramen ovale as left atrial pressure rises. If intra-atrial pressures are abnormal, shunting can occur in either direction through the foramen ovale. Thus left-to-right shunting may occur in babies with an increase in left atrial pressure (due to left-to-right shunting through a ductus arteriosus or to obstruction to flow of blood through the left heart) and right-to-left

Table 10.62 Drug therapy of apnea

Drug	Route	Loading dose (mg/kg)	Maintenance dose (mg/kg)	Frequency	Therapeutic range
Caffeine	Oral, i.v.	10	2.5	24-hourly	5–20 mg/L
Aminophylline	Oral, rectal, i.v.	6	1–2	8- to 12-hourly	5–20 mg/L
Theophylline	Oral, i.v.	5–6	1–2	8- to 12-hourly	5–15 mg/L (28–84 μmol/L)
Doxapram	i.v.	–	1–2.5	1-hourly	< 5 mg/L

Table 10.63 Situations associated with delay in or reversal of postnatal fall in pulmonary vascular resistance

Factor	Comment
Acidosis, hypoglycemia, hypoxemia, hypercapnia, polycythemia	Wide range of neonatal diseases
High altitude	Mediated via lower oxygen tension
Cardiac disease	See Table 10.71
Respiratory disease	Any cause
Ductal closure in utero	Maternal prostaglandin synthetase inhibitor ingestion
Obstructed middle or upper airway	Any cause

Table 10.64 Duct dependent congenital heart lesions

Obstruction to flow through right heart
Pulmonary atresia with intact ventricular septum
Critical pulmonary stenosis
Severe tetralogy of Fallot
Pulmonary atresia with VSD and no aortopulmonary communicating arteries
Tricuspid atresia (unless with large VSD and without pulmonary stenosis)
Obstruction to flow through left heart
Aortic atresia
Critical aortic stenosis
Hypoplastic left heart syndrome
Interrupted aortic arch
Severe coarctation

shunting can occur in persistent pulmonary hypertension or mechanical obstruction to flow through the right heart giving desaturated blood access to the systemic arterial circulation.

Ductus venosus

Blood flow through the ductus venosus falls dramatically when umbilical venous return ceases and functional closure occurs within a few days; however an umbilical venous catheter can sometimes be passed through it into the inferior vena cava and right atrium until at least a week after birth. Clinical relevance of patency of the ductus venosus relates to its usefulness as a route to the heart for central venous pressure monitoring or cardiac catheterization and also to the fact that when it closes, obstruction to pulmonary venous drainage becomes severe in total anomalous pulmonary venous return to the portal vein, causing marked deterioration in cyanosis and respiratory distress.

CARDIOVASCULAR EXAMINATION OF THE NEWBORN

The present history, perinatal and family histories may all give valuable clues to a diagnosis. Routine examination of well babies should include an assessment of the presence or absence of central cyanosis, an evaluation for evidence of heart failure and observations about pulse rate, regularity and character with special reference to the nature of the femoral pulses when compared simultaneously to the right brachial pulse. If the femoral pulses cannot be satisfactorily palpated or are markedly different from right arm pulses, a more thorough cardiovascular assessment including four-limb blood pressure reading, ECG and chest X-ray should be performed. Auscultation of the heart should be performed with an attempt to ensure that heart sounds are louder in the left chest than the right. Then attention should be given to whether the second sound is single or fixedly split and then to murmurs. The presence or absence of murmurs is only part of the neonatal cardiovascular examination. Some murmurs are innocent and many severe lesions have unimpressive murmurs or even none.

If cardiac disease is suspected, the precordium, suprasternal notch and subxiphoid region should be palpated for thrills or abnormal impulses, the skull auscultated for bruits, and a more detailed cardiac auscultation for added sounds and full murmur characterization carried out. Reliable blood pressure measurement in newborn infants requires a quiet and relaxed infant and a cuff of appropriate size (a cuff which covers two-thirds of the length of the upper arm and in which the bladder either encompasses the entire circumference of the arm or is positioned in such a way as to have the center of the bladder over the brachial artery). Detection of pulse reappearance can be by palpation but a Doppler probe is more sensitive, auscultation is very difficult. Oscillometric devices need to be watched whilst recording to ensure that the infant remains peaceful and are second best to direct invasive continuous monitoring of ill infants. The same cuff can be used on the calf with detection of posterior tibial or dorsalis pedis pulses for lower limb systolic pressures. Normal values for systolic pressures in term babies measured non-invasively are given in Table 10.65.[601] Acceptable values in ill preterm babies are different and less clearly defined (Table 10.65).[602,603] A reading up to 20 mmHg systolic higher in the arm than the leg can be normal; discrepancies between arm pressures may give clues as to the site of an aortic arch interruption. Significant coarctation may occasionally be associated with an aberrant right subclavian artery arising distal to the left subclavian, in which case upper to lower limb pulse discrepancy will not exist. Upper limb pressures may be raised in coarctation but in sick infants poor left ventricular function may prevent hypertension.

Table 10.65 Non-invasive (indirect) arm systolic blood pressures (mmHg) with pulse detected by Doppler probe. All infants 38 weeks' gestation or more (from de Swiet et al[601]) Reproduced from Rennie JM & Roberton NRC. Textbook of Neonatology, 3rd edn. Edinburgh: Churchill Livingstone; 1999

Age (days)	3	4	5	6	7	8–10
Awake						
Mean ± SD	72 ± 6	74 ± 9	77±10	77 ± 10	82 ± 9	88 ± 17
Number of infants	4	71	44	42	9	4
Asleep						
Mean ± SD	68 ± 7	70 ± 8	72 ± 8	72 ± 9	72±9	75 ± 9
Number of infants	72	681	426	322	47	18

Table 10.66 Systemic blood pressure in the neonatal period. Healthy LBW infants (no inotropes, no positive pressure ventilation). Some recordings direct intra-arterial, some oscillometric.[602,603] Reproduced from Rennie JM & Roberton, NRC. Textbook of Neonatology, 3rd edn. Edinburgh: Churchill Livingstone. 1999

Day 1			
Birth weight (g)	Number	Systolic range (mmHg)	Diastolic range (mmHg)
501–750	18	50–62	26–36
751–1000	39	48–59	23–36
1001–1250	30	49–61	26–35
1251–1500	45	46–56	23–33
1501–1750	51	46–58	23–33
1751–2000	61	48–61	24–35
Day 1			
Gestation (weeks)	Number	Systolic range (mmHg)	Diastolic range (mmHg)
<24	11	48–63	24–39
24–28	55	48–58	22–36
29–32	110	47–59	24–34
>32	68	48–60	24–34
Week 1			
Day	Number	Systolic range (mmHg)	Diastolic range (mmHg)
1	183	48–63	25–35
2	121	54–63	30–39
3	117	53–67	31–43
4	85	57–71	32–45
5	76	56–72	33–47
6	59	57–71	32–47
7	48	61–74	34–46

CARDIOVASCULAR INVESTIGATION OF THE NEWBORN

Chest X-ray

A systematic approach to the chest X-ray allows maximum information to be obtained; the particular points of relevance to cardiovascular diagnosis are listed in Table 10.67. Immediate management of a baby with a cardiac lesion may be greatly influenced by deciding whether lung blood flow is increased (plethoric lung fields, Fig. 10.35) or decreased (oligemic lung fields, Fig. 10.36). Pulmonary venous obstruction produces X-ray appearances often hard to distinguish from respiratory pathology. Clinical conditions associated with each of these abnormalities are given in Table 10.68.

Electrocardiography

This can provide important diagnostic information when significant heart disease is suspected. A detailed consideration of the subject will be found in Chapter 19. It is important to recognize the normal evolution of the ECG in the newborn and to have access to reference information[604] (Table 10.69).

Hyperoxia (nitrogen washout) test

If cyanosis is due to a cardiac cause, high concentrations of inspired oxygen rarely relieve it significantly, although there are exceptions, for example some common mixing conditions. If respiratory disease is the cause there is often relief from increasing inspired oxygen, although this will not be the case in severe respiratory disease and

Table 10.67 Chest X-ray: points to look for with reference to the cardiovascular system

Bronchial situs	
Lung fields	Oligemia Plethora Venous engorgement Lung pathology
Heart	Position, apex side Size Contour Aortic arch side
Abdomen	Visceral situs
Skeleton	Abnormalities

persistent pulmonary hypertension. This is the basis for the hyperoxia test. If a baby is put in 85% or more inspired oxygen for 15–20 min, a right radial arterial blood or right upper trunk transcutaneous oxygen tension should rise to well above 20 kPa. Failure to do so supports a desaturating cardiac abnormality. Transcutaneous oxygen tension monitors placed on the right upper thorax can give similar information to right radial artery samples but pulse oximetry can be misleading in that elevation of saturation to

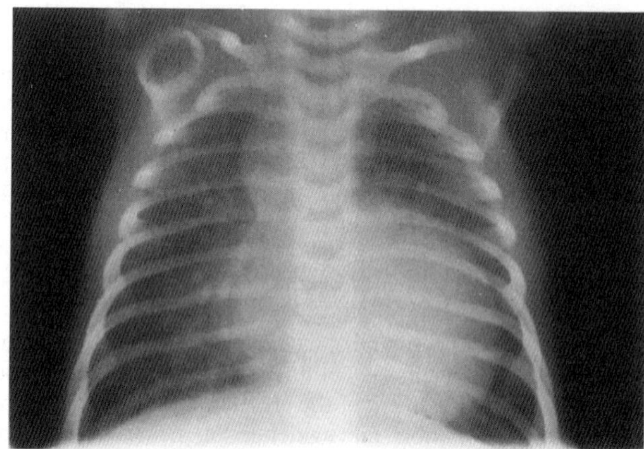

Fig. 10.35 Chest X-ray on cyanotic newborn infant. Lung fields are plethoric (double inlet left ventricle).

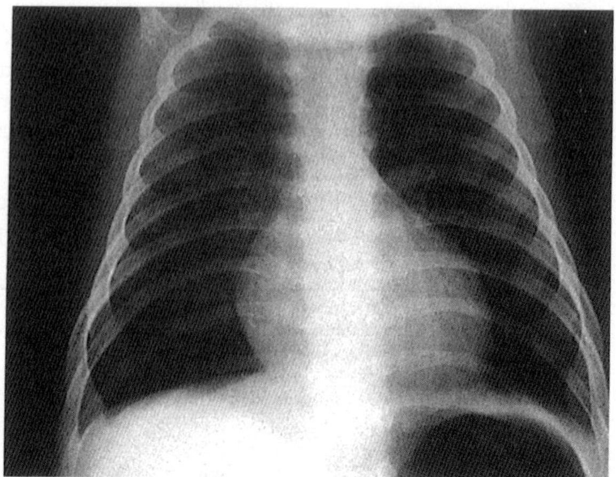

Fig. 10.36 Chest X-ray on cyanotic newborn infant. Lung fields are oligemic (tetralogy of Fallot).

Table 10.68 Lung vascularity on chest X-ray

Oligemia	Tricuspid atresia (unless large VSD) Ebstein's anomaly Pulmonary atresia or critical stenosis
Plethora	Any left-to-right shunt Common mixing without pulmonary stenosis Transposition of great arteries
Venous congestion	Obstruction to flow into or through left heart

normal, even to 100%, would not necessarily mean that arterial oxygen tension had risen above 20 kPa. Theoretical fears about precipitating ductal closure mean that the baby should be closely observed during the test; however, the risk of precipitating a problem is extremely small. Marked prematurity is a contraindication because of the possible consequence of retinopathy.

Echocardiography

Clinical evaluation should always precede echocardiography. Resuscitation and stabilization must always be achieved before transfer to another unit for evaluation. Ultrasound imaging and Doppler assessment allow a precise anatomical and functional diagnosis in the majority of symptomatic neonates with cardiac disease, so that surgery, be it palliative or definitive, is frequently not preceded by cardiac catheterization. The increasing expertise in echocardiography of neonatal pediatricians and the advent of telemedicine are altering transfer patterns of infants with actual or suspected heart lesions.

Cardiac catheterization

Although echocardiography has made neonatal diagnostic cardiac catheterization uncommon, there has been an increase in the number and scope of interventional therapeutic catheterizations in neonates. Good neonatal care is required throughout the procedure. The heart can be approached via umbilical vessels, femoral vessels percutaneously or by cut-down, or rarely by axillary vessel cut-down. The procedure has mortality and morbidity, though these have been greatly reduced by good general neonatal care and by anatomical information obtained from prior echocardiography.

PATTERNS OF CARDIOVASCULAR DISEASE IN THE NEWBORN

Congenital disease accounts for most cardiac disease in the newborn but acquired disease can occur as a result of birth asphyxia, viral infections and other severe postnatal illnesses. Congenital heart disease presents in the newborn period in approximately 4 per 1000 live births. Congenital heart disease may be structural or functional, the latter group being conditions such as conduction disturbances and dysrhythmias where a structural defect as an underlying cause or associated problem usually needs to be carefully excluded.

PRESENTATION AND MANAGEMENT OF CARDIOVASCULAR DISEASE IN THE NEWBORN

Fetal diagnosis[605]

Detailed fetal echocardiography may show cardiac abnormalities from 16 to 18 weeks' gestation onwards. Investigation is performed when a factor increasing the risk of heart disease is identified such as an abnormal view of the heart at a general anomaly scan, an extracardiac abnormality being detected in the fetus, certain parental illnesses or drug therapies or a previously affected infant. Detailed fetal echocardiography of all pregnancies is too resource consuming to be practiced in many places especially as evidence for improved postnatal outcomes after prenatal cardiac diagnosis is conflicting.[606–609] When a baby is born in whom a fetal diagnosis has been made, this must be confirmed by postnatal echocardiography. A normal fetal cardiac scan should not prevent postnatal echocardiography being performed if clinical features point to the possibility of cardiac disease in the newborn.

Cyanosis

To be certain of clinical cyanosis in a newborn infant is not always easy. Factors which complicate the assessment include a high hematocrit, traumatic petechiae on the face, racial pigmentation and acrocyanosis. A plethoric newborn infant may be normally saturated

Table 10.69 Selected ECG measurements in normal pediatric patients

	0–3 days	3–30 days	1–6 months	6–12 months	1–3 years	3–5 years	5–8 years	8–12 years	12–16 years
Heart rate (/min)	90–160	90–180	105–185	110–170	90–150	70–140	65–135	60–130	60–120
PR (msec) lead II	80–160	70–140	70–160	70–160	80–150	80–160	90–160	90–170	90–180
QRS (msec) lead V_5	25–75	25–80	25–80	25–75	30–75	30–75	30–80	30–85	35–90
QRS axis (degrees)	60–195	65–185	10–120	10–100	10–100	10–105	10–135	10–120	10–130
QRS V_1									
Q (mV)	0	0	0	0	0	0	0	0	0
R (mV)	0.5–2.6	0.3–2.3	0.3–2.0	0.2–2.0	0.2–1.8	0.1–1.8	0.1–1.5	0.1–1.2	0.1–1.0
S (mV)	0–2.3	0–1.5	0–1.5	0–1.8	0.1–2.1	0.2–2.1	0.3–2.4	0.3–2.5	0.3–2.2
QRS V_6									
Q (mV)	0–0.2	0–0.3	0–0.25	0–0.3	0–0.3	0.02–0.35	0.02–0.45	0.01–0.3	0–0.3
R (mV)	0–1.1	0.1–1.3	0.5–2.2	0.5–2.3	0.6–2.3	0.8–2.5	0.8–2.6	0.9–2.5	0.7–2.4
S (mV)	0–1.0	0–1.0	0–1.0	0–0.8	0–0.6	0–0.5	0–0.4	0–0.4	0–0.4
TV_1 (mV)	−0.4→0.4	−0.5→0.1	−0.6→0.1	−0.6→0.1	−0.6→0.1	−0.6→0	−0.5→0.2	−0.4→0.3	−0.4→0.3

Reproduced from Emmanouilides et al 1995, as adapted from Davignon A, Rautaharju P, Barselle E, Soumis F, Megelas M. Normal ECG standards for infants and children. Pediatric Cardiology 1979/80; 1:123–124

Values reported as 2–98% (approximate).

but still have enough deoxygenated Hb to look centrally cyanosed. Occasionally non-invasive monitoring or even blood gas sampling will be needed for confirmation. Some 'cyanotic' congenital heart disease may not produce recognizable cyanosis in a newborn baby (unobstructed total anomalous pulmonary venous drainage, double inlet and double outlet ventricles with high lung blood flow and good mixing, and tetralogy of Fallot in which right ventricular outflow obstruction progresses through infancy and is often only mild in the newborn period). Once central cyanosis is identified the immediate priority is to assess that airway and respiration are adequate, regardless of suspected cause. Detailed review of history and a complete physical examination are then important. Features of the different groups of causes and management pathways for a suspected cardiac cause are given in Tables 10.71 and 10.72, respectively. In an ill infant with cyanosis from cardiac disease, the most important specific management issue is whether or not ductal patency needs to be secured with prostaglandin; if in doubt, a trial of the drug is appropriate. Prostaglandin E_1 or E_2 may be given intravenously; prostaglandin E_2 may be given orally or nasogastrically, hourly in the first instance. Doses are given in Table 10.72.

Oxygenation is improved by prostaglandin in conditions with obstructed right heart flow (oligemic lungs on X-ray) and in many cases of transposition of the great arteries. Short-term side-effects of prostaglandin include pyrexia, apnea, jitteriness, convulsions, flushing and diarrhea. These often improve with dosage reduction without loss of therapeutic effect. The drug should be stopped if no benefit is seen after 1–2 h. Persistent pulmonary hypertension in the newborn (PPHN, see below) can at times be difficult to distinguish from cardiac disease even with echocardiography and the two may coexist (Table 10.73).

Heart failure

Features of heart failure include respiratory distress, sweating, hepatomegaly and in severe cases (particularly where failure has been present antenatally) ascites, generalized edema, pleural and pericardial effusions. Tachycardia, gallop rhythm and clinical features of the cause should also be looked for. Structural heart disease (particularly severe left ventricular outflow obstruction), rhythm disturbances, myocardial diseases (cardiomyopathy of any sort, myocarditis and myocardial ischemia or infarction) and non-cardiac diseases may all cause heart failure. Intracerebral and more rarely other arteriovenous malformations, generalized viral and bacterial infections, non-cardiac hypoxemia, severe anemia, marked polycythemia and excessive fluid administration may all precipitate cardiac decompensation.

Table 10.70 Clinical features and investigations which help rapid differentiation of causes for central cyanosis

Causes of cyanosis	Clinical features	Investigations
Respiratory	Marked respiratory distress (unless PPHN in addition) Color improves in oxygen usually	Abnormal lung fields on X-ray Hypercapnia Hyperoxia test (pass)
Cardiac	May have other cardiac signs May have little or no respiratory distress	X-ray may help, lung pathology absent Normo- or hypocapnia Hyperoxia test (fail) ECG abnormal
Neurological (respiratory depression)	Slow respiration Color improves on stimulation and in oxygen. May have other neurological or syndrome features	X-ray normal Hypercapnia Hyperoxia test (pass)
Hematological (methemoglobinemia)	Black mucous membranes, not typical cyanosis, usually very well	Blood gas normal Hyperoxia test (pass)

In all groups history may provide valuable clues. PPHN, persistent pulmonary hypertension in the newborn.

Table 10.71 Management approach to cyanosis due to a suspected cardiac cause

1. General measures	Temperature control, avoid hypoglycemia, ensure ventilation adequate
2. Arterial blood gas	Treat respiratory acidosis Treat metabolic acidosis Ventilate if necessary (hypoxemia alone not indication to ventilate) Consider value of hyperoxia test
3. Chest X-ray	Diagnostic clues may be present Management Oligemia – trial of prostaglandin Plethora – trial of prostaglandin if very hypoxemic or metabolic acidosis
4. ECG	May help with specific diagnosis
5. Drugs	Prostaglandin (see above) Alkali Diuretics if heart failure/pulmonary congestion Antibiotics if significant risk of serious infection
6. Echocardiography	Precise diagnosis often possible (transfer if necessary when stable)

Cyanosis and heart failure

Cyanosis is only a feature of very severe heart failure and heart failure does not develop in many conditions which cause severe cyanosis. Thus, if both cyanosis and heart failure are present, this may be a useful diagnostic aid (Table 10.74).

Collapse

This may be a feature of duct dependent systemic circulation (Table 10.64). Such lesions are also characterized by respiratory distress, massive hepatomegaly, cardiomegaly with congested lung fields on X-ray, right ventricular dominance on ECG and metabolic acidosis. Differential diagnosis includes septicemia and metabolic disorders but if any doubt exists, resuscitation should include prostaglandin, which will almost invariably produce rapid improvement if the diagnosis is cardiac.

Arrhythmia

Tachyarrhythmias may produce collapse, although supraventricular tachycardia (SVT) may produce no symptoms or may cause heart failure. Ventricular tachycardia may be life threatening or asymptomatic with a benign natural history and eventual spontaneous resolution. It is an indication for urgent cardiological referral. Complete heart block may be well tolerated especially if the ventricular rate is above 55/min and rises on activity.

Table 10.72 Drug dosage table

Drug	Route	Dose	Frequency
Prostaglandin			
E_1	i.v.	0.005–0.1 μg/kg/min	–
E_2	i.v.	0.005–0.05 μg/kg/min	–
E_2	Nasogastric	25 μg/kg/h	Hourly initially
Indometacin	i.v.	0.2 mg/kg over 30 min	8- to 12-hourly×3
Tolazoline	i.v.	0.5 mg/kg over 5 min then 0.5 mg/kg/h	–
Prostacyclin	i.v.	2–20 ng/kg/min	–
Dopamine	i.v.	2–20 μg/kg/min	–
Dobutamine	i.v.	2–20 μg/kg/min	–
Captopril	Oral/nasogastric	0.1–0.5 mg/kg/dose Start with lowest dose	8-hourly

Although Stokes–Adams attacks may occur, cardiac failure is the more usual problem in the neonate with complete heart block and both are indications for pacemaker insertion as is a heart rate below 55/min even in the absence of symptoms. Chronotropic drugs rarely have much effect on ventricular rate. The association of rhythm disturbances with structural heart disease must be remembered and the majority of babies with complete heart block without structural heart disease have mothers with serological evidence with or without clinical features of lupus erythematosus or other collagen vascular diseases.[610,611] Supraventricular ectopics (SVEs) are common in normal fetuses and newborns; they are not always conducted to the ventricles (blocked SVEs) in which case they result in a slow and or irregular pulse. In the absence of other cardiovascular signs or ECG abnormalities SVEs do not point to the presence of structural heart disease and resolve within 3 months of birth. There would appear to be an increased risk of SVT in infants with SVEs although clear information on the incidence is not available. Ventricular ectopics (VEs) are found in more than 30% of normal newborn infants and usually resolve rapidly. However if they are a sign of structural heart disease, heart muscle disease or a congenital long QT syndrome there is a risk of serious ventricular dysrrhythmias. A variety of acute metabolic disturbances can precipitate rhythm disturbances but do not require detailed cardiac investigation if rhythm and ECG return to normal when plasma biochemistry is corrected.

Cardiac murmur

Murmurs are often heard at routine examination of newborn infants. Symptoms or any other sign of cardiac disease must be sought as the presence of a murmur is associated with cardiac disease in up to 50% of cases in one recent large study.[612] Asymptomatic murmurs with no other abnormal features may be innocent and have been found in up to 2% of term infants in the first few days after birth;[613] Table 10.75 lists features of innocent neonatal murmurs. If doubt exists, normal blood pressure measurement, ECG and chest X-ray may still allow early discharge and outpatient follow-up. Some cardiac abnormalities can be associated with asymptomatic murmurs without any other physical signs and with normal ECG and chest X-ray. Tricuspid regurgitation and VSD may produce similar pansystolic murmurs at the lower left sternal edge. Tricuspid regurgitation producing a murmur in an otherwise well baby is of no long term significance; a VSD heard in the early neonatal period may never cause symptoms and has a high chance of spontaneous resolution.[614] Aortic and pulmonary valve stenosis (including tetralogy of Fallot) will produce a murmur at birth; evaluation including ECG, chest X-ray and if possible echocardiography is necessary before allowing a baby home if significant outflow tract obstruction is suggested by a loud murmur at the base. The normal murmur from pulmonary artery branches in the newborn is not as loud or as harsh as that from semilunar valve stenosis and radiates laterally.

Table 10.73 Structural cardiac lesions which may be associated with persistent pulmonary hypertension in the newborn infant

Pulmonary venous hypertension	Pulmonary vein stenosis Obstructed total anomalous pulmonary venous drainage Absent left atrioventricular connection with restrictive foramen ovale Left ventricular dysfunction (any cause) Left ventricular outflow obstruction (any cause)
Left-to-right shunts independent of pulmonary vascular resistance	Atrioventricular septal defect Cerebral arteriovenous malformation Coronary arteriovenous fistula
Severe tricuspid regurgitation	Ebstein's anomaly

Hypertension

Neonatal hypertension is usually only identified in infants with other cardiovascular signs or in those known to be at increased risk such as those with chronic lung disease or the infants of cocaine-using mothers. Treatment of neonatal hypertension is only

Table 10.74 Structural cardiac lesions characteristically showing both heart failure and arterial desaturation in the newborn period. Such lesions with pulmonary stenosis in addition are unlikely to have heart failure

Transposition	(i) with large VSD and PDA (ii) with coarctation
Truncus arteriosus	
Tricuspid atresia	(i) with large VSD (ii) with TGA and coarctation
Double inlet ventricle	
Total anomalous pulmonary venous drainage with obstructed pulmonary veins	
Hypoplastic left heart syndrome	
Cerebral arteriovenous malformation (vein of Galen aneurysm)	

PDA, persistent ductus arteriosus; TGA, transposition of the great arteries; VSD, ventricular septal defect.

Table 10.75 Features of innocent neonatal murmurs: in all groups the remainder of the examination is normal

Source/type	Features of murmur	Other points
Pulmonary arteries	Bilateral, base of heart, also over scapulae and lateral chest High pitched mid-systolic	Gone by 6 months
Ductus arteriosus	Pulmonary area rarely diastolic	Gone by 2–3 days
Tricuspid regurgitation	Same as VSD, heard day 1	May be perinatal asphyxia Goes in a few days–weeks
Still's innocent murmur	Vibratory Mid-systolic Between LLSE and apex	Rarely heard in newborn May last years

LLSE, lower left sternal edge.

occasionally necessary, but attention to the underlying cause is always appropriate (Table 10.76).

Association with other abnormalities

Many syndromes include cardiac abnormalities; in some the cardiac malformation may be a major determinant of length or quality of life. Any infant with a congenital abnormality should at very least have a full physical examination of the cardiovascular system. Babies undergoing major surgery on congenital abnormalities which may be associated with cardiac problems should have cardiovascular evaluation to identify possible management problems, as well as to allow comprehensive information to be passed to the family.[615]

CARDIOVASCULAR ASPECTS OF NEONATAL DISEASES

Respiratory distress syndrome

Persistent ductus arteriosus (PDA)

Patency of the ductus arteriosus is associated with worse RDS and delayed closure of the ductus can result in the need for continuing ventilation but clear evidence of reduced long term morbidity or mortality from prophylactic or therapeutic intervention is not available.[616] Antenatal prostaglandin synthetase inhibitor administration predisposes to postnatal delayed closure of the ductus and makes the ductus less responsive to indometacin.[617] The efficacy of antenatal steroid administration in reducing incidence and severity of RDS may in part be due to increasing ductal sensitivity to postnatal constricting influences. Cautious fluid regimes in babies with RDS are associated with a lower incidence of PDA. Etamsylate[618] given to reduce intraventricular hemorrhage has been found in a number of small studies to reduce symptomatic PDA. Prophylactic duct closure with indometacin reduces but does not abolish the occurrence of later symptoms;[619] a similar prophylactic action has been described for ibuprofen.[620] The failure to demonstrate better outcomes following prophylactic use of indometacin[621,622] rightly indicates the need for caution but long term outcome information following treatment only of babies at increased risk of symptomatic PDA is not currently available.

Prediction in the first 3 days of life of high risk of future symptomatic PDA is possible if a duct more than 1.5 mm in diameter is seen on color flow Doppler[623]or low velocity continuous left-to-right shunting is demonstrated by pulsed wave Doppler.[624] The typical clinical features PDA may be hard to detect in a baby with respiratory disease and PDA may cause no murmur or more usually just a systolic one. Other features of PDA in the context of the preterm include apnea, hypotension, heart failure, NEC and metabolic acidosis. When ventilator requirements are increasing after apparently passing the peak of RDS and a continuous murmur is present, the diagnosis is easy; when features are less obvious, the possibility of left-to-right shunting through a PDA must be remembered. The ECG is not usually helpful, and chest X-ray is often non-contributory. If there is clinical doubt, echocardiography imaging, M mode[625] and Doppler examination are required.[626]

Symptomatic PDA should be vigorously treated with fluid restriction and correction of anemia. Digoxin is not widely used and regular furosemide (frusemide) has disadvantages including electrolyte imbalance and possible antagonism of ductal closure. If conservative measures do not rapidly control the situation, indometacin has long been known to be effective in closing the ductus in approximately 70% of premature infants.[627] Intravenous indometacin (0.2 mg/kg) for three doses 8–24 h apart should be used; an infusion over at least 30 min is preferable to a bolus injection because of effects on blood pressure and cerebral circulation[628] although even slow infusions reduce cerebral oxygen delivery.[629] Less than three doses may be used if the Doppler velocity across the ductus can be shown to evolve to a closing pattern after the initial dose.[630] It is possible that ibuprofen may be less active on the cerebral circulation and just as effective at closing the ductus.[631,632] There are problems with commercial availability of a suitable ibuprofen preparation. Fluid retention and elevation of creatinine are temporary adverse effects of indometacin; thrombocytopenia is usually considered a contraindication to its use, as are renal failure and NEC. A repeat course may be used if the beneficial effect is transient although an asymptomatic murmur which reappears after natural or pharmacological ductal closure is more likely to be arising from the pulmonary artery branches than from the ductus.[633] A 5-day course of indometacin[634] or a 6-day low dose course[635] is effective at closing the ductus with a lower relapse rate. Biochemical evidence of renal dysfunction is less on the low dose regimen. The effect on cerebral hemodynamics of prolonged indometacin treatment has not been studied. Two unsuccessful short courses, unacceptable side-effects or a definite contraindication, mean that surgical ligation or clipping of the ductus should be

Table 10.76 Causes of hypertension in the newborn

Renal	Renal vein thrombosis Renal arterial emboli/thrombosis Dysplastic renal disease Polycystic renal disease Urinary tract obstruction Renal infection Renal failure (any cause)
Cardiovascular	Coarctation
Endocrine	Congenital adrenal hyperplasia Hyperaldosteronism Hyperthyroidism Pheochromocytoma Neuroblastoma
Respiratory disease	Bronchopulmonary dysplasia (mechanism unknown)
Neurological disease	Raised intracranial pressure (any cause)
Drugs	Corticosteroids Methylxanthines Phenylephrine (in eyedrops)

carried out. This can be done in the neonatal nursery with low mortality and morbidity. Whether or not echocardiography is regarded as mandatory before using prostaglandin synthetase inhibitor drugs, it certainly is before surgical ligation to confirm the diagnosis and to rule out structural congenital heart disease and systemic to pulmonary collateral arteries which can be found in preterm infants[636] and which cause a continuous murmur.

Persistent pulmonary hypertension of the newborn (PPHN)

Pulmonary hypertension may complicate a variety of neonatal respiratory illnesses (Table 10.63). Diagnosis is helped by recognizing risk factors and by excluding structural heart disease. Lower saturations in the feet than the right hand are characteristic if the ductus arteriosus is open.

Management in general consists of treating predisposing and aggravating factors aggressively, ensuring adequate alveolar recruitment and systemic blood pressure and normalizing acid–base balance. Consideration should then be given to the use of vasodilators. Oxygen and inhaled nitric oxide[637] are the only specific pulmonary vasodilators. Optimum dosage of nitric oxide is unclear but may be 20 parts per million (p.p.m.)[638] and there may be disadvantages to initiating therapy at a lower dose.[639] There are benefits in tailoring ventilatory modes to the individual patient which may be additive to the effects of nitric oxide.[640] Plasma expansion and inotropes may both be needed. ECMO is effective in PPHN but exact indications for its use are unclear, as newer treatment protocols are more effective than those used when ECMO was first introduced. Intravenous magnesium sulfate, prostacyclin and tolazoline may be effective and the latter drug has also been used by inhalation. These treatments have not been extensively evaluated in randomized controlled trials. All infused drugs will lower systemic as well as pulmonary vascular resistance, so blood pressure must be invasively and continuously monitored when they are used. Modest hyperventilation to a carbon dioxide tension of 3–4 kPa or administration of alkali may lower pulmonary vascular resistance but these maneuvers may have adverse effects on the cerebral circulation and are seldom used.

Asphyxia

Persistent pulmonary hypertension

This may also be a feature of perinatal asphyxia, with or without meconium aspiration pneumonitis (see above).

Myocardial ischemia and infarction

Electrocardiographic[641] and pathological[642] studies indicate that myocardial ischemia is common in neonates stressed by asphyxia. Even in mild cases there may be the murmur of tricuspid regurgitation which may be associated with ischemic ECG changes. In severely asphyxiated infants, hypotension from myocardial dysfunction may need inotrope support and any type of arrhythmia can occur. Discrete areas of myocardial infarction can occur secondary to thromboembolic phenomena pre- or postnatally; this is rare but has a high mortality.[643]

Infection

Generalized and pulmonary bacterial and viral infections in the newborn may predispose to PPHN. Myocarditis is a feature of disseminated viral infections and heart failure, shock and arrhythmias may result. Shock may also be caused by peripheral vasodilation and capillary leakage in severe bacterial sepsis. Endocarditis is increasingly being recognized in already sick newborn infants.[644] Clinical features are non-specific. There is rarely underlying structural heart disease. The diagnosis is suggested by multiple septic lesions appearing over time or recurrent bacteremia or fungemia, particularly in the presence of intravenous long lines. Ultrasound scanning can make, but not exclude, the diagnosis. Masses within the heart chambers or in great vessels can be vegetations in association with infection, non-infected thrombus (usually related to presence of an indwelling catheter at that site at some time) or tumors. Prolonged appropriate multiple antimicrobial therapy is indicated for endocarditis.

Metabolic diseases

There are many inborn errors of metabolism and storage diseases which may be associated with cardiomyopathy. Hypertrophic cardiomyopathy seen in the newborn infants of diabetic mothers is worth specific mention because although it is frequently asymptomatic it may cause severe heart failure with gross cardiomegaly and ECG changes. The role of cardiac dysfunction in the respiratory problems encountered in some infants of diabetic mothers needs careful individual assessment, as in some it will be a major contributory factor. This cardiomyopathy is self-limiting, resolving completely in 6–12 months.[645] Digoxin, other inotropes and vasodilators should be avoided in this condition because they may aggravate left ventricular outflow obstruction. Dilated cardiomyopathy may present symptomatically in the newborn period and a vigorous search for familial, infective and metabolic causes is indicated.

GENERAL MANAGEMENT OF NEONATAL HEART DISEASE

All the principles for care of the newborn infant apply to the baby with definite or suspected cardiac disease. These principles should not be neglected because of a desire to get the correct diagnosis or to transfer the infant elsewhere.

Ductal manipulation

The major resuscitative decision with respect specifically to heart disease is whether or not to use prostaglandin. In an unwell baby with poor systemic perfusion the possibility of critical left heart obstruction must always be borne in mind and unless it can be confidently excluded a trial of prostaglandin is appropriate. A cyanosed infant who is well does not need prostaglandin urgently but if there is metabolic acidosis or respiratory distress for which no primary respiratory cause is apparent prostaglandin should be commenced. Pharmacological duct closure with indometacin is never as urgent and if any doubt exists about the diagnosis, echocardiography is essential, as indeed it is before surgical intervention.

Heart failure

Fluid restriction in the short term, optimal oxygenation and the treatment of anemia are important. Digoxin use is time honored but controversial in the treatment of heart failure when associated with left-to-right shunt. Diuretics, usually furosemide (frusemide) with or without a potassium sparing diuretic, are particularly effective in relieving symptoms. Vasodilators in neonatal heart failure are relatively untried, although angiotensin-converting enzyme inhibitors are widely used in infants.[646,647] Aggressive drug therapy for heart failure is appropriate in order to allow adequate nutrition.

Hypotension/low output states

There is no single objective method of assessing clinically the adequacy of the circulation in a newborn infant. Decisions to provide circulatory support are not based on any one parameter alone. Normal ranges for blood pressure can be derived from healthy infants but they do not determine what is an adequate or beneficial blood pressure and there are no randomized trials assessing the outcomes of sick infants treated with different target ranges for blood pressure.

Clinical assessment of end organ perfusion is just as important as aiming at a particular blood pressure.[648] If the urine output is good, there is no metabolic acidosis and there is good peripheral perfusion, the circulation is likely to be adequate whatever the blood pressure. However, preterm infants with higher blood pressure tend to have better clinical outcomes than those with lower blood pressure and, perhaps because it is easily measured, treatment decisions are strongly influenced by blood pressure measurements.

Broad concensus is that if the mean arterial blood pressure is around the gestational age in weeks then it is likely to be adequate;[649] ensuring optimal circulating volume should precede or accompany inotrope support.[650] However, in the majority of cases hypovolemia is unlikely to be the explanation and repeated boluses of colloid for hypotension in preterm infants may be harmful. Early intervention with dopamine or dobutamine[651,652] should be considered. Echocardiography is helpful if doubt about the need for inotrope support exists and central venous pressure measurements may help.

A small number of infants remain hypotensive despite maximal inotropic support and volume replacement. Some of these infants respond well to small doses of hydrocortisone. It is not clear to what extent newborn infants can increase cardiac output by increasing myocardial contractility rather than heart rate. Bradycardia, be it sinus or due to atrioventricular block, resulting in circulatory compromise should be treated by identifying and removing the cause, aided if necessary by drugs such as atropine and isoprenaline or by pacing. Primary tachyarrhythmias such as atrial flutter and atrioventricular re-entry tachycardia (see Ch. 19) can be hard to distinguish from reactive sinus tachycardia but must be recognized and treated if compromising cardiac output. The rare cases of cardiac tamponade from pericardial fluid or air require drainage.

Arrhythmias

Management of these in newborn babies is governed by the same principles as throughout infancy and is discussed in Chapter 19.

Drug therapy

Recommended drugs and dosages for the treatment of neonatal cardiovascular disease are given in Table 10.72.

Interventional cardiac catheterization

Rashkind balloon atrial septostomy still forms part of the emergency management of a number of conditions, particularly transposition of the great arteries (TGA). If diagnostic catheterization is not needed, a balloon atrial septostomy can be performed by an experienced operator under ultrasound control in the neonatal nursery. Balloon valvuloplasty is used in some centers for both critical aortic and critical pulmonary valve stenosis.[653] Balloon dilation of neonatal coarctation is generally not as effective as surgery. The role of ductal stenting in duct-dependent lesions is being explored.[654] Transcatheter ductal closure is not yet feasible in premature newborns.

Surgery

Cardiac surgery in the newborn can be palliative or corrective, closed or open. Surgical treatment for particular conditions is discussed in Chapter 19 and it must be remembered that local practices vary a great deal. In general there is a trend towards performing corrective open procedures at increasingly younger ages. Whatever approach is taken results are better when infants come to operation well resuscitated and stable.

STRUCTURAL HEART DISEASE IN THE PRETERM INFANT

Respiratory pathology and infective processes are so common in the preterm infant that cardiac disease can be forgotten or masked. It is extremely important to bear in mind the possibility of structural and functional cardiac disease as the cause of or a contributory factor to symptoms and signs in the premature infant. In many cases pharmacological or surgical management is possible with ultimate good outcome. Preterm babies may go into heart failure at an earlier postnatal age with a given condition, such as VSD, than a term baby for reasons that are not entirely clear.

CARDIOVASCULAR ASPECTS OF CHRONIC PULMONARY DISEASE IN THE NEWBORN

The role of PDA in prolonging acute respiratory failure in RDS has been discussed above. Chronic lung disease will make clinical features of a left-to-right shunt of any sort very hard to recognize but treatment of the cardiac abnormality may help the respiratory condition. Chronic respiratory failure may cause right heart failure; it is important to avoid hypoxemia in such infants and to treat intercurrent infections and secretion retention vigorously.

GASTROINTESTINAL PROBLEMS AND JAUNDICE OF THE NEONATE

EMBRYOLOGY AND MALFORMATIONS

The gut is derived from the embryonic yolk sac which differentiates in early life into the fore-, mid- and hindgut. The foregut gives rise to the pharynx, thyroid, thymus, parathyroid glands, respiratory tract, esophagus, stomach, upper duodenum, liver and pancreas. The midgut gives rise to the lower half of the duodenum, small intestine and large intestine as far as the distal third of the transverse colon. The rest of the large bowel arises from the hindgut. Agenesis of a complete segment is rare; rather, constriction (atresia) of a small portion is more common, and can occur at any level, because normal development includes luminal obliteration by mucosal growth, followed by recanalization.[655] Atresia is more common at sites where the development of the gut is complex, like the respiratory diverticulum of the foregut (see below).

Between 4 and 6 weeks of fetal life the cranial portion of the foregut differentiates into a complicated branchial arch system which is transitory and obliterated by 7 weeks. Failure of obliteration may result in a persistent sinus, fistula or epithelial lined cyst (e.g. neurenteric cyst). The partitioning of the foregut into the pharynx and trachea may also be incomplete and various types of tracheoesophageal fistula with or without esophageal atresia will result. Abnormal development of the lower end of the foregut may result in a diaphragmatic hernia whilst failure of esophageal differentiation causes achalasia of the cardia or more rarely an esophageal web.

The stomach is relatively immune to embryological malformation. However, the terminal portion of the foregut and cranial end of the midgut undergo major growth in length with consequent herniation from the umbilical cavity (Fig. 10.37).[656] As it returns to the abdomen there is a complex counterclockwise rotation (ultimately 270 degrees) resulting in the fixation of the cecum in the right iliac fossa and the passage of the transverse

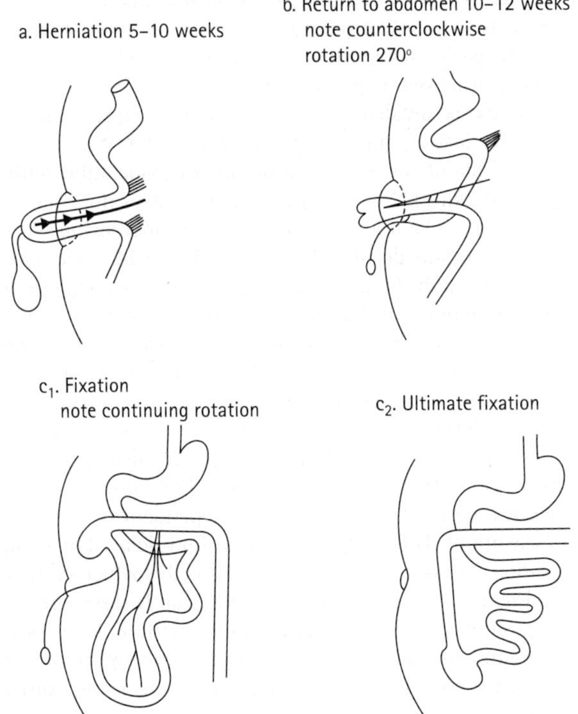

Fig. 10.37 The course of events leading to fixation and final position of the gut within the abdomen. (From Lebenthal et al 1988[656])

colon and mesentery over the second and third parts of the duodenum. The first possible failure is that of the endoderm of the yolk sac to separate from the notochord during the third week which results in a variety of reduplications of the intestine. Incomplete failure of the vitellointestinal duct to regress in the fifth week results in a Meckel's diverticulum and complete failure results in an umbilical fistula. Finally failure in herniation return and fixation of the intestine between the fifth and twelfth weeks may cause major defects such as exomphalos and malrotation.

The cloaca is divided by a membrane at 6 weeks into the sagittally oriented rectum posteriorly and the urogenital sinus anteriorly. Anomalies in rectal differentiation cause a variety of defects ranging from imperforate anus and rectovaginal fistulae to sacral sinus formation. Because rectal differentiation is contemporaneous with that of esophageal differentiation, defects in both structures are often found in the same patient.

The liver is derived from an outpouching of the ventral portion of the duodenum at 4 weeks and defects in its development are rare (Fig. 10.38).[656] Defects in the development of the biliary tree from the cystic duct are more common with either cystic dilation (choledochal cyst) or failure of canalization (biliary atresia) being the commonest disorders. Defects in pancreatic development are also rare but because the final gland is produced by the fusion of a dorsal pancreas from an outpouching of the duodenum just cranial to the hepatic diverticulum and a ventral pancreas from an outpouching in the caudal angle between the gut and hepatic diverticulum (Fig. 10.38) failure of this fusion process may result in an annular pancreas. Cellular differentiation of all the organs of the gut occurs early and is complete in most cases by the end of the first trimester. Intestinal epithelial cells of the first trimester human fetus resemble immature crypt cells of the adult intestine. Morphogenesis of the intestinal epithelium (including differentiation of crypts and villi as well as the intracellular organelles) is completed by about 22 weeks' gestation. Thus, the anatomical development of the gut is complete by the birth of even the 24 week infant and the limiting factor in feeding is the maturation of functional activity.

ONTOGENY OF GUT FUNCTION

Carbohydrate absorption

The absorption of carbohydrates seems to pose no problem even for premature neonates. Human milk and most formula milks usually contain only lactose, thus pancreatic digestion is relatively unimportant and the low levels of amylase detected in the duodenal juice of premature and term infants do not matter. More modified milks contain such elements as corn syrup, amylose or maltodextrins in order to reduce their osmolality; however, glucoamylase and sucrase-isomaltase activity should be adequate for their digestion. The disaccharidases develop in close association with the enterocyte itself and disaccharidase activity first appears with the villus formation. Lactase, however, develops later in comparison with sucrase-isomaltase activity (8–10 months' gestation) but lactose intolerance is very rarely seen in the VLBW infant, presumably because of enzyme induction.

Intestinal absorption of nutrients and electrolytes is dependent on the development of appropriate cellular active transport processes. Studies of everted fetal intestinal sacs have shown that cotransport of glucose/galactose by the sodium-glucose linked transporter (SGLT1) is present as early as 10 weeks and there is a threefold increase in the uptake by 18 weeks. Studies of glucose-evoked potential difference across the duodenum in neonates have confirmed the presence of active glucose transfer in premature neonates, although the number of monosaccharide transporters is reduced in the premature compared with the term infant. Thus carbohydrate digestion/absorption is adequate in the premature infant.

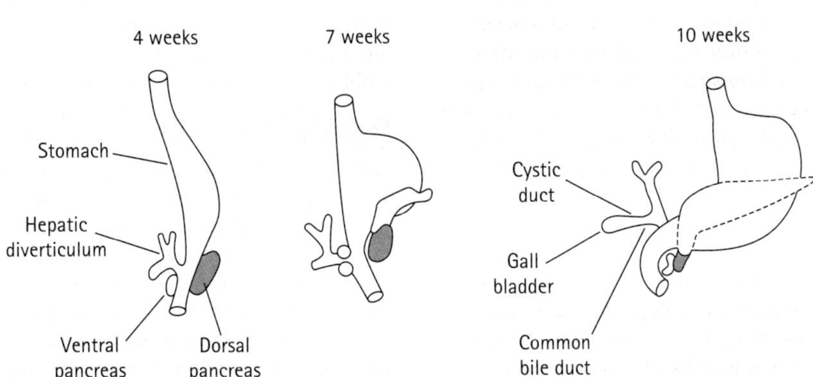

Fig. 10.38 The development of the liver/pancreas from an outpouching of the ventral portion of the duodenum. (From Lebenthal et al 1988[656])

Protein absorption

Protein digestion is initiated in the stomach and gastric peptic activity increases rapidly after birth (from 2 to 50% adult reference levels by 2 months in term infants). Gastric acid secretion (which is necessary for full peptic activity, the pH optima of pepsin being 4–5) does not occur at maximal activity in the preterm infant for about 1 month. It is, however, rapidly buffered by milk because of the overall decreased secretory mass in these infants.

Although tryptic activity is low at birth, pancreatic enzyme induction results in high levels by the first week of life in term and preterm infants. Brush border oligopeptidase activity is similar to that found in adults by the early part of the second trimester and protein digestion appears adequate. Active absorption of L-alanine and L-leucine has also been demonstrated in everted sacs from both 10- and 18-week fetuses. Peptides as well as amino acids can be absorbed by the enterocyte which further enhances the efficiency of protein absorption.

Fat absorption

Lipid digestion is more complex and requires more adaptive mechanisms to ensure maximal absorption of this major source of energy by preterm infants. Four major lipases exist:

1. lingual lipase – this is often bypassed by nasogastric tubes although non-nutritive sucking may increase the contribution of this enzyme;
2. gastric lipase (first demonstrated as having a role in the gastric aspirates of infants with esophageal atresia);
3. pancreatic lipase (this shows rapid substrate induction);
4. bile salt-stimulated lipase (present in high quantities in human milk, irrespective of prematurity and milk volume).

These contribute more than sufficient lipolytic activity even in the preterm infant. Unfortunately, bile salt production in such infants barely reaches the critical micellar concentration and this becomes the rate-limiting factor in fat digestion. However, the palmitic acid of human milk fat is predominantly esterified at the triglyceride 2 position which matches the stereospecificity of pancreatic lipase reducing the need for bile salts. Milk manufacturers tend to compensate for the inefficient fat absorption of their milks by supplementing them with medium chain triglycerides (at the expense of increasing osmolality). The products of fat digestion are absorbed, resynthesized as triglycerides and secreted into the lymphatic system as chylomicrons. Medium chain triglycerides (8–10 carbon chain length) are absorbed without bile salts, and pass to the liver in the portal system.

Salt and water absorption

Salt and water absorption by the enterocyte is present in the early stages of cellular differentiation. It has been shown that adenylate cyclase and Na/K ATPase activities, both closely related to the electrolyte transport processes, develop concomitantly with the brush border translocation mechanisms. Equilibrium dialysis studies of colonic transport mechanisms in the premature infant have demonstrated that the sodium chloride exchange mechanisms are highly active (presumably under the influence of the high levels of aldosterone seen in these infants). Basic transport processes clearly function in early life.

Intestinal motility

The limiting factor in feeding premature infants is intestinal motility, the ontogeny of which lags behind digestion and absorption. The ability to suck is not present until about 34 weeks' gestation (although it can occur earlier) but this can be bypassed by tube feeding. Gastric emptying although poor at birth, is fully functional by 24 h postnatally. It is controlled by duodenal receptors in similar fashion in both premature and mature infants by nutrient density and specific constituents of the meal and is inhibited by pathological processes (e.g. RDS and asphyxia). Small intestinal motor activity is divided into fasting and postprandial motor patterns. The fasting migrating motor complex does not fully develop until about 34 weeks' gestation (in association with the onset of the sucking).[657] Postprandial activity does not occur until later and seems to be a learned phenomenon increasing with the increasing nutritional density of the feeds. Before 34 weeks a highly propulsive activity, the fetal motor complex, is seen which allows the intestine to function and feeding to be effective. Before 26 weeks, only small non-propagated contractions are seen and so enteral feeds may not be tolerated initially. More mature motor function may be induced by feeding, allowing many infants of lower gestation to tolerate enteral feeding. The development of colonic motility has not been studied but appears to be adequate although regular glycerin suppositories may be needed initially. It is also clear that the gut motor function is critically dependent upon the well-being of the infant. Thus, sick infants will show delayed maturation (or regression) of gut motor activity and it is this which causes the functional ileus seen in such infants. More rarely disorders of the nervous system of the gut may present with a true pseudo-obstruction and disordered distal migration of the myenteric nerves can give rise to aganglionic segments as in Hirschsprung's disease.

Postnatal development

There are three elements of postnatal development of the gastrointestinal tract that are of fundamental importance in the consideration of neonatal and later childhood intestinal disease.[658] First is the huge capacity for postnatal growth of small and large intestine. The small intestine increases in length from 4 mm at 4 weeks' gestation to 250–300 cm at term, and the colon is 30–40 cm at term. The postnatal growth of the intestine is at least tenfold, with the small intestine reaching 4–6 m, and the colon 1.5–2.0 m.[659] Secondly, there is increasing evidence that postnatal modelling events, either as part of normal growth or as a response to injury or inflammation, may proceed under very similar regulation to embryonic development.[658] This will soon be the source of therapeutic development. Lastly is the central role of the intestinal immune system – the intestine is the largest immune organ in the body. Very recent environmental and cultural changes in human life have resulted in changes in tolerance to dietary antigens and the enteric flora, and may be the cause of the rapid rise in inflammatory bowel diseases and atopic diseases.[658]

PROBLEMS

The common problems of feeding intolerance, feeding difficulties, vomiting, diarrhea, constipation and gastrointestinal bleeding in the neonatal period will be considered, and then the specific problems of NEC and short bowel syndrome.

Feeding intolerance (Table 10.77)

This is a common problem in the neonatal nursery becoming manifest as increasingly large aspirates and failure to tolerate milk in the tube-fed infant. Care must be taken to check for blood or bile in the aspirate. The former suggests a gastritis and the latter functional or surgical obstruction. Prematurity is the usual cause for failure to tolerate feeds although most infants even as early as 25/26 weeks' gestation will tolerate continuous tube feeds which are started gradually at 1 ml/h and increased, as tolerated, to full requirements over the course of the first week.

Table 10.77 Feeding disorders

Etiology	Investigations
a. 'Feeding intolerance'	
Prematurity	History and examination
Ileus	Nursing observation
Sepsis	Abdominal distention
Major clinical deterioration	Septic screen
Necrotizing enterocolitis	Distention – abdominal wall crepitus, tenderness Abdominal X-ray Proctoscopy
Asphyxia	
Drugs	
All causes of vomiting	
b. 'Feeding difficulties'	
Maternal factors	History and examination
Poor milk supply	Nursing observation
Cracked nipples/ breast abscess	
Tension/anxiety	
Poor ability to suck	
Tachypnea/RDS	
Anatomical abnormality	
Micrognathia	
Macroglossia	
Cleft palate	
Asphyxia	
Bulbar/suprabulbar palsy	Jaw jerk positive
Moebius' syndrome	
Myopathies	Absent reflexes Electromyogram nerve conduction studies
Familial dysautonomia	Jewish race Histamine prick test Pupillary response to metacholine

In their Cochrane review of 10 randomized trials, Premji & Chessell[660] concluded that the evidence to date could not reliably discern between the clinical benefits and risks of continuous versus intermittent milk feeding of preterm infants. A further Cochrane review concluded that the ideal rate of advancement of feeds for preterm infants remains unclear.[661] Hourly intermittent bolus feeds are then introduced and by about 34 weeks' gestation, with the onset of suckling, the infant will tolerate 3- to 4-hourly feeds and is ready for the introduction of orogastric feeding. Attempts to introduce these steps too quickly will result in an increase in the volume of stomach contents aspirated before the next feed (or hourly if continuously fed). Experienced nurses are normally able to distinguish such an increase in aspirate from that occurring unexpectedly and indicating pathology in the gastrointestinal tract. A recent Cochrane review of 14 randomized trials concluded that non-nutritive sucking by preterm infants aided the transition to bottle feedings.[662] Most of the causes of vomiting in the neonatal period can present at this stage with increasing gastric residues but most commonly such an increase in aspirate heralds the onset of ileus secondary to sepsis, a major deterioration in the child's general condition or NEC. Asphyxia may be complicated by gastric stasis and is the commonest organic cause of poor feeding postnatally in the term infant. Failure of initiation of oral feeding for more than 1 week in an asphyxiated term infant indicates a poor prognosis. Drugs used postnatally, especially phenobarbital and diazepam, can delay gastric emptying and enteral feeding may not be possible in the ventilated and paralyzed infant. Other drugs have been assessed in randomized trials for improvement of motility in preterm infants with feeding intolerance, but some, such as erythromycin,[663] do not have current evidence to support such use, and others, such as cisapride,[664] have been withdrawn from use due to side-effects.

Feeding difficulties (Table 10.77)

It may be difficult to establish feeding even in the term infant. Breast problems such as cracked nipples or a breast abscess may prevent breast-feeding, the gold standard route of feeding for both preterm and term infants, but the baby will quickly accept bottle-feeding. Maternal anxiety may also prevent the establishment of breast-feeding and can also lead to clumsy or inappropriate methods of bottle-feeding (resulting usually in overfeeding and vomiting but occasionally in inadequate feeding and failure to thrive). A recent Cochrane review evaluated 20 eligible randomized controlled trials, and concluded that there was clear evidence that professional support and lay support could prolong duration of breast-feeding and promote exclusive breast-feeding respectively.[665]

Disorders of sucking and swallowing can occur. Anatomical abnormalities such as micrognathia, macroglossia and cleft palate often result in poor sucking and slow feeding. Neurological conditions other than asphyxia tend to present with uncoordinated sucking and swallowing causing oral or nasal regurgitation, sometimes accompanied by the signs of a suprabulbar palsy with tongue thrust and a positive jaw jerk. The rare congenital Moebius' syndrome with bilateral facial palsy (and other cranial nerve palsies) due to congenital agenesis of the cranial nerves also results in a poor suck and uncoordinated swallowing. Unilateral nerve lesions do not usually cause problems and where present should be distinguished from myopathies such as mitochondrial myopathy which may cause dysphagia in the neonatal period. The Riley–Day syndrome (familial dysautonomia) may also present in the neonatal period with disorders of swallowing but usually dysphagia occurs later in childhood. Where there is excessive drooling of saliva in association with swallowing difficulties a tracheoesophageal fistula should be considered although the usual clinical picture (coughing, excessive saliva, cyanotic and apneic spells) is quite distinctive and is rapidly diagnosed within a few hours of birth by a plain X-ray with a nasogastric tube inserted.

Vomiting

Vomiting is common in newborn infants. Assessment should always include the overall clinical condition and other symptoms and signs, as well as the volume, frequency and contents of the vomitus (causes and investigations in Table 10.78).

Posseting

Posseting (the regurgitation of small amounts of milk after feeds) is common in the neonatal period and is easily distinguished from pathological vomiting by experienced mothers and midwives. Regurgitation and vomiting both indicate underlying disorders in the newborn period (vomiting is a more serious problem). Rumination is a rare disorder, possibly familial. The baby regurgitates small amounts of food into the mouth which is then chewed with apparent self-gratification. It usually presents after the neonatal period.

Feeding disorders

Feeding disorders are the commonest cause of vomiting in the first month of life after leaving hospital. Greedy babies swallow air. This leads to excessive posseting or vomiting and can usually be recognized by experienced health visitors. Overfeeding or the improper preparation of the bottles is more difficult to spot and commonly presents as vomiting to casualty departments. A careful history of type, amount and constitution of feed is vital in every case of vomiting. With correction of mother's mistakes the symptoms rapidly resolve. However, maternal anxiety or depression is often a coexistent factor in such cases and contributes to the fussy eating and vomiting in these babies. Evidence of affective disorder or postnatal depression in the mother should be sought during history taking and a full family history often reveals predictable stressors such as death of a sibling or other close relative, or a previous stillbirth or neonatal death.

Organic causes of vomiting

Vomiting in the first week of life. Vomiting at this time may be due to difficulties in establishing appropriate feeding. However, more specific organic causes must be excluded by appropriate means. All causes of vomiting (Table 10.78) may present at any time, but in this early period, consideration of the vomitus and baby together with an abdominal X-ray (AXR) can narrow the differential diagnosis. For example:

1. Vomitus
   - Frothy
     - tracheoesophageal fistula
   - Blood
     - maternal – swallowed
     - hemorrhagic disease
     - gastric erosions/stress ulcers
   - Bile
     - intestinal obstruction
     - intestinal perforation/peritonitis
     - intestinal pseudo-obstruction
   - Milk only
     - feeding disorder
     - gastroesophageal reflux
     - food allergy
2. Baby well: abdomen normal
   - AXR – fluid level
     - duodenal/intestinal atresia
     - meconium ileus
     - large bowel obstruction/Hirschsprung's disease
   - AXR – no fluid levels
     - gastroesophageal reflux
     - milk allergy
3. Baby sick
   - Abdomen normal: AXR – no or occasional fluid levels + watery diarrhea
     - sepsis/urinary tract infection
     - increased intracranial pressure/meningitis
     - renal tract disorders
     - metabolic disorders
   - Abdomen distended/tender: AXR – fluid levels (watery diarrhea or bloody diarrhea)
     - NEC
     - obstruction/perforation
     - volvulus
     - intussusception

The commonest cause for vomiting in the first 2 days of life is undoubtedly a neonatal gastritis due to irritation from swallowed liquor and debris from the birth canal. One or two stomach washouts usually suffice to identify the debris (and the altered maternal blood) and to cure the problem. The baby remains well throughout. If the baby is sick, other signs are present or the vomiting persists, then fuller investigations are required. Clearly a septic screen (comprising FBC [full blood count], clotting studies, blood cultures, MSSU [mid stream specimen urine] and possibly LP [lumbar puncture]) are indicated in a baby who is unwell and all vomiting babies need urea and electrolytes checked. Hematemesis may require transfusion and treatment with vitamin K or fresh frozen plasma (FFP) as indicated. Stress ulceration is rare but usually settles with intravenous ranitidine.

Table 10.78 Vomiting

Etiology	Investigations
Feeding disorders	
Overfeeding	Feeding history and observation
Air swallowing	
Maternal stress	Family history
Esophageal disorders	
Tracheoesophageal fistula/frothy vomit day 1	CXR/AXR with large nasogastric tube
Hiatus hernia	Barium swallow/pH study
Gastric disorders	
(Gastritis)	
Maternal debris	Stomach washout
Blood – hemorrhagic disease of the newborn	Clotting screen
Maternal stress illness	History
Pyloric stenosis	Test feed
	Ultrasound/barium meal
Small intestinal disorders	
Congenital	
Duodenal atresia	AXR
Extrinsic duodenal obstruction	AXR
Malrotation	AXR
Volvulus	AXR
Meconium ileus	AXR (calcification)
Intestinal duplication	AXR
Acquired	
Pseudo-obstruction/sepsis	Full blood count, septic screen
NEC	AXR – free or intramural gas
Proctocolitis	Stool cultures
Food allergy	Dietary manipulation
Incarceration/strangulation	Inspection
Inguinal herniae	AXR
Extraintestinal disorders	
Intracranial lesions	
Asphyxia, meningitis	
Intracranial hemorrhage	
Hydrocephalus/SOL	
Renal disorders	
Urinary tract infection	MSU/bag urine
Obstructive uropathy	Renal ultrasound
Metabolic disorders	
Galactosemia	Urine sugar
Hyperammonemias	Urine amino acids
Phenylketonuria	Urine amino acids
Organic acidemias	pH urine
Congenital adrenal hyperplasia	Electrolytes
Drugs	Theophylline

AXR, abdominal X-ray; CXR, chest X-ray; MSU, mid stream urine; NEC, necrotizing enterocolitis; SOL, space occupying lesion.

Bile-stained vomiting is a more sinister sign and usually indicates NEC, obstruction or some other surgical condition. Request for a surgical opinion should always be considered. The higher the obstruction, the earlier the presentation; thus duodenal atresia, jejunal atresia, malrotation and volvulus and high duplications all present in the first 2 days of life with marked vomiting and intolerance of feeds. Low obstructions due to Hirschsprung's disease, milk plug functional obstruction and anal atresia may present more insidiously with a period of obstipation or constipation before the vomiting starts towards the end of the first week. Meconium ileus due to cystic fibrosis presents at any time in the first week (usually in the first few days). Acquired obstruction obviously tends to present later but one should always examine the abdomen carefully for signs of strangulated herniae and intussusception and the presence of anal atresia. These conditions are discussed in more detail elsewhere.

The AXR is pivotal in making the initial diagnosis. Fluid levels indicate both the obstruction and the level of obstruction. Duodenal atresia causes a classic double bubble whilst high obstructions reveal small bowel fluid levels with no gas in the rectum. Colonic disorders may have many fluid levels but often require contrast enemas to distinguish between long segment Hirschsprung's disease, meconium ileus of cystic fibrosis (although abdominal calcification may be seen following intrauterine perforation) and the even more rare true pseudo-obstruction (visceral myopathy or neuropathy). Free abdominal gas indicates an intestinal perforation usually due to NEC but occasionally spontaneous or associated with an atretic segment. Volvulus secondary to malrotation is dramatic with large dilated loops (the American football sign) or may be inferred from the abnormal distribution of the bowel gas in malrotation (although this usually requires upper gut contrast studies for accurate delineation). When fluid levels are less marked and the infant is sick or jaundiced, pseudo-obstruction due to sepsis is likely.

Surgical disorders when identified will require prompt transfer to a unit specializing in neonatal surgery. An intravenous infusion of 10% dextrose should be started and the infant kept warm in the incubator. The stomach should be aspirated hourly and the aspirate replaced as normal saline intravenously. If the infant is shocked, resuscitation with 10–20 ml/kg of plasma is required. If the infant is sick, parenteral antibiotics must be started whilst awaiting the result of the septic screen. In cases of tracheoesophageal fistula, a large bore double lumen tube (raplogal tube) is passed into the proximal pouch. Air is passed into one lumen and aspirated with any secretions from the other. Continuous drainage in this way prevents apnea and aspiration episodes. The infant is nursed prone with a slight head tilt.

General disorders. Non-gastrointestinal causes for vomiting must always be borne in mind. Sepsis will cause an ileus, as already described. Urinary tract infection without bacteremia, however, has long been recognized to present with gastrointestinal symptoms, most commonly with vomiting. (Obstructive renal disease, e.g. ureteral valves, may also present in this way in the absence of infection.) Urine culture microscopy must always be performed. Plasma urea and electrolytes are also important to identify acidosis (renal and metabolic disease) and alkalosis (pyloric stenosis occasionally presents early in the neonatal period). Intracerebral asphyxial insults may cause vomiting acutely due to raised intracranial pressure, and meningitis may present as vomiting at any age. Other cerebral causes of vomiting such as hydrocephalus, space-occupying lesions and the diencephalic syndrome rarely present in this fashion in the neonatal period. Metabolic disorders are a cause of vomiting in the neonatal period and should always be considered if metabolic acidosis (and/or hypoglycemia) is present, or if a baby appears septic but has a metabolic alkalosis (urea cycle disorders). Galactosemia may present as early as the first day and the urine must always be tested for reducing substances. Usually the infants with metabolic disorders start vomiting after milk feeding has been established and they have been exposed to a reasonable protein load (e.g. the hyperammonemias, disorders of amino metabolism and the non-ketotic hypoglycemias). The presence of constipation as well as vomiting in a dysmorphic infant may alert one to the presence of idiopathic hypercalcemia and vomiting with dehydration and electrolyte disturbance to congenital adrenal hyperplasia which may also present with diarrhea. The organic acidemias must be excluded by specific assays (dicarboxylic aciduria) on acute phase urines collected when the patient is symptomatic and, where possible, acidotic. After the first week of life acquired metabolic disorders such as diabetic ketoacidosis and Munchausen syndrome by proxy may rarely have to be considered.

Persisting vomiting/vomiting after the first week of life. Babies presenting after the first week of life tend to have acquired problems although lower intestinal obstructions, malrotation and in the VLBW baby, NEC may present later. Vomiting is one of the commonest presentations to a pediatric unit and consideration of the baby's clinical state again allows a fairly rapid differentiation.

- Baby well: abdomen normal
  - posseting
  - feeding disorder
  - gastroesophageal reflux
  - gastrointestinal food allergy
  - pyloric stenosis
  - urinary tract infection
- Baby unwell: abdomen distended
  - late obstruction
  - peritonitis/appendicitis
  - intussusception
  - NEC

Persistent vomiting even in a relatively well baby, especially if accompanied by poor growth, may indicate a more serious underlying disorder. If investigations are normal, a feeding disorder is excluded and the vomiting still persists then the differential diagnosis usually rests between a dietary food intolerance and gastroesophageal reflux.

Gastroesophageal reflux (*GOR*). GOR may present with vomiting in the first month of life. It must be remembered that GOR is a physiological condition, associated with transient relaxation of the lower esophageal sphincter, and should only be investigated and treated if there is GOR-associated disease present (GORD) – esophagitis, strictures, chronic aspiration, failure to thrive. In the term baby, GORD can be investigated with upper gastrointestinal endoscopy, pH meter or radiolabelled milk scan, although many would use an empirical trial of treatment first. The role of contrast studies is to rule out anatomical lesions (malrotation) or strictures. Infants at risk of GORD include those with repaired esophageal atresia, those with bronchopulmonary dysplasia, and those with severe neurodevelopmental problems. In the premature infant recurrent consolidation due to aspiration from GOR may lead to a disorder indistinguishable from bronchopulmonary dysplasia. GOR may also be a major cause of apneic spells resistant to methylxanthine therapy. Esophageal pH studies may confirm this, although they undoubtedly underestimate postprandial reflux in the preterm baby where the decreased acid production of the stomach is readily buffered for prolonged periods by the milk feed. Sometimes again it is more practical to treat such infants empirically. Treatment includes pharmacological, surgical and non-pharmacological, non-surgical options such as positioning and feed thickeners.

The role of the last group of measures has recently been systematically reviewed, and it was concluded that commonly used conservative measures do not have any proven efficacy in GORD in infancy.[666] Positioning at 60 degree elevation in seats was found to increase reflux compared to prone positioning, and thickened formulas reduced vomiting but not reflux.[666] The supine position is currently recommended for infants due to reduced risk of SIDS. There are no high quality randomized trials of drug or surgical therapy confined to infancy with GOR as a primary outcome, so systematic review is currently unhelpful. Antacids and alginates, prokinetic agents such as domperidone, antisecretory agents such as ranitidine, and proton pump inhibitors such as omeprazole are all used in the treatment of GORD in infancy, although few are licensed for this. Fundoplication, increasingly by the laparoscopic route, is reserved for persisting and severe GORD.

Gastrointestinal food allergy. Food allergy is becoming increasingly common in children, and may present in the first weeks of life, even in solely breast-fed babies.[667] Sensitization can occur due to minute doses of antigens (usually glycoproteins) passing into breast milk. Symptoms such as vomiting follow food ingestion, due to an abnormal immunologically mediated reaction within the gastrointestinal tract. These reactions can be type I immediate hypersensitivity, which will present with vomiting, or type IV delayed hypersensitivity, which presents with poor growth, diarrhea and rectal bleeding. For acute allergy, careful history will reveal the ingestion of an allergen, such as cows' milk protein, followed by vomiting, and occasionally pallor, diarrhea and rarely acute anaphylaxis. The best investigation is exclusion, causing relief of symptoms, and challenge, which may need to be in a controlled environment. The presence of specific IgE antibodies and positive skin-prick tests are valuable, especially in breast-fed babies, but are not invariable. Treatment is elimination of cows' milk, usually by substitution with a protein hydrolysate or amino-acid based feed (Neocate, SHS, Liverpool).

Neonatal diarrhea (Table 10.79)

Diarrhea is a relatively uncommon symptom in the neonatal period although most breast-fed children will have loose yellow seedy stools. Mothers and midwives are very clear when the stools are pathological, usually because they are watery with little or no solid matter, are increased in frequency or contain blood and mucus. The commonest cause of loose stools is phototherapy but this causes no harm as long as the fluids are increased appropriately. The loose stools due to nasojejunal tube feeding are similarly of little importance and usually pass unnoticed by nursing staff. The commonest serious causes of diarrhea are gastroenteritis and NEC and the latter should always be considered in infants with diarrhea. Usually, however, the characteristic bloody/mucusy stool together with the abdominal extension and X-ray signs give the diagnosis.

Outbreaks of viral gastroenteritis are not unknown in the neonatal unit and the infants respond to the normal management of such infections. Stools should be sent for cultures and electron microscopy for viruses. A full infection screen should be performed to exclude systemic causes of diarrhea. Diarrhea always causes loss of water and electrolytes, and dehydration can rapidly occur; the newborn are more susceptible to this, due to gut immaturity. The baby should be rehydrated with oral rehydration therapy (ORT) or intravenous fluids as necessary. Once replacement of deficit has occurred, re-institution of feeds should occur, with maintenance fluids and ongoing losses replaced with ORT or intravenous fluids. Complications of diarrhea include electrolyte disturbance with acidosis, nosocomial spread of the disease (the infants should be isolated), secondary lactose intolerance (check for stool pH and reducing sugars), and secondary cows' milk protein intolerance.

Table 10.79 Neonatal diarrhea

Etiology	Investigations
Iatrogenic	
Phototherapy	
Nasojejunal tube feeding	
Narcotic withdrawal	Drug history – maternal, neonatal
Infective	
Gastroenteritis	
Viral	Stool electron microscopy
Bacterial	Culture
Systemic infection	Infection screen
Surgical	
Necrotizing enterocolitis	Abdominal X-ray
Appendicitis	
Hirschsprung's disease	Rectal examination, biopsy
Congenital enteropathy	
Lactase deficiency	Stool sugars – Clinitest, chromatography
Sucrase-isomaltase deficiency	Biopsy
Glucose-galactose malabsorption	
Congenital Na/H exchange deficiency	
Congenital chloridorrhea	Stool electrolytes/osmolality
Congenital microvillus atrophy	
Tufting enteropathy	
Abetalipoproteinemia	Fasting cholesterol/lipids + biopsy
Acrodermatitis enteropathica	Plasma zinc
Acquired enteropathy	
Food allergy	Family history, eosinophilia on biopsy
Immunodeficiency (SCID)	Immunoglobulins, lymphopenia
Metabolic disorders	
Congenital adrenal hyperplasia	Electrolytes
Dicarboxylic aciduria	Venous pH, urine organic acids
Drugs	
Antibiotics	
Prostaglandins	
Theophylline	
Pancreatic insufficiency	
Cystic fibrosis	
Schwachman–Diamond syndrome	

SCID, Severe combined immunodeficiency.

Other causes of diarrhea are all rare[668] and may present as intractable diarrhea, defined as watery diarrhea for more than 2 weeks. They are often associated with malabsorption and undernutrition. Many of these infants eventually will be found to have a specific diagnosis, but a group remains in which no primary cause can be determined. Congenital disorders of the enterocyte usually cause loose stools in the neonatal period although they may present later with intractable diarrhea since the pathological nature of the stools is not always appreciated initially. An antenatal ultrasound may have shown distended fluid-filled bowel loops. Food allergy, particularly the delayed type, may present as diarrhea. The more specific entity of cows' milk colitis, however, presents with bloody diarrhea and must be differentiated from NEC and other conditions (intussusception, Meckel's diverticulitis and volvulus). Diagnosis rests on the resolution of the symptoms after appropriate substitution of the feed. Where the infant's size and condition permit, a rectal biopsy may show eosinophils in the inflammatory infiltrate. Immunodeficiency, especially severe combined immunodeficiency, may present with diarrhea and often a protein-losing enteropathy in the neonatal period. Lymphopenia on the blood film and other coexistent signs of infection (such as an interstitial pneumonia on chest X-ray) should alert one to this diagnosis. Similarly, abnormalities of the urea and electrolytes or a marked acidosis should suggest the possibility of a metabolic disorder and one should always inquire jointly of the mother's and baby's drug history.

Nutritional management remains the cornerstone of treatment of intractable diarrhea, and the majority require parenteral nutrition, with very careful and slow introduction of enteral feeds.[668] In many cases, home parenteral nutrition or intestinal transplantation are the only long term therapeutic options.

Neonatal constipation (Table 10.80)

The failure to pass meconium in the first 24 h in a term baby is a significant symptom and should prompt a search for the underlying cause. In a preterm baby, however, failure to open the bowels is not uncommon and many neonatal units use glycerin suppositories (chips) from day 1 to encourage bowel actions and facilitate tolerance of enteral feeds. After prematurity, the most common organic cause of constipation in the first weeks of life is Hirschsprung's disease and this must be excluded by rectal examination followed by suction biopsy in all term infants when constipation follows on failure to pass meconium within the first 48 h. Hirschsprung's disease has an incidence of 1 in 5000 live births, and has complex inheritance; to date, eight different genes have been found to be involved.[669] Neonatal constipation should always be taken seriously; failure to open the bowels at least every other day is outside the range of normality. Clinical findings and simple investigations as outlined in Table 10.80 should allow one to identify most organic causes.

Overfeeding is a common cause of constipation in older neonate infants. In this situation either the baby is very greedy or mother mistakes thirst for hunger and the baby is offered, and takes, more and more milk. (It is almost unknown as a cause of constipation in the breast-fed infant when autoregulation of the maternal milk allows a more diluted milk to be provided for the baby as the volume of milk taken increases.) An accurate feeding history soon identifies this problem. It is, however, rare in the early neonatal period.

The management of simple constipation in the neonatal period is similar to that at an older age. Correction of a feeding disorder and provision of an adequate amount of extra water to slake thirst (especially in hot weather) will correct most cases. If this proves insufficient, intermittent suppositories are occasionally successful but more usually infants will need a stool softener (lactulose 2.5 ml b.d.) for a period of time to regularize the bowel habit. Rarely a bowel stimulant such as Senokot is needed.

Table 10.80 Neonatal constipation

Etiology	Investigation
1. Ileus	
Prematurity	Abdominal X-ray
Major insult – sepsis	Abdominal X-ray
Asphyxia	Abdominal X-ray
2. Pseudo-obstruction	
Neuropathy	Abdominal X-ray, barium meal and follow through
Myopathy	Rectal biopsy
3. Meconium plug	
4. Low bowel obstruction	
Meconium ileus/ cystic fibrosis	Immunoreactive trypsin
Hirschsprung's disease	Rectal examination, barium enema
Colonic atresia	
5. Anorectal anomalies	
Imperforate anus – anal atresia, anorectal atresia	Rectal examination
Rectal atresia	
Anal stenosis/stricture	
Rectal stenosis/stricture	
6. Metabolic disorder	
Hypothyroidism	Thyroxin, thyroid stimulating hormone
Hypercalcemia	Calcium
Salt- and water-losing states	Urea and electrolytes
Renal tubular acidosis	Urine pH
7. Overfeeding	

Gastrointestinal bleeding

Gastrointestinal bleeding in the newborn is a potentially serious problem.[670] It can present in four ways – hematemesis, hematochezia (bright red blood passed per rectum), melena or occult bleeding. The initial assessment should rapidly address the need for resuscitation, and whether bleeding is ongoing. Recognition of shock should not rely on hypotension, a late and ominous finding in infancy. Differentiation of upper from lower gastrointestinal bleeding will guide the order of investigations and the therapy. Hematemesis is a clear guide of upper bleeding, melena suggests a source far from the rectum, and hematochezia can occur with small intestinal or colonic bleeding. Diagnostic techniques include upper and lower gastrointestinal endoscopy using neonatal endoscopes, scintigraphy (Meckel's scan), ultrasonography, other imaging, and rarely laparoscopy or laparotomy.

Swallowed maternal blood explains about 30% of bleeding in the newborn.[670] Small amounts of fresh blood or coffee-ground material in vomitus is not rare, and if self-limiting the prognosis is good. The common sources of upper gastrointestinal bleeding in the newborn are nasopharyngeal bleeding, swallowed maternal blood, esophagitis, gastritis and stress ulcer; rarer causes include bleeding disorders, duplication cyst, trauma from tubes, and vascular malformations. The common sources of lower gastrointestinal bleeding in the newborn are anal fissure, enteritis, intussusception, NEC, food allergy and an upper source; rarer causes include pseudomembranous colitis, duplication cyst, Meckel's diverticulum, Hirschsprung's enterocolitis, ischemia and vascular malformations. Treatment of all moderate and severe cases includes assessment, resuscitation, appropriate venous access, consultation with a pediatric surgeon, then identification and treatment of the cause.

Necrotizing enterocolitis (NEC)

NEC is a much feared condition in every neonatal unit, and has a much higher incidence in the VLBW infant, with an incidence of 2–5%. In the UK, a survey by the British Paediatric Surveillance Unit to the end of 1994 reported over 300 new cases, with a total mortality of 22%.[671] The etiology is unknown but is likely to be multifactorial with superinfection by gas-forming bacteria and failure of the mucosal barrier in the immature gut, playing important roles. Precipitating factors include hyperosmolar feeds, perinatal asphyxia, polycythemia and umbilical vessel catheterization. A clear association has emerged between the presence of reversed end-diastolic flow in the umbilical artery in utero in the severely growth retarded infant and the development of NEC in the first weeks of life.[672] Breast milk is partly protective.[673]

The disease presents with increasing aspirates (usually bile-stained) or vomiting (usually bilious but occasionally bloodstained). Diarrhea follows (or occasionally precedes) the failure to tolerate feeds and may be watery or contain mucus and visible blood and pus. The baby is often unwell, lethargic and having apneic episodes. Examination reveals a tense distended tender abdomen which is quiet (or silent if perforation has taken place). Tenderness and/or guarding suggest peritonitis has supervened and in the later stages there may be edema and inflammation of the abdominal wall (producing a 'peau d'orange' appearance in the skin) or an underlying abdominal mass. Blood cultures are positive in 18–60% of cases and septic or hypovolemic shock may be a complication and the infant may collapse and die. Diagnosis is classically made on the plain abdominal X-ray. This initially shows separation of the bowel loops due to ascites with fluid levels. Then the periluminal tramlines indicating intramural gas appear (Fig. 10.39a) especially in the cecum, ascending and descending colon and sigmoid. Later signs include gas in the portal tree (Fig. 10.39b) and gas under the diaphragm following perforation. In the early stages the diagnosis may also be suggested by the presence of a proctocolitis using an auroscope as a proctoscope.

A pancolitis is usually found at postmortem. The histology reveals a characteristic hemorrhagic inflammatory infiltration. The differential diagnoses include generalized sepsis, meconium ileus, malrotation and volvulus, hemorrhagic disease of the newborn, cows' milk colitis and intussusception and the even rarer neonatal appendicitis. The other causes of abdominal distention (Table 10.81) must also be considered especially spontaneous perforation of the gut and other causes of ascites.

The prevention of NEC has been addressed in six Cochrane reviews.[649,650,674–677] None of those concerning feeding strategies[660,661,674,675] contains enough high quality randomized trials of sufficient power to demonstrate superiority of one feeding regime over another. Five randomized trials (involving 2095 newborn) of oral immunoglobulin usage were reviewed by Foster & Cole[676] who concluded that the evidence did not currently support this strategy. Five randomized trials (involving 456 infants) of enteral antibiotic prophylaxis were reviewed by Bury & Tudehope[677] who concluded that a larger single randomized trial was needed to assess benefit and harm. Management is initially medical and conservative.[678] Oral feeds should be stopped and the stomach placed on free drainage. A septic screen is performed and it is customary to give triple intravenous antibiotics (e.g. a penicillin such as benzyl penicillin or amoxicillin, an aminoglycoside such as gentamicin and metronidazole) to cover the bacteremia. Oral vancomycin may be a valuable adjunct to treatment. Blood counts, clotting screen, urea and electrolytes and albumen are checked and appropriate supportive management given as indicated. Most surgeons insist that intravenous feeding through a central line should be instituted for 10 days and the bowel rested. Afterwards feeds should be introduced slowly. Expressed breast milk or a preterm formula are used, although a protein hydrolysate may be needed as lactose and cows'

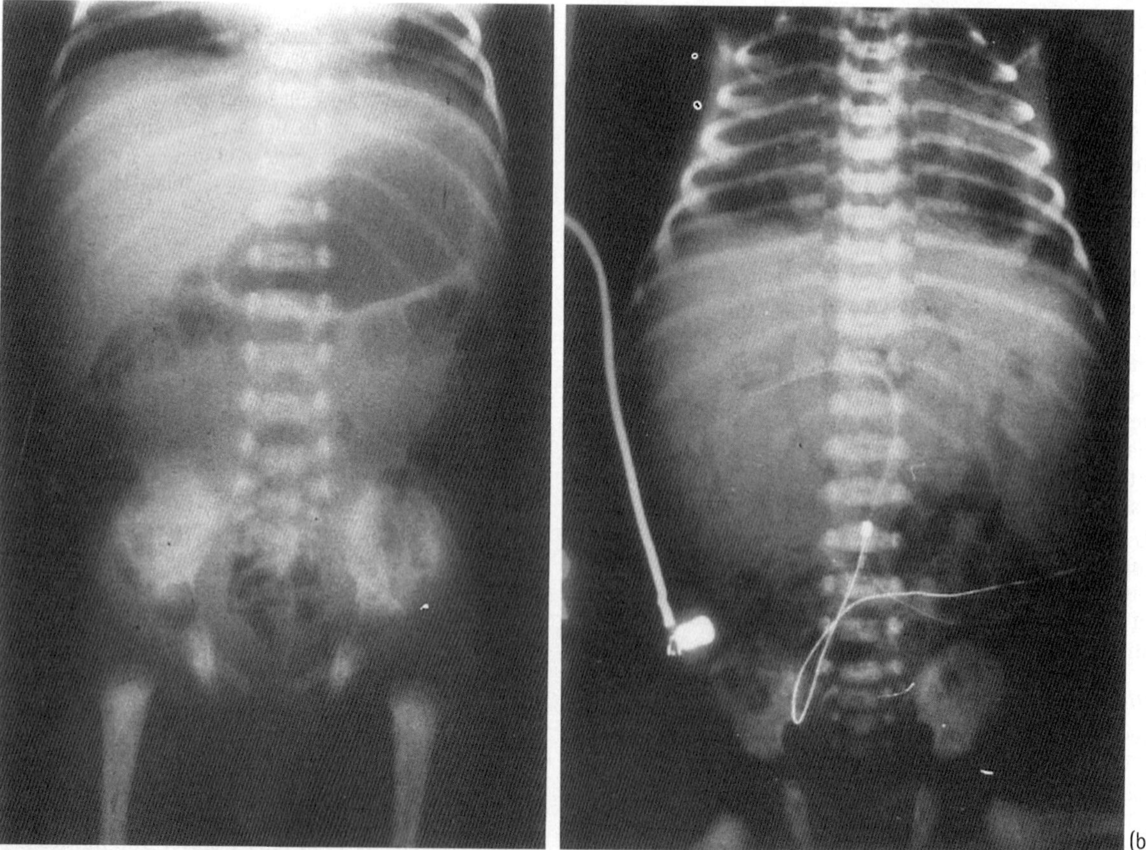

Fig. 10.39 (a) Necrotizing enterocolitis. Double lumen to the colon can be seen clearly at the hepatic flexure and triple lumen in the descending colon – both effects caused by intramural gas. (b) Gas tracts ramifying throughout the liver in portal vessels and periportal tissue. Arterial catheter is adequately sited. The venous catheter passes into the right hepatic vein.

Table 10.81 Cause of abdominal distention

1. Intestinal obstruction
2. Ileus and intestinal pseudo-obstruction
3. Intestinal perforation - Congenital/spontaneous - Acquired
4. Ascites - Congestive cardiac failure/hydrops fetalis - Peritonitis/necrotizing enterocolitis - Hypoalbuminemia/nephrotic syndrome - Urinary/ruptured urinary tract with urethral valves - Biliary/spontaneous rupture of bile duct - Chylous/disordered lymphatic drainage
5. Mass - Hydronephrosis - Congenital malignancy, Wilms'/neuroblastoma - Reduplication - Ovarian

milk protein intolerance are often seen in the recovery phase in these infants. Surgery is required for the acute complications of perforation and sometimes bleeding, or if there is failure to improve with medical therapy. Later complications (stricture formations with subacute small bowel obstruction, blind loop syndrome and rectal bleeding) may also require surgery, as may a recurrence which occurs in 10% of patients. Short bowel syndrome (see below) may occur.

Short bowel syndrome

Short bowel syndrome is defined functionally, rather than anatomically; it exists where there is malabsorption in the presence of a shortened small intestine. The development and refinement of parenteral nutrition, techniques and equipment for prolonged central venous access, new enteral formula development and the back-up of intestinal and/or liver transplantation have changed this from a fatal disorder 30 years ago, to one where most infants can have a prolonged life span into adult life.[679] Given that it is a rare and highly complex problem, assessment and management must involve tertiary center pediatric gastroenterologists and pediatric surgeons; this review will only briefly cover etiology, pathology, physiology and management.

There are marked differences in regional function throughout the gastrointestinal tract. The stomach acts as a reservoir, and the jejunum is the site of greatest nutrient absorption. It is also leaky, allowing bidirectional flow of fluid and electrolytes between luminal and vascular spaces. The ileum is the site of maximal fluid and electrolyte absorption, with less nutrients absorbed. Vitamin B_{12} and bile salts are specifically absorbed in the terminal ileum. The ileocecal valve acts as a barrier to colonic bacteria, and the colon absorbs sodium and water, with a salvage capacity to absorb some carbohydrate and fat. The relative degree of jejunal, ileal and colonic loss in this syndrome determines the pathophysiological effects, and thus the management. By far the commonest cause of short bowel syndrome is NEC, but many other prenatal (vascular accidents, atresias, volvulus, abdominal wall defects) and postnatal (volvulus, thrombosis, Hirschsprung's disease, neuropathies and myopathies causing pseudo-obstruction) etiologies exist.

The management of short bowel syndrome is a complex and multistage process,[668] which initially involves restoration and maintenance of fluid and electrolyte balance, with appropriate parenteral nutritional support to allow the process of intestinal adaptation to begin. In this process, hyperplasia of the mucosal epithelium occurs, with resulting increase in absorptive area, and later of functional capacity. Enteral feeding is slowly begun once the baby has stabilized, usually with an elemental formula. The aim is to increase enteral feeds within the limits of tolerance until weaned from TPN. There are few randomized trials of components of management of short bowel syndrome. Other medical management includes treating hypergastrinemia, cycling TPN, and treatment of small bowel bacterial overgrowth. Surgical management includes stricturoplasties, tapering procedures, and consideration of small bowel and/or liver transplant if vascular access or chronic liver disease become problematic. Complications include macro- and micronutrient deficiency, TPN-associated cholestasis, central venous catheter thrombosis and infection, and small bowel bacterial overgrowth. Prognosis depends upon presence of ileocecal valve, length and quality of remaining bowel, number of anastomoses, and small bowel bacterial overgrowth. The overall survival from diagnosis to 5 years of age is now over 90%, and more than 50% will come off parenteral nutrition.

BILIRUBIN METABOLISM[680]

Bilirubin is one of the end products of heme catabolism and in normal circumstances has to be processed by the liver for its excretion. In early neonatal life there is a much greater production of bilirubin. The Hb mass at birth is high (and further increased by such factors as delayed clamping of the cord) and contains approximately 80% fetal Hb. This is replaced within 4 months by adult Hb. This obligatory red cell turnover is the major factor in the excess bilirubin production (each 1 g Hb produces 600 μmol of bilirubin). To this must be added the bilirubin produced by bruising, cephalhematoma and shunt bilirubin (bilirubin produced by heme pigments in the reticuloendothelial system that are never incorporated into Hb: approximately 20% of the total bilirubin production).

Heme is metabolized to biliverdin by heme oxygenase (Fig. 10.40)[681] which is found in the liver, spleen and macrophages and whose activity is increased manyfold in the face of such an increased substrate load. The biliverdin is rapidly reduced to bilirubin by biliverdin reductase using NADPH as a proton donor. The end product, bilirubin XIIa, is insoluble because of the hydrogen bonding between the two pyrrole rings (a process facilitated by the ionization of the molecule that occurs below pH 7.4) (Fig. 10.41).[682] The insoluble bilirubin is bound to albumin (binding capacity 0.5–1.0 mmol bilirubin/mol albumin). At a bilirubin concentration of 340 μmol/L the molar ratio exceeds 1:1 and dissociation of the bilirubin occurs readily. Because of its fat solubility (increased at low pH) this bilirubin is readily deposited in the tissues.

Bilirubin is transported through the hepatocyte membrane by a carrier-mediated process (Fig. 10.42)[682] and is then carried to the smooth endoplasmic reticulum by ligandin or Y protein. This has a low concentration at birth but increases to adult levels by 5–10 days of age. In the smooth endoplasmic reticulum the bilirubin is conjugated with a uridine moiety to bilirubin monoglucuronide by the enzyme glucuronyltransferase. This too has a low activity at birth but following induction by the high bilirubin load, adult levels are reached by 14 days of age irrespective of gestation (i.e. it is a birth-related event). The activity of this enzyme can be induced by phenobarbital or other microsomal enzyme-inducing drugs. The bilirubin monoglucuronide is converted to bilirubin diglucuronide by glucuronyltransferase (requiring UDP glucuronic acid) and then transported across the canalicular membrane by an energy-dependent carrier-mediated system.

The excretory mechanisms described above result in a high concentration of bilirubin in the bile. In the adult this consists mostly of bilirubin IXa, a pigment which cannot be excreted without

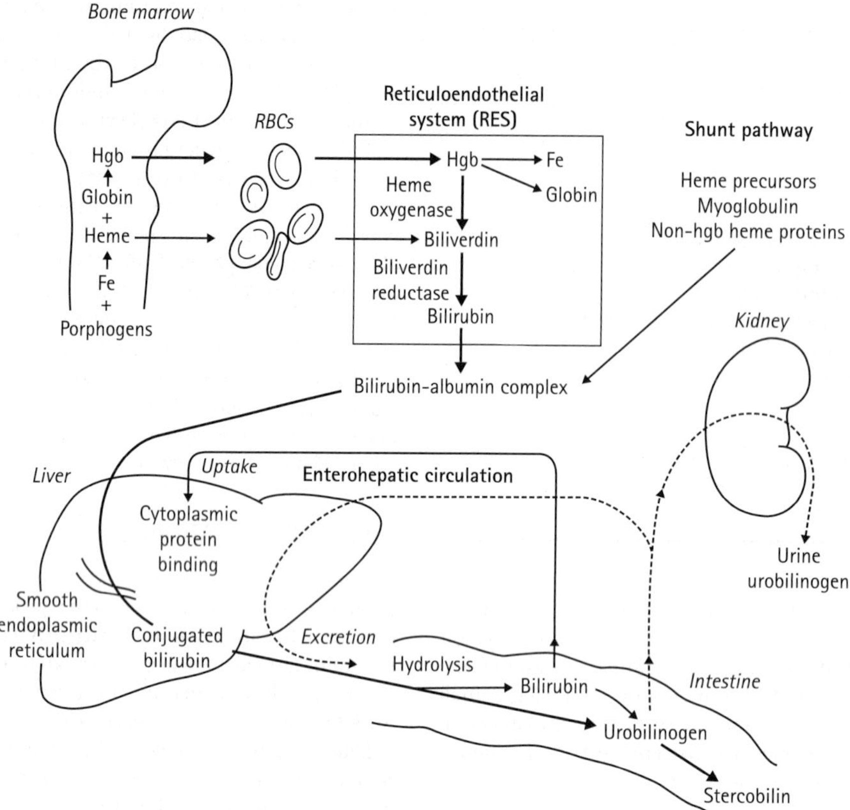

Fig. 10.40 The pathway of bilirubin production, transport and metabolism. (From Garcia 1972[681] with permission.)

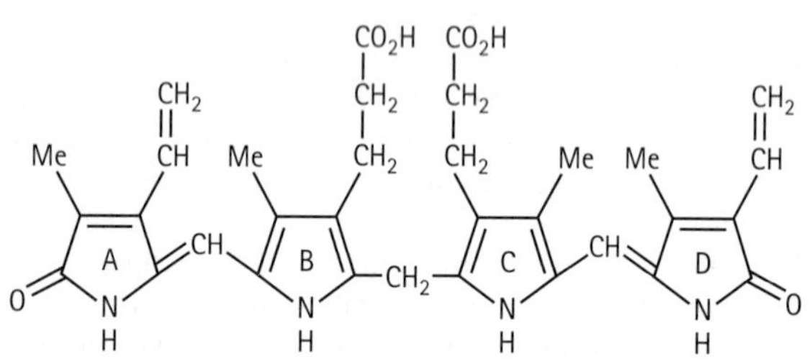

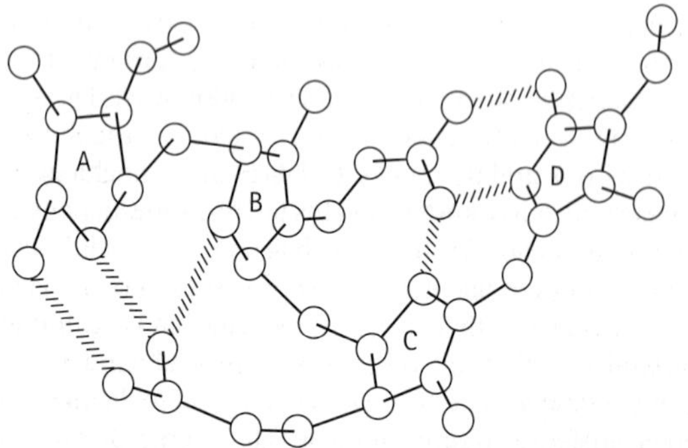

Fig. 10.41 Primary structure of bilirubin above, and below tertiary structure with hydrogen bonds shown as shaded lines. This folded structure serves to mask the polar carboxyl residues and renders the bilirubin molecule water insoluble/fat soluble. (From Schmidt 1978[682])

conjugation which alters its involuted hydrogen-bonded conformation. However, the other bilirubin isomers can be excreted directly in the bile since they are naturally water soluble. The major photochemical effect of phototherapy makes use of this fact. Under blue light (420–480 nm) bilirubin IXa is converted by photoisomerization to Z-lumirubin (Fig. 10.43).[683] There is a 180 degree rotation of a terminal pyrrole which prohibits intramolecular hydrogen bonding, thus disrupting the tertiary structure of the bilirubin IXa isomer, and exposes the carboxyl radical, thus creating a polar water-soluble pigment which can be excreted in the bile.

It is clear from the above that the neonate arrives in the world unable to cope with the normal bilirubin load and thus a degree of jaundice is to be expected. This is recognized by the phrase *physiological jaundice of the newborn*. Postnatally there is a rapid rise in the bilirubin due to a combination of high bilirubin load and decreased hepatic excretion. Following the initial rise there is a slow fall due to the slow development of hepatic carrier proteins (induction of ribosomal enzyme complexes). The maximum allowable level of physiological jaundice is not clear. A level as low as 210 μmol/L by the third day of life has been claimed to indicate the need for further investigation but, in practice, most clinicians probably would not investigate the cause of jaundice unless the patient required phototherapy or other clinical features were present, the most important of which is the postnatal age of patient.

NEONATAL JAUNDICE (Table 10.82)

Early jaundice (< 10 days)

First 24 h (hemolytic disease of the newborn, HDN)

This is by far the most dangerous form of jaundice in the newborn as the bilirubin levels can rise rapidly into the toxic range. The most

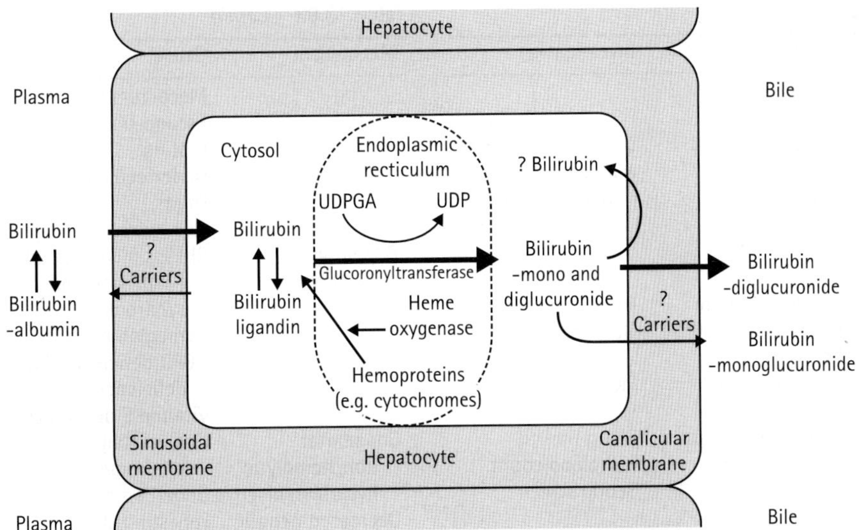

Fig. 10.42 Bilirubin handling by the liver. For explanation see text. (Modified from Schmidt 1978[682])

common cause is rhesus hemolytic disease although with current obstetric management it is now rare in the developed world. Sensitization of the mother (usually by small fetomaternal transfusions in previous pregnancies and particularly deliveries) will result in the production of anti-D IgM and IgG. The latter is responsible for rhesus disease in the neonate which is characterized by a (often highly) positive Coombs' test and extravascular hemolysis in the spleen. ABO incompatibility, now the most common cause for HDN (mother usually blood group O, infant blood group A or B) in the UK occurs in 15% of pregnancies. It is particularly common in Negros. Again the IgG antibody is the important hemolysin but in this case the Coombs' test is often negative (possibly due to the decreased number of A and B sites on the fetal erythrocyte). Laboratory investigation is notoriously unreliable at predicting infants at risk from ABO hemolytic disease but microspherocytosis on the blood film is a useful diagnostic pointer to the condition.[684] Red blood cell destruction occurs primarily by extravascular mechanisms and is more rapid in ABO incompatibility with the antibody disappearing within 2–3 days. Occasionally minor blood group antibodies (anti-Kell, anti-Duffy) cause hemolytic disease and these are usually Coombs' positive.

Hemolysis also occurs in the absence of blood group incompatibility. Sepsis is said to cause jaundice at this age and should always be excluded. In fact, it rarely turns out to be responsible for such early jaundice but congenital infections, e.g. rubella, syphilis and toxoplasmosis, can present in this way. The most common non-immunological cause of hemolytic jaundice within 24 h is congenital hemolytic anemia due to a red cell metabolic defect (e.g. glucose-6-phosphate dehydrogenase (G6PD) deficiency or pyruvic kinase (PK) deficiency) or structural defect (congenital spherocytosis, elliptocytosis and pyknocytosis). In these cases there is often a family history. G6PD deficiency occurs more commonly in patients of Mediterranean, African or Oriental origin. Appropriate hematological investigations and enzyme assays usually provide a rapid diagnosis.

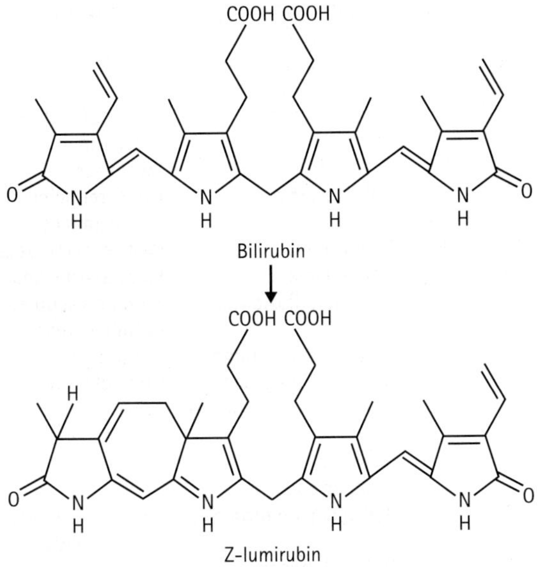

COOH COOH

Bilirubin

COOH COOH

Z-lumirubin

Fig. 10.43 Photoisomerization by light converts the stable isomer of bilirubin to the thermodynamically unstable Z-lumirubin (From McDonagh et al 1982[683])

After 24 h

Of normal neonates 65% exhibit clinical jaundice (85 μmol/L or 5 mg/dl). In most patients excessive jaundice at this stage is due to exacerbation of the normal physiological jaundice of the newborn. The 95th percentile for term infants is 190 μmol/L (11.5 mg/dl) for bottle-fed and 240 μmol/L (14.5 mg/dl) for breast-fed infants. The more premature the infant the more immature the liver although this may be balanced by decreased bilirubin production since exchange transfusion is rarely required despite the almost obligatory use of phototherapy in infants of less than 30 weeks' gestation. Excessive production of bilirubin from severe bruising or cephalhematomata, polycythemia or ingestion of maternal blood commonly causes jaundice in this period.

The most important cause to consider is acquired bacterial infection or rarely congenitally transmitted infections (CMV, rubella, toxoplasmosis, syphilis). Direct involvement of the liver by the infective process is one reason for the jaundice, as is increased bilirubin breakdown with disseminated intravascular coagulation. However, it is likely that the nature of the hyperbilirubinemia is multifactorial.

Inadequate calorie intake and decreased glucose production will lead to a reduction in glycogen and energy available for the production and conversion of the uridine diphosphoglucuronic acid required for the conjugation by the bilirubin glucuronyltransferase.

Table 10.82 Neonatal jaundice

Mechanism	Cause	Investigation
1. Early jaundice (<10 days)		
a. *First 24 h*		
Immune hemolysis	Rhesus disease	Direct Coombs' test
	ABO incompatibility	Maternal/infant blood group
	Rare blood group antibodies	
Non-immune hemolysis	Glucose-6-phosphate dehydrogenase (G6PD) deficiency	Family history G6PD assay
	Pyruvate kinase (PK) deficiency	PK assay
	Congenital spherocytosis	Blood film
Sepsis		Full blood count Septic screen
b. *After 24 h*		
Physiological jaundice	Prematurity	
	Hypoglycemia	
	Hypoxia	
	Dehydration intestinal stasis	
Excess bilirubin production	Bruising	
	Cephalohematoma	
	Disseminated	
	Intravascular coagulation	
	Intraventricular hemorrhage	
	Polycythemia	Full blood count
	Ingestion maternal blood	
	(Melena)	
Infection	Sepsis	Septic screen
	Intrauterine infection	IgM, torch screen
Congenital non-hemolytic hyperbilirubinemia	Crigler–Najjar syndrome	
	Gilbert's syndrome	
Metabolic	Galactosemia	Urine-reducing substances
Congenital hemolytic anemia		
2. Prolonged jaundice (> 10 days)		
a. *Prolonged unconjugated hyperbilirubinemia*		
Breast milk	Breast milk jaundice	Trial of formula milk
	Inhibitor of glucuronyl transferase	
Sepsis	New/persisting	Full blood count, septic screen
Metabolic	Hypothyroidism	Thyroxine, TSH
	Aminoacidemias	Plasma/urine amino acids
	Galactosemia	Urine-reducing substances
	Fructosemia	Liver function tests
	Cystic fibrosis	Immunoreactive trypsin
Increased enterohepatic circulation	Intestinal obstruction	Abdominal X-ray
	Pyloric stenosis	
	Atresia	
	Hirschsprung's disease	
	Meconium ileus	
	Meconium plug	
	Pseudo-obstruction	
	Fasting	
	Underfeeding	
	Drugs	
Persisting hemolysis	Rhesus incompatibility (inspissated bile syndrome)	
	Hemoglobinopathy	
	G6PD deficiency, PK deficiency	
	Vitamin E deficiency	
Congenital non-hemolytic hyperbilirubinemia	Crigler–Najjar syndrome	
	Gilbert's syndrome	
Decreased hepatic uptake	Persisting shunt through ductus venosus	
b. *Prolonged conjugated hyperbilirubinemia*		
Intrahepatic cholestasis		
Infections		
Acquired	Septicemia/bacteremia	Septic screen, chest X-ray
	Urinary tract infection	MSU
	Listeriosis	
	Tuberculosis	
Congenital	Syphilis	
	Malaria	
	Toxoplasmosis	Torch screen
	Hepatitis B, C	Hepatitis B antigen, DNA hepatitis A IgM, HCV RNA
	Epstein–Barr virus	Viral titers
	Rubella	Viral titers
	Coxsackie B, A9	Viral titers
	Cytomegalovirus	Viral titers
	Varicella-zoster	Viral titers
	Herpes simplex	Viral titers
	ECHO virus, adenovirus	Viral titers
	HIV infection	Maternal HIV titers
	Parvovirus B19	
Metabolic disorders	Alpha1-antitrypsin deficiency	alpha1-antitrypsin
	Cystic fibrosis	Immunoreactive trypsin Sweat test
	Galactosemia	Urine-reducing substances
	Fructosemia	WBC enzyme assay
	Tyrosinemia	Plasma/urine amino acids
	GM1 gangliosidosis	Storage vacuoles Lymphocytes
	Gaucher's syndrome	WBC enzyme assays
	Nieman–Pick disease	Urine oligosaccharides
	Mucopolysaccharidosis	Urine mucopolysaccharides
	Sialosis	
	Wolman's disease	
	Zellweger syndrome	Serum catalase/VLC fatty acids
	Dubin–Johnson syndrome	

Table 10.82 Cont'd

Mechanism	Cause	Investigation
	Rotor's syndrome	
	Glutaric aciduria Type II	Urine organic acids
	Bile acid synthesis disorders	
Endocrine	Hypothyroidism	Thyroxine, TSH
	Hypoadrenalism	Urea and electrolytes, 17-OH-progesterone, cortisol, aldosterone
	Hypopituitarism	ACTH
	Diabetes insipidus	Plasma/urine osmolality
	Hypoparathyroidism	
Vascular	Veno-occlusive disease	Ultrasound liver
	Poor perfusion syndromes	
	Budd–Chiari syndrome	
	Hemangioendothelioma	
	Lymphatic defects, familial cholestasis with lymphedema	
Miscellaneous	Infantile polycystic disease	Ultrasound kidney and liver
	Toxins	
	Parenteral nutrition	
	Drugs	
	Halothane	
	Chromosomal disorders – trisomies 21, 18, 13	Chromosomes
	Biliary duct paucity (Alagille's syndrome, non-syndromic)	
	Progressive familial intrahepatic cholestasis (Byler's syndrome)	
	Posthemolytic hepatic dysfunction	
	Neonatal lupus	
Idiopathic neonatal hepatitis		
Extrahepatic cholestasis	Extrahepatic biliary atresia	
	Choledochal cyst	Ultrasound liver
	Bile duct stenosis	
	Spontaneous perforation of bile duct	Abdominal X-ray, ascites
	Gallstones	
	Ascending cholangitis	

ACTH, adernocorticotropic hormone; HCV, hepatitis C virus; MSU, mid stream urine; TSH, thyroid stimulating hormone; VLC fatty acids, very long chain fatty acids; WBC, White blood Cells.

Acidosis may increase bilirubin levels but, more importantly, increases bilirubin toxicity due to the alteration of the equilibrium between free bilirubin and its acid salt, thus decreasing the maximum tolerable level of bilirubin. Dehydration probably increases the bilirubin levels by prolonging gut transit and therefore increasing the enterohepatic circulation. In such conditions as failure to pass meconium, pyloric stenosis and cystic fibrosis with meconium ileus, there will be an increase in the hydrolysis of the conjugated bilirubin by the alkaline duodenal juices and the mucosal beta-glucuronidases of the small intestine, thus increasing the bilirubin returned to the blood via the enterohepatic circulation.

In most cases of neonatal jaundice, the bilirubin levels will fall below the phototherapy range before the end of the second week of life. However, in the premature infant phototherapy may be required for longer. One group of patients that presents with severe early neonatal jaundice that continues beyond the first 10 days (and may also present later) is the rare patient with congenital non-hemolytic hyperbilirubinemias. The most important of these, Crigler–Najjar syndrome, presents as two variants:

1. the autosomal recessive type I with absence of uridine diphosphoglucuronyltransferase (UDPGT) in the liver, characterized by persistent severe unconjugated hyperbilirubinemia;
2. the autosomal dominant type II with defective rather than absent UDPGT activity in which the bilirubin levels are lower (< 340 μmol /L).

This latter variant (known also as Arias syndrome) may present much later in life and for this reason is said to merge diagnostically into the commonest of the unconjugated hyperbilirubinemias, Gilbert's syndrome, which is more common in men and usually presents after puberty. The other familial conjugated hyperbilirubinemias (Dubin–Johnson and Rotor's syndrome) hardly ever present at birth.

Management of early jaundice

Investigation and treatment of cause. It is important that the etiology of the hyperbilirubinemia should be established. A careful obstetric and family history (e.g. spherocytosis) is important. A full blood count, direct Coombs' test, grouping of mother and baby and testing the urine for reducing substances are the usual minimum of investigations required. If infection is suspected a septic and *t*oxoplasmosis, *o*ther infections, *r*ubella, CMV and *h*erpes simplex (TORCH) (congenital infection) screen can be added. Where the hemolysis remains unexplained further hematological investigation (e.g. enzyme assays for G6PD deficiency and PK deficiency) will be needed. In most cases no treatment for the cause of the hemolysis will be available though it behooves the pediatrician to ensure that the mother is given anti-D globulin where indicated. Advice on drugs to be avoided in the future must be made available to the patients with G6PD deficiency. Infection should be treated as indicated.

Treatment of jaundice. *Phototherapy*. The aim of therapy is to keep the level of bilirubin below the toxic level. Phototherapy must be started early enough to prevent the expected rise in bilirubin but not at a level which causes unnecessary work for the nursing staff and, more importantly, an unnecessary separation of mother and baby. Most units have their own chart for plotting bilirubin levels and action lines to indicate the levels at which phototherapy (and exchange transfusion) are indicated. Where a rapidly rising bilirubin is expected such as hemolytic disease and jaundice at less than 24 h, phototherapy should be started straight away and the sequential bilirubin results should be graphed. At a later stage the need for phototherapy is more debatable. As a general rule the more premature the infant the lower the levels of bilirubin that are tolerated and thus a good guiding figure is that phototherapy is indicated when the bilirubin rises above a level given by the formula: birth weight in kg × 100. In term babies phototherapy should be given when the bilirubin rises above 300 μmol/L.

There are many potential complications to phototherapy:

1. Equipment failure/design drawbacks: the lamps must produce radiation in the blue range of 450–460 nm with a minimum irradiance of flux of 4 $\mu W/m^2/nm$. The new generation of phototherapy units are much more efficient than the old (although the blue light is off-putting for the parents). It seems prudent to protect the eyes since changes of premature aging

have been induced by phototherapy in newborn monkeys but no detrimental effect is recorded in the human infant.

2. Dehydration: this is by far the most important complication and is the result of increased insensible water loss through the skin and increased stool water content. Increasing the fluid intake of infants under phototherapy by 15 ml/kg/day will correct this.
3. Loose stools: Z-lumirubin excreted in the bile is a highly polar, non-physiological substance which has a direct secretory effect on intestinal mucosa leading, inevitably, to loose stools. These are not troublesome and frank diarrhea never results. The increased fluid intake is the only therapeutic manipulation required. (Lactose intolerance, however, may also occur.)
4. Parental anxiety: the separation of mother and baby and the terrible color given to the infant by the effective blue lamps are naturally upsetting to parents and a sympathetic explanation of what is happening is mandatory. The best way of minimizing this anxiety is to pay scrupulous attention to the need for phototherapy and to minimize the duration of such therapy.
5. Other effects have been noted experimentally (copper retention, abnormal porphyrin metabolism and damage to DNA in cell cultures) but they do not seem relevant in clinical practice. Bronzing or discoloration of the skin can also occur when phototherapy is used in patients with a cholestatic element to their jaundice.

Exchange transfusion. The exchange transfusion of blood via an umbilical artery or vein is the most efficient way of removing bilirubin (and other noxious substances). It is employed when bilirubin levels reach the toxic range determined both by the gestational age and the clinical state of the baby. Sicker babies with their attendant metabolic derangements such as acidosis are transfused at lower levels. Acceptable criteria for exchange transfusion would be a serum bilirubin of 340 μmol/L (term babies), 300 μmol/L (infants < 2500 g), 250 μmol/L (infants < 1500 g) and 170 μmol/L (infants < 1000 g). In practice, however, most exchange transfusions in the smaller infants (< 1500 g) are performed for reasons other than jaundice (usually a septic child in extremis or for DIC). Most physicians would not immediately exchange an asymptomatic term baby even with severe physiological jaundice greater than 340 μmol/L assuming there was a fairly prompt response to phototherapy (usually given with double lamps in such situations). The commonest indication for exchange transfusion is a rapidly rising bilirubin in the first 24 h of life in babies with hemolytic disease of the newborn (p. 288). The technique is described on page 300. The complications are listed in Table 10.83 together with suitable avoiding action.

Other methods. Attention to clinical detail (for example the correction of acidosis, treatment of infection and maintenance of hemodynamic stability) is valuable. In the small premature infant judicious use of 20% albumen (4–5 ml/kg) will buy time under phototherapy and often obviate the need for a formal exchange transfusion. In the rarer congenital non-hemolytic disorders (Crigler–Najjar type II and Rotor's syndrome) hepatic enzyme inducers such as phenobarbital (1–8 mg/kg/24 h) are used in addition to prolonged daily phototherapy to control the bilirubin levels.

Prolonged jaundice

Any jaundice beyond 10 days in a term infant is pathological but preterm infants (especially VLBW infants) often have jaundice that persists beyond this time for which no cause is found. It is probably wise, however, to investigate all these patients in the same way so that rarer conditions presenting in premature infants are not missed. The basic investigation is the estimation of the percentage of conjugated bilirubin; the majority of patients will have an unconjugated hyperbilirubinemia (conjugated bilirubin < 25% of total). Conjugated hyperbilirubinemia (> 25% of total) is an indication of intra- or extrahepatic cholestasis and is accompanied by bilirubinuria and dark urine (conjugated bilirubin > 25 μmol/L). Early diagnosis, supportive care and specific therapy is mandatory.[687]

Table 10.83 Complications of exchange transfusion

Infection	Sepsis	Strict aseptic technique Fresh blood
	CMV	Appropriate screening donors
	Hepatitis	
Hypothermia		Warm blood/baby
Cardiovascular instability	Transient hypovolemia Hypervolemia	Small aliquots (10–20 ml) Meticulous recording of exchanges
	Cardiac dysrhythmia	Cardiac monitoring
Electrolyte disorders	Hyperkalemia	Monitor electrolytes and blood sugar before and after exchange
	Hypoglycemia	
	Hypocalcemia	Check citrate concentration of donor blood
	Acidosis	
Complications of catheter	Embolic	Minimize duration of catheterization
	Hemorrhage (late portal vein thrombosis)	
Inadequate exchange		Use 170–200 ml/kg over 100 min for full exchange

Prolonged unconjugated hyperbilirubinemia

Breast milk jaundice. The usual cause of such prolonged jaundice is breast milk jaundice but to diagnose this without estimating the percentage of conjugated bilirubin would be negligent. The bilirubin is usually less than 200 μmol/L, but can rise to values up to 400 μmol/L (usually less than 20% conjugated); the patient, however, is well and no treatment is necessary.[685–686] The jaundice usually settles by about 6 weeks although it may occasionally continue up to 4 months. Discontinuation of breast-feeding leads to a rapid fall in the bilirubin. The etiology of this condition long remained obscure and was thought to be due to various constituents of the milk. Breast milk consists of milk constituents which are parceled in maternal breast milk membrane prior to their secretion from the acini of the gland. This membrane is a protein structure and has a functional activity in its own right, e.g. enzymatic (breast milk lipase) and transport (membrane-bound iron). Both of these greatly increase the nutritional efficiency of milk. In patients with breast milk jaundice a beta-glucuronidase has been shown to be present in mother's milk and in the infant's feces (the activity in the stool disappearing with the cessation of breast-feeding coincident with a fall in unconjugated hyperbilirubinemia). It seems likely, therefore, that breast milk jaundice is due to the breast milk beta-glucuronidase causing deconjugation of the bilirubin diglucuronide and intestinal absorption of the fat-soluble bilirubin through the intestinal mucosa, increasing the enterohepatic circulation of bilirubin (Fig. 10.40) and thus increasing the level of unconjugated bilirubin in the blood.[681] It is relevant at this point to contrast this with the mechanism seen in the very rare Lucy Driscoll syndrome in which there is a definite inhibitor of bilirubin glucuronide in mother's milk (recoverable in the infant's serum) and which results in the development of jaundice in all of the mother's offspring (despite her apparent good health). This entity may present in the first few days of life and is occasionally severe enough to require exchange transfusion.

Hypothyroidism. It is mandatory to exclude hypothyroidism as a cause of persistent unconjugated hyperbilirubinemia although in countries with a neonatal screening program for hypothyroidism this is hardly ever a presenting symptom.

Intestinal stasis. The second most common cause now for persistent unconjugated jaundice is an increased enterohepatic circulation of bilirubin. In the normal situation 25% of the conjugated bilirubin reaching the duodenum is deconjugated and reabsorbed. This may be increased in situations of stasis where the alkaline intestinal juices and the mucosal bilirubin diglucuronidases (together with bacterial organisms in conditions of overgrowth) have longer to act on this substrate. Thus surgical conditions such as Hirschsprung's disease, intestinal atresia, pyloric stenosis and the meconium ileus of cystic fibrosis are often complicated by jaundice. Cystic fibrosis may also cause unconjugated jaundice due to hepatic involvement, and such involvement may explain why other conditions can present in this fashion (i.e. sepsis, galactosemia and fructosemia).

Hemolytic causes. Finally, the hemolytic anemias, especially rhesus hemolytic disease and more consistently the rare hemolytic congenital hyperbilirubinemias, will be a cause of prolonged unconjugated jaundice. The management of all such jaundice is the identification and treatment of the underlying disorder as indicated in Table 10.82.

Prolonged conjugated hyperbilirubinemia

This discussion will center on the presentation of the child with prolonged conjugated jaundice to the general pediatrician. The more complicated perspective of the specialist referral center will be dealt with in the section on liver disease (Ch. 17). The main aim of the general pediatrician is to recognize that a cholestatic syndrome is present. The signs listed in Table 10.84, should alert the physician to the presence of such a syndrome. Whilst jaundice is the usual presenting symptom other complications, especially bruising and other evidence of defective hemostasis, hypoalbuminemia or hypoglycemia may also be presenting features. (One should never diagnose hemorrhagic disease of the newborn, especially in a jaundiced child, without checking the liver function tests and percentage conjugated bilirubin.) Clues that suggest an underlying disorder are shown in Table 10.84.

The management of prolonged cholestatic jaundice is aimed at identifying conditions requiring immediate treatment and supportive therapy and then distinguishing between intra- and extrahepatic cholestasis. Blood cultures and a septic screen together with a screen for intrauterine infections (TORCH, Venereal Disease Research Laboratories; VDRL) should be sent in all infants. Parenteral antibiotics should be started if the infant appears unwell. Urine should be tested for reducing substances and sent for sugar chromatography to exclude galactosemia and fructosemia. It is also sensible to exclude galactose and fructose from the diet until the results of this are known. It should be remembered that all infants less than 2 weeks of age (and babies with renal tubular disorders, e.g. Lowe's syndrome) can have reducing substances in the urine. Furthermore, infants with liver disease can both have sugar in the urine and present with septicemia. Initial investigations should include urine for amino acid chromatography to identify particularly tyrosinemia and to send blood for alpha1-antitrypsin phenotyping and serum immunoreactive trypsin (if available), or fecal elastase. Endocrinological disorders and other rare metabolic disorders should be considered and investigated as seems appropriate to the infant. Liver function tests are not discriminatory but serum alpha-fetoprotein is particularly raised in tyrosinemia. A hemorrhagic diathesis should be treated with vitamin K (1 mg i.v.) and fresh frozen plasma if bleeding continues. Other supportive measures for liver failure may be needed.

The next step is to distinguish between intra- and extrahepatic cholestasis. The color of the stool is a useful guide (Table 10.84). Incomplete stool pallor together with evidence of IUGR suggests a prenatal hepatitis causing intrahepatic cholestasis. Complete stool pallor lasting longer than 2 weeks, especially if accompanied by a large hard liver or a conjugated bilirubin level of > 80%, suggests extrahepatic biliary obstruction and referral to a specialist to exclude biliary atresia is required without delay. Where the

Table 10.84 Clinical features that alert one to the presence of conjugated hyperbilirubinemia

a. *Evidence of hepatic disease*	
Jaundice	Urine – Yellow, not colorless from birth. Dark later with bilirubin++ on Clinistix Stools – Pale yellow to white (may be green)
Hepatomegaly	
Pruritus	
Splenomegaly, ascites, edema	
Evidence of bleeding tendency	– Bruising Bleeding
Failure to thrive	
Investigations	– Increased bilirubin, conjugated bilirubin > 80% Increased alanine aminotransferase Increased aspartate transaminase Increased γ-glutamyltransferase Increased α-fetoprotein Prolonged prothrombin time Low albumin Low blood sugar
b. *Features of underlying etiology*	
Maternal history, skin lesions	– Congenital infections
Purpura, choroidoretinitis	– Congenital infections
Cataracts	Galactosemia (urine positive for reducing substances) Lowe's syndrome (aminoaciduria)
Multiple congenital abnormalities	– Trisomy 13, 18, 21
Ascites, bile-stained hernia	– Spontaneous perforation of bile ducts
Cystic mass below the liver	– Choledochal cyst
Situs inversus, midline, liver	– Extrahepatic biliary atresia
Malposition of the viscera	– Biliary hypoplasia
Systolic murmur, dysmorphic facies	
Cutaneous hemangioma	– Hepatic/biliary hemangiomata
Marked splenomegaly	– Lysosomal storage disorder
Hypoglycemia	– Pituitary deficiency
c. *Features indicating the nature of the cholestasis*	
Incomplete stool pallor	– Intrahepatic cholestasis plus low birthweight, moderate hepatomegaly
Complete stool pallor: <10 days transient	– Intrahepatic cholestasis
>10 days permanent	– Extrahepatic cholestasis Plus normal birth weight, firm hard hepatomegaly

diagnosis is less clear cut or delay in referral is experienced, a hepatobiliary ultrasound (to exclude a choledochal cyst) and technetium-99m dimethyl iminodiacetic acid (HIDA) cholescintography (to demonstrate hepatic uptake and functional bile flow) may all be considered. The gold standard for the diagnosis of intra- and extrahepatic cholestasis remains, however, the percutaneous liver biopsy (see Table 10.85). This will also provide for the differentiation between neonatal hepatitis syndrome and bile duct paucity. Paucity of the bile ducts may be further differentiated into syndromic (Alagille's syndrome – characteristic facies, butterfly wing vertebrae, peripheral pulmonary artery stenosis and retinopathy) and non-syndromic. Neonatal hepatitis is the end result of many hepatic insults. In some cases, however, no cause can be found and the final diagnosis is idiopathic neonatal hepatitis. These entities are discussed further in Chapter 17.

Management of neonatal liver disease is supportive and, where possible, definitive.[687] Nutritional support aims to provide sufficient energy and nutrients to combat maldigestion and malabsorption, and specialized formulas are used. Fat soluble vitamin supplementation is required for all cholestatic infants. Management is discussed further in Chapter 17.

HEMATOLOGICAL PROBLEMS OF THE NEWBORN

DEVELOPMENTAL HEMOPOIESIS

Hemopoietic stem cells and hemopoiesis

Hemopoiesis is the process by which life-long production of cells of all the hemopoietic lineages is maintained. The principal cell lineages and current views of the organization of this process are shown in Figure 10.44.

The most primitive, undifferentiated cells in this process are the pluripotent hemopoietic stem cells. These pluripotent stem cells are characterized by their astonishing capacity to choose between one of two destinies depending on the genes they express: they either undergo self-renewal (i.e. they maintain exactly the same pluripotent characteristics after cell division) or alternatively they differentiate. At an early stage in this process of differentiation stem cells commit themselves, via a distinct pattern of gene expression, to producing cells of the lymphoid lineage (lymphoid stem cells) or non-lymphoid lineage (myeloid stem cells).

Myeloid stem cells are able to further differentiate into hemopoietic progenitor cells of all the remaining lineages (erythroid, megakaryocyte, eosinophil, granulocyte, monocyte and basophil) as shown in Figure 10.44. All of these immature stem and progenitor cells look very nondescript and similar by light microscopy but by coordinated expression of many genes in response to a range of stimuli, including hemopoietic growth factors, these nondescript cells develop the appearance and function of the easily recognized mature peripheral blood cells. The process of hemopoiesis outlined here is broadly similar in adults, children, neonates, the fetus and the embryo. However, there are fascinating differences in the regulation of this process and its cellular components during ontogeny which contribute to the nature and management of the neonatal hematological problems described in this section.

Table 10.85 Laboratory investigations of suspected extrahepatic cholestasis (EHC)

1. Conjugated bilirubin	>80% – EHC
2. Liver function/ clotting disorders	γ-glutamyltransferase : aspartate transaminase = 2 : 1 – EHC
3. Ultrasound scan liver/ gallbladder	Cystic dilation – choledochal cyst
4. ^{131}I Rose Bengal excretion test	<10% in stool in 72 h – EHC
5. ^{99m}Tc HIDA scan	
6. Liver biopsy:	
Neonatal hepatitis	Hepatocellular necrosis, giant cell transformation, disorganized/ inflammatory infiltrate of portal tracts, cholestasis, bile duct proliferation
Extrahepatic biliary atresia	Widened portal tracts with prominent distorted angulated bile ducts. Increased fibrosis with inflammatory cell infiltrate. Cholestasis with bile lakes. Giant cell transformation
Alagille's syndrome biliary hypoplasia	Paucity of interlobular ducts compared with portal areas. Mild fibrosis
Non-syndromic biliary hypoplasia	Paucity of interlobular ducts with variable portal fibrosis

Sites of hemopoiesis

While virtually all hemopoiesis in children and adults takes place in the marrow, the principal sites of hemopoietic activity change during ontogeny. The first recognizable signs of hemopoiesis in humans occur in the third week of gestation in the yolk sac. Yolk sac hemopoiesis continues at a low level but by 5 weeks' gestation the majority of stem cells responsible for maintaining hemopoiesis throughout life arise from the embryonic dorsal aorta in the aorto-gonad-mesonephros (AGM) region.[688] Soon afterwards these hemopoietic stem cells migrate to the liver which by 6–8 weeks' gestation becomes the primary site of blood cell production. Most hemopoietic cells produced in the fetal liver are erythroid but small numbers of B-lymphocyte, megakaryocyte and granulocyte/monocyte progenitors are also produced. By the eleventh week, hemopoiesis begins in the bone marrow although the fetal liver remains the principal site of hemopoiesis until the end of the third trimester.

Erythropoiesis

Fetal erythropoiesis

Erythropoiesis is the first hemopoietic lineage to become established. In the very early embryo, when hemopoiesis is mainly taking place in the yolk sac, erythropoiesis is primitive and 'megaloblastic', resembling that in pernicious anemia. By the sixth week of gestation erythropoiesis has become normoblastic and the erythrocytes smaller, though still larger than adult erythrocytes; this is known as definitive erythropoiesis and corresponds to the time when hemopoiesis becomes established in the liver.

Erythropoiesis in the neonate

There are a number of distinct characteristics of erythropoiesis in the newborn relevant to our understanding both of the normal changes in Hb during this period and to identifying significant acquired or inherited abnormalities of erythropoiesis in neonates.

Production of new red blood cells and the rate of Hb synthesis fall dramatically after birth and remain low for the first 2 weeks of life. The exact mechanisms for these changes are unknown but probably reflect the sudden increase in tissue oxygenation at birth and downregulation of erythropoietin production. Although erythropoiesis begins to increase after the first 2 weeks, this starts at the erythroid progenitor stage of differentiation and the rise in Hb and

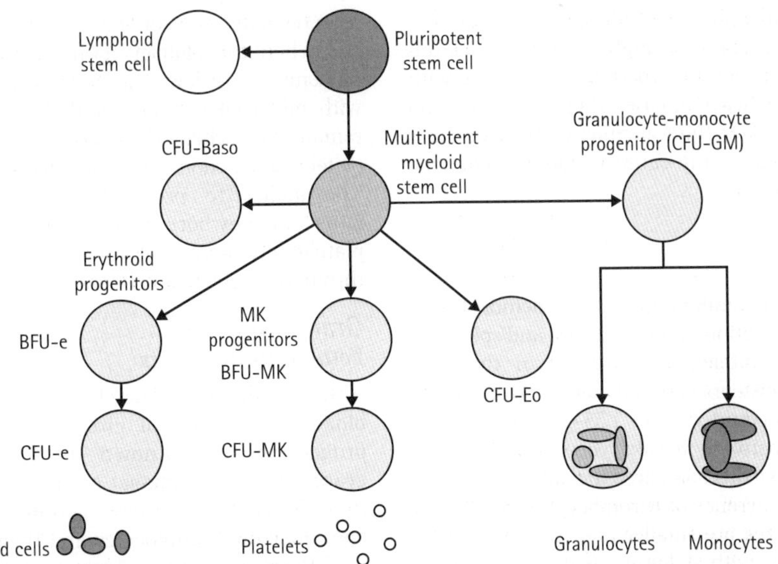

Fig. 10.44 Hemopoiesis: a schematic outline. BFU-e, burst-forming unit erythrocyte; BFU-MK, burst-forming unit megakaryocyte; CFU-baso, colony-forming unit badophil; CFU-e, colony-forming unit erythrocyte; CFU-Eo, colony-forming unit eosinophil; CFU-MK, colony-forming unit megakarocyte; MK, megakaryocyte.

production of mature red cells is not apparent until many weeks later and reaches a maximum only by 3 months of age when a healthy infant should be able to produce up to 2 ml packed red cells/day. Studies in preterm neonates have suggested that over the first 2 months of life the maximal rate of red cell production is ≤1 ml/day since preterm babies receiving erythropoietin are unable to maintain their Hb if > 1 ml of blood/day is venesected for diagnostic purposes.

Neonatal red cells, particularly from preterm babies, have a reduced life span compared to adult red cells. Calculated actuarial red cell life spans for preterm infants are 35–50 days compared to 60–70 days for term infants and 120 days for healthy adults.[689] The reasons are unclear and are likely to predominantly reflect changes in the red cell membrane.

Differences in the red cell membranes of neonates include: increased resistance to osmotic lysis, increased mechanical fragility, presence of vacuoles and internal structures just below the red cell membrane, increased total lipid content and an altered lipid profile, increased insulin-binding sites and reduced expression of blood group antigens such as A, B and I.[690]

There are also numerous differences in red cell metabolism between neonatal and adult red blood cells both in the glycolytic and pentose phosphate pathways which lead to an increased susceptibility to oxidant-induced injury, although the clinical implications of these differences remain unclear.

Globin chain synthesis and Hb production in the fetus and newborn

Knowledge of the normal evolution of embryonic, fetal and 'adult' Hbs during ontogeny is essential to our understanding of the hemoglobinopathies and how they present in neonates. The composition and names of these Hbs are shown in Table 10.86. The first globin chain produced is epsilon globin, encoded on the ε-globin gene cluster, followed almost immediately by alpha- and gamma-globin gene production. HbF ($\alpha2\gamma2$) is therefore produced from very early in gestation (4–5 weeks) and is the predominant Hb until after birth. Adult Hb (Hb A: $\alpha2\beta2$) is also produced from an early stage (6–8 weeks' gestation) but remains at low levels (10–15%) until 30–32 weeks. After this time the rate of HbA production increases at the same time as HbF production falls resulting in an average HbF level at birth of 70–80%, HbA of 25–30%, small amounts of HbA2 and sometimes a trace of Hb Barts ($\beta4$).

Table 10.86 Composition of embryonic, fetal and adult Hbs

Hb	Globin chains: Chromsome 16 α-gene cluster	Globin chains: Chromsome 11 β-gene cluster	Gestation
Embryonic			
Hb Gower 1	ξ2	ε2	From 3 to 4 weeks
Hb Gower 2	α2	ε2	
Hb Portland	ε2	γ2	From 4 weeks
Fetal			
HbF	α2	γ2	From 4 weeks
Adult			
Hb A	α2	β2	From 6 to 8 weeks
HbA2	α2	δ2	From 30 weeks

After birth and over the first year of life HbF falls in healthy term and preterm babies (to < 2% at age 12 months) with a corresponding increase in HbA. In term babies there is little change in HbF in the first 15 days after birth but it declines steeply thereafter as neonatal erythropoiesis starts. In preterm babies who are not transfused HbF may remain at the same level for the first 6 weeks of life before HbA production starts to increase. It is this delay in HbA production (i.e. the switch from the gamma-globin of HbF to the beta-globin of HbA) which can make the diagnosis of beta-globin disorders difficult in the neonatal period. By contrast, the fact that alpha-globin chains are absolutely essential for the production of both HbF and HbA, means that alpha-thalassemia major causes severe anemia from early in fetal life.

Regulation of erythropoiesis in the fetus and newborn: role of erythropoietin

The principal cytokine regulating erythropoiesis in the fetus and newborn is erythropoietin. In the fetus the liver is the main site of erythropoietin production. Since erythropoietin does not cross the placenta, erythropoietin-mediated regulation of fetal erythropoiesis is predominantly under fetal control. The only known stimulus to erythropoietin production under physiological conditions is hypoxia with or without anemia. This explains the high erythropoietin levels in fetuses of mothers with diabetes or hypertension or those with IUGR or cyanotic congenital heart disease where the fetus and newborn are polycythemic rather than anemic; erythropoietin is also increased in fetal anemia of any cause including hemolytic disease of the newborn.[691]

Megakaryocytopoiesis

Fetal megakarytopoiesis

Megakaryocytes and their progenitors have been demonstrated in the yolk sac by 5 weeks' gestation and in the liver and spleen by 10 weeks gestation.[692,693] Platelets first appear in the fetal circulation at 5–6 weeks postconceptional age.[694] During the second trimester the platelet count rises to 175–250 × 10^9/L.[695] There are several differences between megakaryocytopoiesis and its regulation in the fetus and newborn compared to adults which may contribute to the frequent occurrence of thrombocytopenia in sick neonates. Fetal megakaryocytes are smaller and more immature than those in adult marrow with a lower ploidy and reduced formation of proplatelets.[696,697]

Megakaryocytopoiesis in the neonate

In both term and preterm neonates megakaryocytopoiesis proceeds via the same pathway as in adults. Megakaryocytes are derived from mature megakaryocyte progenitors (known as colony-forming units megakaryocyte; CFU-MK) which are present in large numbers in neonatal blood as well as bone marrow. CFU-MK are derived from more primitive megakaryocyte progenitor cells, BFU-MK (burst-forming units megakaryocyte) which are present in 10-fold lower numbers. Quantitation of circulating megakaryocyte progenitors is a useful way of assessing megakaryocytopoiesis in term and preterm neonates and has allowed the common mechanisms of neonatal thrombocytopenia to be elucidated (see p. 308).[698] Platelet counts at birth in term and preterm neonate are within the normal adult range.

Regulation of megakaryocytopoiesis in the fetus and neonate

The principal cytokine regulating platelet production in the fetus and newborn is thrombopoietin, as in adults.[699] Thrombopoietin stimulates megakaryocyte progenitors and mature megakaryocytes both in term and preterm neonates. The major site of fetal and neonatal thrombopoietin production is the liver.[700] Circulating thrombopoietin is detectable in all healthy neonates; preterm neonates have marginally higher thrombopoietin levels compared to term neonates. In neonatal thrombocytopenia thrombopoietin levels rise when the platelet count and/or circulating megakaryocyte progenitors are low (e.g. early-onset thrombocytopenia associated with maternal PET and/or IUGR),[699] while thrombopoietin levels remain low where thrombocytopenia is secondary to increased platelet destruction (e.g. idiopathic thrombocytopenic purpura; ITP). The ability to produce thrombopoietin is reduced in the fetus and newborn which limits their capacity to up-regulate platelet production at times of increased demand, e.g. during thrombocytopenia in neonatal sepsis.[699,701]

Granulopoiesis

Fetal granulopoiesis

Although there are few circulating neutrophils in first trimester blood (around 1% of circulating nucleated cells), neutrophil progenitor cells (known as CFU-GM, colony-forming unit granulocyte-macrophage) are present from 25 days' gestation in the yolk sac and 4.5 weeks' gestation in the fetal liver.[692,693] In the bone marrow granulocytes and their progenitors are not evident until the eleventh week of gestation. The number of granulocytes in fetal blood remains low (0.1–0.2 × 10^9/L) throughout the second trimester and the ratio of immature band forms to mature neutrophils is normal. After the second trimester circulating neutrophils gradually rise to reach over 2 × 10^9/L by term, with slightly lower numbers in preterm neonates (Table 10.87).

Granulopoiesis in the newborn

The principal difference between granulopoiesis in the newborn and later in infancy is the diminished size of the neutrophil storage pool, particularly in preterm infants and most markedly so in those with IUGR or exposure to maternal hypertension.[702,703] The neutrophil storage pool reflects the available reserve of neutrophils which the fetus or neonate can mobilize in response to infection. This may explain the frequency of bacterial infection in such infants. The neutrophil storage pool is defined as the numbers of segmented neutrophils, band neutrophils and metamyelocytes in the bone marrow and so is usually inferred (by the leukocyte response to bacterial sepsis) since bone marrow examination is rarely indicated in the newborn.

In healthy term and preterm neonates the ratio of immature band forms to mature neutrophils is normal. This has led to widespread use of 'I/T' (immature/total) ratios as an indicator of neonatal sepsis. However, there are several important limitations to their value. Preterm infants frequently have markedly increased numbers of all types of immature granulocytic cells on their blood

Table 10.87 Representative normal hematological values at birth and over the first 2 months of life in term babies

	Birth	2 weeks	2 months
Hb (g/dl)	14.9–23.7	13.4–19.8	9.4–13
Hematocrit	0.47–0.75	0.41–0.65	0.28–0.42
Mean cell volume (fl)	100–125	88–110	77–98
Reticulocytes (x10^9/L)	110–450	10–85	35–200
White blood cells (x10^9/L)	10–26	6–21	5–15
Neutrophils (x10^9/L)	2.7–14.4	1.5–5.4	0.7–4.8
Monocytes (x10^9/L)	0–1.9	0.1–1.7	0.4–1.2
Lymphocytes (x10^9/L)	2.0–7.3	2.8–9.1	3.3–10.3
Eosinophils (x10^9/L)	0–0.85	0–0.85	0.05–0.9
Basophils (x10^9/L)	0–0.1	0–0.1	0.02–0.13
Nucleated red blood cells (x10^9/L)	< 5	< 0.1	< 0.1
Platelets (x10^9/L)	150–450	150–450	150–450

These data are obtained from a number of sources and have been chosen to represent data most useful for interpreting the significance of hematological results.

film including metamyelocytes, myelocytes, promyelocytes and blast cells. This appearance in the first few days of life is not usually indicative of sepsis, instead reflecting the normal hematological response of a neonate to preterm delivery; the most useful diagnostic clue to the coincident presence of sepsis is a marked peak in the numbers of band forms compared to other granulocytic cells.

Regulation of granulopoiesis in the fetus and newborn

The regulation of granulopoiesis is not fully understood. Various cytokines stimulate granulocyte production in vitro and in vivo but their exact physiological role is unclear. The principal cytokines which act directly on the granulocyte-macrophage lineage are granulocyte colony-stimulating factor (G-CSF) and granulocyte-macrophage colony-stimulating factor (GM-CSF).[703] Despite unequivocal evidence of their ability to increase neutrophil production in the newborn, their therapeutic role is unclear and may be evident once trials still underway are complete.[704]

Other leukocytes

All types of leukocyte found in adult blood are also seen in the fetus and the newborn:[695] monocytes circulate from 4–5 weeks' gestation and eosinophils and basophils from 14–16 weeks' gestation, each cell type being present in low numbers and increasing slowly to the normal values at term (Table 10.87).

Lymphopoiesis

There are few studies of lymphopoiesis in the human fetus. There appears to be no lymphopoiesis in the yolk sac, but both T lymphocytes and B lymphocytes are found in fetal liver at 7 and 8 weeks' gestation respectively, where they constitute less than 1% of the total nucleated hemopoietic cell population.[694] Shortly thereafter T lymphocytes are detectable in fetal blood and thymus, with marrow T lymphocyte production established during the second trimester.[705] By term T lymphocytes form 40–45% of circulating mononuclear cells with a CD4:CD8 ratio of around 5.0, slightly higher than in adult blood (3.1:1). B lymphocytes are found in fetal blood and bone marrow from around 12 weeks' gestation and constitute 4–5% of circulating mononuclear cells by term.[694]

HEMATOLOGICAL VALUES AT BIRTH

Practical issues: establishing normal values and identifying artefacts

One of the most important aspects of neonatal hematology is knowledge of what is normal in the neonatal period and the factors that impact upon the importance of a laboratory result. These include:

1. *Site of sampling*: capillary or skin puncture samples yield higher Hb levels (2–4 g/dl higher) and hematocrits (up to 20% higher) than venous or arterial samples collected simultaneously.[706]
2. *Quality of the blood sample*: common problems include clotted or partially clotted samples particularly when the baby is polycythemic; and poorly preserved white cell morphology due to excess ethylenediaminetetraacetic acid (EDTA) if there is undue delay in samples reaching the laboratory or a high blood: anticoagulant ratio.
3. *Gestational age-related changes in hematological values*: while there are no significant differences in Hb, hematocrit, white blood cell (WBC) count or platelet count with gestational age from 24 weeks to term, the normal mean cell volume (MCV) is higher in preterm infants (a mean of 135 fl at 24 weeks' gestation, 127 fl at 30–31 weeks and 119 fl at term; Tables 10.87 and 10.88); the number of reticulocytes is twice as high in preterm compared to term infants (6% at 24–25 weeks versus 3.2% at term); and the numbers of circulating nucleated red cells in healthy preterm infants are around twice as high ($\leq 20 \times 10^7$/L) as in term babies.
4. *Postnatal changes in hematological values*: the marked changes after birth in almost all hematological parameters and also in the blood film over the first few weeks of life make it essential to know the postnatal age of a baby to make a sensible interpretation of the hematological results.
5. *Effect of timing of cord clamping and other aspects of delivery on hematological values in the newborn:* Since the placental blood vessels in a term baby contain 50–200 ml of blood, delaying clamping of the cord and holding the baby below the level of the placenta to allow emptying of this blood into the baby's circulation can increase the blood volume by 50–60% with a consequent increase in Hb (to >19 g/dl versus 15–16 g/dl with early clamping of the cord); similar differences are seen in preterm babies.[707]

Normal values for red blood cells and blood volume

Normal values at birth for Hb, hematocrit and MCV are shown in Tables 10.88 and 10.89 for term and preterm babies respectively. In term babies the Hb, hematocrit and red cell indices fall slowly over the first few weeks reaching a mean Hb of 13–14 g/dl at 4 weeks of age and 9.5–11 g/dl at 7–9 weeks of age with a lower limit of normal for the MCV and mean corpuscular Hb (MCH) of 77 fl and 26 pg respectively. For preterm infants changes in Hb, hematocrit and red cell indices in the first few weeks of life are often difficult to interpret because of their variable clinical course and transfusion requirements. However, studies of well preterm infants carried out in the 1970s show a more rapid and steeper fall in Hb reaching a mean of 6.5–9 g/dl at 4–8 weeks postnatal age.[690] The reticulocyte count and numbers of nucleated red cells also fall rapidly after birth as erythropoiesis is suppressed. The reticulocyte count starts to increase in term babies at 7–8 weeks of age to reach $35–200 \times 10^9$/L (1–1.8%) at 2 months of age and in preterm babies at 6–8 weeks of age.

Normal blood volume at birth varies with gestational age as well as the timing of the clamping of the cord. In healthy term infants average blood volume is around 80 ml/kg with a range of

Table 10.88 Representative normal hematological values at birth in preterm babies

	24–25 weeks	26–27 weeks	28–29 weeks	30–31 weeks
Hb (g/dl)	19.4 ± 1.5	19.0 ± 2.5	19.3 ± 1.8	19.1 ± 2.1
Hematocrit	0.63 ± 0.04	0.62 ± 0.08	0.60 ± 0.07	60 ± 0.08
Mean cell volume (fl)	135 ± 0.02	132 ± 14.4	131 ± 13.5	127 ± 12.7
Reticulocytes ($\times 10^9$/L)	279 ± 23	454 ± 15	347 ± 12	278 ± 10
Platelets ($\times 10^9$/L)	150–450	150–450	150–450	150–450

Data adapted from Oski 1993.[690]

50–100 ml/kg. The blood volume is higher in preterm infants with an average of 106 ml/kg and a range of 85–143 ml/kg.[708,709] Term and preterm babies have adequate stores of iron, folic acid and vitamin B_{12} at birth. However, stores of both iron and folic acid are lower in preterm infants and are depleted more quickly, leading to deficiency after 2–4 months if the recommended daily intakes are not maintained (see p. 181 and Ch. 14). In general even term neonates with a normal Hb at birth will have depleted their iron stores by the time they have doubled their birth weight.

Normal values for white cells

The neutrophil and monocyte count vary over the first few days of life even in healthy babies. For the first 12 h they increase then fall to a nadir at 4 days of age. Normal values for neutrophils at birth are also affected by other factors including antenatal history, perinatal history, ethnic origin, site of blood sampling and whether or not the baby has been crying. The neutrophil count is higher in capillary samples and after vigorous crying; it is lower in neonates with IUGR, those born to mothers with hypertension or diabetes and in neonates of African origin.[691,703] All of the other types of white blood cell found in adult blood and also present in the newborn are shown in Table 10.87. Some cell types not found in healthy adults are seen in healthy preterm babies – these include blast cells, other early myeloid cells, nucleated red cells and even occasional megakaryocytes.

Normal platelet count and platelet function

Blood platelet counts at birth in term and preterm neonates are within the normal adult range.[710] Many studies have found impaired function of neonatal platelets in vitro in term and preterm infants; the most consistent abnormalities are reduced aggregation in response to epinephrine (adrenaline), ADP and thrombin. However, these abnormalities do not appear to be of major clinical significance: there is no increased bleeding tendency in neonates with normal platelet counts and coagulation parameters and the bleeding time tested with adult and neonatal devices is normal in term and preterm infants (≤ 135 s).[711]

Normal values and appearance of the neonatal bone marrow

Bone marrow examinations are rarely indicated in the newborn. Nevertheless, some normal data are available. Marrow cellularity is normally high around birth and is higher in preterm compared to term babies. The relative cell proportions for term babies do not differ from those of term babies.[694]

RED CELL DISORDERS

Anemia: introduction and definition

Anemia is the commonest hematological abnormality in the newborn. The cause is often multifactorial. Nevertheless a logical approach and appropriate use of straightforward investigations, as outlined below and summarized on page 302, reveal the cause in most babies. Treatment options are limited and focused on sensible use of blood transfusion and prevention of anemia. The general management of neonatal anemia, including red cell transfusion, is outlined on page 302.

Definition

Anemia is generally defined as a Hb concentration below the normal range for a population of age- and sex-matched individuals. Normal values for term and preterm infants at birth are shown in Tables 10.88 and 10.89; from this it can be seen that, regardless of gestation, any neonate with a Hb of < 14 g/dl at birth on a properly taken blood sample would be considered anemic.

Physiological impact of anemia in the neonate

Anemia is one of the main factors, together with cardiopulmonary function and the position of the Hb–oxygen dissociation curve, which influences tissue oxygenation. The clinical significance of anemia in the newborn does not therefore depend solely upon the Hb concentration. The two most important factors determining the position of the Hb–oxygen dissociation curve are the HbF and 2,3-DPG concentrations within the red blood cells: a high HbF and low 2,3-DPG both cause the curve to be shifted to the left, i.e. the affinity of Hb for oxygen is increased so less oxygen is released to the tissues. This is the situation just after birth and will be more marked in preterm babies with higher HbF concentrations. Over the first few months of life 2,3-DPG levels rise and HbF levels fall so the Hb–oxygen dissociation curve gradually shifts to the right, i.e. the oxygen affinity of Hb falls and oxygen delivery to the tissues increases. This increase in oxygen delivery ameliorates the effects of the falling Hb over the first months of life.

Pathogenesis and causes of neonatal anemia

Anemia in the neonatal period has distinct physiological features compared to older children and a distinct pathogenesis. Interpretation of diagnostic investigations has to be made on a background of ontogeny-related changes in the red cell membrane, red cell enzymes and Hb production which vary with gestational and postnatal age. Furthermore, anemia in the neonate may be attributable to pregnancy-related or pre-existing disorders in the mother. Anemia results from one or more of the following mechanisms:

1. inappropriately reduced red cell production (p. 298);
2. increased red cell destruction/reduced red cell life span (p. 300);
3. blood loss (p. 301);
4. a combination of these mechanisms (anemia of prematurity, p. 302).

Using this approach the principal causes of anemia in the term and preterm neonate are shown in Table 10.89 and a diagnostic approach to identifying these causes is shown in Figure 10.45.

Anemia due to reduced red cell production

The main diagnostic clues are a combination of a low reticulocyte count (< 20 × 10^9/L) together with a negative direct antiglobulin test (Coombs' test). The most important causes are congenital infections (particularly parvovirus) and genetic disorders. Where failure of blood cell production is confined to the red cell series, as with Diamond–Blackfan anemia and most episodes of parvovirus infection, the anemia is said to be due to red cell aplasia but reduced red cell production may also be part of a global failure of hemopoiesis, e.g. in CMV infection or congenital leukemias (see p. 304).

Anemia and congenital infection

Infections which cause anemia due to reduced red cell production include: CMV, toxoplasmosis, congenital syphilis, rubella, herpes simplex, GBS and parvovirus B19. Appropriate tests for these organisms should be carried out wherever there is clinical suspicion which is often prompted by well recognized associated findings such as chorioretinitis, jaundice, pneumonitis, skin lesions, IUGR and hepatosplenomegaly. Maternal infection with parvovirus B19 causes fetal anemia when it occurs in the first or second trimester. The diagnosis of fetal/neonatal parvovirus B19 may be very difficult to make and should be considered in every 'unexplained' case of fetal hydrops (Table 10.90) or neonatal red cell aplasia.[712,713] The reticulocytopenia is severe (usually < 10 × 10^9/L) and thrombocytopenia may also occur. In infection due to CMV,

Table 10.89 Causes of neonatal anemia

A. Impaired red cell production
- Congenital infection, e.g. CMV, rubella
- Diamond–Blackfan anemia
- Pearson's syndrome
- Congenital dyserythropoietic anemia
- Transient erythroblastopenia of childhood (rare in neonates)
- Congenital leukemia

B. Increased red cell destruction (hemolysis)
- Alloimmune: hemolytic disease of the newborn (Rh, ABO, Kell, other)
- Autoimmune, e.g. maternal autoimmune hemolysis
- Infection, e.g. bacterial, syphilis, malaria, CMV, toxoplasma, herpes simplex
- Red cell membrane disorders, e.g. hereditary spherocytosis
- Infantile pyknocytosis
- Red cell enzyme deficiencies, e.g. pyruvate kinase deficiency
- Some hemoglobinopathies, e.g. alpha-thalassemia major, HbH disease
- Macro/microangiopathy, e.g. cavernous hemangioma, DIC
- Galactosemia

C. Blood loss
- Occult hemorrhage before birth, e.g. twin-to-twin, fetomaternal
- Internal hemorrhage, e.g. intracranial, cephalhematoma
- Iatrogenic: due to frequent blood sampling

D. Anemia of prematurity:
- Impaired red cell production plus reduced red cell life span

CMV, cytomegalovirus; DIC, disseminated intravascular coagulation.

Table 10.90 Hematological causes of hydrops fetalis

A. Reduced red cell production
   Parvovirus B19
   Diamond–Blackfan anemia
   Congenital dyserythropoietic anemia
   Congenital leukemia

B. Increased red cell destruction (hemolysis)
   Pyruvate kinase deficiency
   Alpha-thalassemia major
   Hemolytic disease of the newborn – Rhesus, Kell, ABO (rare)

C. Blood loss
   Twin-to-twin transfusion
   Fetomaternal hemorrhage

toxoplasma or herpes simplex the reticulocytopenia is less and may be increased and the blood film often shows abnormal 'viral' lymphocytes, thrombocytopenia and/or neutropenia.

Management. Underlying infection should be treated together with red cell transfusion as indicated following conventional transfusion guidelines (see p. 302). Neonates with red cell aplasia secondary to parvovirus B19 who fail to recover, i.e. their reticulocyte count remains low and they are transfusion-dependent, should be given IVIG to help eradicate persistent viral infection.[714]

Inherited disorders

The principal cause of congenital red cell aplasia is Diamond–Blackfan anemia.[714,748] The incidence is 5–7 cases/million live

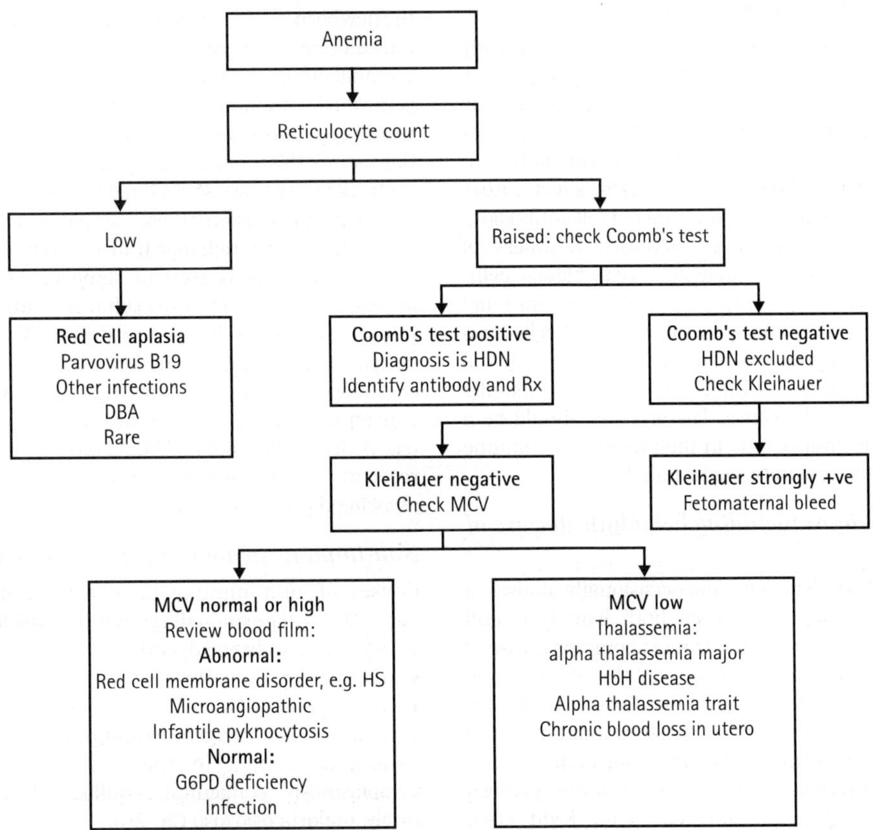

Fig. 10.45 Diagnostic approach to neonatal anemia. G6PD; glucose-6-phosphate dehydrogenase; DBA, Diamond–Blackfan anemia; HDN, hemolytic disease of the newborn; HS, hereditary spherocytosis; MCV, meal cell volume.

births. There is a clear family history in 20% of cases; the remaining 80% are sporadic.[737] Mutations of the RPS gene on chromosome 19 are implicated in some familial and sporadic cases. Most diagnoses are not made until 2–3 months of age when transfusion-dependent anemia becomes apparent but around 25% of cases present at birth and it is a rare cause of mid-trimester fetal anemia and hydrops.[715]

Other inherited/congenital disorders which may present with anemia due to reduced red cell production include Pearson's syndrome and congenital dyserythropoietic anemia (CDA). Pearson's syndrome, which is caused by mutations in mitochondrial DNA, is suggested in neonates who are SGA and thrive poorly in the first few weeks of life, the anemia is normocytic and associated thrombocytopenia and neutropenia are common; abnormal leukocyte vacuolation may be seen in the peripheral blood and highly characteristic vacuolation of early erythoid cells on the marrow aspirate should prompt blood to be sent for mitochondrial DNA analysis to establish the diagnosis. A number of neonates with CDA presenting at birth have been reported. Most affected babies are normally grown with no dysmorphic features, have a normocytic anemia with normal white cells and platelets but a low reticulocyte count and transfusion-dependent anemia. The genetic basis is unknown but most cases are autosomal recessive. The other inherited bone marrow failure syndromes, e.g. Fanconi's anemia, rarely present at birth.

Management. Management of these disorders is discussed in detail in Chapter 21. In the neonatal period the main issues are making the diagnosis and judicious use of red cell transfusion following conventional guidelines (see p. 302). Steroids are rarely used for Diamond–Blackfan anemia in the neonatal period as they are only indicated in transfusion-dependent children.

Anemia due to increased red cell destruction/reduced red cell life span (hemolytic anemia)

Recognition of neonatal anemia due to hemolysis is clinically extremely important even if the anemia is mild and apparently trivial. This is because transient or mild hemolysis in the neonatal period may be the clue to an underlying problem with more serious manifestations later on in childhood (e.g. red cell enzymopathies or hemoglobinopathies) or to problems which might affect future siblings (e.g. alloimmune anemia due to maternal red cell antibodies).

The principal diagnostic clues are: increased numbers of reticulocytes and/or circulating nucleated red blood cells, unconjugated hyperbilirubinemia, a positive Coombs' test (if immune) and characteristic changes in the morphology of the red cells on a blood film (e.g. hereditary spherocytosis). The main types of neonatal hemolytic anemia are listed in Table 10.89. It is usually straightforward to distinguish the cause. The first step should be a Coombs' test which will be positive only in the presence of immune hemolytic anemia and not in non-immune hemolysis.

Immune hemolytic anemias including hemolytic disease of the newborn (HDN)

Maternal autoimmune hemolytic anemia occasionally causes a positive Coombs' in the neonate; however, both hemolysis and anemia in the baby are extremely rare. The most common cause of Coombs'-positive hemolysis is hemolytic disease of the newborn due to transplacental passage of maternal IgG alloantibodies to red cell antigens. Modern Coombs' reagents are so sensitive that a negative Coombs' test virtually excludes neonatal alloimmune hemolysis.

Alloantibodies which can cause hemolytic disease of the newborn include anti-D, anti-c, anti-E, anti-Kell, anti-Kidd (J^k), anti-Duffy (F^y) and antibodies of the MNS blood group system, including anti-U. Anti-D remains the most frequent alloantibody to cause significant hemolytic anemia; it affects 1 in 1200 pregnancies and still causes around 50 deaths per year in the UK. Anti-Kell antibodies also cause severe fetal and neonatal anemia since they inhibit erythropoiesis as well as causing hemolysis. ABO hemolytic disease occurs in offspring of women of blood group O and is confined to the 1% of such women with high-titer IgG antibodies: hemolysis due to anti-A is more common (1 in 150 births) than anti-B. Hemolysis due to IgG anti-A or anti-B rarely causes anemia although the hyperbilirubinemia may be severe; where there is significant anemia it is usually associated with anti-B antibodies. Hemolytic disease of the newborn is a rare cause of 'blueberry muffin' baby.

Management of HDN due to Rh or Kell alloantibodies. The antenatal diagnosis and management of pregnancies affected by red cell alloimmunization are discussed in Chapter 9. Close cooperation between obstetric, pediatric and hematology teams is essential for good management.[716,717] All neonates at risk of hemolytic disease of the newborn should have cord blood taken for Hb, bilirubin and a Coombs' test and should remain in hospital until hyperbilirubinemia and/or anemia have been properly managed. Phototherapy should be given to all Rhesus-alloimmunized infants from birth as the bilirubin can rise steeply after birth and this expectant approach will prevent the need for exchange transfusion in some infants.

Exchange transfusion is required for:

1. severe anemia (Hb < 10 g/dl at birth) or;
2. severe and/or rapidly increasing hyperbilirubinemia as indicated by standard graphs.

Blood for exchange transfusion should be Group O, Rh D-identical with the neonate, Kell-negative and < 5 days old. Current recommendations state that the blood should be CMV-negative but universal leukocyte depletion in the UK means that CMV-untested blood is likely to be of equivalent safety to CMV-negative blood even in the newborn.[718] The blood should be irradiated *if* the baby has received intrauterine transfusion; irradiation of blood for exchange is not essential otherwise but may be carried out in some centers if it can be performed without delay. The ideal product for exchange transfusion would be plasma-reduced whole blood with a hematocrit of 0.45–0.55; this is not currently available in the UK but may become so in the next few years. Packed red blood cells are available for neonatal exchange transfusion: these should have a hematocrit of < 0.6. The technique for exchange transfusion is described on page 292.

'Late' anemia is seen in some babies with milder hemolytic disease who do not require exchange transfusion and in babies who have had earlier exchange transfusion. This presents at a few weeks of age and is due to ongoing hemolysis and postnatal suppression of erythropoiesis. Such babies may require 'top-up' transfusion; conventional guidelines for neonatal transfusion can be followed (see p. 302) but irradiated blood must be used for infants previously receiving intrauterine transfusion to prevent the risk of transfusion-associated graft-versus-host disease.

Non-immune hemolytic anemia presenting in neonates

Causes of non-immune hemolysis in neonates are shown in Table 10.89. The main diagnoses to consider are:

- red cell membrane disorders;
- red cell enzymopathies;
- hemoglobinopathies.

A number of congenital and primary infections can also cause hemolytic anemia in the neonatal period including: CMV, toxoplasmosis, congenital syphilis, rubella, herpes simplex and, rarely, malaria (see also Ch. 26).

Red cell membrane disorders. Red cell membrane disorders can usually be identified by the characteristic shape of red cells on a blood film. Hereditary spherocytosis occurs in 1 in 5000 births. Its usual presentation in the neonate is with unconjugated hyperbilirubinemia. Most affected neonates are not anemic but a small proportion have anemia severe enough to require transfusion. The blood film in hereditary spherocytosis shows moderate numbers of spherocytes; the appearance is identical to that of ABO hemolytic disease but the two disorders are distinguishable by the negative Coombs' in hereditary spherocytosis. Hereditary elliptocytosis is a more complex disorder caused by mutations in the genes for spectrin, ankyrin or Band 4.1. In the common, autosomal dominant form heterozygotes have no clinical manifestations (i.e. no anemia and no jaundice) apart from elliptocytes on the blood film. More important clinically are neonates who have more than one mutation in a red cell membrane protein (they may be homozygous or compound heterozygotes) as they present with the disease hereditary pyropoikilocytosis (HPP). In HPP hemolytic anemia is severe in the neonatal period and many infants require transfusion. The diagnosis of HPP should be easily made by examining blood films from the baby and both parents; a useful diagnosic clue is the low MCV at birth (< 70 fl).

Management. Babies with chronic hemolysis secondary to red cell membrane abnormalities should be given folic acid (i.e. all affected babies except hereditary elliptocytosis heterozygotes who have no significant hemolysis). Red cell transfusion may be required in the neonatal period and, especially in HPP, sometimes indefinitely until the child is old enough to undergo splenectomy. It is important to carry out definitive diagnostic investigations (red membrane studies) on pretransfusion blood samples to minimize diagnostic confusion due to transfused cells.

Red cell enzymopathies. Red cell enzymopathies present in neonates with unconjugated bilirubinemia with or without anemia and, unlike the membrane disorders, usually do not have characteristic changes on the blood film. The most common is G6PD deficiency, which has a high prevalence in individuals from central Africa (20%) and the Mediterranean (10%). G6PD deficiency, which is X-linked, predominantly affects boys though female carriers may have milder symptoms. In neonatal G6PD deficiency jaundice usually presents within the first few days of life and is often severe; anemia is extremely rare and the blood film is completely normal and so the diagnosis must be made by assaying G6PD on a peripheral blood sample.[719] The second most common red cell enzymopathy in neonates, pyruvate kinase deficiency, is more heterogeneous clinically varying from anemia severe enough to cause hydrops fetalis to a mild unconjugated hyperbilirubinemia; the blood film is sometimes distinctive but often shows non-specific changes of non-spherocytic hemolysis. An important point is that neonatal hemolytic anemia may be the only presenting feature of triosephosphate isomerase deficiency, the devastating neurological features of this disorder only becoming apparent 6–12 months later. Persistent hemolysis should therefore always be investigated.

Management. The most important management issues in these disorders are making the diagnosis and issuing parents of babies with G6PD deficiency with the appropriate information about which medicines, chemicals and foods may precipitate hemolysis (Table 10.91). If transfusion is required, conventional guidelines for neonatal transfusion can be followed. Folic acid supplements are not required in G6PD deficiency but are necessary in any baby with chronic hemolysis, e.g. pyruvate kinase deficiency.

Hemoglobinopathies. Hemoglobinopathies, with the exception of alpha-thalassemia major, do not usually present in the neonatal period. Alpha-thalassemia major (all four alpha-globin genes deleted) occurs predominantly in families of south-east Asian origin and presents with mid-trimester fetal anemia or hydrops fetalis, which is fatal within hours of delivery. The only long term survivors of alpha-thalassemia major received intrauterine transfusions. The diagnosis is made by Hb electrophoresis (which shows only Hb Barts); the blood film shows hypochromic, microcytic red cells with vast numbers of circulating nucleated red cells. Symptoms and signs of the major beta-globin hemoglobinopathies (sickle cell disease and beta-thalassemia major) are rare in neonates although modern techniques [e.g. high performance liquid chromatography (HPLC), isoelectric focusing] allow the diagnosis to be made on neonatal blood samples where family studies indicate that both parents are carriers. Many countries and regions with a high prevalence of hemoglobinopathies, including much of the UK, have neonatal screening programs to facilitate early diagnosis which is particularly important in sickle cell disease in order to start penicillin prophylaxis as soon as possible.

Management. Transfusion for hemoglobinopathies is rarely required in the neonatal period. It is important to carry out diagnostic investigations on pretransfusion samples and analysis of parental samples is also essential. Folic acid should be given, until transfusion dependence occurs, as all patients have chronic hemolysis and penicillin prophylaxis should be commenced in babies with all forms of sickle cell disease.

Table 10.91 Drugs and chemicals associated with hemolysis in patients who are G6PD deficient

A. Antimalarials
Primaquine
Pamaquine
(Quinine)*
(Chloroquine)*
B. Antibiotics
Nitrofurantoin
Sulfones, e.g. dapsone
Sulfonamides,**e.g. sulfamethoxazole (Septrin)
Quinolones, e.g. nalidixic acid, ciprofloxacin
(Chloramphenicol)†
C. Analgesics
Aspirin (in high doses)
Phenacetin
D. Chemicals
Naphthalene (mothballs)
Divicine (broad beans)
Methylene blue

* acceptable in acute malaria.
** some sulfonamides do not cause hemolysis in most G6PD deficient patients, e.g. sulfadiazine.
† to be avoided in some types of G6PD deficiency (can be taken by patients with the common, African A- form of G6PD deficiency).

Anemia due to blood loss

Anemia due to blood loss may occur during fetal life, at the time of delivery or postnatally (Table 10.89). In neonates admitted to hospital the most common cause of anemia is blood loss secondary to iatrogenic blood letting.

Blood loss prior to birth, including twin-to-twin transfusion

This usually follows twin-to-twin transfusion or trauma but may be spontaneous. The degree of anemia is variable and the clinical presentation depends on the amount and rate of blood loss. The most useful diagnostic tests are a blood film and a Kleihauer test on maternal blood to quantitate the number of HbF-containing fetal red blood cells in the maternal circulation. Where there is chronic blood loss the baby is often well but may present with cardiac failure; the blood film is hypochromic/microcytic. Where the baby has bled acutely just prior to delivery, they will have signs of circulatory shock and the maternal Kleihauer will show a large fetomaternal bleed; in this situation the Hb may be normal at delivery but fall rapidly as hemodilution occurs and the blood film is normochromic/normocytic with large numbers of nucleated red cells. Twin-to-twin transfusion occurs only in monochorionic twins with monochorial placentas. In this situation fetal–fetal transfusion may occur in up to one third of cases producing a difference in Hb at birth of >5 g/dl. Chronic twin-to-twin transfusion can cause a marked difference in birth weight between twins and evidence of chronic blood loss on the blood film of the donor twin.

Blood loss at or after delivery

This is usually due to obstetric complications, such as placenta previa, placental abruption or incision of the placenta during cesarean section. Such babies are often extremely unwell with circulatory shock, anemia worsening rapidly after birth, large numbers of circulating nucleated red cells and disseminated intravascular coagulation. Similar hematological changes occur after massive internal bleeding in the baby, e.g. subarachnoid or retroperitoneal bleeding, and may be particularly severe where there is damage to the liver. While most cases of internal bleeding will be associated with traumatic delivery, it is important to search for any underlying bleeding diathesis in such babies. Inherited coagulation disorders which may present with bleeding at birth or during the neonatal period are discussed on p. 305.

Anemia of prematurity

The normal physiological fall in Hb after birth is greater in preterm compared to term neonates and has been termed 'physiological anemia of prematurity' since it does not appear to be associated with any abnormalities in the baby. The pathogenesis is not fully elucidated but contributory factors include:

- reduced red cell life span;
- inappropriately low erythropoietin;
- nutritional deficiency (iron and folic acid);
- rapid growth rate.

The nadir of Hb in a well term infant is as low as 9.4–11 g/dl at 8–12 weeks of age (Table 10.87); for a preterm infant the nadir in Hb occurs earlier (4–8 weeks of age) and is lower (6.5–9 g/dl). The diagnosis is usually straightforward – a well preterm baby has a slowly falling Hb with a completely unremarkable blood film showing normochromic/normocytic red cells, slightly low reticulocytes (20×10^9/L) and no nucleated red cells.

Management. This is discussed in detail below. The most important aspects are minimizing the severity of anemia and judicious use of red cell transfusion. Erythropoietin may have a role in some babies (see p. 303).[720]

A simple diagnostic approach to neonatal anemia

Red cell disorders associated with anemia present in three main ways: with a low Hb (anemia), with jaundice and with hydrops. A diagnostic algorithm to help in identifying the cause of neonatal anemia and the most useful investigations is shown in Figure 10.45. Hematological causes of neonatal jaundice and of hydrops are shown in Tables 10.91 and 10.93.

Management of neonatal anemia

There are two facets to management:

1. identifying the underlying cause of the anemia where possible; and
2. deciding whether or not to transfuse.

A brief summary of the indications for red cell transfusion is outlined page. Management of neonatal anemia associated with specific hematological disorders is discussed in the relevant sections (Ch. 21). With increasing recognition of potential transfusion hazards, prevention of neonatal anemia has become extremely important and is discussed on page 303.

Red cell transfusion for neonatal anemia

The threshold levels of anemia which should trigger red cell transfusion in neonates remain controversial. There are several useful reviews and guidelines produced by professional bodies; almost none are evidence based. Nevertheless, compliance with transfusion guidelines reduces transfusion requirements and donor exposure.[721–723] A pragmatic approach is to use the published guidelines to produce local, consensus-based neonatal transfusion protocols which can be enforced and monitored to maintain a consistent and sensible transfusion policy for all neonates (Table 10.93). The red cells used should be packed cells (hematocrit 0.5–0.7) which are ABO and Rh D-compatible with the mother and the baby and which are < 35 days old (if stored in suitable medium, e.g. 'SAG-M'). Specially prepared satellite packs should be used wherever possible to allow multiple-transfused neonates to receive blood from the same donor.

Table 10.92 Hematological causes of neonatal jaundice

A. Red cell membrane disorders
Hereditary spherocytosis
Hereditary pyropoikilocytosis
Other: e.g. homozygous hereditary elliptocytosis
B. Red cell enzymopathies
G6PD deficiency
Pyruvate kinase deficiency
Other: e.g. glucose phosphate isomerase deficiency
C. Hemoglobinopathies
Alpha-thalassemias
Gamma-thalassemias
Other: sickle cell syndromes (occasionally)
D. Immune
Hemolytic disease of the newborn
Maternal autoimmune hemolytic anemia
Drug induced
E. Infection
Bacterial
Viral, e.g. CMV, rubella, herpes simplex
Protozoal, e.g. toxoplasma, malaria, syphilis

Table 10.93 Indications for 'top up' red cell transfusion in preterm infants: based on a summary of national consensus-based guidelines

1. Severe pulmonary disease (babies on mechanical ventilation) Hb < 13 g/dl
2. Acute blood loss with shock
3. Stable newborn with clinical signs of anemia (e.g. tachycardia, poor weight gain) Hb 8–10.5 g/dl (threshold varies in different national guidelines)
4. Stable newborn without signs of anemia Hb < 7 g/dl

These guidelines can be used as the basis to produce more specific local neonatal transfusion protocols which may specify different thresholds for transfusion depending upon other important clinical variables, e.g. the postnatal age of the infant, the FiO_2, whether the baby is on CPAP, whether there are associated major complications, e.g. septic shock, NEC, planned surgery.

Prevention of neonatal anemia, including the role of erythropoietin and hematinics

Approaches to preventing or minimizing neonatal anemia include:

1. limiting iatrogenic blood loss by appropriate use of blood tests;
2. iron and folate supplementation for all preterm infants;
   - iron 3 mg/kg/day from 4 to 6 weeks of age (a pragmatic approach is to give 1 ml of sodium ironedetate –'Sytron' – once daily)
   - folic acid 15 μg daily or 500 μg once weekly;
3. judicious use of erythropoietin.

There have been many controlled trials of erythropoietin for prevention of neonatal anemia. The subject has been extensively reviewed[720] and is only briefly summarized here. Recombinant erythropoietin undoubtedly stimulates erythropoiesis in all preterm infants (i.e. there is no evidence of erythropoietin insensitivity). Erythropoietin is also able to reduce red cell transfusion requirements in preterm infants. However, in most studies only the relatively well infants with low transfusion requirements benefit from this as, even in high doses, the erythropoietin-mediated increase in red cell production is unable to increase sufficiently to cope with the need for frequent phlebotomy and multiple transfusions in sick preterm infants. Despite its marginal role in reducing transfusion requirements, erythropoietin may become more important again if worries over the safety of blood transfusion lead to reduced availability and parental acceptance of red cell transfusion. Erythropoietin also has a useful role where red cell transfusions cannot be used (e.g. preterm babies of Jehovah's witnesses). It is important to know that the Hb does not start to rise until about 10–14 days after erythropoietin has been commenced and iron supplements should be started as soon as possible to prevent the rapid development of iron deficiency in erythropoietin-treated infants.

Polycythemia

For both term and preterm infants polycythemia can be defined as a central venous hematocrit of >0.65; above this level there is an exponential rise in blood viscosity. Clinical manifestations include lethargy, hypotonia, hyperbilirubinemia and hypoglycemia. Polycythemia may also be a contributory factor in neonatal seizures, stroke, renal vein thrombosis and NEC. Causes of polycythemia include:

- IUGR;
- maternal hypertension;
- maternal diabetes;
- endocrine disorders: thyrotoxicosis, congenital adrenal hyperplasia;
- chromosomal disorders – trisomy 21, 18 or 13;
- twin-to-twin transfusion;
- delayed clamping of the cord.

Treatment of neonatal polycythemia is controversial. Most of the evidence supports active management of symptomatic infants by exchange transfusion using a crystalloid solution such as normal saline, while asymptomatic infants should be observed.[691] The aim of exchange transfusion is to reduce the hematocrit to 0.55. There is no evidence to support the use of fresh frozen plasma or albumin for this procedure, both of which carry the risk of transfusion-transmitted infection.

WHITE CELL DISORDERS

Neutropenia

Definition and causes of neonatal neutropenia

Neutropenia is fairly common in preterm neonates but is uncommon in term infants. Since normal values are age and gestational age-dependent, a pragmatic approach is to consider a neutrophil count at birth of $<2 \times 10^9$/L as abnormal and worth monitoring and a neutrophil count during the first month of life of $< 0.7 \times 10^9$/L as significant enough to merit further investigation. Causes of neonatal neutropenia are shown in Table 10.94. In preterm neonates the commonest cause is neutropenia in association with IUGR and/or maternal hypertension. The second most frequent cause in preterm infants, and the most common cause in term infants, is neutropenia secondary to bacterial or viral infection.

Immune neutropenias

Although uncommon, immune neutropenia may be severe in the newborn. Both autoimmune and alloimmune neutropenia occur. Autoimmune neutropenia is secondary to maternal autoimmune disease [e.g. systemic lupus erythematosus (SLE)] and is self-limiting. Alloimmune neutropenia occurs where fetal neutrophils express paternally derived neutrophil-specific antigens not present on maternal neutrophils and against which she produces IgG neutrophil alloantibodies. The causative antibodies are usually anti-NA1 or anti-NA2. It is said to occur in 3% of all deliveries but it seems likely that most cases are so mild they do not present to medical attention. The more severe cases present in the first few days of life with fever and infections of the respiratory tract, urinary tract and skin, particularly due to *Staphylococcus aureus*. The neutropenia is self-limiting, usually resolving within 1–2 months, and the mainstay of treatment is antibiotics.

Non-immune neutropenias

The commonest non-immune cause in preterm infants is neutropenia secondary to IUGR and/or maternal hypertension; it may also occur in infants of diabetic mothers. The exact pathogenesis is unknown. Neutrophil production secondary to reduced numbers of neutrophil progenitors (CFU-GM) is found and most affected neonates have associated thrombocytopenia and increased erythropoiesis (polycythemia and/or increased circulating nucleated red cells).[691] The hematological abnormalities appear secondary to fetal tissue hypoxia. Increased erythropoietin is

Table 10.94 Causes of neonatal neutropenia

1. Immune
   - Alloimmune
   - Autoimmune
2. Infection
   - Acute, perinatal bacterial infection, e.g. group B streptococcus
   - Congenital infections, e.g. CMV
   - Postnatal bacterial infections
   - Postnatal viral infections, e.g. CMV
3. Necrotizing enterocolitis
4. Placental insufficiency
   - Maternal hypertension
   - Intrauterine growth restriction
   - Maternal diabetes
5. Genetic
   - Trisomies: 21, 13 and 18
   - Kostmann's syndrome
   - Schwachman's syndrome
   - Pearson's syndrome
   - Reticular dysgenesis
   - Metabolic disorders, e.g. hyperglycinemia; isovaleri, propionic and methylmalonic acidemia
6. Marrow replacement
   - Congenital leukemia

likely to play a role, perhaps by enhancing erythropoiesis at the expense of neutrophil and platelet production. Neutropenia secondary to IUGR/maternal hypertension reaches its nadir on day 2/3 of life and recovers spontaneously by day 7–10. The severity is directly related to the severity of the IUGR/maternal hypertension. Treatment with recombinant (r) G-CSF or rGM-CSF has not been shown to be helpful.[724,725] Prevention of neutropenia in such infants by prophylactic rGM-CSF is currently being investigated.[704]

Other non-immune causes of neutropenia are listed in Table 10.94. The most important is neutropenia secondary to infection. Any bacterial infections cause acute neutropenia – where this is short lived (6–12 h) it is a normal response, but neutropenia lasting > 12 h in the setting of acute bacterial infection is a poor prognostic sign. Examination of the blood film is often helpful in differentiating neutropenia secondary to infection from that due to viral infection or IUGR. The classical signs of acute bacterial infection are the presence of an increased percentage of band neutrophils and toxic granulation of immature and mature neutrophils followed after 1–2 days by a mature neutrophilia and after 3–5 days by eosinophilia. By contrast, there is no increase in band cells or toxic granulation in viral infections; instead atypical 'viral' lymphocytes are seen. Rare causes of neonatal neutropenia include Kostmann's disease and bone marrow failure syndromes. These should be sought where the neutropenia is prolonged, there is a relevant family history, there is consanguinity or if the baby has typical dysmorphic features (e.g. thumb/radial abnormalities in Fanconi's anemia).

Hemopoietic stem cell disorders including leukemias and myeloproliferative disorders

Congenital leukemias

Congenital leukemia is rare but the diagnosis is usually straightforward. The most common types are acute monoblastic leukemia and acute megakaryoblastic leukemia; around 25% of cases occur in babies with Down syndrome (see Ch. 12). Both have similar presentations but can be differentiated by detailed cytogenetic and immunophenotypic studies on bone marrow and blood leukemia cells. The usual presentation is with clinical signs of anemia and skin lesions caused by focal infiltration by leukemic cells. Congenital leukemia may present as 'blueberry muffin' baby or hydrops fetalis. The prognosis is extremely poor; few are cured by chemotherapy and bone marrow transplantation may be the best option.[726]

Hematological abnormalities in neonates with Down syndrome and other trisomies

Hematological abnormalities are more common in neonates with chromosomal disorders, including Down syndrome, trisomy 13 and trisomy 18, all of which may be associated with pancytopenia. Most babies with Down syndrome have a normal blood count; the remaining 10% have one of three hematological presentations:

1. acute leukemia (see p. 000);
2. transient abnormal myelopoiesis (TAM);
3. mild pancytopenia with subtle myelodysplastic changes.

TAM presents with leukocytosis and an abnormal blood film with circulating blast cells. No treatment is indicated and TAM almost always resolves by the age of 2–3 months.[727]

Abnormal leukocytes in neonatal systemic disease

The blood film often provides clues to other underlying disorders in the newborn. As well as classical features of acute bacterial and viral infections (see p. 349), characteristic changes can be seen in fungal infection where vacuolation of the neutrophils and monocytes may be prominent and fungi may be seen within the phagocytic cells. In NEC neutrophil and monocyte vacuolation are also common. A number of metabolic and storage disorders produce changes in the appearance of leukocytes which can be seen on carefully examined blood films:

- leukocyte vacuolation in Pearson's syndrome (see p. 000);
- giant neutrophil granules in Chediak–Higashi syndrome;
- Alder Reilly leukocyte granules in Hunter's syndrome, Hurler's syndrome and Sanfilippo's syndrome;
- lymphocyte vacuolation in Wolman's disease, alpha-mannosidosis, sialidosis and Sanfilippo's syndrome.

HEMOSTASIS AND THROMBOSIS

Normal hemostasis

Hemostasis involves a complex balance between activators and inhibitors of the coagulation cascade and a system to break down and limit clot size (fibrinolysis).[728] There are five main components: blood vessels, platelets, coagulation factors, coagulation inhibitors and fibrinolysis.

Blood vessels

Vascular endothelium plays a key role in initiation and control of coagulation. Intact endothelium secretes prostaglandin I_2 and nitric oxide which promote vasodilatation and inhibit platelet aggregation. Local damage leads to release of tissue factor and exposure of procoagulants in the subendothelium including collagen and von Willebrand factor. This results in platelet adhesion followed by tissue factor-mediated coagulation. Key inhibitors of coagulation are also present on the endothelial surface including thrombomodulin, antithrombin and protein S. Hence endothelium is responsible for directing coagulation to the site of injury and then limiting the extent of thrombus formation via inhibitors.

Platelets

Platelets aggregate at sites of injury and are vital for primary hemostasis. They also provide a phospholipid surface essential for the coagulation cascade. Both quantitative and qualitative defects can lead to bleeding disorders.

Coagulation factors

Traditional versions of the coagulation cascade based on in vitro clotting tests delineated intrinsic and extrinsic pathways and sequential activation of coagulation factors. It has become clear that the process in vivo is quite different from this and a new pathway has been proposed (Fig. 10.46). Clotting factors generally exist as inactive precursors and require activation to take part in coagulation. The key initiating event is exposure of tissue factor in response to endothelial damage. Tissue factor activates factor VII to form a complex, TF-VIIa, which cleaves factor X to its active form Xa. Xa can convert prothrombin to thrombin with low efficiency but this generation of small amounts of thrombin then activates feedback loops to increase coagulation factor activation. Factor VIII (activated by thrombin) and factor IX (activated by TF-VIIa and factor XI) form a complex VIIIa-IXa known as tenase. Tenase generates activated factor X with great efficiency. Thrombin also activates factor V and a Xa-Va complex is formed which cleaves prothrombin to form thrombin. Thrombin generation leads to conversion of fibrinogen to fibrin with subsequent crosslinking by factor XIII.

Inhibitors of coagulation

Widespread coagulation throughout the body is prevented by inhibitors. Protein C is activated by thrombin. Thrombomodulin, an integral endothelial cell membrane protein, greatly enhances the rate of protein C activation. Once activated protein C forms a complex with

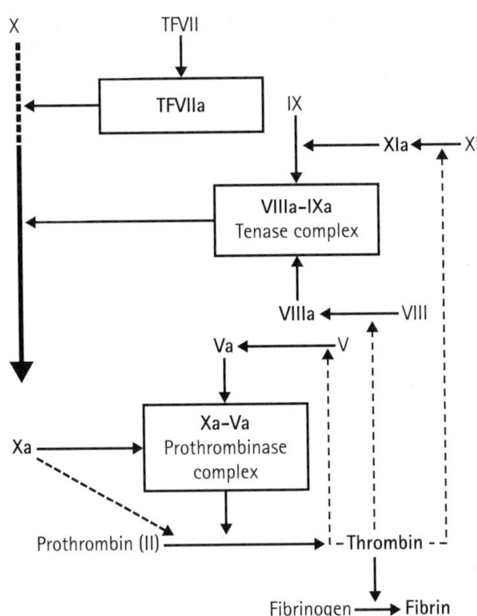

Fig. 10.46 Coagulation cascade. Thick dashed arrows indicate low efficiency pathways. Thin dashed arrows indicate feedback activation loops. Boxes indicate complexes on phospholipid surface.

protein S which increases its activity 10-fold. The activated protein C complex cleaves and inactivates factors V and VIII. A mutation in factor V at the cleavage site, preventing factor V inactivation (factor V Leiden), is associated with thrombophilia. Antithrombin and heparin cofactor II are both potent direct inhibitors of thrombin; levels of these proteins are low at birth but rarely cause thrombosis.[729] Tissue factor pathway inhibitor limits tissue factor-induced initiation of coagulation; deficiency states have not been characterized.

Fibrinolysis

Fibrinolysis limits fibrin deposition at the site of injury. The key enzyme is plasmin. This is produced by the action of tissue plasminogen activator whose activity is catalysed by fibrin itself. Fibrin breakdown is accompanied by the production of degradation products (FDPs) and D-dimers.

Coagulation in the fetus and newborn

Coagulation proteins are synthesized from the fifth week of gestation onwards and do not cross the placenta.[729] Levels gradually rise towards birth but many do not attain adult values during the neonatal period. Birth may cause activation of coagulation; hence levels in preterm infants may be significantly higher than those found in fetuses of the same gestational age. Normal values vary with gestational and postnatal age (Table 10.95).[730–732]

Diagnostic approach to bleeding in neonates

Clinical presentation of bleeding disorders

Neonates exhibit patterns of bleeding distinct from those in older children. Bleeding from the umbilical cord stump, intracranial hemorrhage, cephalhematomas after vacuum extraction, bleeding from venepuncture sites and pulmonary hemorrhage can occur. Bleeding post circumcision is a relatively common presentation of hemophilia but hemarthroses are extremely rare. The most likely cause of bleeding in neonates depends on gestational age and whether the child is sick or well. A thorough clinical assessment is essential and should include sites and severity of bleeding, predisposing factors, drug history (infant and maternal) including vitamin K and a family history of possible coagulation disorders.

Screening tests for bleeding disorders

Initial screening tests should comprise:

1. *prothrombin time* (PT) – measures activity of factors II, V, VII and X;
2. *activated partial thromboplastin time* (APTT) – measures factors II, V, VIII, IX, X, XI and XII;
3. *thrombin time* (TT) – prolonged by quantitative and qualitative disorders of fibrinogen, the presence of inhibitory factors such as fibrin/FDPs and the presence of heparin;
4. fibrinogen level;
5. platelet count.

Results of these tests along with clinical history can guide subsequent investigation. A *reptilase time* (so named because snake venom is used in the test) can also be very helpful; it assesses the same components as a TT but is unaffected by heparin. Bleeding times are generally unhelpful. A diagnostic algorithm is shown in Figure 10.47.

Interpretation of laboratory coagulation tests

Coagulation testing in neonates is often difficult. Since testing is done on plasma, the high hematocrit in many neonates means blood volumes required for testing are relatively large even when using specially adapted microtechniques. Activation of coagulation during sampling is common when venepuncture is difficult and invalidates results. Samples from indwelling lines are frequently heparin contaminated (a marked prolongation of the thrombin time together with a normal reptilase time is the most useful marker of this). Finally, in coagulation factor assays, the lower limit of the normal range in neonates often overlaps with those seen in deficiency states (especially seen with factor II, factor X and factor XI). In such circumstances demonstrating heterozygote levels of factor activity in parents is useful.

Inherited coagulation disorders

Inherited coagulation disorders are rare but often present in the neonatal period hence a high index of suspicion is needed. The commonest are factor VIII (hemophilia A) and factor IX (hemophilia B) with a frequency of 1 in 10 000 and 1 in 60 000 male births respectively. Most other factor deficiencies are autosomal recessive. All produce prolongation of coagulation screening tests with the exception of factor XIII deficiency and, rarely, von Willebrand's disease (vWD). Hence a normal coagulation screen in a child with unexplained bleeding does not exclude all inherited coagulation disorders and further specialized tests may be needed.

This section addresses neonatal aspects of inherited coagulation abnormalities. A comprehensive discussion of these conditions is provided elsewhere (Ch. 21).

Factor VIII deficiency

Clinical presentation. This may be diagnosed or suspected antenatally in families with a history of hemophilia. One-third of cases represent new mutations and are therefore unsuspected at birth. They may present with intracranial hemorrhage, subgaleal or cephalhematomas, bleeding postcircumcision or from venous or arterial puncture sites. Prolonged bleeding from the umbilical cord is less common. The hemorrhage may be life threatening. Large bruises may occur and the diagnosis to be made during investigations of possible non-accidental injury.[733]

Diagnosis. Coagulation tests show a very prolonged APTT with normal PT, TT, platelets and fibrinogen. The definitive diagnosis is made by measurement of factor VIII clotting activity which is $< 50\%$; all other factors, including von Willebrand antigen, are normal. Disease severity is classified according to factor VIII activity with levels $< 1\%$ indicative of severe disease.

Management. Adequate family support is vital and early liaison with a hemophilia center is essential. Treatment should be with

Table 10.95 Reference values for (a) healthy full-term infants and (b) preterm infants during the neonatal period

a) Full term infants

Coagulation Tests	Full-Term Day 1 Mean (95% limits)	Full-Term Day 5 Mean (95% limits)	Full-Term Day 30 Mean (95% limits)
PT(s)	13.0 (10.1–15.9)	12.4 (10.0–15.3)	11.8 (10.0–14.3)
APTT(s)	42.9 (31.3–54.5)	42.6 (25.4–59.8)	40.4 (32.0–55.2)
TT(s)	23.5 (19.0–28.3)	23.1 (18.0–29.2)	24.3 (19.4–29.2)
Fibrinogen (g/L)	2.83 (1.67–3.99)	3.12 (1.62–4.62)	2.70 (1.62–3.78)
Factor V (u/ml)	0.72 (0.34–1.08)	0.95 (0.45–1.45)	0.98 (0.62–1.34)
Factor VII (u/ml)	0.66 (0.28–1.04)	0.89 (0.35–1.43)	0.90 (0.42–1.38)
Factor VIII (u/ml)	1.00 (0.50–1.78)	0.88 (0.50–1.54)	0.91 (0.50–1.57)
Factor IX (u/ml)	0.53 (0.15–0.91)	0.53 (0.15–0.91)	0.51 (0.21–0.81)
Factor X (u/ml)	0.40 (0.12–0.68)	0.49 (0.19–0.79)	0.59 (0.31–0.87)
Factor XI (u/ml)	0.38 (0.10–0.66)	0.55 (0.23–0.87)	0.53 (0.27–0.79)
Factor XII (u/ml)	0.53 (0.13–0.93)	0.47 (0.11–0.83)	0.49 (0.17–0.81)
Factor XIIIa (u/ml)	0.79 (0.27–1.31)	0.94 (0.44–1.44)	0.93 (0.39–1.47)
vWF (u/ml)	1.53 (0.50–2.87)	1.40 (0.50–2.54)	1.28 (0.50–2.46)
Antithrombin (U/ml)	0.63 (0.39–0.87)	0.67 (0.41–0.93)	0.78 (0.48–1.08)
Protein C (U/ml)	0.35 (0.17–0.53)	0.42 (0.20–0.64)	0.43 (0.21–0.65)
Protein S (U/ml)	0.36 (0.12–0.60)	0.50 (0.22–0.78)	0.63 (0.33–0.93)

b) Preterm infants

Coagulation Tests	Premature 30–36 weeks Day 1 Mean (95% limits)	Premature 30–36 weeks Day 5 Mean (95% limits)	Premature 30–36 weeks Day 30 Mean (95% limits)	Premature 30–36 weeks Day 90 Mean (95% limits)	Premature 24–29 weeks Day 1 Mean (95% limits)
PT(s)	13.0 (10.6–16.2)	12.5 (10.0–15.3)	11.8 (10.0–13.6)	12.3 (10.0–14.6)	14.5 (11.7–21.6)
APTT(s)	53.6 (27.5–79.4)	50.5 (26.9–74.1)	44.7 (26.9–62.5)	39.5 (28.3–50.7)	69.5 (40.6–101)
TT(s)	24.8 (19.2–30.4)	24.1 (18.8–29.4)	24.4 (18.8–29.9)	25.1 (19.4–30.8)	
Fibrinogen (g/L)	2.43 (1.50–3073)	2.80 (1.60–4.18)	2.54 (1.50–4.14)	2.46 (1.50-3.52)	1.35 (0.62-4.21)
Factor V (u/ml)	0.88 (0.41-1.44)	1.00 (0.46-1.54)	1.02 (0.48-1.56)	0.99 (0.59-1.39)	
Factor VII (u/ml)	0.67 (0.21-1.13)	0.84 (0.30-1.38)	0.83 (0.21-1.45)	0.87 (0.31-1.43)	
Factor VIII (u/ml)	1.11 (0.50-2.13)	1.15 (0.53-2.05)	1.11 (0.50-1.99)	1.06 (0.58-1.88)	
Factor IX (u/ml)	0.35 (0.19-0.65)	0.42 (0.14-0.74)	0.44 (0.13-0.80)	0.59 (0.25-0.93)	
Factor X (u/ml)	0.41 (0.11-0.71)	0.51 (0.19-0.83)	0.56 (0.20-0.92)	0.67 (0.35-0.99)	
Factor XI (u/ml)	0.30 (0.08-0.52)	0.41 (0.13-0.69)	0.43 (0.15-0.71)	0.59 (0.25-0.93)	
Factor XII (u/ml)	0.38 (0.10-0.66)	0.39 (0.09-0.69)	0.43 (0.11-0.75)	0.61 (0.15-1.07)	
Factor XIIIa (u/ml)	0.70 (0.32-1.08)	1.01 (0.57-1.45)	0.99 (0.51-1.47)	1.13 (0.71-1.55)	
vWF (u/ml)	1.36 (0.78-2.10)	1.33 (0.72-2.19)	1.36 (0.66-2.16)	1.12 (0.75-1.84)	
Antithrombin(U/ml)	0.38 (0.14-0.62)	0.56 (0.30-0.82)	0.59 (0.37-0.81)	0.83 (0.45-1.21)	
Protein C (U/ml)	0.28 (0.12-0.44)	0.31 (0.11-0.51)	0.37 (0.15-0.59)	0.45 (0.23-0.67)	
Protein S (U/ml)	0.26 (0.14-0.38)	0.37 (0.13-0.61)	0.56 (0.22-0.90)	0.76 (0.40-1.12)	

recombinant factor VIII concentrate for bleeding episodes.[734] The best mode of delivery is controversial; there is no evidence that elective cesarean section eliminates bleeding; spontaneous vaginal delivery is acceptable but vacuum extraction should be avoided due to the high rate of subgaleal bleeds and cephalhematomas.[733] There is debate as to whether known hemophiliac newborns should be given prophylactic factor VIII following difficult delivery to reduce the risk of intracranial bleeding. In known or suspected hemophiliac newborns cord blood should always be taken for a coagulation screen and factor VIII level. Vitamin K should be given at birth but the intramuscular route avoided because of hematoma formation.

Factor IX deficiency

This has an identical clinical phenotype to factor VIII deficiency and can only be distinguished by specific factor assays. Unlike factor VIII, factor IX is vitamin K dependent and hence its activity also falls in liver disease and vitamin K deficiency. However there is seldom diagnostic confusion as the latter diseases produce prolongation of other screening tests and characteristic clinical features. Treatment of bleeding is with recombinant factor IX concentrate.

Von Willebrand's disease

This is a complex group of conditions caused by quantitative or qualitative defects in von Willebrand factor (vWF). Neonatal presentation is rare as levels of vWF are elevated at birth.[729] However, one of the most severe forms, type 3 vWD, may present in the neonatal period. In this case factor VIII levels are very low, vWF is virtually absent and the patient presents in a similar way to hemophilia A. Clues to the diagnosis are the absence of X-linked inheritance (it is autosomal recessive) and poor response to factor VIII concentrates. Quantification of vWF makes the diagnosis. Treatment of bleeding is with vWF concentrates (plus factor VIII if severe bleeding) or intermediate purity factor VIII.

Factor XIII deficiency

Factor XIII deficiency presents with umbilical stump bleeding and/or intracranial hemorrhage. Routine coagulation screens are

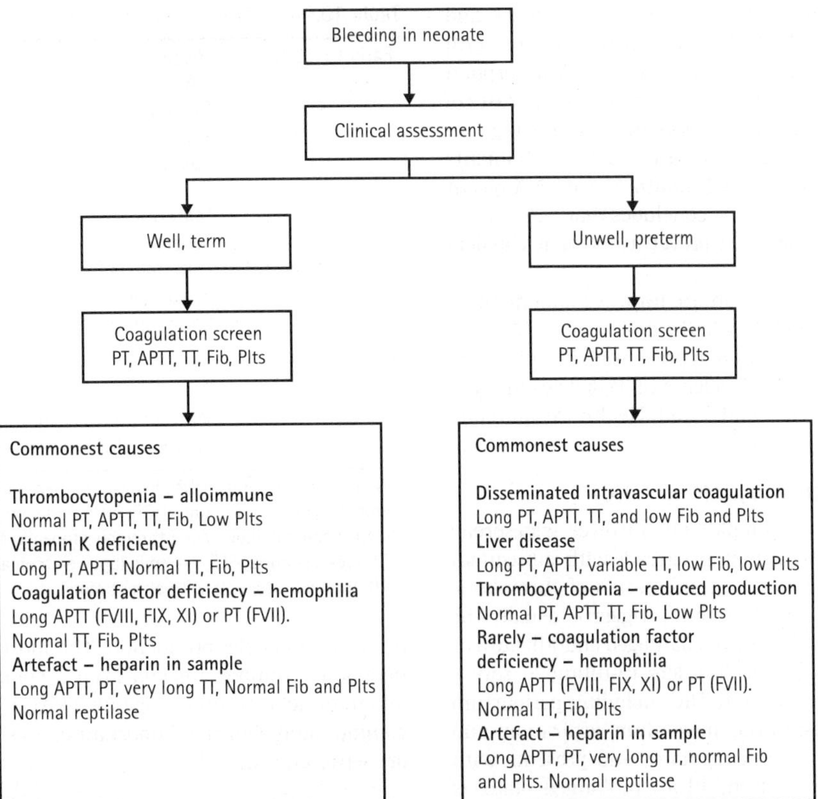

Fig. 10.47 Diagnostic algorithm for bleeding in neonates. APTT, activated partial thromboplastin time; Fib, fibrinogen; Plts, platelets; PT, prothrombin time; TT, thrombin time.

normal. Diagnosis is made by measuring clot solubility in 5 M urea solution; molecular tests for the common mutations are also available. Treatment is with factor XIII concentrate.

Other rarer inherited coagulation factor deficiencies

These can present in the neonatal period with bleeding or unexplained prolongation of coagulation tests. The majority are autosomal recessive. Factor XI deficiency can produce hemophiliac type bleeding and is common in Ashkenazi Jews. Factor VII deficiency can produce a very severe bleeding disorder with a high incidence of intracranial hemorrhage. Recombinant factor VII concentrate can be used but is very expensive and has a very short half-life. Factor XII deficiency produces a markedly prolonged APTT but no clinically apparent bleeding disorder. Dysfibrinogenemias are rare and can produce both hemorrhage and thrombosis.

Acquired disorders of coagulation

Vitamin K deficiency (Hemorrhagic disease of the newborn)

Vitamin K is essential for the production of active forms of factors II, VII, IX, X and protein C and S. Placental transfer of vitamin K occurs but is insufficient to build up adequate stores in the neonate and without supplementation levels fall during the first few days of life.[735] Untreated vitamin K deficiency can lead to hemorrhagic disease of the newborn. It can be classified according to age of onset into classical, early and late.

Classical. Classical presents at 2–7 days old generally in breast-fed term healthy infants. The incidence in babies not receiving supplementation is 0.4–1.7/100 births. Causes include: low vitamin K content in breast milk (< 5 μg/L compared to 50–60 μg/L in formula milk), poor oral intake and a sterile gut. It can be prevented by vitamin K supplementation at birth.

Early. Early presents within the first 24–48 h and is associated with severe vitamin K deficiency in utero. The usual cause is maternal medication that interferes with vitamin K, e.g. anticonvulsants (phenobarbital, phenytoin), antituberculous therapy and oral anticoagulants. It cannot be prevented by vitamin K supplementation at birth.

Late. Late occurs from 2 weeks to 6 months of age. It is usually associated with disorders that reduce vitamin K absorption, e.g. alpha-1 antitrypsin deficiency, biliary atresia, liver disease and malabsorptive states. Breast-fed babies are also at risk. It is prevented by repeated doses of oral vitamin K at birth and in the first weeks of life. Prolonged vitamin K supplementation should be given to all babies with chronic liver disease or other risk factors.

Bleeding manifestations include gastrointestinal, cutaneous and intracranial bleeding. Gastrointestinal bleeding in newborns can be differentiated from melena secondary to swallowed maternal blood by the Apt test. Clotting studies show a prolonged PT with normal platelets and fibrinogen. Low levels of vitamin K dependent factors are seen, and inactive forms (proteins induced by vitamin K absence: PIVKAs) can be measured. Treatment: vitamin K subcutaneously or intravenously (not i.m. due to risk of hematoma); fresh frozen plasma (FFP) may be given for life threatening bleeding prior to vitamin K taking effect.

Vitamin K supplementation at birth. Vitamin K supplementation prevents classical and late vitamin K deficiency bleeding. Controversy surrounds the best mode of administration. Studies by Golding et al[736] suggested a link between intramuscular vitamin K at birth and later childhood malignancies. These studies have been criticized on methodological grounds.[737] Seven further studies failed to confirm the link with malignancy but two produced equivocal results and were unable to rule out a link with early onset (age 1–6 years) acute lymphoblastic leukemia. No link between oral vitamin K and malignancy has been reported but disadvantages of oral vitamin K include unnoticed regurgitation, unpredictable absorption and the need for repeated dosing. In one study there were no cases of vitamin K deficiency bleeding in 320 000 infants given 1 mg i.m. vitamin K at birth, but 32 cases of late disease in 1 200 000 infants given 1 mg orally at birth, 1 week and 1 month of age.[738] A recent Cochrane database systematic review[739] concludes that:

1. intramuscular vitamin K has been proven to prevent classical disease;
2. oral vitamin K has been proven to improve biochemical parameters of vitamin K deficiency in the first week of life;
3. the efficacy of oral supplementation in preventing late disease is unproven. Both The American Academy of Pediatrics and the Royal College of Paediatrics and Child Health recommend vitamin K supplementation at birth.

Disseminated intravascular coagulation (DIC)

The pathophysiology of DIC is complex but involves widespread uncontrolled activation of the coagulation cascade with subsequent consumption of clotting factors and a combination of thrombotic and hemorrhagic manifestations. The initial trigger is usually the release of tissue factor and cytokines from damaged endothelium or monocytes. A number of neonatal disorders resulting in severe hypoxia and/or acidosis can precipitate DIC including peripartum hemorrhage, severe birth asphyxia, meconium aspiration and sepsis. Clinically DIC is seen in sick neonates and presents with generalized bleeding. The PT, APTT and TT are prolonged; platelets and fibrinogen are low. Although D-dimers are of some use in monitoring DIC they should be interpreted with caution as they are not specific and can be found in healthy neonates with no evidence of coagulopathy.[740] The mainstay of management is treatment of the underlying cause. In the presence of uncontrolled bleeding platelet infusion and FFP or cryoprecipitate may be needed. Platelets should be maintained above 50×10^9/L and fibrinogen > g/L.

Other acquired coagulation disorders

Serious liver disease can cause a severe coagulopathy compounded by hepatocyte immaturity, vitamin K deficiency and DIC. Platelets may be low due to impaired production, increased consumption and splenic sequestration. Severe coagulopathy can be seen with amino acid defects, e.g. hyperammonemia. Extracorporeal membrane oxygenation often causes coagulation and platelet disturbances due to consumption of clotting factors and platelets and heparinization. Consumptive coagulopathy with thrombocytopenia can be seen with giant hemangioendotheliomas (Kasabach–Merritt syndrome).

Neonatal thrombocytopenia

Incidence of neonatal thrombocytopenia

Thrombocytopenia (platelets < 150×10^9/L) is found in 1–5% of all newborns and severe thrombocytopenia (platelets < 50×10^9/L) in 0.2%. In neonates admitted to NICUs, thrombocytopenia develops in 22–35% of all admissions and in up to 50% of those neonates who are preterm and sick.[710]

Causes and natural history of neonatal thrombocytopenia

Neonatal thrombocytopenia usually presents in one of two distinct patterns: early thrombocytopenia (within 72 h of birth) and late thrombocytopenia (after 72 h of life). Early thrombocytopenia is more common; the principal causes are shown in Table 10.96. The most frequent cause of early thrombocytopenia in preterm infants is 'placental insufficiency'; this is self-limiting, usually within 10 days, and is rarely severe except in neonates with severe IUGR. It is caused by reduced platelet production. The most important cause of early neonatal thrombocytopenia from a clinical viewpoint is neonatal alloimmune thrombocytopenia (NAITP) (see below). The most common and clinically important causes of late thrombocytopenia are sepsis and NEC.[710]

Table 10.96 Causes of neonatal thrombocytopenia

Early (< 72 h)	*Placental insufficiency (PET, IUGR, diabetes)* NAITP Birth asphyxia Perinatal infection (group B strep, *Escherichia coli, Listeria*) Congenital infection (CMV, toxoplasmosis, rubella) Maternal autoimmune (ITP, SLE) Severe rhesus HDN Thrombosis (renal vein, aortic) Aneuploidy (trisomy - 21, 18, 13) Congenital/inherited (TAR, Wiskott–Aldrich)
Late (> 72 h)	*Late-onset sepsis and NEC* Congenital infection (CMV, toxoplasmosis, rubella) Maternal autoimmune (ITP, SLE) Congenital/inherited (TAR, Wiskott–Aldrich)

CMV, cytomegalovirus; HDN, hemolytic disease of the newborn; ITP, idiopathic thrombocytopenic purpura; IUGR, intrauterine growth restriction; NAITP, neonatal alloimmune thrombocytopenia; NEC, necortizing enterocolitis; PET, pre-eclampsia; SLE, systemic lupus erythematosus; strep, streptococcus; TAR, thrombocytopenia with absent radii.

Neonatal alloimmune and autoimmune thrombocytopenia

NAITP is the platelet equivalent of hemolytic disease of the newborn and alloimmune neutropenia. Fetal and neonatal thrombocytopenia result from transplacental passage of maternal platelet-specific antibodies; in 80% of cases these are anti-HPA-1a antibodies and in 10–15% anti-HPA-5b. Although NAITP is uncommon, affecting 1:1000 pregnancies, it is frequently severe and occurs in the first pregnancy in almost 50% of cases. Intracranial hemorrhage occurs in 10% of cases with long term neurodevelopmental sequelae in 20% of survivors. Diagnosis is made by demonstrating platelet antigen incompatibility between mother and baby; most, but not all mothers, have detectable anti-HPA antibodies. Therapy for NAITP remains controversial (reviewed in Ouwehand et al[741]). Antenatal management may include fetal blood sampling, fetal transfusion with HPA-compatible platelets and/or maternal IVIG therapy; each approach has evidence to support it. All severely affected babies should receive HPA-compatible platelets until a stable platelet count > 50×10^9/L is achieved.

Neonatal autoimmune thrombocytopenia occurs secondary to transplacental passage of maternal platelet autoantibodies, usually maternal ITP. Thrombocytopenia affects the infants of 10% of affected mothers; thrombocytopenia is usually mild and intracranial hemorrhage occurs in 1% or less. In affected babies with severe thrombocytopenia treatment with IVIG is usually effective.

Management of neonatal thrombocytopenia

Management of immune thrombocytopenias is described on page 173. For other forms of neonatal thrombocytopenia therapy mainly depends upon the appropriate use of platelet transfusion. Evidence-based guidelines for neonatal platelet transfusion therapy are yet to be defined; consensus guidelines are available (Hume,[723] discussed in Roberts & Murray[710]). Most of these guidelines recommend platelet transfusion for sick neonates where the platelet count is < 50×10^9/L; for stable, relatively well preterm and term infants platelet counts of 30–50 $\times 10^9$/L do not appear to be associated with an increased risk of hemorrhage;[742] this approach conforms to the current UK guidelines.[721] Since platelet underproduction underlies the majority of neonatal thrombocytopenias, recombinant hemopoietic growth factors, including thrombopoietin and interleukin-11, may be useful future therapies.[710]

Thrombosis in neonates

Neonates have an increased rate of thrombotic problems (2.4 per 1000 hospital admissions). Most thromboses occur in sick neonates and are due to acquired risk factors but inherited deficiencies of coagulation inhibitors can also lead to dramatic thrombosis in otherwise healthy neonates.

Inherited thrombotic disorders

Protein C deficiency. The mode of presentation depends on residual protein C activity. Heterozygotes rarely present as neonates unless there are additional prothrombotic factors. Infants born with undetectable protein C frequently present with neonatal purpura fulminans. DIC occurs with a rapidly progressive hemorrhagic necrosis of the skin accompanied by dermal vessel thrombosis. This is most pronounced in the extremities, leads to skin necrosis and is usually fatal if left untreated. Babies may also show evidence of intrauterine thrombosis with cerebral and ophthalmic damage. Diagnosis is made by the characteristic clinical picture in conjunction very low levels of protein C in the patient and heterozygote levels in the parents. Molecular analysis can be used to confirm the diagnosis retrospectively and may be helpful in prenatal diagnosis in future pregnancies.[743]

Treatment is with FFP or protein C concentrate if available. Heparin and antiplatelet agents do not appear to be effective. Oral anticoagulation is used in the medium to long term to prevent recurrence but its introduction must be covered by infusion of a source of protein C and very careful monitoring is needed to prevent subtherapeutic levels which are associated with recurrence of thrombosis. Other long term treatment strategies include protein C replacement therapy or liver transplantation.

Protein S deficiency. This presents in a similar way to protein C deficiency. Treatment is with FFP or protein S concentrate.

Antithrombin deficiency. This is very rare in the homozygous state. Myocardial infarction, aortic thrombosis and cerebral thrombosis have all been reported in neonates. Antithrombin concentrate is commercially available.

Other inherited thrombotic disorders. The more recently discovered prothrombotic mutations such as factor V Leiden and the prothrombin 202010A promoter mutation have not yet been reported to cause neonatal thrombotic problems in isolation. They may play a role in the presence of other acquired risk factors.

Acquired thrombotic problems

The International Registry of Neonatal Thrombotic Disease has greatly expanded knowledge in this area.[744] Risk factors for thrombosis include the presence of a vessel catheter, shock syndromes (septic, hypoxemic or hypovolemic) and the presence of maternal lupus anticoagulant.

Catheter-related thrombosis. This is the commonest cause of neonatal thrombosis being responsible for > 80% of venous and > 90% arterial thrombosis. Symptomatic thrombosis occurs in 1% of neonates with indwelling vascular catheters, but postmortem studies suggest rates of asymptomatic thrombosis up to 20–30%. Arterial thrombosis can lead to peripheral gangrene and renal hypertension. Venous thrombosis can cause portal hypertension and varices. Diagnosis is made by contrast venography or Doppler ultrasound.[745] Treatment depends on the severity and extent of thrombosis. The first step is prompt removal. If signs progress or have not resolved by 24 h, heparin is the drug of choice but requires a dosing regimen adapted for neonates.[746] Local and systemic thrombolysis with urokinase or tissue plasminogen activator (tPA) can cause high rates of bleeding including intracranial hemorrhage and need specialist advice and monitoring. Prevention of thrombosis is paramount, e.g. correct catheter positioning, prompt removal once unnecessary. Prophylactic low dose heparin prolongs catheter patency but its role in preventing thrombosis is unproven.

Non-catheter-related thrombosis. The commonest non-catheter-related thrombosis is renal vein thrombosis. Nearly 80% present in the neonatal period and thrombosis may even occur in utero. One-quarter are bilateral. Presentation is with a flank mass, hematuria, proteinuria, thrombocytopenia and reduced function of the involved kidney. Predisposing factors include reduced renal blood flow, increased viscosity, hyperosmolar states and hypercoagulability. Hence risk factors are sepsis, maternal diabetes, polycythemia, dehydration and prothrombotic mutations. Treatment is supportive. Heparin and thrombolysis are reserved for extensive bilateral cases. A thrombophilia screen should be performed. Long term outlook is variable.

Neonatal stroke. Neonatal stroke is rare. Causes include bacterial meningitis, hypoxic–ischemic damage and birth trauma. Many cases are idiopathic. Some studies show an increased prevalence of thrombophilia in affected neonates, particularly factor V Leiden.[747] Maternal or neonatal anticardiolipin antibodies have also been linked to neonatal stroke; these are often transient and their causal role is not yet established.This is a rapidly evolving field. It is likely that thrombophilia plays a role in neonatal stroke but additional risk factors are probably also needed.

NEONATAL NEUROLOGY

NEUROLOGICAL ASSESSMENT

Introduction

Clinical examination of the neonatal nervous system is, of necessity, dominated by assessment of motor function. The following description is based on the work of pediatric neurologists such as Saint-Anne Dargassies,[749] Amiel-Tison & Grenier,[750] Prechtl & Bientema,[751] Prechtl,[752] Brazelton[753] and Dubowitz & Dubowitz.[754] Gestational age and drugs can affect tone and reflex response so that an accurate maternal and neonatal history is essential. In term babies the best time to perform a neurological examination is when the baby is quiet and alert having awakened spontaneously after a feed.

State

Normal babies show different states of alertness (Table 10.97).[751,753] The fetus exhibits similar states, apart from crying.[755] Babies born before 36 weeks' gestation spend a great deal of time asleep and fall asleep easily when awakened. Preterm sleep states are less easily characterized than at term. Term babies spend about 50 min of each hour asleep, 50% of the time in quiet sleep. Babies who are continually in one state may be abnormal. One example is the baby who is 'hyperalert' due to withdrawal symptoms after maternal drug abuse, who spends little time asleep and more time crying than is usual. Inability to rouse a baby from sleep is pathological and a baby who is persistently in state 1 is in a coma.

Crying and consolability

During an examination most babies will cry but are consolable. Soundless or hoarse crying results from damage to the larynx from

Table 10.97 Normal neonatal states of Prechtl and Brazelton

Prechtl & Bientema[751]	
State 1	Eyes closed, regular respiration, no movements
State 2	Eyes closed, irregular respiration, no movements
State 3	Eyes open, no gross movements
State 4	Eyes open, gross movements, no crying
State 5	Crying
Brazelton[753]	
State 1	Deep sleep, regular breathing, no movements
State 2	Light sleep, irregular respiration, rapid eye movements, eyes closed
State 3	Drowsy, eyes open or closed, some activity – smooth
State 4	Alert, minimal motor activity
State 5	Eyes open, considerable motor activity
State 6	Crying

intubation or a congenitally abnormal larynx. High pitched crying is more than just a subjective phenomenon: spectral analysis of the sound frequencies contained in cries reveals patterns which can predict outcome. Asymmetrical crying facies is often due to facial palsy.

Posture, spontaneous movement and tone

Normal muscle offers a resistance to stretch felt by the examiner as tone. Tone increases with gestational age and is high in term babies. Term babies lie with their limbs flexed and adducted, unlike preterm babies who adopt an extended posture (Fig. 10.48). Asymmetrical tone does not always indicate asymmetrical pathology in the newborn period. A pattern of mixed change in tone with hypertonia in the limbs and hypotonia in the trunk is abnormal. Tone can alter considerably in relation to feeds and sleep state, and repeated examinations are required to confirm physical signs. Passive tone matures from below upwards, and this forms the basis of several methods of assessing gestational age. This type of assessment is not suitable for ill babies.

A term newborn makes smooth, spontaneous symmetrical limb movements which stop when the baby's attention is diverted.[756] Finger movements are elegant and varied, involving the thumb which can be abducted away from the palm by term.[757] In general, the movements of the newborn have a writhing quality which changes to fidgety after 1 month of age. The repertoire of movement is varied and not stereotyped. A persistently adducted thumb (cortical thumb) is abnormal, and brain damaged babies often have fisted hands and a paucity of fine finger movements.

Jitteriness

The normal term newborn is in a state of hypertonicity, with brisk reflexes tending to clonus. This 'transient spasticity' gradually relaxes over the first 8–10 months in a caudocephalad direction. The high tone can lead to the clinical sign of jittering. Jittering is a high frequency, generalized, symmetrical tremor of the limbs which is stilled by flexion or by inducing the baby to suck on a finger. Jittering is common in the first 2 or 3 days in term babies but if it is excessive or persistent deserves investigation. Repetitive chewing movements or tongue thrusting are not part of jitteriness and imply seizures. Jitteriness is stimulus-sensitive whereas seizures are not. In seizure the movement has a fast and slow component whereas in jittering the tremor is symmetrical. Jittering is never accompanied

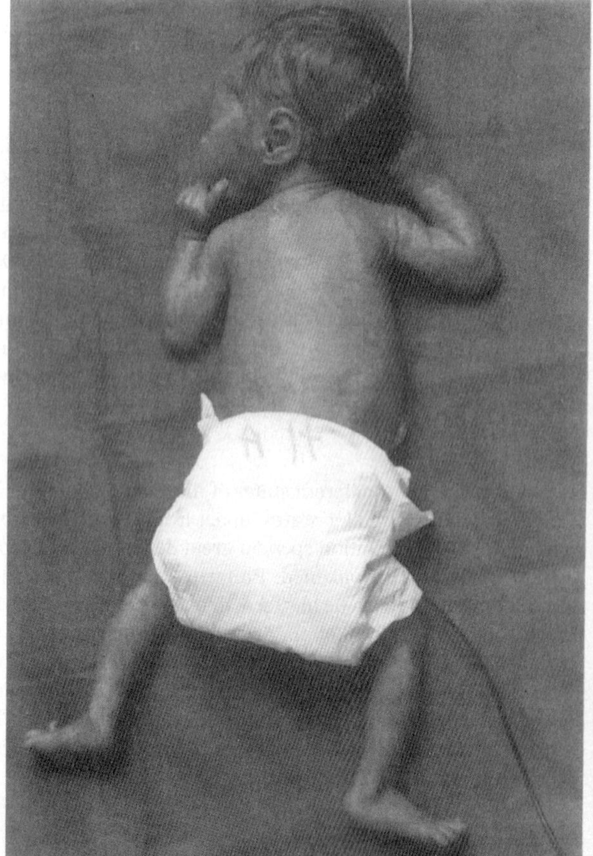

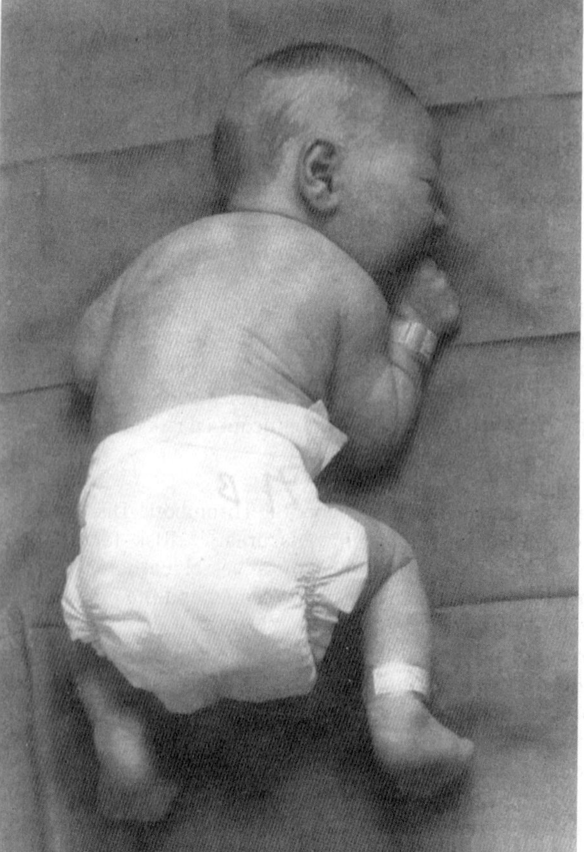

Fig. 10.48 Comparison between low tone in preterm baby (normal) (left) and the high flexor tone of a healthy term baby (right).

by physiological changes due to the autonomic nervous system such as tachycardia, hypertension or apnea.

Limb tone and power

Before passive movements are used to assess tone it may be possible to observe spontaneous movements of the limbs against gravity. Failure to move part or whole of a limb may be due to pain or paralysis. Limb tone is influenced by the tonic neck reflex in newborns which means it is important to have the head in the midline before beginning to elicit passive movements. These involve gentle flexion of the upper and lower limbs, then rapid extension and observation of recoil. A summary is contained within the protocol suggested by Dubowitz & Dubowitz[754] (Fig. 10.49). This examination system, like that of Amiel-Tison,[758] involves assessing angles made by bending and manipulating the limbs. These include the popliteal angle, the foot dorsiflexion angle, the square window and the scarf sign. A reduced popliteal angle and clusters of abnormal signs have been shown to be a sensitive indicator of later outcome.

Trunk and neck tone and power

Normal term babies have sufficient power in their neck muscles to lift their heads slightly when prone or supine. Preterm babies can manage to turn their heads from side to side but have much less power with complete head lag when pulled to sit. In order to judge tone in the neck and trunk, babies should be pulled to sit by holding them at the shoulders and then allowed to fall back again to the couch. If the head is unsupported it will gradually fall forwards or backwards: normal term babies will be able to raise their heads to the vertical again from either direction. There is balance between the neck flexors and extensors during pull-to-sit and back-to-lying maneuvers at term so that the head is held in line with the body during both phases. Immature babies usually have better control in back-to-lying. To assess truncal tone, lie the child on his back and try to push his bottom towards his head using his thighs (Fig. 10.50).[758] With the baby lying on his side, hold the lumbar region and pull both legs backwards with the other hand grasping the ankles. Trunk flexion should always exceed extension. Arching of the trunk is abnormal; backwards arching of the whole back and neck is called opisthotonos.

Reflexes

Tendon and Babinski reflexes

Eliciting tendon reflexes is of less value in the newborn period than later in childhood. Knee and biceps jerks can usually be obtained. Reflexes at term are very brisk due to the high tone, and a few beats of clonus at the ankle are usual. The plantar reflex of Babinski is always extensor and is best omitted as the stimulus often results in a withdrawal response.

Primary neonatal reflexes

Whilst the multiplicity of these responses and the timing of their appearance and disappearance is fascinating it is only necessary to have a working knowledge of a few. The reflexes have parallels in animals; the Moro reflex enables young primates to hold on to their mothers. Primitive reflexes normally habituate after repeated performance: this 'conditioning' is apparent even in fetal life. Persistence of neonatal reflexes can considerably inhibit normal movement in children with cerebral palsy.

Moro

This reflex is elicited by allowing the previously supported head of a baby to fall backwards slightly, whereupon the baby extends and adducts both upper limbs, opening the hands (Fig. 10.51). Babies of greater than 33 weeks' gestation subsequently abduct their arms. The Moro response is present from 28 weeks of gestation and usually disappears by 4 months. Persistence beyond 6 months is always abnormal.

Asymmetric tonic neck reflex

Starting with the baby supine and the head in the midline the head is slowly turned to one side. This results in increased extensor tone in the arm on the side to which the head is turned and increased flexor tone in the arm on the opposite side (fencing posture).

Symmetric tonic neck reflex

This reflex helps the baby to push up on his arms later; when the head is extended on the neck tone increases in the upper limbs and when it is flexed tone reduces.

Placing and stepping

By stimulating the dorsum of the foot, usually by bringing it into contact with the edge of the couch, a mature baby can be induced to 'step' over the edge. With the feet in contact with a solid surface the baby will 'walk'.

Rooting, sucking and swallowing

Stroking the upper lip of a baby of 28 weeks' gestation and above results in the baby searching for the nipple and tests the sensation in the distribution of the 5th cranial nerve. Sucking involves the motor activity of cranial nerves V, VII, XII; swallowing involves IX and X. The sensory input for the sucking reflex comes from the hard palate, not the tongue or cheek. Coordination between sucking and swallowing exists from 28 weeks' gestation but the strength to sustain it and to synchronize breathing is only adequate after 32–34 weeks' gestation. Sucking gradually builds up from bursts of three at a time to eight or more, with a reduction in the interburst interval. If sucking is absent test the gag reflex by gently stroking the soft palate with a cotton bud.

Palmar and plantar

The palmar reflex results from stroking the palmar surface of the hand, eliciting a grasp that is often strong enough to lift the baby from the crib. It is present from 26 weeks' gestation and persists up to 4 months. Stroking the ball of the foot results in curling of the toes in a similar manner to the palmar response.

Special senses

Examination of the eyes and vision

Babies can usually be induced to open their eyes by holding them face to face and spinning them round, or they often open their eyes when sucking. The eyes are in alignment, although a slightly dysconjugate horizontal position is not abnormal in the first 6 weeks. Vertical or skew deviation is always abnormal and has been seen in association with periventricular hemorrhage.[759] Sunsetting (Fig. 10.52) should be noted although it is not as reliable a sign of raised intracranial pressure as later in childhood. The 'doll's eye' maneuver induced by rotating the head from side to side results in reflex deviation of the eyes to the opposite side. It is normally present even in preterm babies, and absence of this reflex indicates severe brainstem damage. Pupil reactions to light are present after 31 weeks' gestation. Visual fixation of a suitable target such as a red woolly ball or a target of broad concentric rings is present from 32 weeks' gestation, and by 34 weeks babies track briefly. By term babies can reliably fix and track an object held 20–30 cm away from the face, and persistent failure to follow a suitable object should give rise to concern. Blinking in response

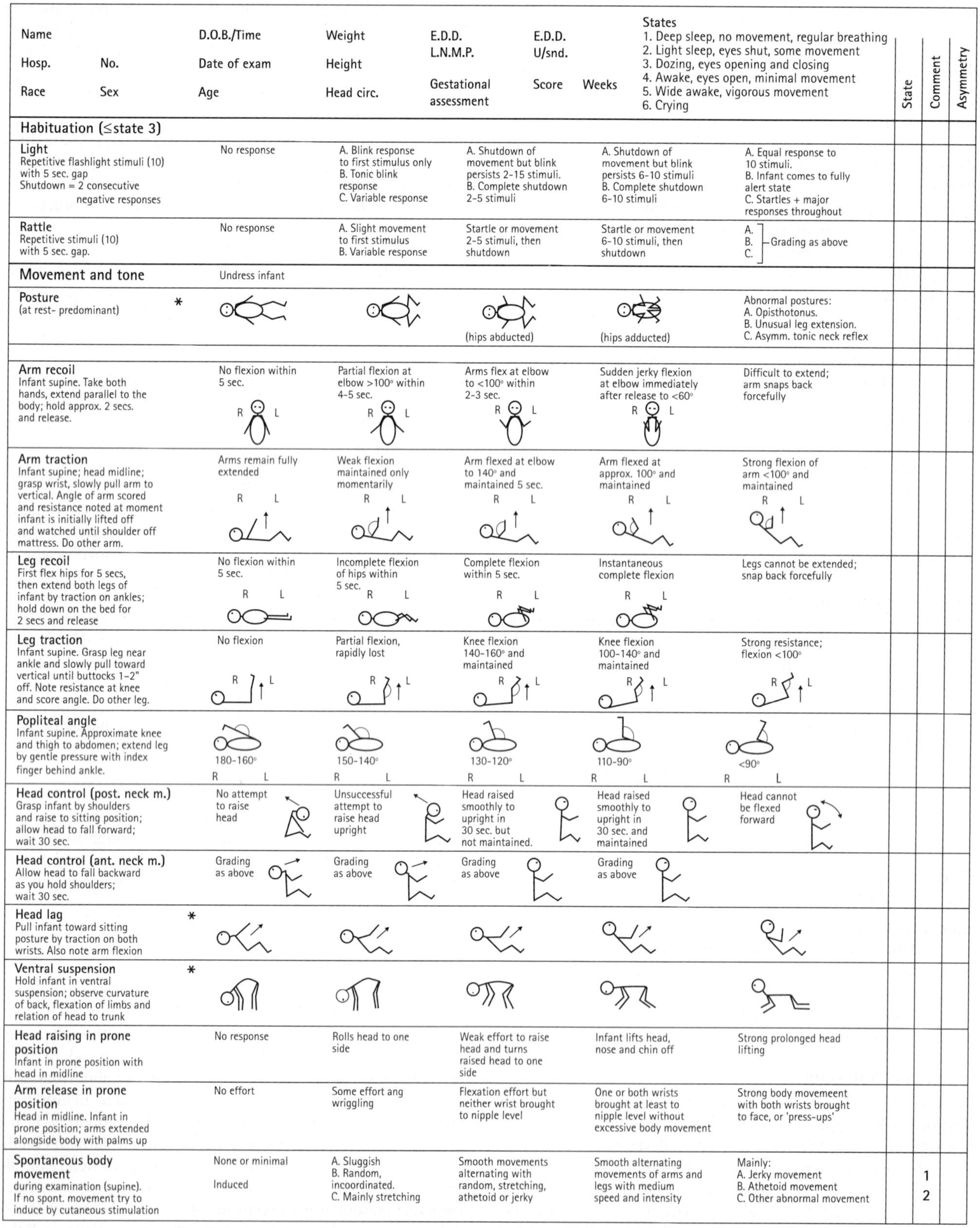

Name		D.O.B./Time	Weight	E.D.D. L.N.M.P.	E.D.D. U/snd.	States		
Hosp.	No.	Date of exam	Height			1. Deep sleep, no movement, regular breathing 2. Light sleep, eyes shut, some movement 3. Dozing, eyes opening and closing 4. Awake, eyes open, minimal movement 5. Wide awake, vigorous movement 6. Crying		
Race	Sex	Age	Head circ.	Gestational assessment	Score / Weeks			

						State	Comment	Asymmetry
Habituation (≤state 3)								
Light Repetitive flashlight stimuli (10) with 5 sec. gap Shutdown = 2 consecutive negative responses	No response	A. Blink response to first stimulus only B. Tonic blink response C. Variable response	A. Shutdown of movement but blink persists 2-15 stimuli. B. Complete shutdown 2-5 stimuli	A. Shutdown of movement but blink persists 6-10 stimuli B. Complete shutdown 6-10 stimuli	A. Equal response to 10 stimuli. B. Infant comes to fully alert state C. Startles + major responses throughout			
Rattle Repetitive stimuli (10) with 5 sec. gap.	No response	A. Slight movement to first stimulus B. Variable response	Startle or movement 2-5 stimuli, then shutdown	Startle or movement 6-10 stimuli, then shutdown	A. B. C. – Grading as above			
Movement and tone	Undress infant							
Posture (at rest- predominant) *			(hips abducted)	(hips adducted)	Abnormal postures: A. Opisthotonus. B. Unusual leg extension. C. Asymm. tonic neck reflex			
Arm recoil Infant supine. Take both hands, extend parallel to the body; hold approx. 2 secs. and release.	No flexion within 5 sec. R L	Partial flexion at elbow >100° within 4-5 sec. R L	Arms flex at elbow to <100° within 2-3 sec. R L	Sudden jerky flexion at elbow immediately after release to <60° R L	Difficult to extend; arm snaps back forcefully			
Arm traction Infant supine; head midline; grasp wrist, slowly pull arm to vertical. Angle of arm scored and resistance noted at moment infant is initially lifted off and watched until shoulder off mattress. Do other arm.	Arms remain fully extended R L	Weak flexion maintained only momentarily R L	Arm flexed at elbow to 140° and maintained 5 sec. R L	Arm flexed at approx. 100° and maintained R L	Strong flexion of arm <100° and maintained R L			
Leg recoil First flex hips for 5 secs, then extend both legs of infant by traction on ankles; hold down on the bed for 2 secs and release	No flexion within 5 sec. R L	Incomplete flexion of hips within 5 sec. R L	Complete flexion within 5 sec. R L	Instantaneous complete flexion R L	Legs cannot be extended; snap back forcefully			
Leg traction Infant supine. Grasp leg near ankle and slowly pull toward vertical until buttocks 1-2" off. Note resistance at knee and score angle. Do other leg.	No flexion R L	Partial flexion, rapidly lost R L	Knee flexion 140-160° and maintained R L	Knee flexion 100-140° and maintained R L	Strong resistance; flexion <100° R L			
Popliteal angle Infant supine. Approximate knee and thigh to abdomen; extend leg by gentle pressure with index finger behind ankle.	180-160° R L	150-140° R L	130-120° R L	110-90° R L	<90° R L			
Head control (post. neck m.) Grasp infant by shoulders and raise to sitting position; allow head to fall forward; wait 30 sec.	No attempt to raise head	Unsuccessful attempt to raise head upright	Head raised smoothly to upright in 30 sec. but not maintained.	Head raised smoothly to upright in 30 sec. and maintained	Head cannot be flexed forward			
Head control (ant. neck m.) Allow head to fall backward as you hold shoulders; wait 30 sec.	Grading as above	Grading as above	Grading as above	Grading as above				
Head lag Pull infant toward sitting posture by traction on both wrists. Also note arm flexion *								
Ventral suspension Hold infant in ventral suspension; observe curvature of back, flexation of limbs and relation of head to trunk *								
Head raising in prone position Infant in prone position with head in midline	No response	Rolls head to one side	Weak effort to raise head and turns raised head to one side	Infant lifts head, nose and chin off	Strong prolonged head lifting			
Arm release in prone position Head in midline. Infant in prone position; arms extended alongside body with palms up	No effort	Some effort ang wriggling	Flexation effort but neither wrist brought to nipple level	One or both wrists brought at least to nipple level without excessive body movement	Strong body movemeent with both wrists brought to face, or 'press-ups'			
Spontaneous body movement during examination (supine). If no spont. movement try to induce by cutaneous stimulation	None or minimal Induced	A. Sluggish B. Random, incoordinated. C. Mainly stretching	Smooth movements alternating with random, stretching, athetoid or jerky	Smooth alternating movements of arms and legs with medium speed and intensity	Mainly: A. Jerky movement B. Athetoid movement C. Other abnormal movement		1 2	

Fig. 10.49 The Dubowitz score. (From Dubowitz & Dubowitz[754] courtesy of Spastics International Publishers Ltd)

to a bright light is a subcortical response and has been recorded in anencephalic and holoprosencephalic babies. Tracking in infancy is not a guarantee of later intact visual function and may be subcortically mediated.[760] Optokinetic nystagmus is present from 36 weeks and preferential looking towards gratings of varying thickness can be used to assess acuity. Visual cortical function is achieved by 6 weeks.[761] Visual evoked potentials are discussed below in the investigation section.

Tremors Mark: Fast (>6/sec.) or Slow (<6/sec.)	No tremor	Tremors only in state 5-6	Tremors only in sleep or after Moro and startles	Some tremors in state 4	Tremulousness in all states			
Startles	No startles	Startles to sudden noise. Moro, bang on table only	Occasional spontaneous startle	2-5 spontaneous startles	6+ spontaneous startles			
Abnormal movement or posture	No abnormal movement	A. Hands clenched but open intermittently. B. Hands do not open with Moro	A. Some mouthing movement. B. Intermittent adducted thumb	A. Persistently adducted thumb. B. Hands clenched all the time	A. Continuous mouthing movement B. Convulsive movements			
Reflexes								
Tendon reflexes Biceps jerk Knee jerk Ankle jerk	Absent		Present	Exaggerated	Clonus			
Palmar grasp Head in midline. Put index finger from ulnar side into hand and gently press palmar surface. Never touch dorsal side of hand	Absent	Short, weak flexion	Medium strength and sustained flexion for several secs.	Strong flexion; contraction spreads to forearm	Very strong grasp. Infant easily lifts off couch			
Rooting Infant supine; head midline. Touch each corner of the mouth in turn (stroke laterally)	No response	A. Partial weak head turn but no mouth opening B. Mouth opening, no head turn	Mouth opening on stimulated side with partial head turning	Full head turning, with or without mouth opening	Mouth opening with very jerky head turning			
Sucking Infant supine; place index finger (pad toward palate) in infant's mouth; judge power of sucking movement after 5 sec.	No attempt	Weak sucking movement: A. Regular B. Irregular	Strong sucking movement, poor stripping A. Regular B. Irregular	Strong regular sucking movement with continuing sequence of 5 movements. Good stripping	Clenching but no regular sucking			
Walking (state 4, 5) Hold infant upright, feet touching bed, neck held straight with fingers	Absent		Some effort but not continuous with both legs	At least 2 steps with both legs	A. Stork posture; no movement. B. Automatic walking			
Moro One hand supports infant's head in midline, the other the back. Raise infant to 45° and when infant is relaxed let his head fall through 10°. Note if jerky. Repeat 3 times	No response, or opening of hands only	Full abduction at the shoulder and extension of the arm	Full abduction but only delayed or partial adduction	Partial abduction at shoulder and extension of arms followed by smooth adduction A. Abd>Add B. Abd=Add C. Abd<Add	A. No abduction or adduction; extension only B. Marked adduction only		J S	
Neurobehavioural items								
Eye appearences	Sunset sign Nerve paisy	Transient nystagmus. Strabismus. Some roving eye movement	Does not open eyes	Normal conjugate eye movement	A. Persistent nystagmus B. Frequent roving movement C. Frequent rapid blinks			
Auditory orientation (state 3, 4) To rattle. (Note presence of startle)	A. No reaction B. Auditory startle but no true orientation	Brightens and stills; may turn toward stimuli with eyes closed	Alerting and shifting of eyes; head may or may not turn to source	Alerting; prolonged head turns to stimulus; search with eyes	Turning and alerting to stimulus each time on both sides		S	
Visual orientation (state 4) To red woollen ball	Does not focus or follow stimulus	Stills; focuses on stimulus; may follow 30° jerkily; does not find stimulus again spontaneously	Follows 30-60° horizontally; may lose stimulus but finds it again. Brief vertical glance	Follows with eyes and head horizontally and to some extent vertically, with frowning	Sustaioned fixation; follows vertically, horizontally, and in circle			
Alertness (state 4)	Inattentive; rarely or never responds to direct stimulation	When alert, periods rather brief; rather variable response to orientation	When alert, alertness moderately sustained; may use stimulus to come to alert state	Sustained alertness; orientation frequent, reliable to visual but not auditory stimuli	Continuous alertness, which does not seem to tire, to both auditory and visual stimuli			
Defensive reaction A cloth or hand is placed over the infants face to partially occlude the nasal airway	No response	A. General quietening B. Non-specific activity with long latency	Rooting; lateral neck turning; possibly neck stretching.	Swipes with arm	Swipes with arm with rather violent body movement			
Peak of excitement	Low level arousal to all stimuli; never > state 3	Infant reaches state 4-5 briefly but predominantly in lower states	Infant predominantly state 4 or 5; may reach state 6 after stimulation but returns spontaneously to lower state	Infant reaches state 6 but can be consoled relatively easy	A. Mainly state 6. Difficult to console, if at all B. Mainly state 4-5 but if reaches state 6 cannot be consoled			
Irritability (states 3,4,5) Aversive stimuli: Uncover, Undress, Pull to sit, Prone, Ventral susp., Moro, Walking reflex	No irritable crying to any of the stimuli	Cries to 1-2 stimuli	Cries to 3-4 stimuli	Cries to 5-6 stimuli	Cries to all stimuli			
Consolability (state 6)	Never above state 5 during examination, therefore not needed	Consoling not needed, Consoles spontaneously	Consoled by talking, hand on belly or wrapping up	Consoled by picking up and holding; may need finger in mouth	Not consolable			
Cry	No cry at all	Only wimpering cry	Cries to stimuli but normal pitch	Lusty cry to offensive stimuli; normal pitch	High pitched cry, often continuous			

Notes * If asymmetrical or atypical, draw in on nearest figure
Record any abnormal signs (e.g. facial palsy, contractures, etc.)

Fig. 10.49 (*Continued*)

Hearing

Babies from 28 weeks' gestation onwards can be shown to respond to noise, usually by turning the head or increased body movements. For electrophysiological methods of assessing the auditory pathway, see investigation section below.

Smell

There is no doubt that babies, including preterm babies, can detect smells. Babies of all gestations have been found to respond to odors such as peppermint, or breast pads soaked in their own mother's breast milk.

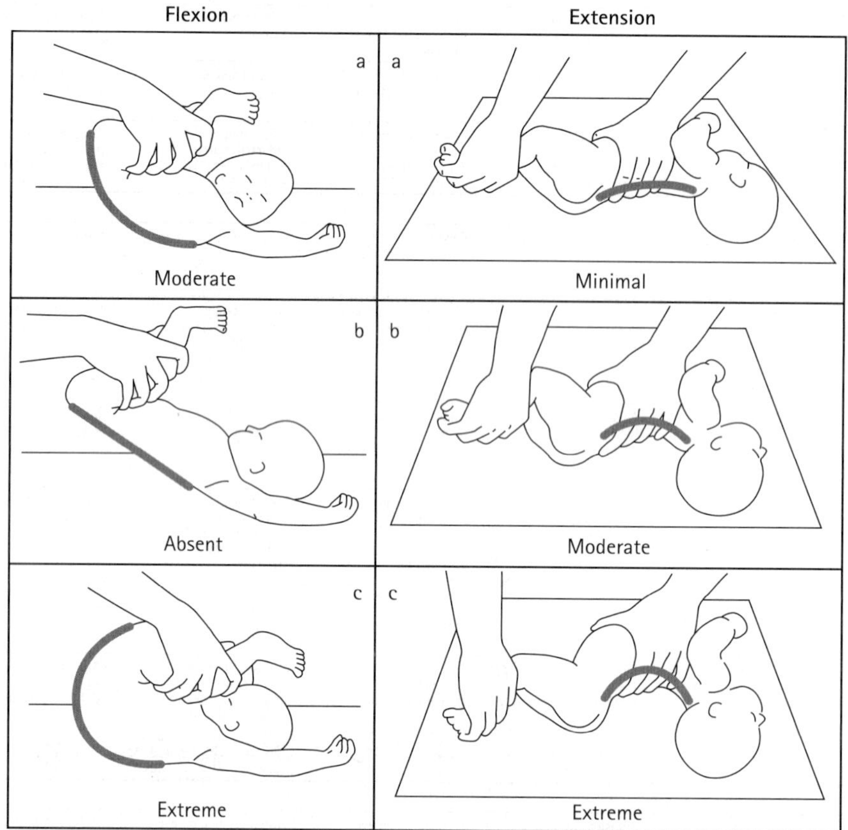

Fig. 10.50 Amiel-Tison system for assessing truncal tone. (From Amiel-Tison 1995[758] with permission)

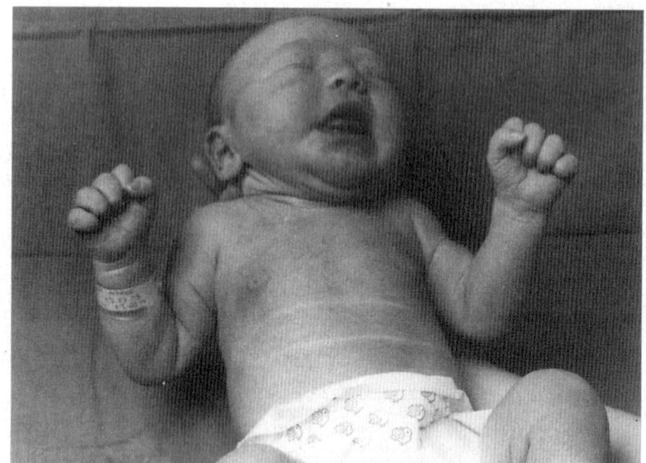

Fig. 10.51 The fully developed Moro reflex, abduction phase.

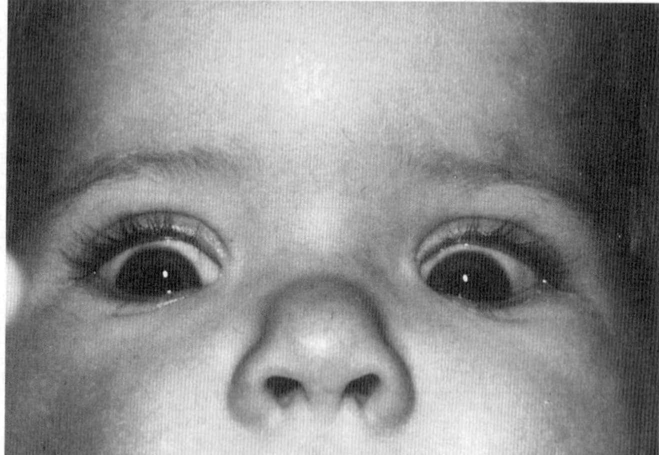

Fig. 10.52 Sunsetting in a baby with raised intracranial pressure.

Sensory testing

Withdrawal

Babies respond to pinprick stimuli with gross body movements or grimacing and there is no doubt that even very preterm babies feel pain. The classical withdrawal response of flexion of the lower limb and extension of the opposite leg in response to pricking the sole of the foot requires motor integrity also, and habituates easily.

Occipitofrontal head circumference and fontanels

Examination is not complete without measuring and charting the occipitofrontal circumference and noting the presence and tension of the fontanels. An extremely large anterior fontanel can indicate hypothyroidism, a non-existent fontanel can mean craniosynostosis. Useful information can be obtained by palpation of the sutures which can be widely spaced (diastasis) or overlapping. During the first 3 months of life the head grows at least 0.5 cm a week, and insufficient head growth is an ominous sign.

INVESTIGATION OF THE NEWBORN NERVOUS SYSTEM

Imaging

Ultrasound is the imaging procedure of first choice in the newborn. The method is relatively cheap, portable and safe enabling repeated examination even of babies in an incubator. Periventricular and other forms of hemorrhage can be identified fairly reliably. The cystic lesions of periventricular leukomalacia can be imaged down to a resolution of 1–2 mm although ultrasound detects only about a third of cases of periventricular leukomalacia when compared to MRI. The method is insensitive for the detection of lesions of the extracerebral space and in the posterior fossa. Several excellent atlases of cranial ultrasound pictures exist.[762,763]

CT scanning provides better information about the posterior fossa and the subdural space than ultrasound, with the disadvantages of X-ray exposure and the need for the baby to travel. MRI appears entirely safe but brings its own problems relating to ferrous metals in life support and monitoring devices. The improved detail, the ability to distinguish gray and white matter and to combine imaging with spectroscopic information means that MRI is preferred where there is access to the equipment. For those who wish to learn more about MRI images the book by Rutherford[764] is a useful resource.

Examination of CSF

Lumbar puncture is often easier with the baby sitting up in the newborn period, and this position results in a more stable oxygen level. The spinal cord of the newborn extends to L_3 so that the L_3/L_4 space is the best one to choose. A blood sample for plasma glucose estimation should be collected before performing the lumbar puncture as the stress response raises the blood sugar level. The CSF glucose value is usually 70–80% of the plasma glucose and should be at least 50% of it. A proper styleted lumbar puncture needle should be used as there have been cases of epidermoid tumors resulting from the implantation of a tiny core of skin during neonatal lumbar puncture with an unstyleted needle. In the neonatal period CSF may be xanthochromic because of jaundice or old intraventricular hemorrhage. The cell count is higher than later in childhood. In preterm neonates the red and white cell counts can each be up to 30/mm^3 (Table 10.98). A recent study with careful documentation showed that the mean value was seven white cells/mm^3 with two standard deviations from the mean being 21.[765] A white cell count of more than 30/mm^3 with neutrophils more than 66% of the total is suspicious. Although in cases of meningitis the white cell count is usually more than 100/mm^3, there is a degree of overlap with the (very) occasional normal baby having a white cell count this high.[765] Seizures do not influence the results. Red cell counts of more than 1000/mm^3 make the interpretation of CSF results impossible: applying correction factors using the ratio of white cells to red cells has been shown to be inaccurate. The only course of action is to repeat the lumbar puncture after 12 h.

Estimation of intracranial pressure (ICP)

ICP usually refers to pressure within the CSF space, and when subtracted from the arterial pressure gives the cerebral perfusion pressure. Rising ICP results in a reduction in cerebral perfusion unless the usual reflex elevation in systemic blood pressure occurs (the Cushing response). The Cushing response may be inadequate in the newborn.[766]

Normal value of ICP in the newborn

Measured directly with accurate pressure transducers at lumbar puncture the pressure is 0–5.5 mmHg.[767] Non-invasive devices designed to be stuck to the fontanel are numerous: the Ladd monitor works using light and a mirror and pneumatic devices working within a plastic blister[768] can give good correlations when used with care, but are not accurate enough for clinical decision making.

Electroencephalography

Conventional multichannel EEG recordings are difficult to obtain in newborn babies. The montage of electrodes is hard to apply and maintain and many babies requiring investigation are in ICUs which are electrically noisy. Short recordings are of less value than prolonged ones as the EEG shows wide variability and changes not only with sleep state but also with the length of the preceding sleep epoch.[769] Continuous monitoring is possible with either a cerebral function monitor, which displays the amplitude of one or two channels of processed EEG, or the Oxford Medilog system which records two channels of EEG on audio tape requiring later analysis. The output can be displayed on a laptop computer at the cot side.

Maturation of EEG

The EEG of very preterm babies is markedly discontinuous (Fig. 10.53) with a pattern of high voltage slow activity with suppressed EEG activity termed 'trace alternant'. This pattern can still be seen during normal sleep in mature babies, but with increasing gestation there is a reduction in amount and duration of trace alternant activity. There is also a pattern, called 'delta brush', of fast waves superimposed on delta waves which can be misinterpreted as convulsive activity. Abnormal background EEG activity correlates well with later adverse outcome in both preterm and asphyxiated term babies.[770–772]

Investigation of the visual pathway

Visual evoked potentials (VEP) are produced within the occipital cortex as a result of repeatedly applying an appropriate visual stimulus so that the minute electrical response to it, which will be identical each time, can be extracted from the random background electrical noise (EEG) by computerized averaging. Stroboscopic or flashing red lights are used which can penetrate closed eyelids. The electrical response 'matures' with advancing gestation and can be detected from 25 weeks. Study of VEPs has been found to be of value in predicting outcome after birth asphyxia,[773] and is a sensitive test for the integrity of the visual pathway. Absent VEPs predicted cortical blindness in preterm babies with extensive cystic leukomalacia.[774]

Investigation of the auditory pathway

Neural pathways for hearing are established and can be tested within hours of birth. The fetus responds to low frequency sounds applied to the maternal abdomen from 19 weeks of gestation, with

Table 10.98 Normal values for CSF in neonates

Type of baby	Red cell count (per cubic mm)	White cell count (per cubic mm)	Protein (g/L) (mmol/L)	Glucose
Preterm < 7 days	30 (0–333)	9 (0–30)	1 (0.5–2.9)	3 (1.5–5.5)
Preterm > 7 days	30	12 (2–70)	0.9 (0.5–2.6)	3 (1.5–5.5)
Term < 7 days	9 (0–50)	7 (0–21)	0.6 (0.3–2.5)	3 (1.5–5.5)
Term > 7 days	< 10	3 (0–10)	0.5 (0.2–0.8)	3 (1.5–5.5)

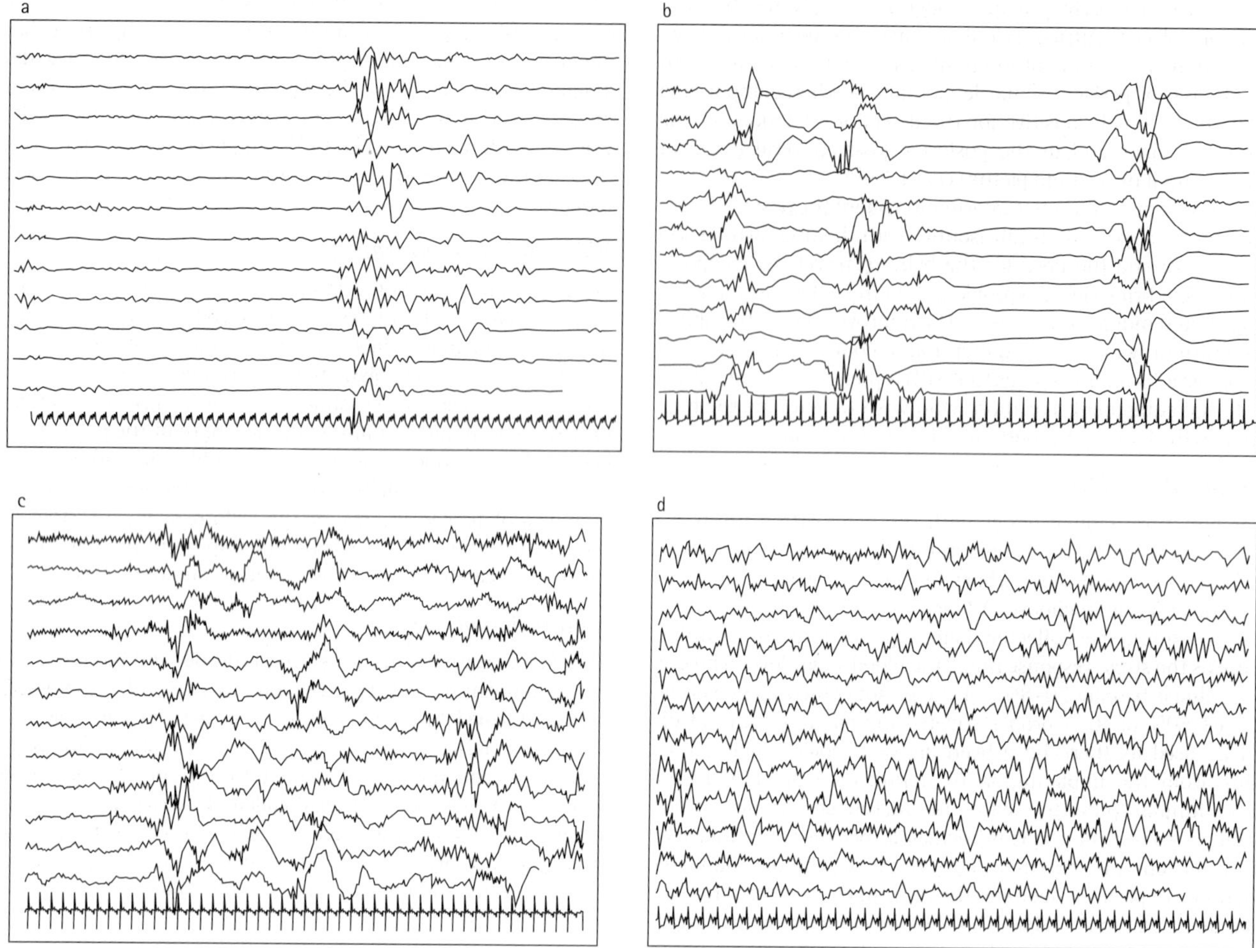

Fig. 10.53 Maturation of the normal EEG in preterm babies: (a) 25 weeks; (b) 29 weeks; (c) 35 weeks; (d) 40 weeks.

a gradual increase in the range of frequency response and sensitivity.[775] Young children who are fitted with hearing aids early have an excellent chance of developing normal speech, but the current average age for the acquisition of hearing aids is often almost 2 years.[776] Bilateral sensorineural deafness occurs in about 1.5 per 1000 children. This has led to the suggestion that all newborns, and certainly those at high risk of deafness by virtue of a positive family history, neonatal illness, cleft palate or LBW should be screened for hearing loss.[777,778] The latter approach will identify 40% of the hearing-impaired children for the work of screening about 10% of the whole population. A successful universal neonatal screening program has been established in north London,[779] and is being developed in the USA but is not supported by all.[780] Neonatal screening programs will never eliminate the need to monitor hearing with distraction testing at 7–9 months because many cases of infant hearing loss are conductive and acquired later due to secretory otitis media. The poor performance of the current distraction testing program is providing a stimulus for discussion regarding a different approach to hearing screening in the UK.[781] A combination approach using screening for high-risk newborns, dissemination of information for parents derived from McCormick,[782] and training of health visitors led to a reduction in the median age at which hearing aids were fitted in one district.[783] There are three main ways in which hearing can be assessed in the neonatal period. These are the auditory response cradle, automated auditory evoked brainstem potentials and otoacoustic emissions.

Auditory response cradle

This test involves placing the baby in a special crib which monitors body movement, respiration and head turning via a pressure-sensitive mattress. The baby is exposed to sounds with a threshold of 90 dB. 1.7% of 6000 babies failed this test in one west London hospital; 20% of these were subsequently confirmed to have significant hearing loss.[784] Seven children who passed the test in the neonatal period were found to be deaf subsequently; five had a progressive hereditary condition or definite postnatal factors. The test also had a high false positive rate in a group of babies tested in Nottingham, and has not been widely adopted. The US equivalent, the Crib-O-Gram, has not proved a success either.

Brainstem auditory evoked potential

These indicate electrical events generated in the brainstem auditory pathway in response to sound (usually a click) presented at the ear. The electrical signals are recorded with EEG electrodes on the scalp. The results of many click stimulations are summed by a computer which uses coherent averaging to eliminate the background noise generated by the local EEG signal. The mature pattern consists of seven waves, but these are poorly developed with increased latency and require a larger stimulus in order to elicit them in babies, in whom the response is present from 24 weeks. Prolongation of brainstem auditory evoked potentials have been described with hyperbilirubinemia and gentamicin toxicity. Automated brainstem response equipment eliminates the need for extensive operator training and is the most widely used method of hearing screening.

Ex-preterm babies are tested as near to term as possible in order to reduce the false positive failure rate to a minimum.

Otoacoustic emissions

Otoacoustic emissions were discovered in 1978. They are low amplitude sound waves which are produced by the inner ear; they occur spontaneously as well as in response to a click stimulus. The automated method depends on the fact that a click stimulus, when presented to an intact hearing ear, evokes an otoacoustic emission which can be detected by a probe lying in the ear canal. Programmable software for measuring otoacoustic emissions has been developed (POEMS) and the system evaluated as a screening method in high-risk newborn babies in Sheffield and Southampton.[778,785] POEMS was quicker to administer than the automated evoked brainstem response method (no scalp electrodes) but there were more false positive results. It has been proposed that POEMS should be used for the first screen with automated brainstem evoked potentials available for those who fail.

CONVULSIONS IN THE NEWBORN

Diagnosis and incidence

Convulsions are more frequent on the first day of life than at any other time, although the diagnosis is easily missed because their manifestations can be extremely subtle.[786] Subtle seizures were the most common type seen in several surveys, occurring in 75% of the cases described by Scher et al.[787] Repetitive lip smacking, cycling or swimming movements, deviation of the eyes and apnea can all be convulsive in origin but are sometimes difficult to distinguish from normal movements or jittering (see Table 10.99).

Continuous monitoring has shown that electrical seizures occur more frequently in the newborn than clinically suspected seizures, and conversely that stereotyped repetitive activity which looks like a seizure is not always associated with EEG change.[788,789] There is as yet no evidence that treating clinical and electrically manifest seizures to electrical silence improves the outcome. There is also controversy about whether the lack of surface EEG activity truly confirms that a suspicious clinical event is not a seizure. There may be EEG change in 'hidden' electrical sites in the hippocampus or brainstem with poor transmission to the scalp because of the reduced myelin content of the neonatal brain. Recognition of seizure activity may be particularly important in babies who are paralyzed as prolonged seizures (>30 min in animals) are accompanied by an increase in cerebral metabolic rate which outstrips the available energy supply and leads to cerebral damage. Changes in cerebral energy metabolites and cerebral blood flow velocity have been seen even in the brief seizures characteristic of the human neonate.[790]

The incidence of seizures in term babies is reported at between 1.6 and 14 per 1000 deliveries. Higher incidences were reported prior to the introduction of low-phosphate milks and half the babies in early series were hypocalcemic. More recent series give an estimate of around 5 per 1000; in most a quarter of the cases are amongst babies of less than 30 weeks' gestation and a half are less than 37 weeks.[791] The incidence of clinically diagnosed seizures in VLBW babies varies from 50 to 60 per 1000[792,793] and 90–130 per 1000 (personal observations).[793]

Table 10.99 Types of seizure in the newborn (adapted from Volpe[759])

Type	Clinical manifestation
Subtle	Eye signs – eyelid fluttering, eye deviation, fixed open stare, blinking Apnea. Cycling, boxing, stepping, swimming movements of limbs Mouthing, chewing, lip smacking, smiling. Often no EEG changes – most likely with ocular manifestations
Tonic	Stiffening. Decerebrate posturing. EEG variable
Clonic	Repetitive jerking, distinct from jittering. Usually EEG change Can be focal or multifocal
Myoclonic	Rapid single repetitive contraction of muscle groups. Rare, but sleep myoclonus is benign EEG often normal, although background EEG can be abnormal

Etiology

Intracranial injury

The majority of cases of seizures in term babies are associated with hypoxic–ischemic encephalopathy (HIE) (Table 10.100).[786,794–799] Newer imaging methods reveal middle cerebral artery infarction (stroke) to be more common than previously suspected.[800] This condition often accompanies perinatal asphyxia but also occurs in association with hypertension and polycythemia. Focal seizures are particularly likely to be caused by arterial infarction and MRI should be requested in these cases, with a repeat scan at 2 weeks if an early result is negative. A thrombophilia screen (looking for disorders such as factor V Leiden) should be carried out in cases of neonatal stroke. Intracranial hemorrhage was diagnosed in 17% of Levene & Trounce's series[794] which included cranial ultrasound but not MRI amongst the investigations. These workers were unable to assign a cause in only 8% of cases.

Maternal drug withdrawal

Methadone withdrawal is more likely to produce seizures than heroin, but modern treatment for neonatal abstinence syndrome is aimed at preventing seizure which has now become rare.

Metabolic causes

The metabolic causes of hypocalcemia, hypoglycemia, hyponatremia and hypomagnesemia now account for less than 10% of cases of neonatal seizure but remain important because they are readily treatable. Hypomagnesemia coexists with hypocalcemia about half the time, and recognition is important because administration of calcium can cause the serum magnesium to drop further. Pyridoxine dependency can be a difficult diagnosis to make; the disorder is autosomal recessive and the fits are intractable until an infusion of 100 mg pyridoxine is given, ideally under EEG monitoring. The response may take up to half an hour. Pyridoxine is necessary for the manufacture of gamma-aminobutyric acid, which is the major inhibitory neurotransmitter, and hence in the familial form of the disease replacement needs to be life long. Temporary deficiency has also arisen following vomiting and incorrectly designed formula baby milks. Inborn errors of metabolism such as non-ketotic hyperglycinemia can cause seizure and these should be suspected if the onset is late and related to milk feeds. Preterm babies can develop transient hyperammonemia and hyperlactemia causing seizures. 'Fifth day fits' were commonly reported in the 1970s and 1980s, but recent reports have failed to identify any cases.

Infection

Infection accounts for about 8% of neonatal fits and evidence of bacterial or viral infection should always be sought, including congenital infections such as CMV.

Table 10.100 Causes of neonatal convulsions (%)

Published series	1	2	3	4	5*	6+	7
Number of cases in report			71	131	100	40	100
Hypoxic–ischemic encephalopathy	53	16	49	30	49	37	32
Intracranial hemorrhage	17		14		7	12	16
Cerebral infarction (stroke)					12	17	7
Meningitis	8	3	2	7	5	5	14
Maternal drug withdrawal			4				
Hypoglycemia	3	2	0.1	5	3		2
Hypocalcemia, hypomagnesemia					22		4
Rapidly changing serum sodium							
Congenitally abnormal brain		8		4	3	17	3
Fifth day fits		52					
Benign familial neonatal seizures							1
Benign neonatal sleep myoclonus							1
Pyridoxine dependent seizures							
Hypertensive encephalopathy				1.4			
Kernicterus					1		
Inborn errors of metabolism					3		3

* This series included > 31 weeks' gestation infants only.
+ This series was limited to cases presenting in the first 48 h of life.
Blanks occur where no cases were recorded in a particular study.
Data in column 1 are from Levene & Trounce,[794] column 2 from Goldberg,[795] column 3 from Andre et al,[796] column 4 from Bergman et al,[797] column 5 from Estan & Hope,[798] column 6 from Lien et al,[799] column 7 from Mizrahi & Kellaway.[786]

Inherited and congenital disorders

Benign familial convulsions are dominantly inherited, and occur in the first 3 weeks of life. The fits can be very frequent but they are usually brief and the prognosis is excellent. The diagnosis rests on excluding other causes and the presence of a positive family history. The chromosomal defect has recently been mapped to the long arm of chromosome 20. Benign neonatal sleep myoclonus may give rise to dramatic manifestations in otherwise entirely healthy newborns who have a normal prognosis.

Sometimes neonatal seizures are the first manifestation of a congenital neurological disorder and these are more likely if the fits are intractable. The condition called 'early infantile epileptic encephalopathy' presents as severe tonic spasms and many of these babies have cerebral malformations. Cases of Aicardi's syndrome (female children with infantile spasms, agenesis of the corpus callosum and a characteristic EEG) would also fall into this group. The phakomatoses occasionally present in the neonatal period, and syndromes like Zellweger's or Smith–Lemli–Opitz can cause neonatal seizures.

Investigations

These follow from the possible causes listed above. Information regarding the delivery is vital to exclude HIE. Essential laboratory investigations include estimation of calcium, magnesium, glucose, acid–base balance and sodium in the blood together with a full infection screen including a lumbar puncture, specimens for virology and a congenital infection screen. A cranial ultrasound scan should be included. If the cause is not revealed second line investigations include MRI, samples to look for maternal 'street' drugs, urinary and blood amino acid estimation, chromosomal analysis, blood ammonia, measurement of organic acids and consideration of a trial of pyridoxine. The value of an EEG examination has already been discussed. An early background interictal EEG is useful in prognosis.[801]

Treatment

General guidelines

Treatment is best given intravenously as intramuscular absorption is erratic and the neonate has little muscle mass. Facilities to site and maintain intravenous lines and to institute artificial ventilation are necessary as many of the available drugs depress respiration and ventilation can become inadequate due to frequent convulsions. The high total body water of the neonate means a large volume of distribution hence the relatively large loading doses suggested in Table 10.101. Many of the drugs are protein bound and can interact with other drugs and bilirubin. Probably the best advice is to use phenobarbital in an adequate dose with an early blood level, and to follow with intravenous phenytoin, then sodium valproate or rectal paraldehyde. Thiopental coma did not improve the outcome in a controlled clinical trial[802] and in resistant cases lidocaine (lignocaine) may be the best alternative.[803]

Phenobarbital

Note the large loading dose, and it is reasonable to give 30 mg/kg if the patient is already ventilated, otherwise use 15–20 mg/kg. Gilman et al[804] achieved seizure control with phenobarbital alone in 77% of cases using a rapid sequential method in which they gave 15–20 mg/kg initially then further doses of 5–10 mg/kg every 30 min up to a maximum of 40 mg/kg and serum level of over 40 mg/L. The half-life is very long and there have been concerns about toxic effects on the developing brain. Nevertheless the drug has other actions, reducing cerebral metabolic rate and acting as a free radical scavenger, which make it a good choice as the first line anticonvulsant. EEG response to anticonvulsant treatment is disappointing.[805,806]

Phenytoin

There is some suggestion that more rapid control of seizures can be achieved with this agent, although its usefulness is limited by the myocardial depressant effect in some babies. Long term treatment is not suggested because of the side-effects and unpredictable metabolism.

Table 10.101 Anticonvulsant drugs in the newborn

Drug	Initial dose	Route	Maintenance dose	Route	Therapeutic level	Half-life	Mode of excretion
Phenobarbital	15–30 mg/kg	i.v.	5 mg/kg/24 h – single dose	i.v./oral	14–40 mg/L 60–180 micromol/L	100–200 h	Hepatic P_{450} cytochrome oxidase
Phenytoin	20 mg/kg in two doses 1 h apart	i.v.	8 mg/kg/24 h in two doses	i.v./oral	10–20 mg/L 40–80 micromol/L	20 h (75 prems)	Liver glucuronidation
Paraldehyde	0.1 mg/kg	p.r.	150 mg/kg/h as dilute 5% solution	i.v.		10 h	Lungs and liver
Diazepam	0.2 mg/kg	i.v.	0.2 mg/kg/h	i.v.		20–60 h	Liver glucuronidation
Clonazepam	0.2 mg/kg	i.v.	0.01 mg/kg/h	i.v.		30 h	Liver glucuronidation
Valproate	20–25 mg/kg	i.v.	5–10 mg/kg/day	Oral	40–50 mg/L 275–350 micromol/L	26–47 h	Hepatic
Lidocaine (lignocaine)	1–2 mg/kg	i.v.	2 mg/kg/h	i.v.	2.4–6 mg/L in adults	200 min	Liver and kidney

Paraldehyde

Rectal administration of paraldehyde has been used for many years with safety and the drug is a useful second line anticonvulsant. There is some experience with intravenous infusions which can be inconvenient as the drug must be light-protected. Concern has been raised regarding pulmonary edema and hepatic necrosis. Intramuscular administration often leads to sterile abscess formation and should be abandoned.

Sodium valproate

Hepatotoxic effects, hyperammonemia and hyperglycinemia may limit the use of this drug in the newborn. Valproate proved effective in six intractable cases of neonatal seizure.[807] The oral solution is apparently absorbed from the rectum.[808]

Duration of treatment

Concern about the effects of anticonvulsant treatment on the developing brain means that most neonatologists would only discharge a baby on maintenance phenobarbital if the neurological examination was abnormal, discontinuing treatment before discharge in those who were neurologically normal.[759] As many as 56% of babies developed subsequent epilepsy in one series[809] although 30% is probably a more realistic figure.[786,787] For babies who are discharged on anticonvulsants consider discontinuation of treatment if the baby is seizure-free at 9 months.

Prognosis

This is related to the cause of the seizures. Following hypoxic–ischemic encephalopathy at term about 25% of those who fit will have sequelae (p. 000). Of 70 cases of clinical seizure in VLBW babies followed in Cambridge, 43 (59%) died, 16 (22%) had a major handicap and 11 (15%) were normal at 18 months. These data are remarkably similar to those of Watkins et al[793] (n = 65, 1988), Van Zeben et al[792] (n = 72, 1990), and Scher et al[787] (n = 62, 1993) although in earlier series as many as 90% of the preterm babies died. The prognosis after hypocalcemic seizure and in familial neonatal seizure is excellent. Symptomatic hypoglycemia and meningitis have a 50% chance of sequelae in the survivors. A normal background interictal EEG at term is a good prognostic factor, with fewer than 10% of such babies experiencing sequelae. The value of a normal neurological examination at discharge in providing early reassurance should not be underestimated either; in one series 11 of 14 babies with seizures who were normal at 4 years were assessed as normal at this stage. However, this apparently normal group of Oxford children then had problems with spelling and memory in adolescence.[810]

INFECTION OF THE NERVOUS SYSTEM IN THE NEWBORN

Neonatal meningitis

Incidence and cause

Meningitis is more common during the first month of life than at any other time: the incidence has been estimated as 0.25–0.5 per 1000 in normal weight babies and 1–2 per 1000 in those below 2.5 kg at birth. Gram negative organisms are more often implicated than later in childhood. The commonest causative organisms are *Escherichia coli* and Group B streptococcus (GBS), the latter reflecting the association with septicemia. *Listeria monocytogenes* is becoming less frequent in the UK since the Government issued advice to pregnant women about avoiding soft cheese and carefully reheating cook–chill food. A wide variety of different organisms have been reported, particularly in the LBW baby. Staphylococci have a predilection for ventriculoperitoneal shunts. Table 10.102 lists 10 important causative bacteria.

Clinical signs and diagnosis

The diagnosis can be difficult and if infection is considered as a cause for a baby's symptoms then a lumbar puncture must be performed. Examples include babies who are shocked and with respiratory distress early in life in whom GBS infection or hyaline membrane disease (or both) could be the cause, and babies

Table 10.102 Bacterial causes of neonatal meningitis

Organism	Incidence (%)
Escherichia coli	34
Group B streptococci	30
Other Gram negative bacilli	8
Listeria monocytogenes	6
Staphylococci	4.5
Other streptococci	4
Pneumococcus	3
Pseudomonas	3
Haemophilus	2
Meningococcus	2

presenting later with subtle signs such as apnea, lethargy or regurgitation of milk. Babies developing hydrocephalus deserve one lumbar puncture even if the etiology is thought to be posthemorrhagic as ventriculomegaly can result from low-grade staphylococcal infection. Cerebral ultrasound scans may reveal intraventricular strands. The difficulty in distinguishing GBS infection from RDS at birth has led to the practice of performing a routine lumbar puncture in all such babies who require artificial ventilation. The yield of positive cultures in this situation is low, and the practice has been abandoned. The white blood cell count and the C reactive protein are raised and the platelet count may be low.

Treatment

Antibiotics alone do not treat meningitis, and the importance of supportive treatment must not be underestimated. Babies are often shocked requiring measures such as artificial ventilation, inotropic support, frequent monitoring of their acid–base state, careful fluid balance and maintenance of nutrition. There is no convincing evidence that adjunctive therapy such as steroid or immunoglobulin administration, exchange transfusion or monoclonal antibody treatment helps in neonatal meningitis.

Most treatment is started without knowledge of the infecting organism. Third generation cephalosporins offer excellent penetration into CSF with wide spectrum of activity including Gram negative organisms. Of those available cefotaxime is probably the best choice with 100% survival reported in one small study though treatment failures and rapid development of resistance have occurred with cefuroxime. Antibiotics should be continued for 3 weeks after the CSF is sterilized. A repeat lumbar puncture should be carried out if there is a failure of clinical response and/or a failure of the laboratory indices of infection to return to normal. An intraventricular tap may be required if the ventricles are seen to enlarge on serial ultrasound scans, and intraventricular therapy should be considered via a surgically implanted reservoir in this situation.

Prognosis

The probability of survival relates mainly to the infecting organism and the gestational age of the baby. Gram negative meningitis now has a 70% survival rate, a considerable improvement on the previous figures of 40–75% mortality. Neurodevelopmental sequelae in the survivors continue to be a problem with approximately one-third of the survivors sustaining an impairment of which deafness is the most frequent.

Viral and protozoal infections

These may be acquired in utero or postnatally and can cause severe neurological impairment. The acronym TORCH has been used to summarize the infections *Toxoplasma*, rubella, CMV and herpes to which should be added human immunodeficiency virus and varicella zoster.

Rubella

Rubella infection in the first 16 weeks of pregnancy can result in a severely damaged baby with cataracts, sensorineural deafness, congenital heart disease, microcephaly, hepatosplenomegaly and thrombocytopenia. The condition is preventable by achieving high immunization coverage.

CMV

CMV can present in a dramatic form with jaundice and petechiae, the 'blueberry muffin' baby. Most babies who are symptomatic at birth will be handicapped. Only 1% of babies born with congenital CMV infection are symptomatic, however, most babies being clinically unaffected by the infection. Perhaps 6% have significant hearing loss at follow-up.[811]

Varicella zoster

Varicella zoster can result in severe damage with cicatricial skin scarring, cataracts and seizures. Sequelae are more likely following infection in the first trimester when the risk was 1/11 in one study.[812] Transmission later in pregnancy can result in zoster or chickenpox in the newborn. If the maternal infection occurs within – 5 to + 5 days of delivery, the fetus will be unprotected by maternal antibody and should be treated with aciclovir and zoster immune globulin.

Herpes simplex virus

Herpes simplex virus can result in severe illness in newborns. There is a high incidence of meningitis and encephalitis. The infection should be treated with aciclovir. Herpes can be difficult to diagnose but the virus can be identified on electron microscopy. There have been case reports of congenitally infected neonates presenting like congenital varicella.

Human immunodeficiency virus

This retrovirus can cause meningitis and encephalopathy. Vertical transmission occurs in 13–45% of cases, a risk which can be reduced by zidovudine[813] and possibly by cesarean section delivery. About one-third of infected children will present in the first year of life. Neurological manifestations include encephalopathy and microcephaly.

Toxoplasma gondii

This protozoan can cause neurological sequelae when acquired in uterine life and the diagnosis is important because the condition is treatable. The organism is mainly acquired from cat litter or consumption of undercooked meat, and the infection may produce only mild symptoms in the mother. Birth prevalence is about 0.5 per 1000 in the UK. The classic triad of hydrocephalus, chorioretinitis and intracranial calcification is extremely rare, with four such cases in the UK between 1975 and 1980. Specific IgM antibody can be demonstrated in the baby who should be treated with pyrimethamine + sulfadiazine followed by spiramycin. The prognosis of symptomatic congenital toxoplasmosis is poor, with 50% suffering impaired vision and 85% mental retardation.

Spirochetal and fungal infections

The incidence of congenital syphilis is rising commensurate with the rise in the use of crack cocaine. All babies with suspicion of congenital syphilis should receive penicillin, and this is also the drug of choice for neonatal Lyme disease. Fungal meningitis and abscess formation is mainly a problem of the VLBW baby requiring intensive care, in whom the mortality from this complication is high.

DEVELOPMENTAL ABNORMALITIES

See Chapter 20 for further information about these conditions.

METABOLIC AND ENDOCRINE DISORDERS

Introduction

Whilst adequate energy is essential to sustain adequate growth of the brain, nutrients also need to be in the appropriate concentrations and supported by the correct hormonal milieu. Inborn errors of metabolism can alter the relative concentrations of amino acids and many of these conditions present in the newborn period with neurological symptoms. High ammonia levels are toxic to the nervous system so that disorders of the urea cycle also present with severe derangement of neurological function. Lack of thyroid hormone causes failure of neurological maturation which rapidly results in permanent damage; the prevention of cretinism by early identification of such individuals with screening and replacement therapy has been a significant advance. Preterm babies have low thyroxine in early postnatal life; two studies suggest a correlation between low levels of thyroid hormones and adverse neurodevelopmental outcome.[814,815]

Urea cycle defects

Hyperammonemia may present with severe neurological disturbance in the newborn period. Recognition is important because many of the conditions are inherited and the babies often succumb without the correct diagnosis being made. There may be lethargy, vomiting and convulsions. Plasma ammonia concentrations above 200 mg/L are toxic and can result from liver failure, enzyme defects of the urea cycle or other disorders of amino acid metabolism such as propionic acidemia and lysine intolerance. Further investigation consists of enzyme assay using leukocytes or liver cells.

Hyperbilirubinemia

Unconjugated bilirubin is lipid soluble and hence able to cross the blood–brain barrier. The classical neurological syndrome of kernicterus presented with opisthotonic posturing and fits is now rare. Such babies were subsequently severely damaged. Damage to the auditory pathways can be demonstrated with prolongation of auditory evoked potentials which return to normal with exchange transfusion, and a reduced incidence of hearing loss in preterm survivors has been claimed to be due to adoption of a policy attempting to prevent high bilirubin levels (above 200 μmol/L).

Hypoglycemia

Prolonged low glucose levels damage the newborn nervous system which is unable to utilize alternative energy sources. There has been some debate recently regarding the degree of hypoglycemia which is required to inflict permanent damage with the suggestion that for preterm babies below 2.6 mmol/L was associated with a reduction in Bayley motor and mental development scores at 18 months.[816] Much more evidence is needed before definite guidelines can be formulated regarding moderate hypoglycemia. The damage which can result from severe reduction in glucose levels is not in doubt, however, and is highlighted by the incidence of impairment in survivors of nesidioblastosis of the pancreas who often have intractable hypoglycemia. Symptomatic hypoglycemia has at least a 50% chance of sequelae in the survivors.

NEONATAL CEREBRAL INJURY

Perinatal stress such as hypotension or trauma can result in cerebral injury. The preterm brain is particularly vulnerable, as are the brains of more mature babies who have been subjected to in utero insults. Neonatal brain injury is best considered as a spectrum with the end result depending on the type and degree of insult, the gestational age of the baby and any underlying factors. The problem is an important one because there is a relationship with later handicap.[817–819]

Periventricular hemorrhage (PVH)

The preterm brain contains a unique structure, the germinal matrix, containing actively dividing neuroblasts and glioblasts. The blood supply is via a capillary bed supplied by Heubner's artery, which is a branch of the anterior cerebral artery. The region of the germinal matrix which is situated at the head of the caudate nucleus is prone to bleeding, and this is the most common form of intracranial hemorrhage in preterm babies. The incidence of intracranial hemorrhage diagnosed with ultrasound in VLBW babies has reduced from around 40% to 15–20% since the widespread introduction of antenatal steroids and postnatal surfactant.[820,821] Rates as low as 13% have been reported from some centers, although one Canadian study found a wide range of incidence.[822]

The term PVH is often used as a generic one, encompassing several different types of hemorrhage in preterm babies. The mildest form is germinal matrix or subependymal bleeding alone. This is often abbreviated to GMH or SEH and is equivalent to Grade 1 PVH in the classification of Levene & De Crespigny[823] and Grade 1 in the classification of Papile et al.[824] Bleeding into the ventricular system, or intraventricular hemorrhage (IVH) was classified by Levene in 1983 as Grade 2 PVH and was subdivided by Papile into Grade 2 when the ventricle is not distended and Grade 3 where it was. Finally, bleeding into the parenchyma of the brain (ParH) was Levene Grade 3 PVH in 1983 and Grade 4 in the Papile classification. A parenchymal hemorrhagic lesion is illustrated with the ultrasound scan appearance in Figure 10.54. Because few now believe that parenchymal hemorrhage represents direct extension of intraventricular bleeding, and because it is now clear that all echodense lesions diagnosed with ultrasound are not certain to be hemorrhagic an alternate new classification has been proposed. This suggests that the term GMH-IVH is used to describe bleeding into the germinal matrix and the ventricle. All other intracranial hemorrhage should be documented as carefully as possible and classified as IPL (intraparenchymal lesion). Parenchymal echodense lesions visualized with ultrasound can represent various forms of pathological lesion including hemorrhagic lesions. One explanation for the frequent association of unilateral hemorrhagic parenchymal lesions with the presence of a germinal matrix hemorrhage is that the latter reduces the perfusion to the adjacent white matter by obstructing venous drainage, causing an infarction.[825] The ultrasound scan appearance of this lesion is that the shape is triangular with the apex at the lateral border of the lateral ventricle. The lesion is often preceded by an ipsilateral GMH-IVH. Distinction is important as the prognosis is different from hemorrhagic periventricular leukomalacia.

Repeated ultrasound scanning of cohorts of VLBW babies has revealed that the incidence and degree of hemorrhage relates to the birth weight and gestational age. The complication develops in early postnatal life, with as many as 36/47 (77%) of lesions present by 6 h in one study and all by 72 h in another. There are several undisputed risk factors. These are:

- gestational age;
- birth weight;
- RDS;
- artificial ventilation;
- hypercarbia;
- pneumothorax.

Less conclusive evidence exists for variables such as the mode and place of delivery, use of beta-sympathomimetics during labor, presence of coagulopathy, acidosis, bicarbonate administration, low blood pressure, fluctuating cerebral blood flow velocity and the administration of vasodilators such tolazoline. The main problem is in distinguishing antecedent from associate. The best 'unifying hypothesis',[826] is that GMH-IVH results from a disturbance of cerebral blood flow in babies who are poor at cerebral autoregulation, and in whom there is often a bleeding tendency.

Attempts to prevent PVH have included administration of agents such as fresh frozen plasma, phenobarbital in nine trials,

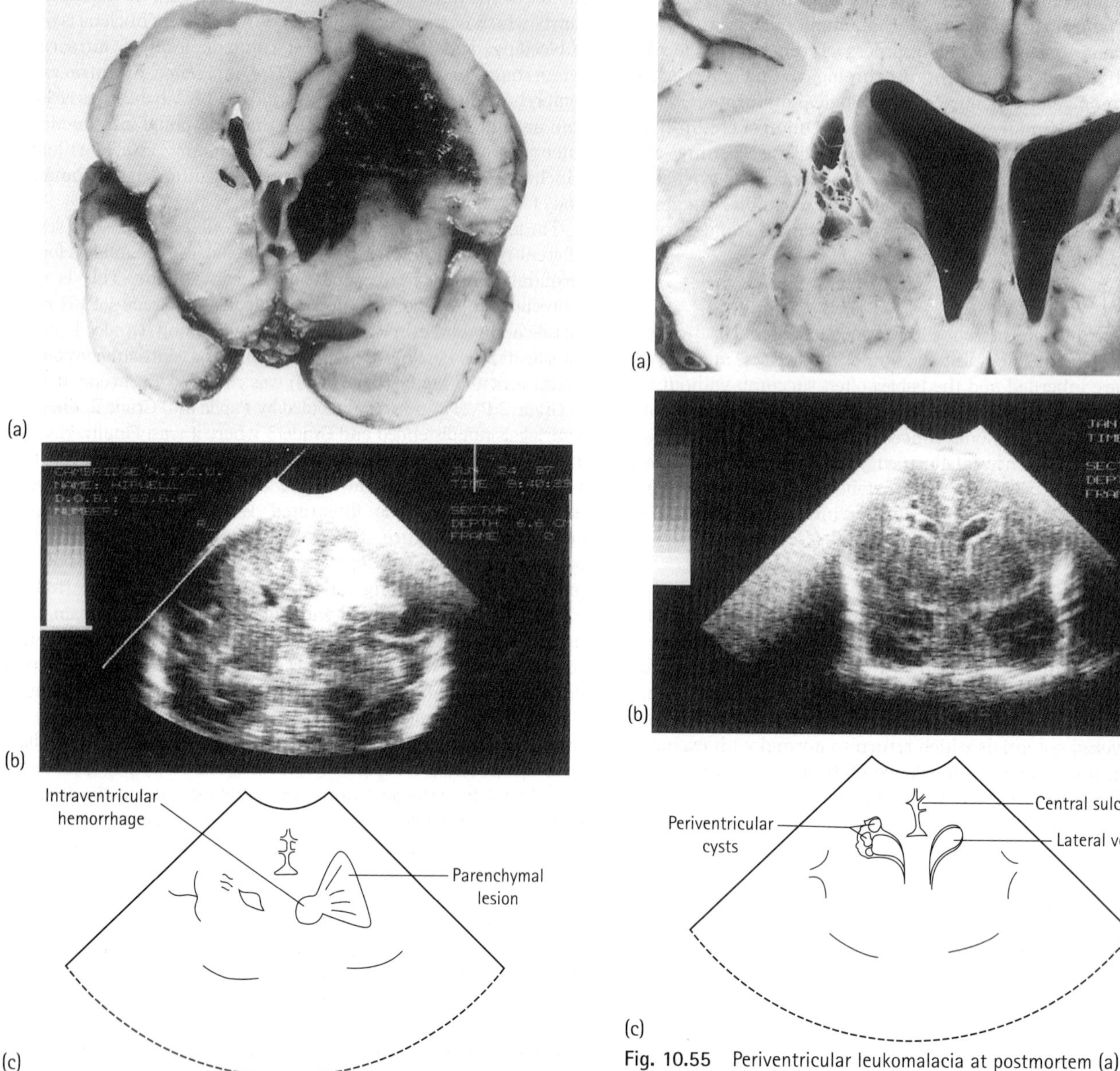

Fig. 10.54 Periventricular hemorrhage, at postmortem (a) and imaged with ultrasound in life [(b), with diagrammatic representation (c)].

Fig. 10.55 Periventricular leukomalacia at postmortem (a) and imaged with ultrasound in life [(b), with diagrammatic representation (c)].

indometacin six trials,[827] tranexamic acid, etamsylate,[828] vitamin E, and pancuronium. A useful reduction can also be obtained with surfactant and antenatal steroids.[829,830]

Periventricular leukomalacia

Periventricular leukomalacia (PVL) was first recognized by pathologists. The 'white spots' appear at the boundary zone of the cerebral circulation in the immature brain and it seems likely that a period of low cerebral blood flow is often exacerbated by flow–metabolism uncoupling. Small cysts can now be diagnosed during life with ultrasound (Fig. 10.55). Cysts can be imaged in between 8 and 17% of babies less than 1500 g. Some series include parenchymal echodense lesions persisting for more than 2 weeks but not evolving into cysts, with a higher incidence of 25%.[831] There can be some difficulty in distinguishing this type of 'flare' from the normal peritrigonal 'blush' described by Di Pietro et al[832] which is normal. It is very important to describe the ultrasound appearances in detail; an echodense lesion in a 1-day-old preterm baby is a long way from the pathological identification of cystic change in the white matter and should not be confidently diagnosed as PVL. Paneth et al[833] found white matter damage at postmortem in preterm babies with cerebral echodensity during life, but in very few were the lesions typical of classical periventricular leukomalacia. In many the white matter damage, with liquefactive necrosis and perivascular hemorrhage, was not restricted to the periventricular region. They suggest that the lesion seen in today's very preterm population differs from that originally described. Cysts disappear after a few months and are replaced by a thinning of the myelin layer. Magnetic resonance imaging confirms reduction in myelin content of the brain.

No agreement has yet been reached on the precise definition of the ultrasound appearances of a 'flare' but follow-up suggests that they are predictive of outcome and hence represent injury.[834,835] These early echodense lesions appear 24–48 h after an insult and are often followed in 2–4 weeks by appearance of cystic change. Studies are still emerging regarding the antecedents: antepartum hemorrhage, asphyxia and surgery particularly for NEC have been suggested.[836,837] Hypocarbia and hyperbilirubinemia are others.[836,838,839] The outlook for the survivors has so far proved extremely poor: of 82 babies reported in several series almost all have severe cerebral palsy. Bilateral cysts greater than 1 cm diameter in the occipital cortex have the worst prognosis.

Intracerebellar hemorrhage

Cerebellar blood can occur as an extension from intraventricular or subarachnoid bleeding or as an isolated event in premature babies. It has been described in association with tight bands around the head. Management is usually conservative and a good outcome has been described at term although preterm babies often succumb as the condition forms part of more extensive PVH.

Thalamic hemorrhage

This type of intracranial bleeding may be primary or secondary to extension from germinal matrix bleeding. Term babies with this condition may present aged about 10 days of age with eye signs (deviation and sunsetting) and fits. 18-month follow-up has revealed no abnormality, in contrast to the babies with 'bright thalamus' described by Shen et al[840] who were all suffering from severe birth asphyxia and subsequently developed cerebral palsy.

Subdural hemorrhage

The incidence of this complication has fallen with more careful obstetric practice, and usually results from tearing of the bridging veins. Babies may present with shock, bradycardia and are frequently asphyxiated. Ultrasound is poor at detecting subdural hemorrhage and suspicion of the diagnosis is an indication for CT scan.

Subarachnoid hemorrhage

Like cerebellar and thalamic bleeding blood in the subarachnoid space is often secondary to PVH, but primary subarachnoid hemorrhage has been described in cases of vitamin K deficiency. Convexity subarachnoid hemorrhage has been diagnosed with ultrasound in a group of babies who had undergone exchange transfusion for rhesus disease.

HYDROCEPHALUS AND VENTRICULOMEGALY

For more information on these conditions see Chapter 20. The following discussion is limited to preterm posthemorrhagic hydrocephalus and the outcome after an in utero diagnosis of ventriculomegaly.

Etiology

Important causes to consider in the newborn period include:

1. cerebral malformations – Arnold–Chiari malformation, Dandy–Walker cysts, aqueduct stenosis, arachnoid cysts;
2. craniosynostosis, e.g. Apert's syndrome;
3. obstruction by a mass – vein of Galen aneurysm, tumors;
4. posthemorrhagic hydrocephalus, particularly in preterm babies;
5. postmeningitic hydrocephalus;
6. X-linked congenital hydrocephalus.

Posthemorrhagic hydrocephalus in preterm babies

This is now the most frequent cause of acquired hydrocephalus in babies and occurs secondary to periventricular hemorrhage. The distance from the midline to the lateral border of the ventricle in a coronal ultrasound view should be measured and plotted on a centile chart – the ventricular index. A ventricular size greater than the 97th centile occurred in 15 of 68 survivors with periventricular hemorrhage from a cohort of 202 VLBW babies. The risk relates to the degree of hemorrhage.

The natural history of ventricular dilation secondary to PVH is that at least half the cases will not progress to require shunting, an important consideration when assessing uncontrolled studies claiming effective 'cures'.[841] The percentage of babies of birth weight less than 1500 g who required ventriculoperitoneal shunt insertion was 1.8% in Liverpool.[842]

Treatment

There is now no place for compressive head wrapping, glycerol or isosorbide in the treatment of hydrocephalus in babies. The definitive treatment is surgical placement of a ventriculoperitoneal shunt and this will be required in most cases of congenital hydrocephalus. The difficulty usually occurs in the cases of posthemorrhagic dilation as some will spontaneously arrest and in some cases the babies are too ill to permit surgery. Suggestions that shunt placement could be avoided by early intervention have not been borne out by a multicenter study in England, Eire and Switzerland enrolling 157 babies with posthemorrhagic hydrocephalus.[843,844] Repeated percutaneous drainage of cerebrospinal fluid did not reduce the eventual requirement for shunt surgery nor improve the neurodevelopmental status at 18 months except in the subgroup with parenchymal lesions. Management of this condition should therefore include a single diagnostic lumbar puncture in order to establish the intracranial pressure, whether the ventriculomegaly is of the communicating type and to exclude infection, and then a wait-and-see policy should be adopted with intervention planned if the head growth is more than twice the usual rate or the baby develops symptoms of raised intracranial pressure. Intervention should be surgical if the baby is fit enough. Acetazolamide and spironolactone were not of any benefit in a randomized controlled trial.[845]

Ventriculoperitoneal shunts

These can be inserted in babies as small as 1500 g. There is a high complication rate in such babies, 30% in some series, with frequent episodes of blockage. Many surgeons like to wait until the cerebrospinal fluid protein is below 1.5 g/L before insertion, particularly in posthemorrhagic hydrocephalus when blood in the CSF makes it viscous. Ventriculoatrial shunting is no longer the method of choice, as the complications specific to this route are serious; these include shunt nephritis, systemic sepsis and pulmonary hypertension.

Prenatally diagnosed ventriculomegaly

Pediatricians are increasingly asked for help in counseling parents whose fetus has enlarged ventricles diagnosed on an antenatal ultrasound scan. The usual basis is a ventricle/hemisphere ratio more than 0.5. More than 50% will have other problems, and a search should be made for intrauterine infection, chromosomal abnormality and spina bifida. Even in the best hands some important associated cerebral malformations can be missed antenatally. The outlook for this group is generally poor and many couples choose termination of pregnancy after counseling if the diagnosis is made early enough. Of those diagnosed later, the differentiation between progressive and non-progressive enlargement needs to be made. If the hydrocephalus is progressive and the pregnancy past 32 weeks' gestation then delivery is probably the best option. Fetuses with non-progressive enlargement without associated abnormality have the best chance of a normal outcome although most were eventually shunt dependent in one series.[846] This selected subgroup also did well in a series from London[847] but these formed only 7% of the total of 267 cases. The chance of chromosomal malformation was 3% if the ventriculomegaly was isolated and 36% when another abnormality, such as syndactyly, was present.

Prognosis

This depends on the underlying condition, and is worse for posthemorrhagic hydrocephalus than the congenital syndromes. Surgery has radically improved the outlook for some children with hydrocephalus, who can now expect to survive and attend normal school. Overall about 86% now survive and two-thirds will have normal intelligence. For preterm babies the prognosis relates to the severity of the associated periventricular hemorrhage and the presence of fits in the neonatal period.[819] About half of these children will have significant neurodevelopmental delay.

RENAL DISEASE IN THE NEONATE

DEVELOPMENT OF THE RENAL TRACT

The human kidney derives from the metanephros, the third and final excretory organ to be formed from the embryonic mesoderm. During the fifth week of embryonic development the ureteric diverticulum develops as an outgrowth of the mesonephric duct from a point near to the cloaca. Growing headwards into the nephrogenic cord the ureteric bud becomes surrounded by the mesodermal tissue which will give rise to the metanephros. Whether the bud induces nephron formation or whether the reverse is the case, primitive nephrons differentiate in close proximity to it.[848]

Nephrogenesis involves:

- ureteric bud induction;
- collecting system development with branching tubulogenesis;
- metanephric mesenchyme conversion to epithelium;
- glomerulogenesis.

The ureteric bud in turn divides and subdivides while growing towards the periphery of the metanephros. Thus the first nephrons to be formed are those most deeply situated in the kidney. As each branch of the duct is surrounded by nephrogenic tissue, the fetal kidney assumes a lobulated appearance which generally disappears before birth in mature infants but may persist longer as an innocent abnormality.

New nephrons continue to form in the human infant until the 34th week of gestation; thereafter, increase of nephron mass is by increase in tubular length and glomerular size. Kidney length increases from a mean of 27 mm at 24 weeks' gestation to 37 mm at 32 weeks and 44 mm at term (Fig. 10.56).[848]

Histological examination of the kidney of a newborn infant commonly reveals a small proportion of sclerosed glomeruli, especially in the subcapsular zone of the cortex. This 'fetal sclerosis' occurs in the youngest glomeruli when their tubules fail to communicate with the ureteric bud as its growth ceases in the later stages of fetal life. In addition, other glomeruli show signs of immaturity varying from unvascularized clumps of epithelial cells to occasional cuboidal epithelium and limited lobulation of the tufts. Microdissection studies have shown that tubular immaturity is probably even more profound than that of the glomeruli, for the ratio of glomerular surface area to tubular volume is much greater than in later childhood.

The ureteric bud, by a process of subdivision followed by coalescence, gives rise to the renal pelvis, calyces and collecting ducts. During this process the oldest, deepest nephrons are lost, although occasionally glomeruli in 'aberrant' positions beneath the pelvic mucosa or within the arterial walls will survive.

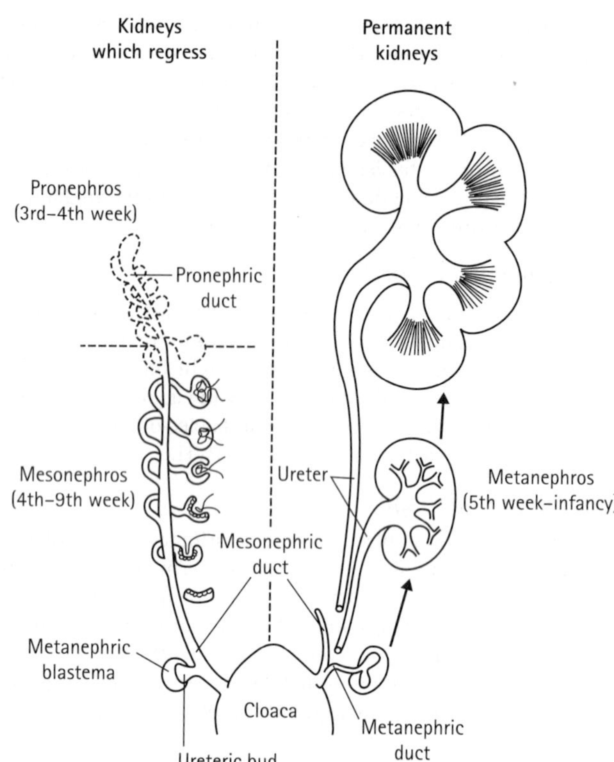

Fig. 10.56 Mammalian renal development. On the left the initial events of pronephric and mesonephric development are illustrated. These structures involute early in gestation. The definitive kidney results from a series of reciprocal interactions between the ureteric bud and the mesonephric blastema or mesenchyme. (From Evan & Larsson 1992[848] with permission)

The urinary bladder is formed from the ventral and cephalic portion of the cloaca after this has been separated from the rectum by the urorectal septum. Into this are incorporated the caudal ends of the mesonephric tubes and ureteric buds. Together these form the bladder and urethra.

Renal function in utero

Urine production increases throughout fetal life until an abrupt decline which occurs just before term. Urine is initially an ultrafiltrate of plasma. The volume varies from 4.5 ml/kg/h at 20 weeks to 6 ml/kg/h at 32 weeks and to 8 ml/kg/h at 39 weeks. Up to 600 ml of amniotic fluid is swallowed daily, 10% of which is derived from non-renal sources including gut, skin, lungs and amniotic membrane. An adequate volume of amniotic fluid is necessary for the normal development of the lungs, facial morphology and limbs.

The kidney is in a state of water diuresis. Sodium is resorbed increasingly with maturation. Its content in amniotic fluid decreases from 120 mmol/L at 20 weeks to 50 mmol/L at term. Glomerular tubular imbalance is present due to the reabsorptive capacity of the relatively smaller and more immature tubules being exceeded by the glomerular filtrate delivered to them. This is a developmental feature and the absence of glucose, phosphate and amino acid in amniotic fluid by term is indicative of tubular maturation.

Postnatal renal function

The anatomical evidence of renal immaturity at birth is reflected physiologically by the markedly diminished glomerular filtration rate (GFR) and renal bicarbonate and glucose reabsorption even when corrected for body size. The GFR of term infants at birth is approximately one-quarter of that of normal adults at 25 ml/min/1.73 m^2 (Table 10.103).[849] The GFR of a 31 weeks' gestational age infant may be 10–20 ml/min/1.73 m^2 and remains low for the first 2–3 weeks after delivery but undergoes a rapid increase at a postconceptional age of 34 weeks when nephrogenesis is completed. The GFR of term infants increases 50–100% in the first week of life after which the rate of increase diminishes and only reaches adult levels (corrected for body surface area) by the second year of life. This point is of crucial importance when considering the renal excretion of many drugs that are administered.

After an initial diuresis the neonate is in a state of positive sodium balance which is a component of normal growth. Term infants are capable of sodium conservation during sodium deprivation but an infant of <35 weeks' gestational age may develop negative sodium balance with resultant hyponatremia. This apparent tubular imbalance may be due to proximal or distal tubular immaturity. The postnatal enhancement in sodium conservation is brought about by increasing responsiveness of the distal tubule to aldosterone and by an increase in the abundance of Na^+K^+ATPase and transporter proteins.

Although preterm infants are able to achieve similar minimal urine osmolalities to adults (values of 50 mOsmol/kg or less) the maximum urine osmolality is about 600–800 mOsmol/kg compared to twice this in older children. This difference is due both to shorter loops of Henle and to reduced tonicity of the medullary interstitium resultant from low urea concentrations in the rapidly growing, anabolic infant. Given a diluting and concentrating capacity that extends from 50 to 600 mOsmol/kg and a renal solute load of approximately 10–50 mOsmol/kg, the maximum and minimum urine flow rates that preterm infants can achieve are 300 and 25 ml/kg/24 h respectively. The latter value, which represents the minimum urine flow rate beyond which sodium retention would result, approximates to 1 ml/kg/h and is the justification for the use of this figure as a clinical indication of renal failure (a lower solute load allows < 0.5 ml/kg/h urine output to be accepted).

In summary, the neonate is capable of rapid adaptation in the extrauterine environment so that homeostasis is normally maintained. The label of poor function or immaturity 'of the newborn kidney' was the result of inappropriate comparison of renal function with that of the adult who has quite different body composition and homeostatic mechanisms. However, while the newborn infant is readily adapting to the extrauterine environment, renal adaptation may be inadequate in the face of stress or inappropriate fluid electrolyte administration.

Table 10.103 Glomerular filtration rates and plasma creatinine (PCr) values

Weeks		After 1 week	1 month	After 2 months
25–28	GFR (ml/min/1.73 m^2)	11	15	50
	GFR (ml/min)	0.6	0.9	6
	PCr (μmol/L)	123	80	35
29–34	GFR (ml/min/1.73 m^2)	15	30	50
	GFR (ml/min)	1.2	2.5	11
	PCr (μmol/L)	80	62	35
38+	GFR (ml/min/1.73 m^2)	41	66	96
	GFR (ml/min)	5	11	21
	PCr (μmol/L)	44	35	35

Figures for GFR derive from creatinine clearance. For routine clinical purposes a reasonable guide to GFR is available from the formula:
GFR (ml/min/1.73 m^2) = k x length (cm)/Pcreatinine (μmol/L)
Values for k of 30 for infants of 25–34 weeks' gestation and 40 for term infants are applicable for the rest of the first year. (Data from Schwartz et al 1987.[849] Average surface areas are 0.1 m^2 at 1.0 kg body weight and

CONGENITAL ABNORMALITIES OF THE KIDNEY AND URINARY TRACT

There are a large number of abnormalities which can occur in the developing urinary tract. Traditionally these have been classified according to morphological criteria. Recent advances in basic cellular and molecular biology studies of kidney and upper urinary tract development in both rodents and humans have suggested that future classifications may be based upon correlation of morphology with pathogenic mechanisms.[850]

Such congenital abnormalities are of importance because they may lead to either: urinary obstruction with increase of pressure in the pelvis and renal tubules and so interfere with renal function; or retention of urine which predisposes to recurrent prolonged infection. By a combination of these factors there is a risk that the renal parenchyma, perhaps already malformed, may be further damaged and so lead to chronic progressive renal failure.

Antenatal detection

Many abnormalities of the urinary tract are now recognized prenatally because of detailed fetal scans at approximately 20 weeks' gestation. In a study of 105 542 total births in two Nottingham hospitals between January 1984 and December 1993, 201 abnormalities of the urinary tract were detected.[851] Between the years 1984 and 1988 the incidence was 1 in 964 compared to 1 in 364 total births in the years 1989–1993 when detailed fetal scanning was introduced. It should be appreciated that a normal ultrasound scan at 20 weeks does not rule out problems such as posterior urethral valves which can produce late hydronephrosis and will only be detected on scans carried out for obstetric reasons. Some urinary tract abnormalities may accompany other congenital abnormalities and be associated with chromosomal disorders, but most of the abnormalities detected affected only one kidney and the infant is entirely symptom free.

Very rarely is intervention provided antenatally and this would only be contemplated in a situation such as a male infant with obstructive uropathy due to posterior urethral valves where there is evidence of bilateral renal involvement and falling liquor volume.[852] Such problems require very detailed assessment in fetal medicine units with joint counseling including the pediatric nephrologist or urologist. If the pregnancy proceeds then delivery should take place in a regional center where immediate nephrourology support is available.

The natural history of many of these antenatally detected urinary tract abnormalities is becoming clearer with time but it is important that parents are given appropriate information and counseling.[853] It is particularly important that there is communication between neonatal and pediatric staff in the postnatal period so that appropriate investigations are arranged.

It is noteworthy that 14% of the 201 abnormalities in our series were labeled as transient hydronephrosis (Table 10.104). This means that although there was significant pelvic dilatation noted antenatally in the fetus, postnatal ultrasound failed to reveal an abnormality. The exact degree of antenatal dilatation is still being evaluated in those fetuses in which there is a renal pelvic dilatation >5 mm at 20 weeks. A repeat ultrasound is usually performed at 36 weeks. Pelvic dilatation > 7 mm on this scan will

Table 10.104 Antenatally detected urinary tract abnormalities – spectrum of conditions in 201 fetuses, Nottingham 1984–1993 (%)

Condition	%
Pelviureteric junction obstruction	26
Multicystic dysplastic kidney	18
Vesicoureteric junction obstruction	8
Vesicoureteric reflux	7
Duplex systems	6
Posterior urethral valves	5
Others, e.g. renal agenesis, single kidney	16
'Transient'	14

usually result in a postnatal ultrasound. If this scan shows no significant pelvic (less than 10 mm dilatation with no calyceal dilatation) or ureteric dilatation and both kidneys appear equal in size then further investigations are not carried out in our unit. There is a slight possibility of missing vesicoureteric reflux (VUR) in this situation but unless there is a strong family history a routine micturating cystourethrogram (MCUG) is not advocated. The child should be referred back for investigation if there is any suspicion of a urinary tract infection or other problems.

Investigation of infants postnatally

The scheme for investigation of antenatally detected urinary tract abnormalities is shown in Figure 10.57. After the initial ultrasound it may be appropriate to discuss management with a pediatric nephrologist or urologist if conditions that require drainage (posterior urethral valves or single hydronephrotic kidney) are recognized. If there are no palpable masses at birth and the child is passing urine and otherwise well then we would usually defer the ultrasound for the first few weeks of life. Certainly it should not be performed before 48 h unless there is strong indication.

Although all children currently undergo MCUG there are increasing concerns about the radiation exposure, expressed both by parents and radiologists. It may be that an MCUG should be performed if there is any suspicion of ureteric or renal dilatation which may represent VUR but its routine use in patients with multicystic dysplastic kidneys or simple hydronephrosis without ureteric dilatation is becoming increasingly questionable. An important practice point is that if a child is found to have gross VUR on MCUG, there should be immediate cover with 3 days of an alternative antibiotic to trimethoprim prophylaxis such as a full course of a cephalosporin. Cases of septicemia have arisen from early MCUG investigations.

Specific congenital abnormalities of the urinary tract will be discussed in Chapter 16.

SYMPTOMS AND SIGNS ASSOCIATED WITH RENAL DISEASE IN THE NEONATE

If not alerted to a renal problem by the antenatal ultrasound then the features of renal disease in the newborn (Table 10.105) can be very non-specific and indistinguishable from illness due to a large number of neonatal disorders.

Malformations of the urinary tract are frequently associated with anomalies of other organs. Bilateral renal agenesis is a classic cause of Potter's syndrome with facial dysmorphism, pulmonary hypoplasia and abnormality of the limbs which result from a lack of amniotic fluid during the second and third trimesters of pregnancy. However, the same physical appearances can be seen in association with any cause of severe bilateral renal malformation resulting in oliguria such as bilateral cystic kidney disease. It is the pulmonary hypoplasia that will determine the outcome of children as infants with milder degrees of pulmonary hypoplasia who survive ventilation in the newborn period and who can be considered for long term dialysis and renal replacement therapy. In recent years oligohydramnios sequence has been reported with the maternal use of angiotensin-II-receptor antagonists.[854]

A palpable abdominal mass in the newborn period may represent severe hydronephrosis due to pelviureteric or vesicoureteric junction obstruction, cystic renal disease, renal vein thrombosis or tumor (most commonly benign mesoblastic nephroma). *Prune belly syndrome* is easily recognizable and involves lax skin, hypoplastic abdominal musculature, undescended testes and dilatation of the urinary collecting system.

Branchio-oto-renal syndrome should be considered when there are obvious branchial arch and ear abnormalities but the clinical spectrum is wide.

Imperforate anus may be part of anomalies such as the Vater association and since renal and cardiac defects are present in nearly 75% of reported cases an ultrasound evaluation of the urinary tract (USS) is justified in all affected infants. USS should also be routine in any child with myelomeningocele. In the presence of other abnormalities, renal tract ultrasound is suggested in infants with a single umbilical artery and also whenever there are urinary tract symptoms in children with chromosomal disorders such as Down and Turner's syndrome.

Renal tubular disorders

These are rare but important causes of failure to thrive in newborns and infancy and should be considered whenever there are persistent electrolyte abnormalities. They are discussed further in Chapter 16.

Hematuria

Macroscopic hematuria is rare in infants but microscopic hematuria is not uncommon in the critically ill preterm infant usually in association with sepsis or hypoxia. There are a number of possible causes as shown in Table 10.106. The presence of a palpable abdominal mass in association with macroscopic hematuria and thrombocytopenia is a powerful pointer to *renal vein thrombosis* (RVT). Urgent ultrasound examination is justified to define the extent of the thrombus formation in this condition which often starts peripherally in the kidney and extends into the major renal veins and inferior vena cava. Risk factors include fetal distress, maternal diabetes, traumatic birth, pre-eclampsia, postnatal respiratory distress, heart disease and polycythemia. The prognosis has improved with the more frequent use of anticoagulants and thrombolysis. In those who have suffered from RVT in utero, tests should be performed for factor V Leiden deficiency.

Renal artery embolization may result from umbilical artery catheterization and should be suspected in any infant with hematuria and hypertension. Renal cortical necrosis can occur after reduction of either the arterial or renal venous circulation and may be patchy and not discernable on ultrasound examinations. In this instance, radionuclide scans may be necessary to define the degree of renal damage.

Drugs which may result in hematuria include aminoglycosides, penicillin, heparin, anticonvulsants, aminophylline and diuretics. Long term furosemide (frusemide) use has been associated with hypercalciuria and secondary gross hematuria. The urinary calcium:creatinine ratio can be as high as 2 mmol/mmol in the normal term infant and 4 in the preterm infant.

Hypercalciuria was not a prominent feature in a recent report of *nephrocalcinosis* in preterm infants but was only measured at term.[855] 16% of babies born at less than 32 weeks' gestation

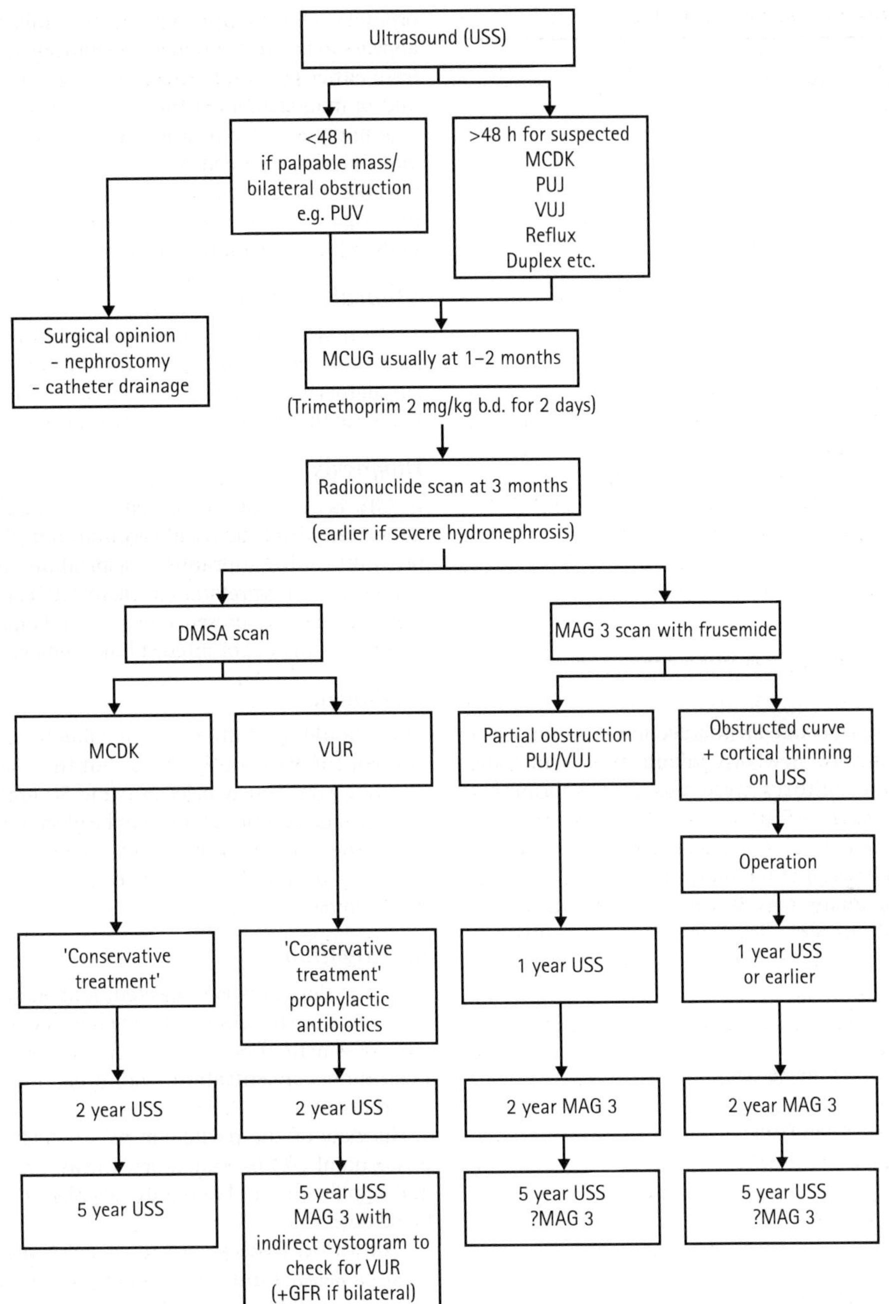

Fig. 10.57 Postnatal scheme for management of antenatally detected urinary tract abnormalities. MCDK, multicystic dysplastic kidney; MCUG, micturating cystourethrogram; PUJ, pelviureteric junction obstruction; PUV, posterior urethral valve; VUJ, vesicoureteric junction obstruction; VUR, vesicoureteric reflux.

developed nephrocalcinosis. The main associations were with extreme prematurity, severe respiratory distress coupled with male sex, frequency and duration of gentamicin use and high urinary oxalate and urate excretion at term.

Proteinuria

The presence of protein is physiological in neonatal urine averaging 500 mg/L on the first day of age and falling to an average of 175 mg/L at 5 days. It will be found in small quantities in all cases of hematuria. Heavy isolated proteinuria is rare and its persistence suggests the possibility of a neonatal glomerulopathy (Table 10.105) or congenital nephrotic syndrome (see Ch. 16).

Pyuria and bacteriuria

Uncentrifuged urine from neonates contains < 5 leukocytes/ml. Pyuria is suggestive of urinary tract infection but its presence is non-specific and can be due to drug reactions, hypercalciuria or inflammation.

Urinary tract infection (UTI)

Asymptomatic or covert bacteriuria occurs more frequently than symptomatic UTI at all ages. Edelman et al[856] reported asymptomatic bacteriuria in 2.9% of 206 premature infants and 0.7% of 836 full-term infants. The true incidence of symptomatic bacteriuria in the neonatal period is difficult to assess because the

Table 10.105 Signs of urinary tract disease in newborns

General features
Lethargy, poor feeding and vomiting
Vomiting
Oliguria
Hypertension
Seizures
Edema and ascites
Hypo/hyperthermia
Jaundice
Physical abnormalities
'Potter's facies'
Pulmonary hypoplasia
Palpable abdominal mass
Absent abdominal muscles
Single umbilical artery
Spinal abnormality
Imperforate anus
Urinary abnormalities
Hematuria
Proteinuria
Pyuria
Bacteriuria

non-specific symptoms are associated with infection in a number of organ systems. In a study of newborn infants with symptoms suggestive of UTI where cultures were taken by suprapubic aspiration, UTI was proven in 65 (0.5%) of 12 942 consecutive live-born infants, 14 of whom were < 37 weeks' gestation.[857] Again, it should be noted that 54 (84%) of 64 infants were male.

Although the young infant may be the most vulnerable to damage associated with urinary tract infection or reflux, in ordinary clinical practice the recognition of symptomatic UTI appears to be uncommon with relatively few patients being referred from either neonatal nursery or primary care for the investigation and/or management of their UTI.[858] The infecting organism is most commonly *E. coli* but other Gram negative bacteria may be found and may have spread hematogenously rather than by ascending infection in the urinary tract. Nevertheless, if UTI is diagnosed the investigations need to be comprehensive in order to exclude underlying congenital obstructive uropathy or VUR.

Table 10.106 Neonatal hematuria

1. Coagulation disorders
   a. Hemorrhagic disease of the newborn
   b. Thrombocytopenia
   c. Disseminated intravascular coagulation
2. Urinary tract infection
3. Acute tubular necrosis
4. Renal vascular disease
   a. Renal vein thrombosis
   b. Renal arterial embolization
   c. Renal cortical necrosis
5. Neonatal glomerulopathy
   a. Syphilis
   b. Toxoplasmosis
   c. Cytomegalovirus
6. Drugs
   a. Antibiotics
   b. Anticoagulants
   c. Diuretics
   d. Anticonvulsants
7. Obstructive uropathies
   a. Hydronephrosis
   b. Posterior urethral valves
8. Cystic diseases
9. Renal tumors
10. Urethral and meatal abnormality

Clinical features

These may be entirely non-specific with irritability, reluctance to feed, vomiting and fever but can proceed to septicemia and circulatory collapse. Less severe cases may present with vomiting, failure to thrive and prolonged or severe jaundice.

Diagnosis

If UTI is strongly suspected a suprapubic aspirate should be attempted, ideally under ultrasound control. Any organism obtained on culture by suprapubic aspiration should be regarded as pathogenic. Interpretation of clean catch or bag urines may be more troublesome. The presence of pyuria, hematuria or proteinuria on dipstick testing are of interest but not diagnostic.

Treatment

This should be initiated immediately with a non-nephrotoxic antibiotic intravenously in any but the mildest case. Co-amoxiclav 30 mg/kg 12-hourly or cefotaxime 50 mg/kg 12-hourly would be appropriate. Antibiotics need to be given for 7–10 days and until at least the initial ultrasound imaging has been performed. Prophylactic antibiotics will need to be maintained until the MCUG has been performed.

Investigation

Once the diagnosis is suspected, immediate investigation includes estimation of Hb, white cell and platelet counts and a blood culture. An assessment of overall renal function is best delivered by plasma creatinine concentration and urea and electrolytes including bicarbonate.

In view of the particular risks associated with VUR, imaging in neonatal UTI is mandatory. Ultrasound will reveal obstruction and significant renal anomaly. Doppler ultrasound will show renal blood flow.

An MCUG is necessary to establish the presence of VUR, but must be delayed until the urine is sterile. Other forms of imaging, e.g. radionuclide scans such as DMSA can be deferred for the first few months unless there is obstruction that needs to be assessed by a dynamic radionuclide scan, e.g. MAG 3 with furosemide (frusemide).

MANAGEMENT OF VESICOURETERIC REFLUX AND REFLUX NEPHROPATHY (see Ch. 16)

Acute renal failure

Almost 100% of newborns void within the first 24 h regardless of gestational age. The majority of term infants void during the first 8 h. Any infant who remains anuric beyond the first day should be carefully examined for abdominal masses or palpable bladder followed by renal function tests and ultrasound of the renal tract.

Diagnosis of acute renal failure (ARF) is made when electrolyte and water homeostasis cannot be sustained. In the majority of instances this is associated with oliguria, although polyuria can be associated with worsening renal insufficiency in patients following relief of obstructive uropathy.

Based on the average dietary solute load and the renal concentrating ability of the newborn infant the very minimum urine output is approximately 1 ml/kg/h. However, critically ill newborns are often administered a low osmotic load in the first few days of life and a more stringent criteria for oliguria of 0.5 ml/kg/h may be more appropriate in these patients.

The incidence of ARF in the newborn nursery is difficult to define and is partly dependent on the population served by the unit reporting the findings.[859] The definition of what constitutes acute renal failure is also difficult but the general agreement is a plasma creatinine >133 μmol/L 2 days after delivery.[860] The plasma creatinine concentration should not rise significantly after birth and a daily increase of 44–88 μmol/L indicates a falling filtration rate regardless of urine output. Blood urea is a less reliable marker of renal function, being more dependent upon protein catabolism and hydration.

Causes of ARF

Recognized causes are indicated in Table 10.107. It is useful to think of causes in terms of prerenal failure, intrinsic renal failure or postrenal or obstructive failure. Postrenal or obstructive failure should be detected from clinical signs and urgent ultrasound. It is often more difficult to differentiate prerenal from intrinsic renal failure. This has often been done on the basis of the amount of fractional excretion of sodium (FE^{Na}).[861] A value > 2.5% is generally taken to indicate established acute renal failure as opposed to prerenal failure where the FE^{Na} is < 2.5%. However, FE^{Na} levels may be more variable in sick preterm infants and the measurement may also be inaccurate if fluids or diuretics have already been administered.

In practice, in those patients without evidence of congestive heart failure a fluid load of 10–20 ml/kg saline or 4.5% albumin can be administered over 1 h with 2 mg/kg of furosemide (frusemide). If the patient is catheterized a continuing lack of urine will confirm a diagnosis of intrinsic renal failure.

In many instances there may have been a single cause contributing to the acute renal failure or it may be due to a summation effect related to previous hypoxia, hypotension and/or sepsis and the use of nephrotoxic drugs. With the low levels of GFR already in these newborn infants, it is important that drugs are very carefully monitored.

Management of established renal failure

Meticulous attention to a number of parameters is essential (Table 10.108). Urinary output is best measured with a urinary catheter which should be removed as soon as practicable because of infection risks.

A central venous presure (CVP) line is rarely practicable in newborn infants but should be considered in neonatal surgical patients undergoing emergency procedures where renal insufficiency is present and access could be placed at the time of operation.

Inotropic agents such as dopamine and dobutamine are frequently used in neonatal intensive care and Seri et al[862] showed that dopamine at a dose of 2 μg/kg/min induced maximal diuresis and natriuresis in sick preterm infants if systemic blood pressure was within the normal range. However, a recent multicenter placebo controlled trial of inotropic support in adult ICU patients[863] showed no benefit and has questioned the use of low dose dopamine in early renal dysfunction in all patients.

Particular problems in the management of ARF relate to the following.

Table 10.107 Renal failure in the neonate

1. Prerenal
   a. Hypotension, poor perfusion
      (i) Respiratory distress syndrome
      (ii) Antepartum hemorrhage
      (iii) Fetomaternal transfusion
      (iv) Twin-to-twin transfusion
   b. Cardiac surgery
   c. Heart failure
   d. Asphyxia
   e. Dehydration
2. Intrinsic renal failure
   a. Congenital abnormalities
      (i) Polycystic kidneys
      (ii) Dysplasia
      (iii) Hypoplasia
   b. Vascular
      (i) Renal cortical necrosis
      (ii) Renal venous thrombosis
      (iii) Renal arterial thrombosis
      (iv) Disseminated intravascular coagulation
   c. Acute tubular necrosis
      (i) RDS
      (ii) Asphyxia
      (iii) Dehydration
      (iv) Poor perfusion
      (v) Cardiac surgery
   d. Interstitial nephritis
   e Infections
      (i) Urinary tract infection
      (ii) Congenital infections
3. Postrenal
   a. Hydronephrosis
   b. Neurogenic bladder
   c. Posterior urethral valves
   d. Ureterocele
   e. Urethral obstruction
   f. Meatal/foreskin obstruction
   g. External pressure
      (i) Sacrococcygeal tumor

Hydration. Many newborns have substantial edema by the time diagnosis of ARF is made yet treatment for associated conditions may lead to continued fluid administration. Conservative fluid management requires the administration of fluids of an appropriate sodium concentration to replace the urinary losses, and as 10% dextrose to replace insensible water losses. These can be quite substantial in premature infants with fever and radiant heaters for phototherapy but losses are decreased in ventilated infants.

Fluid overload, particularly if it is associated with pulmonary edema, may be one of the indications for using peritoneal dialysis or extracorporeal hemofiltration.

Hyperkalemia. This can be a medical emergency if evidence of cardiac toxicity is present with high peaked T-waves and widening of the QRS complex on ECG monitoring. However, newborns appear to be more resistant to hyperkalemia and there may be sufficient time to correct matters using intravenous calcium gluconate, sodium bicarbonate and salbutamol (4 μg/kg i.v. over 20 min). Calcium resonium 1 g/kg inserted rectally is a messy procedure and if hyperkalemia is confirmed and persists then the above measures are only a temporary stopgap until peritoneal dialysis or hemofiltration has been arranged. Insulin and dextrose infusions are potentially lethal in newborns because of hypoglycemia.

Table 10.108 Parameters to be monitored in the neonate with acute renal failure

1. Twice daily or daily body weight
2. Urine output 12-hourly (6-hourly in polyuric patients)
3. Blood pressure and central venous pressure (rarely available)
4. Plasma electrolytes, creatinine, calcium, phosphate, albumin
5. Fluid, sodium, potassium, protein and energy intakes

Acidosis. This can be treated by i.v. infusion of 8.4% sodium bicarbonate using the formula – base deficit × 0.3 × body weight in kg. Half of this dose is usually given initially with careful clinical monitoring.

Hypocalcemia and hyperphosphatemia. Phosphate levels are high in newborn infants (1.6–2.8 mmol/L) but extreme hyperphosphatemia and hypocalcemia may result in convulsions. Calcium carbonate can be used as a phosphate binder to lower plasma phosphate levels but this is another contributory factor to considering dialysis. Dietetic advice should be sought if fluid balance allows intake of milk feeds.

Hypertension. Reference should be made to appropriate blood pressure levels for gestational age.[864] The objective should be to maintain blood pressure below the 95th centile levels for gestational age. Hypertension may be associated with fluid volume overload and may be another indication for dialysis. Intravenous labetalol or hydralazine may be given if urgent treatment is required. If treatment is less urgent, oral propranolol or nifedipine may be used. Severe neonatal hypertension associated with renal artery stenosis or thrombosis can cause cardiac failure in the newborn period.[865]

Drug dosages

These need to be carefully adjusted in renal failure, especially with the background of existing renal insufficiency. The sodium content of administered drugs needs also to be considered.

Dialysis and hemofiltration

Acute renal failure itself is always treatable, particularly if early referral is made. However, there are some newborns such as those with severe HIE or extreme prematurity and multiple organ failure, in whom aggressive intervention is not justified. In order for dialysis to be commenced there should be a reversible cause for the renal failure and no major comorbidities. The decision to treat needs to be made on an individual basis and indications for dialysis are shown in Table 10.109.

Peritoneal dialysis is the treatment of choice in newborns and can be accomplished in the short term even in VLBW infants.[866] The catheters (e.g. Cohen acute peritoneal catheter 5FR 5.5 cm [Cook®]) are inserted using the Seldinger technique but all catheters are prone to leaks and blockage.[867] If a long spell of anuria is anticipated a conventional silastic cuffed Tenckhoff-type catheter can be placed surgically. Peritoneal dialysis is very efficient at removing potassium and sodium but phosphate and creatinine require longer dwell times. Fluid can be removed using 1.36% glucose dialysis solution, which is hypertonic because of the other electrolytes it contains. A 2.27% glucose dialysis solution may be needed. The efficiency of dialysis depends upon the child's overall physical state and the blood pressure which perfuses the peritoneal membrane. Most dialysis fluids contain lactate as the buffer and in newborns it is preferable to use bicarbonate-containing solutions instead.

Table 10.109 Indications for dialysis in neonatal acute renal failure

Sustained potassium > 7 mmol/L
Hyponatremia and fluid overload
Persistent metabolic acidosis
Other electrolyte disturbances
Creation of 'nutritional space'

Although intraperitoneal surgery is not an absolute contraindication to peritoneal dialysis it is often wise to consider an alternative route such as extracorporeal hemofiltration. This requires vascular access which may be obtained via umbilical or femoral vessels. Unlike peritoneal dialysis which can be run by neonatal nurses, hemofiltration requires supervision from renal nurses trained in extracorporeal circuits.[868]

Prognosis

Acute renal failure associated with acute tubular necrosis can recover within a few days but persistent oliguria arouses suspicion that substantial damage such as cortical necrosis may have ensued or the problem may be one of acute on chronic renal failure. Initial ultrasounds may suggest kidneys of good size with loss of cortical medullary differentiation and it is only with time that involution of one or both kidneys may be noted. The prognosis for each individual newborn infant therefore depends partly upon the initial insult. As in older children, ARF associated with multisystem failure has a very poor prognosis.

Chronic renal failure

Infants with presumed ARF not recovering after several weeks as well as those with obstructive uropathies and hypoplastic/dysplastic kidneys may have irreversible renal failure. Renal ultrasound and radionuclide scanning may define the problem but in some it may be necessary to perform a renal biopsy to establish a more accurate diagnosis and prognosis. Chronic peritoneal dialysis is now feasible in most newborn infants but its undertaking requires a great deal of hard work by the carers and extensive renal team involvement. The majority of such newborn infants will also require nasogastric or gastrostomy feeding with close attention to electrolyte, calcium and phosphate balance if normal growth is to ensue. These management issues are discussed in Chapter 16.

EYE PROBLEMS IN THE NEWBORN

A normal visual input is important for a child's development. This section will be concerned with the developing visual system, and the various problems which may befall it in the neonatal period.

THE DEVELOPING VISUAL SYSTEM

Ocular growth

The eye of the infant born at term is at a relatively advanced stage of development as it grows only three times in volume, to reach adult size, compared to the rest of the body's 20 times. While the length of the globe does not reach its adult value of approximately 24 mm until the second decade, the anterior segment of the eye is further advanced, and the cornea is fully grown within a month after birth. Thus, most of the postnatal growth of the eye takes place in its posterior segment, particularly in the peripheral regions of the retina.

Between 6 months' gestational age (GA) and term, at a time when many preterm babies are already born, ocular growth is particularly active, as retinal surface area doubles during this period. Over the ensuing 2 years it increases by a further 50%.[869]

Vascular development

Transient vascular systems. In fetal life there are two transient vascular systems – the hyaloid vascular complex which fills the vitreous cavity and extends forwards and also contributes to the second system, the tunica vasculosa lentis, a vascular structure which surrounds the lens. The hyaloid artery has disappeared by 7 months and the tunica vasculosa lentis regresses between 28 and 34 weeks' GA. As the latter can easily be visualized by direct ophthalmoscopy the degree of regression can be used as a crude estimate of GA.

Retinal vasculature. Until the fourth month of gestation the retina is avascular, relying entirely on the underlying choroidal circulation for its nutrients. From this time the mesenchymal precursors of the retinal vessels grow out from the optic disc and reach the periphery of the nasal retina around 8 months' GA, whilst in the temporal retina, which is the last area to be vascularized, this process is not complete until around term. The stimulus for vasculogenesis is tissue hypoxia mediated through retinal astrocyctes and Muller cells, which secrete vascular endothelial growth factor (VEGF). VEGF is a vascular survival factor which by downregulation results in endothelial apoptosis and capillary retraction. Hence VEGF is vital to the formation and maintenance of a normal retinal circulation.

Visual pathway development

The retina has its full complement of cells by 6 months' GA, but retinal maturational changes continue, particularly in the fovea, for another 4 years. Myelination between the globe and the lateral geniculate nucleus commences at about 6 months' GA and is complete by 2 years. In the posterior visual pathway dendrite formation and synaptogenesis both lead to an increase in volume of the lateral geniculate nucleus and the visual cortex over the first 6 or so months of postnatal life.

Ocular growth, the maturational changes within the eye and the posterior sections of the visual system, are all dovetailed so that they proceed at a predetermined and relatively unimpeded rate to a successful functional outcome in most infants and children. This is even more remarkable for the baby born before term, who is reared in a hostile, often brightly lit environment.[870]

Ophthalmia neonatorum

This is defined as conjunctivitis developing within the first 4 weeks of life (Fig. 10.58). It is a notifiable condition as in the past ophthalmia neonatorum was one of the most important causes of childhood visual disability. Fortunately the situation has now changed, but even today permanent ocular damage can result and treatment must be prompt and appropriate. Although the clinical features of the various types of ophthalmia neonatorum are suggestive of a particular diagnosis they are not sufficiently characteristic to make a definitive diagnosis. A large number of organisms have been implicated and in order of frequency these are *Chlamydia trachomatis*, *Staph. aureus*, *Neisseria gonorrhoeae*, *Streptococcus viridans*, *Haemophilus* group, *E. coli*, and less frequently a number of other organisms including *Pseudomonas aeruginosa* and the herpes simplex virus.

Chlamydia trachomatis. This is the commonest cause of ophthalmia neonatorum (developing in 18–50% of those infants exposed) and although the clinical picture may be mild, subclinical infections are unusual. The incubation period is 7–28 days with a peak incidence in the second week. The condition can be unilateral or bilateral and may range from a mild erythematous response to a severe pseudomembranous conjunctivitis (streptococci are another cause of a pseudomembranous reaction). Only in the most severe infection is the discharge copious and purulent. Even mild disease can cause corneal scarring (pannus), but the risk of this complication is lessened by prompt treatment.

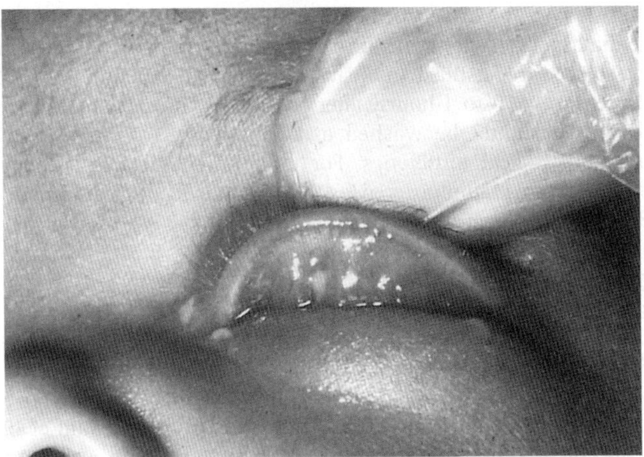

Fig. 10.58 Ophthalmia neonatorum.

Neisseria gonorrhoeae. This infection is acquired during passage down the birth canal of the mother who has either untreated or partially treated gonorrhea. The incubation period is 4–7 days. Characteristically it causes a marked inflammatory reaction with lid and conjunctival edema, and there is a copious purulent, greenish, sometimes bloodstained, discharge held under pressure by the swollen eyelids. This organism is particularly virulent as it alone can penetrate the intact cornea, hence its propensity to cause blindness.

Herpes simplex virus. When ophthalmia neonatorum is caused by this virus it is usually as part of a generalized infection. In addition to the conjunctivitis, corneal clouding and dendritic ulceration occur. In contrast to herpes simplex infections developing at other times of life, neonatal herpes has a propensity to affect both eyes.

Other organisms. These do not individually give rise to distinctive clinical features, although in general a purulent discharge indicates bacterial origin or secondary involvement.

Chemical conjunctivitis. In those countries where prophylaxis against ophthalmia neonatorum is still practiced a chemical conjunctivitis with 1% silver nitrate drops is the rule, occurring 24 h after treatment. This subsides spontaneously within 2–3 days.

Diagnosis and treatment

As the clinical features are at best suggestive but not pathognomonic, accurate diagnosis rests with laboratory tests. No topical antibiotic should be administered until swabs have been taken. Culture media (blood and chocolate agar) should be inoculated at the cot-side. A further specimen which must contain epithelial cells is applied directly to microscope slides and stained by Gram and Giemsa stains, looking in the latter for the intracytoplasmic inclusions of chlamydia (or preferably by direct immunofluorescent antibody assay) and multinucleated giant cells and intranuclear inclusions of herpes simplex. Impression cytology of conjunctival cells is a rapid technique for diagnosing chlamydia.

In several countries, but not the UK, prophylaxis is routinely performed using silver nitrate 1%, tetracycline ointment 1%, or erythromycin ointment 0.5%. Recently povidone iodine 2.5% has been used and may prove more effective.[871] Whichever preparation is used it is applied once to both eyes soon after birth.

All cases of ophthalmia neonatorum should be managed as though they are contagious. Treatment must be started immediately, guided by clinical findings and the results of the histological stains. If there is any evidence of systemic involvement topical and systemic therapy are necessary and all cases of gonococcal and chlamydial infections are so treated. Gonococcal infections are treated with systemic and topical penicillin. In cases of resistance, topical erythromycin and a systemic third generation cephalosporin (ceftriaxone 30–50 mg/kg/day in divided doses); the eye drops are instilled intensively, initially at 15 min intervals decreasing to 3- to 4-hourly after about 6 h. The copious purulent discharge should be washed away by saline irrigation before instilling topical antibiotics. For chlamydial infection systemic erythromycin is administered for 2 weeks; as efficacy of treatment is 80% a second course may be required. Topical tetracycline or sulfacetamide ointment is also used.

Birth trauma

Eyelids and orbit

Ecchymosis of the eyelids is common but is of no long term consequence. Dislocation of the globe from the orbit has been reported rarely and is particularly prone to occur in certain of the craniofacial anomalies such as Apert's syndrome. Although alarming to all, replacement can be achieved by gentle pressure on the globe. Orbital hemorrhage causing proptosis occurs occasionally and is usually the consequence of a prolonged and difficult labor.

Ocular hemorrhages

Hemorrhages onto various ocular tissues are frequent with all types of delivery. Conjunctival hemorrhages resolve rapidly and without sequelae. It is not uncommon for the iris blood vessels to be markedly engorged following birth and on occasion bleeding occurs causing a hyphema, which also settles spontaneously.

The retina is the most frequent site of hemorrhage (up to 50% of all births). Frequently, but not invariably bilateral, most resolve spontaneously without trace over the ensuing days and weeks. If the hemorrhage is large and has a preretinal or vitreous extension this process may take up to 2–3 months, but even so does not result in adverse sequelae. Neonatal retinal hemorrhages do not cause amblyopia. Sometimes it can be difficult to differentiate between retinal hemorrhages due to the birth process or a later acquired non-accidental injury. The distinction, which can be extremely difficult, rests on the history, and whether the features of the hemorrhage are compatible with the history.

Cornea

The cornea may be damaged by forceps injury. This is usually unilateral and causes a cloudy cornea. Although this clears over the ensuing few weeks, in the long term astigmatism, amblyopia and strabismus are likely sequelae. It is important but not always simple to distinguish corneal cloudiness due to injury and infantile glaucoma (Fig. 10.59). Although in glaucoma the corneae are characteristically enlarged, in the neonatal period this may be yet to develop and it is essential to measure the intraocular pressure, which can usually be done at this age without sedation. The following features may also help: history and signs of trauma and the direction of fine lines in the deeper corneal layers. These are breaks in Descemet's membrane and are vertically directed in forceps injury whilst in glaucoma they are almost horizontal.

Cranial nerve palsies

Palsy of one of the ocular motor nerves is not rare, and has in the past often been attributed to birth trauma – almost certainly incorrectly.

Cornea

The normal cornea is hazy until about 27 weeks' GA. Slight haze in preterm and term infants is not rare and clears rapidly, depending on the degree of immaturity. The following causes of a cloudy cornea must also always be considered: infantile glaucoma (see above), a corneal dystrophy, malformation of the anterior segment (Fig. 10.60), and rarely congenital rubella causes a self-limiting cloudy cornea due to keratitis.

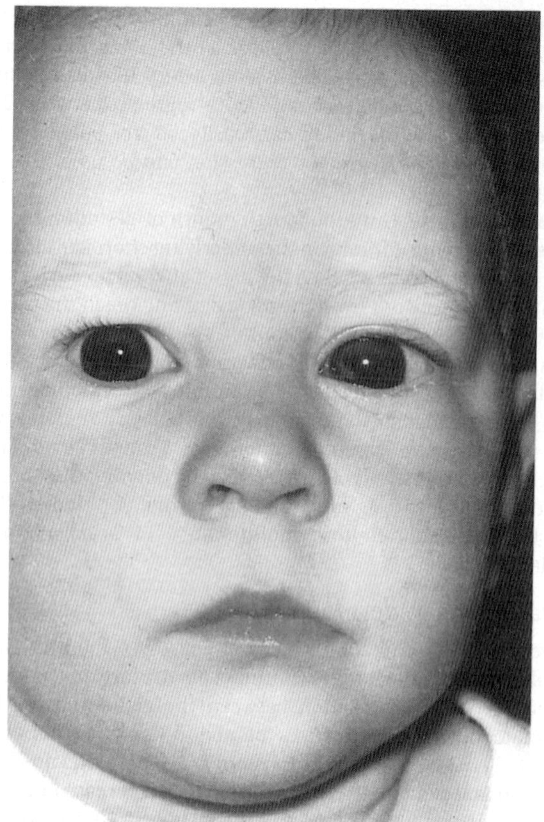

Fig. 10.59 Congenital glaucoma in the left eye. This eye is larger than its fellow, and the cornea is also slightly hazy (dulled corneal light reflex).

Lens

Subtle lens opacities are quite common in preterm neonates. These are in the form of vacuoles and are best seen using the direct ophthalmoscope. They are transient, of no long term significance and their etiology is unknown. Congenital cataract is considered elsewhere (Ch. 29).

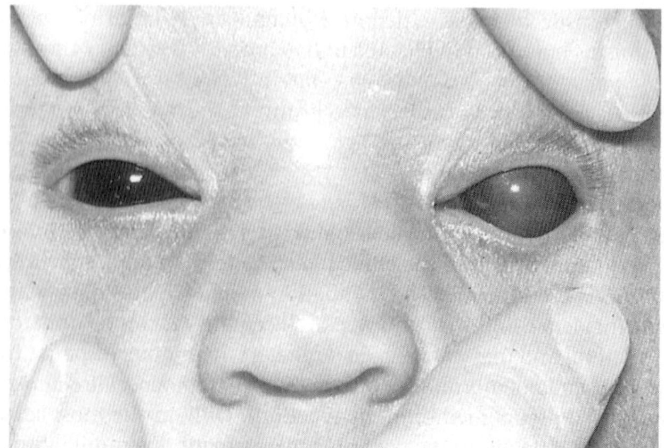

Fig. 10.60 Left cloudy cornea due to malformation of the anterior segment, the so-called anterior cleavage syndrome.

RETINOPATHY OF PREMATURITY

Retinopathy of prematurity (ROP) is a potentially blinding disorder affecting infants born prematurely. Described first in the 1940s there was an epidemic of retrolental fibroplasia (RLF) as it was then known which was brought to an end in the early 1950s by the discovery that the high concentrations of oxygen being given at that time were important in its production. Concomitant with the increased survival of the extremely immature neonate in recent years the incidence of ROP has again risen.

Pathogenesis

ROP is a condition of the immature retinal vasculature and does not develop after the retina is fully vascularized. Retinopathy develops at the junction of the vascularized and yet to be vascularized retina. There are three theories. According to the first classic theory[872,873] the retinal vessels constrict and their endothelial cells are damaged due to raised (i.e. above normal for the fetus) PaO_2 levels. This leads to the production of angiogenic factors and subsequent vasoproliferation. The second theory[874] also postulates the production of angiogenic factors but proposes that this is not induced by vasoconstriction but by direct oxidative insult to the mesenchymal precursors (spindle cells), which then synthesize and secrete angiogenic factors generating the vasoproliferative response by the retinal vessels.

Both theories invoke an oxidative insult, which might be due to a direct cytotoxic action of oxygen itself,[872] indirectly due to ischemia consequent upon the vasoconstriction,[873] or indirectly by oxygen-generated free radicals.[874] The most recent theory invokes growth factors and apoptosis.[875,876] As mentioned, the maintenance of the retinal vascular tree depends on a continuous supply of survival factor (VEGF) which can be downregulated by oxygen. Thus hyperoxia induces a shutdown of VEGF so inducing endothelial apoptosis and excessive capillary regression. The resultant retinal ischemia which follows, generates an upregulation of VEGF, which induces angiogenesis, and the vasoproliferative response of ROP.[876]

All theories concur that oxygen is implicated directly or indirectly in the initiation of ROP. However, once ROP has developed the retina is rendered ischemic and it is this ischemia which contributes to the vasoproliferative response of severe disease. A trial to reduce the severity of the retinal ischemia associated with severe ROP, by oxygen administration was unsuccessful.[877]

Risk factors

ROP is not a totally preventable condition and recently clinicians have tended to regard severe ROP as an inevitable, albeit unpredictable, consequence of extreme prematurity. By far the most powerful ROP risk factor is the degree of immaturity. However many other risk factors have been implicated of which the best known is supplemental oxygen administration. Interest in the role of oxygen in its pathogenesis has reawakened with the finding that oxygen administration in the first few weeks of life is a risk factor for ROP incidence and severity. Fluctuations, even within the normal range, can increase the risk of severe ROP, and PaO_2 monitoring – being intermittent – may mask important variations.[878] These findings have major implications for neonatal care. Nevertheless, it has not been possible to define a concentration, or duration, of oxygen which is, or is not, associated with ROP. The current consensus is that hyperoxia can be important in ROP initiation. Hypoxia on the other hand may increase the severity of established ROP, which is known to be ischemic. Other possible risk factors include blood transfusions, apneic episodes, hypercarbia, low pH, intraventricular hemorrhage and periventricular leukomalacia. A randomized controlled trial showed that early exposure to light is not a factor in ROP development.[879]

Classification

Clinically, ROP is classified by the International Classification of Retinopathy of Prematurity.[880,881]

Acute phase ROP (Fig. 10.61). This is described by four parameters: severity by stage (1–5), location by zone (1–3), extent [clock hours of the retinal circumference (Fig. 10.62)], and the presence of 'plus' disease (Fig. 10.63).

Severity –

Stage 1 – demarcation line, lying within the plane of the retina at the junction of the vascularized and avascular retina. The demarcation line is the accumulation of the mesenchymal precursors of the retinal vessels.

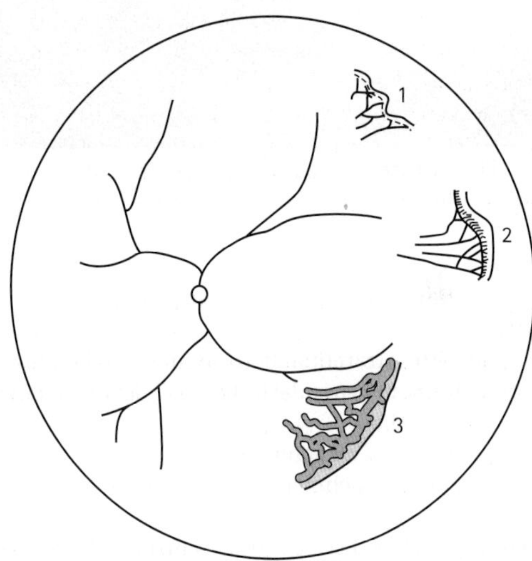

Fig. 10.61 Acute ROP: the first three stages of acute ROP presented for diagrammatic purposes on one retina. Each is shown as a short segment, but can extend over 360°. Stage 1, demarcation line; stage 2, ridge; and stage 3, ridge with extraretinal fibrovascular proliferation. Note abnormal peripheral vascular arborization in all stages, but in stage 3 the vessels are engorged and the lesion is more posteriorly located. Note also that the retina is not fully vascularized.

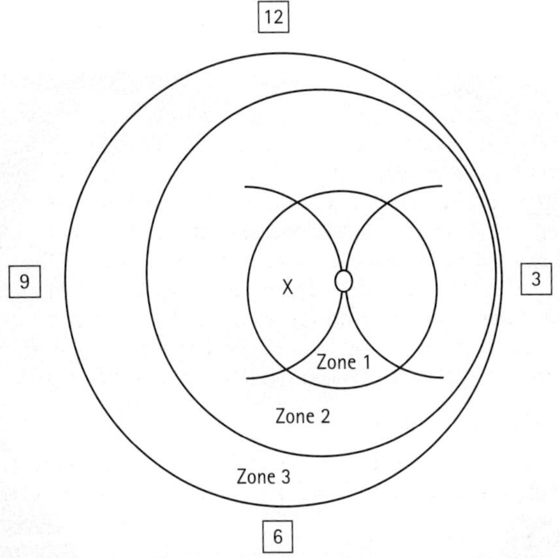

Fig. 10.62 Acute ROP: diagram of the retinal zones. Acute ROP develops at the advancing edge of the growing blood vessels. Numbers on the periphery denote the hours of the clock which are used to describe ROP extent.

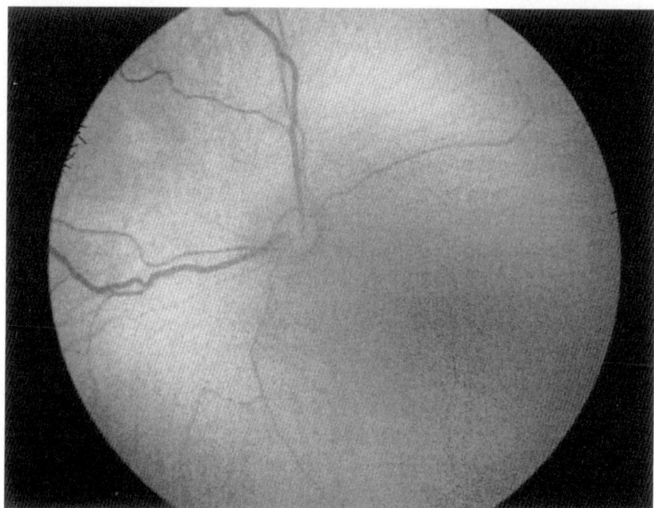

Fig. 10.63 Plus disease – venous congestion. The pattern reflects ROP asymmetry, the engorged vessels point to the active lesion.

Stage 2 – ridge; the demarcation line extends out of the plane of the retina (Fig. 10.64).
Stage 3 – ridge with extraretinal fibrovascular proliferation. This is the stage of frank neovascularization, i.e. definitive new vessels are formed (Fig. 10.65).
Stage 4 – subtotal retinal detachment.
Stage 5 – total retinal detachment.

Location – retinal blood vessels grow centrifugally from the optic disc to zone 3. ROP in zone 1 is far more likely to become severe, and even if treated there is a far greater likelihood of a poor outcome than ROP in zone 3.[882]

Extent – the extent of ROP around the circumference is described in clock hours and this is one of the parameters used to indicate treatment.

'Plus' disease – signs of activity, which in order of severity include: congestion of the retinal vessel of the posterior pole, congestion of the iris vessels so that the pupil does not dilate readily with mydriatics (iris rigidity), and vitreous haze. While this sign cannot be sensibly quantified, it is an important indicator of impending, or current, severe ROP.

Regressed ROP. Not all ROP undergoes complete resolution. Signs in the fundus which signify previous acute ROP are described according to their location – posterior or peripheral – and according to the structures involved, thus:

Vascular – tortuosity, abnormal branching and arcades, and the straightening ('dragging') of the vessels around the disc (Fig. 10.66).

Retinal – pigmentation, folding, stretching, detachment and vitreoretinal membranes.

Incidence. The incidence and severity of acute ROP rises with decreasing birth weight and GA. Quoted figures vary widely, probably due more to examination technique and frequency than neonatal factors. About 30–60% of babies weighing less than 1500 g develop some ROP. Severe disease is virtually confined to those infants $<$ 1500 g birth weight and affects about 6% infants $<$ 1250 g birth weight.[883]

Natural history

As the temporal retina is the last area to be vascularized, most acute ROP develops in that region, although in extremely immature babies it often starts in the nasal retina. The age at onset of acute ROP is governed by the postmenstrual age (PMA) of the baby rather than neonatal events. Thus contrary to expectation, ROP develops later postnatally in the smaller, very immature baby who is ill, compared to his larger, usually fitter more mature counterpart. Retinopathy of prematurity infrequently starts before 31 weeks' PMA, and never after complete retinal vascularization. Stage 3 acute ROP affects almost exclusively infants $<$ 32 weeks' GA, and $<$ 1500 g and develops between about 33 and 41 weeks' PMA.[884]

Outcome

Spontaneous and complete regression is the rule for all stage 1 and 2 acute ROP. Some babies with stage 3 also undergo resolution, but at this stage the likelihood of significant sequelae is very high and some babies become blind – hence the use of the term severe to describe stage 3 and above. All stage 4 and 5 ROP have a poor visual outcome.

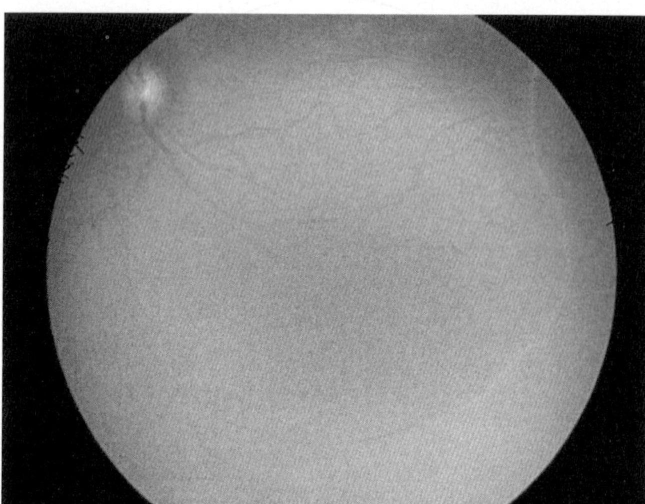

Fig. 10.64 Stage 1 and 2 ROP. Lower end of line is stage 1, but towards its upper end the line becomes more prominent and stands out from the retina as stage 2.

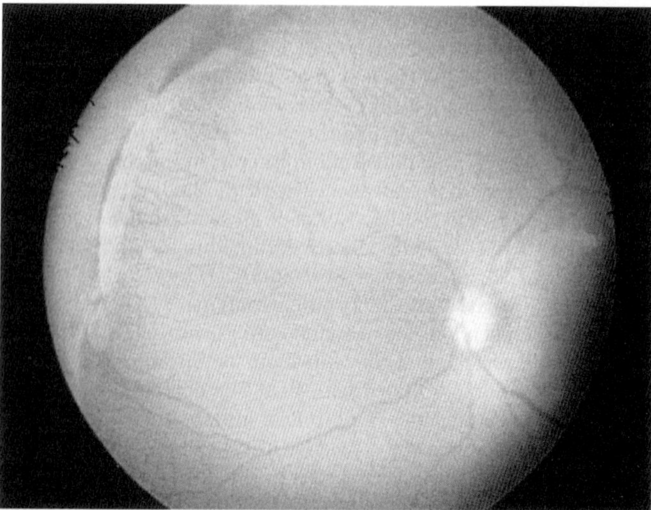

Fig. 10.65 Stage 3 ROP. Ridge with fibrovascular proliferation, and here hemorrhage disconnects a portion of the ROP lesion from the ridge.

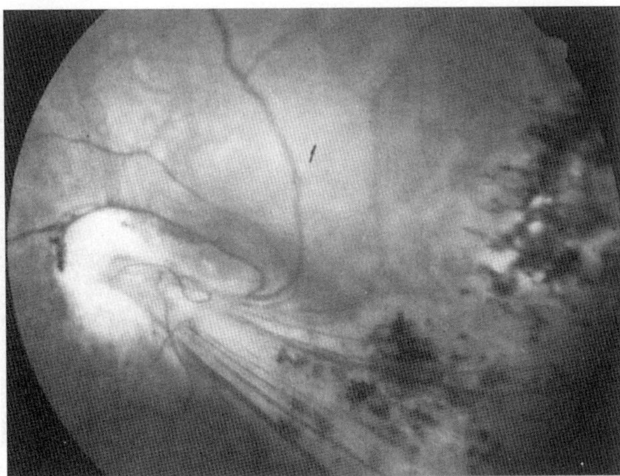
Fig. 10.66 Signs of regressed ROP. Retinal fold extending from the 'dragged' optic disc. Peripheral pigmentation corresponds to the site of the acute lesion. (Reproduced with permission, Editor of the Practitioner.)

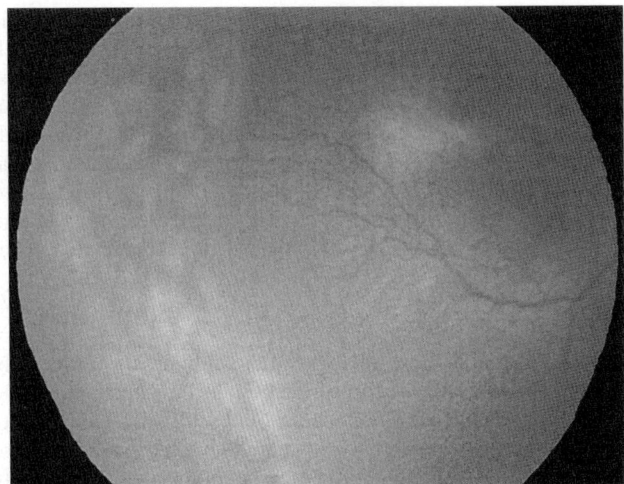
Fig. 10.67 Laser treatment for relatively mild stage 3 ROP. Laser is applied to the avascular retina just anterior to the ROP and not to the lesion itself.

Treatment

As mild ROP spontaneously resolves and the outcome for stages 4 and 5 is dismal, therapeutic intervention can only be considered at stage 3. The current indication for intervention is 'threshold' at which stage the untreated risk of blindness is 50%.[885] 'Threshold' is defined as stage 3 ROP in zone 1 and 2 which extends over 5 or more continuous, or 8 or more cumulative, clock hours of the retinal circumference in the presence of 'plus' disease. It is important to emphasize that the time available for treatment once 'threshold' ROP has been reached is short, and ideally treatment should be undertaken within 2–3 days.[886]

Cryotherapy and laser. Until recently ROP could neither be prevented nor treated. This changed in 1988 when the US-based Multicenter Trial of Cryotherapy for ROP demonstrated that cryotherapy reduced the unfavorable outcome of 'threshold' stage 3 ROP by about 50%[885] and maintained 10 years on.[887] This single study has changed clinical practice worldwide and now cryotherapy is recommended for babies reaching this stage.

More recently laser, delivered via an indirect ophthalmoscope, has been used to treat severe ROP. Both modalities have their indication, but laser is, in most instances, the modality of choice. Either cryotherapy or laser is applied to the peripheral retina anterior to the ridge (Fig. 10.67) – over the full circumference of the globe. The procedure can be performed either under general anesthesia or sedation. Not all babies respond to treatment and there is a recent tendency for zone 1 ROP that carries such a poor prognosis to undertake treatment at a slightly earlier stage,[877] i.e. for zone 2, the presence of dilatation/tortuosity in at least two posterior pole quadrants and stage 3 ROP for at least 5 continuous of 8 cumulative clock hours. For zone 1 ROP: any stage of ROP with posterior pole dilatation/tortuosity in at least two quadrants, or stage 3 ROP, with or without plus disease.

ROP screening

Screening is now recommended[883,886,888] and has the aim of identifying babies at risk of developing stage 3 ROP – these babies require either treatment or, because of sequelae, continued ophthalmic surveillance. UK guidelines specify that all babies of birth weight < 1500 g and < 32 weeks' GA are screened at least fortnightly, commencing at 6–7 weeks' postnatal age and continuing until retinal vascularization is into zone 3 (i.e. peripheral).

Treatment for end-stage disease

Not all ROP responds to treatment and retinal detachment surgery and vitrectomy have been used for end-stage ROP. Vitrectomy is technically well within the scope of many surgeons but to date the visual results have been so poor that it is not recommended. Acute glaucoma sometimes develops in advanced disease. Removal of the lens may be helpful although there is a risk of globe shrinkage.

Differential diagnosis

For the preterm neonate this question hardly ever arises but there are a number of conditions simulating ROP, which may present in the full-term baby or in later life. These include autosomal dominant familial exudative vitreoretinopathy, fetal ischemia (porencephaly, anencephaly), and Coats' disease. The distinction may be impossible on ophthalmological criteria alone, and the family history and systemic aspects must be taken into account.

Ophthalmic sequelae of preterm birth

Sequelae of ROP

All mild ROP (stages 1 and 2) regresses without significantly affecting eye growth and visual function. Severe disease, even after treatment, generates sequelae which include refractive errors (myopia, astigmatism), strabismus, and visual deficits ranging from the very mild to complete blindness. A serious late complication of ROP is retinal detachment, which can develop at any age, even in adulthood.[887]

Sequelae of prematurity

Visual development proceeds according to postmenstrual age rather than postnatal age and failure to appreciate this can result in unnecessary concern about visual functions. Infants and children who were born prematurely, even after ROP has been accounted for, are more prone to suffer visual pathway defects.[889–891] In reality the effects of ROP and neurological insults cannot be differentiated as the proportional effect of neurological damage suffered in the perinatal period compared to that due to prematurity per se is unknown. Neurological insults can vary in location and severity and not surprisingly result in a range of neuro-ophthalmic defects including reduced vision, eye movement disorders, refractive errors and optic atrophy. The causes of reduced vision depend on the nature of the insult (see elsewhere), and the severity of the deficit can range from minimal to severe (cortical visual impairment).[892]

Eye movement disorders include strabismus, gaze and saccadic palsies, and nystagmus. These are commonly associated with neurological insult; indeed the last three mentioned are almost certainly its direct consequence. The incidence of squint ranges from 11% to over 30%.[893] and is particularly high in those with neurological damage such as cystic periventricular leukomalacia, especially if the lesion is posteriorly located. Myopia can be due to ROP,[894] but even in the absence of ROP the ex-preterm child and teenager is more likely to be myopic than his ex-full-term counterpart.[895]

Routine neonatal eye examination

Every baby should have an eye examination in the very early neonatal period before discharge from hospital or equivalent.[896] The following aspects need to be included and although the list looks formidable at first glance each examination need not take more than a minute or so. The neonatal eye examination while seemingly simple is not that easy to perform (puffy eyelids, etc.) and only 50% of congenital cataracts are diagnosed by 10 weeks of age, while 30% remain unidentified until after the first year.[897]

Look for conditions affecting both eyes, but be especially suspicious of asymmetry between the eyes.

Signs of significant birth trauma

These have already been covered, and the word significant is included so that the pediatric resident performing this examination does not feel obliged to dilate pupils in order to look for retinal hemorrhage. Using the direct ophthalmoscope as torchlight, the anterior segment of the eye can be examined for corneal cloudiness, hyphema, etc.

Ocular malformation

With the ophthalmoscope the following are examined:

- *Lids* – ptosis, hemangioma, dermoids;
- *Globe size*
  - microphthalmos
  - macrophthalmos, most important as this could be infantile glaucoma, but in the neonatal period the eyes may still be of normal size as the process is at an early stage;
- *Conjunctiva* – injection or dermoid;
- *Cornea* – cloudiness, consider infantile glaucoma (Fig. 10.59). Opacities may be part of a malformation (Fig. 10.60);
- *Iris* – coloboma.

Leukocoria (white pupil)

This is an important clinical sign, which may signify a condition that is potentially lethal or may have severe consequences for vision. The red reflex is looked for by viewing the undilated pupil, viewing through a direct ophthalmoscope which is held at 33 cm from the eye (without a correction dialed in), or with + 10 dialed in and held close to the infant's eye. This writer prefers the former as it provides a better 'feel', and the location of an opacity can be better determined. The absence of a red reflex must always be taken seriously and it requires *urgent* specialist referral.

Causes of leukocoria (Fig. 10.68) include: cataract, malformations (persistent hyperplastic primary vitreous, coloboma, retinal dysplasia as in Norrie's disease and lissencephaly), tumors (retinoblastoma), myelinated nerve fibers, and inflammations (endophthalmitis). Conditions such as end-stage ROP, Coats' disease and toxocariasis also can give a white pupil but always after the neonatal period.

Ophthalmic family history

It is important to examine the eyes if there is a family history of a serious ophthalmic problem. In some conditions, for example dominantly inherited retinitis pigmentosa, the eyes at this time will be normal and it is not possible to determine whether or not the baby will be affected later. Certain fears can only be eliminated by a detailed examination and the diplomatic effect of this early examination is considerable and provides a good start to any subsequent involvement. A positive family history of infantile glaucoma and retinoblastoma even in the presence of a *normal* neonatal eye examination requires urgent referral and continued ophthalmological review.

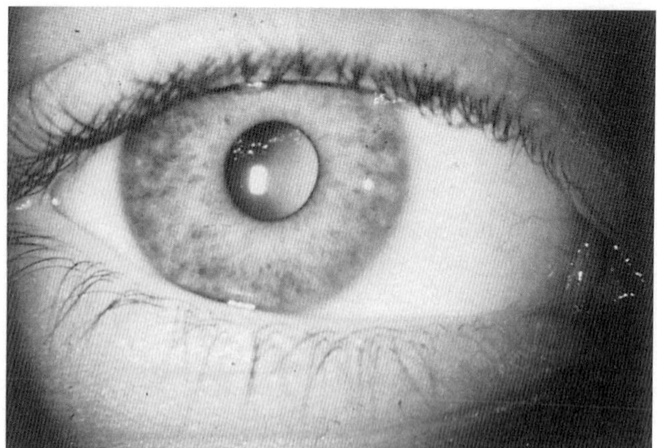

Fig. 10.68 Leukocoria, a frequent presenting sign of retinoblastoma.

INFECTION AND IMMUNITY IN THE NEWBORN

EPIDEMIOLOGY

The incidence of serious neonatal sepsis is uncertain. Under-reporting is common.[898] Rates between 0.22 and 11.2% have been reported from the developed world with mortality rates between 9 and 15%.[899,900] From the developing world rates of 10–30% are reported with mortality between 30 and 45%.[901] The incidence in babies requiring intensive care is much greater and a mortality of around 20% has been recorded over the past 20 years.[902,903] This mortality rises further in VLBW babies undergoing prolonged intensive care.[904]

Recent evidence suggests that perinatal sepsis is also important in the pathogenesis of neurodevelopmental impairment. Infants born at term following maternal infection are nine times more likely to develop cerebral palsy than controls.[905] In preterm infants, sepsis is also associated with adverse neurodevelopmental outcome.[906] Infection remote from the brain may cause cerebral white matter damage leading to poor neurodevelopmental outcome.[907]

The most frequent organisms causing neonatal infection in the UK are shown in Table 10.110.

Gram positives are now the most frequent pathogens because of the increasing importance of coagulase negative staphylococci (CONS). Despite the indolent behavior of CONS and the frequent belief that they are contaminants, they undoubtedly produce virulence factors like toxic exoproteins, hemolysins, DNAse, slime and adhesins.[908]

Newborn babies are colonized with bacteria within a few days of birth and with *Candida* within the first 5 days. Other organisms in the vaginal flora such as *Ureaplasma urealyticum* and *Mycoplasma hominis* have a high vertical transmission rate and are thought to play a role in chronic lung disease and congenital pneumonia.

Many factors predispose newborn infants to infection. Some infections are caused by organisms which colonize the genital tracts of healthy women. Prolonged rupture of membranes (more than 24 h), amnionitis and maternal urinary tract infection are all

Table 10.110 Common organisms causing neonatal infection

	Organism	%
Early onset sepsis (0–4 days)	Group B streptococcus	55
	Escherichia coli	14
	Other streptococci	10
	Haemophilus influenzae	8
Late onset sepsis (5–30 days)	*Staphylococcus epidermidis*	30
	Escherichia coli	21
Late, late-onset sepsis (> 30 days)	*Staphylococcus epidermidis*	66
	Fungi	9

associated with increased risk. The mother's race, socioeconomic status, and her susceptibility to certain pathogens (e.g. rubella, CMV) may increase the risk of transmission of microorganisms through the placenta. Premature and LBW infants have a 3 to 10-fold greater risk of sepsis and/or meningitis than term infants. Male infants may be more susceptible than females but this is controversial. IUGR, excessive manipulation during birth, resuscitation with endotracheal intubation, umbilical catheterization, insertion of long lines, hyperbilirubinemia, iron therapy, total parenteral nutrition (especially lipid infusion), bottle feeding and poor hand washing all predispose to neonatal infection.

Babies may be infected by contact with infected adults or contaminated equipment. Perhaps the only way to prevent nosocomial infection is to reduce these two factors. Good hand washing is the most important measure.[909] Although surveillance of the pattern of infection in individual units is important, routine superficial swabbing of all babies admitted to neonatal units is unwarranted, as is the use of prophylactic antibiotics or antifungal creams for preterm babies. Wide use of broad spectrum antibiotics should be curtailed as it encourages the growth of multiresistant organisms.

HOST DEFENCES

The first defence against infection is the mucosal barrier. This is frequently breached by cutting the umbilical cord, setting up intravenous infusions and breaking the skin for blood tests. Once a bacterium enters the body, it is attacked and lysed by the cellular component of the immune system. During lysis, Gram positives release peptidoglycans whilst Gram negatives release lipopolysaccharide-A (LPS-A) or endotoxin. These substances can initiate a cascade of events that lead to the sepsis syndrome, septic shock, multiple organ failure and death (Fig. 10.69).

Bacterial fragments and endo- or exotoxins stimulate monocytes and neutrophils to produce inflammatory mediators. They also activate the complement, coagulation and fibrinolytic cascades leading to the formation of vasoactive and proinflammatory agents such as prostaglandin E_2, nitric oxide and platelet activating factor (PAF). Macrophages and other cells produce many cytokines, of which tumor necrosis factor-alpha (TNF-alpha), interleukin-1 (IL-1), IL-6, IL-8 and IL-10 have been identified as important in sepsis. Most of these mediators can inhibit or stimulate the release of themselves or other mediators.

Inflammatory mediators, either singly or in concert, lead to chemical and electrical change in the microvascular endothelium and release of adhesion molecules which first trap and then facilitate diapedesis of polymorphonuclear leukocytes (PMNs) into the tissues. This results in the clinical features of sepsis syndrome and septic shock.

Cells in host defense

Phagocytes

Monocytes, macrophages and PMNs phagocytose pathogens, antigens and cell debris and break them down. To combat invading microorganisms adequately, PMNs must arrive at the site of infection within a critical period (2–4 h). Chemotaxis occurs due to factors released by the bacteria or from the complement system (C5a). In the newborn, PMNs exhibit less chemotaxis than in adults. This may be due to markedly decreased membrane deformability of newborn PMNs and to deficiency of C3 and C5. Other factors like Ca^{2+}, zinc and cyclic AMP may also be involved.

Prior to phagocytosing microbes, PMNs or macrophages must attach and opsonize them. This is assisted by factors such as immunoglobulins (mainly IgM) and complement (C3, C5 and C3PA)

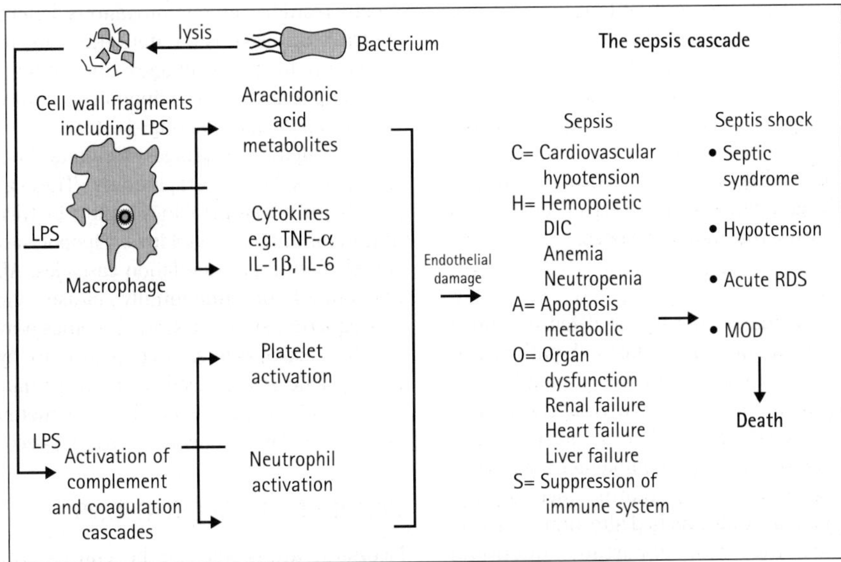

Fig. 10.69 The 'sepsis cascade': DIC, disseminated intravascular coagulation; IL, interleukin; LPS, lipopolysaccharide; MOD, multiple organ dysfunction; RDS, respiratory distress syndrome; TNF, tumor necrosis factor. (Modified from Endotoxin and Septic Shock – the Antibiotic Connection 1994) (Published with permission and courtesy of Dr S K Jackson and Bayer plc UK from their publication)

and is reduced in the newborn. This may be due in part to decreased expression of the complement receptor CR3 (about 60% of adult values) and a relative inability to generate Ca^{2+} ions. For killing bacteria, toxic oxygen products (superoxide, hydroxyl radicals and hydrogen peroxide) are generated. The cationic proteins, lactoferrin and a lysosomal enzyme (myeloperoxidase) interact with hydrogen peroxide to form hypochlorite ions, which are bactericidal. Killing is depressed in newborn phagocytes because of poor production of hydroxyl radicals. All these essential functions are depressed further when an infant is stressed by infection.

Lymphocytes

Lymphocytes control the immune response. B lymphocytes produce antibodies. T lymphocytes have multiple functions including:

- helping B cells to make antibodies;
- recognizing and destroying infected cells;
- activating phagocytes to destroy the pathogens which they have ingested; and
- controlling the level of the immune response.

Other important cells

Eosinophils have a role in killing parasites and controlling inflammation. Basophils, mast cells and platelets release various inflammatory mediators. Platelets release platelet activating factor which is responsible for the increased vascular permeability frequently seen in severe sepsis. Several cell types present antigen to lymphocytes. All these cells interact to generate an effective immune response.

Humoral factors in host defense

Antibodies/immunoglobulins

Antibodies are produced by B lymphocytes and plasma cells. In addition to directly reacting with antigens, antibodies appear to play a significant role in chemotaxis, phagocytosis and the release of mediators.

The production of immunoglobulins by the fetus is limited. Only minute amounts of IgM are produced from 8 weeks' gestation onwards. IgM and IgA do not cross the placenta and thus do not appear in the term infant to any significant extent. IgG, however, is actively transported through the placenta from 30 to 32 weeks' gestation onwards so that the term infant has an IgG level equal to or slightly greater than the maternal levels. Unfortunately, not all subclasses of IgG are transferred equally across the placenta. IgG2 and IgG4 are transferred in very small amounts. Preterm infants born prior to 30 weeks' gestation are deficient in all classes of IgG.

Secretory IgA inhibits the adherence of bacteria to mucosal surfaces and is present in large amounts in colostrum and breast milk. IgE and IgD have no known role in host defense.

Complement

The complement system has a major role in the defense against bacterial, viral and fungal infections. The classical pathway is activated mainly by antigen–antibody complexes or aggregated immunoglobulins. The alternative (properdin) pathway is activated by endotoxins or complex polysaccharides. There is no transfer of complement from mother to fetus. Though complement synthesis begins early in the first trimester, term infants have slightly diminished classical and significantly diminished alternate pathway levels. C3, C4 and C5 are the most important functional components of the system and are approximately 50% of adult levels in term infants. Much lower levels are seen in preterm infants, leading to markedly reduced opsonizing capacity. The receptor for C3b1 on neonatal PMNs is decreased, leading to depressed cell adherence, phagocytosis, mobility and activation of adhesion reactions.

Cytokines

These glycoproteins are secreted by a variety of cells, particularly macrophages, and act as self-regulating inflammatory mediators. Cytokines also modulate immune responses by acting as molecular messengers between cells. The production of interferons in newborn T cells is 10-fold less than in adults. TNF-alpha production is also around 50% of adult levels. These deficiencies, plus a reduced capacity to produce interleukins lead to reduced expression of adhesion molecules on both endothelial and phagocytic cells. Levels of TNF-alpha and IL-6 are increased in sepsis.

Adhesion molecules

These are glycoproteins, which mediate cell to basement membrane and cell to cell attachment. There are several groups. Some are constitutively expressed by cells and others may be induced by cytokines or cellular activation. Adhesion molecules are responsible for trapping rolling leukocytes, leading to their diapedesis into the tissues.

PATHOGENESIS OF NEONATAL SEPSIS

Maternal factors like chorioamnionitis and urinary tract infection increase the risk of infection in the baby by three- to fourfold. Prematurity and LBW increase the risk 20-fold. There is considerable debate about the risk of infection following prolonged rupture of membranes (PROM). Factors which predispose to infection after PROM include chorioamnionitis, premature birth and repeated vaginal examination.[910,911] There is a significant increase in the incidence of early-onset Group B streptococcus (GBS) infection after a brief period of PROM. Though antibiotics are frequently prescribed in cases when meconium aspiration is suspected, there is little evidence to suggest that this is necessary (except in preterm infants where presence of meconium may indicate listeriosis). There is however, evidence that traumatic delivery or presence of perinatal asphyxia and resuscitation at birth are associated with an increased incidence of infection. Neonatal meningitis is infrequent with a reported incidence between 0.25 and 0.5 cases/1000 births[912] and mostly results from hematogenous dissemination.

Once an organism enters the body, it is quickly recognized and taken up by macrophages and other phagocytes and is lysed, releasing toxins such as lipopolysaccharide A. This activates the so-called 'sepsis cascade' (Fig. 10.69).

Activated macrophages stimulate the release of arachidonic acid metabolites like prostaglandins. They also initiate the release of proinflammatory cytokines which in turn switch on the release of anti-inflammatory cytokines. Lipopolysaccharides also activate the complement and coagulation cascades. All the above events working in concert or individually cause endothelial damage. As a consequence, systemic sepsis becomes a multisystem disorder. Effects on the cardiovascular system lead to hypotension. Effects on the hemopoietic system lead to neutropenia, anemia and disseminated intravascular coagulation. There are metabolic effects and apoptosis is accelerated. Left unchecked, sepsis proceeds to septic shock and death.

CLINICAL MANIFESTATIONS

Neonatal infections can be caused by a number of organisms (Table 10.110) and can present in many different ways. It is useful to classify them as early onset sepsis (EOS) and late onset sepsis (LOS). The advantage of such a classification is that it helps in determining the most probable organism, mode of transmission and thus treatment. Whilst most clinicians use this classification there is no consensus as to the precise definition. Some define EOS as occurring between birth and 48 h, others between birth and 72 h and others as after first 24 h and up to 7 days of life. It is however, generally agreed that EOS is caused by organisms acquired from the mother (vertical transmission) whilst LOS is caused by organisms from the environment (nosocomial).

Maternal chorioamnionitis, PROM and urinary tract infection may provide important clues to early diagnosis of sepsis in the newborn. Signs and symptoms of sepsis in the newborn are often non-specific (Table 10.111) and may evolve over time. Sepsis may be fulminant leading to death in several hours from multiorgan failure or may be more protracted. The most frequent indicators are lethargy, poor feeding, abdominal distention, prolonged capillary filling time, glucose intolerance with or without glucosuria and unexplained persistent acidosis. It should be remembered however that many infants with NEC or pneumonia do not have septicemia.

Physical examination may not be very helpful as signs and symptoms of neonatal sepsis are very non-specific but it may help identify congenital infection. Of particular note should be the baby's responsiveness, the color of the umbilicus and the respiratory and heart rates. Unexplained tachycardia may indicate sepsis.[913]

LABORATORY INVESTIGATIONS

There is no single reliable test for neonatal sepsis. Ultimate proof rests on recovering an infecting organism from a normally sterile body fluid, e.g. blood, CSF, urine or aspirate from an infected lesion or tissue. The list of tests which may suggest infection is large (Table 10.112).[914–918]

Microbiological tests

Every unit should monitor its infection patterns as these constantly change. *E. coli* (Table 10.113) continues to be the most important Gram negative organism while GBS and *Staphylococcus epidermidis* are the two most frequent Gram positives. *Staph. aureus* is also frequently seen in NICUs. GBS most frequently presents early with signs and symptoms mimicking RDS. The high incidence of GBS sepsis in the newborn may be due to lack of maternal GBS III serotype antibody. *Staph. epidermidis* is most frequently isolated from more immature babies with indwelling catheters or long lines and usually presents after the first few days of life.

Table 10.111 Most frequent signs and symptoms in neonatal sepsis

Symptoms	Signs
Lethargy	Temperature instability
Poor feeding	Prolonged capillary filling time (hypotension)
'Does not look well'	
Apnea	Widening toe-core temperature difference
Respiratory distress	Hepatomegaly
Pallor	Splenomegaly
Mottling	Full fontanel
Cyanosis	Abnormal neurological reflexes
Abdominal distention	Glucose intolerance
Vomiting/increasing gastric residue	a. Hyper/hypoglycemia b. Glucosuria
Jaundice	Persistent acidosis
Petechiae, purpura, bleeding from prick sites	Painful bones/joints
Irritability	
Seizures	
Sclerema	

Table 10.112 Sensitivity and specificity of various laboratory tests for early diagnosis of neonatal sepsis[914–918]

Test	Sensitivity %	Specificity %	Reference
CRP > 10 mg/L*	75	86	914
Leukopenia < 5000 mm^3*	67	90	914
I/T ratio > 0.2	78	73	914
Thrombocytopenia < 100 000 mm^3	65	57	914
Toxic granulations IL-6 > 32 pg/ml*	44	94	914
TNF-alpha > 12 pg/ml IL-8 > 53 pg/ml*		98.5	915
CRP > 10 mg/L*	93	80	916
Procalcitonin > 2 ng/ml*	92.6	97.5	917
GM-CSF > 120 pg/ml	95	73	918

* Tests we would recommend. CRP, C reactive protein; GM-CSF, granulocyte-macrophage colony-stimulating factor; I/T ratio, immature/total ratio.

Blood culture

Although essential for diagnosis and appropriate management, blood culture results are not immediately available and their yield is low (6–32%). The yield depends on skin disinfection, sample volume and sampling site. Ideally 3 ml of blood is collected for both aerobic and anaerobic cultures. Samples less than 1 ml may produce false negative results.[919] A Gram stain on buffy coat smear may give earlier information, as may sending several blood cultures.

CSF culture

Because meningitis may accompany neonatal sepsis in up to one-third of cases a lumbar puncture should rarely be omitted from the

Table 10.113 Most frequently infecting organisms

From the mother (pre/perinatal)	From the environment (postnatal)
1. *Escherichia coli*	1. *Staphylococcus aureus*
2. Group B streptococci	2. *Staphylococcus epidermidis*
3. *Staphylococcus aureus*	3. *Pseudomonas aeruginosa*
4. *Streptococcus pneumoniae*	4. *Serratia* species
5. *Haemophilus influenzae*	5. Hemolytic streptococci
6. *Neisseria gonorrhoeae*	6. *Citrobacter* species
7. *Proteus* species	7. *Enterobacter* species
8. *Ureaplasma ureolyticum*	8. *Salmonella*
9. *Listeria monocytogenes*	9. Enterococci
10. *Mycoplasma hominis*	10. *Proteus* species
11. *Clostridium perfringens*	11. *Clostridium* species
12. *Mycobacterium tuberculosis*	
13. Other streptococcal species	
14. *Chlamydia trachomatis*	
15. *Treponema pallidum*	
16. *Candida albicans*	
17. TORCH organisms	
18. Malaria	
19. Viruses: vaccinia, Coxsackie, ECHO virus, varicella, herpes, adenovirus, respiratory syncytial, hepatitis, polio, rota and Western equine encephalitis	

TORCH = *Toxoplasma gondii*, rubella, CMV and herpes/hepatitis.

'septic screen'. Some question the wisdom of routine lumbar puncture with septic screens[920] but if CSF examination is omitted the diagnosis of meningitis may be delayed or missed.[921] There is no consensus on this. Interpretation of cerbrospinal fluid tests in the newborn differs from that in older children (Table 10.114).[922,923]

Urine culture

Uncontaminated urine is difficult to obtain. The best method is suprapubic aspiration. Infection should be considered present if there are more than 10 leukocytes/mm^3 in uncentrifuged well-shaken urine or when more than 10^5 CFU/ml of urine are cultured. Urine examination becomes more sensitive when illness occurs after the third day of life and may be positive early in fungal infections. Sensitivity and specificity of routine urine culture is poor.

Superficial and other cultures

Routine cultures from the umbilicus, skin, nose, rectum, etc. demonstrate colonization rather than invasive disease and should not be done. Positive culture from trachea, joints and abscesses may be more relevant. Tips of catheters, long lines and endotracheal tubes should always be sent for culture.

Hematological tests

Neutrophil counts are more valuable than total white cell counts. The early 'band' (metamyelocyte and myelocyte) count and its ratio with total neutrophils (I:T ratio) are more important. An I:T ratio greater than 0.2 suggests infection but still has poor positive predictive value. Other characteristics seen in adults, e.g. toxic granulation, vacuolation, Dohle bodies and decreased leukocyte alkaline phosphatase activity are not reliable in neonatal sepsis. There may be coagulation factor abnormalities but these are not specific. A platelet count less than 150×10^9/L with increased platelet size, carries a poor prognosis. Erythrocyte sedimentation rate (ESR) is a sensitive but non-specific index of infection; it is usually very low in the first days of life and is inversely related to the hematocrit. A micro-ESR (done using a hematocrit tube) greater than 15 mm in the first hour is suggestive of sepsis.

Other tests

The methodological quality of studies assessing diagnostic tests is poor and reported accuracy varies enormously.[924] C-reactive protein (CRP) has been extensively studied as a marker of sepsis and different predictive values have been reported.[925] CRP is unreliable during the first 48 h after birth but sensitivity improves after this period. Other tests for early diagnosis are given in Table 10.112.[915] Procalcitonin may be a useful marker of bacterial infection in all age groups.[926] More recently measures of proinflammatory cytokines have been studied as early diagnostic tests.[927,928] Sensitivities and specificities are given in Table 10.112.

Table 10.114 CSF values in high-risk infants without meningitis

	Term	Preterm
Protein		
Mean (range)	0.9 g/L (0.2–1.7)	1.15 g/L (0.65–1.5)
Cells		
Mean (range)	8.2/mL (0–32)	9.0/mL (0–29)
Glucose		
As percentage of blood glucose level	81%	74%

Adapted from Sarff et al[922] by Davies & Gothefors.[923]

Counter-immune-electrophoresis can be used, particularly for GBS infection, to detect bacterial antigen in blood, urine and CSF. False negative rates are high. Antibody tests are more useful for diagnosing congenital and viral infection. Blood, CSF and urine specimens along with cord blood IgM levels should be taken for virology and serology whenever intrauterine TORCH infections or syphilis are considered. A bone marrow aspirate may help to confirm the diagnosis of tuberculosis. Placental histology is useful in the diagnosis of congenital infections, especially syphilis and listeriosis.

Chest X-ray is often included in a septic screen but X-rays are probably of greater help if there are respiratory symptoms or in the follow-up of infection rather than in making an early diagnosis.

Candida can be diagnosed rapidly by detection of its circulating cell wall or cytoplasmic antigens. *Candida* fragments may be seen in the urine and fungal balls may be detected on renal ultrasound. Polymerase chain reaction (PCR) analysis may improve diagnosis but there is often crossreactivity which reduces specificity.

MANAGEMENT

Prompt, effective therapy is important as babies with infection may deteriorate rapidly. Supportive care, antimicrobial therapy and host defense modulation are all important. As highlighted in Figure 10.69, the cascade of sepsis, cytokine, and inflammatory cell interaction at the endothelial level leads to CHAOS (*c*ardiovascular instability, *h*ematological abnormalities, increased *a*poptosis, *o*rgan dysfunction and *s*uppression of immunity). Along with antibiotics, efforts should be made to correct this chaos.

Septic babies may rapidly lose fluid into the extravascular space (*third spacing*). Meticulous attention to fluid balance and blood pressure is required to maintain tissue perfusion. Increased fluids may be necessary as may blood transfusion to maintain an adequate hematocrit. Inotropic support should be started sooner rather than later. Acid–base balance should be maintained. It is important to maintain tissue oxygenation and nutrition by providing adequate oxygen and calories. Frequently, clinicians stop feeding babies with sepsis. There is no evidence that feeding is harmful in babies with sepsis without intestinal pathology. Calories should be provided parenterally if enteral feeding is not possible. There is little evidence that lipid is harmful during sepsis but it may be prudent to reduce/limit the lipid load during the acute phase of the illness. Single or multiorgan failure in sepsis is not uncommon and this should be treated symptomatically.

ANTIMICROBIAL THERAPY

Because neonatal pharmacokinetics are different, most antimicrobial drugs require modification of dose, dose intervals and duration in the newborn (Table 10.115). For detailed information about individual antimicrobials the reader should refer to a specialized text such as Medicines for Children, Royal College of Paediatrics and Child Health.[929] Slower metabolism and delayed excretion of drugs in the newborn may prolong their half-life, particularly in the very premature. Other factors include the larger volume of extracellular fluid, the amount of serum protein available for binding and drug competition with bilirubin at protein binding sites.

The specific agent(s) chosen to treat infection are determined by knowledge of local pathogens and their susceptibilities, the nature of the illness and the unit policy. Since initial empirical treatment in suspected sepsis cannot cover all possible pathogens, value judgments have to be made. Routine use of cephalosporins as first line therapy is discouraged due to the emergence of resistance. Third

Table 10.115 Antibiotics commonly used in the newborn (in alphabetical order)

	First week of life or preterm			Term infant, more than 7 days old			
Drug	Dosage (mg/kg/day)	Route	Frequency (h)	Dosage (mg/kg/day)	Route	Frequency (h)	*Comment*
1. Amikacin	10–15	i.v./i.m.	8–12	22.5	i.v./i.m.	8	Infuse over 30 min
2. Ampicillin	100	i.v./i.m.	8–12	150–300	i.v./i.m.	6–8	Use higher dose for meningitis
3. Cefotaxime	100–150	i.v./i.m.	12	150–200	i.v.	6–8	Use higher dose for meningitis
4. Ceftazidime	50–100	i.v./i.m.	12	50–100	i.v.	12	
5. Ceftriaxone	50–100	i.v.	12–24	50–100	i.v.	12–24	
6. Chloramphenicol*	25	i.v.	8–12	50	i.v.	6–8	
7. Erythromycin	40–60	i.v.	6	40–60	i.v./p.o.	6–8	Infuse over 60 min
8. Gentamicin*	4–5	i.v./i.m.	18–24	7.5	i.v./i.m.	12–24	Infuse over 30 min
9. Kanamycin*	15	i.v./i.m.	12–18	25	i.v./i.m.	8–12	
10. Methicillin	100	i.v./i.m.	8	200	i.v./i.m.	6–12	
11. Metronidazole	20	i.v.	8	20	i.v.	8	
12. Moxalactam	100	i.v./i.m.	12	100–200	i.v./i.m.	8–12	Do not use as a single drug in neonatal sepsis
13. Netilmicin*	5	i.v./i.m.	12	5	i.v./i.m.	12	
14. Nystatin	2–400 000	p.o. or local	6	2–400 000	p.o. or local	12	
15. Penicillin	30–50	i.v./i.m.	12	40–60	i.v./i.m.	8	
16. Tobramycin*	4.5	i.v./i.m.	12	5–7.5	i.v./i.m.	6–8	Infuse over 30 min
17. Vancomycin*	20–40	i.v.	12	30–60	i.v.	6–8	Infuse over 60 min

* Monitor concentration levels.

generation cephalosporins are particularly useful in the treatment of meningitis due to their excellent penetration into the CSF.

Most antibiotics should be administered intravenously. Intramuscular injections are painful and should be avoided. Absorption after oral therapy in the newborn is erratic and cannot be relied upon. Transdermal application is being studied in preterm infants. Drug levels of some antibiotics must be carefully monitored.

There is no consensus on the duration of therapy.[930] If the baby is well, antibiotic therapy should be stopped as soon as negative culture results are available. However, if the cultures are positive or the clinical picture of sepsis is strong in face of negative cultures, 5–7 days' treatment is recommended. Shorter courses of antibiotics may be equally efficient but less likely to induce resistance.[931] Bacterial meningitis requires 14–21 days of therapy. Osteomyelitis should be treated for at least 4–6 weeks, with the initial 2 weeks of antibiotic therapy being given parenterally.

ADJUNTIVE THERAPIES

Many therapies have significant effects on the inflammatory process but the evidence for their clinical efficacy is lacking.

FFP

There is no evidence that infusion of FFP has any beneficial effect on the humoral immunity of the newborn. Its routine use in sepsis is unjustified.[932]

White cell transfusion

Some have suggested benefit from granulocyte transfusion.[933] Overall experience does not support its use.

Exchange transfusion

Exchange transfusion with adult whole blood has not been shown to be beneficial.

Pentoxifylline

This methylxanthine derivative inhibits TNF-alpha production, preserves microvascular blood flow, inhibits neutrophil deformability and increases the respiratory burst. Two randomized controlled trails of 140 preterm infants show an 86% reduction in mortality.[934,935] Larger studies are required before this therapy can be recommended.

G-CSF and GM-CSF

In several studies involving newborn babies G-CSF and GM-CSF have been shown to increase neutrophils and granulocyte counts and enhance their functional activity. No reduction in mortality from neonatal sepsis has been demonstrated.[936–938]

IVIG

IVIGs have multiple mechanisms of action which promote host defenses. IVIGs bind to cell surface receptors, provide opsonic activity, activate complement, promote antibody dependent cytotoxicity, improve neutrophil chemiluminescence and phagocytosis and can improve neutropenia by enhancing the release of stored neutrophils.[939–941] A Cochrane systematic review[942] suggested that IVIG was safe and was associated with a 50% reduction in relative risk of mortality from suspected neonatal sepsis but confidence intervals were wide (Table 10.116).[941–944] Another systematic review[945] indicated 83% lower odds for mortality and recommended the use of IVIG in the treatment of neonatal sepsis. A Cochrane systematic review on the use of IVIG for sepsis and septic shock in all age groups[946] suggested a beneficial

Table 10.116 IVIG vs placebo or no intervention for suspected neonatal sepsis

Study	Study group Mortality/n	Control group Mortality/n	Relative risk (95% CI)	Weight
Haque[943]	1/30	6/30	0.17 (0.02, 1.30)	42.3%
Christensen et al[941]	0/11	0/11	not estimable	0
Erdem et al[944]	6/20	9/24	0.80 (0.34, 1.86)	57.7%

Mortality from any cause. Table excludes quasi randomized trials. Cochrane review 1999.[942]

effect on all cause mortality (Table 10.117).[946] Amongst all the interventions currently reviewed in the Cochrane Library, IVIG therapy in neonatal sepsis is associated with one of the largest reductions in odds of death.

Table 10.118 lists the non-antimicrobial modalities which have been used to treat sepsis and grades the evidence to support them.

COMPLICATIONS

Complications from neonatal sepsis may result directly from the inflammatory process or from concomitant problems like thrombocytopenia, DIC, fluid and electrolyte or acid–base imbalance. Direct complications like abscess formation, septic embolism and endocarditis are rare but jaundice is frequent and bone destruction following osteomyelitis is not unusual. Secondary *Candida* infection should be actively looked for.

PROGNOSIS

Mortality from neonatal sepsis ranges between 10 and 40% (mean 20%) and has not fallen for many years. Serious morbidity can also result. Dammann & Leviton[907] have shown that infection remote from the brain can cause white matter damage and cerebral palsy in preterm infants. Mortality rate is between 25 and 30% in early onset GBS infection and between 20 and 25% following bacterial meningitis. Long term sequelae like deafness, developmental delay and seizure disorders are seen in 40–80% of survivors following neonatal meningitis.

PREVENTION

The role of hand washing in decreasing nosocomial infections cannot be overemphasized.[947,948] Studies have shown that the quality of the antiseptic agent is more important than the duration of hand cleansing. Preparations containing alcohol gel with emollients are recommended. Infection rates should be monitored following changes in routine practice, hand washing soap or antiseptic. It is important to monitor personnel, the environment, unit overcrowding, visitors and to practice judicious use of antibiotics. Duration of empiric antibiotic therapy should be limited and use of third generation cephalosporins and vancomycin carefully restricted.

Table 10.117 Comparison between polyclonal IVIG or placebo or no intervention in treating sepsis and septic shock

Study	Study group Mortality/n	Control group Mortality/n	Relative risk (CI)	Weight
De Simone et al[16]	7/12	9/12	0.78(0.44, 1.39)	10.8%
Grundmann & Hornung[18]	15/24	19/22	0.72(0.51, 1.03)	23.8%
Dominioni et al[17]	11/29	22/33	0.57(0.34, 0.96)	24.8%
Weisman et al[953]	2/14	5/17	0.49(0.11, 2.13)	5.4%
Chen et al[22]	2/28	1/28	2.00(0.19, 20.82)	1.2%
SUBTOTAL	37/107	56/112	0.68(0.51, 0.89)	66.1%
IgM-enriched IVIG vs placebo or no intervention				
Haque[943]	1/30	6/30	0.17(0.02, 1.30)	7.2%
Wesoly et al[21]	8/18	13/17	0.58(0.33, 1.04)	16.1%
Schedel et al[20]	2/27	9/28	0.23(0.05, 0.97)	10.6%
SUBTOTAL	11/75	28/75	0.38(0.22, 0.67)	33.9%
TOTAL (95%CI)	48/182	84/187	0.58(0.45, 0.74)	100.0%

Mortality from all causes. Cochrane review.[946]

Table 10.118 Non-antimicrobial therapies in neonatal sepsis

Therapy	Recommendation for use	Grade of evidence
1. Anti-inflammatory agents:		
Corticosteroids	No	A
Ibuprofen/indometacin	No	B
Prostaglandin E1	No	B
Pentoxifylline	Yes	A
Naloxone	No	C
2. Drugs modifying coagulation:		
Antithrombin III	No	B
3. Oxygen scavengers:		
N-acetylcysteine	No	C
Selenium	No	C
Nitric oxide	No	C
4. Drugs enhancing host defenses:		
Interferon-gamma	No	C
Immunonutrition	No	C
G-CSF/GM-CSF	No	B
IVIG	Yes	A
5. Other drugs:		
Growth hormone	No	C
Polymyxin B	No	C
Tauroldine	No	C
Fresh frozen plasma	No	B
Granulocyte transfusion	No	A
Exchange transfusion	No	A
Hemofiltration	No	C
Catacholamines	No	C

Evidence has been graded as follows:
Grade A: requires at least one positive randomized clinical trial (RCT) of good quality and consistency as part of the body of literature overall.
Grade B: requires availability of well-conducted clinical trials but no RCT evidence.
Grade C: requires evidence from expert committee reports or opinions and/or clinical experience of respected authorities. Indicates absence of directly applicable studies of good quality.

NEONATAL INFECTIONS

Early onset infection is usually acquired from the mother and frequently causes severe disease in the form of septic shock, pneumonia or meningitis. Risk factors include chorioamnionitis, prolonged rupture of membranes, premature birth and maternal urinary tract infection.

The incidence of early onset infection is around 2–3/1000 live births.[899] The most frequent etiological agents are GBS, *E. coli*, and *Staph. aureus*. *L. monocytogenes* also causes early onset disease but its incidence in the UK is low. The clinical presentation for all organisms is very similar therefore only GBS, which is the most frequent and severe, will be described in detail.

GBS infection

Epidemiology

In Europe and North America, but not in Afro-Asian countries, GBS is the commonest Gram positive bacterium causing neonatal septicemia.[948] The reason for this difference is unclear. The incidence of GBS sepsis in the USA is around 1.4/1000 live births whilst in the UK and Ireland it is 0.6/1000 live births.[949] About 12–23% of female genital tracts are colonized by GBS.[950] Although the vertical transmission rate is approximately 50–70%, neonatal infection occurs in less than 1%. The majority of cases (66%) present during the first 48 h.

Risk factors include exposure to a heavy inoculum of GBS and to a strain with a high potential to invasiveness, preterm delivery, maternal chorioamnionitis, rupture of membranes more than 18 h prior to delivery, intrapartum pyrexia, GBS bacteriuria during the current pregnancy and a previous baby with GBS infection. There is a clear correlation between neonatal disease and low levels of maternal antibody to the capsular polysaccharide of the colonizing strain of GBS at the time of delivery.[951]

Serotype Ia is responsible for 38% of early-onset disease and type III for 31%. Serotype III is responsible for 90% of cases of GBS meningitis and is the main serotype causing late onset GBS infection. Serotype V usually causes infection in adults though it can affect the newborn too.

Clinical features

Almost 90% of infants with early onset disease have signs of infection within the first 4–6 h of birth.[952] The signs are those of sepsis but frequently mimic RDS, birth asphyxia or cyanotic congenital heart disease. If not treated, the baby may rapidly deteriorate and die within hours or days. Hypotension and persistent acidosis carry a poor prognosis.

Late onset GBS disease occurs between 7 and 90 days. It has a wider spectrum of presentation with meningitis being the most common but cellulitis, abscesses, otitis media, arthritis, osteomyelitis, ethmoiditis, fasciitis and conjunctivitis also occur.

Cultures are diagnostic; rapid diagnosis may be made using antigen detection assays but may be unreliable.

Treatment

Penicillin or ampicillin combined with gentamicin is recommended as initial empirical therapy. Once GBS is culture-proven, penicillin remains the drug of choice. Penicillin alone is sufficient. Treatment is usually given for 7–10 days though shorter courses may be adequate. For GBS meningitis it is recommended to use higher doses of penicillin for a minimum of 14 days. Cephalosporins are potential alternatives but the minimal inhibitory concentration (MIC) at which 90% of GBS strains are inhibited by cefotaxime is twice that of penicillin. In a small study, improved results have been obtained using GBS specific (hyperimmune) gamma globulins intravenously. Monoclonal antibody therapy may be another beneficial technique but is currently experimental.

Mortality from GBS infection remains high at 27% in LBW babies with EOS. In term babies it is between 5 and 15%.[953] For LOS the mortality is 3% or less[954] but morbidity data are difficult to access.

Prevention

Since the implementation of intrapartum antibiotic prophylaxis the incidence of early onset GBS disease has fallen by over 65%.[952] Risk based intrapartum prophylaxis appears to be more cost effective than universal intrapartum prophylaxis. Pregnant women with preterm labor (< 35 weeks), prolonged rupture of membranes, known GBS carriage, chorioamnionitis, urinary tract infection or previous history of a baby with GBS infection should be given either penicillin or ampicillin as soon as labor starts and continue to receive the antibiotics until delivery. If the mother receives antibiotics at least 4 h before delivery and the baby is not born prematurely no further intervention is required for the baby. However, if the baby is born prematurely or appears unwell then a full septic screen including a lumbar puncture should be done and the baby started on antibiotics until culture results are available.

Listeriosis

L. monocytogenes is a short Gram positive bacillus which causes EOS and LOS. EOS is predominantly due to serotypes Ia and Ib. It is frequently associated with signs of maternal infection, which can result in abortion, stillbirth or preterm delivery. Affected infants are likely to have pneumonia. LOS is usually due to serotype IVb and is likely to present with meningitis or with signs and symptoms of septicemia. Microabscesses, skin granulomas, hepatosplenomegaly and passage of meconium by preterm infants should arouse the suspicion of *L. monocytogenes* infection.

Diagnosis is based on culture and ELISA (enzyme-linked immunosorbent assay). Ampicillin is very effective and gentamicin acts synergistically. Third generation cephalosporins are ineffective. Mortality from early onset infection is around 15%.

Neonatal meningitis (see also p. 319)

Incidence

A systematic review of 36 studies from developing countries estimated that there are 126 000 cases of neonatal meningitis annually with over 50 000 deaths.[955] In the developed world the incidence is much lower at 0.25–0.5 per 1000 births,[899] though under-reporting is common. It is estimated that meningitis complicates 20% of early onset and 10% of late onset sepsis.[899]

Babies with myelomeningocele, congenital dermal sinus, infected cephalhematoma, osteomyelitis of the skull and otitis media are at increased risk.

Microbiology

Any of the organisms listed in Table 10.113 may cause meningitis. The most frequent organisms are *E. coli* carrying the K1 capsular antigen; GBS type III and *L. monocytogenes* serotype IVb. More recently, *Staph. aureus* and *Staph. epidermidis* have become common organisms causing ventriculitis in infants with ventricular shunt placement for posthemorrhagic hydrocephalus.

Aseptic or viral meningitis is uncommon in the newborn, though Coxsackie B, adeno- and herpes viruses have been implicated.

Pathogenesis and pathology

Generalized inflammation, brain swelling and vasculitis along with cortical thrombophlebitis may cause brain damage and poor outcome. Thrombosis and infarction may occur. Recent evidence suggests that increased cytokine and Th2 cell trafficking into the developing white matter during the inflammatory process may be responsible for the brain white matter injury.[956] At autopsy, subarachnoid inflammatory exudate is more prominent at the base of the brain than over the cortex. Damage to the choroid plexus and ventriculitis may lead to encephalopathy and blockage of the foramena and aqueduct resulting in hydrocephalus. Hemorrhagic cerebral necrosis is most characteristic of *Proteus* infection.

Clinical manifestations

Any of the clinical signs and symptoms listed in Table 10.111 may be present in meningitis. Temperature instability, lethargy, feed intolerance, recurrent apnea and bradycardia, sugar intolerance and unexplained hyponatremia are more frequent in VLBW babies. Bulging or full fontanel and neck stiffness are late manifestations and occur in only 28 and 15% of cases, respectively.[957]

Diagnosis

Diagnosis requires careful evaluation of the CSF with isolation of the infecting organism. A Gram stain of CSF must always be made. The cell count and the protein content are raised while the glucose may be reduced. Specific reference ranges for the newborn should be used (Table 10.114). Countercurrent immunoelectrophoresis or latex agglutination tests may permit an etiological diagnosis within minutes but are not reliable. Blood culture may grow the organism, though as many as 15% of babies with positive CSF culture have negative blood culture.

Any baby suspected of having meningitis should have a cranial ultrasound. This would detect ventriculitis and ventriculomegaly. Further neuroimaging like CT or MRI scans should be done if there are concerns on the ultrasound or complications are suspected. EEG is useful to detect seizures.

Treatment

Treatment consists of antibiotic therapy and supportive care. It is important to maintain blood pressure because this affects cerebral perfusion. Fluctuations in the latter may predispose to ischemic injury or hemorrhage. Convulsions should be controlled with phenobarbital. Fluid restriction may be necessary if there is hyponatremia due to inappropriate secretion of antidiuretic hormone.

Antibiotic therapy should achieve adequate drug levels to sterilize the CSF. Until a definitive diagnosis has been made, a combination of a third generation cephalosporin or ampicillin and an aminoglycoside (gentamicin) should be started intravenously immediately after cultures have been drawn. Third generation cephalosporins are recommended because of the good CSF penetration and safety profile. This regimen does not effectively treat *Listeria* infection. In the UK most clinicians use a combination of cefotaxime and ampicillin/penicillin as empirical therapy.[930] Controlled trials have failed to show any benefit of intraventricular or intrathecal therapy over systemic therapy.[958] Once a specific pathogen has been isolated and its susceptibilities identified, the best drug or combination of drugs should be employed. Benzyl penicillin is the drug of choice for GBS infection. A combination of ampicillin and gentamicin, which have synergistic action, is preferred in infections with *Listeria*, *Proteus mirabilis* and enterococci. A combination of an aminoglycoside with either a ureidopencillin (azlocillin or piperacillin) or a cephalosporin such as ceftazidime should be chosen for meningitis due to *Ps. aeruginosa* or *Serratia marcescens*. Cefotaxime is preferred to other third generation cephalosporins because it is not excreted in the bile and there is more clinical experience with this drug in the newborn. Until recently chloramphenicol was the antibiotic of choice in neonatal meningitis due to its superior penetration into CSF. Despite its well-known toxicity, if serum concentrations are kept between 15 and 25 mg/L, toxicity from this drug is extremely rare. However, with the advent of third generation cephalosporins, chloramphenicol is now not recommended for use in neonatal meningitis.

Whichever drugs are used, careful monitoring of levels in both the serum and perhaps the CSF is essential for effective treatment. Antimicrobial therapy should be continued for a minimum of 14 days for Gram positive organisms and 21 days for Gram negative organisms.[959] The indications for repeat lumbar puncture are controversial. It is probably unnecessary during or after treatment unless the baby does not appear to be responding. With appropriate antibiotic therapy the CSF becomes sterile very quickly and CSF chemistry also normalizes but pleocytosis may continue for some weeks making later CSF results difficult to interpret.

Complications

Hydrocephalus develops during the second week in some cases. Ventricular index should be regularly monitored using ultrasound and head circumference measurements should be taken. In some cases the hydrocephalus arrests but in cases where it is progressive a neurosurgical opinion should be sought.

Meningitis is the commonest cause of acquired sensorineural deafness in children. All infants should have audiological tests and follow-up after meningitis.

Cerebral abscess may occur in babies who respond poorly to antibiotics or who have *Citrobacter* or *Proteus* infection.

Prognosis

Children who develop neonatal meningitis are at significantly greater risk of disability across a large range of health, developmental and behavioral categories, particularly in learning and neuromotor domains. Preterm babies have a much higher frequency of disability, especially neuromotor disabilities and seizure disorders. Severe disability is also significantly more common in infants with meningitis associated with GBS.[960]

Mortality ranges between 20 and 40% depending on gestational age, causative organism and the duration between the onset of the disease and initiation of therapy. Moderate disability occurs in about 30% whilst conditions like blindness, deafness, epilepsy and spastic cerebral palsy occur in another 30%. Only 40% of survivors escape sequelae.

Mycoplasma and *Ureaplasma* are rare causes of meningitis as part of septicemia. The antibiotics of choice are azithromycin or erythromycin.

NOSOCOMIAL INFECTIONS

Stoll and colleagues[902,903] demonstrated that nosocomial infection in VLBW babies is common and carries significant mortality and morbidity. They reported rates between 2 and 25%. Variation in reported rates occurs because of different definitions of nosocomial infection, variable neonatal intensive care facilities and different patient mixes.

The Gram positive organisms most likely to cause nosocomial infections are coagulase negative *Staph. epidermidis*, *Staph. aureus* and *Enterococcus*. The most frequent Gram negative agents are *E. coli*, *Enterobacter* and *Pseudomonas* species.

Risk of nosocomial infections is inversely proportional to birth weight. Intubation, indwelling catheters, parenteral nutrition (in particular lipid infusion) and antibiotic induced overgrowth of resistant flora increase the risk. Gaynes et al[961] showed that 88% of infections in NICUs were associated with umbilical or central catheters.

Late onset sepsis

Coagulase negative Staphylococcus sepsis

Most infants are colonized with *Staphylococcus* by the fifth day of life. Although they may sometimes be culture contaminants there is clear evidence that CONS are also pathogens. Their virulence factors include toxic exoproteins, hemolysins, DNAse, slime and adhesins. Mittendrof et al[962] have shown that CONS infection of the chorioamnion may be associated with subsequent development of cerebral palsy. There are numerous species of CONS but the majority (80%) of infections are due to *Staph. epidermidis*. Slime producing strains are the most frequent because this viscous extracellular polysaccharide helps the organism adhere to catheters etc., and also inhibits phagocytosis and neutrophil chemotaxis.

Clinical features. Presentation is usually subtle rather than acute. Episodes of apnea or bradycardia, low-grade acidosis, pyrexia and increased oxygen requirements may be observed. Acute sepsis syndrome and NEC have also been recorded.[963] The usual site of infection is a catheter or other intravascular device. The main risk factors for catheter related sepsis are catheter hub colonization, exit site colonization, duration of total parenteral nutrition, ELBW (< 1000 g) at the time of catheter insertion and postnatal age (> 1 week) at the time of insertion.[964] Rate of sepsis is related to duration of catheter insertion[965] (Table 10.119). High rates of CONS infection have been reported with ventriculoperitoneal/atrial shunts.

Table 10.119 Incidence of catheter related coagulase negative staphylococcal infection by duration of catheter insertion (Gray et al[965])

Duration of insertion	Incidence (%)
0–7 days	5
8–14 days	15
15–21 days	41
22 days or more	58

Interpretation of positive blood culture results is difficult because of the possibility that they may represent contaminants. Multiple site cultures do not help nor do cultures taken from the lines themselves. CONS lead to leukocytosis, increase in platelet numbers and size and increased CRP. A combination of clinical signs, blood count and CRP may give the best indication of CONS infection.

Treatment. Intravascular catheters should be removed if at all possible. Low dose vancomycin therapy through the line is not recommended. Initial antibiotic therapy for LOS should provide cover for Gram negative bacilli and CONS. For Gram negative organisms either an aminoglycoside or a third generation cephalosporin should be chosen. Following the report by Stoll et al[903] it has become common practice to include vancomycin in empiric therapy. Liberal use of vancomycin carries the risk of selection of vancomycin resistant enterococci. Alternative choices are flucloxacillin or teicoplanin but resistance to these agents is encountered. Careful monitoring of serum vancomycin concentration is advised. There is no consensus about duration of antibiotic therapy. Antibiotics should be stopped if the baby is clinically well, has a normal white cell count and a CRP level of < 10 mg/dl.

Staphylococcus aureus

Staph. aureus infections were common in the 1950s and 1960s but the prevalence fell with improved hygiene and hand washing. Infections are becoming more common again. Systemic infections remain uncommon (less than 1%) and usually take the form of osteomyelitis, and scalded skin syndrome (Ritter's disease) due to phage group II (3A, 3C, 55, 71). Staphylococcal pneumonia is characterized by the formation of pneumatoceles, pyopneumothoraces, or empyema. Superficial infections include conjunctivitis and paronychia. Typical skin lesions are crops of pustules with golden centers surrounded by erythema, which may be seen on any part of the body.

It is important to recognize osteitis due to *Staph. aureus*. The head of the femur is often involved but any bone may be affected. The infant is usually pyrexial, lethargic and may have a pseudoparalysis of the involved limb. There is usually localized swelling with or without discoloration of the overlying skin.

Treatment. For umbilical cord infection, cleaning with alcohol or with chlorhexidine solution may be enough. Systemic infection is best treated with antistaphylococcal penicillins like flucloxacillin.

Gram negative bacilli

Gram negative bacilli account for 30% of LOS in developed countries.[966] The incidence is much higher in developing countries.[901] The commonest organisms are *E. coli, P. aeruginosa, Klebsiella pneumoniae* and *Enterobacter cloacae*. These cause fulminating sepsis due to endotoxin release (LPS-A). Mortality rates between 50 and 70% have been reported.[967,968] However, with addition of IVIG therapy mortality may be lower.[943] For treatment an aminoglycoside or a third generation cephalosporin should be used. IVIG may be beneficial.

Pneumonia (p. 257)

At autopsy, 35% of newborn infants are found to have significant pneumonia.[898] Pneumonia may be acquired in utero (congenital), during birth or nosocomially. Congenital pneumonia may be caused by TORCH group organisms, or be secondary to chorioamnionitis. GBS, *E. coli, Treponema pallidum, M. hominis* and *L. monocytogenes* may all cause congenital pneumonia. Most infants swallow material during birth but few develop pneumonia. It usually presents within the first 24–48 h of life. The most common organisms are *Staph. aureus*, GBS, *E. coli, H. influenzae, Klebsiella* spp. and *Strep. pneumoniae*. The role of *C. trachomatis* and *U. urealyticum* is controversial but these should be looked for in babies who do not improve on conventional therapy.[969]

Nosocomial pneumonia

Common organisms involved are *Staph. aureus, Staph. epidermidis*, and rarely *Ps. aeruginosa*. In babies who have chronic lung disease or are on long term ventilation the incidence of pneumonia may be as high as 35%[970] and additional infecting organisms include fungi, mycoplasma, chlamydia and viruses, particularly RSV during the winter season.

Clinical manifestations

Clinical features include tachypnea, tachycardia, cyanosis and expiratory grunt. Distinction from RDS may be difficult. Symptoms and signs are non-specific. Babies may show signs of cerebral irritation or be hypotonic and lethargic. They do not feed well and may go into heart failure. *C. trachomatis* infection may produce a staccato cough.

Diagnosis

This is based on history, blood culture, and Gram stain and culture of the tracheal aspirate. Early chest radiographs may be unhelpful but they may be confirmatory if taken 48–72 h after onset of symptoms. Serology may also be helpful.

Treatment

Initial therapy should be with ampicillin/penicillin and an aminoglycoside. Flucloxacillin should be used for *Staph. aureus* but vancomycin is preferred for *Staph. epidermidis* and methicillin-resistant *Staphylococcus*. Azithromycin or erythromycin is the drug of choice for *Ureaplasma* and *Mycoplasma* infection. There is no consensus regarding duration of therapy but shorter courses may be as effective as prolonged courses.[931] Supportive therapy with oxygen, intravenous fluids, suction and physiotherapy is also required. Drainage of pleural effusion or empyema may be necessary. Overall prognosis is good.

Gastroenteritis

This is uncommon in the newborn but may occur in epidemics. Rota-, ECHO- and adenovirus infections are the commonest cause. *E. coli, Salmonella, Shigella, Campylobacter* and *Yersinia* are the commonest bacterial agents. There may be vomiting, diarrhea, feed intolerance, dehydration and pyrexia. The mainstay of management is correction of dehydration. Antibiotics should be given if the infection is considered to be invasive.

Necrotizing enterocolitis (NEC) (see also p. 285)

NEC is a major contributor to morbidity and mortality, particularly in small preterm infants. The precise role played by bacteria remains uncertain but NEC has occurred in endemic and epidemic forms. Predisposing factors include LBW, hypoxia, persistent ductus arteriosus, umbilical catheterization, rapid advancement of feeding (particularly with hyperosmolar milk), Hirschsprung's disease, hyperviscosity syndromes and infective diarrhea. Antenatal Doppler studies showing absent/reversed end-diastolic flow in the umbilical artery may also indicate increased risk. In the majority of cases no organism is isolated. Organisms reported in the literature include *E. coli*, *K. pneumoniae*, *Clostridium butyricum*, *Clostridium perfringens*, *Clostridium difficile*, *Salmonella*, *P. mirabilis* and *Ps. aeruginosa*. Viruses such as adeno type 19, Coxsackie, corona and enterovirus have also been implicated.

Clinical manifestations

NEC commonly presents in the first 10 days of life in babies weighing less than 1500 g. There is no sex predisposition. Signs include abdominal distention, increasing gastric residue (may become bile stained), absent bowel sounds, vomiting and passage of blood in the stools. X-ray of the abdomen may show bowel wall edema in the early stages followed by pneumatosis intestinalis, perforation and in severe cases gas in the portal tract.

Treatment

Medical management consists of withdrawal of enteral feeds, gastric suction and administration of intravenous fluids and parenteral nutrition. Empirically a combination of ampicillin, an aminoglycoside (gentamicin) and metronidazole are given for 7–10 days. Some question the routine use of metronidazole in NEC and do not use it routinely. The use of oral aminoglycosides is not recommended. Indications for surgery are debatable and are discussed on page 285. Mortality varies from 0 to 25% and morbidity from 12 to 37%.

Osteomyelitis and septic arthritis

During the first year of life, capillaries perforate the epiphyseal plate providing communication between the joint space and the metaphysis. Thus, septic arthritis and osteomyelitis may often occur together. The source of infection is usually hematogenous but direct trauma during arterial or venous puncture has also been implicated. The commonest organism is *Staph. aureus*. GBS, *Klebsiella* and *E. coli* are also prominent. In underdeveloped countries, *Salmonella osteitis* is frequent. *Staph. epidermidis* and *Candida albicans* are emerging as important etiological agents in extremely preterm infants.

Clinical manifestations

Most cases present insidiously. There may be non-specific symptoms such as poor feeding, lethargy, decreased activity and low-grade fever. Mild unexplained acidosis may be a pointer. Local signs include swelling over the affected area or joint, pseudoparalysis of the limb, and irritability on handling the affected body part.

Diagnosis

Diagnosis is based on radiological confirmation although changes are not seen for 10–14 days. Technetium-99m scan is highly sensitive. Conventional radiographs may miss early lesions. MRI imaging can be helpful. Whole body scanning is advisable as there may be more than one focus of infection. Repeated cultures should be taken.

Treatment

Flucloxacillin and a third generation cephalosporin (cefotaxime) should be started until culture and sensitivity results are available. Therapy should be continued for at least 6 weeks (at least 3 weeks intravenously). There is evidence that surgical aspiration and instillation of antibiotic at the site of the lesion is superior to parenteral therapy alone. Orthopedic consultation should always be sought. Mortality is low; however, reports have indicated a 25% morbidity particularly if hip or knee joints are involved.

Urinary tract infection (see also p. 327)

Urinary tract infection occurs in 3% of preterm and 1% of term infants. It is more common in males and in infants with kidney or renal tract abnormalities, e.g. obstructive uropathy. It is also seen more frequently in babies whose renal parenchyma may have been damaged, e.g. from asphyxia or dehydration.

The most frequent infecting organism is *E. coli* but *Klebsiella* spp. account for 7–11% of infections. In very preterm LBW babies who have received long courses of antibiotics, *C. albicans* is also an important etiological agent.

Clinical manifestations and diagnosis

Clinical signs and symptoms include poor weight gain, jaundice, hepatomegaly, and palpable kidneys. There may be generalized septicemia. Diagnosis is confirmed by urine culture (greater than 100 000 CFU/ml) and >10 white cells/ml in freshly voided or aspirated urine.

Further investigation with ultrasound, micturating cystourethrogram (MCUG) and isotope scanning (DMSA) is advisable as in up to 45% of cases abnormalities have been detected.

Treatment

Empirical therapy with ampicillin and gentamicin is usually adequate but antibiotics must be changed according to urine culture reports. There is a recurrence rate of up to 10%, so follow-up is essential. With current therapy, prognosis is excellent where there has been no renal parenchymal damage and there are no congenital abnormalities. If there is evidence of reflux uropathy then antibiotic prophylaxis with trimethoprin should be initiated.

Conjunctivitis (see p. 331)

The incidence of conjunctivitis varies between 7 and 20%. The higher figure comes mainly from premature infants nursed on NICUs.

Clinical manifestations

In the UK the most common pathogens are *Staph. aureus*, *Strep. pneumoniae*, and *Strep. viridans*. Conjunctivitis usually presents within the first week. *Chlamydia* infections usually, but not always present later. *N. gonorrhoeae* infection is now rare in the UK but if untreated it may lead to corneal ulceration and perforation, iridocyclitis, anterior synechiae and panophthalmitis. *Chlamydia* infection produces a similar clinical picture but only involves the tarsal aspect of the conjunctiva, sparing the cornea.

Diagnosis

This is based on the clinical history, timing, and site of the lesion and on cultures of the discharge. *Chlamydia* infection may be diagnosed by obtaining scrapings from the tarsal conjunctiva and staining with Giemsa stain for intracytoplasmic inclusions.

Treatment

For gonococcus the eye should be cleaned with frequent eye washes of normal saline or water (every 15–30 min at first) followed by instillation of penicillin drops. Penicillin should also be given intravenously for a few days.

For chlamydial infection, 0.5% erythromycin ophthalmic ointment is used with systemic erythromycin therapy for 7–14 days. Chloramphenicol and sulfacetamide ophthalmic preparations may be useful for staphylococcal colonization. The instillation of 1% silver nitrate drops to newborns led to the decline in gonococcal conjunctivitis, but this treatment has generally been abandoned as it leads to significant chemical conjunctivitis.

Otitis media

Examination of the eardrum, particularly in preterm infants, should be a mandatory part of the routine examination of infants with suspected sepsis. The incidence of otitis media in the newborn is 0.6–2.4%. A shorter, widely patent and horizontally placed eustachian tube predisposes to infection. Other factors include chorioamnionitis, asphyxia, prematurity, ventilatory support, cleft palate and Down syndrome. *Strep. pneumoniae* and *H. influenzae* are the commonest organisms involved, although *Staph. epidermidis*, *Branhamella catarrhalis* and *M. tuberculosis* have also been recorded. Presentation is non-specific. Otoscopic examination reveals a dull tympanic membrane which is bulging and has reduced or absent mobility on pneumatic otoscopy. Treatment includes tympanocentesis and appropriate antibiotics. Outcome is usually favorable but the recurrence rate is high and up to 33% develop chronic otitis media.

Umbilical infection

Staph. aureus and *E. coli* are the most frequent organisms causing infection of the umbilicus. The incidence is between 0.5 and 2%. Periumbilical erythema is usually the only clinical feature though severe omphalitis has been reported from developing countries. Simple cleaning with an antiseptic like chlorhexidine is sufficient but for more significant infection broad spectrum systemic antibiotics should be given.

SPECIFIC INFECTIONS

The possible clinical involvement and the infecting organisms are shown in Table 10.120.[971] Only a few specific infections will be discussed in detail.

Table 10.120 Lesions that may be caused by prenatally acquired non-viral infections

Possible clinical involvement	Infecting organisms
Central nervous system	
Meningitis, meningoencephalitis (manifestations may include microcephaly, hydrocephaly, and hydranencephaly, abnormal CNS signs, convulsions, and cerebral calcification)	*Candida albicans, Cryptococcus neoformans, Escherichia coli,* Group B streptococcus, *Listeria monocytogenes, Staphylococcus aureus, Streptococcus pneumoniae, Toxoplasma gondii, Treponema pallidum*
Special sensory organs	
Eye	
Cataracts	*Cryptococcus neoformans, Toxoplasma gondii, Treponema pallidum*
Choroidoretinitis*	*Cryptococcus neoformans, Toxoplasma gondii, Treponema pallidum*
Acute iritis, chronic iridocyclitis, vitritis, glaucoma	*Treponema pallidum*
Optic atrophy	*Toxoplasma gondii, Treponema pallidum*
Uveitis	*Toxoplasma gondii*
Endophthalmitis	*Cryptococcus neoformans*
Conjunctivitis	*Chlamydia trachomatis, Neisseria gonorrhoeae,* and other bacteria
Ear	
Eighth nerve damage	*Toxoplasma gondii, Treponema pallidum*
Otitis media	*Mycobacterium tuberculosis* and other bacteria
Cardiovascular system	
Pericarditis	*Mycoplasma hominis* and other bacteria
Myocarditis	*Toxoplasma gondii, Trypanosoma cruzi*
Respiratory system	
Pneumonia/pneumonitis	*Candida albicans, Chlamydia trachomatis, Cryptococcus neoformans, Mycobacterium tuberculosis, Toxoplasma gondii, Treponema pallidum,* and many other bacteria
Pleural effusion	*Coccidioides immitis,* Group B streptococcus
Skeletal system	
Periostitis and/or defective mineralization and growth disturbances	*Toxoplasma gondii, Treponema pallidum*
Septic arthritis	*Viridans* streptococci and other bacteria
Gastrointestinal system	
Hepatosplenomegaly with or without jaundice	*Cryptococcus neoformans,* Group B streptococcus, *Escherichia coli, Mycobacterium tuberculosis, Plasmodium, Toxoplasma gondii, Treponema pallidum*
Enteritis	Enteropathogenic *Escherichia coli, Listeria monocytogenes, Salmonella, Shigella*
Genitourinary system	
Nephritis, nephrotic syndrome	*Plasmodium, Toxoplasma gondii, Treponema pallidum*
Miliary abscesses	*Coccidioides immitis, Cryptococcus neoformans, Listeria monocytogenes, Neisseria gonorrhoeae*
Vulvovaginitis	*Trichomonas vaginalis*
Balanitis	*Chlamydia trachomatis*
Hematopoietic system	
Anemia, sometimes hemolytic, with jaundice	*Toxoplasma gondii, Treponema pallidum*
Petechiae or purpura, with or without disseminated intravascular coagulation. (Some hemorrhagic skin nodules are erythropoietic in nature)	*Toxoplasma gondii, Treponema pallidum,* and other bacteria
Lymphatic system	
Enlarged lymph glands	*Coccidioides immitis, Mycobacterium tuberculosis, Toxoplasma gondii, Treponema pallidum*
Skin and mucous membranes	
Vesicular lesions, single, grouped or scattered, sometimes unilateral	*Treponema pallidum*
Macular or maculopapular lesions	*Listeria monocytogenes, Toxoplasma gondii, Treponema pallidum,* and other bacteria
Maculopapular, vesicular, or scaling lesions	*Candida albicans*
Pustules, abscesses	*Staphylococcus aureus*
Erythema gangrenosum	*Pseudomonas aeruginosa*
Intrauterine growth retardation	*Plasmodium, Treponema pallidum*

Adapted from Davies et al[971]
Infecting organisms are listed alphabetically and not in order of likelihood.
* The choroidoretinitis caused by *Toxoplasma gondii* and *Treponema pallidum* has been confused with the Aicardi syndrome, in which the lesions are always bilateral, rarely peripheral, and lack pigments, in contrast to that due to these two organisms.

Syphilis

Congenital syphilis is now uncommon in the developed world with only eight confirmed cases in the UK between 1993 and 1995.[972] *T. pallidum* is the etiological agent. Transplacental infection rarely occurs before 18 weeks' gestation as the Langhans' layer of the chorion prevents the passage of the *Treponema*. The fetus is not immunocompetent to mount a response to infection until 20–25 weeks' gestation. Treatment of the mother before the 18th week of gestation will almost always completely protect the fetus. The chances of the fetus remaining uninfected are negligible if the mother is not treated. If the mother has early or latent syphilis the fetus has a 20–70% chance of being infected.

Clinical manifestations

Hematogenous spread in prenatal life determines which fetal organs and tissues are involved. Abortion, stillbirth and hydrops occur in 40% of pregnancies. There may be severe anemia, hepatosplenomegaly or pneumonia soon after birth. 1–3 weeks later the stigmata of congenital syphilis become evident, e.g. nasal obstruction with serosanguineous discharge, copper-colored maculopapular rash, perianal condylomata, rhagades (fissures at mucocutaneous junctions), loss of hair, exfoliation of the nails, iritis and choroiditis. Poor feeding and fever may be accompanied by jaundice, generalized lymphadenopathy and signs of pancreatitis or hepatitis. Bone lesions are seen in nearly all infants beyond the neonatal period.

Diagnosis

This is based on either the visualization of *T. pallidum* by dark ground microscopy or complement fixation (Wasserman) or flocculation tests (Kahn, VDRL). The *T. pallidum* immobilization (TPI) test and direct fluorescent *Treponema* antibody absorption IgM test [fluorescent treponemal antibody absorption (FTAABS), IgM] are more specific. These are positive in the blood and CSF. PCR is highly sensitive.

Treatment

Symptomatic or CNS syphilis should be treated with aqueous crystalline penicillin G 50–100 000 units/kg/day i.m. in two divided doses for at least 10 days. For asymptomatic syphilis, benzathine penicillin G 50–100 000 units/kg given as a single intramuscular injection should be given. If maternal treatment was given during the last 4 weeks of pregnancy or the treatment was not with penicillin or treatment was inadequate or status is unknown, the infant should be treated. Penicillin-allergic patients can be given cephalosporins.

Tetanus

This is very unusual in developed countries but in some parts of the world neonatal tetanus is responsible for 30–40% of all neonatal deaths. *Clostridium tetani* is a Gram positive anaerobic spore-forming bacillus which produces a toxin, tetanospasmin, that causes muscle spasms and convulsions. The toxin, once fixed to the nervous tissue, cannot be neutralized by antitoxins. Mothers who are immunized protect the fetus by actively transporting antitoxins across the placenta.

Clinical manifestations

The incubation period is between 3 days and 3 weeks. Most neonatal cases occur between 3 and 10 days after birth. The umbilicus is the main route of entry. The infant usually presents with difficulty in sucking (due to upper lip spasm), excessive irritability and trismus. This is followed very soon by generalized muscle spasms, convulsions, rigidity and fever. There may also be cardiorespiratory difficulties.

Diagnosis

This is usually easy but meningitis, metabolic disorders and ingestion of phenothiazines must be considered in countries where tetanus is unusual.

Treatment

This is based on the provision of an adequate airway and ventilation, neutralization and elimination of toxins, prevention of spasms and convulsions and maintaining hydration and nutrition. Diazepam, either as a bolus (0.1–2 mg) or as a continuous infusion (10–140 mg/kg/day) is useful in reducing muscular spasm. Paraldehyde or barbiturates may also be used. Human tetanus immune globulin (500–3000 IU) should be given if possible as a single dose but equine tetanus antitoxin may also be used (50 000–80 000 IU). Parenteral penicillin 100 000–150 000 IU should be given for at least 10 days. Fluid, electrolytes and nutrition should be maintained. Where facilities are available, mechanical ventilation and neuromuscular blockade have improved the outcome, which remains gloomy in developing countries.

Tuberculosis

It is rare to see tuberculosis during the first month of life. The mother may transmit the disease through the placenta or the baby may acquire it by aspiration of infected amniotic fluid or vaginal secretions. Symptoms include poor weight gain, lethargy, jaundice, lymphadenopathy and hepatosplenomegaly. The diagnosis may be suspected from seeing a primary focus or hilar lymphadenopathy on a chest X-ray, or on the basis of maternal history. Placental histology and culture of gastric washings or bone marrow aspiration from the infant may help.

If the mother does not have an active lesion, the infant should be given isoniazid (INH 10 mg/kg/day) for 4–6 weeks after which a tuberculin test should be done. If this is negative bacille Calmette–Guérin (BCG) should be given. If the mother has active lesions, the infant should be separated from the mother until a BCG-induced tuberculin (Mantoux) response has been demonstrated. In situations where it is difficult to separate the infant from the mother, the infant should be given isoniazid-resistant BCG and started on isoniazid. The infant can then remain with the mother provided that she is receiving adequate antituberculous therapy.

Current recommendations in the UK are that newborn babies, even if they are contacts, need to be tested for tuberculin sensitivity before being given BCG except in ethnic groups who have a high risk of this disease.

FUNGAL INFECTIONS

Up to 33% of pregnant women have vaginal colonization with *Candida* species. Systemic fungal infection occurs in 3–4% of VLBW infants. Around 27% of VLBW infants are colonized soon after birth and invasive infection develops in around 8% of colonized infants.[973] Risk factors for fungal infection include prematurity (due to maturity dependent immunocompromised state), fungal colonization, antibiotic therapy, intravenous alimentation with fat emulsions and use of postnatal steroids. The commonest fungal pathogens are *C. albicans, Candida parapsillosis, Aspergillus* and *Malassezia furfur*.

Infection in the newborn may be congenital or late onset and may be local or disseminated. Congenital candidal infections are acquired in the birth canal and usually present within the first 24 h of life as an intense desquamating rash. Pustules and satellite lesions are common, and may be confused with scalded skin syndrome (staphylococcal infection). In late onset infection skin lesions appear between the 7th and 10th day as a rash of small papules which coalesces to form cheesy white patches in the mouth, diaper (nappy) area, groin or axillae. Occasionally oral thrush may extend to cause esophagitis.

VLBW babies and those who require prolonged intensive care or have central lines in situ frequently develop line sepsis due to *Candida*. Clinical signs and symptoms are indistinguishable from bacterial sepsis. Affected infants often develop hyperglycemia and thrombocytopenia. There is a high incidence of renal (57%) and central nervous system (59%) involvement in systemic candidiasis.[974,975] There may be endophthalmitis and the eyes should be examined for white fluffy retinal deposits which can progress to involve the vitreous humor, resulting in blindness. Occasionally *Candida* may cause skin abscesses, osteomyelitis and pneumonia.

Diagnosis

The diagnosis of local disease can be confirmed by microscopy and culture of scrapings from the margins of lesions. Systemic candidiasis is diagnosed by growing fungi from blood, CSF or urine, but cultures may be negative even when multisystem disease is seen at autopsy. Urine microscopy may show yeasts or hyphae. Candida antigen or antibody detection tests are useful but not always available. Ultrasound of the kidneys may reveal fungal balls.

Treatment

Local lesions may be treated by nystatin, 100 000 IU four times a day for 5 days, or with miconazole gel (orally) or cream (for the perineum and buttocks). Nystatin with corticosteroid ointment may be used in severe cases of candida dermatitis.

Systemic candidiasis is best treated by removing all central lines and indwelling catheters and starting the infant on intravenous antifungal agents. Amphotericin B has a long half-life and good penetration into the CSF. Starting dose is between 0.5 mg/kg and 1 mg/kg per day given as an infusion over 4–6 h. The infusion syringe and tubing should be protected from light. Principal adverse effects are nephrotoxicity, marrow suppression and hepatotoxicity. Liposomal amphotericin B, where the drug is encapsulated in unilamellar liposomes, is less toxic. The dose of liposomal amphotericin B is 1 mg/kg/day to a maximum of 3–5 mg/kg/day. Treatment should be given for 4–6 weeks. 5-Flucytosine (5-FC) is synergistic with amphotericin and some recommend combined treatment whilst others only add 5-FC if cultures remain positive despite adequate treatment with amphotericin B. There is 4% primary resistance to these drugs and secondary resistance is also emerging. Fluconazole is a broad spectrum antifungal agent that is well absorbed enterally and has shown promising results. Side-effects include hepatotoxicity, skin rashes and thrombocytopenia.

A mortality of 54% and morbidity of 25% have been reported following systemic candida infection in VLBW infants.

Other fungi

Aspergillus and *Tricophyton* species may cause cutaneous disease. *M. furfur* is responsible for intralipid induced fungemia, since it is a lipophilic fungus that often colonizes skin. Treatment consists of removal of lines, discontinuing lipid infusion and instituting antifungal therapy, with any of the above antifungal drugs.

VIRAL INFECTIONS

Other than CMV, serious viral infections in the fetus and newborn are uncommon. Virus infections may cause abortion, stillbirth, congenital malformations, acute neonatal disease, or manifest only after a prolonged period. Most virus infections of the neonate are transmitted from the mother.

Rubella

Rubella vaccination has made congenital rubella syndrome an uncommon disorder in the UK. However, there has been a small resurgence of cases reported to the British Paediatric Surveillance Unit over the period 1996–2000, possibly due to falling vaccine coverage and immigration of non-vaccinated women.[976,977] The risk of both fetal infection and sequelae vary with the gestation when maternal infection occurs. Transmission of the virus to the fetus occurs in 90% in the first 11 weeks, 50% from 11 to 20 weeks' gestation, 37% 20–35 weeks, and 100% during the last month of pregnancy.[978] Serious sequelae in the fetus are seen in 90% if infection occurs before 11 weeks, 30% at 12–20 weeks and none thereafter, aside from some mild growth retardation.[978] The majority of infants with congenital rubella disease result from primary maternal rubella infection, although maternal reinfection may rarely result in an infant with anomalies.[979]

Clinical manifestations

The common manifestations of congenital rubella infection are shown in Table 10.121. Important clinical manifestations are disorders of the eye (microphthalmia, cataract, congenital glaucoma, retinitis), congenital heart disease (PDA, peripheral pulmonary artery stenoses), and neurological sequelae (mental retardation, behavioral disorders, meningoencephalitis, convulsions). There may also be IUGR, microcephaly, thrombocytopenia, hepatosplenomegaly, purpuric skin lesions, pneumonitis and linear bone lesions. Only 68% of infected infants show signs at birth and up to 20% of these may die in infancy. A number of manifestations, however, present much later in life. These include hearing loss (87%), congenital heart disease (46–60%), mental or psychomotor retardation (30–50%), cataract or glaucoma (30–40%), diabetes mellitus, and thyroid dysfunction.

Diagnosis

Virus isolation, either from nasopharyngeal washing, urine or CSF is the most direct method of diagnosis, but may take many weeks. A positive rubella-specific IgM in a neonate and/or the detection of rubella RNA in urine or nasopharyngeal secretions by PCR usually indicates recent postnatal or congenital infection, although false positive results do occur. Rising or persistently stable levels of IgG

Table 10.121 Clinical features of rubella, cytomegalovirus and toxoplasmosis

	Cytomegalovirus	Rubella	Toxoplasmosis
CNS			
Hydrocephaly	+	-	+++
Microcephaly	+	+++	-
Calcification	+++	+	++
Deafness	++	+++	++
Encephalitis	-	-	+
Eyes			
Microphthalmia	+	+	+++
Cataracts	-	++	+
Chorioretinitis	+	+	+++
Intrauterine growth retardation	+	+++	+
Cardiac lesion	-	++	+
Purpuric rash	++	+++	-
Pneumonia	+++	++	++
Hepatospenomegaly	++	+++	++++
Lymphadenopathy	-	-	+
Bony lesion	+	+++	-

from the newborn period to beyond 9 months of age confirm perinatal or congenital infection.

Management

There is no specific treatment for rubella infection. Seronegative women of child-bearing age should be offered vaccination either after a pregnancy test or immediately postpartum. Rubella immunization of 13-year-old girls, which started in the UK in 1970, reduced the incidence considerably and the use of MMR vaccine in the UK from 1988 has made congenital rubella rare.[976] Most new reports of congenital rubella in the UK are of infants born to mothers who were born abroad and came to the UK after the age of schoolgirl immunization.

Cytomegalovirus (CMV)

This member of the herpes group of viruses is the commonest congenital infection in Europe with a prevalence of 3–4/1000 births. CMV is ubiquitous in the community and, although not highly infectious, it may be transmitted transplacentally or through genital secretions, saliva, breast milk or blood transfusion. Maternal infection may be primary or represent a reactivation of latent past infection.

About 50% of women of child-bearing age in the UK remain susceptible to CMV infection and 1% of those susceptible at the beginning of pregnancy will have a primary infection during pregnancy. The greatest risk of fetal damage occurs after primary maternal infection during pregnancy. The fetus will be infected in about 50% of primary maternal infections, but only 10% of the infants will display signs of infection. With reactivated maternal CMV infection, the risk of transmission to the infant or sequelae is <1%.[980] However, cases of severe congenital CMV due to maternal reinfection with a new CMV strain or reactivation of latent CMV have been reported.[981] Unlike rubella, fetal damage may follow primary infection or recurrent infection at any stage of pregnancy.

Clinical manifestations

Most infants with congenital CMV infection are asymptomatic. When symptomatic, the main clinical features are as shown in Table 10.122. The risk of neurological sequelae and IUGR in the fetus is greatest after infection in the first 20 weeks of pregnancy. Effects include microcephaly, chorioretinitis, mental retardation, sensorineural hearing loss and intracerebral periventricular calcification. Infection in the second half of pregnancy usually results in visceral disease such as hepatitis, purpura, hyperbilirubinemia and thrombocytopenia. Other effects include dental abnormalities and inguinal hernias. Pneumonitis is a common feature of postnatally acquired CMV, especially in premature infants, but rarely follows true congenital infection. Infants who have symptoms in the newborn period nearly always have subsequent handicap. Recently, it has been identified that the presence of microcephaly at birth is the strongest predictor of poor cognitive outcome in later life.[982] Up to 10% of the infected infants who are asymptomatic at birth will have CMV-related problems by 3 years of age, the most common problem being sensorineural hearing loss.[983]

Perinatal CMV infection

Many infants acquire CMV infection through breast-feeding, or by contact with infected secretions or blood products in the first weeks of life. This is usually asymptomatic except in premature infants or infants with cellular immunodeficiency in whom CMV infection may result in pneumonitis, hepatitis, thrombocytopenia, neutropenia and uncommonly gastroenteritis. In general, postnatal CMV infection does not result in long term sequelae, with the possible exception of babies less than 2000 g.[984]

Table 10.122 Lesions that may be caused by prenatally acquired viral infections

Pathogen	Clinical sequelae
1. Coxsackie virus	Abortion, mild febrile disease, rash, meningitis, hepatitis, gastroenteritis, myocarditis, congenital heart disease and neurological deficits
2. Cytomegalovirus	Microcephaly, hydrocephaly, microphthalmia, retinopathy, cerebral calcification, deafness, psychomotor retardation, anemia, thrombocytopenia, hepatosplenomegaly, jaundice and encephalopathy
3. ECHO virus	Same as Coxsackie virus
4. Hepatitis B virus	Low birth weight, asymptomatic hepatitis carrier, acute hepatitis, chronic hepatitis
5. Herpes simplex virus	Abortion, microcephaly, cerebral calcification, retinopathy, encephalitis, multiple organ involvement
6. Human immune deficiency virus	Abortion, hydro/microcephaly, limb deformities, intrauterine growth retardation, failure to thrive, rash, hepatosplenomegaly, pneumonia
7. Influenza virus	Abortion
8. Measles virus	Abortion, congenital measles
9. Polio virus	Abortion, congenital poliomyelitis with paralysis
10. Rubella virus	Abortion, microcephaly, cataract, microphthalmia, congenital heart disease, deafness, low birth weight, hepatosplenomegaly, petechiae, osteitis
11. Vaccinia virus	Abortion, congenital vaccinia
12. Varcella-zoster virus	Abortion, limb, cerebral and skin malformation Stillbirth, low birth weight, chorioretinitis, congenital chickenpox, or disseminated neonatal varicella or zoster
13. Variola virus	Abortion, congenital variola

In alphabetical order and not in order of frequency or seriousness.

Diagnosis

Diagnosis is based on isolation of the virus in the throat washings or urine. Cultures must be obtained within the first 3 weeks of life to distinguish congenital CMV infection from perinatally acquired infection. Demonstration of CMV-specific IgM antibody in neonatal serum is also suggestive of congenital infection, but it can only be detected in about 70% of patients. Later in infancy, in the absence of clinical features of congenital infection, laboratory methods alone will not make the distinction between congenital CMV and postnatal infection. Detection of CMV pp65 antigen in blood, or viral DNA by PCR are newer sensitive methods of diagnosis, but are usually not required for the diagnosis of congenital infection.

Treatment and prevention

Intravenous ganciclovir has been used in small trials.[985,986] No firm conclusions about efficacy can be drawn due to small sample sizes.

Ganciclovir may be used to treat infants with life threatening CMV-related organ disease or retinitis involving the macula. Work is in progress towards production of a vaccine.

CMV is spread by intimate contact with infected secretions. Pregnant caregivers and hospital personnel should employ careful hand washing after exposure to the secretions of a CMV-infected infant.

Varicella-zoster virus (VZV) (chickenpox)

Congenital infection

Maternal varicella zoster infection during the first 20 weeks of pregnancy may result in spontaneous abortion, fetal death or in embryopathy characterized by dermatomal skin scarring and limb hypoplasia. There may also be disorders of the central nervous system (microcephaly, cortical atrophy), eyes (cataracts, chorioretinitis), gastrointestinal tract and genitourinary tract. It is hypothesized that the damage results from in utero reactivation of VZV or disseminated fetal infection. Maternal infection in the second half of pregnancy may result in an asymptomatic primary fetal infection followed by herpes zoster in the first years of life in about 1% of exposed infants. A large prospective study from the UK and Germany of the effects of maternal VZV infection in pregnancy estimated the overall risk of embryopathy during the first 20 weeks of pregnancy to be 1%, with the highest risk of transmission of 2% being in the period 13–20 weeks.[987] Occasional cases resulting from maternal infection out to 23 weeks have been reported.[988] Administration of varicella zoster immunoglobulin (V-ZIG) to the mother may modify the course of chickenpox, but it has not been shown to alter the risk of transmission to the fetus.[989]

Perinatal infection

Maternal varicella that occurs in the period 5 days before delivery to 2 days after delivery may result in life threatening, disseminated VZV infection in the infant due to transplacental passage of the virus in the absence of maternal antibody. If the onset of maternal infection is more than 7 days prior to delivery, there is usually sufficient passive transfer of antibody, unless the infant is less than 28 weeks' gestation.

Administration of V-ZIG to the infant has been shown to prevent or modify the course of the illness in most cases. However, as a significant number of infants will develop systemic VZV despite the administration of V-ZIG,[990] all infants with perinatal VZV exposure should be monitored closely for systemic disease, with prompt initiation of intravenous aciclovir should vesicles appear. Hospitalized infants with chickenpox should be placed in respiratory and contact isolation until the lesions have crusted, but breast-feeding can continue.

Herpes simplex virus (HSV)

Neonatal HSV infection is invariably symptomatic and carries a high mortality if untreated. The incidence of disease ranges from 1:2500 live births in some parts of the USA[991] to 1:60 000 live births in the UK.[992] In the past, up to 75% of cases of neonatal infection were due to HSV type 2 and the rest due to type l. More recently, the proportion of cases due to neonatal HSV-1 infection is increasing in the UK and elsewhere around the world possibly due to an increase in genital HSV-1 disease.[992] The infection is acquired from passage through an infected birth canal in 85% of cases, and is postnatally acquired from the oral lesions of an infected caregiver in 10–15% of cases. A true congenital syndrome is seen in < 5% of cases. The greatest risk for transmission (about 50%) is from a primary maternal infection when there has been insufficient time for seroconversion and transplacental transfer of antibody.[993] If a woman with a recurrent infection is shedding virus at delivery, the risk may be 5% or less. Cesarean delivery is not completely effective in preventing transmission to the infant.

Clinical manifestations

Neonatal HSV disease may manifest as lesions localized to the skin, eye or mouth (SEM), as encephalitis, as pneumonitis or as a disseminated multiorgan infection with or without central nervous system involvement. The age of presentation varies with the category of disease. In general, neonatal HSV disease usually presents in the first 3 weeks of life, but it may manifest at any time from day 1 to 4 weeks of life. About 50% of cases now present as SEM disease, possibly due to better awareness of the condition. The typical vesicular, ulcerative lesion usually occurs on the presenting part. Up to 70% of SEM disease will spread to the CNS or elsewhere without treatment, but it is rarely fatal. Infants with SEM disease have 10% long term morbidity, with higher rates seen if there are frequent cutaneous recurrences in early life. The disseminated form typically commences at about 1 week of age with a shock-like syndrome in the absence of positive bacterial cultures with thrombocytopenia, disseminated intravascular coagulation, hepatitis, jaundice, and sometimes encephalitis and seizures. Skin lesions appear in 50% of these cases. Disseminated HSV infection may also present as an interstitial pneumonitis, usually presenting about day 3 of life. The mortality in this group is as high as 50% even with treatment, and over half of the survivors are left with long term sequelae (mental retardation, blindness, seizures, learning defects). The third group present with CNS symptoms such as poor feeding, apnea, lethargy and seizures without visceral involvement, typically in the second to third week of life. It has been hypothesized that this group represents reactivation of an earlier asymptomatic infection. They have a 15% mortality, with severe long term CNS effects seen in 65%.[994]

Congenital infection

Intrauterine HSV infection may manifest as the presence of vesicles or scarring at birth, chorioretinitis, microphthalmia, microcephaly, hydranencephaly or cerebral atrophy on CT scan in the first week of life, organ calcification or organomegaly. The majority of reported cases are due to HSV-2. There is a high rate of early neonatal death and long term central nervous system sequelae.

Diagnosis

If neonatal HSV disease is suspected, viral swabs of skin vesicles, eyes, nasopharynx, and rectum should be sent for HSV culture and immunofluorescence or HSV PCR. CSF should be collected for routine examination, HSV PCR and culture and blood sent for liver function tests, platelet count and coagulation screen. Empirical therapy with systemic intravenous aciclovir should be commenced promptly. A chest radiograph may be indicated if respiratory distress is present. Imaging of the head by ultrasound or CT scan should be performed. Serological assays are usually not helpful in the acute diagnosis of neonatal HSV disease.

Treatment and prevention

Mothers with primary lesions should be delivered electively by cesarean section while mothers with recurrent lesions, if they have a negative culture and do not have lesions or prodrome of infection, may be delivered vaginally. The use of invasive fetal monitoring and vacuum delivery should be avoided where possible in women with known genital HSV disease. Some suggest that the infant should be screened for infection by surface viral swabs at 48 h of life.

Intravenous aciclovir 60 mg/kg/day in three divided doses should be commenced as soon as neonatal HSV disease is suspected.

Many suggest it should be commenced empirically in the offspring of women with known primary genital HSV infection due to the high attack rate. The duration of therapy is 14 days for SEM disease and 21 days for all other categories or where a lumbar puncture could not be performed.[995] Topical therapy may be given in addition to systemic therapy for HSV eye disease under the direction of an ophthalmologist. The prognostic significance of persistence of HSV DNA at the end of therapy is currently under evaluation.

Enteroviruses (non-polio)

Intrauterine, perinatal and postnatal transmission of enteroviruses (coxsackieviruses group A and B, ECHO viruses, enteroviruses 68–71) have been documented, although there are no data on the risks of transmission to the fetus or sequelae. While maternal enterovirus infection during pregnancy has not been conclusively proven to cause an embryopathy, there have been links between some specific enteroviral infections and anomalies in the infant (Coxsackie B virus infection with urogenital anomalies, Coxsackie B3 and B4 viruses with cardiac anomalies, Coxsackie A9 with digestive anomalies).

Perinatal enteroviral infections generally cause asymptomatic infection or mild, non-specific illness, particularly if the baby acquires infection 'horizontally' from other babies. However, if a woman is infected just before or after delivery, severe disease may develop in the 'vertically' infected newborn in the first week after birth. The mother may present with severe abdominal pain mimicking abruption or with respiratory or gastrointestinal symptoms. The baby may present with a sepsis-like syndrome (fever or hypothermia, anorexia, vomiting, lethargy, disseminated intravascular coagulation), gastroenteritis (vomiting, diarrhea, fulminant hepatitis, pancreatitis), a neurological illness (aseptic meningitis, encephalitis or paralysis), a respiratory illness (pneumonitis, pharyngitis, laryngotracheobronchitis), skin or mucosal manifestations (erythematous, maculopapular rash, herpangina, hemorrhagic conjunctivitis), or cardiac disease (myocarditis, pericarditis). Some specific enteroviruses are associated with particular syndromes (see enteroviruses, Ch. 26). Severe ECHO virus infections are more likely to cause hepatitis with massive hepatic necrosis, DIC and death, while coxsackieviruses are more likely to cause myocarditis and meningitis. Neonatal outbreaks of enterovirus 71 (EV 71) have recently been associated with neurological manifestations such as encephalitis, Guillain–Barré syndrome and neurogenic pulmonary edema.[996,997]

Diagnosis

Enteroviruses may be cultured from the nasopharynx, throat swab or feces. Serology is rarely helpful due to poor sensitivity. Detection of enterovirus nucleic acid in the CSF by PCR can be useful in the diagnosis of enteroviral meningitis.

Treatment

The new antiviral agent, pleconaril has been shown to have in vitro activity against a number of enteroviruses, but not EV 71.[998] In a small case series, treatment of severe neonatal enterovirus infection with oral pleconaril was associated with both virological and clinical improvement, but the sample size was too small to determine if this outcome was significant. IVIG has also been used to treat life threatening disease, but its efficacy is unproven for this use.

Parvovirus B19

B19 is a small non-enveloped single-stranded DNA virus. Though associated with many conditions, it primarily affects the fetus and the newborn by lytic infection of the human erythroid progenitor cell. B19 infection is the most important cause of non-immune hydrops in the fetus and the newborn. Treatment is symptomatic but commercial IVIG preparations have been used with benefit.[999]

PARASITIC INFECTIONS

Malaria

Placental transmission of malaria is extremely rare but transfusion-induced malaria is increasingly recognized. Clinical presentation may be indistinguishable from sepsis, or the infant may present with jaundice due to hemolysis.

Diagnosis is made on identifying malarial parasites in the blood film. Treatment should be chloroquine 5–10 mg/kg/day in divided doses for 3–5 days.

Toxoplasmosis

Toxoplasmosis is a worldwide disease. In the UK between 20 and 40% of the population have been infected with this protozoan by adult life. The incidence of congenital toxoplasmosis in Europe is 1–10 in 10 000 newborns.[1000]

Congenital toxoplasmosis infection usually occurs as a result of placental infection after a primary infection in a pregnant woman. Parasites form small focal lesions in the placenta, proliferate and are released as active forms into the fetal bloodstream. Rare cases of fetal transmission have been reported after preconception maternal infection in immunocompetent women,[1001] presumably due to myometrial infection. It is generally accepted that women who bear a congenitally infected child do not have infected children in subsequent pregnancies. However, exceptions to this rule occur and it is suggested that persistence of *Toxoplasma gondii* as cysts in the myometrium with liberation of active forms during pregnancy is one of the main infectious causes of repeated abortion. Congenital toxoplasmosis has been reported following reactivation in women with human immunodeficiency virus (HIV) infection, although it is a rare event, as shown by a European Collaborative Study.[1002]

The risk of transmission and the clinical outcome after maternal toxoplasmosis infection vary with the trimester of pregnancy.[1000] Infection in early pregnancy carries a low risk of transmission which rises to 6% by 13 weeks, 40% at 26 weeks, and 72% at 36 weeks. If a fetus is infected, the risk of developing clinical signs (and the severity of disease) is greatest the earlier in pregnancy the infection occurs, falling from 61% at 13 weeks, to 25% at 26 weeks and 9% at 36 weeks.[1000]

Clinical manifestations

Infection of the fetus with virulent strains early in pregnancy may produce fetal death and abortion. Later infection may cause severe fetal damage or stillbirth and later still, a live-born infant with stigmata of congenital toxoplasmosis. However, up to 70% of infants with congenital toxoplasmosis are asymptomatic at birth. The commonest presenting feature is chorioretinitis. Both eyes are involved in 40% of cases. Other important clinical features are given in Table 10.123. They include hydrocephalus, intracranial calcification, hepatosplenomegaly, jaundice, thrombocytopenia and a maculopapular rash. Clinical sequelae of congenital infection, including visual disturbance, seizures and mental retardation may not manifest until later in life. The prognosis for patients with CNS involvement must be extremely guarded.

Diagnosis

This is usually based on *Toxoplasma* IgM and/or *Toxoplasma* IgA antibody tests. The sensitivity of the IgM-ISAGA test is probably the highest. Persistently elevated *Toxoplasma* IgG beyond 12 months of age, and detection of *Toxoplasma* DNA by PCR in the placenta,

Table 10.123 Comparative frequencies of neonatal neoplasms in different series

	Barson[1008] UK (dates variable)[1]	Davis et al[1009] Glasgow, UK (1955–1988)	Broadbent[1010] Oxford, UK (1970–1977)	Campbell et al[1011] Toronto (1922–1982)	Bader & Miller[1012] USA (1969–1971)[2]	Bader & Miller[1012] Deaths, USA (1960–1969)	Fraumeni & Miller[1013] Deaths, USA (1960–1964)
Leukemia	17	Not surveyed	17	8[3]	5	101	44
Teratoma	67	19	16 (malig.)	Not surveyed (regarded benign)	Not surveyed (regarded benign)	11	9
Neuroblastoma	64	7	27	48 (44%)	21	70	27
Soft tissue sarcoma (rhabdo-, leio-, fibro-)	22	8	13	12 (17%)	4	29	12
Wilms' and mesoblastic nephroma	20	9	8	4 (75%)	5	21	9
CNS	17		12	9 (11%)	1	12	7
Hepatoblastoma		3	3	1	0	15	10
Retinoblastoma		4		7 (76%)	0	1	
Others	78[4]	1	5	3 (100%)	3	35	12
Total	285	51	101	102[5] (42%)	39	295	130[6]
Sex incidence	–	–	1:1	1.7:1	–	–	–

[1] Benign and malignant.
[2] Third National Cancer Study (10% US population surveyed); overall incidence neonatal malignancy USA = 130 cases/year.
[3] Long-term survival
[4] Unclear from report.
[5] Represents 1.9% of all childhood malignancy.
[6] Represents 0.6% childhood deaths from malignancy.

neonatal blood or CSF may also be used to make the diagnosis. In the infant with suspected congenital toxoplasmosis, ophthalmological examination, hearing assessment, and central nervous system examination and imaging should be performed.

Treatment

Infants diagnosed with congenital toxoplasmosis infection should be treated to reduce the incidence of long term sequelae such as chorioretinitis. Two synergistic antimicrobials, either sulfadimidine or sulfadiazine together with pyrimethamine are used. Prolonged treatment for up to 12 months is required to reduce the risk of late reactivation in the eye.[1003] Corticosteroids should be used in the presence of chorioretinitis or raised CSF protein. Many advise treatment of pregnant women with primary toxoplasmosis. A recent systematic review suggests that there are still insufficient data on whether this treatment is effective in preventing neonatal infection.[1004]

Pregnant women should be educated to avoid ingestion of *Toxoplasma* cysts by adequate cooking of meat, washing of garden produce, and washing hands after contact with soil.

NEONATAL NEOPLASIA

Of those rare tumors that present at birth or in the neonatal period less than half will be malignant. It is important to know the natural history as even huge tumor masses or apparently disseminated disease may regress completely and spontaneously. As survival from childhood cancer has improved, death certificate data have become progressively less accurate as an indicator of frequency. Estimates of incidence vary because most reports are referral center rather than population based and some exclude benign tumors. In the USA the best estimate of different malignancies is based on an analysis of 10% of the total population over a 3-year period. This suggests an overall incidence of 1 per 27 000 live births (Table 10.124,[1008–1013] column 5 for proportions of different tumors). In the UK a prevalence of 1 per 12 500–17 500 has been found but this included benign neoplasia (Table 10.124, column 1). Approximately 2% of childhood malignancy will present in the first 28 days of life:[1014] 43% of these will present on the first day; 66% by the end of 1 week;[1011] and 0.6% of pediatric malignant deaths will occur during this period.

ETIOLOGY

1. Transplacental metastases of maternal choriocarcinoma, melanoma and leukemia are well described but very rare.
2. Transplacental carcinogenesis. This is definite for the use of maternal stilbestrol which leads to vaginal adenocarcinoma – the latent period is 10–15 years – it has not been reported neonatally. Transplacental carcinogenesis is also probable for infantile neuroblastoma in the fetal phenytoin syndrome and it is possible for hepatoblastoma when the mother has been taking estrogens in the first trimester.
3. Genetic
   A. Chromosomal
   (i) Down syndrome 21X3 – acute myelogenous and occasionally acute lymphoblastic leukemia presents neonatally. Leukemoid reactions are comparatively common in the neonatal period; they are difficult to distinguish and 15% will go on to develop leukemia later.
   (ii) Klinefelter's syndrome XXY – breast cancer (not reported neonatally), and recent reports of a higher incidence of leukemia.
   (iii) Gonadal dysgenesis 46XY, 45X/46XY, other mosaics – dysgerminomas (not reported neonatally).
   (iv) 13q (retinoblastoma) – may present neonatally. This is the only known inheritable malignancy.
   (v) Fanconi's anemia – leukemia (not reported neonatally).
   (vi) Bloom's syndrome – leukemia (not reported neonatally).
   (vii) Ataxia telangiectasia – lymphoma and gastric carcinoma (not reported neonatally).
   B. Malformation syndromes
   (i) Aniridia – nephroblastoma (possible neonatally).
   (ii) Hemihypertrophy syndrome – nephroblastoma and hepatoblastoma (not recorded neonatally).

(iii) Beckwith–Wiedemann syndrome – nephroblastoma and hepatoblastoma (not recorded neonatally).
(iv) Cryptorchidism – testicular tumors (not recorded neonatally).
(v) Other syndromes – chondrosarcoma (not recorded neonatally).

GENERAL MANAGEMENT

The variety of neonatal neoplasia makes it extremely important that all patients are referred to recognized specialist centers with facilities for diagnostic imaging, expert pediatric and molecular pathology, surgery, radiotherapy, chemotherapy and hematology. Tumor markers have an increasingly important role in both diagnosis and monitoring the response to treatment (Table 10.125).[1015–1025] Large tumors may be problematic more from their size interfering with organ function rather than because of tumor load. Surgery can frequently be more conservative than is generally appreciated and may be curative. Back-up with postoperative intensive care is essential. Neonatal tissue (especially brain, bone, lungs, liver and kidneys) is very sensitive to radiotherapy and the anxieties of infection secondary to immune suppression, or the development of second malignancies means that this therapy should be avoided if possible. Cytotoxic chemotherapy may reduce the infant's effective immune response with in consequence a higher incidence of complications and particularly infection. Chemotherapy can potentially affect a child's subsequent development but will often reduce tumor size very significantly even when used at 50% of the dose recommended in older children. Centralization of referral also allows more realistic parental and family support.

Table 10.124 Features of tumors presenting in the neonatal period

Tumor	Presentation	Investigations	Markers	Treatment	Incidence per 100 000 live births in UK	Notes
Teratoma a. Sacrococcygeal b. Head and neck	1. Prenatal ultrasound 2. Obvious mass a. On buttocks: may be so large as to obstruct delivery b. On neck: may lead to airway obstruction	1. Lateral abdominal X-ray for anterior displacement of rectum ± calcification 2. Neck X-ray 3. Chest X-ray – pulmonary metastases	1. Alpha-fetoprotein: raised malignant; normal benign 2. Beta human chorionic gonadotropin often raised	1. Benign – surgery (remove coccyx or local recurrence common) 2. Malignant – surgery then chemotherapy, radiotherapy	0.27	1. At birth 90% benign, 10% malignant (if present after 2 years 90% malignant) 2. 4:1 females:males 3. 20% of those with intra-abdominal extension are malignant (Altman et al[1018]) 4. Alpha-fetoprotein raised in 70% of malignant variety 5. Solid tumors are more likely to have malignant elements 6. Teratoma rarely present as retroperitoneal (abdominal) mass
Leukemia a. Acute myelogenous (non-lymphocytic)	1. Hepatosplenomegaly 2. Petechiae + bruising 3. Skin infiltration (nodules) 4. Respiratory distress (infiltration) 5. Bone pain 6. Meningeal involvement	1. WBC variable blasts ++ platelets reduced 2. Bone marrow ± biopsy 3. Biopsy skin plaque	1. Enzymes 2. Monoclonal membrane markers 3. Chromosomes (Burmeister & Thiel,[1015] Robinson[1016])	Invariably fatal despite modern chemotherapy ± intrathecal methotrexate	0.29	1. 25% of cases are Down syndrome 2. Differential = hemolytic disease, congenital infection, disseminated neuroblastoma 3. Skin lesions may suggest monocytic leukemia 4. Null acute lymphoblastic leukemia may rarely present neonatally
b. (Leukemoid reactions)	1. Down syndrome child with leukemoid blood reaction	1. WBC 2. Marrow		Spontaneous remission, support with platelets, blood ± antibiotic	–	1. Down syndrome frequent but may be normal karyotype + phenotype

Table 10.124 *(Cont'd)*

Tumor	Presentation	Investigations	Markers	Treatment	Incidence per 100 000 live births in UK	Notes
						2. Indistinguishable from leukemia but regresses over 1–3 months
Neuroblastoma	1. Abdominal mass 2. SVC obstruction 3. Respiratory obstruction 4. Leukoerythroblastic anemia 5. Bluish s.c. nodules 6. Spinal cord compression with pain and paraplegia 7. Horner's syndrome from cervical chain involvement	Stage i confined to structure of origin ii, local unilateral spread iii, bilateral spread iv, remote disease ivs i or ii, with remote disease 1. 24h catecholamines VMA-HVA excretion 2. Calcification on X-ray 3. US 4. IVP 5. bone marrow 6. skel. survey or bone scan	1. VMA } in up 2. HVA } to 95% 3. Vasointestinal peptide (serum) 4. Neurone specific enolase (serum) (Kintzel et al[1017])	Stage i, total excision ii, maximal excision ± chemotherapy iii, chemotherapy plus excision iv, chemotherapy ivs, spontaneous regression usual	0.45	1. 1:40 neonatal autopsies (Guin et al[1019]) 2. Spontaneous regression common (Bolande[1020]) 3. 60% occur in the abdomen or pelvis 4. Prognosis excellent (cf. later in childhood, 5. Accounts for 30–50% neonatal malignancy 6. Mostly stage ivs 7. Associated congenital abnormalities are common (Isaacs[1021])
Soft tissue sarcomas Fibro-, spindle cell leio-, myo-, rhabdomyo-, hemangiopericytomas	1. Mass – particularly in head, neck, extremities	1. Biopsy		1. Excision if possible 2. ± cytotoxics at a reduced dose	0.3	1. If benign soft tissue sarcomas (fibromatosis and myofibromatosis) are included, the incidence is greater than either leukemia or neuroblastomas 2. Locally aggressive 3. Metastases rare (compare older age groups)
Renal a. Nephroblastoma (Wilms') (rare)	1. Prenatal US 2. Postnatal abdominal mass 3. Hematuria – rare	1. US 2. Chest X-ray (pulmonary metastases) 3. Staging – almost always local I or II	1. ↑Inactive renin (Carachi et al[1023])	a. Stage I, surgery + vincristine. II, surgery + vincristine + actinomycin (chemotherapy at 50% dose)	0.13	1. A neonatal renal mass is not likely to be malignant 2. True Wilms' tumors are associated with hemihypertrophy, aniridia, Beckwith's, UG abnormalities 3. Nephroblastomatosis is present in 1:400 autopsies (Machin[1024])
b. Congenital mesoblastic nephroma (more common) (Bolande[1022])	1. Prenatal (US) 2. Postnatal abdominal mass 3. Hematuria – rare	1. US 2. CXR (pulmonary metastases) 3. Staging – almost always local I or II	1. ↑Inactive renin (Carachi et al[1023])	b. Stage I, surgery II, surgery		1. Commoner than Wilms' and do not metastasize 2. Outlook extremely good
CNS Astrocytomas, teratomas, ependymomas oligodendrogliomas, craniopharyngiomas	1. Prenatal US 2. Hydrocephalus cephalopelvic disproportion bulging fontanel	1. US 2. CT 3. NMR		1. Surgery 2. Probably not radiotherapy 3. ±shunt 4. Chemotherapy	0.2	1. High incidence of teratomas 2. Predominantly supratentorial (astrocytomas)

Table 10.124 (*Cont'd*)

Tumor	Presentation	Investigations	Markers	Treatment	Incidence per 100 000 live births in UK	Notes
medulloblastomas	suture separation 3. Increased intracranial pressure with vomiting 4. Convulsions					3. Often large at diagnosis with high incidence of hemorrhage 4. Prognosis poor 5. Best to avoid RT until ≥2 years
Hepatoblastoma						
+ hemangio-endotheliomas (rare)	1. Hepatomegaly 2. ±Respiratory distress 3. ±GI symptoms	1. US	1. Alpha-fetoprotein	1. Surgery 2. ±Preop. chemotherapy 3. ±Low dose radiotherapy preoperative 4. Postop. chemotherapy in low dose	0.05	1. A neonatal liver mass is *not* likely to be malignant, it is more likely to be a hemangioma or mesenchymal hamartoma and may present with cardiac failure or DIC 2. Secondary neuroblastoma or leukemia is a commoner cause of hepatomegaly than is hepatoblastoma 3. Associated with hemihypertrophy and Beckwith's syndrome
Retinoblastoma	1. White eye and squint 2. Heterochromia iridis 3. Abdominal mass	1. CT 2. Chest X-ray 3. Abdominal US	1. Operation - enucleation 2. If bilateral – laser photocoagulation ± RT			1. Family history in 25% and this usually bilateral 2. Abnormality of chromosome 13 common 3. Orbital mass may be an orbital teratoma
Langerhans' cell histiocytosis (no longer considered a neoplastic process) (Huang & Arceci[1025])	1. Skin rash, particularly groins, axillae, neck and behind ears. Occasionally trunk. Usually brown-red raised macules which may coalesce or even ulcerate in skinfolds 2. A 'cradle cap' like skin lesion on the scalp 3. Respiratory distress from infiltration 4. Hepatosplenomegaly 5. Lymphadenopathy 6. Usually little systemic upset	1. Skin biopsy 2. Chest X-ray 3. Skeletal survey for punched-out bone lesions 4. Osmolality of urine for diabetes insipidus		1. Spontaneous remissions 2. If systemic upset/ progression steroids ± vincristine or vinblastine ± VP16		1. Proliferation of tissue macrophages. T-suppressor lymphocytes normally control the macrophages – these are deficient tissue macrophages: liver histiocytes, Kupffer cells lung alveolar histiocytes skin Langhans' cells pleura + peritoneum lymph nodes gut microglia osteoclasts

CT, computerized tomography; HVA, homovanillic acid; IVP, intravenous pyelogram; NMR, nuclear magnetic resonance; RT, radiotherapy; SVC, superior vena cava; UG, urogenital; US, ultrasound; VMA, vanillylmandelic acid.

Table 10.125 Causes of neonatal hypoglycemia

Transient hypoglycemia	Persistent hypoglycemia
Intrauterine growth retardation	Hyperinsulinism Nesidioblastosis Insulinoma
Prematurity	Inborn errors of metabolism Glycogen storage disease
Birth asphyxia	GSD types I, III, IV Galactosemia
Neonatal sepsis	Hepatic gluconeogenic deficiencies Fructose-1,6-diphosphatase
Neonatal cold injury	Pyruvate carboxylase Phosphoenolpyruvate carboxylase
Starvation	Defects in amino acid metabolism Maple syrup urine disease
Congenital heart disease	Methylmalonic acidemia HMG-CoA lyase deficiency
Hyperinsulinism	Beckwith–Wiedemann syndrome
Infant of diabetic mother	Propionic acidemia
Erythroblastosis fetalis	Tyrosinemia type I
Maternal drugs	Mitochondrial fatty acid oxidation defects
Maternal glucose infusions	MCAD deficiency
Idiopathic hyperinsulinism	LCAD deficiency
	Electron transport defects MAD-S deficiency MAD-M deficiency RR-MAD deficiency
	Hormonal deficiencies Congenital hypopituitarism Cortisol deficiency Congenital glucagon deficiency

LCAD, long chain acyl-CoA dehydrogenase; MAD-M, mild multiple acyl-CoA dehydrogenase; MAD-S, severe multiple acyl-CoA dehydrogenase; MCAD, medium chain acyl-CoA dehydrogenase; RR-MAD, riboflavin responsive multiple acyl-CoA dehydrogenase.

NEONATAL METABOLIC DISORDERS

HYPOGLYCEMIA

Glucose homeostasis in the fetus and newborn

The fetus receives a constant supply of glucose across the placenta and this largely determines blood glucose concentrations. Fetal metabolism is directed towards synthesis with insulin as the principal anabolic hormone. Hepatic glycogen accumulates during the third trimester and mobilization of this reserve is the principal source of glucose for the first postnatal hours. At delivery, the constant transplacental glucose supply is interrupted, blood glucose falls and the processes of glycogenolysis and gluconeogenesis are activated mainly by a rise in glucagon, catecholamines and cortisol and a concomitant decrease in insulin levels. Active gluconeogenesis is required for the first few postnatal days to maintain glucose homeostasis until milk feed intakes increase to levels where this is the main source of glucose precursors.

The maintenance of normoglycemia during the newborn period is dependent on adequate fetal glycogen reserves, effective glycogenolysis and gluconeogenesis, an appropriate balance of insulin:glucagon and an increasing postnatal nutritional intake. Hypoglycemia will result if any of these processes are inadequate.

Neuropathology

Glucose is an essential primary fuel for the brain and as this is large in relation to total mass, cerebral glucose consumption is proportionately high. It seems likely that the brain of the term infant can utilize ketones, lactate or amino acids as an alternative to glucose. This may explain the apparent vulnerability of infants with non-ketotic hypoglycemia to cerebral damage. Neurones and glial cells are susceptible to hypoglycemia and vulnerable areas are the cerebral cortex, particularly posteriorly in the parieto-occipital region. Less commonly involved are neurones of the hippocampus, caudate nucleus and putamen but any level of the central nervous system may be involved including anterior horn cells of the spinal cord. Glial injury may relate to subsequent disturbances of myelination.

Definitions of hypoglycemia

Hypoglycemia was defined as a glucose concentration less than two standard deviations below the mean for a particular population; for example, hypoglycemia in the preterm was defined as < 1.1 mmol/L during the first week of life. In full-term infants the corresponding value was < 1.7 mmol/L for the first 72 h of life with a value of < 2.2 mmol/L after 72 h of age. These criteria imply that preterm infants compared to term are less prone to neurological impairment secondary to hypoglycemia and that resistance to hypoglycemia is greatest in the immediate postpartum period. A more satisfactory approach is to define hypoglycemia in the context of acute or chronic neurological dysfunction. For example, moderate hypoglycemia, <2.6 mmol/L, in preterm infants is associated with reduced mental and motor developmental scores.[1026]

The *symptomatic* response of the neonate to low blood glucose is variable with non-specific clinical features including pallor, feeding difficulties, hypotonia, tachypnea, abnormal cry, jitteriness, apnea, irritability, coma and convulsions. This lack of symptomatic specificity can make the interpretation of biochemical hypoglycemia difficult such as the intensively cared for infant where comorbidities can cause similar clinical features or where symptomatic responses may be masked with therapeutic muscle paralysis, severe birth asphyxia or extreme prematurity. Hypoglycemia may be intermittent and it is important to check blood glucose at times of vague but suspicious symptoms.

Some otherwise well infants with low blood glucoses are *asymptomatic* suggesting that alternative metabolic substrates are available for brain metabolism. Such infants in general have a favorable prognosis. However, acute cerebral dysfunction, as measured by auditory and somatosensory evoked potentials, occurs in the majority of neonates when blood glucose levels fall below 2.6 mmol/L even though 50% of them were still asymptomatic.[1027]

As a consequence of these relationships between blood glucose levels and acute and chronic neurological dysfunction, *blood glucose levels < 2.6 mmol/L are accepted as indicating hypoglycemia* which requires treatment regardless of gestation or postnatal age.

On a practical basis, hypoglycemia can be sub classified into two main groups: *transient* and *persistent* hypoglycemia.[1028]

Transient neonatal hypoglycemia

IUGR

Infants with asymmetric growth retardation are particularly prone to both in-utero and postnatal hypoglycemia. The etiology of the hypoglycemia can be multifactorial with metabolic demands of a relatively large brain, depleted glycogen, fat and protein reserves as well as limited gluconeogenic and ketogenic responses which in some are secondary to poorly coordinated counter-regulatory mechanisms.[1029,1030] The presence of prematurity, birth asphyxia or polycythemia can compound the problem.

Birth asphyxia should be avoided (p. 148) and polycythemia corrected (p. 303). Enteral feeds should start within an hour of birth. Blood glucose should be monitored frequently, usually hourly, until normoglycemia is attained when the interval can be extended to 2- then 4-hourly. If normoglycemia cannot be established, then a background intravenous infusion of dextrose is required, starting around 5 mg/kg/min but increasing if necessary the volume per kg and dextrose concentration. Enteral feeds are gradually increased in volume with reciprocal decreases in intravenous dextrose if normoglycemia is maintained. With the discontinuation of intravenous dextrose, the frequency of enteral feeds can be sequentially reduced to 2-, 3- and 4-hourly if normoglycemia is established. In a minority of infants where sustaining normoglycemia is problematic and intravenous glucose requirements are high or prolonged, despite established enteral nutrition, concurrent pathology should be considered. Hypoglycemia in growth restricted infants may produce psychomotor delay[1031] and the problems of persistence of hypoglycemia beyond the neonatal period may be underdiagnosed in asymptomatic infants.[1032]

Prematurity

The immaturity of gluconeogenesis, glycogenolysis and limited glycogen and fat reserves make this group vulnerable to hypoglycemia. Early hypoglycemia, within 1 h of delivery, occurs in up to 70% of infants < 30 weeks' gestation before intravenous dextrose infusions are established and thereafter glucose homeostasis can be unstable in sick premature infants.[1033] Hypoglycemia is usually transient and correctable with dextrose infusions of 5 mg/kg/min but a higher caloric intake to meet energy demands, either parenterally or enterally, should also be established early. Preterm infants will only partially suppress endogenous glucose production with glucose infusions[1034,1035] but also fail to inhibit proteolysis[1036] and early introduction of complete parenteral nutrition (day 1) improves not only energy–nitrogen balance but reduces the frequency of hypoglycemic episodes.[1037] Hypoglycemia in preterm infants is common and this may impair the early detection of underlying metabolic abnormalities or genetic disorders affecting glucose homeostasis.[1038,1039]

Birth asphyxia

Perinatal stress will deplete glycogen reserves and mitochondrial damage may uncouple oxidative phosphorylation with subsequent anaerobic glycolysis and generation of lactate. Hypoglycemia is usually transient and correctable with an intravenous infusion of dextrose at around 5 mg/kg/min. Hyperglycemia should be avoided as it may exacerbate existing metabolic acidosis and compound the hyperosmolar state. Prematurity, IUGR, adrenal hemorrhage and transient hyperinsulinism are common associations.

Neonatal sepsis

Hypoglycemia and sepsis are commonly associated. Pyrexia may increase the metabolic rate, caloric intake may be decreased and insulin sensitivity may be increased.

Neonatal hypothermia

Hypoglycemia is a common feature and glucose homeostasis should be established as part of the resuscitative measures.

Starvation

Failure to establish adequate enteral intake in full-term infants can result in hypoglycemia and this effect is exaggerated by IUGR, prematurity or birth asphyxia.

Congenital heart disease

Hypoglycemia per se can result in transient cardiomegaly. An association exists between hypoglycemia and acute congestive cardiac failure; the etiology of this may be multifactorial with decreased caloric intake, increased metabolic rate, decreased hepatic perfusion or even focal hepatic necrosis. Hypoglycemia has also been observed in children with severe congenital heart disease without cardiac failure. Management consists of restoration of normoglycemia with intravenous glucose and in the longer term adequate caloric intake.

Transient hyperinsulinemia

Infant of diabetic mother

Fetal blood glucose uptake is directly related to maternal blood glucose levels and fetal hyperglycemia results in hyperplasia of the islets of Langerhans, increased peripheral insulin receptors, a decreased glucagon response to postnatal hypoglycemia and delayed evocation of hepatic gluconeogenic pathways. Meticulous control of maternal diabetes in pregnancy and labor can prevent or reduce the severity and frequency of neonatal hypoglycemia and the incidence of macrosomia, RDS, hyperbilirubinemia, polycythemia and hypocalcemia. The incidence of congenital malformations is higher and includes congenital heart disease, central nervous system abnormalities, vertebral anomalies and the caudal regression syndrome which may present in various forms including sacral agenesis, femoral hypoplasia or sirenomelia. Careful control of maternal diabetes preconceptually and in the early weeks of pregnancy reduces the incidence of malformations.

In the majority of infants, postnatal hypoglycemia is transient, < 6 h, and asymptomatic. Blood glucose is usually monitored at birth, 1, 2, 4 and 6 h. Enteral feeds are established within the first hour and thereafter 2-hourly until normoglycemia is established. In the minority of infants hypoglycemia may be more prolonged, up to 3 days, and if normoglycemia is not maintained the infants may become symptomatic. In asymptomatic infants who fail to establish normoglycemia with enteral feeds, a single dose of glucagon (0.03–0.1 mg/kg) may prevent recurrence. In the sick infant, or those intolerant of enteral feeds or where hypoglycemia is prolonged, normoglycemia should be maintained by intravenous infusions of dextrose (4–8 mg/kg/min). Symptomatic hypoglycemia requires an initial bolus of intravenous dextrose (0.25–0.5 g/kg) and thereafter a constant intravenous infusion. Enteral feeds are introduced when appropriate with reciprocal reduction in intravenous infusion rates maintaining normoglycemia and avoiding abrupt changes which can result in reactive hypoglycemia. Rarely, in prolonged hypoglycemia unresponsive to the above measures, hydrocortisone 5 mg/kg 12-hourly has been used.

Erythroblastosis fetalis

An association exists between moderate to severe erythroblastosis fetalis and hypoglycemia secondary to hyperinsulinism. It is estimated that around 20% of infants with cord Hbs < 10 g/dl will have significant hypoglycemia. It is important to monitor blood glucose regularly particularly during and after exchange transfusions.

Beckwith–Wiedemann syndrome

Affected infants may have exomphalos, macroglossia, visceromegaly, giantism, parallel creases on the ear lobes, hyperinsulinemic hypoglycemia and an increased risk of Wilms' tumor and other malignancies.[1040] All features may not be present and infants with only giantism or exomphalos should have blood glucose levels monitored.

The majority of cases are sporadic with a female predominance but in familial forms possible patterns include autosomal dominant, multifactorial and autosomal dominant sex-dependent inheritance.

This multigenic disorder is caused by dysregulation of the expression of imprinted genes in the 11p15 chromosomal region with close associations to insulin-like growth factor (IGF)-II and tumor suppressor genes[1041] and genes implicated in regulation of insulin release.[1042]

Hypoglycemia is usually transient but may be prolonged and severe and occasionally persists into adulthood. Symptomatic hypoglycemia is estimated to occur in around 50% of individuals and may contribute to the mental deficiency recognized as part of this syndrome. The management of persistent hyperinsulinemia is discussed below.

Maternal drugs

Beta-mimetic agents used in the management of premature labor stimulate the fetal pancreas to produce insulin and also reduce fetal hepatic glycogen deposition. Maternal administration of beta-mimetics is usually discontinued when preterm delivery is planned as these agents can also have profound effects on neonatal cardiorespiratory function.

Neonatal hyperinsulinemic hypoglycemia has been reported after maternal administration of chlorpropamide. Thiazide diuretics probably stimulate beta-cell function. Maternal valproate has recently been associated with infant hypoglycemia and features of withdrawal.[1043]

Intrapartum glucose infusion. Fetal insulin secretion can be induced by intrapartum maternal glucose infusions. The incidence of resultant neonatal hypoglycemia is related to maternal blood glucose levels particularly when above 6.6 mmol/L or when maternal glucose infusions are greater than 20 g/h.

Idiopathic transient neonatal hyperinsulinism

The etiology of hypoglycemia in growth retarded infants is multifactorial but in some infants where normoglycemia is not established by 72 h, in spite of adequate nutrition, the possibility of hyperinsulinism should be considered and investigated. This syndrome also occurs in full-term, appropriate for gestational age infants after normal pregnancies and deliveries, without maternal diabetes or drug ingestion. The resolution of transient hyperinsulinemia may take days, weeks or in some instances months, and on occasions diazoxide is required to control hypoglycemia. The etiology of transient hyperinsulinism is unknown and is regarded as a temporary imbalance in the regulatory development of insulin secretion.

Persistent hypoglycemia

Persistent hyperinsulinemia

Recurrent or persistent hyperinsulinemia is the commonest cause of prolonged severe hypoglycemia during the first year of life. The majority present with early neonatal hypoglycemia and are recognized causes of neonatal death and sudden infant death. Fetal hyperinsulinism results in a phenotype similar to that of the infant of the diabetic mother. The physiology of insulin release is being unravelled as are defects in these processes which results in hyperinsulinism (see Shepherd et al[1044] for review). The molecular etiology and the mechanisms responsible for clinical heterogeneity are becoming more clear. Mutations in four different genes have been identified in patients with both autosomal recessive and dominant inheritance. Most cases are caused by mutations in either of the two subunits of the beta cell ATP sensitive K channel (K_{ATP}), whereas others are caused by mutations in glucokinase and glutamate dehydrogenase. However, no genetic etiology has yet been determined for as many as 50% of the cases.[1045] In the neonatal group, the underlying pathology is usually diffuse hyperplasia of the endocrine pancreas whereas in older children solitary islet cell adenomas predominate. However, congenital islet cell adenomas are described in neonates and hyperinsulinemic hypoglycemia, whilst the features of diffuse hyperplasia have also been described in adults. Histological features vary widely. In most instances there is an increase in pancreatic beta cells either organized in groups or as individuals. Somatostatin cells are usually decreased.

Diagnosis of hyperinsulinism

Normoglycemia, > 2.6 mmol/L, may only be attained in infants with hyperinsulinism with increased glucose infusion rates (> 8 mg glucose/kg/min and in individual cases sometimes > 20 mg glucose/kg/min). Insulin secretion is inappropriately high in comparison to simultaneously measured blood glucose. In normal, fasted individuals, insulin levels are low or undetectable, but in organic hyperinsulinism they remain elevated even in the presence of hypoglycemia. Insulin prevents ketogenesis by inhibiting lipolysis and in hyperinsulinism there is no increase in blood ketones. Plasma levels of branched chain amino acids are decreased in hyperinsulinemia. Insulin increases hepatic glycogen reserves and liver size may increase due to glycogen deposition. The measurement of blood ammonia is essential with the description of the syndrome of hyperammonemic hyperinsulinemia.[1046]

Management

Immediate management is to attain normoglycemia by intravenous infusion of dextrose, and this may require rates > 15 mg/kg/min, and the establishment of a normal feed volume in content and volume for age. Hypostop and/or glucagon may be useful as a temporary measure, e.g. resiting intravenous sites. Diazoxide inhibits insulin release, increases epinephrine (adrenaline) secretion and activates glycogenolysis. The therapeutic effects are variable and unpredictable, some infants showing initial benefit with a subsequent return to hypoglycemia. Diazoxide in oral dosage up to 5–20 mg/kg/day orally 8-hourly is usually combined with chlorothiazide 7–10 mg/kg/day in two divided doses, which potentiates its effects and reduces the associated water retention. Both these agents activate potassium channels by different mechanisms, the diuretic also being given concurrently for its ability to overcome the fluid retaining effects of diazoxide. Other complications of diazoxide therapy include edema, non-ketotic–hyperosmolar coma, blood dyscrasias and generalized hypertrichosis. Nifedipine 0.25–2.5 mg/kg/day may be of value as an adjuvant therapy but the precise role of calcium channel blockers has not been defined. The advantages of the above treatments is that they can be given orally and second line drugs require intravenous or subcutaneous infusions. Glucagon infusions at rates between 5 and 10 μg/kg/h in isolation, or at 1.0 μg/kg/h combined with the synthetic somatostatin analog octreotide 10 μg/kg/h may be useful. Surgery may have to be considered in infants where hypoglycemia is still a significant problem despite adequate medical treatment. There is no diagnostic metabolic or endocrine test to distinguish a diffuse pancreatic disorder from an adenoma in a newborn or infant. In older children distinguishing an adenoma from diffuse hyperplasia is now potentially possible using percutanous transhepatic pancreatic venous sampling for insulin, glucose and C-peptide to identify 'hot spots' of insulin hypersecretion. Where no tumor is localized pre- or perioperatively, subtotal or total pancreatectomy may have to be considered, balancing the detrimental effects of hypoglycemia against postpancreatectomy diabetes. The management recommended above is consistent with the consensus view of the European network for research into hyperinsulinism (for further details see Aynsley-Green et al[1047]).

Inborn errors of metabolism

Glycogen storage disease (p. 1206)

Type I glycogen storage disease, glucose-6-phosphatase deficiency and associated transporter defects, may present in its severest form in the neonatal period with hepatomegaly, profound hypoglycemia and lactic acidosis.[1048]

Hepatic gluconeogenic enzyme deficiencies

Fructose-1,6-diphosphatase (p. 1204) deficiency causes a similar biochemical profile to glucose-6-phosphatase deficiency with fasting hypoglycemia, lactic acidosis, ketosis, hyperuricemia and hyperlipidemia. Hepatomegaly in this condition is secondary to lipid accumulation.

Phosphoenolpyruvate carboxykinase converts oxaloacetic acid to phosphoenolpyruvate. Defects of the enzyme restrict the utilization of lactate and gluconeogenic amino acids and this results in hypoglycemia, lactic acidosis and hyperalaninemia.

Pyruvate carboxylase converts pyruvate to oxaloacetic acid and deficiency will limit gluconeogenesis from lactate and alanine. Hypoglycemia may not be a prominent feature as other gluconeogenic amino acids can enter the tricarboxylic acid cycle and be converted through oxaloacetic acid to glucose.

Galactosemia (p. 1202)

Galactosemia commonly presents in the neonatal period with vomiting, diarrhea, failure to thrive, cataracts, hyperbilirubinemia and hypoglycemia.

Defects in amino acid metabolism

Maple syrup urine disease (p. 1185) in neonates may present with vomiting, failure to thrive, a characteristic odor and hypoglycemia with a rapid progression to severe neurological symptoms.

3-hydroxy-3-methylglutaryl-CoA lyase deficiency (HMG-CoA lyase deficiency) (p. 1200) is usually classified as a disorder of leucine metabolism with biochemical features of hypoglycemia, hyperammonemia and metabolic acidosis without ketonuria. Initial presentation may be in infancy, early childhood or the neonatal period.

Methylmalonic acidemia (p. 1186) and proprionic acidemia (p. 1186) can present in the neonatal period with hypoglycemia and metabolic ketoacidosis.

Mitochondrial defects of fatty acid oxidation

Medium chain or general acyl-CoA dehydrogenase (MCAD) deficiency (p. 1198). This is the commonest of the inborn errors of mitochondrial fatty acid catabolism and crises are commonly precipitated by infectious episodes with fever, diarrhea, vomiting, poor feeding, lethargy and coma. Hepatomegaly is inconsistently found but if biopsy is performed shows fatty infiltration. Hypoglycemia is always present. Plasma ammonia may be normal or slightly elevated. Ketonuria is classically absent or inappropriately low. MCAD deficiency has been reported as a cause of sudden and unexpected death in infants. The diagnosis of MCAD deficiency can be made by DNA molecular analysis (90% have a common allelic variant) and/or plasma acylcarnitines.[1049] The severity of clinical symptoms can be prevented by frequent meals, additional carbohydrate intake during stress and supplements of carnitine if required.

Long chain acyl-CoA dehydrogenase (LCAD) deficiency (p. 1199). Attacks of hypoglycemia and hypotonia occur with hepatocardiomegaly during episodes of exacerbation. In a few infants a sensorimotor neuropathy or pigmentary retinopathy has been described.[1049] The earliest presentation of LCAD deficiency was thought to be 2 months until the case report of Chalmers et al[1050] who described a sudden neonatal death at 31 h in a full-term infant who was appropriately grown and without dysmorphic features. Liver, kidneys and muscle showed fatty infiltration.

Hormone deficiencies

Congenital hypopituitarism. Early hypoglycemia may be a presenting feature. Infants are usually at term, normally grown and without other central nervous system defects but there may be a conjugated or unconjugated hyperbilirubinemia. In affected males external genitalia may be small with micropenis. A few infants have associated midline defects including cleft lip and palate or septo-optic dysplasia. Pituitary hormone deficiencies may be partial or complete and are usually multiple. Cortisol and thyroid replacement may be required from the newborn period.

Cortisol deficiency states. Hypoglycemia may be seen in congenital adrenal hyperplasia, bilateral adrenal hemorrhage and congenital adrenal hypoplasia.

Congenital glucagon deficiency. Two cases have been reported and hypoglycemia described in both.

Investigation of hypoglycemia

The majority of infants will have transient hypoglycemia associated with a clinical risk factor (Table 10.126) and do not require extensive investigation. If hypoglycemia persists or is recurrent the infant should be investigated. The priority of investigations may be determined by clinical features or a family history of inborn errors of metabolism or sudden infant death syndrome.

Hypoglycemia should always be confirmed by formal laboratory analysis using a method specific for glucose. Fluoride oxalate tubes should be used to inhibit glycolysis. Glucose requirements of the infant should be calculated in mg/kg/min.

Investigations include a full blood count to exclude polycythemia, a blood gas to determine the presence of a metabolic acidosis and plasma electrolytes, essential if adrenal dysfunction is suspected.

Plasma should be collected at the time of hypoglycemia for insulin, C-peptide, ketone bodies (usually beta-hydroxybutyrate), amino acids, lactate, growth hormone, cortisol and ACTH levels. Blood for insulin and ACTH should be collected into lithium heparin tubes, immediately stored on ice and plasma separated within 20 min. Prior discussion with the investigating laboratory is essential.

Urine should be collected at around the time of hypoglycemia and screened for pH, reducing compounds (Clinitest), ketones and keto acid with 2,4-dinitrophenylhydrazine and for the variety of compounds that react with ferric chloride. Urine should also be analyzed directly for amino acid and organic acids.

Table 10.126 Causes of neonatal hypocalcemia

Neonatal hypocalcemia
Early
Late (neonatal tetany)
Primary hypoparathyroidism
Sporadic
X-linked, autosomal dominant or recessive
DiGeorge syndrome
Maternal hyperparathyroidism
Vitamin D deficiency
Vitamin D dependency
Rickets/osteopenia of prematurity
Primary hypomagnesemia

These investigations may yield the definitive diagnosis or guide to further more specific investigation or analysis. Acylcarnitine profiles using tandem mass spectrometry on dried blood spots are increasingly being used as a diagnostic tool for disorders of intermediate metabolism. Complete characterization of a metabolic defect may require provocation or loading tests or enzyme studies on fibroblasts, leukocytes or tissue biopsies or analysis of DNA.

HYPERGLYCEMIA

Hyperglycemia in the newborn is defined as a blood glucose > 7 mmol/L after a 4 h fast and this value may be used in the diagnosis and subsequent management of the rare phenomenon of transient neonatal diabetes mellitus.

Hyperglycemia in preterm infants

Hyperglycemia is commonly seen in non-fasting preterm infants where blood glucose concentrations >10 mmol/L are not uncommon, may occasionally exceed 20 mmol/L and are most frequently associated with either dextrose infusions or parenteral nutrition. The pathogenesis of this hyperglycemia is uncertain and may include failure to suppress endogenous glucose production, an attenuated insulin release or a decrease in end-organ sensitivity to insulin.[1051] Some regimens for parenteral nutrition include insulin to control not only the hyperglycemia but to improve anabolism and activate lipid clearance.

The adverse effects of hyperglycemia include osmotic diuresis and dehydration, an increase in plasma osmolality and generation of a metabolic acidosis through lactate production.

Blood glucose values which constitute hyperglycemia in preterm infants are not well defined. Most consider it desirable to maintain blood glucose < 10 mmol/L either by decreasing the amount of dextrose infused or prescribing insulin 0.05–0.1 IU/kg. Careful monitoring of blood glucose at least hourly is essential and intermittent doses of insulin are often preferred to a continuous infusion. Whether to control moderate hyperglycemia, 5–10 mmol/L, depends on clinical circumstances. Renal glucose thresholds can be as low as 5 mmol/L in extremely preterm infants and a glucose-induced osmotic diuresis might be an indication to treat with insulin.

Hyperglycemia is also associated with infection, intracranial hemorrhage, severe RDS, NEC, or with pain. Aminophylline and dexamethasone may exacerbate hyperglycemic tendencies.

Hyperglycemia in full-term infants

Early postnatal hyperglycemia has been described in association with compensatory responses to birth asphyxia. The mechanism is thought to involve rapid mobilization of hepatic glycogen by a combination of glucagon and epinephrine (adrenaline) secretion and suppression of insulin release. Early hypoglycemia is much more common in this group although late hyperglycemia and instability of glucose homeostasis is seen in severely birth asphyxiated infants who often have associated hepatic damage.

Transient diabetes mellitus

The onset of permanent diabetes mellitus is rare in infants less than 6 months of age. A transient form of diabetes mellitus may present as early as the first postnatal day or as late as 6 weeks of age. The infants are usually small for gestational age and present, in spite of adequate nutrition, as failure to thrive with wasting and dehydration but with a characteristic 'alert appearance'. Blood glucose levels are variable and may be as low as 13 mmol/L or as high as 110 mmol/L. Glycosuria leads to dehydration which may be rapid in onset and severe. Ketonuria is absent or minimal, in contrast to later-onset permanent diabetes mellitus. Insulin levels are inappropriately low for blood glucose concentrations. Management consists of correction of the dehydration and insulin to achieve normoglycemia. A few infants can be managed without continuation of insulin but the majority require regular insulin in dosage varying from 1 to 3 IU/kg/day for periods as short as 14 days or as long as 18 months. These infants are extremely insulin sensitive. After initial correction of dehydration and establishment of enteral feeds they can usually be managed on a once or twice daily insulin regimen. In the majority, the dose of insulin can be tapered slowly before completely stopping.

In most instances, the condition is sporadic in occurrence although familial cases are reported with a few infants born to diabetic mothers. The etiology of transient diabetes mellitus is thought to be a temporary delay in maturation of beta cell function and control. A few infants have been reported where there was an initial period of hypoglycemia, but within 3–14 days this gave way to hyperglycemia and transient diabetes mellitus. Permanent diabetes mellitus or later recurrence has been reported in a few individuals.

Leprechaunism. A constellation of mutations in the insulin receptor gene give rise to this syndrome of IUGR with minor dysmorphic features and characterized by insulin resistance, elevated plasma insulin levels and glucose intolerance. Infants usually die in the first year of life.

DISORDERS OF CALCIUM AND MAGNESIUM METABOLISM

Normal fetal and neonatal calcium homeostasis

In utero, there is an active movement of calcium from mother to fetus such that by term the concentrations of total and ionized calcium in fetal blood are approximately 10% higher than maternal values. This relatively hypercalcemic state suppresses fetal parathormone secretion and stimulates calcitonin release, conditions which favor fetal mineral deposition. After birth, the infant parathyroid remains suppressed and this transient hypoparathyroid state results in a fall in plasma calcium. In the normal term infant, the plasma calcium decreases during the first 24–72 h after birth, reaching values as low as 1.75–2.0 mmol/L. This state of relative hypocalcemia stimulates parathormone release and suppresses calcitonin secretion. Calcium levels gradually increase to within the normal range for infants by 4–5 postnatal days. This transition in calcium metabolism is usually without clinical features but symptomatic hypocalcemia develops if these mechanisms are delayed or exaggerated.

Hypocalcemia

Mild functional asymptomatic hypocalcemia occurs normally within the first few days of life but levels which constitute biochemical hypocalcemia can be defined as a corrected plasma calcium < 1.75 mmol/L or an ionized calcium < 0.625 mmol/L. Such infants are at risk of symptomatic hypocalcemia.

Calcium is present in plasma in three fractions: (a) protein bound (30–50%); (b) diffusible non-ionized calcium chiefly in complexes with citrate or phosphate (5–15%); and (c) in an ionized state. The ionized state is the metabolically active form but dynamic equilibrium and interchange occurs between calcium in the various plasma fractions. Approximately 80% of protein-bound calcium is attached to albumin and the remaining 20% to globulin. Changes in pH influence calcium binding to albumin and acidosis results in an increased ionized calcium and alkalosis a decrease in ionized calcium.

Clinical assessment of ionized calcium can be made by electrocardiographic observations of the corrected QT interval

(QTc interval) measuring the time from the origin of the Q wave to the origin of the T wave; it is prolonged > 0.19 s in full-term infants and > 0.20 s in preterm infants who have a low ionized calcium value.

There are a number of clinical conditions where hypocalcemia is the presenting feature (Table 10.127) but the commonest of these is early neonatal hypocalcemia.

Early neonatal hypocalcemia

The onset of early neonatal hypocalcemia is typically in the first few days of life and most often between 24 and 48 h. At greatest risk are LBW infants, both premature and growth retarded, birth asphyxiated infants and the infant of the diabetic mother.

Pathogenesis. The etiology of early neonatal hypocalcemia is usually multifactorial. Most symptomatic infants will have had suboptimal postnatal calcium intake. The postnatal rise in parathormone may be delayed in preterm infants, and indeed most infants with early neonatal hypocalcemia have low or undetectable levels of immunoreactive parathormone. Calcitonin levels are normally elevated in the early newborn period but exaggerated concentrations have been documented in premature as well as in asphyxiated hypocalcemic infants. Hyperphosphatemia as a result of hypoxemic tissue damage or excessive catabolism releasing phosphate may lead to hypocalcemia. An intracellular movement of calcium can occur after hypoxic cell injury with depression of plasma calcium levels. Acute respiratory alkalosis can occur in ventilated infants resulting in reduced ionized calcium. Sodium bicarbonate administration or the use of citrated blood in exchange transfusions may create a metabolic alkalosis. Elevated plasma fatty acids generated from intravenous lipid infusions have been reported to lower ionized calcium levels.

Insulin-dependent diabetic mothers tend to have lower plasma magnesium levels throughout pregnancy, and infants have lower cord and 24 h postpartum plasma levels of calcium and parathormone. Chronic maternal hypomagnesemia may cause relative hypoparathyroidism in both mother and fetus. The majority of infants of diabetic mothers are asymptomatic but may show biochemical evidence of hypocalcemia and/or hypomagnesemia. In symptomatic infants with both biochemical abnormalities, the hypocalcemia and hypomagnesemia can be corrected with magnesium treatment.

Table 10.127 Inborn errors of metabolism which may present as acute illness in the newborn period – see also Table 10.126 for metabolic diseases where hypocalcemia is a prominent feature

Disorders of amino acid metabolism
Maple syrup urine disease
Phenylketonuria
Tyrosinemia type I
Non-ketotic hyperglycinemia
Hyperbeta-alaninemia
Sulfite oxidase deficiency
5,10-Methylene tetrahydrofolate reductase deficiency
Methylmalonic acidemia
Propionic acidemia
Isovaleric acidemia
Beta-methylcrotonylglycinuria
Multiple carboxylase deficiency
Hydroxymethylglutaryl-CoA lyase deficiency
Beta-ketothiolase deficiency
2-Methylacetoacetyl-CoA thiolase deficiency
Urea cycle defects
N-acetylglutamate synthase deficiency
Carbamyl phosphate synthetase deficiency
Ornithine transcarbamylase deficiency
Citrullinemia
Argininosuccinic aciduria
Arginase deficiency

Clinical features and course. The symptoms and signs of early neonatal hypocalcemia occur when the calcium falls to < 1.75 mmol/L and can be difficult to differentiate from those of associated pathologies, e.g. HIE or intraventricular hemorrhage, or those of other metabolic abnormalities such as hyponatremia or hypoglycemia.

Management. Early enteral calcium supplementation has been shown to prevent early neonatal hypocalcemia in preterm infants. Gastrointestinal irritation and increased stool frequency are the only significant side-effects. The vitamin D metabolites, 25-hydroxycholecalciferol and 1,25-dihydroxycholecalciferol, are also effective in raising plasma calcium levels but are rarely used.

Infants whose only pathology is early neonatal hypocalcemia and who have neurological symptoms should be treated as described for late neonatal hypocalcemia. Measurement of the Q_0Tc interval can be a useful screening procedure to determine whether low ionized calcium is present in a particular infant. Calcium gluconate 10% (1 ml/kg) can be given intravenously but cautiously over 10 min with ECG monitoring. Decreases in heart rate require slowing of the intravenous infusion or discontinuation. Maintenance calcium gluconate can be given continuously intravenously or orally (75 mg/kg/day). Peripheral intravenous infusions if they extravasate may result in skin slough, tissue necrosis and calcification. The preferred method of maintenance, where there is no central line, is by the enteral route and calcium gluconate 10% 1–2 ml/kg 4- or 6-hourly is usually tolerated.

Late neonatal hypocalcemia (neonatal tetany)

Late neonatal tetany can be regarded as a form of transitory hypoparathyroidism but usually symptomatic hypocalcemia and tetany are only problematic in infants subsequently exposed to high phosphorus intake.

Pathogenesis. Primary maternal hyperparathyroidism complicating pregnancy is rare but a temporary maternal hyperparathyroid state, secondary to vitamin D deficiency, may be more common. That this type of neonatal hypocalcemia is related to maternal vitamin D deficiency is supported by nutritional studies and a seasonal incidence in spring and early summer in the northern hemisphere related to low sunshine exposure in the later months of pregnancy, with low levels of 25-hydroxycholecalciferol in both mothers and infants. Enamel hypoplasia is frequently found in affected infants and is indicative of disordered enamel formation during the last trimester of pregnancy. The mothers of infants with late hypocalcemia tend to be older, of higher parity and of lower social class than mothers of non-hypocalcemic infants.

Occurrence of neonatal tetany in a susceptible population is largely determined by the nature of the milk feed in the newborn period. Cows' milk contains three to four times as much phosphorus as human milk. Partially modified cows' milk formulae (particularly tinned evaporated milks), which still had a high phosphorus content, were used routinely until the mid-1970s when the incidence of neonatal tetany was as high as 1% of formula-fed infants. With the introduction of feeds with a calcium and phosphorus content approximating to that of human breast milk, neonatal tetany is now rare.

Clinical features. Late neonatal tetany usually occurs from the second half of the first week up to several weeks, classically in full-term infants born after a normal labor and delivery who are artificially fed. Although affected infants may have appeared a little jittery or tremulous with increasing tactile irritability of muscles, usually they have been otherwise well, feeding normally, responding normally and with a normal cry, before the sudden onset of convulsions.

Fits are usually transitory lasting for a few seconds and usually focal in nature and between convulsions the infant is alert. Jitteriness is evident on stimulation, the tendon reflexes are increased and increased muscle tone with extension, in the legs particularly, is usual. Trousseau's sign is seldom positive and Chvostek's sign, which can be elicited freely in the newborn infant, is of little value. Recovery may occur spontaneously, but in others fits may continue for several weeks unless treated.

Diagnosis. The diagnosis is based on a low serum calcium, < 1.75 mmol/L, and a high serum phosphorus, > 2.6 mmol/L. Occasionally the serum calcium is not markedly lowered and the raised phosphorus level is probably a more important diagnostic criterion. There is usually an associated hypomagnesemia but this is moderate in degree, in the range 0.5–0.6 mmol/L.

The differential diagnosis of neonatal tetany from other types of convulsions usually rests on the absence of an abnormal birth history, the normal behavior of the infant between the attacks, apart from muscular irritability, the absence of other signs which would indicate intracranial birth injury and the presence of normal or increased deep tendon reflexes.

Treatment. Treatment consists of calcium intravenously or orally usually in the form of calcium gluconate 10% solution 5 ml/kg/day. Vitamin D has also been used in a dosage of 5000 IU/day orally. Although hypocalcemia is the most obvious biochemical abnormality, the most effective treatment is intramuscular magnesium sulfate (0.2 ml/kg 50% solution per dose), particularly when convulsions are occurring; this can be followed with a further one or two doses at 12-hourly intervals. Intramuscular magnesium controls hypocalcemic tetanic fits more effectively than calcium, and calcium more effectively than phenobarbital.

Prognosis. The prognosis of neonatal tetany per se is good, most cases making full recovery without sequelae. Where the hypocalcemia is secondary to an underlying disorder, the prognosis will be of that disorder.

Hypoparathyroidism

Primary hypoparathyroidism is a rare cause of hypocalcemia in the newborn. The diagnosis is confirmed by absent or low parathormone levels in the presence of hyperphosphatemia, hypomagnesemia and low alkaline phosphatase. Sporadic cases occur but most have a genetic basis, usually X-linked recessive, but autosomal recessive and dominant forms have been described.

DiGeorge syndrome is usually sporadic in occurrence and results from an embryological defect of the 4th branchial arch and derivatives of the 3rd and 4th pharyngeal pouches. The pattern of defects includes hypoplasia or absence of the parathyroids, hypoplasia or absence of the thymus and cardiovascular anomalies including aortic and truncal abnormalities with minor facial anomalies. The severity of the congenital heart disease usually determines the early prognosis and the degree of hypoparathyroidism may be variable and transient forms have been described. The etiology is heterogeneous. Several different chromosomal abnormalities have been described but deletions at 22q11.2 are most frequent. Teratogenic causes including retinoic acid and fetal alcohol syndrome are also described. Treatment of hypoparathyroidism consists of supplementation with vitamin D_2 or its analogs 1alpha-hydroxycholecalciferol or 1,25-dihydroxycholecalciferol.

Maternal hyperparathyroidism

Primary maternal hyperparathyroidism is a rare complication of pregnancy with parathyroid adenomas usually responsible but carcinoma has been described. The maternal diagnosis depends on the demonstration of persistently high plasma calcium, elevated plasma parathormone and low urinary calcium and phosphorus. Complications in pregnancy include hyperemesis gravidarum, weakness, renal calculi, spontaneous abortion and late fetal death. The most common neonatal complication is hypocalcemic tetany, observed in around 50% of infants born to mothers with untreated disease. The unexpected occurrence of neonatal tetany may provide the initial clue to the diagnosis of unsuspected maternal hyperparathyroidism. The etiology of neonatal hypocalcemia is thought to reflect prolonged parathyroid suppression from the chronic hypercalcemic state of mother and fetus. However, some infants have normal or elevated parathormone levels and the etiology may be more complex.

The clinical features are those of neonatal tetany. Hypomagnesemia is a frequent occurrence. Most cases of neonatal hypocalcemia secondary to primary maternal hyperparathyroidism are transient but long term congenital hypoparathyroidism has been described.

Maternal medullary carcinoma of the thyroid

Maternal medullary carcinoma of the thyroid is associated with high calcitonin levels. In the one reported case of this disease, several children born prior to maternal diagnosis exhibited radiological features of osteopetrosis.

Hypercalcemia

Plasma calcium levels > 2.75 mmol/L (corrected) are generally regarded as constituting hypercalcemia. Clinical manifestations include weakness, irritability, hypotonia, poor feeding, weight loss, polyuria, polydypsia, constipation and vomiting. The major causes are idiopathic infantile hypercalcemia, hyperparathyroidism, benign familial hypercalcemia, and vitamin D intoxication, and hypercalcemia associated with inadequate phosphorus intake in extremely immature infants.[1052]

Hypomagnesemia

Plasma magnesium levels in the newborn infant are relatively constant through the first week of life (range 0.59–1.15 mmol/L). Hypomagnesemia, < 0.6 mmol/L, does not usually occur during the first few days of life, nor in association with asphyxia, but most commonly occurs towards the end of the first week and later.

Isolated hypomagnesemia can occur as a primary cause of convulsions but is usually associated with concomitant lowering of the plasma calcium as in late neonatal hypocalcemia. Milk formulae with high phosphorus loads predispose to hypocalcemia and also to hypomagnesemia. Neonatal hypomagnesemia is also associated with maternal malabsorption, to parathormone deficiency in the infant, to a primary defect of magnesium absorption in the infant (p. 000) or to magnesium binding by citrate in exchange transfusions.

Treatment of hypomagnesemia is by intramuscular injection of magnesium sulfate 50% 0.2 ml/kg dose. This can be repeated for one or two further doses at 12-hourly intervals. If both hypomagnesemia and hypocalcemia are present, treatment with calcium alone may be ineffective. Improvement may only be achieved after magnesium is prescribed and this often results in the spontaneous rise in serum calcium level. The role of magnesium in relieving the symptoms of hypocalcemia may be due to its capacity to release ionized calcium for effective parathyroid function.

METABOLIC BONE DISEASE IN PRETERM INFANTS

Defective bone mineralization has been recognized in preterm infants for many years but the terminology used to describe this is confusing. The terms *rickets of prematurity* or *osteopenia of prematurity* have been used synonymously. *Osteopenia of prematurity* refers to skeleton hypomineralization of the preterm infant compared to that resulting from in utero accretion of minerals.[1053] *Rickets of prematurity* implies the presence of radiologically detectable abnormalities, appearances which are historically related to vitamin D deficiency in children, but similar appearances can occur in preterm infants with severe metabolic bone disease. The term osteoporosis has been used to describe radiological rarefaction of bone and where this occurs without obvious rachitic changes represents a less advanced stage of metabolic bone disease. Substantial demineralization, quantified sensitively by means of photon absorptiometry or dual energy radiographic densitometry, can occur before radiological changes are obvious.

Pathogenesis

Bone formation is a complex process integrated by hormonal and growth factors and is dependent on an adequate supply of calcium, phosphorus, magnesium, trace metals such as copper, and vitamin D. Matrix formation is as critical as that of subsequent mineralization, and deficiencies at any stage of bone formation may give rise to the common final presentation of disordered bone growth. The etiology of metabolic bone disease in preterm infants is probably multifactorial but a major component is as a consequence of a deficiency of calcium and phosphorus.

The vitamin D status of the infant at birth is largely dependent on the adequacy or otherwise of maternal vitamin D metabolism. In humans, 25-hydroxycholecalciferol crosses the placenta with a close correlation between maternal and cord blood levels both in term and preterm infants. Term infants approximate maternal values but preterm infant levels of 25-hydroxycholecalciferol may be significantly lower. Serum 1,25-dihydroxycholecalciferol levels show no correlation between maternal and cord blood samples, consistent with the concept that the fetoplacental unit is its own source of 1,25-dihydroxycholecalciferol in utero.

The preterm infant may not have full expression of hepatic 25-hydroxylation of vitamin D but the majority of studies would support the concept that this ability appears to be achieved very early in postnatal life. Adequate serum levels can be achieved using vitamin D supplements as low as 400–500 IU/day for the first 1–3 months of life. Preterm infants are also capable of 1alpha-hydroxylation of vitamin D, based on serum estimation of 1,25-dihydroxycholecalciferol, which rises sharply during the first week of life when infants are supplemented with very high vitamin D intakes. On more physiological dosage regimens of vitamin D, 500 IU/day, lower increments of 1,25-dihydroxycholecalciferol are seen over the first week of life but gradually reach maximal values around 3–4 weeks postnatal age. The absorption of vitamin D is dose related and facilitated by bile salts; a low bile salt pool in preterm infants and a diet high in polyunsaturated fatty acids might predispose to a degree of malabsorption of vitamin D. The evidence of significantly increasing hydroxylated derivatives of vitamin D in vitamin D-supplemented preterm infants suggests that this ability is not significantly impaired.

Calcium, unlike phosphorus, is not well absorbed from formula milks. The higher bioavailability in human milk can result in 70% absorption provided that phosphorus and vitamin D contents are adequate. In term milks, the absorption of calcium is in the range of 30–60%, and 80–95% of this absorbed calcium can be retained. Calcium absorption increases with both gestational age and postnatal age. Postnatal age effects may be a reflection of gastrointestinal adaptation to calcium adequacy or deficiency. Absolute calcium retention increases with the amount of calcium ingested and with higher calcium intakes can be greater in preterm infants than occurs in utero. The concentration of calcium in the formula is therefore important, as is the quantity of milk consumed.

Preterm infants absorb phosphorus very efficiently (86–97% of intake) independent of the type of milk or the calcium or phosphorus concentration of that milk. Retention of absorbed phosphorus appears to be directly related to the rates of calcium and nitrogen retention. Calcium and phosphorus absorption are relatively independent. The renal absorption of phosphorus can be almost complete in preterm infants but fractional phosphorus excretion can be increased if phosphorus is supplied in excess, either in absolute terms or in conditions of relative excess, if calcium is deficient.

The in utero accretion of calcium rises exponentially in the last trimester from 114 to 125 mg/kg/day (2.89–3.12 mmol/kg/day) at 26 weeks to 119–151 mg/kg/day (2.97–3.77 mmol/kg/day) at 36 weeks' gestation. Phosphorus accretion over this gestational age range is 60–85 mg/kg/day (1.94–2.74 mmol/kg/day).

The calcium and phosphorus contents of human milk or term formulae cannot meet the requirements of the preterm infants if accretion of these elements is to continue at intrauterine rates. For example, an extreme preterm infant fed a commercial term formula at 150 ml/kg/day would have a calcium intake of 65 mg/kg/day (1.6 mmol/kg/day) and a phosphorus intake of 40 mg/kg/day (1.6 mmol/kg/day). If the infant typically absorbed 50% of the calcium intake and 90% of the phosphorus intake, then this would give an absorbed calcium of only 32 mg/kg/day (0.8 mmol/kg/day) and a phosphorus of 36 mg/kg/day (1.2 mmol/kg/day) available for retention. Comparison of these figures with the in utero accretion rates shows how wide the deficits can be between prenatal and postnatal life.

Histological studies have shown that metabolic bone disease in neonates differs from that of classical vitamin D deficiency rickets with markedly reduced matrix formation and decreased osteoblastic activity perhaps suggesting contributions from other deficiencies. However, more recent histomorphometric studies suggest increased bone resorption rather than impaired formation underlies the development of metabolic bone disease in preterm infants.[1054] Copper deficiency in preterm infants can easily be confused where the radiological findings are of osteoporosis, flaring of anterior ribs, cupping and flaring of metaphyseal regions of long bones and subperiosteal new bone formation. It is equally possible that deficiencies in other nutrients may contribute to metabolic bone disease in preterm infants and, for example, when preterm infants are supplemented with calcium, magnesium absorption and retention decreases, with phosphorus having an additive effect. In these infants, magnesium supplementation can increase absorption and retention and dietary magnesium intakes may have to be higher (10–20 mg/kg/day) than those previously recommended (5–6 mg/kg/day).[1055]

Clinical features

The largest number of reports of metabolic bone disease are in extreme preterm infants. Skeletal mineralization may be compromised by prolonged intravenous nutrition with its inherent limitation of mineral intake as well as concerns about aluminum contamination, fluid restriction resulting in decreased intakes of calcium and phosphorus, prolonged immobility, chronic acidosis, treatment with dexamethasone or furosemide (frusemide) and the use of non-supplemented human breast milk. Many of these factors are common to infants receiving prolonged intensive care and defective mineralization is not specific or more severe in groups with bronchopulmonary dysplasia as was thought in the past.

In the majority of infants with metabolic bone disease there are no overt findings on clinical examination and the diagnosis is dependent on the results of investigation. Occasionally, clinical features are present in preterm infants with well-established and severe rachitic disease (Fig. 10.70). Metabolic bone disease in preterm infants can be associated with impairment of linear growth, spontaneous fractures and chronic respiratory distress.

Investigation and monitoring

Bone mineral content, usually of the forearm, can be measured directly with photon absorptiometry and when specifically calibrated for small infants, can be precise and accurate.[1057] Bone mineralization is assessed relative to body weight or ulnar length and compared to a gestational age curve which represents in utero mineralization. Until recently, photon absorptiometry, although primarily a research tool, has been the only viable technique for the accurate assessment of the state of bone mineralization.[1058]

Photon absorptiometry is both sensitive and precise but it is expensive and the equipment bulk makes it impractical for routine use. Dual energy radiographic densitometry overcomes these difficulties.[1059] Radiographic densitometry has the advantage that bone mineral content can be assessed along the length of a bone or comparison easily made between bones. This may be important as bone mineralization is not uniform and wider assessment of the state of mineralization could be a major advantage.[1060]

The radiological changes of rickets in preterm infants are cupping and fraying of the metaphyses together with the loss of the

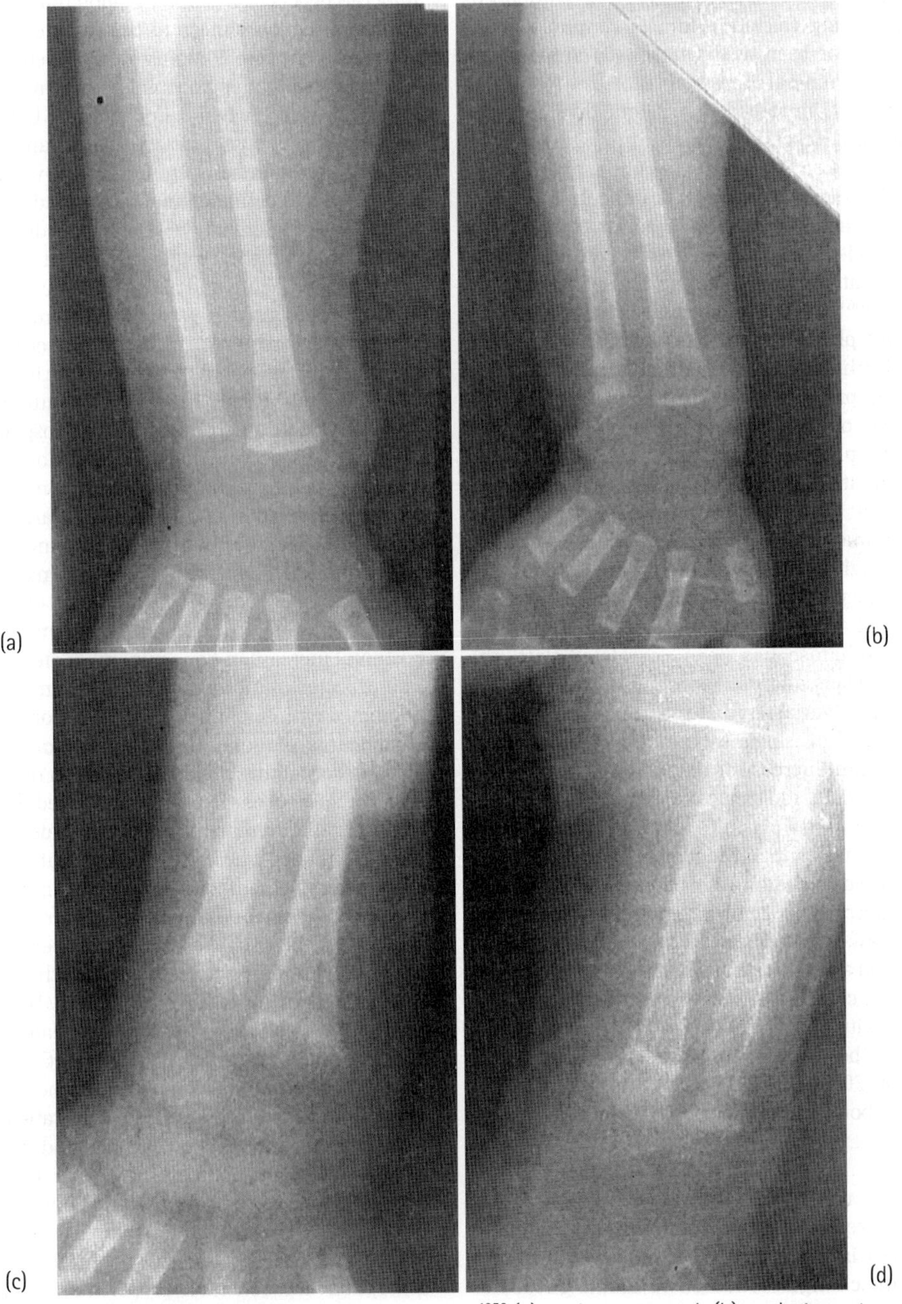

Fig. 10.70 X-ray grading of changes of rickets of prematurity at the wrist:[1056] (a) grade 0 = normal; (b) grade 1 = osteopenia only; (c) grade 2 = cupping and fraying of ulnar metaphysis; (d) grade 3 = spontaneous fracture in association with grade 2 changes. (X-rays by kind permission of Professor N. McIntosh.)

provisional zone of calcification (Fig. 10.70). Periosteal reactions and fractures of bone may also occur. Substantial demineralization has to occur before radiological changes become apparent and a dependence solely on radiological methods will seriously underestimate the extent of the spectrum of metabolic bone disease. Measurement of cortical thickness as a means of studying bone formation similarly lacks precision in the study of bone mineralization.

In formula-fed infants, plasma calcium and phosphorus values are not good indicators of early metabolic bone disease with plasma calcium only falling significantly in the most severely affected infants with overt radiological rickets and phosphorus values often remaining unchanged. In infants fed human milk, phosphorus depletion is commonly recognized and characterized by hypophosphatemia, hypercalcemia, hypercalciuria, hypophosphaturia and elevated levels of plasma alkaline phosphatase. Prolonged absence of phosphorus from the urine with persisting calcinuria implies continued tissue phosphorus depletion and has been used sequentially in individual infants to assess the need for mineral supplementation.

Measurement of vitamin D metabolites has limited value in the diagnosis or management of rickets of prematurity.

The use and interpretation of plasma alkaline phosphatase activity as a marker of bone metabolism can be difficult in preterm infants. Reference values have been established for total plasma alkaline phosphatase activity in cord blood from preterm and term infants and it appears that the bone alkaline phosphatase is the predominant isoenzyme.[1061] The liver isoenzyme is undetectable in preterm and term infant plasma. Plasma fetal intestinal alkaline phosphatase is low at birth both in term and preterm infants but increases dramatically in preterm infants in the postnatal period, peaking at around 2 weeks of age when it may contribute up to 30% of the total activity in plasma. Thereafter peak plasma fetal intestinal alkaline phosphatase activity declines to negligible levels by 6–7 weeks' postnatal age. The postnatal rise is related to gestational age and is marked in infants less than 34 weeks' gestation but rises only slightly in term infants. In preterm infants, total plasma alkaline phosphatase activity in the third trimester decreases with gestational age in infants 5–10 days postnatal age and total alkaline phosphatase has been correlated with the radiological features of rickets and used to monitor the effects of metabolic studies. The wide variability between individual infants makes its usefulness limited on single samples[1062] but sequential measurements from an infant increase its diagnostic value.

In spite of these constraints, radiological appearances of rickets crudely correlate with total plasma alkaline phosphatase measurements although not with osteopenia[1062] or with bone mineral content as measured by photon absorptiometry. Equally high total plasma alkaline phosphatase activity, representing metabolic bone disease in preterm infants, has been related to slower growth rates in the neonatal period and to a significant reduction in attained length at 12 years.[1063] A combination of the criteria serum total alkaline phosphatase activity above 900 IU/L and serum inorganic phosphate concentrations below 1.8 mmol/L yields a sensitivity of 100% at a specificity of 70%. This is probably the best available screening method for low bone mineral density in preterms.[1064]

Management

The key to management of this disorder must be prevention, with a sufficient nutritive intake from early postnatal life to allow mineralization to proceed in a manner which avoids clinical and overt radiological rachitic changes. Whether we should go further than this goal and attempt to achieve 'normal' mineralization in all preterm infants using in utero mineral accretion rates is an unresolved question.[1065]

Although vitamin D deficiency is not a major factor in the etiology of metabolic bone disease of preterm infants, it facilitates normal mineralization and should be supplemented to around 500–1000 IU/day. In established metabolic bone disease, modest increases in vitamin D intake, 1000–2000 IU/day, are still used for short periods in conjunction with mineral supplementation. Regular monitoring is essential to avoid hypercalcemia, a particular problem with the hydroxylated derivatives of vitamin D – 1alpha-hydroxycholecalciferol and 1,25–dihydroxycholecalciferol.

Metabolic balance studies have shown that with calcium and phosphorus supplementation of term formulae, which have a mineral composition similar to that of human milk, postnatal retention of calcium and phosphorus can approximate intrauterine accretion.[1066] Comparison of intrauterine accretion and postnatal retention of minerals depends on the assumption that the chemical growth of the preterm infant is similar to that of the fetus in utero. This is not necessarily the case. Photon absorptiometric studies have shown that the preterm infant approaching term may have a bone mineral deficit as much as 30% when compared with full-term infants. Long term studies have shown that preterm infants have a rapid phase of mineral accretion between 40 and 60 weeks' postconceptional age which reduces perinatal mineralization deficits that might otherwise persist into childhood.[1058] Ziegler[1067] discusses this dilemma and emphasizes that the avoidance of overt bone disease should be the criterion for calcium and phosphorus need, rather than the necessity to achieve fetal accretion rates or in utero rates of mineralization. On this basis the requirement of the preterm infant for calcium and phosphorus is probably greater than the intake from human milk but less than that needed to achieve intrauterine accretion rates. The problem is how much calcium and phosphorus is required to avoid overt bone disease and how this need should be assessed.

The calcium and phosphorus concentrations in milk from mothers of preterm and term infants are similar and a premature infant fed 150 ml/kg/day receives an intake of around 55 mg/day (1.3 mmol/day) of calcium and 22 mg/day of phosphorus (0.5 mmol/day). Sequential measurements of bone mineral content in preterm infants fed human breast milk have shown that the postnatal increase in bone mineral content is significantly less than that expected in utero. Supplementation of maternal milk has been attempted with calcium or phosphorus or both, addition of skimmed components of donor human milk, mixing maternal milk with formula containing high concentration of calcium and phosphorus and the use of proprietary powdered fortifiers. Indiscriminate fortification of human milk is to be avoided and reserved for extreme preterm infants where this type of nutrition is the major dietary source. Supplementation with calcium or phosphorus, salts or sugars may result in increased osmolality, dilution of other constituents if mineral solutions are used, precipitation of salts and potentially undesirable intakes of other nutrients. Phosphorus supplements of up to 9 mg/dl (13 mg/100 cal) have been used to maintain the plasma phosphorus greater that 1.5 mmol/dl and avoiding excess urinary calcium losses. Calcium supplements should not be given without a proportionate amount of phosphorus in order to maintain the calcium : phosphorus ratio in the range of 1.4–2.0. Simultaneous additions of calcium and phosphorus salts to milks may result in precipitation. This can be avoided by adding the phosphorus first (usually disodium phosphate) and then calcium (usually calcium gluconate/glubionate). Diverse salts of calcium and phosphorus have been used to supplement preterm feeds and the absorption and retention properties vary. Mineral solubility may limit absorption and retention and absolute mineral content of the feeds cannot be the sole criterion on which selection is made and more attention should be focused on bioavailability.

The American Academy of Pediatrics,[1068] on the basis of estimated fetal requirements, has advised enteral intakes of calcium 185–210 mg/kg/day (4.6–5.2 mmol/kg/day) and phosphorus 123–140 mg/kg/day (4–4.6 mmol/kg/day) for infants between 26 and 31 weeks' gestation. To achieve these intakes, assuming a fluid intake of 150 mg/kg/day, milk formulae would have a calcium content of 126–140 mg/dl (3.1–3.5 mmol/dl) and phosphorus 82–93 mg/dl (2.7–3.1 mmol/dl). A more cautious approach has been adopted by ESPGAN Committee on Nutrition,[1065] representing European opinion, where recommended calcium content of formulae would be between 56 and 112 mg/dl (1.4–3.8 mmol/dl) with a phosphorus content 40–72 mg/dl (1.3–2.3 mmol/dl). LBW formulae currently available in the UK have calcium contents in the range 70–110 mg/dl (1.7–2.7 mmol/dl) and phosphorus 35–60 mg/dl (1.2–2.0 mmol/dl), compositions not optimal to meet mineral requirements if intrauterine accretion rates are to be attained but levels which should avoid overt bone disease. The number of studies using calcium- and phosphorus-supplemented milks, to the levels recommended by the American Academy of Pediatrics, are still small and they have only given limited information as to their efficacy, desirability or potential drawbacks. Excess dietary calcium can cause supermineralization in preterm infants, impede fat absorption as well as that of other minerals and lead to the risk of nephrocalcinosis.

Parenterally fed preterm infants are at particular risk of inadequate supply of calcium and phosphorus.[1069] The solubility and stability of mineral substrate in parenteral solutions depends on a number of factors and precipitation of salts can occur readily, resulting in blocked lines and the potential for microembolization of crystalline particles. Most parenteral nutrition regimens can routinely achieve intakes of calcium of 1.5 mmol/kg/day and phosphorus 1.0 mmol/kg/day. By prescribing increased amounts of calcium and phosphorus only when fluid and amino acid intakes are appropriate, avoiding prolonged standing times, using the more soluble calcium gluconate rather than the chloride and only adding calcium and phosphorus to already diluted parenteral solutions, precipitation can be avoided and intakes of calcium around 2.0 mmol/kg/day and phosphorus 1.7 mmol/kg/day can be achieved.

NEONATAL PRESENTATION OF INBORN ERRORS OF METABOLISM

Major advances have been made in the recognition and understanding of many inborn errors of metabolism. Prenatal diagnosis is available for a number of conditions allowing parents to avoid recurrence of serious disease or early management and treatment to avoid deleterious effects on the developing fetus or neonate. Increasingly successful treatment regimens are being devised but the outcome may depend on the earliest possible recognition and institution of therapy. Only a minority of inborn errors of metabolism are routinely screened for in the newborn and early recognition is often dependent on maintaining a high index of clinical suspicion and a low threshold for sometimes basic and sometimes complex biochemical investigations. This is particularly true where inborn errors can present as acute and serious illness in the newborn period.[1070]

The aim of this review is to consider what inborn errors of metabolism can present in the newborn period and their clinical features. Although investigation and management will be discussed, details of individual inborn errors of metabolism will be found in Chapter 24 and will be cross-referenced.

Acute metabolic disorders

A number of metabolic disorders can present with acute overwhelming symptoms in the newborn period particularly the urea cycle defects, organic acidemias and certain aminoacidopathies (Table 10.128). The majority of these disorders have no detrimental effects on fetal development because placental perfusion can correct the disordered metabolic accumulation. As a consequence, the majority of infants are full term, of normal growth, without dysmorphic features and asymptomatic at birth. An exception to this generalization is where the primary defect is in cerebral metabolism as occurs in non-ketotic hyperglycinemia (p. 000). These infants may be born with established brain damage and have clinical features of hypertonia, lethargy, poor feeding and seizures, both grand mal and myoclonic. Other similar conditions include primary lactic acidosis, pyridoxine dependent seizures and primary molybdenum deficiency.

Fetal disorders of fatty acid oxidation can predispose the mother to acute fatty liver of pregnancy and the HELLP syndrome of hemolysis, elevated liver enzymes, and low platelet count (see e.g. Matern et al[1071]).

Many of the disorders are inherited as autosomal recessives and there may be a family history of consanguinity, previous perinatal loss or sudden and unexpected death in infancy. Autopsy findings may have been non-specific and unrevealing unless specific biochemical investigations were done. A few inborn errors of metabolism have other patterns of inheritance, for example X-linked recessive in ornithine transcarbamylase deficiency (p. 1179).

Clinical features

The initial symptoms are usually non-specific with lethargy, poor feeding, poor weight gain and vomiting. Diarrhea is less common but occurs in galactosemia (p. 1202) and hereditary tyrosinemia (p. 1174).

In the case of the infant who is well at birth, the onset of symptoms may be within a few hours of the first milk feed or may be delayed several weeks. The relationship to milk feeds and protein load may be further emphasized when the initial symptoms resolve with a period of intravenous fluids to recur again when milk feeds resume.

Progressive accumulation of intermediate metabolites may have neurotoxic effects and encephalopathic symptoms may accompany the presentation with apnea, periodic respirations, hypotonia, hypertonia, decerebrate rigidity, seizures and coma.

The clinical features may mimic the presentation of an acute neonatal infection. Indeed sepsis is a common accompaniment of acute exacerbations of metabolic disease as occurs in maple syrup

Table 10.128 Metabolic storage disorders which may be suspected in neonates

Glycogen storage diseases
Type I, glucose-6-phosphatase system deficiencies
Type II, Pompe's disease, alpha-1,4-glucosidase deficiency
Type III, debrancher deficiency
Type IV, brancher deficiency
Lipid storage diseases
GM1 gangliosidosis type I
Gaucher's disease
Niemann–Pick disease
Wolman's disease
Farber's disease
Mucolipidoses
Type I, sialidosis
Type II, I-cell disease
Mucopolysaccharidoses
Type VII, beta-glucuronidase deficiency
Glycoprotein storage disease
Fucosidosis

urine disease (p. 1185), galactosemia (p. 1202) or the mitochondrial disorders of fatty acid oxidation (p. 1221). Certain metabolic disorders may predispose to the risk of infection, for example infants with type I glycogen storage disease (p. 1201).

Clinical examination may be unrevealing. Tachypnea may indicate an underlying metabolic acidosis. Hepatomegaly, if present, classically occurs in the glycogen storage disorders, galactosemia and fructose-1,6-diphosphatase deficiency (p. 1204), but has been described in some infants with urea cycle defects, disorders of mitochondrial fatty acid oxidation and some aminoacidopathies. Cataracts can occur in newborn infants with galactosemia. Dislocated lens, characteristic of homocystinuria (p. 1175) and sulfite oxidase deficiency (p. 1177), have been described in the first month of life. Abnormal hair fragility can be present in some infants with argininosuccinic aciduria (p. 1179).

The majority of infants with acute metabolic disease do not have congenital anomalies but dysmorphic features are characteristic of some metabolic disorders such as multiple acyl-CoA dehydrogenase deficiency. Ambiguous genitalia occur in association with congenital adrenal hyperplasia.

Abnormal urinary odors may accompany metabolic disorders: phenylketonuria, mousy or musty; maple syrup urine disease, maple syrup or burnt sugar; isovaleric acidemia and glutaric acidemia type II, sweaty feet and beta-methylcrotonylglycinuria of cat urine.

Initial laboratory investigations

Infants suspected of acute metabolic disease require basic investigations not only for clinical management and resuscitation but to begin to determine the nature of the inborn error. Initial investigations should include blood gases, plasma electrolytes, plasma calcium and magnesium, blood glucose and lactate, blood ammonia and a full blood count. Valuable information can be gained by urine screening tests for pH, glucose (Clinistix), reducing compounds (Clinitest), ketones and keto acids with 2,4-dinitrophenylhydrazine and for the variety of compounds that react with ferric chloride. Urinary creatinine may be useful for standardization of subsequent investigations. These basic investigations should be available in all laboratories and be completed rapidly.

The differential diagnosis and the diseases which may be detected by Clinitest, ferric chloride and 2,4–dinitrophenylhydrazine testing of urine are discussed in Chapter 24.

Metabolic acidosis. This is frequently present in acutely ill infants with galactosemia, gluconeogenic disorders, glycogen storage disease and particularly the organic acidemias (Tables 10.127 and 10.128). Infants with organic acidemias may have a significant anion gap. Secondary lactic acidosis is common seen in neonatal medicine secondary to infection, hypoperfusion syndromes, or indeed secondary to other metabolic disorders such as the organic acidemias, urea cycle disorders and fatty acid oxidation defects. Primary lactic acidoses occur in disorders of pyruvate metabolism and mitochondrial respiratory chain disorders (p. 1219).

Hyperammonemia. A high blood ammonia is present in the primary enzyme defects of the urea cycle (Table 10.127) and is exacerbated by high protein loads whether this is from milk or endogenous catabolism. Secondary hyperammonemia is often seen in the defects of mitochondrial fatty acid oxidation and the organic acidemias and recently described in hyperinsulinemia (p. 1248). Delayed ontogeny of the urea cycle in preterm infants, particularly those receiving high protein loads, may result in severe hyperammonemia. Blood urea may be inappropriately low in the presence of defects of the urea cycle.

Hypoglycemia. This is the predominant feature of the primary defects of carbohydrate metabolism and of mitochondrial fatty acid oxidation but can be present in disorders of amino acid metabolism or organic acidemias. Hypoglycemia is frequently present as part of the acute metabolic derangements in maple syrup urine disease, methylmalonic acidemia, glutaric acidemia type II and hydroxymethylglutaryl-CoA lyase deficiency (Tables 10.127 and 10.128). The list is not exhaustive but illustrates the overlap in presentations and the importance of blood glucose estimations in the investigation, monitoring and treatment of suspected metabolic disease.

Liver transaminases and direct hyperbilirubinemia. Elevated plasma alanine or aspartate aminotransferases are secondary to hepatotoxicity and may be found in galactosemia, type III glycogen storage disease, disorders of mitochondrial fatty acid oxidation and in the urea cycle defects (Tables 10.127 and 10.128). Indirect hyperbilirubinemia is a common accompaniment to a wide range of newborn illnesses. A direct hyperbilirubinemia occurs in those diseases which damage the liver, in particular galactosemia, fructose intolerance and tyrosinemia, but is also seen in the later stages of the presentation of urea cycle defects, mitochondrial respiratory chain disorders, and alpha$_1$ antitrysin deficiency.

Thrombocytopenia and neutropenia. These can be features of methylmalonic acidemia, propionic acidemia, isovaleric acidemia and lysinuric protein intolerance. In addition neutropenia has been described in carbamyl phosphate synthetase deficiency and non-ketotic hyperglycinemia and glycogen storage disease type Ib. Defective platelet function and bleeding may be a feature of type I glycogen storage disease (Tables 10.127 and 10.128). The presence of neutropenia and or thrombocytopenia can be indices of sepsis in the newborn infant without an underlying inborn error of metabolism.

Anemia. Anemia can be found in association with methylmalonic aciduria and some of the aminoacidopathies.

Detailed laboratory investigation

If hyperammonemia, unexplained metabolic acidosis, or hypoglycemia is present then it must be assumed that the symptoms are secondary to an inborn error of metabolism and the infant thoroughly investigated.[1072] This may require urine and plasma samples to be sent to a specialist laboratory. In general the full range of tests described below may have to be performed, but a priority order of investigations can be made on the basis of clinical features and the results of initial laboratory investigations, e.g. in the case of a vomiting infant with hypoglycemia and a urine positive for reducing substances, urine sugar chromatography will be the first priority to exclude galactosemia. Collaboration and discussion with personnel in a specialist center or laboratory is essential and investigations can be organized for each specific patient. Not all sick newborn infants with metabolic disease need have hypoglycemia, metabolic acidosis or hyperammonemia. For example infants with non-ketotic hyperglycinemia may have severe encephalopathic features but unrevealing initial investigations. Detailed metabolic investigation can be worth pursuing even when initial laboratory results are unsupportive.

Semiquantitative analysis of urinary amino acids can be made relatively rapidly by thin layer or paper chromatography. A complete quantitative amino acid analysis of plasma, CSF or urine is made by automated ion exchange chromatography and may take 12–24 h. Thin layer chromatography of sugars is semiquantitative but rapid and usually diagnostic. Urinary organic acids may initially be analyzed by gas–liquid chromatography but preferably by gas chromatography–mass spectrometry which can analyzed from a dried blood spot. Lactate and pyruvate are generally measured in plasma but urinary lactate measurements have been advocated for the differentiation of a primary from a secondary lactic acidosis. Acylcarnitine profiles using tandem mass spectrometry on dried blood spots are increasing being used as a diagnostic tool.

These investigations may give a definitive diagnosis or one where there is a high index of suspicion of a known inborn error to allow specific treatment to begin. Complete characterization of an inborn error of metabolism may require enzyme studies on fibroblasts, leukocytes or tissue biopsies including DNA analysis.

Acute management of severe metabolic disease

Cardiorespiratory homeostasis and the correction of biochemical abnormalities are the priorities. The extent of resuscitative measures will depend on the clinical state of the infant and often must be instituted before a definitive diagnosis has been established.

Intravenous fluids are given as 10% dextrose solutions, the volume/kg/h will depend on the state of hydration and the presence of renal dysfunction. Hypoglycemia and hypocalcemia should be corrected. Hyperglycemia can potentiate the generation of lactate and should be avoided. This is particularly important for patients with pyruvate dehydrogenase complex defects where a high carbohydrate load can dramatically accentuate the acidosis.

If the infant has a metabolic acidosis with no respiratory acidosis or a compensatory respiratory alkalosis, the metabolic acidosis should be corrected with sodium bicarbonate initially with boluses to raise the pH to around 7.25 and then maintained if necessary by a slow intravenous infusion. If the infant has a combined respiratory and metabolic acidosis with hypoventilation secondary to cerebral depression, the respiratory component is firstly corrected by ventilatory support and then the metabolic acidosis corrected. During this resuscitative phase, a mild respiratory alkalosis (PCO_2 4.0–4.5 kPa) can be induced by hyperventilation, which may assist in correcting a very low pH as well as having beneficial effects on the control of cerebral edema. Oxygen should be given as required to maintain normal arterial saturation. Muscle paralysis with ventilatory support may have a specific role in severe lactic acidosis reducing the peripheral production. Blood gases and electrolytes should be monitored frequently.

Good tissue perfusion and oxygenation is essential to avoid secondary lactic acidosis. In correction of hypotension it may be more appropriate to use an inotropic agent such as dopamine rather than a high protein load of plasma or blood. As perfusion improves, the metabolic acidosis may worsen as peripheral lactate is brought into the circulation. Convulsive episodes may accentuate anaerobic metabolism and should be treated initially with intravenous phenobarbital.

Vitamins are essential cofactors for some enzymes and in certain conditions where cofactor function is abnormal reduced enzyme activity will result. Enzyme activity in some instances can be increased by prescribing vitamins in doses approximately 10–100 times the daily requirement. In the situation of the critically ill infant without as yet a specific diagnosis, the empirical use of multivitamins is justified and should include thiamin (50–500 mg), riboflavin (20–50 mg), biotin (10–100 mg), nicotinamide (400–600 mg), pyridoxine (10–100 mg), vitamin B_{12} (1–2 mg), folic acid (15–30 mg), ascorbic acid (300–3000 mg), pantothenic acid (30–50 mg). Multivitamin preparations for intravenous use are available. Secondary carnitine deficiency is common in many metabolic disorders especially fatty acid oxidation defects and organic acidemias and should be given 100–200 mg/kg/day intravenously by continuous infusion or in divided doses orally.

Protein catabolism can exacerbate most of these disorders and once the infant's condition is stable and the acute metabolic derangements have been corrected, calories can be increased by gradual increments of intravenous 20% dextrose. Hyperglycemia is to be avoided as it may exacerbate metabolic acidosis and insulin 0.05–0.1 IU/kg can be used to maintain blood glucose <10 mmol/L. Insulin may also increase anabolism and can be used regularly 4- to 6-hourly. Once the infant is stabilized on this regimen and to maintain anabolism, protein and lipids are introduced either by the enteral or parenteral route. Protein can be commenced at 0.25–0.5 g protein/day and if tolerated increased by the same amount daily to reach 1.5 g/kg/day with an aimed caloric intake of 120 kcal/kg/day.

Specific treatments

Where investigations have led to a definitive diagnosis or where there is a high index of suspicion of an inborn error, specific treatment can be instituted. In urea cycle defects a combination of dietary therapy and the use of drugs to provide alternative pathways for nitrogen excretion can be successful. Arginine functions as an essential amino acid and supplementation will allow excretion of additional nitrogen. Amino acid nitrogen can be excreted as hippuric acid if sodium benzoate is given or as phenylbutylglutamine after administration of phenylbutyrate. The use of medications alone may be sufficient, but dialysis may also be necessary. Hemodialysis and hemodiafiltration are more effective than peritoneal dialysis, and the methods of choice in the initial treatment of urea cycle defects, maple syrup urine disease, and the organic acidemias. Exchange transfusion should be reserved for exceptional circumstances.[1073]

Dietary modifications have been particularly successful in phenylketonuria (p. 1172) and galactosemia (p. 1202). Supplementations of vitamin B_{12} in methylmalonic aciduria (p. 1186), carnitine in organic acidemias (p. 1183), biotin in carboxylase deficiencies (p. 1188) and pyridoxine in homocystinuria (p. 1175) have been successful in some individuals. Alteration of the ratio of fat : carbohydrate : protein in the diet or the frequency of feeding have been used in the management of type I glycogen storage disease (p. 1206), fructose-1,6-diphosphatase deficiency (p. 1204) and the mitochondrial disorders of fatty acid oxidation[1049] (p. 1219).

Investigations where death is inevitable

The situation may arise where death is inevitable but the exact definitive diagnosis of an inborn error of metabolism has not been conclusively established. In these circumstances it is important that the fullest information be obtained to advise parents of the risks of recurrence in subsequent pregnancies. An autopsy is vital and should preferably be performed soon after death. The majority of parents, with skilled counseling, will give postmortem permission before the infant dies. At autopsy liver, kidney, skeletal muscle, cardiac muscle and areas of brain thought to be involved should be fixed for light and electron microscopy. Duplicate frozen tissue samples suitable for cryostat sections should be obtained. Skin or pericardial fibroblast cultures should be established. A substantial amount of each tissue should be snap frozen as 0.5 cm^3 cubes in liquid nitrogen and stored at –70°C for subsequent enzyme analysis. Certain disorders particularly those of membrane associated enzymes where there is a transport function or where the membrane is important for regulatory function or where the enzyme itself is sensitive to freeze–thaw may best be analyzed on fresh tissue. Specialist advice should be sought. Some parents will agree only to a limited postmortem, for example wedge biopsy or needle biopsy of liver with skin samples for culture from the incision site. In these circumstances all available urine and plasma should be frozen and stored at –70°C. Blood should be taken into EDTA tubes for subsequent DNA extraction, and a blood spot on a screening card for tandem mass spectrometry.

Suspected metabolic storage disorders

Metabolic storage disorders which may present in the newborn period are shown in Table 10.128 but often symptoms and a diagnosis may be delayed into infancy or childhood depending on the severity of the enzyme deficiency or the rate of expression of pathognomonic features. Infants with glycogen storage disease may have hepatomegaly with or without obvious hypoglycemic symptoms. Pompe's disease, type II glycogen storage disease (p. 1243), is not associated with hypoglycemia but infants may have macroglossia, hypotonia, hepatomegaly and cardiomegaly with cardiac failure. In addition to type II glycogen storage disease, cardiac failure and cardiomyopathy may suggest a mitochondrial respiratory chain defect, or a long chain fatty acid oxidation disorder, and Barth syndrome in the presence of neutropenia.[1074]

The clinical features of the mucopolysaccharidoses (p. 1239) are rarely fully expressed in the newborn period and a Hurler-like phenotype with coarse facies, macroglossia, limited growth and skeletal abnormalities is more likely to be a lipid or mucolipid storage disorder particularly GM1 gangliosidosis type I (p. 1244) or I-cell disease (p. 1242).

The acute infantile variant of Niemann–Pick disease (p. 1237), Gaucher's disease (p. 1235) and Wolman's disease (p. 1239) may present in the newborn period with hepatosplenomegaly, feeding difficulties, vomiting, choking, cyanotic episodes, failure to thrive and disorders of tone. Gastrointestinal symptoms are particularly marked in Wolman's disease with diarrhea and abdominal distention in addition to vomiting.

Congenital disorders of glycosylation are rare and involve abnormal glycosylation of certain glycoproteins. The features are variable with cardiomyopathy, pericardial effusions, failure to thrive, abnormal fat distribution and facial dysmorphism.

Metabolic disorders associated with dysmorphic features

Inborn errors of metabolism may be associated with dysmorphic features suggesting that metabolic derangements in utero have disrupted normal fetal ontogeny, for example congenital adrenal hyperplasia in females is associated with ambiguous genitalia.

Peroxisomal disorders

Disorders of peroxisomal biogenesis as well as deficiencies in peroxisomal enzymes may present in the newborn period.[1075]

***Zellweger syndrome* (cerebrohepatorenal syndrome).** This autosomal recessive condition has a number of characteristic clinical features. Craniofacial abnormalities may include a high forehead, flat occiput, wide sutures and fontanel, absent orbital ridges, micrognathia, redundant neck skin folds, external ear abnormalities and a high arched palate. The neurological features include hypotonia, poor feeding, nystagmus, hypo- or areflexia, psychomotor retardation and seizures. The brain is abnormal with disordered neuronal migration. Hepatomegaly is characteristic with prolonged jaundice, elevated transaminases and a progression to cirrhosis. The kidneys may show multiple cysts. Ocular abnormalities include cataracts, retinal pigmentation, optic disc pallor and Brushfield spots. Radiologically stippled calcification of the patella or acetabulum may be present. The clinical expression includes milder forms of the disorder (for review see Lazarow et al[1075]).

Neonatal adrenoleukodystrophy. The clinical syndrome and symptoms may be indistinguishable from Zellweger syndrome.[1075] The presence of skeletal stippling or renal cysts at autopsy have not been encountered in neonatal adrenoleukodystrophy.

Infantile Refsum's disease. This condition was originally described as an association between elevated plasma phytanic acid in infants with craniofacial dysmorphism, ocular abnormalities, hepatomegaly and psychomotor retardation with peroxisomes absent or deficient.

Rhizomelic chondrodysplasia punctata. This condition is inherited as an autosomal recessive and is characterized by short stature, symmetrical rhizomelia with marked shortening of the humerus and femur and punctate calcification around the epiphysis with coarse irregularity of the metaphyses. Severe psychomotor retardation, hepatomegaly and craniofacial dysmorphism with cataracts and corneal changes complete the clinical picture.[1075]

Hyperpipecolic acidemia. This syndrome is characterized by elevated pipecolic acid in plasma, minor dysmorphic features, optic disc pallor, retinal pigmentation, psychomotor retardation and hepatomegaly with abnormal liver function progressing to cirrhosis. The postmortem findings show adrenal abnormalities, renal cysts, normal neuronal migration in the brain and normal peroxisomes in liver but a disturbance in multiple peroxisomal function.

Zellweger-like phenotype with structurally intact peroxisomes. The biochemical defect in this group is confined to disorders of very long chain fatty acid oxidation or bile salt metabolism but with intact peroxisomes and include peroxisomal 3-oxoacyl-CoA thiolase deficiency peroxisomal acyl-CoA oxidase deficiency and peroxisomal bifunctional enzyme deficiency.

Mitochondrial electron transport chain defects

Multiple acyl-CoA dehydrogenase deficiencies (MAD) or glutaric acidemia type II. MAD deficiency is classified into two variant forms, a severe (MAD-S) neonatal form or glutaric aciduria type II and a mild (MAD-M) variant with later onset.

In the severe neonatal form (MAD-S) two subgroups have been identified, those with congenital abnormalities and those without congenital abnormalities. In MAD-S deficiency with congenital abnormalities, characteristically the infants are born prematurely and may be growth retarded but develop a metabolic acidosis in the first 24 h of life with a characteristic odor of 'sweaty feet'. All patients have died in the first week of life. Neonatal MAD-S deficiency is associated with congenital abnormalities including facial dysmorphism, polycystic kidneys or some form of cystic dysplasia, cerebral abnormalities including disorders of migration, pulmonary hypoplasia, hypospadias and minor abnormalities of nail or palmar creases. At autopsy fatty infiltration of the liver, heart and kidneys is present. In MAD-S deficiency without congenital abnormalities the clinical course is similar with acidosis, hypoglycemia and odor with death occurring rapidly. Both types are a result of deficiencies of electron transport chain flavoprotein or its oxidoreductase. In MAD-M deficiency the clinical presentation is heterogeneous with first symptoms in the neonatal period, childhood or adulthood and characterized by vomiting, acidosis and hypoglycemia.

Riboflavin responsive defects of beta-oxidation or riboflavin responsive multiple acyl-CoA dehydrogenase deficiencies (RR-MAD). Some patients presenting with a Reye-like syndrome or hypoglycemia in the first years of life with defects in beta-oxidation have been shown to be responsive to riboflavin. The biochemical etiology remains to be confirmed but a therapeutic trial with riboflavin should be attempted in all patients presenting with an organic aciduria suggesting a MAD deficiency.

Disorders of cholesterol biosynthesis

Smith–Lemli–Opitz syndrome. Smith–Lemli–Opitz syndrome is a syndrome of mental retardation and multiple congenital malformations. The defect is thought to be in the gene coding for the enzyme 3beta-hydroxysteroid-delta^7-reductase with the consequence of reduced conversion of 7-dehydrocholesterol to cholesterol and a reduction in plasma and tissue levels of cholesterol with an increase in 7-dehydrocholesterol. The common dysmorphic features are hypospadias, ambiguous genitalia, syndactyly of the toes, microcephaly, blond hair, anteverted nares, low set ears, palatal abnormalities, mignognathia, congenital heart disease and renal abnormalities. Severe feeding problems are common requiring nasogastric or gastrostomy feeding. Cholesterol supplementation of the diet may increase plasma cholesterol and in some has beneficial effects. Other disorders of cholesterol biosynthesis can result in dysmorphic features but are not as well characterized as Smith–Lemli–Opitz syndrome.[1076]

Miscellaneous conditions with newborn presentations

Crigler–Najjar syndrome; cystic fibrosis, alpha$_1$-antitrypsin deficiency; Menkes' kinky hair syndrome, hypophosphatasia; hereditary orotic aciduria; glucose-6-phosphate dehydrogenase deficiency; pyruvate kinase deficiency; pyridoxine-dependent convulsions; congenital erythropoietic porphyria; aminolevulinate dehydratase porphyria (Ch. 24).

REFERENCES (* Level 1 evidence)

DEFINITIONS – WORLD HEALTH ORGANIZATION

1 Human Embryo and Fertilisation Act 1990. London: HMSO; 1990.

EPIDEMIOLOGY AND EVIDENCE BASED NEONATAL CARE

2 Platt MJ. Child health statistics review. Arch Dis Child 1998; 79:523–527.

3 Liu JM, Li S, Lin Q, et al. Prevalence of cerebral palsy in China. Int J Epidemiol 1999; 28:949–954.

4 Pharoah PO, Cooke T, Johnson MA, et al. Epidemiology of cerebral palsy in England and Scotland 1984–9. Arch Dis Child Fetal Neonatal Ed 1998; 79:F21–F25.

5 Hagberg B, Hagberg G, Beckung E, et al. Changing panorama of cerebral palsy in Sweden. VIII. Prevalence and origin in the birth year period 1991–94. Acta Paediatr 2001; 90:271–277.

6 Kavcic A, Perat MV. Prevalence of cerebral palsy in Slovenia: birth years 1981–1990. Dev Med Child Neurol 1998; 40:459–463.

7 Robertson CM, Svenson LW, Joffres MR. Prevalence of cerebral palsy in Alberta. Can J Neurol Sci 1998; 25:117–122.

8 Stanley FJ, Watson L. Trends in perinatal mortality in Western Australia 1967 to 1985. BMJ 1992; 304:1658–1663.

9 Donoghue D. The report of the Australian and New Zealand Neonatal Network, 2000. Sydney: Aust N Z Network Neurol; 2002.

10 Tin W, Milligan DW, Pennefather P, et al. Pulse oximetry, severe retinopathy, and outcome at one year in babies of less than 28 weeks gestation. Arch Dis Child Fetal Neonatal Ed 2001; 84:F106–F110.

11 International Neonatal Network, Scottish Neonatal Consultants, Nurses Collaborative Study Group. Risk adjusted and population based studies of the outcome for high risk infants in Scotland and Australia. Arch Dis Child Fetal Neonatal Ed 2000; 82:F118–F123.

*12 Kenyon SL, Taylor DJ, Tarnow-Mordi W; ORACLE Collaborative Group. Broad-spectrum antibiotics for preterm, prelabour rupture of fetal membranes: the ORACLE I randomised trial. ORACLE Collaborative Group. Lancet 2001; 357:979–988.

*13 Early versus delayed neonatal administration of a synthetic surfactant – the judgment of OSIRIS. The OSIRIS Collaborative Group (open study of infants at high risk of or with respiratory insufficiency – the role of surfactant. Lancet 1992; 340:1363–1369.

14 Peto R, Baigent C. Trials: the next 50 years. Large scale randomised evidence of moderate benefits. BMJ 1998; 317:1170–1171.

*15 The Cochrane Library. http://www.update-software.com/cochrane/default.HTM. accessed 12/4/02.

16 De Simone C, Delogu G, Corbetta G. Intravenous immunoglobulins in association with antibiotics: a therapeutic trial in septic intensive care unit patients. Crit Care Med 1988; 16(1):23–26.

17 Dominioni L, Dionigi R, Zanello M, et al. Effects of high-dose IgG on survival of surgical patients with sepsis scores of 20 or greater. Arch Surg 1991; 126(2):236–240.

*18 Grundmann R, Hornung M. Immunoglobulin therapy in patients with endotoxemia and postoperative sepsis – a prospective randomized study. Prog Clin Biol Res 1988; 272:339–349.

*20 Schedel I, Dreikhausen U, Nentwig B, et al. Treatment of gram-negative septic shock with an immunoglobulin preparation: a prospective, randomized clinical trial. Crit Care Med 1991; 19(9):1104–1113.

21 Wesoly C, Kipping N, Grundmann R. [Immunoglobulin therapy of postoperative sepsis. Z Exp Chir Transplant Kunstliche Organe 1990; 23(4):213–216.

22 Chen JY. Intravenous immunoglobulin in the treatment of full-term and premature newborns with sepsis. J Formos Med Assoc 1996; 95:839–844.

23 Erdem G, Yurdakok M, Tekinalp G, Ersoy F. The use of IgM-enriched intravenous immunoglobulin for the treatment of neonatal sepsis in preterm infants. Turk J Pediatr 1993; 35(4):277–281.

24 Haque KN, Zaidi MH, Bahakim H. IgM-enriched intravenous immunoglobulin therapy in neonatal sepsis. Am J Dis Child 1988; 142(12):1293–1296.

*25 Shenoi A, Nagesh NK, Maiya PP, et al. Multicenter randomized placebo controlled trial of therapy with intravenous immunoglobulin in decreasing mortality due to neonatal sepsis. Indian Pediatr 1999; 36(11):1113–1118.

26 Weisman LE, Cruess DF, Fischer GW. Current status of intravenous immunoglobulin in preventing or treating neonatal bacterial infections. Clin Rev Allergy 1992; 10(1-2):13–28.

*27 Alejandria MM, Lansang MA, Dans LF, et al. Intravenous immunoglobulin for treating sepsis and septic shock (Cochrane Review). In: The Cochrane Library, Issue 1, 2002. Oxford: Update Software.

28 Richardson DK, Gray JE, McCormick MC, et al. Score for neonatal acute physiology: a physiologic severity index for neonatal intensive care. Pediatrics 1993; 91:617–623.

29 The International Neonatal Network. The CRIB (clinical risk index for babies) score: a tool for assessing initial neonatal risk and comparing performance of neonatal intensive care units. Lancet 1993; 342:193–198.

30 Maier RF, Rey M, Metze BC, et al. Comparison of mortality risk: a score for very low birthweight infants. Arch Dis Child Fetal Neonatal Ed 1997; 76:F146–F150.

31 Richardson D, Tarnow-Mordi WO, Lee SK. Risk adjustment for quality improvement. Pediatrics 1999; 103(1 suppl E):255–265. (Review)

32 Parry GJ, Gould CR, McCabe CJ, et al. Annual league tables of mortality in neonatal intensive care units: longitudinal study. International Neonatal Network and the Scottish Neonatal Consultants and Nurses Collaborative Study Group. BMJ 1998; 316(7149): 1931–1935.

33 UK Neonatal Staffing Study Collaborative Group. Patient volume, staffing, and workload in relation to risk-adjusted outcomes in a random stratified sample of UK neonatal intensive care units: a prospective evaluation. Lancet 2002; 359:99–107.

34 Mant J, Hicks N. Detecting differences in quality of care: the sensitivity of measures of process and outcome in treating acute myocardial infarction. BMJ 1995; 311:793–796.

35 Scottish Neonatal Consultants' Collaborative Study Group and International Neonatal Network. Trends and variations in use of antenatal corticosteroids to prevent neonatal respiratory distress syndrome: recommendations for national and international comparative audit. Br J Obstet Gynaecol 1996; 103:534–540.

THE ECONOMICS OF NEWBORN CARE

36 Macfarlane A, Mugford M. Birth counts: statistics of pregnancy and childbirth, 2nd edn. London: The Stationery Office; 2000.

37 Gennaro S. Leave and employment in families of preterm low birthweight infants. Image – The Journal of Nurse Scholarship 1996; 28:193–198.

38 Ladden M. The impact of preterm birth on the family and society: transition to home. Part 2. Pediatr Nurs 1990; 16:620–622, 626.

39 Warner KE, Luce BR. Cost-benefit and cost-effectiveness analysis in health care:

principles, practice and potential. Ann Arbor, Michigan: Health Administration Press; 1982.
40 Finkler SA. The distinction between costs and charges. Ann Intern Med 1982; 96:102–109.
41 Broughton PMG, Hogan TC. A new approach to the costing of clinical laboratory tests. Ann Clin Biochem 1981; 18:330–342.
42 Drummond MF, Jefferson TO on behalf of the BMJ Economic Evaluation Working Party. Guidelines for authors and peer reviewers of economic submissions to the BMJ. BMJ 1996; 313:275–283.
43 Chalmers I, Enkin M, Kierse MJNC. Effective care in pregnancy and childbirth: a synopsis for guiding practice and research. In: Chalmers I, Enkin M, Kierse MJNC, eds. Effective care in pregnancy and childbirth. Oxford: Oxford University Press; 1989:1465–1477.
44 Rosser RM, Kind P. A scale of valuations of states of illness: is there a social consensus? Int J Epidemiol 1978; 7:347–358.
45 Torrance GW, Feeny D. Utilities and quality-adjusted life years. Int J Technol Assess Health Care 1989; 5:559–575.
46 Mehrez A, Gafni A. Quality-adjusted life years, utility theory, and healthy-years equivalents. Med Decis Making 1989; 9:142–149.
47 Nord E. An alternative to QALYs: the saved young life equivalent (SAVE). BMJ 1992; 305:875–877.
48 Boyle MH, Torrance GW, Sinclair JC, et al. Economic evaluation of neonatal intensive care of very-low-birthweight infants. N Engl J Med 1983; 308:1330–1337.
49 Kitchen WH, Bowman E, Callanan C, et al. The cost of improving the outcome for infants of birthweight 500–999 g in Victoria. J Paediatr Child Health 1993; 29:56–62.
50 Walker DB, Feldman A, Vohr BR, et al. Cost-benefit analysis of neonatal intensive care for infants weighing less than 1000 grams at birth. Pediatrics 1984; 74:20–24.
51 Walker DB, Vohr BR, Oh W. Economic analysis of regionalized neonatal care for very low-birth-weight infants in the state of Rhode Island. Pediatrics 1985; 76:69–74.
52 Briggs A, Sculpher M. Sensitivity analysis in economic evaluation of health care technologies: the role of sensitivity analysis. Health Econ 1995; 4:355–372.
53 Petrou S, Mugford M. Predicting the costs of neonatal care. In: Hansen TN, McIntosh N, eds. Current topics in neonatology. Vol. 4. London: WB Saunders; 2000:149–174.
54 Briggs AH, Gray AM. Handling uncertainty when performing economic evaluation of healthcare interventions. Health Technol Assess 1999; 3(2):1–134.

THE NORMAL FETAL–NEONATAL TRANSITION

55 Bisset WM, Watt JB, Rivers JPA, et al. Postprandial motor response of the small intestine to enteral feeding in pre-term infants. Arch Dis Child 1989; 64:1356–1361.
56 Smith CA, Nelson NM. Physiology of the newborn, 4th edn. Springfield: Charles C Thomas; 1976.

EXAMINATION OF THE NEONATE

57 Wren C, Richmond S, Donaldson L. Presentation of congenital heart disease in infancy: implications for routine examination. Arch Dis Child 1999; 80:F49–F53.
58 Ward-Platt MP. Newborn screening examination (excluding congenital dislocation of the hip). Semin Neonatol 1998; 3:61–66.
59 Hall DMB, ed. Health for all children, 3rd edn. Oxford: Oxford University Press; 1996.
60 National Screening Committee. First report of the national screening committee. Health Departments of the United Kingdom. London: Department of Health; 1998. Also www.open. gov.uk/doh/nsc/nsch.htm
61 Wilson JMG, Jungner G. Principles and practice of screening for disease. Public Health Paper No 34. Geneva: World Health Organization; 1968.
62 Cochrane AL, Holland WW. Validation of screening procedures. Br Med Bull 1971; 27:3–8.
63 Taylor D, Rice NSC. Congenital cataract, a cause of preventable child blindness. Arch Dis Child 1982; 57:165–167.
64 Taylor D. Congenital cataract: the history, the nature and the practice. Eye 1998; 12:9–36.
65 Rogers GL, Tishler CL, Tsou BH, et al. Visual acuities in infants with congenital cataracts operated on prior to 6 months of age. Arch Ophthalmol 1981; 99:999–1003.
66 Rahi JS, Dezateux C. National cross sectional study of detection of congenital and infantile cataract in the United Kingdom: role of childhood screening and surveillance. BMJ 1999; 318:362–365.
67 Silove ED. Assessment and management of congenital heart disease in the newborn by the district paediatrician. Arch Dis Child 1994; 70:F71–F74.
68 Richmond S, Wren C. Early diagnosis of congenital heart disease. Semin Neonatol 2001; 6:27–35.
69 Wren C, Richmond S, Donaldson L. Temporal variability in birth prevalence of cardiovascular malformations. Heart 2000; 83:414–419.
70 Ainsworth SB, Wyllie JP, Wren C. Prevalence and significance of cardiac murmurs in neonates. Arch Dis Child 1999; 80:F43–F45.
71 Abu-Harb M, Hey E, Wren C. Death in infancy from unrecognised congenital heart disease. Arch Dis Child 1994; 71:3–7.
72 Leck I. Congenital dislocation of the hip. In: Wald N, Leck I, eds. Antenatal and neonatal screening. Oxford: Oxford University Press; 2000.
73 Standing Medical Advisory Committee. Screening for the detection of congenital dislocation of the hip in infants. London: Department of Health and Social Security; 1969.
74 Godward S, Dezateux C. Surgery for congenital dislocation of the hip in the UK as a measure of outcome of screening. Lancet 1998; 351:1149–1152.
75 Chan A, Cundy PJ, Foster BK, et al. Late diagnosis of congenital dislocation of the hip and presence of a screening programme: South Australian population-based study. Lancet 1999; 354:1514–1517.
76 Gardiner HM, Dunn PM. Controlled trial of immediate splinting versus ultrasonographic surveillance in congenitally dislocatable hips. Lancet 1990; 336:1553–1556.
77 Langkamer VG, Clarke NMP, Witherow P. Complications of splintage in congenital dislocation of the hip. Arch Dis Child 1991; 66:1322–1325.
78 Committee on Quality Improvement and Subcommittee on Developmental Dysplasia of the Hip. Clinical practice guideline: early detection of developmental dysplasia of the hip. Pediatrics 2000; 105:896–905.
79 Lehmann HP, Hinton R, Morello P, et al. Developmental dysplasia of the hip practice guideline: technical report. Committee on Quality Improvement, and Subcommittee on Developmental Dysplasia of the Hip. Pediatrics 2000; 105:e57.
80 Scorer CG, Farrington G. Congenital deformities of the testis and epididymis. London: Butterworths; 1971:15–27.
81 Lee PA, O'Leary LA, Songer NJ, et al. Paternity after bilateral cryptorchidism. A controlled study. Arch Pediatr Adolesc Med 1997; 151:260–263.
82 Swerdlow AJ, Higgins CD, Pike MC. Risk of testicular cancer in a cohort of boys with cryptorchidism. BMJ 1997; 314:1507–1511.
83 Colodny AH. Undescended testes – is surgery necessary? N Engl J Med 1986; 314:510–511.
84 Hadziselimovic F. Pathogenesis of cryptorchidism. In: Kogan SJ, Hafez ESE, eds. Pediatric andrology. Vol 7. The Hague: Martinus Nijhoff; 1981:147–162.
85 Lee TWR, Skelton RE, Skene C. Routine neonatal examination: effectiveness of trainee paediatrician compared with advanced neonatal nurse practitioner. Arch Dis Child 2001; 85:F100–F104.

LABOR WARD ROUTINES

*86 Wiswell TE, Gannon CM, Jacob J, et al. Delivery room management of the apparently vigorous meconium-stained neonate: results of the multicenter, international collaborative trial. Pediatrics 2000; 105:1–7.
87 Lundström KE, Pryds O, Greisen G. Oxygen at birth and prolonged cerebral vasoconstriction in preterm infants. Arch Dis Child Fetal Neonatal Ed 1995; 73:F81–F86.
88 Mercer JS. Current best evidence: a review of the literature on umbilical cord clamping. J Midwifery Womens Health 2001; 46:402–414.

POSTNATAL WARD ROUTINES

89 Danielson B, Castles AG, Damberg CL, et al. Newborn discharge timing and readmissions: California 1992–1995. Pediatrics 2000; 106:31–39.
90 Laing IA, Wong CM Hypernatraemia in the first few days: is the incidence rising? Arch Dis Child Fetal Neonatal Ed. 2002; 87:F158–162.
91 Ebbesen F. Recurrence of kernicterus in term and near-term infants in Denmark. Acta Paediatr 2000; 89:1213–1217.
*92 Zupan J, Garner P. Topical umbilical cord care at birth. Cochrane Database Syst Rev 2000; 2:CD001057.

FEEDING THE FULL-TERM NEWBORN

93 Howie PW, Forsyth JS, Ogston SA, et al. Protective effect of breastfeeding against infection. BMJ 1990; 300:11–16.

94 Gillman MW, Rifas-Shiman SL, Camargo CA Jr, et al. Risk of overweight among adolescents who were breastfed as infants. JAMA 2001; 285:2461–2467.
95 Thompson NP, Montgomery SM, Wadsworth ME, et al. Early determinants of inflammatory bowel disease: use of two national longitudinal birth cohorts. Eur J Gastroenterol Hepatol 2000;12(1):25–30.
96 Corrao G, Tragnone A, Caprilli R, et al. Risk of inflammatory bowel disease attributable to smoking, oral contraception and breastfeeding in Italy: a nationwide case-control study. Cooperative Investigators of the Italian Group for the Study of the Colon and the Rectum (GISC). Int J Epidemiol 1998; 27(3):397–404.
97 Ivarsson A, Hernell O, Stenlund H, et al. Breast-feeding protects against celiac disease. Am J Clin Nutr 2002; 75(5):914–921.
98 Peters U, Schneeweiss S, Trautwein EA, et al. A case-control study of the effect of infant feeding on celiac disease. Ann Nutr Metab 2001; 45(4):135–142.
99 Plagemann A, Harder T, Franke K, et al. Long-term impact of neonatal breast-feeding on body weight and glucose tolerance in children of diabetic mothers. Diabetes Care 2002; 25(1):16–22.
100 Alm B, Wennergren G, Norvenius SG, et al. Breast feeding and the sudden infant death syndrome in Scandinavia, 1992–95. Arch Dis Child 2002; 86(6):400–402.
101 McVea KL, Turner PD, Peppler DK. The role of breastfeeding in sudden infant death syndrome. J Hum Lact 2000; 16(1):13–20.
102 Hamlyn B, Brooker S, Oleinikova K, et al. Infant feeding 2000. London: The Stationery Office; 2002.
103 World Health Organization. Protecting, promoting and supporting breatfeeding: The special role of maternity services (a joint WHO/UNICEF statement). Geneva: World Health Organization; 1989.
*104 Simmer K. Long chain polyunsaturated fatty acid supplementation in infants born at term (Cochrane review). In: The Cochrane Library, Issue 2, 2002. Oxford: Update Software.

BIRTH TRAUMA
105 Hoeksma AF, Wolf H, Oei SL. Obstetrical brachial plexus injuries: incidence, natural course and shoulder contracture. Clin Rehabil 2000; 14:523–526.
106 Mills JF, Dargaville PA, Coleman LT, et al. Upper cervical spinal cord injury in neonates: the use of magnetic resonance imaging. J Pediatr 2001; 138:105–108.

BIRTH ASPHYXIA
107 Bax M, Nelson KB. Birth asphyxia: a statement. Dev Med Child Neurol 1993; 35:1023–1024.
108 Levene MI. Birth asphyxia. In: David TJ, ed. Recent advances in paediatrics. Edinburgh: Churchill Livingstone; 1995:13–27.
109 Curtis PD, Matthews TG, Clarke TA, et al. Neonatal seizures: The Dublin Collaborative Study. Arch Dis Child 1988; 63:1065–1068.
110 Nelson KB, Ellenberg JH. Obstetric complications as risk factors for cerebral palsy or seizure disorders. JAMA 1984; 251:1843–1848.
*111 Thacker SB, Stroup D, Change M. Continuous electronic heart rate monitoring for fetal assessment during labor. Cochrane Database Syst Rev 2001; 2: CD000063.
*112 Neilson JP, Mistry RT. Fetal electrocardiogram plus heart rate recording for fetal monitoring during labour. Cochrane Database Syst Rev 2000; 2:CD00016.
113 Casey BM, McIntire DD, Leveno KJ. The continuing value of the Apgar score for the assessment of newborn infants. N Engl J Med 2001; 344:467–471.
114 Nelson KB, Ellenberg JH. Apgar scores as predictors of chronic neurological disability. Pediatrics 1981; 68:36–44.
115 Perlman JM, Risser R. Can asphyxiated infants at risk for neonatal seizures be rapidly identified by current high-risk markers? Pediatrics 1996; 97:456–462.
116 Pasternak JF, Gorey MT. The syndrome of acute near-total intrauterine asphyxia in term infants. Pediatr Neurol 1998; 18:391–398.
117 Phelan JP, Ahn MO, Korst L. Intrapartum fetal asphyxial brain injury with absent multiorgan system dysfunction. J Matern Fetal Med 1998; 7:19–22.

HYPOXIC–ISCHEMIC ENCEPHALOPATHY
118 Sarnat HB, Sarnat MS. Neonatal encephalopathy following fetal distress. Arch Neurol 1976; 33:696–705.
119 Levene MI, Kornberg J, Williams TH. The incidence and severity of post-asphyxial encephalopathy in full-term infants. Early Hum Dev 1985; 11:21–26.
120 Nelson KB, Leviton A. How much of neonatal enceophalopathy is due to birth asphyxia? Am J Dis Child 1991; 145:1325–1331.
121 Adamson SJ, Alessandra LM, Badawi B. Predictors of neonatal encephalopathy in full term infants. BMJ 1995; 311:598–602.
122 Amiel-Tison C. Birth injury as a cause of brain dysfunction in full-term newborns. In: Korobkin R, Guilleminault L, eds. Advances in perinatal neurology. Vol 1. New York: Spectrum; 1979.
123 Hull J, Dodd KL. Falling incidence of hypoxic–ischaemic encephalopathy in term infants. Br J Obstet Gynaecol 1992; 99:386–391.
124 Windle WF. An experimental approach to prevention or reduction of the brain damage of birth asphyxia. Dev Med Child Neurol 1966; 8:129–140.
125 Myers RE. Two patterns of perinatal brain damage and their conditions of occurrence. Am J Obstet Gynecol 1972; 112:246–276.
126 Levene MI, Evans DH. Continuous measurement of subarachnoid pressure in the severely asphyxiated newborn. Arch Dis Child 1983; 58:1013–1015.
127 Levene MI, Evans DH, Forde A, et al. Value of intracranial pressure monitoring of asphyxiated newborn infants. Dev Med Child Neurol 1987; 29:311–319.
128 Perlman JM, Tack ED, Martin T, et al. Acute systemic organ injury in term infants after asphyxia. Am J Dis Child 1989; 143:617–620.
129 Van Bel F, Walther FJ. Myocardial dysfunction and cerebral blood flow velocity following birth asphyxia. Acta Paediatr Scand 1990; 79:756–762.
130 Perlman JM, Tack ED. Renal injury in the asphyxiated newborn infant: relationship to neurological outcome. J Pediatr 1988; 113:875–879.
131 Fernandez F, Barrio V, Guzman J. Beta-2-microglobulin in the assessment of renal function in full term newborns following perinatal asphyxia. J Perinat Med 1989; 17:453–454.
132 Roberts DS, Haycock GB, Dalton RN, et al. Prediction of acute renal failure after birth asphyxia. Arch Dis Child 1990; 65:1021–1028.
133 Wirrell EC, Armstrong EA, Osman LD, et al. Prolonged seizures exacerbate perinatal hypoxic–ischemic brain damage. Pediatr Res 2001; 50:445–454.
134 Gilman JT, Gal P, Duchowny MS, et al. Rapid sequential phenobarbital treatment of neonatal seizures. Pediatrics1989; 83:674–678.
135 Hall RT, Hall FK, Daily DK. High-dose phenobarbital therapy in term newborn infants with severe perinatal asphyxia: a randomised, prospective study with three year follow up. J Pediatr 1998; 132:345–348.
*136 Evans DJ, Levene MI. Anticonvulsants for preventing mortality and morbidity in full term newborns with perinatal asphyxia (Cochrane Review). In: The Cochrane Library, Issue 1, 1998. Oxford: Update Software.
137 Mujsce DJ, Stern DR, Vannucci RC, et al. Mannitol therapy in perinatal hypoxic–ischemic brain injury. Ann Neurol 1988; 24:338.
138 Levene MI, Evans DH. Medical management of raised intracranial pressure after severe birth asphyxia. Arch Dis Child 1985; 60:12–16.
139 Vannucci RC, Towfighi J, Heitjan DF, et al. Carbon dioxide protects the perinatal brain from hypoxic–ischemic damage: an experimental study in the immature rat. Pediatrics 1995; 95:868–874.
140 De Vries LS, Levene MI. Cerebral ischemic lesions. In: Levene MI, Chervenak FA, Whittle MJ, eds. Fetal and neonatal neurology and neurosurgery. London: Churchill Livingstone; 2001:373–404.
141 Rosenberg AA. Response of the cerebral circulation to hypocarbia in postasphyxial newborn lambs. Pediatr Res 1992; 32:537–541.
142 Hagberg H, Blomgren K, Mallard C. Neuroprotection of the fetal and neonatal brain. In: Levene MI, Chervenak FA, Whittle MJ, eds. Fetal and neonatal neurology and neurosurgery. London: Churchill Livingstone; 2001:505–520.
143 Gunn AJ, Gluckman PD, Gunn TR. Selective head cooling in newborn infants after perinatal asphyxia: a safety study. Pediatrics 1998; 102:885–892.
144 Azzopardi D, Robertson NJ, Cowan FM, et al. Pilot study of treatment with whole body hypothermia for neonatal encephalopathy. Pediatrics 2000; 106:684–694.
145 Battin MR, Dezoete JA, Gunn TR, et al. Neurodevelopmental outcome of infants treated with head cooling and mild hypothermia after perinatal asphyxia. Pediatrics 2001; 107:480–484.
146 Pourcyrous M, Leffler CW, Bada HS, et al. Brain superoxide anion generation in asphyxiated piglets and the effect of indomethacin at therapeutic dose. Pediatr Res 1993; 34:366–369.

147 Palmer C, Towfighi J, Roberts RL, et al. Allopurinol administered after inducing hypoxia–ischemia reduces brain injury in 7-day-old rats. Pediatr Res 1993; 33:405–411.
148 Van Bel F, Shadid M, Moison RM. Effect of allopurinol on postasphyxial free radical formation of cerebral hemodynaemics, and electrical brain activity. Pediatrics 1998; 101:185–193.
149 Casey BM, McIntire DD, Leveno KJ. The continuing value of the Apgar score for the assessment of newborn infants. N Engl J Med 2001; 344:467–471.
150 Nelson KB, Ellenberg JH. Apgar scores as predictors of chronic neurological disability. Pediatrics 1981; 68:36–44.
151 Thomson AJ, Searle M, Russell G. Quality of survival after severe birth asphyxia. Arch Dis Child 1977; 52:620–626.
152 Levene MI, Sands C, Grindulis H, et al. Comparison of two methods of predicting outcome in perinatal asphyxia. Lancet 1986; i:67–69.
*153 Peliowski A, Finer NN. Birth asphyxia in the term infant. In: Sinclair JC, Bracken MB, eds. Effective care of the newborn infant. Oxford: Oxford University Press; 1992:249–279.
154 Levene MI. The asphyixated newborn infant In: Levene MI, Chervenak FA, Whittle MJ, eds. Fetal and neonatal neurology and neurosurgery. London: Churchill Livingstone; 2001:471–504.
155 Robertson CMT, Finer NN, Grace MGA. School performance of survivors of neonatal encephalopathy associated with birth asphyxia at term. J Pediatr 1989; 114:753–760.
156 Rutherford MA, Pennock JM, Counsell SJ. Abnormal magnetic resonance signal in the internal capsule predicts poor neuro-developmental outcome in infants with hypoxic ischemic encephalopathy. Pediatrics 1998; 102:323–329.
157 Rutherford MA, Pennock J, Schwieso J. Hypoxic–ischaemic enceophalopathy: early and later magnetic resonance imaging findings in relation to outcome. Arch Dis Childhood 1996; 75:F145–F151.
158 Barkovich AJ, Hajnal BL, Vigneron D. Prediction of neuromotor outcome in perinatal asphyxia: evaluation of MR scoring systems. Am J Neuroradiol 1998; 19:143–149.
159 Levene MI, Fenton AC, Evans DH, et al. Severe birth asphyxia and abnormal cerebral blood-flow velocity. Dev Med Child Neurol 1989; 31:427–434.
160 Eken P, Toet MC, Groenendaal F, et al. Predictive value of early neuroimaging, pulsed Doppler and neurophysiology in full term infants with hypoxic–ischaemic encephalopathy. Arch Dis Child 1995; 73:F75–F80.
161 Liao HT, Hung KL. Anterior cerebral artery Doppler ultrasonography for prediction of outcome after perinatal asphyxia. Chung Hua Min Kuo Hsiao Erh Ko I Hsueh Tsa Chih 1997; 38:208–212.
162 Ilves P, Talvik R, Talvik T. Changes in Doppler ultrasonography in asphyxiated term infants with hypoxic–ischaemic encephalopathy. Acta Paediatr 1998;87:680–684.
163 Wertheim D, Mercuri E, Faundez JC. Prognostic value of continuous electroencephalographic recording in full term infants with hypoxic ischaemic encephalopathy. Arch Dis Child 1994; 71:F97–F102.
164 Selton D, Andre M. Prognosis of hypoxic–ischaemic encephalopathy in full term newborns – value of neonatal electroencephalography. Neuropediatrics 1997; 28: 276–280.
165 Hellstrom-Westas L, Rosen I, Svenningsen NW. Predictive value of early continuous amplitude integrated EEG recordings on outcome after severe birth asphyxia in full term infants. Arch Dis Child 1995; 72:F34–F38.
166 Al Naqeeb N, Edwards AD, Cowan FM, et al. Assessment of neonatal encephalopathy by amplitude-integrated electroencephalography. Pediatrics 1999; 103:1263–1271.
167 Toet MC, Hellstrom-Vestas L, Groenendaal F. Amplitude integrated EEG 3 and 6 hours after birth in full-term neonates with hypoxic–ischaemic encephaloopathy. Arch Dis Child Fetal Neonatal Ed 1999; 81:F19–F23.
168 Ferrari F, Biagioni E, Cioni G. Neonatal electroencephalography. In: Levene MI, Chervenak FA, Whittle MJ, eds. Fetal and neonatal neurology and neurosurgery. London: Churchill Livingstone; 2001:155–180.

RESUSCITATION IN THE NEWBORN
169 Palme-Kilander C. Methods of resuscitation in low-Apgar-score newborn infants – a national survey. Acta Paediatr Scand 1992; 81:739–744.
*170 Resuscitation at birth. The newborn life support provider course manual. London: Resuscitation Council; 2001.
*171 International guidelines for neonatal resuscitation: an excerpt from the guidelines 2000 for cardiopulmonary resuscitation and emergency cardiovascular care: International Consensus on Science 2000. Pediatrics 2000; 106:1–16.
*172 Zideman DA, Bingham R, Beattie T, et al. Recommendations on resuscitation of babies at birth. Resuscitation 1998; 37:103–110.
173 Cross KW. Resuscitation of the asphyxiated infant. Brit Med Bull 1966; 22:73–78.
174 Dawes GS. Foetal and neonatal physiology. Chicago: Year Book Medical Publishers; 1968:141–159.
175 Levene MI, Tudehope D, Thearle J. Essentials of neonatal medicine. Oxford: Blackwell Scientific; 1987.
176 Milner A. The importance of ventilation to effective resuscitation in the term and preterm infant. Semin Neonatol 2001; 6:219–224.
177 Moreland TA, Brice JEH, Walker CHM, Parija AC. Naloxone pharmacokinetics in the newborn. Brit J Clin Pharmacol 1980; 9(6): 609–612.
*178 Cochrane Injuries Group Albumin Reviewers. Human albumin administration in critically ill patients: systematic review of randomised controlled trials. BMJ 1998; 317:235–240.
179 Saugstad OD. Resuscitation of newborn infants with room air or oxygen. Semin Neonatol 2001; 5:233–239.
180 Ramji S, Ahuja S, Thirupuram S, et al. Resuscitation of asphyxic newborn infants with room air or 100% oxygen. Pediatr Res 1993; 34:809–812.
*181 Saugstad OD, Rootwelt T, Aalen O. Resuscitation of asphyxiated newborn infants with room air or oxygen: an international controlled trial: the Resair 2 study. Pediatrics 1998; 102:e1.
182 Vento M, Asensi M, Sastre J, et al. Resuscitation with room air instead of 100% oxygen prevents oxidative stress in moderately asphyxiated term neonates. Pediatrics 2001; 107:642–647.
183 Wiswell TE, Bent RC. Meconium staining and the meconium aspiration syndrome: unresolved issues. Pediatr Clin North Am 1993; 40:955–981.
184 Cleary GM, Wiswell TE. Meconium-stained amniotic fluid and the meconium aspiration syndrome. An update. Pediatr Clin North Am 1998; 45:511–529.
185 Carson B, Losey RW, Bowes WA. Combined obstetric and pediatric approach to prevent meconium aspiration syndrome. Am J Obstet Gynecol 1976; 126:712–717.
*186 Wiswell TE. Handling the meconium-stained infant. Semin Neonatol 2001; 6:225–231.

THE SMALL FOR GESTATIONAL AGE INFANT
187 Jones RAK, Roberton NRC. Small for dates babies: are they really a problem? Arch Dis Child 1986; 61:877–880.
188 Koh THHG, Aynsley-Green A, Tarbit M, et al. Neural dysfunction during hypoglycaemia. Arch Dis Child 1988; 63:1353–1358.
189 McIntosh N, Kempson C, Tyler RM. Blood counts in extremely low birthweight infants. Arch Dis Child 1988; 63:74–76.

DEVELOPMENTAL CARE
190 Volpe JJ. Brain injury in the premature infant – from pathogenesis to prevention. Brain Dev 1997; 19:519–534.
191 Wolke D. Annotation: supporting the development of low birthweight infants. J Child Psychol Psychiatry 1991; 32(5):723–741.
192 Wolke D. Environmental and developmental neonatology. J Reprod Infant Psychol 1987; 5:17–42.
*193 Symington A, Pinelli J. Developmental care for promoting development and preventing morbidity in preterm infants. Cochrane Database Syst Rev 2001; 3.
194 Lotas MJ. Effects of light and sound in the neonatal intensive care unit environment on the low-birth-weight infants. NAACOG's Clin Issues Perinat Women's Health Nurs 1992; 3(1):34–44.
195 Blackburn S. Environmental impact of the NICU on developmental outcomes. J Pediatr Nurs 1998; 13(5):279–289.
*196 Mann NP, Haddow R, Stokes L, et al. Effect of night and day on preterm infants in a newborn nursery: randomized trial. BMJ 1986; 293(6557):1265–1267.
*197 Slevin M, Farrington N, Duffy G et al. Altering the NICU and measuring infants' responses. Acta Paediatr 2000; 89(5):501–502.
198 Peters KL. Infant handling in the NICU: does developmental care make a difference? An evaluative review of the literature. J Perinat Neonat Nurs 1999; 13(3):83–109.
199 Gorski PA, Huntington L, Lewkowicz DJ. Handling preterm infants in hospitals: stimulating controversy about timing of stimulation. Clin Perinatol 1990; 17:103–112.
200 King JA, Barkley RA, Barrett S. Attention-deficit hyperactivity disorder and the stress response. Biol Psychiatry 1998; 44:72–74.

201 Thomas KA. Biorhythms in infants and role of the care environment. J Perinat Neonat Nurs 1995; 9:61–75.
202 Anand KJS. Long-term effects of pain in neonates and infants. In: Jensen TS, Turner JA, Wiesenfeld-Hallin Z, eds. Procedings of the 8th World Congress on Pain, Progress in Pain Research and Management. Seattle: IASP Press; 1997:881–892.
203 McIntosh N. Pain in the newborn, a possible new starting point. Eur J Pediatr 1997; 56:173–178.
204 Updike C, Schmidt RE, Macke C, et al. Positional support for premature infants. Am J Occup Ther 1986; 40(10):712–715.
*205 Downs J, Edwards A, McCormick D, et al. Effect of intervention on the development of hip posture in very preterm babies. Arch Dis Child 1991; 66:797–801.
206 Whitely S, Cowan M. Developmental interventions in the newborn intensive care unit. NAACOG's Clin Issues Perinat Women's Health Nurs 1991; 2(1):84–110.
*207 Pinelli J, Symington A. Non-nutritive sucking for promoting physiologic stability and nutrition in preterm infants. Cochrane Database Syst Rev 2001; 3:CD001071.
*208 Stevens B, Johnston C, Franck L, et al. The efficacy of developmentally sensitive interventions and sucrose for relieving procedural pain in very low birth weight neonates. Nurs Res 1999; 48(1):35–43.
*209 Stevens B, Yamada J, Ohlsson A. Sucrose for analgesia in newborn infants undergoing painful procedures. Cochrane Database Syst Rev 2001; 4:CD001069.
210 Corff KE, Seiderman R, Venkataraman PS, et al. Facilitative tucking: a non-pharmocologic comfort measure for pain in preterm infants. J Obstet Gynecol Neonatal Nurs 1995; 24(2):143–147.
*211 Taquino L, Blackburn S. The effects of containment during suctioning and heelstick on physiological and behavioral responses of preterm infants. Neonatal Network – J Neonatal Nurs 1994; 13(7):55.
212 Padden T, Glenn S. Maternal experiences of preterm birth and neonatal intensive care. J Reprod Infant Psychol 1997; 15(2):121–139.
213 Harrison H. The principles of family-centred neonatal care. Pediatrics 1993; 92:643–650.
214 Meyer EC, Coll CTG, Lester BM, et al. Family-based intervention improves maternal psychological well-being and feeding interaction of preterm infants. Pediatrics 1994; 93:241–246.
215 Als H, Lawhon G, Brown E, et al. Individualized behavioral and environmental care for the very low birth weight preterm infant at high risk for bronchopulmonary dysplasia: Neonatal intensive care unit and developmental outcome. Pediatrics 1986; 78(6):1123–1132.
*216 Als H, Lawhon G, Duffy F, et al. Individualized developmental care for the very low-birth-weight preterm infant: medical and neurofunctional effects. JAMA 1994; 272(11):853–858.
217 Becker PT, Grunwald PC, Moorman J, et al. Outcomes of developmentally supportive nursing care for very low birthweight infants. Nurs Res 1991; 40(3):150–155.
*218 Fleischer BE, Vandenberg K, Constantinou J, et al. Individualized developmental care for very-low-birth-weight premature infants. Clin Pediatr 1995; 10:523–529.
*219 Westrup B, Kleberg A, von Eichwald K, et al. A randomized controlled trial to evaluate the effects of the newborn individualized developmental care and assessment program in a Swedish setting. Pediatrics 2000; 105:66–72.
*220 Stevens B, Petryshen P, Hawkins J, et al. Developmental versus conventional care: a comparison of clinical outcomes for very low birth weight infants. Can J Nurs Res 1996; 28(4):97–113.
221 Ariagno RL, Thoman EB, Boedikker MA, et al. Developmental care does not alter sleep and development of premature infants. Pediatrics 1997; 100:1–7.
*222 Buehler DM, Als H, Duffy FH, et al. Effectiveness of individualized developmental care for low-risk preterm infants: behavioral and electrophysiologic evidence. Pediatrics 1995; 96:923–932.
223 Kleberg A, Westrup B, Sternqvist K. Developmental outcome, child behaviour and mother–child interaction at 3 years of age following newborn individualized developmental care and intervention program (NIDCAP) intervention. Early Hum Dev 2000; 60(2):123–135.
224 Silverman WA. Overtreatment of neonates? A personal retrospective. Pediatrics; 1992;90:971–976.

SPECIAL CARE – FLUID BALANCE

225 Simpson J, Stephenson TJ. Regulation of extracellular fluid volume in neonates. Early Hum Dev 1993; 34:179–190.
226 Stephenson TJ, Broughton Pipkin F, Elias-Jones AC. A study of factors influencing plasma renin and renin substrate concentrations in the premature human newborn. Arch Dis Child 1991; 66:1150–1154.
227 Tarnow-Mordi W, Shaw JCL, Liu D, et al. Iatrogenic hyponatraemia of the newborn due to maternal fluid overload: a prospective study. Br Med J 1981; 283:639–642.
228 Gill A, Yu WYH, Bajuk B, et al. Postnatal growth in infants born before 30 weeks' gestation. Arch Dis Child 1986; 61:549–553.
229 Hamilton CM, Shaw JCL. Changes in sodium and water balance, renal function and aldosterone excretion during the first seven days of life in very low birth weight infants. Pediatr Res 1984; 18:91.
230 Rees L, Shaw JCL, Brook CGD, et al. Hyponatraemia in the first week of life in preterm infants. Part II. Sodium and water balance. Arch Dis Child 1984; 59:423–429.
231 Keen DV, Pearse RG. Birthweight between 14 and 42 weeks' gestation. Diagn Histopathol 1985; 6:89–111.
232 Shaw JCL. Growth and nutrition of the very preterm infant. In: Whitelaw A, Cooke RWI, eds. The very immature infant less than 28 weeks' gestation. London; Churchill Livingstone; 1988.
233 Riesenfeld T, Hammerlund K, Sedin G. Respiratory water loss in fullterm infants on their first day after birth. Acta Paediatr Scand 1987; 76:647–653.
234 Hammarlund K, Sedin G, Stromberg B. Transepidermal water loss in newborn infants. VIII Relations to gestational age and post-natal age in appropriate and small for gestational age infants. Acta Paediatr Scand 1983; 72:721–728.
235 Stephenson TJ, Marlow N, Watkin S, et al. Pocket neonatology. Edinburgh: Churchill Livingstone; 2000:426.
236 Costarino A, Baumgart S. Modern fluid and electrolyte management of the critically ill premature infant. Pediatr Clin North Am 1986; 33:153–178.
*237 Kavvadia A, Greenough A, Dimitriou G, et al. Randomised trial of fluid restriction in ventilated very low birthweight infants. Arch Dis Child 2000; 83:F91–F96.
238 Wilkins BH. Renal function in sick very low birthweight infants: 1. Glomerular filtration rate. Arch Dis Child 1992; 67:1140–1145.
*239 Bell EF, Acarregui MJ. Restricted versus liberal water intake for preventing morbidity and mortality in preterm infants (Cochrane Review). In: The Cochrane Library, Issue 3, 2000. Oxford: Update Software.
240 Von Stockhausen HB, Struve M. Die Auswirkungen einer stark unterschiedlichen parenteralen Flussigkeitszufuhr bei Fruhund Neugeborenen in den ersten drei Lebenstagen. Klin Padiatr 1980; 192:539–546.
241 Lorenz JM, Kleinman LI, Kotagal UR, et al. Water balance in very low-birth-weight infants: relationship to water and sodium intake and effect on outcome. J Pediatr 1982; 101:423–432.
242 Tammela OKT, Koivisto ME. Fluid restriction for preventing bronchopulmonary dysplasia? Reduced fluid intake during the first weeks of life improves the outcome of low birthweight infants. Acta Paediatr 1992; 81:207–212.
243 Bell EF, Warburton D, Stonestreet BS, et al. Effects of fluid administration on the development of symptomatic patent ductus arteriosus and congestive heart failure in premature infants. N Engl J Med 1980; 302:598–604.
*244 Schierhout G, Roberts I. Fluid resuscitation with colloid or crystalloid solutions in critically ill patients: a systematic review of randomised trials. Br Med J 1998; 316: 961–964.
*245 Dixon H, Hawkins K, Stephenson TJ. Comparison of albumin versus bicarbonate treatment for neonatal metabolic acidosis. Eur J Pediatr 1999; 158:414–415.
*246 Osborn DA, Evans N. Early volume expansion versus inotrope for prevention of morbidity and mortality in very preterm infants (Cochrane Review). In: The Cochrane Library, Issue 2, 2001. Oxford: Update Software.
247 Cartlidge PHT, Rutter N. Serum albumin concentration and oedema in the newborn. Arch Dis Child 1986; 61:657–660.
248 Obladen M, Sachsenweger M, Stahnke M. Blood sampling in very low birth weight infants receiving different levels of intensive care. Eur J Pediatr 1988; 147:399–404.
249 Jones RWA, Rochefort MJ, Baum JD. Increased insensible water loss in newborn infants nursed under radiant warmers. BMJ 1976; 2:1347–1350.
250 Wilkins BH. Renal function in sick very low birthweight infants: 2. Urea and creatinine excretion. Arch Dis Child 1992; 67:1146–1153.

251 Slater JE. Retention of nitrogen and minerals by babies 1 week old. Br J Nutr 1961; 15:83–97.
252 Flood RG, Pinelli RW. Urinary glycocyamine, creatine and creatinine. 1. Their excretion by normal infants and children. Am J Dis Child 1949; 77:740–745.
253 Barlow A, McCance RA. The nitrogen partition in newborn infants' urine. Arch Dis Child 1948; 23:225–230.
254 Tuck S. Fluid and electrolyte balance in the neonate. In: Roberton NRC, ed. Textbook of neonatology. London: Churchill Livingstone; 1986:162–177.
255 Greenough A, Greenall F, Gamsu HR. Selective paralysis of neonates – effects of fluid balance, catecholamine levels and heart rate variability. Abstracts of Paediatric Research Society 1986; September.
256 Kavvadia V, Greenough A, Dimitriou G, et al. Comparison of the effect of two fluid input regimes on perinatal lung function in ventilated very low birthweight infants. Eur J Pediatr 1999; 158:917–922.
257 Modi N. Development of renal function. Br Med Bull 1988; 44:936–956.
258 Wilkins BH. Renal function in sick very low birthweight infants: 3. Sodium, potassium and water excretion. Arch Dis Child 1992; 67:1154–1161.
259 Tuck S. Fluid and electrolyte balance in the neonate. In: Robertson NRC, ed. Textbook of neonatology. London: Churchill Livingstone, 1986; 162–177.
260 Stephenson TJ, Broughton Pipkin F, Hetmanski D, et al. Atrial natriuretic peptide in the preterm newborn. Biol Neonate 1994; 66(1): 22–32.
261 Kojima T, Hirata Y, Fukuda Y, et al. Plasma atrial natriuretic peptide and spontaneous diuresis in sick neonates. Arch Dis Child 1987; 62:667–670.
262 Rascher W, Seyberth HW. Atrial natriuretic peptide and patent ductus arteriosus in preterm infants. Arch Dis Child 1987; 62:1165–1167.
263 Andersson S, Tikkanen I, Pesonen E, et al. Atrial natriuretic peptide in patent ductus arteriosus. Pediatr Res 1987; 21:396–398.
264 Wilkinson AR. Cardiovascular adaptation in the very immature infant. In: Whitelaw A, Cooke RWI, eds. The very immature infant less than 28 weeks' gestation. London: Churchill Livingstone; 1988.

SPECIAL CARE – SODIUM AND POTASSIUM
265 Modi N. Sodium intake and preterm babies. Arch Dis Child 1993; 69:87–91.
266 Rees L, Shaw JCL, Brook CGD, et al. Hyponatraemia in the first week of life in preterm infants. Part II. Sodium and water balance. Arch Dis Child 1984; 59:423–429.
267 Broughton Pipkin F, Stephenson TJ. Plasma renin and renin substrate concentrations in the very premature human baby. Early Hum Dev 1989; 19:71.
268 Ito Y, Matsumoto T, Ohbu K, et al. Concentration of human atrial natriuretic peptide in cord blood and the plasma of the newborn. Acta Paediatr Scand 1988; 77:76–78.
269 Stephenson TJ, Broughton Pipkin F. Atrial natriuretic factor: the heart as an endocrine organ. Arch Dis Child 1990; 65:1293–1294.
270 Modi N. Development of renal function. Br Med Bull 1988; 44:936–956.
271 Wilkins BH. Renal function in sick very low birthweight infants: 3. Sodium, potassium and water excretion. Arch Dis Child 1992; 67:1154–1161.
272 Moniz CF, Nicolaides KH, Bamforth FJ, et al. Normal reference ranges for biochemical substances relating to renal, hepatic and bone function in fetal and maternal plasma throughout pregnancy. J Clin Pathol 1985; 38:468.
273 Guignard JP, John EG. Renal function in the tiny premature infant. Clin Perinatol 1986; 13:377–401.
274 Wilkins B. The renal effects of aminophylline in very low birth weight neonates. Early Hum Dev 1986; 15(3):184–185.
275 Shortland D, Trounce JCQ, Levene MI. Hyperkalaemia, cardiac arrhythmias and cerebral lesions in high risk neonates. Arch Dis Child 1987; 62:1139–1143.
276 Lorenz M, Kleinman LI, Markarian K. Potassium metabolism in extremely low birth weight infants in the first week of life. J Pediatr 1997; 131:81–86.
277 Vasarhelyi B, Tulassay T, Ver A, et al. Developmental changes in erythrocyte Na^+, K^+ -ATPase subunit abundance and enzyme activity in neonates. Arch Dis Child 2000; 83:F135–F138.

SPECIAL CARE – THERMOREGULATION
278 Rutter N. Temperature control and its disorders. In: Rennie JM, Roberton NRC, eds. Textbook of neonatology, 3rd edn. Edinburgh: Churchill Livingstone; 1999:289–303.
*279 Sarman I, Tunell R. Providing warmth for preterm babies by a heated, water filled mattress. Arch Dis Child 1989; 64:29–33.
*280 Sarman I, Can G, Tunell R. Rewarming preterm infants on a heated, water filled mattress. Arch Dis Child 1989; 64:687–692.
281 Hey EN. Thermal neutrality. Br Med Bull 1975; 31:69–74.
282 Sauer PJJ, Dane HJ, Visser HK. New standards for neutral thermal environment of healthy very low birthweight infants in week one of life. Arch Dis Child 1984; 59:18–22.
*283 Flenady VJ, Woodgate PG. Radiant warmers versus incubators for regulating body temperature in newborn infants. Cochrane Database Syst Rev; 2002; 2:CD000435.

SPECIAL CARE – ENTERAL NUTRITION
*284 Lucas A, Morley R, Cole TJ, et al. A randomised multicentre study of human milk versus formula and later development in preterm infants. Arch Dis Child Fetal Neonatal Ed 1994; 70:F141–F146.
285 Kelly EJ, Newell SJ. Gastric ontogeny: clinical implications. Arch Dis Child 1994; 71:F136–F141.
286 Bisset WM, Watt JB, Rivers JPA, et al. Ontogeny of fasting small intestinal motor activity in the human infant. Gut 1988; 29:483–488.
287 Newell SJ, Sarkar PK, Durbin GM, et al. Maturation of the lower oesophageal sphincter in the preterm baby. Gut 1986; 29:167–172.
288 McClean P, Weaver LT. Ontogeny of human pancreatic exocrine function. Arch Dis Child 1993; 68:62–65.
289 Hamosh M. Digestion in the newborn. Clin Perinatol 1996; 23:191–210.
290 Schmitz J. Digestive and absorptive function. In: Walker WA, Durie PR, Hamilton JR, et al, eds. Pediatric gastrointestinal disease. Philadephia: BC Decker; 1996:263–279.
291 Jakobsson I, Lindberg T, Lothe L, et al. Human alpha lactalbumin as a marker of macromolecular absorption. Gut 1986;27: 1029–1034.
292 McClure RJ, Chatrath MK, Newell SJ. Changing trends in feeding policies for ventilated preterm infants. Acta Paediatr 1996; 85: 1123–1125.
293 Malcolm G, Ellwood D, Devonald K, et al. Absent or reversed end diastolic flow velocity in the umbilical artery and necrotising enterocolitis. Arch Dis Child 1991; 66:805–807.
294 Karsdrop VHM, Van-Vugt JMG, Van-Geijn HP, et al. Clinical significance of absent or reversed end diastolic velocity waveforms in umbilical artery. Lancet 1994; 344:1664–1668.
295 Ewer AK, McHugo JM, Chapman S, et al. Fetal echogenic gut: a marker of intrauterine gut ischaemia. Arch Dis Child 1993; 69:510–513.
296 Newell SJ. Enteral feeding in the micropremie. Clin Perinatol 2000; 27:221–234.
*297 McClure RJ. Trophic feeding of the preterm infant. Acta Paediatr 2001; 90(suppl):19–21.
298 Hughes CA, Dowling RH. Speed of onset of adaptive mucosal hypoplasia and hypofunction in the intestine of parenterally fed rats. Clin Sci (Colch) 1980; 59:317–327.
299 Goldstein RM, Hebiguchi T, Luk GD, et al. The effects of total parenteral nutrition on gastrointestinal growth and development. J Pediatr Surg 1985; 20:785–791.
300 Berseth CL, Nordyke C. Enteral nutrients promote postnatal maturation of intestinal motor activity in preterm infants. Am J Physiol 1993; 264:G1046–1051.
*301 McClure RJ, Newell SJ. Randomised controlled trial of trophic feeding and gut motility. Arch Dis Child Fetal Neonatal Ed 1999; 80:F54–F58.
*302 Schanler RJ, Shulman RJ, Lau C, et al. Feeding strategies for premature infants: randomized trial of gastrointestinal priming and tube-feeding method. Pediatrics 1999; 103:434–439.
*303 McClure RJ, Newell SJ. Randomised controlled trial of clinical outcome following trophic feeding. Arch Dis Child Fetal Neonatal Ed 2000; 82:F29–F33.
304 Lucas A, Bloom SR, Aynsley Green A. Gut hormones and 'minimal enteral feeding'. Acta Paediatr Scand 1986; 75:719–723.
*305 McClure RJ, Newell SJ. Randomized controlled study of digestive enzyme activity following trophic feeding. Acta Paediatr 2002; 91(3):292–296.
*306 Shulman RJ, Schanler RJ, Lau C, et al. Early feeding, feeding tolerance, and lactase activity in preterm infants. J Pediatr 1998; 133:645–649.
*307 Tyson JE, Kennedy KA. Minimal enteral nutrition for promoting feeding tolerance and preventing morbidity in parenterally fed infants. Cochrane. Database Syst Rev 2000; 2:CD000504.
308 Tsang RC, Lucas A, Uauy R, et al. Nutritional needs of the preterm infant: scientific

basis and practical guidelines. In: Tsang RC, Lucas A, Uauy R, et al, eds. Baltimore: Williams & Wilkins; 1993.
309 ESPGAN. Nutrition and feeding of preterm infants. Acta Paediatr Scand 1987; 336:1–14.
*310 Lucas A, Morley R, Cole TJ, et al. Breast milk and subsequent intelligence quotient in children born preterm. Lancet 1992; 339: 261–264.
*311 Lucas A, Gore SM, Cole TJ, et al. Multicentre trial on feeding low birthweight infants: effects of diet on early growth. Arch Dis Child 1984; 59:722–730.
312 Ewer AK, Durbin GM, Morgan ME, et al. Gastric emptying in preterm infants. Arch Dis Child 1994; 71:F24–F27.
*313 Lucas A, Cole TJ. Breast milk and neonatal necrotising enterocolitis. Lancet 1990; 336:1519–1523.
314 Wilson AC, Forsyth JS, Greene SA, et al. Relation of infant diet to childhood health: seven year follow up of cohort of children in Dundee infant feeding study. BMJ 1998; 316:21–25.
*315 Lucas A, Brooke OG, Morley R, et al. Early diet of preterm infants and development of allergic or atopic disease: randomised prospective study. BMJ 1990; 300:837–840.
*316 O'Connor DL, Hall R, Adamkin D, et al. Growth and development in preterm infants fed long-chain polyunsaturated fatty acids: a prospective, randomized controlled trial. Pediatrics 2001; 108:359–371.
317 Standing Committee on Nutrition of the British Paediatric Association. Is breast feeding beneficial in the UK? Arch Dis Child 1994; 71:376–380.
318 Barker DJ. Childhood causes of adult disease. Arch Dis Child 1988; 63:867–869.
*319 Singhal A, Cole TJ, Lucas A. Early nutrition in preterm infants and later blood pressure: two cohorts after randomised trials. Lancet 2001; 357:413–419.
320 Zeigler JB, Cooper DA, Johnson RO, et al. Postnatal transmission of AIDS-associated retrovirus from mother to infant. Lancet 1985; i:896–897.
*321 McClure RJ, Newell SJ. Effect of fortifying breast milk on gastric emptying. Arch Dis Child Fetal Neonatal Ed 1996; 74:F60–F62.
*322 Ewer AK, Yu VY. Gastric emptying in preterm infants: the effect of breast milk fortifier. Acta Paediatr 1996; 85:1112–1115.
*323 Lucas A, Fewtrell MS, Morley R, et al. Randomized outcome trial of human milk fortification and developmental outcome in preterm infants. Am J Clin Nutr 1996; 64:142–151.
324 Schanler RJ, Abrams S. Postnatal attainment of intrauterine macromineral accretion rates in low birth weight infants fed fortified human milk. J Pediatr 1995; 126:441–447.
*325 Porcelli P, Schanler R, Greer F, et al. Growth in human milk-fed very low birth weight infants receiving a new human milk fortifier. Ann Nutr Metab 2000; 44:2–10.
*326 Lucas A, Morley R, Cole TJ, et al. Early diet in preterm babies and developmental status at 18 months. Lancet 1990; 335:1477–1481.
*327 Lucas A, Bishop NJ, King FJ, et al. Randomised trial of nutrition for preterm infants after discharge. Arch Dis Child 1992; 67:324–327.
*328 Cooke RJ, Griffin IJ, McCormick K, et al. Feeding preterm infants after hospital discharge: effect of dietary manipulation on nutrient intake and growth. Pediatr Res 1998; 43:355–360.
*329 Book LS, Herbst JJ, Atherton SO, et al. Necrotizing enterocolitis in low birth weight infants fed an elemental formula. J Pediatr 1975; 87:602–605.
330 McKeown RE, Marsh TD, Amarnath U, et al. Role of delayed feeding and of feeding increments in necrotizing enterocolitis. J Pediatr 1992; 121:764–770.
*331 Fast C, Roseggar H. Necrotising enterocolitis prophylaxis: oral antibiotics vs oral immunoglobulins. Acta Paediatr 1994; 396(suppl):86–90.
*332 Premji S, Chessell L. Continuous nasogastric milk feeding versus intermittent bolus milk feeding for premature infants less than 1500 grams. Cochrane Database Syst Rev 2001; 1:CD001819.
*333 Steer PA, Lucas A, Sinclair JC. Feeding the low birthweight infant. In: Sinclair JC, Bracken MB, eds. Effective care of the newborn infant. Oxford: Oxford University Press; 1992:94–140.
*334 Bishop NJ, King FJ, Lucas A. Increased bone mineral content of preterm infants fed with a nutrient enriched formula after discharge from hospital. Arch Dis Child 1993; 68:573–578.
335 Newell SJ, Booth IW, Morgan ME, et al. Gastro-oesophageal reflux in preterm infants. Arch Dis Child 1989; 64:780–786

ORGANIZATION OF NEONATAL INTENSIVE CARE SERVICES
336 British Association of Perinatal Medicine. Standards for hospitals providing neonatal intensive and high dependency care (second edition) and categories of babies requiring neonatal care. Published by the BAPM August 2001. Available: http://www.bapm-london.org/publications/hosp_standards.pdf

PRACTICAL PARENTERAL NUTRITION
337 Wilson DC. Nutrition of the preterm baby. Br J Obstet Gynaecol 1995; 102:854–860.
338 Heird WC. Parenteral feeding. In: Sinclair JC, Bracken MB, eds. Effective care of the newborn infant. Oxford: Oxford University Press; 1992:141–160.
*339 McClure RJ, Newell SJ. Randomised controlled study of clinical outcome following trophic feeding. Arch Dis Child 2000; 82:F29–F33.
340 Wilson DC, McClure G. Energy requirments in sick preterm babies. Acta Paediatr 1994; 405(suppl):60–64.
341 Wilson DC, McClure G, Halliday HL, et al. Nutrition and bronchopulmonary dysplasia. Arch Dis Child 1991; 66:37–38.
*342 Wilson DC, Cairns P, Halliday HL, et al. Randomised controlled trial of an aggressive nutritional regimen in sick very low birthweight infants. Arch Dis Child 1997; 7:F4–F11.
343 Young VR, El-Khoury AE. The notion of nutritional essentiality of amino acids, revisited, with a note on the indispensable amino acid requirment in adults. In: Cynober LA, ed. Amino acid metabolism and therapy in health and nutritional disease. Boca Raton: CRC Press; 1995:191–232.
*344 McIntosh N, Mitchell V. A clinical trial of two parenteral nutrition solutions in neonates. Arch Dis Child 1990; 65:612–699.
345 Cairns PA, Wilson DC, Jenkins J, et al. Tolerance of mixed lipid emulsion in neonates: effect of concentration. Arch Dis Child 1996; 75:F113–F116.
*346 Cairns PA, Stalker DJ. Carnitine supplementation of parenterally fed neonates (Cochrane Review). In: The Cochrane Library Issue 2, 2002,Oxford: Update Software.
347 Wilmore DW, Dudrick SJ. Growth and development of an infant receiving all nutrients exclusively by vein. JAMA 1968; 203:860–868.

BLOOD GASES AND RESPIRATORY SUPPORT
348 Tremblay LN, Slutsky AS, Dreyfuss D, et al. Ventilator-induced lung injury. Mechanisms and correlates. In: Marini JJ, Slutsky AA, eds. Physiological basis of ventilatory support. New York: Marcel Dekker; 1999.
349 Clark RH, Gerstmann DR, Jobe AH, et al. Lung injury in neonates: causes, strategies for prevention, and long term consequences. J Pediatr 2001; 139:478–484.
350 Groneck P, Speer CP. Inflammatory mediators and bronchopulmonary dysplasia. Arch Dis Child Fetal Neonatal Ed 1995; 73:F1–F3.
*351 The Acute Respiratory Distress Syndrome Network. Ventilation with lower tidal volumes as compared with traditional tidal volumes for acute lung injury and the acute respiratory distress syndrome. N Engl J Med 2000; 342:1301–1308.
352 Ranieri VM, Suter PM, Tortorella C, et al. Effect of mechanical ventilation on inflammatory mediators in patients with acute respiratory distress syndrome: a randomized controlled trial. JAMA 1999; 282:54–61.
353 American Thoracic Society, European Respiratory Society. Respiratory mechanics in infants: physiologic evaluation in health and disease. Am Rev Resp Dis 1993; 147:474–496.
354 McLain BI, Evans J, Dear PRF. Comparison of capillary and arterial blood gas measurements in neonates. Arch Dis Child 1989; 63:743–747.
355 Morgan C, Newell SJ, Ducker DA, et al. Continuous neonatal blood gas monitoring using a multiparameter intra-arterial sensor. Arch Dis Child Fetal Neonatal Ed 1999; 80:F93–F98.
356 Bohnhorst B, Peter CS, Poets CF. Pulse oximeters' reliability in detecting hypoxemia and bradycardia: comparison between a conventional and two new generation oximeters. Crit Care Med 2000; 28:1565–1568.
357 Mok JYQ, McLaughlin FJ, Pintar M, et al. Transcutaneous monitoring of oxygenation: what is normal? J Pediatr 1986; 108:365–371.
358 Mok JYQ, Hak H, McLaughlin FJ, et al. Effect of age and state of wakefulness on transcutaneous oxygen values in preterm infants: a longitudinal study. J Pediatr 1988; 113:706–709.
359 Prendiville A, Schulenberg WE. Clinical factors associated with retinopathy of prematurity. Arch Dis Child 1988; 63:522–527.

*360 The STOP-ROP Study Group. Supplemental therapeutic oxygen for prethreshold retinopathy of prematurity (STOP-ROP), a randomized, controlled trial. I: primary outcomes. Pediatrics 2000; 105:295–310.
361 Tin W, Milligan DW, Pennefather P, et al. Pulse oximetry, severe retinopathy, and outcome at one year in babies of less than 28 weeks gestation. Arch Dis Child Fetal Neonatal Ed 2001; 84:F106–F110.
362 Trounce JQ, Shaw DE, Levene MI, et al. Clinical risk factors and periventricular leukomalacia. Arch Dis Child 1988; 63:17–22.
363 Calvert SA, Hoskins EM, Fong KW, et al. Etiological factors associated with the development of periventricular leukomalacia. Acta Paediatr Scand 1987; 76:254–259.
364 Ikonen RS, Janas MO, Koivikko MJ, et al. Hyperbilirubinemia, hypocarbia and periventricular leukomalacia in preterm infants: relationship to cerebral palsy Acta Paediatr Scand 1992; 81:802–807.
365 Graziani LJ, Spitzer AR, Mitchell DG, et al. Mechanical ventilation in preterm infants: neurosonographic and developmental studies. Pediatrics 1992; 90:515–522.
366 Collins MP, Lorenz JM, Jetton JR, et al. Hypocapnia and other ventilation-related risk factors for cerebral palsy in low birth weight infants. Pediatr Res 2001; 50:712–719.
367 HIFI Study Group. High frequency oscillatory ventilation compared with conventional mechanical ventilation in the treatment of respiratory failure in preterm infants. N Engl J Med 1989; 320:90–93.
368 Rhodes PG, Graes GR, Patel DM, et al. Minimizing pneumothorax and bronchopulmonary dysplasia in ventilated infants with hyaline membrane disease. J Pediatr 1983; 103:634–637.
369 Wung JT, James S, Kilchevsky E, et al. Management of infants with severe respiratory failure and persistence of the fetal circulation without hyperventilation. Pediatrics 1985; 76:488–494.
370 Avery ME, Tooley WH, Keller JB, et al. Is chronic lung disease preventable? A survey of eight centres. Pediatrics 1987; 79:26–30.
371 Kraybill EN, Runyan D, Bose CL, et al. Risk factors for chronic lung disease in infants with birth weights of 751–1000 grams. J Pediatr 1989; 115:115–120.
*372 Woodgate PG, Davies MW. Permissive hypercapnia for the prevention of morbidity and mortality in mechanically ventilated newborn infants (Cochrane Review). Cochrane Database Syst Rev 2001; 2:CD002061.
373 Skoutelli HN, Dubowitz LMS, Levene MI, et al. Predictors associated with survival and normal neurodevelopmental outcome in infants weighing less than 1001 grams at birth. Dev Med Child Neurol 1985; 27:588–595.
*374 Crowley P. Prophylactic corticosteroids for preterm birth. Cochrane Database Syst Rev 2000; 2:CD000065.
375 Scottish Neonatal Consultants Collaborative Study Group and International Neonatal Network. Trends and variations in use of antenatal corticosteroids to prevent neonatal respiratory distress syndrome: recommendations for national and international comparative audit. Br J Obstet Gynaecol 1996; 103:534–540.
*376 Davis PG, Henderson Smart DJ. Nasal continuous positive airways pressure immediately after extubation for preventing morbidity in preterm infants. Cochrane Database Syst Rev 2000; 3:CD000143.
377 Van Marter LJ, Allred EN, Pagano M, et al. Do clinical markers of barotrauma and oxygen toxicity explain interhospital variation in rates of chronic lung disease. Pediatrics 2000; 105:1194–1201.
378 Verder H, Robertson B, Greisen G, et al. Surfactant therapy and nasal continuous positive airway pressure for newborns with respiratory distress syndrome. N Engl J Med 1994; 331:1051–1055.
379 Verder H, Albertsen P, Ebbesen F, et al. Nasal continuous positive airway pressure and early surfactant therapy for respiratory distress syndrome in newborns of less than 30 weeks' gestation. Pediatrics 1999; 103:e24.
380 Herman S, Reynolds EOR. Methods of improving oxygenation in infants mechanically ventilated for severe hyaline membrane disease. Arch Dis Child 1973; 48:612–617.
381 Stewart AR, Finer NN, Peters KL. Effects of alterations of inspiratory and expiratory pressures and inspiratory/expiratory ratios on mean airway pressure, blood gases and intracranial pressure. Pediatrics 1981; 67:474–481.
382 Oxford Region Controlled Trial of Artificial Ventilation (OCTAVE) Study Group. A multicentre randomised controlled trial of high against low frequency positive pressure ventilation. Arch Dis Child 1991; 66:770–775.
*383 Greenough A, Milner AD, Dimitriou G. Synchronized mechanical ventilation for respiratory support in newborn infants (Cochrane Review). Cochrane Database Syst Rev 2001; 1:CD000456.
384 Field D, Milner AD, Hopkin IE. Inspiratory time and tidal volume during intermittent positive pressure ventilation. Arch Dis Child 1985; 60:259–261.
385 Bartholomew KM, Brownlee KG, Snowden S, et al. To PEEP or not to PEEP? Arch Dis Child 1994; 70:F209–F212.
386 Simbruner G. Inadvertent positive end expiratory pressure in mechanically ventilated newborn infants: detection and effect on lung mechanics and gas exchange. J Pediatr 1986; 108:589–595.
387 Stenson BJ, Glover RM, Laing IA, et al. Life threatening inadvertent positive end expiratory pressure. Am J Perinatol 1995; 12:336–338.
388 Tarnow-Mordi WO, Griffiths P, Wilkinson AR. Low inspired gas temperature and respiratory complications in very low birth weight infants. J Pediatr 1989; 114:438–442.
389 Tarnow-Mordi WO, Sutton P, Wilkinson AR. Inadequate humidification of respiratory gases during mechanical ventilation of the newborn. Arch Dis Child 1986; 61:698–700.
390 O'Hagan M, Reid E, Tarnow-Mordi WO. Is neonatal inspired gas humidity accurately controlled by humidifier temperature? Crit Care Med 1991; 19:1370–1373.
391 Prendiville A, Thomson A, Silverman M. Effect of tracheobronchial suction on respiratory resistance in intubated preterm babies. Arch Dis Child 1986; 61:1178–1183.
392 Simbruner G, Coradello H, Fodor M, et al. Effect of tracheal suction on oxygenation, circulation, and lung mechanics in newborn infants. Arch Dis Child 1981; 56:326–330.
393 Perlman JM, Volpe JJ. Suctioning in the preterm infant: effects on cerebral blood flow velocity, intracranial pressure, and arterial blood pressure. Pediatrics 1983; 72:329–334.
394 Greenough A, Greenall F, Gamsu H. Synchronous respiration: which ventilator rate is best? Acta Paediatr Scand 1987; 76:713–718.
395 Bernstein G, Knodel E, Heldt GP. Airway leak size in neonates and autocycling of three flow-triggered ventilators. Crit Care Med 1995; 23:1739–1744.
396 Chan V, Greenough A. Comparison of weaning by patient triggered ventilation or synchronous intermittent mandatory ventilation. Acta Paediatr Scand 1994; 83:335–337.
397 Bernstein G, Heldt GP, Mannino FM. Increased and more consistent tidal volumes during synchronised intermittent mandatory ventilation in newborn infants. Am J Respir Crit Care Med 1994; 150:1444–1448.
398 Cleary JP, Bernstein G, Mannino FL, et al. Improved oxygenation during synchronised intermittent mandatory ventilation in neonates with respiratory distress syndrome: a randomised, crossover study. J Pediatr 1995; 126:407–411.
399 Govindaswami B, Bejar R, Bernstein G, et al. Reduction in cerebral blood flow velocity (CBFV) variability in infants <1500 gm during synchronised intermittent mandatory ventilation. Pediatr Res 1993; 33:1258–1260.
*400 Bernstein G, Mannino FL, Heldt GP, et al. Randomized multicentre trial comparing synchronized and conventional intermittent mandatory ventilation in neonates. J Pediatr 1996; 128:453–463.
*401 Beresford MW, Shaw NJ, Manning D. Randomised controlled trial of patient triggered and conventional fast rate ventilation in neonatal respiratory distress syndrome. Arch Dis Child Fetal Neonatal Ed 2000; 82:F14–F18.
*402 Baumer JH. International randomised controlled trial of patient triggered ventilation in neonatal respiratory distress syndrome. Arch Dis Child Fetal Neonatal Ed 2000; 82:F5–F10.
*403 Greenough A, Wood S, Morley CJ, et al. Pancuronium prevents pneumothoraces in ventilated premature babies who actively expire against positive pressure ventilation Lancet 1984; i:1–3.
*404 Shaw NJ, Cooke RWI, Gill AB, et al. Randomised trial of routine versus selective paralysis during ventilation for neonatal respiratory distress syndrome. Arch Dis Child 1993; 69:479–482.
405 Bhutani VK, Abassi S, Sivieri EM. Continuous skeletal muscle paralysis: effect on neonatal pulmonary mechanics. Pediatrics 1988; 81:419–422.
406 Froese AB, Bryan AC. High frequency ventilation Am Rev Respir Dis 1987; 135:1363–1374.
407 Boynton BR, Hammond MD, Fredburg JJ, et al. Gas exchange in healthy rabbits during

high-frequency oscillatory ventilation. J Appl Physiol 1989; 66:1343–1351.
408 Chan V, Greenough A, Milner AD. The effect of frequency and mean airway pressure on volume delivery during high frequency oscillation. Pediatr Pulmonol 1993; 15:183–186.
409 Chan V, Greenough A. The effect of frequency on carbon dioxide levels during high frequency oscillation. J Perinat Med 1994; 22:103–106.
*410 Henderson-Smart DJ, Bhuta T, Cools F, et al. Elective high frequency oscillatory ventilation versus conventional ventilation for acute pulmonary dysfunction in preterm infants (Cochrane Review). Cochrane Database Syst Rev 2001; 3:CD000104.
411 Carter JM, Gerstmann DR, Clark RH, et al. High-frequency oscillatory ventilation and extracorporeal membrane oxygenation for the treatment of acute neonatal respiratory failure. Pediatrics 1990; 85:159–164.
412 Clark RH, Yoder BA, Sell MS. Prospective, randomized comparison of high-frequency oscillation and conventional ventilation in candidates for extracorporeal membrane oxygenation. J Pediatr 1994; 124:447–454.
*413 HIFO Study Group. Randomized study of high-frequency oscillatory ventilation in infants with severe respiratory distress syndrome. J Pediatr 1993; 122:609–619.
414 Gerstmann DR, DeLemos RA, Clark RH. High-frequency ventilation: issues of strategy. Clin Perinatol 1991; 18:563–580.
415 Carlo WA, Chatburn RL, Martin RJ. Randomized trial of high frequency jet ventilation in respiratory distress syndrome. J Pediatr 1987; 110:275–282.
*416 Bhuta T, Henderson-Smart DJ. Elective high frequency jet ventilation versus conventional ventilation for respiratory distress syndrome in preterm infants. Cochrane Database Syst Rev 2000; 2:CD000328.
*417 UK Collaborative ECMO Trial Group. UK collaborative randomised trial of neonatal extracorporeal membrane oxygenation. Lancet 1996; 348:75–82.
418 Ignarro LJ. Biological actions and properties of endothelium derived nitric oxide formed and released from artery and vein. Circ Res 1989; 65:1–21.
419 Miller OI, Celermajer DS, Deanfield JE, et al. Guidelines for the safe administration of inhaled nitric oxide. Arch Dis Child 1994; 70:F47–F49.
*420 Finer NN, Barrington KJ. Nitric oxide for respiratory failure in infants born at or near term (Cochrane Review). Cochrane Database Syst Rev 2001; 4:CD000399.
*421 Barrington KJ, Finer NN. Inhaled nitric oxide for respiratory failure in preterm infants (Cochrane Review). Cochrane Database Syst Rev 2001; 3:CD000509.
422 Davidson D, Barefield ES, Kattwinkel J, et al. Safety of withdrawing inhaled nitric oxide therapy in persistent pulmonary hypertension of the newborn. Pediatrics 1999; 104(2 part 1):231–236.
423 Dworetz AR, Moya FR, Sabo B, et al. Survival of infants with persistent pulmonary hypertension without extracorporeal membrane oxygenation. Pediatrics 1989; 84:1–6.
424 Schreiber MD, Heymann MA, Soifer SJ. Increased arterial pH, not decreased pACO2, attenuates hypoxia-induced pulmonary vasoconstriction in newborn lambs. Pediatr Res 1986; 20:113–117.
425 Greenspan JS, Wolfson MR, Rubenstein SD, et al. Liquid ventilation of human preterm neonates J Pediatr 1990; 117:106–111.
426 Leach CL, Greenspan JS, Rubenstein SD, et al. Partial liquid ventilation with Liquivent: a pilot safety and efficacy study in premature newborns with severe respiratory distress syndrome (RDS). Pediatr Res 1995; 37:220.

NEURODEVELOPMENTAL OUTCOME

427 Escobar GB, Littenberg B, Pettiti DB. Outcome among surviving very low birthweight infants: a meta-analysis. Arch Dis Child 1991; 66:204–211.
428 Ens-Dokkum MH, Johnson A, Schrender M, et al. Comparison of mortality and rates of cerebral palsy in two populations of VLBW infants. Arch Dis Child 1997; 66:204–211.
429 Pharoah POD, Cooke RWI. Effects of birthweight, gestational age, maternal obstetric history on birth prevalence of cerebral palsy. Arch Dis Child 1987; 62:1035–1040.
430 Pharoah POD, Cooke RWI. Birthweight specific trends in cerebral palsy. Arch Dis Child 1990; 65:602–606.
431 Stanley FJ, Watson F. Trends in perinatal mortality and cerebral palsy in Western Australia 1967–1985. BMJ 1992; 304:1658–1663.
432 Cummins SK, Nelson KB, Grether JK, et al. Cerebral palsy in four northern Californian counties: births 1983 through 1985. J Pediatr 1993; 123:230–237.
433 Evans DJ, Levene MI. Evidence of selection bias in preterm survival studies: a systematic review. Arch Dis Child 2001; 84:F79–F84.
*434 Wood NS, Marlow N, Costeloe K, et al. Neurologic and developmental disability after extremely preterm birth. N Engl J Med 2000; 363(6):378–384.
435 Huddy CLJ, Johnson A, Hope PL. Educational and behavioural problems in babies of 32–35 weeks' gestation. Arch Dis Child 2001;85(1):F23–F28.
436 Kramer MS, Demissie K, Yang H, et al. The contribution of mild and moderate preterm birth to infant mortality. JAMA 2000; 284:843–849.
437 Pharoah POD, Adi Y. Consequences of in-utero death in a twin pregnancy. Lancet 2000; 355:1597–1602.
438 Wu YW, Colford JM. Chorioamnionitis as a risk factor for cerebral palsy. JAMA 2000; 284(11):1417–1424.
439 Tin W, Fritz S, Wariyar U, et al. Outcome of very preterm birth: children reviewed with ease at 2 years differ from those followed up with difficulty. Arch Dis Child 1998; 79:F83–F87.
440 Morley R, Brooke OG, Cole TJ, et al. Birthweight ratio and outcome in preterm infants. Arch Dis Child 1990; 65:30–34.
441 Cooke RWI. Factors affecting survival and outcome. Arch Dis Child 1994; 71:F28–F33.
442 Synnes AR, Ling EW, Whitfield MF, et al. Perinatal outcomes of a large cohort of extremely low gestational age infants (23–28 completed weeks of gestation). J Pediatr 1994; 125:952–960.
*443 Fanaroff AA, Wright LL, Stevenson DK, et al. Very low birth weight outcomes of the National Institute of Child Health and Human Development Neonatal Research Network, May 91 to December 92. Am J Obstet Gynecol 1995; 173:1423–1431.
444 Bottoms SF, Paul RH, Mercer BM, et al. Obstetric determinants of neonatal survival: antenatal predictors of neonatal survival and morbidity in extremely low birth weight infants. Am J Obstet Gynecol 1999; 180:665–669.
445 McCarton CM, Wallace IF, Divon M, et al. Cognitive and neurologic development of the premature, small for gestational age infant through age 6: comparison by birth weight and gestational age. Pediatrics 1996; 98: 1167–1178.
446 Rennie JM. Perinatal management at the lower margin of viability. Arch Dis Child 1996; 74:F214–F218.
*447 Costeloe K, Hennessy E, Gibson AT, et al. The Epicure Study: outcomes to discharge from hospital for infants born at the threshold of viability. Pediatrics 2000; 106(4):659–671.
448 Doyle LW. Outcome at 5 years of age of children 23 to 28 weeks' gestation: refining the prognosis. Pediatrics 2001; 108(1):134–141.
*449 Draper ES, Manktelow B, Field DJ, et al. Prediction of survival for preterm births by weight and gestational age: retrospective population based study. BMJ 1999; 319: 1093–1097.
*450 Cartlidge PHT, Stewart JH. Survival of very low birth weight and very preterm infants in a geographically defined population. Acta Paediatr 1997; 86:105–110.
451 Lefebvre F, Glorieux J, St-Lauren-Gagnon T. Neonatal survival and disability rate at age 18 months for infants born between 23 and 28 weeks of gestation. Am J Obstet Gynecol 1996; 174:833–838.
*452 Tin W, Wariyar U, Hey E. Changing prognosis for babies of less than 28 weeks gestation in the north of England between 1983 and 1994. BMJ 1997; 314:107–111.
453 Stewart A, Reynolds EOR, Lipscomb AP. Outcome for infants of very low birth weight. Lancet 1981; 1:1038–1039.
454 Emsley HCA, Wardle SP, Sims DG, et al. Increased survival and deteriorating developmental outcome in 23 to 25 week old gestation infants, 1990–4 compared with 1984–9. Arch Dis Child 1998; 78:F99–F104.
455 Wariyar U. Pregnancy outcome at 24–31 weeks gestation mortality. Arch Dis Child 1989; 64:670–677.
456 Saigal S, Szatmari P, Rosenbaum P, et al. Intellectual and functional status at school entry of children <1000 g at birth. J Pediatr 1990; 116:409–416.
457 Aylward GP. Outcome studies of VLBWI: meta-analysis. J Pediatr 1989; 115:515–520.
458 Olsen P, Myrman A, Rantakallio P. Educational capacity of low birthweight children up to age 24. Early Hum Dev 1994; 36:191–203.
459 Skuse D. Survival after being born too soon, but at what cost? Lancet 1999; 354:354–356.
460 Ng PC, Dear PRF. The predictive value of a normal ultrasound scan. Acta Paediatr Scand 1990; 79:286–291.

461 Rennie JM. Neonatal cerebral ultrasound. Cambridge: Cambridge University Press; 1997.
462 Ventriculomegaly Trial Group. Randomised trial of early tapping in neonatal periventricular dilatation. Arch Dis Child 1994; 70:F129–F136.
463 Graham M, Levene MI. Predicition of cerebral palsy in very low birthweight infants by ultrasound. Lancet 1987; ii:593–594.
464 Appleton RE, Lee REJ, Hey EN. Neurodevelopmental outcome of transient neonatal echodensities. Arch Dis Child 1990; 65:27–29.

NEONATAL DEATH
465 Wilson RE. Parents' support of their other children after a miscarriage or perinatal death. Early Hum Dev 2001; 61:55–65.
466 SANDS. After stillbirth and neonatal death: what happens next? London: Stillbirth and Neonatal Death Society; 1986.
467 Porter HJ, Keeling JW. Value of perinatal necropsy examination. J Clin Pathol 1987; 40:180–184.

PULMONARY DISORDERS AND APNEA
468 Taeusch HW, Boncuk-Dayanikli P. Respiratory distress syndrome. In: Yu VYH, ed. Pulmonary problems in the perinatal period and their sequelae. London: Baillière Tindall; 1995.
469 Rubaltelli FF, Bonafe L, Tangucci M, et al and the Italian Group of Neonatal Pneumology. Epidemiology of neonatal acute respiratory disorders. A multicenter study on incidence and fatality rates of neonatal acute respiratory disorders according to gestational age, maternal age, pregnancy complications and type of delivery. Biol Neonate 1998; 74:7–15.
*470 Crowley P. Prophylactic corticosteroids for preterm birth. Cochrane Database Syst Rev 2001; 3:CD000065.
*471 ACTOBAT Study Group. Australian collaborative trial of antenatal thyrotropin releasing hormone (ACTOBAT) for prevention of neonatal respiratory disease. Lancet 1995; 345:877–882.
472 Crowther CA, Hiller JE, Haslam RR, et al. Australian collaborative trial of antenatal thyrotropin releasing hormone: adverse effects at 12 month follow up. Pediatrics 1997; 99:311–317.
473 Sweet DG, Halliday HL. Current perspectives on the drug treatment of neonatal respiratory distress syndrome. Pediatr Drugs 1999; 1:19–30. (Review article with 104 references)
474 Jobe AH. Pulmonary surfactant therapy. N Engl J Med 1993; 328:861–868.
475 Halliday HL, Speer CP. Strategies for surfactant therapy in established neonatal respiratory distress syndrome. In: Robertson B, Taeusch HW, eds. Surfactant therapy for lung disease. New York: Marcel Dekker; 1995.
*476 Soll RF. Prophylactic natural surfactant extract for preventing morbidity and mortality in preterm infants. Cochrane Database Syst Rev 2001; 3:CD000511.
*477 Soll RF. Prophylactic synthetic surfactant for preventing morbidity and mortality in preterm infants. Cochrane Database Syst Rev 2001; 3:CD001079.
*478 Soll RF. Synthetic surfactant for respiratory distress syndrome in preterm infants. Cochrane Database Syst Rev 2001;3: CD001149.
*479 Ainsworth SB, Beresford MW, Milligan DWA, et al. Pumactant and poractant alfa for treatment of respiratory distress syndrome in neonates born at 25–29 weeks' gestation: a randomised trial. Lancet 2000; 355:1387–1392.
*480 Halliday HL. Natural vs synthetic surfactants in neonatal respiratory distress syndrome. Drugs 1996; 51:226–237.
*481 Soll RF, Blanco F. Natural surfactant extract versus synthetic surfactant for neonatal respiratory distress syndrome. Cochrane Database Syst Rev 2001; 3:CD 000144.
482 Dechant KL, Faulds D. Colfosceril palmitate: a review of the therapeutic efficacy and clinical tolerability of a synthetic preparation (Exosurf©) in neonatal respiratory distress syndrome. Drugs 1991; 42:877–894.
*483 Ho JJ, Subramanuam P, Henderson-Smart DJ, et al. Continuous distending pressure for respiratory distress syndrome in preterm infants. Cochrane Database Syst Rev 2001; 3:CD002271.
*484 Verder H, Robertson B, Greisen G, et al for the Danish-Swedish Multicenter Study Group. Surfactant therapy and nasal continuous positive airway pressure for newborns with respiratory distress syndrome. N Engl J Med 1994; 331:1051–1055.
*485 Verder H, Albertsen P, Ebbesen F, et al. Nasal continuous positive airway pressure and early surfactant therapy for respiratory distress syndrome in newborn infants of less than 30 weeks' gestation. Pediatrics 1999; 103:e24.
486 Morley C. Continuous distending pressure. Arch Dis Child Fetal Neonatal Ed 1999; 81:F152–F156.
487 Courtney SE, Pyon KH, Saslow JG, et al. Lung recruitment and breathing during variable versus continuous flow nasal continuous positive airway pressure in premature infants: an evaluation of three devices. Pediatrics 2001; 107:304–308.
*488 Lee K-Y, Dunn MS, Fenwick M, et al. A comparison of underwater bubble continuous positive airway pressure with ventilator-derived continuous positive airway pressure in premature neonates ready for extubation. Biol Neonate 1998; 73:69–75.
489 South M, Morley C. Synchronous mechanical ventilation of the neonate. Arch Dis Child 1986; 61:1190–1195.
490 Greenough A, Greenall F, Gamsu H. Synchronous respiration: which ventilator rate is best? Acta Paediatr Scand 1987; 76:713–718.
*491 Barrington KJ, Finer NN. Inhaled nitric oxide for respiratory failure in preterm infants. Cochrane Database Syst Rev 2001; 3:CD000509.
*492 Henderson-Smart DJ, Davis PG. Prophylactic methylxanthine for extubation in preterm infants. Cochrane Database Syst Rev 2001; 3:CD000139
*493 Baumer JH. International randomised controlled trial of patient triggered ventilation in neonatal respiratory distress syndrome. Arch Dis Child Fetal Neonatal Ed 2000; 82:F5–F10.
*494 Davis PG, Henderson-Smart DJ. Nasal continuous positive airways pressure immediately after extubation for preventing morbidity in preterm infants. Cochrane Database Syst Rev 2001; 3:CD000143.
*495 Halliday HL. Towards earlier neonatal extubation. Lancet 2000; 355:2091–2092. (Review article based upon results of Cochrane Reviews)
496 Halliday HL. Neonatal patent ductus arteriosus. Pediatr Rev Commun 1988; 3:1–17. (Review article with 97 references)
497 Lipscomb AP, Thorburn RJ, Reynolds EOR, et al. Pneumothorax and cerebral haemorrhage in preterm infants. Lancet 1981; i:414–416.
*498 McCord FB, Curstedt T, Halliday HL, et al. Surfactant treatment and incidence of intraventricular haemorrhage in severe respiratory distress syndrome. Arch Dis Child 1988; 63:10–16.
499 Ogata ES, Gregory GA, Kitterman JA, et al. Pneumothorax in the respiratory distress syndrome: incidence and effect on vital signs, blood gases and pH. Pediatrics 1975; 58:177–183.
500 Halliday HL. Other acute lung disorders. In: Sinclair JC, Bracken MB, eds. Effective care of the newborn infant. Oxford: Oxford University Press; 1992.
501 Northway WH, Rosan RC, Porter DY. Pulmonary disease following respirator therapy of hyaline membrane disease. Bronchopulmonary dysplasia. N Engl J Med 1967; 276:357–368.
502 Jobe AH, Ikegami M. Mechanisms initiating lung injury in the preterm. Early Hum Dev 1998; 53:81–94. (Review article with 66 references)
503 Speer CP. New insights into the pathogenesis of pulmonary inflammation in preterm infants. Biol Neonate 2001; 79:205–209. (Review article with 89 references)
504 Corcoran JD, Patterson CC, Thomas PS, et al. Reduction in the risk of bronchopulmonary dysplasia from 1980–1990: results of a multivariate logistic regression analysis. Eur J Pediatr 1993; 152:671–681.
505 Gonzalez A, Sosenko IRS, Chandar J, et al. Influence of infection on patent ductus arteriosus and chronic lung disease in premature infants weighing 1000 grams or less. J Pediatr 1996; 128:470–478.
506 Giacoia GP, Neter E, Ogra P. Respiratory infections in infants with idiopathic apnea. Pediatrics 1981; 63:537–542.
507 Goodwin SR, Graves SA, Haberkern CM. Aspiration in the intubated premature infant. Pediatrics 1985; 75:85–88.
508 Dammann O, Leviton A. Maternal intrauterine infection, cytokines, and brain damage in the preterm newborn. Pediatr Res 1997; 42:1–8. (Review article)
509 Dammann O, Leviton A. Role of the fetus in perinatal infection and neonatal brain damage. Curr Opin Pediatr 2000; 12:99–104. (Review article)
510 Lee K-S, Khoshnood B, Wall SN, et al. Trend in mortality from respiratory distress syndrome in the United States, 1970–1995. J Pediatr 1999; 134:434–440.
511 Avery ME, Gatewood O, Brumley G. Transient tachypnea of newborn. Possible delayed resorption of fluid at birth. Am J Dis Child 1966; 111:380–385.

512 Morrison JJ, Rennie JM, Milton PJ. Neonatal respiratory morbidity and mode of delivery at term: influence of timing of elective caesarean section. Br J Obstet Gynaecol 1995; 102:101–106.

513 Walters DV, Olver RE. The role of catecholamines in lung liquid absorption at birth. Pediatr Res 1978; 12:239–242.

514 Halliday HL, McClure G, Reid MMcC. Transient tachypnoea of the newborn: two distinct clinical entities? Arch Dis Child 1981; 56:322–325.

515 Tudehope DI, Smyth MJ. Is 'transient tachypnoea of the newborn' always a benign disease? Report of 6 babies requiring mechanical ventilation. Austr Paediatr J 1979; 15:160–165.

516 Madar J, Richmond S, Hey E. Surfactant-deficient respiratory distress after elective delivery at 'term'. Acta Paediatr 1999; 88:1244–1248.

517 Wiswell TE, Rawlings JS, Smith FR, et al. Effect of furosemide on the clinical course of transient tachypnea of the newborn. Pediatrics 1985; 75:908–910.

518 Halahakoon CH, Halliday HL. Other acute lung disorders. In: Yu VYH, ed. Pulmonary problems in the perinatal period and their sequelae. London: Baillière Tindall; 1995.

519 Webber S, Wilkinson AR, Lindsell D, et al. Neonatal pneumonia. Arch Dis Child 1990; 65:207–211.

520 Hemming VG, Overall JC, Brett MR. Nosocomial infections in a newborn intensive-care unit. N Engl J Med 1976; 294:1310–1316.

521 Naeye RL, Peters EC. Amniotic fluid infections with intact membranes leading to perinatal death: a prospective study. Pediatrics 1978; 61:171–177.

*522 Boyer KM, Gotoff SP. Prevention of early-onset neonatal group B streptococcal disease with selective intrapartum chemoprophylaxis. N Engl J Med 1986; 314:1665–1669.

*523 Kenyon SL, Taylor DJ, Tarnow-Mordi W. Broad-spectrum antibiotics for preterm, prelabour rupture of fetal membranes: the ORACLE 1 randomised trial. Lancet 2001; 357:979–988.

524 Mifsud A, Seal D, Wall R, et al. Reduced neonatal mortality from infection after introduction of respiratory monitoring. BMJ 1988; 296:17–18.

525 Herting E, Gefeller O, Land M, et al. Surfactant treatment of neonates with respiratory failure and group B streptococcal infection. Pediatrics 2000; 106:957–964.

526 Gregory GA, Gooding CA, Phibbs RH, et al. Meconium aspiration in infants – a prospective study. J Pediatr 1974; 85:848–852.

*527 Cardozo L, Fysh J, Pearce JM. Prolonged pregnancy: the management debate. BMJ 1986; 292:1059–1063.

*528 Crowley P. Interventions for preventing or improving outcome of delivery at or beyond term. Cochrane Database Syst Rev 2001; 3:CD000170.

529 Halliday HL, Hirata T. Perinatal listeriosis – a review of twelve patients. Am J Obstet Gynecol 1979; 133:405–410.

*530 Linder N, Aranda JV, Tsur M, et al. Need for endotracheal intubation and suction in meconium-stained neonates. J Pediatr 1988; 112:612–615.

*531 Wiswell TE, Gannon CM, Jacob J, et al. Delivery room management of the apparently vigorous meconium-stained neonate: results of the multicenter, international collaborative trial. Pediatrics 2000; 105:1–7.

*532 Halliday HL. Endotracheal intubation at birth for preventing morbidity and mortality in vigorous meconium-stained infants born at term. Cochrane Database Syst Rev 2001; 3:CD000500.

*533 Findlay RD, Taeusch HW, Walther FJ. Surfactant replacement for meconium aspiration syndrome. Pediatrics 1996; 97:48–52.

534 Wiswell TE, Tuggle JM, Turner BS. Meconium aspiration syndrome: have we made a difference? Pediatrics 1990; 85:715–721.

535 Macfarlane PI, Heaf DP. Pulmonary function in children after neonatal meconium aspiration syndrome. Arch Dis Child 1989; 63:368–372.

536 Goldberg RN. Sustained arterial blood pressure elevation associated with small pneumothoraces: early detection via continuous monitoring. Pediatrics 1981; 68:775–777.

537 Madansky DL, Lawson EE, Chernick V, et al. Pneumothorax and other forms of pulmonary air leaks in the newborn. Am Rev Respir Dis 1979; 120:729–737.

538 Swischuk LE. Two lesser known but useful signs of neonatal pneumothorax. Am J Roentgenol 1976; 127:623–627.

539 Van Gelderen WFC. Ultrasound diagnosis of an atypical pneumomediastinum. Pediatr Radiol 1992; 22:469–470.

540 McIntosh N, Prakesh P, Smith A. Air leaks and vasopressin release. Arch Dis Child 1990; 65:1259–1262.

541 Berger JT, Gilhooly J. Fibrin glue treatment of persistent pneumothorax in a premature infant. J Pediatr 1993; 122:958–960.

*542 Greenough A, Wood S, Morley CJ, et al. Pancuronium prevents pneumothoraces in ventilated premature babies who actively expire against positive pressure ventilation. Lancet 1984; i:1–3.

*543 Heicher DA, Kasting DS, Harrod JR. Prospective clinical comparison of two methods for mechanical ventilation of neonates: rapid rate and short inspiratory time versus slow rate and long inspiratory time. J Pediatr 1981; 98:957–961.

544 Fujimura M, Kitajima H, Nakayama M. Increased leukocyte elastase of the tracheal aspirate at birth and neonatal pulmonary emphysema. Pediatrics 1993; 92:564–569.

545 Speer CP, Ruess D, Harms K, et al. Neutrophil elastase and acute pulmonary damage in neonates with severe respiratory distress syndrome. Pediatrics 1993; 91:794–799.

546 Rettwitz-Volk W, Scholosser R, Von Loewenich V. One sided high frequency oscillatory ventilation in the treatment of neonatal unilateral pulmonary emphysema. Acta Paediatr 1993; 82:190–192.

547 Dear PRF, Conway SP. Treatment of severe bilateral interstitial emphysema in a baby by artificial pneumothorax and pneumotomy. Lancet 1984; i:273–277.

548 Clark RH, Gerstmann DR, Null DM, et al. Pulmonary interstitial emphysema treated by high frequency oscillatory ventilation. Crit Care Med 1986; 14:926–930.

549 Hart SM, McNair M, Gamsu HR, et al. Pulmonary interstitial emphysema in very low birthweight infants. Arch Dis Child 1983; 58:612–615.

550 Fenton TR, Bennett S, McIntosh N. Air embolism in ventilated very low birthweight infants. Arch Dis Child 1988; 63:541–543.

551 Kogutt MS. Systemic air embolism secondary to respiratory therapy in the neonate: six cases including one survivor. Am J Roentgenol 1978; 131:425–429.

*552 Raju TNK, Langenberg P. Pulmonary hemorrhage and exogenous surfactant therapy: a metaanalysis. J Pediatr 1993; 123:603–610.

553 Kluckow M, Evans N. Ductal shunting, high pulmonary blood flow, and pulmonary hemorrhage. J Pediatr 2000; 137:68–72.

*554 Stevenson DK, Walther F, Long WA and the American Exosurf Neonatal Study Group. 1. Controlled trial of a single dose of synthetic surfactant at birth in premature infants weighing 500–699 grams. J Pediatr 1992; 120:S3–S12.

555 Van Houten J, Long W, Mullet M, et al. Pulmonary hemorrhage in premature infants after treatment with synthetic surfactant: an autopsy evaluation. J Pediatr 1992; 120:S40–S44.

556 Pandit PB, Dunn MS, Colucci EA. Surfactant therapy in neonates with respiratory deterioration due to pulmonary hemorrhage. Pediatrics 1995; 95:32–36.

557 Pandit PB, O'Brien K, Asztalos E, et al. Outcome following pulmonary haemorrhage in very low birthweight neonates treated with surfactant. Arch Dis Child Fetal Neonatal Ed 1999; 81:F40–F44.

558 Wigglesworth JS, Desai R. Is fetal respiratory function a major determinant of perinatal survival? Lancet 1982; i:264–267.

559 Wigglesworth JS, Desai R. Use of DNA estimation for growth assessment in normal and hypoplastic fetal lungs. Arch Dis Child 1981; 56:601–605.

560 McIntosh N. Dry lung syndrome after oligohydramnios. Arch Dis Child 1988; 63:190–193.

561 Tubman TRJ, Halliday HL. Surfactant treatment for respiratory distress following prolonged rupture of membranes. Eur J Pediatr 1990; 149:727–729.

*562 UK Collaborative ECMO Trial Group. UK collaborative randomised trial of neonatal extracorporeal membrane oxygenation. Lancet 1996; 348:75–82.

563 Milner AD, Fox G. Congenital abnormalities of the respiratory system. In: Yu VYH, ed. Pulmonary problems in the perinatal period and their sequelae. London: Baillière Tindall; 1995.

564 Stocker JT, Drake RM, Madewell JE. Cystic and congenital lung disease in the newborn. Perspect Pediatr Pathol 1978; 4:93–154.

565 Blau H, Barak A, Karmazyn B, et al. Postnatal management of resolving fetal lung lesions. Pediatrics 2002; 109:105–108.

566 Stocker JT. Sequestrations of the lung. Semin Diagn Pathol 1986; 3:106–121.

567 Shennan AT, Dunn MS, Ohlsson A, et al. Abnormal pulmonary outcomes in premature infants: prediction from oxygen requirements in the neonatal period. Pediatrics 1988; 82:527–532.
568 Wilson ME, Mikity TG. A new form of respiratory disease in premature infants. Am J Dis Child 1960; 99:489–499.
569 Tremblay LN, Slutsky AS. Ventilator-induced injury: from barotrauma to biotrauma. Proc Assoc Am Physicians 1998; 110:482–488.
570 Rojas MA, Gonzalez A, Bancalari E, et al. Changing trends in the epidemiology and pathogenesis of neonatal chronic lung disease. J Pediatr 1995; 126:605–610.
571 Philip AGS. Oxygen plus pressure plus time: the etiology of bronchopulmonary dysplasia. Pediatrics 1975; 55:44–50.
572 Yu VYH, Ng PC. Chronic lung disease. In: Yu VYH, ed. Pulmonary problems in the perinatal period and their sequelae. London: Baillière Tindall; 1995.
573 Thurlbeck WM. Morphologic aspects of bronchopulmonary dysplasia. J Pediatr 1979; 95:842–843.
*574 Halliday HL, Ehrenkranz RA. Early postnatal (<96 hours) corticosteroids for preventing chronic lung disease in preterm infants. Cochrane Database Syst Rev 2001; 3:CD001146.
*575 Halliday HL, Ehrenkranz RA. Moderately early (7–14 days) postnatal corticosteroids for preventing chronic lung disease in preterm infants. Cochrane Database Syst Rev 2001; 3:CD001144.
*576 Halliday HL, Enrenkranz RA. Delayed (> 3 weeks) postnatal corticosteroids for chronic lung disease in preterm infants. Cochrane Database Syst Rev 2001; 3:CD001145.
*577 Barrington JK. The adverse neuro-developmental effects of postnatal steroids in the preterm infant: a systematic review of RCTs. BMC Pediatr 2001; 1:1. (Available: http://www.biomedcentral.com/1471-2431/1/1)
*578 Halliday HL, Patterson CC, Halahakoon CWNL on behalf of the European Multicenter Steroid Study Group. A multicenter, randomized open study of early corticosteroid treatment (OSECT) in preterm infants with respiratory illness: comparison of early and late treatment and of dexamethasone and inhaled budesonide. Pediatrics 2001; 107:232–240.
*579 Tyson JE, Wright LL, Oh W, et al. Vitamin A supplementation for extremely-low-birth-weight infants. N Engl J Med 1999; 340:1962–1968.
*580 Sweet DG, Halliday HL. A risk–benefit assessment of drugs used for neonatal chronic lung disease. Drug Saf 2000; 22:389–404. (Review article based upon Cochrane Reviews)
581 Pandit PB, Dunn MS, Kelly EN, et al. Surfactant replacement in neonates with early chronic lung disease. Pediatrics 1995; 95:851–854.
582 Whitley RJ, Brasfield D, Reynolds DW, et al. Protracted pneumonitis in young infants associated with perinatally acquired cytomegalovirus infection. J Pediatr 1976; 89:16–22.
583 Stagno S, Brasfield DM, Brown MB, et al. Infant pneumonitis associated with cytomegalovirus, chlamydia, pneumocystis and ureoplasma: a prospective study. Pediatrics 1981; 68:322–329.
584 Strome M, Donahoe PK. Advances in management of laryngeal and subglottic stenosis. J Pediatr Surg 1982; 17:591–596.
585 Cotton R, Seid AB. Management of the extubation problem in the premature child. Anterior cricoid split as an alternative to tracheotomy. Ann Otorhinolaryngol 1980; 89:508–511.
586 Henderson-Smart DJ. Recurrent apnoea. In: Yu VYH, ed. Pulmonary problems in the prenatal period and their sequelae. London: Baillière Tindall; 1995.
587 Arad-Cohen N, Cohen A, Tirosh E. The relationship between gastroesophageal reflux and apnea in infants. J Pediatr 2000; 137:321–326.
588 Milner AD, Boon AW, Saunders RA, et al. Upper airways obstruction and apnoea in preterm babies. Arch Dis Child 1980; 55:22–25.
589 Howell J, Clozel M, Aranda JV. Adverse effects of caffeine and theophylline in the newborn infant. Semin Perinatol 1981; 5:359–369.
*590 Scanlon JEM, Chin KC, Morgan MEI, et al. Caffeine or theophylline for neonatal apnoea? Arch Dis Child 1992; 67:425–428.
*591 Steer PA, Henderson-Smart DJ. Caffeine versus theophylline in preterm infants. Cochrane Database Syst Rev 2001; 3:CD000273.
592 Barrington KJ, Finer NN, Peters KL, et al. Physiologic effects of doxopram in idiopathic apnea of prematurity. J Pediatr 1986; 108:125–129.
*593 Henderson-Smart DJ, Steer PA. Doxapram treatment for apnea in preterm infants. Cochrane Database Syst Rev 2001; 3:CD000074.
*594 Henderson-Smart DJ, Steer PA. Doxapram versus methylxanthine for apnea in preterm infants. Cochrane Database Syst Rev 2001; 3:CD000075.
595 Kimball AL, Carlton DP. Gastroesophageal reflux medications in the treatment of apnea in premature infants. J Pediatr 2001; 138:356–360.
596 Koons AH, Mjoica N, Jadeja N, et al. Neurodevelopmental outcome of infants with apnea of infancy. Am J Perinatol 1993; 10:208–211.
597 Liu LMP, Cote CJ, Goudsouzian NG, et al. Life-threatening apnea in infants recovering from anesthesia. Anesthesiology 1983; 59:506–510.
*598 Henderson-Smart DJ, Bhuta T, Cools F, et al. Elective high frequency oscillatory ventilation versus conventional ventilation for acute pulmonary dysfunction in preterm infants. Cochrane Database Syst Rev 2001; 3:CD000104.
*599 Halliday HL. Which interventions for neonatal respiratory failure are effective? Croat Med J 1998; 39:165–170. (Review article based upon results of Cochrane)

NEONATAL CARDIOVASCULAR DISEASE

600 Evans NJ, Archer LNJ. Postnatal circulatory adaptation in healthy term and preterm neonates. Arch Dis Child 1990; 65:24–26.
*601 de Swiet M, Fayers P, Shinebourne EA. Systolic blood pressure in a population of infants in the first year of life: the Brompton study. Pediatrics 1980; 65:1028–1035.
*602 Hegyi T, Carbone MT, Anwar M, et al. Blood pressure ranges in premature infants: 1. The first hours of life. J Pediatr 1994; 124:627–633.
*603 Hegyi T, Anwar M, Carbone MT, et al. Blood pressure ranges in premature infants: 2. The first week of life. Pediatrics 1996; 97:336–342.
*604 Davignon A, Rautaharju P, Barselle E, et al. Normal ECG standards for infants and children. Pediatr Cardiol 1979/80; 1:123–124.
605 Wyllie J, Wren C, Hunter S. Screening for fetal cardiac malformations. Br Heart J 1994; 71(suppl):20–27.
*606 Allan LD, Apfel HD, Printz BF. Outcome after prenatal diagnosis of the hypoplastic left heart syndrome. Heart 1998; 79:371–374.
607 Kumar RK, Newburger JW, Gauvreau K, et al. Comparison of outcome when hypoplastic left heart syndrome and transposition of the great arteries are diagnosed prenatally versus when diagnosis of these two conditions is made only postnatally. Am J Cardiol 1999; 83:1649–1653.
*608 Tworetzky W, McElhinney DB, Reddy V, et al. Improved surgical outcome after fetal diagnosis of hypoplastic left heart syndrome. Circulation 2001; 103:1269–1273.
*609 Franklin O, Burch M, Manning N, et al. Prenatal diagnosis of coarctation of the aorta improves survival and reduces morbidity. Heart. 2002; 87(1):67–69.
*610 Press J, Uziel Y, Laxer RM, et al. Long-term outcome of mothers of children with complete heart block. Am J Med 1996; 100:328–332.
611 Eronen M, Siren M-K, Ekblad H, et al. Short and long-term outcome of children with congenital complete heart block diagnosed in utero or as a newborn. Pediatrics 2000; 106:86–91.
*612 Ainsworth SB, Wyllie JP, Wren C. Prevalence and clinical significance of cardiac murmurs in neonates. Arch Dis Child 1999; 80:F43–F45.
*613 Arlettaz R, Archer N, Wilkinson AR. Natural history of innocent heart murmurs in newborn babies: controlled echocardiographic study. Arch Dis Child 1998; 78:F166–F170.
*614 Roguin N, Du Z-D, Barak M, et al. High prevalence of muscular ventricular septal defect in neonates. J Am Coll Cardiol 1995; 26:1545–1548.
615 Tulloh RMR, Tansey SP, Parashar K, et al. Echocardiographic screening in neonates undergoing surgery for selected gastrointestinal malformations. Arch Dis Child 1994; 70:F206–F208.
*616 Knight DB. The treatment of patent ductus arteriosus in preterm infants. A review and overview of randomised trials. Semin Neonatol 2001; 6:63–73.
617 Norton ME, Merrill J, Cooper BAB, et al. Neonatal complications after the administration of indomethacin for preterm labor. N Engl J Med 1993; 329:1602–1607.
618 Rosti L, Piva D, Rosti D. Ethamsylate in the prevention of patent ductus arteriosus. Arch Pediatr Adolesc Med 1994; 148:1103–1104.

*619 Cotton RB, Haywood JL, Fitzgerald GA. Symptomatic patent ductus arteriosus following prophylactic indomethacin. Biol Neonate 1991; 60:273–282.

*620 Varvarigou A, Bardin CL, Chemtob S, et al. Early ibuprofen administration to prevent patent ductus arteriosus in premature newborn infants. JAMA 1996; 275:539–544.

*621 Fowlie PW. Prophylactic indomethacin: systematic review and meta-analysis. Arch Dis Child 1996; 74:F81–F87.

*622 Schmidt B, Davis P, Moddemann D, et al. Long-term effects of indomethacin prophylaxis in extremely low birth weight infants. N Engl J Med 2001; 344:1966–1972.

623 Kluckow M, Evans N. Early echocardiographic prediction of symptomatic patent ductus arteriosus in preterm infants undergoing mechanical ventilation. J Pediatr 1995; 127:774–779.

*624 Su B-H, Watanabe T, Shimizu M, et al. Echocardiographic assessment of patent ductus arteriosus shunt flow pattern in premature infants. Arch Dis Child 1997; 77:F36–F40.

625 Iyer P, Evans N. Re-evaluation of the left atrial to aortic root ratio as a marker of patent ductus arteriosus. Arch Dis Child 1994; 70:F112–F117.

626 Evans N. Diagnosis of patent ductus arteriosus in the preterm newborn. Arch Dis Child 1993; 68:58–61.

*627 Gersony WM, Peakham GJ, Ellison RC, et al. Effects of indomethacin in premature infants with patent ductus arteriosus; results of a national collaborative study. J Pediatr 1983; 102:895–906.

*628 Colditz P, Murphy D, Rolfe P, et al. Effect of infusion rate of indomethacin on cerebrovascular responses in pre term neonates. Arch Dis Child 1989; 64:1–12.

629 Edwards AD, Wyatt JS, Richardson C, et al. Effects of indomethacin on cerebral haemodynamics in very pre term infants. Lancet 1990; 335:1491–1495.

*630 Su BH, Peng C-T, Tsai C-H. Echocardiographic flow pattern of patent ductus arteriosus: a guide to indomethacin treatment in premature infants. Arch Dis Child 1999; 81:F197–F200.

631 Patel K, Marks KA, Roberts I, et al. Ibuprofen treatment of patent ductus arteriosus. Lancet 1995; 346:255.

*632 Van Overmeire B, Follens I, Hartmann S, et al. Treatment of patent ductus arteriosus with ibuprofen. Arch Dis Child 1997; 76:F179–F184.

*633 Arlettaz R, Archer N, Wilkinson AR. Closure of the ductus arteriosus and development of pulmonary branch stenosis in babies less than 32 weeks gestation. Arch Dis Child 2001; 85:F197–F200.

*634 Hammerman C, Aramburo MJ. Prolonged indomethacin therapy for the prevention of recurrences of patent ductus arteriosus. J Pediatr 1990; 117:771–776.

*635 Rennie JM, Cooke RWI. Prolonged low dose indomethacin for persistent ductus arteriosus of prematurity. Arch Dis Child 1991; 66:55–58.

636 Shaughnessy CD, Reller MD, Rice MJ, et al. Development of systemic to pulmonary collateral arteries in premature infants. J Pediatr 1997; 131:763–765.

*637 Roberts JD, Fineman JR, Morin FC, et al. Inhaled nitric oxide and persistent pulmonary hypertension of the newborn. N Engl J Med 1997; 336:605–610.

*638 Tworetzky W, Bristow J, Moore P, et al. Inhaled nitric oxide in neonates with persistent pulmonary hypertension. Lancet 2001; 357:118–120.

*639 Cornfield DN, Maynard RC, deRegnier RA, et al. Randomized controlled trial of low dose inhaled nitric oxide in the treatment of term and near term infants with respiratory failure and pulmonary hypertension. Pediatrics 1999; 104:1089–1094.

*640 Kinsella JP, Truog WE, Walsh WF, et al. Randomized multicenter trial of inhaled nitric oxide and high frequency oscillatory ventilation in severe, persistent pulmonary hypertension of the newborn. J Pediatr 1997; 131:55–62.

641 Jedeikin R, Primhak A, Shennan AT, et al. Serial electrocardiographic changes in healthy and stressed neonates. Arch Dis Child 1983; 58:605–611.

642 Setzer E, Ermocilla R, Tonkin I, et al. Papillary muscle necrosis in a neonatal autopsy population: incidence and associated clinical manifestations. J Pediatr 1980; 96:289–294.

643 Tillett A, Hartley B, Simpson J. Paradoxical embolism causing fatal myocardial infarction in a newborn infant. Arch Dis Child 2001; 85:F137–F138.

644 Opie GF, Fraser SH, Drew JH, et al. Bacterial endocarditis in neonatal intensive care. J Paediatr Child Health 1999; 35:545–548.

645 Way GL, Woolfe RR, Eshaghpour E, et al. The natural history of hypertrophic cardiomyopathy in infants of diabetic mothers. J Pediatr 1979; 95:1020–1025.

646 Shaw NJ, Wilson N, Dickinson DF. Captopril in heart failure secondary to left to right shunt. Arch Dis Child 1988; 63:360–363.

647 Leversha AM, Wilson NJ, Clarkson PM, et al. Efficiency and dosage of enalapril in congenital and acquired heart disease. Arch Dis Child 1994; 70:35–39.

648 Kluckow M, Evans N. Low systemic blood pressure in the preterm infant. Semin Neonatol 2001; 6:75–84.

649 Joint Working Party of British Association of Perinatal Medicine and the Research Unit of the Royal College of Physicians. Development of audit measures and guidelines for good practice in the management of neonatal respiratory distress syndrome. Arch Dis Child 1992; 67:1221–1227.

650 Keeley SR, Bohn DJ. The use of inotropic and afterload reducing agents in neonates. Clin Perinatol 1988; 15:467–489.

*651 Gill AB, Weindling AM. Randomised controlled trial of plasma protein fraction versus dopamine in hypotensive very low birth weight infants. Arch Dis Child 1993; 69:284–287.

652 Seri I. Circulatory support of the sick preterm infant. Semin Neonatol 2001; 6:85–95.

*653 Hanley FL, Sade RM, Freedom RM, et al. Outcomes in critically ill neonates with pulmonary stenosis and intact ventricular septum: a multi institutional study. J Am Coll Cardiol 1993; 22:183–192.

654 Salmon AP, Keeton BR, Sethia B. Developments in interventional catheterisation and progress in surgery for congenital heart disease: achieving a balance. Br Heart J 1993; 69:479–480.

PROBLEMS AND JAUNDICE OF THE GASTROINTESTINAL NEONATE

655 Dyball REJ, Navaratnam V, Tate PA. Basic embryology and the embryological basis of malformation syndromes. In: Rennie JM, Roberton NRC, eds. Textbook of neonatology, 3rd edn. Edinburgh: Churchill Livingstone; 1999:121–132.

656 Lebenthal E, Heitlinger L, Milla PJ. Prenatal and perinatal development of the gastrointestinal tract. In: Milla JP, Muller DPR, eds. Harries paediatric gastroenterology, 2nd edn. Edinburgh: Churchill Livingstone; 1988: 3–29.

657 Bisset WM, Watt JB, Rivers JPA, et al. Ontogeny of fasting small intestinal motor activity in the human infant. Gut 1988; 29:483–488.

658 Walker-Smith J, Murch S, eds. Diseases of the small intestine in childhood, 4th edn. Oxford: Isis Medical Media; 1999:1–10.

659 Weaver LT. Anatomy and embryology. In: Walker WA, Durie PR, Hamilton JR, et al, eds. Pediatric gastrointestinal disease, 2nd edn. St Louis: Mosby; 1996:9–30.

*660 Premji S, Chessell L. Continuous nasogastric milk feeding versus intermittent bolus milk feeding for premature infants less than 1500 grams (Cochrane Review). In: The Cochrane Library, Issue 2, 2002. Oxford: Update Software.

*661 Kennedy KA, Tyson JE, Chamnanvanakij S. Rapid versus slow rate of advancement of feedings for promoting growth and preventing necrotizing enterocolitis in parenterally fed low-birth-weight infants (Cochrane Review). In: The Cochrane Library, Issue 2, 2002. Oxford: Update Software.

*662 Pinelli J, Symington A. Non-nutritive sucking for promoting physiologic stability and nutrition in preterm infants (Cochrane Review). In: The Cochrane Library, Issue 2, 2002. Oxford: Update Software.

*663 Ng E, Shah V. Erythromycin for feeding intolerance in preterm infants (Cochrane Review). In: The Cochrane Library, Issue 2, 2002. Oxford: Update Software.

*664 McClure RJ, Kristensen JH, Grauaug A. Randomised controlled trial of cisapride in preterm infants. Arch Dis Child 1999; 80:F174–F177.

*665 Sikorski J, Renfrew MJ, Pindoria S, et al. Support for breastfeeding mothers (Cochrane Review). In: The Cochrane Library, Issue 2, 2002. Oxford: Update Software.

*666 Carroll AE, Garrison MM, Christakis DA. A systematic review of nonpharmacological and nonsurgical therapies for gastroesophageal reflux in infants. Arch Pediatr Adolesc Med 2002; 156:109–113.

667 Walker-Smith J, Murch S, eds. Diseases of the small intestine in childhood, 4th edn. Oxford: Isis Medical Media; 1999:205–234.

668 Walker-Smith J, Murch S, eds. Diseases of the small intestine in childhood, 4th edn. Oxford: Isis Medical Media; 1999:279–298.

669 Amiel J, Lyonnet S. Hirschsprung disease, associated syndromes, and genetics: a review. J Med Genet 2001; 38:729–739.

670 Faubion WA Jr, Perrault J. Gastrointestinal bleeding. In: Walker WA, Durie PR, Hamilton JR, et al, eds. Pediatric gastrointestinal disease, 3rd edn. Hamilton: BC Decker; 2000:164–178.
671 British Paediatric Surveillance Unit. Annual Report. London: Royal College of Paediatrics and Child Health; 1997.
672 Hackett GA, Campbell S, Gamsu H, et al. Doppler studies in the growth retarded foetus and prediction of necrotising enterocolitis, haemorrhage and neonatal morbidity. BMJ 1987; 294:13–16.
673 Lucas A, Cole TJ. Breast milk and neonatal necrotising enterocolitis. Lancet 1990; 336:1519–1523.
*674 Kennedy KA, Tyson JE, Chamnanvanakij S. Early versus delayed initiation of progressive enteral feedings for parenterally fed low birth weight or preterm infants (Cochrane Review). In: The Cochrane Library, Issue 2, 2002. Oxford: Update Software.
*675 Tyson JE, Kennedy KA. Minimal enteral nutrition for promoting feeding tolerance and preventing morbidity in parenterally fed infants (Cochrane Review). In: The Cochrane Library, Issue 2, 2002. Oxford: Update Software.
*676 Foster J, Cole M. Oral immunoglobulin for preventing necrotizing enterocolitis in preterm and low birth weight infants (Cochrane Review). In: The Cochrane Library, Issue 2, 2002. Oxford: Update Software.
*677 Bury RG, Tudehope D. Enteral antibiotics for preventing necrotizing enterocolitis in low birth weight or preterm infants (Cochrane Review). In: The Cochrane Library, Issue 2, 2002. Oxford: Update Software.
678 Israel EJ, Morera C. Necrotizing enterocolitis. In: Walker WA, Durie PR, Hamilton JR, et al, eds. Pediatric gastrointestinal disease, 3rd edn. Hamilton: BC Decker; 2000:665–676.
679 Vanderhoof JA. Necrotizing enterocolitis. In: Walker WA, Durie PR, Hamilton JR, et al, eds. Pediatric gastrointestinal disease, 3rd edn. Hamilton: BC Decker; 2000:583–602.
680 Weinberg RP. Gastroenterology. I. Bilirubin physiology. In: Roberton NRC, ed. Textbook of neonatology. London: Churchill Livingstone; 1986:383–393.
681 Garcia LM. Disorders of bilirubin metabolism. In: Assali NS, ed. Pathophysiology of gestation. Vol III. New York: Academic Press; 1972:457.
682 Schmidt R. Bilirubin metabolism: the state of the art. Gastroenterology 1978; 74:1307–1312.
683 McDonagh AF, Palmer LA, Lightner DA. Phototherapy for neonatal jaundice. J Am Chem Soc 1982; 104:6867.
684 Brouwers HAA, Ertbruggen I, Alsbach GPJ, et al. What is the best predictor of the severity of ABO-haemolytic disease of the newborn? Lancet 1988; ii:641–643.
685 Roberts EA. The jaundiced baby. In: Kelly DA, ed. Diseases of the liver and biliary system in children. Oxford: Blackwell Science; 1999:11–45.
686 Gartner LM, Herschel M. Jaundice and breastfeeding. Pediatr Clin North Am 2001; 48(2):389–399.
687 Gourley CR, Arend RA. Beta-glucuronidase and hyperbilirubinaemia in breast fed and formula fed babies. Lancet 1986; i:644–646.

HEMATOLOGICAL PROBLEMS OF THE NEWBORN
688 Marshall CJ, Thrasher AJ. The embryonic origins of human haematopoiesis. Br J Haematol 2001; 112:838–850.
689 Pearson HA. Life span of the fetal red blood cell. J Pediatr 1967; 70:166.
690 Oski FA. The erythrocyte and its disorders. In: Nathan A, Oski FA, eds. Hematology of infancy and childhood. New York: WB Saunders; 1993:18.
691 Watts TL, Roberts IAG. Haematological abnormalities in the growth-restricted infant. Semin Neonatol 1999; 4:41–54.
692 Huyhn A, Dommergues M, Izac B, et al. Characterization of hematopoietic progenitors from human yolk sacs and embryos. Blood 1995; 86:4474–4485.
693 Campagnoli C, Fisk N, Overton T, et al. Circulating hematopoietic progenitor cells in first trimester fetal blood. Blood 2000; 95:1967–1972.
694 Hann IM. The normal blood picture in neonates. In: Hann IM, Gibson BES, Letsky EA, eds. Fetal and neonatal haematology. London: Baillière Tindall; 1991.
695 Forestier F, Daffos F, Galacteros F. Haematological values of 163 normal fetuses between 18 and 30 weeks of gestation. Pediatr Res 1986; 20:342–346.
696 Hegyi E, Nakazawa M, Debili N, et al. Developmental changes in human megakaryocyte ploidy. Exp Hematol 1991; 19:87–94.
697 de Alarcon PA, Graeve JL. Analysis of megakaryocyte ploidy in fetal bone marrow biopsies using a new adaptation of the feulgen technique to measure DNA content and estimate megakaryocyte ploidy from biopsy specimens. Pediatr Res 1996; 39:166–170.
698 Murray NA, Roberts IAG. Circulating megakaryocytes and their progenitors in neonatal thrombocytopenia. Pediatr Res 1996; 40:1–8.
699 Watts TL, Murray NA, Roberts IAG. Thrombopoietin has a primary role in the regulation of platelet production in preterm babies. Pediatr Res 1999; 46:28–32.
700 Wolber E-M, Bame C, Fahnenstich H, et al. Expression of the thrombopoietin gene in human fetal and neonatal tissues. Blood 1999; 94:97–105.
701 Albert TSE, Meng G, Simms P, et al. Thrombopoietin in the thrombocytopenic term and preterm newborn. Pediatrics 2000; 105:1286–1291.
702 Ohls RK, Li Y, Abdel-Mageed A, et al. Neutrophil pool sizes and granulocyte colony-stimulating factor production in human mid-trimester fetuses. Pediatr Res 1995; 37:806–811.
703 Christensen RD, Calhoun DA, Rimsza LM. A practical approach to evaluating and treating neutropenia in the neonatal intensive care unit. Clin Perinatol 2000; 27:577–601.
704 Modi N, Carr R. Promising strategems to reduce the burden of neonatal sepsis. Arch Dis Child Fetal Neonatal Ed 2000; 83:F150–F153.
705 Pahal G, Jauniaux E, Kinnon C, et al. Normal development of human fetal hematopoiesis between eight and seventeen weeks' gestation. Am J Obstet Gynecol 2000; 183:1029–1103.
706 Thurlbeck SM, McIntosh N. Preterm blood counts vary with sampling site. Arch Dis Child 1987; 62:74–87.
707 Linderkamp O, Nelle M, Kraus M, et al. The effect of early and late cord-clamping on blood viscosity and other hemorheological parameters in full-term infants. Acta Paediatr 1992; 81:745–750.
708 Usher R, Lind J. Blood volume of the newborn premature infant. Acta Paediatr Scand 1965; 54:419.
709 Sisson TRC, Lund CJ, et al. The blood volume of infants. I The full term infant in the first year of life. J Pediatr 1959; 55:163.
710 Roberts IAG, Murray NA. Neonatal thrombocytopenia: new insights into pathogenesis and implications for clinical management. Curr Opin Pediatr 2001; 13:16–21.
711 Stuart MJ, Graeber JE. Normal hemostasis in the fetus and newborn: vessels and platelets. In: Polin RA, Fox WM, eds. Fetal and neonatal physiology. Philadelphia: WB Saunders; 1998:1834–1848.
712 Gratacos E, Torres PJ, Vidal J, et al. The incidence of human parvovirus B19 infection during pregnancy and its impact on perinatal outcome. J Infect Dis 1995; 171:1360–1363.
713 Lallemand AV, Doco-Fenzy M, Gaillard DA. Investigation of nonimmune hydrops fetalis: multidisciplinary studies are necessary for diagnosis – review of 94 cases. Pediatr Dev Pathol 1999; 2:432–439.
714 Fisch P, Handgretinger R, Schaefer H. Pure red cell aplasia. Br J Haematol 2000; 111:1010–1022.
715 Brown K. Haematological consequences of parvovirus B19 infection. Bailliere's Best Pract Res Clin Haematol 2000; 13:245–259.
716 Stockman JA, de Alarcon PA. Overview of the state of the art of Rh disease: history, current clinical management, and recent progress. J Pediatr Hematol Oncol 2001; 23:385–393.
717 Grant SR, Kilby MD, Meer L, et al. The outcome of pregnancy in Kell alloimmunisation. Br J Obstet Gynaecol 2000; 107:481–485.
718 Williamson LM. Leucocyte depletion of the blood supply – how will patients benefit? Br J Haematol 2001; 110:256–272.
719 Luzzatto L. Glucose-6-phosphate dehydrogenase deficiency. In: Nathan A, Oski FA, eds. Hematology of infancy and childhood, 4th edn. New York: WB Saunders; 1993:674–695.
720 Ohls RK. The use of erythropoietin in neonates. Clin Perinatol 2000; 27:681–696.
721 Voak D, Cann R, Finney RD, et al. Guidelines for administration of blood products: transfusion of infants and neonates. Transfus Med 1994; 4:63–69.
722 Hume H. Red blood cell transfusions for preterm infants: the role of evidence-based medicine. Semin Perinatol 1997; 21:8–19.
723 Hume H. Blood components: preparation, indications and administration. In: Lilleyman J, Hann I, Blanchette V, eds. Pediatric hematology, 2nd edn. London: Churchill Livinstone; 1999:709–739.

*724 Miura E, Procianoy RS, Bittar C, et al. A randomised, double-masked, placebo-controlled trial of recombinant granulocyte colony-stimulating factor administration to preterm infants with the clinical signs of early-onset sepsis. Pediatrics 2001; 107:30–35.

*725 Cairo MS, Agosti J, Ellis R, et al. A randomized, double-blind, placebo-controlled trial of prophylactic recombinant human granulocyte-macrophage colony-stimulating factor to reduce nosocomial infections in very low birth weight neonates. J Pediatr 1999; 134:64–70.

726 Bajwa RP, Skinner R, Windebank KP, et al. Chemotherapy and marrow transplantation for congenital leukaemia. Arch Dis Child Fetal Neonatal Ed 2001; 84:F47–F48.

727 Lange B. The management of neoplastic disorders of haematopoiesis in children with Down's syndrome. Br J Haematol 2000; 110:512–524.

728 Hutton RA, Laffan MA, Tuddenham EGD. Normal haemostasis. In: Hoffbrand AV, Lewis SM, Tuddenham EGD, eds. Postgraduate haematology, 4th edn. Oxford: Oxford University Press; 1999:550–580.

729 Andrew M. The relevance of developmental haemostasis to haemorrhagic disorders of newborns. Semin Perinatol 1997; 21:70–85.

730 Andrew M, Paes B, Johnston M. Development of the human coagulation system in the healthy premature infant. Blood 1988; 72:1651.

731 Andrew M, Paes B, Johnston M. Development of the hemostatic system in the neonate and young infant. Am J Pediatr Haematol Oncol 1990; 12:95.

732 Seguin JH, Topper WH. Coagulation studies in very low-birthweight infants. Am J Perinatol 1994; 11:27–29.

733 Kulkarni R, Lusher J. Perinatal management of newborns with haemophilia. Br J Haematol 2001; 112:264–274.

734 Smith PS. Congenital coagulation protein deficiencies in the perinatal period. Semin Perinatol 1990; 14:384–392.

735 Zipursky A. Prevention of vitamin K deficiency bleeding in newborns. Br J Haematol 1999; 104:430–437.

736 Golding J, Greenwood R, Birmingham K, et al. Childhood cancer, intramuscular vitamin K, and pethidine given during labour. BMJ 1992; 305:341–346.

737 Brousson MA, Klein MC. Controversies surrounding the administration of vitamin K to newborns: a review. Can Med Assoc J 1996; 154:307–315.

738 Cornellison M, von Kries R, Loughnan P, et al. Prevention of vitamin K deficiency bleeding: efficacy of different multiple oral dose schedules of vitamin K. Eur J Pediatr 1997; 156:126–130.

*739 Puckett RM, Offringa M. Prophylactic Vitamin K for Vitamin K deficiency bleeding in neonates. Cochrane Database Syst Rev 2000; 4:CD002776.

740 Karpatkin M. Coagulation problems in the newborn. Semin Neonatol 1999; 4:1–7.

741 Ouwehand WH, Smith G, Ranasinghe E. Management of severe alloimmune thrombocytopenia in the newborn. Arch Dis Child Fetal Neonatal Ed 2000; 82:F173–F175.

742 Murray NA, Howarth LJ, McMcloy M, et al. Platelet transfusion in the management of severe thrombocytopenia in neonatal intensive care unit (NICU) patients. Transfus Med 2002; 12(1):35–41.

743 Marlar RA, Montgomery RR, Broekmans AW. Diagnosis and treatment of homozygous Protein C deficiency. Report of the working party on homozygous protein C deficiency. International Committee of Haemostasis and Thrombosis. J Pediatr 1989; 114:528–534.

744 Schmidt B, Andrew M. Neonatal thrombosis: report of a prospective Canadian and international registry. Pediatrics 1995; 96:939–943.

745 Alkalay AL, Mazkereth R, Santulli T, et al. Central venous line thrombosis in premature infants: a case management and literature review. Am J Perinatol 1993; 10:323–326.

746 Andrew M, de Veber G. Paediatric thromboembolism and stroke protocols. Hamilton: BC Decker; 1997.

747 Mercuri E, Cowan F, Gupte G, et al. Prothrombotic disorders and abnormal neurodevelopmental outcome in infants with neonatal cerebral infarction. Pediatrics 2001; 107:1400–1404.

748 Vlachos A, Klein GW, Lipton JM. The Diamond Blackfan Anemia Registry: tool for investigating the epidemiology and biology of Diamond–Blackfan anemia. J Pediatr Hematol Oncol 2001; 23:377–382. (Review)

NEONATAL NEUROLOGY

749 Saint-Anne Dargassies S. Neurological development in full term and premature neonates. North Holland: Elsevier; 1977.

750 Amiel-Tison C, Grenier A. Neurological assessment within the first year of life. New York: Oxford University Press; 1986.

751 Prechtl HFR, Bientema D. The neurological examination of the full term newborn infant, Clinics in developmental medicine. No 12. London: SIMP/Heinemann; 1964.

752 Prechtl HFR. The neurological examination of the full term newborn infant, 2nd edn. Clinics in developmental medicine. No 63. London: SIMP/Heinemann; 1977.

753 Brazelton TB. Neonatal behavioural assessment scale. Clinics in developmental medicine. No 50. London: SIMP/Heinemann; 1973.

754 Dubowitz L, Dubowitz LMS. The neurological assessment of the preterm and full term newborn infant. Clinics in developmental medicine. No 79. London: SIMP/Heinemann; 1981.

755 Prechtl HRF. Ultrasound examination of human fetal behaviour. Early Hum Dev 1985; 12:91–98.

756 Prechtl HFR. Qualitative changes of spontaneous movements in fetus and preterm infant as a marker of neurological dysfunction. Early Hum Dev 1990; 23:151–158.

757 Ferrari F, Cioni G, Prechtl HFR. Qualitative changes of general movements in preterm infants with brain lesions. Early Hum Dev 1990; 23:193–231.

758 Amiel-Tison C. Clinical assessment of the infant nervous system. In: Levene MI, Lilford RJ, eds. Fetal and neonatal neurology and neurosurgery, 2nd edn. Edinburgh: Churchill Livingstone; 1995:83–104.

759 Volpe JJ. Neurology of the newborn, 4th edn. Philadelphia: WB Saunders; 2001:103–133.

760 Dubowitz LMS, Mushin J, de Vries L, et al. Visual function in the newborn infant: is it cortically mediated? Lancet 1986; i:1139–1140.

761 Braddick O, Wattam-Bell J, Atkinson J. Orientation-specific cortical responses develop in early infancy. Nature 1986; 320:617–619.

762 Govaert P, De Vries LS. An atlas of neonatal brain sonography. Clinics in developmental medicine. No 141–142. Cambridge: MacKeith Press; 1997.

763 Rennie JM. Neonatal cerebral ultrasound. Cambridge: Cambridge University Press; 1997.

764 Rutherford M. MRI of the neonatal brain. London: WB Saunders; 2002.

765 Ahmed A, Hickey S, Ehrett S, et al. Cerebrospinal fluid values in the term neonate. Pediatr Infect Dis J 1996; 15:298–303.

766 Kaiser AM, Whitelaw AGL. Hypertensive response to increased intracranial pressure in infancy. Arch Dis Child 1988; 63:1461–1465.

767 Kaiser AM, Whitelaw AG. Cerebrospinal fluid pressure during post haemorrhagic ventricular dilatation in newborn infants. Arch Dis Child 1985; 60:920–924.

768 Rochefort MJ, Rolfe P, Wilkinson AR. New fontanometer for continuous estimation of intracranial pressure in the newborn. Arch Dis Child 1987; 62:152–155.

769 Eyre JA, Nanei S, Wilkinson AR. Quantification of changes in normal neonatal EEGs with gestation from continuous 5 day recordings. Dev Med Child Neurol 1988; 30:599–607.

770 Hellstrom-Westas L, Rosen I, Svenningsen NW. Predictive value of early continuous amplitude integrated EEG recordings on outcome after severe birth asphyxia in full term infants. Arch Dis Child 1995; 72:F34–F38.

771 Eken P, Toet MC, Groenendaal F, et al. Predictive value of early neuroimaging, pulsed Doppler and neurophysiology in full term infants with hypoxic–ischaemic encephalopathy. Arch Dis Child 1995; 73:F75–F80.

772 Holmes GL, Lombroso CT. Prognostic value of background patterns in the neonatal EEG. J Clin Neurophysiol 1993; 10:323–352.

773 Taylor MJ, Murphy WJ, Whyte HE. Prognostic reliability of SEPs and VEPs in asphyxiated newborn infants. Dev Med Child Neurol 1992; 34:507–515.

774 De Vries LS, Connell J, Dubowitz LMS, et al. Neurological, electrophysiological and MRI abnormalities in infants with extensive cystic leukomalacia. Neuropediatrics 1987; 18:61–66.

775 Hepper PG, Shahidullah BS. Development of fetal hearing. Arch Dis Child 1994; 71:F81–F87.

776 Robertson C, Aldridge S, Jarman F, et al. Late diagnosis of congenital sensorineural hearing impairment: why are detection methods failing? Arch Dis Child 1995; 72:11–15.

777 Stapells DR, Kurtzberg D. Evoked potential assessment of auditory system integrity in infants. Clin Perinatol 1991; 18:497–518.

778 Kennedy CR, Kimm L, Caferelli Dees D, et al. Otoacoustic emissions and auditory brainstem responses in the newborn. Arch Dis Child 1991; 66:1124–1129.

779 Watkin PM. Neonatal otoacoustic emission screening and the identification of deafness. Arch Dis Child 1996; 74:F16–F25.

780 Bess FH, Paradise JL. Universal screening for infant hearing impairment: not simple, nor risk-free, and not presently justified. Pediatrics 1994; 93:330–334.

781 Haggard MP. Hearing screening in children – state of the art(s). Arch Dis Child 1990; 65:1193–1198.

782 McCormick B. Screening for hearing impairment in young children. London: Chapman & Hall; 1988.

783 Scanlon PE, Bamford JM. Early identification of hearing loss: screening and surveillance methods. Arch Dis Child 1990; 65:479–485.

784 Tucker SM, Battacharya J. Screening of hearing impairment in the newborn using the auditory response cradle. Arch Dis Child 1992; 67:911–919.

785 Stevens JC, Webb HD, Hutchinson J, et al. Click evoked otoacoustic emissions compared with brain stem electrical response. Arch Dis Child 1989; 64:1105–1111.

786 Mizrahi EM, Kellaway P. Diagnosis and management of neonatal seizures. New York: Lippincott Raven; 1998.

787 Scher MS, Aso K, Beggarly ME. Electrographic seizures in preterm and full term neonates: clinical correlates, associated brain lesions and risk for neurologic sequelae. Pediatrics 1993; 91:128–134.

788 Weiner SP, Painter MJ, Geva D, et al. Neonatal seizures: electroclinical dissociation. Pediatr Neurol 1991; 7:363–368.

789 Boylan GB, Pressler RM, Rennie JM, et al. Outcome of electroclinical, electrographic, and clinical seizures in the newborn infant. Dev Med Child Neurol 1999; 41:819–825.

790 Boylan GB, Panerai RB, Rennie JM, et al. Cerebral blood flow velocity during neonatal seizures. Arch Dis Child 1999; 80:F105–F110.

*791 Lanska MJ, Lanska DJ, Baumann RJ, et al. A population based study of neonatal seizures in Fayette County, Kentucky. Neurology 1995; 45:724–732.

792 Van Zeben-Van der Aa DM, Verloove-Vanhorick SP, den Ouden L, et al. Neonatal seizures in very preterm and very low birthweight infants: mortality and handicaps at two years of age in a nationwide cohort. Neuropediatrics 1990; 21:62–65.

793 Watkins A, Szymonowicz W, Jin X, et al. Significance of seizures in very low birthweight infants. Dev Med Child Neurol 1988; 30:162–169.

794 Levene MI, Trounce JQ. Neonatal convulsions: towards more precise diagnosis. Arch Dis Child 1986; 61:78–87.

795 Goldberg JH. Neonatal convulsions – a ten year review. Arch Dis Child 1983; 58:976–978.

796 Andre M, Matisse M, Vert P, et al. Neonatal seizures – recent aspects. Neuropaediatrics 1988; 19:201–207.

797 Bergman I, Painter MJ, Hirsch RP, et al. Outcome in neonates with convulsions treated in ICU. Ann Neurol 1983; 14:642–657.

798 Estan J, Hope PL. Unilateral neonatal cerebral infarction in full term infants. Arch Dis Child 1997; 76:F88–F93.

799 Lien JM, Towers CV, Quilligan EJ, et al. Term early-onset neonatal siezures: obstetric characteristics, etiologic classifications and perinatal care. Obstet Gynecol 1995; 85:163–169.

800 Koelfen W, Freund M, Varnholt V. Neonatal stroke involving the middle cerebral artery in term infants: clinical presentation, EEG and imaging studies. Dev Med Child Neurol 1995; 37:203–212.

801 Watanabe K, Miyazaki S, Hara K, et al. Behavioural state cycles, background EEGs and prognosis of newborns with perinatal hypoxia. Electroencephalogr Clin Neurophysiol 1980; 49:618–625.

802 Goldberg PN, Moscoso P, Bauer CR. Use of barbiturate therapy in severe perinatal asphyxia. J Pediatr 1986; 109:851–856.

803 Hellstrom-Westas L, Westergren U, Rosen I, et al. Lidocaine for treatment of severe seizures in newborn infants. Acta Paediatr Scand 1988; 77:79–84.

804 Gilman JT, Gal P, Duchowny MS, et al. Rapid sequential phenobarbital treatment of neonatal seizures. Pediatrics 1989; 83:674–678.

805 Painter MJ, Scher MS, Stein AD, et al. Phenobarbital compared with phenytoin for the treatment of neonatal seizures. N Engl J Med 1999; 341:485–489.

806 Boylan GB, Rennie JM, Pressler RM, et al. Phenobarbitone, neonatal seizures and video-EEG. Arch Dis Child 2002; 86:F165–F170.

807 Gal P, Oles KS, Gilman JT, et al. Valproic acid efficacy, toxicity, and pharmacokinetics in neonates with intractable seizures. Neurology 1988; 38:467–471.

808 Steinberg SA, Shalev RS, Amr N. Valproic acid in neonatal status convulsivus. Brain Dev 1986; 8:278–280.

809 Ledigo A, Clancy RR, Berman PH. Neurologic outcome after electroencephalographically proven neonatal seizures. Pediatrics 1991; 88:583–596.

810 Temple CM, Dennis J, Carney R, et al. Neonatal seizures: long term outcome and cognitive development among 'normal' survivors. Dev Med Child Neurol 1995; 37:109–118.

811 Peckham CS, Johnson C, Aden A, et al. The early acquisition of cytomegalovirus infection. Arch Dis Child 1987; 62:708–785.

812 Paryani SG, Arvin AM. Intrauterine infection with varicella zoster virus after maternal varicella. N Engl J Med 1986; 314:1542–1546.

813 Editorial. Zidovudine for mother, fetus and child: hope or poison? Lancet 1994; 344:207–209.

814 Lucas A, Rennie JM, Baker BA, et al. Low plasma triiodothyronine concentrations and outcome in preterm infants. Arch Dis Child 1988; 63:1201–1206.

815 Den Ouden AL, Kok JH, Verkerk PH, et al. The relation between neonatal thyroxine levels and neurodevelopmental outcome at age 5 and 9 years in a national cohort of very preterm and/or very low birthweight infants. Pediatr Res 1996; 39:142–145.

816 Lucas A, Morley R, Cole TJ. Adverse neurodevelopmental outcome of moderate neonatal hypoglycaemia. BMJ 1988; 297:1304–1308.

817 Stewart AL, Reynolds EOR, Hope PL, et al. Probability of neurodevelopmental disorders estimated from ultrasound appearance of the brains of very preterm infants. Dev Med Child Neurol 1987; 29:3–11.

818 De Vries LMS, Dubowitz LMS, Dubowitz V, et al. Predictive value of cranial ultrasound in the newborn baby: a reappraisal. Lancet 1985; i:137–140.

819 Cooke RWI. Determinants of major handicap in post haemorrhagic hydrocephalus. Arch Dis Child 1987; 62:504–507.

820 Szymonowicz W, Yu VYH, Bajuk B, Astbury J. Neurodevelopmental outcome, periventricular haemorrhage and leukomalacia in infants 1250 g or less at birth. Early Hum Dev 1986; 14:1–7.

821 Strand C, Laptook AR, Dowling S, et al. Neonatal intracranial haemorrhage: I. Changing pattern in inborn low-birth-weight infants. Early Hum Dev 1990; 23:117–128.

822 Synnes AR, Chien L-Y, Peliowski A, et al. Variations in intraventricular hemorrhage incidence rates among Canadian neonatal intensive care units. J Pediatr 2001; 138:525–531.

823 Levene MI, De Crespigny L. Classification of intraventricular haemorrhage. Lancet 1983; i:643.

824 Papile L, Burstein J, Burstein R, et al. Incidence and evolution of subependymal and intraventricular haemorrhage: a study of infants of birth weight less than 1500 g. J Pediatr 1978; 92:529–534.

825 Gould SJ, Howard S, Hope PL, et al. Periventricular intraparenchymal cerebral haemorrhage in preterm infants: role of venous infarction. J Pathol 1987; 151:197–202.

826 Levene MI. Neonatal neurology. Current reviews in paediatrics. No 3. Edinburgh: Churchill Livingstone; 1987.

*827 Ment LR, Oh W, Ehrenkranz RA, et al. Low dose indomethacin therapy and prevention of intraventricular hemorrhage: a multicenter randomized trial. Pediatrics 1994; 93:543–550.

*828 EEC Working Group. EEC trial of ethamsylate in prophylaxis against periventricular haemorrhage. Arch Dis Child 1994; 70:F201–F205.

*829 Crowley PA. Prophylactic steroids for preterm delivery (Cochrane Review) In: The Cochrane Library, Issue 2, 1999. Oxford: Update Software.

*830 Soll RF, Morley CJ. 1999 Prophylactic versus selective use of surfactant for prevention of morbidity and mortality in preterm infants (Cochrane Review). In: The Cochrane Library, Issue 2, 1999. Oxford: Update Software.

831 Trounce JQ, Fagan D, Levene MI. Intraventricular haemorrhage and periventricular leucomalacia: ultrasound and autopsy correlation. Arch Dis Child 1986; 61:1203–1207.

832 Di Pietro MA, Brody BA, Teele RL. Peritrigonal echogenic 'blush' on cranial sonography: pathologic correlates. Am J Radiol 1986; 146:1067–1072.

833 Paneth N, Rudelli R, Kazam E, et al. Brain damage in the preterm infant. Clinics in developmental medicine. No 131 London: MacKeith Press; 1994:119–137.
834 Graham M, Levene MI, Trounce JQ, et al. Prediction of cerebral palsy in very low birthweight infants. Lancet 1987; ii:593–596.
835 Appleton RE, Lee RE, Hey EN. Neurodevelopmental outcome of transient neonatal intracerebral echodensities. Arch Dis Child 1990; 65:27–29.
836 Calvert SA, Hoskins EM, Fong KW, et al. Etiological factors associated with the development of periventricular leucomalacia. Acta Paediatr Scand 1987; 76:254–259.
837 Trounce JQ, Shaw DE, Levene MI, et al. Clinical risk factors and periventricular leucomalacia. Arch Dis Child 1988; 63:17–22.
838 Ikonen RS, Janas MO, Koivikko MJ, et al. Hyperbilirubinemia, hypocarbia and periventricular leukomalacia in preterm infants: relationship to cerebral palsy. Acta Paediatr 1992; 81:802–807.
839 Fujimoto S, Togari H, Yamaguchi N, et al. Hypocarbia and cystic periventricular leukomalacia in premature infants. Arch Dis Child 1994; 71:F107–F110.
840 Shen EY, Huang CC, Chyou S, et al. Sonographic findings of the bright thalamus. Arch Dis Child 1986; 61:1096–1099.
841 Whitelaw A, Rivers RPA, Creighton L, Gaffney P. Low dose intraventricular fibrinolytic treatment to prevent posthaemorrhagic hydrocephalus. Arch Dis Child 1992; 67:12–14.
842 Cooke RWI. Early and late ultrasonographic appearance and outcome in very low birthweight infants. Arch Dis Child 1987; 62:931–937.
*843 Ventriculomegaly Trial Group. Randomised trial of early tapping in neonatal posthaemorrhagic ventricular dilatation. Arch Dis Child 1990; 65:3–10.
*844 Ventriculomegaly Trial Group. Randomised trial of early tapping in neonatal posthaemorrhagic ventricular dilatation: results at 30 months. Arch Dis Child 1994; 70:F129–F136.
*845 Kennedy CR, Ayers S, Campbell MJ, et al. Randomized, controlled trial of acetazolamide and furosemide in posthemorrhagic ventricular dilation in infancy: follow-up at 1 year. Pediatrics 2001; 108:597–607.
846 Hudgins RJ. Natural history of fetal ventriculomegaly. Pediatrics 1988; 82:692–697.
847 Nicolaides KH, Berry S, Snijders RJM, et al. Fetal lateral cerebral ventriculomegaly: associated malformations and chromosomal defects. Fetal Diagn Ther 1990; 5:5–14.

RENAL DISEASE IN THE NEONATE

848 Evan AP, Larsson L. Morphological development of the nephron. In: Edelman CM, ed. Pediatric kidney disease. Boston: Little, Brown: 1992:19–48.
849 Schwartz GJ, Brion LP, Spitzer A. The use of plasma creatinine concentration for estimating the glomerular filtration rate in infants, children and adolescents. Pediatr Clin North Am 1987; 40:1005–1022.
850 Pohl M, Bhatnagar V, Mendoza SA, et al. Toward an etiological classification of developmental disorders of the kidney and upper urinary tract. Kidney Int 2002; 61:10–19.
851 James CA, Watson AR, Twining P, et al. Antenatally detected urinary tract abnormalities: changing incidence and management. Eur J Pediatr 1998; 157:508–511.
852 Quintero RA, Arias F, Cotton DB, et al. In-utero percutaneous cystoscopy in the management of fetal lower obstructive uropathy. Lancet 1995; 346:537–540.
853 Watson AR. Management of antenatally detected urinary tract abnormalities. Curr Paediatr 1999; 9:232–236.
854 Martinovic J, Benachi A, Laurent N, et al. Fetal toxic effects and angiotensin-II-receptor antagonists. Lancet 2001; 358:241–242.
855 Narenda A, White MP, Rolton HA, et al. Nephrocalcinosis in preterm babies. Arch Dis Child 2001; 85:F207–F213.
856 Edelman CM, Ogwo JE, Fine BP, et al. The prevalence of bacteriuria in full-term and premature newborn infants. J Pediatr 1973; 82:125–132.
857 Drew JH, Acton C. Radiological findings in newborn infants with urinary infection. Arch Dis Child 1976; 51:628–630.
858 Watson AR. Urinary tract infection in early childhood. J Antimicrob Chemother 1994; 34(suppl A):53–60.
859 Karlowicz MG, Adelmann RD. Nonoliguric and oliguric acute renal failure in asphyxiated term neonates. Pediatr Nephrol 1995; 9:718–722.
860 Chevalier ZL, Campbell F, Brenbridge AAG. Prognostic factors in neonatal acute renal failure. Pediatrics 1984; 74:265–272.
861 Mathew OP, Jones AS, James E, et al. Neonatal renal failure: usefulness of diagnostic indices. Pediatrics 1980; 65(1):57–59.
862 Seri I, Rudas G, Bors Z, et al. Effects of low dose dopamine infusion on cardiovascular and renal functions, cerebral blood flow and plasma catecholamine levels in sick, preterm neonates. Pediatr Res 1993; 34:742–749.
*863 Australia and New Zealand Intensive Care Society (ANZICS) Clinical Trials Group. Low-dose dopamine in patients with early renal dysfunction: a placebo-controlled randomised trial. Lancet 2000; 356:2139–2143.
864 Archer N. Neonatal blood pressure: normal values (Appendix 4). In: Rennie JM, Robertson NRC, eds. Textbook of neonatology, 3rd edn. Edinburgh: Churchill Livingstone; 1999:1403.
865 Hawkins KC, Watson AR, Rutter N. Neonatal hypertension and cardiac failure. Eur J Pediatr 1995; 154:148–149.
866 Coulthard MG, Vernon B. Managing acute renal failure in very low birthweight infants. Arch Dis Child 1995; 73:F187–F192.
867 Kohli HS, Bhalla D, Sud K, et al. Acute peritoneal dialysis in neonates: comparison of two types of peritoneal access. Pediatr Nephrol 1999; 13:241–244.
868 Haycock GB. Acute renal failure in the newborn infant. Care Crit Ill 1993; 9(6):250–254.

EYE PROBLEMS IN THE NEWBORN

869 Fielder AR, Moseley MJ, Ng YK. The immature visual system and preterm birth. In: Hull D, Cooke R, Whitelaw A, eds. The very immature infant. Br Med Bull 1988; 44:1093–1118.
870 Fielder AR, Moseley MJ. Environmental light and the preterm infant. Semin Perinatol 2000; 24:291–298.
*871 Isenberg SJ, Wood LM. A controlled trial of povidone-iodine as prophylaxis against ophthalmia neonatorum. N Engl J Med 1995; 332:562–566.
872 Ashton N. Oxygen and retinal blood vessels. Trans Ophthalmol Soc UK 1980; 100:359–362.
873 Patz A. Retrolental fibroplasia (retinopathy of prematurity). Trans Ophthalmol Soc N Z 1980; 32:49–54.
874 Kretzer FL, Hittner HM. Retinopathy of prematurity: clinical implications of retinal development. Arch Dis Child 1988; 63:1151–1167.
875 Alon T, Hemo I, Itin A, et al. Vascular endothelial growth factor acts as a survival factor for newly formed retinal vessels and has implications for retinopathy of prematurity. Nat Med 1995; 1:1024–1028.
876 Pierce EA, Foley ED, et al. Regulation of vascular endothelial growth factor by oxygen in a model of retinopathny of prematurity. Arch Ophthalmol 1996; 114:1219–1228.
*877 STOP-ROP Multicenter Study Group. Supplemental therapeutic oxygen for prethreshold retinopathy of prematurity (STOP-ROP), a randomized, controlled trial. I: Primary outcomes. Pediatrics 2000; 105:295–310.
878 Cunningham S, Fleck BW, Elton RA, et al. Transcutaneous oxygen levels in retinopathy of prematurity. Lancet 1995; 346:1464–1465.
*879 Reynolds JD, Hardy RJ, Kennedy KA, et al. For the Light Reduction in Retinopathy of Prematurity (LIGHT-ROP) Cooperative Group. Lack of efficacy of light reduction in preventing retinopathy of prematurity. N Engl J Med 1998; 338:1572–1576.
880 Committee for the Classification of Retinopathy of Prematurity (CCRoP). The international classification of retinopathy of prematurity. Br J Ophthalmol 1984; 68:690–697.
881 Committee for the Classification of Retinopathy of Prematurity (CCRoP). An international classification of retinopathy of prematurity. II The classification of retinal detachment. Arch Ophthalmol 1987; 105:906–912.
882 Kivlin JD, Biglan AW, Gordon RA, et al Early retinal vessel development and iris vessel dilatation as factors in retinopathy of prematurity. Cryotherapy for Retinopathy of Prematurity (CRYO-ROP) Cooperative Group. Arch Ophthalmol 1996; 114:150–154.
883 Fielder AR, Levene MI. Screening for retinopathy of prematurity. Arch Dis Child 1992; 67:860–867.
*884 Palmer EA, Flynn JT, Hardy RJ, et al. The Cryotherapy for Retinopathy of Prematurity Cooperative Group. Incidence and early course of retinopathy of prematurity. Ophthalmology 1991; 98:1628–1640.
*885 Cryotherapy for Retinopathy of Prematurity Cooperative Group (CRPCG). Multicenter trial of cryotherapy for retinopathy of prematurity: preliminary results. Arch Ophthalmol 1988; 106:471–479.

886 Royal College of Ophthalmologists and British Association of Perinatal Medicine Joint Working Party. Retinopathy of prematurity: guidelines for screening and treatment. London: BPA; 1995.
*887 Cryotherapy for Retinopathy of Prematurity Cooperative Group. Multicenter trial of cryotherapy for retinopathy of prematurity: ophthalmological outcome at 10 years. Arch Ophthalmol 2001; 119:1110–1118.
888 American Academy of Pediatrics, American Association for Pediatric Ophthalmology and Strabismus, American Academy of Ophthalmology. Screening examination of premature infants for retinopathy of prematurity. Pediatrics 2001; 108:809–811.
889 Fielder AR, Foreman N, Moseley MJ, et al. Prematurity and visual development. In: Simons K, ed. Early visual development, normal and abnormal. New York: Oxford University Press; 1993:485–504.
890 Crofts BJ, King R, Johnson A. The contribution of low birth weight to severe vision loss in a geographically defined population. Br J Ophthalmol 1998; 82:9–13.
891 Burgess P, Johnson A. Ocular defects in infants of extremely low birthweight and low gestational age. Br J Ophthalmol 1991; 75:84–87.
892 Pike MG, Holmstrom G, de Vries LS, et al. Patterns of visual impairment associated with lesions of the preterm infant brain. Dev Med Child Neurol 1994; 36:849–862.
*893 Bremmer DL, Palmer EA, Fellows RR, et al. Strabismus in premature infants in the first year of life. Cryotherapy for Retinopathy of Prematurity (CRYO-ROP) Cooperative Group. Arch Ophthalmol 1998; 116:329–333.
894 Quinn GE, Dobson V, Siatkowski M, et al for the Cryotherapy for Retinopathy of Prematurity Cooperative Group. Does cryotherapy affect refractive error? Ophthalmology 2001; 108:343–347.
895 Fledelius HC. Pre-term delivery and subsequent ocular development. A 7–10 year follow-up of children screened 1982–84 for ROP. 3. Refraction. myopia of prematurity. Acta Ophthalmol Scand 1996; 74:297–300.
896 Blair M. The need for and the role of a coordinator in child heath surveillance promotion. Arch Dis Child 2001; 84:1–5.
897 Rahi JS, Dezateux C for The British Congenital Cataract Interest Group. Measuring and interpreting the incidence of congenital ocular anomalies: lessons from a national study of congenital cataract in the UK. Invest Ophthalmol Visual Sci 2001; 42: 1444–1448.

INFECTION AND IMMUNITY IN THE NEWBORN
898 Barton L, Hodgmann JE, Pavalova Z. Causes of death in extremely low birth weight infants. Pediatrics 1999; 103(2):446–451.
899 Isaacs O, Barfield CP, Grimwood K, et al. Systematic bacterial and fungal infection in infants in Australian Neonatal Units. Australian Study Group for Neonatal Infections. Med J Austr 1995; 162:178–201.
900 Beck Sague CM, Azimi P, Fonseca SN, et al. Blood stream infections in neonatal unit patients: results of a multicentre study. Pediatr Infect Dis J 1994; 13:1110–1116.
901 Bhutta ZA. Neonatal infections. Curr Opin Paediatr 1997; 9:133–140.
902 Stoll BJ, Gordon T, Korones SB, et al. Early onset sepsis in VLWB infants: a report from the NICHD Neonatal Research Network. J Pediatr 1996; 129:72–80.
903 Stoll BJ, Gordon T, Korones SB, et al. Late onset sepsis in VLBW neonates: a report from NICHD Neonatal Research Network. J Pediatr 1996; 129:63–71.
904 Phillips AGS. The changing face of neonatal infections: experience at a regional medical centre. Pediatr Infect Dis J 1994; 13:1098–1102.
905 Grethers JK, Nelson KB. Maternal infection and cerebral palsy in infants in normal birth weight. JAMA 1997; 278(3):207–211.
906 Murphy DJ, Sellers S, Mackenzie IZ, et al. Case control study of ante natal and intra partum risk factors for CP in very preterm singleton babies. Lancet 1995; 346(8988):1449–1454.
907 Dammann O, Leviton A. Infections remote from the brain, neonatal white matter damage and CP in preterm infants. Semin Pediatr Neurol 1998; 5(3):190–201.
908 Rupp ME, Archer GL. Coagulase negative staphylococci: pathogens associated with medical progress. Clin Infect Dis 1994; 19:231–245.
909 Haque KN, Chagla AH, Shaheed MM. Half a decade of neonatal sepsis at King Khalid University Hospital, Riyadh, Saudi Arabia. J Trop Med 1989; 35:31–34.
910 Haque KN. Indications for antimicrobial therapy in babies born after PROM: the Saudi experience. Postgrad Doc 1993; 16(9):342–347.
*911 Seaward PG, Hannah ME, Myhr TL, et al. International muticentre term prelabour rupture of membrane study: evaluation of predictors of clinical chorio-amnionitis and postpartum fever in patients with prelabour rupture of membranes. Am J Obstet Gynecol 1997; 177:1024–1029.
912 Synott MB, Morse DL, Hall SM. Neonatal meningitis in England and Wales: a review of routine national data. Arch Dis Child 1994; 71:75–80.
913 Griffin MP, Moormann JR. Abnormal heart rate characteristics predict sepsis in newborns. Pediatrics 2001; 107:97–104.
914 Berger C, Uehlinger J, Ghelfi D, et al. Comparison of CRP and white blood cell count with differential in neonates at risk of septicemia. Eur J Paed 1995; 154(2):138–144.
915 Silverra RC, Procianoy RS. Evaluation of IL-6, TNF alpha and IL-1 beta for early diagnosis of neonatal sepsis. Acta Paediatr 1999; 88(6):647–650.
916 Franz AR, Steinback C, Kron M et al. Reduction of unnecessary antibiotic therapy in newborn infants using IL-8 and CRP as markers of bacterial infection. Pediatr 1999; 104(3):447–453.
917 Chiesa C, Panero A, Rossi N et al. Reliability of procalcitonin concentration for the diagnosis of sepsis in critically ill neonates. Clin Infect Dis 1998; 26(3):664–672.
918 Kennon C, Overturf G, Bessman S et al. GM-CSF as marker of bacterial infection in neonates. J Pediatr 1996; 128:765–769.
919 Schelonka RL, Chai MK, Yoder BA, et al. Volume of blood culture required to detect common neonatal pathogens. J Pediatr 1996; 129(2):275–278.
920 McMohan AH, Jewes L, deLouvois J. Routine lumbar puncture in the newborn – are they justified? Eur J Pediatr 1990; 149:797–799.
921 Wiswell TE, Baumgart S, Gannon CM, et al. No lumbar puncture in the evaluation of early neonatal sepsis: will meningitis be missed? Pediatrics 1995; 96(6):803–806.
922 Sarff LD, Platt LH, McCracken GH Jr. Cerebrospinal fluid evaluation in neonates; comparison of high risk infants with and without meningitis. J Pediatr 1976; 99:873–879.
923 Davies PA, Gothefors LA. Bacterial infection in the fetus and newborn infant. Philadelphia: WB Saunders; 1984.
*924 Fowlie PW, Schmidt B. Diagnostic tests for bacterial infection from birth to 90 days. Arch Dis Child 1998; 78(2):F92–F98.
925 Berger C, Uehlinger J, Ghelfi D, et al. Comparison of CRP and white blood cell count with differential in neonates at risk of septicaemia. Eur J Pediatr 1995; 154(2):138–144.
926 Chiesa C, Panero A, Rossi N, et al. Reliability of procalcitonin concentration for the diagnosis of sepsis in critically ill neonates. Clin Infect Dis 1998; 26(3):664–672.
927 Franz AR, Steinbach G, Kron M, et al. Reduction of unnecessary antibiotic therapy in newborn infants using IL-8 and CRP as markers of bacterial infections. Pediatrics 1999; 104(3):447–453.
928 Kennon C, Overturf G, Bessman S, et al. GM-CSF as a marker of bacterial infection in neonates. J Pediatr 1996; 128:765–769.
929 Royal College of Paediatrics and Child Health. Medicines for children. London: RCPCH Publications; 1999.
930 Haque KN. Management of neonatal sepsis in the UK: a national audit of practice. J Clin Excell 2000; 2(2):81–86.
931 Escobar G, Zukin T, Usatin M, et al. Early discontinuation of antibiotic treatment in newborns admitted to rule out sepsis, a decision rule. Pediatr Infect Dis J 1994; 13:860–866.
*932 Northern Neonatal Network Nursing Initiative. Randomised trial of prophylactic early FFP or gelatine or glucose in preterm babies: outcome at two years. Lancet 1996; 348(9022):229–232.
*933 Cairo MS, Worcester CC, Rucker RW. Randomised trial of granulocyte transfusion versus intravenous immunoglobulin therapy for neutropenia and sepsis. J Pediatr 1992; 120(2):281–285.
934 Krause PJ, Maderoza EG, Contrino J, et al. Modulation of neonatal neutrophils function by Pentoxifylline. Pediatr Res 1991; 2:123–127.
*935 Lauterbach R, Pawlik D, Kowalczyk D, et al. Effect of immunomodulatory agent, Pentoxifylline in the treatment of sepsis in prematurely delivered infants: a placebo controlled double blind trial. Crit Care Med 1999; 27(4):807–814.
936 Bedford-Russell AR, Davies GE, Ball SE, et al. G-CSF treatment for neonatal neutropenia. Arch Dis Child 1995; 72:53–54.
*937 Gillian ER, Christensen RD, Suen Y, et al. A randomised placebo controlled trial of recombinant human G-CSF administration in newborn infants with presumed sepsis: significant

induction of peripheral and bone marrow neutropenia. Blood 1994; 84:1427–1433.

*938 Carr R, Modi N, Dore J, et al. Randomised controlled trial of prophylactic GM-CSF in human newborns less than 32 weeks of gestation. Pediatrics 1999; 103:796–802.

939 Baley JE. Neonatal sepsis: the potential for immunotherapy. Clin Perinatol 1988; 15(4):755–771.

940 Fujiwara T, Tanichi S, Hattori K, et al. Effect of IVIG on phagocytosis by PMN in whole blood of neonates. Clin Exp Immunol 1997; 107(3):435–439.

941 Christensen RD, Brown MS, Hall DC, et al. Effect of neutrophils kinetics and serum opsonic capacity of IVIG to neonates with clinical signs of early-onset sepsis. J Pediatr 1991; 118(4):606–614.

*942 Ohlsson A, Lacey J. IVIG in suspected or subsequently proved neonatal infection (Cochrane Review). In: The Cochrane Library, 1999. Oxford: Update Software.

943 Haque KN. IgM-enriched IVIG therapy in neonatal sepsis. Am J Dis Child 1988; 142:1293–1296.

944 Erdem G, Yurdakok, Tekinalp G, Ersoy F. The use of IgM-enriched intravenous immunoglobulin for the treatment of neonatal sepsis in preterm infants. Turkish J Pediatr 1993; 35:277–281.

*945 Jenson HB, Pollock BH. Meta-analysis of the effectiveness of IVIG for prevention and treatment of neonatal sepsis. Pediatrics 1997; 99(2):E2.

*946 Alejandria M, Lansang M, Dans L, et al. IVIG for treating sepsis and septic shock (Cochrane Review). In: The Cochrane Library, 1999. Oxford: Update Software.

947 Boyce JM. It is time for action: improving hand hygiene in hospitals. Ann Intern Med 1999; 130:153–155.

948 Haque KN, Chagla AH. Do gowns prevent infection in neonatal intensive care units? J Hosp Infect 1989; 14:159–162.

949 Heath P. Group B streptococcus disease. In: 15th Annual report (2000–2001) of British Paediatric Surveillance Unit. London: Royal College of Paediatrics and Child Health. 2001: 17–19.

950 Fernandez M, Baker CJ. Group B streptococcal infections. Semin Pediatr Infect Dis 1999; 10:104–110.

951 Klegerman ME, Boyer KM, Papierniak CK, et al. Estimation of the protective level of human IgG antibody to the type-specific polysaccharide of GBS type Ia. J Infect Dis 1983; 148:648–655.

952 Boyer KM, Gotoff SP. Antimicrobial prophylaxis of GBS sepsis. Clin Perinatol 1988; 15:831–850.

953 Weisman LE, Stoll BJ, Cruess DF. Early-onset GBS disease: a current assessment. J Pediatr 1992; 121:428–433.

954 Schrag SJ, Zywicki S, Farley MM, et al. GBS in the era of intrapartum antibiotic prophylaxis. N Engl J Med 2000; 342:15–20.

955 Stoll BJ. The global impact of neonatal infection. Clin Perinatol 1997; 24:1–21.

956 Dammann O, Leviton A. Brain damage in preterm newborns: might enhancement of developmentally regulated endogenous protection open a door for protection? Pediatrics 1999; 104:541–550.

957 Siegal JD. Neonatal sepsis. Semin Perinatol 1985; 9(1):20–28.

958 McCraken GH, Nelson JD. Antimicrobial therapy for newborns, 2nd edn. New York: Grune and Stratton; 1983.

959 Volpe JJ. Neonatal meningitis. In: Volpe JJ, ed. Neurology of the newborn, 3rd edn. Philadelphia: WB Saunders; 1995:730–768.

960 Bedford H, deLouvois J, Halket S, et al. Meningitis in infancy in England and Wales: follow up at age 5 years. BMJ 2001; 323:533–536.

961 Gaynes RP, Edwards JR, Jarvis WR, et al. Nosocomial infection amongst neonates in high-risk nurseries in United States. National nosocomial infection surveillance systems. Paediatrics 1996; 98:357–361.

962 Mittendrof R, Covert R, Kohn J, et al. The association of CONS isolated from chorioamnion at delivery and subsequent development of cerebral palsy. J Perinatol 2001; 21:3–8.

963 Scheifele DW. Role of bacterial toxins in neonatal necrotising enterocolitis. J Pediatr 1990; 117:544–551.

964 Mahieu LM, DeMuynck AO, Ieven MM, et al. Risk factors for central vascular catheter associated blood stream infections among patients in a neonatal intensive care unit. J Hosp Infect 2001; 48:108–116.

965 Gray RP, Richardson DK, McMcormick MC, et al. CONS bacteraemia among VLBW infants: relation to admission, illness severity, resource use and outcome. Pediatrics 1995; 95:225–230.

966 Gladstone IM, Ehrenkranz RA, Edberg SC, et al. A ten year review of neonatal sepsis and comparison with previous fifty years experience. Pediatr Infect Dis J 1990; 9:819–825.

967 Leigh L, Stoll JB, Rahman M, et al. *Pseudomonas aeruginosa* infection in the VLBW infants: a case controlled study. Pediatr Infect Dis J 1995; 14:367–371.

968 Koutouby A, Habibullah J. Neonatal sepsis in Dubai, United Arab Emirates. J Trop Pediatr 1995; 41:177–180.

*969 Wang EE, Ohlsson A, Kellner JD. Association of *Ureaplasma urealyticum* colonisation with CLD of prematurity: result of a meta-analysis. J Pediatr 1995; 127:640–644.

*970 Halliday HL, McClure G, Reid M, et al. Controlled trial of artificial surfactant to prevent RDS. Lancet 1984; i:476–478.

971 Davies PA, Robinson RJ, Scopes JW, et al. Medical care of newborn babies. Clinics in developmental medicine nos 44/45. Spastics International Medical Publications. London: Heinemann; 1972.

972 British Paediatric Association Surveillance Unit. 10th annual report. London: BPA; 1995.

973 Baley JE, Kliegman RM, Boxerbaum F, et al. Fungal colonisation in VLBW infants. Pediatrics 1986; 78:225–232.

974 Noe HN, Tonkin ILD. Renal candidiasis in the neonate. J Urol 1982; 127:517–519.

975 Faix RG. Systemic Candida infections in infants in intensive care nurseries: high incidence of central nervous system involvement. J Pediatr 1984; 105:616–622.

976 Tookey PA, Peckham CS. Surveillance of congenital rubella in Great Britain, 1971–96. BMJ 1999; 318:769–770.

977 Rahi J, Adams G, Russell-Eggit I, et al. Epidemiological surveillance of rubella must continue. BMJ 2001; 323:112.

978 Miller E, Cradock-Watson JE, Pollock TM. Consequences of confirmed maternal rubella at successive stages of pregnancy. Lancet 1982; 2:781–784.

979 Best JM, Banatvala JE, Morgan-Capner P, et al. Fetal infection after maternal reinfection with rubella: criteria for defining reinfection. BMJ 1989; 299:773–775.

980 Boppana SB, Fowler KB, Britt WJ, et al. Symptomatic congenital cytomegalovirus infection in infants born to mothers with pre-existing immunity to cytomegalovirus. Pediatrics 1999; 104:55–60.

981 Boppana SB, Rivera LB, Fowler KB, et al. Intrauterine transmission of cytomegalovirus to infants of women with pre-conceptional immunity. N Engl J Med 2001; 344:1366–1371.

982 Noyola DE, Demmler GJ, Nelson CT, et al. Early predictors of neurodevelopmental outcome in symptomatic congenital cytomegalovirus infection. J Pediatr 2001; 138:325–331.

983 Fowler KB, McCollister FP, Dahle AJ, et al. Progressive and fluctuating sensorineural hearing loss in children with asymptomatic congenital cytomegalovirus infection. J Pediatr 1997; 130:624–630.

984 Paryani SG, Yeager AS, Hosford-Dunn H, et al. Sequelae of acquired cytomegalovirus infection in premature and sick term infants. J Pediatr 1985; 107:451–456.

985 Whitley RJ, Cloud G, Gruber W, et al. Ganciclovir treatment of symptomatic congenital cytomegalovirus infection: results of a phase II study. National Institute of Allergy and Infectious Diseases Collaborative Antiviral Study Group. J Infect Dis 1997; 175:1080–1086.

986 Nigro G, Krzysztofiak A, Bartmann U, et al. Ganciclovir therapy for cytomegalovirus-associated liver disease in immunocompetent or immunocompromised children. Arch Virol 1997; 142:573–580.

987 Enders G, Miller E, Cradock-Watson J, et al. Consequences of varicella and herpes zoster in pregnancy: prospective study of 1739 cases. Lancet 1994; 343:1548–1551.

988 Chant KG, Sullivan EA, Burgess MA, et al. Varicella-zoster virus infection in Australia. Austr N Z J Publ Health 1998; 22:413–418.

989 Heuchan AM, Isaacs D. The management of varicella-zoster virus exposure and infection in pregnancy and the newborn period. Australasian Subgroup in Paediatric Infectious Diseases of the Australasian Society for Infectious Diseases. Med J Aust 2001; 174:288–292.

990 Reynolds L, Struik S, Nadel S. Neonatal varicella: varicella zoster immunoglobulin (VZIG) does not prevent disease. Arch Dis Child Fetal Neonatal Ed 1999; 81:F69–F70.

991 Gutierrez KM, Falkovitz HM, Maldonado Y, et al. The epidemiology of neonatal herpes simplex virus infections in California from 1985 to 1995. J Infect Dis 1999; 180:199–202.

992 Tookey P, Peckham CS. Neonatal herpes simplex virus infection in the British Isles. Pediatr Perinatal Epidemiol 1996; 10:432–442.

993 Brown ZA, Selke S, Zeh J, et al. The acquisition of herpes simplex virus during pregnancy. N Engl J Med 1997; 337:509–515.
994 Whitley RJ. Neonatal herpes simplex virus infections. Clin Perinatol 1988; 15:903–916.
995 American Academy of Pediatrics. Herpes simplex. In: Pickering L, ed. 2000 Red Book Report of the Committee on Infectious Diseases, 25th edn. Elk Grove Village: American Academy of Pediatrics; 2000:309–318.
996 McMinn P, Stratov I, Nagarajan L, et al. Neurological manifestations of enterovirus 71 infection in children during an outbreak of hand, foot, and mouth disease in Western Australia. Clin Infect Dis J 2001; 32:236–242.
997 Ho M, Chen ER, Hsu KH, et al. An epidemic of enterovirus 71 infection in Taiwan. Taiwan Enterovirus Epidemic Working Group. N Engl J Med 1999; 341:929–935.
998 Rotbart HA, Webster AD. Treatment of potentially life-threatening enterovirus infections with pleconaril. Clin Infect Dis J 2001; 32:228–235.
999 Schwarz TF, Roggendrof M, Hottentrager B, et al. Immunoglobulins in the prophylaxis of parvovirus B19 infection. J Infect Dis 1990; 162:1214–1216.
***1000** Dunn D, Wallon M, Peyron F, et al. Mother-to-child transmission of toxoplasmosis: risk estimates for clinical counselling. Lancet 1999; 353:1829–1833.
1001 Vogel N, Kirisits M, Michael E, et al. Congenital toxoplasmosis transmitted from an immunologically competent mother infected before conception. Clin Infect Dis 1996; 23:1055–1060.
1002 Dunn D, Gilbert R, Newell ML, et al. Low incidence of congenital toxoplasmosis in children born to women infected with human immunodeficiency virus. European Collaborative Study and Research Network on Congenital Toxoplasmosis. Eur J Obstet Gynecol Reprod Biol 1996; 68:93–96.
1003 McAuley J, Boyer KM, Patel D, et al. Early and longitudinal evaluations of treated infants and children and untreated historical patients with congenital toxoplasmosis: The Chicago Collaborative Treatment Trial. Clin Infect Dis J 1994; 18:38–72.
***1004** Peyron F, Wallon M, Liou C. Treatments for toxoplasmosis in pregnancy. Cochrane Database Syst Rev 2000; 2:CD001684.

NEONATAL NEOPLASIA
1008 Barson AJ. Congenital neoplasia; the society's experience. Abstract. Arch Dis Child 1978; 53:436.
1009 Davis CF, Carachi R, Young DG. Neonatal tumours: Glasgow 1955–1986. Arch Dis Child 1988; 63:1075–1078.
1010 Broadbent VA. Malignant disease in the neonate. In: Roberton NRC, ed. Textbook of neonatology. Edinburgh: Churchill Livingstone; 1986.
1011 Campbell AN, Chan HSL, O'Brien A, et al. Malignant tumours in the neonate. Arch Dis Child 1987; 62:19–23.
1012 Bader JL, Miller RW. US cancer incidence and mortality in the 1st year of life. Am J Dis Child 1979; 133:157–159.
1013 Fraumeni JF Jr, Miller RW. Cancer deaths in the newborn. Am J Dis Child 1969; 117:186–189.
1014 Halperin EC. Neonatal neoplasms. Int J Radiat Oncol Biol Phys 2000; 47:171–178.
1015 Burmeister T, Thiel E. Molecular genetics in acute and chronic leukemias. J Cancer Res Clin Oncol 2001; 127:80–90.
1016 Robinson DL. Childhood leukaemia: understanding the significance of chromosomal abnormalities. J Pediatr Oncol Nurs 2000; 18:111–123.
1017 Kintzel K, Sonntag J, Strauss E, et al. Neuron-specific enolase: reference values in cord blood. Clin Chem Lab Med 1998; 36:245–247.
1018 Altman RP, Randolph JG, Lilley JR. Sacrococcygeal teratomata. American Academy of Pediatrics Surgical Section Survey 1973. J Pediatr Surg 1974; 9:389–398.
1019 Guin GH, Gilbert EG, Jones B. Incidence of neuroblastoma in infants dying of other causes. Am J Clin Path 1969; 51:126–136.
1020 Bolande RP. Benignity of neonatal tumors and concept of cancer repression in early life. Am J Dis Child 1971; 122:12–14.
1021 Isaacs H. Perinatal (congenital and neonatal) neoplasms: a report of 100 cases. Pediatr Pathol 1985; 3:165–216.
1022 Bolande RP. Congenital and infantile neoplasia of the kidney. Lancet 1974; ii: 1497–1499.
1023 Carachi R, Lindop GBM, Leckie BJ. Inactive renin: a tumour marker in nephroblastoma. J Pediatr Surg 1987; 22:278–280.
1024 Machin GA. Persistent renal blastoma (nephroblastometosis) as a frequent precursor to Wilms tumour: a pathophysiological and clinical review. Am J Pediatr Hematol Oncol 1980; 2:353–362.
1025 Huang F, Arceci R. The histiocytoses of infancy. Semin Perinatol 1999; 23:319–331.

NEONATAL METABOLIC DISORDERS
1026 Lucas A, Morley R, Cole TJ. Adverse neurodevelopmental outcome of moderate neonatal hypoglycaemia. BMJ 1988; 297:1304–1308.
1027 Koh THHG, Eyre JA, Tarbit M, et al. Neurophysiological dysfunction in relation to the concentration of glucose in the blood. Early Hum Dev 1988; 17:287.
1028 Aynsley-Green A, Soltesz G. Hypoglycaemia in infancy and childhood. In: Aynsley-Green A, Chambers TL, eds. Current reviews in paediatrics. Edinburgh: Churchill Livingstone; 1985.
1029 Hawdon JM, Ward-Platt MP. Metabolic adaptation in small for gestational age infants. Arch Dis Child 1993; 68:262–268.
1030 Hawdon JM, Weddell A, Aynsley-Green A, et al. Hormonal and metabolic response to hypoglycaemia in small for gestational age infants. Arch Dis Child 1993; 68:269–273.
1031 Duvanel CB, Fawer C-L, Cotting J, et al. Long-term effects of neonatal hypoglycaemia on brain growth and psychomotor development in small for gestational age preterm infants. J Pediatr 1999; 134:492–498.
1032 Hume R, McGeechan A, Burchell A. Failure to detect preterm infants at risk of hypoglycaemia prior to discharge home. J Pediatr 1999; 134:499–502.
1033 Lyall H, Burchell A, Howie PW, et al. Early detection of metabolic abnormalities in preterm infants impaired by disorders of blood glucose concentration. Clin Chem 1994; 40:526–530.
1034 van-Goudoever JB, Sulkers EJ, Chapman TE, et al. Glucose kinetics and glucoregulatory hormone levels in ventilated preterm infants on the first day of life. Pediatr Res 1993; 33:583–589.
1035 Tyrala EE, Chen X, Boden G. Glucose metabolism in the infant weighing less than 1100 grams. J Pediatr 1994; 125:283–287.
1036 Hertz DE, Karn-CA, Liu-YM, et al. Intravenous glucose suppresses glucose production but not proteolysis in extremely premature newborns. J Clin Invest 1993; 92:1752–1758.
***1037** Murdock N, Crighton A, Nelson LM, et al. Low birthweight infants and total parenteral nutrition immediately after birth. II. Randomised study of biochemical tolerance of intravenous glucose, amino acids, and lipid. Arch Dis Child 1995; 73:F8–F12.
1038 Hume R, Lyall H, Burchell A. Impairment of the activity of the microsomal glucose-6-phosphatase system in premature infants. Acta Paediatr 1992; 81:580–584.
1039 Hume R, Burchell A. Abnormal expression of glucose-6-phosphatase in preterm infants. Arch Dis Child 1993; 68:202–204.
1040 Elliott M, Bayly R, Cole T, et al. Clinical features and natural history of Beckwith–Wiedemann syndrome: presentation of 74 new cases. Clin Genet 1994; 46:168–174.
1041 Mannens M, Hoovers JM, Redeker E, et al. Parental imprinting of human chromosome region 11p15.3-pter involved in the Beckwith–Wiedemann syndrome and various human neoplasia. Eur J Hum Genet 1994; 2:3–23.
1042 Fournet JC, Mayaud C, de Lonlay P, et al. Unbalanced expression of 11p15 imprinted genes in focal forms of congenital hyperinsulinism– association with a reduction to homozygosity of a mutation in ABCC8 or KCNJ11. Am J Pathol 2001; 158:2177–2184.
1043 Ebbesen F, Joergensen A, Hoseth E, et al. Neonatal hypoglycaemia and withdrawal symptoms after exposure in utero to valproate. Arch Dis Child 2000; 83:F124–F129.
1044 Shepherd RM, Cosgrove KE, O'Brien RE, et al on behalf of the EU funded European Network for Research into Hyperinsulinism in Infancy (ENRHI). Hyperinsulinism of infancy: towards an understanding of unregulated insulin release. Arch Dis Child 2000; 82:F87–F97.
1045 Glaser B, Thornton P, Otonkoski T, et al. Genetics of neonatal hyperinsulinism Arch Dis Child 2000; 82:F79–F86.
1046 Stanley CA, Lieu YK, Hsu BYL, et al. Hyperinsulinism and hyperammonemia in infants with regulatory mutations of the glutamate dehydrogenase gene. N Engl J Med 1998; 338:1352–1357.
1047 Aynsley-Green A, Hussain K, Hall J, et al. Practical management of hyperinsulinism in infancy. Arch Dis Child 2000; 82:F98–F107.
1048 Chen Y-T, Burchell A. Glycogen storage diseases. In: Scriver CR, Beaudet AL, Sly WS, et al, eds. The metabolic bases of inherited disease, 7th edn. New York: McGraw Hill; 1995:935–965.
1049 Roe CR, Coates PM. Mitochondrial fatty acid oxidation disorders. In: Scriver CR, Beaudet

AL, Sly WS, et al, eds. The metabolic bases of inherited disease, 7th edn. New York: McGraw Hill; 1995:1501–1533.

1050 Chalmers RA, English N, Hughes EA, et al. Biochemical studies on cultured skin fibroblasts from a baby with long-chain acyl-CoA of dehydrogenase-deficiency presenting as sudden neonatal death. J Inher Metabol Dis 1987; 10:260–262.

1051 Hawdon JM, Aynsley-Green A, Bartlett K, et al. The role of pancreatic insulin secretion in neonatal glucoregulation. II. Infants with disordered blood glucose homeostasis. Arch Dis Child 1993; 68:280–285.

1052 Lyon AJ, McIntosh N, Wheeler K, et al. Hypercalcaemia in extremely low birth-weight infants. Arch Dis Child 1984; 59:1141–1144.

1053 Greer FR. Osteopenia of prematurity. Annu Rev Nutr 1994; 14:169–185.

1054 Beyers N, Alheit B, Taljaard JF, et al. High turnover osteopenia in preterm babies. Bone 1994; 15:5–13.

1055 Giles MM, Laing IA, Elton RA, et al. Magnesium metabolism in preterm infants: effect of calcium, magnesium, postnatal and gestational age. J Pediatr 1990; 117:147–154.

1056 Koo NNI, Gupta JM, Nayanar VV, et al. Skeletal changes in preterm infants. Arch Dis Child 1982; 57:447–452.

1057 Greer FR, MacCormick A. Improved bone mineralisation and growth in premature infants fed fortified own mother's milk. J Pediatr 1988; 112:961–966.

1058 Horsman A, Ryan SW, Congdon PJ, et al. Bone mineral content and body size 65 to 100 weeks postconception in preterm and full term infants. Arch Dis Child 1989; 64:1579–1586.

1059 Lyon AJ, Hawkes DJ, Doran M, et al. Bone mineralisation in preterm infants measured by dual energy radiographic densitometry. Arch Dis Child 1989; 64:919–923.

1060 Tsukahara H, Sudo M, Umezaki M, et al. Measurement of lumbar spinal bone mineral density in preterm infants by dual-energy X-ray absorptiometry. Biol Neonate 1993; 64:96–103.

1061 Crofton PM, Hume R. Alkaline phosphatase isoenzyme in the plasma of preterm and term infants: serial measurements and clinical correlations. Clin Chem 1987; 33:1783–1787.

1062 Nassir DK, Mcintosh N, Lyon A, et al. Ultrasonic diagnosis and monitoring of rickets in immature infants. Br J Radiol 1987; 60:618.

1063 Fewtrell MS, Cole TJ, Bishop NJ, et al. Neonatal factors predicting childhood height in preterm infants: evidence for a persisting effect of early metabolic bone disease? J Pediatr 2000; 137:668–673.

1064 Backstrom MC, Kouri T, Kuusela AI, et al. Bone isoenzyme of serum alkaline phosphatase and serum inorganic phosphate in metabolic bone disease of prematurity. Acta Paediatr 2000; 89:867–873.

1065 ESPGAN Committee of Nutrition. Nutrition and feeding of preterm infants. Acta Paediatr Scand 1987; 336(suppl):9–10.

1066 Giles MM, Fenton MH, Shaw B, et al. Sequential calcium and phosphorus balance studies in preterm infants. J Pediatr 1987; 110:591–598.

1067 Ziegler EE. Nutrient requirements of the preterm infant: an overview. In: Tsang RC, ed. Vitamin and mineral requirements in preterm infants. New York: Marcel Decker; 1985:203–212.

1068 American Academy of Pediatrics. Pediatric nutrition handbook. National Health and Safety performance standards. Oak Grove Village, Illinois. 1985:66–87.

1069 Koo WW. Parenteral nutrition-related bone disease. J Parenter Enteral Nutr 1992; 16:386–394.

1070 Saudubray J-M, Charpentier C. Clinical phenotypes: diagnosis/algorithms. In: Scriver CR, Beaudet AL, Sly WS, et al, eds. The metabolic bases of inherited disease, 7th edn. New York: McGraw Hill; 1995:327–400.

1071 Matern D, Hart P, Murtha AP, et al. Acute fatty liver of pregnancy associated with short-chain acyl-coenzyme A dehydrogenase deficiency. J Pediatr 2001; 138:585–588.

1072 Burton BK. Inborn errors of metabolism: the clinical diagnosis in early infancy. Pediatrics 1987; 79:359–369.

1073 Chakrapani A, Cleary MA, Wraith JE. Detection of inborn errors of metabolism in the newborn. Arch Dis Child 2001; 84:F205–F210.

1074 Barth P, Wanders RJ, Vreken P. X-linked cardioskeletal myopathy and neutropenia (Barth syndrome–MIM 302060). J Pediatr 2000; 135:273–276.

1075 Lazarow PB, Moser HW. Disorders of peroxisome biogenesis. In: Scriver CR, Beaudet AL, Sly WS, eds. The metabolic bases of inherited disease, 7th edn. New York: McGraw Hill; 1995:2287–2324.

1076 Clayton PT. Disorders of cholesterol biosynthesis. Arch Dis Child 1998; 78:185–189.

11

Infant feeding

Anthony F Williams

Infant feeding practices not only affect growth rate and morbidity during infancy but have implications for health during later childhood and adult life. Promoting optimal nutrition is thus an important aspect of child health. Changing behavior requires not only an understanding of physiological and biochemical facets but an appreciation of the strong social and cultural influences underlying variation between and within countries.

BREAST-FEEDING

INCIDENCE OF BREAST-FEEDING

Over the past 10 years the proportion of mothers initiating breast-feeding in the UK has risen steadily (Table 11.1), particularly in areas with historically low uptake such as Scotland and Northern Ireland. However the UK still has far to go to match trends in many other industrialized nations, for example Scandinavia, Australia and New Zealand where initiation rates exceed 90%. Factors consistently shown to affect the incidence of breast-feeding in the UK are shown in Table 11.2. Social class, educational and geographical gradients are particularly marked. In England and Wales in 1995 91% of social class I mothers versus 50% in social class V chose to breast-feed their baby. Moreover, in London and South-East England 76% initiated breast-feeding, but only 50% in Scotland. The chosen method of infant feeding is therefore a strong marker of social and educational inequality: group education and peer counseling programs have been identified as effective methods of increasing the incidence of breast-feeding,[1] and require further study in the UK.

Table 11.1 Incidence of breast-feeding in the UK, 1975-2000

	England & Wales	Scotland	Northern Ireland
1975	51	n/a	n/a
1980	67	50	n/a
1985	65	48	n/a
1990	64	50	36
1995	68	55	45
2000	70	63	54

Table 11.2 Factors affecting the incidence of breast-feeding in the UK

Favor breast-feeding
Social class I
Mother educated beyond 18 years of age
Mother over 24 years of age
Live in South-East England
First baby
Breast-fed previous baby
Hinder breast-feeding
Smoking

DEFINITION AND PREVALENCE OF 'BREAST-FEEDING'

Because breast-fed babies may receive other fluids and foods it is necessary for monitoring and research purposes to define carefully the meaning of 'breast-feeding'. World Health Organization terminology has now been widely adopted[2] (Table 11.3). Accuracy of definition is particularly important when considering studies of the effect of breast-feeding on maternal and infant health because exclusively breast-fed babies have, for example, significantly lower prevalence of gastrointestinal infection and lower blood pressure at school age than those who were only partially breast-fed[3].

Table 11.3 World Health Organization definitions of 'breast-feeding'

Breast-feeding
Infant has received *any* breast milk, expressed or from breast

Exclusive breast-feeding
Infant has received *only* breast milk and no other liquids or solids except vitamin/mineral supplements and medicines

Predominant breast-feeding
Breast milk the predominant source of nourishment but other drinks (e.g. water, herbal drinks, teas, etc.) may have been given

Full breast-feeding
Exclusive or predominant breast-feeding

Complementary feeding
Infant has received breast milk and solid or semi-solid foods

Bottle feeding
Infant has received liquid or semi-solid food from a bottle with a teat

In the UK the term 'prevalence' has been used in national surveys to describe the proportion of babies partially or exclusively breast-fed at specified ages. A consistent trend has been the rapid decline observed during the first 6 weeks of life, particularly the first 2. Mothers who are socially and educationally disadvantaged are more likely to give up early. About 80% who stop in the first 2 weeks say that they wanted to breast-feed for longer, the commonest reasons given being 'insufficient milk/baby hungry' (44%), 'sore nipples or breasts' (36%), 'baby would not suck' (20%). As such symptoms probably arise through errors of technique and failure to recognize the normal feeding pattern of the breast-fed baby, better professional education on the management of breast-feeding could prove helpful.[4]

IS BREAST-FEEDING IMPORTANT?

Breast milk is anatomically a connective tissue, consisting of cells (including lymphocytes and macrophages) suspended in a biochemically complex matrix. The function of many breast milk constituents is still not understood and it can reasonably be asked whether there is proof of biological benefit to the baby, or whether the presence of these substances is an accident of nature.

Breast-feeding and infection

Breast-feeding is crucial to survival in less-developed countries: infants fed formula are more likely to *die* of diarrheal disease than those breast-fed. The contribution of breast-feeding to maternal and child health in industrialized countries has been harder to confirm: randomized controlled trials are clearly unethical and most evidence comes from case-control and cohort studies. Methodological problems include: the variable duration of breast-feeding, poor definition of the term 'breast-feeding' (Table 11.3), confounding by sociocultural factors (Table 11.2), 'ascertainment bias' and inadequate definition of disease outcomes. A literature review concluded that most studies were methodologically flawed but more recent studies have taken account of these criticisms. For example, a prospective cohort study in Scotland concluded that bottle-fed infants were more likely to develop gastroenteritis, respiratory symptoms, and to be admitted to hospital than those breast-fed for 13 weeks or more, even after adjustment for confounding factors. Partially breast-fed infants derived less benefit.[5] Several recent comprehensive literature reviews have reiterated the evidence that breast-feeding protects against these conditions and others, including *Haemophilus influenzae* b infection, otitis media and necrotizing enterocolitis.

Breast-feeding and allergy

Studies of breast-feeding and allergic disease have yielded conflicting evidence. The notion that artificial feeding caused eczema was introduced over 60 years ago but subsequent studies have not all substantiated this, one even suggesting eczema was commoner in breast-fed infants. This disparity may be attributable to several factors: firstly, those with a history of allergy probably self-select for breast-feeding. Secondly, *exclusive* breast-feeding for as long as 6 months is uncommon in most industrialized countries and partial breast-feeding may not be effective. Thus, although breast-feeding is commonly believed to protect against allergic disease the evidence is inconsistent.

Breast-feeding and long term morbidity

Some case-control and ecological data suggest that the incidence of juvenile-onset, insulin-dependent diabetes mellitus (IDDM) is slightly decreased in children who were breast-fed. Immunological mechanisms linking cows' milk and diabetes have been proposed but current evidence is inconclusive.[6,7] More recently some evidence has emerged that breast-fed babies are less likely to develop obesity in childhood, and have lower systolic blood pressure at school age.[3]

Breast-feeding and neurological development

Numerous studies have found a statistically significant association between breast-feeding and mental development in infancy and childhood but potential confounding influences are numerous, e.g. parental alcohol intake, smoking behavior and intelligence. The differences seem most marked in infants prematurely born and in the majority of studies persist even after adjustment for identifiable confounding influences.[8] Although it has been suggested that they may be explained by differences in the fat composition of formula and breast milk this is currently unproven.

Breast-feeding and the mother's health

Exclusive breast-feeding contributes to child spacing through induction of lactational amenorrhea. Globally this may be its most important benefit to maternal health.[9] Many studies have shown that breast-feeding also significantly reduces a mother's risk of premenopausal breast cancer though data are inconsistent, possibly because tumor type influences the relationship. There is no evidence that breast-feeding adversely influences long term bone mineralization in the mother.[10] Although bone turnover increases during lactation and some demineralization occurs there is compensatory remineralization on weaning. These events appear endocrinologically mediated and are not preventable by calcium supplementation.[11]

ESTABLISHING AND MAINTAINING BREAST-FEEDING

Breast milk production

Progesterone, prolactin and human placental lactogen induce hyperplasia and hypertrophy of the ducts and secretory structures of the breast during pregnancy. In the second half of pregnancy the breast is capable of secreting small amounts of milk. This is known as lactogenesis, stage 1. At birth the inhibitory influence of maternal progesterone is removed and milk production is stimulated by prolactin released in response to sucking. Sucking is therefore the primary stimulus to milk production and the means by which infant demand increases breast milk supply. Pregnancy is not an essential prerequisite to lactation which can be induced even after adoption by allowing the infant to suck (*'adoptive lactation'* or *'relactation'*).

During the first 3–5 days of life the volume of milk produced increases.[12] This is known as stage 2 of lactogenesis. Early milk ('colostrum') is rich in protein, particularly secretory immunoglobulin A. As the volume increases the protein and electrolyte content fall and the carbohydrate and fat content increase. By the fifth day the breasts typically produce more milk than the infant chooses to take at a feed. It was found that 5-day old babies took significantly less milk from the second breast than the first when the breasts are presented in random order (left/right or right/left) at a feed. This confirmed the breasts were not actually 'empty' and the baby chooses to leave milk behind.[13]

Many other experiments have confirmed that the *yield* (or volume of milk obtainable by expressing the breasts over a 24 h period) usually exceeds the baby's *intake.* In one study it was 7% greater than average intake measured by test weighing and in another an average 'residual volume' of over 100 ml/day (range 0–457 ml/day) could be extracted from the breast in addition to the baby's normal intake. Regular pumping increases yield further and an increment of 20% over intake was achieved in one study.

These observations make it hard to understand why most UK mothers who abandon breast-feeding in the early weeks of life believe they have 'insufficient milk'. They (and sometimes health professionals) probably fail to recognize differences in the feeding patterns of breast- and bottle-fed babies. Breast-fed babies tend to feed frequently, particularly during the early weeks of life when milk production is rapidly increasing, effectively reaching a plateau between 1 and 3 months of age. This must not be interpreted as undersupply. The amount of time a baby spends sucking gives no useful information about the baby's intake as there is very pronounced variation between individual mother–baby pairs.

Breast-feeding management

Important features of breast-feeding management are shown in Table 11.4.[14] Evidence for the 'Ten Steps' has recently been published in an extensive literature review.[15] They form the basis for accrediting health care facilities as *'Baby Friendly'* (there are currently 42 such maternity hospitals and four primary care facilities in the UK). The effectiveness of the *'Baby Friendly Hospital Initiative'* as an intervention has been confirmed in a cluster randomized trial performed in Belarus, part of the former Soviet Union.[16] Babies born in Baby Friendly Hospitals were significantly more likely to be exclusively breast-fed at 3 months and 6 months; moreover they were at significantly reduced risk of diarrheal disease and atopic eczema. Scottish audit data have also shown that babies born in Baby Friendly Hospitals are more likely to be breast-fed at the end of the first week of life.[17]

Table 11.4 Steps which help to establish breast-feeding in hospital

Every facility providing maternity services and care for newborn infants should:

1. Have a written breast-feeding policy that is routinely communicated to all health care staff.
2. Train all health care staff in skills necessary to implement this policy.
3. Inform all pregnant women about the benefits and management of breast feeding.
4. Help mothers initiate breast-feeding as soon as possible after delivery.
5. Show mothers how to breast-feed and how to maintain lactation even if they should be separated from their infants.
6. Give breast-fed newborn infants no food or drink *unless medically indicated.*
7. Practice rooming-in – allow mothers and infants to remain together – 24 hours a day.
8. Encourage breast-feeding on demand.
9. Give no artificial teats or dummies (pacifiers) to breast-feeding infants.
10. Foster the establishment of breast-feeding support groups and refer mothers to them on discharge from the hospital.

Modified from WHO/UNICEF 1989[14].

Early feeding, positioning and attachment

Babies should be given an opportunity to breast-feed as soon as possible after birth when they are alert and active. New mothers may need to be taught that babies do not always cry when hungry, but show other signs such as rooting activity. Early feed supervision will help to ensure that the baby is both correctly *positioned* (i.e. head and shoulders facing the breast) and *attached.*

The mechanics of breast-feeding (Fig. 11.1)[18] must be understood if the importance of correct *attachment* (relationship between baby's mouth and mother's breast) is to be appreciated. As the baby attaches the nipple is drawn into the mouth, retained by suction, and elongated to about three times its former length. The lateral margins of the tongue curve upwards to enclose it in a cup formed by tongue and hard palate. Milk is then stripped by a peristaltic wave running anteroposteriorly along the tongue. In this way milk is ejected from the lactiferous sinuses under the positive pressure created by nipple compression; negative pressure retains the nipple in the mouth and draws milk into the stripped lactiferous sinuses. This process is frictionless and the nipple should not be traumatized if the baby attaches correctly.[18] The mechanics of breast- and bottle-feeding are different and many believe babies may develop 'nipple confusion' if switched from one to the other (see below).

Incorrect attachment is a common cause of feeding problems.[19] The mother may say that her baby seems fretful and hungry yet is reluctant to suck, or that the nipple is sore, even bleeding. Such symptoms should prompt observation of a feed to check the physical signs of correct attachment which include:

- baby's chin touching breast;
- baby's lower lip turned out;
- mouth wide open;
- cheeks rounded, not drawn in;
- swallowing seen or heard;
- slow, rhythmical jaw movements with few pauses, not bursts of rapid sucking.

Doubts about technique should prompt expert midwifery assessment of feeding technique rather than resort to ineffective remedies such as creams, sprays or nipple shields. The last may even exacerbate the problem by hindering milk flow. The midwifery skills necessary to resolve this problem are outside the scope of this chapter.

Supplementary feeds

Supplementary feeds of formula or water are unnecessary for healthy, term breast-fed babies. There is no evidence that supplementary water or dextrose feeds accelerate resolution of neonatal jaundice in breast-fed babies. If anything they *increase* the incidence of early jaundice.

Healthy breast-fed term babies do not require routine blood glucose monitoring. Blood glucose concentrations of such babies may fall below 2 mmol/L without clinical signs of neuroglycopenia, probably because ketone bodies are effectively mobilized and act

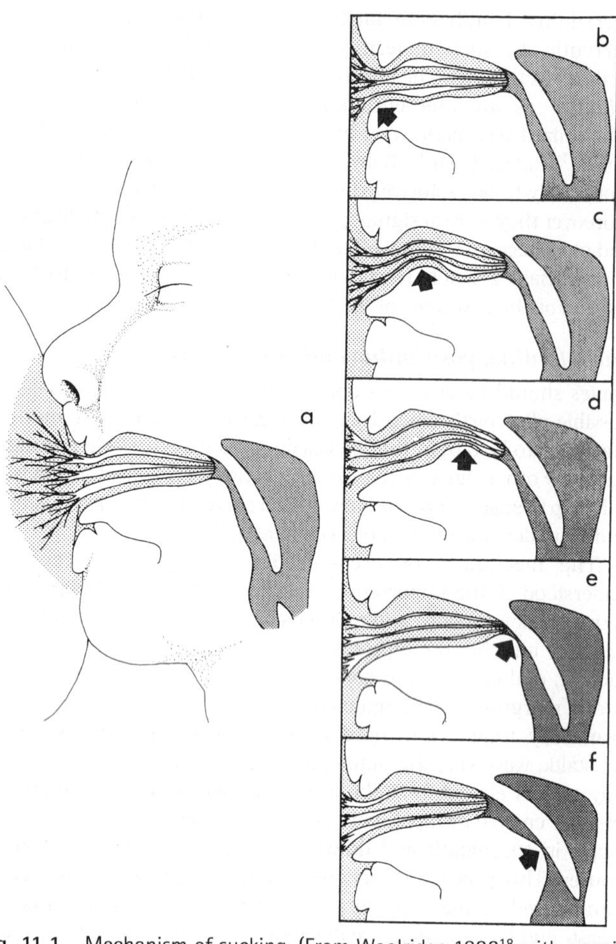

a. 'Teat' is formed from the nipple and much of the areola, with the lacteal sinuses, which lie behind the nipple, being drawn into the mouth with the breast tissue. The soft palate is relaxed and the nasopharynx is open for breathing. The shape of the tongue at the back represents its position at rest, cupped around the tip of the nipple.

b. The suck cycle is initiated by a welling up of the anterior tip of the tongue. At the same time the lower jaw, which had been momentarily relaxed (not shown), is raised to constrict the base of the nipple, thereby 'pinching off' milk within the ducts of the teat (these movements are inferred as they lie outside the sector viewed in ultrasound scans).

c. The wave of compression by the tongue moves along the underside of the nipple in a posterior direction, pushing against the hard palate. This roller-like action squeezes milk from the nipple. The posterior portion of the tongue may be depressed as milk collects in the oropharynx.

d, e. The wave of compression passes back past the tip of the nipple and pushes against the soft palate. As the tongue impinges on the soft palate the levator muscles of the palate contract raising it to seal off the nasal cavity. Milk is pushed into the oropharynx and is swallowed if sufficient has collected.

f. The cycle of compression continues and ends at the posterior base of the tongue. Depression of the back portion of the tongue creates negative pressure drawing the nipple and its milk contents once more into the mouth. This is accompanied by a lowering of the jaw which allows milk to flow back into the nipple.

Fig. 11.1 Mechanism of sucking. (From Woolridge 1986[18] with permission) The figure shows a complete 'suck' cycle; the baby is shown in median section. The baby exhibits good feeding technique with the nipple drawn well into the mouth, extending back to the junction of the hard and soft palate (the lactiferous sinuses are depicted within the teat though these cannot be visualized on scans). In ultrasound scans it appears that compression by the tongue, and negative pressure within the mouth, maintain the tongue in close conformation to the nipple and palate. Events are portrayed here rather more loosely to aid clarity.

as alternative cerebral fuels. 'Symptomatic' hypoglycemia in a breast-feeding baby should never be attributed to starvation alone; there is likely to be an underlying illness such as infection. Simple supplementary feeding is not therefore the solution.[20]

In some cultures (e.g. south Asian) it is believed that colostrum is detrimental, and 'prelacteal' feeds (e.g. teas, or formula in the UK) are used. There is a common misconception that this practice has a religious basis: it is in fact contrary to Islamic teaching and to be discouraged.[21]

Demand feeding

Babies should be allowed to feed until satiated whenever they are hungry. Limiting sucking time does not reduce the incidence of nipple trauma which is more likely to be attributable to poor attachment (see above). It is impossible to make rules about the frequency of feeds because babies vary greatly. They may feed only on a few occasions in the first 24 h becoming more active and hungry on the second and third days.

The duration of a breast-feed bears little relationship to the amount of milk consumed. Although a cross-sectional study suggested that, *on average*, 90% of the feed is consumed in the first 4 min, subsequent studies have shown that this conceals pronounced interindividual variation. It is therefore impossible to formulate a rule applicable to all mothers and babies.

It is not necessary for babies to take both breasts at every feed. Babies adjust their milk intake to allow for variation in its fat (i.e. energy) content. When mothers were instructed to offer only one breast rather than both at each feed babies extracted more hindmilk, thereby consuming more fat and maintaining a constant total daily energy intake.[22] Moreover, if the mother curtails feeding at the first breast in order to offer both routinely there is a theoretical risk that the baby will consume excessive volumes of low energy foremilk, leading to lactose overload with explosive, watery stools and 'colic'.

Maintaining lactation

Well babies should be with their mothers continuously (i.e. 'rooming-in'; Table 11.4) in the postnatal period. All breast-feeding mothers should be taught how to express milk by hand, though many prefer to use an electric pump. If so there is good evidence that pumping both breasts simultaneously (rather than sequentially), coupled with breast massage, increases yield.[23] A mother should express milk at least six times each day if separated from her baby, commencing as soon as possible after the birth. Expressed milk can be given by gavage, bottle or cup, the last being practicable for some babies of 30 weeks' gestation upwards. It has been claimed that cup feeding causes less 'nipple confusion' than using a bottle though controlled studies have not been performed.

CONTRAINDICATIONS TO BREAST-FEEDING

There are few absolute contraindications to breast-feeding. Galactosemia is one, and disorders of long chain fatty acid oxidation another, though with phenylketonuria it is usually possible to continue, supplementing with a low phenylalanine formula according to blood concentrations. Infant formula supplements may also be prescribed in medium chain acyl co-A dehydrogenase deficiency to prevent fasting hypoglycemia. Maternal infections such as hepatitis B and tuberculosis do not contraindicate breast-feeding though in both cases the baby should be immunized and treated with appropriate prophylaxis. Currently there is no consensus on maternal hepatitis C.

Human immunodeficiency virus (HIV) infection

Transmission of HIV to the baby of a breast-feeding mother was first described in a mother known to have been postnatally infected by blood transfusion, but other similar cases have since been described. In mothers infected antenatally the additional risk of vertical transmission attributable to breast-feeding has been estimated as about 15% rising to about 30% if the mother is infected postnatally. Mothers in the UK known to be HIV antibody positive and those at risk of infection are counseled not to breast-feed as part of a package of measures designed to reduce perinatal transmission rates. Appropriate strategies for countries with high infant mortality attributable to malnutrition or infectious disease in which the risk of bottle-feeding outweighs the risk of vertical transmission are currently being researched. Adequate breast-feeding support may be particularly important for such women as there is some evidence that mastitis (including 'subclinical mastitis') significantly increases HIV transmission risk.

Drugs in breast milk

There are very few instances in which maternal drug therapy need prevent breast-feeding; the decision should be based upon the toxicity of the drug, the quantity which the infant is likely to ingest, and the capacity of the infant to detoxify or excrete. Helpful, regularly updated texts are available to give specific guidance.[24,25] The balance of benefit and risk must also be considered: thus highly toxic drugs such as anti-mitotic agents and some retinoids contraindicate breast-feeding even though the amount ingested may be small. The quantity of any drug passed into milk may either be measured or calculated from consideration of its lipid solubility and the drug's pKa. The more ionized the drug, the less likely it is to pass into milk (pH 7.2): thus passage of drugs with higher pKa is more limited. A helpful general guideline to reduce infant exposure is to choose drugs with a shorter half-life and advise that they be taken immediately after a feed: as milk and plasma concentrations are in equilibrium, peak milk concentration will have declined by the next feed.[24]

GROWTH OF BREAST-FED BABIES

Growth references in common use [such as The National Center for Health Statistics (NCHS) and Tanner datasets] do not describe accurately the natural trajectory of the breast-fed infant who, in both industrialized and developing countries, grows rapidly in the first 2 months, slowing thereafter (Fig. 11.2).[26] This deceleration in weight velocity was once described as 'growth faltering' and speculatively attributed to a shortfall in energy intake from breast milk though estimated energy requirements then (and even now) were then set too high.

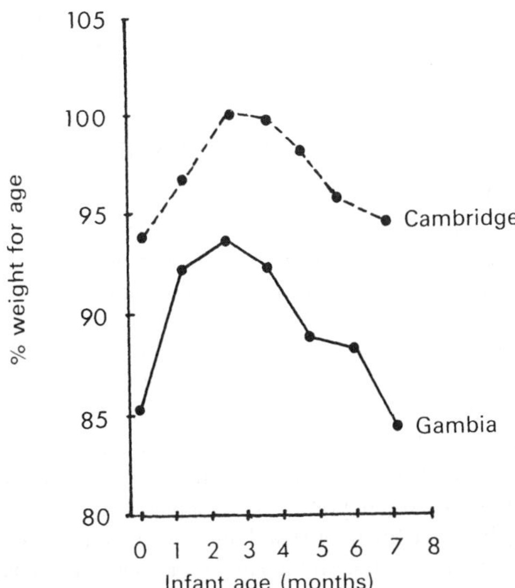

Fig. 11.2 The weight trajectory of breast-fed infants showing the normal acceleration relative to standard growth charts in the early months of life. (From Whitehead & Paul 1984[26], with permission)

It is very important that the early weight spurt apparent on such charts should not be interpreted as evidence of 'overfeeding'. Equally the deceleration after 2 months is not 'growth faltering' attributable to inadequate breast milk supply. These deviations from centile lines reflect inadequacies of the charts, not suboptimal growth patterns. The UK 1990 growth references may better reflect the early growth of breast-fed babies (being based on Cambridge infants) but a chart based on the growth pattern of healthy babies fed according to World Health Organization recommendations is in preparation at present.[27]

COMPLEMENTARY FEEDING OF BREAST-FED BABIES

Following systematic review of the evidence an expert consultation by the World Health Organization recently recommended exclusive breast-feeding for the first 6 months of life (with introduction of complementary foods and continued breast-feeding thereafter). This was associated with reduced incidence of diarrheal disease, increased maternal postpartum weight loss, and a prolonged duration of lactational amenorrhea with respect to breast-feeding exclusively for the first 4 months of life only. There have been few randomized studies of the appropriate timing of complementary feeding among breast-fed babies. One performed in Honduras showed that *total* daily energy intake and growth rate were comparable in early and late weaned infants, though breast milk intake simply fell in those given solid food intake earlier.[28]

It is important to recognize that this recommendation applies to *populations*, within which there may be subgroups (such as those of low birth weight) at potential risk of iron or trace mineral deficiency resulting from low stores at birth. As such it is not intended to apply to all individuals: indeed differences in the social and cultural preferences of mothers from country to country mean that complementary foods are used for many reasons other than nutritional ones (for example the need to return to work). There seems no reason, however, that any mother need be concerned that her milk supply is insufficient for at least the first 4 months

(17 weeks) of life. The observation that 91% of UK mothers had introduced solid foods by this stage in 1995 stands in stark contrast to the available evidence.

SUPPLEMENTS FOR BREAST-FED BABIES

Vitamin K

Dietary deficiency of vitamin K may result in hemorrhagic disease of the newborn (HDN) (Ch 10, Gastrointestinal problems and jaundice of the neonate). Human milk contains less vitamin K than cows' milk or formula (Tables 11.5[29] and 11.6[30]) and supplementation from birth has been recommended for many years. An intramuscular injection of vitamin K (1 mg phytomenadione) offers the most effective prophylaxis but was associated in one study with an increased incidence of later childhood malignancy. Although several other studies have not confirmed this association, many parents still prefer the option of oral supplementation. In England and Wales the Department of Health has recommended that parents be offered this choice, and an information leaflet is available to help them. A preparation licensed for oral administration to healthy term babies (*Konakion MM Paediatric,* Roche) is now available. The same preparation may be given parenterally (i.m./i.v.) to preterm babies or to those with other risk factors (for example instrumental delivery, mother taking anticonvulsants). Some ill babies (for example those with liver disease, malabsorption or on prolonged broad spectrum antibiotic therapy) may require continued supplementation in higher doses. If an oral dose (2 mg) is given at birth it will need to be repeated: the datasheet advises a second 2 mg dose at 4–7 days and further monthly doses during the period of exclusive breast-feeding. However, experts have recommended alternative schedules for subsequent doses, including 25 μg daily as practised in The Netherlands.[31] Unfortunately there are no comparative data yet on safety or efficacy.

Table 11.5 Composition of mature human milk

Total nitrogen	2.1 g/L
Protein	10.7 g/L
Casein	41% of total protein
α-lactalbumin	28% of total protein
Lactoferrin	14% of total protein
Serum albumin	2% of total protein
Lysozyme	1% of total protein
Secretory IgA	14% of total protein
Non-protein nitrogen	0.4 g/L
Fat	42 g/L
Cholesterol	0.42 mmol/L
Carbohydrate	74 g/L
Total energy	700 kcal/L
Sodium (23)	6.5 mmol/L
Potassium (39)	15.4 mmol/L
Calcium (40)	8.8 mmol/L
Magnesium (24)	1.2 mmol/L
Phosphorus (31)	4.8 mmol/L
Chloride (35)	12.3 mmol/L
Iron (56)	13.6 μmol/L
Copper (64)	6 μmol/L
Zinc (65)	45 μmol/L
Vitamin A (retinol)	600 μg/L
Vitamin D	0.1 μg/L
Vitamin E	3500 μg/L
Vitamin K	15 μg/L
Thiamin (B_1)	160 μg/L
Riboflavin (B_2)	310 μg/L
Nicotinic acid	2300 μg/L
Pyridoxine (B_6)	59 μg/L
Vitamin B_{12}	0.1 μg/L
Folic acid	52 μg/L
Pantothenic acid	2600 μg/L
Biotin	7.6 μg/L
Vitamin C	38 mg/L

(After DHSS 1977[29]). Atomic weights of minerals in parentheses.

Table 11.6 Composition of cow's milk and infant formula

Major nutrients	Cow's milk	Infant formula
Protein	33	15–20* g/L
Casein:whey	79:21	80:20 or 40:60
Carbohydrate	48	48–100 g/L
Fat	38	23–50 g/L
Linoleic and linolenic acid		>1% of total energy
Minerals		
Sodium	59 (35–90)	15–35 mg/dl
Potassium	150 (110–170)	50–100 mg/dl
Chloride	95 (90–110)	40–80 mg/dl
Calcium	120 (110–130)	30–120 mg/dl
Phosphorus	95 (90–100)	15–60 mg/dl
Ca:P ratio	1.2:1	1.2–2.2:1
Magnesium	12 (9–14)	2.8–12 mg/dl
Iron	50 (30–60)	70–700 μg/dl
Zinc	350 (200–600)	200–600 μg/dl
Copper (see text)	20 (10–60)	10–60 μg/dl
Vitamins		
A (retinol)	31 (27–36)†	40–150 μg/dl
D	0.02	0.7–1.3 μg/dl
E (α-tocopherol)	0.09	>0.3 mg/dl
K	1–8.5	>1.5 μg/dl
C	2	>3 mg/dl
Thiamin (B_1)	40 (30–60)	>13 μg/dl
Riboflavin (B_2)	190 (150–230)	>30 μg/dl
Nicotinaminde (B_3)	80 (60–130)	>230 μg/dl
Pyridoxine (B_6)	40 (21–72)	>5 μg/dl
B_{12}	0.3	>0.01 μg/dl
Pantothenic acid	0.35 (0.2–0.5)	>200 μg/dl
Biotin	2 (1.0–1.3)	>0.5 μg/dl
Folic acid	5	>3 mg/dl

Data from DHSS 1980[30].
*May be <1.5 if casein:whey ratio 40:60.
†Summer–winter range for vitamins.

Vitamin D

Breast milk contains less calcium, phosphate and vitamin D than cows' milk or infant formula. Young babies meet their vitamin D requirements from stores at birth and sunshine exposure but nutritional rickets is occasionally seen. It is particularly associated with late introduction of complementary foods, Asian or black ethnic minority origin, and iron deficiency.[32] A relatively high proportion of such young children (between 20 and 35% in a national study of Asian infants and toddlers) have low plasma 25-OH-vitamin D concentrations particularly during the winter months.[33]

Pregnant and breast-feeding women should take 10 μg of vitamin D daily, as the reference nutrient intake (RNI) set for these groups is most unlikely to be met from food. Breast-fed babies should be given a supplement of 280 iu (7 μg/day) from 6 months onwards, though it may be started earlier in groups considered at increased risk by virtue of their ethnic origins or cultural background. Other babies should commence vitamin D supplements when no longer receiving infant formula, usually from about 12 months of age.

Iron

Breast milk contains little iron though its bioavailability is high. Birth stores are the principal source of iron in young infants. Thus breast-fed babies do not require iron supplements unless additional risk factors are present, such as low birth weight. There may be adverse effects of iron supplements in babies who do not need them. In one study weight gain was impaired.[34] Moreover iron, copper and zinc compete for absorption across the intestinal mucosa, so other trace mineral deficiencies (particularly zinc) may be precipitated.

Water

It is well established that breast-fed babies do not need supplements of water: the solute load of breast milk is low enough to permit free water availability even in tropical climates.

Fluoride

See Dental health, page 402.

BREAST-FED BABIES WHO FAIL TO THRIVE

Physiological failure of milk supply is rare. Faulty breast-feeding technique more often underlies poor weight gain and expert midwifery counseling is essential. A history of early feeding difficulty or nipple pain may be obtained, the baby eventually becoming undemanding and sleepy. Breast engorgement or mastitis may have occurred, again indicating ineffective drainage. Physical illness in the baby needs to be excluded, particularly if change has been recent. Otherwise attention to technique and increasing the frequency of feeds, sometimes combined with expression may help to increase supply. There is no evidence that metoclopramide, domperidone or other galactogogues more effectively increase supply than the physiological approach suggested.

Test weighing using mechanical scales underestimates intake and is of no clinical value at all. Electronic scales can improve weighing precision but may still undermine the mother's confidence and raise problems of interpretation. Firstly, test weighing must proceed for *at least* 48 h to take account of day-to-day and circadian variation. Secondly, the range of normal is very wide and the baby's milk consumption less than the mother's potential yield; the intake of one group of 3 month old babies varied from 523–1124 g/day but, on average, a further 100 g could be obtained by expression. Finally, the baby's energy intake cannot be derived from weighed milk intake as the fat content of breast milk varies so much and tends to be inversely proportional to the volume of milk consumed. For all these reasons test weighing is of very limited value in the clinical context; it is much more important to diagnose problems with breast-feeding technique (p. 395) and refer to a professional competent in breast-feeding management.

INFANT FORMULA FEEDING

An *'infant formula'* is legally defined as a product that by itself meets the nutritional requirements of normal healthy infants in the first 4–6 months of life. The composition of infant formula is controlled by European Community and UK legislation. *'Follow-on formula'* is intended for use by normal healthy infants over 6 months of age as 'the principal liquid element in a progressively diversified diet'. It is not legally required to meet by itself the infant's entire nutritional needs.

Unmodified milks from cows, sheep, goats and other animals are unsuitable for feeding infants. Amongst other things they generate a high *renal solute load* (p. 400), have inappropriate calcium: phosphorus ratio, and are low in iron and vitamin content. Some years ago a Department of Health & Social Security report set compositional guidelines for infant formula manufacturers. The philosophy underlying these was that the nutrient content of infant formula should match as closely as possible that of mature human milk, unless significant differences in nutrient bioavailability existed between breast milk and formula (as is the case, for example, with iron and protein; see below).

Although this principle has continued to influence formula manufacture a more recent report has proposed that innovations should not merely focus on composition but seek demonstrable benefit in *outcome*, matching as closely as possible the nutritional optimum of the healthy breast-fed infant. This change has been stimulated by increasing appreciation of the molecular complexity of human milk and by the application of novel processes (such as recombinant DNA technology) to produce in vitro human milk constituents for addition to formula. It is essential to demonstrate that such developments will be both effective and safe.

COMPOSITION OF HUMAN MILK

The composition of expressed human milk has been extensively studied in view of its relevance to formula manufacture. Table 11.5 is based on a study of the composition of mature human milk expressed by UK mothers.[35] It is worth noting briefly the factors that affect milk composition and some important qualitative nutritional differences between human milk and formula (e.g. protein, fat, minerals and vitamins).

Factors affecting milk composition

Gestation of baby

Most studies have found milk of mothers delivering prematurely to be higher in protein and sodium content but lower in lactose. Some of the differences can be explained by reduced milk output (similar changes happen again at weaning) but serum leakage due to immaturity of mammary epithelial integrity might also be relevant.

Maternal diet and nutritional state

The effect of energy intake on the output and macronutrient content of breast milk has been overstated in the past. Lactational efficiency is relatively unaffected by maternal body mass index (BMI). The fat content does, however, reflect qualitatively the amount and type of fat the mother consumes in her diet.

Stage of lactation

Stage of lactation affects all milk constituents. Early milk is arbitrarily classified as *colostrum* (0–5 days) or *transitional* milk (5–10 days). Thereafter it is termed *mature.* Protein concentration changes greatly in the early stages, mainly because the immunoglobulin content of colostrum falls about 50-fold in the first week. The total output of immunoglobulin A nevertheless changes little because the volume of milk produced increases. Sodium concentration similarly falls in early lactation as the lactose concentration rises. Amongst the micronutrients, iron and copper concentrations fall slowly during lactation but zinc drops about 10-fold over a year. The changes in protein, lactose and sodium content reverse at weaning so that colostrum, weaning milk and 'preterm milk' are very similar in composition.

Changes within a feed

Fat concentration changes most, more than doubling during a feed. This may be a simple physical effect as it can be mimicked simply by squeezing milk from a sponge.

Time of day

Fat concentration shows most change and is inversely related to the time which has elapsed since the last feed: the longer the interval the lower the foremilk fat. Variation in nursing patterns considerably affects circadian changes in fat concentration for this reason.

Protein and non-protein nitrogen

Estimates of human milk protein concentration vary between 0.8 and 1.3 g/day for methodological reasons. The *crude protein* content is total nitrogen (g) × 6.38 which is always higher than the true figure as 25% of total nitrogen is *'non-protein nitrogen'*. Some of this, including urea, is incorporated into body protein together with the principal nutritional proteins, alpha-lactalbumin and casein. Many milk proteins (e.g. secretory immunoglobulin A, lactoferrin) do not primarily function as nutrients and can be recovered from the stool though their digestibility increases with age. This difference in the digestibility of human and cows' milk proteins is one reason that the protein content of an infant formula does not straightforwardly equate with that of human milk.

A further reason is the difference in *protein quality*, i.e. the relative match between the amino acid content of a dietary protein and the requirement for growth and metabolism. Protein quality can be expressed numerically either by essential 'amino acid score' or 'net protein utilization', the proportion of ingested protein which is retained. Human milk is used as a reference protein in both cases, e.g.:

$$\text{Amino acid score} = \frac{\text{mg limiting essential amino acid in 1 g test protein} \times 100\%}{\text{mg limiting essential amino acid in 1 g human milk protein}}$$

By regulation an infant formula must be based on soya or cows' milk protein. The latter has broadly two classes: whey (or acid-soluble) proteins and caseins (acid-precipitable curd). As whey and casein differ in amino acid composition the quality of cows' milk protein can be manipulated by changing the whey : casein ratio from 20 : 80 to 60 : 40, closer to that of human milk. Such formulae are known as *whey dominant*. The claim that casein dominant formula 'satisfies hungry babies' has no justification, though UK babies commonly change to these within the first 6 weeks.[4]

The plasma amino acid concentrations of babies fed cows' milk protein based formula containing 1.25 or 1.3 g/100 ml cows' milk protein as opposed to the usual 1.5–2.0 g/dl (Table 11.6) more closely approximate those of breast-fed babies. The whey:casein ratio also has less effect at these intakes. Thus the protein content of current formulae might be higher than necessary. It is possible that the higher protein intake of formula fed babies, through increasing insulin secretion, explains the differences in growth and body composition observed particularly in the second half of infancy. However breast-fed babies also self-regulate energy intake at lower levels, and have lower levels of energy expenditure.

Fat

Breast milk contains long (LCT) and medium chain triglycerides (MCT). The fat composition of milk varies extensively with maternal diet. In recent years it has been speculated that provision of the polyunsaturated fatty acid (PUFA) precursors linoleic (C_{18}–2ω6) and linolenic acid (C_{18}–3ω3) in formula is insufficient to meet the demands of the growing nervous system for the long chain polyunsaturated fatty acid (LCPUFA) docosohexaenoic acid (C_{22}–6ω3). In support of this, significant differences in the brain lipid composition of breast-fed and formula fed babies have been observed.[36] There is, however, no conclusive evidence that the addition of LCPUFAs to formula is of significant short or long term health benefit for term infants.[37]

Iron

Cows' milk contains less iron than human milk and, furthermore, cows' milk iron is less bioavailable. Formulae are therefore enriched with iron salts, usually ferric ammonium citrate. Formulae sold in the USA vary widely in iron content; so-called 'regular' formula contains 1 mg/L iron whereas 'iron-fortified' formulae contain > 10 mg/L. A US randomized trial showed superior iron status and psychomotor development among infants fed 'iron-fortified' formula.[38] However those sold in the UK contain 5–7 mg/L iron and it is not possible to extrapolate the results of the US study to UK practice. If the mother is not breast-feeding, continued use of infant formula or follow-on formula to at least 12 months of age is nevertheless important in building iron stores and preventing iron deficiency in the toddler years.[39] There is no evidence that 'follow-on' formulas promote better iron status than normal infant formulas, though either is preferable to cows' milk.

Manufacture of infant formula

Manufacture of infant formula in simple terms changes the composition of cows' milk (Table 11.6) as follows:

1. The protein and electrolyte content of cows' milk (see 'solute load' below) are reduced.
2. The whey:casein blend may be altered to improve protein quality and digestibility.
3. The calcium and phosphorus content is reduced and the Ca:P ratio altered.
4. The carbohydrate content is increased by addition of lactose or maltodextrins (glucose polymers).
5. The fat blend is changed using vegetable oil to reduce saturated fat intake and increase intake of polyunsaturated fat, thus improving fat absorption.
6. Trace minerals are added, particularly iron and copper
7. Vitamins are added.

'RENAL SOLUTE LOAD'

Both glomerular filtration rate and tubular concentrating power are reduced in the newborn (Ch. 10, Special care–sodium and potassium). This limits the clearance and elimination of urea produced if protein intake exceeds growth demands. The *renal solute load* of a feed is the total quantity of unutilized dietary solute that must be eliminated in available water. It can be calculated by summing urea production and sodium and potassium chloride intake surplus to growth and non-urinary losses. (In urea production each gram of dietary protein over growth and maintenance requirements generates a solute load of 4 milliosmoles) Human milk generates a solute load of 79 milliosmoles/L and unmodified cows' milk 221 milliosmoles/L. Thus, an infant with maximal tubular concentrating power of 600 milliosmoles/L of urine will require at least 370 (or 221/600 × 1000) ml of water for the safe elimination of the solute load generated by a liter of cows' milk. A high insensible water loss caused by diarrhea or fever may restrict water available for solute excretion and therefore give rise to hypernatremia. Energy density also has a bearing on solute load because it affects milk intake, and thus water available for urine formation.

MILK CONSUMPTION

The normal intake of both breast- and bottle-fed babies is extremely variable and the oft-quoted requirement of 150 ml/kg/day is merely a guideline. In fact the intakes of healthy formula fed infants 0–2 months old fed *ad libitum* were 169 ± 25 [1 standard deviation (SD)] ml/kg/day (boys) and 157 ± 22 ml/kg/day (girls).[40] Similarly, although the average breast milk intake of 3 month old infants is 700–800 ml/day, there is approximately 100% difference between the extremes of the normal range.

Consequently one cannot specify a 'normal' milk intake for any individual infant. Acceptable intake is reflected in satisfactory growth but, if the baby is not growing, the baby may be fed *ad libitum* or formula intake increased to the upper end of the normal range (mean + 2 SD) before investigating other causes.

GROWTH OF FORMULA FED BABIES

Several recent prospective studies have measured protein:energy intakes and growth during infancy. Bottle-fed infants consumed 66–70% more protein in the first 6 months than those exclusively breast-fed and, unlike breast-fed infants,[41] did not reduce their milk intake when weaning foods were introduced. At 1 year of age bottle-fed infants were heavier and fatter than breast-fed though length and head circumference were similar.[41] These growth differences are consistent with a recent cross-sectional observation that breast-fed babies may be less likely to become obese as children,[42] and that weaning later (beyond 13 weeks) is associated with reduced body mass index at school age.[3]

SOYA FORMULA AND OTHER MILKS

Soya formula is overused. It is suitable for the infants of vegan mothers who choose not to breast-feed but has a dubious role in the prophylaxis or treatment of cows' milk protein allergy because cross-sensitivity to soya protein occurs in 15–43% of affected children. A formula based on cows' milk protein hydrolysate is preferable both in proven cows' milk protein intolerance (CMPI) and post gastroenteritis lactose intolerance because CMPI often coexists. Another concern is the very high phytoestrogen content of soya formula: although there are no long term data on the effects of these compounds on young infants consensus advice is that soya formulas should not be used unnecessarily. They can be used in the management of galactosemia (Ch. 24) because they are lactose free.

COMPLEMENTARY FEEDING – 'WEANING'

The term 'weaning' is commonly used to describe the gradual introduction of foods (or 'solids') other than breast milk or formula, though it more correctly describes a reduction in the number of breast-feeds. The phrase 'complementary feeding' is therefore preferred, because it indicates the important role played by continued breast-feeding, particularly in resource-poor countries.

Complementary feeding functions nutritionally to increase the energy, vitamin and mineral density of the diet as demands begin to outstrip milk supply. However it has broader functions in infant development helping, for example, to encourage tongue and jaw movements in preparation for speech, introducing new tastes and textures, and increasing social interaction with carers. It is important that complementary feeding is paced to accord with developmental changes in gross, fine motor and oral motor function if later 'behavioral' eating problems are to be avoided. From about 6 months relatively bland (unseasoned), single ingredient foods (such as thinly puréed rice, fruit or vegetables can be offered once- or twice-daily from a spoon after breast-feeds. As the spoon is accepted thicker purées may be offered, with progression to lumps and small finger foods as fine motor skills progress. In some cultures there may be more dependence on hand feeding at this stage, with little use of the spoon.[21] By about 1 year of age the infant should be receiving (chopped) family foods at about three main meals with intervening snacks. Breast milk should remain the principal source of fluid, though formula (in amounts of no more than 500–600 ml/day) may now be replaced by pasteurized whole cows' milk.

WEANING PROBLEMS

The largest share of weaning problems is borne by infants in less-developed countries placed at risk of gastrointestinal infection and energy dilution. Traditional gruels may be less nutritious than milk; programs encouraging use of locally produced bean/flour mixes have effectively reduced the incidence of childhood malnutrition.

Vegetarian and ethnic minority diets

Certain minority groups (e.g. vegans, Rastafarians) have limited choice of weaning foods. Protein quality, zinc, iron and vitamin B_{12} intake may be low. Phytates may reduce mineral availability (especially calcium and iron) and increase dietary bulk, compromising energy intake. Suggestions for a suitable vegetarian weaning diet are summarized in Table 11.7.[43]

Asian babies in the UK tend to be weaned later than white ones, particularly those of Bangladeshi and Pakistani background.[44]

Table 11.7 Suggestions for vegetarian weaning diets (After Poskitt 1988[43])

Nutrient	Problem	Solution
Energy	Energy density reduced by water absorption and fiber content. Most fruit low in energy	Use oils in cooking and spreading fats on food. Cereals, pulses, bananas and avocados are energy dense
Protein	Quality variable	Mix complementary food groups to achieve balanced intake, i.e. milk (dairy), legumes, grains, green vegetables
Vitamins	Low B_{12}, D and riboflavin	Use eggs, vitamin D-supplemented margarine or fish oils (if permissible). Consider oral B_{12} supplement
Minerals	Phytates reduce availability (especially of iron). Zinc and calcium intakes may be low	Green leaf vegetables rich in iron. Vitamin C increases uptake. Dairy products important as calcium/zinc source

They are more likely to be breast-fed initially, but also more likely to receive cows' milk in the first year of life, often with complementary foods such as rusk added to the feeding bottle. Amongst children of Indian background 38% of 9-month olds in a national survey had never eaten meat. These dietary habits help to explain the higher incidence of iron deficiency anemia amongst Asian toddlers in the UK.[45] A significant proportion of Asian toddlers also show hypovitaminosis D[33] and sometimes frank rickets.[46] Early supplementation with vitamin D, coupled with supplementation for the mother during pregnancy and breast-feeding could help prevent this. Although more Asian mothers (> 50% at 9 months) than white ones (20%) give vitamins there is still room for improvement.

There has been no comparable national study of black, Afro-Caribbean babies in the UK but they are also likely to be at increased risk of vitamin D deficiency also, particularly if Rastafarian.

Iron deficiency

Iron deficiency has its roots in progressive depletion of iron stores during infancy though it may not be present until the second year of life. The most effective prophylactic measures are prolonged breast milk or formula feeding (preferably into the second year of life[39]) with avoidance of cows' milk, provision of heme iron (as meat or fish), vitamin C with meals (as vitamin drops or fruit), and prescription of iron supplements for babies of low birth weight. Tea is an unsuitable drink for infants as tannins complex iron and reduce availability.

VITAMIN SUPPLEMENTS

Formula is fortified with vitamins, and supplementation is unnecessary until cows' milk is introduced at about 1 year of age. Breast-fed babies should receive vitamin supplements. (e.g. Department of Health vitamin ACD drops, *Abidec™*, *Dalivit™*) from 6 months of age or in some cases earlier (Ch. 14). Vitamin supplements should be continued until 2 years of age, and preferably until 5. Department of Health vitamin drops contain (per ml): 5000 units vitamin A, 2000 units vitamin D, 150 mg vitamin C. Dose = five drops/day.

DENTAL HEALTH

Water fluoridation reduces the incidence of dental caries but fluoride supplementation (0.25 mg/day from 6 months of age) is desirable if the supply is unfluoridated and the risk of caries high. Excessive supplementation causes enamel mottling and must be avoided. Teeth should be brushed after eating or drinking, initially without toothpaste but later with only a small (less than pea-sized) amount. Fluoride supplements should be reduced to take account of intake from toothpaste. Minimizing intake of non-milk extrinsic sugars without sacrificing diet palatability, and using a cup from about 6 months, rather than a bottle, for liquids also help to prevent caries.

DRINKS AND WATER

Boiled tap water is sufficient if required for bottle-fed babies under 6 months of age. Flavored drinks are unnecessary. Natural mineral water, or water drawn through a domestic softener is of unsuitable electrolyte content and should not be given to babies.

Displacement of milk with flavored drinks during weaning is a common cause of failure to thrive. Moreover it may increase non-milk extrinsic sugar (e.g. sucrose) intake to exceed the recommended maximum of 10% of energy intake.

PASTEURIZED COWS' MILK

Pasteurized whole cows' milk should not be given to infants under 1 year of age (Ch. 14) and semi-skimmed milk should be avoided in children under 2 years. Other milk products, such as cheese and yoghurt, may be used from 6 months onwards.

REFERENCES (* Level 1 evidence)

1 NHS Centre for Reviews and Dissemination. Promoting the initiation of breast-feeding. Effective Health Care 2000; 6(2):1–12.

2 World Health Organization DoDaARDC. Indicators for assessing breast-feeding practices. WHO/CDD/SER/91 1991; 14:1–14.

3 Wilson AC, Forsyth JS, Greene SA, et al. Relation of infant diet to childhood health: seven year follow up of cohort of children in Dundee infant feeding study. BMJ 1998; 316:21–25.

4 Foster K, Lader D, Cheesbrough S. Infant feeding 1995. London: The Stationery Office; 1997:1–174.

5 Howie PW, Forsyth JS, Ogston SA, et al. Protective effect of breast feeding against infection. BMJ 1990; 300:11–16.

6 Harrison LC. Cow's milk and IDDM. Lancet 1996; 348:905–906.

7 Ellis TM, Atkinson MA. Early infant diets and insulin-dependent diabetes mellitus. Lancet 1996; 347:1464–1465.

8 Anderson JW, Johnstone BM, Remley DT. Breast-feeding and cognitive development: a meta-analysis. Am J Clin Nutr 1999; 70:525–535.

9 Ramos R, Kennedy KI, Visness CM. Effectiveness of lactational amenorrhoea in prevention of pregnancy in Manila, the Philippines: non-comparative prospective trial. BMJ 1996; 313:909–912.

10 Eisman J. Relevance of pregnancy and lactation to osteoporosis. Lancet 1998; 352:504–505.

11 Abrams SA. Editorial. Bone turnover during lactation – can calcium supplementation make a difference? J Clin Endocrinol Metab 1998; 83(4):1056–1058.

12 Neville MC, Keller R, Seacat J, et al. Studies in human lactation: milk volumes in lactating women during the onset of lactation and full lactation. Am J Clin Nutr 1988; 48:1375–1386.

*13 Drewett RF, Woolridge MW. Milk taken by human babies from the first and second breast. Physiol Behav 1981; 26:327–329.

14 WHO/UNICEF. Protecting, promoting and supporting breast-feeding. The specific role of maternity services. Geneva: WHO; 1989.

15 Vallenas C, Savage F. Evidence for the Ten Steps to successful breast-feeding. WHO/CHD/ 98.9. Geneva: World Health Organization; 1998:1–111.

*16 Kramer MS, Chalmers B, Hodnett ED, et al. Promotion of breast-feeding intervention trial (PROBIT). JAMA 2001; 285:413–420.

17 Tappin DM, Mackenzie JM, Brown AJ, et al. Breast-feeding rates are increasing in Scotland. Health Bulletin 2001; 59(2):102–113.

18 Woolridge MW. The 'anatomy' of infant feeding. Midwifery 1986; 2:164–171.

19 Woolridge MW. The aetiology of sore nipples. Midwifery 1986; 2:172–176.

20 Williams AF. Hypoglycaemia of the newborn: a review. Bull World Health Organ 1997; 75(3):261–290.

21 Gatrad A, Sheikh A. Muslim birth customs. Arch Dis Child, Fetal Neonatal Ed 2001; 84(1):F6–F8.

*22 Woolridge MW, Ingram JC, Baum JD. Do changes in pattern of breast usage alter the baby's nutrient intake? Lancet 1990; 336:395–397.

*23 Jones E, Dimmock PW, Spencer SA. A randomised trial to compare methods of milk expression after preterm delivery. Arch Dis Child, Fetal Neonatal Ed 2001; 85(2):F91–F95.

24 Hale TW. Medications and mothers' milk, 9th edn. Amarillo, TX: Pharmasoft; 2000.

25 Briggs GG, Freeman RK, Yaffe SJ. Drugs in pregnancy and lactation, 5th edn. Baltimore: Williams and Wilkins, 1998.

26 Whitehead RG, Paul AA. Growth charts and the assessment of infant feeding practices in the western world and in developing countries. Early Hum Dev 1984; 9:187–207.

27 de Onis M, Habicht J-P. Anthropometric reference data for international use: recommendations from a World Health Organization Expert Committee. Am J Clin Nutr 1996; 64:650–658.

*28 Cohen RJ, Brown KH, Canahuati J, et al. Effects of age of introduction of complementary foods on infant breast milk intake, total energy intake, and growth: a randomised controlled study in Honduras. Lancet 1994; 344:288–293.

29 Department of Health and Social Security. The composition of mature human milk. Report on health and social subjects 12. London: HMSO; 1977.

30 Department of Health and Social Security. Artificial feeds for the young infant. Report on health and social subjects 18. London: HMSO; 1980.

31 Tripp JH, McNinch AW. The vitamin K debacle: cut the Gordian knot but first do no harm. Arch Dis Child 1998; 79:295–299.

32 Wharton BA. Low plasma vitamin D in Asian toddlers in Britain. Br Med J 1999; 318:2–3.

33 Lawson M, Thomas M, Hardiman A. Dietary and lifestyle factors affecting plasma vitamin D levels in Asian children living in England. Eur J Clin Nutr 1999; 53:268–272.

34 Idradjinata P, Watkins WE, Pollitt E. Adverse effects of iron supplementation on weight gain of iron-replete young children. Lancet 1994; 343:1252–1254.

35 Committee on Medical Aspects of Food Policy (COMA). The composition of mature human milk. Report on health and social subjects 12. London: HMSO; 1977.

36 Farquharson J, Cockburn F, Patrick WA, et al. Infant cerebral cortex phospholipid fatty-acid composition and diet. Lancet 1992; 340:810–813.

*37 Simmer K. Long chain polyunsaturated fatty acid supplementation in infants born at term. (Cochrane Review). Cochrane Library; 2001.

*38 Moffatt MEK, Longstaffe S, Besant J, et al. Prevention of iron deficiency and psychomotor decline in high-risk infants through use of iron-fortified infant formula: a randomised clinical trial. J Pediatr 1994; 125:527–534.

*39 Williams J, Wolff A, Daly A, et al. Iron supplemented formula milk related to reduction in psychomotor decline in infants from inner city areas. BMJ 1999; 318:693–698.

40 Fomon SJ, Thomas LN, Filer LJ, et al. Food consumption and growth of normal infants fed milk based formulas. Acta Paediatr Scand Suppl 1971; 223:1–36.

41 Heinig MJ, Nommsen LA, Peerson JM, et al. Energy and protein intakes of breast-fed and formula-fed infants during the first year of life and their association with growth velocity: the DARLING study. Am J Clin Nutr 1993; 58:152–161.

42 von Kries R, Koletzko B, Sauerwald T, et al. Breast feeding and obesity: cross sectional study. BMJ 1999; 319:147–150.

43 Poskitt EME. Vegetarian weaning. Arch Dis Child 1988; 63:1286–1292.

44 Thomas M, Avery V. Infant feeding in Asian families. London: The Stationery Office; 1997.

45 Lawson MS, Thomas A, Hardiman A. Iron status of Asian children aged 2 years living in England. Arch Dis Child 1997; 78:420–426.

46 Mughal MZ, Salama H, Greenaway T, et al. Lesson of the week: florid rickets associated with prolonged breast feeding without vitamin D supplementation. BMJ 1999; 318(7175):39–40.

Section 3

The specialties

Section 3

The specialties

12

Genetics

Michael A Patton

INTRODUCTION

There have been many advances in the understanding of human genetics in the last 10–20 years and the purpose of this chapter is to present some of the basic concepts of genetics in relation to pediatric practice. Rather than becoming polarized in an argument about which disorders are due to 'nature' and which are due to 'nurture', it is more fruitful to consider human disease as a spectrum from those conditions like Duchenne muscular dystrophy and Down syndrome, which are purely genetic, through to those which are purely environmental such as scurvy and tuberculosis (Fig. 12.1).[1] Between the two extremes are many common diseases like diabetes mellitus, ischemic heart disease and congenital malformations in which both genetic and environmental factors are involved. Such conditions may be referred to as multifactorial. Disorders which are at the genetic end of the spectrum are either due to changes in a single gene or to visible changes in the chromosomes.

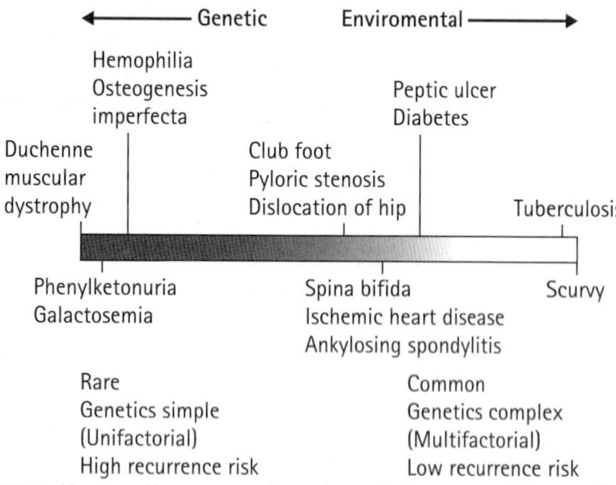

Fig. 12.1 Human disease may be seen as being on a spectrum from those diseases which are exclusively genetic to those which are exclusively environmental. (From Emery & Mueller 1988[1])

EPIDEMIOLOGY

The frequency of genetic disorders has not increased, but they have become relatively more important with the decline in mortality from infectious diseases that has resulted from vaccination, improved living standards and antibiotic therapy. The relative importance of genetic disease is also increasing for other reasons. There is rapidly increasing knowledge in the field of medical genetics. The number of human chromosomes was only established in 1956 and since then our knowledge of genetics has advanced at an exponential rate with the first draft of the human genome being completed in 2001. Prenatal diagnosis has offered the opportunity of preventing an increasing number of serious handicaps, and the developments in DNA technology have meant that many of the genes that predispose to common adult disorders such as heart disease and cancer are now being identified and may play a major role in identifying the predisposition in these disorders, and developing strategies for their prevention.

Genetic disorders are a major component in childhood mortality with up to half of childhood deaths in hospital having a genetic or partly genetic cause. In addition to mortality, genetic disorders produce a substantial morbidity. They often require frequent hospital admissions or complex surgery and this is reflected in a number of studies on the incidence of genetic disorders amongst pediatric inpatients; the incidence of genetic or partially genetic disease amongst pediatric inpatients has been found to be between 11 and 27%.[2] It should also be noted that many chronic genetic disorders may place a considerable financial strain on health resources, e.g. the average annual cost of a patient with cystic fibrosis in 1990 was £8000 and the lifetime cost of continual nursing care for a severely handicapped individual may be over £1 000 000.

In the field of mental handicap the genetic contribution is even greater. With the recognition of chromosomal disease it has been found that around one-third of mental handicap is due to chromosomal abnormality and future studies which include analysis for fragile X and molecular abnormalities are likely to find an even greater contribution from genetic causes. Overall more than 50% of mental handicap is due to genetic factors, and many of these could be prevented by genetic counseling and prenatal diagnosis (Table 12.1).[3]

The same situation applies in visual handicap and profound childhood deafness. In previous generations retrolental fibroplasia and ophthalmia neonatorum contributed significantly to childhood blindness but the frequency of these disorders is declining with improved medical care. One survey[4] conducted in a national school for children who are registered blind has shown that about 50% of childhood blindness has a genetic basis and that this is largely due to single gene disorders (Table 12.2).[4] In studies on congenital deafness around 30% has been attributed to genetic factors and once again many of these are due to single gene disorders (Table 12.3).

Table 12.1 Causes of severe mental retardation

Etiology	Frequency (%)
Chromosomal	33
Single gene disorder	15
Malformation syndrome	13
CNS malformation	7
Perinatal factors	15
Infections, trauma	3
Unknown	14

(Based on a regional study of mentally handicapped children in Hertfordshire, Laxova et al 1977[3])

Even before birth chromosome abnormalities are a major cause of fetal wastage with between 15 and 30% of all human conceptions having an abnormal karyotype and being spontaneously aborted or failing to implant.

The incidence of genetic disorders is roughly comparable in different parts of the world, but the frequency of specific disorders may vary for reasons such as inbreeding, selective advantage and genetic isolation.[5] The frequency of sickle cell disease mirrors the frequency of malaria since carriers of sickle cell trait have a greater resistance to *Plasmodium falciparum* malaria. This frequency has taken many generations to develop from a relatively small selective advantage and will remain in those racial groups for a very considerable number of generations even after they have moved to countries without malaria. Cystic fibrosis is one of the most frequent single gene disorders in Western Europe, and although this is probably attributable to a selective advantage in gene carriers, the mechanism has yet to be demonstrated. For other recessive disorders in small isolated communities the frequency of affected children may be increased by inbreeding, e.g. oculocutaneous albinism in the Hopi Indians, congenital adrenal hyperplasia in the Yupik Eskimos and Ellis–van Creveld syndrome in the Amish community (Table 12.4). It should be noted that genetic disease may pose a major health problem even in underdeveloped countries where infections are still a major cause of childhood deaths, e.g. in Thailand up to 500 000 children suffer from variable degrees of chronic ill health due to the interaction of different thalassemia genes.

MITOSIS AND MEIOSIS

Chromosomes are the means whereby the genes are transmitted from one cell generation to the next. This transmission of genetic

Table 12.2 99 Children in blind school, Edinburgh (1988)

Genetic = 50%	Non-genetic = 50%
Congenital cataract	Birth asphyxia
Anophthalmos	Optic nerve hypoplasia
Leber's amaurosis	Cortical blindness
Laurence–Moon–Biedl	Retrolental fibroplasia
Retinitis pigmentosa	Hydrocephalus
Retinal dystrophy	Non-accidental injury

(Modified from Philips et al 1987[4])

Table 12.3 Causes of severe childhood deafness

Etiology	Frequency (%)
Genetic	30
Acquired	40
Unknown	30

information must be precise and accurate and is achieved via one of the two mechanisms of cell division, either mitosis which is the division of somatic cells resulting in the growth of specific organs or the overall body, or meiosis which is the specialized cell division resulting in gamete formation, and may be referred to as 'reduction division' since it involves the reduction of the original *diploid* (2n) complement of 46 chromosomes to the *haploid* (n) complement of 23 chromosomes.

MITOSIS: CELL DIVISION

Somatic cell division is a cyclical procedure, the length of the total cycle varying from organism to organism and between cell types. Essentially the cycle can be divided into the *interphase* stage during which DNA synthesis and hence chromosome replication occurs, and the mitotic stage during which the actual division process takes place. During interphase the chromosomes are not condensed and are invisible other than as a mass of chromatin, but the mitotic phase is characterized by the gradual condensation of the chromatin through *prophase* into recognizable chromosomes, each comprising two sister chromatids held together at the centromere and aligned on the equatorial plate of the cell. This stage of the cell division is known as *metaphase* and is the stage at which the chromosomes are usually visualized. The centromere divides longitudinally and under the influence of the 'spindle apparatus' homologous daughter chromatids move to opposite cell poles (*anaphase*), where they are included in separate daughter nuclei (*telophase*). The products of mitotic division, therefore, are two daughter cells identical in all respects with the parent cell from which they have arisen.

MEIOSIS: PRODUCTION OF GAMETES

Meiosis comprises a single replication of the genetic material in interphase followed by two successive nuclear divisions.

As chromosomes begin to condense into the prolonged prophase characteristic of this type of division, homologous chromosomes pair closely with one another (*synapsis*) to form bivalents, and exchange segments of genetic material in a process known as *meiotic recombination* (Fig. 12.2). This recombination ensures the individuality of the offspring in much the same way as shuffling a pack of cards ensures that in each game the players will receive a different combination of cards. As condensation of chromatin continues the centromeres of the paired chromosomes repel one another, and eventually two daughter chromosomes of differing genetic constitution are formed from each bivalent (*metaphase I*). These daughter chromosomes each contain a mixture of genetic material from both parents of the individual concerned and they segregate at random (but in equal numbers) into the daughter nuclei formed at this stage in the cycle (*anaphase I*), thus completing the first stage of the process. The second stage is a straightforward mitotic division in which the centromeres of the daughter chromosomes divide and homologous centromeres with their attached chromatids travel to opposite cell poles.

The outcome of this two-stage division process is a quartet of nuclei, each with half (n) the original number (2n) of chromosomes, and with new combinations of parental genes.

Table 12.4 Racial and geographic differences in the frequency of genetic disease

Disease	Racial/geographic group	Birth incidence
Sickle cell disease	African	1 in 50
Thalassemia	Mediterranean	1 in 100
Oculocutaneous albinism	Hopi Indians	1 in 250
	N. Europeans	1 in 40 000
Congenital adrenal hyperplasia	Yupik Eskimos	1 in 500
	N. Europeans	1 in 10 000
Cystic fibrosis	N. Europeans	1 in 2000
	Orientals	Very rare
Tay-Sachs disease	Ashkenazi Jews	1 in 3600
Neural tube defects	N. Ireland	1 in 300
Ellis-van Creveld syndrome	Amish	1 in 200
	N. European	1 in 60000

Spermatogenesis and oogenesis

The basic pattern of chromosome behavior is the same during meiosis in both male and female gametogenesis, but there are differences in timing of the various stages. Spermatogenesis begins around puberty, and continues throughout life, with spermatozoa produced by continuing meiotic division of primary spermatocytes. On the other hand, oogenesis commences in intrauterine life but is arrested at a very early stage in meiosis I, with completion of the cycle only when ovulation occurs, anything up to 50 years later.

Spermatogenesis and oogenesis also differ in that, while the former gives rise ultimately to four functional sperm, the latter normally yields only a single functional ovum, with the other three products of the division process forming 'polar bodies', each with its

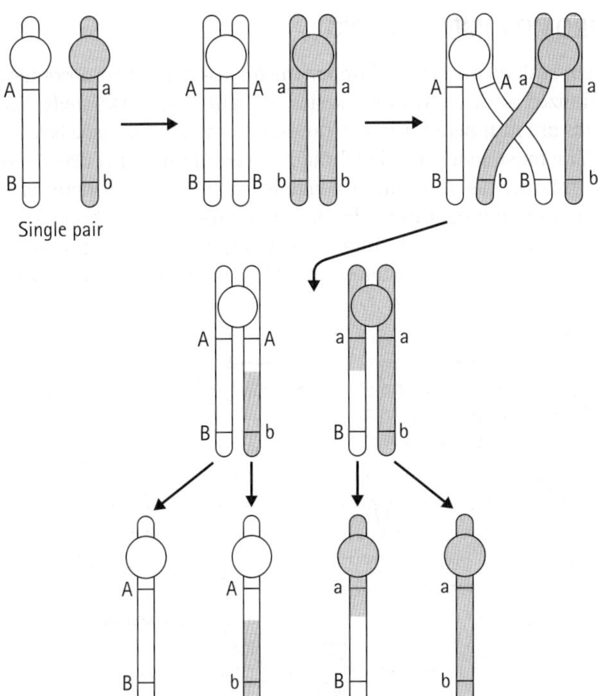

Fig. 12.2 'Crossing over' – the exchange of genetic material between homologous chromosomes.

haploid chromosome constitution, but with only a relatively small amount of cytoplasm. The polar bodies are non-functional and do not contribute to the future offspring.

CHROMOSOMES

PREPARATION OF BLOOD CHROMOSOMES

The original demonstration that there are 46 chromosomes in the human cell was made using fibroblast cultures from fetal lung.[6] In routine clinical practice, however, it is human lymphocytes that are used for the standard chromosome analysis since a blood sample is convenient to obtain and relatively easy to prepare.

The standard preparation of chromosomes from a blood sample is illustrated in Figure 12.3. The first stage of the process (i) is to separate the white cells from the rest of the blood sample. This is done by centrifugation using a medium such as Ficoll, which leaves the lymphocytes in a buffy coat at the top of the tube. The second stage (ii) is to cultivate the lymphocytes in vitro. The lymphocyte rarely divides in circulation but when a *mitogen* (a chemical which stimulates mitosis or cell division) such as phytohemagglutinin is added the lymphocytes undergo a cell division in about 48 to 72 h. The third stage (iii) is to arrest the cell division in metaphase when the chromosomes are at their most contracted and are best visualized. This is done by adding colchicine to the culture at 69–70 h. The fourth stage (iv) is to release the chromosomes from the nucleus and spread them on a microscope slide. This is carried out by placing the cultured cells in hypotonic saline and dropping the solution carefully onto a microscope slide from a sufficient height to give a reasonable spread of chromosomes. The fifth stage (v) is to fix and stain the spread for microscopic analysis (Fig. 12.4). Most of the analysis is carried out under the microscope, but a photograph of the spread may be taken and a mounted karyotype prepared as a permanent record or for further analysis. It is usual to analyze several cells in preparing a report.

CHROMOSOME BANDING

When stained and viewed under the microscope, chromosomes are visualized as a continuous series of light and dark *bands*. These bands are numbered using a standard nomenclature (see below).

The most widely used technique is G-banding. This uses Giemsa dye mixture as the staining agent, following treatment of the chromosome preparations by one of a variety of methods, among which are included incubation at various temperatures, denaturation of the chromosomal DNA or treatment with various proteolytic enzymes, e.g. trypsin (Fig. 12.4). Such techniques result in the production of a large number of dark- and pale-staining bands and allows the identification of individual chromosomes.

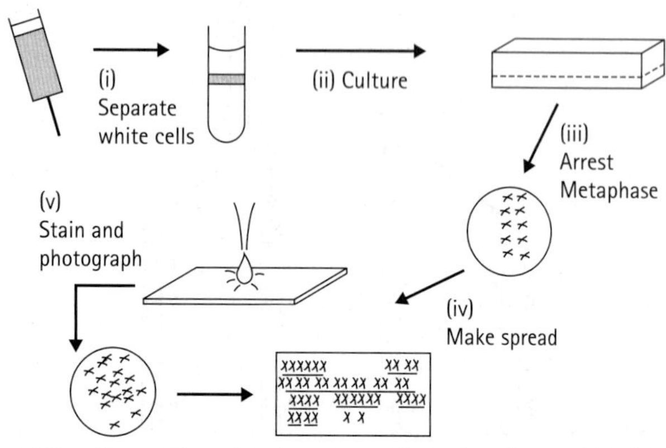

Fig. 12.3 Preparation of a chromosome karyotype from a blood sample.

BONE MARROW

Bone marrow contains many rapidly dividing cells and thus it is possible to locate cells that are already in metaphase. When the marrow preparation is appropriately spread it is possible to obtain a direct preparation in this way for analysis. However, short term culture is generally used. Marrow analysis is used in leukemias where chromosome abnormalities may be present in the marrow but not in the peripheral blood. It is of value both for diagnosis and prognosis.

FIBROBLASTS

Culture of connective tissue in vitro will result in the growth of fibroblasts, which may be used for chromosome culture. In the live patient the most common source of fibroblasts is in the skin. At postmortem connective tissue may be obtained from many different sources, but usually it is adequate to take a sample of skin under sterile conditions for culture.

Fibroblast cultures are obtained in about 2 weeks when they have formed a monolayer over the base of the culture flask. It is possible to disperse the monolayers into cell suspensions by adding trypsin and subculture again on several occasions. Such cultures may also be used for metabolic studies and may be stored long term at −70°C.

AMNIOCENTESIS

Fluid taken at amniocentesis between 12 and 16 weeks' gestation contains skin cells shed from the fetus and amniotic membranes. These cells are not very numerous in the sample but may be cultured up in a similar way to fibroblasts. It takes 2–3 weeks to culture and analyze the cells.

CHORIONIC VILLUS SAMPLES

Another approach to prenatal diagnosis is to obtain a sample of chorionic villi from the membranes surrounding the fetus at 9–11 weeks' gestation. This material is fetal in origin, but has to be separated from maternal tissue under the dissecting microscope before analysis. Chorionic villi are rapidly dividing and it is possible to obtain direct preparations without culture. However, because of the possibility of maternal contamination and mosaicism most diagnostic laboratories prefer to wait until culture is also available at 1–2 weeks before giving a definitive result.

FLUORESCENT IN SITU HYBRIDIZATION (FISH)

There has been a considerable gap between cytogenetic analysis at the microscopic level and molecular genetics at the gene level, but it is now possible to combine a gene specific probe with a fluorescent dye and to demonstrate the location of that gene on the chromosome spread.

The FISH technique has wide applications. It has been very valuable in looking for small chromosome deletions such as in Williams syndrome and DiGeorge syndrome (Fig 12.5) and has greatly extended the ability to make such diagnoses. It has also been used with chromosome specific probes on the uncultured cells to get

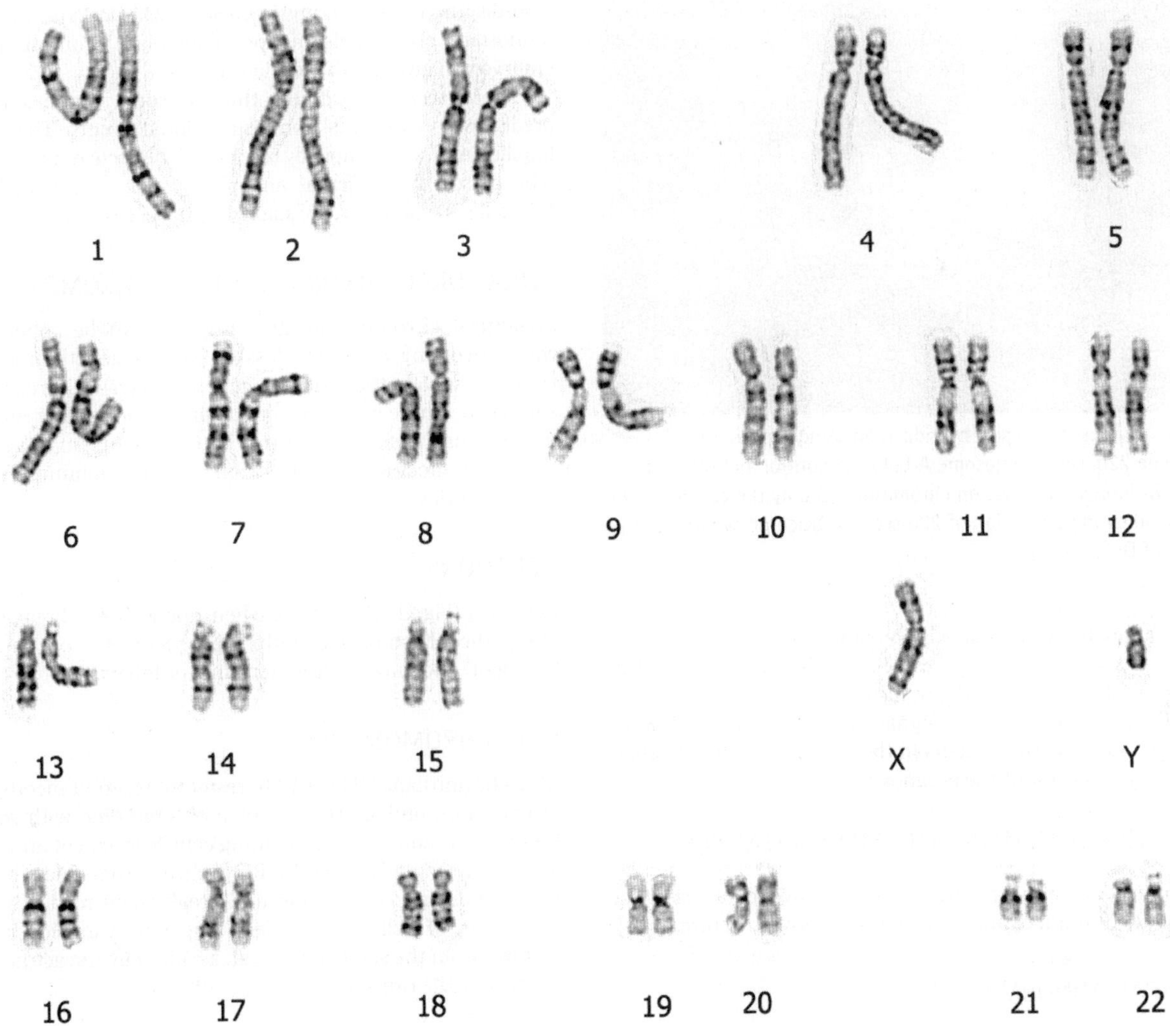

Fig. 12.4 Standard chromosome karyotype.

rapid chromosome diagnosis, e.g. in prenatal diagnosis or for a rapid diagnosis of chromosome abnormalities in the neonatal unit. Another role has been to develop 'chromosome paints' with fluorescent gene probes specific to individual chromosomes. Initially this technique was limited by the relatively small number of fluorescent dyes but by using the spectral division of color and computer enhancement it is now possible to assign a separate color to each chromosome and make the analysis of complex chromosomal translocations easier.

One area of the chromosome that is relatively difficult to visualize is the end or telomere and as a consequence chromosome deletions at the telomeres may be missed on conventional analysis. Knight & Flint [7] developed a range of telomeric gene probes that have in clinical practice allowed the identification of chromosome abnormalities in another 7% of children with mental retardation and apparently normal chromosomes on routine analysis.

FISH techniques also have an important role in gene mapping and the identification of chromosome imbalance in malignancy.

INDICATIONS FOR CHROMOSOME STUDIES

Chromosome analysis can be a most valuable diagnostic test, allowing precise clinical diagnosis and offering the opportunity for prevention of serious handicap by prenatal diagnosis. However, as cytogenetic investigations require highly skilled scientific staff and are very time consuming, the clinician will have to exercise some discretion in requesting these investigations. It will often be helpful to discuss the need for genetic testing with the clinical geneticist or laboratory concerned.

The indications for chromosome studies in pediatric practice include:

1. Mental retardation especially if there is a family history of mental retardation or when associated with physical abnormalities. It should be borne in mind that there are specific tests now for some forms of mental handicap, e.g. fragile X, Prader–Willi syndrome, Williams syndrome, and these will need to be requested separately with appropriate samples.
2. Multiple congenital abnormalities. It should be remembered that even if the diagnosis of Down syndrome is obvious clinically, it is still important to determine whether it is a standard trisomy 21 or not.
3. Intersex conditions manifesting as the presence of ambiguous genitalia in the newborn, inguinal herniae in a girl or the failure of development of secondary sexual characteristics at adolescence. Cryptorchidism or minor degrees of hypospadias alone are unlikely to be manifestations of a chromosome abnormality.
4. Congenital lymphedema may be a manifestation of Turner's syndrome and Noonan's syndrome, and part of the investigation should include chromosome analysis.

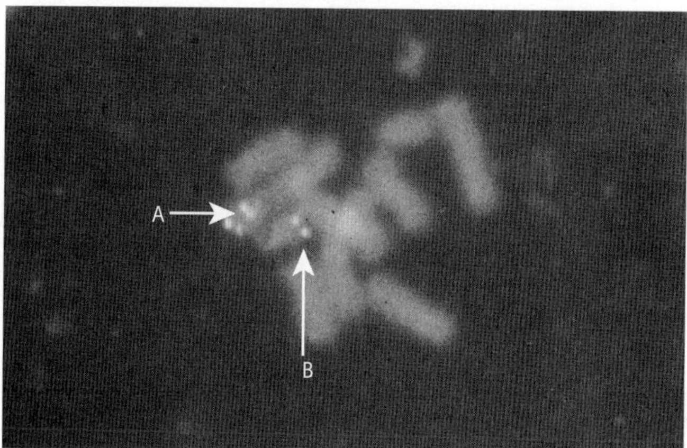

Fig. 12.5 Fluorescent in situ hybridization using probes for chromosome 22q. On chromosome A both the control and the 22q probe show fluorescence, but on chromosome B only the control probe shows up indicating a deletion of 22q seen in DiGeorge syndrome. (Courtesy of Dr J. Taylor)

5. Gross failure to thrive, which is prenatal in origin may be due to a chromosome abnormality especially when accompanied by minor physical abnormalities or mental handicap.
6. Childhood leukemias and malignancies will often reveal major chromosomal rearrangements in the cancerous cells and these may be an indicator of the prognosis.

TYPES OF CHROMOSOME ABNORMALITY

The chromosome abnormalities fall into two categories: (a) abnormalities of number and (b) abnormalities of structure.

NUMERICAL ABNORMALITIES

Numerical abnormalities may be euploid or aneuploid and arise from errors in cell division.

Euploidy describes chromosome constitutions which are multiples of the haploid (n) number (23 in man), thus diploid, 2n = 46, triploid, 3n = 69, or tetraploid, 4n = 92. Multiples greater than 2n are designated by the general term *polyploid. Aneuploidy* refers to those karyotypes in which the chromosome complement is not an exact multiple of the haploid number and includes both the trisomic and monosomic states.

Polyploids (other than triploids) usually result from the occurrence of nuclear division without simultaneous cell division, so that the chromosome complement of a single cell is doubled. Triploidy usually arises from the fertilization of a single ovum by two spermatozoa (*dispermy*).

Mixoploidy is divided into *mosaicism* where there are two or more genetically different cell lines in an individual derived from a single zygote and *chimerism* where an individual has arisen from the fusion of two zygotes or exchange of cells between two zygotes. Chimerism is extremely rare and not usually of clinical significance whereas mosaicism is relatively frequent and may be a cause of diagnostic difficulty.

Non-disjunction is the term used to describe the failure of homologous chromosomes or sister chromatids to separate and migrate to opposite poles of the nucleus during cell division and is the major mechanism by which monosomic and trisomic states originate. The consequences of non-disjunction vary depending on whether the event occurs during meiosis, or mitosis. Non-disjunction occurring in meiosis will give rise to trisomy or monosomy, but non-disjunction taking place in mitosis in the early embryo will give rise to mosaicism.

There seems no doubt that in some families there is a predisposition towards non-disjunctional events. The number of families in which aneuploidy recurs and the occurrence of individuals who possess two different aneuploidy states, e.g. both Down and Klinefelter's syndromes, are suggestive evidence of this predisposition.

STRUCTURAL ABNORMALITIES IN CHROMOSOMES

Structural chromosome abnormalities can be subdivided into those involving a definite loss or gain of genetic material, and those in which the existing genetic material is rearranged in some way. These rearrangements arise from one or more breaks in the chromosomes. Figure 12.6 presents in diagrammatic form the mechanisms of origin of the common structural abnormalities.

DELETIONS

Deletions (Fig. 12.6a) result when one or more breakages occur along the chromosome with subsequent loss of the resulting fragment, and may be either terminal or interstitial.

RING CHROMOSOMES

Ring chromosomes (Fig. 12.6b) result from simultaneous breakage in both long and short arms of a chromosome with subsequent fusion of the ends of the remaining centric fragment and loss of the acentric terminal segments. Ring chromosomes are notoriously unstable during cell division and break down readily so that the proportion of cells with a clear ring may vary considerably in cultures from the same individual, as also may the actual form and number of the rings observed.

INVERSIONS

Inversions (Fig. 12.6c), as their name suggests, result from a reversal of the sequence of genes in a segment of chromosome lying between two points of breakage. Inversions may be either *paracentric* involving double breakage in only one arm of a chromosome without any alteration in arm ratio, or *pericentric* involving breakage on either side of the centromere. While paracentric inversions can be identified only by the use of banding techniques, pericentric inversions frequently result in an alteration in arm ratio such that the abnormality is easily identifiable in mitotic chromosomes even without banding.

The clinical significance of inversions is a subject for debate. If there is no loss of genetic material then the significance may be minimal, provided only that the rearrangement in sequence of the genes on the inverted segment does not, per se, result in abnormal expression of those genes. The vast majority of paracentric inversions are likely to be harmless; however, the risk of having an unbalanced rearrangement in offspring would be increased if there is a family history of recurrent miscarriage or congenital malformations. Small pericentric inversions, including the relatively common pericentric inversions of chromosomes 2 and 9, also seem to be associated with a relatively small risk of unbalanced chromosome arrangements in offspring, and in some cases might be regarded as normal variants. However, the effects of inversions can be unpredictable and the risks in the individual case should be assessed in the light of the family history and cumulative experience from the medical literature.

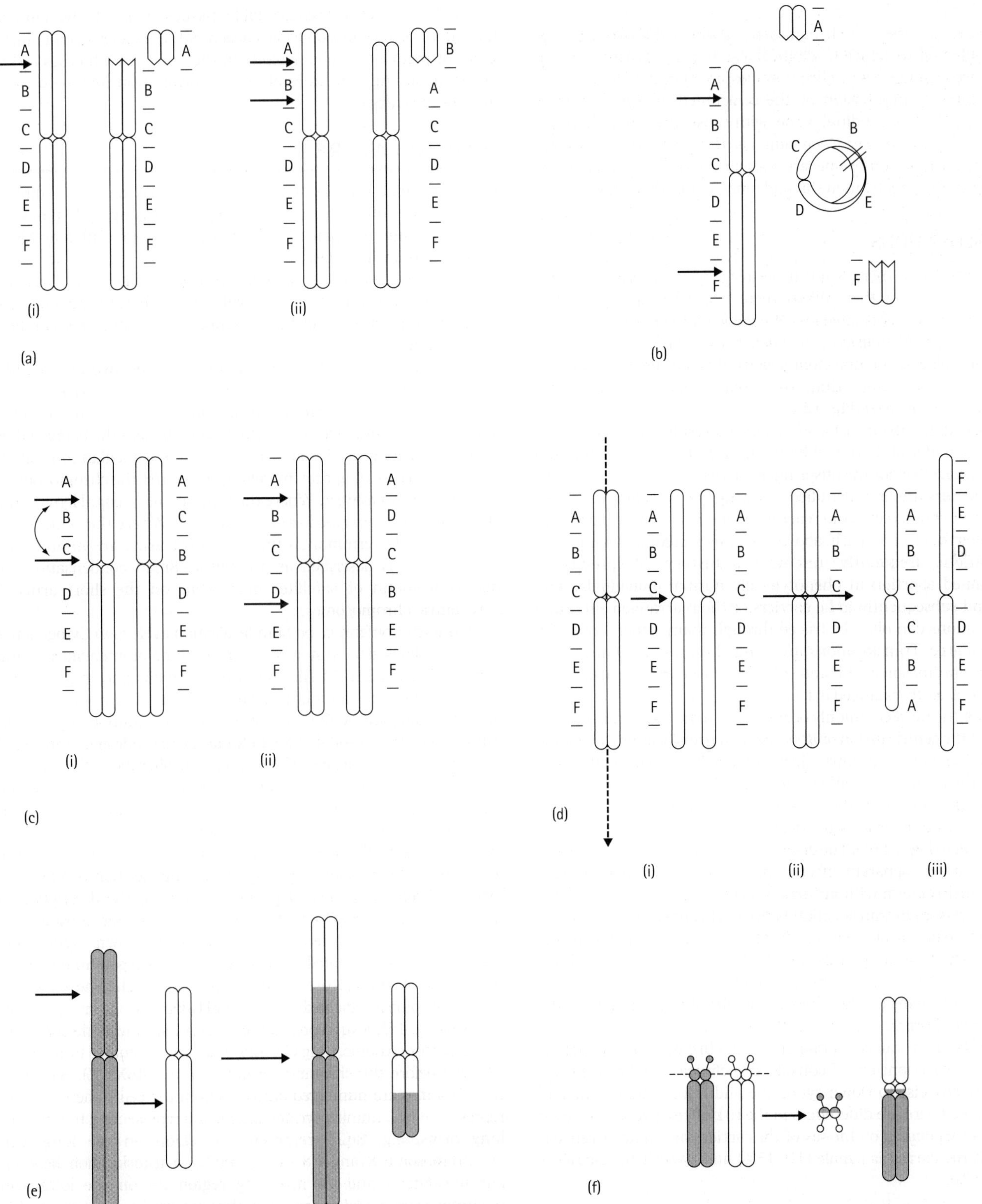

Fig. 12.6 Structural rearrangements in chromosomes. (a) Deletions may be (i) terminal or (ii) interstitial. (b) Ring chromosome. (c) Inversions may be (i) paracentric or (ii) pericentric. (d) Isochromosome formation: (i) normal mitosis with longitudinal division of the centromere; (ii) misdivision of the centromere in the transverse plane leading to the products (iii) of either isochromosome of the short arm. (e) Balanced reciprocal translocation. (f) Robersonian or centric fusion translocation.

ISOCHROMOSOMES

An isochromosome is a chromosome in which the two arms are genetically and structurally identical, e.g. two short arms from the same chromosome. Such chromosomes are thought to arise as a direct result of misdivision of the centromere in the transverse rather than the longitudinal plane, with subsequent reunion of the centric elements of sister chromatids (Fig. 12.6d). Individuals carrying an isochromosome are therefore effectively trisomic for one part of the genetic material and monosomic for another.

TRANSLOCATIONS

In a translocation there is a transfer of genetic material from one chromosome to another. When there is a mutual exchange of segments with no associated loss of genetic material this is termed a *balanced reciprocal translocation*. Such translocations may involve either homologous or non-homologous chromosomes and can be the result of no more than two breaks, one in each of the chromosomes involved (Fig. 12.6e).

Provided that the translocation does not result in the loss or gain of genetic material there will be no harm to the carrier, although the potential effect for the offspring of carriers may be considerable. Many carriers are first identified following the detection of one or other product of a reciprocal rearrangement in an abnormal infant, in a stillbirth, or in an early abortus. Family studies following such observations frequently uncover a history of previously unexplained abortion in phenotypically normal individuals, who are found subsequently to be carriers of the rearrangement. Such translocations can often be traced through many generations of a large pedigree. Translocations involving chromosome 9 and those between chromosomes 11 and 22 appear to carry a particularly high risk of an unbalanced defect.

One of the most commonly occurring structural rearrangements in man is the centric fusion or Robertsonian translocation, involving, by definition, only acrocentric chromosomes. The break points occur close to the centromere, either one in the short arm and one in the long arm, in which case the metacentric chromosome formed has a single centromere, or in both short arms with a resultant dicentric chromosome (Fig. 12.6f). The deleted short arm material is generally lost without any apparent effect on phenotype, presumably because it is heterochromatin without structural genes.

A Robertsonian translocation between chromosomes 13 and 14 is thought to be one of the most common structural rearrangements in man, with a frequency of 0.05–0.08% in the newborn population. This rearrangement usually functions more or less normally during meiosis but there is a small risk of trisomy 13 in the offspring of carriers.

Robertsonian translocations involving chromosome 21 such as 14,21 translocations are of considerable clinical significance since they may give rise to Down syndrome and have a high chance of recurrence. There are differences in the risk of recurrence of Down syndrome depending on the sex of the carrier parent. Recurrence is higher if the carrier is female (10–15%) and lower if the carrier is male (<5%).

MOSAICISM

Significant levels of mosaicism are reasonably easy to demonstrate. The examination of 30 metaphases will be sufficient to demonstrate mosaicism at the 10–15% level, but many more metaphases would be needed to exclude lower levels of mosaicism. It may be difficult to exclude mosaicism as a diagnosis, and failure to demonstrate mosaicism in blood need not necessarily exclude the diagnosis as a possibility in other less available tissues. One of the clinical indicators of chromosome mosaicism is the appearance of linear areas of pigmentary abnormality in the skin. In such cases a skin biopsy including both normal and abnormal skin may be used to look for mosaicism.

NOMENCLATURE

In the normal human somatic cell nucleus there is a diploid complement of 46 chromosomes comprising 22 pairs of autosomes, and one pair of *sex chromosomes*, represented as XX in females and XY in males.

Chromosomes can be arranged in pairs on the basis of certain morphological features. Such morphological features include size, centromere position, and the presence of satellites or secondary constrictions.

The *centromere* is the point of union of the two chromatids. The position of the centromere in relation to the *telomeres* (or chromosome ends) determines the actual shape of the chromosome and divides it into two *arms* which vary in length, being either short (p), or long (q). Where the centromere is median in position and the arms are of approximately equal length, the chromosome is described as *metacentric*. Where the arms are of unequal length, the chromosome is described as *submetacentric*. Where the centromere is more nearly terminal so that the short arms are minute, the chromosome is described as *acrocentric*. Small condensations of heterochromatin or satellites may occur on the short arms of acrocentric chromosomes.

The Paris Conference on Standardization in Human Cytogenetics in 1971 devised a system of chromosome nomenclature and symbols (Table 12.5).[8,9] The conventions which apply in use of this nomenclature are as follows. The number of chromosomes is given first followed by the sex chromosome constitution, e.g. 45X in Turner's syndrome and 47XXY in Klinefelter's syndrome. Autosomal aneuploidies are indicated by a numerical alteration, the extra or deficient chromosome being designated by a + or – before the chromosome involved, e.g. 47XX,+21, a female with Down syndrome, or 45XX,–21, a female missing a 21 chromosome. When placed after a symbol a + or – means an increase or decrease in the length of a chromosome, e.g. 18p– represents deletion of the short arm of chromosome 18. Diagonals are used in the description of mosaicism, e.g. 45XO/46XX represents a Turner mosaic and 46XX/47XX,+21 a female with mosaic Down syndrome. Translocation is designated by the letter t followed in parentheses by an indication of the nature of the translocated chromosome. An isochromosome is indicated by the letter i before the chromosome arm involved, e.g. 45X,i(Xq) represents an isochromosome for the long arm of one X chromosome. Ring chromosomes are designated by the letter r placed before the chromosome involved, e.g. 46X,r(X). Bands on chromosomes are numbered outwards from the centromere and are represented by a number written after p or q representing the short or long arms, e.g. 8q24 represents a region on the long arm of chromosome 8 and t(8;14) (q24;q32) a translocation between chromosome 8 and 14 involving region 24 on the long arm of chromosome 8 and region 32 on the long arm of chromosome 14.

CHROMOSOMAL SYNDROMES

DOWN SYNDROME

Incidence

Since the original description of the condition by Langdon Down in 1866, this disorder has been recognized to be the commonest single

Table 12.5 Table of nomenclature symbols[8,9]

1–22	The autosome numbers
X, Y	The sex chromosomes
Diagonal (/)	Separates cell lines in describing mosaicism
Plus sign (+) or minus sign (–)	When placed immediately before the autosome number or group letter designation indicates that the particular chromosome is extra or missing; when placed immediately after a symbol it means an increase or decrease in length of the chromosome
Asterisk (*)	Designates a chromosome or chromosome structure explained in text or footnote
cen	Centromere
dic	Dicentric (presence of two centromeres)
h	Secondary constriction or negatively staining region
i	Isochromosome
inv	Inversion
inv (p+q) or inv (p–q+)	Pericentric inversion
mar	Marker chromosome
mat	Maternal origin
p	Short arm of chromosome
pat	Paternal origin
q	Long arm of chromosome
r	Ring chromosome
s	Satellite
t	Translocation
del	Deletion
der	Derivative chromosome
dup	Duplication
ins	Insertion
inv ins	Inverted insertion
rep	Reciprocal translocation
rec	Recombinant chromosome
rob	Robertsonian translocation ('centric fusion')
ter	Terminal or end (pter = end of short arm; qter = end of long arm)
:	Break (no reunion, as in a terminal deletion)
: :	Break and join
-	From–to

All symbols for rearrangements are placed before the designation of the chromosome or chromosomes involved and the rearranged chromosome or chromosomes should always be placed in parentheses.

cause of mental handicap occurring in approximately 1 in 700 of all live births in all populations. However, the incidence varies with the age of the mother: the incidence for mothers aged 25 years is 1 in 1400 and increases to reach an incidence of 1 in 46 for mothers aged 45 years (see Fig. 12.7).

Clinical features

In most instances Down syndrome is recognizable at birth by the craniofacial features (Fig. 12.8). The head circumference is small with a brachycephalic skull. The neck is short and thick. The palpebral fissures slope upwards (i.e. the outer canthus is higher than the inner canthus) and there may be marked epicanthic folds. Brushfield's spots (whitish spots scattered round the periphery of the iris) are found more frequently in Down syndrome than in the general population. There is an increased incidence of lens opacities. The ears are small with an overfolding helix. The nasal bridge is flat. The tongue appears large and may protrude because the mouth is relatively small. Eruption of the teeth is frequently delayed with abnormalities in dental positioning. The hair may be fine and sparse.

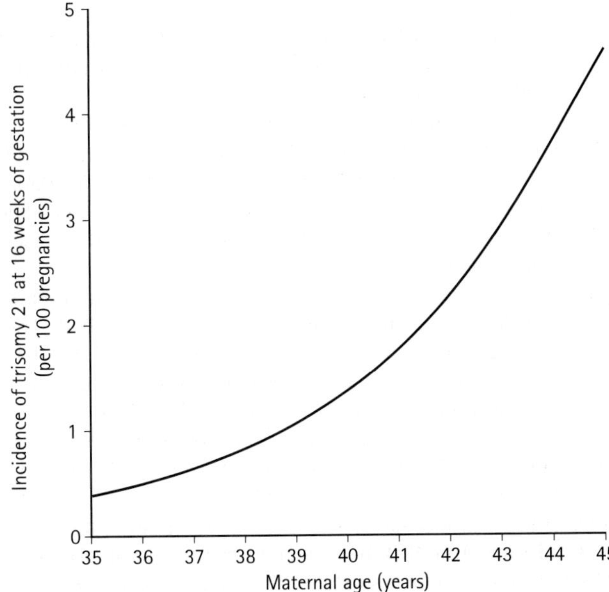

Fig. 12.7 The frequency of Down syndrome increases with maternal age.

The hands are short and broad. The fifth finger is short and incurved (clinodactyly). Radiologically this feature is accompanied by shortening of the shaft of the middle phalanx. A single transverse palmar crease (or simian crease) is seen in both hands in at least 50% of children with Down syndrome. A unilateral transverse palmar crease may be demonstrated in 2–5% of chromosomally normal infants. A deep plantar crease ('sandal gap')

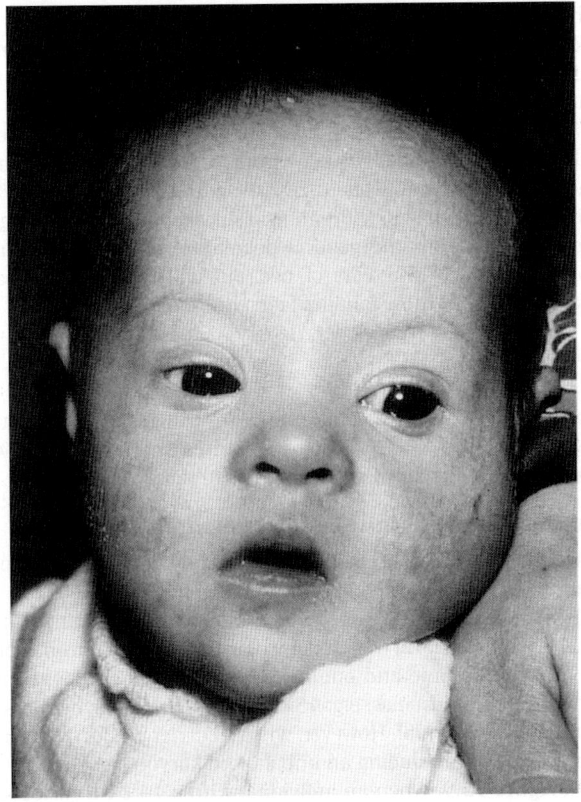

Fig. 12.8 Facial features of Down syndrome.

between the first and second toe may also be a helpful diagnostic sign. The other dermatoglyphic features noted in Down syndrome include an increase in ulnar loops, a single flexion crease on the fifth finger and a distal axial triradius.

Congenital heart disease occurs in between 40 and 60% of infants with Down syndrome. Atrioventricular canal and ventricular septal defects are the commonest types of cardiac lesion seen. Intestinal atresia, in particular duodenal atresia, is also considerably more common in Down syndrome. One-third of cases of congenital duodenal atresia occur in Down syndrome.

Initially a child with Down syndrome may be hypotonic, but the early developmental milestones are eventually reached. The ultimate IQ ranges from 20 to 75 with a mean around 50. The earlier assessment of development tends to be more favorable than the formal measurement of IQ in later childhood. Children with Down syndrome are often affectionate and good humored but like all stereotypes this tends to underestimate the range of personality and behavioral traits seen in a defined group.

Intellectual function shows a decline with age in adults with Down syndrome and this has been attributed to a presenile dementia. It is, therefore, particularly interesting to note the relationship between Down syndrome and Alzheimer's disease.[10] The neuropathology of both conditions is very similar with senile plaques and neurofibrillary tangles; however, while there is a generalized depletion of all neurotransmitters in Down syndrome, in Alzheimer's disease it is more specifically a depletion of the cholinergic neurotransmitters. Gene mapping studies have found mutations in the amyloid precursor protein gene on chromosome 21 in some early onset familial cases of Alzheimer's disease.

The development of secondary sexual characteristics is delayed in Down syndrome. Adult males with Down syndrome are infertile and in females there is delayed puberty but they will usually be fertile. The incidence of leukemia, but not other malignancies, is greater in Down children. A transient leukemoid reaction may occur in newborns with Down syndrome. In the first year of life acute non-lymphoblastic leukemia predominates, but in older children it is predominantly acute lymphoblastic leukemia. Overall the incidence is 10–18 times greater than that in the general childhood population.

A generation ago two-thirds of children with Down syndrome died in early childhood usually from the associated congenital abnormalities. Now only about 20% die in the first year and 45% of individuals with Down syndrome will survive to 60 years of age.[11] This is less than in the general population where 86% can be expected to live to 60 years of age, but will represent a greater burden of care for those families facing the diagnosis today.

Cytogenetics

Full trisomy 21

Approximately 95% of children with Down syndrome have 47XX,+21 or 47XY,+21. Trisomy 21 arises as a result of meiotic non-disjunction usually from the maternal side.

Translocation as a cause of Down syndrome

A number of different translocations may give rise to Down syndrome. They account for 2–3% of Down individuals.

The most frequent is a Robertsonian 14,21 translocation (Fig. 12.9). In this form the carrier would have one 14 chromosome, one 21 chromosome and one fused 14,21 chromosome giving a total of 45 chromosomes, e.g. 45XX, –14, –21 complement, and is phenotypically normal. However, when a carrier produces offspring there is a risk of producing an unbalanced karyotype.

In Figure 12.9, when an individual with a 14,21 translocation produces offspring with an individual with a normal karyotype then three viable chromosome arrangements may be produced: (i) a normal karyotype, (ii) a balanced translocation and (iii) an unbalanced translocation giving 46 chromosomes with trisomy 21. Other arrangements can be produced, but these will be non-viable or lead to early miscarriage, e.g. monosomy 21, monosomy 14 or trisomy 14. While in theory it may appear that one-third of pregnancies would produce an unbalanced translocation with trisomy 21, this does not take into account the selective disadvantage that acts on gametogenesis, fertilization or the early zygote. From analysis of pooled family data the likelihood of a female carrier producing an unbalanced trisomic child is 15%, and the likelihood of a male carrier producing an unbalanced trisomic child is 2.5%. The different risks may be explained by selective disadvantage in the sperm carrying the extra 21 chromosome.

A 21,22 Robertsonian translocation may also give rise to Down syndrome in a similar way. Very rarely a 21,21 translocation may arise. Carriers of this 21,21 translocation can only produce zygotes that are either monosomic or trisomic for chromosome 21, and since monosomy 21 would almost always be lethal their risk of producing a child with trisomy 21 is virtually 100%.

Mosaic trisomy 21

In about 2.5% of individuals with Down syndrome there is a mosaic combination of cells with a normal karyotype and cells with trisomy 21. The phenotypic variation produced may range from apparently normal individuals to those with typical Down syndrome. Occasionally unsuspected low grade maternal mosaicism (at the level of 2–3% trisomic cells) may be uncovered when more than one child with trisomy 21 is born into a family.

Genetic counseling and screening

It is essential to determine the chromosome karyotype in the affected child prior to genetic counseling, since the recurrence risks are different for standard trisomy 21 and translocation trisomy 21.

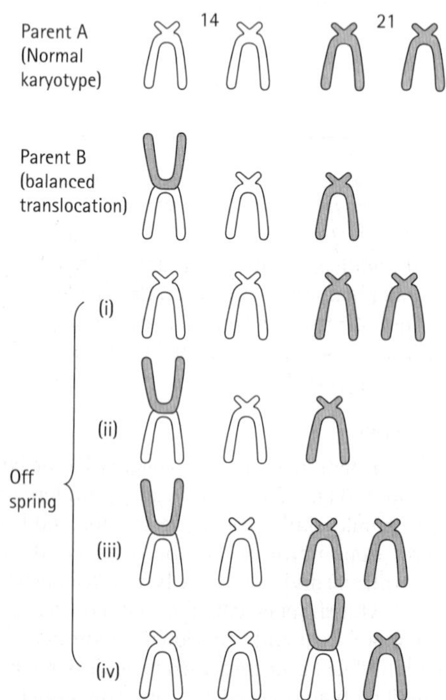

Fig. 12.9 Segregation of a 14,21 translocation. Four combinations may be produced: (i) normal karyotype; (ii) balanced translocation; (iii) unbalanced trisomy 21; (iv) unbalanced trisomy 14 (lethal).

In the case of a child with a standard trisomy 21 the chance of recurrence in further children is 1% in mothers under 35 years and twice the maternal age risk in mothers over 35 years. Since the trisomy has not arisen as a result of a translocation and a chromosome test will be offered in further pregnancies, it is not necessary to examine the parents' chromosome karyotype.

When Down syndrome has arisen as a result of an unbalanced translocation, it is necessary to check both parents' chromosomes and if one is found to be a carrier, then further family studies are necessary to determine if other members of the family are also carriers. The recurrence risks for carriers of a 14,21 translocation carrier are given above. In some instances neither parent is found to be a translocation carrier and the unbalanced translocation has arisen de novo. In such situations the chance of recurrence in further pregnancies is equivalent to the population risk.

Since Down syndrome is a major cause of mental handicap, pregnancy screening and chromosome analysis have been incorporated into various public health programs. Since the incidence of Down syndrome increases with increasing maternal age, amniocentesis has been offered to mothers aged 35 and above. This approach, if fully taken up by all mothers, would diagnose 30% of all pregnancies with Down syndrome, and the remaining 70% would occur in younger mothers. It should be remembered that the vast majority of pregnancies occur in mothers under 35 years, and to offer amniocentesis to all mothers irrespective of age would be unacceptable because of the small but significant risk of miscarriage.

Another approach to screening in pregnancy is to look at the level of alpha-fetoprotein in maternal serum (MSAFP) from blood samples taken around 12 weeks' gestation. Higher levels of MSAFP are associated with an increased risk of neural tube defects. This work has been expanded to look not simply at one parameter in maternal serum but three. It has been shown that by combining the levels of MSAFP, estriol and human chorionic gonadotrophin with maternal age, it is possible to predict those pregnancies at greater risk of having trisomy 21 in all ages and to diagnose 60% of pregnancies with Down syndrome without increasing the amniocentesis rate.

Increasingly ultrasound scanning in the first trimester is being used to screen for Down syndrome. If there is an increased amount of thickening over the back of the neck this is referred to as increased nuchal translucency. Increased nuchal translucency can be measured and the greater risk of chromosome abnormalities can be calculated. If there is an increased risk then a definitive test using chorionic villus sampling can be carried out. This approach will diagnose up to 80% of Down syndrome in the early stages of pregnancy.

TRISOMY 18 (EDWARDS' SYNDROME)

This was first described by Edwards.[12] Although much rarer than Down syndrome, it is the second commonest autosomal trisomy with an incidence between 1 in 3500 and 1 in 7000. It is also associated with increased maternal age. Of the affected infants some 80–90% die within the first week usually from cardiopulmonary failure. A few cases have been reported surviving into the teens, but they have all been profoundly retarded.[13]

There is often polyhydramnios and intrauterine growth retardation. The cranium is long and narrow with a prominent occiput. The ears are low set and frequently underdeveloped. The facies characteristically shows micrognathia and narrow sloping palpebral fissures. The hands are clenched with the second and fifth fingers overlapping the third and fourth fingers (Fig. 12.10a). There may be other flexion deformities. The nails are hypoplastic. The feet show a 'rocker bottom' appearance like the shape of the runners of a rocking chair (Fig. 12.10b).

A variety of congenital malformations are present. Anomalies of the gastrointestinal tract are particularly common, e.g. intestinal atresias, malabsorption and exomphalos. Around one-third of cases of exomphalos detected prenatally on ultrasound have trisomy 18. Renal abnormalities are also frequent with renal hypoplasia or cystic dysplasia being one of the commoner and more serious abnormalities. Congenital heart defects, ocular abnormalities and neural tube defects can also occur.

In the past a number of conditions which clinically appeared similar to trisomy 18 but showed normal karyotypes were described as pseudotrisomy 18. Some of these cases were probably Pena–Shokier syndrome[14] which is autosomal recessive. It presents with a combination of microcephaly, joint contractures, pulmonary hypoplasia and cataracts, and should be considered in the differential diagnosis when the karyotype is normal.

The vast majority of cases arise as a result of primary non-disjunction and have a regular trisomy 18. Like trisomy 21, it is

(a)

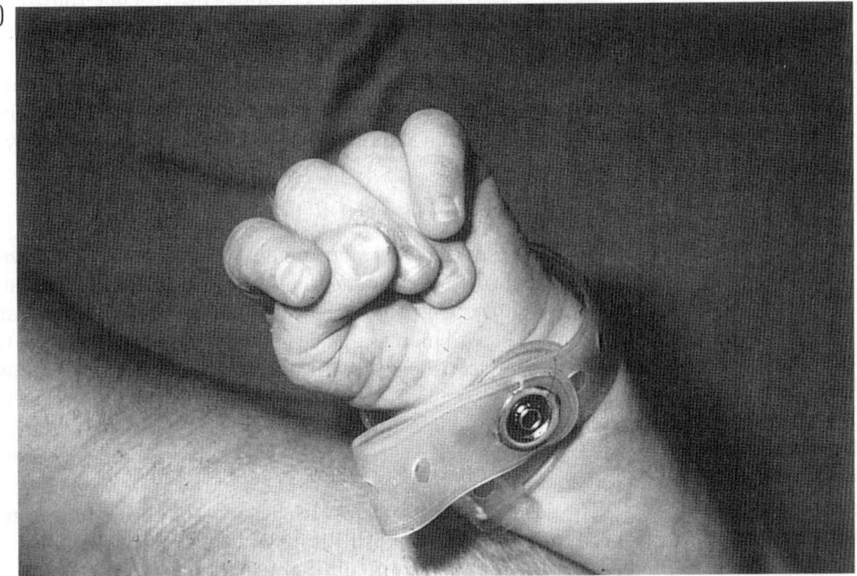

(b)

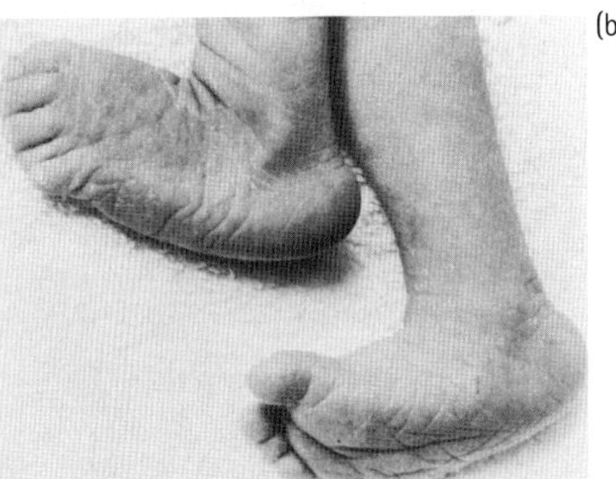

Fig. 12.10 The typical appearance of the hands (a) and feet (b) in trisomy 18 (Edwards' syndrome).

associated with increased maternal age and thus may be diagnosed on screening prenatally. After the birth of one affected child, the chance of recurrence is 1% in younger mothers.

A partial trisomy 18 may arise in the offspring of carriers of reciprocal translocations involving chromosome 18. Available data suggest it is the proximal region of the long arm (pter to q21) that primarily determines the phenotypic features of Edwards' syndrome.

TRISOMY 13 (PATAU'S SYNDROME)

This syndrome has an incidence around 1 in 6000.[15] The majority of affected children have multiple malformations and die shortly after birth. The few cases reported with longer survival have all been severely retarded. There is some maternal age effect, but probably not as significant as that seen in trisomy 21 or trisomy 18.

The affected children show intrauterine growth retardation. There may be marked microcephaly. Structural malformations of the brain are common and this may alter facial development. Instead of two cerebral hemispheres with lateral ventricles, a single forebrain with a single ventricle may form. This malformation sequence is known as holoprosencephaly (Fig. 12.11). The process alters the development and separation of optic vesicles from the forebrain and the migration of the median process from the forehead to form the nose. In its most extreme form the optic vesicles may fuse to give cyclopia. More usually (Fig. 12.12) there is marked hypotelorism with a small nose and cleft lip and palate. Ocular abnormalities such as microphthalmos are common, often reflecting the underlying cerebral abnormality.

In the hands, postaxial polydactyly is frequent. Flexion contractures and 'rocker bottom' feet may also be present. Scalp defects may be helpful diagnostically as they rarely appear in other abnormalities. Internally, in addition to cerebral malformations, renal and cardiac abnormalities are also frequent.

The majority of cases of trisomy 13 arise as a result of primary non-disjunction.

It may occasionally arise from an unbalanced chromosome translocation t(13q,14q). In the vast majority of cases carriers of a t(13q,14q) do not produce unbalanced progeny. In 230 pregnancies to carriers of a t(13q,14q) studied in a European collaborative study there were no cases of unbalanced progeny, but in practice it is appropriate to counsel such carriers with a small recurrence risk and offer amniocentesis.

Normal development

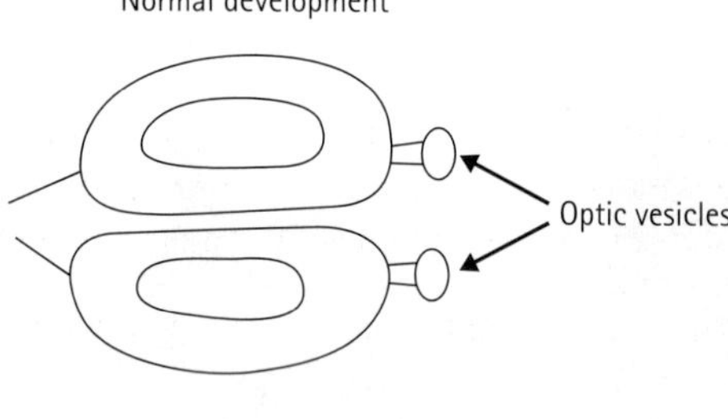

Holoprosencephaly

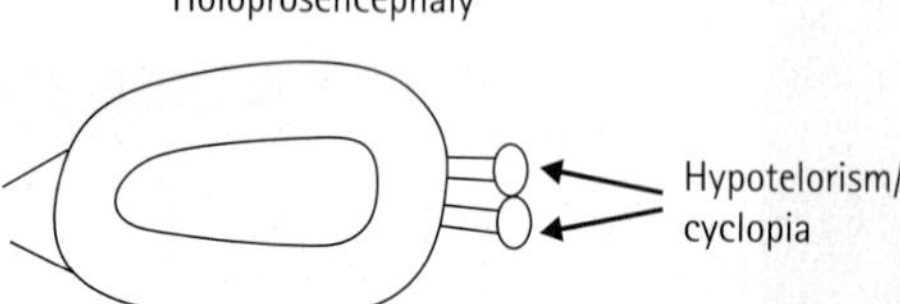

Fig. 12.11 Holoprosencephaly sequence. The forebrain divides into two hemispheres and the optic vesicles develop from these to form the eyes. In holoprosencephaly the forebrain divides incompletely and the optic vesicles develop in close proximity, leading to hypotelorism or cyclopia.

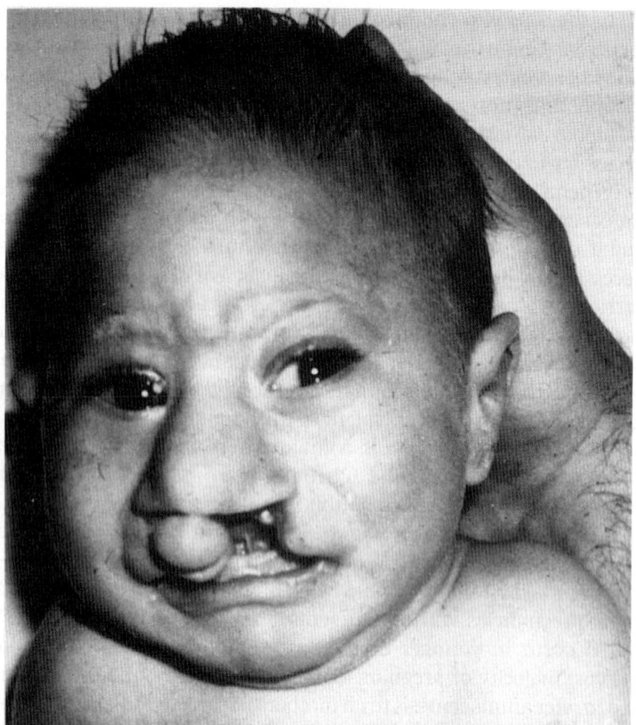

Fig. 12.12 Facial features of trisomy 13 (Patau's syndrome).

4p⁻ (WOLF–HIRSCHHORN) SYNDROME

This syndrome gives a clearly recognizable phenotype. The features include microcephaly, hypertelorism, low set simple ears, coloboma (25%), cleft palate (30%), renal abnormalities, heart defects (50%) and intrauterine growth retardation. The facial features (Fig. 12.13) are described as resembling a Greek helmet since the flat nasal bridge appears to run in continuity from the glabella in much the same way that the protective nose piece is incorporated into a Greek helmet.

Death usually occurs in early childhood (at least one-third die in the first year of life) and survivors invariably show profound mental retardation with seizures. As 10% arise from balanced translocations it is important to examine the parents' chromosomes. The deletion required to produce this syndrome may be very small and may require specific cytogenetic tests to identify it.

5p⁻ (CRI DU CHAT) SYNDROME

This was one of the first autosomal deletions to be recognized. The syndrome derives its name from the striking cat-like cry that is heard in infancy. This cry is related to the hypoplastic larynx and tends to lessen with increasing age and growth of the larynx. In the newborn the face is round with microcephaly, micrognathia and down-slanting palpebral fissures. With further growth the microcephaly remains but the face becomes long and narrow. Survival into adult life with severe mental retardation has frequently been described.

The deletion may involve a variable amount of the short arm of chromosome 5 but band 5p15 is invariably involved.[16] About 15% of cases arise from a balanced reciprocal translocation.

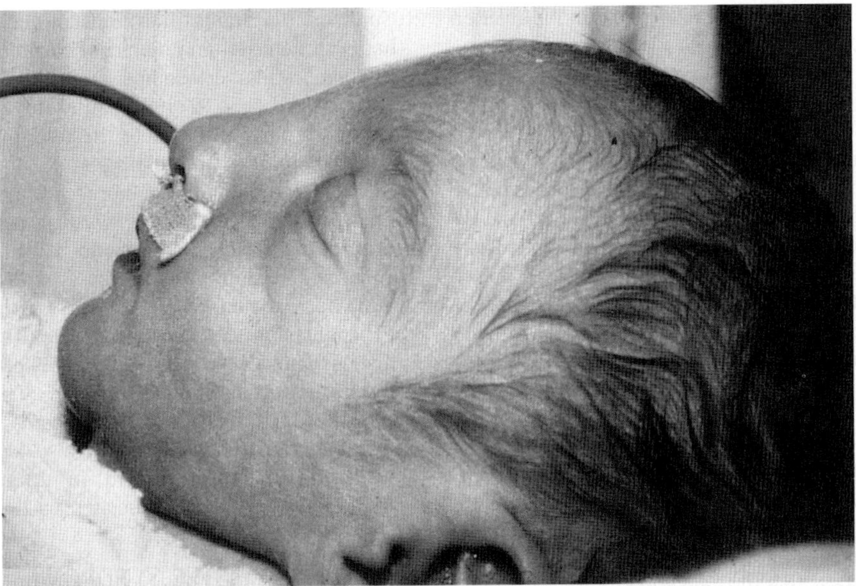

Fig. 12.13 Facial features of $4p^-$ (Wolf–Hirschhorn) syndrome.

$18q^-$ SYNDROME

The cardinal features of this syndrome are intrauterine growth retardation, profound mental retardation and a 'carp-shaped mouth'. Cleft palate, heart defects and ocular defects are also common. Genital hypoplasia may occur. Serum immunoglobulin A (IgA) is decreased in about half the affected individuals.

Survival to adult life has been reported although with severe mental handicap. The majority of cases arise de novo.

DELETIONS OF 13q

Deletions of 13q14 (Fig. 12.14) are associated with retinoblastoma. The dysmorphic features associated with this deletion are variable. Further genetic analysis of the interstitial 13q14 deletions has led to a recognition that this chromosomal region contains an anti-oncogene responsible for inhibiting the proliferation of embryonic retinal cells.[17] In the presence of a homozygous deletion or a deletion in one allele with a mutation in the other allele, retinal cells continue to proliferate in a malignant fashion producing a retinoblastoma. Inherited forms of retinoblastoma are usually bilateral whereas isolated cases of retinoblastoma are usually unilateral and are the result of a somatic mutation in the retinoblastoma gene that has arisen in one eye.

Terminal deletions of 13 may also produce eye abnormalities but not retinoblastoma. They also characteristically have hypoplastic thumbs and anal atresia. Most die in the neonatal period.

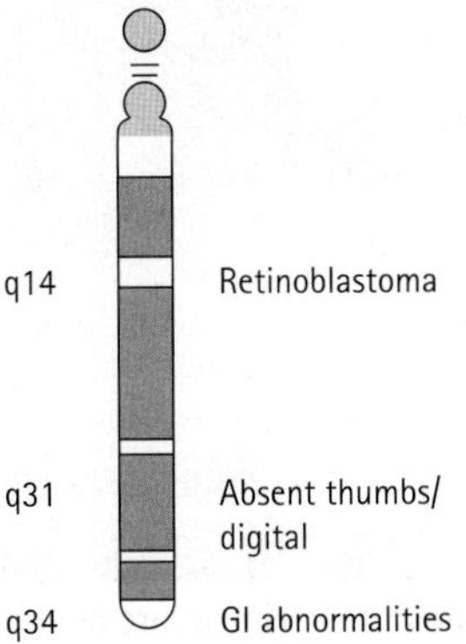

Fig. 12.14 Deletions of the long arm of chromosome 13.

DiGEORGE SYNDROME (22q11 DELETION)

Prior to the discovery of the underlying chromosome defect this disorder was described with different emphasis and with different names, e.g. velocardiofacial syndrome, Sphrintzen syndrome or CATCH 22. With the advent of fluorescent gene probes this has become one of the commonest chromosomal microdeletion syndromes.

About 75% of patients with 22q11 deletion will have significant congenital heart defects.[18] The range of defects is wide but tetralogy of Fallot and abnormalities in the main arteries are most frequently seen. About 50% of patients will have defects of the palate. This is often velopharyngeal insufficiency rather than overt cleft palate. Hypocalcemia may also occur and is a cause for fits. Developmental delay tends to be mild and a significant number of affected children have normal development. In the original description of this syndrome there was severe immunodeficiency with T cell depletion[19] but this now appears to be relatively rare.

The main indication for requesting a 22q deletion test is the presence of congenital heart defect or facial clefting but it is appropriate to consider it with any feature of the syndrome. The facial features include a long bulbous nose and a small mouth but the facial features are relatively subtle. When a deletion is identified it is important to carry out testing in the parents as around 30% of cases are inherited.

By dissecting out the critical region of the deletion it has been possible to identify a T box developmental gene as the primary cause of heart defects in the syndrome.[20]

WILLIAMS SYNDROME

Williams syndrome was initially referred to as infantile hypercalcemia as the biochemical change was the usual presentation. It is now recognized to be a more generalized syndrome with 'elfin facies', short stature, supravalvular aortic stenosis, hyperacusis and developmental delay.[21] After autosomal dominant supravalvular aortic stenosis was recognized to be due to a defect in elastin, it was found that there is a deletion of elastin and contiguous genes in Williams syndrome. It is now easily diagnosed by a FISH probe for elastin on chromosome 7, but obviously the features such as learning difficulties and the characteristic behavior are due to the adjacent genes in the deletion rather than elastin alone.[22]

ANIRIDIA–WILMS

The relationship between bilateral aniridia and Wilms tumor is associated with deletions of chromosome 11p13. It is a good example of a contiguous gene deletion in which gene involved in eye development (Pax 6) is deleted together with an oncogene WT1. There is often developmental delay and growth retardation as well due to deletion of other genes in the area. This concept of a contiguous gene deletion syndrome will probably be found to be a cause of many other apparently unrelated features in malformation syndromes.

ANGELMAN SYNDROME AND PRADER–WILLI SYNDROME

Although these are very different clinical disorders it is important to consider these two syndromes together as they can both be due to deletions of chromosome 15 and illustrate an important biological principle known as genetic imprinting.

Prader–Willi syndrome usually presents with neonatal hypotonia with feeding difficulties and in males undescended testes.[23] As the affected child becomes older the muscle tone and feeding difficulties improve but the child develops a voracious appetite (hyperphagia) and becomes obese. Affected children will also have developmental delay and in later life may suffer from the complications of obesity. Angelman syndrome presents with severe developmental delay, inappropriate laughter and complex seizures. There may be a characteristic electroencephalogram (EEG) in early life[24] and later absence of speech and ataxia.

The commonest cause of these syndromes are deletions of 15q11–13 but it was found that Prader–Willi syndrome was due to paternal deletions and Angelman syndrome was due to maternal deletions. This phenomenon would not be predicted by Mendelian inheritance where the paternal origin of a mutation does not usually matter and is an example of genetic imprinting. It appears that both paternal and maternal chromosome 15s are required in early embryonic development and that paternal and maternal chromosome 15q12 have different functions. Thus genetic imprinting may be defined as the determination of gene expression depending on the parental origin.

The situation became more complex with analysis of other cases. In some cases there was no deletion but two copies of chromosome 15 from the same parent, which is referred to as uniparental disomy.[25] In the case of Prader–Willi syndrome this would have started with trisomy 15 in which there were two copies of the maternal 15 and one of paternal 15 and then if the paternal chromosome 15 is lost the child effectively has two maternal chromosome 15s and no paternal 15. The net effect is the same as a deletion of the paternal chromosome 15. The situation is now more complicated as there can also be mutations affecting the imprinting mechanism and in Angelman syndrome point mutations in the UBE3A gene at 15q12.

KILLIAN–PALLISTER SYNDROME

Most chromosomal disorders can be diagnosed on blood analysis. However this is not the case in the Killian–Pallister syndrome. It is unusual in that a mosaic cell line containing tetrasomy 12p is found in the skin fibroblasts but not in the blood. Although the mosaicism is relatively tissue specific the effects are generalized.[26] There is severe mental retardation with coarse facial features and a characteristic bitemporal loss of hair growth (Fig. 12.15).

OTHER AUTOSOMAL ABNORMALITIES

Many other aberrations involving the autosomes have been described. As a general rule they are associated with low birth weight, mental retardation and physical malformations. In many instances a specific phenotype cannot be delineated because gene

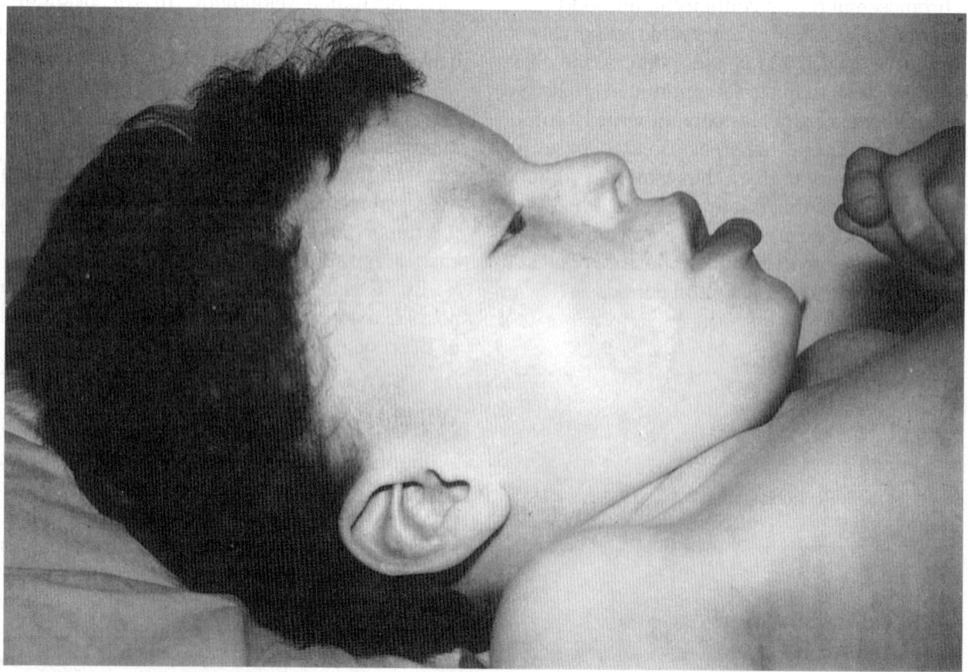

Fig. 12.15 The Killian–Pallister syndrome is caused by a mosaic isochromosome 12p, which is present in skin culture but not in blood culture. The syndrome has a characteristic coarse facies.

dosage will depend on the exact breakpoints and in the case of unbalanced translocations, which other chromosome is involved. It is recommended that the reader refers to a chromosomal atlas such as de Grouchy & Turleau,[27] Gardner & Sutherland[28] or Schnizel[29] for details of other autosomal abnormalities.

SEX CHROMOSOME ABNORMALITIES

TURNER'S SYNDROME

The syndrome was first described in 1938 and subsequently became the first disorder recognized to have a chromosomal basis. It is a frequent finding in first trimester abortions, but, as many 45X conceptuses are non-viable, the frequency at birth is 1 in 3000 live-born females.

Clinical features

At birth there is lymphedema (Fig. 12.16) especially in the dorsum of the hand and there may be redundant skin over the back of the neck. Hydrops and cystic hygroma are seen in utero and may occasionally be present in the neonate.

In childhood, Turner's syndrome may present with short stature. There is a short webbed neck with low posterior hairline. The chest is shield shaped with widely spaced nipples. The carrying angle at the elbow is increased (cubitus valgus). Pigmented nevi and a tendency to keloid scarring are frequently found. Coarctation of the aorta may also be present. Around 60% will have renal tract abnormalities, which include horseshoe kidneys and duplex ureters, but these do not usually compromise renal function. Mental development is normal although detailed psychometric testing may demonstrate a minor defect in spatial perception.

At puberty Turner's syndrome may present for the first time with primary amenorrhea and failure of secondary sexual development. Streak gonads are found with ultrasound and at laparotomy. The patients are almost invariably sterile, but menstruation and secondary sexual development may be induced by estrogen replacement (see Ch. 13, Physical growth and development).

Girls with Turner's syndrome have a normal life span. It is now recognized that hypertension may be a complication in adult life, and in the absence of hormone replacement osteoporosis may also develop.

Cytogenetics

Although 60% of patients with Turner's syndrome have a 45X karyotype, a variety of chromosome abnormalities are seen with the syndrome (Table 12.6).

Mosaic cell lines arise from mitotic non-disjunction in early embryogenesis. On the whole the phenotype with mosaicism is similar to the classical features of Turner's syndrome. When the mosaicism involves an XY cell line there is an increased risk of gonadoblastoma, and the streak ovaries should be removed. In the rare situation of an unbalanced X:autosome translocation and in some cases of ring X, mental retardation may occur.

Turner's syndrome is not associated with increased maternal age and as it usually arises from mitotic rather than meiotic error is not associated with an increase of recurrence in further pregnancies.

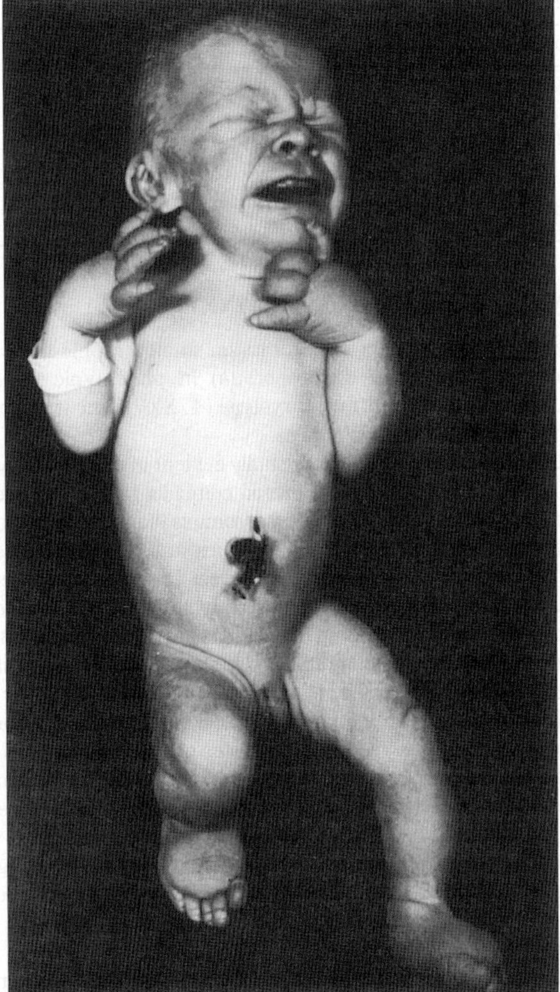

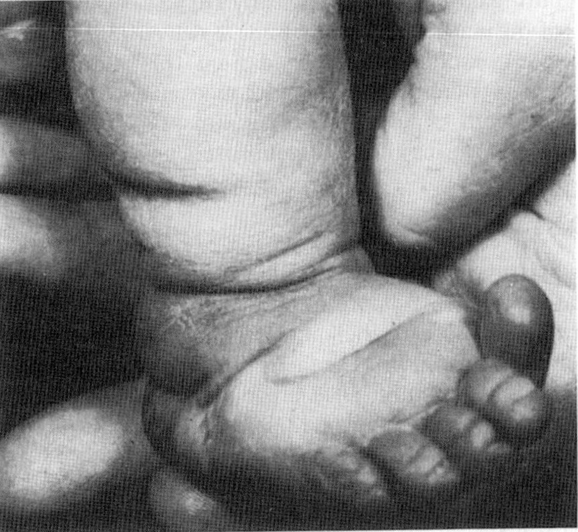

Fig. 12.16 Turner's syndrome in the neonate may present with edema of the hands and feet.

47XXX

The majority of girls with triple X (47XXX) will not have been brought to medical attention and have had their chromosomes tested. However prospective studies have identified some potential differences. Their height tends to be greater than average and in statistical terms there is a slight lowering of mean IQ, but no specific abnormal behavioral patterns. Fertility is normal. In theory there should be an increased risk of sex chromosome aneuploidy in the offspring of these girls, but in practice the risk appears to be insignificant.

Table 12.6 Chromosome abnormalities in Turner's syndrome

Chromosome abnormality	Percentage
45XO	60
Mosaic XX/XO	20
Isochromosome Xq or Xp	5
46X del (X)	5
46X ring (X)	5
With Y chromosome	5

KLINEFELTER'S SYNDROME (47XXY)

Klinefelter's syndrome of gynecomastia, small atrophic testes and absent spermatogenesis (azoospermia) in phenotypic males is associated with an abnormal karyotype (47XXY). The incidence is around 1 in 1000 live-born males.

The clinical features are not usually evident in the first few years of life although it may be discovered coincidentally in apparently normal male infants. When the syndrome is diagnosed early there are often considerable parental anxieties and careful counseling will be required. At puberty, however, the secondary sexual characteristics develop poorly and body fat tends to take on a feminine distribution with gynecomastia in 50% of cases. Beard growth is minimal and in adult life patients will rarely need to shave more than twice a week. The testes remain small and infertility may be the presenting feature in adult males. Sexual function is normal although the libido is reduced. The testosterone levels are low and the gonadotrophin levels elevated and testosterone replacement may be helpful. Testicular histology shows an increase in Leydig cells and interstitial fibrosis. Height is usually increased with relatively long limbs. The mean intelligence is on average slightly reduced in Klinefelter's syndrome, but this rarely poses a problem.

Cytogenetics

About two-thirds of XXY males are the result of disjunctional errors either during oogenesis or in the early zygote cleavage having two copies of the maternal X chromosome as detected by chromosomal markers. As would be predicted from this the incidence of Klinefelter's syndrome increases with maternal age. In about 15% of patients with Klinefelter's there is a mosaic XY/XXY form but even in mosaic forms infertility would usually occur.

48XXXY AND 49XXXXY

These karyotypes produce more clinical disturbance than 47XXY. Mental retardation is more frequent and there may be skeletal abnormalities, especially radioulnar synostosis (leading to inability to supinate the forearm). The facies may also be dysmorphic with hypertelorism, epicanthic folds, broad nose and large open mouth. As they are very different from Klinefelter's syndrome it is better to describe them by their karyotypes.

XX MALES

Very rarely patients have been identified who have an essentially male phenotype with an apparently normal 46XX karyotype. This has lead to further basic research into the embryological determination of sex. On molecular analysis these males will almost invariably be found to have the SRY gene. This gene is now known to be the main genetic switch in determining whether a fetus becomes male or female. After the SRY gene has been expressed there may still be other hormonal and genetic factors which will modify the sexual phenotype. Amongst the hormonal factors are congenital adrenal hyperplasia in which an overproduction of androgens will lead to virilization and testicular feminization in which the absence of testosterone receptors prevents the development of the external genitalia. There are also other modifying genes on the autosomes found through the analysis of malformation syndromes, e.g. the gene responsible for sex reversal in camptomelic dysplasia is the SRY related gene SOX9[30] and the gene responsible for ovarian dysgenesis in blepharophimosis–ptosis syndrome is the forkhead transcription factor FOXL2.[31] A good review of the role of SRY in sexual differentiation is given by Goodfellow & Lovell-Badge.[32]

XYY SYNDROME

The initial reports of males with 47XYY came from studies of males in institutions for mentally ill criminals and this biased ascertainment initially distorted the understanding of this chromosomal abnormality.

It is relatively common with an incidence of 1 in 1000 males. In order to obtain a truer picture of the syndrome a number of prospective studies have been carried out looking for example at the karyotypes of all newborn children in a particular area and following those with sex chromosome abnormalities through childhood.[33] The XYY karyotype is associated with a normal birth weight but increased growth in early to mid-childhood. About a third are in the 90th centile for height. Intelligence is not significantly different from their chromosomally normal siblings. Detailed psychological testing does reveal a tendency to compulsive behavior, which in certain settings may lead to socially deviant behavior, but in the presence of a stable family background this can be more appropriately channeled. It should be remembered that the vast majority of males with 47XYY remain undetected in the community.

FRAGILE X MENTAL RETARDATION

It has long been recognized that there is a considerable excess of males in the mentally handicapped population, and it is now realized that this is due to a considerable number of X-linked forms of mental retardation.[34] The most significant of these is mental retardation associated with the Xq27 folate-sensitive fragile site.

In 1969 Lubs demonstrated a fragile site on the X chromosome in a family with mental retardation, but it was initially regarded as an isolated curiosity. Around the same time Dr Gillian Turner studied a number of X-linked mental retardation families in a mental handicap institution and described their relatively 'normal looking' appearance together with large testes. Lubs had described the cytogenetic finding and Turner the phenotypic appearance of fragile X mental retardation. Several years later connection between the clinical and laboratory findings was firmly established[35] and the condition is now recognized as the second commonest cause of mental handicap in males after Down syndrome. The incidence of fragile X mental retardation is 1 per 1000 males. In a study of autism 5% of the male patients were found to have fragile X mental retardation.

Clinical features

The phenotype of fragile X mental retardation is not as striking as that of Down syndrome, but with experience can be recognized (Fig. 12.17). Fragile X males have a large forehead, large head, long nose, prominent chin and long ears. The facial phenotype, however, becomes more obvious with age and is not easily recognizable in younger children.

Fragile X males tend to be larger at birth and taller than other children, but do not achieve the full growth predicted by the centile chart. In adult life fragile X males tend to be short. The head

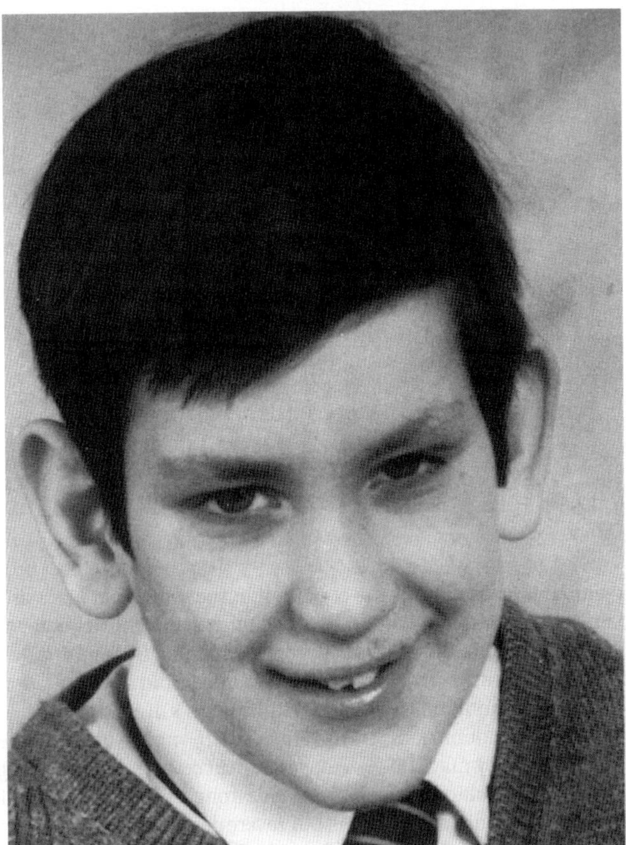

Fig. 12.17 Facial features of fragile X mental retardation (reproduced with permission).

circumference is increased with many having a head circumference greater than the 97th centile. Similarly the ear length is increased. This is an extremely useful clinical sign and may be measured and compared with a centile chart prepared from a normal population.[14]

Macro-orchidism is present in 80% of adult fragile X males and 15% of prepubertal fragile X boys. The size of the testes may be considerably enlarged. In one series the range was 15–127 ml (the Prader orchidometer can only be used for testicular volumes up to 25 ml!). The large testes are functionally normal and the increased size may be due to an increase in interstitial edema or connective tissue. Large testes are a relatively rare feature in other syndromes with mental handicap.

It has been suggested that there may be a connective tissue abnormality in fragile X. There is a slight increase in the frequency of mitral valve prolapse, aortic root dilatation and hernias. More striking clinically is the soft skin and joint hypermobility, which may be helpful diagnostically.

The range of intellectual handicap in fragile X males varies but most are moderately to severely retarded. Females tend to be more mildly affected. There is also a suggestion that intelligence may decline with age. Speech development is particularly affected in fragile X males and behavioral changes and seizures may occur. The level of intellectual deficit can, to some extent, be determined by the molecular testing. Medical treatment with folate therapy has been suggested to improve behavior and improve IQ, but it does not appear to be effective in properly controlled trials.

Molecular genetics

The fragile site in the X chromosome was initially used to diagnose this disorder but in affected males only 5–20% of cells will demonstrate the fragile site and in female carriers only half of the carriers could be detected by the cytogenetic test. It is now recognized that the fragile site is a marker for the disease rather than its cause.

The diagnostic difficulties were resolved by the identification of the FMR-1 gene at Xq27.[36] The gene has within it a repeating sequence of three nucleotides CGG. Normal individuals have up to 50 copies of the nucleotide repeat. If the number of repeats is greater than 50 it becomes unstable in meiosis and can then increase in repeat number. The initial increase to between 50 and 150 repeats is referred to as the *premutation*. It may be found in intellectually normal males and female carriers. However, after passing through meiosis in the female the size of the repeats increases to the *full mutation* of greater than 150 repeats and can then produce learning difficulties in both males and females. In a male with the premutation the repeat length is not significantly increased in spermatogenesis. Repeat number may increase or decrease in the full mutation during somatic cell division and therefore somatic mosaicism can be detected in some affected individuals. The full mutation affects the methylation of the DNA and this in turn switches off the FMR-1 gene and will affect both intellectual function and the cytogenetic fragility. At present the exact function of the gene is not clear but the gene product has been identified and a transgenic mouse model is available for further research.[37]

In terms of inheritance therefore it appears very similar to X-linked recessive inheritance as the condition is passed through females and will affect males, but daughters may also be affected with a degree of learning difficulties and the mutation can arise from unaffected males.

The discovery of the FMR-1 gene has meant that accurate follow-up and counseling of families is possible (Fig. 12.18). Prenatal diagnosis using chorionic villus sampling (CVS) and molecular analysis is possible in the first trimester of pregnancy.

SINGLE GENE DISORDERS: INHERITANCE

Distributed amongst the 46 chromosomes, there are approximately 50 000 structural genes, which code for specific proteins. The position at which the structural gene lies on the chromosome is referred to as the *locus*. At the locus there is a pair of alleles. If an

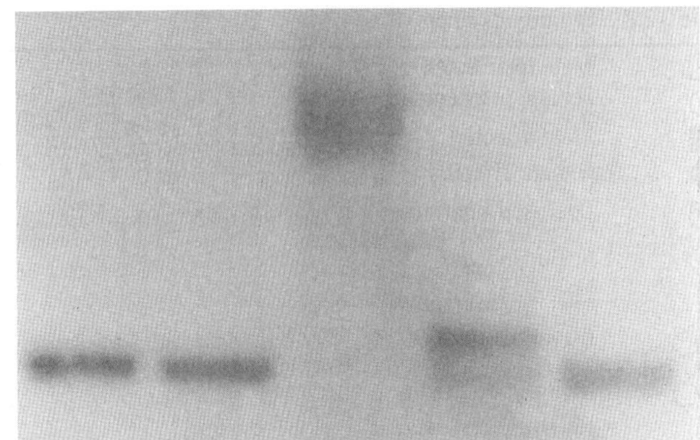

Fig. 12.18 Autoradiograph of Southern blot looking for fragile X. The DNA has been digested by the restriction enzyme Eco R1 and probed with FMR-1 probe OX1.9. The normal fragment size is seen in lanes 1, 2 and 5. In lane 3 there is an expanded fragment (< 500 repeats) indicating an affected boy. In lane 4 there is a female with a normal band and a slightly larger band above, indicating a carrier of a premutation. (Courtesy of R. Taylor).

individual possesses two alleles that are the same, the individual is said to be *homozygous* for that particular trait. If the two alleles are different, the individual is said to be *heterozygous*. A gene which is manifest in the heterozygote is *dominant*, whereas a gene which is only manifest in the homozygote is *recessive*. These terms do not refer to the characteristics of the genes, but only to their manifestations. It is, therefore, more correct to refer to a 'dominant disorder' rather than a 'dominant gene'.

A trait or disorder which is determined by a gene on an *autosome* is said to be inherited as an autosomal trait and may be dominant or recessive. A trait or disorder that is determined by a gene on one of the *sex chromosomes* is said to be sex linked and may also be either dominant or recessive.

DRAWING THE PEDIGREE

The first stage in analyzing the pattern of inheritance in a family is to draw up a pedigree. This is a shorthand method of putting all the relevant family information together in a systematic way. The symbols used in drawing up a pedigree are illustrated in Table 12.7. Each individual in a pedigree is identified from his generation (Roman numerals) and his location in the generation (Arabic numerals). Thus the index case or proband in Figure 12.19 is IV.4. It is usually necessary to ask specifically about consanguinity and miscarriages as most patients will not realize that these details are relevant.

AUTOSOMAL DOMINANT INHERITANCE

In an autosomal dominant disorder an affected individual possesses the abnormal (mutant) gene and its normal allele. When an affected individual marries a normal person, on average half their children will be affected. This is because an affected person produces gametes that have either the mutant allele for the disorder or the normal allele. If the normal allele is represented as 'a' and the abnormal allele as 'A' then the various combinations are illustrated in Table 12.8.

Classically an autosomal dominant disorder can be traced back through several generations, but if the condition is severe, affected individuals may not survive to have children and transmit the disease to subsequent generations. In such cases the affected individual is 'sporadic', as the condition in the individual has arisen as a new mutation and they will not live to reproduce. The frequency of new mutations arising varies from condition to condition, e.g. about 50% of cases of neurofibromatosis arise from new mutations whereas new mutations are rare in Huntington's disease.

Table 12.7 Pedigree symbols

Symbol	Meaning
□	Male unaffected
○	Female unaffected
■	Male affected
●	Female affected
⊠	Deceased unaffected
◇	Sex unknown
	Miscarriage or termination
	Dizygotic twins
	Monozygotic twins
	Heterozygote
	Propositus or index case
	Consanguineous marriage
	Illegitimate or adopted
	Female without offspring
②	Two unaffected females

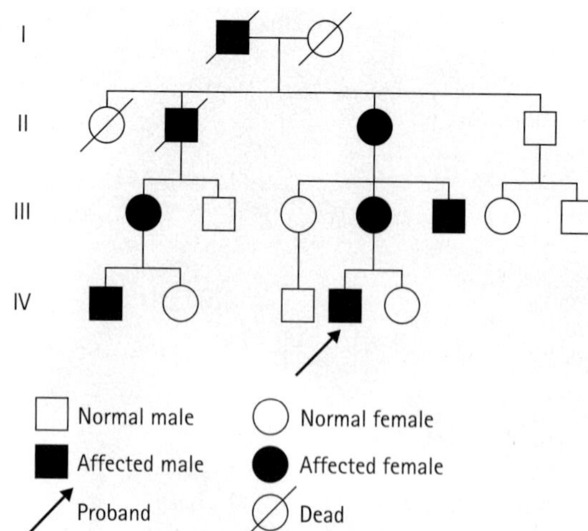

Fig. 12.19 Pedigree pattern of an autosomal dominant trait.

Autosomal dominant traits affect both males and females (Fig. 12.19). They may show great variation in severity (= *expressivity*) as in neurofibromatosis, which may range from being a relatively mild pigmentary skin disorder to a cause of severe deformity. Sometimes the gene may not express itself at all in which case it is said to be non-penetrant. This phenomenon explains apparent skipped generations in certain pedigrees. The *penetrance* of the trait is the proportion of heterozygotes who express a trait.

Some autosomal genes are expressed more frequently in one sex than in the other. This is referred to as sex-influenced inheritance or, in the extreme case in which only one sex is affected, as *sex-limited inheritance*. Possible examples of sex-influenced autosomal traits include hemochromatosis, gout and male pattern baldness. The underlying difference in expression may be due to the different hormonal background.

In myotonic dystrophy it was suggested that the severity of the condition tended to increase with each generation, e.g. the grandparent could have had cataracts only, while the mother had myotonia and muscle weakness and the affected child had the disorder in its congenital form with developmental delay. This was referred to as *anticipation*. It was initially thought that the cause of this was a bias in ascertainment but it is now clear that the underlying mutation is a triplet repeat in the myotonin kinase gene. Triplet repeats within a gene may become unstable at a critical size and at

Table 12.8 Autosomal dominant inheritance

		Affected parent (Aa) ↓ gametes	
		A	a
Normal parent (aa) → gametes	a	Aa affected	aa normal
	a	Aa affected	aa normal

this point there may be an increase in the repeat size number during meiosis leading to an increasing severity in the next generation.

Occasionally it is known that a particular disorder is autosomal dominant and fully penetrant, and yet an unaffected parent will have two affected offspring. It is very unlikely that this was due to two independent de novo mutations and the most likely explanation is *germinal* or *gonadal mosaicism*. In this situation the unaffected parent carries the mutation only in the testis or ovary and not in the other tissues of the body.

AUTOSOMAL RECESSIVE INHERITANCE

Autosomal recessive traits affect both sexes and only homozygotes are affected. The affected individuals in a family are all in one sibship, i.e. they are brothers and sisters (Fig. 12.20). The parents of an affected child or children are both heterozygotes, and are perfectly healthy. It is, therefore, not possible to trace the disease through several generations unless there is complex inbreeding. With rare recessive traits the parents of affected individuals are often related, the reason being that cousins are more likely to carry the same genes because they inherited them from a common ancestor.

When parents have a child affected by an autosomal recessive disorder the likelihood of the next pregnancy being similarly affected is 1 in 4. The risk remains 1 in 4 for each successive pregnancy no matter how many children may be affected in the family. If the normal allele is represented as 'A', and the abnormal allele as 'a', then the possible combinations are illustrated in Table 12.9.

Nowadays, since families tend to be small, it frequently happens that an autosomal recessive condition appears sporadic with only one affected person in the family.

The majority of inborn errors of metabolism are due to deficiencies of specific enzymes and are inherited as autosomal recessive traits. In some instances it may be possible to demonstrate that individuals are heterozygotes in these disorders by finding an intermediate level of enzyme activity.

Where a number of different mutant alleles exist it is occasionally possible to find an individual who is heterozygous for two different mutant alleles. An example of this is seen in the hemoglobinopathies. An individual may be heterozygous for both HbS and HbC. Such double heterozygotes or 'genetic compounds' have a disease intermediate in severity between sickle cell disease and HbC disease.

CODOMINANCE

Codominance is the term used for two traits, which are both expressed in the heterozygote. An example of codominance is the inheritance for the blood groups A and B. An individual with both alleles will have the blood group AB.

Table 12.9 Autosomal recessive inheritance

		Normal heterozygous parent (Aa) gametes ↓ gametes	
		A	a
Normal heterozygous parent (Aa) → gametes	A	AA normal	Aa unaffected heterozygote
	a	Aa unaffected heterozygote	aa affected

X-LINKED RECESSIVE INHERITANCE

In theory sex-linked inheritance could be either X-linked or Y-linked, but as there are no structural genes other than those determining sexual development on the Y chromosome, sex linkage is effectively the same as X linkage.

An X-linked recessive trait is one which is due to a mutant gene on the X chromosome, and is carried by females to affect males (Figs 12.21 and 12.22). The affected males are *hemizygous* (with the mutant gene on their single X chromosome) while the carrier females are heterozygous and are usually perfectly healthy. X-linked disorders may also be transmitted by affected males through their daughters unless the disorder is so severe that affected males do not survive to have children (e.g. Duchenne muscular dystrophy). Hemophilia is an X-linked recessive disorder where improvements in medical treatment and surgical techniques have led to affected males often surviving into adult life. If an affected male marries a normal female and if the hemophilia gene is represented as X^h and the normal gene as X, then the various gametic combinations that can occur are represented in Table 12.10. Thus, all daughters of an affected male are carriers and all his sons are normal. In the case of a woman who is a carrier (XX^h) and who marries a normal male then half her sons will be affected and half her daughters will be heterozygote carriers (Table 12.11).

Quite often in serious X-linked conditions there is only one affected boy in a family. Such a sporadic case may be the result of a new mutation in the affected boy's X chromosome and in such cases

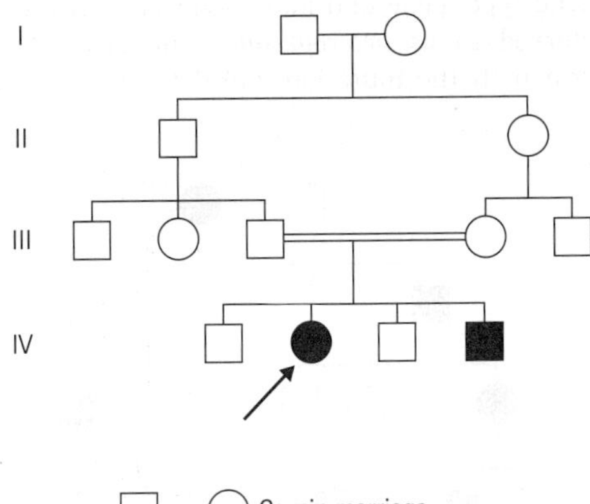

Fig. 12.20 Pedigree pattern of an autosomal recessive trait.

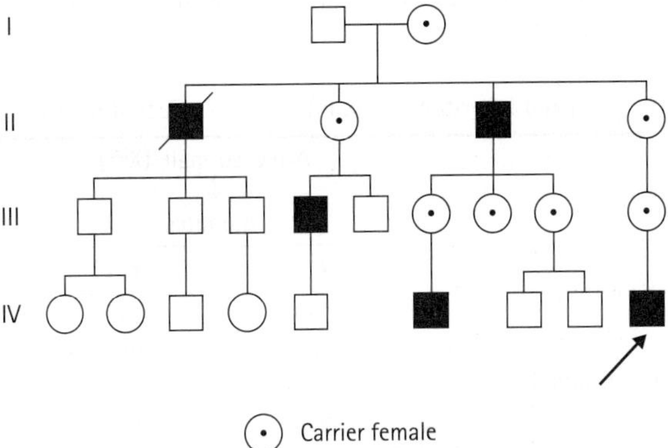

Fig. 12.21 Pedigree pattern of an X-linked recessive trait in which affected males reproduce.

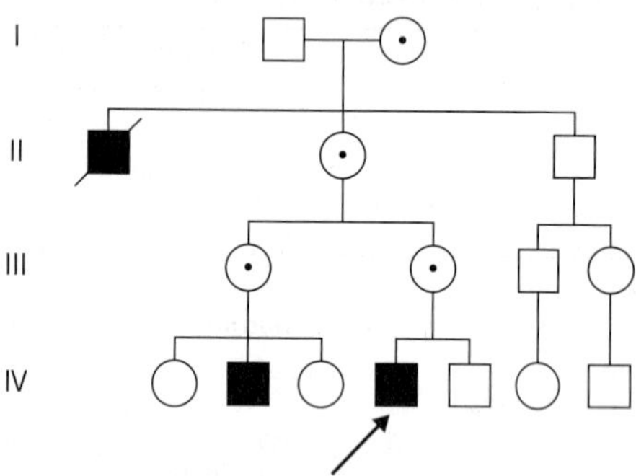

Fig. 12.22 Pedigree pattern of a severe X-linked recessive trait in which affected males do not survive to have children.

Table 12.11 X-linked inheritance: the offspring of affected females

		Normal male (XY) ↓ gametes	
		X	Y
Carrier female (XX^h) → gametes	X	XX normal daughter	XY normal son
	X^h	XX^h carrier daughter	X^hY hemophiliac son

recurrence would not occur in the family. It is also possible that the mother might be a carrier, and by chance the mutant gene has not been transmitted to any of her other male offspring. In families with predominantly female offspring an X-linked mutation may be inherited through the female line for a few generations without affected males. In one-third of isolated cases of Duchenne muscular dystrophy the mutation occurs in the affected boy, and in two-thirds of cases the mother is a carrier. It is obviously of vital importance to determine if the mother is a carrier in order to provide accurate information about recurrence risks. The probability of the mother being a carrier can be calculated using knowledge of the numbers of unaffected males in the family (the more unaffected males the less chance the mother is a carrier), the level of creatine kinase (female heterozygotes have slightly higher levels than female controls from the general population) and using information from DNA studies. This analysis is well reviewed in Emery.[38]

In a number of special circumstances a female may exhibit manifestations of an X-linked recessive trait. It may occur as a result of random inactivation or lyonization of the X chromosome. In early embryogenesis in the female zygote one of the X chromosomes is inactivated in each cell. This process is random so that on average half the cells in a female will have one X chromosome inactivated and half will have the other X chromosome inactivated. However, occasionally by chance the majority of cells will have the X chromosome with the normal allele inactivated and the mutant allele will be partially expressed. This situation is seen in female carriers of Duchenne muscular dystrophy where about 5% of female carriers may show some muscle weakness. It may also occur in the rare situation when a female is both a carrier of an X-linked mutation and has a 45X karyotype (Turner's syndrome). Finally it can also occur in common X-linked disorders such as red–green color blindness where an affected male marries a female heterozygote and produces a daughter in whom both X chromosomes possess the mutant allele.

Table 12.10 X-linked inheritance: the offspring of affected males

		Affected male (X^hY) ↓ gametes	
		X^h	Y
Normal female (XX) → gametes	X	XX^h carrier daughter	XY normal son
	X	XX^h carrier daughter	XY normal son

X-LINKED DOMINANT INHERITANCE

An X-linked dominant disorder is one which is manifest in the heterozygous female as well as in the hemizygous male. The pedigree pattern superficially resembles that of autosomal dominant inheritance, but in an X-linked dominant disorder an affected male transmits the disease to all his daughters and to none of his sons. Affected females transmit the disease equally to sons and daughters half of whom, on average, will be affected (Fig. 12.23).

There are relatively few X-linked dominant disorders. One example is vitamin D-resistant rickets (hypophosphatemia). In some X-linked dominant disorders the condition is lethal in males and so only females are affected (e.g. incontinentia pigmenti).

MITOCHONDRIAL INHERITANCE

While the vast majority of genes are located in the nuclear genome there are a small number of genes located on the mitochondrial DNA (mtDNA). The mitochondrial DNA consists of 16.5 kb of circular DNA and accounts for 1% of the total DNA. MtDNA encodes for the proteins essential for aerobic respiration and defects in mtDNA reflect abnormalities in this function.[39] Each cell contains between 1000 and 100 000 copies of mtDNA. In the vast majority of cells the functional mtDNA will be identical. This is referred to as *homoplasmy*. However where there is a mutation in the mtDNA it will not usually be present in all mitochondria and cells will have a mixture between mitochondria with the 'wild type' gene and mitochondria with the mutation. This is referred to as *heteroplasmy*. The proportion of the mitochondria with the mutation will determine whether there

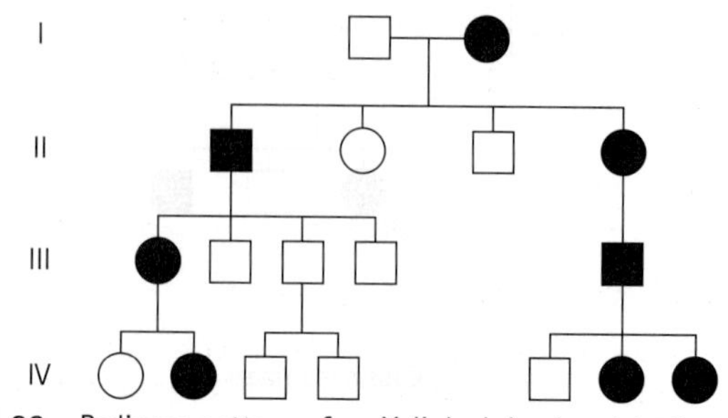

Fig. 12.23 Pedigree pattern of an X-linked dominant trait.

is a phenotypic effect from the mutation. In practice over 85% of the mitochondria would need to have the mutation before there was a phenotypically significant defect in the enzymes of the respiratory chain.

In mitochondrial diseases there may also be variation among tissues on the body. This may have considerable practical implications in diagnosis since a blood sample may not give an accurate reflection of abnormalities in other tissues. For this reason muscle biopsy is the mainstay of diagnosis of mitochondrial diseases rather than blood sampling. In many mitochondrial diseases there will be characteristic 'ragged red fibers' on Gomori staining and a non-specific elevation of the lactate and pyruvate in the blood. It also follows from these tissue differences that prenatal diagnosis may be difficult as the proportion of a mitochondrial mutation in a chorionic villus sample may not reflect the proportion of the mutation in other parts of the fetus.

The segregation of mitochondrial genes does not follow Mendelian inheritance. Mitochondrial genes are not passed paternally as the mitochondria are in the tail of the sperm and only the nucleus of the sperm penetrates the ovum at fertilization. The ovum on the other hand has a relatively large volume of cytoplasm and thus contains many mitochondria. The exact proportion of offspring affected will depend on the proportion of mitochondria containing the specific mutation in the fertilized ovum. It is thus very difficult to give accurate recurrence risks for mitochondrial disorders and the best guide at present is to rely on the statistical data from family studies.

Another complication in mitochondrial disease is that some of the enzymes in the respiratory chain and hence some of the mitochondrial functions are not coded for in the mtDNA but are coded for in the nuclear DNA. Mutations in these genes affecting mitochondrial function are inherited in a Mendelian pattern. One example of such a disorder is Barth syndrome (endocardial fibroelastosis, neutropenia and muscle weakness) which is due to a mutation in the G-45 gene on the X chromosome and is therefore inherited as an X-linked recessive disorder.[40]

There are a number of characteristic mitochondrial disorders which are important in clinical practice :

- Kearns–Sayre syndrome: this is a progressive external ophthalmoplegia with ptosis and muscle weakness.
- MERRF: myoclonic epilepsy with ragged red fibers.
- MELAS: mitochondrial encephalomyopathy with lactic acidosis and stroke-like episodes.
- Leber's hereditary optic neuropathy (LHON) which presents as acute or subacute visual failure in the second or third decade.[41]

However in many cases the clinical phenotype will not fit into a characteristic presentation and the possibility of mitochondrial disease should be considered in cases of lactic acidosis, muscle weakness, cardiomyopathy, deafness or pigmentary retinopathy.

In clinical practice pathological mutations are most significant, but there is also a wide range of harmless variation in the mtDNA. Such genetic variations are similar to the variation seen in blood groups and are known as *polymorphisms*. The mitochondrial polymorphisms have been used to study human evolution and the spread of different populations.[42]

DNA AND GENE ACTION

STRUCTURE AND FUNCTION OF GENES

The genetic material that is capable of providing a perfect replica in cell division is in the form of a molecule of DNA. While it is possible to study chromosomes at a microscopic level, the genes are well below the resolution of the microscope. Looking at the chromosomes under the microscope is rather like looking at the wrapping around the genes. In rough terms a 5 cm length of DNA is compressed into a chromosome 10 000 times smaller by tight coiling and packing with proteins called *histones*.

DNA consists of long chains of molecules called *nucleotides*. Each nucleotide consists of a nitrogenous base (*adenine, thymine, guanine* or *cytosine*), a pentose sugar and a phosphate group. The pentose sugar in DNA is deoxyribose. The DNA (unless denatured) is in the form of two polynucleotide chains arranged in a double helix (Fig. 12.24a).[43,44] The arrangement of the bases in the double helix is not random since adenine in one chain always pairs with thymine, and in the other cytosine always pairs with guanine. Thus the arrangement of nucleotides in the two chains is *complementary*, and in cell division using one chain a complementary chain may be synthesized, thus preserving the sequence of bases in each daughter cell.

The sequence of bases is important, because the arrangement of the bases provides the genetic code from which proteins may be made (Fig. 12.24b). The genetic information in the DNA is first *transcribed* with messenger ribonucleic acid (mRNA) and this in turn is *translated* into the synthesis of a polypeptide chain. RNA is very similar to DNA in structure except (i) the thymidine is replaced by uracil, (ii) the deoxyribose is replaced by ribose and (iii) it is a single-stranded rather than a double-stranded polynucleotide chain.

The DNA, which is responsible for the synthesis of specific proteins, forms the structural genes. The information is in the form of a *triplet code*, a sequence of three bases or a *codon* determines one amino acid. Since there are four bases involved the possible combination that could be provided is $4^3 = 64$. Since there are only 20 amino acids this code is said to be degenerate and most amino acids can be coded for by more than one triplet sequence. The code also provides codons to initiate and terminate synthesis.

In the first stage of protein synthesis the DNA sequence between the initiation codon and the stop codon is transcribed into mRNA. The mRNA then moves from the nucleus to the ribosomes in the cytoplasm. Here the second stage takes place, viz. the translation of mRNA into a polypeptide chain. The ribosome binds to the initiation site on the mRNA and for each codon an amino acid is added on using transfer RNA (tRNA). Transfer RNA is another form of RNA, which because of its molecular configuration is able to carry an amino acid and match it to the appropriate codon.

It has become apparent that the majority of DNA does not code for proteins and is not transcribed at all. The total amount of human DNA is 3 billion bases and if each gene were around 2000 bases in length this would allow for 1.5 million genes. Instead it is estimated that there are around 50 000 structural genes and 90% of the genome is DNA which does not code for proteins. Much of this is highly repetitive in its sequences and may have some as yet undefined function in the control of gene action. There are various classes of non-coding DNA. One form of the highly repetitive DNA known as microsatellite DNA is widely distributed throughout the genome and also because it is variable between individuals it can be used by researchers in mapping genes in family linkage studies. In another form there are also copies of genes which are non-functional and are known as pseudogenes. There are also inactivated DNA sequences known as transposable sequences which resemble the sequence found in retroviruses and indeed may have entered the human DNA from viral infection.

The structural gene has an ordered sequence that is illustrated in Figure 12.25. Upstream of the structural gene there is highly repetitive DNA and within this there are two promoter regions which regulate gene transcription. The beginning of the structural gene is marked by an initiation codon AUG which indicates where

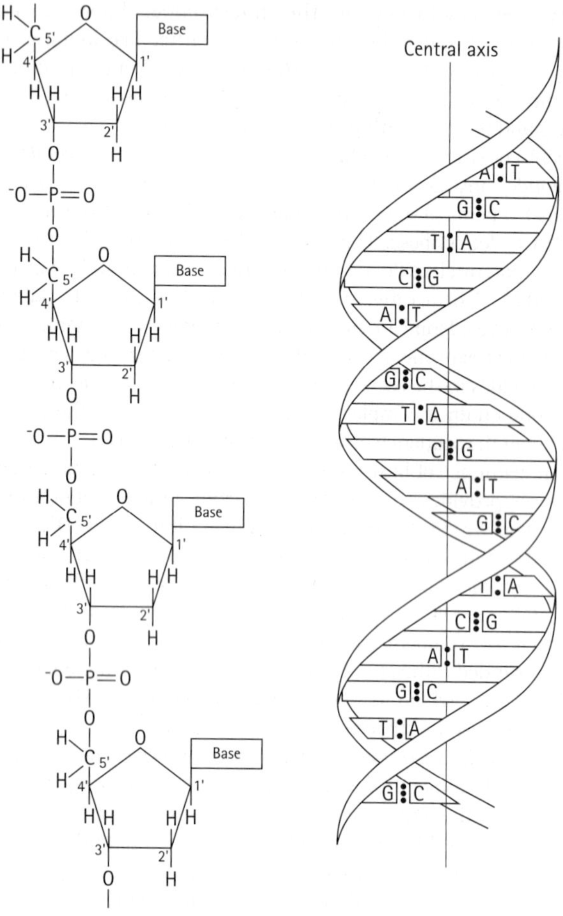

Fig. 12.24 (a) The structure of DNA. (From Weatherall 1986[43] with permission)

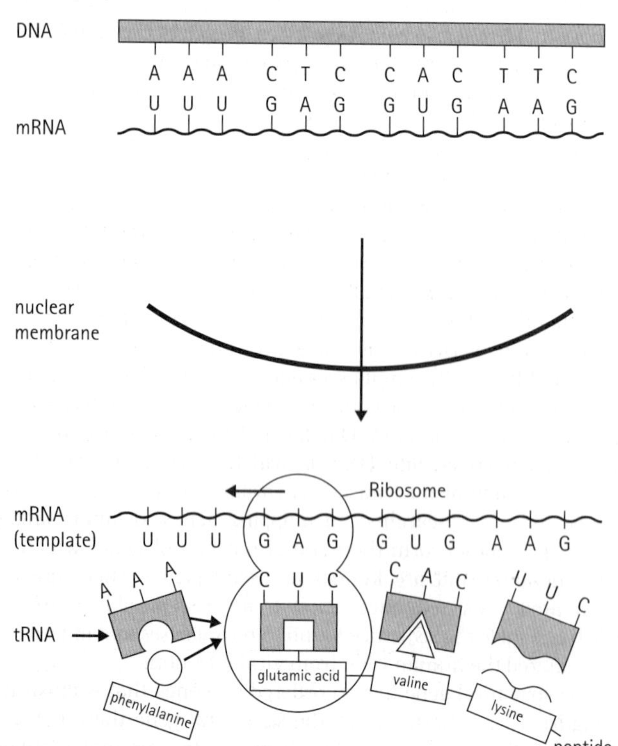

Fig. 12.24 (b) The production of proteins from DNA. (Modified from Emery 1983[44] with permission)

transcription begins. Within the region that is transcribed, the DNA may be divided into *exons* and *introns*. The exons mark the regions of DNA that code for the amino acids in the translated protein, whereas the introns or intervening sequences are spliced out of the processed RNA before it migrates to the cytoplasm as mRNA. The introns probably have a role in gene regulation. The complexity of genes varies, e.g. insulin has two introns, whereas some collagen genes may have as many as 50 introns. At the end of the transcribed gene there is a stop codon and further downstream an AATAAA sequence that allows the release of the RNA.

This description of one gene producing one protein has been derived from biochemical studies in bacteria and it is often more complex than this in human genetics. In some cases such as the hemoglobin genes or some developmental genes there is a cluster of genes closely positioned together and the genes will work together to produce a complex protein or sequence of changes. In the case of the muscle protein dystrophin involved in Duchenne muscular dystrophy there is a very large gene measuring 2.5 million bases and within this gene there are several tissue specific promoters which produce different forms of dystrophin in different tissues. With immunoglobulins there is enormous diversity that comes from the alternative splicing of the RNA and DNA. With insulin the gene produces a precursor protein preproinsulin which is subsequently cleaved enzymatically after protein translation leaving the physiologically active insulin and its protein precursors.

At a disease level there are now many examples of one gene being associated with more than one disease. Most mutations in the androgen receptor gene will cause differing degrees of androgen insensitivity, but a CAG repeat mutation in the same gene produces X-linked spinomuscular atrophy and gynecomastia. Similarly different mutations in the cystic fibrosis transmembrane receptor (CFTR) gene may produce the classical features of cystic fibrosis at one end of the spectrum and bilateral absence of the vas deferens without respiratory disease at the other end of the spectrum.

MUTATIONS AT A MOLECULAR LEVEL

A *mutation* represents a change in the genomic material. Mutations may occur in somatic cells or germinal cells. Somatic cell mutation may predispose to malignancy, but will not be inherited. Mutations in the germinal cells, on the other hand, may be transmitted in the form of genetic disease. Mutations may be in the form of large chromosomal rearrangements as described in the earlier part of the chapter or may occur at molecular level in a single gene.

At a molecular level the main types of structural mutation are:

1. Single base substitutions ('point mutations') – These involve the substitution of one base for another but may have different effects. A full nomenclature for describing these may be found in Antonarkis.[45]
   - Missense mutations: the replacement of one amino acid for another in the gene product. A good example of such a mutation is sickle cell disease in which an A to T substitution in the 6th codon of the globin gene changes GAG to GTG and hence leads to the substitution of valine for glutamic acid and the subsequent physiological effects on the hemoglobin molecule.
   - Nonsense mutations: the replacement of an amino acid codon with a stop codon (UAA or UAG or UGA) which leads to a truncation of the gene product.
   - Splice site mutations: a single base substitution which creates or destroys an intron–exon splice site.
2. Deletions – Deletions may vary in size from single bases to megabase lengths of DNA. There are many examples of

Fig. 12.25 The structural gene consists of promoter and terminator sequences that are located at either end of the gene. The coding sequence of the gene is made up of exons and introns (the mRNA of which will eventually be spliced out before translation into a protein).

molecular deletions, e.g. over 60% of mutations in Duchenne muscular dystrophy are due to deletions in the dystrophin gene. One specific type of deletion is that which occurs in the promotor sequence of the gene as these will affect the rate of synthesis of the gene product rather than its structure, e.g. promoter deletions have been reported in thalassemia.

3. Insertions and duplications – These mutations may arise from unequal crossing over at meiosis and can disrupt the gene.
4. Frameshift mutations – These can be produced by deletions or single base substitution and as a result all the subsequent codons in the gene are misread as the nucleotides must be read in 'threes'.
5. Dynamic mutations – When there are trinucleotide or triplet repeats in a gene the transmission of the exact number of repeats may become genetically unstable and may increase further in subsequent generations, e.g. fragile X mental retardation, myotonic dystrophy and Huntington's disease.

In addition to the structural classification for mutations it is possible to classify mutations in functional terms. Some mutations will produce no change in the function of the gene and thus will not be selected against in evolutionary terms. These non-pathological changes become variations or polymorphisms in the population. When a new change is found in a gene it is important to determine whether it is pathological or simply a polymorphism.

Mutations may produce loss of function. In many cases this loss of function is not critical unless both alleles have a loss of function and then the level of the gene product becomes critically low. This is the situation in autosomal recessive disorders. Other genes may serve a more critical role and the loss of function in one allele will be sufficient to produce an effect. This is referred to as haploinsufficiency and is the situation that is found in autosomal dominant inheritance. If a chromosome deletion in the same area produces the phenotype then haplosufficiency of critical genes is likely to be the molecular mechanism.

Collagen is made up of three strands of procollagen polypeptides in a triple helix. The procollagen polypeptides are produced by several collagen genes. A heterozygous mutation in one of these collagen genes may produce serious abnormalities in collagen because the abnormal procollagen polypeptide produced binds abnormally with the other procollagen polypeptides and leads to major disruption in the final collagen product. The effect of this mutation has been described as 'protein suicide' or a dominant negative effect. This is the underlying molecular pathology in some forms of osteogenesis imperfecta.

Mutations can produce a gain of function. The gain of function may be due to the overproduction of a protein such as the peripheral myelin protein (PMP22) in Charcot–Marie–Tooth disease or the accumulation of protein aggregates in Huntington's disease. It may also be due to a receptor being switched on permanently as the GNAS subunit of the G protein in McCune–Albright syndrome.

Genetic heterogeneity underlies much of the complexity of inherited disease. The term may be used to describe how similar conditions may have different patterns of inheritance, e.g. Noonan's syndrome and Turner's syndrome both have short stature and a webbed neck but Noonan's syndrome is autosomal dominant and Turner's syndrome is chromosomal. It may also apply at the molecular level. *Locus heterogeneity* describes the situation where the same disease may be caused by mutations in different genes, e.g. osteogenesis imperfecta may be caused by mutations in either the COL1A1 on chromosome 17 or the COL1A2 gene on chromosome 7. *Allelic heterogeneity* describes the situation where the same disease may be caused by different mutations in the same gene, e.g. there are now over 700 recognized mutations in the CFTR gene causing cystic fibrosis.

Mutations usually produce a permanent change in the gene, but DNA has some ability to repair itself. This has been studied largely from disorders where DNA damage leads to malignancy. Ultraviolet exposure leads to the formation of pyrimidine dimers binding the nucleotide bases. In the rare skin disorder xeroderma pigmentosum such abnormal dimers cannot be repaired because of an enzyme deficiency and ultimately skin tumors develop. The stages in the normal repair are illustrated in Figure 12.26.[46] Firstly, the single strand of DNA with the dimer formation is excised and removed, then using a DNA replicase a new strand is synthesized using the complementary strand as a template; finally the new strand is fixed into strands of the original using a DNA ligase. Some of the other inherited disorders leading to premature aging are also due to defects in DNA repair.

THE HUMAN GENOME MAPPING PROJECT

One of the most important events in human biology has been the mapping of genes to their chromosome location which started in the mid-1980s and by February 2001 the first draft of the human genome was published.[47,48] To understand the process it is necessary to look at the classical approaches to gene mapping and also the more automated approach.

TRADITIONAL GENE MAPPING

Gene mapping has depended on finding gene loci that are linked. When two genetic loci are close together on the same chromosome they are said to be *linked*. If two loci are at different ends of the chromosome then it is very likely that they will be separated during meiosis since there are two or three crossovers for each chromosome (see Fig. 12.2). The closer together they are the less likely that they will be separated during meiosis. Thus a measure of how close gene loci are to each other is the frequency of recombination. This is measured in *map units* or *centiMorgans* where 1 centiMorgan is equivalent to a 1% chance of recombination.

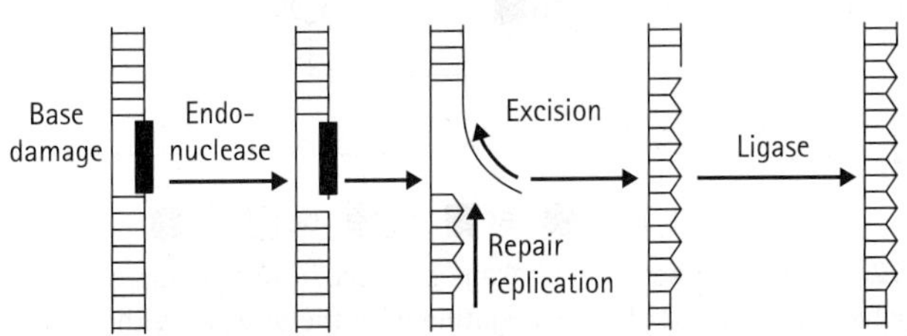

Fig. 12.26 DNA may be damaged but has a capacity to repair itself (From Bundey 1985[46] with permission)

Gene mapping has been of considerable practical value in medical genetics. There are a large number of single gene disorders in which the underlying biochemical abnormality and gene mutation are unknown, but because the location of the disorder on the gene map is known, it is possible to track the disease through a family using linked polymorphic markers and offer prenatal diagnosis or, in the case of adult disorders, presymptomatic diagnosis. It has also been possible to progress from gene localization to sequencing the gene and to identifying the gene product. A good example of this was the research that led to the discovery of dystrophin as the altered gene product in Duchenne muscular dystrophy.[49] This approach is known as *reverse genetics*, since it reversed the traditional approach of identifying the gene mutation from the enzyme or protein abnormality.

Genes may be mapped in a number of ways:

1. *Pedigree analysis*: if the pattern of inheritance conforms with X-linked inheritance, then the gene in question is on the X chromosome. This simple approach has made the X chromosome the most fully mapped chromosome.
2. *Chromosome rearrangement*: if an association is found between a disorder and a specific chromosome rearrangement, then the gene for that disorder may be located at the chromosome breakpoints. For example, patients were found with retinoblastoma and deletions of 13q14 and further research has identified the gene responsible for retinoblastoma to be located in this region.
3. *In situ hybridization*: if the amino acid structure of a protein is known then it is possible to predict which codons would code for it and therefore to synthesize a short oligonucleotide gene probe from it and label that probe with an isotope. The gene probe is then added to a chromosome spread and will hybridize to the complementary DNA in the chromosome. The localization of the gene is thus identified by an increased uptake of isotope at a specific site on the karyotype.
4. *Somatic cell hybridization*: using a virus it is possible to fuse human and mouse cells into a single hybrid cell. With subsequent cell divisions the human chromosomes are gradually lost, until there are cell lines with just one or two human chromosomes. By comparing the biochemical activity of a specific enzyme with the chromosome complement in each hybrid cell line, it is possible to deduce which chromosome the gene for the specific enzyme is on.
5. *Linkage analysis*: if a specific genetic marker segregates in a family with a single gene disorder, then the gene for that disorder will be located on the same chromosome as the marker and the position of two genes can be estimated from the frequency of crossovers. For example, in Figure 12.27, a large family with an autosomal dominant disorder is studied with a DNA polymorphism which gives four alleles, A, B, C and D. In the first generation the disease is inherited with the B allele from the grandfather (I.1) to his son (II.1). In other words the DNA polymorphism B and the disease allele are on the same particular chromosome and the linkage phase is established. In the third generation it is possible to see if any recombination takes place. In all but one of the eight children the B polymorphism segregates with the disease and the D polymorphism segregates with the normal allele. The exception is III.7 in whom there has been a recombination. Thus there has been one recombination out of eight meioses and the recombination rate is 12.5% or 0.125. Obviously not all families are so obligingly large and informative, but it is still possible to carry out linkage analysis with smaller families because the number of meioses may be added together.

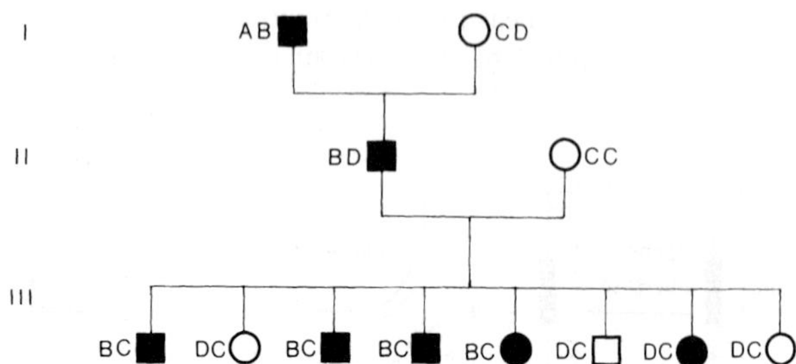

Fig. 12.27 Gene mapping by linkage analysis. In this pedigree the polymorphic marker B is segregating with the disease, with the exception of III.7 where a meiotic recombination between the polymorphic marker and the disease has occurred.

The usual way of expressing linkage is as the log of the odds of linkage or the *lod score* and this is expressed in terms of genetic distance by the recombination fraction θ. A recombination fraction of 0.05 represents a 5% chance of recombination. A lod score of 3 or over, for a recombination fraction of 0.05 or less, is significantly close linkage for prenatal diagnosis.

AUTOMATED APPROACH

While the traditional approaches have continued to prove useful in mapping diseases it was realized that a more industrialized approach using banks of automated gene sequencers could be used for systematically identifying all the genes. The DNA is basically cut into small sections and cloned and then the fragments are sequenced. The order of the fragments can be worked out if they have overlapping sequences and eventually all the DNA in the human genome can be sorted into these overlapping fragments. The structural genes can be identified by relating the DNA to expressed sequences (ESTs) and from this the total number of genes can be identified. One of the first surprises from the Human Genome project was the finding that humans did not have 100 000 genes as had been previously predicted but probably only have about 35 000 genes. This gives us only twice as many genes as the nematode worm and might be taken to indicate we are not as complex or advanced in evolutionary terms as we had thought. It is however probably not correct to equate biological complexity with the number of genes. An analogy could perhaps be taken from literature. Everyone writes with the same number of letters in the alphabet but that does not stop Shakespeare from writing great sonnets. In the same way it may be the complexity of gene expression that distinguishes humans from other species. One of the most challenging questions that comes from the genome project is the fact that the difference between some primates and humans comes down to a mere 1% of genes. Perhaps determining what this makes difference will help to define the essential qualities that make the human species different and define the biological basis of humanity.

At present there is only a draft of the genome available and many gaps to fill in with further sequencing. At the time of writing about 14 000 genes have been identified. This is just a beginning and there will need to be an enormous amount of research to determine the clinical significance of the genes in relation to disease and normal function.

Already there are a number of new developments in human genetics which will develop the discoveries of the human genome:

- Bioinformatics – The amount of information that has to be analyzed is staggering and making sense of the interrelationship between genes will be even more challenging. This has lead to the development of new information technology systems to handle the data.

- Comparative genomics – The genome mapping project is not confined to analyzing the human genome and the genomes of other species are being analysed using the same technology. This has already meant that location of human diseases can be identified by finding a similar defect in the mouse and working back from the knowledge of the position of the defect on the mouse chromosomes to the homologous position on the human chromosome.[50]
- Transgenic animals – It is often necessary to test out treatments in animals but difficult to find the appropriate animal model. Now it is possible to take a gene mutation causing human disease and to insert the mutated human gene into a mouse embryo and construct a transgenic mouse model that matches the human disease very accurately.
- Gene expression and proteomics – Having found a disease causing gene it is then necessary to see how that gene is expressed and what the protein it produces is like. The studies will therefore move from the gene (genomics) to the protein (proteomics).
- Pharmacogenomics – At present it costs about £250 million to develop a new drug and along the way there will be many potential drugs which might be effective but cannot be used because a small number of people will develop severe side-effects from the potential drug. It has been discovered that many of these side-effects are determined by genetic variation. Therefore if those who might develop side-effects could be identified genetically before the drug was used then it would be possible to bring many new drugs safely to the market and possibly to reduce the enormous cost of development. Another approach that might be used in pharmacogenomics is to define the heterogeneity within a disease and to target drug treatment more specifically, e.g. rather than treating all individuals with high blood pressure with the same drugs it might be possible by genetic analysis to identify those with abnormal salt metabolism from those with abnormal vascular responses.
- Gene therapy – Although gene therapy is the ultimate aim for genetic research it is likely to take some time for this to be more widely successful. There are many technical problems to solve. At present the correct gene is usually introduced into the patient using a viral vector, but this is relatively inefficient and even when it does correctly enter the disease tissue it is lost rapidly. There are also problems about using a virus even when it has been biologically inactivated and the use of a viral vector would probably never be acceptable in the treatment of neurological disease since it might well cause serious complications. There is considerable knowledge of the genetic defect in cystic fibrosis and a number of attempts have been made to use gene therapy to treat cystic fibrosis with rather disappointing results so far.[51] Because of the risks involved it may well be malignant disease rather than chronic genetic disease where the first major successes take place.

THE USE OF MOLECULAR GENETICS IN DIAGNOSIS

The recent rapid advances in medical genetics have come about largely because of the development of DNA technology. Some knowledge of the technology is helpful in understanding its practical application in the diagnosis of genetic disease. A more detailed review of the laboratory techniques may be found in Strachan & Read[52] and Elles.[53]

DNA extraction

DNA may be extracted from many different tissues. In most clinical work blood samples will be used as a source of DNA but in population studies buccal scrapes or mouthwashes may be useful for limited DNA testing. It may also be possible to extract DNA from the dried blood spots used for neonatal screening and this may be a source of archival DNA from a child who has subsequently died. Pathology samples are more difficult to analyze as the DNA is often broken down in the fixation process and only short DNA sequences may be analyzed. In prenatal diagnosis chorionic villi provide the best source of DNA.

The DNA is obtained by lyzing the cells, digesting the proteins by a proteinase and purifying the DNA by serial extractions with phenol and chloroform. The purity of the DNA obtained is then determined by spectroscopy and running an electrophoretic gel. Extracted DNA may be stored for many years at –80°C.

The preparation of gene probes and gene library

A *gene probe* is a single-stranded segment of DNA which can be used to determine whether a particular DNA sequence is present or absent in an individual's genome. Gene probes may be prepared in three ways:

1. If the DNA sequence is fully known, then a small oligonucleotide probe may be synthesized in vitro.
2. If there is a ready source of mRNA such as the mRNA for alpha- and beta-globin in reticulocytes then complementary DNA (cDNA) may be made using reverse transcription.
3. If the DNA sequence is not known, then an isolated segment of DNA which is known to be situated very close to the same region of the chromosome may be selected and used to track the inheritasnce of a specific structural gene within a family.

In practice most gene probes used in clinical work have been isolated from individual chromosomes sorted by their differential fluorescence, and prepared as a gene library by cloning the smaller fragments into bacterial plasmids. Once in this form the probes can be multiplied up by growing the bacteria and will be available for repeated use. In order to use the probe in analysis of a patient's DNA it must be labeled either with an isotope such as P32 or often more conveniently with a non-isotopic method.

To illustrate how a gene probe could be used in diagnosis a simple example is illustrated in Figure 12.28. If it is necessary to determine whether a blood sample is from a male or female, DNA is extracted from the sample and denatured to make it single stranded.

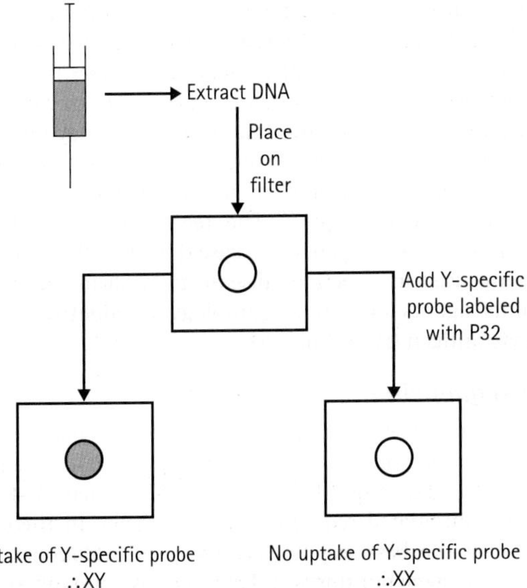

Fig. 12.28 Dot blotting using a Y-specific probe.

This DNA is then put on a filter and an isotope labeled Y-specific probe is added to the filter. The Y-specific probe is a DNA sequence derived from the Y chromosome and only found on the Y chromosome. If the individual is male, the Y-specific probe with the isotope will bind on to the individual's DNA and when this is exposed to an X-ray plate, it shows up as a 'hot dot'. If the individual is female then the Y-specific probe will not find a complementary sequence to bind to and is washed off the filter, so that when the filter is exposed to radiographic plate, no dot shows up.

Southern blotting

The first widespread use of DNA hybridization was Southern blotting, but is now being superceded by new techniques. The DNA is extracted and cut into small fragments with a *restriction enzyme* which will recognize specific DNA sequences and cleave the DNA at these points. The DNA may then be separated by electrophoresis so that the smallest fragments move fastest through the gel. If this is compared to a control sample the specific size of the DNA fragment may be estimated. Throughout the genome there will be variations or polymorphisms in the cutting sites for the restriction enzymes [*restriction fragment length polymorphisms* (RFLPs)] and therefore it will be possible to study the pattern of inheritance of these RFLPs within a family. If a particular RFLP is located close to a disease gene locus, it will be possible to follow the segregation through the family and make use of this in predicting whether or not a disease has been passed on within the family. The main disadvantages of using Southern blotting are that it takes relatively large amounts of DNA and involves the use of radioisotopes, which require some days to develop on the X-ray plate.

It should be noted that this technique is named after its originator (Southern[54]), but rather confusingly a geographical nomenclature has been applied to other techniques, e.g. a DNA–RNA blot is known as a Northern blot, and a protein–monoclonal antibody analysis is known as a Western blot!

Polymerase chain reaction

The polymerase chain reaction (PCR) is now the most frequently used technique in molecular biology. It basically is used to study a specific area of DNA using short complementary sequences of DNA (*oligonucleotides*) from both the 3' and the 5' ends of the DNA to be studied. These oligonucleotides build copies of the DNA using a *heat stable polymerase* (Taq 1). It is then possible to heat the mixture and the DNA strands will separate. On cooling, the DNA can once more be duplicated and the process repeated again and again leading to an exponential increase in the copies of the two fragments. The main advantages of this technique are that it is very quick, highly sensitive and very robust and it can be used to study mRNA as well as DNA. It can also be used to study very small amounts of almost any tissue, e.g. the blood spots on a Guthrie card or the cells found in a mouth wash sample.[55] The technique is widely used in molecular diagnosis of genetic disease (Figs 12.29 and 12.30). It is also being used in infectious disease to confirm the presence of infectious agents and in immunology to identify the human leukocyte antigen (HLA) haplotype.

Gene sequencing

There are a number of techniques available to decode or sequence a gene into its component nucleotide bases. Originally the process of sequencing a gene might have taken a PhD student 3–4 years but now semi-automated sequencers are available. In theory it may appear that the best way to identify gene mutations is to fully sequence the gene but this is still a major task and full exclusion of mutations causing the disease will still be very difficult, expensive and time consuming. Figure 12.31 illustrates the use of a gene sequencer in identifying a mutation in the ROR2 gene in a patient with Robinow syndrome and shows a point mutation in the gene sequencer printout.

A different strategy is to take a two step approach and to carry out a screen for mismatch between the known DNA sequence and the patient's DNA first and then to look at any areas of mismatch with full sequencing. A number of techniques have therefore been evolved to screen for mismatching between the known gene sequence and the patient's DNA. Single stranded conformation polymorphism (SSCP) analysis is relatively inexpensive but has limited sensitivity. Another technique known as denaturing high performance liquid chromatography (HPLC) requires relatively expensive equipment but is very sensitive and can be used with a high throughput of samples. A protein truncation test may be used

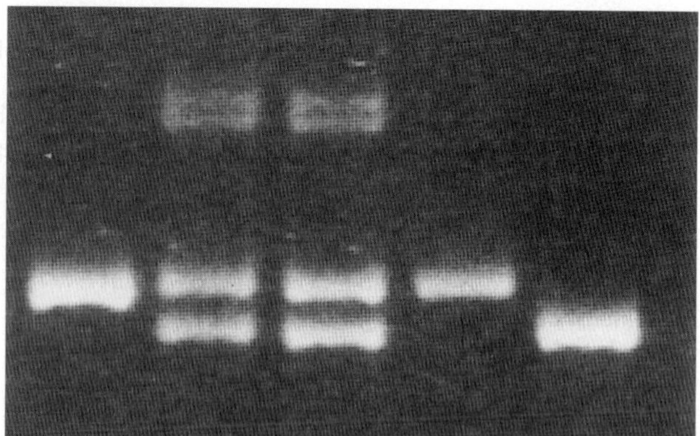

Fig. 12.29 PCR of exon of CFTR gene. Lanes 1 and 4 show homozygous normal individuals. Lanes 2 and 3 show heterozygous carriers of the ΔF508 mutation and lane 5 shows an affected homozygous ΔF508 individual. (Courtesy of R. Taylor)

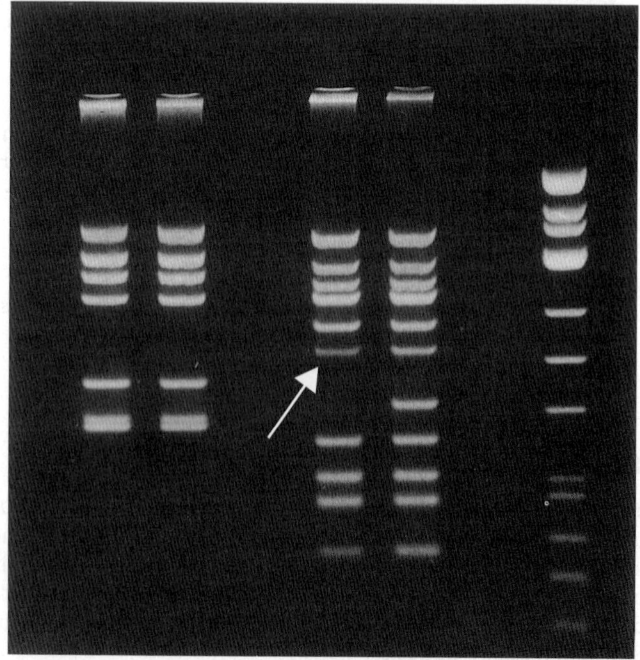

Fig. 12.30 Multiplex PCR testing for deletions in the dystrophin gene. The third lane from the left shows a band missing in amplifying exons from the 3' end of the gene, indicating a patient affected with Duchenne muscular dystrophy. (Courtesy of R. Taylor)

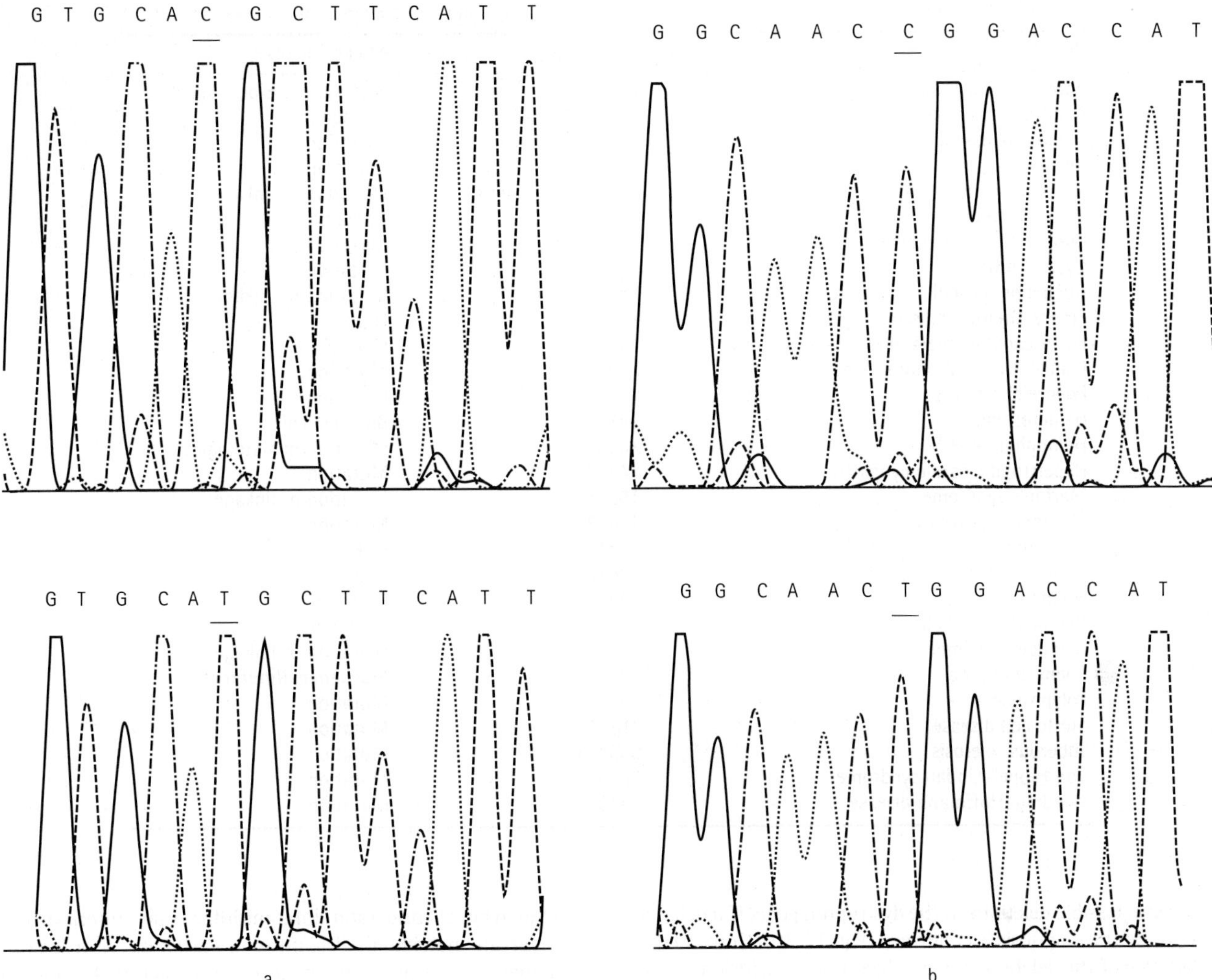

Fig. 12.31 Gene sequencing of the ROR2 gene in Robinow syndrome. The bases are labelled fluorescently and scanned. The upper printout shows the normal sequences and the lower printout shows two point mutations (a) is a 550C → T and (b) is a 565C → T change (Courtesy of Dr Afzal).

to screen for mutations that lead to terminating mutations which shorten the gene product.

Some researchers have looked to the computer industry for inspiration and have tried to develop a DNA chip consisting of a microarray of literally thousands of individual DNA hybridization reactions on a small silicon wafer. Each reaction would cause a color change and the whole chip would be read by an automated scanning microscope. By further analogy with the computer industry further development may increase the number of reactions per chip and bring the cost per test down.

The techniques of molecular genetics have moved out of the research laboratory into the diagnostics laboratory. There are now many diseases in which gene analysis may help in diagnosis, but it is still necessary to recognize the limitations of the present technology. A summary of these is given in Table 12.12. The tests roughly fall into three groups:

1. Fully diagnostic – In these diseases there is only one mutation and analysis of this will give a clear and conclusive result which may be used to confirm or exclude the disorder. Examples of these are sickle cell disease where the only mutation is the point mutation in position 6 of the beta-globin chain and in myotonic dystrophy and fragile X where there is an expansion of a triplet repeat sequence.
2. Partially diagnostic – In these disorders there is more than one mutation that may cause the disorder and while it may be possible to make a clear positive diagnosis it is more difficult to exclude the diagnosis without fully sequencing the whole gene. There are many examples of this, but two will illustrate the point.
   - In cystic fibrosis around 70–80% of patients have a deletion of the codon for phenylalanine at position 508 (ΔF508) and if a patient is found to be homozygous for this mutation the diagnosis is confirmed (Fig. 12.29). If, however, the patient without a family history of cystic fibrosis is tested for ΔF508 and is found not to have it, the diagnosis is not completely excluded as it is possible to have any one of several hundred other mutations. Rather than trying to test for such a large number of mutations it is possible to test for the commonest 20 mutations using a multiplex PCR test and this will give a 95% exclusion which is sufficient in most cases. The problem also exists if the patient is found to be heterozygous for ΔF508. The patient might be an unaffected heterozygote carrier or could be an affected homozygote with another rarer mutation on the other chromosome 7.
   - The other example is Duchenne muscular dystrophy. By using a combination of gene probes it is possible to look for

Table 12.12 Single gene disorders with their chromosome locations and approaches to diagnostic testing

Disease	Location(s)	Molecular tests
Adrenoleukodystrophy	Xq27	Mutation or biochemical
Adult polycystic kidney disease	16p13, 4q13	Linkage
Alpha-thalassemia	16p13	Mutation
Beta-thalassemia	11p15	Mutation
Charcot–Marie–Tooth disease	17p11, 1q21, Xq13	Mutation or linkage
Color blindness	Xq27	Research
Congenital adrenal hyperplasia	6p21	Mutation
Cystic fibrosis	7q31	Mutation
Duchenne muscular dystrophy	Xp21	Mutation or linkage
Emery–Dreifuss muscular dystrophy	Xq27	Linkage
Facioscapulohumeral muscular dystrophy	4q34	Linkage
Fragile X mental retardation	Xq27	Mutation
Friedreich's ataxia	9q13	Mutation
Galactosemia	9p13	Biochemical
Hemophilia A & B	Xq28	Mutation/hematological
Hypertrophic cardiomyopathy	14q12	Mutation
Marfan's syndrome	15q21	Mutation or linkage
Myotonic dystrophy	19q13	Mutation
Neurofibromatosis type 1	17q11	Linkage
Neurofibromatosis type 2	22q11	Mutation
Noonan's syndrome	12q23	Research
Oculocutaneous albinism	11q14	Research
Osteogenesis imperfecta	7q21, 17q21	Mutation or linkage
Phenylketonuria	12q24	Biochemical/mutation
Polyposis coli	5q21	Mutation
Sickle cell disease	11p15	Mutation
Tuberous sclerosis	9q34, 16p13	Mutation
Von Hippel–Lindau syndrome	3p25	Mutation
Werdnig–Hoffmann disease	5q13	Mutation

several possible deletions in the dystrophin gene. If a deletion is found the diagnosis is confirmed (Fig. 12.30). However, the absence of the deletion only provides a 60% exclusion of the diagnosis.

In both these examples the molecular test has to be used in conjunction with the other clinical information and the accuracy and limitations of the tests must be appreciated.

3. Genetic linkage tests – In these cases the location of the gene is known but not the specific mutation. By using linked genetic polymorphisms it is possible to follow the inheritance of the disease through the family and make a prediction of whether other members of the family may be carriers or become affected. These tests will have a small chance of error (usually about 3–5%) due to the possible recombination between the disease gene and the genetic polymorphism. As these are indirect tests it is also important to be certain of the diagnosis and whether there is more than one gene locus causing the disorder. The family structure and the ability to collect sufficient samples from the relevant members of the family may limit the use of this approach.

MULTIFACTORIAL INHERITANCE

Many common disorders including congenital malformations show some increase in frequency within families, but follow no simple Mendelian pattern of inheritance. In these disorders the condition becomes manifest when there is a sufficient combination of genetic predisposition and environmental factors. These disorders are, thus, referred to as multifactorial.

One way of understanding multifactorial inheritance is to consider an individual's *liability* to a particular disorder to be a combination of genetic and environmental factors. Liability in the general population will have a normal distribution and it is only those whose liability goes beyond a certain threshold who will show the disease or malformation (Fig. 12.32). This would be a relatively small proportion of the general population. First degree relatives of those who manifest the disorder will have half the genes in common with their affected relatives and therefore have a greater proportion of the genetic predisposition than the general population. If one then looked at the distribution of liability in first degree relatives it would be shifted away from the distribution in the general population, so that a greater proportion of first degree relatives would be affected than in the general population (Fig. 12.32).

While the mathematical model of liability may be helpful in understanding the principles of multifactorial inheritance it is not of practical value in providing information on recurrence risks for genetic counseling. These are best provided by the statistical analysis of family studies. For example the recurrence of neural tube defects in those families who have already had an affected child is around 5% or 15 times the risk for the general population. Similar studies looking at the offspring of those affected by spina bifida have shown a 5% risk for their offspring. Table 12.13[44] gives some of the empiric risks for common disorders calculated from family studies. With new techniques in molecular biology it may become possible to identify the genetic factors in multifactorial disorders. This has to some extent already been achieved in ischemic heart disease where many of the genes involved in lipoprotein metabolism have been identified.

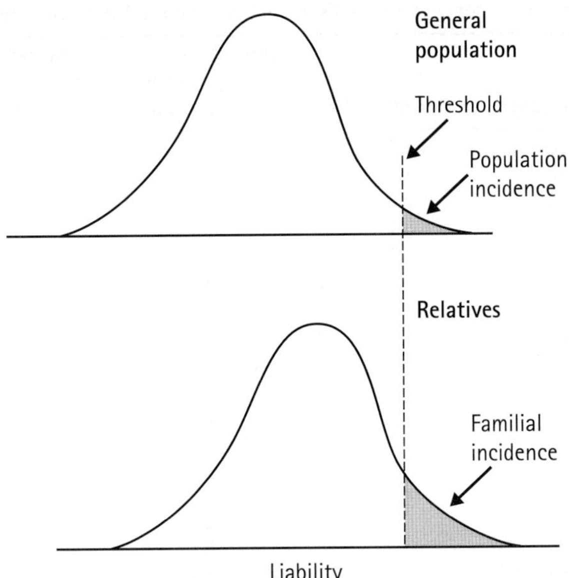

Fig. 12.32 Hypothetical curve of liability in the general population and in relatives for a hereditary disorder in which the genetic predisposition is multifactorial.

With multifactorial inheritance there are some general rules which are helpful.

1. The risk for sibs is approximately equal to the risk for offspring. On the whole the risks are lower than those for Mendelian inheritance.
2. The risks for second degree relatives (uncles, aunts, nephews and nieces) is considerably smaller than those for first degree relatives. The risks for third degree relatives (cousins) are for practical purposes more or less the same as those for the general population.
3. If the frequency of a multifactorial disorder is q, then the risk for first degree relatives is approximately the square root of q, e.g. esophageal atresia occurs in 1 in 10 000 births; the risk for further offspring is the square root of 0.0001 = 1/100.
4. If there is a sex difference in the frequency of the disorder, then the risks are greater for further relatives of the rarer sex. For example, with pyloric stenosis males are affected five times as frequently as females. After an affected male the risk of further affected children is 2%, but after an affected female the risk is 9%.
5. The risks increase with the number of affected individuals in the family. The risk after a second affected child is more than twice the risk after a single affected child. For example after one child with a cleft lip and palate the risk is 4%, but after two affected children it is 10%.
6. In theory the recurrence data collected from family studies are only relevant for the same racial group and geographical area. If there are differences in the incidence of a disorder in different racial groups and countries, then care must be taken in applying the data, e.g. the recurrence risk for anencephaly and spina bifida is less in blacks than whites.

The epidemiological studies in neural tube defects have shown the value of looking at both the environmental and genetics aspects of multifactorial disease. The studies looked at the geographic variation of spina bifida and also looked at environmental factors, which might explain this variation. It was suspected that dietary factors and especially vitamin intake was important. Eventually trials with periconceptual supplementation of folic acid to pregnant mothers at higher risk of having a child with a neural tube defect demonstrated the predicted rate of the malformation could be reduced by 60%. This together with the use of rubella vaccination are excellent examples of the primary prevention of congenital abnormalities.

MALFORMATION SYNDROMES

The majority of single congenital malformations have a multifactorial inheritance and a relatively low risk of recurrence. In the case of multiple malformations or the combination of mental handicap and congenital abnormalities, then considerable care needs to be exercised, since a proportion of such cases are caused by single gene mutations and consequently have a high risk of recurrence.

Another reason why it is important to recognize when a malformation is part of a syndrome is that it may give a better indication of the ultimate prognosis or likelihood of subsequent complications. For example, the Stickler syndrome is an autosomal dominant disorder with variable expression. It may present in the newborn with a cleft palate and micrognathia and a characteristic facial appearance with a flat nasal bridge (Fig. 12.33). There is often severe myopia and possibly retinal detachment; by anticipatory follow-up the retinal detachment can be prevented by early treatment.

The clinical approach to the diagnosis and study of malformations and birth defects is known as *dysmorphology*.[14] There are a number of concepts that are useful in delineating patterns of malformation.

1. A *syndrome* is a recognized pattern of clinical abnormalities that have a single cause, e.g. the Meckel syndrome is an autosomal recessive disorder in which postaxial polydactyly, encephalocele, cystic dysplastic kidneys and hepatic fibrosis occur together.

Table 12.13 Recurrence risks (%) for some common disorders (From Emery 1983[44] with permission)

Disorder	Incidence	Sex ratio M:F	Normal parents having a second affected child	Affected parent having an affected child	Affected parent having a second affected child
Anencephaly	0.20	1:2	5*	–	–
Asthma	3–4	1:1	10	26	–
Cleft palate only	0.04	2:3	2	7	15
Cleft lip ± cleft palate	0.10	3:2	4	4	10
Club foot	0.10	2:1	3	3	10
Congenital heart disease (all types)	0.50	–	1–4	1–4	–
Diabetes mellitus (early onset)	0.20	1:1	8	8	10
Dislocation of hip	0.07	1:6	4	4	10
Epilepsy ('idiopathic')	0.50	1:1	5	5	10
Hirschsprung's disease	0.02	4:1		–	–
Male index			2	–	–
Female index			8	–	–
Mental retardation ('idiopathic')	0.30–0.50	1:1	3–5	–	–
Profound childhood deafness	0.10	1:1	10	8	–
Pyloric stenosis	0.30	5:1			
Male index			2	4	13
Female index			10	17	38
Renal agenesis (bilateral)	0.01	3:1			
Male index			3	–	–
Female index			7	–	–
Schizophrenia	1–2	1:1	10	16	–
Scoliosis (idiopathic, adolescent)	0.22	1:6	7	5	–
Spina bifida	0.30	2:3	5*	3*	–

*Anencephaly *or* spina bifida.

2. An *anomalad* is a recognized pattern of congenital abnormalities that may have several different causes, e.g. the Robin anomalad of micrognathia, cleft palate and posteriorly displaced tongue may be a feature of Stickler's syndrome, fetal compression, cerebrocostal syndrome and others.
3. An *association* is a combination of congenital abnormalities that occur together at a frequency greater than by chance alone, but do not appear to recur in families, e.g. the VATER association is a combination of Vertebral abnormalities, Anal atresia, TracheoEsophageal fistula, Radial and Renal abnormalities. The combination of abnormalities might represent an insult at a specific point in embryonic development which affects all systems developing at that particular time in embryogenesis.
4. A *sequence* is a series of malformations that arise secondary to one specific developmental incident, e.g. in the prune belly sequence urethral or bladder neck obstruction leads to bladder distension which in turn leads to abdominal distension, hydronephrosis and possibly interference with testicular descent and the iliac blood supply. When the pressure is sufficient to overcome the obstruction the bladder may deflate leaving the characteristic wrinkled prune belly appearance.
5. A *deformation* arises not from an error in embryological development but because normal fetal growth is restricted, e.g. the low set ears, micrognathia and joint contractures seen with oligohydramnios in utero.

THE CLINICAL APPROACH TO THE DIAGNOSIS OF A DYSMORPHIC SYNDROME

With the exception of radiological and cytogenetic investigations the diagnosis of a dysmorphic syndrome rarely depends on laboratory investigations. It is primarily a clinical diagnosis based on the assessment of the clinical signs and knowledge of the pattern of abnormalities seen in the dysmorphic syndromes.

In trying to weigh up the significance of specific dysmorphic features it is helpful to consider whether they are relatively common or rarely seen outside the context of a dysmorphic syndrome. Abnormalities such as a single palmar crease or partial syndactyly between the second and third toes are commonly seen in the general population and therefore are relatively minor clinical signs. Features like retinitis pigmentosa, cleft lip and polydactyly are rare in the general population as single abnormalities, and are frequently a feature of syndromes and therefore are relatively major clinical signs. Occasionally there is a specific feature that is diagnostic such as the 'hitchhiker thumb' seen in the autosomal recessive diastrophic dwarfism (Fig. 12.34).

In trying to describe dysmorphic features, in particular facial characteristics, everyday language may be very imprecise and subjective so it is helpful to use defined terms (Table 12.14) as far as possible and to keep photographic records. The objectivity may also be improved by anthropometric measurements. There is a

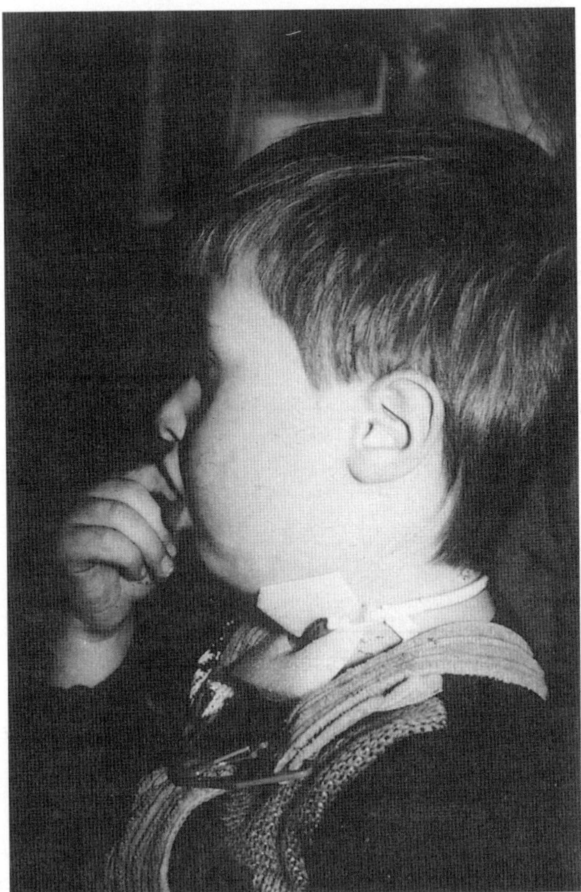

Fig. 12.33 Stickler's syndrome.

Table 12.14 Descriptive terms used in dysmorphology

Hypertelorism	Increased distance between the eyes
Hypotelorism	Decreased distance between the eyes
Blepharophimosis	Narrowed palpebral fissures
Synophyris	Medial fusion of the eyebrows
Nasal bridge	Upper part of nose between eyes
Alae nasi	Lateral border of nostril
Columella	Medial part or septum of nostril
Philtrum	Vertical folds on upper lip
Pterygium	Webbing, e.g. webbing of neck = pterygium colli
Syndactyly	Fusion of digits
Preaxial polydactyly	Extra digit(s) on lateral border of limb
Postaxial polydactyly	Extra digit(s) on medial border of limb
Clinodactyly	Incurving usually of 5th digit
Brachydactyly	Short fingers or toes
Camptodactyly	Bent and contracted digits
Ectrodactyly	Cleft hand or foot
Symphalangism	Fusion of phalanges
Phocomelia	Absence of limb
Rhizomelia	Shortening of proximal segment of limb
Mesomelia	Shortening of middle segment of limb
Acromelia	Shortening of distal segment of limb
Dysplasia	Generalized abnormality of development, e.g. skeletal dysplasia

considerable literature on the use of anthropometric measurements in dysmorphology but some of the more useful measurements are listed in Jones.[14]

The diagnosis of a dysmorphic syndrome depends primarily on pattern recognition and knowledge. The task has been helped by the publication of some excellent photographic atlases.[14,56] As there are now over 2000 malformation syndromes described, a computerized database is a great asset in the recognition of rare syndromes which may have been described on only a few occasions.[57,58]

The subject of dysmorphology has proven itself in identifying the genes that control normal development. Genetic studies in Waardenburg syndrome which is deafness, heterochromia and depigmentation have lead to the identification of a developmental gene responsible for the migration of cells from the neural crest.[59] Studies on craniosynostosis syndromes such as Pfieffer's and Apert's syndrome have identified a group of genes such as fibroblast growth factor or fibroblast growth factor receptor which play a very significant part in skeletal development.[60]

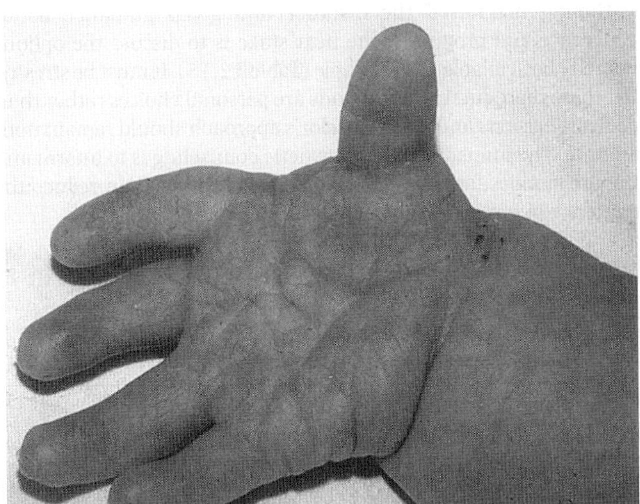

Fig. 12.34 'Hitchhiker thumb' in diastrophic dwarfism.

COUNSELING AND GENETIC SERVICES

ORGANIZATION OF SERVICES

While all pediatricians and other doctors will be involved in providing some genetic information and counseling to their patients, the increasing complexity of medical genetics has led to the development of a new specialty which links the clinical and laboratory aspects. In England each regional health authority (population 1.5–4.5 million) has a regional genetic service, which combines clinical and laboratory skills. One of the important aspects of such a service is that it is orientated towards the extended family rather than the individual, and as such can provide the follow-up required for chromosome translocations or single gene disorders. Separate family records are kept on a long term basis as opposed to the relatively short periods individual records are kept in most general hospitals. In addition to this, DNA may be 'banked' from family blood samples and be available for family studies in the future. Coordinating this may require a computerized follow-up or genetic register. The philosophy of family orientated screening can provide a highly personalized

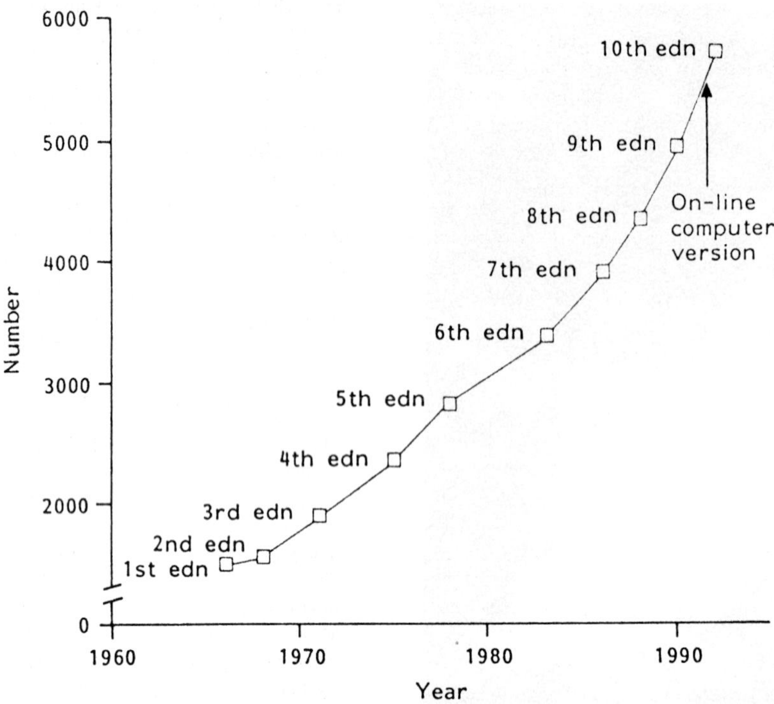

Fig. 12.35 Numbers of confirmed gene loci given in McKusick's catalogs from 1966 to 1992. Including unconfirmed loci the total number of disorders listed by 1992 was 5710. (From Emery & Malcolm 1995[62] with permission)

service which is very cost effective in terms of preventing handicap.

APPROACHES TO GENETIC COUNSELING

As in all areas of medicine the first stage of genetic counseling is to establish an accurate diagnosis. Without accurate diagnosis the counseling may be erroneous. There are a number of problems in establishing a diagnosis which are unique to medical genetics. The first is the enormous number of genetic disorders which have now been described. There are over 10 000 single gene traits or disorders.[61] In addition to this, there are many chromosomal abnormalities and malformation syndromes, and the number of disorders described is increasing exponentially (Fig. 12.35).[62] The second problem is that the disorders are often very rare and thus even a specialist covering a relatively large population cannot rely solely on his own personal experience, but must be familiar with the medical literature. A third problem is heterogeneity. *Heterogeneity* may be at the clinical or molecular level. At the clinical level it means that two or more disorders may have the same phenotype, e.g. both Marfan's syndrome and homocystinuria have dislocation of the lenses with a similar physical habitus, but Marfan's syndrome is autosomal dominant, whereas homocystinuria is autosomal recessive. At a molecular level it means that a number of different allelic mutations can cause the same disease. This point is of considerable practical significance if a specific DNA diagnosis is to be made. Fourthly, the individuals who come to the genetic clinic may not themselves have any clinical features of the genetic disorder in question and so clinical examination will not necessarily provide the appropriate diagnosis. It is essential before seeing the individual in the clinic to obtain as much background medical information about the family as possible. This may mean a careful search of hospital records and considerable ingenuity in tracking the results of autopsies or laboratory investigations.

Having established the correct diagnosis it is then necessary to discuss the prognosis and likelihood of recurrence. It is particularly important to discuss the prognosis in the case of parents whose experience of a disorder may be limited because, for example, the disease has not yet progressed to any significant extent in their affected child. It should also be remembered that some conditions, such as neurofibromatosis, may show a considerable range of expression and this should be taken into account in giving advice. The risk of passing on the gene for neurofibromatosis is 1 in 2, but as only about one-third of patients have serious medical complications from the disease the risk of serious complications in offspring is $1/2 \times 1/3$ or 1 in 6.

Having diagnosed the disorder and given guidance about recurrence and prognosis, the next stage is to discuss the options that may be available to the couple (Table 12.15). It must be stressed that these reproductive discussions are personal choices rather than medical decisions and the counselor's approach should remain non-directive. The immediate aim of genetic counseling is to inform and support families faced with genetic disease rather than reduce the frequency of genetic handicap per se.

Table 12.15 Options which may be available for couples receiving genetic counseling

No further action
Restrict family size
Adoption
Artificial insemination by donor
Ovum donation or preimplantation diagnosis

With advances in technology accurate prenatal diagnosis can be offered for most genetic disorders and malformations. This may be by ultrasound or by an invasive test such as amniocentesis or chorionic villus sampling. For severe handicaps the option of termination of pregnancy is welcomed by many couples but in some cases prenatal diagnosis may also be used to guide and improve early neonatal treatment such as corrective surgery. In these instances it is very helpful for the couple to have the opportunity to discuss the surgical management with the pediatric surgeon when a diagnosis is made during pregnancy.

Choosing the right time for genetic counseling is very important. The couple whose child has just died from a major congenital malformation will usually want to come to terms with their loss before considering the recurrence in further pregnancies. On the other hand, leaving genetic counseling until pregnancy is advanced may produce an emotional crisis which could have been avoided by anticipation. It is to the advantage of the family and the geneticist if the initial referral is made before pregnancy.

While the above description outlines one approach to genetic counseling, it is important that the counselor's approach should be flexible. It is important to allocate sufficient time for the counseling session and to be able to elucidate the couple's feelings with open ended questions. It should be noted that a report from a working party of the Clinical Genetics Society in the UK (endorsed by the Royal College of Paediatrics and Child Health) regarded genetic screening of children for late-onset disorders when there is no treatment for the disorder screened (e.g. Huntington's disease) to be unethical.[63]

It has been shown that a patient's comprehension of the genetic information is limited by anxiety and the counselor must ensure that the patient is given every opportunity to express feelings and be put at ease as far as possible. It is often helpful to follow the session with a letter to the family outlining the important pieces of information and give them the opportunity of a further session or sessions to discuss the matter further. The consequences of genetic counseling can be profound and far reaching and so such advice should not be given lightly. Further information on genetic counseling is given elsewhere.[64]

GENETIC SCREENING IN THE POPULATION

The usual provision of genetic services is on an individual or family basis. The follow-up in families may be extended to the wider family and may be on a long term basis. This approach is difficult using the normal hospital record systems and a computerized genetic register may be developed. The genetic register can program follow-up for screening tests and make appointments for counseling when children grow up and want to make their own decisions.

It has also been recognized that genetic testing might be very effective for public health screening and the prevention of inherited disease. The development of genetic services for population screening requires a different approach (Ch. 4. Ethical aspects of genetic testing). The development of a population screening program should meet certain criteria:

1. The screening test should allow a useful outcome either because early diagnosis will improve treatment or because genetic testing allows reproductive choice.
2. The testing should be socially and ethically acceptable which means that issues of consent and discrimination need to have been fully considered.
3. The screening test must be accurate with a high sensitivity and specificity.
4. The screening program should be cost effective with the benefits outweighing the costs.

In many inherited diseases the rarity of the condition will not justify specific screening in the population but there is the possibility of adding many other tests on to the present neonatal blood spots as many different PCR tests can be undertaken with the same sample. Such an approach would widely increase the opportunity for screening but would require a great deal more information to be given with a consent process. There is considerable debate at present about the possibility of neonatal screening for cystic fibrosis. It is relatively easy to include on the Guthrie card but as explained the genetic tests only pick up 95% of the known mutations which limits the accuracy of the test. There is also a debate about whether the outcome of testing should be early treatment or the detection of heterozygote carriers to offer prenatal testing. Neonatal screening for cystic fibrosis is being piloted in a number of limited studies at present (see also Ch. 18).

There are several screening tests routinely used in pregnancy (see also Ch. 9). Screening for rubella, venereal disease and rhesus incompatibility have long been established. The screening for Down syndrome is also widely used although different approaches may be taken. The use of fetal ultrasound has also allowed many fetal malformations to be recognized at an early stage, but there may be difficulties in considering this as a screening test. The test is usually used to monitor normal fetal growth and formal consent for screening for malformations is not always requested. This may be a problem for couples who would not consider the option of termination of pregnancy. Similarly some of the ultrasound findings are also difficult to interpret and unnecessary anxieties may be raised.

With carrier screening for genetic disorders there is often a difficulty in knowing which stage of life is best for screening. The neonatal period may be relatively easy from the organization point of view but the knowledge of carrier status is not needed at that stage and results will often be lost before the individual starts a family. Premarital counseling and testing may seem to be the best option but not all pregnancies are planned and such programs have had very low levels of recruitment. Testing in pregnancy may also seem relatively easy as all mothers come to the antenatal clinic but it may be a very emotional time to test and puts a great time pressure on the laboratory for rapid test results.

Many genetic screening programs will take a two stage approach. One example of this would be to take a family history asking about bowel cancer and only to offer screening to those with a first degree relative whose cancer came on before the age of 45 years. The family history is easy to take and only identifies those with a 10% or greater risk of bowel cancer and then the use of resources for colonoscopy or gene testing is only concentrated on those with highest risk. A similar approach in screening for Down syndrome in pregnancy is to use maternal age as the first risk stratification and then use biochemical or ultrasound screening as a second risk stratification with chromosome testing only offered to those at highest risk.

In some populations the risk of genetic disease may be confined to specific ethnic groups and knowing ethnic origin may be the first stage in screening. Such programs need to be carefully designed to avoid discrimination issues. Often the best approach is to make screening 'bottom up' rather than 'top down'. Rather than impose a program with government directives it is better to provide the screening resources to the specific ethnic group so that they may organize their own program. This approach has worked very successfully in screening for Tay–Sachs disease in the Ashkenazi Jewish populations.

Another two stage approach is *cascade screening*. This is effectively a systematic follow-up from the procedure already used in the genetic clinic. For example children with cystic fibrosis are identified and genotyped and counseling is offered to their immediate family. From this the screening can be offered to members of the extended family out to cousins. This means that the population that is screened is at high risk of being carriers and there is already knowledge of the disorder within the population screened. It obviously falls short of comprehensive population screening but can still be very economic and effective.[65]

REFERENCES (* Level 1 evidence)

1 Emery AEH, Mueller RF. Elements of medical genetics, 7th edn. Edinburgh: Churchill Livingstone; 1988.

2 Emery AEH, Rimoin DL, eds. Principles and practice of medical genetics, 2nd edn. Edinburgh: Churchill Livingstone; 1990.

3 Laxova R, Ridler MAC, Bowen-Bravery M. An etiological survey of the retarded Hertfordshire children who were born between January 1 1965 and December 1967. Am J Med Genet 1977; 1:75–86.

4 Philips CI, Levy AM, Newton M, et al. Blindness in schoolchildren: importance of heredity, congenital cataract and prematurity. Br J Ophthalmol 1987; 71:578–584.

5 Mueller RF, Young ID. Emery's elements of medical genetics 8th edn. Edinburgh: Churchill Livingstone; 1995.

6 Tijo JH, Levan A. Chromosome number in man. Hereditas 1956; 42:1–6.

7 Knight SJ, Flint J. Perfect endings: a review of subtelomeric probes and their use in clinical diagnosis. J Med Genet 2000; 37:401–409.

8 Chicago Conference. Standardization in human genetics. Birth Defects 1966; ii, no. 2.

9 Paris Conference. Standardization in human cytogenetics. Birth defects: original articles series, viii, 1972 & Supplement 1975 xi, 9. New York; 1971.

10 Lott IT, Head E. Down syndrome and Alzheimer: a link between development and aging. Ment Retard Dev Disabil Rev 2001; 7:172–178.

11 Baird PA, Sadovnick AD. Life expectancy in Down syndrome adults. Lancet 1988; ii:1354–1356.

12 Edwards JH, Harnden DG, Cameron AH, et al. A new trisomic syndrome. Lancet 1960; i:787–790.

13 Mehta L, Shannon RS, Duckett DP, et al. Trisomy 18 in a 13 year old girl. J Med Genet 1986; 23:256–278.

14 Jones KL. Smith's recognisable patterns of human malformation, 5th edn. Philadelphia: WB Saunders; 1997.

15 Patau K, Smith DW, Therman E, et al. Multiple congenital anomaly caused by an extra autosome. Lancet 1960; i:790–793.

16 Mainardi PC, Perfumo C, Cali A, et al. Clinical and molecular characterisation of 80 patients with 5p deletion: genotype– phenotype correlation. J Med Genet 2001; 38:151–158.

17 Knudson AG. Hereditary cancer: two hits revisited. J Cancer Res Clin Oncol 1996; 122:135–140.

18 Ryan AK, Goodship JA, Wilson DA, et al. Spectrum of clinical features associated with interstitial chromosome 22q11 deletions: a European collaborative study. J Med Genet 1997; 34:798–804.

19 DiGeorge AM. Congenital absence of the thymus and its immunologic consequences: concurrence with congenital hypothyroidism. In: Good RA, Bergsma D, eds. Birth defects. New York:. 1968:116–121.

20 Merscher S, Funke B, Epstein JA, et al. TBX1 is responsible for cardiovascular defects in velo-cardio-facial/DiGeorge syndrome. Cell 2001; 104:619–629.

21 Burn J. Williams syndrome. J Med Genet 1986; 23:389–395.

22 Donnai D, Karmiloff-Smith A. Williams syndrome: from genotype through to the cognitive phenotype. Am J Med Genet 2000; 97:164–171.

23 Butler MG, Meaney FJ, Palmer CG. Clinical and cytogenetic survey of 39 individuals with the Prader–Labhart–Willi syndrome. Am J Med Genet 1986; 23:793–809.

24 Boyd S, Harden A, Patton MA. The EEG in early diagnosis of the Angelman (Happy Puppet) syndrome. Eur J Pediatr 1988; 147:508–513.

25 Malcolm S, Clayton-Smith J, Nichols M, et al. Uniparental paternal disomy in Angelman's syndrome. Lancet 1991; 337:694–697.

26 Reynolds JF, Daniel A, Kelly T, et al. Isochromosome 12p mosaicism (Pallister mosaic aneuploidy of Pallister–Killian syndrome): report of 11 cases. Am J Med Genet 1987; 27:257–274.

27 Grouchy J, Turleau C. Clinical atlas of human chromosomes, 2nd edn. Chichester: John Wiley; 1984.

28 Gardner RJM, Sutherland GR. Chromosome abnormalities and genetic counseling, 2nd edn. Oxford: Oxford University Press; 1996.

29 Schnizel A. Catalogue of unbalanced chromosome aberrations in man, 2nd edn. Berlin: Walter de Gruyter; 2001.

30 Foster JW, Dominguez-Sterglich MA, Guioli S, et al. Campomelic dysplasia and autosomal sex reversal caused by mutations in an SRY related gene. Nature 1994; 372:525–530.

31 Crisponi L, Deiana M, Loi A, et al. The putative forkhead transcription factor FOXL2 is mutated in blepharophimosis/ptosis/ epicanthus inversus syndrome. Nat Genet 2001; 27:159–166.

32 Goodfellow PN, Lovell-Badge R. SRY and sex determination in mammals Ann Rev Genet 1993; 27:71–92.

33 Ratcliffe SG, Paul N. Prospective studies on children with sex chromosome aneuploidy. Birth defects: original articles series. Vol 22, No 3. New York: Alan Liss; 1985.

34 Glass IA. X-linked mental retardation. J Med Genet 1991; 28:361–371.

35 Sutherland GR, Hecht F. Fragile sites on human chromosomes. Oxford: Oxford University Press; 1985.

36 Hirst MC, Suthers GK, Davies KE. X-linked mental retardation: the fragile X syndrome. Hospital Update 1992; 18:736–742.

37 Hergersberg M, Matuso K, Gassmann M, et al. Tissue specific expression of a FMR-1/beta galactosidase gene in transgenic mice. Hum Mol Genet 1995; 4:359–366.

38 Emery AEH. Duchenne muscular dystrophy (revised edn). Oxford: Oxford University Press; 1987.

39 Chinnery PF, Howell N, Andrews RM, et al. Clinical molecular genetics. J Med Genet 1999; 36:425–436.

40 D'Adamo P, Fassone L, Gedeon A, et al. The X-linked gene G4.5 is responsible for different infantile dilated cardiomyopathies. Am J Hum Genet 1997; 61:862–867.

41 Riordan-Eva P, Harding AE. Leber's hereditary optic neuropathy: the clinical relevance of different mitochondrial DNA mutations. J Med Genet 1995; 32:81–87.

42 Cavalli-Sforza LL, Cavalli-Sforza F. The great human diasporas : the history of diversity and evolution. Massachusetts: Addison-Wesley; 1995.

43 Weatherall DJ. The new genetics and clinical practice, 2nd edn. Oxford: Oxford University Press; 1986.

44 Emery AEH. Principles and practice of medical genetics. Edinburgh: Churchill Livingstone; 1983.

45 Antonarakis SA. Recommendations for a nomenclature system for human gene mutations. Hum Mutat 1998; 11:1–3.

46 Bundey S. Genetics and neurology. Edinburgh: Churchill Livingstone; 1985.

47 The human genome. Nature 2001; 409:813–957.

48 The human genome. Science 2001; 1291:1145–1434.

49 Witkowski JA. The molecular genetics of Duchenne muscular dystrophy: the beginning of the end. Trends Genet 1988; 4:27–30.

50 Afzal AR, Rajab A, Fenske CD, et al. Recessive Robinow syndrome – allelic to dominant brachydactyly type B is caused by mutations in ROR2. Nat Genet 2000; 25:419–422.

51 Griesenbach U, Alton EW. Recent progress in gene therapy for cystic fibrosis. Curr Opin Mol Ther 2001; 3:385–389.

52 Strachan T, Read AP. Human molecular genetics, 2nd edn. Oxford: BIOS Publications; 1999.

53 Elles R. Molecular diagnosis of genetic diseases. New Jersey: Humana Press; 1996.

54 Southern EM. Detection of specific sequences among DNA fragments separated by gel electrophoresis. J Mol Biol 1975; 98:503–517.

55 Lancet Editorial. DNA diagnosis and the polymerase chain reaction. Lancet 1988; i:1372–1373.

56 Baraitser M, Winter RM. A colour atlas of clinical genetics. London: Wolfe Medical Publications; 1983.

57 Winter RM, Baraitser M, Douglas JM. A computerized database for the diagnosis of rare dysmorphic syndromes. J Med Genet 1984; 21:121–124.

58 Patton MA. A computerized approach to dysmorphology. MD Computing 1987; 4:33–39.

59 Tassabehji M, Read AP, Newton VE, et al. Waardenburg's syndrome patients have mutations in the human homologue of the Pax 3 paired box gene. Nature 1992; 355:635–636.

60 Park WJ, Bellus GA, Jabs EW. Mutations in the fibroblast growth factor receptors: phenotypic consequences during eukaryotic development. Am J Hum Genet 1995; 57:748–754.

61 McKusick VA. Mendelian inheritance in man. Catalogs of autosomal dominant, autosomal recessive and X linked phenotypes, 10th edn. Baltimore: Johns Hopkins University Press; 1992. Online. Available: www.ncbi.nlm.gov/Omim.

62 Emery AEH, Malcolm S. An introduction to recombinant DNA in medicine, 2nd edn. Chichester: John Wiley; 1995.

63 Clarke A. The genetic testing of children – Report of a working group of the Clinical Genetics Society – Chairman, Dr Angus Clarke. March 1994. J Med Genet 1994; 34:785–797.

64 Harper PS. Practical genetic counselling, 5th edn. Oxford: Butterworth Heineman; 1996.

65 Super M, Schwarz MJ, Malone G, et al. Active cascade testing for carriers of cystic fibrosis gene. BMJ 1994; 308:1462–1467.

13

Endocrine gland disorders and disorders of growth and puberty

Christopher J H Kelnar, Gary E Butler

MECHANISMS OF HORMONE ACTION

DEFINITION

Hormones are chemical substances secreted directly into the bloodstream which affect the specific functioning of a cell or system in some other part of the body. They are produced from endocrine glands. The integration of hormone activity is of vital importance for the maintenance of a stable and appropriate internal environment and for the response to external environmental changes. Few hormones have unique actions and few bodily processes are determined by one hormone.

TYPES OF HORMONE

Hormones can be divided into four distinct broad categories in terms of glands of origin, basic chemical nature, mode of synthesis, transport in the circulation, half-life, mode of action, metabolism and excretion. The properties of these groups, peptides, steroids, iodothyronines and catecholamines, are summarized in Table 13.1. Actions at cellular level are summarized in Figures 13.1 and 13.2.

ORGANIZATION OF ENDOCRINE SYSTEM

The biological effects of hormones are regulated within well-defined physiological limits by a complex system of stimulation, inhibition and feedback control – secretion, delivery to target cells, recognition by receptors, exertion of a specific biological action, appropriate degradation and feedback to secretory cells to inhibit further production. Control mechanisms are complex and may involve other hormones (facilitative, additive or antagonistic), neurotransmitters and metabolic substrates. The principles are summarized schematically in Figure 13.3.

Interrelationships between environment and endocrine and central nervous systems are close. Physiological states, such as sleep, are important in the hypothalamic control of growth and sex steroids modify behavior at puberty. The hypothalamus, situated between brain and pituitary gland, has an important integrative and regulatory role, exerting effects on the pituitary adenohypophysis via a series of small peptides secreted from the ventromedial nucleus near the median eminence. Their synthesis and release is determined by neurotransmitters such as dopamine, serotonin and noradrenaline, and others such as acetylcholine, melatonin and gamma-aminobutyric acid (GABA) may also be important. Some peptides have stimulatory and some inhibitory activity in terms of pituitary hormone secretion.

Neurosecretory cells producing neurotransmitters are in close anatomical relationship with hypothalamic secretory neurones whose axons anastomose with portal blood vessels traversing the pituitary stalk and transporting hypothalamic peptides to the pituitary. Blood-borne anterior pituitary hormones in turn control secretion by a number of glands – thyroid, adrenals and gonads – as well as physiological processes such as growth and lactation. The ontogeny of fetal pituitary hormone secretion and brain–hypothalamo–pituitary connections is discussed on pp. 449–452. Other endocrine systems are independent of hypothalamo–pituitary axis control – serum calcium is the major controlling mechanism for parathyroid hormone (PTH) secretion as is plasma glucose for pancreatic insulin secretion.

Laboratory-based advances are making an important and relevant impact on the endocrine practice – protein chemistry is increasing understanding of how growth hormone (GH) regulates growth, differentiation and metabolism; transmembrane signaling

Table 13.1 Categories of hormone

	Peptides	Steroids	Iodothyronine	Catecholamines
Synthesis	From large precursors (prohormones) via enzymatic reactions	From common precursor (cholesterol) via enzymatic reactions	In thyroid gland from iodine and tyrosine via enzymatic reactions	In adrenal medulla and in sympathetic and central nervous tissues and chromaffin tissue from phenylalanine and tyrosine via enzymatic reactions
Storage (gland of origin)	High proportion	Very little	High proportion	Very little
Solubility	Aqueous	Lipid	?	?
Circulation	Unbound	Plasma protein bound	Plasma protein bound	Unbound
Half-life	Minutes	Hours	Days	? (short)
Periphery	Little transformation	Transformation ++ increasing biological activity	Little transformation	Little transformation
Action	Via specific plasma membrane receptors and cyclic AMP (cAMP)	Via binding to cytoplasmic receptors and stimulating nuclear messenger ribonucleic acid (mRNA) and protein synthesis	As steroids (no cytoplasmic receptor for T3)	Via alpha-, beta- and dopaminergic cell surface receptors

cAMP, cyclic adenosine monophosphate.

can now 'explain' such pediatric endocrine disorders as McCune–Albright syndrome, pseudohypoparathyroidism (PHP) type 1, acromegaly, and many thyroid, adrenocortical and ovarian granulosa cell tumors as disorders of heterotrimeric 'G' (Gs alpha) proteins which are important for the GTP binding and hydrolysis that amplifies hormonal signals. In particular, two G proteins have been identified which are susceptible to naturally occurring mutations: Gsalpha, the activator of adenylyl cyclase and Gi2alpha, involved in adenylyl cyclase inhibition and ion channel modulation. The gene encoding Gsalpha (GNAS1) may be altered by functional loss or gain mutations. Thus, heterozygous inactivating germline mutations cause PHP type 1a in which physical features of Albright's hereditary osteodystrophy (AHO) are associated with resistance to several hormones, i.e. PTH, thyroid stimulating hormone (TSH) and gonadotrophins, that activate Gs-coupled receptors, or pseudopseudohypoparathyroidism in which AHO is the only clinical manifestation.[1]

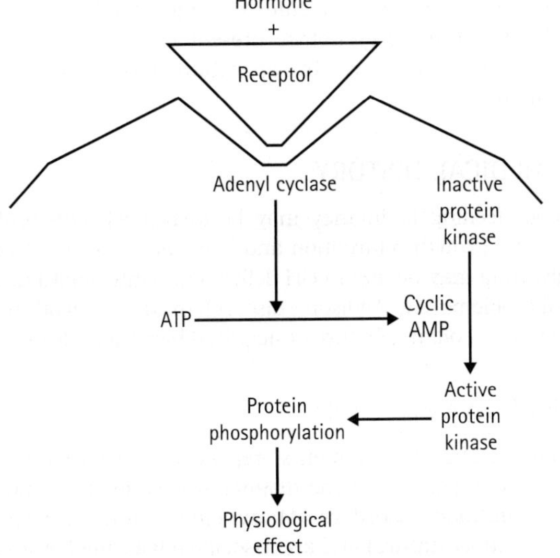

Fig. 13.1 Cellular mechanism of action of peptides.

Rapid molecular genetics advances are enabling recognition of the genetics and biochemistry of sex determination [e.g. targeted mutagenesis of the Sf1 (FtzF1) gene prevents gonadal and adrenal development and causes male-to-female sex-reversal].[2] New disease mechanisms are being described – mosaicism in pseudoachondroplasia and McCune–Albright syndrome; placental mosaicism in some forms of intrauterine growth retardation (IUGR); imprinting (parental origin effects) in Prader–Willi and Angelman syndromes, PHP, Beckwith–Wiedemann syndrome, and, possibly, Silver–Russell syndrome. The mapping of the human genome will undoubtedly lead to advanced strategies for disease screening and gene therapy.

In addition, it is becoming recognized that fetal and childhood growth may have important implications not only for the child but also for adult health and disease (see pp. 452).

A working classification of pediatric endocrine disorders is now available.[3]

HISTORY TAKING AND EXAMINATION

Clinical manifestations of endocrine disorders are diverse and subtle. A full history and comprehensive clinical examination can yield important clues.

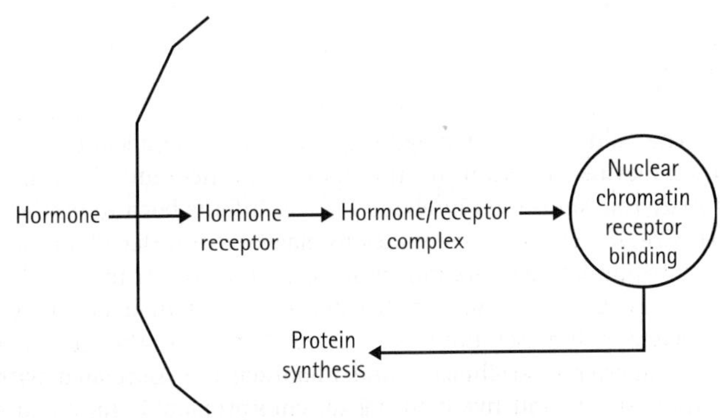

Fig. 13.2 Cellular mechanism of action of steroids.

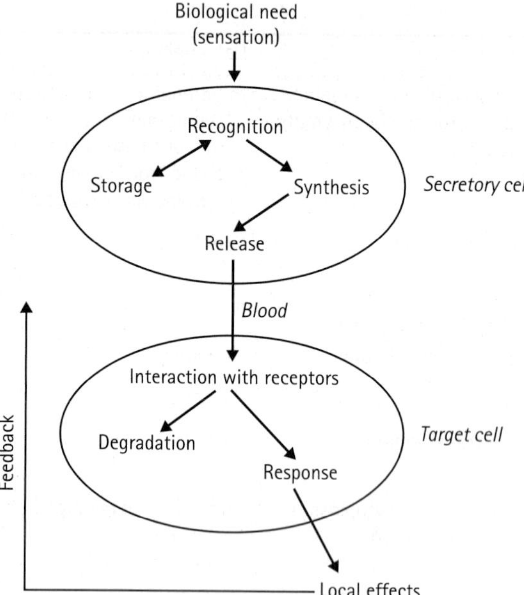

Fig. 13.3 Organization of the endocrine system.

FAMILY HISTORY

Some endocrine disorders are familial. Autosomal recessively inherited conditions include congenital adrenal hyperplasia. A history of unexplained neonatal deaths may be significant in this context, particularly in parts of the world where neonatal pediatric services are poorly developed.

Inheritance in other conditions is less clear: the human leukocyte antigen (HLA) identical sibling of a child with insulin dependent diabetes mellitus has about a 90-fold increased risk of developing the disease before 15 years yet less than 1% of genetically susceptible children will ever develop diabetes. Autoimmune processes are important in its pathogenesis and a family history of autoimmune disease (e.g. moniliasis, pernicious anemia, alopecia or vitiligo) should alert the clinician to disorders such as diabetes mellitus, Addison's disease, hypothyroidism or hypoparathyroidism. Growth hormone (GH) deficiency can be familial.

A family history of early or late puberty may be relevant (ask about age of menarche in mother and older girl siblings; ask fathers whether they were growing fast after they left school and when they started shaving) but there is considerable variation in the timing of puberty amongst normal family members.

Sometimes a child of normal stature is short for the parents (e.g. a girl with Turner syndrome and tall parents). An unusually short parent can have an undiagnosed disorder (e.g. GH deficiency, skeletal dysplasia or pseudohypoparathyroidism; Fig. 13.4) which the child has inherited.

PREGNANCY

Maternal illness during pregnancy may have significant effects on endocrine function in the fetus and neonate. Neonatal hyperthyroidism is seen in about 1.5% of infants born to mothers with Graves' disease. This relates to placental transfer of human thyroid-stimulating immunoglobulins. In the first trimester, 19-norprogestogens (e.g. norethisterone) for recurrent abortion are associated with masculinization of a female fetus. In the second or third trimesters, carbimazole and thiouracil are associated with neonatal goiter and hypothyroidism; chlorpropamide may cause neonatal hypoglycemia.

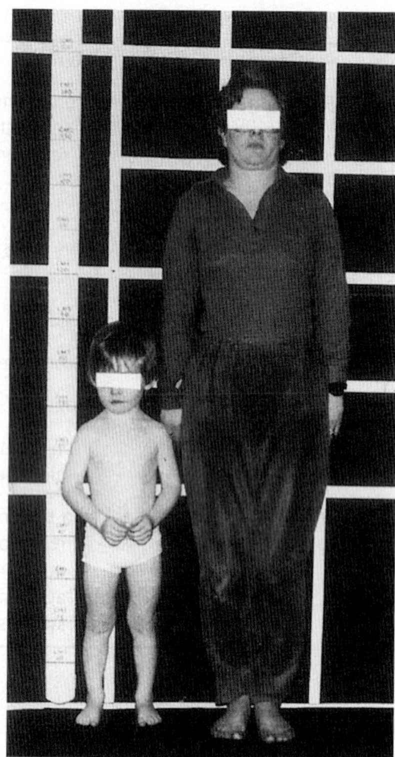

Fig. 13.4 Pseudohypoparathyroidism in mother and child (see also Fig. 13.6).

NEONATAL HISTORY

Breech delivery, micropenis, hypothermia and hypoglycemia are all commoner in infants with GH insufficiency or panhypopituitarism. Birth asphyxia may be associated with subsequent precocious puberty.

Ambiguous genitalia suggest congenital adrenal hyperplasia (CAH, most commonly 21-hydroxylase deficiency in a genotypic female) or an androgen biosynthetic defect (in a phenotypic male). Severe vomiting, hyponatremic dehydration and excessive urinary sodium loss suggest a form of CAH, hypoplasia or pseudohypoaldosteronism (or renal disease). Hypertension can develop in the 11 beta-hydroxylase form of CAH.

Prolonged jaundice is a clue to congenital hypothyroidism. Other clinical signs may not be present until later. Even where screening programs are in operation false negatives can occasionally occur.

PAST MEDICAL HISTORY

Very poor feeding in infancy may be associated with prolonged intrauterine growth retardation and later short stature. Recurrent hypoglycemia may be due to GH deficiency, panhypopituitarism or adrenal problems (e.g. Addison's disease). Insidious fall off in school performance is often a feature of acquired hypothyroidism.

CLINICAL EXAMINATION

Accurate height measurements, repeated to determine growth velocity, are important in the diagnosis of endocrine (and many other) childhood disorders. Many cause slow growth (and, ultimately, short stature) and are associated with mild or moderate obesity – best assessed using skinfold calipers (Fig. 13.5) in addition

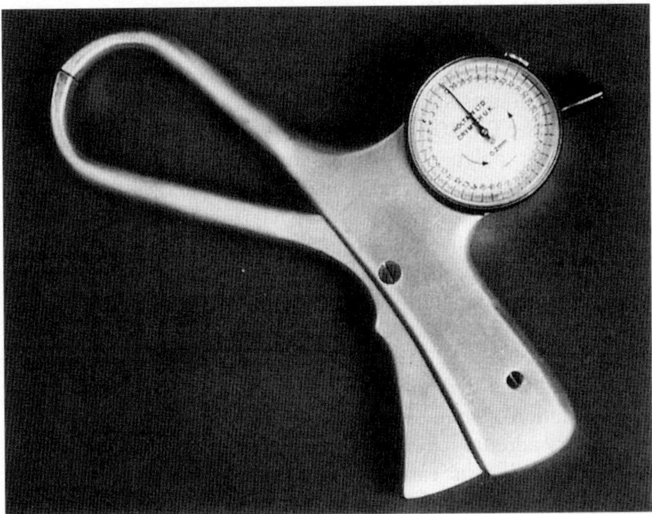

Fig. 13.5 Skinfold calipers.

to weighing to calculate body mass index (BMI). In contrast, obesity due to an excessive food intake causes rapid growth and tall stature in childhood. Endocrine causes of abnormally rapid growth in childhood include precocious puberty, thyrotoxicosis and gigantism.

Disproportionate stature (abnormal body proportions) is seen in longstanding panhypopituitarism, hypothyroidism and GH deficiency, skeletal dysplasias and some inborn metabolic errors. Short fourth and fifth metacarpal bones are characteristic of pseudohypoparathyroidism (Fig. 13.6) and Turner syndrome.

Delayed puberty in girls may be due to Turner syndrome. Primary amenorrhea may be associated with CAH, Turner syndrome or rarer disorders of sexual differentiation.

Hirsutism may be due to CAH or Cushing's syndrome. The latter is often associated with temporarily rapid growth, truncal obesity, striae, and moon face. Secondary hypertension can be due to endocrine disease (usually adrenal cortical mineralocorticoid excess).

Fundal examination and visual fields assessment are vital in any child with abnormal growth or recurrent headache. Craniopharyngioma commonly presents in this way. Dysmorphic features (especially midline abnormalities) may be associated with hypothalamo–pituitary or other endocrine disorders.

ENDOCRINE TESTS

Diagnosis can often be suspected on the basis of history and clinical findings. In puberty, clinical staging of secondary sexual characteristics is an excellent 'bioassay' of hormone function. A girl of 14 years with stage 2 breast development[4] can be reassured that puberty is underway, without measuring estradiol or luteinizing hormone (LH) – indeed a 'random' clinic measurement would suggest the opposite (see below).

Nevertheless, biochemical assessment is often necessary, either to confirm or refute a diagnosis or to assess the appropriateness and effectiveness of treatment[5] but the information obtained must be assessed critically if misleading conclusions are not to be drawn.

Many hormones are secreted episodically in pulses or may vary diurnally. A single measurement may therefore be meaningless or misleading. Dynamic tests to assess maximum secretory capacity will give different normal values to physiological secretory profiles.

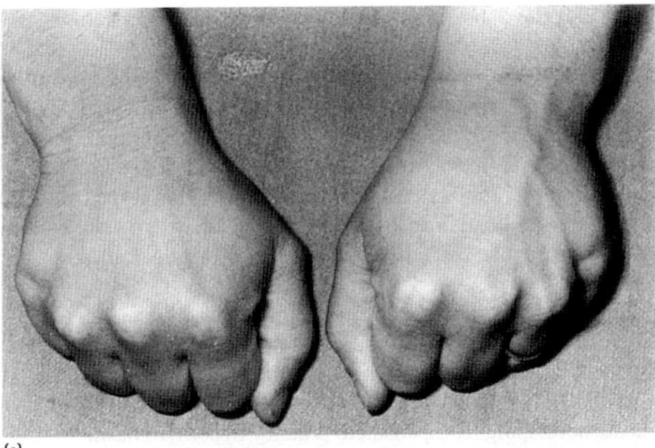

(a)

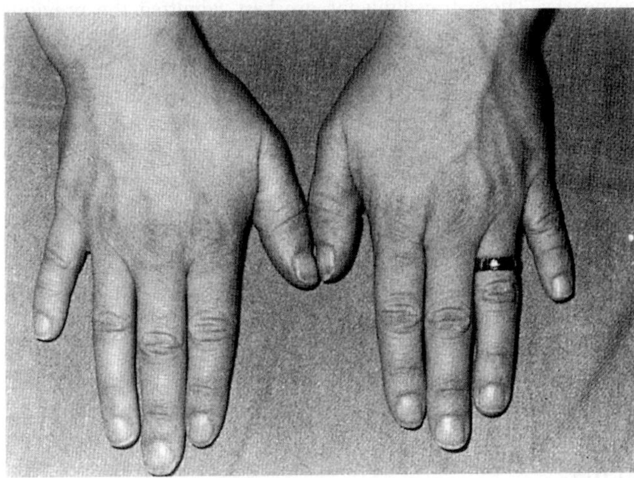

(b)

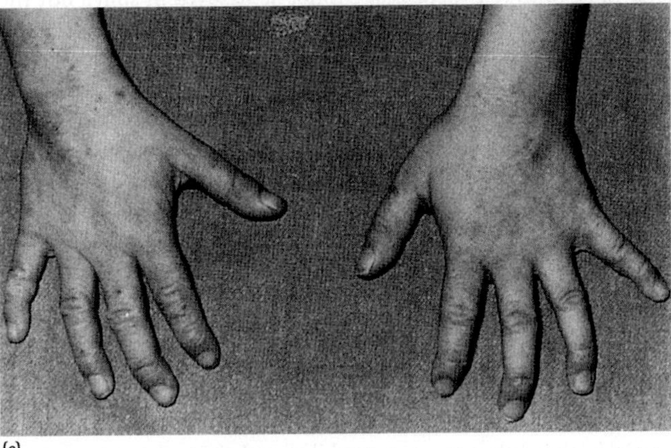

(c)

Fig. 13.6 Short fifth metacarpal in a mother (a, b) and child (c) with pseudohypoparathyroidism (see also Fig. 13.4).

Needless tests provide irrelevant information, waste laboratory time and resources and cause unnecessary discomfort to the child.

BLOOD

A single, random blood test for hormone assay may give insufficient information. Dynamic tests requiring serial samples in children can be difficult or dangerous. There must be no errors in patient preparation (e.g. fasting), request forms, specimen collection, transport to and receipt by the laboratory, and reporting, communication and interpretation of results.

Stress from cannulation (or the thought of it) will affect levels of hormones such as cortisol, GH and prolactin (PRL). Baseline samples must be obtained before suppression or stimulation tests commence. A sample 30 min before baseline may, for example, help to quantify and reduce stress effects or indicate that a spontaneous pulse of growth hormone has just been secreted which will result in a blunted response to a stimulus because of the lack of a readily releasable GH pool.

It may be necessary to measure simultaneously hormones at both ends of a feedback system – adrenocorticotropic hormone (ACTH) levels will be inappropriately high for the normal cortisol levels in untreated CAH; raised TSH levels with normal thyroxine (T4) levels indicate developing (compensated) primary hypothyroidism.

Overnight fasting does not preclude day case tests if the family live nearby. Those travelling far are best admitted the previous evening. Fasting from midnight (water only allowed) is generally safe in the older child provided testing starts before 9 a.m. but is dangerous in a child with GH deficiency or panhypopituitarism. If this is suspected blood glucose levels should be checked at regular intervals overnight. Younger children are particularly vulnerable to fasting hypoglycemia.

URINE

Urine sampling is atraumatic in children (less so in infants). 24-h collections can reflect overall production of (e.g.) steroids more accurately than isolated plasma samples but can be difficult to obtain, even in hospital. Expressing results per 24 h per gram excreted creatinine may not control for this and even distort results.

SALIVA

Many hormones (e.g. peptides) cannot be assayed in saliva but the technique is useful for steroids, e.g. cortisol, progesterone and testosterone.[6] Most children over about 6 years can produce saliva. Specimens can be collected easily and non-invasively, serially or during dynamic tests. Wash the mouth out with water and wait a few minutes before allowing saliva to dribble into a plain tube. Sialogogues (e.g. citric acid or a lemon sweet) may be helpful but are usually unnecessary.

ERRORS

Specimen collection, labeling, transport

Ensure that an adequate volume sample is obtained in the correct tube at the appropriate time. Ensure, particularly during serial/dynamic tests that the collection time is marked on each container, that tubes are not muddled and that adequate, correct information is on the request form. Liaise with the laboratory beforehand if samples need special handling, e.g. ACTH assay samples into cooled lithium heparin tubes, centrifuged immediately at 4°C and plasma stored at 20°C until assay.

Reporting

Laboratory transcription errors can occur. Incorrect comments may be added about the normality or otherwise of a result if the child is of different age or sex to that recorded on the form (first names can be ambiguous), if a sample is thought to have been at a different time or is stimulated rather than basal. Reports may be delayed, lost or misfiled. Verbal reports may be misheard.

Interpreting results

Units can be misunderstood. The Systeme International has simplified and standardized the reporting of many hormones in molar amounts (SI units) but is still not used universally (e.g. USA). (See Ch. 40.)

For larger polypeptides, including many hormones (whose structure cannot be physicochemically characterized), values are reported in terms of 'units' calibrated in terms of 'standards' derived from specific assays from material that may have different biological or immunological properties.

Laboratories sometimes report with spurious accuracy, e.g. to too many decimal places. Standard errors are seldom quoted and may be difficult to define as concentrations of many hormones are not normally distributed and skewed towards higher values. Log transformation often normalizes clinical, e.g. weight, and laboratory, e.g. urinary adrenal steroid metabolites, data.

Hypersecretion is easier to diagnose than hyposecretion – a concentration half the mean of values in the normal population is more likely to fall within the 'normal range' than a concentration that is twice normal (Fig. 13.7)[487] and it is more difficult analytically to measure low hormone levels.

This is important for screening tests (e.g. T4 or TSH for congenital hypothyroidism) or choosing particular assay techniques – TSH immunoradiometric assays (IRMA) give added precision at low levels compared to radio immunoassay (RIA) (helpful in managing thyroxine replacement). LH and follicle stimulating hormone (FSH) IRMA and ultrasensitive immunofluorometric assays (IFA) are providing insights into the evolution of the hypothalamo–pituitary–gonadal axis during childhood and puberty control mechanisms for puberty (see pp. 485–489).

The prevalence of a condition is important in determining the likely significance of an abnormal result in individual patients. Screening for congenital hypothyroidism (1 in 4000) with a TSH assay with 0.1% false positive rate will yield 4 out of 5 positive results in babies without the disease.

Quoted normal ranges may be based on an inappropriate 'normal' population (e.g. of adults) or taken over inappropriately from a laboratory using a different assay technique. Many clinicians underestimate the magnitude of change in laboratory values

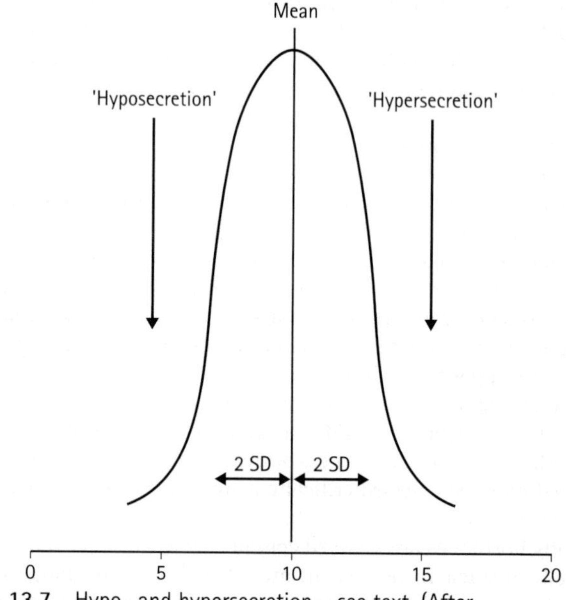

Fig. 13.7 Hypo- and hypersecretion – see text. (After Jeffcoate 1981[487])

necessary before that change is significant in clinical terms – before two consecutive glycosylated hemoglobin results can be said to be significantly different a change of > 21% is likely to be required.

WHAT DO RESULTS MEAN?

Results are interpreted within pre-existing diagnostic frameworks which may be based on current concepts of disease classification rather than clear ideas of pathogenesis. Such preconceptions may lead to misinterpretation, e.g. the differential diagnosis of precocious puberty and the categorization of GH secretion into 'normal', 'partial deficiency' or 'deficiency'.

HORMONE ACTION AND MEASUREMENT

Many assays measure total hormone plasma levels of which only a small amount may be free, unbound and metabolically active. Direct measurement of the free, active hormone is of more value in diagnosis and treatment, and abnormal hormone levels due to abnormalities of the binding protein can be more easily detected. It is invalid to extrapolate from isolated plasma samples to overall secretion or production rates. Circulating hormone levels may not reflect activity at tissue level. Many hormones have paracrine activity locally at tissue level and are not released in measurable quantities into the peripheral circulation.

Many laboratory assays are based on immunoassay techniques. These have, in many areas, replaced pre-existing bioassay (in vivo) techniques. One assay type is not intrinsically 'better' than another – that preferable in particular circumstances will depend on the information sought.

What is measured in an immunoassay may not always have biological significance. For example, in mild acromegaly GH levels as measured by RIA may be very high, suggesting that GH molecular forms with low biological activity may be present.

CIRCULATING HORMONE LEVELS AND RECEPTORS

Endocrine disorders may not only result from hormone under- or over-production but also from lack of tissue response to normal circulating concentrations. Receptor or postreceptor defects ('end-organ unresponsiveness') may be important, e.g. bone or renal unresponsiveness to PTH in pseudohypoparathyroidism, pseudohypoaldosteronism, partial insensitivity of androgen-dependent structures causing incomplete masculinization in some genotypic males or, as seems increasingly possible, in some children with 'idiopathic' growth failure.

Receptor assays, when available, may provide an indicator of biological activity. However structural and functional properties of receptors may not be the same: in a given disorder they could be abnormal in number, function or both. In clinical practice, many defects must be inferred from finding functional inadequacy in clinical term with abnormally high circulating levels of the hormone(s) that stimulate that tissue activity.

LIAISON WITH LABORATORY STAFF, FAMILIARITY WITH TECHNIQUES

Pediatricians investigating potential endocrine disorders should establish good working relationships with their laboratory colleagues. In this way many potential pitfalls can be avoided. In addition, the clinician should try to become familiar with at least some basic principles of common and important assay techniques. Two-way interchange of information between clinician and laboratory staff increases knowledge and understanding in both and provides a more appropriate and efficient service to patients.

FETAL ENDOCRINOLOGY

FETAL ENDOCRINE FACTORS

Profound perinatal changes occur in many endocrine glands. Progress in understanding fetal endocrine functioning has come from increased access to wide ranges of abortus material from normal pregnancies, animal studies (which must be interpreted carefully in applying results to man), tissue culture experiments, advances in non-invasive (ultrasound) assessment of fetal growth and techniques such as fetoscopy.

Although fetal growth is ultimately controlled by genetic endowment, it is influenced by a number of fetal factors (including hormones and growth factors), uterine environment and other environmental factors. Control of fetal growth is by complex interaction between an evolving central nervous system, endocrine maturation, local tissue (paracrine) growth factors and placental and maternal hormone secretion – within environmental constraints which may impair fetal growth (Table 13.2).

Organogenesis occurs at a variety of times and tempos – organ embryogenesis and functional cell differentiation during the first trimester; rapid growth largely due to cell hyperplasia during the second; further functional maturation during the third. It is likely that endocrine factors, fetal, maternal and placental, are more involved with non-specific growth stimulation or maturation[7] and that specific stimuli to growth in individual cells and cell systems result from paracrine peptide growth factors derived locally. Positive and negative feedback loops are important in the dynamic regulation of developmental signaling and feedback failure can cause disease.[8] Measurable hormone levels in fetal circulation do not necessarily indicate a functional role at that time; target organ receptors may only appear later.

ONTOGENY OF FETAL HORMONE SECRETION

Anterior pituitary

The anterior pituitary is of ectodermal origin arising from Rathke's pouch, an evagination from the roof of the primitive buccal cavity

Table 13.2 Factors reducing fetal growth

Maternal illness during pregnancy
Chronic maternal disease
Maternal age (less than 20, over 35 years)
Increased parity
Maternal short stature
Ethnic group
Birth weight of other family members
Lower social class
Smoking
Poor nutrition
Alcohol
Poor weight gain
Multiple pregnancy
High altitude
Genetic factors
Fetal disease
Fetal abnormalities

appearing from about 3 weeks postconception. After 2 months, pouch anterior wall cells proliferate and differentiate to form the pituitary anterior lobe. Growth hormone (GH) is found in the fetal pituitary and circulation by 10 weeks' gestation and levels are very high (greater than 200 mU/L) by mid-pregnancy.[9]

Extrinsic and intrinsic signaling gradients determine expression patterns of pituitary-specific factors in the developing anterior pituitary gland. Rpx is a factor required for early differentiation of the anterior pituitary.[10]

In man, no anterior pituitary hormone crosses the placenta in physiologically significant amounts. Fetal growth continues relatively normally with absent GH secretion – anencephalics are only slightly small for gestational age (SGA).[11] However there is a small reduction in birth length for weight in babies with congenital GH deficiency[12] although postnatal growth failure is more marked. GH receptors do not appear before the second trimester in man (not before birth in rat or sheep). In vitro, GH stimulates insulin-like growth factor 1 (IGF-1) release from isolated fetal hepatocytes by 12 weeks' gestation[13] but has no effect on fetal muscle growth. GH promotes beta cell replication and insulin release in pancreatic islet cell cultures from 12- to 25-week fetuses[14] and any effects of GH in utero may be via insulin (see below). Nevertheless, the human growth hormone (hGH)/human placental lactogen (hPL) gene family, which consists of two GH and three PL genes, is important in the regulation of maternal and fetal metabolism and the growth and development of the fetus.[15] However it seems that prenatal IGF-1 production is largely independent of GH and that IGF-1 (and not GH) is the major factor in intrauterine growth regulation.

PRL [198 amino acids structurally related to GH, molecular weight (MW) 22 500] is synthesized by the fetal anterior pituitary from about 7 weeks postmenstrual age[16] and the pituitary content increases subsequently. Fetal plasma levels rise during the third trimester to peak just before term. Cord blood levels are higher than maternal and normal in anencephalics (cf. GH). Its physiological role in man (other than in the initiation and maintenance of lactation in women) is unknown.

ACTH is present in fetal pituitary by 10 weeks and responsible for adrenal cortical steroidogenesis and growth.[17]

LH and FSH may be present from as early as 5 weeks.[18] At each stage, gonadotrophin (GT) levels are higher in female than male fetuses. They are probably more important for later gonadal development than for early sexual differentiation.

The cytokine receptors for GH, prolactin and leptin probably have a critical role in regulating embryo, placental and fetal development.[19]

Posterior pituitary

In the 6-week embryo, a downward extension of neural tissue from the floor of the diencephalon has formed the infundibulum. This gives rise to the stalk and neurohypophysis (posterior pituitary). From 12 weeks, nine amino acid peptides – vasopressin and oxytocin – are synthesized in and secreted from the supraoptic and paraventricular hypothalamic nuclei and transported via axons in the supraopticohypophyseal tract to capillaries drained by inferior hypophyseal veins. They have no known fetal function. Vasotocin seems to be concerned with water shifts across fetal membranes.

Thyroid

The fetal thyroid is active from mid-gestation and develops autonomously from the mother. Thyroxine (T4) is present at low but increasing levels from about 20 weeks but the more physiologically active metabolite tri-iodothyronine (T3) is present only in persisting low levels from about 30 weeks. Reverse T3 (rT3) levels are high due to active conversion from T4 in fetal liver, and placenta which also deiodinates T4 and T3 to inactive rT3 and T2 respectively.

T4, T3 and TSH were thought not to cross the placenta significantly. Thyroid hormones were also thought inessential for normal fetal somatic (and brain) growth (c.f. other primate species). Recent research suggests that maternal thyroid hormones do reach the developing embryo and fetus throughout gestation and exert important developmental effects on the fetal brain. Thus thyroid hormones are important in human fetal development and maternal–fetal transfer protects the human fetus from adverse effects of fetal thyroid hormone deficiency.[20] Maternal thyroxine plays a crucial role in the development of the fetal brain in early pregnancy,[21] especially through regulation of gene expression for aspects of CNS development. This has implications for limitations to effectiveness of screening programs in preventing adverse neurological sequelae in every case even with early throxine substitution.[22]

Adrenal

During the second month adrenal cortical tissue differentiates into peripheral neocortex and active inner fetal zone. Rapid fetal zone hyperplasia and hypertrophy occurs[23] to comprise 85% of total adrenal size and is the major site of dehydroepiandrosterone sulphate (DHAS) and 16-hydroxy DHAS production. As there is little fetal zone 3beta-hydroxysteroid dehydrogenase (3betaOHSD) activity, these compounds are produced in large quantities (equal to cortisol production) and placentally aromatized to estrogen, especially estriol. Fetal cortisol synthesis is maintained from placental progesterone and, possibly under the influence of progesterone, increased fetal zone 11beta-hydroxylase and 21-hydroxylase activity leads to considerable cortisol production. Progesterone and PRL, as well as estrogens, are implicated in fetal 3betaOHSD inhibition and thus fetal zone maintenance.

A high rate of DHAS secretion is an intrinsic property of human adrenocortical cells and ACTH is the only hormone required for its synthesis. In tissue culture, even fetal zone cells increase 3betaOHSD activity in response to ACTH to levels of definitive zone cells and distinction between zonae fasciculata and reticularis is lost. ACTH stimulation increases intra-adrenal blood flow leading to enhanced zonae fasciculata and reticularis activity but has no effect on zona glomerulosa function. Zonal differences in blood flow may therefore have important consequences on zonal function – adrenarche may be a by-product of the need of the inner cells of the fetal adrenal to respond to the hormonal milieu of pregnancy by developing an androgen (i.e. estrogen precursor) synthesizing zone.

It is speculated that fetal adrenal steroidogenic patterns, which could reflect placental and fetal growth (see below), might provide a link with the development of adult hypertension.[24]

Within a few days of birth the fetal zone rapidly begins to atrophy. By 3 months the adrenal weight has halved and the weight at birth is not regained until puberty.

Gonads

Primitive gonads appears in the fourth week as a longitudinal ridge of proliferating celomic epithelium and underlying mesenchyme between mesonephros and dorsal mesentery. Primordial germ cells appear in the yolk sac wall by 3 weeks and migrate towards and enter the ridges by 6 weeks until when male and female human fetal gonads are morphologically identical. Primitive, undifferentiated gonads will develop in a female manner unless directed towards male differentiation by the presence of the sex-determining region of the Y chromosome – SRY (see below).

In females, proliferating epithelial cords surround primordial germ cells in the mesenchyme. These cords subsequently degenerate and are replaced by others which remain near the surface of the gland whilst the surface epithelium thickens. Germ cells develop into oogonia surrounded by follicular cells derived from surface epithelium.

From the third month, oogonia undergo meiosis to form primary oocytes which, by birth, have completed prophase of the first meiotic division and entered a resting stage. At sexual maturity, they complete the first meiotic division to form secondary oocytes which are extruded into the Fallopian tube at ovulation. Primary oocytes are surrounded by a layer of flat epithelial cells, later to form the granulosa cells – the complex is known as the primordial follicle. This is surrounded by a basal lamina and, externally, a layer of thecal cells. In the maturing follicle there is oocyte enlargement, granulosa cell proliferation and thecal differentiation into inner vascular and outer fibrous layers. Some 6–7 million oogonia are present by 6 months postconception but only 2–4 million primordial follicles at birth and less than half a million by menarche. Most follicles degenerate – only a few are lost by ovulation during reproductive life.

In males, in the presence of a Y chromosome carrying a testis determining gene – sex-determining region of the Y chromosome (SRY) – on its short arm and cell membrane histocompatability (H-Y) antigen, normally the primitive sex cords proliferate and differentiate to form testis cords. These become separated from surface epithelium by a layer of dense fibrous connective tissue (tunica albuginea) which, with the degeneration of the surface epithelium, forms the testis outer surface (capsule).

The testis cords differentiate to form the rete testis and straight and convoluted tubules. They remain solid until puberty when they develop a lumen and form seminiferous tubules. In the fetus they comprise primitive germ cells surrounded by supporting cells which will eventually develop into Sertoli (sustentacular) cells. Leydig (interstitial) cells develop from mesenchyme.

The major hormonal stimulus for fetal Leydig cells is testosterone, and for primitive seminiferous tubule, germ cell and Sertoli cell formation is placentally derived human chorionic gonadotrophin (HCG). At this stage, there is little pituitary GT secretion – anencephalic male genital tract development is normal.

Before gonadal differentiation, Wolffian ducts have already developed (by 4 weeks). Müllerian ducts appear at about 7 weeks. In males, in the presence of a testis, degeneration of Müllerian structures occurs by 9 weeks under the influence of Müllerian inhibiting hormone (MIH), a high molecular weight glycoprotein secreted by the Sertoli cells. MIH is a member of the transforming growth factor beta (TGFbeta) family (like the inhibins and activins). The human MIH gene has been cloned and mapped to the short arm of chromosome 19. There is a critical period during which Müllerian tissue is sensitive to inhibition by MIH – although MIH is now known to be produced by Sertoli cells until puberty, no postnatal physiological effects have been identified.

Leydig cell testosterone secretion is responsible for persistence of the Wolffian ducts and their differentiation into epididymis, vas deferens, seminal vesicles and ejaculatory ducts. Male external genitalia are sensitive to dihydrotestosterone (DHT) rather than testosterone and the enzyme which converts the latter to the former, 5-alpha-reductase, is present in high concentrations in these tissues. DHT is responsible for fusion of labia, growth of the phallus and formation of the scrotum.

In females, in the absence of Leydig cell testosterone secretion, Wolffian ducts virtually completely disappear. The Müllerian system, in the absence of Sertoli cell MIH secretion, differentiates into upper vagina, uterus and Fallopian tubes.

In humans, it now seems that testis development depends on a regulated genetic hierarchy initiated by the Y-linked SRY gene. Several components of the testis determining pathway have recently been identified but it seems that early gonadal development is the result of a network of interactions instead of the outcome of a linear cascade.[25] Targeted mutagenesis of the Sf1 (FtzF1) gene prevents gonadal and adrenal development and causes male-to-female sex-reversal[2] and accumulating evidence suggests that testis formation in man is sensitive to gene dosage.[26]

Development of a fetus into a phenotypic male thus depends, first, on testis formation and second, on hormone production by the fetal testis. Disorders of testicular hormone production or action can lead in severe cases to phenotypic abnormalities or can predispose towards impaired reproductive health. There is evidence, of variable quality, for deteriorating human male reproductive health, including an increase in testicular cancer and falling sperm counts. It seems likely that sperm production in adulthood is susceptible to 'hormonal' disruption in fetal and neonatal perhaps in relation to estrogenic and (especially) anti-androgenic environmental chemicals.[27]

Parathyroid

The fetus accumulates calcium rapidly. Maternal PTH and 1,25-dihydroxycholecalciferol (1,25-DHCC) levels are high during pregnancy and there is active calcium (and phosphate) transfer to the fetus. 25-HCC crosses the placenta and preterm infants have lower levels than term infants by when levels are comparable to those in the mother. PTH and 1,25-DHCC levels are low at birth but calcitonin levels are high. Calcitonin reduces fetal bone resorption; low PTH levels aid bone calcification.

Pancreas

Insulin is present in fetal pancreas by 8 weeks and plasma by 12 weeks and is an important anabolic factor in response to maternal glucose concentrations with major, particularly in the last trimester, influence on somatic size and growth. Fetal hyperinsulinemia causes adiposity and has little effect on lean body mass but there is a permissive effect on protein synthesis and hepatic glycogen deposition. Insulin does not cross the placenta in physiologically significant amounts. In normal pregnancy, fetal plasma glucose levels are modulated by maternal homeostatic mechanisms. The fetus of a poorly controlled diabetic mother has greatly increased adipose tissue stores, organomegaly and increased birth size.[28] Other disorders associated with hyperinsulinism [e.g. nesidioblastosis (PHHI) and Beckwith–Wiedemann syndrome] are associated with fetal overgrowth. Monogenic diseases that impair glucose sensing, lower insulin secretion or increase insulin resistance are associated with impaired fetal growth.[29] Insulin appears to have no direct action on release of IGF from human fetal connective tissue or hepatocytes in tissue culture and may act through stimulation of nutrient uptake and utilization.[7]

Glucagon is present in human fetal pancreatic tissue from 10 weeks and cannot cross the placenta. Its fetal metabolic role is still largely unknown but there is a high overall circulating insulin: glucagon ratio in the fetus favouring anabolism.[30]

Human pancreatic polypeptide (HPP) secreting cells are present in the pancreatic head by 18 weeks but sparse in the adult organ. HPP may have a role in liver glycogenolysis. The physiological role of pancreatic D (somatostatin secreting) cells, present from 10 weeks, is unknown.

Growth factors

By the second trimester, insulin-like growth factors are present in many fetal tissues including liver, kidneys, gut, lung, cardiac and skeletal muscle, fetal zone adrenal, hemopoietic cells and dermis. They are regulated independently of GH and are important for fetal growth regulation. Both IGF-1 and IGF-2 are mitogenic and also cause tissue differentiation. IGF-1 is particularly important in muscle fiber, ovarian granulosa cells (causing LH receptor and sex steroid accumulation) and brain astrocyte differentiation. IGF-2, like IGF-1, increases extracellular connective tissue matrix synthesis, especially in chondrocytes. It synergizes with nerve growth factor in promoting neurite outgrowth from sensory and sympathetic ganglia.[9] Indeed, the primary fetal axis involved in the regulation of fetal growth is the glucose–insulin–IGF-1 axis.[31]

Epidermal growth factor (EGF) (and its probable fetal form, transforming growth factor alpha (TGFalpha)) influences the growth, differentiation and function of epithelial cells, including lung and gut. It modulates trophoblast differentiation and function in tissue culture with release of human placental lactogen (HPL) and human chorionic gonadotrophin (HCG) via placental receptors[32] and may be important in fetal growth retardation.[33]

Overall late gestational fetal growth is primarily determined by the functional status of the pathways by which nutrients are transferred from the mother across the placenta and taken up by fetal tissues. Both maternal and fetal endocrine systems can influence this pathway at several levels, including regulation of placental metabolism.[31]

LONG-TERM IMPLICATIONS OF FETAL GROWTH

Most small for gestational age (SGA) babies are appropriately grown for their small parents, and maternal size, in particular, is an important determinant of birth weight. Some babies seem small because the expected date of delivery is incorrect. However, at any gestational age, babies can also be born small either because of (1) underlying pathology in the fetus (chromosomal or other genetic factors) or (2) intrauterine starvation due to abnormal placental function causing intrauterine growth retardation (IUGR). This uteroplacental insufficiency may relate to reduced maternal and placental perfusion and is associated with low pO_2, low pH and raised lactate levels in the fetus and neonate and redistribution of fetal blood flow from the thoracic aorta to the middle cerebral artery to protect, as far as possible, the growing and maturing fetal brain.[34]

IUGR is now thought to be important not just in the short (e.g. neonatal hypoglycemia) or medium term (e.g. difficult feeding in infancy and poor growth) but because of possible long term (adulthood) consequences. Epidemiological evidence suggests that small fetuses are more likely in adulthood to develop premature adrenarche,[35] hypertension and other cardiovascular diseases and type 2 diabetes mellitus[36] and, in girls, ovarian hyperandrogenism and polycystic ovarian syndrome.[35] Babies most at risk of subsequent hypertension are those born small with large placentae[37] and it is not yet clear how this relates to a pathophysiological classification of small babies nor whether, for example, 'normal' birth weight babies lighter than they should have been for their tall parents (and thus also starved in utero) are at risk.

A suggested explanation for the association between low birth weight and hypertension, coronary artery disease, and insulin resistance, and type 2 diabetes is thus intrauterine programing in response to maternal malnutrition. Such infants could have been exposed to excessive cortisol in utero due to relative placental 11betaOHSD deficiency.[24] However it is possible that the link could be genetically determined insulin resistance resulting in impaired insulin-mediated growth in the fetus associated with insulin resistance in adult life.[29]

Early nutrition is undoubtedly important for long term outcomes – i.e. it has biological as well as nutritional effects – and fetal malnutrition is likely to result in life-long metabolic dysregulation.[36]

PLACENTAL HORMONE SECRETION

The placenta is the source of a hormone structurally similar to pituitary GH (differing from pituitary GH by 13 amino acids) coded by a variant GH gene (human growth hormone V) inactive in the pituitary. Placental GH appears to be secreted into the maternal circulation in large amounts towards full term but has disappeared within 1 h of delivery.[38] Thus during pregnancy, pituitary GH (hGH-N) expression in the mother is suppressed and hGH-V, the GH variant expressed by the placenta, becomes the predominant GH in the mother.

hPL is also structurally similar to GH (85% homology). HPL may be an important (necessary or permissive) fetal growth factor. By the second trimester, levels are comparable to those promoting DNA synthesis and cellular anabolism in isolated human connective tissues and hepatocytes. Actions on DNA synthesis are via paracrine IGF release. Specific HPL receptor binding sites are present in fetal liver and skeletal muscle in increasing numbers from 12 weeks.

hPL, which is the product of the hPL-A and hPL-B genes, is secreted into both the maternal and fetal circulations after the sixth week of pregnancy. hGH-V and hPL act in concert in the mother to stimulate insulin-like growth factor (IGF) production and modulate intermediary metabolism, resulting in an increase in the availability of glucose and amino acids to the fetus. In the fetus, hPL acts via lactogenic receptors and possibly a unique PL receptor to modulate embryonic development, regulate intermediary metabolism and stimulate the production of IGFs, insulin, adrenocortical hormones and pulmonary surfactant.

The placenta secretes HCG (structurally similar to thyrotrophin but with significant thyroid stimulating activity), which is more likely than fetal pituitary derived LH to be the important stimulus to fetal Leydig cell testosterone production.

MATERNAL DISEASE AND ENDOCRINE FUNCTION

Maternal thyrotoxicosis occurs in about 1 in 2000 pregnancies but hyperthyroid women seldom become pregnant unless treated and abortion commonly occurs. After the first trimester there is relative independence of fetal and maternal pituitary–thyroid axes. Iodine, antithyroid drugs and human thyroid stimulating immunoglobulins (TSI) cross the placenta from mother to fetus. Neonatal thyrotoxicosis occurs in about 1.5% of infants born to mothers with Graves' disease (see later). The risk relates more to the presence of TSI than to disease activity and the disease may have been inactive for many years.

Hypocalcemia used to occur in full-term infants fed with high phosphate load cows' milk preparations. The same problem occurring in some babies on low phosphate milks suggests that maternal factors such as osteomalacia due to vitamin D deficiency (or rarer conditions such as pseudohypoparathyroidism with maternal hypocalcemia) may be important.

Fetal effects from poor maternal diabetic glycemic control are described above. Fetal hyperinsulinism causing neonatal hypoglycemia is seen there and in hyperinsulinemic hypoglycemia of infancy (PHHI – nesidioblastosis).

MATERNAL DRUGS AND ENDOCRINE FUNCTION

In second and third trimesters, substances of MW < ~ 600 cross the placenta including most drugs which are often more toxic to fetus than mother. Examples of drugs affecting endocrine function include iodides (cough mixtures, radiographic contrast media) which cause hypothyroidism with neonatal goiter, carbimazole and thiouracil (similar effects), and glucocorticoids.

NEONATAL ENDOCRINOLOGY

By late gestation, the fetus has developed significant endocrinological autonomy. Nevertheless, profound hormonal changes occur during and shortly after birth. This has implications for newborn screening: transient abnormalities may be misinterpreted as permanent, or vice versa.

Important endocrine disorders may present in the newborn. In this section, clinical and biochemical clues and general principles are discussed.

HYPOGLYCEMIA

Hypoglycemia is a common finding in the neonate although the definition of clinically significant hypoglycemia remains controversial. Pragmatic recommendations for blood glucose levels at which clinical interventions should be considered are given by Cornblath et al.[39] Fetal metabolism is essentially anabolic: enzymes concerned with formation of glycogen, fat and protein are increasingly active with advancing gestation in mammalian liver – glycogenolytic and gluconeogenic enzymes appear relatively inactive before birth. At delivery, transplacental glucose ceases. Full-term infants experience falls in blood glucose during the early hours after birth to about 2.5 mmol/L. Normal feeding is important for the subsequent rise in blood glucose levels as are hormonal changes stimulating liver glycogenolysis and gluconeogenesis and lipolysis. Glucagon levels rise, GH levels are high and there is a surge in TSH, T3 and T4 secretion.

Birth asphyxia is an important cause of neonatal hypoglycemia causing rapid depletion of glycogen stores. Glucose is the most important substrate for brain metabolism. The large neonatal brain: body mass ratio largely explains the increased susceptibility to hypoglycemia – prolonged or recurrent hypoglycemia is a preventable cause of long-term neurological damage and mental retardation.

Neonatal hypoglycemia may be an important clue to endocrine disorders such as PHHI or insulinoma, congenital hypopituitarism (panhypopituitarism or isolated ACTH or GH deficiency) and adrenal disease causing glucocorticoid deficiency (e.g. congenital adrenal hypoplasia, hyperplasia or following bilateral adrenal hemorrhage). It is important to remember that hypoglycemia, at any age, is not a diagnosis in itself.

MICROPENIS

Small penis and under-developed genitalia without hypospadias are characteristic findings in a male infant with pituitary disease – generalized, GT deficiency or GH deficiency – or rudimentary testes. The association with hypoglycemia is characteristic of hypothalamo–pituitary disorders; hypotonia and feeding difficulties suggest Prader–Willi syndrome. Other congenital abnormalities may suggest other syndromes in which hypogonadism is a feature.

AMBIGUOUS GENITALIA

The cause of ambiguity, and sex of the infant, cannot be identified by clinical examination alone (see Fig. 13.52) – an urgent karyotype must be obtained. If both gonads are palpable in the labioscrotal folds the baby is likely to be a male with XY karyotype in whom there is a defect in testosterone biosynthesis or tissue insensitivity to androgen. If no gonads are palpable the most likely diagnosis is congenital adrenal hyperplasia (CAH) – watch for possible salt loss in the commonest type (21-hydroxylase deficiency). Rarely hypertension will develop (11beta-hydroxylase deficiency).

Fetal androgen deficiency in a male may result in appearances anywhere between severe hypospadias to a 'normal female'. Exposure of a female fetus to androgen may result in appearances between clitoromegaly and 'normal male'. It is important, therefore, to try to classify disorders etiologically rather than descriptively.

Gender depends on a number of features which are normally self-consistent in any one individual: genetic sex – XX or XY; gonadal sex – presence of ovaries or testes; phenotypic sex – internal and external genital structures. Sex of rearing usually depends more on functional possibilities than on genetic or gonadal sex.

PROLONGED JAUNDICE

Primary hypothyroidism was a common cause of prolonged jaundice in the UK before universal screening but even now, no screening program can identify every case and TSH levels should always be repeated if there is clinical suspicion of the diagnosis.

SALT WASTING

Vomiting, diarrhea and dehydration in the early days or weeks of life is seldom due to endocrine disease; sodium and water loss in the stool from gastroenteritis or vomiting associated with pyloric stenosis are much commoner. Sodium loss in the urine is due to renal or adrenal disease. In renal disease, aldosterone levels will be high but generally low in adrenal disease (CAH or corticosterone methyl oxidase deficiency). In pseudohypoaldosteronism, aldosterone levels will be very high. If appropriate and prompt treatment is not given, symptoms can rapidly progress to vascular collapse with severe hyperkalemia and hyponatremia, hypoglycemia, metabolic acidosis, coma and death.

HYPOTHERMIA

Preterm babies are at particular risk of hypothermia. The SGA infant is also at increased risk because of high surface area and lack of subcutaneous fat. Suspect hypothalamo–pituitary disease with persisting hypothermia, particularly in association with hypoglycemia or micropenis.

THE-SMALL-FOR-GESTATIONAL-AGE (SGA, LOW BIRTH LENGTH) BABY

Some SGA babies have grown slowly for much of pregnancy while others only more recently. These situations can be distinguished by serial ultrasound measurements of biparietal diameter and lower thoracic circumference. The prognosis for growth and development varies with the time of onset of poor growth. Babies who have grown slowly before ~ 35 weeks are increasingly likely to be not only light- but also short-for-gestational age at birth and to have a low head circumference. They characteristically feed extremely poorly in infancy and later may show characteristic dysmorphic features: body asymmetry, clinodactyly, triangular 'elfin' facies – the Silver–Russell syndrome – and present in childhood with short stature.

Some SGA babies have specific reasons for slow intrauterine growth, e.g. congenital rubella, chromosome disorders or major congenital abnormalities. Suspect Turner syndrome in a SGA female baby with peripheral edema.

UNDESCENDED TESTES

Cryptorchidism, in the context of otherwise normal external male genitalia, is much less common than normally retractile testes. Normal testes have usually descended by 36 weeks' gestation due to GT-induced testosterone. They will not do so if there is GT deficiency, defective testicular testosterone production or anatomical impediment in the line of descent (much more commonly a unilateral problem). Even in cases of unilateral cryptorchidism, the contralateral (descended) testis is now known to be frequently abnormal and cryptorchidism to be usually due to an endocrine abnormality at pituitary or testicular level or both. Karyotype and endocrine investigation should be undertaken and hormonal treatment and, if necessary, orchidopexy during the early months of life are now thought to be essential to optimize fertility.[40] Environmental and genetic causes for the increasing frequency of the problem are a current area of scientific interest.

SCREENING

Few infants show diagnostic features of hypothyroidism at birth. Screening programs in the USA and Europe have suggested an incidence of about 1 in 4000, double that expected from results of retrospective surveys.

Congenital hypothyroidism is an excellent disease for which to screen – it is common, unreliably diagnosed clinically until too late, detectable with simple and cheap biochemical tests on small amounts of easily stored blood, and prompt and adequate treatment prevents significant neurodevelopmental deficit. It is generally thought that adequate treatment within 4 weeks leads to normal overall development although subtle perceptual and hearing/speech deficits may remain.[41] There are two alternative strategies for the screening program. If T4 alone is used, there is too much overlap between normal and hypothyroid values at the end of the first week. TSH must be measured in addition in those babies where the T4 is 'low'.

In many countries (including the UK) TSH is measured as the primary test – there is no overlap between normal and high levels, high levels are easier to interpret as abnormal (a level twice normal is less likely to fall within the 'normal range' – see p. 448) and are easier to measure reliably. Hypothyroidism due to pituitary or hypothalamic disease is missed (TSH levels are low) but these babies usually have clinical features associated with other pituitary hormone deficiencies (e.g. micropenis, hypoglycemia) and thyroid function is usually sufficiently preserved to prevent neurological and intellectual problems even with later diagnosis.

Screening has shown transient abnormalities, previously unrecognized, to be almost as common in many countries. In particular, preterm infants may have temporary functional abnormalities and clear-cut diagnosis may be difficult. Any abnormal screening result must be confirmed by definitive tests before diagnosis commitment to long-term therapy but the results should not be awaited before treatment is started. Generally good results (normal mental and psychomotor development) are achieved in congenital hypothyroidism following prompt detection (by newborn screening) and early postnatal thyroxine treatment in adequate dosage.

It is possible to screen newborn babies for 21-hydroxylase deficiency for raised 17OH progesterone levels using the 'Guthrie' test filter paper. The incidence is between 1 in 5000 and 1 in 23 000 (gene frequency in Europe and USA ~ 1 in 100). Boys do not have significant abnormalities at birth and there may be significant morbidity or even mortality if they present without warning with salt wasting. The non-salt losing boy (around 50% in the UK) presents late with pseudoprecocious puberty, rapid growth and tall stature but a short final height prognosis. Despite severe consequences of late diagnosis and newborn screening programs in most countries of the developed world, in the UK it is generally considered unnecessary or 'uneconomical' to screen even though this would only add a small additional unit cost in the screening laboratory already measuring TSH and phenylalanine.

Selective screening ('at risk' populations) has been suggested as an alternative approach, particularly in countries where blood steroid assays are not readily available.[42]

DISORDERS OF SEXUAL DIFFERENTIATION[43]

It is increasingly possible to determine underlying pathophysiological processes which have led to inappropriate virilization or its inappropriate lack.[25] Nevertheless descriptive terms are sometimes of value (if they are not used simply to hide ignorance).

Abnormal external genitalia may be found in many dysmorphic syndromes. Specific disorders of fetal sexual differentiation have been descriptively categorized on the basis of gonadal (dys)morphology into the following three groups:

FEMALE PSEUDOHERMAPHRODITISM

There is virilization of external genitalia with XX karyotype and normal ovaries and Müllerian structures. Important causes are summarized in Table 13.3. Virilization may be due to excessive fetal androgen production or exposure to increased transplacental androgen (maternal or iatrogenic). Some remain idiopathic.

Preterm female infants have underdeveloped labia mimicking 'clitoromegaly'. Clitoromegaly is found in some rare dysmorphic syndromes (e.g. Beckwith, Seckel and Zellweger).

Virilization by fetal androgens

Virilizing congenital adrenal hyperplasia

21-Hydroxylase (P-450_{c21}) deficiency is the commonest cause of virilization in the genotypic female. The degree of intrauterine virilization may depend on the completeness of the block, but the degree of salt loss, when present, correlates poorly with the degree of virilization.

Some females have relatively normal looking genitalia at birth but in the majority there is clitoromegaly and variable labial fusion. There may be a urogenital sinus with common opening for urethra and vagina. In severely affected cases, appearances are 'normal male' with a 'penile' urethra but with no testes in the 'scrotum'. Ovarian and Müllerian development (upper vagina, cervix, uterus

Table 13.3 Causes of female pseudohermaphroditism

Virilization by:
1. Fetal androgens – congenital adrenal hyperplasia (21-hydroxylase, 11beta-hydroxylase, 3beta-hydroxysteroid dehydrogenase deficiencies)
2. Maternal androgen-secreting tumor
3. Iatrogenic (progestational abortifacients)
4. Miscellaneous (see text)
5. Idiopathic

and Fallopian tubes) is normal. Most males appear normal at birth – the scrotum may occasionally appear pigmented and the penis large.

In 11beta-hydroxylase (P-450_{c11}) deficiency, virilization is variable but seems more often severe enough for females to be brought up as males.[44] It is much less common than 21-hydroxylase deficiency but relatively common in the Middle East. Hypertension, which occurs in some, takes time to develop. Males appear normal at birth.

In contrast, in 3beta-hydroxysteroid dehydrogenase deficiency,[45] ambiguous genitalia occur in either sex. Males are incompletely virilized (see below). Females are virilized by excessive production of the (weak) adrenal androgen dehydroepiandrosterone (DHA). There is usually severe associated salt wasting in early infancy.

Other causes of fetal androgen overproduction, for example adrenal adenoma or congenital nodular adrenal hyperplasia, seem excessively rare.

Transplacental virilization

Maternal androgens

Variable fetal virilization from maternal ovarian and adrenal tumors has been described.[46]

Iatrogenic

During the 1950s recurrent spontaneous abortion was treated with natural (progesterone, 17OH progesterone) and synthetic (medroxyprogesterone, norethynodrel) progestogens with androgenic properties resulting in significant virilization of female fetuses. Such treatment is now almost never used.

MALE PSEUDOHERMAPHRODITISM

There is incomplete virilization of the external genitalia, XY karyotype and normally differentiated testes for one of three reasons (see Table 13.4): abnormality of MIH secretion or action, deficient fetal testosterone synthesis due to Leydig cell hypoplasia or an inborn metabolic error, or impaired peripheral androgen metabolism. There is an association with other abnormalities in rare dysmorphic syndromes (e.g. Meckel, Opitz and Smith–Lemli–Opitz). The genetics of undermasculinization is reviewed by Ahmed & Hughes.[47]

Persistent Müllerian structures

This is a rare familial condition. The original patient presented as a 'normal male' with an inguinal hernia, found at surgery to contain Müllerian structures (Fallopian tubes and uterus). External genitalia generally look normally male although cryptorchidism is common.[48]

Table 13.4 Causes of male pseudohermaphroditism

Impaired Leydig cell activity
Leydig cell hypoplasia
Inborn errors of testosterone biosynthesis (see Fig. 13.8)
Impaired peripheral tissue androgen metabolism
5alpha-reductase deficiency
Receptor defects
Testicular feminization (complete)
Testicular feminization (incomplete)
Reifenstein's syndrome
Infertile male syndrome
Postreceptor defects
Abnormal secretion or action of MIH (persistent Müllerian duct syndrome)
Associated with dysmorphic syndromes (e.g. Opitz, Smith–Lemli–Opitz)

Deficient fetal testosterone biosynthesis

Leydig cell hypoplasia

This is another rare disorder, probably autosomal recessive (but obviously male limited) with defective Leydig cell differentiation[49] and testosterone response to HCG. Phenotype is female but Müllerian structures are absent because of normal Sertoli cell MIH production.

Inborn errors of testosterone biosynthesis (see Fig. 13.8)

These result in defective virilization of the male's internal and external genitalia. Adrenocortical steroid biosynthesis is affected when the defect is at an early stage in the pathway so that hypoglycemia and salt loss may occur. MIH synthesis is unaffected; Müllerian structures are absent.

Cholesterol desmolase deficiency ((P-450_{scc}) cholesterol side chain cleavage deficiency, lipoid adrenal hyperplasia)

This is due to deficiency of any of the microsomal enzymes 20alpha-hydroxylase, 20,22-desmolase (the rate limiting step) or 22alpha-hydroxylase converting cholesterol to pregnenolone, causing defective androgen, glucocorticoid (GC) and mineralocorticoid (MC) biosynthesis with cholesterol accumulation in the gland. The P-450_{scc} gene is located in the q23 to q24 region of chromosome 15. In surviving cases, genitalia appear female and there is severe salt loss and hypoglycemia, often with fatal outcome – prompt treatment may be life saving.

3beta-hydroxysteroid dehydrogenase deficiency (3beta-HSD)

Two genes encode for 3beta-HSD – type I (placental) and type II (adrenal and gonadal). Patients with classical 3beta-HSD deficiency have type II gene point mutations. Genotypic males are incompletely (variably) virilized. Wolffian structures are normal. Salt loss and hypoglycemia are generally severe with high mortality.

17alpha-hydroxylase deficiency (P-450_{c17})

This results in GC and androgen deficiency (hypoglycemia and complete lack of virilization) plus mineralocorticoid excess due to ACTH drive (Fig. 13.8) resulting in hypokalemic alkalosis and hypertension. At puberty there may be virilization with gynecomastia.

17,20-desmolase (P-450_{c17} 17,20-lyase deficiency)

This is characterized by inadequate virilization and excessive urinary pregnanetriolone excretion. Gluco- and mineralocorticoid pathways are intact. Nevertheless, a single gene encoding cytochrome P-450_{c17} controls both 17alpha-hydroxylase and 17,20-desmolase activities – combined defects have been reported regardless of phenotype.

17beta-hydroxysteroid dehydrogenase deficiency

There is defective conversion of androstenedione to testosterone and estrone to estradiol. Adrenal steroidogenesis is normal. In most cases, male infants are sufficiently poorly virilized to be reared as females but there is significant virilization at puberty.

Impaired peripheral androgen metabolism[43]

There are three types, which collectively constitute the commonest group of male pseudohermaphrodite patients:

1. 5alpha-reductase deficiency
2. X-linked abnormalities of the androgen receptor (including complete or incomplete androgen insensitivity, Reifenstein and the infertile male syndromes)

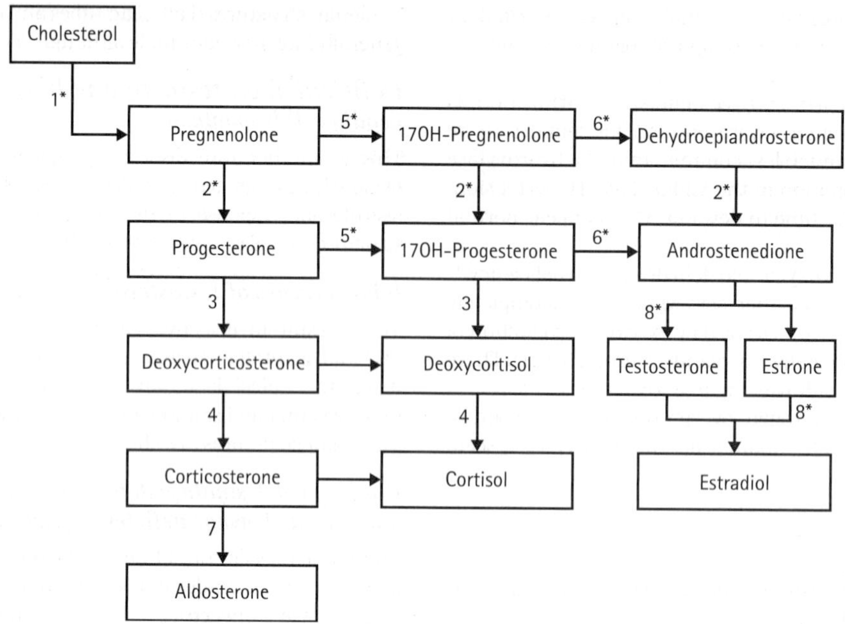

Fig. 13.8 Inborn errors of testosterone biosynthesis – marked with an asterisk (compare with Fig. 13.50). 1* – cholesterol side chain cleaving system (20alpha-hydroxylase, 20,22-desmolase, 22alpha-hydroxylase); 2* – 3beta-hydroxysteroid dehydrogenase; 3 – 21-hydroxylase; 4 – 11beta-hydroxylase; 5* – 17alpha-hydroxylase; 6* – 17,20-lyase (desmolase); 7 – 18-hydroxylase and 18-hydroxysteroid dehydrogenase; 8* – 17beta-hydroxysteroid dehydrogenase.

3. postreceptor (receptor-positive) resistance (a similar clinical spectrum to 2 but normal receptor function).

5alpha-reductase deficiency

Virilization of external genitalia in the male fetus requires testosterone and dihydrotestosterone (DHT). DHT is formed from testosterone by the action of 5alpha-reductase type 2 (5alphaR-2). Two human cDNA clones for 5alpha-reductase have been isolated and the 5alpha-reductase 2 gene mapped to band 23 of the short arm of chromosome 2 (2p23). Mediation of androgenic effects requires a functional androgen receptor (AR) located in the cytoplasmic compartment of target cells. Any event which impairs DHT formation (mutation within the 5alphaR-2 gene or 5alphaR-2 inhibitors) or normal function of the AR (mutation in the AR gene, anti-androgens) may result in insufficient androgen action in the male fetus and in subsequent undervirilization in the newborn.[50]

5alpha-reductase deficiency is an autosomal recessive defect. The biochemical defect is in the conversion of testosterone to dihydrotestosterone (DHT) in the androgen target cell characterized by a high plasma testosterone : DHT ratio (after HCG stimulation in prepuberty). Definitive diagnosis is by finding diminished 5alpha-reductase activity in genital skin fibroblast cultures. Newborn external genitalia appear female (fetal DHT deficiency produces a very small phallus and perineal hypospadias) but the testosterone-dependent internal (Wolffian) genital structures develop normally with testes capable of spermatogenesis.

At puberty considerable, but incomplete, virilization occurs spontaneously with male body habitus, psychosexual orientation and gender conversion. External genitalia remain small but large testosterone doses may produce cosmetic improvement. DHT therapy has proved disappointing.

Androgen receptor defects

These may result either from major structural abnormalities of the androgen receptor (AR) gene or point mutations altering either AR messenger RNA or single amino acids causing a spectrum of appearance from 'female' (complete and incomplete testicular feminization) to 'male' (Reifenstein syndrome and infertile male syndrome). The AR gene has been cloned and is located on the q11–12 region of the X chromosome. Mutations in exon 2 and 3 code for the DNA region have been identified in patients with 'receptor positive' androgen insensitivity. However most mutations are in exons 4–8 which code for the steroid binding domain – 'receptor negative' androgen insensitivity.

As well as natural mutations in the 5alphaR-2 gene and AR gene, recent attention is being focused on environmental endocrine disruptors that are able to mimic steroid 5alpha-reductase deficiency or partial androgen insensitivity syndrome. Any event which impairs DHT formation (mutation within the 5alphaR-2 gene or 5alphaR-2 inhibitors) or normal function of the AR (mutation in the AR gene, anti-androgens) may result in insufficient androgen action in the male fetus and in subsequent undervirilization in the newborn. Hypospadias may be due to a defect in androgen action due to mutation of the 5alphaR-2 or of the AR gene and mutation of unidentified genes may underlie displacement of the urethral meatus from the tip to the ventral side of the phallus. An etiological role for environmental industrial and agricultural chemical products has also been postulated, since ethnic as well as geographical differences in the incidence of hypospadias have been noted. Thus cryptorchidism and micropenis may represent an intersex phenotype, even if they are isolated, and etiological factors include 5alpha-reductase 2 gene, AR gene mutation or environmental hormonal disruptors (chemicals or phytoestrogens).[27,50]

Complete testicular feminization: patients generally present after puberty with primary amenorrhea but normal breast development, scanty pubic and axillary hair, and female body habitus and psychosexual orientation. There is a short blind ending vagina as Müllerian structures have regressed. Gonads show Leydig cell hyperplasia with defective spermatogenesis and may undergo malignant change if they are not removed. In *incomplete testicular feminization* there is more virilization with prepubertal clitoromegaly and variable labial fusion. There may be a mixture of virilization and feminization at puberty.

In *Reifenstein's syndrome* appearance is generally male but with severe (perineal) hypospadias. Virilization at puberty may be significant but still inadequate and associated with gynecomastia. There is male psychosexual orientation and infertility. In the *infertile male syndrome* there is a normal prepubertal male appearance although penis and testes may be rather small. Gynecomastia develops at puberty and there is oligospermia and infertility.

ABNORMAL GONADAL DIFFERENTIATION

This is a clinically heterogeneous group, including true hermaphroditism and syndromes of dysgenetic gonadal development. In most there is ambiguity of external genitalia in the newborn.

True hermaphroditism usually presents with abnormal external genitalia (e.g. phallus with urogenital sinus at the base). Testicular and ovarian tissue are present, more commonly as ovotestes than as separate gonads. The commonest karyotype is 46XX (58%), 10% are XY and the remainder mosaics, of which the commonest is 46XX/46XY (13%). If the diagnosis is made neonatally, testicular tissue should be removed, and gender assignment should be female – there is good feminization at puberty with menstruation and fertility is possible.

XX males usually present with hypogonadism as adults but genital ambiguity may occur. H-Y antigen is present.[51]

Klinefelter's syndrome may be suspected in a neonate with hypospadias, small testes and extension of the scrotal skin onto the shaft of a small penis or found by serendipity at antenatal screening but is seldom diagnosed before the time of puberty.

Mixed gonadal dysgenesis: generally there is a testis with Wolffian (and absent Müllerian) structures on one side, with streak gonad and Müllerian (but poorly developed Wolffian) development on the other. Karyotype is generally 46XY or 45XO/46XY mosaic – the latter associated with clinical features and the growth pattern of Turner syndrome. Bilaterally dysgenetic testes are less common. In both groups there is a high risk of malignant change in the gonads.

Turner syndrome

Pure gonadal dysgenesis seldom presents before puberty. There are normal female external genitalia but the karyotype may be 46XX or 46XY. Gonadal malignant change is common.

Agonadism presents in a variety of clinical guises depending on the timing of testicular involution. There may be normal female appearances with absent Müllerian and Wolffian structures, micropenis with rudimentary testes or anorchia in an otherwise normal male.

CLINICAL MANAGEMENT

Initial assessment

Uncertainty as to the sex of their newborn baby is extremely distressing to parents. Emphasize that their baby's sex will be swiftly determined, the baby is either male or female (and not 'somewhere in between') and that the cause of the problem will be discovered. Birth should not be registered until sex of rearing is decided. Appearance of external genitalia is important in this decision – an adequately functional phallus cannot be created out of very little tissue – but is unhelpful in reaching an etiological diagnosis.

Check the family history and for any hormone treatment during the pregnancy. Look for associated abnormalities or dysmorphic features. The most important aspect of clinical examination is for the presence of gonads – a clinical classification based on their number is useful for planning immediately relevant investigations:

In *all* patients, an urgent karyotype is indicated.

If *no* gonads are palpable: the most likely diagnosis is 21-hydroxylase deficiency in a genotypic female – salt loss may occur. Measurement of plasma 17OH progesterone will confirm the diagnosis; urinary pregnanetriol levels are high. 11-deoxycortisol levels are high in 11beta-hydroxylase deficiency. Male pseudohermaphroditism with intra-abdominal testes is much less common and true hermaphroditism very rare.

If *one* gonad is palpable mixed gonadal dysgenesis (usually with XO/XY karyotype) is least uncommon. Pelvic ultrasound and genitogram, HCG test, gonadal biopsy and exploratory laparotomy may be necessary.

If *two* gonads are palpable, male pseudohermaphroditism is likely. An HCG test measuring testosterone, DHT, DHA and androstenedione will help distinguish 5alpha-reductase deficiency, testosterone biosynthetic disorders and androgen receptor or postreceptor defects. In vitro androgen binding studies and measurement of 5alpha-reductase activity in genital skin fibroblast cultures may be necessary. A genitogram may be helpful in imaging internal genitalia and lower urinary tract.

MANAGEMENT: CHOICE OF GENDER/GENDER IDENTITY

Choice should normally be based on appearance of external genitalia and functional possibilities in the context of information (cytogenetic, biochemical and radiological) about the nature of the underlying defect and implications for pubertal development. The decision should be made jointly by parents (whose ethnic background may be important in determining their views), pediatric endocrinologist and surgeon. Karyotype is usually irrelevant. In cases where the phallus seems inadequate but there are pressures for male gender assignment, information about likely growth of the phallus in response to androgen can be predicted with depot testosterone (50 mg once monthly i.m. for 3 months).

It used to be thought that psychosexual orientation was dependent on sex of rearing but some of the early work in this area has been discredited[52] (for a journalistic but interesting account see Colapinto[53]). Observations in the 'natural history' of patients with 5alpha-reductase deficiency and those with 17beta-hydroxysteroid dehydrogenase deficiency suggest that the role of the fetal testis and androgens in 'imprinting' male gender identity is crucially important.[54]

Nevertheless, ideally, sex of rearing should be decided as early as possible. Conventionally, surgery has been carried out so as to achieve cosmetically acceptable external genitalia by 2 years. However parent/patient organizations (such as the Intersex Society of North America) have been outspoken in their view that surgery should be carried out only if and when the intersexed person requests it, and then only after she/he has been fully informed of the risks and likely outcomes. Guidelines have been published by the British Association of Pediatric Surgeons *(http://www.baps.org.uk)*.

Sometimes, because of late presentation or late diagnosis in the older child, or if there is spontaneous 'inappropriate' feminization or virilization at puberty, gender reassignment is indicated. With expert psychiatric support and counseling this can be satisfactorily achieved but cultural considerations may again be important.

The status of the empirical evidence for the development of gender and sexuality in 46XX persons with classical CAH and its implications for clinical practice has been reviewed by Meyer-Bahlburg.[55]

INCIDENCE OF TUMORS IN INTERSEX DISORDERS

Patients with a Y chromosome but androgen insensitivity or a disorder of gonadal differentiation are at increased risk of neoplasia in an intra-abdominal gonad by adolescence or early adulthood. The risk with scrotal gonads is probably much less, particularly with regular clinical and ultrasound follow-up.

Carcinoma in situ, benign hamartomas and seminomas are reported in complete gonadal dysgenesis patients. In them, therefore, testes should be removed, but some argue that this should be done after spontaneous feminization has taken place at puberty. In contrast, virilization at puberty will occur in incomplete testicular feminization (incomplete androgen insensitivity) or an androgen biosynthetic defect and the testes should be removed in childhood.

Tumors are common in dysgenetic gonads. Benign gonadoblastomas may be endocrinologically functional and malignant seminomas, dysgerminomas, choriocarcinomas or yolk sac tumors are reported.[56] Unless there can be careful observation of scrotal gonads through childhood and puberty (with subsequent removal), they are best removed in childhood.

PHYSICAL GROWTH AND DEVELOPMENT

ASSESSMENT

Historical aspects

Within the last century it has been appreciated that assessment of a child's growth is the best marker of their well-being. Measuring of groups of children or particular populations over time, it has been possible to pass comment about the influence of social changes on the health of children as this is reflected directly in growth of stature and the timing of sexual maturation. The average height of populations in the developed world is increasing generation upon generation but in the developing world inadequate nutrition with its intermittent supply still has a profound adverse effect on physical growth and on the health of children. Growth velocity remains one of the most useful indices of public health and economic well-being in both developing and socially heterogeneous developed countries.[57]

Much has been written on historical, social and international aspects of growth and the following sources could be considered for those who wish to explore this field further, Eveleth & Tanner[58] and Ulijaszek et al.[59]

The normal pattern of growth

The normal pattern of expected growth is traditionally displayed on a growth chart. Growth charts or standards reflect the pattern of growth of a population under study and consequently do not describe exactly the growth curve of any individual child. Nevertheless they are important tools, but it must be remembered that each child has their own individual pattern of growth and timing of the events of puberty. This is called their 'tempo' of growth.

Choice of growth chart

Two types of growth chart each with different form of construction are available within the United Kingdom. The UK1990 standards[60] are recommended for general use (Royal College of Pediatrics and Child Health Working Party[61]). These are cross-sectional charts based largely on single measurements of many thousands of children at different ages and the LMS statistical method[62] is employed to produce the mean and multiples of the standard deviation at each age and thus the smooth curves found on the growth charts (Figs 13.9–13.12). The nine centile bands are equally spread, interval 0.67 standard deviations (SD), and range between − 2SD (2nd centile) and +2SD (98th centile). In an attempt to quantify extremes of variation, two further centile lines (0.4th and 99.6th which is +/− 2.67 SD) are provided with shaded areas above and below respectively. The measurements of 1 in 250 normal children lie above and below these lines but the chances of finding a pathological cause for abnormal growth in a child is greater outwith these boundaries. The Buckler–Tanner charts are of the tempo-conditional type; they are constructed based largely on longitudinal data, i.e. serial measurements from the same child and the shape of the curve reflects the growth pattern of an individual child more closely.[63] These charts are only recommended for height measurements beyond the age of 2 years, weight standards already being outmoded for the UK population. Consequently they are best reserved for the longitudinal follow-up of the growth in height of an individual child. The variations in growth particularly at puberty can be followed more easily, and the additional colored lines assist in determining whether the growth of an adolescent with onset of puberty not at the 50th centile is normal or otherwise (Figs 13.13, 13.14).

Racial, ethnic and national factors

UK growth charts have mainly been constructed from measurements from the indigenous white population, whereas today the population is multiracial. There are differences in body proportions between the main three human races. People of African origin have longer legs, with the opposite being true for those of Mongolian racial origin. The pattern and tempo of growth are similar across mankind. Although African origin and Mongolian origin children start puberty and mature earlier than Caucasian children, these differences are not outwith expected norms. Even if standards particular to each racial group were available, with social integration they would be little use in practice. Standard UK1990 charts are valid both before and during puberty for all children irrespective of ethnic background. It is the calculation of a child's target height which needs to be considered in determining whether the child is of abnormal stature not their ethnic background per se.

Decimal ages and decimal charts

The year time scale on a growth chart may be divided according to weeks or months, or can have a decimal scale (i.e. thousandths of a year, usually rounded to two decimal places). For routine use the standard weekly or monthly subdivisions are preferable as this helps with accurate plotting. Decimal ages are advantageous when the calculation of height velocity is required and when more precise plotting of the growth chart is necessary, for example in long term follow-up. Decimal ages are calculated according to the following example (see Table 13.5 for decimal age conversion):

a. Date of examination:	12th May 2003	Decimal date from Table: 2003.359
b. Date of birth:	23rd September 1997	Decimal date 1997.726
Subtracting *b* from *a*:		Decimal age: 5.633 year

Height velocity can be calculated as the height increment (cm) divided by interval between measurements in decimal years:

c. Decimal age at examination:	5.633 years
d. Decimal age at previous examination:	4.876 years
Height increment over interval *c* – *d* 0.757 years:	4.2 cm
Height velocity (annualized, see below):	5.5 cm/year

Plotting growth charts

Mis-plotting is a common error even by experienced personnel, so care should be taken and the plot reviewed with reference to previous plots when available. A precise dot, uncircled, provides

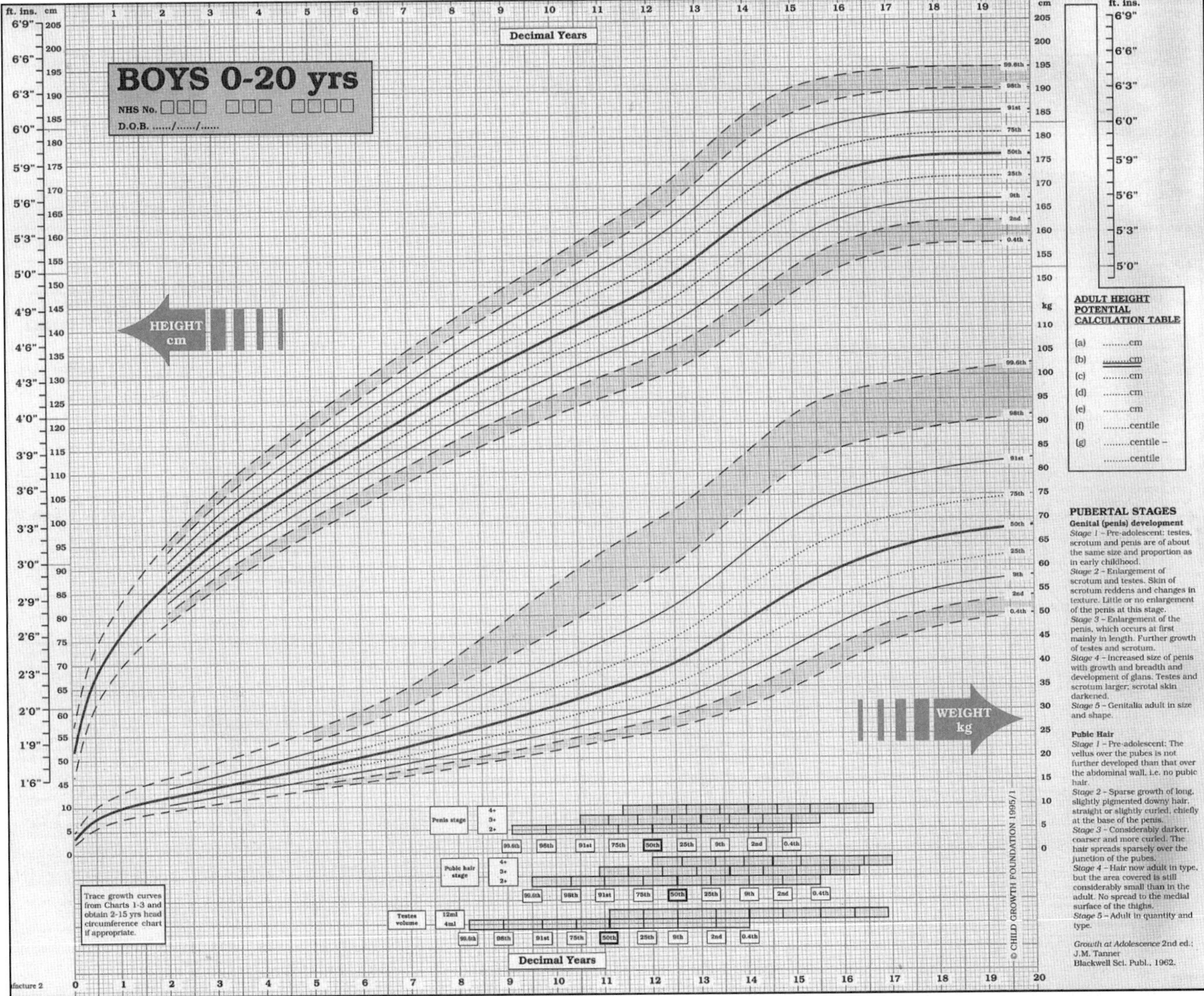
BOYS 0-20 yrs
NHS No.
D.O.B. ....../....../......
Decimal Years
HEIGHT cm
WEIGHT kg
ADULT HEIGHT POTENTIAL CALCULATION TABLE
(a) ....cm
(b) ....cm
(c) ....cm
(d) ....cm
(e) ....cm
(f) ....centile
(g) ....centile – ....centile
PUBERTAL STAGES
Genital (penis) development
Stage 1 – Pre-adolescent: testes, scrotum and penis are of about the same size and proportion as in early childhood.
Stage 2 – Enlargement of scrotum and testes. Skin of scrotum reddens and changes in texture. Little or no enlargement of the penis at this stage.
Stage 3 – Enlargement of the penis, which occurs at first mainly in length. Further growth of testes and scrotum.
Stage 4 – Increased size of penis with growth and breadth and development of glans. Testes and scrotum larger; scrotal skin darkened.
Stage 5 – Genitalia adult in size and shape.
Pubic Hair
Stage 1 – Pre-adolescent: The vellus over the pubes is not further developed than that over the abdominal wall, i.e. no pubic hair.
Stage 2 – Sparse growth of long, slightly pigmented downy hair, straight or slightly curled, chiefly at the base of the penis.
Stage 3 – Considerably darker, coarser and more curled. The hair spreads sparsely over the junction of the pubes.
Stage 4 – Hair now adult in type, but the area covered is still considerably small than in the adult. No spread to the medial surface of the thighs.
Stage 5 – Adult in quantity and type.
Growth at Adolescence 2nd ed.: J.M. Tanner Blackwell Sci. Publ., 1962.
Penis stage
Pubic hair stage
Testes volume
Trace growth curves from Charts 1-3 and obtain 2-15 yrs head circumference chart if appropriate.
© CHILD GROWTH FOUNDATION 1995/1

Fig. 13.9 UK1990 standard centile chart for height, weight and pubertal staging in boys (© Child Growth Foundation).

maximum clarity on the chart as this will not overlap with previous or subsequent points.

Screening for growth disorders in the community (growth monitoring)

Screening for growth and other disorders by height and weight measurement assists in the diagnosis of problems which would otherwise be missed or come to light at a later stage where the outcome of treatment may be less favourable. Many hormones influence skeletal and somatic growth in childhood including GH, thyroxine, glucocorticoids, androgens and estrogens, insulin and polypeptide growth factors. Growth *monitoring* is important in the early detection of disease in children and of particular value in detecting a wide variety of endocrine abnormalities in which poor growth may be the earliest, or only, sign of a problem.

Measurements must be conducted by trained staff using reliable and calibrated equipment. Regular updates on training are required. No clear scientific evidence exists as to the cost-effectiveness of screening or for the most efficient schedule. The British Society for Paediatric Endocrinology and Diabetes endorses universal growth assessment for all children in the UK, which should be at the very minimum on one occasion, possibly combined with a school entry assessment. With the proposed introduction of a single measurement at school entry policy[64] scientific evidence needs to be accumulated to determine whether this is indeed the optimal approach. In the meantime, it is recommended that those areas which conduct a more intensive growth monitoring policy should not make any strategic changes until any decisions can be taken based on such evidence.

Which measurement?

Standard measurements include supine length and weight with head circumference up until 2 years of age (no reliable head circumference charts exist beyond this point at the present time). Beyond that height and weight are the norm. The British Society for Paediatric Endocrinology and Diabetes recommends that recording and plotting of a child's height and weight at every encounter is an example of best clinical practice. Body mass index charts (weight in kg/height in meters squared) are now available and can be used to assess a child's body composition and follow any changes (Figs 13.11 and 13.12). However as an approximation, a child's weight centile should not be more than 2 centile bands above

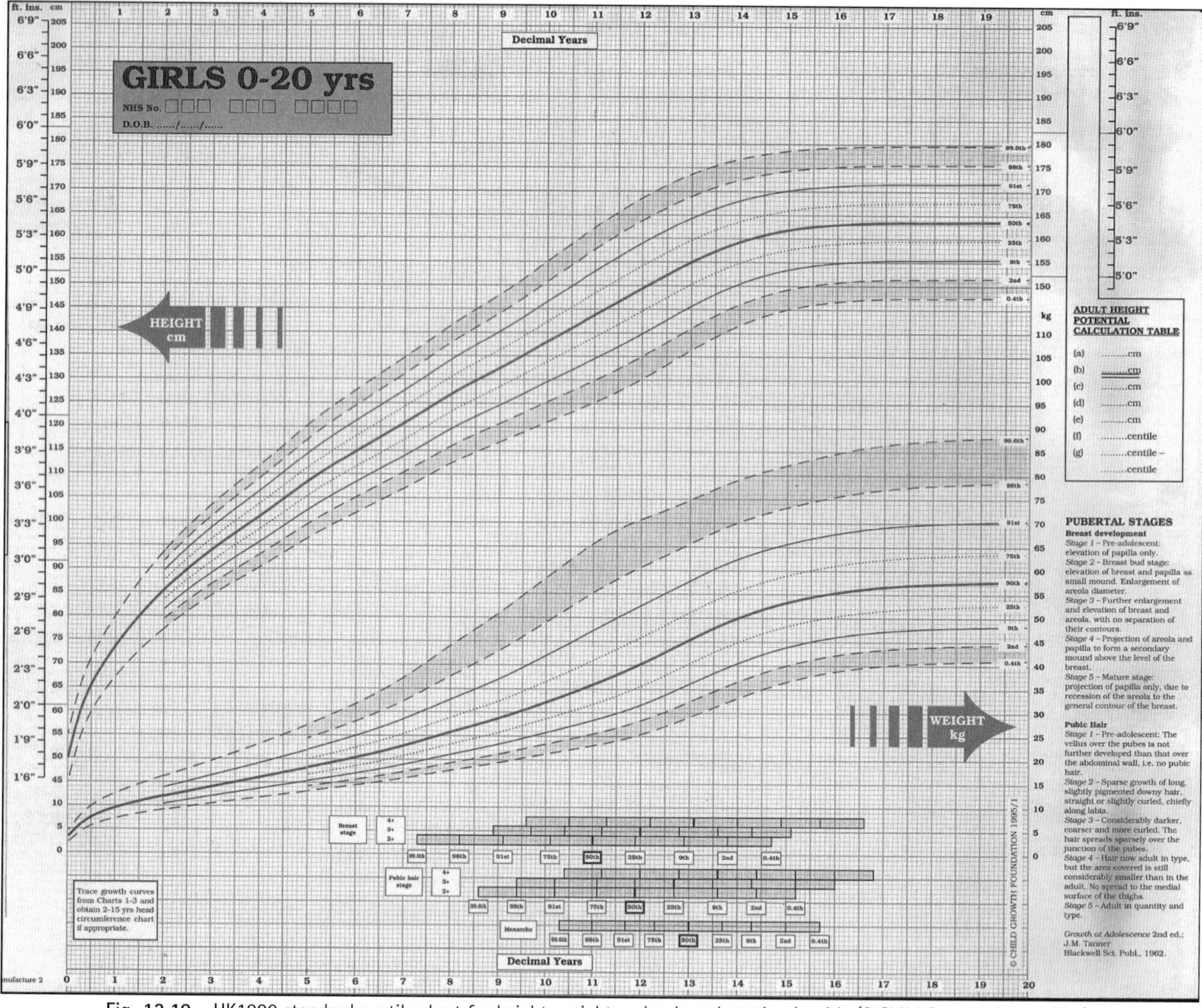
GIRLS 0-20 yrs
NHS No.
D.O.B. ....../....../......
Decimal Years
HEIGHT cm
WEIGHT kg
ADULT HEIGHT POTENTIAL CALCULATION TABLE
PUBERTAL STAGES
Breast development
Stage 1 – Pre-adolescent: elevation of papilla only.
Stage 2 – Breast bud stage: elevation of breast and papilla as small mound. Enlargement of areola diameter.
Stage 3 – Further enlargement and elevation of breast and areola, with no separation of their contours.
Stage 4 – Projection of areola and papilla to form a secondary mound above the level of the breast.
Stage 5 – Mature stage: projection of papilla only, due to recession of the areola to the general contour of the breast.
Pubic Hair
Stage 1 – Pre-adolescent: The vellus over the pubes is not further developed than that over the abdominal wall, i.e. no pubic hair.
Stage 2 – Sparse growth of long, slightly pigmented downy hair, straight or slightly curled, chiefly along labia.
Stage 3 – Considerably darker, coarser and more curled. The hair spreads sparsely over the junction of the pubes.
Stage 4 – Hair now adult in type, but the area covered is still considerably smaller than in the adult. No spread to the medial surface of the thighs.
Stage 5 – Adult in quantity and type.
Growth at Adolescence 2nd ed.; J.M. Tanner Blackwell Sci. Publ., 1962.
Breast stage
Pubic hair stage
Menarche
Trace growth curves from Charts 1-3 and obtain 2-15 yrs head circumference chart if appropriate.
© CHILD GROWTH FOUNDATION 1995/1

Fig. 13.10 UK1990 standard centile chart for height, weight and pubertal staging in girls (© Child Growth Foundation).

or below their height centile. This approximates to the 98th and 2nd centiles for body mass index (BMI) respectively. Skinfold thickness may be assessed to determine the degree and pattern of obesity and to calculate body composition (percentage body fat). They can also be measured serially on a child to monitor response to a treatment or intervention but current standards are outdated and should not be used. Mid-arm circumference may be a useful simple measure of the degree of nutrition in young children, particularly in developing countries (see Ch. 14).

Sitting height and subischial leg length (which is height – sitting height) are useful measures to investigate body disproportion, e.g. in skeletal dysplasia, or following interventions which affect spinal growth. A sitting height stadiometer and training in measurement technique are required (see below and Fig. 13.15c) and new population standards are available.[65] Crown–rump measurement is the equivalent to sitting height in children less than 2 years. Arm span is usually similar to standing height and therefore is a useful measure in the investigation of disproportion and also in the follow-up of children who are developing deformity, e.g. from a scoliosis, and when height measurement is not possible, e.g. in spastic diplegia. Useful reference manuals of normal physical measurements and characteristics are Buckler[66] and Hall et al.[67]

Knemometry is the technique of choice for studying short term growth as it allows precise, reproducible, non-invasive measurements of lower leg length in growing children, such that daily (or even within-day) and weekly fluctuations in leg length can be documented, e.g. during intercurrent illness or when daily[68] or alternate day[69] steroids are administered therapeutically. Knemometry ignores spinal growth and may be influenced by the hydration of soft tissues overlying bone. As a research technique it has provided valuable insights into the factors inhibiting growth.

Which equipment?

The most accurate height measuring equipment is the Harpenden Stadiometer, which reads to 0.1 cm (Fig. 13.15a). This is precision equipment but is not robust and the counter breaks easily with careless use. The Raven Magnimeter is the most suitable for routine clinic use. Portable equipment such as the Leicester Height Measure or the Minimeter are suitable for community or field measurements. The latter needs to be recalibrated on each occasion.

Referral guidelines

Consider referral for any boy whose BMI falls above the 99.6th centile/below the 0.4th centile as significantly over/underweight even on the basis of a single measurement. It is possible that a boy whose BMI falls in the tinted areas should also be referred. However, during infancy large but transient changes in centile may occur due to the shape of the charts, and these changes are normal. It should be remembered that the earlier the age of the second rise, the greater the risk of future obesity. Remember also that while BMI has a high correlation with relative fatness or leanness it is actually assessing the weight-to-height relationship: **this may give misleading results in boys who are very stocky and muscular who might appear obese on the BMI alone.**

BOYS

BMI CHART

(BIRTH - 20 YEARS)

United Kingdom cross-sectional reference data : 1995/1

Name...

NHS No. □□□ □□□ □□□□

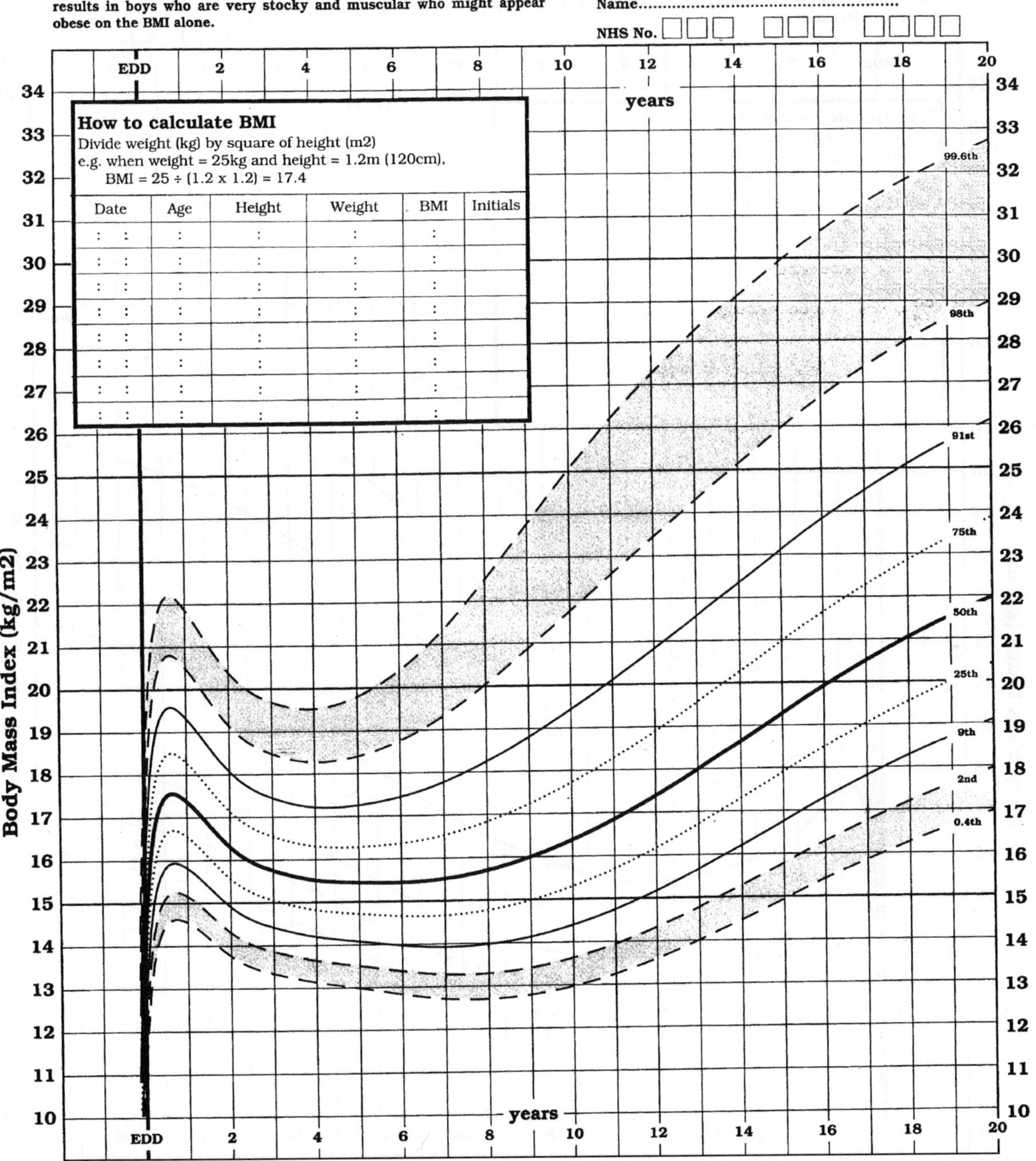

How to calculate BMI
Divide weight (kg) by square of height (m2)
e.g. when weight = 25kg and height = 1.2m (120cm),
BMI = 25 ÷ (1.2 x 1.2) = 17.4
Date
Age
Height
Weight
BMI
Initials
Body Mass Index (kg/m2)
EDD
years
99.6th
98th
91st
75th
50th
25th
9th
2nd
0.4th

Reference

Body Mass Index reference curves for the UK, 1990 (TJ Cole, JV Freeman, MA Preece) *Arch Dis Child* 1995; **73**: 25-29

Fig. 13.11 Body mass index reference centile chart for boys (© Child Growth Foundation).

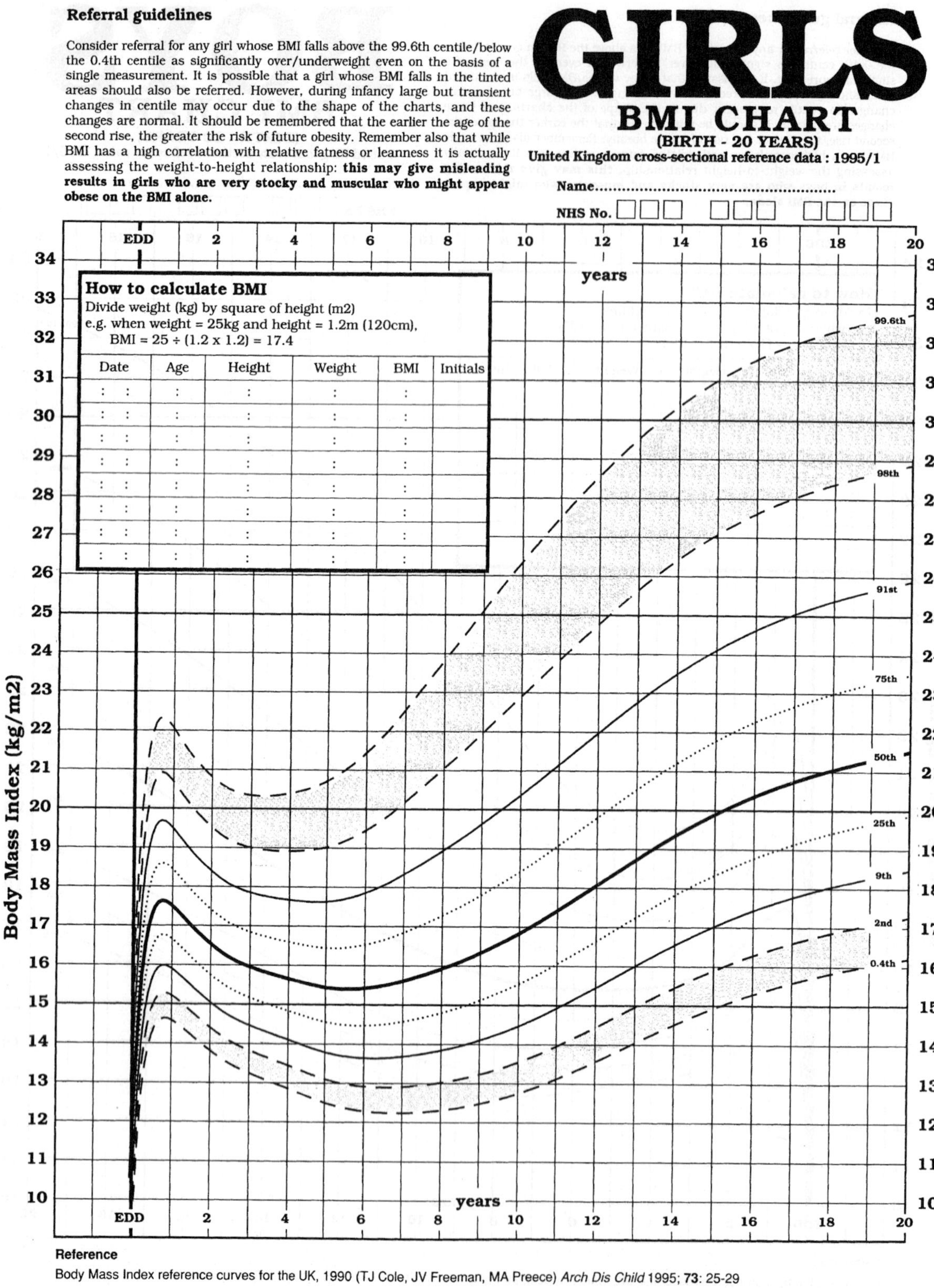

Referral guidelines

Consider referral for any girl whose BMI falls above the 99.6th centile/below the 0.4th centile as significantly over/underweight even on the basis of a single measurement. It is possible that a girl whose BMI falls in the tinted areas should also be referred. However, during infancy large but transient changes in centile may occur due to the shape of the charts, and these changes are normal. It should be remembered that the earlier the age of the second rise, the greater the risk of future obesity. Remember also that while BMI has a high correlation with relative fatness or leanness it is actually assessing the weight-to-height relationship: **this may give misleading results in girls who are very stocky and muscular who might appear obese on the BMI alone.**

BMI CHART

(BIRTH - 20 YEARS)

United Kingdom cross-sectional reference data : 1995/1

Name...

NHS No. ☐☐☐ ☐☐☐ ☐☐☐☐

How to calculate BMI

Divide weight (kg) by square of height (m2)

e.g. when weight = 25kg and height = 1.2m (120cm),

BMI = 25 ÷ (1.2 x 1.2) = 17.4

Date	Age	Height	Weight	BMI	Initials
: :	:	:	:	:	
: :	:	:	:	:	
: :	:	:	:	:	
: :	:	:	:	:	
: :	:	:	:	:	
: :	:	:	:	:	
: :	:	:	:	:	
: :	:	:	:	:	

Body Mass Index (kg/m2)

EDD 2 4 6 8 10 12 14 16 18 20 years

99.6th 98th 91st 75th 50th 25th 9th 2nd 0.4th

Reference

Body Mass Index reference curves for the UK, 1990 (TJ Cole, JV Freeman, MA Preece) *Arch Dis Child* 1995; **73**: 25-29

Fig. 13.12 Body mass index reference centile chart for girls (© Child Growth Foundation).

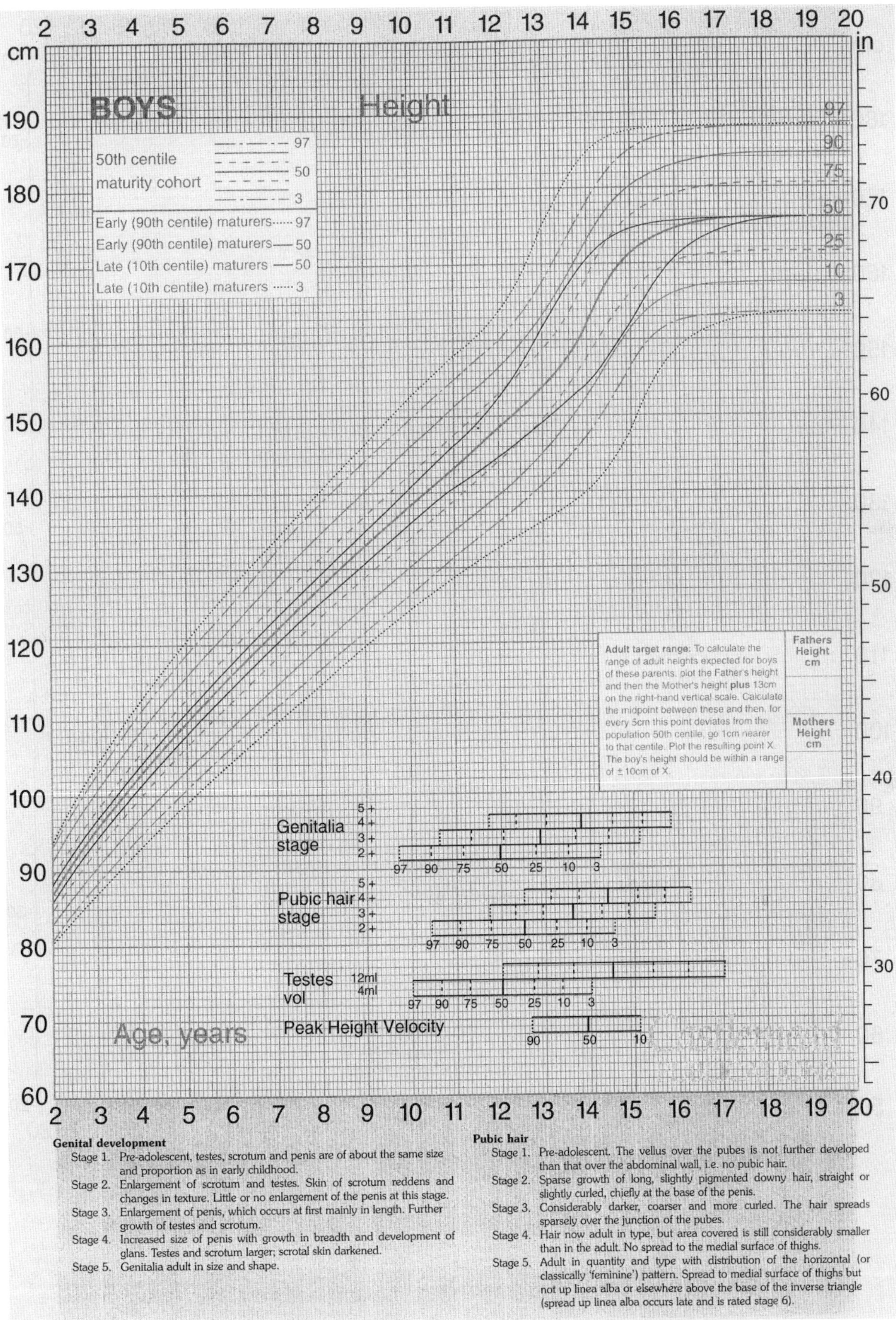
BOYS
Height
cm
in
50th centile maturity cohort
97
50
3
Early (90th centile) maturers······ 97
Early (90th centile) maturers— 50
Late (10th centile) maturers — 50
Late (10th centile) maturers ······ 3
Adult target range: To calculate the range of adult heights expected for boys of these parents, plot the Father's height and then the Mother's height plus 13cm on the right-hand vertical scale. Calculate the midpoint between these and then, for every 5cm this point deviates from the population 50th centile, go 1cm nearer to that centile. Plot the resulting point X. The boy's height should be within a range of ± 10cm of X.
Fathers Height cm
Mothers Height cm
Genitalia stage
Pubic hair stage
Testes vol
12ml
4ml
Peak Height Velocity
Age, years
Genital development
Stage 1. Pre-adolescent, testes, scrotum and penis are of about the same size and proportion as in early childhood.
Stage 2. Enlargement of scrotum and testes. Skin of scrotum reddens and changes in texture. Little or no enlargement of the penis at this stage.
Stage 3. Enlargement of penis, which occurs at first mainly in length. Further growth of testes and scrotum.
Stage 4. Increased size of penis with growth in breadth and development of glans. Testes and scrotum larger; scrotal skin darkened.
Stage 5. Genitalia adult in size and shape.
Pubic hair
Stage 1. Pre-adolescent. The vellus over the pubes is not further developed than that over the abdominal wall, i.e. no pubic hair.
Stage 2. Sparse growth of long, slightly pigmented downy hair, straight or slightly curled, chiefly at the base of the penis.
Stage 3. Considerably darker, coarser and more curled. The hair spreads sparsely over the junction of the pubes.
Stage 4. Hair now adult in type, but area covered is still considerably smaller than in the adult. No spread to the medial surface of thighs.
Stage 5. Adult in quantity and type with distribution of the horizontal (or classically 'feminine') pattern. Spread to medial surface of thighs but not up linea alba or elsewhere above the base of the inverse triangle (spread up linea alba occurs late and is rated stage 6).

Fig. 13.13 Buckler Tanner height centile chart for boys (© Castlemead Publications).

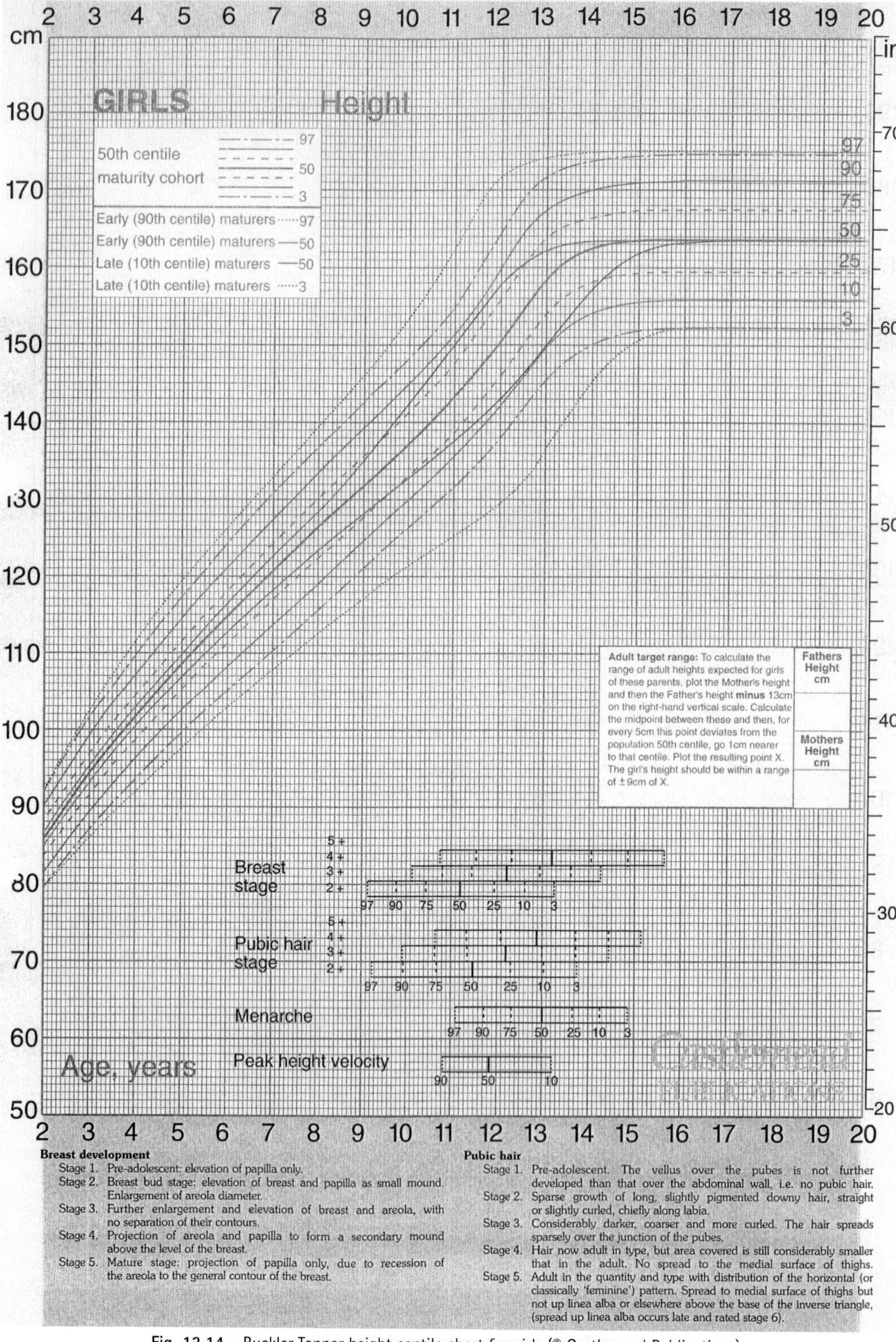
GIRLS
Height
cm
in
2 3 4 5 6 7 8 9 10 11 12 13 14 15 16 17 18 19 20
180 170 160 150 140 130 120 110 100 90 80 70 60 50
70 60 50 40 30 20
50th centile maturity cohort 97 50 3
Early (90th centile) maturers ······97
Early (90th centile) maturers —50
Late (10th centile) maturers —50
Late (10th centile) maturers ······3
97 90 75 50 25 10 3
Adult target range: To calculate the range of adult heights expected for girls of these parents, plot the Mother's height and then the Father's height minus 13cm on the right-hand vertical scale. Calculate the midpoint between these and then, for every 5cm this point deviates from the population 50th centile, go 1cm nearer to that centile. Plot the resulting point X. The girl's height should be within a range of ±9cm of X.
Fathers Height cm
Mothers Height cm
Breast stage
5+ 4+ 3+ 2+
97 90 75 50 25 10 3
Pubic hair stage
5+ 4+ 3+ 2+
97 90 75 50 25 10 3
Menarche
97 90 75 50 25 10 3
Peak height velocity
90 50 10
Age, years
Castlemead Publications
Breast development
Stage 1. Pre-adolescent: elevation of papilla only.
Stage 2. Breast bud stage: elevation of breast and papilla as small mound. Enlargement of areola diameter.
Stage 3. Further enlargement and elevation of breast and areola, with no separation of their contours.
Stage 4. Projection of areola and papilla to form a secondary mound above the level of the breast.
Stage 5. Mature stage: projection of papilla only, due to recession of the areola to the general contour of the breast.
Pubic hair
Stage 1. Pre-adolescent. The vellus over the pubes is not further developed than that over the abdominal wall, i.e. no pubic hair.
Stage 2. Sparse growth of long, slightly pigmented downy hair, straight or slightly curled, chiefly along labia.
Stage 3. Considerably darker, coarser and more curled. The hair spreads sparsely over the junction of the pubes.
Stage 4. Hair now adult in type, but area covered is still considerably smaller that in the adult. No spread to the medial surface of thighs.
Stage 5. Adult in the quantity and type with distribution of the horizontal (or classically 'feminine') pattern. Spread to medial surface of thighs but not up linea alba or elsewhere above the base of the inverse triangle, (spread up linea alba occurs late and rated stage 6).

Fig. 13.14 Buckler Tanner height centile chart for girls (© Castlemead Publications).

Table 13.5 Decimal year calculation

	1	2	3	4	5	6	7	8	9	10	11	12	13	14	15	16	17	18	19	20	21	22	23	24	25	26	27	28	29	30	31
JAN	000	003	005	008	011	014	016	019	022	025	027	030	033	036	038	041	044	047	049	052	055	058	060	063	066	068	071	074	077	079	082
FEB	085	088	090	093	096	099	101	104	107	110	112	115	118	121	123	126	129	132	134	137	140	142	145	148	151	153	156	159			
MAR	162	164	167	170	173	175	178	181	184	186	189	192	195	197	200	203	205	208	211	214	216	219	222	225	227	230	233	236	238	241	244
APR	247	249	252	255	258	260	263	266	268	271	274	277	279	282	285	288	290	293	296	299	301	304	307	310	312	315	318	321	323	326	
MAY	329	332	334	337	340	342	345	348	351	353	356	359	362	364	367	370	373	375	378	381	384	386	389	392	395	397	400	403	405	408	411
JUN	414	416	419	422	425	427	430	433	436	438	441	444	447	449	452	455	458	460	463	466	468	471	474	477	479	482	485	488	490	493	
JUL	496	499	501	504	507	510	512	515	518	521	523	526	529	532	534	537	540	542	545	548	551	553	556	559	562	564	567	570	573	575	578
AUG	581	584	586	589	592	595	597	600	603	605	608	611	614	616	619	622	625	627	630	633	636	638	641	644	647	649	652	655	658	660	663
SEP	666	668	671	674	677	679	682	685	688	690	693	696	699	701	704	707	710	712	715	718	721	723	726	729	731	734	737	740	742	745	
OCT	748	751	753	756	759	762	764	767	770	773	775	778	781	784	786	789	792	795	797	800	803	805	808	811	814	816	819	822	825	827	830
NOV	833	836	838	841	844	847	849	852	855	858	860	863	866	868	871	874	877	879	882	885	888	890	893	896	899	901	904	907	910	912	
DEC	915	918	921	923	926	929	932	934	937	940	942	945	948	951	953	956	959	962	964	967	970	973	975	978	981	984	986	989	992	995	997

Weight is best measured on accurate electronic scales (e.g. Seca) but regularly calibrated and checked balance scales may also be appropriate in certain circumstances (e.g. when electrical power is not available). Head circumference is best measured using specially constructed tape (Lasso-o, Child Growth Foundation, Fig. 13.15d) but a disposable paper tape folded or cut in half lengthways to reduce its breadth to reduce the inaccuracy can be used.

How to measure

The following simple steps can ensure accurate and reproducible measurements.

Height

Remove the child's shoes and position the child with the heels and back touching the backboard; instruct the child to stand erect. Position the child in the 'Frankfurt position' so that the lower border of the orbit is in the same horizontal plane as the external auditory meatus (Fig. 13.15a). The horizontal moveable part of the equipment is then lowered onto the child's head and the reading taken to the nearest 0.1 cm. Some observers prefer to stretch the child gently under the mastoid processes while the child takes a breath in and then exhales, noting the maximum measurement. Others prefer the unstretched technique but whichever technique is employed, consistency is required. Children with unequal leg length should be measured on the longest leg and this fact entered into their record. Diurnal variation in height may show as much as a 2 cm drop from rising in the morning to the afternoon. Where accurate determination of height velocity is required, the child should be measured at the same time of the day, preferably in the afternoon, and by the same observer where possible.

Supine length

Infants and children under 2 years, or those with a handicap can be measured supine. This technique requires at least two people, one being the child's parent if available (Fig. 13.15b). One person should hold the child's head against the headboard in the Frankfurt plane as above, whilst the other straightens the legs and moves the footboard up against both heels firmly. The measurement can then be taken. Children with unequal leg length should be measured on the longest leg, but the frequent practice of measuring one leg only can give inaccurate readings because of pelvic tilt.

Sitting height

The child is positioned on the sitting height table as upright as possible with the legs fully in contact with the table. (Fig. 13.15c) Back and foot supports are adjusted to support the child. Head positioning and measurement technique is the same as for height (see above). Sitting height may also be measured by placing a flat-topped stool of known height below the stadiometer, and subtracting this amount from a measurement of the child sitting on the stool.

Weight

Infants should be weighed naked. Older children can be weighed in light underclothes and with shoes removed. Uncooperative toddlers can be weighed with an adult, subtracting the adult's weight measured separately.

Head circumference

This measurement is the maximum occipitofrontal circumference with the reading taken on three occasions (Fig. 13.15d). A thin specially constructed tape measure is required (see above).

Height velocity

Much has been written on the use of height velocity as part of the assessment of the growth of a child. Appreciation of the total amount grown at each age for any child is important as part of their assessment. However the individual pattern of growth of any child can show daily, weekly and seasonal variations. Height velocity is

(a)

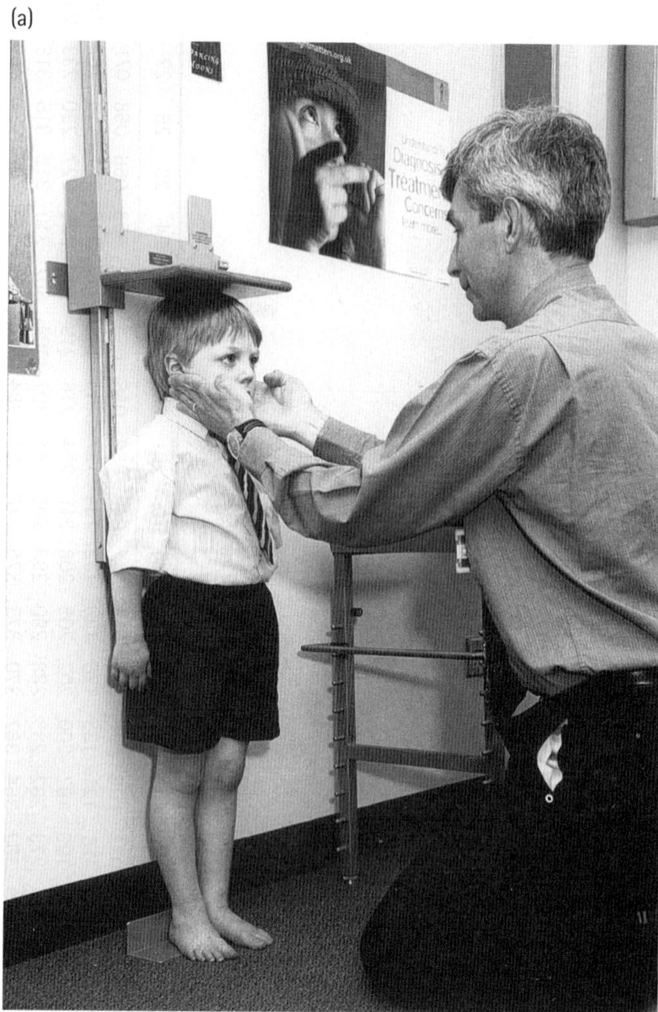

(b)

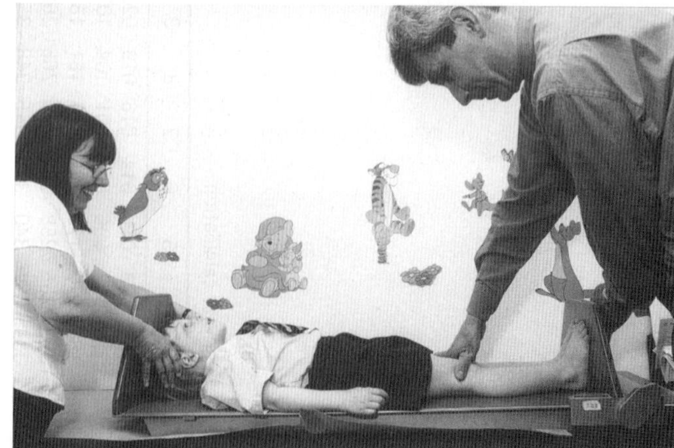

Fig. 13.15 Correct positioning and technique for accurate measurement of (a) height, (b) supine length, (c) sitting height, (d) head circumference. For description see text.

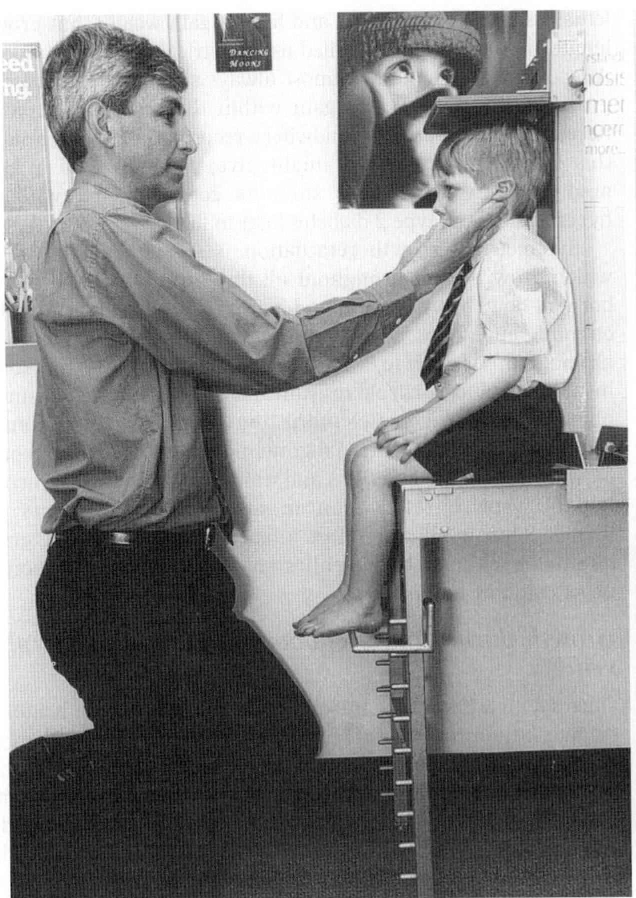

(c)

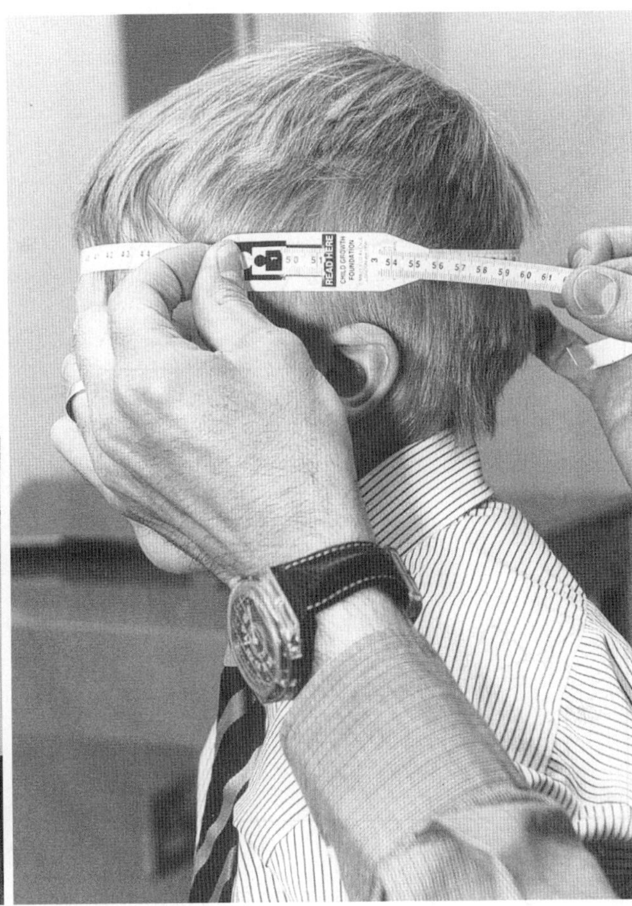

(d)

Fig. 13.15 Continued

usually assessed over periods of not less than 1 year to avoid the seasonal effects and to minimize the effect of measurement error, but increments of less than 1 year can be 'annualized' for comparative purposes and this is often sufficient to recognize growth problems quickly. For the method of calculation of height velocity see 'decimal ages' above. Even so, annual height velocity tends to oscillate with the periodicity of approximately 2 years[70] and this needs to be taken into consideration during interpretation of growth patterns (Fig. 13.16). Rhythms of growth are reviewed by Wales & Gibson.[71] Measurement of height velocity is an accurate, cheap and non-invasive contribution to assessing the appropriate dose of endocrine replacement therapy. This must be combined with a regular assessment of skeletal maturation (bone age). Otherwise, for example, rapid growth due to over-replacement with thyroxine in the management of acquired hypothyroidism may be mistaken for desirable 'catch-up' growth.

Biochemical markers of growth

In certain circumstances, carefully chosen biochemical markers of growth may overcome some of these disadvantages. Biochemical markers are free from observer bias and their precision is independent of frequency of sampling. Bone alkaline phosphatase (BALP) is found in hypertrophic chondrocytes of the epiphyseal growth plate, in matrix vesicles associated with bone mineralization and in mature osteoblasts. There is a close quantitative relationship between serial measurements of BALP and height velocity in short normal children undergoing GH treatment.[72]

Procollagen type I C-terminal propeptide (PICP) is released into the circulation by proliferating osteoblasts during collagen biosynthesis; the crosslinked telopeptide of type I collagen (ICTP) is released by collagen breakdown during bone modelling; procollagen type III N-terminal propeptide (P3NP) is released during soft tissue growth but is not present in bone. These markers are useful as early predictors of height velocity responses to growth promoting therapies,[72] and in evaluation of therapies with potentially adverse effects on growth.

In the assessment of a child's growth potential calculation of mid-parental height is essential. The difference between the male and female 50th centile heights is 14 cm. For a boy, mid-parental height is calculated as the simple average of parents height + 7 cm, for a girl average of parents heights – 7 cm. The mid-parental height (MPH) can be plotted on the growth chart (Fig. 13.9) and 90% of children will achieve an adult height within + or – 10 cm of that value (the target centile range). Caution needs to be exercised when predicting adult height if one parent is of extreme stature. A chart to help assess whether a child's short stature is of familial origin or not is also available.[73]

Standard deviation scores

Standard deviation scores (SDS) have traditionally been used to monitor individual and group variations in height or any other growth parameter over time, as the function of age is excluded, and this makes statistical analysis possible. Height measurements are normally distributed and SDS can be estimated from the UK1990 charts, each centile band being equally spaced 0.67 SD apart. For more accurate calculation and for measures such as weight and body mass index which are in a positively skewed distribution, the methodology of Cole[62] should be used.

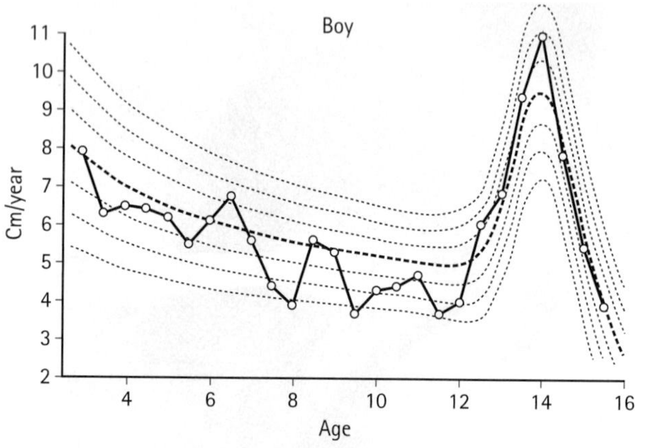

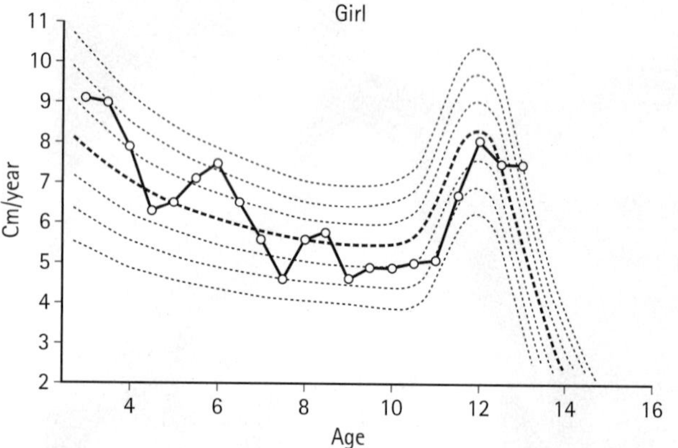

Fig. 13.16 Height velocity standards for boys and girls (redrawn from Tanner 1976) showing a height velocity curve for a typical normal boy and girl, both demonstrating the cyclical nature of growth. (From Butler et al 1990[70])

VARIATIONS IN GROWTH

Postnatal adjustment

Weight at birth generally reflects the intrauterine environment and nutrition and most if not all infants will show a degree of tracking, i.e. a shift across centiles for height, weight and head circumference within the first 6 months after birth. The challenge here is to differentiate between a normal growth variant and failure to thrive or another pathological process. However, normal variation, i.e. adjustment to the genetic growth pattern, will show a shift upwards or downwards by as much as 2 centile bands, followed by stabilization of growth, and subsequent following of the child's genetically determined centile band. Abnormal growth patterns will continue to show centile change beyond the first 6 months, and further investigation should take place. Weight gain is more susceptible to the influence of feeding problems and intercurrent illnesses. The regular and accurate assessment of supine length in an infant will help distinguish between normal variation and true failure to thrive and as length in the normal situation will demonstrate less fluctuation than weight.

Intrauterine growth retardation and catch-up growth

Low birth weight (below 2nd centile for gestational age) may originate as a result of poor fetal growth throughout pregnancy or just in the last trimester. Both are of different causality and produce a different outcome. The latter arises as a result of maternal factors such as placental failure or pre-eclampsia. An otherwise normal fetus is starved of nutrients and fails to gain weight, but grows in length near normally, so-called asymmetrical growth retardation. After birth, these infants almost always show complete catch-up growth with rapid weight gain within the first 6–12 months.[74] Recent research based on midwifery record archives suggests that this rapid gain in weight might give the individual a higher predisposition to diseases such as coronary artery disease, hypertension and type 2 diabetes later in life.[36]

Symmetrical growth retardation is shown by those fetuses which grow poorly throughout all three trimesters and who are born at low birth weight and with reduced length and head circumference. The etiology is fetal rather than maternal and although this is likely to be multifactorial, endocrine factors such as insulin and glucocorticoid resistance have been implicated, and the phenomenon of genetic imprinting may also be responsible. Imprinting of certain paternal growth genes appears to be required for normal growth. Deletions and uniparental disomy can account for the growth retardation in about 10% of infants with Russell–Silver syndrome. Most infants with this form of growth retardation either catch up either very slowly (3 years or more), or never catch up fully.

Growth during the prepubertal years and referral criteria

Once set on a particular trajectory, a child's growth in height will deviate little from its centile band until the onset of puberty. So predictable is this pattern, that concern should be raised if height drifts up or down by as little as one height centile band, even within the designated normal range (i.e. 2nd–98th centiles), and an explanation sought. This is the basis of the advice given to those conducting community growth screening programs.

Syndrome specific charts

The pattern of growth is so reproducible in certain conditions that specific growth charts are available, e.g. for Down[75] and Turner[76] syndromes. They serve a very useful purpose in allowing correct judgments to be made about the growth of children with these conditions, and whether other external factors such as poor nutrition or ill health are affecting a child's growth adversely. In addition they assist with the prediction of adult height and in quantifying the effect of any treatments, such as the use of growth hormone in Turner syndrome.

Medical conditions which affect growth

Previously, chronic ill health from conditions such as cystic fibrosis, diabetes mellitus, inflammatory bowel disease, chronic renal failure and asthma could be associated with poor growth and weight gain and a delay in the onset of puberty, although with modern treatment regimens and much more careful attention to nutrition, this is rarely seen. However, poor growth can still be associated with severe forms of inflammatory bowel disease, juvenile chronic arthritis, chronic renal failure and congenital adrenal hyperplasia, even when the associated glucocorticoid therapy is reduced to a minimum. The most frequently seen cause of iatrogenic growth failure is in the survivors of childhood malignancy. Treatment regimens including cranial and total body irradiation, and high dose chemotherapy, often with stem cell rescue or bone marrow transplant usually cause growth and thyroid hormone deficiencies, and steroidogenesis from the adrenals and gonads is frequently impaired. Hormone replacement may restore growth, but the success of treatment depends on how much primary damage is caused to the tissues of the body by the oncological regimens.

BONE AGE

The bone age is a useful guide to an individual child's growth potential but the value of this investigation as a diagnostic tool is frequently overestimated, its main place being in adult height prediction. A bone age radiograph when scored according to current techniques gives a value (the 'Bone Age') which represents the 50th centile for a child of that age with that degree of skeletal maturation. This result can be interpreted in the same way as any measurement plotted on a reference chart. The 3rd and 97th bone age centiles correspond to approximately plus or minus 2 years of the child's chronological age. Whether a bone age is 'advanced' or 'delayed' its main value is estimating the growing time remaining.

Conventionally X-rays of the left wrist are used because there is a large aggregation of long and round bones in this single area which can be imaged at minimal radiation dose. The Greulich & Pyle system[77] provides pictorial standards for direct comparison with the individual child's X-ray and the best fit determines the bone age. The Tanner–Whitehouse system (currently TW3)[78] requires the scoring of epiphyseal maturation of 13 individual bones (radius, ulna, 1st, 3rd and 5th metacarpals and phalanges) which is more accurate and more suitable for longitudinal follow-up of the individual child. Bone ages can be performed serially, especially when monitoring response to treatment or an intervention, but as the rating system imposes artificial stages on a continuous biological process, it is not recommended to perform the investigation at less than 6-monthly intervals.

Epiphyseal fusion and growth cessation are now known to be related to estrogen secretion in both sexes. Thus estrogen deficiency due to mutations in the aromatase gene (CYP19) and estrogen resistance due to disruptive mutations in the estrogen receptor gene have no effect on normal male sexual maturation in puberty. However, these mutations result in an absent pubertal growth spurt, delayed bone maturation, unfused epiphyses, continued growth into adulthood and very tall adult stature in both sexes.[79]

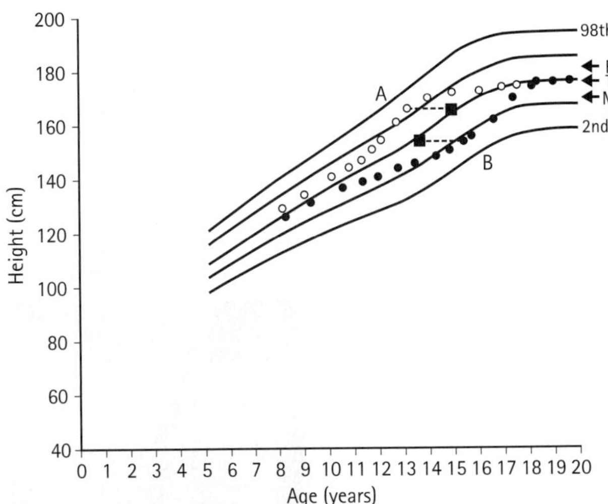

Fig. 13.17 Examples of the use of mid-parental height and bone age in the prediction of adult height in an early maturing (A) and a late maturing (B) boy. For details see text. circle = height plot for chronological age, square = height plot for bone age, F = father's height, M = mother's adjusted height, T = target height.

PREDICTION OF ADULT HEIGHT

It is helpful to plot the child's height for bone age on the height chart and following the bone age/height centile through to maturity can give a reasonable approximation of the child's projected adult height. Figure 13.17 gives examples of height for chronological age and height for bone age plots in two boys, one early maturing and one late maturing, both however achieving 50th centile adult height. Although adult height prediction can be used for children with parents within the population norms it is far less reliable in extremes of stature. Predicted adult height can be estimated based on the two principal bone age rating systems, TW3[78] and Greulich & Pyle,[77] with a margin of error of approximately + or – 4 cm. Mathematical description of growth and growth curves has frequently been undertaken, but the Infant–Childhood–Puberty model of Karlberg et al[80] provides the best description of growth during the three postnatal phases: infantile – principally under nutritional influence; childhood – growth being predominantly controlled by growth hormone secretion; and puberty – where both sex steroids and growth hormone drive growth. More recently, mathematical models have been derived to predict the response to an intervention, e.g. growth hormone treatment.[3]

ASSESSMENT OF PUBERTY

The adolescent years are manifested by fundamental changes to the physical and psychological functioning of a person. To a pediatrician the process of puberty may influence the pathological process or management of some conditions and conversely a number of chronic conditions influence, usually adversely, the process of puberty, either in a consonant way (the normal pattern of development but accelerated or delayed in time) or in a dissonant way (disruption of the normal pubertal process). Consequently an assessment of pubertal staging should be part of the clinical examination of any adolescent patient. The universally accepted method of pubertal staging is according to Tanner.[4]

Clinical staging of puberty

Boys

In the male, ratings are expressed as stages of genital (penis) development, pubic hair development and testicular volume. Knowledge of these standards is extremely important when assessing growth in adolescents. They are shown in Figures 13.19–13.21 and are described below.

Genitalia (penis) development stages (Fig. 13.18)

Stage G1: Preadolescent. Testes, scrotum and penis are about same size and shape as in early childhood.

Stage G2: Scrotum slightly enlarged, with reddening of the skin and changes in the texture. Little or no enlargement of the penis at this stage.

Stage G3: Penis slightly enlarged, at first mainly in length. Scrotum further enlarged than in stage G2.

Stage G4: Penis further enlarged, with growth in breadth and development of glans. Further enlargement of scrotum and darkening of scrotal skin.

Stage G5: Genitalia adult in size and shape.

Testicular volume. Testicular volumes are assessed by palpation in comparison with a string of plastic models of testicular shape known as the Prader orchidometer (Fig. 13.19). Although this principally measures spermatic tubular growth, testicular volume correlates closely with testosterone secretion. The models are marked according to their volumes in milliliters.

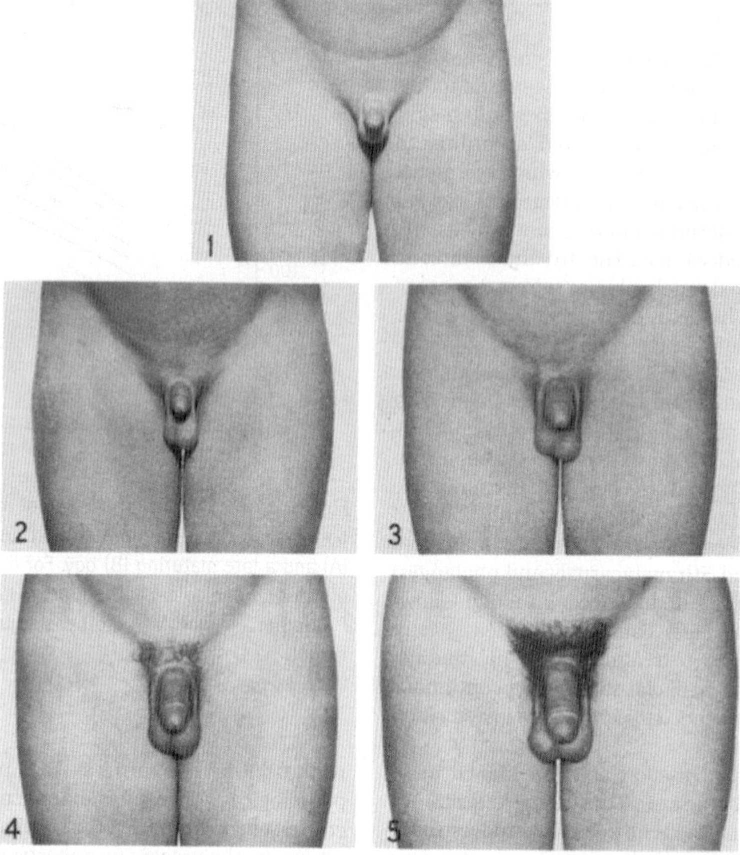

Fig. 13.18 Standards for genital (penis) development. (From Tanner 1962[4] with permission)

1–2 ml are prepubertal;
3–4 ml mark the beginning of puberty;
8–10 ml are associated with the beginning of height acceleration in mid-pubertal boys, usually at stage G3;
12–15 ml coincide with the maximum growth velocity, usually at stage G4;
20 ml (usually at stage G5) signifies that most boys have passed the peak of their growth spurt and are beginning to fuse their epiphyses on account of higher levels of testosterone secretion.

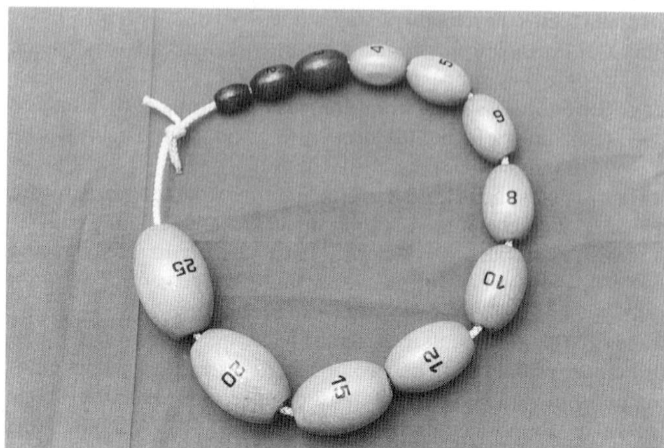

Fig. 13.19 The Prader orchidometer for the assessment of testicular volume.

The majority of adult males reach volumes of 15–25 ml. Testicular volumes of less than 12 ml in adulthood may be associated with reduced fertility.

Pubic hair stages for boys and girls (Fig. 13.20)

Stage PH1: Preadolescent. The vellus over the pubes is not further developed than that over the abdominal wall, i.e. no pubic hair.

Stage PH2: Sparse growth of long, slightly pigmented downy hair, straight or slightly curled, chiefly at the base of the penis or along labia.

Stage PH3: Considerably darker, coarser and more curled. The hair spreads sparsely over the junction of the pubes.

Stage PH4: Hair now adult in type, but area covered is still considerably smaller than in adults. No spread to medial surface of thighs.

Stage PH5: Adult in quantity and type with distribution of the horizontal (or classically 'feminine') pattern. Spread to medial surface of thighs, but not up the linea alba.

Stage PH6: Spread upwards along the linea alba (the typical male escutcheon).

Girls

In girls it is the development of the breast which provides the best marker as to girls' progress through puberty (Fig. 13.21).

Breast development

Stage B1: Preadolescent: elevation of papilla only.

Stage B2: Breast bud stage: elevation of breast and papilla as small mound. Areolar diameter enlarged over stage B1.

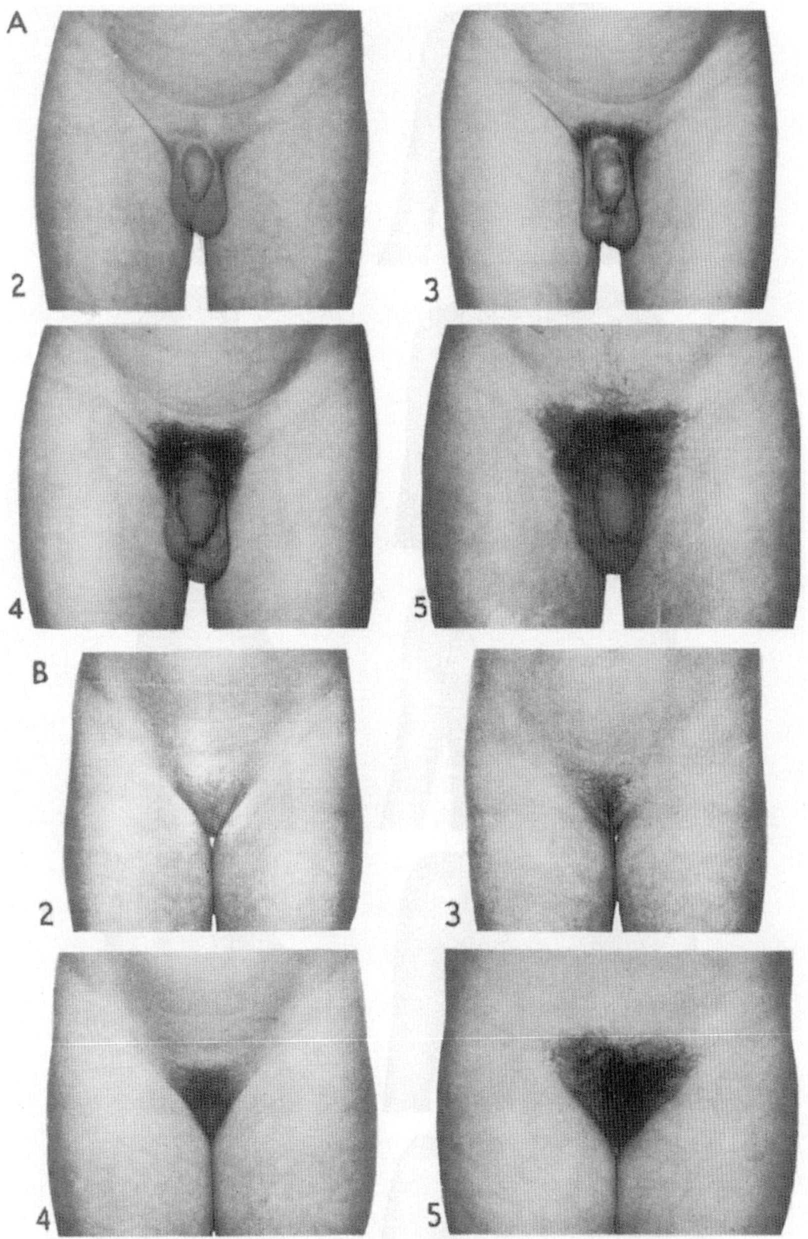

Fig. 13.20 Standards for pubic hair development in boys and girls. (From Tanner 1962[4] with permission)

Stage B3: Breast and areola both enlarged and elevated more than in stage B2, but with no separation of their contours.

Stage B4: The areola and papilla form a secondary mound projecting above the contour of the breast.

Stage B5: Mature stage: papilla only projects, with the areola recessed to the general contour of the breast.

The timing of puberty

In almost all children the pattern of progress through puberty is constant but the timing of attainment of each stage can be considerably variable. Centile bands for boys and girls at each stage of puberty are found beneath the weight curves on standard growth charts (see Figs 13.9 and 13.10). The onset of puberty G2 in boys occurs at the mean age of 12.0 years (range 98th centile 9.8 years to 2nd centile 14.2 years) and in girls, the mean age at B2 is 11.0 years (range 98th centile 8.2 years to 2nd centile 13.8 years). The mean age at menarche is 13.0 years (range 98th centile 11.0 years to 2nd centile 15.0 years). The duration of puberty (stage G/B2 to stage G/B5) may unusually take less than 2 years and more than 5 years, but on average is 3.0 years (2.3 years B2 – menarche in girls). A very rapid, delayed or halted passage through puberty especially with an attenuated adolescent growth spurt should be of major concern and a search for systemic or intracranial pathology should be conducted.

Other markers of puberty

Often it is not possible to perform a formal Tanner pubertal staging due to inappropriate circumstances or refusal. Adolescents may be prepared to self-rate themselves if provided with line diagrams and simple descriptions or an orchidometer for boys. Axillary hair begins to appear 2 years after pubic hair. Facial hair grows initially above the upper lip (moustache area) at about G4. By the time sideburns begin to appear, a boy will have reached G5. The voice begins to break at G3–4. The timing of the first conscious

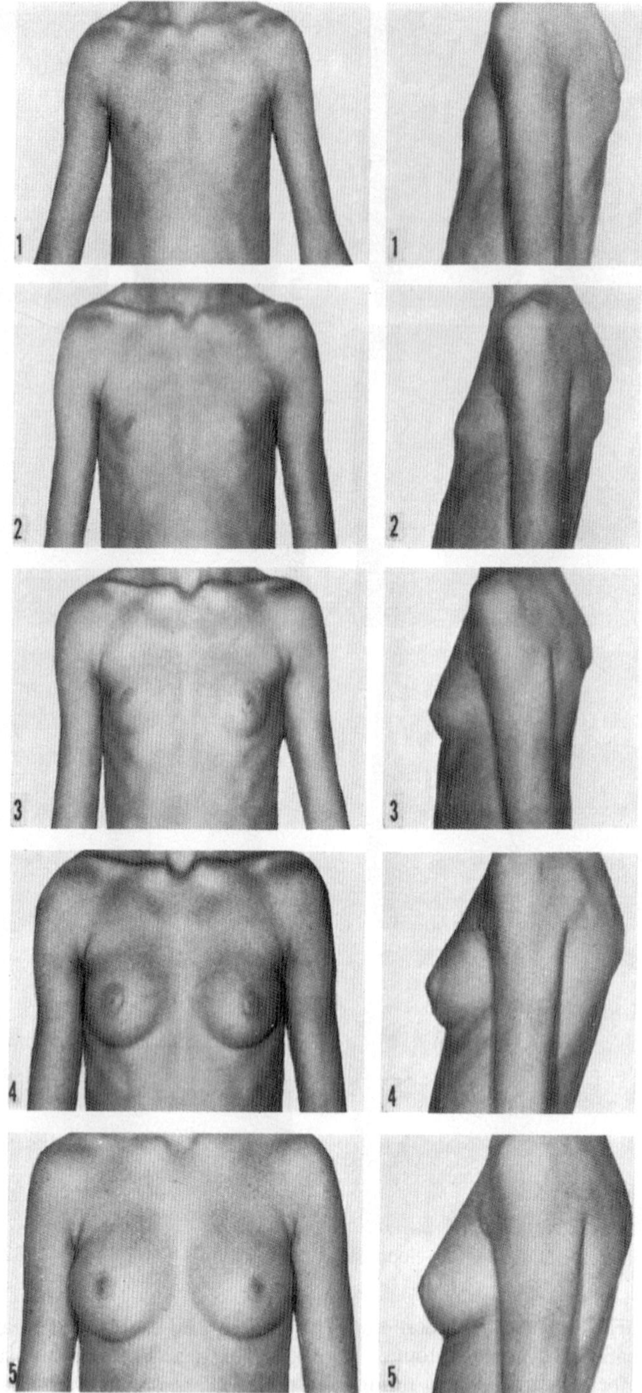

Fig. 13.21 Standards for breast development. (From Tanner 1962[4] with permission)

ejaculation is very variable, but occurs in 90% boys by age 14 years. Sperm can be detected in early morning urine samples as early as 12 years of age and in early puberty (G2) before any other clinical features are apparent. Menarche occurs by the time 90% of girls have reached B4 and PH4.

GROWTH DURING PUBERTY

Prior to the onset of puberty height velocity gradually declines to between 4–6 cm/year (the prepubertal growth lag) and this is much more marked in boys than in girls, especially when the onset of puberty is delayed (constitutional or maturation delay). The endocrinology of puberty gives a different tempo in boys compared with girls (Fig. 13.22). As soon as puberty begins with breast development in girls height acceleration occurs and body shape changes become apparent. Maximal growth (peak height velocity) is achieved 1 year after the onset of puberty (mean 8 cm/year, range 6–10 cm/year) but the intensity of the spurt, i.e. maximal velocity achieved, is greater in early maturers and lower in later maturers. Menarche occurs 2.3 years (mean) subsequently when growth is on its decline. Girls gain on average 20–25 cm during puberty and average growth post menarche is 6 cm.

In boys peak height velocity is attained usually 2 years after the onset of puberty with maximum strength spurt following this. Peak

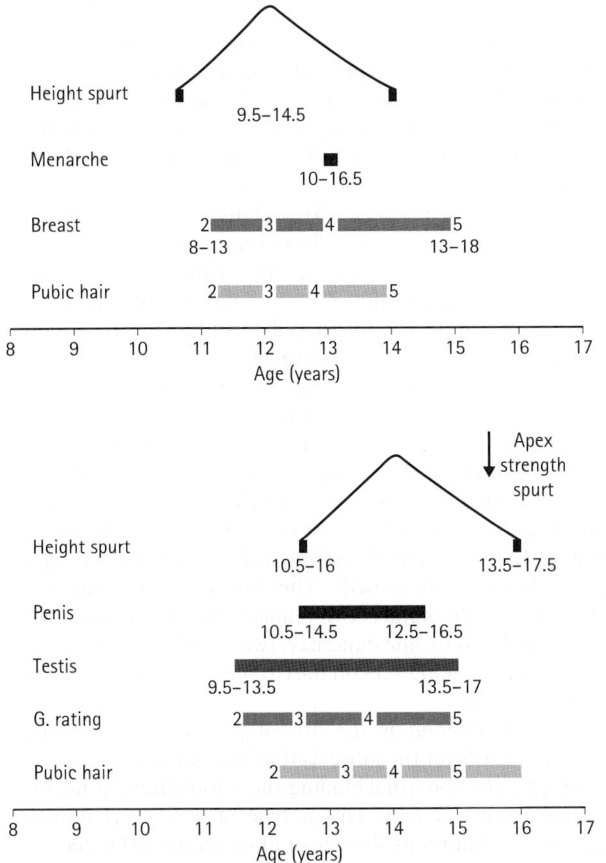

Fig. 13.22 Diagram of sequence of events in normal male and female puberty. Numbers indicate age ranges of each landmark stage. (From Marshall & Tanner 1970[488] with permission of the BMJ Publishing Group)

height velocity is on average 9 cm/year ranging from 6 to 13 cm, the later maturers growing less intensely. Boys grow on average between 25 and 30 cm although the total growth during puberty is unpredictable and is the principal source of error of height prediction methods.

COMMON ERRORS IN PUBERTAL ASSESSMENT

The method of construction of the UK1990 growth charts reflects average population growth in children of average age at puberty (see above) so it is normal to see crossing of centile lines during the teenage years. This should not cause alarm and can be interpreted by knowing the adolescent's pubertal stage. The onset of puberty in boys is frequently missed as early scrotal and testicular changes are subtle and require careful inspection. Accurate documentation of pubertal stages is important, as 'false starts' can be common. Testicular volume is often overestimated, the orchidometer representing testicular size only, and not accessory structures such as the epididymis and scrotal skin.

PUBERTAL VARIATIONS

Precocious adrenarche

Adrenarche, the awakening of the adrenal cortex to produce adrenal androgens, commences from around the age of 6 years and can be more pronounced in some children causing the appearance of pubic and axillary hair, greasiness of the skin and adult body odor. This proceeds only very slowly and in general is felt to be a variant of normal, although links have been made in girls with hyperinsulinism and polycystic ovarian syndrome later on in life. For more detail see adrenarche (below).[35]

Isolated menarche

Rarely an apparently prepubertal girl may present with a vaginal bleed of a few days' duration which sometimes can be repeated at monthly intervals. Exclusion of intrapelvic pathology is necessary by pelvic ultrasound and measurement of estradiol and gonadotrophins, after which this feature can be regarded as a variant of normal. A thin endometrial echo may be seen on the pelvic ultrasound scan. A single isolated vaginal withdrawal bleed (dark blood) in an otherwise prepubertal girl may be due to involution of a dominant follicular ovarian cyst.

Adolescent gynecomastia

Gynecomastia, either unilateral or bilateral, occurs in 40% of normal boys as a result of a testosterone/estrogen imbalance and the commonest time of onset is between Tanner stages G3 and G4, and it usually disappears 1 to 2 years later when testosterone levels rise (Tanner stage G4 to G5). In most situations no treatment, only reassurance, is required. Persistent discs of breast tissue may require surgical removal for cosmetic reasons (see below – gynecomastia).

GROWTH REGULATION AND DISORDERS OF GROWTH

THE GROWTH HORMONE (GH) AXIS AND GROWTH

GH, a 191 amino acid anterior pituitary polypeptide, is secreted episodically throughout 24 h, but predominantly at night during slow wave sleep during which there are usually three to five discrete pulses and is of cardinal importance in the control of growth. Release is mediated by the two hypothalamic peptides: GH releasing hormone (GHRH) – stimulatory, and somatostatin – inhibitory. Dopaminergic, serotonergic and noradrenergic pathways impinge on the GH regulatory neurone system, but cholinergic neurotransmitter pathways seem particularly important in controlling GHRH and somatostatin release. Hippocampal impulses, perhaps sleep-related, are stimulatory whilst impulses from the amygdala may be either stimulatory or inhibitory. Somatostatin secretion is mediated via the hypothalamic ventromedial nucleus.

A number of drugs induce changes in GH secretion via specific neurotransmitter pathways: clonidine is stimulatory via alpha-adrenergic and diazepam via GABA pathways; bromocriptine, propranolol and cholinergic agents probably inhibit somatostatin release. This is relevant in understanding pharmacological stimulation tests and, potentially, for therapy to stimulate GH secretion.

GH releasing hormone was first identified from the pancreas of a woman with Turner syndrome who developed acromegaly which failed to resolve after transsphenoidal pituitary surgery. Full bioactivity resides in its first 29 amino acids. Recently, a long-recognized family of potent small synthetic GH releasing peptides, GH releasing hexapeptide (GHRP) and its analogues, have become important for their potential future therapeutic roles. GHRPs are active given by intravenous, subcutaneous, intranasal and oral routes releasing GH via a specific, non-opiate, non-GHRH pituitary receptor – GHRPs do not interact with GHRH and somatostatin (SRIH) receptors. An additional, hypothalamic, site of action is possible as they require intact GHRH secretion to be effective. Continuous GHRP administration leads to pulsatile GH release.

Analogues such as GHRP6 (hexarelin) and GHRP2 are currently under investigation as are non-peptide orally active mimetics such as L–692,429. At equivalent (near-maximal) intravenous doses, hexarelin is a more potent GH secretogogue than GHRH but acts synergistically with GHRH when administered synchronously to healthy adult male volunteers.[81] Intranasal hexarelin is also a potent GH secretogogue in prepubertal children with constitutional short stature.[82] GHRPs given intravenously and orally are currently under investigation in a variety of groups of short stature children. Their potent ability to stimulate GH synthesis and release plus their effectiveness when given orally make them potentially useful, both as diagnostic agents in the evaluation of pituitary disorders and as oral GH secretogogues in 'short normal' children and those in whom 'GH deficiency' is largely hypothalamic rather than pituitary in origin (e.g. post-radiotherapy). They are ineffective in children with organic pituitary disease. For a review see Huerta & Rogol.[83]

Recently, ghrelin, a 28 amino acid peptide, has been identified as the natural ligand of the GH secretogogue receptor in the hypothalamus and pituitary.[84,85] In humans, the serum GH response to intravenous ghrelin is greater than that observed with GHRH, and when ghrelin and GHRH are co-administered, the response is augmented. Ghrelin has been isolated from the arcuate nucleus, but the GI tract, and particularly the stomach, appears to be a major site of production. Plasma ghrelin-like immunoreactivity is increased by fasting, reduced by feeding and correlates negatively with BMI.[86] Ghrelin is probably involved in integrating the hormonal and metabolic responses to fasting, producing an increase in GH secretion, increased drive to eat, inhibition of insulin secretion and activation of mechanisms directed at maintaining blood glucose levels.[87]

The effective therapeutic use of GHRH itself, potentially a physiological way of treating GH deficiency when the pituitary is intact, has been hampered by the lack of a depot preparation. However subcutaneous GHRH (given twice daily) has been shown to be effective at stimulating growth, e.g. in children treated with cranial irradiation-induced GH deficiency.[88]

Yet other peptides are also important in the regulation of GH secretion: endorphins, neurotensin and vasoactive intestinal peptide (VIP) are stimulatory whilst substance P and central thyrotrophin-releasing hormone (TRH) pathways are inhibitory. VIP may have an important role in the release of GH and prolactin in health and disease (e.g. obesity, anorexia nervosa).[89,90]

GH is unusual in being species specific. Two forms are present in man and it is secreted as a heterogeneous molecular species. The predominant, and presumably more bioactive, form is of MW 22 000 (22K). An approximately 20K form is present in smaller amounts. Structurally abnormal GH variants with varying bioactivity could be important in the etiology of growth failure in certain rare conditions but are unlikely to be common reasons for poor growth in the population as a whole.

GH is not inhibited by feedback from peripheral endocrine glands although thyroxine and glucocorticoids influence its secretion. Regulation is by GH itself (at hypothalamic and pituitary levels), peripheral GH-dependent growth factors (e.g. IGF-1), GHRH and somatostatin and metabolic factors such as free fatty acids and glucose. The physiological role of GHRPs is still unclear. The integration of this control with physiological states – sleep, exercise, appetite and nutrition – is via the monoaminergic and peptide systems described above.

The plasma half-life of exogenously administered GH is 20–25 min; that of endogenous GH is thought to be similar or shorter although this remains controversial. GH affects linear growth directly by stimulating early epiphyseal growth plate precursor cell differentiation but it is uncertain whether it has anabolic effects independent of IGF-1. Paracrine IGF-1, produced locally in proliferating chondrocytes of the growth plate, is more important than liver-derived circulating IGF-1 in stimulating epiphyseal cartilage growth.

In the interaction between GH and tissue growth, the GH receptor is of crucial importance. The GH receptor was cloned from rabbit liver based on amino acid sequence data and from human liver by cross hybridization and consists of a 620 amino acid (AA) peptide situated astride the target cell membrane with a single transmembrane domain. The extracellular hormone-binding domain consists of approximately 245 AAs and there is a cytoplasmic region of 350 residues (Fig. 13.23).

Eighty-five per cent of the cytoplasmic domain is unnecessary for signal transduction. Overall there is 24% homology with the PRL receptor – some sections are strikingly similar. Defects in the gene encoding the receptor have been identified in GH insensitivity syndrome (GHIS, Laron-type dwarfism) indicating that the receptor is required for normal growth. The extracellular component circulates as a high affinity GH binding protein (GHBP). One molecule of GH binds to, and dimerizes, two molecules of receptor – thus there are two binding sites on the GH molecule with the second near the N terminus.

Receptor dimerization is the first step in the GH signaling pathway. A prediction of the model is that high levels of circulating GH, or GH with one abnormal binding site, should have antagonist rather than agonist activity. This is true of site 2 GH mutants although site 1 GH mutants show poor antagonism. GH to receptor concentrations of 1:1 show antagonism as predicted.

Laron dwarfism[91] is the classical form of GHIS resulting from molecular defects in the GH receptor caused by gene deletions or point mutations.[92] Evidence[93] that heterozygous expression of GH receptor mutations may be associated with growth failure, raises questions not only as to whether heterozygotic expression of Laron dwarfism results in a clinically important phenotype but also whether a significant minority of children with 'idiopathic short stature' could be heterozygous for mutations of the GH receptor with abnormal receptor signaling.[94] This also has implications for investigation and diagnosis of short stature and GH 'deficiency'.

Current GH signal transduction models[95] involve activation by GH of a GH receptor-associated tyrosine kinase (GHRTK), an important early (and perhaps initiating) step in signal transduction. GHRTK, stimulated within less than 30 s of GH binding to the receptor by very low GH concentrations, is likely to have a role in stimulation by GH of a variety of cellular responses including kinase activity and gene expression. In particular, GH stimulates tyrosyl phosphorylation and kinase activity of a GH dependent GH

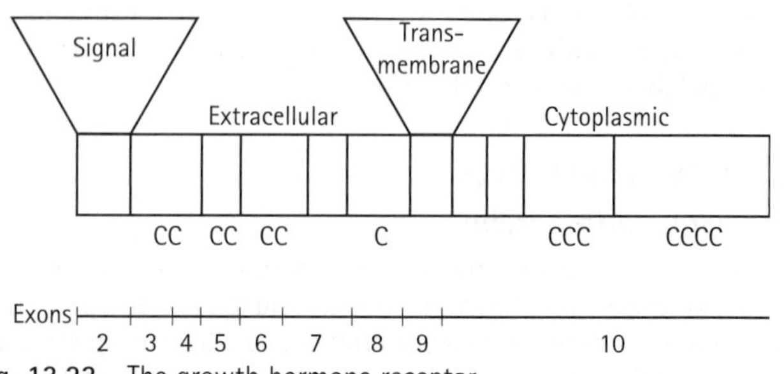

Fig. 13.23 The growth hormone receptor.

receptor-associated kinase JAK 2 (one of a family of Janus kinases). JAK 2 probably serves as a signaling molecule for multiple members of a cytokine/hematopoietin family which includes GH, PRL, erythropoietin, interleukin-3, etc. GHRTK functions both to activate other proteins by phophorylation and to phosphorylate tyrosyl residues in itself and the GH receptor. These phosphorylated tyrosines may serve as docking sites for proteins in other signaling pathways. Such studies should lead to the identification of new cellular actions for GH.

GH receptors in sheep hepatocytes turn over rapidly (every 30–90 min); their number is regulated by, for example, nutritional factors and estrogens as well as GH itself.[96] It is likely that acuteness or chronicity of GH exposure profoundly influences GH receptor turnover rates. GHBP levels also vary diurnally and do not correlate with GH peaks. Human GHBP and GH receptor are encoded by a single species mRNA.[97] Proteolysis is probably the major mechanism for GHBP production in man – GHBP blood levels probably do not represent GH receptor status in functional terms.

Thus to be biologically active, GH must bind to a transmembrane receptor, which must dimerize and activate an intracellular signal transduction pathway causing IGF-1 synthesis and secretion. However, IGF-1 which, in blood, is itself bound to members of a family of binding proteins (IGFBPs), must bind to the IGF-1 receptor, in turn activating its own signal transduction pathways producing mitogenic and anabolic responses and tissue growth. Thus GH effects its action on target tissues by binding to specific receptors expressed both in the liver and other target tissues throughout the body. This activates genes which include those which code for IGF-1 which stimulates tissue growth by endocrine and (largely) paracrine and autocrine activity. The complexity of these pathways (together with the vagaries of GH assays and the pulsatile nature of GH release) help to explain the difficulties in measuring 'GH secretory ability' in many short stature children.

The clinical phenotypes of GH insensitivity reflect the effects of postnatal IGF deficiency and are broadly identical to the phenotype of complete congenital GH deficiency. This phenotype differs somewhat from that of defects of the IGF-1 gene[98,99] indicating that prenatal IGF-1 production is largely independent of GH and that IGF-1 (and not GH) is a major factor in intrauterine growth regulation.

GROWTH REGULATION

The determination of the somatotroph cell line is dependent on various transcription factors: Lhx3, Prop-1, and Pit-1. Pit-1 also plays a role in the activation and regulation of the somatotroph gene product, GH. Additional factors such as CREB and the GHRH receptor, may be important for somatotroph determination, while Zn-15 and Pitx2 are thought to be involved in GH gene activation.[10]

A gene thought to be critical for normal growth, the 'short stature homeobox-containing gene' (SHOX), has been identified[100,101] on the pseudoautosomal region of the sex chromosomes (a region of the X chromosome which normally escapes X inactivation). A SHOX mutation was described in 1 of 91 children with idiopathic short stature[100] and has been found to be common in Leri–Weill dyschondrosteosis – an autosomal dominant form of mesomelic dysplasia which has a number of features in common with Turner syndrome (e.g. wide carrying angle, scoliosis and palatal abnormalities).[102,103] SHOX mutations are implicated in both the short stature and skeletal dysplastic abnormalities of Turner syndrome.[100,101,104]

Mechanisms by which physiological states, GH regulation and genetic determination of growth potential are integrated to achieve appropriate stature are largely unknown. Tanner[105] has proposed that the CNS contains a 'sizostat' – the rate of synthesis or release of a specific molecule could decrease as maturity increases and another molecule could be synthesized in proportion to the amount of growth. A 'mismatch' would be sensed by the sizostat and growth adjusted accordingly. This concept, and 'catch-up'[106] and 'catch-down' growth made it uncertain that exogenous hormone therapy in various categories of short children would necessarily increase final height significantly and this has, generally, been found to be the case in practice in recent years.

'Catch-up' growth, rather than CNS-dependent, is more likely intrinsic to the growth plate. Baron et al[107] infused dexamethasone phosphate into one proximal tibial growth plate of 5 week old rabbits over 4 weeks and inactive vehicle into the contralateral growth plate. Growth plate growth velocity was determined radiologically. Dexamethasone significantly decreased growth velocity in the growth plate compared to the contralateral control causing significant growth deficit. After the end of the infusion, growth velocity in the dexamethasone-treated growth plate rebounded above that of the control, ultimately correcting approximately half the deficit suggesting that 'catch-up' growth is, at least in part, intrinsic to the epiphyseal growth plate and cannot be explained by central mechanisms alone.

Mathematical models of human growth were descriptive[108] but those relating to possible underlying dynamics of hormonal (and other) control have since been proposed.[80] This 'infancy–childhood–puberty' model of growth suggests that the infancy component (which is a continuation of fetal growth) is primarily determined by nutritional factors, the childhood component by GH and the puberty component by sex steroids. The infancy component is initially rapid but decelerates as the influence of GH appears by the end of the first year. The effect of GH is sustained but in the absence of adequate sex steroid secretion the pubertal growth spurt is blunted or absent. The combined input of the three components results in the normal pattern of growth to final height. Such a model, simplistic if control mechanisms are seen as 'all or none' phenomena, does potentially enable effects of different insults which may affect growth and different treatment modalities to be studied more effectively. Tall children secrete more GH than their short peers[109] and GH secretory pulse amplitude correlates with growth velocity although not very strongly.

'Growing pains' appear to be a frequent form of pain in otherwise healthy schoolchildren. However, they probably have little to do with growth. The pain or ache is usually bilateral, commonly situated in the front of the thighs, in the calves and behind the knees and never situated at or near any joints. There is never any limp, tenderness, redness or swelling. The groin is sometimes affected. Discomfort may come on suddenly or gradually and does not usually occur every day and usually occurs late in the day and in the evening. When the child wakes in the morning, the pain has usually disappeared. It was once said that emotional growth can be painful but physical growth is not. Perhaps it is simply best to admit ignorance about the cause(s) of 'growing pains' and recognize that they are harmless and self-limiting. They may also be part of the migraine/periodic syndrome spectrum (see migraine in Ch. 20).

THE SHORT OR SLOWLY GROWING CHILD

The 'normality' of a child's height is determined by reference to growth charts showing population norms. Ideally each country and ethnic group should have its own growth standards. In practice, UK charts serve well even in developing countries and for ethnic minorities within the UK because differences in final stature reflect minor differences in growth velocity over the whole growing period. Introduction in the UK of nine centile growth charts, based on seven largely cross-sectional local growth surveys between 1978 and 1990[60] should help to facilitate the appropriate referral of children with growth disorders following community height *screening* (see above). The lowest centile is the 0.4 line – only one normal child in 250 will fall below that line which is a clear indicator for referral. The interval between each provided pair of centile lines is the same – two-thirds of a standard deviation. Two per cent of the normal population will have a height below the second centile. It is recommended that any child between the 2nd and 0.4 centiles is monitored to see whether their growth is normal. Versions are available for community and hospital use.

Revised charts based on the Tanner–Whitehouse growth standards (determined in a longitudinal study of South of England children in the 1960s) have been produced – the Buckler–Tanner 1995 longitudinal standards.[63] Height revision is adjusted to take account of the recent cross-sectional studies and of Buckler's longitudinal study of adolescent growth.[110] For *monitoring* the growth pattern in an individual child such charts are preferable. Three per cent of normal children will, by definition, be below the third centile on a distance (height for age) chart yet a child with a growth disorder of recent onset will be of normal stature. Only serial measurements and calculation of growth velocity will distinguish normality from abnormality.

Parental genetic contributions reduce the population standard deviation of height by about 30%. Ninety-five per cent of the children of given parents will have a height prognosis within ±10 cm of the mid-parental *centile*. Children also 'inherit' an environment from their parents. A child's shortness, whilst 'appropriate' for his short parents, may reflect poor nutrition or emotional deprivation continuing down the generations with no family member achieving their true genetic height potential. The mean height of children from lower social class IV and V families remains significantly less than that of those from higher social classes I and II in Britain in the 1980s as it did in the 1870s despite the secular trend to increasing height in both groups.[57]

The possibility of an unrecognized and untreated growth disorder in an unusually short parent must be excluded before attributing a child's shortness to constitutional reasons – pathology, e.g. GH deficiency, a skeletal dysplasia or pseudohypoparathyroidism, may also be genetically transmitted.

The differential diagnosis of short stature or slow growth is summarized in Table 13.6. Whatever their ultimate height prognosis, some short children may suffer emotionally and underachieve. 'Western' society views tallness as a positive attribute and the social consequences of short stature are not dependent on the presence of underlying pathology, which must be sought if growth velocity is inadequate. Without diagnostic clues from history or examination, the screening test for a child presenting with short stature is calculation of growth velocity.

A small child who is growing normally may have small parents (constitutional short stature, but see above), growth (and likely maturational) delay, a previous period of poor growth (e.g. due to prolonged IUGR, e.g. Silver–Russell syndrome – see Fig. 13.24) or a combination of these factors.

There are currently many children who are short without a recognized cause. These children, with so-called idiopathic short stature (ISS), can be considered either as part of the continuum between complete growth hormone deficiency (GHD) and normality, or as short stature in the absence of a demonstrable abnormality of the GH–IGF-1 axis.[111] Synonyms of the condition have included normal short stature, primary or constitutional short stature, normal-variant short stature, constitutional delay of growth and adolescence (CDGA) and familial short stature (FSS).

Table 13.6 Differential diagnosis of short stature and slow growth

Short with currently normal growth velocity
Constitutional short stature, short normal parent(s)
Previous problem affecting growth, now cured or no longer operative
Prolonged intrauterine growth retardation – light for gestational age, low birth length and head circumference, difficult feeders in infancy, including Silver–Russell syndrome – triangular facies, clinodactyly, facial and limb length asymmetry
Congenital heart disease
Physiological growth delay (delayed bone age, normal height prognosis)
Growing slowly (whether already short or still of normal stature)
With increased skinfold thicknesses
Endocrine disease (e.g. panhypopituitarism, severe growth hormone insufficiency – idiopathic or secondary to tumor or irradiation, hypothyroidism, pseudohypoparathyroidism, Cushing's syndrome)
Disproportionate
Short limbs for spine (the dyschondroplasias) (e.g. achondroplasia, hypochondroplasia, multiple epiphyseal dysplasia)
Short limbs and spine (spine relatively shorter) (e.g. mucopolysaccharidoses, metatropic dwarfism)
Often without other obvious signs of disease (see text)
Chromosomal abnormalities (e.g. Turner syndrome – other signs variable)
Unrecognized asthma (may be misdiagnosed)
Malabsorption due to celiac disease, ulcerative colitis, Crohn's disease (bowel habit may be normal)
Psychosocial deprivation
Malnutrition
Cardiovascular or renal disease

The definition of ISS cannot be refined until we have an adequate definition of GHD. An agreed current working definition is that ISS is a heterogeneous state that encompasses individuals of short stature, including those with FSS, for which there is no currently recognized cause.

Many children referred to as having ISS will undoubtedly have some undiagnosed underlying pathology within the GH–IGF-1 axis and increasing understanding of the pathophysiology of growth disorders will reduce the number of children categorized as having ISS.[111,112]

The relatively poor sensitivity and specificity of GH stimulation tests[113] (see below) means that many patients currently labeled as having idiopathic GHD would probably be better categorized as having ISS. Many of these 'misdiagnosed' patients are currently responding well to GH therapy. Significant increases in final height have been reported after treatment of ISS with GH, although many of the studies have involved small numbers of patients and have suffered from significant methodological faults. Whilst patients with ISS may show psychological stress, they do not appear to have clinically significant behavioral or emotional problems, and it needs to be established whether being taller produces measurable psychological benefit. There is no strong evidence that GH therapy improves psychological adaptation in children with ISS. From a socioeconomic perspective, more evidence of the effectiveness of GH therapy in individual patients with ISS is required before the use of pooled funds can be justified.[111] However, any treatment recommendations based on socioeconomic considerations should be

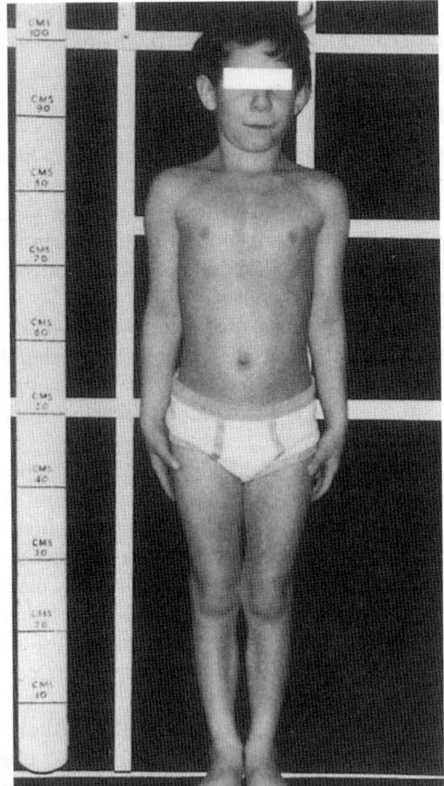

(a)

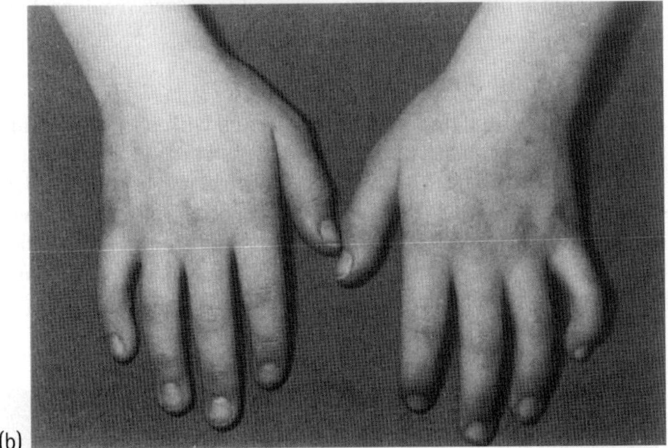

(b)

Fig. 13.24 A child with prolonged intrauterine growth retardation (Silver–Russell) syndrome presenting with short stature. Note the triangular facies, low-set ears, asymmetry (a) and clinodactyly (b).

tempered by the fact that it is still not possible to discriminate clearly between partial GHD, subtle abnormalities of the GH–IGF-1 axis and many cases of ISS.[111]

The differential diagnosis of causes of slow growth, whatever the current height, is wide (see Table 13.6). Genetic and dysmorphic syndromes of short stature are reviewed by Borochowitz & Rimoin.[114]

Endocrine causes

Impaired GH secretion

A few children lack the gene for making GH, demonstrate prenatal GH deficiency, respond to GH therapy with the major antibody response expected to a foreign protein and cannot be treated with any form of GH. Otherwise there is a wide spectrum of GH and IGF-1 secretory ability, which, within the normal population, is likely to be largely genetically determined (see above). At one end of the spectrum are children, perhaps 1 in 4000,[115] with severe GH insufficiency ('GH deficiency'). They grow slowly (Fig. 13.25) and demonstrate characteristic clinical features – truncal obesity with characteristic fat 'marbling' (Fig. 13.26), crowding of mid-facial features with immature appearance and small genitalia with micropenis in boys – and show an inadequate (< 7 mU/L) response to a pharmacological stimulus to GH secretion.[116]

There is a continuum from ISS (see above) through moderate GH insufficiency (so-called 'partial' GH deficiency with GH responses in the 7–15 mU/L range), short normal, averagely tall to tall normal individuals and those with gigantism (Fig. 13.27). Some short, slowly-growing children have what is considered to be an abnormal pattern of GH pulsatile release but normal GH responses to stimulation tests – 'neurosecretory dysfunction'.[117] It is possible that genetic polymorphism for the GH or IGF-1 receptor, IGF-1 or IGFBP3, could also underlie the spectrum of height seen in a normal population. Heterozygosity for classical autosomal recessive disorders could, speculatively, explain growth abnormalities in many children with 'idiopathic' short stature.

Severe GH insufficiency may be congenital, acquired, isolated or associated with other pituitary hormone deficiencies. Many children with 'idiopathic isolated GH deficiency' have a hypothalamic disorder of GHRH release responding to a GHRH bolus by secreting GH normally (see below). In others, high resolution CT or MR scanning demonstrates abnormalities ranging from absent septum pellucidum associated with other midline defects (septo-optic dysplasia) to pituitary hypoplasia.

Acquired GH 'deficiency' may result from intracranial tumor (e.g. craniopharyngioma) or from cranial irradiation for medulloblastoma or acute lymphoblastic leukemia. The effects of chemotherapy on growth (and endocrine function) are increasingly recognized. Temporary GH deficiency is seen in children with

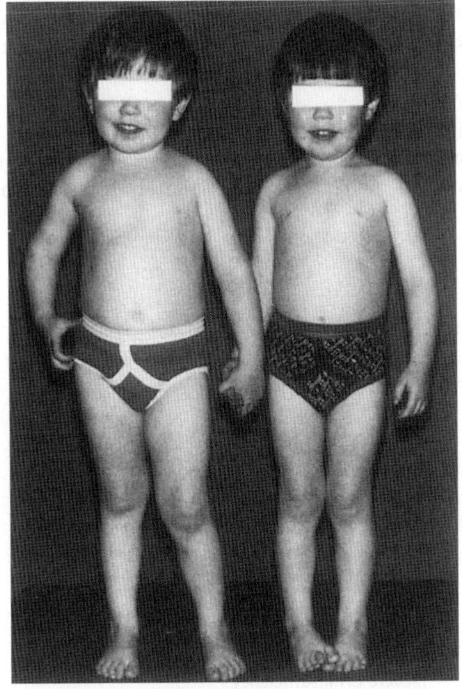

Fig. 13.25 A boy with severe GH insufficiency (right) who is shorter than his 2 years younger brother. Triceps and subscapular skinfold measurements were 97th centile.

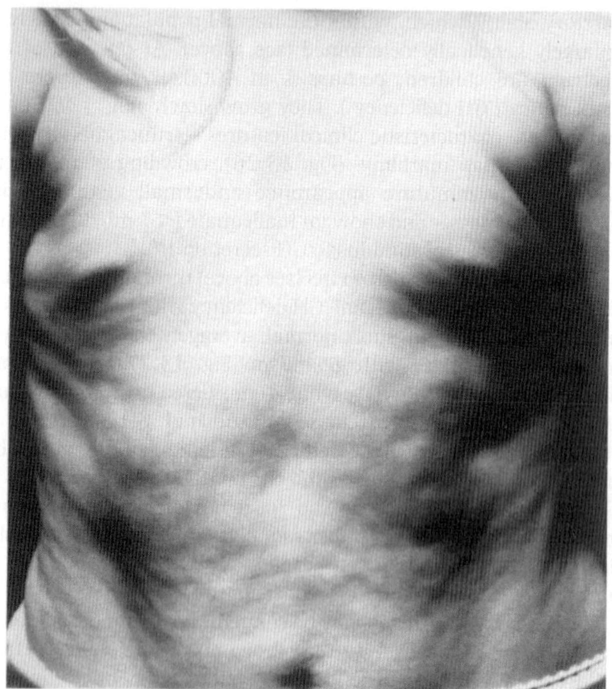

Fig. 13.26 Characteristic 'marbling' of fat in severe GH insufficiency.

psychosocial deprivation (see below) and occurs physiologically in late prepuberty and early male puberty. GH biosynthesis and release is also impaired in other conditions (e.g. primary hypothyroidism or celiac disease) – secretion normalizes with treatment of the underlying disorder.

Hypothyroidism

Acquired primary hypothyroidism is usually autoimmune (Hashimoto thyroiditis). Poor growth velocity and school performance often precede the well-known symptoms and signs by many months. Abnormal growth in thyroid disorders is reviewed by Grüters.[22]

Steroids

Growth failure from glucocorticoids is usually iatrogenic (excessive medication) rather than due to pituitary dependent Cushing's disease (excess ACTH secretion), adrenal tumor (benign or malignant) or ectopic tumor ACTH production which are all rare in children. Alternate day steroid regimens seem less growth suppressing.

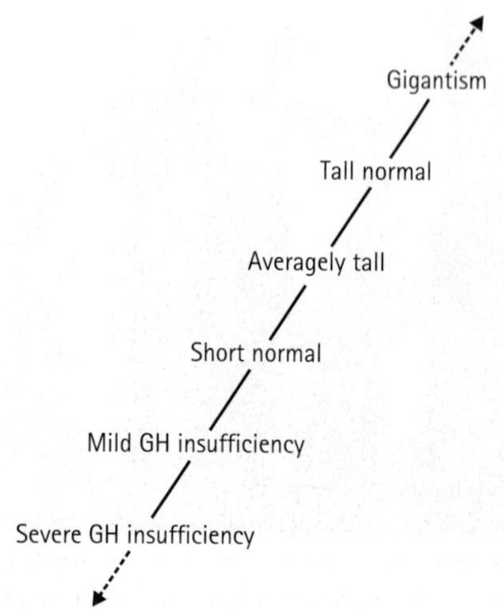

Fig. 13.27 The spectrum of growth hormone secretory ability.

Disproportionate short stature

Most constitutional disorders of bone involve long bones and spine to a different extent leading to disproportionate short stature. This may be obvious clinically when there is gross disproportion but may need to be specifically identified from sitting height measurements (subischial leg length equals standing height minus sitting height) and reference to standard charts.

The most important group of skeletal dysplasias affecting cartilage and/or bone growth and development are the osteochondrodysplasias. Those affecting tubular or spinal bone growth or both are known as chondrodystrophies. It is increasingly possible to classify skeletal dysplasias on a pathophysiological basis.[118]

It is important to recognize disproportionate short stature so that accurate diagnosis can be made without unnecessary investigation. In general, biochemical investigation is unhelpful other than when a mucopolysaccharidosis or disorder of calcium metabolism is suspected and bone biopsy is rarely diagnostic. A full or selective skeletal survey generally yields most helpful diagnostic information and must be interpreted by a radiologist with particular expertise. Even so, radiological changes in many conditions only become diagnostic in older children.

In general specific therapy is unavailable (although there can be a short term response to GH therapy) but accurate diagnosis is necessary for genetic counseling and accurate prognosis. Limb lengthening orthopedic procedures are reviewed by Saleh et al.[119]

Chromosomal abnormalities

Many chromosomal disorders are associated with poor growth and short stature, particularly absence, partial deletion or translocations of the X chromosome (Turner syndrome and its mosaic forms – Fig. 13.28; see below). Turner syndrome girls with tall parents may not become conspicuously short until puberty fails to start. Growth charts for Turner syndrome[76] and Down syndrome[75] are available.

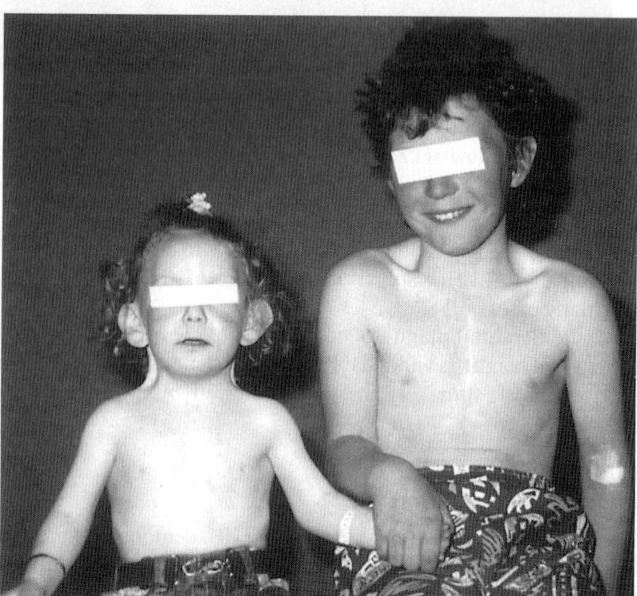

Fig. 13.28 Two unrelated girls with Turner syndrome.

Inheritance of two maternal alleles from the same parent (uniparental disomy), in this case on chromosome 7, may be a feature in some patients with severe IUGR (Silver–Russell syndrome or primordial dwarfism). There are several potentially relevant genes which map to the long arm of chromosome 7, e.g. those for IGFBP1, IGFBP3 and the EGF receptor. Whether any are influenced by the disomy, and thus involved in the pathogenesis of Silver–Russell syndrome remains to be determined. Some children with postnatal short stature following IUGR appear to have alterations in IGF-1 receptor (IGF-1R) binding.[120]

Chronic disease

Differential diagnosis of the short but not fat child covers virtually the whole field of chronic disorders. Some may be suspected from history or clinical findings but poor growth is often the major diagnostic clue to psychosocial deprivation (see below), unrecognized or undertreated asthma, renal tubular acidosis and malabsorption syndromes such as celiac disease and chronic inflammatory bowel disease, Crohn's disease or ulcerative colitis. Worldwide, protein/calorie deprivation is the commonest cause of growth failure; GH levels are high but peripheral growth factor synthesis and IGF-1 levels are low.

Psychosocial deprivation

Psychosocial deprivation often causes poor growth, may mimic idiopathic hypopituitarism in terms of GH responses to conventional stimuli[121,122] and abnormal overnight GH secretory profiles may return to normal rapidly following admission to hospital.[123] Any child growing poorly at home who thrives in hospital or when fostered (Fig. 13.29) should be suspected of being emotionally deprived. Accurately maintained growth data are increasingly accepted as evidence in British courts. Severe growth failure may result from Munchausen syndrome by proxy (child abuse).[124]

Laron dwarfism [91,125]

This is an autosomal recessively inherited syndrome associated with molecular defects in the GH receptor caused by gene deletions or point mutations.[126] These children, whose GH is active in in vitro GH receptor assays, characteristically demonstrate severe postnatal growth failure, secrete abundant GH (with normal or elevated serum levels) but have markedly reduced serum concentrations of IGF-1 and IGFBP3 and do not respond to GH therapy. In clinical trials, some respond well to IGF-1 therapy[127] but its future availability is now in doubt.

Early cases demonstrated low serum GHBP concentrations indicating abnormalities of the extracellular domain of the GH receptor, i.e. circulating GHBP. Many may have deletions or point mutations of the GH receptor gene (nine coding regions – exons – occupying an 87 kilobase segment of chromosome 5) coding for the GH-binding domain. However, it now seems that a minority of the several hundred cases identified worldwide have normal circulating GHBP levels suggesting a degree of heterozygosity and defects in either the portion of the extracellular domain of the GH receptor molecule needed for dimerization or intracellular defects affecting signal transduction.

INVESTIGATION OF POOR GROWTH

This is summarized in Table 13.7. Random determination of serum GH levels is unhelpful – pulsatile release and short serum half-life

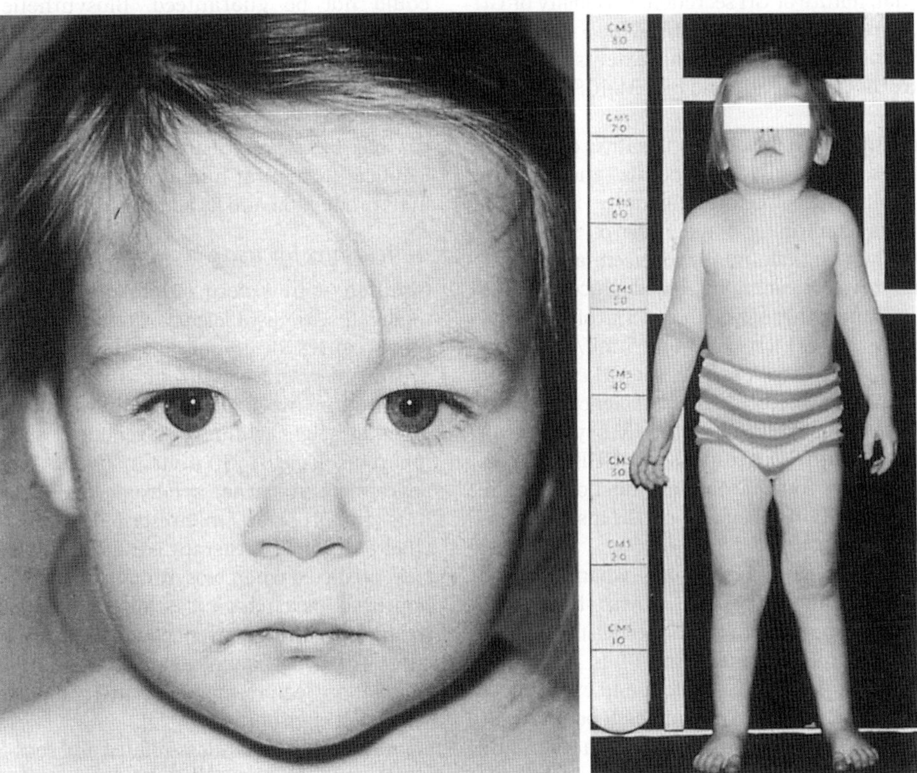

Fig. 13.29 An emotionally abused child (note the characteristic expression of 'frozen watchfulness'), photographed on the day of admission to hospital. In the ward environment she showed remarkable 'catch-up' growth and growth hormone secretion normalized. She has since been successfully adopted.

Table 13.7 Investigation of poor growth

Full medical and social history
Accurate measurement of the child and his parents
Thorough clinical examination (including measurement of blood pressure, fundi, visual fields)
Bone age
Karyotype (girls)
Specific investigation (when indicated)
Hematological (e.g. Hb, FBC, ESR)
Biochemical (e.g. Ca, PO_4, alkaline phosphatase, urea and electrolytes)
Cardiac
Respiratory
Renal
Gastrointestinal including jejunal biopsy
Endocrine (e.g. T4, prolactin, GnRH, TRH tests, growth hormone provocation test*)
Skeletal (e.g. radiograph of pituitary fossa, skeletal survey)

* Growth hormone 'provocation' tests (see text):
post-exercise, 3–4 h postprandial, 1 h after sleep onset } 'screening'
clonidine, ITT, arginine, glucagon } 'pharmacological'
physiological sleep studies
urinary GH.

often result in low levels in normal children. Establishing a reasonable assessment of GH secretory ability or a firm diagnosis of GH deficiency can be difficult because of the pulsatile, and predominantly nocturnal, nature of GH secretion, variability of GH assays (monoclonal, polyclonal, RIA, IRMA which recognize different circulating forms of GH to varying extents) and the complexity of the control of GH secretion and the GH–IGF-1-growth metabolic pathways.

All GH provocation tests may give false negative or positive responses. Screening tests are difficult to standardize and response is variable.[113] The insulin hypoglycemia (tolerance) test (ITT) remains the standard for confirming a diagnosis of severe GH insufficiency. Adequate (symptomatic) hypoglycemia must be obtained if results are to be meaningful (blood glucose < 2.2 mmol/L). Following adequate hypoglycemia, 85% of 'normal' children will produce a serum GH level of over 15 mU/L (usually after 30–60 min). In conjunction with an ITT, the GH response to GHRH is useful for determining whether 'GH insufficiency' is due to a pituitary defect or hypothalamic disorder of GHRH synthesis or release.[128] In the latter case the GH response to GHRH will be normal indicating that pituitary somatotrophs are functional, e.g. in many children with 'isolated GH insufficiency' or 'GH insufficiency' secondary to cranial irradiation.[129]

Tests of GH secretion must be performed only when indicated (and when other possible causes of poor growth have been considered). They should only be undertaken in specialist endocrine units experienced with their performance. An ITT is potentially dangerous and requires supervision by competent and experienced junior pediatric staff working from clear and understood protocols and guidelines. These should ensure that glucose and hydrocortisone are drawn up in readiness, there is checking of insulin and glucose dosages, continual presence of a dedicated and experienced member of nursing staff present throughout for monitoring of blood glucose and conscious level, adequate and secure venous access established before insulin is administered and detailed instruction for management of hypoglycemia.

Some centers measure spontaneous nocturnal pulsatile GH release to provide greater insight into secretory control mechanisms. Their relevance to short stature assessment or as a predictor of response to therapy remains controversial, though there may be a relationship between the amplitude of GH pulses and growth velocity. Such tests are impracticable for 'screening' large numbers of children.

Urinary GH measurement could become a useful, non-invasive, repeatable and cheap way of assessing physiological GH secretion but urinary GH levels vary considerably day by day, are approximately 1000-fold lower than in plasma and until recently, accuracy and reproducibility were poor.[130]

Measurements of serum IGF-1 and IGFBP3 (and, perhaps, urinary GH) may be useful screening tests for identifying short children who need more complex investigations of GH secretory ability.[131]

TREATMENT OF POOR GROWTH

Treatment aims to correct the underlying problem where possible (e.g. gluten-free diet in celiac disease, thyroxine in hypothyroidism) and can only maximize remaining growth potential. The sooner poor growth is recognized, its cause diagnosed and treated, the better the height prognosis.

Growth hormone

Preparations

From 1958 to 1985, pituitary derived GH was available in limited quantities for children with GH 'deficiency'. These preparations were withdrawn because some batches could have been contaminated with Creutzfeldt–Jakob disease (CJD) 'prion' and current purity could not be guaranteed. Biosynthetic GH, *Escherichia coli* synthesized and produced by recombinant DNA technology, became available in the UK by late 1985. This was initially with an additional amino-terminal methionine (192 amino acids). Since December 1988, natural sequence 191 amino acid biosynthetic GH has been prescribable in the UK. This is physicochemically identical to natural human hormone. No brain tissue is involved in its production and its administration cannot transmit CJD.

Indications for use

Children with severe GH insufficiency (GH 'deficiency') and moderate GH insufficiency should be treated with GH provided other causes of impaired GH secretion have been excluded. Treatment with a physiological replacement dose of 15–21 units (5–7 mg)/m^2/week in daily s.c. doses will result in > 90% achieving an adult height within their genetic target height range.[132] Larger (pharmacological – 30 units/m^2/week, 10 mg/m^2/week) doses are appropriate in Turner syndrome and chronic renal failure.[133,134] It is inappropriate to prescribe GH indiscriminately to short children[135] and GH therapy is indicated in fewer situations than had been predicted when biosynthetic GH first became available.[136] The improved psychological state resulting from knowledge that treatment is being given could itself have a growth-stimulating effect via hypothalamic pathways – children with psychosocial deprivation secrete more GH and grow better when in a normal emotional environment.

Although a social class-related and socially desirable attribute in 'developed' societies, tall stature does not confer innate biological advantage in all societies. In disadvantaged environments (e.g. the Peruvian Andes), small mothers have more surviving offspring;[137] in an agricultural peasant economy, a small man is more efficient than a tall one, requiring to do less work to feed himself.[138,139] Even if GH therapy increases the height of a normally growing short child, will taller stature in itself contribute to academic or material success or psychological contentment? Leaving aside methodological problems in assessing possible psychological disadvantage from short stature in childhood,[140] it seems probable that there are genuine cultural differences in the psychological effects of short stature even between 'developed' countries (e.g. USA and UK).[141,142]

GH therapy seems to be of particular benefit to children with Turner syndrome and could also benefit those with prolonged IUGR (who often remain short despite normal postnatal growth). The variable outcomes of studies of GH in IUGR probably reflect their heterogeneity of etiology of growth retardation.[143] There is controversy over whether catch-up growth in SGA children has adverse metabolic consequences (e.g. insulin resistance) particularly if high GH doses are used.[144] There is encouraging medium-term growth improvement in children with chronic renal failure treated with GH[133,134] and a product licence for this use of GH is now available in a number of countries. Infants with chronic renal failure have also been found to benefit in the short term.[145]

GH is being evaluated in the treatment of some skeletal dysplasias.[146] In these groups, surgical limb lengthening may be indicated once the postpubertal patient is able to decide whether they wish to undergo these major and prolonged procedures.

Due to the shortage of available GH over many years, the dose used in severe GH insufficiency was the most 'cost effective' (in terms of increase in growth velocity achieved per unit GH given) rather than that which would maximally stimulate growth so that, even now, the optimal treatment regimen is not clearly established. A GH dose of 6–8 mg (18–24 units)/m^2/week divided into daily (bedtime) subcutaneous injections may be most effective. Higher (pharmacological) doses [~ 10 mg (30 units) /m^2/week] are more effective in chronic renal disease, Turner syndrome[147] and IUGR. Optimal regimens during puberty have not been established although there is some evidence that mimicking the increase in endogenous GH secretion at the pubertal growth spurt produces a better height outcome.[148] The role of short bursts of GH therapy in a variety of situations remains to be evaluated.

GH antibodies could result in severe growth restriction in a previously normal child but antibodies of sufficient specificity and binding capacity to produce growth attenuation are rare. Potential metabolic side-effects include glucose intolerance, hyperinsulinism, hyperlipidemia, and hypertension. Reports of an increased risk of type 2 diabetes[149] are controversial. Benign intracranial hypertension[150] and slipped capital femoral epiphysis are associations but the latter is found in GH deficient children prior to GH treatment. Leukemia may be more common in GH deficient children treated with GH but there is no evidence causally linking GH treatment itself with leukemia. GH is best avoided in syndromes with chromosomal fragility, e.g. Fanconi syndrome. Psychological harm could result if treatment expectations are not fulfilled.

GHRH therapy may be appropriate in many 'GH insufficient' children when the problem is at hypothalamic, rather than pituitary, level but optimal treatment regimens are unclear.[151] Although it is possible that future growth-promoting treatment modalities could include intranasal GH,[152] intranasal GHRH, depot (intramuscular) GHRH, and IGF-1 in particular circumstances, with several of these preparations bioavailability, practical production difficulties and costs or possible side-effects remain problematic. The most promising developments in the therapeutic application of growth stimulating compounds seems currently to be in the use of depot GH preparations and GH releasing peptides which may impinge significantly on the management of certain types of growth disorder in the future.

Anabolic steroids

Synthetic steroids with enhanced anabolic but little androgenic activity are valuable in growth delay, increasing (normal) slow growth in early male puberty and in Turner syndrome. As with GH therapy, the decision to use these preparations should generally be the province of the specialist in growth disorders.[153]

Emotional support

Emotional support is particularly important for short stature children and their families. Specific treatment may not be available, may be of unproven benefit or may start too late to achieve adequate stature. Any child physically different from his or her peers will attract attention: a short child has to cope with an identity which is determined primarily (and seen by others) in terms of their size.[154] Growth related changes in body shape and size are important determinants of perceived age and adult care-giving responses.[155] Short children must be treated appropriately for their chronological age, emotionally, intellectually and practically. Teasing, bullying and expectations based on physical size rather than on intrinsic abilities will cause immature behavior, underperformance at school and may impair growth further.[156] They are likely to be aggressive to siblings and peers and more anxious and depressed than controls.[157] Poor examination results cause the small school-leaver to have particular difficulties finding employment.

Children treated with GH should not routinely stay on GH therapy once they reach adulthood. Nevertheless, there is evidence that untreated GH deficiency in adulthood is associated with reduced muscle strength and increased fatigue, a high fat to muscle ratio, reduced bone mineral content with increased risk of osteoporosis and fractures and adverse cardiovascular risk factors (dyslipidemia and increased fibrinogen levels). All children who have received GH replacement therapy should have their GH status reassessed in young adulthood. Patients with clear structural lesions of the hypothalamus/pituitary (organic GHD secondary to a mass lesion, pituitary surgery or radiotherapy) are likely to remain GH deficient and should be considered for GH treatment in adulthood, but others (e.g. with 'idiopathic isolated' GH deficiency) frequently have a normal GH secretory capacity on retesting.[158]

THE TALL OR RAPIDLY GROWING CHILD (Table 13.8)

Tall stature presents less often than short – syndromes causing tallness are rare[159] whereas poor growth is a common result of childhood disease, and childhood tallness, unless extreme, is socially advantageous. Nevertheless, a tall child is often taken for older and expectations may be greater than can be met. Clumsiness and gangliness may result from neurological immaturity for size.

Advanced skeletal maturation may be associated with tallness in childhood (and a normal growth velocity) but this rarely results in problems or medical help being sought (c.f. growth delay).

Constitutional tall stature infrequently presents but tall mothers sometimes worry about their normal daughters' heights. In this situation, drug treatment – attempting to limit GH secretion whilst allowing normal sex steroid mediated skeletal maturation [e.g. with bromocriptine,[160] somatostatin analogue (octreotide) or anticholinergic drugs such as pirenzapine or rapidly advancing skeletal maturation (using sex steroids)] – is generally unsatisfactory.

Table 13.8 Differential diagnosis of tall stature or rapid growth

Tall with currently normal growth velocity
Constitutional tall stature (tall normal parent(s))
Previous rapid growth (usually due to overeating)
Physiological growth advance

Currently rapid growth (whether already tall or still of 'normal' stature)
Associated with precocious puberty
Idiopathic (physiological)
Pathological
- Intracranial space-occupying lesions
- Gonadal tumors
- Ectopic gonadotropin-producing tumor (e.g. hepatoblastoma)
- Adrenal
  - Congenital adrenal hyperplasia (21-hydroxylase deficiency, 11beta-hydroxylase deficiency)
  - Cushing's syndrome
  - Neoplasia
- Estrogen ingestion (e.g. mother's oral contraceptives)
- Primary hypothyroidism
- Undefined mechanisms
  - Birth asphyxia
  - Mental retardation, including tuberous sclerosis
  - Neurofibromatosis, McCune–Albright syndrome

Not associated with signs of puberty
Hyperthyroidism
Growth hormone excess (gigantism)

With obesity: currently excessive food intake

With dysmorphic features or disproportion
Marfan's syndrome
- Long, narrow limbs (dolichostenomelia)
- Arachnodactyly
- Scoliosis
- Aortic incompetence – dissecting aneurysm
- Myopia, retinal detachment, upward lens dislocation
- Autosomal dominant (often new mutation)

Homocystinuria
- Marfanoid body habitus
- Mental retardation
- Stiff joints with knock knee
- Downward lens subluxation
- Urine positive for homocystine
- Autosomal recessive

Congenital contractural arachnodactyly
- Kyphoscoliosis
- Joint contractures
- No ocular or CNS problems
- Autosomal dominant

Sotos' syndrome (cerebral gigantism)
- Large size at birth
- Hypertelorism, downslanting palpebral fissures, prominent forehead
- Large hands and feet
- Large male external genitalia
- Mental retardation ±, hypotonia, ataxia

Klinefelter's syndrome
- Disproportionately long legs
- Small firm testes
- Hypogonadism, infertility, with or without gynecomastia

Estrogen therapy causes an initial increase in growth velocity and potential side-effects from the high doses necessary, both short term (headaches and nausea) and long term (diabetes mellitus, hyperlipidemia, hypertension, endometrial carcinoma),[161] limit its usefulness. It cannot be used much earlier than normal pubertal onset and treatment after the growth spurt is underway (early in female puberty) will have only a small effect on reducing final height.

When height prognosis remains unacceptably high to child and family, surgical epiphysiodesis, an established procedure for reducing moderate leg length discrepancy, may be indicated. Surgical management of tall stature is reviewed by Macnicol.[162]

Tall stature syndromes

These are outlined in Table 13.8. Gigantism due to excessive GH secretion is extremely rare in pediatric practice (c.f. acromegaly after epiphyseal closure).

Tallness and obesity

Tallness in childhood is commonly associated with food intake which is, or has been, excessive for growth and energy requirements. In wealthy societies, eating is a social as well as a nutritional activity and moderate fatness in a baby may be seen as proof of mother love. Fat babies tend to be placid and little trouble. Once a child is overweight, calorie intake need not be excessive to maintain the situation. Continuing overeating causes rapid growth, skeletal maturational advance and early epiphyseal closure – adult height is not increased. If overeating stops but calorie reduction is insufficient to lose weight, growth velocity is normal but the child is tall and bone age remains advanced.

Rapid growth and precocious puberty

If nutrition has been normal, rapid growth is most commonly due to precocious puberty. Final height may be significantly short (depending on etiology and duration) due to early epiphyseal closure in pathological precocious puberty but in children with constitutional advance of growth and puberty their genetic adult height potential will be reached.[163]

Endocrine causes of rapid growth

These are either uncommon (thyrotoxicosis) or rare (gigantism, excess androgen secretion from an adrenal tumor).

OBESITY AND THINNESS

Malnutrition leading to obesity or thinness is discussed in Chapter 14. Discussion here is limited to some general comments and consideration of endocrine disorders which may be associated with each nutritional state.

Mechanisms of body mass regulation include genetic, environmental and behavioral factors. Genetic studies in obese mice have revealed the ob gene, its products leptin and the leptin receptor to be important factors in the regulation of both appetite and energy expenditure.[164] Leptin is a 16 kD adipocyte-derived hormone which circulates in the serum in free and bound forms. Initial models of leptin action included leptin-deficient ob/ob mice and leptin-insensitive db/db mice. Peripheral or central administration of leptin reduces body weight, adiposity, and food intake in ob/ob mice but not in db/db mice. Leptin acts through the leptin receptor (part of the cytokine receptor family). In rodents as well as in humans, homozygous mutations in genes encoding leptin or the leptin receptor cause early-onset morbid obesity, hyperphagia and reduced energy expenditure.[165]

Leptin concentrations correlate with adipose tissue mass, and are regulated by feeding and fasting, insulin, glucocorticoids, and other factors. Leptin acts via CNS to reduce food intake and increase energy expenditure. Most obese humans are not leptin deficient, but have a leptin concentration raised in proportion to their fat mass. In the human, leptin deficiency or insensitivity now seems unlikely to be a major cause of obesity.

Leptin is thought to play a role as an endocrine mediator in sexual development and reproduction (see below).

Weight in itself is a poor guide to nutrition – the interpretation of a high weight for a child's height as 'obesity' may be seriously misleading at times when growth and fatness are varying in opposite directions: a normal early pubertal boy is growing slowly but increasing body fat rapidly. Poor weight gain in a baby may be normal if the mother is tall and the father short as the maternal environment (in addition to genetic factors) is important in determining birth weight. In infancy weight gain largely reflects fluid flux; in the older child differences between normal and abnormal rates of weight gain are smaller than the reproducibility of weight measurements obtained some months apart even on sophisticated (and well-maintained and balanced) weighing scales.

The use of body mass index (BMI) – weight (kg)/height $(m)^2$ – provides a practical clinical tool for identification of adults with different degrees of obesity which carry particular adverse risks, for example hypertension, hypercholesterolemia and type 2 diabetes. However use of a stable height as a basis for calculation, inapplicable to growing children, had limited its usefulness in pediatric practice. Age related curves are necessary and UK pediatric standards are now available,[62] showing that BMI changes substantially in children, rising steeply in infancy, falling during preschool years (from around 2 years of age) and rising again (between 5 and 8 years – the 'adiposity rebound') and into adulthood.

Children accumulate fat free mass as they grow and muscle is denser than fat. Thus BMI underestimates the percentage of lean body mass by taking no account of variations in muscularity: particularly fit and muscular individuals will have a relatively high BMI.

In normal and underweight individuals, between one-quarter and one-half of total body fat is subcutaneous – most excess fat in the obese is deposited there. Thus the adequacy, inadequacy or overadequacy of nutrition is effectively assessed from skinfold measurements using calipers (see Fig. 13.5)[166] comparing results with available standards for age.[167] Measurement of limb circumference assesses muscle and bone as well as fat. Measurements of triceps and subscapular skinfolds are representative of total body fat[168] and show least between observer error.[169]

Care must be taken in interpretation: standards will depend on racial, maturational and genetic factors as well as age and change as nutritional recommendations and feeding policies vary. British children were fatter in 1975[167] than in 1962[4] and there is evidence that this trend is continuing.[170] Standards reflect what is present in the 'normal' population, not necessarily what is optimally physiological. Despite this, skinfold measurements provide quick, easy and reproducible estimates of nutritional state and are particularly useful in longitudinal assessment of an individual child.

OBESITY

A standard definition of 'overweight' and obesity' in children and young people is desirable. In adults, cut-off points for overweight and obesity are based on morbidity and mortality associated with excessive weight. In the absence of such data in children, the International Obesity Task Force defined the cut-offs for young people by back-extrapolating from the BMI centile corresponding to values of > 25 kg/m^2 (overweight) and 30 kg/m^2 (obese) at age 18.[171] Simply defining overweight as > 85th BMI centile and obesity as > 95th centile means that as standards are updated the nature of any secular trend to increasing obesity is obscured (15% and 5% will always be overweight or obese respectively) and international comparisons are obscured.[172]

The prevalence of overweight and obesity amongst children has trebled in 20 years[173] and is now a global epidemic.[174] The increase is not only in industrialized but also in developing countries. Overeating is the commonest cause of childhood obesity. Energy intake surplus to requirements for growth, thermogenesis, basal metabolism and activity results in fat deposition (Fig. 13.30). It is likely that some, but not all, obese individuals eat, or have been eating, excessively. Nevertheless, observed variation between individuals in energy intake necessary to achieve normal fat deposition is likely to reflect genetic factors as well as differences in energy expenditure. Relative contributions of environmental and genetic factors remain poorly understood and certainly differ between different obese individuals.

It is no longer thought that there is a necessary progression from the fat infant to fat child with ultimate adult obesity. The first year of life is not critical for determining adipocyte numbers which are related to the degree and duration of obesity rather than age at onset. Fat infants are two to three times likelier to become obese children than their normal peers but progression from childhood to adult obesity is not inevitable: 80% will be of normal weight by primary school[175] and there is scope for therapeutic interventions. A childhood BMI > 85th centile, an obese parent and an early recurrence of the adiposity rebound (at about 5 years) may predict adult obesity.[176,177]

Mild overweight seems unlikely to be associated with short- or long-term ill-health. Nevertheless, childhood obesity may affect educational attainment and interpersonal relationships adversely, especially in boys.[178] Obesity may persist into adulthood and is associated with an increased risk of hypertension, stroke, myocardial infarction or type 2 diabetes mellitus, osteoarthritis, breast and

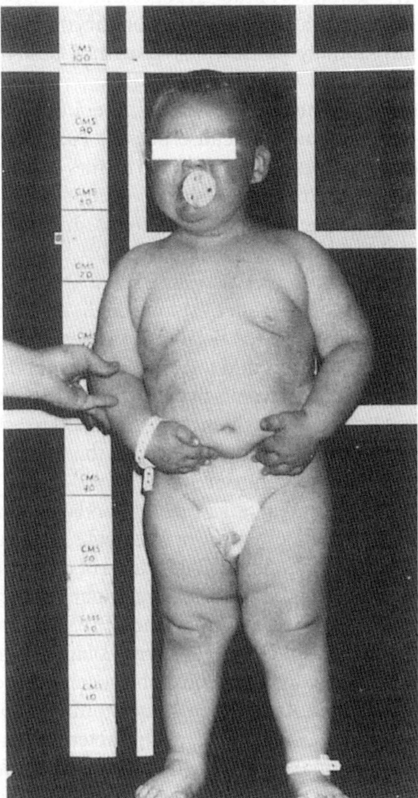

Fig. 13.30 Gross obesity in a toddler due to excessive food intake.

bowel cancers, skin disorders and asthma and other respiratory problems. Hypertension, dyslipidemia and hyperinsulinemia are increasingly found in obese children with two or more risk factors found in 58% of obese children[179] with significantly increased odds ratios for raised diastolic BP (2.4), raised low density lipoprotein (LDL) cholesterol (3.0), raised high density protein (HDL) cholesterol (3.4), raised systolic BP (4.5), raised triglycerides (7.1) and high fasting insulin (12.6).

The most important treatment goal is sustainable healthy eating (rather than 'dieting') and habitual reasonable levels of physical activity (e.g. walking and cycling). Young obese children should aim to maintain their weight (which they will 'grow into') rather than lose weight. Interventions involving parents and behavior modification may be effective.[180] Advice is only likely to be successful if the child and whole family are involved and motivated. Evidence-based management of childhood obesity is summarized by Edmunds et al[181] and a Scottish Intercollegiate Guideline Network[182] guideline for obesity in children and young people is due to be published in 2003.

Obesity can be genetic or endocrine in origin. Height measurement is an important screening test. Overeating causes an increase in growth velocity and these children are generally tall for age with bone age advance. There is early epiphyseal closure and usually no final height increase. Some adolescent boys, in particular, may present with obesity, below average height and delayed puberty. Acceleration of height velocity is seen with rapid weight gain and strict dieting is associated with slowing of linear growth. Thus if overeating stops but there is insufficient reduction in calorie intake to lose weight, growth velocity may be normal but the child is tall and bone age remains advanced.

In contrast, virtually all endocrine and hypothalamic causes of obesity are associated with poor linear growth, short stature and bone age delay. Endocrine causes include excessive corticosteroid administration, GH insufficiency, hypopituitarism, hyper- or hypogonadotrophic hypogonadism, hypothyroidism, pseudohypoparathyroidism and craniopharyngioma. Cushing's syndrome may initially cause rapid growth. Obesity also occurs with hyperinsulinism.

Hypothalamic damage from tumors, meningitis, encephalitis, radiotherapy or trauma may cause obesity. Possible mechanisms underlying the obesity include endocrine factors (hyperinsulinism – but this could be cause or effect), hyperprolactinemia, GH deficiency (but suppressed GH secretion may also be due to obesity) and nutritional and psychological factors.

Hypothalamic syndromes associated with mental retardation and obesity include Laurence–Moon–Biedl and Prader–Willi. Craniopharyngioma may be associated with obesity after surgery or radiotherapy even if vision and activity are normal, food intake is appropriate and endocrine replacement therapy optimal. It seems likely that 'Fröhlich syndrome' (one case of blindness, short stature, obesity and pubertal failure with a cyst in the region of the sella turcica) was due to craniopharyngioma.

The obesity of Down and other mental handicap syndromes may relate both to underlying genetic or metabolic abnormalities and physical inactivity – the latter is a major cause of obesity in physically handicapped children (e.g. spina bifida, muscular dystrophy).

Diagnosis of Prader–Willi syndrome (PWS) is based on the characteristic history and clinical features . Diagnosis may often be made at birth from the association of characteristic facial features with history of poor fetal movements, hypotonia and poor feeding. Abnormalities on chromosome 15 are characteristic and molecular genetic techniques make the diagnosis more certain. Genomic imprinting (differential expression of genetic material depending on whether it originates from father or mother) occurs in the majority: if the 15q deletion (15q11q13) is paternally inherited, PWS results; when it is maternal, Angelman syndrome. 20–25% of PWS have normal chromosomes due to maternal uniparental 15 disomy.

Endocrine features of PWS include hypogonadism (micropenis, hypoplastic scrotum and bilateral cryptorchidism in males), normal or increased GT secretion, poor secondary sexual development and delayed menarche, insulin resistance and diabetes mellitus and growth failure. Energy requirements are abnormally low and appetite insatiable. Growth may be particularly poor when appetite is most successfully controlled and during adolescence. Scoliosis may impair spinal growth and, with gross obesity, predisposes to respiratory failure and death. There is a suggestion from uncontrolled cohort studies that GH therapy is effective in stimulating growth if started in the young child and can result in a height within the parent-based target range within 3 years of treatment. It seems beneficial in metabolic terms (body composition, fat utilization) and clinically in improving muscle tone and power[183,184] and the response is dose-related.[185]

'Simple' obesity (due to large appetite and excessive food intake) is associated with a number of minor (secondary) endocrine abnormalities. Increased adrenal androgen secretion for chronological (but not for bone) age could be a factor influencing the early onset of puberty in such children[186] but increased GC metabolite excretion may reflect increased liver cortisol metabolism. There is frequently hyperinsulinemia, more marked in girls, older children and longstanding obesity, and unrelated to adipocyte size.[187] It is thought to be related to both insulin resistance (with a fall in the concentration of adipocyte insulin receptors) and excessive carbohydrate intake[188] leading to a vicious cycle. A low sex hormone binding globulin (SHBG) level for age is a useful biochemical marker for insulin resistance.[189] A low calorie diet results in a rapid fall in insulin levels (before there are changes in weight, body fat mass or adipocyte size) with a rapid rise once dieting ceases, again preceding these other changes.[190] The risk of developing overt type 2 diabetes mellitus increases with age and the degree of obesity but is an uncommon complication.

THINNESS

Skinfold measurements, not weight, are best guides to thinness and undernutrition. A healthy child who is offered appetising food in adequate amounts and variety in an emotionally supportive environment will eat enough to enable him to grow normally. This may be much less than mother (or granny) feels should be eaten. A thin child who is growing normally and not getting thinner should not be investigated or treated; one who is growing slowly or getting thinner needs investigation, diagnosis and treatment.

Recognizable syndromes (e.g. lipodystrophy, Marfan syndrome) and malignancies are rare, but unrecognized organic disease (e.g. asthma, malabsorption due to celiac disease, ulcerative colitis or Crohn's disease) may present with few overt signs and commonly cause poor growth and thinness. Calories may be too few but some children are on inadequate diets for ethnic or cultural reasons and some mothers are so concerned to prevent obesity that calorie intake is deficient. In the UK, emotional problems are common causes of thinness and poor growth. Anorexia nervosa may be life-threatening in an adolescent.

Acute malnutrition causes loss of fat and muscle; chronic malnutrition causes stunting but thinness may be masked by fat deposition.[191] Secondary endocrine responses to malnutrition result from the need to conserve the limited energy intake available. Cortisol, TSH, T3, GT and IGF-1 levels are low.

IGF-1 is controlled to a major extent by nutrition. In kwashiorkor and marasmus growth slows because of end-organ unresponsiveness to the action of GH – GH levels are high[192] and IGF-1 levels low.[193]

Acute fasting in the human is associated with a reduction in GH receptor numbers and a low protein diet in the rat has the same effect. Receptor loss can be prevented with GH infusion suggesting that resistance is at the post-receptor level.[194] Amino acid deprivation has a direct effect on IGF-1 gene expression. Protein restriction in very young rats leads to longer term resistance to the growth promoting effects of exogenous IGF-1. Zinc deficiency in children is associated with reduced IGF-1 levels[194] and zinc supplementation may stimulate catch-up growth.

Anorexia nervosa patients have normal cortisol production but decreased clearance rates[195] due to low liver 11betaOHSD activity. 5alpha-reductase levels are also reduced[196] – this enzyme is also present in the liver. With gas liquid chromatography of urine, rises to normal in 5alpha androgen and GC metabolites are seen during recovery from cachexia in anorexia nervosa. The secretory pattern of LH is immature[197] and pubertal development either does not begin, halts (and may regress) or there is amenorrhea, depending on age at onset of anorexia and its degree. GH responses to stimulation are blunted.[198] Estrogen deficiency is likely to reduce GH pulsatile release – induction of puberty with low dose gonadotrophin releasing hormone (GnRH) causes marked changes in GH pulsatility[199] – this may be an additional mechanism by which growth slows. Multicystic ovaries (a normal phase in ovarian maturation) are seen during recovery.[200] Vomiting, hypotension and cachexia may suggest Addison's disease but are generally much more severe in anorexia nervosa (although the vomiting may be concealed) – hirsutism may also occur in both.

The battle to get a healthy child to eat more than necessary is one that parents are likely to lose and can produce emotional problems in both child and parents then or later. Reassurance that a thin child is healthy and growing normally will often, in itself, defuse an emotionally strained family situation. In other circumstances, treatment of the underlying cause of the thinness is necessary but may be easier with an organic than an emotional disorder.

ENDOCRINOLOGICAL ASPECTS OF PUBERTY AND ADOLESCENCE

THE GONADS

Ovaries and testes have two main functions: development and maintenance of secondary sexual characteristics and reproductive capability. Sex steroidogenic pathways in adrenals and gonads are identical – relative differences in types and quantities of individual androgens and estrogens reflect different enzymic activities.

PHYSIOLOGY

The ovary

Endocrine functions reside in ovarian follicles. Luteinizing hormone (LH) binds to theca cells to stimulate androstenedione and testosterone biosynthesis from cholesterol. These diffuse into granulosa cells which convert them to estrone (E1) and estradiol (E2) respectively (aromatization) under the influence of follicle stimulating hormone (FSH). E1 and E2 interconversion also takes place in the granulosa cells. E1 is largely albumin bound; E2 is also bound to a specific globulin which also binds testosterone.

Estrogens stimulate secondary sex character development and, in the sexually mature, estrogens and progestogens ensure fertility by releasing ova and regulating the menstrual cycle. Estrogens are responsible for growth of vagina, uterus and Fallopian tubes, and have a major role in normal pubertal growth spurt and fusion of epiphyses at the end of puberty. They are metabolized in liver and excreted in urine.

The mechanism by which the dominant follicle suppresses others in both ovaries is unclear. Inhibin[201,202] is found in follicular fluid, is thought to be secreted by granulosa cells and may have local effects as well as affecting feedback inhibition of FSH.

The testis

Both LH and FSH are required for spermatogenesis. FSH is necessary for initial establishment of mature germinal epithelium and initiation of spermatogenesis. LH effects are mediated through Leydig cells testosterone secretion. Spermatogenesis duration is approximately 74 days. Thus testosterone has both endocrine (secondary sexual characteristics and libido development) and paracrine effects (a permissive effect on spermatogenesis in the presence of FSH).

Two per cent of testosterone in the mature male is in free active form, one-third is bound to a specific beta-globulin – sex hormone binding globulin (SHBG) and the remainder to albumin. In the target organs which require dihydrotestosterone (DHT) (scrotum, phallus, prostate), testosterone is converted to DHT by 5alpha-reductase; in other tissues (e.g. bone, muscle, internal genitalia) testosterone acts directly.

Testosterone exerts negative feedback on LH secretion mainly at hypothalamic level but has little effect on FSH. However FSH levels are high in the castrate. There is also a family of gonadal peptides which have inhibitory ('inhibin') and stimulatory ('activin') feedback effects at pituitary level and important gonadal (paracrine) effects. Modulation of FSH secretion at pituitary level is by mechanisms distinct from the GnRH receptor on the pituitary gonadotroph.[202] Inhibins are now known to be secreted in a variety of forms from the testis (Sertoli cells), placenta and ovary (granulosa cells).

The inhibins (A and B) are heterodimeric glycoproteins, consisting of two dissimilar subunits,[201] alpha and either alphaA (inhibin-A) or betaB (inhibin-B), defined on the basis of the property of GT secretion, preferentially FSH, suppression[203] and are similar to other glycoproteins such as TGFbeta, erythroid differentiation factor and MIH. Activin consists of two inhibin alpha subunits.

Recent development of assays with sufficient sensitivity and specificity to distinguish different inhibin forms has led to important physiological insights. In women there is a characteristic pattern of changes in inhibin concentration during the menstrual cycle – inhibin-B is predominant during the follicular phase, inhibin-A during the luteal phase and early pregnancy.[204,205] In men, there is no inhibin-A but inhibin-B concentrations reflect Sertoli cell function with an inverse relationship between FSH and inhibin-B suggesting a critical role for inhibin-B in FSH secretion regulation.[206] The inhibins may be important in normal puberty (see below).

The adrenals produce quantitatively more androgens than testes and these are of importance in childhood in physiological and pathological situations. In puberty and subsequently the role of the testes is qualitatively paramount because testosterone is much more potent than androstenedione or dehydroepiandrosterone (DHA) – testicular failure causes hypogonadism despite normal adrenal function. Small quantities of estrogen are produced by normal testes by Sertoli cell aromatization of androgen. Testosterone is also metabolized to estrogen in some peripheral tissues (notably adipose cells) and the liver prior to urinary excretion.

ENDOCRINE BACKGROUND TO NORMAL PUBERTY

Physical changes of puberty are discussed elsewhere. Individual secondary sexual characteristics result from different hormonal events and must be assessed independently. Over the last century, children have tended to become taller and reach physical and sexual maturity earlier[57] but whether this process is continuing is more contentious.[207,208]

Reports of and recommendations based on data which purport to show that African–American and White American girls are showing secondary sexual development respectively 2 years and 1 year earlier than was the case a generation ago[209,210] may well be the result of methodological (selection and observer) bias. Early breast development may be mimicked superficially by obesity which will bias self-reported data.

Although an increasing prevalence of obesity in the population might be an explanation for a genuine advance in the timing of puberty onset, the age of menarche (a much more robust maturational marker) does not seem to be lowering comparably further in industrialized nations.[211] This implies either significant methodological flaws in the study of Herman-Giddens et al[209] [and in unpublished UK data from the Avon Longitudinal Study of Parents and Children (ALSPAC)] or that the tempo of pubertal progression is slower than was previously the case (for which there is no evidence or obvious physiological explanation at a population, as opposed to individual, level).[207,208]

In this context, the recent claim that similar differences in the timing of male puberty (onset of genital and pubic hair growth) have been occurring[212] must be treated with caution.

Although puberty timing and duration are very variable between normal individuals, pubertal development is an harmonious process: marked discrepancies from the normal sequence of events (loss of consonance) should lead to suspicion of pathology. In contrast, adolescence is sometimes far from harmonious – social pressures may be particularly marked in many who are sexually mature but still growing emotionally and intellectually, and emotional problems seen in those with the timing of puberty at either end of the normal spectrum.

CHANGES IN FETUS, INFANT AND CHILD AND THEIR RELEVANCE TO PUBERTY INITIATION

Fetal GT production occurs from the fifth week, rising until 20 weeks. Levels are higher in females perhaps because of feedback inhibition by fetal testosterone in males. Placental human chorionic gonadotrophin (HCG) is secreted from implantation onwards and is the major stimulus for fetal Leydig cell testosterone and it seems unlikely that the fetal hypothalamo–pituitary–gonadal axis is fully functional by postpubertal standards. After delivery, a rise in GT levels persists for several months in both sexes. Total testosterone levels are high in males. During the first year, the axis becomes quiescent. There is little evidence for the existence of specific inhibitory hormones (see pineal, p. 505) although CNS inhibitory influences could be important – precocious puberty is common following cranial irradiation for acute lymphoblastic leukemia (ALL).

Pulsatile GnRH secretion is of paramount importance in primate sexual maturation but puberty initiation does not result from sudden hypothalamic GnRH activation – there is increasing biochemical and ultrasound evidence for activity well before the onset of clinical gonadarche. During childhood, there is gradual amplification of GnRH signals with pulses of low frequency and amplitude[213] in the young child. From well before the clinical onset of puberty, around adrenarche, nocturnal pulsatile GnRH secretion is detectable with increasing pulse frequency[214] associated with multicystic prepubertal ovaries on ultrasound (Fig. 13.31). This normal stage of development (characterized by the presence of > 6 follicles of diameter > 4 mm) is associated with activation of the axis resulting in nocturnal pulsatile GnRH secretion[215] without (as yet) estrogen-mediated positive feedback.[216]

Modulation of pituitary LH secretion resulting from increased GnRH pulse frequency is an important characteristic of transition between juvenile and peripubertal stages in man (Fig. 13.32).[214] Biochemical assessment in prepuberty has been helped by the development of sensitive LH radiometric assays[214] although the bioactivity of what is measured is not beyond question. Using an ultrasensitive immunofluorometric assay (IFA), pulsatile LH and FSH fluctuations can be seen even in Kallmann syndrome patients[213,217] but, in contrast to normal late prepubertal children, there is poor synchronization between LH and FSH pulses and absence of entrainment to sleep. A crucial condition for normal pubertal development may involve organization of neuronal circuits which not only maintain synchronized pulsatile GnRH release but enable their incorporation into the daily sleep–wake rhythm.[213,218] It is likely that continuing pubertal transition to adult pituitary–gonadal function involves gradual further recruitment, organization and synchronization of GnRH neuronal discharge over an increasing proportion of the evening/night and resetting of gonadal negative feedback.[213] Clinically, an early morning testosterone measurement is a useful predictor of the imminence of puberty.[219]

Thus the prepubertal testis is not quiescent.[220] Corroborative evidence for activity of the prepubertal testis has come from studies in the cebus monkey[221] and, more recently the marmoset. The latter is an excellent primate model surrogate for man for studying testicular maturation[222] in which there is evidence of functional (and largely GnRH-dependent) activation of Sertoli, Leydig and germ cells in the prepubertal testis.[223]

Data,[224] using sensitive and specific assays to distinguish different inhibin forms, have shown that in normal boys testicular production of inhibin-B increases as puberty progresses and that the initiation of puberty is accompanied by a dramatic switch from a positive to a negative relationship between inhibin-B and FSH. Inhibin-B may also be a more sensitive predictor than testosterone of clinical pubertal onset. The two peaks of inhibin-B (during infancy and early puberty) appear to reflect the two periods of Sertoli cell proliferation in normal human males. During mid-childhood a relatively constant amount of inhibin-B is secreted.

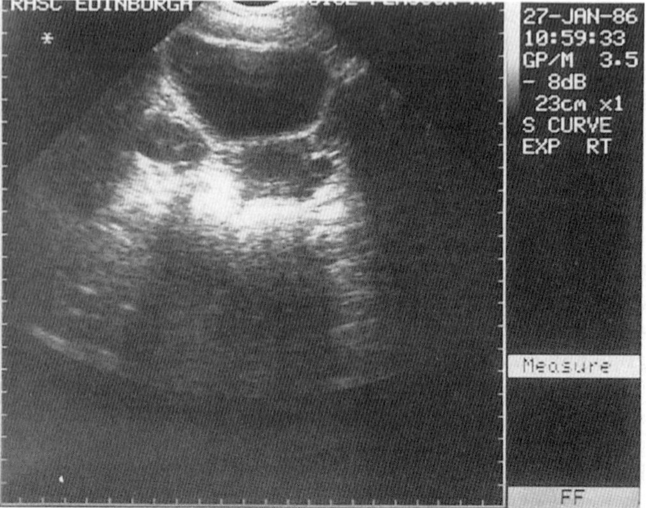

Fig. 13.31 The multicystic appearance of late prepubertal ovaries.

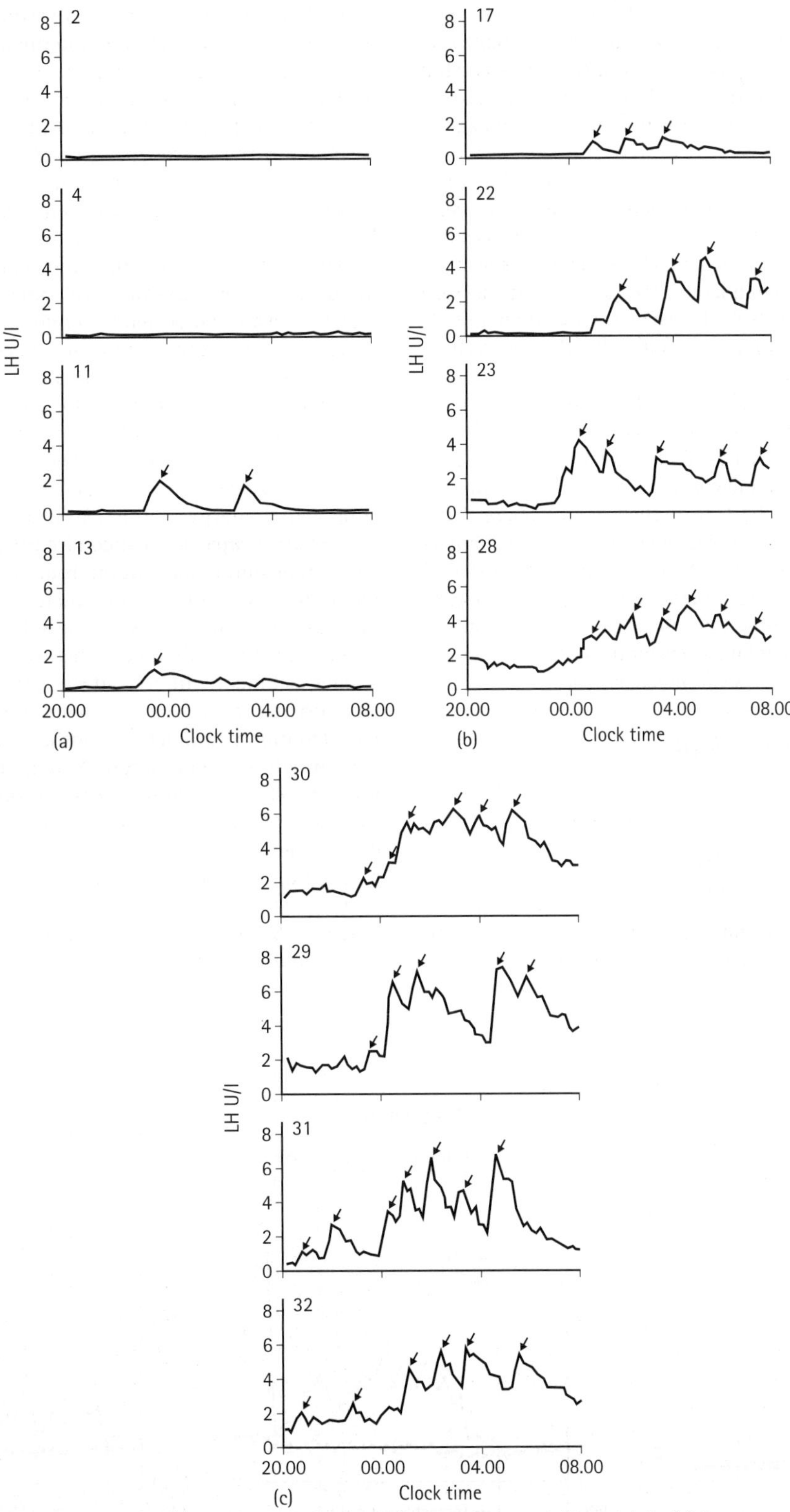

Fig. 13.32 Evolution of GT secretory profiles (1). Profiles of plasma LH between 20.00 and 08.00 h in (a) four young prepubertal subjects (G1 PH1 testicular volume = 2 ml); arrowheads indicate a significant LH pulse; none of these patients progressed into puberty during the following 12 months; (b) four prepubertal subjects: two with G1 PH1 testicular volume = 2 ml at time of study, but progression into puberty with testicular volume = 4 ml within 12 months (subjects 15 and 13); two in earlier puberty at study (G1 PH1–2 testicular volume 3–4 ml); (c) four pubertal subjects (G2–3 PH1–3 testicular volume 6–10 ml). (From Wu et al 1990[214])

The early FSH-independent increase in inhibin-B that precedes clinical puberty and continues to stage G2[4] may be stimulated by testosterone or other Leydig cell factors. The inverse relationship between inhibin-B and FSH that develops from mid-puberty onwards is consistent with the establishment of the negative feedback loop at this stage.[225]

Although median levels of inhibins-A and -B remain low until after age 10 years in girls, there is evidence, from sporadically increased levels in normal prepubertal girls and their positive correlation with FSH levels, of sporadic FSH-dependent follicular development in infancy and childhood.[226] In puberty, the increase in inhibins-A and -B and their lack of positive correlation with FSH from stage B3[4] onwards, suggests that follicular growth is dependent more on the duration of FSH elevation above a critical threshold than the levels per se.[226] Normal ranges for inhibins-A and -B in childhood and puberty are now available.[225, 226]

As puberty progresses, GnRH (and thus GT) pulse frequency remains at about 2 h but there is increasing amplitude and daytime as well as nocturnal pulses (Fig. 13.33).[227] In the follicular phase of the menstrual cycle, GnRH pulse frequency increases to approximately hourly and falls to 3 hourly in the luteal phase. Increasing sex steroid secretion resulting from increasing pulsatile GnRH secretion produces the physical changes of puberty and all pubertal events can be induced by pulsatile administration of exogenous GnRH[228,229] – even if this is a cumbersome way to do so in clinical practice.

ADRENARCHE AND GONADARCHE

See p. 521

CHANGES OF BODY COMPOSITION AND METABOLIC SIGNALS FOR PUBERTY ONSET

Although in pathological situations (e.g. anorexia nervosa, excessive exercise) nutritional factors are important for pubertal development and menarche, there is no evidence for the hypothesis that menarche depends on attainment of a critical weight for height. For a given body weight, the proportion of girls reaching menarche increases with age and the relative weight (weight as a percentage of standard weight) at 11 years explains less than 5% of variation in the age of menarche.[230] It is likely that in normally nourished populations genetic factors are of paramount importance for the timing of menarche – this is probably true of pubertal onset and events in general.

This does not mean that metabolic factors and signals are unimportant for pubertal development.[231] From animal studies and circumstantial evidence in man, it appears that brain (rather than pituitary) maturation is of primary importance for puberty onset. Are there simply genetically determined biological clocks which, in the absence of pathological modulators, trigger puberty or could there be metabolic or other cues which signal into the CNS? In anorexia nervosa or severe malnutrition there are low GT levels, menstruation ceases and puberty regresses as a way of conserving energy – the likely outcome of maintenance of reproductive capacity in such circumstances would be disastrous for mother and fetus. Although anorexics who regain ~ 75% of ideal body weight resume menstrual cycling with normal pituitary responsiveness to GnRH,[232] leanness alone cannot account for the reproductive disturbances: sustained exercise (in female distance runners) affects GnRH pulse amplitude[233] and amenorrheic ballet dancers who stop training resume normal menstruation within a few months without detectable changes in body weight or composition[234] suggesting that metabolic signals are important in controlling reproductive function in these situations and, speculatively, in the control of normal pubertal development.

Indeed, the discovery of leptin, the ob gene product, has now provided a molecular basis for the lipostatic theory of the regulation of energy balance. In ob/ob mice leptin treatment restores fertility. Leptin interacts with many messenger molecules in the brain.

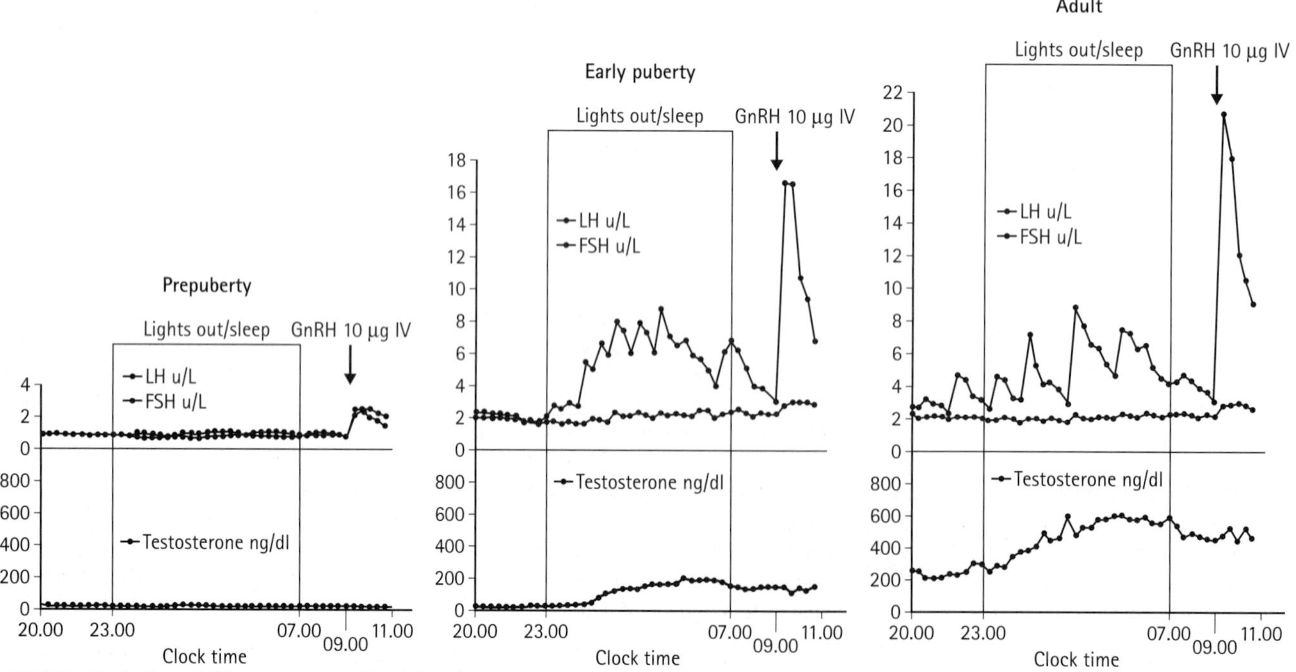

Fig. 13.33 Evolution of GT secretory profiles (2) and response to exogenous GnRH at different stages of pubertal development. (Data by courtesy of Dr FCW Wu[214])

Leptin suppresses neuropeptide Y (NPY) expression in the arcuate nucleus. Increased NPY activity has an inhibitory effect on the gonadotrophin axis and represents a direct mechanism for inhibiting sexual maturation and reproductive function in conditions of food restriction and/or energy expenditure. By modulating the hypothalamo–pituitary–gonadal axis both directly and indirectly, leptin may serve as an important signal from fat to the brain about the adequacy of fat stores for pubertal development and reproduction. Normal leptin secretion is necessary for normal reproductive function to proceed and leptin may be a signal allowing for the point of initiation of and progression toward puberty.[235]

Although there are pubertal increases in basal insulin levels which may be secondary to changes in GH, insulin also enhances basal and GnRH-stimulated GT release by pituitary cells in vitro[236] and affects brain neurotransmitter activity by regulating precursor availability. Thus both direct humoral stimuli and metabolic factors could influence the GnRH pulse generator and leptin is an important link between fat and brain.

ABNORMAL PUBERTY

As with other normally distributed characteristics (e.g. height or IQ) there is no absolute age at which pubertal timing becomes abnormal. Pubertal onset at an 'average' time does not necessarily exclude a pubertal disorder. The mean UK age of onset is such that 3% of boys and girls will have started puberty by 9 and 8 years respectively and only 3% will have no pubertal signs by 13.8 and 13.4 years, respectively. A useful clinical rule is that puberty should be investigated if there is an abnormal sequence of pubertal changes (i.e. loss of consonance), any abnormal sign or symptom of underlying pathology and if signs have or have not (respectively) appeared outwith the above age limits.

Children with precocious puberty may simply have early onset of normal (central) mechanisms (which may be idiopathic or secondary to underlying pathology) or may have an abnormal mechanism causing development (pseudopuberty). Children with no signs by 14 years may have delay in maturation (on a background of constitutional growth delay) but may permanently lack ability to develop spontaneously. Investigations, potential outcomes and management are different in each situation and depend on not only presence or absence of underlying pathology but also emotional and psychological consequences. A clinical classification of disorders of puberty or its timing is given in Table 13.9.

Table 13.9 A simplified classification of disorders of puberty (see text)

Precocious puberty
Consonance:
Idiopathic central precocious puberty
Central precocious puberty due to, e.g.
Intracranial tumors
Cranial irradiation
Raised intracranial pressure
Gonadotropin-independent precocious puberty (GIPP, testotoxicosis)
Loss of consonance (pseudopuberty)
Isolated premature thelarche
Thelarche variant
Adrenal causes
Premature pubarche
Congenital adrenal hyperplasia
Cushing's syndrome
Adrenocortical tumors
Gonadal causes
Ovarian cysts
Ovarian or testicular tumors
Ingestion of sex steroid (accident or child abuse)
Primary hypothyroidism
McCune–Albright syndrome
Extrapituitary tumors (e.g. hepatoblastoma)
Delayed puberty
Consonance
Constitutional delay of growth and puberty
Chronic systemic disease
Idiopathic hypogonadotropic hypogonadism
Hypogonadotropic hypogonadism due to, e.g.
Kallmann's syndrome
Craniopharyngioma
Cranial irradiation
Panhypopituitarism
Primary hypothyroidism
Loss of consonance
Turner syndrome
Ovarian agenesis with normal karyotype
Polycystic ovaries
Anorchia (primary or secondary to testicular irradiation)

PRECOCIOUS SEXUAL MATURATION

It was conventionally considered that there were only two distinct conditions resulting in premature sexual maturation from a gonadal axis etiology: central precocious puberty and isolated premature thelarche, of which the latter is a benign condition and not requiring treatment. However, there is no pathognomonic endocrinological distinction between these two conditions; LH and FSH secretion represent a complete spectrum with girls with isolated premature thelarche (see below) having predominant FSH secretion and those with central precocious puberty predominant LH secretion.[237]

The concept of loss of consonance is particularly useful in the differential diagnosis of precocious puberty[238] but initiation of normal pubertal events can be due to underlying pathology and gonadotrophin-independent precocious puberty (GIPP, an important but rare cause of precocious puberty in boys) may be clinically identical to 'consonant' precocious puberty.

Pseudopuberty (loss of consonance)

Isolated premature thelarche

This presents with breast development in the absence of any other pubertal signs although vaginal bleeding may occur. Onset is usually in the first year and uncommon after 2 years. There is usually cyclical waxing and waning of mild breast development (stage < B3) which may have persisted from postnatal breast enlargement (potentially in both sexes) due to placental maternal estrogen transfer. In contrast to true precocious puberty, pubic and axillary hair does not develop, growth velocity is normal for age and skeletal maturation is not advanced.

There is evidence for increased estrogen production,[239] high basal and GnRH-stimulated FSH levels[240] and pulsatile nocturnal GT, predominantly FSH, secretion.[241] Ultrasound may show several ovarian cysts whose size changes with breast size and moderate uterine enlargement.

A primary abnormality in GnRH pulse generation resulting predominantly in FSH secretion is unlikely as there is no response to GnRH analogues. The activin/inhibin system may be important for pathogenesis – inhibin-B as well as FSH levels are high[242] – potentially exerting effects both at pituitary level, on FSH independently of the gonadotroph GnRH receptor,[202] and at gonadal level by paracrine regulation.

There is waxing and waning of breast enlargement with gradual disappearance over months or years. Puberty generally takes place normally at appropriate age. Treatment consists of explanation and reassurance. Pelvic ultrasound and measurement of GTs basally and following a low dose (0.25 mcg/kg i.v.) GnRH test may be helpful in doubtful cases. Occasionally, particularly in girls presenting after 2 years, there may be confusion with early true precocious puberty and a 'non-classical' variant[243] which has a high incidence of progression to central precocious puberty.

An intermediate syndrome, 'thelarche variant', has been described[244] with GT independence and postulated ovarian lesion of folliculogenesis (see below). It is now clear that the variation in gonadotrophin secretion in this situation represents a spectrum of disorders of gonadal maturation which have received different names depending on the countries in which they were reported, including unsustained central sexual precocity, slowly progressive precocious puberty, thelarche variant and exaggerated thelarche. It is probable that all four conditions are identical. However, patients with the condition, which is mid-way between isolated premature thelarche and central precocious puberty, have a normal height prognosis and, indeed, do not respond to gonadotrophin releasing hormone analogue treatment.[244]

Adrenal causes

The normal rise in adrenal androgens in mid-childhood (adrenarche, see p. 521) sometimes manifests with appearance of pubic (and less commonly axillary) hair – 'premature pubarche' – without breast development but with increased height velocity. Such children are particularly sensitive to adrenal androgens or at the upper end of a secretory spectrum. The timing of true pubertal onset is generally unaffected. In occasional children with true precocious puberty, pubic hair development may be the first sign. Other causes of adrenal androgen secretion must be considered in the differential diagnosis and excluded.

Congenital adrenal hyperplasia (CAH), specifically non-salt-losing 21-hydroxylase deficiency in boys, is the commonest cause of precocious pseudopuberty. There is virilization in early childhood but testes classically remain prepubertal – adrenals are the androgen source. Occasionally ACTH-responsive adrenal rests will cause some testicular growth but significant enlargement signifies secondary central precocious puberty (Fig. 13.34) – a common consequence of GC therapy on the pre-existing advanced skeletal maturation. Mild or late-onset forms of 21-hydroxylase or 3beta-hydroxysteroid dehydrogenase deficiencies may present with pubic hair growth in girls mimicking premature pubarche.

Cushing's syndrome and adrenocortical tumors

(see p. 526)

Gonadal causes

Testicular tumors are uncommon in children and (usually benign) Leydig cell androgen-secreting lesions are rare. Clinically, presentation may be with normal pubertal development but the affected testis is enlarged and the contralateral small and atrophic from suppression of the hypothalamo–pituitary–gonadal axis. Enlargement may be uniform or with a palpable nodule causing confusion with enlargement due to ACTH-responsive adrenal rests in CAH. Rapid onset of true pubertal onset may follow surgical removal.

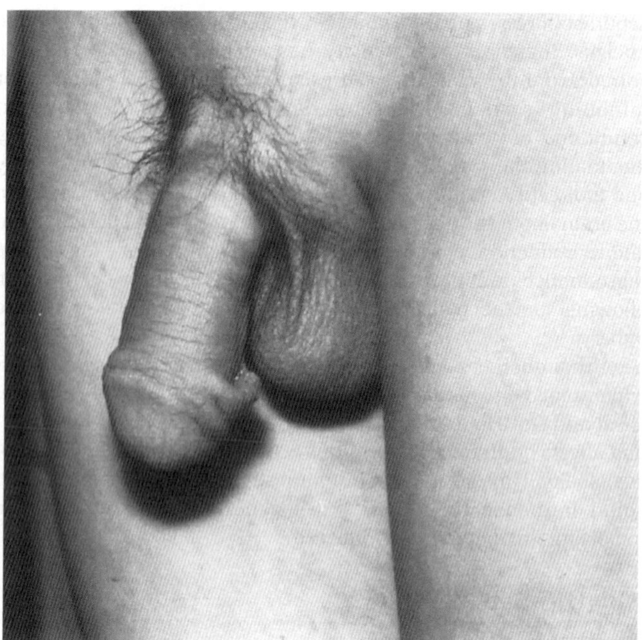

Fig. 13.34 True precocious puberty following glucocorticoid treatment of congenital adrenal hyperplasia. Note the testicular enlargement (same child as Fig. 13.53).

Ovarian tumors are also rare causes of precocious pseudopuberty, accounting for only around 1% of all cases. Least uncommon is the rare granulosa-theca cell tumor[245] and presentation is rarely before 4 years. Distinguishing features include early (in context of other pubertal signs) irregular vaginal bleeding or regular anovulatory cycles, marked areolar pigmentation and abdominal pain. A pelvic or abdominal mass is usually palpable.

Ovarian cysts are found in normal and precocious puberty. Multicystic appearances of late prepubertal and early pubertal ovaries are described above. Isolated follicular cysts may cause breast development, can be a feature of isolated premature thelarche and may regress spontaneously with conservative management.[246] Chronic estrogen secretion and large size may necessitate surgical removal. Polycystic ovaries may be common in puberty and late prepuberty and can be associated with pubertal delay.

Ingestion of sex steroid

Most commonly there is accidental ingestion of mother's contraceptive pills and estrogen will cause slight breast enlargement and, often, an estrogen withdrawal bleed.

Child abuse

Sex steroids may be administered deliberately and chronically as a form of child abuse.[247] Sexual abuse (and pelvic neoplasia) must be excluded when vaginal bleeding is the presenting feature of precocious pseudopuberty. Factitious vaginal bleeding may be caused by presentation of mother's menstrual blood as though it came from the child. The laboratory can determine its origin.

Thyroid disease

Primary hypothyroidism may be associated both with delayed and precocious puberty. Unusually (in the context of precocity) growth velocity will not have been rapid, stature may be short and bone age is characteristically delayed. It is usually seen in girls (in whom autoimmune hypothyroidism is commoner). Breast development is the main feature (sometimes with galactorrhea) but there is usually little (androgen dependent) pubic or axillary hair development. In boys enlarged testes consisting of seminiferous tubules without Leydig cells has been described.[248] Pulsatile FSH release is common in primary hypothyroidism[249] but only results in precocious pseudopuberty in a few. Follicular cysts are seen on ovarian ultrasound in association with FSH predominance and suppressed GH pulsatility.[250] The latter may contribute to slower height velocity.

The child may be clinically euthyroid at presentation in puberty with normally maintained TSH and thyroid hormone levels. The pituitary fossa may be enlarged (Fig. 13.35) due to pituitary hyperplasia[251] – the pituitary gland shrinks rapidly on thyroxine therapy. Ultimately, secondary pituitary failure may result, with an empty but still enlarged fossa on CT or MRI scan. Menarche may occur early while growth is still accelerating (cf. normal puberty and central precocious puberty). Treatment is with thyroxine.

McCune–Albright syndrome

This syndrome is the association of hyperpigmented macules, precocious sexual development and thinning and sclerosis of bone with fractures in young children without systemic disease.[252,253] The syndrome comprises macular brown skin hyperpigmentation with characteristic ragged edges, areas of rarefaction, commonly in long bones and elsewhere (polyostotic fibrous dysplasia – Fig. 13.36) and multiple endocrinopathies with glandular hyperfunction (thyrotoxicosis with goiter, GH hypersecretion, Cushing's syndrome, hyperprolactinemia, hyperparathyroidism, precocious puberty and hyperphosphaturic rickets).

Endocrine hyperfunction is autonomous and not secondary to central trophic hormone stimulation. There are analogies with endocrinopathies in multiple endocrine neoplasia syndromes (see Ch. 20).[254] They are due to an activating missense mutation in the gene encoding the Gsalpha subunit of the G protein that stimulates cyclic AMP formation. The mutation is variably expressed in different tissues consistent with a mosaic distribution of aberrant cells from a somatic cell mutation.[255]

Precocious puberty is the usual presentation, sometimes with early vaginal bleeding (cf. central precocious puberty). Bone lesions

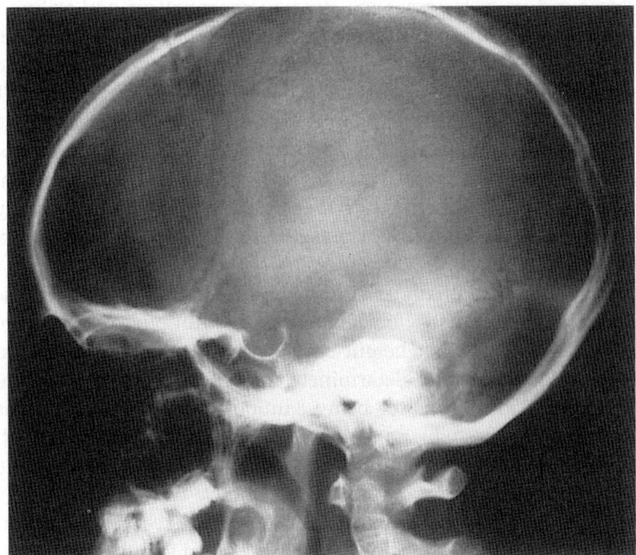

Fig. 13.35 Enlarged pituitary fossa due to pituitary (thyrotroph) hyperplasia in a child with primary hypothyroidism presenting with precocious puberty.

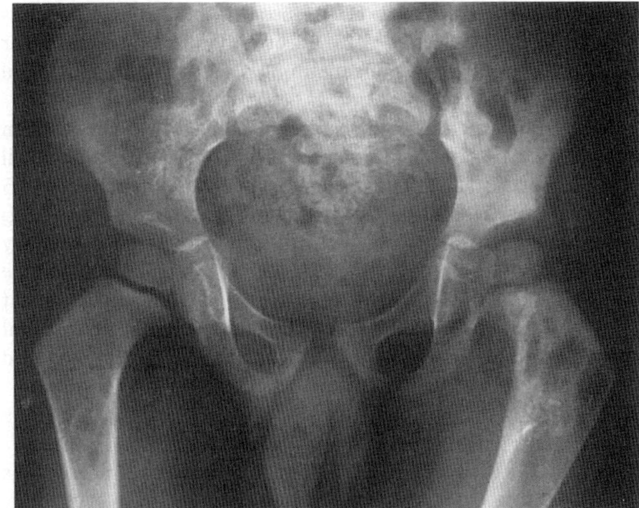

Fig. 13.36 Polyostotic fibrous dysplasia of bone in the McCune–Albright syndrome.

may not develop for many years and the skin pigmentation is inconstant. In girls, ovaries may be asymmetrically enlarged by isolated follicular cysts. The GT response to exogenous GnRH is 'prepubertal' with absent GT pulsatility and, as would be expected, suppression of puberty with GnRH agonists is ineffective.[256] Cyproterone acetate or medroxyprogesterone are drugs of choice.

Extrapituitary tumors

These tumors may cause precocious puberty as a result of the ectopic secretion of GT-like substances. Least uncommon are hepatoblastomas in boys and ovarian chorionepitheliomas and teratomas in girls; extrapituitary intracranial malignant teratoma and pineal choriocarcinoma have been reported. In boys testicular enlargement is rapid and vaginal bleeding often occurs early in girls.

Central precocious puberty

Normal activation of the hypothalamo–pituitary–gonadal axis may occur abnormally early, secondary to an underlying disorder or idiopathically. The pattern of secondary sexual characteristic development and endocrine findings are as in puberty developing at a more average time ('consonance') except that growth acceleration may occur relatively early in boys. This, plus more rapid epiphyseal maturation in boys in early puberty, may compromise final height more than expected in boys even with early presentation. In general, early age at onset and short parents imply worse height prognosis but accurate individual prediction is difficult – predictive equations are most accurate for children of 'average' height developing normally at an 'average' time – and will tend to underestimate adult height in this context.[163]

Mechanisms initiating normal pubertal development are still not clearly understood, perturbations in timing even less so. Central precocious puberty presents much more frequently in girls (female: male ratio of about 10:1) and in the majority (> 80%) of girls no sinister underlying cause is found. With high resolution neuroradiological scanning, hypothalamo–pituitary hamartomas have been reported[257] but their incidence in the normal population at equivalent age is unclear. In boys, however, there is a high incidence of intracranial pathology, especially tumors such as teratomas, astrocytomas or gliomas causing pineal destruction – neuroradiological investigation is necessary even without abnormal signs. The sex difference in incidence of idiopathic precocious puberty may relate to lower GT release thresholds to endogenous pulsatile GnRH in girls. GIPP (see below) may account for precocious puberty in a significant number of boys in whom normal central mechanisms had previously been implicated.

In girls, investigation is necessary to confirm the mechanism and to exclude an underlying cause. Ovarian ultrasound, which will show characteristic multicystic appearances, and low dose (0.25 mcg/kg i.v.) GnRH test (more practical than overnight GT profiling) will confirm central precocious puberty and exclude primary ovarian pathology. Neuroradiological investigation may be necessary (mandatory in boys). In addition to tumors, important central pathologies include CNS infection, raised intracranial pressure, trauma (during birth or childhood head injury) and previous cranial irradiation.

Silver-Russell syndrome [258,259]

Abnormalities of sexual development, including precocious puberty, can be associated with this prolonged IUGR syndrome. Elevated urinary and serum GTs have been reported but the etiology is unclear.

Gonadotrophin-independent precocious puberty (GIPP, testotoxicosis) [260]

Incidence, importance and classification are still controversial[261] – characteristically there are normal somatic consequences (consonance) from abnormal mechanisms (pseudopuberty). Diagnostic criteria are absent GT spontaneous pulsatility on bioassay and by RIA, poor but variable GT response to GnRH, no clinical response to GnRH analogue therapy and cyclical steroidogenesis. In reported studies there is a strong family history of precocious puberty but the etiology is unknown. Nearly all cases have been boys – girls may have the McCune–Albright syndrome. Maturation of testicular steroidogenesis and spermatogenesis is normal but GnRH/GT-independent. An LH receptor mutation resulting in increased cAMP and autonomous Leydig cell activity has been found in some.[262] Treatment with medroxyprogesterone or ketoconazole[263] has been reported but in view of the latter's toxicity it cannot be generally recommended.

Investigation and diagnosis

In summary it is reasonable to investigate any girl < 8 and boy < 9 years with secondary sexual characteristics. Where a girl's development is harmonious and proceeds at a normal tempo (consonance) and clinical examination is normal, invasive investigation to exclude pathology is unnecessary but basal TSH, estradiol and PRL measurement with skull X-ray, low dose GnRH test and pelvic ultrasound will give valuable information about the mechanism and underlying pathology. Overnight profiling of GT secretion is essentially a research tool. If no underlying cause is found which itself requires treatment, the need to suppress GT secretion and further development is considered below. Adrenal or intracranial pathology must be actively sought in boys by steroid profiling and neuroradiological (CT or MRI) investigation. GIPP must be considered in boys, particularly if there is a family history of precocious puberty, as there is no response to GnRH analogue therapy.

Clinical consequences and management

Management of precocious pseudopuberty is of the underlying cause. In central precocious puberty, an underlying cause requires treatment and pubertal suppression may be necessary also. In idiopathic cases, suppression may be indicated on social and psychological (rather than medical) grounds (see below).

Treatment of central precocious puberty has traditionally been with progestogen-like drugs such as cyproterone acetate and medroxyprogesterone. Cyproterone has been widely used in the UK for many years and is generally effective and free from significant side effects in a dose of 75–100 mg/m^2/day given twice daily. It has progestational, anti-androgenic, anti-gonadotrophic and adrenal suppressive activities – the precise mechanism by which GT secretion is suppressed is unclear. It may predominantly directly inhibit ovarian steroidogenesis.[216] Treatment is continued until such time as further pubertal progression is more appropriate – its actions reverse when treatment ceases.

Problems with cyproterone relate to adrenal suppression and treated children must carry a steroid 'card' or talisman and need steroid cover during major stress, illness or surgery. Cortisol deficiency in other situations is uncommon unless high doses are used. Adults treated with cyproterone (for prostatic carcinoma) have altered lipid metabolism which may be of concern if childhood treatment is prolonged. Taking the natural history of central precocious puberty into account, there is no evidence for improvement in height prognosis. Although still widely used, it has been replaced as treatment of choice by GnRH analogues (see below). It remains important for treatment of GIPP and is used to cover the initial (stimulatory) phase of GnRH analogue therapy (see below).

GnRH analogues (GnRHa) are specific and effective in suppressing central precocious puberty. Although licensed in the UK for management of adults with prostatic carcinoma, the D-serine-6 analogue has been widely used in precocious puberty given intranasally although it is also effective subcutaneously. The D-tryptophan-6 analogue is effective given once monthly subcutaneously and is available as a depot preparation which is administered about every 10 weeks.[264]

Although they act by desensitizing the pituitary to GnRH and inhibiting pulsatile GnRH secretion, analogues have an initial stimulatory effect (lasting several weeks) on sex steroid secretion. This is of most practical relevance in a girl sufficiently advanced for a menstrual bleed to occur. In this situation, particularly, additional treatment with cyproterone for the first 4 weeks of analogue therapy is appropriate. Height velocity may initially increase further due to the effect of sex steroids on spinal growth.

Effectiveness of therapy is best assessed by serial pelvic ultrasound in girls (assessing ovarian morphology and volume, uterine cross-sectional area and endometrial thickness), by clinical assessment of testicular volume in boys, plasma estradiol and testosterone measurements (respectively) and (if necessary) GT responsiveness to GnRH (0.25 mcg/kg i.v.). There is no effect on the adrenal axis (cf. cyproterone) but (as with cyproterone) probably no effect on improving height prognosis. Slowing of epiphyseal maturation on treatment is mirrored by a slowing of height velocity (perhaps due to reduced GH pulsatile secretion secondary to sex steroid suppression).

In the absence of underlying pathology, there is no *prima facie* reason why those who, for genetic or constitutional reasons, are destined to reach adult height earlier than average should fail to reach their genetically determined adult height. There are also methodological reasons for being cautious about the conclusions from many studies which purport to show that interventions with GnRHa increase adult height. Many studies include patients in the 'precocious puberty' group who probably have thelarche variant[163] (see above). In addition, most studies fail to recognize that in comparing adult height achieved with predicted adult height (PAH) at the start of treatment, skeletal maturational (bone age) estimations on the same individual repeated through puberty do not show increments of 1 'year' bone age (BA) per year chronological age (CA) because BA accelerates and deviates from a cross-sectional-based centile in a way similar to that for height. BA standards[77,265] are based on those with puberty at an average age, thus in those entering puberty at an age younger than average, a rapid acceleration and progressive advancement of BA occurs – at peak height velocity BA velocity can be up to 2.5 'years' per year.[110,266] As a result, predicted adult height at the start of treatment is misleadingly low and any treatment effect on adult height (e.g. from GnRHa treatment) will be overestimated.[163]

It is on this theoretical background that specific growth stimulation using GH therapy in addition to pubertal suppression is being assessed[267] but is best reserved for those in whom final height is particularly reduced due to underlying pathological causes of precocious puberty.[163]

Whatever the therapy, secondary sexual development will seldom diminish significantly and families must be warned not to expect dramatic cosmetic improvement. GnRH analogues may allow further long-term progression of pubic and axillary hair. There is evidence in girls for reversibility of inhibition[268] and for recovery of hypothalamo–pituitary–gonadal function and ovarian activity occurring from the pretreatment stage of puberty.[269] There is little experience of long-term outcomes of GnRH analogue therapy in boys – observed effects on inhibition of seminiferous tubule activity could impair subsequent fertility if irreversible.

Emotional problems are often considerable in these children who are already tall for age. They appear clumsy and, in association with precocious puberty, may be more aggressive with undesirable social consequences. They feel different both because of size and precocious development and are often ill-equipped to cope with psychological aspects of adolescence, particularly if parents and teachers are uncomprehending or embarrassed. Ultimate short stature may be particularly emotionally disabling against this background. However the indication for suppressing puberty with gonadotrophin releasing hormone analogues is for psychological or psychosocial reasons and not to achieve an improvement in final stature.[163]

The decision to treat idiopathic central precocious puberty thus depends on age at onset, rate of progression, level of emotional support provided by parents and other social and psychological factors. Menarche in primary school can cause additional psychological problems. In every case emotional support must be given.

DELAYED SEXUAL MATURATION

Late puberty, particularly when accompanied by short stature and delayed skeletal maturation, is the commonest reason for referral to a pediatric endocrinologist. This 'constitutional delay of growth and puberty' (CDGP) is seen more commonly in boys who are also more stressed by it as growth deceleration continues until puberty is well advanced. Pathological causes of late puberty are much commoner in girls (e.g. Turner syndrome) – central causes are equally common in both sexes. A karyotype is an important early investigation in any slowly growing girl and mandatory if puberty is delayed even without any syndromic 'stigmata'. Virtually any chronic systemic disease may be associated with both growth retardation and pubertal delay.

Constitutional delay of growth and puberty (CDGP)

This is the likely diagnosis in a healthy adolescent short for the family but not for pubertal stage and skeletal maturation, giving a normal height prognosis. There is often a family history of CDGP in parents or siblings but its presence does not make the diagnosis and absence does not exclude it. CDGP is commoner and often more stressful in boys. Emotional, psychological and social consequences may be severe despite absence of underlying pathology. Aspects of treatment which require consideration are puberty induction, growth stimulation and emotional support. Individual treatment modalities interact with each other in terms of their psychological and physical effects.

Chronic systemic disease

Chronic systemic disease may cause slowing of growth which may or may not be reversible and is often associated with subsequent maturational delay or pubertal failure. Anorexia nervosa results in secondary endocrine disturbances whilst pubertal delay causes secondary psychological disturbances. A sympathetic clinical psychologist or child psychiatrist is helpful in providing evidence of underlying emotional disturbance and managing primary or secondary emotional problems.

Causes of growth and maturational delay or failure in these conditions may be explicable in nutritional, secondary hormonal, metabolic or therapeutic (e.g. glucocorticoid treatment) terms. However in many conditions the etiology is both multifactorial and poorly understood.

Malnutrition and weight loss

Undernutrition is the commonest worldwide cause of growth failure and pubertal delay and may occur in 'developed' countries, for example with inappropriate 'faddish' diets or emotional deprivation. Whatever the specific relevance of metabolic signals for the onset of puberty, it is likely that growth retardation and pubertal delay or failure are a secondary adaptation to the need to conserve energy and to prevent reproduction in suboptimal circumstances.

Exercise

Intensive training (e.g. in female gymnasts) can be associated with delayed sexual maturation and amenorrhea with intensive exercise such as in distance runners. Amenorrheic ballet dancers who stop training may resume normal menstruation within a few months without detectable changes in body weight or composition.[270]

Hypothalamo–pituitary disorders

Hypogonadotrophic hypogonadism may cause pubertal delay, arrest or infertility depending on age at onset and severity. The cause is usually a hypothalamic disturbance in GnRH pulsatile release. To date, four genes have been identified as causes of 'idiopathic' hypogonadotrophic hypogonadism (IHH) in the human accounting for 20% of cases described: KAL, the gene for X-linked Kallmann syndrome (IHH and anosmia), DAX1, the gene for X-linked adrenal hypoplasia congenita (IHH and adrenal insufficiency), GNRHR (the GnRH receptor), and PC1 (the gene for prohormone convertase 1, causing a syndrome of IHH and defects in prohormone processing).[271]

Primary GT deficiency is usually associated with pituitary tumors (e.g. craniopharyngioma) and other pituitary hormone deficiencies. Cranial irradiation is associated with (hypothalamic) GT deficiency. Prolactinomas are rarely associated with delayed puberty – moderately elevated PRL levels are due to stress.

In contrast to CDGP, a child with hypogonadotrophic hypogonadism is generally normal or tall for the family and bone age is arrested at around 13 'years' in the older child. A family history of delay with hypogonadism (cryptorchidism or micropenis) and anosmia suggests *Kallmann's syndrome* – inherited as an autosomal dominant with relative male limitation. Features may include color blindness, other midline craniofacial abnormalities, nerve deafness, mental retardation and renal anomalies. Differentiation from CDGP[213] is generally possible at presentation and molecular genetic abnormalities (in the KAL gene) have now been described.[271]

Mental retardation syndromes associated with GT deficiency and obesity include Laurence–Moon–Biedl (with polydactyly and retinitis pigmentosa) and Prader–Willi.

Hypothyroidism

Acquired hypothyroidism is often associated with pubertal delay but may cause precocious puberty.

Gonadal

Disorders of ovarian function

These may relate to defective estrogen secretion or action (hypogonadism), androgen overproduction (hirsutism, amenorrhea or virilization), ovulatory failure (infertility) or menstrual abnormalities (amenorrhea and infertility).

Turner syndrome (TS). Primary gonadal dysgenesis is much commoner in girls because of the high incidence of Turner syndrome. Although diagnosis is usually possible well before the age when puberty should occur, even in those with no dysmorphic features, few children are now measured regularly and accurately by primary carers so that presentation with delayed puberty is common. There is a poor correlation between physical manifestations (Figs 13.37, 13.38) – neonatal lymphedema, broad ('shield') chest with widely spaced nipples, webbed neck, high arched palate, low posterior hair line, wide carrying angle, short fourth metacarpals and hypoplastic or malformed (spoon-shaped) nails (Fig. 13.39), cardiac and renal abnormalities – and the precise genetic abnormality.

One to two per cent of all conceptuses have TS but rates of early spontaneous miscarriage are very high so the birth prevalence is about 1 in 2500. About half have a single X chromosome and the remainder have one normal X and one abnormal because of partial deletions, ring formation or short or long arm isochromosomes. At least 10% have mosaicism (different proportions of abnormal cells in different tissues). In children with mixed karyotypes, there is an equal abnormal genetic contribution from mother and father whereas in the 45X karyotype the missing chromosome is paternal in origin. The presence of Y chromosomal material can also be detected by karyotype and molecular genetic techniques. If it is found, gonads should be removed to prevent possible malignant change (e.g. gonadoblastoma).

Short stature homeobox-containing (SHOX) gene mutations have been implicated in both the short stature and skeletal dysplastic abnormalities of Turner syndrome.[104] Genomic imprinting (differential expression of genetic material depending on whether it originates from father or mother) is important in several disorders (e.g. Prader–Willi/Angelman syndromes,). It is important in determining some aspects of the TS phenotype (e.g. cardiac abnormalities, neck webbing) when the normal X chromosome is maternal in origin.

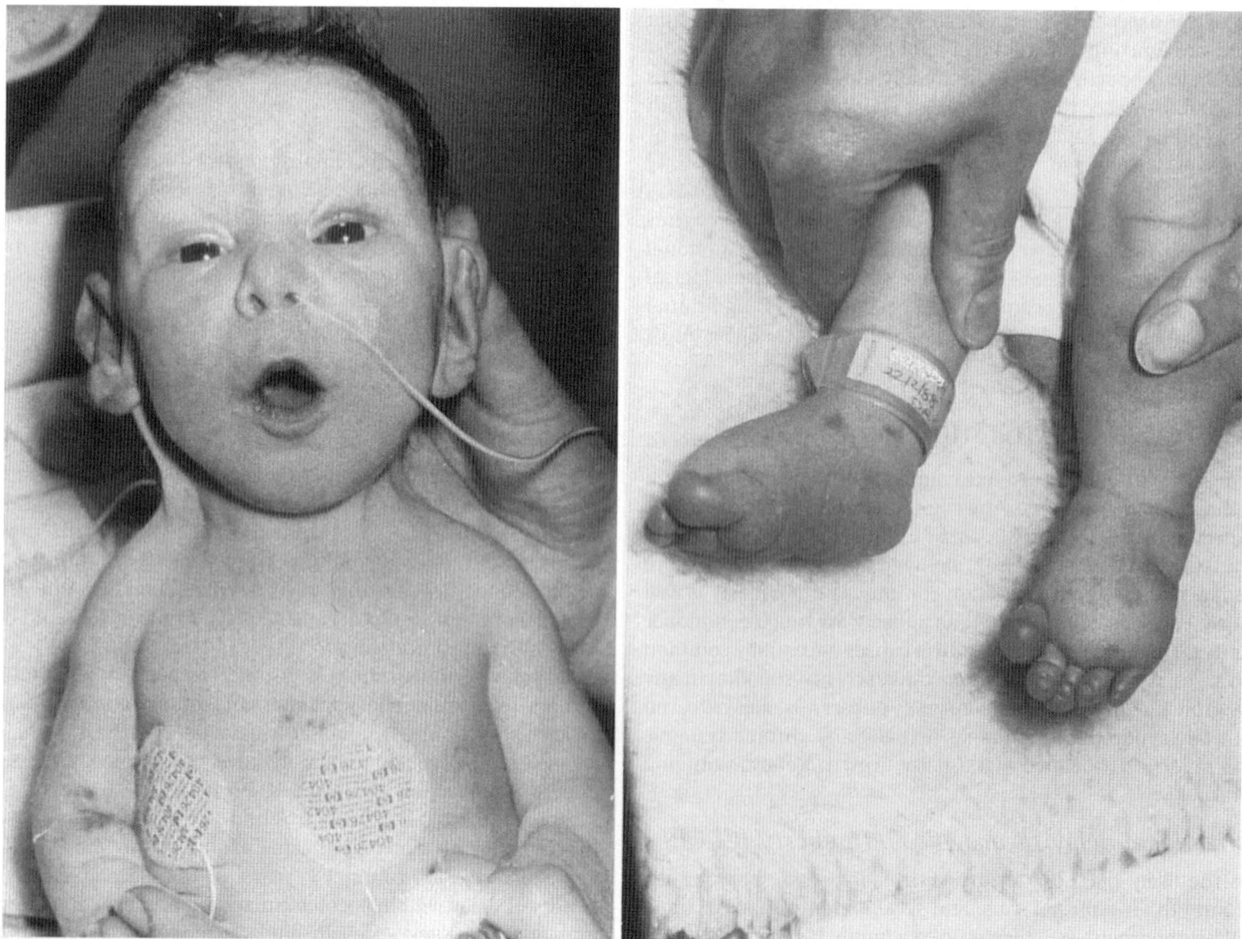

Fig. 13.37 Turner syndrome diagnosed at birth – note the peripheral edema in a small for gestational age infant.

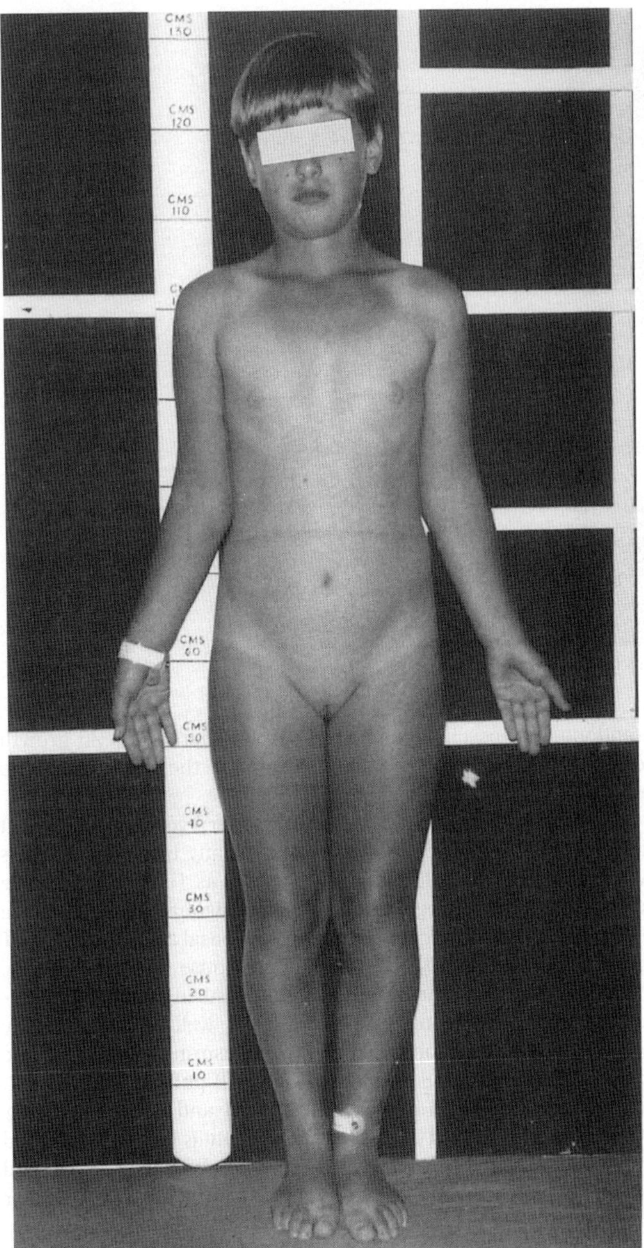

Fig. 13.38 Turner syndrome presenting with pubertal delay in a 14-year-old girl.

The fetal ovary forms normally and germ cell numbers are normal until the end of the second trimester. These then decline to birth and subsequently at a variable but increased rate so that a 'menopause' occurs before puberty in the majority. Some will enter puberty spontaneously – commoner with 'mosaicism' (but see above). With partial deletions, long arm preservation may be important for ovarian function and short arm deletions are associated with the growth deficit.

There is defective end organ responsiveness to growth factors at cartilage and collagen level and a spectrum of GH secretory insufficiency. Intrauterine growth is poor, growth velocity declines progressively after infancy and the pubertal growth spurt is absent. As the height relationship with parents is maintained, TS girls with tall parents (or, more specifically, a tall parent from whom their normal X chromosome has been inherited) may not become conspicuously small until they fail to enter puberty when their normal peers are growing rapidly. Approximately 20 cm in height is lost compared to relevant population means – the mean adult UK height is about 143.0 cm although it may be a little more in 'mosaics' and when short arm material is present. Thus about 20% of TS girls will achieve a spontaneous final height above the 3rd centile for the normal population. Specific growth charts for Turner syndrome are available.[76] Significant deviation from syndrome specific centiles necessitates a search for additional pathology (e.g. hypothyroidism or Crohn's disease).

Mean IQ is 95 and the majority have IQs within the normal range. Many have specific difficulties with visiospacial perception and full psychometric assessment will allow specific remedial help. Autoimmune disease is commoner in TS – autoimmune thyroiditis[272] is an increasing risk with age and particularly by adolescence.[273] The frequency of antithyroid antibodies also increases with age as it does in the normal population – elevated antibody titers indicate the need for regular evaluation of thyroid function.

The nature of the dysplastic bone abnormality is unclear. However bone mineralization is important in TS girls – it is uncertain whether absence of estrogen during early and mid-childhood compromises eventual acquisition of a healthy skeleton.

Ideally estrogen replacement must be initiated to keep the TS girl in line with her peers and increased at a physiological rate. An appropriate regimen is described below. This produces good cosmetic breast appearances and allows normal psychological maturation. Oral estrogen enters the portal circulation and exposes the liver to high levels – transdermal natural estrogen patches will be preferable in the future. Estrogen replacement therapy is necessary at least until menopausal age and probably beyond. Ultra-low dose estrogen in early childhood cannot be recommended on present evidence. Delaying estrogen therapy much beyond 13 years may risk increased social isolation, stigmatization and psychological distress and reduced life-long bone mineralization.

Growth-promoting therapy with GH with, or without additional anabolic steroid (oxandrolone) has been widely studied in TS,[274–277] but many questions remain unanswered. Current knowledge may be summarized as follows: pharmacological doses of GH produce a dose-related increase in height to socially acceptable levels in many TS girls; most gain is during the first 3 years of therapy; individual responses are variable and unpredictable; combining GH with oxandrolone increases the tempo of growth, thus shortening the duration of GH therapy to final height, and may contribute extra height gain – androgenic side-effects of oxandrolone are dose related whereas the growth promoting effect is not and thus very low doses (0.0625 mg/kg daily) are optimal.

TS women are candidates for in vitro fertilization using donated ova. In future, they, and perhaps women with acquired gonadal dysgenesis who have had abdominal irradiation in childhood, will be candidates for cryopreservation and ovarian autografts, although the latter group, unlike TS women, will have compromised uterine function.[278]

Rarely ovarian agenesis occurs with a normal female karyotype. Stature is normal and there are no dysmorphic features. The presence of an XY cell line necessitates removal of dysgenetic gonads.

Disorders of testicular function

These are uncommon. Anorchia is usually detected prepubertally but may be secondary to testicular irradiation in the treatment of ALL or follow suboptimal management of testicular torsion.

Polycystic ovarian syndrome

Menstrual disturbances in many adult women presenting with polycystic ovarian syndrome (hirsutism, obesity and menstrual

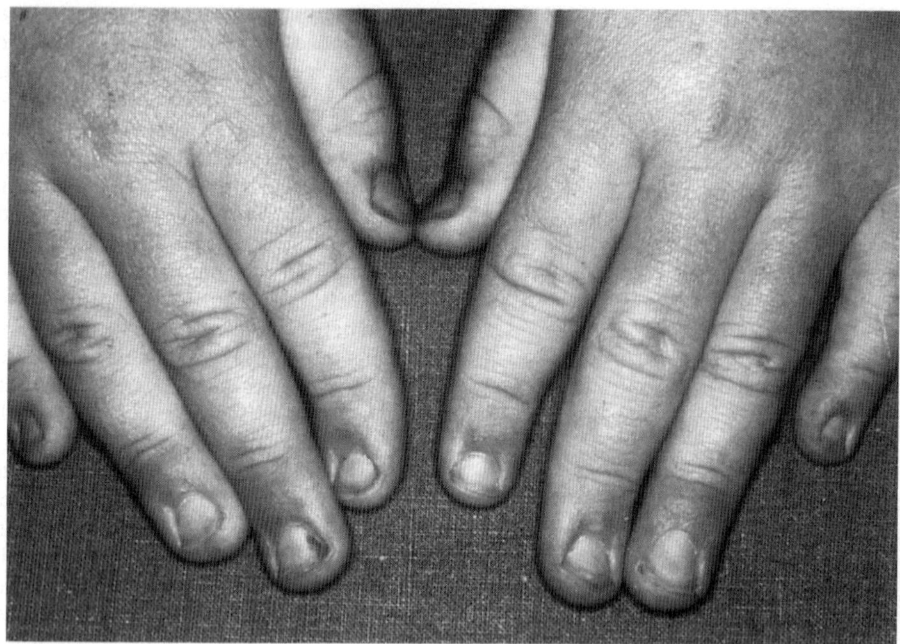

Fig. 13.39 The nails in Turner syndrome (the same girl as in Fig. 13.38).

irregularities) had been thought to date from puberty but ultrasonic appearances (enlarged ovaries with many small circumferential cysts surrounding increased stromal tissue) may be common in prepuberty and an important pathological cause of pubertal delay. The primary abnormality may be ovarian hyperandrogenism with secondarily raised LH levels, LH:FSH ratios and normal FSH levels.[279]

It now seems that there is an association with premature pubarche and prepubertally detectable hyperinsulinemia and dyslipidemia. Birth weight SD scores have been found to be lower in premature pubarche girls than in controls, and particularly so in those with hyperinsulinemia and subsequent ovarian hyperandrogenism. This suggests that these associations may result, at least in part, from a common prenatal origin.[35]

Investigation

Distinguishing physiological from pathological delay may be impossible clinically. Assessment must include physical examination (nutritional state, fundal and visual field assessment) and calculation of height velocity. Loss of 'consonance' – tall stature for the family associated with pubertal delay and delayed bone age is incompatible with CDGP and may be due to Klinefelter's syndrome, hypogonadism or GT deficiency; marked pubic or axillary hair growth in a girl with absent breast development suggests Turner syndrome. The appropriateness or otherwise of height velocity can only be determined in the context of pubertal stage – e.g. growth should be accelerating in a girl with stage 2 breast development but slow growth is normal in a boy until 8–10 ml testicular volumes. Assessment of skeletal maturity may indicate likely delay before puberty starts spontaneously (if it will do so) but seldom distinguishes pathology from physiological delay.

Children with loss of consonance should be investigated at any age as should those with signs or symptoms attributable to an underlying pathological process. Where height and degree of skeletal maturational delay seem appropriate for the family in terms of final height prediction, delay is probably physiological. Three per cent of normal boys and girls will have no signs of puberty by 13.8 and 13.4 years respectively and it is reasonable to investigate those presenting after this. Even if delay is physiological it is unkind (in emotional and psychological terms) and inappropriate (in growth terms) to allow too much delay in relation to the child's peers and pubertal induction may be indicated.[153]

Raised GT levels are diagnostic of primary gonadal failure but are not elevated before about 10 years. At any age, normal testes will respond to stimulation by LH (given as HCG) by secreting testosterone. In hypogonadotrophic hypogonadism there is a presumed lack of LH receptors in the testis, basal and stimulated GT levels will be low and the testosterone response to HCG is absent. Pubertal imminence can be assessed by measuring nocturnal GTs – pulsatile nocturnal GnRH release occurs well before clinically detectable signs – or more practically by measuring the GT response to a small (0.25 mcg/kg i.v.) dose of GnRH. If puberty is imminent, LH responsiveness will exceed that of FSH and rise significantly. Where available, skilled ultrasound assessment is helpful in girls and non-invasive. An 8 a.m. plasma testosterone level may be a useful simple guide in boys but inhibin-B may be a more sensitive predictor than testosterone of clinical pubertal onset.[225]

Moderately raised basal PRL levels may be due to stress but higher levels are a sensitive indicator of reduction in its dopaminergic inhibitory control secondary to hypothalamic lesions or those causing portal compression (e.g. craniopharyngioma, radiotherapy, histiocytosis X). Hyperprolactinemia is itself a cause of delayed puberty. Prolactinomas are rare in children – PRL levels are generally very high (> 3000 mU/L). A significantly elevated PRL is thus a sensitive indicator of intracranial pathology as a cause of delayed puberty and an indication for neuroradiological investigation which is important if an evolving endocrinopathy is suspected – hypogonadotrophic hypogonadism may be the first sign of panhypopituitarism.

There is physiological blunting of GH secretion in late prepuberty in both sexes and in early male puberty so that, if pharmacological testing of GH secretion is deemed necessary and is to be interpreted correctly, sex steroid priming is necessary. Diethylstilbestrol was originally studied in both sexes but depot testosterone or oral estrogen is used in boys and girls respectively.

If pathology is suspected, investigations should be carried out urgently (treatment of underlying pathology may be necessary) and puberty induced at normal time and tempo. Otherwise, although much can be learnt by several months' observation of growth and for early signs of puberty, the psychological pressures on some can be considerable.[153] The short, undeveloped and poorly qualified 16-year-old school leaver may find it particularly hard to obtain employment. It is inappropriate to induce puberty late to maximize prepubertal growth because continuing late prepubertal growth deceleration is leading to a lower point from which to accelerate and the magnitude of the pubertal growth spurt in a late developer is generally smaller. It is also unkind to subject a child to unnecessary social and emotional pressures.

With optimal treatment, puberty can be started at an appropriate time and progressed at a physiological tempo. In girls, too large a starting dose and too rapid escalation of estrogen therapy will reduce the magnitude of the growth spurt, produce cosmetically unattractive 'cylindrical' breasts and potential difficulties in important emotional and psychological aspects of adolescent development. A boy may have 2 years or more from early testicular enlargement until he notices height acceleration. Meanwhile his more average peers are both more developed and growing three- to fourfold faster. Stimulation of growth during early male puberty is thus of considerable potential psychological benefit. Possible therapies (anabolic steroid, androgen or GH) are reviewed by Kelnar.[153]

Clinical consequences and management

Emotional and psychological consequences of delay are not dependent on the presence of underlying pathology – the commonest group, boys with CDGP, may suffer considerably yet are entirely normal. Where an underlying non-endocrine condition is responsible, diagnosis and optimal management may facilitate spontaneous development. When pubertal induction is necessary, it should mimic closely normal pubertal progression to optimize growth, cosmetic appearances and psychological maturation. Too rapid induction is disadvantageous, and is unnecessary if induction is not unduly delayed.

Puberty induction

Induction in girls is with estrogen whatever the precise nature of pubertal failure. An appropriate starting regimen is ethinylestradiol 1–2 mcg orally daily, increasing to 10 mcg over 18–24 months. At that dose, or before if breakthrough bleeding occurs, a progestogen (e.g. norethisterone 350 mcg) should be added for 5 days every 4 weeks. Unopposed estrogenic endometrial stimulation otherwise increases risks of endometrial or breast carcinoma. Full secondary sexual development will generally occur with ethinylestradiol 20–30 mcg – a low estrogen combined contraceptive pill may then be conveniently substituted. If hypogonadism is permanent, estrogen/progestogen therapy must be maintained to enable sexual intercourse to be enjoyed without discomfort, prevent osteoporosis and, perhaps, early atherosclerosis. Transdermal natural estrogen, when available in low enough dosage for pubertal induction, will be preferable.

Many different regimens are used for hormone replacement therapy (HRT) in young women, and it is likely that optimal HRT in young women (in terms of bone strength, cardiovascular protection, feminization, etc.) is different from that appropriate for older women who are 'conventionally' postmenopausal. Certainly, transdermal estradiol combined with vaginal progesterone is a highly satisfactory combination for establishing a physiological endometrium in women with premature ovarian failure.[280]

In boys, physiological sex steroid replacement is even more difficult. Conventionally, depot preparations of testosterone esters (e.g. Sustanon 50–100 mg i.m. once every 6 weeks increasing gradually over 2 years to 250 mg i.m. twice weekly) are used. Oral testosterone (undecanoate, TU) was considered too variably and excessively absorbed for pubertal induction but recent experience suggests that resulting high total testosterone levels reflect changes in SHBG on treatment, and that appropriate free (active) testosterone levels for pubertal induction are achievable with TU 40 mg alternate daily – TU may be the treatment of choice for the short, sexually immature adolescent boy where explanation and reassurance alone are not enough.[153] Long term androgen replacement will probably be best given using testosterone implants or transdermally – patches are now available in the UK and suitably low-dose regimens for pubertal induction need evaluation.

Human chorionic gonadotrophin (HCG) therapy is an alternative in boys – in girls it may cause abdominal pain, ascites and hemorrhagic rupture of ovarian cysts. HCG (i.e. LH) is started alone (500 units i.m. weekly, increasing to 2000 units over 2 years) and then in combination with human menopausal gonadotrophin (HMG, i.e. FSH) to induce spermatogenesis. Optimal fertility in both sexes requires eventual low dose pulsatile GnRH therapy.

The physician will need to assess carefully individual underlying psychological and social pressure before deciding on the optimal management of CDGP which might comprise anabolic steroid (oxandrolone) or testosterone therapy.[153] Emotional support is always important whatever other treatment modalities are used but the morale boost from an increase in growth velocity in early male puberty is often dramatic with improvement in school attendance and performance.

OTHER DISORDERS RELATED TO FEMALE AND MALE REPRODUCTION

AMENORRHEA

Amenorrhea may be secondary (absent menstruation with previously normal menstrual history) – causes include pregnancy, anorexia nervosa, intense training or chronic underlying disease – or primary (menstrual bleeding has never occurred). Primary amenorrhea may be a consequence of abnormal GnRH pulsatile secretion or release – a middle stage between GnRH deficiency causing delayed or arrested puberty or infertility due to anovulatory cycles. Other important causes include primary ovarian failure (often in Turner syndrome), gonadal dysgenesis with absent uterus (e.g. the XY girl) or imperforate hymen. Hypertension suggests 17alpha-hydroxylase deficiency.

NOONAN SYNDROME (MIM163950)

In this syndrome, which is thought to have an incidence of 1 in 1000 to 1 in 2500 live births, there is frequently variable hypogonadism associated with characteristic features such as pulmonary valvular stenosis, a broad forehead with hypertelorism, epicanthic folds, ptosis and downward slanting palpebral fissures, abnormal or low-set ears, neck webbing, low posterior hair line, shield chest or kyphoscoliosis, deafness, visual problems, clotting disorders and short stature (Fig. 13.40). However, as in Turner syndrome, all these are inconstant and diagnosis has been clinical, with the typical facial features and at least two other features as key elements. The phenotype changes with age.

Cryptorchidism is found in about two-thirds of boys but sexual development generally occurs spontaneously but is delayed. Infertility is usual. In girls (whose karyotype is normal) puberty and menarche can be delayed (presentation may be with primary amenorrhea) but fertility seems common. Mean adult height is approximately 162.5 cm (males) and 153 cm (females) although standards are based on relatively small numbers and largely cross-sectional data. GH treatment improves medium term height velocity and theoretical adverse effects on cardiac ventricular wall thickness (potentially leading to hypertrophic obstructive cardiomyopathy) have not been seen.[281,282]

Noonan syndrome has recently been found to be caused by mutations in the PTPN11 gene which encodes the protein tyrosine phosphatase SHP-2 (a protein that controls cardiac semilunar valvulogenesis) on the long arm of chromosome 12 (12q24.1).[283] Discovery will facilitate both knowledge of the true incidence and phenotypic diversity and the design of appropriately controlled studies of the efficacy of GH therapy with sufficiently large numbers of subjects defined on a molecular genetic basis and followed to final height.

KLINEFELTER'S SYNDROME (47XXY)

There is tall stature for the family with disproportionately long legs from childhood (Fig. 13.41), small testes for apparent virilization (Fig. 13.42) and azoospermia. Presentation is usually with tall stature, hypogonadism (often with marked pubertal gynecomastia) or infertility. The incidence is about 1 in 500 to 1000 live births. Extremely tall ultimate height with increasingly disproportionately long legs relates to testosterone secretion inadequate for conversion to estrogen and epiphyseal closure at the appropriate time or for normal rapid late pubertal spinal growth – GH predominantly stimulates long bone growth. Spontaneous pulsatile GT secretion in pre- and peripubertal 47XXY boys may be normal (c.f the usual GT elevation in adults). Pubertal onset is generally not delayed. Mean IQ is below the population mean, but most are within the normal range. If the diagnosis is made sufficiently early, excessive stature can be prevented, or at least reduced, by high dose testosterone treatment or epiphysiodesis.

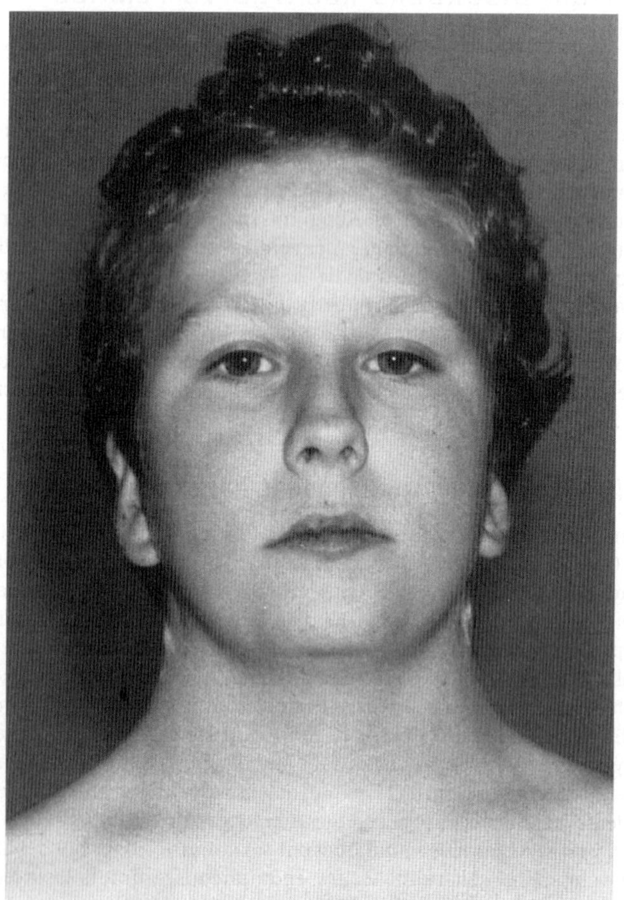

Fig. 13.40 Noonan's syndrome.

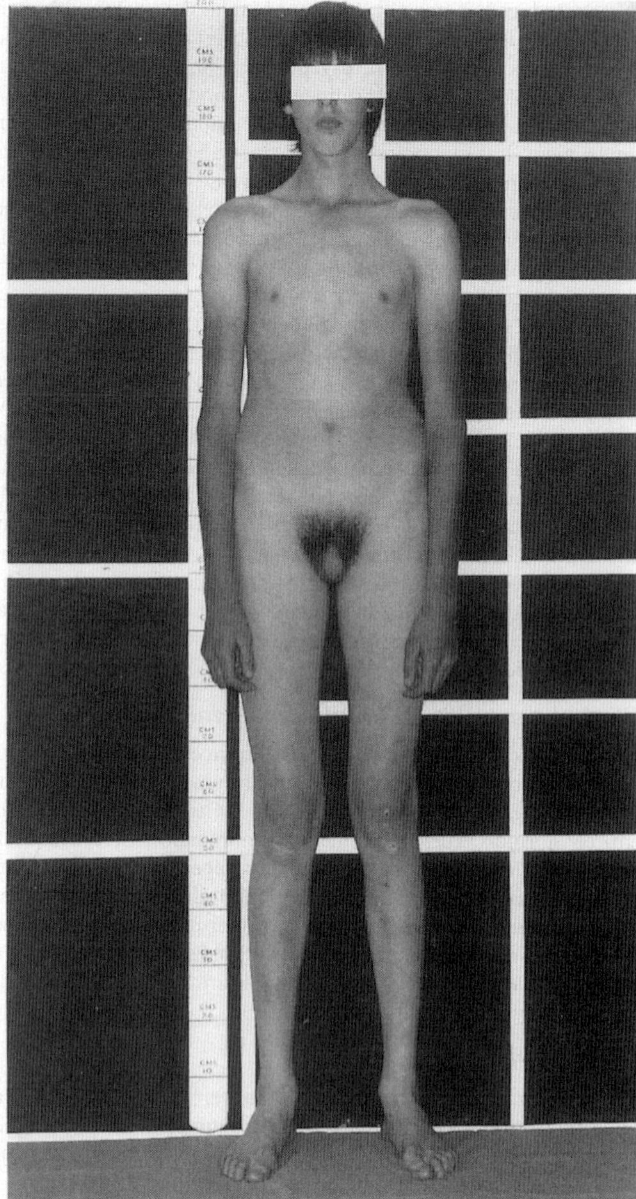

Fig. 13.41 Klinefelter's syndrome – note the disproportionately long legs in this 202 cm 18-year-old.

GYNECOMASTIA

Hormonal effects on breast structures are complex. In males androgens are important in inhibiting stimulatory estrogenic effects on breast tissue; breast development occurs in pubertal girls at estrogen levels comparable to those in adult males. It also occurs in androgen insensitivity syndromes, where testosterone is inactive because of androgen receptor deficiency, at normal male estradiol levels.

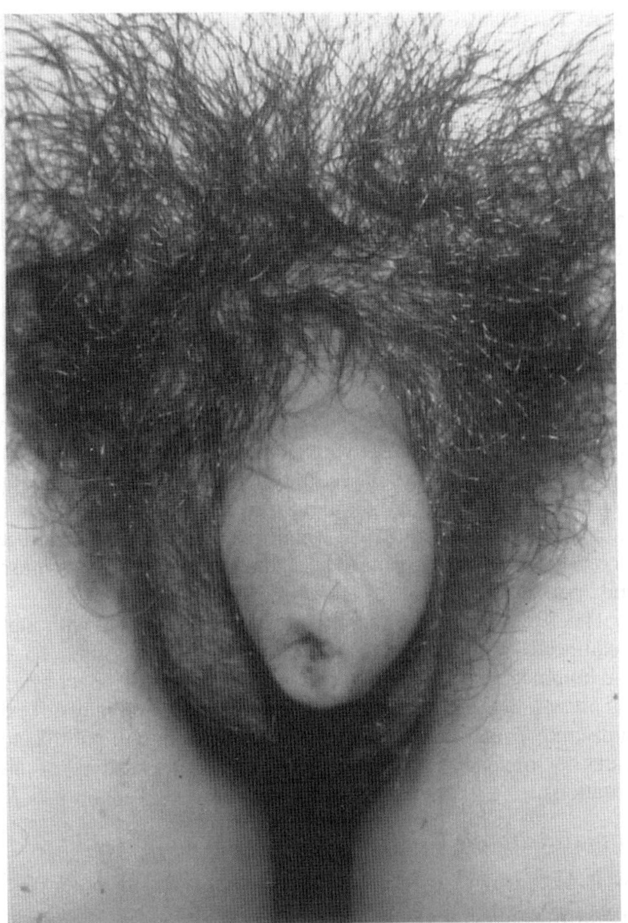

Fig. 13.42 Genitalia in Klinefelter's syndrome – note the small testes for the degree of virilization (the same subject as in Fig. 13.41).

Thus a degree of gynecomastia occurs in < 50% of normal boys during early to mid-puberty when estrogen levels are high in relation to androgens. It is usually mild, resolving spontaneously within 12–18 months, but sometimes subareolar mastectomy is necessary if the condition is distressing and persistent. Gynecomastia is a particular feature of Klinefelter's syndrome (see above). Gross pubertal gynecomastia, prepubertal gynecomastia or persistence in late puberty requires investigation.

Prepubertal gynecomastia may be unilateral, can cause discomfort and is usually benign, self-limiting and idiopathic. Exposure to exogenous estrogen or endogenous production by adrenal, testicular or other tumors must be excluded and drugs such as digoxin, methyldopa, ketoconazole and cannabis and amfetamine abuse have been associated.

UNDESCENDED TESTES

This common problem is considered elsewhere. Many 'undescended' testes are simply retractile, can be manipulated into the scrotum and will descend (and stay in the scrotum) at puberty. Hypogonadotrophic hypogonadism is the commonest cause of cryptorchidism which is now known to be an important cause of infertility secondary to impaired hormonal priming in infancy and genetic defects have been described in a minority of subjects.[271] In bilateral cryptorchidism fertility is likely to be severely compromised. Cryptorchidism and micropenis may represent an intersex phenotype, even if they are isolated and a karyotype should always be checked. In unilateral cryptorchidism the undescended testis fails to establish an adequate adult stem cell pool by 2–3 months of age and similar (if less severe) changes occur in the contralateral (descended) testis. To enhance the chance of adult fertility, hormonal treatment (GnRH analogue, e.g. buserelin 400 mcg intranasally tds for 4 consecutive weeks) should start by 6 months of age. If there is no response HCG should be given (500 units i.m. weekly for 3 consecutive weeks). If there is still no response, orchidopexy and testicular biopsy should be carried out. The biopsy will identify those with a germ cell count < 0.2/tubule and/or no adult dark (Ad) spermatogonia. They should be treated with a further course of a GnRH analogue (10 mcg every other day for 6 months) – GnRHa has been shown to induce increased numbers of germ cells and their differentiation from gonocytes into Ad spermatogonia which improves the chance of fertility.[40]

Scrotal testes are thus necessary functionally (testosterone biosynthesis, spermatogenesis/fertility), cosmetically and because of the (difficult to quantify) risk of malignant change in functional intra-abdominal testes. A testis which is not in the scrotum by infancy is now thought unlikely to show adequate spermatogenesis. Functional but ectopic tissue which cannot be brought into the scrotum surgically is probably best removed unless it is easily accessible to clinical examination and follow-up can be assured. Non-functioning intra-abdominal testicular tissue is probably best left – it carries extremely low risk of malignant change and may be impossible to locate at laparotomy or laparoscopy.

THE HYPOTHALAMO–PITUITARY UNIT

CONNECTIONS/ANATOMY/PHYSIOLOGY

Ontogeny of fetal hypothalamo–pituitary hormone biosynthesis is described on p. 449. By 15 weeks' gestation, the hypothalamus is anatomically mature and functionally active and by 18 weeks, pituitary vascularization is complete. The hypothalamo– pituitary axis is functional by 20 weeks with development of the portal system.

Functional maturity is important for normal development of thyroid (secondary to TSH secretion), external genitalia in the male (GH and GTs) and adrenal (ACTH and related peptides).

The pituitary gland is situated within the pituitary fossa, directly below and in close relationship with the hypothalamus. Laterally are the cavernous sinuses, the internal carotid arteries, the 3rd, 4th and 6th cranial nerves and temporal lobes. Above lie arachnoid and subarachnoid spaces and above them the optic chiasma and hypothalamus.

The hypothalamus has afferent connections with frontal cortex, thalamus, amygdala, hippocampus and anterior thalamic (autonomic) nuclei and can integrate and respond to a wide range of physiological and behavioral inputs. Efferent pathways also connect with midbrain, pons, medulla, amygdala and hippocampus and there are specific pathways to adenohypophysis via the portal system and to neurohypophysis via the supraopticohypophyseal tract.

Neuroendocrine control of hypothalamic secretion is by CNS neurotransmitters including dopamine, noradrenaline, serotonin, acetylcholine, gamma-aminobutyric acid (GABA), melatonin and histamine. Anterior pituitary hormone secretion is directly controlled by hypothalamic factors (regulatory peptides) which affect hormone synthesis and release (Table 13.10).

Table 13.10 Hypothalamic regulatory peptides and their properties

Regulatory peptide	Amino acids	Molecular weight
Growth hormone releasing hormone	40/44	4545/5040
Somatostatin (growth hormone release inhibiting hormone)	14	1638
Gonadotropin releasing hormone/ luteinizing hormone releasing hormone	10	1182
Thyrotropin releasing hormone	3	362
Corticotropin releasing hormone/factor	41	4758

ANTERIOR PITUITARY HORMONES

Corticotrophin (ACTH)

ACTH is a single chain 39 amino acid polypeptide. The first 24 N-terminal amino acids are identical in most species and produce the biological (adrenocortical) activity. However ACTH is one of a group of related pituitary peptides which originates from a common large molecular weight (31 000) glycosylated precursor molecule, pro-opiomelanocortin (POMC). Glycosylation accounts for basophil staining of pituitary corticotrophs.

The bovine precursor protein (Fig. 13.43)[284] consists of 265 amino acids encoding three peptides: ACTH, beta-lipotrophin (beta-LPH) and a 105 amino acid N-terminal sequence N-POMC. Human N-POMC is a 76 amino acid peptide of molecular weight 11 200. All three POMC-derived peptides are found in the same secretory granules within the cell, are released concomitantly into the circulation in equal concentrations, become undetectable after hypophysectomy and their plasma concentrations rise after adrenalectomy. Secretion is stimulated by median eminence extracts containing CRF activity and suppressed by dexamethasone. Plasma concentrations of N-POMC and ACTH correlate closely, reflecting coordinated synthesis and secretion.

No clearly defined physiological role for beta-LPH and N-POMC has yet been identified although species similarity of the three POMC constituents makes this likely. Met-encephalin (the first five residues of beta-endorphin, beta-LPH 61–65) has opiate agonist activity but no circadian secretory rhythm and may originate from the adrenal medulla rather than the pituitary.

The principal modulator of ACTH secretion is CRF but vasopressin also has a stimulatory effect on ACTH secretion, directly and by potentiating the actions of CRF. Neurotransmitter pathways important in ACTH secretion are alpha-adrenergic (perhaps most important), cholinergic, serotoninergic and histaminergic (all excitatory) and via GABA (inhibitory).

ACTH release is circadian resulting in the early morning peak of ACTH and cortisol in association with more frequent ACTH pulses. Factors modulating its secretion are cortisol (by negative feedback at hypothalamic (mainly) and pituitary levels via fast and slow feed back loops) and ACTH itself at pituitary level.

ACTH stimulates adrenal growth and cortisol synthesis and release. Plasma half-life is about 10 min. Mechanisms stimulating adrenocortical steroidogenesis are complex: ACTH binds to its adrenal cell membrane receptor, in the presence of calcium ions, to generate cyclic AMP; cyclic AMP activates, by phosphorylation, enzymes which stimulate hydrolysis of cholesterol esters (first steps in adrenal steroidogenesis). Rapid steroid production follows (Fig. 13.50). There is also a slower, chronic effect on protein synthesis in the cytochrome P-450 dependent enzyme systems (11beta-, 17alpha- and 21-hydroxylases).

ACTH acutely stimulates aldosterone release from zona glomerulosa cells – this has important practical implications for managing of salt-losing CAH – and modulates adrenal androgen secretion. It stimulates amino acid and glucose uptake by muscle and lipolysis in adipose cells and inhibits thymic growth.

The 13 ACTH N-terminal amino acids are identical with alpha melonocyte stimulating hormones (alpha-MSH) (see Fig. 13.43) and homologous with amino acids 7–13 of beta-MSH. Beta-MSH is not present in the pituitary or circulation in man and may not exist in discrete form. The etiology of skin pigmentation in pathological states is unclear – ACTH itself is probably causative in some situations.

Somatotrophin (GH)

See p. 475.

Gonadotrophins (GTs – LH, FSH)

LH and FSH are glycoproteins (MW 30 000 and 32 000 respectively), each with identical A but different B chains and possibly stored within the same secretory granules in pituitary gonadotrophs. Release is controlled by a single hypothalamic hormone, GnRH (see Table 13.10). GnRH is released in a pulsatile manner.

In men, LH stimulates testicular Leydig cell testosterone secretion and FSH stimulates spermatogenesis. In women, LH induces ovulation, maintains the corpus luteum and stimulates it to produce progesterone and estrogens. Ovarian follicles secrete estrogens in response to FSH and endometrial gland growth and secretion result from estrogen and progesterone secretion, respectively. In men, LH secretion is under negative feedback control from testosterone and FSH secretion is regulated by inhibin-B secreted by testicular Sertoli cells. In the female, estrogens exert either positive feedback at pituitary level (before ovulation) or

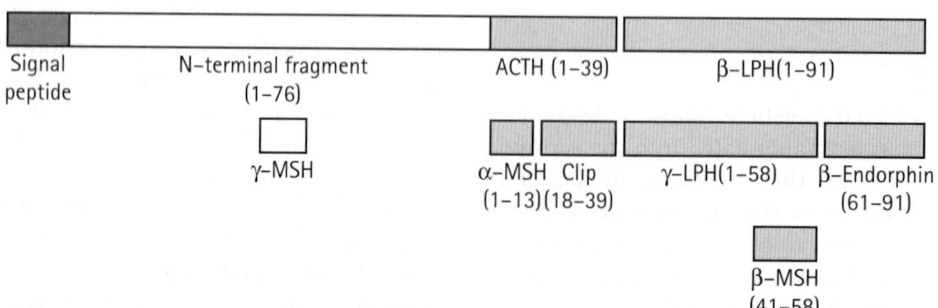

Fig. 13.43 Structure of bovine pro-opiomelanocortin (POMC). (After Nakanishi et al 1979[284]) (The connecting peptide N-POMC 79–109 has been omitted.)

negative feedback (at other times). For further details on the inhibins see p. 485.

Prolactin (PRL)

PRL (198 amino acids, MW 22 500) is strikingly homologous with GH. Its major role is in initiation and maintenance of lactation. Its role in childhood, when levels are low and constant, is unknown although it rises in response to stress. There is no evidence that slight rises during normal puberty are important in pubertal onset or control. Transiently high levels in neonates secondary to feto-placental estrogen may cause galactorrhea ('witch's milk') from engorged breasts in either sex.

PRL is predominantly under inhibitory dopaminergic control and hyperprolactinemia is an important early non-specific sign of neuroendocrine disturbance and intracranial pathology. A PRL inhibiting factor (PIF) has been postulated but has not been characterized. GABA may also have some inhibitory effect but TRH and VIP are stimulatory.

Thyrotrophin (TSH)

TSH is a glycoprotein, MW 26 600. It shares a common A chain with LH and FSH. TRH stimulates TSH synthesis and release which increases thyroid vascularity and stimulates follicular cell hypertrophy. TSH stimulates iodine uptake, organification, coupling of tyrosines and the synthesis and release of thyroxine (T4) and tri-iodothyronine (T3). Feedback inhibition is by T3, both directly and via deiodination of T4 within the pituitary. In man dopaminergic inhibition may occur at the level of the thyrotroph; the inhibitory role of somatostatin is unclear in normal physiology. Glucocorticoids inhibit TSH release at hypothalamic level.

After birth, there is a large rise in TSH release followed by a more gradual rise in circulating T4 and T3 levels. TSH levels return to normal by the end of the first week but thyroid hormone levels may be elevated for up to several weeks.

Melanocyte-stimulating hormones (alpha- and beta-MSH)

See above under ACTH.

POSTERIOR PITUITARY HORMONES

Arginine vasopressin (antidiuretic hormone, AVP) and oxytocin

Vasopressin and oxytocin are 9 amino acid peptides differing from each other at two sites (amino acids 3 and 8). They are synthesized in the supraoptic (mainly vasopressin) and paraventricular (mainly oxytocin) hypothalamic neurones bound to proteins (neurophysins I and II) whose function is unknown. Both hormones reach the posterior pituitary, where they are stored in secretory granules, via the supraopticohypophyseal tract.

The principal stimulus to vasopressin (AVP) release is rising plasma osmolality but plasma volume and blood pressure may exert independent effects. Some physiological states (e.g. pain, stress, sleep) also stimulate vasopressin release. The most important physiological action is to cause water reabsorption by renal distal tubules and collecting ducts – water is reabsorbed in excess of sodium resulting in concentrated urine. Plasma osmolality is normally kept within the range 275–290 mosmol/kg throughout life.

The principal stimulus to oxytocin release is suckling. Oxytocin stimulates the 'let-down' reflex during lactation and uterine contractility. It has weak antidiuretic activity. Except in pregnancy and the puerperium, its physiological role in man is unknown. Neither excess nor deficiency is associated with any syndrome in children (or adults).

DISEASES OF THE HYPOTHALAMO-NEUROHYPOPHYSEAL UNIT

Diabetes insipidus (DI)

Hypothalamic AVP deficiency leads to voiding of inappropriately large volumes of dilute urine (polyuria). If thirst sensation is normal, fluid lost is replaced and there is excessive drinking (polydipsia) to maintain normal plasma osmolality. Nocturia is invariable and may present as secondary enuresis in older children. If thirst recognition is defective (usually due to extensive hypothalamic damage to both AVP and thirst osmoreceptors) or there is no access to adequate or appropriate fluid (e.g. in neonate or infant), hypernatremic dehydration may result in fever, irritability, vomiting and failure to thrive, and polyuria may be absent.

Polyuria and polydipsia may result from renal unresponsiveness to AVP (nephrogenic DI, see Ch. 16). Sometimes primary polydipsia ('compulsive water drinking') may develop in children (leading to secondary polyuria). Both these situations must be considered in the differential diagnosis as must other causes of polyuria (e.g. urinary tract infection, diabetes mellitus). Defects in AVP release are usually due to hypothalamic dysfunction – more than 75% of secretory capacity must be lost before symptoms develop. Removal of, or damage to, the neurohypophysis does not cause DI.

DI is rare in childhood – with an incidence in Caucasian populations of 5 per million per year. Causes are listed in Table 13.11.[285–288]

Primary DI may be familial or sporadic and families with dominant or X-linked inheritance have been described.

Familial AVP deficiency (DI) is of variable severity which increases with age and may not manifest itself clinically until adolescence. It is probably due to a degenerative process in the cells of the hypothalamus that produce antidiuretic hormone (AVP). As there is high redundancy of function (more than 75% of secretory capacity must be lost before symptoms develop) it is not surprising that, despite being inherited, the condition may take many years to develop.

AVP deficiency is found in 25–50% of children with Langerhans' cell histiocytosis and may precede other evidence of the disease by months or years (see Ch. 21). Other rare infiltrative causes include Hodgkin's disease, leukemias and sarcoidosis but transient DI is common after head injury and pituitary surgery. It may complicate severe neonatal infections and may be associated with autoimmune states with AVP antibodies.

Differential diagnosis of polyuria depends on history, examination and laboratory tests. Osmotic diuresis (e.g. due to salt or glucose) is readily excluded from the history and by testing the urine

Table 13.11 Causes of diabetes insipidus (data from Crawford & Bode 1975, Czernichow et al 1985, Niaudet et al 1985, Perheentupa 1995)[285–288]

Hypothalamic tumor 38% – craniopharyngioma 23% (usually postoperative); germinoma 6.5%; optic neuroma rarely
Idiopathic 23% – autoimmune factors may be important
Congenital renal 23%
Histiocytosis X 8%
Cerebral malformations 3%
Primary polydipsia 3%
Traumatic 2%

for glucose. Habitual polydipsia most often develops in response to fluids being offered to pacify a demanding infant or young child. Such primary polydipsia of 'psychogenic' origin is suggested by fluctuating symptoms, evidence of psychological difficulties in the child or family, and a refusal of water (as opposed to juice) if waking thirsty at night. A morning plasma osmolality in the normal range (cf. in DI) often contrasts with a low value in the evening.

History of head injury, meningitis or encephalitis should be sought. Poor growth suggests either inadequate appetite or food intake relating to the polydipsia or an associated anterior pituitary lesion with TSH, GH, GT or ACTH deficiencies. TSH or ACTH deficiency may temporarily conceal DI until thyroxine or cortisol replacement is given. Headaches, vomiting and visual disturbances indicate raised intracranial pressure secondary to tumor.

Synchronous measurements of plasma and urinary osmolality are valuable provided accurate assays are available. If not, plasma sodium (not specific gravity) should be substituted. Inappropriately low urinary osmolality with raised plasma osmolality confirms DI – charts aiding interpretation have been produced for children.[289] To achieve this mismatch a water deprivation test may be necessary. Plasma AVP assays are increasingly available but their value in diagnosis of central DI in children is not established (high, diagnostic values are found in nephrogenic DI).

Water deprivation tests are potentially both dangerous and misleading if inadequately supervised and a strict protocol should be followed. Specific additional endocrine and neuroradiological investigations may be necessary.

Provision of adequate water with free access to solute-free fluid at all times is vitally important. Treatment with AVP has been much simplified by the availability of a synthetic AVP analogue 1-desamino-8D-arginine vasopressin (DDAVP, desmopressin) which has a longer duration of action than AVP itself. It can be administered intranasally – a reasonable starting dose is 0.25 mcg (in neonates), 0.5–1.0 mcg (infants) and 2.5 mcg (children). Therapeutic effect is seen within 1 h. The 2 or 3 times daily dose is adjusted to provide an antidiuretic effect for 8–12 h and may need increasing during rhinitis. DDAVP, like other small peptides, is orally active and can now be given orally – initially 100 mcg tds; maintenance 200–600 mcg per day in divided doses as above.

Special care must be taken with infants who do not have free access to water and children with an impaired sense of thirst. Water intoxication is a risk with overdosage or if water is given inappropriately. A talisman detailing the disease and its therapy should be carried or worn at all times.

Poor control of DI is associated with nocturia, enuresis, irritability and poor behavior and school performance. Appetite and growth velocity may be poor. Polyuria may lead to secondary enuresis. If treatment is optimal, prognosis reflects the underlying condition in secondary DI; in treated primary DI growth and development should be normal.

DI, diabetes mellitus, optic atrophy, deafness syndrome ('DIDMOAD' syndrome, Wolfram syndrome)

See p. 546.

Syndrome of inappropriate secretion of antidiuretic hormone (SIADH)

Causes are listed in Table 13.12. Excessive AVP secretion results in water retention, hypo-osmolality and dilutional hyponatremia. Inhibition of aldosterone with continuing AVP secretion leads to paradoxically high urinary sodium levels and concentrated urine. AVP levels may not be supranormal but are inappropriately high for the expanded extracellular volume and hypo-osmolality.

Table 13.12 Causes of inappropriate ADH secretion

CNS disease/disorder
Meningitis/encephalitis
Trauma
Tumor
Hemorrhage
Hypoxia
Ischemia
Malformation
Guillain–Barré syndrome
Obstructed ventriculoatrial shunt
Lung disease
Pneumonia
Tuberculosis
Pneumothorax*
Asthma*
Cystic fibrosis*
Ventilation
Postoperative (including mitral valvotomy,* ductus arteriosus ligation*)
Drugs (e.g. analgesics, sedatives, anesthetics)
Malignancy
Trauma/burns
Endocrine/metabolic
Hypothyroidism
Adrenocortical failure
Hypoglycemia
Idiopathic

* May be secondary to reduced left atrial filling.

In pediatric practice, SIADH is usually seen either in neonates following birth asphyxia, hyaline membrane disease or intraventricular hemorrhage, or in older children in association with meningitis, encephalitis or CNS tumors. It occasionally complicates pneumonia or pulmonary tuberculosis, vincristine or cyclophosphamide therapy, and is a common, temporary (up to several days) complication of surgery requiring general anesthesia. It may be a particular problem in burns and trauma patients. SIADH may be iatrogenic, due to inappropriate intravenous fluid therapy.

The first signs and symptoms are often masked by, or taken as manifestations of the underlying problem – anorexia, confusion, headaches, muscle weakness and cramps. Eventually, there is vomiting, convulsions or coma. There is no edema. Diagnosis depends on clinical suspicion and the above biochemical findings.

Treatment is by water restriction to between 30 and 50% maintenance and sodium replacement to compensate for secondary sodium losses. Correction should be gradual (over several days). In situations where this cannot be achieved drug therapy may be indicated. Lithium and demethylchlortetracycline have serious side-effects in children and should not be used. Furosemide (frusemide) (with slow infusion of hypertonic saline) may be indicated – AVP antidiuretic analogues which, it was hoped, would become the treatment of choice, have all had significant vasopressor activity.[290]

DISEASES OF THE ADENOHYPOPHYSIS

GH insufficiency and excess

See p. 527.

ACTH excess

Hypercortisolism in children usually results from excessive GC medication. Endogenous adrenocortical overactivity is rare, whether due to adrenal tumor (benign or malignant), hyperplasia, ectopic tumor ACTH production or to pituitary dependent ACTH secretion (Cushing's disease). Cushing's syndrome includes all pathological states secondary to excessive GC production. Cushing found a basophil pituitary adenoma in only six of his original 12 patients[291] – it is now thought that bilateral adrenal hyperplasia secondary to excessive ACTH secretion of pituitary origin is not a single entity and may be due to a variety of hypothalamic, pituitary or even CNS (neurotransmitter) abnormalities.

Classical clinical features of hypercortisolism (hypertension, striae, truncal obesity, moon face, osteoporosis) are less obvious in children than in adults. Growth failure is usually marked but there can be temporary adrenal androgen-mediated acceleration. Investigation with low and high-dose dexamethasone suppression tests and the human corticotrophin-releasing hormone (hCRH) test will identify the etiology[292] – Cushing's disease itself is probably the commonest cause in children and adolescents.

The aim in treating Cushing's disease is to control cortisol overproduction (if appropriate by removing the source of ACTH hypersecretion) whilst avoiding permanent endocrine deficiencies and dependence on replacement therapy. In practice, treatment of Cushing's syndrome in children is still controversial given its poorly understood and diverse etiological basis. Options include surgery to adrenals or pituitary, pituitary irradiation (conventional or with radioactive implants), or medical management with dopaminergic agents or serotonin antagonists – collaboration between pediatric and adult endocrinologists, an experienced neurosurgeon and a radiotherapist is essential for a successful therapeutic outcome.[292]

ACTH deficiency

ACTH deficiency is usually associated with other anterior pituitary hormone deficiencies which may be congenital, idiopathic, due to brain malformations or pituitary hypoplasia or to tumors such as craniopharyngioma (especially following surgery and/or radiotherapy). Hypothalamic CRF/pituitary ACTH secretion is more resistant to irradiation than the GH or GnRH axes.

Isolated ACTH deficiency is rare, may be congenital and can be associated with primary hypothyroidism – thyroxine therapy precipitates adrenal insufficiency by increasing cortisol clearance.

Congenital panhypopituitarism (see Fig. 13.44) is associated with severe neonatal hypoglycemia but isolated ACTH deficiency does not usually produce as severe adrenal hypofunction as in primary adrenal insufficiency. GC and adrenal androgen secretion are impaired; aldosterone secretion is normal. Collapse with salt loss may occur during severe intercurrent illness or general anesthesia. Treatment is with appropriate GC replacement.

TSH deficiency

Congenital hypothyroidism due to decreased TSH stimulation of thyroid hormone secretion may be due to abnormalities of hypothalamic or pituitary development, isolated TRH or TSH deficiency (familial or idiopathic) or panhypopituitarism. Congenital primary hypothyroidism is 15- to 30-fold commoner.

TSH deficiency may present in later childhood, usually in association with other anterior pituitary hormone deficiencies and secondary to tumors (especially craniopharyngioma), cranial irradiation (to which the thyroid axis is relatively resistant) or meningitis. Symptoms and signs due to associated deficiencies usually predominate.

Differential diagnosis of primary, secondary (pituitary) and tertiary (hypothalamic) hypothyroidism and management is discussed below.

Gonadotrophin (GT) deficiency

Isolated GT deficiency may occur without underlying anatomical abnormality. Usually congenital abnormalities of brain

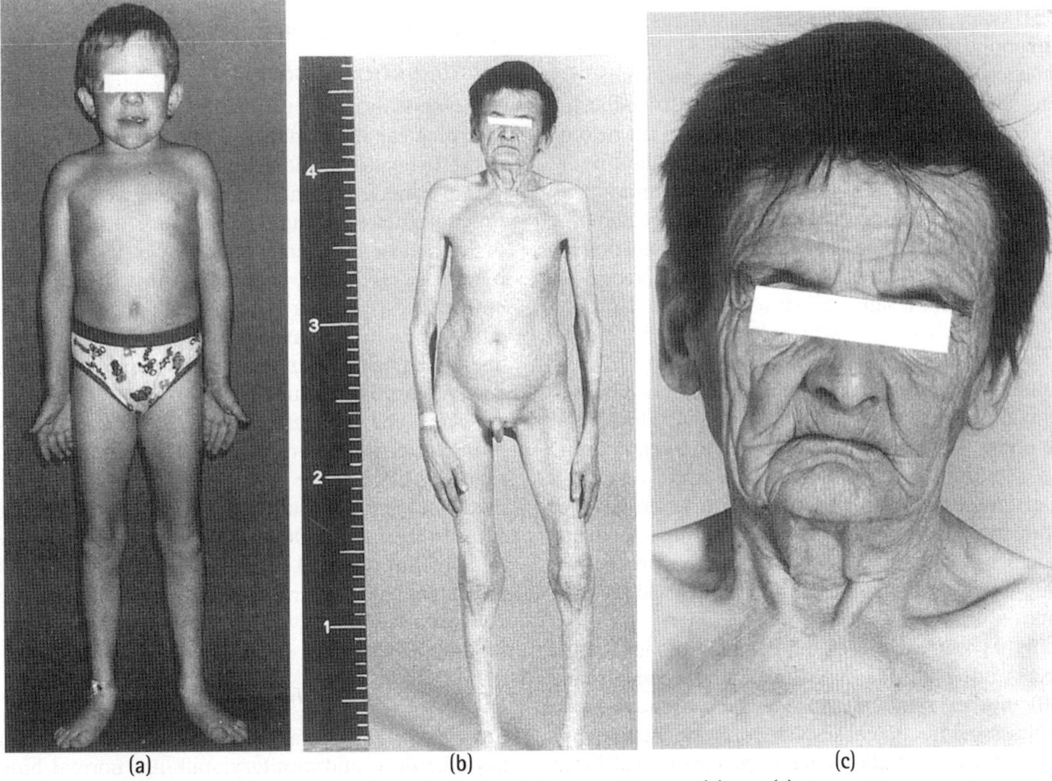

Fig. 13.44 Untreated panhypopituitarism (a) at age 11 years, (b) and (c) at age 71 years.

development give rise to hypothalamic GnRH deficiency, either isolated (e.g. Kallmann's syndrome) or associated with other hypothalamic disturbances. GT deficiency may be associated with other pituitary hormone deficiencies in pituitary aplasia or hypoplasia, craniopharyngioma, etc.

Hyperprolactinemia

Moderately raised PRL levels are an early non-specific sign of neuroendocrine disturbance and particularly of suprasellar or hypothalamic space-occupying lesions. Stress causes a rise in PRL levels and serial sampling at half hourly intervals from an indwelling cannula may be necessary to distinguish the two. Very high levels result from PRL-secreting micro- or macroadenomas but these are extremely rare in children. They may cause delayed puberty. Raised PRL in association with raised GT (and especially FSH) levels cause precocious puberty in primary hypothyroidism.

Intracranial space-occupying lesions

These are the second commonest neoplasms in children (after leukemia) accounting for 20% of the total. Endocrine aspects are of practical importance in a variety of ways:

As 'early warning' signs of intracranial pathology

1. Moderately raised PRL levels in the absence of stress (see above).
2. Slow growth or signs of precocious or delayed puberty resulting from endocrine dysfunction may precede more specific clinical manifestations by many months.

In pre-, peri- and postoperative management

1. Hydrocortisone cover must be adequate for the stress of surgery, irradiation or radioactive implant.
2. Transient DI is common after surgery to the pituitary area but temporary inappropriate ADH secretion may occur (management is reviewed by Albanese et al[293]).

Permanent hormone replacement therapy after surgery and/or radiotherapy

1. The need for therapy should be reassessed in terms of adeno- and neurohypophyseal function after these procedures – variable deficiencies of any or all hormones may be found.
2. Some tumors are particularly associated with endocrine dysfunction. These include craniopharyngiomas (see below), hypothalamic and optic nerve gliomas, third ventricular tumors and pituitary adenomas. Third ventricular tumors and hamartomas and other tumors of the pituitary stalk region may result in hypofunction, but may, like many pituitary adenomas, be functional. They seem commoner in boys and precocious puberty may be the earliest sign.

Craniopharyngioma

This is the commonest tumor affecting the hypothalamo–pituitary region in childhood and accounts for 8–13% of all intracranial tumors in those under 14 years of age. It results from embryonic, slowly growing remnants of Rathke's pouch and is initially suprasellar in origin. Expansion posterosuperiorly erodes the dorsum sellae causing hypothalamic and midbrain displacement. Nearly all contain areas of calcification but the tumors are usually cystic (containing cholesterol, cell debris and altered blood) with solid components.

Although benign, progressive local enlargement into important surrounding tissues, often late diagnosis (during the second decade of life) and difficulty of removal cause serious consequences. Regular growth assessment, clinical suspicion in a slowly growing child and fundal examination with recurrent headache or delayed puberty would all help reduce delay from first symptoms or signs to diagnosis. Obvious visual field defects, visual acuity impairment or neurological signs (cranial nerve palsies, optic atrophy, papilledema, effortless vomiting due to raised intracranial pressure) indicate a large tumor.

Plain lateral skull X-ray is often diagnostic revealing a mass containing calcification eroding the clinoid processes and an abnormally enlarged sella. CT or MR scanning will confirm the diagnosis and determine any degree of suprasellar extension.

If the lesion is small (15% are still intrasellar at diagnosis) and adequate follow-up can be ensured with neuroradiological (CT or MR) facilities, observation alone is justifiable. The endocrine situation is never improved by surgery or radiotherapy (usually it is made worse) and endocrine disturbance alone is not an indication for either form of treatment. When surgery is indicated, and it is urgent when there are visual or neurological disturbances, complete surgical excision without causing other damage is seldom possible because of the hardness of the tumor and its size (particularly if diagnosis is late). Subtotal excision is often inevitable whatever the preoperative intent and, although the tumors are not very radiosensitive, postoperative irradiation is thought to reduce recurrence risk.

Pre-, peri- and postoperative management and fluid balance must be meticulous. Pre-existing hormone deficiency should be corrected but hydrocortisone to cover the stress of the procedure must always be given even if ACTH reserve seems adequate. The need for long-term replacement therapies should be assessed several weeks postoperatively. DI may only become obvious after cortisol replacement. Occasional damage to the thirst center causes major management problems. In many cases, GH, thyroxine, hydrocortisone (certainly to cover stress and sometimes regularly), DDAVP and pubertal induction will be necessary. Despite appropriate hormone replacement, obesity can be a major long-term problem in many patients. The prognosis is improved with early diagnosis and careful initial management.

OTHER DISORDERS

Septo-optic dysplasia

Septo-optic dysplasia (SOD) is a condition characterized by midline neurological abnormalities associated with pituitary and optic nerve hypoplasia. The abnormalities and their manifestations are variable but a presentation may be with disturbed hypothalamic function and resulting hypopituitarism (usually GT, GH and AVP deficiencies) in infancy with hypothermia, hypoglycemia and blindness. CT or MR scanning shows variable hypoplasia of the optic nerves, chiasma and hypothalamic infundibular region, often with an absent septum pellucidum. Similar endocrine consequences are sometimes seen in other midline developmental abnormalities such as corpus callosum agenesis.

The homeobox gene Hesx1/HESX1 was initially implicated in pituitary development through loss-of-function studies in the mouse. Although the etiology of SOD is unknown, a homozygous missense point mutation in the gene resulting in a single amino acid substitution, Arg160Cys (R160C), is associated with a heritable form of human SOD.[294] Hesx1/HESX1 gene mutatations may be important in providing a genetic basis for more general midline defects associated with an undescended or ectopic posterior pituitary.[295]

Empty sella syndrome

Pituitary hypoplasia is associated with a small fossa. The infundibulum and pituitary stalk are normal but the chiasmatic cistern may extend into the small sella and appear empty with the stalk outlined by CSF. Enlargement of the sella and pituitary has been found in some cases of primary hypothyroidism.[251] Decreasing pituitary size on thyroxine replacement may give the appearance of an empty sella with the small pituitary gland situated posteroinferiorly within the enlarged fossa.

Diencephalic syndrome

This is usually due to an anteriorly growing hypothalamic glioma which presents in infancy or early childhood with excessive alertness and hyperexcitability, pallor, vomiting, gross wasting and failure to thrive. CSF protein levels are raised and tumor cells may be present. CT or MR scanning will confirm the diagnosis.

Sotos' syndrome (cerebral gigantism)[296]

Prenatal overgrowth occurs in several syndromes, including the Sotos' and Weaver syndromes which are probably closely related. Birth weight and length are high reflecting the rapid intrauterine growth. This continues until by middle childhood growth velocity is normal. As puberty occurs early, final stature is seldom excessive. Mental retardation is common but may be mild or absent. Associated cardiac defects are common and there are increased malignancy risks. There are also similarities with another tall stature syndrome, Beckwith–Wiedemann, and excessive secretion of fetal growth factors could be etiologically important.

THE PINEAL GLAND

The pineal, like the hypothalamus, develops from the diencephalon. Ependymal cells and vascular mesenchyme from the anterior part of the diencephalic roof plate form the choroid plexus. Caudally, the roof plate of the diencephalon thickens, evaginates by about 7 weeks and forms an ultimately cone-shaped solid organ, the pineal, attached by a peduncle to the posterior border of the third ventricle. It lies in the quadrigeminal cistern between the superior colliculi covered by the splenium of the corpus callosum and is innervated by postganglionic sympathetic superior cervical ganglionic nerve fibers. Pinealocytes form a mosaic pattern around capillaries, astrocytes and ganglion cells.

At one time thought to be the seat of the soul, seen as guiding the cerebral hemispheres or, more mundanely, being important in the control of the onset of human puberty, the pineal role remains speculative. Pinealocytes convert tryptophan via serotonin to melatonin which is primarily produced by the pineal gland during the dark period of the light–dark cycle.

It had been conjectured that endocrine pubertal events are inhibited prepubertally by melatonin following reports that its concentration falls abruptly between pubertal stages G1 and G2 from age 11.5 to 14 years and that melatonin inhibits gonadal development in some males. However, there appears to be no inhibitory effect of melatonin on GT secretion and 24-h melatonin profiles are similar in prepuberty, puberty and adulthood (low day-time levels, high nocturnal levels). Levels in precocious puberty are similar to those in normal puberty implying that melatonin has no major role in normal or precocious puberty, although blindness, which would upset the pineal circadian clock, is associated with early menarche.

Melatonin may have a role in inhibiting gonadal development – using a sensitive and specific assay, with frequent night-time sampling, nocturnal melatonin levels decrease significantly with sexual maturation and age.[297] However the greatest fall in mean nocturnal melatonin levels was between prepubertal children under and over 7 years which does not support the hypothesis that it is that fall which triggers pubertal onset. There is evidence for a decline in the day to night increment of serum melatonin concentrations from infancy to childhood, that children with early puberty have lower melatonin day to night increments than age matched controls, and that those with constitutionally delayed puberty show increments comparable to those of preschool children.[298]

This implies a relationship between maturation and the mechanisms controlling pineal gland secretion whether or not melatonin plays any significant role in the onset of puberty. Certainly, in seasonal breeders melatonin regulates reproductive physiology and influences the age of sexual maturation in laboratory rodents. In the human, melatonin rhythms are closely related to those of reproductive hormones during infancy and reciprocally correlated during puberty. There are melatonin receptors in the brain and gonads, and sex hormone receptors in the pineal gland but functional relationships have not been demonstrated.

In pediatric practice, the pineal is important in two, sometimes related, contexts: rare pineal tumors and precocious puberty. Pineal tumors comprise $< 1\%$ of all intracranial tumors, are associated with precocious, delayed or absent puberty, but classically cause precocious puberty in boys. Lesions can be multifocal. About half are radiosensitive germinomas; astrocytomas, gliomas, germ cell teratomas and carcinomas also occur. Pineal destruction is usually associated with precocious puberty. Germinomas sometimes secrete HCG and alpha-fetoprotein and secreting pineoblastomas and pineocytomas (pinealomas) occur.

Signs of raised intracranial pressure are common due to aqueduct compression. Visual loss, paresis of upward gaze and hypothalamic dysfunction (obesity, loss of temperature control, DI) may occur. Surgery is hazardous. Most pineal tumors recur after radiotherapy but germinomas are curable.

The pineal normally calcifies to varying extent with age. It is rarely seen radiographically before 6 years, is found in 2% by 8 years and 10% by 15 years (30% on CT scan). CT or MR scanning is indicated if calcification is seen on skull radiographs up to about 10 years and in any boy with central precocious puberty.

THE THYMUS

The thymus comprises cells of two origins. The epithelial component derives from 3rd and 4th pharyngeal pouches, the same embryological origin as the parathyroids. Thymic migration to the thorax from about 6 weeks is associated with parathyroid migration and branchial (pharyngeal) arch organization to form the aortic arch and other structures. Abnormal thymic stromal differentiation results in DiGeorge syndrome.

T-lymphocyte progenitors travel from fetal liver and, postnatally, from bone marrow and undergo maturation within the thymus to form T-lymphocytes – the lymphoid component. Thymic stromal cells manufacture humoral substances, thymosin and thymopoietin, thought to be important in this maturational process. The thymus is the major site of production of immunocompetent T lymphocytes from their hematopoietic stem cells. Thymic hormones induce in situ T-cell marker differentiation, expression and functions. These polypeptide hormones localize in the reticulo-epithelial (RE) cells of the thymic cellular microenvironment. Thymosin derivatives have been detected as products of neoplastically transformed cells and employed in the early diagnosis of neoplasms. In clinical trials, thymic hormones strengthen the effects of immunomodulators in immunodeficiencies, autoimmune diseases, and neoplastic malignancies.[299]

Thymus and other lymphoid tissues reach their greatest proportion of body weight at birth, and by puberty are nearly twice their size in the young adult. The decline to adult size is probably sex steroid mediated. Adrenalectomy delays involution and severe infection or stress hasten it. In addition to its central role in immune regulation, the thymus may influence non-immunological components of the body, including the neuroendocrine system.

Cellular immune deficiencies of aging correspond to decline in function of the hypothalamic–pituitary–endocrine axis. Recent studies point to important roles for the pituitary, the pineal, and the autonomic nervous system as well as the thyroid, gonads and adrenals in thymus integrity and function. Thymic function at the local level requires complex cellular interactions among thymic stromal cells and developing thymocytes, involving paracrine and autocrine mediators including interleukins and interferon-gamma. An important endocrine function of the thymus is to package zinc in zinc-thymulin for delivery to the periphery.[300]

Thymic tumors are rare, but may arise from either tissue component. There is an association with myasthenia gravis and tumors secreting an ACTH-like substance causing Cushing's syndrome are described.

THE THYROID GLAND

EMBRYOLOGY

The thyroid gland develops as an epithelial proliferation in the pharyngeal gut floor at 17 days between what will become the body and root of the tongue – the foramen cecum. It descends as a bilobed diverticulum in front of the pharyngeal gut, still connected to it by a canal – the thyroglossal duct. This normally disappears but cystic remnants may persist – a thyroglossal cyst. Migration continues in front of hyoid bone and laryngeal cartilages to the definitive position in front of the trachea by 7 weeks.

PHYSIOLOGY

By 30 min postdelivery, TSH levels surge, perhaps reacting to the cooler extrauterine environment. In response, within 28 h, total and free T3 and T4 levels rise – thyroxine-binding globulin (TBG) levels do not change. High rT3 levels fall gradually over weeks. The importance of 'physiological neonatal hyperthyroidism' is not known, but animal data suggest a role in catecholamine-mediated brown fat and non-shivering thermogenesis.

Normal thyroid function is crucial in infancy and childhood because of its importance for normal somatic and brain growth and development. Thyroid hormone actions include protein synthesis, cholesterol turnover, water and ion transport and thermogenesis. There are direct and indirect (growth factor synthesis) effects on growth and CNS and skeletal development.

The thyroid concentrates iodide from blood (as do other tissues – salivary and mammary glands, placenta, uterus, stomach and small bowel) and (uniquely) combines it with tyrosine to form metabolically active derivatives. Endemic dietary iodine deficiency is the commonest cause of hypothyroidism and affects some 300 million people worldwide.

Steps in thyroid hormone biosynthesis are summarized in Figure 13.45. Inborn errors of each step are described and comprise about 10% of neonates with congenital non-endemic hypothyroidism. Transport of iodide into thyroid cells is rate-limiting. Iodide oxidation (activation) is followed by peroxidase-catalysed tyrosine iodination and iodotyrosine coupling to form T3 and T4. Thyroglobulin (TG), a high molecular weight iodinated glycoprotein, provides tyrosyl residues for iodotyrosine synthesis (any other physiological role is speculative) and reaches the circulation via thyroid lymphatics. Mono- and di-iodotyrosines (MIT and DIT), T3 and T4 are stored as extracellular colloid. Thyroid hormone secretion involves formation of intracellular colloid droplets, fusion with lysosomes, proteolytic digestion and hydrolysis of thyroglobulin to form free MIT, DIT, T3 and T4. T3 and T4 are released into the circulation; MIT and DIT are deiodinated and free iodide is reutilized for hormone synthesis.

Physiological thyroid hormone action at cellular level is by binding to a specific nuclear plasma membrane and mitochondrial receptors. T3 binding to nuclear receptors seems most important.

For many years it was believed that maternal thyroid hormones did not reach the developing embryo and fetus throughout gestation. More recent research has shown that this is not the case and that these hormones, derived from the mother, probably do exert important developmental effects on the fetal brain.

There is increasing evidence from animal (largely rat) experiments that if the fetal thyroid gland is underactive (congenital hypothyroidism), the transfer of normal amounts of maternal thyroxine (T4) is crucial and protects the fetal brain until birth.[20] Most of the results from animal experiments seem relevant in man, and some, such as the transfer of maternal hormones from mother to fetus during pregnancy and their protective effects on the fetal brain of infants with congenital hypothyroidism, have also been directly demonstrated in man.[301]

Specifically, current evidence suggests that if fetal thyroid secretion is impaired (congenital hypothyroidism), transfer of maternal thyroid hormone (thyroxine, T4) is normally sufficient to enable the fetal brain to convert this thyroxine to tri-iodothyronine (T3) upon which fetal brain growth and development is dependent, and thus to avoid major subsequent neurodevelopmental problems until birth. The protective effect of normal maternal circulating T4 concentrations ends at birth and cerebral T3 deficiency in the newborn follows, which is why treatment with thyroxine must be started in the congenitally hypothyroid baby within a few weeks of birth.[302]

In some parts of the world, severe iodine deficiency is endemic amongst the population and can result in low maternal T4 levels during early pregnancy. In that situation even prompt treatment of the congenitally hypothyroid baby with thyroxine following birth does not prevent subsequent neurological problems and cognitive and intellectual impairment. This emphasizes the crucial role of maternal thyroxine in the development of the fetal brain in early pregnancy.[21]

Thus the effects of congenital hypothyroidism alone on fetal brain growth and development do not result in significant or irreversible neurodevelopmental abnormalities. The central nervous system damage in congenital hypothyroidism is preventable by adequate early postnatal thyroxine treatment provided maternal thyroid status has been adequate during the pregnancy. This is also demonstrated by the generally good results (normal mental and psychomotor development) achieved in this condition following prompt detection (by newborn screening) and early postnatal thyroxine treatment in adequate dosage (see below).

REGULATION OF FUNCTION

Plasma iodide and circulating TSH levels regulate thyroid follicular cell function. Circulating FT4 exerts negative feedback on TSH release. 75 to 80% of circulating FT3 is produced by deiodination of T4 in peripheral tissues. The control mechanism for production of T3 in non-thyroidal tissue is poorly understood but during many disease states or fasting T4 conversion to T3 is reduced and

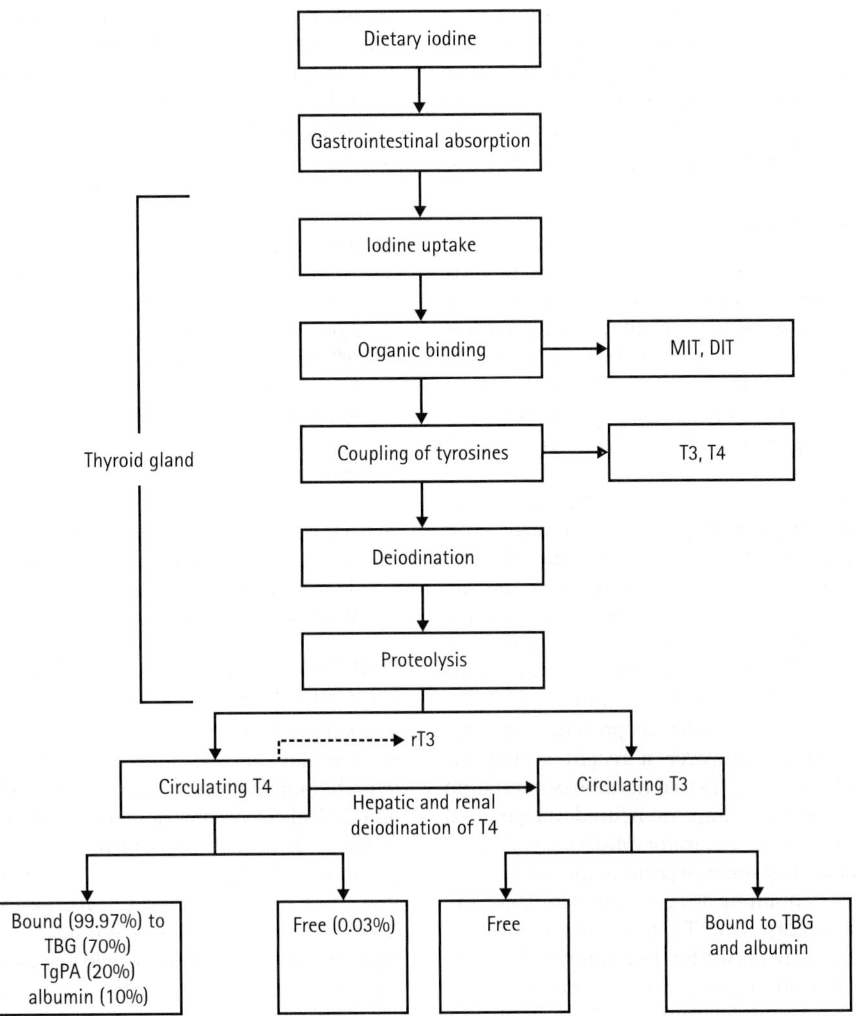

Fig. 13.45 Thyroid hormone biosynthesis. DIT, di-iodo tyrosine; MIT, mono-iodo tyrosine; TBG, thyroxine binding globulin; TgPA, thyroglobulin antibody by passive agglutination.

(inactive) rT3 accumulates. T3 has three to four times the potency of T4 and binds to cell membrane receptor proteins with 10-fold greater affinity.

THYROID FUNCTION TESTS (TFTs)

Normal ranges for TFTs are age related and vary between laboratories. The most sensitive single test of primary thyroid disease is plasma TSH immunoradiometric assay (IRMA). In primary hypothyroidism levels are raised; in hyperthyroidism (or overtreatment of hypothyroidism) levels are suppressed, usually to below the assay detection limit (< 0.1 mU/L). RIA TSH measurement will not reliably distinguish appropriate from excessive replacement.

Total T3 (TT3) and T4 (TT4) levels reflect TBG levels; free (active) hormone measurements (FT3, FT4) reflect functional thyroid status more accurately. T3 may be a more sensitive guide to developing thyrotoxicosis than T4 if TSH IRMA assays are unavailable, but diagnosis on clinical examination is seldom problematic.

It is good practice to measure TSH and FT4 simultaneously to assess the whole axis. TRH tests are useful in assessing hypothalamo–pituitary function: in hypothalamic or pituitary disease, basal TSH levels will be inappropriately low for the T4 levels; in pituitary disease, TSH levels will fail to rise in response to TRH (7 mcg/kg i.v. over several minutes); in hypothalamic disease there is an exaggerated and delayed TSH response (60 min levels higher than at 20 min) as TSH must be synthesized before its release, but this is not always seen and can occur in normal children.

Most specific situations where non-thyroidal illness, pregnancy or drug treatment cause abnormal TFTs (e.g. malnutrition, anorexia nervosa) are uncommon in pediatric practice provided tests are not performed during severe intercurrent illness. During the acute phase of such illnesses (e.g. severe burns or trauma, diabetic ketoacidosis, liver or renal failure), TT3, TT4 and FT3 levels are often low, FT4 may be low or normal (depending on assay methodology); TSH may also be low or normal. During recovery, thyroid hormone levels gradually normalize, but persisting low levels, even with raised TSH levels, do not necessarily indicate hypothyroidism.

Drugs affecting TFTs include estrogens, salicylates, phenytoin, carbamazepine, glucocorticoids and propranolol. Iodide (in expectorants) can cause clinical, as well as biochemical, hypothyroidism.

Apparent thyroid disorders in euthyroid patients due to abnormal carrier proteins will not cause confusion if free hormone and IRMA TSH assays are available. Children with hereditary TBG deficiency (X-linked dominant inheritance, incidence 1 in 10 000, males:females 9:1) will have low TT4 and TT3 levels; high levels of TBG, and thus of TT4 and TT3, are seen during estrogen therapy. In both situations, FT4, FT3 and TSH levels are normal and the patient is clinically euthyroid.

Raised TSH levels with normal FT4 levels in treated hypothyroidism may indicate poor compliance (other than just before a clinic visit). TFTs must always be considered in the context of growth velocity and skeletal maturation and not in isolation (see earlier). Clinical examination alone for signs of hypothyroidism or thyrotoxicosis is a very insensitive guide.

FUNCTION IN PRETERM INFANTS

TT4 and FT4 levels increase with gestation – ~ 25% of preterm infants have low levels by term standards (50% at less than 30 weeks). FT4 levels are never as low as in congenital hypothyroidism. There is presumed hypothalamic immaturity: TSH levels may be normal or low; TSH and T4 levels rise normally following TRH. T4 levels correct spontaneously with maturation over 4–8 weeks, postnatal growth and development are normal and treatment is unnecessary.

There are babies (term or preterm), however, with significantly reduced FT4 levels (into the congenital hypothyroidism range). This seems much commoner in Europe than the USA (perhaps reflecting relative iodine availability).[303] Cord blood T4 and TSH levels are normal for gestation – transient hypothyroidism develops during the first 2 weeks with important implications for screening. In many, thyroid function quickly normalizes; in others, recovery may take 1–2 months and treatment has been thought to be necessary (based on observational studies) in order to prevent abnormal neurodevelopmental outcomes. However a recent systematic review[304] does not support the use of thyroid hormones in preterm infants to reduce neonatal mortality, improve neurodevelopmental outcome or to reduce the severity of respiratory distress syndrome.

Transient hypothyroidism may occur in preterm infants exposed in utero to maternal iodine-containing drugs or following injection of radiographic contrast agents. Low T3 levels are commonly seen in preterm infants and may persist for 1–2 months. They are due to the lower T3 postnatal surge and reduced conversion of T4 to T3 in peripheral tissues resulting from, e.g. birth asphyxia, hypoglycemia, hypocalcemia and relative malnutrition. FT4 and TSH levels are usually normal for gestational age and no treatment is necessary.

HYPOFUNCTION

Congenital

Thyroid dysgenesis

The commonest cause of congenital hypothyroidism is aplastic, hypoplastic or ectopic thyroid tissue – thyroid dysgenesis – occurring with consistent prevalence worldwide: 1 in 3500 to 4500 births. Females are twice as commonly affected but familial cases are rare – nearly all occur sporadically and idiopathically although there is increased incidence in Down syndrome babies and seasonal variation. In ~ 50% there is some functioning thyroid tissue resulting in a spectrum of severity of hypothyroidism. There is generally no relationship with maternal thyroid function, treatment with thyroxine or thyroid autoimmune status. A role for immunoglobulins which block TSH-stimulated thyroid cell growth in vitro in pathogenesis remains speculative.

Dyshormonogenesis (inborn errors of thyroid hormone biosynthesis)

Autosomal recessively inherited defects in thyroid hormone biosynthesis are the second commonest causes of congenital hypothyroidism, accounting for about 10% of those identified on screening (i.e. about 1 in 40 000 births). Presence of a goiter at birth is strongly suggestive but may not develop for months or years. There is a spectrum of hypofunction but it is generally less severe than in the dysgenetic group. Sex incidence is equal.

A defect may occur at any biosynthetic step (Fig. 13.45):

1. Decreased TSH responsiveness – very rare.
2. Decreased trapping of iodide: thyroid enlargement and reduced (or virtually absent) radioiodine (RAI) uptake by thyroid and tissues such as salivary glands and gastric mucosa.
3. Defective organification: peroxidase deficiency (defective oxidation of thyroidal iodide to reactive iodine). The association with high tone or complete nerve deafness (Pendred syndrome, 2 per 100 000 children of school age) is not due to peroxidase deficiency – the precise etiology of the thyroid biosynthetic defect (and deafness) is unknown. Together, these are the commonest dyshormonogenetic defects. In peroxidase deficiency (and most Pendred patients) there is a rapid fall in thyroid radioactivity with thiocyanate or perchlorate after radioiodine administration.
4. Defective iodotyrosine coupling or deiodination: non-deiodination of MIT and DIT leads to their leakage from the gland, urinary excretion and iodine loss.
5. Abnormal thyroglobulin synthesis, storage or release.

Hypothalamo–pituitary (tertiary/secondary) congenital hypothyroidism

Congenital hypothyroidism due to TRH or TSH deficiency may be familial or sporadic, isolated or associated with other hypothalamo–pituitary deficiencies and can be associated with anatomical defects (e.g. absent pituitary or sella turcica). Prevalence is about 1 in 100 000 births. Associated hypothyroidism will be missed by TSH screening. This is not critically important – there are often associated features (dysmorphism, micropenis, hypoglycemia) drawing attention to the differential diagnosis. Hypothyroidism is generally mild and treatment can be unnecessary for some months.

Clinical and laboratory features

During the early weeks of life babies are usually asymptomatic and early clinical signs are non-specific (Fig. 13.46): even in 'developed' countries only about 5% are diagnosed before the positive screening result and only ~ 50% can be diagnosed reliably before 3 months, by when subsequent neurodevelopmental problems are much more likely. No screening program is totally reliable – there must still be clinical suspicion in certain circumstances. Important features include: umbilical hernia, wide posterior fontanelle or goiter at birth, a placid, sleepy, 'good' baby, poor feeding, constipation, hypothermia, peripheral cyanosis, edema, prolonged physiological jaundice. More specific features such as the coarse facies, large tongue, hoarse cry, dry skin and low hair line are late signs.

Biochemically, both dysgenetic and dyshormonogenetic groups have low T4 and high TSH levels after neonatal changes have settled. About 1 in 6 will have T4 levels in the lower part of the normal range.

Screening

Although clinical detection of congenital hypothyroidism is unreliable, no screening program is 100% specific and sensitive: there may be laboratory error, communication breakdown between laboratory and clinician and there is a minority of affected babies in whom the screening result will be normal. Up to 10% of babies with congenital hypothyroidism will not have grossly elevated screening TSH values. Where TSH is used for screening, hypothyroidism due to hypothalamic or pituitary disease will be missed; where T4

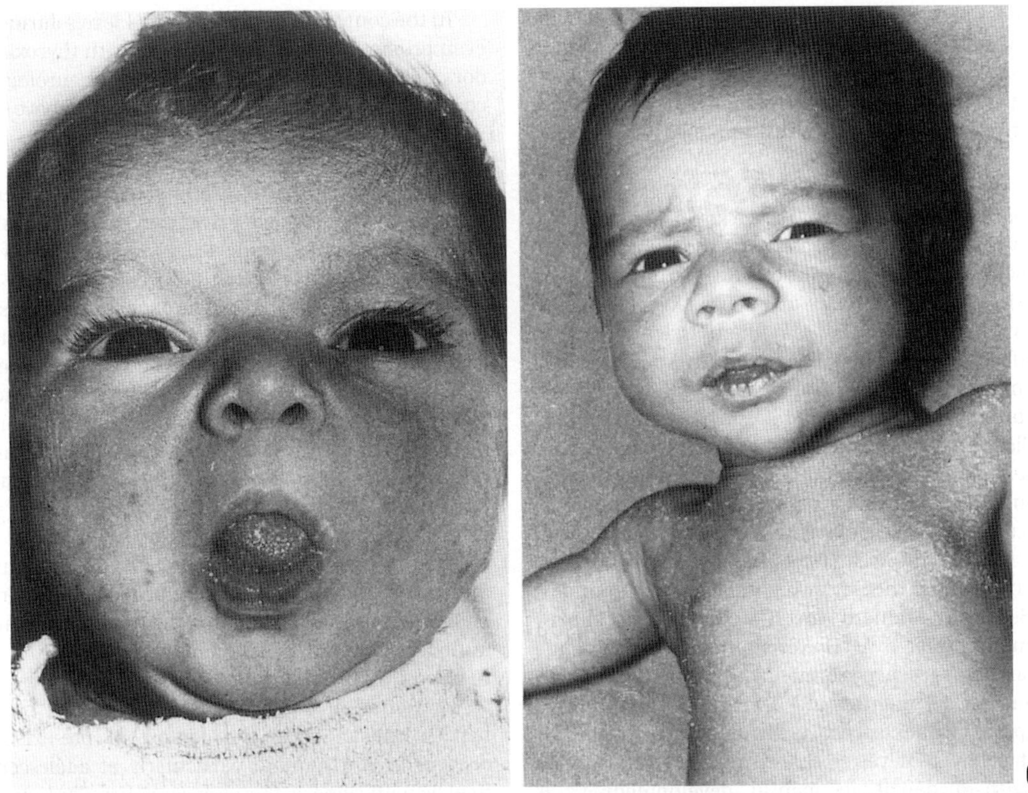

Fig. 13.46 Congenital hypothyroidism presenting (a) at 3 months in 1978 (prior to UK screening) and (b) at 10 days following a raised level of TSH screening (1983).

(followed by TSH for the lower range of T4 values) is used, a 10th centile or absolute T4 level of 130–140 nmol/L cut-off is used as < 20% of affected babies have low normal (90–140 nmol/L) T4 levels.

All abnormal or suspicious screening results must be confirmed before the infant is committed to long-term therapy but it is safer to start thyroxine whilst definitive results are awaited. If they are normal, full reassessment is necessary.

Scanning

Thyroid scans using ^{99m}Tc-pertechnetate or ^{123}I-labeled sodium iodide (the latter has the advantage of shorter half-life and better concentration in the thyroid) are no longer routinely recommended in the newborn for detection and anatomical localization of functioning thyroid tissue and to exclude the commonest dyshormonogenetic defect (organification). Results are unreliable, especially when tests are performed by inexperienced investigators, and misleading results can result from maternal blocking immunoglobulins or perinatal iodine contamination. Ultrasound can reveal whether thyroid tissue is present in the normal position. If no gland is detectable with normal T3 but low T4 levels and measurable levels of thyroglobulin, an ectopic rest of thyroid tissue is likely.

Following ^{123}I-labeled sodium iodide scanning, most dyshormonogenetic defects (other than of iodide trapping) will show high or normal isotope uptake and normal thyroid position and anatomy. In the commonest defect (peroxidase deficiency) there is discharge of 60–70% of radioactive iodide within 1 h following perchlorate. If organification is normal, less than 5–10% is discharged within 1 h. Frequencies of different possible biosynthetic defects are unknown although molecular genetic studies have revealed mutations in the thyroid peroxidase (TPO) and thyroglobulin genes in some familial cases.[305]

Treatment

Once the diagnosis is suspected, treatment is urgent and should be started immediately blood has been taken for definitive testing without waiting for those results. Sodium-l-thyroxine (l-T4) is the treatment of choice as it is reliably absorbed and its peripheral endogenous conversion to T3 allows automatic 'fine tuning' of function. In infancy, T4 levels should be in the upper normal range and T3 levels normal. TSH levels must not be used as a guide to treatment efficacy in infancy – in > 50% the feedback set point is abnormal and TSH levels remain high in the presence of adequate replacement and normal T4.

Starting dose of l-T4 is 10–15 mcg/kg orally once daily and is usually appropriate throughout infancy. A retrospective, non-randomized study[306] has shown higher full scale and verbal IQ results at 7–8 years on this dose compared with lower doses, but the higher-dose group were also treated earlier. Prospective randomized studies are needed. Subsequently, the required daily dose is ~ 100 mcg/m^2/24 h. Overtreatment will cause symptoms and signs of thyrotoxicosis but clinical assessment alone only detects significant under- or over-replacement. Marginal over-replacement can generally be compensated for by endogenous deiodination but under-replacement may result in significant long-term neurological impairment.

Growth, TFTs, bone age maturation and clinical progress (including psychomotor development) should be checked regularly during the first year. Assessment should be at 1 month and then every 3 months. It is essential that parents know the importance of giving the l-T4 regularly and do not forget or stop treatment because their baby seems normal.

By the third year of life, briefly interrupting medication will have no long-term effects on brain growth and development and is necessary to assess the need for permanent treatment. So as to minimize the time off treatment, T3 (with its shorter half-life) can be substituted for l-T4 therapy (100 mcg l-T4 is equivalent to 20 mcg T3) for 2 weeks, all treatment stopped for 7 days, thyroid function checked (and an isotope scan performed if indicated) and the previous l-T4 dose restarted immediately whilst results are awaited and assessed. Alternatively l-T4 can simply be discontinued for 2 weeks.

Outcome

'Not the magic wand of Prospero or the brave kiss of the daughter of Hippocrates ever effected such a change as that which we are now enabled to make in these unfortunate victims, doomed heretofore to live in hopeless imbecility, an unspeakable affliction to their parents and their relatives' – William Osler[307] on the transforming effects of the then recently introduced thyroid replacement therapy. However although gross physical manifestations of congenital hypothyroidism are abolished by treatment, significant neurodevelopmental and intellectual deficits remain unless treatment is started during the early weeks of life.[302]

With screening programs, sufficiently early diagnosis is almost always possible and neurodevelopmental prognosis good. At 2 years, children adequately treated before 4 weeks show no differences from controls on the Bayley mental development index, and at 3, 4 and 5 years, in Stanford Binet IQ assessment in contrast to those inadequately treated.[308] However, there may be subtle deficiencies in hearing/speech performance scales at 1 year and practical reasoning at 18 months and 3 years and, possibly, in motor and perceptual abilities, speech, behavior and personality.[302]

It seems that a low T4 level (< 30–40 nmol/L) at diagnosis is associated with a deficit in mental development.[309] A comprehensive UK survey[310] has demonstrated a discontinuous effect of severity of congenital hypothyroidism with a risk of a 10 point IQ deficit with initial thyroxine level of < 40 nmol/L. Lower social class (perhaps also associated with poorer compliance) may also adversely affect outcome.

Acquired

Hypothyroidism may develop, usually insidiously, at any age. Important causes are summarized in Table 13.13.

Endemic iodine deficiency

Worldwide, ~ 300 million people have endemic goiter. Simple iodine deficiency is generally responsible but genetic factors may predispose and environmental goitrogens (e.g. *Brassica* vegetables) potentiate the effects. Iodine deficiency leads to deficient thyroid hormone production, TSH hypersecretion and increased iodide trapping with goiter and raised T3:T4 ratio. Such compensatory mechanisms can result in euthyroidism with goiter or varying degrees of goitrous hypothyroidism. In endemic areas < 8% of the population may be affected.

The problem is still common in some areas of Europe, Scandinavia and the Middle East including Switzerland, Finland, Austria, Germany, Italy, Spain, Greece, Lebanon and Iraq. In Switzerland and Finland iodination of salt can effectively reduce the prevalence of endemic cretinism to very low levels.[303]

Table 13.13 Important causes of acquired hypothyroidism in childhood

Autoimmune thyroiditis
Thyroid dysgenesis
Endemic iodine deficiency
Exposure to goitrogens
Hypothalamopituitary disease (TRH/TSH deficiency)

In the context of low maternal T4 levels during early pregnancy, even prompt treatment of the baby with thyroxine following birth does not prevent the child from having neurological problems and cognitive and intellectual impairment (see above).

Autoimmune (Hashimoto) thyroiditis

This commonest cause of acquired hypothyroidism in non-endemic areas of iodine deficiency was described by Hashimoto. Girls are much more commonly affected; a family history of thyroid disorders is found in about one-third.

The gland, infiltrated by lymphocytes and plasma cells (delayed hypersensitivity) with fibrosis and degeneration, is generally irregularly enlarged and firm. There is prominence of normal architecture but usually no nodules. Acinar regeneration can occur – growth immunoglobulins and TSH may be important for this. One or more of several possible types of circulating antithyroid antibodies are found in about 95% at presentation but such antibodies also occur in up to 20% of the 'normal' population (some of whom may eventually develop thyroiditis). The commonest antibodies are against thyroglobulin and microsomes but antiperoxidase (now commonly available), TSH-receptor blocking or stimulating, colloid and thyroid growth inhibiting or stimulating antibodies may occur. Antinuclear factor (ANF) is particularly likely to be positive in children.

Presentation may be with euthyroid goiter, goiter with hypothyroidism or in the context of pre-existing autoimmune disease. In < 10%, and particularly at adolescence, presentation may be with signs of thyrotoxicosis. Usually, however, onset is with insidious hypothyroidism – classical myxedema may not occur for many months (Fig. 13.47). School performance frequently deteriorates but can be attributed to other problems. Height velocity slows but this may not be recognized if children are not measured regularly – slow growth must be prolonged before a single measurement or simple observation detects conspicuous short stature.

In a still euthyroid child, diagnosis can be made on the basis of goiter, increased antiperoxidase, antithyroglobulin or antimicrosomal antibody titers, abnormal thyroid scan with positive perchlorate discharge test and biochemical signs of compensated hypothyroidism.

Associated multiple endocrine deficiency disease includes diabetes mellitus with or without adrenal insufficiency (Schmidt syndrome), hypoparathyroidism, moniliasis, pernicious anemia and thrombocytopenia. Fewer than 30% of children with type 1 diabetes mellitus will have detectable thyroid antibodies and 10% will have raised TSH levels. There is an association between autoimmune thyroid disease and a variety of cytogenetic disorders including Down, Turner, Klinefelter and Noonan syndromes. All children with diabetes mellitus or cytogenetic disorders should be screened regularly for thyroid disease.

There is usually progressive thyroid atrophy and treatment, once started, is generally life-long. If there is initial hyperfunction, euthyroidism and eventual hypothyroidism will probably develop. Spontaneous remission is said to occur in < 30% of adolescents. Nodules in Hashimoto thyroiditis are due to lymphoid or thyroid hyperplasia and only rarely indicate malignancy.

Diffuse goiter in a euthyroid adolescent occurs commonly in non-endemic areas. Some have Hashimoto thyroiditis but in others aspiration biopsy shows a colloid goiter with no evidence of the characteristic lymphocytic infiltration and there may be autosomal dominant transmission. Although, in the medium term, the goiter usually regresses untreated, the common finding of thyroid-stimulating immunoglobulins (TSI), and the fact that a significant

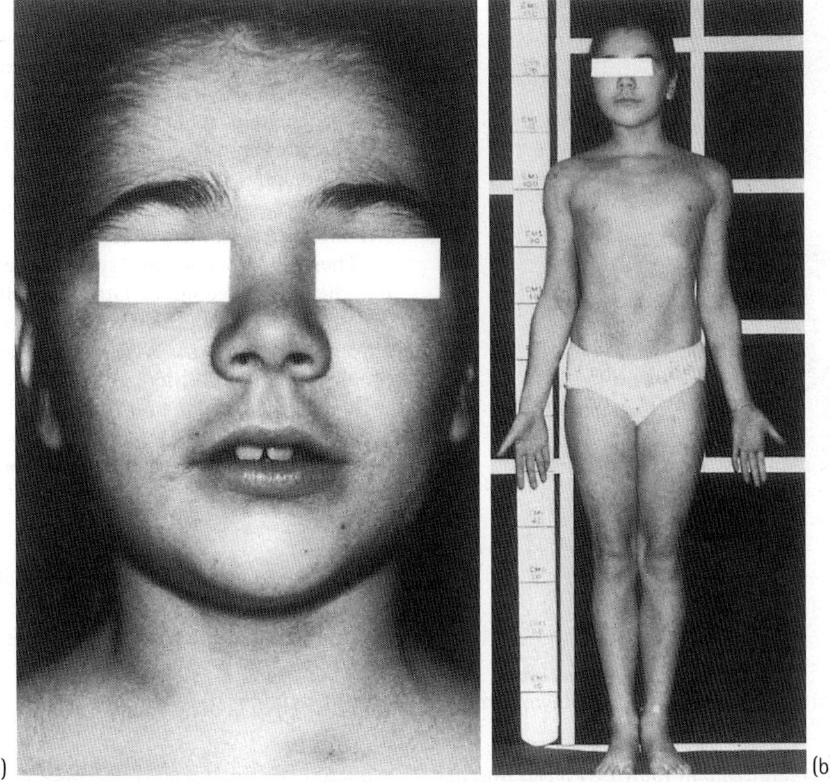

Fig. 13.47 The result of insidious development of hypothyroidism over several years.

number of adults presenting with nodular goiters have a history of diffuse adolescent goiter, suggest that autoimmune mechanisms are important for pathogenesis.

Thyroid dysgenesis

Most inborn errors of biosynthesis present in the newborn or by infancy. However, if defects are mild and compensated, goiter develops slowly and hypothyroidism may not develop until childhood. There is an increased incidence of thyroid dysgenesis in Down syndrome.

Ectopic and inadequately functional thyroid may present as an enlarging mass at the base of the tongue or along the course of the thyroglossal duct ('cryptothyroidism'). Removal of a 'thyroglossal cyst' may result in severe hypothyroidism if that is the only functional thyroid tissue present.

Thyroid destruction due to infiltration with cystine crystals may cause eventual hypothyroidism in children with cystinosis.

Exposure to goitrogens

Foods interfering with thyroid hormone biosynthesis include cabbage, cassava and soybeans. Ingestion of goitrogen in the context of a genetically predisposed population or iodine deficiency is more likely to result in frank hypothyroidism. Drugs acting similarly include iodide (in proprietary expectorants), perchlorate and thiocyanate, lithium, amiodarone, phenylbutazone, aminoglutethemide, aminosalicylic acid and the specifically antithyroid drugs, carbimazole and propylthiouracil.

Hypothalamo–pituitary dependent hypothyroidism

Slowing of linear growth due to TSH or associated GH deficiency is the usual presentation with a history of head injury, cranial irradiation for leukemia or medulloblastoma, meningitis or granulomatous disease. Craniopharyngioma must be excluded. There may be associated neurological signs, and symptoms or signs relating to underlying disease, or hypothalamo–pituitary dysfunction. Latent hypothalamo–pituitary hypothyroidism may develop in 'isolated' GH deficiency treated with GH and may prevent growth acceleration.

Thyroid hormone unresponsiveness

Families with goiter and variable thyroid hormone unresponsiveness have been described with possible autosomal dominant or recessive inheritance. The defect may be at receptor or postreceptor level.

Presentation and diagnosis

Slowing of height velocity is the earliest sign. Retrospectively, growth data (or holiday photographs) will help pinpoint age at onset. Skinfold measurements are usually increased and bone age delayed but both are common in many childhood endocrinopathies. Very delayed skeletal maturation (> 3 years over chronological age) is a particular feature. Muscle weakness is common on testing but is seldom a presenting complaint. Muscle atrophy, hypertrophy and dysfunction have been described. Classical signs of myxedema develop gradually with infiltration of many tissues (including skin) by mucopolysaccharides, hyaluronic acid and chondroitin sulfate (Fig. 13.47). Skin becomes yellow from high carotene levels and there may be tiredness (with poor school performance), cold intolerance and characteristically slow relaxation of tendon reflexes. Hypertrichosis with low hair line may occur as may hair loss with alopecia (Fig. 13.48).

Classically pubertal delay occurs, but a significant minority develop precocious puberty and this may occur whilst the child is still clinically euthyroid. A failing thyroid gland causes

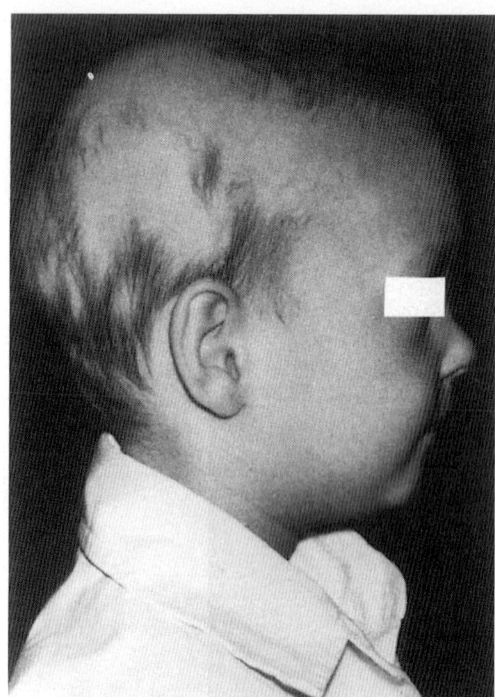

Fig. 13.48 Alopecia associated with autoimmune hypothyroidism.

hypothalamic release of TRH; consequent high TSH levels initially maintain euthyroidism but TRH also stimulates PRL and GT (LH and FSH) release causing ovarian estradiol secretion and breast development in girls and testicular (and sometimes penile) enlargement in boys. PRL may cause inhibition of gonadal stimulation by LH but not FSH resulting in sustained gonadal stimulation. A direct effect of TSH on the HCG receptor has also been described.[311] Clinically there is loss of consonance with breast development with or without galactorrhea in girls. Testicular (with or without penile) enlargement occurs in boys due to the FSH-dependent seminiferous tubule development. LH-dependent Leydig cell development does not occur and there is little (androgen-dependent) pubic or axillary hair development. There is no increase in height velocity, short stature and (pathognomonic) BA delay. The sella turcica may be enlarged. Why a minority of children with acquired hypothyroidism develop sexual precocity rather than pubertal delay is unexplained. On thyroid replacement therapy pubertal development arrests and there may be some regression until puberty recommences at a time appropriate to bone age maturity.

Clinical diagnosis of acquired hypothyroidism must be confirmed biochemically before treatment is started. Low total or free T4 or T3 levels confirm hypothyroidism, raised TSH levels that the defect is at thyroid level. A goiter necessitates thyroid and other autoantibody measurement. If there is no goiter, or no evidence of autoimmune disease, thyroid scanning to exclude dysgenesis is valuable.

Inappropriately low (i.e. low or normal) TSH levels for low T3 or T4 levels suggest hypothalamic or pituitary disease. A TRH test may be helpful. With acquired TSH deficiency, pituitary function and neuroradiological tests are necessary to identify other pituitary hormone deficiencies and exclude a pituitary tumor.

Treatment

The drug of choice is sodium-1-thyroxine (l-T4) – usually ~ 100 mcg/m^2/24 h once daily but precisely adjusted individually. Catch-up growth usually follows onset of treatment and height prognosis is favourable in comparison with most growth disorders. However, it is important to interpret height velocity on treatment in the context of accurate assessment of rate of bone age maturation. Inappropriately rapid skeletal maturation for height velocity indicates overtreatment and will result irretrievably in stunting due to early epiphyseal fusion. IRMA TSH levels are sensitive markers of over-replacement, under-replacement or non-compliance (except in hypothalamo–pituitary disease).

There is still controversy about whether to treat euthyroid patients with compensated autoimmune hypothyroidism. Treatment does not alter the natural progression of the disease and chronic oversecretion of TRH/TSH is not generally associated with problems (although there are theoretical risks in children treated with radiotherapy for brain tumors), but enlarged pituitary fossa and secondary pituitary failure have been described. Often free T4 levels are low and treatment should certainly start if so or growth velocity is slow.

Outcome

Mental retardation does not occur in late onset hypothyroidism. School performance and growth improve on appropriate replacement therapy. Final height is normal for the family.

HYPERFUNCTION

Neonatal

Neonatal thyrotoxicosis is rare and usually due to transplacental passage of TSI from a mother with active or inactive Graves' disease or Hashimoto thyroiditis. High maternal antibody titers are strong predictors of neonatal disease in a clinically euthyroid mother whose disease has been inactive for many years. Only ~ 1.5% of mothers with thyrotoxicosis due to Graves' disease will have affected babies. Thyrotoxicosis is nevertheless rare in pregnancy – autoimmune disease tends to remit during pregnancy and anovulatory cycles are common in thyrotoxic women.

Goiter may be present at birth and an irritable infant rapidly develops tachycardia, dysrhythmias, flushing, hypertension and weight loss (until cardiac failure supervenes) despite ravenous hunger. There may be associated jaundice, hepatosplenomegaly and a bleeding tendency due to thrombocytopenia and low prothrombin levels. In some, symptoms and signs are delayed for 7–10 days either because of transplacental passage of maternal antithyroid drugs or postnatal T4 to T3 conversion.

Total and free T4 and T3 levels are high and TSH suppressed within a few days – cord blood levels may be normal. The half-life of TSI is 2–3 weeks and clinical resolution of the disorder mirrors their degradation – the condition is generally self-limiting over 4–12 weeks. In severely affected babies, mortality may be as high as 25% due to cardiac arrhythmias or high output failure. Propranolol (1–2 mg/kg/24 h) with carbimazole (0.5–1 mg/kg/24 h) and Lugol's iodine (5% iodine, 10% potassium iodide, 8 mg tds) to inhibit thyroid hormone synthesis and secretion may be life-saving. Satisfactory response is usually seen within 24–36 h. As thyrotoxicosis comes under control, iodine and propranolol can be gradually withdrawn and carbimazole gradually discontinued from about 6 weeks. Rarely, persisting hyperthyroidism suggests early onset Graves' disease.

Graves' disease

In children, thyrotoxicosis is nearly always due to Graves' disease, is much rarer than hypothyroidism and rarer than in adults – only about 5% of patients with Graves' disease present in childhood or adolescence, usually in the second decade. It is three- to five-fold commoner in girls. As in Hashimoto thyroiditis, there is evidence of an autoimmune disorder on a background of genetic (HLA A1, B8, DR3) predisposition and positive family history of thyroid disease in about 60%.

The thyrotoxicosis is due to thyroid follicular cell TSH receptor IgG antibodies – thyroid stimulating immunoglobulins (TSI) – which bind to the extracellular receptor domain stimulating thyroid hormone release analogously to TSH via the adenyl cyclase cAMP system. They do not cause the eye signs although these too are immunologically mediated. The TSH receptor is a 744 amino acid, single chain, polypeptide glycoprotein member of the guanine-nucleotide binding (G) protein-coupled receptor family and represents the primary target antigen for autoantibodies mediating the hyperthyroidism and goiter of Graves' disease. Glycosylation is necessary for receptor expression and hormone-receptor interactions.

Clinical features

The onset may be insidious and is usually well established before presentation to a physician. As in hypothyroidism, poor school performance may be marked, but usually from poor concentration, tiredness and behavior disturbances with temper tantrums and emotional lability. There is marked weight loss despite rapid growth and enormous appetite. The gland is usually diffusely enlarged and often with a bruit. Many systemic (tachycardia, tremor and sweating) and eye (staring due to lid retraction, wide palpebral aperture and lid lag) signs reflect sympathetic overactivity. Periorbital puffiness, exophthalmos, chemosis and squint due to infiltration of the orbit, lacrimal glands and ocular muscles occur less commonly and severely than in adults, but exophthalmos in particular may persist once euthyroidism is established. Pretibial myxedema characteristic of adults is rare in children.

Diagnosis

In children, a clinical diagnosis can usually be made confidently, but there must be biochemical confirmation and hyperthyroidism secondary to TSH hypersecretion must be excluded. Usually free and total T4 levels are high (occasionally they are normal but T3 levels are raised) and TSH is suppressed even using a sensitive (IRMA) assay. TSI are positive. Skeletal maturity is generally advanced disproportionately for the rapid growth.

Treatment

Treatment aims to reduce excessive thyroid hormone secretion and blunt the somatic consequences (largely mediated via beta-adrenergic pathways). The former may be achieved with antithyroid drugs (e.g. carbimazole or propylthiouracil), surgery (subtotal thyroidectomy) or radioactive iodine (^{131}I). In childhood, in most centers, antithyroid drugs are the initial treatment of choice. These inhibit di-iodotyrosine and iodothyronine formation and, to some extent, tyrosine iodination. Thyroid function normalizes by 3–4 weeks. The initial dose of carbimazole in childhood is 0.5 mg/kg/24 h and of propylthiouracil 5 mg/kg/24 h, both in three divided doses.

Skin rashes occur in ~ 2–3% on either drug, are usually transient and a change of therapy is not usually necessary, particularly if antihistamine is used symptomatically. More seriously, agranulocytosis may occur idiosyncratically, unpredicted from serial blood counts. Full recovery usually occurs on stopping treatment and the alternative generally substituted as cross-reactivity is rare. Progressive neutropenia can also occur and symptoms such as sore throat must be taken seriously and blood count checked regularly.

Once clinical and biochemical euthyroidism is achieved, it is probably beneficial (in terms of reducing both the goiter and necessity for frequent monitoring of thyroid function for developing hypothyroidism) to add l-thyroxine to an appropriate (usually half to one-third of initial dose) antithyroid medication. Combination therapy has also been reported to decrease production of TSI and the frequency of thyrotoxicosis recurrence in adults.[312]

Although antithyroid drugs do not alter the natural disease process, they do, in most children, allow maintenance of euthyroidism until spontaneous remission occurs (usually after about 2 years). Signs that this is not the case include persisting goiter and continuing presence of TSI. In any case there is a high relapse rate (50–70% within 2 years).

Beta-blockers (e.g. propranolol) are valuable during the first 2–3 weeks of treatment in providing symptomatic relief of tachycardia, nervousness and tremor and can then be discontinued as the specific antithyroid drug becomes clinically effective.

Subtotal thyroidectomy is the treatment of choice in young adults in whom hyperthyroidism has returned after > 2 years of medical treatment or if compliance with treatment is poor – and, because of high relapse rates on medical treatment, is the primary treatment of choice in some centers with a surgeon experienced in thyroid surgery. Patients must be made euthyroid before surgery in which case morbidity and mortality are comparable to other major procedures. Specific complications include laryngeal nerve palsy (transient or permanent), transient hypocalcemia (~ 10%) and permanent hypoparathyroidism (~ 1%). One year postsurgery, 80% are euthyroid, 15% have permanent hypothyroidism (easily treated with thyroxine) and 5% are still thyrotoxic. Either thyrotoxicosis or hypothyroidism may develop many years after surgery in a previously euthyroid patient.

Radioactive iodine (^{131}I iodide) is the treatment of choice if judged by ease of administration, efficacy, short-term safety and cost. UK use has traditionally been restricted to adults > 40 years because of fears (based on few data) that risks of congenital malformations in subsequent pregnancies are increased or if used in younger patients, leukemia or thyroid cancer could result – radiation is an important cause of thyroid cancer in children as the short-lived radioactive fallout caused by the 1986 Chernobyl nuclear power plant accident demonstrated.[313]

A lower age cut-off of 17 years is still recommended in the USA.[314] Generally, use in UK pediatric practice has been restricted to poorly compliant adolescents who cannot be rendered euthyroid for surgery, but with increasing long term experience practice may change. There is a high incidence of hypothyroidism (25% in the first year, a subsequent annual rate of 24% and an incidence of 80% by 15 years post-treatment).

Hashimoto thyroiditis

About 5–10% of children, particularly adolescents, present with hyperthyroidism. Occasionally Graves' disease and Hashimoto thyroiditis coexist: there are clinical and laboratory features of the latter with TSI antibodies present. Treatment is as for Graves' disease.

TSH hypersecretion

This is a rare cause of thyrotoxicosis, described either with a pituitary TSH-secreting tumor or a defect in TSH feedback inhibition by T3 causing goitrous hyperthyroidism associated with high TSH levels – an indication for neuroradiological evaluation.

Autonomous functioning nodules

These are uncommon in children and adolescents, usually occurring after ~ 35 years. Occasionally, single nodules of follicular adenoma (diameter > 3 mm) are found in association with thyrotoxicosis. Diagnosis is by isotope scanning. Carcinoma occurs in less than 1% of functional nodules (see below).

NEOPLASIA (Table 13.14)

A history of head and neck irradiation was common in children presenting with thyroid cancer and is so following Chernobyl[313] (see above). Palpable thyroid nodules must be taken seriously – the prevalence of malignancy in childhood thyroid nodules is probably less than 15–20% but still higher than in adults.

Thyroid neoplasia may arise from follicular epithelium (follicular adenoma and carcinoma, papillary carcinoma, anaplastic carcinoma) or other tissue (medullary carcinoma, lymphoma, teratoma, metastatic tumor). More than 50% of solitary thyroid nodules in childhood are cystic lesions or benign adenomas. Hyperfunctioning adenomas are rare and 90% of malignant nodules consist of well-differentiated follicular carcinomas. In this group, prognosis is better than for rarer types.

Features suggestive of malignancy include history of head and neck irradiation, a hard or rapidly enlarging nodule, lymphadenopathy, hoarseness, dysphagia or metastases. Nodules in Hashimoto thyroiditis rarely represent carcinomatous change. In other situations, radioisotope and ultrasound scanning are valuable for differential diagnosis. Ultrasound identifies cystic lesions (usually benign); if iodide is concentrated by the nodule(s), carcinoma is rare. Small needle aspiration biopsy[315] may aid further diagnosis of cystic lesions and distinguish benign from malignant lesions.

Treatment (where possible following needle biopsy histology) is surgical removal of the affected thyroid lobe and subsequent total thyroidectomy if frozen sections reveal malignancy. Radioiodine treatment postoperatively is reserved for metastatic disease or distant lymph node involvement. Prognosis is excellent even with metastatic well-differentiated follicular carcinoma. TSH must be fully suppressed chronically by adequate thyroxine therapy so as not to stimulate tumor growth or regrowth. Life expectancy is normal with follicular carcinoma but not with rarer carcinomas despite radical surgery, radiotherapy and chemotherapy.

An important rare thyroid carcinoma [medullary thyroid carcinoma (MTC), accounting for < 10% of thyroid carcinomas] arises from parafollicular (C) cells, nearly always secretes calcitonin and sometimes other hormones (e.g. ACTH, serotonin, prostaglandins). Although often sporadic, they are associated with syndromes involving tumors of neuroectodermal origin (multiple endocrine neoplasia – MEN) inherited autosomal dominantly.

Table 13.14 Types of thyroid neoplasia

Follicular (epithelial) tumors
Follicular adenoma
Follicular carcinoma
Papillary carcinoma
Anaplastic carcinoma
Non-follicular tumors
Medullary carcinoma
Lymphoma
Teratoma
Miscellaneous

MEN type 2 (MEN 2) comprises three syndromes, with medullary thyroid carcinoma alone (familial MTC), MTC, pheochromocytoma and hyperparathyroidism (MEN 2A) or MTC, pheochromocytoma, ganglioneuromatosis and a Marfanoid habitus (MEN 2B). (MEN 1 comprises hyperparathyroidism, pancreatic islet cell tumors and pituitary adenomas.)

These familial endocrine neoplasia syndromes (MEN 1, MEN 2 and von Hippel–Lindau) can now be diagnosed genetically in childhood. The MEN1 gene is on chromosome 11, the MEN2 gene on chromosome 10, and children with a mutation and all offspring of affected subjects where the mutation is unknown should be screened on a regular basis.[316]

In a family with MEN 2 cases, molecular techniques, detecting the predisposing gene abnormality on chromosome 10, indicate whether a child (at 50% risk) has inherited the condition. The aggressive nature of the thyroid lesion, which may develop in childhood or adult life (usually before pheochromocytoma), has led to a search for markers of its presence whilst still microscopic. Calcitonin levels are usually normal at this stage but may rise significantly following pentagastrin infusion. Currently, annual stimulation tests provide the best monitor in affected children – rising levels with time as well as raised absolute values may be suspicious. Prophylactic thyroidectomy may be justified – therapy (as well as diagnostic) consensus guidelines for MEN 2 (and MEN 1) have recently been published.[316]

PARATHYROID GLANDS AND CALCIUM METABOLISM

There are two pairs of parathyroid glands, superior and inferior, although two, five or six glands may be present in normal individuals. Paradoxically, the inferior pair originates (at ~ 5 weeks) from 3rd pharyngeal pouch (endodermal) tissue, the superior pair from the 4th pouch. The inferior pair are pulled medially and caudally by the migrating thymus to the thyroid; the superior attach higher on its dorsal surface. There are two cell types: chief cells secrete parathyroid hormone (PTH) and oxyphil cells (function unknown).

Although the major function is contributing to calcium and phosphate homeostasis by PTH production, its role in health and disease must be considered in conjunction with other hormones and metabolic factors.

PHYSIOLOGY OF CALCIUM HOMEOSTASIS

Calcium must be accumulated by a growing child – 99% of total body calcium is present in the skeleton. Nevertheless, as well as for bone mineralization, calcium is important for normal endocrine and neuromuscular function at plasma membrane level, enzymatic reactions and blood coagulation, so that the 1% in extra- and intracellular fluids must be closely regulated within narrow concentration limits. Thus homeostatic control mechanisms are inevitably complex. Serum calcium concentration is maintained within normal limits by the interaction of vitamin D, PTH and calcitonin acting at three target tissues: bone, kidneys and gastro-intestinal tract. Unlike calcium, normal serum inorganic phosphate levels are age-related during childhood (declining from high levels in infancy).

Calcium is present in serum in three fractions in dynamic equilibrium: 50% ionized (metabolically active), 40% protein bound (inactive), the remainder complexed to phosphate, citrate, etc. The proportion of ionized calcium is controlled by vitamin D, PTH and calcitonin but is affected by acid–base changes (acidosis increases and alkalosis decreases ionized calcium levels as hydrogen ions compete with calcium for albumin binding sites). Vitamin D itself is biologically inactive and must be hydroxylated to active metabolite.

Total serum calcium is measured routinely – ionized levels may be measured directly using ion-selective electrodes. Indirect estimation of biologically active calcium using a formula may be misleading if serum protein concentrations are low. In hypoproteinemic states total calcium may be low but ionized calcium normal. Diet and diurnal variation will influence many indices of mineral and bone metabolism.

Although hypo- or hypercalcemia may be associated with disorders of vitamin D metabolism or parathyroid disease, non-endocrine disorders (e.g. chronic renal failure) may be etiologically important. Specific disorders of mineral and bone metabolism occur in infants, occasionally secondarily to maternal hyperparathyroidism.

Peak bone mass accumulation and mineralization occurs during puberty, continues into early adult life and is influenced by genetic (racial) factors, body mass, adequate calcium intake during growth and physical activity. Vitamin D receptor genotypes may be diagnostically useful in selecting adults with osteoporosis at increased fracture risk. Reduced peak bone mass occurs in GH deficiency, GT deficiency, male hypogonadism, Turner syndrome and delayed puberty. Bone mass is also reduced by malnutrition, chronic illness and anorexia nervosa. Appropriate management of these conditions will reduce risks of clinically significant osteoporosis from middle-age.

CALCIUM REGULATION IN THE FETUS AND NEONATE

Normal fetal bone mineralization requires considerable net calcium and phosphorus transfer from mother to fetus. There is active placental transport of calcium and some 80% of the total accumulates in the third trimester. Fetal blood total and ionized calcium levels exceed those in the mother by about 0.5 and 0.25 mmol/L respectively and absolute values have doubled from mid-gestation to a mean of 2.75 mmol/L at term.

PTH and calcitonin do not cross the placenta but it is not clear whether active vitamin D metabolites do. Both fetal kidney and placenta can synthesize the active metabolite 1,25-dihydroxy vitamin D. Although their importance compared with that of the maternal kidney is uncertain, it seems likely that fetal 1,25-dihydroxy D is the major stimulus to placental calcium transfer perhaps analogously to its effect on intestinal calcium absorption.

To accommodate fetal transfer, there is increased maternal intestinal calcium absorption – calcium loss to the fetus stimulates maternal PTH secretion and maternal 1,25-dihydroxy vitamin D levels are raised. In the fetus, conversely, PTH levels are suppressed and calcitonin levels high encouraging bone mineralization.

At birth, cessation of transplacental calcium and these hormonal changes cause significant lowering of serum calcium. Lowest levels are reached, in the term neonate, between 24 and 48 h after birth; by 5 days rising PTH and falling calcitonin levels have established 'normal' serum calcium levels. Intestinal absorption of calcium and phosphate (very low in the fetus) is, suddenly, the sole mechanism and source – 1,25-dihydroxy vitamin D_3 secretion increases sharply.

As with other physiological changes from fetal to extrauterine life (e.g. circulatory, respiratory, bilirubin metabolism), these complex adaptations lead potentially to a variety of neonatal disorders especially in the preterm.

Vitamin D

Vitamin D (calciferol) is a collective term for two steroid-related, cholesterol-derived, naturally occurring compounds: vitamin D_2 (ergocalciferol) – derived from the plant sterol ergosterol, and vitamin D_3 (cholecalciferol) – produced in skin by the effect of ultraviolet irradiation on a precursor (7-dehydrocholesterol) in the epidermal Malpighian layer (Fig. 13.49). In man D_2 and D_3 are equally active biologically. Serum D_3 levels are higher in summer than winter (reflecting differences in sunlight exposure). Pigmented skin synthesizes it less efficiently.

Plant and animal foods (e.g. fish, eggs, butter and margarine) are important sources of D_2 and D_3 respectively. Absorption is via upper small intestine and lymphatic system in chylomicrons. Normal bile salt secretion is necessary – absorption is impaired by steatorrhea. In blood, ~ 98% is bound to a high MW liver-derived protein which also transports and binds active vitamin D metabolites and acts as a buffer against vitamin D toxicity.

The first step in vitamin D activation (Fig. 13.49) is 25-hydroxylation in liver microsomes but bowel and kidney may contribute. 25-hydroxy D is the major circulating metabolite but is metabolically inactive and converted in mitochondria of the proximal renal tubule to two major metabolites, the proportions depending on physiological requirements: active 1,25-dihydroxy D and 24,25-dihydroxy D (some, but much less, biological activity). Other metabolites of uncertain pathophysiological significance and with varying biological activities can be formed. Placenta and bone can also hydroxylate at C l.

1,25-dihydroxy D has major effects on intestinal villus and crypt cells, osteoblasts and osteoclasts and distal renal tubular cells. The net effect is to increase serum calcium and phosphate by stimulating intestinal absorption and mobilization from bone, and reducing renal excretion. Calcium mobilization from bone is also PTH dependent.

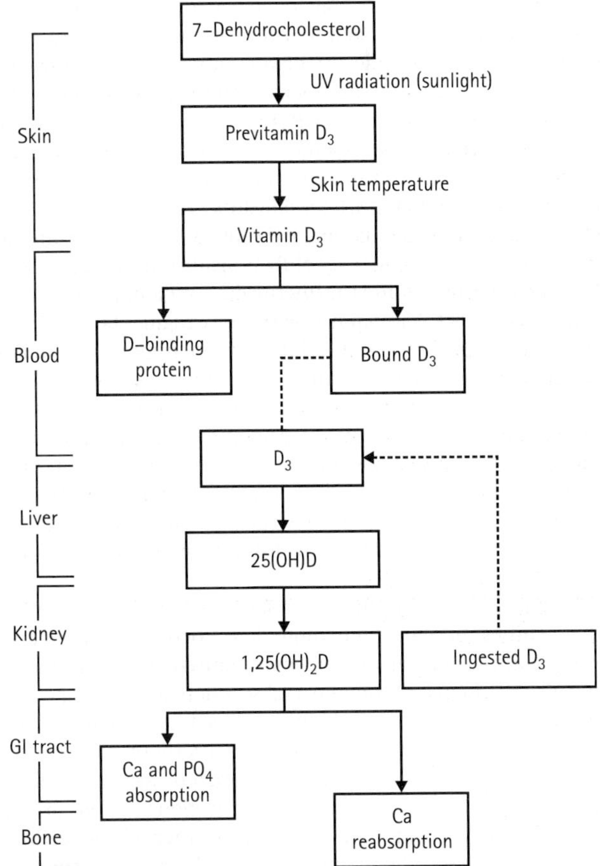

Fig. 13.49 Vitamin D metabolism and its regulation.

Average total serum concentrations of 1,25-dihydroxy D are 1000-fold lower than of 25-hydroxy D but there is only a 10-fold difference in relative concentrations of the free (metabolically active in the case of 1,25-dihydroxy D) components.

Parathyroid hormone (PTH)

PTH is an 84 amino acid peptide MW 9500. 34 amino acids at the amino- (N-) terminal are essential for receptor binding and activation and thus biological activity. The PTH gene is close to the insulin gene on the short arm of chromosome 11. PTH is synthesized by parathyroid chief cells and cleaved from higher molecular weight biologically inactive precursors which are not released into the circulation. Both intact PTH and carboxy- (C-) terminal fragments are released into the circulation and the proportion of the latter is increased in primary hyperparathyroidism. Intact PTH is metabolized by liver (predominantly) and kidney and fragments returned to the circulation. Intact PTH and N-terminal fragments are cleared rapidly (< 10 min); C-terminal fragments (mainly metabolized by kidney) are cleared more slowly (2 h). Thus circulating PTH is a heterogeneous mixture of intact hormone together with N-, C-terminal and intermediate fragments.

Serum calcium concentration is the major regulator of PTH synthesis and release. There is a greater response to evolving hypocalcemia than to falling levels within the normal range. Hypercalcemia suppresses PTH secretion. Catecholamines, vitamin D metabolites and cortisol increase PTH secretion but their physiological function is doubtful.

The major role of PTH is prevention of hypocalcemia by three main mechanisms: calcium resorption from bone, renal calcium reabsorption and, indirectly, increasing intestinal calcium absorption by stimulating renal 1,25-dihydroxy D synthesis.

In bone, it both regulates calcium movement between bone fluid surrounding surface and lacunar osteocytes and extracellular fluid, and influences remodelling. Osteoblasts (not osteoclasts) have PTH receptors and it is presumably release of an osteoblast factor which promotes osteoclast activation. PTH has several effects on renal tubules, acting distally to promote calcium and inhibit phosphate and bicarbonate reabsorption and proximally to stimulate hydroxylation at C1 to form 1,25-dihydroxy D.

Heterogeneity of circulating PTH forms makes measurement difficult. There is cross reactivity of RIAs against the intact molecule, the N- and C-terminals and the intermediate region. Because serum half-lives of intact PTH and N-terminal fragments are shorter than those of the C-terminal or intermediate fragments, the latter account for ~ 80% of immunoreactive material measured and better reflect PTH secretion rates. Except in chronic renal failure (where C-terminal and intermediate fragments accumulate because of impaired glomerular filtration), assays specific for C-terminal or intermediate fragment PTH provide better discrimination between normal and raised PTH levels. Some PTH RIAs (and bioassays) are too insensitive to distinguish between normality and hyposecretion.

There is diurnal circadian variation in serum PTH secretion – higher values in early morning. For correct interpretation, simultaneous serum calcium and phosphate concentrations should be measured. Renal phosphate reabsorption and urinary cyclic adenosine monophosphate (cAMP) may need assessment. The ratio of tubular maximal rate of phosphate reabsorption to glomerular filtration rate is calculated from simultaneous fasting serum and urinary phosphate and creatinine concentrations – ratios are high in hypoparathyroidism, low in hyperparathyroidism. cAMP is important in PTH release into the circulation in response to hypocalcemia; measurement is useful for indirectly assessing circulating active PTH, evaluating the renal response to exogenous PTH and distinguishing pseudohypo- from hypoparathyroidism.

Calcitonin

Calcitonin is synthesized in and secreted by thyroid parafollicular (C) cells of neuroectodermal origin. It is discussed here because of its importance in calcium metabolism.

As for insulin and PTH, the gene encoding calcitonin is on the short arm of chromosome 11. Calcitonin is a 32 amino acid peptide, MW 3500, derived from a polypeptide precursor by loss of N- and C-terminal fragments. Species differences derive from mid-molecule amino acid sequences. The entire sequence is required for biological activity. Calcitonin-like bioactive material has been identified in thymus, lung, adrenal medulla, brain and parathyroid glands but none is a major source of circulating calcitonin.

As with PTH, serum calcium concentration is the major regulator of calcitonin secretion but with opposite effect: hypercalcemia stimulates and hypocalcemia suppresses calcitonin secretion. Gastrointestinal hormones such as gastrin, glucagon and cholecystokinin stimulate calcitonin secretion as do estrogens, beta-adrenergic agonists and 1,25-dihydroxy D, but none seems physiologically important. Pentagastrin (a synthetic gastrin derivative) is used to stimulate calcitonin secretion in the diagnosis of medullary thyroid carcinoma.

More sensitive assays are helping to define calcitonin changes with age and deficiency states. In children, monomeric calcitonin (the major active circulating form) is present in very low concentrations – levels are higher in infancy.

Like PTH, calcitonin influences serum calcium levels by action on bone, kidneys and bowel. It inhibits bone resorption by reducing osteoclast cytoplasmic motility. In kidney it binds to specific receptors to increase calcium, phosphate, magnesium, sodium and potassium excretion and stimulates 1-hydroxylation in the proximal tubule to produce 1,25-dihydroxy D. This promotes intestinal calcium reabsorption indirectly but it may also have a direct, but inhibitory, effect.

The importance of calcitonin for physiological calcium metabolism regulation remains uncertain. Neither thyroidectomy nor calcitonin hypersecretion from medullary thyroid carcinoma affects serum calcium levels. Its major inhibitory effect on bone resorption is directly antagonistic to PTH and 1,25-dihydroxy D and its role in that context may be prevention of excessive resorption. It is secreted in response to eating calcium-rich food secondarily to secretion of various gastrointestinal and pancreatic hormones which it itself inhibits. The net effect is delayed calcium absorption which may be important in preventing postprandial hypercalcemia and hypercalciuria.

A major physiological role may be in situations (fetal life, infancy, pregnancy and lactation) with extra needs for calcium and when calcitonin and 1,25-dihydroxy D levels are high – calcitonin may prevent unwanted bone resorption whilst allowing the stimulatory effect of vitamin D on intestinal calcium absorption.

DISORDERS OF CALCIUM AND BONE METABOLISM

Metabolic and hormonal interactions in many of these disorders are complex. Advances in understanding the molecular pathogeneses of disorders of calcium, vitamin D and bone, including the roles of the extracellular calcium sensor, the vitamin D receptor, and new factors for bone cell embryogenesis and function, are reviewed by Langman.[316a]

Significant diagnostic pointers can be obtained from a full history (including family history) and specific abnormalities found on examination. To minimize effects of food and diurnal changes, blood is ideally taken in the fasting state in the morning and, when possible, without compression of the arm (venous stasis also influences calcium levels).

The important basic laboratory measurements are of serum calcium (Ca), phosphate (P) and alkaline phosphatase (ALP) which should be interpreted in the context of simultaneously estimated serum total protein and albumin, electrolytes, creatinine, magnesium and pH. Urine measurements (early morning or 24-h collections) of calcium, phosphate, creatinine and hydroxyproline (a measure of bone turnover) may be valuable. If significant abnormalities are found, more complex investigations can be instigated assessing aspects of parathyroid function, vitamin D metabolism and bone turnover as indicated.

INFANCY

Important problems in infancy are:

1. Hypocalcemia: early and late neonatal hypocalcemia
2. Hypercalcemia
   a. Idiopathic infantile hypercalcemia (see below)
   b. Familial hypocalciuric hypercalcemia (see below)
   c. Neonatal primary hyperparathyroidism
   d. Hypervitaminosis D (see below)
   e. Other associations: fat necrosis; phosphate deficiency
3. Metabolic bone disease in the preterm infant.

ABNORMAL 1,25-DIHYDROXY VITAMIN D SECRETION OR ACTION

Increased intake (hypervitaminosis D)

Vitamin D intoxication usually results from excessive treatment of hypoparathyroidism, rickets, renal osteodystrophy, etc. with concentrated preparations – it is available in proprietary multivitamin preparations without prescription in many countries and may also be prescribed inappropriately. 'Stoss therapy' – administration of 600 000 units for the prevention of rickets – is not now used but was formerly a cause. Toxicity may persist for many weeks because of adipose tissue storage. Despite its potency, an advantage of the synthetic analogue of 1,25-dihydroxy D (1alpha-hydroxy D) is its short half-life with more rapid return to normocalcemia after inadvertent overdose.

Clinical signs reflect hypercalcemia from excessive intestinal calcium absorption and bone resorption. Initially, there is nausea and vomiting with anorexia, constipation and polyuria. Infants fail to thrive and become irritable. Ultimately, there may be nephrocalcinosis with renal insufficiency and ectopic calcification. Investigation confirms hypercalcemia with hypercalciuria; serum PTH will be suppressed – normal or elevated PTH with hypercalcemia indicate hyperparathyroidism.

Treatment is by withdrawing the vitamin D preparation and calcium supplements (if any), saline infusion and furosemide (frusemide) (to increase urinary calcium loss) and glucocorticoids (e.g. hydrocortisone 4 mg/kg/24 h 6-hourly) which gradually reduces intestinal calcium absorption.

Idiopathic hypercalcemia of infancy was though to be due to excessive vitamin D administration. This is unlikely to be the case, although it remains a heterogeneous and poorly understood condition. The fall in incidence of the mild form observed in the UK preceded the reduction in vitamin D supplementation of artificial infant feeds. Incidence of the severe form[317] often associated with mental retardation, cardiovascular abnormalities (supravalvar aortic stenosis or peripheral pulmonary stenosis) and facial and other dysmorphic features[318] has not changed. The mild form is now rarely seen. The severe form (Williams syndrome) may be due to a defect in calcitonin synthesis or release resulting from a neural crest developmental anomaly affecting face, heart and thyroid C-cell (calcitonin-producing) precursors which would explain the variable relationship between somatic developmental abnormalities and degree of calcium homeostatic disturbance (calcium levels may be normal). The molecular genetic defect in Williams syndrome is now known to be a deletion of the elastin gene and other contiguous genes at 7q11.23.[319]

Increased synthesis

Hypercalcemia from raised 1,25-dihydroxy D levels (with suppressed PTH) is seen in granulomatous disease (sarcoidosis, tuberculosis, etc.) due to conversion of 25-hydroxy D into the active metabolite by 1-hydroxylation in granulomatous cells. Similar findings in some patients with lymphoma are unusual – most patients with hypercalcemia due to malignant disease have low 1,25-dihydroxy D levels and reduced intestinal calcium absorption and other mechanisms are presumably involved.

Increased secretion and/or responsiveness (absorptive hypercalciuria)

This specific type of 'idiopathic' hypercalciuria is thought to be due to a primary abnormality of secretion of, or responsiveness to, 1,25-dihydroxy D. It may be transmitted autosomal dominantly and cause renal stones or hematuria. A form secondary to a renal tubular defect is also found (see renal hypercalciuria below) and may share a common pathogenesis.

Rickets (Table 13.15) is caused by defective growth plate mineralization and may be due to decreased calcium and phosphate availability in extracellular fluid at those sites (deficiency or malabsorption of vitamin D, defective formation or action of 1,25-dihydroxy D – calciopenic rickets; increased renal phosphate excretion or decreased intake – phosphopenic rickets). Phosphopenic rickets is usually due to renal phosphate loss (see below) but hypophosphatemia, commonly seen in low birth weight preterm infants, is due to inadequate phosphate intake – see also Chapters 10, 14 and 16.

ABNORMAL PTH SECRETION OR ACTION

Increased PTH secretion may be a normal physiological compensatory response to hypocalcemia (secondary hyperparathyroidism). Primary hyperparathyroidism is due to abnormally increased secretion

Table 13.15 Classification of rickets

'Classical': lack of sunshine, diet deficient in vitamin D	Immigrants (pigmented skin); during rapid growth (infancy/puberty)
Malabsorption	Celiac disease; giardiasis; hepatobiliary disease (biliary atresia/fistula; cirrhosis; neonatal hepatitis)
Hereditary renal (mainly tubular)	Hypophosphatemic; vitamin D dependency; fibrous dysplasia/neurofibromatosis (with hypophosphatemia); Fanconi's syndrome (including cystinosis, tyrosinemia, Lowe's syndrome, Wilson's disease); distal renal tubular acidosis
Acquired renal (mainly tubular)	Chronic renal failure (glomerular); hypophosphatemia; hypercalciuria

of PTH, is rare in childhood and uncommon even by adolescence with an overall prevalence of 25 per 100 000.

The etiology is unknown but cases may be sporadic (nearly always associated with a solitary adenoma, rarely with carcinoma) or familial (usually due to hyperplasia of all four glands). Familial cases may be isolated (autosomal dominant and recessive forms are reported), but may be associated with autosomal dominant multiple endocrine neoplasia syndromes – MEN1 (see below), in association with pancreatic tumors or gastrinoma and pituitary adenomas; MEN2, with medullary thyroid carcinoma and pheochromocytoma. There is also an association with autosomal dominant hypocalciuric hypercalcemia syndrome where there is defective renal calcium excretion (see below).

Heterozygous germline mutations of the tumor suppressor gene MEN1 (on chromosome 11) are responsible for multiple endocrine neoplasia type 1 (MEN1), a dominantly inherited familial cancer syndrome characterized by the combined occurrence of pituitary, parathyroid, and enteropancreatic tumors.[320] It typically presents with clinical signs or symptoms in the middle decades of adult life but intractable peptic ulceration (Zollinger–Ellison syndrome due to a gastrin secreting pancreatic tumor) is reported by adolescence and raised gastrin and calcium levels may be found in asymptomatic family members by then. Hypercalcemia occurs in about 97% and the serial fasting serum calcium measurement is a valuable screening test.

The clinical spectrum of primary hyperparathyroidism ranges from asymptomatic to lethal. There may be fatigue, anorexia, constipation, polyuria, polydipsia, renal stones, bone pain and pathological fractures. Diagnosis depends on demonstration of inappropriately high PTH levels for hypercalcemia on three separate occasions. This is found otherwise only in familial hypocalciuric hypercalcemia (see below) where urinary calcium excretion is low for the hypercalcemia. Antibody against the C-terminal or intermediate PTH fragments is more sensitive to high PTH levels. Radiographically, there is usually generalized bone demineralization, osteolysis and subperiosteal bone resorption especially of the phalanges and, occasionally, cysts.

Once diagnosis is secure, surgical parathyroid exploration by an experienced surgeon is necessary. Preoperative localization of the responsible gland is unreliable (although ultrasound may detect enlargement < 1 cm) – hyperplasia of all four is common. In this situation total parathyroidectomy with autotransplantation of tissue into the forearm is the treatment of choice. Other family members should be screened for hypercalcemia.

Decreased secretion (hypoparathyroidism – HP)

HP is much commoner than hypersecretion but less common than decreased peripheral hormone action ['end-organ resistance' due to receptor or postreceptor abnormalities – pseudohypoparathyroidism (PHP)].

Cases may be sporadic or familial. Presentation can be in the neonate and may be transient, permanent (autosomal dominant, recessive, sex-linked recessive and sporadic forms have all been described), or part of DiGeorge syndrome – see Chapter 25. Post-neonatal onset may be idiopathic or occur secondarily to neck surgery, irradiation, hemosiderosis, hypomagnesemia, etc.

A familial (autosomal recessive) form may be associated with autoimmune disease affecting other endocrine glands (especially Addison's disease) and mucocutaneous candidiasis [polyglandular autoimmune disease (PGAD) type 1]. Presentation is with severe candidiasis (due to a defect in cellular immunity) followed, successively, by HP and Addison's disease (rarely before mid-childhood). Other autoimmune manifestations include alopecia, vitiligo, thyroiditis, chronic hepatitis and pernicious anemia. Parathyroid antibodies cause glandular destruction.[321]

Clinical signs and symptoms of HP are from hypocalcemia due to decreased renal calcium reabsorption, bone resorption and, indirectly, decreased intestinal calcium absorption. Manifestations depend on age, severity and speed of onset and relate to the neuromuscular system (latent tetany – positive Chvostek and Trousseau signs; overt tetany – paresthesiae, muscle cramps, carpopedal spasm), brain (focal or grand mal convulsions, papilledema, basal ganglia calcification, eventual mental retardation), heart (prolonged QT interval), eyes (lenticular cataracts), ectodermal changes (dry skin, coarse hair, brittle nails, tooth enamel hypoplasia).

Treatment aims to correct hypocalcemia and prevent recurrence (treatment of associated problems may also be indicated). A vitamin D preparation is currently the long-term treatment of choice – PTH is expensive and must be given parenterally daily.

Acute hypocalcemia is treated with 10% calcium gluconate (9.4% calcium by weight) 1–2 ml/kg by slow i.v. injection repeated, as necessary, 6 hourly or carefully and slowly infused (in dilute form). Oral calcium supplements (e.g. calcium gluconate) and a vitamin D analogue (e.g. 1alpha-hydroxy D 25–50 ng/kg/24 h) should be started and serum and urinary calcium levels checked 3 monthly. Vitamin D will not correct renal calcium loss – although there is reduced urinary calcium excretion, there is relative hypercalciuria due to deficient (PTH mediated) renal tubular calcium reabsorption and thus serum calcium levels should be maintained in low normal range to avoid nephrocalcinosis and renal stones. Treatment with a thiazide diuretic and sodium restriction may be necessary.

Decreased peripheral action (pseudohypoparathyroidism – PHP)

Uncommon causes of PTH-resistant HP include severe hypomagnesemia (which causes resistance to and decreased secretion of PTH) and calciopenic rickets (due to low 1,25-dihydroxy D levels). Receptor or postreceptor defects of response to PTH at the target organ (especially the renal tubule) are commoner, first described by Albright et al – pseudohypoparathyroidism.[322] This heterogeneous condition has been divided into several types:

Type1 (originally described by Albright)

There is often symptomatic hypocalcemia in mid-childhood on a background of variable mental retardation and characteristic (but inconstant) somatic features ('Albright's hereditary osteodystrophy', AHO) including short stature, obesity, round face, short neck and marked metacarpal and metatarsal shortening (especially 4th and 5th – see Figs 13.4 and 13.6). There is no phosphaturic response to PTH administration and a blunted urinary cyclic AMP increase in comparison with both normals and patients with HP. This type has been further subdivided on the basis of decreased (Type 1a) or normal (Type 1b) amounts of a protein membrane component that couples the PTH receptor to the catalytic unit of the adenylate cyclase.

Type 2

In this rarer form the defect is thought to be due to an intracellular defect beyond cyclic AMP generation – cyclic AMP responses to PTH are normal but the phosphaturic response is defective.

These differences do not entirely explain the very variable clinical manifestations (see below). Some patients with somatic features show no renal resistance to PTH – pseudopseudohypoparathyroidism (pPHP). In some families, PHP Type 1 and pPHP coexist and individuals may fluctuate between normo- and hypocalcemia.

PTH activates the adenylate cyclase system via the Gs alpha member of the 'G' protein family, a heterotrimeric guanine nucleotide binding protein. The gene encoding Gs alpha is GNAS1. The Gs alpha protein membrane component is deficient in PHP Type 1a/pPHP.[323] Numerous GNAS1 mutations have been identified in PHP-1a and pPHP.[324] Patients with either disorder show skeletal and developmental defects (AHO). Owing to paternal imprinting with inactivation of the paternal allele, which may be tissue- or cell-specific, resistance toward PTH and, often, other hormones is only observed in patients with PHP-1a, i.e. the variable and tissue-specific hormone resistance observed in PHP-1a may result from tissue-specific imprinting of the GNAS1 gene.[1] Patients with PHP-1b show PTH-resistant hypocalcemia and hyperphosphatemia but no AHO. The abnormal regulation of mineral ion homeostasis, such as in PHP-1a/pPHP kindreds, is paternally imprinted. Recent linkage studies have mapped the genetic defect responsible for PHP-1b to chromosome 20q13.3, making it likely that mutations in distinct regions of the GNAS1 gene are the cause of at least three different forms of PHP.[325]

The G protein family mediates numerous transmembrane hormone and sensory transduction processes in eukaryotic cells including LH, GH and TSH synthesis and release.[1] Unsurprisingly, therefore, abnormalities of other peptide hormones, particularly thyroid and GT, have been described in these patients. It is likely that abnormalities of GH secretion also occur – the growth hormone-releasing factor (GRF)/receptor complex on the somatotroph activates a similar coupling ('G') protein to stimulate adenylate cyclase and hence GH synthesis and release. Thus in PHP there could be a defect in GRF binding and/or activation of its regulatory protein similar to that postulated for the defect in PTH regulatory protein.

Although these individuals are a heterogeneous group, some grow better on GH treatment.[326] Treatment of hypocalcemia in PHP is analogous to treatment in HP (see above).

ABNORMAL CALCITONIN SECRETION

Increased

Hypocalcemia is almost never a feature of calcitonin excess. High calcitonin levels are seen in *medullary thyroid carcinoma* (sporadic or in MEN2), and a variety of non-thyroid tumors in adults but have not been described in children. Levels are high in the rare autosomal recessive condition pycnodysostosis and may be raised in pancreatitis. High levels, presumably due to a normal physiological response, are described in hypercalcemic states and renal insufficiency.

Decreased

A number of congenital and acquired hypocalcitoninemic conditions are described, including primary hypothyroidism or post-thyroidectomy, anticonvulsant treatment (phenytoin or primidone) and Williams syndrome. Hypercalcemia does not occur.

ABNORMALITIES OF PHOSPHATE EXCRETION

Increased

Phosphopenic rickets result from excessive urinary phosphate excretion with resulting hypophosphatemia (Table 13.15) and only rarely from inadequate intake (other than in the preterm infant; see above and Ch. 10). Familial forms of primary hypophosphatemia secondary to renal phosphate loss have been described including X-linked (dominant) hypophosphatemic rickets (Albright's vitamin D resistant rickets) and autosomal dominant and recessive forms. Phosphopenic rickets is a feature of Fanconi syndrome (sporadic or familial, idiopathic or secondary to a number of inborn metabolic errors), has been described in rare (usually benign mesenchymal) tumors and is a feature of distal renal tubular acidosis (sporadic and familial).

Decreased

Decreased renal phosphate excretion is important in the pathogenesis of *renal osteodystrophy* – other factors such as altered vitamin D metabolism become increasingly important as renal failure worsens (see Ch. 16). *Tumor calcinosis* (deposition of calcium phosphate around large joints due to increased phosphate reabsorption) is rarely seen outside Africa and may be familial or sporadic.

ABNORMALITIES OF CALCIUM EXCRETION

Increased

Hypercalciuria may be associated with hypercalcemia (e.g. vitamin D intoxication, primary hyperparathyroidism), normocalcemia [e.g. distal renal tubular acidosis, following corticosteroid, furosemide (frusemide) or immobilization] or may be 'idiopathic'. Absorptive (see above) and renal forms (renal hypercalciuria) of this last group occur but may share a common pathogenesis.

Decreased (familial hypocalciuric 'benign' hypercalcemia)

There are inappropriately raised (normal or high) PTH levels with hypercalcemia (see above). Inheritance is autosomal dominant. Hypercalcemia results from increased tubular calcium reabsorption, but there are no consequent symptoms of chronic hypercalcemia. There is a presumed abnormal set point for calcium mediated PTH suppression but no abnormalities of vitamin D metabolism, calcitonin secretion or parathyroid histology have been found. Parathyroid surgery is ineffective and contraindicated.

PRACTICAL DIFFERENTIAL DIAGNOSIS

Rickets

Initial clinical assessment, characteristic radiographic changes and raised ALP, decreased P and normal (especially in phosphopenic rickets) or decreased Ca in serum usually make diagnosis straightforward. It is important to determine etiology (Table 13.15) and further tests will usually be necessary.

Normal PTH and cyclic AMP levels are characteristic of phosphopenic rickets (usually familial X-linked hypophosphatemic, but associated hypercalciuria suggests the rarer autosomal recessive type unless there is inadequate phosphate intake in, for example, the preterm infant). Tumor rickets should be considered in sporadic cases presenting in late childhood or adolescence. Renal function must be assessed to exclude primary renal causes such as chronic renal failure and Fanconi syndrome (which may be secondary to other inborn metabolic errors) and is characterized by glycosuria and aminoaciduria .

Secondary hyperparathyroidism (i.e. secondary to calcium malabsorption) with raised PTH levels suggests calciopenic rickets, usually due to lack of vitamin D or impaired synthesis or action of the active metabolite 1,25-dihydroxy D. Further differential diagnosis necessitates measurement of individual vitamin D metabolites: low levels of 25-hydroxy D are found in all acquired forms (nutritional, liver disease, malabsorption, anticonvulsants). If 25-hydroxy D levels are normal, low 1,25-dihydroxy D levels indicate vitamin D deficient rickets type 1 and high levels indicate end-organ resistance to its action (type 2).

Hypocalcemia

In the presence of normal total protein, albumin and magnesium levels and renal function, repeated fasting early morning hypocalcemia is interpreted in the context of serum phosphate levels. If these are high, HP or PHP is likely and can be differentiated on the basis of PTH and cyclic AMP measurements: in PHP, PTH levels are high and, in type 1 – the common form – there is blunted cyclic AMP response to PTH infusion; in HP, PTH levels are low and the cyclic AMP response is normal.

Low or normal serum phosphate levels suggests calciopenic rickets; elevated ALP and PTH levels will confirm the diagnosis which should be further elucidated as above.

Hypercalcemia

Confirmed raised fasting early morning hypercalcemia on at least three occasions with normal renal function and serum protein and albumin levels is uncommon in childhood. Raised or even detectable PTH levels in the presence of hypercalcemia are inappropriate and indicate primary hyperparathyroidism. MEN syndromes should be excluded and family members screened for hypercalcemia. Detectable PTH levels with hypercalcemia but hypocalciuria are characteristic of familial hypocalciuric hypercalcemia.

Suppressed PTH levels suggest vitamin D intoxication (most commonly), idiopathic infantile hypercalcemia, malignancy, sarcoidosis or Addison's disease.

HP from PHP

Hypomagnesemia, because of its dual effect on PTH secretion and resistance to PTH action, may produce features of both HP and PHP – serum magnesium must be checked in hypocalcemia. Somatic features of Albright's hereditary osteodystrophy (see above) and radiographic changes of hyperparathyroidism indicate PHP. In HP, PTH levels are inappropriately low for hypocalcemia; PTH levels are high in PHP. Deficient cyclic AMP generation after PTH infusion is characteristic of PHP. Measurement of plasma cyclic AMP has replaced the older tests which measured urinary cyclic AMP excretion.

THE ADRENAL GLANDS

The adrenal glands are formed from mesodermal and ectodermal components which form cortex and medulla respectively. During the fifth week, mesothelial cells migrate and proliferate to form large acidophilic cells which comprise the fetal cortex. These become surrounded by smaller cells which later make up the definitive cortex. Meanwhile, sympathetic neural crest neuroblasts invade the medial aspect of the fetal cortex forming the adrenal medulla rather than nerve processes and known as chromaffin cells.

For ontogeny of fetal adrenal steroidogenesis see p. 449. The neonatal adrenals are comparable in size to the kidneys. After birth, there is rapid atrophy of the fetal zone of the cortex and adrenal weight at birth is only regained by late puberty. The definitive cortex secretes glucocorticoids (GC) affecting carbohydrate metabolism, mineralocorticoids (MCA) affecting electrolyte balance and androgens (which are also estrogen precursors). The medulla secretes catecholamines (adrenaline and noradrenaline).

THE ADRENAL CORTEX

Morphology and steroidogenesis

The cortex comprises three histologically distinct zones but cells appear to migrate through them changing function as they do so. This has important implications for control of steroidogenesis. The outer (subcapsular) zone, the zona glomerulosa, consists of balls of small cells and overlies the radially arranged cord-like bundles of larger cells of the zona fasciculata. The innermost area, the zona reticularis, consists of a network of short cords with capillaries and only gradually becomes a distinct zone from ~ 6 years and largely accounts for the pubertal adrenal size and weight spurt. In contrast, there is relatively little change in postnatal morphological glomerulosa and fasciculata appearances.

In tissue culture, fasciculata and reticularis cells differ functionally as well as histologically preferentially synthesizing GC (cortisol) and androgens respectively. Dehydroepiandrosterone (DHA) is a marker of zona reticularis function. Increasing production of androgens by reticularis from about 5 or 6 years and peaking around 12 or 13 years – 'adrenarche' – is synchronous with morphological and functional reticularis development. Aldosterone, the main MC, is uniquely produced in the zona glomerulosa.

Plasma measurements of adrenal steroids reflect one moment in time, but many steroids are released episodically in relation to circadian rhythms and to environmental stimuli, often in sudden bursts at intervals.

Cortisol is secreted intermittently in response to pulsatile ACTH release. Most secretory activity occurs during sleep but there are, on average, about nine episodes of cortisol secretion through a 24-h period in adults under basal conditions. The circadian diurnal cortisol rhythm results from maximal duration and number of ACTH secretory episodes between 3 a.m. and 8 a.m. Circadian cortisol rhythm is present by ~ 6 months and is abolished in Cushing's syndrome.

ACTH binds to receptors on the adrenal cell membrane, activating adenylate cyclase (a calcium dependent step); cyclic AMP activates enzymes (mainly intracellular protein kinases) which stimulate hydrolysis of cholesterol esters. Steroidogenesis is initiated in mitochondria by cholesterol binding to a C27 side chain cleavage enzyme which starts its stepwise conversion to pregnenolone, a necessary step in biosynthesis of all three groups of adrenal cortical hormones.

There are acute and chronic responses to ACTH in terms of GC biosynthesis. In contrast, the glomerulosa only seems to produce aldosterone acutely – chronic ACTH stimulation is not generally associated with sustained hyperaldosteronism. ACTH is probably the most, and perhaps only, important adrenal androgen modulator. It is likely that changes in adrenal androgen production with age (c.f. unchanging cortisol levels for surface area) result from ACTH-mediated intrinsic local vascular and morphological changes and children with familial glucocorticoid deficiency demonstrate diminished adrenal androgen secretion implicating a significant role for ACTH, rather than a specific, unidentified, pituitary adrenal androgen stimulating hormone, in the induction of adrenarche.

Physiological ACTH levels regulate acute aldosterone fluctuations – ACTH is important in the pathogenesis of GC-suppressible hyperaldosteronism. Although the primary control mechanism is the renin–angiotensin system (see Ch. 16), this ACTH role is important in managing salt losing CAH.

GCs such as cortisol and corticosterone are fast feedback antagonists of ACTH secretion; other steroids [e.g. deoxycorticosterone (DOC), deoxycortisol (S) and synthetic GCs] show delayed feedback inhibition. The relative importance of these responses in normal physiological control of ACTH is unclear.

Simplified steroidogenic pathways are summarized in Figure 13.50. For the clinician, working knowledge of the pathways will aid understanding of physical and biochemical consequences of various types of congenital hyperplasia.

Approximately 70% of circulating cortisol is bound to a 52 000 molecular weight alpha-2 globulin, transcortin (corticosteroid binding globulin – CBG) and ~ 20% albumin-bound. Aldosterone, other GCs and precursors are less strongly bound to CBG and synthetic steroids only weakly. CBG is synthesized in liver; levels are increased by estrogen and decreased in cirrhosis. Binding sites are saturated when total plasma cortisol levels exceed about 600 nmol/L; at normal concentrations very little free cortisol is in plasma or excreted in urine. Urinary free cortisol is thus a sensitive screening test for Cushing's syndrome Cortisol plasma half-life is 60–90 min; that of aldosterone is only ~ 20 min because proportionately much less is protein-bound. Important adrenal androgens include DHA and its sulfated form (DHAS) which is also synthesized by the gland. DHAS half-life is 10–20 h; DHA secretion is episodic and concurrent with cortisol. Aldosterone levels show marked circadian changes which follow cortisol but are significantly influenced by posture.

Normal values for individual steroids and urinary metabolites in infancy, childhood and puberty are available[327] based on cross-sectional and mixed longitudinal studies.

Urine sampling is atraumatic and 24-h collections are more likely than isolated plasma samples to reflect accurately overall steroid production. However such collections may be difficult and unreliable in infants and young children. In general steroids are present in urine in about 1000 times their plasma concentrations. However, because of the complexity of metabolic pathways via which adrenal (and gonadal) steroids are excreted (and influences of disease or drugs) there can be uncertainty about clinical significance, relationship to gland of origin or even specific steroid from which they derive. Nevertheless, steroid profiles are valuable in complementing plasma steroid assays, e.g. studying normal children longitudinally to determine changes with age and the mechanism of adrenarche, detecting abnormal metabolites (e.g. secreted by tumors), metabolite ratios (e.g. in 5alpha-reductase deficiency), differential diagnosis of rarer or less clear-cut forms of CAH and differential diagnosis of salt losing states in infancy due to aldosterone biosynthetic defects.

Adrenarche

During the early months of life the fetal zone rapidly atrophies so that high fetal and neonatal DHAS levels [reflecting low 3beta-hydroxysteroid dehydrogenase (3betaOHSD) fetal zone activity] fall and remain low for ~ 6 years. During mid-childhood adrenal androgen secretion rises steeply ('adrenarche') (Fig. 13.51)[328] – coincident with zona reticularis development.

Adrenarche is important because of (1) its role in precocious sexual (pubic and axillary) hair development in mid-childhood; (2) possible relevance to triggering normal puberty, although underlying mechanisms and relationship to subsequent rises in GT and gonadal steroids at clinical puberty onset ('gonadarche') are controversial; (3) the association between premature adrenarche and subsequent functional ovarian hyperandrogenism, polycystic ovarian syndrome, and insulin resistance in later life ('syndrome X') but which may present by childhood or adolescence, and an association with previous intrauterine growth retardation; (4) potential etiological relevance to concomitant steep rise in normal blood pressure (BP) centiles and the mid-childhood growth spurt.

The adrenal androgen rise is not accompanied by significant increases in intermediate metabolites in cortisol or corticosterone

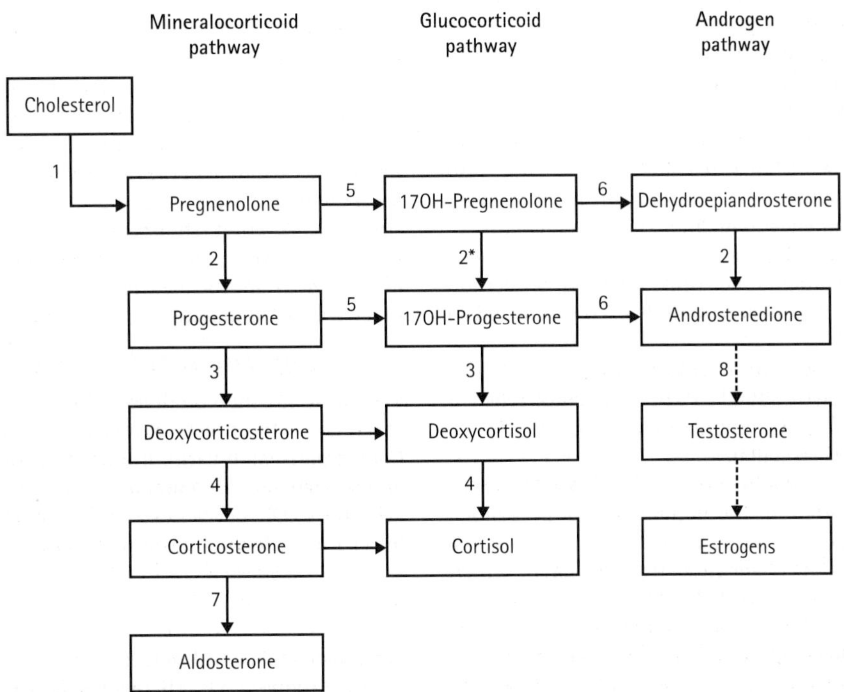

Fig. 13.50 Pathways of adrenal biosynthesis. 1 – cholesterol side chain cleaving system (20alpha-hydroxylase, 20,22-desmolase, 22alpha-hydroxylase); 2 – 3beta-hydroxysteroid dehydrogenase; 3 – 21-hydroxylase; 4 – 11beta-hydroxylase; 5 – 17alpha-hydroxylase; 6 – 17,20-lyase; 7 – 18-hydroxylase and 18-hydroxysteroid dehydrogenase; 8 – 17beta-hydroxysteroid dehydrogenase.

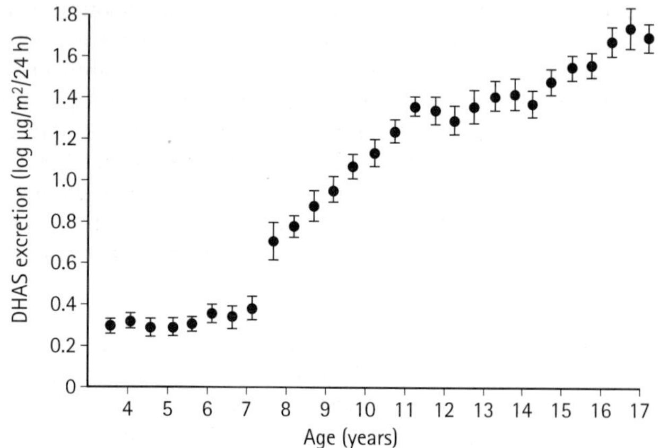

Fig. 13.51 Urinary excretion of dehydroepiandrosterone sulfate (DHAS) in childhood. (From Kelnar 1985[328])

biosynthesis for body surface area. It is likely that this disassociation reflects changes in adrenal steroidogenesis with age in response to ACTH-mediated changes in adrenal blood flow and cell morphology rather than a separate adrenal androgen stimulating hormone.

In some children, predominantly girls, the rise manifests as appearance of pubic, and sometimes axillary, hair ('premature pubarche'). These children probably represent one end of a spectrum of adrenal androgen secretion or perhaps of sensitivity to its action as plasma levels are not always high for age. It must be distinguished from non-classical, late onset or missed CAH and (rare) adrenal tumors (in which, in contrast, androgens are not dexamethasone-suppressible) as well as from true precocious puberty. Although 'exaggerated' pubarche per se is probably physiological and has no adverse effect on the onset and progression of gonadarche and final height (puberty timing is normal or slightly early), hirsutism or polycystic ovarian disease may develop at puberty. Thus 'exaggerated' adrenarche can be a forerunner of syndrome X in some children (see above).[35] The association of these endocrine-metabolic abnormalities with reduced fetal growth and their genetic basis remain to be elucidated.[35]

The role of adrenarche in man remains controversial – it is difficult to extrapolate from pathological situations to normal gonadarche control. Adrenarche may be delayed in children with CDGP and isolated GH deficiency but not in hypergonadotrophic hypogonadism (e.g. Turner syndrome). Children with Addison's disease enter puberty normally and in diabetic adolescents gonadarche may proceed normally despite delayed adrenarche. Children with congenital adrenal hypoplasia all have hypogonadotrophic hypogonadism and do not enter puberty normally.

Adrenarche is coincident with the preadolescent fat spurt[167] and with the mid-childhood growth spurt.[4,329] The latter could reflect a bone and muscle response to adrenal androgens, directly or indirectly by influencing GH secretion.

Adrenarche could simply be a by-product of the need of inner fetal adrenal cells to respond to the hormonal milieu of pregnancy by developing an androgen (i.e. estrogen-precursor) synthesizing zone. Other than man, only the chimpanzee has adrenarche which therefore occurs in two species which have the most prolonged interval between birth and puberty. Adrenarche may merely be revealed by such an interval. However the more complex the organism the greater the advantage in prolonging the period between birth and reproductive activity to allow brain growth and childhood learning. If during that period androgens are required for continuing skeletal and muscular growth, this could be achieved by transferring androgen biosynthesis from gonad to adrenal – adrenarche.

Congenital adrenal hyperplasia (CAH)

CAH describes collectively a group of autosomal recessively inherited disorders of adrenal corticosteroid biosynthesis due to deficiency of one of five enzymes in the cholesterol to cortisol biosynthetic pathway – 21-hydroxylase (21OH, P-450$_{c21}$), 11beta-hydroxylase (11betaOH, P-450$_{c11}$), 3beta-hydroxysteroid dehydrogenase (3betaOHSD), 17alpha-hydroxylase (17alphaOH, P-450$_{c17}$) and cholesterol desmolase (P-450$_{scc}$) (see Fig. 13.50). Deficiencies of other enzymes such as 17,20-desmolase (P-450$_{c17}$ 17,20-lyase), 17beta-hydroxysteroid dehydrogenase (17betaOHSD) and 5alpha-reductase have effects limited to the adrenal androgen (and gonadal) biosynthetic pathway.

The steroidogenic block due to a specific enzyme deficiency will have potential clinical effects by two types of mechanism: (1) distal hormone deficiency and (2) the effect of ACTH drive, a compensatory response in CRF–ACTH release secondary to the defect in cortisol biosynthesis and reduced feedback inhibition of ACTH, leading to a) proximal metabolite accumulation and b) abnormal production of steroids whose biosynthesis is unaffected by the primary enzyme deficiency (Table 13.16).

Thus in the commonest form of CAH (21OH deficiency, P-450$_{c21}$ deficiency) there is, potentially, cortisol deficiency (in practice unstressed cortisol levels are normal as the enzyme deficiency is seldom complete), aldosterone deficiency and salt loss (when the defect is also present in the zona glomerulosa); plasma 17-hydroxyprogesterone (17OHP), and its principal urinary metabolite, pregnanetriol, levels are raised (and conveniently measured to confirm the diagnosis) and ACTH hypersecretion results in excess adrenal androgen and virilization (by birth in females, during early childhood in undiagnosed males).

Inappropriately raised plasma ACTH levels for plasma cortisol are pathognomonic of CAH – measuring cortisol alone is useless for diagnosis. Although the clinical picture may suggest the specific underlying enzyme defect, definitive diagnosis is dependent on detecting raised plasma levels of precursors in plasma by RIA or IRMA and characteristic urinary metabolites. Occasionally, measurement following ACTH stimulation may be necessary if the situation is not clear-cut. Pointers to the possibility of CAH include ambiguous genitalia in the newborn, vomiting with dehydration and urinary salt wasting during early days or weeks of life, collapse during stress (e.g. severe intercurrent illness or general anesthesia) at any age, hypertension, hirsutism or inappropriate virilization, primary amenorrhea, unexplained previous neonatal death (particularly if parents are consanguineous) and a family history of CAH.

21-Hydroxylase (21OH, P-450$_{c21}$) deficiency

This is by far the commonest form of CAH worldwide although there are considerable ethnic differences. The frequency of the homozygous state varies from 1 in 5000 (Europe) to 1 in 23 000 and is particularly common in Alaskan Eskimos (1 in 700). Non-classical 21OH deficiency (see below) seems commoner and may affect 1 in 30 Jews of Eastern European (Ashkenazi) origin and 1 in 100 other whites.[330]

Genetics

Molecular genetic techniques have localized two genes encoding the 21OH enzyme, CYP21B (active) and CYP21A (inactive), to the short arm of chromosome 6 either side of the genes for the fourth component of complement – there is close linkage with the HLA complex. Deletion of CYP21B is associated with severe, salt wasting disease and the HLA B47, DR7 haplotype; deletion of CYP21A seems not to cause any hormonal abnormality.[331] Most affected individuals are compound heterozygotes. HLA associations with non-classical 21OH deficiency vary between ethnic groups.

The presence of salt wasting in association with virilization was thought to breed true in affected families because of separate genetic regulatory control of glomerulosa and fasciculata – only salt wasters have an additional glomerulosa 21OH defect. Although there are separate control mechanisms for 21OH activity in these zones and simple virilizing and salt-wasting forms have different HLA associations, families who do not breed true are reported.[332] Obligate heterozygote parents of salt losing and simple virilizing patients show identical sodium, aldosterone and renin responses to a low sodium diet and some infants with aldosterone biosynthetic defects subsequently develop normal glomerulosa 21OH activity suggesting that other (non-HLA linked) mechanisms are involved in enzyme expression.

The importance of these molecular genetic developments lies in the practical ability to confirm (pre- or postnatally) whether family members are affected or unaffected and in advancing understanding of pathogenesis.

Prenatal diagnosis of 21OH deficiency was first reported in 1965[333] on the basis of elevated 17-ketosteroids and pregnanetriol levels in amniotic fluid (i.e. dilute fetal urine) of an affected fetus. Raised 17OHP and androstenedione levels have since been found in many studies and HLA genotyping of amniotic cells was used in addition. Chorionic villus sampling, and molecular typing for restriction fragment length polymorphisms of the chromosome 6 loci, 21-hydroxylase gene and HLA, is now possible by 8–11 weeks' gestation and has replaced HLA genotyping of amniotic cells. Rapid early prenatal diagnosis by direct assay of specific mutations using DNA amplification by polymerase chain reaction (PCR) is now feasible.

Antenatal diagnosis (AND) and treatment

Where there has been a previously affected female child, the possibility of prenatal treatment to reduce or prevent significant neonatal virilization in a second affected female fetus and obviate the need for surgery in infancy and beyond is potentially attractive. Dexamethasone (which crosses the placenta) can be used in a dose not exceeding 20 mcg/kg/day of the prepregnancy weight in two to three divided doses) to suppress the excessive ACTH/androgen induced virilization. Fetuses in whom therapy would be appropriate are affected females – a one in eight possibility with each pregnancy. However dexamethasone must be started very early in pregnancy, because sexual differentiation starts at 6 weeks' gestation and significantly before antenatal diagnosis is possible. Thus seven out of eight infants will have treatment unnecessarily for a number of weeks. In affected female infants treatment is continued to term.

Although data from uncontrolled studies are now available concerning prenatal diagnosis and dexamethasone therapy,[334,335] the degree of benefit (reduced virilization) compared to potentially significant maternal side-effects is unclear – possible long-term childhood side-effects have not been studied. At present, therefore, there seems insufficient evidence regarding the safety of mother and fetus to recommend general dexamethasone use outwith controlled scientific studies.[335] However some consider it effective and safe.[334]

Heterozygote detection and neonatal screening

Stimulated 17OHP levels after ACTH will distinguish classical 21OH deficiency patients from heterozygotes for classical or non-classical disease and from HLA-typed normal family members but HLA typing cannot be used on a population basis to detect heterozygosity (e.g. in the spouse of a potential carrier).

Newborn screening is highly desirable. Male infants (with normal genitalia) may give no warning of a salt losing crisis with higher morbidity and mortality.[336] Females may be sufficiently virilized to be thought normal males leading to later gender reassignment or hysterectomy and sterility. Non-salt losing males may be late diagnosed by when secondary true precocious puberty and ultimate short stature may be inevitable. In a retrospective study covering the last 30 years in five middle European countries there was a fourfold higher mortality amongst siblings and salt wasting males in the first year of life compared with the general population. It was calculated that 2–2.5 salt-wasting and up to 5 simple virilizing infants stay undiagnosed, out of 40 expected CAH patients per year in the countries investigated. Both clinical detection and treatment of CAH patients, at least in males, were insufficient.[336]

Classical 21OH deficiency is commoner than phenylketonuria and, in Europe, is nearly as common as congenital hypothyroidism. A reliable and cheap (in centers already providing a neonatal screening service) screening test is available[337] using heel-prick capillary blood samples taken onto filter paper to measure 17OHP, easily done as part of the 'Guthrie test' procedure.

Significant mortality and serious physical and emotional morbidity consequent on late diagnosis has led to many screening programs worldwide, e.g. Italy, France, Japan, Ireland, New Zealand and a number of USA states. Experience from screening more than 1 million neonates in over 13 screening programs in six countries confirms that screening improves detection of salt wasting newborns whose diagnosis is otherwise delayed or missed and in whom there is significant mortality and morbidity.[338] Morbidity in non-salt losing males presenting in mid-childhood is also considerable.

Genotyping may be a helpful diagnostic tool and a good complement to neonatal screening, especially in confirming or discarding the diagnosis in cases with slightly elevated 17OHP levels. It also provides information on disease severity, which reduces the risk of overtreatment of mildly affected children.[339]

In the UK it is generally considered unnecessary or 'uneconomical' to screen the whole newborn population even though this would add only small additional unit cost in screening laboratories already measuring TSH and phenylalanine. There may be insufficient acknowledgement of considerable potential morbidity and concentration on mortality statistics. There are, to date, few published data on improvements in morbidity resulting from early detection and treatment.

Clinical presentation

Classical simple virilizing 21OH deficiency in a karyotypic female results in masculinization generally leading to ambiguous external genitalia recognized at birth (Fig. 13.52) but occasionally so severe that the infant is thought to be a normal male. Internal female structures including ovaries, Fallopian tubes and uterus are normal (there are no testes to elaborate MIH) but there is variable labioscrotal fold fusion with a urogenital sinus, genital pigmentation and clitoromegaly. Males usually appear normal at birth but present with penile enlargement, rapid growth (and tall stature) and advanced skeletal maturation (leading to eventual short stature) within a few years (Fig. 13.53). Finding small testes with clinical signs of precocious puberty suggests the adrenals as the androgen source but skeletal maturational advance can be so marked that true precocious puberty develops when treatment starts (see Fig. 13.34).

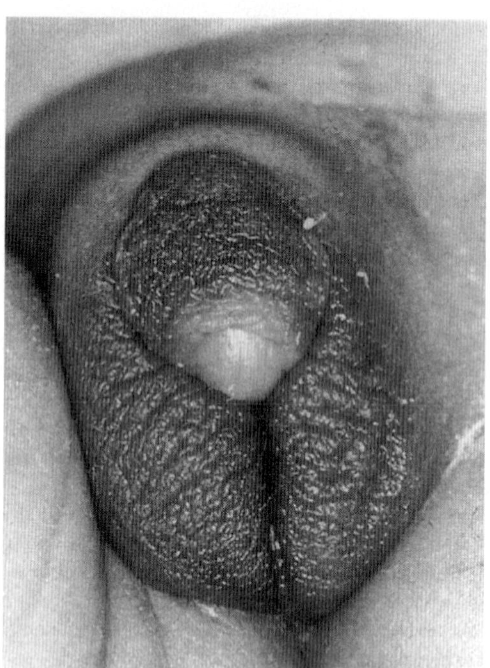

Fig. 13.52 Ambiguous genitalia in a 10-day-old genotypic female due to 21-hydroxylase deficiency.

In the classical salt wasting form (50–75%) there is an additional defect in mineralocorticoid biosynthesis with aldosterone deficiency due to an inability to convert progesterone to deoxycorticosterone in the glomerulosa. Presentation in both sexes is with severe renal wasting of sodium, dehydration and vomiting within a few days or weeks of birth – this should be foreseen as a possibility in a baby with ambiguous genitalia.

Non-classical ('mild, late-onset') 21OH deficiency was suspected in women presenting with hirsutism and infertility and family studies in classical 21OH deficiency characterized it as having different (and differing) HLA associations from classical forms but also autosomal recessive.[340] It may present as early as 6 months or later with premature pubarche, rapid growth (and reduced height prognosis), acne, male-type baldness in the female, delayed menarche or secondary amenorrhea. There is an association with polycystic ovarian disease[35] – infertility may result and respond to GC therapy.

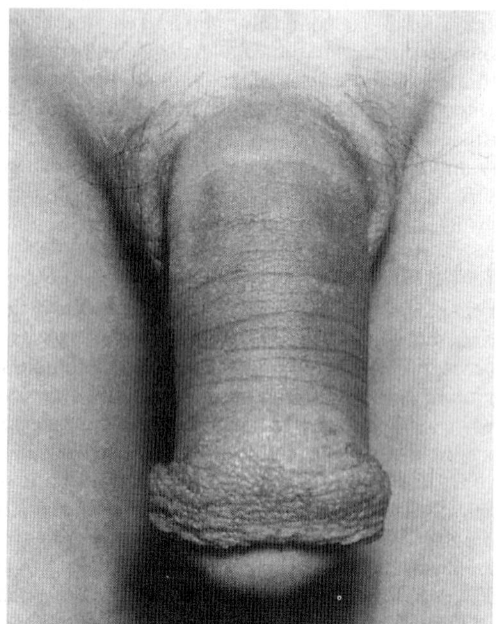

Fig. 13.53 Precocious pseudopuberty – a boy with non-salt-losing 21-hydroxylase deficiency at presentation at 5 years – testicular volume 2 ml (see also Fig. 13.34).

Laboratory diagnosis

17OHP measurement in the newborn is reliable for screening and diagnosis but false positives are reported in preterm or sick neonates. Plasma ACTH, androstenedione and urinary pregnanetriol levels will also be raised. In the salt wasting form, there is urinary sodium loss (cf. the gut in gastroenteritis); aldosterone levels are low for the high renin levels (cf. renal disease). Clinical and laboratory features of this and the other least uncommon forms of CAH are summarized in Table 13.16. Management is discussed below.

11beta-hydroxylase (11betaOH, P-450$_{c11}$) deficiency

This accounts for some 5% of CAH. There is no HLA association (cf. 21OH deficiency). Clinical manifestations are, as predicted from biosynthetic pathways (Fig. 13.50), identical to 21OH deficiency from the virilizing point of view – in some affected individuals there is restriction of the defect to the glucocorticoid pathway. In over 50%, however, the glomerulosa is also affected but the consequences differ from 21OH deficiency (Table 13.16) because there is accumulation of deoxycorticosterone (DOC) which has significant MC (salt-retaining) properties and, in excess, causes hypertension. DOC may not be directly responsible for hypertension in all cases as some patients with 11betaOH deficiency with raised DOC levels are normotensive and others are hypertensive with normal or only slightly raised DOC levels. Other DOC metabolites such as 18-hydroxy DOC have been implicated.

18-hydroxylation (the next step in the aldosterone biosynthetic pathway) is a function of the same mitochondrial enzyme – a defect in 18-hydroxylase is often seen with 11betaOH deficiency. Milder (late onset) forms and even salt wasting patients have been reported – clinically 11betaOH deficiency is as heterogeneous as 21OH deficiency.

Hypertension, when present, is characteristic and may be extreme; hypokalemic alkalosis is common. Virilizing effects are as described under 21OH deficiency above. DOC and deoxycortisol (S) levels are raised, as are their respective urinary tetrahydro (TH) metabolites (THDOC and THS), and rise further following ACTH, but their proportional elevations vary between subjects. Prenatal diagnosis has been carried out using a combination of amniotic fluid studies and maternal urinary THS measurement. Management is discussed below.

3beta-hydroxysteroid dehydrogenase (3betaOHSD) deficiency[45]

This is also associated with ambiguous genitalia in newborns but the site of the block (Fig. 13.50) results in potential ambiguity both in genotypic males and females (Table 13.16): high levels of DHA and its peripheral conversion to potent androgens result in variable clitoromegaly in females but are insufficient to fully masculinize a male infant, resulting in variable hypospadias (often the severe perineoscrotal form) with palpable testes. The defect in MC biosynthesis usually causes severe salt wasting. Mild defects are important causes of hirsutism presenting in young adult women so that, as in 21OH deficiency, mild, late-onset forms are apparently commoner than the classical severe type.[341] There is

Table 13.16 Clinical and laboratory features in the commonest forms of congenital adrenal hyperplasia

Enzyme deficiency	Sexual ambiguity in newborn	Salt-wasting	Hypertension	Blood	Urine
21-hydroxylase (simple virilizing)	Female	–	–	17OHP ++ An ++ DHA n/+ Renin n/+	PT ++ Aldo n
21-hydroxylase (salt-wasting)	Female	+	–	17OHP ++ An ++ DHA n/+ Renin ++	PT ++ Aldo –
11beta-hydroxylase	Female	–	+	17OHP + An ++ DHA + Renin ––	PT + THS ++ Aldo –
3beta-hydroxysteroid dehydrogenase	Male and female	+	–	17OHP n/+ An ++ DHA +++ Renin +	PT n/+ Aldo –

17OHP = 17alpha-hydroxyprogesterone, An = delta-4-androstenedione, DHA = dehydroepiandrosterone, THS = tetrahydrodeoxycortisol, Aldo = aldosterone, PT = pregnanetriol
+++ = very high, ++ = high, + = moderately high, n = normal, – = low, –– = very low.

no HLA association and neither ethnic nor geographical clustering. Prenatal diagnosis is impossible because of low 3betaOHSD fetal zone activity.

17 alpha-hydroxylase (17OH, P-450$_{c17}$) deficiency

Mineralocorticoid biosynthesis is intact (Fig. 13.50) and ACTH drive may result in neonatal hypertension and hypokalemic alkalosis. Deficient adrenal (and gonadal) sex steroid secretion means that karyotypic females usually present with failure of puberty and primary amenorrhea; males have ambiguous genitalia or virilize inadequately at puberty with gynecomastia. No HLA linkage has been demonstrated – the gene for 17OH is on chromosome 10.[342]

Cholesterol desmolase deficiency (P-450$_{scc}$, cholesterol side chain cleavage deficiency, lipoid adrenal hyperplasia)[343]

This was originally described as lipoid adrenal hyperplasia because of adrenal accumulation of cholesterol. Pregnenolone is the precursor of all MCs, GCs and androgens (Fig. 13.50) and complete deficiency is presumably incompatible with life. In contrast to congenital adrenal hypoplasia (see below) gonadal steroids are also deficient. The P-450$_{scc}$ gene has been located in the q23 to q24 region of chromosome 15.

Management of CAH

The basic defect (in cortisol biosynthesis) has wide repercussions including survival itself, sexual differentiation, growth, pubertal development and adult sexual functioning. Management potentially involves sex assignment, hormone therapy, surgery and psychological and emotional support with attention to growth and puberty and not merely adrenal steroid levels.

Hormone replacement is aimed at appropriately suppressing excessive ACTH drive rather than simply replacing cortisol – cortisol levels are often normal in the unstressed situation. In a baby with salt loss, titration of the appropriate GC replacement dose (against ACTH, adrenal androgen or 17OHP levels) is misleading until there is sodium balance (evidenced by normal plasma renin and plasma and urinary sodium). In the older child also, raised ACTH levels may be due to inadequate MC replacement.

The normal cortisol production rate is lower than originally thought: approximately 6–7 mg/m^2/day.[344,345] Appropriate GC replacement will allow normal growth, skeletal maturation and puberty – hydrocortisone (HC) 12–15 mg/m^2/day in two to three divided doses is usually appropriate. However larger doses (< 20–25 mg/m^2/day) may be necessary to suppress androgen levels and a combination regimen of physiological GC replacement with anti-androgens or aromatase inhibitors has been suggested[346] as has carbenoxolone as an 11betaOHSD inhibitor[347] – or bilateral laparoscopic adrenalectomy for difficult to control cases.[348]

To mimic normal diurnal rhythms, approximately two-thirds of the total HC dose is usually given first thing in the morning and the last dose at bedtime. In some it is necessary to give a longer acting steroid (e.g. prednisone or dexamethasone) at bedtime if early morning ACTH and 17OHP levels are not to be too high – once-daily dexamethasone may be appropriate for adolescents and adults and may also improve ovarian function in women.

The correct GC dose must be determined for each individual. Too low a dose will allow androgen-mediated excessively rapid growth, disproportionate bone age advance and eventual stunting. Too much will cause slowing of linear growth, delay (but not comparable delay) in bone maturation, also resulting ultimately in short stature. Swinging from one extreme to the other causes cumulative deficits in height prognosis.

Monitoring is by accurate growth and bone age assessment supplemented by home finger-prick blood spot 17OHP profiles four times daily approximately monthly. Abnormally rapid growth and bone age maturation is associated with non-suppressed 17OHP levels (> 40 nmol/L), whereas GC over-replacement, evidenced by pathologically slow growth, is associated with levels < 10 nmol/L.

GC therapy must be increased two- to threefold during stress such as significant infection or general anesthesia which could otherwise precipitate hypoglycemia and collapse. The family should be provided with, and instructed in the use of home blood glucose monitoring strips, and injectable hydrocortisone in case the child is vomiting or becomes rapidly ill at home. A MedicAlert bracelet or talisman should be worn – as with other patients on steroid medication.

Mineralocorticoid (MC) replacement is necessary in salt losing forms of CAH, given as the synthetic analogue 9alpha-fluorocortisol (fludrocortisone) 0.1–0.15 mg/m^2/day in one or two daily doses. However the salt losing crisis cannot be treated with fludrocortisone (nor with hydrocortisone which has limited MC activity) – emergency treatment with sodium replacement and i.v. normal or even hypertonic saline will be necessary as the total body sodium deficit is considerable. Once sodium balance is restored, fludrocortisone is introduced (and GC dose titration can begin) but oral sodium supplements (initially 2 mmol/kg/day) may also be required during infancy. Regular BP and urinary electrolyte measurements are sufficient check that MC replacement is appropriate. Renin and aldosterone clinic measurements may not be very meaningful. After infancy, children can adjust their salt intake and theoretically do not require long-term MC replacement. In practice, health and growth seem better if MC therapy is continued. The hypertension found in some forms of 11betaOH and 17OH deficiencies responds to GC suppression of ACTH/MC over-production.

Sex assignment seldom poses problems but for a review of the development of gender and sexuality in 46XX persons with classical CAH and its implications for clinical practice see Meyer-Bahlburg.[55] In 21OH and 11betaOH deficiencies karyotypic females with ambiguous genitalia should normally be reared as girls – internal sexual organs are normal female and with appropriate therapy there is a significant chance of fertility. Clitoral reduction is sometimes appropriate for cosmetic reasons (see below). Assignment in rarer forms (3betaOHSD, 17OH and cholesterol desmolase deficiencies) where males may be very poorly virilized depends on functional possibilities after potential reconstructive procedures.

In severely virilized females, clitoral reduction is widely felt to be best undertaken before 6 months. The vascular and neural supply to the glans is maintained to aid later sexual functioning and pleasure. Labial separation, if necessary, may be carried out simultaneously. Vaginal reconstruction has been thought best delayed until after puberty – often simple stretching will allow estrogen-mediated development at puberty obviating the need for major surgery. However contrary views in favour of early one stage reconstructive surgery have recently been expressed.[349] Fertility prospects are generally good in males, but the presence of adrenal rests within the testes of adult males with classic CAH are more frequent in the salt wasting form and are associated with a higher risk for infertility.[350] Infertility is reduced in affected women.

Emotional support is necessary for families of children with ambiguous genitalia particularly in the neonatal period and adolescence. Reports of high rates of homosexuality in female CAH patients may reflect inadequate vaginoplasty and difficult heterosexual relationships but effects of high androgen levels on the female fetal cerebral cortex could be important. Psychosexual outcomes in individuals treated prenatally will help to resolve the question but are not yet available.

Hyperadrenocorticism

Adrenal hypercorticism is commonly secondary to trophic hormone stimulation causing adrenal hyperplasia and hypersecretion and rarely primary (usually due to adrenal tumor). Clinical features are mimicked by (and in practice much more commonly due to) excessive GC administration (iatrogenic Cushing's syndrome – see below). Causes are listed in Table 13.17.

Cushing's syndrome[291]

Cushing's syndrome – disorders due to chronic excessive GC production – is uncommon in childhood – only 5–10% of reported cases – and rare in young children. It may be due to: (1) benign or malignant adrenal tumor; (2) pituitary ACTH hypersecretion (Cushing's disease); (3) ACTH or CRF hypersecretion from malignant extrapituitary tumors (ectopic ACTH syndrome); (4) supraphysiological parenteral, oral, nasal or topical GC or ACTH therapy for other medical conditions – most frequently.

Table 13.17 Important causes of adrenocortical hyperfunction

Glucocorticoids	Iatrogenic (glucocorticoid therapy); Cushing's syndrome; carcinoma/adenoma; bilateral hyperplasia (Cushing's disease/pituitary tumor/ ectopic ACTH-secreting tumor)
Mineralocorticoids	Primary hyperaldosteronism; Conn's syndrome (adenoma); Bartter's syndrome; congenital adrenal hyperplasia (17alpha-hydroxylase and 11beta-hydroxylase deficiencies); deoxycorticosterone- (DOC) or corticosterone-secreting tumors
Sex steroids	*Androgens* Congenital adrenal hyperplasia (21-hydroxylase and 11beta-hydroxylase deficiencies); 'premature' adrenarche (pubarche); virilizing carcinoma/adenoma *Estrogens* Feminizing carcinoma/adenoma

Clinical features are due to cortisol excess resulting in protein catabolism, increased carbohydrate production, fat accumulation and potassium wasting. In children, classical signs and symptoms (hypertension, truncal obesity, moon face, striae, proximal muscle weakness, osteoporosis, psychiatric symptoms) are usually less clear-cut than in adults and combined growth effects of hypercortisolism and excess adrenal androgen secretion may cause growth failure or temporarily rapid growth. The former is commoner, however, and hirsutism, progressive truncal obesity and growth failure (cf. obesity due to overeating), make up the most common presenting triad. Hypertension is usually only moderate and of multifactorial pathogenesis.

Iatrogenic disease must be specifically sought. ACTH is used to treat hypsarrhythmia and oral GC is used for a variety of chronic renal and connective tissue disorders (now less commonly for asthma). Large doses of inhaled steroids can be associated with significant adrenal suppression and growth failure[351] as can nasal drops[352] and topical steroids, depending on the extent of surface treated, frequency of application, potency of drug, use of occlusion and the age of patient.[353,354] Infants, treated for seborrheic dermatitis/eczema, and adolescents are relatively sensitive to topical steroid side-effects – an infant's (wet and occluded) napkin area has relative absorption 42-fold higher than the forearm; adolescents' increasing fat deposits and muscle mass inducing dermal remodelling makes them particularly susceptible to striae particularly around breasts and buttocks. If the hypothalamo–pituitary–adrenal axis is suppressed, treatment must be withdrawn gradually if acute adrenal insufficiency (see below) is not to be precipitated.

No single screening test is reliable in detecting Cushing's syndrome at an early stage or in differentiating it from exogenous obesity. A normal plasma cortisol diurnal rhythm, with normal urinary free cortisol levels and a normal short (overnight) dexamethasone suppression test (0.3 mg/m^2 orally at midnight measuring 8 a.m. plasma cortisol) will reasonably exclude the diagnosis. A 2-day low dose (6 mg/kg every 6 h) dexamethasone suppression test measuring plasma cortisol at 48 h, or urinary free cortisol corrected for creatinine, is necessary if results are equivocal.

Once the diagnosis is established, further differential diagnosis of the cause may also be difficult. Rapidly evolving symptoms, palpable abdominal mass and virilization at any age make adrenal carcinoma most likely and this is relatively common in infancy, but generally diagnosis depends on imaging techniques (e.g. adrenal ultrasound, pituitary and adrenal CT scanning, adrenal iodocholesterol scintigraphy) and further dynamic hormone tests (e.g. response to metyrapone, high dose dexamethasone, CRF). Diagnostic algorithms are available[292] although investigation should be carried out in specialist centers.

Treatment depends on the cause and may be medical, surgical (to pituitary or adrenals), radiotherapy or radioactive implants. Medical treatment (e.g. with drugs blocking cortisol biosynthesis or GC antagonists) is of value in many patients prior to surgery, if inoperable lesions are found and in Cushing's disease. In virtually all situations, however, treatment is urgent because of the progressive and severe natural course untreated.

Hyperaldosteronism

Primary mineralocorticoid (MC) hypersecretion is very rare in childhood and usually due to a zona glomerulosa adenoma (Conn syndrome)[355] or bilateral hyperplasia. There is sodium retention and hypertension with hypokalemia, renin suppression and hyperaldosteronism which fails to suppress with dexamethasone. In addition to hypertension, there may be muscle weakness, polyuria and impaired growth. Treatment is medical (long-term spironolactone) in hyperplasia and surgical in adenoma.

Familial forms of hyperaldosteronism

Dexamethasone-suppressible hyperaldosteronism is clinically and biochemically indistinguishable from primary hyperaldosteronism but aldosterone levels suppress rapidly on dexamethasone. Hypertension can be controlled by GC therapy. Autosomal dominant inheritance (not HLA linked) has been proposed.[356] *Bartter's syndrome*[357] is discussed in Chapter 16. *Apparent mineralocorticoid excess (AME) syndrome* is often familial – aldosterone levels are low and there is no evidence for over-production of other MCs. The pathogenesis is now known to be primary *11beta-hydroxysteroid dehydrogenase (11betaOHSD) deficiency* resulting in defective cortisol metabolism to cortisone. The resulting prolongation of cortisol half-life and bioactivity may result in sufficient MC activity to cause hypertension. Diagnosis depends on the finding of a raised (> 1) ratio of the main urinary metabolite of cortisol (tetrahydrocortisol, THF) to that of cortisone (THE) on gas chromatography, in association with low renin hypertension and normal or low aldosterone levels.

11betaOHSD is a widely distributed enzyme which exists in two types – type II is found in the placenta and distal renal nephron, is NAD dependent and converts the (active) glucocorticoid cortisol (F) to (inactive) cortisone (E) (Fig. 13.54). The mineralocorticoid receptor (MR) has little affinity for E whereas aldosterone cannot be inactivated in this way and retains full access to the MR. Increased availability and binding of cortisol at the MR at the renal distal tubule is the currently accepted pathophysiological mechanism underlying AME.

11betaOHSD may be of wider importance than simply in the etiology of AME. It is plentiful in the placenta and could be important in protecting the fetus from maternal cortisol. Epidemiological evidence suggests that small fetuses are more likely in adulthood to develop hypertension and other cardiovascular diseases and type 2 diabetes mellitus.[36,37,358] There is also epidemiological evidence that babies most at risk of subsequent hypertension are those born small with large placentae.[37] In rats, increased 11betaOHSD activity is associated with increased fetal

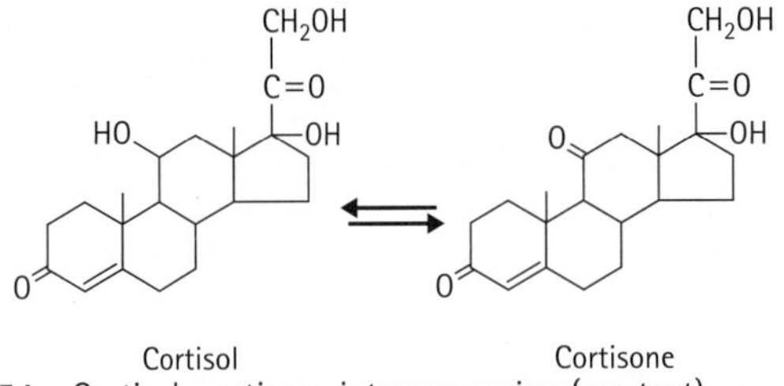

Fig. 13.54 Cortisol–cortisone interconversion (see text).

weight, decreased activity with large placentae. It is speculated that the growth-retarded human fetus has been exposed to excessive cortisol in utero due to relative placental 11betaOHSD deficiency which could reflect placental and fetal growth and that this has long lasting effects (e.g. adult hypertension) by imprinting via brain receptor or neurochemical mechanisms.[24]

Secondary hyperaldosteronism may be due to various causes, most importantly renin-secreting tumors either of the juxtaglomerular apparatus or from ectopic sites such as pancreatic adenocarcinoma. Renin levels are very high.

Pseudohypoaldosteronism due to end-organ resistance to aldosterone is characterized by high levels of urinary aldosterone metabolites which distinguish it from 18-hydroxylase and dehydrogenase deficiencies. Clinical presentation is identical and it is discussed under sodium losing states (see below).

Insufficiency

Adrenocortical hypofunction may result from primary adrenal disorders or may be secondary to hypothalamo–pituitary disorders. Hypofunction may be complete or affect specific functions – GC, MC or androgen biosynthesis. Chronic conditions may present with dramatic symptoms relating to acute adrenal insufficiency ('Addisonian crisis') but may remain asymptomatic and diagnosis may be long delayed. Causes are listed in Table 13.18.

Congenital adrenal hypoplasia

After CAH, this is the commonest neonatal cause of adrenal hypofunction. Sporadic cases are associated with anencephaly or other congenital (e.g. renal and cardiac) malformations and maternal pre-eclampsia. Familial forms are sex-linked or autosomal recessive. Adrenocortical failure presents with adrenal hypoplasia or atrophy – combined adrenal autopsy weight < 1g or < 1% of total body weight is characteristic. It is a rare cause of low maternal estriol levels during pregnancy.

Histological findings are heterogeneous but of three main types: (1) primary (cytomegalic) – a rare form in males, with poorly differentiated cortex, disordered architecture and giant cells; (2) secondary (anencephalic) – the commonest in sporadic and familial cases – the fetal zone is reduced or absent but definitive cortex is well differentiated, mimicking the appearance in anencephalics; (3) miniature, comprising about one-third of cases – the glands are small but normally differentiated.

All three types occur sporadically.

Two hereditary forms have been characterized: (1) autosomal recessive, usually associated with the miniature histological type; (2) X-linked, usually associated with the cytomegalic form and affecting boys. This type is now known to be due to mutations in the DAX-1 gene – DAX-1 is a member of the orphan nuclear hormone receptor family expressed in the adrenal gland, gonads, ventromedial hypothalamus and pituitary gonadotrophs.[2,359] There is an association with hypogonadotrophic hypogonadism and with X-linked glycerol kinase deficiency.[360]

Table 13.18 Important causes of adrenocortical hypofunction

Cause
Primary complete (glucocorticoids/mineralocorticoids/androgens)
Congenital adrenal hypoplasia
Lipoid adrenal hyperplasia (cholesterol desmolase deficiency)
Addison's disease
Adrenal apoplexy (Waterhouse–Friderichsen syndrome)
Adrenal hemorrhage/cysts
Adrenoleukodystrophy
Autoimmune multiple endocrinopathy syndromes
Primary selective – glucocorticoids
Congenital adrenal hyperplasia (21-hydroxylase, 17alpha-hydroxylase and 11beta-hydroxylase deficiencies)
Iatrogenic
Hereditary unresponsiveness to ACTH
Primary selective – mineralocorticoids
Pseudohypoaldosteronism
Aldosterone biosynthetic defect (18-hydroxylase and 18-dehydrogenase deficiency)
Primary selective – androgens
17,20-desmolase deficiency
Secondary
Iatrogenic (glucocorticoid therapy)
Hypothalamopituitary dysfunction
Panhypopituitarism
Isolated ACTH deficiency
Craniopharyngioma
Structural midline defects

In all types and forms, clinical presentation is within the first few hours or days of life with vomiting, diarrhea, apnea, hypoglycemia with convulsions, hyponatremic dehydration, hyperkalemia and metabolic acidosis. Plasma cortisol and aldosterone levels are very low with high renin. ACTH levels are very high (c.f. adrenal failure secondary to pituitary disorders but not differentiating it from CAH). In karyotypic females it is indistinguishable from cholesterol desmolase deficiency but other forms of CAH can be identified as described above. Treatment is analogous to that of salt losing CAH. Prognosis was poor but is now much improved, particularly in those surviving the first few days.

Familial GC deficiency (hereditary unresponsiveness to ACTH)

Onset is after the first year, sometimes with recurring hypoglycemia but often merely with a history of prostration during intrinsically mild intercurrent illness. There is hyperpigmentation and tall stature is common.[361] Inheritance is probably autosomal recessive. Pathogenesis is unknown but may be degenerative – the glomerulosa is broad but fasciculata and reticularis are reduced to a fibrous band.

There is a defect in cortisol production with high ACTH levels, and also diminished adrenal androgen secretion implicating a significant role for ACTH in the control of adrenal androgen secretion. MC production is normal under basal conditions but may not remain so, making the distinction from Addison's disease particularly difficult. Treatment is with GC which must be increased during severe intercurrent illness.

Addison's disease[362]

This primary chronic form of adrenal insufficiency is rare in childhood affecting ~ 1 in 10 000. Hypoadrenalism much more commonly results from corticosteroid medication suppressing the pituitary–adrenal axis (see below). Variations in incidence – historically, geographically and in age of onset – probably represent changes in the epidemiology of the primary causes of adrenal damage and failure: until the 1950s, tuberculosis was overwhelmingly the commonest cause but 20 years later accounted for only about 1 in 5 UK cases.

The commonest cause is now autoimmune (AI) adrenal disease. As with other AI diseases there is a familial incidence and female preponderance. Adrenalitis is characterized by lymphocyte infiltration and adrenal microsomal and mitochondrial autoantibodies are found. The medulla is unaffected. There are associations with other autoimmune conditions including hypoparathyroidism (in about 1 in 3 cases) and mucocutaneous candidiasis [polyglandular autoimmune disease (PGAD) type 1], thyroid disease and/or diabetes mellitus (PGAD type 2) and a range of other autoimmune endocrinopathies (PGAD type 4).[321] Antibody titers are generally low, decrease further with age and do not correlate with the severity of the endocrinopathies. Cell-mediated (T-lymphocyte) processes are more likely to be responsible for the adrenal cortical destruction. Familial (autosomal recessive) occurrence probably relates to the inheritance of the underlying tendency to AI disease – there is an association with HLA-A1, -A3 or -B8.

There is GC and MC deficiency which may not develop simultaneously. In childhood, presenting features are usually hypoglycemia, progressive lassitude and muscle weakness, gastrointestinal disturbances (including constipation or diarrhea, vomiting and abdominal pain), associated with mild hyperpigmentation (classically of buccal and vaginal mucosa, nipples and palmar creases and pressure areas – axillae and groin, due to pituitary beta-lipotropin secretion). In practice, pigmentation may simply appear as excellent suntan or 'dirt' over extensor surfaces exposed to friction (e.g. knees, knuckles, elbows).

Major symptoms result from cortisol deficiency and consequent high plasma ACTH elevation. Glycogen stores are low – severe hypoglycemia may occur during fasting or intercurrent stress or illness. Hyponatremia results from aldosterone deficiency and reduced plasma volume induced vasopressin secretion causing water retention.

Characteristic laboratory findings are hyponatremia, hyperkalemia, raised urea, fasting hypoglycemia and anemia. Basal cortisol, aldosterone and adrenal androgen levels are commonly normal but with raised ACTH levels. Cortisol levels do not rise 60 or 120 minutes after a 'short' ACTH test (i.v. 1,24-ACTH 500 ng/1.73 m^2) – although the sensitivity of this test is debatable[354,363] – or after i.m. ACTH 25 mg/m^2 (8-hourly for 3 days). Low T4 with raised TSH levels may be found but often correct rapidly with GC treatment without thyroxine. Adrenal autoantibodies are characteristically present even before clinical onset and should lead to regular testing of adrenal function in patients with other AI disorders or siblings of affected individuals.

Acute *'Addisonian' crisis* may occur as the presenting feature in a previously unsuspected case precipitated by intercurrent illness or stress. There is hypotension (otherwise uncommon in children with Addison's disease), dehydration, prostration and collapse, with hypoglycemia and the classical electrolyte disturbances described above, superimposed on symptoms and signs of the precipitating cause. Treatment with intravenous hydrocortisone and plasma or normal saline with 5 or 10% dextrose is urgent. Intravenous or intramuscular hydrocortisone must be continued whilst oral GC replacement is started. With adequate sodium replacement, MC treatment is not usually necessary acutely.

GC therapy must be increased two- to threefold during stress such as significant infection or general anesthesia which could otherwise precipitate hypoglycemia and collapse. Instruction should be given in the use of home blood glucose monitoring strips and injectable hydrocortisone provided for home use in case the child is vomiting or becomes rapidly ill at home. A MedicAlert bracelet or talisman should be worn.

Long-term treatment is with oral hydrocortisone, usually 10–15 $mg/m^2/24$ h – the dose individually adjusted based on disappearance of symptoms, normal growth and skeletal maturation and normal diurnal ACTH levels. MC dosage (fludrocortisone 0.1–0.15 $mg/m^2/24$ h) is less critical provided it is adequate and assessed as in salt losing CAH. Treatment must be life-long. Adrenal androgen therapy is unnecessary in childhood but a mild androgenic preparation may improve libido and pubic hair growth in adolescent and adult women. It is usually considered that puberty is normal in timing and progression (cf. congenital adrenal hypoplasia). Prognosis is normal in terms of health and life span presupposing optimal prevention and treatment of acute crises.

Sodium losing states

These may be due to renal disease (e.g. dysplasia, tubular disease, Bartter's syndrome), or adrenal insufficiency. Adrenal urinary sodium wasting is characterized by hyperkalemia and due to defective aldosterone biosynthesis (congenital adrenal hypoplasia, salt wasting forms of CAH – see above – or isolated aldosterone biosynthetic defects) or impaired action at the renal tubule (pseudohypoaldosteronism).

Isolated defects of aldosterone biosynthesis may result from defective 18-hydroxylation or 18-dehydrogenation in conversion of corticosterone to aldosterone (see Fig. 13.50). Both are due to deficiency of corticosterone methyloxidase (CMO) which converts corticosterone to 18-hydroxycorticosterone – defective hydroxylation is known as CMO I, defective dehydrogenation as CMO II.

Inheritance is autosomal recessive. Presentation is with marked salt wasting, hyperkalemia and failure to thrive usually in early infancy. GC and androgen function are normal. Although, as in 21OH deficiency, there can be self-regulation of salt intake and proximal renal tubular maturation, the salt wasting tendency is life-long and MC replacement should be for life.

Pseudohypoaldosteronism is due to a primary renal tubular sodium/potassium ATPase defect. The effects of aldosterone are mediated largely through activation of the epithelial sodium channel, and inactivating mutations of this channel lead to pseudohypoaldosteronism with signs of mineralocorticoid deficiency. Clinical presentation is identical to the 18-oxidation (CMO) defects (see above) but aldosterone is markedly elevated and MC therapy ineffective as the proximal renal tubule is unresponsive to its action. Treatment is with sodium supplements. Transient pseudohypoaldosteronism has been reported with the renal tubular resistance to aldosterone secondary to renal disease.[364]

Adrenoleukodystropy (ALD)

Various uncommon associations between chronic adrenal insufficiency and progressive brain demyelinization are described with differing inheritance[365] but have in common the abnormal accumulation of saturated unbranched or monosaturated very long chain fatty acids due to a defect in their catabolism. The ALD gene has been identified and maps to the long arm of the X chromosome (Xq28).[366] Adrenal insufficiency is secondary to cortical destruction – treatment is with GC and MC. The neurological disorder is progressive – these and related conditions (e.g. Zellweger syndrome) are further discussed in Chapter 20.

Other causes of acute adrenal insufficiency include adrenal destruction, e.g. hemorrhage due to birth trauma (see Ch. 10), and Waterhouse–Friderichsen syndrome (sepsis and collapse, often associated with meningococcemia).

Steroid withdrawal

Most commonly, adrenal crisis results from abrupt withdrawal of GC medication when the axis is suppressed from chronic GC administration (oral, inhaled, intranasal or topical) or failure to increase GC during severe intercurrent illness or stress (see above). Alternate day GC causes less hypothalamo–pituitary–adrenal axis suppression and appears more growth sparing.[69] ACTH treatment is associated with more rapid current growth than is high dose GC, but this probably results from additional secondary adrenal androgen secretion and, if bone age advances disproportionately rapidly, ultimate stature may be just as impaired.

Tumors

Adrenal cortical tumors are rare in children. Virilizing tumors[367] are relatively commoner than feminizing or non-secreting tumors and are usually carcinomas rather than adenomas although their malignancy can be difficult to determine. They are histologically identical to those causing Cushing's syndrome but differ in secretory pattern and thus clinical manifestations. Predominantly androgen hypersecretion produces pseudoprecocious puberty – tall stature with growth acceleration and precocious pubic and axillary hair; in boys growth of the penis with prepubertal size testes, in girls clitoromegaly and labial enlargement. Treatment other than by surgical removal is disappointing and the prognosis often poor in any case.

THE ADRENAL MEDULLA

The medulla comprises cells of neuroectodermal origin which synthesize and secrete catecholamines, hormones containing a dihydroxylated phenolic ring. The most active compounds, adrenaline and noradrenaline, are both secreted by the medulla and noradrenaline is also produced in sympathetic ganglion cells.

Catecholamine biosynthesis

Catecholamines are synthesized (Fig. 13.55) from dietary tyrosine and tyrosine converted from phenylalanine by liver hydroxylation. Tyrosine is converted to dihydroxyphenylalanine (DOPA) in brain and sympathetic tissue as well as adrenal medulla. There is then conversion to dihydroxyphenylethylamine (dopamine) and to noradrenaline and, only in the adrenal medulla and the organ of Zuckerkandl at the aortic bifurcation, to adrenaline. Catabolism and excretion (Fig. 13.55) is via vanillylmandelic acid (VMA) and homovanillic acid (HVA), urinary markers for catecholamine hypersecretion. Hypoglycemia, hypoxia, hypovolemia and exercise stimulate catecholamine release. Adrenaline has alpha- and beta-adrenergic effects but noradrenaline is mainly alpha-adrenergic. Vasoconstriction is alpha receptor mediated; cardiac stimulation is via the beta receptor. Dopaminergic effects also occur.

Hypofunction

Adrenomedullary hypofunction is seldom important clinically. Adrenomedullary unresponsiveness is a rare cause of hypoglycemia in children but might be found less infrequently if catecholamines were measured more often during hypoglycemia. Sweating and pallor do not occur. The disorder may be of primarily hypothalamic origin as adrenocortical responsiveness may also be impaired and there is an association with perinatal problems.

In familial dysautonomia (Riley–Day syndrome), an autosomal recessive condition commonest in Ashkenazi Jews, there is

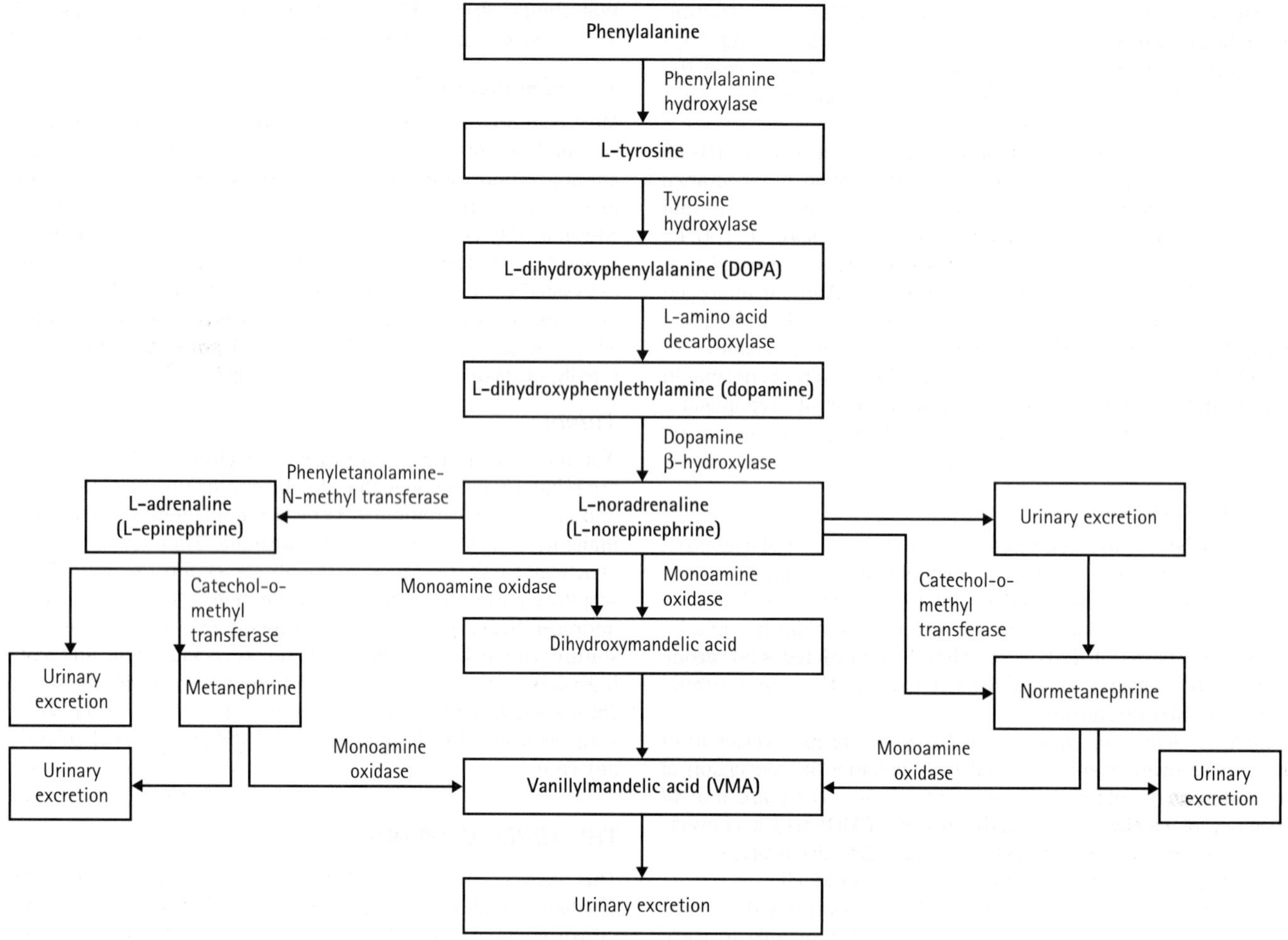

Fig. 13.55 Catecholamine biosynthesis and metabolism.

disturbed autonomic function due to dopamine-beta-hydroxylase deficiency resulting in impaired noradrenaline biosynthesis. Urinary VMA is decreased and urinary levels of HVA, a dopamine metabolite, are high. There is impaired swallowing in infancy with aspiration pneumonia, excessive sweating and salivation, defective lacrimation, labile BP, indifference to pain, loss of taste buds and corneal insensitivity and ulceration. Treatment is symptomatic and the majority die in childhood.

Hyperfunction

Catecholamine hypersecretion is usually associated with hypertension due to a neural crest catecholamine-secreting tumor – pheochromocytoma, neuroblastoma, ganglioblastoma or ganglioneuroma, although the mechanism of hypertension in neuroblastoma patients may be renovascular in origin – and is discussed below.

ENDOCRINE HYPERTENSION

IMPORTANCE OF HYPERTENSION IN CHILDHOOD

The majority of children with higher than average blood pressure (BP) for age are part of a normal spectrum and those above the 95th centile will, in general, come within the category of essential hypertension although many will simply be obese.[368] BP tracking occurs from an early age in normal children – there are steeper rises in normal levels from ~ 7 years of age. The pathogenesis of essential hypertension is poorly understood – primary endocrine abnormalities seem unlikely to be of paramount significance. Until pathogenesis is clearer, preventive measures aimed at children in the upper BP centiles will remain controversial. Mass BP screening of children is probably unjustified.[369]

In contrast, children with sustained and very high BP are likely to have hypertension secondary to specific, and treatable, causes – overwhelmingly (~ 90%) renal disease (see Ch. 16). Diagnosis and treatment are urgent because, in this group, there is high morbidity and mortality from untreated hypertension. Too few ill children have BP measured. Regular measurements should be made in those with renal disease or diabetes and if previously high BP has been found.[369]

Endocrine hypertension usually results from corticosteroid excess (with low renin levels, c.f. renal causes) or, less commonly, from catecholamine excess.

ENDOCRINE CAUSES OF HYPERTENSION

Corticosteroid excess

Congenital adrenal hyperplasia (CAH)

Some patients with 11betaOH deficiency and all with 17OH deficiency are hypertensive from ACTH-stimulated mineralocorticoid overproduction secondary to impaired cortisol biosynthesis. In both, excessive DOC levels are generally thought to be responsible for the hypertension (but see above). Appropriate GC treatment returns BP to normal.

Primary and familial forms of hyperaldosteronism

Although rare, their study has increased understanding of mechanisms which may have much wider significance (see above).

Cushing's syndrome

Hypertension is common in children with Cushing's syndrome but BP may be only moderately elevated. Its etiology is multifactorial including the significant mineralocorticoid effect of excessive cortisol secretion, increased renin substrate and, perhaps, increased vascular reactivity to vasoconstrictors (see above).

Exogenous excessive administration of glucocorticoid is a much commoner cause of hypertension than any of the above.

Catecholamine excess

Pheochromocytomas are rare causes of secondary childhood hypertension which develop from chromaffin cells. Two-thirds are from the adrenal medulla but they can also arise from the sympathetic chain in the abdomen, the mediastinum or the neck. They are usually sporadic but may be familial and associated with MEN1 and MEN2 and von Hippel–Lindau syndrome (pheochromocytoma, retinal hemangioblastoma, renal cysts and carcinoma) or neurofibromatosis. The tumors can be bilateral and multiple. In childhood, hypertension is nearly always sustained rather than paroxysmal and headaches, sweating, nausea and vomiting common. There may be visual disturbances, abdominal pain, polydipsia and polyuria, convulsions and acrocyanosis.

Diagnosis depends on raised plasma catecholamine levels and increased urinary excretion of catecholamines and their metabolites (metanephrines, VMA and HVA). Repeated collections and estimations may be necessary. Localization of the tumor(s) may be possible by non-invasive techniques [ultrasound, CT scan, ^{131}I- or ^{23}I-metaiodobenzylguanidine (MIBG) scintigraphy].

If invasive techniques (e.g. arteriography or vena caval catecholamine sampling) are planned there must be full alpha- and beta-sympathetic blockade, careful BP monitoring and drugs which will acutely lower BP should be immediately available. Blockade is necessary preoperatively to prevent severe hypertension, hypotension and dysrhythmias during definitive surgical removal. Complete surgical removal results in BP normalization and, usually, 'cure' – only 5–10% are malignant. Analogous pharmacological blockade is necessary in children with hypertension associated with neuroblastoma.

ENDOCRINE CONSEQUENCES FOR SURVIVORS OF CANCER

Long-term effects of radiotherapy (RT) and chemotherapy (CT) on growth and endocrine function have become more obvious and important as survival following childhood cancers has improved. The incidence of childhood cancer is 100–130 per 10^6 per annum and 1 in 600 children under the age of 15 years will develop cancer which is now curable in 65–70%. One in 1000 young adults is now a childhood cancer survivor. Leukemia (predominantly lymphoblastic) makes up approximately one-third of childhood cancers and brain and spinal tumors about one-quarter. Treatment-induced late effects are potentially manifested in a number of areas including growth and puberty, endocrine dysfunction, infertility, cognitive dysfunction and the risk of second tumors.

The risk relates to treatment modality and the challenge remains to further improve survival rates whilst reducing the incidence and severity of treatment-induced late effects. These can be anticipated and monitored to optimize prevention and treatment – ideally through multidisciplinary follow-up involving pediatric oncologist, pediatric endocrinologist, pediatric neurologist, radiation oncologist, pediatric neurosurgeon, clinical psychologist and social worker.

Adverse effects on growth may result from radiation-induced hormone deficiencies, impaired spinal growth from spinal RT (and from CT), hypothyroidism from spinal RT, precocious or delayed puberty from abnormal GT secretion, gonadal failure (puberty/fertility) from RT or CT, and problems with nutrition or obesity.[370]

At diagnosis of acute lymphoblastic leukemia (ALL), there is already low bone turnover with reduced levels of collagen formation and resorption markers (PICP, PIIINP and ICTP). In remission, there is further bone synthesis suppression (low levels of PICP and PIIINP) and growth suppression[371,372] which probably relates to glucocorticoid (prednisolone) and high dose methotrexate therapies. This suggests that there may be an increased risk of long term osteoporosis and fractures. Comparison between countries suggests that the degree of growth impairment is proportional to the intensity of the CT regimen. CT has a disproportionate effect on spinal growth impairment perhaps because of the large numbers of spinal epiphyses. High dose cranial irradiation is associated with a significant potential height deficit because of the combined effects of precocious puberty and an impaired pubertal growth spurt (see below).

The hormone deficiency effects of RT will depend on the site of irradiation, total dose of irradiation, fractionation schedule and the child's age at treatment. Growth impairment will result from RT to the hypothalamo–pituitary axis (the hypothalamus is more radiosensitive than the pituitary and the GH axis the most radiosensitive followed by the gonadal axis). RT to the spine (in the treatment of medulloblastomas, ependymomas, germinomas) will result in late pubertal growth failure (the spinal growth spurt occurs towards the end of secondary sexual development) and primary hypothyroidism due to a direct effect on the thyroid gland. CT (glucocorticoids, methotrexate) will also impair growth (see above). Tumor recurrence should always be considered as a cause of growth failure in these patients.

RT doses of > 24 Gy will be associated with precocious (especially in young girls) or delayed puberty and GH deficiency within 5 years. Very RT high doses (e.g. ~ 54 Gy used in craniopharyngioma) will cause GH deficiency within 2 years. Lower doses (< 24 Gy) may be associated with precocious puberty, an impaired pubertal growth spurt due to relative GH insufficiency in that context and reduced pubertal spinal growth. Total body irradiation (TBI) used as preparation for bone marrow transplantation (~ 7.5–15.75 Gy) may also be associated with pubertal GH insufficiency, thyroid dysfunction and a radiation-induced skeletal dysplasia.

The same total dose of RT given in several fractions minimizes GH deficiency and growth impairment and fractionated TBI produces less damage to normal tissues. Younger children (especially girls) are more likely to develop precocious puberty and a pubertal growth spurt can be mistaken for 'catch-up' growth. Obesity can normalize growth at the expense of disproportionate BA advance and reduced height prognosis.

Clinical growth assessment should consist of the regular measurement of sitting and standing height, skinfolds, weight and calculation of BMI, and puberty staging. Laboratory assessment (baseline free thyroxine, cortisol, testosterone/estradiol, IGF-1, etc.), physiological profiles (GH, GTs, cortisol, etc.) and dynamic tests (insulin hypoglycemia, GnRH, HCG, TRH, synacthen, etc.) will be relevant. Integrating the information as a prelude to appropriate investigation and treatment is an important role for the pediatric endocrinologist in the multidisciplinary team. Much information can be gleaned from careful anthropometry and pubertal assessment in the context of knowledge about the anticancer treatment received so as to minimize investigations in children who have already been through many unpleasant treatments and investigations.

Available treatment modalities include the use of GH for growth failure, pubertal suppression and thyroxine, glucocorticoid and sex steroids as indicated.

If a child has a good prognosis from the underlying condition 2 years from treatment, GH therapy should be given when indicated on biochemical and anthropometric grounds. There is no evidence that GH is associated with reactivation of the primary lesion.[373]

The majority of childhood cancer survivors are fertile. There are low risks of infertility following chemotherapy for Wilms' tumor and ALL and following cranial RT < 24 Gy. Infertility or subfertility is common after CT for Hodgkin's disease RT (TBI, testicular or pelvic). Thus ovarian failure after TBI is common with the risk relating to age at treatment (younger children are at lower risk). Physiological sex steroid replacement therapy improves uterine function (blood flow, endometrial thickness) so that these women could potentially benefit from assisted reproductive technologies. However they have reduced uterine distensibility with increased risk of IUGR and miscarriage or preterm delivery.

In boys, the germinal epithelium is much more sensitive to radiation than Leydig cells – 1.2 Gy to the testis will result in azoospermia, whereas > 20 Gy (in prepuberty) or > 30 Gy (post-puberty) is necessary before Leydig cell function is damaged significantly. Thus spontaneous progression through puberty does not necessarily indicate subsequent fertility.

As part of their monitoring, childhood cancer survivors should have routine assessment of gonadal function. The majority will be fertile and the risk of infertility relates to the treatment received. In some situations hormonal manipulation may restore fertility. Counseling is necessary for young people at high risk of infertility and sperm cryopreservation is available for postpubertal boys. Ovarian cortical strip cryopreservation is one current research technique in girls. Strategies to protect the prepubertal testis from damaging effects of CT or RT are under investigation.

An evidence based guideline for the long term follow-up of child and adult survivors of childhood cancer has been developed.[373a]

THE PANCREAS AND CARBOHYDRATE METABOLISM

PANCREATIC MORPHOLOGY

The pancreas forms by proliferation of endodermal duodenal epithelium at the end of the fourth week of development as separate dorsal and ventral pancreatic buds. The ventral bud migrates posteriorly from a position close to the primitive liver bud and bile duct to lie in close contact with the dorsal bud. The duct systems and parenchyme subsequently fuse and the definitive (common) pancreatic duct is formed by the distal part of the dorsal and entire ventral duct. Failed fusion is a common normal variant. The pancreas is supplied by the splenic and superior mesenteric arteries and drained by the splenic and superior mesenteric veins into the portal vein. The islets of Langerhans, the pancreatic endocrine units, develop from the parenchymatous pancreatic tissue during the third month, are scattered throughout the gland and secrete insulin by about 5 months. There is a rich blood supply to and rich sympathetic and parasympathetic (vagal) innervation in contact with the islet cells.

Exocrine pancreatic function is discussed in Chapter 17. The main endocrine secretions, insulin and glucagon, are intimately concerned in glucose homeostasis. Insulin is secreted from islet beta cells, glucagon from alpha cells. There are also delta cells (thought to secrete somatostatin and perhaps gastrin) and a fourth cell type, F cells, which secrete pancreatic polypeptide (PP). The physiological importance of PP is unclear although it is secreted in response to food. Somatostatin's role in this context is in downregulating the rate of entry of nutrients from the gut by delaying gastric emptying, decreasing duodenal motility, altering splanchnic blood flow, suppressing pancreatic exocrine and endocrine (insulin and glucagon) secretion and gastrin and secretin production from the gut. Thus integration of islet cell hormone and portal vein hormonal secretions is influenced by nutritional state, extrapancreatic hormones (especially gastro-intestinal inhibitory polypeptide – GIP) and autonomic input.

INSULIN

Insulin is formed in beta cells from a 9000 molecular weight precursor, proinsulin, itself derived from a larger polypeptide precursor, preproinsulin. Proinsulin is an 86 amino acid linear molecule with three peptide chains – A, B and (intermediate) C (Fig. 13.56). A and B peptides are joined by two disulfide bonds. C peptide is cleaved in Golgi apparatus by proteolytic enzymes leaving the covalently bonded A and B peptides (chains) – the definitive insulin molecule (MW 6000) (Fig. 13.56) – stored in cytoplasmic granules. Insulin and C peptide are thus present in granules in equimolar concentrations and expelled together into the draining capillary (emiocytosis). Circulating C peptide is a marker for endogenous insulin secretion, disappearing at the end of the partial remission ('honeymoon') period of diabetes mellitus.

Insulin is the major metabolic hormone. Factors modulating secretion include glucose, amino acids, glucagon, secretin, gastrin and GIP. During feeding, rising blood glucose and amino acid concentrations stimulate release – there are two phases in the response, a short-lived burst as preformed insulin is released and a slower and more sustained phase of de novo synthesis.

Insulin stimulates glucose uptake by muscle and fat cells, its conversion to glycogen and triglycerides and amino acid incorporation into muscle protein. Lipolysis, glycogenolysis, gluconeogenesis and muscle breakdown are inhibited and hepatic glycogen synthesis stimulated. The net effect is a fall in blood glucose associated with low circulating levels of free fatty acids, ketone bodies and branched chain amino acids. As plasma glucose levels fall below normal (e.g. during starvation), insulin secretion diminishes and secretion of glucagon and other hormones which increase blood glucose levels (catecholamines, GH, glucocorticoids) is stimulated ('counter-regulation') leading to stabilization of blood glucose levels. Insulin is mainly degraded in liver and kidney but also in pancreas and other tissues.

GLUCAGON

Glucagon is a single chain 29 amino acid polypeptide (MW 3485) secreted by islet alpha cells. Plasma levels increase during starvation – falling blood glucose levels are probably the major release stimulus but protein ingestion stimulates secretion through release of gut hormones such as pancreozymin. Anxiety and exercise increase secretion via sympathetic pathways. Somatostatin suppresses secretion.

Glucagon increases glucose levels by liver glycogenolysis and gluconeogenesis, stimulates fat cell lipolysis (increasing free fatty acids and ketones) and insulin, catecholamine, GH and calcitonin

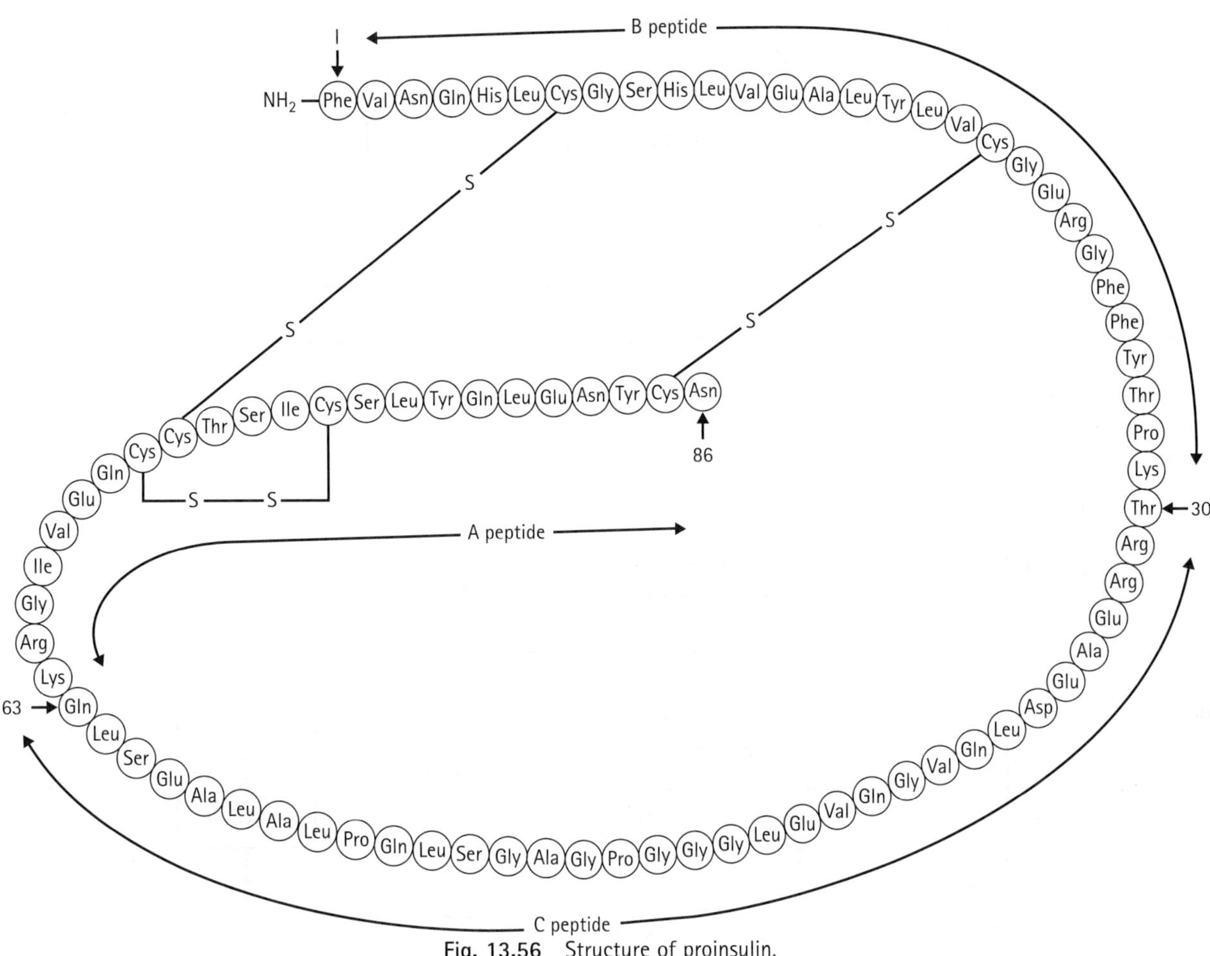

Fig. 13.56 Structure of proinsulin.

release. Circulatory half-life is only about 10 min – degradation is mainly in liver and kidney.

Integration

Interaction between insulin, glucagon and other counter-regulatory hormones is crucial in glucose and protein homeostasis, to provide sufficient and constant supply of glucose substrate to brain and for growth and energy requirements in infancy and childhood. The liver is particularly important for glucose homeostasis – liver gluconeogenesis, glycogenolysis and glycogen synthesis are summarized in Figure 13.57.

During *starvation*, two-thirds of daily glucose production is directly utilized by the brain as an energy source, insulin secretion falls and counter-regulation follows. This produces increased proteolysis, lipolysis, glycogenolysis and gluconeogenesis with reduced tissue glucose uptake resulting in increasing blood glucose levels. There are increased plasma fatty acids (used as an additional energy source), glycerol, ketone bodies and branched chain amino acids associated with high levels of glucagon, cortisol, GH and catecholamines and low or undetectable insulin levels (Fig. 13.58).

In the *fed* state, circulating glucose stimulates insulin secretion and suppresses counter-regulation. Proteolysis, lipolysis, glycogenolysis and gluconeogenesis are suppressed, tissue glucose uptake increases and blood glucose levels fall (Fig. 13.58).

Understanding glucose homeostasis is necessary for rational differential diagnosis, investigation and treatment of hypoglycemia.

Surprisingly little is known about overnight blood glucose levels in normal children. Cyclical variation, periodicity 80–120 min, has been observed with a gradual fall until wakening with no evidence of a dawn blood glucose rise. Maintenance of normoglycemia is likely to be mediated through free fatty acid metabolism with glycogen stores being relatively protected overnight and available for any acute hypoglycemic crisis.

DIABETES MELLITUS (DM)

DM is defined as a metabolic disorder of multiple etiology characterized by chronic hyperglycemia with disturbances of carbohydrate, protein and fat metabolism resulting from defects in insulin secretion, insulin action, or both. Consensus guidelines discussing the epidemiology, classification and management details have been published by the International Society for Pediatric and Adolescent Diabetes (ISPAD)[374] and evidence-based guidelines, with a section on diabetes in children and young people, have been published by the Scottish Intercollegiate Guidelines Network.[375]

HISTORICAL CONTEXT

DM was first mentioned (though not by name) in the 'Ebers' papyrus (about 1550 BC). 'Diabetes' (siphon or diuresis) was first used by the Turkish physician Aretaeos of Capadokia (AD 130–200): 'Diabetes is an awkward affection melting down the flesh and limbs into the urine ... patients never stop making water ... life is short and painful ... they

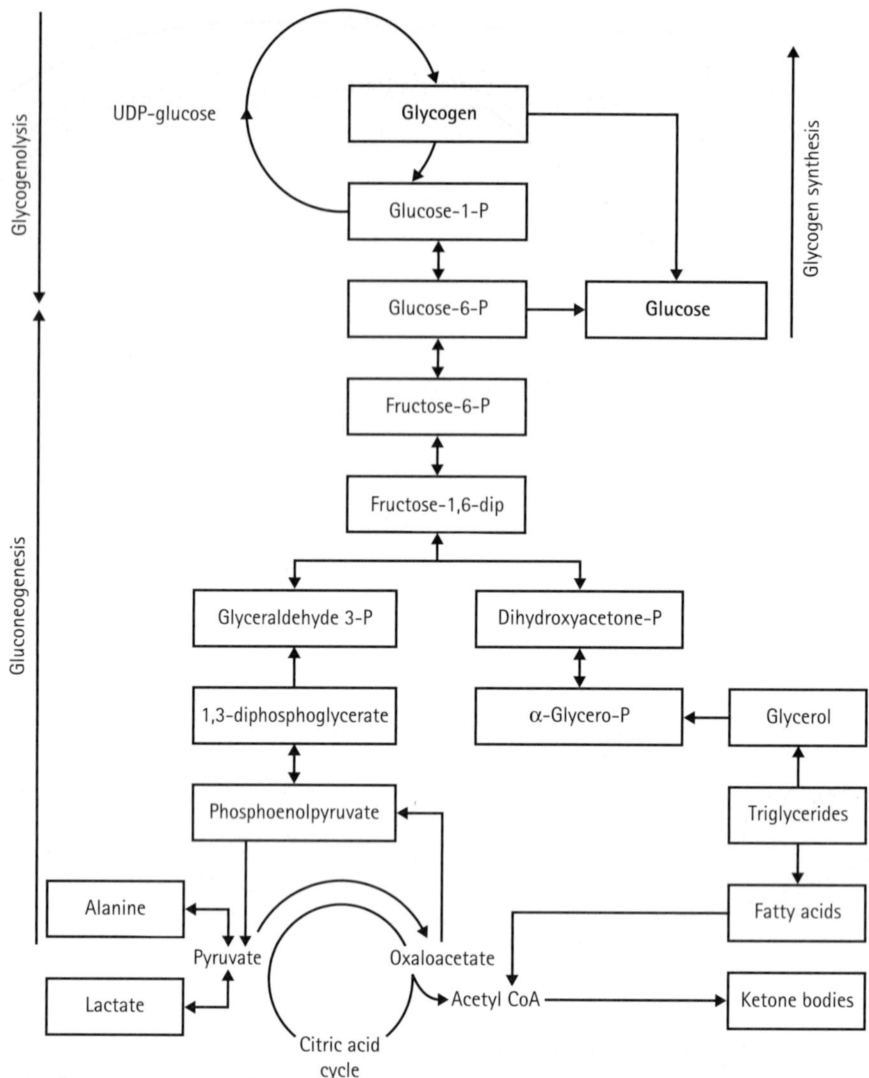

Fig. 13.57 Metabolic pathways of liver gluconeogenesis, glycogenolysis and glycogen synthesis.

are affected with nausea, restlessness and a burning thirst and at no distant term they expire.' (Aretaeos AD 130–200). The sweetness of diabetic urine ('mellitus' = sweet), first mentioned in sixth century AD Indian Vedic literature was rediscovered by Thomas Willis (1684).[376] Matthew Dobson (1776) showed that the sweet taste was due to sugar and that serum also tasted sweet.[377]

For 1500 years it was thought that the kidney's inability to retain water caused diabetes. Von Mering & Minkowski[378] showed that total pancreatectomy in dogs resulted in diabetes mellitus and, within 10 years, islet function was becoming understood and fasting and dietary treatment introduced. The discovery of insulin by Banting et al[379] led to early development of insulin for treatment of human diabetes.

Recognition of the spectrum of diabetes and its manifestations led to a WHO classification: primary diabetes mellitus is insulin dependent (IDDM) – type 1, or non-insulin-dependent (NIDDM) – type 2, irrespective of age of onset.

DM is the commonest metabolic or endocrine disorder in children and adolescents and is almost invariably type 1. In the past, the diagnosis (as opposed to the management) of DM in children and adolescents has not been complex. However the current etiological diversity of DM in the young makes their differential diagnosis very important for determining prognosis and appropriate treatment.[380]

Non-insulin-dependent DM occurs temporarily in the partial remission ('honeymoon') phase of type 1 DM and permanently in type 2 DM, genetic syndromes accompanied by DM, and maturity onset diabetes in the young (MODY). The overall UK prevalence in young people of non-type 1 DM is currently around 3% of the total with type 2 making up less than 0.5%. In a largely Caucasian population, MODY is over 10 times commoner than type 2 DM. However, type 2 DM predominates in areas with large ethnic minority (e.g. Asian Indian) populations.[380]

Typical phenotypic features in type 1, type 2 DM and MODY are summarized in Table 13.19[489] – based on referrals to a specialist genetics of diabetes unit in Exeter, UK,[380] and ISPAD.[374] There is no single phenotypic marker that is pathognomonic for non-type 1 DM making both diagnosis in individual patients and epidemiological study difficult.[380]

TYPE 2 DM

Type 2 DM has become very much commoner in adolescents and children in association with the dramatically rising prevalence of obesity in these age groups. Intrauterine exposures may increase the risk of type 2 DM[36] and a recent further possible intrauterine

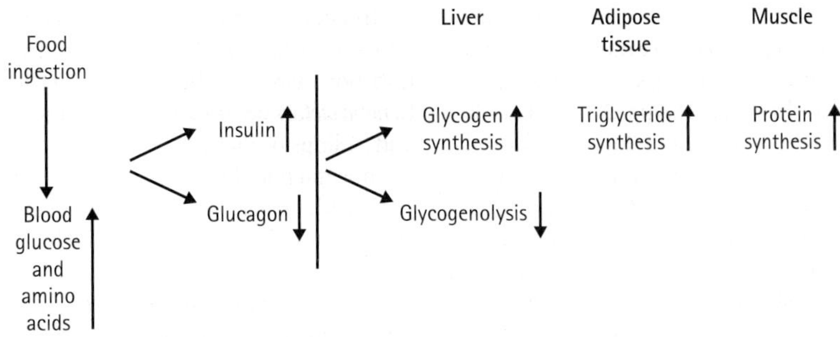

Effects: nitrogen sparing; triglycerides saved for future needs; low circulating levels of ketone bodies, free fatty acids and branched chain amino acids

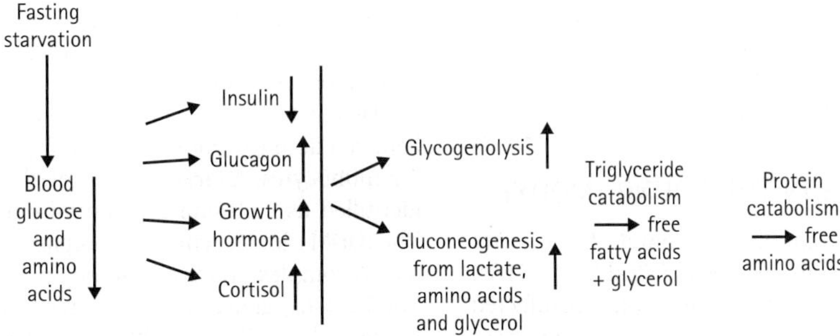

Effects: free fatty acids as energy source; ketone bodies generated from fatty acids; amino acids released by proteolysis for hepatic gluconeogenesis

Fig. 13.58 Metabolic and endocrine characteristics of fed and fasted states.

environmental association is maternal smoking during pregnancy.[381] It is likely that many genes are involved in the etiology of type 2 DM, each contributing a small amount to the overall risk.[382] Certain ethnic indigenous populations seem particularly at risk of type 2 DM (e.g. Pima Indians, Australian Aboriginals, Tonga Islanders). Among 15- to 19-year-old North American Indians, the prevalence of type 2 diabetes per 1000 is now 50.9 for Pima Indians, 4.5 for all US American Indians. From 1967–1976 to 1987–1996, the prevalence increased sixfold for Pima Indian adolescents. Among African–Americans and whites aged 10–19 years in Ohio, USA, type 2 diabetes accounted for 33% of all cases of DM.[383]

Table 13.19 Characteristics of pediatric DM patients (After Hattersley 2000[380], 2001[489])

	Type 1	MODY GCK	MODY HNFalpha-1	Type 2	Diabetes + syndromes
Age of diagnosis in pediatric clinic	11 (0–16)	5 (0–16) = age of testing	15 (4–16)	15 (10–16) usually post-pubertal females	Variable
Severity of glycemia	Progressive 11–50 mmol/L	Mild 5.5–14 mmol/L	Variable, progressive 5–25 mmol/L	Variable 5–25 mmol/L	Variable 5–25 mmol/L
Ketosis	Ketosis prone, insulin dependent by 5 yrs post diagnosis	No ketoacidosis, not insulin dependent	Ketoacidosis rare, not insulin dependent	Ketoacidosis rare, not insulin dependent	Ketosis in DIDMOAD, not in others
Optimal treatment	Insulin	Diet	Sulphonylureas	Metformin	Variable
Parents affected	0–1	1 (often not diagnosed)	1	1–2	Rarely
Obesity	+/-	+/- (5% BMI > 30)	+/- (5% BMI > 30)	++++	Variable + to +++
Acanthosis nigricans	-	-	-	++	Variable
Racial	Low type 2 prevalence	Low type 2 prevalence	Low type 2 prevalence	High type 2 prevalence	All
Islet antibodies	++++	-	-	-	-
Biochemical features		Small increment OGTT	Large increment OGTT, high HDL, low renal threshold	Variable	Low HDL, high TG
Genetic test specificity	+	++++	++++	-	+++

BMI, body mass index; DIDMOAD, DIDMOAD syndrome; GCK, glucokinasel; HDL, high density lipoprotein; HNF, hepatic nuclear factor; MODY, maturity onset diabetes in the young; OGTT, oral glucose tolerance test; TG, thyroglobulin.

In Japanese adolescents, type 2 DM is four times commoner than type 1. In the USA, young people with type 2 DM are most commonly obese girls from minority populations with insulin resistance, acanthosis nigricans and a family history of type 2 DM. This is becoming a major health problem with < 45% of children diagnosed with DM in parts of the USA now having type 2. Currently, in the UK, type 2 DM is also becoming much commoner, especially in early post-pubertal obese girls. There is seldom ketosis at presentation, fasting insulin levels are raised (with low SHBG level[189] – a marker of insulin resistance), and there is often dyslipidemia and hypertension. Chronic microvascular complications are at least as severe and occur as early and rapidly as in type 1 DM.

There can be diagnostic confusion with type 1 and maturity onset diabetes in the young (MODY – see below), but there is, in contrast with type 1, obesity and a stronger family history (an 80% chance of one or both parents having type 2 DM). The obesity and family history do not help the differential diagnosis from MODY where there is a similar family history and age of onset.

MATURITY ONSET DIABETES IN THE YOUNG (MODY)

MODY is a heterogeneous group of autosomal dominantly inherited, young-onset beta-cell disorders (Table 13.19). Characteristically, two or more consecutive generations are affected with individuals diagnosed before 25 years of age. MODY comprises two discrete clinical syndromes (Table 13.19): glucokinase MODY [caused by mutations in the glucokinase (GCK) gene on chromosome 7p, MODY 2] and transcription factor MODY [caused by mutations in the genes encoding hepatocyte nuclear factor (HNF)-1alpha (chromosome 12q, MODY 3 – the commonest form), HNF-1beta (MODY 5), HNF-4alpha (chromosome 20q, MODY 1) and insulin promoter factor (IPF)-1 (MODY 4)].[380]

MODY should be particularly suspected if there are three consecutive generations with DM, insulin requirements persistently < 0.5 U/kg/day and no tendency to ketosis. GCK MODY is mild and non-progressive with hyperglycemia caused by a resetting of the pancreatic glucose sensor. It is treated with diet, and complications are rare. In contrast, transcription factor MODY results in a progressive beta-cell defect with a high incidence of diabetic complications.[384] Sulphonylureas are the treatment of choice for patients with HNF-1alpha mutations and very good control is achievable.[385] HNF-1beta mutations are associated with DM and renal cysts and HNF-1beta has a critical role in renal development.[386] Diagnostic molecular genetic testing is available for the more common MODY genes.

TYPE 1 DM

The remainder of this section refers to type 1 DM unless otherwise stated.

Incidence and Pathogenesis

Prevalence (sum of patients related to total age-related population) and incidence (age-related annual manifestations) show wide variation. A 400-fold variation exists in worldwide incidence rates for type 1 DM – and have yielded intriguing findings: annual incidence rates broadly increase with distance (north and south) from the equator both within Europe (3.7 per 100 000 in France, 45 per 100 000 in Finland) and within quite small distances within countries (about 2-fold higher in Scotland than England and higher in northern Scotland than south).[387] Within individual areas, incidence is higher in whites than non-whites, in boys (M:F ratio about 1.1:1) and increases with age, peaking at adolescence. In many studies in geographically disparate countries an increasing incidence of between 2 and 5% per annum is reported (a rise in 50% over 10 years).

Incidence and prevalence differences reflect the complex interaction of genetic and environmental factors (e.g. temperature, nutrition, viruses, chemical toxins) in the development of diabetes. *Genetic factors* are important: there is an increased incidence in parents and siblings of diabetics – the risk to a sibling is 15- to 50-fold that in the normal population. 12–15% of young people under the age of 15 years with diabetes mellitus have an affected first degree relative[388] and children are three times more likely to develop diabetes if their father has diabetes rather than their mother.[389] Inheritance is likely to be polygenic or multifactorial rather than Mendelian (monogenic). Such genetic factors ('susceptibility genes') modify the risk of diabetes but are neither necessary nor sufficient for disease to develop.

Monozygotic twins are concordant for diabetes five times more frequently than dizygotic twins but the rate is much lower than in type 2 diabetes and a discordance rate of nearly 50% over a 30-year follow-up suggests the importance of environmental factors in clinical manifestation of the genetically determined predisposition.

Type 1 DM is a T cell mediated autoimmune disease involving beta cell damage from inflammatory cytokines and autoaggressive T lymphocytes. A large number of chromosomal regions have been identified as containing potential diabetes susceptibility genes.[390] The IDDM1 locus, which encompasses the major histocompatibility (HLA) complex on chromosome 6p, is the major genetic risk factor. The HLA-DQ genes are the primary susceptibility genes within this region – loci DR3 and DR4 have particularly strong associations and increase the relative risk for developing diabetes between three-fold (DR3) and 14-fold (DR3/DR4 heterozygosity). The IDDM2 locus maps to a variable number of tandem repeats in the insulin gene region on chromosome 11.[390]

Molecular epidemiological studies have demonstrated that DNA sequences coding for the presence of an amino acid other than aspartic acid in the 57th position of the DQB1 gene (non-ASP-57) is highly associated with IDDM susceptibility (much more strongly than for DR3/DR4) in most, but not all racial or ethnic groups.

The HLA identical sibling of a child with type 1 diabetes has about a 90-fold increased risk of developing the disease before 15 years. The risk is hardly increased at all if the sibling is HLA non-identical. Of all type 1 diabetics, 90–98% express DR3, DR4 antigens or both, but less than 1% of healthy subjects with such markers will ever develop diabetes.

Environmental factors are crucial for disease expression and clinical diabetes development and may be either causative or protective.[391] Epidemiological data indicate that such factors operate from early in life. The search for preventable environmental triggers for autoimmune destruction and acute decompensation precipitating clinical diabetes onset (by when > 90% of beta cell function is destroyed) continues.

Viruses can cause diabetes in animals; in humans there is seasonal variation of clinical onset in association with high viral prevalence and a particular association with Coxsackie B4.[392] However, it is known that beta cell destruction, ultimately leading to decompensation and clinical onset of diabetes, has been occurring over many years. A virus or other 'insult' (early exposure to cows' milk protein, chemical toxin, food or cooking product or even stressful life events have been postulated) may, therefore, be responsible for triggering autoimmune (AI) beta cell destruction in genetically susceptible individuals. Relatively acute decompensation, up to many years later, leading to clinical presentation is often due to an intercurrent infection when insulin requirements rise and cannot, by then, be met.

Histopathological studies indicate that AI mechanisms are paramount in diabetes pathogenesis which has implications for its prevention or modification by immunosuppression.

Glutamic acid decarboxylase (GAD) catalyzes the formation of gamma-aminobutyric acid (GABA), which is a major transmitter in the central nervous system but also exerts functions in peripheral organs. Molecular analyses have revealed roles for GAD isoforms in autoimmune human diseases including type 1 DM.[393] Other pancreatic islet cell autoantigens associated with type 1 DM include protein tyrosine phosphatase-like molecules IA-2 (a 979 amino acid transmembrane protein on human chromosome 2q35) and IA-2beta (a 986 on chromosome 7q36). Autoantibodies to IA-2 are detected in 60–80% of newly diagnosed type 1 patients and in less than 2% of controls. In first degree relatives of type 1 patients, the presence of autoantibodies to IA-2 is predictive of type 1 DM and in combination with autoantibodies to glutamic acid decarboxylase the positive predictive value is in the 50% range.[394]

Almost 80% of prediabetic and newly diagnosed patients with type 1 DM are positive for anti-GAD and over 90% of children with newly diagnosed type 1 DM have an autoimmune response to GAD, islet cell autoantibodies (ICA) or IA antibodies, singly or in combination.[395] Thus the presence of ICA at a high titer (> 20 JDF units) predicts a 40–60% risk of developing type 1 DM within the next 5 to 7 years. The presence of multiple autoantibodies increases the risk still further. There is strong association between type 1 diabetes and other AI disease (e.g. thyroid, adrenal, parathyroid).

Recognition of specific genetic, immune and metabolic markers offers prediction of development of diabetes in high risk groups sufficiently early for the prospect of intervention to prevent ongoing beta cell destruction and clinical disease. However, as yet, there is no evidence for effective methods of prevention of type 1 DM.[396] Screening (whether in the general population or in high risk children and young people) is considered unethical and is not recommendable except in the context of randomized trials of prevention therapies strategies (e.g. with specific immunotherapy, oral insulin or nicotinamide) which are currently in progress.[375]

Clinical onset and diagnosis[397]

Although, in retrospect, parents may feel their newly diagnosed diabetic child has not been 'right' for several months with poor appetite and malaise, the clinical onset in most children is usually relatively acute: increasing polyuria (due to osmotic glucose load), secondary polydipsia, weight loss, anorexia and fatigue develop over days or weeks.[374] Some children present particularly acutely with rapid onset of ketoacidosis and coma. This may be commoner in DR3/DR4 heterozygotes,[398] with DR3 patients presenting less acutely.[399] More acute onset has also been reported in younger children[400] perhaps because of lack of awareness by parents or health professionals, or pre-existing enuresis. The urine of any child with secondary enuresis should therefore be tested for glucose.

Once suspected diagnosis is not usually difficult, but too often there is delay because urine is not tested (for glucose and ketones) when a child presents with non-specific symptoms or signs – anorexia, vomiting, abdominal pain, tachypnea (assumed to be 'pneumonia'), vaginal candidiasis, fatigue or irritability, recurrent skin infections.[374] Finding glycosuria or hyperglycemia (random level = 11.1 mmol/L) is an emergency – the child should preferably be seen the same day and certainly within 24 h and never simply referred by letter to an outpatient clinic. If diagnosis and treatment are not prompt, further catabolism may rapidly cause increasing ketosis and acidosis (Fig. 13.59) with coma and death. There is a significant morbidity and mortality in children who present with severe ketoacidosis and dehydration and coma at presentation carries a 12-fold higher risk of death.

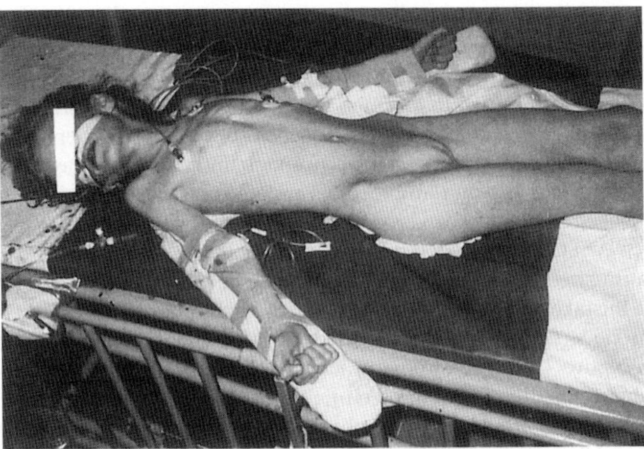

Fig. 13.59 A newly (and 'late') diagnosed diabetic with severe ketoacidosis and dehydration.

If the diagnosis is in doubt, criteria are the same in children as for adults:[401,402]

- symptoms (polyuria, polydypsia or unexplained weight loss) plus random venous plasma glucose = 11.1 mmol/L, *or*
- fasting venous plasma glucose = 7 mmol/L [impaired fasting glycemia (IFG) is indicated by a level = 6.1 and < 7 mmol/L], *or*
- plasma glucose = 11.1 mmol/L at 2 hours after a 75 g oral glucose load (impaired glucose tolerance is indicated by levels of 7.75 mmol/L up to 11.1 mmol/L).

Normal values 2 hours following the glucose load are < 7.75 mmol/L.

In asymptomatic patients, the diagnosis should only be made on the basis of at least two abnormal measurements of significant hyperglycemia on separate days.

Improvements in health education (of parents and professionals) and prompt access to a specialist pediatric unit will help reduce the incidence of severe ketoacidosis. The introduction of an educational poster to primary and secondary schools and private practices in Parma, Italy reduced the incidence of diabetic ketoacidosis (DKA) at presentation from 78 to 12.5%.[403]

Morbidity and mortality could be reduced if specific well-tried, well-understood and adequately supervised management guidelines are followed. An integrated care pathway (ICP) for management of DKA[404] heightens awareness of optimal diabetes management, increases confidence in management by staff and reduces inappropriate treatment variation leading to improvements in clinical practice (see below). Such ICPs are also of potential benefit in other areas of diabetes management (e.g. the management of the newly diagnosed child without ketoacidosis, hypoglycemia, or children undergoing emergency or elective surgery).

Initial management of the child without ketoacidosis

Most children who have developed diabetes have only mild symptoms and are not ketoacidotic. With a network of primary carers (e.g. diabetes community nurses) nearly all such children can be successfully managed at home.

This approach is being increasingly adopted in many UK centers and is cost-effective but may be inappropriate for socially deprived families, rural settings a long way from the hospital or, particularly, in areas where adequate personnel with specialist training are unavailable in the community. Some parents are so distressed at diagnosis that admission is desirable. A home-based program of management and education for children and their families is an appropriate alternative to a hospital-based program[375] but potential benefits of home management – greater acceptance by the family and a quick return to 'normal' family life – can also be achieved if the child's hospital admission is sensitively handled. There is no evidence that either home or hospital initial management and education is superior and the appropriate choice should depend on local circumstances and resources.

Whatever strategy is adopted, several days will be necessary for unhurried education of child and family in basic diabetic care. It is a mistake to try to impart too much early information – upset, anxious, grieving or frightened parents and children are not receptive learners. Simple practical information and instruction about insulin, injection techniques and dietetic principles are important with a positive emphasis that, provided simple guidelines are followed, the child will soon be feeling better than for some weeks and will be able to take part in all the activities enjoyed. Availability of a personal diabetes handbook with written information is helpful. In some centers, before the child leaves hospital, hypoglycemia is induced in the parents' presence (morning insulin is given, breakfast omitted and the child exercised until symptoms occur) so that all can experience the symptoms for the first time in a controlled and supportive environment.

Recognition and treatment of ketoacidosis

A child with ketoacidosis and severe dehydration (Fig. 13.59) is dangerously ill and requires emergency treatment. Vomiting and abdominal pain with tenderness and guarding may mimic an acute abdomen whilst hyperventilation may be misdiagnosed as pneumonia. There may be circulatory collapse, oliguria and coma. Salicylate poisoning should be considered in the differential diagnosis.

In children known to have type 1 DM on insulin, ketoacidosis is usually precipitated by intercurrent infection (fever is not part of DKA), but may occur if too little insulin is given (perhaps because of fear of hypoglycemia), insulin is omitted altogether (e.g. by an emotionally disturbed adolescent) or with menstruation or severe emotional upset. In this group, there may not be pronounced hyperglycemia particularly if insulin has been (correctly) continued or increased but vomiting has led to inadequate carbohydrate (CHO) intake. For this reason, urinary ketones should always be tested for by the established diabetic when there is significant hyperglycemia on home blood glucose testing as metabolic decompensation may be more severe than realized. Near patient blood ketone testing is becoming available and may prove valuable in monitoring the adequacy of treatment[405] and, for example, 'sick day' management at home.

DKA management is facilitated by the use of an integrated care pathway to reduce inappropriate treatment variation leading to improvement in clinical practice.[404] The priority is appropriate *volume repletion* – rehydration is more crucial than insulin in the early stages. Initial fluid should be isotonic (0.9%, 150 mmol/L) saline, or PPS if there is circulatory collapse or unconsciousness – 10–20 ml/kg within the first 30–60 min for initial volume expansion. A rapid history, clinical examination and blood glucose (by indicator stick) will confirm the diagnosis and a sample for true blood glucose, urea and electrolytes, plasma osmolality and arterial blood gas estimation should be obtained as the infusion is set up. Full blood count, hematocrit, platelets and an infection screen (blood culture, urine microscopy and culture, viral cultures, swabs) should be obtained and the ECG monitored.

Dehydration should be assessed clinically – mild (3–5%): dry mucous membranes, reduced skin turgor; moderate (6–8%): the above plus sunken eyes and poor capillary return; severe (≥ 9%): shock with poor perfusion, hypotension, thready pulse, tachycardia – and, if possible, by weighing and comparing with average weights for age or previous records. PPS should be given if there is severe dehydration and/or marked acidosis.

Whilst hypernatremia is due to severe water loss (exceeding sodium loss), hyponatremia is usually factitious – high glucose levels increase extracellular tonicity and draw water out of cells thereby diluting the extracellular sodium content – and often associated with hyperlipidemia. Empirically derived equations have been developed to calculate the 'true' sodium value which results when all excess glucose is removed from the extracellular fluid: either the plasma [glucose] (mmol/L) is divided by 4 and the result added to the measured plasma [Na] (mmol/L) or subtract 5 from the plasma [glucose] mmol/L, divide the result by 3 and add this figure to the plasma [Na] (mmol/L). It can be helpful to apply one or other when managing DKA with initial hyponatremia to identify the [Na] which will be reached with approaching normoglycemia a number of hours later. Plasma sodium levels should rise as ketoacidosis is corrected. (If levels are > 150 mmol/L, 0.45% saline should be substituted for 0.9% saline.) If the plasma sodium is falling rapidly, fluid replacement should be recalculated to be given over 48 h.

Creatinine levels may be spuriously high due to assay interference by acetoacetate and hematocrit may be falsely elevated by osmotic swelling of erythrocytes in the Coulter counter.

Dehydration should generally be corrected over 24 h with 0.9% saline. The deficit (ml) is calculated as % dehydration × weight (kg) × 10. Normal fluid requirements are calculated as 100 ml/kg for the first 10 kg body weight, 50 ml/kg for the second 10 kg and 20 ml/kg for the remainder. The hourly infusion rate is then calculated as

$$\frac{\text{maintenance requirement} + \text{deficit}}{24}$$

The volume of any albumin that may have been given during resuscitation should be ignored.

Indications for correcting over 48 h are pH < 7.1, initial plasma [Na] < 128 or > 150 mmol/L or any child aged 5 years or less.

A short acting *insulin* must be used and is best given as a continuous intravenous infusion by syringe pump at a rate of 0.03 to 0.05 units/kg/h (50 units of a short-acting insulin in 50 ml of 0.9% saline produces a solution containing 1 unit/ml of insulin). The aim is to decrease the blood glucose gently (by about 2–3 mmol/L/h) and the rate of insulin infusion adjusted in aliquots of 0.1 ml (= 0.1 units)/hour (0.03 units/kg/h should be the minimum infusion rate). This regimen results in a smooth and steady fall whilst being sufficient to switch off ketone production. The infusion should be changed 12 hourly.

Acidosis will almost always correct with correction of fluid balance. Correction should not be too rapid and as pH is a log scale small changes are significant. If the acidosis is not correcting, resuscitation may have been inadequate and more PPS may need to be given.

Bicarbonate should be considered only with severe acidosis (pH < 7.0), impending circulatory collapse (requiring inotrope support) or respiratory depression and used only on advice of senior medical staff as a slow i.v. infusion. In less severe ketoacidosis it may increase the risk of cerebral edema (due to the large sodium load) and hypokalemia (more rapid shift of potassium into cells) with increased morbidity and mortality. It must be infused slowly intravenously (over 30–60 min) and separately. The amount needed is derived from the formula:

$$\begin{aligned}&\text{mmol bicarbonate (ml of 8.4\% } NaCO_3\text{) required}\\&= \text{wt (kg)} \times \text{base deficit (mmol/L)} \times 0.1\end{aligned}$$

Once blood glucose levels are ≤ 13 mmol/L, 0.45% saline/5% dextrose is substituted for 0.9% saline. The insulin infusion rate is then adjusted to maintain blood glucose levels between 7 and 13 mmol/L. If blood glucose levels fall to 7 mmol/L or less, 10% dextrose and 0.45% saline should be substituted without decreasing the rate of insulin infusion further as adequate insulin is necessary to switch off ketosis.

Potassium. There is always substantial depletion of total body potassium whatever the initial plasma level, which will fall once insulin is commenced. KCl (20 mmol/500 ml saline) should be added once the child has passed urine (or in the knowledge that urine has been passed in the previous 4 hours). Potassium replacement can be adjusted to maintain normal plasma levels. A cardiac monitor (observing for T wave changes) is important if levels are abnormal.

If no urine is passed by 4 hours, catheterization may be necessary. Inappropriate ADH secretion may develop (low urine output, high urinary and falling plasma osmolalities) necessitating fluid restriction to prevent cerebral edema. Low plasma sodium levels may be factitious (see above) – plasma osmolality is a better hydration guide. All urine passed should be tested for glucose and ketones.

Neurological observations should be as frequent as indicated and changes or development of headache reported to medical staff immediately. A nasogastric tube should be passed if there is vomiting or drowsiness (the stomach will be dilated and aspiration can be fatal), aspirated hourly, and gastric losses included in an accurate fluid balance record. Intravenous ranitidine (1 mg/kg tds) should be given if the aspirate is positive for blood. Antibiotics may be necessary if infection is suspected once bacteriology specimens are obtained. Fluid balance should be calculated hourly and near patient blood glucose should be monitored hourly using a strip test read on a glucose meter. Capillary or venous blood gas measurements, plasma glucose (measured in the laboratory) and urea and electrolytes should be checked 4 hourly until the pH reaches 7.3. The aim should always be to correct metabolic abnormalities slowly – too rapid changes are thought to contribute the risk of cerebral edema (see below) with significant morbidity and mortality.

Once the fluid deficit is corrected, maintenance requirements should be recalculated and given. The nasogastric tube is removed when bowel sounds are present. Oral fluids can be started gently as tolerated from 12 to 18 h onwards once pH > 7.3 and urinary ketones are moderate or less. Intravenous fluids are discontinued when the child is rehydrated, drinking, eating a light diet and ketone free. Intravenous insulin is continued until ketones are absent and just prior to a meal. If the insulin infusion is stopped prematurely, ketonuria and anorexia will take longer to resolve and acidosis may persist.

A suitable initial s.c. insulin regimen is 0.8 units/kg/day given as two-thirds daily dose pre-breakfast [of which one-third as short acting (soluble) insulin and two-thirds as intermediate-acting (isophane) insulin], and one-third total daily dose split as short acting insulin pre-tea (evening meal) and one-third as intermediate-acting insulin pre-bed. 30–60 min after s.c. insulin is given the i.v. insulin infusion is discontinued and the child fed. Potassium should be given orally (as KCl 1 mmol/kg/24 h) for 2 days. Children with DKA are best managed on a high dependency unit and high quality, appropriately experienced nursing care is essential. After recovery, diabetes education begins.

Cerebral edema

Cerebral edema is the main cause of morbidity and mortality and single commonest cause of death in children with diabetes.[406] It is a feared complication of DKA often developing several hours after starting treatment in a context of apparent biochemical and clinical improvement. Over a 3-year period in the mid to late 1990s in the UK, the calculated risk of developing cerebral edema was 6.8 per 1000 episodes of DKA. The risk is higher in new (11.9 per 1000 episodes) as opposed to established (3.8 per 1000) diabetes. Within childhood, there are no sex or age differences but children are more susceptible than adults. Little is known of the etiology of cerebral edema in DKA – over-rapid fluid replacement and insulin infusion, hypoxemia and injudicious bicarbonate use[407] may increase its likelihood, but it is unlikely to be due solely to management factors – changing management practices have not been associated with a drop in the incidence – and biological patient variables may be important. There may be an association with low arterial partial pressures of carbon dioxide and high urea levels (reflecting the degree of dehydration) at presentation.[407]

Signs and symptoms of cerebral edema consist of headache, irritability, decreasing conscious level (falling Glasgow Coma Score, GCS) and convulsions. Danger signs are a falling plasma sodium concentration, poor urine output, bradycardia and hypertension. Papilledema is a late sign. Hypoglycemia should be excluded. Diagnosis and treatment are urgent. 0.5 g/kg of 20% (2 g in 10 ml) mannitol should be given i.v. over 30–60 min but needs to be started within a few minutes of the diagnosis of cerebral edema if it is to be effective. Mannitol may need to be repeated and there should be urgent discussion with senior medical and ITU/anesthetic staff about the need for intubation and hyperventilation. Any child with a GCS falling below 12 should be observed carefully where there are facilities and expertise for intubation. A GCS of less than 8 will need urgent elective intubation and ventilation which may be life saving. MR scanning is helpful if available. Fluid should be restricted to two-thirds maintenance and the fluid deficit corrected over 48–72 (rather than 24) hours. Unfortunately, cerebral edema occurs even when management of DKA follows current 'best practice' guidelines and mortality (24%) and morbidity (35% of survivors) rates remain high.[408]

Long-term management[409]

Sir Derrick Dunlop opening a 1965 diabetes mellitus symposium in Edinburgh asked 'is the occurrence of these complications [retinopathy, nephropathy, neuropathy, coronary and peripheral angiopathy] to be regarded fatalistically as something inherent in the diabetic process ... or can they be postponed by care and trouble directed to the control of the metabolic disturbance?'

It took nearly another 30 years to provide the answer. Perhaps observation of the effects of poor maternal diabetic control on her fetus[28] should have alerted pediatricians earlier to likely long term consequences of poor metabolic control and chronic hyperglycemia in childhood, but there is now irrefutable epidemiological evidence (at least in those aged 13 years or over) from the American 10 year prospective Diabetes Control and Complications Trial[410] that if good long term glycemic control is achieved, risks of microangiopathic complications (retinopathy, nephropathy and neuropathy) are greatly reduced. The question is not now 'why' or 'whether' to maintain good glycemic control but 'how'.

Other questions remain. Pediatricians seldom see complications silently bequeathed with their patients to adult diabetologists. What level of childhood or adolescent glycemic control constitutes 'sufficiently good' or 'optimal' control? Is prevention of complications by establishment of good control in childhood and adolescence a realistic goal? How is it to be achieved in the context of normal physical and emotional growth and normal daily activities and family lifestyle? Will it be at expense of more hypoglycemia? If so, how frequent or severe must it be in children of different ages before it affects cognitive function long term? Does more education or new or improved skills in family or clinician necessarily produce better control? Risks for macrovascular disease seem unaffected by tight glycemic control. The St Vincent and ISPAD declarations seek to achieve maximum quality of life for patients with diabetes through efficient use of available resources. How is this to be attained with health care resources dwindling in many 'developed' countries, let alone in parts of the world (including even Eastern Europe) where insulin itself is unavailable?

There is now no doubt that better metabolic control is associated with fewer and delayed microvascular complications.[410] This applies to younger children and suboptimal metabolic control at all ages is likely to be associated with higher risks of acute (DKA, severe hypoglycemia) and long-term complications. In very young children, the achievement of very tight glycemic control must be balanced against the increased risks of severe, and potentially damaging, hypoglycemia.

Optimal control must also be achieved in the context of normal family and school life and normal physical and emotional growth. Diabetes is a largely self (child and family) managed condition and successful care models need to focus on strategies that promote and maintain improved self-care behaviors. Children, young people and their families need to be empowered to control diabetes.[411,412] Specific attempts to increase the effectiveness of education in diabetes care are beneficial in improving short- and perhaps long-term control. Focuses need increasingly to be on insulin regimens that are flexible and fit the demands of school and social life. New technologies [continuous subcutaneous insulin infusion (CSII), inhaled insulin, continuous glucose monitoring systems, etc.][413] have the potential to allow young people with type 1 DM to take control of their diabetes.[414]

Motivation derives from encouragement and explanation, not coercion and arbitrary rules. Diabetes must not be ignored but should not need to preoccupy the child or family. Goals need to be framed from the perspective of the person with diabetes and their family. Education (instruction) is a partnership between health care professionals and families which attempts to achieve this through increased understanding of diabetes, empowerment and self-confidence in management.[415] Specific management aims and decisions will reflect the child's age, the family's diverse abilities, motivation and psychosocial backgrounds and personnel and resources available in hospital and community. A consistent approach by all members of the team is vital and will do much to create an environment in which the quality of control can improve.

Normoglycemia is dependent on an appropriate balance between calorie (carbohydrate, fat and protein) intake necessary for normal growth and energy expenditure and insulin. Diverse uncontrollable or unpredictable factors affect glycemia, e.g. intercurrent infection, a birthday party, attending the clinic, exams, GH, puberty, menstruation. Living with diabetes may require support which can be derived from involvement with self-help organizations.

Achieving 'tight' glycemic control in the context of a 'normal' lifestyle remains difficult for many families – in many children control is inadequate – but is helped by the multidisciplinary approach of the pediatric diabetes clinic: doctors have specialist knowledge of pediatrics, growth and diabetes; there is a dietitian present with expertise in pediatric diatetics and diabetes; a psychologist or child psychiatrist may sit in or be readily available. Family emotional problems may be precipitated by diabetes impacting on parents or other siblings; the child's and family's emotional responses to diabetes will themselves have major effects on glycemic control. Omission of insulin, simulating hypoglycemia or making up test results is common and an understandable response in many situations either to gain reward or avoid reprimand. This does not represent severe underlying psychopathology but should prompt a re-evaluation of management and a consistent parental and professional approach with proactive psychological involvement (see below).

Diabetes nurse specialists (DNS) are important assets to a clinic as key members of the multidisciplinary diabetes team linking family, home, school, community and hospital in a way that other health professionals cannot. They provide specific support in hospital and at home at diagnosis and at times of crisis, visit schools to talk to teachers, provide continuing support, advice and education, by telephone and through home and school visits and discuss specific problems with the hospital-based team.

Insulin regimens

Insulin is vital for glucose transport, storage and disposal. Glucose transport into cells provides energy, conversion to glycogen provides storage in liver and muscle, excess glucose is converted into fat and protein catabolism is inhibited. The body's insulin requirements are continually fluctuating. In normal individuals, glucose is the main stimulus to insulin release from pancreatic beta cells; insulin is secreted into the portal vein and is immediately physiologically available. Insulin levels thus rise rapidly after meals and snacks with equally rapid falls to basal secretory rates between meals and at night. The main aim in type 1 DM management is to reproduce physiological insulin secretion with the aim of optimizing glycemic control. Most current practicable regimens do so relatively poorly, but modern molecular engineering techniques – leading to the development of extremely short acting and extended action (true basal background) insulin analogues, together with developments in continuous subcutaneous insulin infusion (CSII) pump technology – are providing opportunities for young people with type 1 DM to take more informed control of their diabetes and achieve improved glycemic control[413] – and see below. In the UK, financial constraints (rather than clinical needs) are currently limiting the use of CSII therapy in children and adolescents (as well as adults) with type 1 DM.

The regimen chosen must be individualized for child and family. Examples are shown in Figure 13.60. Conventional therapy for type 1 diabetes has consisted of twice daily soluble and isophane insulin regimens with support from a multidisciplinary health care team and regular diabetes and health monitoring. Such twice daily regimens are still frequently used by many children and young people and are simple but inflexible (meals need to be eaten on time and have a relatively fixed carbohydrate content). A relatively physiological split is 30% soluble/70% isophane but other proportions (10–50% soluble) are available. The insulins can either be premixed and injected using an insulin 'pen' or mixed by the patient (necessitating use of a syringe and needle). Such regimens are associated with variable results.[388,416]

Alternatively, a generally more satisfactory regimen consists of the pre-breakfast insulin given as above (either free mixing or premixed) but the evening soluble and isophane insulins split with soluble insulin given before the evening meal (supper, Scottish 'tea') and the isophane before bed. This reduces the risk of nocturnal hypoglycemia and early morning hyperglycemia and there are limited data supporting an improvement in glycemic control using three rather than two daily injections.[388,417,418] Short acting analogue insulin can be substituted for soluble insulin in these regimens and may be valuable in managing some patients – e.g. toddlers whose appetite is unpredictable can be injected after the meal.[419] Lente insulin is far from ideal as a 'background' – it has a peak in action between 2 and 6 hours

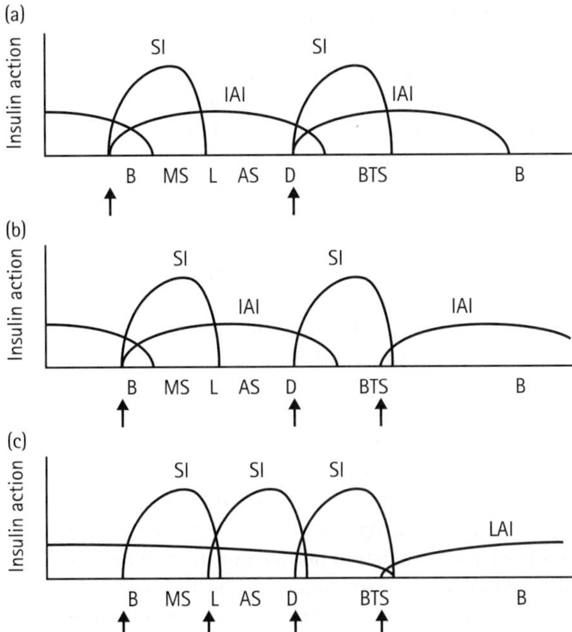

Fig. 13.60 Examples of insulin regimens: (a) two daily doses of short- and intermediate-acting insulins; (b) as (a) but the evening intermediate-acting insulin delayed until bedtime; (c) insulin pen regime – combination of preprandial short-acting insulin with long-acting insulin at bedtime. Key: B = breakfast; MS = midmorning snack; L = lunch; AS = afternoon snack; D = dinner (Scottish tea); BTS = bedtime snack; SI = short-acting insulin; IAI = intermediate-acting insulin; LAI = long-acting insulin; ↑ = insulin injection.

after s.c. injection and even ultralente has a significant peak at 18–12 h.[420]

More intensive multiple daily injection (MDI) basal–bolus regimens are also used. In one regimen, soluble insulin is given preprandially (i.e. before meals) and isophane insulin at bedtime. The soluble insulin provides sufficiently sustained action over the day to provide basal as well as bolus (mealtime) insulin availability. The main disadvantage is the need for four injections daily but this is compensated for by flexibility of lifestyle, meal sizes and times and exercise. Alternatively, boluses of rapid acting insulin analogues (see below) can be given up to five times daily preprandially with isophane at bedtime. The analogue can be given immediately before (or even during or immediately after) a meal (obviating the need to wait 20–30 min with soluble insulin). Basal (isophane) insulin generally needs to be given twice daily. There may be a reduced risk of nocturnal hypoglycemia and improved postprandial control with analogue[421–423] rather than soluble insulin[410] regimens with the added potential for improved glycemic control.

CSII regimens deliver insulin via an indwelling subcutaneous (usually abdominal) fine cannula, powered by microprocessor controlled pump devices which allow variable and programmable basal infusion rates between meals and overnight together with boluses of insulin when food is taken. This is undoubtedly the regimen which currently approximates most closely to physiological insulin delivery in people who do not have diabetes, with the potential for optimal glycemic control and reduced risk of hypoglycemia. Missing a meal or unexpected exercise can be adjusted for much more readily.

In contrast to the situation when insulin pump therapy was first introduced in the 1970s,[424,425] current CSII and pumps seem well tolerated by children and young people because of their small size, and flexible programmability which puts them in control of their diabetes – sporting activities without hypoglycemia, flexible meals in keeping with their peer group and less nocturnal hypoglycemia. However there are still few published randomized trial data on the efficacy and safety of CSII versus MDI regimens. Evidence regarding the impact of an intensive insulin regimen (four or more injections or CSII) on long term control is derived principally from the Diabetes Control and Complications Trial (DCCT) which also involved a comprehensive patient support element (diet and exercise plans, monthly visits to the health care team, etc.).[410] Thus although intensive insulin therapy (MDI or CSII) significantly improved glycemic control over a sustained period compared with conventional insulin therapy (two injections per day), DCCT did not include children aged less than 13 years and, due to the study design, it is impossible to separate the benefits of intensive insulin therapy from intensive support.

In any case, intensive insulin therapy should only be delivered as part of a comprehensive support package.[375] Thus CSII has resource implications – not only are insulin pumps and their consumables expensive (approximately £3000 for a pump, which has an expected life of about 7 years, and over £1000 per annum for consumables per patient) but intensive support is necessary from diabetes teams (increased patient and family contact and support at least in the early stages, continuous blood glucose monitoring downloading and advice, etc.). At the time of writing there are approximately 600 CSII pumps in use in the UK compared to approximately 20 000 in Germany and 81 000 in the USA. Pump therapy is widely used in Scandinavia where in some clinics over 40% of patients receive CSII. CSII pump technology will shortly be appraised in England by the National Institute for Clinical Excellence (NICE) (and subsequently by the Health Technology Board for Scotland) to determine whether it should be made generally available on the UK National Health Service.

The insulin regimen should be tailored to the individual child to achieve the best possible glycemic control without disabling hypoglycemia.[375] The number of daily insulin injections does not necessarily correlate with excellence of glycemic control. In Sweden, Nordfeldt & Ludvigsson[426] consistently achieve mean HbA_{1c} levels of 7% with a low incidence of severe hypoglycemia, but in Belgium, Dorchy et al[416] achieve similar results using a twice daily insulin regimen. Other important factors for good glycemic control include continuing support from the health care team, psychosocial factors or dedicated home blood glucose self-monitoring.

There are currently two rapid acting insulin analogues available: lispro insulin (reversed proline and lysine at positions B29 and B30) and aspart insulin (aspartate substituted for proline at B28). Plasma insulin concentrations peak more rapidly and higher and decrease more rapidly than following soluble s.c. insulin. The peak action is approximately 1 h after injection and there is no activity by 3–4 h. A virtually peakless long acting insulin analogue (glargine insulin) has recently become available[427] – there is C terminal elongation of the insulin beta chain by two arginines and replacement of asparagine by glycine in position A21. There are as yet few data in children and adolescents but hypoglycemia risks may be reduced using glargine compared to NPH (lente) insulin.[428]

About 30–60% of children and adolescents demonstrate a partial remission ('honeymoon') phase (insulin requirements < 0.5 units/kg/day) for up to 6 months (sometimes longer) after diagnosis. Subsequently average insulin requirements are in the order of 0.6–0.8 units/kg/day although considerably higher doses are necessary during the adolescent growth spurt (early in female and late in male puberty).

Insulin requirements will vary according to activity levels, intercurrent illness, etc. Insulin resistance will develop when blood glucose levels have been high over a period of days or weeks (perhaps due to injecting into lipohypertrophic sites, eating inappropriately, intercurrent infection or omitting insulin). Increased insulin doses may be necessary for several weeks but it is important then to reduce the dose once more to avoid a vicious cycle of eating more to prevent hypoglycemia resulting in weight gain and further increased insulin requirements and appetite.

Insulin adjustments are ideally based on home self-monitoring of blood glucose. With consistent abnormalities at a particular time of day the appropriate insulin is adjusted up or down by child or parent, if necessary after consultation by phone with a member of the diabetes team – development of skills in independent adjustment of insulin varies considerably between individuals and their families. Written information should be given for 'sick day' management. Adjustment only every few months in clinic is very unsatisfactory.

Subcutaneously injected insulin bioavailability is very variable.[429] Rates vary with injection site – fastest from the abdomen and slower from the thigh than the arm – and with exercise (see below) or if the site is rubbed after injection. If the same injection site is used repeatedly (because the injection becomes painless) lipohypertrophy (Fig. 13.61) is likely and injecting into lipohypertrophic injection sites is an extremely common cause of poor and unpredictable insulin absorption and erratic glycemic control amongst children and young people with type 1 DM .

Of all the continuing developments in alternative insulin delivery routes (including oral, transdermal, intranasal),[429] inhaled insulin, absorbed across the alveolar surface of the lungs, is closest to widespread practical application. Both liquid and dry powder formulations have been developed. There is a rapid onset and early peak action (similar to the time course of s.c rapid acting analogue insulin) but with a longer period of action (more comparable to s.c. soluble insulin).[430] Insulin could be given by inhalation as often as necessary as preprandial boluses – injections would still be required for basal insulin administration. The relative efficiency of insulin delivery by aerosol, compared to s.c. injection, has been estimated as between 8 and 25%.[431] Initial studies in children and adolescents seem promising.[413]

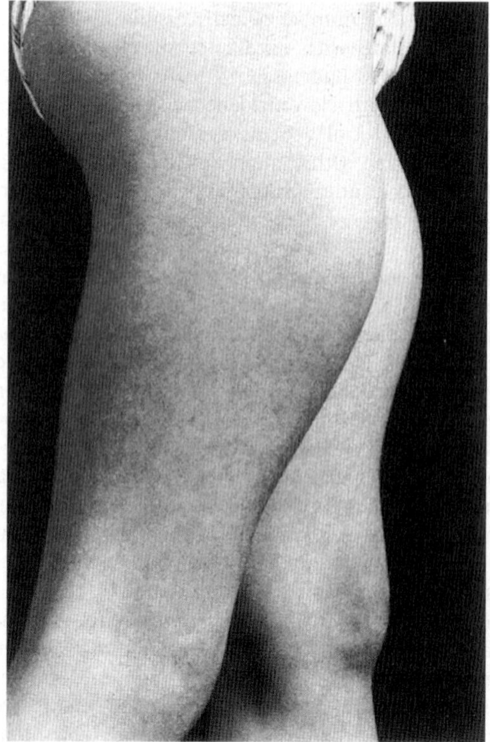

Fig. 13.61 Severe lipohypertrophy in a diabetic child on human insulin who was not adequately rotating the injection sites.

If a child with type 1 DM requires emergency or elective surgery, clear protocols or an integrated care pathway should be in place to facilitate safe management. In the perioperative period, additional metabolic demands contributing to unstable glycemic control potentially include preoperative fasting and dehydration, the stress response to surgery and anesthesia and postoperative calorie and fluid deficits. With careful management, mortality and morbidity should be no higher than in children without diabetes.

By clinical presentation more than 90% of beta cell function is already destroyed. Non-specific immunosuppressive therapy at diagnosis, with toxic drugs such as ciclosporin A, were shown to prolong the partial remission period, but no case of total remission or with normal glucose tolerance has been reported[432] and renal toxicity was common. Nevertheless, less toxic immunosuppressive agents have been developed and the possibility of a potential 'cure' for diabetes by pancreatic islet cell transplantation to secrete insulin physiologically in response to endogenous metabolic signals is an extremely attractive proposition.

However, despite the successful reversal of diabetes in many small animal models, insulin independence after islet allotransplantation has been very difficult to achieve in the human: the use of diabetogenic immunosuppressive agents to suppress both islet alloimmunity and autoimmunity, the critical islet mass to achieve insulin independence and the detrimental effects of transplanting islets in an ectopic site and loss of graft function with time.[433]

Promising new research approaches to these problems, including xenogeneic sources of cells, engineering islet cells with genes that induce expression of immunoprotective molecules, and neogenesis factors that may sustain populations of transplanted beta cells, are demonstrating that islet allotransplantation still has great potential to become an established treatment option for diabetic patients in the future.[434]

The development of human beta cell lines derived for pancreatic tissue obtained from infants with persisting hyperinsulinemic hypoglycemia of infancy (PHHI), and which respond to physiological glucose levels, are of potential use both in gene therapy for PHHI and in cell transplantation studies for administering insulin for the treatment of diabetes mellitus.[435]

Diet

If it is to be acceptable to child and family and followed in practice, diet should be closely related to recommendations for non-diabetics, but is inevitably tempered by the family's eating habits which may fall short of that ideal. Rigid and dogmatic rules encourage non-compliance. In the past, diets have involved 'quantitative' advice with a 'stable' carbohydrate intake at regular intervals – breakfast, mid-morning snack, lunch, mid-afternoon snack, evening meal, bedtime snack.

A regimen which includes dietary management has been shown to improve glycemic control[410] and is recommended.[375] Specialist dietetic advice should be given by a dietitian with expertise in childhood diabetes wherever possible. Until the 1980s, counting of carbohydrate exchanges was recommended. The carbohydrate (CHO) exchange system (one exchange = 10 g CHO) has the virtue of dogmatic simplicity allowing a wide variety of foods to be eaten, but all nutrients can, of course, be converted directly or indirectly to glucose. The previously conventional guide to CHO intake (100 g per day for a 1 year old plus an extra 10 g per day for each additional year of age) needed to be varied considerably to meet growth and energy requirements of the individual. The proportion of CHO was high enough (40–50%) to enable fat intake to be reasonably low – less than 35% of calories should be from fat which should be polyunsaturated to reduce long-term risks of hyperlipidemia and cardiovascular disease.

In more recent years, the recognition that not all types of carbohydrate have the same effect on blood glucose levels and of the potentially restrictive nature of counting CHO exchanges has led to a change in focus to 'healthy eating'.[436] Although there is little evidence to recommend either a 'qualitative' or 'quantitative' approach as the most effective mode of dietary therapy, newer insulin regimens (MDI or CSII) require CHO intake assessment if short or rapid acting insulin is to be given in appropriate dosage.

CHO type remains important: concentrated, rapidly absorbed, sugary food taken in significant and regular amounts precludes stable glycemic control and should be confined to occasional treats before exercise, or at the end of a meal. Starchy, low fiber foods are acceptable, but starchy high fiber foods (Table 13.20) are best, because of their gradual absorption and metabolism. With education of the general population towards 'healthy eating' these foods are now more socially accepted and more easily obtainable cheaply.

Dietary management is therefore the 'art of the possible' and involves educating the whole family's eating habits. A pediatric dietician with an interest in diabetes is a crucial part of the management team. A sensible approach to 'treats', fast foods and reasonable flexibility over timing is more likely to lead to co-operation; psychological benefit (not being different to family and friends) is likely to benefit lifestyle and control.

Exercise

Exercise has major effects and in children is variable and capricious. Regular exercise allows participation in peer group activities and improves self-confidence and physical fitness. Strenuous exercise usually results in rapid but unpredictable falls in blood glucose (increased insulin mobilization results from increased blood flow and muscular activity). Energy stores (and particularly muscle glycogen) are depleted during medium to long duration exercise and hypoglycemia can occur up to many hours afterwards. Before activity, an extra 10–30 g CHO may be necessary depending on age, blood glucose level and the intensity of exercise planned (best taken as pure fruit juice or an isotonic sport drink). Such drinks are best taken during and after exercise as well rather than loading with carbohydrate before the exercise starts. It is sensible to have a snack within an hour of completing the activity and post- (as well as pre-) exercise insulin doses may need to be reduced.

On a background of under-insulinization, exercise results in counter-regulation and hyperglycemia with ketosis.[437] It is important not to exercise in the presence of ketones – exercise is not a replacement for insulin. On activity holidays it is often sensible to cut insulin by < 50% if severe hypoglycemia is not to result on the first day even with additional snacks.

Table 13.20 Some high fiber foods

Wholemeal bread
Wholemeal spaghetti
Wholemeal cereals
Weetabix
Jacket potatoes
Ryvita
Oatcakes
Dried beans
Lentils
Fruits
Apples
Bananas
Blackberries
Pineapple
Strawberries
Vegetables
Brussels sprouts
Cabbage
Peas
Sweetcorn

Psychological intervention

In the past, there has sometimes been a tendency to expect children with diabetes to take on too much responsibility for their diabetes management at too young an age.[438] As they grow older, children with diabetes pass through a stage of 'interdependence' (between total dependence on parents and full independence) where they know what to do and how to do it, in terms of the practicalities of, for example, drawing up and injecting insulin and self blood glucose monitoring (SBGM), but are not ready to take responsibility for injections or monitoring. Maintaining parental involvement improves glycemic control.[439,440]

Managing diabetes is inevitably stressful at times, both for the children with diabetes themselves and for their families. Factors contributing to an increased risk of young people with diabetes developing psychological problems include: too much responsibility being placed on the child; avoidance coping[438] – never coming to terms with diabetes emotionally or developing conscious or unconscious strategies which do not address the problem faced; family conflict or lack of communication both within the family and with the diabetes team; low socioeconomic status or a non-traditional family structure; poor maternal health, especially depression.[441]

Eating disorders are commoner in adolescents with diabetes compared with non-diabetic peers, adversely affect glycemic control and can be difficult to treat.[442] Regular assessment for psychological problems, especially maladaptive coping strategies and eating disorders is desirable.[375]

Psychological or educational interventions have positive effects on psychological outcomes, knowledge about diabetes and glycemic control[443] – interventions which promote diabetes-specific coping skills are effective and add to the effectiveness of intensive management. Thus the use of cognitive coping strategies targeted at diabetes-specific problems is recommended[375] and parental support and family communication should be encouraged, with targeted psychological treatment of family disruption and related stress factors.[375] Education programs, computer-assisted packages and telephone prompting should be considered as part of a multidisciplinary lifestyle intervention program.[375] It is desirable that health care professionals should receive training in patient-centered interventions in diabetes.[375]

Glycemic control and its assessment

Many children with type 1 DM enjoy active and healthy lives but some are poorly controlled requiring frequent hospital admissions for ketoacidosis, hypoglycemia or stabilization. Poor control may reflect unhappiness or instability in the family (see above), particularly if there has never been emotional (as opposed to intellectual) acceptance of diabetes.

'Brittle' diabetes[444] is now accepted to be insulin omission and is almost invariably due to such problems – injection sites should be checked for lipohypertrophy, but fruitless searches for underlying metabolic abnormalities is counterproductive. Long-term poor control causes severe stunting of growth and pubertal development and may be associated with 'Cushingoid' obesity and hepatomegaly (Mauriac syndrome). Gross abnormalities are now seldom seen and assessment of physical and emotional growth and well-being while essential are, in themselves, insufficient – normal growth and no reported symptoms of hypo- or hyperglycemia may be found even when glycemic control is far from ideal.

Insulin adjustments are ideally based on home self blood glucose monitoring (SBGM). Checking for glycosuria gives limited retrospective information about likely previous blood glucose levels (has the level been high enough to exceed the renal threshold for glucose since the bladder was last emptied?), do not warn of impending hypoglycemia, and are useless with normoglycemia as the optimal therapeutic goal. Even early morning glycosuria may be misleading, reflecting early morning hyperglycemia (excessive insulin the previous evening with counter-regulation, the Somogyi effect[445]), too little insulin, or the 'dawn phenomenon' – decreased insulin sensitivity due to nocturnal GH peaks.[446]

Immediate knowledge of blood glucose levels is only of practical benefit if child and parents understand their significance and relevance and are motivated to take appropriate action on the basis of consistent abnormalities. That SBGM monitoring does not, in itself, lead to better control[447] is not surprising in this context. Blood tests done in rotation once or twice daily just before main meals and at bedtime, and occasionally 60–90 min after main meals, an acceptable regimen for many, will provide most information from fewest tests. Blood glucose estimation is of particular value during illness or symptoms that could relate to hypoglycemia. Nevertheless blood tests are uncomfortable and a chore. Education and motivation will reduce the number omitted, done inaccurately or of results made up to 'keep the doctor happy'. Intensive treatment of type 1 DM (using MDI or CSII) requires more frequent measurements (post- as well as pre-prandially) for optimal glycemic control.

Conventional SBGM makes information about nocturnal (hypo)glycemia hard to obtain.[448] The recent development and availability of a continuous glucose monitoring system (CGMS) is a major advance. In one system, the glucose sensor is inserted (via a needle which is then withdrawn) into s.c. tissue, usually of the anterior abdominal wall. An electrical signal is generated by the oxidation (catalysed by glucose oxidase in the sensor) of glucose in the interstitial fluid. Data are analyzed every 10 s and average 5 min values (288 per day) are stored for subsequent downloading (usually by a diabetes team nurse or doctor). Values are, unfortunately, not available to the patient in 'real-time' but are in other systems which are becoming available. Sensor readings have to be calibrated against regular conventional SBGM. The patient enters event markers (e.g. for times of insulin doses, food intake, exercise). Patterns of hypo- and hyperglycemia not detectable by conventional SBGM will become apparent in young people using CGMS[449] and improvement in glycemic control can be expected. As with conventional SBGM, the relative error of the measurements is likely to increase at levels in the hypoglycemia range and the relative importance of pressure or temperature changes (especially overnight) remains to be determined.[413]

Amongst available technologies, the combination of CSII therapy with glucose sensor data from CGMS currently provides the nearest approach to mimicking physiological insulin secretion and allowing motivated children and young people to achieve and maintain optimal control of their diabetes whilst minimizing hypoglycemia (not least at night).

Hemoglobin forms a non-enzymatic link with glucose – percentage of glycosylated hemoglobin (HbA_{1c}) is an objective measure of integrated glycemic control over the previous 6–8 weeks.[450] Assessed in this way, the majority of diabetic children are less than ideally controlled,[388,451] and in some control is abysmal. Identifying this group is easier than improving the situation. There has been doubt as to the appropriateness of some laboratory quoted normal ranges for HbA_{1c} and the 'target range' (6–8% with a DCCT equivalent method) is lower than previously considered desirable. It is likely that the risk of microvascular complications rises sharply above mean HbA_{1c} levels > 9%.[452] This has implications for children at greater risk of hypoglycemia and its consequences, when 'tight' glycemic control is the aim[448] (see below). Finding high values is helpful when home monitoring results apparently indicate excellent control – either monitoring technique is faulty or, commonly, there is deliberate manipulation due to emotional disturbance.[453]

HbA_{1c} values will reflect average blood glucose levels over the previous 6 to 8 weeks. The ideal HbA_{1c} value (between 6 and 8% with a DCCT equivalent method) reflects average blood glucose levels since the last HbA_{1c} estimation of approximately 6.5 mmol/L and 10.5 mmol/L respectively. A 1% increase in HbA_{1c} values reflects an average increase in blood glucose levels of 2 mmol/L – a mean HbA_{1c} value of (say) 10% will result from mean blood glucose levels of around 14.5 mmol/L, i.e. very poor control.

HbA_{1c} estimation is much more valuable if the current result is available in clinic so that appropriate discussion can take place with the child and parent(s) and appropriate advice given. In many clinics, portable or fixed analysers are available to provide such a service; if that is not the case, capillary blood samples on filter paper or in special containers can be obtained at home shortly before the next clinic visit and posted to the laboratory. Shorter term indices of glycemic control – e.g. plasma proteins such as fructosamine – may be useful when assessing, for example, the efficacy of a specific therapeutic intervention.

Hypoglycemia[454,455]

Parents, and many children, worry particularly about 'hypos' and, especially, nocturnal hypoglycemia which is likely to be commoner with the quest for tighter glycemic control.

There are few long-term neurophysiological and psychometric studies of effects of frequent mild hypoglycemia.[456] Children's hypoglycemic symptoms differ from adults'. In very young children, neuroglycopenic symptoms (dizziness, poor concentration, drowsiness, weakness) and non-specific symptoms (tearfulness, confusion, tiredness, irritability, aggression) are reported more frequently than autonomic symptoms (hunger, trembling, pallor). Sweating is absent during the early stages of hypoglycemia in prepubertal children with type 1 DM and other symptoms may be minimal. This is despite the fact that children (with and without diabetes) have a much more pronounced catecholamine response to hypoglycemia than do adults. However the prolonged nature of nocturnal hypoglycemic episodes in children may be explained in part by defective counter-regulation.[457] Weakness is the symptom most commonly reported by children and the sign most frequently reported by their parents is pallor.

Children diagnosed before 3 years appear to have particular problems with hypoglycemia.[458] This relates both to the common occurrence of hypoglycemia in children with type 1 DM (the normal young child has a relative inability to maintain normoglycemia during even periods of 6–12 h without food) and to the increased sensitivity to hypoglycemia of the still maturing brain.

Occasional mild hypoglycemia – a feeling of hunger with faintness, headache or belligerency if a meal is delayed – indicates tight control and seems harmless. Hypoglycemia is usually caused by delayed or missed food, unexpected (or unexpectedly strenuous) exercise or excess insulin administration (by mistake, or, more rarely, deliberately). There is particular risk soon after diagnosis when endogenous insulin secretion is temporarily partially re-established.[459]

Both stress and early stages of an intercurrent viral illness can cause hypo- rather than hyperglycemia. Severe hypoglycemia can be associated with transient hemiparesis.[460] Children and young people with diabetes should always carry extra glucose: 3 glucose tablets should be taken at early signs of hypoglycemia (alternatives are 50 ml of lucozade or 2 teaspoons of glucose powder added to juice) and followed by food.

A child having a moderate or severe hypo will require assistance. A semiconscious or uncooperative child who cannot coordinate swallowing a sweet drink should be given 'hypostop' gel. This is available on prescription in the UK and is rubbed into the inside of the cheek but should not be given to an unconscious child unless by a health care professional. In the unconscious or fitting child at home, glucagon (available as a glucagen kit, 1 mg i.m. or s.c.) should be given. Both will improve neuroglycopenia and the conscious level sufficiently for oral sugary carbohydrate (e.g. sugary juice plus toast and jam) to be given. If it is not, glucose levels will fall again – sometimes a problem with glucagon as it can induce vomiting. Blood glucose levels should be checked at home every 15 min for an hour to ensure that they return to normal. The next dose(s) of insulin may need to be reduced depending on the cause.

Prolonged severe hypoglycemia resulting in cerebral edema is seen following deliberate and massive insulin overdose and in adolescents after significant alcohol intake and can cause death or permanent brain damage.

ADOLESCENCE

Adolescence is characterized by major changes in energy intake, growth and hormonal maturation as well as by profound changes in cognitive function, lifestyle, mood and coping. In non-diabetic adolescents, fasting insulin levels increase in both sexes through puberty until Tanner stages 3 or 4, with higher levels in girls reflecting their earlier growth spurt and marginally earlier pubertal maturation. These increases in both basal and stimulated insulin levels reflect and compensate for decreased insulin sensitivity during puberty which is partly due to the significant increase in growth hormone (GH) secretion.

Optimal glycemic control may be particularly difficult to achieve in adolescents: rapid growth necessitates a high calorie intake and must be paralleled by sufficient increases in insulin at that pubertal stage. Many adolescents are underinsulinized on conventional regimens and the daily insulin dose may need to be increased to around 1.5 units/kg during the pubertal growth spurt. Menstruation may precipitate ketoacidosis; important exams cause stress; emotional lability may cause rebelliousness against dietary restrictions, the need for monitoring control or insulin injections. Eating disorders (anorexia nervosa, bulimia) are common[442] (see above).

Standard insulin regimens through puberty will not correct all the metabolic abnormalities or maintain optimal glycemic control. However, in practical terms these considerations are overshadowed for many young people by lifestyle and behavior which characterize adolescence and militate against good glycemic control in adolescents with type 1 diabetes. Adolescents develop through stages of dependence and interdependence before becoming independent. They develop psychologically and emotionally at different rates and may regress at times. It is a time of testing out and experimentation. It can be a very confusing and frightening time for adolescents and their parents particularly if there is the added stress of diabetes.

Any chronic illness in adolescents complicates their developmental problems and may jeopardize their autonomous development. It can also make it difficult for parents to give up their parental role. Changes occur in the adolescent's self-concept and body image, and in their relationships with parents, friends, partners and the medical team. The self-care demands of diabetes are often in conflict with the experiences of adolescence.

Psychological transition from childhood to adolescence and beyond requires new approaches to motivation and education, flexible diet, insulin regimens and lifestyle. Maintaining parental involvement through the adolescent stage of 'interdependence' (see above) improves glycemic control[439,440] and improved control leads to better quality of life.[461]

Seeking excitement and involvement in risk-taking behaviors is the norm during adolescence. This extends from music and dance to sexual behavior and the use of drugs. The impact of drug use on diabetes is relatively unknown with most of the evidence anecdotal, apart from information on alcohol and tobacco. Cigarette smoking greatly increases the microvascular risks to the diabetic. Alcohol use, in particular binge drinking which is common in adolescents, potentiates hypos. Adolescents must be aware of these risks and how to avoid the dangers and pitfalls. Health professionals should avoid being judgmental and encourage their patients to discuss these issues openly so that appropriate advice can be given. Drug taking should always be taken into consideration when trying to identify reasons for admission with DKA or severe hypos in this age group. Young female patients need to be very aware of the risks of unplanned pregnancy and health professionals should seek opportunities to discuss contraception and preconception care with adolescent girls with diabetes.

Coping strategies adopted by adolescents with diabetes range from obsessional control to denial of diabetes. Those using denial will generally come to the attention of health professionals reasonably quickly but those who are obsessional may never be recognized and may be seen as 'good diabetics'. Chronic insulin omission ('brittle diabetes') will be reflected in weight loss and is associated with episodes of DKA and poor glycemic control.

Glycemic control is generally better in adolescents who have supportive families although the adolescent with diabetes may feel isolated and not know anyone else with the condition. Many adolescents appear to benefit from sharing experiences with others in a variety of contexts – diabetes holiday camps and UK Youth Diabetes projects can help overcome this problem and UK health professionals should encourage families to join Diabetes UK.

Special adolescent needs are often poorly met. Specific adolescent clinics, jointly staffed by pediatricians and adult diabetologists with empathy for the adolescent and his or her 'world-view' may be the ideal – a paternalistic approach is doomed to failure. Annual screening should be carried out to pick up early manifestations of complications (see below). Psychological care should be an integral part of the support offered particularly in view of the fact that psychological problems are more common where chronic illness exists. There is probably no 'right' time for transition or transfer and the timing must both be individualized and determined by local arrangements and resources.[374]

Clinics should ideally be run at a convenient time for the patients outwith school time and completely separate from other diabetes clinics. There are some adolescents who do not attend clinic and refuse support in the community. It is important that these patients are identified and some form of contact, no matter how minimal, should be maintained – ideally with a diabetes nurse specialist with specific responsibilities for the adolescent service.

The overall aims of a service for young people with diabetes should be to ensure normal growth and development, minimize episodes of DKA and hypoglycemia, screen for and minimize the risks of complications (see below), promote social and psychological well-being, reduce risk-taking behavior and give support and education to empower the patient to become independent and in control of their diabetes.

Complications

Complications are seldom seen before puberty even in long-standing diabetes. Sex steroid secretion at puberty could be important in their development and progression but pathogenesis is still poorly understood. Their relevance to the pediatrician is that – extrapolating from the results of the DCCT[410] – optimal childhood glycemic control is extremely important in the prevention of microvascular disease and that very early changes can be detected by screening techniques.

Early abnormalities in children and adolescents (e.g. microalbuminuria, background retinopathy) predict later development of long term microvascular complications[410,462] and maintaining glycemic control to as near normal as possible significantly reduces the long term risk of microvascular diseases.[410] An HbA_{1c} > 10% over time in young people with diabetes increases the risk of the development of retinopathy by approximately eightfold.[410] Thus with the aim of management of type 1 DM to reduce the risk of long term microvascular complications, the target for all young people with diabetes is the optimizing of glycemic control towards a normal level.[375]

Microalbuminuria is a marker for early nephropathy. Using the first morning urine sample[463] and relating concentration to creatinine is probably appropriate but its presence is likely to be related to such factors as acute glycemic control, posture, exercise, hydration and BP. It remains unclear how persistent and at what level it must be to cause concern or how justifiable is long-term antihypertensive therapy in a child with a raised diastolic BP and microalbuminuria. BP rises concurrently with the onset of microalbuminuria and is also closely related to BMI.[464]

The literature is unclear about the timing of commencing screening in young people with diabetes – age and puberty are reported without any strict definition. For clarity and simplicity 12 years of age in both boys and girls has been suggested.[375] However early microvascular abnormalities may occur before puberty, which then appears to accelerate these abnormalities.[465]

The following can be detected and should be screened for in young people with diabetes: retinopathy (by ophthalmoscopy or fundal photography); microalbuminuria [by albumin excretion rate (AER) or albumin/creatinine ratio (ACR)] and hypertension.[464] Young people with diabetes from the age of 12 years should annually receive examination of the retina, have their urine tested for microalbuminuria (overnight AER or first morning ACR) and have their blood pressure measured.[375]

Every effort should be made to optimize glycemic control in young people with diabetes who have abnormal levels of microalbuminuria or elevated blood pressure for age so as to minimize the chance of progression to microangiopathic disease (retinopathy, nephropathy and neuropathy). There is no evidence that routine screening for autonomic neuropathy or hyperlipidemia is of benefit.[375]

In type 1 diabetes, preproliferative retinopathy has been identified within 3.5 years of diagnosis in postpubertal patients[466] and within 2 months of the onset of puberty – screening for diabetic retinal disease is effective at detecting unrecognized sight-threatening retinopathy.[467] Ideally retinal photography or slit lamp biomicroscopy utilized by trained individuals should be employed in a program of systematic screening for diabetic retinopathy, with dilated direct ophthalmoscopy used for opportunistic screening.[375]

ASSOCIATIONS – THYROID DISORDERS AND CELIAC DISEASE

Both thyroid[468] and celiac[469] disease are commoner in young people with type 1 DM compared with non-diabetic subjects – both may occur with minimal or no symptoms and thus be missed during routine care. It is recommended that young people with diabetes should be screened for thyroid and celiac disease at diabetes onset and at intervals throughout their lives.[375] Screening for other autoimmune endocrine disorders has also been suggested. Standard blood tests exist to screen for thyroid and celiac disease, but there are limited data to support the specific frequency of screening. There are also few data as to which screening tests should be used, but it is our practice to check TSH levels (by capillary sample at the same time as an HbA_{1c} check) as part of the annual review.

Dietary management in young people with type 1 DM and celiac disease is complex and can be difficult for the family, but the potential benefits of treatment with a gluten-free diet include control of symptoms, stabilization of diabetes and prevention of complications (infertility, osteoporosis and malignancies such as small bowel lymphoma) associated with celiac disease.[470]

OTHER DIABETIC SYNDROMES IN CHILDHOOD[471]

Secondary diabetes mellitus

Diabetes may occur with islet damage secondary to other factors [e.g. pancreatitis and pancreatic disease in cystic fibrosis (see below); thalassemia; certain drug or poison ingestion]. It may occur in association with individually rare genetic syndromes (e.g. Prader–Willi, Down, Alstrom, DIDMOAD – see below) or with abnormalities of insulin or its receptors. It may be secondary to other endocrine disorders (e.g. Cushing's syndrome, pheochromocytoma).

DIDMOAD (diabetes insipidus, diabetes mellitus, optic atrophy and deafness) syndrome, Wolfram syndrome[472]

Optic atrophy (OA) and diabetes insipidus (DI) usually present on a background of established diabetes mellitus. The bilateral progressive OA is present in nearly all by young adulthood causing eventual blindness. DI occurs in about one-third and the (high tone) deafness is usually not severe. Inheritance is autosomal recessive and a nuclear gene at chromosome 4p16.1 (WFS1/wolframin) has been identified that segregates with disease status. Mutation analysis of the WFS1 gene in Wolfram syndrome patients has identified mutations in 90% of patients but the biological or clinical significance is not yet established.[473]

Cystic fibrosis (CF) and diabetes

Longer survival is resulting in diabetes being seen increasingly in CF patients: 20% will develop secondary diabetes by the age of 20, and the incidence increases to 80% by age 35.[474] Limited data suggest that clinical symptoms deteriorate when diabetes develops in cystic fibrosis although no evidence exists that the presence of diabetes or its treatment affects long term survival. It is recommended that patients with CF should be screened annually for diabetes (testing for hyperglycemia, glycosuria and/or a raised HbA_{1c}) from 10 years of age.[375] Insulin therapy will help prevent catabolic weight loss. A high energy intake (high fat and high complex carbohydrate) is recommended.[374]

Neonatal diabetes mellitus

Transient neonatal diabetes mellitus is a rare condition – the UK national incidence is 1 in 400 000 live births[475] generally seen in SGA infants. Presentation is with rapid weight loss, severe dehydration, fever and vomiting without diarrhea. Thirst and polyuria are usually unnoticed. Babies appear pale and lively. Blood glucose is very high with glycosuria but only mild (if any) ketonuria and acidosis. There is extreme insulin sensitivity – treatment is with 0.01 unit/kg/h continuous infusion and normal saline initially. The condition is self-limiting, resolving before 1 year of age (median 3 months). Subsequent glucose tolerance is normal but there is a predisposition to type 2 diabetes in later life, perhaps because of reduced beta cell functional capacity. Seventy-five per cent of cases are associated with either paternal uniparental disomy of chromosome 6 or an unbalanced duplication of paternal chromosome 6 – the imprinted gene responsible maps to chromosome 6q24 and may be important for normal pancreatic development.[476]

Occasionally permanent diabetes presents at this age. Distinction from the transient form can only be made on follow-up but cerebellar hypoplasia and Walcott–Rallison syndrome are associations, again suggesting an autosomal recessive inheritance pattern. A mutation in the gene insulin promoter factor 1 has been identified as a cause of the pancreatic agenesis.[476]

HYPOGLYCEMIA

Hypoglycemia is a common, but often poorly investigated and managed, metabolic abnormality in infancy and childhood but not a diagnosis in itself. If prolonged or recurrent it can result in severe neuroglycopenia, potentially irreversible brain damage and long-term mental handicap particularly in the very young.

Blood glucose regulation and the metabolic consequences of starvation are discussed above (and see Figs 13.57 and 13.58).

Normal neonates and young children tolerate fasting less well than adults – blood glucose levels may start to fall after periods as short as 6–12 h which has implications for the preoperative management of children requiring surgery. Glucose levels appear to fall in a cyclical fashion overnight in normal children, some falling into the 'hypoglycemic' range before compensation.

The principal metabolic substrate for energy production in the fetus is glucose provided continuously via the placenta. After delivery the neonate must adapt to alternating periods of enteral milk feeding and starvation. After the first 24 h normal babies fed on demand feed frequently (even twice an hour to begin with) taking small quantities with each feed. Until feeding is established, the neonate is dependent on glycogenolysis and gluconeogenesis to maintain normoglycemia. SGA babies (who have low liver glycogen stores but high glucose requirements) and those with sepsis or birth asphyxia are at particular risk of hypoglycemia (see also Ch. 10).

Neonatal symptoms are non-specific and include 'jitteriness', hypotonia, feeding difficulties, pallor, apnea, tachypnea, convulsions and coma. In older children, symptoms and signs are attributable to neuroglycopenia (confused or bizarre behavior, bad temper, irritability, headache, visual disturbances, hunger, abdominal pain, convulsions, coma) or to counter-regulation (pallor, sweating, nausea, vomiting).

Blood glucose levels below which there is arbitrarily defined hypoglycemia (e.g. 2.2 mmol/L) are controversial – it is unclear whether 'low' but asymptomatic blood glucose levels cause short or long term problems in different age groups. Prolonged or recurrent symptomatic hypoglycemia is undoubtedly associated with permanent neurological damage.

ETIOLOGY

There are many potential causes of hypoglycemia – the most important are classified by age at presentation in Table 13.21.[289] Endocrine causes are discussed in the section relating to the relevant gland; causes of hyperinsulinism are discussed below.

Persistent neonatal hypoglycemia is usually due to hyperinsulinism, deficiency of a counter-regulatory hormone or of a gluconeogenic or glycogenolytic enzyme. Recent onset recurring hypoglycemia is most commonly due to hyperinsulinism, 'accelerated starvation', defective hepatic gluconeogenesis or GH and/or glucocorticoid deficiency. Accidental or non-accidental administration of hypoglycemic agents must be considered and hypoglycemia anticipated in any child who has ingested alcohol.

DIFFERENTIAL DIAGNOSIS

History and examination may provide diagnostic clues, for example a family history of neonatal death or acidosis in an inherited metabolic disorder, short stature with micropenis in hypopituitarism, hepatomegaly in galactosemia or gluconeogenic or glycogenolytic disorders, macroglossia and transverse ear lobe creases in Beckwith–Wiedemann syndrome.

Essential diagnostic information is obtained from blood and urine samples taken *when there is hypoglycemia* and before treatment commences. Blood glucose, ketone bodies, lactate, free fatty acids, branched chain amino acids, insulin, GH, cortisol and catecholamines and urinary ketone bodies, catecholamine metabolites and reducing substances should ideally be measured. If sampling is difficult the most important assays are for blood glucose, plasma insulin and cortisol and urinary ketone bodies and samples should be deep frozen for future analysis.

The metabolic consequences of starvation with counter-regulation are increased plasma fatty acids, glycerol, ketone bodies, and branched chain amino acids associated with high levels of cortisol, GH and catecholamines. Insulin levels will be low or undetectable. Significant ketosis excludes hyperinsulinism as the cause for hypoglycemia but 'ketotic hypoglycemia' is not a diagnosis in itself and requires further elucidation to find the cause. Important endocrine causes of ketotic hypoglycemia include deficiencies of counter-regulatory hormones (GH and ACTH deficiencies, CAH – especially during intercurrent stress or infection – Addison's disease, familial glucocorticoid deficiency and adrenomedullary unresponsiveness).

Hyperinsulinism results in hypoglycemia without ketonuria because insulin inhibits lipolysis. Plasma insulin levels may not be

Table 13.21 Causes of hypoglycemia by age

Transient neonatal
Decreased glucose production
Birth asphyxia
Small for gestational age
Sepsis
Starvation
Hypothermia
Hyperinsulinism
Infant of diabetic mother
Erythroblastosis
Beckwith–Wiedemann–syndrome (usually)
Maternal glucose infusions
Idiopathic
Persistent neonatal and infancy
Hyperinsulinism
PHHI (nesidioblastosis)
Islet cell adenoma/hyperplasia/leucine sensitivity
Beckwith–Wiedemann syndrome (sometimes)
Hormonal
Growth hormone deficiency
Hypopituitarism
Glucocorticoid
Congenital adrenal hyperplasia
ACTH deficiency
Glucagon deficiency
Hypothyroidism (?)
Inborn errors of metabolism (enzyme deficiency – see Fig. 13.57)
Glucose-6-phosphatase – glycogen storage disease (GSD) Type I*
Amylo-1,6-glucosidase (GSD III)*
Debrancher*
Phosphorylase (GSD VI)*
Phosphorylase kinase*
Glycogen synthetase*
Fructose-1,6-diphosphatase*
Phosphoenolpyruvate carboxykinase*
Pyruvate carboxylase*
Galactose-1-phosphate uridyl transferase (galactosemia)
Beta-oxidation defects*
Fructose intolerance
Maple syrup urine disease
Later childhood
Accelerated starvation
Hormonal
As above
Addison's disease
Familial glucocorticoid deficiency
Enzyme deficiency
Those marked* above
Adrenomedullary hyporesponsiveness
Liver disease
Fulminant hepatitis
Reye's syndrome
Jamaican vomiting sickness
Hyperinsulinism
Insulin administration (including Munchausen by proxy syndrome)
Oral hypoglycemics (including Munchausen by proxy syndrome)
Ingestion
Alcohol
Salicylates

elevated but will be high for plasma glucose; plasma ketone bodies may be detectable but will be low for the glucose level.

Further differential diagnosis may necessitate 24 h metabolic profiles, calculation of the glucose infusion rate necessary to maintain normoglycemia, assessment of glycogen reserve by glucagon provocation tests and of gluconeogenesis.

After exclusion of other causes of ketotic hyperglycemia, there remains a group of children who regularly develop hypoglycemia during periods of fasting 'accelerated starvation'. Jewish children are absolved from fasting on Yom Kippur (Day of Atonement) until they are 'adult' (13 years). More severe hypoglycemia with convulsions may occur during intercurrent infection (particularly with vomiting), after pronounced physical activity or during preoperative starvation. There is often a history of difficult delivery or intrauterine growth retardation and the child (usually a boy) may be underweight. The hypoglycemic tendency is usually outgrown by later childhood. It is likely that they represent one end of a normal distribution of ability to maintain normoglycemia during fasting.

Defects in beta oxidation of fatty acids are increasingly recognized as important causes of hypoglycemia in previously 'idiopathic' groups. Ketone levels are low (cf. ketotic hypoglycemia including 'accelerated starvation'), plasma fatty acid levels are high (cf. hyperinsulinism). Medium-chain acyl CoA dehydrogenase (MCAD) deficiency may now be specifically diagnosed by molecular genetic studies and by measuring urinary phenylpropionyl glycine levels which are high following an oral phenylpropionic acid load due to inability to convert phenylpropionic acid to hippuric acid, an essential step in fatty acid oxidation. A newborn screening program could be greatly beneficial but has still not been properly evaluated.[477,477a]

ENDOCRINE PANCREATIC ABNORMALITIES CAUSING HYPOGLYCEMIA

These are almost always due to hyperinsulinism – glucagon deficiency seems very rare. Transient neonatal hypoglycemia due to hyperinsulinism is seen in the infant of a poorly controlled diabetic mother (fetal hyperinsulinism secondary to maternal hyperglycemia) and is found in erythroblastosis fetalis (cause unknown) and Beckwith–Wiedemann syndrome (see Ch.10).

In a minority of infants of diabetic mothers hypoglycemia is delayed, but persisting neonatal hypoglycemia is usually associated with an underlying structural pancreatic abnormality. These conditions may not present until later in the first year, making hyperinsulinism the commonest cause of persistent hypoglycemia in infants below 1 year of age or even in childhood.

It is likely that the spectrum of histological findings, from discrete beta cell adenoma(s) through diffuse beta cell hyperplasia, microadenomatosis and nesidioblastosis to functional beta cell disorder alone, and perhaps also 'leucine sensitive hypoglycemia', all result from the same pathological process, probably in the control of pancreatic endocrine secretion.[478]

PERSISTENT HYPERINSULINEMIC HYPOGLYCEMIA OF INFANCY (NESIDIOBLASTOSIS)

Persistent hyperinsulinemic hypoglycemia of infancy (PHHI) is a rare disorder which may be familial or sporadic, and which is characterized by unregulated secretion of insulin and profound hypoglycemia in the neonate. Unregulated insulin release in focal beta cell abnormalities (comprising about 40% of patients) is due to the somatic loss of the maternal allele from chromosome 11p15 leading to hemi- or homozygosity of a paternally inherited mutation of the gene controlling the sulphonylurea receptor (SUR1).[479] It is thought that unregulated insulin release from diffuse pancreatic beta cell abnormalities is caused by mutations in the genes encoding the sulphonylurea receptor, the inward rectifier potassium channel (Kir6.2), the glucokinase gene (dominantly inherited), or the glutamate dehydrogenase gene.

It has been established that human beta cells can be developed from PHHI tissue removed at surgery (see below) and stably repaired using genetic engineering with cDNAs encoding the above two components of potassium ATP channels (SUR1 and Kir6.2) together with PDX1 (a regulator of beta cell development and insulin synthesis).[479,480] This development of human beta cell lines that respond to physiological glucose levels may be of use in gene therapy for PHHI and in cell transplantation studies for administering insulin for the treatment of diabetes mellitus.[435]

The term nesidioblastosis ('germ islands'), first used[481] to describe abnormal differentiation of isolated pancreatic islet cells from blastic duct cells, was associated with severe hypoglycemia in infancy by Yakovac et al.[482]

The majority of infants present neonatally with symptoms (including convulsions) of intractable hypoglycemia. Occasionally presentation is later in the first 6 months. There may be a positive family history.[483] They are obese, resembling the infant of the poorly controlled diabetic mother (hyperinsulinism is common to both). There may be a history of maternal glucose intolerance during previous pregnancies.

Diagnosis is dependent on demonstrating hyperinsulinemic hypoglycemia without significant ketosis. Very high glucose infusion rates (> 15 mg/kg/min) may be necessary to maintain normoglycemia – rates above 6–9 mg/kg/min are highly suggestive of hyperinsulinism. The demonstration, when hypoglycemic, of a glycemic response to glucagon, low branched chain amino acid levels, and insulin suppression following somatostatin infusion will confirm the diagnosis.

The management priority is to correct hypoglycemia but this can be difficult because of the high glucose infusion rates necessary and technical problems with siting infusion lines. Glucagon (0.1 mg/kg) has only transient effects in mobilizing glucose from glycogen stores, but can be invaluable to cover re-siting. Long acting somatostatin analogues may aid longerterm maintenance of normoglycemia but GH may be as effective and have fewer potential side-effects. Conventionally, medical treatment is with diazoxide (< 25 mg/kg/24 h), and its effect is potentiated by thiazide diuretics, but adequate control is seldom achieved without the need for continuing high rates of glucose infusion and side-effects (including hypertrichosis) are common. More recently, calcium channel blockers (e.g. slow release nifedipine) have been found to be effective.[484]

If medical therapies are unsuccessful, surgery is urgently indicated. Preoperative imaging (ultrasound and CT scanning) may not discriminate between a diffuse process and a discrete lesion (and the biochemical consequences are identical). If a discrete adenoma is found it should be resected – this may be curative; if not, subtotal (95%) pancreatectomy (more effective than less radical removal) is performed. This may, commonly, result in 'cure' – normoglycemia without medical therapy, or normoglycemia on diazoxide, diabetes mellitus or still unstable glycemic control. In this last situation, or if the infant remains on glucose infusion-dependent, total pancreatectomy is performed. Post-pancreatectomy diabetes is generally easy to manage on small doses of insulin (e.g. once daily intermediate acting) because of associated alpha cell loss causing glucagon deficiency and altered CHO absorption secondary to pancreatic exocrine deficiency.

Current views on the management of PHHI, derived from a Consensus Workshop held by the European Network for Research into Hyperinsulinism (ENRHI) in 1999, are summarized by Aynsley-Green et al[485] and Hussain & Aynsley-Green.[486]

Maintenance of normoglycemia, optimal medical management and, where necessary, early recourse to surgery, prevents previously common permanent neurological damage and mental retardation.

ACKNOWLEDGMENT

Dr. Butler is grateful to the Child Growth Foundation for permission to reproduce the centile charts in Figures 13.9–13.12. Decimal and duodecimal versions of the charts may be purchased from Harlow Printing, Maxwell Street, South Shields NE33 4PU. The Child Growth Foundation, 2 Mayfield Avenue, Chiswick, London W4 1PW may be contacted for sources of growth measuring equipment, training and information. He is also grateful to Castlemead publications, Raynham House, Broadmeads, Ware, Hertfordshire SG12 9HY for permission to reproduce the Buckler–Tanner centile charts in Figures 13.13–13.14.

REFERENCES (* Level 1 evidence)

1 Lania A, Mantovani G, Spada A. G protein mutations in endocrine diseases. Eur J Endocrinol 2001; 145:543–559.

2 Achermann JC, Meeks JJ, Larry Jameson J. Phenotypic spectrum of mutations in DAX-1 and SF-1. Mol Cell Endocrinol 2001; 185:17–25.

3 Ranke MB, Wit J-M, Kelnar CJH, eds. Classification system for pediatric endocrine diseases (Version 1.1) Edition J & J Palatium Verlag. Mannheim: 2000.

4 Tanner JM. Growth at adolescence 2nd edn. Blackwell Oxford; 1962.

5 Ranke M, ed. Diagnostics of endocrine function in children and adolescents, 2nd edn. Heidelberg: Barth Verlag; 1996.

6 Butler GE, Walker RF, Walker RV, et al. Salivary testosterone levels and the progress of puberty in the normal boy. Clin Endocrinol 1989; 30:587–596.

7 Milner RDG, Hill DJ. Fetal growth signals. Arch Dis Child 1989; 64:53–57.

8 Freeman M. Feedback control of intercellular signaling in development. Nature 2000; 408:313–319.

9 Kaplan SL, Grumbach MM, Shepard TH. The ontogenesis of human fetal hormones. 1. Growth hormone and insulin. J Clin Invest 1972; 51:3080–3093.

10 Cohen LE. Genetic regulation of the embryology of the pituitary gland and somatotrophs. Endocrine 2000; 12:99–106.

11 Honnebier WJ, Swaab DF. The influence of anencephaly upon intrauterine growth of the fetus and placenta and upon gestation length. Br J Obstet and Gynaecol 1973; 80:577–588.

12 Gluckman PD, Gunn AJ, Wray A, et al. Congenital idiopathic growth hormone deficiency associated with prenatal and early postnatal growth failure. J Pediatr 1992; 121:920–923.

13 Strain AJ, Hill DJ, Swenne I, Milner RDG. The regulation of DNA synthesis in human fetal hepatocytes by placental lactogen, growth hormone and insulin-like growth factor 1/somatomedin C. J Cell Physiology 1987; 132:33–40.

14 Sandler S, Andersson A, Korsgren O, et al. Tissue culture of human fetal pancreas:growth hormone stimulates the formation and insulin production of islet-like cell clusters. J Clin Endocrinol Metab 1987; 65:1154–1158.

15 Handwerger S, Freemark M. The roles of placental growth hormone and placental lactogen in the regulation of human fetal growth and development. J Pediatr Endocrinol Metab 2000; 13:343–356.

16 Siler-Khodr TM, Morgenstern LL, Greenwood FC. Hormone synthesis and release from human fetal adenohypophysis in vitro. J Clin Endocrinol Metab 1974; 39:891–905.

17 Kahri AI, Huhtaniemi F, Salmenpetra M. Steroid formation and differentiation of cortical cells in tissue culture of human fetal adrenals in the presence and absence of ACTH. Endocrinol 1976; 98:33–41.
18 Kaplan SL, Grumbach MM, Aubert ML. The ontogenesis of pituitary hormones and hypothalamic factors in the human fetus: maturation of central nervous system regulation of anterior pituitary function. Recent Prog Horm Res 1976; 32:161–234.
19 Symonds ME, Mostyn A, Stephenson T. Cytokines and cytokine receptors in fetal growth and development. Biochem Soc Trans 2001; 29:33–37.
20 Calvo R, Obregon MJ, Ruiz de Oña C, Escobar del Rey F. Congenital hypothyroidism as studied in rats. Crucial role of maternal thyroxine but not of 3,5,3'-triiodothyronine in the protection of the fetal brain. J Clin Invest 1990; 86:889–899.
21 Morreale de Escobar G, Obregón MJ, Escobar del Rey F. Is neuropsychological development related to maternal hypothyroidism or maternal hypothyroxinemia? J Clin Endocrinol Metab 2000; 85:3975–3987.
22 Grüters A. Growth and thyroid disorders. In: Kelnar CJH, Savage MO, Stirling HF, Saenger P, eds. Growth disorders – pathophysiology and Treatment. London; Chapman & Hall; 1998:565–574.
23 Idelman S. The structure of the mammalian adrenal cortex. In: Chester Jones I, Henderson IW, eds. General, comparative and clinical endocrinology of the adrenal cortex. London: Academic Press; 1978: vol 2:1–199.
24 Seckl JR, Cleasby M, Nyirenda MJ. Glucocorticoids, 11beta-hydroxysteroid dehydrogenase, and fetal programming. Kidney Int 2000; 57:1412–1417.
25 Migeon CJ, Wisniewski AB. Human sex differentiation: from transcription factors to gender. Horm Res 2000; 53:111–119.
26 Veitia RA, Salas-Cortes L, Ottolenghi C, et al. Testis determination in mammals: more questions than answers. Mol Cell Endocrinol 2001; 20:179:3–16.
27 Sharpe RM. Hormones and testis development and the possible adverse effects of environmental chemicals. Toxicol Lett 2001; 120:221–232.
28 Farquhar JW. The child of the diabetic woman. Arch Dis Child 1959; 34:76–96.
29 Hattersley AT, Tooke JE. The fetal insulin hypothesis: an alternative explanation of the association of low birthweight with diabetes and vascular disease. Lancet 1999; 353:1789–1792.
30 Aynsley-Green A. Metabolic and endocrine interrelations in the human fetus and neonate. Am J Clin Nutr 1985; 41:399–417.
31 Gluckman PD. Endocrine and nutritional regulation of prenatal growth. Acta Paediatr 1997; 423(Suppl):153–157.
32 Morrish DW, Bhardwaj D, Dabbagh LK, et al. Epidermal growth factor induces differentiation and secretion of human chorionic gonadotrophin and placental lactogen in normal human placenta. J Clin Endocrinol Metab 1987; 65:1282–1290.
33 Lawrence S, Warshaw JB. Increased binding of epidermal growth factor to placental membranes in IUGR fetal rats. Pediatr Res 1989; 25:214–218.
34 Soothill P, Holmes R. Normal fetal growth. In: Kelnar CJH, Savage MO, Stirling HF, Saenger P, eds. Growth disorders – pathophysiology and treatment. London: Chapman & Hall; 1998:143–157.
35 Ibanez L, Dimartino-Nardi J, Potau N, Saenger P. Premature adrenarche – normal variant or forerunner of adult disease? Endocr Rev 2000; 21:671–696.
36 Barker DJ, Hales CN, Fall CH, et al. Type 2 (non-insulin-dependent) diabetes mellitus, hypertension and hyperlipidemia (syndrome X): relation to reduced fetal growth. Diabetologia 1993; 36:62–67.
37 Barker DJP, Bull AR, Osmond C, Simmonds SJ. Fetal and placental size and risk of hypertension. BMJ 1990; 301:259–262.
38 Frankenne F, Closset J, Gomez F, et al. The physiology of growth hormone in pregnant women and partial characterisation of the placental GH variant. J Clin Endocrinol Metab 1988; 66:1171–1180.
39 Cornblath M, Hawdon JM, Williams AF, et al. Controversies regarding definition of neonatal hypoglycemia: suggested operational thresholds. Pediatrics 2000; 105:1141–1145.
40 Hadziselimovic F. Cryptorchidism, its impact on male fertility. Summary of the 4th International Symposium on Pediatric Andrology. Basel, Switzerland, November 10–11 2000. Horm Res 2001; 55:55.
41 Simons WF, Fuggle PW, Grant DB, Smith I. Intellectual development at 10 years in early treated congenital hypothyroidism. Arch Dis Child 1994; 71:232–234.
42 Solyom J, Hughes IA. Value of selective screening for congenital adrenal hyperplasia in Hungary. Arch Dis Child 1989; 64:338–342.
43 Danon M, Friedman SC. Ambiguous genitalia, micropenis, hypospadias and cryptorchidism. In: Lifshitz F, ed. Pediatric endocrinology. New York: Marcel Dekker; 1996;281–304.
44 Zachmann M, Tassinari D, Prader A. Clinical and biochemical variability of congenital adrenal hyperplasia due to 11-beta-hydroxylase deficiency. A study of 25 patients. J Clin Endocrinol Metab 1983; 56:222–229.
45 Bongiovanni AM. The adrenogenital syndrome with deficiency of 3beta-hydroxysteroid dehydrogenase. J Clin Invest 1962; 41:2086–2092.
46 Verhoeven ATM, Mostblum JL, Van Lonsden HAIM, et al. Virilization in pregnancy coexisting with an ovarian mucinous cystadenoma: a case report and review of virilizing ovarian tumors in pregnancy. Obstet Gynecological Surv 1973; 28:597–622.
47 Ahmed SF, Hughes IA. The genetics of male undermasculinization. Clin Endocrinol 2002; 56:1–18.
48 Josso N, Fekete C, Cachin O, et al. Persistence of Mullerian ducts in male pseudohermaphroditism and its relationship to cryptorchidism. Clin Endocrinol 1983; 19:247–258.
49 Berthezene F, Forest MG, Grimaud JA, et al. Leydig cell agenesis. New Engl J Med 1976; 295:969–972.
50 Sultan C, Paris F, Terouanne B, et al. Disorders linked to insufficient androgen action in male children. Hum Reprod Update 2001; 7:314–322.
51 Kofman-Alfaro S, Valdes E, Teran J, et al. Endocrine and immunogenetic evaluation of an XX male infant with perineoscrotal hypospadias. Acta Endocrinol 1985; 108:421–427.
52 Diamond M, Sigmundson HK. Sex reassignment at birth. Long-term review and clinical implications. Arch Pediatr Adolesc Med 1997; 151:298–304.
53 Colapinto J. As nature made him: the boy who was raised as a girl. New York: HarperCollins; 2000.
54 Imperato-McGinley J, Peterson RE, Gautier T, Sturla E. Androgens and the evolution of gender identity among male pseudohermaphrodites with 5-alpha-reductase deficiency. N Engl J Med 1979; 300:1233–1237.
55 Meyer-Bahlburg HF. Gender and sexuality in classic congenital adrenal hyperplasia. Endocrinol Metab Clin North Am 2001; 30:155–171.
56 Savage MO, Lowe DG, Ransley PG, et al. Germ cell neoplasia in patients with abnormal sexual differentiation. Pediatr Res 1986; 20:1183 (A131).
57 Floud R, Gregory A, Wachter K. Height, health and history: nutritional status in the United Kingdom Cambridge: Cambridge University Press; 1990:1750–1980.
58 Eveleth PB, Tanner JM. World-wide variation in human growth, 2nd edn. London: Cambridge University Press; 1990.
59 Ulijaszek SJ, Johnston FE, Preece MA, eds. The Cambridge encyclopedia of human growth and development. Cambridge: Cambridge University Press; 1998.
60 Freeman JV, Cole TJ, Chinn S, et al. Cross-sectional stature and weight reference curves for the UK, 1990. Arch Dis Child 1995; 73:17–24.
61 Wright CM, Booth IW, Buckler JMH, et al. Growth reference charts for use in the United Kingdom. Arch Dis Child 2002; 86:11–14.
62 Cole TJ, Freeman JV, Preece MA. Body mass index reference curves for the UK 1990. Arch Dis Child 1995; 73:25–29.
63 Tanner JM, Buckler JM. Revision and update of Tanner–Whitehouse clinical longitudinal charts for height and weight. Eur J Pediatr 1997; 156:248–249.
64 Hall DMB, Elliman D, eds. Health for all children. 4th edn Oxford: Oxford Medical Publications (in press); 2002.
65 Dangour AD, Schilg S, Hulse JA, Cole TJ. Sitting height and subischial leg length centile curves for boys and girls from Southeast England. Ann Hum Biol 2002; 29:290–305.
66 Buckler JMH. A reference manual of growth and development, 2nd edn. Oxford; Blackwell; 1997.
67 Hall JG, Froster-Iskenius UG, Allanson JE. Handbook of normal physical measurements. Oxford: Oxford Medical Publications; 1989.
68 Wolthers OD, Pedersen S. Short term linear growth in asthmatic children during treatment with prednisolone. BMJ 1990; 301:145–148.
69 Wales JKH, Milner RDG. Variation in lower leg growth with alternate day

steroid treatment. Arch Dis Child 1988; 63:981–983.
70 Butler GE, McKie M, Ratcliffe SG. The cyclical nature of prepubertal growth. Ann Hum Biol 1990; 17:177–198.
71 Wales JKH, Gibson AT. Short term growth: rhythms, chaos or noise? Arch Dis Child 1994; 71:84–89.
72 Crofton PM, Stirling HF, Schönau E, Kelnar CJH. Bone alkaline phosphatase and collagen markers as early predictors of height velocity response to growth-promoting treatments in short normal children. Clin Endocrinol 1996; 44:385–394.
73 Cole TJ. A simple chart to identify non-familial short stature. Arch Dis Child 2000; 82:173–176.
74 Karlberg J, Albertsson-Wikland K. Growth in full-term small-for-gestational-age infants: from birth to final height. Pediatr Res 1995; 38:733–739.
75 Styles ME, Cole TJ, Dennis J, Preece MA. New cross sectional stature, weight and head circumference rederences for Down's syndrome in the UK and the Republic of Ireland. Archives of Disease in Childhood 2002; 87:104–108.
76 Lyon AJ, Preece MA, Grant DB. Growth curve for girls with Turner syndrome. Arch Dis Child 1985; 60:932–935.
77 Greulich, WW, Pyle, SI. Radiographic atlas of skeletal development of the hand and wrist, 2nd edn. Stanford: Stanford University Press; 1959.
78 Tanner JM, Healy MJR, Goldstein H, et al. Assessment of skeletal maturity and prediction of adult height (TW3 method). London: Academic Press; 1983.
79 MacGillivray MH, Morishima A, Conte F, et al. Pediatric endocrinology update: an overview. The essential roles of estrogens in pubertal growth, epiphyseal fusion and bone turnover: lessons from mutations in the genes for aromatase and the estrogen receptor. Horm Res 1998; 49(suppl 1):2–8.
80 Karlberg J, Engstrom I, Karlberg P, Fryer JG. Analysis of linear growth using a mathematical model. Acta Pediatr Scand 1987; 76:478–488.
81 Massoud AF, Hindmarsh PC, Matthews DR, et al. The GHRP hexarelin is capable of releasing GH after two successive IV doses and acts synergistically with GHRH. Horm Res 1995; 44(suppl 1):23 (A89).
82 Laron Z, Frenkel J, Silbergeld A. Biochemical and growth promoting effects of a growth hormone releasing peptide – hexarelin – (HEX) in children. Horm Res 1995; 44 (suppl 1):20 (A76).
83 Huerta MG, Rogol AD. Treatment of growth disorders: growth hormone-releasing hormone and other growth hormone secretagogues. In: Kelnar CJH, Savage MO, Stirling HF and Saenger P, eds. Growth disorders – pathophysiology and treatment. London: Chapman & Hall; 1998:701–720.
84 Kojima M, Hosoda H, Date Y, et al. Ghrelin is a growth-hormone-releasing acylated peptide from stomach. Nature 1999; 402:656–660.
*85 Toogood AA, Thorner MO. Ghrelin, not just another growth hormone secretagogue. Clin Endocrinol 2001; 55:589–591.
86 Ariyasu H, Takaya K, Tagami T, et al. Stomach is a major source of circulating ghrelin, and feeding state determines plasma ghrelin-like immunoreactivity levels in humans. J Clin Endocrinol Metab 2001; 86:4753–4758.
87 Broglio F, Arvat E, Benso A, et al. Ghrelin, a natural GH secretagogue produced by the stomach, induces hyperglycemia and reduces insulin secretion in humans. J Clin Endocrinol Metab 2001; 86:5083–5086.
88 Ogilvy-Stewart AL, Stirling HF, Kelnar CJH, et al. Treatment of radiation-induced growth hormone deficiency with growth-hormone releasing hormone (GHRH). Clin Endocrinol 1997; 46:571–578.
89 Baranowska B, Radzikowska M, Wasilewska-Dziubinska E, et al. The role of VIP and somatostatin in the control of GH and prolactin release in anorexia nervosa and in obesity. Ann N Y Acad Sci 2000; 921:443–455.
90 Fazekas I, Bacsy E, Varga I, et al. Effect of vasoactive intestinal polypeptide (VIP) on growth hormone (GH) and prolactin (PRL) release and cell morphology in human pituitary adenoma cell cultures. Folia Histochem Cytobiol 2000; 38:119–127.
91 Laron Z, Pertzelan A, Mannheimer S. Genetic pituitary dwarfism with high serum concentration of growth hormone. A new inborn error of metabolism? Isr J Med Sci 1966; 2:152–155.
92 Rosenfeld RG, Rosenbloom AL. Guevarra-Aguirre J. Growth hormone (GH) insensitivity due to primary GH receptor deficiency. Endocr Rev 1994; 15:369–390.
93 Goddard AD, Covello R, Luoh S-M, et al. Mutations of the growth hormone receptor in children with idiopathic short stature. N Engl J Med 1995; 333:1093–1098.
94 Salerno M, Balestrieri B, Matrecano E, et al. Abnormal GH receptor signaling in children with idiopathic short stature. J Clin Endocrinol Metab 2001; 86:3882–3888.
95 Baumann G. Growth hormone binding protein. J Pediatr Endocrinol Metab 2001; 14:355–375.
96 Gluckman PD, Breier BH, Sauerwein H. Regulation of the cell surface growth hormone receptor. Acta Pediatr Scand 1990; 366(suppl):73–78.
97 Mullis PE, Holl RW, Lund T, Brickell PM. Regulation of growth hormone-binding protein production by r-hGH in a hepatoma cell line. Horm Res 1995; 44(suppl 1):3 (A9).
98 Woods KA, Fraser NC, Postel-Vinay M-C, et al. A homozygous splice site mutation affecting the intracellular domain of the growth hormone (GH) receptor resulting in Laron syndrome with elevated GH-binding activity. J Clin Endocrinol Metab 1996; 81:1686–1690.
99 Woods KA, Camacho-Hubner C, Savage MO, Clarke AJL. Intrauterine growth retardation and postnatal growth failure associated with deletion of the insulin-like growth factor-I gene. N Engl J Med 1996; 335:1363–1367.
100 Rao E, Weiss B, Fukami M, et al. Pseudoautosomal deletions encompassing a novel homeobox gene cause growth failure in idiopathic short stature and Turner syndrome. Nat Genet 1997; 16:54–63.
101 Ellison JW, Wardak Z, Young MF, et al. PHOG, a candidate gene for involvement in the short stature of Turner syndrome. Hum Mol Genet 1997; 6:1341–1347.
102 Belin V, Cusin V, Viot G, et al. SHOX mutations in dyschondrosteosis (Leri–Weill syndrome). Nat Genet 1998; 19:67–69.
103 Shears DJ, Vassal HJ, Goodman FR, et al. Mutation and deletion of the pseudoautosomal gene SHOX cause Leri–Weill dyschondrosteosis. Nat Genet 1998; 19:70–73.
104 Clement-Jones M, Schiller S, Rao E, et al. The short stature homeobox gene SHOX is involved in skeletal abnormalities in Turner syndrome. Hum Mol Genet 2000; 9:695–702.
105 Tanner JM. The regulation of human growth. Child Dev 1963; 34:817–847.
106 Prader A, Tanner JM, von Harnack GA. Catch-up growth following illness or starvation. J Pediatr 1963; 62:646–659.
107 Baron J, Klein KO, Colli MJ, et al. Catch-up growth after glucocorticoid excess: a mechanism intrinsic to the growth plate. Endocrinology 1994; 135:1367–1371.
108 Preece MA, Hendrich I. Mathematical modelling of individual growth curves. Br Med Bull 1981; 37:247–252.
109 Albertsson-Wikland K, Rosberg S, Isaksson O, Westphal O. Secretory pattern of growth hormone in children of differing growth rates. Acta Endocrinol 1983; 103 (suppl 256):72.
110 Buckler JMH. A longitudinal study of adolescent growth. London: Springer Verlag; 1990.
111 Kelnar CJH, Albertsson-Wikland K, Hintz RL, et al. Should we treat children with idiopathic short stature? Horm Res 1999; 52:150–157.
112 Pasquino AM, Albanese A, Bozzola M, et al. Idiopathic short stature. J Pediatr Endocrinol Metab 2001; 14(suppl 2):967–974.
113 Hindmarsh PC. Endocrine assessment of growth. In: Kelnar CJH, Savage MO, Stirling HF, Saenger P, eds. Growth disorders – pathophysiology and treatment. London: Chapman & Hall; 1998:237–250.
114 Borochowitz ZU, Rimoin DL. Genetic and dysmorphic syndromes of short stature. In: Kelnar CJH, Savage MO, Stirling HF, Saenger P, eds. Growth disorders – pathophysiology and treatment. London: Chapman & Hall; 1998;297–322.
115 Vimpani GV, Vimpani AF, Lidgard GP, et al. Prevalence of severe growth hormone deficiency. BMJ 1977; ii:427–430.
116 Argente J, Abusrewil SAS, Bona G, et al. Isolated growth hormone deficiency in children and adolescents. J Pediatr Endocrinol Metab 2001; 14(suppl 2):1003–1008.
117 Spiliotis BE, August GP, Hung W, et al. Growth hormone neurosecretory dysfunction. A treatable cause of short stature. J Am Med Assoc 1984; 251:2223–2230.
118 Shohat M, Rimoin DL. The skeletal dysplasias. In: Lifshitz F, ed. Pediatric endocrinology. New York: Marcel Dekker; 1996; 131–148.
119 Saleh M, Bomd J, Fletcher S. Limb-lengthening techniques. In: Kelnar CJH, Savage MO, Stirling HF, Saenger P, eds. Growth disorders – pathophysiology and treatment. London: Chapman & Hall, 1998:721–744.

120 Ducos B, Cabrol S, Houang M, et al. IGF type 1 receptor ligand binding characteristics are altered in a subgroup of children with intrauterine growth retardation. J Clin Endocrinol Metab 2001; 86:5516–5524.
121 Powell GF, Brasel A, Blizzard RM. Emotional deprivation and growth retardation simulating idiopathic hypopituitarism. I. Clinical evaluation of the syndrome. N Engl J Med 1967; 276:1271–1278.
122 Powell GF, Brasel, Raiti S, Blizzard RM. Emotional deprivation and growth retardation simulating idiopathic hypopituitarism. II. Endocrinologic evaluation of the syndrome. N Engl J Med 1967; 276:1279–1283.
123 Stanhope R, Adlard P, Hamill G, et al. Physiological growth hormone secretion during the recovery from psychosocial dwarfism: a case report. Clin Endocrinol 1988; 28:335–340.
124 Lyall EGH, Crofton PM, Stirling HF, Kelnar CJH. Albuminuric growth failure. A case of Munchausen syndrome by proxy. Acta Pediatr1992; 81:373–376.
125 Laron Z. Laron syndrome: from description to therapy. Endocrinologist 1993; 3:21–28.
126 Amselem S, Duquesnoy P, Duriez B, et al. Spectrum of growth hormone receptor mutations and associated haplotypes in Laron syndrome. Hum Mol Genet 1993; 2:355–359.
127 Ranke MB, Savage MO, Chatelain PG, et al. Long-term treatment of growth hormone insensitivity syndrome with IGF-I. Results of the European Multicentre Study. The Working Group on Growth Hormone Insensitivity Syndromes. Horm Res 1999; 51:128–134.
*128 Grossman A, Savage MO, Wass JA, et al. Growth-hormone-releasing factor in growth hormone deficiency: demonstration of a hypothalamic defect in growth hormone release. Lancet 1983; ii:137–138.
129 Grossman A, Lytras N, Savage MO, et al. Growth hormone releasing factor: comparison of two analogues and demonstration of hypothalamic defect in growth hormone release after radiotherapy. Br Med J (Clin Res Ed) 1984; 288:1785–1787.
130 Girard J, Celniker A, Price DA, et al. Urinary measurement of growth hormone secretion. Acta Pediatr Scand 1990; 366(suppl):149–154.
131 GH Research Society. Consensus guidelines for the diagnosis and treatment of growth hormone (GH) deficiency in childhood and adolescence: summary statement of the GH Research Society. J Clin Endocrinol Metab 2000; 85:3990–3993.
132 Thomas M, Massa G, Bourguignon JP, et al. Final height in children with idiopathic growth hormone deficiency treated with recombinant human growth hormone: the Belgian experience. Horm Res 2000; 55:88–94.
*133 Vimalachandra D, Craig JC, Cowell C, Knight JF. Growth hormone for children with chronic renal failure (Cochrane Review) Cochrane Database Syst Rev 2001; 4:CD003264.
*134 Vimalachandra D, Craig JC, Cowell CT, Knight JF. Growth hormone treatment in children with chronic renal failure: A meta-analysis of randomized controlled trials. J Pediatr 2001; 139:560–566.
135 Kelnar CJH. Growth hormone therapy in Noonan syndrome. Horm Res 2000; 53(suppl 1):77–81.
136 Paterson WF, Donaldson MDC, Greene SA et al. The boom that never was: results of a 10 year audit of pediatric growth hormone prescribing in Scotland. Health Bull 2000; 60:457–466.
137 Frisancho AR, Sanchez Z, Pollardel D, Yanez L. Adaptive significance of small body size under poor socioeconomoic conditions in southern Peru. Am J Phys Anthropol 1977; 39:255–262.
138 Malcolm LA. Growth and development in New Guinea. Monograph no. 1. Madang Institute of Human Biology 1971.
139 Stini WA. Malnutrition, body size and proportion. Ecology Food Nutr 1972; 1:121.
140 Kranzler JH, Rosenbloom AL, Proctor B. Is short stature a handicap? A comparison of the psychosocial functioning of referred and nonreferred children with normal short stature and children with normal stature. J Pediatr 2000; 136:96–102.
141 Stabler B, Clopper RR, Siegel PT, et al. Academic achievement and psychological adjustment in short children. The National Cooperative Growth Study. J Dev Behav Pediatr 1994; 15:1–6.
142 Skuse DH, Gilmour J, Tian CS, Hindmarsh PC. Psychosocial assessment of children with short stature:a preliminary report. Acta Paediatr Scand 1994; 406:11–16.
143 Albanese A, Stanhope R. Growth and metabolic data following growth hormone treatment of children with intrauterine growth retardation. Horm Res 1993; 39:8–12.
144 Cianfarani S, Germani D, Branca F. Low birthweight and adult insulin resistance: the 'catch-up growth' hypothesis. Arch Dis Child (Fetal Neonatal Ed) 1999; 81:F71–73.
145 Maxwell H, Rees L. Recombinant human growth hormone treatment in infants with chronic renal failure. Arch Dis Child 1996; 74:40–43.
146 Burren CP, Werther GA. Skeletal dysplasias: response to growth hormone therapy. J Pediatr Endocrinol Metab 1996; 9:31–40.
147 Donaldson MDC. Growth hormone therapy in Turner syndrome – current uncertainties and future strategies. Horm Res 1997; 48 (suppl 5):35–44.
148 Mauras N, Attie KM, Reiter EO, et al. High dose recombinant human growth hormone (GH) treatment of GH-deficient patients in puberty increases near-final height: a randomized, multicenter trial. Genentech, Inc., Cooperative Study Group. J Clin Endocrinol Metab 2000; 85:3653–3660.
149 Cutfield WS, Wilton P, Bennmarker H, et al. Incidence of diabetes mellitus and impaired glucose tolerance in children and adolescents receiving growth-hormone treatment. Lancet 2000; 355:610–613.
150 Malozowski S, Tanner LA, Wysowski DK, et al. Benign intracranial hypertension in children with growth hormone deficiency treated with growth hormone. J Pediatr 1995; 126:996–999.
151 Smith PJ, Brook CGD. Growth hormone releasing hormone or growth hormone treatment in growth hormone insufficiency? Arch Dis Child 1988; 63:629–634.
152 Hedin L, Diczfalusy M, Olsson B, et al. Nasal delivery of human growth hormone: a new route of administration. Acta Pediatr Scand 1989; 367(suppl):158.
153 Kelnar CJH. Does the short, sexually immature adolescent boy need treatment and what form should it take? Arch Dis Child 1994; 71:285–287.
154 Skuse DH. The psychological consequences of being small. J Child Psychol Psychiatry 1987; 28:641–650.
155 Alley TR. Growth produced changes in body size as determinants of perceived age and adult care giving. Child Dev 1983; 54:241–248.
156 Gordon M, Crouthamel C, Post EM, et al. Psychosocial aspects of constitutional short stature: social competence, behavior problems, self-esteem and family functioning. J Pediatr 1982; 101:477–480.
157 Mussen PH, Jones MC. Self-conceptions, motivations and interpersonal attitudes of late- and early-maturing boys. Child Dev 1957; 28:243–256.
158 Nicolson A, Toogood AA, Rahim A, shalet SM. The prevalence of severe growth hormone deficiency in adults who received growth hormone replacement in childhood. Clin Endocrinol (Oxf). 1996; 44:311–316.
159 Donaldson MDC, Kelnar CJH. Tall stature. In: Ranke MB, Wit J-M, Kelnar CJH, eds. Classification system for pediatric endocrine diseases, Edition J & J. Mannheim: Palatium Verlag; 2000:12–13 & 42–49.
160 Schwartz HP, Joss E, Zuppinger K. Bromocriptine treatment in adolescent boys with familial tall stature. A pair-matched controlled study. J Clin Endocrinol Metab 1987; 65:136–140.
161 WHO. Collaborative study of neoplasia and steroid contraceptives. Invasive cervical cancer and combined oral contraceptives. Br Med J 1985; 290:961–965.
162 Macnicol MF. Surgical management of tall stature. In: Kelnar CJH, Savage MO, Stirling HF, Saenger P, eds. Growth disorders – pathophysiology and treatment. London: Chapman & Hall; 1998:791–799.
163 Kelnar CJH, Stanhope R. Height prognosis in girls with central precocious puberty treated with GnRH analogues (invited commentary). Clin Endocrinol 2002; 56:295–296.
164 Halaas JL, Gajiwala KS, Maffei M, et al. Weight-reducing effects of the plasma protein encoded by the obese gene. Science 1995; 269:543–546.
165 Janeckova R. The role of leptin in human physiology and pathophysiology. Physiol Res 2001; 50:443–459.
166 Tanner JM, Whitehouse RH. The Harpenden skinfold caliper. Am J Phys Anthropol 1955; 13:743–746.
167 Tanner JM, Whitehouse RH. Revised standards for triceps and subscapular skinfolds for British children. Arch Dis Child 1975; 50:142–145.
168 Parizkova J, Roth Z. The assessment of depot fat in children from skinfold thickness measurements by Holtain (Tanner–Whitehouse) caliper. Hum Biol 1972; 44:613–620.

169 Womersley J, Durnin JV. An experimental study on variability of measurements of skinfold thickness on young adults. Hum Biol 1973; 45:281–292.

170 Hughes JM, Li L, Chinn S, Rona RJ. Trends in growth in England and Scotland, 1972 to 1994. Arch Dis Child 1997; 76:182–189.

171 Cole TJ, Bellizzi MC, Flegal KM, et al. Establishing a standard definition for child overweight and obesity worldwide: international survey. BMJ 2000; 320:1240–1243.

172 Jebb SA, Prentice AM. Single definition of overweight and obesity should be used. BMJ 2001; 323:999.

173 Chinn S, Rona RJ. Prevalence and trends in overweight and obesity in three cross sectional studies of British children, 1974–94. BMJ 2001; 322:24–26.

174 WHO. Obesity: preventing and managing the global epidemic. Geneva: WHO; 1998.

175 Poskitt EME, Cole TJ. Do fat babies stay fat? BMJ 1977; i:7–9.

*176 Parsons TJ, Power C, Logan S, Summerbell CD. Childhood predictors of adult obesity: a systematic review. Int J Obes Relat Metab Disord 1999; 23(suppl 8):S1–107.

177 Whitaker RC, Wright JA, Pepe MS, et al. Predicting obesity in young adulthood from childhood and parental obesity. N Engl J Med 1997; 337:869–873.

178 Gortmaker SL, Must A, Perrin JM, et al. Social and economic consequences of overweight in adolescence and young adulthood. N Engl J Med 1993; 329:1008–1012.

179 Freedman DS, Dietz WH, Srinivasan SR, Berenson GS. The relation of overweight to cardiovascular risk factors among children and adolescents: The Bogalusa Heart Study. Pediatrics 1999; 103:1175–1182.

*180 Campbell K, Waters E, O'Meara S, Summerbell C. Interventions for preventing obesity in children (Cochrane Review). Cochrane Database Syst Rev 2001; 3:CD001871.

*181 Edmunds L, Waters E, Elliott EJ. Evidence based management of childhood obesity. BMJ 2001; 323:916–919.

*182 SIGN Guideline. Childhood obesity (in press) Scottish Intercollegiate Guidelines Network; 2003, http://www.sign.ac.uk/.

183 Eiholzer U, l'Allemand D. Growth hormone normalises height, prediction of final height and hand length in children with Prader–Willi syndrome after 4 years of therapy. Horm Res 2000; 53:185–192.

184 Eiholzer U, l'Allemand D, van der Sluis I, et al. Body composition abnormalities in children with Prader–Willi syndrome and long-term effects of growth hormone therapy. Horm Res 2000; 53:200–206.

185 Carrel AL, Myers SE, Whitman BY, Allen DB. Sustained benefits of growth hormone on body composition, fat utilization, physical strength and agility, and growth in Prader–Willi syndrome are dose-dependent. J Pediatr Endocrinol Metab 2001; 14:1097–1105.

186 Savage DCL, Forsyth CC, Cameron J. Excretion of individual adreno-cortical steroids in obese children. Arch Dis Child 1974; 49:946–954.

187 Lestradet H, Deschamps I, Giron B, Ostrowski ZL. Relationship between the size of the adipocytes, blood glucose, plasma insulin, NEFA and the degree of obesity in children In: Howard A, ed. Recent Advances in obesity research. London: Newman Publishing; 1975:167–169.

188 Grey N, Kipnis DM. Effect of diet composition on hyperinsulinemia of obesity. N Engl J Med 1971; 285:827–831.

189 Galloway PJ, Donaldson MD, Wallace AM. Sex hormone binding globulin concentration as a prepubertal marker for hyperinsulinemia in obesity. Arch Dis Child 2001; 85:489–491.

190 Brook CGD, Lloyd JK. Adipose cell size and glucose tolerance in obese children. Arch Dis Child 1973; 48:301–302.

191 Cutting WAM, Elton RA, Campbell JL. Stunting in African children. Arch Dis Child 1987; 62:508–509.

192 Pimstone B, Barberazat G, Hansen J, Murray P. Studies on growth hormone secretion in protein-calorie malnutrition. Am J Clin Nutr 1968; 21:482–487.

193 Mohan PS, Rao KSJ. Plasma somatomedin activity in protein calorie malnutrition. Arch Dis Child 1979; 54:62–64.

194 Ketelslegers JM, Maiter D, Maes M. Nutrition and growth. In: Kelnar CJH, Savage MO, Stirling HF, Saenger P, eds. Growth disorders – pathophysiology and treatment. London: Chapman & Hall; 1998:79–96.

195 Boyar RM, Hellman LD, Roffward H, et al. Cortisol secretion and metabolism in anorexia nervosa. N Engl J Med 1977; 296:190–193.

196 Bradlow HL, Boyar RM, O'Connor J, et al. Hypothyroid-like alterations in testosterone metabolism in anorexia nervosa. J Clin Endocrinol Metab 1976; 43:571–574.

197 Boyar RM, Katz J, Finkelstein JW, et al. Anorexia nervosa: immaturity of the 24 hour luteinizing hormone secretory pattern. N Engl J Med 1974; 291:861–865.

198 Huseman C, Johanson A. Growth hormone deficiency in anorexia nervosa. J Pediatr 1975; 87:946–948.

199 Stanhope R, Pringle PJ, Brook CGD. Alteration in the nocturnal pulsatile release of GH during the induction of puberty using low dose pulsatile LHRH: a case report. Clin Endocrinol 1985; 22:117–120.

200 Treasure JL, Gordon PAL, King EA, Wheeler M, Russell GFM. Cystic ovaries: a phase of anorexia nervosa. Lancet 1985; ii:1379–1382.

201 Ling N, Shao-Yao SY, Ueno N, et al. Pituitary FSH is released by a heterodimer of the beta-subunits from the two forms of inhibin. Nature 1986; 321:779 –782.

202 Vale W, Rivier J, Vaughan J, et al. Purification and characterisation of an FSH releasing protein from porcine ovarian follicular fluid. Nature 1986; 321:776–779.

203 Burger HG, Igarashi M. Inhibin: definition and nomenclature, including related substances. J Clin Endocrinol Metab 1988; 66:885–886.

204 Groome NP, Illingworth PJ, O'Brien M, et al. Measurement of dimeric inhibin-B throughout the human menstrual cycle. J Clin Endocrinol Metab 1996; 81:1401–1405.

205 Illingworth PJ, Groome NP, Duncan WC, et al. Measurement of circulating inhibin forms during the establishment of pregnancy. J Clin Endocrinol Metab 1996; 81:1471–1475.

206 Illingworth PJ, Groome NP, Byrd W, et al. Inhibin-B: a potential candidate for the principal bioactive inhibin form in plasma in men. J Clin Endocrinol Metab 1996; 81:1321–1325.

207 Rosenfield RL, Bachrach LK, Chernausek SD, et al. Current age of onset of puberty. Pediatrics 2000; 106:622–623.

208 Viner R. Splitting hairs. Is puberty getting earlier in girls? Arch Dis Child 2002; 86:8–10.

209 Herman-Giddens ME, Slora EJ, Wasserman RC, et al. Secondary sexual characteristics and menses in young girls seen in office practice: a study from the Pediatric Research in Office Settings network. Pediatrics 1997; 99:505–512.

210 Kaplowitz PB, Oberfield SE. Reexamination of the age limit for defining when puberty is precocious in girls in the United States: implications for evaluation and treatment. Drug and Therapeutics and Executive Committees of the Lawson Wilkins Pediatric Endocrine Society. Pediatrics 1999; 104:936–941.

211 Whincup PH, Gilg JA, Odoki K, et al. Age of menarche in contemporary British teenagers: survey of girls born between 1982 and 1986. BMJ 2001; 322:1095–1096.

212 Herman-Giddens ME, Wang L, Koch G. Secondary sexual characteristics in boys: estimates from the national health and nutrition examination survey III, 1988–1994 Arch Pediatr Adolesc Med 2001; 155:1022–1028.

213 Wu FCW, Butler GE, Kelnar CJH, et al. Patterns of pulsatile luteinizing hormone and follicle stimulating hormone secretion in prepubertal (midchildhood) boys and girls and patients with idiopathic hypogonadotrophic hypogonadism (Kallmann's syndrome): a study using an ultrasensitive time-resolved immunofluorometric assay. J Clin Endocrinol Metab 1991; 72:1229–1237.

214 Wu FCW, Butler GE, Kelnar CJH, Sellar RE. Patterns of pulsatile LH secretion before and during the onset of pubertty in boys – a study using an immunoradiometric assay. J Clin Endocrinol Metab 1990; 70:629–637.

215 Boyar RM, Finkelstein J, Roffwarg H, et al. Synchronisation of augmented luteinising hormone secretion with sleep during puberty. New Engl J Med 1972; 287:582–586.

216 Stanhope R, Pringle PJ, Adams J, et al. Spontaneous gonadotrophin pulsatility and ovarian morphology in girls with central precocious puberty treated with cyproterone acetate. Clin Endocrinol 1985; 23:547–553.

217 Brown DC, Kelnar CJH, Wu FCW. Energy metabolism during human male puberty II: Use of testicular size in predictive equations for basal metabolic rate. Ann Hum Biol 1996; 23:281–284.

218 Wu FCW, Butler GE, Kelnar CJH, et al. Ontogeny of pulsatile gonadotrophin releasing hormone (GnRH) secretion from midchildhood through puberty to adulthood in the human male: a study using deconvolution analyses and an ultrasensitive immunofluorometric assay. J Clin Endocrinol Metab 1996; 81:1798–1805.

219 Wu FCW, Butler GE, Brown DC, et al. Early morning testosterone is a useful predictor of the imminence of puberty. J Clin Endocrinol Metab 1993; 76:26–31.

220 Chemes HE. Infancy is not a quiescent period of testicular development. Int J Androl 2001; 24:2–7.
221 Rey RA, Campo SM, Bedecarras P, et al. Is infancy a quiescent period of testicular development? Histological, morphometric and functional study of the seminiferous tubules of the Cebus monkey from birth to puberty. J Clin Endocrinol Metab 1993; 76:1325–1331.
222 Millar MR, Sharpe RM, Weinbauer GF, et al. Marmoset spermatogenesis: organisational similarities to the human. Int J Androl 2000; 23:266–277.
223 Kelnar CJH, McKinnell C, Walker M, et al. Testicular changes during infantile 'quiescence' in the marmoset and their gonadotrophin dependence: a model for investigating susceptibility of the prepubertal human testis to cancer therapy? Hum Reprod 2002; 1:1367–1378.
224 Crofton PM, Illingworth PJ, Groome NP, et al. Changes in dimeric inhibin A and B during normal early puberty in boys and girls. Clin Endocrinol 1997; 46:109–114.
225 Crofton PM, Evans AEM, Groome NP, et al. Inhibin B in boys from birth to adulthood: relationship with age, pubertal stage, follicle stimulating hormone and testosterone. Clin Endocrinol 2002; 56:215–221.
226 Crofton PM, Evans AEM, Groome NP, et al. Dimeric inhibins in girls from birth to adulthood: relationship with age, pubertal stage, follicle stimulating hormone and oestradiol. Clin Endocrinol 2002; 56:223–230.
227 Penny R, Olambiwannu NO, Frasier SD. Episodic fluctuations of serum gonadotrophins in pre- and post-pubertal girls and boys. J Clin Endocrinol Metab 1977; 45:307–311.
228 Stanhope R, Brook CGD, Pringle PJ, et al. Induction of puberty by pulsatile gonadotrophin-releasing hormone. Lancet 1987; ii:552–555.
229 Wu FCW, Feek CM, Glasier A. Long-term pulsatile GnRH therapy in males with idiopathic hypogonadotrophic hypogonadism (IHH). J Endocrinol 1987;112(suppl):A37.
230 Stark O, Peckham CS, Moynihan C. Weight and age at menarche. Arch Dis Child 1989; 64:383–387.
231 Brown DC, Kelnar CJH, Wu FCW. Energy metabolism during human male puberty I: Changes in energy expenditure during the onset of puberty in boys. Ann Hum Biol 1996; 23:273–279.
232 Warren MP, Jewelewicz R, Dyrenfurth I, et al. The significance of weight loss in the evaluation of pituitary responsiveness to LH-RH in women with secondary amenorrhea. J Clin Endocrinol Metabol 1975; 40:601–611.
233 Veldhuis JD, Evans WS, Demers LM, et al. Altered neuroendocrine regulation of gonadotrophin secretion in women distance runners. J Clin Endocrinol Metab 1985; 61:557–563.
234 Warren MP, Vande Wiele RL. Clinical and metabolic features of anorexia nervosa. Am J Obstet Gynecol 1973; 117:435–449.
235 Kiess W, Muller G, Galler A, et al. Body fat mass, leptin and puberty. J Pediatr Endocrinol Metab 2000; 13 (suppl 1):717–722.
236 Adashi EY, Hsueh AJ, Yen SS. Insulin enhancement of luteinizing hormone and follicle-stimulating hormone release by cultured pituitary cells. Endocrinology 1981; 108:1441–1449.
237 Pescovitz OH, Hench KD, Barnes KM, et al. Premature thelarche and central precocious puberty: the relationship between clinical presentation and the gonadotrophin response to luteinizing hormone-releasing hormone. J Clin Endocrinol Metab 1988; 67:474–479.
238 Bridges NA, Christopher JA, Hindmarsh PC, Brook CGD. Sexual precocity: sex incidence and etiology. Arch Dis Child 1994; 70:116 –118.
239 Radar NK, Ansusingha K, Kenny FM. Circulating bound and free oestradiol and oestrone during normal growth and development in premature thelarche and isosexual precocity. J Pediatr 1976; 89:719–723.
240 Ilicki A, Prager-Lewin R, Kauli R, et al. Premature thelarche – natural history and sex hormone secretion in 68 girls. Acta Pediatr Scand 1984; 73:756–772.
241 Stanhope R, Abdulwahid NA, Adams J, Brook CGD. Studies of gonadotrophin pulsatility and pelvic ultrasound distinguish between isolated premature thelarche and central precocious puberty. Eur J Pediatr 1986; 145:190–194.
242 Crofton PM, Evans AEM, Groome N, et al. Plasma inhibin in healthy girls and in girls with disorders of puberty. Horm Res 2000; 53(suppl 2):P1-269 80.
243 Stanhope R. Premature thelarche: clinical follow-up and indication for treatment. J Pediatr Endocrinol Metab 2000; 13:827–830.
244 Stanhope R, Brook CGD. Thelarche variant: a new syndrome of precocious sexual maturation? Acta Endocrinol 1990; 123:481–486.
245 Zangeneh F, Kelly VC. Granulosa-theca-cell tumor of the ovaries in children. Am J Dis Child 1968; 115:494–508.
246 Lyon AJ, DeBruyn R, Grant DB. Transient sexual precocity and ovarian cysts. Arch Dis Child 1985; 60:819–822.
247 Meadow R. Munchausen syndrome by proxy. Arch Dis Child 1982; 57:92–98.
248 Laron Z, Karp M, Dolberg L. Juvenile hypothyroidism with testicular enlargement. Acta Pediatr Scand 1970; 59:317–322.
249 Buchanan CR, Stanhope R, Jones J, et al. Gonadotrophin, growth hormone and prolactin secretory dysfunction in primary hypothyroidism. Pediatr Res 1988; 23:A133.
250 Pringle PJ, Stanhope R, Hindmarsh PC, Brook CGD. Abnormal sexual development in primary hypothyroidism. Clin Endocrinol 1988; 28:479–486.
251 Floyd JL, Dorwart RH, Nelson MJ, et al. Pituitary hyperplasia secondary to thyroid failure: CT appearance. Am J Neurol Radiol 1984; 5:469–471.
252 McCune DJ, Bruch H. Osteodystrophia fibrosa: report of a case in which the condition was combined with precocious puberty, pathological pigmentation of the skin and hyperthyroidism, with a review of the literature. Am J Dis Child 1937; 54:806–848.
253 Albright F, Butler AM, Hampton AO, et al. Syndrome characterized by osteitis fibrosa disseminata, areas of pigmentation and endocrine dysfunction with precocious puberty in females, report of five case. N Engl J Med 1937; 216:727–746.
254 Di George A. Albright syndrome: is it coming of age? J Pediatr 1975; 87:1018–1020.
255 Shenker A, Weinstein LS, Moran A, et al. Severe endocrine and non-endocrine manifestations of the McCune–Albright syndrome associated with activating mutations of stimulatory G protein Gs. J Pediatr 1993; 123:509–518.
256 Foster CM, Comite F, Pescovitz OH, et al. Variable response to a long-acting agonist of luteinizing hormone-releasing hormone in girls with McCune–Albright syndrome. J Clin Endocrinol Metab 1984; 59:801–805.
257 Cacciari E, Frejauille E, Cicognani A, et al. How many cases of true precocious puberty in girls are idiopathic? J Pediatr 1983; 102:357–360.
258 Russell A. A syndrome of 'intrauterine' dwarfism recognizable at birth with craniofacial dysostosis, disproportionately short arms and other anomalies (5 examples). Proc R Soc Med 1954; 47:1040–1044.
259 Silver HK, Kiyasu W, George J, Daemer WC. A syndrome of congenital hemihypertrophy, shortness of stature and elevated urinary gonadotrophins. Pediatrics 1953; 12:368–375.
260 Rosenthal SN, Grumbach MM, Kaplan SL. Gonadotrophin independent sexual precocity with premature Leydig and germinal cell maturation (familial testotoxicosis): effects of a potent luteinising hormone-releasing factor agonist and medroxyprogesterone acetate therapy in four cases. J Clin Endocrinol Metab 1983; 57:571–579.
261 Lee PA. Disorders of puberty. In: Lifshitz F, ed. Pediatric endocrinology. New York: Marcel Dekker; 1996:175–196.
262 Shenker A, Laue L, Kosugi S, et al. A constitutively activating mutation of the luteinizing hormone receptor in familial male precocious puberty. Nature 1993; 365:652–654.
263 Holland FJ, Fishman L, Bailey JD, Fazekas ATA. Ketoconazole in the management of precocious puberty not responsive to LHRH-analogue therapy. N Engl J Med 1985; 312:1023–1028.
264 Paterson WF, McNeill E, Reid S, et al. Efficacy of Zoladex LA (goserelin) in the treatment of girls with central precocious or early puberty. Arch Dis Child 1998; 79:323–327.
265 Tanner JM, Whitehouse RH, Cameron N, et al. Assessment of skeletal maturity and prediction of adult height, 2nd edn. London: Academic Press; 1983.
266 Buckler JMH. Growth at adolescence. In: Kelnar CJH, Savage MO, Stirling HF Saenger P, eds. Growth disorders – pathophysiology and treatment. London: Chapman & Hall; 1998; 179–193.
267 Pucarelli I, Segni M, Ortore M. Combined therapy with GnRH analog plus growth hormone in central precocious puberty. J Pediatr Endocrinol Metab 2000; 13(suppl 1):811–820.
268 Ward PS, Ward I, McNinch AW, Savage DCL. Reversible inhibition of central precocious

puberty with a long-acting GnRH analogue. Arch Dis Child 1986; 60:872–874.
269 Stirling HF, Butler GE, Glasier A, et al. Hypothalamo-pituitary-ovarian function after D-ser LHRH agonist (Buserelin) treatment for central precocious puberty. J Endocrinol 1989; 121(suppl):A153.
270 Roemmich JN, Richmond RJ, Rogol AD. Consequences of sport training during puberty. J Endocrinol Invest 2001; 24:708–715.
271 Seminara SB, Oliveira LM, Beranova M, et al. Genetics of hypogonadotropic hypogonadism. J Endocrinol Invest 2000; 23:560–565.
272 Kelnar CJH. Thyroid disturbances in cytogenetic diseases. Dev Med Child Neurol 1989; 31:400–404.
273 Pai GS, Leach DC, Weiss L, et al. Thyroid abnormalities in 20 children with Turner syndrome. J Pediatr 1977; 91:267–269.
274 Sas TC, de Muinck Keizer-Schrama SM, Stijnen T, et al. Normalization of height in girls with Turner syndrome after long-term growth hormone treatment: results of a randomized dose-response trial. J Clin Endocrinol Metab 1999; 84:4607–4612.
275 Bramswig JH. Long-term results of growth hormone therapy in Turner syndrome. Endocrine 2001; 15:5–13.
276 Johnston DI, Betts P, Dunger D, et al. A multicentre trial of recombinant growth hormone and low dose estrogen in Turner syndrome: near final height analysis. Arch Dis Child 2001; 84:76–81.
277 Betts PR, Butler GE, Donaldson MD, et al. A decade of growth hormone treatment in girls with Turner syndrome in the UK. UK KIGS Executive Group. Arch Dis Child 1999; 80:221–225.
278 Bath LE, Critchley HOD, Chambers SE, et al. Ovarian and uterine characteristics after total body irradiation in childhood and adolescence: response to sex steroid replacement. Br J Obstet Gynaecol 1999; 106:1265–1272.
279 Rebar R, Judd SL, Yen SSC, et al. Characterisation of the inappropriate gonadotrophin secretion in polycystic ovary syndrome. J Clin Invest 1976; 57:1320–1325.
280 Critchley HOD, Buckley CH, Anderson DC. Experience with a 'physiological' steroid replacement regimen for the establishment of a receptive endometrium in women with premature ovarian failure. Br J Obstet Gynaecol 1990; 97:804–810.
281 Macfarlane CE, Brown DC, Johnston LB, et al. Growth hormone therapy and growth in children with Noonan syndrome: results of 3 years' follow-up. J Clin Endocrinol Metab 2001; 86:1953–1956.
282 Kirk JMW, Betts PR, Donaldson MDC, et al. Short stature in Noonan syndrome: response to growth hormone therapy. Arch Dis Child 2001; 84:440–443.
283 Tartaglia M, Mehler EL, Goldberg R, et al. Mutations in PTPN11, encoding the protein tyrosine phosphatase SHP-2, cause Noonan syndrome. Nat Genet 2001; 29:465–468.
284 Nakanishi S, Inove A, Kita T, et al. Nucleotide sequence of cloned cDNA for bovine corticotrophin–lipoprotein precursor. Nature 1979; 278:423–427.
285 Crawford JD, Bode HH. Disorders of the posterior pituitary in children. In: Gardner LI, ed. Endocrine and genetic diseases of childhood and adolescence, 2nd edn. Philadelphia: Saunders; 1975:126–158.
286 Czernichow P, Pomerade R, Brauner R, Rappaport R. Neurogenic diabetes insipidus in children. In: Czernichow P, Robinson AG, eds. Diabetes insipidus in man. Basel: Karger; 1985:190–209.
287 Niaudet P, Dechaux M, Lercy D, Broyer M. Nephrogenic diabetes insipidus in children. In: Czernichow P, Robinson AG, eds. Diabetes insipidus in man. Basel: Karger; 1985:224–231.
288 Perheentupa J. The neurohypophysis and water regulation. In: Brook CGD, ed. Clinical paediatric endocrinology, 3rd edn. Oxford: Blackwell; 1995:560–615.
289 Aynsely-Green A. Hypoglycaemia. In: Brook CGD, ed. Clinical paediatric endocrinology, 2nd edn. Oxford: Blackwell; 1989:618–637.
290 Hofbauer KG, Marr SC. Vasopressin antagonists: present and future. Kidney Int 1987; 31:521.
291 Cushing H. Basophil adenomas of the pituitary body and their clinical manifastations (pituitary basophilism). Bull Johns Hopkins Hosp 1932; 50:137–195.
292 Weber A, Trainer PJ, Grossman AB, et al. Investigation, management and therapeutic outcome in 12 cases of childhood and adolescent Cushing's syndrome. Clin Endocrinol (Oxf) 1995; 43:19–28.
293 Albanese A, Hindmarsh P, Stanhope R. Management of hyponatremia in patients with acute cerebral insults. Arch Dis Child 2001; 85:246–251.
294 Dattani ML, Martinez-Barbera J, Thomas PQ, et al. Molecular genetics of septo-optic dysplasia. Horm Res 2000; 53 (suppl 1):26–33.
295 Brickman JM, Clements M, Tyrell R, et al. Molecular effects of novel mutations in Hesx1/HESX1 associated with human pituitary disorders. Development 2001; 128:5189–5199.
296 Sotos JF, Dodge PR, Muirhead D, et al. Cerebral gigantism in childhood: a syndrome of excessively rapid growth with acromegalic features and non-progressive neurologic disorder. N Engl J Med 1964; 271:109–116.
297 Waldhauser W, Weiszenbacher G, Frisch H, et al. Fall in nocturnal serum melatonin during prepuberty and pubescence. Lancet 1984; i:362–365.
298 Attanasio A, Borelli P, Marina R, et al. Serum melatonin in children with early and delayed puberty. Neuroendocrinol Lett 1983; 5:387–392.
299 Bodey B, Bodey B Jr, Siegel SE, Kaiser HE. Review of thymic hormones in cancer diagnosis and treatment. Int J Immunopharmacol 2000; 22:261–273.
300 Hadden JW. Thymic endocrinology. Ann NY Acad Sci 1998; 840:352–358.
301 Darras VM, Hume R, Visser TJ. Regulation of thyroid hormone metabolism during fetal development. Mol Cell Endocrinol 1999; 25:37–47.
302 Bongers-Shokking JJ, Koot HM, Verkerk PH, et al. Influence of timing and dose of thyroid hormone replacement on development in infants with congenital hypothyroidism. J Pediatr 2000; 136:292–297.
303 Delange F, Henderson P, Bourdoux P, et al. Regional variations of iodine nutrition and thyroid function during the neonatal period in Europe. Biol Neonate 1986; 49:322–330.
***304** Osborn DA. Thyroid hormones for preventing neurodevelopmental impairment in preterm infants (Cochrane Review). Cochrane Database Syst Rev 2001; 4:CD00107.
305 Bikker H, Vulsma T, Baas F, de Vijlder JJM. Identification of five novel inactivating mutations in the human thyroid peroxidase gene by denaturing gradient gel electrophoresis. Hum Mutat 1995; 6:9–16.
306 Rovet J, Ehrlich RM. Longterm effects of l-thyroxine treatment for congentital hypothyroidism. J Pediatr 1995; 126:380–386.
307 Osler W. Sporadic cretinism in America. Transactions of the Congress of American Physicians and Surgeons 1897; 4:169–206.
308 New England Congenital Hypothyroidism Collaborative. Characteristics of infantile hypothyroidism discovered on neonatal screening. J Pediatr 1984; 104:539–544.
309 Fuggle PW, Grant DB, Smith I, Murphy G. Intelligence, motor skills and behavior at 5 years in early treated congenital hypothyroidism. Eur J Pediatr 1991; 159:570–574.
310 Tillotson SL, Fuggle PW, Smith I, et al. Relation between biochemical severity and intelligence in early treated congenital hypothyroidism: a threshold effect. BMJ 1994; 309:440–445.
311 Hidaka A, Minegishi T, Kohn LD. Thyrotropin, like luteinizing hormone (LH) and chorionic gonadotrophin (CG) increases cAMP and onositol phosphate levels in cells with recombinant human LH/CG receptor. Biochem Biophys Res Commun 1993; 196:187–195.
312 Hashizume K, Icikawa K, Sakurai A, et al. Administration of thyroxine in treated Graves' disease. N Engl J Med 1991; 324:947.
313 Shibata Y, Yamashita S, Masyakin VB, et al. 15 years after Chernobyl: new evidence of thyroid cancer. Lancet 2001; 358:1965–1966.
314 Wartofsky L. Radioiodine therapy for Graves' disease: case selection and restrictions recommended to patients in North America. Thyroid 1997; 7:213–216.
315 Corrias A, Einaudi S, Chiorboli E, et al. Accuracy of fine needle aspiration biopsy of thyroid nodules in detecting malignancy in childhood: comparison with conventional clinical, laboratory, and imaging approaches. J Clin Endocrinol Metab 2001; 86: 4644–4648.
316 Brandi ML, Gagel RF, Angeli A, et al. Guidelines for diagnosis and therapy of MEN type 1 and type 2. J Clin Endocrinol Metab 2001; 86:5658–5671.
316a Langman C. New developments in calcium and vitamin D metabolism. Curr Opin Pediatr 2000; 12:135–139.
317 Martin NDT, Snodgrass GJAI, Cohen RD. Idiopathic infantile hypercalcemia – a continuing enigma. Arch Dis Child 1984; 59:605–613.
318 Williams JCP, Barratt-Boyes BG, Lowe JB. Supravalvular aortic stenosis. Circulation 1961; 24:1311–1318.

319 Morris CA Mervis CB. Williams syndrome and related disorders. Annu Rev Genomics Hum Genet 2000; 1:461–484.

320 Tsukada T, Yamaguchi K, Kameya T. The MEN1 gene and associated diseases: an update. Endocrinol Pathol 2001; 12:259–273.

321 Betterle C, Dalpra C, Greggio N, et al. Autoimmunity in isolated Addison's disease and in polyglandular autoimmune diseases type 1, 2 and 4. Ann Endocrinol (Paris) 2001; 62:193–201.

322 Albright F, Burnett CH, Smith PH. Pseudohypoparathyroidism: an example of 'Seabright-Bantam syndrome'. Endocrinology 1942; 30:922–932.

323 Levine MA, Jap T-S, Mauseth RS, et al. Activity of the stimulating guanine nucleotide-binding regulatory protein in erythrocytes from patients with pseudohypoparathyroidism and pseudopseudohypoparathyroidism: biochemical, endocrine and genetic analysis of Albright's hereditary osteodystrophy in six kindreds. J Clin Endocrinol Metab 1986; 62:497–502.

324 Ahmed SF, Dixon PH, Bonthron DT, et al. GNAS1 mutational analysis in pseudohypoparathyroidism. Clin Endocrinol 1998; 49:525–532.

325 Bastepe M, Juppner H. Pseudohypoparathyroidism. New insights into an old disease. Endocrinol Metab Clin North Am 2000; 29:569–589.

326 Stirling HF, Barr DGD, Kelnar CJH. Familial growth hormone releasing factor deficiency in pseudopseudohypoparathyroidism. Arch Dis Child 1991; 66:533–535.

327 Honour JW, Kelnar CJH, Brook CGD. Urine adrenal steroid excretion rates in childhood reflect growth and activity of the adrenal cortex. Acta Endocrinol 1991; 124:219–224.

328 Kelnar CJH. Adrenal steroids in childhood. MD thesis, University of Cambridge; 1985.

329 Molinari L, Largo RH, Prader A. Analysis of the growth spurt at age seven (mid-growth spurt). Helv Pediatr Acta 1980; 35:325–334.

330 Speiser PW, Dupont B, Rubinstein P, et al. High frequency of nonclassical steroid 21-hydroxylase deficiency. Am J Hum Genet 1985; 37:650–667.

331 White PC, Grossberger D, Onufer BJ, et al. Two genes encoding steroid 21-hydroxylase are located near the genes encoding the fourth component of complement in man. Proc Natl Acad Sci USA 1985; 82:1089–1093.

332 Stoner E, DiMartino J, Kuhnle U, et al. Is salt-wasting in congenital adrenal hyperplasia genetic? Clin Endocrinol 1986; 24:9–20.

333 Jeffcoate TNA, Fliegner JRH, Russell SH, et al. Diagnosis of the adrenogenital syndrome before birth. Lancet 1965; ii:553–555.

334 New MI, Carlson A, Obeid J, et al. Prenatal diagnosis for congenital adrenal hyperplasia in 532 pregnancies. J Clin Endocrinol Metab 2001; 86:5651–5657.

335 Kelnar CJH. Antenatal treatment of a mother bearing a fetus with congenital adrenal hyperplasia. Arch Dis Child (Fetal Neonatal Ed) 2000; 82:F176–F181.

336 Kovacs J, Votava F, Heinze G, et al. Lessons from 30 years of clinical diagnosis and treatment of congenital adrenal hyperplasia in five middle European countries. J Clin Endocrinol Metab 2001; 86:2958–2964.

337 Pang S, Hotchkiss J, Drash AL, et al. Microfilter paper method for 17alpha-hydroxy progesterone radioimmunoassay: its application for rapid screening for congenital adrenal hyperplasia. J Clin Endocrinol Metab 1977; 45:1003–1008.

338 Pang S, Dobbins RH, Kling S, et al. Worldwide newborn screening update for classical congenital adrenal hyperplasia. In: Schmidt BJ, ed. Current trends in infant screening. Amsterdam: Elsevier Science; 1989:307–312.

339 Nordenström A, Thilén A, Hagenfeldt L, et al. Genotyping is a valuable diagnostic complement to neonatal screening for congenital adrenal hyperplasia due to steroid 21-hydroxylase deficiency. J Clin Endocrinol Metab 1999; 84:1505–1509.

340 Rosenwaks Z, Lee PA, Jones GS, et al. An attenuated form of congenital virilizing adrenal hyperplasia. J Clin Endocrinol Metab 1979; 49:335–339.

341 Pang S, Lerner A, Stoner E, et al. Late onset adrenal steroid 3beta HSD deficiency: a cause of hirsutism in pubertal and postpubertal women. J Clin Endocrinol Metab 1985; 60:428–429.

342 Chung BC, Picado-Leonard J, Hanio M, et al. Cytochrome P450 c17: cloning of human adrenal and testis cDNA indicates the same gene is expressed in both tissues. Proc Natl Acad Sci USA 1987; 84:407–411.

343 Richmond EJ, Flickinger CJ, McDonald JA, et al. Lipoid congenital adrenal hyperplasia (CAH): patient report and a mini-review. Clin Pediatr (Phila) 2001; 40:403–407.

344 Linder BL, Esteban NV, Yergey AL, et al. Cortisol production rate in childhood and adolescence. J Pediatr 1990; 117:892–896.

345 Kerrigan JR, Veldhuis JD, Leyo SA, et al. Estimation of daily cortisol production and clearance rates in normal pubertal males by deconvolution analysis. J Clin Endocrinol Metab 1993; 76:1505–1510.

346 Cutler GB Jr, Laue L. Congenital adrenal hyperplasia due to 21-hydroxylase deficiency. N Engl J Med 1990; 323:1806–1813.

347 Irony I, Cutler GB. Effect of carbenoxolone on the plasma renin activity and hypothalamic–pituitary–adrenal axis in congenital adrenal hyperplasia due to 21-hydroxylase deficiency. Clin Endocrinol (Oxf) 1999; 51(3):285–291.

348 Meyers RL, Grua JR. Bilateral laparoscopic adrenalectomy: a new treatment for difficult cases of congenital adrenal hyperplasia. J Pediatr Surg 2000; 35:1586–1590.

349 Schnitzer JJ, Donahoe PK. Surgical treatment of congenital adrenal hyperplasia. Endocrinol Metab Clin North Am 2001; 30:137–154.

350 Cabrera MS, Vogiatzi MG, New MI. Long term outcome in adult males with classic congenital adrenal hyperplasia. J Clin Endocrinol Metab 2001; 86:3070–3078.

351 Patel L, Wales JK, Kibirige MS, et al. Symptomatic adrenal insufficiency during inhaled corticosteroid treatment. Arch Dis Child 2001; 85:330–334.

352 Findlay CA, Macdonald JF, Wallace AM, et al. Childhood Cushing's syndrome induced by betamethasone nose drops, and repeat prescriptions. BMJ 1998; 317:739–740.

353 Massarano AA, Hollis S, Devlin J, David TJ. Growth in atopic eczema. Arch Dis Child 1993; 68:677–679.

354 Patel L, Clayton PE, Addison GM, et al. Adrenal function following topical steroid treatment in children with atopic dermatitis. Br J Dermatol 1995; 132:950–955.

355 Conn JW. Primary aldosteronism and primary reninism. Hosp Pract 1974; 9:131–140.

356 New MI, Oberfield SE, Levine LS, et al. Demonstration of autosomal dominant transmission and absence of HLA linkage in dexamethasone suppressible hyperaldosteronism. Lancet 1980; i:550–551.

357 Bartter FC, Pronove P, Gee JR, et al. Hyperplasia of the juxtaglomerular complex with hyperaldosteronism and hypokalaemic alkalosis. Am J Med 1962; 33:811–828.

358 Osmond C, Barker DJP, Winter PD, et al. Early growth and death from cardiovascular disease in women. BMJ 1993; 307:1519–1524.

359 Tabarin A. Congenital adrenal hypoplasia and DAX-1 gene mutations. Ann Endocrinol (Paris) 2001; 62:202–206.

360 Bartly JA, Miller DK, Hayford JT. Concordance of X-linked glycerol kinase deficiency with X-linked congenital adrenal hypoplasia. Lancet 1982; ii:733–736.

361 Elias LL, Huebner A, Metherell LA, et al. Tall stature in familial glucocorticoid deficiency. Clin Endocrinol (Oxf) 2000; 53:423–430.

362 Addison T. On the constitutional and local effects of disease of the suprarenal capsule. London: Highley D; 1855.

363 Crowley S, Hindmarsh P, Honour JW, et al. Failure of the short synacthen test to detect adrenal insufficiency in children on inhaled steroids. J Endocrinol 1992; 132:95.

364 Bulchmann G, Schuster T, Heger A, et al. Transient pseudohypoaldosteronism secondary to posterior urethral valves – a case report and review of the literature. Eur J Pediatr Surg 2001; 11:277–279.

365 Migeon CJ, Lanes RL. Adrenal cortex: hypo- and hyperfunction. In: Lifshitz F, ed. Pediatric endocrinology. New York: Marcel Dekker; 1996:321–346.

366 Mosser J, Douar AM, Sarde C-O, et al. Putative X-linked adrenoleukodystrophy gene shares unexpected homology with ABC transporters. Nature 1993; 361:726–730.

367 Wolthers OD, Cameron FJ, Scheimberg I, et al. Androgen secreting adrenocortical tumors. Arch Dis Child 1999; 80:46–50.

368 de Swiet M, Dillon MJ. Hypertension in children. BMJ 1989; 299:469–470.

369 de Swiet M, Dillon MJ, Littler W, et al. Measurement of blood pressure in children. BMJ 1989; 299:497.

370 Shaw MP, Bath LE, Kelnar CJH, Wallace WHB. Obesity in leukemia survivors – the familial contribution. Pediatr Hematol Oncol 2000; 17:231–232.

371 Ahmed SF, Wallace WHB, Crofton PM, et al. Short-term changes in lower leg length in children treated for acute lymphoblastic leukemia. J Pediatr Endocrinol Metab 1999; 12:75–80.

372 Crofton PM, Ahmed SF, Wade JC, et al. Bone turnover and growth during and after continuing chemotherapy in children with acute

lymphoblastic leukemia. Pediatr Res 2000; 48:490–496.
373 Swerdlow AJ, Reddingius RE, Higgins CD, et al. Growth hormone treatment of children with brain tumors and risk of tumor recurrence. J Clin Endocrinol Metab 2000; 85:4444–4449.
373a SIGN Guideline. Long term survivors of childhood cancer. Scottish Intercollegiate Guidelines Network; 2003, http://www.sign.ac.uk/
374 ISPAD. Consensus Guidelines for the management of type 1 diabetes in children and adolescents. Swift PGF, ed. Zeist, Netherlands: Medical Forum International; 2000.
*375 SIGN Guideline 55. Children and young people with diabetes. Scottish Intercollegiate Guidelines Network; 2001. http://www.sign.ac.uk/
376 Willis T. Practice of physick. London; 1684.
377 Dobson M. Experiments and observations on the urine in diabetes. Medical observations and enquiries 5. London; 1776.
378 Von Mering J, Minkowski O. Diabetes mellitus nach Pankreasextirpation. Archiv für experimentalische Pathologie und Pharmacologie 1890; 26:371–387.
379 Banting FG, Best CH, Collip JB, et al. Pancreatic extracts in the treatment of diabetes mellitus. Can Med Assoc J 1922; 12:141–146.
380 Hattersley AT. Diagnosis of maturity-onset diabetes of the young in the pediatric diabetes clinic. J Pediatr Endocrinol Metab 2000; 13(suppl 6):1411–1417.
381 Montgomery SM, Ekbom A. Smoking during pregnancy and diabetes mellitus in a British longitudinal birth cohort. BMJ 2002; 324:26–27.
382 Permutt MA, Hattersley AT. Searching for type 2 diabetes genes in the post-genome era. Trends Endocrinol Metab 2000; 11:383–393.
383 Fagot-Campagna A, Pettitt DJ, Engelgau MM, et al. Type 2 diabetes among North American children and adolescents: an epidemiologic review and a public health perspective. J Pediatr 2000; 136:664–672.
384 Owen K, Hattersley AT. Maturity-onset diabetes of the young: from clinical description to molecular genetic characterization. Best Pract Res Clin Endocrinol Metab 2001; 15:309–323.
385 Pearson ER, Liddell WG, Shepherd M, et al. Sensitivity to sulphonylureas in patients with hepatocyte nuclear factor-1alpha gene mutations: evidence for pharmacogenetics in diabetes. Diabetic Med 2000; 17:543–545.
386 Kolatsi-Joannou M, Bingham C, Ellard S, et al. Hepatocyte nuclear factor-1beta: a new kindred with renal cysts and diabetes and gene expression in normal human development. J Am Soc Nephrol 2001; 12:2175–2180.
387 Rangasami JJ, Greenwood DC, McSporran B, et al. Rising incidence of type 1 diabetes in Scottish children, 1984–93. The Scottish Study Group for the Care of Young Diabetics. Arch Dis Child 1997; 77:210–213.
388 DIABAUD. Factors influencing glycemic control in young people with type 1 diabetes in Scotland: a population-based study (DIABAUD2). Diabetes Care 2001; 24:239–244.
389 Gale EA, Gillespie KM. Diabetes and gender. Diabetologia 2001; 44:3–15.
390 Kelly MA, Mijovic CH, Barnett AH. Genetics of type 1 diabetes. Best Pract Res Clin Endocrinol Metab 2001; 15:279–291.
391 Chowdhury TA, Mijovic CH, Barnett AH. The etiology of type I diabetes. Best Pract Res Clin Endocrinol Metab 1999; 13:181–195.
392 Banatvala JE, Bryant J, Scherntaner G, et al. Coxsackie B, mumps, rubella and cytomegalovirus-specific IgM responses in patients with juvenile-onset insulin-dependent diabetes in Britain, Austria and Australia. Lancet 1985; i:1409–1412.
393 Leslie RD, Atkinson MA, Notkins AL. Autoantigens IA-2 and GAD in type I (insulin-dependent) diabetes. Diabetologia 1999; 42:3–14.
394 Notkins AL, Lan MS, Leslie RD. IA-2 and IA-2beta: the immune response in IDDM. Diabetes Metab Rev 1998; 14:85–93.
395 Zimmet P. Antibodies to glutamic acid decarboxylase in the prediction of insulin dependency. Diabetes Res Clin Pract 1996; 34(suppl):S125–31.
396 Rosenbloom AL, Schatz DA, Krischer JP, et al. Therapeutic controversy: prevention and treatment of diabetes in children. J Clin Endocrinol Metab 2000; 85:494–522.
397 Brink SJ. Presentation and ketoacidosis. In: Kelnar CJH, ed. Childhood and adolescent diabetes. London: Chapman & Hall; 1995:213–240.
398 Knip M, Ilonen J, Mustonen A, Akerblom HK. Evidence of an accelerated beta-cell destruction in HLA-DW3/DW4 heterozygous children with type 1 (insulin-dependent) diabetes. Diabetalogia 1986; 29:347–351.
399 Ludvigsson J, Samuelsson V, Beauforts C, et al. HLA-DR3 is associated with a more slowly progressive form of type 1 (insulin-dependent) diabetes. Diabetalogia 1986; 29:207–210.
400 Jefferson IG, Smith MA, Baum JD. Insulin dependent diabetes in under 5 year olds. Arch Dis Child 1985; 60:1144–1148.
401 American Diabetes Association. Report of the Expert Committee on the diagnosis and classification of diabetes mellitus. Diabetes Care 1997; 20:1183–1197.
402 WHO. Definition, Diagnosis and classification of diabetes mellitus and its complications. Geneva: WHO; 1999 (Available from http://whqlibdoc.who.int/hq/1999/WHO_NCD_NCS_99.2.pdf)
403 Vanelli M, Chiari G, Ghizzoni L, et al. Effectiveness of a prevention program for diabetic ketoacidosis in children. An 8-year study in schools and private practices. Diabetes Care 1999; 22:7–9.
404 Noyes KJ, Henderson A, Hughes H, et al. An integrated care pathway for the management of diabetic ketoacidosis. J Pediatr Endocrin Metab 2001; 14(suppl 3):PP-120 1064.
405 Wallace TM, Meston NM, Gardner SG, Matthews DR. The hospital and home use of a 30-second hand-held blood ketone meter: guidelines for clinical practice. Diabetic Med 2001; 18:640–645.
406 Scibilia J, Finegold D, Dorman J, et al. Why do children with diabetes die? Acta Endocrinol 1986; 113(suppl 279):326–333.
407 Glaser N, Barnett P, McCaslin I. Risk factors for cerebral edema in children with diabetic ketoacidosis. The Pediatric Emergency Medicine Collaborative Research Committee of the American Academy of Pediatrics. N Engl J Med 2001; 344:264–269.
408 Edge JA, Hawkins MM, Winter DL, Dunger DB. The risk and outcome of cerebral edema developing during diabetic ketoacidosis. Arch Dis Child 2001; 85:16–22.
409 Shield JPH, Baum JD. Long term management: scope and aims. In: Kelnar CJH, ed. Childhood and adolescent diabetes. London: Chapman & Hall; 1995:241–252.
410 Diabetes Control and Complications Trial Research Group. Effect of intensive diabetes treatment on the development and progression of long term complications in adolescents with insulin-dependent diabetes mellitus. J Pediatr 1994; 125:177–188.
411 Wolpert HA, Anderson BJ. Management of diabetes: are doctors framing the benefits from the wrong perspective? BMJ 2001; 323:994–996.
412 Wolpert HA, Anderson BJ. Metabolic control matters: Why is the message lost in the translation? The need for realistic goal-setting in diabetes care. Diabetes Care 2001; 24:1301–1303.
413 Tamborlane WV, Bonfig W, Boland E. Recent advances in treatment of youth with type 1 diabetes: better care through technology. Diabetic Med 2001; 18:864–870.
414 Scott A, Donnelly R. Improving outcomes for young people with diabetes: use of new technology and a skills-based training approach is urgently needed. Diabetic Med 2001; 18:861–863.
415 Ross LA, Frier BM, Kelnar CJH, Deary IJ. Child and parental mental ability and glycemic control in children with type 1 diabetes. Diabetic Med 2001; 18:364–369.
416 Dorchy H, Roggemans MP, Willems D. Glycated hemoglobin and related factors in diabetic children and adolescents under 18 years of age: a Belgian experience. Diabetes Care 1997; 20:2–6.
417 Hinde FRJ, Johnston DI. Two or three insulin injections in adolescence? Arch Dis Child 1986; 61:118–123.
418 Bougneres PF, Landais P, Mairesse AM, et al. Improvement of diabetic control and acceptability of a three-injection insulin regimen in diabetic adolescents. A multicenter controlled study. Diabetes Care 1993; 16:94–102.
419 Tupola S, Komulainen J, Jaaskelainen J, Sipila I. Post-prandial insulin lispro vs. human regular insulin in prepubertal children with type 1 diabetes mellitus. Diabetic Med 2001; 18: 654–658.
420 Lepore M, Pampanelli S, Fanelli C, et al. Pharmacokinetics and pharmacodynamics of subcutaneous injection of long-acting human insulin analog glargine, NPH insulin, and ultralente human insulin and continuous subcutaneous infusion of insulin lispro. Diabetes 2000; 49:2142–2148.
421 Gale EA. A randomized, controlled trial comparing insulin lispro with human soluble insulin in patients with type 1 diabetes on intensified insulin therapy. The UK Trial Group. Diabetic Med 2000; 3:209–214.
*422 Brunelle BL, Llewelyn J, Anderson JH Jr, et al. Meta-analysis of the effect of insulin lispro on severe hypoglycemia in patients with type 1 diabetes. Diabetes Care 1998; 10:1726–1731.

423 Mohn A, Matyka KA, Harris DA, et al. Lispro or regular insulin for multiple injection therapy in adolescence. Differences in free insulin and glucose levels overnight. Diabetes Care 1999; 1:27–32.
424 Pickup JC, Keen H, Parsons JA, Alberti KG. Continuous subcutaneous insulin infusion: an approach to achieving normoglycemia. BMJ 1978; 1:204–207.
425 Tamborlane WV, Sherwin RS, Genel M, Felig P. Reduction to normal of plasma glucose in juvenile diabetes by subcutaneous administration of insulin with a portable infusion pump. N Engl J Med 1979; 300:573–578.
426 Nordfeldt S, Ludvigsson J. Severe hypoglycemia in children with IDDM. A prospective population study, 1992–1994. Diabetes Care 1997; 20:497–503.
427 McKeage K, Goa KL. Insulin glargine: a review of its therapeutic use as a long-acting agent for the management of type 1 and 2 diabetes mellitus. Drugs 2001; 61:1599–1624.
428 Schober E, Schoenle E, Van Dyk J, Wernicke-Panten K. Comparative trial between insulin glargine and NPH insulin in children and adolescents with type 1 diabetes. Diabetes Care 2001; 24:2005–2006.
429 Danielsen GM, Drejer K, Langkjær L, Plum A. New routes and means of insulin delivery. In: Kelnar CJH, ed. Childhood and adolescent diabetes. London; Chapman & Hall; 1995:571–584.
430 Heinemann L, Traut T, Heise T. Time-action profile of inhaled insulin. Diabetic Med 1997; 14:63–72.
431 Patton JS, Bukar J, Nagarajan S. Inhaled insulin. Adv Drug Deliv Rev 1999; 35:235–247.
432 Rubenstein AH, Pyke DA. Immunosuppression in the treatment of insulin-dependent (type 1) diabetes. Lancet 1987; i:436–437.
433 White SA, James RF, Swift SM, et al. Human islet cell transplantation – future prospects. Diabetic Med 2001; 18:78–103.
434 Warnock GL. Frontiers in transplantation of insulin-secreting tissue for diabetes mellitus. Can J Surg 1999; 42:421–426.
435 Macfarlane WM, Chapman JC, Shepherd RM, et al. Engineering a glucose-responsive human insulin-secreting cell line from islets of Langerhans isolated from a patient with persistent hyperinsulinemic hypoglycemia of infancy. J Biol Chem 1999; 274:34059–34066.
436 British Diabetic Association. Dietary recommendations for people with diabetes: an update for the 1990s. Diabetic Med 1992; 9:189–202.
437 Vranic M, Berger M. Exercise and diabetes mellitus. Diabetes 1979; 28:147–173.
438 Reid GJ, Dubow EF, Carey TC, et al. Contribution of coping to medical adjustment and treatment responsibility among children and adolescents with diabetes. J Dev Behav Pediatr 1994; 15:327–335.
439 Satin W, La Greca AM, Zigo MA, Skyler JS. Diabetes in adolescence: effects of multifamily group intervention and parent simulation of diabetes. J Pediatr Psychol 1989; 14:259–275.
440 Anderson BJ, Brackett J, Ho J, Laffel LM. An office-based intervention to maintain parent–adolescent teamwork in diabetes management. Impact on parent involvement, family conflict, and subsequent glycemic control. Diabetes Care 1999; 22:713–721.
441 Blankfield DF, Holahan CJ. Family support, coping strategies and depressive symptoms among mothers of children with diabetes. J Fam Psychol 1996; 10:173–179.
442 Jones JM, Lawson ML, Danman D, et al. Eating disorders in adolescent females with and without type 1 diabetes: cross sectional study. BMJ 2000; 10:1563–1566.
*443 Hampson SE, Skinner TC, Hart J, et al. Effects of educational and psychosocial interventions for adolescents with diabetes mellitus: a systematic review. Health Technol Assess 2001; 5:1–79.
444 Tattersall RB. Brittle diabetes. Clin Endocrinol Metab 1977; 6:403–419.
445 Gerich J, Cryer P, Rizza R. Hormonal mechanisms in acute glucose counterregulation: the relative roles of glucagon, epinephrine, norepinephrine, growth hormone and cortisol. Metabolism 1980; 29:1164–1175.
446 Schmidt MI, Ndjii-Georgopoulos A, Rendell M, et al. The dawn phenomenon, an early morning glucose rise: implications for diabetic instability. Diabetes Care 1981; 4:579–585.
447 Hermansson G, Ludvigsson J, Larsson Y. Home blood glucose monitoring in diabetic children and adolescents. A 3 year feasibility study. Acta Pediatr Scand 1986; 75:98–105.
448 Davis EA, Keating B, Byrne GC et al. Hypoglycemia: incidence and clinical predictors in a large population-based sample of children and adolescents with IDDM. Diabetes Care 1997; 20:22–25.
449 Kaufman FR, Gibson LC, Halvorson M. A pilot study of the continuous glucose monitoring system: clinical decisions and glycemic control after its use in pediatric type 1 diabetic subjects. Diabetes Care 2001; 24:2030–2034.
450 Jovanovic L, Peterson CM. The clinical utility of glycosylated hemoglobin. Am J Med 1981; 70:331–338.
451 Danne T, Mortensen HB, Hougaard P, et al. Persistent differences among centers over 3 years in glycemic control and hypoglycemia in a study of 3,805 children and adolescents with type 1 diabetes from the Hvidore Study Group. Diabetes Care 2001; 24:1342–1347.
452 Krolewski AS, Laffel LM, Krolewski M. Glycosylated hemoglobin and the risk of microalbuminuria in patients with insulin-dependent diabetes mellitus. N Engl J Med 1995; 332:1251–1255.
453 Citrin W, Ellis GJ, Skyler JS. Glycosylated hemoglobin: a tool in identifying psychological problems. Diabetes Care 1980; 3:563–564.
454 Gold AE, Frier BM. Hypoglycaemia – practical and clinical implications. In: Kelnar CJH, ed. Childhood and adolescent diabetes. London: Chapman & Hall; 1995:351–367.
455 McAulay V, Deary IJ, Frier BM. Symptoms of hypoglycemia in people with diabetes. Diabetic Med 2001; 18:690–705.
456 Northam EA, Anderson PJ, Jacobs R, et al. Neuropsychological profiles of children with type 1 diabetes 6 years after disease onset. Diabetes Care 2001; 24:1541–1546.
457 Matyka KA, Crowne EC, Havel PJ, et al. Counterregulation during spontaneous nocturnal hypoglycemia in prepubertal children with type 1 diabetes. Diabetes Care 1999; 22:1144–1150.
458 Matyka KA, Wigg L, Pramming S, et al. Cognitive function and mood after profound nocturnal hypoglycemia in prepubertal children with conventional insulin treatment for diabetes. Arch Dis Child 1999; 81:138–142.
459 Fainmesser P, Laron Z, Feiman G, et al. The incidence of hypoglycemia in newly diagnosed diabetic children during the first year of disease. International Study Group of Diabetes in Children and Adolescents Bulletin 1986; 13:39–40.
460 Spallino L, Stirling HF, O'Regan M, et al. Transient hypoglycemic hemiparesis in children with IDDM. Diabetes Care 1998; 21:1567–1568.
461 Hoey H, Aanstoot HJ, Chiarelli F, et al. Good metabolic control is associated with better quality of life in 2,101 adolescents with type 1 diabetes. Diabetes Care 2001; 24:1923–1928.
462 Holl RW, Lang GE, Grabert M, et al. Diabetic retinopathy in pediatric patients with type-1 diabetes: effect of diabetes duration, prepubertal and pubertal onset of diabetes, and metabolic control. J Pediatr 1998; 132:790–794.
463 Cowell CT, Rogers S, Silink M. First morning urine albumin concentration is a good predictor of 24-hour urinary albumin excretion in children with type 1 (insulin-dependent) diabetes. Diabetologia 1986; 29:97–99.
464 Schultz CJ, Neil HA, Dalton RN, et al. Blood pressure does not rise before the onset of microalbuminuria in children followed from diagnosis of type 1 diabetes. Oxford Regional Prospective Study Group. Diabetes Care 2001; 24:555–560.
465 Schultz CJ, Konopelska-Bahu T, Dalton RN, et al. Microalbuminuria prevalence varies with age, sex, and puberty in children with type 1 diabetes followed from diagnosis in a longitudinal study. Oxford Regional Prospective Study Group. Diabetes Care 1999; 22:495–502.
466 Bonney M, Hing SJ, Fung AT, et al. Development and progression of diabetic retinopathy: adolescents at risk. Diabetic Med 1995; 12:967–973.
*467 Hutchinson A, McIntosh A, Peters J, et al. Effectiveness of screening and monitoring tests for diabetic retinopathy – a systematic review. Diabetic Med 2000; 17:495–506.
468 Radetti G, Paganini C, Gentili L, et al. Frequency of Hashimoto's thyroiditis in children with type 1 diabetes mellitus. Acta Diabetol 1995; 32:121–124.
469 Carlsson AK, Axelsson IE, Borulf SK, et al. Prevalence of IgA-antiendomysium and IgA-antigliadin autoantibodies at diagnosis of insulin-dependent diabetes mellitus in Swedish children and adolescents. Pediatr 1999; 103:1248–1252.
470 Holmes GK. Celiac disease and type 1 diabetes mellitus – the case for screening. Diabetic Med 2001; 18:169–177.
471 Batch JA, Werther GA. Unusual diabetes and diabetes in the context of other disorders. In: Kelnar CJH, ed. Childhood and adolescent diabetes. London: Chapman & Hall; 1995:397–418.

472 Cremers CW, Wijdeveld PG, Pinckers AJ. Juvenile diabetes mellitus, optic atrophy, hearing loss, diabetes insipidus, atonia of the urinary tract and bladder, and other abnormalities (Wolfram syndrome). A review of 88 cases from the literature with personal observations on 3 new patients. Acta Paediatr Scand 1977; 264(suppl):1–16.

473 Khanim F, Kirk J, Latif F, Barrett TG. WFS1/wolframin mutations, Wolfram syndrome, and associated diseases. Hum Mutat 2001; 17:357–367.

474 Lanng S, Hansen A, Thorsteinsson B, et al. Glucose tolerance in patients with cystic fibrosis: five year prospective study BMJ 1995; 311:655–699.

475 Shield JP, Gardner RJ, Wadsworth EJ, et al. Aetiopathology and genetic basis of neonatal diabetes. Arch Dis Child (Fetal Neonatal Ed) 1997; 76:F39–42.

476 Shield JP. Neonatal diabetes: new insights into etiology and implications. Horm Res 2000; 53(suppl 1):7–11.

477 Leonard JV, Dezateux C. Screening for inherited metabolic disease in newborn infants using tandem mass spectrometry. BMJ 2002; 324:4–5.

477a Tanner S, Sharrard M, Cleary M, et al. Screening for medium chain acyl-CoA dehydrogenase deficiency has still not been evaluated. BMJ 2001; 322:112.

478 Aynsley-Green A, Soltesz G. Hypoglycaemia in infancy and childhood. Edinburgh: Churchill Livingstone; 1985.

479 Macfarlane WM, Cragg H, Docherty HM, et al. Impaired expression of transcription factor IUF1 in a pancreatic beta-cell line derived from a patient with persistent hyperinsulinemic hypoglycemia of infancy (nesidioblastosis). FEBS Lett 1997; 413:304–308.

480 Macfarlane WM, O'Brien RE, Barnes PD, et al. Sulfonylurea receptor 1 and Kir6.2 expression in the novel human insulin-secreting cell line NES2Y. Diabetes 2000; 49:953–960.

481 Laidlaw GF. Nesidioblastosis: islet tumor of pancreas. Am J Pathol 1938; 14:125–134.

482 Yakovac WC, Baker L, Hummeler K. Beta cell nesidioblastosis in idiopathic hypoglycemia of infancy. J Pediatr 1971; 79:226–231.

483 Woo D, Scopes JW, Polak JM. Idiopathic hypoglycemia in sibs with morphological evidence of nesidioblastosis of the pancreas. Arch Dis Child 1976; 51:528–531.

484 Lindley KJ, Dunne MJ, Kane C, et al. Ionic control of beta cell function in nesidioblastosis. A possible therapeutic role for calcium channel blockade. Arch Dis Child 1996; 74:373–378.

485 Aynsley-Green A, Hussain K, Hall J, et al. Practical management of hyperinsulinism in infancy. Arch Dis Child (Fetal Neonatal Ed) 2000; 82:F98–107.

486 Hussain K, Aynsley-Green A. Management of hyperinsulinism in infancy and childhood. Ann Med 2000; 32:544–551.

487 Jeffcoate SL. Efficiency and effectiveness in the endocrine laboratory. London: Academic Press; 1981.

488 Marshall WA, Tanner JM. Variations in the pattern of pubertal changes in boys. Arch Dis Child 1970; 45:13–23.

489 Hattersley AT. Transcribing diabetes. J Pediatr Endocrinol Metab 2001; 14(suppl 3): 1025.

14

Nutrition

Lawrence Weaver, Christine Edwards, Barbara Golden, John Reilly

NUTRITION, GROWTH, DEVELOPMENT AND DISEASE

Optimal nutrition is the foundation of good health. In pediatrics, health, growth and development are all aspects of a single process, which is dependent in large part, on the provision of appropriate diet and the effective ingestion, digestion, absorption and metabolism of its energy and nutrients. Nutrition is concerned with how food is used by the body, and the changing composition of the body is an index of nutritional status and a reflection of what is eaten.

Malnutrition implies both under- and overnutrition and is a consequence of disturbance of energy and nutrient balance, between supply and demand. Undernutrition is often manifest as growth failure, which may be due to insufficient energy or nutrient intake, disordered digestion, absorption or metabolism, or excessive losses.[1] Foods deficient in specific nutrients may cause specific diseases (such as scurvy or anemia). Overeating causes obesity. Chronic disease is frequently associated with undernutrition and nutrient deficits. However nutrient deficiencies lead to depletion of tissue stores, derangement of normal biochemistry and disordered tissue function before they are manifest as anatomical changes, and may easily go unrecognized. Awareness of poor nutrition is critical to the effective management of many childhood diseases, particularly those that are chronic, and there is growing evidence that undernutrition in early life may play a part in the genesis of chronic adult disease.

This chapter aims to summarize the knowledge required to evaluate the nutritional needs of normal and sick children and to provide them with a healthy diet or nutritional support. We provide a summary of nutrient requirements, how they are defined and how they should be properly used. Nutritional assessment is an essential prerequisite to the provision of nutritional support and the principal methods used are outlined. Healthy diets for the infant, toddler, child and adolescent are then described. The next section summarizes how nutritional support can be provided to the sick child and is followed by an account of some of the main causes of over- and undernutrition. A trained nutrition team should work together in the clinic, ward and community to provide nutritional support for sick children. The basic science of nutrition (composition of food, metabolic pathways, gastrointestinal physiology, body composition, etc.) is not covered in this chapter.

NUTRITIONAL REQUIREMENTS

BACKGROUND AND DEFINITIONS

Figures for nutrient requirements set by expert committees emphasize the avoidance of nutrient deficiency. They do not concern themselves with the safety of excess intake (Table 14.1). Underlying the concept of requirement is the assumption that, for most nutrients, need is approximately normally distributed (Fig. 14.1) in any population. To determine requirements of nutrients that are sufficient to meet the needs of whole populations, they have been set 'high' in the distribution, at approximately two standard deviations (SD) above the mean requirement. With the exception of energy (excess energy intake leads to obesity) consumption of a nutrient in excess of requirements of this magnitude is not harmful and setting a high value as a reference nutrient intake (RNI) or recommended daily allowance (RDA) entails minimal risk for most nutrients.

In the UK, the term 'dietary reference values' (DRVs) is used rather than 'recommendations'.[2] The basic approach to defining requirements remains the same, but up to three reference values are set for each nutrient. These values reflect the range of nutrient requirements (low, medium and high) (Fig. 14. 1) rather than just one reference value. The three DRVs are:

1. the 'estimated average requirement' (EAR), or the mean requirement;
2. the 'reference nutrient intake' (RNI), or the mean requirement +2 SD; and
3. the 'lower reference nutrient intake' (LRNI), or the mean requirement – 2 SD.

For some nutrients the 1991 UK report set a 'safe intake' if there were insufficient data upon which to set DRVs. This was judged to be an intake at which there was no risk of deficiency and below a level where there was a risk of adverse effects.

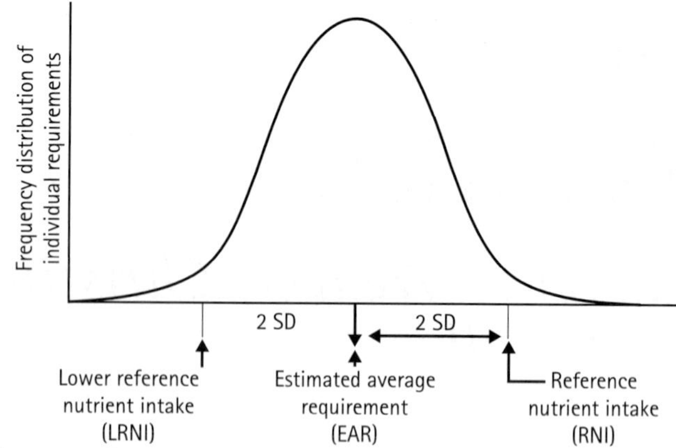

Fig. 14.1 Relations between various reference values for nutritional requirements. SD, standard deviation.

APPLICATIONS AND LIMITATIONS OF DIETARY REFERENCE VALUES

There are three main applications of DRVs:

1. To assess the adequacy of the dietary intake of individuals or groups. For example, if a hospital population of children consume a diet below the LRNI for a particular nutrient, their diet is probably deficient in that nutrient.
2. As a guide to prescribing or designing the diet of individuals or groups. The DRVs (often the EAR) can be a useful starting point in setting a diet prescription, in the absence of any other information on the requirements of the patient, and DRVs are also used in the design of infant milk formulae.
3. Food labeling. A food might be described as containing x% of the EAR for iron, for example.

When applying DRVs, their limitations must be borne in mind. In childhood estimates of requirement are usually based on limited data. They change over the years and DRVs should be regarded as best estimates at the time that they were set. They are often reviewed in the light of new information. For example, the 1979 UK estimates of energy requirements during infancy have subsequently been shown to be too high.[3] In this chapter RNI is used in place of the formerly used RDA. The use of RNI or RDA to set requirements rather than EAR will produce higher estimates of deficiency and higher prescriptions for diet. This means that the recommended intakes may be very different in countries where RDA is used and not EAR. There are also variations in the values agreed for the RNI or RDA between different national committees.

Table 14.1 Criteria used for setting nutrient requirements

- Amount taken by a group of people without deficiency developing
- Amount needed to cure deficiency
- Amount needed to maintain enzyme saturation
- Amount needed to maintain blood or tissue concentration
- Amount associated with an appropriate biological marker of adequacy

NUTRITIONAL REQUIREMENTS DURING INFANCY AND CHILDHOOD

ENERGY

Energy is required for physical activity, thermogenesis, tissue maintenance and growth. Dietary energy is consumed in the form of fat, protein and carbohydrate. Dietary protein does not simply build new tissue but is also oxidized to provide energy. In the UK and in most Western countries dietary surveys of children of school age show that they consume about 35–40% of dietary energy in the form of fat, 10–15% as protein and 40–50% as carbohydrate.[4,5] These figures are very similar to those of adults in the same countries and imply that the characteristic macronutrient composition of the diet is 'set' at a relatively young age. The main food sources of dietary fat are milk and milk products, fried foods and meat products (Table 14.2).[6–10] In developing countries and in vegetarian children the contribution to energy intake of carbohydrate is much higher and the contribution of fat is generally much lower.

In infants and children, the energy requirement is the amount of dietary energy needed to balance energy expended and energy deposited in new tissue (growth). Energy expenditure can be subdivided into basal (BMR) or resting metabolic rate [RMR around 65% of total energy expenditure (TEE) in most healthy children]; energy expended on physical activity (around 25% of TEE in most healthy children) and thermogenesis (approximately 8% of TEE) (Fig. 14.2). BMR or RMR can be considered to be a 'maintenance' cost since it is the energy cost of biosynthesis, turnover, cellular ion pumps, physical work (respiratory and cardiac function). The energy expended on physical activity varies widely between children and is generally reduced when they are sick. The energy expended in thermogenesis is primarily the cost of digesting, absorbing and

Table 14.2 Sources of dietary protein, fat and carbohydrate

Nutrient	Main sources in UK diet	Alternative good sources
Protein	Meat products, cereal products, milk products, vegetables, savoury snacks *Milk, cereals, meat*	
Fat		
Saturated	Milk products, cereal products, meat products, vegetables and savoury snacks (incl. chips), confectionery *Milk and milk products, cereals, meat, vegetables*	
PUFA n-3	Chips, cereals, meat, nuts. *Vegetables, cereal products, fish, meat, milk products*	Fish oils
PUFA n-6	Vegetables, cereal products, fat spreads, meat products *Vegetables, cereal products, fat spreads, meat products*	Vegetable oils
Mono-unsaturated	Chips and savoury snacks, meat products, cereal products, milk products *Milk and milk products, meat products, cereal products, vegetables*	Olive oil
Trans	Cereal products, meat products, meats, fat spreads, confectionery *Cereals, cereal products, milk, meat fat spreads*	
Total	Meat products, cereal products, milk products, chips, savoury snacks, confectionery *Milk products, cereals, meat products and vegetables*	
Carbohydrate		
Starch	Cereals, potatoes *Cereals, vegetables*	
Sugars	Cereal products, sucrose, confectionery, beverages, milk products *Beverages, milk and milk products, confectionery, cereals*	
Dietary fiber	Cereals (bread, breakfast cereals), vegetables, fruit and nuts *Cereals, vegetables*	

In descending order of contribution to diet. *Sources of nutrients for infants are shown in italics.* PUFA, polyunsaturated fatty acid.
From National Diet & Nutrition Survey 1990, 1995, 2000 [6–9] and Garrow et al 2000[10]

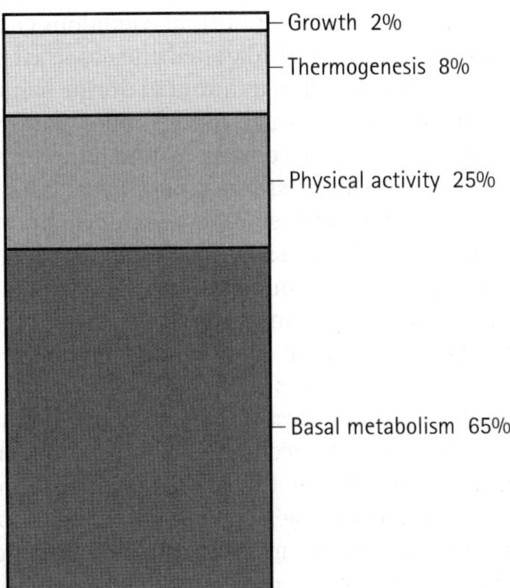

Fig. 14.2 Components of total energy expenditure in childhood.

resynthesizing nutrients ('diet-induced thermogenesis'). Growth demands some energy expended on biosynthesis and the energy content of newly synthesized tissue. This represents up to about 35% of energy intake in rapidly growing infants, but falls for the rest of childhood (to about 2% of energy intake) because growth rate is so much slower thereafter.

The 1991 UK committee[2] recommended an EAR for energy (Table 40.17) but no RNI or LRNI. In clinical or dietetic use the EAR can provide a basis for estimating the energy requirements of individual infants and children. Alternatively a more considered approach involves estimating BMR (Table 14.3)[2] from equations based on age, weight and gender and multiplying this by a factor to take into account physical activity. In most children 1.5–2 times BMR will cover TEE. Estimation of minimum energy requirements using this approach, though better than depending on the EAR, can lead to large errors for individual children. However, although ideal, *measurement* of RMR and/or TEE is not usually a practical option in clinical practice and the former is therefore often the more widely used estimate.

Broadly dietary recommendations fall into two time periods; those for children under and over 5 years. The high demand for

Table 14.3 Equations for predicting basal metabolic rate (MJ/d) from body weight (kg)

	Age (years)	Equation
Boys	0–3	0.249w – 0.127
	4–10	0.095w + 2.110
	11–18	0.074w + 2.754
Girls	0–3	0.244w – 0.130
	4–10	0.085w + 2.33
	11–18	0.056 + 2.898

Adapted from Schofield 1985[2a]

energy in the under-5s necessitates a more energy-dense diet with less complex carbohydrate and a greater proportion of energy from fat. Recommendations for children over 5 years in general mirror those for adults based on a desire to encourage healthy eating habits in later life rather than specific needs for childhood.

PROTEINS AND AMINO ACIDS

Proteins are essential components of every living cell and subserve numerous biological functions. Dietary protein is essential to maintain nitrogen balance in the body and to provide sources of sulfur. Protein intake is particularly important in childhood where rapid growth requires amino acids to provide the building blocks for new muscle and other structural proteins. All amino acids provide nitrogen for synthesis of human proteins but some dietary amino acids are 'essential' as they cannot be synthesized de novo. Adequate intake of these essential amino acids is achievable only with a diet containing a wide variety of protein sources. Average requirements increase with age in absolute terms (EAR at 4 months is 10.6 g/day and at 18 years is 46.1 g/day) but decrease per kg body weight (EAR is 120 mg N/kg/day at 1 year and 96 mg N/kg/day in adults; Table 40.17). If energy intake is below requirements protein stores will be used for energy, yielding approximately 17 kJ (4 kcal)/g. In the UK most diets contain protein well in excess of the daily requirements.

FATS

Fats are a major calorie source with an energy density of approximately 37 kJ (9 kcal)/g and they are also essential for the formation of membranes and neural tissue. Different types of fat play particular roles in the structure and function of cell membranes and neural tissue and the quality as well as the quantity, of fat intake is very important. Dietary fats (lipids) are mostly triglycerides containing a wide variety of fatty acids. Where a fatty acid is replaced with phosphate a phospholipid is produced and substitutions with other compounds produce other structural and functional lipids such as sphingolipids and glycolipids.

Fats from animal produce tend to contain saturated fatty acids with no double bonds and those from plants and fish tend to contain mono- or polyunsaturated fatty acids (PUFAs). This is not universally true: some plants, such as coconut, produce saturated fat. High saturated fat diets have been implicated in the development of coronary heart disease (CHD) in the adult whereas there is evidence that diets high in polyunsaturated or monounsaturated fats protect against CHD.[11] To encourage good eating habits in adolescents and adults, it is recommended that children over 5 years should adopt a diet with a similar fat content to that recommended for adults. Thus 10% of daily energy needs should be from saturated fat, 12% from monounsaturated fats, 6% from polyunsaturated, with a mixture of n-6 and n-3 fatty acids (with at least linoleic 1%, alpha-linolenic 0.2%) and trans fatty acids 2%, giving a total fatty acid intake of 30% dietary energy or 33% including dietary glycerol. For children under 5 years a higher energy requirement makes these recommendations unsuitable and a fat intake providing up to 50% of daily needs is recommended.

There are two essential fatty acids – linoleic (C18:2n-6) and alpha-linolenic (C18:3n-3) – which the human body cannot synthesize. These are precursors of phospholipids, prostaglandins, thromboxane, leukotrienes and arachidonic (AA), eicosapentanoic (EPA) and docosahexaenoic (DHA) acids. Young infants have limited ability to transform linolenic acid to DHA and linoleic to AA, which are both present in human milk. Many infant formulae do not contain DHA and the membrane phospholipids in the brain of infants whose intake of DHA is deficient have substituted saturated fatty acids for DHA.[12] While some infant formulas have been supplemented with PUFAs their impact on neurodevelopment, except in the preterm, is unproven.[13]

CARBOHYDRATES

Carbohydrates in the diet provide energy of approximately 17 kJ (4 kcal)/g and are also an important component of structural and functional glycoproteins and glycolipids. Glucose is an essential fuel for the brain, which cannot metabolize fat for energy. It can be synthesized by the liver from amino acids and propionic acid, but a minimum amount of dietary carbohydrate is necessary to inhibit ketosis and to allow complete oxidation of fat. In adults this is likely to be about 50 g/day, a figure based on theoretical models, and the amounts needed in childhood are not known.

Carbohydrates can be divided into sugars (up to three residues), oligosaccharides (up to 10 residues) and complex carbohydrates (polysaccharides) on the basis of chain length. It is recommended that intake of extrinsic sugar is restricted to less than 10% of energy intake to prevent dental caries. There is very little evidence that excessive sugar intake plays a major role in the development of obesity. Indeed, diets high in sugar are often low in fat and in adults are associated with a low body mass index (BMI).[14]

Some oligosaccharides are undigestible in the human small intestine. These include fructo-oligosaccharides such as raftilose from inulin, and galactosyl-oligosaccharides such as raffinose in beans. Similar oligosaccharides are present in human milk. These pass to the colon where they are rapidly fermented to short chain fatty acids (SCFA) and gases and may produce flatulence if eaten in excess. These oligosaccharides are believed to have 'prebiotic' properties: that is they promote the growth of beneficial bacteria, mainly bifidobacteria and lactobacilli, in the colon.

Complex carbohydrates include starch and dietary fiber. Starch is found in several forms in food, some of which are less digestible than others. Starch cooked under normal conditions can be rapidly or slowly digestible, but is mostly digested and absorbed in the small intestine, whereas raw starches, as found in unripe bananas or raw potato and some processed starches (retrograded amylose) such as in some cornflakes or cooked cooled potatoes, may be resistant to human enzymes (resistant starch) and pass into the colon undigested.[15] Other modified starches, included in many foods during manufacture and processing, are also resistant to digestion. More starch may escape small intestinal digestion in young children than in adults, owing to immaturity of digestion in early life, and this will influence colonic function and the energy absorbed from food.

Non-digestible carbohydrates iclude on-strach polysaccharides and lignin. Dietary fiber polysaccharides are undigested in the small intestine and are fermented by the colonic microflora to SCFA and gases. These SCFA are rapidly absorbed resulting in an average energy value of 8.4 kJ (2 kcal)/g for dietary fiber. The calorific value of SCFA is closer to that of glucose, but some dietary fiber is poorly fermented and if it escapes fermentation it can cause increased fecal output with increased loss of nitrogen and energy, and even some micronutrients.

Because diets high in dietary fiber are less energy dense and more satiating than the converse, it is not recommended that infants and young children consume high-fiber diets. Nevertheless dietary fiber plays an important part in normal large bowel function (see Ch. 17) and is an essential constituent of the healthy diet from an early age. Older children, however, who do not need such an energy-dense diet, should be encouraged to eat foods rich in complex carbohydrates. There are no recommendations for childhood fiber intake in the UK diet but the American Academy of Pediatrics[16] has recommended in intake of 0.5 g/kg body weight of fiber for children, which may not be appropriate for older teenagers. Also in the USA, a dietary fiber intake in grams according to age in years plus five has been advocated from 3 years onwards, aiming to progressively reach the levels recommended for adults.[17]

VITAMINS AND MINERALS

Vitamins are a group of naturally occuring organic nutrients that have little in common except that they are essential in the diet. They can be divided into water-soluble and fat-soluble vitamins. Water-soluble vitamins are easily absorbed, sometimes by active transport, and are not stored in the body to any great extent. Excessive intake normally results in excretion of the excess in the urine. Fat-soluble vitamins, on the other hand, are absorbed with fat and thus any factor reducing the amount of fat digested and/or absorbed will reduce their absorption. Fat-soluble vitamins are also stored in the body and thus deficiencies in the diet may take some time to affect nutritional status, but they are more likely to have toxic effects if eaten in excess.

Minerals are the inorganic elements (other than carbon, hydrogen and nitrogen) that are found in the body and which are essential constituents of diet. They include the 'trace elements' which are required in very small, but vital amounts. Minerals serve many different biological functions ranging from structural (calcium in bone), transport (iron in hemoglobin), energy metabolism [phosphorus in adenosine triphosphate (ATP)], endocrine (iodine in thyroid), neurotransmission (magnesium) and enzyme action (molybdenum).

The dietary sources, function and requirements of vitamins and minerals are shown in Tables 14.4–14.7 of this chapter and of Chapter 40. Deficiency diseases associated with these micronutrients are summarized below.

NUTRITIONAL ASSESSMENT

Nutritional assessment is the evaluation of an individual's nutritional status and requirements. It is a means by which the undernourished (or overnourished) child can be identified, the nutritional effects of therapy and the efficacy of nutritional interventions monitored, and the prevalence of under- or overnutrition in a group determined. Undernutrition is common, particularly among sick children in hospital,[17] and evidence that it has important clinical consequences has led to increasing interest in methods for assessing nutritional status in children.[18]

There are five principal approaches to nutritional assessment: anthropometric; dietary; biochemical; clinical; functional. Each evaluates a different aspect of nutritional status. All have limitations, and there is still much debate over choice of methods, reference values, and interpretation of measurements. Functional assessment, the use of functional deficits (e.g. deficits in immune function or muscle function) to identify or measure undernutrition, is not discussed here since it is so rarely used in children and remains experimental.[19] Assessment of growth is an integral part of the anthropometric assessment of nutritional status, but because growth assessment is dealt with in detail in Chapter 13 it will not be considered in depth here.

ANTHROPOMETRIC NUTRITIONAL ASSESSMENT

Anthropometry is the measurement of physical dimensions of the human body at different ages. Typically, the measurements are compared with population reference data to identify abnormalities that may result from nutrient (usually energy or protein) deficiencies or excess.

Table 14.4 Dietary sources of vitamins

Vitamin	Food sources
Thiamin	Cereals (breakfast cereals, bread), vegetables (potatoes), milk and milk products, meat and meat products, cereal products
Vitamin B_{12}	Milk and milk products, meat and meat products, cereals (Alternative source: yeast extract for vegetarians)
Folic acid	Cereals, vegetables, milk products, liver *Breakfast cereals, bread, vegetables, milk products*
Vitamin B_6	Vegetables, cereal products, milk products, meat products *Milk and milk products, vegetables, breakfast cereals* (Alternative sources: poultry, fish, eggs, nuts)
Niacin	Cereal products (bread, breakfast cereals), meat products, milk and milk products. vegetables
Riboflavin	Milk products, cereal products (bread, breakfast cereals), meat products. *Cereals, milk*
Biotin	(Good sources: liver, egg, cereals, yeast)
Pantothenic acid	(Good sources: widely distributed, meat, cereals, legumes)
Vitamin C	Beverages (fruit juice), vegetables (potatoes), fruit and nuts, *Vegetables, beverages*
Vitamin A	Retinol: vegetables, milk products, fat spreads, cereal products. *Milk products, meat products, vegetables* Beta-carotene: vegetables, meat and meat products. *Vegetables*
Vitamin D	Cereal products, fat spreads, meat products (Alternative source: oily fish) *Fat spreads, breakfast cereals, milk and milk products*
Vitamin E	Vegetables, fat spreads, cereal products *Fat spreads, vegetables, meat and meat products, cereal products*
Vitamin K	(Good sources: vegetables, margarines, but synthesized in colon)

Sources of nutrients for infants are shown in italics
From National Diet and Nutrition Survey 1990, 1995, 2000[6–9] and Garrow et al 2000[10]

Table 14.5 Structure, function and mode of absorption of water soluble vitamins

Vitamin	Chemical structure	Functions	Absorption
Thiamin	Pyrimidine ring joined to thiazole ring	Thiamin pyrophosphate coenzyme for many reactions in carbohydrate metabolism	Active transport or passive transport at concentration > 1μmol or 5 mg/day
Vitamin B_{12}	Cobalamin, porphyrin like ring containing cobalt; 5-deoxyadenosylcobalamin, methyl cobalamin, hydroxycobalamin	Cofactor for methionine synthetase, methylmalonyl-CoA mutase	Absorbed bound to various carrier proteins; R protein in stomach, IF protein in small intestine. Transcobalamin in basolateral membrane, 70% efficient
Folic acid	Folate, substituted pteridine ring linked to p-aminobenzoic acid. Exists as polyglutamated reduced or substituted forms of folic acid	Coenzyme for several reactions, transfer of single carbon units in reactions essential to metabolism of several amino acids and nucleic acid synthesis	Various dietary forms need to be hydrolysed before absorption as monoglutamyl folate by active transport
Vitamin B_6	Pyridoxine, pyridoxal, pyridoxamine, pyridoxine HCl	Pyridoxal phosphate coenzyme for reactions related to protein metabolism, amino transferase decarboxylase and for amine synthesis, e.g. 5HT, heme synthesis, glycogen metabolism, sphingolipid and niacin synthesis	Hydrolysed and absorbed passively
Niacin	Nicotinamide	NAD, NADP for oxidoreductases	Absorbed as nicotinic acid, nicotinamide, NMN
Riboflavin	Isoalloxazine ring with ribityl side chain. Flavin mononucleotide, flavin adenosine dinucleotide	Flavoprotein enzymes in oxidative reductive reactions, in metabolic pathways and cellular respiration	By sodium-dependent saturable proteins
Biotin	Imidazole ring fused to tetrahydrothiophene ring with valeric acid side chain	Cofactor for carboxylases in fatty acid synthesis, metabolism, gluconeogenesis branched chain amino acid metabolism	Actively absorbed as free biotin in small intestine
Pantothenic acid	Dimethyl derivative of butyric acid linked to beta-alanine	Constituent of CoA and esters essential for lipid and carbohydrate metabolism	Ingested as part of CoA released by intestinal phosphatase absorbed as pantothenic acid
Vitamin C	Ascorbic acid	Essential for hydroxylation of proline and lysine in collagen synthesis, needed for carnitine and noradrenaline synthesis	Active sodium linked absorption

IF, intrinsic factor; NAD, nicotinamide adenine dinucleotide; NADP, nicotinamide adenine dinucleotide phosphate; NMN, nicotinamide mononucleotide.

Table 14.6 Structure, function and mode of absorption of fat soluble vitamins

Vitamin	Chemical structure	Functions	Absorption
Vitamin A	Retinol, beta-carotene, six beta-carotene = one retinol	Cellular differentiation, vision, fetal development, immune system, spermatogenesis, appetite, hearing, growth	With fat 80% absorbed
Vitamin D	Calciferol, ergocalciferol, cholecalciferol. Metabolized in skin, liver and kidneys to active forms	Essential for calcum absorption, regulates calcium metabolism, involved in immune system	With fat 80% absorbed
Vitamin E	Tocopherols, tocotrienols; 8 naturally occurring forms	Antioxidant prevents lipid peroxidation	With fat absorption
Vitamin K	2 metholnaphthoquinone rings, with side chains. Phylloquinone, menaquinone, menadione	Needed for gla-proteins. Catalyses synthesis of prothrombin in liver for clotting factors VII, IX and X	With fat 50–80% absorbed

Three basic measurements (body height, weight and age) are used to derive the following indices: height-for-age (low height-for-age, 'stunting', is an index of chronic undernutrition); weight-for-age; weight-for-height (low weight-for-height, 'wasting', is an index of acute undernutrition). A detailed description of how to perform these measurements and interpret the calculations is found in Gibson[19] and their use in the classification of childhood malnutrition is described below.

The BMI – weight (kg)/height $(m)^2$ – is a simple and useful tool for assessing or monitoring overweight and underweight. Many countries have population reference data for BMI from birth to adulthood, and these are available as BMI charts for clinical use. BMI can be expressed as a SD score or as a centile, and a cut-off is often used to define over- or undernutrition. For example, the UK[20] and the USA[21] have reference data and charts for screening in primary care. In the UK it is suggested that children who cross two centile 'spaces' or who are below the 2nd or above the 98th centile should be considered as likely to require further assessment. It is important to note that using cut-off points in this way carries the risk of misclassifying individual children, but this is reduced if there is other (e.g. biochemical or clinical) evidence of nutritional abnormalities, or if serial measures of BMI are available.

In clinical practice these whole-body anthropometric indices are useful, but can be limited, as for instance, when a child has ascites, fluid retention, or a large solid tumor. Such conditions can confound weight-based anthropometric indices, and the most useful and widely used alternatives are mid upper arm circumference (MUAC – related to muscle mass and fat mass, an index of 'protein/energy' status), skinfold thickness (notably over the triceps: an index of fatness), and indices derived from these (arm muscle area or arm muscle circumference), which are more

Table 14.7 Dietary sources of minerals

Minerals	Food sources of major minerals	Alternative good sources
Iron	Cereal products (bread, breakfast cereals), vegetables, meat/meat products. *Cereals, meat, vegetables*	
Calcium	Milk and milk products, cereal products *Milk, milk products, cereals*	
Phosphorus	Milk products, cereal products, meat products, vegetables *Milk and milk products, cereal products, meat*	
Potassium	Vegetables, milk products, cereal products, meat products *Milk and milk products, vegetables, cereal products*	
Copper	Cereal products, vegetables, milk products, fruit *Cereal products, meat and meat products, vegetables*	
Iodine	Milk products, cereal products *Milk and milk products, cereal products*	Shellfish, legumes, cereals, liver, seafood, seaweeds, iodized salt
Zinc	Meat and meat products, milk, cereal products, vegetables	
Selenium	(Good sources: cereals, meat, fish)	Amount in foods depends on soil quality Deficiency may occur where soil is poor
Magnesium	Cereals, milk products, vegetables, meat products *Cereals, milk products*	
Chromium	(Good sources: yeast, meat, cereals, legumes, nuts)	

Sources of nutrients for infants are shown in italics.
From National Diet & Nutrition Survey 1990, 1995, 2000[6–9] and Garrow et al 2000[10]

specific indices of muscle bulk and are particularly useful in measuring small changes.[19]

When reporting and interpreting raw or derived anthropometric indices (e.g. BMI, weight-for-height, height-for-age) relative to a reference population there are three principal approaches: classification with reference to centiles; use of percentage of reference median; use of SD or 'Z' scores. While the first two approaches are most commonly used in clinical nutritional assessment, there is now a consensus that the third approach, the calculation of SD scores, is more clinically informative, and should be adopted more widely. Detailed discussion and demonstration of this point is provided in Krick.[22]

DIETARY NUTRITIONAL ASSESSMENT

Assessment of nutritional status based on dietary intake should take into account current and past food intake. Dietary assessments should be done by a pediatric dietitian who has the skills to ensure that all aspects of intake are considered, including assessment of the quantities of food eaten. Specific foods which appear to cause vomiting, diarrhea, malabsorption, etc. must also be identified, and 'food' should not only refer to that taken at meals but also include snacks eaten.

Weighed intakes should provide the most accurate record of food intake. However, the dietitian has to rely on the patient or family recording all food and drink taken (taking into account any wastage), and that the foods eaten reflect usual dietary habits rather than particular foods which are easy to weigh and record. Alternatively a diet history, based on 'typical' or 'usual' food intake, can be recorded. For this purpose 3-, 5- or 7-day food record diaries are used. The longer duration has the advantage of more clearly reflecting variations in food habits, but the disadvantage of the recording becoming onerous and thus more inaccurate. Assessment of dietary intake based on a recall method is dependent on the parent and/or child remembering all food and drink taken during the previous 24 h, and this being a typical day. A food frequency questionnaire presents the respondent with a list of foods that should be scored, in terms of the number of times that they are eaten each day, week or month. Food composition tables or computer programs are used to estimate intake of individual nutrients.

In children and adolescents all methods of dietary assessment have limited accuracy and the data obtained should always be interpreted with caution. Dietary assessment in children is best viewed as a means of explaining or solving a nutritional problem, rather than definitively identifying or confirming it. For example, an apparently low vitamin C intake might explain vitamin C deficiency, but should not be used to diagnose vitamin C deficiency (that would require biochemical assessment).

For nutritional assessment of infants (excluding those who are exclusively breast-fed), dietary assessment methods are more accurate, since much food is provided by milk feeds and most mothers can readily provide a fairly accurate record of the number and volume of feeds and the amount of solids taken. The dietitian must include bottles taken during the night, as well as other fluids (types used, frequency and volumes taken). The accuracy of the history can often be verified by checking the number of tins, bottles or cartons of formula powder used each week. Intake of vitamin and mineral supplements can be calculated from how regularly they are taken and the type of preparation used. Dietary assessment of an infant of less than 6 months should include assessment of the mother's nutritional status while pregnant, and her lactational performance if she is breast-feeding. This may require weighing the infant before and after a feed (see Ch. 11).

BIOCHEMICAL NUTRITIONAL ASSESSMENT

Biochemical nutritional assessment requires measurement of nutrient concentrations in the blood, urine, other fluids or tissues. There is an optimal concentration of nutrients within the body, below and above which deficiency and toxicity can occur (Fig. 14.3). However circulating concentrations of nutrients are not an accurate measurement of tissue stores and reflect the immediate availability of particular nutrients. In the blood some nutrients are found 'free' (e.g. vitamin C), some 'bound' (e.g. calcium, iron) to carrier proteins, and some as 'precursors' (e.g. beta-carotene). Each nutrient has its own site of storage and function and so universally applicable statements about biochemical nutritional assessment are not possible.

In pediatric practice, measurements of nutrient concentrations or biochemical markers of nutritional status and/or growth are made most commonly in the blood or urine. In certain nutritional deficiency or toxicity states, and in some metabolic diseases, measurements of concentrations of particular nutrients in specific tissues should be made. Changes in circulating concentrations of many nutrients occur only when tissue stores have been depleted and normal blood concentrations do not necessary indicate normal nutritional status (Fig. 14.3). The nutrients that are commonly measured in the blood are discussed here. Interpretation of the concentrations of those measured in other tissues will be found in relevant chapters.

Blood urea reflects not only renal function but also protein intake. It can be low in rapidly growing neonates and in children with hepatic failure. High blood urea can be a marker of the infant or toddler with a high cows' milk intake. Low serum albumin can be an indicator of inadequate protein intake or excessive protein loss in inflammatory bowel disease, for instance, but because of compensatory mechanisms that maintain circulating protein concentrations, it is not an early or sensitive sign of undernutrition. Plasma amino acids measured quantitatively may show low glutamine. In the fasting state, hepatic uptake of alanine for gluconeogenesis causes blood levels of this amino acid to fall. In patients on vegan diets or where severely reduced protein intake limits lysine availability for its synthesis, carnitine deficiency may develop. In these circumstances clinical effects are rare.

Alkaline phosphatase is a sensitive indicator of nutritional rickets and osteomalacia. Measurement of vitamin D level is not

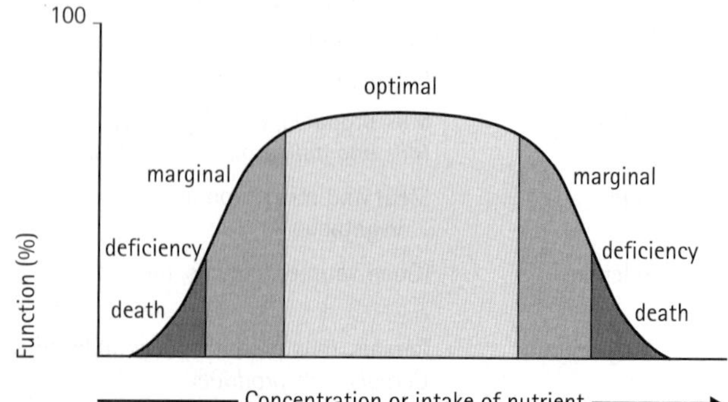

Fig. 14.3 Relations between low, optimal and high concentrations of nutrients and hypothetical physiological and biochemical functions.

indicated in the presence of normal calcium and phosphate. Prevalence studies have shown how difficult it is to make absolute definitions of iron deficiency. Hemoglobin and red cell indices may not fully reflect iron stores. Ferritin reflects total body iron stores but is also an acute phase protein and concentrations may be falsely high in acute infection. Serum iron, total iron binding capacity (TIBC) and free erythrocyte protoporphyrin (FEP) may be measured: iron falls, and TIBC and FEP rise in iron deficiency anemia.

Deficiency of water-soluble vitamins is rare in developed countries, athough this may develop rapidly in patients who are receiving inadequately supplemented intravenous fluids or total parenteral nutrition. Red cell transketolase activity gives an indirect indication of thiamine deficiency which can occur because of the demands of a high glucose intake for thiamine pyrophosphate cofactor. Deficiency of vitamin B_{12}, vitamin A or vitamin E develops late because of large tissue stores. Prothrombin time reflects vitamin K status if liver function is normal.

Circulating concentrations of trace elements (copper, zinc, selenium) decrease late in deficiency. Zinc or magnesium deficiency occurs in Crohn's disease and other causes of chronic diarrhea. Low glutathione peroxidase activity in red cells indirectly indicates selenium deficiency but a direct selenium assay may be preferable.

The sections below contain an account of the major features of macronutrient and micronutrient deficiencies.

CLINICAL NUTRITIONAL ASSESSMENT

Clinical nutritional assessment is limited by its subjectivity, even when performed by specialists.[23] Signs of 'pure' or single nutrient deficiencies rarely occur alone and physical signs, such as glossitis or angular stomatitis are relatively non-specific. Physical examination should therefore be interpreted in association with anthropometric, dietary and biochemical nutritional assessment.

The 'classical' physical signs of protein-energy malnutrition, some vitamin and mineral deficiencies are described below and in relevant chapters of this textbook. It should be remembered, however, that physical signs are a late manifestation of nutrient deficiency, occurring after tissue stores have been depleted, and adaptive changes have failed to maintain normal nutrient homeostasis and function (Fig. 14.3).

HEALTHY DIET: INFANCY, CHILDHOOD AND ADOLESCENCE

INFANT

Milk is the sufficient and sole source of energy and nutrients for the first 6 months of life. Current World Health Organization (WHO) recommendations are that term infants should be exclusively breast-fed from birth until about 6 months.[24,25] Complementary (non-milk, weaning) foods should be introduced at around this time, to fill the gap between the energy and nutrient needs provided by milk and those that the infant requires to maintain normal growth and development (Fig.14.4).

Human milk

Human milk is a complex blend of nutrients and immunological and other bioactive substances. The former provide the energy, macronutrients (carbohydrates, fats and proteins) and micronutrients (vitamins and minerals) that the baby needs to grow, develop and function (physical activity, thermogenesis, essential organ function – BMR) (Fig.14.2). The latter confer protection from bacterial and viral infections and assist adaptation

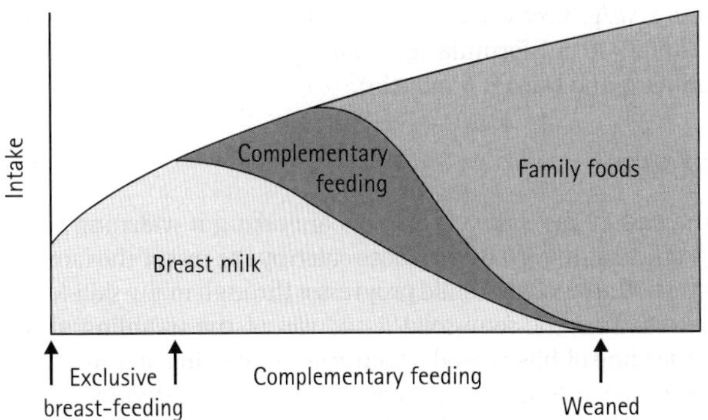

Fig. 14.4 Contributions of milk, complementary and family foods to energy and nutrient needs in infancy.

to life outside the womb. The composition of human milk changes both during the course of lactation and during a single feed to both anticipate and meet the nutritional needs of the growing infant.

Formula milk

Approved infant formulas provide safe alternatives to breast milk. They broadly resemble human milk in terms of their chemical composition but lack the enzymes, immunological or other bioactive substances found in human milk. The majority of formulas are based on cows' milk and are either whey or casein predominant. The former have a protein content based on demineralized whey with a whey:casein ratio similar to breast milk (60% whey:40% casein). The protein source of casein-predominant formulas is skimmed cows' milk with a ratio of 80% casein:20% whey. Ideally infants should remain on the formula first used until the end of the first year of life but a follow-on formula may be used from the age of 6 months. Whole cow's milk should not be used as the main milk drink for infants until the age of 1 year.

Soya formulas should be used only for infants with proven intolerance to cows' milk formulas or lactose (see Ch. 11) and for infants of vegetarian mothers who have elected not to breast-feed. Although satisfactory growth has been achieved in babies fed formulas based on cows' milk and soya, their nutritional composition differs from that of human milk, for example in their essential fatty acid contents, non-nutritional factors, and bioavailability of some micronutrients such as iron. Short and long term studies on risk of infection, growth and neurological outcome of children who have received these formulas suggest that human milk is preferable to 'artificial' formulas for the infant.[24] The feeding of the normal newborn infant is considered in greater detail in Chapter 11.

Complementary foods

At about 6 months of age complementary foods (non-milk, 'solids') should be introduced into the diet (Fig. 14.4). The infant's iron stores are becoming depleted, chewing needs to be developed, and milk alone is insufficient to meet the growing nutritional requirements of the infant.[24,25] In addition to a non-milk diet, infants should continue to receive a minimum of 500–600 ml of breast or formula milk daily. Non-wheat cereals, fruit, vegetables and potatoes are all suitable first weaning foods. Between 6 and 9 months of age, meat, fish, all cereals, pulses, fish and eggs can be introduced. No salt should be added to home-prepared foods, and only enough sugar used to make sour fruits palatable. Complementary foods should aim to have an energy density of at least 1 kcal/g. Breast-fed and artificially-fed infants that consume less than 500 ml formula feed daily should have supplements of vitamins A and D from 6 months.[11]

TODDLER

By the end of the first year infants are taking a widening range of foods and beginning to share those eaten by the rest of the family. The feeding of the preschool child progresses through many skill-learning processes, from the semi-solid/liquid diet of the weanling, through finger-feeding of bits of food which require chewing at around 1 year of age, to spoon-feeding by the age of 2 years, to mastering child-sized cutlery and adult-type food by the age of 5 years.

Nutritionally, toddler foods bridge the gap between the energy-dense diet of the infant, which provides around 50% of energy from fat, and that of the adult, where around 35% of energy should be derived from fat. Toddlers, however, have smaller gastric capacities than adults, and a balance must be struck between the gradual reduction of energy-dense, fat-containing foods and the introduction of lower fat foods.[25a] Surveys of nutritional intakes for this age group show that the energy intake from fat declines with increasing age.[7] Non-digestible carbohydrates ('fiber') should be a part of complementary foods. Infants are at risk of iron deficiency and care should be taken that foods containing adequate iron are used. In both cases the use of 'whole' foods that are rich in these substances is preferred to supplements or fortified foods.

The toddler should continue to consume around 500 ml of milk daily (or equivalent from other foods such as yoghurt and cheese). Full-fat milk should be used from 1–2 years of age. Thereafter, as long as growth and energy intake are satisfactory, semi-skimmed milk can be given from the age of 2–5 years of age. After 2 years of age other lower fat dairy products such as yoghurt, spreads and cheese may be used. Many toddlers become fussy and difficult with meals and it may be more appropriate to follow a feeding regimen based on three small meals and three snacks daily. Some young children begin to prefer easily assimilated liquids, particularly if given from bottles, for solid food, which requires chewing and the use of cutlery. 'Bottle caries' is a result of continual ingestion of sweetened liquids from a teated bottle.[8] After the first year all drinks taken during the day should be taken from a cup.

SCHOOLCHILD

After the age of 5 years the diet can change towards that advised for adults.[26] Fiber intake should increase with generous consumption of fruits, vegetables and high fiber cereals such as wholemeal bread, pasta and breakfast cereals. Saturated fat intake should be moderated by the use of skimmed or semi-skimmed milk, low fat or polyunsaturated spreads, low fat dairy products and eating fish, poultry and lean meats. The intake of non-milk extrinsic sugar should be avoided because of its association with dental caries. A reduction in energy intake from a lowering of fat intake should be compensated for by a commensurate increase in starch intake.[27] Compositionally, the diet should reflect the DRVs shown in the tables above.[2] National surveys have shown that some toddlers and young children are at risk of inadequate energy, vitamin A, iron and zinc intakes.[7] There has also been concern of the risk of rickets in Asian children,[28] who should receive vitamin D supplementation up to the age of 5 years.

ADOLESCENT

Energy intake in adolescence should meet the demands needed to achieve peak growth velocity and that required for high physical activity. The timing of the adolescent growth spurt varies between individuals so that nutrient requirements should be related to weight and height rather than age.[2] Weight gain in girls is mainly due to fat deposition whereas boys accumulate more muscle and skeletal tissue.

Eating habits show a trend to persist with time and a healthy adolescent diet should anticipate and minimize the long term risks of chronic cardiovascular diseases,[29] obesity, diabetes and other adult conditions associated with a poor diet.[30] Many teenagers adopt a 'grazing' eating pattern, consuming snacks and 'fast food' meals. Concern about body image may lead to abnormal eating and exercise patterns. In extreme cases anorexia nervosa and bulimia may result, but these disorders are primarily psychiatric not nutritional (Ch. 33).

Studies of childhood teenage eating habits show that many children consume diets low in various nutrients, in particular iron, calcium, thiamine and riboflavin.[5] Although weights and heights are generally within the normal ranges, on average children consume < 90% of EAR for energy, and some teenage girls considerably less. This may reflect the sedentary lifestyles of many children and female concern for body image. Bread, milk, meat products, chips, cakes and puddings are reported as the main sources of energy, and at all ages children consume about 35% of food energy as fat. An increasing proportion takes in excess of food energy from saturated fat. In association with insufficient physical exercise this may contribute to overweight and obesity, which are growing problems, as described below. A significant number of children do not meet their RNI for vitamin A, riboflavin, iron, zinc, magnesium and calcium, and teenage girls fare worse than boys, with > 40% having iron intakes below the LRNI.

Many adolescents will experiment with different diets. 'Vegetarian' diets, which include some animal foods such as milk, cheese or eggs, usually achieve adequate nutrient intakes. Teenagers who elect to follow a vegan regimen should take supplements of vitamin B_{12}, calcium, vitamin D, iron and zinc. Avoidance of specific foods on religious or cult grounds may result in severe nutrient deficiencies unless the dietary regimen has been based on long established traditional practices.

PRINCIPLES OF NUTRITION SUPPORT

Poor nutrition is not only a consequence of many diseases, particularly of the digestive system[30a] (Table 14.8), but is also a common feature of chronic illnesses, follows major surgery and occurs when patients are unable to eat or make proper use of their diet.[31] Malnutrition can be detected in a significant number of children admitted to hospital.[17] Children can also become malnourished for non-medical reasons, such as inappropriate or missed hospital meals (Table 14.9) and whatever the cause, the effect is a disturbance of energy and nutrient balance (Fig. 14.5).

The skills required to deal with assessment, prescription, administration and monitoring of treatment increasingly fall outside the expertise of a single practitioner. Nutrition support should be provided by a team, led by a pediatrician trained and experienced in clinical nutrition, comprising dietitians, nutrition nurse specialists, a pharmacist in charge of the preparation and prescription of parenteral solutions, a biochemist responsible for monitoring biochemical outcome and a surgeon with experience of gastrostomies and insertion of intravenous long lines for parenteral nutrition (PN) (Table 14.10). Introduction of nutrition teams is associated with a reduction of mechanical, metabolic

Table 14.8 Diseases of childhood associated with malnutrition

Low birth weight
Short bowel syndrome
Cystic fibrosis
Mucosal diseases of the gastrointestinal tract
Celiac disease
Persistent diarrhea syndromes
Cows' milk protein enteropathy
Soy protein enteropathy
Tropical sprue
Allergic gastroenteritis
Persistent diarrhea syndromes
Immune deficiency disorders
Inflammatory bowel disease
Chronic liver disease
Juvenile chronic arthritis
Chronic renal disease
Congenital heart disease
Burns and trauma
Anorexia nervosa
HIV infection and AIDS
Childhood cancers

and infection-related complications of PN, shorter duration in hospital and decline in the cost of nutrition support.[32] Nutrition support may be provided either enterally or parenterally. Before starting nutrition support it is essential to properly assess the patient's nutritional status and nutritional needs (see before and Bresson et al[33]).

ENTERAL TUBE FEEDING

Enteral feeding should be used if the gastrointestinal tract is accessible and functional. PN should be reserved for conditions where enteral nutrition cannot meet energy and nutrient requirements via the gut alone. There are many indications for enteral tube feeding (Table 14.11).

Delivery routes and systems

Enteral feeding is a means by which nutrients can be delivered to the gastrointestinal tract by tube or enterostomy. This can be done continuously, as bolus feeds or as intermittent continuous feeds (Table 14.12). In continuous feeding the enteral feed is infused over a period of hours (usually from 8–24 h) using a pump, which regulates the volume administered. Bolus feeding simulates the usual pattern of feeding, generating a postprandial metabolic response that is greater than that when continuous feeds are given. Feeds can be given at intervals from hourly to 4 hourly. Intermittent continuous feeding combines the feeding techniques of bolus and continuous feeds.

The choice of mode of delivery can be made using the algorithm shown in Figure 14.6. Nasogastric tubes are easy to introduce and have fewer complications than nasojejunal tubes. Nasogastric tube feeding is also more 'physiological' in that the defence and digestive functions of the stomach are utilized, but gastroesophageal reflux and aspiration are more likely to occur. Nasojejunal tubes are used when these risks are high, such as in children with neuromuscular disease, severe neurological handicap and gastrointestinal motility disorders.

Enterostomies offer a means of delivering enteral feeds directly into the stomach or jejunum, bypassing proximal mechanical, surgical or pathological obstructions. They are also preferred when

Table 14.9 Principal reasons why children get malnourished

Social and psychological factors
- 'Faddy' and inappropriate diets
- Poverty and disadvantage of family
- Chronic pain, depression or apathy

Medical reasons
- Disease-related anorexia, maldigestion and absorption
- Increased energy needs
- Altered taste perception
- Reduced ability to suck, chew or swallow
- Physical or mental disability

Hospital specific factors
- Meals missed due to investigation or treatment
- Food served that takes no account of disability
- Lack of nursing supervision at meal times
- Reduced absorption following surgery

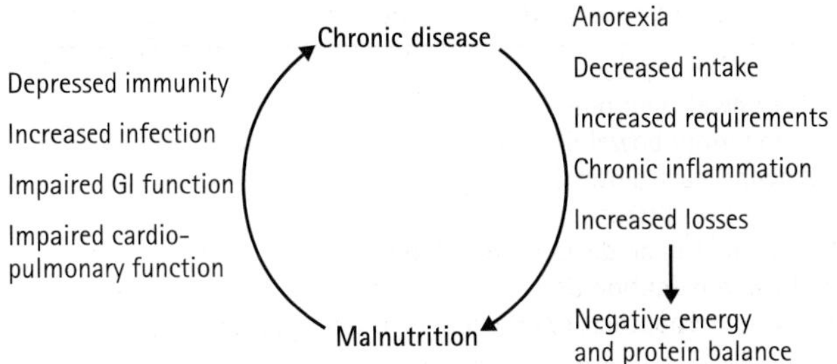

Fig. 14.5 Vicious cycle of chronic disease and malnutrition: disturbance of energy and nutrient balance.

Table 14.10 Composition and functions of members of nutrition support team

Member	Functions
Dietitian	Assesses nutritional status Calculates nutritional requirements Designs enteral or parenteral feeding regimes
Nurse specialist	Acts jointly with clinician, dietitian and pharmacist in practical aspects of nutrition support Patient and community care training Care of enterostomy tubes and central venous lines
Clinician	Overall responsibility for nutritional care Monitors outcome and liaises with medical/surgical team Diagnosis and management of underlying conditions and of complications of nutritional support
Pharmacist	Responsible for provision of enteral and parenteral nutrition solutions Advises on compatibility and drug interactions
Surgeon	Fashions enterostomies and inserts intravenous catheters
Biochemist	Monitors biochemical indices of nutritional status
Bacteriologist	Detection and advice on treatment of intravenous line infections

Table 14.11 Condition in which nutrition support may be indicated

Gastrointestinal disease
- Short bowel syndrome
- Inflammatory bowel disease
- Following gastrointestinal surgery
- Chronic liver disease
- Glycogen storage disease types I and III
- Fatty acid oxidation defects
- Severe enteropathies and disorders of digestion

Neurological disease
- Coma and severe facial and head injury
- Severe mental retardation and cerebral palsy
- Dysphagia secondary to cranial nerve palsy, muscular dystrophy, myasthenia gravis

Malignant disease
- Obstruction of esophagus and upper gut
- Head and neck
- Abnormality of deglutition following surgical intervention
- Gastrointestinal side-effects from chemotherapy and/or radiotherapy
- Terminal support care

Pulmonary disease
- Bronchopulmonary dysplasia
- Cystic fibrosis
- Chronic lung disease

Congenital anomalies
- Tracheoesophageal fistula
- Esophageal atresia
- Cleft palate
- Pierre Robin syndrome

Other
- Primary malnutrition
- Anorexia nervosa
- Cardiac failure
- Chronic renal disease
- Severe burns
- Severe sepsis
- Severe trauma

pharyngeal discomfort is intolerable or the risk of aspiration high. Percutaneous endoscopic gastrostomy (PEG) is an increasingly popular technique of tube placement, and the gastrostomy button is a useful innovation for long term feeding. Flush with the skin the button can be connected to a feeding tube at the child's convenience and avoids a long tube protruding from the abdomen (Fig. 14.7) Many children who require long term enteral nutrition have gastrostomies, including many who receive home enteral feeding (see below). For children with neurological handicaps, particularly those with difficulty swallowing, gastrostomies greatly facilitate both feeding and nursing. In some children a fundoplication may be required to prevent gastric regurgitation. The advantages and disadvantages of enterostomies are listed in Table 14.13.

Enteral formulas

There is a range of enteral feeds available for children. Many are based on cows' milk and are suitable for children with an intact and functional gastrointestinal tract. These whole protein formulas are used to provide full or partial nutrition support and can be supplemented with extra energy (in the form of a glucose polymer or fat emulsion) and protein. Specialized formulas are designed to meet the altered nutrient needs and gastrointestinal and/or metabolic problems of children with different diseases. These include elemental formulas based on amino acids, vegetable oils (composed of a mixture of medium chain and long chain triglycerides) and glucose, designed for children with protracted diarrhea and severe enteropathies; protein hydrolysates for children with sensitivity to food proteins; formulas that are lactose-free by substitution of lactose with another carbohydrate, and feeds based on soya, which are free of lactose and cows' milk protein. Modular feeds allow each macronutrient to be combined in amounts and source appropriate for the special needs of the child. There are also special feeds for children with hepatic, renal and metabolic diseases, which are discussed in Chapters 16, 17 and 24. Almost all clinical needs can be met by ready-prepared, commercially-available formulas, and the reader should consult the literature produced by the manufacturers for full details of their composition and indications (see Table 40.16).

Table 14.12 Advantages and disadvantages of enteral feeding methods

Feeding method	Advantages	Disadvantages
Continuous infusion	Larger volumes of feed can be administered Smaller bore tubes can be used Less gastric distension Less 'dumping' so that feeds with higher nutrient densities can be given	Tube may become dislodged during feed administration with risk of aspiration Electric feeding pumps, reservoirs and giving-sets are expensive Some feeds containing insoluble substances cannot be given
Bolus feeds	Mimics the normal feeding gut hormonal response Position of feeding tube can be checked prior to each feed Simple procedure only: a syringe required for feed to be administered Contact with child at each feed time	Gastric distension and vomiting A wider-bore feeding tube may be required which may cause discomfort in nasopharynx if nasogastric feeding route used 'Dumping' may be experienced especially if high nutrient dense feeds given Adequate fluid requirement may be difficult to achieve
Intermittent continuous feeds	Larger volumes can be tolerated Fine bore tubes can be used The feeding tube position can be checked prior to each feed Nutrient-dense feeds can be administered	Requires a great deal of supervision Electric feeding pumps, reservoirs and giving-sets are expensive

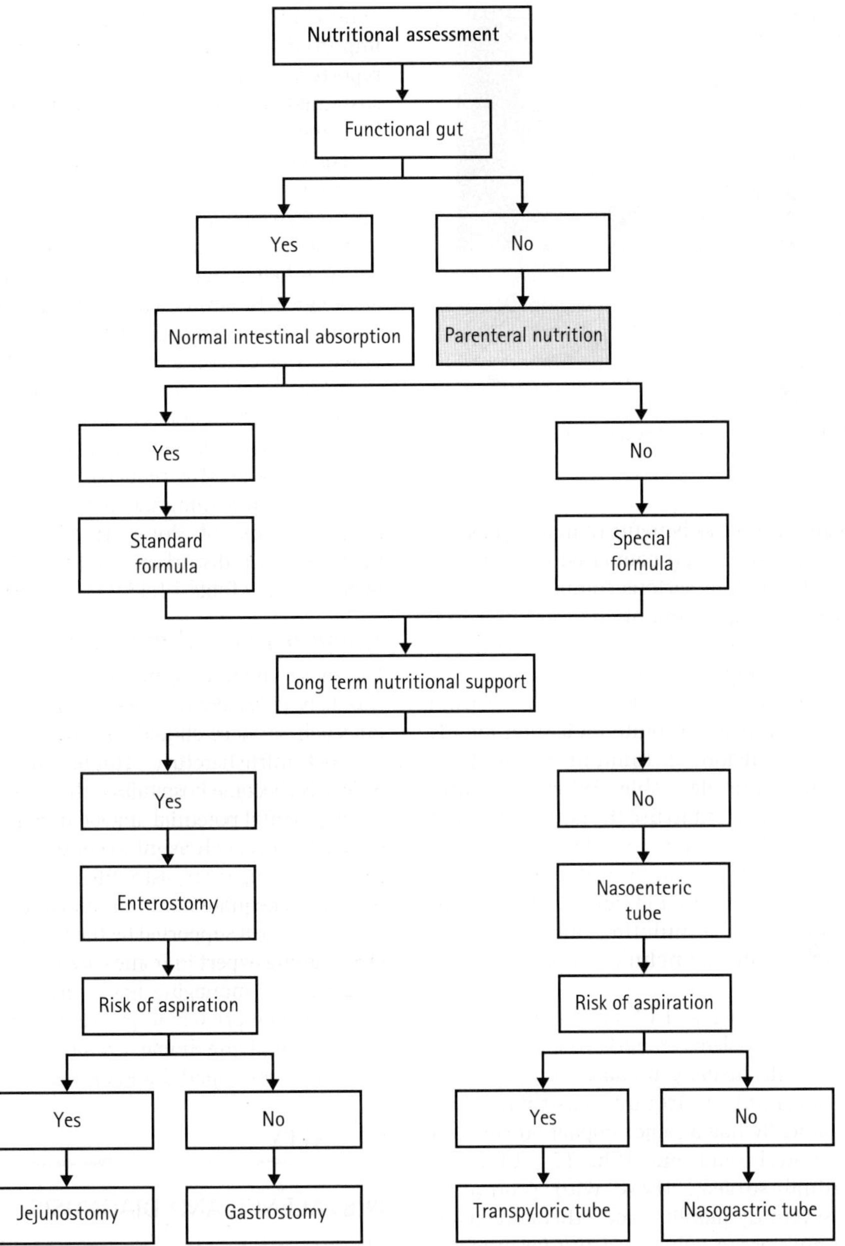

Fig. 14.6 Algorithm for choice of route of delivery of enteral feeds.

Home-prepared feeds and liquidized foods should not be used for enteral nutrition of children because of uncertain nutrient quality, a risk of bacterial contamination and of the feeding tube becoming blocked with food particles. During the first year of life infants who require enteral feeding and have a normal functioning gastrointestinal tract and require no nutrient modification, should receive one of the standard infant formulas (Ch. 11).

Home enteral tube feeding

Home enteral feeding (HEF) should be considered when the sole reason for the child being in hospital is enteral nutritional support.[34] It has been estimated that the expense and effort (of providing equipment, feeds and training) is justified by a minimum of 10 days of HEF. Children with chronic diseases, such as cystic fibrosis, neuromuscular disorders, malignant disease and renal failure, can greatly benefit from HEF: some have received it for more than 10 years, and its use is growing.[35] Many children, who are happy and able to pass their own nasogastric tubes, prefer night-time HEF. Children with enterostomies may also receive HEF.

PARENTERAL NUTRITION

PN is a means by which nutrients are delivered to the patient via the vein. It may provide complete nutritional support – total parenteral nutrition (TPN) – or be combined with enteral feeding. The administration and monitoring of PN is complex and should be undertaken by the nutrition support team. The process by which energy and nutrient requirements are calculated, techniques of delivery and assessment of PN are well described in a number of reviews.[18]

Indications and complications of PN

The principal indications for PN are shown in Table 14.14. Although sometimes life-saving, PN has been subjected to few

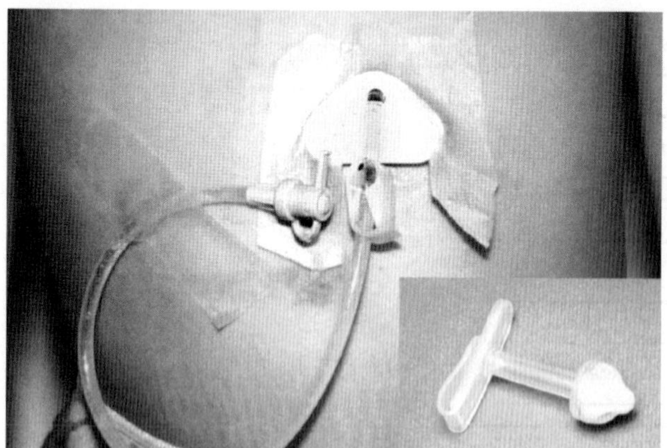

Fig. 14.7 Gastrostomy feeding tube in situ. Inset: gastrostomy button.

controlled clinical trials and its precise benefits remain unclear.[36] PN is both complex and expensive when compared with enteral nutrition, and because of the risk of serious complications and evidence that enteral nutrition helps to maintain gastrointestinal structure and function, there has been a reappraisal of its use in some groups of patients, for example in those receiving intensive care. Whilst there can be little doubt that gastrointestinal 'failure' (from whatever cause) is an absolute indication for PN (Table 14.14), complete exclusion of luminal nutrients is frequently neither essential nor desirable. When planning nutritional intervention it is important to use the gastrointestinal tract if possible. Total enteral nutrition may be feasible if a transpyloric or jejunostomy tube is used. Even if only minimal volumes of enteral feed can be given in addition to PN, this can help to prevent cholestasis by stimulating bile flow and pancreatic secretions, maintain splanchnic blood flow and provide mucosal nutrition.

Overall, the most frequent recipients of PN are preterm infants (Ch. 10). Infants with surgical problems comprise the next largest group, and are fed parenterally usually because of gut failure following surgery for congenital or acquired gastrointestinal disease, and PN has undoubtedly had a major impact on survival in children with short bowel syndrome (Ch. 17). Children undergoing gastrointestinal surgery, those with protracted diarrhea (see before) or severe dysmotility, and others receiving intensive care often with multiorgan failure account for much of the remaining PN usage.

Ethical dilemmas arise in relation to the care of children in whom there is little or no prospect of establishing full enteral feeding at any time in the future, such as those with congenital enteropathies (Ch. 17). The prognosis in short bowel syndrome has improved considerably over the past 20 years[37] and in some reported cases less than 20 cm of small bowel has ultimately sustained normal growth. Small bowel transplantation offers hope for some children who are chronically dependent on TPN.[38]

For children receiving PN for more than a few weeks, cyclical nutrition should be considered. This involves a gradual decrease in the time over which it is given, so that eventually the PN can be infused overnight and the central venous line left clamped for 12 h during the day. This helps to encourage mobility and psychomotor development and reduce the adverse effects of prolonged hospitalization. Oromotor skills should be promoted with comforters and, when possible, small amounts of enteral feed by mouth. The expert advice of a speech therapist should be sought at an early stage. Cyclical PN may help protect against cholestasis and hepatic dysfunction.

Catheter-related sepsis is a serious complication of PN and its incidence is greatly reduced by scrupulous attention to sterile procedures and minimal handling of intravenous lines.[32] Other complications of long term PN include electrolyte and micronutrient disturbances, thromboembolism and pulmonary hypertension (Table 14.15).

Home parenteral nutrition

For those children committed to long term PN, home treatment should be considered.[34] The nutritional support industry and hospital outreach services should together provide the organizational and support infrastructure. Home PN offers children who would otherwise become hospitalized the possibility of realizing growth and developmental potential, a good quality of life, and a reduced risk of complications such as intravenous line sepsis. Suitable patients are those with long term gastrointestinal failure who are medically stable and have adequate home circumstances. The carers must be highly motivated, well supported by the nutrition support team and capable of becoming expert in home care including sterile technique, setting up infusions, managing lines, setting pumps, and recognizing and reacting appropriately to problems. The most frequent diagnoses in children receiving home PN are short bowel, severe dysmotility, congenital enteropathy, and Crohn's disease.[39]

OBESITY

PREVALENCE AND DIAGNOSIS

Obesity is now a major pediatric health problem in the developed world. For example, in England in 1996 11% of 6-year-olds and 17% of 15-year-olds were obese (BMI > 95th percentile;[40]). Childhood obesity prevalence has also increased markedly in many developing countries.[41]

Table 14.13 Advantages and disadvantages of enterostomies

Type	Advantages	Disadvantages
Gastrostomy	Gastric digestive and anti-infective properties retained Intermittent bolus regimens possible Percutaneous endoscopic placement or interventional radiology Conversion to transpyloric route possible	Risk of aspiration and gastroesophageal reflux Dumping syndrome
Jejunostomy	Low risk of reflux and aspiration	Continuous infusion necessary Gastric functions bypassed Risk of upper GI intussusception

Table 14.14 Common indications for parenteral nutrition

	Neonates	Older infants and children (relative)	
Absolute indications	Intestinal failure (e.g. functional immaturity, short bowel, pseudo-obstruction) Necrotizing enterocolitis	Gastrointestinal failure	Short bowel syndrome Protracted diarrhea Chronic pseudo-obstruction Postoperative gastrointestinal surgery Radiation/cytotoxic drug therapy (e.g. bone marrow transplantation)
Relative indications	Respiratory failure requiring IPPV Promotion of growth in preterm infants	Intensive care and multiorgan failure	Severe IBD Acute pancreatitis Acute renal failure Acute liver failure Extensive burns Severe trauma

IBD, inflammatory bowel disease; IPPV, intermittent positive pressure ventilation.

Obesity must be assessed using objective measurements.[42] Measuring body weight alone is inadequate: weight must be adjusted for height. This adjustment is best done by calculating BMI.[42] Since BMI changes with age and differs between the sexes, interpretation of a single value requires a comparison to population reference data, i.e. a cut-off point in the BMI distribution must be applied to define overweight and obesity. Use of the 95th percentile to define obesity is recommended and has a number of advantages.[42] First, it identifies the fattest children with moderate sensitivity and high specificity (low false positive rate). Second, the definition has clinical/biological significance: children with BMI above the 95th percentile have a high probability of remaining obese, and of experiencing the morbidity associated with obesity.[43]

CLINICAL CONSEQUENCES

Childhood obesity causes morbidity in childhood, and increases morbidity and mortality in adulthood.[43] Psychosocial morbidity is common, and a range of other problems (respiratory, metabolic, hepatic, orthopedic) less common. In adolescents and young adults, obesity has adverse 'social' effects. These include reduced educational attainment and income in both the UK and the USA.[43] Cardiovascular risk factors are associated with obesity, even in childhood and they tend to 'cluster' in the obese child.[44] Childhood obesity has a strong tendency to persist after the age of about 3 years,[45] and it increases morbidity and premature mortality in adult life, particularly from cardiovascular disease and diabetes.[46,47]

Table 14.15 Complications of parenteral nutrition

Phlebitis
Infection
Hypo- and hyperglycemia
Electrolyte disturbance
Fluid overload, dehydration
Hypophosphatemia
Anemia
Platelet and neutrophil dysfunction
Trace element deficiencies
Trace element excess
Vitamin deficiencies
Hyperammonemia
Essential fatty acid deficiency
Cholestasis and hepatic dysfunction
Metabolic acidosis
Hypercholesterolemia
Hypertriglyceridemia
Air and thromboembolism

CAUSES

Obesity is a disorder of energy balance. Excess dietary (food) energy is stored as fat *and* lean tissue, so that obese children have both a larger fat mass and lean body mass than their non-obese peers. Larger fat-free mass and body mass means that the energy requirements of the obese child are considerably *higher* than those of the non-obese child. Obese patients tend to report low food intakes, implying reduced metabolic rate as a cause. This is rarely the case and most obese children and adolescents substantially under-report their true dietary intake.[48] One consequence is that dietary intakes reported by obese patients/their families must be viewed with caution, and can only provide a crude estimate of eating habits.

TREATMENT

Detailed descriptions of therapeutic strategies for treating childhood obesity are provided elsewhere,[42] and a comprehensive but non-systematic review of the pediatric obesity treatment literature is provided by Epstein et al.[49] The focus of therapy is modest dietary restriction and 'healthy eating' (to reduce energy intake), usually with behavioral modification and parent training, often with an exercise prescription (to increase energy expenditure). As in adults, childhood obesity is often resistant to treatment so therapy should be offered only where the child/family perceive the need to make lifestyle changes, or where there is severe obesity related comorbidity (such as sleep apnea). Therapy should usually involve the family, and focus on lifestyle changes. Three high quality randomized controlled trials have shown that training children and families in altered eating behavior, in combination with increased physical activity, and/or decreased sedentary behavior is beneficial.[50–52] This need not involve structured exercise, and a focus on diet plus reduced TV viewing has been successful. A target of less than 14 h TV viewing/computer use per week is an appropriate adjunct to dietary therapy.

SECONDARY OBESITY

Careful history and examination will usually differentiate between simple obesity and any underlying pathology which may be responsible (Table 14.16). The child with simple obesity often has relatively tall stature. In contrast children with Cushing's syndrome and hypothyroidism have relative or short stature, and growth failure. Hyperphagic dysmorphic syndromes include the Prader–Willi and Laurence–Moon–Biedl syndromes, but many dysmorphic syndromes with mental handicap can be associated with voracious appetite. Some chromosomal abnormalities (Down and Klinefelter's syndromes) are associated with obesity. Recurrent headaches with recent increases in severity and frequency may indicate a hypothalamic or pituitary tumor. Severe mood disturbance, unstable temperature, polyuria and polydypsia and visual disturbance support this diagnosis. It is vital to identify causes of secondary obesity early. Management of secondary obesity involves treatment of the underlying disease.

MALNUTRITION

The term 'primary malnutrition' is used to describe conditions that result from a diet that does not satisfy nutritional requirements. 'Secondary malnutrition' refers to that associated with underlying disease or trauma, such as inflammatory bowel disease, severe burns or after major bowel surgery.[1] Primary malnutrition, which accounts for the vast majority of cases, is associated with poverty, inadequate food, lack of hygiene, recurrent infections, and lack of health care. It is extremely common, affecting around a third of the world's children because so many live in poverty in the 'developing' world.[53] It is 'an accomplice in at least half of the 10.4 million childhood deaths each year' (http://www.who.int/nut/pem.htm). Lack of effective prevention and treatment accounts for almost all of these unnecessary deaths. In the survivors, malnutrition leads to permanent suboptimal physical and mental development affecting billions of adults mainly in south and south-east Asia, Africa and South America. Fortunately, in most of the world except Africa, the prevalence of malnutrition is falling slowly.

CLASSIFICATION OF MALNUTRITION

Malnutrition in children is the outcome of abnormally slow and sometimes negative weight gain, development and physiological functions. It is characterized by shortness and thinness and there is often evidence of specific nutrient deficiencies. Nutritional edema is a less common complication. It is associated with marked abnormalities of metabolism and its cause is not clear.

Malnutrition is most easily diagnosed and classified using anthropometry; by measuring the child's dimensions and weight, and relating them to what would be expected normally, based on reference data, as outlined in the section on Anthropometric nutritional assessment. Various reference data have been compiled, mostly from cross-sectional surveys in the USA, UK and other countries, and several classifications of malnutrition have been proposed (Table 14.17). The Wellcome and Waterlow classifications are useful together as they identify which children need which treatment and the degree of urgency. The most recent WHO manual on malnutrition[53] uses a new classification, defining it as the presence of significant wasting (weight < –2 SD of reference weight-for-height), equivalent to approximately 80% weight-for-height.[54] Severe malnutrition means severe wasting (weight < –3 SD of reference weight-for-height) or/and nutritional edema. Without intervention, children with severe malnutrition usually deteriorate rapidly until they are at high risk of imminent death. Stunted children (height < –2 SD of reference height-for-age, approximately 90% height-for-age) are also at increased risk of death but to a lesser extent.

Wasting and edema can develop rapidly and resolve rapidly: measurable stunting develops slowly and, even with intervention, usually carries on until puberty in a poor environment. Although puberty tends to be delayed, final height is less than predicted. This applies to whole populations living in poverty. It is associated with less than expected IQ. The combination reduces the chances of good employment, prosperity, normal birth weights and improved life opportunities in the next generation.

CLINICAL FEATURES

Clinical features of malnutrition vary enormously and none distinguishes primary from secondary malnutrition. In an infant, because head size is better preserved than length or weight, the trunk and limbs often appear relatively small. Abdominal girth is variable and sometimes relatively large due to gaseous distension. The older child, on the other hand, may appear well-proportioned and healthy but diminutive. This implies predominant stunting and thus mild to moderate problems over a long period. However, an acute severe problem in a previously well-nourished child may be visible first as wasting alone. Severely malnourished children are usually wasted and stunted.[1]

In general, edema is less common in very young infants. It often arises over a few days, when a child, already compromised nutritionally and failing to thrive, develops an infection like measles or gastroenteritis. If beyond the walking stage, oedema is first noted on both feet; if younger, it may first be seen in the hands or around the eyes. The child is obviously ill, apathetic, irritable and anorexic. Skin lesions tend to be more common and more severe in the edematous child. Typically, they start as a darkening and thickening of the keratin layer which when damaged, splits or flakes off leaving patches of hypopigmented thin skin and sometimes oozing sores that refuse to heal. Such skin damage tends to occur round the orifices (mouth, perianal and perineal), over joints and on the extremities. It also occurs where edema stretches the skin, as on the foot and lower leg. Firm, smooth hepatomegaly, associated sometimes with vast deposits of lipid, is also frequent in the edematous child. However, abdominal distension, which is common, is usually mainly gaseous. Stool frequency tends to be increased but volume is reduced and consistency and appearance variable, often loose, green and mucusy.

Table 14.16 Causes of obesity

Functional	
Simple obesity	Excessive dietary intake Lack of exercise/mobility (spina bifida, muscular dystrophy)
Organic	
Hypothalmic disturbance	Pituitary tumors
Hyperphagic syndromes	Prader–Willi syndrome Lawrence–Moon–Biedl syndrome
Corticosteroid excess	Cushing's (iatrogenic, pituitary, adrenal)
Hypothyroidism	Thyroid failure
Chromosomal	Down syndrome Klinefelter's syndrome
Cerebral disease	Tumors, infection, hydrocephalus

Table 14.17 Classifications of childhood malnutrition

Classification	Definition	Grade	Nutritional edema
WHO	Weight-for-height/length[1,2]		
	< −2 SDS	Malnourished	Absent
	< −3 SDS	Severely malnourished	Absent
	Any	Severely malnourished	Present
	Height/length-for-age		
	< −2 SDS	Stunted	
	< −3 SDS	Severely stunted	
Wellcome	Weight-for-age %		
	80–60	Undernourished/kwashiorkor	Absent/Present
	< 60 (≈ −4 SDS)	Marasmus/marasmic-kwashiorkor	Absent/Present
Waterlow	Weight-for-height/length %		
	89–80	Mild wasting	
	79–70	Moderate wasting	
	< 70 (≈−3 SDS)	Severe wasting	
	Height/length-for-age %		
	94–90	Mild stunting	
	89–85	Moderate stunting	
	< 85 (≈−3 SDS)	Severe stunting	

[1]SDS = standard deviation score or number of standard deviations from median of reference data (NCHS/WHO (WHO 1999[54]))
[2]'height', for standing children, 'length' for supine infants. Standing reduces height by approximately 5 mm.

Other clinical features include depigmentation, thinning and straightening of the hair associated with increased fragility and pluckability. In contrast, in longstanding malnutrition, eyelashes tend to be long and silky and in some children, lanugo hair grows luxuriantly. Many of these clinical signs can be recognized in Figures 14.8 and 14.9, which show infants with kwashiorkor (edematous malnutrition) and marasmus (severe wasting) respectively. Clinical features of specific nutrient deficiencies are often present, such as rickets, scurvy, keratomalacia, etc. (see below). When a child is severely malnourished, he or she may develop any or all of the following: extreme apathy, hypotonia, pallor, hypothermia, cold extremities with prolonged capillary refill time, a weak pulse, dyspnea, petechiae, purpura and jaundice. They are, in their various ways, evidence of septicemia, cardiac and hepatic failure and eventually, loss of cell homeostasis which, untreated, is fatal.

LABORATORY INVESTIGATIONS

Laboratory investigations are generally unhelpful. Hemoglobin falls but serum ferritin tends to rise and there is anisocytosis. Severely malnourished children, with their damaged skin and mucosae, prolonged intestinal transit time and reduced secretions, are very susceptible to infection. They also have impaired resistance to

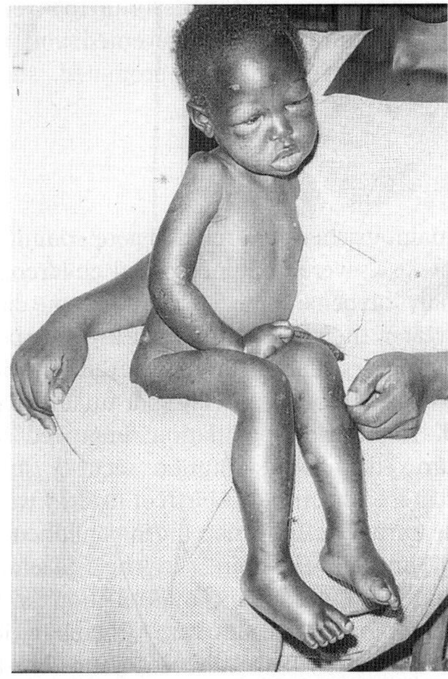

Fig. 14.8 Child with kwashiorkor. (With permission of R.G. Whitehead)

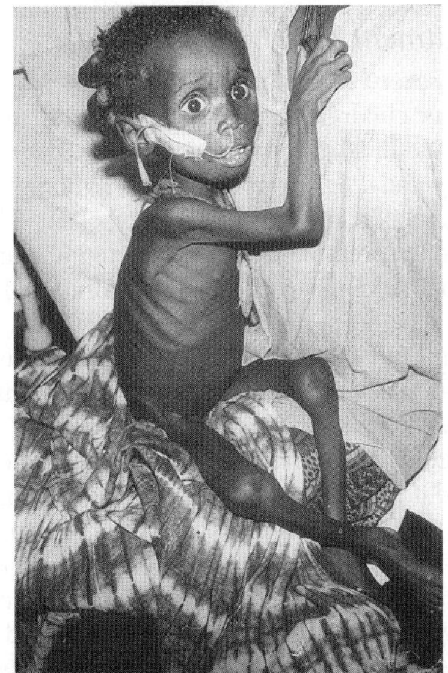

Fig. 14.9 Child with nutritional marasmus. (With permission of R.G. Whitehead)

infection, in particular, depressed cell mediated immune responses. Fever and the cardinal signs of local inflammation tend to be slight or absent. White cell counts and C-reactive protein (CRP) rise little. In very ill children, neutropenia may occur, with hypothermia and hypoglycemia when feeding has been withheld for only a few hours. Serum electrolytes do not reflect body content, only circulating concentrations. Thus, high serum potassium masks intracellular potassium deficiency, and in hospital it is most likely due to intravenous delivery and impaired cellular uptake. A low serum sodium masks sodium overload and the only useful interpretation is that the child is very ill. Magnesium deficiency occurs. Serum urea tends to be low, reflecting low protein intake and reduced catabolism. Serum albumin is almost invariably low in edematous children. This finding led the way to the protein deficiency theory of development of nutritional edema in some children. However, edema is not due to low serum albumin alone, protein deficient diets are not limited to those children who develop edema and dietary protein repletion does not cure it.[55] At present, the most likely pathogenesis of edematous malnutrition involves extensive membrane dysfunction due to lipid peroxidation, a product of antioxidant deficiency in the face of acute pro-oxidant stress.[56] Associated with this, red blood cell glutathione and plasma zinc, copper, selenium and glutathione peroxidase, vitamin E and carotene are all particularly low in edematous children while free iron, a major pro-oxidant, circulates because transferrin concentrations are very low.

MANAGEMENT

Successful management of malnutrition should mean complete catch-up followed by sustained normal growth, health and development. This is rarely achieved. Effective home management should be widely implemented for children with less than severe malnutrition (weights-for-height between −2 and −3 SD of WHO reference values) and stunting in order to prevent growth faltering. This is also rarely achieved. It requires education and practical help to ensure exclusive breast-feeding to 6 months; continued breast-feeding to 2 years; good hygiene; more energy-dense diets, containing all essential nutrients, taking into account their bioavailability; regular monitoring of body weight; and early, appropriate treatment of complications like infections.

Phases of treatment

Management of severe malnutrition, that is, of severely wasted and/or edematous children, is described in detail in the WHO manual.[54] It is best divided into three phases. Following clinical evaluation, the *Initial Phase* involves resuscitation, treatment of infection and correction of disordered metabolism. This requires prevention, and often treatment, of electrolyte imbalance, specific deficiencies, hypoglycemia, hypothermia, dehydration, heart failure and shock. This can be performed most safely in a well-staffed specialized hospital unit. Bacterial infection must be assumed and treated with broad spectrum antibiotics unless and until a specific infection is diagnosed which requires specific therapy.

Intravenous fluids pose a major risk of iatrogenic stress and should be avoided if possible. Oral rehydration is recommended for dehydration (Ch. 35). However, compared with the standard WHO oral rehydration solution (ORS), the solution should contain less sodium but more potassium and magnesium, zinc and copper, all of which are grossly deficient in the malnourished child with acute diarrhea. Such a solution is available commercially (ReSoMal) but can also be prepared from WHO ORS. Frequent breast-feeding is encouraged. Instead of or in addition to this, a special cows' milk based formula with relatively low protein, fat and sodium contents and osmolarity is recommended, to provide minimal stress. A commercial product, 'F-75', is available for major emergencies but recipes, from ingredients likely to be available, are also provided in the WHO manual. In this initial phase, every effort is made to ensure that children receive sufficient intake for maintenance of body weight (0.42 MJ (100kcal)/kg/day) but not growth. This sometimes requires very frequent, small tube-feeds because anorexia and vomiting are major problems especially in edematous children. It is very important to feed regularly throughout the night as this is when hypothermia and hypoglycemia tend to occur. F-75 contains extra minerals and vitamins but further supplements of vitamin A and folic acid are also recommended. Iron is contraindicated because of its potential toxicity and aggravation of infection.

Usually within a week, the second or *Rehabilitation Phase* is heralded by increased appetite and improvement of major abnormalities including loss of edema. The principles of management change to include feeding to appetite, stimulating emotional and physical development and preparing for home. The child can be moved to a rehabilitation unit in the community. At this stage, the formula feed is changed to one that provides more energy and protein for growth. Commercially available 'F-100' contains 0.42 MJ/100 ml, 12% energy from protein and 53% from fat. Like F-75, it also provides extra minerals and vitamins but not iron. However, supplementary iron is necessary during this phase for new hemoglobin synthesis. Like F-75, F-100 can also be prepared from usually available ingredients but both 'home-prepared' feeds benefit from the addition of extra minerals and vitamins. These are best provided as a commercial preparation. During this rehabilitation phase, provided there are no setbacks, the child's dietary intake increases steadily, the frequency of feeding is reduced and weight gain is rapid, up to 20 times normal, on average 10 g/kg/day. The child's mother or closest carer must be taught how to make home as conducive as possible to normal growth and development of her child. This includes teaching of nutrition and food preparation, hygiene and the value of play for mental and physical development.

When the child has reached −1 SD weight-for-length or height, equivalent to 90% of WHO reference, he or she is ready for home and the final *Follow-Up Phase* commences. Ideally, the child is recalled or visited at increasing intervals for up to 3 years to ensure that recurrence of malnutrition is prevented and that healthy physical and mental development is promoted, supported and achieved.

PREVENTION

A few severely malnourished children in a poor community imply a large number of less severely malnourished children. If they are ignored, as usually happens, some deteriorate, some die and all are blighted for the rest of their lives by not realizing their potential. The ideal solution to primary malnutrition is prevention. However, this requires what we are presently unwilling or unable to provide to a large section of the world's population, improved standards of living: health care, education, sanitation, security, sufficient good quality food and more, to permit the birth of healthy well-nourished infants, tolerable burdens of infection during childhood and hence, normal growth and development. In the 'developed' world, however, prevention of secondary malnutrition is achieved to varying extents within good health care systems in, for example, children with inflammatory bowel disease, cystic fibrosis and those with various inborn errors of metabolism (Chs 17, 18 and 24).

MICRONUTRIENT DEFICIENCY AND EXCESS

Micronutrients are generally recognized as the vitamins and essential trace elements. Vitamins are preformed organic compounds required in the diet within a given physiological range to ensure optimal health (Table 14.4). The same requirement applies to the 10–17 essential trace elements.[57] They comprise about 0.03% of body weight. The most abundant and best known is iron while one of the least abundant but also well known, is iodine. Cobalt, a less obvious essential trace element, is required at only one hundred-thousandth the intake of iron and, in humans but not ruminants, has to be supplied within vitamin B_{12}.

Nutrients essential for optimal health can be divided into two types related to their roles: type I and type II nutrients.[57] Type I nutrients include all of the vitamins and essential trace elements except zinc. Each has a limited number of specific functions and most have body stores. After they are depleted, specific signs of deficiency appear, which makes specific diagnosis relatively easy. Type II nutrients include major body elements such as potassium, sodium, sulfur and nitrogen and the essential amino acids. Zinc, a micronutrient, is also a classic type II nutrient. These are required for maintenance and growth of all cells and they tend not to have effective stores. Deficiency limits, first and foremost, cell hyperplasia and hypertrophy. In childhood, the consequence is growth failure. This, in turn, reduces the requirement of all nutrients. Thus, deficiencies of type II nutrients are difficult to diagnose and often overlooked. However, they are no less important than type I nutrient deficiencies and should be considered as possible contributors to growth failure, particularly when the diet is monotonous or specialized.

Interactions among nutrients and the other components within diets influence the final balance of nutrients absorbed. This is particularly important when therapeutic diets, enteral feeds and food supplements are prescribed, or when the diet is monotonous. For example, a diet with a high phytate content (the storage form of phosphate in plants) reduces the availability of nutrients such as zinc, iron and copper; a diet high in ascorbic acid content increases iron but decreases copper absorption; and many trace elements interfere with one another's absorption. Thus, the intake of a particular micronutrient does not necessarily reflect its bioavailability. Important characteristics of a few of the essential micronutrients are summarized below and fuller information can be found elsewhere.[57,58]

IRON

For body iron, 70% is contained within heme where it is intimately involved in O_2 carriage. Iron is a highly reactive element as ferrous ion releases an electron to become ferric ion. The freed electron takes part in many normal metabolic events such as electron transfer in the mitochondrial respiratory chain and free radical production which, on the one hand, is used to kill pathogens but on the other, may result in peroxidation of membrane lipids, a highly dangerous complication. This hazard is reduced by an elaborate system of iron binding proteins, the main ones being heme which holds ferrous iron, ferritin which binds stored ferric iron, and transferrin which carries ferric iron between cells.[59]

Iron deficiency causes a microcytic, hypochromic anemia after iron stores are depleted. This is a particular hazard of preterm birth because iron stores accumulate first in the fetal liver in late gestation. Iron deficiency anemia in infants also occurs when they are fed largely cows' milk because it is a poor source of iron[60] and it can cause gastrointestinal blood loss. Appropriate advice is to introduce heme-containing foods like meat and liver, replace cow's milk with breast milk or formula and, if necessary, provide iron supplements. Iron deficiency is also relatively common in teenage boys and girls. Vegetarians are at higher risk than omnivores because non-heme iron is less bioavailable than heme iron and their phytate intake tends to be high. Iron deficiency is also associated with reduced exercise tolerance, with impaired resistance to infection and poor mental development. It is likely that anemia is a late manifestation and that the other more subtle features occur earlier, at least in infants.

Iron excess is at least as damaging as iron deficiency. Acute iron poisoning is less common than it used to be, hemochromatosis and multiple blood transfusions are also relatively rare but malnutrition, particularly edematous malnutrition, is commonly complicated and aggravated by iron excess.[59] In edematous malnutrition, although anemia is usual, plasma ferritin and hepatic iron content are high while plasma transferrin, but not plasma iron, is low. This leads to an increased risk of free iron circulating which, together with antioxidant deficiencies, may lead to membrane lipid peroxidation and therefore to some of the features of edematous malnutrition. Iron supplementation can also increase the risk of infection. Although infections in malnutrition are hard to diagnose because of the paucity of clinical signs of the host response, they tend to be more severe. This is partly due to free circulating iron, which is available to the invading microbial pathogens. Thus, although the treatment of anemia with iron is usually effective, it is not always so and may be deleterious in children with malnutrition.

Iron status can be measured in different ways, some more specific than others. For example, anemia is a non-specific measure, which may be due to many nutrient deficiencies in addition to iron or other non-nutritional causes. In contrast, low plasma ferritin and low transferrin receptor concentrations are quite specific, each for a different aspect of iron status: the former implies low iron stores, the latter, low uptake of iron for heme synthesis.

COPPER

Though the dietary requirement for copper is only about one-tenth that of iron or zinc, it is also crucial to normal metabolism. Copper shares several features with iron. It is reactive, cuprous copper releasing an electron to become cupric copper and vice versa. It circulates bound largely to caeruloplasmin, otherwise known as ferroxidase I which catalyzes the oxidation of ferrous to ferric iron. Thus, copper deficiency interferes with iron metabolism. Located at the active site of several other oxidases, copper is also involved in the crosslinking of connective tissue proteins such as collagen and elastin and responsible for end oxidation in the respiratory chain. Thus, the main features of copper deficiency are hypochromic, microcytic anemia indistinguishable from that of iron deficiency, neutropenia, tortuous dilatations of blood vessels, herniae, osteoporosis clinically not unlike infantile rickets, skin and hair hypopigmentation and neurological problems.

Like iron, copper stores accumulate in the fetal liver in late gestation. Similarly, cows' milk is a poor source of copper. Thus, copper deficiency commonly occurs in preterm infants and infants fed largely cows' milk. It tends to accompany malnutrition, particularly edematous malnutrition and its role in the enzyme, superoxide dismutase, may be important in this respect.

Copper toxicity is usually insidious, most commonly from chronic ingestion associated with copper piping or utensils carrying relatively acidic fluids. The excess copper ends up in the liver and cirrhosis ensues. Two inherited inborn errors of metabolism involve copper transporting ATPases, Wilson's disease and Menkes syndrome. Wilson's disease, an autosomal recessive defect, usually presents in adolescence with cirrhosis associated with excessive hepatic copper. High concentrations of copper in the brain, eye and kidneys also occur but low biliary excretion of copper and low plasma caeruloplasmin (Ch. 24). Treatment with copper chelators or zinc, which inhibits copper absorption, is partially effective in controlling copper accumulation. Menkes, or steely hair syndrome, is also autosomal recessive in origin but more like copper deficiency in presentation in that progressive anemia, hypopigmentation, hypothermia, osteoporosis, cardiovascular abnormalities and mental deterioration occur from infancy and plasma copper is low. However, the syndrome is unresponsive to copper (Ch. 24).

Copper status is usually assessed as plasma copper in clinical practice. However, this is limited in its ability to define status because it follows closely plasma caeruloplasmin, which is an acute phase protein whose concentration depends primarily on whether an acute phase response is operating. Erythrocyte superoxide dismutase level reflects copper status more accurately.

IODINE

Iodine plays its major role in the hormone, thyroxine, whose function and disorders are covered in Chapter 13. Iodine deficiency disorders are of worldwide importance accounting for stunting and suboptimal mental development in many millions of children and, subsequently, adults in developing regions with low iodine water supplies. Selenium deficiency, which is also widespread, may influence the response to iodine deficiency, particularly in regions within China.[57] Iodine excess also impairs thyroid function in communities with a high intake of food of marine origin.

ZINC

The dietary requirement for zinc is similar to iron and its body content is about half as much. However, unlike iron or copper, zinc is relatively unreactive. About 60% of plasma zinc is bound loosely to albumin, about 25% is bound to alpha-2 macroglobulin and the rest to amino acids and other small molecules. Zinc is a classic type II nutrient without an effective store. Its presence in association with over 200 ubiquitous enzymes, including those necessary for DNA, RNA and protein syntheses, means that it is necessary for normal cell metabolism, hyperplasia and hypertrophy. Intracellular zinc concentration remains more or less normal in simple zinc deficiency: when low, it signifies the presence of other disease. Zinc deficiency decreases cell turnover and growth until the demand for zinc meets the supply. Clinically this means that zinc deficiency in childhood is associated, primarily, with growth failure. This is followed by skin lesions in areas subject to trauma, poor wound healing, impaired cell mediated immunity and diarrhea associated with intestinal mucosal atrophy.

Conditions in which zinc deficiency is common include poverty and thus, inadequate, monotonous, relatively low protein, low zinc diets; increased zinc loss from burns or protein losing enteropathies; increased zinc demand for healing or for rapid growth. The autosomal recessive inherited disease, acrodermatitis enteropathica, is associated with, apparently, reduced zinc absorption only. Its clinical features are those of simple zinc deficiency as described above. It can be treated successfully with zinc supplements thereby overcoming the intestinal block (see Chapters 17 and 28).

Zinc status is particularly difficult to define or measure because intracellular concentrations are controlled within narrow limits and there is no store to sample. In zinc deficiency, hair and plasma zinc tend to decline. However, hair zinc is hard to measure reproducibly and it may even rise in severe zinc deficiency as hair growth ceases. Low plasma zinc often implies an ongoing acute phase response rather than zinc deficiency. Thus, its interpretation requires an independent measure of the acute phase response; and knowledge of zinc intake and demand are also useful. In practice, a trial of zinc supplementation is usually the most helpful provided that its endpoint is defined at the outset. Thus, if zinc deficiency is present, the child should respond within a month by, for example, gaining weight more rapidly than before supplementation.

Zinc toxicity is very unusual in childhood because homeostatic mechanisms prevent excess intestinal absorption. A new syndrome featuring hyperzincemia with clinical features of gross inflammation has been described. There is no evidence however that zinc excess causes the clinical features.[61]

VITAMIN A

The vitamin A family is headed by all-*trans* retinol and includes all naturally occurring compounds with the biological activity of retinol, as well as the provitamin A carotenoids, such as beta-carotene. Preformed vitamin A is found in liver, dairy products and oily fish and over 80% may be absorbed (Table 14.4). The carotenoids are present in many plant foods and absorption varies from 5 to 50%. They act as anti-oxidants themselves and are also converted to vitamin A by oxidative cleavage. The vitamin A family members are fat soluble and bound in plasma to specific retinoid-binding proteins (RBP) which protect them from oxidation. They are also stored mainly in the liver.

In childhood, vitamin A is best known for its roles in vision, in immunity and in cell differentiation. Vitamin A deficiency is a major public health problem, affecting at least 200 million of the world's children, particularly malnourished children.[62] Only a small proportion has overt clinical signs. These start with night blindness and Bitot's spots on the conjunctivae which result from squamous metaplasia, then xerophthalmia, keratomalacia and eventually blindness. At the same time children suffer increased severity of infections and mortality is high. Prevention is possible using a 'massive dose' approach, which depends on the ability of vitamin A to be stored and used slowly. A large oral dose is also used for xerophthalmia.

Vitamin A toxicity can occur, which can be acute or chronic. Both are usually iatrogenic, resulting from gross overdoses of vitamin preparations. Typically, the former resolves completely but the latter, which is more common, occasionally causes permanent damage to liver, muscle, vision and bones.

Vitamin A status is assessed by different methods in different situations, often by serum retinol in hospital; and by presence or absence of Bitot's spots or conjunctival impression cytology in populations. Serum retinol is depressed in the acute phase response and affected by protein and zinc intake: therefore, relative dose response tests are becoming more popular wherein serum retinol is measured before and after a supplement of vitamin A.

VITAMIN D

This comprises vitamins D_2 and D_3, which are both fat soluble. D_3 is hydroxylated in the liver to 25-hydroxyvitamin D, which is further hydroxylated in the kidney to 1,25-dihydroxyvitamin D, which acts as a hormone and the most biologically active form of the vitamin. This stimulates calcium absorption in the small intestine and calcium resorption from bone. It also promotes cell maturation within the intestine and it increases bone formation and growth plate mineralization by providing sufficient circulating calcium. It increases resistance to infections through effects on several cell types involved in immune responses. The vitamin is stored within fat depots.

Egg yolk, fortified margarines and spreads and especially cod liver oil are rich in vitamin D (Table 14.4): breast milk is a poor source. By far the major source is photoconversion of 7-dehydrocholesterol, through exposure of the skin to ultraviolet B light. This means that breast-fed infants in the UK who are mostly indoors or covered up are at risk of deficiency. Daily supplementation is recommended. Very preterm infants are also prone to deficiency signs but other factors contribute as well as vitamin D deficiency. Fat malabsorption, for any reason, is associated with vitamin D deficiency.

Vitamin D deficiency in early life results in rickets, which is characterized by failure of linear growth, poor bone mineralization and muscle weakness. In infancy, frontal bossing, craniotabes and rachitic rosary are typical: later, short stature, bowed legs and swollen wrists are more distinctive. Bone pain, anemia and respiratory infections are common. Plasma alkaline phosphatase is high but this is not specific for vitamin D deficiency: plasma 25-hydroxyvitamin D is also low. Radiological changes include poor mineralization, delayed epiphyseal development and marked metaphyseal changes including cupping, fraying and splaying (Fig. 14.10).

Vitamin D toxicity usually results from injudicious supplementation and is associated first with failure to thrive and gastrointestinal features including constipation, and later, urinary tract features with nephrocalcinosis and eventually renal failure. Hypercalcemia and increased bone mineralization occur. Therapy includes glucocorticoids and a low calcium diet.

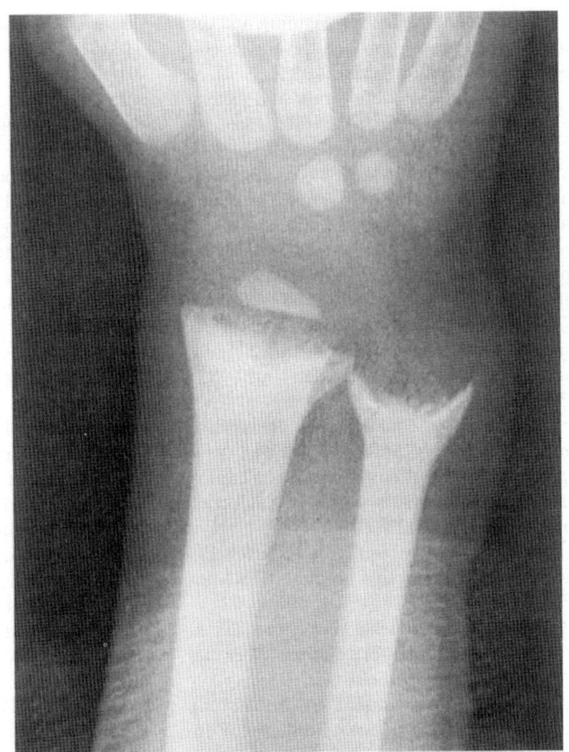

Fig. 14.10 Rickets: X-ray of wrist showing frayed radial and ulnar metaphyses with slight expansion.

FOLATE

Folate comprises the double aromatic ring of a pteridine linked to para-aminobenzoate and glutamate. It is water soluble and functions as a coenzyme receiving and donating single carbon fragments. It provides methylene groups for pyrimidine synthesis and formyl groups for purine synthesis for DNA and RNA biosynthetic cycles. It also participates in methylation of a variety of substrates, for example, DNA, myelin and phospholipids.[10] Over half of natural folates are in the 5-tetrahydrofolate form attached to a polyglutamyl chain. The best dietary source is liver (Table 14.4). Synthetic folic acid is twice as bioavailable as natural folates.

Marginal folate deficiency is very common but the extent to which this contributes to suboptimal health is not yet clear. However high folate status during the first few weeks after conception reduces the risk of neural tube defects in the offspring: women liable to become pregnant are advised to take folate supplements (Ch. 9). Folate deficiency accompanies malnutrition and also occurs as a complication of increased requirements for growth or erythropoiesis, malabsorption syndromes, impaired utilization due to vitamin B_{12} deficiency and as a result of treatment with methotrexate, trimethoprim and some anticonvulsants. Overt folate deficiency is characterized by megaloblastic anemia with thrombocytopenia, leukopenia and increased segmentation of nuclei in polymorphs.

The risk of folate toxicity has become an important issue since recognition of the need for relatively high doses of folic acid to prevent neural tube defects. High doses may mask vitamin B_{12} deficiency allowing the neuropathy induced by the latter to progress. They *may* also interfere with anticonvulsive therapy and with antifolate therapy for malignancies.

Folate status is best estimated as erythrocyte folate concentration but, due to the long life of erythrocytes, this does not change quickly in response to deficiency or excess. In contrast, serum folate falls quickly when folate absorption falls but this is not necessarily associated with folate deficiency.

REFERENCES (* Level 1 evidence)

1 Doherty CP, Reilly JJ, Paterson WF, et al. Growth failure and malnutrition. In: Walker WA, et al, eds. Pediatric gastrointestinal disease, 3rd edn Hamilton, Ontario: Decker; 2000:12–27.

2 Department of Health. Dietary reference values for food energy and nutrients for the UK. Report on health and social subjects No. 41. London; HMSO:1991.

2a Schofield C. Predicting basal metabolic rate, new standards and review of previous work. Hum Nutr Clin nutr Clin Nutr 1985; 39C(Suppl 1):5–42.

3 Prentice AM, Lucas A, Vasquez-Velasquez L, et al. Are current dietary guidelines in young children a prescription for overfeeding? Lancet 1988; ii:1066–1069.

4 Department of Health. The diets of British school children. Reports on health and social subjects No. 36. London: HMSO; 1989.

5 TSO. National diet and nutrition survey: young people aged 4–18 years. London: HMSO; 2000.

6 Gregory J, Foster K, Tyler H, Wiseman M, eds. National diet and nutrition survey London: HMSO, 1990.

7 National Diet and Nutrition Survey. Children aged 1½ to 4½ years. Vol 1. Report of the diet and nutrition survey. London: HMSO; 1995.

8 National Diet and Nutrition Survey. Children aged 1½ to 4½ years. Vol 2. Report of the dental survey. London: HMSO; 1995.

9 Gregory J, Lowe S, eds. National diet and nutrition survey 2000. London: The Stationery Office, 2000.

10 Garrow JS, James WPT, Ralph A, eds. Human nutrition and dietetics, 10th edn. Edinburgh: Churchill Livingstone; 2000.

11 Department of Health. Weaning and the weaning diet. Report on health and social subjects No. 45. London: HMSO;1994.
12 Cockburn F. Neonatal brain and dietary lipids. Arch Dis Child 1994; 70:F1–F2.
13 Koletzko B, Agostoni C, Carlson SE, et al. Long chain polyunsaturated fatty acids and perinatal development. Acta Paediatr 2001; 90:460–464.
14 Bolton-Smith C, Woodward M. Dietary composition and fat to sugar ratios in relation to obesity. Int J Obes 1994; 18:820–828.
15 Englyst HN, Kingman SM, Cummings JH. Classification and measurement of nutritionally important starch fractions. Eur J Clin Nutr 1992; 46:S33–S50.
16 American Academy of Pediatrics. Conference on dietary fiber in childhood, New York, May 24, 1994. A summary of conference recommendations on dietary fiber in childhood. Pediatrics 1995; 96:1023–1028.
17 Hendrikse WW, Reilly JJ, Weaver LT. Malnutrition in a children's hospital. Clin Nutr 1997; 16:13–18.
17 Williams CL, Bollella M, Wynder EL. A new recommendation for dietary fiber in childhood. Pediatrics 1995; 96:985–988.
18 Goulet O. Assessment of nutritional status in clinical practice. Baillieres Clin Gastroenterol 1998; 12:647–669.
19 Gibson RS. Principles of nutritional assessment. Oxford: Oxford University Press. 1990.
20 Cole TJ, Freeman JV, Preece MA. Body mass index reference curves for the UK 1990. Arch Dis Child 1995; 73:25–29.
21 CDC 2001 www.cdc.gov/nchs/about/major/nhanes.growthcharts/datafiles.htm.
22 Krick J. Using the Z score as a descriptor of discrete changes in growth. Nutr Supp Serv 1986; 6:14–21.
23 Cross JH, Holden C, Macdonald A, et al. Clinical examination compared with anthropometry in evaluating nutritional status. Arch Dis Child 1995; 72:60–61.
24 Michaelsen KF, Weaver LT, Branca F, et al. Feeding and nutrition of infants and young children. Copenhagen: WHO; 2000.
25 Dewey KG. Nutrition, growth and complementary feeding of the breastfed infant. Pediatr Clin N Am 2001; 48:87–104.
25a MAFF, Healthy diets for infants and young children; a guide for professionals, London: The Stationery Office, 1997.
26 HEBS. Eating for health. Edinburgh: The Stationery Office; 1999.
27 MAFF. The national food survey. London: The Stationery Office; 1997.
28 Lawson M, Thomas M. Vitamin D concentrations in Asian children aged 2 years living in England: population survey. BMJ 1999; 318:28.
29 Aggett PJ, Haschke F, Heine W, et al. ESPGAN Committee on Nutrition. Childhood diet and prevention of coronary heart disease. J Pediatr Gastroenterol Nutr 1994; 19:261–269.
30 World Health Organization. Diet, nutrition and chronic disease. Technical Support Series No. 79. WHO; 1990.
30a Goulet O. Nutritional support in malnourished pediatric patients. Baillieres Clin Gastroeneterol 1988; 12:843–876.
31 Lennard-Jones JE, ed. A positive approach to nutrition as treatment. London: King's Fund Centre; 1992.
32 Silk DBA, Cottam TK, Nielsen MS. Organisation of nutritional support in hospitals. Kent: British Association for Parenteral and Enteral Nutrition 1994.
33 Bresson JL. Protein and energy requirements in healthy and ill paediatric patients. Baillieres Clin Gastroenterol 1998; 12:631–645.
34 Elia M, Cottee S, Holden C. Enteral and parenteral nutrition in the community. Kent: British Association for Parenteral and Enteral Nutrition; 1994.
35 McCarey D, Buchanan E, Gregory M, et al. Home enteral feeding of children in the West of Scotland. Scot Med J 1996; 41:147–149.
36 Souba WW. Nutritional support. N Engl J Med 1997; 336:41–48.
37 Booth IW, Lander AD. Short bowel syndrome. Baillieres Clin Gastroenterol 1998; 12:739–773.
38 Beath SV, Protheroe SP, Brook GA, et al. Early experience of paediatric intestinal transplantation in the United Kingdom 1993 to 1999. Transplant Proc 2000; 32:1225.
39 Colomb V, Goulet O, Ricour C. Home enteral and parenteral nutrition in children. Baillieres Clin Gastroenterol 1998; 12:877–894.
40 Reilly JJ, Dorosty AR. Epidemic of obesity in UK children. Lancet 1999; 354:1874–1875.
41 Martorell R, Khan L, Hughes ML, et al. Overweight and obesity in preschool children from developing countries. Int J Obes 2000; 24:959–967.
42 Barlow SE, Dietz WH. Obesity evaluation and treatment: expert committee recommendations. Pediatrics 1998; 102:E29.
43 Dietz WH. Health consequences of obesity in youth: childhood predictors of adult disease. Pediatrics 1998; 101:518–525.
44 Morrison JA, Sprecher DL, Barton BA, et al. Overweight, fat patterning, and cardiovascular disease risk factors in black and white girls. J Pediatr 1999; 135:458–464.
45 Must A, Jacques PF, Dallal GE, et al. Long term morbidity and mortality of overweight adolescents. N Engl J Med 1992; 327:1350–1355.
46 Whitaker RC, Wright JA, Pepe MS, et al. Predicting obesity in young adulthood from childhood and parental obesity. N Engl J Med 1997; 337:869–873.
47 Vanhala M, Vanhala P, Kumpusalo E, et al. Relative weight gain and obesity as a child predict metabolic syndrome as an adult. Int J Obes 1999; 23; 656–659.
48 Maffeis C, Schutz Y, Zaffanello M, et al. Elevated energy expenditure and reduced energy intake in obese children: paradox or poor dietary reliability in obesity. J Pediatr 1994; 124:348–354.
49 Epstein LH, Myers MD, Raynor HA, et al. Treatment of pediatric obesity. Pediatrics 1998; 101:554–570.
*50 Mellin LM, Slinkard CE, Irwin CE. Adolescent obesity intervention: validation of the SHAPEDOWN program. J Am Diet Assoc 1987; 87:333–338.
*51 Epstein LH, Valoski AM, Vara LS. Effects of decreasing sedentary behaviour and increasing activity on weight change in obese children. Health Psychol 1995; 14:109–115.
*52 Epstein LH, Palluch RA, Gordy CC, et al. Decreasing sedentary behaviour in treating pediatric obesity. Arch Pediatr Adolesc Med 2000; 154:220–226.
53 de Onis M, Monteiro C, Akré J et al . The worldwide magnitude of protein-energy malnutrition: an overview from the WHO Global Database on Child Growth. Bull World Health Organ 1995; 71:703–712.
54 World Health Organization. Management of severe malnutrition: a manual for physicians and other senior health workers. Geneva: WHO; 1999.
55 Golden MH. Protein deficiency, energy deficiency and the oedema of malnutrition. Lancet 1982; i:1261–1265.
56 Golden MH. Oedematous malnutrition. Br Med Bull 1998; 54:433–444.
57 Hallberg L, Sandstrom B, Ralph A, et al. Iron, zinc and other trace elements. In: Garrow JS, James WPT, Ralph A, eds. Human nutrition and dietetics, 10th edn. London: Harcourt; 2000:177–205.
58 Golden MHN. The nature of nutritional deficiency in relation to growth failure and poverty. Acta Paediatr Scand (suppl) 1991; 374:95–110.
59 Ramdath DD, Golden MHN. Non-haematological aspects of iron nutrition. Nutr Res Rev 1989; 2:29–49.
60 Lawson M. Infancy and childhood. In: Task Force Report of the British Nutrition Foundation, eds. Iron: nutrition and physiological significance. London: Chapman & Hall; 1995:93–105.
61 Sampson B, Richmond P, Golden BE, et al. Identification of the zinc binding protein in a child with hyperzincaemia as calprotectin (MRP8/ MRP14). In: Roussel AM, Anderson RA, Favrier AE, eds. Trace element metabolism in man and animals – 10. London: Plenum; 2000:1031–1034.
62 World Health Organization. Indicators for assessing vitamin A deficiency and their application in monitoring and evaluating intervention programmes. Micronutrient Series. Geneva: WHO; 1996.

15

Fluid, electrolyte and acid–base disturbances

Gale A Pearson

INTRODUCTION

Disturbances of the 'internal milieu' are common in pediatric illness. This chapter will focus mainly upon the background (i.e. the reasons why they are so common) and the associated clinical issues that arise as a consequence. Two appendices are also provided as references for the less clinical material. The 'Physical and physiological influences on the internal distribution of water and electrolytes' and 'Acid–base chemistry and blood gas measurement' are nonetheless essential knowledge for the clinician. Otherwise the layout of the chapter is intended to provide the reader with the information required to deal with clinical situations of increasing complexity as the chapter proceeds. Wherever possible, generic descriptions have been favored over specific diseases since the intended focus is not upon the differential diagnosis of deranged laboratory results. This is because in the first instance and to a large extent, abnormalities of fluid balance, electrolytes and acid–base can be characterized, assessed and treated on their own merits. Clinical situations often arise where this approach is necessary whilst the diagnosis is still being determined. Nevertheless the best clinical solution will always involve treatment of the cause both in terms of the diagnosis and pathophysiology.

Careful assessment is an essential prerequisite to proper handling of fluid, electrolytes and acid–base in children. In this respect clinical judgment and laboratory assessment are complementary to each other. Therapeutic decisions should not be made on laboratory findings alone but in the hospital situation, patients cannot be managed to modern clinical standards without appropriate measurement and monitoring.

The first priority when a patient presents, is a rapid assessment of the need for resuscitation following an 'ABC' approach (see Ch. 35). Then a comprehensive history of the disorder should be taken and skilled clinical examination performed to determine the speed and extent of investigation and the intensity of treatment. The patient should be weighed at this point. Biochemical investigation also forms part of the assessment and should be performed whenever fluid therapy is contemplated, particularly if by the intravenous (i.v.) route. Baseline investigations should include the determination of serum urea, creatinine, electrolytes, osmolality and some indication of acid–base status such as serum bicarbonate along with the hematological profile. Patients with abnormalities of acid–base detected by this screening and those with significant respiratory problems should be further investigated with arterial blood gases. Urine electrolyte content, urea, pH and osmolality should be measured if there is a clinical suspicion of an abnormality of fluid balance or renal function. During the subsequent care of acutely unwell babies and children, the volume of urine production should be monitored, with repitition of laboratory urinary analysis where relevant. Whilst it is helpful if accurate urine collections can be obtained to calculate electrolyte excretion, measurements performed on casual urine specimens can be interpreted by relating sodium and potassium concentrations to the urinary creatinine content (see 'Fractional sodium excretion' below). Further assessment both clinically and biochemically should be made as soon as the response to treatment can be assessed.

The body content and internal distribution of fluid and electrolytes are subject to tight physiological controls and are conveniently interpreted using 'compartment' models. The most important distinction for fluid, electrolyte and acid–base is between the intra- and extracellular environment, which is preserved by the cell membrane. Likewise the composition of the various extracellular fluids depends heavily on the integrity and function of epithelia and the vascular endothelium. The extracellular fluid (ECF) consists of intravascular fluid (plasma) and extravascular fluid. The latter includes 'tissue' or 'interstitial' fluid as well as specialized collections of transcellular fluids formed by secretory activity which include gastrointestinal (GI) secretions, synovial fluid, ocular and cerebrospinal fluids. Body compartments can also be conceptualized if not defined anatomically, by the behavior/ distribution of solutes within them. This latter approach is more commonly applied in pharmacology than physiology but it usefully defines some aspects of the behavior of the body as a compartmentalized vessel. In a 'one-compartment' model the drug, once administered, is assumed to instantly distribute homogeneously throughout the volume of distribution. In a two-compartment model the drug distributes rapidly through a small volume, central compartment that usually corresponds to blood and the extracellular fluid of highly vascular organs and more slowly through a larger compartment, which usually includes adipose tissue and intracellular fluid (ICF).

Both total ECF volume and the distribution of fluid between extracellular compartments can vary widely in disease. Furthermore, one of the main consequences of ECF changes is corresponding or consequential change within the ICF. These changes are dictated by the interplay of hydrostatic, oncotic and osmotic forces, endothelial and cell membrane permeability and the integrity of active homeostatic systems such as membranous Na^+/K^+ ATPase.

DIFFERENCES AMONG BABIES, CHILDREN AND ADULTS

The physiological differences between premature and term neonates and among babies, older children and adults are extreme. From a constitutional perspective, neonates have proportionally the greatest water content and obese adults the least. The 'total body water' accounts for 80% of mass at birth and this percentage falls to 60% by 1 year of age. The change is the result of a disproportionate increase in cell mass (due to growth) compared to the volume of ECF. The percentage of water in postpubertal females is lower than males due largely to their higher percentage of body fat. In both sexes, throughout adulthood, the body water content falls with advancing age.

Children need higher water and electrolyte intakes than adults making them more susceptible to dehydration. Their increased water losses are due to the:

- caloric expenses of a high metabolic rate;
- high insensible loss (high minute ventilation, high surface area:volume ratio, immature epidermis in premature babies);
- decreased ability to concentrate urine.

The distribution of water between the 'compartments' also differs between infants and adults (Table 15.1). During the first few days of life there is a transfer of water from ICF to ECF. This mechanism, which may protect the infant against the effects of dehydration, increases the already large ECF volume and could be a factor in the occurrence of edema sometimes observed at this time. The ICF accounts for an increasing percentage of total body water up to 1 year of age but this is mostly a reflection of the reduction in ECF volume. The ratio of ICF:ECF volume increases from unity, nearing the adult value of 2:1 some time after the age of 1 year.

The sodium content per kilogram body weight is 35–50% higher in the infant than in the adult due to the greater amount of extracellular fluid. With the relative reduction of ECF with growth, adult values are reached at about 2 years of age. Neonatal calcium and phosphate levels are higher than maternal levels, the former as a result of placental function and the latter as a consequence of the resulting fetal parathyroid hormone levels. Intracellular calcium stores are lower however making muscle function (particularly myocardium) more dependent upon the serum ionized calcium.[1] The average plasma concentration of chloride is also higher in babies, like the phosphate levels. Anion/cation balance must exist for there to be electroneutrality and both are balanced by a lower bicarbonate level. Age and gender-related reference ranges should be available from the laboratory for each electrolyte being measured.

As already stated, babies have a higher obligatory urinary water loss than older children and adults, a consequence of a higher urinary solute load and a decreased concentrating ability (to about 600 mosm/L).[2] These features are a consequence of tubular immaturity, one aspect of which is that fewer nephrons have loops which extend into the renal medulla. The result is a much higher flux of water and electrolytes. A term infant exchanges about one-half of his ECF in the day whilst an adult exchanges only one-seventh. Renal immaturity is accentuated in the premature infant.[2] It manifests in a number of ways including a tubular leak of bicarbonate creating a tendency towards metabolic acidosis and an almost unique ability to develop genuine sodium depletion through urinary losses even in the absence of diuretics.

Babies also have a reduced ability to deal with a water load,[2] a consequence of a low glomerular filtration rate (GFR). The GFR subsequently increases over the first 6 months of life.

Table 15.1 Partition of body fluids (average figures)

	Adult (70 kg; 1.85 m^2)			Infant (3 kg; 0.2 m^2)		
	% Body weight	Liters	Liters/m^2	% Body weight	Liters	Liters/m^2
Intracellular	40	28	15.2	38	1.14	5.70
Extracellular						
Interstitial*	16	11.2	6.0	33	0.99	4.95
Plasma	4	2.8	1.5	5	0.15	0.75
Total	60	42	22.7	76	2.28	11.4

* Includes transcellular fluids.

MAINTENANCE FLUID AND ELECTROLYTE REQUIREMENTS

The prescription of fluids for children has three components:

1. meeting maintenance requirements;
2. coping with ongoing losses;
3. correcting fluid and electrolyte deficits.

The first two components will be dealt with here. The correction of fluid and electrolyte deficits is covered under 'Fluid and electrolyte disturbances' below.

Normal water requirement is closely linked to energy requirements, both on account of the associated heat production and the urinary solute load resulting from the diet. A normal infant requires 110 cal/kg body weight/day and, it is claimed, approximately 150 ml fluid (i.e. solution) per 100 cal expended. For babies an enteral food source is available which balances calories and volume perfectly. A breast-fed term newborn drinks approximately 150 ml/kg/day. This gives the baby 100 kcal/kg/day of energy (the creamatocrit of breast milk increases during a feed but on average it contains 67 kcal/100 ml or 20 kcal/ounce). This ratio of water to energy promotes optimum growth. However 150 ml of milk does not contain 150 ml of water and the volume requirement of enteral milk (150 ml/kg/day) does not transpose to the prescription of parenteral fluids.

In contrast to fats, carbohydrates and salts have low volumes in solution and when parenteral fluids and nutrition are limited to a few days in a previously healthy child, a calorie intake of 20–35% of the average normal requirement will suffice. Thereafter a more comprehensive approach is required. Catabolism due to illness is unresponsive to hyperalimentation and feeding in excess of metabolic requirements during illness increases morbidity.[3,4] Fluid provision needs to be adapted to the circumstances. Even when water intake is zero during illness, appreciable quantities of water are being produced by the oxidation of the hydrogen content of tissues undergoing catabolism and water is preserved by increased antidiuretic hormone (ADH) levels. Baseline 'maintenance' fluids are a considerable overestimation of water requirement for most hospitalized patients. Indeed unrestricted fluid regimes should only be allowed in enterally fed patients when relying on satiety. Mandatory reductions to baseline fluids apply for patients receiving i.v. fluids, nursed in bed, paralyzed, breathing humidified gases or being nursed in a humidified environment. All fluids administered must be taken into account in the fluid balance including drugs, flushes for i.v. and intra-arterial (i.a.) lines etc. A regime for making interactive decisions about fluid management is summarized in Table 15.2.

For example, using this regime, a 10 kg child being ventilated for bacterial pneumonia might be prescribed an i.v. fluid regime of 100 ml/kg × 0.75 (for breathing humidified gases) × 0.7 (if paralyzed) × 0.7 (for the risk of high ADH levels) = 37 ml/kg/day. Subsequent provision would be judged in the light of fluid balance (weight), plasma urea and electrolytes and urinalysis.

A normal dietary sodium intake ranges between 1 and 4 mmol (23–2 mg)/kg body weight/day. The normal daily dietary potassium intake ranges between 1 and 3 mmol (39–117 mg)/kg body weight. A 500 ml bag of 4% dextrose and 0.18% saline with 10 mmol of potassium added to each bag when infused at 100 ml/kg/day provides; 16 calories/kg/day, 3 mmol/kg/day of sodium and 2 mmol/kg/day of potassium. 10% dextrose infused at the same rate provides 40 calories/kg/day which is 6.9 mg/kg/min of glucose which satisfies the normal immediate calorie requirement for babies.

ONGOING LOSSES

Stipulated 'normal' maintenance requirements include an allowance for natural sensible and insensible losses. To prospectively compensate for abnormal fluid and electrolyte losses, the volumes involved must be measured and recorded and the composition of the fluid determined (Table 15.3). The primary fluid loss is always from the extracellular compartment and its composition can often be anticipated according to its origin. Acute losses from the intravascular compartment can be replaced directly. Furthermore equilibration of fluid and electrolytes occurs between compartments (particularly between the ICFs and ECFs). The ICF is not directly accessible and replacement regimes devised to compensate for previous (as opposed to current) losses are

Table 15.2 Volume of intravenous fluid administered. (From Shann 1999[5] with permission)

		Fluid regime / adjustment
Baseline	1 Day of age	50 ml/kg/day
	2 Days of age	75 ml/kg/day
	3+ Days of age	100 ml/kg/day
	< 10 kg	100 ml/kg/day
	10–20 kg	1000 ml/day + 50 ml/kg/day for every kg > 10 kg
	> 20 kg	1500 ml/day + 20 ml/kg/day for every kg > 20 kg
Decreases	Humidified gases	× 0.75
	Paralyzed	× 0.7
	High ADH (e.g. IPPV or coma)	× 0.7
	Hypothermia	– 12% per °C core temp is < 37
	High ambient humidity	× 0.7
	Renal failure	× 0.3 (+ urine output)
Increases	Full activity and oral feeds	× 1.5 / free fluids
	Fever	+ 12% per °C core temp is > 37
	Room temp > 31°C	+ 30% per °C
	Hyperventilation	× 1.2
	Preterm neonate (< 1.5 kg)	× 1.2
	Radiant heater	× 1.5
	Phototherapy	× 1.5
	Burns day 1	+ 4% per 1% of body surface area affected
	Burns day 2 +	+ 2% per 1% of body surface area affected

ADH, antidiuretic hormone; IPPV, intermittent positive pressure ventilation

Table 15.3 Composition of solutes in body fluids

	Na^+ (mmol/L)	K^+ (mmol/L)	Cl^- (mmol/L)	HCO_3^- (mmol/L^{-1})
Plasma	135–145	3.5–5	98–110	18–25
Interstitial fluid	145	4.1	117	27
Intracellular fluid	10	159	3	7
Saliva	10–25	20–35	10–30	2–10
Gastric	20–80	5–20	100–150	0
Jejunal	130–150	5–10	100–130	10–20
Ileal	50–150	3–15	20–120	30–50
Diarrheal	10–90	10–80	10–110	20–70
Sweat (normal)	10–30	3–10	10–35	0
Sweat (cystic fibrosis)	50–130	5–25	50–110	0
Burn exudate (includes 30–50 g/L of protein)	140	5	110	20

CF, cellular fluid

considered in more detail below under 'Fluid and electrolyte disturbance'.

MONITORING

The intensity with which patients are monitored in respect of fluid electrolytes and acid–base is, like other aspects of their care, based primarily on the clinical impression of illness severity. At the highest levels of intensity, intake and sensible losses may be monitored to allow fluid balance to be determined several times per hour. Electrolyte levels and acid–base status may also be measured as frequently. At the other end of the spectrum an experienced clinician, given a good history of a child with reasonable renal function, can treat the majority of cases effectively with limited resources and little or no laboratory help. On a normal pediatric ward, the sickest patients and those exclusively dependent upon i.v. fluids should have their weight, fluid balance and serum urea electrolytes and bicarbonate determined daily.

Monitoring fluid balance by means of daily weight measurements is considered the practical standard when issues of fluid balance are of importance. It has the advantage that it includes the impact of abnormal insensible losses, which are otherwise difficult to quantify. Clearly strict attention to technique should be maintained to provide interpretable results. Patients should not be clothed during measurement and the weight of any medical kit that is attached to them should be the same at each measurement. The results should be graphed with particular attention to the accuracy of the plot. The relationship between total body water and body weight is linear over short time scales within an individual but there is considerable variation between individuals. This is largely accounted for by variation in the amount of adipose tissue (which contains < 10% water). Hence at the point of clinical presentation with significant illness, the patient's weight must be measured and recorded so that subsequent changes can be correctly interpreted.

TOTAL BODY WATER AND SODIUM BALANCE

As already stated, the proportion of body weight that is attributable to its water content varies with age, sex and the amount of adipose tissue present. Total body water can be measured by indicator dilution methods (e.g. deuterium) or bioimpedance. For dilution methods the results differ between the chosen solutes according to their true distribution and the relative truth of the assumption that the material will diffuse rapidly throughout the water of the body before significant metabolism or excretion occurs. The results obtained from bioimpedance measurements are also dependent upon scrupulous technique. Water loss from the body occurs by various routes such as insensible perspiration, transpiration from lungs, and loss in urine, feces and sweat. Normally losses in feces and sweat are minimal. Insensible perspiration is essential to dissipate heat generated by metabolism and is augmented as required by sweating.

Of the sensible water losses, the principal physiological control is over the volume and content of urine production. This is reduced by ADH, which works on the collecting duct and increased by atrial natiuretic peptide (ANP), which is released from the heart when the ECF is expanded. ANP inhibits sodium reabsorption in the distal nephron and increases GFR by increasing blood pressure and the filtration fraction. There are however obligatory water losses in the urine – the volume required to excrete the solute load – which are higher in babies. ADH release occurs in response to osmoreceptors in the hypothalamus and baroreceptors (really stretch receptors) in the circulation. The osmoreceptors are by far the more sensitive, enabling fine control over plasma osmolality but the ADH response that they initiate is muted compared to that caused by a fall in plasma volume. Strong releases of ADH occur in response to reduced plasma volume irrespective of the tonicity of the plasma. Water balance naturally fluctuates with the dictates of sodium balance (renin–angiotensin system). The urine sodium content can be used to differentiate oliguric states since it is a reasonably reliable predictor of extracellular fluid volume. If renal perfusion pressure falls to levels short of those that produce acute renal failure, the kidneys produce good 'quality' concentrated urine (osmolality > 300 mosm/L, urine:plasma urea ratio > 5) with a urine sodium < 20 mmol/L. The fractional sodium excretion = (urinary sodium × plasma creatinine)/(plasma sodium × urinary creatinine) is also low ≈0.4. These findings are ablated by diuretic therapy. In acute tubular necrosis the urine 'quality' is poor, urine sodium is > 40 mmol/L and fractional sodium excretion is ≥ 7.

Most of the sodium excretion from the body occurs via the kidney which can compensate within wide limits for variation in the dietary intake. Normal glomerular filtrate has an osmolality of 300 mosmol/kg but the osmolality of the urine excreted by adolescents and adults may range from 30 to 1200 mosmol/kg (specific gravity 1.001–1.035). The infant kidney is unable to form such concentrated or dilute urine, a more realistic range being 100–600 mosmol/kg (specific gravity 1.003–1.023). Sodium depletion (unlike water depletion) does not occur under conditions of reduced intake but requires some abnormal loss – in sweat, alimentary secretions or urine.

The regulation of body sodium is closely linked to water.[6] Control of the osmolality of the extracellular fluid through changes in thirst and renal water excretion would otherwise lead to large changes in body volume in the face of sodium imbalance. Control over absorption and excretion of sodium is mediated primarily by the renin–angiotensin system. Adequacy of circulating blood volume and blood pressure affect perfusion of the juxtaglomerular apparatus which if inadequate leads to the production of renin and thus aldosterone. The principal site of sodium control by alsosterone is the distal nephron (after the essential resorption of the majority of the sodium in the glomerular filtrate which occurs in the proximal tubule). In hypervolemia, renin production is decreased and atrial natriuretic peptide is released. The GFR increases supplying more sodium (and water) to the distal convoluted tubule where it passes on into the urine.

COMPARTMENTAL DISTRIBUTION OF WATER AND ELECTROLYTES

The physical and physiological influences on the internal distribution of water and electrolytes are covered in Appendix 1. Figure 15.1 highlights the difference in composition between various ECFs and ICF. In essence, ECF is rich in sodium and chloride with relatively small amounts of potassium. The reverse applies to ICF where potassium, protein and phosphate predominate. Indeed the internal distribution of potassium is related to cell mass, about 70% of the total body content being found in muscle. The concentration of magnesium is also greater in ICF, with 50% of the body's content being in the cells of soft tissue and most of the remainder in bone. The sum of anions and cations in ICF is greater than that in ECF. Normal osmotic equilibrium *is* present however because there is an excess of divalent and polyvalent anions in ICF each contributing several electrical charges but only one osmotic particle. Secondly, some intracellular univalent ions (especially potassium) are not in free ionic form, but in combination with anions.

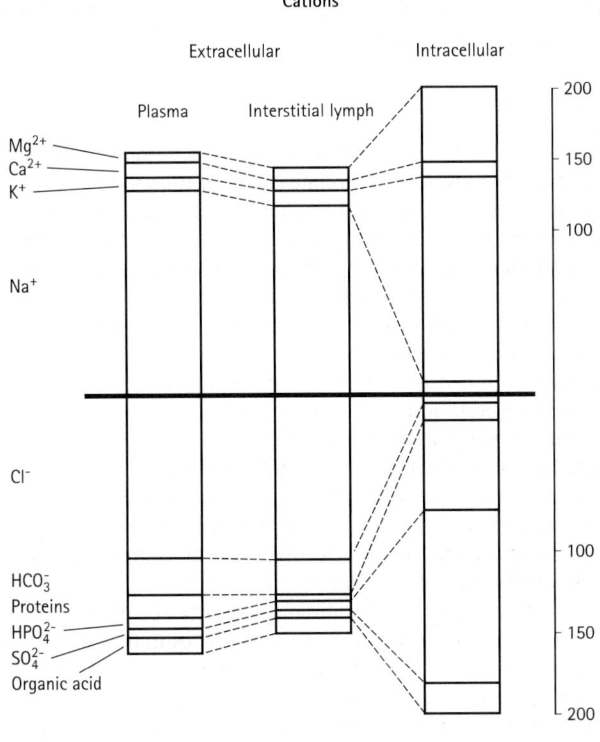

Fig. 15.1 Ionic composition of body fluids. The ionic composition of intra- and extracellular fluids. Cations are displayed above the dark horizontal line and anions below it. (From Ichikawa 1990[7] with permission)

The two divisions of ECF most frequently involved in the understanding of disease states are plasma and interstitial fluid. Normally, plasma water accounts for approximately 93% of the plasma volume. The remaining 7%, although predominantly proteins, includes lipids, electrolytes, glucose and urea. The plasma volume occupied by electrolytes is always insignificant.

ACID–BASE

Most disturbances of fluid and electrolyte metabolism are associated with changes in the acid–base state of the blood. For example reduction in ECF volume leads to circulatory failure or 'shock'. The associated cellular hypoxia causes acidosis predominantly by the production of lactate. Some relevant details of acid–base chemistry and blood gas measurement are contained in Appendix 2.

Hydrogen ion concentration ($[H^+]$) within the body is closely controlled under normal conditions but the extreme concentrations that can arise during illness can range from 40 to 400% of the normal mean. Thus the body can be considered tolerant of changes in hydrogen ion concentration even if these conditions are not favored. The normal $[H^+]$ is 37–48 nmol/L in babies corresponding to pH 7.43–7.32. The normal $[H^+]$ range in infants and children is 37–46 nmol/L corresponding to a pH of 7.43–7.34. Values higher than the upper limit of normal $[H^+]$ (lower pH) are acidotic and values lower than the lower limit (higher pH) are alkalotic.

For there to be long term stability of $[H^+]$, metabolic production of acid must be balanced by respiratory and renal excretion. Respiration controls $[H^+]$ by clearing carbon dioxide. The kidney controls urinary excretion of $[H^+]$, the resorption of bicarbonate and the excretion of the non-volatile acids that are produced during metabolism. The latter are derived principally from the sulfur contained in the methionine and cysteine of protein and form the titratable acid and ammonium in the urine.

Fluctuations in acid–base are tempered by:

- dilution of any acid produced;
- buffering;
- regulation of respiratory rate to control plasma CO_2 tension;
- renal resorption of filtered bicarbonate, and excretion of excess hydrogen ion (Fig. 15.2).[8]

Derangements of acid–base that are due primarily to fluctuations in $PaCO_2$ (and hence carbonic acid) are termed 'respiratory', all others are 'metabolic'. These acid–base fluctuations have a variety of consequences:

- Serum potassium levels change: Acute rises in $[H^+]$ (acidosis) equilibrate across the cell membrane. An efflux of intracellular potassium ions preserves the transmembrane electrical potential but results in hyperkalemia. Similarly alkalosis from any cause results in an influx of potassium into the cells and hypokalemia. These changes occur without perturbing the whole body potassium. The relationship between acid–base and potassium flux is complicated if insulin is being administered since it promotes potassium movement into cells along with glucose.
- Albumin binding is affected: For example alkalosis increases the ratio of bound to unbound (ionized) Ca^{2+} and can lead to tetany.
- Hemoglobin dissociation is affected: Acidosis increases the P50 of the hemoglobin dissociation curve creating potential problems with oxygen delivery and alkalosis decreases it creating potential problems with oxygen uptake.
- Regional blood flow may change: $[H^+]$ fluctuations (especially those caused by CO_2) affect vascular tone. Hypercapnic acidosis causes cerebral vasodilatation and pulmonary vasoconstriction.[9]

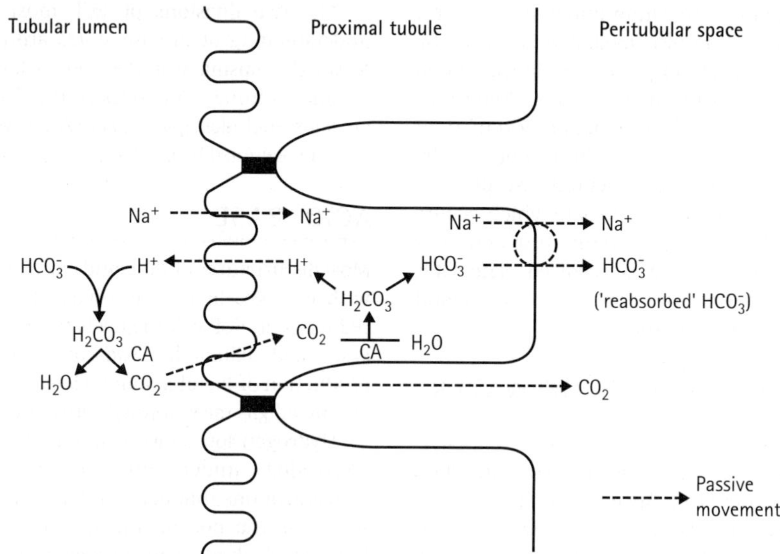

Fig. 15.2 Reabsorption of filtered bicarbonate. Reabsorption of filtered bicarbonate is achieved via H^+ secretion. The secreted H^+ (derived from carbonic acid) reacts with bicarbonate in the tubular fluid to reform carbonic acid which dissociates into carbon dioxide and water. Hence a bicarbonate anion is lost from the tubular fluid. But since the hydrogen ion came from a reaction which also generated a bicarbonate anion in the peritubular fluid, the net result is bicarbonate reabsorption. This figure illustrates the situation in the proximal convoluted tubule where 90% of filtered bicarbonate is reabsorbed. CA, carbonic anhydrase. (From West 1989[5] with permission)

- Pharmacodynamic and pharmacokinetic effects occur: For a variety of drugs, e.g. weak acids and alkalis, tissue penetration is affected by ionization.

Most importantly a level of compensation is achieved via the alternate mechanism (changing levels of CO_2 or bicarbonate respectively). The rapid respiratory compensation for metabolic derangements is mediated by changes in respiratory drive and is effected as altered minute ventilation controls the $PaCO_2$. Metabolic compensation for respiratory acidosis is much slower and is effected by renal conservation of bicarbonate. In either case, full compensation is unusual but would bring the $[H^+]$ right back into the normal range if it worked.

DISTURBANCE OF ACID–BASE

RESPIRATORY ALKALOSIS

Hyperventilation causes a reduction in $PaCO_2$ and acute changes in $PaCO_2$ have a linear effect on $[H^+]$ (1 kPa to 5.5 nmol/L). Thus $[H^+]$ is low and $PaCO_2$ is low. Common causes include excessive mechanical ventilation, central hyperventilation associated with encephalopathy, central nervous system (CNS) infection, trauma, etc. Acutely hypoxic and acidotic patients can hyperventilate. In the latter case some degree of compensation for the high $[H^+]$ is achieved. One would expect the calculated bicarbonate and base excess from the blood gas machine to be normal. Treatment is directed at the specific cause.

RESPIRATORY ACIDOSIS

Hypoventilation causes a rise in $PaCO_2$. Acute changes in $PaCO_2$ have a linear effect on $[H^+]$ (1 kPa to 5.5 nmol/L). Thus $[H^+]$ is high and $PaCO_2$ is high. Common causes include respiratory depression, obstructive and restrictive respiratory diseases, terminal exhaustion, inadequate mechanical ventilation, etc. Similar derangements may be caused by muscle weakness and increased CO_2 production (malignant hyperthermia, seizures ...). One would expect the calculated bicarbonate and base excess to be normal. Treatment is directed at improving respiratory function/support and to a lesser extent minimizing CO_2 load, e.g. by lowering the metabolic rate and providing fat as a metabolic substrate. If it is unsuccessful then compensation occurs over several days through renal conservation of bicarbonate. A compensated respiratory acidosis therefore has a near normal (but high) $[H^+]$ and a high $PaCO_2$ and one would expect the bicarbonate level calculated by the blood gas machine to be high.

METABOLIC ALKALOSIS

An acute fall in hydrogen ion concentration without a fall in CO_2 may be due to a rise in bicarbonate concentration or less commonly a loss of [H+] ions. Some compensatory CO_2 retention may occur and reduced respiratory drive should be anticipated, for example if one is attempting to wean mechanical ventilation. The calculated base excess would be expected to be high (see below) but under most circumstances confusion should not occur with a compensated respiratory acidosis because the $[H^+]$ will be near normal (but low). If the patient is being mechanically ventilated to a low $PaCO_2$ then the true interpretation of the blood gas may only be possible when placed in the wider clinical context.

During potassium deficiency renal conservation of K^+ occurs at the expense of H^+ which creates a metabolic alkalosis with a paradoxically acid urine. The problem is aggravated by hyponatremia. Intracellular acidosis occurs by a similar mechanism (lost K^+ replaced by H^+ and Na^+).

Chloride depletion is a common consequence of loop diuretic therapy but can also occur from gastrointestinal losses or as a secondary consequence of chronic respiratory acidosis. It is associated with increased sodium reabsorption in the proximal convoluted tubule and excess H^+ and K^+ loss, the former resulting in increased bicarbonate absorption from the filtrate. Chloride sensitive causes of metabolic alkalosis are associated with low urinary chloride (< 20 mmol/L) and chloride insensitive forms with higher urinary chloride. The former include diuretic therapy, vomiting and chloridorrhea and the latter, citrate poisoning. Diminished ECF volume will perpetuate a metabolic alkalosis because it is associated with an obligatory increase in proximal tubular Na^+ reabsorption.

By analogy, a metabolic alkalosis can be produced by the loss of hydrogen ion by vomiting, or by the introduction of bicarbonate-containing material into the body. In either event the blood pH tends to increase. In the former case an increase in total buffer base occurs and a reduction in H_2CO_3. In the latter an increase in total buffer base occurs but with an increase in H_2CO_3. Renal compensation corrects both imbalances.

In the rare circumstances where a metabolic alkalosis requires treatment it is important to treat the cause rather than the effect. Treat hypokalemia with potassium supplements and hypochloremia with saline infusion. Acid loads can be delivered where necessary however in the form of ammonium chloride (avoid in liver failure in favor of dilute hydrochloric acid 200 mmol/L in 5% dextrose).

METABOLIC ACIDOSIS

An acute rise in $[H^+]$ with a normal or even reduced $PaCO_2$ (attempted compensation) results from an abnormal bicarbonate loss or a non-carbonic source of excess H^+. The calculated base deficit (negative base excess) would be expected to be high and the calculated bicarbonate would be expected to be low. Treatment must be directed at the cause. Routine investigation of a metabolic acidosis in order to determine the cause includes measurement of urine pH, anion and osmolar gaps and measurement of the serum lactate and/or arteriovenous oxygen difference as markers of the adequacy of tissue perfusion/oxygen delivery.

The anion gap is calculated according to the formula:

$$[Na^+] - ([Cl^-] + [HCO_3^-])$$

An anion gap greater than 12 implies the presence of a 'non-Henderson–Hasselbalch' source of acid. The osmolar gap is the difference between measured and calculated osmolality. If measured osmolality is > 15 mosm/L higher than calculated then this implies the presence of additional osmotically active solutes.

Under certain circumstances it is justifiable to attempt to compensate a metabolic acidosis therapeutically by administering exogenous base such as sodium bicarbonate, for example to supplement recognized bicarbonate losses (e.g. urine, ileostomy fluid) or to treat drug overdoses involving agents that are weak acids. Bicarbonate can also be used as emergency therapy if there is associated symptomatic hyperkalemia or an inadequate response to inotropic support in the context of severe acidosis ($[H^+] > 63$ nmol/L, pH < 7.2). This bicarbonate rapidly forms CO_2 because of the prevailing pH. It thus creates a respiratory load. Furthermore although CO_2 diffuses fairly freely across the various membranes in the body, the bicarbonate ion may take several hours to attain access to all phases. It is possible therefore for exogenous bicarbonate to aggravate intracellular acidosis and similarly to lower the pH of cerebrospinal fluid. This latter effect explains the persistent respiratory alkalosis which occurs when metabolic acidosis is artificially corrected rapidly by administration of exogenous bicarbonate.

MIXED DISTURBANCES

A number of mixed acid–base disturbances are worthy of mention. For example mixed metabolic and respiratory acidosis is common in critical illness. Disease processes that cause combined effects such as these inevitably limit or curtail physiological compensation causing more severe and persistent increases in $[H^+]$. Similarly the combination of heart failure (hence diuretic therapy) and chronic respiratory disease can cause hypokalemic/hypochloremic metabolic alkalosis and compensated respiratory acidosis. In which case $[H^+]$ levels fall, bicarbonate levels rise and CO_2 retention may be exacerbated.

Severe vomiting (e.g. in pyloric stenosis) causes loss of hydrogen and chloride ions causing hypochloremic alkalosis. Concurrent hypokalemia can lead to production of a paradoxically acid urine. In diabetic ketoacidosis complicated by severe vomiting the concurrent loss of hydrogen ions may lead to an apparent discordance with the severity of hyperglycemia and dehydration.

In salicylate poisoning the initial upset is usually respiratory alkalosis, partly compensation for the acid load but mostly from direct stimulation of respiratory drive. The supervening metabolic acidosis is due to uncoupled oxidative phosphorylation and increased metabolism of lipid, carbohydrate and amino acids. Blood gases show a high anion gap metabolic acidosis due to the salicylic acid, ketones, free amino acids and lactate. Respiratory alkalosis which is commonly associated with low ionized calcium levels gives way to respiratory acidosis as the conscious level is reduced. Hyperglycemia is common and may mimic diabetic ketoacidosis. Hypoglycemia may occur in small children.

CAUTIONARY NOTES ON LABORATORY TESTS OF FLUID AND ELECTROLYTES

The diagnosis of dehydration is essentially a clinical one. Body water content is not measured reliably under clinical as opposed to laboratory conditions. The total body water is not a particularly useful measurement under most circumstances since it is hard to standardize between individuals. The common assumption in clinical practice is that uremia indicates dehydration (and usually a contraction of the ECF volume) or renal failure. There are other causes of uremia however such as excessive protein catabolism and the metabolism of ingested blood. In water depletion, the packed cell volume (PCV) tends to remain normal, whilst the concentrations of hemoglobin and plasma proteins show only slight increases. Unfortunately these observations are often obscured because the predehydration figures are not known.

In hyperlipidemia, uremia or diabetes mellitus, the amount of lipids, urea or glucose may be large enough to produce a reduction in sodium concentration per unit volume. In hyperlipidemia the amount of water in plasma may be reduced to 75% of the norm and consequently the concentration of sodium apparently reduced. Nevertheless when expressed per liter of water (rather than solution) it is normal.

Serum potassium measurements must be interpreted in context since levels may not reflect total body levels. Beta-adrenergic stimuli, alkalosis or insulin therapy all lower serum potassium. However confidence that total body levels have not changed should not translate to a reticence to treat the serum level whether it is high or low because of the physiological consequences.

Serum phosphate levels like those of potassium are poor predictors of body levels since it is principally an intracellular anion. Plasma levels fluctuate as the result of shifts between ECF and ICF, they are also closely linked to ionized calcium levels. False low values/assay interference occur after mannitol administration or in the presence of lipemia, free hemoglobin (hemolysis) or bilirubinemia.

Calcium and magnesium homeostasis are closely linked to phosphate levels. Interpretation of total calcium levels must also be put into context with the serum albumin although it is more physiological to look directly at the ionized (free) component. Albumin binding of all species (drugs, bilirubin, calcium....) changes radically with acid–base. Respiratory alkalosis is capable of inducing tetany.

FLUID AND ELECTROLYTE DISTURBANCE

EDEMA

Edema is common in a variety of clinical situations particularly in the severely ill and malnourished. It is a common manifestation of a systemic inflammatory response and is therefore not necessarily a manifestation of fluid overload. Indeed in many clinical situations the edematous patient has a reduced intravascular volume. Indicators of hypervolemia such as hepatomegaly, high pulmonary blood flow and pulmonary edema make the clinical diagnosis of fluid overload more likely. However water intoxication causes hyponatremia long before significant edema occurs. Diuretic-resistant edema may occur in renal or cardiac failure: the implication is that renal excretion is impaired in spite of the possible presence of an increased ECF volume. The total body sodium under these circumstances may be increased but water retention is even more marked, resulting in hyponatremia.

Where capillary endothelial damage has occurred, for example as a consequence of a systemic inflammatory response then the resultant edema may again be resistant to treatment with diuretics and fluid restriction. The latter leads to hypernatremia due to the associated leak of protein into the interstitial fluid. Treatment with supplemental i.v. infusion of albumin under such circumstances contributes to the interstitial albumin load unless endothelial repair has occurred. The sequence of events leading to this syndrome is complicated and involves excessive secretion and/or diminished inactivation of aldosterone and ADH together with the changes in capillary permeability. The outcome is an increase in the volume of interstitial fluid but a decrease in plasma volume. This results in prerenal uremia which is further aggravated by sodium restriction. Hypoalbuminemia such as occurs in nephrosis causes edema by altering the balance between hydrostatic and colloid osmotic pressures.

CLINICAL SIGNS OF DEHYDRATION

A history of increased thirst and oliguria implies dehydration, the clinical signs of which include reduced skin turgor, dry mucous membranes, sunken eyes and a sunken fontanelle. In the extreme case, signs of shock are present such as poor peripheral perfusion (prolonged capillary refill), cold peripheries, poor peripheral pulses, Kussmaul respiration (from metabolic acidosis) and ultimately hypotension and prostration. The clinical severity of dehydration can be matched to a pragmatic scale (mild, moderate, severe) (Table 15.4). This can then be used as a guide to the proportion of the premorbid weight that has been lost as fluid (e.g. 3%, 6%, 9%) and subsequently the fluid deficit that needs to be replaced (30 ml/kg, 60 ml/kg or 90 ml/kg). Dehydration severe enough to cause weight loss of 15% of the premorbid weight (as water), can reputedly occur and does not preclude successful salvage. However there is good evidence that even relatively experienced pediatricians overestimate the degree of dehydration during clinical examination. The danger is that this overestimate will then lead to excessive fluid administration. Furthermore individual clinical signs such as dry mucous membranes and a sunken fontanelle, prove to be remarkably poor objective predictors of dehydration as determined retrospectively.[10]

DEHYDRATION

Water and electrolyte losses occur in tandem but not always in strict proportion depending upon the source of the fluid loss and the nature of intake or replacement at the time. Thus the result may leave the plasma isotonic with respect to normal values, hypertonic or hypotonic. The loss of water and sodium in proportion leads to isotonic dehydration. An excess loss of water or the use of hypertonic fluids as intake leads to hypertonic dehydration. An excess loss of electrolyte or the use of hypotonic fluids as intake leads to hypotonic dehydration.

Hyperosmolar dehydration can result from the provision of incorrectly reconstituted feed or hyperosmolar (e.g. sugary) drinks. The infant's inability to handle the solute load causes an osmotic diuresis and the hyperosmolar intake compounds the situation. Water is lost initially from the extracellular fluid but the hyperosmolal plasma equilibrates with the intracellular environment. ECF volume is hence relatively preserved and the ICF experiences a greater fluid loss than in other forms of dehydration. Thus more of the total body water is lost for the same degree of hemodynamic compromise. Thrombosis, most notably of intracranial venous sinuses and renal veins, may occur. More importantly, rehydration involves re-expansion of the ICF volume and carries a high risk of cerebral swelling. It should therefore be performed slowly (over at least 48 h). Hyperosmolality is usually but not exclusively recognized by hypernatremia. It is also present in hyperglycemic dehydration due to diabetic ketoacidosis.

By contrast in hypo-osmolar dehydration the predominant water loss is from the extracellular (hence including the vascular) space and so hypotension and shock occur earlier and are more severe for a given amount of water loss. Relative preservation of intracellular turgor may increase the risk of cerebral ischemia during hypotension.

Table 15.4 Fluid loss in dehydration

		L		
	% Body weight	Adult (70 kg)	Infant (6 kg)	Signs and symptoms
Mild	3	2.0	0.18	Thirst; oliguria; dry mucous membranes
Moderate	6	4.0	0.36	Thirst; oliguria; restlessness; weakness and tachycardia
Very severe	7–14	5–10	0.42–0.84	Collapse, convulsions, blood pressure low; sunken eyeballs and fontanelle; loss of skin turgor with 'doughy' feeling; plasma sodium, urea and osmolality all raised

In all forms of dehydration, shock, acidosis and hypoglycemia are treated aggressively but rehydration should be more controlled, using normal saline initially irrespective of the serum sodium.

Thus salt is replaced in hypo-osmolal dehydration and in hyperosmolal dehydration the serum osmolality is sustained during the early stages of rehydration – reducing the risk of cerebral edema. A policy of aiming to replace water deficit over at least 48 h in all forms of dehydration protects against the common tendency to overestimate the water deficit. Replacement of potassium stores may take days as the rate of administration has to be limited to allow time for redistribution into the ICF. The associated protein calorie deficit may take weeks to correct.

ENTERAL REHYDRATION

When dehydration complicates illness in children, hospital admission is reserved for the younger patients and the more severe cases. There is therefore a tendency towards i.v. rehydration regimes for these patients. This may not always be appropriate. For example, from a wider perspective oral rehydration regimes for diarrhea are appropriate in over 90% of cases and most do not require hospitalization. The therapeutic effects of oral rehydration solutions (ORS) include facilitation of sodium transport across the bowel wall driven by glucose. A variety of proprietary preparations are available. Those intended for pre-emptive use contain less sodium than those designed specifically for rehydration of the dehydrated patient. Preference should be given to those in which the carbohydrate content is provided as monosaccharides (glucose) since disaccharidases are brush border enzymes which may be depleted by the illness. Loss of brush border lactase is the cause of postenteritic lactose intolerance which, when present, causes osmotic diarrhea if dairy products are introduced too early during recovery.

The principles of enteral fluid management in treating diarrhea are:

1. It is usually wrong to interrupt breast-feeding.
2. Supplemental water is allowed during treatment with ORS provided sufficient ORS has been administered.
3. A guide to the required volume of ORS is that it should normally equal the volume of stool produced.

When dehydration is evident at presentation as much as 50–100 ml/kg of ORS can be given enterally over 4–6 h depending upon its severity. Subsequent treatment with as much as 200–300 ml/kg/day is usually well tolerated, if faced with equivalent losses.

HYPONATREMIA

Hyponatremia causes ileus, listlessness and ultimately cerebral edema and convulsions, the extent of the symptoms being more closely related to the rapidity of change in serum sodium than the absolute value. There are some patients whose plasma sodium concentrations remain below the lower limit of the normal range (e.g. 132 mmol/L) without symptoms and who excrete supplemental sodium to maintain this 'new' steady state.

Hyponatremia can occur in the face of normal total body sodium [syndrome of inappropriate secretion of antidiuretic hormone (SIADH), glucocorticoid deficiency, water overload...], raised total body sodium with greater retention of water (heart failure, cirrhosis, nephrotic syndrome and sequestration) or decreased total body sodium (increased losses – particularly enteral, diuretic therapy or inadequate intake). Sodium loss is usually associated with a concomitant water loss and, as described above, the resultant serum sodium depends upon the balance between the two. Hyponatremia is common in preterm infants because of their high urinary losses. Breast milk on its own contains inadequate amounts of sodium for their needs.

Hyponatremia occurs as the result of water intoxication in a variety circumstances including:

- the prescription of hypotonic i.v. fluids particularly if too much fluid is prescribed (see Table 15.2);
- SIADH;
- missed cases of acute renal failure, e.g. in hemolytic uremic syndrome.

Babies are susceptible to water intoxication because of their relatively low GFR. Clinical manifestations may appear when water amounting to as little as 5% of body weight is retained. The excess water is widely distributed between both ECF and ICF.

SIADH is well recognized but it is frequently a misnomer. ADH secretion can be considered an appropriate evolutionary physiological response to injuries/illnesses which are of sufficient severity to preclude drinking for several days. The most common causes are CNS injury and bacterial pneumonia. The retained water however often does not come from a physiological source but from a prescription to administer fluid in quantities that did not anticipate the ADH secretion.[11] In any case the clinical picture of water intoxication (hyponatremia) develops. The diagnosis is made by proving that urine osmolality exceeds that of a hypo-osmolar plasma (i.e. inappropriate retention of water by the kidney) and the treatment is usually fluid restriction (see below and Table 15.2).

Two 'salt wasting' syndromes are worthy of individual mention because of the extraordinary scale of the sodium loss involved. In the salt losing forms of congenital adrenal hyperplasia, deficiency of cortisol and aldosterone leads to natriuresis in the neonatal period. The clinical presentation however is with vomiting and weight loss. 'Cerebral salt wasting' is a condition which can appear in the first week after brain injury and spontaneously resolves in 2–4 weeks. It is characterized by natriuresis and subsequent hyponatraemic dehydration. It can be confused with SIADH in its early stages. Both conditions display coincident urine hyperosmolarity and hypo-osmolar plasma. The distinction is made by 24 h urinary sodium content which is high in salt wasting and normal in SIADH. The pathogenesis is unclear but it may prove to be a dopaminergic phenomenon or related to other circulating natriuretics such as atrial natriuretic peptide.[12] The treatment is to supply adequate salt *and water* (as opposed to fluid restriction in SIADH) but fludrocortisone may also be required.

Euvolemic hyponatremia with or without hyperkalemia can occur in a variety of critical illness states in the absence of renal dysfunction. Known precipitants include anoxia, septicemia and malnourishment. Pragmatically these should be assumed to be Addisonian crises (i.e. they should prompt the administration of steroids) but some may be due to failure of the Na^+/K^+ ATPase, the so called 'sick cell syndrome'.[13]

Rapid correction of hyponatremia is justified in circumstances where severe symptoms have resulted from a rapid fall in serum sodium. If a good history is not available, symptoms are severe and serum Na^+ is < 120 mmol/L a rapid initial correction is justifiable to values of 125 mmol/L. To increase the serum sodium by 2 mmol/L/h (maximum safe rate):[14]

$$\text{Infusion rate (ml/h)} = 8 \times \text{wt (kg)}/(\%\ \text{saline being used}).$$

Further increase in serum sodium is best achieved more gradually with fluid restriction. In all other circumstances slow correction is advisable by fluid restriction alone and the provision of normal rather than increased sodium supplements.[15]

The neurological symptoms associated with acute hyponatremia are in part due to cerebral edema and may improve with the hypertonic saline as the brain shrinks.[16] The adult medical literature contains references to 'central pontine myelinosis' which can lead to quadriplegia and may occur in association with the rapid correction of chronic hyponatremia.

HYPERNATREMIA

Hypernatremia can occur in association with low total body sodium, in which case the salt loss has occurred in the context of a greater water loss (e.g. osmotic diuresis, vomiting/diarrhea). When losses are predominantly water, total body sodium balance may be close to normal (e.g. fever, radiant heater, phototherapy, diabetes insipidus) as is the case when the interstitial fluid space expands at the expense of the plasma volume (e.g. capillary leak). True excess of sodium can also occur (e.g. when i.v. sodium bicarbonate is used to repeatedly correct metabolic acidosis without treating the cause or when malreconstituted formula is fed to a baby).

In all hyperosmolar states, water moves from ICF to ECF and so the ICF is dehydrated. Neurological symptoms predominate (irritability, seizures and coma). The loss of volume of brain cells can even cause cerebrovascular disruptions and bleeding. Treatment of hypernatremia should be aimed at the primary cause and any necessary rehydration should be slow because of the risks of cerebral edema. These risks are compounded by the formation of idiogenic osmoles within the cell. This term is used to describe additional osmotically active substances formed apparently in response to the hyperosmolal ECF that serve to counter the shrinkage of the cell volume. The term 'idiogenic' has persisted since it was originally coined, despite the fact that at least some of the molecular species concerned have been established.[17]

True sodium overload without dehydration requires removal with loop diuretics or renal replacement therapy as required. [Renal replacement therapy now includes hemofiltration (both low and high flow), hemodiafiltration, plasma filtration, plasmapheresis, peritoneal dialysis and hemodialysis.]

There is no such thing as pure water depletion; however excessive fluid losses from very high in the GI tract (saliva) and diabetes insipidus can lead to severe water depletion in the face of trivial sodium losses. Diabetes insipidus describes a situation where there is inadequate ADH resulting from injuries to the neurohypophysis or alternatively there is resistance to the effects of ADH on the kidney (nephrogenic). The diagnosis is usually made when polyuria is recognized in association with hypernatremia. If necessary a dehydration test exaggerates the discrepancy between urine and plasma tonicity. Central causes can be treated with vasopressin (1 unit/kg in 50 ml at 1 ml/h). Nephrogenic causes necessitate treatment with dietary sodium restriction and if necessary deliberate sodium depletion induced by thiazide diuretics (presumed to enhance sodium and therefore water absorption in the proximal convoluted tubule).

HYPOKALEMIA

Hypokalemia without a true deficit in potassium can result from redistribution into the cells in response to a beta-adrenergic stimulus, alkalosis, excess insulin or rarer causes like familial hypokalemic periodic paralysis. Since the body potassium level is closely linked to muscle mass, reduction in muscle mass is associated with reduction in total body potassium but the relative amount of potassium and nitrogen remains constant. Hypokalemia with a deficit in potassium can result from inadequate intake, or increased renal (diuretic) or GI losses introducing a host of potential diagnoses including endocrine disturbances such as Cushing's syndrome and primary hyperaldosteronism. One situation that requires clinical caution is where i.v. therapy is employed to correct severe dehydration and associated acidosis (e.g. diabetic ketoacidosis). The patient's initial plasma potassium concentration is artificially elevated due to compartment shifts that have occurred as a consequence of the acidosis. A whole body potassium deficit means that, in the absence of renal failure, hypokalemia is inevitable during rehydration unless potassium supplements are included in the regime.

Irrespective of the cause, hypokalemia has cardiovascular, neuromuscular and metabolic consequences including a propensity for dysrhythmias, ileus, muscle weakness and effects on carbohydrate and protein metabolism. Electrocardiograph (ECG) changes include the effects on ST depression, flattening or inversion of the T wave, prolonged Q–T interval and prominent or even bifid U waves. Potassium replacement has to be given into the ECF even though the principal destination is the ICF. Infusion rates should never exceed 0.5 mmol/kg/h for fear of deranging the myocardial membrane potential and hence causing lethal arrhythmia. The ECG changes associated with serum potassium levels reflect the cell membrane potential and so hyperkalemic changes may be seen with a normal serum potassium if correction of hypokalemia is performed too rapidly. Adequate replacement may take days where there is whole body depletion. Potassium supplements/replacement should not be given in the presence of oligo/anuria without regular monitoring of serum levels.

HYPERKALEMIA

Hyperkalemia without true overload (or even deficit) may result from measurement error (e.g. hemolysis in the sample), acidosis, insulin deficiency, or drugs such as digoxin, beta blockers and depolarizing muscle relaxants. There is also a hyperkalemic form of familial periodic paralysis. High serum potassium occurs in instances of increased load (e.g. iatrogenic infusion, tissue destruction, GI bleed and tumor lysis syndrome) usually in combination with decreased excretion (e.g. renal failure or mineralocorticoid deficiency). Significant elevation of the whole body potassium:nitrogen ratio is rare since fatal hyperkalemia occurs early. Hyperkalemia is dangerous because of its effects upon cell membrane potential and therefore upon cardiac rhythm (sinus arrest and ventricular fibrillation). The point at which such rhythm supervenes is unpredictable but depends upon the rate of rise of the serum level and the age/maturity of the patient. Neonates are far more tolerant of hyperkalemia than older children and adults, particularly in relation to the propensity for ventricular dysrhythmias. The normal range of serum level extends higher in preterm babies.

The principal recognizable ECG changes, where rhythm is preserved, are tall peaked T waves and prolonged p waves.

In acute renal failure hyperkalemia may be dramatic and easily aggravated by simultaneous injury to other organs and tissues increasing the load. In chronic renal failure GFR has to get down to 5–10% before hyperkalemia results although the 'renal reserve' for potassium excretion is reduced before this. The most severe consequence of hyperkalemia is cardiac arrest, which can occur at any point in the progression of the ECG abnormalities and arrhythmias. If the problem is detected before cardiac arrest then possible emergency therapeutic measures cause compartment shifts from ECF to ICF:

- correction of acidosis (mild acidosis 1 mmol/kg, severe acidosis 2–3 mmol/kg of $NaHCO_3$);

- salbutamol administration (2.5–5 mg nebulized or i.v. 1–5 µg/kg/min);
- glucose and insulin (2 ml/kg of 50% dextrose and 0.1 U/kg of soluble insulin).

A slower response can be obtained using ion exchange resins such as calcium polystyrene sulfonate (Resonium) 0.5 g/kg dose per rectum. An i.v. bolus of calcium (0.1 mmol/kg to a max of 5 mmol) can temporarily stabilize the heart rhythm whilst other treatments are initiated. Renal replacement therapy (dialysis) is indicated if the hyperkalemia is recalcitrant (as it will be if it is due to renal failure).

CALCIUM AND MAGNESIUM

Parathormone (PTH) increases calcium by promoting bone resorption, increasing calcium reabsorption from the renal tubule and increasing activation of vitamin D, which increases enteral absorption of calcium and phosphate. Calcitonin is secreted by the thyroid and thymus in response to hypercalcemia and lowers both calcium and phosphate levels.

Hypocalcemia is common in sick infants due to high levels of PTH antagonists like glucocorticoids and calcitonin. It may also be due to i.v. bicarbonate therapy or the use of citrated blood products. If persistent in the newborn it may be due to DiGeorge syndrome, maternal vitamin D deficiency, cow's milk feeding or magnesium deficiency. It causes jittery symptoms in babies, multifocal clonic convulsions and rarely ECG abnormalities, dysrhythmias or heart failure. Normal requirements are 0.3 mmol/kg/day increased to 1 mmol/kg/day when treating deficiency. Calcium infusion has vasoconstrictive and inotropic effects of greater significance in children than in adults. Vasoconstriction predominates in hypomagnesemic states. Calcium opposes the negative inotropic effects of hyperkalemia.

Hypomagnesemia usually occurs in the context of parenteral nutrition because of solubility problems caused by the concurrent administration of phosphate. Clinical problems are rare until levels fall below 0.5 mmol/L but do include lethal arrhythmias such as ventricular fibrillation/ventricular tachycardia (VF/VT) and torsade de pointes. Deficiency also reduces cardiac contractility but during infusion, magnesium salts are reasonably potent vasodilators and will drop the blood pressure. Magnesium has also been used to treat pulmonary hypertension and asthma. Hypocalcemia and hypokalemia may not respond to supplementation if concurrent hypomagnesemia is uncorrected.

Hypercalcemia is rare but occurs in the recovery phase of acute renal failure, a variety of endocrine diseases, hypervitaminosis D and granulomatous disorders. Idiopathic hypercalcemia is a feature of Williams syndrome. Most cases of hypercalcemia are iatrogenic. Symptoms include neurological problems (hypotonia, seizures and coma), cardiovascular problems (tachyarrhythmias) and in chronic cases hypertension. Severe cases are treated with renal replacement therapy (dialysis).

Hypermagnesemia occurs when excessive administration (cathartics or enemas) coincides with renal failure. Symptoms are similar to hypercalcemia but include bradyarrhythmias with first degree block and broad QRS. Treatment is again focused upon enhanced excretion. Serious arrhythmias may respond to calcium.

PHOSPHATE

Phosphate excretion involves free filtration at the glomerulus with passive reabsorption of 80% in the proximal convoluted tubute (PCT) as a symport with sodium. [A symport is a membrane carrier that combines the movement of more than one type of molecule (species) in a given direction. Both species bind on one side of the membrane and are then translocated to the other side.] Although PTH results in phosphate release from bone and increased phosphate absorption from the gut, its net effect at high levels is to decrease plasma phosphate because it inhibits its renal tubular reabsorption. The fetus is relatively hypoparathyroid in response to active calcium influx across the placenta.

Hypophosphatemia occurs from:

- inadequate intake: e.g. breast-fed preterm infants;
- impaired GI absorption: e.g. as a consequence of antacids containing calcium, magnesium or aluminum (such as sucralfate);
- cellular redistribution: e.g. alkalosis, therapy for diabetic ketoacidosis, beta 2-adrenergic stimulation;
- carbohydrate infusions and other forms of hyperalimentation which can lead to hypophosphatemia by stimulating insulin release (phosphate moves into cells with glucose in response to insulin) (successful stimulation of an anabolic state after critical illness can be associated with a profound and symptomatic hypophosphatemia);
- excessive losses: e.g. as a consequence of diuretics, steroids, cytotoxic regimes or paracetamol poisoning;
- trauma (including burns);
- hereditary hypophosphatemic rickets.

The most important feature of phosphate physiology is the formation of adenosine triphosphate (ATP). Symptomatic hypophosphatemia occurs in severe depletion and causes muscle weakness that can aggravate respiratory failure and reduce myocardial contractility. When necessary, phosphate supplementation should aim to provide a dose of up to 1 mmol/kg/day (max 20 mmol) (beware some proprietary supplements frequently have a high potassium content).

Hyperphosphatemia occurs in neonates fed cows' milk or inadequately adjusted formula feed, tumor lysis syndrome and renal failure, severe hemolysis, hyperthyroidism, acromegaly, hypoparathyroidism and phosphate poisoning. Symptoms are those of the consequent hypocalcemia and deposition of hydroxyapatite crystals in cornea, lungs, heart, etc. Treatment includes resuscitation to restore ECF volume. In the absence of renal failure, phosphate binders and alkaline diuresis may be used.

CONCLUSION

The intention of this chapter has been to cover fluid, electrolyte and acid–base from a clinical perspective. This has necessarily led to the omission of some essential basic science, some of which is contained in the following two appendices. However the key point is that whilst fluid, electrolyte and acid–base disturbances can and should be evaluated and treated on their own merits they should be considered as effects of illness. To 'cure' them the cause must be treated.

APPENDIX 1: PHYSICAL AND PHYSIOLOGICAL INFLUENCES ON THE INTERNAL DISTRIBUTION OF WATER AND ELECTROLYTES

MEMBRANE PROPERTIES AND FUNCTION

The homeostasis of body fluids is intricately related to the integrity and function of their adjacent membranes. An 'ideal' membrane permits only water to pass through, and is impermeable to dissolved substances. Membranes resemble molecular sieves with the added influence of the solubility of substances in the membrane lipids. Isolated cellular membranes are partially permeable. They are fully permeable to water and small crystalloid molecules but will not permit the passage of larger molecules such as proteins and mucopolysaccharides. The metabolic activity of the cell maintains differences between the intracellular and extracellular concentrations of various ions. This ability decreases if the cell is cooled or poisoned. Cell membranes carry negative internal and positive external charges and the membrane potential is governed by the ratio of internal to external concentration of ions.

Substances cross membranes in several ways. Water or solutes may simply flow through pores. Solutes may also dissolve in the membrane and diffuse through it in solution or they may be actively transported from one side to the other. Potassium penetrates cells more rapidly than sodium, probably in part due to the smaller diameter of the potassium ion. At equilibrium the rate of movement of any material across a membrane is equal in both directions.

Under normal circumstances exchange between physical compartments in the body is tightly regulated by both steroid hormones (cortisol, aldosterone) and peptide hormones (ADH and thyroxine). Water and small solutes pass freely through intercellular pores in endothelium and in and out of cells through a facilitative transport mechanism in the cell membrane mediated by specialized transmural proteins – 'aquaporins'. The expression of aquaporins within a membrane may provide a mechanism for physiological control of the movement of small solutes as well as water.[18] The nature of such transcellular transport mechanisms, which also include epithelial sodium channels (ENaC), and their role in health and disease is only now becoming apparent.

The structure of the capillary endothelium varies according to site but there are common features in the basic structure that persist throughout. A layer of thin endothelial cells, one cell thick, lines the luminal surface of a basement membrane. The luminal surfaces of these cells bear a negative charge, imparted by a layer of glycosaminoglycans. These species restrict the permeability of the membrane with regard to negatively charged molecules such as albumin. The cellular lining may be fenestrated (depending upon the site) and there are numerous clefts between cells and tubular channels that traverse the epithelial cells themselves. Endothelial cells may change shape with changes in pressure and have physiological responses to blood flow and shear stress, which include the release of vasoactive mediators and anticoagulants.

For the diffusion of small water-soluble molecules (e.g. sodium, chloride and glucose) across capillary endothelium, the size and number of the pores (which vary depending upon the site) is not rate limiting and movement is dictated by blood supply, i.e. is 'flow limited'. These movements are dictated by the Fick equation (diffusion rate = blood flow/arteriovenous concentration difference) and Fick's law of diffusion which relates the diffusion rate:

- directly to the diffusion coefficient of the solute (related to molecular size and therefore weight);
- directly to the area of the capillary membrane;
- directly to the concentration gradient;
- inversely to the thickness (and hence permeability) of the membrane.

Capillary diffusion gradients depend on capillary size. As intercapillary distances increase, there will be islands of tissue where supply or removal of solutes becomes inadequate.

In addition to solute diffusion, bulk movement of fluid across membranes (filtration) also carries solutes across the membrane or through its pores. This occurs irrespective of whether it is initiated by hydrostatic or osmotic influences. The anatomical variation in the size and number of clefts between endothelial cells is related to their filtration properties. By far the most important homeostatic mechanism controlling this process is the vasomotor control of precapillary vessels. Glomeruli are specialized exceptions where control is exerted over pre- and postcapillary vessels. The filtration of fluid is a passive process proceeding at a rate dictated by:

- the filtration coefficient of the membrane (influenced by its surface area and permeability);
- the hydrostatic pressure gradient (greater within the arterial end of the capillary but consistent across a glomerulus);
- the colloid osmotic pressure gradient,

in a relationship described by Starling's law of ultrafiltration. The net filtration is out of the capillary at the arterial end and into the capillary at the venous end.

Epithelial and endothelial function are profoundly affected by the processes of acute inflammation in which both cell destruction and damage to basement membranes occur. Endothelial damage can be initiated and/or aggravated by activated neutrophils, which degranulate releasing proteolytic enzymes such as elastase, and reactive oxygen species in addition to cationic proteins. Activated platelets also contribute. Further endothelial cell destruction involves the stripping of glycosaminoglycans from the luminal surface of capillaries. The loss of their negative luminal charge increases the permeability of the endothelium to albumin. An interstitial edema of relatively protein rich fluid results.

The physical factors that govern transport across all membranes (cell membrane, capillary endothelium, etc.), include total osmotic pressure, hydrostatic pressure, colloidal (oncotic) pressure of proteins, Donnan equilibrium and the law of electroneutrality. (Properties that are determined by the number rather than the nature of the particles present are termed 'colligative'. One of the most important points about colligative properties is that they are interrelated. They include such characteristics as the lowering of vapor pressure, the elevation of boiling point, the reduction of freezing point and osmotic pressure.)

The equivalent weight (gram equivalent) of an electrolyte

$$= \frac{\text{molecular weight in grams}}{\text{valency}}$$

e.g. sodium $\frac{23}{1} = 23$, calcium $\frac{40}{2} = 20$.

In the SI system (Système International d'Unités) the preferred unit for chemical measurement is the mole (the amount of a substance with a mass equal to its molecular weight expressed in grams). According to this system concentrations are expressed in millimoles/liter (mmol/L) rather than as milliequivalents/litre. The relationship between the numerical values is:

$$\frac{\text{mEq/L}}{\text{valency}} = \text{mmol/L}$$

therefore for monovalent species $\text{mEqL}^{-1} = \text{mmolL}^{-1}$

MOLARITY

Molarity is defined as the gram molecules (moles) of solute *per liter of solution.*

MOLALITY

Molality is defined as the gram molecules (moles) of solute *per kilogram of solvent.*

At all body temperatures 1 kg of water is regarded as occupying 1 liter.

The terms molarity and molality should not be confused. For dilute aqueous solutions they are approximately equal, but in the body the distinction is marked.

OSMOLARITY

One liter of solution containing 1 mole of undissociated solute represents an osmolarity of 1 osmol/L or 1000 mosmol/L. An aqueous solution of such concentration will exert an osmotic pressure of 22.4 atmospheres under ideal conditions and with an ideal membrane.

OSMOLALITY

Osmolality is applicable when the concentration of solute is molal. This term, unlike osmolarity, takes account of the solute volume.

For undissociated non-electrolyte solutions the molarity (molality) and osmolar (osmolal) concentrations are identical. For a substance dissociating fully into ions, however, each ion has the same osmotic effect as an undissociated molecule (i.e. dissociation increases the osmotic effect beyond that expected in terms of the molar content of the undissociated solute). A molar solution of sodium chloride (Na^+Cl^-) has, therefore, an ideal osmotic pressure of 2 × 22.4 atmospheres (2 osmoles). Calcium chloride ($Ca^{2+}2Cl^-$) yields three osmotically active ions if fully dissociated. In practice it is only with very dilute solutions that full dissociation occurs and the appropriate correction factor (osmotic coefficient) must be applied to calculate the osmolality when only the molality is known. Conversely association of macromolecules will result in a lowering of the theoretical osmotic pressure.

Solutions with the same osmotic pressure are termed isosmotic, and if separated by an 'ideal' membrane are termed isotonic when no net transfer of water occurs between them. Naturally most compartments in the body are in osmotic equilibrium although this does not apply to fluids such as urine and saliva. It is most convenient to determine osmolality by using an osmometer which actually measures the freezing point of plasma. Normal plasma osmolality is approximately 285 mosmol/kg body water.

Plasma and extracellular osmolality are closely related to the concentration of the major cation, sodium. A similar relationship exists between the osmolality of ICF and intracellular potassium concentration. The polyvalent protein anions contribute about 16 electrical milliequivalents per liter of plasma water but they only represent approximately two osmotically active particles per liter.

PHYSIOLOGICAL MOVEMENTS OF WATER AND ELECTROLYTES

When a solute is added to a solution on one side of a membrane there is a potential difference in concentration between the phases. Equilibrium can be established by:

- free distribution of the solute on both sides of the membrane (this is possible only with a diffusible solute and permeable membranes);
- passage of water through the membranes, thereby eliminating the potential difference by equalizing the number of water molecules per unit area on each side of the membrane;
- by applying pressure to the solution to increase the potential again to that of pure water.

The addition of a diffusible solute to one compartment thus results in an increase of total osmolality in both compartments without net water transfer. A non-diffusible solute increases the effective as well as total osmolality and results in a transfer of water from one compartment to the other (Fig. 15.3).

Physiologically, urea may be regarded as being a freely diffusible (penetrating) solute, and increasing the concentration of urea in the body causes no transfer of water between the phases. An exception is when urea is rapidly removed from the plasma by hemodialysis, when water moves into the ICF before outward diffusion of intracellular urea can occur. In diabetes mellitus the elevated plasma glucose concentration causes intracellular water loss, because glucose is not a diffusible solute in the absence of insulin.

Although sodium, potassium and chloride are freely diffusible, the fact that most of the sodium and chloride are found in the ECF and that the potassium is mainly intracellular demonstrates the presence of an active transport mechanism. The distribution of potassium between the ICF and ECF is heavily dependent upon the action of the Na^+/K^+ ATPase. This latter enzyme imports 2 × K^+ from the ECF and exports 3 × Na^+ from the ICF. Electrical neutrality may be preserved by the efflux of a Cl^-, which adds to the osmotic effect leading to a reduction of the ICF volume. The balance of potassium across the cell membrane otherwise contributes to the resting membrane electrical potential. Acid–base status, insulin and

Diffusible solute and permeable membrane

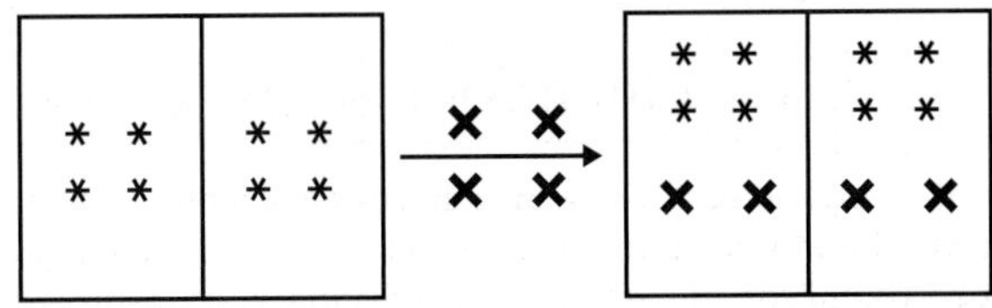

Non-diffusible solute

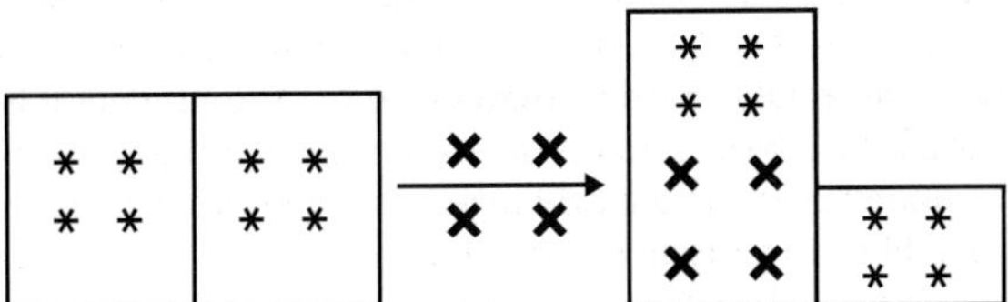

Fig. 15.3 Water distribution in response to changes in tonicity. In each example two fluid spaces are separated by a membrane which is permeable to water. The effect of adding solute to the left hand compartment is displayed on the right. Relative changes in volume accompany the movement of water.

catecholamines all exert effects upon the distribution of potassium across the cell membrane. Acidosis causes an efflux of potassium from the cell and alkalosis the reverse. The greatest effect occurs with mineral acids rather than lactic or keto acids where the cell is more permeable to the accompanying anions and the effects on potassium levels lag behind those of pH.

The fixed intracellular anions (protein and phosphate) are unable to traverse the membrane and their concentrations will largely determine the concentration of potassium in the ICF. Inhibiting cellular metabolism by cooling or by enzyme inhibitors results in the disappearance of the sodium and potassium gradients normally present. The maintenance of a high intracellular potassium content by cells in a saline medium requires the presence of oxygen, glucose and L-glutamate. The absence of any one of these materials results in entry of sodium into the cell and diffusion of potassium into the ECF. Thereafter, application of Donnan equilibrium (see below) allows entry of water and further sodium ions, causing swelling, and finally rupture of the cell.

The diffusion of chloride ions into or out of the cell is intimately related to the membrane potential.

Membrane potential

The cell membrane may be regarded as being permeable to water, potassium and chloride, but impermeable to protein, phosphate and sodium. An electrochemical potential difference exists between the two sides of the membrane, referred to as the membrane potential. This has been measured in various cells and within experimental error the relationship for calculating its value depends upon the relative concentrations of diffusible ions in the ECF and in the ICF.

A potential difference also exists across the membrane separating the intravascular phase of ECF (plasma) from the extravascular phase (interstitial fluid). This E_m is small since the gradients exhibited by sodium, potassium and chloride are not great. This is because sodium ions can penetrate capillary membranes freely, there being no active transport, and the electrolyte gradients result only from the presence of non-diffusible protein anions in plasma.

Donnan membrane equilibrium

When a diffusible solute is added to water on one side of a partially permeable membrane, rapid diffusion of the solute and water occurs between the phases. Small electrolyte differences occur when a non-diffusible ion (e.g. a plasma protein with anionic charge) is present on one side of the membrane. The drive to maintain electrical neutrality then causes movement of diffusible ions (Na^+ in our example) against their own concentration gradient. The number of diffusible ions that move increases disproportionately as the concentration gradient of protein rises and the result is a greater concentration of osmotically active particles in the phase containing the non-penetrating protein ion. The movement of protein itself across capillary membranes is resisted by a negative charge on the luminal surface of the vascular endothelium largely generated by glycosaminoglycan molecules. The osmotic effect exerted by colloids (colloid osmotic pressure or oncotic pressure) is quantitatively small but nevertheless it may be crucial in the fine balance of fluid movement across capillary beds.

These conditions exist even in the absence of active transport such as between plasma and interstitial fluid but can be magnified or opposed by active transport, which can maintain an intracellular ion at a constant concentration as though it were a non-penetrating ion. Unless opposed, there is a tendency for water to move into the compartment containing the constrained anion. The metabolic process preventing the entry of water into cells is directly related to the extrusion of sodium (Na^+/K^+ ATPase).

Hydrostatic and colloid osmotic pressure

Equilibrium in plasma is established between the formation and the reabsorption of interstitial fluid by the interplay of hydrostatic and colloid osmotic pressures.

The total osmotic pressure of plasma (285 mosmol/kg body water) is equivalent to about 6.5 atmospheres (5000 mmHg), but the proportion due to the colloid osmotic pressure of the proteins is small, being less than 30 mmHg. Since the interstitial fluid contains only small amounts of protein, the difference in colloid osmotic pressure (oncotic pressure) is equivalent to about 25 mmHg.

Although it is small, this figure is of fundamental physiological importance in controlling the flow of water between plasma and tissue fluids.

Since albumins have smaller molecular weights than globulins, approximately 80% of the plasma protein osmotic effect is due to albumin. Thus hypoalbuminemia predisposes to the formation of increased amounts of interstitial fluid, causing clinically detectable edema.

APPENDIX 2: ACID–BASE CHEMISTRY AND BLOOD GAS MEASUREMENT

An 'acid' is any molecule or ion which tends to donate a proton (H^+) and a 'base' is any molecule or ion which tends to accept a proton. Hence (as implied) the acidity of a solution is its hydrogen ion concentration.

	acid	proton	base
In general:	HB	H^+	B^-

B^- is referred to as the conjugate base of the acid HB (conjugate acid).

The more readily an acid donates a proton the stronger it is. The more readily a base accepts a proton the stronger it is. The dissociation of a conjugate acid to produce a proton occurs as part of an equilibrium described by an equilibrium constant 'K'

$$\text{where } K = \frac{[H^+]\,[B^+]}{[HB]}$$

K is large for strong acids and small for weak acids. Hence pK [the negative logarithm (to base 10) of K] is low for strong acids and high for weak acids. Biological acids may be neutral molecules, cations or anions. Biological bases may be anions or neutral molecules. Water is amphoteric (i.e. acts either as an acid or a base).

Sorensen introduced the term pH, which is the negative logarithm (to base 10) of the molal hydrogen ion activity. The term simplifies the appreciation of hydrogen ion concentration in relation to the behavior of buffers. Its use however can be misleading in clinical situations and the hydrogen ion concentration is the preferred nomenclature (see below).

Hydrogen ion activity $(H^+) = [H^+] \times f$, where f = activity coefficient.

In dilute aqueous solution f tends to 1.0 and (H^+) tends to $[H^+]$. It is, therefore, justifiable to derive the equation

$$pH = pK + \log \frac{[\text{conjugate base}]}{[\text{conjugate acid}]}$$

In clinical practice acid–base discussions are conducted using a shorthand based upon the carbonic acid/bicarbonate system which is quantitatively the most important buffer in plasma and whole blood. All the buffer systems are however in equilibrium so the approach may have some shortcomings. With these provisos the Henderson–Hasselbalch equation applies:

$$pH = pK + \log \frac{[HCO_3^-]}{[H_2CO_3]}$$

When considering the roles of respiratory and renal physiology on acid–base the equation may be considered as:

$$pH = pK + \log \frac{\text{renal component}}{\text{respiratory component.}}$$

'Buffers' are substances which tend to prevent a change in pH occurring within a system when either an acid or a base is added. Biological buffer systems are composed of a solution of weak acids together with their conjugate bases. Increases in the $[H^+]$ of the system cause conjugation of the buffer and vice versa. For any given addition of acid or base the change in ratio will be least (most efficient buffering) when:

$$[\text{conjugate base}] = [\text{conjugate acid}],$$

i.e. when $\log \frac{[\text{conjugate base}]}{[\text{conjugate acid}]} = 0$ and pH = pK

Chemically, the carbonic acid bicarbonate buffer system is not ideal for maintaining pH = 7.40, since the pK ≈ 6.1 and the ratio of buffer base:buffer acid is 20:1.

Fortunately the respiratory center is extremely sensitive to changes both in the CO_2 tension and the pH of plasma. This is the main reason why the system is effective physiologically in conserving blood pH within narrow limits.

BIOLOGICAL BUFFER SYSTEMS (Table 15.5)

The relative importance of the various buffers depends both upon their concentrations in the body compartments concerned and on the prevailing pH values. The bicarbonate system is the most important in plasma, with proteins and phosphate making smaller contributions. Hemoglobin is the most important buffer within erythrocytes, whilst within other cells the major buffers are phosphates and proteins.

Blood gas machines measure pH, PCO_2 and PO_2 and it is best to limit one's interpretation to these parameters. The machines however can perform calculations using assumptions (that may be erroneous) to derive other parameters such as the base excess. The sort of assumptions made in these calculations are: the relevant hemoglobin concentration (if it has not been measured), the solubility coefficient of carbon dioxide in plasma (which is assigned a designated value whereas it may vary) and constancy of the pK of the Henderson–Hasselbalch equation (which again may vary significantly. Given these assumptions, the following parameters may be presented:

- Base excess. The difference between the observed buffer base and the normal buffer base. The base excess is a measure of the metabolic contribution to the hydrogen ion concentration. It is an empirical expression which approximates (by calculation) the amount of acid (or base for a 'base deficit') which would be needed to titrate one liter of blood to a $[H^+]$ of 40 nmol/L (pH 7.4). The base excess of blood with a $[H^+]$ of 40 nmol/L, $PaCO_2$ 40 mmHg (5.33 kPa), total [Hb] 15 g/dl at 37°C is zero. In a metabolic acidosis where non-volatile acids such as lactic acid have accumulated, a negative base excess or base deficit results. Conversely, in a metabolic alkalosis the buffer base may increase, giving a positive base excess. In respiratory acidosis, for each moiety of H^+ produced, a corresponding increase in HCO_3^- occurs and total buffer base remains unaltered. A comparable situation occurs in respiratory alkalosis. Respiratory acidosis and alkalosis thus produce no change in the base excess unless renal compensation occurs.
- Standard bicarbonate. This is another index of the metabolic component. It is the calculated concentration of plasma bicarbonate in fully oxygenated blood at a PCO_2 of 40 mmHg and at 37°C. Normal range = 22–26 mmol/L plasma.
- Actual bicarbonate (mmol/L plasma) is the calculated bicarbonate content of the plasma.
- Total CO_2 content = actual bicarbonate + (PCO_2 mmHg × 0.03). This parameter is by definition a measure of both the metabolic and respiratory components of blood acid–base status. It is of interest to consider the possible effect of PCO_2 on the actual bicarbonate and total CO_2 content values, and to compare these with the unaltered standard bicarbonate.

Table 15.5 Biological buffer systems

Approximate % contribution to buffering of whole blood	Buffer acid (HB)	H^+	+	Buffer base⁻ (B^-)
64	H_2CO_3	H^+	+	HCO_3^-
1	$H_2PO_4^-$	H^+	+	HPO_4^{2-}
6	HPr	H^+	+	Pr^- (Pr = protein)
29	HHB	H^+	+	Hb^- (Hb = hemoglobin)

The strong ion theory has been proposed as a more comprehensive approach towards interpretation of acid–base.[19–21] The term 'strong ion' is used to describe species which are almost entirely dissociated at physiological pH (Na^+, K^+, Ca^{2+}, Mg^{2+}, Cl^-, lactate). The 'strong ion difference' is essentially a more comprehensive 'anion gap' calculated as the charge difference between the sum of measured strong cations and that of strong anions. It is regarded as an independent variable determining $[H^+]$ and as such is comparable to the 'buffer base' (the sum of the buffer anions in the blood). Hence falls in strong ion difference have an acidifying effect. The two other independent variables regarded as affecting $[H^+]$ are the PCO_2 and the charge from weak acids, increases of which also increase $[H^+]$. All three effect their influence on $[H^+]$ by altering the degree of dissociation of water (which is amphoteric) into hydrogen ions and hydroxyl groups. Other variables such as the concentration of bicarbonate ions are regarded as dependent variables to be in essence, ignored. Changes in dependent variables are impossible without changes in independent ones. Thus if PCO_2 and the charge from weak acids remain constant, hydrogen ion and bicarbonate can only be changed by altering the concentration of strong ions. The latter maneuver requires their movement between compartments or out of the body.[20,21]

To use the strong ion difference as an analytical approach in clinical practice requires more extensive laboratory activity. It has been asserted to be useful in some acid–base derangements such as hyperchloremic acidosis.[22]

PH VERSUS [H⁺]

Hydrogen ion concentration ([H^+]) has been used in place of pH in this chapter because in clinical practice physiological measurements and therapeutic influences create changes that are linear in [H^+] (as opposed to inverse logarithmic in pH) and therefore more easily interpreted.[23] For example, acute changes in $PaCO_2$ affect [H^+] in the ratio 1 kPa to 5.5 nmol/L. Tracking the [H^+] is intuitively easier and makes it easier to monitor the effect of therapeutic interventions, which have their effects primarily on the molar [H^+].

A change of 0.3 pH units is equivalent to a twofold change in the concentration of hydrogen ion because $\log_{10}2$ is 0.3. A pH of 7.4 corresponds to a [H^+] of 40 nmol/L. An increase of 40 nmol/L reduces the pH to 7.1. A similar numerical change in pH towards alkalosis (pH 7.7) involves a reduction in [H^+] of only 20 nmol/L (to halve the concentration). A drop in pH from 7.4 to 6.8 involves a sixfold increase in [H^+].

There is a counter to this argument which is becoming less relevant as the technology of blood gas machines improves. It is again linked to the linear versus logarithmic nature of the variables. When using ion specific electrodes (like a pH electrode) a precise value for the potential difference being measured is necessary to minimize error in the calculation of ionic concentration. The logarithmic transformation hides the errors in measurement of the potential difference in the decimal places of the pH. For example each millivolt error in measurement creates a 4% error in the calculated [H^+]. Whereas an error of more than 5 millivolts creates a change of only 0.1 pH units. Thus, when using [H^+] for clinical decisions, greater technical precision may be required and therefore better performance of the electrode in terms of drift and other errors.

FURTHER READING

Ganong WF. Review of medical physiology. Los Altos: McGraw Hill; 1999.

Halperin MLG. Fluid, electrolyte, and acid–base physiology: a problem-based approach. Philadelphia: WB Saunders; 1999:

REFERENCES (* Level 1 evidence)

1 Anderson PA. Maturation and cardiac contractility. Cardiol Clin 1989; 7(2):209–225.

2 Aperia A, Broberger O, Herin P, et al. Postnatal control of water and electrolyte homeostasis in pre-term and full-term infants. Acta Paediatr Scand Suppl 1983; 305:61–65.

3 Jaksic T, Shew SB, Keshen TH, et al. Do critically ill surgical neonates have increased energy expenditure? J Pediatr Surg 2001; 36(1):63–67.

4 Shew SB, Jaksic T. The metabolic needs of critically ill children and neonates. Semin Pediatr Surg 1999; 8(3):131–139.

5 Shann F. Paediatric fluid and electrolyte therapy. In: Oh TE, ed. Intensive care manual. Hong Kong: Butterworth-Heinemann; 1999.

6 Carlotti AP, Bohn D, Mallie JP, et al. Tonicity balance, and not electrolyte-free water calculations, more accurately guides therapy for acute changes in natremia. Intensive Care Med 2001; 27(5):921–924.

7 Ichikawa I. Pediatric textbook of fluids and electrolytes. Philadelphia: Williams & Wilkins; 1990.

8 West JB. Best and Taylor's physiological basis of medical practice. Philadelphia: Williams & Wilkins; 1989.

9 Domino KB, Swenson ER, Hlastala MP. Hypocapnia-induced ventilation/perfusion mismatch: a direct CO_2 or pH-mediated effect? Am J Respir Crit Care Med 1995; 152(5 pt 1):1534–1539.

10 Mackenzie A, Barnes G, Shann F. Clinical signs of dehydration in children. Lancet 1989; 2(8663):605–607.

11 Halberthal M, Halperin ML, Bohn D. Lesson of the week: Acute hyponatraemia in children admitted to hospital: retrospective analysis of factors contributing to its development and resolution. BMJ 2001; 322(7289):780–782.

12 Maesaka JK, Gupta S, Fishbane S. Cerebral salt-wasting syndrome: does it exist? Nephron 1999; 82(2):100–109.

13 Gill G, Leese G. Hyponatraemia: biochemical and clinical perspectives. Postgrad Med J 1998; 74(875):516–523.

14 Shann F. Drug doses 10th edn. Melbourne: Collective Pty; 1998.

15 Gross P, Reimann D, Neidel J, et al. The treatment of severe hyponatremia. Kidney Int Suppl 1998; 64:S6–11.

16 Porzio P, Halberthal M, Bohn D, et al. Treatment of acute hyponatremia: ensuring the excretion of a predictable amount of electrolyte-free water. Crit Care Med 2000; 28(6):1905–1910.

17 Arieff AI, Kleeman CR. Studies on mechanisms of cerebral edema in diabetic comas: effects of hyperglycemia and rapid lowering of plasma glucose in normal rabbits. (J Clin Invest 1973; 52:571–583). J Am Soc Nephrol 2000; 11(9):1776–1788.

18 Cooper GJ, Boron WF. Effect of PCMBS on CO_2 permeability of Xenopus oocytes expressing aquaporin 1 or its C189S mutant. Am J Physiol 1998; 275(6 pt 1):C1481–1486.

19 Kellum JA. Metabolic acidosis in the critically ill: lessons from physical chemistry. Kidney Int Suppl 1998; 66:S81–86.

20 Wooten EW. Strong ion difference theory: more lessons from physical chemistry. Kidney Int 1998; 54(5):1769–1770.

21 Wooten EW. Analytic calculation of physiological acid–base parameters in plasma. J Appl Physiol 1999; 86(1):326–334.

22 Kellum JA, Bellomo R, Kramer DJ, et al. Etiology of metabolic acidosis during saline resuscitation in endotoxemia. Shock 1998; 9(5):364–368.

23 Hooper J, Marshall WJ, Miller AL. Log-jam in acid–base education and investigation: why make it so difficult? Ann Clin Biochem 1998; 35(pt 1):85–93.

16

Disorders of the urinary system

Alan R Watson, C Mark Taylor, Mary McGraw

RENAL PHYSIOLOGY

The main function of the kidney is the regulation of water and electrolyte homeostasis, and excretion of nitrogenous and other waste products. Hormonal function is also important and includes the regulation of erythropoiesis, vitamin D and parathyroid hormone, as well as arterial blood pressure through the renin and angiotensin system. Water homeostasis is achieved by the nephrons and for simplicity their function can be considered in four parts:

1. ***Glomerular filtration.*** This refers to the bulk flow of plasma water across the glomerular capillary wall into Bowman's capsule. The process is rapid so that an amount of water equivalent to the entire plasma volume is cleared every 25–30 min. Filtration is passive and is driven by the glomerular intracapillary pressure, the work for which is generated by the left ventricle. The glomerular filtration rate (GFR) is closely regulated by adjusting intracapillary pressure through afferent and efferent arteriolar tone. Autoregulation keeps the GFR constant over a wide range of blood pressure. Superimposed on this there is also a circadian rhythm, which has an amplitude of about 25%. GFR also responds to physiological events, such as a high protein meal and pregnancy. In early infancy, the GFR, whether standardized for body surface area or for weight, is a fraction of that in older children and adults. Outside of the neonatal period it is conventional to express GFR per body surface area as this relationship holds constant from about 3 years of age until late adulthood, the normal being between 85 and 140 ml/min/1.73 m^2.

2. ***Isosmotic salt and water reabsorption.*** At least 80% of the filtered salt and water is recovered in the proximal tubule in the cortex of the kidney. Although this requires energy expenditure through Na^+-K^+-ATPase, the process is facilitated by the fact that plasma in the peritubular capillaries has a high oncotic pressure. Glomerular filtration is a selective process and proteins such as albumin are retained in the circulation. The plasma leaving the glomerulus, which goes on to supply the peritubular capillaries, is hyperoncotic and contributes an additional driving force for water reabsorption.

The active export of sodium from the basolateral surface of the proximal tubular cells by Na^+-K^+-ATPase creates an ionic and sodium gradient across the epithelium. This gradient is responsible for the cotransport systems, which recover glucose, phosphate and amino acids. Hydrogen ion secretion by the proximal epithelium is essential for the recovery of filtered bicarbonate. In the presence of apical carbonic anhydrase, H^+ and HCO_3 combine to form carbonic acid. This dissociates to carbon dioxide, which can readily enter the cell and is converted back to bicarbonate. The essential luminal hydrogen ion secretion, which permits this process, also depends on the sodium gradient. Failure of the sodium gradient for any reason gives rise to the Fanconi syndrome of impaired proximal tubular reabsorption of bicarbonate, glucose, phosphate and amino acids (see Fanconi's syndrome).

3. ***Urine dilution.*** In the thick ascending limb of the loop of Henle sodium is actively pumped into the renal interstitium. However, owing to the water proofing effect of Tamm–Horsfall protein, uniquely secreted into the lumen of this part of the nephron, water cannot follow. Nascent urine flowing along this section of the nephron therefore becomes increasingly dilute, achieving an osmolality of < 80 mOsm/kg. Meanwhile the renal interstitium becomes hyperosmolar, reaching 1400 mOsm/kg in the renal papillae, the deepest part of the medulla (Fig. 16.1).

An important anatomical feature is that at the end of the diluting section, the nephron is reflected back to pass by the hilum of its own glomerulus. Here the specialized tubular cells of the macula densa relate intimately with the juxtaglomerular apparatus and both the afferent and efferent arterioles. At this site tubular performance is policed, and filtration regulated by a process referred to as tubuloglomerular feedback. If there is a major failure of tubular reabsorption upstream of the macula densa there will be increased sodium chloride delivery to this site which in turn signals for downregulation of filtration. The kidney fails safely. One can appreciate that the low GFR observed in infancy is an appropriate response to the smaller capacity for salt and water recovery by the relatively short proximal tubules. Newborns are much more dependent on the distal nephron for electrolyte reabsorption. This is one of the reasons why mineralocorticoid deficiency has such profound effects in the newborn compared to older subjects.

4. ***Urine concentration.*** Beyond the macula densa the distal nephron, derived originally from the ureteric bud, has two special properties. One is the presence of epithelial sodium channels (EnaC). These are the rate-limiting step for sodium recovery and are synthesized in response to aldosterone. This system allows fine tuning of sodium balance by reabsorbing sodium in exchange for hydrogen ion and potassium. Healthy children exposed to salt restriction can almost fully recover sodium in the nephron. However, newborns commonly have a fractional excretion of 1%, and in preterm infants as much as 5% of the filtered sodium load. Aldosterone is stimulated not only by the renin–angiotensin system but also directly by the plasma potassium concentration, a feature which assists in excretion of a potassium load. The second feature is

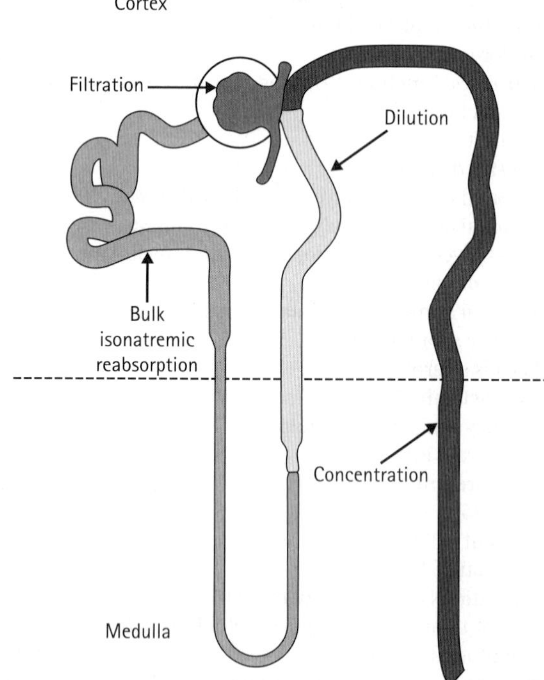

Fig. 16.1 Simplified drawing of a nephron. Isonatremic reabsorption of tubular fluid takes place in the proximal tubule in the cortex. The thick ascending limb of the loop of Henle is a diluting segment in which sodium chloride is avidly recovered but water does not follow. All the distal nephron can be regarded as a functional whole. It is derived from the original ureteric bud. It is responsive to hormones that regulate volume osmolality and potassium concentrate. Note that the junction between the diluting and concentrating segments meets at the juxtaglomerular apparatus of the self-same nephron providing a point at which tubular performance regulates the rate of glomerular filtration.

the presence of aquaporins, membrane bound molecules which under the influence of vasopressin permit the passage of water. In this case, water moves down an osmotic gradient from the dilute urine arriving in the distal nephron to the hyperosmolar medullary interstitium surrounding the collecting ducts. The maximum urine concentration capacity thus depends on the presence of vasopressin, the integrity of vasopressin-2 receptor and aquaporin assembly, as well as a high medullary interstitial solute (sodium and urea). In breast-fed infants, whose dietary protein is efficiently used for anabolism, there is proportionately less for urea generation. Thus the maximal medullary concentration and urine concentration capacity is reduced. In health, and with adequate protein intake, children over 6 months of age can generate urine concentration > 870 mOsm/kg and figures approaching this can be achieved from the early weeks of life.

At least 80% of the filtered salt and water is recovered in the proximal tubule

Over 6 months of age urine concentrations of > 800 mosmol/kg can be generated and this concentration would be the end point in a water deprivation test for diabetes insipidus

Predicted GFR ml/min/1.73m² = 40 × ht(cm)/plasma creatinine μmol/L

ASSESSMENT OF RENAL FUNCTION

MEASUREMENT OF GFR

There is no direct way to measure the bulk flow of plasma water into Bowman's capsule. However, by assuming that small molecules traverse the capillary wall as easily as water, and using a low molecular weight marker substance which is neither absorbed nor excreted by the tubule, nor bound to proteins or lipids, one can calculate GFR. A time-honored marker is inulin, an inert sugar with a molecular weight of 5500 which can be measured with accuracy in plasma and urine. After an intravenous loading dose, an infusion is maintained to provide a constant plasma concentration of inulin (P). One then needs to know either the mass of inulin excreted over a fixed time (urine volume × urine concentration, UV), or, assuming a steady state the dose of inulin infused, which should be the same, one can then deduce the theoretical volume of plasma that contains the mass of inulin excreted per minute using the formula: (UV)/P. The volume of plasma cleared of its inulin can then be regarded as the net volume of water that has been filtered; the glomerular filtration rate. It is convention to express this rate per 1.73 m^2, the average body surface area of an adult man. This allows comparison of rate between individuals of different stature and holds true down to 3 years of age.

In clinical practice, one seldom requires the precision of inulin clearance methods and such tests are best reserved for specialist departments. The same can be said for slope clearance methods, although they have the important advantage that timed urine collections are not required. In slope clearance methods, a bolus of a marker (inulin, ^{51}Cr edetic acid, or ^{99m}Tc DTPA) is injected rapidly into a vein. Following this there is a complex distribution into the extracellular fluid space, as well as clearance from the circulation by glomerular filtration. After approximately 1 h, the plasma concentration falls exponentially. Two or more plasma samples are then taken over the next few hours and from the slope of the declining concentration one can estimate the theoretical volume of distribution at the moment of injection and the half-time when 50% of the marker has been cleared. From this information, GFR can be estimated. Precision of this method is excellent except at very high filtration rates.

Endogenous creatinine is a useful, although imperfect, marker with which to measure clearance. Formal creatinine clearance studies relying on timed urine samples have poor precision, probably because children are unable to void to completion on demand. There is *no* place for such tests in routine pediatric practice. More accurate, reproducible and user friendly is the interpretation of plasma creatinine in relation to a child's height. In the steady state creatinine excretion (UV creatinine) is matched by creatinine synthesis in muscle and is thus related in turn to muscle mass and body weight. Body weight and height also feature in the calculation of surface area in the denominator of the GFR expression. Although the logic is tortuous this conveniently resolves to the formula:

GFR/body surface area = (body height/plasma creatinine) × constant

Much hinges on the accuracy of plasma creatinine measurement, especially at the low concentrations of normal range. New automated methods overcome errors from drugs or non-creatinine chromogens. Using these methods, and with the child's height in cm and plasma creatinine expressed in μmol/L, the constant in the above equation is approximately 40. Put another way, in children outside infancy, if the body height/creatinine ratio is > 2cm/μmol/L, GFR is likely to be normal; if < 1.5 it is certainly reduced and there is uncertainty between these two ranges. The formula performs well when used sequentially to follow GFR in an individual.

Given that tubular performance upstream of the macula densa governs filtration rate by tubular glomerular feedback mechanisms, clinicians are able to use estimates of GFR as a guide to whole kidney performance. It is not surprising that some of the most abrupt and severe reductions of GFR are caused by interstitial or tubular injury rather than isolated glomerulonephritis. The corollary of this is that extensive glomerular destruction may occur with little, if any, change in plasma creatinine. In a disorder, which gives a progressive loss of nephrons over time, surviving nephrons will exhibit hyperfiltration. Thus considerable nephron loss has to occur before there is any downward trend in GFR; renal impairment is a late indicator. It is helpful to correlate impaired GFR with kidney size as determined, for example, by ultrasound. If kidney size is normal, or perhaps increased, while GFR is impaired, it is likely that the nephron population is intact but parenchymal injury has induced a shutdown of filtration. The causes may be inflammatory, drug induced, metabolic as in hypoxia or recent ischemia, or secondary to malignant infiltration. By contrast, if both kidneys are small it is likely that the nephron population is reduced because of some previous destructive process. Small echobright kidneys with normal contours might suggest a previous glomerulonephritis. Small kidneys with an irregular outline are seen following the coarse scarring of pyelonephritis or secondary to renal dysplasia.

PROXIMAL TUBULAR FUNCTION

Glucose is not normally detected by conventional glucose oxidase strip reagent until the plasma glucose concentration exceeds 10 mmol/L, the renal threshold for glucose. Glycosuria occurring at a lower threshold may indicate an isolated transport defect, idiopathic renal glycosuria. If this occurs in conjunction with other markers of proximal tubular dysfunction it implies either renoparenchymal injury, chronic renal failure or the Fanconi syndrome.

Amino acids are readily filtered in the glomerulus and extensively reabsorbed in the proximal tubule by five separate cotransport systems:

1. basic amino acids and cystine
2. glutamic and aspartic acids
3. neutral amino acids
4. imino acids
5. glycine.

At very high plasma concentrations an amino acid may overspill into the urine. With normal plasma concentrations, newborns frequently have mild generalized aminoaciduria as a transient event. Otherwise, generalized aminoaciduria with normal plasma concentrations indicates tubulopathy in exactly the same way as glycosuria (above). Specific patterns of aminoaciduria imply isolated transport defects, e.g. cystinuria.

Phosphate is extensively recovered in the proximal tubule. However, the amount of phosphate filtered is close to the maximum rate of recovery, so that small changes in recovery rate govern plasma phosphate concentrations. Under normal conditions phosphate reabsorption will exceed 80% and the fractional excretion will therefore be less than 20% of filtered load. The fractional excretion can be calculated easily for any compound freely filtered at the glomerulus by comparing its clearance with that of creatinine:

Fractional excretion of x (%) = (urine x/plasma x) ÷ (urine creatinine/plasma creatinine) × 100

Calcium is partly bound to protein and only the ionised fraction, about 50% of the total, is available for filtration. In the proximal tubule calcium reabsorption is proportionate to salt and water reabsorption. Thereafter there is both passive and active reabsorption in the loop of Henle. Ten per cent of the filtered calcium then reaches the distal nephron and of this two-thirds will be reabsorbed. Hypercalciuria can be readily diagnosed by urine calcium/creatinine ratio. The normal upper limit in children is given below:

Age range	*Urine calcium/creatinine (molar)*
0–6 months	< 2.4 mmol/mmol
7–18 months	< 1.7 mmol/mmol
1½ > –6 years	< 1.2 mmol/mmol
7 years–adult	0.7 mmol/mmol

DISTAL TUBULAR FUNCTION

Although the ability to excrete a water load can be tested, it has little clinical relevance. Impairment of water excretion occurs in the syndrome of inappropriate antidiuretic hormone (ADH) secretion and an extremely rare familial condition that mimics it in which ADH is not the cause. These conditions are suggested by a low plasma sodium concentration in the absence of dehydration.

T*ests of urine concentration capacity*, by contrast, are important. A simple screening test is to measure the urine osmolality on the first urine sample voided in the morning after fluids are restricted at bedtime. A urine osmolality value of 600 mosmol/kg is generally taken as excluding significant impairment of urinary concentration. However, in a recent study in 318 apparently healthy children with a median age of 9.8 years the median osmolality was 845 mOsm/kg (range 275–1344). Only 82% of males and 75% of females had an osmolality of 600 mosmol or more.[1]

If the diagnosis of diabetes insipidus is entertained, a water deprivation test should only be undertaken in hospital with close observation of hydrational status. The end point is either a urine concentration capacity > 800 mosmol/kg or a 3% body weight loss, by which time the plasma osmolality should be rising and in excess of 295 mOsm/kg. If the latter, the final urine osmolality would be accepted as the *concentration capacity*. In fully expressed diabetes insipidus a urine osmolality will remain lower than that of plasma. As well as the obvious risks, young children find water deprivation disagreeable. A screening test for the ability to concentrate urine is to administer DDAVP 20 μg nasally (10 μg for infants) in the normally hydrated state. At 1 h children are asked to void and that urine sample is discarded. Between 1 and 5 h after DDAVP normal children will produce a urine osmolality in excess of 800 mOsm/kg (infants < 600 mosml/kg). Patients with pituitary diabetes insipidus will respond to this test either normally or they will achieve osmolalities close to normal. Failure to respond implies either nephrogenic diabetes insipidus, in which case the urine osmolality will be below that of plasma, or chronic renoparenchymal disease, where the urine osmolality will be similar to plasma concentrations. Normality and fully expressed diabetes insipidus are easy to distinguish. Problems arise when the urine osmolality falls between 300 and 870 mOsm/kg. Often this is because the water deprivation study has not been conducted rigorously. Also habitual water drinkers, especially those with poor dietary protein intake, have a reduced medullary solute concentration and underachieve for this reason. Reductions in maximal urine concentration capacity may be seen in any renoparenchymal disorder, including recent upper urinary tract infection. As chronic renal failure progresses, concentrating and diluting capacity is lost and urine osmolality approaches that of plasma.

TESTS OF RENAL TUBULAR ACIDOSIS

The kidney is responsible for the excretion of a small proportion of the total acid production of the body, this being those acids which cannot be metabolized to carbon dioxide and water and eliminated by respiration. Thus in severe renal failure patients develop a moderate acidosis with an *increased* anion gap. The acidosis of chronic renal failure is readily corrected by 1–2 mmol/kg/day of administered bicarbonate. Renal tubular acidosis describes the hyperchloremic acidemia with a *normal* anion gap, (Na + K) – (Cl + HCO_3) = < 20 mmol/L, which occurs with normal glomerular function. There is either a failure to recover filtered bicarbonate, an inability to secrete hydrogen ion or both.

In the proximal tubule H^+ is buffered by bicarbonate and leads to net bicarbonate recovery via the formation of carbon dioxide. Less than 10% of the filtered bicarbonate is presented to the distal nephron. In the distal nephron, where luminal bicarbonate is at a low concentration, two other buffering systems are proportionately more important. One is the tubular secretion of ammonia (NH_3) generated by the deamination of glutamine. In the presence of H^+ an ammonium (NH_4^+) ion forms which is unable to diffuse back across the tubular epithelium. The second is the conversion of filtered alkaline phosphate HPO_4^{2-} to acid phosphate $H_2PO_4^-$. These buffers allow the urine to 'carry' more hydrogen ion. In health, the actual H^+ gradient becomes apparent in that the urine can be made acid with a pH as low as 4.5.

Complex tests of *urine* acidification are seldom required in clinical practice. A simple overnight fast would be a sufficient stimulus in most people to induce a urine pH < 5.5 in the first voided urine in the morning. However, a recent study in healthy schoolchildren demonstrated that only eight children had a urine pH of 5.4 or less on the first morning sample.[1] To test the maximum H^+ gradient delivered by the distal nephron it may be necessary to induce a metabolic acidemia by administration of ammonium chloride enterically. In distal renal tubular acidosis (*type 1 RTA*) urine pH remains above 6.5 even if the plasma bicarbonate is reduced to < 22 mmol/L. This test is seldom required as type 1 RTA patients typically present with sufficient systemic acidosis to observe the inappropriately alkaline urine. Moreover, correction of acidosis occurs at modest doses of sodium bicarbonate such as 3–5 mmol/kg body weight per day.

90% of bicarbonate is recovered in the proximal tubule, and the remainder distally, so that the threshold at which bicarbonate normally starts to appear in the urine is a plasma concentration of 25–26 mmol/L. In infants this threshold is rather lower at approximately 22 mmol/L. In patients presenting with hyperchloremic acidosis in whom proximal renal tubular acidosis is suspected, sodium bicarbonate is infused intravenously to lift the plasma concentration of bicarbonate. The bicarbonate concentrations in paired plasma and urine samples are plotted, thus determining the renal threshold. Note that while the plasma bicarbonate concentration is below the threshold for bicarbonate recovery it is possible for normal distal mechanisms of urinary acidification to produce an acid urine. A simple clue to proximal renal tubular acidosis is the very large requirement for replacement bicarbonate to improve the acidemia. Often this amounts to more than 10 mmol/kg/day which is quite unlike that required to control the acidemia of chronic renal failure or distal (type 1) renal tubular acidosis.

RENAL TUBULAR DISORDERS

Defects in renal tubular transport may result in marked derangements in electrolyte and mineral homeostasis with significant morbidity. Recent advances in molecular genetics and biology have provided exciting new insights into the function of specific transport proteins and the physiology of renal tubular handling of solutes for many of these inherited disorders.[2]

FANCONI'S SYNDROME

The Fanconi syndrome consists of a generalized failure of proximal tubular reabsorption. That is to say that all cotransport systems fail together suggesting a primary problem in the cells maintaining their polarized state. This leads to glycosuria, phosphaturia, calciuria, bicarbonaturia and generalized hyperaminoaciduria. Proximal sodium reabsorption also fails and the distal nephron, driven by aldosterone, attempts to recover sodium, but only at the expense of potassium and hydrogen ion secretion. Hypokalemia results and is often severe. The salt and water wasting gives rise to polyuria, polydipsia and failure to thrive. Usually children exhibit a metabolic acidosis secondary to the urinary loss of bicarbonate (type 2 renal tubular acidosis). However, distal hydrogen ion secretion in most forms of Fanconi's syndrome is normal, and during periods of hypovolemia and reduced glomerular filtration, the pH of urine may actually fall below 5.5. In states of extreme dehydration hypokalemic alkalosis may be seen. At other times hypokalemia with *acidosis* is a strong pointer to a proximal tubular lesion. The hypokalemia itself may aggravate the proximal tubular nephropathy as well as giving rise to muscle weakness, growth retardation and constipation. The glycosuria and aminoaciduria, in themselves have little in the way of clinical sequelae. The hypercalciuria is not associated with urinary stone formation, probably because of the very high urine flow rate. Plasma calcium concentrations tend to be normal. By contrast hypophosphatemia is the principal cause of the osteopenia and rickets of the Fanconi syndrome.

In clinical practice Fanconi's syndrome is rare. The causes are legion and include primary disorders, sometimes familial with a variety of inherited patterns. Some of these are likely to prove to be secondary to respiratory chain defects and one type has been described in which the brush border of the proximal tubular cell is absent. The condition can arise secondarily due to intoxication by heavy metals or drugs and in relation to other inborn errors of metabolism (see Table 16.1). However, by far the commonest single cause of the Fanconi syndrome is *nephropathic cystinosis* and this condition is therefore dealt with in more detail.

Cystinosis

Cystinosis is a rare metabolic disorder inherited as an autosomal recessive trait. The gene responsible for the condition lies on chromosome 17p, and codes for cystinosin, a lysosomal transmembrane protein essential for the transport of cystine.[3] In the disorder cystine is stored intracellularly in lysosomes and there is a defect in the ability to transport cystine back into the cytoplasm. How this disrupts tubular function is unknown at present. Various patterns of cystinosis have been described. In the benign adult form cystine crystals are deposited only in the cornea, bone marrow and leukocytes; there appears to be no renal involvement. A juvenile form of the disorder includes a slowly progressive nephropathy, which becomes manifest in the second decade of life. By contrast, infantile nephropathic cystinosis is the most severe form. These infants appear normal at birth and the disorder becomes apparent at around 6 months of age with failure to thrive, polyuria, polydipsia, episodes of dehydration and unexplained fever. Rickets occurs early.

Over the first few years the glomerular filtration rate remains normal, and it is during this early stage that abrupt episodes of dehydration and electrolyte disturbance precipitated by intercurrent infective illnesses can prove fatal. The GFR declines with time so that end-stage renal failure is reached in untreated patients within 10 years of diagnosis. There is profound growth retardation and photophobia is a universal complaint due to cystine deposition in the eye. In later childhood, children have biochemical evidence of hypothyroidism and hypercholesterolemia.

The diagnosis is confirmed by the positive identification of cystine deposition. In the first months of life the kidneys look histologically normal, but later the birefringent crystals of cystine can be seen in the interstitial tissue between tubules. Interstitial fibrosis then occurs so that the kidneys in time become small and contracted. Crystals can be seen in the cornea by slit lamp examination of the eye. The cystine concentration of leukocytes can be measured, and this test can be applied shortly after birth. Antenatal diagnosis is also possible, cystine measurements being made on fibroblasts obtained from amniotic fluid or chorionic villus sampling.

Cystinosis patients are difficult to manage and require careful electrolyte supplementation. Many need tube feeding to ensure an adequate salt, water and calorific intake.[4] Attempts to reduce the

Table 16.1 Associations with Fanconi's syndrome

Inborn errors of metabolism
Nephropathic cystinosis
Lowe's syndrome (oculocerebrorenal dystrophy)
Glycogen storage
Galactosemia
Fructose intolerance
Tyrosinemia type 1
Wilson's disease (hepatolenticular dystrophy)
Tubulotoxic events
Drugs, e.g. tetracycline, ifosfamide
Heavy metals, e.g. lead, cadmium, uranium, mercury, thallium
Maleic acid (experimental)

glomerular filtration rate, and thus the electrolyte loss, using indometacin are advocated. Cysteamine treatment can mobilize intralysosomal cystine and deplete cystine in cells. Cysteamine has a foul taste and compliance with this therapy is often poor. However, where cysteamine therapy or phosphocysteamine therapy has been given early with rigid compliance, children have retained kidney function longer than expected.[5]

Once end-stage renal failure is reached, renal transplantation is an effective treatment. The transplant may become colonized by host cells, which will store cystine, but the tubular cells of the donor do not have the underlying biochemical defect and long term kidney function is satisfactory. Concern is raised, however, that long term survivors risk previously unrecognized complications such as corneal degeneration, diabetes mellitus, and cerebral atrophy.

Renal tubular disorders are rare but important causes of failure to thrive and electrolyte disturbances

Cystinosis is the commonest cause of a Fanconi syndrome

Nephrocalcinosis is an early complication of type 1 renal tubular acidosis but does not occur in type 2 proximal RTA

RENAL TUBULAR ACIDOSIS

Renal tubular acidosis refers to conditions in which there are defects in the tubular reabsorption of bicarbonate, the excretion of hydrogen ion or both.[6] They can be primary disorders, or secondary to a wide range of pathogenic insults to the tubular cells. Four types are described (see also Table 16.2).

Type 1 renal tubular acidosis

Permanent distal renal tubular acidosis (*type 1 RTA*) is more often a sporadic disease, although families with autosomal dominant inheritance are well described. The nature of the cellular defect is known. For example, an autosomal recessive form with accompanying sensorineural deafness is caused by a mutation in the beta subunit of H^+-ATPase located in the apical membrane of intercalated cells of the distal nephron.[7] A mutation of a 116 kDa subunit of H^+-ATPase is found in autosomal recessive type 1 RTA without hearing loss.[8] The resulting functional defect prevents active hydrogen ion secretion. Defects in anion exchange mechanisms have been found in autosomal dominant forms of type 1 RTA.[9] Infants present with growth retardation, vomiting, polydipsia, constipation and dehydration, although these symptoms may be mild and in sporadic or autosomal dominant cases the diagnosis is often not made until the child is more than 2 years of age. Osteomalacia and rickets do not occur, with the exception of the autosomal recessive form with normal hearing, but nephrocalcinosis is an early complication secondary to the accompanying hypercalciuria and hypocitraturia. Treatment demands life-long therapy with bicarbonate or citrate. While the acidosis is readily correctable with modest doses of bicarbonate, 3–5 mmol/kg body weight per day, higher doses of 5–7 mmol/kg and good compliance with therapy is essential if progressive nephrocalcinosis is to be avoided. The long term stability of renal function depends on control of nephrocalcinosis.

Table 16.2 Classification of renal tubular acidosis (RTA)

Type 1 – Distal RTA
Primary
– sporadic, familial (autosomal dominant)
– transient infantile
Secondary
– interstitial nephritis, hypergammaglobulinemia, transplant rejection
– hypercalciuria, nephrocalcinosis
– drugs, lithium, amphotericin
Type 2 – Proximal RTA
Primary
Secondary – Fanconi's syndrome
Type 3 – Mixed proximal and distal RTA
Type 4 – Hyperkalemic RTA
Hypoaldosteronism, Addison's disease, congenital adrenal hyperplasia
Pseudohypoaldosteronism
Distal tubular dysfunction, e.g. obstructive uropathy
Hyperreninemia, hypoaldosteronism in chronic renal failure
Angiotensin-converting enzyme inhibitors
Early childhood hyperkalemia RTA (transient)

Type 2 renal tubular acidosis

Proximal renal tubular acidosis (*type 2 RTA*) occurs because of failed bicarbonate reabsorption in the nephron. As a primary disorder both autosomal recessive and autosomal dominant inheritance patterns have been described. The molecular mechanisms are less well understood than in type 1 RTA, but abnormalities in the Na/HCO_3 cotransporter have been found in a case with ocular lesions. A transient form of type 2 RTA occurs in infants. In any child suspected of having type 2 RTA it is important to look for other evidence of proximal tubular dysfunction as bicarbonate wasting occurs as part of the Fanconi syndrome. Patients with type 2 RTA present with growth retardation and vomiting. Because they have normal urine acidification mechanisms in the distal nephron nephrocalcinosis does not occur. The low bicarbonate threshold means that the more one increases the plasma concentration therapeutically, the greater the urine loss. Thus massive bicarbonate replacement is needed to control the acidemia, often more than 10–15 mmol of bicarbonate/kg body weight/day.

Type 3 renal tubular acidosis

The term *type 3 RTA* is used to describe a mixed picture of both proximal and tubular defects and can occur with almost any renoparenchymal injury.

Type 4 renal tubular acidosis

Type 4 RTA is probably the most common subtype in children. In this there is hyperchloremic acidosis with hyperkalemia and usually an acid urine during acidosis. The pathogenesis is linked to $H^+/K^+/Na^+$ exchange in the collecting duct. It is therefore seen in states of mineralocorticoid deficiency such as congenital adrenal hyperplasia and Addison's disease. Similarly it is seen in pseudohypoaldosteronism in which there is end organ unresponsiveness to aldosterone, for example with mutations causing loss of function of the epithelial sodium channel, or occasionally in conditions where there is direct damage to the renal medulla as in obstructive uropathy. In all these cases there is accompanying salt wasting which is most evident in the very young child who relies heavily on the distal nephron for physiological sodium reabsorption. Type 4 RTA can also occur with hyporeninism and hypoaldosteronism in chronic renal failure patients who are not volume depleted. An isolated early childhood form of type 4 RTA has been described. This occurs without salt wasting and the condition resolves by 5 years of age. Both sexes are affected and the disorder appears in siblings. High dose alkaline therapy may be required (up to 20 mmol/kg/day), but this dose independently corrects the hyperkalemia. Nephrocalcinosis does not occur and the underlying nature of the defect is not known.

HYPOKALEMIC ALKALOSIS

Severe potassium chloride wasting can occur from either the gastrointestinal tract or from the kidney. Examples of the first include pyloric stenosis, laxative abuse or familial chloride diarrhea. In these situations the kidney will initially respond appropriately by avid electrolyte conservation and a reduction in urine output. However, if potassium deficiency is severe enough, proximal tubular cells become vacuolated and lose their ability to reabsorb salt and water. In this situation, there can be an additional proximal tubular defect causing inappropriate salt and water loss – hypokalemic nephropathy.

Renal potassium wasting occurs in covert diuretic abuse, notably with furosemide (frusemide), or as a group of primary disorders generally referred to as *Bartter's syndrome*. The hypokalemic alkalosis of all of the above disorders is accompanied by various degrees of *extracellular fluid volume depletion*. It is this feature that distinguishes them from the hypokalemia and alkalosis of actual or apparent mineralocorticoid excess, in which there is enhanced sodium and water reabsorption in the distal nephron giving rise to *extracellular sodium expansion* and hypertension (see below).

Bartter's syndrome

Bartter's syndrome is a rare disorder, either familial or sporadic, which can affect both children and adults. The pathogenesis is best explained by a failure of chloride reabsorption in the thick ascending limb of the loop of Henle, thus resembling the pharmacological effect of furosemide (frusemide). Three subtypes have been described with loss of function mutations in the furosemide (frusemide)-sensitive Na-K-2 Cl cotransporter (type 1), the potassium channel regulator ROMK (type 2) or the basolateral chloride channel CLCNKB (type 3).[10–12] However there are cases where the molecular abnormality has not been found. As a secondary response to salt wasting, there is activation of the renin–angiotensin–aldosterone pathway in an attempt to recover sodium chloride in the distal nephron. This is achieved at the expense of increased potassium and hydrogen ion secretion, which largely explains the hypokalemic alkalosis.

Children present with failure to thrive, hypotonia, lethargy, poor feeding, polydipsia and polyuria. There is a wide spectrum of disease expression with a severe form presenting in the neonatal period. Such infants are usually born prematurely after a pregnancy complicated by polyhydramnios. In early life they may become so volume depleted as to experience secondary oliguric renal failure, during which time the hypokalemic alkalosis is masked. Dehydration also gives rise to episodes of fever and developmental delay. In this group, there is hypercalciuria and bone demineralization, which may be secondary to the increased production of prostaglandins PGE_2 and PGI_2, which are found in this and other forms of Bartter's syndrome. Nephrocalcinosis is a serious and early complication except in type 3. The neonatal form of Bartter's syndrome, first described by Fanconi in 1971, has at times been inappropriately titled calcium losing tubulopathy, or primary hyperprostaglandin E syndrome.

Management consists of potassium, sodium and chloride replacement. Prostaglandin inhibitors such as indometacin 3 mg/kg daily in divided dose are indicated, and angiotensin-converting enzyme inhibitors such as captopril may give additional control.

Bartter's syndrome presenting in older children may run a relatively mild course without hypercalciuria or nephrocalcinosis. Simple potassium supplementation may be all that is required.

Gitelman's syndrome

Gitelman's syndrome is a distinct autosomal recessive disorder in which there is renal loss of both potassium and magnesium so that hypokalemia and hypomagnesemia are combined with metabolic alkalosis and hypocalciuria. If Bartter's syndrome is analagous to the effects of furosemide (frusemide), Gitelman's syndrome mimics the effects of thiazide diuretics, and mutations have been confirmed in the thiazide sensitive cotransporter gene (NCCT). These patients present with muscle weakness, particularly after exercise. Many patients come to medical attention incidentally when they are investigated for intercurrent illnesses.[13] The salt wasting is mild in comparison to Bartter's syndrome and growth and renal function are unaffected. Potassium and/or magnesium supplements help to ameliorate symptoms.

Hypokalemic alkalosis with extracellular sodium expansion

Hypokalemic alkalosis, with volume expansion and hypertension, can occur because of increased sodium recovery by the epithelial sodium channel with consequent secretion of potassium and hydrogen ions. An obvious cause of this is mineralocorticoid excess, as in *Conn's syndrome*; vanishingly rare in childhood. However, there are other conditions with similar dynamics of increased distal sodium recovery in which plasma aldosterone concentrations are suppressed or normal. These are referred to as disorders of *apparent mineralocorticoid excess*. One of these is 11beta-hydroxysteroid dehydrogenase deficiency, a rare inherited disorder in which the conversion of cortisol to cortisone at the site of the mineralocorticoid receptor is defective. As a result, physiologically normal amounts of cortisol can directly operate the mineralocorticoid receptor in the collecting duct, thus driving distal sodium reabsorption. Children present with severe labile hypertension and failure to thrive. Hypercalciuria and nephrocalcinosis occur. The condition is inherited as an autosomal recessive. Another is *Liddle syndrome*. In this, mutations in the beta or gamma subunit of the amiloride-sensitive epithelial sodium channel give rise to a constitutive gain of function; the opposite of pseudohypoaldosteronism type 1. The syndrome is familial and can present clinically either in childhood or adult life. Treatment of both these disorders consists of amiloride to reverse the salt and water retention. This controls blood pressure and normalizes plasma potassium.

Renal tubular hyperkalemia

This refers to the failure of the tubules to secrete potassium in conditions other than chronic renal failure. This can occur if there is a failure in the renin–angiotensin–aldosterone pathway. Examples would include treatment with angiotensin-converting enzyme inhibitors such as captopril and the failure to synthesize mineralocorticoid in the salt-losing forms of congenital adrenal hypoplasia. In these situations, there will also be reduced ability to secrete hydrogen ion resulting in type 4 renal tubular acidosis (see above).

Primary pseudohypoaldosteronism type I is an autosomal dominant disorder with variable penetrance. There is loss of function of the epithelial sodium channel in the distal tubule leading to salt wasting, volume contraction, hyperkalemia and metabolic acidosis (type 4 renal tubular acidosis). Aldosterone is appropriately elevated both by the high potassium and via the activated renin–angiotensin pathway. Infants present in the neonatal period with failure to thrive, vomiting and dehydration. As they do not respond to synthetic mineralocorticoids, they are dependent on sodium supplements. Once past 2 years of age the salt wasting improves as the kidney becomes less dependent upon the distal nephron for sodium recovery, but sodium replacement is still needed to optimize growth.

Early childhood hyperkalemia describes a transient disorder in infants presenting with hyperkalemia and type 4 renal tubular acidosis, and thus similar initially to pseudohypoaldosteronism type I. They present with failure to thrive and vomiting. Salt wasting is variable being absent in some cases, and blood pressure is normal. There appears to be end organ unresponsiveness to aldosterone as plasma concentrations of aldosterone may be elevated. Treatment consists of bicarbonate and, if necessary, a controlled potassium intake or even potassium ion exchange resins. Growth appears to normalize by 6 months and therapy can be discontinued at about 5 years of age.

Gordon's syndrome *(pseudohypoaldosteronism type II, or 'chloride shunt' syndrome)* is a rare disorder of hyperkalemia, hyperchloremic metabolic acidosis, volume expansion and hypertension. Plasma renin activity and aldosterone concentrations are suppressed. Patients may also have hypercalciuria and a tendency to stone formation. The mechanism of the disorder at a cellular level is unknown beyond the concept that there is unregulated chloride reabsorption. Treatment is with thiazide diuretic.

Cystinuria causes renal calculi and is associated with excess excretion of cystine, ornithine, lysine and arginine ('cola') amino acids

Severe primary hyperoxaluria may require liver and kidney transplantation

Nephrogenic diabetes insipidus can cause hypernatremia and mental retardation if not recognized

Cystinuria

Cystinuria is a complex genetic disorder involving at least three alleles governing dibasic amino acid (lysine, orthnithine, arginine) and cystine transport.[14] It is more common in Japanese and Caucasians, with an incidence of 1:18 000 in Japan and 1:20 000 in the UK. Defects are seen in both renal tubular and intestinal epithelial transport. Nutritional disturbances probably do not arise because amino acids are absorbed from the gut as oligopeptides rather than free amino acids. Renal tubular cells demonstrate an inability to take up cystine from their brush border, but can do so from the basolateral surface. Because the excretion of cystine can exceed the amount filtered, there is evidence of net cystine secretion by the tubule.

The clinical manifestations are confined to individuals in whom the cystine concentration in urine exceeds its solubility product and leads to calculus formation. This occurs in homozygotes, and in those heterozygous for the type II allele.[15] Family studies show that heterozygotes excrete different amounts of cystine depending on the allele type (see below). Almost all untreated homozygotes will experience calculi at some time in their lives, a quarter of them before 20 years of age. Obstruction and infection cause lasting damage to the urinary tract. Patients present with renal colic or episodes of hematuria. The stones are radiopaque because of their high sulfur content. Ultrasound is a good way of identifying calculi in both the renal collecting system and the bladder but often misses calculi in ureters. Microscopy of the urine reveals flat hexagonal birefringent crystals under polarized light, and the nitroprusside test for urinary disulfides is positive. Confirmation is by quantification of urinary cystine secretion:

Cystine excretion as urinary cystine/creatinine ratio

Normal		< 12 mmol/mmol (< 24 mg/g)
Heterozygote	type I	< 1 mmol/mmol
	type II	35–140 mmol/mmol
	type III	12–70 mmol/mmol
Homozygous cystinuria		> 120 mmol/mmol (> 240 mg/g)

The mainstay of treatment is to keep the urine volume sufficiently high that cystine is kept below its solubility maximum of 1.25 mmol/L (300 mg/L). This necessitates fluid loading, especially at night to overcome the normal night-time antidiuresis. The solubility maximum of cystine increases to 2.0 mmol/L (500 mg/L) where the urine pH exceeds 7.5. A second line of treatment, additional to and not a substitute for the first, is to prescribe bicarbonate or citrate to ensure that the early morning urine pH is alkaline.

Family members should be screened so that presymptomatic, affected members can be treated early. It is easier to prevent stone formation than to dissolve existing stones. In difficult cases with existing calculi a further increase in cystine solubility can be achieved by forming a thiol-cysteine disulfide with agents such as D-penicillamine.

Hyperoxaluria

Hyperoxaluria is a rare but important metabolic disorder to consider in a child with renal calculi or nephrocalcinosis. The majority of urine oxalate is derived from the hepatic metabolism of glyoxalate and ascorbate with a small proportion being ingested with diet. Oxalate is a metabolic end product, which is excreted via the kidneys, and its relative insolubility may lead to nephrocalcinosis or stone formation.

Enteric hyperoxaluria can occur in patients with chronic diarrhea due to short gut syndromes or other enteropathy.

Primary hyperoxaluria is a rare autosomal recessive disorder of oxalate metabolism due to a deficiency of hepatic alanine glyoxylate transferase (AGT) (type 1) or glycerate reductase/D-glycerate dehydrogenase (type 2). Both types lead to excessive urine oxalate excretion. In type 1 there is excess urinary glycolic acid, whereas type 2 is characterized by increased urinary L-glycerate.

Random urine samples for urine oxalate:creatinine ratio is part of the standard workup for children with renal stones but the normal ranges vary considerably with age and it is important to consult the laboratory for age-specific reference data. Normal results require measurement of 24 h urinary oxalate and glycolate excretion and organic analysis of urine (for L-glycerate).

Treatment of hyperoxaluria includes high fluid intake, crystal inhibitors such as citrate, orthophosphate, magnesium and pyridoxine to act as a co-factor for AGT deficient type 1 patients. Dietary advice should aim to avoid high oxalate foods and beverages such as black tea or cocoa as part of a high fluid intake. Patients with obstructing stones require urgent urological assessment to avoid renal damage due to obstruction and infection.

Anyone with significant renal impairment, i.e. GFR < 75 ml/min/1.73 m^2 should undergo specialist review. Oxalosis is a term used to describe the final stage of primary hyperoxaluria when reduction of glomerular filtration rate produces systemic oxalate excretion, with crystals being deposited in bone, muscles, artery walls, eyes, skin and nerves. Isolated renal transplantation has now been replaced by combined liver and kidney transplantation with good results.[16]

Oculocerebrorenal (Lowe's) syndrome

Oculocerebrorenal (Lowe's) syndrome describes a rare syndrome of mental retardation, excess aminoaciduria, cataract and glaucoma. It is transmitted as an X-linked recessive trait mapped to Xp24-24. Most carriers are normal, or at worst have early onset of cataract, but several female cases have been reported. The gene appears to code for a phosphatidyl inositol biphosphate phosphatase localized in the Golgi complex.

Clinical features

Boys present from 2 months of age with the facial features of large ears, prominent forehead, flattened nasal bridge and prominent scalp veins in a pale skin. Cataract is typical and in the early stages may only be detected by slit lamp examination. The severity of the cataract varies, as does its distribution. Buphthalmos and congenital glaucoma may be present.

Intermittent pyrexia and failure to thrive are usual, and growth retardation, osteoporosis and rickets often occur. The mental deficiency is usually severe, with loss of muscle tone, hypermobility of joints and absent or greatly diminished tendon jerks. The eyes often roll in pseudonystagmus and it is commonly noted that children press on their eyeballs with their fingers to produce visual 'hallucinations'. The EEG may show the fast 24 cycle per second general activity. The blood pressure is normal and ultrasound of the kidneys is often normal. Proteinuria occurs with complex tubular dysfunction, which may not manifest itself until the second year of life. Tubular acidosis, usually of classical 'distal type' is present and there is hyperphosphaturia with hypophosphatemia, normocalcemia and elevated levels of alkaline phosphatase.

Treatment

Treatment is supportive with adequate replacement of bicarbonate, potassium, phosphate and vitamin D metabolites. As with all rare conditions, parents may obtain benefit from contact with other families.

Hereditary hypophosphatemic rickets (vitamin D-resistant rickets)

Hypophosphatemic rickets is a rare dominantly transmitted X-linked disease, for which the affected gene (PHEX, phosphate regulating gene), has recently been identified.[17] Hypophosphatemia is due to a urinary leak of phosphate, which is itself secondary to a defect of proximal tubular sodium/phosphate cotransport.

Clinical signs are rickets in a child, and sometimes osteomalacia or bone deformities in the adult. Hypophosphatemia is associated with hyperphosphaturia, elevated serum alkaline phosphatase but with normal plasma calcium, calcitriol and PTH levels. No other tubular defects can be found and there is never the aminoaciduria associated with nutritional rickets or Fanconi's syndrome.

Treatment is with phosphate supplements which, if given on a regular basis, should improve bone mineralization and prevent bony deformities. Oral neutral phosphate (Phosphate Sandoz) should be pushed to the limit of tolerability in a dose of 50–100 mg/kg/day given as at least four, preferably five, doses. High doses produce diarrhea and compliance with the medication must be constantly encouraged. Alfacalcidol is also introduced in an initial dose of 20–40 ng/kg/day but a careful watch must be kept for hypercalcemia and hypercalciuria.[18]

Nephrogenic diabetes insipidus

Nephrogenic diabetes insipidus (NDI) is the isolated inability of the kidney to concentrate urine in response to circulating arginine vasopressin. Although acquired forms exist, the disorder mostly occurs in infants and is congenital. At a molecular level, two disease mechanisms have been found.[19] In 90% of congenital cases NDI is an X-linked disorder so that the full expression of the disease is confined to males. Mutations can occur in the arginine vasopressin-2 receptor (AVP2R) encoded at Xq28. AVP2R is normally located in the basolateral membrane of the collecting duct epithelial cell. On recognizing AVP the receptor signals to the cell nucleus through cyclic AMP leading to synthesis of the water channel aquaporin-2 and its insertion into the apical membrane. In this way, vasopressin regulated the ability of water to flow down the osmolar gradient from the dilute tubular fluid to the hyperoncotic medullary interstitium. Among the remaining families with autosomal nephrogenic diabetes insipidus, mutations have been found in the gene coding for aquaporin-2 on 12q13. It appears that the aquaporin molecule is synthesized, but not routed to its apical destination, resulting in a loss of water transport. It is possible to distinguish between these forms, in that those with an aquaporin-2 defect show a rise in urinary cyclic AMP with vasopressin stimulation, while those with the receptor defect do not.

Clinical features

The condition usually presents in infancy but a late recognition can occur. Polyuria and polydipsia are prominent features but difficult to recognize in infancy, although a preference for water rather than milk feeds may be evident. Water loss leads to recurring episodes of hypernatremic dehydration, fever, constipation and vomiting. Episodes of dehydration can seriously compromise intellectual development, and many cases exhibit growth retardation. The renal defect is permanent, but with increasing age water intake spontaneously increases to compensate for the persistent polyuria so that patients learn to avoid episodes of dehydration.

Diagnosis and differential diagnosis

Plasma sodium and chloride concentrations are increased and, when dehydration is severe, renal plasma flow falls leading to raised blood urea and serum creatinine levels. The osmolality of the urine is commonly less than 100 mOsm/kg. If a paired plasma and urine osmolality is obtained as soon as an infant presents with a dehydrational state, this is often sufficient to lead to the diagnosis. Always ensure that the kidneys are structurally normal by ultrasound. Renal dysplasia and reflux nephropathy may present with a water losing crisis in infancy. In apparently normally hydrated children fluid restriction to test renal concentrating ability must be carried out with very careful inpatient supervision, as severe dehydration may rapidly ensue. DDAVP has no effect on urine concentration and this forms the basis for the diagnosis.

Treatment

Replacement of urinary water losses, by increasing the fluid intake, is the basis of treatment. This may need to be by nasogastric tube feeding in the very young, although most infants will readily drink extra water given between milk feeds, even when appetite is poor. Paradoxically, thiazide diuretics have been shown to decrease free water clearance and urine flow rate in this condition. This action depends on the induction of a state of salt depletion, which causes an increase in proximal tubular reabsorption, and therefore diminished excretion of sodium and water to the distal nephron. The effect can be maintained by a low-salt diet, when thiazide diuretics are stopped. Unfortunately, the urine volume may decrease only by about one-third. The addition of prostaglandin synthetase inhibitors such as indometacin to this treatment causes a further fall in urine volume. It does not enhance urine concentration but, by reducing GFR and enhancing tubular sodium reabsorption, restricts salt (and thus water) delivery to the collecting duct, reducing total water losses. Provided adequate supplies of water are maintained from early infancy, mental development is preserved but physical growth often remains a problem. The prognosis depends on making the diagnosis early and fastidious parental supervision of hydration.

In later childhood it is often preferable to discontinue the thiazide/indometacin therapy because it carries significant hazards, particularly peptic ulceration and hemorrhage, and interstitial renal fibrosis. Most older children adapt well to the inconvenience of polydipsia and polyuria. Therapy can be reintroduced for longer or shorter periods as needed – for example during a holiday to a hot climate where excessive thirst could be a serious problem.

CONGENITAL ABNORMALITIES OF THE URINARY TRACT

Development of the renal tract has been described in Chapter 10. The increasing use, and accuracy, of obstetric ultrasound has added considerably to our recognition of urinary tract abnormalities (see neonatal renal). Some of these are obviously important to recognize, because of their potential for causing considerable renal damage, e.g. posturethral valves in a male infant, but others produce no symptoms in infancy or childhood and their natural history is still being defined, e.g. unilateral multicystic dysplastic kidney.

RENAL AGENESIS

Bilateral renal agenesis is incompatible with prolonged life, due to the associated pulmonary hypoplasia and oligohydramnios sequence.

Unilateral renal agenesis occurs in about 0.1% of the infant population, is more common in males and has been described in association with abnormalities of the external ear on the ipsilateral side. Atresia of the corresponding ureter is frequent and supports the view that unilateral renal agenesis is commonly the result of failure of formation of the ureteric bud or its inability to stimulate differentiation of the nephrogenic mesoderm. There is now a strong suspicion that many cases of unilateral renal agenesis are due to multicystic dysplastic kidneys, which have become involuted in utero.

Ultrasound and dimercaptosuccinic acid (DMSA) scan, including views of the whole abdomen to exclude ectopic location, should be undertaken. The presence of a normal hypertrophied kidney on the contralateral side should lead to reassurance and there is no need for long-term follow-up unless there are associated abnormalities.

RENAL FUSION AND ECTOPIA

The metanephric blastema is originally sited in the pelvis and ascends to its subdiaphragmatic position during early fetal life. During the ascent, some rotation occurs, so that the renal pelvis, which originally lies anterior to the disc-shaped pelvic metanephros, comes to lie medial to the lumbar kidney. Moreover, the kidney assumes its reniform shape by virtue of its lumbar position and the rotation it undergoes. An ectopic non-ascended kidney is therefore likely to be non-reniform in shape, being usually discoid, and to have a pelvis and ureter arising anteriorly. The ureter may have a normal vesical opening but may also open in an ectopic position in the bladder, bladder neck, urethra or vaginal vault. The blood supply is derived from nearby arteries such as the common iliac. A frequent site for the ectopic kidney is in the pelvis but it may be higher up the posterior abdominal wall or crossed to the opposite side. Such 'crossed' ectopia is more often than not fused with the normal kidney – 'crossed fused ectopia'. Fusion of normally placed kidneys may also occur – commonly at the lower poles – and gives rise to the 'horseshoe kidney' (Fig. 16.2). The fusion of such kidneys prevents normal medial rotation, and the ureters arise from an anterior or lateral, rather than medial, position relative to the renal parenchyma.

The site of an ectopic kidney may render it more vulnerable to trauma or liable to obstruct the delivery of an infant (although most pelvic kidneys do not). The usual route of the ureter may impede urinary drainage and lead to stasis and dilatation with subsequent infection. Dysplastic tissue is not infrequently also found, increasing the risk of infection. An ectopic ureteric orifice in the bladder may lead to vesicoureteric reflux. If the ureter opens into the urethra or vagina there may be incessant urinary incontinence. Despite these problems many malpositioned or fused kidneys function well and are quite unproductive of symptoms.

Diagnosis is made by appropriate radiological investigations, particularly ultrasound and radionuclide imaging.

DUPLEX SYSTEMS

Varying degrees of duplication occur. Double and completely separate pelves may occur (on one or both sides), draining via separate ureters to separate ureteric orifices in the bladder. There may be two pelves and one ureter or the two ureters may unite in Y fashion during the descent to the bladder. Such duplication is sometimes associated with vesicoureteric reflux or other abnormalities and this gives rise to problems such as recurrent infection.

However, duplex kidneys is probably one of the commonest abnormalities detected on imaging of the urinary tract and in the

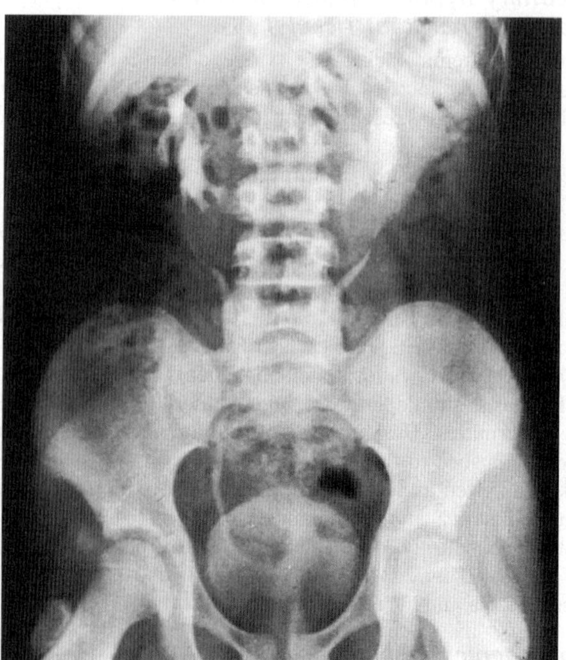

Fig. 16.2 Horseshoe kidney. Intravenous urogram showing rotated kidneys with calyces overlying pelves and ureters running inferiorly and then medially to produce 'flower vase' configuration.

absence of other urinary tract disease requires no treatment. Occasionally one of the ureters is associated with a ureterocele (cystic dilatation of the intravesical portion of the ureter) which can lead to obstruction and hydronephrosis (Fig. 16.3).

The ureter leading from the lower pelvis to the upper ureteric orifice is most often the abnormal one. Either ureteric orifice may open ectopically elsewhere in the bladder, urethra or vagina. It can give rise to the problem of continued wetting and is one of the conditions to consider when a child is referred with a wetting problem and has never apparently had a dry day.

(a)

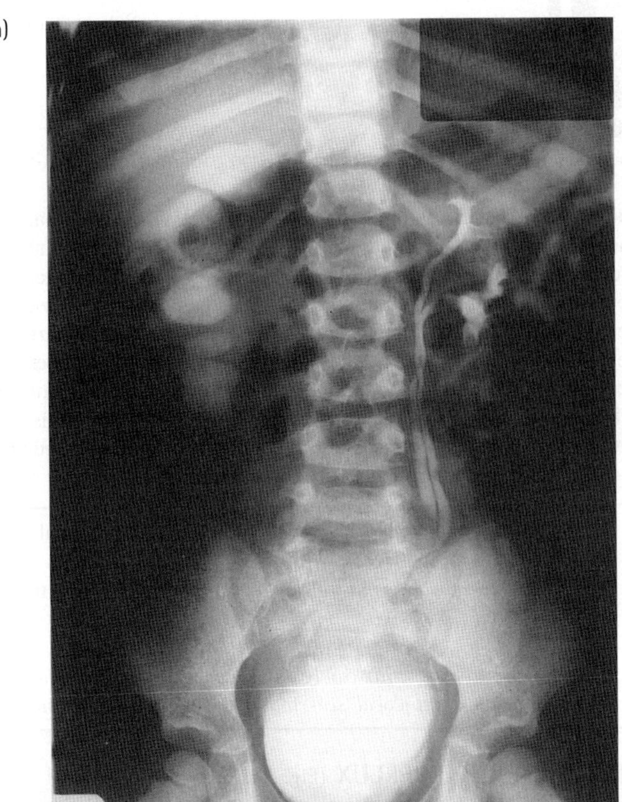

(b)

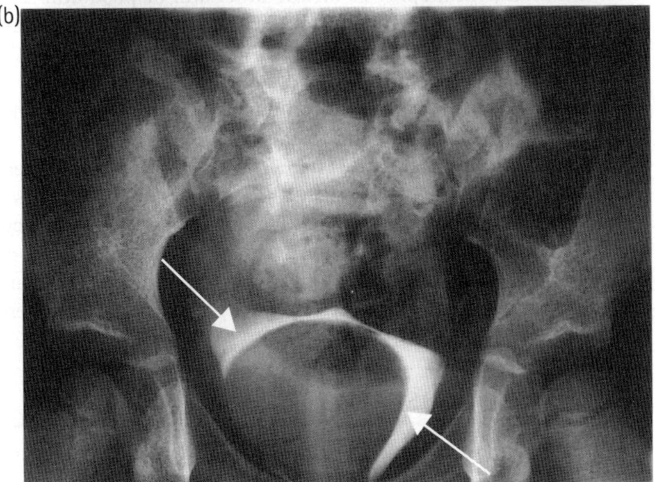

Fig. 16.3 (a) IVU in a 3-year-old girl with urinary tract infection, duplex system of left side and gross hydronephrosis on right side. (b) Hydronephrosis associated with large ureterocele seen as filling defect in bladder.

RENAL DYSPLASIA AND HYPOPLASIA

It is difficult to know whether these two conditions should be separated. True hypoplasia (i.e. a normally developed but unduly small kidney) is rare. It is best identified by its small size and diminution of the number of papillae and calyces present. Most cases are associated with some degree of dysplasia as well. Renal dysplasia may produce diminution or increase in total renal size, but its characteristic is the presence of pluripotent undifferentiated mesenchyme which may give rise to aberrant tissue such as cartilage and smooth muscle within the kidney. Cyst formation is common and has been attributed to premature cessation of branching by the ureteric bud which, being unable to induce nephron formation, degenerates and becomes cystic. Obstruction to the ureter in fetal life is also a factor in pathogenesis, and causes well marked dilatation of Bowman's capsule in some cases. The dysplasia may be unilateral when the opposite kidney functions normally, or may be bilateral.

Renal hypoplasia and dysplasia contribute significantly to the causes of chronic renal failure in childhood, especially now that dialysis and transplantation are possible, even for small infants. Many children may go undetected but progress into chronic renal failure at the end of the first decade when their body size begins to outgrow their kidney reserve.

Oligomeganephronia is one form of dysplastic kidney when there is a reduced number of very large nephrons, which undergo progressive focal sclerosis.

MULTICYSTIC DYSPLASTIC KIDNEY

The most common cystic lesion recognized antenatally is a multicystic dysplastic kidney (MCDK) disease (Fig. 16.4). In this disorder renal dysplasia is associated with a variable number of cysts and is believed to result from failed coordination development of the metanephros and the branching ureteric bud. Al-Khaldi et al[20] reported 44 fetuses with MCDK disease. In 14 fetuses the disease was bilateral and there were associated lethal abnormalities or syndromes. All 30 surviving infants had unilateral disease, 6 (20%) having significant reflux into the normal contralateral kidney. Although there have been occasional reports of sepsis, hypertension and even malignancy in association with cystic dysplastic kidneys, current management is conservative as many MCDK kidneys involute with time.[21]

POSTERIOR URETHRAL VALVES

This affects male infants with an incidence of approximately 1 in 12 000 pregnancies.[22] Even with antenatal detection and, occasionally, intervention with vesicoamniotic shunts in utero, many fetuses do not survive to term, or die in the neonatal period, because of the associated oligohydramnios and the severe lung abnormalities. However, posterior urethral valves represent a spectrum of disorders, with some neonates presenting with bladder outflow obstruction, infection and acute renal failure (ARF) in the newborn period in association with urosepsis (Fig. 16.5). Other children present later with apparently minor symptoms. Most cases are managed in conjunction with a pediatric urologist and the prognosis will depend upon the degree of associated renal dysplasia and bladder abnormality.

PELVIURETERIC JUNCTION (PUJ) AND VESICOURETERIC JUNCTION OBSTRUCTION (VUJ)

These two conditions cause hydronephrosis antenatally and have provided some of the biggest dilemmas in respect of

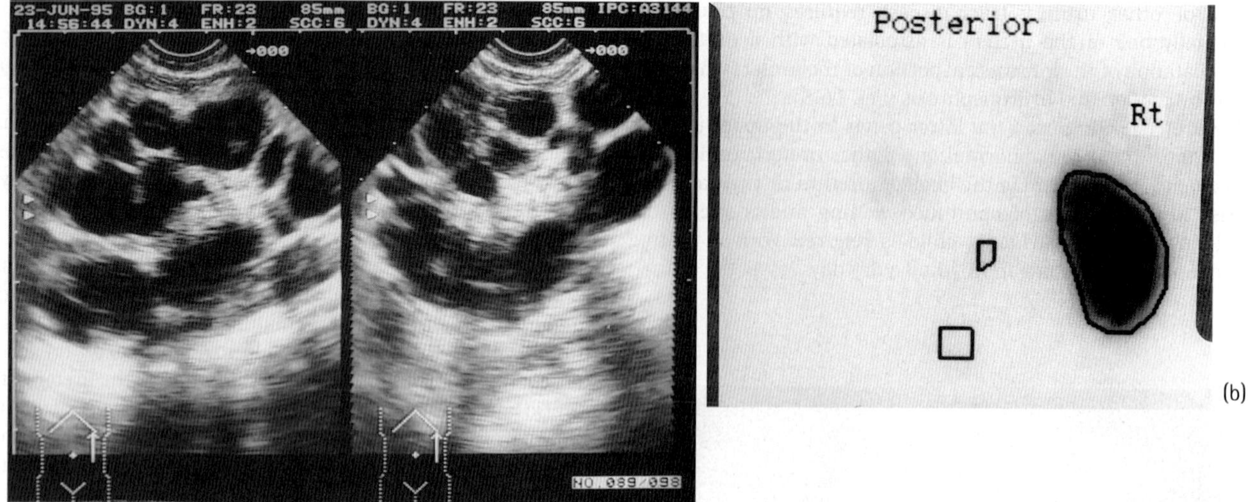

Fig. 16.4 (a) Postnatal ultrasound of infant with left MCDK showing numerous cysts in enlarged kidney. (b) Non function confirmed on DMSA scan.

postnatal management. PUJ and VUJ can occur at any time of life in association with intermittent abdominal pain, hematuria, urinary tract infection and asymptomatic flank mass. Such symptoms or signs are justification for a pyeloplasty or reimplant operation.

However, most infants with antenatally detected hydronephrosis have little in the way of signs or symptoms postnatally. In the rare instances, where there is a large tense kidney, with very diminished function, then an initial nephrostomy is undertaken. Most infants are assessed by a combination of ultrasound, micturating cystourethrogram (MUCG) (to exclude associated reflux) and a radionuclide scan, which is preferably MAG 3 (^{99m}Tc-labeled mercaptoacetyltriglycine), rather than DTPA (^{99m}Tc-labeled diethylenetriamine-pentaacetic acid) (Fig. 10.2). The general consensus is that a combination of significant calyceal, as well as pelvic, dilatation, accompanied by a reduction of differential function below 40% on the radionuclide scan, are indicators for an operative approach (Fig. 16.6).[23] There are no controlled trials to guide us and information concerning patients with significant dilatation is best reviewed by pediatric nephrologists, pediatric urologists and pediatric radiologists in combined nephrouroradiology meetings.

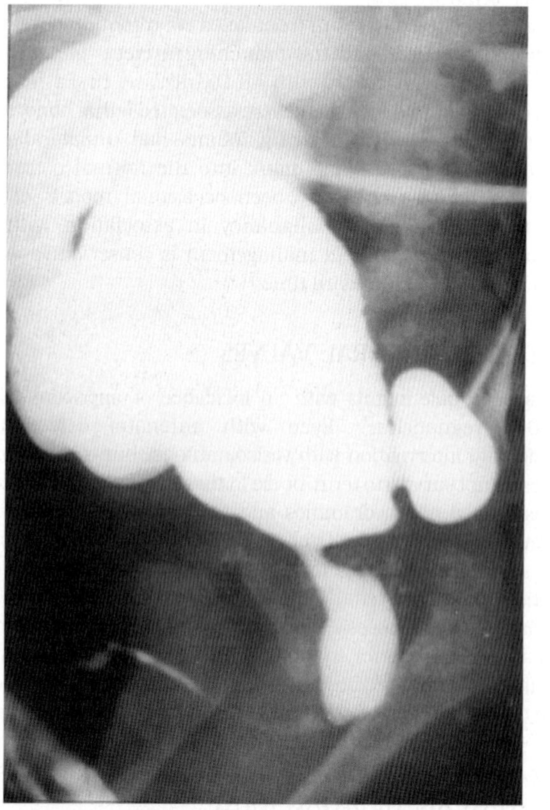

Fig. 16.5 Micturating cystourethrogram in a male infant presenting with septicemia and acute renal failure. Gross dilatation of posterior urethra, bladder diverticulum and reflux into dilated ureter.

Multicystic dysplastic kidney (MCDK) is usually a unilateral condition and most involute with time

Posterior urethral valves must always be considered in a male infant with urosepsis

Severe vesicoureteric reflux can be associated with small dysplastic kidneys and apparent global 'scarring' in the absence of infection

VESICOURETERIC REFLUX (Fig. 16.12)

Even minimal hydronephrosis on the antenatal or postnatal scan may be associated with gross degrees of reflux on the MCUG. Care should be taken in neonates, where gross reflux is detected on the MCUG, to ensure that a 5-day course of full dose antibiotics is prescribed before recommencing prophylactic antibiotics, as fatal urosepsis has occurred after this investigation.

It is now obvious that many children with gross reflux at a very early age already have very poorly functioning kidneys at the outset, even in the absence of infection (Fig. 16.7).[24] Many of these kidneys are already probably severely dysplastic. Although there is no controlled trial in this young age group, the management of infants with reflux is generally conservative (see Urinary tract infections below).

RENAL CYSTIC DISEASE

There are a number of disorders that share renal cysts as a common feature (Table 16.3).

These disorders may be inherited or acquired in the clinical context and associated systemic manifestations may help distinguish cystic disorders one from another. A solitary cyst in a young child may indicate a calyceal diverticulum rather than a simple cyst,

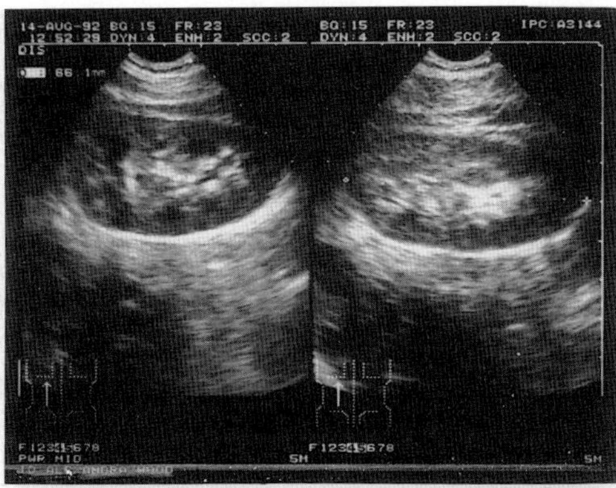

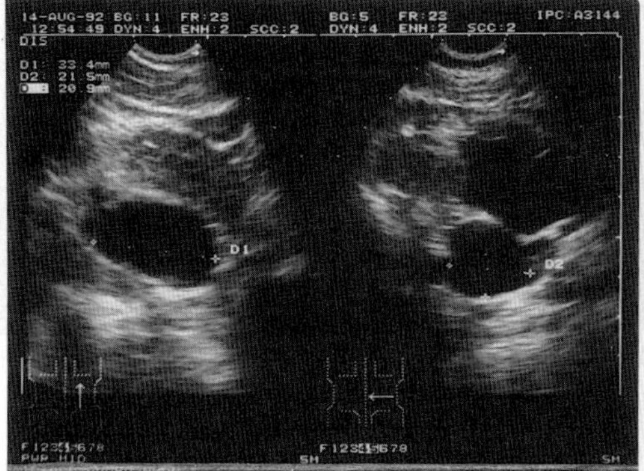

(a)

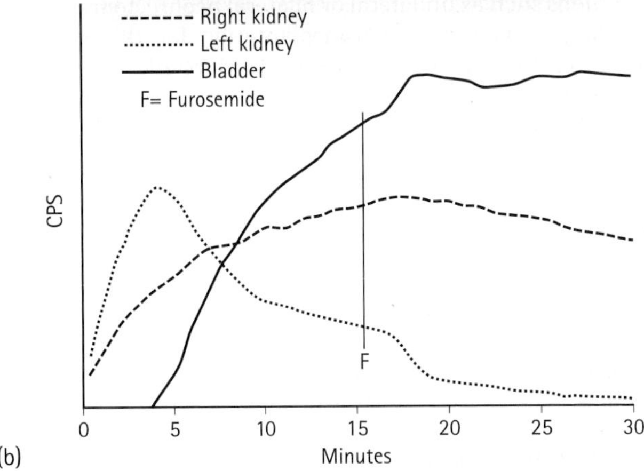

(b)

Fig. 16.6 (a) Ultrasound of 1-month-old infant with antenatally detected right hydronephrosis showing normal left kidney and dilatation of pelvis and calyces on right side. (b) Excretion curves of MAG 3 scan in the same infant showing normal excretion left kidney and delayed excretion right side with poor response to furosemide (frusemide). Differential function: right 36%, left 64%.

which is more common in adult life. Bilateral enlarged kidneys in a neonatal infant would raise the suspicion of autosomal recessive polycystic kidney disease, which is more likely in this context than of autosomal dominant polycystic kidney disease or tuberous sclerosis complex. Renal insufficiency in an adolescent might suggest juvenile nephronophthisis or autosomal recessive polycystic kidney disease as possible etiologies.

AUTOSOMAL RECESSIVE POLYCYSTIC KIDNEY DISEASE (ARPKD)

ARPKD is an inherited malformation complex with varying degrees of renal collecting duct dilatation and biliary ectasia.[25] There is an estimated incidence of 1 in 20 000 live births and it appears to occur more frequently in Caucasians than in other ethnic populations.

Etiology and pathogenesis

The ARPKD locus has now been mapped to the short arm of chromosome 6 (6p21–12) and to date all phenotypic variants appear to result from mutations in the single gene.[26]

Late in the 1970s ARPKD was subdivided into four distinct phenotypes according to the age of presentation and the proportion of dilated renal collecting ducts. However, the process typically begins in utero and the renal cystic lesions appear to be superimposed on a normal developmental sequence. The tubular abnormality primarily involves fusiform dilatation of the collecting ducts. The early liver lesion appears to involve defective remodelling of the ductal plate in utero such that primitive bile duct configurations persist and progressive portal fibrosis evolves.

Clinical features

The clinical spectrum of ARPKD is variable and depends on the age at presentation.[27] Most patients are identified either in utero or at birth. The most severely affected fetuses present in pregnancies

(a)

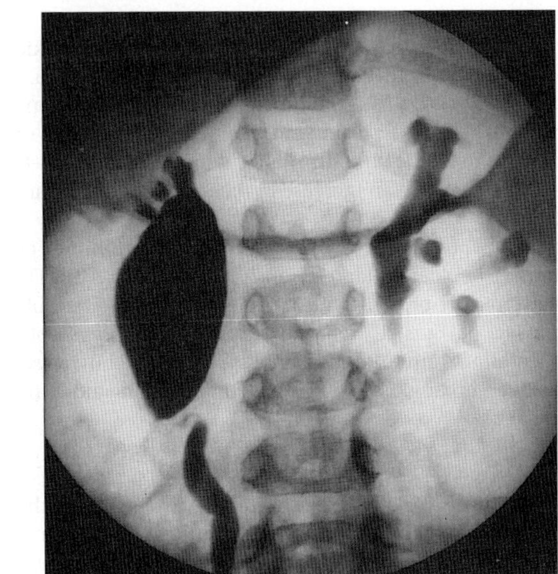

(b)

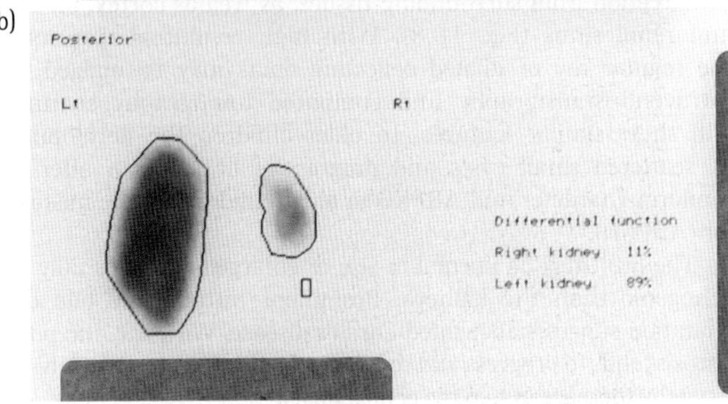

Fig. 16.7 (a) Postnatal MCUG on infant with antenatally detected hydronephrosis showing gross reflux bilaterally with pseudo PUJ appearance on right side. (b) DMSA scan in same infant showing very poor function on right side suggesting dysplastic kidney (no history of infection).

Table 16.3 Renal cystic disorders

Genetic disorders
Autosomal dominant
Autosomal dominant polycystic kidney disease (ADPKD)
Von Hippel–Lindau disease (VHL)
Tuberous sclerosis complex (TSC)
Adult-onset medullary cystic disease

Autosomal recessive
Autosomal recessive polycystic kidney disease (ARPKD)
Juvenile-onset nephronophthisis
Other rare syndromes associated with multiple malformations

X-linked
Orofaciodigital syndrome type 1

Nongenetic disorders
Developmental
Medullary sponge kidney
Renal cystic dysplasia; multicystic dysplasia; cystic dysplasia associated with lower urinary tract obstruction, diffuse cystic dysplasia (syndromal and non-syndromal)

Acquired
Simple cysts
Hypokalemic cystic disease
Acquired cystic disease (in advanced renal failure)

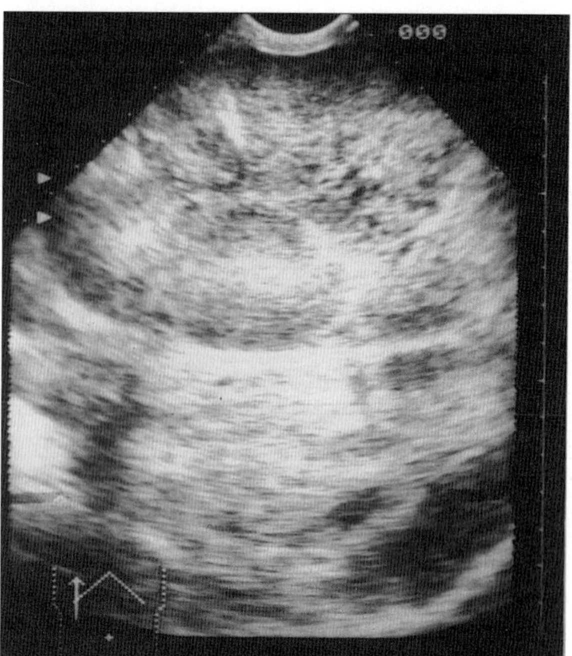

Fig. 16.8 Ultrasound showing diffuse increase in echogenicity. Bilateral enlargement in newborn with ARPKD.

with oligohydramnios and have enlarged echogenic kidneys. They may die at birth because of pulmonary hypoplasia. Those infants who survive the perinatal period have hypertension, renal failure and portal hypertension. Renal hypertension usually develops in the first few months and ultimately affects 70–80% of patients. There is also an increase in the incidence of urinary tract infections.

Portal hypertension can be the predominant clinical abnormality in older children and adolescents with ARPKD. These children typically present with hepatosplenomegaly and bleeding esophageal or gastric varices as well as hypersplenism. Hepatocellular function is usually preserved but ascending suppurative cholangitis is a serious complication and can cause hepatic failure.

Diagnosis

In the antenatal period, oligohydramnios or enlarged echogenic kidneys suggest ARPKD. Postnatally, ultrasound can reveal symmetrically enlarged diffusely echogenic kidneys, with poor demarcation from surrounding tissues, as well as cortex, medulla and renal sinus (Fig. 16.8). With high resolution ultrasound the regular ray of dilated collecting ducts may be imaged and intravenous urography and computed tomography scanning will show similar features. In older children the development of scattered small cysts and progressive fibrosis can alter the reniform character and ARPKD in older children can be mistaken for (ADPKD).

The liver may be normal in size or enlarged and is usually less echogenic than the kidneys. Prominent intrahepatic bile duct dilatation suggests associated Caroli's disease. With age, the portal fibrosis tends to progress and there may be hepatosplenomegaly and a patchy increase in hepatic echogenicity.

Outcome

The estimated perinatal mortality is 30–50%. For those who survive the first month of life the reported mean 5 year patient survival rate is 80–95%.[28] The prognosis outside the perinatal period is improved, because of the availability of aggressive interventions such as unilateral or bilateral nephrectomy, and the availability of dialysis and transplantation for this group of children. For those with end-stage renal failure and severe portal hypertension, combined liver and kidney transplantation may be indicated.

AUTOSOMAL DOMINANT POLYCYSTIC KIDNEY DISEASE (ADPKD)

ADPKD is a multisystem disorder characterized by multiple bilateral renal cysts and associated with cysts in other organs such as liver, pancreas and arachnoid membranes. It is one of the most common hereditary diseases affecting approximately 1 in 400 to 1 in 1000 individuals.

Etiology and pathogenesis

The genes responsible for ADPKD have provided a major breakthrough in the study of the disease. PKD1 is the gene on chromosome 16 and is responsible for 85% of clinically detected cases and PKD2 has been identified in the long arm of chromosome 4 and there is likely to be a third gene. Proteins encoded by PKD1 and PKD2 have been named polycystin 1 and polycystin 2 respectively. Molecular genetic work has stimulated a great deal of research into variation in disease progression between patients and this appears to depend upon underlying mutations, modifying genes, somatic mutations and environmental factors.[29]

Clinical features

It is very rare for ADPKD to manifest clinically in childhood, but an occasional child may have significant renal enlargement with hypertension. Urinary tract infections are also known to exacerbate kidney disease in adults. Although ADPKD may be recognized incidentally on renal ultrasound scans done for urinary tract infection (UTI) investigation etc., there is a general consensus that asymptomatic children from affected families should not be routinely screened for this condition either by ultrasound or genetic studies. They should be free to make their own autonomous decision as to whether they want to be investigated when they reach adulthood.

FAMILIAL JUVENILE NEPHRONOPHTHISIS AND MEDULLARY CYSTIC DISEASE COMPLEX

Juvenile nephronophthisis (NPH) and medullary cystic disease complex are histologically similar diseases differing in their mode of transmission and age of onset.

Recent studies have mapped a gene (NPHP1) for juvenile NPH to the chromosome region 2q13. Approximately 85% of purely renal NPH involves defects in NPHP1, which involves a novel protein product called nephrocystine.[30] Large homozygous deletions have been detected in 80% of affected members of NPH families and in 65% of sporadic cases.

Radiologically the disease is characterized by chronic sclerosing tubular interstitial nephropathy with sparse inflammatory cell infiltration and the development of medullary cysts late in the disease course. There is an irregular thickening of the tubular basement membrane (TBM) with the absence of certain TBM components and the novel expression of alpha-5 integrin in tubular epithelial cells.

Clinical features

Reduced urinary concentrating capacity is common in patients with NPH and this usually precedes a decline in renal function. The mean age of onset is 4 years. Polyuria and polydipsia are common symptoms and the patients may be anemic, even before the onset of renal insufficiency. Growth retardation, out of proportion with the degree of renal insufficiency, is a common finding.[31] A gradual decline in renal function is typical and end-stage renal failure usually develops by adolescence. The disease is not known to recur in renal allografts.

In 10–15% of NPH there is an association with retinitis pigmentosa caused by retinal degeneration (Senior–Loken syndrome) and presents with coarse nystagmus and early blindness. NPH associated with ocular motor apraxia and coexisting retinal degeneration (Cogan's syndrome) has been reported in several kindreds and a subset of these patients have also had mental retardation. Congenital hepatic fibrosis occurs occasionally in patients with NPH.

AUTOSOMAL DOMINANT MEDULLARY CYSTIC KIDNEY DISEASE

This nephropathy is histologically indistinguishable from recessive NPH and has been reported with male to male transmission in successive generations, suggesting an autosomal dominant mode of inheritance. Progression to end-stage renal failure occurs in the third to fourth decade of life.

MEDULLARY SPONGE KIDNEY

Again this condition more commonly comes to light in adult life, when calcification in the renal pyramids may give rise to calculi, abdominal pain and hematuria. It is occasionally identified in childhood for the same reasons, but more often because of the urographic appearance of streaky opacification in the renal pyramids.

TUBEROUS SCLEROSIS COMPLEX (TSC)

TSC is an autosomal dominant disorder in which tumor-like malformations, called hamartomas, develop in multiple organ systems. This affects 1 in 10 000 individuals but spontaneous mutations appear to occur at high frequency and are estimated to account for 60% of new cases.

Renal cystic disease is the earliest finding in TSC and may be the presenting manifestation in infants and children before even the seizures and mental retardation have become manifest alongside the facial angiofibromas, hypomelanotic macules and periungual fibromas.

The principal hamatomas in TSC are angiomyolipomas. They rarely occur before 5 years of age but increase in frequency and size and give rise to hemorrhage or mass effects leading to severe hypertension and progressive decrease in renal function. Malignant tumors, found in TSC patients, were originally thought to be a renal cell carcinoma but are now regarded as malignant epitheloid angiomyolipomas.[32]

URINARY TRACT INFECTIONS

FREQUENCY AND DYSURIA SYNDROMES

Although frequency and dysuria are commonly associated with urinary tract infection, only 25% of children who have these symptoms have significant bacteriuria, based on 10^5 organisms/ml ($> 10^8$/L), which is the diagnostic standard for voided specimens of urine. Viral infections may play a part and acute vulvitis or balanitis may be associated with poor hygiene, perineal candidiasis or contact sensitivity to nylon pants. Attention should be paid to the possibility of pin worm infestation or constipation.

There is a small group of children where pathological causes, such as infection or stone, have been excluded and frequency persists. It is possible that emotional factors are at work and generally the condition is self-limiting. Occasionally anticholinergic drugs such as oxybutynin may be required to improve bladder stability. Recurrent urinary tract symptoms associated with anogenital signs may be a pointer to sexual abuse.

URINARY TRACT INFECTION (UTI)

UTI is invasion of the urinary tract (bladder and/or kidneys) with bacteria, which often causes inflammatory response and symptoms. UTI is important because of its association with:

1. *morbidity* such as septicemia and failure to thrive, enuresis and poor school attendance;
2. unsuspected *congenital abnormalities* of the urinary tract such as posterior urethral valves, pelviureteric junction obstruction, ureterocele and other obstructive uropathy;
3. *vesicoureteric reflux* (VUR) with its potential for renal scarring, hypertension and chronic renal failure in later life.

Obstructive anomalies are found in 0–4%, and vesicoureteric reflux in 8–40%, of children being investigated for their first UTI. A systematic overview of diagnostic imaging in UTI concluded that there was no direct evidence that children who have routine diagnostic imaging after their first UTI are better off than those who do not.[33] Increasing concern about radiation exposure, the potential distress of the investigations and their cost have all added to the continued debate about appropriate investigations and management of UTI in children.

There is a strong association between urinary tract infection and vesicoureteric reflux, with subsequent scarring of the kidneys, termed *reflux nephropathy* or chronic pyelonephritis. This condition has been quoted as causing up to 25% of cases of end-stage renal failure in children and adults. These children are also at risk of developing hypertension, with a reported risk of between 10 and

23%.[34] Obviously these adverse outcomes are of concern and have long term implications for monitoring of blood pressure and future pregnancies.[35] However the risk of such adverse outcomes may have been overstated as:

1. Many children had VUR as a cause of their end-stage renal failure (ESRF) in *association* with obstructive uropathy and other abnormalities of the urinary tract.[36] In a recent analysis of causes of ESRF in 686 UK children reflux nephropathy accounted for 7.2% of cases.[37]
2. The postnatal investigation of neonates (mostly boys) with antenatally recognized hydronephrosis has shown that gross vesicoureteric reflux can result in dramatic reduction in renal function on isotope renography in the *absence* of infection in such infants, suggesting underlying dysplasia.[39] These children, with 'congenital' reflux nephropathy, need to be distinguished from those whose kidneys were originally normal and where vesicoureteric reflux and infection resulted in acquired scars.
3. The incidence of hypertension in association with renal scars may be overstated as the reports are from specialist centers. Although hypertension may develop during long term follow-up and the rare child with renal scarring has malignant hypertension, Wolfish et al[34] *no* hypertension in a retrospective study of 146 children with renal scarring and primary vesicoureteric reflux.[40]

So, although it is accepted that UTI is associated with reflux nephropathy, it must be remembered that in some children the damage has already occurred prenatally and reflux need not always be or have been present to achieve renal damage.

Young age at first infection appears to be an important risk factor with a higher prevalence of vesicoureteric reflux and potential for damage in the growing kidney.[41] Older children being followed for VUR can have progression of, but rarely new scar formation. Such new scars appear mostly in children who have suffered further UTIs or in those with a history of delayed diagnosis and treatment.[42,43]

It would appear that we should concentrate more of our efforts on the detection and treatment of UTI in *infants* and those with *recurrent infections*. Over-zealous investigation should be avoided and the imaging procedure(s) selected properly (see later).

Epidemiology

It is estimated that at least 1% of boys and 3% of girls experience a UTI during their first decade. The true prevalence is uncertain, as urine collection methods are still inadequate. It is only during the first 12 months of life that both symptomatic UTI and asymptomatic bacteriuria affect males more than females.[44] Nosocomial urinary tract infections, associated mainly with urinary catheters, are an important cause of hospital morbidity.

Circumcision and urinary tract infection

A number of studies have suggested an association between UTI and the uncircumcised state, but these studies have been criticized on methodological grounds. A more recent case control study, in the setting of a large ambulatory pediatric service in 144 boys < 5 years of age who had a microbiologically proven symptomatic UTI, has shown that circumcision was associated with a decreased risk of symptomatic UTIs.[45] This is not a strong indication for circumcision, but it does emphasize that particular care should be taken with the foreskin in male infants who are known to have obstructive uropathy or an anatomical abnormality which might predispose to UTI.

Urinary tract infection and breast-feeding

There is a strong suggestion that breast-feeding may reduce the risk of UTI.[46] The mechanism by which breast milk may be protective is unclear but a preliminary report suggests that neutral oligosaccharides found in breast milk inhibit bacterial adhesion to uroepithelial cells.

Asymptomatic bacteriuria (ABU)

There is no evidence that screening for bacteriuria in healthy children is of value in preventing renal disease and general screening programs are not advocated.[47] It should be ascertained that the child with ABU is truly asymptomatic with a negative family history and normal examination. The prevalence of ABU in schoolgirls has been reported to be 1.2–1.8%. Studies during the 1980s indicated that treatment increased the risk of complications.[48] It would appear that bacteria of low incidence in the urinary tract prevent invasion by other bacteria.

CLINICAL PRESENTATION OF UTI

The younger the child the more non-specific the symptoms:

1. Prolonged *neonatal* jaundice is a classical association of bacteriuria in the newborn. A high index of suspicion should be maintained in any baby 'going off', or who has abdominal distension, disturbance of temperature regulation, changing ventilation requirements or metabolic disturbance.
2. *Infants* may present with vomiting, diarrhea, poor feeding and failure to thrive or fever. UTI should be excluded in any infant with an unexplained temperature. The pooled prevalence of UTI in febrile infants and young children is about 5%.[49] Suprapubic aspiration of urine should always be attempted in children presenting as sick and septicemic as part of the 'septic workup'.
3. Young infants can present with *ARF* and gross electrolyte abnormalities when infection occurs in an abnormal urinary tract.
4. *Cystitis-like* symptoms such as frequency and dysuria are common symptoms in the older child. There may be mild lower abdominal discomfort and hematuria. Such symptoms do not exclude involvement of the upper urinary tract.
5. *Acute pyelonephritis*. The classical symptoms of high fever, abdominal or loin pain and rigors in the child who is very unwell is an uncommon clinical presentation in children. The presence of such symptoms, or septicemia, in a young infant does influence subsequent management and intensity of the investigations. A raised ESR, white blood count and C-reactive protein levels along with reduced renal concentrating capacity have been used to distinguish upper from lower tract involvement, but there is no certain diagnostic test.

Examination

This should include palpation for renal masses and fecal loading as there is a strong association between UTI and constipation. A palpable bladder combined with a poor urinary stream suggests obstructive uropathy due to posturethral valves in a male infant or neurogenic bladder. Examination of the spine and lower limb reflexes should be included. Examination of the anal and genital areas might suggest signs of sexual abuse in a female infant. A rare abnormality such as ureterocele may even be noticed at the vaginal introitus. There are a number of syndromes associated with urinary tract abnormalities such as prune belly and anorectal anomalies.

Diagnosis of urinary tract infection

The classical definition of significant bacteriuria [10^5 organisms per ml (10^8/L) of urine] is still applied in childhood with the proviso that any bacteriology reports should always be interpreted in the clinical context. It is important to remember that the original criteria were based upon midstream urine collections in adult females, when two such samples increased the probability to 96%. It is possible that a lower colony count, especially with a pure growth on repeated samples, is clinically important, but bacteriology labs still apply the same diagnostic criteria. Any growth obtained on a suprapubic urine sample is regarded as significant.

Urine collection

Since there is a large focus on infants with UTI, greater attention needs to be given to *urine collection methods* in this group of infants, both in primary care and hospital practice:

Different types of *urine collection bags* are now available but are prone to provide contaminated specimens if not applied properly and not removed as soon as the urine is passed. Recent work has suggested that urine could be collected from infants using a urine collection pad and removing the urine by syringe from the pad.[50] This method needs to be assessed further before it can be recommended for general use.

Clean catch urine. In some young infants micturition occurs as a reflex action stimulated by bladder fullness. Micturition can be encouraged by tapping in the suprapubic region, stroking alongside the spine or even exposure to cold while undressing. Sterile trays should always be to hand and parents should be encouraged to participate in this method of urine collection.

Midstream urine collection. The older continent boy can easily introduce a sterile container into the urinary stream and there is no need for specific cleansing of the glans or withdrawal of the prepuce. Similarly the vulva does not require cleansing (antiseptics are to be avoided) in older girls, but cleaning with sterile water may be required in younger girls where a sterile container placed inside a potty is usually employed. Using the child's own potty is not satisfactory and is a common reason for erroneous results in general practice.

Suprapubic aspiration of urine (SPA) is a safe and reliable method of obtaining urine in infants and young children in whom the distended bladder is an abdominal organ. The procedure should be taught to the junior staff and an important practice point is to aspirate while advancing the needle rather than on withdrawal to minimize the risk of contamination. If an ultrasound machine is available then bladder size can be checked before attempting the procedure.

Catheter specimen of urine. Catheterization is only resorted to if there has been a failed SPA or in a sick older child where urine cultures need to be obtained before commencing antibiotics. Instrumentation of the lower urinary tract does carry the risk of introducing infection or traumatizing the urethra.

Microscopy

Although the finding of pyuria is good supportive evidence of UTI, up to 50% of patients with significant bacteriuria will not demonstrate a significant number of white cells (> 5 white cells per high powered field) in the centrifuged urine specimen. A recent study confirmed that pyuria may occur in 9% of febrile children *without* a urinary tract infection.[51] We no longer request routine microscopy of urine for white cells on children referred to outpatients, but it may still have a role in the child admitted to hospital acutely unwell. In this situation, the presence of bacteria and white cells on a fresh urine specimen is strong evidence to support the diagnosis of a UTI and to commence appropriate antibiotic therapy.

Dipsticks

Urine dipsticks, which incorporate strips for the detection of white blood cells (leukocyte esterase), or the production of nitrite by reduction of nitrate, are increasingly favored for the diagnosis of UTI (Table 16.4). The nitrate might not be reduced to nitrite if there is frequent bladder emptying, dilute urine, inadequate dietary nitrate or infection with enzyme deficient bacteria giving the test a low sensitivity rate. The meta-analysis by Gorelick & Shaw[52] found the summary estimate of sensitivity for nitrite or leukocyte esterase positive to be 88% and the sensitivity of positive Gram stain (on an unspun specimen) to be 93%. Tests with a high specificity have a low rate of false positive results and the specificity of leukocyte esterase is 84% and nitrite 98%. Hence a urine specimen obtained in an asymptomatic child in the outpatient department, which is clear and negative on dipstick, does not need laboratory assessment and culture. A positive nitrite and leukocyte result is an indication for urine culture and empirical treatment with antibiotics, while awaiting culture, if the child is symptomatic.

Dip slides

Dip slides for transmitting urine specimens or bottles containing boric acid have been promoted as a means of collecting specimens at home where there are transport difficulties to the laboratory.

Table 16.4 Interpretation of urine dipsticks in renal disease

Feature	Method	Comment
pH	Methyl red Bromothymol blue	Normal range 4.5–8; typically in early morning urine pH 8: renal tubular acidosis, infection with urea-splitting organisms
Hemoglobin	Ortholidine + peroxidase	Detects hemoglobin and myoglobin; does not distinguish hemoglobinuria from hematuria False negative: ascorbic acid, rifampin (rifampicin) False positive: iodine, hypochlorite
Protein	Protein binding to tetrabromophenol blue	Only detects albumin, does not detect light chains False positive: alkaline urine
Glucose	Glucose oxidase peroxidase	Also detects fructose, lactose, galactose False negative: ascorbic acid
Leukocyte esterase	3-Hydroxy-5-phenolpyrrole + leukocyte esterase Griess's test	Detects intact or lysed leukocytes; sensitivity/specificity contentious False positive: vaginal contamination
Nitrite		Some organisms do not reduce nitrate Urine in bladder > 4 hours for accurate result

However, technical failures with dip slides may be disappointingly high and if the container with boric acid is not filled with urine to the appropriate level then growth may be inhibited.[53]

Handling of urine culture specimens

Since we are so reliant upon urine culture to confirm the UTI, it is important that all urine cultures should be submitted to the laboratory with the minimum delay. If there is any delay, storage at 4°C will still permit accurate diagnosis for 24 h and possibly longer.

Guidelines published by the Royal College of Physicians for the management of acute urinary tract infection in childhood[54] emphasized the importance of urine culture methods and this is still a key factor. A recent study in our unit of 257 referrals to the children's clinic from primary care showed that only 66% of urine cultures had been taken by appropriate methods, and only 39% of parents had been given appropriate instructions on how to collect the urine sample. If we are to stress the importance of investigating *every* child with a first UTI, then we must pay attention to obtaining the proof that such an infection has occurred.

Table 16.5 Antibiotics used in the treatment and prophylaxis of urinary tract infections

	Treatment (dose in mg/kg/day)	Dose interval (h)	Prophylaxis (dose in mg/kg/day)
Co-amoxiclav	75 mg i.v.	8	NR
	20–40 oral amox content	8	NR
	25–45 oral amox content	12 (duo suspension)	NR
Amoxicillin	25 oral	8	NR
Trimethoprim	8 oral	12	2
Nalidixic acid	50 oral	6	12.5
Nitrofurantoin	3–5 oral	6	1
Cefotaxime	100 i.v.	12	NR
Cefradine	25–50 oral	8–12	NR
Cefuroxime	60 mg i.v.	8	NR
	6.25–25 oral	12	NR
Gentamicin	2 mg/kg/dose i.v.	Depends upon renal function and levels	NR

NR, not recommended for prophylaxis

MICROBIOLOGY

Escherichia coli is responsible for at least 80% of UTIs in childhood. Other organisms that commonly cause infection include *Proteus*, *Enterococcus*, *Pseudomonas* and *Klebsiella* species. *Staphylococcus aureus* and *Staphylococcus epidermidis* are urinary pathogens in small children. Any organism may cause sepsis in this young age group, with the kidney and urinary tract becoming involved by hematogenous spread from a generalized septicemia.

Pathophysiology

A symptomatic or covert bacteriuria occurs more frequently than symptomatic UTI at all ages. It must be remembered that many young infants are sitting in nappies filled with feces. Infection of the urinary tract must be related to both the characteristics of the invading bacteria and those of the host urinary tract. Virulence factors have been well studied in *E. coli* and most strains isolated from patients with suspected upper UTIs have pili or fimbriae, which are polypeptides with tubular receptors specific for glycolipid components of human cell membranes. Such fimbriae allow attachment to the receptors, which are expressed on uroepithelial cells. Over 90% of *E. coli* isolated from children with a first episode of pyelonephritis expressed P. fimbriae compared with 19.2% of isolates of children with cystitis. The roles of other virulence factors are reviewed elsewhere.[55]

TREATMENT

Parenteral antibiotic therapy is required in any child with systemic symptoms. Initial therapy in neonates is usually intravenous ampicillin and gentamicin, and in the older child, a cephalosporin, such as cefotaxime.[56] The duration of intravenous therapy is always controversial: a minimum of 5 days is generally recommended but it would depend upon the child's symptoms, such as fever, and whether obstructive uropathy is suspected. If intravenous therapy is used it should be continued until the child is apyrexial for 24 h and a total of 10–14 days therapy should be completed with a switch to oral antibiotics as appropriate. A check should always be made that the follow-up urine culture is sterile.

Suitable oral antibacterial drugs used in the treatment of UTI are shown in Table 16.5. Information should be available from the local microbiology laboratory about changing pattern of *antibiotic resistance* locally. 50% of *E. coli* isolates locally are resistant to ampicillin and the level of trimethoprim resistance is approximately 20%. The recent prescription of broad spectrum antibiotics to a child may dramatically alter the bowel flora and select resistant organisms such as *Klebsiella*. Although not generally recommended for children, ciprofloxacin (8–15 mg/kg/day) has proven to be a useful oral antibiotic for the treatment of *Pseudomonas* infections and avoids the need for parenteral therapy. The dosage of all drugs should be carefully checked in children with known renal impairment.

The duration of treatment for a child with an uncomplicated urinary tract infection treated by the oral route should be for 5–7 days. In children under 1 year of age, those who require intravenous therapy or who have an abnormal initial ultrasound, prophylactic therapy should be continued until investigations are completed. In both groups, urine culture should be taken to ensure resolution of the infection.

Single doses or short courses of antibiotics are not advised in any child presenting with a first febrile infection on an uninvestigated urinary tract. However, a recent meta-analysis found that a 2–4 day course of oral antibiotics is as effective as 7–14 days in eradicating lower tract UTI in children.[57]

Treatment and investigation of UTI go hand in hand. Children with obstructive uropathy such as posterior urethral valves should be managed in centers where there is both nephrology and urology expertise.

PREVENTION OF UTI

Recurrence of UTI is common in children, with about 30% of girls having another UTI within 1 year.[58] This may be due to abnormal Gram negative colonization of the introitus and periurethral areas in girls. Enquiries should be made about voiding habits (school toilets are often a problem!) and constipation, which has a strong association with voiding dysfunction and recurrent UTI.[59] It is important to provide the child and family with information about trying to reduce the number of urine infections and part of the outpatient consultation should be the provision of an information sheet such as the example below:

Prevention of urinary tract infections

When your child has a urinary tract infection, the doctor will prescribe antibiotics. As well as the antibiotics, there are also some things you can do to help the infection to get better and also prevent another infection.

1. *AVOID CONSTIPATION. You can do this by giving your child a high fiber diet to include wholemeal bread, whole-wheat cereals and fresh fruit and vegetables. Ensure that your child drinks a lot and has regular exercise. The doctor may also give your child a medicine to soften the stools.*
If your child has any problems with WORMS let the doctor know.

2. *In young girls the tube to the bladder is very close to the back passage. WIPING should be done in a front to back direction.*

3. *It is better to take a shower rather than a bath. Always avoid irritating soaps and bubble baths. CLEANLINESS is very important to help prevent infection.*

4. *EMPTYING THE BLADDER PROPERLY IS VERY IMPORTANT. Encourage your child to use the toilet regularly and empty the bladder every 2–3 hours. Sometimes we ask that your child will double empty the bladder. The child will pass water then wait a few minutes before trying to pass water again.*

5. *Always encourage your child to DRINK as much as possible during the day, and to EMPTY THE BLADDER PROPERLY LAST THING AT NIGHT.*

6. *CORRECT UNDERWEAR. Avoid tight underpants or pantyhose. They prevent air from circulating freely and encourage the warm, moist environment which favors infection. Soft cotton briefs, changed daily, are a far better choice. Consider changing the washing powder you use for the panties if irritation persists.*

7. *When taking antibiotics the full course must be taken at the time required. Any PROBLEMS such as burning when passing water, going to the toilet often, or blood in the water SHOULD BE REPORTED to the doctor.*

We hope that these ideas will help you to help your child. Please do not hesitate to ask questions or contact us if you are worried.

Cranberry juice has been advocated as a treatment for reducing the recurrence rate for UTI. A recent randomized trial in adult women showed a 20% reduction in absolute risk in those taking 50 ml of cranberry–lingonberry juice concentrate daily for 6 months compared to the control group.[60]

INVESTIGATIONS OF CHILDREN WITH UTI

At present the consensus is that all children, boys and girls, should undergo appropriate investigations after the *first* proven urinary tract infection. However, opinions differ about appropriate investigations at different ages, especially when children are referred for investigation and urine cultures have been taken by dubious methods. This is particularly relevant to one of the high risk groups, namely infancy. The nature and extent of investigations depend, to a large extent, upon the age of the child, clues from the history and the examination, and the availability of local imaging facilities and expertise. One is more inclined to investigate more fully a child who presents with a septicemic illness than a child referred to the outpatient department with dysuria and frequency with a culture taken inappropriately. The following imaging techniques are employed for the investigation of children with proven UTI.

Ultrasound (US) (all age groups)

Ultrasound will reveal anatomical information, even in the kidney without function. It will give basic information on the structure of the urinary tract, and kidney sizes should be recorded with reference to centile charts based on the child's height. US will also reveal problems of obstruction and bladder abnormality as well as stones. It is relatively cheap and requires no radiation (Fig. 16.9).

However, US is operator-dependent and is difficult in uncooperative children. It may only show gross scarring. Significant vesicoureteric reflux may be present with a normal ultrasound especially in the newborn period.[61]

Initially it was suggested that a *plain abdominal X-ray* was always required with the ultrasound. However, unless stones are suspected from the history, or there is the suggestion of a spinal abnormality on abdominal examination, a plain X-ray is now not *routinely* performed. We did originally use it to highlight to the child and the family the presence of fecal masses implying constipation, but there is a poor correlation between clinical and X-ray features of constipation and children are now not routinely reviewed in the clinic if they have had an uncomplicated UTI and the US is normal. In skilled hands the ultrasound may suggest renal scarring.

Intravenous urogram (IVU)

This has been superseded by the US, but may be requested if there is an ill defined abnormality on the ultrasound examination, if DMSA is not readily available, or if detailed upper tract imaging is required prior to surgery (Fig. 16.3).

Although intravenous urography is widely available it does require an intravenous injection and the radiation dose can be high unless the number of films is limited. It also gives poor visualization of scars in infants.

Micturating cystourethrogram

A micturating cystourethrogram (MCUG) is still routine in children under one year of age with a proven UTI, as this is the major risk period for scarring from vesicoureteric reflux. This examination is only required in those *over* one year of age who have recurrent infections or abnormalities on the ultrasound (or IVU) or a strong family history of vesicoureteric reflux and/or renal scarring. An MCUG is requested more readily in boys, particularly if there are any reported difficulties with the urinary stream.

The MCUG is the most traumatic of the imaging investigations for UTI.[62] It is important that experienced radiologists perform the technique. This should avoid the need to repeat the procedure in referral centers because of failure to visualize problems, such as the posterior urethra, in male infants. A study performed in our department has shown the benefit of proper preparation of the child and family for this procedure using stories and play preparation.[63] At least 48 h antibiotic cover should be prescribed to cover the MCUG (usually trimethoprim twice a day) and, if the child is discovered to have reflux, then s/he should be immediately commenced on antibiotic prophylaxis if s/he is not already on it.

Direct isotope cystography

Direct isotope cystography (technetium pertechnetate) gives lower radiation dose than contract cystography but still requires catheterization and the bladder structure and urethra are not visualized.

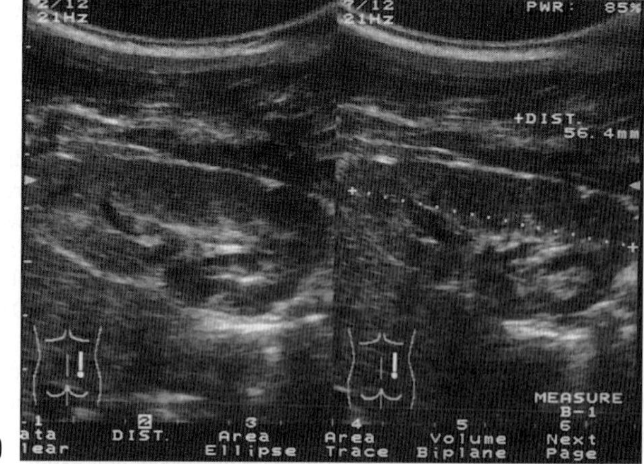

(a)

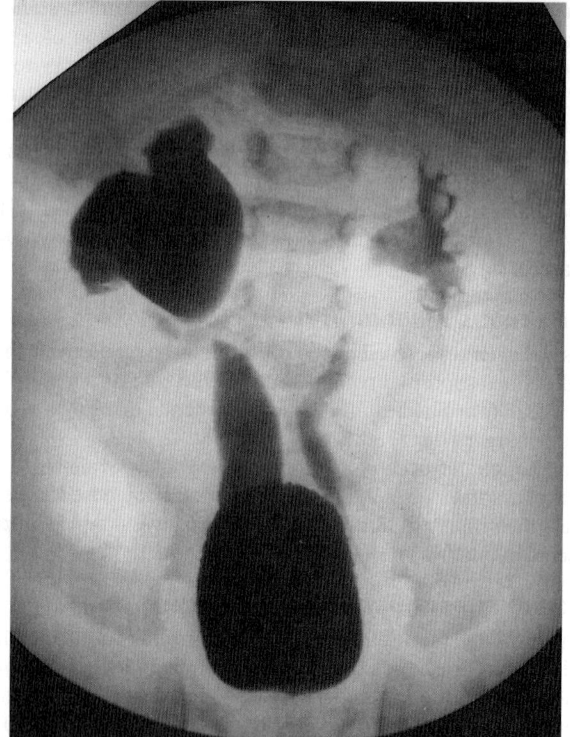

(b)

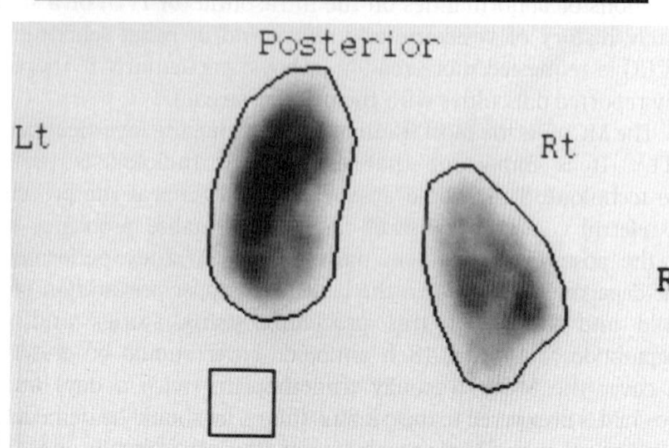

(c)

Fig. 16.9 Investigation in a 2-year-old boy with proven UTI: (a) ultrasound revealed normal left kidney (6.6 cm) with right kidney (shown) 5.6 cm and extensively scarred, especially at lower pole; (b) MCUG showed bilateral vesicoureteric reflux, gross right side; (c) DMSA shows scarring at both poles laterally of right kidney (40% of differential function).

Dimercaptosuccinic acid scan

Dimercaptosuccinic acid (DMSA) scan demonstrates acute renal involvement in UTIs and is the best technique for detection of scars and determining differential renal function (Fig. 16.9). A DMSA scan performed during or soon after the acute illness may show acute defects of the renal parenchyma, which do not necessarily result in permanent scars (Fig. 16.10)[64] and should therefore be delayed 3–6 months after the infection if using this technique to determine permanent renal damage.

Isotope renography (MAG 3 or DTPA)

These isotopes are good for confirming obstruction and calculation of differential kidney function as the radionuclide is taken up by the kidney and excretion curves are generated (Fig. 16.6b). Initial curves are not comparable to DMSA for definition of renal cortical anatomy or scarring, although the resolution is better with the MAG 3 scan which is now favored. The technique does require intravenous injection.

In the cooperative child, over 4–5 years of age, the scanning can continue as the child empties his or her bladder. This is the basis of *indirect micturating cystography*, which obviously has a lower radiation dose than the direct MCUG (Fig. 16.11). Although catheterization is avoided, the technique still requires intravenous injection of isotope. Improvements in the technique have reduced the number of false negative results in comparison with a direct MCUG and the indirect method is preferred for follow-up studies.

CHOICE OF IMAGING TECHNIQUES IN CHILDREN WITH SYMPTOMATIC UTI

It should be stressed that the decision to initiate investigations in any child should take note of the clinical history and examination, proof of the urine infection, age of the child and availability of local imaging techniques. Clinical history may not be closely related to radiological findings but nevertheless one is more inclined to investigate a child presenting with symptoms suggestive of acute pyelonephritis rather than a child referred to the outpatient department with frequency and dysuria. In a prospective study of 257 children referred to our *outpatient* clinic by primary care physicians the incidence of significant radiological findings in a high risk group (symptoms suggesting upper tract involvement, recurrent urinary infections, less than 2 years old, family history of renal tract anomaly, macroscopic hematuria) was 7.5% compared to 1% in a low risk (mainly lower tract symptoms) group (Savill & Watson 1996, unpublished observations).

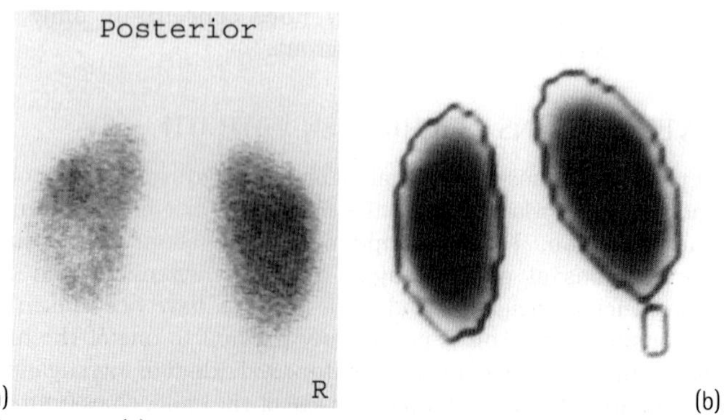

(a) (b)

Fig. 16.10 (a) DMSA scan showing parenchymal defects in left kidney of 3-year-old with pyelonephritis. (b) DMSA scan in the same child 4 months later showing resolution of acute changes.

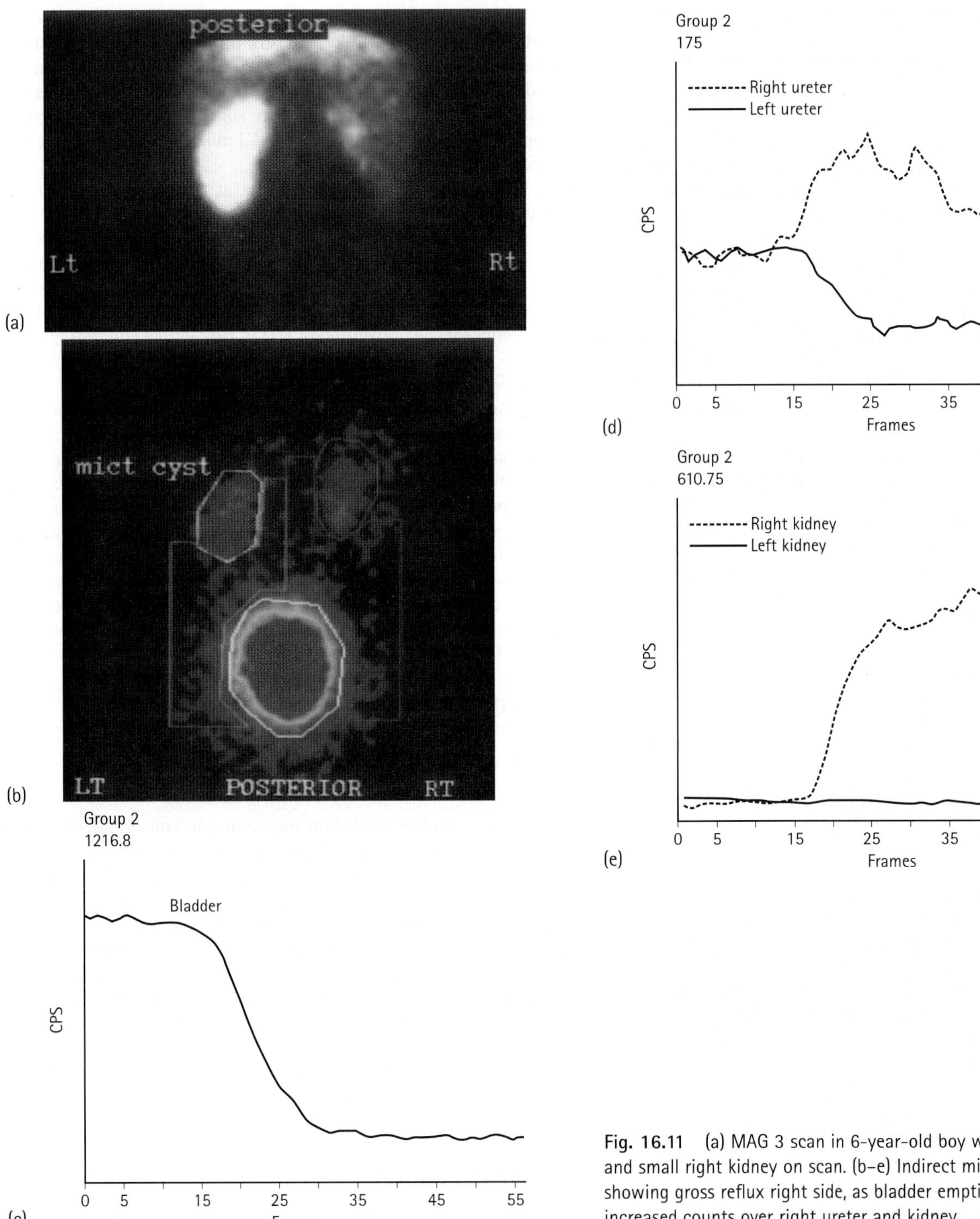

Fig. 16.11 (a) MAG 3 scan in 6-year-old boy with history of UTI and small right kidney on scan. (b–e) Indirect micturating cystogram showing gross reflux right side, as bladder empties, reflected in increased counts over right ureter and kidney.

Since it is generally agreed that younger children are more vulnerable to renal damage and that obstructive uropathy, although uncommon, should be detected, the regimen set out in Table 16.6 is suggested. Crucial to this plan of investigation is the quality of the ultrasound examinations available at each hospital. Some authors have advocated routine DMSA scans because of the poor correlation with ultrasound of the urinary system (USS) for detection of scars. However, USS performed by experienced radiologists using good equipment has shown very good detection of most abnormalities and comparable to DMSA.[65,66]

FURTHER MANAGEMENT OF CHILDREN WITH UTI

Further management depends mainly on the results of investigations but also on the previous and family history. This includes: relief of obstruction; prevention of further infection; and investigation of siblings.

Relief of obstruction

In the unusual situation, where a child presents with an obstructive uropathy or stones, a surgical consultation will be required. Children with suspected neurogenic bladder require further

Table 16.6 Investigation of children with proven UTI – choice of imaging techniques

0–1 year of age	
a	Ultrasound of the urinary system (USS) (kidneys, ureters and bladder)
b	Direct micturating cystourethrogram (MCUG) (catheterization should be delayed until the urine is free from infection but delay for up to 6 weeks is not necessary)
c	DMSA scan
Caveats	
i	If the USS is normal and performed by a reliable operator and the child was not febrile and hospitalized one could consider omitting the MCUG and waiting
ii	If there is significant hydronephrosis on the ultrasound in the absence of reflux on the MCUG then a pediatric nephrology or urology opinion should be sought to plan the need for further imaging such as isotope renography with MAG 3 or DTPA
iii	DMSA scan should be delayed for 6 months if vesicoureteric reflux (VUR) and child on prophylactic antibiotics to give acute changes time to resolve
iv	If presentation is with a febrile episode and the diagnosis of UTI is uncertain, then acute DMSA during hospital admission will show parenchymal involvement
v	If outpatient referral and USS and MCUG normal (reliable operator) then DMSA not necessary
1–5 years	
a	USS of the urinary system
b	MCUG only if USS/DMSA shows abnormality, or if there are recurrent proven infections and/or strong family history. The detection of VUR will warrant prophylactic antibiotics for 1–2 years
c	DMSA scan if the child has had suspected pyelonephritis, abnormal USS or if the MCUG shows evidence of severe reflux (to better define scarring)
Caveats	
i	MAG 3 with indirect micturating cystography may be attempted in children over 3 years who are cooperative
ii	USS with bladder emptying should be performed in those with daytime wetting symptoms
iii	In some centres USS can provide as accurate an evaluation of scars and differential volume as DMSA
Over 5 years	
a	USS of the urinary system
b	DMSA scan if abnormal ultrasound or severe systemic symptoms (during acute hospitalization)
c	Isotope renography with indirect micturating cystography to define reflux if scarring present on ultrasound/DMSA
d	Direct MCUG only if surgery contemplated or recurrent symptoms despite negative indirect micturating cystography

imaging, such as MRI scans of the spine and urodynamic evaluation of the bladder.[67]

Prevention of further infection

Even in the child presenting with a first UTI, it is important to stress preventive measures (see above). It is particularly important to stress a normal bladder emptying routine and to treat constipation. Dietary advice should be given on increasing fiber in the diet and the use of mild laxatives such as lactulose (occasionally stronger ones such as Senokot may be required for short periods).

There is a significant group of children with dysfunctional voiding patterns (see under Wetting problems) who are prone to recurrent infections. Such children may require assessment of bladder emptying by ultrasound and stressing the importance of double or triple voiding. In addition, some are best managed with prophylactic antibiotics given for 6–12 months to break the vicious cycle of reinfection.

Antibiotics given as a single dose at night reduce the risk of recurrent UTI compared to placebo or no treatment. However, a recent systematic review suggests that most published studies to date have been poorly designed with biases known to overestimate the true treatment effect. Large, properly randomized, double-blinded trails are still needed to determine the efficacy of long-term antibiotics for the prevention of UTI in susceptible children.[68]

Investigation of siblings

Vesicoureteric reflux is known to occur in 20–30% of siblings[69] and VUR behaves as an autosomal dominant condition with variable penetrance. In any family where VUR is detected, the parents are advised to keep a close eye out for UTI in other children and obstetric staff should be alerted in future pregnancies. When moderate to gross reflux is noted in one child, an ultrasound should be requested on siblings, and if abnormal, an MCUG or indirect radionuclide cystogram may be considered. Although others have advocated an MCUG on all, it is felt that this more conservative approach is a useful compromise, in view of the potentially traumatic nature of the MCUG and radiation dose.

VESICOURETERIC REFLUX (Fig. 16.12)

MANAGEMENT OF CHILDREN WITH VESICOURETERIC REFLUX

In recent years the pendulum has swung to conservative medical management for this condition. Surgical reimplantation of the ureters is reserved for those children with obstructive uropathy or recurrent symptomatic urine infections despite prophylaxis. This approach has been confirmed by both the Birmingham and International study comparing conservative versus operative management, where the incidence of new scars, progression of existing scars, overall kidney function and frequency of breakthrough urinary tract infections was no different in the two groups.[70,71] Even with children with severe bilateral VUR and nephropathy, the group thought to have the highest risk of developing end-stage renal failure, surgical correction had no discernible benefit.[72]

MEDICAL REGIMEN

This includes repeated discussion with the child and family about general preventive measures, including regular, frequent repeat-voiding and avoidance of constipation. Low dose antibiotic prophylaxis should be taken in a single evening dose and urine cultures should be taken if the child has any symptoms. We no longer encourage the *routine* culture of urine samples from asymptomatic children but emphasize the need for cultures if *symptomatic*. Urine specimens obtained at the clinic that are negative on dipstick are also not routinely cultured. An explanatory booklet is given to the family and they are asked to record details of any positive urine culture results taken in the primary care setting. When the child is taking prophylactic antibiotics we stress to the family:

1. Try to avoid *missing* any doses.

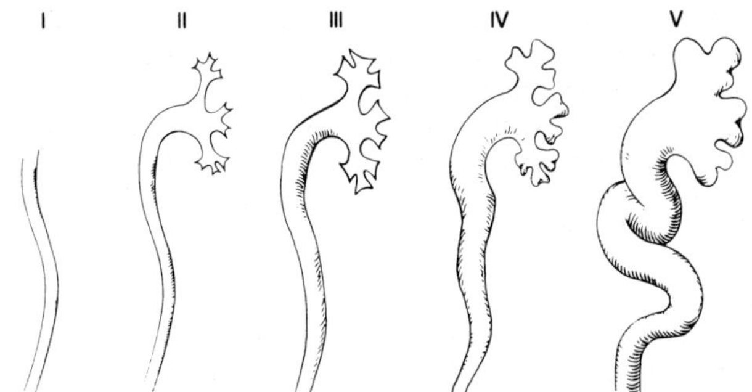

Fig. 16.12 International classification of grades of reflux: I ureter only; II ureter, pelvis and calyces, no dilatation; III mild or moderate dilatation and/or tortuosity of the ureter and mild or moderate dilatation of renal pelvis but no, or only slight, blunting of the fornices; IV moderate dilatation and/or tortuosity of the ureter and moderate dilatation of renal pelvis and calyces. Complete obliteration of sharp angle of fornices but maintenance of capillary impression in majority of calyces; V gross dilatation and tortuosity of ureter, gross dilatation of renal pelvis and calyces, capillary impressions are no longer visible in majority of cases.

2. Do *not* double up the dose if your child has a suspected urine infection. *Do* obtain a urine culture and take it to your doctor or clinic.
3. If your child is given another antibiotic for an infection such as a sore throat, then *continue* the prophylactic antibiotic.

The duration of antibiotic prophylaxis is debatable, but in our unit it is given for a 2-year period. After such time it is appropriate to reassess kidney growth and evidence of scarring by ultrasound and DMSA scans. This will determine the planning of long-term follow-up. Urinary prophylaxis is discontinued after the 2-year period if the child has been free of infections and if there is:

1. No evidence of scars on DMSA/ultrasound. Discharge to primary care and see again if recurrent infections.
2. Scarring in *one* kidney. Review annually and reinstigate prophylaxis if further documented infection. May repeat ultrasound and/or DMSA in further 2 years. If child remains normotensive after 10 years of age refer to general practitioner for blood pressure measurements yearly.
3. *Bilateral renal scarring.* These children are at greater risk of chronic renal insufficiency and/or hypertension and should be under long-term follow-up by a pediatric nephrologist. Further assessment may include annual blood pressure checks and a MAG 3 scan with indirect cystography combined with ^{51}Cr EDTA GFR measurement at 5-year follow-up.

From the above regimen it should be noted that the direct MCUG is *not* repeated without good reason, as we know from previous studies that a great deal of reflux resolves and the damage is done early. The exception is in the child with recurrent *symptomatic* infections where surgery may be contemplated. There may be an element of non-compliance, resulting in recurrent infections, or the antibiotic sensitivity of the local organisms may have changed.

SURGICAL REGIMEN

Difficult cases with complex anomalies of the urinary tract and those children with recurrent symptomatic infections are best referred to a unit where there is joint discussion between a pediatric urologist, nephrologist and radiologist. The standard reimplantation procedure is the Cohen or Leadbetter Politano technique, which involves changing the intramural segment of ureter through the bladder wall. Operative success rates are 90–95% in centers with pediatric urological expertise.

There has been a great deal of interest recently in the 'sting' procedure, with the submucosal injection of substances such as polytetrafluoroethylene paste or, more recently, microsilicone particles alongside the ureter. This can be done as a day case procedure. Although there may be good success rates in experienced hands there have been concerns raised about long-term consequences of injection of foreign material and the need in some cases for repeated injection and cystograms to check the effectiveness of the procedure.

Urinary tract infection is defined by symptoms and a positive urine culture (> 10^5 organisms/ml in specimens passed per urethra)

Investigations for UTI depend upon the age of the child, upper or lower tract symptoms and availability of imaging techniques

The management of vesicoureteric reflux is predominantly conservative with prophylactic antibiotics

WETTING PROBLEMS

This is a common symptom, which can cause much distress and anxiety to the child and parents. *Enuresis* can be defined as the involuntary voiding of urine in a child over 5 years of age without structural or neurological disease of the bladder or urinary tract, whereas *incontinence* is the leakage of urine in a child with structural or neurological disease of the bladder or urinary tract.

Enuresis is far more common than incontinence and the two should be distinguished from the history, physical examination and limited investigations, as shown in Table 16.7.

IDIOPATHIC (PRIMARY) NOCTURNAL ENURESIS

This can affect up to 10% of 7-year-old children and there is usually a family history in close relatives. Epidemiological studies show that if one parent has a history of nocturnal enuresis, his/her children are five to seven times more likely to have the disorder than those

Table 16.7 Differential diagnosis of enuresis

Diagnosis	Clinical indicators
Urinary tract infection	Other urinary tract symptoms, secondary onset wetting
Detrusor instability	Daytime symptoms of urinary frequency, urgency and urge incontinence usually with a minor degree of wetness and worse in the afternoons
Neuropathic bladder	Constant severe daytime wetting, soiling, lumbosacral dimple or nevus, abnormal gait, abnormal perianal or lower limb neurology, palpable bladder
Ectopic ureter	Constant dribble of urine between voidings
Posterior urethral valves	Poor urinary stream, daytime wetting, palpable bladder
Chronic renal disease	Chronic ill health, hypertension, palpable kidneys or bladder, anemia, polydipsia
Diabetes mellitus	Recent illness with weight loss, thirst and polydipsia

without an affected parent. Recent genetic studies in families with nocturnal enuresis have located two markers known as ENUR1 which flank the enuresis gene on chromosome 13.[73]

As well as the inherited tendency, physiological disturbances such as nocturnal polyuria, small functional bladder capacity and decreased arousal response to the full bladder have been identified. The history should attempt to identify any environmental factors such as stress and emotional disturbances; potential physical disorders that may lead to wetting should be excluded on thorough physical examination and urinalysis.

Spontaneous resolution of nocturnal enuresis occurs at the rate of 15% per annum. If the child is distressed by the wetting, or it is leading to distress within the family, then treatment should be considered. An interested and sympathetic health care professional can certainly help to support the family. In children aged between 5 and 7 years, the strategy of explanation, reassurance, star charts and praise or small rewards for dry nights is usually all that is necessary. For older children conditioning therapy with an enuresis alarm is the most effective treatment.[74] However, it is hard work and the child and family need to be closely supervised and supported.[75]

The role of medication remains controversial but may give some short-term relief. Desmopressin, a synthetic analogue of antidiuretic hormone, can be given as a nasal spray or tablet but relapse is usual when treatment finishes.[76] Imipramine is also effective but has a higher incidence of side-effects and is potentially lethal to children in accidental overdose.[77] There may be benefit from combining desmopressin with an alarm but again there are significant relapse rates.[78]

DIURNAL ENURESIS DUE TO BLADDER INSTABILITY

This problem is usually classified as enuresis because there is no structural or neurological deficit. The wetting results from a functional disturbance of the detrusor muscle, which intermittently contracts during the filling/storage phase of the bladder at a time when the muscle is normally relaxed. The child has difficulty suppressing these contractions (normally an involuntary reflex), which therefore results in leakage of urine and urgency/urge incontinence before the child contracts the pelvic floor to stop micturition. The condition has a strong association with urinary tract infection and constipation, and emotional stresses may precipitate the problem in some children.

Treatment is again aimed at providing information and support along with establishing a routine of complete and regular emptying of the bladder to restore the child's confidence. Star charts and rewards may be helpful. Constipation must be vigorously treated and urine infection eradicated. If infections are proven, then the child will justify an ultrasound of the urinary tract with a check on bladder emptying. Day case assessment by experienced urology nurses may help to promote biofeedback training and promote compliance. An anticholinergic drug such as oxybutynin is usually effective but more conservative measures should be tried first. Some families require the support of a psychologist.

NEUROPATHIC BLADDER

Myelomeningocele is the main cause of neuropathic bladder in the pediatric population. Although children with myelomeningocele are usually born with normal kidneys, the function of the obstructed neuropathic bladder can result in chronic kidney damage if unrecognized.[79] Neuropathic bladder/sphincter dysfunction is complex and these children require careful assessment in specialist centers with expertise in urodynamics. The detrusor and/or striated pelvic floor muscles may lack spinal motor innovation (inactivity); with lesions above the level of the spinal motor neuron pelvic floor muscles are overactive during filling and voiding. This dyssynergic pelvic floor activity constitutes a functional infravesical obstruction during voiding, implying a high risk of kidney damage because of high emptying pressures.

Clean intermittent catheterization has been the major advance in the management of children with neuropathic bladders. It provides a means of both promoting continence as well as safeguarding kidney function. Oxybutynin to inhibit detrusor overactivity is often combined with intermittent catheterization.

Small capacity bladders may require augmentation procedures using the patient's own ureter or bowel. At the same time, the appendix can be used to fashion a Mitrofanoff channel to the umbilicus or laterally for intermittent catheterization. Patients and families derive great benefit from close support by a specialist nurse.

Ectopic ureter is a rare cause of day and night-time wetting and is suggested by a history of never having been dry in the day and dribbling of urine

Conditioning therapy with an enuresis alarm is the most effective treatment for nocturnal enuresis in older cooperative children

Clean intermittent catheterization is the mainstay of treatment for neuropathic bladders

HEMATURIA

Children may present with gross (or macroscopic) hematuria, in which case they are usually quickly brought to medical attention, or they may be found to have microscopic hematuria on routine urinalysis using one of the many types of urinary testing strips (dipsticks). The degree of hematuria is a poor guide to the severity of any underlying disease, but careful examination of the urine is an important non-invasive diagnostic tool.

Urinary dipsticks are very sensitive for blood and it is important that the manufacturer's instructions are followed closely and the test repeated on further samples. Microscopic hematuria may be transient and can occur in the context of exercise or stress. Urine could also be contaminated with blood from the external genital area, urethral meatus or menstrual blood.

Gross hematuria may be described as coke- or tea-colored due to the oxidized heme pigment, but it may also be bright red, suggesting an extrarenal or lower urinary tract source. Inquiry should be made of other possible causes of red urine, such as foods (beetroot, berries and food dyes) and drugs (e.g. rifampicin). Hemoglobinuria and myoglobinuria should also be considered (Table 16.4). Urate crystals may give the urine a pinkish tinge when present in high concentration, particularly in young infants.

URINE MICROSCOPY

Microscopy of fresh urine should be performed in all cases of hematuria to confirm the presence of red blood cells. Red cells hemolyze in standing urine, and fresh urine is also better for the identification of red cell or heme granular casts which are a strong pointer to a renal source for the hematuria (Fig. 16.13). Microscopy may also reveal pyuria and/or motile bacteria (suggesting infection) or crystals (using contrast microscopy). It may be possible to differentiate glomerular bleeding, when the red cells appear

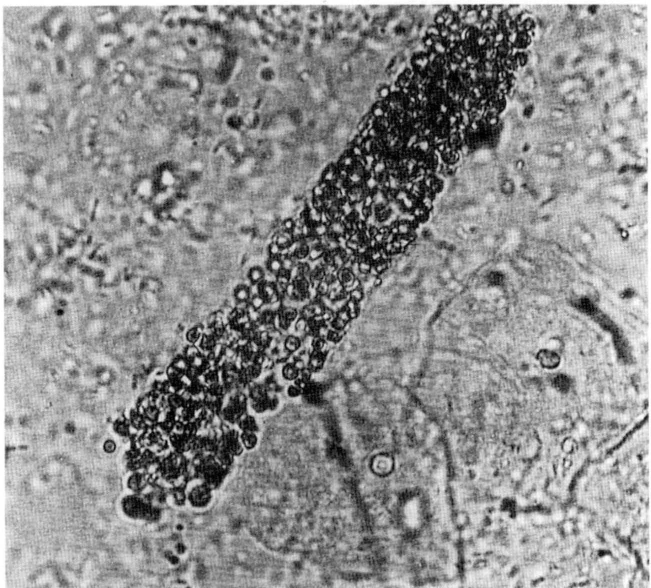

Fig. 16.13 Red cell granular cast. The outlines of many erythrocytes can still be made out clearly. (x 400)

dysmorphic, from bleeding originating from the lower urinary tract, when the red cells tend to be of uniform shape and size.[80]

Table 16.8 Causes of hematuria

1. Infection	a. Bacterial b. Viral c. Schistosomiasis d. Tuberculosis
2. Glomerular diseases	
3. Stones	a. Urolithiasis b. Idiopathic hypercalciuria
4. Trauma	
5. Anatomic abnormalities	a. Congenital abnormalities, e.g. pelviureteric junction obstruction b. Polycystic kidneys c. Tumor
6. Vascular	a. Arteritis b. Infarction and thrombosis c. Loin pain–hematuria syndrome
7. Hematological	a. Coagulopathies b. Sickle-cell disease
8. Drugs	e.g. Cyclophosphamide
9. Exercise-induced	
10. Factitious	

CAUSES OF HEMATURIA

The causes of hematuria are listed in Table 16.8. Many of the causes can be differentiated on the basis of the history, examination and urinalysis. If gross hematuria is reported, then the child or observer should be asked if it is more prominent in the initial or terminal parts of the urinary stream. Initial hematuria suggests a urethral cause, but this line of questioning is unlikely to be as relevant as it is in the adult patient, where bladder tumors and stones are much more prominent causes of hematuria.

Infection

Hematuria associated with dysuria, frequency, enuresis and suprapubic discomfort suggests a hemorrhagic cystitis, while systemic upset, fever, abdominal pain or loin tenderness suggest pyelonephritis. Urinary tract infection, either proven or suspected, remains a common cause of hematuria. Since other symptoms and signs may be minimal, it is essential that appropriate urine cultures are taken before treatment is initiated.

Viral infections can result in acute hemorrhagic cystitis, particularly adenovirus types 11 and 21. This is usually a self-limiting illness with resolution towards the end of the first week.

Persistent dysuria, hematuria and sterile pyuria would suggest tuberculosis, in the right clinical context, but this would be a very rare cause of hematuria in children in Western countries. Infection with *Schistosoma haematobium* is an important cause of hematuria in endemic areas such as the Middle East and Africa. The ova can cause a granulomatous reaction in the bladder wall and lower ureter, and prompt treatment is essential (see Ch. 26).

Glomerulonephritis

The history of an upper respiratory tract or other infection, particularly if associated with gross hematuria, is suggestive of some form of acute postinfectious glomerulonephritis. Recurrent macroscopic hematuria in the older child raises the suspicion of IgA nephropathy.

A positive family history of renal disease with or without deafness suggests the possibility of hereditary nephritis.

Renal calculi

Incidence

The incidence of urinary tract calculi in children is approximately 1–5/100 000 in developed countries. It is much higher in areas of the world where stone disease is endemic, e.g. Middle East. In these areas, there are more likely to be urate calculi, whereas in Europe most children with stones will have them as a result of infective causes. These are more likely to occur in the presence of obstruction to the urinary flow combined with infection, reduced fluid intake and episodes of dehydration. Stone formation may also occur due to underlying genetic factors such as hyperoxaluria or tubular transport problems such as cystinuria and hypercalciuria syndromes.

Clinical features

The classical presentation of renal colic, common in adult patients, is rare in childhood. More often calculi are recognized as a result of investigations in children for urinary tract infection or hematuria. Many children are diagnosed incidentally when imaging techniques such as ultrasound are carried out for investigation of abdominal pain. Certain children are at high risk of renal calculi and these include ex-premature babies, those who are immobilized or who have a neuropathic bladder. A family history of renal calculi should always be sought.

Investigation

Most stones are associated with infection and magnesium/ammonium phosphate complex. However, screening investigations, as listed in Table 16.9, are necessary, as hypercalciuria and hyperoxaluria may both need treatment, and the amino acid profile should define cystinuria.[81] Rare inborn errors of purine metabolism, xanthinuria and 2,8-dihydroxyadenine due to adenine phosphoribosyl transferase deficiency need to be remembered.

Table 16.9 Investigations for children with renal calculi

1. Urinalysis including pH and urine for amino acids
2. Urine culture
3. Plasma biochemistry including creatinine, chloride, bicarbonate, calcium, phosphate, urate, magnesium levels
4. Second morning urine sample for calcium:creatinine and oxalate: creatinine ratios (24 h urine collections to confirm hypercalciuria or hyperoxaluria in older children)
5. Analysis of calculus if available

Management

This will depend upon the severity of the presentation, but percutaneous nephrostomy to treat an obstructed kidney, due to stones, is rarely required. Renal ultrasound is the most sensitive method for identifying stones within the kidney or renal pelvis, as these will show as echo-bright densities casting acoustic shadows. Occasionally, ultrasound will miss ureteric calculi in a child with acute renal colic with or without hematuria. A plain abdominal X-ray and IVU will possibly be required.

Extracorporeal shockwave lithotripsy (ESWL) can be successfully performed under general anesthesia in children, but may be less successful if the stone is very hard (e.g. cystine), if it is located at the lower pole calyx or if it is very large and fragments are likely to obstruct the ureter. There is some evidence that ESWL causes a short term of reduction in renal function and may have long-term effects on developing kidneys.

Direct nephrolithotomy may be required for a large staghorn calculus in the renal pelvis. Other urological techniques such as percutaneous nephrolithotomy and ureteroscopy may be attempted in some children.

Trauma

Hematuria is associated with an obvious history of a damaging event. There is often bruising and other signs of external injury. With increasing recognition of the spectrum of sexual abuse, it is important that a careful history be taken if the injury involves the anogenital region.

Anatomic abnormalities

Although it is sometimes hard to equate abnormalities on X-ray with hematuria, there is no doubt that problems such as hydronephrosis, due for example to pelviureteric junction obstruction, can be a cause of hematuria. Although autosomal dominant polycystic kidney disease is increasingly recognized in childhood by the use of ultrasound scanning, it very rarely results in hematuria in the pediatric population.

The major kidney tumor of childhood is nephroblastoma (Wilms' tumor), and this usually presents as an abdominal mass, with one-third of patients having associated hematuria, mainly microscopic. Bladder tumors are very rare in childhood[82] and so cystoscopy is rarely indicated, unlike the case in the adult population.

Vascular and hematological causes

Hematuria may occur in the context of any child with a problem such as hemophilia, leukemia or sickle-cell disease. The hematuria in the latter condition is presumably due to sickling of erythrocytes in the hypertonic, hypoxemic medulla, with resulting local papillary infarcts. It is unlikely to be the initial presentation.

Gross hematuria, associated with a palpable mass, in a newborn infant, would suggest renal vein thrombosis. Hematuria may be part of the symptom complex in a multisystem disorder such as polyarteritis.

The loin pain–hematuria syndrome, which predominantly affects young women, is rare in childhood and requires renal angiography in suspected cases.

Drugs

There is an extensive list of drugs, poisons and ingested substances, which can give rise to hematuria.[83] Cyclophosphamide is a well-recognized cause of a sterile hemorrhagic cystitis, and a high fluid intake should be maintained during the use of this drug. Other drugs such as sulfonamides can cause crystalluria.

Exercise-induced

Hematuria may occur after severe exercise and has usually disappeared within 48 h. It would appear to have a glomerular origin and is an accentuation of the small amount of blood excreted by a number of people after heavy exercise.

Factitious hematuria

This may be part of the spectrum of Munchausen syndrome by proxy, where the child's carer (usually the mother) adds blood to the urine sample after it has been passed. There may be other pointers in the history or behavioral observations, which suggest this diagnosis.[84] A forensic laboratory may be able to determine whether the origin of the blood is from the parent or child.

INVESTIGATIONS IN A CHILD WITH HEMATURIA

The tests performed will depend upon the information provided from the history, examination and urinalysis. Again, it should be stressed that *microscopy* on a fresh urine sample can be invaluable, as identification of dysmorphic red cells and heme granular or red cell casts (the urine should be centrifuged for 3 min at 3000 rev/min) strongly suggests a nephritic process and the child will be investigated accordingly. A *familial* condition may be detected by testing the urine of all immediate family members, particularly in cases of persistent microscopic hematuria.

Urine culture

A proven bacterial infection will lead to the appropriate investigations. Urine is rarely cultured for viruses, but should be considered in epidemics.

Hematology

Full blood count and film. Coagulation tests if appropriate.

Biochemistry

1. Plasma urea, electrolytes, creatinine, calcium, phosphate, alkaline phosphatase, albumin, total protein.
2. Urine calcium/creatinine ratio on second morning sample (if > 0.7 mmol/mmol confirm with a 24-h collection).

Radiology

1. An ultrasound of the urinary tract in experienced hands should define any hydronephrosis, masses, renal calculi, etc. A plain abdominal X-ray is not required routinely.
2. An intravenous urogram may be ordered to confirm any suspicion raised on the initial screening ultrasound or to define the level of obstruction if ureteric stones are suspected.
3. A micturating cystourethrogram or cystoscopy is *rarely* necessary in childhood, but may be indicated based on the history. If there is recurrent or persistent gross unexplained hematuria then cystoscopy during an episode may localize the bleeding to one

kidney (in which an anatomic abnormality is probably present) or to both kidneys (making glomerulonephritis more likely).
4. Further radiological investigations may include CT scanning or MRI for renal masses, radionuclide scans to define parenchymal masses or rarely renal arteriography.

Further tests for glomerulonephritis

Glomerulonephritis should be suspected if there are characteristic urinary changes or if the hematuria is persistent and no other cause can be found. The appropriate investigations will be discussed in detail later but should include:

1. throat swab for bacteria and viruses;
2. antistreptolysin O titer and other streptococcal antigens;
3. complement studies;
4. autoantibody screen including antinuclear factor antibody;
5. viral titers including screening for hepatitis B surface antigen.

Hearing test

In cases of suspected familial nephritis.

Renal biopsy

This is never routine and is only performed when there are indications of a more serious and potentially progressive disease, such as: progressive or persistent renal impairment; hypertension; persistent hypocomplementemia; heavy proteinuria; a familial disease that has not been characterized; a systemic disorder where therapy may be influenced by the histopathological findings, e.g. Systemic lupus erythematosus (SLE). Renal biopsies are also carried out in children with persistent microscopic hematuria (usually of greater than 1 year's duration), often because of the family's request to know a specific diagnosis and prognosis (Fig. 16.14).

Only nephrologists experienced in the technique should carry out a renal biopsy. They should have access to expert pathology advice, based on light and electron microscopy as well as immunofluorescence (or immunohistochemistry). In most instances, the biopsy is performed under ultrasound (or IVP) guidance in the sedated child. The biopsy can be carried out as a day case procedure with appropriate preparation of the child and family.[85] An open renal biopsy under general anesthetic is only necessary in the very young child. In expert hands the morbidity associated with renal biopsy is low.

The commonest cause of hematuria in childhood is infection

Children with macroscopic hematuria and persistent microscopic hematuria should undergo a renal tract ultrasound but rarely need cystoscopy

Hypercalciuria can cause hematuria and can be screened for by a second morning urine calcium/creatinine ratio

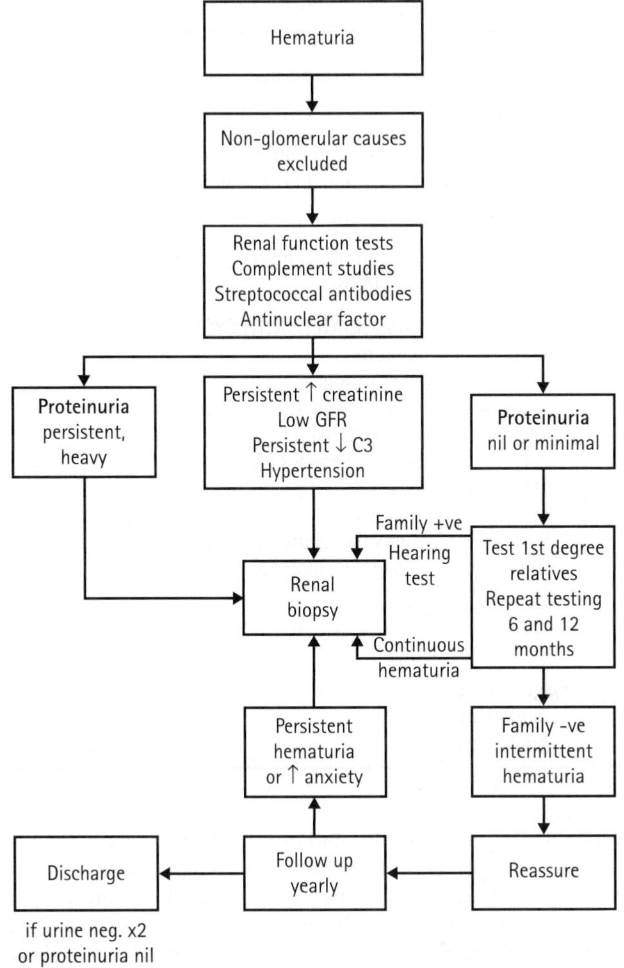

Fig. 16.14 A scheme for the management of children with hematuria.

GLOMERULONEPHRITIS

Glomerulonephritis, or more simply nephritis, is both a generic term for several diseases, and a histopathological term signifying inflammation and proliferation of cells within the glomerulus. In many instances the inflammatory changes are initiated by immunological mechanisms, but in others the pathogenesis is unknown.

Injury may be limited to the kidney alone, or the immune or non-immune mechanisms may be part of a systemic disorder (Table 16.10).

We still understand very little of the specific events involved with glomerulonephritis, and so when therapy has been employed it has tended to be 'blunderbuss' in nature, with broad spectrum immunosuppressive drugs such as corticosteroids, azathioprine and cyclophosphamide, or other therapies such as plasma exchange.

PATHOLOGY

Many of the categories of so-called primary glomerulonephritis (Table 16.10) are based on histopathological descriptions obtained from renal biopsy specimens. The terminology is derived from changes that are found on light, electron and immunofluorescent microscopy (Figs 16.15 and 16.16).

CLINICAL PATTERNS OF GLOMERULONEPHRITIS

Patients with glomerulonephritis may present with:

1. Asymptomatic *hematuria* and/or proteinuria.
2. *Acute nephritic syndrome* characterized by hematuria, oliguria, edema and hypertension. The hematuria is heavy with red cell casts on microscopy. Proteinuria is variable.
3. *Nephrotic syndrome* characterized by heavy proteinuria leading to hypoalbuminemia and edema with hyperlipidemia. The urinalysis shows heavy proteinuria (+++ or > 5 g/L) with variable hematuria. Microscopy may show fatty casts and free fat droplets.

It is important to appreciate that there is a spectrum of clinical presentation and patients may have a mixed picture of nephritis/

Table 16.10 Classification of glomerular disorders

PRIMARY GLOMERULONEPHRITIS
1. Immune complex glomerulonephritis
a. Postinfectious acute glomerulonephritis
b. IgA nephropathy (Berger's disease)
c. Membranoproliferative glomerulonephritis (types I to III)
d. Membranous glomerulonephritis (idiopathic)
2. Anti-GBM-antibody-mediated glomerulonephritis
3. Uncertain etiology, e.g. minimal lesion glomerulonephritis, focal segmental glomerulosclerosis
GLOMERULONEPHRITIS ASSOCIATED WITH SYSTEMIC DISORDERS
1. Immunologically-mediated
a. Henoch–Schönlein purpura
b. Systemic lupus erythematosus and other collagen disorders, e.g. scleroderma
c. Polyarteritis nodosa, Wegener's granulomatosis and other vasculitides
d. Mixed cryoglobulinemia
e. Systemic infections (subacute bacterial endocarditis, shunt nephritis, syphilis, malaria, hepatitis B, HIV)
2. Hereditary disorders
a. Familial nephritis, e.g. Alport syndrome
b. Sickle cell anemia
3. Other conditions
a. Diabetes mellitus
b. Amyloidosis

nephrosis. For example, the majority of children with Henoch–Schönlein purpura have nephritis with asymptomatic hematuria and/or proteinuria, which usually resolves, but may progress into a nephritic syndrome. If the proteinuria is so heavy that hypoalbuminemia results, then the patient may have the clinical picture of nephrotic syndrome.

ACUTE GLOMERULONEPHRITIS

Acute glomerulonephritis is associated with dark urine, diminished urine output, edema, hypertension and varying degrees of renal insufficiency, i.e. an acute nephritic syndrome. Some of the family contacts may exhibit a milder form with asymptomatic hematuria.

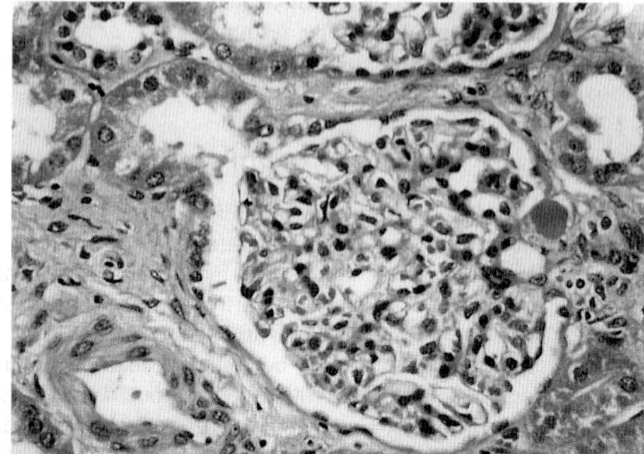

Fig. 16.15 Light microscopy of a normal glomerulus. Part of the proximal tubule at upper left hand corner and hilum on the right.

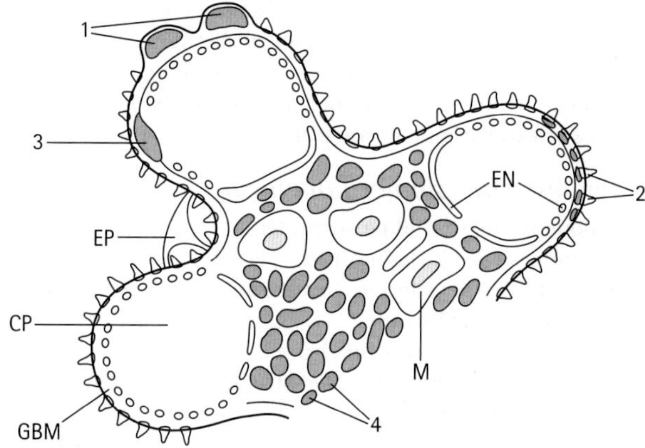

Fig. 16.16 Schematic depiction of the anatomy of the glomerulus and possible sites of immune complex deposition (CP, capillary space; EN, endothelial; EP, epithelial; GBM, glomerular basement membrane; M, mesangial cell). Deposits are in the following locations: 1, subepithelial lumps; 2, intramembranous; 3, subendothelial; 4, mesangial.

In children, the majority of cases will be postinfectious, with group A beta-hemolytic streptococcus being the organism most commonly implicated. Acute poststreptococcal glomerulonephritis (APSGN) may follow nasopharyngeal or skin infection.

Although the disease is now uncommon in Western countries, it is still very prevalent in many parts of the world where overcrowding, poor nutrition and widespread skin sepsis (particularly following scabies) still prevail. As APSGN has diminished in developed countries, other postinfectious causes of acute nephritis are being recognized. These include infection with staphylococcal, pneumococcal, salmonella and mycoplasma species, as well as viral infections such as Coxsackie, ECHO, Epstein–Barr, chickenpox, hantavirus and influenza viruses.

Clinical features

Poststreptococcal glomerulonephritis is most common in the younger school-age child but can occur at any age. The acute nephritis typically develops 1–2 weeks after an upper respiratory tract infection with sore throat (Fig. 16.17). The latent period associated with pyoderma-related APSGN is more variable. The severity of renal involvement may vary from asymptomatic hematuria with normal renal function to ARF.

Facial swelling may be the first symptom, and is often attributed to oversleeping or allergic problems. However, increasing edema or the occurrence of gross hematuria will bring the child to medical attention earlier.

There may be a variety of non-specific symptoms, such as malaise, abdominal pain, anorexia, headaches and weakness. Oliguria may only be revealed on direct questioning.

Edema and hypertension may be noted on physical examination. The degree of hypertension is variable and not proportional to the degree of edema, which may be sufficient to cause pleural effusions and, rarely, congestive cardiac failure. The rare patient may also develop hypertensive encephalopathy, with headaches, alteration of mental state, convulsions and coma.

Diagnosis

Urinalysis will show heavy hematuria and variable proteinuria, with microscopy revealing numerous dysmorphic red cells and heme granular casts in the florid case. Casts may only be found on centrifuged urine in the mild case. Blood should be taken for full

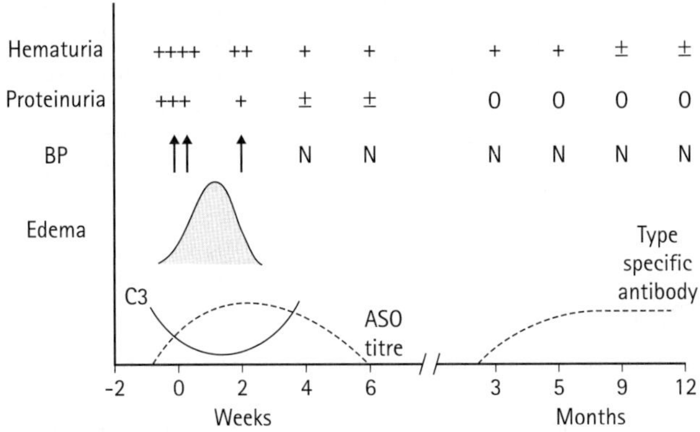

Fig. 16.17 Course of acute poststreptococcal glomerulonephritis.

blood count and platelets (a mild normochromic normocytic anemia due to dilution is usually present) and renal function tests, which will include plasma electrolytes, bicarbonate, urea, creatinine, serum albumin and total protein levels.

The diagnosis is confirmed by finding evidence of recent streptococcal infection, along with hypocomplementemia. Throat swabs from both the patient and family should be cultured, and the patient's blood is sent for antibody titers to streptococcal antigens. Since the antistreptolysin O (ASO) titer may not rise after streptococcal skin infection, a request should be made for anti-DNase B and antihyaluronidase titers which may show a significant rise in this context. Total hemolytic complement and the components C3 and C4 should also be measured, along with antinuclear antibodies (to exclude lupus nephritis). Other immunological tests may include viral, antineutrophil cytoplasmic antibody (ANCA), antiglomerular basement (anti-GBM), immunoglobulin and cryoglobulin titers, as appropriate.

The very edematous child may justify a chest X-ray (pleural effusions and cardiomegaly), and a renal ultrasound should be performed.

The combination of an acute nephritic syndrome, evidence of recent streptococcal infection and a low C3 level are sufficient evidence to support the diagnosis of APSGN. A renal biopsy is indicated *when* there is evidence of: worsening renal failure; development of nephrotic syndrome; a normal C3 level in the acute phase; or the persistence of marked hematuria and proteinuria with hypocomplementemia for several weeks.

The complications of APSGN are those of any child with ARF (see p. 638), and include hypertension, fluid overload, hyperkalemia, uremia, hypocalcemia, hyperphosphatemia, acidosis and seizures.

Treatment

A 10-day course of penicillin is prescribed to the patient and any culture-positive family members. There is no evidence that it affects the natural history of glomerulonephritis but it is known to limit the spread of the nephritogenic strains. Activity need not be restricted, and dietary and drug management will depend upon the degree of renal function and the need to control hypertension. Fortunately, in most children with APSGN, the illness is mild and manageable by conservative treatment without resort to acute dialysis.

Prognosis

Complete recovery occurs in over 95% of children with poststreptococcal glomerulonephritis.[86] In a small minority, there may be a rapid progression of the renal disease with extensive crescent formation ('rapidly progressive glomerulonephritis') leading to glomerular hyalinization and chronic renal insufficiency. There is little evidence that progression to a chronic glomerulonephritis occurs following APSGN. However, some patients with a pre-existing chronic glomerulonephritis may have an exacerbation precipitated by a streptococcal illness. Second attacks of APSGN are very rare, and there is no indication for penicillin prophylaxis or tonsillectomy. Children with APSGN can usually be quickly discharged from hospital if their renal function is satisfactory or improving and there is no hypertension. Repeat blood tests will be required to check that the complement levels have returned to normal and to confirm a significant rise in ASO titers. Microscopic hematuria may persist for 1–2 years, but if the urinalysis, blood pressure and creatinine are normal then the patient can be discharged from long-term follow-up.

IgA NEPHROPATHY

IgA nephropathy (IgAN) is a mesangial proliferative glomerulonephritis, which is unique among glomerular diseases in being defined by an immunohistochemical finding, i.e. mesangial deposition of IgA, rather than by light microscopy. This clinical/pathological entity is now recognized as being probably the commonest cause of recurrent, symptomless, macroscopic hematuria and persistent microscopic hematuria in children and young adults.[87] There appears to be a marked geographical variation in its incidence, being commoner in Southern Europe, South East Asia and Japan. This may reflect both the more frequent use of biopsies in patients with persistent microscopic hematuria in some units, as well as possible dietary factors.[88]

There is a 2:1 male predominance for IgA nephropathy, with the peak incidence in late childhood through early adult life.

Clinical features

The major modes of presentation are macroscopic hematuria or the incidental finding of hematuria and proteinuria on routine urinalysis. The blood pressure, creatinine and complement levels are typically normal, and less than 50% of patients are reported to have raised serum IgA levels. The clinical diagnosis is further supported by episodes of *recurrent* macroscopic hematuria occurring 1–3 days after an upper respiratory tract infection. This is in contrast to APSGN, where the latent period is usually 7 days. Microscopic hematuria usually persists in IgA nephropathy between the episodes of macroscopic hematuria. Rarely, the presentation is with a nephrotic syndrome or a picture of acute glomerulonephritis with hypertension, acute renal insufficiency and crescents on renal biopsy indicative of a rapidly progressive glomerulonephritis.

Diagnosis

The condition is often recognized from the clinical pattern and after other causes of hematuria and postinfectious nephritis have been ruled out.

The renal biopsy usually reveals focal and segmental mesangial proliferation and increased mesangial matrix, with occasional patients showing diffuse disease with crescents and scarring. The electron microscopic finding, of mesangial deposits, is non-specific, but the diagnosis is supported by immunofluorescent deposits of mesangial IgA and lesser amounts of IgG, C3 and, less commonly, IgM.

Mesangial deposits of IgA also occur in Henoch–Schönlein purpura, but this is usually distinguishable from the clinical features. However, it has been well documented for IgA nephropathy and a Henoch–Schönlein syndrome to occur in the same patient, separated in time by several years, suggesting the two conditions have a common immunopathological basis.

Normal levels of C3 complement and anti-DNA antibodies will distinguish IgA nephropathy from poststreptococcal glomerulonephritis and lupus nephritis respectively.

Treatment

No therapy has been shown to alter the course of IgA nephropathy. Patients with recurrent macroscopic hematuria should ensure good hydration and antibiotics if bacterial infection is proven. Tonsillectomy is unproven. Although IgAN may cause a rapidly progressive course there are no evidence based recommendations for treatment, although pulse corticosteroids and cyclophosphamide used in other necrotizing glomerulonephritis has been used.[89] In patients with significant proteinuria and/or progressive renal disease, angiotensin-converting enzyme (ACE) inhibitors and rigorous control of hypertension are advocated.[90] The use of long term azathioprine, prednisolone, 4 weeks of intravenous heparin and warfarin versus heparin and warfarin alone was evaluated in children with severe IgAN proteinuria but normal renal function.[91] Renal function remained normal but proteinuria diminished in the group treated with immunosuppressants. Long term results are awaited as are trials of other immunosuppressants and fish oil.

Prognosis

IgAN is generally a benign disease in childhood, but some children may have a progressive course and in adult series, up to 25% of patients have ultimately developed renal failure, and the process may also occur in transplanted kidneys. Neither the number of episodes of gross hematuria nor the persistence of microscopic hematuria between episodes correlates with the likelihood of progressive disease.

Activity need not be restricted. Patients will need to be monitored in the outpatient clinic for signs such as hypertension, diminished renal function and heavy proteinuria, which might portend progressive disease.

Since the prognosis of IgA nephropathy is generally so good, and there is no specific treatment, routine renal biopsy may be deferred, unless there is a suggestion of progressive disease. However, some would advocate a renal biopsy in any child with persistent hematuria after 12–24 months of observation, even if the renal function remained normal. The biopsy will help to establish a diagnosis on which a firmer prognosis may be based. It should help to allay child and parental anxiety even though no specific treatment may be available. The information may be relevant for future employment counseling, particularly with respect to the Armed Forces.

HENOCH–SCHÖNLEIN PURPURA NEPHRITIS

Henoch–Schönlein purpura is one of the commonest systemic diseases with renal involvement encountered in children. It is a vasculitis of the smallest blood vessels (capillaries, arterioles and venules), with characteristic skin involvement, gastrointestinal symptoms and joint manifestations in a large percentage of patients.

Renal involvement is present in 70% of children, and is usually manifest within the first months, but can be delayed up to 3 months after the rash. It is mainly mild and asymptomatic, with microscopic hematuria and low grade proteinuria. Renal biopsy would only be undertaken if there were signs of persistent or progressive renal impairment or the development of heavy proteinuria or nephrotic syndrome. The histological appearances may vary from mild mesangial proliferation through to diffuse proliferation with a large percentage of crescents or membranoproliferative changes. Immunofluorescence reveals mesangial IgA deposits, and presumably the process is of an immune-complex-mediated disease, but the precise etiology is unclear.

Rapidly progressive glomerulonephritis, with crescents, is commoner than with IgA nephropathy and justifies immunosuppressive therapy but there are no conclusive studies. Children with persistent urinary abnormalities following Henoch–Schönlein purpura should continue to be followed in the outpatient clinic to detect the late development of hypertension and renal impairment.[92]

MEMBRANOPROLIFERATIVE GLOMERULONEPHRITIS (MPGN)

This type of chronic glomerulonephritis was first recognized in 1965, and was originally described as chronic lobular glomerulonephritis, mesangiocapillary glomerulonephritis, or chronic hypocomplementemic glomerulonephritis. MPGN, in children and young adults, is usually idiopathic and presents as a primary kidney disease without systemic manifestations. The disease is often associated with nephritic factors, which are autoantibodies that bind to and stabilize the C3 convertase of the alternative or classical pathways, thus resulting in continued complement activation. Three histological types have been described.

Type 1 MPGN

This is the most common form, with the glomeruli revealing an accentuation of the lobular pattern due to a generalized increase in mesangial cells and matrix. The glomerular capillary walls appear thickened and in some areas duplicated or split due to interposition of mesangial cytoplasm and matrix between the endothelial cells and glomerular basement membrane. Crescents may be present, and MPGN is one form of a rapidly progressive glomerulonephritis. Deposition of C3 and a lesser amount of immunoglobulin is shown on immunofluorescence, and electron microscopy confirms the presence of deposits in the subendothelial and mesangial regions.

Type 2 MPGN

In this type, the capillary walls demonstrate irregular, ribbon-like thickening due to dense deposits. Electron microscopy reveals extensive homogeneous electron-dense material in the glomerular basement membrane in the region of, but distinct from, the lamina densa.

Type 3 MPGN

In type 3 disease there are contiguous subepithelial and subendothelial deposits associated with disruption of the basement membrane.

Clinical features

MPGN is most common in the second decade of life. The clinical onset is variable with, gross hematuria, nephrotic syndrome or asymptomatic proteinuria and microscopic hematuria. In about one-third of patients, hypertension and an elevated serum creatinine are evident at presentation.

Both MPGN and acute poststreptococcal glomerulonephritis may present with a nephritic syndrome, low C3 and elevated ASO titer levels (coincidental in MPGN). The distinction may have to be made on natural history grounds.

Most patients with APSGN recover within 4 weeks, with return of complement levels to normal. A persistently low C3 with a nephrotic state or heavy hematuria would be an indication for renal biopsy to exclude MPGN.

There is an association between partial lipodystrophy, low concentrations of C3, the presence of a C3 nephritic factor and type 2 MPGN.

Treatment and prognosis

Evaluating therapeutic regimes in a chronic disease with such a variable course as MPGN has been difficult. Success may depend upon the degree of histopathological change and the stage at which treatment is initiated.[93] Success in stabilizing the clinical course has been reported in patients receiving long-term alternate-day prednisolone therapy or inhibitors of platelet function. The actuarial kidney survival curves have shown 50% of patients to be in end-stage disease at approximately 10 years with renal failure more likely in patients with type 2 MPGN.

Membranoproliferative glomerulonephritis associated with systemic disease

The features of MPGN can be seen in the renal biopsies of patients with a number of systemic conditions, such as SLE, polyarteritis nodosa and Henoch–Schönlein purpura.

MPGN features may also accompany chronic infections such as subacute bacterial endocarditis, infected ventricular–atrial shunts, syphilis, hepatitis C, hepatitis B, candidiasis and malaria. The infecting organisms usually have low virulence and the host is chronically seeded with foreign antigen. The combination with host antibodies results in complexes being deposited in the glomerular mesangium, producing mesangial proliferation and interposition. Immune deposits are subendothelial and in the mesangium. Hence, the disease is like type 1 MPGN with hypocomplementemia. If elimination of the infecting agent is achieved, then the lesion may heal, but with scarring, and there is the possibility of progression to end-stage renal failure.

Chronic infections may also produce the pathological changes of membranous glomerulopathy, focal glomerulosclerosis, and focal and segmental proliferative glomerulonephritis.

MEMBRANOUS GLOMERULONEPHRITIS

Membranous glomerulonephritis (MGN) is the commonest cause of nephrotic syndrome in adults, but is uncommon in childhood, accounting for less than 5% of pediatric patients undergoing biopsy for nephrotic syndrome. It very rarely causes hematuria alone. Membranous glomerulonephritis is defined by the histological appearances on light microscopy of diffuse thickening of the glomerular basement membranes without significant proliferative changes. On silver staining, the continuous subepithelial deposits give a spike appearance to the glomerular basement membrane, and immunofluorescent microscopy demonstrates granular deposits of IgG and C3, which can be also identified by electron microscopy.

Clinical features

The disease can occur at any age, but is most common in the second decade of life. The presentation may be covert, with disease discovered at routine urinalysis, or it may present with nephrotic syndrome and, less often, macroscopic hematuria. The blood pressure and C3 levels are normal.

It is usual practice to biopsy children who present with nephrotic syndrome over 10 years of age, because of the likelihood of finding a condition other than minimal lesion glomerulonephritis, such as MGN. This type of glomerulonephritis may occasionally be seen in association with SLE, drug therapy, such as gold or penicillamine, syphilis, hepatitis B virus infection and some cancers.

Treatment and prognosis

Spontaneous remission is quite common with this pathology, and the present consensus is that children who are not clinically nephrotic are at only slight risk of developing renal failure in the long term and do not require treatment. However, children with a prolonged nephrotic syndrome may have a poor prognosis and alternate-day steroid therapy has been suggested. The nephrotic state is best controlled with salt restriction, diuretics, lipid lowering drugs and ACE inhibitors.

SYSTEMIC LUPUS ERYTHEMATOSUS

Systemic lupus erythematosus (SLE) is a multisystem immune-complex-mediated disorder, which has a wide spectrum of clinical manifestations. Lupus is rare before puberty, although onset in the first year of life has been recorded. The female:male ratio rises from 2:1 in prepubertal children up to 4.5:1 in adolescents and 8–12:1 in adults. Renal involvement may vary from microscopic hematuria and mild proteinuria through to renal insufficiency and nephrotic syndrome. Since the overall prognosis of childhood and adult SLE is closely correlated with the nature of the pathological renal lesions, it has been recommended that a kidney biopsy be performed on all patients presenting with renal involvement to establish the severity of the histological changes. These may vary from normal to mesangial lupus, proliferative (focal and diffuse) and membranous appearances.

Treatment and prognosis

Clinical symptoms, such as malaise, skin rash and arthritis, are controlled with the lowest doses of corticosteroids possible. Laboratory monitoring of parameters such as complement levels and anti-DNA antibody titers are also useful. More aggressive therapy is prescribed for major organ involvement with renal, cardiac or central nervous complications, and may include high dose methylprednisolone or cyclophosphamide pulses.[94] Plasma exchange therapy has also been advocated but should be reserved for patients with severe cryoglobulinemia or vasculitis. Azathioprine has been used as a steroid-sparing agent, in the long term, to prevent steroid toxicity and a meta-analysis has shown a additional clinical benefit of cytotoxic agents, when used in combination with corticosteroids, in the maintenance phase.[95]

The prognosis for survival in patients with SLE has improved considerably over the past two decades. The 10-year survival figure is approximately 90%. The object is to achieve a balance between suppressing the disease process without invoking complications of the therapy itself. The majority of patients with lupus nephritis can be successfully treated and will maintain normal renal function. In a few patients, the active renal disease progresses and irreversible renal involvement with glomerular scarring and interstitial fibrosis may result. Renal transplantation can be quite successful in this group.

Rapidly progressive glomerular nephritis

Rapidly progressive glomerular nephritis (RPGN) is a description of the clinical course of several forms of nephritis where there is acute renal insufficiency associated with the presence of extensive crescents on the renal biopsy. Such crescents may be found in poststreptococcal, membranoproliferative, lupus and Henoch–Schönlein purpura nephritis, as well as the glomerulonephritis of Goodpasture's disease.

After the above forms of glomerular nephritis have been excluded, there remains a small group of patients with so called idiopathic rapidly progressive disease. Often there is no evidence for immunological mechanisms and the C3 level is normal. All forms of RPGN have crescents, which are found on the inside of Bowman's capsule, and are composed of fibrin, proliferating epithelial cells of the capsule, basement-membrane-like material and macrophages.

The stimulus for crescent formation is believed to be the deposition of fibrin in Bowman's space as a result of necrosis or disruption of the glomerular capillary wall.

Severe crescentic nephritis is associated with ARF in association with a nephritic or nephrotic syndrome. Although there have been well-documented spontaneous recoveries of renal function with poststreptococcal and Henoch–Schönlein purpura nephritis, many patients will progress to end-stage renal failure within weeks or months after onset. With such a rare condition it is hard to mount a controlled trial, but some patients have improved with aggressive therapy combining immunosuppressive agents with anticoagulation and plasma exchange.

GOODPASTURE'S AND GOODPASTURE-LIKE SYNDROME

This refers to a combination of pulmonary hemorrhage and glomerulonephritis associated with antibodies against lung and glomerular basement membrane. It is one form of a rapidly progressive glomerulonephritis, with immunofluorescence showing a continuous linear pattern of IgG along the glomerular basement membrane. Goodpasture's syndrome is extremely rare in childhood but a similar clinical picture of pulmonary hemorrhage and glomerulonephritis may occur in association with SLE, anaphylactoid purpura, polyarteritis nodosa and Wegener's granulomatosis.

Hemoptysis is the usual presenting complaint and pulmonary hemorrhage can result in death. Antiglomerular basement antibodies (Goodpasture's) or antineutrophil cytoplasmic antibodies (C-ANCA in Wegener's) support the diagnosis.

As well as ameliorating the renal injury, a combination of plasma exchange and immunosuppressive therapy, with prednisolone and cyclophosphamide early in the disease may even be life saving.[96]

HEREDITARY NEPHRITIS (ALPORT SYNDROME)

Hereditary nephritis is not a homogeneous entity, as the clinical expression of the disease and the mode of inheritance can vary widely between families. The classic description of Alport syndrome was of a progressive hematuric nephritis associated with sensorineural deafness and ocular abnormalities such as anterior lenticonus and cataracts. The gene in Alport has been located to X chromosome (Xq21.2–q22.2) and it is hypothesized that the basic genetic defect lies in the gene for the alpha-5 chain of type IV collagen of basement membranes.[97] Two forms of Alport syndrome (AS) have been established, on a molecular genetic basis: an X-linked dominant form resulting from mutations at the COL4A5 locus, primarily affecting the alpha-5 (IV) chain and an autosomal recessive form arising from mutations at the COL4A3 locus or the COL4A4 locus. There is also the possibility of an autosomal dominant form.

The condition is generally more severe in male members of the family, with most (but not all) females remaining in good health throughout life. The prognosis is best based upon the progress of other affected family members, as there appears to be a correlation between deafness, ocular abnormalities, proteinuria and chronic renal failure.

Renal biopsy in the early stages of Alport syndrome shows only focal mesangial hypercellularity. There is progressive glomerular sclerosis, tubular atrophy, interstitial inflammation and foam cells (non-specific lipid-laden tubular or interstitial cells). Immunofluorescence is unrewarding, but electron microscopy may reveal irregular thickening, thinning, splitting and layering of the basement membrane of the glomeruli, with a lattice work appearance described as 'basket weave' (Fig. 16.18). These findings are very suggestive of Alport syndrome of the classical type but may occur in patients without an abnormal family history, suggesting a new mutation.

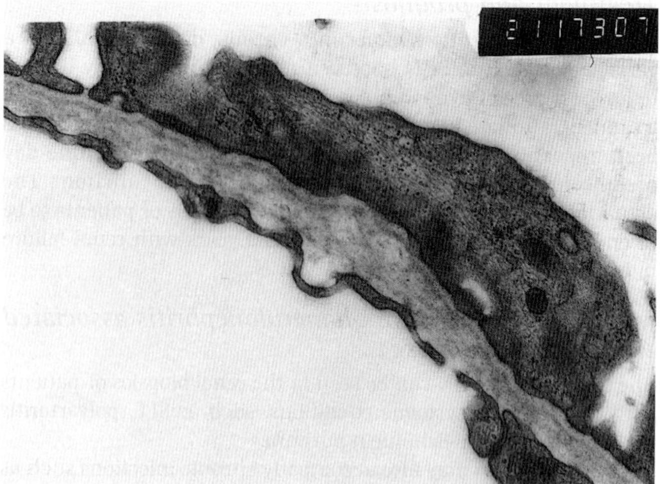

Fig. 16.18 Electron microscopy of basement membrane in a child with Alport syndrome. Lattice work appearance.

Clinical features

The disease is characteristically silent during childhood, but microscopic hematuria and proteinuria may be identified in affected family members after the first few years of life. There is progression in the second decade of life, as sclerosis proceeds, and the proteinuria becomes heavier, with hypertension and renal failure. Nephrotic syndrome can occasionally occur at presentation, or late in the disease process. There is no effective treatment, and dialysis and transplantation will be required as early as the second or third decade of life. Antiglomerular basement membrane nephritis is a rare but dramatic manifestation occurring in 3–4% of Alport syndrome transplanted patients.

The deafness is initially high frequency, but is progressive and may ultimately be quite profound, especially in males. It is wise to carefully assess the hearing of children with any type of inherited nephritis. This may be of more initial importance than the renal disease.

A pattern of painless recurrent macroscopic hematuria after infections and persistent microscopic hematuria suggests IgA nephropathy

Partial lipodystrophy is associated with membranoproliferative glomerulonephritis

A family history of chronic renal failure and deafness strongly suggests Alport syndrome

---

BENIGN HEMATURIA: SPORADIC AND FAMILIAL

In any child with persistent microscopic hematuria it is important to test the urine of all first degree family members even though there is no clear history of familial nephritis. A familial recurrent hematuria syndrome is generally inherited as an autosomal dominant trait, but recessive examples may occur. The microscopic hematuria may sometimes be accompanied by shortlived episodes of frank hematuria with mild proteinuria. However, there is usually no impairment of renal function.

The condition is generally regarded as benign (synonym: benign familial hematuria) and hence not all children have been subjected to renal biopsy. Part of the reluctance to do so is because of the absence of therapeutic measures and the lack of a history of progressive nephritis.

However, even if the biopsy is normal on light microscopy and immunofluorescence, it may be possible to demonstrate changes in the glomerular basement membrane (GBM) on electron microscopy.[98] Basement membrane nephropathy has been grouped into:

1. Group 1. Lamellation type, with features indistinguishable from Alport syndrome.
2. Group 2. Extensive thinning, commonly found in children with mild microscopic hematuria (thin glomerular basement membrane disease).[99]
3. Group 3. Idiopathic hematuria, with minimal basement membrane alteration.

The long-term outcome for types 2 and 3 is still uncertain but in the absence of a positive family history is usually regarded as benign. However, cases of renal insufficiency have been described, even with minor GBM changes and so follow-up every 1–2 years with urinalysis, blood pressure and creatinine measurements is justified.

Children with hematuria *and* proteinuria have renal parenchymal disease until proven otherwise. However, the child with asymptomatic, low degree, isolated hematuria and a negative family history is likely to have a favorable prognosis, and a renal biopsy is not initially warranted.[100] However, prolonged clinic supervision can generate its own anxiety and a suggested approach is shown in Figure 16.14.

FABRY DISEASE (ANDERSON–FABRY DISEASE)

Fabry disease is an X-linked disorder associated with deficiency of the enzyme alpha-galactosidase A, resulting in the intracellular accumulation of neutral glycosphingolipids with terminal alpha-linked galactosyl moieties. Fabry coined the term 'angiokeratoma corporis diffusum'. The angiokeratomas usually appear during the second decade of life presenting as dark red macules or papules of various size.

The nephropathy of Fabry disease typically manifests as mild to moderate proteinuria, sometimes with microhematuria, and end-stage renal failure usually develops by the fourth or fifth decade of life. Fabry disease is a multisystem disorder with involvement of the heart, kidneys, skin, peripheral and central nervous systems. Enzyme replacement therapy with intravenous agalsidase beta appears to control symptoms but also potentially reverses the disease process.

NAIL–PATELLA SYNDROME

Nail-patella syndrome is an autosomal dominant disorder consisting of hypoplasia or absence of the patellae, dystrophic nails, dysplasia of the elbows and iliac horns, and renal disease.

The nephropathy is usually benign and includes microhematuria and mild proteinuria, which usually appear in adolescence or young adulthood. Some patients develop nephrotic syndrome and mild hypertension and are at risk of progression to end-stage renal failure.

OTHER SYSTEMIC DISORDERS ASSOCIATED WITH GLOMERULAR DISEASE

Scleroderma

Scleroderma, or progressive systemic sclerosis, is a rare multisystem disorder in children. Renal involvement is unusual at the outset, but can occur with progression of the disease, and is characterized by proteinuria, hypertension and renal insufficiency. Scleroderma renal crisis occurs, with the abrupt onset of malignant hypertension and oliguric renal failure. The angiotensin-converting enzyme inhibitor, captopril, has been used successfully in its treatment.

Vasculitis

Vasculitis is characterized by inflammation of medium or small blood vessels. Classification is difficult because of the heterogeneous nature of many of these conditions and the overlapping clinical features. Vasculitis of small vessels occurs with Henoch–Schönlein purpura and conditions such as serum sickness, whereas vasculitis with granuloma formation is found in Wegener's granulomatosis. Vasculitis of medium and large arteries with giant cells is characteristic of systemic or temporal arteritis and also Takayasu's arteritis.

Polyarteritis nodosa

This is a necrotizing vasculitis of small and medium-sized muscular arteries. There is multiple organ involvement with angiographic features of aneurysms in hepatic, renal and abdominal vessels. Elevated antineutrophil cytoplasmic antibodies (P-ANCA) are present in 80% of patients with 'pauci-immune' vasculitis. The prognosis will depend upon the organ systems involved, and can be improved with the use of corticosteroid and immunosuppressive therapy such as cyclophosphamide.

Diabetic nephropathy

Diabetic nephropathy is a leading cause of end-stage renal failure (ESRF) in adult patients in Western societies and is characterized by persistent albuminuria (> 300 mg/24 h), on at least two occasions, 3 months apart. Diabetes mellitus in childhood is rarely associated with significant clinical manifestations of renal disease. However, the highest long term incidence of nephropathy is found in those who develop type 1 diabetes between the ages of 11 and 20 years. The median time between the onset of proteinuria and ESRF is 14 years, for those diagnosed under the age of 12, and 8 years for those diagnosed between the ages of 12 and 20. Mogensen[101] described five distinct stages of renal dysfunction: renal hypertrophy and hyperfiltration; microalbuminuria; incipient nephropathy; overt nephropathy and ESRF. Tight glycemic control will prevent the mild physiological derangements of increased glomerular filtration rate and microalbuminuria, but established diabetic nephropathy with extensive basement membrane thickening cannot be reversed.

Amyloidosis

Juvenile idiopathic arthritis (JIA) has become a common cause of secondary amyloidosis in children following the eradication of tuberculosis and chronic osteomyelitis in Western countries. However, it is very rare in childhood and only occurs after many years of severe disease. Renal vein thrombosis is a well-documented complication of renal amyloidosis. Confirmation of the diagnosis requires biopsy material. Immunosuppressive agents such as busulfan may be of benefit.

PROTEINURIA

Although proteinuria is one of the cardinal features of renal disease, and a risk factor for deterioration in most renal conditions, its isolated occurrence may be a transient finding in healthy children. Proteinuria combined with hematuria is much more significant.

In the normal individual, minimal protein is filtered, because of the change and size selectivity of the glomerular capillary wall.

Proteins are negatively charged and are repelled to the glomerular capillary wall, which contains sialoproteins and proteoglycans, such as heparan sulfate, that are negatively charged. In addition, the tight collagen meshwork within the glomerular basement membrane, and the overlying visceral glomerular epithelial cells with their interdigitating foot processes, act as an effective size barrier, with little protein passing through the filtration slit diaphragms. Proteinuria may result from increased glomerular permeability due to:

1. loss of the negative charges in the basement membrane;
2. an increase in the effective pore size or number due to direct damage to the basement membrane, or possibly a change in the structure of the basement membrane resulting from loss of the anionic proteins;
3. the hemodynamic effects of angiotensin II and other vasoactive amines, which may explain the mild proteinuria seen with heart failure.

Albumin (MW = 69 000) is the predominant protein lost in the urine, but globulin excretion may also be increased.

Another type of proteinuria, *tubular* proteinuria, occurs when there is increased excretion of the normally filtered low-molecular weight proteins, such as immunoglobulin light chains and beta$_2$-microglobulin (MW < 50 000). Tubular proteinuria occurs when proximal tubular reabsorption is impaired, as in the Fanconi syndrome, or when the production is increased to a level exceeding tubular reabsorption capacity, e.g. in multiple myeloma.

NORMAL VALUES

Most of the filtered protein is reabsorbed, and the normal daily protein excretion in a child is < 4 mg/h/m^2, or < 150 mg/24 h in an adult. Albumin accounts for about 25% of the normal protein excretion, and after severe exercise, proteinuria may increase several fold, with the albumin excretion representing up to 80% of total urinary protein. 40% of normal urinary protein is of tissue origin, and the major protein in this group is uromucoid or Tamm–Horsfall protein, which is produced in the distal tubule.

DETECTION

Testing for proteinuria has been simplified by the use of dipsticks, which are impregnated with a dye, tetrabromophenol blue, which changes color according to the quantity of protein present. The strips detect predominantly albuminuria, but a negative dipstick does not exclude the presence in the urine of low concentrations of globulins, hemoglobin, Bence Jones protein or mucoproteins. These would be detected by 3% sulfosalicylic acid, which detects all proteins. However, dipsticks predominate in clinical practice. It is important to appreciate that false negative results can also occur with very acid or dilute urine, whereas false positive results may occur in the presence of highly concentrated or alkaline urine (pH > 8) along with gross hematuria, pyuria and contamination with antiseptics, such as chlorhexidine.

Dipsticks are highly sensitive and cannot accurately measure protein excretion, which is best quantified using timed (preferably 24 h) urine collections. However, obtaining accurate 12- or 24-h urine collections in children can be difficult to accomplish. Single voided urine samples, which relate the concentration of both the protein and creatinine in the same sample, have a high correlation with 24-h urine excretion rates. The urine protein:creatinine ratio can be used to estimate the severity, and follow the progress, of proteinuric patients. The normal urine protein:creatinine ratio is < 20 mg/mmol in the early morning urine sample.[102]

Protein selectivity index

This has usually been measured by comparing the clearances of small and large molecular weight proteins, on the basis that diseases such as glomerulonephritis, which cause severe histological change to the glomeruli, are more likely to result in the urinary loss of large plasma proteins than are diseases such as minimal change nephrotic syndrome, in which there is no obvious glomerular injury. However, there is considerable overlap in the results and the test is no longer performed routinely. It is preferable to rely on clinical features and/or the response to corticosteroids in children with nephrotic syndrome.

The causes of proteinuria are listed in Table 16.11.

INTERMITTENT PROTEINURIA

Transient proteinuria may be found in patients with high fevers in excess of 38.5°C. The mechanism is unknown and the proteinuria usually resolves as the fever abates.

Proteinuria, like hematuria, may also follow vigorous exercise and usually resolves within 48 h of rest.

Postural or *orthostatic* proteinuria is important because it is a relatively frequent cause of referral to pediatric clinics. It is suggested by finding normal protein excretion (< 20 mg/mmol) in the first morning urine after being supine overnight and increased protein excretion in the upright collection. Long-term follow-up has suggested that orthostatic proteinuria, as an isolated finding, is benign. These patients do not need prolonged follow-up in the clinic, if the history and examination and other urinary findings are normal. However, it is important to note that patients with glomerular disease will often have an orthostatic component to their proteinuria, so that true orthostatic proteinuria should not be diagnosed unless the urine collected in the supine position has no protein detectable by routine methods.

PERSISTENT PROTEINURIA

In these patients, the amount of protein present in the individual samples may vary considerably, but is persistent, unless it resolves as in acute glomerulonephritis. If the proteinuria is associated with additional evidence for renal disease, e.g. microscopic hematuria, then these patients are most likely to have significant pathology in the kidney or urinary tract.

GLOMERULAR PROTEINURIA

In the majority of cases, persistent proteinuria is of glomerular origin. The degree of proteinuria may range from > 4 mg/h/m^2, to < 400 mg/h/m^2, when it is usually associated with altered levels of protein in the plasma and nephrotic syndrome. Acute and chronic glomerulonephritis are believed to produce proteinuria as a result of damage to the glomerular basement membrane, which increases the permeability to plasma proteins to a degree which overwhelms the tubular absorptive mechanisms. In conditions such as minimal change or congenital nephrotic syndrome, it is usually a highly selective loss of albumin as a result of loss of the glomerular anionic charge for reasons still to be elucidated.

There has been a great deal of interest in recent years in patients who develop proteinuria with a reduced renal mass. Evidence has accumulated that the remaining nephrons, in such patients, are subject to hyperfiltration damage, which produces progressive glomerulosclerosis.[103] Hence several long-term studies are evaluating the use of ACE inhibitors or angiotensin II, receptor antagonists to ameliorate the progression of renal disease.

Table 16.11 Causes of proteinuria

INTERMITTENT PROTEINURIA
1. Postural (orthostatic)
2. Non-postural
   a. Exercise
   b. Fever
   c. Anatomic abnormalities, e.g. urinary tract
   d. Glomerular lesions, e.g. IgA nephropathy
   e. Random finding; no known cause

PERSISTENT PROTEINURIA
1. Glomerular
   a. Isolated asymptomatic proteinuria
   b. Damage to glomerular basement membrane, e.g. acute or chronic glomerulonephritis
   c. Loss or reduction of basement membrane anionic charge, e.g. minimal change and congenital nephrosis
   d. Increased permeability in residual nephrons, e.g. chronic renal failure
2. Tubular
   a. Hereditary, e.g. cystinosis, Wilson's disease, Lowe's syndrome, proximal tubular acidosis, galactosemia
   b. Acquired, e.g. interstitial nephritis, acute tubular necrosis, post renal transplantation, pyelonephritis, vitamin D intoxication, penicillamine, heavy metal poisoning (gold, lead, mercury, etc.), analgesic abuse, drugs

TUBULAR PROTEINURIA

The amount of protein in the urine resulting from tubular damage is usually not as great as with glomerular disease but it has occasionally been sufficient to result in a nephrotic syndrome. Transient overflow proteinuria may occur after repeated blood or albumin infusions, and increased secretion of tubular proteins may occur with urinary tract infection or transiently in the neonatal period. Many hereditary causes of tubular proteinuria are part of a Fanconi-type syndrome.

PERSISTENT ASYMPTOMATIC PROTEINURIA

This is defined as proteinuria, in apparently healthy children, occurring without hematuria, but persisting on repeated testing over 3 months. Significant proteinuria (Uprot/Ucr > 20 mg/mmol) is usually an indication for proceeding with further investigations. These would include urine culture, full blood count, blood chemistry including electrolytes, urea, creatinine, albumin and an accurate measurement of glomerular filtration rate. The serological tests are performed at the same time and will include antistreptolysin O, antinuclear antibodies, immunoglobulins and complement studies. A renal tract ultrasound and plain abdominal X-ray will usually exclude any significant urinary tract pathology. A renal biopsy will only be considered in those with confirmed proteinuria or when there are other abnormal tests, such as a decreased GFR, abnormal urinary sediment, hypocomplementemia or evidence of generalized vascular disease.

NEPHROTIC SYNDROME

The nephrotic syndrome is characterized by:

1. heavy proteinuria (> 40 mg/h/m^2 or protein/creatinine ratio > 200 mg/mmol);
2. hypoalbuminemia (< 25 g/L);
3. edema.

The incidence of all forms of nephrotic syndrome in childhood is 2–4 per 100 000 population, but this figure will vary according to the ethnic mix of the population. For instance, the incidence amongst Asian children in two cities in the UK was reported as ranging from 9–16 per 100 000 respectively.[104]

The predominant pathology is minimal change disease (MCD), with contributions from other pathologies such as focal segmental glomerulosclerosis (FSGS) and MPGN. This applies only in Caucasian populations, as around the world the pathology varies. For instance, the predominant lesion in West Africa is quartan malaria nephropathy, with schistosomiasis being responsible for the majority of the cases in South America.

Nephrotic syndrome could be subdivided into congenital, idiopathic (primary) or secondary. Many of the secondary causes have already been mentioned, and include Henoch–Schönlein purpura nephritis; connective tissue disorders (e.g. SLE); toxic causes (e.g. drugs and heavy metal poisoning); sickle-cell disease; and amyloidosis.

IDIOPATHIC NEPHROTIC SYNDROME

Minimal change disease accounts for approximately 85% of cases presenting in childhood but only 10% of cases in adults. The other histological types of mesangial proliferative and FSGS may well represent the spectrum of a single disorder with varying histological features. There are familial cases of MCD, but these appear to be very rare in the UK. The gene locus for steroid sensitive idiopathic nephrotic syndrome appears to be distinct from the NPH52 gene, located on chromosome 1q25 that has been mapped in a subgroup of autosomal recessive steroid resistant nephrotic syndrome.[105]

The cause of minimal change nephrotic syndrome (MCNS) remains unknown. It is more prevalent in families with an atopic history, and some studies have suggested an abnormality of T cell function. Although broad spectrum immunosuppressive drugs have been used to control the disease, there is lack of evidence for classical mechanisms of immunological injury.

In minimal change disease, the glomeruli appear normal or show a minimal increase in mesangial cells and matrix. The immunofluorescence studies are negative, and electron microscopy reveals gross epithelial cell (podocyte) foot process fusion, which is a non-specific finding in any patient with heavy proteinuria.

Clinical features

Minimal change nephrotic syndrome is more common in boys than girls (2:1) and usually occurs between the ages of 2 and 6 years. There may be an antecedent history of an upper respiratory tract infection and, certainly, these are well known to precipitate relapses in this condition. The presenting feature is usually edema, which is first noticed around the eyes (Fig. 16.19). Since the condition is so uncommon in general practice, many children are treated for allergic conditions before the true nature of the condition is appreciated. The edema may become generalized, with swollen limbs, ascites and pleural effusions with, diminishing urine output. There may be lethargy, poor appetite, mild diarrhea and, sometimes, abdominal pain.

Investigations

The diagnosis is suggested by simple urinalysis, which will show heavy proteinuria (+++ or > 5 g/L). About 30% of patients will have transient microscopic hematuria, but gross hematuria is rare. Heavy proteinuria can be confirmed by timed urine collections or by early morning urine protein/creatinine ratio (> 200 mg/mmol).

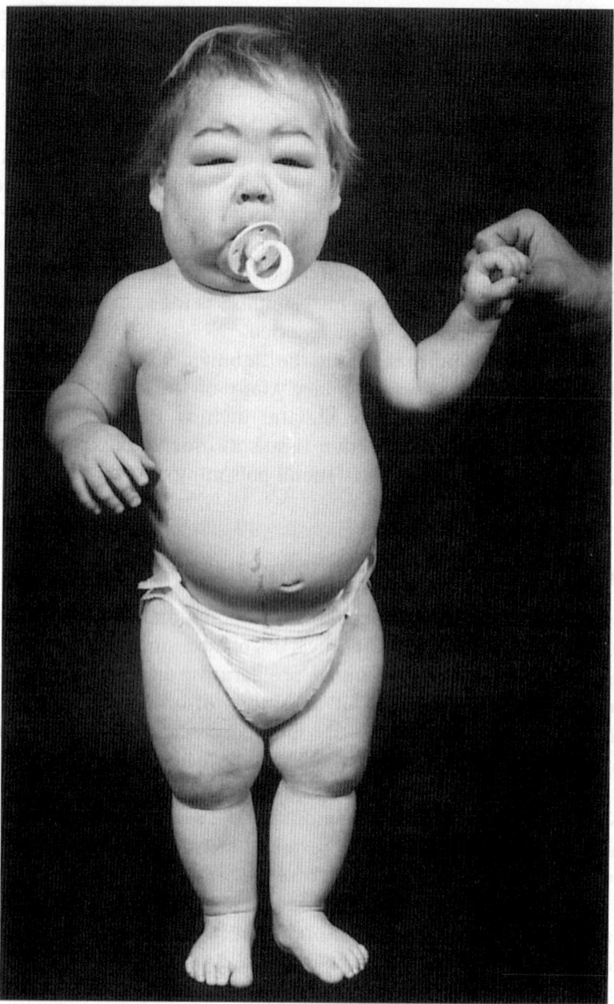

Fig. 16.19 17-month-old male infant with nephrotic syndrome and gross generalized edema (anasarca).

Renal function is usually normal, but there will be a low serum albumin (< 25 g/L), with raised serum cholesterol and triglyceride levels. Swabs should be taken from the throat and any skin lesions, as well as a urine culture. Overt or covert infection can be the cause of steroid resistance. Serological tests such as complement studies, an ASO titer, hepatitis B surface antigen and antinuclear factor antibodies need only be measured in patients when there is a mixed nephritic/nephrotic picture. The traditional urine protein selectivity index can be omitted, because in terms of prognosis, the response to corticosteroids is more important.

Children between the ages of 1 and 10 years are very likely to have *steroid-responsive minimal change disease* and so prednisolone therapy is usually initiated without a renal biopsy. This latter procedure is recommended *before* treatment with corticosteroids when the nephrotic syndrome occurs:

1. onset at less that 6 months of age (congenital nephrotic syndrome types);
2. evidence of a mixed nephritic/nephrotic picture with hypertension and/or low plasma C3 (pathology other than MCD more likely);

A biopsy may be *considered* in children with nephrotic syndrome and:

1. onset between 6 and 12 months of age;
2. onset over 12 years of age (other pathology may be more likely);
3. persistent hypertension, microscopic hematuria, or low plasma C3;
4. renal failure – persistent and not attributable to hypovolemia.

Complications

Children with nephrotic syndrome still have a 1–2% mortality rate. The two major complications are infection and thrombosis.

Peritonitis is the most frequent type of infection and *Streptococcus pneumoniae* is the most common organism. Gram negative bacteria are also encountered. The reasons for the susceptibility may be multifactorial and include decreased immunoglobulin levels, ascitic fluid acting as culture medium and immunosuppressive therapy. While on corticosteroids the clinical findings may be masked, and so any child with nephrotic syndrome and abdominal pain should be carefully evaluated in conjunction with a surgeon. Although there are instances where an unnecessary laparotomy has been carried out on a child with primary peritonitis, before the edema and nephrotic state has been recognized, there are also instances of children with nephrotic syndrome and appendicitis. In the very edematous state, penicillin prophylaxis may be considered, but antibiotics to cover Gram negative organisms should be used for any suspected peritonitis, until the cultures and sensitivities are known. Some authors have advocated polyvalent pneumococcal vaccine when the child is in remission, but this does not appear to be fully effective, as not all the serotypes are covered.

Chickenpox and measles are major threats to the immunocompromised child. It is likely that the child has received MMR, but if not, measles and varicella immunity status should be checked as part of the routine evaluation. Zoster immune globulin should be given if there is chickenpox exposure while taking high dose prednisolone or alkylating agents and aciclovir given promptly if the condition develops.

Nephrotic children also have a tendency to arterial and venous thrombosis. The nephrotic syndrome is a hypercoagulable state with high levels of fibrinogen, factor VIII: R: AG and alpha-2-macroglobulin with a decrease of both functional and immunological antithrombin III.[106] The greatest risk of thrombosis appears to be when the albumin level is very low. Children with nephrotic syndrome should be seen for prompt assessment if they have a potentially dehydrating state such as vomiting and diarrhea.

Treatment

Hospitalization should only be required for the initial attack, when the diagnosis can be established, treatment initiated and the response evaluated. It will also give an opportunity to educate the patient and the family in what may be a frustrating chronic illness. Good education and efficient communication should enable further problems to be assessed and treated on an outpatient basis.

Bed rest does not need to be enforced, as the child will determine their appropriate activity level.

Dietary advice

The traditional high-protein, no-salt-intake diet should be abandoned in favor of trying to maintain the recommended daily allowances of calories and protein in a child whose appetite is likely to be markedly diminished until on steroids.[107] When edema is present, a no-added-salt diet is advised, with avoidance of foods known to be high in sodium, particularly snack or processed foods.

Diuretics

A moderate fluid restriction of 750–1000 ml is advocated in the edematous state. Diuretics should be used with caution in plasma-volume-depleted nephrotic patients, as they may be predisposed to fluid and electrolyte disturbances. Thiazide diuretics have little effect. Cautious use of loop diuretics such as furosemide (frusemide) (1–2 mg/kg per 24 h), in combination with an aldosterone antagonist such as spironolactone 0.5–5 mg/kg per 24 h (which may take several days to act), can be used to control the edema, until there is a diuretic response to the corticosteroids. Occasionally, metolazone (0.2–0.4 mg/kg per 24 h), in combination with furosemide (frusemide), may be needed to induce a diuresis, but careful biochemical monitoring is required.

If there are signs of hypovolemia, such as abdominal pain (due to a contracted plasma volume), hypertension, oliguria or evidence of renal insufficiency, then an intravenous salt-poor 20% albumin infusion (1 g/kg) given over 1–2 h with careful monitoring and followed by furosemide (frusemide) (1–2 mg/kg) may reverse the situation. Albumin infusions are both expensive and potentially hazardous, as pulmonary edema could be precipitated if the volume status has been misjudged. Since most of the infused albumin is rapidly lost in the urine, there is little place for their routine use. Mannitol (5 ml/kg of 20% solution) and furosemide (frusemide) (2 mg/kg/dose) have also been used to treat diuretic-resistant edema.[38]

Corticosteroid therapy

Corticosteroid therapy has been used in childhood nephrotic syndrome since the 1950s. Of those children who present with a typical illness, 95% will respond to steroid therapy within the first 4 weeks. Nephrotic syndrome is potentially a chronic disease with about 70% of patients suffering a relapsing course and therefore being at risk of adverse effects of repeated steroid treatment.

A number of steroid regimens have been suggested. The consensus regimen proposed by the British Association for Paediatric Nephrology[108] was prednisolone 60 mg/m^2/day until the urine was protein-free for 3 days, followed by 40 mg/m^2 for 4 weeks. In a national audit conducted in the UK in 1998, this was found to be associated with a high relapse rate.

The current consensus on management is shown in Figure 16.20, the major change being that daily prednisolone is now given in a dose of 60 mg/m^2 (maximum 80 mg) for a full 28 days followed by a further month of alternate day therapy at 40 mg/m^2 (maximum 60 mg). The increase in the initial steroid dose acknowledges the evidence that the relapse rate is reduced with increased duration of initial therapy.[109] However, it falls short of the 3 month duration of initial prednisolone therapy recommended by Hodson et al[110] in a meta-analysis of randomized controlled trials. Nephrologists remain concerned about the possibility of steroid side-effects, with this large initial dosage, and their effect on the hypothalamic pituitary axis. Trials are being proposed of regimens comparing a standard therapy with one involving the use of alternate day steroids over 6 weeks.

Surprisingly, there is usually little gastric upset from the use of soluble prednisolone in children, and the more expensive enteric coated forms or drugs to control gastric acidity are not routinely prescribed. Children who have problems with vomiting or diarrhea should receive intravenous methylprednisolone in an equivalent dose to the oral prednisolone dosage and additional care should be taken to monitor blood pressure. It is important to exclude occult infection such as UTI as a cause of steroid resistance.

The parents should be told daily steroids may well alter the child's behavior as well as increasing the appetite. General dietary advice about avoiding excess consumption of snacks, etc. should be given. A steroid warning card should be issued, and the parents should report if the child is exposed to infections such as measles or chickenpox, while on daily steroids. Immunization using live vaccines should be avoided until the child has been off daily steroids for at least 3 months, but are permissible if the child is on alternate day steroids (< 0.5 mg/kg body weight/day). Overall, vaccines are best given when the child has been in remission for some months and inactivated, rather than live, polio should be utilized.

Steroid-responsive patients

The family are instructed in the use of dipsticks for recording the first morning urine protein results, which should be carefully logged in a diary. This can serve as an individual record of the child's condition over a number of years.

When there is a relapse of proteinuria [three consecutive days of heavy proteinuria (++ or greater)], treatment may be withheld for up to 5 days (or possibly 10 if variable proteinuria) unless the child becomes edematous. This is because some children will spontaneously remit during this period. If proteinuria persists, then remission is induced with daily steroids as before until the urine is protein free for 3 days, and then alternate day corticosteroids are continued for 28 days. More than 75% of children with minimal change nephrotic syndrome will have at least one relapse.

Frequent relapses or steroid dependency

If the child has two or more relapses within 6 months of initial treatment, or four or more relapses within any 12-month period (frequent relapser), then a slow weaning dose of alternate day prednisolone may be considered, after inducing remission with daily steroids as above. The prednisolone may be weaned off over 6 months, and by this means steroid toxicity may be minimized.

Steroid dependency may be defined as those who relapse on two consecutive occasions as prednisolone is being decreased, or within 2 weeks of it being discontinued. If a child requires more than 0.5 mg/kg of prednisolone on alternate days to remain protein free, and particularly if there are signs of steroid toxicity, then alternative therapy should be considered. Such steroid side-effects would include stunting of growth, cataracts, obesity and behavioral changes, but alternative therapy to corticosteroids and/or the advice of a pediatric nephrologist will, preferably, have been sought before many of these side-effects are manifest. Alternative therapy consists of levamisole, cyclophosphamide, chlorambucil and ciclosporin (Fig. 16.20) which all reduce the risk of relapse in children with relapsing steroid sensitive nephritis compared with prednisolone alone.[111]

Cyclophosphamide

When cyclophosphamide was originally used in MCNS it was prescribed for 6–12 months and achieved 90% long-term remission. However, this was before gonadal toxicity was appreciated, and many young men were subsequently rendered oligo- or azoospermic. Consequently, the course of cyclophosphamide has been restricted to 8 weeks and is given after remission has been induced with daily steroids, which are then usually tapered off over 4–6 weeks. The restriction to shorter courses of 8 weeks means the remission rate has been reduced to approximately 50% at 2 years.

The potential toxic effects of bone marrow depression, hemorrhagic cystitis and mild alopecia can be minimized by close monitoring of weekly blood counts and clinic visits. Although there is no firm guarantee of future fertility, restriction of therapy to less than 16 weeks or 300 mg/kg body weight appears to be safe.[112,113] Nevertheless, this point needs to be discussed at length with the parents, as a prolonged remission cannot be guaranteed and there may still be long-term effects from the use of this drug. Chlorambucil does not appear to be superior to cyclophosphamide and its use has been more limited.

It was once customary to perform a renal biopsy on all nephrotic children *prior* to cyclophosphamide therapy. However, this is

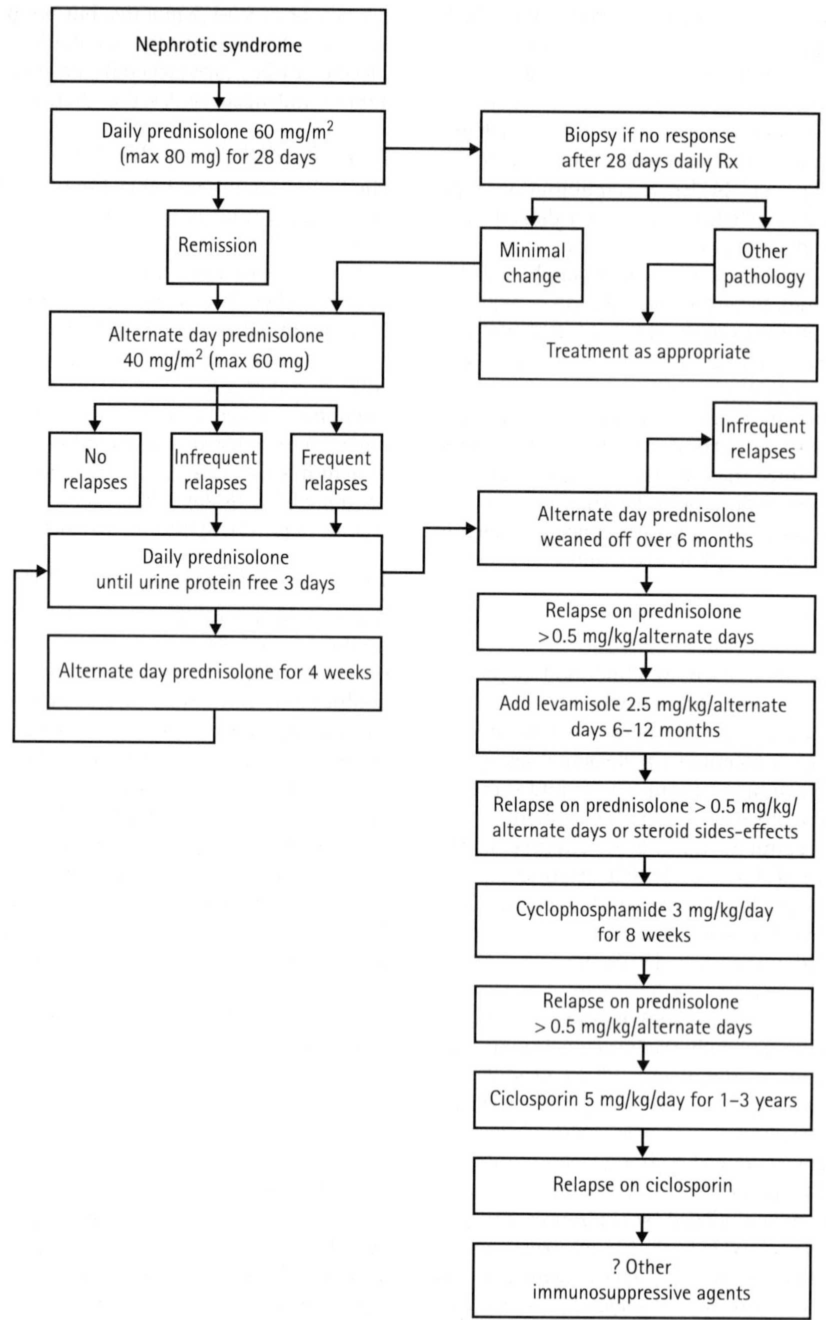

Fig. 16.20 Scheme for the management of children with nephrotic syndrome.

probably no longer justifiable if the patient is still *steroid responsive*. Even if FSGS changes are found on biopsy, the best prognostic indicator remains *steroid responsiveness*.

Psychosocial

We have found it helpful to provide the family of a child with nephrotic syndrome with an information booklet about the condition, as a great deal of anxiety can result with the clinical course of relapse and remission. In addition, the parents have benefited from attending a local parents' group, where they can discuss and share many of their anxieties.[114]

If a nephrotic child has been free of relapses for 5 years, then there is a strong chance of a long-term remission. However, some children may continue to relapse into adult life, and those who develop nephrosis earlier in life are likely to relapse more often.[115] With a decreasing relapse rate the urine tests can be performed less frequently, but the family should be cautioned to test urine at times of stress such as incidental infection.

FOCAL SEGMENTAL GLOMERULOSCLEROSIS (FSGS)

This is characterized on light microscopy by sclerosis or hyalinosis of glomeruli in a focal and segmental distribution. The involved area obliterates Bowman's space and is adherent to the capsule without epithelial cell proliferation. Epithelial foot process fusion is similar to that seen in MCD and electron microscopy should confirm the sclerosing nature of the lesion. There may be non-specific deposition of

IgM and C3 in the affected segments. Tubular atrophy and interstitial fibrosis are proportional to the extent of glomerular damage.

The typical features of FSGS may be missed if the renal biopsy is too superficial, as the changes are more likely to be seen in the juxtamedullary region. FSGS usually carries with it an entirely different prognosis from minimal lesion, especially if the patient is steroid resistant. Again, the important practice point is that, if the patient responds to steroids, then whether the histology shows MCD and FSGS is generally irrelevant as long as steroid resistance does not develop. Even when the patient is steroid resistant, some authors have advocated the use of immunosuppressive agents such as cyclophosphamide.[116] This agent may reduce the proteinuria sufficiently for the patient to remain edema free, with all its attendant benefits.

Orthostatic (postural) proteinuria should be proven by finding no significant protein in the first morning compared to the afternoon sample

Steroid responsiveness not the underlying pathology suggests a better outcome in idiopathic nephrotic syndrome

Children with nephrotic syndrome are susceptible to life threatening events such as thrombosis and infection

---

CONGENITAL NEPHROTIC SYNDROME

Nephrotic syndrome is very rare during the first year of life, and an onset before 3 months of age implies an inborn basis for this disorder. Congenital nephrotic syndrome was predominantly described in children of Finnish extraction (hence 'Finnish type') and is an autosomal recessive disorder. The major pathological feature is dilatation of the proximal convoluted tubules (microcystic disease), but this is very variable. The glomeruli may initially appear quite normal by light microscopy, but later show mesangial hypercellularity with an increase in matrix. Most glomeruli are immature. Both sexes are equally affected, and prematurity, with a placenta which weighs more than 25% of the infant's birth weight, is typical. Proteinuria is usually present at birth, and a frank nephrotic syndrome is usually apparent within 3 months of life. The clinical course is one of persistent edema and recurrent infections.

This condition was previously almost invariably fatal before 2 years of age. However, more aggressive feeding regimes with unilateral or bilateral nephrectomy and the appropriate management for end-stage renal disease has resulted in increasing numbers of children being successfully transplanted with normal growth and development.[117] Genetic counseling is very important, as antenatal diagnosis is possible by measuring the alpha-fetoprotein level in the amniotic fluid, as early as 15 weeks of gestation. The gene for the Finnish type has been mapped to the long arm of chromosome 19.

Other histological types have been described in association with nephrotic syndrome in the first year of life (Table 16.12). Diffuse mesangial sclerosis is a steroid-resistant lesion with progressive loss of renal function, and renal replacement therapy may be required in the second year of life. Patients with the histological appearances of FSGS and minimal change have also been described in very young patients. Biopsy is therefore essential, because minimal change may respond to a course of steroids.

In any female infant with early-onset nephrotic syndrome, chromosome analysis should be considered, as there is an association between nephrotic syndrome, pseudohermaphroditism and Wilms' tumor (Drash syndrome). There appears to be a distinctive kidney lesion characterized by fibrillar sclerosing of the mesangium, thickening of the glomerular capillary walls and mesangial deposits of IgM.

Secondary causes of infantile nephrotic syndrome are shown in Table 16.12. Syphilis can cause a membranous type of glomerular nephropathy, while cytomegalovirus and toxoplasmosis may be coincidental rather than causative agents. Mercury intoxication can cause a nephrotic syndrome, which usually responds to withdrawal of the toxic agent.

RENAL HYPERTENSION

The prevalence of hypertension in childhood is not clearly defined but is believed to be between 1 and 3%. About 10% of such children will have a secondary cause for their hypertension.[118] Reference needs to be made to appropriate centile charts of blood pressure for the child's sex and height when deciding whether a child is hypertensive.[119] Sustained hypertension, especially if severe, is likely to be due to renal disease.

CAUSES

The causes of renal hypertension are listed in Table 16.13.

Renal parenchymal disease is the largest category. The hypertension may occur acutely, as with acute renal failure from any cause (particularly hemolytic uremic syndrome), acute glomerulonephritis and Henoch–Schönlein nephritis. Hypertension, in these situations is often accentuated by fluid overload, but in many other cases the renal parenchymal disease is associated with the excess production of renin. The most important cause in this category is scarring associated with reflux nephropathy (formerly called chronic pyelonephritis) or obstructive uropathy. One of the reasons for following children for coarse renal scarring associated with reflux, either in the clinic or in general practice, is to detect the 8–10% who may well develop hypertension.[34] The onset of hypertension in such children can be quite explosive, with the first manifestation being headaches, central nervous disturbance and convulsions. Hypertensive retinopathy may even progress after control of the hypertension and result in blindness.[120]

INVESTIGATIONS

In moderate (blood pressures consistently above the 95th centile for age and sex) and severe hypertension, investigations will include urinalysis, urine culture, full blood count, electrolytes, creatinine, calcium, phosphate and a peripheral vein renin and aldosterone measurement. The chest X-ray, ECG (preferably echocardiogram) and 24-h urine for vanillylmandelic acid (VMA) and catecholamines (or urine VMA:creatinine ratio) should also be considered. However, investigations must include imaging of the renal tract, which

Table 16.12 Causes of infantile nephrotic syndrome

Primary	a.	Congenital nephrotic syndrome – 'Finnish' microcystic disease
	b.	Diffuse mesangial sclerosis
	c.	Minimal change nephrotic syndrome
	d.	Focal segmental glomerulosclerosis
	e.	Drash syndrome
Secondary	a.	Syphilis
	b.	Toxoplasmosis
	c.	Cytomegalovirus
	d.	Mercury
	e.	Nail–patella syndrome

Table 16.13 Causes of renal hypertension

1. Chronic renal failure and post renal transplant
2. Renal parenchymal disease
   a. Scarring due to reflux nephropathy or obstructive uropathy
   b. Acute or chronic glomerulonephritis
   c. Hemolytic uremic syndrome
   d. Renal dysplasia
   e. Polycystic kidneys
3. Renovascular disease
   a. Renal artery stenosis
   b. Renal artery thrombosis
   c. Renal artery aneurysm
   d. Arteriovenous fistula
   e. Vasculitis, e.g. polyarteritis nodosa
4. Renal tumors
   a. Nephroblastoma
   b. Hamartoma
   c. Hemangiopericytoma

initially will be with an ultrasound scan. Further imaging may include radionuclide imaging such as ^{99m}Tc dimercaptosuccinic acid (DMSA) scanning and further investigation of a renal mass may include computed tomographic scanning. If renal vascular disease is considered, then angiographic investigation in a specialist center will be required (Fig. 16.21). If a small shrunken kidney is found on investigation, then its removal may be considered if it contributes less than 10% to the overall kidney function and it is proven, by measuring the renin levels from both renal veins, to be the source of excess renin production.

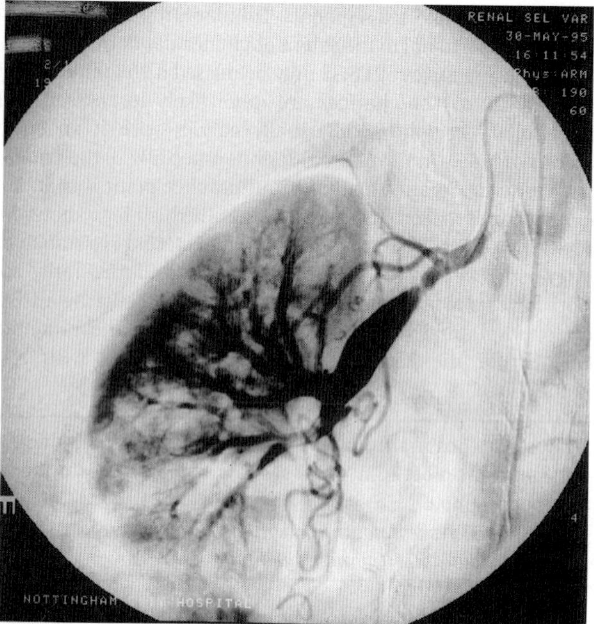

Fig. 16.21 Renal angiogram in 13-year-old female with sustained hypertension and abnormal spectral Doppler flow on ultrasound. 33% stenosis of the mid portion of the main renal artery.

TREATMENT

The list of hypertensive agents is shown in Tables 16.14 and 16.15. The pharmacokinetics and exact dosing schedules of many of these drugs have not been fully evaluated in children, as many drugs are not licensed for use in children. It is important to consider compliance, particularly in the long term with adolescent patients. The favored combination is a beta adrenergic blocker, such as propanolol, in two to three divided doses or once daily atenolol (if renal function is adequate) with a vasodilator such as slow-release nifedipine. The angiotensin-converting enzyme inhibitor, captopril, has proved very useful in patients with renin-dependent hypertension and, again, the equivalent once daily enalapril should help with long-term compliance and ease of administration.

Nephrectomy or heminephrectomy may be considered in some instances. Success has been achieved by percutaneous balloon angioplasty or direct vascular surgery in patients with renal artery stenosis.

ACUTE RENAL FAILURE

Acute renal failure (ARF) is a sudden decrease in renal function resulting in an accumulation of nitrogenous wastes and associated with fluid and electrolyte imbalance. A urine output of 300 ml/m^2/24 h (or 1.0 ml/kg/h) is required to excrete the daily solute output. ARF is therefore usually associated with oliguria, although it may be associated with polyuria, particularly in the neonate. The incidence of ARF in children varies according to the population studied. In the UK, data from children referred to regional nephrology units for further management, suggested an incidence of 7.5 children per million population per year.[121]

PATHOGENESIS

Prerenal

If renal perfusion pressure falls, renal blood flow and glomerular filtration rate (GFR) decline but there is excretion of good quality urine (see Table 16.16). Causes include:

1. excess losses
   — gastroenteritis
   — diabetes
   — burns
   — ileus
   — hemorrhage

Table 16.14 Drug therapy of hypertensive crisis

Drug	Administration	Onset of effect	Side-effects
Nifedipine	Sublingual hourly p.r.n. 0.2–0.5 mg/kg	Minutes	Headaches, tachycardia
Sodium nitroprusside	0.5–10 mcg/kg/min as infusion	Seconds/minutes	VERY rapid effect, titrate dose, cyanide accumulates after 48 h of use
Labetalol	1–3 mg/kg/hr	10–30 min	Postural hypotension
Hydralazine	Slow i.v. 0.1–0.5 mg/kg	10–30 min	Tachycardia, flushing, headaches
Phentolamine	0.02–0.1 mg/kg	Minutes	Use in catecholamine excess states

Table 16.15 Maintenance oral therapy for treatment of hypertension

Vasodilators		
Nifedipine	0.25–2 mg/kg per 24 h	2 divided doses
Hydralazine	1–8 mg/kg per 24 h	2–3 divided doses
Prazosin	0.05–0.4 mg/kg per 24 h	2–3 divided doses
Minoxidil	200 µg–1.0 mg/kg	Single dose
Beta-blockers		
Propanolol	1–10 mg/kg per 24 h	2–3 divided doses
Atenolol	1–4 mg/kg per 24 h	Once/day if adequate renal function
Diuretics		
Frusemide	1–5 mg/kg per 24 h	1–2 divided doses
Spironolactone	1–3 mg/kg per 24 h	1–2 divided doses
ACE inhibitors		
Captopril	0.5–5 mg/kg per 24 h	2–3 divided doses
Enalapril	0.1 mg–1 mg/kg per 24 h	Single dose

These children appear dehydrated with signs including sunken fontanel, poor peripheral perfusion with wide peripheral core temperature gap, tachycardia, and hypotension.

2. impaired cardiac output
   — congestive heart failure
   — pericardial tamponade
   — sepsis/shock
3. hypoalbuminemic states
   — nephrotic syndrome
   — liver failure

These children are often edematous but have intravascular volume depletion with signs including poor peripheral perfusion with wide peripheral core temperature gap and tachycardia. Blood pressure, particularly in nephrotic syndrome, is variable.

Renal

Intrarenal causes of renal failure may be vascular, glomerular or tubular. These children are more likely to present with oliguria and signs of fluid overload, although those with tubular damage may present with polyuric renal failure. Causes include:

1. vascular
   — renal vein thrombosis
   — arterial occlusion
   — arteritis
   — hemolytic uremic syndrome
2. glomerular
   — acute glomerulonephritis
3. tubular
   — nephrotoxins (especially drugs)
   — acute interstitial nephritis
   — myoglobinuria
   — hemoglobinuria
   — crystal nephropathy
   — secondary to prerenal failure.

Postrenal

Many children with obstructive causes present acutely with infection associated with obstruction and have signs of septicemia. A poor urinary stream or a palpable bladder is highly suggestive of bladder outflow obstruction. Causes include:

— posterior urethral valves
— pelviureteric junction obstruction
— vesicoureteric junction obstruction
— neuropathic bladder
— nephrolithiasis.

Table 16.16 Biochemical urine indices in renal failure

	Prerenal	Renal
Urine osmolality (mOsm/kg)	> 500	< 350
Urine Na (mmol/L)	< 20	> 40
U/P creatinine	> 40	< 20
U/P urea	> 15	< 5
FeNa+ $= \frac{\text{UNa x PCr}}{\text{PNa x UCr}}$	< 1%	> 3%

AGE AT PRESENTATION

The cause of renal failure varies according to the age group of the child.

Neonates

The commonest cause in neonates is perinatal asphyxia. The frequency of ARF in association with asphyxia is unclear, as this depends on the definitions used and the population studied. Although up to 60% of severely asphyxiated infants, in one study, were shown to have renal failure, none of these required dialysis.[122] Renal failure, in association with asphyxia, is usually polyuric renal failure, which can be managed conservatively with appropriate fluid management. Other common causes include posterior urethral valves and cardiac surgery.

Infants and older children

The commonest cause at all other ages is hemolytic uremic syndrome, which is responsible for between 150 and 200 cases of ARF per annum in the UK. This usually presents with diarrhea and thus may need to be differentiated from prerenal failure due to diarrhea losses. Cardiac surgery and congenital obstructive uropathy remain important causes of renal failure, particularly in infancy.

HISTORY AND EXAMINATION

Often the diagnosis may be clear, e.g. after cardiac bypass surgery, burns, or in association with multiorgan failure as in septicemia. In less obvious cases important clues in the history may include a history of diarrhea and vomiting, a poor urinary stream or exposure to drugs. Important features to note on examination include the state of hydration, blood pressure and other features including the presence of enlarged kidneys or a palpable bladder.

INVESTIGATIONS

Initial investigations should include full biochemical indices, including renal function and acid–base status together with hematological indices, including a blood film, and in many cases a blood culture. Dipstick urinalysis for blood and protein, microscopy and culture of the urine should also be performed and in some cases urine electrolytes may be helpful in differentiating prerenal and renal failure (see Table 16.16). A renal tract ultrasound will give information on renal size and will exclude obstruction.

All other investigations ordered will depend on these initial screening results. If the ultrasound suggests bladder outflow obstruction a micturating cystogram will be necessary to demonstrate the presence of urethral valves. If the ultrasound suggests pelviureteric obstruction a percutaneous nephrostomy together with a nephrostogram (or antegrade pyelogram) will be both therapeutic and diagnostic.

If the clinical picture is that of acute glomerulonephritis then further serological investigations and a renal biopsy will help to elucidate the cause and also guide further management with respect to immunosuppressive therapy (see Glomerulonephritis).

MANAGEMENT

Fluids and circulation

Volume depletion with a low blood pressure, low central venous pressure and a wide peripheral core temperature gap requires resuscitation with either volume expanders, e.g. isotonic saline, or 4.5% albumin 20 ml/kg. Low dose dopamine was commonly administered to critically ill patients because it increased renal blood flow and induced diuresis in healthy volunteers. However, a recent randomized placebo-controlled trial in adult intensive care unit patients did not confer clinically significant protection from renal dysfunction.[123] If poor peripheral perfusion remains, i.e. a wide peripheral core temperature gap, despite an adequate circulating volume and perfusion pressure, a vasodilator, hydralazine 0.2 mg/kg, may reverse the peripheral vasoconstriction.

Volume overload with hypertension, raised central venous pressure and edema may be treated with a diuretic such as furosemide (frusemide) 1–5 mg/kg/intravenously. If there is no response dialysis is indicated.

Maintenance fluids should be calculated as insensible losses together with continuing losses. Daily fluid requirements are directly related to energy expended. In practice, insensible losses are calculated as approximately 400 ml/m^2 body surface area. Modifications are required in the presence of fever (an increase of 12% of calculated insensible losses per degree above 37.5°C), tachypnea (an increase of 20–25%), or in neonates nursed under radiant heaters (an increase of 25%).

Electrolyte disturbances

Hyperkalemia

- Salbutamol (alpha-2 adrenoceptor stimulant) as the first choice treatment.[124] Salbutamol can be given intravenously (4 mcg/kg in 10 ml of water over 10 min) or by nebulizer (2.5 mg < 25 kg body weight or 5 mg > 25 kg body weight).
- 10% calcium gluconate 0.5 ml/kg over 5–10 min antagonizes the effect of hyperkalemia on cells and is useful for prevention, or treatment of cardiac dysrhythmias.
- 8.4% sodium bicarbonate 1–2 mmol/kg may lower serum potassium in the presence of acidosis.
- Glucose 0.5 g/kg/h with insulin 0.1 u/kg/h intravenously acts rapidly (within 1 h) to lower potassium but has been superseded by salbutamol.
- Calcium resonium 1 g/kg orally or rectally acts more slowly.

Salbutamol, the correction of acidosis and insulin shift potassium intracellularly, should only be regarded as temporary measures until dialysis can be established.

Hyponatremia

Hyponatremia may be associated with neurological disturbances and convulsions particularly with values less than 120 mmol/L. This is often due to fluid overload and therefore treatment should be aimed at fluid removal. However, excess losses, particularly gastrointestinal, are associated with true sodium deficits, which should be replaced. Sodium deficit may be calculated as follows:

mmol sodium deficit = (140 – actual serum sodium) × 0.6 × body weight in kg.

Half the deficit should be replaced in the first 24 h and the situation reviewed.

Hypocalcemia

Symptomatic patients may be given a bolus of 10% calcium gluconate 0.5 ml/kg intravenously over 5–10 min. Slower correction may be achieved by an infusion of 10% calcium gluconate, 0.1 mmol/calcium/kg body weight/h. The dose should be adjusted by frequent blood monitoring at least 6-hourly. Reduction of high phosphate levels may also improve plasma calcium levels.

Hypomagnesemia

50% magnesium sulfate 0.1 ml/kg intramuscularly.

Acidosis

Sodium bicarbonate 2 mmol/kg should be given intravenously as immediate treatment. The total deficit may be calculated as follows:

(24 – the actual bicarbonate) × 0.6 × body weight in kg.

Half this amount may be given as an infusion over 4–6 h, and the acid–base status rechecked. Sodium bicarbonate needs to be given with caution, particularly in neonates and infants, as it may cause sodium, and thus fluid, overload as well as precipitating hypocalcemic symptoms.

Hyperuricemia

Uric acid levels are elevated in ARF and no specific treatment is usually given. Tumor lysis syndrome with grossly elevated uric acid levels can occur in the treatment of lymphomas and leukemia and a high fluid intake, allopurinol and an alkali therapy are usually employed.[125] However, the production of uric acid may be switched to that of xanthine and hypoxanthine, which can also cause a crystalline nephropathy.

Convulsions

Convulsions may be due to electrolyte disturbances, uremia, hypertension, or the underlying disease such as hemolytic uremic syndrome. Many anticonvulsants tend to accumulate in renal failure. The safest emergency treatment is diazepam 0.25 mg/kg intravenously.

Hypertension

Hypertension may be due to fluid overload, which should be treated appropriately. Severe hypertension should be treated with labetalol 1–3 mg/kg/h as an intravenous infusion, which will lower blood pressure in a controlled manner. Nitroprusside 0.5–0.8 mcg/kg/min intravenously is a suitable alternative although cyanide levels need to be monitored after 24 h. If intravenous access is difficult, sublingual nifedipine 0.25 mg/kg is an effective alternative. For sustained moderate hypertension a suitable regimen is a beta-blocker (e.g. propranolol) with or without a vasodilator (e.g. hydralazine) and/or calcium channel blocker (e.g. nifedipine).

Nutrition

Adequate nutrition is essential to prevent catabolism and the child should receive at least the estimated average requirement (EAR) for energy for chronological age. Energy is best provided as a combination of carbohydrate and fat, often using glucose polymers exclusively or in combination with fat emulsions. Protein intake will depend upon whether the child is being managed conservatively or is on dialysis.[126] Enteral feeding should be used whenever possible, although intravenous feeding may on occasions be necessary. Fluid restriction may limit the amount of nutrition that can be administered and this may be an indication to institute dialysis or increase ultrafiltration on dialysis. Specialized renal feeds often contain a high energy density and may need to be introduced gradually to prevent gastrointestinal intolerance. The protein, phosphate, sodium and potassium content of feeds need to be analyzed carefully as many are unsuitable for use in renal failure.

Anemia

This is inevitable in ARF but transfusion is only indicated if there are symptoms or the hemoglobin concentration is less than 6 g/dl or falling rapidly. Caution is required in transfusing a child who is not on dialysis as hyperkalemia and fluid overload may be precipitated.

Dialysis

The need for dialysis will in part be guided by the anticipated prognosis for recovery. If a quick return of renal function seems likely then the child may be managed conservatively. However, if a prolonged period of oliguria seems likely it is better to dialyze earlier and be able to ensure adequate nutrition as well as maintain metabolic balance. Guidelines on the indications for dialysis may be:

1. uncontrollable fluid overload/hypertension;
2. uncontrollable acidosis;
3. symptomatic electrolyte disturbances not controlled by above measures;
4. symptomatic uremia;
5. presence of a dialyzable toxin;
6. established anuria, even if 1–5 not present, provided obstruction excluded.

Peritoneal dialysis

Peritoneal dialysis is the preferred option for most patients and is particularly useful in the hemodynamically unstable patient, who may tolerate hemodialysis, or even hemofiltration, poorly.

A soft Silastic or a more rigid polyethylene catheter is inserted percutaneously into the abdomen using a Seldinger technique. Commercially available dialysis solutions containing electrolytes, and glucose as an osmotic agent, are then introduced into the abdominal cavity. The volume and duration of the cycles of fluid are adjusted according to the ultrafiltration and clearance requirements of the patient.

Hemodialysis

Hemodialysis may be used in patients in whom there are technical difficulties encountered in running peritoneal dialysis, for example catheter blockage or leakage. It may also be used in those children in whom peritoneal dialysis is contraindicated, for example children with intra-abdominal sepsis, major intra-abdominal pathology or following recent abdominal surgery. Vascular access is usually obtained via a venous catheter inserted percutaneously into a large vessel (either subclavian or femoral vein), to permit the necessary rapid blood flow rates required. Commercially available filters and lines are available to enable hemodialysis to be undertaken even in neonates, but such children need to be managed in specialist nephrology centers where nephrology nursing expertise is available.

Hemofiltration

Hemofiltration is an alternative therapy in the critically ill, immobile child as it is usually well tolerated.[127] It involves an extracorporeal procedure whereby plasma is ultrafiltered by hydrostatic pressure across a highly permeable hemofilter. In conventional continuous arteriovenous hemofiltration (CAVH), hydrostatic pressure is generated by the patient's own arteriovenous gradient (Fig. 16.22).

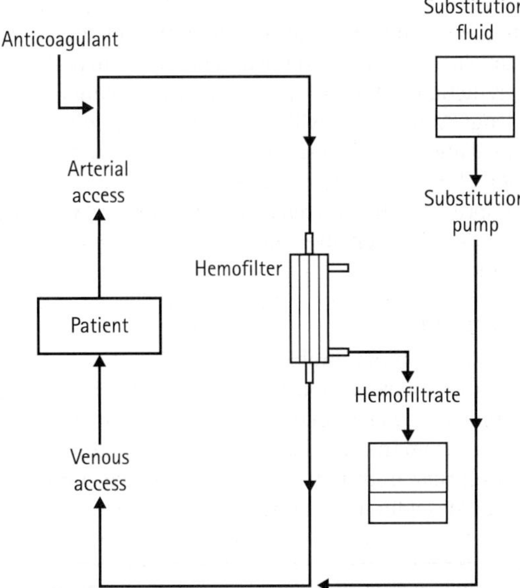

Fig. 16.22 Schematic diagram of continuous arteriovenous hemofiltration (CAVH).

However, if there is difficulty in obtaining arterial access then continuous venovenous hemofiltration (CVVH) can be undertaken, often using the standard double lumen catheters used for hemodialysis. A blood pump is then required in the exit venous line. The most important use of hemofiltration is for safe removal of fluid often from unstable critically ill patients. Convective transport of solutes does however also occur and can be increased by running dialysis fluid countercurrent across the filter, a procedure known as continuous hemodialfiltration (Fig. 16.23). CAVH does not require the use of specialized equipment and can therefore be run by most trained intensive care staff. CVVH or hemodialfiltration (CVVHD), however, require the expertise of hemodialysis trained staff.

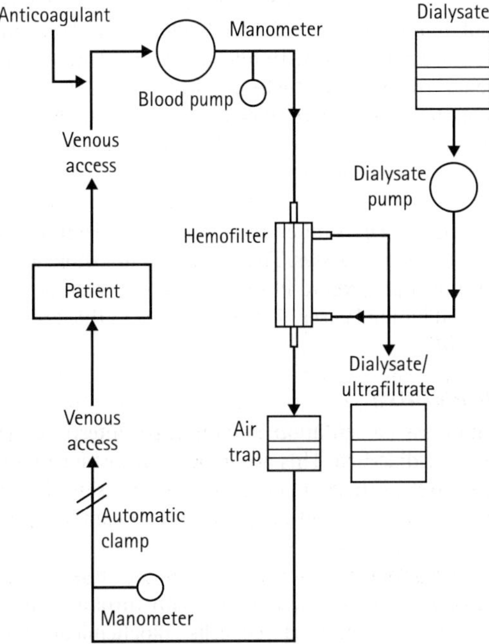

Fig. 16.23 Schematic diagram of continuous venovenous hemodiafiltration (CVVHD).

Drugs

The kidney is the major route of elimination of many drugs and their metabolites. Decreased renal function leads to both predictable and unpredictable changes in the pharmacokinetic profiles of various drugs. Many drugs will also be removed by dialysis although as peritoneal and hemodialysis remove different sized molecules, the elimination of drugs may be different with the two forms of dialysis. It is therefore essential to refer to either drug data sheets or a reference text[128] to ensure the correct dosages of drugs are administered.

Family support

ARF is an uncommon problem in developed countries. When dialysis is anticipated or a biopsy is necessary the child is transferred to a designated pediatric nephrology center, which can be some distance away from the patient's home, and this adds to the family's stress. Appropriate information and psychosocial support from the center's multidisciplinary team are very necessary.

Hyperkalemia is a medical emergency if ECG changes are present
Intravenous labetalol or sodium nitroprusside is required for hypertensive encephalopathy but blood pressure reduction should be gradual

Peritoneal dialysis is favored in renal-only acute renal failure but hemofiltration is increasingly used in intensive care units, especially with multiorgan failure

---

HEMOLYTIC UREMIC SYNDROME

The hemolytic uremic syndromes (HUS) comprise a heterogeneous group of disorders in which a triad of features, microangiopathic hemolytic anemia, thrombocytopenia and ARF occur together. They are a major cause of ARF in childhood responsible for around 150–200 cases per annum in the UK and can be classified into two categories, the epidemic and sporadic forms.

The epidemic form occurs most commonly in the summer months, affects younger children and is associated with a prodromal illness usually of bloody diarrhea. The majority of these cases are associated with infections, the commonest etiologic agent being the verocytotoxin producing *E. coli*. A variety of other bacteria, viruses and *Rickettsiae* have also been described in association with the syndrome. The prognosis for a full recovery in this group is excellent and 75% can be expected to make a full recovery.

The sporadic form is much more rare and accounts for only 5% of the total number of cases. This form does not show any seasonal variation, nor a prodromal illness. This group includes those rare relapsing and familial cases. 70% of patients in this group progress to renal failure.

Clinical features

The commonest presentation is with gastrointestinal symptoms, usually bloody diarrhea. This prodrome may last for up to 2 weeks before the onset of the triad of features comprising the syndrome. Increasing pallor and mild jaundice due to hemolysis are noted, together with decreasing urine output. Typical hematological features are then present, the blood film revealing a microangiopathic hemolytic anemia, with thrombocytopenia and the presence of fragmented red cells. Biochemical changes are indicative of renal dysfunction together with macroscopic or microscopic hematuria and variable proteinuria. There is often no correlation between the severity of the hemolysis and the renal failure. Other non-renal features include:

Gastrointestinal

Colitis is a feature of the disease and it may be difficult to distinguish between the prodrome and the onset of the disease itself. The presence of abdominal pain, and the passage of blood and mucus per rectum may lead to misdiagnosis as intussusception, ulcerative colitis or even Henoch–Schönlein syndrome. The acute colitic phase is usually self-limited although, when severe, complications such as rectal prolapse, bowel necrosis with perforation, or intussusception can occur.

Cardiorespiratory

Most of the cardiovascular manifestations are due to volume overload. However, there are reports of cardiac involvement with thrombotic microangiopathy resulting in myocarditis, cardiomyopathy and cardiac failure.

Neurological

Minor neurological disturbances of irritability, drowsiness, myoclonic jerks and tremor or ataxia are common. These may be due to metabolic derangements, or accelerated hypertension as well as a result of neurological involvement in the disease. More major neurological involvement such as coma, focal neurological deficit or decerebrate rigidity occurs less frequently although seizures may occur in up to 30% of patients.[129] Early regional EEG abnormalities, especially those in the occipital and temporal areas, are potentially useful in identifying those who might subsequently develop visual problems and epilepsy.[130]

Pathogenesis

The endothelial cell is the main site of injury in hemolytic uremic syndrome and a variety of mechanisms have been postulated.[131]

Verocytotoxins

The association of a verocytotoxin producing *E. coli* (VTEC), most commonly serotype O157: H7, with the epidemic form of HUS, was first described in 1983. Verocytotoxin has been shown to be cytopathic to cultured endothelial cells. Around 5% of individuals with VTEC will develop hemolytic uremic syndrome, with higher rates in younger children. The role of antibiotics in influencing the clinical course are conflicting with studies showing both an increase and a decrease in the incidence of HUS in VTEC infections.[132,133]

Observations have suggested that neutrophils may also have an important role in this pathogenesis. This magnitude of a peripheral blood neutrophilia indicates both the likelihood of developing HUS and the severity of HUS once it has occurred.[134] A high neutrophil count, $> 20 \times 10^9$, is associated with an adverse prognosis.[135] 93% of patients with a neutrophil count $< 20 \times 10^9$ have a good outcome compared to 33% of those with a neutrophil count $> 20 \times 10^9$. Neutrophils from patients with HUS have been shown to have increased adhesion to endothelium and are able to induce endothelial injury in vitro. It is postulated that these activated neutrophils degranulate onto endothelium causing damage by local release of proteases such as elastase, which has been found to be elevated in patients with HUS.

Verocytotoxin also causes the release of von Willebrand factor (factor VIII related antigen), which mediates platelet adhesion to the endothelium and promotes the formation of platelet thrombi. Raised factor VIII related antigens, together with an abnormal multimer pattern have been shown in HUS. These abnormalities return to normal on recovery but have been shown to persist in patients with recurrent episodes or in patients with progressive disease.

Prostacyclin

Prostacyclin is produced by normal endothelial cells and is a powerful inhibitor of platelet aggregation. Its precise role in the pathogenesis of HUS remains controversial, although prostacyclin activity has been shown to be low, either due to accelerated prostacyclin degradation or due to a reduction in production of prostacyclin in some patients with HUS.

Neuraminidase

Neuraminidase is an enzyme produced by a number of microorganisms, although in many it is cell bound and not released. It removes sialic acid from erythrocytes, platelets and glomeruli exposing the hidden Thomsen–Friedenreich antigen (T-cryptantigen). Anti-T, an IgM antibody present in most adult plasma, can then react with this exposed antigen leading to all the clinical manifestations of HUS. This phenomenon has been described in association with sporadic HUS in association with, most commonly, *Streptococcus pneumoniae* but also other infections including influenza, parainfluenza, *Clostridium perfringens*, and *Bacteroides fragilis*.

Factor H and the complement pathway

There are many reports of decreased C3 levels in children with HUS, and in some cases, this is permanent, suggesting primary complement activation. Some cases are linked to abnormalities of complement Factor H, an important regulator of the alternative complement pathway. Following the observation of Warwicker et al,[136] several studies have linked mutations in the Factor H gene with familial or sporadic HUS. Complement levels should be checked in all children with atypical HUS, but normal levels still do not rule out the possibility of factor H related HUS which may need diagnosis by molecular genetic means.[137]

Management

Many children with hemolytic uremic syndrome can be successfully managed with supportive therapy and careful attention to fluid balance, without the need for dialysis. However, it is essential to arrive at the diagnosis as soon as possible, as much morbidity can be induced by inappropriate fluid therapy, in patients whose renal function is compromised. Therefore the diagnosis should be suspected in any child with acute bloody diarrhea, and biochemistry, hematology and fluid balance monitored appropriately. Children with deteriorating renal function, oliguria/anuria or poor prognostic features should be referred early to a pediatric nephrology center. Poor prognostic features would include older children without a diarrheal prodrome, evidence of non-renal involvement including encephalopathy or cardiomyopathy, or those children with a high neutrophil count $> 20 \times 10^9$/L. A prospective study of children with HUS showed that 57% of children received dialysis.[138] Treatments other than careful supportive therapy together with dialysis should be reserved for those children with the more severe disease who would be predicted to have a poorer outcome.

A wide variety of treatments have been used in HUS but none has been shown by controlled studies to affect prognosis, with the exception of the use of plasma infusion in a multicenter study.[139] Unfortunately this study is disadvantaged by the inclusion of children with epidemic HUS, who would be expected to have a good prognosis, together with those with sporadic HUS, who would be expected to have a poorer prognosis. The benefits of plasma, therefore, need to be weighed against the disadvantages. Such disadvantages would include the risk of volume overload, the transmission of blood-borne viral diseases and the worsening hemolysis that may be seen in those patients with neuraminidase associated HUS. Plasma exchange has also been advocated and although it has been shown to be of benefit in thrombotic thrombocytopenic purpura in both the acute illness and in patients with recurrent episodes, there are insufficient data on children with HUS. There are theoretical reasons why it may be beneficial and its use may therefore be justified in the child with a severe deteriorating course, particularly with neurological involvement.

The observed abnormalities of prostacyclin metabolism, seen in some patients with HUS, have led also to the use of prostacyclin infusions. Studies have produced conflicting results, although again it may be justified in the patient with a severe deteriorating course.

Influencing long term outcome

The acute mortality of HUS is around 5% in most series. The long term consequences are, however, less well documented and although the majority of survivors recover completely, a small proportion do develop a secondary decline in renal function. Evidence of hypertension or impaired glomerular filtration rate is seen in between 11 and 25% of patients. Although children who remain on dialysis longer have a higher risk of long term renal problems, the long term sequelae cannot however be reliably predicted by the acute clinical course. Persistent proteinuria is associated with a less good prognosis. A positive correlation between microalbuminuria and systolic blood pressure and a negative correlation between microalbuminuria and glomerular filtration rate[140] suggests that those children with albuminuria should receive longer and closer follow-up to identify occult nephropathy earlier. A recent study has suggested that long term follow-up should be carried out on all children with proteinuria, hypertension, abnormal ultrasound or an impaired GFR at one year.[141] The full implications of the long-term sequelae of HUS may not yet have been realized, as a study on renal functional reserve demonstrated that all patients who had apparently made a complete recovery presented abnormalities in their renal functional reserve similar to that seen in children with a single kidney. However, the patients with HUS showed in addition an increase in microalbuminuria after a protein load, which may imply a poorer long-term prognosis.[142]

Hemolytic uremic syndrome associated with verocytotoxin producing *E. coli* is a major cause of acute renal failure in childhood

Atypical or familial HUS has a poorer prognosis and may be associated with mutations in Factor H associated with the alternative complement pathway

Persistent proteinuria, hypertension and/or reduced GFR are poor prognostic features after any acute or chronic renal insult

---

CHRONIC RENAL FAILURE

Data on the prevalence of chronic renal failure are uncertain, at least in part as a result of the differing definitions of the level of renal dysfunction.

European data[121] suggest a prevalence of between 25 and 50 children per million child population with a glomerular filtration rate (GFR) less than 25–50 ml/min/1.73 m^2.

End-stage renal failure is defined as the stage at which dialysis and renal transplantation are required (Table 16.17). There is no absolute level of renal function at which this is required although in practice it is usually a GFR < 10 ml/min/1.73 m^2. There are national and international renal registries for end-stage renal failure, which are important for identifying changes in incidence, treatment modalities and outcome. The European Dialysis Transplant Association (EDTA) register of children under 15 years of age accepted for renal replacement therapy each year suggests an incidence increasing from 4.6 per million child population in 1971 to 7–8 per million child population per annum in 1991.[143] In the UK, the national renal registry reveals a take-on rate of at least 1.7 per million total population, with a prevalence of at least 12.2 per million total population.[37] The number of patients receiving treatment is increasing as the treatment criteria broaden and, in particular, younger children being now accepted for renal replacement therapy.

The etiology of renal failure varies according to the child's country of origin, and age at presentation. In the UK the four commonest causes are currently renal dysplasia and related conditions, obstructive uropathy, glomerulonephritis and reflux nephropathy.[37]

CLINICAL PRESENTATION

In many children, chronic renal failure will be the end result of known progressive renal disease. More recently, antenatal diagnosis has led to detection of renal tract malformations before symptoms develop. Other children may present with signs and symptoms associated with renal failure. These may be non-specific symptoms, including lethargy, poor appetite and nausea, together with urinary symptoms, including polyuria or enuresis.

Growth

Growth failure is a major problem for children with chronic renal failure. The severity of the growth failure is related to the age at presentation: 50% of children with renal failure since infancy have growth failure, with a height of > 2 SD below the mean height for age, in contrast to 10% of those with acquired disease. Important factors contributing to the growth failure include: acidosis, salt depletion, other biochemical abnormalities, renal osteodystrophy, and energy malnutrition. Estimation of renal function would be a routine investigation in a child presenting with unexplained growth failure.

Renal osteodystrophy

Phosphate retention, secondary hyperparathyroidism and skeletal resistance to parathyroid hormone, intestinal malabsorption of calcium leading to hypocalcemia and altered vitamin D metabolism all contribute to the disturbances in bone and mineral metabolism associated with renal osteodystrophy. The severity of the bone disease is related to age at onset and underlying renal disease, together with the level of renal function and duration of renal failure. It is more common with the congenital and obstructive uropathies and rarely manifests clinically with a GFR of above 25 ml/min/1.73 m^2 although biochemical abnormalities are seen with a GFR between 50 and 80 ml/min/1.73 m^2.[144] Symptoms may include poor growth, bone pain, skeletal deformities, and slipped epiphyses.

Table 16.17 Stages of chronic renal failure

	GFR (ml/min/1.73 m^2)	
Mild	50–75	Asymptomatic
Moderate	25–50	Metabolic abnormalities
Severe	< 25	Progressive growth failure
End-stage renal failure	< 10	Require renal replacement therapy

Anemia

Anemia secondary to a lack of erythropoietin is also a well recognized complication of renal failure and may be the presenting feature of the condition.

Hypertension

Renin dependent hypertension is the commonest cause of hypertension in childhood and may be associated with renal failure. The presentation of renal failure may therefore be with the symptoms of hypertension including headache, visual disturbances or hypertensive encephalopathy.

MANAGEMENT

Fluid and electrolyte therapy

Many children with congenital renal diseases, in particular dysplasia, obstructive uropathy and nephronophthisis, have poor renal concentrating capacity with polyuria and salt loss. Salt supplementation is often necessary and salt deficiency is an important cause of poor growth in these infants. Children with acquired diseases, in particular focal glomerulosclerosis and other forms of glomerulonephritis, may have salt and water retention and therefore require salt restriction. Acidosis is common and should be corrected with sodium bicarbonate.

Infection

Urine cultures should be checked, especially in those with abnormalities of the urinary tract, as repeated infection may hasten progression of CRF.

Renal osteodystrophy

The impairment of renal production of 1,25-dihydroxycholecalciferol is a major factor in the development of renal osteodystrophy. Pharmacological replacement, with 1-alpha-hydroxycholecalciferol, should be commenced when there are biochemical features of altered mineral metabolism (hypocalcemia, hyperphosphatemia, rising alkaline phosphatase or hyperparathyroidism) or if the GFR falls below 25 ml/min/1.73 m^2. An initial dose would be 10 ng/kg/per 24 h, increasing according to clinical and biochemical parameters, up to dosages of 50 ng/kg/per 24 h. Hyperphosphatemia also plays an important role in the development and maintenance of secondary hyperparathyroidism. Initially, dietary phosphate restriction may be sufficient to control hyperphosphatemia, although this can be difficult in young infants on a predominantly milk diet. Phosphate binders may become necessary and calcium carbonate would be the drug of choice. Aluminum hydroxide, although an effective phosphate binder, is best avoided in children because of its potentially neurotoxic effects.

Erythropoietin

The production of human erythropoietin (rhEPO), by recombinant DNA techniques, has made possible the treatment of the anemia of chronic renal failure and significantly improved the quality of life for many patients. The use of rhEPO, usually given subcutaneously, has been shown to be effective in raising the hematocrit of children with end-stage renal failure. It is also effective in predialysis patients. There is, however, concern that administration of rhEPO may increase the blood viscosity, causing glomerular hypertension and glomerular hyperfiltration with acceleration in functional renal decline. RhEPO may result in hypertension and it is not known if effects on renal function are independent or consequent upon changes in blood pressure. Despite these concerns, rhEPO should be considered for all patients with severe anemia. Blood pressure and renal function should be monitored closely.

Growth hormone

Short stature is a serious problem for children with chronic renal failure. Endogenous growth hormone secretion is normal, as are serum levels of insulin like growth factors I and II. However, exogenous growth hormone has been shown to increase the height velocity in a number of conditions in which growth hormone secretion is not impaired. More recently its efficacy in children with chronic renal failure has been studied. It has been shown that growth hormone does increase the short term growth velocity of prepubertal children with chronic renal failure and is now licensed for use. A study in children treated with growth hormone for up to 9 years showed persistent catch up growth and an improvement in final height compared with untreated children.[145]A further study[146] suggested that the improvement in height, obtained after a limited course of growth hormone, was maintained after discontinuation of treatment. The optimal treatment regimen of growth hormone therefore remains unknown. Of most concern is that growth hormone may accelerate renal functional decline by increasing renal plasma flow and glomerular hyperfiltration. In view of the possible side-effects its use should be restricted to children who are below the third centile for height and in whom all other abnormalities such as electrolyte and acid–base balance, renal osteodystrophy and nutritional deficiencies have been corrected.

Nutrition

General recommendations for children with chronic renal failure suggest that children should have at least the EAR for chronological age for energy, although many will need additional energy to promote growth. Protein intake should be based on the reference nutrient intake (RNI) for height age. However, individual dietary and biochemical assessment will determine requirements, as well as the stage of management.[147] Large reliance is placed upon nutritional supplements to achieve nutritional goals in infants and children with chronic renal failure and the assistance of an experienced pediatric dietitian is essential. In many infants and young children the supplements are delivered either nasogastrically or preferably via the gastrostomy route, if long term feeding is required.[148]

Phosphate restriction naturally follows protein restriction but the majority of children require phosphate binders, in the form of calcium carbonate, to control serum phosphate and parathyroid hormone levels in advancing chronic renal failure. Each child will also need assessing individually, with respect to fluid and electrolyte needs, along with adequacy of micronutrient intake. These children require frequent and repeated assessments of their dietary prescriptions, if growth is to be maintained or promoted.

Over the last decade considerable attention has focused on dietary modifications to retard the progression of chronic renal failure. Of particular interest has been the role of restriction of dietary phosphate and protein in retarding the progression of chronic renal failure. Both the efficacy and safety of severe protein restriction in growing children requires evaluation, because of the concern regarding the effect of protein restriction on growth. The results from trials using protein restriction of 1 g/kg/day have shown conflicting results in the effect on GFR, although no adverse effect on growth has been demonstrated.[149] Compliance with dietary manipulations in childhood is often poor and in the European study on protein restriction only 76% of children adhered to their dietary prescription. Further studies are needed before such treatments are recommended for widespread clinical use in children.

Renal dysplasia/hypoplasia is the commonest category of conditions causing chronic renal failure (CRF) in childhood

Recombinant erythropoietin by subcutaneous or intravenous injections can correct the anemia of CRF

Renal transplantation is the treatment of choice for children with end-stage renal failure and is increasingly performed before dialysis is necessary

---

Dialysis

Dialysis does achieve satisfactory control of fluid and biochemistry, but is an incomplete form of renal replacement therapy, and is therefore considered a stepping stone to renal transplantation in most children. The two main forms of dialysis are chronic peritoneal dialysis and hemodialysis. The choice between peritoneal dialysis and hemodialysis will depend on patient preference, geographical and practical considerations.

Chronic peritoneal dialysis (CPD)

Access to the peritoneal cavity is by way of a surgically implanted permanent Silastic catheter.[150] When CPD was first introduced, children underwent continuous ambulatory peritoneal dialysis (CAPD), where the dialysis fluid was exchanged three or four times via 'bag changes'. The advent of automated peritoneal dialysis (APD), in the 1980s, meant that children could receive most of their dialysis overnight (nocturnal intermittent peritoneal dialysis, NIPD) or mostly overnight with daytime dwell as well (continuous cycling peritoneal dialysis, CCPD). APD is now the preferred modality in many Western countries, with the obvious benefit of freedom from daytime exchanges at school.

The disadvantages of CPD are the risk of peritonitis and other abdominal complications such as hernias.

Hemodialysis

Hemodialysis requires adequate vascular access either via an arteriovenous fistula, or more commonly, via an indwelling vascular catheter, usually in the subclavian or jugular vein. Although the technical principles of hemodialysis are similar in adults and children, because of the challenges presented by the smaller intravascular volumes of children and the potential hemodynamic instability, together with the psychological issues it is recommended that children be treated in units with pediatric expertise. Difficulties with vascular access, including infection, are a disadvantage of the technique.

Transplantation

Renal transplantation is the best mode of renal replacement therapy for children and adolescents.[151,152] In the UK, 76% of children with end-stage renal failure have a functioning graft. At all ages pediatric renal transplant recipients have better survival than do dialysis patients of the same age. Moreover, successful transplantation confers a degree of physiological and psychological rehabilitation not seen with any form of dialysis. Some patients may be fortunate enough to receive a transplant without dialysis with pre-emptive transplant rates of around 10% in Europe and over 20% in North America.

Graft survival

Graft survival rates in the UK suggest 1-year graft survival of 80% for cadaveric renal transplantation, with over 90% survival for live donor grafts. Longer term follow-up results need to be interpreted with caution as treatment modalities and immunosuppressive regimens have changed considerably over the last decade.

However, 10- and 13-year survival rates of 52% and 61% have been reported. The use of live donor grafts between countries is very variable. In the UK less than 10% of grafts are from live donor, in North America 50% and in Scandinavia as high as 70%.

Graft success rates are dependent on a wide variety of factors including tissue matching, donor age, storage time of the kidney, immunosuppression regimens, previous transplantation and original and associated diseases. There was concern about outcomes in the younger renal transplant recipient, as early European and North American data tended to suggest that graft survival was lower in children under 2 years compared to older children, but more recent reports are more encouraging.[153,154]

Table 16.18 Primary renal disease causing end-stage renal failure in 686 patients in the UK[37]

		%
1.	Primary renal dysplasia	27.7
	Renal dysplasia	20.4
	Multicystic dysplastic kidneys	2.2
2.	Prune belly syndrome	2.2
	Renal hypoplasia	1.9
3.	Others	1.0
	Obstructive uropathy	20.2
	Posturethral valves	15.4
4.	Neuropathic bladder	2.0
	Others	2.8
5.	Glomerular disease	17.3
	Primary focal segmental glomerulosclerosis	6.4
6.	D+ hemolytic uremic syndrome	2.9
	Henoch–Schönlein nephritis	1.6
7.	Alport syndrome	1.2
	Other	5.2
8.	Reflux nephropathy and CRF of uncertain etiology	9.2
	Reflux nephropathy	7.2
9.	Chronic renal failure – uncertain etiology	2.0
	Primary tubular and interstitial disorders	7.3
10.	Nephronophthisis	5.3
	Primary interstitial nephritis	1.2
	Others	0.8
	Congenital nephrotic syndrome	6.9
	Congenital nephrotic syndrome (Finnish)	2.6
	Other types	4.3
	Renal vascular disorders	4.5
	Cortical necrosis	1.9
	Renal vein thrombosis	1.5
	Others	1.1
	Metabolic diseases and drug nephrotoxicity	3.1
	Cystinosis	2.0
	Primary hyperoxaluria type 1	0.4
	Others	0.7
	Polycystic kidney disease	2.2
	Autosomal recessive PKD	1.8
	Polycystic kidney disease (other)	0.4
	Malignant and related diseases	1.6
	Wilms' tumour	1.2
	Other	0.4

Results from live donation are consistently superior and comparable with other age groups.[155,156] In cadaveric transplantation there is a tendency to use young donors in young recipients and when stratified for donor age, recipient age does not seem to influence outcome. It is anticipated that policies involving not using organs from young donors in young recipients will improve the outcome of this group. More recent concern has focused on the outcome of renal transplantation in adolescents[157] in whom long term outcome lags significantly behind that of younger children. Poor compliance is a major contributory factor in these young people.

Immunosuppression

All transplanted children will remain on immunosuppressive therapy with a calcineurin inhibitor, either ciclosporin or tacrolimus, usually with steroids and, in some, also azathioprine. It is important to consider the side-effects of these medications, including risk of infection, hypertension, hirsutism and other cosmetic side-effects which may influence compliance, particularly in adolescents. There are a number of newer immunosuppressive medications available and under development so that in future it may be possible to provide immunosuppression with greater specificity and fewer toxic effects.

Rehabilitation

Growth is improved after renal transplantation, with a significant increase in growth velocity in prepubertal children. However, perhaps one of the most important issues when considering the quality of life following renal transplantation is the neurodevelopmental and the psychological outcome.

Early reports of children with chronic renal failure, particularly those who had had renal failure since infancy, showed a worrying proportion of those children having significant developmental delay.[158] The etiology was felt to be multifactorial, including: poor biochemical control; inadequate nutrition; the use of aluminum-containing phosphate binders; and psychosocial factors. However, recent studies have been more encouraging, with the authors suggesting that the marked improvement in neurodevelopmental outcome was due to a shift in emphasis in renal failure management, with a more aggressive approach to nutrition and biochemical parameters.[159,160]

Studies on older children with renal failure have demonstrated effects on cognitive development, but despite these deficits there is no difference in grades achieved at school. Studies on the psychosocial adjustment of adult survivors of pediatric dialysis and transplant programs have shown that although the educational and employment achievements of those with renal disease are less than those of controls, two-thirds of the patients leave school with qualifications and two-thirds are in employment.[161]

In conclusion, therefore, dialysis and transplantation enable the majority of children with end-stage renal failure to enter adulthood in good physical health and well adjusted socially. However, the burden for families caring for children with renal failure, as with many other chronic illnesses is considerable. It is essential that such families have the benefits of support from an experienced multidisciplinary team which includes nursing and medical staff, dietitians, social workers, teachers, play leaders, psychologists and psychiatrists, who are able to work not only in hospital but also support the families in their own communities.[162]

REFERENCES (* Level 1 evidence)

1 Skinner R, Cole M, Pearson ADJ, et al. Specificity of pH and osmolality of early morning urine sample in assessing distal renal tubular function in children: results in healthy children. BMJ 1996; 312:1337–1338.

2 Zelikovic I. Molecular pathophysiology of tubular transport disorders. Pediatr Nephrol 2001; 16:919–935.

3 Town M, Jean G, Cherqui S, et al. A novel gene encoding an integral membrane protein is mutated in nephropathic cystinosis. Nat Genet 1998; 18(4):319–324.

4 Coleman JE, Watson AR. Gastrostomy buttons for nutritional support in children with cystinosis. Pediatr Nephrol 2000; 14:833–836.

5 Van't Hoft WG, Gretz N. The treatment of cystinosis with cysteamine and phosphocysteamine in the United Kingdom and Eire. Pediatr Nephrol 1995; 9:685–689.

6 Rodriguez-Soriano J, Vallo A. Renal tubular acidosis. Pediatr Nephrol 1990; 4(3):268–275.

7 Karet FE, Finsberg KE, Nelson RD, et al. Mutations in the gene encoding beta 1 subunit of H^+-ATPase cause renal tubular acidosis with sensorineural deafness. Nat Genet 1999; 21:84–90.

8 Smith AN, Skaug J, Choate KA, et al. Mutations in the ATP6NIB, encoding a new kidney vacuolar proton pump 116-kD subunit, cause recessive distal renal tubular acidosis with preserved hearing. Nat Genet 2000; 26:71–75.

9 Bruce LJ, Cope DL, Jones GK, et al. Familial distal renal tubular acidosis is associated with mutations in the red cell anion exchanger (band 3, AE1) gene. J Clin Invest 1997; 100:1693–1707.

10 Simon DB, Karet FE, Hamdan JM, et al. Bartter's syndrome, hypokalaemic alkalosis with hypercalciuria, is caused by mutations in the Na-K-2Cl cotransporter NKCC2. Nat Genet 1996; 13:183–187.

11 Simon DB, Karet FE, Rodriguez-Soriano J, et al. Genetic heterogeneity of Bartter's syndrome revealed by mutations in the K+ channel, ROMK. Nat Genet 1996; 14:152–155.

12 Simon DB, Bindra RS, Mansfield TA, et al. Mutations in the chloride channel gene CLCNKB cause Bartter's syndrome type III. Nat Genet 1997; 17:171–177.

13 Cruz DN, Shaer AJ, Bia MJ, et al. for the Yale Gitelman's and Bartter's Syndrome Collaborative Study Group. Gitelman's syndrome revisited: an evaluation of symptoms and health-related quality of life. Kidney Int 2001; 59:710–717.

14 Byrd DJ, Lind M, Brodehl J. Diagnostic and genetic studies in 43 patients with classic cystinuria. Clin Chem 1991; 37:68–73.

15 Goodyer P, Saadi I, Ong P, et al. Cystinuria subtype and the risk of nephrolithiasis. Kidney Int 1998; 54:56–61.

16 Cochat P. Primary hyperoxaluria type 1. Kidney Int 1999; 55:2533–2547.

17 The Hyp Consortium. A gene (PEX) with homologics to endopeptidases is mutated in patients with X-linked hypophosphataemic rickets. Nat Genet 1995; 11:130–136.

18 Reusz GS, Hoyer PF, Lucas M, et al. X-linked hypophosphataemia: treatment height gain and nephrocalcinosis. Arch Dis Child 1990; 65:1125–1128.

19 Morelo JP, Bichet DG. Nephrogenic diabetes insipidus. Annu Rev of Physio 2001; 63:607–630.

20 Al-Khaldi N, Watson AR, Zuccollo J, et al. Outcome of an antenatally detected cystic dysplastic kidney disease. Arch Dis Child 1994; 70:520–522.

21 Sukthankar S, Watson AR on behalf of the Trent and Anglia Paediatric Nephrourology Group. Unilateral multicystic dysplastic kidney disease: defining the natural history. Acta Paediatr 2000; 89:811–813.

22 James CA, Watson AR, Twining P, Rance CH. Antenatally detected urinary tract abnormalities: changing incidence and management. Eur J Pediatr 1998; 157:508–511.

23 Ulman I, Jayanthi VR, Koff SA. The long-term follow up of newborns with severe unilateral hydronephrosis initially treated nonoperatively. J Uro 2000; 164(3 Pt 2): 1101–1105.

24 Anderson PAM, Rickwood AMK. Features of primary vesicoureteric reflux detected by prenatal sonography. Br J Uro 1991; 67:267–271.

25 Guay-Woodford LM. Autosomal recessive disease: clinical and genetic profiles. In: Torres V, Watson M, eds. Polycystic kidney disease. Oxford: Oxford University Press; 1996:237–267.

26 Guay-Woodford LM, Muecher G, Hopkins SD, et al. The severe perinatal form of autosomal recessive polycystic kidney disease (ARPKD) maps to chromosome 6p21.1–p12: implications for genetic counselling. Am J Hum Genet 1995; 56:1101–1107.

27 Jamil B, McMahon LP, Savige JA, et al. A study of long-term morbidity associated with autosomal recessive polycystic kidney disease. Nephrol Dial Transplantation 1999; 14:205–209.

28 Roy S, Dillon M, Trompeter R, Barratt T. Autosomal recessive polycystic kidney disease: long-term outcome of neonatal survivors. Pediatr Nephrol 1997; 11:302–306.

29 Peters DJM, Breuning MH. Autosomal dominant polycystic kidney disease: modification of disease progression. Lancet 2001; 358:1439–1444.

30 Konrad M, Saunier S, Heidet L, et al. Large homozygous deletions of the 2q13 region are a major cause of juvenile nephronophthisis. Hum Mol Genet 1996; 5:367–371.

31 Ala-Mello S, Kivivuori S, Ronnholm K, et al. Mechanism underlying early anemia in children with familial juvenile nephronophthisis. Pediatr Nephrol 1996; 10:578–581.

32 Torres V. Tuberous sclerosis complex. In: Torres V, Watson M, eds. Polycystic kidney disease. Oxford: Oxford University Press; 1996: 283–308.

*33 Dick PT, Feldman W. Routine diagnostic imaging for childhood urinary tract infections: a systematic overview. J Pediatr 1996; 128:15–22.

34 Goonasekera CDA, Shah V, Wade AM, et al. 15-year follow-up of renin and blood pressure in reflux nephropathy. Lancet 1996; 347:640–643.

35 Jacobsson SH, Eklof O, Eriksson CG, et al. Development of hypertension and uraemia after pyelonephritis in childhood. 27 year follow up. BMJ 1989; 299:703–706.

36 Alexander SR, Arbus GS, Butt KMH, et al. The 1989 Report of the North American Pediatric Renal Transplant Cooperative Study. Pediatr Nephrol 1990; 4:542–553.

37 Lewis M, Watson AR, Clark G, et al. Report of the paediatric renal registry 1999. In: The UK Renal Registry: Second Annual Report. London: Renal Association; 1999:175–187.

38 Lewis MA, Awan A. Mannitol and frusemide in the treatment of diuretic resistant oedema in nephrotic syndrome. Arch Dis Child 1999; 80:184–185.

39 Farhat W, McLorie G, Geary D, et al. The natural history of neonatal vesicoureteral reflux associated with antenatal hydronephrosis. J Urol 2000; 164:1057–1060.

40 Wolfish NM, Delbrouck NF, Shanon A, et al. Prevalence of hypertension in children with primary vesicoureteral reflux. J Pediatr 1993; 123:559–563.

41 Watson AR. Urinary tract infection in early childhood. J of Antimicrob Chemother 1994; 34(A):53–60.

42 South Bedfordshire Practitioners' Group. Development of renal scars in children: missed opportunities in management. BMJ 1990; 301(6760):1082–1084.

*43 Smellie JM, Ransley PG, Normand ICS, et al. Development of new renal scars: a collaborative study. BMJ 1985; 290:1957–1960.

44 Wettergren B, Jodal U, Jonasson G. Epidemiology of bacteriuria during the first year of life. Acta Pediatr Scand 1985; 74:925–933.

45 Craig JC, Knight JF, Sureshkumar P, et al. Effect of circumcision on incidence of urinary tract infection in preschool boys. J Pediatr 1996; 128:23–27.

46 Pisacane A, Graziano L, Mazzarella G, et al. Breast-feeding and urinary tract infection. J Pediatr 1992; 120:87–89.

47 Kemper KJ, Avner ED. The case against screening urinalyses for asymptomatic bacteriuria in children. Am J Dis Child 1992; 146:343–346.

48 Hansson S, Jodal U, Noren L, et al. Untreated bacteriuria in asymptomatic girls with renal scarring. Pediatrics 1989; 84:964–968.

49 Moyer VA, Craig J. Acute urinary tract infection. In: Moyer VA, Elliott EJ, Davis RL, et al, eds. Evidence based pediatrics and child health London; BMJ Books: 2000; 35:318–325.

50 Vernon S. Urine collection from infants: a reliable method. Paediatr Nurs 1995; 7(6):26–27.

51 Turner GM, Coulthard MG. Fever can cause pyuria in children. BMJ 1995; 311:924.

*52 Gorelick MH, Shaw KV. Screening tests for urinary tract infection in children: a meta-analysis. Pediatrics 1999; 104:54.

53 Jewkes FEM, McMaster DJ, Napier WA, et al. Home collection of urine specimens – boric acid bottles or dipslides? Arch Dis Child 1990; 65:286–289.

54 Royal College of Physicians. Guidelines for the management of acute urinary tract infection in childhood. Report of a

working group of the Research Unit, Royal College of Physicians. J R Coll Physicians 1991; 25:36–42.

55 Stull TL, LiPuma JJ. Epidemiology and natural history of urinary tract infections in children. Med Clin North Am 1991; 75:287–297.

56 Sherbotie JR, Cornfeld D. Management of urinary tract infections in children. Med Clin North Am 1991; 75:327–338.

57 Michael M, Hodson EM, Craig JC, et al. Short compared with standard duration of antibiotic treatment for urinary tract infection; a systematic review of randomised controlled trials. Arch Dis Child 2002; 87:118–123.

58 Hansson S, Jodal U. Urinary tract infection. In: Barratt MT, Avner ED, Harmon WE eds. Pediatric nephrology, 2nd edn. Boston: Little, Brown; 1999:1943–1991.

59 Dohil R, Roberts E, Verrier Jones K, Jenkins HR. Constipation and reversible urinary tract abnormalities. Arch Dis Child 1994; 70:56–57.

60 Kontiokari T, Sundqvist K, Nuutinen M, et al. Randomised trial of cranberry-lingonberry juice and Lactobacillus GG drink for the prevention of urinary tract infections in women. BMJ 2001; 322:1571–1573.

61 Tibballs JM, De Bruyn R. Primary vesicoureteric reflux – how useful is postnatal ultrasound? Arch Dis Child 1996; 75:444–447.

62 Phillips D, Watson AR, Collier J. Distress and radiological investigations of the urinary tract in children. Eur J Pediatr 1996; 155(8):684–687.

63 Philips DA, Watson AR, MacKinlay D. Distress and the micturating cystourethrogram: does preparation help? Acta Paediatr 1998; 87:175–179.

64 Jakobsson B, Svensson L. Transient pyelonephritic changes on 99m Technetium-dimercaptosuccinic acid scan for at least five months after infection. Acta Paediatr 1997; 86:803–807.

65 Barry BP, Hall N, Cornford E, et al. Improved ultrasound detection of renal scarring in children following urinary tract infection. Clin Radiol 1998; 53:747–751.

66 Morin D, Veyrac C, Kotzki PO, et al. Comparison of ultrasound and dimercaptosuccinic acid scintigraphy changes in acute pyelonephritis. Pediatr Nephrol 1999; 13:219–222.

67 O'Donnell PD. Pitfalls of urodynamic testing. Urol Clin of North Am 1991; 18:257–268.

68 Williams GL, Lee A, Craig JC, et al. Cochrane Review. The Cochrane Library, 4. Oxford: Update Software; 2002.

69 Aggarwal VH, Verrier-Jones K. Vesicoureteric reflux – screening of the first degree relatives. Arch Dis Child 1989; 64:1538–1541.

*70 Birmingham Reflux Study Group. Prospective trial of operative versus non-operative treatment of severe vesico-ureteric reflux in children: five years' observation. BMJ 1987; 295:237–241.

*71 International Reflux Study in Children: European Group. Five year study of medical and surgical treatment in children with severe reflux: radiological renal findings. Pediatr Nephrol 1992; 6:223–230.

72 Smellie JM, Barratt TM, Chantler C, et al. Medical versus surgical treatment in children with severe bilateral vesicoureteric reflux and bilateral nephropathy: a randomised trial. Lancet 2001; 357:1329–1333.

73 Eiberg H, Berendt I, Mohr J. Assignment of dominant inherited nocturnal enuresis to chromosome 13q. Nat Genet 1995; 10:354–356.

*74 Lister-Sharpe D, O'Meara, Bradley M, Sheldon TA. A systematic review of the effectiveness of interventions for managing childhood nocturnal enuresis (CRD report 11). NHS Centre for Reviews. York: University of York; 1997.

75 Evans JHC. Evidence based management of nocturnal enuresis. BMJ 2001; 323:1167–1169.

*76 Glazener CMA, Evans JHC. Desmopressin for nocturnal enuresis in children (Cochrane review). The Cochrane Library, 2. Oxford: Update Software; 2000.

*77 Glazener CMA, Evans JHC. Tricyclic and related drugs for nocturnal enuresis in children (Cochrane review). The Cochrane Library, 2. Oxford: Update Software; 2000.

78 Bradbury MG, Meadow SR. Combined treatment with enuresis alarm and desmopressin for nocturnal enuresis Acta Paediatr 1997; 84:1014–1018.

79 Borzykowski M, Mundy AR. The management of neuropathic bladder in childhood. Pediatr Nephrol 1988; 2:56–66.

80 Shichiri M, Oowada A, Nishio Y, et al. Use of autoanalyser to examine urinary-red-cell morphology in the diagnosis of glomerular haematuria. Lancet 1986; I:781–782.

81 Hulton S. Evaluation of urinary tract calculi in children. Arch Dis Child 2001; 84:320–323.

82 Rayner RJ, Watson AR, Bishop MC. Haematuria in an adolescent due to bladder carcinoma. Eur J Pediatr 1988; 147:328–329.

83 Meadow R. Haematuria. In: Postlethwaite RJ, ed. Clinical paediatric nephrology. Oxford: Butterworth Heineman; 1994:6.

84 Rinaldi S, Strologo LD, Montecchi F, Rizzoni G. Relapsing gross haematuria in Munchausen syndrome. Pediatr Nephrol 1993; 7:202–203.

85 Tomsett A, Watson AR. Renal biopsy as a day case procedure. Paediatr Nurs 1996; 8(5):14–15.

86 Clark G, White RHR, Glasgow EF, et al. Poststreptococcal glomerulonephritis in children: clinicopathological correlations and long-term prognosis. Pediatr Nephrol 1988; 2:381–388.

87 Donadio JV Jr, Grande JP. Immunoglobulin A nephropathy: a clinical perspective. J Am Soc of Nephrol 1997; 8:1324–1332.

88 Takebayashi S, Yanase K. Asymptomatic urinary abnormalities found via the Japanese school screening program: a clinical, morphological and prognostic analysis. Nephron 1992; 61:82.

*89 Nolin L, Courteau M. Management of IgA nephropathy: evidence based recommendations. Kidney Int 1999; 70(suppl): S56-S62.

90 Floege J, Feehally J. IgA nephropathy: recent developments. J Am Soc Nephrol 2000; 11:2395–2403.

91 Yoshikawa N, Ito H. Combined therapy with prednisolone, azathioprine, heparin-warfarin, and dipyridamole for paediatric patients with severe IgA nephropathy: is it relevant for adult patients? Nephrol Dial Transplantation 1999; 14:1097–1099.

92 Berg UB, Widstam-Attorps UC. Follow-up of renal function and urinary protein excretion in childhood IgA nephropathy. Pediatr Nephrol 1993; 7:123–129.

93 McEnery PT, Coutinho MJ. Membranoproliferative glomerulonephritis. In: Holliday MA, Barratt TM, Avner ED, eds. Pediatric nephrology, 3rd edn. Baltimore: Williams & Wilkins; 1994:739–753.

94 Balow JE, Boumpas DT, Fessler BJ, Austin II HA. Management of lupus nephritis. Kidney Int 1996; 49(53):S88–S92.

*95 Bansal VI, Betow JA. Treatment of lupus nephritis: a meta-analysis of clinical trials. Am J Kidney Dis 1997; 29:193–199.

96 Turner AN, Rees AJ. Anti-glomerular basement membrane antibody disease. In: Brady HR, Wilcox N, eds. Therapy in nephrology and hypertension: a companion to Brenner and Rector's 'The Kidney'. Philadelphia: WB Saunders; 1999:152–157.

97 Tryggvason K, Zhou J, Hostikka SC, Shows TB. Molecular genetics of Alport syndrome. Kidney Int 1993; 43:38–44.

98 Lang S, Stevenson B, Risdon RA. Thin basement membrane nephropathy as a cause of recurrent haematuria in childhood. Histopathology 1990; 16:331–337.

99 Monnens LAH. Thin glomerular basement membrane disease. Kidney Int 2001; 60:799–800.

100 Vehaskari VM. Asymptomatic haematuria: a cause for concern? Pediatr Nephrol 1989; 3:240–241.

101 Mogensen CE. How to protect the kidney in diabetic patients with special reference to IDDM. Diabetes 1997; 46(suppl 2): 104–111.

102 Elises JS, Griffiths PD, Hocking MD, et al. Simplified quantification of urinary protein excretion in children. Clin Nephrol 1988; 30:225–229.

103 Fogo A, Kon V. Pathophysiology of progressive renal disease. In: Holliday MA, Barratt TM, Avner ED, eds. Pediatric nephrology, 3rd edn. Baltimore: Williams & Wilkins; 1994: 1228–1240.

104 Sharples PM, Poulton J, White RHR. Steroid responsive nephrotic syndrome is more common in Asians. Arch Dis Child 1985; 60:1014–1017.

105 Fuchschuber A, Gribouval O, Ronner V, et al and members of the APN Study Group. Clinical and genetic evaluation of familial steroid-responsive nephrotic syndrome in childhood. J Am Soc Nephrol 2001; 12:374–378.

106 Hoyer PF, Gonda S, Barthels M, et al. Thromboembolic complications in children with nephrotic syndrome. Acta Pediatr Scand 1986; 75:804–810.

107 Watson AR, Coleman JE. Dietary management in nephrotic syndrome. Arch Dis Child 1993; 69:179–180.

108 Consensus statement on management and audit potential for steroid responsive nephrotic syndrome. Report of a workshop by the British Association for Paediatric Nephrology and Research Unit, Royal College of Physicians. Arch Dis Child 1994; 70:151–157.

*109 Bargman JM. Management of minimal lesion glomerulonephritis: evidence-based recommendations. Kidney Int 1999; 55(Suppl 70):S3-S16.

110 Hodson EM, Knight JF, Willis NS, Craig JC. Corticosteroid therapy in nephrotic syndrome: a meta-analysis of randomised controlled trials. Arch Dis Child 2000; 83:45–51.

111 Durkan AM, Hodson EM, Willis NS, Craig JC. Immunosuppressive agents in childhood nephrotic syndrome: a meta-analysis of randomized controlled trials. Kidney Int 2001; 59:1919–1927.

112 Watson AR, Rance CP, Bain J. Long term effects of cyclophosphamide on testicular function. BMJ 1985; 291:1457–1460.

113 Watson AR, Taylor J, Rance CP, Bain J. Gonadal function in women treated with cyclophosphamide for childhood nephrotic syndrome: a long-term follow-up study. Fertil Steril 1986; 46(2):331–333.

114 Moore EA, Collier J, Evans JHC, Watson AR. Information needs of parents of children with nephrotic syndrome. Child Health 1994; 2(4):147–149.

115 Lewis MA, Baildom EM, Davis N, et al. Nephrotic syndrome: from toddlers to twenties. Lancet 1989; I:255–259.

116 Cortes L, Tejani A. Dilemma of focal segmental glomerular sclerosis. Kidney Int 1996; 49(53):S57–S63.

117 Holmberg C, Laine J, Ronnholm K, et al. Congenital nephrotic syndrome. Kidney Int 1996; 49(53):S51–S56.

118 Dillon MJ. Investigation and management of hypertension in children. Pediatr Nephrol 1987; 1:59–69.

119 de Man SA, Andrea JL, Bachmann H, et al. Blood pressure in childhood: pooled findings in six European studies. J Hypertension 1991; 9:109–114.

120 Browning AC, Mengher LS, Gregson RM, Amoaku WM. Visual outcome of malignant hypertension in young people. Arch Dis Child 2001; 85:401–403.

121 British Association for Paediatric Nephrology. Report of a Working Party: the provision of services in the United Kingdom for children and adolescents with renal disease. BAPN; 1991.

122 Karlowicz MG, Adelman RD. Nonoliguric and oliguric renal failure in asphyxiated term neonates. Pediatr Nephrol 1995; 9:718–722.

*123 Australia and New Zealand Intensive Care Society (ANZICS) Clinical Trials Group. Low dose dopamine in patients with early renal dysfunction: a placebo-controlled trial. Lancet 2000; 356:2139–2143.

124 McClure RJ, Prasad VK, Brocklebank JT. Treatment of hyperkalaemia using intravenous and nebulised salbutamol. Arch Dis Child 1994; 70:126–128.

125 Jones DP, Mahmoud H, Chesney RW. Tumour lysis syndrome: pathogenesis and management. Pediatr Nephrol 1995; 9:206–212.

126 Watson AR. Nutrition in renal disease. In: Davies D, ed. Nutrition in child health. London: Royal College of Physicians; 1995: 133–142.

127 Kierdorf H, Sieberth HG. Continuous treatment modalities in ARF. Nephrol Dial Transplantation 1995; 10:2001–2008.

128 Wong AF, Bolinger AM, Gambertoglio JG. Pharmacokinetics and drug dosing in children with decreased renal function. In: Holliday MA, Barratt TM, Avner ED, eds. Pediatric nephrology, 3rd edn. Baltimore: Williams & Wilkins; 1994;1305–1314.

129 Gallo GE, Gianantonio CA. Extrarenal involvement in diarrhoea associated haemolytic uraemic syndrome. Pediatr Nephrol 1995; 9:117–119.

130 Eriksson KJ, Boyd SG, Tasker RC. Acute neurology and neurophysiology of haemolytic-uraemic syndrome. Arch Dis Child 2001; 84:434–435.

131 Kaplan BS, Cleary TG, Obrig TG. Recent advances in understanding the pathogenesis of the hemolytic uremic syndromes. Pediatr Nephrol 1990; 4:276–283.

132 Shiomi M, Togawa M, Fujita K, Murata R. Effect of early oral fluoroquinolones in hemorrhagic colitis Escherichia coli O157:H7. Pediatr Nephrol 1999; 41(2):228–232.

133 Wong CS, Jelacic S, Habeeb RL, et al. The risk of hemolytic-uremic syndrome after antibiotic treatment of O157:H7 infections. New Eng J Med 2000; 342(26):1930–1931.

134 Buteau C, Proulx F, Chaibou M, et al. Leukocytosis in children with E. coli O157:H7 enteritis developing the haemolytic-uremic syndrome. Pediatr Infect Dis 2000; 19(7):642–647.

135 Coad NAG, Marshall T, Rowe B, Taylor CM. Changes in the postenteropathic form of hemolytic uremic syndrome in children. Clin Nephrol 1991; 35:10–16.

136 Warwicker P, Goodship THJ, Donne RL, et al. Genetic studies into inherited and sporadic haemolytic uraemic syndrome. Kidney Int 1998; 53:836–844.

137 Taylor CM. Complement factor H and the haemolytic uraemic syndrome. Lancer 2001; 358:1200–1202.

138 Milford DV, Taylor CM, Guttridge B, et al. Haemolytic uraemic syndromes in the British Isles 1985–8: association with verocytotoxin producing *E. coli*. Part 1: clinical and epidemiological features. Arch Dis Child 1990; 65:716–721.

139 Loirat C, Sonsino E, Hinglais N, et al. Treatment of the childhood haemolytic uraemic syndrome with plasma. Pediatr Nephrol 1988; 2:279–285.

140 Fitzpatrick MM, Shah V, Trompeter RS, et al. Long term renal outcome of childhood haemolytic uraemic syndrome. BMJ 1991; 303:489–492.

141 Small G, Watson AR, Evans JHC, Gallagher J. Hemolytic uremic syndrome: defining the need for long-term follow-up. Clin Nephrol 1999; 52(6):352–356.

142 Perelstein EM, Grunfield BG, Simsolo RB, et al. Renal functional reserve in haemolytic uraemic syndrome and single kidney. Arch Dis Child 1990; 65:728–731.

143 Broyer M, Chantler C, Donckerwolke R, et al. The paediatric registry of the European Dialysis and Transplant Association: 20 years' experience. Pediatr Nephrol 1993; 7:758–768.

144 Norman LJ, Coleman JE, Macdonald IA, et al. Nutrition and growth in relation to severity of renal disease in children. Pediatr Nephrol 2000; 15:259–265.

*145 Haffner D, Schaeffer F, Nissel R, et al. Effect of growth hormone treatment on adult height of children with chronic renal failure. N Engl J Med 2000; 343:923–930.

146 Rees L, Ward G, Rigden S. Growth over 10 years following a one year trial of growth hormone therapy. Pediatr Nephrol 2000; 14:309–314.

147 Coleman JE. The kidney. In: Shaw V, Lawson M, eds. Clinical paediatric dietetics 2nd edn. Oxford: Blackwell Science; 2001:158–182.

148 Coleman JE, Watson AR, Rance CH, Moore EA. Gastrostomy buttons for nutritional support in children on dialysis. Nephrol Dial Transplantation 1998; 13:2041–2046.

149 Wingen AM, Fabian-Bach C, Mehls O. Low protein diets in children with chronic renal failure. Pediatr Nephrol 1991; 5:496–500.

150 Watson AR, Gartland C on behalf of the European Paediatric Peritoneal Dialysis Working Group. Guidelines by an ad hoc European committee for elective chronic peritoneal dialysis in pediatric patients. Peritoneal Dial Int 2001; 21:240–244.

151 Watson AR. Renal transplantation in children. Curr Paediatr 1993; 3:151–155.

152 Warady BA, Alexander SR, Watkins S, et al. Optimal care of the pediatric end stage renal disease patient on dialysis. Am J Kidney Dis 1999; 33:567–583.

153 Vester U, Offner G, Hoyer PF, et al. End stage renal failure in children younger than 6 years: renal transplantation is the therapy of choice. Eur J Paediatr 1998; 157:239–242.

154 Dall'Amico R, Ginevri F, Ghio L, et al. Successful renal transplantation in children under 6 years. Pediatr Nephrol 2001; 16(1):1–7.

155 Tyden G, Berg U, Bohlin AB, Sandberg J. Renal transplantation in children less than 2 years old. Transplantation 1997; 63:554–558.

156 Kari JA, Romagnoli J, Duffy P, et al. Renal transplantation in children under 5 years of age. Pediatr Nephrol 1999; 13:730–736.

157 Gjertson DW, Cecka JM. Determinants of long-term survival of pediatric kidney grafts reported to the United Network for organ sharing kidney transplant registry. Pediatr Transplantation 2001; 5(1):5–15.

158 Geary DF, Haka-Ikse K. Neuro-developmental progress of young children with

chronic renal disease. Pediatrics 1989; 84:68–72.
159 Becker N, Brandt JR, Sutherland TA, et al. Improved neurological outcome of young children on nightly automated peritoneal dialysis. Pediatr Nephrol 1997; 11:676–679.
160 Warady BA, Belden B, Kohaut E. Neurodevelopmental outcome of children initiating peritoneal dialysis in early infancy. Pediatr Nephrol 1999; 13:759–765.
161 Reynolds JM, Garralda ME, Postlethwaite RJ, Goh D. Changes in psychosocial adjustment after renal transplantation. Arch Dis Child 1991; 66:508–513.
162 Watson AR. Strategies to support families of children with end-stage renal failure. Pediatr Nephrol 1995; 9: 628–631.

17

Disorders of the alimentary tract and liver

W Michael Bisset, Susan V Beath, Huw R Jenkins, Alastair J Baker

INTRODUCTION

Optimum growth and development is dependent on the normal functioning of the gastrointestinal tract and of the liver. When this activity is deranged the child will develop symptoms of gastrointestinal disease and as a consequence will frequently fail to thrive.

The gastrointestinal tract extends from the mouth to the anus and is structurally and functionally divided into the mouth, oropharynx, esophagus, stomach, small intestine and colon (Table 17.1). Following the ingestion of food by the mouth the bolus is moved by the oropharynx into the esophagus which acts as a conduit for the transfer of food to the stomach where it is stored and mixed prior to its controlled passage into the small intestine. In the small intestine the food is digested and absorbed before moving on into the large intestine where salt and water are conserved prior to excretion. This simplified view of gastrointestinal function disguises the very complex nature of the many systems which interact to give normal intestinal function.

Table 17.1 The function of the gastrointestinal tract

Section of gut	Function
Mouth	Grinding of food by teeth Lubrication by salivary secretions
Oropharynx	Move food into esophagus Protect airway
Esophagus	Propulsive conduit for food Clearance of regurgitated food Prevention of reflux
Stomach	Store for food Gastric acid production Pepsin production
Small intestine	Digestion of food Absorption of food Immune tolerance
Terminal ileum	Absorption of vitamin B_{12} Absorption of bile salts
Pancreas	Digestive enzyme production Bicarbonate production
Colon	Reabsorption of luminal fluid Storage and excretion of feces

GASTROINTESTINAL FUNCTION

DIGESTION

Ingested food consists almost exclusively of large macromolecules which the intestinal tract is unable to absorb without prior digestion. Complex carbohydrates are broken down into their component monosaccharides, fats with the help of the emulsifying activity of bile salts are digested to free fatty acids and monoacylglycerol and proteins are dismantled into dipeptides and amino acids. The digestive enzymes act mainly within the lumen of the stomach and small intestine although the process is completed for carbohydrate by small intestinal brush border disaccharidases.

TRANSPORT

Discrete transport processes are present within the epithelial cells of the intestinal tract to promote the absorption of nutrients, salts and water by some cells and the excretion of salt and water by others. Many of these processes are dependent on the electrochemical gradient across the cell wall created by the Na^+/K^+ ATPase ion pump. This generates a low Na^+ concentration and a negative charge within epithelial cells, which facilitate the movement of specific ions and solutes through transmembrane proteins which traverse the lipophilic cell membrane.

MOTILITY

The movement of food along the gut is integrated with, and related to, the function of each section of the intestine. The rate of emptying of nutrients from the stomach is closely controlled to prevent overloading of the small intestine. Specific patterns of fasting motor activity have developed in the small intestine to clear the lumen of food debris after meals and highly developed control mechanisms are present to facilitate the controlled emptying of the distal colon and rectum at the time of defecation.

IMMUNITY

The gastrointestinal tract serves as the interface between ingested elements from the external environment and the internal milieu of the individual. By a combination of immunological and non-immunological mechanisms the entry of noxious substances such as bacteria, viruses and undigested food protein is prevented. The development of tolerance to the foreign proteins of commonly ingested food is vital to the normal functioning of the gut.

ENDOCRINE

The gastrointestinal tract is a major endocrine organ and many regulatory peptides with endocrine, paracrine and neurocrine functions are released along the length of the intestine. The function of many of these peptides is poorly understood although it is clear that they have an important role in modulating intestinal secretion, growth and motor function.

A more detailed description of the anatomy and physiology of the intestinal tract[1] is given in subsequent sections of this chapter.

THE NATURE OF GASTROINTESTINAL DISEASE

Normal intestinal function requires the combined action of each of the functional systems described above and if any one should break down intestinal function will be compromised. An understanding of the basic physiology of these systems is important when one is interpreting symptoms of gastrointestinal disease and planning the rational investigation of these problems.

Diarrheal disease will develop if, as a consequence of maldigestion or active secretion, there is an increased effluent of fluid passing into the colon from the small intestine or if the absorptive capacity of the colon is compromised by disease.[2] Loss of normal intestinal motility will result in the development of symptoms of obstruction and where a defect of mucosal immunity is present recurrent enteric infection is likely to occur. Damage to the digestive or absorptive capacity of the small intestine will result in failure of the patient to grow adequately.

THE MOUTH

The mouth is responsible for the grinding of food into small fragments, through the voluntary action of the tongue and jaw, prior to its passage into the esophagus. In addition, the fragments are mixed with salivary secretions which help lubricate the food and initiate digestion, through the action of salivary amylase and lingual lipase. Any disease of the mouth which makes feeding painful or compromises the normal process of deglutition is likely to lead to difficulties with feeding.

While most oral lesions are the result of local disease, both gastrointestinal and systemic disease may result in abnormalities within the mouth.[3] It is therefore important to look closely at the mouth in all children undergoing physical examination.

THE LIPS

Unilateral or bilateral clefts of the upper lip are among the most common of congenital malformations and are frequently found in combination with a cleft of the palate (see Ch. 36). Dryness of the lips with cracking may be due to mouth breathing, and fissure formation at the angle of the mouth may result from chronic drooling in children with swallowing disorders. Nutritional deficiencies of iron, zinc and riboflavin may all produce an angular stomatitis.

Edema of the lips may occur as part of an immediate hypersensitivity reaction following the direct contact of the lips with a sensitized protein or as part of the systemic response in anaphylaxis. In Crohn's disease intermittent swelling of the lips may be associated with cobblestone ulceration of the buccal mucosa.

THE ORAL MUCOSA

Ulceration to the buccal mucosa occurs most commonly in healthy individuals as a result of recurrent aphthae. These may be precipitated by local trauma and heal spontaneously within 2 weeks. More persistent ulcers may occur in chronically debilitated patients, children with poor dental hygiene and as mentioned above in inflammatory bowel disease (IBD). Extensive ulceration of the oral mucosa in association with lesions on the perineum are seen in Stevens–Johnson syndrome and less commonly in Behçet's syndrome.

Abnormal pigmentation may be seen in Addison's disease and Albright's syndrome; in Peutz–Jeghers syndrome there is freckling of the lips and buccal mucosa and in lead, mercury and bismuth poisoning pigmented lines are sometimes seen near the dental margin of the gums. Koplik's spots are characteristically present in measles, palatal petechiae may be seen in rubella and oral vesicles in chickenpox can make feeding very uncomfortable.

The most common infections involving the mucosa are herpes stomatitis and thrush. Primary herpes infection occurs most commonly in children between the ages of 1 and 3 years and presents with pyrexia, lymphadenopathy and the eruption of vesicular lesions on the buccal mucosa, lips and on the skin below the mouth. The vesicles burst forming painful ulcers making the ingestion of solids and liquids very uncomfortable. Although the condition is self-limiting, with a course of 7–10 days, this may be shortened by treatment with oral aciclovir.[4]

Oral candidiasis or thrush commonly occurs in young babies who become infected in the neonatal period but may also develop in patients on broad spectrum antibiotics, inhaled steroids or in patients who are immunosuppressed. Gut carriage may also lead to infection of the napkin area. Treatment is with a topical antifungal such as nystatin.

THE GUMS

Infection of the gums in children most commonly results from poor oral hygiene and leads to inflammation of the free margin of the gingiva. Hypertrophy of the gums is a common side-effect of phenytoin treatment and may also be rarely seen in Langerhans' cell histiocytosis (see Ch. 22). Bleeding of the gums may be secondary to local infection but will also occur in children with bleeding diatheses and in nutritionally compromised patients who are vitamin C deficient.

THE TONGUE

Macroglossia occurs in hypothyroidism, as part of generalized visceral enlargement in Beckwith's syndrome and in glycogen storage disease type II. A normal-sized tongue may appear to be enlarged if the oral cavity is small as in children with Down syndrome. The tongue can also be enlarged by a lymphangioma or a hemangioma and a mass in the region of the foramen cecum may be due to a lingual thyroid.

The surface of the tongue becomes coated in children with poor oral hygiene and in patients with dehydration. In scarlet fever the tongue is first white and coated and then becomes red, hence the name 'strawberry tongue'. In familial dysautonomia the tongue is smooth due to the absence of papillae and in congenital familial telangiectasia the vascular abnormality may be clearly seen. The focal loss of papillae leads to the so-called 'geographical tongue', a benign self-limiting condition.

THE TEETH

The primary dentition usually erupts at about 6 months but in hypothyroidism, hypopituitarism, rickets, congenital syphilis and cleidocranial dysostosis this can be delayed. Premature shedding of these teeth is likely to occur in hypophosphatasia and in mercury poisoning. The enamel of the teeth will become hypoplastic as a result of such insults as prematurity, kernicterus, vitamin D deficiency and from congenital infections such as rubella and syphilis. Similarly the shape of the teeth may be abnormal as a consequence of congenital infection (notched incisors in congenital syphilis) or in ectodermal dysplasias where the teeth may be peg shaped.

A black staining of the teeth can occur with oral iron, a brown discoloration occurs with congenital defects of enamel and dentine, in congenital porphyria the teeth are a purplish brown and in neonatal unconjugated hyperbilirubinemia a green staining may be left. The administration of tetracycline to a mother after the fourth month of pregnancy or to the infant in the first year of life will result in yellow discoloration of the primary dentition and administration up to the age of 7 years will affect the permanent dentition.

THE SALIVARY GLANDS

With the exception of mumps, inflammation or enlargement of the salivary gland is uncommon in childhood. Acute bacterial parotitis may occur in the neonate or debilitated child and is characterized by a unilateral swollen tender parotid gland. Infection with *Staphylococcus aureus* is generally responsible and treatment with flucloxacillin is required.

Recurrent parotitis either uni- or bilateral may occur where the symptoms are generally mild and not associated with systemic upset. Treatment with parotid massage and stimulants of salivary flow such as chewing gum along with oral penicillin are generally helpful. The condition is self-limiting and generally resolves by puberty. Less commonly, recurrent pain and infection may be precipitated by salivary stones.

THE ESOPHAGUS

STRUCTURE AND FUNCTION

The esophagus is a long narrow muscular tube which connects the oropharynx and stomach providing a conduit for the passage of food. The lumen of the esophagus is lined by a stratified squamous epithelium and is encircled by an inner circular and an outer longitudinal layer of muscle. The muscle of the upper third of the esophagus is striated and is dependent on extrinsic innervation from the vagus nerve while the muscle in the lower third is smooth muscle and is under the influence of both intrinsic and extrinsic controls. The muscle of the middle third forms a transitional zone. Two high pressure zones are found along the length of the esophagus, one at the proximal end forms the upper esophageal sphincter and the other at the distal end forms the lower esophageal sphincter.

Deglutition

After food has been chewed and mixed with saliva a bolus of food is isolated and pushed back, between the tongue and the hard palate, towards the pharynx at the same time as the soft palate is raised to close off the nasopharynx. As the food enters the oropharynx an involuntary reflex is initiated whose afferent limb is transmitted along the glossopharyngeal nerve and the superior laryngeal branch of the vagal nerve to the medulla. Efferent impulses from the facial, glossopharyngeal, vagus, accessory and hypoglossal nerves result in contraction of the pharyngeal muscles and relaxation of the upper esophageal sphincter with movement of the bolus of food onward into the upper esophagus. Entry of food into the larynx is prevented by cessation of respiration, elevation of the larynx and closure of the glottis.

Given the very complicated nature of this reflex and its reliance on many cranial nerve nuclei within the brainstem it is perhaps not surprising that central nervous system disorders which result in the development of bulbar or pseudobulbar palsies will disturb the swallowing reflex; similarly any anatomical disorder of the pharyngeal apparatus (i.e. Pierre Robin or cleft palate) will disrupt normal feeding (Table 17.2). Disordered deglutition is also likely to result in the nasopharyngeal regurgitation of food and the aspiration of ingested food into the lungs. This reflex develops in the neonate at approximately 34 weeks' gestation.

Oromotor coordination develops throughout the first year of life to accommodate the many food consistencies and textures experienced by the child after weaning. If inappropriate foods are given, which fail to match the child's oromotor development, feeding may become difficult and lead to the development of behavioral problems at meal times.

Esophageal peristalsis

During primary peristaltic activity pressure waves of 50–80 mmHg (7–11 kPa) propagate down the esophagus, pushing the bolus of food at a velocity of 2–5 cm/s. A marked reduction in magnitude and propagation velocity of this activity is seen in cerebral palsied children with severe gastroesophageal reflux. Secondary peristaltic activity which develops in response to distension of the esophagus and plays an important role in clearing regurgitated gastric contents back into the stomach is also compromised in children with neurological disease. Tertiary peristaltic activity occurs spontaneously and may be responsible for the pain induced by esophageal spasm.

Lower esophageal sphincter

The lower esophageal sphincter is a zone of raised pressure (20 mmHg; 3 kPa), just proximal to the gastroesophageal junction which has a central role in the control of the reflux of gastric contents into the esophagus.[5] The lower esophageal sphincter shows maturational changes with pressures rising from as low as 5 mmHg (0.7 kPa) at 30 weeks' postconceptual age up to the adult level of 20 mmHg (3 kPa) by the first year of life.[6]

The effectiveness of the lower esophageal sphincter as an antireflux barrier depends also on a number of anatomical factors which assist the sphincteric smooth muscle. A length of intra-abdominal esophagus potentiates the high pressure zone of the sphincter, the acute angle between the esophagus and fundus of the

Table 17.2 A list of the causes of dysphagia

1. Anatomical abnormalities
   a. Cleft palate
   b. Micrognathia (Pierre Robin)
   c. Macroglossia
   d. Cysts, tumors and diverticulae of the pharynx
   e. Esophageal atresia
   f. Esophageal stricture
      (i) Anastomotic
      (ii) Corrosive
      (iii) Reflux esophagitis
   g. Esophageal compression
      (i) Aortic arch anomaly
      (ii) Mediastinal tumor
      (iii) Esophageal duplication
2. Neuromuscular
   a. Prematurity
   b. Cerebral palsy of any type
   c. Bulbar or pseudobulbar palsies
   d. Isolated cranial nerve paralysis or agenesis
   e. Familial dysautonomia (Riley–Day syndrome)
   f. Achalasia
   g. Esophageal dysmotility (i.e. spasm)
   h. Myasthenia gravis or dystrophia myotonica
3. Inflammatory/trauma
   a. Stomatitis
   b. Acute tonsillopharyngitis
   c. Esophagitis
      (i) Reflux
      (ii) Corrosive
      (iii) Infective (i.e. candida)
   d. Foreign body
4. Behavioral
   a. Rumination
   b. Globus hystericus

stomach forms a flap valve which closes as the intragastric pressure rises and the crura of the diaphragm press on the lower esophagus. These mechanisms are illustrated in Figure 17.1. Loss of the normal anatomy of the gastroesophageal junction as occurs in patients with sliding hiatus hernias severely disrupts these mechanisms and increases the likelihood of gastroesophageal reflux.

DYSPHAGIA

Diagnosis

The diagnosis of dysphagia can be made by taking a detailed clinical history and by careful observation of the child feeding. Nasal

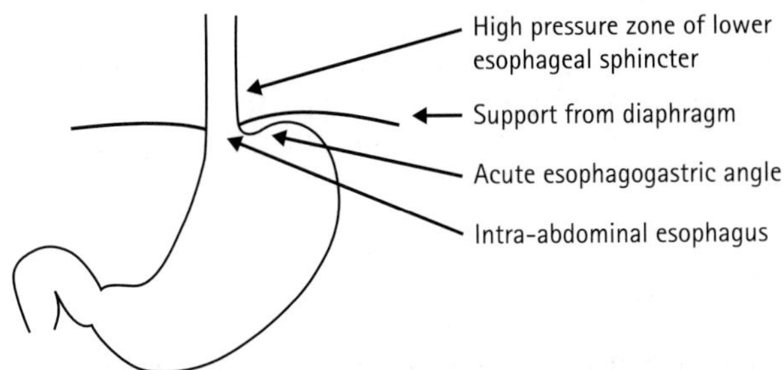

Fig. 17.1 The factors contributing to the normal function of the lower esophageal sphincter.

regurgitation of liquids in the absence of vomiting is suggestive of nasopharyngeal reflux and coughing and choking during feeding is very suggestive of aspiration into the larynx. As a consequence the child may develop recurrent chest infections due to aspiration or, because of the difficulty in ingesting an adequate calorie intake, the child may fail to thrive.

Many of the anatomical abnormalities will be obvious on inspection (Table 17.2) and most neuromuscular disorders will be associated with other neurological sequelae such as cerebral palsy. Inspection of the mouth by a speech therapist will give insight into the level of oromotor coordination; video fluoroscopy (except esophageal atresia) will define the degree of pharyngeal coordination during swallowing and the motility of the esophagus and will determine whether aspiration or nasopharyngeal regurgitation has occurred. A chest X-ray will show signs of an aspiration pneumonia or mediastinal space occupation and laryngoscopy and esophagoscopy will allow direct visualization of any motor incoordination, foreign bodies or strictures that may be present.

Treatment

The management of dysphagia depends very much on the underlying cause. Great care and attention is needed with feeding technique but in some patients the airway has to be protected by instituting nasogastric or gastrostomy feeding. Neuromuscular disorders of swallowing are also frequently associated with severe gastroesophageal reflux and in conditions such as cerebral palsy and familial dysautonomia an antireflux procedure such as a Nissen fundoplication is frequently required in addition to a gastrostomy.

GASTROESOPHAGEAL REFLUX

Gastroesophageal reflux is the passive regurgitation of gastric contents into the esophagus and should not be confused with vomiting, which is an active process and requires the contraction of the diaphragm and abdominal muscles to initiate the event.[7] Gastroesophageal reflux will result if there is incompetence of the sphincteric mechanisms at the gastroesophageal junction or if raised intragastric or intra-abdominal pressures are able to overcome this mechanism. It is clear that the lower esophageal sphincter is poorly developed in the very young infant and that the formation of a sliding hiatus hernia severely limits the competence of the sphincter. Similarly in conditions where gastric emptying is delayed or in chronic respiratory diseases, such as cystic fibrosis, where coughing increases intra-abdominal pressure, gastroesophageal reflux is exacerbated. In atopic children, dietary protein intolerance may be a significant factor in the development of reflux symptoms.[8]

With prolonged ambulatory recordings of intraesophageal pH (Fig. 17.2) it has become clear that gastroesophageal reflux is a physiological phenomenon which occurs in most children for between 1 and 5% of any 24 h period with the majority occurring in the postprandial periods. Whether gastroesophageal reflux is deemed to be trivial or pathological is dependent on many factors of which the parents' perception of the problem, the absolute level of reflux and the development of any complicating sequelae are important.[9] It has been shown that in normal individuals reflux most commonly occurs as the child is swallowing and the lower esophageal sphincter is relaxing to allow the passage of food into the stomach.[10] During these brief 'unguarded moments' ingested food and acid pass into the lower esophagus where a secondary peristaltic wave promptly clears the food back into the stomach. If, however, esophageal peristalsis is deranged the contact time of gastric acid on the esophageal mucosa will be prolonged.

In a patient with very severe reflux, spontaneous relaxations of the lower esophageal sphincter occur throughout the day leading to many more 'unguarded moments'. The most troublesome reflux occurs in patients with cerebral palsy or previous esophageal surgery where disordered innervation of the esophagus leads to increased spontaneous relaxation of the sphincter and poor peristaltic clearing mechanisms.

Clinical features

The passive regurgitation of milk occurs in up to half of newborn babies[11] and is accepted by most mothers as being a normal feature of infancy. With time the problem steadily improves and with the introduction of solids and the development of a more upright posture the problem clears in almost all cases.[12,13] Problems, however, develop where the mother is inexperienced or stressed and has difficulty coping with the problem or where complications such as esophagitis, aspiration or failure to thrive occur.

In most children with reflux the volume of milk which is lost with each regurgitation is insignificant but in some children the intake is severely compromised and as a consequence weight gain is poor. With the prolonged contact of gastric acid on the esophageal mucosa an esophagitis may develop. This may present clinically as blood in the vomit or more insidiously with the development of anemia or stricture. Older children may complain of heartburn with reflux while smaller infants may develop feeding difficulties due to esophageal discomfort.

Aspiration in cerebral palsied children is very common, due to an inability to protect the upper airway from food during both swallowing and regurgitation. When considering the differential diagnosis for children with recurrent cough or respiratory tract infections, one must include gastroesophageal reflux. Aspiration is thought to be a cause of 'near miss episodes' and in some circumstances may present with the sudden death of the infant. A bizarre presentation of gastroesophageal reflux has been described (Sandifer syndrome) where reflux episodes are associated with dystonic movements of the neck.[14] The clinical clue is that these episodes occur after meals and it has been postulated that stimulation of vagal afferents by the falling esophageal pH results in reflex stimulation of the spinal accessory nerve with the resulting contraction of the sternomastoid.

Although most children with reflux present in the first year of life there are some who present later with symptoms of heartburn or vomiting and a small group who though apparently symptom free through most of their lives present with a peptic stricture of the esophagus (Fig. 17.3). Chronic irritation by acid reflux may lead to replacement of the esophageal mucosa with a columnar epithelium (Barret's esophagus). This metaplastic change can lead to increased risk of adenocarcinoma in later life. There is also the occasional child who will present outwith the first 2 years of life with the precipitous development of severe gastroesophageal reflux in whom detailed investigation may reveal the presence of a posterior fossa tumor.

In children with reflux there may also be longer term behavioral sequelae which can frequently lead to major management problems. Some children are reluctant to eat, particularly solids, and as a consequence feeding problems develop which may last long after the reflux has apparently cleared. Other children who find it easy to reflux are able to regurgitate at will and use this as a powerful attention-seeking tool. A small number of children develop the ability to ruminate, a condition which is generally associated with prolonged periods of reflux.

Diagnosis

In the majority of cases the diagnosis is made clinically from the history of effortless vomiting occurring after meals and no further investigations are required. Where the clinical picture is unclear or where symptoms suggest a more severe problem, further investigation is required. Unfortunately no single investigation provides all the information which is required. A 24 h pH study will quantify the degree of acid reflux (Fig. 17.2), a barium meal will tell you if there is a hiatus hernia or more distal obstruction (i.e. malrotation) but it has poor sensitivity and frequently misses short reflux episodes. If esophagitis is suspected an endoscopy is required and a full blood count may show evidence of anemia secondary to blood loss. The presence of fat-laden macrophages in the sputum may help in the detection of aspiration. A fuller discussion of esophageal investigations is given later in this section.

Treatment (Table 17.3)

Although it is possible to differentiate between physiological and pathological reflux by using 24 h pH studies, it is likely that in most children treatment decisions will be determined largely on clinical grounds. In an otherwise well baby who is growing adequately and who is free of any complicating features it is likely that the condition will follow a benign course and will resolve spontaneously. The mother should be reassured and advised of simple measures to help with the problem. If the infant is being overfed this should be stopped and if over 3 months of age the introduction of solids should be encouraged. There is generally no need to alter the child's feed but where there is a strong family history of atopy or signs of eczema the introduction of a hypoallergenic feed may be indicated.

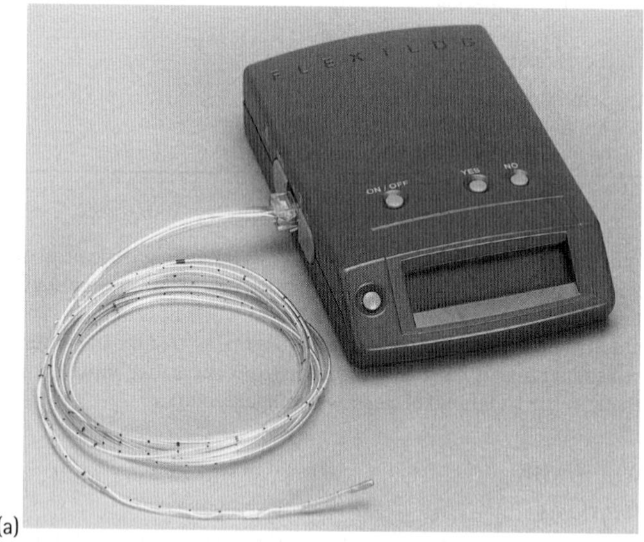

(a)

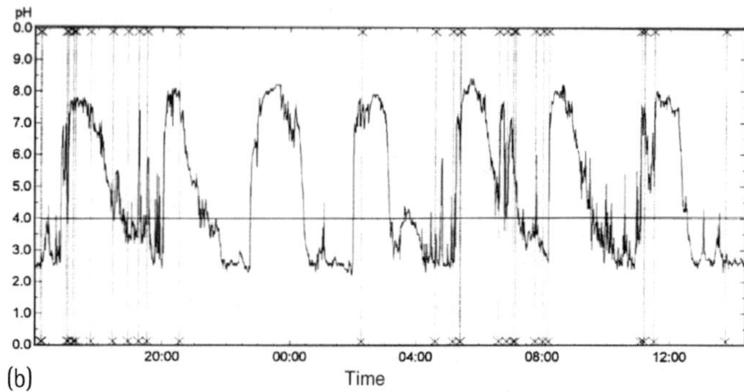

(b)

Fig.17.2 (a) A solid state 24 h pH recorder with recording electrode. (b) A trace from a 24 h pH recording showing prolonged reflux episodes (pH < 4) after feeds. The time is shown on the horizontal axis.

Table 17.3 Treatment for children with gastroesophageal reflux (see text for details)

Clinical condition	Treatment
Very mild reflux	Mother reassured Simple feeding advice
Mild reflux	Thickened feeds
Moderate reflux	Prokinetic drugs (consider risk v benefit)
Reflux with esophagitis	Add histamine 2 blockers Proton pump inhibitor
Severe reflux	Consider continuous nasogastric tube feeding in children less than 1 year as an alternative to fundoplication
Failure of medical treatment	Fundoplication
Esophagitis with stricture	Fundoplication with dilatation

As the consistency of the feed seems to influence the degree of reflux, thickening agents are found to be helpful in many babies. Alginate compounds are sometimes also found to relieve symptoms.

Traditionally it was advised that children with reflux should be kept sitting upright in a chair but it is likely that this may increase intra-abdominal pressure and exacerbate the problem. The left lateral position has also been suggested but maintaining a small child for any length of time in any given position is likely to be very difficult.

Where these simple measures fail to reduce reflux, the use of prokinetic agents should be considered. Unfortunately cisapride,[15] which was previously widely used for this purpose, has been withdrawn from most markets, because of cardiotoxic effects, and is only now available on a limited basis. Domperidone and metoclopramide are alternatives but the former is not licensed to treat reflux in children and the latter can be associated with extrapyramidal side-effects. They act by increasing the rate of gastric emptying and it has been postulated that they also increase the lower esophageal sphincter pressure. They do, however, have to be taken continuously to be effective.

In patients with esophagitis, measures in addition to those described above have to be taken.[16] Histamine 2 (H_2) blocking drugs such as cimetidine or ranitidine, or proton pump inhibitors such as omeprazole, will raise the pH of the regurgitated food and seem to help in the healing of esophagitis. It is, however, unclear how long and in what dose this treatment should be continued as suitable controlled trials have yet to be carried out. Antacids have no place in the treatment of esophagitis as the amount required to adequately alkalinize the gastric juices would be likely to lead to salt overload.

In young children with reflux there is an expectation that spontaneous clinical improvement is likely up to about 18 months of age. Continuous nasogastric feeding significantly reduces the amount of reflux and in some children with severe symptoms, may be preferable to fundoplication. Although this treatment needs a high degree of motivation from the parents it may adequately control symptoms until they spontaneously improve.

Where medical management fails to control complications and gastroesophageal reflux persists, a surgical antireflux procedure is indicated.[17] Where stricture formation has already occurred this should be combined with dilatation of the stricture. It is important that an experienced pediatric surgeon carries out these procedures as the operation may be complicated by retching or gas bloat syndromes. Careful preoperative assessment of patients is required to try and minimize subsequent complications.[18]

A suggested plan of treatment for patients with gastroesophageal reflux is shown in Table 17.3.

ACHALASIA

Achalasia of the cardia results from a failure of the lower end of the esophagus to relax with swallowing with the development of dysphagia, aspiration, retrosternal discomfort and weight loss. This functional obstruction is caused by neurodegenerative changes in the enteric nerves of the esophagus.

The condition is very uncommon in childhood and may be confused with a peptic stricture in young children and anorexia nervosa in older children. An autosomal recessive form occurs which is associated with hypoadrenalism and absent tear production.

The diagnosis is confirmed by the barium swallow appearance of esophageal dilatation with a funnel-shaped narrowing at the lower end and by esophageal manometry which demonstrates disturbed peristaltic activity in the body with increased basal tone and failure of relaxation of the lower esophageal sphincter.

The condition is generally progressive and is treated either by pneumatic dilatation of the lower esophageal sphincter or by Heller's cardiomyotomy.[19] Dilatation procedures frequently have to be repeated more than once and effective treatment of the achalasia may lead to the development of gastroesophageal reflux. For this reason a myotomy and fundoplication procedure are frequently combined.

ESOPHAGEAL INVESTIGATIONS

A number of esophageal investigations are available but unfortunately no single test is likely to give all the information that is required to resolve a clinical problem.[20] Each test gives information on a specific aspect of esophageal structure or function and it is necessary for tests to be combined for an overall picture to be obtained (Table 17.4).

Barium studies

Traditionally the barium swallow has been the investigation of choice in children with gastroesophageal reflux. While it is true that contrast studies give good information on the anatomy of the esophagus and the gastroesophageal junction it is a very insensitive test for reflux and the mucosal changes of esophagitis will only show if they are well advanced (see Fig. 17.3). Video studies are useful in detecting abnormalities of swallowing and motility

Table 17.4 Investigations of esophageal structure and function

Test	Uses
Barium studies	Define anatomy of upper GI tract
Scintiscanning	For the detection of reflux and aspiration (not as sensitive as pH studies)
Manometry	Detect achalasia or esophageal spasm
pH monitoring	Most sensitive test for acid reflux
Esophagoscopy	Detects esophagitis and allows mucosal biopsy
Trial of NG feeding	Unmasked reflux in patients with poor oral intake

GI, gastrointestinal; NG, nasogastric

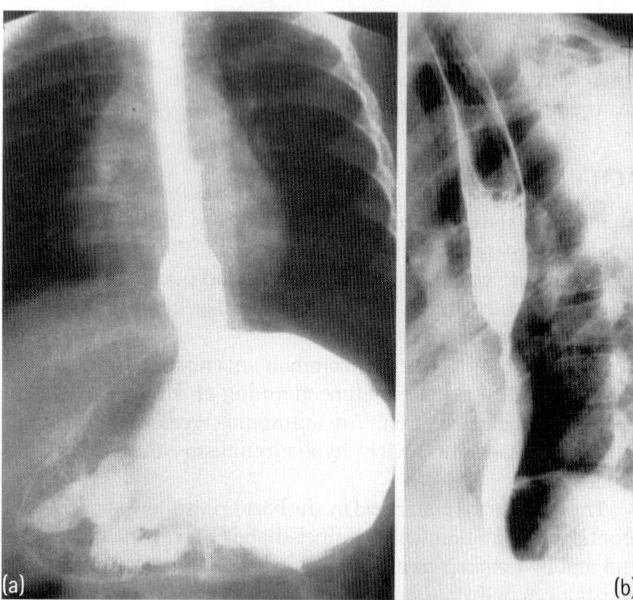

Fig. 17.3 (a) A barium meal showing gross gastroesophageal reflux. (b) A lateral view of the esophogus showing a peptic stricture with proximal dilatation.

disturbances of the body of the esophagus. It is important that screening is continued until contrast has passed into the jejunum as abnormalities of gastric emptying or malrotation will otherwise be missed.

Gastroesophageal scintigraphy

Scintiscanning using technetium-99m-labeled milk has been shown to be more sensitive in detecting reflux than barium studies and with prolonged scans gastric emptying can be measured and bronchial aspiration of the milk can be detected. The method, however, requires the patient to remain still for up to 30 min on a gamma camera and gives very little anatomical information.

Esophageal manometry

This technique is presently available in only a few pediatric centers and its clinical uses are limited to the diagnosis of the less common conditions such as achalasia and esophageal spasm. The measurement of lower esophageal sphincter pressure is a very insensitive indicator of gastroesophageal reflux.

Esophageal pH monitoring

The prolonged ambulatory recording of esophageal pH using catheter-mounted electrodes is a very sensitive means of quantifying acid gastroesophageal reflux (Fig. 17.2). Modern computerized systems allow the length of time and the number of episodes of acid reflux to be measured and their division between awake, asleep, postprandial and fasting periods can be derived. Unfortunately it fails to detect non-acid reflux and with the realization that up to 50% of reflux in some patients may be non-acid, the potential limitations of this investigation are becoming clear.

Esophagoscopy

If significant reflux is found or esophagitis is suspected it is important that an esophagoscopy is carried out. This is the only method which allows accurate assessment of esophagitis both visually and histologically and mucosal inflammation can be detected at a very early stage long before any radiological changes are found. With modern pediatric endoscopes the procedure can be carried out as a day case under sedation or a short general anesthetic.

Trial of nasogastric tube feeding

The assessment of children with cerebral palsy is often compromised by the fact that their oral intake is significantly reduced and reflux may not be seen during barium studies. The passage of a nasogastric tube and the administration of appropriate feed volumes often unmasks symptoms of reflux and facilitates the administration of contast during barium studies.

THE STOMACH AND DUODENUM

STRUCTURE AND FUNCTION

The stomach is a J-shaped organ which lies obliquely across the midline in the upper abdomen. It is covered by an inner oblique, middle circular and outer longitudinal layer of smooth muscle and is lined by a columnar epithelium which is indented with gastric pits. The muscular layer is thickened at the pylorus which acts as a valve to control the rate of emptying from the stomach. The columnar epithelium produces mucus which forms a protective layer over the mucosa. The pits in the antrum, body and distal fundus are short and contain the parietal cells which produce hydrochloric acid and intrinsic factor, the chief cells which synthesize and secrete pepsinogen, endocrine cells and mucus-producing cells which are located at the neck of the glands. The pyloric glands which also contain endocrine cells are more tortuous and secrete large amounts of mucus.

Gastric motility

Following the ingestion of food, the body and fundus distend greatly and act as a reservoir for the storage of food. In contrast the antrum is a more muscular organ which, working in concert with the pylorus, produces propagative, segmenting and retrograde activity to break the food down into small, easily digested pieces.

Liquids generally empty very rapidly from the stomach with the rate being determined by the pressure gradient across the pylorus. A typical half emptying time for a drink of orange squash is 15 min. Solids in contrast empty much more slowly with a half emptying time being more typically between 90 and 120 min. The rate of emptying is very closely controlled by mechanoreceptors in the antrum and chemorecepters in the duodenum which feed back to the gastric smooth muscle to limit the rate of emptying. As a consequence of this a homogenized meal will empty more rapidly than a solid meal and a low energy meal will empty faster than a more energy dense meal. The rate of emptying is also inhibited by the presence of undigested fat in the ileum and by distension of the rectum due to fecal loading. The non-gastrointestinal factors which influence gastric emptying are discussed further in the section on vomiting.

Digestion

Pepsinogen is released from zymogen granules in the chief cells of the gastric glands in response to the ingestion of food. Under the influence of hydrochloric acid and then by the autocatalytic action of free pepsin the active pepsin is formed. This enzyme has a pH optimum of 1.0–1.5 and initiates proteolysis in the stomach by hydrolyzing peptide bonds at the amino groups of aromatic or acidic amino acids.

It is also likely that triglyceride hydrolysis starts in the stomach with the activation of the acid-stable lingual lipase and possibly also by the action of gastric lipase. In the preterm infant, because of the very low activity of pancreatic lipase it is likely that this mechanism is of some importance.

Gastric acid production

Hydrochloric acid is actively secreted by the parietal cells of the gastric glands maintaining the pH of the stomach at approximately 1. The rate of acid production is modulated by circulating levels of the gut hormone gastrin which is produced by G cells within the antrum of the stomach. The acid environment of the stomach has an important defensive role against ingested pathogens and as mentioned above provides the optimal environment for activity of the gastric digestive enzymes. The low pH facilitates the absorption of inorganic iron by preventing its precipitation. Excessive acid production, however, is likely to lead to an increasing incidence of duodenal ulceration.

The parietal cells are also responsible for the secretion of the glycoprotein intrinsic factor which stabilizes vitamin B_{12} during intestinal transit and binds to specific receptors in the terminal ileum prior to absorption. In autoimmune gastritis where the parietal cells are destroyed, hydrochloric acid and intrinsic factor production cease, resulting in achlorhydria and vitamin B_{12} deficiency.

GASTRITIS

Acute gastritis

Acute inflammation of the stomach may arise from conditions as diverse as irritation from non-steroidal anti-inflammatory drugs (NSAIDs), chemical ingestion or the duodeno gastric reflux of bile. Many of these conditions are self-limiting and may resolve spontaneously if the insult is removed. If the cause of the mucosal irritation persists the gastritis may become chronic and in the case of continued NSAID ingestion, may proceed to peptic ulceration.

Chronic gastritis

There are two main form of chronic gastritis, atrophic and non-atrophic. The former is usually associated with autoimmune disease and leads to loss of glandular tissue with resulting achlorhydria and loss of intrinsic factor production. This condition is very rare in childhood.

Non-atrophic gastritis is most commonly caused by *Helicobacter pylori* although less common causes include Crohn's disease and eosinophilic gastroenteritis.[21] Diagnosis is made by histological examination of mucosal biopsies from the antrum, incisura and body of the stomach. The Syndey classification of gastitis[22] has been devised primarily for adults but it is likely that the general principles also apply to children. In *Helicobacter pylori* infection, the gastric antrum frequently has a nodular appearance and histologicaly, acute infection is associated with an increase in intraepithelial neutrophils which progresses to chronic inflammatory changes with associated increase in lymphoid follicles.

PEPTIC ULCERATION

Acute ulcers

Peptic ulceration can occur acutely in response to stress or the administration of ulcerogenic drugs. Stress ulcers can occur in either the stomach or duodenum and are most common in the neonatal period in response to birth asphyxia or respiratory distress but they can also occur in later childhood following severe burns, meningitis or other major stresses. In patients receiving NSAIDs for conditions such as juvenile arthritis or corticosteroids for severe asthma or IBD, acute ulcers can also occur. It is unlikely that *Helicobacter pylori* plays a significant role in acute ulceration.

A stress ulcer is likely to present with intestinal bleeding or acute pain and should be treated with an H_2 blocker or proton pump inhibitor but where perforation occurs, surgery is required. In situations where stress ulceration is likely, prophylaxis with gastroprotective drugs should be considered.

Chronic ulcers

Chronic peptic ulceration occurs most commonly in children over the age of 5 years but unlike acute ulcers which affect the stomach and duodenum equally, chronic ulcers occur 10 times more frequently in the duodenum. As in adulthood there is very frequently a family history of peptic ulcer disease with a slight (3:2) male to female preponderance.

In many older children the classical ulcer symptoms of localized epigastric discomfort, nocturnal wakening and relief of symptoms with food or antacids are present. However, in younger children more non-specific symptoms such as vague abdominal pain, vomiting and nausea may make the diagnosis less clear. Some children may present with an occult anemia or more acutely with a hematemesis or melena. Because of the vague nature of many of these symptoms it is very important to differentiate between peptic ulcer disease and the far more common 'non-organic' recurrent abdominal pain of childhood. The presence of epigastric pain, nocturnal wakening, a progressive worsening of symptoms, an iron deficiency blood picture or a family history should alert one to the possibility of duodenal ulceration.

While the diagnosis can be made on a barium meal, carried out by an experienced radiologist, the relatively poor sensitivity of this test (50%) means that where a peptic ulcer is suspected upper gastrointestinal endoscopy should be the investigation of first choice.[23] In addition to visualizing the ulcer, endoscopy allows one to look for *Helicobacter pylori* infection in mucosal biopsies. Although the measurement of gastric acid output is a very insensitive way of diagnosing peptic ulcer disease, in the rare situation where multiple ulcers refractory to treatment are present it is important to measure fasting serum gastrin and basal and stimulated gastric acid output levels to exclude the possibility of a gastrin-secreting pancreatic tumor (Zollinger–Ellison syndrome).

Treatment

Much of the advice for treatment of peptic ulceration has been extrapolated from the adult experience as clinical trials in children have been limited by the small number of patients and by ethical constraints. It is likely, however, that one is dealing with a similar condition in both groups of patients as the clinical experience of therapeutic regimes is similar in each.

The treatment of chronic peptic ulcer disease is primarily aimed at reducing excess gastric acid production and eradicating *Helicobacter pylori* infection which is invariably present. A 6 week course of treatment with acid suppressive therapy will provide symptomatic relief of dyspeptic symptoms within 1–2 weeks in most patients and by the end of the 6-week course the ulcers will have healed in over 80% of patients. Recurrence of ulcer symptoms is likely to develop unless attempts are made to eradicate *Helicobacter pylori* and a course of triple therapy using one of the regimes outlined in the section on anti-*Helicobacter* therapy, is indicated at the time of initial treatment. If symptoms recur after treatment it is likely that the *Helicobacter pylori* has not been completely eradicated.

HELICOBACTER PYLORI

Since the identification of *Helicobacter pylori* in the mucosa of the gastric antrum[24] there has been an explosion of interest in the role of this small spiral organism and its causal relationship to gastritis, duodenal ulcer, recurrent abdominal pain, lymphoproliferative disorders and gastric cancer.

While *Helicobacter pylori* is undoubtedly a causal factor in the pathogenesis of peptic ulcer disease in both children and adults, the presence of infection need not imply the presence of active disease. Up to half of the world's population are infected with *Helicobacter pylori*, the majority of whom will have no recognizable disease. Similarly in children the presence of an active gastritis may not lead to the development of any symptoms and the priority when investigating a child is to determine the cause of their symptoms and not whether they are or are not infected with *Helicobacter pylori*. Our present understanding remains incomplete and many questions remain unanswered. There have however been consensus statements in recent years from both Europe and North America which begin to answer questions such as, who should be screened for infection, how they should be tested, who should be treated and what is the optimal method of eradicating *Helicobacter pylori*?[25–27] (see Table 17.5)

Pathogenesis

This organism is recognized as the most important cause of non-autoimmune gastritis in both children and adults. It may colonize either the antrum of the stomach, leading to increased acid production, or the body of the stomach where inflammation may lead to the development of an atrophic gastritis. Normal duodenal mucosa is not colonized unless gastric metaplasia has developed. *Helicobacter pylori* lies deep within the mucus layer which covers the gastric mucosa and through the action of the enzyme urease, which produces ammonia and the release of cytotoxins, the underlying mucosa becomes damaged and inflamed. During endoscopy a nodular inflammation of the antrum may be seen and hypertrophy of the gastric mucosal folds has been reported.

Epidemiology

Helicobacter pylori is acquired in early childhood and, once infected, children are likely to remain colonized, despite the mounting of a host response, for the rest of their life unless they are inadvertently treated with antibiotics. The incidence of *Helicobacter pylori* infection in industrialized countries is approximately 0.5% of the susceptible population per year compared to a rate of 3–10% in developing countries. Spread occurs though close physical contact either by oral–oral or fecal–oral routes with the prevalence increasing where there is social deprivation or institutionalization.

Table 17.5 Agreed points from consensus statements on *Helicobacter pylori*

1. The aim of diagnosis is to find the cause of the symptoms rather than the presence of *Helicobacter pylori*
2. Testing all children and treating those positive for *Helicobacter pylori* is not recommended
3. Antibody tests of blood, serum or saliva are not recommended
4. Upper gastrointestinal endoscopy and biopsy is the best test for a child with chronic upper abdominal pain or suspected peptic ulcer disease
5. A child diagnosed with peptic ulcer disease by barium study should undergo endoscopy if symptoms recur
6. The urea breath test is not a satisfactory alternative to endoscopy for *Helicobacter pylori* diagnosis because of the wide differential diagnosis. It can be used for confirming success of treatment
7. Screening for *Helicobacter pylori* in asymptomatic individuals is not indicated
8. Treatment should be given when *Helicobacter pylori* is causing active disease (i.e. duodenal ulcer). When it is present without associated disease (i.e. asymptomatic child) the need for treatment should be discussed with the parents

Diagnosis of Helicobacter pylori

Biopsy and histopathology

Endoscopy and biopsy is the most reliable method for diagnosing infection. Multiple biopsies from antrum, incisura and body of the stomach allow the location and severity of inflammation to be defined and the presence of small spiral organisms on specially stained tissue sections confirms the presence of infection. In patients with infection that is resistant to treatment, biopsy allows culture and antimicrobial sensitivity to be determined.

The advantages of high sensitivity and specificity and the ability to examine the esophagus and duodenum at the same time have to be balanced against the invasiveness, availability and cost of the procedure.

Rapid urease (CLO) test

A single gastric biopsy is placed in the well of a CLO test slide. If *Helicobacter pylori* is present, its urease activity will cleave urea to produce ammonia which will turn the pH indicator red if left at room temperature for 24 h (see Fig. 17.4). This test gives indirect evidence of infection but because of a relatively poor positive predictive value cannot be relied upon in isolation to make a diagnosis.

Serology

This test is based on the detection of specific IgG to *Helicobacter pylori* in serum samples. The tests are cheap and relatively easy to set up. In children however the humoral immune response to infection may be slow to develop and this test is most unreliable in children under 5 years. The accuracy of serum based kits in symptomatic patients is between 60 and 70%. These tests cannot be used to confirm eradication after treatment as antibodies may remain positive for many months despite successful therapy. The recent consensus reports do not recommend the use of serological testing as the primary means of diagnosing *Helicobacter pylori* infection.

Tests using salivary antibodies are not presently recommended but stool tests for *Helicobacter pylori* antigens appear a little more promising.

C^{13} urea breath test

This non-invasive test involves the patient taking a small oral dose of C^{13}-enriched urea following a test meal which delays gastric emptying. If *Helicobacter pylori* is present within the stomach the urea is cleaved, releasing C^{13}-enriched CO_2 which is then exhaled in the breath. By collecting two breath samples, one before and the other 30 min after taking the oral urea, a rise in C^{13} levels in the breath signifies infection. This test has a sensitivity of 95% and a specificity of almost 100%. The sensitivity is reduced if antibiotics or acid suppressing drugs are not discontinued for 1 month prior to the test. The breath collection may also be technically difficult in young children.

The primary role of breath testing is confirming successful eradication after a course of treatment.

Symptoms

It is likely that the majority of children infected with this organism have no symptoms but, conversely, in children with evidence of

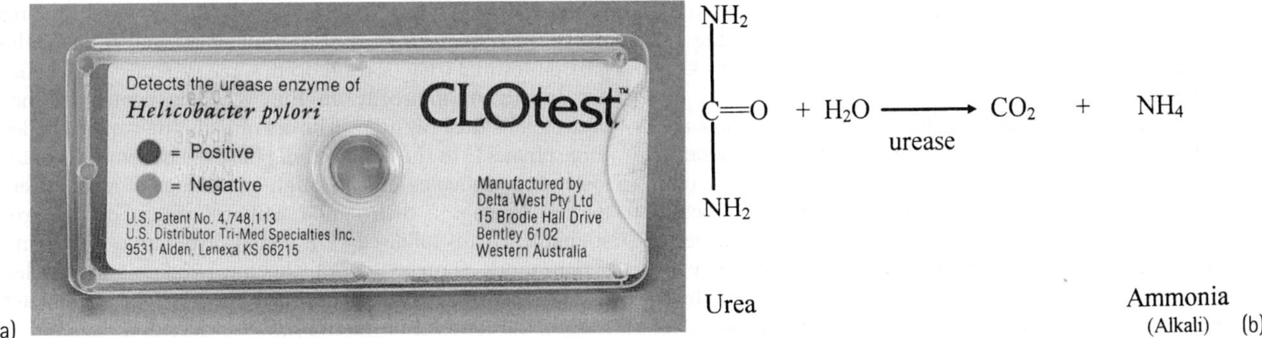

Fig. 17.4 (a) The CLO test used to detect *Helicobacter pylori* in mucosal biopsies. (b) The action of urease.

chronic peptic ulceration, *Helicobacter pylori* is likely to have an important role in its pathogenesis. Why the majority of children have no symptoms and only a small minority develop peptic disease remains unclear. It is not possible to differentiate infected from non-infected patients on the basis of history alone and in infected patients only those with proven ulceration responded well to eradication therapy.[28] This would suggest that *Helicobacter pylori* gastritis does not in isolation cause symptoms.

It was initially thought that *Helicobacter pylori* infection might be a significant cause of recurrent abdominal pain in childhood. While 5–17% of such children may be infected, it has been found that 5–29% of children without pain also had evidence of infection. It is therefore quite clear that this infection is not a significant factor in children with recurrent abdominal pain and current recommendations are that such children should not be screened for infection.

Treatment

Who to treat?

Eradication therapy is recommended where *Helicobacter pylori* infection and symptoms due to that infection are both present. However because infection with *Helicobacter pylori* is so common many children in whom infection is found will either be asymptomatic or will have symptoms not directly attributable to the infection. In this latter group the decision to treat is less clear-cut as it may not be of any benefit to the child and may carry the risk of side-effects from treatment.

Treatment is indicated for children with *Helicobacter pylori* infection and gastric or duodenal ulcer. In the rare patient with mucosa-associated lymphoid tissue (MALT) lymphoma or atrophic gastritis with intestinal metaplasia eradication therapy is also indicated.

Many children with *Helicobacter pylori* infection have evidence of gastritis without either gastric or duodenal ulceration. Under such circumstances treatment is unlikely to benefit the child. There is at present no convincing evidence that eradication therapy will reduce the risk of later peptic ulceration, adenocarcimoma or lymphoma. The clinician should discuss the pros and cons of treatment with the child and his/her parents before making a decision on whether to treat or not.

At present there is no evidence that children with recurrent abdominal pain or asymptomatic children benefit from eradication therapy.

Drug therapy

No properly controlled trials of *Helicobacter pylori* eradication therapy in children have been carried out and most of the available information is extrapolated from adult studies. A number of factors however are clear. Firstly the most important determinant of the success of therapy is compliance with treatment and secondly it is recommended that three medications are given twice daily for 1–2 weeks.[29] The use of one or two medicines is likely to be ineffective and will increase the risk of drug resistance developing. The recommended first line treatment for *Helicobacter pylori* eradication is given in Table 17.6.[26] It is suggested that successful eradication is confirmed by C^{13} breath testing and where reinfection occurs the use of alternative antibiotics such as tetracycline (over 12 years) or bismuth salts should be considered.

UPPER GASTROINTESTINAL BLEEDING

Bleeding from the upper gastrointestinal tract may present either as a hematemesis or melena depending on the site and severity of the bleeding. In the majority of cases the bleeding has little hemodynamic effect but major bleeds warrant urgent treatment. It is important, however, when taking a history to be sure that the child has in fact passed blood. The swallowing of bloodstained liquor, sucking on a cracked nipple, a recent nose bleed and the recent ingestion of beetroot can all mimic an intestinal hemorrhage.

Diagnosis

The most likely cause for a bleed can be determined from the age of the child and by searching for clues from the history and examination.[30,31] A history of previous gastrointestinal symptoms, recent drug ingestion, umbilical catheterization as a neonate, stigmata of chronic liver disease or a bleeding diathesis, or evidence

Table 17.6 Recommended first-line eradication therapy for *Helicobacter pylori* in children. (From Gold et al 2000[26])

Medication		Dose
Omeprazole (or equivalent proton pump inhibitor)		1 mg/kg/day up to 20 mg twice a day
Give two of three antibiotics	amoxicillin	50 mg/kg/day up to 1 g twice a day
	metronidazole	20 mg/kg/day up to 500 mg twice a day
	clarithromycin	15 mg/kg/day up to 500 mg twice a day
Treatment should be as a twice-daily regimen (to aid compliance) for 7–14 days		

of subcutaneous or cutaneous hemangioma should be sought (Table 17.7). In children with forceful vomiting due to gastroenteritis, Mallory–Weiss tears are the likely cause if specks of blood are present in the vomitus.

A full blood count will give an indication of the duration and severity of the bleed but may be misleading in the acute situation. A clotting screen will define the nature of any bleeding disorder that may be present. Direct visualization of the upper gastrointestinal tract by endoscopy should be carried out within 24 h of the bleed or whenever the patient is hemodynamically stable. This investigation will allow the detection of esophagitis, esophageal varices, gastric and duodenal ulcers and vascular malformations of the intestine proximal to the third part of the duodenum. If bleeding persists and these initial investigations are negative, a small bowel meal should be carried out to exclude intestinal polyps and where vascular malformation is suspected a selective angiogram should be carried out. If bleeding persists and no cause can be found a laparotomy may be indicated.

At times it can be very difficult to distinguish between upper and lower tract bleeding and it is suggested that this section is read in conjunction with the section on rectal bleeding (see p. 691).

Treatment

The initial treatment of the shocked patient is resuscitation, ensuring the patient has a secure airway and is breathing adequately with maintenance of the circulation by the rapid infusion of 10–30 ml/kg initially of saline and then whole blood when available. Any bleeding diathesis should be corrected and attempts should be made to define the underlying cause. If varices are found the patient should be treated by a team experienced with this type of problem. A description of the management of a variceal bleed is given in the section on liver disease (see p. 710). Most patients stop bleeding with simple medical management, and treatment should be aimed at the underlying cause of the bleeding.

VOMITING

Vomiting is a very common symptom of disease in childhood and should not be confused with the regurgitation of food which occurs in conditions such as gastroesophageal reflux. The vomiting reflex is the body's response to noxious stimuli, which may reside within the gastrointestinal tract or result from some systemic disturbance and act directly or indirectly on the 'vomiting center' in the area postrema of the brainstem. The act of vomiting can be divided into three phases.[32] In the pre-ejection phase the patient feels nauseous, looks pale, salivates and through the action of visceral efferent nerves develops a tachycardia with relaxation of the proximal stomach. This is followed by a period of retching and then, with synchronous contractions of the intra-abdominal muscles and diaphragm with an open glottis, upper esophageal sphincter and mouth, the contents of the stomach are ejected.

In the neonate, vomiting may be the first symptom of an intestinal obstruction, although any infection, metabolic disturbance or cerebral insult may present in an identical manner. The presence of bile in the vomit would suggest an obstruction distal to the duodenum. As the child becomes older the range of conditions causing obstructive and metabolic problems will change and in addition dietary indiscretions or intolerances may develop. The possibility of idiopathic hypertrophic pyloric stenosis should be considered in any baby of 1–4 months of age who develops projectile vomiting. In the older child drugs taken either accidentally or therapeutically may result in vomiting. A history of recurrent episodes of severe vomiting punctuated by asymptomatic periods should alert one to the possibility of cyclical vomiting. The symptoms of vomiting and diarrhea are frequently combined during enteric infections and it is likely that on a worldwide scale this is the most common cause of vomiting.

Table 17.7 Causes of upper gastrointestinal bleeding

1. Hemorrhagic disease of the newborn
2. Stress peptic ulcer
3. Blood dyscrasia
4. Esophagitis
   a. peptic
   b. caustic
5. Esophageal varices
6. Mallory–Weiss tear
7. Chronic ulcers
   a. gastric
   b. duodenal
8. Gastric erosions
   a. salicylates
   b. non-steroidal anti-inflammatory drugs
   c. corticosteroids
9. Infantile hypertrophic pyloric stenosis
10. Foreign body
11. Vascular malformations
12. Intestinal polyps

Diagnosis

A good history and examination will often give strong pointers to the most likely cause for the vomiting. A pyloric tumor or the mass of an intussusception may be palpable on abdominal examination. In some patients, particularly the very young, clues may be few and far between, and it must also be remembered that the differential diagnosis varies greatly depending on the age of the patient and on whether any associated features such as diarrhea are present (Table 17.8).

An erect and supine abdominal X-ray will show multiple air–fluid levels in intestinal obstruction but it must also be remembered that a functional obstruction due either to some intrinsic abnormality of the gut or to the toxic effect of sepsis or metabolic derangement may also give a similar picture. Barium contrast studies will define the nature of surgical causes of vomiting which are not clear from plain films. Where appropriate, detailed infection and metabolic screens should be carried out and signs of raised intracranial pressure should be sought. The serum electrolytes will give information on the extent of the vomiting and may even, as in the case of the hypochloremic hypokalemic alkalosis of pyloric stenosis, give clues to the underlying cause.

If a non-organic cause for the vomiting is suspected or if a behavioral element is thought to be present, referral to a psychiatrist or psychologist for a diagnostic assessment should be considered.

Treatment

The treatment should be aimed at the resuscitation of the patient in the first instance and then more specifically at the underlying cause of the vomiting. Electrolyte losses should be corrected and oral fluids should be stopped. If vomiting persists a nasogastric tube should be passed and where an obstructive lesion seems likely a pediatric surgeon should be consulted. As an adjunct to the treatment of the underlying problem antiemetic drugs may be

Table 17.8 Causes of vomiting in infancy

Cause	First week of life	After first week
Alimentary tract	Duodenal atresia Jejunal atresia Malrotation/volvulus Duplication of bowel Diaphragmatic hernia Meconium ileus Hirschsprung's disease Anal atresia Functional obstruction	Malrotation/volvulus Hirschsprung's disease Intussusception Strangulated hernia Pyloric stenosis Functional obstruction Peptic ulceration Appendicitis Bezoar Crohn's disease
Metabolic	Galactosemia Organic acidemia Hyperammonemia Hypercalcemia Hypoadrenalism	Organic acidemia Hyperammonemia Hypoadrenalism Diabetic ketoacidosis Drug intoxication Reye's syndrome Uremia
Dietetic	Cow's milk intolerance	Cow's milk intolerance Celiac disease Overeating
Infection	Any infection	Gastroenteritis Tonsillitis Otitis media Urinary infection Meningitis Septicemia
Cerebral	Birth trauma Hydrocephalus	Head injury Cerebral tumor Encephalitis Increased intracranial pressure
Others		Motion sickness Cyclical vomiting

useful in modifying the emetic response. Given the wide variety of stimuli which can produce vomiting and the varying mode of actions of these drugs it is perhaps not surprising that these agents are not universally effective.

INFANTILE HYPERTROPHIC PYLORIC STENOSIS

Pyloric stenosis develops in approximately 3 per 1000 live births with a male to female preponderance of 4:1. The cause of the condition is unclear although a reduced number of cases occur in babies with blood group A and there is also a strong familial pattern of inheritance. A thickening of the pyloric muscle results in gastric outlet obstruction with resulting vomiting.

Symptoms of projectile vomiting occurring 10–20 min after a feed, develop between the second and fourth week of life, although they can occasionally occur either sooner or at up to 4 months of age. With progressive vomiting the infants loose weight and may eventually become dehydrated and alkalotic. On clinical examination gastric peristaltic activity may be seen, and palpation of the right upper quadrant of the abdomen during a test feed will reveal the pyloric tumor in most cases. If the mass cannot be felt diagnosis can be aided by a barium meal which will show a narrow elongated pyloric canal or by ultrasound which should also define the mass.

The initial management of the patient after the diagnosis has been confirmed is intravenous rehydration and correction of any acid–base disturbance. The patient should then undergo a Ramstedt's pyloromyotomy where the pyloric muscle is split down to the mucosa. Oral feeds can be restarted 24 h after surgery (see Ch. 36).

Other surgical causes of vomiting are discussed more fully in Chapter 36.

PSYCHOGENIC VOMITING

Recurrent episodes of vomiting, sometimes referred to as cyclical vomiting, occur in children who are generally of school age.[33] The attacks, which can occur as frequently as once a week in some children and as infrequently as every 6 months in others, are generally preceded by a prodromal phase when the child is pale and withdrawn with the attack lasting anything from 12 to 72 h. The vomiting may also be associated with features of the periodic syndrome such as abdominal pain or headache.

The vomiting may be exacerbated by the child's desire to drink large amounts of fluid; persistent vomiting can lead to Mallory–Weiss tears, dehydration, electrolyte imbalance and eventually coma. It is frequently difficult to define the factors which precipitate each attack but a careful history may reveal stress factors, the most common being marital conflicts and school-based problems. The children require a full blood count, the measurement of serum electrolytes and a urine culture; a barium meal examination will exclude a hiatus hernia or a malrotation. If gastroesophageal reflux is clinically suspected a 24 h pH study should be considered. Rare metabolic problems such as medium chain acyl CoA dehydrogenase deficiency (MCAD) or ornithine transcarbamylase deficiency in girls need to be considered and excluded. In a small number of children an intercurrent viral infection may appear to initiate the episode.

If left untreated the majority of children will grow out of the problem but this may take many years. In others, headache may become a prominent feature and a picture of migraine may develop later.[34] If stress factors have been revealed from the history, psychological therapy may be of benefit in preventing further attacks while in those with migraineous features, dietary exclusion of cheese, chocolate, caffeine or citrus fruits should be considered. During acute attacks the child may require hospital admission for intravenous fluids and a careful physical examination should be carried out to exclude any organic cause for the vomiting. Antiemetic drugs may be of limited use during acute attacks but the administration of psychotropic drugs long term is not helpful.

FOREIGN BODIES

Children between the ages of 1 and 4 are particularly liable to swallow foreign bodies. The majority of these cause very few problems and simply pass straight through the intestine but long pointed objects such as fish bones or needles can become lodged in the pharynx, esophagus or occasionally in the duodenal loop. If the foreign body becomes lodged in a high position, coughing and choking may occur but frequently there may be no initial symptoms. Perforation of the mucosa will result in the development of a mediastinitis or peritonitis and where a battery becomes lodged a caustic stricture or mucosal erosion may develop.

Bezoar

The repeated ingestion of hair or paper or fibers from clothing or blankets can result in the formation of a large non-opaque foreign body in the stomach. These masses can grow to quite a large size but frequently there are very few symptoms other than vague abdominal pain or halitosis. The bezoar may be felt by abdominal palpation or outlined on a contrast study where the barium adheres to the fibrous mass.

Treatment

Small foreign bodies without sharp edges should be left to pass through the intestine. If they do not appear within 72 h a plain X-ray should be taken to check on their position. Sharp foreign bodies should be removed endoscopically under direct vision. If endoscopic removal from the stomach is not possible a laparotomy will be required.

GASTRIC INVESTIGATIONS

Barium studies

In patients with chronic nausea and vomiting a barium meal will define the anatomy of the stomach and detect the presence of a hiatus hernia, reflux, if it occurs during the examination, malrotation or any space occupation due to a bezoar. Although duodenal ulcers may be detected, endoscopy is the investigation of choice where a mucosal lesion is suspected.

Gastroscopy

Fiberoptic endoscopy is the preferred investigation for detecting duodenal or gastric ulcers or the antral gastritis associated with *Helicobacter pylori* infection. The method can be used in infants of all ages allowing histological and microbiological confirmation of the suspected diagnoses.[35]

THE SMALL INTESTINE

STRUCTURE OF THE SMALL INTESTINE

In man the small intestine occupies the major length of the gastrointestinal tract and is the major organ of digestion and absorption. In the adult the small intestine varies in length from 3 to 5 m depending on the state of contraction, while in the term infant the length is probably nearer 1.5 m. The small intestine is divided into the duodenum which extends from the pylorus to the duodenal–jejunal flexure at the ligament of Treitz; and the remaining small intestine is arbitrarily divided into the jejunum and ileum which represent the proximal two-fifth and distal three-fifths respectively.

In cross-section the structure of the small intestine is grossly similar throughout. The inner circular lumen is lined by a highly convoluted mucosa which exposes a large surface area for the absorption of nutrients. Underneath the surface epithelium lies the submucosa which in turn is encircled by the muscularis which comprises an inner circular and an outer longitudinal layer. The outermost layer is the serosa which is in continuity with the peritoneum. The mesentery of the small intestine is inserted diagonally across the posterior abdominal wall from the ligament of Treitz to the cecum. When this mesentery is shortened by malrotation of the small intestine it becomes unstable and is liable to twist.

Mucosa

The mucosa consists of the surface epithelium and the lamina propria. The mucosal surface is covered by villi which project into the lumen and greatly increase the surface area and by the crypts of Lieberkühn which lie between the villi and form a depression in the mucosa (Fig. 17.5).[36] In the jejunum the villous:crypt ratio is 3:1 but this decreases more distally to 1–2:1 in the ileum. Underneath the surface epithelium lies the lamina propria which contains a connective tissue core for the villi along with the vascular, lymphatic and neural networks which serve the nutrient and transport needs of the surface epithelium.

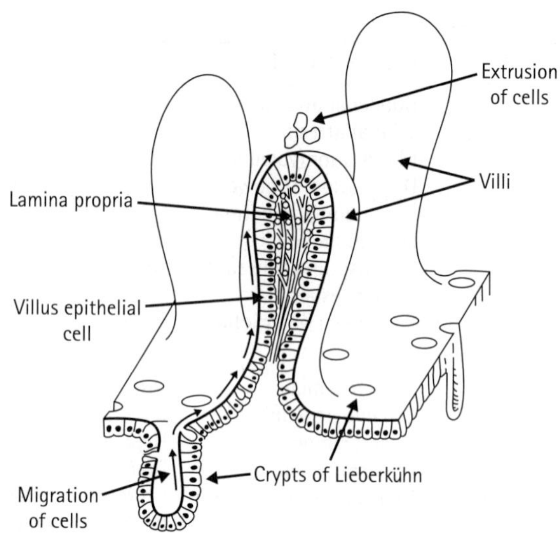

Fig. 17.5 A diagrammatic view of the surface of the small intestine. (Reproduced from *Harries' paediatric gastroenterology*[36] by kind permission of the publisher.)

The surface epithelium

The crypts and villi should be thought of as the functional unit of the surface epithelium. The crypts contain paneth, goblet, endocrine and undifferentiated cell types. Goblet cells which lie on the lateral wall of the crypts produce large amounts of protective mucus and the endocrine cells, which are neuroectodermal in origin, synthesize and secrete gastrointestinal hormones. Rapidly dividing undifferentiated cells migrate up the length of the crypts and on to the villi where they transform into mature villus cells (Fig. 17.5). The rate of division of these cells and their speed of migration is under the control of the trophic effect of enteral nutrients and a number of gut hormones. When enteral nutrients are removed as a result of starvation or the prolonged use of parenteral nutrition, mucosal hypoplasia results while in the adaptation to small intestinal resection the rate of cell turnover increases resulting in mucosal hypertrophy and increased villous length.

As the epithelial cells reach the villous tip they degenerate and fall off into the lumen. This rapid turnover of the villous epithelium takes between 4 and 6 days and explains both why the intestinal mucosa is on the one hand very susceptible to the toxic effects of ionizing radiation and chemotherapeutic drugs and why on the other its rate of repair and recovery from serious insult can be very rapid. The enterocytes have a well-developed brush border which further increases the surface area of the mucosa to luminal nutrients and supports the enzymes responsible for the final digestion of nutrients prior to absorption.

The cells in the crypts play an important role in the secretion of water and electrolytes into the lumen in contrast to the villous cells which largely absorb water, electrolytes and nutrients. In health the small intestine is a net absorber of water but in situations where the villous structure is damaged (i.e. celiac disease) or where mucosal inflammation stimulates the activity of the secretory crypt cells (i.e. Crohn's disease) this situation is reversed leading to active mucosal secretion. A similar situation occurs in rotavirus gastroenteritis where the rapid turnover of regenerative cells results in villi populated with immature cells which have yet to develop significant absorptive capacity.

The muscularis

The motor activity of the small intestine is provided by the inner circular and outer longitudinal muscle layers which are present along the whole length of the small intestine. Nerve fibers freely travel between these layers with extension distally onto the mucosa and proximally through afferent and efferent fibers which project both to and from the brainstem and cerebral cortex.

DIGESTION[37]

Digestion of carbohydrates

Starch, the main form of ingested carbohydrate, is a mixture of long chains of glucose units linked at the alpha-1,4 position (amylose), and shorter chains of alpha-1,4-linked glucose units connected by alpha-1,6 links to give a branched structure (amylopectin). As the intestine is only able to absorb monosaccharide units these large molecules require digestion by hydrolytic enzymes.

This digestion takes place in two steps; the first, occurring within the lumen of the gut, breaks the starch into oligosaccharides and the second, which occurs on the brush border of the small intestine, further digests these carbohydrates to their component monosaccharides. The luminal digestion is carried out by amylase from the salivary glands and the pancreas, which hydrolyzes alpha-1,4 bonds, breaking the amylose into maltose (two glucose units) and maltotriose, and amylopectin into limit dextrins with on average eight glucose units and one or more alpha-1,6 branching points. In the adult approximately 15% of duodenal amylase activity is salivary in origin but in the newborn infant, where pancreatic exocrine function is very poorly developed, this may increase to 50%.

Dietary disaccharides and the products of amylase digestion are further hydrolyzed by the enzymes of the enterocyte brush border membrane. These include the alpha-glucosidases sucrase, isomaltase, maltase and trehalase, the latter having no functional significance in the human. The beta-galactosidase lactase is also present. The substrate and product of each of these enzymes is outlined in Table 17.9. These enzymes are all high molecular weight glycoproteins which are synthesized in the endoplasmic reticulum, processed in the Golgi and inserted into the plasma membrane. The sucrase and isomaltase activities originate from a large molecule which is synthesized in continuity and subsequently split, after insertion in the brush border, into two separate functional units. Damage to the villi results in loss of disaccharidase activity with lactase being the most susceptible enzyme.

Undigested carbohydrate is fermented by colonic bacteria and salvaged as short chain fatty acids. If however the carbohydrate load is large, the osmotic pull will draw fluid into the lumen causing diarrhea.

Table 17.9 Carbohydrate digestion by the brush border

Enzyme	Substrate	Product
Lactase	Lactose	Glucose Galactose
Sucrase	Sucrose	Glucose Fructose
Maltase	Maltose	Glucose
Isomaltase	Isomaltose Limit dextrins	Glucose Glucose
Glucoamylase	Maltose Glucose oligomers	Glucose Glucose

Digestion of proteins

Ingested proteins are all very large molecules which require to be broken down to their constituent amino acids or di- and tripeptides before absorption can occur. The process of protein digestion involves the initial extraction of protein from food due to mastication and the mechanical activity of the stomach and denaturation of the protein which is promoted by the low pH of the stomach. The subsequent hydrolysis of the denatured protein is brought about by four major groups of enzymes: the pepsins secreted by the chief cells of the gastric glands and trypsins, elastase and chymotrypsins which are all secreted by the acinar cells of the pancreas. All four enzymes are secreted as proenzymes with hydrogen ions promoting the activation of pepsin and the enzyme enterokinase and trypsin activating the other three. The presence of enterokinase, which is found on the brush border membrane of the proximal small intestine, is vital for the activation of these pancreatic proteinases. Luminal digestion is completed by the action of amino- and carboxypeptidases which cleave the terminal amino acids of the peptides. This results in a mixture of small peptides and free amino acids being presented to the brush border membrane. The larger peptides are further hydrolyzed by brush border-bound peptidases leaving free amino acids, dipeptides and tripeptides for absorption.

Digestion of lipids

Dietary lipids are mainly in the form of triglycerides but phospholipids and cholesterol esters are also present in smaller amounts. Lipid digestion occurs mainly in the small intestine under the influence of bile salts which form an emulsion of the ingested fat and of pancreatic lipase which hydrolyzes the ester links at the 1 and 3 position of the triacylglycerol to yield monoacylglycerol and free fatty acid.

The presence of an adequate concentration of bile salts in the lumen of the small intestine (> 2 mmol/L) is of vital importance, as a failure to form a fat emulsion with small micelles (approx. 1 μm in diameter) severely reduces the surface area of contact between the lipase and the fat with resulting maldigestion. Inadequate bile salt concentrations can occur where there is an obstruction to biliary flow, deconjugation by luminal bacteria or where the total bile salt pool is depleted by bile salt malabsorption due to ileal resection.

Pancreatic lipase is quantitatively the most important enzyme in the digestion of triacylglycerols but lingual and gastric lipase are also present. Gastric lipase may be important in the hydrolysis of lipids with short and medium chain fatty acids, and in the preterm and newborn infant where pancreatic exocrine function is very poorly developed it is likely that lingual and gastric lipase are the major enzymes of lipid digestion, helped in breast-fed babies by breast milk lipase. Ingested phospholipids are hydrolyzed by pancreatic phospholipase and cholesterol esters are hydrolyzed by pancreatic cholesterol esterases.

The resulting monoacylglycerols, free fatty acids and cholesterol are absorbed by the epithelial cells of the small intestine. The fat-soluble vitamins A, D, E and K are absorbed from micelles and where the production of micelles is compromised by low bile salt concentrations, fat-soluble vitamin malabsorption is likely to occur.

Following the digestion and absorption of the lipid from the micelles the bile salts are reabsorbed by the terminal ileum and recycled through an enterohepatic circulation.

INTESTINAL ABSORPTION

The absorptive surface area of the small intestinal mucosa is greatly enhanced by the mucosal folds and by the presence of villi. The differentiated villous cells are responsible for the absorption of electrolytes and the products of the luminal and brush border digestion of food. Water is transported passively and moves down its osmotic gradient through a paracellular path. The epithelial cells are polarized with a brush border membrane facing the lumen of the intestine, a tight junction joining the lateral border of adjacent enterocytes and a basolateral membrane which is in close contact with the vasculature of the villi (Fig. 17.6).

The membranes of cells are very rich in lipid and thus while free fatty acids and monoacylglycerols can readily pass into epithelial cells, water-soluble compounds such as monosaccharides, amino acids, dipeptides and electrolytes all require specific transport processes to facilitate absorption.[38]

Electrolyte absorption

The direction of movement of an electrolyte across a cell membrane is determined by the electrical and chemical gradient which exists across that membrane. In the villous cells of the small intestine there is a strong electrochemical gradient for Na^+ across the brush border membrane with the inside of the cell –40 mV relative to the luminal surface and the intracellular Na^+ concentration being much lower than that found externally (Fig. 17.6). This gradient is maintained by the activity of the basolateral membrane Na^+/K^+ ATPase which pumps Na^+ out of the cell at the expense of the hydrolysis of ATP.

Sodium absorption may be either electroneutral when the absorption of Na^+ and Cl^- is coupled, or electrogenic when it is linked to the absorption of a solute such as glucose or an amino acid. Once absorbed the Na^+ is actively pumped out of the cell by Na^+/K^+ ATPase and the Cl^- is able to leave down its electrochemical gradient. K^+ is transported across the small intestine by a passive process while HCO_3^- is absorbed across the jejunum by a Na^+ dependent process.

Solute absorption

The absorption of glucose and galactose across the brush border membrane occurs by a carrier-mediated process which is driven by the Na^+ gradient across the cell, while fructose is absorbed by a Na^+-independent mechanism. Similarly group-specific active Na^+-coupled cotransport is responsible for the absorption of free amino acids and unhydrolyzed short peptides.

The presence of a luminal solute enhances the absorption of Na^+ and water by the small intestine. This explains the success of glucose electrolyte solution in the oral rehydration of children with diarrheal disease.

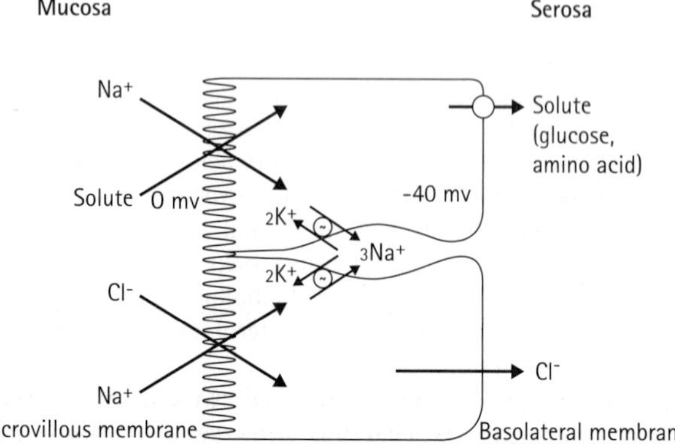

Fig. 17.6 A diagrammatic view of the Na^+, Cl^- and solute absorption across the enterocyte of the small intestinal villi. Water moves passively between the cells down an osmotic gradient.

SMALL INTESTINAL MOTILITY

In the fasting state small intestinal motor activity is characterized by a highly organized band of propagative activity, which moves down the intestine from the stomach to the ileum, called the migrating motor complex.[39] This activity develops between 2 and 4 h after a meal and recurs, every 25 min in the term infant and every 90 min in the older child, until disrupted by the next meal. The exact role of the migrating motor complex is uncertain but it has been postulated that it helps clear the small intestine of undigested food debris between meals and this may in part explain the very high incidence of bacterial overgrowth in patients where this activity is absent.

Following the ingestion of food the rate of transit through the small intestine is slowed to allow the complete digestion and absorption of the luminal contents. The rate of slowing is dependent on the energy density of the meal with lipids exerting a greater inhibitory effect than carbohydrates or protein. If undigested lipid reaches the ileum a powerful entero-entero reflex called the 'ileal brake' reflexly decreases the rate of gastric emptying and the degree of propagated intestinal motor activity, a situation which might pertain in patients with cystic fibrosis. Mouth to cecal transit time as measured by the breath hydrogen method is increased from 60 to 90 min in the fasting state to 3–4 h postprandially.

IMMUNE DEFENCES

The gastrointestinal tract, as with other mucosal surfaces, acts as an important interface between the external environment and the internal milieu of the individual. On the one hand it has to allow the uninterrupted passage of nutrients while on the other it acts as a major barrier to the entry of toxic macromolecules derived from the microbiological flora of the gut or from ingested food. (Table 17.10).

Non-immunological mechanisms

Gastric acid has an important role in initiating the digestion of ingested protein and in activating the intraluminal proteases.

Table 17.10 Gastrointestinal defense mechanisms

1. Non-immunological mechanisms
    a. Intraluminal
        (i) Gastric acid
        (ii) Pancreatic proteases
        (iii) Intestinal motility
    b. Mucosal
        (i) Mucin
        (ii) Microvillous membrane
        (iii) Lysozyme
2. Immunological mechanisms
    a. Mucosal immune system
        (i) Secretory antibody production
        (ii) Cellular immunity
    b. Systemic antibody production

The colonization of the small intestine by bacteria may be enhanced by reduced gastric acidity and the failure to fully digest large macromolecules may facilitate the absorption of large unaltered proteins. Normal peristaltic small intestinal motor activity is required to clear the small intestine of food debris between meals and to prevent colonization by bacteria. The mucosal surface which comprises the microvillous membrane and overlying mucus acts as a physical barrier to the attachment and uptake of luminal antigen and bacteria.

Immunological mechanisms

The specific immunological response to absorbed antigen is expressed by the production of secretory antibodies, systemic antibodies and by activation of the cellular immune system.

The secretory response is initiated by the absorption of antigen across specialized epithelial cells (M cells) which over lie lymphoid aggregates in the small intestine. This antigen is then passed to the underlying lymphoid tissue where, with the help of T lymphocytes, B lymphocytes are activated to become IgA producing cells. These cells initially proliferate and then migrate through the thoracic duct into the systemic circulation. The plasma cells then move back into the lamina propria where dimeric IgA, and to a lesser extent IgG, is produced prior to processing by the epithelial cells and secretion into the lumen in their secretory form. Secretory IgA is also produced by the salivary and mammary glands. A systemic immune response will occur in response to some antigens with the production of IgG, IgE and IgD.

T cells are also activated by the absorption of foreign antigen and these follow a path similar to that described above, back into the lamina propria. Along with these activated lymphocytes, mast cells and macrophages are also available to initiate a cell mediated response within the intestinal mucosa.

A failure of activation or conversely an overactivation of these immune defences will result in the development of gastrointestinal disease.

MALABSORPTION

Malabsorption may result either from a failure of the intraluminal digestion of food or from a defect of mucosal function which prevents the absorption of nutrients. The range of conditions which can cause malabsorption is extensive and is listed in Table 17.11. The presenting signs and symptoms are also very variable and may include diarrhea, vomiting, abdominal distension and weight loss. Some children, however, do not have symptoms directly referable to the gastrointestinal tract and may present with evidence of nutritional or other deficiency states.

A good history, with particular reference to the dietary and family history, it vital in assessing any child with suspected malabsorption. The age of the child is also important as food allergy is most likely to present in the first 6 months of life while celiac disease can only develop after gluten products have been introduced into the diet. One might expect diarrhea to be a universal feature in a child with malabsorption but such is the reserve capacity of the small intestine and the ability of the colon to absorb fluids and electrolytes, that this is not always the case. Failure to thrive, anemia and non-gastrointestinal symptoms such as chest problems in cystic fibrosis should be sought. The sections below outline the major causes of malabsorption along with a guide to diagnosis and treatment.

Table 17.11 Causes of malabsorption

Disorders of intraluminal digestion

1. Congenital
   a. Pancreatic
      (i) Cystic fibrosis
      (ii) Shwachman's disease
   b. Hepatic
      (i) Neonatal hepatitis
      (ii) Hepatocellular failure
      (iii) Cholestasis
   c. Intestinal
      (i) Enterokinase deficiency
2. Acquired
   a. Pancreatic
      (i) Chronic pancreatitis
   b. Hepatic
      (i) Neonatal hepatitis
      (ii) Hepatocellular failure
      (iii) Cholestasis
   c. Intestinal
      (i) Bacterial overgrowth

Disorders of intestinal mucosal function

1. Congenital
   a. Carbohydrate absorption
      (i) Glucose–galactose malabsorption
      (ii) Sucrase–isomaltase deficiency
      (iii) Alactasia
   b. Amino acid absorption
      (i) Cystinuria
      (ii) Hartnup disease
   c. Fat absorption
      (i) Abetalipoproteinemia
      (ii) Lymphangiectasia
   d. Electrolyte absorption
      (i) Chloride-losing diarrhea
      (ii) Primary hypomagnesemia
      (iii) Acrodermatitis enteropathica
   e. Enteropathies
      (i) Microvillous atrophy
      (ii) Idiopathic
2. Acquired
   a. Enteropathies
      (i) Celiac disease
      (ii) Food allergic
      (iii) Autoimmune
      (iv) Postgastroenteritis
   b. Infections
      (i) Tuberculosis
      (ii) Giardiasis
      (iii) Hookworm
   c. Infiltrations
      (i) Crohn's disease
      (ii) Reticuloses
   d. Anatomical
      (i) Intestinal fistulae
      (ii) Short gut syndrome
   e. Drugs
      (i) Chemotherapeutic agents

CELIAC DISEASE

Although first described in children over 100 years ago it was only in 1950 that Dicke noticed the association between celiac disease and the dietary protein gluten, and it was still later in 1957 that the enteropathy associated with this condition was first described following peroral jejunal biopsy. The enteropathy associated with celiac disease involves predominantly the proximal small intestine and following the removal of gluten from the diet it resolves completely.

In the last decade there has been a dramatic change in our understanding of celiac disease brought about largely by the introduction of screening tests which have unmasked a large population with lesser symptoms or sometimes none at all.[40]

Pathophysiology

Celiac disease is a multifactorial condition where environmental, genetic and immunological factors interact to produce damage to the mucosa of the proximal small intestine.

Genetic

The human leukocyte antigen (HLA) DQw2 is found in 95% of patients with celiac disease against only 20% in the general population. HLA DR5/DR7 is found in the remaining 5% of patients. Siblings who share for the above HLA types have 40% concordance for celiac disease while in monozygotic twins there is 70% concordance. Of particular interest is the increased prevalence of celiac disease in approximately 6% of first degree family members.

Environmental

The exposure of the small intestine to gluten from wheat, barley or rye is a prerequisite for the development of celiac disease. The small amount of gluten found in oats may also cause problems for some patients. The amount of gluten in the diet is also a factor in the time of presentation and the type of symptoms the patient may experience.[41] In Sweden where the weaning diet contains large amounts of gluten, children with celiac disease present most commonly with classical symptoms of diarrhea and failure to thrive between the age of 1 and 2 years. In contrast in Denmark where the weaning diet has much less gluten, children present between 7 and 9 years with milder symptoms such as anemia or abdominal pain.

Immunological

The contact of gluten with the small intestinal mucosa activates a cellular immune response in which T cells are activated and cytokines are released. The net result of this is that the mucosa is damaged and heavily infiltrated with inflammatory cells. The villus structure is completely lost and the crypts hypertrophy in an attempt to repair the damage. This transformation is outlined in Figure 17.7. There is also a humoral immune response which leads to the production of antibodies against grain peptides (antigliadin) and connective tissue autoantigens (antiendomysial, antireticulin). It is unlikely that these play a part in the tissue damage.

Presenting symptoms

The classical form of celiac disease presents with severe diarrhea, abdominal distension, weight loss, anemia and a general debilitation. This is most commonly found in younger patients while in older children there is a tendency for symptoms to be milder. Such symptoms might include abdominal pain, mild anemia, linear growth failure or pubertal delay. The older child is often free of diarrhea.

Celiac disease can be present in association with dermatitis herpetiformis, an itchy vesicular rash of the skin. There is now an irrefutable association between celiac disease and other autoimmune conditions such as type 1 diabetes mellitus[42] and hyperthyroidism and with genetic abnormalities such as Down syndrome[43] and Turner's syndrome[44]. Frequently it is the associated condition that is diagnosed first and it has been suggested that patients with the above conditions should all be screened for celiac disease at diagnosis.

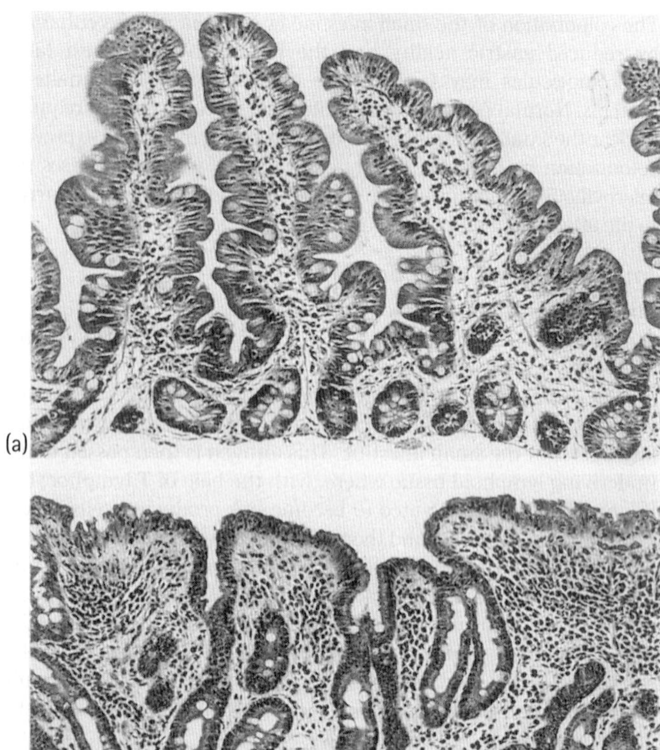

Fig. 17.7 A light micrograph (magnified x 240, stain hematoxylin and eosin) of a jejunal biopsy in (a) a normal child and (b) a child with untreated celiac disease. (Reproduced by kind permission of G Anderson)

Epidemiology

Generally celiac disease is uncommon in black African, Japanese and Chinese populations. Previously it was thought that the prevalence of celiac disease in Europe was about 1 in 3000. With the possibility of screening populations for celiac antibodies it is now being realized that the true prevalence is probably 10 times higher at approximately 1 in 300. This situation has been described as the 'celiac iceberg' in which only a small percentage of patients are diagnosed and 'visible above the waterline' while the majority are undiagnosed and 'hidden' from view.[45] This is illustrated schematically in Figure 17.8. Silent celiac patients will have positive celiac antibodies and histological evidence of celiac disease but will not have overt symptoms. These children are often labeled asymptomatic but when diagnosed and started on treatment, many feel better and only report symptoms in retrospect. Other children, so-called latent celiacs, have positive celiac antibodies but have a normal or near normal duodenal mucosa. If followed, many of these children go on to develop classical histological changes in their small intestine in subsequent years.

Screening tests

The starting point is either with a patient in whom there is a clinical suspicion of celiac disease or with a patient diagnosed as having a condition which is associated with a greatly increased risk of developing celiac disease (see Table 17.12). The former group all

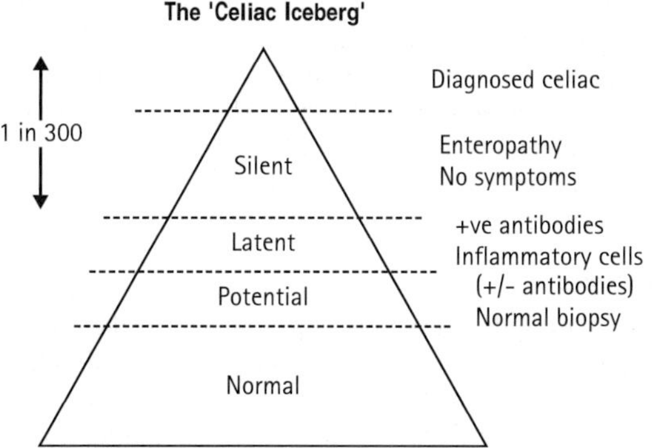

Fig. 17.8 The 'celiac iceberg'. Approximately 90% of people with celiac disease are presently undiagnosed.

require further investigation while screening of the latter group is presently the subject of debate. There has been reluctance by some to offer screening to the patient groups listed in Table 17.12 because of the concern that yet another diagnosis in a patient who is 'asymptomatic' may be unhelpful. It is however becoming increasingly clear that up to 50% of patients identified in screening programs are indeed symptomatic and receive benefit in terms of improved symptoms and quality of life from treatment of their celiac disease.

The most sensitive and specific screening test for celiac disease, in common use at present, is the measurement of serum IgA antiendomysial antibodies (AEA). Antireticulin and antigliandin IgA antibodies are also present in most patients and in children under 2 years of age the latter antibody may be of more value than the antiendomysial antibody. The yield from screening can be increased slightly by measuring all three antibodies with the downside being the increased cost. The antigen recognized by the antiendomysial antibody is tissue transglutaminase (tTG) and the development of an enzyme linked immunosorbent assay (ELISA) to antihuman tTG is proving in trials to be more sensitive and equally specific as AEA measurement. A dot blot test based on the measurement of antihuman tTG offers potential as an easy and accurate method to non-invasively screen for celiac disease.[46] Measurement of IgA AEA in suspected celiac patients is limited by the small but significant association of IgA deficiency. This limits the sensitivity of the test to 90–95% while the measurement of both IgA and IgG antihuman tTG overcomes this problem and gives sensitivities approaching 100%. Presently the use of the antihuman tTG assay is restricted to research laboratories.

Diagnosis

The main diagnostic test for celiac disease is small intestinal biopsy and until the screening tests described above have a sensitivity and specificity of 100% this will remain the case. From the time of their introduction in the 1950s biopsies of the jejunum were carried out using Crosby or Watson capsules. This technique, which required the capsules to be swallowed and the child sedated, was very unpleasant for the child and due to problems with the capsule firing, was not always successful. In recent years most pediatric centers have adopted upper intestinal endoscopy as the primary method for intestinal biopsy. This is a relatively rapid and reliable method of collecting mucosal samples from the distal duodenum and if three or four biopsies are taken the diagnostic yield is comparable to the traditional capsule biopsy.

The last published criteria for celiac disease were produced by the European Society for Paediatric Gastroenterology and Nutrition (ESPGAN) in 1990.[47] Although they were written before the introduction of widespread screening for celiac disease, the general principles still apply today.

The primary criterion for making a diagnosis of celiac disease is the presence of characteristic small intestinal mucosal abnormalities on biopsy (see Fig. 17.7b). The second requirement is a clear-cut clinical remission on starting a gluten free diet. Antibody testing is seen as a back up, rather than a replacement for intestinal biopsy. It can however be very helpful in determining compliance to treatment as the antibodies should become negative in patients adhering to a strict diet. In patients where there is diagnostic doubt or no initial biopsy has been taken, a gluten challenge is required. This ideally should be carried out after at least 2 years of treatment and not before the age of 6 years. A 'control' intestinal biopsy is taken before challenge and a further biopsy 3–6 months after starting on gluten or sooner if the patient relapses. It is recommended that patients who were truly asymptomatic at diagnosis should undergo a control biopsy. With an increasing number of asymptomatic patients picked up because of screening it is likely that compliance by parents and patients with this recommendation will be poor.

Table 17.12 Conditions associated with an increased prevalence of celiac disease

Condition	Percentage
Type 1 diabetes	1–10
Autoimmune thyroid disease	
Children	8
Adult	3
Turner's syndrome	8
Down syndrome	4–12
1st degree relative of known celiac	6
General population	0.2–1

Treatment

The treatment of celiac disease is with life-long exclusion of gluten from the diet. This essentially means avoiding all wheat, barley and rye products. Tolerance of oats is variable and a number of patients need to also exclude this. The education of the child and their parents in this diet, needs the expert help of a pediatric dietitian. Many gluten free products are commercially available and this goes some way to making what is essentially a very restrictive diet, a little easier to tolerate.

Some newly diagnosed children, particularly those with a classical presentation, may be severely malnourished at the time of diagnosis. Addition nutritional supplementation will be required and in the very lethargic child, short term nasogastric feeding may be required until the child is able to feed. Because of the risk of osteoporosis, all patients with celiac disease require a good calcium intake and often require calcium supplements.

Consequences of untreated celiac disease

Because most patients with celiac disease are presently undiagnosed and many may have little in the way of symptoms, it has been argued that there is little point in screening at risk groups. Untreated celiac disease however can lead to anemia, osteoporosis, reproductive problems and worryingly an increased risk of intestinal malignancy. In children who do not comply with their gluten free diet school performance is poorer. In studies where patients without apparent intestinal symptoms are screened for celiac disease, up to 50% in whom a diagnosis is ultimately confirmed feel that they benefit from gluten exclusion in terms of reduced intestinal symptoms (i.e. pain or stool frequency) or increase in general well-being.

Untreated celiac disease is clearly linked to an increased rate of malignancy. In a study of 210 adults celiacs over an 11 year period, in those not adhering to a gluten free diet the rate of all malignancy was increased 2.6-fold, mouth, pharynx and esophagus neoplasm 22-fold and non-Hodgkin's lymphoma of the intestine 77-fold.[48] In patients newly diagnosed with small intestinal lymphoma 12% have celiac disease against an incidence of celiac disease in the general population of 0.5%.

FOOD ALLERGY

Food allergy most commonly develops in the first few months of life with the most common allergens being cow's milk protein, although soya protein and a wide range of other dietary proteins may also be responsible. This sensitization develops most commonly in atopic individuals with a family history of food allergy or clear evidence of another atopic symptoms such as eczema, asthma or urticaria. In many of these children, although their intolerance generally resolves between the age of 18 months and 5 years, symptoms of asthma and hay fever frequently follow. In older patients sensitization may follow an enteric infection leading to persistent intestinal symptoms long after the pathogen has been cleared.

In healthy individuals oral tolerance to dietary protein develops through the suppression of lymphocytes within the intestinal mucosa.[49] This occurs when a large antigen load is presented to the immune system by the epithelium without costimulation and in the case of low dose antigen, processing by the M cell from the Peyer's patches leads to the production of suppressor lymphocytes which home in on the lamina propria. Where mucosal integrity is compromised these mechanisms break down and sensitization to food allergens may develop. Mucosal integrity will be disrupted by enteric infection but it is clear that a close interaction between the epithelial cell and the gut flora is also important in maintaining integrity. It has recently been shown that the administration of the probiotic *Lactobacillus* GG, which promotes the colonization of the gut by 'healthy bacteria', to the mother before and the infant after birth, reduced the subsequent development of atopic disease.[50]

Cow's milk protein intolerance

This condition develops most commonly within the first 6 months of life and occurs predominantly in formula-fed babies or babies receiving cow's milk in weaning foods. Breast-fed babies are also at risk as cow's milk protein is secreted at lactation if the mother's diet contains cow's milk. The most common symptoms at presentation are of vomiting, diarrhea and poor weight gain with eczema frequently present in babies and asthma or hay fever in older children.[51] Rectal bleeding due to an allergic colitis may be a presenting symptom in some infants.

Diagnosis

The diagnosis is made from the history and from the characteristic improvement in symptoms with exclusion of cow's milk protein from the diet. Jejunal biopsy is likely to reveal a patchy partial villous atrophy with eosinophilic infiltrate, although in some patients the enteropathy may be more severe and be difficult to distinguish pathologically from celiac disease. Jejunal biopsy however is not required in most patients as the condition usually responds well to an exclusion diet and is self-limiting, but if there is severe failure to thrive or a failure to respond to a cow's milk-free diet a jejunal biopsy is essential to exclude any other more serious pathology. A full blood count may reveal evidence of a peripheral eosinophilia, serum immunoglobulins may show a raised IgE and a low IgA and skin test or radioallergosorbent testing (RAST) may reveal positive reactions to food and environmental allergens. These latter tests are all non-specific with a high false negative rate and in many patients who are quite clearly food allergic they may still be negative.

Management

It is usual to exclude cow's milk protein from the diet and as many atopic children also react to egg protein a combined milk and egg exclusion is frequently required. It is essential that the diet is supervised by a dietitian to ensure that adequate calories and calcium remain in the diet. A complete milk substitute based on a whey or casein hydrolysate should be prescribed, and where the infant has been weaned the mother should be instructed on a diet containing milk- and egg-free solids. The use of soya formula can lead to problems as 30% of children allergic to cow's milk protein also react to soya. A small number of patients will even fail to tolerate a hydrolyzed formula and an elemental feed may be substituted. Some older children refuse to take these milk substitutes because of the taste and under such circumstances, if the diet is otherwise adequate, an oral calcium substitute should be prescribed. Alternatively if the intake is poor, the feed can be given by nasogastric tube.

Most children will improve quickly after starting their diet but it may take many months for full catch-up growth to occur in children who have been failing to thrive. The natural history of this condition is one of spontaneous remission but in some children further intolerances may develop.

Multiple food intolerances

Although cow's milk protein, soya and egg are most commonly responsible for food intolerances in children, wheat, colorings, preservatives and sugar have all been implicated. In the very atopic child almost any dietary intolerance is possible. In addition to the gastrointestinal and atopic symptoms described above for cow's milk protein intolerance, behavior disturbance and hyperactivity may occur in some children.

It should be possible to discover which foods are responsible for the symptoms by taking a good dietary history, and an appropriate exclusion diet should be devised. In some children, however, it is difficult to isolate which foods are causing the problem and under these circumstances two options are available. One can either put the child on a diet limited to just five or six foods and if this settles the symptoms then add one new food at a time, or alternatively the mucosal allergic reaction can be suppressed by drug therapy. Oral sodium cromoglycate, antihistamines or systemic steroids may be helpful in some patients. Drugs are not however a substitute for proper dietary management and if serious symptoms persist the use of more hypoallergenic amino acid based feeds should be considered.

Eosinophilic gastroenteritis

It is likely that a fair degree of overlap exists between the allergic conditions described above and eosinophilic gastroenteritis. The condition is characterized by an eosinophilic infiltrate which can involve the stomach and/or small intestine and which appears to be triggered by the presence of dietary antigens. Three forms of the condition, each involving a different layer of the intestine, have been described.

The mucosal form is characterized by protein loss with hypoalbuminemia and edema. Damage to the antral and duodenal mucosa will result in blood loss and anemia while jejunal damage leads to an enteropathy with malabsorption. Where the muscle layer is involved symptoms of intestinal obstruction occur and in the serosal form of the condition an eosinophilic ascites may develop. Most patient are likely to have the markers of atopy which are outlined above.

Diagnosis will be suggested by the history of atopy with abdominal pain, diarrhea, vomiting, weight loss and edema. Some patients, however, may have no abdominal symptoms. Barium contrast studies may show evidence of inflammation in the mucosal form or luminal obstruction in cases involving the enteric smooth muscle. Upper gastrointestinal endoscopy is invaluable for detecting antral and duodenal lesions and for confirming the diagnosis by mucosal biopsy. Jejunal biopsy will define the involvement of the small intestine but if the disease is patchy, inflamed areas may be missed. Protein loss from the intestine may be detected by measuring the excretion of chromium-51-labeled albumin in the stool over a 5-day period or by measuring the stool alpha-1 antitrypsin.

Treatment with dietary exclusion is frequently all that is required in the mucosal form but where there is transmural or serosal inflammation, oral corticosteroids may also be required in addition. The level of therapy required will vary from patient to patient but those with mucosal disease are likely to be the most responsive to therapy. Where intestinal obstruction occurs surgery with local resection is likely to be required.

POSTENTERITIS ENTEROPATHY

While most enteric infections are self-limiting and are free of long term sequelae, some organisms damage the mucosal surface of the gut resulting in a persistence of symptoms long after the original infective organism has been cleared. This postenteritis syndrome can be caused by viruses such as adenovirus or by bacterial pathogens such as the enteropathogenic *Escherichia coli* which totally denude the mucosa of villi. The consequences of acute enteric infections and their management are discussed more fully later in this chapter (see p. 679).

CONGENITAL ENTEROPATHIES

Intractable diarrhea presenting from the time of birth may be caused by inborn errors which result either in a disruption of enterocyte absorptive or secretory function, or where structural genes are damaged, leading to an enteropathy of the small intestinal mucosa. Microvillus inclusion disease (microvillus atrophy) is the best characterized of these congenital enteropathies but other forms include intestinal epithelial dysplasia (tufting enteropathy) and syndromic forms which are associated with dysmorphic features.[52]

Microvillus atrophy is characterized by a hypoplastic villous atrophy associated with depletion and shortening of the microvilli over the villous epithelium.[53] This condition can be differentiated from other congenital enteropathies by the presence of smudging of stains which outline the microvillous membrane and by electron micrographs which show the presence of characteristic microvillous inclusions in the villous enterocytes. Patients who survive with this condition are likely to remain dependent on parenteral nutrition as no specific treatment is known.

For children with the other forms of congenital enteropathy the lack of understanding of the underlying cause makes treatment and prognostication difficult. Nutritional support with predigested hypoallergenic feeds and intravenous alimentation can greatly prolong life but will frequently not alter the underlying disorder.

AUTOIMMUNE ENTEROPATHY

In a small number of patients with intractable diarrhea and an enteropathy the presence of autoantibodies to the cytoplasm of enterocytes has been described. Autoimmune enteropathy presents with intractable watery and sometimes bloody diarrhea between 3 months and 2 years of age.[54] In some of these patients other organ-specific autoantibodies or autoimmune diseases have also been found, making it likely that the intestinal disease is caused by an autoimmune process. Treatment of these children with hypoallergenic diets, steroids and immunosuppressive drugs, such as azathioprine, ciclosporin or tacrolimus, is successful in some cases.

PROTEIN-LOSING ENTEROPATHY

Small amounts of albumin pass into the gut each day and under the influence of pancreatic enzymes are digested and reabsorbed. In response to an increased loss into the gut the liver is able to compensate by increasing the rate of albumin synthesis by up to a factor of two. Above this level, however, the patient becomes increasingly hypoproteinemic.[55] Those proteins with the longest half-lives (albumin and IgG) are the first to fall and in severe protein-losing enteropathies between 10 and 50% of the plasma albumin pool may be lost into the gut each day.

Etiology

Protein-losing enteropathy may arise either as a consequence of the increased permeability of the intestine to plasma proteins or as a result of disordered intestinal or mesenteric lymph flow which leads to the loss of lymphocytes and fat, in addition to protein, into the intestine. Protein loss owing to increased permeability is most marked in hypertrophic gastritis, eosinophilic gastroenteritis and in some forms of intestinal polyposis but any condition which results in severe damage or inflammation to the lining of the gut is likely to result in increased luminal protein loss. Lymphangiectasia is the most common cause of disordered lymph flow. The conditions associated with protein-losing enteropathy are listed in Table 17.13

Clinical features and diagnosis

The clinical features are of peripheral edema and ascites, when the serum albumin falls below 20 g/L, in addition to those of the underlying condition. The diagnosis of a protein-losing enteropathy is confirmed by the detection of increased amounts of protein in the stool in the face of a low serum albumin. The increased losses can be shown by the presence of > 4% loss of chromium-51-albumin in the stool over a 5-day period and by increased levels of fecal alpha-1 antitrypsin. The cause of the protein loss, which may be from the stomach, small intestine or large intestine, can best be defined by endoscopy and biopsy.

The treatment is that of the underlying condition but 20% albumin infusion may be required in the short term to correct the hypoalbuminemia and edema.

INTESTINAL LYMPHANGIECTASIA

The lymphatics of the small intestine play a vital role in the absorption of fat, being responsible for the transport of chylomicrons from the mucosal cells, via the thoracic duct to the venous system. This lymphatic fluid is also rich in protein and in

Table 17.13 Causes of protein-losing enteropathy

1. Increased mucosal permeability to protein
   a. Hypertrophic gastritis
   b. Eosinophilic gastroenteritis
   c. Polyposis
   d. Inflammatory disease
      (i) Crohn's disease
      (ii) Ulcerative colitis
      (iii) Enterocolitis
      (iv) Pseudomembranous colitis
      (v) Radiation enteritis
      (vi) Graft-versus-host disease
      (vii) Autoimmune enteropathy
   e. Celiac disease
   f. Nephrotic syndrome
   g. Esophagitis
2. Altered lymph flow
   a. Primary intestinal lymphangiectasia
   b. Secondary intestinal lymphangiectasia
      (i) Congestive cardiac failure
      (ii) Constrictive pericarditis
      (iii) Lymphoma
      (iv) Tuberculous adenitis
      (v) Volvulus

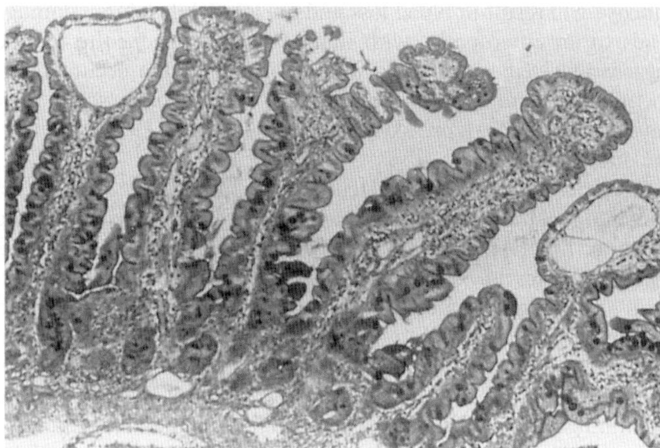

Fig. 17.9 A jejunal biopsy from a patient with lymphangectasia showing lymphatic vacuolation of the villi (magnified x 240, stain hematoxylin and eosin). (Reproduced by kind permission of PJ Milla)

lymphocytes. In intestinal lymphangiectasia these lymphatic channels become blocked and as a consequence protein and lymphocytes are lost into the gut while fat and fat-soluble vitamins are malabsorbed.

The condition may be either congenital when it is frequently associated with other abnormalities of lymphatic development, such as peripheral lymphedema, or it may arise secondary to acquired lymphatic obstruction from congestive cardiac failure, constrictive pericarditis, malrotation or infiltration of the lymphatics by neoplastic processes. Examination of the jejunal mucosa under a dissecting microscope reveals pale villi of normal length. On higher magnification the lymphatics of the lamina propria and submucosa are distended and filled with lipid staining material (Fig. 17.9).

Patients are likely to present with diarrhea, abdominal distension with hypoproteinemia leading to edema and ascites. The loss of lymphatic cells will result in lymphopenia and an increased susceptibility to infections. Fat-soluble vitamin deficiencies are likely to lead to rickets and clotting abnormalities. The diagnosis is confirmed by the characteristic jejunal biopsy findings in a patient with lymphopenia and a protein-losing enteropathy.

If the primary cause of the lymphangiectasia cannot be remedied treatment involves the use of a high protein diet to compensate for the large stool losses. The substitution in the diet of long chain by medium chain fats which are absorbed directly into the portal venous circulation reduces the protein loss. In some patients regular albumin infusions may be required to control hypoproteinemia.

IMMUNE DEFICIENCY AND GUT DISEASE

The normal immune function of the small intestine plays a major part in preventing both the absorption of foreign proteins and the penetration of enteric pathogens across the lining of the gut. While the immunodeficiencies themselves very rarely cause any primary damage to the gut, the consequences of the sensitization of the gut to foreign proteins or of recurrent enteric infections can lead to structural damage to the small intestinal mucosa with the development of malabsorption and diarrhea and as a consequence, failure to thrive.[56] The immunodeficiencies which can lead to compromised intestinal function are listed in Table 17.14

While the majority of children with IgA deficiency may have no symptoms, the incidence of food allergy and of celiac disease is increased as is infection with *Giardia lamblia*. In agammaglobulinemia and common variable immundeficiency (CVI), as well as giardiasis, bacterial overgrowth and non-specific colitis can occur. Where T cell function is compromised in CVI, chronic fungal infection and a non-specific enterocolitis may develop. Granulomatous disease can cause liver and perianal abscesses, and an enterocolitis which can mimic Crohn's disease; a granulomatous narrowing of the gastric antrum has also been reported.

In both Wiskott–Aldrich and DiGeorge syndrome there is T cell dysfunction, the former associated with severe eczema and thrombocytopenia and the latter associated with esophageal, parathyroid and cardiac defects. Acquired immunodeficiency syndrome frequently presents with opportunistic intestinal infection with *Cryptosporidium*, *Candida*, *Salmonella* or cytomegalovirus.

The diagnosis and treatment of these immune deficiencies is more fully described in Chapter 25. When gut disease occurs, therapy should be aimed at the primary disorder, at treating the enteric infection and at supporting nutrition with elemental feeds or even parenteral nutrition.

Immunodeficiencies may themselves occur as a consequence of primary gastrointestinal disease and this in turn can feed back to

Table 17.14 Immune deficiency leading to gastrointestinal disease

1. Antibody defect
   a. X-linked agammaglobulinemia
   b. IgA deficiency
2. Combined immunodeficiency
   a. Common variable immunodeficiency
   b. Severe combined immunodeficiency
3. Defect of phagocytosis
   a. X-linked chronic granulomatous disease
4. Immunodeficiency as part of a syndrome
   a. Wiskott–Aldrich syndrome
   b. DiGeorge syndrome
5. Acquired immunodeficiency syndrome

potentiate the initial disorder. This can occur in any severely malnourished child, in patients where gut protein loss results in hypoproteinemia and hypogammaglobulinemia and in acrodermatitis enteropathica where zinc deficiency suppresses immune function.

SHORT GUT SYNDROME

Resection of part of the small intestine is not uncommonly required in neonates who develop an acute surgical problem (Table 17.15). Similarly in the older child intestinal resection may be required following trauma or volvulus formation. The consequences of such a resection depend very much on the length of gut resected, the part of the small intestine resected, whether the ileocecal valve and colon are still present and on the nutritional state of the patient.[57] Loss of more than 30 cm of intestine is likely to have nutritional consequences to the infant. The remaining bowel, however, has great powers of adaptation and it is possible for as little as 20 cm of small intestine with an intact ileocecal valve to adapt adequately to support life by enteral nutrition.

Clinical features

As a consequence of the loss of intestinal surface area the child develops diarrhea and the absorption of all nutrients, minerals and vitamins is reduced. This is likely to lead to weight loss and the development of specific nutritional deficiencies.

Loss of the terminal ileum will lead to malabsorption and depletion of the bile salt pool and failed vitamin B_{12} absorption will over a period of years lead to the development of a deficiency state. If duodenal bile salt concentration falls below 2 mmol/L micelle formation may be inhibited leading to malabsorption of long chain fats, and the passage of bile salts into the colon will result in intestinal secretion which will compound the diarrhea. The ileum is also rich in enteroglucagon, a potent trophic factor in intestinal adaptation, and where the ileum has been resected the adaptive response may be further delayed or blunted.

The ileocecal valve has a vital role in preventing the reflux of colonic flora into the small intestine and when the valve is resected bacterial overgrowth of the small intestine is an almost inevitable sequela. This leads to mucosal damage and the deconjugation of bile salts with resulting disruption of lipid solubilization and intestinal secretion. Without an ileocecal valve the length of gut that is needed to support life is probably more than doubled and this is further increased if the colon has also been extensively resected.

The small intestine also has an important role in the metabolism of gastrin and where a large length of jejunum is resected hypergastrinemia with increased gastric secretion can occur. This not only increases the fluid load on the intestine but also lowers the duodenal pH and as a result reduces bile salt solubility and the activity of the digestive enzymes.

Table 17.15 Causes of the short bowel syndrome in the neonate

1. Small intestinal malrotation with volvulus
2. Jejunal and ileal atresias
3. Meconium ileus
4. Omphalocele or gastroschisis with volvulus
5. Internal hernias
6. Necrotizing enterocolitis
7. Congenital short small bowel

Management

During the period of adaptation which follows an intestinal resection the turnover of regenerative cells in the crypts of the small intestine increases and as a consequence the length of villi increases. With time this leads to an increase in the absorptive capacity of the residual small intestine. This process, however, may take many months and the mainstay in management is the promotion of the adaptive response and the nutritional support of these patients during this period.

One of the most potent trophic factors in promoting adaptation is the presence of food within the gastrointestinal tract. Starvation is known to produce a partial villous atrophy which is reversed by refeeding. In the short gut syndrome it is therefore most important that enteral feeding is maintained at a level which is able to stimulate the adaptive response while at the same time not causing torrential diarrhea. Because of the reduced digestive and absorptive capacity of the small intestine it is usual to feed these infants with a predigested feed, synthetic elemental feed or a modular feed to which carbohydrate and fat can be added individually as tolerated.

There is also a need to control the many complications of the short gut syndrome in order to further increase the absorptive and digestive capacity of the gut. These treatments are listed in Table 17.16. In some infants where very little small intestine remains, or where the adaptive response has been blunted by loss of the ileum and ileocecal valve, the child may remain dependent on parenteral nutrition and under such circumstances efforts should be made to institute this therapy at home. These most severe patients may also be candidates for intestinal transplantation (see p. 686).

INBORN ERRORS OF DIGESTION AND ABSORPTION

Although most causes of gastrointestinal disease are acquired, there are a number of specific inborn errors of intestinal function which interfere with the normal digestion and absorption of nutrients. Although these disorders are generally uncommon it is important to be aware of their existence as failure to recognize their signs and symptoms may have severe consequences for the child. A knowledge of normal intestinal physiology is important if the clinical consequences of these defects are to be understood.

CARBOHYDRATE MALABSORPTION

Carbohydrates will be malabsorbed if there is a failure of luminal or brush border digestion or a defect in the transport proteins which facilitate the absorption of monosaccharides. The most common inborn error involving carbohydrate digestion is cystic fibrosis in which luminal levels of pancreatic amylase are markedly reduced. Of the disaccharidases outlined in Table 17.9, specific defects of

Table 17.16 Complications in short gut syndrome and their treatment

Complications	Treatment
Bacterial overgrowth	Antibiotics Resect stricture or stagnant loop
Gastric hypersecretion	Histamine 2 blockers
Rapid transit	Loperamide
Malabsorption of fats	Medium chain triglycerides in feeds
Bile salt diarrhea	Bile salt chelator: colestyramine
Poor growth	Increase parenteral nutrition

lactase, sucrase–isomaltase and trehalase have all been reported although the latter defect is of no clinical significance.

The presence of increased concentrations of disaccharides in the lumen of the small intestine leads to an osmotic diarrhea that results in abdominal distension with large water and electrolyte losses which can be life threatening in young infants.

Lactase deficiency

Primary lactase deficiency is very uncommon and presents with profuse watery diarrhea soon after the introduction of milk feeds. The diagnosis can be suspected from the clinical history and the response to a lactose-free diet, although it can only be confirmed by the measurement of brush border lactase activity. The condition is thought to be inherited in an autosomal recessive fashion.

In many African and Asian races, adult levels of lactase activity fall far below those found in European races. This has previously been labeled 'late onset lactase deficiency', but given that most of these individuals do not have any symptoms, it is probably incorrect to say that they are deficient. Transient lactase deficiency commonly occurs as a result of damage to the intestinal mucosa from a primary infective agent.

Sucrase–isomaltase deficiency

The incidence of this deficiency is probably very low although it is said to affect up to 10% of Greenland Eskimos. The condition probably occurs in a number of distinct genetic forms and this may in part explain the variability in its clinical presentation. Symptoms of diarrhea and failure to thrive usually develop following the introduction of sucrose or complex carbohydrate into the diet, but in some children the symptoms may be very mild and the condition goes undiagnosed. As sucrase also contributes to a large part of the brush border maltase activity the use of refined formula feeds which all contain glucose polymer invariably results in an increase in the diarrhea.[58]

In response to an oral sucrose load, exhaled breath hydrogen rises and sucrose can be detected by sugar chromatography of the loose stools. Jejunal biopsy will show normal mucosal morphology but histochemical studies reveal low or absent enzyme activity. Dietary removal of sucrose and complex carbohydrate results in an immediate symptomatic recovery.

Glucose–galactose malabsorption

The condition results from a defect in the transport protein which is responsible for sodium–glucose and sodium–galactose linked cotransport.[59] Diarrhea develops shortly after the first feed and persists until glucose and galactose are removed from the diet. In contrast fructose absorption is normal and sodium–amino acid cotransport is preserved. In some children the degree of glucose intolerance decreases with increasing age. The inheritance is autosomal recessive and is treated with the fructose-containing feed, Galactamin 19.

LIPID MALABSORPTION

Lipid malabsorption with steatorrhea will result from failed luminal solubilization and digestion of triglycerides, as occurs in pancreatic insufficiency, biliary disease and the short gut syndrome, and from failure of mucosal fat transport as occurs in abetalipoproteinemia and hypobetalipoproteinemia.

Abetalipoproteinemia

This autosomal recessive condition which was first described in 1950 is characterized by the presence from birth of steatorrhea, acanthocytosis on the peripheral blood film and failure to thrive; if diagnosis is delayed signs of ataxia and retinopathy may develop in the second decade.

Failure to synthesize apoprotein B means that chylomicrons cannot be manufactured and exported into the lymphatics. Lipid electrophoresis reveals absent serum low density lipoprotein (LDL), very low density lipoprotein (VLDL) and chylomicrons and as a consequence serum triglyceride and cholesterol levels are low. Jejunal biopsy reveals fat-laden enterocytes.

There is now strong evidence that the neurological signs result from chronic vitamin E deficiency and if treatment is started promptly with a low fat diet, large oral supplements of vitamin E (100 mg/kg/24 h) along with supplements of the other fat-soluble vitamins the development of ataxic symptoms and mental deterioration can be prevented.

PROTEIN MALABSORPTION

The digestion of proteins is dependent on the action of proteases which are secreted by the stomach, pancreas and the intestinal mucosa. Inborn errors of these enzymes are very uncommon although specific deficiencies of trypsinogen and enterokinase have been reported. Both these conditions result in failure to thrive, hypoproteinemia, edema, anemia and neutropenia, and following the introduction of a protein hydrolysate feed with oral pancreatic supplements there is a marked improvement in symptoms.

Defects of brush border amino acid absorption tend to have few clinical consequences as the particular amino acid can still be absorbed as part of a dipeptide. This explains why cystinuria and iminoglycinuria do not result in the development of any nutritional deficiencies and why in Hartnup disease symptoms tend to develop only when the diet is otherwise compromised. Defects of basolateral transport appear, however, to have more severe clinical consequences.

Hartnup disease

A defect in the transport of free neutral amino acids across the brush border of the small intestine and the proximal renal tubules of the kidney leads to a pellagra-like skin rash in areas exposed to sunlight with associated diarrhea and a dementing psychiatric illness. These features are the result of low levels of tryptophan leading to the decreased production of nicotinamide. Treatment with nicotinamide supplementation controls the symptoms of pellagra which spontaneously become less severe with increasing age.

Lysinuric protein intolerance

In this disorder there is impaired absorption by the small intestine, liver and kidneys of the dibasic amino acids lysine, ornithine and arginine. Because peptide-bound lysine absorption is absent the patients present with severe failure to thrive, diarrhea, hepatosplenomegaly and mental retardation within the first 6 months of life. Hyperammonemia occurs following a protein load owing to the low level of urea cycle intermediates, and as a consequence treatment is with oral citrulline.

DISORDERS OF ELECTROLYTE AND MINERAL ABSORPTION

Congenital chloride diarrhea

This condition is characterized by severe watery diarrhea with hypochloremia, hypokalemia and metabolic alkalosis.[60] This autosomal recessive condition is characterized by a defect in Cl^-/HCO_3^+ transport in the ileum and colon with the resulting loss of large amounts of Cl^- in the stool. Na^+ is also lost in the stool and as a consequence the patients develop secondary hyperaldosteronism with urinary sparing of Na^+ and loss of K^+. This secretion starts in utero and is associated with maternal polyhydramnios which frequently results in premature delivery. In the neonatal period the presence of diarrhea may be missed leading to confusion with Bartter's syndrome in which the Cl^- loss is primarily renal and not intestinal. If the salt losses are not corrected the infant will become increasingly dehydrated and may die. Alkalosis is not present at birth and only develops over the subsequent weeks. Those infants who survive without adequate electrolyte replacement are invariably growth retarded with hypotonia and developmentally delayed as a consequence of chronic salt depletion.

The diagnosis is made from the high Cl^- content of the stool with levels > 90 mmol/L exceeding the sum of the Na^+ and K^+ concentrations. Blood gases will show a metabolic alkalosis, serum Cl^- and K^+ are low while the Na^+ level is likely to be normal. Urinary electrolytes will show very low or absent Na^+ and Cl^- excretion with markedly raised K^+ losses in the face of hypokalemia.

Treatment is with oral electrolyte supplements in the form of both NaCl and KCl given in amounts large enough to suppress the hyperaldosteronism, maintain urinary Cl^- excretion and correct the electrolyte deficiency. This treatment does not influence the diarrhea but results in the normal growth and development of the child.

Congenital sodium diarrhea

Diarrhea secondary to a defect of Na^+/H^+ exchange can present in newborn babies in a manner very similar to congenital chloride diarrhea.[61] The watery stools however contain more sodium than chloride and the child will develop a metabolic acidosis. Treatment with sodium citrate and oral rehydration solutions maintains fluid and electrolyte balance.

Acrodermatitis enteropathica

This is an autosomal recessive condition characterized by a specific defect in the absorption of zinc by the histologically normal small intestinal mucosa. The resulting zinc deficiency leads to a florid rash over the perineum (Fig. 17.10), buttocks and oral region with associated diarrhea, infection, alopecia and behavioral disturbance. The clinical features are reversed promptly by treatment with oral zinc supplements, which need to be taken life-long.

Primary hypomagnesemia

This autosomal recessive condition results from the defective absorption of magnesium by the small intestine and leads in the first few weeks of life to tetany and generalized convulsions associated with hypomagnesemia and hypocalcemia. On a normal diet the patient is in negative magnesium balance but this can be reversed by giving oral magnesium supplements. These supplements increase serum levels of both magnesium and calcium but unfortunately frequently induce diarrhea.

INVESTIGATION OF THE SMALL INTESTINE

A wide range of tests are available to look at the structure and function of the small intestine. Each test has its own specific indications and limitations and with the correct choice of investigations the maximum relevant information can be obtained with the minimum of invasive investigations.

RADIOLOGY

Plain abdominal X-ray is of value in detecting intestinal obstruction and the presence of free gas will also be seen if perforation has occurred. The barium follow-through or small bowel enema is the investigation of choice to define the anatomy of the small intestine and to demonstrate the gross mucosal pattern. This examination will define the rotation of the small intestine and allow the detection of blind loops, strictures and duplication cysts. Contrast studies are also invaluable in detecting small bowel involvement in Crohn's disease, intestinal polyps and infiltrative lesions of the small bowel such as non-Hodgkin's lymphoma.

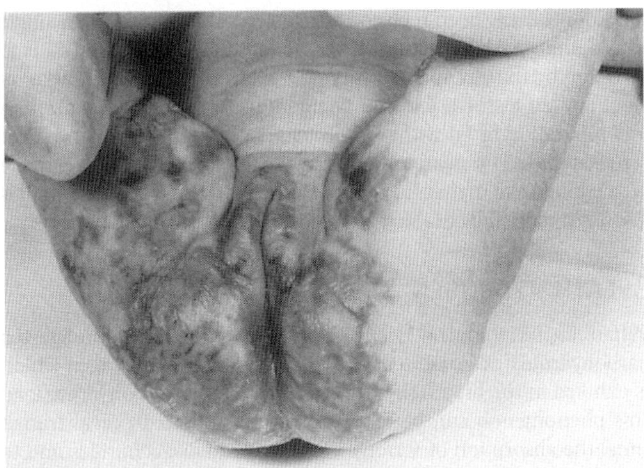

Fig. 17.10 The napkin area of a child with acrodermatitis enteropathica. (Reproduced by kind permission of PJ Milla)

The ectopic gastric mucosa in Meckel's diverticulum can be outlined with a technetium-99m pertechnetate scan and mucosal inflammation can be detected with the autologous labeling of leukocytes with technetium-99m hexametazime (HMPAO).

Celiac axis angiography is only very rarely required to define the site of intestinal hemorrhage from a vascular malformation.

SMALL INTESTINAL BIOPSY

The development of peroral small intestinal biopsy using the Watson or Crosby capsule in the late 1950s led to major advances in the diagnosis and management of small intestinal disease. This method has now been largely superceded by the use of upper gastrointestinal endoscopy for small bowel biopsy. Biopsies need to be taken from the distal second or third part of the duodenum in order to avoid the presence of Brunner's glands, which are found more proximally. This technique has the advantage that the area for biopsy can be directly visualized, other pathologies may be detected at endoscopy and with the development of small instruments, biopsies in preterm infants are now possible. A limitation is that biopsies tend to be small and more difficult to orientate but this problem can be largely overcome by taking multiple biopsies.

If the biopsy material is correctly stored it is possible to carry out the quantitative measurement of brush border disaccharides by histochemical methods, to characterize the infiltrate in the lamina propria with immunostaining, and with electron microscopy the characteristic lesion of microvillous atrophy can be seen.

Serial mucosal biopsy is also valuable in monitoring the therapeutic response to therapy.

NUTRIENT LOSS IN STOOL

Traditionally the loss of protein and fat in feces has been quantified by 5-day stool collections. Loss of protein labeled with chromium-51 albumin can be quantified by the measurement of radioactivity in the stool and the fat content can be directly measured. These techniques have now largely been replaced by simpler tests which rely on single stool samples. Alpha-1 antitrypsin is a protein which is resistant to digestion by the gut and excretion in the feces is a reliable marker of stool protein loss. Fat loss can be quantified by the homogenization and separation of fat within fecal material by centrifugation of spot stool samples. The steatocrit refers to the fat content as a percentage of the total solid matter in the stool. Carbohydrate loss in the stool is discussed more fully in the section on stool chromatography.

BREATH HYDROGEN

When bacteria in the colon come in contact with undigested carbohydrate it is fermented with the production of hydrogen which is exhaled in the breath. By the use of a suitable carbohydrate load this phenomenon can be used to measure mouth to cecal transit time, the absorption of a range of mono- and disaccharides and to detect colonization of the small intestine by bacteria.

Lactulose is a naturally occurring carbohydrate which is not absorbed or digested by the human small intestine but is readily fermented by colonic bacteria to produce hydrogen. Therefore the time between an oral dose (250 mg/kg) and a rise in the basal level of breath hydrogen is an indication of mouth to cecal transit time. If an oral load of glucose (2 g/kg) is given to a healthy fasting subject the monosaccharide should be completely absorbed by the small intestine and no breath hydrogen peak will occur. In a patient with glucose–galactose malabsorption the glucose will pass straight into the colon causing a large peak in breath hydrogen along with abdominal pain and diarrhea. Finally, in a patient with bacterial overgrowth the glucose will be fermented almost immediately it leaves the stomach producing a very brisk and early rise in breath hydrogen.

STOOL CHROMATOGRAPHY

Whenever a patient has osmotic diarrhea it is likely that the stool will contain sugars. While reducing sugars can be crudely detected using clinitest tablets, the quantification and characterization of these sugars by stool chromatography can be very useful, when taken along with the carbohydrate content of the child's feed or a specific oral load, in defining the cause of the underlying disorder. Two classic examples are the child with sucrase–isomaltase deficiency who, following the ingestion of complex carbohydrate, has loose stool containing limit dextrins, maltotriose and maltose and the baby with glucose–galactose malabsorption who, following a milk feed, has diarrhea containing glucose and galactose.

Specimens require immediate transport to the laboratory so that further digestion of sugars by colonic bacteria is prevented.

DUODENAL INTUBATION

When bacterial overgrowth is suspected, intubation with aspiration of duodenal juices is essential to confirm the diagnosis and define the sensitivities of the organisms present. Aspiration will similarly allow the concentration and pattern of luminal bile salts to be measured. The technique used to measure pancreatic function is described in the section on the pancreas.

GASTROINTESTINAL TUMORS

JUVENILE POLYPS

The most common polyp found in childhood is the juvenile polyp. These inflammatory lesions are found most frequently in the rectosigmoid but may develop more proximally and in 50% of cases more than one may be found. They present most frequently with painless rectal bleeding, in children between the ages of 2 and 5, although rarely they may present with recurrent abdominal pain and intussusception. These polyps do not undergo malignant change although if more than 10 lesions are seen, juvenile polyposis coli should be suspected. This condition can be differentiated from familial polyposis coli by the earlier age of onset and the presence of inflammatory, rather than adenomatous, polyps.

The diagnosis can be confirmed by flexible colonoscopy and at the same examination the polyps can be diathermied and removed for histological examination.

FAMILIAL ADENOMATOUS POLYPOSIS (FAP)

This autosomal dominant condition is characterized by multiple adenomatous polyps throughout the large intestine and is likely to present insidiously with diarrhea, blood and mucus in the stools. The polyps which generally appear after puberty, slowly enlarge with time until they invariably undergo malignant change.[62] The children of affected adults should be offered genetic screening and with the recognition of mutations in the FAP gene on chromosome 5q21 and the association with congenital hypertrophy of the retinal pigment epithelium (CHRPE), patients at high risk of developing the condition can be detected. Those at high risk require regular colonoscopic screening from the age of 12 years. Although the rate of polyp growth may be slowed by non-steroidal anti-inflammatory drugs, for the majority of individuals total colectomy in early adulthood is still the treatment of choice.

In Gardner's syndrome adenomatous polyps are seen throughout the gut in association with bone osteomas and epidermoid cysts.

PEUTZ–JEGHERS SYNDROME

In this autosomal dominant condition multiple hamartomatous polyps are distributed throughout the jejunum, ileum and large intestine of children in association with pigmentation of the oral mucosa and the skin of the perioral region, the digits and the anus. The condition presents with anemia owing to blood loss or with obstruction secondary to intussusception. Malignant change is thought not to occur.

PSEUDOPOLYPS

In response to any inflammatory reaction the intestinal mucosa may become swollen and a polyp-like structure will be formed. As a result of enteric infections or allergy, lymphoid hyperplasia of the ileum may occur and in conditions such as ulcerative colitis and Crohn's disease exuberant mucosal inflammation leads to pseudopolyp formation. The true nature of the lesions can be defined by mucosal biopsy.

HEMANGIOMAS

Intestinal hemangiomas which are frequently multiple are a well-recognized cause of rectal bleeding. Small colonic lesions can be sclerosed during endoscopic examination but laparotomy may be required for large angiomas and small intestinal lesions.

MALIGNANT TUMORS

Fortunately, malignant tumors of the intestine are very rare in childhood and in particular colonic and gastric neoplasms, which are so common in adult life, are hardly ever seen.

Small intestinal lymphoma of the non-Hodgkin's type is, however, occasionally seen. These tumors may be unifocal and present with obstruction or intussusception of the ileocecal region, or more commonly they are multifocal and present with ascites. Lymphoma is more likely to occur in children with immunodeficiency or following infection with the Epstein–Barr virus while in adults there is a clear association with untreated celiac disease. If a laparotomy is required for intestinal obstruction the diagnosis can be made from the histology of the resected specimen but under other circumstances bone marrow aspiration and cytological examination of ascitic fluid is required.

THE PANCREAS

CYSTIC FIBROSIS

Cystic fibrosis is an autosomal recessive condition which affects approximately 1 in every 2000 live Caucasian births.[63] The underlying defect results from one of a number of possible mutations, in a chloride transporter protein which lines ductular epithelium. This results in inspissation of mucus in the ducts of the pancreas and in the bronchial and biliary trees with the resulting development of pancreatic insufficiency, chronic respiratory disease and biliary cirrhosis. In this section discussion will be confined to the effects of cystic fibrosis on the pancreas and intestine[64] (Table 17.17) as the pulmonary (see Ch. 18) and hepatic (see p. 711) consequences are discussed elsewhere.

Pancreatic insufficiency

The inspissated concretions result in distension of the ducts and acini of the pancreas which with time progress to the formation of small cysts with destruction and fibrosis of the exocrine tissue. As a consequence of this the output of pancreatic enzymes and bicarbonate falls, leading to pancreatic insufficiency. In some patients endocrine pancreatic tissue is also damaged with the development of diabetes mellitus. Approximately 85% of patients with cystic fibrosis have pancreatic insufficiency with resulting malabsorption and steatorrhea, while in the remaining 15%, although not normal, the pancreas has adequate reserve capacity. Signs of pancreatic insufficiency are usually present within the first 2 years of life with the passage of foul, bulky pale stools. In the majority of untreated children, growth is abnormal and fat-soluble vitamin deficiencies are likely to develop.

Table 17.17 Gastrointestinal manifestations of cystic fibrosis

1. Pancreas
   a. Pancreatic insufficiency
   b. Pancreatitis
   c. Diabetes mellitus
2. Hepatobiliary
   a. Biliary cirrhosis
   b. Lobular cirrhosis
   c. Cholelithiasis
   d. Biliary obstruction
3. Intestinal
   a. Meconium ileus
   b. Rectal prolapse
   c. Intussusception
   d. Esophageal reflux
   e. Esophageal varicies
   f. Distal intestinal obstruction syndrome

As a consequence of chronic steatorrhea, bile salts are lost in the stool leading to depletion of the bile salt pool which may be further compounded if liver disease reduces the rate of synthesis. The resulting reduction in bile salt concentration will not only reduce the solubilization of lipids in the duodenum but may also reduce the solubilization of cholesterol and predispose to the formation of gallstones.

Meconium ileus

Cystic fibrosis may present in the first day or two of life with vomiting and abdominal distension due to meconium ileus. This obstruction to the small intestine with thick tenacious meconium may be complicated by volvulus, atresia or peritonitis. Plain abdominal X-ray will show dilated loops of intestine with meconium, outlined by trapped air, present in the obstructed segment of bowel and gastrografin enema will reveal a microcolon distal to the obstruction. The enema may be of benefit in the non-surgical clearance of the meconium (see Ch. 36).

Difficulty in passing stool may also lead to rectal prolapse.

Distal intestinal obstruction syndrome

This condition, which is sometimes also referred to as meconium ileus equivalent, is a common problem known to occur in up to 15% of patients with cystic fibrosis. It is most common in adolescence and is characterized by recurrent episodes of subacute or occasionally acute obstruction with abdominal pain, vomiting and anorexia. Marked fecal loading may be detected by abdominal palpation or plain abdominal X-ray. If treatment with laxatives fails, the use of mucolytic drugs or balanced intestinal lavage should be considered.

Diagnosis of cystic fibrosis

The main diagnostic test for cystic fibrosis is the sweat test which measures the increased sodium content found in the sweat of children with cystic fibrosis. The vast majority of healthy children have a sweat sodium less than 45 mmol/L while in cystic fibrosis it is greater than 74 mmol/L in 99% of cases. A modification of this test measures the sweat osmolality which is greater than 125 mOsmol/L in cystic fibrosis.

Many mutations have been described of the cystic fibrosis gene. If the patient's DNA is tested against the most common 20 mutations for the study population, it is possible to get a diagnostic accuracy of about 99%. Screening for cystic fibrosis in newborn babies can be carried out by heterozygote screening of mothers using genetic techniques or by immunoreactive trypsin measurement of a blood spot from a Guthrie card after birth.

Treatment

As far as the intestinal complications of cystic fibrosis are concerned the main treatment for pancreatic insufficiency is with oral pancreatic supplements. Although only 10% of normal lipase activity is required to prevent steatorrhea, the majority of ingested supplements are inactivated by the low pH of the stomach and as a consequence symptoms may persist. This may be overcome by incorporating the pancreatic supplements within a pH-sensitive microsphere. The dose required by each patient is likely to vary greatly, although an inadequate dose will result in a failure to relieve symptoms while an excessive dose may lead to perianal excoriation or some children may develop thickening of the colonic mucosa with the development of obstruction.

The nutritional intake of patients with cystic fibrosis is frequently less than recommended for their age and given that their requirements may be up to 40% above average, it is perhaps not surprising that many children grow poorly. With improved dietary advice and the use of nutritional supplements children with cystic fibrosis are now growing better and as a consequence they are surviving longer. Where supplements cannot be given enterally, nasogastric or gastrostomy feeding may be helpful. Oral fat-soluble vitamin supplements, in particular vitamin E, are also required.

SHWACHMAN'S SYNDROME

After cystic fibrosis, Shwachman's syndrome is probably the next most common cause of pancreatic insufficiency in childhood.[63] This autosomal recessive condition is characterized by the presence of neutropenia with impairment of neutrophil function. The neutropenia may occur cyclically as may the thrombocytopenia which is seen in two-thirds of patients. Arrest in proliferation of the myeloid series may be seen on bone marrow aspiration and leukemic transformation has been reported in a number of patients. Bony abnormalities with metaphyseal chondrodysplasia are frequently seen with involvement of the femoral neck.

The diagnosis should be considered in any child with pancreatic insufficiency, a normal sweat test and neutropenia. Treatment is with pancreatic supplements and fat soluble vitamins and where symptomatic neutropenia persists, the use of human granulocyte colony stimulating factor should be considered. The patients are particularly prone to recurrent infections and antibiotic prophylaxis may be of some benefit.

ACUTE AND CHRONIC PANCREATITIS

Pancreatitis is uncommon in childhood and frequently when it does occur no obvious precipitating cause can be found. Obstruction to the pancreatic duct, loss of vascular integrity and a direct insult to the parenchymal cells are all factors which can lead to the development of pancreatitis. Trauma, frequently as a consequence of child abuse, is one of the commonest causes of acute pancreatitis[65] while hereditary causes are the most common reason for chronic pancreatitis.[66] Some hereditary cases may be due to a defect which prevents the inactivation of pancreatic trypsin with resulting autodigestion. The causes of pancreatitis are listed in Table 17.18

Table 17.18 Causes of pancreatitis

1. Acute
   a. Trauma
   b. Infections
      (i) Mumps
      (ii) Coxsackie
      (iii) Leptospira
      (iv) Ascaris
   c. Gallstones
   d. Drugs
      (i) Valproic acid
      (ii) Cytosine arabinoside
      (iii) L-asparaginase
   e. Inflammatory bowel disease
   f. Metabolic
      (i) Reye's syndrome
      (ii) Refeeding malnutrition
      (iii) Parenteral nutrition
   g. Vasculitis
   h. Duodenal ulcer
   i. Idiopathic
2. Chronic
   a. Hereditary
   b. Metabolic
      (i) Hyperlipidemia
      (ii) Hyperparathyroidism
      (iii) Cystic fibrosis
   c. Duct malformations
   d. Idiopathic

Presentation

Attacks of pancreatitis are characterized by severe epigastric or umbilical pain which tends to be constant rather than colicky and which can radiate to the back or shoulders. The pain is exacerbated by food and is not relieved by antacids. The patient will find abdominal movement uncomfortable and if the pancreatitis is severe, hemorrhagic bruising of the flanks with a paralytic ileus may develop. When the course is prolonged the condition may be complicated by circulatory collapse, hyperglycemia, hypocalcemia or by the formation of pleural effusions and pancreatic pseudocysts. The diagnosis is confirmed by markedly raised levels of serum amylase.

Treatment

The management of acute pancreatitis is conservative. All oral feeds should be stopped and intravenous fluids should be given to correct any fluid losses and to provide normal requirements. Acute pancreatitis can be very painful requiring adequate analgesia and where the patient is vomiting a nasogastric tube should be passed. An acute attack will normally last for between 3 and 5 days but if the attack is more prolonged total parenteral nutrition should be started and treatment with a somatostatin analogue should be considered. The patient should be monitored for the development of complications and serial abdominal ultrasounds will allow fluid collections to be detected at an early stage. Pseudocysts which fail to resolve spontaneously require to be drained.

In both acute and chronic pancreatitis if an underlying cause has been defined, this should be appropriately treated. Where a duct abnormality has been isolated reconstructive surgery may be of benefit and if a localized area of the pancreas is responsible for recurrent attacks, a partial pancreatectomy should be considered.

INVESTIGATION OF THE PANCREAS

The most commonly used indirect measure of pancreatic function in childhood is the sweat test which was discussed in the section on cystic fibrosis (see p. 677). The remaining investigations can be divided into blood tests which measure the level of pancreatic enzymes (i.e. amylase), tests which measure fecal fat or enzyme activity, more direct measures of pancreatic function and radiological imaging methods.

Pancreatic function tests

These tests can be divided into the traditional tests which require duodenal intubation and the newer tubeless function tests. The traditional tests remain the most accurate although they are also the most invasive. They involve the collection of duodenal juice during a basal fasting period followed by the stimulation of the pancreas with cholecystokinin (1–2 IU/kg) and then secretin (1–2 IU/kg) with the further collection of duodenal juice. In pancreatic insufficiency the stimulated levels of lipase and trypsin are reduced and the juice fails to alkalinize following stimulation with secretin. The tubeless tests rely on the pancreatic enzymes cleaving an ingested compound (bentiromide or fluorescein dilaurate) and the amount subsequently collected in the urine is a measure of pancreatic function.

Stool elastase activity is a non-invasive measure of pancreatic function which although not as accurate as the intubation technique described above, is easy to carry out. Pancreatic lipase activity can also be indirectly measured by the labeling of a fatty substrate with C^{13} and measuring the appearance of the stable isotope in the breath.

Radiology

Ultrasound is a very useful non-invasive imaging method in pancreatitis as it will show pancreatic edema during the acute attack, outline any fluid collections and allow gallbladder disease to be excluded. Where more detailed imaging is required of the structure of the pancreas, computerized tomographic (CT) techniques using X-ray and magnetic resonance imaging (MRI) may be used. In chronic pancreatitis where imaging of the pancreatic ducts is required to exclude a malformation or stricture, endoscopic retrograde cholangiopancreatography (ERCP) or magnetic resonance cholangiopancreatography (MRCP) can be used. Any abnormality of the structure of the duodenum will be seen on a barium study.

DISORDERS OF GASTROINTESTINAL MOTILITY

Disorders of gastrointestinal motility are very common in childhood and are responsible for such diverse conditions as gastroesophageal reflux, the irritable bowel syndrome and chronic constipation.[67] Normal contractile activity relies on the coordinated action of the intestinal smooth muscle, its enteric and central neural connections and the humoral environment of the gut. Diseases exist in which damage to the enteric nervous system (Hirschsprung's disease) or smooth muscle (familial visceral myopathy) severely compromises the luminal transit of food and present with the symptoms of intestinal obstruction. The central nervous system has an important role in the modulation of intestinal motility with central insults commonly resulting in vomiting or even paralytic ileus. Lesser disturbances such as stress may lead to vomiting, abdominal pain and diarrhea.

ESOPHAGUS AND STOMACH

Motility disorders of the esophagus and stomach have already been discussed in their respective sections (pp. 657 and 662).

INTESTINAL PSEUDO-OBSTRUCTION

Intestinal pseudo-obstruction is a clinical syndrome characterized by the signs and symptoms of intestinal obstruction in a patient without any evidence of an obstructing lesion. Pseudo-obstruction occurs most commonly as a primary disorder in childhood; it may be familial, but may occasionally present in adolescence as a secondary manifestation of some other disease such as diabetes mellitus. The disorder tends to be generalized, involving either the smooth muscle or the enteric nerves of the entire length of the intestine.

A quarter of children present at birth and by 1 year two-thirds have developed symptoms of abdominal distension, vomiting, constipation and failure to thrive. Frequently it is only after laparotomy that the condition is diagnosed. Associated abnormalities of the urinary tract such as megacystis and megaureter are found in some patients and an association with malrotation of the small intestine has been reported. Diagnosis can be made from the history and from intestinal manometry which shows either a disruption or loss of cyclical fasting motor activity. A full thickness biopsy is required for a definitive diagnosis.

The condition is complicated by bacterial overgrowth of the small intestine and is punctuated by repeated episodes of obstruction. In some patients this can be significantly improved by the formation of a defunctioning ileostomy. Nutrition is frequently compromised and in the most severe cases survival without total parenteral nutrition may not be possible.

LARGE INTESTINE

Colonic motility disorders will present in the neonatal period with the delayed passage of meconium and symptoms of intestinal obstruction if severe, or may be delayed for many months or years when they are more likely to present with chronic constipation. Hirschsprung's disease (see Ch. 36), hypo- and hyperganglionosis are now all well-recognized entities but unfortunately the nature of the structural or functional disorder in children with chronic constipation due to other causes is less well defined.

Treatment is symptomatic with oral laxatives in milder cases. In more severe cases, regular enemas may be required and in some patients the use of regular intestinal lavage through a continent cecostomy is effective. Where these techniques fail a defunctioning stoma or resection of the affected bowel may be required.

ACUTE INFECTIVE DIARRHEA

Acute infective diarrhea is one of the major causes of morbidity and mortality in childhood in the world today, killing up to 3 million children each year. In developed countries each child under 5 years has one to two episodes each year and over 10% of all hospital admissions in this age group are with acute diarrhea. In developing countries the much higher incidence of diarrheal illness is a consequence of the combined effect of contaminated water supplies, the preparation of bottle feeds under unhygienic conditions and from malnutrition which frequently occurs in these children at the time of weaning.

Most acute diarrheal illnesses in well-nourished children are self-limiting and resolve within a few days. However, when frequent reinfection occurs, the child may develop a state of chronic diarrhea which will inevitably result in further malnutrition and an increased susceptibility to recurrent infection. It is this vicious cycle of events which along with the acute effects of dehydration leads to the significant mortality from this condition in developing countries.

ETIOLOGY AND PATHOGENESIS

The infective agent in acute diarrhea cannot always be isolated but with improvements in diagnostic techniques a pathogen can be isolated in up to 80% of cases. Viral agents are the most common cause of acute infective diarrhea in childhood, followed by bacteria and then protozoal infection. The causes of acute infective diarrhea are shown in Table 17.19.

In the young infant who is most at risk from the complications of acute diarrhea a number of protective mechanisms exist to limit the effect of infective pathogens. The acid content of the stomach and IgA secreted by the small intestine and in breast milk will limit the growth of bacteria in the upper small intestine and the resulting predominance of bifidobacteria in feces may inhibit colonization by enteric pathogens. These factors all lead to a reduced incidence of

Table 17.19 Causes of acute infective diarrhea

Viruses
Rotavirus
Astrovirus
Adenovirus
Parvovirus-like (i.e. Norwalk agent)
Coronavirus
Bacteria
Campylobacter sp.
Salmonella sp.
Escherichia coli
Shigella sp.
Yersinia enterocolitica
Vibrio cholerae
Clostridium difficile
Protozoa
Giardia lamblia
Cryptosporidium
Entamoeba histolytica

acute enteric infection in breast-fed infants. Modification of the intestinal flora with probiotics may be of benefit both in preventing and reducing the severity of acute infective diarrhea.[68]

Viral infection

The agent most commonly responsible for acute infantile gastroenteritis is the rotavirus. The rotavirus selectively attacks the mature enterocytes at the tips of the small intestinal villi which are killed and shed into the lumen. This leads to the increased production of immature crypt-like cells with shortening of the villi. These cells have greatly reduced absorptive and disaccharidase activity and this loss of normal small intestinal function combined with the active secretion of fluids and electrolytes, leads to the production of diarrhea. Following the clearance of the viral pathogen the functional mucosal abnormalities resolve.

Bacterial infection

Four major mechanisms are responsible for the effects of bacterial pathogens. Organisms such as *Vibrio cholerae* and some strains of *Escherichia coli* synthesize proteins called enterotoxins which are able to promote intestinal secretion. The preservation of electrogenic sodium-linked solute cotransport in these patients is exploited by the use of sodium- and glucose-containing oral rehydration solutions (ORS) which are able to promote net intestinal absorption in the face of active secretion.

Enteropathogenic organisms such as some strains of *E. coli* adhere to the brush border membrane of the small intestine causing severe mucosal damage which may take many weeks to recover and such children may require parenteral nutritional support during the intervening period. *Shigella* species and *E. coli* serotypes O124 and O164 possess enteroinvasive properties leading to the development of watery diarrhea and dysentery with bacterial invasion of the colonic mucosa, while some bacteria, such as *Clostridium difficile* also produce cytotoxins, which have a direct toxic effect on enterocytes.

CLINICAL FEATURES

Acute infective diarrhea characteristically results in a combination of nausea, vomiting, abdominal pain and diarrhea. In some children the symptoms may be relatively trivial while in others dehydration and metabolic disturbances may be life threatening. Symptoms appear generally to be most severe in younger and in malnourished infants who also run the risk of becoming septicemic with some bacterial pathogens. Bloody diarrhea frequently occurs in *Shigella, Salmonella, Campylobacter* and *E. coli* O157 infection. In children infected with *E. coli* O157 monitoring for signs of hemolytic uremic syndrome (HUS) and renal failure are required, particularly those under the age of 5 years who are most vulnerable to this complication. Diarrhea and vomiting may also occur in a number of other medical conditions and it is important to consider systemic infection, metabolic disorders, surgical problems and other gastrointestinal disorders in the differential diagnosis of such patients.

The most serious consequence of acute diarrhea and vomiting is dehydration. The severity of the dehydration (see Table 17.20), which can be assessed clinically, determines the best treatment for the child. Children on high solute diets, who develop diarrhea, may develop hypernatremic dehydration in which case the signs of dehydration are less obvious although lethargy and irritability may develop earlier.

Loss of bicarbonate and potassium in the stool, poor tissue perfusion, hypoglycemia, ketosis and renal failure may all lead to severe metabolic derangement. Symptoms of lethargy and irritability are particularly marked in hypernatremic dehydration and its rapid correction with i.v. fluids may lead to cerebral edema as a result of fluid shifts across the blood–brain barrier. This can result in convulsions or even death.

MANAGEMENT

The management of children with acute infective diarrhea hinges upon the treatment of their dehydration. The treatment required depends very much on the severity of their dehydration and on the facilities which are available. Most mild cases can be treated at home by their family practitioner with ORS but where dehydration is more severe, social circumstances are poor or where other complicating medical factors are present, hospital admission is required. Even in moderate dehydration, ORS remains the treatment of choice although this therapy is underused in developed countries, where intravenous therapy is often used inappropriately.[69] Additionally one has to consider how best to feed these infants during both the acute and recovery phase of their illness. Generally drug therapy has no role in the management of acute diarrhea.

Oral rehydration therapy

The management of acute diarrhea was revolutionized by the introduction of ORS over 30 years ago. This treatment continues to be the mainstay of therapy and by preventing the patient becoming dehydrated, it has greatly reduced the morbidity and mortality. While most children with acute diarrhea will have active intestinal secretion, their ability to absorb fluid and electrolytes is largely preserved.

Table 17.20 Assessment of the severity of dehydration

	No dehydration	5% Dehydration	10%+ Dehydration
Condition	Well, alert	Restless, irritable	Lethargic, unconscious
Eyes	Normal	Sunken	Very sunken and dry
Tears	Present	Absent	Absent
Mouth and tongue	Moist	Dry	Very dry
Thirst	Not thirsty	Thirsty, drinks eagerly	Drinks poorly
Skin pinch	Goes back quickly	Goes back slowly	Goes back very slowly

As outlined in Figure 17.6, the absorption of sodium and glucose across the luminal surface of the enterocyte is facilitated by a transmembrane cotransport system. Solutions containing sodium and glucose in an optimum concentration are absorbed at an accelerated rate and where this is greater than the fluid losses incurred by the diarrheal process, dehydration can be prevented. It must be remembered that ORS does not stop the diarrhea and this is probably one of the reasons why its acceptance in developed countries is sometimes poor, as parents want any treatment to be a 'quick fix' to their child's problems.

The main recommendations for the treatment of acute diarrhea have come from the World Health Organization (WHO).[70] Their oral rehydration solution contained 111 mmol/L of glucose and 90 mmol/L of sodium (see Table 17.21). There has however been concern that in developed countries where cholera is an uncommon cause of diarrhea, this sodium concentration is too high and a concentration of 60 mmol/L has been suggested by the European Society for Pediatric Gastroenterology and Nutrition.[71] It has also recently been shown that the traditional ORS which has a slightly hyperosmolar osmolality of 311 mOsmol/L may not be as effective as solutions with a lower osmolality of 210–260 mOsmol/L. This has resulted in revised recommendations by the WHO suggesting that rehdration solutions should contain 75 mmol/L of sodium and 75 mmol/L of glucose with a resulting osmolality of 245 mOsmol/L.[72] It must be remembered that fruit juices and colas are entirely unsuitable as ORS as they contain large amounts of sugar and very small amounts of electrolytes.

Fluid replacement therapy

When assessing how best to treat a child with infective diarrhea one should first assess the severity of the patient's dehydration (see Table 17.20). The majority of children presenting for medical attention in developed countries are not yet dehydrated and the aim of treatment should be to prevent this occurring. Such children are often reluctant to take ORS and normal age appropriate diet should be continued. Unweaned infants should continue either with breast-feeding or undiluted formula feed. The diet of older children should contain complex carbohydrate and meat but large amounts of fat or simple sugars should be avoided. There is increasing evidence that not only is the continued use of diet safe in children with infective diarrhea but through the trophic effect on the intestinal mucosa, a more rapid recovery of symptoms is promoted.[73]

Children who are dehydrated and not shocked should be rapidly rehydrated with ORS. They should receive 50 ml/kg in the first 4 h with an additional 10 ml/kg for each stool and supplements for any vomiting. In the more severely dehydrated child up to 100 ml/kg can be given in the first 4 h. By giving frequent small sips, vomiting can be reduced. If the child will not take adequate volumes of ORS administration by nasogastric tube is preferable to intravenous administration in the non-shocked child who is not vomiting. Once the child is rehydated, normal diet should be resumed as for the non-dehydrated child.

Intravenous rehydration is required if the patient is shocked or where repeated vomiting prevents adequate oral rehydration. The shocked patient should receive 20–40 ml/kg boluses of normal saline until the signs of shock resolve. ORS should be introduced at the earliest opportunity to continue the rehydration of the patient and food intake should be started as soon as it is likely to be tolerated. If continued intravenous rehydration is required, a 5% deficit should be corrected over 24 h and a 10% deficit (Table 17.20) over 48 h with a 0.45% saline/dextrose solution.

Other therapies

Generally antibiotics have no place in the management of acute infective diarrhea, the exception being *Shigella, Vibrio cholerae, Clostridium difficule* and *Giardia*. Similarly antimotility drugs, many of which are opiate derivatived, should not be given. There is now increasing evidence that probiotic therapy is beneficial in the treatment of acute infective diarrhea. A large European multicenter study has shown that *Lactobacillus rhamnosus* strain GG given with ORS, reduces the length of diarrhea and the time of hospital stay.[68]

Complications

Acute infective diarrhea may be complicated by the extraintestinal spread of the infection with the development of intestinal perforation, abscess formation, septicemia and meningitis. If dehydration is pronounced acute renal failure may develop and if hypernatremia is corrected too rapidly cerebral edema with convulsions is likely to occur. This complication is less common when ORS is used as fluid shifts occur more slowly. In some children severe damage to the intestinal mucosa will lead to the development of diarrhea which persists long after the original pathogen has been cleared.

CONCLUSIONS

There have been many changes and advancements in the management of acute infective diarrhea in the last 10 years. There is clear agreement that ORS is the preferred method of rehydration, that diet should be introduced at an early stage and that drugs have very little role in the treatment of this problem.[74] These points are summarized in Table 17.22.

PROTRACTED DIARRHEA IN EARLY INFANCY

Protracted diarrhea may be defined as the passage of four or more watery stools per day persisting for at least 2 weeks.[2] This definition

Table 17.21 Major constituents of appropriate oral rehydration solutions (mmol/L) compared to inappropriate preparations

	Glucose (or other sugar)	Sodium	Potassium	Base	Osmolality
WHO (original)	110	90	20	30	311
ESPGHAN	74–111	60	20	10	225–260
WHO (revised 2001)	75	75	20	10	245
Solution **NOT** *suitable for ORS*					
Cola	700	2	0	13	750
Apple Juice	690	3	32	0	730

WHO, World Health Organization; ESPGHAN, European Society for Paediatric Gastroenterology, Hepatology and Nutrition.

Table 17.22 Principles of treatment of acute gastroenteritis (Adapted from Szajewska et al 2000[74])

1. Use of ORS for dehydration
2. Use hypotonic ORS, Na 60–75 mmol/L (see Table 17.21)
3. Fast oral rehydration, over 3–4 h
4. Rapid realimentation with normal feeding thereafter
5. Use of special formula is unjustified
6. Use of diluted formula is unjustified
7. Continuation of breast-feeding at all times
8. Supplementation of ORS for ongoing losses
9. No unnecessary medications

ORS, oral rehydration solution

encompasses a wide variety of disorders (Table 17.23) and a definitive diagnosis may only be made in approximately 70% of cases. In most instances, the protracted diarrhea appears to follow an episode of acute gastroenteritis in early infancy, although by the time of presentation to hospital it may be impossible to isolate an infective agent from the stool. Furthermore, unless the situation is managed effectively at an early stage, a cycle of malabsorption and malnutrition may result which will further compromise intestinal function and perpetuate the diarrhea.

One proposed sequence of events is that an acute infective insult may sensitize the intestine to foreign proteins (usually cow's milk protein), and subsequent ingestion of the offending food antigen causes further damage to the intestinal mucosa thus continuing the diarrhea (see also Ch. 31). Although the resulting enteropathy may be caused primarily by the protein content of the milk feed, disaccharide intolerance (particularly lactose) may also develop and the institution of an appropriate exclusion diet will often result in resolution of the diarrhea. In this situation, an exclusion diet may be necessary only for 2 or 3 months after which a normal weaning diet can be reintroduced. In some cases, particularly in the developing world, bacterial overgrowth of the small intestine may be an added complication and bacterial toxins themselves may impair mucosal function.

Celiac disease, cystic fibrosis, selective inborn errors of absorption and immunodeficiency states may all present with intractable diarrhea of infancy. These conditions are discussed elsewhere in this chapter.

Table 17.23 Causes of protracted diarrhea in early infancy

1. Food sensitivity/postenteritis syndrome
2. Cystic fibrosis
3. Celiac disease
4. Microvillus inclusion disease
5. Congenital chloride losing diarrhea
6. Congenital short bowel
7. Inborn error of carbohydrate absorption
   a. Sucrase–isomaltase deficiency
   b. Glucose–galactose malabsorption
8. Immunodeficiency
9. Hormone-secreting tumor (i.e. VIPoma)
10. Autoimmune enteropathy
11. Bacterial overgrowth
12. Non-accidental injury (laxative administration)
13. Idiopathic

Less common causes include autoimmune enteropathy while in some children there may be a family history suggesting an inborn error as a causative factor. A proportion of these infants may suffer from congenital chloride losing diarrhea or intestinal microvillus inclusion disease.[52] Where intestinal secretion is present in utero there may be a history of polyhydramnios or premature labor.

INVESTIGATIONS

Collection and examination of the stool is vital and a careful search for intestinal pathogens (bacteria, viruses, parasites) should be undertaken at an early stage. The stools should be analyzed for the presence of reducing substances (> 1%) and stool electrolytes and osmolality should be measured to determine whether the diarrhea is osmotic or secretory in nature (Table 17.24). Chromatography of a fresh stool specimen may help in the diagnosis of inborn errors of carbohydrate absorption and in determining the osmotically active substances within the stool. Valuable information may also be obtained by fasting the child as this is likely to result in a marked diminution of osmotic diarrhea with little change in secretory diarrhea. It is essential to collect and measure the volume of all stools as this will influence the amount and the nature of fluid replacement therapy.

Jejunal biopsy is invaluable in detailing the morphology of the small intestinal epithelium and a sweat test can rule out cystic fibrosis. Blood tests are of limited value although peripheral blood eosinophilia may be present in children with food protein sensitivity and investigation of immune function may reveal specific abnormalities in the child with diarrhea due to immunodeficiency. Measurement of electrolytes and acid–base balance is important in the day-to-day management of fluid balance and may be abnormal in children with congenital chloride-losing diarrhea. If the cause of the diarrhea is not immediately evident serum should be sent for gut-autoantibody estimation to exclude gut autoimmune disease, and circulating gut hormones should be measured to exclude a hormone-secreting tumor. Serum and urine toxicology should be checked if laxative abuse by the mother is suspected.

Radiological studies are rarely informative but barium meal and follow-through will exclude malrotation and may occasionally demonstrate a blind loop. Endoscopic evaluation of the upper and lower gastrointestinal tract is often helpful and multiple biopsies may be taken for examination by light and electron microscopy in addition to obtaining fluid from the lumen of the gut, which should be screened for the presence of pathogens.

TREATMENT

The management of the infant with protracted diarrhea depends on the cause and the severity of the condition. In many cases dietary manipulation is the mainstay of management as appropriate exclusion diets often reduce the volume of diarrhea. A variety of hypoallergenic feeds may be appropriate either as a complete feed (e.g. Nutramigen, Mead Johnson, and Neocate, Scientific Hospital

Table 17.24 Stool analysis in osmotic and secretory diarrhea

	Osmotic	Secretory
Osmolality (mOsmol/L)	400	290
Na^+ (mmol/L)	30	105
K^+ (mmol/L)	30	40
$(Na^+ + K^+) \times 2$	120	290
Solute gap (mmol/L)	280	0

Supplies) or as a modular feed (e.g. comminuted chicken, Cow & Gate) when the protein, carbohydrate and fat contents of the diet can be varied independently. The assistance of an experienced pediatric dietitian is essential in the management of any infant with protracted diarrhea. Those infants who are severely malnourished or who do not respond to enteral feeding and dietetic management may, in addition, need a period of intravenous feeding. If this fails to resolve the problem, long-term parenteral nutrition or even gut transplantation need to be considered.

In certain situations drug therapy may be beneficial. If there is evidence of bacterial overgrowth and bile salt degradation, colestyramine and antibiotics may help the situation. Antisecretory agents such as chlorpromazine, octreotide and loperamide may be beneficial in some cases where the primary pathology is not reversible.

In general terms, for those children who present several weeks or months after birth the prognosis is good, while for those who present at birth with an intractable secretory diarrhea the prognosis is poor and the mortality high.

INTESTINAL FAILURE

DEFINITION AND PREVALENCE

Intestinal failure is defined as the inability of the alimentary tract to digest and absorb sufficient nutrients to maintain normal growth and health. Acute intestinal failure is relatively common and self-limiting as in, for example, surgical treatment for an ileal atresia, or an episode of rotavirus gastroenteritis. Chronic intestinal failure resulting in dependence on intravenous feeding/parenteral nutrition is less common and is variously defined as intestinal failure persisting for 4 or 6 or 8 weeks. A survey by the British Paediatric Surveillance Unit (BSPU) of the UK in 1995 identified 54 children who had been on parenteral nutrition (PN) for more than 8 weeks. The annual incidence of children dependent on PN for up to 4 weeks in order to recover from major illness or surgery is likely to be 10 times larger since the pharmacy records at one large regional English hospital (Birmingham Children's Hospital) showed that over 200 infants and children received PN for at least 7 days during 1995 when the BPSU survey was carried out. Whatever the precise number of children affected, the prevalence of treated intestinal failure appears to be increasing as illustrated by the year 2000 report of the British Artificial Nutrition Survey (BANS) in which 80 children from 14 centers were identified as being managed at home on PN. The administration of PN either at home or in hospital is complex with many potential, even life threatening, complications, which means that patients with intestinal failure benefit from early referral to a multidisciplinary team experienced in the management of this highly technical therapy.[75–77]

ETIOLOGY

The vast range in functions and huge physical dimensions of the gastrointestinal system, mean that the possible causes of intestinal failure are numerous and often overlap with disorders in other systems. Broadly, there are three categories of intestinal failure: disorders related to reduced surface area or intestinal mass (e.g. short gut syndrome), disorders of motility (e.g. Hirschsprung's disease) and disorders of the mucosa (e.g. microvillus inclusion disease) (Table 17.25). Intestinal failure may be caused by a primary disease of the gastrointestinal tract or it may be secondary to disease in other systems (e.g. immunodeficiency).

Clinical presentation at different ages

Congenital

Intestinal failure may present antenatally or in the neonatal period where it tends to have a congenital cause. Polyhydramnios is an important sign common in conditions in which the gastrointestinal tract produces excess secretions as in microvillus inclusion disease or in a glucose/galactose transporter defect. The antenatal ultrasound may show distended loops of bowel as early as 20 weeks' gestation in babies who develop features of pseudo-obstruction, and gastroschisis can be diagnosed from 12 to 14 weeks' gestation. Antenatal diagnosis is important as it allows the parents to be prepared and for delivery to take place in a unit with rapid access to a neonatal surgical facility.

The cardinal symptoms of intestinal failure are vomiting (with or without bile), abdominal distension, protracted diarrhea, and constipation. These symptoms will be rapidly followed by dehydration, weight loss, shock and renal failure (Table 17.26). Perhaps the most sinister symptom in babies is that of a secretory diarrhea such as occurs in microvillus inclusion disease. In this condition large volume watery diarrhea is uninfluenced by restricted intake. Such diarrhea which has the appearance of water, can be mistaken for urine, with the result that the severity of illness is not recognized until renal failure develops. Another diagnostic pitfall is when the symptoms are intermittent as can occur in midgut malrotation and which may present at any age with pain and vomiting with spontaneous remissions when the associated volvulus untwists and frees the mesenteric blood supply. Once a midgut volvulus is recognized it is usual to proceed to a laparotomy

Table 17.25 Causes of intestinal failure. Examples in brackets (also see Table 17.23)

	Primary gastrointestinal disorders	Secondary gastrointestinal disorders
Reduced surface area or mass	Gastroschisis, small bowel atresia Mid-gut volvulus, necrotizing enterocolitis Crohn's disease	Gardener's syndrome Meconium ileus equivalent (cystic fibrosis) Vascular accident (mesenteric artery thrombosis)
Motility disorder	Aganglionosis (Hirschsprung's disease) Megacystis microcolon syndrome	Tumors secreting vasoactive substances (VIPoma) Inappropriate use of purgatives (Munchausen by proxy)
Mucosal lesion	Microvillus inclusion disease Abnormal electrolyte or solute transporters Congenital disaccharidase deficiency Lymphangiectasia Enteropathies (celiac disease, autoimmune) Crohn's disease	Postgastroenteritis viral disease (rotavirus) Ischemia reperfusion injury after cardiac bypass Mucositis secondary to chemotherapy Graft-versus-host disease Immune deficiency (see also Table 17.14)

Table 17.26 Symptoms and signs of intestinal failure

Early	Late
Polyhydramnios	Weight loss
Vomiting	Malabsorption (see also Table 17.11)
Diarrhea	Food aversion
Perineal ulceration	Micronutrient deficiency including zinc
Abdominal distension (and pain)	Water and fat soluble vitamin deficiency
Weight loss	Abdominal pain (colicky)
Electrolyte imbalance	Edema
Convulsions	Opportunistic infection

and Ladds procedure which fixes the bowel and prevents future volvulus and ischemia of the midgut.

Malabsorption may be the predominant problem in children with short gut or mucosal disorders; this is manifested by diarrhea which is exacerbated by feeding. Clinical signs of malabsorption include: excoriated perineum secondary to carbohydrate malabsorption; edema secondary to protein losing enteropathy and bulky offensive stools secondary to fat malabsorption.

The presence of opportunistic infections such *Candida* species and *Cryptosporidium parvum* should raise the possibility of immune deficiency either primary or acquired as a result of infection by human immunodeficiency virus. Granulomas may be present on mucosal biopsy which may suggest an autoimmune enteropathy if Crohn's disease and mycobacterial infection have been excluded.

Acquired

During infancy and childhood the causes of intestinal failure are usually of an acquired nature such as trauma and food antigen intolerance (celiac disease usually presents from 9 months of age and older). Munchausen's by proxy is an important diagnosis to consider in a child whose symptoms were not apparent until months or years after birth and in whom the disease appears to be relentlessly progressive despite visits to more than one expert center. Usually such cases do not have a clear diagnosis, but have been labeled 'atypical pseudo-obstruction' or 'protracted diarrhea'.

INVESTIGATIONS

A detailed history and examination including height, weight, midarm circumference, triceps skin fold and head circumference should be carried out. Blood and urine tests should be done with the aim of identifying the extent of illness, devising a management plan and to make a diagnosis (Table 17.27). In addition radiology, histopathology and evaluation of intestinal motility[78] are key investigations in arriving at a diagnosis.

Table 17.27 Investigations in intestinal failure: acute (less than 4 weeks old); chronic (more than 4 weeks old)

		Acute (less than 4 weeks old)	Chronic (more than 4 weeks old)
Key clinical facts to be elicited		Vomiting related to feeding or not Bile present in vomitus? Presence of pain Nature of diarrhea: watery, offensive, blood present?	Symptoms are static, improving worsening? Which is the dominant symptom? Does the diarrhea reduce when nil by mouth (osmotic), or is it similar in fasting and fed state (secretory)
Biochemistry	Blood	Electrolytes, chloride, acid base, amylase	Liver function tests, parathyroid hormone
	Urine	Acidification, laxative screen	Urinary sodium : potassium ratio
	Stool	Microscopy including electron microscopy Culture, ELISA test for rotavirus Reducing substances, electrophoresis Chymotrypsin, steatocrits	Stool electrolytes (? sodium losing diarrhea; see also Table 17.24) Intestinal transit time by the appearance of orally administered pigment in stool (e.g. Carmine red) Fecal alpha-1 antitrypsin concentration
Hematology		Full blood count (polycythemia ?dehydrated) blood film (?fragmented cells as in hemolytic uremic syndrome)	Full blood count, anemia, also note neutropenia (Shwachman's syndrome), lymphopenia (lymphangiectasia) Coagulation profile (? vitamin K malabsorption)
Radiology		Plain abdominal X-ray (gas pattern, intramural gas?, calcification) Abdominal ultrasound to identify cystic lesions, e.g. pancreatic pseudocyst	Small bowel contrast study (provides information about malrotation, reflux, motility disorders) Scintiscanning (gastric emptying) Venogram if difficulty with central venous access
Manometry			Esophageal, upper small bowel and rectal manometry, depending on likely site of lesion
Histopathology		Mucosal biopsy Full thickness biopsy of large bowel and proximal bowel if indicated	Duodenal or jejunal tissue for dissacharidase measurement Liver biopsy, repeat intestinal mucosal biopsy

MANAGEMENT

Multidisciplinary team

Children with intestinal failure will require urgent resuscitation, initially rehydration with saline and glucose and usually followed by PN if it is clear that intestinal failure is either life threatening or likely to persist for some weeks. Most hospitals have guidelines for prescribing PN which should avoid over- and underprovision of calories since both can cause fatty liver and liver dysfunction. After initial resuscitation a team consisting of dietitian, specialist nurse, pharmacist, pediatric gastroenterologist, radiologist and surgeon should establish the diagnosis, prognosis and plan treatment. For patients with a purely medical cause for intestinal failure, the role of the surgeon will be limited to careful placement of central venous feeding catheters to minimize trauma to major veins and the superior vena cava in particular. However, patients with short gut will require frequent review by the multidisciplinary team as the maturing and adapting intestine becomes capable of greater volumes of feed which may need to be enhanced with trophic agents (e.g. pectin, *Sacromyces boulardii*). If intestinal adaptation does not occur, the presence of strictures, blind ending loops and dilated non-propulsive bowel should be considered, since well timed surgery will facilitate reduced dependency on parenteral nutrition.[79]

Dietetic management

There are several excellent monographs on this topic.[80] In brief four main themes can be identified:

1. Establish oral feeding including sucking and chewing as soon as practical. Even if the quantity of nutrition consumed is negligible, the positive effects on development in speech, social skills and physiology of the upper intestinal tract are great. When it is available, breast milk is ideal, otherwise a hydrolysate is frequently used initially (e.g. Peptijunior, Pregestimil, Neocate) for neonates who have immature pancreatic function and an intestinal mucosal barrier which is still highly permeable to foreign proteins.
2. Initiate continuous nasogastric tube feeding in short gut patients in order to promote intestinal adaptation. In this situation some oral feeding is also important and the usual compromise is to offer bottle or bolus feeds during the day and feed by infusion pump for 12–18 h overnight.
3. If feed tolerance is poor consider the use of a modular feed in which the carbohydrate, fat and protein components can be varied independently of each other to achieve a more digestible feed (e.g. less carbohydrate for infants with short gut, medium chain fat for children with lymphangiectasia). Pharmaceutical agents to improve gastric emptying (e.g. domperidone, and even cisapride where the risk: benefit ratio favors its use), or to slow transit time (e.g. loperamide 50–200 μg per kg per dose, two to four times per day) can be used in conjunction with manipulations to the feed.
4. Keep micronutrient balance (e.g. fat soluble vitamins and trace elements) and sodium balance under regular review in case supplements to the feed are necessary.

Avoidance of complications

Infection

The child with intestinal failure is susceptible to serious infections mainly via the intravenous feeding catheter. Skin organisms which have colonized the catheter via the hub and access ports and which are normally considered to be of low pathogenicity, can cause major systemic upset in the presence of the PN solutions which are a good growth medium for bacteria. Less frequently bacteria from the bowel appear to translocate to the circulation. Infection from any source however, is a risk factor for hepatic impairment especially in the preterm infant who will become chronically cholestatic after two or three infections when such infections occur within months of birth.[81] Sepsis at any age diminishes transport of bile from hepatocytes into bile canaliculi leading to retention of bile salts which itself leads to disruption of hepatocyte function.[82] Other risk factors include overprovision of nutrients which is associated with depletion of glutathione, induction of steatosis, and lipids which are occasionally associated with macrophage activation syndrome. The latter complication may also be enhanced by infection. Avoiding sepsis depends on good hygiene and restricting the number of individuals who have access to the feeding catheter.[76] In France it has been shown that patients discharged home on PN had one-tenth the incidence of central line infections compared to hospitalized patients.[83]

Hepatic

In patients fed by the intravenous route, purified nutrients consisting of simple glucose, essential amino acids, and triglyceride (derived from soya oil) are delivered to the hepatic sinusoids via the hepatic artery without the benefit of intestinally derived growth factors. This may explain the frequently observed phenomenon of fatty liver in parenterally fed patients (see also Table 17.28). Patients who are fed exclusively by the parenteral route are more likely to experience cholestasis. Total enteral starvation deprives the liver of intestinally derived growth factors and hormones including cholecystokinin and is associated with reduced portal blood flow. The effect is to reduce bile secretion at canalicular level and also to reduced motility of the large bile ducts related lack of cholecystokinin, which itself is produced in response to fat in the duodenum. Other risk factors for cholestasis include:

1. Prematurity since the immature liver is unsuited structurally (paucity of bile ductules) and physiologically (detoxification and conjugation pathways are inadequate) to handle nutrients which have not been passaged through the placenta or gastrointestinal tract. The majority of babies less than 28 weeks' gestation who receive PN become cholestatic.
2. Emergency abdominal surgery especially if it leads to short gut syndrome.[82,84]
3. Other chronic disease, e.g. low cardiac output states, thalassemia (iron overload).
4. Lack of a multidisciplinary care team.[77]

Avoiding liver damage therefore depends on establishment of oral feeding as soon as possible, rigorous hand washing routine[85] and a low threshold for suspecting and treating infection.

Thromboembolism and thrombosis

This is more commonly a complication of long term PN, although there are case reports of extensive thrombosis of the inferior vena cava occurring a few days after insertion of a femoral line. A review of patients at Great Ormond Street Hospital, England

Table 17.28 Complications of parenteral nutrition upon the liver

Biliary sludge, gallstones and occasionally cholecystitis
Steatosis which may be intense and leading to hepatomegaly and fibrosis
Fibrosis which may be portal and within the parenchyma ('pericellular fibrosis')
Cirrhosis and portal hypertension

showed a prevalence of 30% of their patients on long term PN had evidence of pulmonary embolus,[86] and in a group of patients referred for consideration of small bowel transplantation, 50% had indirect evidence of pulmonary hypertension by electrocardiogram (ECG) criteria.[87] Around 10% of children referred for small bowel transplantation have superior vena cava thrombosis (Intestinal Transplant Registry) and most such children have a history of 10 or more insertions of the feeding catheter (unpublished observation, SV Beath, 2001). Strategies for avoiding this complication are not agreed, but the following treatments are used: oral warfarin, oral aspirin, heparin added to the vamin compent of the PN solution. Avoidance of infection which renders blood more coagulable and the designation of a senior surgeon to be responsible for line insertion are generally considered helpful.

Social insolation

The nursing skills which parents are obliged to learn and the need to protect their child from accidental damage to his feeding catheter mean that some families are disinclined to travel outside their home except for hospital visits. In order to avoid this, the involvement of a social worker, specialist nurse and play specialist are vital in encouraging the child and family to integrate in society, to benefit from education and to make adequate developmental progress despite the restrictions of PN. Contact with self-help groups such as PINNT (Patients on Intravenous and Nasogastric Nutrition Therapy, who have a children's section, Half-PINNT) and the Children's Liver Disease Foundation (CLDF) can be encouraged (see Charities and Organizations, p. 712).

Surgical

Non-transplant surgery

This consists of a range of surgical operations ranging from those which are consequent on the primary procedure such as closure of a stoma previously created to treat a bowel perforation, to identification and repair of strictures, to reconstruction of residual intestine. The indications and timing for reconnection surgery are usually clear, but intestinal lengthening and tapering operations remain somewhat controversial. Since some poor early experiences in which prolonged surgery was carried out in infants already experiencing hepatic complications, it is now recognized that longitudinal intestinal lengthening and tapering operations (the Bianchi procedure) are more successful in children with dilated non-propulsive bowel who are at least 12 months old and in whom intestinal adaptation appears to be static. Non-transplant surgery for short gut is likely to proliferate as innovative surgeons describe techniques such as the creation of artificial strictures and reverse segments for expanding the residual bowel prior to lengthening and tapering.[88,89] Patients who have been referred for possible small bowel transplantation may be suitable for this kind of non-transplant surgery, so it is important for specialist teams to network even when operating in different institutions.

Small bowel transplantation

This operation was first performed in the 1950s in the dog, but it did not become accepted into clinical practice in humans until the availability of the potent immune suppressant tacrolimus in 1990, when two groups in North America (in London, Ontario and Pittsburgh) were able to achieve a 1-year survival of 70%.[90,91] Although tacrolimus has been essential in allowing small bowel allografts to be tolerated, there is a higher rate of opportunistic infection because of the necessary increased exposure to immunosuppression. The 3- and 5-year survival reported from the Intestinal Transplant Registry remains at 50%; however, results are somewhat better in the busier centers (Pittsburgh, Omaha, Miami) where 15–30 transplants per center are performed annually and in which 3-year survival is 65%.[92] Nevertheless, this still means that the transplant option is generally reserved for patients with life threatening complications such as PN related liver disease or recurrent line sepsis.[93]

Indications for referral. The precise indications for referral for consideration for small bowel transplantation continue to be debated. Most centers are prepared to review patients with intestinal failure at any stage, but recommend early referral if the child is becoming progressively jaundiced (i.e. if plasma bilirubin is in excess of 100 μm/L) or if there are complications associated with intravenous cannulation. Patients who have developed a thrombosis of the superior vena cava may become impossible to cannulate safely and if stenting of the superior vena cava[94] is contraindicated this group of patients will be considered for isolated bowel transplant provided their liver function is satisfactory. Failure to progress with intestinal adaptation and tolerance of enteral feeds in patients with short gut may also prompt a referral.

Types of intestinal transplants (see Fig. 17.11). Of the 696 intestinal transplants carried out in 656 individuals and reported to the Intestinal Transplant Registry (http://www.intestinaltransplantregistry.org/),[95] 426 were children. Two-thirds were combined procedures with liver and bowel, one-quarter isolated small bowel transplants and about 10% multivisceral involving variously stomach, colon, pancreas, kidney combined with small bowel and liver grafts. In infants for whom small donors are very scarce, a technique to cut down the size of organs from donors up to five times the size of the patient has been developed[96] (see Fig. 17.11c). The survival after isolated bowel transplant is better in the first 12 months (90% compared with 70% for combined liver and bowel transplants), but the long term complications of rejection and opportunistic infections are similar resulting in 3–5-year graft survival which is no different when compared to combined liver and bowel grafts.

Complications. The complications related to small bowel transplantation are numerous. Early complications, that is within 7 days, are generally related to the surgery and the consequences of organ preservation and reperfusion. These include perforation of native bowel and transplanted bowel (30% in pediatric series), bile leaks, pancreatitis, stomal prolapse, ileus and translocation of enteric bacteria to the liver and systemically via the portal vein. Unlike isolated liver transplantation, thrombosis of the splanchnic vasculature (i.e. portal vein, hepatic artery) is almost unheard of because the anastomoses are large usually being made between the aorta on the arterial side and inferior vena cava on the venous side.[97]

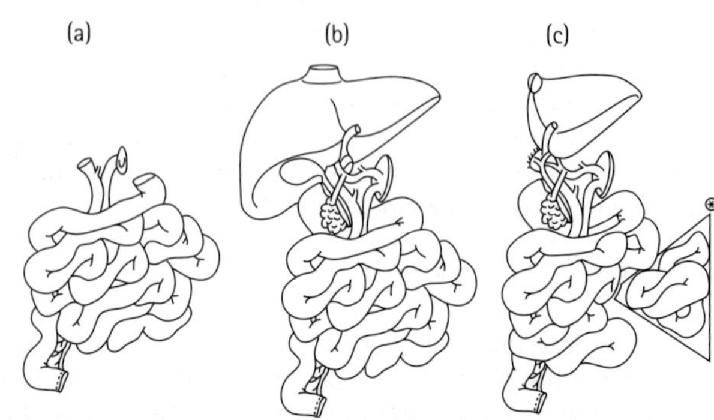

Fig. 17.11 Anatomical sketch of (a) isolated small bowel allograft; (b) combined liver and small bowel allograft; (c) reduced en-bloc liver and small bowel allograft. (Line drawing by J de Ville de Goyet)

Early medical complications include generalized edema secondary to fluid retention, ileus secondary to morphine and acute cellular rejection of the small bowel allograft and infection by enteric bacteria. Rejection of the small bowel is very common and occurs in 90% of recipients and can be identified by fever, deterioration in absorption of feed and changes in the morphology of the mucosa in which the lamina propria becomes infiltrated with a mixed population of neutrophils and lymphocytes and the villous crypts become disrupted by invading lymphocytes inducing apoptosis. Rejection is easily treated by increasing the immune suppression provided it is detected early. Untreated rejection in the immediate postoperative period may progress rapidly to severe rejection in 12–48 h and can be life threatening as the inflammatory process leads to ulcer formation, some of which are full thickness lesions which perforate causing a peritonitis and systemic sepsis from escaping enteric bacteria. The occurrence simultaneously of rejection and infection is a paradox peculiar to small bowel transplantation which requires increased immunosuppression rather than less and is one of the reasons that this form of transplantation still has a relatively high early mortality.

The long term complications are mainly related to opportunistic infections including cytomegalovirus, cryptosporidiosis, mucosal fungal infections and Epstein–Barr virus (EBV). EBV is a particularly important complication for children after intestinal transplantation in whom it is often a primary infection. In the context of selective T lymphocyte inhibition induced by tacrolimus treatment, the B lymphocytes infected with the EBV proliferate greatly and may become malignant resulting in post-transplant lymphoproliferative disease (PTLD). Up to 30% of small bowel transplant recipients in the transplant program in Pittsburgh developed PTLD within 2 years of transplantation with half (15% overall) eventually dying from this complication.[98] Optimal management requires early detection and the use of antiviral agents such as ganciclovir and antitumour therapy such as cyclophosphamide and anti-CD20 antibody which destroys B lymphocytes (e.g. Rituximab). Chronic rejection appears to be partly a vascular phenomenom in which the mesentery of the distal bowel in particular becomes infiltrated with inflammatory cells leading to occlusion and ischemia. The early symptoms are subtle resembling an intermittent distal ileal obstruction syndrome. Small bowel transplant recipients also experience the usual childhood infections such as otitis media and viral gastroenteritis; the latter can be severe and necessitate a temporary resumption of PN to hasten recovery.

Outcome. One in five small bowel transplant recipients do not survive the early postoperative period, generally reflecting their poor condition at the time of surgery. Those children who are discharged from hospital do well, with 70% completely independent of PN. In one small dietetic study over half the recipients had moved onto an ordinary family diet and had either maintained normal growth or some had demonstrated catch-up growth.[99] The number of appliances such as Broviac lines, nasogastric tubes, gastrostomy tubes, stoma bags reduces steadily in the 3 years after transplant. Most families report a sense of greater freedom and improved quality of life compared with that which they experienced with intravenous feeding before the transplant.

INTESTINAL FAILURE AND QUALITY OF LIFE

Measurement tools for quality of life are numerous,[100,101] but the most commonly used ones appear to be questionnaires in which the subject chooses one of five possible choices in response to questions about emotions (hopes and fears), physical function, pain, relationships (e.g. The General Health Questionnaire GHQ, The Nottingham Short Form-36, The Euro-Qol Questionnaire), and semistructured questionnaires which allow a more individualized response by the subject. Semistructured questionnaires may give a more accurate picture of the subject's quality of life but suffer from lack of validity and it is not usually possible to generalize the data to other subject groups. Disease specific questionnaires are being developed (e.g. IBD).[102] These difficulties have not prevented researchers attempting to measure quality of life for individuals on PN using the generic questionnaires such as the GHQ and SF-36 and proxy markers for quality of life.[103] In the case of children on PN, the results have reflected their parents' views but it is clear that families cope with the demands of home PN by developing obsessive/neurotic traits and that there is a high incidence of depression compared with the general population. A small study using the SF-36,[190] compared families with children who were clinically stable on home PN with small bowel transplant recipients, and found very little difference between the two groups. Both groups also completed developmental assessments (The Bayley Scale and Wechsler Tests) and achieved similar but rather low scores especially in the children who had been dependent on PN from birth.

PROGNOSIS

Although chronic intestinal failure is a disabling condition with long term implications for the child's development and carers, medical advances have allowed such children to be kept alive and even discharged home with good quality of life. In children without major complications the 5–10 year survival is around 80%.[85]

In contrast children who develop serious complications especially cholestasis are at risk of early death from overwhelming sepsis. Of 44 children assessed at Birmingham Children's Hospital (England) and considered to fulfill criteria for intestinal transplantation, 23 died before organs became available. Children with intestinal failure who are experiencing complications related to the administration of PN should be referred for assessment to allow them to have the opportunity to have their intestinal failure treated by intestinal transplantation.

THE COLON

STRUCTURE

The colon is a long hollow tube which, with the exception of the sigmoid which has a short mesentery, lies retroperitoneally. Along its length from the ileocecal valve to the anus the mucosa is lined by a cuboidal epithelium which is indented with crypts. The mature colon has no villi and no brush border disaccharidase activity. Submucosal and myenteric nerve plexuses are present, similar to those in the small intestine, but the smooth muscle layers differ in that the longitudinal layer is incomplete forming three tenia coli.

FUNCTION

The large intestine fulfills both storage and salvage functions. The colon stores the intestinal contents prior to excretion, but it is also an organ of conservation which reduces liquid ileal effluent to solid feces excreted via the anus. It plays an important role in the salvage of electrolytes and water, and in addition, the salvage of nutrients in the form of short chain fatty acids.

Absorption

Although it is clear that the majority of water and electrolyte absorption occurs in the small intestine, it is often the adequacy of colonic function which determines whether the child experiences diarrhea, and whether or not there is net loss of water and electrolytes from the body. In small intestinal disease there is an increase in the volume of fluid arriving at the ileocecal valve but the colon has a reserve reabsorptive capacity which can adequately absorb the excess ileal effluent. When there is massive small intestinal secretion, the reserve reabsorptive capacity of the colon may be overwhelmed, resulting in diarrhea. In addition, in disorders which compromise colonic function such as IBD, diarrhea may occur as a result of either reduced colonic absorptive capacity or frank colonic secretion.[104]

The importance of the colonic sodium absorptive mechanism is demonstrated clinically by the high rate of sodium supplementation necessary for normal growth in infants with ileostomies. The majority of sodium absorption occurs via an active, electrogenic mechanism, while chloride is absorbed down its electrochemical gradient. Potassium is secreted into the lumen largely in response to electrochemical gradients and, in older children, bicarbonate is secreted into the colonic lumen via an exchange mechanism with chloride. Recently it has been shown that colonic sodium absorptive processes are already highly efficient in preterm infants and there is evidence that circulating aldosterone levels may be important in the regulation of these mechanisms.[105] In addition to its role in the absorption of water and electrolytes, the colon may also salvage extra nutrient energy from the contents of the gastrointestinal tract via the absorption of short chain fatty acids such as acetate, butyrate and propionate. These are produced by colonic bacterial fermentation of unabsorbed dietary carbohydrate and studies have shown that they are rapidly absorbed from the large intestine, providing a significant additional source of energy, and also that they promote further colonic salt and water absorption.

The salvage of electrolytes, water and nutrients requires sophisticated integration of the functions of bacterial digestion, epithelial transport and motor activity of the colonic muscle layers. Details of colonic motility patterns are scanty in childhood, although a major proportion of the total mouth to anus transit time occurs in the large intestine.

INFLAMMATORY BOWEL DISEASE

Although infective agents are the commonest cause of IBD in a worldwide context, the term will be used in this section to describe chronic inflammation of the gastrointestinal tract in the absence of a detectable pathogenic agent. Included in this definition in descending order of importance are Crohn's disease, ulcerative colitis and allergic colitis. In addition, the term 'indeterminate colitis' has been employed to describe children with colitis which is impossible to precisely categorize at presentation: the final diagnosis may often only become evident in these patients with the lapse of time and further, or repeated, investigation.

EPIDEMIOLOGY

The prevalence of Crohn's disease in both Wales and Scotland[106,107] appears to have increased in the 1980s and 1990s, with the incidence of Crohn's being at least twice as common as ulcerative colitis. In Sweden, the incidence of pediatric IBD has also increased over a 10 year period,[108] although in contrast to the UK this was primarily an increase in ulcerative colitis. A recent prospective study of pediatric IBD in the British Isles, from the British Paediatric Surveillance Unit (BPSU), has suggested an estimated incidence of IBD of 5.3 per 100 000 children under the age of 16, equivalent to about 700 new cases per annum in the UK, with Crohn's disease again being twice as common as ulcerative colitis.[109] This study suggests that 10% of patients may be of Asian origin (an over-representation compared with the overall population) with some 5% of patients from the Afro-Caribbean population. There is a slight male preponderance (58%). In childhood the peak in incidence is between 11 and 13 years, although 13% of cases in the recent BPSU study developed in children aged less than 10 years. Although Crohn's disease and ulcerative colitis may present in early childhood, it seems likely that many cases of colitis presenting in the first 2 years of life may be related to food allergy that responds to an appropriate exclusion diet, and with a favorable long term prognosis.[110]

ETIOLOGY/PATHOPHYSIOLOGY

The etiology and pathogenesis of Crohn's disease and ulcerative colitis are unknown despite many theories and much painstaking research work.[111] There is no doubt that there is a genetic preponderance for both diseases and twin studies suggest a much higher concordance in monozygotic than in dizygotic twins. It is likely that Crohn's disease and ulcerative colitis are related polygenic diseases,[112] and gene linkage studies have identified a number of possible susceptibility genes,[113] thus HLA correlations are HLA DR3 and DQ2 in determining the extent of the disease, and HLA DR103 in predicting severity. Susceptibility genes for IBD also appear to be located on chromosomes 3, 7 and 12 with Crohn's disease specifically on chromosome 16 and ulcerative colitis on chromosomes 2 and 6. However, many of the findings require replication in different populations.

Multiple immunological abnormalities have been described in patients with IBD but none has convincingly been shown to be a primary pathogenetic event. Environmental factors such as bacterial pathogens or their products, dietary components and intercurrent infections appear necessary to trigger and maintain the diseases and may well interact with specific genes.[111] The basic problem appears to be an overstimulation or over-reaction of the mucosal immune system to a particular antigenic stimulus in genetically susceptible individuals although the antigenic stimulus, such as a microorganism or food antigen, may vary from case to case. Though there has been controversy over the role of the measles virus, and indeed the measles mumps rubella (MMR) vaccine, there is no convincing evidence that this is related to the development of IBD. Infectious agents have been postulated as playing a major role but so far the evidence is inconclusive. There is no conclusive evidence for causal associations for any environmental exposure in the etiology of Crohn's disease or ulcerative colitis, although there is strong evidence incriminating dietary allergens, particularly dairy produce and soya milk, in the pathogenesis of allergic colitis in younger children.[114]

Studies have, however, shown that intestinal permeability may be increased in Crohn's disease and it is conceivable that this could result in an increase in absorption of antigens from the gut, which may be important in the pathogenesis of the disease. Finally, it has been suggested that psychosomatic factors may be important and a 'colitis personality' was previously defined. However, several studies have not supported this concept and it is hardly surprising that there may be a higher incidence of emotional problems and depression found in sufferers and their families as a consequence of their chronic, debilitating disease. Thus adequate psychological and emotional support from health care staff is of paramount importance in the management of children with IBD. Adequate communication is vital, and several self-help groups publish helpful booklets and can provide additional support and information for the child and family (see Charities and Organizations, p. 712).

CROHN'S DISEASE

Pathology

The disease may involve any part of the gastrointestinal tract from the lips to the perianal area, and normal bowel may be found in between affected areas. The inflammation is transmural, often extending from the mucosa to the serosal surface, resulting in sinus tracts or fistulae formation. In childhood disease, terminal ileitis is common with variable involvement of the colon in 50–70%[115] and the recent UK British Paediatric Surveillance Unit study[109] suggested that one-third of patients have small intestinal disease, one-third ileocolitis and one-third colitis, with total colitis being more common (50%) than segmental colitis or isolated proctitis. Macroscopically, the bowel mucosa may look inflamed, and small shallow, aphthoid or linear ulcers may be present. Later on in the disease, deeper fissures may occur leading to the classic 'cobblestone' appearance of the mucosa, as well as stricturing of the bowel. Histologically, there is transmural inflammation and the diagnostic hallmark is the finding of non-caseating epithelioid granulomata with giant cells which may not be present in all affected tissues.

Clinical features

The insidious onset and subtle nature of the symptoms and signs of Crohn's disease often result in a considerable delay in diagnosis with left-sided colonic disease being usually diagnosed more rapidly than diffuse small intestinal disease. The manifestations of the disease depend upon the site of involvement but periumbilical, colicky abdominal pain, diarrhea with or without blood and growth failure are the commonest forms of presentation. Occasionally more subtle manifestations, such as oropharyngeal disease, perianal skin tags and fissuring or growth failure, may be the first signs of the disorder in the absence of overt gastrointestinal symptoms. The diarrhea in Crohn's disease is likely to be due to a combination of several factors which may include mucosal dysfunction, bile acid malabsorption, bacterial overgrowth and protein exudation from inflamed bowel.

On examination, it is important to ascertain whether extraintestinal manifestations of Crohn's disease are present. Thus there may be intermittent pyrexia, clinical anemia, arthralgia and arthritis, uveitis, finger clubbing, perianal disease (skin tags, bluish discoloration, fissures, fistulae), oral ulceration, skin manifestations (erythema nodosum and pyoderma gangrenosum), signs of liver dysfunction and evidence of growth failure and delayed sexual maturation. Examination of the abdomen may reveal generalized or localized tenderness and occasionally an ill-defined palpable mass. The importance of growth retardation and pubertal delay must be emphasized as it may occur in up to 30% of children with Crohn's disease and may be present well before the diagnosis is made.[116] There is little evidence that this is due to a primary endocrine disturbance and the most likely reason for growth failure is nutritional deprivation or a direct effect of inflammatory molecules such as cytokines on the growing skeleton. Growth failure must be detected earlier as there is evidence that this can be successfully reversed by prompt treatment.[117,118]

Osteopenia has recently been recognized and is an important complication of IBD, particularly in children with Crohn's disease, and although the mechanisms are not yet fully elucidated, the cause appears to be a combination of both the disease itself and drug treatment with steroids.[119]

Diagnosis

Laboratory assessment involves the search for infective agents in the stools of patients with Crohn's disease presenting with diarrhea. Hematological investigation often reveals iron-deficiency anemia and acute phase reactants such as erythrocyte sedimentation rate (ESR) and C reactive protein (CRP) may be elevated, although not universally. Thrombocytosis and hypoalbuminemia may also be present and these appear to be more reliable markers of disease activity. Plasma zinc levels are frequently low and liver function tests may be abnormal. It should, however, be remembered that alkaline phosphatase is a zinc-dependent enzyme which may be spuriously depressed in the presence of zinc deficiency. Recent studies also suggest that measurement of stool calprotectin, a protein secreted into the gut by lymphocytes, is a reliable indicator of intestinal inflammation.[120]

Radiological assessment is important and plain abdominal X-rays may reveal evidence of intestinal obstruction or bowel dilatation. A barium meal and follow-through is vital in order to assess the small bowel and, although a small bowel meal (via a transpyloric tube) is the most sensitive technique, this is not always acceptable as it may be particularly uncomfortable for the child. The presence of skip lesions, with narrowing of the lumen, thickening and fissuring ('rose-thorn ulcers') of the bowel wall and fistulae formation are all highly suggestive of Crohn's disease (Fig. 17.12). Technetium white cell scanning has been suggested as a useful investigation for initial screening/follow-up but there is continued debate about the sensitivity and specificity of this investigation.[121]

Endoscopy remains the most important tool for assessing both the upper gastrointestinal tract and colon (Fig. 17.13), and colonoscopy has superceded the barium enema as the primary investigation of the lower bowel. Several authors have suggested that upper intestinal endoscopy should be performed at the same time as colonoscopy, as a majority of patients with IBD may show histological abnormalities in the upper gastrointestinal tract, which may be useful in diagnosis.[122]

Treatment

The goal of therapy is both to induce and maintain a remission of active disease and also to correct malnutrition and promote growth.

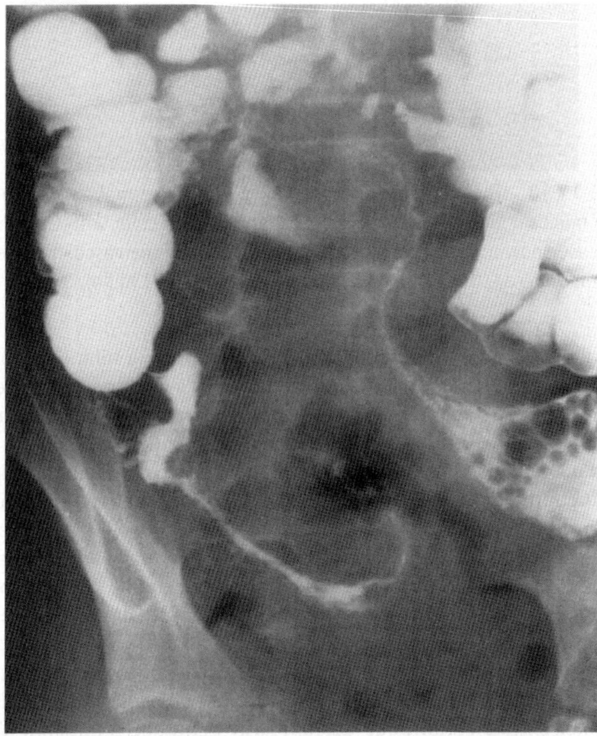

Fig. 17.12 Extensive narrowing of the ileum in a child with small intestinal Crohn's disease. (Reproduced by kind permission of PJ Milla)

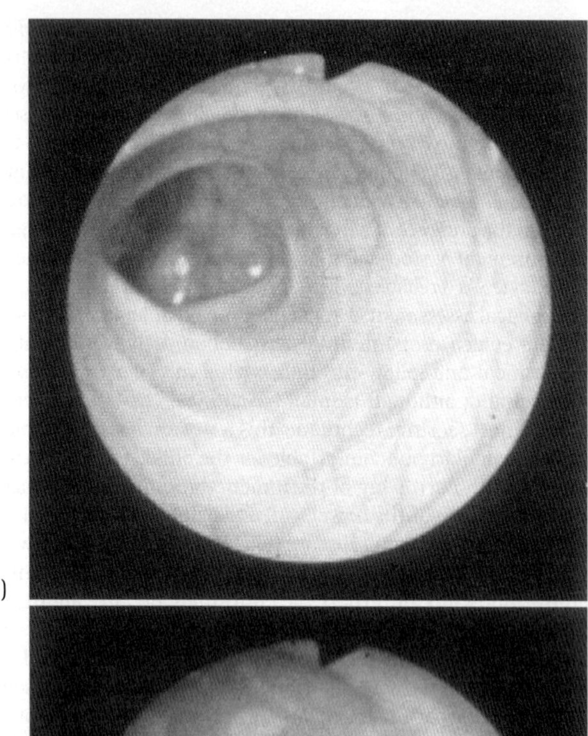

(a)

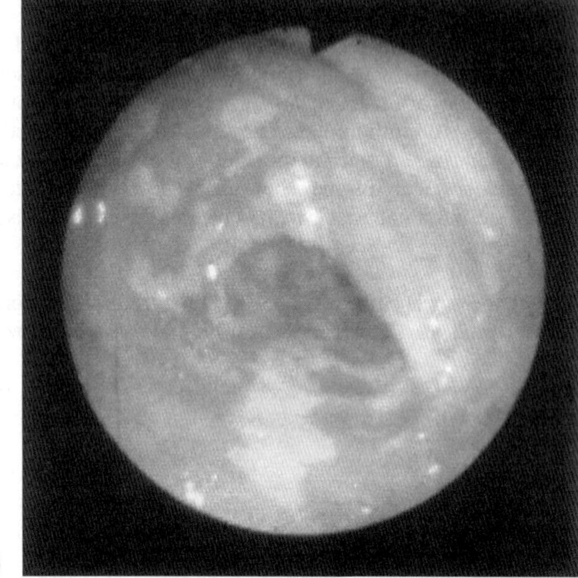

(b)

Fig. 17.13 The colonoscopic appearance in (a) a normal child with the mucosal blood vessels clearly seen and (b) in a child with Crohn's disease showing 'snail tract' ulceration and loss of the vascular pattern of the mucosa. (Reproduced by kind permission of PJ Milla)

There is no convincing evidence that any drug alters the long term natural history of Crohn's disease, but several agents have a place in the treatment of the disorder. Steroids may induce remission in over 70% of patients and prednisolone should be given in an initial dose of 2 mg/kg/day (max. 40 mg) with a gradual reduction after 2–4 weeks, preferably to an alternate-day regimen in order to minimize the growth-suppressive side-effects. There is no good evidence that low dose steroid therapy can maintain remission and, if possible, steroid therapy should be gradually reduced over a further 6–8 weeks and stopped if the disease is quiescent.

Sulfasalazine (50–80 mg/kg/day) is useful in the treatment of active Crohn's colitis in inducing remission, although there is little evidence that continuous therapy will maintain remission. The active moiety of sulfasalazine is 5-aminosalicylic acid and new preparations containing this drug may be effective alternatives in the future in those patients who experience side-effects related to sulfasalazine.[123] There is an increasing use of immunomodulatory drugs, such as azathioprine and 6-mercaptopurine, which may allow reduction or cessation of steroids and also help to maintain remission.[124] However, although very useful, such drugs are potentially hazardous and their use should be monitored carefully. Metronidazole may be effective in colonic and particularly perianal disease although peripheral neuropathy may develop with its long term use. In children who are acutely toxic and systemically unwell on presentation, it is reasonable to start intravenous broad spectrum antibiotics, including metronidazole, in addition to intravenous steroids until the disease begins to remit.

There are potential advances in the use of new biological drugs such as anti-TNF alpha monoclonal antibody; inflammatory cytokines (such as TNF alpha) tend to be consistently elevated in the mucosa and the anti-TNF alpha monoclonal antibody shows promise as an agent which might block TNF activity, and thus provide a normal form of therapy for Crohn's disease. However, its place in the treatment of children with Crohn's disease is not yet established.

Nutritional therapy has recently been recognized as a very important therapeutic modality in Crohn's disease, not only in the correction of specific nutrient deficiencies, but also in the reduction of disease activity and the reversal of growth failure. Patients may need specific therapy with iron, folate, vitamin B_{12} and zinc in addition to ensuring an adequate energy intake via the oral or nasogastric route or indeed via intravenous feeding. Furthermore, nutritional therapy has been shown to be effective in inducing remission of active disease[125] and both enteral and parenteral routes may be used. Over the last decade, there has been increasing use by pediatric gastroenterologists (though less use by adult gastroenterologists) of enteral nutrition as a primary therapy to induce remission.[126] An analysis of five randomized clinical trials comprising 147 children showed that enteral nutrition was as effective as corticosteroids in inducing remission;[127] however there is still debate as to the appropriate place of enteral therapy in the treatment of Crohn's disease and randomized trials involving large numbers of patients are necessary. Several questions remain unanswered, i.e. how the enteral therapy works, whether a polymeric diet is as effective as an elemental diet, whether or not large intestinal disease is treated as effectively as small intestinal disease and the role of on-going maintenance – there is some evidence that intermittent periods of enteral feeding may maintain remission, but these results need to be confirmed.[128] The indications for surgical intervention in Crohn's disease include intestinal obstruction, fistula formation, hemorrhage and perforation, and a failure of medical therapy, particularly where there is growth failure. The surgical results in Crohn's disease are most encouraging in children with localized ileal disease,[129] although children with both large and small bowel disease may require reoperation at a later date. Elective surgery is perhaps most important in children nearing puberty with specific growth problems and it is very important to use as an option when the disease is not too extensive and it is feasible to resect the diseased bowel.[118] The early use of surgery can be vital during the narrow window of therapeutic opportunity before the pubertal growth spurt is complete. Although colectomy in ulcerative colitis is curative, in Crohn's disease, although surgery may modify the immediate outcome, it does not appear to prevent recurrence.

Prognosis

The prognosis for childhood Crohn's disease is reasonably optimistic and, although the morbidity is relatively high, the mortality is low.[130] Psychosocial aspects particularly those influencing quality of life are being investigated in the childhood IBD population.

The risk of colorectal carcinoma in childhood with Crohn's colitis is not well defined although there is a suggestion that the incidence is slightly increased when compared with a control population. Long term follow-up studies are needed to clarify this point and in the meantime the large intestine in patients with colitis should be inspected regularly by colonoscopy.

ULCERATIVE COLITIS

Pathology

Ulcerative colitis is an inflammatory disease of the large intestinal mucosa and the abnormal changes are seen most commonly in the rectum and distal colon, although the whole colon may be affected. Indeed, pancolitis is the most common form (62%) while disease of the left colon (22%) or rectum (16%) occurs less frequently. Unlike Crohn's disease, the inflammation is continuous and it is usually limited to the colonic mucosa. Macroscopically the mucosa is friable and granular, and ulceration may be present in association with a bloody or mucopurulent exudate. The ulceration, which is often patchy, may be interspersed with areas of regenerating epithelium, resulting in pseudopolyp formation. In addition, there may be an inflammatory reaction in the distal ileum, so-called 'backwash ileitis'. The characteristic histological features are an acute and chronic inflammatory cell infiltrate in the lamina propria, distortion of crypt architecture, the presence of crypt abscesses and goblet cell depletion.

Clinical features

The commonest presenting features are diarrhea, often associated with blood and mucus, and tenesmus with lower abdominal pain which is relieved by defecation. Attacks may be graded as mild, moderate or severe depending upon stool frequency, abdominal tenderness, fever and the degree of anemia and hypoalbuminemia. It is important to recognize that 5–10% of patients with ulcerative colitis may present with fulminating colitis associated with toxic megacolon, and a plain abdominal X-ray should be performed to look for the presence of a dilated colon (usually exceeding 6 cm in diameter).

On examination the only positive findings may be minimal lower abdominal tenderness, although in severe disease the child may be pyrexial, dehydrated, anemic and profoundly toxic. It is important to look carefully for evidence of extraintestinal manifestations which are similar to those of Crohn's disease, although growth retardation occurs less frequently in ulcerative colitis and affects less than 20% of patients at presentation.

Diagnosis

Infective agents such as *Shigella, Salmonella, Campylobacter, Yersinia* and *Entamoeba* may cause an acute or chronic colitis, and it is vital to look carefully for pathogens in the stool and perform appropriate serological tests. Further laboratory assessment may reveal anemia, raised levels of ESR and CRP, leukocytosis and hypoalbuminemia which may reflect the disease activity. Radiological investigations should include plain abdominal X-ray, in patients with severe disease, and a good colonoscopy examination makes barium enema examination unnecessary. Endoscopic evaluation of the whole colon is very useful in assessing both the severity and extent of inflammation. However, the procedure should be deferred, or at least limited, in patients with acute severe colitis because of the risk of toxic megacolon and perforation.

Treatment

Therapy is directed towards inducing and maintaining remission in mild or moderate disease and may be life saving in fulminating colitis. Patients with mild disease are best treated with sulfasalazine (50–80 mg/kg/day) and, in those children with disease confined to the distal colon, a topical steroid preparation may be useful. Moderately severe disease (bloody diarrhea five times/day, abdominal pain, fever) may require the addition of oral steroids (prednisolone 1–2 mg/kg/day, max. 40 mg) in order to induce remission, and this dose should be gradually reduced after 2 weeks if the child's condition is improving. Antispasmodic medication and agents which decrease gut motility should not be given as they may precipitate the development of toxic megacolon.

Severe, fulminating colitis is a medical emergency which is easily underestimated. The child should receive nothing by mouth and intravenous therapy is always indicated. The patient will usually need rehydration and blood transfusion, and regular albumin infusions are often required. All children should receive intravenous hydrocortisone (10 mg/kg/day) and broad spectrum antibiotics (penicillin, gentamicin, metronidazole) and, if malnourished, parenteral nutrition should be instituted at an early stage. Many children with severe colitis will respond to this aggressive medical therapy within 7–10 days, but if by this time there is no improvement, or the child develops a complication such as toxic megacolon, colonic hemorrhage or perforation, then surgery is necessary. In addition to emergency surgery for complications of acute disease, elective surgery may be required if there is a failure of medical therapy, severe growth retardation unresponsive to improved nutrition or severe colonic dysplasia with the risk of adenocarcinoma formation in long-standing colitis. The surgical procedures available for the child include a proctocolectomy with ileostomy or ileal reservoir, or a colectomy with rectal mucosectomy and endorectal pull-through.[131]

As regards the maintenance of remission, there is good evidence that continued therapy with sulfasalazine (or its derivatives) is superior to placebo in preventing relapse although, in some patients, alternate-day steroids may also be required. Immunosuppressive drugs are proving to be useful in patients with intractable disease.

In contrast to Crohn's disease, there is little evidence that aggressive nutritional therapy alone, either enteral or parenteral, is effective in inducing remission in ulcerative colitis, although the correction of malnutrition and specific nutritional deficiencies is mandatory in all patients.

Prognosis

Approximately 90% of patients with ulcerative colitis presenting in childhood or adolescence will experience one or more relapses of their disease after initial treatment. The majority will be able to lead a relatively normal life despite chronic disease but some 20% will be chronically incapacitated. The prognosis is best for isolated, distal colitis, with only 10% progressing to pancolitis; overall, approximately 30% of patients will eventually require colectomy. There is an increased risk of developing large intestinal adenocarcinoma in patients with long-standing ulcerative colitis, although the risk is probably considerably less than previously thought.[132] The advent of flexible endoscopy has made possible careful, regular surveillance of the colonic mucosa and colonoscopy and biopsy should be performed at regular intervals in older patients with long-standing colitis.

RECTAL BLEEDING

The passage of small amounts of blood per rectum is not uncommon in childhood and is rarely of sinister significance, being often due to a simple anal fissure or self-limiting infective colitis. It is important to determine whether it is bright red blood that has been passed, around, after or mingled with the stool as in the case of bleeding from the colon, or whether the blood is altered, or indeed melena, which may signify a more proximal source of bleeding. It is also helpful to determine whether there is mucus or slime in the stool or if there is associated diarrhea or constipation, abdominal pain or perianal pain on defecation.

Clinical examination should attempt to assess the degree of blood loss and whether anemia is present. Adequate visualization of the perianal region is mandatory and the use of a pediatric proctoscope may yield important diagnostic clues. General examination includes a detailed examination of the skin for evidence of purpura and telangiectases, circumoral pigmentation, and evidence of arthritis and renal abnormalities should be sought. Although direct visualization of the stool may reveal fresh blood or melena, chemical testing may be required when occult bleeding from a more proximal source is present. A number of kits are available for the testing of occult fecal blood, although most are highly sensitive and are likely to give false positive results, particularly if the child is receiving vitamin C supplements or food high in peroxidase activity such as uncooked vegetables.

Etiology

Table 17.29 outlines some of the commoner causes of rectal bleeding in childhood. It is important at any age (particularly in the neonatal period) to exclude swallowed blood as a cause of rectal bleeding. The etiology of bleeding per rectum is influenced by the age of the patient and also by the mode of clinical presentation. Thus, a child with chronic constipation who passes bright red blood on the surface of the stool may have an associated anal fissure, while the infant with intussusception may present with colicky abdominal pain, shock and the passage of 'red currant jelly stools'. Acute vomiting and bloody diarrhea may herald the onset of intestinal infection and the presence of hematuria and proteinuria may suggest Henoch–Schönlein purpura or the hemolytic uremic syndrome. Chronic blood loss with the painless passage of bright red blood is suggestive of a colonic polyp or hamartoma and a detailed family history may be helpful.

Table 17.29 Causes of rectal bleeding in childhood

1. Anal fissure
2. Infective colitis
   a. *Shigella*
   b. *Salmonella*
   c. *Campylobacter*
   d. *Escherichia coli* O157
3. Allergic colitis
4. Intestinal polyps
   a. Juvenile polyps
   b. Familial polyposis coli
   c. Peutz–Jeghers syndrome
   d. Gardner's syndrome
5. Generalized bleeding diathesis
6. Inflammatory bowel disease
7. Rectal prolapse
8. Intussusception
9. Meckel's diverticulum/gut duplication
10. Henoch–Schönlein purpura
11. Hemangioma/angiodysplasia/telangiectasia
12. Upper gastrointestinal bleeding

Investigation and treatment

The pattern of investigation will depend upon the urgency of the clinical presentation. Thus an infant who is shocked and passing bright red blood per rectum will need resuscitation and an urgent plain abdominal X-ray and possibly a contrast enema to exclude intussusception. Usually the presentation is less acute and initial laboratory assessment should include a full blood count, ESR, serum iron and ferritin estimation, serum electrolytes and clotting studies. In cases of bloody diarrhea, stool culture is mandatory and plain abdominal X-ray may be helpful. The most useful investigation is colonoscopy, which after scrupulous bowel preparation will provide direct visualization of the colonic mucosa and allow multiple biopsies to be obtained for histology. Furthermore, the procedure may be therapeutic as smaller polyps may be removed at colonoscopy by diathermy.

Isotope scanning using technetium may identify ectopic gastric mucosa in either a Meckel's diverticulum or in a duplication of the intestine, and labeling of red blood cells with the isotope may also be useful in detecting the site of active, but occult, gastrointestinal blood loss. In the last resort, in selected cases of severe chronic unexplained iron-deficiency anemia associated with positive fecal occult blood, it may be necessary to perform angiography to localize the source of bleeding and rarely laparotomy and intraoperative endoscopy is indicated.

CHRONIC GASTROINTESTINAL SYMPTOMS

RECURRENT ABDOMINAL PAIN

Recurrent abdominal pain is a relatively common pediatric problem, occurring primarily in older children and adolescents. The term generally describes recurrent and moderately severe episodes of abdominal pain over a period of at least 3 months which may lead to absence from school and may affect the child's lifestyle. Typically the pain is non-specific although most children describe colicky, periumbilical discomfort. Most importantly the child is healthy in between these episodes and physical examination is normal. 10–20% of schoolchildren are affected.[133]

Etiology and pathogenesis

Although early studies showed that in only 7% of cases is an organic cause found to explain the pain,[133] it is increasingly recognized that many conditions may cause such pain, such as constipation, abdominal migraine,[134] gastritis and peptic ulcer associated with *Helicobacter pylori* and the irritable bowel syndrome[135] (Table 17.30). As clinical examination is usually normal, it is vital to take a detailed and comprehensive history which may provide clues as to the etiology of the pain.

Although organic disease can cause recurrent abdominal pain, when investigations are normal, psychological disturbances including over-reaction to normal life events and family dysfunction have often been considered important in the pathogenesis of the symptoms. However, studies have failed to show any psychological differences among children with recurrent abdominal pain compared with control subjects, although a proportion of these children and their families may benefit from psychological or family therapy.

Management

Blanket investigation is no substitute for a careful history and examination although selective laboratory and radiological testing

Table 17.30 Organic causes of recurrent abdominal pain in childhood

1. Gastrointestinal
   a. Constipation
   b. Peptic ulceration/gastritis
   c. Gastroesophageal reflux
   d. Anatomical abnormalities
      (i) Meckel's diverticulum
      (ii) Malrotation
   e. Inflammatory bowel disease
   f. Food intolerance
   g. Infection (e.g. *Yersinia ileitis*)
   h. Pancreatitis
   i. Hepatobiliary disease
2. Others
   a. Migraine
   b. Urinary tract disorder
      (i) Chronic infection
      (ii) Hydronephrosis
      (iii) Calculi

may be necessary, based on the pediatrician's clinical assessment. Routine urine testing and culture is mandatory and a full blood count and ESR may be helpful in excluding anemia and inflammatory conditions. If the child's symptoms are suggestive of pancreatitis, then a serum amylase may be useful when the child is experiencing pain, and liver function tests may be abnormal in children with pain due to hepatobiliary disease. Radiological investigations are usually unhelpful although a plain abdominal film will reveal calcification and gross constipation which may not be evident clinically. An abdominal ultrasound can be of use, particularly if urinary symptoms are suspected, but only rarely is it necessary to perform barium studies in order to exclude malrotation and IBD. Screening for *Helicobacter pylori* infection (see p. 660) may not be helpful in children with generalized abdominal pain but where symptoms suggest peptic ulcer disease, upper gastrointestinal endoscopy and biopsy will be required.

Treatment will depend on the clinical assessment and on the results of investigations undertaken. It is important to exclude constipation as therapeutic intervention may cure the child's pain. In children where there is a typical history of abdominal migraine,[134] a trial of antimigraine prophylaxis such as pizotifen and/or the exclusion of cheese, chocolate, citrus fruit and caffeine (the 4Cs) is sometimes justified, particularly if the child is missing a substantial amount of schooling. In the majority of cases, however, none of these measures is indicated and the most important therapeutic maneuver is to reassure the child and his parents that there is no serious organic disease present. It is often helpful to emphasize that the disorder is common in childhood and that the symptoms are likely to improve with age. It is important also to explain that although there is no obvious organic cause for the pain, it is not suggested that the pain is imaginary; rather it can be useful to admit that we as physicians do not understand why the pain is occurring, but do know that stress and emotional upheaval will tend to exacerbate the symptoms. In some children who present with intractable symptoms it is helpful to enlist the services of either a child psychologist or psychiatrist at an early stage so that a joint approach can be made in the exclusion of organic and non-organic causes for the recurrent abdominal pain.

Prognosis

Prospective follow-up studies have been undertaken in children with recurrent abdominal pain and these suggest that a substantial proportion of children may continue to suffer in adult life from the symptoms of irritable bowel syndrome. Furthermore it has been suggested that in children who develop symptoms at an early age and in whom treatment is delayed, the prognosis may be worse. It is tempting to speculate that recurrent abdominal pain in childhood and the irritable bowel syndrome found in later life are manifestations of the same condition, although further large prospective studies are needed to clarify this point.

INFANTILE COLIC

Infantile colic is a condition which is difficult to classify and define. It is used to describe the baby who, in the first few weeks of life, has frequent spells of inconsolable crying, usually occurring in the evening, and often associated with excessive flatus. The infant appears to be suffering abdominal pain although the 'colic' is intermittent and usually self-limiting, often subsiding after 3 months of age. The disorder occurs equally in boys and girls and may occur in up to 20% of all babies in the first few months of life. The pathogenesis of the disorder is still unclear and several etiologic theories have been proposed including psychosocial factors, a failure of parent–infant interaction and milk allergy.[136]

Although the pathogenesis of the disorder is unclear, all the evidence points to an intestinal origin for the discomfort, and fundamental physiological and clinical research needs to be undertaken in order to understand the phenomenon more clearly.

As regards management, the most important therapeutic maneuver is to carefully examine the baby and reassure the parents that colic is common, self-limiting and without harmful long term effects. Many remedies have been tried but the sheer number of treatment options testifies to the fact that none works particularly well. However, for the parents who are at the end of their tether, it may be worth a trial of simple measures such as gripe or peppermint water, and where a child is clearly atopic a cow's milk exclusion may be of benefit; a whey-based hydrolysate formula is the feed of choice.[137] Counseling and support of the parents, however, remains the mainstay of management.[138]

Although the condition is usually self-limiting by 3 months of age, some children continue to experience colic throughout the first year of life and go on to develop recurrent abdominal pain and the irritable bowel syndrome in later life.

CHRONIC CONSTIPATION

Although often regarded as a less than glamorous and rather insignificant problem by many physicians, chronic constipation is of great importance to the child and his family. It should be stressed that early accurate assessment and prompt treatment of constipation is vital to the child's well-being and lifestyle, as delays in management will only exacerbate the problem and perpetuate the child's lack of self-esteem and feelings of hopelessness. Furthermore it has been shown that constipation may cause reversible urinary tract abnormalities that may predispose the child to urinary tract infection and enuresis.[139]

The term constipation is used to describe difficulty or delay in the passage of stools, which may progress to a chronic state where defecation is infrequent and the bowel motions passed are hard pellets or firm and very bulky; in addition there may be leakage of fecal liquid around the hard compacted stools in the dilated rectum causing soiling, which is distressing for the child and may result in inappropriate referral to a child psychiatrist. It is important to distinguish chronic constipation and associated overflow incontinence from true encopresis, which is the voluntary passage of normal stools in an inappropriate fashion or place. Normal bowel frequency varies widely although the average baby passes three to six stools per day in the neonatal period, one to two stools per day at 1 year of life and approximately one stool per day, or every other day, in the preschool years.[140]

Pathophysiology and clinical features

Although the vast majority of children presenting with constipation have no serious underlying organic pathology, it is generally true that the younger the child, the more likely it is that the problem is due to a congenital abnormality of the lower bowel. It is particularly important to diagnose Hirschsprung's disease (see Ch. 36) at an early stage, as the infant is at risk from developing an associated and severe life-threatening enterocolitis. Such children almost always have symptoms of constipation dating from before 3 months of age with the majority presenting in the first few days of life. Most children with chronic constipation, however, present in the preschool years with symptoms that may have been present for several months and sometimes several years. In these children it is unlikely that organic disease is present although the organic pathologies shown in Table 17.31 should be considered. A careful history and examination, particularly of the perianal region, is crucial in the evaluation of the problem, and the need for further investigation is dictated by the clinical assessment.

By the time most children present to the pediatrician, an enlarged megacolon full of hard feces is present. The child is usually otherwise well although abdominal pain and occasionally nausea and vomiting may be associated with chronic constipation. The original genesis of the constipation is often difficult to pinpoint and several initiating factors may have been involved such as a loss of appetite during an acute illness, the prescription of constipating medications following a bout of diarrhea, pain from an anal fissure, a stressful life event, difficult toilet training made worse by inadequate facilities at school or aggressive management by parents determined to see their child toilet trained at a very early age. It has also become clear that chronic constipation may be a manifestation of food intolerance and this should be considered in a child or family with a strong history of atopy.

Chronic constipation is most often the end result of a sequence of events which starts with an episode of acute constipation which is inadequately treated. Adequate bowel evacuation relies on the child experiencing the urge to defecate consequent on the distension of the rectum with feces. If this urge is suppressed, for whatever reason, retained feces become hard and painful to expel, the rectum becomes distended, reducing rectal sensation and the urge to defecate is diminished. A consequence of this chain of events is persistent fecal loading, a capacious rectum and frequent overflow soiling caused by fluid stool passing around the hard feces and staining the child's pants. As a result of these symptoms the parents may adopt a punitive approach towards the child which may compound an already unfortunate situation.

The problem of chronic constipation in children with neurological disability such as cerebral palsy, or spinal cord abnormalities such as myelomeningocele, is especially intractable due to a combination of reduced sensation, weakness of the muscles of the pelvic floor and abdominal wall, and also particular abnormalities of gastrointestinal motility in these patients. These difficulties should be anticipated and appropriate measures taken at an early stage.

Table 17.31 Organic causes of constipation

1.	Dietary
2.	Dehydration
3.	Intestinal obstruction
4.	Anal fissure/stenosis
5.	Hirschsprung's disease
6.	Hypo/hyperganglionosis
7.	Cerebral palsy
8.	Spinal cord lesion
9.	Cystic fibrosis
10.	Food allergy
11.	Hypothyroidism
12.	Hypercalcemia
13.	Hypokalemia
14.	Lead poisoning
15.	Renal failure

Management

Prompt management of children with acute constipation may prevent the development of chronic constipation and the vicious cycle outlined above. In the baby with delayed passage of meconium and continuing constipation, Hirschsprung's disease should be excluded by rectal suction biopsy at an early stage. Investigation of older children and exclusion of the rare organic causes of chronic constipation will depend on the clinical features following a careful history and examination. Laboratory assessment is usually not warranted, but a plain abdominal film may be very helpful in assessing the degree of constipation and the size of the rectum, and also to demonstrate the fact to the child and his parents.[141] General measures such as ensuring an adequate fluid and fiber intake are important and the advice of a pediatric dietitian is helpful in this regard. If anal stenosis is present, then repeated gentle anal dilatation, or an anal stretch under anesthesia, may be of benefit. It is important to carefully examine the perianal region for the presence of an anal fissure as the application of local anesthetic preparations may encourage the child to open his bowels.

It is important to explain to the child and his parents the sequence of events leading to chronic constipation and to outline the aims of therapy which are designed to clear the enlarged rectum and distal colon of feces, and subsequently keep it empty. It should be stressed that the situation is not the child's or family's fault and that treatment may involve many months of therapy. It is vital to provide a reassuring approach that the situation will improve, although setbacks and further bouts of constipation may be encountered during this period. It is not adequate to prescribe a 2-week course of laxatives and tell the family that the situation will improve with time. In practical terms, the initial therapeutic goal is to empty the rectum and distal colon and this usually can be achieved only with daily, or twice-daily pediatric enema preparations. This may be undertaken on an outpatient basis if the general practitioner or health visitor is enthusiastic, but frequently it is necessary to admit the child to hospital for 1 or 2 days and establish that the bowel is empty with an abdominal radiograph prior to starting laxative therapy. Once the large intestine is empty, oral laxatives should be prescribed in adequate doses to ensure that the child's bowels are open at least once a day. It is usual to combine a stool softener such as lactulose with a stimulant aperient such as senna. If the initial dose of laxatives is inadequate, it should be increased; if the laxatives result in diarrhea the dose should be reduced. With time, however, sensation will return to the rectum as its size decreases, and the amount of laxative medication can eventually be decreased and finally stopped.

In addition to medical therapy, it is usually beneficial to institute a behavioral program based on simple rewards such as a modified star chart, where the child is rewarded for a normal, daily bowel action. This is coupled with advice that the child should be able to visit the toilet in a relaxed atmosphere at regular times and it is helpful to see the child regularly in the outpatient clinic, initially at fortnightly intervals, to provide continuing support and encouragement. The child should be encouraged to drink plenty of fluid and to eat a good balanced diet containing fruit and vegetables.

Treatment of children with chronic neurological disease and spinal cord lesions poses particular difficulties and early institution of regular suppositories and oral laxative therapy may be helpful. Furthermore, the development of an enema continence catheter (Cardiomed catheter, Cambmac Instruments Ltd), whereby the colon is emptied on a regular basis, is providing a useful adjunct in patients with constipation and fecal incontinence who experience little or no rectal sensation.

Overall the long term prognosis for functional chronic constipation is excellent and this should be emphasized to both the child, the parent and the physician.

Short segment Hirschsprung's disease

In a small proportion of children who present in childhood with a history of chronic constipation dating from birth and associated with the delayed passage of meconium, a diagnosis of short segment Hirschsprung's disease is made. In these children anorectal manometry is abnormal but rectal biopsy may be unremarkable. The term 'internal sphincter spasm' may be a more appropriate term for this condition with treatment involving a full anal sphincter stretch and internal sphincterotomy performed under general anesthesia.

In some children with chronic constipation rectal biopsy may show either an increase or decrease in the number of ganglion cells. Such hypo- or hyperganglionosis undoubtedly can result in altered colonic motility which leads to chronic constipation and the development of a megacolon.

CHRONIC NON-SPECIFIC DIARRHEA (CNSD)

The syndrome of CNSD (previously known as toddler diarrhea or irritable colon of childhood) is now recognized to be by far the commonest cause of diarrhea without failure to thrive in early childhood; the mechanisms underlying the disorder are largely unknown and speculative, thus making it difficult to advise with confidence about management. It has been suggested that CNSD is self-limiting in 90% of cases, although others have reported a high incidence of constipation on follow-up and a significant history of functional bowel disorders in close family members.[142] Indeed it seems likely that CNSD may be merely part of a spectrum of gastrointestinal motility disorders that includes colic in infancy, recurrent abdominal pain in older children and the irritable bowel syndrome in adults.

Clinical features

Children with CNSD present with loose stools usually between the ages of 6 months and 5 years. The condition is commoner in boys and a careful history will usually elicit the characteristic features of a variable pattern of stool consistency and frequency, often following an initial episode of acute gastroenteritis, with firmer stools passed in the morning and decreasing in consistency later in the day. Occasionally there may be a history of alternating diarrhea and constipation and the presence of undigested foods (especially peas and carrots), with or without mucus, is typical of the disorder. The diarrhea is often exacerbated by a high roughage diet, fruit and sugary drinks. The absolute characteristic of the condition is the absence of failure to thrive, and it is of paramount importance to carefully document the child's height and weight on presentation and at subsequent follow-up. If the child is failing to thrive, the diagnosis must be suspect and further investigation is then warranted.

Etiology and pathogenesis

Although the precise pathophysiological mechanisms operating in CNSD are unknown, several possible etiological factors have been suggested. It is important to exclude excessive intake of fruit juices as a cause of diarrhea. Food allergy can cause similar symptoms in childhood and, although circumstantial evidence for this may be present in the form of a strong personal or family history of atopy, the most important diagnostic test is the response to an elimination diet and challenge. It has been suggested that a low dietary fat intake is a possible cause of CNSD as gastric emptying and gut transit time may be slowed by increasing dietary fat intake. It is thus conceivable that a diet low in fat causes rapid gastric emptying with increased propagative motor activity resulting in the formation of loose stools.

Abnormal intestinal secretion has been implicated in the causation of CNSD as has a primary motility disturbance. It has been suggested that some children with CNSD may demonstrate a significantly higher incidence of environmental indicators of personal or family stress compared with matched controls,[143] which is in keeping with the anecdotal experience of many clinicians.

Diagnosis

CNSD is primarily a diagnosis of exclusion although there are certain positive clinical features, already described, which may provide a pointer to the diagnosis. The prime feature is that the child is healthy and growing normally. In some children there may be a family history of functional bowel disorders, or indeed a personal or family history of food intolerance. It is important to exclude both urinary and enteric infection although food intolerance and the postenteritis syndrome are the main differential diagnoses. Any evidence of malabsorption, atypical clinical features or failure to thrive should prompt further investigation.

Treatment

In the majority of cases, simple reassurance is all that is required. It is important to explain to the parent that, apart from the loose stools, the child is otherwise well and thriving, and the problem is likely to improve. It is also useful to explore the probable etiology of the disorder which may be explained in terms of deranged motility which will improve with time. It is very important to emphasize that growth and general health will be normal in the future, and there will be no delay in achieving continence. Most parents will accept with relief the fact that their child has no serious disease, but for parents who feel that the problem is too difficult to manage, further measures may be necessary.

It is important to advise the parents to avoid giving an excessive intake of fruit juices or squash. Dietary treatment may be beneficial and, in those children with a strong personal or family history of atopy or in whom chronic diarrhea was manifested following an episode of acute gastroenteritis, a trial of an exclusion diet (usually cow's milk and egg free) may be helpful. The services of an experienced pediatric dietitian are invaluable, and the diet must be adhered to for at least 1 month before any decisions are taken about its efficacy. If there is an improvement in symptoms, the diet is continued for at least 3 months before trying to gradually reintroduce the excluded foods. Some pediatricians have achieved success by increasing the child's fat intake so that 50% of the calories are derived from fat.

Although aspirin has previously been shown to be of benefit in some children with CNSD, it should not now be routinely used in view of the possible association with the development of Reye's syndrome. There is evidence that loperamide may provide symptomatic improvement and it can be used intermittently. All drugs, however, have significant side-effects and they should be prescribed only in carefully selected cases. Recent reports of the benefits of stress reduction and environmental management in children with toddler diarrhea are intriguing and highlight that support and parental training in consistent, effective management of their child's behavior can alleviate some of the symptoms of CNSD.

Prognosis

Overall parents can be reassured that the prognosis for their child with CNSD is very good. In the past, the condition has been described as benign and self-limiting and although it is known that diarrhea may persist after toilet training, it usually becomes less obvious to the parents who no longer have to change dirty nappies. It is possible that a proportion of children who manifest CNSD may represent one end of a spectrum of familial functional bowel disorders which will re-emerge as continuing gastrointestinal complaints as they become older.

INVESTIGATION OF THE COLON

Investigation of colonic anatomy and physiology has in the past been difficult, largely owing to the relative inaccessibility of the large intestine and the fact that investigation has involved the use of invasive techniques and exposure to radiation. Those investigative techniques in most common usage are described below.

Radiology

The plain abdominal film (supine and/or erect) can be very useful in the investigation of acute and chronic gastrointestinal disease. Thus the presence of fluid levels may indicate intestinal obstruction, and free gas in the peritoneal cavity may represent intestinal perforation. Repeated plain abdominal films are an essential part of the management of toxic megacolon associated with colonic inflammatory disease such as fulminant ulcerative colitis.

Barium enema examination is now used much less frequently to study colonic anatomy since the advent of colonoscopy, although it may yield useful diagnostic information as well as being potentially therapeutic in cases of intussusception. The indications for barium enema examination include neonatal intestinal obstruction, intussusception and, in some centers where colonoscopy is not available, it may be of help in patients with rectal bleeding or suspected IBD. The use of double contrast barium enema technique is preferable for demonstrating colonic polyps or subtle mucosal disease, although it can be an uncomfortable examination for the child. The need for barium enema examination in Hirschsprung's disease has largely been superseded by the use of rectal suction biopsy.

Radioisotopic scanning after injection of technetium-labeled leukocytes may have a part to play in the diagnosis of the site and extent of inflammatory disease[144] and occasionally patients with unexplained lower gastrointestinal blood loss may require investigation by a technetium-99m-labeled red blood cell scan or selective angiography of the inferior mesenteric artery.

Rectal suction biopsy

Biopsy of the rectal mucosa and submucosa is the most useful technique for diagnosing Hirschsprung's disease but it also may be helpful in the diagnosis of neural lipidoses and amyloidosis. The technique is usually carried out under sedation, and multiple biopsies at varying intervals from the anal margin can be taken. The biopsies are studied for the presence or absence of ganglion cells and for the activity of cholinesterase.[145]

Colonoscopy

The use of flexible endoscopy in pediatric practice has revolutionized the investigation of large intestinal disease in childhood.[146] Using the technique it is possible to traverse and visualize the whole colon and also to obtain multiple biopsies for histological assessment.

Proctoscopy can be performed easily at the bedside in older children and the use of an auroscope may be useful in neonates. Rigid sigmoidoscopy is uncomfortable for the child and this technique has been superseded by the use of small diameter flexible pediatric colonoscopes. Colonoscopy may be performed under sedation using a combination of pethidine and midazolam given intravenously immediately prior to the procedure. Alternatively a short general anesthetic may be more comfortable for the patient, easier for the operator and reduce recovery time. For an adequate inspection of the colon to be undertaken, it is vital that bowel preparation is effective and this may require the administration of 'clear fluids' for 24 h before the examination in addition to generous doses of laxatives and occasional recourse to rectal washouts. The procedure is generally well tolerated and the experience of centers using the technique in childhood has been that the complication rate is minimal.

Motility studies

Anorectal manometry is a useful technique for distinguishing the different causes of constipation and is particularly helpful in the diagnosis of short segment Hirschsprung's disease where the characteristic abnormality of failed internal sphincter relaxation is seen. Large bowel transit can be measured by the ingestion of multiple radio-opaque markers followed by a plain abdominal film at 48 and 72 h. More detailed investigation of colonic motility is at present only available in research centers.

FAILURE TO THRIVE

DEFINITION

A child is said to be failing to thrive when his or her rate of growth fails to meet the potential expected for a child of that age (see also Ch. 13). The absolute height or weight for any one child depends on many factors including the child's age, ethnic origins and the mid-parental height. As intrauterine nutrition also has a major influence on the birth weight, the weight of a child at 6–8 weeks is often taken as a baseline for the subsequent measurement of growth. Because the growth rate of a child is at its greatest during the first 2 years of life, it is at this time that children most commonly fail to thrive.

Standard growth charts are commonly used to define how the growth of a child compares to the norm (see Fig. 17.14). It must be remembered that these charts are constructed using a group of children, living in a given area at a given time and may not be appropriate for all populations. A single plot on a centile chart is of limited value and it should be possible with most children to obtain detailed information about weight gain over the first 2 years of life from their child health clinic book. The definition of 'failure to thrive' should be based on a downward trajectory through the centiles rather than on a single measurement. Children born at the

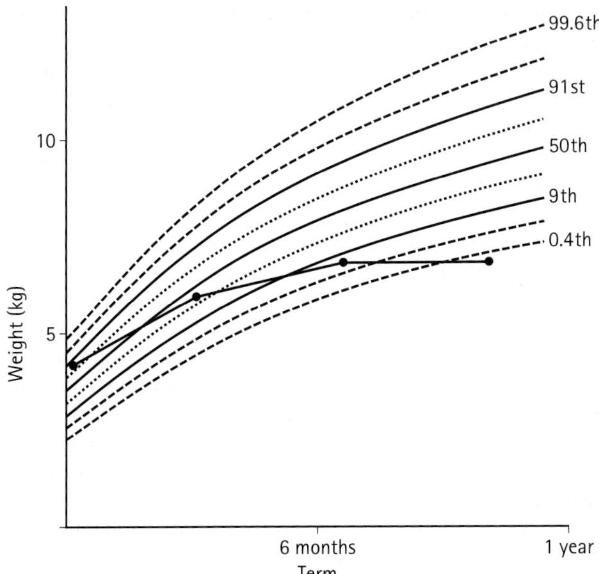

Fig. 17.14 A growth chart showing the weight of a child with failure to thrive crossing down the centiles.

Table 17.32 Classification of failure to thrive

1.	Reduced intake of nutrients a. Feeding difficulties (MOST COMMON CAUSE) b. Neglect and withholding of food c. Anorexia d. Mechanical and coordination problems with swallowing
2.	Inability to digest or absorb nutrients a. Pancreatic insufficiency b. Small intestinal disease
3.	Excessive loss of nutrients a. Vomiting b. Protein-losing enteropathy c. Chronic diarrhea
4.	Increased nutrient requirements due to underlying disease a. Chronic cardiac or respiratory failure b. Chronic infection
5.	Unable to fully utilize nutrients a. Metabolic disorder b. Dysmorphic syndrome

extremes (very large or very small) of weight will tend over time to move toward the average, thus a child with above average weight falling down the centiles is likely to be of less significance than a child of below average weight who has fallen by a similar amount. Changes in centile position over time can best be represented by a standard deviation score (SDS).[147] Population studies have shown that less than 5% of children will fall in weight by 1.4 standard deviations and that less than 1% will fall by 1.9 standard deviations in the first 18 months of life. Children growing at rates below the 5% population norm can be considered to be failing to thrive. When children fail to gain weight for only a few months, height and head circumference will continue to increase at a normal rate slowing when the nutritional insult is more prolonged and when linear growth and brain growth may both be compromised.

ETIOLOGY

Failure to thrive is not a diagnosis but simply a term, which collectively describes the end result of a great number of different events (see Table 17.32). It is now clear that the vast majority of children with failure to thrive are not suffering from organic disease and are not the subject of neglect. In a population study carried out in Newcastle, England social class, breast-feeding and deprivation were no more common among children failing to thrive than in a control population.[148,149] In contrast, where children were referred for further investigation of failure to thrive by their health visitor, there was an excess of non-breast-fed babies from lower socioeconomic groups and deprived households. This suggests that there is bias among health professionals when the referral of such children is considered.

Further study of nutritional intake in children failing to thrive suggests that up to 50% have either moderate or strong evidence of undernutrition and that inadequate intake of nutrients is the single most important cause. Other characteristics in this population were late weaning, the presence of an immature feeding pattern, higher rates of early feeding difficulty and less interest in food.

Organic conditions probably account for about 5% of children with failure to thrive and should be suspected in the child with chronic diarrhea or vomiting. Child neglect or abuse are probably relevant in a further 5% (see Ch. 5).

DIAGNOSIS AND TREATMENT

It should be possible to identify the cause of a child's failure to thrive by taking a clear history. Information about diet, the timing of weaning, the time taken to feed, the variety of feeds and the presence or absence of gastrointestinal symptoms is vitally important. With appropriate training this is something that community pediatric nurses and health visitors can be trained to do and the detection and treatment of failure to thrive is something that under most circumstances can be carried out completely in the community. The gastrointestinal causes of failure to thrive are outlined in the following section.

Advice from a health visitor or dietitian should be aimed at giving advice to improve the child's nutrient intake.[150,151] Higher energy foods should be encouraged and food textures and consistency should be appropriate for the child's oromotor skills. Many feeding problems result from difficulties in the interaction between the child and his/her parents at the time of feeding. Correct positioning of the child, the use of appropriate feeding utensils and trying to make meal times enjoyable for both the child and the parent are all essential. It is only when these methods fail to improve growth that referral for further specialist opinion should be sought.

GASTROINTESTINAL CAUSES OF FAILURE TO THRIVE

Gastrointestinal disease can result in failure to thrive if the child's nutritional intake is compromised, if nutrients fail to be absorbed or digested, or if there are excessive losses of nutrients from the gut (Table 17.33).

Children with a cleft palate, neuromuscular incoordination of the pharynx or disordered esophageal function will have difficulty swallowing and may aspirate feeds. Anorexia is a common feature of IBD, enteric infection and disorders of the stomach and duodenum. This may be further compounded by therapeutic diets which are frequently unpalatable. Patients who are severely malnourished as a consequence of chronic anorexia and who have normal digestive and absorptive function are likely to show a marked rise in weight in response to enteral tube feeding.

Table 17.33 Gastrointestinal causes of failure to thrive: expanded from sections 1c, 1d, 2 and 3 of Table 17.32

1. Anorexia
   a. Inflammatory bowel disease
      (i) Crohn's disease
      (ii) Ulcerative colitis
   b. Food allergic disease
   c. Gastroduodenal disease
      (i) Duodenal ulcer
      (ii) Idiopathic gastroparesis
      (iii) Gastritis
   d. Chronic enteric infection
      (i) Stagnant loop syndrome
      (ii) Small bowel colonization in malnutrition
   e. Iatrogenic
      (i) Therapeutic diets
      (ii) Drugs
2. Mechanical disorder of ingestion (see Table 17.2)
   a. Absent sucking
      (i) Neurodevelopmental delay
   b. Oral malformation
      (i) Cleft palate
      (ii) Pierre Robin syndrome
   c. Defective swallowing
      (i) Neuromuscular incoordination
      (ii) Cerebral palsy
      (iii) Brainstem tumor
   d. Dysphagia
      (i) Neuromuscular incoordination
      (ii) Esophagitis and stricture
3. Inability to digest or absorb nutrients (see Table 17.11)
   a. Pancreatic insufficiency
      (i) Cystic fibrosis
   b. Small intestinal disease
      (i) Celiac disease
      (ii) Food-sensitive enteropathy
      (iii) Inborn error of digestion or absorption
      (iv) Short gut syndrome
4. Excessive losses of nutrients
   a. Recurrent vomiting
      (i) Gastroesophageal reflux
      (ii) Pyloric stenosis
   b. Protein-losing enteropathy (see Table 17.13)

Pancreatic exocrine insufficiency, which is most commonly due to cystic fibrosis, and disorders of the digestive and absorptive apparatus of the small intestine will result in poor weight gain in the face of an adequate nutritional intake. Recurrent vomiting resulting from severe gastroesophageal reflux may limit the amount of nutrients entering the small intestine and nutrient losses in the stool may occur in patients with chronic diarrhea.

Investigations

When it is felt that a child's failure to thrive is due to gastrointestinal disease it is important that the nature of the disease and any nutritional consequences are clearly defined.

Fall-off in weight and height in children with gastrointestinal disease is the main indication of significant malnourishment. Malabsorption of iron, calcium, zinc and vitamins will lead to anemia, poor bone mineralization, blood clotting abnormalities and an increased susceptibility to infection. A falling albumin level indicates either decreased protein synthesis as a result of lack of substrate or excessive losses into the gut. The measurement of the indices mentioned above will give an idea of the severity of the nutritional problem.

When the child is vomiting, barium studies will allow the anatomy of the upper gastrointestinal tract to be defined, a 24 h pH study will allow the degree of gastroesophageal reflux to be quantified and endoscopic examination will allow mucosal abnormalities to be defined. When pyloric stenosis is suspected a test feed should be carried out and where bilious vomiting is present erect and supine X-rays will ascertain whether the child has an intestinal obstruction.

Diarrhea may be either osmotic or secretory. In the former, which results from the osmotic effect of undigested food, the electrolyte content of the stools is likely to be low while sugars and fat, which can be quantified by stool chromatography or fecal fat measurement, will almost certainly be present in the stool. The pattern of sugars in the stool may also reflect the underlying abnormality and can be of great value in diagnosing inborn errors of digestion and absorption. A fast will stop an osmotic diarrhea while a secretory process will result in the continued loss of electrolyte-rich fluid in the stool (Table 17.24). In any infant with diarrhea who is failing to thrive a sweat test and a jejunal biopsy will allow cystic fibrosis, celiac disease, cow's milk protein intolerance and a range of other disorders which result in an enteropathic process to be diagnosed. Signs of atopy, infection or immune deficiency should be sought if these seem clinically likely. In many conditions the clinical response to treatment is a useful confirmation of the suspected diagnosis. If colonic disease is suspected by the presence of blood or mucus, colonoscopy with biopsy will allow the nature of any inflammatory disorder to be defined.

Abdominal pain and colic are most frequently due to the irritable bowel syndrome which is not associated with failure to thrive. However, when poor growth does occur one must consider the possibility of food allergy, pancreatitis, IBD and in particular Crohn's disease. Endoscopic examination of the stomach and colon along with a barium follow-through study should help localize the problem while a raised amylase will support the diagnosis of pancreatitis and a raised ESR and platelet count will support an inflammatory cause.

Failure to thrive may be the only symptom of gastrointestinal disease in some patients and this frequently results in a long delay between the initiation of the disease process and the eventual diagnosis. When small intestinal disease is present the extensive reserve capacity of the colon allows excessive fluid entering the colon to be reabsorbed with the resulting passage of formed stools. One should be aware that in celiac disease, cow's milk protein intolerance and in older children with Crohn's disease diarrhea is not always present. Without an awareness of these conditions an early diagnosis is unlikely to be made.

Further information on the diagnosis and treatment of the conditions mentioned above can be found elsewhere in this chapter.

NUTRITION IN PATIENTS WITH GASTROINTESTINAL DISEASE

Gastrointestinal disorders in childhood frequently have major nutritional consequences and dietary manipulation plays an important role in the treatment of such patients. An understanding of the nutritional requirements in childhood is of help both in planning the treatment of patients who are malnourished as a result of gastrointestinal disease and also in communicating with the pediatric dietitian who is responsible for the supervision of the child's dietary management.[152] Full details of nutritional requirements and the consequences of malnutrition are given in Chapter 14.

In children who are failing to grow adequately it is important to define whether their nutritional intake is adequate. Where deficiencies exist they should be corrected by giving adequate amounts of food but energy intake can also be boosted by the use of feeds fortified with added glucose polymer or fat. Diets low in vitamins and minerals should also be appropriately supplemented.

Therapeutic diets for the treatment of gastrointestinal disease should be closely supervised by a dietitian.[152] In celiac disease gluten exclusion is required but in food allergic patients multiple exclusions may be needed to prevent the development of symptoms. Elemental diets which may be used in Crohn's disease are frequently administered by nasogastric tube because of their unpalatable taste. Similarly children who require energy supplements because of problems with swallowing will benefit from nasogastric feeds. Whenever possible the enteral route should be used to supplement nutrition and when an oral intake is not possible delivery directly into the stomach or jejunum by nasogastric tube or gastrostomy or nasojejunal tube should be considered. Accurate enteral infusion pumps allow the steady delivery of feeds during the day or night and in many children this treatment can be continued safely at home.

In some of these children the gastrointestinal tract may be too severely damaged to tolerate a full enteral intake and under these circumstances parenteral nutrition will be required. It should be possible to maintain good nutrition in all children and this will invariably require the surgical placement of a tunneled central venous catheter which will guarantee good venous access and allow the use of hyperosmolar solutions. When parenteral nutrition is prolonged it is important to closely monitor for vitamin or trace mineral deficiencies as requirements will frequently be increased in patients with gastrointestinal disease. An enteral intake, with its trophic effect on the gut, should be continued during periods of parenteral nutrition and increased as tolerance improves.

In a few children intestinal function may be so severely compromised that recovery may take many months or be unlikely ever to occur. Under such circumstances home parenteral nutrition should be considered. It is now technically possible to maintain normal growth and development over prolonged periods in children receiving this therapy at home. With improved results, small intestinal transplantation is a treatment that should be considered in selected patients (see p. 686).

The use of a nutrition care team, comprising a doctor, nurse, pharmacist, dietitian and biochemist, is of great help in supervising and monitoring the treatment of children with complicated nutritional problems managed both in hospital and at home.

HEPATIC AND BILIARY DISEASE

ANATOMICAL STRUCTURE AND FUNCTION OF THE LIVER

The anatomical site and structural organization of the liver are designed to maintain close homeostatic control of the constituents of portal blood when returned to the hepatic venous system. Substrates from the portal system are rapidly taken into the liver cells, metabolized, stored and their products transferred as required into the blood and bile. Blood-, bile- and lymph-containing channels transport nutrients, metabolites, antigens, antibodies, hormones and drugs to and from hepatocytes, and also to the other specialized liver cells, the Kupffer cell, the sinusoidal endothelial cell, the stellate cells and to the cells of the biliary tree.

The basic functional unit of the liver is the acinus, being the mass of parenchyma receiving its blood supply from a single portal tract. Blood from terminal branches of the hepatic artery and portal vein in the portal tract enters and traverses the sinusoids, specialized capillaries lined by Kupffer and endothelial cells which contain fenestra allowing ready access of plasma and its contents to the surface of the hepatocyte (Fig. 17.15).[153] The sinusoids drain to the central vein of the hepatic lobule, and ultimately into the inferior vena cava. The hepatocytes near the portal tracts receive more oxygen, nutrients and hormones, have a higher metabolic rate, synthesize more proteins and regenerate more rapidly than those nearer the central vein. Those near the central vein are particularly susceptible to hypoxic and toxic injury. This structure can regain its pristine condition when destroyed by acute toxins such as paracetamol or type A viral hepatitis. Persisting injury with infiltration by migratory cells of the reticuloendothelial system sets in train a complex series of interactions increasing deposition of extracellular matrix components leading ultimately to irretrievable disruption of the acinar relationships by cirrhosis, with consequences for homeostatic function.

CLINICAL ASSESSMENT OF LIVER DYSFUNCTION

Unfortunately, the sensitivity and specificity of many clinical symptoms and signs in liver disease are low so that diseases may be present without detectable signs or symptoms and those present may not be specific to liver disease. Thus, for example, it is possible to have chronic viral hepatitis B for decades proceeding to cirrhosis without any external, or for that matter biochemical, evidence. Features with some degree of sensitivity in established liver disease are:

- Jaundice with dark urine implies cholestatic liver disease. The urine of infants should not contain significant color or stain the napkin and yellow urine strongly suggests obstruction of bile flow. Yellow sclerae suggests cholestatic jaundice but are often difficult to detect in small infants and those with some scleral pigment.
- Liver palms, although not often seen in the first year of life.
- Splenomegaly in portal hypertension, although as children get older a larger spleen can be accommodated beneath the ribs, further reducing the sensitivity of this sign.
- Coagulopathy has particular significance in liver disease. In the context of cholestasis, it may represent failure of absorption of sufficient vitamin K especially in infants where it may present as bleeding diathesis known as hemorrhagic disease of the newborn. Intracranial bleeding is associated with severe long-term morbidity. Infants should not normally suffer spontaneous bleeding and fresh blood from sites such as the umbilicus or nares should always prompt a search for evidence of vitamin K

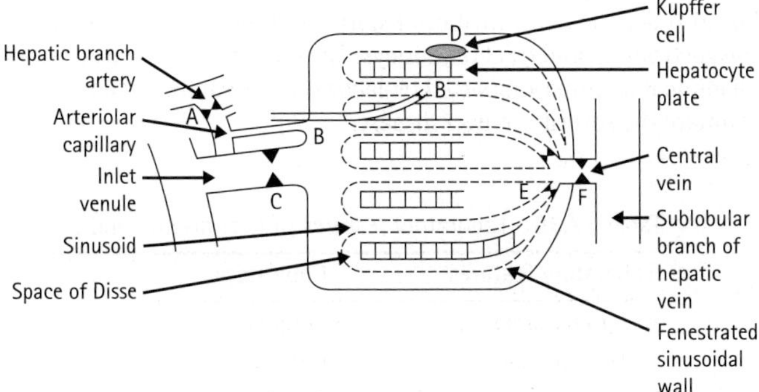

Fig. 17.15 A diagrammatic representation of the liver sinusoids and their blood supply. A–F represent sites of possible sphincters involved in controlling blood flow through the hepatic sinusoids. (From *Liver Disorders in Childhood* 2/e by Mowat.[153] Reprinted by permission of Elsevier Science Ltd.)

malabsorption including due to liver disease. Jaundice may be so mild as to be disregarded in such cases. In cases of coagulopathy not responsive to vitamin K, coagulation factors are being consumed by intravascular consumption or are not being formed. Thus in the patient with liver disease and coagulopathy unresponsive to vitamin K but without consumptive coagulopathy liver synthetic failure must be present. This criterion is the most sensitive for liver failure in children. Others include hypoglycemia and encephalopathy.

- Pale stools in cholestatic liver disease. Particular emphasis should be placed on examining stool and urine, as the history particularly from first-time parents of infants with possible liver disease, can be misleading. White stools, or stools the color of cream cheese or uncooked pastry are clearly abnormal. Those with mild degrees of green pigment or pale yellow or a pale buff brown color may also represent reduced bile flow as for example in the case of developing biliary atresia.
- Hepatomegaly is likely to be associated with liver disease, hepatic mass or cardiac failure. Infants may have up to 2 cm of liver edge palpable below the costal margin but the texture is soft. Riedel's lobe is seldom encountered in practice. Abnormal texture and an irregular inferior margin strongly suggest established liver disease with fibrosis/cirrhosis. Changed liver conformation with prominence in the midline but an impalpable right lobe suggests collapse, regeneration and the development of cirrhosis. A liver of this shape is also found in the Budd–Chiari syndrome as a consequence of caudate hypertrophy. Tenderness of a smooth liver suggests rapid recent increase in liver size for example in acute hepatitis but also cardiac failure.

Severity of liver dysfunction can be considered in three broad categories. These are:

1. cholestasis, implying impairment of bile flow with consequent reduction of intraluminal bile salt concentration, associated conjugated hyperbilirubinemia and raised serum bile acids, the latter causing pruritus;
2. portal hypertension (PHT) with associated hypersplenism and the effects of portosystemic shunting (if present);
3. hepatocellular impairment (cell function) representing evidence of failure of synthetic and homeostatic function.

Clinical and basic laboratory findings can be interpreted according to this classification although some such as ascites are represented in more than one category (Tables 17.34 and 17.35). Transudative ascites can result from a combination of increased portal pressure and low plasma oncotic pressure (implying low serum albumin). Serum albumin reflects liver synthetic function but also depends on nutritional status and losses, for example via the gastrointestinal tract or kidneys. Thus it is necessary to consider all clinical features supported by laboratory parameters in order to evaluate the severity of liver disease.

Table 17.34 The clinical features of liver disease and their significance

Clinical features	Cholestasis	PHT	Cell function
Jaundice	Conjugated	–	Mixed if severe
Pruritus	+	–	–
Leuconychia	+	–	–
Clubbing	+	+	–
Fat soluble vitamin deficiency	+	–	–
Xanthomas	+ but not in PFIC	–	–
Splenomegaly	–	–	+
Cutaneous shunts	–	+	–
Other cutaneous stigmata	–	+	+
Hypersplenism	–	+	–
Cyanosis–hepatopulmonary syndrome	–	+	–
Esophageal varices	–	+	–
Ascites	–	+	+
Encephalopathy	–	+	+
Dependent edema	–	–	+
Malnutrition	+	+	+

PFIC, progressive familial intrahepatic cholestasis; PHT, portal hypertension

Ultrasound

Ultrasonography has become a mainstay in examining liver parenchymal texture, anatomical structures, portal and arterial blood flow and pathological lesions. Particular examples are cysts, abscesses, solid tumors, hemangioendotheliomas, dilatation of the biliary tree from choledochal cysts and tumors. Calculi, sludge and polyps in the gallbladder can be visualized. It is unhelpful in diagnosing biliary atresia other than it may show absence of the gallbladder. Parenchymal echotexture is increased with fatty liver, in storage disorders and in leukemic infiltration.

Other imaging

CT scanning, MRI, cholangiography and angiography, percutaneous transhepatic cholangiography (PTC) and endoscopic retrograde cholangiopancreatography are very informative although their safe and effective use requires specialist diagnostic imaging expertise.

Percutaneous liver biopsy

Skilled histological interpretation, histochemical and biochemical analysis and bacterial, fungal or viral culture of liver biopsy tissue yields results which may be of crucial diagnostic importance. It gives invaluable information on the severity of liver damage and structural change and also in assessing the requirements for therapy in chronic hepatitis. An ultrasound scan, to exclude a focal

Table 17.35 Laboratory features of liver disease and their significance

Laboratory features	Cholestasis	PHT	Cell function
Serum bilirubin	Conjugated	–	Mixed
Serum albumin	N	N (low in severe enteropathy)	Low
Serum cholesterol	High except in familial intrahepatic cholestasis	N	Low
Prothrombin time/ratio	N if vitamin K replete	N*	Prolonged if severe

N, normal; *implies minor prolongation seen in portal vein thrombosis; PHT, portal hypertension liver lesion or bile duct obstruction, is required before a biopsy. Contraindications are: INR (international normalized ratio for prothrombin time) greater than 1.3, platelet count of less than 70×10^9/L, hydatid cyst or abscess in the right lobe of liver, angiomatous malformation of liver and hepatocellular carcinoma but not hepatoblastoma. It should only be undertaken by trained personnel with adequate vascular access and available surgical support.

NEONATAL CHOLESTASIS SYNDROME

Hepatitis in infancy is characterized by clinical and laboratory features of hepatic inflammation with conjugated hyperbilirubinemia. It must be suspected in any jaundiced infant particularly if the urine is yellow rather than colorless, or if jaundice persists beyond 14 days of age. Specimens of stools must be saved in a container that excludes light and examined for pigment by the clinician in person according to the description above (Clinical assessment, pp 699–701). If the stools contain no yellow or green pigment, cholestasis is complete and biliary atresia must be suspected.

Occasionally, infants will present with bleeding diathesis, hypoglycemia, fluid retention or malabsorption. The most important investigation is INR following administration of parenteral vitamin K, which if it remains abnormal indicates acute liver failure (ALF).

The prognosis is that of the associated disorder (see remainder of chapter). Chronic liver disease rarely occurs in cholestasis associated with infection, or when disease remains cryptogenic after full investigation, unless there is a positive family history or consanguinity. Neonatal cholestasis may be complicated by progressive intrahepatic cholestasis particularly those with normal serum gamma-glutamyltranspeptidase (gamma-GT) activity in the presence of liver disease.

Differential diagnosis

Three management priorities can be identified:

1. to prevent complications such as hemorrhagic disease of the newborn and hypoglycemia;
2. to identify treatable bacterial, metabolic, endocrine or hematological disorders and initiate treatment (Tables 17.36 and 17.37);
3. to diagnose biliary atresia as early as possible so as to optimize the surgical outcome.

Evidence of consanguinity or liver disease in siblings suggests the possibility of familial, genetic, metabolic or hemolytic disease. Review of the perinatal case records and past medical history may reveal uterine infection, exposure to toxins and drugs or prolonged parenteral nutrition. Physical abnormalities are occasionally very helpful (Table 17.38).

Coagulopathy due to vitamin K malabsorption (late hemorrhagic disease of the newborn), hypoglycemia, septicemia, urinary tract infection, syphilis and herpes simplex infections, listeriosis and toxoplasmosis all have effective treatments. Galactosemia (galactose-1-phosphate uridyl transferase activity), fructosemia (dietary exposure) and tyrosinemia (urinary succinylacetone excretion) should also be excluded immediately since dietary treatment is available. Inborn errors of bile acid synthesis can respond to primary bile acid treatment. Early diagnosis of alpha-1 antitrypsin deficiency, cystic fibrosis and Niemann–Pick type C clarifies the prognosis and allows genetic counseling. Associated endocrine disorders (Table 17.39) must also be excluded on the basis of the clinical findings and appropriate laboratory investigations. Current subgroups of progressive familial intrahepatic cholestasis (PFIC) appears in Table 17.40.

Table 17.36 Disorders associated with neonatal cholestasis

1. Intrahepatic disorders
   a. Inherited disorders
   b. Endocrine abnormalities
   c. Vascular abnormalities
   d. Severe hemolytic disease
   e. Chronic hypoxia and circulatory abnormalities
   f. Chromosomal anomalies
   g. Intravenous nutrition
   h. Drugs
   i. Alagille syndrome
   j. Sclerosing cholangitis
   k. Maternal systemic lupus erythematosus
   l. Variants of progressive intrahepatic cholestasis
   m. Idiopathic
2. Extrahepatic disorders
   a. Biliary atresia
   b. Choledochal cyst
   c. Spontaneous perforation of the bile duct
   d. Inspissation in the biliary system
      (i) Hemolytic disorders
      (ii) Cystic fibrosis
      (iii) Total parenteral nutrition
      (iv) Congenital infections
   e. Gallstones
   f. Malignant nodes
   g. Tumor of the duodenum or pancreas
   h. Hemangioendotheliomata

A skillfully interpreted percutaneous liver biopsy is usually required for diagnosis. Some of the material obtained must be frozen at −70°C for subsequent biochemical analysis for inherited disorders (Table 17.37) if indicated by the liver histology or other investigations. Outstanding results of investigations for conditions including congenital infections (Table 17.41) should not be allowed to delay diagnosis of biliary atresia or other surgically correctable disorders.

If percutaneous liver biopsy shows increased edema, fibrosis and bile duct reduplication, biliary atresia is highly likely although this appearance can also be found in some genetic and endocrine disorders, in some infants who will ultimately develop bile duct hypoplasia and in some of the conditions within the spectrum of intrahepatic cholestasis shown in Table 17.40.

Table 17.37 Inherited disorders associated with neonatal cholestasis

1. Galactosemia
2. Alpha-1 antitrypsin deficiency
3. Cystic fibrosis
4. Tyrosinemia
5. Niemann–Pick types A and C
6. Gaucher's disease
7. Wolman's disease
8. Zellweger syndrome
9. Polycystic disease [autosomal recessive polycystic kidney disease (ARPKD)]
10. Erythrophagocytic reticulosis
11. Neonatal hemochromatosis
12. Defects in synthesis of primary bile acids
13. Variants of progressive intrahepatic cholestasis (PFIC)

Table 17.38 Helpful physical findings in neonatal cholestasis

Physical signs	Disorder suggested
IUGR, skin lesions, purpura, choroidoretinitis, myocarditis	Congenital infections
Cataracts	Galactosemia, hypoparathyroidism
Multiple and characteristic abnormailties	Trisomy 21, 18, 13, Lawrence-Moon-Biedl, Beckwith-Wiedemann syndromes
Mass beneath liver	Choledochal cyst
Ascites bile stained hernia and umbilicus	Spontaneous perforation of the bile ducts
Murmur, characteristic facies, embryotoxon	Alagille syndrome
Cutaneous hemangioma	Hemangioendothelioma of liver
Situs inversus, cardiac defect 'cor triatrium'	Biliary atresia
Optic nerve hypoplasia, wandering eye movements, micropenis	Hypopituitarism

IUGR, intrauterine growth retardation

Table 17.39 Endocrine disorders associated with hepatitis syndrome in infancy

1. Hypopituitarism (Spray et al 2000[154])
2. Diabetes insipidus
3. Hypoadrenalism
4. Hypothyroidism
5. Hypoparathyroidism
6. Growth hormone deficiency may become evident toward the end of infancy

Paucity of interlobular bile ducts (intrahepatic biliary hypoplasia)

The above diagnosis is based on a decrease in the number of interlobular bile ducts seen in portal tracts (ratio < 0.06) on liver biopsy. It is found in prematurity, occasionally in conditions causing hepatitis in infancy and with right sided cardiovascular anomalies, classically peripheral pulmonary stenosis, skeletal and ocular anomalies defining Alagille syndrome (AS; syndromic paucity of the intrahepatic bile ducts; arteriohepatic dysplasia). Diagnosis is supported by the typical facies: triangular face shape, deep-set eyes, overhanging forehead, a straight nose which in profile is in the same plane as the forehead and a small pointed chin, posterior embryotoxon and vertebral arch defects on spinal radiographs. AS is inherited in an autosomal dominant fashion, with one of a wide variety of Jagged 1 mutations on chromosome 20q shown in most affected families studied. Phenotypic expression is variable. Mild cases may have intermittent pruritus only. Jaundice is usually evident from the neonatal period, which often persists but may clear in puberty. The long-standing cholestasis causes jaundice, pruritus, hypercholesterolemia and xanthelasma. The long term prognosis is uncertain but 30% may progress to cirrhosis and 5–10% die from liver disease.[156,157] In one series 25% died from cardiac involvement or infection. The treatment is that of chronic cholestasis with particular emphasis on adequacy of vitamin E replacement and the control of pruritus. Intolerably low quality of life may be an indication for liver transplantation in AS.

Liver disease associated with parenteral nutrition

Prolonged intravenous nutrition, particularly in early infancy causes cholestasis and hepatocellular damage which may progress to cirrhosis and liver cancer if intravenous feeding cannot be stopped.[158] The mechanism remains unclear. Prevalence increases with the degree of prematurity, growth retardation before birth, the duration of intravenous feeding and the absence of enteral food intake. Sepsis, hypoxia, shock, blood transfusion, intra-abdominal surgery and potentially hepatotoxic drugs may aggravate the liver damage.[159] Inspissated bile syndrome is an important complication.

Clinical features and laboratory findings

The first clinical indication of hepatic involvement is usually the appearance of conjugated hyperbilirubinemia. Biochemical tests of liver function are elevated. It is important to consider other causes of cholestasis in neonates before concluding that it is due to intravenous nutrition. If intravenous nutrition can be withdrawn the jaundice settles, although liver function tests may remain abnormal for 6 months and liver biopsy changes persist for up to 1 year. Ursodeoxycholic acid and cholecystokinin may be beneficial in promoting bile flow.

Table 17.40 Currently recognized variants of progressive familial intrahepatic cholestasis (PFIC) (From Thompson & Strautnieks 2001[155])

Clinical variant	Genetic marker or locus	Features
Byler disease or PFIC1	Ch 18 autosomal recessive	Low gGT, diarrhea, FTT, Byler bile on EM
BSEP deficiency or PFIC2	Ch 2 autosomal recessive	Low gGT
Other low gGT variants	Unknown	29% of low gGT PFIC have no Ch 2 or 18 marker
Aagenes syndrome	Ch 15 autosomal recessive	High gGT, lymphedema, seen in South Norway
American Indian cholestasis	Ch 14 autosomal recessive	High gGT, otitis media, paper money skin
Neonatal sclerosing cholangitis	Unknown	High gGT, clinically similar to biliary atresia
MDR3 deficiency	Ch 7 autosomal recessive	High gGT, bile phospholipid transport defect
With renal polycystic disease ARPKD, Caroli disease	Ch 6 autosomal recessive	High gGT, renal failure

BSEP, bile salt export pump; EM, electron microscopy; FTT, failure to thrive; gGT, gamma glutamyl transferase; MDR3, multidrug resistance 3

Table 17.41 Infections causing hepatitis in infancy

1. Viral infections
   a. Cytomegalovirus
   b. Epstein–Barr virus
   c. Rubella virus
   d. Varicella zoster virus
   e. Hepatitis A
   f. Hepatitis B virus (+ delta virus)
   g. Non-A, non-B hepatitis
   h. Herpes simplex virus
   i. Coxsackie A9, B
   j. Echo virus 9, 11, 14, 19
   k. Adenovirus
   l. Reovirus type III
2. Non-viral infections
   a. Bacterial infection
   b. Psittacosis
   c. *Listeria*
   d. *Treponema pallidum*
   e. *Toxoplasma gondii*
   f. Tuberculosis
   g. Malaria

Disorders requiring urgent surgical treatment

Biliary atresia is a disorder of unknown cause where a destructive sclerosing inflammatory process causes obstruction of the extrahepatic bile ducts and extends into the major intrahepatic bile ducts. If surgery is to be successful it must be performed before complete intrahepatic occlusion occurs. In the liver substance the portal tracts become distended with edema, a mild inflammatory cell infiltrate and increased fibrous tissue deposition. Proliferation of distorted bile ductules occurs around the periphery. By 6–10 weeks of age the portal blood pressure is increased. Cirrhosis rapidly develops. The mean age at death in untreated cases is 11 months with less than 5% surviving beyond 2 years.

Clinical features

The first sign of biliary atresia is prolongation of jaundice. The urine is always yellow. The stools contain no yellow or green pigment, but in up to 30% of infants with biliary atresia stools are pigmented in the first weeks after birth before bile flow is completely obstructed. Biliary atresia must be considered in any infant remaining jaundiced beyond 14 days of age. The incidence in the prematurely born or light-for-gestational age infant is the same as full term. There may be hepatomegaly or splenomegaly. Investigations to confirm the diagnosis must be completed before signs of chronic liver disease develop. All too frequently the infant's apparent well-being causes health workers to overlook biliary atresia in the early weeks when surgery is most likely to be successful.

Laboratory investigations

There is no single test to guarantee a prelaparotomy diagnosis of biliary atresia. Percutaneous liver biopsy showing the features described above in all portal tracts is suggestive of atresia, if alpha-1 antitrypsin deficiency, cystic fibrosis and arteriohepatic dysplasia (Alagille syndrome) have been excluded. Radionuclide studies such as technetium-99m-tagged iminodiacetic acid derivative (IDA) (e.g. methylbromo-IDA) are only of value in excluding biliary atresia when it shows continuity between the biliary system and gastrointestinal tract. ERCP is helpful in diagnosing ambiguous cases.

Diagnosis of biliary atresia is confirmed at laparotomy, which should only be undertaken by a surgeon performing at least five Kasai portoenterostomies per year who can assess changes in the porta hepatis and proceed to portoenterostomy. Currently there are only three such centers in England and Wales. An anastomosis is fashioned between the area of the porta hepatis from which the inflamed bile duct remnants have been resected and a Roux-en-Y loop is fashioned allowing bile to drain from the main hepatic bile ducts directly into the bowel. Good bile flow can be achieved in 70% operated on by 60 days of age but in only 20–30% following later surgery.[160]

Complications

Cholangitis occurs in a significant minority of cases in the first 2 years after surgery. It is characterized by fever, recurrence or aggravation of jaundice and occasionally features of septicemia. Blood culture, ascitic aspirate or liver biopsy, to identify the organism responsible, should precede intravenous antibiotic therapy, which is continued for 7–14 days. Prophylactic antibiotics are of no proven value. Recurrent cholangitis has an adverse effect on liver function, indicating the need for early and aggressive treatment.

Portal hypertension is present in almost all cases of biliary atresia at the time of initial surgery. At 5 years of age approximately 50% will have esophageal varices but only 10–15% will have alimentary bleeding in whom band ligation is the treatment of choice. All patients have a degree of malabsorption in the first year indicating dietary supplements with medium chain triglycerides and glucose polymers. Supplements of fat-soluble vitamins E, D, K and A are essential.

Prognosis

The prognosis of biliary atresia has been transformed by the Kasai operation and with liver transplantation as an option if necessary. Following the Kasai procedure a normal serum bilirubin is found in 65% of patients with a 90% 10-year survival and with a good quality of life into the fourth decade. Overall there is no evidence of portal hypertension in 25%, 10% with normal transaminases and 15% with abnormal transaminases, 40% will have varying degrees of portal hypertension, almost all with good quality of life. Subsequent liver transplantation will be required by 35% and with this combined approach child mortality can be reduced to less than 5% compared with universal mortality 30 years ago.[161]

Choledochal cyst

In this disorder there is enlargement or dilatation of part or all the extrahepatic biliary system. Bile flow may be obstructed with intrahepatic changes similar to those of biliary atresia, progressing to cirrhosis. Cholangitis, cyst rupture, pancreatitis, gallstones and carcinoma of the cyst wall are other important complications. Ultrasound antenatal diagnosis occurs infrequently. In infancy it presents with features of neonatal cholestasis. In older children there may be recurrent upper abdominal pain, recurrent jaundice and/or a palpable cystic mass but the classical triad is rare. Diagnosis is by ultrasonography and percutaneous transhepatic cholangiography. The treatment is surgical removal with biliary drainage via a Roux-en-Y loop. Intrahepatic elements of the cyst are associated with a poorer prognosis with increased risk of developing biliary cirrhosis.

Spontaneous perforation of the bile duct

Perforation occurs at the junction of the cystic duct and common hepatic duct in infants. The etiology is unclear but may represent the consequence of a choledochal malformation. Mild jaundice, acholic stools, failure to thrive and biliary ascites with bile-stained hernia and umbilicus are the clinical features. Treatment entails surgical drainage of the biliary system into a Roux-en-Y loop.

HEPATITIS AND LIVER INFECTIONS

Acute and chronic inflammation of the liver with varying degrees of hepatocellular necrosis may be due to a wide range of causes including viral infections, autoimmunity, drugs and toxins, metabolic and infiltrative conditions. Chronic low-grade hepatitides may progress to cirrhosis despite repeatedly measured normal serum transaminases.

Viral hepatitis (see also Ch. 26)

The term viral hepatitis is usually applied to infections caused by viruses with a high degree of hepatotrophism. Five distinct agents can be identified at present.

Acute viral hepatitis type A (HAV)

Following ingestion of enterovirus type 72 (picorna), the virus becomes established in the liver, spills into the biliary system and is excreted in the stools. Stool virus concentration is highest 7 days before the onset of biochemical hepatitis, falls rapidly but may still be detected months later in patients with an atypical relapsing course. The diagnosis is confirmed by finding specific HAV IgM antibodies appearing as early as 7 days after exposure, reaching peak concentrations at 20–40 days and usually clearing by 60 days. Infection occurs predominantly in early childhood and is related to overcrowding and poor hygiene. In northern Europe only 10–15% become infected in childhood. Children under 2 years are very unlikely to become icteric; the likelihood of severe hepatitis increases with age.

Clinical features

The incubation period varies from 15 to 40 days, followed by a preicteric stage which may be accompanied by anorexia, nausea, vomiting, fever, headache, lassitude, dull intermittent upper abdominal pain and loose stools. The liver may be enlarged and tender, and the spleen enlarged. Jaundice and pruritus may develop with dark urine and pale stools. Jaundice usually lasts for 2 weeks, but may persist for months or follow a relapsing course. Chronic liver disease does not occur although transient liver nodularity with portal hypertension can occasionally persist for up to 1 year. Rare complications include ALF, bone marrow aplasia, pancreatitis, myocarditis and polyneuropathy.

Prevention

The provision of drinking water uncontaminated by fecal pathogens and the safe disposal of sewage is essential in the prevention of this disorder. Person to person spread may be minimized by scrupulous hand washing after defecation and before handling food. Two doses of hepatitis A vaccine 14 days apart provide over 95% protection and are extremely safe.

Viral hepatitis type B (HBV)

Hepatitis B (HBV) is a DNA-containing virus of the hepadna group. HBV DNA can integrate into the hepatocyte genome. In up to 10% of adults, less than 20% of 2–3 year olds, 80% of infants aged 6 months or less and up to 90% of newborns, the immune response to infection is incomplete and a chronic infective carrier state occurs. This carrier state may be associated with normal liver structure and function or a range of pathological abnormalities including chronic hepatitis, cirrhosis and hepatocellular carcinoma. Patients with HBV may be superinfected by the delta virus (HDV).

Serological responses in HBV infection

Viral antigens and antibodies to them may be present so transiently that they are never detected or they may persist in high concentrations indefinitely. The antigens and antibodies used in clinical practice are given in Table 17.42. There may be an interval following the disappearance of an antigen before its antibody becomes detectable or both may be present together. Immunosuppressed children with hepatitis B infection usually have massive viral replication within the liver but may lack serological evidence. HBV DNA may be detectable by very sensitive techniques even after successful anti-e seroconversion occurring spontaneously or induced by interferon treatment.

Table 17.42 Serological markers in viral hepatitis type B

Marker	Clinical significance
HBsAg	Acute or chronic hepatitis B infection
HBsAb	Immunity to hepatitis B, postinfective or with active or passive immunization
HBcAb IgM	High titer: acute hepatitis, recent infection
HBcAb IgG	Past exposure to hepatitis B
HBeAg	Highly infectious state, high risk of progressive liver disease and HCC
HBeAb	Less infective state in the HbsAb-positive patient with low risk of progressive liver disease and HCC
HBV DNA by direct DNA hybridization	Quantification of viral replication

HCC, hepatocellular carcinoma

Clinical features

The acute and chronic responses to HBV infection in childhood are given in Table 17.43. At all ages the carrier rate and risk of serious sequelae are higher in males than in females. Those with anicteric hepatitis with minimal elevation of serum transaminases appear to be at greater risk of becoming chronically infected. The population chronic carrier rate varies from 0.1% in northern Europe and North America to 10% in southern European and Mediterranean countries and as high as 20% in parts of Africa and south-east Asia.

Only 5% of infections in early infancy are symptomatic, as opposed to 40% in later life. The clinical features of acute HBV are similar to those of HAV but the incubation period ranges from 30 to 180 days and often the onset is more insidious. In many instances infection is asymptomatic and the carrier state is only detected by serological testing.

Table 17.43 Clinical expression of hepatitis B virus in childhood

1. Asymptomatic development of HBsAb
2. Acute hepatitis, anicteric or icteric
3. Papular acrodermatitis
4. Acute liver failure
5. Acute hepatitis proceeding to chronic hepatitis or cirrhosis
6. Disorders associated with circulating immune complexes
   a. Glomerulonephritis
   b. Periarteritis
   c. Pericarditis
   d. Arthritis
7. Chronic hepatitis
8. Cirrhosis
9. Hepatocellular carcinoma
10. 'Healthy' carrier state
11. Carrier state with immune disorders
    a. Down syndrome
    b. Malignant disease and its treatment
    c. Renal failure
    d. Immunosuppression with transplantation

Natural history of HBV infection

It has been estimated that 20–25% of those infected in infancy are still positive in the fourth decade. HBe clearance rate varies between 2% per annum for those infected in earlier infancy to 20% of children infected later in life. The conversion to anti-HBs in carriers is much rarer at between 0 and 2% per annum.

Neither the clinical features nor biochemical tests of liver function predict the histological findings. Cross-sectional studies of children with HBV in Europe show chronic aggressive hepatitis (CAH) in over 50%, with chronic persistent hepatitis in 33%, the remainder having chronic lobular hepatitis or minimal changes. Histological diagnosis of cirrhosis is made in approximately 5% but as many as a third may become cirrhotic. Those with active CAH are more prone to develop cirrhosis and its complications, particularly if super-infected by delta virus. Hepatocellular carcinoma, associated with HBV infection, accounted for 13% of childhood cancers in Taiwan seen in children as young as 8 months but has almost disappeared since the introduction of neonatal vaccination against HBV. Children with chronic persistent hepatitis or chronic lobular hepatitis have a good prognosis over a period of 15 years in terms of developing cirrhosis.[162]

Prevention of HBV

All blood and blood-derived products should be screened for hepatitis B. Blood, saliva, urine and other secretions are infectious. Wearing disposable gloves and hand washing after handling blood or excretions appear to minimize the risk of infection to close contacts. Highly immunogenic synthetic vaccines are available and should be used to protect family members where an index case has been identified. Medical and paramedical personnel must be similarly protected. Hyperimmune gamma-globulin to HBV (HBIG) should be administered immediately after accidental inoculation of possibly hepatitis B-positive blood.

The combined use of HBIG in a dose of 200 IU, with active immunization starting within 48 h of delivery with further doses at 1, 2 and 12 months, is very effective in producing high anti-HBs titers. Further doses are recommended later if the anti-HBs titer falls below 100 IU/L. This schedule should be applied to all infants of mothers who are found to be HBsAg positive by screening during pregnancy, including those who are HBe antibody positive. In areas of high prevalence it is likely that the vaccine alone will be used for reasons of cost. It is probably more cost effective to protect all newborns than to set up a system to identify those at risk and this regime has been recommended by the WHO. In Africa and other localities where infection is acquired after the neonatal period, vaccination at 3 months would seem to be cost effective. Instead of the UK recommended dose of 20 mg, doses as low as 2 mg given intradermally or intramuscularly are almost as efficacious.

Therapy of chronic hepatitis

In European children, treatment with interferon alpha 2b, 3 MU/m^2 for 3 months increased anti-HBe seroconversion rates over 12 months from 13% in controls to 40%. Pretreatment with steroids is not beneficial. The long term clinical and histological benefit is assumed but unproven.[163,164] No benefit has been shown of combined lamivudine interferon treatment. Lamivudine may have a role in reducing viral load in patients with abnormal immunity or those who cannot tolerate interferon.

Viral hepatitis delta (HDV)

HDV is a defective RNA virus that requires the presence of HBV core Ag to replicate. It may be transmitted by parenteral inoculation or close body contact. Subjects may be simultaneously infected with HBV or HBV carriers may be superinfected. When acquired simultaneously with HBV it may cause acute hepatitis varying from asymptomatic infection to ALF. Usually a chronic HBV carrier state does not follow. Superinfection of HBV carriers causes a serious exacerbation of the hepatitis with progression to ALF, chronic active hepatitis or cirrhosis. The diagnosis is confirmed by detecting antibodies to the delta virus. There is no effective treatment. HBV vaccination should limit its spread. It is rare in the UK and in children.

Viral hepatitis type C (HCV)

It has been shown that this 9500-RNA-base *Flavivirus* was responsible for up to 90% of post-transfusion hepatitis in North America prior to the screening of blood products. Infection in childhood was almost entirely acquired from unscreened blood products before 1989. It has now become rare with new infections by vertical transmission occurring in 5% of pregnancies of infected mothers. No vaccine is currently available.

The natural history of HCV infection

The consequences of infection for adults are becoming clearer and it is assumed that they are similar for children. A mild hepatitis typically follows infection and an incubation period of about 60 days. Only 30% are icteric and fulminant liver failure occurs exceedingly rarely. Perhaps 30–40% of immunocompetent patients will clear the virus while developing anti-HCV antibodies. The remainder will have chronic infection with anti-HCV antibodies and RNA polymerase chain reaction (PCR) positivity. Of these the majority will have mild liver disease such as minimal change or chronic persistent hepatitis with normal or occasionally abnormal transaminases. Liver disease is slowly progressive with cirrhosis developing over 20 years in 5–25% with one-third taking 50 years or longer to develop cirrhosis.[165] Concomitant liver diseases such as drug induced, iron overload, HBV or alcohol will increase the rate of progression. Genotype 1 tends to progress more quickly and hepatocellular carcinoma occurs in 1–10%. Non immunocompetent patients are more likely to develop chronic infection while antibodies to HCV may remain negative. The presence of HCV RNA can be used to demonstrate infection and the response to treatment.

Treatment

Interferon and ribavirin treatments have been used with benefit in adults, are being evaluated in children and should only be undertaken by specialist services under a research protocol. Sustained virological response (SVR), implying lack of viremia with associated improvement of inflammatory liver damage at least 12 months after completion of treatment, is the current outcome measure. Virus genotype 1 should be treated for 48 weeks and others for 24 weeks. SVR for genotype 1 is 30–40% and for other genotypes 60%+. Side-effects of both drugs are frequent. Pegylated interferon promises even better results.[166]

Prevention of cross infection

HCV is blood borne and despite being less infectious than HBV requires scrupulous antisepsis for spilled blood. Razors and toothbrushes should be separated from others. Counseling of sexual infectious risk, said to be 5% per partner, is required. HCV can also be detected in breast milk but breast-feeding is not contraindicated.

Viral hepatitis E (HEV)

This enterically transmitted 30 nm RNA virus is responsible for epidemics of hepatitis in the Middle East and Asia. Icteric disease occurs in 1–3% of infections. The prognosis is usually good but mortality is recognized in pregnant women and in association with other liver diseases including Wilson's disease. Chronicity has not been documented but a relapsing course may occur.

NON-VIRAL INFECTIONS

Hepatic abscesses

Hepatic abscesses may be caused by almost any bacteria or fungi, in association with any septicemic state, particularly with portal pyemia from appendix abscess and Crohn's disease. Patients at risk include those with primary or secondary immune deficiencies, particularly chronic granulomatous disease. Secondary infection of another hepatic lesion such as bile duct obstruction, or sickle cell infarct may occur.

Clinical features

There are frequently no clinical or biochemical features of liver disease, but high spiking fever is universal and abdominal pain frequent. Diagnosis rests on ultrasonic detection of the lesion but CT scan is necessary to demonstrate possible appendix abscess and exclude associated malignancy. Successful management requires appropriate antibiotics as determined by culture of material aspirated from the lesion together with ultrasonically guided drainage. Surgical drainage is required if there is associated peritonitis, bile duct obstruction or if chronic abscesses with firm walls are present.

Hepatic amebiasis

This disorder has a high prevalence in children in endemic areas. Malaise, fever, rigors and tender hepatomegaly are usual. It is unusual to obtain a history of diarrhea. Secondary bacterial infection may be present. Diagnosis is based on finding living ameba in the stools or gut biopsy and positive serological tests.

Treatment

Metronidazole (50 mg/kg/24 h in three doses for 10 days) is the treatment of choice. Therapeutic needle aspiration or surgical drainage may be necessary when rupture of the abscess seems imminent or the liver lesion enlarges in spite of drug treatment.

Hydatid disease

Hydatid disease is usually caused by the larval stage of the dog tapeworm *Echinococcus granulosus*. Rarely the fox tapeworm, *Echinococcus multilocularis*, may be responsible.

Clinical features

Infection is usually acquired asymptomatically in early childhood. Earlier signs are discomfort in the right hypochondrium or hepatomegaly. Rarely rupture into the biliary system may cause cholangitis; sudden collapse may be precipitated by rupture into the peritoneum. The diagnosis is based on positive serological tests. A secondary bacterial infection may produce a liver abscess. Treatment is surgical resection. Patients with *E. multilocularis* infection or those too ill for surgery may respond to prolonged courses of mebendazole or albendazole.

Schistosomiasis

Hepatic features are firm hepatomegaly, portal hypertension with splenomegaly, ascites and/or hematemesis. Liver disease may occur as early as 2 years after initial infection. The recovery of ova in stools or rectal mucosa proves infection as positive serology does not distinguish past from present infection. The treatment is praziquantel. Alimentary bleeding due to portal hypertension should be treated by injection sclerotherapy or banding, not by portosystemic shunting.

Liver infestations

The liver and biliary system may be damaged by infestation with *Fasciola hepatica* (sheep), *Clonorchis sinensis* (freshwater fish), *Opisthorchis felineus* and *Opisthorchis viverrin* (cat) and by larvae of the roundworm *Ascaris*. All cause cholangitis which may become suppurative and be complicated by bile duct obstruction, calculus formation, bile duct carcinoma, biliary cirrhosis and portal hypertension.

CHRONIC LIVER DISEASES

Chronic liver disease implies evidence of liver damage persisting longer than 6 months likely to lead to irreversible change in the structure of the liver and the complications of cirrhosis. It may develop asymptomatically, insidiously and without the physical signs associated with established cirrhosis. Conversely, the presentation frequently appears acute when features of decompensation appear suddenly or when a relapsing course presents with severe exacerbation. Liver biopsy to aid in etiological diagnosis and assess progress of disease should be performed unless there is a specific contraindication. If there is evidence of hepatitis B infection biopsy should be delayed for 6 months to allow spontaneous remission.

Features suggesting chronicity

Chronic hepatitis should be suspected in the following situations:

1. relapse of an apparent acute hepatitis;
2. clinical or biochemical features of hepatitis persisting beyond 8 weeks;
3. hepatitis occuring after a history of neonatal cholestasis;
4. signs such as a small or hard liver, enlarged left or collapsed right lobe of liver, or others shown in Table 17.34.

Autoimmune liver diseases

Autoimmune chronic active hepatitis (AIH) and sclerosing cholangitis (AISC) are recognized to be part of an overlap syndrome.[167] At presentation, when patients may have aggressive hepatitis, occasionally ALF, or cirrhosis, it may be difficult to distinguish from Wilson's disease. High serum immunoglobulins with IgG commonly greater than 16 g/L, low concentrations of C4, and the presence of one or more non-organ-specific antibodies, particularly antinuclear, antismooth muscle are found in smooth muscle antibody/antinuclear antibody (SMA/ANA) antibody positive AIH and AISC. Antiliver/kidney microsomal antibodies define a subgroup sometimes called type 2 AIH, very rarely associated with AISC and serum IgG level may be normal. IBD may be present in up to 30% of all patients. Presence of antigastric parietal cell antibodies is a marker of possible autoimmune polyendocrinopathy.

Drug treatment

Prednisolone in a dose of 2 mg/kg/day up to a maximum 50 mg/kg/day is given initially and continued until serum transaminase values fall by 80% or to less than 100 IU/L. Over the course of 2–3 months the dose is gradually reduced to that which will have no side-effects whilst maintaining normal transaminases, typically 0.1 mg/kg/day. Ursodeoxycholic acid 15–20 mg/kg/day is given for AISC. If the reduction of the steroid dose is associated with a rise in transaminase level, azathioprine 0.5 mg/kg/day is added and the dose increased gradually to 1.5 mg/kg/day. Weekly full blood counts and platelet counts are essential early in azathioprine therapy. Mycophenolate mofetil is a powerful second-line steroid sparing alternative to azathioprine. Liver–kidney–microsome (LKM) antibody positive patients will require indefinite treatment, while a minority of SMA/ANA positive patients can slowly reduce and stop steroids after years of successful treatment.

The majority of patients have cirrhosis at the time of diagnosis but over 90% can be maintained in biochemical remission by immunosuppressive therapy with stable liver function and without side-effects of medication over a 20 year period. Patients with sclerosing cholangitis have a marginally increased risk of need for liver transplantation during that period.

Sclerosing cholangitis

Sclerosing cholangitis is a chronic obliterative inflammation in the intrahepatic and/or extrahepatic biliary system shown as irregularities in the outline of the ducts with areas of stricturing and dilatation (beading) on cholangiography. The various types are listed in Table 17.44. Modes of presentation include all the manifestations of chronic liver disease including normal biochemical liver function tests.

Treatment

Symptomatic treatment includes adequate replacement of fat-soluble vitamins and colestyramine to relieve pruritus. Ursodeoxycholic acid may be beneficial. Dietary, drug and/or surgical treatment of bowel disease associated with AISC and AIH is necessary but does not influence the biliary pathology.

Wilson's disease

This inborn error of metabolism is characterized by defective biliary copper excretion. The spectrum of mutations causing a defective transport protein, ATP7B has been described.[168] Wilson's disease may simulate virtually any form of liver disease from the age of 4 years onwards but typically presents in adolescence with ALF or severe hepatitis.[169] Coombs negative hemolytic anemia or evidence of renal tubular damage often with hypophosphatemia suggests the diagnosis. In 80% the serum ceruloplasmin value is less than 20 g/dl (1.25 μmol/L). The current gold standard for positive diagnosis is urinary copper excretion requiring both 1.2 mmol/24 h and more than 25 mmol/24 h with 1 g of penicillamine. The liver copper concentration is >250 mg/g of dry weight. Kayser–Fleischer rings may be identified by slit lamp examination in children over the age of 7.

Table 17.44 Classification of sclerosing cholangitis

1.	Autoimmune (with or without chronic inflammatory bowel disease) with high serum immunoglobulins and non-organ-specific autoantibodies, C4 concentration normal and circulating T lymphocytes displaying IL-2R < 5%
2.	Following cholestasis in infancy or with family history or consanguinity (neonatal sclerosing cholangitis)
	Associated with:
3.	Langerhans' cell histiocytosis
4.	Immune deficiency states particularly HIV and CD40 ligand deficiency
5.	Cystic fibrosis
6.	Biliary surgery, or trauma
7.	Ischemia after liver transplantation or in sickle cell disease
8.	Primary (with or without chronic inflammatory bowel disease with normal serum immunoglobulins and no autoantibodies)

Treatment

The prognosis of Wilson's disease at treatment is predicted by the total score according to Table 17.45. A score > 9 is associated with an early death (< 2 months) unless liver transplantation can be arranged. Patients with score < 6 should respond satisfactorily to penicillamine (5 mg/kg/day increased by 5 mg/kg/day at 2-weekly intervals to 20 mg/kg/day) and zinc sulfate 100–300 mg three times a day after meals given at different times from the penicillamine. Patients with scores of 6–9 require close monitoring. Recovery on treatment may take 12 months or longer.

It is *essential* to screen families of patients with Wilson's disease to enable early treatment. Serum transaminases, copper, ceruloplasmin and urinary penicillamine challenge are required for all first-degree relatives. Genetic markers are available, but since more than 100 alleles have been described genetic tests are often not fully informative.

Other copper associated liver diseases

Indian childhood cirrhosis was largely confined to the Indian subcontinent and was characterized by necrosis of hepatocytes containing Mallory's hyaline and orcein-staining copper-associated protein due to accumulation of copper in the liver. Over 80% died within 6 months. Elimination of exposure to dietary copper has resulted in near elimination of the disease. Rare non-Indian cases have been described both with and without excessive environmental exposure to copper but with similar poor prognosis.

Non-alcoholic steatohepatitis (NASH)

This condition, long recognized in adult practice, is becoming increasingly prevalent in children.[170] Presentation is with incidentally discovered raised serum transaminases or fat on liver ultrasound shown as brightness. Children are often obese with a high fat and refined carbohydrate diet and sedentary lifestyle. The diagnosis is by exclusion of other liver disease caused by fat in the liver and by the characteristic liver biopsy features of inflammation, macrovesicular fat and occasional fibrosis. Other causes of fatty infiltration include alpha-1 antitrypsin deficiency, HCV, and milder forms of glycogen storage disease. A glucose tolerance test is mandatory. Treatments suggested have included antibiotics against bacterial translocation, antioxidants and metformin, but dietary and lifestyle changes to reduce weight are the mainstay of management. Progressive liver fibrosis will be found in 5–10%.

ACUTE LIVER FAILURE

The adult terminology 'fulminant liver failure' based on the onset of encephalopathy is not helpful in pediatrics as in infants and small

Table 17.45 Prognostic score in Wilson's disease

Bilirubin (μmol/L)	Aspartate amino-transferase (U/L)	Prothrombin time INR	Prognostic score
N < 20	N < 40	N < 1.3	
< 100	< 100	< 1.3	0
101–150	101–150	1.3–1.6	1
151–200	151–200	1.7–2.0	2
201–300	201–300	2.1–2.5	3
> 300	> 300	> 2.5	4

N, normal; INR, international normalized ratio

children severe liver failure may occur without apparent encephalopathy.[171] 'Acute liver failure' (ALF) is preferred for children with a 'de novo' liver injury causing coagulopathy without disseminated intravascular coagulation or vitamin K deficiency.[172] Two minority subgroups may be defined, one with hyperacute presentation of duration less than 1 week and typically low levels of jaundice, and one with subacute presentation of more than 8 weeks. ALF is a rare, complex, multisystem disorder with a mortality of 30–100%. Life-threatening complications include septicemia especially from fungi, and raised intracranial pressure secondary to encephalopathy proceeding to impaired cerebral blood flow. In ALF, but possibly not the subacute subgroup, if the patient survives, the liver usually regains normal histology and function.

Diagnosis

The differential diagnosis of ALF is shown in Table 17.46. Although no diagnosis is possible in up to 40% of cases the search for a diagnosis should not delay transfer of the patient to a center with facilities and experience of managing ALF.

Clinical features

The grades of hepatic encephalopathy are shown in Table 17.47. Prognostic features for ALF other than paracetamol toxicity and Wilson's disease appear in Table 17.48. The prognosis for ALF from Wilson's disease appears in Table 17.45. Adverse prognostic markers for paracetamol toxicity include metabolic acidosis, renal dysfunction and encephalopathy but not very high transaminases. Unlike ALF of other causes, INR of > 4.0 does not necessarily herald a poor prognosis in paracetamol toxicity.

Indications for liver transplantation

Since the 5 year survival following liver transplantation for children with ALF is approximately 70%, transplantation is indicated when the prognosis of the liver failure is worse than that of transplantation.[173] This assumes no other factors influencing overall prognosis of the underlying condition, for example respiratory chain disorders with central nervous system complications.

Treatment

Intensive care aimed at preventing and treating complications is essential until the liver function recovers or transplantation can be performed. Early arrangements should be made to transfer the child to a pediatric intensive care unit (PICU) with the experience to manage the multisystem complications and to proceed to liver transplantation if indicated. *Sedatives must not be given unless patients are to be ventilated.* Vitamin K is given to optimize coagulation. Hypoglycemia must be prevented by intravenous glucose. Protein intake is restricted to 0.5 g/kg/day. Lactulose may precipitate diarrhea without altering the outcome. Ranitidine given intravenously may prevent bleeding from gastric erosions. Prophylactic antibiotics and antifungals are indicated as 40% of cases have early covert sepsis.

Reye's syndrome and Reye-like ALF

Reye's syndrome is an increasingly rare, acute, frequently fatal encephalopathy of unknown cause occurring in children of any age. It is characterized by a self-limiting abnormality of mitochondrial structure and function with an acute catabolic state. It occurs following an unremarkable viral infection of the respiratory or gastrointestinal tract. Aspirin may play a role although Reye's syndrome has been disappearing in countries where aspirin is still given to children and at a similar rate as in countries where it has

Table 17.46 The causes of acute liver failure

1. Infective
   a. Viral hepatitis
      (i) A, B, B+, delta, C, enteric or blood-borne NANB
      (ii) Parvovirus B19
      (iii) Epstein–Barr virus
      (iv) Cytomegalovirus
      (v) Herpes virus
      (vi) Adenovirus
      (vii) Echovirus
      (viii) Yellow fever
      (ix) Lassa fever
      (x) Ebola
      (xi) Marburg
   b. Leptospirosis
   c. Septicemia
2. Toxic
   a. *Amanita phalloides*
   b. Carbon tetrachloride
   c. Paracetamol
   d. Halothane
   e. Valproate
   f. Carbamazepine
   g. Phenytoin
   h. Isoniazid
   i. Amiodarone
   j. Cytotoxics
   k. Monoamine oxidase inhibitors
   l. Chemotherapy particularly actinomycin D causing veno-occlusive disease
3. Metabolic
   a. Galactosemia
   b. Fructosemia
   c. Tyrosinemia
   d. Familial erythrophagocytic reticulosis (hemophagocytic lymphohistiocytosis)
   e. Neonatal hemochromatosis
   f. Wilson's disease
   g. Niemann–Pick disease type C
   h. Mitochondrial respiratory chain defects
4. Ischemia
   a. Budd–Chiari syndrome
   b. Acute circulatory failure
   c. Septicemia with shock
   d. Heat stroke
   e. Leukemia
5. Cryptogenic in 40%

NANB, non-A non-B

Table 17.47 The grade of hepatic encephalopathy

Grade of encephalopathy	Features
1.	Lethargy, minor reductions in consciousness or motor function, vomiting
2.	Stupor, irrational hyperactivity, combative behavior
3.	Unresponsive to command but responds to pain
4.	Unresponsive to command, extensor posturing and rigidity, brainstem depression with respiratory and vasomotor failure

Table 17.48 Prognostic markers in acute liver failure

Prognostic factor	Risk of mortality (%)
INR ≥ 4.0	93
Serum bilirubin > 235 μmol/L	92
Age < 2 years	96
WBC ≥ 9 × 10^9/L	93
Encephalopathy grade 3 or 4	90+
Drug etiology	90+
Etiology unknown	90+
HBV	70–90
HAV	50–70
3 or more adverse factors	100

been prohibited. Reye's syndrome must be distinguished from an increasing range of inborn errors of metabolism that present in a similar fashion, particularly urea cycle disorders, fatty acid oxidation disorders, e.g. medium chain acyl CoA dehydrogenase deficiency, organic acidemias and mitochondrial respiratory chain disorders, sometimes called Alper syndrome (see Ch. 24). Respiratory chain disorders are increasingly recognized as causing encephalopathy often with fits followed by ALF. They are often distinguished by very high serum transaminases and mild or initially absent jaundice, perhaps precipitated by sodium valproate.[174,175] For some of these conditions there may be specific treatment to prevent relapse, and genetic counseling may be possible. In all these conditions liver transplantation is not usually required despite the severity of the initial coagulopathy and may be contraindicated in view of the neurological sequelae.

In Reye's syndrome encephalopathy with prominent vomiting may proceed over 4–60 h to brain death. Diagnosis of Reye's syndrome or Reye-like conditions must be suspected in any encephalopathy if there is laboratory evidence of liver involvement such as raised serum transaminases, hyperammonemia, hypoglycemia or prolonged INR.

Treatment

Mortality is as high as 40% with a considerable proportion of survivors being left with brain damage or with progressive encephalopathy in those with respiratory chain disorders. The patient should be nursed in a fashion that minimizes increases in intracranial pressure while being transferred to a specialist PICU. At presentation it is essential to collect and store serum (at – 70°C) and urine in order to diagnose Reye-like disorders.

Hemophagocytic lymphohistiocytosis

In this rare condition due to uncontrolled activation of the immune system particularly by viral infection, and that results in aggressive tissue damage by histiocytes and possible liver failure. Lymphadenopathy and hepatosplenomegaly are frequently present. Inflammatory markers particularly triglycerides and ferritin are elevated, fibrinogen is low, and cytopenia is indicative of disseminated intravascular coagulation and bone marrow involvement.[176] Recent work has shown abnormalities of the perforin gene with failure of apoptosis in infected cells the likely primary event.[177] Treatment includes anti-T cell globulin and etoposide. Prognosis is poor and particularly grave in infants.

CIRRHOSIS

The main pathophysiological effects are impaired hepatic function and portal hypertension. Hepatocellular carcinoma may develop. Although the diagnosis of cirrhosis implies an irreversible and usually progressive pathological change, it may be compatible with normal growth and activity for many years.

There are two broad pathological categories, biliary cirrhosis and so-called postnecrotic cirrhosis. Genetic factors contribute to both pathological varieties (Table 17.49).

Clinical and laboratory features

Clinical and non-specific laboratory features are described above. Five disorders may cause particular diagnostic difficulty: extrahepatic portal hypertension, congenital hepatic fibrosis, constrictive pericarditis, sclerosing cholangitis and infiltrative disorders such as reticulosis.

Management

Based on the history, examination findings and standard investigations listed in Table 17.50, a differential diagnosis may be possible prior to performing a liver biopsy. In considering the genetic disorders, principal consideration must be given to those with effective treatment, e.g. Wilson's disease and AIH, and to identify surgically correctable abnormalities of the biliary tree, e.g. choledochal cyst. The further aim of management is to minimize further liver damage by treating the cause of liver disease and preventing or controlling complications (Table 17.51).

Table 17.49 Causes of cirrhosis in childhood

1. Biliary
   a. Biliary atresia
   b. Intrahepatic biliary hypoplasia
   c. Choledochal cyst
   d. Cystic fibrosis
   e. PFIC
   f. Bile duct stenosis or obstruction
   g. Choledocholithiasis
   h. Sclerosing cholangitis
   i. Cholangitis due to
      (i) *Fasciola*
      (ii) *Clonorchis sinensis*
      (iii) *Ascaris*
   j. Pancreatic tumors
   k. Langerhans' cell histiocytosis
2. Postnecrotic
   a. Hepatitis in infancy
   b. Autoimmune chronic active hepatitis
   c. Acute viral hepatitis (viral hepatitis, B, C, delta, non-A non-B)
   d. Hepatitis due to drugs, e.g. actinomycin D, methotrexate
   e. Toxins, e.g. aflatoxin, copper, copper associated liver diseases
3. Genetic disorders
   a. Wilson's disease
   b. Galactosemia
   c. Fructosemia
   d. Glycogen storage disease type IV
   e. Hurler's syndrome
   f. Alpha-1 antitrypsin deficiency
   g. Tyrosinemia
   h. Cystinosis
   i. Gaucher's disease
   j. Wolman's disease
   k. Niemann–Pick disease type C
   l. Defects in fatty acid oxidation
   m. Sickle cell disease
   n. Thalassemia
   o. Hepatic porphyria
   p. Hemochromatosis, idiopathic
   q. Hemochromatosis secondary to chronic hemolytic disease
   r. Defects in primary bile salt synthesis
4. Venous congestion
   a. Constrictive pericarditis
   b. Ebstein's anomaly
   c. Congestive cardiac failure
   d. Budd–Chiari syndrome
   e. Venacaval webs
   f. Veno-occlusive disease
   g. Radiation

PFIC, progressive familial intrahepatic cholestasis

Table 17.50 First line investigations in children with evidence of chronic liver disease

FBC reticulocytes, film, INR, APTT, fibrinogen, cross match, Coombs test
Renal, bone, liver, lipid profiles, amylase, CK, blood glucose, lactate, urate
Blood gases
Ferritin, copper, caeruloplasmin, zinc
Alpha-fetoprotein
Alpha-1 antitrypsin phenotype
CF alleles, sweat test
Immunoglobulins, complement C3 and C4, autoantibody screen
Serology for hepatitis B HBsAg, eAg, HCV Ab, HCV RNA PCR, CMV, EBV
24 h urine copper collection and penicillamine challenge
CXR (cardiac echo if constrictive pericarditis is possible)
Liver and spleen ultrasound

APTT, activated partial thromboplastin time; CF, cystic fibrosis; CK, creatine kinase; CMV, cytomegalovirus; CXR, chest X-ray; EBV, Epstein-Barr virus; HCV, hepatitis C virus; PCR, polymerase chain reaction

Portal hypertension (see below) causes splenomegaly, ascites and alimentary bleeding. Splenomegaly and hypersplenism rarely require intervention. Ascites may respond to spironolactone 4–7 mg/kg/day. If there is hyponatremia, water restriction is essential. It is rarely possible to reduce the sodium intake to less than 0.5 mmol/kg/day. If these measures are unsuccessful albumin infusions with simultaneous furosemide (frusemide) 0.5–1 mg/kg/day may control ascites for 7–21 days. Paracentesis may be necessary if there is severe abdominal distension or respiratory embarrassment, followed by 20% intravenous albumin 5 ml/kg. It is essential to monitor the patient's weight, abdominal girth, urinary output of water and sodium and to measure the serum urea and creatinine when managing ascites.

Treatment of alimentary bleeding

However small the bleed the child should be immediately admitted to the nearest hospital with resuscitation facilities. Following small initial bleeds, shock requiring rapid blood transfusion may occur. Bleeding decreases hepatic perfusion with the possibility of ischemic hepatitis and hepatic encephalopathy. On admission, a baseline assessment of the clinical state should be made, blood crossmatched, and a secure intravenous line established. Intravenous octreotide 25 μg/h is indicated if bleeding does not stop rapidly. A Sengstaken–Blakemore tube of suitable size should be available and chilled to facilitate insertion by an experienced operator. Oral ranitidine and sucralfate reduce the risk of bleeding from gastric erosions. Intravenous vitamin K should be given. As soon as the patient is stable, arrangements should be made to transfer to a unit equipped to manage the causes and complications of portal hypertension. Endoscopy is essential to determine the cause and source of bleeding, which may be gastric erosions or peptic ulceration rather than varices. It should be combined with band ligation or injection sclerotherapy if necessary.[178] Propranolol 1 mg/kg/day in two doses may be helpful in preventing first bleed or reducing the frequency of subsequent bleeds. Emergency portosystemic shunting is rarely required.

Table 17.51 Complications of cirrhosis

1. Portal hypertension and hypersplenism
2. Bleeding diathesis
3. Hypoxemia
4. Increased susceptibility to infection
5. Hyperdynamic circulation (cardiac failure)
6. Ascites
7. Spontaneous bacterial peritonitis
8. Pulmonary hypertension
9. Hepatoma
10. Malnutrition
11. Gallstone formation
12. Renal failure
13. Hepatic encephalopathy
14. Endocrine changes
15. Impaired hepatic metabolism of drugs and hormones
16. Impaired neurodevelopment, particularly gross motor

Spontaneous bacterial peritonitis

This potentially lethal complication occurring in children with ascites requires early diagnosis and an antibiotic regimen effective against *Streptococcus pneumoniae* and Gram negative organisms. It may present with clear signs of peritonitis and fever. Blood culture and diagnostic ascitic tap are essential to identify the pathogen and select appropriate antibiotic therapy.

Chronic hepatic encephalopathy

Chronic hepatic encephalopathy is a complex neuropsychiatric syndrome with major portosystemic shunting and usually cirrhosis.[179,180] It is characterized by intellectual impairment, personality change and clouding of consciousness. Sleep patterns may be disturbed. Causes of hepatic encephalopathy and compounding factors are given in Table 17.52.

Treatment

The objective of treatment is to prevent accumulation of ammonia and other vasoactive or false neurotransmitter substances in the gut, to remove or correct identifiable precipitating factors and to try to improve liver function. Protein intake should be reduced to 0.5–1 g/kg of body weight initially but then increased if tolerated. Sodium benzoate may be beneficial.

Nutritional complications of severe liver disease[181]

Progressive liver disease and portal hypertension are associated with a characteristic habitus having a full abdomen with thin limbs. Body weight underestimates the severity of derangement of body composition. Anorexia complicates management.

Dietary management of cholestasis and cirrhosis

The calorie requirements may be up to 40% above recommended daily intake for weight. The diet must contain sufficient protein (up

Table 17.52 Causes of hepatic encephalopathy

1. End stage chronic parenchymal disease
2. Acute or subacute liver failure
3. Liver disease with severe portosystemic shunting
4. Precipitating factors
a. Sedative medications
b. Hypoglycemia
c. Hypokalemia
d. Hypovolemia
e. Sepsis
f. Gastrointestinal bleeding
g. Hypoxia
h. High protein diet

to 4 g/kg/day), essential fatty acids, minerals, trace elements and vitamins. Anorexia is frequently a problem, which may be aggravated by restricted fluid and/or salt intake. Fat malabsorption of varying severity is usual. Water- and fat-soluble vitamin supplements are frequently required. If hepatic encephalopathy develops, dietary protein intake should be stopped and gradually reintroduced up to the maximum tolerated, while sodium benzoate is given. There is no proven advantage in using branched chain amino acids.

Pulmonary complications

Hepatopulmonary syndrome (HPS) presents insidiously as exertional dyspnea followed by cyanosis.[182] Type 1 HPS implies pulmonary capillary vasodilatation and type 2 new vessel intrapulmonary shunts both with ventilation/perfusion mismatch. The degree of shunting does not correlate with the severity of the liver damage or portal hypertension but may relate to the degree of portosystemic shunting. Hypoxia may be partially relieved by increasing inspired oxygen concentration and is cured by liver transplantation. Portopulmonary hypertension may develop due to pulmonary vasoconstriction, the converse of the dilatation of HPS.[183,184]

Hepatorenal failure

Oliguric renal failure without structural abnormalities in the kidney (functional renal failure) is frequently a terminal event in advanced cirrhosis. There is a slow development of uremia, oliguria, and hyponatremia with a low urinary sodium concentration. Glomerular filtration may show transient improvement with inotropes. Liver transplantation is the definitive treatment.

PORTAL HYPERTENSION

Portal vein obstruction

The portal vein may be obstructed by infective or thrombotic disorders or by a congenital abnormality. The presenting features are asymptomatic splenomegaly, alimentary bleeding with portal hypertension at any age throughout childhood or adult life, and rarely ascites and failure to thrive. The diagnosis is suspected by the finding of portal hypertension or esophageal varices in a patient with splenomegaly and no clinical or biochemical evidence of liver disease. The diagnosis is confirmed by ultrasonography or angiography. The treatment is that of bleeding esophageal or rectal varices.[185] There is an increased frequency of bleeding during adolescence.[186] Hepatic encephalopathy may occur in adult life.

Congenital hepatic fibrosis

The clinical features are those of portal hypertension, hepatomegaly and occasionally cholangitis. Liver function tests are usually normal although the alkaline phosphatase may be elevated. Diagnosis requires an adequate liver biopsy showing wide bands of fibrous tissue linking portal tracts but clearly demarcated from the hepatic parenchyma. The bands contain irregularly shaped clefts lined by bile duct epithelial cells. Portal veins are sparse. There is little inflammatory cell infiltrate unless there is associated cholangitis. There is frequently significant associated renal disease, particularly infantile polycystic disease and renal excretion scans are essential. A wide range of dysmorphic syndromes is associated including Senior–Loken syndrome, Lawrence–Moon–Biedl syndrome and neurofibromatosis. Alimentary bleeding from varices is treated by band ligation, cholangitis with appropriate antibiotics. Rarely liver transplantation is indicated for biliary cirrhosis secondary to chronic cholangitis.

Cystic fibrosis (see Ch. 18)

Clinical syndromes include:

1. prolonged conjugated hyperbilirubinemia in infancy presenting as a hepatitis syndrome sometimes difficult to distinguish from biliary atresia;
2. massive hepatic steatosis which reverses as nutrition improves; and
3. cirrhosis with portal hypertension and variceal hemorrhage, hypersplenism or splenic pain.

Biliary abnormalities take the form of microgallbladder present in up to a third, with gallstones in as many as 12%. Up to 40% of patients with CF have evidence of liver disease.

The treatment is aimed at improving nutrition, particularly deficiency of fat-soluble vitamins, and the management of portal hypertension. Ursodeoxycholic acid (15–20 mg/kg/day) improves transaminases, serum bile acids and ultrasound findings but is of uncertain effect on prognosis.[187] Surgery may be required for symptomatic gallstones. Liver transplantation has also been performed with good results but no large series has clarified indications and outcomes.

LIVER TUMORS

Primary liver tumors are rare and occur at approximately one-tenth of the frequency of neuroblastoma. Malignant tumors include hepatoblastoma and hepatocellular carcinoma, both of which are usually accompanied by a high alpha-fetoprotein level, fibrolamellar hepatoma (accompanied by transcobalamin markers), rhabdomyosarcoma and cholangiocarcinoma. Other tumors appear in Table 17.53.[188] Infantile hemangioendothelioma may present in two forms: 'sump' effect with consumptive features of Kasabach–Merritt syndrome and 'shunt' like with high output cardiac failure. The others present with abdominal distension, hepatomegaly, abdominal pain or rarely complications of the tumor, such as virilization. Diagnosis is supported by the demonstration of a space-occupying lesion within the liver by imaging.

Malignant tumors are treated with appropriate chemotherapeutic agents followed by resection. Hemangioendothelioma is treated by surgical hepatic artery ligation in congestive cardiac failure. Such surgery should be confined to specialist centers.

Table 17.53 Tumors of the liver in childhood

	Benign/malignant
Hepatoblastoma (Stringer et al 1995[188])	M
Hepatoma/HCC including fibrolamellar HCC	M
Small cell tumor of infancy	M
Biliary rhabdomyosarcoma	M
Lymphoma	M
Neuroblastoma (including 4S)	M (spontaneous remission)
Secondary carcinomas/sarcomas	M
Hemangioendothelioma/angiosarcoma	B/M
Mesenchymal hamartoma	B
Adenoma	B
Focal nodular hyperplasia/nodular regenerative hyperplasia	B
Inflammatory pseudotumor	B

HCC, hepatocellular carcinoma.

LIVER TRANSPLANTATION

With 5 year survival rates as high as 90% for chronic liver diseases, orthotopic liver transplantation should be considered in any child with acute or chronic liver disease if death within 1 year is likely, as a consequence of liver disease when the quality of life has deteriorated to unacceptable levels, or if irreversible damage to the central nervous system or other organs is likely as a consequence of liver disease. Transplantation must be considered in acute or subALF and in selected children with an increasing range of metabolic disorders (Table 17.54). Auxiliary transplants may be most suitable for some of these latter indications. Full consideration must be given to other forms of treatment and the presence of relative contraindications. The results are better in children transplanted in a good nutritional state and if the procedure is elective.[189]

Table 17.54 Indications for liver transplantation.

Indications for liver transplantation	Examples
Decompensation of cirrhosis	Uncontrollable ascites Encephalopathy Failure to thrive Coagulopathy unresponsive to vitamin K
Untreatable complications of portal hypertension	Hepatorenal syndrome Hepatopulmonary syndrome
Poor quality of life	Pruritus Lethargy
Life-threatening complications	Varices refractory to all other treatments
Selected liver tumours	Unresectable chemosensitive hepatoblastoma Benign but unresectable tumors
Extrahepatic manifestations of hepatic inborn errors of metabolism	Crigler–Najjar type 1 Primary oxaluria Propionic acidemia
Acute liver failure	INR > 4 Grade 3 or 4 encephalopathy Children under 2 years

Complications

Complications are those of major surgery involving multiple vascular and biliary anastomoses, of rejection and the effects of long term antirejection drugs. Rejection occurs in up to 70% but is resistant to treatment with steroids in about 15%. In patients with poor graft function, opportunistic infections remain a high risk while those on modest doses of antirejection drugs are at risk of infections with community-acquired and gastrointestinal organisms. Between 1 and 6 months, cytomegalovirus, and opportunistic infection with organisms such as *Nocardia* and *Pneumocystis* may occur. EBV infection may lead to post-transplant lymphoproliferative disease particularly but not exclusively in patients who have received exceptional total immunosuppression for rejection. Ciclosporin has reduced the risk of infective complications but has major side-effects including chronic renal dysfunction, neurotoxicity and cosmetic considerations.

The longest survivor to date remains well 25 years after transplant, and the majority of survivors have a good quality of life. Life-long immunosuppressive therapy with expert medical supervision is required. The supply of suitable donor organs remains a major limiting factor in liver transplantation in childhood despite improvements from reducing organs, splitting organs between two recipients and using part of the liver of live related donors. Selecting the appropriate time for surgery can be difficult, being a compromise between early enough to receive a liver while in good condition and not undertaking transplant with its risks of complications before it is clearly necessary. Thus, it is essential that patients who may become candidates for transplantation should be referred at the earliest possible stage to units with the expertise to advise on the optimum timing.

PEDIATRIC GASTROENTEROLOGY AND HEPATOLOGY – CHARITIES AND ORGANIZATIONS

British Society of Pediatric Gastroenterology, Hepatology and Nutrition E-mail: secretary@bspghan.org.uk Website: http://bspghan.org.uk

Children's Liver Disease Foundation, 36 Great Charles Street, Birmingham B3 3JY, United Kingdom. Tel: 0121 212 3839, Fax: 0121 212 4300. E-mail: cldf@childliverdisease.org Website: http://www.childliverdisease.org

Coeliac UK, PO Box 220, High Wycombe, Bucks HP11 2HY, United Kingdom. Tel: 01494 437278, Fax: 01494 474349 E-mail: adminsec@coeliac.co.uk Website: http://www.coeliac.co.uk

Crohn's in Childhood Research Association, Parkgate House, 356 West Barnes Lane, Motspur Park, Surrey KT3 6NB, United Kingdom. Tel: 020 8949 6209, Fax: 020 8942 2044. Email: support@cicra.org Website: http://www.cicra.org

Cystic Fibrosis Trust, 11 London Road, Bromley, Kent BR1 1BY, United Kingdom. Tel: 020 8464 7211, Fax: 020 8313 0472 Website: http://www.cftrust.org.uk

European Society for Paediatric Gastroenterology, Hepatology and Nutrition Website: http://www.meb.uni-bonn.de/espghan/

Gut Motility Disorders Support Network, 7 Walden Road, Sewards End, Saffron Walden CB10 2LE, United Kingdom. Tel: 01799 520580 E-mail: help@gmdnet.org.uk Website: http://www.cafamily.org.uk/Direct/g42.html

Ileostomy and Internal Pouch Support Group, National Secretary, PO Box 132, Scunthorpe, Humberside DN15 9YW, United Kingdom. Tel: 0800 018 4724, Fax: 01724 721601 E-mail: ia@ileostomypouch.demon.co.uk Website: http://www.ileostomypouch.demon.co.uk

National Association for Crohn's and Colitis, 4 Beaumont House, Sutton Road, St Albans, Herts AL1 5HH, United Kingdom. Tel: 01727 844296, Fax: 01727 862550 E-mail: nacc@nacc.org.uk Website: http://www.nacc.org.uk.

The North American Society for Pediatric Gastroenterology, Hepatology and Nutrition NASPGHAN, PO Box 6, Flourtown, PA 19031, USA Tel: (215) 233 0808, Fax: (215) 233–3939 E-mail: naspghan@naspghan.org Website: http://www.naspghan.org/

Patients on Intravenous & Nasogastric Nutrition Therapy, PO Box 3126, Christchurch, Dorset BH23 2XS, United Kingdom. E-mail: pinnt@dial.pipex.com Website: http://www.pinnt.com

REFERENCES (* Level 1 evidence)

1 Johnston LR, Alpers DH, Christensen J, et al. Physiology of the gastrointestinal tract, 3rd edn. Philadephia: Lippincott Williams & Wilkins; 1994.

2 Bisset WM. Understanding diarrhoea. Curr Paediatr 2001; 11:291–295.

3 Porter S, Speight PM. Disorders of the oral cavity. In: Walker WA, Hamilton JR, Watkins JB, et al, eds. Pediatric gastrointestinal disease. Hamilton: BC Decker; 2000:257–265.

4 Amir J, Harel L, Smetana Z, et al. Treatment of herpes simplex gingivostomatitis with aciclovir in children: a randomised double blind placebo controlled study. BMJ 1997; 314:1800–1803.

5 Omari TI, Miki K, Davidson G, et al. Characterisation of relaxation of the lower oesophageal sphincter in healthy premature infants. Gut 1997; 40:370–375.

6 Newell SJ, Sarkar PK, Durbin GM, et al. Maturation of the lower oesophageal sphincter in the preterm baby. Gut 1988; 29:167–172.

7 Orenstein SR, Izadnia F, Khan S. Gastroesophageal reflux disease in children. Gastroenterol Clin North Am 1999; 28:947–969.

8 Kelly KJ, Lazenby AJ, Rowe PC, et al. Eosinophilic esophagitis attributed to gastroesophageal reflux: improvement with an amino acid-based formula. Gastroenterology 1995; 109:1503–1512.

9 Glassman M, George D, Grill B. Gastroesophageal reflux in children. Clinical manifestations, diagnosis, and therapy. Gastroenterol Clin North Am 1995; 24:71–98.

10 Mahony MJ, Migliavacca M, Spitz L, et al. Motor disorders of the esophagus in gastro-oesophageal reflux. Arch Dis Child 1988; 63:1333–1338.

11 Nelson SP, Chen EH, Syniar GM, et al. Prevalence of symptoms of gastroesophageal reflux during infancy. A pediatric practice-based survey. Pediatric Practice Research Group. Arch Pediatr Adolesc Med 1997; 151:569–572.

12 Carre IJ. The natural history of the partial thoracic stomach (hiatus hernia) in children. Arch Dis Child 1959; 34:344–353.

13 Johnston BT, Carre IJ, Thomas PS, et al. Twenty to 40 year follow up of infantile hiatal hernia. Gut 1995; 36:809–812.

14 Sutcliffe J. Tortion spasms and abnormal postures in children with hiatus hernia: Sandifer's syndrome. Prog Pediatr Radiol 1969; 2:190–197.

15 Vandenplas Y, Belli DC, Benatar A, et al. The role of cisapride in the treatment of pediatric gastroesophageal reflux. The European Society of Paediatric Gastroenterology, Hepatology and Nutrition. J Pediatr Gastroenterol Nutr 1999; 28:518–528.

16 Cucchiara S, Franco MT, Terrin G, et al. Role of drug therapy in the treatment of gastro-oesophageal reflux disorder in children. Paediatr Drugs 2000; 2:263–272.

17 Allal H, Captier G, Lopez M, et al. Evaluation of 142 consecutive laparoscopic fundoplications in children: effects of the learning curve and technical choice. J Pediatr Surg 2001; 36:921–926.

18 Richards CA, Milla PJ, Andrews PL, et al. Retching and vomiting in neurologically impaired children after fundoplication: predictive preoperative factors. J Pediatr Surg 2001; 36:1401–1404.

19 Karnak ISM. Achalasia in childhood: surgical treatment and outcome. Eur J Pediatr Surg 2001; 11:223–229.

20 Rudolph CDM. Guidelines for evaluation and treatment of gastroesophageal reflux in infants and children: recommendations of the North American Society for Pediatric Gastroenterology and Nutrition. J Pediatr Gastroenterol Nutr 2001; 32:S1–S31.

21 Blecker U, Gold BD. Gastritis and peptic ulcer disease in childhood. Eur J Pediatr 1999; 158:541–546.

22 Dixon MF, Genta RM, Yardley JH, et al. Classification and grading of gastritis. The updated Sydney System. International Workshop on the Histopathology of Gastritis, Houston 1994. Am J Surg Pathol 1996; 20:1161–1181.

23 Dohil R, Hassall E. Peptic ulcer disease in children. Best Practice Res Clin Gastroenterol 2000; 14:53–73.

24 Marshall BJ, Warren JR. Unidentified curved bacilli in the stomach of patients with gastritis and peptic ulceration. Lancet 1984; 1:1311–1315.

25 Drumm B, Koletzko S, Oderda G. *Helicobacter pylori* infection in children: a consensus statement. European Paediatric Task Force on *Helicobacter pylori*. J Pediatr Gastroenterol Nutr 2000; 30:207–213.

*26 Gold BD, Colletti RB, Abbott M, et al. *Helicobacter pylori* infection in children: recommendations for diagnosis and treatment. J Pediatr Gastroenterol Nutr 2000; 31:490–497.

27 Hassall E. Guidelines for approaching suspected peptic ulcer disease or *Helicobacter pylori* infection: where we are in pediatrics, and how we got there. J Pediatr Gastroenterol Nutr 2001; 32:405–406.

28 Gormally SM, Prakash N, Durnin MT, et al. Association of symptoms with *Helicobacter pylori* infection in children. J Pediatr 1995; 126:753–756.

29 Rowland M, Imrie C, Bourke B, et al. How should *Helicobacter pylori* infected children be managed? Gut 1999; 45(suppl 1):136–139.

30 Fox VL. Gastrointestinal bleeding in infancy and childhood. Gastroenterol Clin North Am 2000; 29:37–66.

31 Treem WR. Gastrointestinal bleeding in children. Gastrointest Endosc Clin North Am 1994; 4:75–97.

32 Andrews PL, Hawthorn J. The neurophysiology of vomiting. Baillieres Clin Gastroenterol 1988; 2:141–168.

33 Andrews PL. Cyclic vomiting syndrome: timing, targets, and treatment—a basic science perspective. Dig Dis Sci 1999; 44:31S–38S.

34 Dignan F, Symon DN, AbuArafeh I, et al. The prognosis of cyclical vomiting syndrome. Arch Dis in Child 2001; 84:55–57.

35 Gershman G, Ament ME. Pediatric upper gastrointestinal endoscopy: state of the art. Acta Paediatr Taiwan 1999; 40:369–392.

36 Milla PJ, Muller DPR. Harries paediatric gastroenterology, 2nd edn. Edinburgh: Churchill Livingstone; 1988.

37 Hamosh M. Digestion in the newborn. Clin Perinatol 1996; 23:191–209.

38 Caspary WF. Physiology and pathophysiology of intestinal absorption. Am J Clin Nutr 1992; 55:299S–308S.

39 Milla PJ. Intestinal motility during ontogeny and intestinal pseudo-obstruction in children. Pediatr Clin North Am 1996; 43:511–532.

40 Murray JA. The widening spectrum of celiac disease. Am J Clin Nutr 1999; 69:354–365.

41 Weile B, Cavell B, Nivenius K, et al. Striking differences in the incidence of childhood celiac disease between Denmark and Sweden: a plausible explanation. J Pediatr Gastroenterol Nutr 1995; 21:64–68.

42 Holmes GK. Coeliac disease and type 1 diabetes mellitus – the case for screening. Diabet Med 2001; 18:169–177.

43 Zachor DA, Mroczek-Musulman E, Brown P. Prevalence of celiac disease in Down syndrome in the United States. J Pediatr Gastroenterol Nutr 2000; 31:275–279.

44 Bonamico M, Bottaro G, Pasquino AM, et al. Celiac disease and Turner syndrome. J Pediatr Gastroenterol Nutr 1998; 26:496–499.

45 Csizmadia CG, Mearin ML, von Blomberg BM, et al. An iceberg of childhood coeliac disease in the Netherlands. Lancet 1999; 353:813–814.

46 Baldas V, Tommasini A, Trevisiol C, et al. Development of a novel rapid non-invasive screening test for coeliac disease. Gut 2000; 47:628–631.

47 Walker-Smith J, Guandalini S, Schmitz J, et al. Revised criteria for diagnosis of coeliac disease. Report of Working Group of European Society for Paediatric Gastroenterology and Nutrition. Arch Dis Child 1990; 65:909–911.

48 Holmes GK, Prior P, Lane MR, et al. Malignancy in coeliac disease—effect of a gluten free diet. Gut 1989; 30:333–338.

49 Murch S. The immunologic basis for intestinal food allergy. Curr Opin Gastroenterol 2000; 16:552–557.

50 Kalliomaki M, Salminen S, Arvilommi H, et al. Probiotics in primary prevention of atopic disease: a randomised placebo-controlled trial. Lancet 2001; 357:1076–1079.

51 Vanderhoof JA. Food hypersensitivity in children. Curr Opin Clin Nutr Metab Care 1998; 1:419–422.

52 Goulet OJ, Brousse N, Canioni D, et al. Syndrome of intractable diarrhoea with persistent villous atrophy in early childhood: a clinicopathological survey of 47 cases. J Pediatr Gastroenterol Nutr 1998; 26:151–161.

53 Davidson GP, Cutz E, Hamilton JR, et al. Familial enteropathy: a syndrome of protracted diarrhea from birth, failure to thrive, and hypoplastic villus atrophy. Gastroenterology 1978; 75:783–790.

54 Hill SM, Milla PJ, Bottazzo GF, et al. Autoimmune enteropathy and colitis: is there a generalised autoimmune gut disorder? Gut 1991; 32:36–42.

55 Proujansky R. Protein-losing enteropathy. In: Walker WA, Hamilton JR, Watkins JB, et al, eds. Pediatric gastrointestinal disease. Hamilton: BC Decker; 2000:89–96.

56 Seidman EG. Gastrointestinal manifestations of primary immunodeficiency disease. In: Walker WA, Hamilton JR, Watkins JB, et al, eds. Pediatric gastrointestinal disease. Hamilton: BC Decker; 2000:525–547.

57 Booth IW, Lander AD. Short bowel syndrome. Baillieres Clin Gastroenterol 1998; 12:739–773.

58 Baudon JJ, Veinberg F, Thioulouse E, et al. Sucrase-isomaltase deficiency: changing pattern over two decades. J Pediatr Gastroenterol Nutr 1996; 22:284–288.

59 Wright EM. I. Glucose galactose malabsorption. Am J Physiol 1998; 275:G879–G882.

60 Kere J, Lohi H, Hoglund P. Genetic disorders of membrane transport III. Congenital chloride diarrhea. Am J Physiol 1999; 276:G7–G13.

61 Booth IW, Stange G, Murer H, et al. Defective jejunal brush-border Na+/H+ exchange: a cause of congenital secretory diarrhoea. Lancet 1985; 1:1066–1069.

62 Hyer W, Beveridge I, Domizio P, et al. Clinical management and genetics of

gastrointestinal polyps in children. J Pediatr Gastroenterol Nutr 2000; 31:469–479.

63 Durie PR. Inherited and congenital disorders of the exocrine pancreas. Gastroenterologist 1996; 4:169–187.

64 Eggermont E. Gastrointestinal manifestations in cystic fibrosis. Eur J Gastroenterol Hepatol 1996; 8:731–738.

65 Sakorafas GH, Tsiotou AG. Etiology and pathogenesis of acute pancreatitis: current concepts. J Clin Gastroenterol 2000; 30:343–356.

66 Dodge JA. Paediatric and hereditary aspects of chronic pancreatitis. Digestion 1998; 59(suppl 4):49–59.

67 Milla PJ. Motility disorders in childhood. Baillieres Clin Gastroenterol 1998; 12:775–797.

68 Guandalini S, Pensabene L, Zikri MA, et al. *Lactobacillus* GG administered in oral rehydration solution to children with acute diarrhea: a multicenter European trial. J Pediatr Gastroenterol Nutr 2000; 30:54–60.

69 Guandalini S. Treatment of acute diarrhea in the new millennium. J Pediatr Gastroenterol Nutr 2000; 30:486.

70 World Health Organization. The treatment of diarrhea: a manual for physicians and other senior health workers. Geneva. 1995. Online: Available: http://www.who.int/child-adolescent-health/New_Publications/CHILD_HEALTH/WHO.CDR.95.3.pdf or http://www.who.int/child-adolescent-health/New_Publications/CHILD_HEALTH/textrev4.htm

71 Booth I, Cunha Ferriera R, Desjeux J. Recommendations for composition of oral rehydration solutions for the children of Europe. Report of an ESPGAN Working Group. J Pediatr Gastroenterol Nutr 1992; 14:113–115.

72 World Health Organization. Expert consultation on oral rehydration salts (ORS) formulation. Geneva. 2001. Online: Available: http://www.who.int/child-adolescent-health/New_Publications/CHILD_HEALTH/Expert_consultation.htm

73 Sandhu BK, Isolauri E, Walker-Smith JA, et al. A multicentre study on behalf of the European Society for Paediatric Gastroenterology and Nutrition Working Group on Acute Diarrhoea. Early feeding in childhood gastroenteritis. J Pediatr Gastroenterol Nutr 1997; 24:522–527.

74 Szajewska H, Hoekstra JH, Sandhu B. Management of acute gastroenteritis in Europe and the impact of the new recommendations: a multicenter study. The Working Group on acute Diarrhoea of the European Society for Paediatric Gastroenterology, Hepatology, and Nutrition. J Pediatr Gastroenterol Nutr 2000; 30:522–527.

75 Bisset WM, Stapleford P, Long S, et al. Home parenteral nutrition in chronic intestinal failure. Arch Dis Child 1992; 67:109–114.

*76 Puntis JWL, Holden CE, Smallman S, et al. Staff training: a key factor in reducing intravascular catheter sepsis. Arch Dis Child 1991; 66:335–337.

*77 Beath SV, Booth IW, Murphy MS, et al. Nutritional care and candidates for small-bowel transplantation. Arch Dis Child 1995; 73:348–350.

78 Milla PJ. The role of gastrointestinal motility studies. Clin Paediatr 1994; 2:689–703.

79 Stringer MD, Puntis JWL. Short bowel syndrome. Arch Dis Child 1995; 73:170–173.

80 Ryan SW. ed. Nutritional support. Clin, Paediatr 1997; 5:177–323.

*81 Beath SV, Davies P, Papadopoulou A, et al. Parenteral nutrition related cholestasis in post surgical neonates: multivariate analysis of risk factors. J Pediatr Surg 1996; 31:604–606.

82 Sax HC, Bower RH. Hepatic complications of total parenteral nutrition. J Parenter Enter Nutr 1988; 12:615–618.

*83 Ricour C, Gorski AM, Goulet O, et al. Home parenteral nutrition in children. 8 years of experience with 112 patients. Clin Nutr 1990; 65–71.

84 Vanderhoof JA, Langnas AN, Pinch LW, et al. Short bowel syndrome. J Pediatr Gastroenterol Nutr 1992; 14:359–369.

85 Puntis JWL. Nutritional support at home and in the community. Arch Dis Child 2001; 84:295–298.

*86 Dollery CM, Sullivan ID, Bauraind O, et al. Pulmonary embolism and long term central venous access for parenteral nutrition. Lancet 1994; 344:1043–1045.

87 Pollard A, Sreeram N, Wright JG, et al. ECG and echocardiographic diagnosis of pulmonary thromboembolism associated with central venous lines. Arch Dis Child 1995; 73:147–150.

88 Georgeson K, Halpin D, Figueroa R, et al. Sequential intestinal lengthening procedures for refractory short bowel syndrome. J Pediatr Surg 1991; 29:316–321.

89 Bianchi A. Longitudinal intestinal lengthening and tailoring: results in 20 children. J R Soc Med 1997; 90:429–432.

90 Grant D, Wall W, Mimerault R. Successful small bowel–liver transplantation. Lancet 1990; 335:181–184.

91 Todo S, Tsakis A, Abu-Elmagd K. Cadaveric small bowel and small bowel–liver transplantation in humans. Transplantation 1992; 53:369–376.

92 Langnas AN, Sudan DL, Kaufman S, et al. Intestinal transplantation: a single-center experience. Transplant Proc 2000; 32:1228.

93 Goulet O, Jan D, Brousse N, et al. Intestinal transplantation. J Pediatr Gastroenterol Nutr 1997; 25:1–11.

94 Peters M, Beath SV, Puntis JWL, et al. Superior vena cava thrombosis causing respiratory obstruction successfully resolved by stenting in a small bowel transplant candidate. Arch Dis Child 2000; 83:163–164.

*95 Intestinal transplant registry. Available: http://www.intestinaltransplantregistry.org/

96 de Ville de Goyet J, Mitchell A, Mayer AD, et al. En-bloc combined reduced-liver and small bowel transplants: from large donors to small children. Transplantation 2000; 69:555.

*97 Sudan DL, Kaufman S, Shaw BW Jr, et al. Isolated intestinal transplantation for intestinal failure. Am J Gastroenterol 2000; 95:1506–1515.

98 Green M, Cacciarelli T, Mazariegos G, et al. Serial measurement of Epstein–Barr viral load in the peripheral blood in paediatric liver transplant recipients during treatment of posttransplant lymphoproliferative disease. Transplantation 1998; 12:1641–1644.

99 Clark S, Hunt J, Daly A, et al. How much are children eating after intestinal transplant? Transplant Proc 2003 (in press).

100 Brook GA. Quality of life issues: parenteral nutrition to small bowel transplantation – a review. Nutrition 1998; 14:813–816.

101 Loonen HJ, Derkx BH, Otley AR. Measuring health related quality of life of pediatric patients. J Pediatr Gastroenterol Nutr 2001; 32:523–526.

102 Richardson G, Griffiths AN, Miller V, et al. Quality of life in inflammatory bowel disease: a cross-cultural comparison of English and Canadian children. J Pediatr Gastroenterol Nutr 2001; 32:573–578.

103 Sudan DL, Iverson A, Weseman RA, et al. Assessment of function, growth and development, and quality of life long term after small bowel transplantation. Transplant Proc 2000; 32:1211–1212.

104 Jenkins HR, Milla PJ. The effect of colitis on large intestinal electrolyte transport in early childhood. J Pediatr Gastroenterol Nutr 1993; 16:402–405.

105 Jenkins HR, Fenton TR, McIntosh N, et al. The development of colonic sodium transport in early childhood and its regulation by aldosterone. Gut 1990; 31:194–197.

106 Cosgrove M, Al-Atia R, Jenkins HR. The epidemiology of inflammatory bowel disease. Arch Dis Child 1996; 74:460–461.

107 Barton JR, Gillon S, Ferguson A. Incidence of inflammatory bowel disease in Scottish children between 1968 and 1989; marginal fall in ulcerative colitis, threefold rise in Crohn's disease. Gut 1989; 30:618–622.

108 Lindberg E, Lindquist B, Holmquist L, et al. Inflammatory bowel disease in children and adolescents in Sweden 1984–1995. J Pediatr Gastroenterol Nutr 2000; 30:259–264.

109 Sawczenko A, Sandhu BK, Logan RFA, et al. Prospective survey of childhood inflammatory bowel disease in the British Isles. Lancet 2001; 357(9262):1093–1094.

110 Hill SM, Milla PJ. Infantile colitis. BMJ 1991; 302:545–546.

111 Fiocchi C. Inflammatory bowel disease; etiology and pathogenesis. Gastroenterology 1998; 115:182–205.

112 Tysk C, Lindberg E, Jarnerot G, et al. Ulcerative colitis and Crohn's disease in selected population of monozygotic and dizygotic twins: a study of heritability and the influence of smoking. Gut 1998; 29:990–996.

113 Satsangi J, Jewell DP, Bell JI. The genetics of inflammatory bowel disease. Gut 1997; 40:572–574.

114 Jenkins HR, Pincott JR, Soothill JF, et al. Food allergy: the major cause of infantile colitis. Arch Dis Child 1984; 59:326–329.

115 Griffiths AM. Crohn's disease. Recent Adv Pediatr 1992; 10:145–152.

116 Motil KJ, Grand RJ, Davis-Kraft L, et al. Growth failure in children with inflammatory bowel disease: a prospective study. Gastroenterology 1993; 105:681–691.

117 Saha MT, Ruuska T, Laippala P, et al. Growth of pre-pubertal children with inflammatory bowel disease. J Pediatr Gastroenterol Nutr 1998; 26:310–314.

118 Walker-Smith JA. Management of growth failure in Crohn's disease. Arch Dis Child 1996; 75:351–354.

119 Cowan FJ, Warner JT, Gregory JW, et al. Osteopenia in childhood inflammatory bowel disease. J Pediatr Gastroenterol Nutr 1996; 22(4):427.

120 Bunn SK, Bisset WM, Main MJC, et al. Faecal calprotectin: non invasive measure of bowel inflammation in childhood inflammatory bowel disease. J Pediatr Gastroenterol Nutr 2001; 33:14–22.

121 Shah DB, Cosgrove M, Rees JIS, Jenkins HR. The technetium white cell scan as an initial imaging investigation for evaluating suspected childhood inflammatory bowel disease. J Pediatr Gastroenterol Nutr 1997; 25:524–528.

122 Ruuska T, Vaajalahti P, Arajarvi P, et al. Prospective evaluation of upper gastro-intestinal mucosal lesions in children with ulcerative colitis and Crohn's disease. J Pediatr Gastroenterol Nutr 1994; 19:181–186.

123 Leichtner AM. Aminosalicylates for the treatment of inflammatory bowel disease. J Pediatr Gastroenterol Nutr 1995; 21:245–252.

124 Kirschner BS. Safety of azathioprine and 6-mercaptopurine in paediatric patients with inflammatory bowel disease. Gastroenterol 1998; 115:813–821.

125 Griffiths AM, Ohlsson A, Sherman PM, et al. Meta-analysis of enteral nutrition as a primary treatment of active Crohn's disease. Gastroenterology 1995; 108:1056–1067.

126 Griffiths AM. Enteral nutrition: the neglected primary therapy of active Crohn's disease. J Pediatr Gastroenterol Nutr 2000; 31:3–5.

*127 Heuschkel RB, Menache CC, Megerin JT, et al. Enteral nutrition and cortosteroids in the treatment of acute Crohn's disease in children. J Pediatr Gastroenterol Nutr 2000; 31:8–15.

128 Wilschanski M, Sherman P, Pencharz P, et al. Supplementary enteral nutrition maintains remission in paediatric Crohn's disease. Gut 1996; 38:543–548.

129 Davies G, Evans CM, Shand WS, et al. Surgery for Crohn's disease in childhood: influence of site of disease and operative procedure on outcome. Br J Surg 1990; 77:891–894.

130 Ferguson A, Sedgwick DM. Juvenile onset inflammatory bowel disease: predictions of morbidity and health status in early adult life. J R Coll Physicians Lond 1994; 28:220–227.

131 Rintala RJ, Lindahl HG. Proctocolectomy and J-pouch ileo-anal anastomosis in children. J Pediatr Surg 2002; 37(1):66–70.

132 Fozard JBJ, Dixon MF. Colonoscopic surveillance in ulcerative colitis – dysplasia through the looking glass. Gut 1989; 30:285–292.

133 Apley J. The child with abdominal pains. Oxford: Blackwell Scientific Publications; 1959.

134 Symon DNK, Russell G. Double-blind placebo controlled trial of pizotifen syrup in the treatment of abdominal migraine. Arch Dis Child 1995; 72:48–50.

135 Hyams JS, Treem WR, Justwich CJ, et al. Characterisation of symptoms in children with recurrent abdominal pain: resemblance to irritable bowel syndrome. J Pediatr Gastroenterol Nutr 1995; 20:209–214.

136 Hill DJ, Hosking CS. Infantile colic and food hypersensitivity. J Pediatr Gastroenterol Nutr 2000; 30(suppl):S67–76.

137 Wade S, Kilgour T. Clinical review: infantile colic. BMJ 2001; 323:437–440.

138 Taubman B. Parental counselling compared with elimination of cows milk or soy milk protein for the treatment of infantile colic syndrome: a randomised trial. Pediatrics 1988; 81:756–761.

139 Dohil R, Roberts E, Verrier Jones K, et al. Constipation as a cause of reversible urinary tract abnormalities. Arch Dis Child 1994; 70:56–57.

140 Weaver LT, Steiner H. The bowel habit of young children. Arch Dis Child 1984; 59:649–652.

141 Blethyn AJ, Verrier Jones K, Newcombe R, et al. Radiological assessment of constipation. Arch Dis Child 1995; 73:532–533.

142 Davidson M, Wasserman R. The irritable colon of childhood (chronic non-specific diarrhea syndrome). J Pediatr 1966; 69:1027–1038.

143 Dutton PV, Furnell JRG, Spiers AL. Environmental stress factors associated with toddler diarrhoea. J Psychosom Res 1985; 29:85–88.

144 Jobling JC, Lindley KJ, Yousef Y, et al. Investigating inflammatory bowel disease – white cell scanning, radiology and colonoscopy. Arch Dis Child 1996; 74:22–26.

145 Qualman SJ, Murray R. Aganglionosis and related disorders. Hum Pathol 1994; 45:1141–1149.

146 Wyllie R, Kay MH. Colonoscopy and therapeutic intervention in infants and children. Gastrointest Endosc Clin North Am 1994; 4:143–160.

147 Wright C, Avery A, Epstein E, et al. New chart to evaluate weight faltering. Arch Dis Child 1998; 78:40–43.

148 Wright C, Loughridge J, Moore G. Failure to thrive in a population context: two contrasting studies of feeding and nutritional status. Proc Nutr Soc 2000; 59:37–45.

149 Wright C, Birks E. Risk factors for failure to thrive: a population-based survey. Child Care Health Dev 2000; 26:5–16.

150 Wright C. A randomised controlled trial of specialist health visitor intervention for failure to thrive. Arch Dis Child 2000; 82:88.

151 Wright CM. Identification and management of failure to thrive: a community perspective. Arch Dis Child 2000; 82:5–9.

152 Shaw V, Lawson M. Clinical paediatric dietetics, 2nd edn. Oxford: Blackwell Science; 2001.

153 Mowat AP. Liver disorders in childhood, 2nd edn. London: Butterworths; 1987.

154 Spray CH, Mckiernan P, Waldron KE, et al. Investigation and outcome of neonatal hepatitis in infants with hypopituitarism. Acta Paediatr 2000; 89:951–954.

155 Thompson RJ. Strautnieks SS. Genetic defects of canalicular transport. In: Arias IM, Boyer JL, Chisari FV, et al, eds. The liver: biology and pathobiology (4). Philadelphia: Lippincott, Williams & Wilkins; 2001:383–388.

156 Emerick KM, Rand EB, Goldmuntz E, et al. Features of Alagille syndrome in 92 patients: frequency and relation to prognosis. Hepatology 1999; 29:822–829.

157 Lykavieris P, Hadchouel M, Chardot C, et al. Outcome of liver disease in children with Alagille syndrome: a study of 163 patients. Gut 2001; 49:431–435.

158 American Gastroenterological Association. Medical position statement: parenteral nutrition. Gastroenterology 2001; 121:966–969.

159 Andorsky DJ, Lund DP, Lillehei CW, et al. Nutritional and other postoperative management of neonates with short bowel syndrome correlates with clinical outcomes. J Pediatr 2001; 139:27–33.

160 Baker A, Dhawan A, Hadzic N, et al. Biliary atresia. In: David TJ, ed. Recent advances in paediatrics. Vol. 16. London: Churchill Livingstone; 1998:25–40.

161 Balistreri WF, Grand R, Hoofnagle JH, et al. Biliary atresia: current concepts and research directions. Summary of a symposium. Hepatology 1996; 23:1682–1692.

162 Fujisawa T, Komatsu H, Inui A, et al. Long-term outcome of chronic hepatitis B in adolescents or young adults in follow-up from childhood. J Pediatr Gastroenterol Nutr 2000; 30:201–206.

163 Bortolotti F, Jara P, Barbera C, et al. Long term effect of alpha interferon in children with chronic hepatitis B. Gut 2000; 46:715–718.

164 Yuen MF, Hui CK, Cheng CC, et al. Long-term follow-up of interferon alfa treatment in Chinese patients with chronic hepatitis B infection: The effect on hepatitis B e antigen seroconversion and the development of cirrhosis-related complications. Hepatology 2001; 34:139–145.

165 Poynard T, Ratziu V, Benmanov Y, et al. Fibrosis in patients with chronic hepatitis C: detection and significance. Semin Liver Dis 2000; 20:47–55.

166 Manns MP, McHutchison JG, Gordon SC, et al. Peginterferon alfa-2b plus ribavirin compared with interferon alfa-2b plus ribavirin for initial treatment of chronic hepatitis C: a randomised trial. Lancet 2001; 22(358):958–965.

167 Gregorio GV, Portmann B, Karani J, et al. Autoimmune hepatitis/sclerosing cholangitis overlap syndrome in childhood: a 16-year prospective study. Hepatology 2001; 33:544–553.

168 Thomas GR, Forbes JR, Roberts EA, et al. The Wilson disease gene: spectrum of mutations and their consequences. Nat Genet 1995; 9: 210-217.

169 Loudianos G, Gitlin JD. Wilson's disease. Semin Liver Dis 2000; 20:353–364.

170 James OF, Day CP. Non-alcoholic steatohepatitis (NASH): a disease of emerging identity and importance. J Hepatol 1998; 29:495–501.

171 Rivera-Penera T, Moreno J, Skaff C, et al. Delayed encephalopathy in fulminant hepatic failure in the pediatric population and the role of liver transplantation. J Pediatr Gastroenterol Nutr 1997; 24:128–134.

172 Bhaduri BR, Mieli-Vergani G. Fulminant hepatic failure: pediatric aspects. Semin Liver Dis 1996; 16:349–355.

173 Durand P, Debray D, Mandel R, et al. ALF in infancy: A 14-year experience of a pediatric liver transplantation center. J Pediatr 2001; 139:871–876.
174 Kayihan N, Nennesomo I, Ericzon BG, et al. Deterioration of neurological disease after orthotopic liver transplantation for valproic acid-induced liver damage. Pediatr Transplant 2000; 4:211–214.
175 Goncalves I, Hermans D, Chretien D, et al. Mitochondrial respiratory chain defect: a new etiology for neonatal cholestasis and early liver insufficiency. J Hepatol 1995; 23:290–294.
176 Hirst WJ, Layton DM, Singh S, et al. Haemophagocytic lymphohistiocytosis: experience at two UK centres. Br J Haematol 1994; 88: 731–739.
177 Stepp SE, Dufourcq-Lagelouse R, Le Deist F, et al. Perforin gene defects in familial hemophagocytic lymphohistiocytosis. Science 1999; 286:1957–1959.
178 Karrer FM, Narkewicz MR. Esophageal varices: current management in children. Semin Pediatr Surg 1999; 8:193–201.
179 Blei AT, Cordoba J. Hepatic encephalopathy. Am J Gastroenterol 2001; 96:1968–1976.
180 Butterworth RF. Complications of cirrhosis III. Hepatic encephalopathy. J Hepatol 2000; 32(suppl 1):171–180.
181 Novy MA, Schwarz KB. Nutritional considerations and management of the child with liver disease. Nutrition 1997; 13:177–184.
182 Gupta D, Vijaya DR, Gupta R, et al. Prevalence of hepatopulmonary syndrome in cirrhosis and extrahepatic portal venous obstruction. Am J Gastroenterol 2001; 96:3395–3399.
183 Yang YY, Lin HC, Lee WC, et al. Portopulmonary hypertension: distinctive hemodynamic and clinical manifestations. J Gastroenterol 2001; 36:181–186.
184 Salvi SS. Liver disease and pulmonary hypertension. Gut 2000; 47:595.
185 Heaton ND, Howard ER. Complications and limitations of injection sclerotherapy in portal hypertension. Gut 1993; 34:7–10.
186 Lykavieris P, Gauthier F, Hadchouel P, et al. Risk of gastrointestinal bleeding during adolescence and early adulthood in children with portal vein obstruction. Pediatrics 2000; 136:805–808.
187 Colombo C, Crosignani A, Battezzati PM. Liver involvement in cystic fibrosis. J Hepatol 1999; 31:946–954.
188 Stringer MD, Hennayake S, Howard ER, et al. Improved outcome for children with hepatoblastoma. Br J Surg 1995; 82:386–391.
189 Goss JA, Shackleton CR, McDiarmid SV, et al. Long-term results of pediatric liver transplantation: an analysis of 569 transplants. Ann Surg 1998; 228:411–420.
190 Protheroe S, de Ville de Goyet J, Kelly DA, et al. Quality of life in children on home parental nutrition and following intestinal transplantation. Arch Dis Child 2002; 86:A23.

18

Respiratory disorders

Edited by Peter Helms, John Henderson

INTRODUCTION AND CONTEXT

Acute respiratory illness is among the most common reasons for admission to medical pediatric beds in industrialized countries and, together with acute gastroenteritis, acute respiratory infections (ARI) remain among the commonest causes of death and serious morbidity in young children in underdeveloped and emerging economies (Fig. 18.1). Despite a high worldwide prevalence of ARI the infective agents differ in that bacterial infections, including tuberculosis, are common in underdeveloped countries while viral infections are more commonly associated with ARI in developed economies. In temperate countries there is also a marked seasonality of ARI with a significant rise in prevalence in the winter months falling to relatively low levels in the summer – so much so that many acute medical pediatric units have low occupancy rates in the summer months. This seasonal pattern of illness is most dramatically seen for respiratory syncytial virus (RSV) bronchiolitis (Fig. 18.2). Whereas serious morbidity and mortality from respiratory disease has fallen to very low levels in developed economies, the total burden of respiratory disease remains high with a shift from life-threatening ARI to an increased incidence of asthma and related atopic disease. The reasons for what has been termed the 'asthma and atopy epidemic' are not yet entirely clear although several environmental risk factors have been proposed including a reduction in the overall burden of infectious disease – the so-called hygiene hypothesis,[1] dietary factors including low antioxidant intake[2,3] and greater intake of processed fats.[4] Whereas in the last decade increased exposure to allergens and particularly those within the internal environment including house dust mite were considered to be major factors, recent work does not support this association.[5,6] Prospective birth cohort studies are currently in progress in order to clarify the relative contribution of the putative risk factors.[7,8]

IN DEVELOPED ECONOMIES

The marked reduction in the prevalence of life-threatening ARI in developed countries in the last 50 years reflects an improved standard of living, immunization against tuberculosis, pertussis, diphtheria, measles and *Haemophilus influenzae* and the introduction of effective antimicrobial drugs and a relatively low rate of HIV infection. For those children with life-threatening disease technological advances in managing respiratory failure have also had their impact. Targets for further reductions in the burden of illness particularly in the youngest age groups would be the elimination of RSV infection by an effective vaccine and a reduction in exposure to cigarette smoke in utero and in early childhood. Whereas the work load for acute asthma in hospitals has been diminishing, the burden in primary care still remains at high levels with the highest annual incidence, in proportion

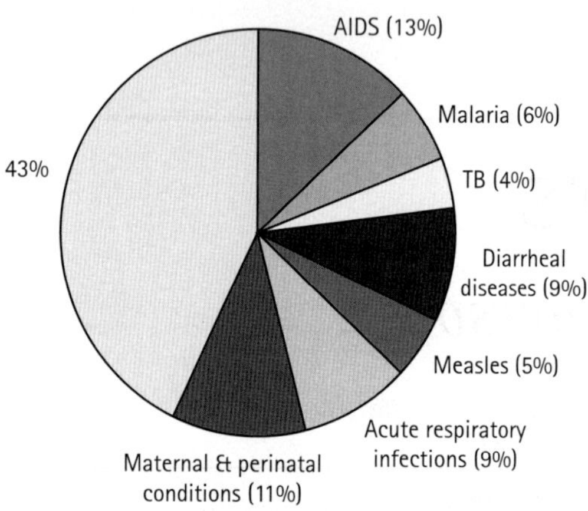

Fig. 18.1 Causes of death in children under 5 years of age in Africa and South East Asia (www.who.int/inf-new/conclu.htm).

to the at-risk population, in the youngest age groups (Fig. 18.3). Ecological analyses have suggested that the early and sustained use of prophylactic therapy, particularly inhaled corticosteroids (ICS), have contributed to this reduction in hospital admissions although this beneficial outcome needs to be balanced by concerns about the possible systemic effects of long term use of ICS.[4]

In developed economies improvements in therapeutic options including age appropriate inhalation delivery devices, antibiotics and organization of care have resulted in increasing actuarial survival for conditions that in previous generations and epochs were invariably fatal in childhood. This increased survival applies to a number of conditions including cystic fibrosis, unusual congenital anomalies such as congenital diaphragmatic hernia and respiratory complications of other conditions such as extreme prematurity (pp. 793 – Chronic lung disease) and neuromuscular disorders (pp. 798 – Long term ventilation and Ch. 20). In cystic fibrosis, for example, a strong cohort effect on actuarial survival, although modulated by socioeconomic factors, has become apparent since the disease was first characterized in the 1940s (Fig. 18.4).[9] The increased survival of children with significant lung disease, or with neuromuscular disorders and associated respiratory impairment, has effectively exported much morbidity and mortality into adult life. These medical 'successes' have placed increased burdens on affected individuals and their families and in order to maintain a satisfactory quality of life more attention is now being given to psychosocial aspects of disease and to palliative care (see Chs 34 and 37). Quality of life instruments are being increasingly used to assess the impact of disease and in assessing therapeutic interventions.[10, 11]

IN UNDERDEVELOPED AND EMERGING ECONOMIES

Respiratory diseases are a significant cause of mortality in developing countries (Fig. 18.1). In a global health context these potentially avoidable causes of death have moved up the political agenda and leaders of the G7 industrialized countries have voiced increasing concerns about the burden of infectious diseases including ARI and have set 10-year targets for their reduction. One such target is to halve tuberculosis incidence and deaths by applying effective interventions such as immunization and making antimicrobial therapy more accessible to vulnerable populations. Although such programs can be effective such interventions require reductions in the prices of effective drugs and vaccines. In Malawi for example, increasing the immunization cover from 50% in 1980 to a figure approaching 90% in 1998 resulted in a dramatic fall in serious morbidity and deaths from measles (Fig. 18.5). Despite the fact that the measles vaccine is safe and effective and costs less than 15p (US$0.26) for a single dose, less than 50% of eligible children are currently immunized in African countries. Deaths from pneumonia can also be significantly reduced if the World Health Organization (WHO) guidelines are fully implemented. The WHO program requires identification of children with clinical evidence of pneumonia followed by early introduction of antibiotics and advice on use of fluids and adequate nutrition. This program can be delivered relatively inexpensively by village health workers who are trained to identify signs of pneumonia including rapid breathing and chest indrawing and who use appropriate antibiotics and discourage the use of commercial cough remedies, some of which contain harmful ingredients. The benefits of such programs can be dramatic (Fig. 18.6).

FETAL PROGRAMMING OF LUNG DISEASE IN CHILDREN AND ADULTS

There is growing evidence that fetal life and early childhood are critical periods of development for many diseases that present during child and adult life. In humans and other long-gestation species, the development of lung architecture occurs during fetal and early postnatal life. A number of epidemiological studies have

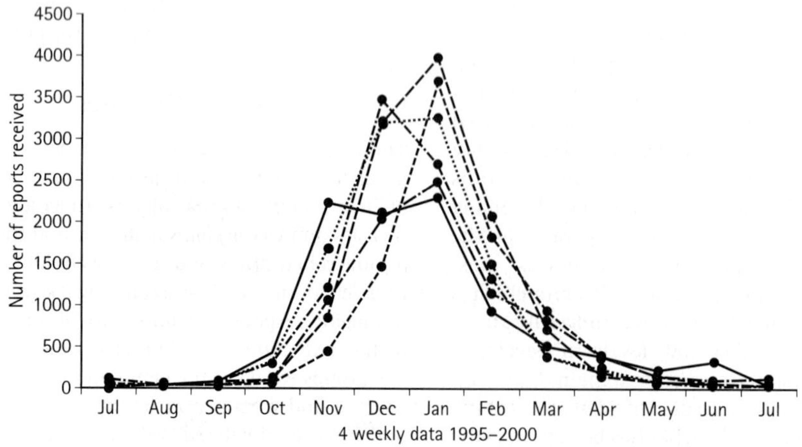

Fig. 18.2 Reports of respiratory syncitial virus (RSV) isolates from 1995 to 2000 (Public Health Laboratory, England and Wales). Data from CDSC (www.phls.co.uk).

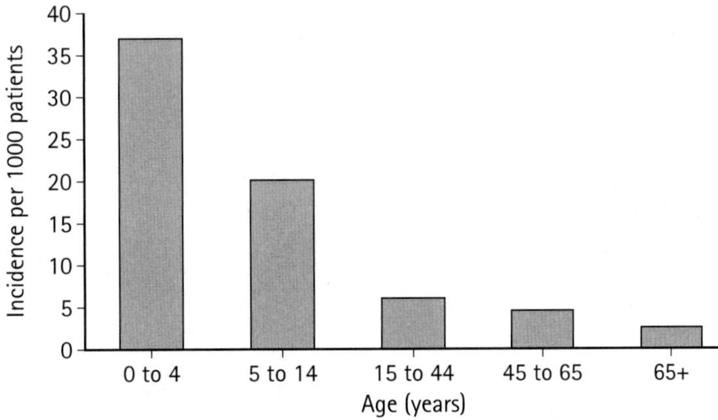

Fig. 18.3 Annual incidence of physician-diagnosed asthma in Scottish General Practices 1998. Data from the General Practice Data Evaluation Project (GDEP) Scotland.

demonstrated associations between prenatal factors that restrict intrauterine growth and respiratory symptoms in infancy. This observation led to speculation that factors which impair fetal growth may also constrain fetal lung development resulting in permanent changes to lung architecture. Work in fetal lambs with imposed growth restriction during late gestation has demonstrated structural and mechanical abnormalities of the lungs but no effects on surfactant protein expression in these animals.[12] Barker et al[13] described an association between low birth weight and lung function decrements in over 5000 adult males. Furthermore, respiratory infection during early childhood was associated with further decrements in adult lung function in this population, suggesting that either impaired lung function at birth was associated with predisposition to pulmonary infections during infancy or that respiratory infections, such as pneumonia and whooping cough, cause airway and lung remodeling which further impairs lung function. A follow-up study of lung function in infancy has demonstrated reduced forced expiratory flows at the age of 2 months in infants who subsequently developed pneumonia[14] supporting a role for predisposition to infections in infants who already have pre-existing lung function impairment. Other epidemiological studies have confirmed an association between respiratory infections during infancy and early childhood and later functional abnormalities consistent with airway obstruction in adults.[15]

GENETIC DETERMINANTS

Pulmonary disease may accompany a number of genetic disorders in children and some pulmonary diseases have a genetic basis, although this is seldom based on simple Mendelian inheritance but may have polygenic or multifactorial etiology. A clear exception to this is cystic fibrosis, which results from a variety of mutations in a single gene located on chromosome 7q that encodes the CFTR protein (see pp. 763 – Cystic fibrosis). Since the CFTR gene was isolated in 1989, more than 900 mutations have been described (www.genet.sickkids.on.ca/CFTR), although only a handful of these are common in populations of patients with cystic fibrosis. A number of other conditions have been associated with increased frequency of CFTR mutations, including asthma, allergic bronchopulmonary aspergillosis (ABPA) in asthma, neonatal transient hypertrypsinemia, chronic pancreatitis and congenital bilateral absence of the vas deferens. Recurrent nasal polyposis has also been described as a 'monosymptomatic' form of cystic fibrosis.

Asthma (see pp. 751) is a complex, polygenic disease that results from the exposure of genetically susceptible individuals to environmental triggers, possibly at critical stages of development, for the disease to be expressed. Linkage studies and genome-wide searches have identified a number of potential candidate genes for asthma and atopy[16] but no single gene accounts for a major part of the expression of the disease. Also, the rate of increase in

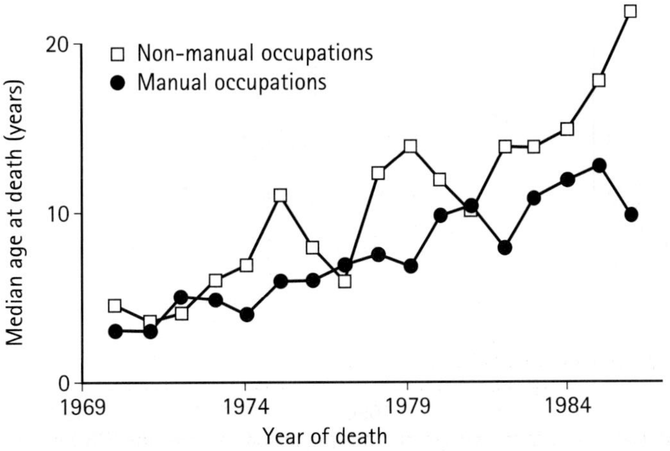

Fig. 18.4 Influence of socioeconomic status on survival in subjects with cystic fibrosis. (From Britton 1989[9] with permission)

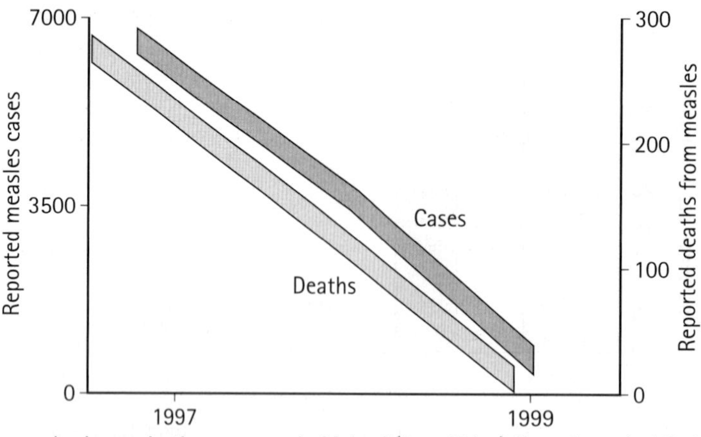

Fig. 18.5 Impact of introducing a measles immunization program in Malawi (East Africa). Data from the World Health Organization (www.who.int/inf-new/child3.htm).

asthma prevalence in the United Kingdom and other Western countries is inconsistent with major shifts in population genetics. Therefore, attention has focused on identification of environmental exposures that may be causally implicated in the etiology of asthma and atopy.

The approach to bronchiectasis in children without cystic fibrosis (non-CF bronchiectasis) has changed in emphasis from the role of childhood infections, such as pertussis, tuberculosis and complicated measles, to the role of intrinsic defects with an inherited basis. Although deficiency of protease inhibitors, primarily alpha-1 antitrypsin, is often included in the work-up of these children, it is not a condition that presents in this way. Primary ciliary dyskinesia however, is increasingly recognized in children with chronic suppurative lung disease and bronchiectasis. Primary ciliary dyskinesia (PCD) is generally observed to follow an autosomal recessive mode of inheritance, although dominant and X-linked inheritances have been described. Linkage studies of separate populations with PCD have mapped loci to a number of chromosomes and a recent genome-wide screen has demonstrated extensive locus heterogeneity in PCD.[17] Candidate genes for the disease include those encoding the intermediate and heavy dynein chains, e.g. DNAI2 and DNAH5. Dynein also has a pivotal role in determining normal left–right axis asymmetry during embryogenesis and, in the mouse model, mutations affecting the function of node monocilia are associated with randomization of situs. Therefore, 50% of subjects with immotile cilia syndrome (Kartagener) have situs inversus.

Immune deficiency (see Ch. 25) is another important risk factor for bronchiectasis. A recent survey of 150 patients, mainly adults, with bronchiectasis, during which systematic investigations for possible heritable causes were performed, identified 12 subjects with abnormalities of immune function, including common variable immune deficiency (CVID), IgM deficiency and isolated IgG subclass deficiencies.[18]

Other pulmonary diseases that have a genetic basis but rarely present during childhood include interstitial lung disease in association with collagen disorders, such as lupus erythematosus, and sarcoidosis. There is increasing interest in the origins of chronic obstructive pulmonary disease (COPD), which has been demonstrated in several studies to cluster within families, independent of smoking status. It is possible that mechanisms such as oxidative lung injury due to deficiencies of components of the antioxidant defenses, such as superoxide dismutase and glutathione-S-transferases, are responsible for respiratory morbidity in childhood that is the antecedent of COPD in adults. Increasing knowledge of the genetic and cellular regulation of pulmonary inflammation and defense is likely to lead to new insights into the origins of pulmonary diseases. The challenge will be to recognize individuals at risk and develop effective interventions to prevent the onset or alter the natural history of some of these conditions.

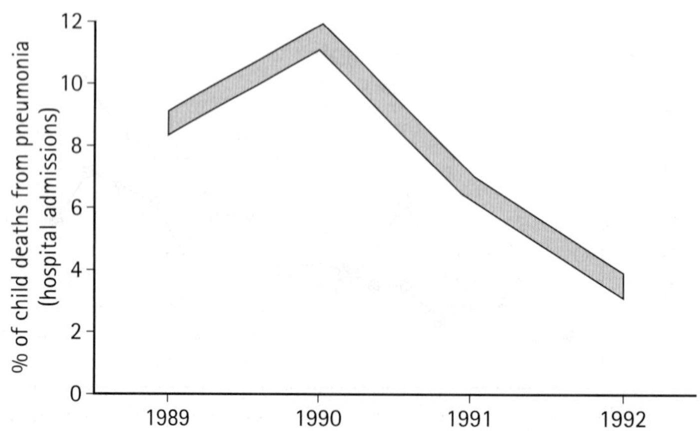

Fig. 18.6 Reduction in hospital deaths attributable to pneumonia after the introduction of the WHO guidelines for identifying and managing acute respiratory infection in childhood (www.who.int/inf-new/child3.htm).

ENVIRONMENTAL RISK FACTORS

Tobacco smoke exposure

A recent systematic review demonstrated a consistent relationship between parents' smoking and respiratory illnesses and symptoms and middle ear disease in children with odds ratios between 1.2 and 1.6.[19] The odds are greater for preschool children and higher for maternal compared with paternal smoking. The latter observation might be explained by increased exposure to maternal rather than paternal smoking among preschool children. Alternatively, a prenatal effect of maternal smoking on the developing (see pp. 722 – Development of the respiratory system) fetal lungs might be responsible. One of the difficulties of disentangling the interrelationships of prenatal and postnatal tobacco smoke exposure on children's respiratory symptoms in epidemiological studies is the observation that prenatal maternal smoking is almost always associated with postnatal tobacco smoke exposure.

Several studies have demonstrated an association between prenatal tobacco smoke exposure and decrements in pulmonary function in infants soon after delivery and before the onset of symptoms. Such decrements appear to be associated with respiratory symptoms during the first year after birth[20–22] and it seems likely that in utero smoke exposure causes growth restraint of fetal airways. The longer term effects of such fetal growth restraint have yet to be determined. Recent studies have attempted to examine the differential effects of intrauterine and postnatal tobacco smoke exposure on the outcomes of asthma and wheezing in later childhood. Gilliland and colleagues[23] have demonstrated associations between in utero exposure and physician diagnosed asthma in later childhood but, although current or past environmental (postnatal) exposure was related to wheezing symptoms, there was not a significant relationship with asthma. The authors speculated that environmental exposure may act as a cofactor for attacks of wheezing but did not appear to be a factor that induced asthma in this population.

Parental smoking has also been demonstrated in several case control and cohort studies[24] to be significantly associated with sudden infant death syndrome (SIDS). Maternal smoking was associated with increased risk and a dose–response effect has been demonstrated in several studies, suggesting a causal relationship, and, although smoking rates vary with socioeconomic status, the risk appears to be consistent across socioeconomic groups. Fleming and colleagues[25] in a study of sudden infant death after the 'Back to Sleep' campaign in the United Kingdom calculated an odds ratio of SIDS for maternal smoking during pregnancy of 2.1 with an additional independent effect of paternal smoking. The mechanisms for this effect have not been elucidated but fetal lung growth restraint or effects of smoking on neurological responses to thermal, hypoxic or hypercapnic stress have been postulated. Recent pathological studies of infants dying of SIDS have demonstrated increased thickness of the airway wall in infants of mothers who smoked compared with infants of non-smoking mothers, suggesting that airway obstruction may be an important mechanism.

Many studies have concentrated on the respiratory health effects of passive exposure to tobacco smoke in children. However, active smoking by children remains a significant health problem. A recent survey of 14–16-year-old children revealed that 30% had been active smokers in the previous 12 months, with 14.1% reporting regular smoking.[26]

Social deprivation (see also Ch. 8)

Using the World Bank definition of $1/person/day, it is estimated that 2.1 billion of the world's population live in conditions of absolute poverty below this threshold. Diseases associated with poverty are primarily infectious diseases, which are linked to inadequate income, lack of access to clean water and sanitation, malnutrition and poor access to medical services. In developing countries, the commonest causes of death in children under 5 years of age are lower respiratory infections, diarrheal illnesses and measles. Acute lower respiratory tract infections account for 2.1 million deaths annually in young children in the developing world with approximately 40% estimated to be related to malnutrition.[27,28] Some developing countries have achieved lower rates of poverty related ill health by government interventions in health, education and social security and also by active programs to increase the levels of female literacy in their populations.

In the United Kingdom, adults and children of lower socioeconomic status have also been demonstrated to be at higher risk of communicable diseases, particularly respiratory infections.[29] A longitudinal study of a UK cohort born in 1946 demonstrated that a poor home environment, parental bronchitis and atmospheric pollution were the best predictors of lower respiratory infections in the first 2 years after birth and these factors together with later smoking and childhood respiratory infections were the best predictors of lower respiratory tract diseases in adults.[30] It is possible that increased infections in socially disadvantaged populations are related to crowding and increased exposure to infectious agents or to alterations in host immunity, possibly related to nutritional status. One of the characteristic diseases of social deprivation, tuberculosis (see Infectious Diseases (Tuberculosis), Ch. 26), has recently shown a reversal of the decline in notified cases in England (Public Health Laboratory Service; http://www.phls.co.uk) with the largest number of cases reported from urban regions, particularly London. The annual incidence of tuberculosis in children in England and Wales is currently around 3.5 per 100 000 with a doubling of cases in London reported between 1993 and 1998.[31] In contrast with the adult population in which the majority of cases occur in males, the sex distribution in children appears to be even. Studies of variations in tuberculosis rates between electoral wards in inner cities have suggested that the country of birth was the single most explanatory variable, with measures of poverty being of only secondary importance.[32,33]

Early respiratory infections

Strachan[1] first proposed the 'hygiene hypothesis' that infections in early childhood prevented the development of allergic diseases. An inverse relationship was observed between family size, particularly the presence of older siblings, and features of allergic disease, including hay fever and positive skin prick test responses, but not with asthma. Recent observations that the prevalence of allergy is reduced in farming communities[34] might also be explained by increased exposure to infections in early life in this setting, although other differences in lifestyle between rural farming and urban communities are possible confounders of this relationship. T cell responses may be central to the mechanisms of these observed associations. Activated T lymphocytes are important in maintaining lung inflammation in adults with asthma and the demonstration of increased concentrations of soluble interleukin 2 (IL-2) receptors in children with asthma suggests that activated T cells are important in this context also. Atopy in children has been proposed to represent persistence of fetal Th2 responses[35] with the production of type 2 cytokines (interleukins 4, 5, 6, 10, 13) in response to allergens. Infections may be important in early childhood by stimulating Th1 predominant responses [IL-2, interferon-gamma, tumor necrosis factor alpha (TNF-alpha)]. Survivors of a measles epidemic in Guinea-Bissau were found to have decreased prevalence of atopy compared with immunized children,[36] although the possibility that children with impaired Th1 responses were more susceptible to dying during the epidemic has been raised. Also, exposure to tuberculosis has been shown to result in lower prevalence of atopy, but not asthma, in a large Finnish study.[37] The potential for immune modulation of T helper response by bowel flora and the effect of antibiotics on bowel colonization has also been studied. These clinical observations together with laboratory studies of T cell sensitization have led to the development of strategies to modulate the switch from Th2 to Th1 predominant responses, either by allergen avoidance from early gestation[38] or by the development of vaccines, Th1 selective adjuvants or immunotherapy.

In addition to potential protective effects on later development of asthma, viral respiratory infections have also been proposed as contributors to the development of obstructive airways disease. A number of studies have reported persistent or recurrent wheezing after RSV bronchiolitis in infants. However, there is still debate about whether RSV causes asthma or whether severe RSV infection is a manifestation of pre-existing risk factors for both bronchiolitis and asthma.[39] It is hoped that randomized controlled trials of RSV prophylaxis will be able to address some of these questions but these are currently restricted to high-risk infants.

Diet

The prenatal effects of maternal famine were studied in a Dutch population exposed to the famine of 1944–45. The prevalence of obstructive airways diseases in the offspring of famine-exposed mothers was higher, particularly when the exposure occurred in early gestation. This effect did not appear to be mediated through increased prevalence of atopic disease in this population, suggesting that impairment of fetal lung development was an important factor.

A number of dietary constituents have been examined in relation to their potential role in the etiology of lung diseases, including fatty acids, antioxidants and sodium intake. The observation that Eskimos had a low prevalence of lung disease and a diet high in oily fish prompted speculation that *n*-3 fatty acids, which competitively inhibit the metabolism of arachidonic acid, may be protective against asthma.[40] However, there is only weak evidence for this and no intervention studies have yet been done.

Oxidative damage to the lungs, mediated through oxygen free radicals, is believed to be important in the pathogenesis of asthma and chronic obstructive pulmonary disease (COPD). Fruit is a major source of antioxidant vitamins and epidemiological associations between fruit intake and lung function in adults have been established. A positive association between fresh fruit consumption and lung function has also been demonstrated in children.[41] Selenium is essential to the activity of glutathione peroxidase enzymes that are involved in the lung's antioxidant defenses. Low serum concentrations of selenium have been demonstrated in subjects with asthma but it is unclear whether selenium deficiency contributes to the development of asthma or if selenium consumption occurs as a consequence of oxidant injury. A recent ecological study of asthma and allergy (ISAAC) did not demonstrate an increased prevalence in countries in which selenium deficiency is endemic[42] compared with areas with abundant dietary selenium sources. Low dose vitamin A supplementation has been examined for its possible protective role in the development of lower respiratory infections in children. Two intervention studies in developing countries have suggested that this effect is strongly related to nutritional status with decreased acute lower respiratory infections observed in underweight children only[43,44] and adverse effects noted in children of normal nutritional status.

Regional differences in asthma mortality have been correlated with table salt purchase, leading to the possibility that dietary sodium may be an important factor in asthma pathogenesis. However, dietary salt intake in children has been associated with increased bronchial responsiveness to methacholine but not with a diagnosis of asthma or with exercise-induced bronchospasm.[45]

Atmospheric pollution

There is clear evidence that atmospheric pollution may exacerbate respiratory symptoms in human subjects but what is less clear is whether specific pollutants have a causal role in the pathogenesis of respiratory diseases. The principal pollutants of the external (outdoor) environment include nitrogen oxides (NO, NO_2), ozone, sulfur dioxide (SO_2) and particulates from the burning of fossil fuels. Hospital admission rates for respiratory diseases, especially pneumonia, have been demonstrated to be correlated with high atmospheric concentrations of particulates (PM_{10}), NO_2 and ozone[46] and effects of NO_2, carbon monoxide (CO) and SO_2 on general practice consultations for asthma have been found to be stronger in children than in adults.[47] The well documented rise in the prevalence of asthma in industrialized countries has coincided with a general increase in the density of road traffic in the majority of these countries. Therefore a number of studies have investigated the possibility that traffic pollution is an exposure that initiates asthma in previously unaffected individuals but with conflicting results. A landmark study of this aspect of lung disease in children was undertaken following the German reunification in 1989. This allowed a study of two genetically similar populations exposed to different levels of atmospheric pollution with higher concentrations of industrial pollutants (SO_2 and particulates) in Leipzig, East Germany compared with Munich, West Germany where traffic density was higher. The results of this study demonstrated a higher lifetime prevalence of asthma and a greater prevalence of sensitization to common aeroallergens in the West German population compared with the East German population, suggesting that prolonged exposure to industrial pollutants was not associated with the development of asthma or allegy.[48] The same group studied the relationships between traffic density and respiratory health of children in several school districts in Munich and, although demonstrating associations between traffic density and small decrements in lung function, found no association between high traffic density and either lifetime prevalence of asthma or bronchial responsiveness to cold air.[49] It should be borne in mind that geographical comparisons such as this are prone to confounding by other differences in exposures between the populations, such as indoor environment and lifestyle variations. The importance of the indoor environment for respiratory diseases has been highlighted in observational studies of populations in developing countries that rely on burning fossil fuels for domestic energy where this practice appears to be associated with increased respiratory infections and obstructive airways diseases in children[50] although no controlled studies have been done and few have measured exposures directly. An association between gas cooking and asthma in children has been described[51] and Burr and colleagues[52] have recently described an increased 12-month prevalence of wheeze in 12–14-year-olds in association with the use of bottled gas, paraffin and other unusual domestic fuels for heating. However, of all the potential indoor pollutants to which children may be exposed it is likely that parental tobacco smoke exposure has the single greatest effect on their respiratory health.

DEVELOPMENT OF THE RESPIRATORY SYSTEM

The links between development and disease are well illustrated in the respiratory system. Although anatomically there is no sudden change at the time of birth, enormous alterations in function occur during subsequent growth and development. The observation that respiratory illness has high prevalences in infancy and early childhood and again in late adult life points to important features of maturation and aging and possible links between early adverse environmental exposures and lifetime respiratory health.[13,53]

FETAL AND PERINATAL DEVELOPMENT

Structural development

Lung growth and development commences in early intrauterine life with the development of the trachea from the primitive esophagus at approximately 5 weeks of gestational age. The right and left lung buds develop at about 7 weeks and the formation of the main lobar structures is already evident by 9 weeks. This process of branching airway development continues through the first trimester of pregnancy and is largely complete by 16 weeks of gestational age. By this time the lungs have a glandular appearance with alveoli emerging over the next 8–10 weeks increasing in complexity and surface area up to and beyond term.[54,55] Arguments concerning the duration of alveolar development have depended on the distinction of saccules and alveoli and on techniques for counting alveolar number in postmortem lungs. Current opinion suggests that about 50% of the final complement of alveoli is present at term with 85% complete by 2–3 years of age. The process of alveolization is accompanied by a reduction in interstitial tissue and the remodeling of capillaries into a single network and with an enormous thinning of the blood gas barrier. A network of elastin strands form the 'skeleton' (likened to a fishnet) between which the new alveoli are formed. Normal fetal breathing movements are important in promoting this growth. Adverse influences on this ordered sequence of development will have important and different consequences for future respiratory health of the individual depending on their timing and duration. Generally the earlier the insult the more profound the long term consequences.

Implications for disease

Many adverse intrauterine influences, for example congenital diaphragmatic hernia[56] and renal agenesis and oligohydramnios[57] can have devastating effects on subsequent lung growth and development. Insults during the early phase of airway development will reduce branching and will inevitably lead to reductions in the number of alveoli that can bud from a reduced number of terminal bronchioles (Fig. 18.7). Indeed this can be inferred from physiological measurements in infants with impairment of intrauterine growth due to diaphragmatic hernia or to reduced fetal breathing movements associated with spinal muscular atrophy of intrauterine origin.[58] The importance of fetal breathing movements has been demonstrated in a series of elegant experiments in laboratory animals in which the relative contributions of fetal breathing and the volume of amniotic fluid have been demonstrated.[59] As pulmonary vascular development follows the development of the airways it is hardly surprising that pulmonary perfusion anomalies have also been observed in the survivors of diaphragmatic hernia repair despite what appears to be satisfactory radiological outcome.[60] Although the intrauterine insults described above are dramatic, they are thankfully relatively rare in population terms. What may be more relevant for population respiratory health are more subtle influences on lung growth and development in utero and in early life. Such associations between early respiratory symptoms and adverse enviromental exposures have been inferred by the association between low birth weight and subsequent respiratory health and in particular chronic respiratory lung disease of adulthood.[13] The most clearly identified adverse exposure at a whole population level is fetal tobacco smoke exposure associated with maternal smoking in pregnancy. Whereas postnatal or environmental tobacco smoke (ETS) exposure has a significant influence on respiratory morbidity in the young,[61] the effects of prenatal exposure are likely to be more long lasting. Studies which have assessed lung function soon after birth, when the effects of ETS would be expected to be small, have shown evidence of reduced airway function.[62,63] Whereas it is clearly not possible to identify the exact mechanisms of these effects in humans animal studies have shown that fetal ETS significantly reduces cell division in the lung as evidenced by reduced DNA, reduces alveolar number and reduces the amount of connective tissue within the lung.[64,65]

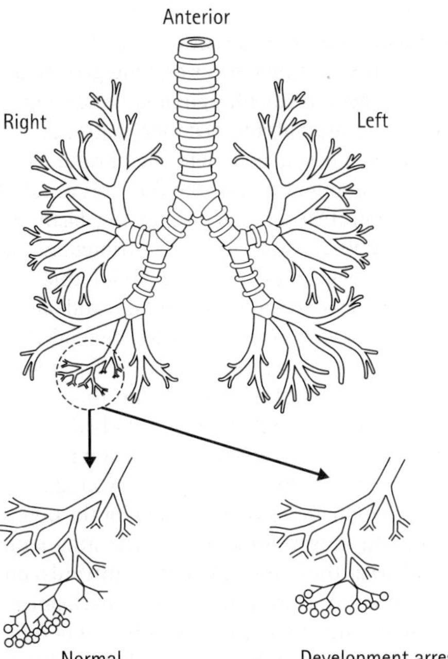

Fig. 18.7 Representation of the bronchial tree in a normal newborn infant and in an infant with intrauterine pulmonary hypoplasia in whom peripheral airway development has been impaired. Note the implication for reduced alveoli.

The structure of the airways themselves also has important functional consequences. Cartilaginous structures appear in segmental bronchi at 10–12 weeks of gestational age but continue to develop in small bronchi until after birth. Generalized bronchomalacia or local disorders affecting the trachea and bronchi are associated with several important disorders including tracheomalacia, stovepipe trachea and lobar emphysema. Airway smooth muscle contrary to popular belief is found at term down to the smallest terminal and respiratory bronchioles and consequently failure of wheezing influence to respond to bronchodilators cannot be ascribed to the absence of smooth muscle at this level. Vascular modeling after birth may be disturbed as a result of widespread perinatal lung damage such as chronic lung disease of prematurity, or in association with congenital heart disease (Ch. 19), leading to persistence of pulmonary hypertension. A number of major developmental defects in the nasopharynx may lead to respiratory obstruction, infection or recurrent aspiration. These include choanal atresia or stenosis, palatal anomalies and, on a cellular level, ciliary dyskinesia. These, as well as mid-facial syndromes, Down syndrome and neuromuscular disorders, can lead to obstructive apnea or sleep-disordered breathing problems (see pp. 746 – Apnea and breathing disorders).

The chest wall

The chest wall is defined as the structures which surround the lung and which have significant influences on lung growth and function. It includes the rib cage, the diaphragm and the abdominal contents together with the paraspinal and accessory muscles of respiration. The diaphragm becomes a complete membrane by 8 weeks of gestation and the abdominal wall is complete at 9 weeks allowing the establishment of effective fetal breathing. At birth however, the proportion of fatigue resistant (type I) striated muscle fibers is approximately 10%, much less than the 50% found in adults. The proportion is even less in preterm infants and along with the instability of the chest wall explains in part the tendency of preterm infants to develop respiratory failure and suffer from apnea. The diaphragm is also inserted more directly into the chest wall with a reduced area of apposition (or alignment with the lower rib cage) than that found in mature subjects and this again results in a relative functional impairment in the infant and very young child. The chest wall has important influences on the function of the underlying lungs both in maintaining lung volume at rest (the lung tends to seek a lower volume whereas the chest wall recoils outwards) and in its role as the 'respiratory pump'. During growth and development important changes occur in the function of the chest wall, not only at rest but also during respiratory efforts that affect underlying lung function.

POSTNATAL DEVELOPMENT

After alveolization is complete at approximately 3 years of age, the lungs grow as a result of stretch, mainly due to the associated growth of the rib cage. This can be seen in the different patterns of growth inferred from postmortem pathological studies and physiological lung volumes measured during respiratory maneuvers (Fig. 18.8). This disparity emphasizes the significant influence of the chest wall on the function of the underlying lung. The stretch and subsequent growth of volume of the lung results in what has been termed 'dysynaptic' growth. In infancy the airways are relatively large in relation to the total lung volume, a ratio which falls progressively during subsequent growth. This feature of physiological lung growth results in a gradual fall in the contribution of peripheral airway resistance to overall airway resistance, a feature which also contributes to the severe nature of lower repiratory illnesses and an increased tendency to develop symptomatic airway obstruction in infancy and early childhood. Another feature during growth and development is that females appear to have more patent airways (lower resistance) than males as seen in physiological measurements[67,68] and in the increased risk of significant respiratory morbidity in boys. This relative female advantage reverses during puberty and is in part explained by the increased stretch of the underlying lung that is associated with increased muscular development and thoracic expansion in males at that time.

Large airways are supported by cartilage in order to resist collapse during expiration whereas smaller peripheral airways within the lung have no such support but rely on the distending pressure within the lung parenchyma to remain patent. In infancy and early childhood this distending pressure is low and in the region of 0.15 kPa at the end of quiet expiration. In the young healthy adult these pressures increase to between 0.5 and 1.0 kPa, differences which can be largely attributed to increasing chest wall recoil associated with maturation. A highly compliant (or floppy) chest wall is an advantage in utero in that the low lung distending pressure reduces the amount of lung liquid that needs to be cleared by lymphatic drainage soon after birth. However, in the transition to air breathing the highly compliant and unstable rib cage has significant functional consequences. Whereas it is the chest wall that determines the distribution of ventilation and airway function, in infancy and early childhood it is the gradual loss of the elastic recoil of structures within the lungs themselves that is associated with increasing peripheral airway closure and reduced airway function in the elderly (Fig. 18.9).

The thoracic configuration is also different in infants and young children in that the ribs are more horizontally placed with less potential for thoracic expasion than in older children and adults.[69] As a consequence infants and very young children rely more on diaphragmatic activity and this in combination with a more direct insertion into the rib cage and a reduced number of type I muscle fibers (slow twitch high oxidative fibers) places the infant and young child at significant risk of developing respiratory failure when presented with an added respiratory loads. Any additional impairment of the chest wall itself, for example in association with scoliosis or neuromuscular disorders, will only augment this relative inefficiency of the respiratory system in early life.

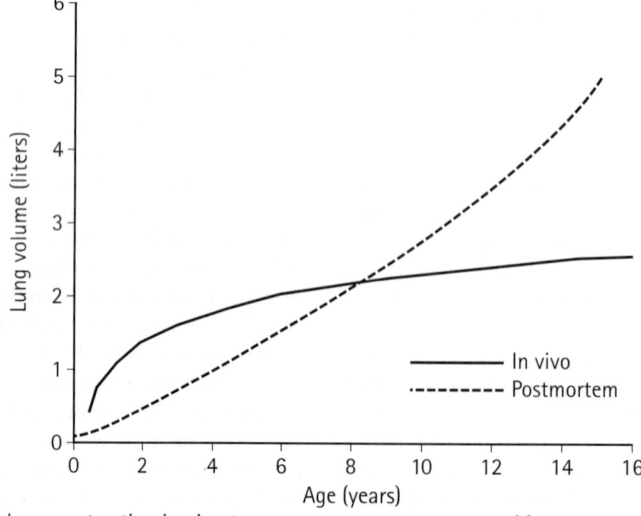

Fig. 18.8 Increase in lung volume in boys contrasting in vivo to postmortem measurements. Measurements in vivo are of total lung capacity (Polgar & Weng1979[67]) and are in influenced by increasing inspiratory effort with age. Measurements postmortem (Thurlbeck 1982[66]) are made at the same distending pressure of 3.3 kPa.

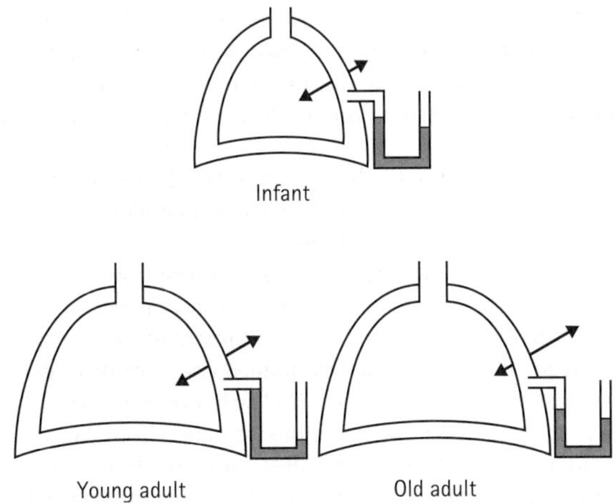

Fig. 18.9 Interaction between outward recoil of chest wall and inward recoil of the underlying lung. The reduced chest wall recoil in the infant results in low transpulmonary pressures whereas in the elderly reduced lung recoil has the same effect. Low transpulmonary pressures result in increasing risks of peripheral (small) airway closure.

The upper airway of the infant and young child is also structurally different from that of the mature child or adult in that the posterior nasopharynx is relatively crowded and therefore vulnerable to obstruction. The immaturity of the facial skeleton, particularly the mid-facial skeleton in the infant and young child, results in the relative backward displacement of the tongue. Together with the hypertrophy of the tonsilar tissue that occurs in early childhood it is hardly surprising that upper respiratory airway obstruction is a common clinical feature in early life (Fig. 18.10).

Gas exchange

Gas exchange is relatively inefficient in early childhood as a consequence of a poor pulmonary support offered by the compliant chest wall and low transpulmonary distending pressure found as a consequence (Fig. 18.8). At the low lung volumes found in infancy and early childhood, airways in the lung bases are more likely to close with subsequent shunting of blood through non-ventilated areas.[71] Remarkably, adequate gas exchange regularly occurs in the human infant after only 0.7 of gestation (28 weeks) has elapsed. The immediate process of adaptation takes about 5 hours. Thereafter a large (A–a) DO_2 (see pp. 729 – Terminology) persists up to term mostly due to intrapulmonary anatomical shunt through non-alveolized vessels while persistence through the first year is largely due to the ventilation/perfusion imbalance described above and very litte to any diffusion limitation. Thus the mean PaO_2 for a term infant for the first week of life is 10 kPa, giving an approximate (A–a) DO_2 of 4 kPa compared with 1 kPa for an adult. Oxygen consumption per kg and hence alveolar ventilation in the newborn is two to three times adult values.

Developmental disorders of gas exchange are not common. Severe lung hypoplasia may impose limits in the newborn period which diminish with growth. Incomplete collateral ventilation (the canals of Lambert are not apparent in lungs from preschool children) may lead to atelectasis and hence impaired gas exchange in disease.

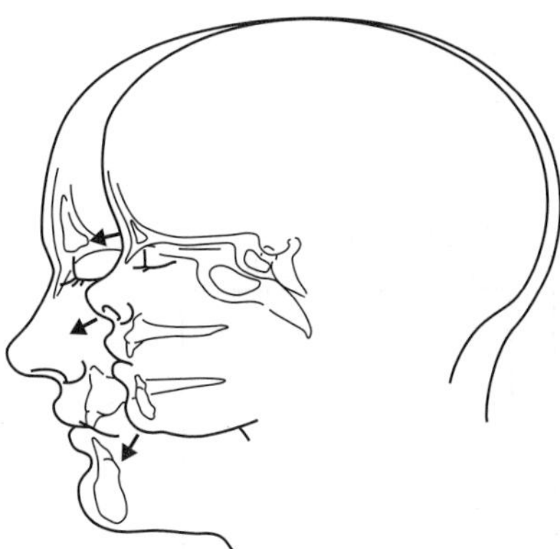

Fig. 18.10 Growth of facial skeleton from childhood to adult life. The relative hypoplasia of the facial skeleton and sinuses renders the infant and very young child prone to upper airway obstruction as a consequence of crowded hypopharynx. (From Proctor 1964[70])

RESPIRATORY PHYSIOLOGY, PATHOPHYSIOLOGY AND THE MEASUREMENT OF RESPIRATORY FUNCTION

The principal function of the respiratory system is gas exchange: oxygenation of the blood and the removal of carbon dioxide. A knowledge of the means whereby this is achieved forms the basis for understanding many of the clinical features of respiratory disease and of lung function tests. The principles of disturbed pathophysiology are no different in children and adults. However growth and development add further dimensions both to the interpretation of data and to the challenge of making the measurements. There are several reference texts and laboratory manuals on applied respiratory physiology.[68,72,73]

RESPIRATORY FUNCTION TESTS

A decision to carry out respiratory function tests will generally have followed clinical assessment and can often usefully be combined with other investigations. The tests should be performed by an operator experienced in dealing with children, who can allay their anxiety and turn natural inquisitiveness and playfulness to advantage. A positive approach, with lots of encouragement and the insight to abandon a session before failure to cooperate turns into panic, are essential virtues.

For most simple procedures the equipment found in any adult lung function laboratory will be adequate. In infancy most measurements can only be made in specialized laboratories and will not be dealt with in this chapter. Preschool children form another difficult group, where specially adapted equipment may be needed and where the repeatability of measurements is not as good as in older children and adults. Spirometric measurements, for example, are rarely reliable below age 5; peak flow can occasionally be measured in 3–4-year-olds and hence the burgeoning interest in tidal breathing techniques in this young age group.[74]

Interpretation

Lung function is most closely related to body length or height but with small additional effects of age and sex, particularly around puberty, and of ethnic group. In the presence of scoliosis, arm span can be substituted directly for length. Body weight is a poor reference standard, since its variation in disease can be extreme. The significance of individual measurements in relation to the population is found by reference to a graph or table of predicted values.[67,68] For sequential measurements in an individual, the confidence limits or coefficient of variation for repeated measurements must be sought. In asthma it is only appropriate to use the 'optimum' or maximum value for an individual rather than the population reference value as the target for home monitoring of peak flow.

AIRWAY FUNCTION

As most lung problems in infancy and childhood relate to obstructive lung disease measurements that reflect airway caliber are of intense interest and relevance.

The conducting airways extend from the tip of the nose to the terminal bronchioles. Although generally envisaged simply as a set of branching tubes, they are physiologically very active, constantly varying their caliber and the nature of their secretions, in response to changing environmental exposures.

The airways condition the inspired air, bringing it up to 37°C at 100% relative humidity by the level of the segmental bronchi during quiet breathing. The volume of the conducting airways constitutes a dead space (i.e. the volume of the lungs which although ventilated does not contribute to alveolar gas exchange, sometimes called wasted ventilation), measuring about 2.2 ml/kg throughout life.[67] Disorders of airway structure such as bronchiectasis lead to an increase in anatomical dead space. In addition, the ventilation of underperfused regions of the lung, such as the apices in the erect posture, leads to another form of wasted ventilation referred to as physiological dead space.

Airway resistance (R_{aw}) is a function of gas flow and pressure drop: airway resistance = pressure drop/flow. The reciprocal of R_{aw}, airway conductance (G_{aw}), is often used, since its relationship with lung volume is linear, rather than curvilinear as with R_{aw}. In peripheral airways, because the total cross-sectional area of the enormous number of airways is large, gas velocity and resistance are low. In the most distal respiratory bronchioles, alveolar ducts and alveolar spaces, gas molecules move by diffusive processes. In the larger central airways, where flow is high, the pattern of gaseous movement is somewhere between ordered laminar flow and freely developed or 'turbulent' flow and as a consequence resistance increases steeply with flow. During nasal breathing in infancy, about 50% of the total resistance is nasal, 25% is in the glottis and large central airways and the remainder in the peripheral airways. This distribution of resistance together with the relatively crowded upper airway renders infants particularly prone to develop upper airway obstruction. The highly compliant chest wall and consequent tendency to peripheral airway closure, particularly at lung bases, (pp. 724 – Postnatal development) also renders the infant prone to small airway diseases (e.g. bronchiolitis) in contrast to older children and adults in whom the small airways represent a clinically 'silent zone'.

Dynamic airway narrowing during forced expiratory effort is important as a cause of airway obstruction in children with a wide variety of obstructive airway diseases.

During forced expiratory maneuvers intrapulmonary airways progressively close as lung volume falls. However if the airways were rigid structures from alveoli to the upper airway, expiratory flow rates during forced efforts would be maintained constant throughout the whole of expiration. However this is clearly not the case as airways progressively lose their cartilaginous support from large central airways to bronchiolar level. Towards the lung periphery the airways rely on the tension within the surrounding connective tissue elements for their support, a tension which in turn is dependent on the stretch or inflation of the lung. When the lung is fully distended the intrapulmonary airways are most widely open. However as the lung empties and transpulmonary pressure falls the airways progressively close from the periphery towards the larger central airways. During forced expiratory maneuvers a point is reached where the pressures within and surrounding the airway reach equality (the so-called equal pressure point or EPP), and at which point expiratory flow becomes effort independent. EPP is usually reached somewhere near the mid-point of a forced expiratory effort whereas in diseases associated with increased lung compliance (reduced lung recoil), or in airway obstruction, the EPP occurs closer to the lung periphery and expired flow rates become limited earlier and earlier during expiration. This produces the concave flow volume curve so characteristic of moderate to severe asthma or cystic fibrosis. (Fig. 18.11). Obstruction in larger airways reduces peak expiratory flow rates, the effort dependent portion of the expiratory flow maneuver, and result in a characteristic appearance (Fig. 18.11). During forced inspiration the airways remain widely patent throughout and as a consequence inspiratory flow is more symmetrical and maintained for longer than during expiration.

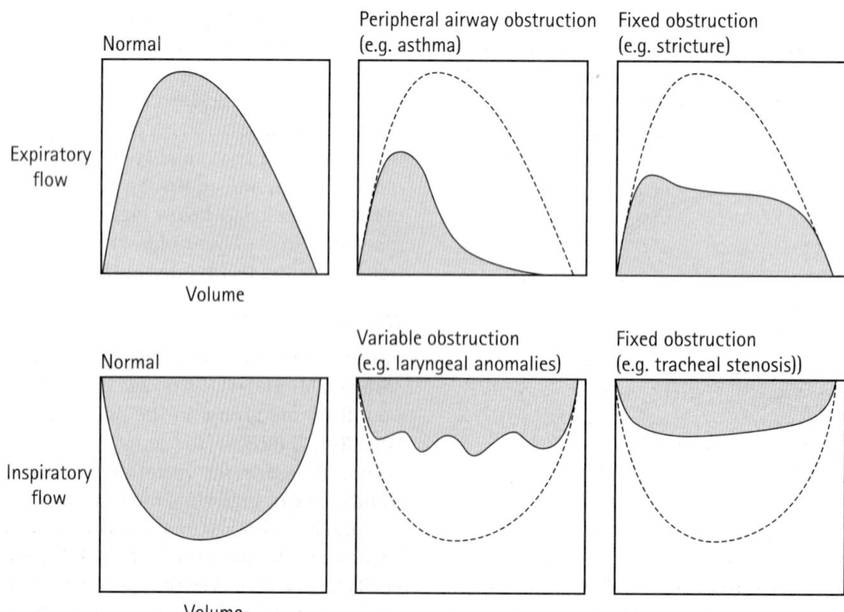

Fig. 18.11 Flow volume curves. Maximum forced expiratory and inspiratory flow volume curves, showing patterns characteristic of airflow obstruction at various sites.

The exceptions to this rule are in fixed large airway obstruction or in profound neuromuscular weakness or where the site of the obstruction is extrathoracic. Variable large airway obstruction such as in obstructive sleep apnea may be associated with characteristic oscillations during inspiration (Fig. 18.11).

Inflammation, excessive mucus secretion and active contraction of airway smooth muscle all lead to increased airflow obstruction. Although these processes may be part of normal defense mechanisms in the lungs, one of the characteristic features of asthma is an exaggerated airway responsiveness (i.e. reversible airway narrowing in response to either allergic or non-immunological irritant factors). The degree of airway responsiveness can be measured by standardized challenge procedures based, for instance, on exercise or inhalation challenge with pharmacological agents such as histamine or methacholine (see pp. 754 – Non-specific hyperreactivity).

Measurement of airflow obstruction

Forced expiratory maneuvers, which require a maximum expiratory effort from total lung capacity, form the basis of the most useful tests of airway obstruction. The peak expiratory flow (PEF), the forced expiratory volume in the first second of expiration (FEV_1) and the indices derived from the maximum expiratory flow volume (MEFV) curve are the most commonly performed. In general, the best of three efforts (after two practice blows for novices) should be recorded, the single most important variable being the completeness of the maximum inspiratory effort at the start of each procedure. Most children from 5 years old can manage to perform a PEF maneuver, although the other forced measurements (FEV_1, MEFV curve) cannot be performed to the recommended adult standards of less than 5% viability in children under 7 or 8 years. In children under 7 years, the whole vital capacity may be exhaled in under 1 s; in this group, the $FEV_{0.75}$ or $FEV_{0.5}$ have been suggested as more sensitive indices of obstruction. Mini-peak flow meters are suitable for home monitoring, in spite of being a rather insensitive measure of airways obstruction.

It is particularly important for quality control to be able to see the spirogram from which forced expiratory indices (the forced vital capacity, FVC and its derivatives) are derived. Its shape bears important information about both the technical quality of a test and the underlying pathophysiology. Airway obstruction is indicated by a reduction in the ratio FEV_1/FVC (or $FEV_{0.75}/FVC$) since airway obstruction will prolong the expiratory time constant of the lungs and reduce the rate of emptying (Fig. 18.12). The FEV_1/FVC ratio normally decreases with age, from over 90% in the youngest children in whom it can be measured to over 75% in young adults. The FEV_1 (or $FEV_{0.75}$), with contributions from the peak flow and the flow-limited sections of the expiratory maneuver, provides the best overall index of airway obstruction.

The shape of the expiratory flow volume curve provides additional information, which is not available from the spirogram (volume against time), concerning the nature and site of obstruction (Fig. 18.11). The disadvantages of numerical analysis of the flow volume curve include very poor reproducibility, even in normal children. Compensatory changes in lung volume with airways disease or its treatment may explain the apparent changes in forced flow expiratory rate as airway caliber is modified by lung stretch. The maximal expiratory procedure itself may induce airway obstruction in asthmatics with very reactive airways although this effect is transient and is responsive to inhaled bronchodilators.

Flow volume curves have another important function, in the assessment of upper (extrathoracic) airflow obstruction. Use is made of the pattern of flow limitation produced on maximum inspiratory effort from residual volume as well as on the actual maximal inspiratory flow rate at midvital capacity (MIF_{50}) in assessing extrathoracic airway obstruction. Normally the ratio MIF_{50}/MEF_{50} is close to or greater than 1.

Methods for measuring airflow obstruction which do not depend on respiratory effort, and which have therefore been adapted for use in infants and young children, include the plethysmographic determination of airway resistance and the measurement of total respiratory system resistance (impedance) by a forced oscillation and interrupter techniques.[74] Like PEF these methods are influenced mainly by large airway function and are especially sensitive to glottic narrowing and (in nose-breathing infants) to nasal obstruction.

Peak flow measurements

Objective evidence of the severity and nature of airway obstruction in wheezy children of school age can be obtained by means of twice-daily peak flow measurements that can easily be made at home using a peak flow meter. Values can be recorded on a diary card and, if necessary, displayed in graphical form to provide information about the variability of airway obstruction. Estimates of peak flow variability have been used in epidemiological studies of asthma but are of little value in the diagnosis of individual children. In contrast, peak flow measurements made at home can be of great value in providing objective evidence of the severity of asthma. A single isolated value of peak flow (or of any other measure of lung function) is of little use in the assessment of severity since variability, even within a 24-h period, is so great.

Measurement of bronchial responsiveness (bronchial provocation tests)

Bronchial provocation tests rarely help in the diagnosis of asthma as they are neither specific nor sensitive for asthma. They may be used in order to assess the importance of airway responsiveness in a patient with atypical symptoms (e.g. chronic cough) or in patients with other forms of airway obstruction (e.g. cystic fibrosis, bronchiectasis). Their main use is as a research tool in whole population studies or in assessing the response to prophylactic anti-asthma therapy. Children under the age of 6 can be tested only under the conditions of a research laboratory. Simple, repeatable measurement techniques (FEV_1, PEF) are the reference norms for bronchial provocation tests but increasingly techniques that reflect airways resistance including specific resistance and interrupter techniques are being employed.[74]

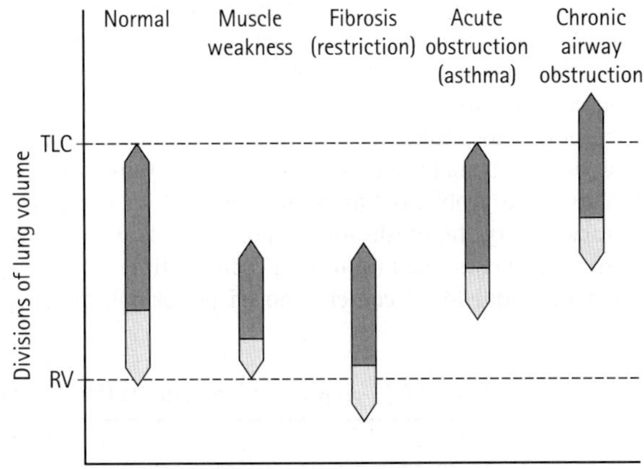

Fig. 18.12 Causes of reduced vital capacity. The length of the arrows indicates the vital capacity and the position indicates the changes in total lung capacity (TLC) and residual volume (RV) for each condition in relation to normal. The horizontal line across each arrow indicates the usual end-expiratory curve (functional residual capacity, FRC).

There are three broad categories of challenge test: pharmacological challenge by aerosol, bronchial provocation with aerosolized antigen and exercise (or isocapnic hyperventilation) challenge. In order to determine the degree of responsiveness, pharmacological or exercise challenges are usually used. Exercise is said to be specific for asthma, whereas a response to pharmacological challenge also occurs in other lung disorders. Antigen provocation is a risky procedure confined to research laboratories.

Pharmacological challenge with solutions of histamine, methacholine or adenosine is performed by administering increasing concentrations of aerosol by jet nebulizer at regular intervals, until at least a 20% fall in PEF or FEV_1 has been produced (or the maximum concentration has been reached). By interpolation on a graph the concentration which provokes a 20% fall in PEF or FEV_1 (PC_{20}) can be calculated. The PC_{20} or the cumulative dose (PD_{20}) is an index of bronchial responsiveness. There is a continuum of values of PC_{20} from the lowest in severe, labile asthma to the highest in normal individuals. Many factors influence asthmatics, such as environmental antigen exposure (pollen, dust mite), time of day and recent medication. In children with other forms of chronic bronchial obstruction (e.g. cystic fibrosis), bronchial responsiveness appears to become greater as their airway obstruction worsens.

Exercise-induced asthma (EIA) can be reproducibly induced by having a child run for 5–6 min at a rate sufficient to produce a heart rate of > 170 beats/min, ideally on a treadmill in an air-conditioned laboratory. The fall in PEF or FEV_1 can be expressed as a percentage of the baseline value, to provide an index of EIA (upper limit of normal about 15%). Again, a number of clinical variables (a recent cold) and laboratory conditions (air temperature and humidity) may affect the result; outdoor tests of a similar type are very poorly repeatable. Used as a diagnostic aid, EIA has poor sensitivity and specificity. Exercise tests can be used to study the protective effects of drugs given before challenge and to demonstrate their value to the child and family. They can also be used to show that some children get 'short of breath' when they exercise not because of EIA but simply because they are unfit!

Normal (reference) values

The choice of reference norms remains controversial. Whereas many equipment manufacturers use composite reference values[67] there may be important racial and regional differences that need to be accounted for. For example, reference values for Caucasian European children may not be appropriate for children of African origin[75] and even within Europe differences in flow rates have been reported between studies from northern and south-eastern Europe.[76] Another particular problem is in predicting expected values in children and adolescents who fall between the published reference norms for children, usually up to 18 years of age, and those of adults, usually starting at about 18 years. A possible solution to these problems has been suggested by the European Respiratory Society Standardisation Report of 1989 which provided all the summary equations up to that point in time.[68] This report suggested that individual centers should perform lung function measurement in a sample of 50–100 normal children from their own population and then identify and use the published norms that most closely fit these local values.

THE AIRSPACES: LUNG VOLUME AND COMPLIANCE

Physiology

As described above (Postnatal development) the elasticity of the lung and chest wall (i.e. compliance: change in volume for a given change in pressure) is such that at high volumes, the respiratory system tends to deflate and at low volumes to expand, reaching equilibrium at the functional residual capacity (FRC) where the outward recoil of the chest wall and inward recoil of the lungs are in equilibrium. Alteration in the balance of forces between lungs and chest wall and airways obstruction will alter the FRC. Since airway dimensions are partly dependent on traction from the surrounding tissues, the basal airways may close completely toward the end of a normal expiration in infants.

In pulmonary fibrosis where the lungs are less compliant (stiffer), the inward recoil forces of the lungs are greater and FRC is low. Conversely in emphysema and chronic asthma (where the lungs are 'stretched') the inward recoil forces are lower and hence FRC is increased. Removing the supporting influence of the chest wall completely, as in pneumothorax, causes the lung to collapse.

Airway closure is a clinically important factor causing an increase in FRC. Obstructed airways tend to close earlier during expiration, leading to true 'gas trapping'.

The other 'static lung volumes', total lung capacity (TLC) and residual volume (RV), depend on several factors: lung compliance, chest wall compliance, the force of the respiratory muscles, and the caliber of the small intrapulmonary airways. These may all be important in relation to changes in the vital capacity (VC) in disease and need to be interpreted together with expiratory flow rates (Table 18.1).

Measurement of lung volume and compliance

Lung volume is most commonly estimated by clinical examination aided by chest radiography. On formal laboratory testing, the distinction is often made between dynamic lung volumes produced by respiratory effort (e.g. vital capacity) and static lung volumes measuring absolute volume (e.g. FRC, RV and TLC). Static lung volumes and lung compliance are less often measured and require a specialized lung function laboratory.[68]

The vital capacity is a most useful, repeatable measurement, although almost any disturbance of lung function will lead to its reduction (Fig. 18.12). Measured on an electronic spirometer (or as part of a flow volume maneuver), it provides a simple means of monitoring progress in a number of rare or chronic disorders. FVC can be reduced by poor or inefficient inspiratory or expiratory efforts due to chest wall disorders such as scoliosis to neuromuscular disorders or as a consequence of premature airway closure resulting in gas trapping and an elevated RV (Table 18.1, Fig. 18.12).

Table 18.1 Lung function patterns (for spirometry)

Setting	FEV/FVC	FVC	MEF_{50}	MIF_{50}	PEFR
Poor effort/weakness	Normal	Reduced	Normal	Reduced	Reduced
Mild asthma/cystic fibrosis	Normal	Normal	Reduced	Normal	Normal
Severe asthma/cystic fibrosis	Reduced	Reduced	Reduced	Reduced	Reduced

Lung volume may also be valuable in following the course of patients with these disorders. There are two methods: by the plethysmographic technique and by dilution of an inert non-absorbable gas such as helium. The former technique measures all the gas in the thoracic cage, whether or not it is in communication with airways, using simple physical principles (Boyle's law) and complex equipment. The latter technique, relying on equilibration between the gas in the lungs and in a bag containing a mixture of air and helium, tends to underestimate the volume of those parts of the lung which are very poorly ventilated (i.e. in the presence of obstructed airways). Both techniques require very cooperative subjects and are rarely reliable in the routine clinic setting under the age of 8.

VENTILATION AND PERFUSION

Physiology

During tidal breathing, air is distributed within the lungs according to local variations in airway resistance and lung compliance. In the upright subject, because of the weight of the lungs (density about 0.2 g/ml), the pleural pressure is more negative near the apex so that the airspaces are relatively overdistended compared with those near the base. The ventilatory turnover is greater near the base, although because of the lower volume of the basal airspaces, the local airways are narrower and more readily close completely in disease. However in infants the low chest wall recoil results in a reversal of the normal apex to base gradient in ventilation (see pp. 724 – Postnatal development). Disease may also affect the regional distribution of ventilation by affecting the chest wall (e.g. spinal muscular atrophy, severe rickets in infancy), the diaphragm (e.g. congenital diaphragmatic hernia, eventration or paralysis), the airways (e.g. bronchiectasis, asthma) or the airspaces (e.g. lobar pneumonia, pulmonary edema).

The matching of alveolar ventilation to pulmonary perfusion takes place at alveolar level. The airways also play a small part in this homeostatic mechanism. Alveolar hypoxia induces local pulmonary arteriolar constriction by a nitric oxide-dependent mechanism, cutting down the local blood supply. The effect is amplified by acidosis. The particular problems of the perinatal period are described in Chapter 10.

In older children, a sustained increase in pulmonary resistance, usually associated with severe chronic and generalized disease (e.g. chronic lung disease of prematurity, terminal cystic fibrosis), may lead to cor pulmonale.

Mismatching of ventilation ($\dot{V}$) and perfusion ($\dot{Q}$) occurs in acute lung disease before adaptation has occurred and in severe chronic disease, beyond the limits of adaptation. Its effects are wasted ventilation (excessive dead-space ventilation) on the one hand, and hypoxemia (due to right-to-left intrapulmonary shunting) on the other. Hypoxemia due to mild $\dot{V}/\dot{Q}$ imbalance, as well as that due to alveolar hypoventilation, is largely corrected by increased inspired oxygen concentrations.

Tests of the distribution of ventilation and perfusion

Regional distribution of ventilation and perfusion can fairly simply be studied in standard nuclear medicine facilities, using X-ray emitting radionuclides and a gamma camera (see pp.733 – Imaging). Other tests remain research procedures.

GAS TRANSFER AND GAS TRANSPORT

Physiology

Within the alveoli, gas movement takes place by diffusion. Transfer of oxygen from alveolus (PaO_2 14 kPa) into the pulmonary capillary and of carbon dioxide in the reverse direction ($PaCO_2$ 5 kPa) take place by passive diffusion down concentration gradients.

The gradient of PO_2 can be thought of as running from alveolus to mitochondrion. Oxygen is transported as oxyhemoglobin. The quantity of oxygen carried depends on the PaO_2 (and its characteristic sigmoid relationship with oxygen saturation), the hemoglobin concentration and the cardiac output: oxygen delivered = oxygen content of blood × cardiac output. Thus oxygen delivery will be reduced by anemia, hypoxemia or diminished cardiac output. Metabolic acidosis (anerobic metabolism leading to lactic acid production) is one consequence of impaired oxygen delivery.

The oxygen dissociation curve is also affected by a number of other factors: the dominant class of hemoglobin (e.g. HbF in the newborn), adaptive variations in intracellular 2,3-diphosphoglycerate (2,3-DPG) concentration with chronic anemia and arterial pH and $PaCO_2$ (the Bohr effect).

The transport of CO_2 is much more robust, since the CO_2 content of blood is almost linearly related to PCO_2 over the clinical range. Respiratory acidosis results from hypercapnia.

Respiratory failure is a general term used to imply a breakdown of the supply of oxygen and removal of CO_2. A single definition which covers the whole pediatric range would be inappropriate, since degrees of acute disturbance of blood gases which may have dire clinical consequences in a preterm neonate may have little effect on a chronically sick older child. In pediatrics, particularly in newborns when the labile fetal circulation shunts through fetal channels, a low PaO_2 may indicate a complex failure of ventilation and circulation which it would be inappropriate to label as 'respiratory' (see Ch. 10).

Terminology

Hypoxemia

Hypoxemia (PaO_2 at sea level in postneonates of less than 12 kPa) may have several causes (Fig. 18.13, Table 18.2). At altitude the oxygen content of inspired air is reduced and the PaO_2 will fall. However acclimatization principally by hyperventilation and the development of polycythemia preserves the oxygen content of arterial blood.

Alveolar hypoventilation may be due to mechanical factors (stiff or obstructed lungs), weakness of respiratory muscles or a defect of the control of breathing. Hypoxemia and hypercapnia result.

Shunt refers to systemic venous blood which effectively bypasses ventilated portions of lung. There are two main varieties of right-to-left shunt: intracardiac shunt and intrapulmonary shunt. In childhood, the main extrapulmonary cause of shunt is cyanotic congenital heart disease. Breathing 100% oxygen for at least 5 min (the nitrogen washout test) is useful for diagnosing this 'central' shunting. In order to understand this test, the shape of the hemoglobin–oxygen dissociation curve should be borne in mind. Even if the PO_2 of pulmonary venous blood is > 55 kPa (400 mmHg) the content of oxygen in that blood will be hardly greater than if the PO_2 is 13 kPa (100 mmHg). When mixed with shunted blood of low oxygen content the PaO_2 will fall dramatically. Even when the lungs are completely normal, the presence of a very small central shunt will prevent a significant rise in PaO_2 when breathing 100% oxygen. A rise in PaO_2 to 20 kPa (150 mmHg) makes cyanotic heart disease an unlikely cause of hypoxemia. On the other hand, if breathing 100% oxygen (for a minimum of 5 min) does successfully elevate the PaO_2 the hypoxemia in air is likely to have been due to intrapulmonary shunting (regions of low $\dot{V}/\dot{Q}$ ratio) or hypoventilation. A specific exception to this rule is the situation of

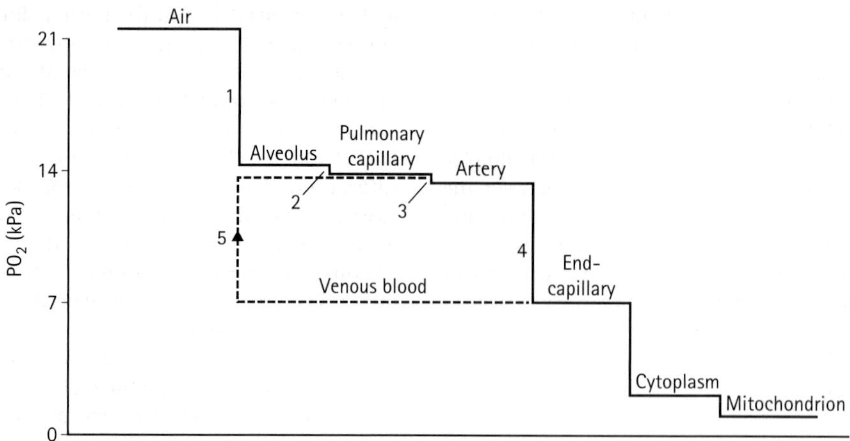

Fig. 18.13 The oxygen 'waterfall' in health and disease. Under normal circumstances oxygen is transported down a gradient between atmospheric air and the mitochondria where it is consumed.

Table 18.2 The oxygen waterfall in disease: hypoxia. Various causes of hypoxemia have their effect at different steps in the waterfall. Increase in inspired oxygen concentration (the hyperoxia test) will usually correct the first two causes of hypoxemia. The level of arterial PCO_2 depends on the degree of compensatory hyperventilation which is possible; in severe lung disease, hypercapnia may develop

Causes of hypoxia	Effect of increase in FiO_2	Value of $PaCO_2$
1. Decreased alveolar ventilation	Correction of hypoxemia	Increase
2. Impaired diffusion	Correction of hypoxemia	Decrease (unless severe imbalance)
3. Right–left shunt and ventilation/perfusion imbalance	No change if pure right–left shunt	Decrease (unless severe shunting)
4. Decreased oxygen delivery*	No change	Decrease (due to metabolic acidosis)
5. Demand for oxygen exceeding supply**	Depends on cause	Increased mixed venous PCO_2

FiO_2 = inspired oxygen concentration
$PaCO_2$ = arterial PCO_2
* PaO_2 may be normal under these circumstances; not true hypoxemia
** Refers to fall in mixed venous (pulmonary artery) PO_2; PaO_2 may be normal

pulmonary hypertension in the newborn, when oxygen therapy, by reducing pulmonary vascular resistance, can abolish the extrapulmonary right-to-left shunt through fetal channels, causing the hypoxemia to resolve for 'vascular' rather than 'pulmonary' reasons.

Ventilation/perfusion ($\dot{V}/\dot{Q}$) mismatching is by far the commonest cause of hypoxemia in pulmonary disease. Blood leaving alveolar units which are underventilated but well perfused will have a low O_2 content and a raised CO_2 content. For the reasons mentioned above the total PaO_2 will fall and hyperventilation results. CO_2 is washed out of the well-ventilated lung units. As the CO_2 content of blood bears an almost linear relationship to $PaCO_2$ the reduction in CO_2 content of blood leaving well-ventilated units offsets the rise in that leaving poorly ventilated alveoli. However, no matter how good the ventilation of healthy alveolar units, the O_2 content of blood leaving them remains the same and does not offset the reduced content of those leaving poorly ventilated alveoli. Hypoxemia due to $\dot{V}/\dot{Q}$ imbalance will therefore be unaltered by hyperventilation, an increased ventilatory drive will persist and the $PaCO_2$ may fall. (This is sometimes referred to as type I respiratory failure.)

This is the situation in the early stages of acute asthma and bronchiolitis. Increasing the inspired oxygen concentration will improve the oxygen content of poorly ventilated areas and the PaO_2 will rise as a result. Patients are able to compensate for the increase in dead space initially by increasing overall minute ventilation but eventually they may become exhausted or, because of worsening disease, the dead space may rise. In either case alveolar hypoventilation results and the $PaCO_2$ will eventually rise (type II respiratory failure).

Alveolar hypoventilation

Alveolar hypoventilation in the presence of normal lungs or severe ventilation/perfusion mismatching, as described under hypoxemia, results in *hypercapnia*, a rise in $PaCO_2$. Hypercapnia should always be taken very seriously. In acute, respiratory disease the $PaCO_2$ may remain normal or low for some time but may eventually rise very quickly. Children in whom this happens are very often exhausted and may well require ventilatory support. With chronic hypercapnia, central insensitivity results as CSF pH is buffered by a rise in bicarbonate. Administration of an oxygen-enriched gas to a patient not receiving assisted ventilation may result in a further dangerous increase in $PaCO_2$ because of removal of the hypoxemic drive to respiration. In practice this is extremely uncommon in children as chronic type II respiratory failure is rare. Oxygen should therefore never be withheld from children with acute disease.

Alveolar–arterial PO_2 difference

(A–a) DO_2 is a measure of the degree of right-to-left shunt (of all types).

In respiratory failure of whatever cause the PaO_2 falls while the patient is breathing air. When accompanied by alveolar hypoventilation the $PaCO_2$ rises. An assessment of respiratory failure may be made by use of the alveolar air equation:

$$P_AO_2 = P_IO_2 - (P_ACO_2/R) + F$$

where P_AO_2 is the partial pressure of oxygen in the alveoli, P_IO_2 is the partial pressure of inspired oxygen (minus water vapor) (partial pressure: 6 kPa at body temperature), P_ACO_2 is the mean alveolar PCO_2, *R* is the respiratory quotient (approximately 0.8 in normal individuals) and F is a small correction factor which for clinical purposes can be omitted. P_ACO_2 in most clinical situations is equal to $PaCO_2$. Normally with a $PaCO_2$ of 5 kPa and a barometric pressure of 100 kPa breathing air (O_2 content = 0.21) and a water vapor pressure of 6 kPa, $P_AO_2 = 0.21\ (100 - 6) - (5/0.8) = 13.5$ kPa.

In a normal child breathing air the difference between the P_AO_2 and the PaO_2 is 1–2 kPa. In pure alveolar hypoventilation this difference does not change or become smaller. In the presence of shunt or $\dot{V}/\dot{Q}$ imbalance the difference rises. Hence the (A–a) DO_2 is an index of severity of mismatching of gas and blood.

Example 1. A baby with severe bronchiolitis may have a PaO_2 of 10 kPa in 70% oxygen and a $PaCO_2$ of 8 kPa. The (A–a) $DO_2 = 0.7\ (100-6)-(8/0.8)-10 = 46$ kPa. He has both $\dot{V}/\dot{Q}$ mismatching, resulting in a rise in (A–a) DO_2, and alveolar hypoventilation, resulting in a rise in $PaCO_2$.

Example 2. A child with infective polyneuritis breathing 30% oxygen has a $PaCO_2$ of 7 kPa and a PaO_2 of 18 kPa. The (A–a) $DO_2 = 0.3\ (100-6)-(7/0.8)-18 = 1.5$ kpa. This child has pure alveolar hypoventilation as the (A–a) DO_2 is normal and the $PaCO_2$ is raised.

In rare disorders which affect the alveolar membrane, where clinical disability is mainly reduced exercise tolerance and airway function is normal, oxygen transport across the membrane may be adequate at rest but not during exercise. The (A–a) DO_2 may become abnormally wide only during exercise.

Acid–base abnormalities

These relate to disturbed hydrogen ion homeostasis in body fluids. The maintenance of a normal blood pH is a function of lung and kidney which together control the buffering capacity of the blood. The most important physiological buffer is bicarbonate, because of its relationship with CO_2 which is excreted through the lungs. The Henderson–Hasselbalch equation describes the relationship:

$$H^+ + HCO_3^- \rightleftharpoons H_2CO_3 \rightleftharpoons CO_2 + H_2O$$

From this

$$H^+ \propto CO_2/HCO_3^-$$

and

$$pH = -\log H^+ \propto \log (HCO_3^-/CO_2)$$

Provided the ratio of HCO_3/CO_2 remains constant, the pH will remain constant.

When the acid–base balance is disturbed and the normal values of pH and PCO_2 are altered it is helpful to know something of the status of the buffering system in the blood in order to try to unravel the sequence of events. The *base excess* is a useful parameter which reflects the metabolic component of the abnormality under steady state conditions (*not* during rapid changes in acid–base status). When the blood gases are analyzed the pH of the sample is determined. The CO_2 electrode is calibrated with gases of high and low CO_2 concentrations and the $PaCO_2$ of the sample determined. Blood pH and log $PaCO_2$ have a linear relationship whose slope varies according to whether there is an excess or deficit of base. The line which describes the relationship when there is neither excess nor deficit is known as the 'normal buffer baseline'. The amount of base which has to be added to or removed from this 'ideal' sample to reach the line which describes the actual sample is referred to as the base excess or deficit (see also Ch. 15).

In *respiratory acidosis* the $PaCO_2$ rises and the pH falls. In order to maintain the ratio HCO_3/CO_2 the kidney conserves bicarbonate.

Metabolic acidosis in pulmonary or cardiac disease reflects tissue hypoxia due to poor oxygen delivery, resulting in an increase in metabolic acid. There are, of course, several other important causes of metabolic acidosis (e.g. renal failure, severe infection, acute diabetic ketoacidosis). Bicarbonate falls as it buffers the rise in hydrogen ions. There is simultaneous increased drive to breathe, with increased CO_2 removal and a return towards normal HCO_3/CO_2 ratio.

Respiratory alkalosis occurs when the $PaCO_2$ falls due to voluntary or artifactual hyperventilation or hyperventilation due to CNS pathology (e.g. meningoencephalitis). The hydrogen ion concentration falls and to conserve the HCO_3/CO_2 ratio and hence the pH, the kidney sheds bicarbonate.

Metabolic alkalosis occurs in children when acid is lost through vomiting, as in pyloric stenosis. Hydrogen ions are lost and the bicarbonate rises. Hypoventilation produces a compensatory rise in CO_2.

Mixed respiratory and metabolic acidosis is a common situation in pediatric practice. Tissue hypoxia results in metabolic acidosis and inadequate ventilation results in respiratory acidosis. The $PaCO_2$ is elevated and the bicarbonate and pH are low. There will be a base deficit.

The administration of bicarbonate in this situation is tempting, particularly when the pH is below 7.2. In order for bicarbonate to correct the metabolic component, CO_2 must be formed and excreted from the lungs. In the presence of respiratory failure with an already elevated $PaCO_2$ this may not be possible. Administration of bicarbonate may elevate the $PaCO_2$ even further. The blood–brain barrier is much more permeable to CO_2 than it is to bicarbonate. Thus the effect on the CSF will be to paradoxically reduce pH and this can precipitate collapse in a child who is not receiving ventilatory support. Even in pure metabolic acidosis (e.g. diabetic ketoacidosis), rapid administration of bicarbonate can have this effect.

The treatment for mixed acidosis is the correction of the respiratory component first of all by increasing ventilation. The metabolic component may respond to better oxygenation, improved circulation or correction of anemia. When the $PaCO_2$ has returned to normal, bicarbonate may be given if the metabolic component persists.

Measurement of gas transfer

Gas transfer at alveolar level can be studied by measuring the diffusing capacity for carbon monoxide (D_{co}). By measuring the FRC by helium dilution simultaneously, the diffusing capacity can be normalized for variation in lung volume (K_{co}). The test has its main use in detecting the response to treatment of interstitial lung diseases (e.g. those associated with connective tissue disorders) in older children.

Measurement of arterial blood gases and acid–base balance

Oximetry has largely replaced arterial blood gas measurement for most children. Blood gas measurements are indicated for worsening acute lung disease where exhaustion (muscle fatigue) suggests the need for mechanical ventilation and in chronic lung disease as a guide to progress. Sampling of arterialized capillary blood (i.e. after warming or application of histamine cream) may be adequate for pH monitoring, but in general arterial sampling is preferable for postneonatal patients.

Blood should be collected from a radial artery cannula or, if impossible to site, by arterial puncture from the radial artery.

This vessel is preferred for three reasons. First, the chance of sampling venous blood in error is small as no major veins lie nearby. Second, there is a good collateral circulation to the hand should circulation be compromised in any way as a result of the procedure. Third, the vessel is accessible. If pulsation is difficult to feel, as in shock, it may be approached blindly. The femoral artery, on the other hand, has a direct medial relation to the femoral vein. Infection may be introduced into the femoral sheath or into the hip joint from the groin. Collaterals will not compensate for femoral artery thrombosis, a particular hazard if the vessel is damaged in the presence of hypovolemia. It is also worth remembering that the femoral vessels may be used for cannulation at cardiac catheterization and it is particularly annoying for the cardiologist if the site has been traumatized.

As the walls of arteries are particularly sensitive and because more than one attempt may be necessary to obtain blood, local anesthetic cream should be applied to the site 30 min before starting and local anesthetic should be injected around the site. As well as being a kindness, this should allow the blood to be collected under conditions which are as stable as possible although admittedly anxiety is not always avoided. Hyperventilation will reduce the $PaCO_2$ and consequently the pH will rise; crying in a child who has a right-to-left intracardiac shunt may increase the shunt and reduce the PaO_2.

Non-invasive methods of measuring oxygenation include the transcutaneous PO_2 electrode, which is at best a trend indicator in postneonatal patients, and the pulse oximeter for monitoring oxygen saturation (e.g. in acute severe asthma and during sleep studies). For PCO_2, transcutaneous measurements again provide trends while end-tidal sampling using an infrared CO_2 meter gives a useful assessment of alveolar breath (and hence arterial) CO_2 only when lung disease is mild and during mechanical ventilation.

BREATHING

Physiology

The principal muscle of inspiration is the diaphragm, innervated by the phrenic nerve (C2–5). As with other skeletal muscles in general, within its usual working range the tension it can generate is proportional to its length. Because the diaphragm adopts a curved shape, when it contracts the pressure difference across it is proportional to the tension developed and inversely proportional to the radius of the curvature. Thus as a pressure generator, the diaphragm works best near its end expiratory position, where its radius of curvature is smallest. Hyperinflation by flattening the diaphragm, and hence increasing the radius of curvature, reduces the effective pressure generated for any particular muscle tension, reduces efficiency and may lead to muscle fatigue. The resulting alveolar hypoventilation, whose onset can be quite sudden, is the major contributory factor to respiratory failure in severe bronchiolitis.

The interaction of the diaphragm with the rest of the chest wall and abdomen is crucial. Because of its tangential insertion, normal diaphragmatic contraction causes the chest wall to expand laterally ('bucket handle' effect) and anteriorly ('pump handle' effect). Scoliosis, for example, disturbs normal integrated movements of diaphragm and chest wall and may lead to respiratory failure, presenting initially during sleep, when the diaphragm may be the sole muscle of breathing.

The phasic action of the intercostal muscles plays a part in stabilizing the chest wall, as illustrated by the indrawing (rib recession) which occurs during inspiration in patients with intercostal weakness (e.g. acute polyneuritis, spinal muscular atrophy) or in normal infants during rapid eye movement (REM) sleep (when the intercostal muscles remain passive). The diaphragm compensates for a floppy chest wall by increasing the amplitude of its contractions. This manifests itself as 'abdominal breathing' (i.e. large amplitude abdominal excursions) and may, if excessive, lead to muscle fatigue and respiratory failure. The intercostal muscles are particularly important in infancy, as the chest is inherently unstable and the expanding action of the diaphragm is less effective because of its less acute more direct insertion into the rib cage and because of the more horizontal arrangement of the ribs.[69]

The distribution of inspired gas depends on regional lung mechanics. In health, posture may affect the distribution of ventilation.

Expiration is normally a passive function, dependent on the elastic recoil of the lungs and chest wall. The elastic work normally carried out by the diaphragm in expanding the lungs and chest is thus almost totally 'recovered' during deflation; the work expended in overcoming frictional forces (the resistance to air flow) is dissipated as heat. However, active expiratory effort, applied mainly by the muscles of the anterior abdominal wall, may be needed if ventilatory demands are great (e.g. during exercise), if there is increased resistance to expiratory airflow (e.g. laryngeal edema) or if the natural recoil of the lungs is reduced (as in emphysema). The diaphragm may be used as a brake during expiration, although when a more effective brake is required (e.g. in neonatal respiratory distress or infantile bronchiolitis), the variable resistance of the glottis may be used, resulting in the characteristic 'grunt'.

From the point of view of the respiratory physician, the brain is part of the respiratory system! Apart from recognized CNS disorders which can affect the respiratory centers (e.g. Leigh's disease) and primary hypoventilation, altered central respiratory drive is especially dependent on sleep state (see pp. 746 – Apnea and breathing disorders during sleep). REM sleep is normally associated with a small drop in PaO_2. However, when upper airway obstruction is present (e.g. due to weakness or to tonsillar or adenoidal hypertrophy) or in the presence of severe lung disease (e.g. cystic fibrosis, severe scoliosis) the degree of hypoventilation may be profound, leading to periods of extreme hypoxia. The consequences may be severe (pulmonary hypertension, hypoxic fits or brain damage) or limited to sleep disturbance as a consequence of repeated waking, leading to excessive somnolence (or paradoxically in children, hyperactivity) the following day.

Control of breathing may become clinically important in chronic respiratory failure with hypercapnia (e.g. terminal lung disease, chronic neuromuscular disorders) when renal compensation for respiratory acidosis leads to an increase in plasma and CSF bicarbonate concentration. This acts as a buffer, blunting the sensitivity of the respiratory center to further rises in PCO_2, again leading to severe hypoventilation during REM sleep, when the metabolic control of breathing is paramount.

Measurement of respiratory muscle strength

The function of the respiratory muscles is best assessed by clinical observations assisted (in the absence of gross lung disease) by comparison of supine and standing vital capacity. Diaphragmatic paralysis will be indicated by a fall in vital capacity of more than 10% accompanied by paradoxical respiratory movements of the rib cage and abdomen in the supine posture. Direct measurements by mouthpiece and transducer of the maximum pressure which can be generated at the mouth during inspiratory effort from residual volume, and expiratory effort from total lung capacity, allow precise quantitations of respiratory muscle strength. Unfortunately, if weakness affects the facial muscles, children find it impossible to maintain an airtight seal around a mouthpiece.

The measurement of breathing pattern, breathing during sleep and control of breathing are dealt with in the section on apnea and breathing disorders during sleep.

SPECIAL INVESTIGATIONS – IMAGING

Despite recent advances in imaging (see also Ch. 39), the plain chest radiograph continues to play a fundamental role in the evaluation of the pediatric respiratory system. Thoracic imaging contributes in various ways to patient management: firstly it helps to establish or substantiate a diagnosis, and decide whether further examinations are required. Radiology also assists in excluding other pathologies, in determining the extent of disease, its natural history and the effects of therapy. Imaging investigations should always be considered in conjunction with the overall clinical picture, respiratory function tests and blood tests if they are to be interpreted correctly.

Apart from ultrasound (US) examination and magnetic resonance imaging (MRI), all imaging techniques involve irradiation. Certain images involve exceedingly low radiation doses, e.g. krypton 81m ventilation lung scan (^{81m}Kr V); others are more invasive with significantly high inherent radiation, e.g. cardiac catheterization, computed tomography (CT) or bronchography. It is therefore important to consider the invasiveness, the radiation dose and the potential discomfort to the patient when planning detailed pulmonary investigations.

The importance of the esophagus in particular cannot be overemphasized when chest disease in young patients is being investigated. Diseases of the upper gastrointestinal (GI) tract, e.g. hiatus hernia, gastroesophageal reflux or recurrent aspiration, may all manifest with chest signs or symptoms.

RADIOGRAPHY OF UPPER AIRWAYS

The lateral neck/postnasal space and sinuses are frequently included on the same lateral radiograph. The palatine tonsils as well as the adenoidal area can be studied on this film. The adenoids may be quite large in normal children making the diagnosis of adenoidal hypertrophy difficult. The relationship of the trachea to the cervical spine as well as the general tracheal caliber should be well visualized. The lateral view has certain technical limitations and it is important to be sure that the projection is adequate, i.e. the floors of the anterior, middle and posterior fossae of the skull are overlapping, and that the cervical spine is truly lateral. The normal space between the trachea and the cervical spine is one vertebral body: an apparent increase in this space may be pathological but may also be due to the radiograph being taken in expiration – in this latter situation the trachea typically shows an acute angle.

The frontal projection visualizes the facial sinuses but in children under 5–6 years of age the relatively small size of the facial bones makes it exceedingly difficult to interpret plain sinus views. Although the antra are usually aerated sufficiently by the age of 18–24 months to be seen on a radiograph, diagnosing sinusitis from plain radiographs is notoriously unreliable. In older children the ethmoid and frontal sinuses, the nasal septum and turbinate bones should be seen.[77] There is a wide age range in the normal development of these sinuses such that when sinusitis needs to be diagnosed or excluded with certainty most radiologists would now recommend CT or MRI in pediatric patients.

CHEST RADIOGRAPHY

For a frontal posteroanterior (PA) chest radiograph [anteroposterior (AP) in younger children], the patient must be straight. This is best evaluated on the film by either the relationship of the medial ends of the clavicles to the pedicle of the vertebral body or by the symmetry of the anterior ribs on each side. Even slight rotation can cause unusual appearances in a normal patient. The medial ends of the clavicles should lie at the level of the fourth vertebral body. Radiographs in inspiration are generally preferred, the degree of inspiration judged by counting either the anterior rib ends in the mid-clavicular line down to the level of the diaphragm (there should be 5–6 ribs present) or counting the posterior aspect of the ribs where one should see down to the 10th rib on inspiration above the hemidiaphragm. An expiration film is often regarded as being of little value although it infers that no overinflation or air trapping is present and this film may permit exclusion of lobar consolidation. The expiration film should not be disregarded but rather carefully reviewed to consider whether it needs to be repeated. Pathological conditions which result in a loss of compliance, e.g. opportunistic infection in the immunosuppressed child, cause repeated 'expiration films' to be obtained. It is worth noting that the normal pediatric cardiothoracic ratio of 60% may be exceeded on an expiratory radiograph in a normal child leading to the erroneous impression of cardiomegaly.

In the infant or sick child, supine AP chest radiographs are commonly carried out. The classic signs of well-known pathological conditions alter, e.g. a pleural effusion may only be seen as an 'apical cap'; a pneumothorax may not appear as a peripheral lung edge and a pneumomediastinum may appear only as a vague transradiancy in the mediastinum. A lateral chest radiograph with a horizontal beam is useful when doubt persists following the AP view.

The normal visualization of the cardiac outline as well as the diaphragm is due to an aerated lung being adjacent to a more solid non-aerated organ. Loss of the normal outlines means that the adjacent lung tissue is no longer aerated; this can occur with consolidation (i.e. fluid in the alveolar spaces due to infection, inflammation or pulmonary edema). If the airway remains patent throughout then consolidation without major collapse may occur. If there is collapse in a lobe of lung, i.e. loss of volume, then bronchial pathology, e.g. foreign body, mucus or extrinsic compression, must be borne in mind. When consolidation occurs first it is not possible for this solid pulmonary parenchyma to lose volume to any major extent. The diagnosis of a collapsed lobe is made by either identifying a displaced fissure or observing a displaced hilum and fewer vessels in the remaining lung parenchyma.

The lateral chest radiograph requires a greater exposure than the frontal film and because the two lungs are superimposed it makes interpretation difficult. This film should not be part of a 'routine' chest radiograph in pediatrics but rather reserved for certain clinical situations. The presence or absence of overinflation may be best assessed on this view. Metastases in children with known solid tumors are less likely to be overlooked when the frontal and lateral films are taken together routinely; however if metastases are to be confidently excluded then a CT is required. In a child with recurrent chest pathology undergoing investigation a lateral film at the time of the first chest radiograph is strongly recommended. In the long-term follow-up of chronic chest disease, e.g. cystic fibrosis, many would recommend that a lateral view is carried out whenever the PA film is obtained. The normal lateral chest radiograph should show progressive transradiancy over the dorsal spine, i.e. the lower vertebral bodies are blacker than the upper ones. The lateral film may detect smaller volumes of pleural fluid than can be seen on the frontal view by revealing obliteration of the posterior costophrenic angle. The trachea is well seen; displacement and narrowing are readily detected on this projection whereas tracheal compression is rarely detected on the frontal view.

A filter view (Figs 18.14b and 18.15b) is a frontal (AP) coned view of the mediastinum using a high voltage (130–140 kV) technique and a copper/tin/aluminum filter very close to the radiograph tube.[78]

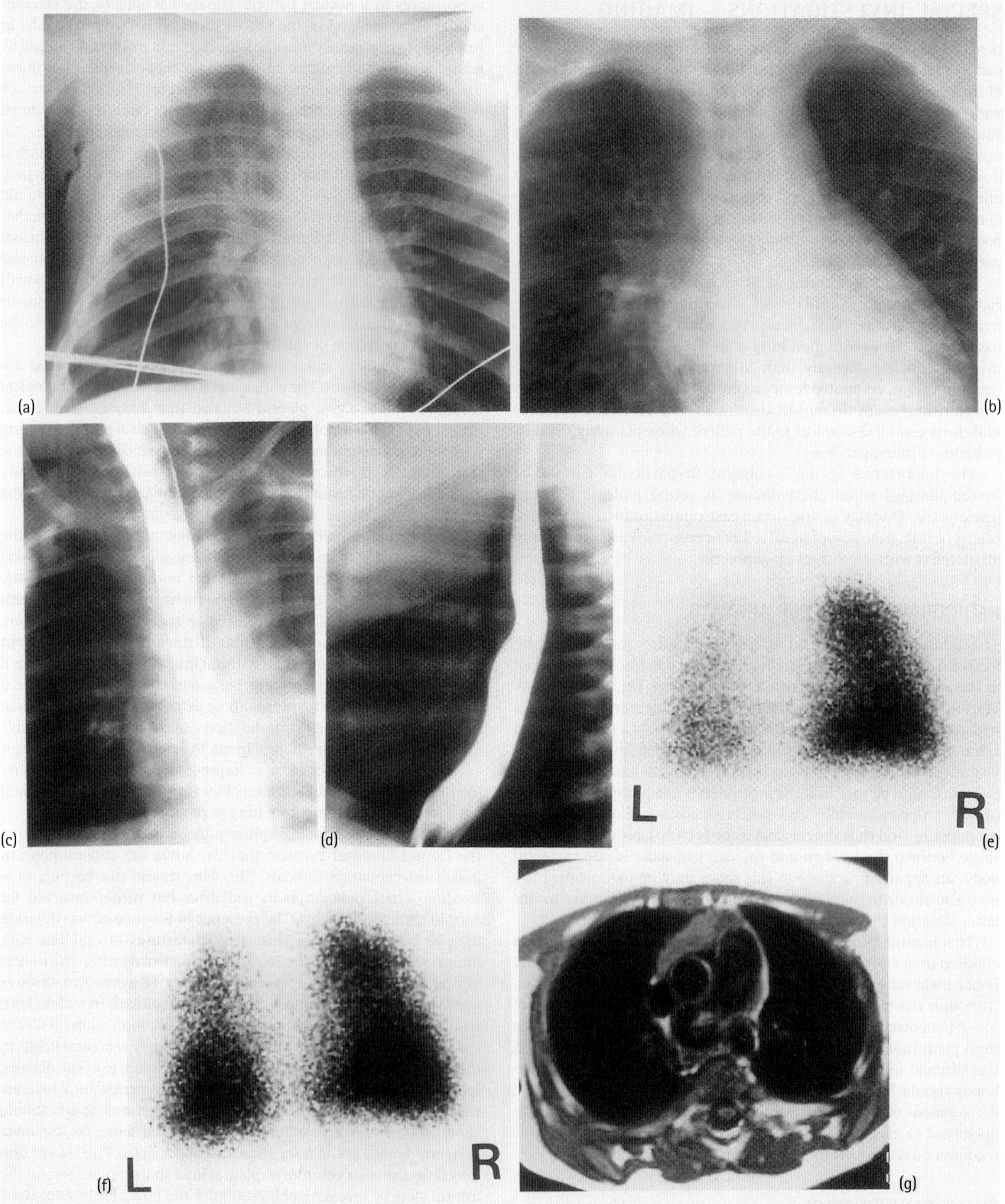

Fig. 18.14 A 6-month-old boy with stridor. (a) The PA chest radiograph shows evidence of overinflation of both lung fields. The left upper zone shows fewer vessels than on the right. There is a deformity of the posterior aspect of the right 7th rib but no previous surgery had been undertaken. (b) High kV filter image. The trachea, carina and major bronchi appear essentially normal. (c) Barium swallow. The frontal projection reveals a normal esophagus. (d) The lateral projection of the barium swallow shows clear indentation on the anterior wall of the esophagus at

Magnification is routinely employed. This gives good visualization of the trachea, carina and main bronchi on a single film although thoracic CT has now become more widely used in the evaluation of airway compression or suspected mediastinal disease.

When the patient is too unwell to sit upright, a horizontal beam radiograph can be useful. For this the patient is placed supine or in a decubitus position and the horizontal X-ray beam allows the effect of gravity to be maximized in order to demonstrate air–fluid interfaces or positional shifts of fluid. Thus either a frontal or a lateral film can be obtained. This technique is useful to demonstrate a small pleural effusion, the presence of pneumomediastinum or pneumothorax and, with intrapulmonary pathology, to demonstrate air–fluid interfaces such as in an abscess.

COMPLEX RADIOGRAPHY

Oblique radiographs to search for rib fractures are generally recommended as part of a skeletal survey in the context of suspected non-accidental injury. Technetium (Tc) methylene diphosphate (MDP) bone scans are also sensitive in detecting rib fractures (see Ch. 39 – Skeletal system). Plain tomography, which is rarely now necessary, allows radiographic sections of the lung fields and mediastinum to be obtained but has been largely superseded by CT.

BRONCHOGRAPHY

This examination is infrequently performed since surgical treatment for bronchiectasis is now uncommon, and regional lung function can be assessed accurately by radioisotopes. As high-resolution CT (HRCT) is very accurate in defining bronchiectasis, bronchography is very rarely necessary prior to surgery. The major indication for bronchography is for suspected localized bronchomalacia. However it is an invasive procedure and should only be undertaken by an experienced pediatric radiologist. Bronchoscopy is also useful in the investigation of localized tracheobronchomalacia (see section on bronchoscopy).

CARDIAC CATHETERIZATION/ PULMONARY ANGIOGRAPHY

This is the most invasive radiological investigation in the cardiorespiratory system and is therefore reserved for those patients in whom the diagnosis is unconfirmed by any other technique. Digital subtraction angiography allows a small volume of contrast to be used and provides high quality imaging with a lower radiation burden to the child (Fig. 18.16d and e). With the use of radioisotope ventilation/perfusion scans, CT and more recently gadolinium-enhanced dynamic MRI, the need for pulmonary angiography continues to decrease. However, certain conditions may still require angiographic intervention and embolization, e.g. arteriovenous malformation and the sequestrated lung segment.

FLUOROSCOPY

Fluoroscopy of the thorax includes evaluation of the lungs, diaphragm, pleura, mediastinum and trachea. Whenever there is a complicated unexplained chest problem, valuable information can be obtained when an experienced radiologist fluoroscopes the thorax. Before beginning any fluoroscopic examination, the clinical questions to be answered should be well formulated and the previous and current chest radiographs reviewed.

Fluoroscopy should occur prior to any barium examination. The information available includes details of the movement of both hemidiaphragms with spontaneous and forced ventilation and the position of the mediastinum and the effect of respiration on both the mediastinum and trachea. If consolidation is present, its exact position, mobility and the presence of calcification can be ascertained. Fluid may be localized on fluoroscopy. If a diagnostic tap is thought necessary with small amounts of fluid, then ultrasound may aid in a successful tap.

ESOPHAGEAL EXAMINATION (Fig. 18.14c and d)

In the vast majority of cases this is simply a barium swallow or esophagogram. A fully distended esophagus is essential for an adequate barium or contrast study. This examination is aimed at showing extrinsic lesions such as a vascular ring pressing on or displacing the esophagus. An aberrant left pulmonary artery (so-called pulmonary sling) may only be visible on the true lateral projection. Intrinsic diseases, e.g. hiatus hernia, gastroesophageal reflux or incoordinate swallowing with aspiration, can also be diagnosed, although the latter requires videofluoroscopy during swallowing.

A dedicated esophagogram is necessary in those patients with a normal barium swallow in whom an H-type tracheoesophageal fistula is suspected. It requires an injection of water-soluble, non-ionic contrast via an esophageal tube which is gradually withdrawn with the child in the prone position. Prone positioning allows the dependent anterior esophagus to be well coated which, with the aid of gravity, helps improve the likelihood of finding a small fistula to the trachea. A video recording in the lateral projection is essential since spot films are too slow to detect a small fistula.

ULTRASOUND (US)

Aerated lung prevents the propagation of an ultrasound beam. Pathology, e.g. pleural fluid or other collection, must lie adjacent to the pleura or heart to be visualized. In the opaque hemithorax on chest radiograph (CXR), i.e. so-called lung white-out, US can easily distinguish between the presence of fluid, a mass or lung collapse and can give a useful guide as to how much fluid is present. When a peripheral lung mass is present then ultrasound can determine if this is predominantly cystic or solid. Occasionally in a child with pneumonia it is difficult both clinically and radiologically to assess how much fluid is present in addition to the consolidation; US is particularly useful if the consolidation is basal in location. Effusion and empyema may require tapping or draining and in this context US is very useful in defining the appropriate site for chest tube insertion. The diaphragm is well visualized by US especially on the right and therefore may be useful when defects are suspected. In addition, in cases of suspected diaphragmatic palsy or paralysis subsequent to surgery US is as accurate as fluoroscopy in assessing

the level of the carina. This is a typical appearance of an aberrant left pulmonary artery which is only seen in the true lateral projection on barium. (e) Krypton 81m ventilation lung scan shows normal ventilation of the right lung with decreased ventilation of the left upper lobe. (f) 99mTc macroaggregate perfusion scan reveals a normal right lung with decreased perfusion of most of the left lung. The left lung contributed 32% to overall perfusion and 39% to overall ventilation. (g) MRI scan of the mediastinum shows the aberrant left pulmonary artery arising from the right pulmonary artery and curling around behind the trachea but in front of the esophagus. This child underwent resection and anastomosis of the left pulmonary artery to the main pulmonary artery. The postoperative V/Q lung scan revealed a normally perfused and ventilated left lung (not illustrated).

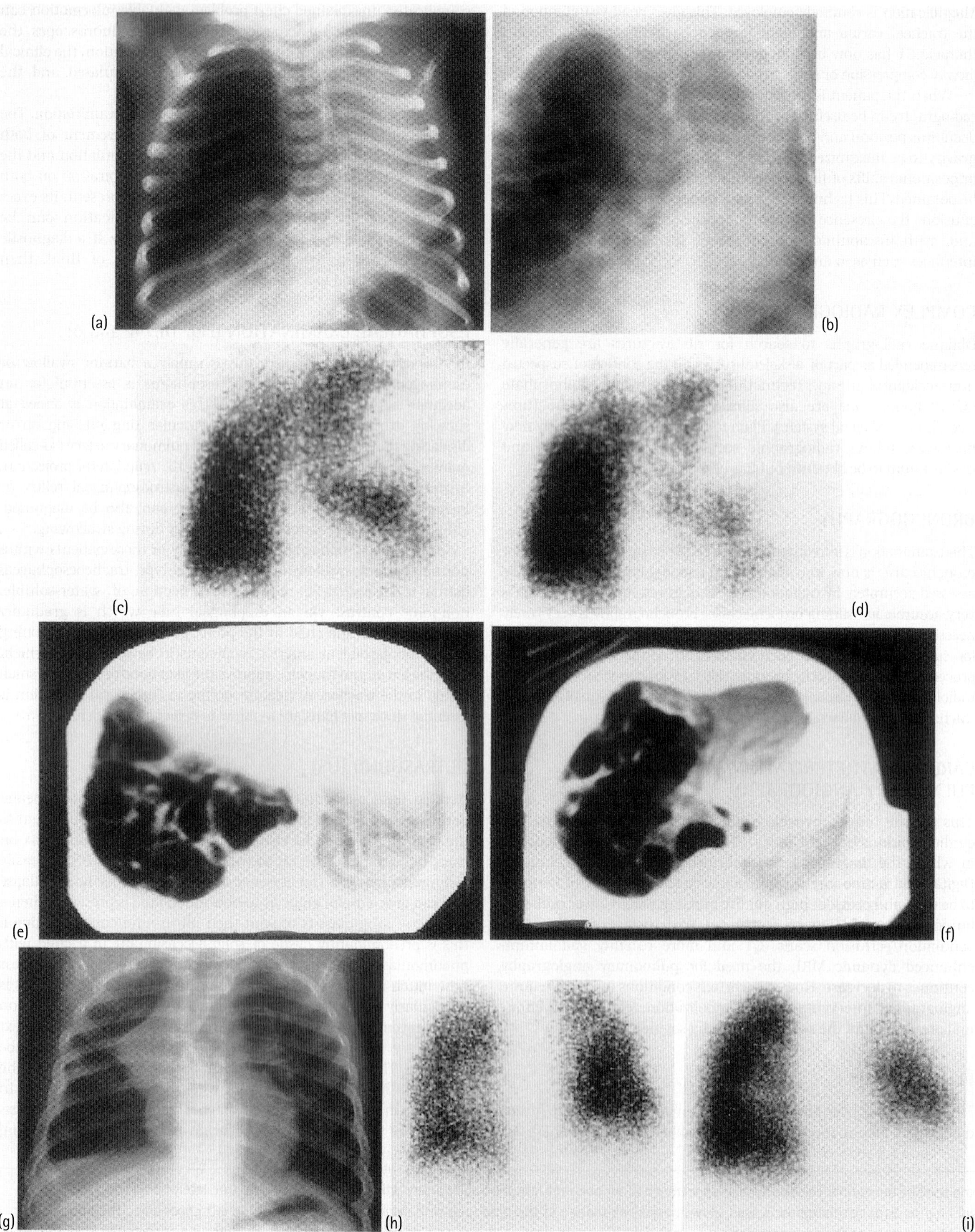

Fig. 18.15 This neonate had progressive respiratory distress at 4 h of age. The pregnancy and labor were uneventful. (a) PA chest radiograph shows the mediastinum deviated to the left with compression of the left lung. The right hemithorax is transradiant. (b) High kV filter radiograph shows numerous opacities through the transradiant right lung. The deviated mediastinum is again clearly demonstrated. These features suggested

diaphragmatic motion and has the advantage that it can be performed in the intensive care setting rather than only in the radiology department. Antenatal diagnosis by US of diaphragmatic hernia, adenomatoid malformations as well as fluid collections in the lungs may alert the pediatrician to the birth of an infant who may require the facilities of a neonatal intensive care team.[79]

Children with stridor in whom the diagnosis of extrinsic compression is being considered should undergo US examination. US in experienced hands can detect the site of the aortic arch and may thus pick up a right-sided aortic arch or double aortic arch. The detection of an aberrant left pulmonary artery arising from the right pulmonary artery and swinging back to the left between the esophagus and trachea may be missed, however, on US/echocardiography.

The normal thymus can have a variety of appearances being particularly prominent in children less than 3 years of age. A large thymus can be mistaken for a mediastinal mass or upper zone pneumonia but when a large normal thymus is found on US corresponding to the apparent abnormality on CXR, more sinister pathology can be ruled out. In cases of suspected sequestrated segment US may show the feeding vessel arising from the abdominal aorta coursing upwards into the chest. US may be used to visualize gastroesophageal reflux but is time-consuming, operator dependent and not widely utilized. The superior extent or level of reflux cannot be assessed on US.

RADIOISOTOPE INVESTIGATION (Figs 18.16c and d, 18.14e and f, 18.15c, d, h and i)

Isotope scans provide a functional image which may be quantified; this contrasts with the anatomical information available from radiology and makes the two examinations complementary.

KRYPTON-81m (^{81m}Kr) VENTILATION/TECHNETIUM (^{99m}Tc) MACROAGGREGATE (MAA) PERFUSION LUNG SCAN (^{81m}Kr $\dot{V}$/^{99m}Tc MAA $\dot{Q}$)

Sequential images of both ventilation and perfusion can be obtained in children of any age. $\dot{V}/\dot{Q}$ scans have been carried out in the newborn. Multiple views are obtained so that a three-dimensional image of the lungs is built up. ^{81m}Kr is an inert radioisotope gas with a half-life of 13 seconds. The inspired air/^{81m}Kr mixture never reaches equilibrium in the alveolar airspaces. The image is therefore of alveolar ventilation and not lung volume. This holds true for all children over 1–2 years but in the neonate/infant the high respiratory rate may invalidate this situation so that the ^{81m}Kr $\dot{V}$ scan may reflect a complex lung volume/specific ventilation situation. Xenon-133 (^{133}Xe) is used in many institutions where Kr is unavailable. The advantages of this gas are its ready availability and relatively long half-life of 5.3 days; the disadvantages are the relatively high radiation dose. It is absorbed when given via intravenous infusion resulting in a high background activity and, most importantly, it requires very good patient cooperation so that it is used with difficulty in the child under 6 years old. Only a single posterior view can be obtained and therefore it is difficult to compare the ^{99m}Tc MAA $\dot{Q}$ scan images with the ^{133}Xe image. In the older cooperative child the ability to carry out a wash-in, equilibrium image and wash-out allows assessment of gas trapping.

The use of labeled particles to monitor mucociliary clearance requires a cooperative child breathing ^{99m}Tc-labeled microspheres. Relatively large particles are required and imaging must take place over some hours. In this circumstance a ^{99m}Tc MAA perfusion scan should be done 48 h preceding the mucociliary study.

^{99m}Tc MAA are injected intravenously and are stopped by the first capillary bed, normally the lungs. This gives images of pulmonary perfusion. In pulmonary hypertension caution should be exercised but a perfusion scan may be undertaken if clinically indicated. In the presence of right-to-left shunts perfusion lung scans have been used without ill effect; the ^{99m}Tc MAA are then seen in the systemic circulation (mainly kidneys and brain).

The $\dot{V}/\dot{Q}$ images reflect regional lung function. There is no other non-invasive method available to assess regional $\dot{V}/\dot{Q}$. Indications for $\dot{V}/\dot{Q}$ scanning include establishing the diagnosis in children with suspected pulmonary artery pathology, e.g. absent pulmonary artery or segmental pulmonary artery stenosis. In the small lung/small hemithorax or a hyperlucent lung the final diagnosis may be made when the chest radiograph is taken in conjunction with the $\dot{V}/\dot{Q}$ scan and fluoroscopy. Conditions such as congenital absence of the pulmonary artery, hypoplastic lung, sequestrated lung segment and Macleod's syndrome (obliterative bronchiolitis) can be distinguished. The diagnoses of bronchiectasis or inhaled foreign body may be excluded by a normal lung scan although radioisotope studies in these conditions are generally used during long-term follow-up to monitor regional lung function. The extent of disease may be established in certain chronic disorders (e.g. cystic fibrosis, post-transplant obliterative bronchiolitis) although CT can provide similar information. The effect of treatment, both medical as in chronic lung disease and surgical for pulmonary arterial pathology, can also be monitored.

The ^{81m}Kr $\dot{V}$ lung scan gives a very small radiation dose so that in a $\dot{V}/\dot{Q}$ scan the majority of the dose is from the ^{99m}Tc MAA. The dose varies with age and is roughly equivalent to 1.5 minutes' screening by fluoroscopy.

RADIOISOTOPE MILK SCAN

This is used for evaluation of gastroesophageal reflux and pulmonary aspiration. ^{99m}Tc sulfur colloid is added to a normal feed

the diagnosis of cystic adenomatoid malformation of either the entire right lung or a lobe. (c) Krypton-81m ventilation lung scan. The left lung is normally ventilated whilst on the right there is a defect in the upper outer portion and also in the inferomedial aspect of this lung but the compressed right upper lobe is well ventilated as is the compressed middle lobe. (d) 99mTc macroaggregate perfusion scan. The left lung is normal. The right lung shows a similar appearance to that seen on the ventilation scan with quite good perfusion of the right upper and middle lobes only. (e) CT scan shows the cystic spaces within the overinflated right lobe to better advantage. (f) A higher CT scan cut shows the relatively normal right upper lobe which is displaced across the midline by the pathological right lower lobe. This child underwent right lower lobe lobectomy. (g) The postoperative chest radiograph at the age of 9 months shows the mediastinum is now central with obliteration of the right costophrenic angle and distortion of the mediastinum presumably by postoperative fibrosis. (h) The krypton-81m ventilation lung scan. The right lung shows good ventilation of the middle and lower zones but when taken in conjunction with the chest radiograph that part of the lung overinflated and lying immediately above the right hemidiaphragm is not participating in ventilation. (i) 99mTc macroaggregate perfusion scan shows the right lung not as well perfused as it is ventilated with the area of compensatory emphysema in the right lower zone being most affected.

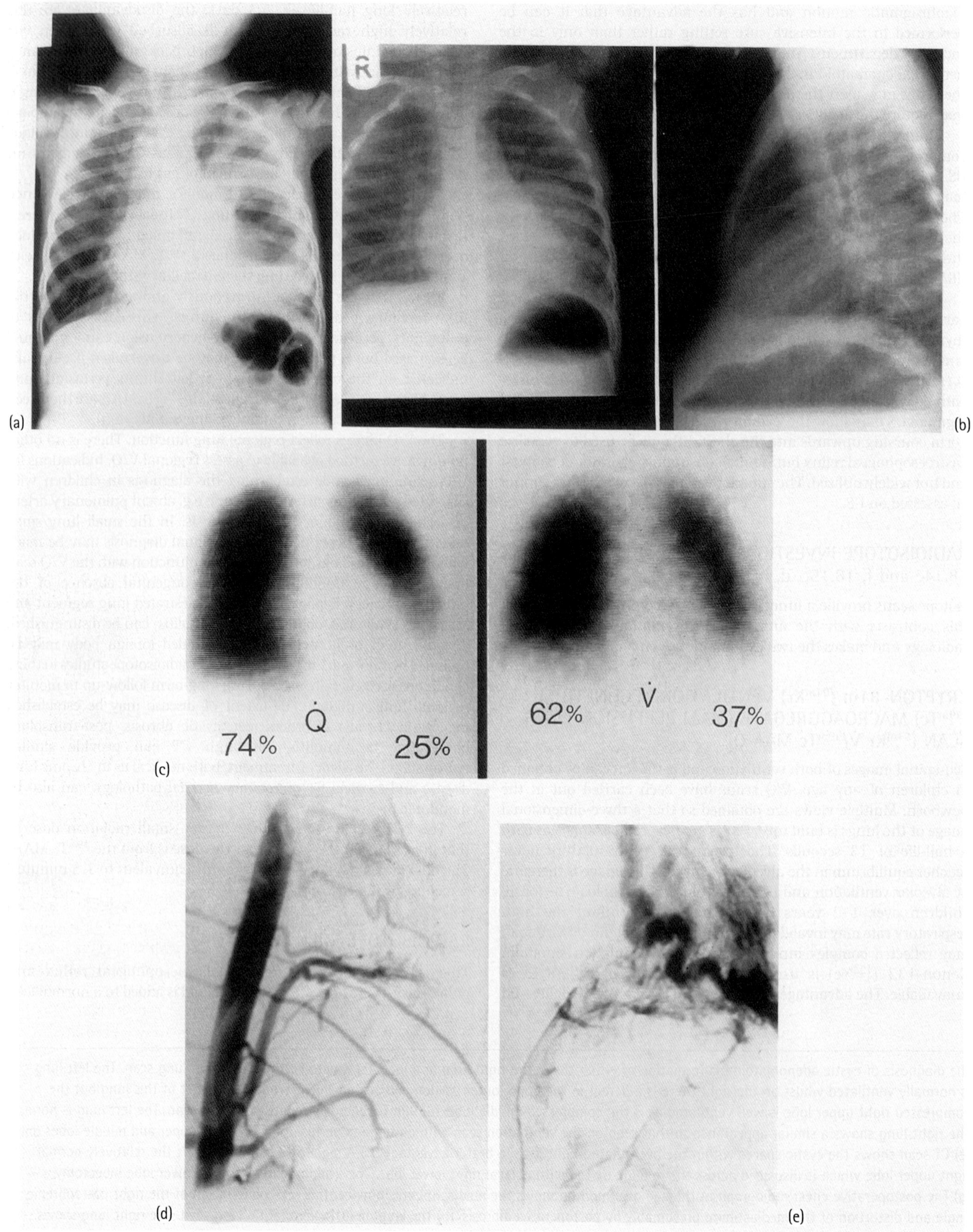

Fig. 18.16 A 3-year-old girl with unresolved pneumonia in the left lower lobe. (a) PA chest radiograph at 3 months of age. (b) Following recovery from the acute episode the routine follow-up chest radiograph 6 months later showed persistent shadowing in the left lower lobe.

(10 MBq/100 ml). Following the feed a small volume of non-radioisotope fluid is given to clear any activity from the esophagus. Infants are cuddled for 5 min; all children are placed supine over the gamma camera. Continuous imaging for 1 h then takes place with delayed images of the lungs 3–5 h after completion of the feed. The Tc-sulfur colloid has a small particle size and is not absorbed by gut mucosa. When aspiration occurs the activity may be seen in the lung. Ciliary movement and bronchial clearance seem to be relatively ineffective in removing the aspirated isotope. One must ensure that the esophagus and lungs are assessed independently of the high activity in the stomach.

This test is more sensitive than a barium swallow in detecting gastroesophageal reflux since the esophagus is studied for up to 60 min continuously rather than intermittently as with barium studies. Quantification of the reflux permits assessment of therapy (see Chapter 17 – Esophageal investigations).

COMPUTED TOMOGRAPHY (Fig. 18.15e and f)

As CT scanning times reduce, the indications for thoracic CT in children increase substantially. CT affords excellent anatomic detail, particularly in older children who can suspend respiration, but CT does unfortunately carry a large radiation burden and so should be used sparingly in young patients. Most pediatric centers now routinely utilize low dose (low mA) techniques to keep radiation to a minimum especially during thoracic CT. There are essentially two approaches or types of chest CT studies generally performed. Standard, contiguous 5–10 mm sections are used when the whole chest or mediastinum is examined in detail. Indications here would include assessment of the pulmonary vasculature, empyema (Fig. 18.17) or suspected adenopathy typically performed after intravenous contrast enhancement. Standard contiguous slices would also be used in staging for suspected lung metastases in children with known solid tumors and this is generally done without contrast administration. So-called high resolution CT (HRCT) involves using fine sections, usually 1 mm slices, at 10 to 20 mm intervals through the lungs to assess for diffuse lung disorders such as an interstitial disease or bronchiectasis.[80] Very fine detail of selected areas of the lung that are achievable with HRCT can help characterize unusual processes, define their extent and in certain cases plan an appropriate area for biopsy. As only selected areas through the lungs are examined, HRCT involves a relatively low radiation dose in comparison to standard CT. HRCT is very accurate in the assessment of bronchiectasis (Fig. 18.18). A normal HRCT essentially excludes this diagnosis assuming the study is of a reasonable quality. Expiratory images in cooperative older children can be very useful in showing air trapping with small airways disease, e.g. obliterative bronchiolitis post-lung transplantation (Fig. 18.19). In other diffuse lung diseases such as cystic fibrosis, the role of CT is not well established.

Virtually all solid tumors with the exception of neuroblastoma (which characteristically metastasizes to bone) require a chest CT at

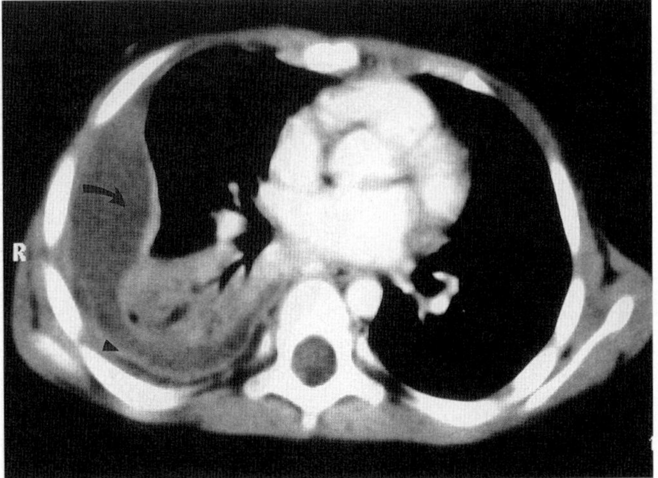

Fig. 18.17 Axial CT after intravenous contrast enhancement showing a moderate sized, low attenuating right-sided pleural effusion (curved arrow), proven to be an empyema at drainage. Note the adjacent area of consolidation, some thickening of the parietal pleura (arrowhead) and edema of the extrapleural space. Intravenous contrast administration has resulted in dense opacification of the cardiac chambers and descending aorta.

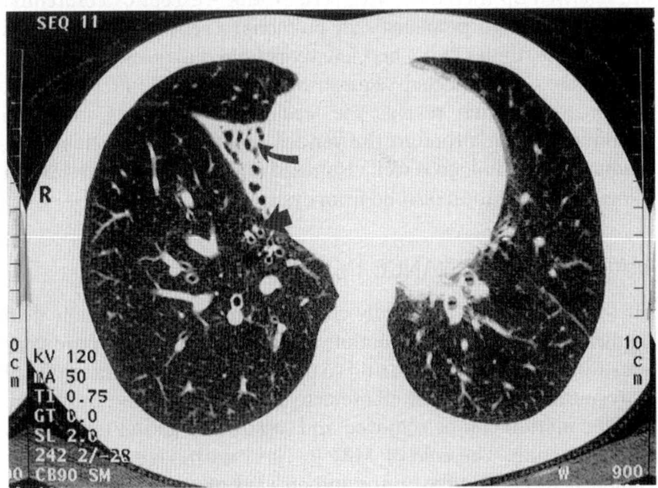

Fig. 18.18 High resolution chest CT image showing chronic right middle lobe collapse with airway dilatation, i.e. bronchiectasis (curved arrow). In addition bronchial wall thickening is seen in the right lower lobe with the classic *signet ring* sign of bronchiectasis, which is due to a dilated airway adjacent to a more normal sized pulmonary artery, also evident (thick arrow). Normal cardiac pulsation has resulted in blurring of the cardiac outline on the left.

(c) A ^{99m}Tc macroaggregate perfusion scan (Q) and a krypton 81m ventilation scan (V) were obtained 1 year following the acute episode. The left lung shows decreased perfusion compared to the right with the left lung only contributing 25% of overall perfusion. On ventilation the left lung contributes 37% and there is a segment in the left lower zone which is relatively well ventilated but not perfused. The diagnosis of a sequestrated segment was suggested. (d) A digital subtraction angiogram was carried out. The arterial phase shows a vessel arising from the abdominal aorta going cranially into the thorax to supply the abnormal area on chest radiograph. (e) The venous phase shows the drainage from the sequestrated segment all going cranially. At surgery a sequestrated segment in the left lower lobe was resected.

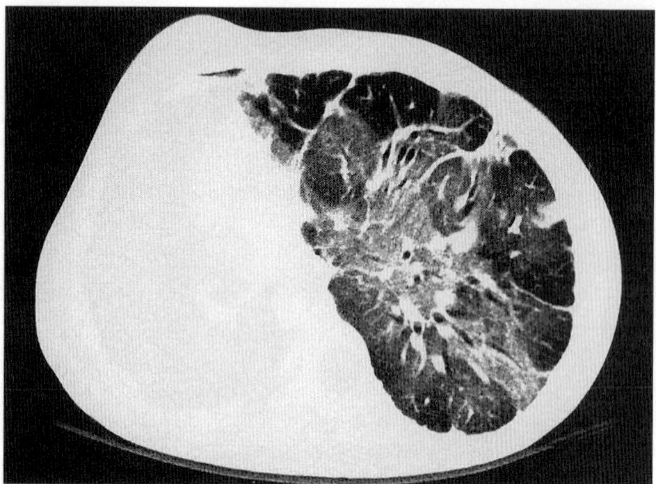

Fig. 18.19 Axial high resolution CT post single lung transplant in a child who had had a previous right pneumonectomy for cystic fibrosis. Obliterative bronchiolitis is evident in the left lung transplant, manifesting as areas of varying attenuation and curvilinear interstitial septal thickening. The peripheral blacker or low density foci represent areas of air trapping which become more conspicuous in older, cooperative patients who can breath-hold for expiratory images.

presentation. If the initial CT is negative for metastases, most cancers are followed up thereafter with serial CXRs – except osteosarcoma which has a high propensity for pulmonary relapse and so merits repeated CT studies in the first few years from diagnosis.

In cases of suspected sequestrated segment CT after contrast enhancement often reveals the feeding vessel arising from the abdominal aorta although the venous drainage is less often seen. Mediastinal pathology is well visualized and tissue characterization allows differentiation of solid from cystic lesions.

MAGNETIC RESONANCE IMAGING (Fig. 18.14g)

MRI creates images by rapidly changing the strong magnetic field applied to the body; no radiation is involved. The images are very sensitive to motion artefact and so normal cardiac pulsation as well as respiratory movement create artefacts. With cardiac gating the cardiac motion can be removed and respiratory gating techniques are improving. The role of MRI in chest pathology is still being established. The mediastinum and airways are well visualized but negative signals from aerated lung preclude good pulmonary imaging for the foreseeable future. The technique is highly accurate in assessing vascular anatomy and so can easily demonstrate a vascular ring or double aortic arch. Recently fast gadolinium-enhanced angiographic sequences have been developed which when more widely available will likely reduce the indications for arteriography of the lungs and great vessels. Imaging times for most MR sequences are still in the order of 2–5 min. A cooperative, still patient is an absolute prerequisite hence there is a continuing need for sedation or anesthesia in smaller children.

ENDOSCOPY (BRONCHOSCOPY)

BACKGROUND

The passage of instruments through the larynx to visualize, sample and manipulate the lower airways is a procedure with applications in many areas of pediatric respiratory medicine.

Bronchoscopy has a long history. It was first developed nearly a hundred years ago for the diagnosis and removal of foreign bodies from the trachea or bronchus. Early instruments were rigid and had a low level of illumination and a limited visual field. With better illumination and improved optics wider applications became possible.

The first flexible fiberoptic bronchoscope was developed in Japan in 1966. This instrument made it possible to see easily parts of the airway that were difficult to visualize using the rigid bronchoscope. It also became possible to perform bronchoscopic examinations without the need for general anesthesia, and with a significant reduction in operative morbidity. This led to a dramatic increase in the usefulness of bronchoscopy as a diagnostic and therapeutic tool. The application of fiberoptic bronchoscopy to pediatrics had to await the development of smaller instruments. Wood and Fink first described the use of the flexible bronchoscope in children in 1978.[82] Fiberoptic bronchoscopes small enough for use in children only became widely available in 1981. With technical progress in production, fiberoptic bundles have become smaller allowing a greater number of bundles per unit space. This has increased the flexibility of the bronchoscope while retaining and even enhancing light transmission. As a result, newer, smaller bronchoscopes with a wider field of vision providing a sharper, less grainy picture are being manufactured. A range of flexible instruments suitable for pediatric use is now available (Table 18.3). These advances in instrumentation have made bronchoscopy an increasingly useful diagnostic and therapeutic tool in infants and children.

The main difference between airway endoscopy in adults and children is that the adult respiratory physician is usually looking for evidence of malignancy while the pediatrician is more commonly looking for anatomical airway abnormalities or inflammatory or infective conditions. In children also, upper airway problems are a common reason for endoscopic evaluation and bronchoscopy almost always involves examination of the upper as well as the lower airway. Indeed, when the flexible bronchoscope is passed through the nose, endoscopic examination of the nose and pharynx becomes a routine part of the examination.

Table 18.3 Examples of flexible endoscopes commonly used in the examination of the pediatric airway

Model	Outer diameter (mm)	Angulation	Suction channel (mm)	Comments
BFN20	1.8	Up 160°; down 90°	None	
BFXP40	2.8	Up 180°; down 130°	1.2	Can pass through a 3.5 mm ET tube
BF3C30	3.5–3.6	Up 180°; down 130°	1.2	Previously, has been the standard flexible instrument used in children
BFP30	4.9–5.0	Up 180°; down 130°	2.2	

All these instruments are manufactured by the Olympus Optical Company, but other manufacturers make instruments of similar specifications.
ET, endotracheal.

TECHNIQUES USED IN PEDIATRICS

Instruments

In order to perform bronchoscopy in children, the bronchoscope must meet some specific technical requirements. Firstly, the instrument must be sufficiently small that it can safely enter the trachea (in a full-term newborn infant the trachea is approximately 5 mm in diameter). Secondly, it must have suitable optical characteristics and provide for illumination of the airway.

Rigid bronchoscopes

Small rigid bronchoscopes meet these criteria and are available in sizes ranging from 2.5 mm (the nominal size of a rigid bronchoscope refers to the smallest internal diameter through which instruments may be passed, not to the outer diameter which may be several millimeters greater because of the thickness of the material). Instruments used in infants are usually 3 mm or the 3.5 mm instruments with an external diameter of 4–5 mm.

Rigid bronchoscopy in children requires general anesthesia. Since the rigid bronchoscope is relatively large in relation to the airway, the bronchoscope functions as an artificial airway during anesthesia allowing good control of the airway for prolonged periods. Ventilation and maintenance of oxygenation are achieved through the bronchoscope, either with positive pressure inflation or with a Venturi jet injection device. With appropriate anesthetic technique, spontaneous respiration through the bronchoscope allows assessment of tracheo- or bronchomalacia.

The optical properties of the rigid bronchoscope alone are poor but when a Hopkins glass rod telescope is passed through the bronchoscope, the optical resolution is unequalled. Rigid bronchoscopy is particularly good at visualizing the posterior wall of the larynx such as when looking for a laryngeal cleft or H-type tracheoesophageal fistula. In children, although angulated telescopes can be used to look into the upper airways, direct access to more distal bronchi and to the upper lobes using a rigid bronchoscope is limited.

The main advantage of the rigid bronchoscope is that it provides complete airway control during the procedure. The excellent view and the extensive range of instruments available mean that a wide variety of therapeutic maneuvers can be carried out. The rigid bronchoscope remains the instrument of choice for foreign body removal, tissue resection, and biopsy where there is a risk of copious hemorrhage.

Flexible bronchoscopes

In the flexible fiberoptic bronchoscope, light to visualize the airway is transmitted via a solid bundle of glass fibers. Flexible bronchoscopes are essentially solid and the child has to breathe around rather than through the instrument. There are now a range of instruments available suitable for use in infants and children (Table 18.3). The distal tip of all these instruments can be flexed by the operator in a single plane. Side to side movement is brought about by rotation of the shaft of the instrument. All but the smallest flexible instruments incorporate a small working channel through which suction can be applied.

Currently, the standard pediatric instrument has an external diameter of 2.9 mm with a 1.2 mm suction channel. The suction channel can be used to perform bronchoalveolar lavage, or to pass small instruments for bronchial brushings or bronchial biopsy. In older children, a small adult bronchoscope with an external diameter of 4.9 mm can be used. This has a larger working channel enabling better suctioning and the use of larger biopsy forceps for epithelial or transbronchial biopsy.

In infants less than 3000 g, a 3.5 mm fiberoptic bronchoscope will nearly totally obstruct the airway. Bronchoscopy can be performed by pre-oxygenating the infant with 100% oxygen and limiting the time below the glottis to 30–40 seconds. Alternatively, the airways of small neonates can be visualized with the 2.2 mm 'ultrathin' bronchoscope which lacks a suction channel. This bronchoscope can be passed through a connector placed between the endotracheal tube and the ventilator allowing uninterrupted ventilation and oxygen delivery during the procedure.

Video recording

Video recording is now an important part of any endoscopic procedure in children. With a video monitor, the operator's assistants can view the findings and anticipate the operator's needs. Video recording improves documentation of endoscopic findings and facilitates communication with other members of the clinical team. Reviewing the video record with a child's parents can be particularly helpful in communicating to them the study findings.

Setting and techniques

There are two general approaches to performing bronchoscopy in children: using either conscious sedation or under general anesthesia.

General anesthesia is not essential for flexible bronchoscopy in children. In many cases, airway endoscopy can be safely performed under conscious sedation and topical anesthesia. Adequate sedation has most frequently been achieved using a combination of an opiate and a short acting benzodiazepine, most commonly midazolam (0.1–0.3 mg/kg^{-1}) and pethidine (1–2 mg/kg^{-1}). Shorter acting opiates such as fentanyl have increasingly replaced pethidine. Solutions of lidocaine (lignocaine) (maximum dose 7 mg/kg^{-1}) delivered directly via the suction channel allow topical anesthesia above the vocal cords and below in the trachea and main bronchi. A topical vasoconstrictor, applied to the nasal passages before the procedure, enlarges the nasal passages and decreases the risk of epistaxis. Bronchoscopy under sedation with topical anesthesia can provide excellent access to the entire airway including the upper airway, allowing examination of the dynamic anatomy of the airway during normal spontaneous respiration. Unfortunately, it is often difficult to be precise about the level of sedation achieved and the child is often sedated to a deeper level than is consistent with conscious sedation.

Rigid bronchoscopy invariably requires general anesthetic. When general anesthesia is employed for flexible endoscopy, or bronchoscopy performed on a ventilated patient, the flexible bronchoscope is passed down an endotracheal tube. In recent years, a laryngeal mask airway has been used as an alternative to endotracheal intubation. A laryngeal mask offers easy access to the airway and permits direct inspection of the vocal cords, larynx and airway. A laryngeal mask has the important additional advantage of allowing the use of a larger diameter bronchoscope with a larger suction channel than could be passed through an endotracheal tube on the same child. This can make direct removal of foreign bodies possible or allow larger biopsies to be obtained through the use of larger instruments or biopsy forceps. The benefits of general anesthesia using a laryngeal mask in terms of child safety and comfort as well as the ease of examination have been increasingly recognized.[83] In many circumstances this is becoming the preferred approach.

Patient monitoring

Above all else, it is absolutely essential that one person other than the endoscopist is solely responsible for observing and monitoring the child during the procedure. Before the procedure, children undergoing endoscopy should have an i.v. line placed. Monitoring during the procedure should always include continuous pulse oximetry as well as monitoring of heart rate, respiration and colour. Access to appropriate suction, supplemental oxygen, resuscitation equipment, and antagonists for sedative agents (naloxone and flumazenil) must be immediately available and staff involved in airway endoscopy must be fully trained in resuscitation.

Contraindications and complications of airway endoscopy

With increasing experience the contraindications to bronchoscopy are largely relative. When performed by properly trained personnel in carefully controlled conditions, bronchoscopy is a low-risk procedure. Nevertheless, bronchoscopy should only be performed if the relative benefits of the procedure outweigh the risks. Complications are more likely in children with:

1. bleeding diatheses that cannot be corrected;
2. massive hemoptysis;
3. severe airway obstruction;
4. severe hypoxia;
5. pulmonary hypertension;
6. lung abscess where there is a risk of pus spreading throughout the lung if the cavity is ruptured. Anklyosis of the jaw or neck may preclude rigid bronchoscopy.

The complications of airway endoscopy can generally be divided into those associated with the medications used before and during the endoscopic procedure and those related to the instrumentation.[85]

Inadequate topical analgesia may lead to reactions such as laryngospasm or other vagally mediated phenomena. Inadequate sedation may lead to patient discomfort while too much sedation may lead to respiratory depression and apnea. Episodes of hypoxemia, bradycardia or apnea are common but usually transient and self-limiting.

Transient high fever is common within 24 h after a bronchoalveolar lavage. Small hemoptyses commonly follow biopsy procedures. The risk of trauma to the oropharynx or airway is greater with the rigid bronchoscope. More serious problems including laryngospasm and pneumothorax can occur but are rare. Airway instrumentation may exacerbate airway narrowing in children with already compromised airways such as for example subglottic stenosis. In these children, nebulized adrenaline (epinephrine) or intravenous corticosteroids may tide the child over. Rarely, intubation may be necessary. The reported incidence of pneumothorax following transbronchial biopsy is up to 8%.[85]

With careful attention to detail, the safety record of airway endoscopy in children is excellent and bronchoscopy can now be performed easily and safely even in small premature neonates.

Infection control

To prevent cross-infection between children or contamination of specimens collected, endoscopes must be scrupulously cleaned and disinfected after each use. Rigid bronchoscopes can be autoclaved. Flexible bronchoscopes require cold sterilization using agents such as activated glutaraldehyde or peracetic acid. Detailed guidelines have been published on the appropriate duration of sterilization particularly for high risk infections such as TB or HIV.[86]

Clinical staff that may be exposed to body secretions during bronchoscopy should use universal precautions.

USES AND INDICATIONS FOR AIRWAY ENDOSCOPY IN CHILDREN

Clinical use of airway endoscopy in children falls into two broad categories.

Diagnostic uses

There are a number of common uses for airway endoscopy (Table 18.4). Nowadays, the flexible bronchoscope is the instrument of choice for most diagnostic purposes.[87]

1. Direct observation of intranasal, laryngeal, intratracheal and intrabronchial abnormalities

Bronchoscopy allows the direct visualization of the nasal passages, pharynx, larynx and vocal cords, glottis, trachea, carina, lobar bronchus and more peripheral bronchi. Abnormalities of airway structure, size or patency including congenital anomalies, stenosis or extrinsic airway compression, and endobronchial masses particularly foreign bodies or mucus plugging, can all be seen. If an obstructing lesion pulsates it may point to the presence of a vascular abnormality such as a vascular ring. In children with tuberculosis, evidence of airway compression or granulation tissue may guide the need for steroid therapy or for the resection of granulation tissue.[88] In children with stridor or persistent wheezing the abnormal airway dynamics can be identified. Areas of inflammation or bleeding may be directly identified.

2. Direct suction and bronchoalveolar lavage

If secretions are profuse, samples may be collected by suction either directly or after lung washings with saline. Bronchoalveolar lavage (BAL) is a method of collecting fluid through the suction channel of a wedged fiberscope after saline has been injected. This method is commonly used for collection of bronchoalveolar material for the analysis of cellular or biochemical components.[89]

Usually, BAL is carried out in the most affected area identified radiologically or by endoscopy. In diffuse lung disease, the right middle lobe is preferred because fluid recovery is better. BAL is carried out using sterile normal saline solution warmed to body temperature. Various protocols for determining the amount of fluid to be lavaged are available but there is limited information on which is optimal. Fluid is instilled in between two and four aliquots. The first aliquot collected is of more bronchial origin; subsequent

Table 18.4 Indications for bronchoscopy

Stridor
Unexplained or persistent wheeze
Unexplained or persistent cough
Unexplained hemoptysis
Possible tracheobronchial foreign body aspiration
Investigation of chest radiograph abnormalities
Persistent/recurrent lobar consolidation or atelectasis
Recurrent or persistent infiltrates
Lung lesions of unknown etiology
Pulmonary infection – to identify pathogens
In infection unresponsive to antibiotics
In a child with cystic fibrosis to identify pathogens
In an immunosuppressed child
Recurrent infection
Intensive care/anesthetic room
Examine for the position, patency or airway damage due to endotracheal or tracheostomy tubes
Facilitate difficult intubations
Airway injury
Assessment of injury from toxic inhalation or aspiration
Other therapeutic and diagnostic indications
Endobronchial stent placement
Sampling and/or removal of airway secretions and mucus plugs
Endobronchial and transbronchial biopsy

aliquots, which are usually pooled, sample more distal airspaces. Generally, the initial fraction is used for culture while the later fraction is submitted for cytological and biochemical analysis. A BAL can be considered technically satisfactory if fluid recovery is greater than 40% of the volume instilled and the lavage fluid (except for the first sample) contains few epithelial cells.

3. Bronchial biopsy

Endoscopic biopsy forceps allow biopsy of abnormal looking areas. This may be useful if there is suspicion of a granulomatous disease (e.g. caseating tuberculosis). However, samples obtained by gastric lavage remain the gold standard in children suspected of TB. In children with poorly controlled asthma, mucosal biopsies have been used to investigate the extent of bronchial inflammation. With infiltrative lung disorders, transbronchial biopsy may provide an alternative to open or percutaneous lung biopsy, although the small samples obtained are not always sufficient to make a diagnosis.

With an endobronchial brush inserted through the suction channel, it is easy to collect ciliated epithelium from the lower airways. However, ciliary dyskinesia can usually be diagnosed from material obtained by nasal brushings without the need for brush biopsy of the lower respiratory tract.

4. Bronchography

Although bronchography has largely been superseded by the development of high resolution CT, it is easy and safe to obtain a precise bronchogram by injection of contrast medium through the suction channel into the desired lobe or segment. This technique can produce very high quality bronchograms while minimizing the volume of contrast material used.

Therapeutic bronchoscopy

1. Endoscopic removal of material

Operative procedures such as the extraction of foreign bodies are difficult with flexible instruments and rigid instruments are almost always used for this purpose. Material obstructing the airway such as a foreign body, mucus plug or tissue mass can all be removed endoscopically. Mucus plugs can usually be aspirated through the suction channel of flexible instruments.

2. Placing of endobronchial stents

Stents have been widely used in adults for palliation of inoperable tracheobronchial malignancies. In children, tracheobronchial stenoses are usually congenital. Surgical treatment has been unsatisfactory, largely because of the occurrence of recurrent stenoses. There is growing experience with the use of balloon-expandable, metal stents especially for the treatment of severe tracheal stenosis, either congenital or after tracheoplasty for congenital tracheal stenosis repair, and for severe tracheobronchomalacia in children as young 2 months.[90,91]

SPECIFIC CLINICAL INDICATIONS FOR AIRWAY ENDOSCOPY[92–94]

STRIDOR[95]

Chronic stridor is the commonest indication for examination of the airway in infants and children. If stridor is mild and/or intermittent then a conservative approach may be appropriate. Even with mild stridor, an endoscopy may be useful if the parents are very anxious. Demonstrating the abnormality on a video recording to the parents may be particularly valuable in helping them understand the basis of the problem and a definite diagnosis can be very reassuring.

When the stridor is severe, persistent, associated with apnea, failure to thrive or an abnormal cry, or is present in a child who has previously been ventilated then chances of a structural abnormality are high and endoscopy is indicated.[94]

The flexible bronchoscope is well suited for the evaluation of stridor. Because the instrument is passed through the nose, the entire airway can be examined. More importantly, a transnasal approach in a spontaneously ventilating sedated child leaves the laryngeal structures in their natural state, without any distorting forces being applied. This allows an evaluation of the 'normal' airway dynamics. If the child has stridor at the time of the examination, then the vibrating structures giving rise to the noise can be identified.

Laryngomalacia

Laryngomalacia is the commonest cause of persistent non-infective stridor accounting for over 75% cases and is easily diagnosed endoscopically.

Stridor is usually evident in the first few days of life but may not be evident until later in the first month. The noise is a fairly characteristic jerky, inspiratory crowing noise which varies in intensity from breath to breath, commonly being loudest when the infant is crying or in the supine position. The noise may disappear when the infant is quiet, asleep or prone. Usually there is no respiratory distress or cyanosis. Stridor may worsen during an upper respiratory tract infection. Feeding difficulties and failure to thrive are very uncommon except in severe cases. The noise usually lessens gradually as the child becomes older and in the majority of children has disappeared by about 2 years.

The endoscopic findings of laryngomalacia are characteristic. The epiglottis is long and omega-shaped (Ω). The tissues of the larynx are floppy so that the epiglottis, arytenoids and aryepiglottic folds can be seen collapsing inwards on inspiration, prolapsing into and narrowing the glottic opening. The floppy tissues vibrate during inspiration causing the stridor while on expiration the positive pressure of air blows them apart. Concomitant lesions below the cord are not uncommon. Accordingly, it is important that bronchoscopy is performed in addition to laryngoscopy.

Subglottic stenosis

Subglottic stenosis may be congenital or acquired. It is characterized by a narrowing in the subglottic region such that a bronchoscope appropriately sized for the child's age and size cannot pass through the subglottic area or passes snugly. Clinically, children may present with stridor, cough or recurrent croup.

Congenital subglottic stenosis is secondary to a small cricoid or thick submucosa. The prognosis is good, with fewer than 50% coming to tracheostomy. Acquired subglottic stenosis is most commonly secondary to prolonged endotracheal intubation in the neonatal period. It may coexist with damage to other parts of the larynx and trachea.

Vocal cord paralysis

Vocal cord paralysis, unilateral or bilateral, is the second most common laryngeal anomaly in neonates. Vocal cord paralysis may be congenital, secondary to central nervous system disorders or iatrogenic after surgical repair of cardiovascular disorders. In iatrogenic cases, unilateral paralysis is more frequent and the paralysis is temporary usually recovering within 2–4 weeks. Children with vocal cord paralysis have a weak or absent cry, respiratory obstruction and difficulty in feeding. The diagnosis is made at laryngoscopy when vocal cord paralysis is observed.

Subglottic hemangiomata

Although rare, subglottic hemangiomata may be life-threatening. Typically, an afebrile infant presents with biphasic inspiratory and expiratory stridor. The voice is typically normal and there is commonly no swallowing difficulty. In most cases, symptoms are present before 16 weeks of age. The initial presentation may mimic croup but rather than resolve stridor is progressive. Diagnosis may be difficult because of the rarity of the lesion and the overlap in presentation with other commoner illnesses such as croup. The presence of skin hemangioma should alert the clinician. An association between extensive hemangioma present in a cervico-facial 'beard' distribution and subglottic hemangioma has been noted. If present, the early evaluation of the airway may be appropriate.[96] Diagnosis is confirmed by the presence of a characteristic red or blue lesion seen at endoscopy. Regression usually begins by 2 years of age and thus a conservative approach is preferred. If the airway is compromised, tracheostomy may be necessary until regression occurs.

PERSISTENT OR UNILATERAL WHEEZING

Persistent wheezing unresponsive to bronchodilators or unilateral wheezing is an important indication for bronchoscopic examination. Lower airway problems were found in 79% of one large series. Tracheomalacia, compression of the left main bronchus usually in association with cardiac anomalies and tracheal compression due to vascular structures were the commonest structural findings. However, previously unsuspected foreign bodies were also surprisingly common.[97]

PERSISTENT COUGH

If persistent cough is unresponsive to treatment, bronchoscopy may be indicated although the diagnostic yield may be low in the absence of other symptoms and signs. It can, however, be reassuring if the airways are normal.

UNEXPLAINED HEMOPTYSIS

Hemoptysis is an unusual symptom in children. If the bleedings is of significant size or is persistent and a careful history and examination, including a careful examination of the mouth and nose, fails to identify a cause then bronchoscopy is indicated. The chances of finding a cause are greater if the bleeding is active at the time of the examination. Rigid bronchoscopy with its better suction is safer if hemoptysis is brisk. Heavily bloodstained BAL fluid raises the possibility of pulmonary hemosiderosis. The demonstration of hemosiderin-laden macrophages in the lavage fluid confirms the diagnosis. If hemoptysis persists after a normal bronchoscopy, a pulmonary origin for the blood is unlikely.[94]

PERSISTENT ATELECTASIS

If atelectasis persists despite adequate treatment, bronchoscopy should be considered to exclude a foreign body, remove mucus plugs and obtain pathological specimens. In one large reported series, around 60% of children with persistent atelectasis had a diagnostic abnormality.[97] While the causes were diverse, the commonest finding was the presence of a central mucus plug. Removal of large plugs by lavage and suction frequently can lead to complete and immediate resolution, particularly in young children with massive atelectasis.

RECURRENT/PERSISTENT PULMONARY INFILTRATES

Bronchoscopy combined with BAL can provide valuable information in the assessment and treatment of a child with pulmonary infiltrates and should be performed in every child suspected of interstitial lung disease.

In an immunocompetent child

When a child with pulmonary infiltrates fails to respond to a broad spectrum antibiotic or where an atypical pneumonia is suspected and other techniques of collecting airways secretions are not practical, bronchoscopy with BAL can be used to collect specimens for microbiological and cytological analysis. However, samples collected by BAL can be contaminated by bacteria normally present in the respiratory tract. Interpretation of cultures, therefore, needs to be based on quantitative cultures with appropriate thresholds and/or identification of intracellular bacteria on direct examination of the sample in conjunction with the clinical picture. Newer molecular techniques are extending the range of organisms that can be detected.

In children with alveolar proteinosis, alveolar hemorrhage and pulmonary histiocytosis, BAL may be diagnostic. In other situations even if not diagnostic, BAL cell profiles may help orientate further investigations.[89] Once a diagnosis of an alveolar inflammatory process has been reached, inflammatory markers in BAL fluid may help monitor disease activity and progression although there is as yet no general consensus on the measurement or interpretation of such markers.

Finally, bronchoscopy and BAL may have a therapeutic role in the removal of material present in the airways resulting from lipoid material in alveolar structures. Several reports have shown that whole lung lavage may be an effective treatment in some children with alveolar proteinosis.[98]

In an immunocompromised child

In the immunocompromised child with pulmonary infiltrates, bronchoscopy and BAL have an even more important role. In children with primary immunodeficiency, or immunodeficiency secondary to chemotherapy for malignancy or following bone marrow or solid organ transplant who develop pneumonitis, BAL should ideally be performed soon after clinical and radiological signs develop, before any antibiotic therapy is started. Where antibiotics are started empirically, bronchoscopy and BAL may be informative in those who do not improve despite adequate antibiotic therapy.

The identification of primary pathogens, such as *Mycobacterium tuberculosis*, *Pneumocystis carinii*, or RSV not usually isolated from BAL fluid, may be diagnostic. Where the organisms may also be present as airway commensals or contaminants (e.g. Aspergillus, atypical mycobacteria, cytomegalovirus), interpretation is more difficult.

Children with HIV can develop a range of respiratory presentations ranging from acute pneumonia to interstitial pneumonitis (Ch. 25 – *Pneumocystis carinii* section of HIV section and Pneumonia in the immunocompromised child). Bronchoscopy and BAL may help differentiate infectious causes such as *P. carinii* from non-infectious pulmonary complications such as lymphoid interstitial pneumonitis.

BAL and transbronchial biopsy (TBB) are frequently used in the monitoring of children after lung transplantation, either routinely or as a result of clinical and/or radiological deterioration.[85,99] TBB is necessary to establish a histological diagnosis of rejection while BAL fluid can be used for microbiological studies to exclude infection.

BRONCHOSCOPY AND INHALATION OF FOREIGN MATERIAL

Foreign body aspiration

Aspiration of a foreign body in a child is amongst the most important indications for bronchoscopy. Indeed, the presence of a foreign body cannot be reliably excluded without a bronchoscopy.

The typical history is of the sudden onset of choking, coughing or wheezing. A careful history will identify a choking episode in most cases. After the initial period, a symptom free interval may follow. Some patients with foreign bodies have chronic or subtle clinical features (atelectasis, recurrent or persisting pneumonia, persistent wheezing unresponsive to bronchodilators, diminished local breath sounds) and radiological changes (hyperinflation or atelectasis of an affected segment) but no history of foreign body aspiration. Others may have no physical or radiological signs.

Peanuts (groundnuts) and other nuts are the most common objects inhaled in the United Kingdom. These are among the most irritating agents to bronchial epithelium and can lead to florid local inflammation and necrosis if not rapidly removed. Grass seeds and seed husks are commoner in other parts of the world and maybe especially troublesome, because their barbed nature prevents expectoration or removal by bronchoscopy. The most common site of impaction of a foreign body is in a segmental bronchus, particularly on the right side. Rarely, laryngeal obstruction may lead to rapid asphyxia.

In most cases, the history, physical examination and radiographic studies produce a high index of suspicion. In these cases, the child should have rigid bronchoscopy without delay.

When there is doubt as to whether a child has aspirated a foreign body, a flexible bronchoscopy may be valuable diagnostically. In some children, foreign body aspiration may be totally unsuspected. Wood found a previously unsuspected foreign body in nearly 1% of children undergoing flexible bronchoscopy.[97] If a foreign body is identified, then the child should have a rigid bronchoscopy to remove it. Occasionally when removal of a foreign body has been unusually delayed, it may be necessary to resect an irretrievably damaged lung segment.

Recurrent aspiration

Bronchoscopy and BAL can be useful in the investigation of a child suspected of recurrent aspiration. Chronic pulmonary aspiration of oral and/or gastric contents occurs when normal airway protective mechanisms are impaired, bypassed or overwhelmed. The resulting airway contamination causes lung injury which may lead to bronchospasm, atelectasis, pulmonary edema, pneumonia or bronchiectasis depending on the frequency and quantity of aspiration, the composition and pH of aspirated material and the efficacy of the lung clearance response. Thus, there may be a range of clinical presentations ranging from wheezing, through recurrent episodes of pneumonia to chronic inflammation with eventual interstitial fibrosis and bronchiectasis. Children with neurodevelopmental problems are particularly susceptible. The predominant site of pathology depends on the patient's habitual posture: upper lobes in infants nursed supine; basal disease for older children propped in a semi-recumbent position.

There are three main groups of pathophysiological processes that interfere with normal airway protective mechanisms and lead to recurrent aspiration (Table 18.5). Anatomical abnormalities such as cleft palate or laryngeal cleft can lead to pooling of food or saliva in the pharynx. Abnormal swallowing coordination occurring in children with neuromuscular disorders such as cerebral palsy or dysautonomia results in aspiration of material with swallowing. In both situations, symptoms are likely to occur during feeding. Esophageal disorders cause aspiration by a number of mechanisms. Fistulous connections will lead to lower airway soiling particularly during feeding. There may be soiling of the lower airway from overspill of contents refluxed from the stomach or more rarely from overspill from a dilated esophagus in conditions such as achalasia.

Table 18.5 Causes of recurrent inhalation

Swallowing disorders
Anatomical abnormalities
Cleft palate
Macroglossia
Laryngeal cleft
Neuromuscular disorders
Cerebral palsy
CNS degenerative disorders
Congenital neuromuscular disorders
Dysautonomia
Esophageal lesions
Obstruction
Stricture or compression
Systemic sclerosis
Achalasia
Tracheoesophageal fistula
Gastroesophageal reflux
Hyperinflation (severe asthma, cystic fibrosis)

The diagnosis of recurrent aspiration can be surprisingly problematic. Associated disorders, varying clinical presentations and lack of specific diagnostic criteria all contribute to frequent diagnostic difficulties. Diagnosis starts with a careful history and examination combined with observation of the child feeding followed by imaging studies including a CXR, barium swallow and video recording of the child swallowing. If a fistula is suspected, specific lateral X-ray views are taken while injecting contrast through a slowly withdrawn gastric tube with side holes. The gold standard for demonstrating gastroesophageal reflux is 24-h pH probe study. Gastroesophageal scintiscans using radiolabeled milk may provide direct evidence of aspiration. While positive studies are highly suggestive of chronic aspiration false positives may occur and none of these tests may rule out aspiration (Ch. 17 – Esophageal investigation).

Bronchoscopy may provide direct evidence of anatomical abnormalities such as the presence of a tracheoesophageal fistula. The semi-quantitative estimation of lipid-laden alveolar macrophages (LLMI) in bronchoalveolar fluid has been used as a marker of chronic aspiration. While more recent studies suggest that LLMI alone cannot be used to diagnose chronic aspiration it may be a useful adjunct when taken in combination with other investigations.[100]

BRONCHOSCOPY IN INTENSIVE CARE AREAS AND ANESTHETIC ROOMS

There are now a number of important uses for airway endoscopy in intensive care units and anesthetic rooms.

Endoscopic intubation is a useful method for performing endotracheal intubation in difficult to intubate children whose larynx is otherwise impossible to visualize. The endotracheal tube is passed over a flexible bronchoscope and then directly positioned in the airway under direct visualization. Using the ultrathin 2.2 mm

chemoreceptor control mechanisms, e.g. congenital central hypoventilation, results in hypoventilation that is most marked, but not confined to, quiet sleep. During REM sleep, infants and children have frequent central apneas. In asymptomatic infants, these have been demonstrated to exceed 20 seconds' duration and to be associated with desaturations to below 81%.[122] Therefore, their clinical significance remains uncertain. The physiological changes occurring during REM sleep also contribute to increased upper airway resistance associated with obstructive sleep apnea syndrome, in which loss of genioglossus tone is an important factor, and to hypoventilation in cases of diaphragmatic paresis or palsy, when ventilation during wakefulness and quiet sleep is maintained by intercostal and accessory muscle activity. Thus, investigation of children with damage to or disorders of any component of the respiratory musculature must include measurements of respiration during sleep, particularly during intercurrent illnesses associated with increased work of breathing, including upper and lower respiratory tract infections. Abnormal respiratory muscles that provide adequate alveolar ventilation when a child is well may not be able to cope under conditions of increased workloads.

In normal infants the diaphragm has a much higher proportion of fast twitch, type II muscle fibers, which are more susceptible to fatigue than the slow twitch type I fibers that predominate in the adult. Thus diaphragmatic fatigue may be a contributory factor to apnea or hypoventilation, particularly during REM sleep, under conditions of increased work of breathing (e.g. upper respiratory tract infection with increased upper airway resistance) (see also pp. 724 – Development of the respiratory system section, The chest wall).

CONGENITAL CENTRAL HYPOVENTILATION SYNDROME

Central hypoventilation in children may occur as a primary congenital abnormality of control of respiration or less commonly it is secondary to one of a number of other conditions outlined in Table 18.7. Congenital central hypoventilation syndrome (CCHS) is usually present from birth but a late-onset form has been described, typically presenting between 2 and 4 years in association with hypothalamic disorders, including endocrinopathies.

In CCHS, there is hypoventilation that is most marked during quiet sleep (during which autonomic chemoreceptor control normally predominates). However, ventilatory control is also abnormal during REM sleep and wakefulness to a variable degree. Proposed diagnostic criteria[123] include:

- persistent evidence of hypoventilation during sleep ($PaCO_2 > 60$ mmHg (8 kPa));
- onset of symptoms usually in the first year after birth;
- absence of primary pulmonary or neuromuscular disease;
- no evidence of primary heart disease.

Table 18.7 Causes of central hypoventilation in children

Primary
Congenital central hypoventilation syndrome
Secondary
Obesity, e.g. Prader–Willi syndrome
Brainstem lesions, e.g. Arnold–Chiari malformation, achondroplasia with foramen magnum compression
Inborn errors of metabolism
Neurodegenerative disorders
Familial dysautonomia
Drugs
Hypothyroidism
Hyperthermia
Myasthenia gravis

Severity may range from mild alveolar hypoventilation during quiet sleep (QS) with adequate alveolar minute ventilation during wakefulness to complete apnea during QS and severe hypoventilation even when awake.

Although the precise pathophysiological mechanisms underlying CCHS remain unclear, it is consistently associated with failure of normal chemoreceptor control of respiration. Children with CCHS have absent ventilatory responses to hypoxia and hypercapnia and there is evidence that these abnormalities are due to dysfunction of central integration of chemoreceptor input[124,125] rather than chemoreceptor insensitivity. Some arousal responses to hypercapnia or hypoxia may be present however, particularly in REM sleep, and some children with CCHS increase ventilation in response to exercise. No consistent structural or functional abnormality of the brainstem has been found in association with CCHS, though abnormalities of the arcuate nucleus have been described in postmortem studies, and functional MRI has shown deficits in cerebellar structures to ventilatory challenges in some affected individuals.[126] Ventilation during wakefulness is maintained by mechanisms associated with arousal, cognitive activities and exercise that are modulated by the reticular activating system, forebrain or mechanoreceptor afferents.

It has been proposed that CCHS may be part of a generalized disorder of the autonomic nervous system. First-degree relatives of subjects with CCHS have been demonstrated to have a greater prevalence of autonomic nervous system dysfunction compared to relatives of control children.[127] There is reduced beat-to-beat variability in the heart rate and some patients have episodes of marked bradycardia during sleep.[128] There is also a well described association between CCHS and a number of other conditions, including Hirschsprung's disease in 16% of cases, ophthalmological abnormalities, and occasionally ganglioneuroma or ganglioneuroblastoma. In cases of CCHS with Hirschsprung's disease, an association with a point mutation in exon 12 of the receptor tyrosine kinase proto-oncogene RET has been described.[129] This gene is believed to be important in the migration of neural crest cells and development of CO_2 sensitivity. Studies of RET knockout mice have demonstrated decreased ventilatory responses to hypercapnia in these animals. However, mutations of the RET proto-oncogene cannot account for the majority of cases of CCHS.

Other clinical associations of CCHS include nocturnal seizures, reversal of the normal circadian pattern of urine production, with a major diuresis occurring at night, fluid retention during even minor intercurrent infections, due to increased antidiuretic hormone (ADH) secretion, and ventilation/perfusion mismatching with severe hypoxemia complicating relatively mild hypoventilation during sleep. Some children with CCHS develop hypothermia rather than pyrexia during infections, and many show abnormalities of the normal diurnal patterns of body temperature change.

Presentation of CCHS is variable and depends on the severity of hypoventilation. Some infants present at birth with apnea requiring positive pressure ventilation. Most presenting in this way do not breathe spontaneously for the first few months after birth but may progress to a pattern of adequate ventilation during wakefulness as a result of normal maturation of the respiratory control system. Other modes of presentation include cyanosis, cor pulmonale or occasionally unexplained apnea or apparent life-threatening events.

Investigations should include evaluation of pulmonary, cardiac and neurological status with chest radiograph and CT if indicated, ECG, echocardiogram, EEG and MRI of the brain and brainstem. If there is significant hypotonia, nerve conduction studies, electromyogram and muscle biopsy should be considered as well as metabolic investigations, including carnitine levels. The definitive diagnosis depends on careful evaluation of ventilation and gas exchange during different behavioral states using polygraphic recordings (PSG) of respiration, sleep state and blood gases. Some authorities recommend also measuring the response to hypercapnia using a rebreathing or steady state challenge. The former is not suitable for use in infants, so the ventilatory response to breathing 3% and 5% CO_2 via a head box can be performed. Although the underlying physiological abnormality does not change in CCHS, physiological maturation of the respiratory control system can lead to alterations in the adequacy of ventilation, particularly outside quiet sleep, so the PSG should be repeated on a regular basis. If there are associated symptoms of constipation, vomiting or abdominal distension, a rectal biopsy should be performed to look for evidence of Hirschsprung's disease.[130]

Management

To date, no clinically acceptable respiratory stimulant has been demonstrated to consistently increase alveolar ventilation in children with CCHS. Theophylline, naloxone, imipramine and chlorpromazine are ineffective. Trials of the respiratory stimulants doxapram and almitrine have been small and have not demonstrated consistent improvements in spontaneous ventilation or gas exchange. Medroxyprogesterone has been used successfully but is limited by pituitary/adrenal suppression.

The treatment of CCHS is lifelong and most children with the condition will require support with positive pressure ventilation during sleep. Positive pressure ventilation can be delivered by tracheostomy, particularly in infants and those requiring daytime and nocturnal ventilation, but there is increasing experience of the use of non-invasive ventilation using a face mask or nasal mask, even in young children, although there are reports of mid-facial growth abnormalities with long term use of tightly applied face masks. Persistent ventilation/perfusion mismatch may require the addition of supplemental oxygen, even when alveolar ventilation is adequate. Negative pressure ventilation has also been used in the treatment of CCHS but the equipment required is generally regarded as being too cumbersome for ease of home ventilation and negative pressure ventilation may lead to upper airway obstruction in association with absent pharyngeal dilator activity during inspiration.

Electrical pacemakers applied to the phrenic nerves have been used to treat CCHS but in the past have been associated with permanent damage to the nerves and diaphragmatic muscle fatigue. Recently phrenic nerve stimulation using bipolar or quadripolar electrodes has been used successfully in children with CCHS with promising long term outcomes, although active children with CCHS had a higher incidence of pacemaker complications than tetraplegic children fitted with the same pacemakers. There is a theoretical risk of nerve damage if nerve stimulation is used for 24 h a day, so most centers recommend their use for a maximum of 16 h per day. In children with CCHS who have the most severe form of the condition, with a need for ventilatory support when awake as well as when asleep, daytime phrenic pacing, combined with night-time non-invasive ventilatory support may allow improved quality of life and greater independence, with no necessity for a permanent tracheostomy. Phrenic nerve stimulation has now been used successfully for up to 20 years in some patients.[131,132]

Outcome

Many children with CCHS lead relatively normal lives and attend mainstream schooling. However, the majority have persisting hypotonia and varying degrees of neurocognitive deficits. Seizure disorders are common in CCHS but whether these are due to the underlying neurological disorder or secondary to unrecognized hypoxemic episodes is not clear. Affected children usually have poor growth and delayed onset of puberty. Long term life expectancy is not clear at present but is likely to be related to the development of pulmonary hypertension and cor pulmonale which are common sequelae a in follow-up studies of children with CCHS.[119,130,133]

OBSTRUCTIVE SLEEP APNEA SYNDROME

Any structural cause of upper airway narrowing can exacerbate the normal reduction of oropharyngeal caliber during inspiration, leading to complete or partial obstruction of the airway. The commonest cause in children is adenotonsillar hypertrophy with a peak incidence between 2 and 8 years of age. Young children are at particular risk because of the relatively crowded hypopharynx at this stage of development (see pp. 726 – Airway function). Episodes of obstruction occur primarily during REM sleep, in contrast with obstructive apneas in adults, which occur in all sleep stages.

Although upper airway obstruction is a fundamental component of obstructive sleep apnea syndrome (OSAS), the symptoms are not simply related to structural narrowing of the airway. Not all children with OSAS associated with adenotonsillar hypertrophy will have their symptoms alleviated by adenotonsillectomy and radiological studies have not shown a correlation between the size of enlarged tonsils and adenoids and the presence of OSAS. Abnormal central control of upper airway activation during inspiration and elevated arousal thresholds to hypercapnia have been demonstrated in children with OSAS. Obstructive apneas are also observed in children with craniofacial abnormalities (e.g. Robin sequence), narrow upper airways in association with Down syndrome, and neuromuscular disorders associated with hypotonia (e.g. muscular dystrophies) or incoordination (e.g. cerebral palsy). Children with Robin sequence may present with severe airway obstruction within hours of birth but often present after an asymptomatic interval of several weeks with obstruction during sleep or apparent life-threatening episodes. OSAS has also been described in association with obesity in children, e.g. Prader–Willi syndrome.

Symptoms commonly described by parents of children with OSAS include snoring, episodes of apnea during sleep, mouth breathing, restless sleep with frequent waking, abnormal sleeping positions and occasionally daytime somnolence. However, the elevated arousal threshold of children with OSAS compared with adults, probably results in less reported daytime somnolence in children with this condition. On the other hand, subcortical arousals and autonomic disturbances seen on polygraphic sleep studies in children with OSAS with a reduction in the proportion of time spent in REM sleep may be associated with adverse effects on behavior and cognitive performance described in these children. Less common symptoms include nocturnal enuresis in older children, morning headaches, attention deficit, hyperactivity, developmental delay, hypertension and poor growth. Although overt failure to thrive is uncommon in children with OSAS, it is not unusual to document a growth spurt after adenotonsillectomy. This may be mediated by insulin like growth factor (IGF-1), which has been demonstrated to increase following adenotonsillectomy for OSAS.[134]

The presentation of OSAS in children with cor pulmonale is now a rare occurrence due to increased recognition and earlier diagnosis of OSAS. However, asymptomatic pulmonary hypertension has been described in over one-third of children with clinically diagnosed OSAS.[135]

The diagnosis of OSAS is strongly suggested by a history of persistent snoring and breathing difficulty during sleep or obstructive apneas observed by parents. However, clinical history in combination with ENT examination has been shown to have low sensitivity and specificity compared with polysomnography for the diagnosis of OSAS. Most pediatric units have the facility to carry out continuous recordings of respiratory motion, oxygen saturation (SpO_2), and some proxy for nasal airflow using either a nasal thermistor or end-tidal CO_2 measurements. Such recordings have relatively high false negative rates and detailed polygraphic studies (polysomnography or PSG) using age-appropriate diagnostic criteria[136] may be required for definitive diagnosis. The typical appearances of an obstructive apnea demonstrated by PSG are shown in Figure 18.20.

The majority of children with OSAS in association with adenotonsillar hypertrophy will have resolution of their symptoms after adenotonsillectomy. For children with persistent OSAS after adenotonsillectomy or those with obstruction in the absence of large tonsils and adenoids, other treatment options include the use of nasopharyngeal airways, particularly helpful for infants with Robin sequence, or nasal continuous positive airway pressure (nCPAP). The latter has been used successfully and is well tolerated by infants and children.[138] For many children, this treatment can be administered safely at home but should be re-evaluated on a regular basis as CPAP requirements are likely to change with growth. Surgical interventions, such as uvulopalatopharyngoplasty, have been used successfully in children with cerebral palsy and hypotonia of the upper airway but have not been studied in otherwise uncomplicated children with OSAS. Severe and persisting OSAS that has not responded to nCPAP may rarely necessitate consideration of tracheostomy.

The long term outcome of OSAS in children is not well described. It is possible that OSAS presents in subjects who are predisposed to airway obstruction at a time when adenotonsillar size is maximal in proportion to airway diameter and one study has documented recurrence of OSAS in 13% of adolescents who had previously undergone adenotonsillectomy.[139]

ASTHMA

WHAT IS ASTHMA?

There is no universally accepted clinical definition of asthma, although several descriptive definitions have been devised for epidemiological studies. These generally include spontaneous variation of airway caliber over time and response to inhaled bronchodilator. Two pathophysiological features of the disease are generally agreed: airway inflammation and increased airway

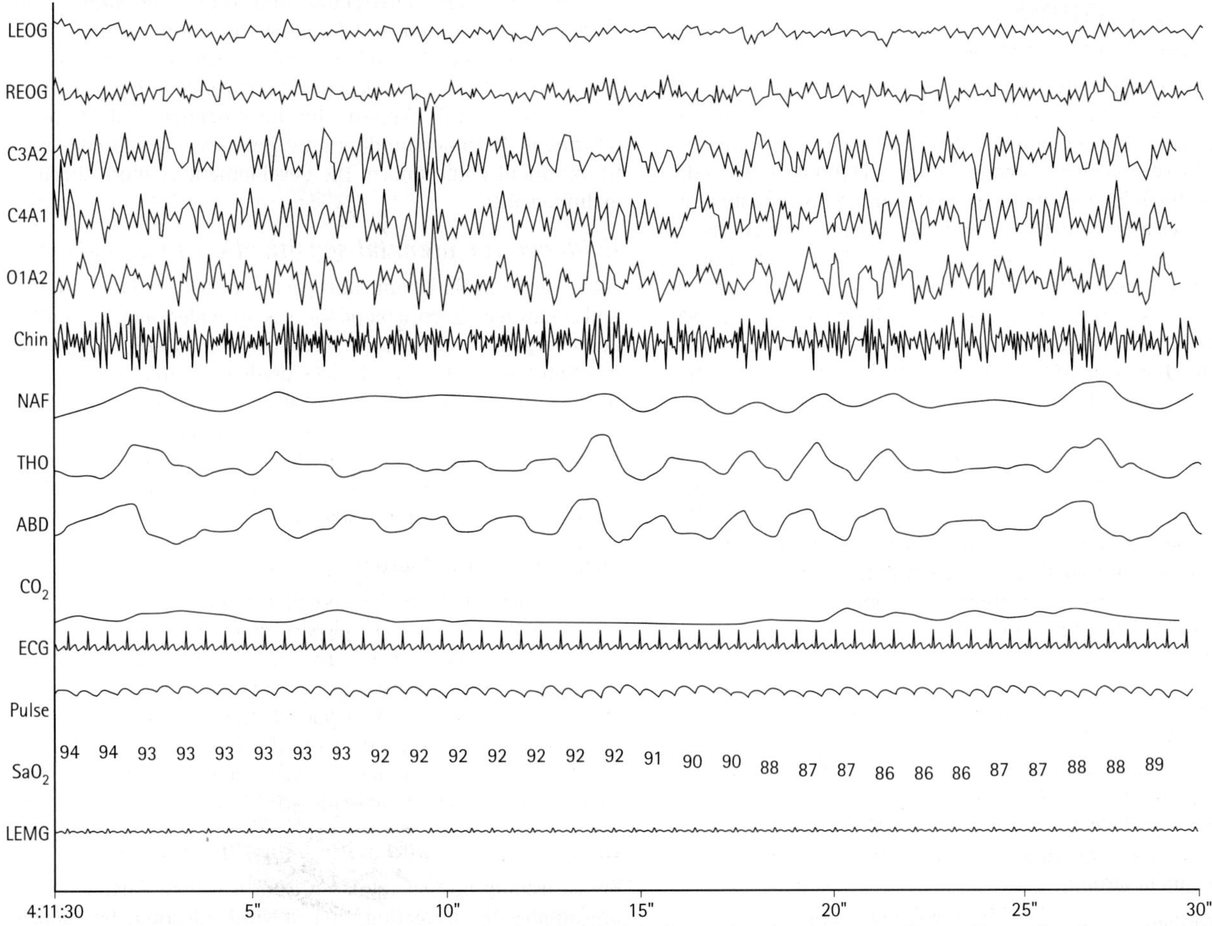

Fig. 18.20 Portion of a polysomnogram from an 18-month-old girl with obstructive sleep apnea syndrome. The patient has a short obstructive apnea of 8 s duration. Despite the brevity of the event, it is associated with significant desaturation (86%). Note also the lack of EEG arousal in response to the obstruction. The SaO_2 at the beginning of the event is slightly low due to a preceding apnea. A second, single-breath obstruction is also seen. The end-tidal PCO_2 channel is partially obstructed and not picking up well in this epoch.
LEOG and REOG, left and right electro-oculograms; C3A2, C4A1, and O1A2, EEG channels; Chin, submental EMG; NAF, oronasal airflow; THO, thoracic movement; ABD, abdominal movement; CO_2, end-tidal PCO_2; Pulse, oximeter pulse waveform; SaO_2, arterial oxygen saturation; LEMG, tibial EMG. (From Marcus 2001[137] with permission)

reactivity. In children there are at least two phenotypes of wheezing disorder, one which affects predominantly preschool children where 60% of children are not atopic and one which is the classic phenotype of atopic asthma developing during childhood and making up 90% of asthma in schoolchildren. Some authorities would reserve the term asthma for this second phenotype.[140] The term atopic as applied to asthma is similarly vague. It is a combination of family history positivity for allergic disease, personal atopic history or skin prick test (SPT) positivity to aeroallergens. In a research context, atopy could be defined as skin prick test positivity to one common aeroallergen with a wheal of > 3 mm in children over 3 years.

The nature of the inflammation in the atopic and non-atopic phenotypes appears to be different (Table 18.8) although there are very few age-matched studies available.[142] In the atopic group, eosinophils and mast cells predominate in bronchoalveolar lavage fluid suggesting eosinophilic inflammation of the mucosa. The neutrophil appears to be the dominant cell type in non-atopic wheeze.[143]

There are many disorders that share some of the features of inflammation and airway reactivity with asthma. These include chronic obstructive airway disease in adults, chronic lung disease of prematurity and bronchiectasis.

WHO DEVELOPS ASTHMA?

Genetics (see also pp. 719 – Genetic determinants)

There is an increased chance of becoming asthmatic if either parent has a history of asthma or atopy although maternal disease appears to confer greater risk. Further analysis of parental influence suggests that maternal asthma affects predominantly preschool wheeze (odds ratio (OR) 5.0) whilst both maternal and paternal asthma increase the risk for later asthma (ORs 4.6 and 4.1). These observations are supported by a study of SPT positive and negative asthma at age 6 years. Both parents contribute to SPT positive asthma but only the mother to SPT negative wheeze. Epidemiological studies suggest family inheritance of lung function, bronchodilator responsiveness and different modes of inheritance for asthma, eczema and hay fever.[144] In industrialized countries with a Western lifestyle, sensitization to perennial aeroallergens is strongly associated with asthma, whereas sensitization to seasonal aeroallergens is closely related to allergic rhinitis. Asthma, allergic rhinitis, and eczema are multifactorial diseases brought about by various familial and environmental influences. Children are more likely to inherit the same allergic disorder that their parents have than a different allergic disorder. Clearly the expression of disease is a reflection of the multifactorial roles of genetics and the environment.

Table 18.8 Wheeze and atopic asthma

Preschool wheeze	Atopic asthma
Maternal influence through genetic effects or intrauterine environment	Possible predominant paternal influence
Smaller airways suggested from lung function at birth*	Normal size airways at birth*
About 40% atopic	About 90% atopic
Large proportion become asymptomatic at school age – 'transient early wheeze'	Symptoms start later - 'late onset wheeze' – or persist from early childhood
Predominantly neutrophil inflammation	Eosinophilic inflammation

* Martinez et al 1991[141]

In addition to the epidemiological evidence, there are many biological studies that have provided evidence for genetic predisposition to asthma.

Genome screens have demonstrated the likely complexity and polygenetic nature of the heritable risk factors of asthma and associated phenotypes of atopy and bronchial hyperresponsiveness (BH).[145,146] Regions of interest that have received particular attention are 5q and 11q. It has been demonstrated that a trait for an elevated level of serum total IgE is coinherited with a trait for BH and that a gene governing BH is located near a major locus that regulates serum IgE levels on chromosome 5q. These findings are consistent with the existence of one or more genes on chromosome 5q31–33 contributing to susceptibility to asthma.[147] In one study of a random group of families, markers on 5q and 11q were related to BH and total IgE.[148] However, the linkage of IgE and BH and chromosome 5q23–33 markers has not been confirmed in other populations or in studies of atopic families. It seems that the identification of a relevant locus or loci for atopy let alone asthma is likely to be some way off. Candidate gene studies are appearing in ever increasing numbers and many of the reported associations are likely to be confounded by geographical and racial variation in allelic frequencies and complex gene/gene and gene/environmental interactions.[149]

Whatever the outcome of the searches for genomic regions of interest and candidate genes and their contribution to the expression of asthma and atopy there is intense interest in the genetic determinants of response to therapy. Beta-2 receptor polymorphisms and glucocorticoid resistance are two such genetic traits that could explain the heterogeneity of response to treatment.[150] Understanding how genetics can influence response to treatment could inform the development of more specific anti-asthma drugs.

Evidence for prenatal sensitization to aeroallergens

Although house-dust mite antigen can be detected in amniotic fluid and cat antigen in cord blood there is no evidence of IgE antibody to aeroallergens in cord blood. Total cord blood IgE does not predict wheezing at 4 years but it does predict eczema and aeroallergen sensitization defined by SPT. There is some evidence of Th2-lymphocyte proliferation in cord blood reflecting activation by specific aeroallergens[38,151] and although small amounts of mRNA to IL-4 and IL-5 have been detected the significance of this observation is unclear (Fig. 18.21).

Other prenatal factors

From studies of lung function at birth and their relationship to wheezing in childhood, it appears that maternal smoking during pregnancy is related to poorer function, probably due to smaller airways, and an increased risk of wheezing illnesses in preschool children.[22,141] There is no evidence that allergen modification of prenatal diet has any effect on the development of asthma.[152] Whether children of mothers who have low antioxidants in their diet have more wheezing is under investigation.

Breast-feeding and wheezing illness

Breast-feeding protects children from transient early wheezing,[153] presumably by protecting against viral infection, but appears to increase the risk of asthma in children over 6 years, but only if the children are atopic and their mothers asthmatic.

The 'hygiene' hypothesis

The type of T cell memory that develops against allergens is currently believed to be the result of complex interactions between environmental and genetic susceptibility factors, which occur postnatally when the naive immune system directly confronts the outside environment. However, Th2-skewed responses to common environmental allergens, comprising IL-4, IL-5, IL-6, IL-9 and IL-13, are present in virtually all newborn infants and are dominated by high level production of IL-10 (Fig. 18.21). Moreover, these responses are demonstrable within 24 h of culture initiation, arguing against a significant contribution from covert in vitro T cell priming and/or differentiation. These findings imply that the key etiologic factor in atopic disease may not be the initial acquisition of allergen-specific Th2-lymphocyte skewed immunity per se, but instead may be the efficiency of immune deviation mechanisms, which in normal (non-atopic) individuals redirect these fetal immune responses toward the Th1 cytokine phenotype.[154] Infection seems to be the most efficient promotor of a Th1-lymphocyte response.

Children who are in nursery in the first 6 months of life suffer more viral illnesses and up to the age of 2 years have more wheezing illnesses, presumably reflecting respiratory viral infections. Despite the increased risk of viral illnesses and wheezing before 2 years, more siblings and early attendance at nursery before 4 months of age are associated with a reduction of wheezing illnesses at age 6 years. This supports the promotion of an immunological balance in favor of Th1 from a very early age. However, if nursery is entered after age 1 year there is no effect on asthma.

Whereas the variations in allergic sensitization with family size and economic status are clear,[155] the relationship between infection and asthma is less clear and it has been difficult to relate specific infections to a reduction in atopy.

Infection with RSV results in more wheezing illness and more bronchial reactivity.[39] In children with mild illness wheezing is greatest in the first 2 years but can last until 11 years.[156] There is not an increased risk of allergic sensitization however. There is likely to be a complex relationship between a genetic influence on the response to RSV and persistent airway reactivity but it does not seem to be related to family history of atopy.

Exposure to house dust mite and pets

In a group of children who had a family history of asthma, house dust mite (HDM) exposure in infancy was related to asthma at 11 years.[157] However, in a longitudinal study of a birth cohort, there was no relationship between early indoor exposure to either cat or HDM antigen and asthma.[7] Although it is possible to reduce exposure to dust mite it remains to be seen whether reduction to exposure reduces symptoms after asthma and house dust mite allergy are established.[158] Although sensitization to HDM is prominent in urbanized Western cultures, sensitization may occur to many other aeroallergens and is probably dependent on their local prevalence. For instance, at high altitudes, where HDM are sparse, asthma is prevalent and the commonest sensitization is to cat allergens. Sensitization to cat allergen may be dependent on the timing of exposure as children exposed to pets during the first year of life have been shown to have a lower frequency of allergic rhinitis at 7–9 years of age and of asthma at 12–13 years. Also, children exposed to cat during the first year of life are less often SPT positive to cat at 12–13 years.[159] Therefore, it seems that early exposure to cats may induce tolerance to cat antigen. However, children who become sensitized to cat allergen are likely to be symptomatic and there remains the problem of how to advise high-risk parents about early allergen exposure. It cannot be said with authority whether exposure is adverse, beneficial or makes no difference to the likelihood of the child developing asthma or atopic disease.

Rural children. Rural dwelling children seem to have much less asthma than urban dwelling children. Perhaps there is reduced atopy in farming families but there are other explanations such as greater exposure to bacterial infection or differences in diet and intestinal microflora in farming populations.[160]

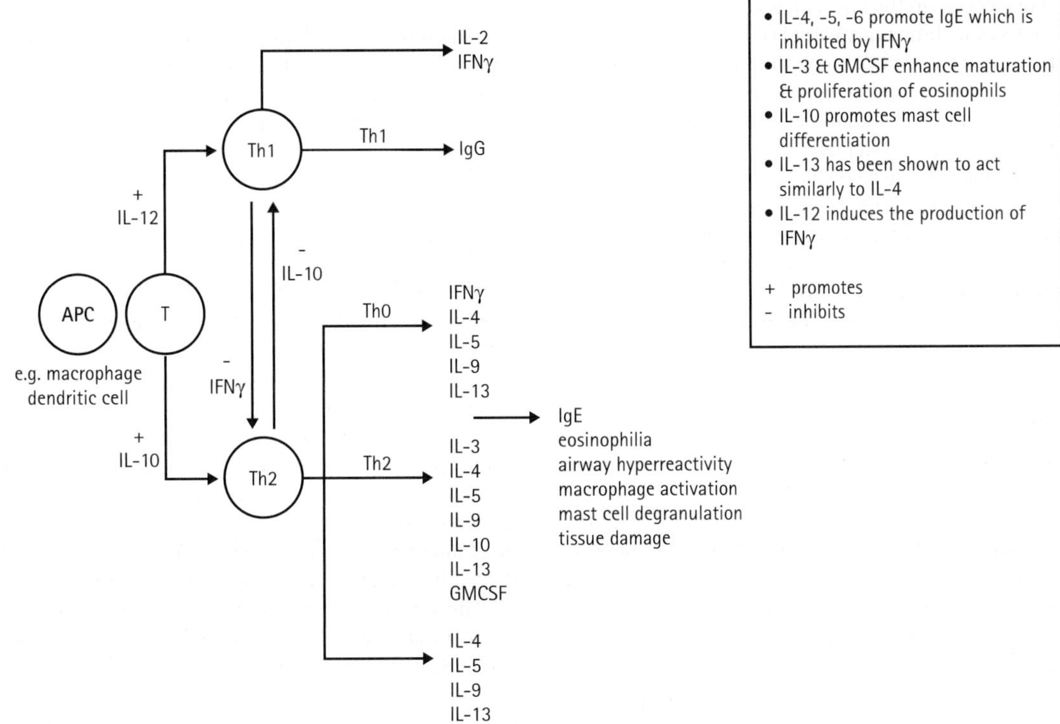

Fig. 18.21 Mechanisms and network of cellular and cytokine responses involved in allergic disease. APC, antigen presenting cell; GMCSF, granulocyte macrophage colony-stimulating factor.

Antibiotics and intestinal flora

The frequent prescription of antibiotics, likely to alter gut flora in young children, has been linked to the observation that gut flora differ between atopic and non-atopic children, with more lactobacilli in the non-atopic group. The lifetime prevalence of asthma is increased four times in children who have had antibiotics in the first year of life and this is related to the number of courses.[161]

HOW COMMON IS ASTHMA?

The prevalence of asthma increased throughout the 1990s but the major increase appears to have been in the reporting of mild symptoms.[162,163] There is some concern about the classification of asthma based on responses to questions about 'current' wheeze or 'ever' wheeze in children because of the potential for recall bias by parents forgetting about symptoms. Currently, about 15% of parents in the United Kingdom report wheeze in their children. There is no doubt there is an increase in atopy.[164] It is difficult to know how much use of medication has prevented an increase in moderate and severe asthma.

The prevalence of asthma has been measured using questionnaires, most notably the International Study of Asthma and Allergies in Childhood (ISAAC) questionnaire[165] but basing the *diagnosis* of asthma on a questionnaire alone has been challenged.[166] Questionnaires have also been used to measure *severity* and it is here that their use is better validated.[167] The use of a symptom diary to assess severity assumes that the diagnosis has been made, including objective measurements.

The prevalence of asthma has been measured by questionnaires that asked about wheeze frequency, cough, other evidence of atopy and severity. There is some evidence that the prevalence of reported wheeze and sensitization to aeroallergens is still increasing in Australia and in Europe. An Australian group has shown that 16% of 8–11 year olds report wheeze in the last year, whereas over 30% have had a doctor diagnosis of asthma and nearly 50% of all children have been prescribed asthma treatment at some time. In epidemiological studies misclassification due to random reporting error is not likely to influence prevalence calculations, although it may influence the care the patient is given. If there is a systematic reporting error – over or under-reporting – this will influence prevalence.

There has been a wide variation in the questions included in asthma questionnaires[168] and it has been suggested that about 20% of respondents who are parents of children who have been labeled wheezy have misunderstood what wheeze is. Parents of different ethnicities describe respiratory sounds differently and so it will be difficult to compare prevalence studies based on questionnaires in different ethnic groups.

Why has asthma increased?

The number of children in families together with the decrease in childhood illnesses, the increase in atopy because of exposure of predisposed children to allergens such as house dust mite, and the use of antibiotics are among the many reasons cited for an increase in asthma and atopy.[155] Whilst overdiagnosis may be partly responsible, the increase in atopy over the last 20 years within the same families suggests a real increase.[169]

BRONCHIAL LABILITY AND AIRWAY INFLAMMATION

Bronchial hyperresponsiveness (BH) refers to the liability of the asthmatic airway to respond to a given stimulus with a greater degree of narrowing than the non-asthmatic airway. It has been suggested that a measure of BH should be made in the diagnosis and monitoring of asthma. No test, whether bronchial challenge (pp. 727 – Measurement of brochial responsiveness) or other testing, will perfectly discriminate between asthmatics and non-asthmatics. The choice of test will depend, among other things, on the sensitivity and specificity profile for diagnosing asthma in the age of the child being tested, the lung function test to be used to measure response, remembering children under 5 years are unlikely to be able to undertake conventional spirometry or peak flow measurements, and the conditions which testing demands. Bronchial challenge testing may be *specific* (allergen-induced) or *non-specific* to variety of physical or chemical stimuli. The former is rarely if ever carried out in children and is potentially hazardous.

Exercise-induced bronchoconstriction

Many children with asthma or with preschool wheeze have exercise-induced wheezing or breathing difficulty. Airway narrowing due to exercise and hyperventilation is mediated both by the alteration of the osmotic environment of the airway and by airway cooling. For testing, free running for 6 min on a treadmill with a slope of 10% and a speed of 5 kph is sufficient exercise. A positive test, as seen in the majority of children with untreated asthma, will result in a fall in peak expiratory flow (PEF) or forced expiratory volume in 1 second (FEV_1) in the majority of children with untreated asthma. A beta-agonist taken before exercise will prevent this decrease in lung function. The balanced sensitivity and specificity profile is 75%/75% for a 9% fall in FEV_1.[170] The theoretical population distribution of bronchial reactivity to exercise is shown in Figure 18.22a. The role of exercise testing in the diagnosis of asthma has been controversial as it is considered by some authorities to have too poor a sensitivity and specificity profile. Nevertheless, if a child who complains of difficulty in breathing with exercise is heard to wheeze on exercise testing, this can be very helpful in confirming symptoms and in determining treatment. There are many recommendations for the conditions in which formal exercise testing should be undertaken – control of laboratory temperature and humidity for example – but these are not practical in the average clinical practice. Cold air challenge can imitate exercise-induced bronchoconstriction but this is even more complicated for day-to-day practice. Some children will hyperventilate but the demonstration of bronchoconstriction in response to hyperventilation has never been recommended in the diagnostic workup of asthma.

Non-specific hyperreactivity

Agents which act directly on airway smooth muscle such as methacholine and histamine have been widely used to measure airway reactivity. These enjoy a balanced sensitivity and specificity profile of greater than 80%/80% for a total provoking dose of methacholine of 5.5 mmol for normal children and asthmatics.[170] In Europe and the USA these tests seem to be more widely used than in the UK. It may become necessary for asthma research to report subjects' BH before they are included in a clinical trial. The USA guidelines for the management of asthma[172] suggest that testing for BH could be part of the asthma investigation.

The most sensitive airways respond to very dilute concentrations of a provocative agent and normal children to the most concentrated (Fig. 18.22b). Asthma treatment should result in airways becoming less responsive. The theoretical distribution of responsiveness in a normal population has been derived from a number of studies that have reported the proportions of normal children who respond to different doses of provoking agent.[171] Bronchodilators block the response to nearly all bronchoconstrictor

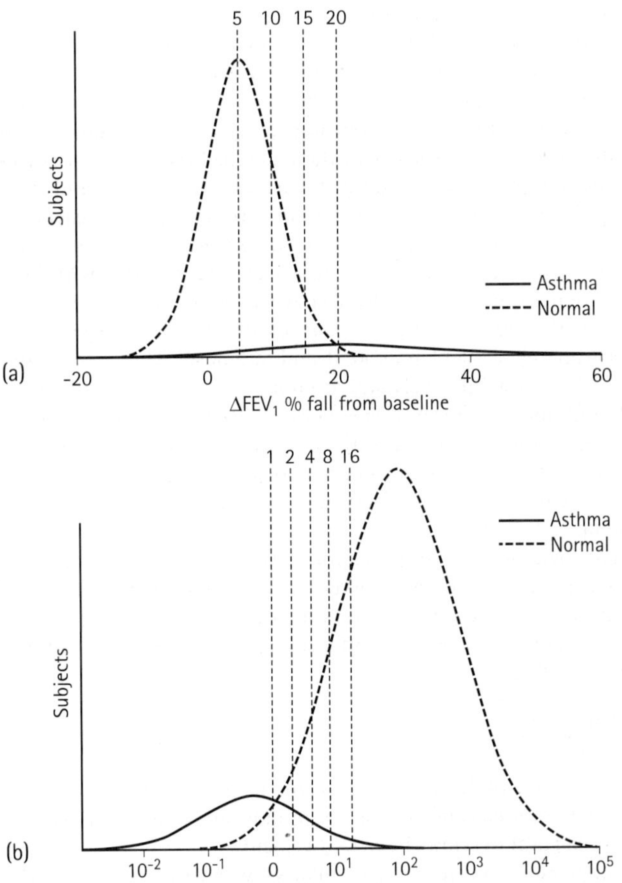

Fig. 18.22 (a) Theoretical population distribution of bronchial reactivity to exercise expressed as fall in FEV_1 based on data for normal children and asthmatics. The height and area under each curve represents the proportional size of the two populations, 90% normal children and 10% asthmatics. The vertical cutoff points represent the numbers of children with falls in FEV_1 5–20% in response to exercise. There is a large overlap between normals and asthmatics. (From Godfrey et al 1999[171] with permission) (b) Theoretical distribution of response to chemical agonist causing a 20% fall in FEV_1. The vertical lines refer to increasing doses of agonist (µmol) causing a 20% fall in FEV_1 (PD20). Children with asthma respond at a lower dose than normals.

challenges by their direct action on smooth muscle. Corticosteroids are less effective at this and take longer to act. Both of these observations explain why beta-agonists are useful immediate protectors of challenge and why lung function and BH may take months to improve following treatment with corticosteroids.

Bronchodilator responsiveness (BDR)

This is also recommended in the USA guidelines for the investigation of asthma. However, unlike testing for BH with non-specific agents, no dose–response effect in children has been evaluated in a population study, something that would be needed if BDR were to be a useful diagnostic test. In the biggest study in children undertaken to date, normal children responded to bronchodilator by an average 2% increase in FEV_1, 9% at most[173] whereas children with moderately severe asthma have an average response of about 9% improvement in FEV_1, 17% at most. The degree of bronchodilation observed in patients is probably related to the test used to measure airway caliber. Measurements of airway resistance are probably more sensitive than forced expiratory maneuvers but it is possible that they are less specific. The real value of BDR as a diagnostic test in children, especially those with mild asthma, has yet to be clarified.

Bronchial inflammation

Examination of bronchial biopsy material and bronchoalveolar lavage fluid are research procedures.[174] Surrogate markers of bronchial inflammation are being developed but these markers relate poorly to measurements of lung function including measurements of BH and do not relate to symptoms. This is not unsurprising, as lung function testing and symptomatology reflect not only airway narrowing due to inflammation but also due to smooth muscle tone. Measurements of BH relate better to symptoms than inflammatory markers. Nitric oxide (NO) is produced in the inflamed airway and concentrations of exhaled NO (eNO) correlate with blood and sputum eosinophils. eNO is increased in asthmatics and responds to treatment with inhaled corticosteroids. Standardized guidelines for the measurement of eNO[175] and standard equipment are available. Sputum eosinophil counts in schoolchildren are only possible in 60% of subjects but this test seems to be more promising, although expensive, as are measurements of serum and urine eosinophil breakdown products (eosinophil cationic protein and eosinophil protein X). The value of surrogate inflammatory markers as either a test for asthma or for monitoring progress in preschool children, 40% of whom do not have atopic asthma, is yet to be described. Children without atopy have lower values than those with positive skin prick tests as might be expected.

WHAT IS NOT ASTHMA?

Bronchiolitis

Whilst the word asthma is still used for preschool non-atopic wheeze, nearly all agree that most wheezing in infants below 1 year old is probably not asthma. The relationship between RSV bronchiolitis and subsequent wheeze remains controversial.[39,156] Children who have more severe symptoms in early life tend to have more atopic illness later,[176] probably because these were children already predisposed to asthma and atopy (see pp. 721 – Early respiratory infections).

Persistent isolated cough (PIC)

This is quite different from asthma. 'Cough-variant' asthma used to be applied to PIC. It seems that, in some children with asthma, cough is dominant but there are usually other features of asthma. Parents of children with asthma do not report cough alone as a symptom.[168] When parents report cough, they are correct[177] and although they can tell when coughing is better or worse they cannot tell by how much. Coughers are no more atopic than normal children.[178] They cough from sleep, are unlikely to sleep less than normal children,[177] benefit very little from high-dose corticosteroids[179] and not at all from bronchodilators.[180]

Shortness of breath

This is not a symptom that defines asthma. Exercise causes shortness of breath – although some parents report that their child is unduly short of breath – and difficulty in breathing at night can be caused by snoring. Obese children complain of difficulty in breathing but have no more bronchial hyperresponsiveness than other children, although girls who become obese between 6 and 11 years do appear to develop bronchial responsiveness. Doctor-diagnosed asthma appears to increase as children become more obese, but this is unrelated to atopy.[181] These two observations question how the diagnosis of asthma was made.

CLINICAL ASTHMA

Children can present at any age. It is acknowledged that asthma is not usually diagnosed in the first year. One way of classifying children who present with wheeze is into transient, persistent and late-onset (Fig. 18.23). Those with transient wheeze are those who are non-atopic and have poorer airway function at birth; those with persistent symptoms are those who have normal airway function at birth and tend to be atopic; those with late-onset asthma are also atopic and have normal airway function at birth.[182]

Diagnosis

The difficulty of the asthma history. The triad of cough, wheeze and difficulty breathing are together the best indicators of childhood asthma. To take only reported wheeze as indicative of asthma risks both under- or overdiagnosing asthma – about 25% of parents with children with asthma do not use what they hear as means of knowing whether their child is wheezy.[168] Some parents call the noise they hear by another name. Difficulty in breathing is how many parents know their child is wheezy, but this symptom is not specific for asthma. Although it is true that older children have night-time symptoms it is unclear in prepubertal children whether night-time respiratory symptoms reflect asthma. A snoring history is rarely taken and the sound of rattly breathing is difficult to convey in language.[183] Isolated cough is a different paradigm. The specificity of exercise-induced wheeze as a reported symptom has not been evaluated for asthma. It is true that most children with asthma will have difficulty in breathing on exercise but so also do unfit and overweight children. Whilst children with atopic asthma are more likely to have parents who have allergic illnesses, the specificity and sensitivity of reported family history is unknown.

It is reasonably easy to agree that a child with recession and wheeze heard on auscultation has asthma, but it is very difficult to be certain in the absence of clinical signs.

Physical examination

In a child on a routine visit to a physician with a history of respiratory symptoms, examination is nearly always normal. Nowadays children usually present and are treated before chest hyperinflation is a problem or growth becomes affected. Other signs of atopy such as eczema may be evident.

Investigations

Other than the measurement of peak expiratory flow (PEF), lung function is rarely undertaken in general practice in the UK.

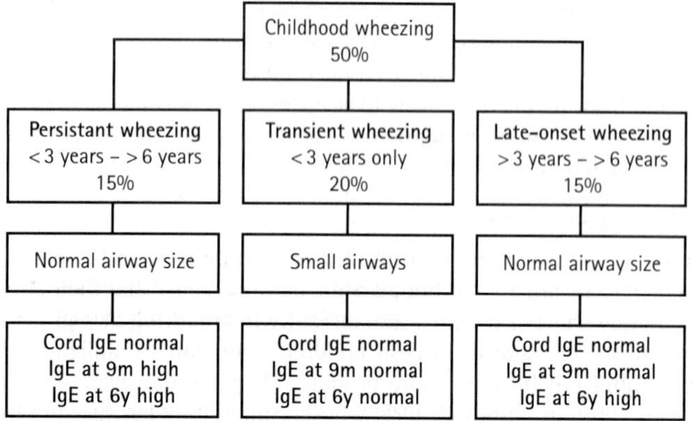

Fig. 18.23 Types of wheezing illness in childhood. Scheme adapted from the Tucson birth cohort (Martinez et al 1995[182]). Note that approximately 50% of children in this whole population study wheezed at some time in their early years. 9m, 9 months; 6y, 6 years.

Although there are new techniques for assessing lung function in preschool children[184] (see also Airway function, p. 726), these are not widely available and are sometimes difficult to interpret. Their place in clinical medicine is still being evaluated. Bronchodilator responsiveness (BDR) of greater than 12% FEV_1 is considered to be highly sensitive for asthma, but there are likely to be false positives in children with chronic lung disease of prematurity and with isolated cough. Routine testing for bronchial responsiveness (pp. 726 – Airway function) for diagnostic purposes is not undertaken routinely in the UK. It is likely that children with high measurements of IgE (> 3000 IU) have asthma but when levels are low (100–400 IU) the measurement has poor specificity. Approximately 10% of persistent and late-onset wheezers are not atopic, have low IgE levels and are not sensitized to aeroallergens. Although most children of school age with significant respiratory symptoms of intermutual breathlessness and wheeze are atopic and have bronchial hyperresponsiveness, objective assessment of these features cannot in themselves confirm or refute the diagnosis of asthma.

The logical approach to diagnosis is to see the child when the carer perceives he/she is symptomatic. It would be reasonable to accept that wheeze on auscultation would merit a bronchodilator and if there was a response then one of the criteria of asthma, airway lability, has been met.

Follow-up

History and examination

A careful plot of height is important in any child with chronic disease. In a disease where corticosteroids are often prescribed it is very important to know the height velocity.

Simple questions to a schoolchild, 'How is your asthma?', 'Have you had difficulty in breathing?', 'Does your asthma stop you doing things?' and 'Does it keep you awake at night?' have been validated with good questionnaire ratings but not against FEV_1.[167] Days missed from school are important and should be recorded as absolute numbers rather than by qualitative answers such as 'a lot' or 'not many' as these mean different things to different parents. Similarly, use of a bronchodilator should be recorded as number of days in the week for actual symptoms, as opposed to prophylactic use.

The keeping of diaries for the recording of symptoms and PEF measurements is only useful if the information recorded is accurate. Asthmatic children and their parents as a group are not good at this and false entries or absent entries are not unusual.[185] Questions such as those outlined above are believed to be more helpful in adults and this could well be the case in children.

Investigations

Traditionally PEF measurements have been used to monitor asthma. These measurements have appeared to be useful because they can be recorded at home. However symptom scoring, PEF measurements and spirometry are poorly concordant and parents and children are not good at recording PEF measurements. PEF may well be useful for individuals however, especially children with poor symptom perception, who may rely on PEF to guide medication.

Spirometry

Measurement of forced expiratory volumes has been considered to be the 'gold standard' for the measurement of lung function. These variables have the best reproducibility of all forced expiratory measurements.[186] Despite this, spirometry is little used in general pediatric practice. There are a number of difficulties. Few pediatricians or family doctors will have been trained in the optimal performance of spirometry and so it is understandable that they should be reluctant to introduce spirometry into their practice. Maintenance and calibration of equipment is also required.

It is important when interpreting repeat measurements to know the day-to-day *repeatability* and the within-occasion repeatability. Within-occasion repeatability, which is considered to reflect repeatability of the measuring instrument, is usually better than between-occasion repeatability, which includes biological variability. In a condition such as asthma, which is characterized by airway lability there are likely to be large between-occasion differences. There is very little information about this in children.[186] A within-occasion repeatability of $< 12\%$ FEV_1 is considered normal. Any change above that, say following a bronchodilator, would be considered abnormal. Within-occasion repeatability can be considered similar for children with no respiratory disease and those with asthma. Between-occasion repeatability measurements for different respiratory function tests in children with and without disease are not readily available. If respiratory function tests are to help with clinical decisions, information about repeatability needs to be readily available. The day-to-day repeatability of FEV_1 is approximately 15% (2 standard deviations of the differences between measurements). If a measurement lies within 15% of the previous measurement, then it cannot be said with 95% certainty that there has been true change.

Spirometry blows should be technically acceptable. The biggest problems are ensuring maximal inspiratory and residual volumes are reached.[187] If they are not, then indices which are referenced to forced vital capacity, such as mid-expiratory flows, cannot be calculated (pp.726 – Airway function).

Adherence to treatment

There is ample evidence that treatment adherence, even in a clinical trial, is poor.[188,189] This is due to poor treatment supervision by parents. Children from poorer socio-economic backgrounds are at greatest disadvantage in this respect. Adolescent asthmatics will readily admit to poor adherence, the reasons given being forgetfulness, belief that the medication is ineffective, denial that they are asthmatic, difficulty using inhalers, inconvenience, fear of side-effects, embarrassment and laziness. Some of these reasons may well apply to parents who are in charge of children's treatment.

Treatment

Guidelines in the USA have been widely ignored[190] and there is little to suggest that the position is different in the UK. Evidence-based medicine is hard to promote. For example, despite a Cochrane review suggesting that there is no evidence for the benefit of inhaled corticosteroids in children with intermittent wheeze,[191] over 60% of preschool boys have been prescribed such treatment.[192] The reason for overprescribing is likely to be a consequence of parental pressure.

Comprehensive evidence-based guidelines for the management of childhood asthma recently became available in the UK.[193]

Education

Recent publications support the role of asthma education and environmental control,[193] although some of this is still controversial. A Cochrane review demonstrated no effect on subsequent admissions of an education program for families of children who had attended an emergency department in the previous 12 months.[194] However, just on the basis of this, it would be illogical not to educate asthmatic families as some will benefit. What then is the best education that can be offered to an average family with a child with asthma? The following statements and educational points are empirical and the education given can be tailored to the family and needs to be given over several consultations.

Allergic asthma (when a child is sensitized to an aeroallergen) will not 'go away' and desensitization to aeroallergens such as pollen is not efficient. Children will always have a tendency to become wheezy if exposed to allergens. Older children will be able to say what upsets them. This is the reason for continuous treatment if allergic children have persistent symptoms.

- Non-allergic asthma – in preschool children – becomes less troublesome in most children after the start of school.
- All children with asthma are likely to become wheezy when they get a cold. There is no place for antibiotics in the treatment of colds because viruses cause these. Please do not ask your doctor for them.
- The mainstay of treatment in children with persistent asthma is prevention with continuous treatment and the dosage will need regular reviewing.
- Early treatment with bronchodilators and oral corticosteroids for children with both intermittent asthma and persistent asthma can prevent hospital admission. Please always make sure you have enough of both.
- No smoking by parents or child.
- Reasonable attempts at reducing damp, mold, house dust mites, cat and dog dander should be made. (There is no evidence yet that this makes any difference[195] although there are many studies which suggest that dampness is an adverse risk factor for asthma.)
- Understanding what drugs are supposed to do and how to take them. Bronchodilators relax the muscle in the airway. They work for 8 h, some longer. They are given via an inhaler. Nebulizers are no more helpful than spacers.
- Prednisolone tablets may take 6 h to work. They take the swelling out of the airways.
- Inhaled corticosteroids reduce airway inflammation in children who have allergic asthma and in a few others. The doses recommended should not produce side-effects but it is important to have growth monitored regularly.

Bronchodilators

It is axiomatic that short-acting bronchodilators are the cornerstone of treatment. In view of the wide choice of devices for inhaled delivery there is little or no place for oral bronchodilators, which can produce significant systemic effects such as tachycardia and tremor. The only exceptions would be in infants and very young children in whom there are genuine difficulties in delivery of drugs by the inhaled route.

Beta-agonists

Inhaled beta-agonists can be given by a metered dose aerosol via a spacer device or in children over 6 years by a breath-actuated inhaler or dry powder device. Spacers should be washed only once a month and air-dried as more frequent washing and friction increase the electrostatic charge on the inside wall and so reduce the amount of the dose delivered. Puffs should be given one at a time with five breaths for each. Tidal breathing is all that is necessary. CFC-free inhalers are now available and should be used in preference. For beta-agonists the dosage need not be altered. There is little to choose between the short-acting beta-agonists available in the UK.

Long-acting beta-agonists

These drugs should be used in conjunction with inhaled corticosteroids (ICS). At present there is no evidence of their value as monotherapy in adults. Long-acting beta 2-agonists are corticosteroid sparing and can help reduce the dosage of ICS by half.[196] In this respect these drugs are particularly helpful in treating difficult asthma.

Sodium cromoglycate

This drug is an anti-inflammatory preparation but its use is no longer fashionable. One major disadvantage of this drug is that it is recommended that it is given four times each day. This is because it blocks exercise-induced wheezing for 4–6 hours. No good trials that include preschool children have been undertaken to investigate whether there is benefit in taking it twice a day. Current evidence suggests that it is of little benefit for the treatment of persistent asthma.[197]

Nedocromil

This drug has been promoted as a treatment for exercise-induced asthma. There is no difference in effect between it and sodium cromoglycate although there is some benefit over ICS given in a moderate dose. In favor of nedocromil is its absence of effect on growth.[198]

Ipratropium

This is an anticholinergic drug and can be used three times a day. It is used mainly in the management of acute severe asthma where together with salbutamol and corticosteroids its use can reduce hospital admission rates.[199]

Inhaled corticosteroids (ICS)

There is ample evidence for the effect of these drugs on atopic asthma. There is however no proven benefit for children with non-atopic asthma. Although preschool children with persistent asthma benefit as a group[200] the analysis of the atopic and non-atopic subgroups in this study has rarely been undertaken. For children with intermittent preschool wheeze benefit was only in the aeroallergen sensitized group.[201] Provided dosages are equipotent, it appears to be unimportant which ICS preparation is prescribed. Doses should be carefully titrated. In children with mild to moderate asthma adverse effects on linear growth are apparent even in dosages of 400 μg/day of either budesonide[198] or beclometasone.[202] It remains unclear whether the decrement in growth is sustained or whether it reverses with 'catch up' after therapy is discontinued. Most of the efficacy of fluticasone in adults and adolescents with moderate to severe asthma is achieved at a dose of 100–250 μg/day, with a maximum effect at around 500 μg/day.[203] This may be the reason that adding a long acting beta-agonist is more efficacious than increasing the dose of fluticasone beyond 500 μg/day.

Since absorption and adrenal suppression in adult patients prescribed ICS are dependent on whether or not they have asthma[204] it seems wise to be certain of the diagnosis first. Although accumulating evidence shows that asthmatic children, even when they have been treated with ICS for years, attain normal adult height, there are individual rare cases where ICS use is associated with clinically relevant growth suppression. Regular and careful measurement and plotting of height is essential. Reports of adrenal suppression emphasize the need for careful evaluation of patient response to ICS. Spacer devices should be used in all children up to 6 years for the delivery of ICS and for older children on dosages over 400 μg/day of beclometasone or equivalent, spacers are recommended. Without spacers there is significant oropharyngeal deposition of the drug.[193]

Antileukotrienes

Currently, the most compelling evidence from published trials suggests that leukotriene receptor antagonists can be used as add-on therapy to inhaled corticosteroids to allow tapering of corticosteroid dose and reduction in beta-agonist use.[205] There may also be a role for these agents as first-line therapy in young children with mild asthma.

Immunotherapy

Although desensitization to allergens has been a long-established procedure, there is little evidence that asthmatic children benefit from desensitization. It is not established management for asthma in the UK.

Anti-IgE monoclonal antibody

This is a promising new treatment for severe allergic asthma. Its place is probably in the treatment of difficult asthma. It appears to be safe and is given every 2–4 weeks as a subcutaneous injection. In a group of children on modest doses of ICS there was a steroid-sparing effect.[206]

Complementary therapy. The Cochrane reviews on the value of breathing exercises, acupuncture, Alexander technique, 'manual' therapies, such as physiotherapy and osteopathy indicate that these have no benefit or no proven benefit because too few acceptable trials have been undertaken.

Inhalers for children[207]

The vast majority (> 90%) of childhood inhaled asthma medication is prescribed and delivered using pressurized metered dose inhalers (pMDIs). The real benefits of pMDIs lie in their relatively low cost and their ease and portability of use. However, due to the need to coordinate the actuation of the device with inhalation, these devices, when used alone, are not suited to children under 5 years. Typically pMDIs are combined with a spacer device, to aid the inhalation of the drug, ensuring a better disposition to the lung. Spacer devices with masks for young children have a typical lifespan of 6–12 months.

Although breath-actuated pMDIs are available, reducing the physical requirements for coordinated inhalation, their use in children is often hampered by the reaction of children to the sound and feel of the device as it activates.

Newer dry-powder inhalation systems (DPIs) are also generally believed to improve drug deposition to the lung (around 30% of dose compared to only 10–20% with pMDIs) and as such suggest both clinical and cost benefits. The portability of DPIs compared to pMDIs + spacers is seen as an attraction, as is the increased ability to monitor closely delivered dosage. However, the relatively low inspiratory flow in younger children can cause problems with their use as DPI systems rely on the patient's own inhalation to disperse the drug. The use of dry-powder systems is generally not advised in children under 5 years, although there may be individual cases where there is a clear justification for their use if it can be shown that the child can operate the system correctly and can receive the correct dosage to the lung.

There is evidence that ICS delivered using DPI devices cause more systemic side-effects than by pMDI (especially with large volume spacer) devices hence the British Thoracic Society guideline recommendations to avoid DPIs for corticosteriod delivery in children. For beta-agonists, dosages delivered by DPI, pMDI and breath-actuated inhalers are equivalent.[207] Beta-agonists delivered by breath-actuated inhalers are preferred by schoolchildren as they are easier to carry and are associated with fewer stigmata.

Nebulizers are significantly more costly to operate than other inhalation devices and thus their use is now largely reserved for the treatment of acute asthma in patients who are so severely affected that they cannot use inhaled pMDI based treatment.[208]

DIFFICULT ASTHMA

The problems of 'difficult' asthmatic children seem to fall into four categories: alternative diagnoses such as laryngeal dysfunction and obliterative bronchiolitis, poor treatment adherence, true corticosteroid unresponsive asthma, over-reporting of symptoms by either children or their parents[174] or exacerbated by other conditions (see Other wheezing illness, p. 759).

The diagnosis of childhood asthma is usually made only on the reporting of symptoms by parents, without any objective evidence of airway disease in the child. Treatment is adjusted according to the reported symptoms. If these are either overestimated or overinterpreted, treatment can be increased and management considered 'difficult'. It might be helpful then to consider difficult asthma as **either** recurrent observed wheezing poorly responsive to treatment with the demonstration of poor lung function where this is possible **or** frequently reported respiratory symptoms consistent with asthma, apparently poorly responsive to treatment.

Deaths from asthma in children

Death is unusual (Fig. 18.24). In the 1980s it was thought to be associated with either poor medical or parental supervision of treatment.[209] Sudden unexpected deaths in children are probably now rare. The impression is that children who die have difficult asthma and either are poorly supervised or have a sudden severe terminal episode on a background of poor lung function.

Brittle asthma or chronic poor lung function?

Severity has traditionally been considered in terms of drug dosage needed to control symptoms. It should be possible in schoolchildren to discover whether lung function is consistently poor with reversibility to beta-agonists or whether attacks are frequent and intermittent with good function in between. 'Difficult' asthma is probably a heterogeneous condition requiring better definition of causation.

Persistent wheezing in infants (<1 year old) and preschool children.

Some infants with so-called post-bronchiolitic wheeze, recurrent wheeze with viral infections, or persistent wheeze, have small airways[182] and like preschool wheezy children the majority are not atopic. In infants this is difficult to be sure about. However unlike their older counterparts, infants and non-atopic preschool children respond poorly to treatment. Unlike older children with difficult asthma, very few of these infants require hospital admission because of hypoxemia but because they are unresponsive to drug treatment they are perceived as 'difficult'.

Definition

The following seems to be a reasonable definition of poor control. A child with difficult asthma is one who requires ≥800 μg/day beclometasone or budesonide or ≥ 400 μg fluticasone or >1 mg/kg/alternate days prednisolone *and* requiring bronchodilators (additional to any long-acting beta-agonists they may already be taking) on 3 days every week for wheezing with related proven poor lung function (< 80% FEV_1) and reversibility *or* one proven episode requiring additional steroids every month *or* school absence > 5 days/term because of asthma.

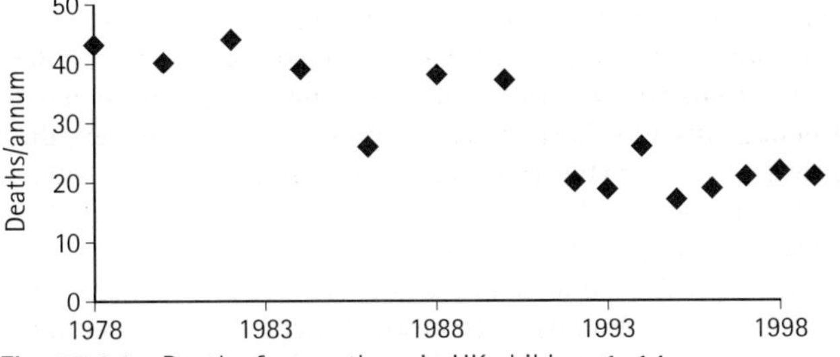

Fig. 18.24 Deaths from asthma in UK children 1–14 years.

Radiographs should be reviewed for evidence of bronchiolitis obliterans, bronchiectasis, bronchogenic cyst and so on. Ventilation/perfusion and CT scans may be needed for clarification.

Vocal cord dysfunction especially in conjunction with asthma can be confusing.[210] This is a condition that is considered psychogenic, can be mistaken as 'difficult' asthma and result in an unnecessary increase in treatment. The so-called wheeze has a large inspiratory element and abnormalities on inspiratory flow volume curves may be apparent on spirometry. If the diagnosis cannot be made by a good history then laryngoscopy may be necessary to look for thickened vocal cords.

Poor treatment adherence is quite common. Supervision of treatment at home, checking of prescribing treatment in the community, the collecting of prescriptions at the chemist can all be checked. It is certainly a matter of opinion, but without objective evidence, that no treatment or too much treatment is given in order to demonstrate 'severity' so that the family can claim disability living allowance. Both practices are child protection issues but because of the difficulty of providing evidence there is little documentation of these practices.

True severe and difficult asthma with frequent school absence, hospital admissions and little response in lung function and/or symptoms causes a lot of morbidity in a few children. These may be children who are highly atopic or who appear to have fixed lung function abnormalities.[174,211] True corticosteroid resistance is fortunately very rare and very difficult to prove. Alternative treatment with ciclosporin has proven benefit in adults and has been used in children.[212] Treatments such as methotrexate and immunoglobulin infusions have not been properly tested. In small open unrandomized studies some children seem to benefit.

OTHER WHEEZING ILLNESSES

Chronic chest infection

Chronic chest infection and the associated inflammation is related to airways hyperreactivity. Cystic fibrosis (p. 763) can present as a wheezing illness, disclosed by RSV or other viral infection. Whether children with persistent wheeze (p. 744 – Persistent wheezing) are all investigated for CF remains a clinical decision. Poor weight gain, isolation of *Staphylococcus aureus* from secretions, prolonged oxygen requirement and persistent patchy changes on the chest radiograph would all suggest that further investigation should be undertaken. Bronchiectasis (p. 783) and ciliary dyskinesia (p. 783) both predispose to wheeze but the clinical feature that predominates is cough and sputum production. Treatment is of the primary problem with antibiotics and physiotherapy with bronchodilators if necessary. Immunoglobulin deficiency (or immunoglobulin subclass deficiency) is often considered as a cause of persistent wheeze but this is rarely the case. Immune deficiencies usually present in the chest with persistent changes suggestive of bacterial infection (p. 784 – Immunodeficiency).

Congenital abnormalities (see p. 787 – Congenital abnormalities)

Rare intrabronchial or mediastinal lesions can cause wheezing in infants by airway narrowing or compression. Abnormal vessels and intrathoracic masses such as bronchogenic cyst, teratoma, neuroblastoma, sequestration and even cardiomegaly can cause extrabronchial compression and tachypnea in early infancy. Isolated wheezing is very unusual. Intrabronchial lesions include bronchomalacia and bronchial stenosis. Some are associated with congenital lobar emphysema. Chest radiography in an infant who has unexplained respiratory symptoms may show focal signs but often the diagnosis can only be made on bronchoscopy. Children with the H-type tracheoesophageal fistula can present with recurrent chestiness. Chest radiographs will demonstrate abnormalities consistent with atelectasis and pneumonia, identical to those in children with recurrent aspiration due to gastroesophageal reflux.

Foreign body inhalation

In children who have a first episode of wheezing over the age of 1 year this is the main differential diagnosis. In 80% there will be a history of wheezing. There are usually, but not always, asymmetric abnormalities on the chest radiograph, most often hyperinflation on the side of the foreign body, about 60% on the right. Decision about bronchoscopy should be made on the history, i.e. of choking with related onset of wheeze. Suspicion of a foreign body should be aroused when wheezing does not respond to treatment with bronchodilators.

Gastroesophageal reflux (GOR)

GOR can contribute to asthma either by a vagally mediated reflex mechanism or, rarely, by aspiration. In infants who wheeze recurrently the question of aspiration arises more frequently. Most children under 18 months with recurrent respiratory symptoms are wheezy. There is no association between indices that describe the amount of acid reflux and measures the degree of abnormality in lung function.[213] What matters may be the individual responsiveness to GOR, not how much GOR there is. Whilst treatment of reflux is associated with improvement in certain groups of patients, particularly those with pneumonia, the evidence is less convincing for asthma and wheezing disorders in infants. Where there is radiographic evidence supporting a diagnosis of aspiration, then appropriate investigations for GOR are justified. There is however no good radiological technique which reliably demonstrates aspiration. There is at present nothing to support the routine investigation for GOR in infants and children with persistent wheezing. In asthmatic children who also have gastroesophageal reflux there is no overall improvement in asthma following treatment for gastroesophageal reflux.[214]

ACUTE ASTHMA

An acute exacerbation of asthma is an episode of increased cough and difficulty in breathing not completely relieved by the usual dose of bronchodilator (Fig.18.25). There are multiple triggers, most commonly intercurrent viral illness, but also exposure to aeroallergens (house dust mite, cat dander, grass pollen), exercise, emotional stress and non-adherence to preventative treatment. Of children attending hospital for acute asthma, about 25% are children with their first episode of severe wheeze. In the UK, between February 1995 and January 1996, 62% of pediatric admissions for acute asthma were < 5 years.[215] In the UK, hospital admissions are less frequent in August, almost certainly reflecting the reduction of viral infections during the holiday season when families are more outdoors.

Since 40% of preschool children with recurrent wheeze are non-atopic, some authorities might prefer to call these children's illnesses 'acute wheezing in a preschool child'. It is likely they will continue to be called asthma, irrespective of age and atopic status.

During an asthma attack, smooth muscle constriction causing bronchial narrowing, inflammation leading to airway mucosal edema and excess mucus secretion contribute to airway obstruction. This causes increased airway resistance. There is reduced ventilation in some areas and absent ventilation in others, because of airway closure. This results in ventilation/perfusion mismatching and hypoxemia, which in turn stimulates ventilation. Carbon dioxide (CO_2) is extremely diffusible and is rapidly washed out of normally ventilated alveoli. As alveolar minute ventilation rises as a result of hypoxemic drive, arterial CO_2 ($PaCO_2$) will fall. However, with continued increased work of breathing, exhaustion sets in and minute ventilation falls, leading to a rise in $PaCO_2$. The treatment of acute asthma is directed at stopping this happening.

Age	Mild/moderate	Severe
1–5 years	SaO_2 > 96% mild SaO_2 93–96% moderate Tachycardia Nasal flare Use of accessory muscles Head retraction Unable to feed	SaO_2 < 93% Confusion and anxiety Fatigue Silent chest
> 5 years	As above plus PEF below 50% of previous best	As above plus PEF below 33% of previous best

Do not compare PEF to predicted values – only compare to child's previous best
Do not use this criterion if it is the child's first ever attempt at PEF

Beware the older child with respiratory rate > 30/min (Tachypnea may reflect pneumothorax or pneumonia)

Fig. 18.25 Assessment of acute asthma.

Postmortem findings demonstrate mucus plugging obstructing airways, widespread epithelial desquamation, subepithelial fibrosis and inflammatory cell infiltration (mainly eosinophils and lymphocytes) in the epithelium, subepithelium and airway lumen. There is also smooth muscle hyperplasia and edema of bronchial walls. A nearly universal finding is hyperinflation due to gas trapping distal to obstructed airways.

Prevention of acute attacks is the cornerstone of asthma treatment. For children < 5 years it is recommended that inhaled medicines are administered from a pressurized metered-dose inhaler (pMDI) and spacer, using a face mask if required.[207]

Home assessment and management of asthma

Written management plans, if followed, can be useful to remind parents that, if required, high doses of bronchodilator inhalers should be used and when to seek medical advice. However, although written plans are frequently provided, they are often not used. Although some asthma management plans rely on measurement of children's peak flow to guide treatment, it has been shown that this does not help prevent or predict acute attack[216] (see pp. 756 – Clinical asthma, Follow-up).

Although it seems sensible to double the dose of inhaled corticosteroids (ICS) if symptoms increase, there is no evidence that this prevents or shortens exacerbations. To treat exacerbations leading to hospital admission parents should be given a short course of oral prednisolone (1–2 mg/day to a maximum of 40 mg/day) with clear instructions about its use. This has been shown to prevent the need for hospital admission and shorten the length of exacerbation.[217,218] Hyperactivity and hyperphagia are sometimes reported by parents, but are transient. If children are vomiting, intravenous hydrocortisone should be used. Often a single dose is effective. Parents need to be instructed when to give this and what dose to give. They should also be aware that if there is worsening or lack of response to therapy at home, they should seek medical advice. Some children with acute severe asthma often do not recognize the severity of the attack.[219]

Emergency assessment and management outside hospital

The trigger is usually a viral infection but, for children who have never wheezed before, inhalation of a foreign body should always be considered. Food allergies can present with wheeze but there is usually evidence of previous eczema.

A brief history should include usual medication, extra medication and outcomes of previous episodes. Physical examination is often of limited value as it is difficult to categorize severity of wheeze according to physical signs. There is poor correlation between the severity of airway obstruction as measured by arterial oxygen saturation and physical signs.[220] Nasal flaring, use of accessory muscles, and sternal recession all reflect an increased work of breathing. A silent chest, reflecting exhuastion, altered conscious level and cyanosis are late signs.

Pulsus paradoxus is not often measured in children as it is technically difficult and not that informative. However, a fall in systolic blood pressure of greater than 25 mmHg on inspiration is indicative of severe airway obstruction.[221]

Measurement of oxygen saturation is helpful in monitoring the severity of an acute exacerbation of asthma and has a prognostic value. An $SaO_2 < 92\%$ indicates hypoxia and the need for supplemental oxygen. Hypoxia can worsen with bronchodilatation if patients are not pre-oxygenated as beta 2-agonists administered without oxygen can lead to pulmonary vasodilatation, reperfusion of poorly ventilated areas and increased cardiac output, causing increased ventilation/ perfusion mismatch.[222] Children should be reassessed frequently for signs of response to treatment or deterioration (Fig. 18.26).

Bronchodilators should be given via MDI and spacer with a facemask if necessary. This has been shown to be as effective as nebulized treatment in preventing the need for hospital admission and additional intravenous therapy[223] and to be associated with shorter hospital stays and reduced readmission rates.[83] As the duration of bronchodilator effect may be only 20–30 min, inhaled beta 2-agonists should be repeated, if necessary continuously, until arrival at hospital. Oral prednisolone should be given following salbutamol to any child with asthma severe enough to warrant attention at hospital, as it is maximally effective some hours after administration. Prednisolone is sometimes vomited and should be replaced with intravenous corticosteroids. Antibiotics are not routinely indicated.[172]

Further management in hospital

Administration of corticosteroids within 1 h of presentation to an accident and emergency department significantly reduces the need for hospital admission in patients with acute asthma. However, there should be no urgency to send an asthmatic child home after apparently successful inhaled treatment. The effect can be short-lived. Observation over several hours after prednisolone may be necessary, either as an inpatient or in an observation area. A measurement of arterial oxygen saturation (SaO_2) should be done at the first assessment. Children who have previously required intravenous therapy or ventilatory support for previous attacks should be admitted immediately and monitored closely. In general, the younger the child, the more easily they will tire. Some children with difficult asthma (p. 758 – Difficult Asthma) have a detailed personal summary so that treatment can be individualized according to previous responses. In severe and life-threatening asthma a calm and structured approach is required (Fig. 18.26b).

More information can be obtained from observation than auscultation. Signs such as sternal recession, use of accessory muscles of respiration and nasal flare signify increased work of breathing and are more usually present than tachypnea. Hyperinflation of the chest is often present. The loudness of wheeze is not a good prognostic sign, as for wheeze to be audible there must

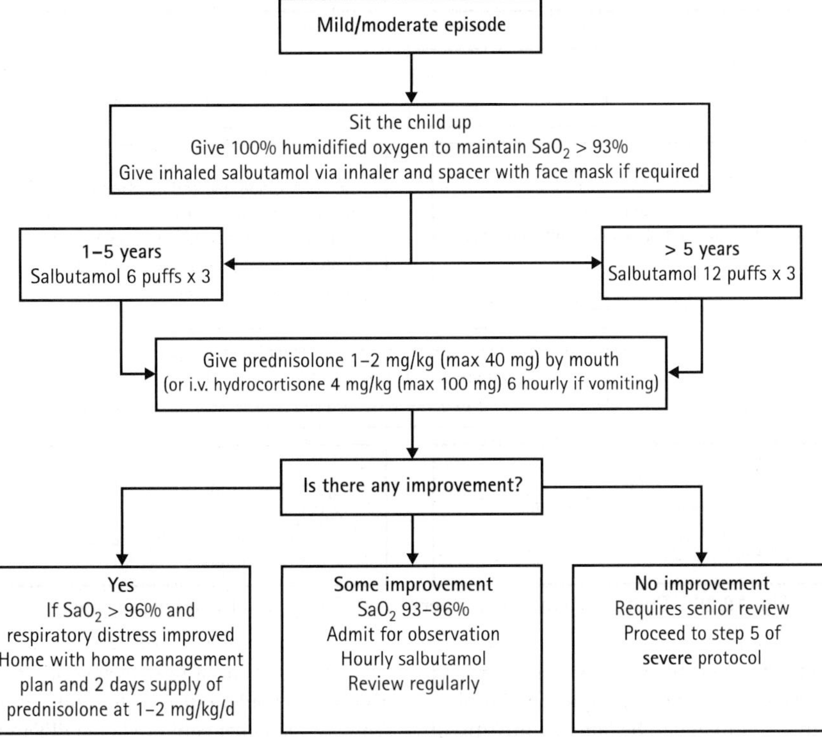

Fig. 18.26 (a & b) Management of acute asthma.

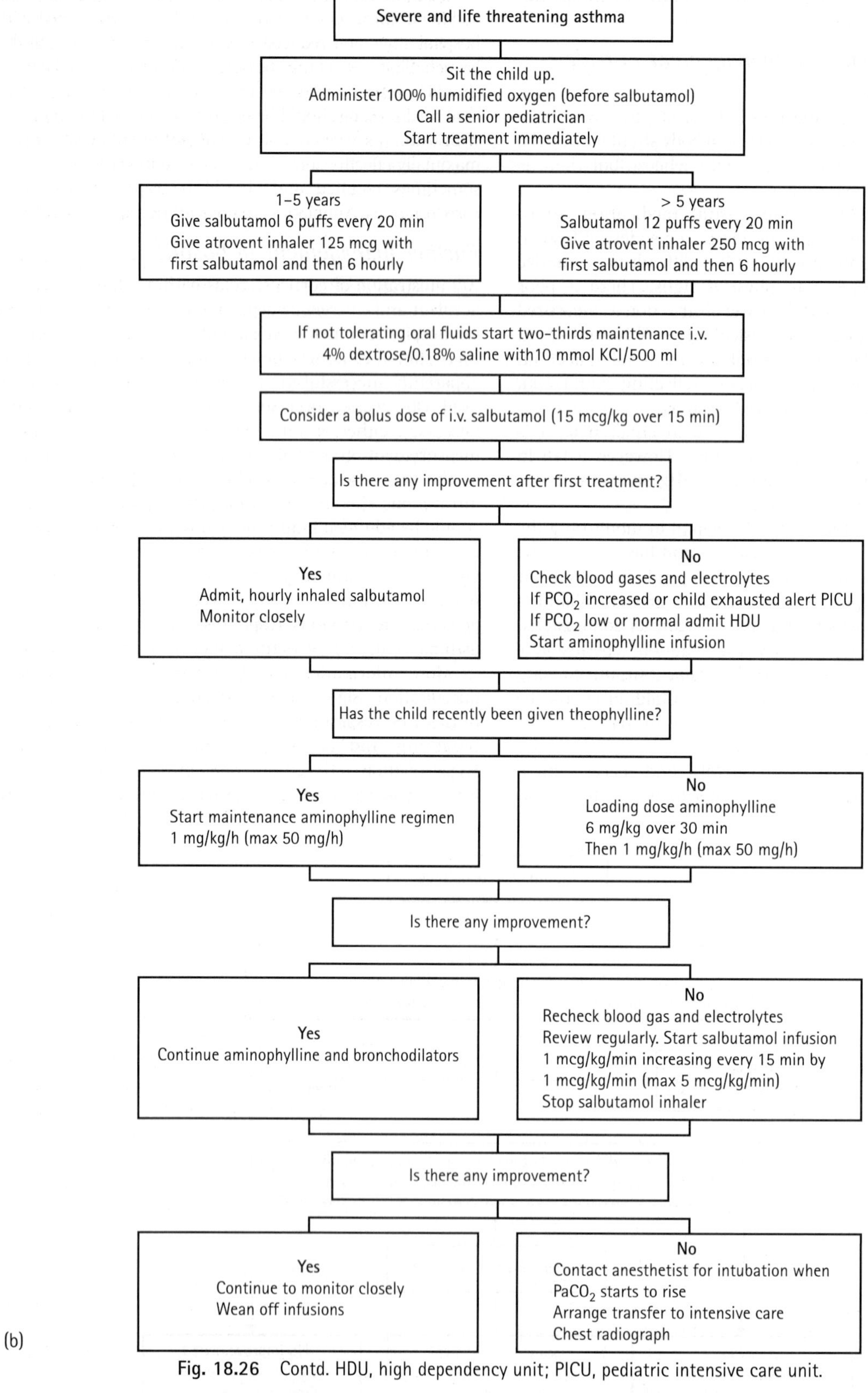

Severe and life threatening asthma
Sit the child up.
Administer 100% humidified oxygen (before salbutamol)
Call a senior pediatrician
Start treatment immediately
1–5 years
Give salbutamol 6 puffs every 20 min
Give atrovent inhaler 125 mcg with
first salbutamol and then 6 hourly
> 5 years
Salbutamol 12 puffs every 20 min
Give atrovent inhaler 250 mcg with
first salbutamol and then 6 hourly
If not tolerating oral fluids start two-thirds maintenance i.v.
4% dextrose/0.18% saline with10 mmol KCl/500 ml
Consider a bolus dose of i.v. salbutamol (15 mcg/kg over 15 min)
Is there any improvement after first treatment?
Yes
Admit, hourly inhaled salbutamol
Monitor closely
No
Check blood gases and electrolytes
If PCO2 increased or child exhausted alert PICU
If PCO2 low or normal admit HDU
Start aminophylline infusion
Has the child recently been given theophylline?
Yes
Start maintenance aminophylline regimen
1 mg/kg/h (max 50 mg/h)
No
Loading dose aminophylline
6 mg/kg over 30 min
Then 1 mg/kg/h (max 50 mg/h)
Is there any improvement?
Yes
Continue aminophylline and bronchodilators
No
Recheck blood gas and electrolytes
Review regularly. Start salbutamol infusion
1 mcg/kg/min increasing every 15 min by
1 mcg/kg/min (max 5 mcg/kg/min)
Stop salbutamol inhaler
Is there any improvement?
Yes
Continue to monitor closely
Wean off infusions
No
Contact anesthetist for intubation when
PaCO2 starts to rise
Arrange transfer to intensive care
Chest radiograph
(b)

Fig. 18.26 Contd. HDU, high dependency unit; PICU, pediatric intensive care unit.

be flow of gas through the airways. A silent chest is a sign of critical airway obstruction. Cyanosis is a worrying sign and implies impending respiratory failure. Agitation can be due to a mixture of fear and hypoxia.

Measurement of peak expiratory flow (PEF) can be carried out if the child is able, but is only really useful if the child's best PEF is known. Using per cent predicted PEF might be misleading as there is a wide range and it is the change from baseline that is informative.

According to the British Thoracic Society (BTS) guidelines, a PEF < 50% is a sign of severe asthma and if < 33% life-threatening.[224]

Chest radiographs do not need to be performed routinely and radiological features of hyperinflation do not correlate with clinical severity. They can be justified on the first or an atypical presentation, if an air leak, foreign body or pneumonia is clinically suspected or if the attack is severe enough to warrant intensive care.

Blood gas analysis should be undertaken when there is severe hypoxemia (SaO_2 < 85% in air) or when there is progressive rise in oxygen requirement despite treatment. $PaCO_2$ levels above normal reflect respiratory failure and alveolar hypoventilation due to exhaustion (Fig. 18.26b). A rising $PaCO_2$ suggests the need for transfer to intensive care and if greater than 10 kPa is an indication for ventilatory support. Some children will need support before this if they are becoming exhausted or for safety during transport to an intensive care unit. Endotracheal intubation should be undertaken immediately in cases of apnea or coma. Rarely, in older children if hypercapnia has developed over several days, renal compensation may occur and the rapid fall in $PaCO_2$ on mechanical ventilation can cause a marked alkalosis, which may provoke tetany.

Nasal oxygen should be given during administration of inhaled bronchodilator when a spacer is used, failing which facial oxygen should be administered before bronchodilatation as hypoxia can worsen.

In severe life-threatening asthma inhaled beta 2-agonists via MDI and spacer (or nebulizer), with face mask if required, should be given continuously.[225] Intravenous access should be secured for further treatment to be administered if there is no response to treatment. Prednisolone should be given orally as described above.

The addition of repeated doses of anticholinergics to beta 2-agonists appears safe, improves lung function and may prevent the need for hospital admission in schoolchildren with acute severe asthma.[226]

Intravenous therapy should be considered if there is a poor response to inhaled treatments, in young children and those who are severely ill. The side-effects of continuous infusion of aminophylline or salbutamol should be considered as well as the benefit gained from not being disturbed for frequent inhaler treatment.

Theophylline has been shown to improve spirometry at 6 h and arterial oxygen saturation in the first 30 h after administration and safely hastened the recovery of children with severe asthma who were also receiving salbutamol, ipratropium, and corticosteroids with no difference in total side-effects between aminophylline and placebo groups.[227] Aminophylline continues to have a place in the management of severe acute asthma in children unresponsive to initial treatment. If a child is on regular theophylline, the usual loading dose of aminophylline should be omitted.

Although inhalation of bronchodilators is the mainstay of treatment for children with acute asthma, mucosal edema and excess secretions may reduce absorption of the drug. In cases of severe obstruction non-responsive to inhaled therapy, intravenous administration of 15 mcg/kg salbutamol over 10 min has been shown to result in more rapid recovery, improvement in oxygenation and earlier discharge from the emergency room with no increase in adverse effects.[228] Infusion of intravenous salbutamol should also be considered in a tiring child to prevent the need for frequent waking for inhaled treatment. Electrolytes should be checked prior to intravenous therapy as aminophylline and salbutamol can cause hypokalemia. Continuous monitoring of pulse rate can be performed using a saturation monitor.

There is some evidence that the addition of intravenous magnesium sulfate to standard treatment with bronchodilators and systemic steroids can provide increased bronchodilatation. Two pediatric randomized controlled studies recruited children who had peak expiratory flows (PEF) < 60% predicted after nebulized therapy. Those who received intravenous magnesium had significantly greater improvement in PEF, FEV_1 and clinical asthma scores, with no effect on blood pressure. A Cochrane review concluded that although there is no support for its routine use in all patients with acute asthma, those with acute severe asthma benefited with no significant adverse effects.[229]

Non-pharmacological aspects of treatment are also important. Parents should be encouraged to remain with their children while in hospital. Vomiting may occur, especially following coughing, but most children are able to tolerate oral fluids. Intravenous fluids are not usually required in older children, but infants and young children may become dehydrated due to increased respiratory rate and evaporative fluid losses and reduced oral intake. Care should be taken to manage fluid balance, especially in infants, as hyponatremia due to inappropriate ADH secretion exacerbated by overzealous fluid administration is a well-documented complication of acute asthma.

When assessing the effect of inhaled beta 2-agonists, time for effect must be allowed for (at least 15 min for salbutamol to have maximal effect). Children should be reviewed regularly following treatment as continuing deterioration despite treatment may lead to the need for ventilatory support. Pulse oximetry should be used to monitor oxygen requirements.

Complications

Air leaks are a very rare complication of acute asthma and do not usually require treatment. Spontaneous pneumomediastinum causes chest pain, dyspnea, and subcutaneous emphysema. The diagnosis is confirmed by chest radiography and generally resolves spontaneously within a few days.[230] Pneumothoraces in spontaneously breathing asthmatics are also rare and similarly most do not require active treatment.

Acute onset of flaccid paralysis has been described following acute asthma, with absent motor action potential and normal sensory responses, which are highly suggestive of motor anterior horn cell disease. It is thought that a combination of immune suppression, stress, and neurotoxic drugs used to treat acute asthma triggered by a viral disease may increase susceptibility to viral invasion of the anterior horn cell with enteroviruses other than poliovirus.

Education

During admission for an acute exacerbation, parents may be more receptive to education about asthma. Parents should be taught at the very least how to administer bronchodilators properly before discharge and be given a self-management plan (pp. 757 – Clinical asthma, Education). It should be ensured that parents have sufficient medication, both to finish a course of oral steroids and to continue prescribed maintenance treatment. Inhaler technique should be checked and the emergency plan reviewed. General practitioners should be informed of the admission and follow-up arranged.

Follow-up

All children who have required hospital admission for acute severe asthma should be seen in clinic after 4–6 weeks. General practitioner and pediatrician should decide further care jointly. It is important to check inhaler technique at each visit and optimise adherence to treatment.

CYSTIC FIBROSIS

Cystic fibrosis (CF) is the most common life-limiting genetic disorder of Caucasian populations. It is a multisystem disorder, with significantly reduced life expectancy, despite recent improvements in management. The CF molecular defect affects salt transport across epithelial cells, and this is reflected in the organs characteristically involved by the condition, that is lungs, pancreas, sweat gland and liver, among others. The majority of morbidity and mortality associated with CF relates to the lung involvement, with an unremitting cycle of infection, inflammation and damage. With a modern team approach to CF care, however, most children with the condition can have fulfilling and relatively healthy school years, and can look forward to full-time employment as adults.

EPIDEMIOLOGY OF CYSTIC FIBROSIS

There are over 6000 patients in the UK with this condition and at least 30 000 in the USA.[231] The prognosis for patients with CF has improved Consistently and substantially in the last four decades. In a study reported in 1991, the median life expectancy of a child with cystic fibrosis, born in 1990, was estimated to be 40 years. This was double the median survival estimated for a child born in 1970.[232] In the UK, there are now more adults than children with CF. In the US,[231] similar trends towards greatly improved survival, with each successive decade, have been observed. Median survival in females is consistently slightly better than for males.

Survival data for birth cohorts from 1947 to 1967 in the UK were published recently.[233] The survival for each successive cohort was better than that of the previous one, but the mortality beyond the age of 20 does not appear to be improving, and averages about 50 per 1000 per year. This suggests that the survivors in each cohort are mainly those with mild disease and the advances in care, which have led to these improvements in survival, have predominately extended survival in patients with moderately severe disease.

GENETICS OF CYSTIC FIBROSIS

Those affected by cystic fibrosis are homozygous for mutations within a gene on the long arm of chromosome 7. This gene codes for a protein known as the cystic fibrosis transmembrane conductance regulator (CFTR). CFTR has many functions, but is primarily involved in salt transport across epithelial cell membranes. It is a regulated anion channel which accounts for the cyclic AMP regulated chloride conductance of the apical membrane of airway epithelial cells. The presence of two abnormal CFTR genes either eliminates or markedly impairs this conductance pathway.[234] Around 1 in 25 people in the UK carry abnormal CFTR genes, resulting in an incidence of the disease of approximately 1 per 2000 children born. To date, over 1000 mutations in the CFTR gene have been associated with a CF disease phenotype. From a molecular biological perspective, the CFTR mutations have been grouped into five classes based on the primary mechanism responsible for reduced CFTR function and this has provided a useful framework for considering genotype/phenotype relationships.[235] Class I mutations (e.g. G542X) are those in which stop codons or frameshift mutations lead to permanent termination of mRNA translation and thus no protein production. Class II mutations disrupt the intracellular processing of CFTR protein, which is degraded by the cell before reaching the cell membrane, where it needs to be located to function. An example of this is ΔF508, the commonest mutation worldwide. Because both Class I and II mutations prevent sufficient CFTR expression at the cell membrane, it might be predicted that these are associated with typical cystic fibrosis including pancreatic insufficiency, progressive pulmonary disease and male infertility. In Class III mutations (e.g. G551D) CFTR reaches the cell membrane but is not functional. These also appear to be associated with a severe disease phenotype. In Class IV mutations (e.g. R117H) CFTR reaches the cell membrane and has some residual function. These mutations appear to result in mild disease and in particular are reported with pancreatic sufficiency.[236] Class V mutations (e.g. 3849 + 10KBC-T) include splice mutations and result in reduced expression of full-length mRNAs and a decrease in the quantity of fully functional CFTR at the cell membrane. Genotype/phenotype correlations in the limited number of patients with these mutations have indicated a mild phenotype for pancreatic disease.[237]

An international CF Genotype/Phenotype Consortium has demonstrated that certain mutations are associated with pancreatic sufficiency.[238] The occurrence or severity of pulmonary disease is not, however, related to known genotypes. A recent longitudinal analysis of pulmonary function in CF patients revealed that ΔF508 homozygous patients had a higher rate of pulmonary function decline than patients who were heterozygous for ΔF508 or who had two no ΔF508 mutations.[239] The wide intra-genotype variation in pulmonary disease has been proposed to reflect environmental factors, the presence of polymorphisms or modifier genes, as well as differences in therapy and/or patient compliance. The impact of polymorphisms such as those which result in mannose binding lectin deficiency have been shown to have a significant effect on severity of lung disease in CF.[240]

Since the identification of the CF gene there has been a growing understanding that the spectrum of disease associated with mutations in CFTR may range from typical cystic fibrosis to that of male infertility (due to bilateral absence of the vas deferens) with no recognizable pulmonary or pancreatic disease. A 50% reduction in CFTR expression is physiologically insignificant, as heterozygotes, or disease carriers, express only 50% of normal CFTR and have no CF disease phenotype. The presence of a mild mutation plus a severe mutation is associated with pancreatic sufficiency but lung and sweat duct dysfunction. Such individuals are estimated to have around 5% of normal CFTR function. With two severe mutations (Class I, II or III) the level of function of CFTR is generally less than 1%. This suggests that while lung and sweat duct dysfunction may occur with expression of CFTR of around 5%, pancreatic disease will only occur when expression of CFTR is less than this, and probably when it is less than 1%.[234]

PATHOPHYSIOLOGY OF CYSTIC FIBROSIS DISEASE

The important role of CFTR in epithelial salt transport accounts for the pathological characteristics of the condition, i.e. primarily affecting organs in which salt transport plays an important role (the lungs, pancreas, liver, vas deferens, sweat gland). Interestingly other organs, such as the kidney, in which CFTR is expressed, are spared. The pathophysiological processes in the main organs involved are considered below.

Sweat produced by CF patients has a higher than normal concentration of salt. In temperate climates, this is only associated with symptoms infrequently. However, a study of patients presenting with heat exhaustion in New York in the late 1940s led to the first description of this characteristic in CF patients.[241] In the CF sweat gland, as in normal individuals, fluid first secreted by the tubule has a similar salt concentration to plasma, i.e. it is relatively salty. As the salt passes through the absorptive duct, in the normal individual NaCl but not water is transported back towards the blood so that the final sweat is mostly water with very little salt remaining. However, as the sweat passes through the CF duct either CFTR is not present or its channel does not function and so chloride cannot enter the duct cell through the apical membrane or leave through the basolateral membrane. Consequently sweat leaves the duct almost as salty as it entered, in marked contrast to what happens in individuals who have got normally functioning CFTR. Measurement of sodium and chloride concentrations in the sweat is the basis of the sweat test, the most frequently used diagnostic test for cystic fibrosis.

In the pancreas, the acini secrete enzymes which digest food. In addition, the pancreatic ducts secrete a large amount of HCO_3^- into the intestine to neutralize the effect of acid from the stomach. Fluid, which is high in HCO_3^-, is rapidly added to the lumen of the pancreatic ducts and dilutes the enzymes as they pass through the duct. In CF, HCO_3^- secretion is barely detectable in pancreatic juice. Until recently it has been thought that it is the lack of a function of the chloride channel Cl^- in CFTR in the duct cells which means that Cl^- cannot recycle and little if any additional fluid and HCO_3^- can be added to the duct lumen. However, it has recently been shown that CFTR can conduct HCO_3^-, and impairment of this transport may be the primary abnormality in the CF pancreas.[242] The end result of the low HCO_3^- concentration in the fluid in the pancreatic ducts is that the enzymes become concentrated in this relatively acid fluid where they form plugs and destroy cells of that part of the pancreas, before being washed into the intestines. The process progresses until little pancreas is left. It is suggested that pancreatic insufficiency does not appear until > 85% of the pancreas is lost. This progresses at a variable rate in CF patients. In some, pancreatic insufficiency develops in utero, but in others it develops over a period of many years.

The precise mechanisms of liver involvement in CF are uncertain, but may relate to the CFTR defect causing abnormal biliary secretion, or an abnormal 'bile acid balance'. This leads to thickening of bile and the formation of plugs within the bile ducts. The resulting ductular obstruction and abnormal bile flow ultimately results in the development of bile duct irregularities inside and outside the liver and cirrhosis in either one or several parts of the liver.

In the airway, the pathophysiological events which lead to persistent infection, airway inflammation and progressive bronchiectasis, are complex. Figure 18.27 is an attempt to summarize current understanding of these pathophysiological processes in the CF airway. Studies of CFTR gene expression in the airway have suggested that it is found at the apical membrane of ciliated surface epithelial cells throughout the airway and in submucosal gland serous cells of cartilaginous airway regions.[234] The significant transport process in this surface epithelium is absorption of Na, Cl, and water. In vitro studies have shown that the rate of Na absorption is enhanced by CFTR deletion and reduced by CFTR expression. It has been known for some time that Na enters the epithelial cell across the apical membrane via amiloride sensitive epithelial Na channels (ENaC). Microelectrode studies have suggested that Cl ions and water passively follow the actively transported Na from the airway to the interstitium. There is now growing evidence that the primary function of CFTR in the airway surface epithelium is not as a cellular Cl conductance, which provides a pathway for Cl flow during NaCl absorption, but that rather one of its roles is to downregulate the activity of ENaC. Therefore in CF, ENaC activity is upregulated relative to normals, and Na absorption across the airway epithelium is increased.

In healthy lungs, the lower airways are kept clear and sterile by a complex interaction of different processes. These include mucociliary transport of a thin layer of airway surface liquid, innate defense mechanisms and acquired immunological processes. Airway surface liquid is composed of two layers: a mucoid upper layer, and liquid periciliary layer. In CF, dehydration of the airway surface liquid, through overactive salt absorption results in derangement of mucociliary transport. However mucus secretion,

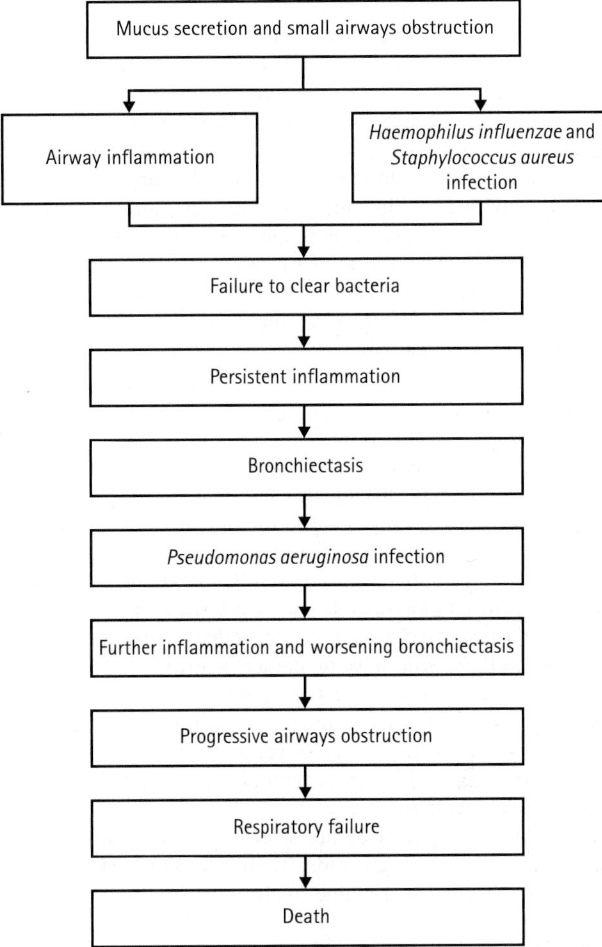

Fig. 18.27 Pathophysiology of cystic fibrosis.

by goblet cells and submucosal glands (which is independent of CFTR), continues unimpaired and the result is the production of mucus plugs. Recently a group of low molecular weight cationic proteins secreted by epithelial and immune cells and known as defensins have been identified. Their activity is diminished at high NaCl concentrations and studies have suggested that a high salt concentration in the airway surface liquid of CF patients leads to an inability of defensins to exert their antimicrobial action.[243] One of the problems in this field is the difficulty of studying the very thin fluid layer of airway surface liquid, so it is still uncertain whether the salt concentration in the airway surface liquid from CF patients is increased. A number of different studies[234] have tried to investigate the mechanisms by which the CF airway is susceptible to colonization with organisms such as *Pseudomonas aeruginosa*, *Staphylococcus aureus* and *Haemophilus influenzae*. There is evidence to suggest that defects in CFTR enhance the adhesion of bacterial pathogens to airway epithelia. Other studies have shown that exoproducts of *Pseudomonas* have enhanced activity in CF airways. Formation of mucus plugs may provide these bacteria with an environment in which to multiply.

Mechanisms of airway inflammation in CF have been investigated extensively and more recently studies involving bronchoalveolar lavage of CF patients have helped elucidate evidence of CFTR related dysregulation in the inflammatory response. In a group of CF infants evidence for lower respiratory tract infection was present in almost 40% with total cell counts and

IL-8 concentrations increased in infected compared with uninfected CF infants and controls.[244] It was concluded that the inflammation occurred secondary to infection. This view was challenged by the findings of two groups of investigators who performed BAL on infants with CF and found evidence of lung inflammation in the BAL in the absence of microbiological evidence of infection.[245,246] Accumulating evidence from the lung and other organs[247] suggests that, in an environment in which CFTR does not function normally, the inflammatory response is deranged, and this may be related to the pathophysiological effects of CF. Deficient production of anti-inflammatory cytokines like IL-10 has been demonstrated and it may be one of the mechanisms by which the inflammatory response in the CF lung is dysregulated.[248]

DIAGNOSIS OF CYSTIC FIBROSIS

CF has a wide spectrum of clinical manifestations and patients may present with a variety of clinical features, to a range of medical specialists. Table 18.9 shows some of the clinical features which may lead to a presentation of CF. CF should be part of the differential diagnosis of individuals who present in this way. The diagnosis can then be confirmed by sweat and/or genetic testing. When a diagnosis of CF is confirmed in a child, it is good practice to investigate all other siblings, even those who have no clinical features of the condition. This may be done by sweat or genetic testing.

In a number of UK regions, screening for CF has been introduced, either in the neonatal period, to detect infants before they develop the disease, or antenatally, so that termination of pregnancy can be offered.

The clinical features of CF are described in detail below. If CF is suspected, on clinical grounds, then a sweat test should be performed. The most reliable technique is the quantitative pilocarpine iontophoresis method. A weak electrical current aids the penetration of positively charged pilocarpine into the skin to induce maximal sweating. Pilocarpine is a sweat gland secretagogue. Sweat is collected onto low sodium filter paper of similar size to the stimulated area, or into macroduct 'Wescor' collectors. Measurements in situ (Orion method) are unreliable. Sweat should be collected for between 20 and 30 min. A sweat rate of less than 1 $g/m^2/min$ indicates a significant problem with sweat stimulation or collections and sweat concentrations failing to meet this rate should not be analysed. Essentially for a 30 min collection on 5.5 cm diameter filter paper, this equates to 71 mg. A study of sweat tests in 725 infants found that the mean (95% CI) normal sweat chloride was 10.6 (9.9–11.3).[248] In CF infants who were ΔF508 homozygotes, ΔF508 compound heterozygotes, or two other mutant alleles, mean sweat chloride levels were 99.9, 98.8 and 96.6 mmol/L. Healthy heterozygotes had a mean chloride concentration of 14.9 (13.4–14.6) mmol/L. The mean +3 standard deviations for the group of heterozygotes was 40 mmol/L. The Genotype/Phenotype Consortium studied 798 patients of a wide age range.[238] ΔF508 homozygotes had a mean (SD) sweat chloride concentration of 106 (22) mmol/L; all ΔF508 heterozygotes apart from R117H had mean sweat chloride concentrations 100 (20) to 110 (18) mmol/L; ΔF508/R117H mean sweat chloride was 82 (19) mmol/L. The upper limit of normal for sweat chloride is considered to be 40 mmol/L. Sweat chloride >60 mmol/L is considered diagnostic of CF. Values of sweat chloride of 40–60 mmol/L are considered highly suggestive of CF, and in this situation the sweat test should be repeated and/or genetic testing conducted. Although, in CF patients there is a fall in sweat chloride with age, the magnitude of this fall is not sufficient to cause diagnostic confusion, if these criteria are used.[249]

Table 18.9 Presentation of cystic fibrosis – indications for a sweat test

Pulmonary
Chronic or recurrent cough, pneumonia or bronchiolitis
Purulent sputum production
'Difficult' asthma
Unexplained hemoptysis
Nasal polyps, chronic sinusitis
Gastrointestinal
Meconium ileus, meconium plug syndrome
Failure to thrive
Steatorrhea, malabsorption
Rectal prolapse
Atypical gastroesophageal reflux
Hypoproteinemia, edema
Neonatal hepatitis syndrome
Other
Pseudo-Bartter's syndrome
Heat exhaustion
Male infertility
Salty taste when kissed
Sibling with cystic fibrosis
Short stature

Other indices, or measurements available from the sweat test have also been evaluated for their diagnostic potential. Some sweat testing systems report only sweat sodium concentrations, which are not, on their own, considered sufficient to differentiate between control and CF populations. Patients with CF usually have a sweat chloride : sodium ratio of greater than 1, but the value of this ratio as a discriminating measure has not been conclusively demonstrated. Some sweat testing systems measure sweat conductivity alone. Again, there are concerns about whether this can discriminate between CF patients and normal individuals. In general a diagnosis of CF should not be based on sweat conductivity measures alone.

Genetic testing for CF

In a child suspected to have CF, DNA testing for the more common CFTR mutations is a valuable diagnostic test. If two CFTR mutations are identified, this confirms the diagnosis of CF. In all children in whom CF has been diagnosed by sweat testing, identification of the CFTR mutations provides more information concerning potential genotype/phenotype correlations and can be used for cascade testing of the extended family (see below). DNA may be obtained from mouthwash samples, buccal scrapes, or white blood cells. Following DNA extraction, samples are usually tested using one of the commercially available kits. These should test sufficient gene mutations to account for a high proportion of known gene mutations in the region, or particular ethnic group of the patient. For example, the Cellmark Diagnostics ARMS Multiplex test kit gives results for the four most common CF alleles in north west England.[250] If only one, or none of the gene mutations is identified, then further testing can be conducted for other common CF genes.

Newborn screening for CF

The improved survival in CF, observed over the last few decades, has been largely attributed to therapeutic interventions. This has led to the hypothesis that therapeutic interventions administered before the onset of clinical signs or symptoms may have greatest benefit in improving life expectancy. Such preventative treatment could only be initiated if infants were identified as having CF by newborn screening. Neonatal screening became feasible with the development, in 1979, of a radioimmunoassay for immunoreactive trypsin (IRT) suitable for use on dried blood spots from newborns.[251] IRT levels are elevated in the first few weeks of life in babies with CF. However, in the first week of life, when most newborn blood samples are routinely taken, specificity of a single elevated IRT is low. Thus two or three stage protocols based on a second IRT test with or without subsequent DNA analyses have been developed to reduce the false positive diagnoses associated with one stage IRT testing.[251] Based on these protocols, sensitivities of between 85 and 90% (conventionally calculated excluding infants with meconium ileus) have been reported but these may be overestimates due to underascertainment of milder cases of CF not detected by screening.

Despite acceptable test performance, there is still controversy in some countries about whether neonatal screening for CF should be introduced nationally.[252] In 1983 the American Cystic Fibrosis Foundation identified a need for further information on the benefits and risks of early diagnosis and treatment before newborn screening could be recommended.[253] Subsequently, a number of studies have been published from different countries. Dankert-Roelse and te Meerman[254] observed that patients identified by neonatal screening had less pulmonary inflammation and less deterioration of lung function than patients detected on clinical symptoms. Farrell et al[255] found that neonatal screening provides the opportunity to prevent malnutrition in infants with CF. A systematic review[256] identified two randomized controlled trials of neonatal screening in CF. A meta-analysis was not possible and the reviewers concluded that there was little evidence of either benefit or harm from neonatal screening. Further information would be obtained from these trials when an individual patient data meta-analysis was conducted. This is now underway. A decision has been taken recently to introduce neonatal screening throughout the UK.

Antenatal screening for CF

There are a number of programs that can be implemented when screening for CF in the antenatal period. Population based antenatal screening aims to identify, firstly, pregnant women and their partners who are both carriers of the CF gene. Strategies to achieve this include testing of all women attending antenatal clinics to detect carrier status, followed by selective testing of their partners when this is found (referred to as 'stepwise screening') or routine testing of both parents (couple screening).[257] Selective screening of families known to be high risk, i.e. have a relative with CF, known as cascade screening, can be offered when a child is diagnosed with CF.[250]

Where both parents are found to be carriers, testing of the fetus is then performed using direct gene analysis. Fetal material is obtained by chorionic villus biopsy at 9–10 weeks, a procedure which is associated with an increased miscarriage rate of 1–4%. If the couple present after the first trimester, fetal material is obtained by amniocentesis, which is associated with a miscarriage rate of 0.5–1.0%. The negative effects, when screening antenatally for CF, relate to the adverse effects of termination, the risk of spontaneous miscarriage caused by the fetal testing procedure, anxiety because of the screening process, and the implications of diagnosing carrier status in well, asymptomatic adults.

Screening programs include not only the testing process, but also counseling of parents regarding the implications of having a child with CF and the option of termination, and the implications for future reproductive plans, in order that informed choices may be made. Recently a National Institutes of Health consensus statement[258] on genetic testing for CF recommended that CF genetic testing should be offered to adults with a positive family history of CF, to partners of people with CF, to couples currently planning a pregnancy particularly those in a high-risk population, and to couples seeking prenatal testing.

CLINICAL FEATURES OF CYSTIC FIBROSIS

CF is a multisystem disorder and clinical progression in an individual patient is unpredictable. With appropriate treatment, the majority of the clinical features, which are evident on presentation, can be corrected or controlled, and most children with CF achieve normal growth with few signs of chest infection and malabsorption.

Gastrointestinal

Meconium ileus causes intestinal obstruction in up to 15% of newborn children with CF (Fig. 18.28). The condition may be detected antenatally by the presence of a 'bright bowel' due to inspissated meconium. After birth, failure to pass meconium, abdominal distension and bile-stained vomiting are characteristic of the condition. Abdominal radiographs reveal distended loops of small bowel and ground glass opacification in the lower abdomen. A Gastrografin enema typically demonstrates the presence of a microcolon and may also soften the meconium mass to relieve obstruction. However, the majority of cases require surgical intervention to remove impacted meconium and resect non-viable bowel. Antenatal meconium peritonitis, neonatal volvulus and ileal atresia are rare complications.

Distal intestinal obstruction syndrome (DIOS), sometimes referred to as 'meconium ileus equivalent' has a similar pathophysiology to meconium ileus and occurs in older children and adults. The terminal ileum becomes occluded with sticky, mucofeculent material causing colicky abdominal pain, vomiting and abdominal distension. Typically, a fecal mass can be palpated in the right iliac fossa. There is some debate concerning the precise mechanisms which contribute to DIOS. Inadequate dosing with pancreatic enzyme supplements has been suggested as a contributory factor but DIOS does occur in CF patients with pancreatic sufficiency. Mild symptoms can be relieved with oral osmotic laxatives, such as lactulose, and adequate hydration. When the abdominal pain is severe and/or accompanied by signs of subacute intestinal obstruction, treatment with Gastrografin,

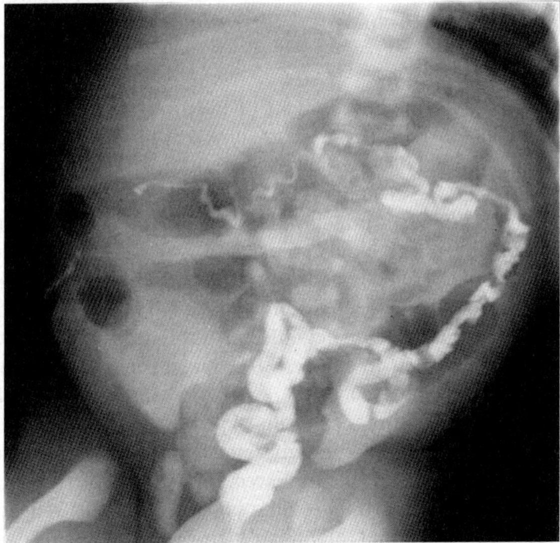

Fig. 18.28 Barium enema showing typical microcolon consequent to meconium ileus intestinal obstruction.

N-acetylcysteine or balanced electrolyte intestinal lavage is necessary. Other causes of abdominal symptoms including constipation, appendicitis, pancreatitis, Crohn's disease, neoplasms and gynecological conditions should be considered. Occasionally a DIOS mass may form the apex of an intussusception.

Malabsorption due to pancreatic insufficiency occurs in around 85% of children with CF. At presentation, affected infants often have a voracious appetite but are slow to gain weight. Malabsorption is exacerbated by abnormal duodenal acidity, intestinal mucosal dysfunction and impaired bile salt excretion. Failure to thrive is accompanied by steatorrhea, manifest by the frequent passage of large, greasy and offensive stools. Distension of the abdomen is a common feature in infants and children who present with CF. A voracious appetite may compensate sufficiently for malabsorption to enable reasonable weight gain in early childhood and diagnosis may be delayed in these children. Recurrent rectal prolapse occurs in up to 10% of undiagnosed children with CF and may be the sole presenting feature. CF should always be considered in children who present with rectal prolapse, even if other features of CF are absent. Inadequate absorption of fat-soluble vitamins has occasionally caused symptoms, including bleeding disorders due to vitamin K deficiency, benign intracranial hypertension, due to vitamin A deficiency and hemolytic anemia or neurological symptoms due to vitamin E deficiency.

Salt deficiency is common at diagnosis and can result in severe hypochloremic metabolic alkalosis. Undiagnosed CF infants with loose stools and poor weight gain are sometimes treated by substitution of cow's milk with a soya-milk based formula. Such children are at risk of developing hypoproteinemic edema, anemia and essential fatty acid deficiencies.

An apparently new CF-specific bowel abnormality was first described in 1994.[259] A cluster of cases, all of them children, presented with subacute bowel obstruction and failed to respond to medical therapy. At surgery they were found to have marked thickening and stenosis, but not inflammation, in the ascending colon. The histology revealed extensive submucosal fibrosis. A large number of other cases have now been identified and there is an association between this condition and treatment with high-strength pancreatic enzyme preparations.[260] In the UK, these findings led the Medicines Control Agency to advise that the dose of pancreatic enzymes should not exceed 10 000 units of lipase per kilogram per day and that certain high strength preparations should not be used in children.[261]

Respiratory

The most troublesome symptoms of CF are those related to the chest and around 97% of deaths in CF are due to pulmonary causes. The age of onset and progression of respiratory symptoms varies considerably among CF patients. A persistent cough, often rattly and exacerbated by viral infections, is often the first symptom. Occasionally the cough is paroxysmal and associated with vomiting, leading to the misdiagnosis of pertussis. Some infants present with a prolonged bronchiolitic type illness and many have recurrent wheezing, suggestive of asthma. In a minority, the wheezing is persistent in the first 1–2 years, gradually improving throughout early childhood. At least 20% of CF children have coexistent atopic asthma. Sputum expectoration is usually only obvious in older children although some infants and young children vomit sputum that has been swallowed. Initially, sputum is relatively clear or creamy but with increasing infection becomes yellow and then green. Occasional blood streaking occurs during acute infections but massive fresh hemoptysis due to rupture of bronchial arteries is rare and confined to patients with more severe disease.

Clinical signs are usually absent in children with CF unless they have advanced disease. In infants with wheezing and hyperinflation there may be Harrison's sulci, an increase in the anterior–posterior diameter of the chest wall and downward displacement of the liver. In older children, persistent hyperinflation leads to a barrel-shaped chest and kyphosis. Finger clubbing develops in parallel with the progression of suppurative lung disease. Chest auscultation may be normal even in the presence of extensive respiratory disease but may reveal an increased expiratory phase, inspiratory and expiratory crackles of varying coarseness and polyphonic wheezing. Central cyanosis is a very late sign of respiratory disease.

Other respiratory complications

Sinus infection occurs in most children with CF. Sinus X-rays invariably show opacifications but acute purulent sinusitis causing symptoms is uncommon. Expanding sinus mucoceles causing bone deformity are a rare complication. Between 10 and 30% of patients develop nasal polyps. These can grow rapidly and often recur after surgical treatment.

Spontaneous pneumothorax is a relatively rare complication in childhood but occurs in up to 20% of adults. It is more common in males than females. Small asymptomatic pneumothoraces can be treated conservatively. Larger pneumothoraces and those causing pleuritic pain or breathlessness require an intercostal chest drain. Surgical treatment, such as pleurectomy or pleurodesis may be considered in cases when conservative measures fail to bring about re-expansion or when pneumothoraces are recurrent. Widespread pleurodesis carries the risk of rendering the patient unsuitable for future heart–lung transplantation.

Mild hemoptysis is common but up to 7% of older patients can have massive, even life-threatening hemoptysis. If significant bleeding occurs after appropriate antibiotic treatment and correction of any underlying coagulopathy, surgical procedures such as angiographic bronchial artery embolization, thoracotomy and bronchial artery ligation have been used. Lobar collapse is rare but occurs more frequently in early childhood. In most cases treatment with aggressive physiotherapy and antibiotics is effective. Microabscesses are inevitable in the advanced stages of the disease. Large abscess formation is relatively rare. Patients with advanced lung disease causing severe hypoxia are at risk of developing pulmonary hypertension and right ventricular hypertrophy. Doppler echocardiography usefully detects the early development of cor pulmonale. Overt signs of pulmonary heart disease do not occur until end-stage disease.

Simple allergy to *Aspergillus fumigatus* is common in CF but up to 10% of patients develop allergic bronchopulmonary aspergillosis. This is characterized by increased respiratory symptoms with wheezing, fleeting pulmonary shadows, blood and sputum eosinophilia, raised total IgE levels, raised IgE and IgG to *A. fumigatus* and positive *A. fumigatus* sputum cultures (Fig. 18.29). Treatment of this condition is considered in the following section. Mycetomas and invasive aspergillosis can occur in CF but are rare.

Investigations used to monitor pulmonary disease

Initial findings on chest radiography are hyperinflation and peribronchial infiltrates. For unknown reasons changes are frequently predominant in the upper lobes and particularly on the right. With disease progression extensive peribronchial thickening is represented by tramline shadows and thick-walled circles in cross-section. Larger infiltrates become more prominent and extensive. Areas of atelectasis or consolidation may occur and peripheral rounded opacities 0.5 cm in diameter appear. These represent abscesses or infected bronchiectatic areas and when drained appear as permanent ring shadows (Fig. 18.30).

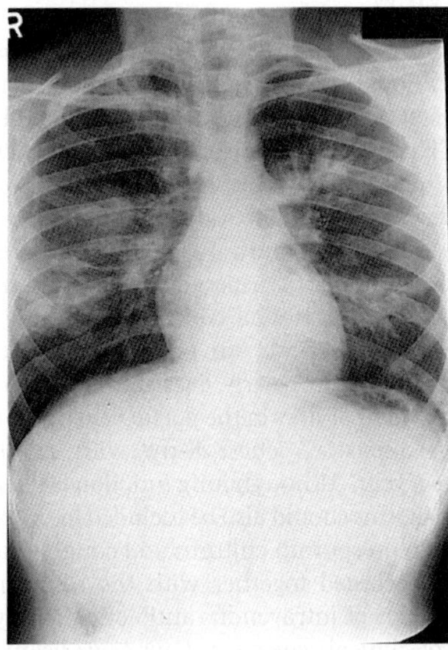

Fig. 18.29 Typical widespread nodular opacities caused by allergic bronchopulmonary aspergillosis.

Children with CF, and their parents, vary in the degree to which they report clinical symptoms, and clinicians may differ in how they respond to individual clinical problems. It is useful therefore to have objective measures of pulmonary disease. These include chest X-ray scoring systems and pulmonary function tests. Chest-X-ray scoring systems in clinical use include the Chrispin–Norman,[262] the Brasfield[263] and the Northern scores.[264] The Northern score is more recent, and unlike the other two, does not require a lateral film, therefore reducing the amount of radiation exposure. It has shown good inter- and intra-observer reproducibility. The lung is divided into four quadrants in the PA film, and a score of four allocated to each quadrant, depending on the degree of change, including bronchial wall thickening, bronchiectasis, lung collapse, etc. A further four points may be added for generalized changes, such as hyperinflation, bringing the total score possible to 20. Scoring systems can provide an overall assessment of the degree of pulmonary disease and can monitor progression of disease.

Most infants with CF identified by neonatal screening programs have normal measurements of lung dynamics at diagnosis. Infant lung volumes can be measured plethysmographically and expiratory flow rates assessed using the 'squeeze' or rapid thoracoabdominal compression technique, but these are not in routine clinical use. From the age of 4–5 years children should be taught to perform maximal forced expiratory maneuvers, so that spirometric measurements can be made from reliably reproduced flow volume loops. Measurements of maximal mid-expiratory flow are most sensitive in detecting the early development of small airways obstruction but measurements have a wide coefficient of variation. Forced expiratory volume in the first second (FEV_1) is most commonly used in determining the need for changes in treatment and for predicting long-term prognosis in children with more advanced disease. Kerem et al[265] have shown that an FEV_1 of less than 30% predicted value is associated with a 50% risk of death within 5 years. Measurement of bronchodilator responsiveness can be used to assess whether, if airways obstruction is present, it may be worsened by coexisting asthma.

In children with moderate to severe lung disease, hypoxia may occur at night, particularly during respiratory exacerbations. This can be assessed by overnight oxygen saturation studies, where cumulative pulse oximetry data are recorded. Normal daytime oxygen saturation measurements are usually sustained until severe lung disease occurs,

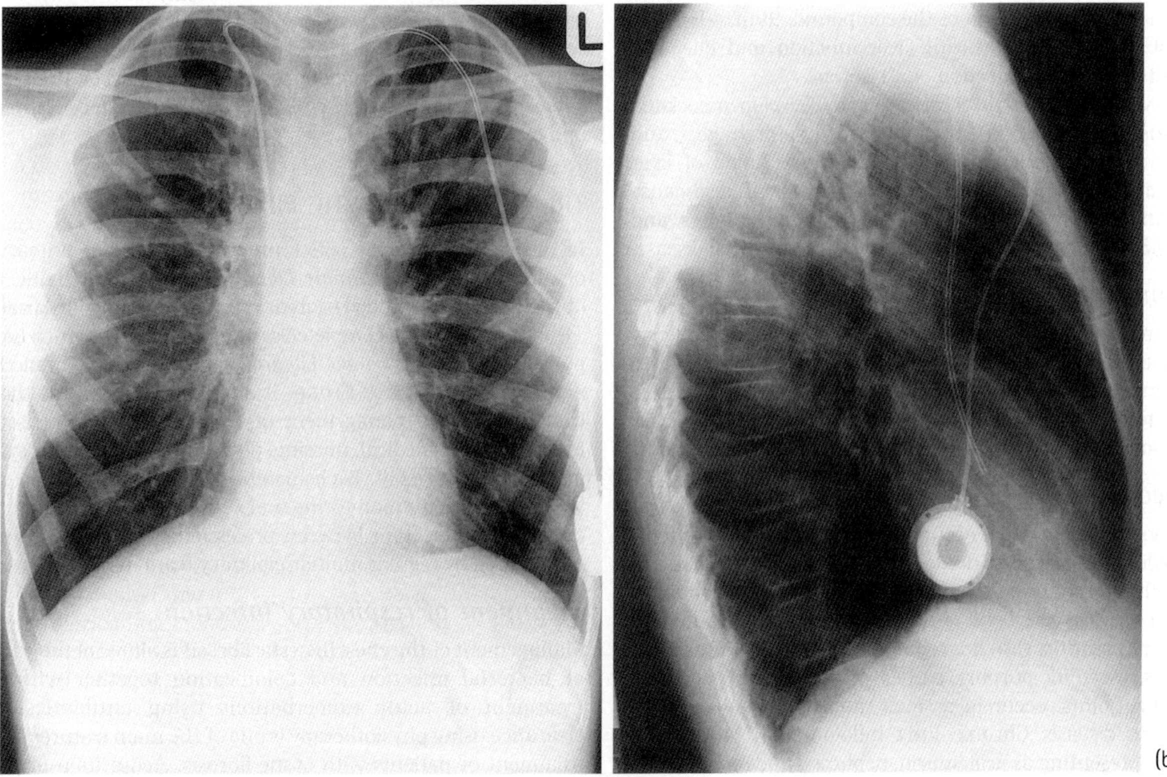

(a) (b)

Fig. 18.30 (a & b) PA and lateral films showing bronchial wall thickening, cyst formation and peripheral small round opacities. The latter represent abscesses or bronchiectatic areas impacted with purulent secretions. A totally implanted venous access device is in situ.

unless the child is acutely unwell. Exercise tolerance can be usefully assessed by graded exercise testing under controlled conditions.

Bronchodilator responsiveness should be assessed regularly to determine the usefulness of bronchodilator therapy and because in some children these drugs can exacerbate airway obstruction.

Liver disease (see also Ch. 11)

A spectrum of liver abnormalities may occur in CF. A few patients with CF have prolonged neonatal jaundice. Neonatal hepatitis is a very rare presenting illness. Hepatomegaly secondary to fatty infiltration is well recognized in malnourished patients but can occur in those who are thriving. Gallstones occur more frequently in people with CF than in the normal population. They are generally asymptomatic and are often an incidental finding on routine ultrasound. Progressive liver involvement, with liver cirrhosis and portal hypertension occurs in a minority. A recent epidemiological study reported that the clinical presentation of cystic fibrosis-related liver disease is relatively uncommon in young children, there is a peak in adolescence (with as many as 20% adolescents developing chronic liver disease) and a fall in prevalence over the age of 20.[266]

Both early detection and assessment of progression of liver disease in CF are relatively difficult. This is because, by the time liver disease is evident, as in a patient with an enlarged liver or spleen, there is often already portal hypertension and liver cirrhosis. Biochemical measures of liver function may not be useful because the level of abnormality does not always correlate with the extent of liver involvement.[267] Abnormalities of these tests may also be due to an effect other than CF liver disease such as an adverse effect of a drug treatment. Ultrasound can be used to assess the presence and progression of liver disease.[268] It can show alterations in liver size and texture and can also be used to assess the size and direction of blood flow in the portal vein. However results may vary with different operators. Another means of identification of liver disease is the use of radioisotope scanning-hepatobiliary scintigraphy.[269] Measuring the hepatic excretion of the compound, 99mTc-HIDA is a method of objectively measuring liver function and bile acid secretion and requires the injection of an isotope.

Children with advanced liver disease may develop associated complications including acute variceal hemorrhage, and hematemesis. Hematemesis may be the first presentation of liver disease and may be confused with hemoptysis. It may also cause aspiration and respiratory deterioration. Jaundice, ascites and encephalopathy occur very rarely in children with advanced disease.

Diabetes mellitus

Endocrine pancreatic insufficiency occurs with increasing frequency after the age of 10 years. Blood glucose, urinalysis and glycosylated hemoglobin measurements do not reliably identify diabetes compared with glucose tolerance tests.[270] Ketoacidosis is rare. Most CF diabetics benefit from insulin therapy but should not change to a diabetic diet.

Miscellaneous

Transient non-specific arthritis occurs in some CF patients and most commonly affects the knee and ankle joints. The condition is possibly related to high levels of circulating immune complexes. It should be distinguished from hypertrophic pulmonary osteoarthropathy and other causes of arthritis. Oral fluoroquinolones cause joint pains in some patients. Vasculitic purpuric rashes, predominantly occurring below the knee joints, occur in a small number of patients with advanced lung disease. Chronic lung inflammation has caused renal amyloid presenting as proteinuria, nephrosis and renal failure. There is an increased incidence of gastrointestinal malignancies among CF patients.

ANNUAL REVIEW

The basis of much of CF care depends on close monitoring for multi-system complications and disease progression. To ensure that this is undertaken systematically, and that important problems are not missed, most CF centers have introduced a detailed clinical review, which is performed once a year, when the child is clinically well. This annual review should include measurement of renal and liver function, full blood count, coagulation and vitamin levels. Allergic bronchopulmonary aspergillus can be screened for by measurement of IgE, eosinophil count and *A. fumigatus* titers. In children aged 10 and above, an oral glucose tolerance test is advised. Many centers use yearly liver ultrasound scanning, with Doppler measurement of flow in the portal vein, to detect changes of CF-related liver disease. A chest X-ray with scoring should be performed once a year. Although lung function is usually measured at each clinic visit, this should also be included in the annual review. Organisms grown on sputum cultures and cough swabs during the year should be recorded together with the numbers of hospital admissions and days of intravenous antibiotic therapy.

A number of clinical scoring systems have been devised for CF patients. The most widely used is the Shwachmann–Kulczycki score.[271] This is divided into four areas, with a maximum of 25 points allocated to each. These areas are general activity, physical examination, nutrition and chest X-ray findings. A score of 85–100 indicates excellent clinical status. The Shwachmann–Kulczycki score has been criticized as it has not been validated by studies of inter- and intra-observer reproducibility and the scores allocated are based on subjective assessment of clinical features.

The annual review also provides an opportunity for professionals such as dietitian, physiotherapist and psychologist to see the child and spend more time reviewing clinical status and management than is normally available during clinic. All the results, conclusions and management changes initiated as a result of the annual review should be communicated to the parents and child, by the clinician, at a detailed interview. A summary should be sent to the family doctor and many centers also send one to the parents. The annual review procedure has never been formally subjected to a randomized controlled trial, but, anecdotally, parents and children seem to value it.

TREATMENT OF CYSTIC FIBROSIS

In this section evidence concerning treatments has primarily been obtained from *The Cochrane Library* as either systematic reviews of randomized controlled trials or randomized controlled trials. Table 18.10 shows a list of completed systematic reviews, which have been published on *The Cochrane Library* by the Cochrane Cystic Fibrosis and Genetic Disorders Group. It should be stressed at the outset that the clinical management of CF involves a multidisciplinary team including medical, nursing, physiotherapy, dietetic, psychology and social work staff. Each member of the team will be involved in the assessment, monitoring and supervision of the child and her care. Communication between professionals is important and can be achieved by regular multidisciplinary team meetings.

Treatment of respiratory infection

Management of the chest in cystic fibrosis is aimed at the prevention of bacterial infection and colonization together with prompt treatment of acute exacerbations using antibiotics. Airway clearance using physiotherapy is one of the main features of regular treatment of patients with cystic fibrosis. Acquisition of strains of antibiotics in children with cystic fibrosis tends to be age related. *Staph. aureus* is usually the first organism to be isolated, followed by

Table 18.10 Systematic reviews published by the Cochrane Cystic Fibrosis and Genetic Disorders Group

Antifungal therapies for allergic bronchopulmonary aspergillosis in people with cystic fibrosis
Bisphosphonates for osteoporosis in people with cystic fibrosis
Chest physiotherapy compared to no chest physiotherapy for cystic fibrosis
Deoxyribonuclease for cystic fibrosis
Elective versus symptomatic intravenous antibiotic therapy for cystic fibrosis
Enteral tube feeding for cystic fibrosis
Home intravenous antibiotics for cystic fibrosis
Inhaled corticosteroids for cystic fibrosis
Macrolide antibiotics for cystic fibrosis
Nebulized anti-pseudomonal antibiotic therapy for cystic fibrosis
Nebulized hypertonic saline for cystic fibrosis
Newborn screening for cystic fibrosis
Once daily versus multiple daily dosing with intravenous aminoglycosides for cystic fibrosis
Oral calorie supplements for cystic fibrosis
Oral steroids for cystic fibrosis
Oral non-steroidal anti-inflammatory drugs for cystic fibrosis
Prophylactic antibiotics for cystic fibrosis
Single versus combination intravenous antibiotic therapy for people with cystic fibrosis
Ursodeoxycholic acid for cystic fibrosis-related liver disease
Vaccines for preventing infection with *Pseudomonas aeruginosa* in people with cystic fibrosis
Vaccines for preventing influenza in people with cystic fibrosis
Non-invasive ventilation for cystic fibrosis
Physical training for cystic fibrosis

H. influenzae and finally *Ps. aeruginosa*. Chronic colonization with this organism occurs in up to 80% of adults with CF,[272] although it is unclear whether acquisition of *Ps. aeruginosa* causes a decline in pulmonary function or is merely a marker of worsening prognosis.[273] Regular microbiological surveillance of sputum provides information about the lower respiratory tract flora, can help define new isolates within the airways and can also be used to define when 'colonization' has occurred. Colonization has various definitions but a frequent one is 'growth of an organism on three occasions in 6 months despite appropriate antibiotic treatment'. Specimens from the lower airways are acquired by various methods, including sputum expectoration and 'cough swab' or 'deep throat swab'. The last two are particularly helpful in children. The cough swab is performed by teaching the child to cough and placing a swab in the oropharynx during the cough.

One strategy for prevention of infection with *Staph. aureus* is to use continuous oral antistaphylococcal treatment from the time of diagnosis. A Cochrane Systematic Review which included three randomized controlled trials of a total of 177 patients, found a reduced prevalence of *Staph. aureus* in the respiratory secretions in children receiving this regimen and one study showed a shorter duration of hospital admissions in the second year of life in this group.[274] The review suggested that antistaphylococcal antibiotic prophylaxis may be of benefit when commenced early in infancy and continued up to 3 years of age but there was insufficient evidence to comment on longer-term effect.

Concern about the association between colonization with *Ps. aeruginosa* and worsening respiratory function has led to strategies to eradicate *Ps. aeruginosa* when it is first identified. In a small randomized controlled trial,[275] Valerius et al showed that chronic colonization can be prevented by treatment with a combination of oral and nebulized antipseudomonal antibiotics. As there are only limited oral antipseudomonal antibiotics available, and development of resistant organisms is an important problem, oral therapy is not an appropriate option for long-term antipseudomonal prophylaxis. An alternative, which has been developed over the last 20 years, is the use of antipseudomonal antibiotics delivered in a nebulized form. A systematic review of nebulized antipseudomonal antibiotics for cystic fibrosis included 10 trials and a total of 758 participants.[276] The review suggested that this therapy was associated with an improvement in lung function and reduced frequency of respiratory exacerbations in cystic fibrosis. There was most information about treatment with tobramycin, which is the most commonly used nebulized antipseudomonal antibiotic in North America, but in Europe colistin is most frequently used.

Cross-infection between CF patients of pathogenic organisms is now widely reported. It was first demonstrated between CF patients colonized with *Burkholderia cepacia*.[277] This was reported to be associated with more rapid deterioration in lung function and some patients experienced an acute severe deterioration and death. Because of this evidence, it is generally accepted within CF clinics and wards that *B. cepacia* positive patients should be segregated from *B. cepacia* negative patients. However recently it has been shown that a more virulent epidemic form of *B. cepacia* can be spread within a *B. cepacia* cohort of CF patients and that this has also been associated with deaths. This has led to recognition that policies to 'cohort' patients may not be adequate and complete segregation of CF patients harboring harmful transmissible organisms is the safest practice.[278]

In 1996 a series of children was reported from one CF center in whom colonization by the same beta-lactam resistant strain of *Ps. aeruginosa* in over 70% of those colonized with *Ps. aeruginosa*.[279] This evidence has led to strategies of segregating patients colonized with *Ps. aeruginosa* from those not colonized both as inpatients and in outpatient clinics. *B. cepacia* and *Ps. aeruginosa* are generally only harmful to other CF patients. However organisms such as methicillin resistant *Staph. aureus* may colonize the airways of CF patients and if transmitted represent a risk, not only to CF patients, but to other groups of patients. Individuals with CF who are colonized with such organisms should be strictly isolated when admitted to hospital and in the outpatient clinic.

Respiratory exacerbations, which are variously defined, but usually associated with increased sputum production, increased respiratory symptoms, a decline in lung function and at times chest X-ray changes, are treated with oral or intravenous antibiotics. The choice of these antibiotics is usually based on recent organisms grown from the sputum and their sensitivities to antibiotics. In the patient not colonized with *Ps. aeruginosa* a supplemental oral antibiotic which is effective against *Staph. aureus* and *H. influenzae* such as a broad spectrum cephalosporin is appropriate. Treatment with such antibiotics needs to use specific doses recommended for CF patients and is usually continued for 10–14 days. Similarly treatment of exacerbations with intravenous therapy is generally for around 2 weeks. There is some controversy about intravenous treatment regimens. In patients colonized with *Ps. aeruginosa* a broad-spectrum antipseudomonal cephalosporin such as ceftazidime has been used in a number of centers. It was speculated that this may have been associated with the emergence of a resistant strain of *Pseudomonas* in the center where widespread cross-infection was reported.[279] A systematic review compared treatment with a single intravenous antipseudomonal antibiotic compared with the same single therapy plus an additional antibiotic.[280] The most frequent comparison studied was that of beta-lactam antibiotic versus a beta-lactam aminoglycoside combination. While the meta-analysis did not demonstrate any significant differences between monotherapy and combination therapy for efficacy, single therapy was associated with in an increase in the number of patients with resistant *Ps. aeruginosa* at follow up. While the authors of the systematic review were cautious in their conclusions and suggested that these preliminary findings needed to be investigated in a randomized controlled trial, such studies have been used as evidence supporting the use of combination antipseudomonal antibiotic regimens. It has been suggested that intravenous aminoglycoside therapy, given as a single daily dose, may be as effective with fewer toxic effects than the conventional three times daily dosing. The results of a systematic review were inconclusive[281] and clinical trials are now in progress.

Aspergillus species (*Aspergillus fumigatus*) may be grown from the sputum of patients with CF. This may be associated with the condition known as allergic bronchopulmonary aspergillosis (ABPA), diagnosed by a number of clinical and laboratory criteria including a history of wheeze and expectoration of plugs of sputum, pulmonary infiltrates shown as shadows on the chest X-ray (Fig. 18.29), raised total serum immunoglobulin E and antibodies to *A. fumigatus*. Corticosteroids in high doses are the main treatment for APBA because they are thought to treat the inflammatory and allergic aspects of the condition. An alternative strategy to treat APBA is to reduce or clear the lung of *A. fumigatus* by antifungal therapy. This has been shown to be of some benefit in patients with asthma but a recent systematic review in cystic fibrosis patients failed to identify any randomized controlled trials in this group.[282]

Physiotherapy

In the CF airway excess mucus and sputum are associated with plugging and airways obstruction. In established disease bronchiectasis is present. Airway clearance with chest physiotherapy has, for many decades, been an integral part of CF management. This generally started at the time of diagnosis and continued throughout life. When the CF patient is well, sessions usually take 20 min twice a day.

A number of different physiotherapy techniques are used.[283] These include postural drainage, percussion and vibration techniques, huffing and directed coughing. The active cycle of breathing technique includes relaxation and breathing control, forced expectoration technique, thoracic expansion exercises and may also include postural drainage or chest clapping. Devices are used in some physiotherapy regimes and include positive expiratory mask therapy or high-pressure positive expiratory masks and oscillating devices such as the flutter/cornet or the oscillator vest.

Physiotherapy techniques are generally taught to patients and/or their families by a specialist CF physiotherapist. These techniques can be regularly reviewed by the physiotherapist in the CF clinic. A meta-analysis of chest physiotherapy in CF using sputum weight and pulmonary function as primary outcomes suggested that standard physiotherapy produces greater sputum expectoration than no physiotherapy and that in addition exercise was associated with improved lung function results.[284] There was no difference demonstrated between the modes of physiotherapy used in the treatment of CF.

Anti-inflammatory therapy

Because persistent inflammation is implicated in the pathophysiology of CF, for many years now strategies for reducing airway inflammation in CF have been investigated. The most powerful anti-inflammatory agents are corticosteroids and a number of trials of long-term oral corticosteroid therapy have been conducted in CF and these have been assessed in a systematic review.[285] This review showed that oral steroids at a dose equivalent to 1 mg/kg of prednisolone on alternate days were associated with a slowing in the progression of lung disease in CF. This benefit, mainly determined by a change in spirometric lung function, needs to be balanced against the adverse effects observed. Linear growth retardation was seen as early as 6 months from the start of treatment in the higher dose (2 mg/kg) group and from 2 years of treatment in the 1 mg/kg alternate day treatment group. Other adverse effects including abnormalities in blood glucose and cataracts resulted in early termination of one of the randomized controlled trials. A long-term follow up study at 10 years showed that catch-up growth started 2 years after treatment with oral steroids was stopped. However, alternate day treatment with oral steroids may have resulted in growth impairment up to adulthood in boys but not in girls.

Because of these long-term adverse effects of oral steroids, other strategies for delivering anti-inflammatory therapy have been explored. A systematic review of inhaled corticosteroids in CF,[286] which included nine trials, found that current evidence from randomized controlled trials was insufficient to establish whether this treatment was beneficial or harmful. The review recommended further trials to determine whether this therapy was effective and there is currently a trial of withdrawal of inhaled steroid treatment in progress in the UK. A systematic review of non-steroidal anti-inflammatory therapy[287] provided preliminary evidence that these drugs may prevent pulmonary deterioration in patients with mild lung disease due to CF. However the review recommended that further trials were required, before this treatment was introduced into clinical practice, to confirm whether their use prevented pulmonary deterioration and was associated with improved nutritional status. Concerns about introducing such therapy into widespread clinical use include the known serious adverse effects of non-steroidal anti-inflammatory drugs including gastrointestinal bleeding and perforation.

Mucolytics

A number of different treatments have been used to try to reduce the viscosity of CF sputum and therefore aid its clearance. Most recently the two treatments that have been studied in clinical trials are recombinant deoxyribonuclease (rhDNase) and hypertonic saline. In 1990 a human recombinant DNase was produced and has been commercially available since 1992. This treatment was studied in a very large (over 900 participants) clinical trial in people with CF.[288] The results produced were exciting because it was the first treatment shown clearly to produce a > 5% improvement in lung function in CF. However, follow-up was for only 6 months, did not include children under 5 years of age and excluded patients with severe lung disease. A systematic review of randomized controlled trials including the large 6 month trial showed this improvement in lung function over the short term, the only adverse effect being hoarseness of the voice.[289] Further studies are in progress to assess whether rhDNase affects lung function in CF over the longer term.

Nebulized hypertonic saline has been proposed to improve sputum clearance by a variety of postulated mechanisms. These include reducing the degree of cross-linking in the thick mucus gel in CF and therefore lowering viscosity and elasticity, inducing osmotic flow of water into the mucus layer and therefore improving mucus rheology and finally increasing the ionic concentration of the mucus and therefore causing conformational changes. A systematic review of 12 randomized controlled trials[290] showed that nebulized hypertonic saline improves mucociliary clearance immediately after administration. However, the maximum time for which data were recorded in these trials was only 3 weeks. This was therefore insufficient for this treatment to be recommended in CF patients. A trial comparing nebulized rhDNase, given daily, with nebulized hypertonic saline and rhDNase given on alternate days in CF has recently reported[291] a significantly greater increase in FEV_1 over 12 months, than hypertonic saline.

Nutritional support

The main aims of nutritional support in CF are to achieve optimal nutritional status, with normal growth and development throughout childhood. This is accomplished in a large majority of CF children. Regular assessment of nutrition, including height and weight measurements by a specialist CF dietitian is recommended. The main strategy is to maximize energy intake from food and to ensure adequate pancreatic enzyme supplementation. Additional support is needed for the minority of children in whom this approach is not successful. There are no precise rules about when nutritional interventions are considered, but the dietitian will consider whether the child is gaining weight and height satisfactorily along the centiles, the pattern of recent weight gain, the body mass index and its centile, and the percentage ideal weight for height.

Nutritional supplements are commercially available products, usually in the form of flavored milkshakes or other drinks. Alternatives are glucose copolymer powders, which are added to normal food. They are frequently introduced during a period of acute weight loss, but are often taken long-term, even if that was not the original intention. These products are expensive if used all the time. There are also concerns that, particularly in young children, they may simply replace food and impair the development of normal eating behavior. A systematic review has highlighted the lack of evidence for the efficacy of oral calorie supplements in CF.[292] A trial, in CF children, is in progress to evaluate this further.

Enteral feeding via nasogastric, orogastric, or gastrostomy tubes is considered for children whose nutritional state is unsatisfactory despite dietary advice and/or nutritional supplements. The feeds are commercially available and the range of products includes elemental, semi-elemental and whole protein feeds. Evidence for the efficacy of these feeds from randomized controlled trials is lacking;[293] however a case series and other reports have described long-term benefits of enteral feeding including improvement in catch-up growth, lung function and positive changes in body composition.[293]

Exocrine pancreatic insufficiency occurs in CF resulting in fat malabsorption. This means that malabsorption of fat soluble vitamins A, D, E and K is likely. Vitamin A deficiency has been documented in CF and is associated with night blindness and xerophthalmia; this responded to treatment with vitamin A supplementation.[294] Vitamin D deficient rickets is very rare in CF. Reduced bone mineral density and osteopenia are now reported, particularly in older children and adults. However, the etiology of this is likely to be multifactorial and it is unclear how much, if any, contribution vitamin D deficiency makes to reduced bone mineralization. Vitamin E levels in the serum are nearly always low in children with CF who do not receive supplementation.[295] Deficiency of vitamin E has been linked to neurological abnormalities in older patients.

Routine supplementation of vitamins A, D and E is recommended for all pancreatic insufficient patients with CF. For children over the age of 1 year, the dose recommended for vitamin A is 4000–10 000 IU daily, vitamin D 400 IU daily and vitamin E 50–100 mg daily. Plasma levels should be measured as part of the annual review and the dose of vitamin adjusted appropriately. Pancreatic sufficient patients should also be monitored by measuring their vitamin levels annually, but generally supplements are not required and should only be used if low plasma levels are detected.

Patients with CF are at an increased risk of developing vitamin K deficiency due to fat malabsorption, bowel salt deficiency, liver disease and antibiotic therapy. Prolonged prothrombin times are indicative of severe vitamin K deficiency and supplementation should be used if this is found. Plasma vitamin K levels are an unreliable assessment of status. Vitamin K is present in many of the multivitamin preparations but additional supplementation can be given in the presence of prolonged prothrombin time, particularly if there is concomitant liver disease.

Pancreatic enzyme replacement therapy

More than 90% of adults with CF have exocrine pancreas insufficiency and require enzyme supplements to aid absorption.[231] Clinical signs of malabsorption include fatty stools and poor weight gain, but steatorrhea should be confirmed by direct microscopy for fat globules or by measuring fecal elastase in the stool.

In babies and infants with CF, enteric coated enzyme granules can be administered via a teaspoon at intervals throughout the feed (mixed with a little milk or pureed fruit). Infants and young children require higher doses of pancreatin/kg/body weight than older children and adults. This reflects their higher fat intake (5 g fat/kg/day compared with the average adult intake of 2 g fat/kg/day). Enzymes have often been prescribed on the basis of one dose for meals and a smaller dose for snacks. However, better control may be achieved by titrating the dose against the fat content of the meal. On this basis most patients require 50–100 units of lipase/g dietary fat/kg/day.

Treatment of liver disease in cystic fibrosis

As described earlier, the early detection and assessment of progression of liver disease in CF are relatively difficult. Therefore by the time liver disease has been diagnosed, there is usually irreversible cirrhosis with portal hypertension. Earlier abnormalities in liver function and liver appearances on ultrasound are less specific and may or may not indicate early liver damage. In the last decade, ursodeoxycholic acid, a naturally occurring hydrophilic bile acid, has been used both for prevention and treatment of liver disease in CF.[296] There has been evidence from clinical trials that improvement in liver transaminases is seen when ursodeoxycholic acid treatment is used. However the effectiveness of this therapy in preventing or treating liver disease in CF has not been demonstrated and further clinical trials are needed. Many clinics are now using ursodeoxycholic acid in patients who show elevated liver transaminases or abnormalities on ultrasound suggestive of early liver disease.

Liver transplantation has been used successfully in some patients with advanced liver cirrhosis due to CF. Referral should be to a specialized liver transplantation unit. Assessment for liver transplantation requires a detailed assessment of the CF patient's respiratory status, as this may deteriorate during the peri- and postoperative periods.

End-stage lung disease and lung transplantation

Since 1985 when the first lung transplants were performed in people with CF, this therapy has become an option for patients with end-stage lung disease. Originally heart/lung transplantation was performed but increasingly double lung transplantation is being performed. Lack of donor organs remains the biggest problem for transplant programs. Survival data in adults following heart/lung transplantation from two UK centers have reported 69% and 72% survival at 1 year and 52% and 58% survival at 2 years.[297] Survival is not reported to be as good in children and data in children have shown a 46% 3-year survival in children over 10 and 42% in those under 10 years of age.[298] If this option is not available or considered appropriate good supportive and palliative care must be provided (see Ch. 37). Although mechanical ventilation is not appropriate, an option that may be considered is non-invasive ventilatory support (pp. 798 – Long term ventilation).

Psychosocial

A long-term chronic illness within a family takes an enormous emotional toll (see also Ch. 34). In the toddler years, there are particular problems over eating and physiotherapy. Whilst there may be a period of relative stability in mid-childhood, these problems commonly recur in adolescence. At this age, there is often a rejection of many of the treatments, leading to anguish on the part of the parents and more rapid deterioration in the children. Needle phobia can be common. The needs of normal siblings in the family must also be considered, particularly when apparently excessive attention is given to the affected child. Schooling problems may occur in relation to medication and particularly pre-meal pancreatic enzyme replacement. In the more severely affected, delayed adolescence with poor growth will have an adverse effect on peer influence and self-confidence. Many multidisciplinary CF teams now include a dedicated CF psychologist, who can help and support families during difficult times. Although death of a CF patient in childhood is now relatively rare, such events can cause considerable distress and anxiety to other patients in the clinic. Other children with CF, as well as the CF team can benefit from psychological support during such difficult times.

RESPIRATORY INFECTIONS

Although mortality from respiratory infections in previously healthy children is now very rare in the UK, respiratory infections still account for a large number of hospital admissions, a half of all illnesses in preschool children and one-third of all GP attendances. The preschool child has, on average, 6–8 respiratory infections per year, ranging from mild colds to severe bronchiolitis. Lower respiratory tract infections are commonest in the first year of life and then fall in incidence in subsequent years.

UPPER RESPIRATORY TRACT INFECTIONS

Upper respiratory tract infections (URTIs) are common and, although rarely fatal are a source of considerable morbidity, especially in young children. URTIs account for 95% of all respiratory infections and include colds, pharyngitis, tonsillitis, otitis media, sinusitis, croup and epiglottitis.

The common cold

The common cold is a short, mild and usually self-limiting illness. There is significant impact in terms of school absence and complicating factors such as secondary bacterial infection and exacerbation of other underlying respiratory conditions including asthma and cystic fibrosis. Children may have up to 12 colds per year, usually acquired from nurseries or from siblings. The causative organisms of the common cold are viruses of which there are more than 200 types. The most common agent is rhinovirus, responsible for up to 40% cases. Adeno-, rota-, myxo-, corona-, ECHO and Coxsackie viruses and *Mycoplasma pneumoniae* are all associated with coryzal symptoms.

Clinical features

The common cold is characterized by rhinorrhea, sore throat, cough, fever and malaise lasting up to 7 days and often a lingering mucopurulent nasal discharge. Otitis media may be a complicating feature, often with secondary bacterial infection. Headache may be troublesome in the older child. In infants colds may be manifest as irritability, snuffles and difficulty with feeding and diarrhea, especially with rotavirus and enteroviral infections. Infants less than 3 months of age are particularly susceptible to rapidly evolving secondary bacterial lower respiratory tract infection.

Differential diagnosis

Other infections such as septicemia, meningitis and pneumonia should be considered in infants with poor feeding. Allergic rhinitis is sometimes difficult to distinguish from the apparent permanent colds of toddlers, but is characterized by a clear watery nasal discharge with a pale nasal mucosa. The discharge associated with a foreign body is unilateral, purulent, foul-smelling and blood-stained. Other diseases may present with a nasal discharge including primary ciliary dyskinesia and immune deficiencies.

Treatment

Many interventions for the treatment and prevention of colds have been studied since the 1940s and the evidence demonstrates no benefit in terms of clinical improvement or number of days missed from school or work from the treatment of upper respiratory tract infections with antibiotics.[299] Intranasal interferons have been shown to prevent and to attenuate the course of experimental and to a lesser extent natural colds, but with a high incidence of adverse effects, for example bloodstained nasal discharge, and therefore have no place in everyday use.[300] Dipyridamole, palmitate, ICI 130 685, Impulsin and Pleocarnil are all antiviral agents that have been shown to prevent the common cold and are well tolerated. Further assessment of antivirals focusing on non-virus-specific compounds needs to be carried out.

Measures such as Echinacea, humidified air, nasal decongestants, vitamin C and zinc have shown some positive results but there is insufficient evidence to recommend any of these measures for the treatment or prevention of colds.

Acute otitis media (see also Ch. 30)

Acute otitis media is one of the most frequent diseases in early infancy and childhood. The peak incidence is between 6 and 15 months. Although for most children, acute otitis media is a disease which resolves spontaneously, it represents a large health problem and a substantial amount of money is spent on antimicrobials to treat this disease. Secondary bacterial infection is common following a viral upper respiratory tract infection. *H. influenzae, Streptococcus pneumoniae, Moraxella catarrhalis, M. pneumoniae* and occasionally Gram negative bacteria, particularly in the neonatal period, are the most likely bacterial pathogens.

Symptoms and signs

Non-specific symptoms such as fever, poor feeding, irritability, diarrhea and vomiting are presenting features of an infant with otitis media. An older child will complain of earache. On examination, a red, dull, bulging tympanic membrane suggests acute suppurative otitis media. Hemorrhagic bullae on the surface of the eardrum suggest *M. pneumoniae* infection. Rupture of the membrane may follow, often with dramatic relief of pain.

Complications

Meningitis and mastoiditis are unusual but important complications. Chronic suppurative otitis media has in the past been attributed to inadequate treatment of the acute infection, but with the lack of evidence to support the increased benefit of antibiotic therapy, this relationship remains unclear. Temporary hearing loss at all sound frequencies is common.

Treatment

Analgesia and antipyretics should be used for symptomatic relief. Despite a large number of published clinical trials, there is no consensus on the use of antibiotic therapy for acute otitis media. The primary considerations are firstly whether treatment with antibiotics is justified and secondly the optimal duration of treatment.

The decline in suppurative complications of otitis media in North America and Europe during the 1940s and 1950s has been attributed to antibiotic therapy and a semi-randomized trial in Sweden of 1365 subjects in 1954[301] reported a rate of mastoiditis of 17% in the untreated group versus none in the penicillin treated group. More recently, evidence suggests that long-term outcomes are similar in antibiotic treated and untreated children with acute otitis media living in developed countries.[302]

A meta-analysis pooling the results of 10 studies suggested that in comparison to placebo, antibiotics provide a small benefit for acute otitis media in children, in terms of a reduction in pain at 2–7 days into the illness.[303] As most cases will resolve spontaneously, this benefit must be weighed against the possible adverse reactions and the emergence of resistant bacteria. A recent systematic review has shown that a short course of antibiotics (less than 7 days) is as effective as a longer course (7 days or greater) for the treatment of uncomplicated acute otitis media in children.[304]

Current evidence does not support the use of decongestants or antihistamines in otitis media. No additional benefit has been demonstrated in terms of symptom relief or prevention of complications and an increased risk of adverse effects was shown.[305]

Pharyngitis and tonsillitis

Sore throat is a common complaint and is usually associated with upper respiratory tract infections. Although it is largely a self-limiting problem, it causes significant morbidity and absence from school and high consultation rate in general practice and again a significant number of antibiotics are prescribed.

Etiology and diagnosis

Most sore throats have a viral etiology, especially in children under the age of 3 years. Viral pathogens include adenovirus, influenza and parainfluenza, Coxsackie A and Epstein–Barr virus (EBV), which are the causes of herpangina and of glandular fever respectively. The primary bacterial etiology is group A beta-hemolytic streptococcus. It is very difficult to distinguish clinically between viral and bacterial causes of sore throat and results of throat swab culture correlate poorly with symptoms. A purulent exudate over the tonsils does not signify a bacterial etiology, but a membrane may be suggestive of EBV or diphtheria. Petechial hemorrhages on the palate and cervical lymphadenopathy are non-specific signs which often accompany pharyngitis. Interpretation of throat swabs is complicated by the 40% asymptomatic carriage rate in the general population. Rapid antigen tests may be used but this test has poor sensitivity and has not significantly changed practice in primary care.[306]

Treatment

The majority of children with sore throats require only symptomatic treatment with simple analgesia. A recent meta-analysis suggested that antibiotic treatment of sore throats reduced the number of complications including glomerulonephritis, rheumatic fever, acute otitis media, acute sinusitis and quinsy.[307] However, the incidence of these complications in the UK is extremely low and the evidence does not support the routine use of antibiotics to prevent complications. Penicillin has been shown to have a small benefit in providing symptomatic improvement in children with severe symptoms of sore throat, but is not recommended for routine use.[308] If group A beta-hemolytic streptococcus has been isolated, a 10 day, four times a day course of penicillin or a shorter course of a cephalosporin or macrolide may be effective. The advantages of the convenience of the once or twice daily cephalosporin regimen should be balanced against the potential for the emergence of resistant stains of streptococcus.

The effectiveness of tonsillectomy in the treatment of recurrent tonsillitis has not been formally evaluated.[309] Tonsillectomy has a significant perioperative complication rate of around 1–2%, but there are suggested benefits for children, not only in reducing the number of sore throats, but for general health including growth. Tonsillectomy is generally considered if the child has had more than 6–7 significant recurrences over 1–2 years despite antibiotic treatment, has significant obstructive sleep apnea, or has had two or more peritonsillar abscesses.

Diphtheria

Diphtheria is an acute, communicable disease caused by *Corynebacterium diphtheriae*. Despite the success of mass immunization in many countries, diphtheria continues to play a major role as a potentially lethal infectious disease. Early, accurate microbiological diagnosis and the identification of contacts and carriers are imperative since delay in specific therapy may result in death. Recent developments have focused upon methods for detection of the lethal and potent exotoxin produced by the causative organism, *C. diphtheriae*. This detection is the definitive test for the microbiologic diagnosis of diphtheria.

Symptoms and signs

The possibility of diphtheria should always be considered in the differential diagnosis of sore throat, especially in patients travelling from Eastern Europe or Bangladesh. The incubation period is 1–6 days and therefore it is possible that travellers may arrive in the early stages of the disease. The disease is generally characterized by local growth of the bacterium in the pharynx with pseudomembrane formation. The membrane becomes greenish-black and firmly adherent and can involve the tonsillar zones, larynx, soft palate, uvula, and nasal cavities. Less commonly, bacterial growth can occur in the stomach or lungs; systemic dissemination of toxin then invokes lesions in distant organs. When the membrane involves only the nasal septum the disease is relatively minor; however, extension to the larynx causes stridor and upper airway obstruction. In the days before immunization, laryngeal diphtheria was the commonest reason for tracheostomy in Britain. The patient presents with a sore throat, stridor, fever and is generally unwell. The clinical features may be indistinguishable from epiglottitis.

Treatment

The child should be isolated and urgent attention should be given to protecting the airway, with a team on standby for tracheostomy if necessary. Treatment is with antitoxin 5000–30 000 units intravenously and systemic penicillin 4 hourly. Erythromycin can be used to treat carriers.

Whooping cough (see also Ch. 26)

Whooping cough, or pertussis, is a respiratory infection caused predominantly by the organism *Bordetella pertussis*, although adenovirus, *M. pneumoniae* and *Chlamydia trachomatis* have also been associated with a whooping cough like illness. *B. pertussis* is transmitted by respiratory droplets and causes disease only in humans. Whooping cough is an uncommon but serious illness, particularly in children under the age of 5 years. Vaccines made from killed whole *B. pertussis* organisms have been available since the 1950s, but even in developed countries with well-funded immunization programs, whooping cough epidemics still occur and children still die from the disease.

Prevention

There appear to be three main reasons for the failure to control pertussis in the developed world. Firstly, neither immunization nor infection confers life-long immunity. Secondly, although pertussis is generally regarded as a disease of children, recent evidence has shown that adults suffer from milder forms of the disease and act as a reservoir for infection. Finally, whole cell pertussis vaccines (WPV) display a level of toxicity that discourages immunization uptake, including a very low but measurable incidence of transient severe reactions such as hypotonic-hyporesponsive episodes, convulsions and acute encephalopathy. In addition, there is a public perception that WPVs may be responsible for serious, permanent neurological disturbances, despite research in the 1980s showing that such events are far less likely to be caused by WPV than by whooping cough itself.

The routine use of whole cell pertussis vaccines was suspended in several countries in the late 1970s and early 1980s, leading to a resurgence of whooping cough. Acellular pertussis vaccines containing purified or recombinant *B. pertussis* antigens instead of intact organisms were developed and have been shown to be as effective and less toxic than the whole cell vaccines.[310]

The current rate of immunization uptake is around 93%. Infants below the age of vaccination are now the population at highest risk.

Symptoms and signs

A catarrhal stage of fever, non-specific cough and nasal discharge for 7–10 days precedes the onset of a hacking cough, which is mainly nocturnal before becoming constant and occurring in paroxysms, classically rising in pitch and terminating with a whoop. Between coughing spasms, the child looks quite well, but the cough may be forceful enough to precipitate vomiting, petechiae, subconjuctival hemorrhages, pneumothorax and subcutaneous emphysema or even rib fractures. After the acute phase of the disease, many patients continue to cough for prolonged periods, sometimes for several months. No significant long term respiratory morbidity has been shown and bronchiectasis is now exceedingly rare in developed countries.

Young infants and neonates. In spite of the accelerated immunization schedule since the late 1970s, there has been a steady increase in the number of reported cases in young unimmunized infants, according to Communicable Diseases Surveillance Centre (England and Wales) statistics. There is little placentally transferred passive immunity to pertussis and, until primary vaccination is completed at 4 months, this age group is vulnerable if exposed. Despite aggressive intensive care treatment, there is still a significant mortality, particularly in those requiring mechanical ventilation. In this age group, presentation is likely to be more severe and atypical and may be confused with more common illnesses such as bronchiolitis. There is very often a household contact with pertussis, often the mother, which may be proven with a positive culture, or careful history taking may reveal a history of concurrent paroxysmal cough. Presenting features in this age group include a non-specific cough, poor feeding, vomiting, cyanosis, apneas and bradycardia, usually with no characteristic paroxysmal cough or whoop, which can make the diagnosis difficult. Apnea may lead to cardiac arrest and indicates the requirement for intubation and ventilation. There is a high rate of major complications such as bacterial pneumonia, pulmonary hypertension, air leaks, seizures and encephalopathy. Pertussis can occasionally be the cause of sudden infant death syndrome.

Diagnosis (see also Ch. 26 – Case definition)

Various diagnostic methods are available to identify *B. pertussis*, including culture from pernasal swab, serology and polymerase chain reaction (PCR). There is a characteristic lymphocytosis and an extreme blood leukocytosis may be an independent predictor of mortality in the neonatal age group.[311] Chest X-rays may demonstrate pulmonary infiltrates, particularly in the perihilar region which may be due to excess secretions, leading to areas of atelectasis with compensatory areas of hyperinflation of other areas of the lung.

Treatment

Pertussis is highly infectious and barrier nursing of hospitalized patients must be carried out. Ventilatory support may be needed for respiratory failure or prolonged apnea.

Erythromycin is the antibiotic of choice for clearance of *B. pertussis* infection on culture; however, it is only effective during the infectious catarrhal stage of the disease. Early phase I clinical trials of an intravenous pertussis immunoglobulin have indicated that this preparation is safe and achieves high levels of pertussis toxin antibody titers in infants.[312] A double blind placebo-controlled study of salbutamol (albuterol) treatment for pertussis showed no benefit.[313]

In view of the high rate of secondary transmission of the organism to household members, an alternative approach is to use erythromycin as chemoprophylaxis for close contacts of the primary case and this may be protective to non-immunized or partially immunized infant contacts, who are at risk of severe disease. A review of the evidence for the use of erythromycin in preventing secondary transmission showed very little benefit, compared to the protection conferred by the vaccine.[314] Further blinded randomized controlled trials of erythromycin prophylaxis should consider shorter courses of erythromycin as well as the newer macrolide antibiotics, which have fewer adverse effects.

INFECTIONS CAUSING UPPER AIRWAY OBSTRUCTION

The major infective causes of upper airway obstruction are croup, epiglottitis and bacterial tracheitis (Table 18.11). Rarer causes include retropharyngeal abscess, cellulitis or severe tonsillitis. Other causes of stridor include foreign body aspiration, angioneurotic edema, vallecular cyst or abscess, inhalational burns, diphtheria, epiglottic hemangiomas or other congenital abnormalities.

Croup

Croup (laryngotracheobronchitis) is a common cause of airway obstruction in children. The term croup refers to a clinical syndrome characterized by a barking cough, inspiratory stridor and hoarseness of the voice. These symptoms are thought to be due to edema of the larynx, trachea and bronchi as a result of a viral infection, hence the term laryngotracheobronchitis. Parainfluenza types 1 and 2 are the most common infecting organisms, but rhinovirus and RSV can also cause croup. Although croup is a self-limiting illness, it causes frequent visits to GPs and hospital emergency departments and often results in hospitalization. Although severe croup occurs infrequently, early recognition of the signs of severe airway obstruction is important.

Symptoms and signs

Coryzal symptoms are followed over 12–24 h by a harsh, barking cough. Stridor is most evident when the child is upset and the

Table 18.11 Clinical presentations of upper airway obstruction due to infections

	Croup	Epiglottitis	Bacterial tracheitis
Age	1–2 years	2–6 years	Throughout childhood
Causative organism	Parainfluenza	*Haemophilus influenzae*	*Staphylococcus aureus* *Streptococcus pneumoniae* *Haemophilus influenzae*
History	Onset 1–2 days Coryza Barking cough	Onset < 24 h Sore throat Dysphagia	Onset < 24 h Rattling cough Sore throat
Signs	Fever < 38.5°C Non-toxic Harsh stridor Hoarse voice	Fever 38–40°C Toxic Upright position Open mouth, drooling Muffled stridor	Fever 38–40°C Toxic Mucopurulent secretions Absent or soft stridor
Course	Resolves 4–10 days Intubation < 3%	All need intubation	Intubation in > 80%, often > 1 week
Treatment	Steroids Adrenaline (epinephrine)	Cephalosporin	Cephalosporin

parents often report that the onset of symptoms is at night, when the child is woken in the early hours of the morning by cough and stridor. Usually, croup resolves spontaneously over a 3–4 day period.

Assessment of severity

Laboratory and radiological investigations are unhelpful. The decision to treat or admit to hospital is based on clinical features and an assessment of the severity of the croup. Signs of a severe episode of croup include restlessness, cyanosis and subcostal and intercostal recession. The intensity of the stridor itself is a poor indicator of severity. Restlessness is a sign of hypoxemia and should not be confused with anxiety. A child that requires oxygen as suggested by the oxygen saturation is likely to have severe upper airways obstruction.

Management

The hospital management of croup has altered significantly over the last decade. Evidence shows that the introduction of the use of steroids has resulted in decreased use of health care services in terms of fewer admissions to hospitals and intensive care units.

Children with mild croup require reassurance. There is no evidence that steroids have a place in the management of this group. No evidence yet supports the effectiveness of mist therapy or nebulized saline, although there are some randomized controlled trials underway to investigate these approaches.

Steroids. A number of randomized controlled trials of glucocorticosteroids have been published and the evidence suggests that all children with croup symptoms who demonstrate increased work of breathing should be treated with steroids.[315] The most commonly studied steroids have been dexamethasone and budesonide. Dexamethasone is a potent steroid with an anti-inflammatory ratio of 5:1 compared with prednisolone. It can be administered either by mouth or i.m. injection. Budesonide is a synthetic glucocorticoid with a significantly lower bioavailability than beclometasone because of its hepatic first-pass clearance. Most of the nebulized dose is deposited to the upper airways, the point of maximal inflammation in croup. No significant difference in efficacy has been demonstrated between oral dexamethasone and nebulized budesonide and both treatments are effective as early as 6 h and for up to at least 12 h after administration. Oral dexamethasone (0.6 mg/kg) may be the best treatment option because of its ease of administration, widespread availability and lower cost. In a child who is vomiting, nebulized budesonide (2 mg) or i.m. dexamethasone may be preferable. Use of steroids is associated with improvement in scores of croup severity, a decrease in time spent in the emergency department, shorter hospital stay and decreased use of co-interventions such as nebulized adrenaline (epinephrine) and endotracheal intubation.

Adrenaline. Adrenaline (epinephrine) is a potent stimulator of alpha- and beta-adrenergic receptors. In patients with croup, it is believed to provide short-term benefit due to its ability to reduce bronchial and tracheal secretions and mucosal edema. Nebulized adrenaline (5 ml of 1:1000 solution) should be considered for children with croup who have moderate to severe respiratory distress. The onset of action has been observed as early as 30 min after treatment and its duration is around 2 h.[316] Because of the relatively short duration of action, patients may have rebound symptoms as the effects of the drug wane. Glucocorticosteroids should therefore be given at the same time as adrenaline to prevent this and patients given adrenaline should be observed carefully for at least 2 h. There is some evidence that it is safe to discharge improved patients after a period of observation.[317]

Epiglottitis

Epiglottitis is an airway emergency with a high risk of acute complete obstruction of the upper airway and is caused primarily by *H. influenzae* type b (Hib). The epiglottis is characteristically swollen, edematous and cherry red. The introduction of the conjugate vaccine in the UK in October 1992 has substantially reduced the incidence of epiglottitis; however there has been a recent resurgence of cases due to vaccine failure[318] and clinicians should continue to have a high index of suspicion, even in a fully vaccinated child. Other pathogens include *Streptococcus*, *Staphylococcus* and *Klebsiella*.

Hib has been shown to be an important cause of life-threatening childhood infections worldwide. Epiglottitis is the second most common Hib disease in industrialized countries and accounts for 10% of Hib infections worldwide with meningitis being the most common (52%). Epidemiological data from 19 countries before introduction of the vaccine showed average incidence rates of epiglottitis of 13 per 100 000 in children aged 0–4 years and 5 per 100 000 in those aged 0–14 years, with higher rates in Sweden and parts of Australia and lower rates in developing countries. Worldwide there were 12 000 cases per year and 400 deaths, i.e. 2.5% mortality.

Prevention

Conjugate vaccines against Hib were introduced in the late 1980s and have been shown to have an efficacy exceeding 90% from the first months of life.[319]

The vaccine has induced a dramatic decline in the incidence of Hib over a short period. This is partly due to the ability of the vaccine to prevent nasopharyngeal Hib colonization. In the UK, children receive three doses at 2, 3 and 4 months of age as part of the standard vaccination program. 90% coverage has been achieved and the incidence of all Hib infections is now 2 per 100 000 or less in children aged 0–4 years, which represents a decline of over 97%.

Clinical features

Differences between the presentation of croup and epiglottitis are presented in Table 18.11. Epiglottitis generally affects slightly older children, usually aged 2–6 years, although it has been reported in infants and is being increasingly recognized in adults. It may occur at any time of year, but more often in spring and winter. Children usually lack a viral prodrome and complain of a sore throat which progresses within hours to a toxic illness in which the child appears irritable, pyrexial and dyspneic. The child has dysphagia and prefers to sit forward with the neck extended and the arms forward for support to optimize the patency of the airway. There is marked intercostal and subcostal recession and use of the accessory muscles of respiration. A soft inspiratory stridor results from edema of the supraglottic mucosa and physical obstruction of the airway results in drooling and muffled voice. Fatigue develops if the obstruction is not relieved and cyanosis and deteriorating conscious level are precursors of impending complete obstruction and respiratory arrest.

Diagnosis

The diagnosis is made on clinical grounds and ensuring an adequate airway takes precedence over all investigations. Airway radiology should never delay definitive diagnosis and management of the airway. The full blood count shows a characteristic immature polymorphonuclear leukocytosis and blood cultures are positive for *H. influenzae* in around 50% cases.[320] The yield of positive culture results from pharyngeal swab is lower than that of blood.

Treatment

As soon as epiglottitis is suspected, preparations should be made to protect the airway and the child should be given 100% humidified oxygen. Any procedure that may cause distress to the child, such as examination of the throat, should be avoided as this may precipitate sudden occlusion of the airway due to intense vagal discharge and laryngeal spasm. Attempts should be made to provide a comfortable environment for the child with the parent present. Observation of the child or radiological confirmation of the diagnosis are not appropriate and can be dangerous, due to rapid progression of the airway occlusion. Intravenous access should be obtained only after stabilization of the airway and fluid resuscitation may be required for the toxic child.

Airway management. Direct examination of the larynx is indicated to exclude other causes of laryngeal obstruction such as abscesses or foreign bodies. This should be carried out under inhalational anesthesia, with a team on standby prepared for immediate airway intervention with either an endotracheal tube or tracheostomy. This team should include a pediatrician, anesthetist and ENT surgeon and preferably the examination is carried out in the anesthetic room with the child breathing spontaneously. Nebulized adrenaline (epinephrine) may provide temporary relief, but should not be used unless measures for protecting the airway are already available and should be abandoned if causing distress to the child. Inhalation of sevofluorane has been described in recent case reports as a safe and effective anesthetic induction agent and is better tolerated than the traditional agent halothane.[321]

Antimicrobial therapy. In addition to airway management, antibiotics are the definitive treatment for epiglottitis. Third generation cephalosporins such as cefotaxime and ceftriaxone are usually recommended to cover the increasing emergence of beta-lactamase producing strains of *H. influenzae* that are resistant to treatment with ampicillin or chloramphenicol. Rifampicin prophylaxis (20 mg/kg daily for 4 days) may be recommended for non-immunized contacts and to the index case to eradicate carriage of the organism.

Complications

Pulmonary edema following relief of the upper airway obstruction is a recognized complication and is probably due to alterations in capillary wall permeability. This can be managed by using a moderate level of CPAP or positive pressure ventilation with positive end expiratory pressure (PEEP). Other manifestations of Hib infection such as exudative tonsillitis, otitis media, pneumonia, meningitis, pericarditis and septic arthritis have been observed to coexist with epiglottitis.

Bacterial tracheitis

Bacterial tracheitis is a severe condition characterized by acute upper airway obstruction and purulent secretions within the trachea. Affected children can present at any age with a fever, sore throat and soft stridor. Prolonged endotracheal intubation is often required and severe septicemia may follow. Mortality and morbidity are significant. *Staph. aureus* is the commonest organism involved, with *Strep. pneumoniae* and *H. influenzae* also significant as causative organisms. There is a suggestion of an epidemiological change in recent years towards a less morbid condition in which children are less toxic and require intubation less frequently, with *M. catarrhalis* and viral causes becoming more common.[322] Diagnosis is usually made at laryngoscopy and secretions are collected for culture. Treatment is with a broad spectrum, intravenous antibiotic.

LOWER RESPIRATORY TRACT INFECTIONS

Lower respiratory tract infections (LRTIs) are a common cause of mortality in developing countries and represent a major cause of morbidity among children worldwide. LRTIs account for 5% of all respiratory infections and include bronchiolitis, pneumonias and bronchiectasis. One in four children has a LTRI in the first year of life. Differential diagnoses include cystic fibrosis, aspiration associated with gastroesophageal reflux or tracheoesophageal fistula.

Bronchiolitis

Bronchiolitis is the commonest cause of lower respiratory tract illness in infants and is an important cause of acute and long-term morbidity. The infecting organism in around 75% cases is respiratory syncytial virus (RSV); others include adenovirus and rhinovirus. RSV causes annual winter epidemics of respiratory disease and can also manifest as pneumonia, otitis media, croup or mild upper respiratory tract infections. During a single epidemic, over 70% of infants become infected with the virus and almost all infants are infected by the end of their second winter.

Thirty per cent of these develop lower respiratory tract symptoms and between 0.5 and 1.5% are admitted to hospital with RSV bronchiolitis.

Infants at high risk of severe RSV bronchiolitis include those born prematurely, and those with cardiovascular disease, chronic respiratory disease including bronchopulmonary dysplasia (BPD) and cystic fibrosis or immunosuppression.

Clinical features

Acute. The peak age of infants hospitalized with RSV bronchiolitis is around 3 months. The clinical features of the illness reflect the plugging of small airways with inflammatory exudates leading to a large increase in airways resistance and a corresponding increase in work of breathing leading to fatigue of the respiratory muscles. Characteristically there is a short prodromal upper respiratory tract illness with coryzal symptoms and low-grade pyrexia, followed by a relatively sudden onset of tachypnea, hypoxia, a moist cough and difficulty with feeding. Increased work of breathing is reflected by suprasternal, subcostal and intercostal recession with head bobbing and nasal flaring. The predominant feature on auscultation is crackles with, or without the presence of wheeze. As the chest becomes hyperinflated, the liver is displaced and is often easily palpable in the abdomen.

Signs of more severe illness include apnea, especially in young and preterm infants, irritability, listlessness, cyanosis and reduced conscious level. Approximately 2% of infants that are hospitalized with RSV bronchiolitis require ventilatory support because of either an obstructive bronchiolitis or, more unusually, a restrictive pneumonia or acute respiratory distress syndrome (ARDS).

Chronic. Lower respiratory tract RSV infections are associated with increased respiratory morbidity in the early years of life. Comparison at 9–10 years of age of previously healthy babies who had RSV infection with carefully matched controls demonstrated that there is a threefold increase in respiratory symptoms and asthma or airways obstruction requiring bronchodilator therapy.[323] The mechanisms contributing to this chronic respiratory morbidity and its associations with atopy are unclear.

Diagnosis

Rapid identification of RSV infection can be confirmed by immunofluorescence on nasopharyngeal aspirate samples, which gives a result within hours, or by viral culture.

Radiology

Chest radiology is unhelpful in typical cases of bronchiolitis and should be avoided unless there is an underlying illness or deterioration in clinical status suggesting the need for intensive care. CXR show hyperinflation with multiple areas of interstitial infiltration. Signs of segmental collapse, representing atelectasis, occurs in 25% and this often leads to the inappropriate use of antibiotics.

Treatment

Current therapy for RSV bronchiolitis is essentially supportive, involving maintenance of hydration and oxygen status. Nasogastric or intravenous feeding is required if the baby is unable to suck. Oxygen saturation monitoring is necessary and oxygen should be administered via nasal prongs or headbox if the oxygen saturation falls below 92%. An increasing oxygen requirement indicates worsening disease with increasing ventilation/perfusion imbalance. Hypercapnia is a sign of exhaustion and alveolar hypoventilation and if this develops the baby should be moved to a high-dependency area or intensive care for ventilatory support.

Overall, the evidence from the results of randomized controlled trials does not support the use of additional therapies. Bronchodilators have not been shown to be helpful for either inpatients or outpatients, except perhaps in reducing a clinical severity score,[324] and desaturations have been reported after salbutamol (albuterol) nebulization.[325] The majority of studies have demonstrated no benefit from inhaled or oral corticosteroid therapy either in the acute phase or in the prevention of post-bronchiolitic wheezing.[326,327] Antibiotics are not indicated except in the case of secondary bacterial infection which is rare in babies that do not need ventilatory support.

Ribavirin inhibits viral replication and is the only antiviral agent available against RSV. Although early studies of the effect of ribavirin found some benefit, a systematic review of 10 trials showed no reliable evidence of a positive outcome.[328] A trial of ribavirin in preterm infants with BPD who had a respiratory deterioration while on the neonatal intensive care unit (NICU) has shown an increased speed of recovery and improved lung function at 6 months[329] and therefore may be considered as adjunctive therapy in this particular group of patients.

For those infants who require respiratory support, particularly infants with chronic lung disease, conventional ventilation alone may be insufficient. Extracorporeal membrane oxygenation (ECMO) has been shown to be associated with a survival of over 50%.[330] Nitric oxide may improve the respiratory status of those infants with restrictive lung disease or pre-existing pulmonary hypertension by improving gas exchange, although its long-term influences remain unproven. Exogenous surfactant can improve oxygenation and may lead to a shorter duration of ventilatory support and ICU care,[331] although further randomized controlled trials to confirm these findings are awaited.

Prevention

RSV is spread by direct contact with infected secretions and contaminated objects and this may be reduced by effective and appropriate hand-washing and cohort nursing. The importance of these measures in the prevention of RSV transmission should not be underestimated. There is as yet no safe and effective vaccine for use in infants. A formalin-inactivated vaccine was introduced in the 1960s but this led to more severe respiratory disease in vaccinated infants during the following season. Until an effective vaccine is developed, alternative prophylactic measures must be optimized.

High-dose RSV immunoglobulin given intravenously has been shown to reduce the number of hospital days and the requirement for intensive care in premature infants with or without BPD, with 17 patients needed to be treated to prevent one hospital admission.[332] This treatment is not safe in infants with congenital heart disease[333] and, because it is given intravenously is expensive to administer.

Palivizumab, a monoclonal RSV antibody has recently been proposed as an alternative immunoprophylactic agent. In a randomized, double-blind controlled multicenter trial,[334] infants were given palivizumab at a dose of 15 mg/kg or placebo by i.m. injection every 30 days for a total of five doses. Palivizumab resulted in a 55% reduction in RSV related hospital admission and was most effective in infants under 6 months born at or before 35 weeks' gestation. The number needed to treat was 17, i.e. 17 patients would need to be given monthly injections to prevent one RSV related hospital admission. There were also fewer admissions to ICU, fewer total hospital days and fewer days with supplementary oxygen. The administration of the product appears to be safe and is easier to administer than intravenous immunoglobulin (IVIG) but it is costly and should therefore be reserved for infants at highest risk of severe RSV infection.

Pneumonia

Lower respiratory tract infections are a common cause of morbidity among children in developed countries and a major cause of mortality in developing countries. Of these infections, pneumonia is the most serious and can still be difficult to diagnose because of lack of reliable diagnostic methods. The epidemiological pattern of pneumonia is constantly altering because of changes in patient characteristics, altered immune status and changes in medical practice. There is an increasing level of resistance to antibiotics by the more common pathogens such as *Streptococcus pneumoniae*. For these reasons, accurate identification and treatment of the individual etiological organisms causing pneumonia is important.

Etiology

Identification of the etiological organism is a challenge because of difficulty in obtaining adequate samples, lack of reliable diagnostic methods and difficulty in differentiating infection from colonization. An organism may be identified in up to 60–70% of pneumonia patients, using serology combined with culture and PCR. Of these, around 40–50% are bacterial causes and 20–25% are viral. Evidence of more than one infectious agent has been found with mixed bacterial, mixed viral or mixed viral–bacterial infections, although these may not be as common as was previously thought.

Community acquired pneumonia

Community acquired pneumonia is defined as pneumonia acquired outside of the hospital setting and its diagnosis and management has been the subject of a recent systematic review.[335] The most commonly encountered pathogen is *Strep. pneumoniae* (pneumococcus), which is recognized as an important cause of pneumonia in children, regardless of age, in both the inpatient and outpatient setting. In developed countries, *Strep. pneumoniae* probably accounts for 25–30% of cases of community acquired pneumonia in children. Viruses are responsible for about 20% of cases overall, although these are the most common cause in younger children. The commonest viral cause is respiratory syncytial virus with others including influenza A, influenza B, parainfluenza, and adenovirus. RSV and influenza viral infections typically peak in late autumn and winter, whereas bacterial pneumonias exhibit less marked seasonal fluctuations. *Chlamydia pneumoniae* and *Mycoplasma pneumoniae* occur commonly in children older than 4–5 years and increase in incidence over the age of 10 years. The introduction of the Hib vaccine has almost eliminated *H. influenzae* type b as a cause of pneumonia. Non-serotypable *Haemophilus* and *M. catarrhalis* were previously considered non-pathogenic for the respiratory tract but do occasionally cause pneumonia. Enterobacteriaceae, Group A *Streptococcus* and *Staphylococcus aureus* are uncommon in the immunocompetent host, but when they occur can cause severe disease including lung abscesses, empyema and pneumatoceles. Atypical organisms such as *Chlamydia* species and *Legionella* species can cause disease of the lower respiratory tract in children although these organisms are seen more commonly in adults.

Clinical features

Community acquired pneumonia is classically characterized by a sudden onset of fever, tachypnea, cough and difficulty with feeding. These symptoms are frequently preceded by a relatively minor upper respiratory tract illness with coryza and low-grade fever. It is often difficult to distinguish those children with viral pneumonia from those with bacterial disease (Table 18.12) and there is considerable overlap in the clinical findings in young children and infants with pneumonia and other LRT illnesses such as bronchiolitis. Guidelines developed by the World Health Organization (WHO) for clinical diagnosis of pneumonia in the developing world emphasize the importance of tachypnea and recessions as the best indicators in young children. On examination, crackles on auscultation are classical, and bronchial breathing is a late sign indicating consolidation. Wheeze may also be present in viral or mycoplasma pneumonia. Symptoms of lower lobe pneumonia in older children may include abdominal pain, reflecting referred pain from the diaphragmatic pleura and can occasionally lead to a paralytic ileus with abdominal distension. Upper lobe consolidation may be associated with neck pain and apparent neck stiffness. Chest pain is common and is due to accompanying pleuritis.

Table 18.12 Features of bacterial and viral pneumonias

	Bacterial	Viral
Fever	>38.5°C	<38.5°C
Respiratory rate	>50/min	Normal or raised
Recession	Present	Marked
Wheeze	Not usually early sign	Often present
CXR	Consolidation	Hyperinflation Segmental collapse in 25%
Coexisting disease	Consider influenza, measles, other viruses; cystic fibrosis, immune problem if recurrent	Consider bacterial infection; aspiration if recurrent

Laboratory investigations

In many cases, no pathogen is identified using routine laboratory investigations and this leads to the uncertainty about the most appropriate antibiotic regimen to prescribe. Because of changing epidemiological patterns and the increasing emergence of antibiotic resistant organisms, there is increasing work looking into the rapid identification of the infecting organism so that appropriate treatment can be initiated early. Newer methods such as serology and PCR have complemented the use of bacterial and viral cultures to assess the etiology of pneumonia.

Blood cultures yield an organism in only around 10–15% of cases. Only a small number of bacterial pneumonias are accompanied by bacteremia and many children receive antibiotics before reaching hospital.

Culture of respiratory specimens is the best method for identifying organisms causing pneumonia on culture. However, small children are unable to expectorate sputum and procedures such as bronchoalveolar lavage are generally regarded to be too invasive to be used routinely, other than on an intensive care unit.

Nasopharyngeal specimens are routinely used for viral culture and should be collected as soon as possible as viral shedding is maximal at the time of onset of symptoms. The presence of a virus in the upper respiratory tract does not necessarily imply that this is the cause of the pneumonia.

Antigen detection is less rewarding in children than in adults, although compared with blood cultures, antigen screening has a better identification rate for *Pneumococcus*. Pneumococcal antigen can be detected in sputum, blood, pleural fluid and urine.

Serology can support a diagnosis, but paired titers with a specimen for convalescent titers at 2–4 weeks are necessary leading to a delay and can be complex due to multiple serotypes. This method is useful for the detection of atypical species such as mycoplasma and chlamydia.

PCR is a technique used to amplify deoxyribonucleic acid from microorganisms in either blood or respiratory secretions.

This technique offers the possibility of a rapid bacteriological diagnosis for clinicians and may be more sensitive than bacterial culture, especially if antibiotics have already been given. The main disadvantage of this technique is its cost.

Other routine investigations include full blood count and C-reactive protein (CRP). A high white cell count and CRP may be more suggestive of bacterial pneumonia, although there is considerable overlap so that confident prediction of the microbiological diagnosis is not possible on these parameters alone.

Radiology

Because the clinical features of pneumonia may be non-specific, chest X-rays are often used to confirm the presence and determine the location of a pulmonary infiltrate. CXRs do not reliably distinguish between bacterial and viral pneumonias, although interstitial shadowing or peribronchial infiltrates are said to be more characteristic of a viral infection and lobar consolidation of pneumococcal disease. The radiological features of segmental consolidation are difficult to distinguish from those of segmental collapse seen in around 25% viral LRTIs. Complete resolution of radiographic changes may take several weeks. CXRs are also used to identify associated air leaks, effusions and abscesses.

Treatment

For the management of pneumonia in children, it is important firstly to grade the severity of the illness and secondly to define the likely etiology and to direct treatment against the identified pathogen. These factors are important in deciding whether to withhold or to prescribe antibiotic therapy, whether the child requires admission to hospital and whether therapy should be given via the oral or intravenous route. As outlined above, definitive information about the causative organism is rarely available, and therefore empirical treatment is often necessary.

The majority of children with community acquired pneumonia can be managed in primary care. In the mildly unwell, ambulatory child, infection is most likely to be viral and therefore antibiotics can be withheld. Children who are feeding poorly, vomiting or in need of supplementary oxygen require hospital admission. Supportive measures include adequate hydration and nutrition. Mobilization of secretions and analgesia may also be required.

Because of increasing concerns about antimicrobial resistance, it is preferable that effective narrow spectrum agents are used wherever possible. Penicillin remains the treatment of choice for *Strep. pneumoniae*, and other beta-lactam agents such as third generation cephalosporins are often recommended as an appropriate first line option in those community acquired pneumonias requiring hospitalization and intravenous treatment. Both mycoplasma and chlamydia are susceptible to macrolides such as erythromycin and the newer agents azithromycin and clarithromycin[336] and these are the treatment of choice in penicillin-resistant strains of *Strep. pneumoniae*. Azithromycin, given once daily for 5 days has been shown to be as effective as erythromycin given three times daily for 10 days, with significantly fewer side-effects, in patients that do not require intravenous therapy.[337] The shorter course of treatment may also aid compliance in this age group. Randomized controlled trial evidence has also shown that an early switch to oral therapy after a short (2 day) course of intravenous therapy, has comparable efficacy to a full week's course of intravenous therapy, and can reduce hospital stay and costs, with no increased adverse patient outcome.[338]

Prevention

The introduction of the Hib vaccination program has dramatically reduced the incidence of pneumonia associated with this organism. In spite of the effectiveness of antibiotic therapy, an effective vaccination against pneumococcus is desirable for those children with underlying illnesses, e.g. sickle cell disease and immune deficiencies, particularly with the increasing emergence of antibiotic-resistant strains. The existing capsular polysaccharide vaccine is neither immunogenic nor protective in children and is not recommended for use in children under 2 years. A recent advance is the development of a conjugate pneumococcal vaccine (see Ch. 6). Such vaccines will only represent a partial solution however due to the complex and varied etiology of the disease.

Atypical pneumonia

Mycoplasma

Mycoplasma is a common cause of pneumonia in schoolchildren and young adults. Epidemics tend to occur in 4–7 year cycles with a peak incidence in autumn, thought to correspond with children returning to school. In early school years it is responsible for about 12% of pneumonia, rising to 20% in older schoolchildren and over 30% in young adults. The incubation period is 2–3 weeks. The symptoms associated with pneumonia are often much worse than the physical signs would suggest. Classically, a dry cough develops over 1–2 days with a low-grade fever. The cough can be debilitating and may be confused with pertussis. Often severe, systemic complaints such as weakness, headache, sore throat and chest or abdominal pain predominate. Signs in the chest are often insignificant but careful auscultation may reveal fine crackles, either localized or multifocal, and wheeze may be present. Chest X-ray changes are non-specific and variable, from multifocal to lobar shadowing, with effusions in 20%. A diagnosis of *M. pneumoniae* is suggested by a positive titer for cold agglutinins and a rise in titer of specific antibodies. Cold agglutinins are neither fully sensitive nor specific for mycoplasma infection and may also occur in cytomegalovirus (CMV) and EBV infection. Culture of the organism takes about 3 weeks and is therefore not of clinical use. PCR can be applied to blood or nasal secretions and may increase diagnostic yield in combination with serology. Erythromycin or one of the newer macrolides such as azithromycin or clarithromycin are effective treatments for mycoplasma.[336]

Chlamydia

Chlamydia is an obligate intracellular parasite. Three species of chlamydia are pathogenic in man.

Chlamydia trachomatis is a cause of pneumonia in the newborn and can be recovered from 25% of infants of mothers who have been identified positive for chlamydial antigen. It can be acquired across intact amniotic membranes and so babies delivered by cesarean section can be infected as well as those delivered vaginally. About 15% of infected infants develop signs of pneumonia, from 4–6 weeks of age, a dry, 'staccato' cough in the neonatal period being a distinguishing feature. Crackles are described more frequently than wheeze. There is a history of sticky eye in 50%. Chlamydia is isolated by cell culture from respiratory secretions or conjunctival scrapings. Chlamydia may also be isolated from high vaginal swab from the mother in whom carriage may be asymptomatic. The respiratory disease is generally mild and responds poorly to erythromycin. Respiratory symptoms can persist for at least 7 years afterwards but it is difficult to know whether this is because chlamydial infection identifies a host susceptibility or because it leads to permanent damage.

Chlamydia pneumoniae, identified in 1986, is a common cause of community acquired pneumonia in school-age children. Symptoms are initially upper respiratory followed by a prolonged hoarse cough which may persist for months after treatment. Treatment is with erythromycin or another macrolide antibiotic.

Chlamydia psittaci is the cause of psittacosis, a rare and potentially fatal zoonosis acquired from birds. Most wild urban birds are infected but the infectivity of birds to man is variable: pigeons are poorly infective but parakeets and budgerigars are highly infective. The symptoms and signs range from a mild 'flu-like' illness to pulmonary involvement with a mild to moderately severe pneumonia. The diagnosis rests on a history of contact with infected birds in the presence of respiratory infection and with rising titers to chlamydial antigen. Treatment is with a macrolide antibiotic, or a tetracycline in children over 12 years. Extrapulmonary manifestations include myocarditis, nephritis, thrombophlebitis and meningoencephalitis.

Legionnaire's disease

Legionnaire's disease is an unusual disorder in childhood. It occurs either sporadically or in epidemics in communities. *Legionnella pneumophila* is a gram negative, aerobic organism. It survives in warm water and is harbored in water supplies and water-cooled air-conditioning systems and transmission is either by inhalation or by ingestion of contaminated water. Infected infants and children suffer from widespread and sometimes life-threatening pneumonia. Serological studies demonstrate raised titers to *L. pneumophila* and the organism can be identified at lung biopsy. Treatment is with macrolides, quinolones or co-trimoxazole.

Q fever

This is caused by infection with the rickettsial organism *Coxiella burnetii* acquired from livestock such as cattle and sheep. Animal to animal transmission is via ticks; however, infection to humans is airborne from contaminated feces, urine and birth products such as placenta. It is a frequent cause of 'flu-like' symptoms and when the organism causes pneumonia, fever is universal and is accompanied by a dry cough. Diagnosis is serological and if erythromycin is ineffective it usually responds to treatment with quinolones or rifampicin.

Fungal infections

Despite the prevalence of fungi in the environment fungal disease is rare. Fungi cause both pathogenic and opportunistic infections and in the United Kingdom the latter, affecting children with altered host defense mechanisms, are by far the most prevalent.

Histoplasmosis, blastomycosis and coccidioidomycosis are exceptionally rare in children outside the United States and South America. All cause illnesses which range from asymptomatic infection to disseminated disease and all have clinical features which are very similar to tuberculosis. In the lung, granulomas associated with hilar lymphadenopathy can progress to pneumonia, cavitating pulmonary lesions and pleural disease. Diagnosis rests on appropriate skin testing and sputum culture. Amphotericin B is used to treat severe blastomycosis and coccidioidomycosis but the treatment of histoplasmosis is extremely difficult.

Aspergillus causes two forms of respiratory disease in childhood: allergic bronchopulmonary aspergillosis caused by hypersensivity in children with underlying lung conditions such as asthma and cystic fibrosis and invasive pneumonitis.

Actinomycosis is due to species of *Actinomyces* which live in the mouth, in dental plaque and calculus. As mouth hygiene has become better actinomycosis, in which organisms reach the chest by inhalation, has become rare.

Parasites

Pulmonary eosinophilia or Loeffler's syndrome is believed to be caused by *Ascaris, Toxocara*, hookworms or *Strongyloides*, although drugs such as aspirin, penicillin and the sulfonamides have been implicated. Pulmonary involvement includes cough, wheezing, shortness of breath, hemoptysis, fever and weight loss. Diagnosis is suggested by migratory pulmonary infiltrations and a high eosinophil count in the peripheral blood. Identification of the offending parasite can be made by stool examination and by serological methods.

Pulmonary tuberculosis (see Ch. 26)

RESPIRATORY DEFENSES AND INFECTION IN THE IMMUNOCOMPROMISED HOST

The lungs are constantly exposed through respiration to a multitude of airborne particles and microorganisms. A complex system of host defense exists for protection against this repeated challenge, but when this breaks down significant and repeated infection can occur.

PULMONARY HOST DEFENSE

There are both physical and immune defenses. Immune defense mechanisms are either innate or specific, although there is much interaction between the two.[339]

Physical and innate immune defense

The upper airway and branching airways in the lung are the first line of defense with airborne particle deposition dependent on particle size, flow rates during inspiration, and age.[340] Large particles (> 10 microns) are usually trapped in the upper airway whereas smaller particles may be able to penetrate beyond the terminal bronchioles. Particulate or chemical stimulation may trigger the neurally mediated protective reflexes of sneeze, cough and bronchoconstriction. Cough is also an adjunct to the normal mechanism of mucociliary clearance and is particularly important when the latter is defective. Laryngeal integrity and competence of airway protective reflexes are important further defense mechanisms.

The bronchial tree down to the 16th bronchial division at the terminal bronchioles is lined by ciliated columnar epithelium. This is covered by a layer of mucus which is propelled by ciliary movement to the oropharynx where it is swallowed or expectorated. Small particles and organisms are thereby cleared from the airways. Each epithelial cell has around 200 cilia composed of nine interconnected doublet microtubules surrounding and joined to two centrally positioned microtubules. Cilia start beating with a slow recovery stroke by bending sideways and backwards, followed by an effective stroke which propels mucus in a cephalad direction.[341] Ciliary beating results from adenosine triphosphate (ATP) driven sliding of microtubules via dynein arms, and is coordinated locally in metachronal waves. Normal ciliary beat frequency is 11–16 Hz.

Tracheobronchial mucus is produced by the submucosal glands, goblet cells, Clara cells, and through transudation from the vascular space and alveolar fluid. It consists of glycoproteins (mucins), proteoglycans, lipid and water. Traditionally the mucus blanket is thought to consist of an inner periciliary layer (sol phase) in which the cilia beat, and an outer gel phase which is viscous and into which the tips of the cilia just penetrate. An alternative model has been proposed with mucins forming a tangled network extending to the epithelial surface.[341]

The lungs however provide an additional chemical defense. Airway surface fluid contains a variety of antimicrobial molecules, including lysozyme, complement, fibronectin, transferrin, lactoferrin, lipopolysaccharide binding protein, defensins, cathelicidins, and collectins.[339] There has been much recent interest in the role of these substances in health and disease states. The collectins include surfactant proteins A and D and mannose-binding lectin, synthesized by the distal airways and alveolar type II cells. The epithelium appears to be able to respond to the presence of pathogens by induction of these antimicrobial factors, as well as by secretion of cytokines for recruitment of inflammatory cells.[342]

Macrophages are present in large numbers throughout the lung, in alveoli, airways, and in the interstitium. They play an important role in defense against agents that have escaped clearance by the above mechanisms, through phagocytosis but also by activating other inflammatory cells. Mast cells and polymorphonuclear leukocytes can also be activated through non-immunological mechanisms. Neutrophils can be recruited and activated in the lung, and kill pathogens by phagocytosis and mechanisms including the respiratory burst. This is more effective if they are opsonized with specific antibody.[343] Some encapsulated organisms are not susceptible unless opsonization occurs.

Specific immune defense

The predominant antibody in respiratory secretions in the upper airway is secretory IgA, which is synthesized locally in the submucosa and is dimeric in structure.[340] IgA can activate the alternative complement pathway and can inhibit viral binding to epithelial cells and neutralize toxins. Conversely IgG relies on transudation from the bloodstream with an increased concentration in the lower airways where it exceeds IgA concentration in bronchoalveolar fluid. IgG activates complement via the formation of immune complexes and acts as an opsonin facilitating phagocytosis. IgM and IgE are also present in respiratory secretions.

Lymphocytes are the main effector cells in the specific immune response, comprising approximately 10% of the cells in bronchoalveolar fluid.[339] Pulmonary macrophages, dendritic cells and B cells act as antigen presenting cells, interacting with CD4+ T cells, leading to secretion of interleukin 1 (IL-1). This activates CD4+ cells further to produce IL-2 which induces proliferation of both CD4+ and CD8+ cells. CD4+ cells can stimulate B cells to produce immunoglobulin and also produce lymphokines such as interferon gamma which activates macrophages and natural killer cells in delayed-type hypersensitivity.[343] CD8+ cells effect cell-mediated cytotoxicity which destroys virus-infected cells.

IMPAIRED HOST DEFENSE

Impairment of any of the above mechanisms can lead to infection. This applies to innate physical defenses as well as to the specific immune pathways. Compromise of the upper airway defenses, such as bypassing the upper airway by tracheostomy or in children with neurological disability associated with impaired cough or laryngeal reflexes, leads to recurrent respiratory infections. Mucociliary clearance is affected by a variety of environmental pollutants as well as by disease states. The former include sulphur dioxide, nitrogen dioxide, and tobacco smoke.[341] It is also impaired in cystic fibrosis, mainly due to abnormal amounts of viscous mucus, asthma, and respiratory infection.[341] Recent viral and bacterial infections can produce a secondary ciliary dysfunction.

PRIMARY CILIARY DYSKINESIA

Cilia line the nasal cavity, paranasal sinuses, middle ear, eustachian tube, and parts of the male and female genital tracts. They are also present in spermatozoa. The term primary ciliary dyskinesia (PCD) refers to all congenital abnormalities of ciliary function. If ciliary beating is slow or uncoordinated then mucociliary clearance will be impaired. The incidence of PCD is at least 1 in 20 000, but there is probably significant underdiagnosis.[344] The clinical features are variable but the main feature is chronic sinopulmonary infections. It can present in the neonatal period with unexplained tachypnea or pneumonia, particularly when there are no other risk factors, or rhinitis. In the older child there may be apparent asthma that responds poorly to treatment, or chronic wet cough with sputum production. There may be a history of chronic secretory otitis media with continuous discharge after grommet insertion.[345] Purulent rhinitis and sinusitis are common. Adult males are usually infertile due to defective sperm motility and there is associated female subfertility. Repeated respiratory infection can lead to bronchiectasis.

Fifty per cent of patients with PCD have malrotation of the internal viscera with dextrocardia or complete mirror image arrangement. The absence of normal ciliary activity is thought to allow random rotation of the thoracic and abdominal viscera early in development. Kartagener's syndrome refers to a triad of situs inversus, sinusitis, and bronchiectasis.[346] Inheritance is generally autosomal recessive through a number of gene mutations that are reflected in the range of structural defects observed.[344]

Guidelines for diagnosis and standards of care have been published.[345] The clinician should have a high index of suspicion and a child should be investigated if there is any combination of the above clinical problems. However it may be appropriate to investigate for other disorders first. Initial screening of suspected cases can be carried out using the saccharin test, which relies on the time taken to taste sweetness after saccharin powder has been placed in the nose. Healthy individuals have a transit time of less than 20 min. The test is not suitable for young children. If it is abnormal or not possible, there should be an assessment of ciliary function. Ideally this should not be performed within 4–6 weeks of an upper respiratory tract infection. Ciliated cells can be obtained from the nasal mucosa using a cytology brush. These should be examined in a center with appropriate equipment and expertise by direct inspection and quantification of ciliary beat frequency (CBF). If CBF is low or the beat pattern is abnormal, ciliary ultrastructure should be examined using electron microscopy.

Ciliary abnormalities in PCD include defects in the dynein arms, radial spokes, microtubules, nexin links between microtubules, and ciliary disorientation.[346] Secondary ciliary abnormalities can occur, mostly with microtubular defects.[344] Unless the ultrastructure is completely diagnostic of PCD, a repeat sample should be taken, ideally from a different site. Exhaled, particularly nasal, concentration of nitric oxide is low in PCD and this has been suggested as an initial screening test.[347]

Daily physiotherapy is recommended with increased frequency during exacerbations of respiratory infection. Exercise should be encouraged and bronchodilator therapy may be useful.[345] There should be regular monitoring of pulmonary function and sputum surveillance. Prolonged oral and, if necessary, intravenous antibiotics should be given early in any respiratory infection.[345] Children should be referred for otolaryngological examination including hearing assessment. Nasal steroids may be helpful. Generally the prognosis is good with appropriate management.

BRONCHIECTASIS

Bronchiectasis is irreversible dilatation of the subsegmental airways.[348] Its incidence in developed countries has decreased over recent decades, having previously followed measles, pertussis and

Table 18.13 Causes of bronchiectasis

Cystic fibrosis
Immunodeficiency
Primary ciliary dyskinesia
Bacterial pneumonia
Foreign body aspiration
Allergic bronchopulmonary aspergillosis
HIV infection
Gastroesophageal reflux
Mycobacteria tuberculosis endobronchitis
Bordetella pertussis
Adenovirus pneumonia
Measles pneumonitis
Alpha-1 antitrypsin deficiency
Marfan syndrome
Ehlers–Danlos syndrome
Autoimmune disorders
Asthma
Young's syndrome
Bronchogenic carcinoma
Williams–Campbell syndrome

pulmonary tuberculosis. It is now mostly associated with an underlying condition. Recognized causes of bronchiectasis are listed in Table 18.13.

The underlying pathophysiology appears to be accumulation of purulent secretions and obstruction of the airway leading to dilatation. There is loss of the ciliated epithelium and the airway elastic tissue together with edema and chronic inflammation. Classification into cylindric, varicose and saccular types has been described but this does not generally correlate with the underlying etiology.[348]

There is a rare congenital form (Williams–Campbell syndrome) in which the airway cartilage is abnormal. Bronchiectasis may follow the right middle lobe syndrome, in which there is chronic atelectasis. Young's syndrome comprises bronchiectasis, sinusitis, obstructive azoospermia, but with normal ciliary function.

Symptoms are chronic cough, purulent sputum, and recurrent respiratory infections. There may be crackles over affecte lobes, wheeze and digital clubbing. Chest radiography may show non-specific changes such as peribronchial thickening, atelectasis, and persistent infiltrates.[349] High resolution CT has replaced bronchography as the investigation of choice. This may show thick walled and dilated bronchi that are larger than their accompanying pulmonary artery (the 'signet ring' sign), and associated lobar or segmental collapse.[349] Pulmonary function tests usually show an obstructive defect with combined obstructive and restrictive patterns in advanced disease.[348]

Underlying conditions should be sought in children without a clear cause.[350] Appropriate investigations are directed towards the conditions listed in Table 18.13, and include sweat test, immune function studies, analysis of mucociliary clearance, esophageal pH monitoring, and serum alpha-1 antitrypsin concentration. Flexible bronchoscopy can be used to look for bronchial stenosis, compression or foreign body, as well as directing antibiotic therapy.

Sputum cultures commonly yield *Staphylococcus aureus*, *Streptococcus pneumoniae*, *Haemophilus influenzae*, and possibly *Pseudomonas aeruginosa* or *Escherichia coli*. Oral and occasionally intravenous antibiotics should be given during exacerbations guided by sputum surveillance. Regular physiotherapy is an important aid to mucus clearance. Treatment should be given for the underlying cause if appropriate. Bronchodilators may be of benefit, as directed by spirometry. Surgical resection may be helpful, especially when bronchiectasis is limited to one lobe.[351]

IMMUNODEFICIENCY (see also Ch. 25)

Respiratory tract infections are common in childhood and most children do not have an immunodeficiency. However if there is a defect in immune defense then respiratory infection can be one of the first and most serious clinical manifestations.

This may be a primary immunodeficiency, an acquired disorder or from immunosuppressant therapy for another condition. Any of the following presentations may be an indicator that there is a problem in the immune system and that investigation may be warranted.[352]

- Recurrent bacterial respiratory infections
- Persistent respiratory infection not responding to appropriate therapy
- Severe infection with an organism of low pathogenicity
- Presence of an opportunistic pathogen
- Unexplained bronchiectasis
- Family history of primary immunodeficiency or unexplained infant deaths
- Features of a syndrome associated with immunodeficiency

It is important to be aware of and to look for other features that are associated with immunodeficiency disorders, for example growth failure, chronic diarrhea, skin infections and rashes, and hepatosplenomegaly.[352] The possibility of more common conditions should be entertained first. Immune function investigations should be conducted in a step-wise fashion, starting with a full blood count, differential white cell count, and serum concentrations of IgG, IgM, IgE and IgA. Depending on these results, the persistence of symptoms and the degree of suspicion, further investigations may include the following: serum concentrations of IgG subclasses, HIV status, quantification of specific antibody responses, e.g. to tetanus toxoid or pneumococcal vaccination, complement studies, lymphocyte phenotype and function, and neutrophil function. The clinical presentation and the organisms involved can be a guide to the most appropriate investigations.

PRIMARY IMMUNODEFICIENCIES

These have been recently classified into broad categories including:[353]

- Predominantly antibody defects
- Combined B and T cell immunodeficiencies
- Congenital defects of phagocyte number and/or function
- Complement deficiencies
- Other well-defined immunodeficiency syndromes (e.g. Wiskott–Aldrich syndrome, DiGeorge syndrome, ataxiatelangiectasia).

Predominantly antibody defects

X-linked agammaglobulinemia usually presents in early childhood with recurrent respiratory infections, with a particular susceptibility to encapsulated bacteria such as *Streptococcus pneumoniae* and *Haemophilus influenzae*. Serum concentrations of IgG, IgA and IgM are absent or very low and there is a decrease in circulating B lymphocytes. Common variable immunodeficiency can present in the second or third decade, usually with recurrent pyogenic respiratory infection. There is a progressive decline in concentrations of IgG, IgA and often IgM. Both conditions should be treated with immunoglobulin replacement. Bronchiectasis can result from recurrent infection.

Selective IgA deficiency is present in 1 in 700 Caucasians but in many individuals it is asymptomatic.[353] However in some it may be related to recurrent sinopulmonary infections and autoimmune disease. Replacement therapy is not usually required.

It is also sometimes difficult to establish the clinical significance of selective IgG subclass deficiency. IgG2 antibodies are primarily directed against polysaccharide-encapsulated bacteria and this response is generally poor in children under the age of 2 years, predisposing this group to infection with these organisms. Some children with IgG subclass deficiency may have recurrent infections, particularly if there is associated IgA deficiency, but others are asymptomatic. Specific antibody response is of greater clinical importance.[352]

Combined B and T cell immunodeficiencies

Severe combined immunodeficiencies (SCIDs) often present in the first 6 months of life with persistent respiratory infections, particularly with viruses, fungi, or intracellular bacteria (see Ch. 25). *Pneumocystis carinii* is the most common respiratory pathogen.[354] Other important features are failure to thrive, recurrent oral candidiasis and persistent diarrhea. The absolute lymphocyte count is usually low. Early diagnosis is extremely important with bone marrow transplantation a potentially curative procedure. In X-linked hyper-IgM syndrome B lymphocytes are unable to switch immunoglobulin production from IgM to IgG, IgA or IgE, due to a deficiency of the CD40 ligand normally found on activated T cells. There is also neutropenia and infants are prone to opportunistic infection.[352]

Congenital defects of phagocyte number and/or function

These give particular susceptibility to *Staphylococcus aureus*, *Pseudomonas aeruginosa*, enteric Gram negative bacteria, and fungi. Neutropenia may be isolated, or part of a wider disorder. Respiratory infection often occurs in association with involvement of the skin and gastrointestinal tract. Chronic granulomatous disease (CGD) results from a deficiency in intracellular killing of ingested microorganisms through a failure of production of superoxide. Chronic infected granulomata may form in the lungs, lymph nodes, liver, urogenital and gastrointestinal tracts. There are X-linked and autosomal recessive forms.[355] Diagnosis is by demonstration of failure of phagocytes to produce a normal respiratory burst, for example with the nitroblue tetrazolium (NBT) test, or by assessment of superoxide production with flow cytometry.[355] Treatment includes prophylaxis with co-trimoxazole and itraconazole, prompt empirical therapy for acute infections, interferon gamma, and potentially bone marrow transplantation.

SECONDARY IMMUNODEFICIENCY (see also Ch. 25)

Acute respiratory infections are a leading cause of death worldwide, with many due to immunodeficiency from malnutrition. All aspects of immune defense may be compromised by malnutrition leading to infection from both common and opportunistic organisms. Infections themselves may cause immunosuppression, for example pneumonia following measles. Many chronic conditions can also lead to a secondary immunodeficiency. Immunoglobulins can be lost in nephrotic syndrome or protein losing enteropathy. Children who have had a splenectomy or who have functional hyposplenism from sickle cell disease are at increased risk of infection with encapsulated organisms.

Respiratory tract infection is one of the main manifestations of HIV infection. Upper and lower respiratory tract infections are common, not only with usual bacteria and viruses such as *Strep. pneumoniae*, *H. influenzae* and RSV, but also opportunistic organisms. *Pneumocystis carinii* pneumonia (PCP) is a common first AIDS indicator illness.[356] The pattern of PCP in HIV infection has changed with prophylactic therapy and highly active antiretroviral therapy, but considerable associated mortality remains.[356] *Mycobacterium tuberculosis* is an extremely important pathogen, especially worldwide. Lymphocytic interstitial pneumonitis (LIP) is a non-infectious complication of HIV, with characteristic diffuse reticulonodular infiltrates on chest radiography. It can present with a gradual onset of cough, tachypnea, and hypoxia, and may respond to systemic corticosteroids.

Cytotoxic therapy in the treatment of malignancy or immunosuppressant therapy for bone marrow or solid organ transplantation is the commonest cause of secondary immunodeficiency. Although its incidence has decreased, infection is a major reason for treatment-related death in childhood leukemia, particularly with bacterial sepsis.[357] The main risk factor is chemotherapy-induced neutropenia, underlying the need for prompt antibiotic treatment in febrile neutropenia, with the use of empirical antifungal therapy if it is prolonged. The causative organisms in respiratory infection following bone marrow transplantation vary with the time period after transplantation. An initial period of neutropenia induced by the conditioning regimen predisposes towards bacterial and fungal pneumonias. With engraftment there is the risk of acute graft-versus-host disease, with the need for immunosuppressive therapy with corticosteroids and ciclosporin, associated with viral (particularly (CMV), fungal and *P. carinii* infection. Late pneumonias (more than 4 months post transplant) are related to humoral defects to encapsulated organisms. Bronchiolitis obliterans can occur during this period. CMV is the major organism causing pulmonary infection in recipients of solid organ transplants.

PNEUMONIA IN THE IMMUNOCOMPROMISED CHILD

(see also Ch. 25)

It is important to have a low threshold for investigation and treatment of immunocompromised children. Similarly a respiratory tract infection that is unusually prolonged or has atypical features should raise the suspicion of an immunodeficiency. Children with significant immunocompromise will often present for the first time with respiratory disease, and common respiratory pathogens can be devastating. Likely organisms can be predicted in a known defect but any infection is potentially possible and microbiological investigation should be conducted carefully in order to obtain a diagnosis. In addition mixed infection is not uncommon. There are also non-infectious processes that may either simulate or complicate infection, including pulmonary edema, atelectasis, hemorrhage, drug- or radiation-induced pneumonitis, and tumor infiltration.

Fever is a sensitive sign of infection, but clinical and other features may vary due to the abnormal host response. An interstitial pneumonitis may present with a dry cough, tachypnea and dyspnea, but there may be few findings on auscultation. Chest radiography can show variable abnormalities and is not specific but there are some recognizable patterns. Diffuse interstitial changes are associated with infection with *P. carinii*, and viral infections such as CMV and adenovirus. Lobar consolidation can be caused by common bacteria, but can also be seen in some fungal infections. A nodular appearance, cavitation or abscess formation occurs in bacterial infection with *Staph. aureus* and anerobes, and fungal infections. Computed tomography, particularly high resolution, can provide extra information, and is a more sensitive investigation for other complications, e.g. bronchiectasis or bronchiolitis obliterans.

Blood cultures should be obtained before empirical treatment is started. Treatment protocols vary between centers and with the clinical setting, but usually include broad-spectrum antibiotic cover of Gram negative and Gram positive organisms. A macrolide may be added to cover *Mycoplasma pneumoniae*, high-dose co-trimoxazole for *P. carinii*, and antifungal therapy may be indicated. Urine or blood can be sent for bacterial antigen detection but serology is rarely helpful due to limited antibody response. Nasopharyngeal aspirates are useful in the younger child with urgent immunofluorescence for respiratory viruses, CMV and *P. carinii*. Sputum collection is often difficult, but in the older child sputum can be induced by the nebulization of hypertonic saline. Gastric aspirates are helpful in the diagnosis of *Mycobacterium tuberculosis*.

Further investigation is necessary when there is failure to respond to empirical therapy and when the causative organism is not identified. Flexible bronchoscopy with bronchoalveolar lavage (BAL) is a safe procedure that is now often used in immunocompromised children and increases the diagnostic yield.[358] However even this technique has limitations in identifying pathogens, particularly after empirical treatment or with the use of prophylactic therapy. If children are intubated, an alternative is non-bronchoscopic bronchoalveolar lavage. Transbronchial biopsy is useful following lung transplantation. Open lung biopsy is generally reserved for both treatment and diagnostic failure despite BAL, and can identify both infection and non-infectious conditions.[359]

PNEUMOCYSTIS CARINII PNEUMONIA

(see also Ch. 25)

P. carinii is now regarded as an atypical fungus and is the leading opportunistic pathogen, particularly in those with impaired cell mediated immunity.[360] It can cause a severe interstitial pneumonitis presenting with non-specific features including cough, tachypnea, fever, hypoxia and often no added sounds on auscultation. It is common in HIV infection when its presentation may be more insidious and it is often the first AIDS indicator disease.[356] Chest radiography typically shows diffuse bilateral infiltrates that spread outwards from the perihilar areas (Fig. 18.31). Two morphologic forms of *P. carinii* are recognized. Cysts contain sporozoites and are identified with most of the traditional staining techniques, whereas the smaller trophozoite forms are more abundant and attach themselves to type I pneumocytes. The host inflammatory response plays a significant part in the lung damage in infection.[360] The organism cannot be cultured but can be identified in sputum, nasopharyngeal aspirate, BAL fluid, or lung biopsy. Immunofluorescent techniques with monoclonal antibodies can be used, and polymerase chain reaction (PCR) methods are still under evaluation. Serum lactate dehydrogenase (LDH) is raised in the majority of HIV infected patients with PCP and can act as a non-specific clue to the diagnosis.[360]

Treatment is high dose intravenous co-trimoxazole (20 mg/kg/day of trimethoprim in four divided doses) for 14–21 days. Intravenous pentamidine is an alternative if there is treatment failure or if co-trimoxazole is not tolerated. Respiratory support may be necessary. Corticosteroids have reduced the need for mechanical ventilation and mortality in non-randomized studies[361] but considerable mortality remains.[356] If corticosteroids are to be used the possibility of coincident CMV infection should be considered and appropriate cover provided (see Ch. 25 – *P. carinii* and CMV). Children at risk of *P. carinii* infection should have prophylaxis with co-trimoxazole, with dapsone or inhaled pentamidine as other options.

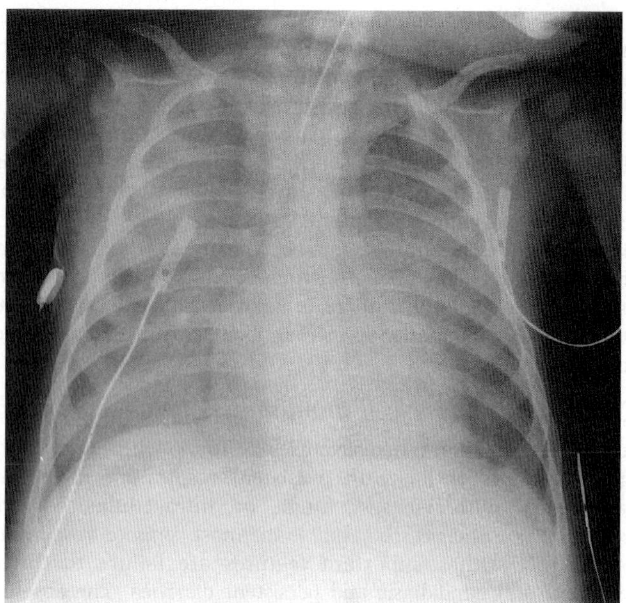

Fig. 18.31 Bilateral interstitial pneumonitis due to *Pneumocystis carinii* in an infant with vertically acquired HIV infection.

VIRAL PNEUMONIAS

Cytomegalovirus

Like other herpes viruses, CMV can become latent following primary infection.[362] Pneumonitis can occur following reactivation in CMV-positive patients with secondary immunodeficiency, or with primary infection. It is particularly a problem in HIV infection, bone marrow, renal and lung transplantation. The clinical features of CMV pneumonitis are similar to PCP with a diffuse reticulonodular pattern on chest radiography. There may be extrapulmonary involvement, such as hepatitis, colitis, or retinitis. CMV can be identified in urine, blood, nasopharyngeal aspirates, and BAL fluid, in association with immunofluorescence and polymerase chain reaction techniques. However these results may need to be interpreted with caution. A definitive diagnosis of CMV pneumonitis is made with lung biopsy, with characteristic intranuclear and intracytoplasmic inclusions and positive immunohistochemistry. Quantitative PCR for CMV plasma viral load can guide treatment and prophylaxis in bone marrow transplantation. Treatment includes intravenous ganciclovir and hyperimmune CMV immunoglobulin, but mortality is significant. Those at high risk can receive prophylaxis with ganciclovir, aciclovir, or CMV immunoglobulin.

Varicella zoster

Primary varicella infection in the immunocompromised, particularly lymphopenic, patient can produce overwhelming disease with visceral dissemination and pneumonitis. There may be cough, dyspnea and chest pain, with bilateral nodular infiltrates on chest radiography that may coalesce. Varicella in the immunocompromised child should be treated promptly with intravenous aciclovir.[363] Varicella-zoster immunoglobulin (VZIG) should be given within 72 h to at-risk patients who have had exposure to varicella.

Herpes simplex

Mucocutaneous herpes simplex infection is common in severe immunodeficiency. More severe infection can progress to involve the upper airway and trachea, and to cause pneumonitis. Prophylaxis and treatment is with aciclovir.

Adenovirus

Adenoviruses commonly cause respiratory infections in immunocompetent children, but can result in a severe pneumonia in the immunocompromised. There may be associated renal or hepatic involvement. There is no specific antiviral therapy but ribavirin may be used.

Measles

Bacterial pneumonia can complicate measles infection and this is a major cause of death of children in developing countries. There is insufficient evidence to support the use of antibiotics in all children with measles to prevent pneumonia.[364] With immunocompromise, measles can cause a progressive giant cell pneumonia that may be fatal. There may be an atypical rash, and coarse nodular infiltrates on chest radiography. Prior exposure to measles or vaccination is usually protective and with good uptake of immunization it is fortunately rare.

FUNGAL INFECTIONS

Aspergillus

Invasive pulmonary aspergillosis, usually due to *Aspergillus fumigatus*, can occur in prolonged neutropenia, bone marrow transplantation and HIV infection. Clinical features include fever, cough, chest pain, tachypnea and rapid deterioration. A chronic necrotizing form also exists. Chest radiography can show nodular changes and cavitation, and CT imaging is sensitive.[365] BAL may be useful but definitive diagnosis is with lung biopsy. Treatment includes high dose amphotericin B or liposomal amphotericin, and itraconazole. Further therapy may include the use of granulocyte colony-stimulating factor and surgery on focal lung lesions.[365]

Candida spp.

Prolonged neutropenia, HIV infection, combined immunodeficiencies, and prolonged presence of a central venous catheter are the major risk factors for deeply invasive *Candida* infection.[365] Pulmonary infection can result from hematogenous spread or aspiration from the oropharynx. Treatment is with amphotericin B or fluconazole.

PARAPNEUMONIC EFFUSIONS AND EMPYEMA

Parapneumonic effusions and empyema are complications of bacterial pneumonia and lie on a continuum. Initially there is pleural inflammation with leakage of fluid and protein. Bacterial invasion ensues, followed by leukocytes and then activation of fibroblasts with the formation of loculations. If the inflammatory process continues, a thick peel is formed on both pleural surfaces with pleural fluid becoming a gelatinous mass. The visceral peel can contract and entrap the underlying lung.[366] There may be fever, cough, chest or abdominal pain and dyspnea. The usual clinical signs are reduced breath sounds and dullness to percussion on the affected side, and children with empyema usually look unwell. There is often anemia, leukocytosis, thrombocytosis and raised inflammatory markers such as C-reactive protein.[367]

The most common bacteria responsible are *Staphylococcus aureus*, *Streptococcus pneumoniae*, *Haemophilus influenzae*, and Group A *Streptococcus*. However in many cases an organism is not identified as children have often had prior antibiotic therapy. Ultrasound is very useful and can identify fibrinous septation, rind formation and also lung mobility. Computed tomography can be used as an additional mode of imaging.

Blood cultures should be taken and appropriate intravenous antibiotics that include activity against *Staph. aureus* started. All but the smallest pleural effusion should be aspirated to guide antibiotic therapy and to help staging. Small uncomplicated effusions may be managed with antibiotic therapy alone. Larger effusions that do not have septation on ultrasound are probably best managed with closed chest tube drainage. Traditionally this has been performed with a large bore drain under general anesthesia with application of negative suction pressure. Drains should be removed once there is minimal drainage over 24 h. The presence of loculations may make drainage difficult and there are additional therapeutic options. The place of intrapleural fibrinolytic therapy in childhood empyema is unclear but has recently been subject to a randomized placebo controlled trial.[368] Treatment with urokinase for 3 days was associated with a shorter hospital stay, particularly if a small percutaneous drain was used.

Imaging can be used to assess response to treatment but should not dictate therapy alone. Multiloculated effusions and organizing empyemas may not resolve with chest tube placement and fibrinolysis and may need operative intervention. Thoracotomy with removal of fibrinopurulent debris and if necessary decortication of thickened parietal pleura to release entrapped lung can produce rapid recovery with a short hospital stay.[369] The use of video-assisted thoracoscopic surgery (VATS) as an alternative method of debridement of the pleural space has increased over recent years. Centers experienced in the technique advocate its use early in the course of the disease.[370] However the relative merits of fibrinolysis, VATS and thoracotomy are still unclear.

Intravenous antibiotics should be continued until there is clinical improvement with defervescence guided by change in inflammatory markers. Oral antibiotics should be given for at least another 2 weeks. Chest radiography may show pleural thickening for several months. With appropriate management most children make a good recovery.

CONGENITAL ABNORMALITIES

Congenital lung malformations have assumed increased importance as a result of routine detailed antenatal ultrasound scanning. Pediatricians may be involved in counseling pregnant women about the prognosis for the fetus, as well as in the postnatal management of an apparently normal baby with a small malformation which in past years would have escaped discovery. It is a field in which there is little evidence base, and in which the nomenclature is confusing, and used differently ante- and post-natally. There is also increasing interest in the longer term consequences of all congenital lung malformations, as greater numbers survive into adult life; follow-up studies have been reviewed recently.[371]

GENERAL PRINCIPLES

It is better to describe the abnormality as seen, in simple English, without speculating as to the embryology, since such speculation will almost inevitably be proved wrong in the future.[372] Table 18.14 illustrates this approach. A detailed justification of this nomenclature can be found elsewhere.[372] Two new terms deserve further elaboration. Congenital large hyperlucent lobe (CLHL) is a factual description of an appearance on a CXR or CT scan, whereas congenital lobar emphysema is a frightening and wrong allusion to a condition of elderly smokers, when in fact the pathology may actually be too many, not too few alveoli. Congenital thoracic malformation (CTM) is used to describe both sequestration and cystic adenomatoid malformation because they are ends of a

Table 18.14 Comparison of new nomenclature with old terms, based on the principles of describing what is seen, in clear language, without embryological speculation

New nomenclature	Old terms superseded
Congenital large hyperlucent lobe (CLHL)	Congenital lobar emphysema Polyalveolar lobe
Congenital thoracic malformation (CTM) – described as solid or cystic; if cystic, the cysts are described as single or multiple, thin or thick walled, and the contents described (either from CXR and other imaging, or from pathological examination of excised specimens)	Cystic adenomatoid malformation Congenital pulmonary airway malformation Malinosculation Sequestration (intra- and extrapulmonary) Bronchogenic cyst Reduplication cyst Foregut cyst
Congenital small lung (CSL)	Pulmonary hypoplasia
Absent lung, absent trachea	Agenesis of lung, tracheal aplasia
Absent bronchus	Bronchial atresia
Narrow bronchus, narrow trachea	Bronchial stenosis, tracheal stenosis
Bilateral right lung, bilateral left lung	Right isomerism, left isomerism

spectrum and not discrete entities. Either may have a systemic arterial supply, and pathological features of both may be found in the same lesion.

A further important principle is to describe the lung systematically. For these purposes, the lung is broken into six trees (bronchial, systemic and pulmonary arterial, systemic and pulmonary venous, and lymphatic). Other relevant systems should be described (chest wall, heart and mediastinum, abdomen) and all other systems reviewed, because, as with other congenital abnormalities, there may be coexistent problems elsewhere.

NASOPHARYNGEAL ABNORMALITIES

Babies are obligate nose breathers, so bilateral choanal stenosis or atresia presents with respiratory distress at birth. Milder forms may present with difficulty feeding. Unilateral disease may present later in childhood, sometimes with a unilateral nasal discharge. Diagnosis is suspected if a nasogastric tube cannot be passed into the pharynx. Management is surgical. Pierre Robin syndrome results in the tongue obstructing breathing secondary to micrognathia. The baby should be nursed prone but if this is unsuccessful a carefully positioned nasopharyngeal tube or tracheostomy may be necessary until the mandible grows sufficiently to accommodate the tongue, usually before the age of 1 year. Babies with congenital syndromes associated with midfacial hypoplasia (e.g. Aperts) should also be considered at risk for obstruction to breathing, at least during sleep. Congenital tumors and cysts, such as teratoma, hemangioma, ectopic thyroid and cystic hygroma, are unusual causes of pharyngeal obstruction, all of which require surgical treatment. Crowding of the pharynx occurs in Down syndrome and in disorders associated with a large or abnormally positioned tongue. Sleep-disordered breathing may result from airway obstruction as muscle tone falls during sleep, and polysomnography is indicated for diagnosis. If obstructive sleep apnea is present, adenotonsillectomy may relieve symptoms (for cleft lip and palate, see Ch. 36).

CONGENITAL STRIDOR

Laryngomalacia

This accounts for over 75% of stridor in infancy. On endoscopy, the arytenoids, epiglottis and aryepiglottic folds are sucked inwards on inspiration; there may be associated pharyngomalacia and tracheomalacia. Presentation is with isolated stridor in an otherwise well baby in the first days of life, but usually not at birth, but may be delayed until over 1 month. The inspiratory stridor is worse during periods of agitation and upper respiratory tract infection.

If the clinical presentation is characteristic, and the infant is improving, no investigation is needed. If there are any atypical features, including growth failure, bronchoscopy should be performed, to exclude other or multiple causes of stridor. This investigation requires skilled anesthesia; the occasional child may require ventilation after the procedure. The stridor usually disappears by the age of 2 years but sometimes goes on until the child starts school.

Laryngeal stenosis

This is the second commonest cause of congenital stridor and may be caused by supraglottic, glottic or subglottic webs or subglottic stenosis. The most severe form of congenital laryngeal disease is absent larynx. This results in normal appearances from above, but intubation is impossible. The lungs are normal or large. Most laryngeal webs are glottic and present with stridor and a poor cry at or shortly after birth. The severity of the symptoms depends on the size of the web, which may indeed cause complete airway obstruction, a condition incompatible with life unless diagnosed and treated within minutes of delivery. Many of these babies have other severe abnormalities. Treatment is surgical.

Subglottic stenosis is usually the result of soft tissue thickening of the subglottic area, usually acquired following prolonged intubation during the neonatal period. Occasionally laser resection of the granulation tissue or tracheostomy is required but most improve as the larynx grows. Localized tracheo- or bronchomalacia resulting from damage in the neonatal period due to ventilatory assistance may also cause stridor with or without wheeze in the first few years of life. These babies are more likely to require hospital admission if they acquire a respiratory infection as they will almost certainly have associated lower respiratory tract damage.

Subglottic hemangiomata

These become obvious before 6 months and 50% of babies have hemangiomata elsewhere, usually on the skin. The diagnosis is confirmed at endoscopy. Most regress during the first 2 years and thus a conservative approach is preferred. If medical treatment is indicated for severe obstruction or complications, prednisolone or interferon may shrink the hemangioma. Severe cases may need laser surgery or even tracheostomy.

Vocal cord paralysis

This can be unilateral or bilateral. Unilateral is more frequent. Paralysis may be associated with other abnormalities especially in the cardiovascular and respiratory systems. In most cases the paralysis is temporary with recovery within 4 weeks. Birth trauma with stretching of the neck and the recurrent laryngeal nerve may be a factor. Bilateral paralysis is usually associated with central nervous system disorders, such as hydrocephalus, which may themselves have a poor prognosis. Diagnosis is made at laryngoscopy.

Laryngeal clefts

Laryngeal clefts are associated with tracheoesophageal fistulae in about 20% and hydramnios in 30%. The infant presents with a toneless cry, choking and cyanosis on feeding, and aspiration pneumonia. Later in childhood a chronic cough or recurrent lower respiratory tract infection may be the only clue. Diagnosis is at laryngoscopy; inexperienced operators may miss a small cleft. Surgical repair can be extremely difficult.

Laryngeal cysts

Laryngeal cyst are very rare and cause stridor and a poor cry in the neonatal period. Endoscopy should be performed cautiously, and no attempt should be made to approach or go past the cyst if the airway is critically narrowed. Laser deroofing of the cyst is curative.

Vascular abnormalities

Vascular abnormalities include abnormalities of the vessels of the aortic arch which cause tracheal compression, usually presenting during the first year of life, but delayed presentation as steroid resistant asthma is not uncommon. Stridor, wheezing and a barking cough are the commonest presenting symptoms. Since the larynx is not involved, the tone of the cry is normal. Excessive secretions, difficulty with feeding and apneic episodes are sometimes associated. Further details are given in the section on lower airway vascular anomalies (below).

TRACHEOESOPHAGEAL FISTULA (see also Ch. 36)

The preoperative pulmonary problems associated with tracheoesophageal fistula (TEF) are related either to aspiration of secretions or food through the larynx if, as is usual, the upper end of the esophagus is blind or to reflux of stomach and duodenal secretions through the distal end of the esophagus into the tracheobronchial tree.

In the rare H-type fistula (4%) aspiration of food may cause recurrent chest infection. The underlying abnormality may even not be diagnosed until adult life. The diagnosis of the H-type TEF is not easy and rests on the demonstration of contrast medium flowing through the fistula (see Ch. 26). Seventy per cent of lesions lie high in the esophagus and since the fistula passes obliquely upwards from the esophagus the procedure should be carried out with the child lying prone. Late presentation may occur with coughing after drinking, hemoptysis, retrosternal pain and recurrent infection.

Prognosis of TEF is related to the gestational maturity of the baby, the presence of pulmonary disease before surgery, the incidence of postoperative pulmonary disease and the presence of associated abnormalities. TEF has a reported association with other congenital abnormalities of 50–70% and 2% of these are associated abnormalities of the respiratory tract.

Long-term follow-up of survivors of surgery suggests that airway disease is common. This may be related to disorders of esophageal motility and repeated small aspirations or they may be related to the severity of the initial respiratory disease. In addition, at the site of the fistula tracheal cartilage is inadequately formed or missing and there is an absence of normally ciliated respiratory epithelium. Tracheomalacia accounts for the brassy cough, worse during upper respiratory tract infections. Apneic episodes following feeding are a problem in a small number of babies and the incidence of sudden unexpected death is increased. Whether this is due to aspiration or associated with the tracheomalacia is debated. A mild restrictive pattern of pulmonary physiology is not uncommon in survivors. Some children develop scoliosis, which is a well described complication of thoracotomy,[373] although probably much less frequent with modern surgical techniques.

LOWER AIRWAY ABNORMALITIES

Trachea

With total or partial absence of the trachea ('tracheal aplasia'), the main bronchi either communicate only with each other or with the esophagus. The trachea may be smaller than normal in both the sagittal and coronal planes in Down syndrome. Congenital intrinsic tracheal narrowing (stenosis) may take the form of a gradual tapering, an isolated segmental narrowing or a membranous web, or be due to a nodule of ectopic esophageal tissue. Congenital extrinsic compression may be due to a vascular ring or pulmonary artery sling (below).

Bronchial tree

Bronchial arrangement and connections

Airway morphology is defined by the number of lobes (three for right sided, two for left) and the length of the main bronchus before the first bifurcation (short for right sided, long for left). The commonest abnormal bronchial arrangement is mirror image, which may be associated with primary ciliary dyskinesia. This must be distinguished from a right sided congenital small lung (CSL), which may have a systemic arterial supply. In 80% of cases, bilateral right lung is associated with asplenia and hence the risk of overwhelming pneumococcal disease, bilateral left lung with polysplenia. Both are associated with abdominal visceral malrotation and complex congenital heart disease.[374,375] Recently, a syndrome of BLL, normal atrial arrangement, and severe tracheobronchomalacia presenting as steroid resistant wheeze has been described.[376] Other variants are indeterminate morphology; bronchi crossing the mediastinum to supply the contralateral lung (crossover) and even a tongue of lung crossing the mediastinum (horseshoe lung).[377]

Congenital absence of a lobe or lung

Absent lung ('aplasia') is not uncommon but absence of a lobe or of both lungs is rare. There may be a rudimentary bronchial stump. In bilateral absent lungs the trachea ends blindly and the pulmonary artery arises from the aorta. Unilateral absent lung is often associated with other ipsilateral malformations.

Congenital small lungs

Small ('hypoplastic') lungs may be normal or abnormal in form. Alveoli are reduced in number or size. Normal right and left lung weights at term are 21 and 18 g respectively; the lungs are small if the lung/body weight ratio is less than 0.012.[378] The reduction in alveoli may be associated with fewer airway generations. Small lungs may be isolated with no underlying cause, but are more usually associated with a variety of other malformations. These include diaphragmatic defects, renal anomalies, extralobar pulmonary parenchymal malformations, and severe neuromuscular and musculoskeletal disorders. Most of these associations have a causal relationship but some, such as that with Down syndrome are puzzling. Lung growth before birth is dependent upon blood supply, availability of space, respiratory movements taking place in utero and fluid filling the airways. The causes of bilateral small lungs (BSL) are summarized in Table 18.15.

Disorders of the bronchial walls

Airway caliber abnormalities may result in all or part of the bronchial tree being too large or too small. Congenital tracheobronchomegaly (Mounier–Kuhn syndrome) is associated with tracheomalacia and bronchiectasis. There are saccular bulges between the cartilages. An autosomal recessive connective tissue defect has been postulated.[379] This is supported by the occasional association of Mounier–Kuhn syndrome with Ehlers–Danlos syndrome, cutis laxa or Kenny–Caffey syndrome.

Localized narrowing and in particular obstruction due to an absent bronchus often results in cystic degeneration of the lobe distal to the obstruction before birth, as fetal lung liquid continues to be secreted and cannot drain into the amniotic cavity. Absent bronchus may be detected radiographically in an asymptomatic individual and presentation may be late. The radiological appearances are virtually diagnostic, consisting of an ovoid hilar opacity, most commonly in the left upper lobe, with branches radiating out into a distal area of hyperlucency. The opacity represents a distended, mucus-filled bronchus that is continuous with the distal airways but has no connection with the more proximal, blind ending airway. The interruption to the airway may take the form of a membrane, a fibrous cord or a gap. The focal opacity seen in absent bronchus is not present in CLHL. The continuity of the cyst with the distal airways and the hyperinflation of the distal lung distinguish absent bronchus from 'bronchogenic cyst'.[380] True congenital bronchiectasis is much rarer than previously thought, but may be found within a CTM.

Congenital bronchomalacia may be isolated, with generally a good prognosis, at least in the short term, and has been described in association with other congenital abnormalities including connective tissue disorders, and Larsen and Fryn's syndrome. Williams and Campbell described a syndrome of generalized bronchomalacia affecting the second to the seventh generations of the bronchial tree. The occurrence in two siblings and the very early onset of symptoms suggests a congenital etiology. Finally, bronchomalacia may be secondary to other congenital abnormalities, such as vascular ring. Fixed bronchial narrowing may be due to defects in the wall (e.g. complete cartilage rings) or extrinsic compression by an abnormal vessel or cyst.

Abnormal bronchial connections

The separation of those parts of the primitive foregut to become esophagus and trachea may be incomplete resulting in TEF (above). Communication between the trachea and a CTM is also recorded.

Alveolar disorders

Counting alveolar numbers requires an open lung biopsy, and is usually of theoretical importance only. CLHL is an example of a disorder of alveoli. CLHL may be diagnosed antenatally, or present with tachypnea and respiratory distress in the newborn period, or be a chance finding on a CXR later in life. In some cases it is due to partial obstruction of the lobar bronchus leading to air trapping. The obstruction may be caused by external compression, for example by a cyst or abnormal blood vessel; alternatively, intrinsic abnormalities such as mucosal flaps, mucus plugs or twisting of the lobe on its pedicle may be responsible.[381] A deficiency of bronchial cartilage is a diagnosis of exclusion; in practice the cause is frequently not identified. Some patients also have congenital cardiac anomalies. CLHL affects the left upper lobe in about half the cases, the right middle and right upper lobes in most of the remainder and the lower lobes in less than 10%. Curiously, it almost never becomes infected; if CLHL is the seat of recurrent infection, suspect that the appearances are secondary to bronchial stenosis. Diagnosis should be confirmed on a CT scan, which distinguishes CLHL from a thin walled cystic CTM. If the infant is symptomatic and fails to thrive, then surgical removal is advised. If the child is well, no treatment is needed; even quite dramatic looking CLHL become less prominent. Another cause of CLHL is a polyalveolar lobe, which is a pathological, not a clinical diagnosis. A polyalveolar lobe has a normal number of conductive airways but an increased number of normal sized alveoli in each acinus.

Solid and cystic thoracic lesions: clinical approach

When assessing patients with a suspected congenital lung malformation, it is more logical to describe abnormalities by their appearance, whether on images (CXR, CT or magnetic resonance imaging, MRI), or pathologically. The use of terms like 'reduplication cyst' and 'bronchogenic cyst' in clinical practice, *prior to the resection of the abnormality*, imply embryology and/or pathology, and should be discarded. A better term to be used in clinical practice, which makes no assumptions, is CTM, some forms of which were previously described as a congenital cystic adenomatoid malformation (CCAM) or congenital pulmonary airway malformation (CPAM). CTM encompasses a spectrum of conditions, clinically described as cystic, intermediate or solid. It will be seen that the clinical definition of CTM includes what the pathologist may previously have described as a CCAM, or a bronchogenic or reduplication cyst, or other more specific term.

Solid and cystic lesions: pathological approach

The same constraints of clarity outlined above should apply to the pathologist. CTM should be used in pathological descriptions,

Table 18.15 Causes of bilateral congenital small lungs. Occasionally no underlying cause can be found

Underlying problem	Example
Abnormal thoracic contents	Diaphragmatic hernia, pleural effusion, large congenital thoracic malformation
Thoracic compression from below	Abdominal tumors, ascites
Thoracic compression from the sides	Amniotic bands, oligohydramnios, asphyxiating thoracic dystrophy, scoliosis
Abnormal vascular supply	Pulmonary valve or artery stenosis, tetralogy of Fallot
Neuromuscular disease	CNS, anterior horn cell, peripheral nerve or muscle disease reducing fetal breathing movements

attaching the term cystic, intermediate or solid as above, and describing the tissue in terms of what is seen down the microscope.

Bronchogenic and other foregut cysts are one type of CTM recognizable by cartilage and glands in their wall and a lining of respiratory epithelium. They are usually situated in the mediastinum close to the carina (51%) but may be found in the right paratracheal region (19%), alongside the esophagus (14%), the hilum of the lung (9%) or a variety of other locations (7%) including the substance of the lungs, and even beneath the diaphragm.[382] Cysts may be lined by respiratory type epithelium but lack cartilage in their walls. Cysts may also have a gastric, intestinal or squamous epithelial lining and a muscle coat. These types of cyst are usually situated in the posterior mediastinum or, as they may be associated with vertebral malformations, even within the spine. They may also be associated with abdominal cysts.

Pathologically, five patterns of 'CPAM' have been recognized, which *clinically* may also be mimicked by other conditions such as pulmonary hamartoma or ectopic tissue (below), which are readily distinguished pathologically. The blood supply may be from either or both of the pulmonary artery and the aorta. Some workers incorporate 'sequestration' into the 'CPAM' spectrum. The fact that 'extralobar sequestrations' may contain tissue identical to CCAM underscores the logic of combining not separating these two conditions and dropping the terms 'sequestration', 'CPAM' and 'CCAM' in favor of the single, catch-all term CTM.[383–385] The five pathological types formerly described as CPAM are overlapping entities. Type 0 ('acinar dysplasia') is incompatible with life. Microscopically, bronchial-type airways that have cartilage, smooth muscle and glands are separated by abundant mesenchymal tissue. Type 1 ('cystic CCAM') is the commonest. The boundary between the lesion and the adjacent normal lobe is sharply delineated but there is no capsule. Radiographically, air-filled cysts that are usually limited to one lobe compress the rest of the lung, depress the diaphragm and cause mediastinal shift. The cysts range in size from 1 to 10 cm. They are lined by pseudostratified ciliated columnar epithelium interspersed with rows of mucus cells of pyloric type. The relevant bronchus is often absent, yet the cysts are usually radiolucent, presumably due to collateral ventilation. Type 2 (intermediate type 'CCAM') is sponge-like, consisting of multiple small cysts as well as solid pale tumor-like tissue. Microscopically the cysts are seen to be dilated bronchioles separated by normal alveoli. Occasional examples contain striated muscle. This type of lesion may be also identified within 'extralobar sequestrations'. Type 3 (solid type 'CCAM') is a large, bulky lesion that typically involves and expands a whole lobe, the others being compressed and the mediastinum displaced. Microscopically, an excess of bronchiolar-like structures are separated by small airspaces which have a cuboidal lining, with no cystic change. Type 4 is characterized by large air-filled cysts which are peripheral and thin walled. They have a simple squamous epithelium composed of alveolar type I cells resting upon loose mesenchymal tissue.

A further type of CTM is 'mesenchymal cystic hamartoma' (MCH). The lesions may be supplied by bronchial, intercostal or phrenic arteries. Pathological examination shows them to consist of multilocular, thin-walled cysts lined by primitive mesenchymal cells that support a ciliated cuboidal epithelium. Muscular hamartomas, which are small focal proliferations of smooth muscle, are occasionally observed incidentally in the lung, sometimes associated with similar lesions in the bowel and liver.

The sequestration spectrum has been used to indicate that a portion of lung exists without appropriate bronchial and vascular connections. Classically, no airway connects the lesion to the tracheobronchial tree and the blood supply is systemic; however in some there may be a normal airway. Alternatively, an 'airway' may connect the sequestration to the esophagus or stomach in a complex 'bronchopulmonary–foregut malformation'. Occasionally, 'sequestration' is associated with duplication of the esophagus, stomach or pancreas. There is therefore a spectrum of abnormalities associated with 'pulmonary sequestration'.[386,387] Conventionally, two forms have been recognized: extralobar, which has its own covering of visceral pleura, and intralobar, which is embedded in otherwise normal lung. Both should be considered part of the CTM spectrum. There is often a defect in the diaphragm and about 15% of 'extralobar sequestrations' are abdominal. The veins leaving an 'extralobar sequestration' generally join the azygos or other systemic veins whereas an 'intralobar sequestration' usually has normal pulmonary venous connections, but as with all CTMs, any combination of arterial supply and venous drainage is possible. The lung tissue in a 'sequestration' is often poorly developed and cystically dilated. The cysts are lined by columnar or cuboidal epithelium, or the 'sequestered' lung may be entirely composed of structures resembling alveolar ducts. Mucus distends the multiple intercommunicating spaces and the lesion appears solid radiographically, unless air enters through a bronchial connection or, in the case of 'intralobar sequestration', by collateral ventilation, when fluid levels are often seen.

Management of CTM

CTM most commonly presents as an antenatal ultrasound finding. Antenatal management is beyond the scope of this chapter. The postnatal management of antenatally diagnosed CTM is fraught with difficulty, because of a lack of good information about natural history. If a baby has had a CTM diagnosed antenatally, then a CXR and a thoracic CT scan should be performed. Even quite large malformations may not be apparent on a CXR alone.[388] If the presence of a CTM is confirmed, there is no evidence base on which to offer advice. Reasons for operative removal would be the (currently unquantifiable) risk of infection; risk of malignancy; and (if there is a large systemic arterial supply) risk of high output heart failure. If operation is contemplated, then it is important to delineate the vascular supply (below) to minimize the risk of severe bleeding. An option for selected malformations with a systemic arterial supply may be coil embolization of the feeding vessels. The author's practice is to offer surgical treatment for all but the smallest CTMs, usually carried out in the second year of life. Others would operate on even the smallest malformation. CTM may also present later in life as a chance finding, with recurrent infection, hemoptysis or steroid unresponsive wheeze due to compression of a large airway. Treatment considerations for the asymptomatic CTM diagnosed later in childhood are largely the same as for antenatally diagnosed ones; symptomatic CTM should be excised. In particular, when once a CTM has become infected, recurrence is inevitable and operation should be advised. Excision may also be needed to confirm the diagnosis and exclude more sinister causes such as a malignancy.

Abnormally placed pulmonary tissue (APPT) and abnormal intrapleural tissue (AIPT)

AIPT of adrenocortical tissue, thyroid (lacking C-cells) and liver has been described in the lung and pancreatic tissue has been noted within so-called 'intralobar sequestrations' with gastrointestinal connections. Rarely, a whole kidney may be found above the diaphragm but outside the lung. There may be ectopic lung tissue in the neck, the abdomen or the chest wall, often associated with skeletal or diaphragmatic abnormalities.

The arterial trees

There are two arterial trees (pulmonary and systemic), which are considered separately. Systemic arterial abnormalities of the great vessels of the mediastinum can be subdivided from those of the bronchial circulation. Finally, the pulmonary capillary bed may be bypassed leading to direct arteriovenous communication; or absent, resulting in minimal pulmonary arteriovenous connections.

Pulmonary arterial abnormalities

In general, the pulmonary arteries and veins follow the bronchial anatomy, and thus pulmonary arterial and venous arrangement mirrors bronchial arrangement. There are important exceptions. The first of these is congenital origin of the left pulmonary artery from the right ('pulmonary artery sling'), sometimes with a crossover arterial segment, with the right upper lobe supplied by a branch from the left pulmonary artery. Surgical repair of a sling with a crossover may result in infarction of the right upper lobe if the abnormal vessel has not been discovered. Isolated crossover pulmonary artery branches in the absence of bronchial crossover are occasionally seen. They cross the mediastinum to supply lung segments which often are abnormal in other ways.

Lobar and segmental vessels as well as the main pulmonary arteries may be narrowed, and there may be multiple constrictions. Unilateral absence of a pulmonary artery leads to the lung on that side receiving only systemic blood, either through anomalous systemic arteries or enlarged bronchial arteries. The defect may be isolated or associated with other cardiovascular anomalies.

Anomalous systemic arteries supplying the lung may be associated with any CTM, or even be an isolated finding.[389] When operation is contemplated for any CTM, it is important that abnormal vasculature is detected. Inadvertent severance of anomalous systemic arteries has led to fatal hemorrhage, whilst ligation of anomalous veins from adjacent non-sequestered lung has led to infarction of normal tissue. They are also found if the pulmonary artery is absent and may also be part of complex arteriovenous malformations. One or both pulmonary arteries may take origin from the aorta. Bilateral origin from the aorta is part of the spectrum of common arterial trunk. Unilateral origin of pulmonary artery from the aorta may be an isolated abnormality.

Congenitally small unilateral pulmonary artery is usually seen in association with an ipsilateral CSL. Normal pulmonary blood flow is needed for normal lung development. Bilateral small or absent pulmonary arteries are usually part of the spectrum of pulmonary valve atresia/tetralogy of Fallot. Very large pulmonary arteries which compress the central airways are seen in absent pulmonary valve syndrome.

Abnormalities of the systemic arteries

Two groups of abnormalities are relevant to the lung. The first group is those producing a vascular ring. There are a number of different variants, which present with stridor, cough, wheeze, and sometimes with recurrent infection or feeding difficulty. Diagnosis is by barium swallow, echocardiogram or bronchoscopy. Treatment is surgical, but prolonged postoperative symptoms due to the chronic effects of airway compression are common. The second group is the collateral vessels which may arise from the aorta and supply all or part of one or both lungs, or a CTM. These may be hypertrophied bronchial arteries or abnormal non-bronchial vessels; there may be multiple collaterals. This last group may be seen in association with direct pulmonary arteriovenous connections ('pulmonary arteriovenous malformations'). Aneurysm of aortopulmonary collateral vessels has been described.

The venous trees

Anomalous pulmonary veins result in blood from the lungs returning to the right side of the heart. The anomalous veins may join the inferior caval vein or hepatic, portal or splenic veins below the diaphragm, or above the diaphragm they may drain into the superior caval vein or its tributaries, the coronary sinus or the right atrium. The anomaly may be total or partial, unilateral or bilateral, and isolated or associated with other cardiopulmonary developmental defects. Anomalous pulmonary venous connections are often narrow and this may cause relatively mild pulmonary hypertension.

A particular clinical problem is the 'scimitar' syndrome; this is characterized by a small right lung, resulting in the heart being in the right chest (cardiac dextroposition), and an abnormal band shadow representing the abnormal venous drainage to the systemic veins, fancifully compared to a scimitar (which in fact is often absent). Initial treatment which may need consideration is coil occlusion of aortopulmonary collaterals and occasionally of an abnormal vein if venous drainage is double-arched (to both caval vein and left atrium). This intervention may be followed by surgical correction. The results are unlikely to be perfect; some blood supply may be restored, but the ultimate functional result will depend on the normality of the underlying lung. In view of evidence in other contexts that normal intrauterine blood supply is essential for normal lung development, it would be naive to suppose that a perfect functional result could be achieved whatever treatment is given. Pulmonary venous obstruction is a not infrequent late complication of surgery, particularly if surgery is carried out in infancy. Occasionally lobectomy or pneumonectomy is performed, usually in the context of severe pulmonary hypertension; this operation should only be a last resort.[390,391]

Absence of the pulmonary veins or narrowing of their ostia into the left atrium similarly results in pulmonary venous obstruction. Partial anomalous pulmonary venous drainage may be obstructed or unobstructed. Unilateral anomalous venous drainage may be part of complex lung malformations; it may also be seen in association with what appears to be a simple lung cyst. This underscores the need for accurate delineation of all abnormalities in even straightforward appearing cases. Minor abnormalities of venous connection, such as of a segment direct to the azygos system, are not uncommon and usually not of practical significance.

No congenital disorders of the systemic (bronchial) venous tree have been described.

Disorders of connection between the pulmonary and venous trees

An important group of abnormalities which potentially involves systemic and pulmonary arterial and venous trees are the various forms of 'pulmonary arteriovenous fistulae'. They range from the diffuse, microscopic to the single or multiple large abnormality. The large connections may have both a systemic and a pulmonary arterial supply. There may be arteriovenous malformations elsewhere in the body, and they may be part of Osler–Weber–Rendu disease. Presentation is with cyanosis, the chance discovery of an asymptomatic mass on CXR, or with a complication such as systemic embolization or abscess. Confirmation of the diagnosis is with contrast echocardiography. Treatment of discrete lesions is with transcatheter embolization.[392] Medium term follow-up has confirmed that the results are good. Multiple diffuse lesions in both lungs cannot be embolized, and may lead to progressive cyanosis and polycythemia. If symptoms are severe, lung transplantation may need to be considered.

Congenital alveolar capillary dysplasia (misalignment of lung vessels) represents a failure of capillaries to extend into the alveolar tissue of the lung, and presents as persistent fetal circulation, which relentlessly progresses to death whatever treatment is given. Histology shows increased septal connective tissue and pulmonary veins accompanying small pulmonary arteries in the centers of the acini rather than occupying their normal position in the interlobular septa (misalignment of lung vessels). The pulmonary arteries are decreased in number and show increased muscularization. Pulmonary lobules are small and radial alveolar counts may be decreased. Alveoli are decreased in complexity, their walls contain few capillaries and there is poor contact of capillaries with alveolar epithelium. The primary fault is poorly understood. The relationship of congenital alveolar capillary dysplasia to a condition previously described as congenital alveolar dysplasia is unclear.

Lymphatic tree

Congenital lymphangiectasia may be isolated, associated with abdominal lymphangiectasia, or found with congenital heart disease. It usually presents with relentlessly worsening respiratory distress which does not respond to any treatment. Rarely, milder localized cases may present in adolescence.[393] Diagnosis is by open lung biopsy.

Congenital chylothorax may be an isolated abnormality, or associated with congenital abnormality of the main lymphatic duct or pulmonary lymphatics. Associations with Noonan, Ullrich, Turner and Down syndrome, fetal thyrotoxicosis, H-type tracheo-esophageal fistula and mediastinal neuroblastoma have been described; familial cases have been reported.

RELEVANT CARDIAC ABNORMALITIES

Cardiac malformations may be coincidental, or a fundamental part of the malformation. They are sufficiently common that echocardiography should be a routine part of the workup of congenital lung disease. Coincidental malformations are seen with, for example, CLHL ('congenital lobar emphysema'). Lung abnormalities in which heart disease is fundamental include those with the pulmonary atresia spectrum (above). By definition, lung blood supply is abnormal. These however usually present to the pediatric cardiologists.

DIAPHRAGM AND CHEST WALL ABNORMALITIES

Diaphragmatic anomalies

Diaphragmatic hernia occurs in about 1:3600 live births. Classification is according to position – 70–90% occur through the left diaphragm, most commonly posterolaterally between the lumbar and costal muscle fibers (the foramen of Bochdalek).

Usually the diagnosis is made antenatally. Postnatally the infant presents with respiratory distress and physical examination suggests displacement of the heart, reduced air entry and bowel sounds in the chest. Bowel is seen in the chest on a chest radiograph. Treatment is surgical and it is the degree of pulmonary hypoplasia and iatrogenic ventilator induced lung damage that largely determines outcome. Both lungs exhibit abnormal airway branching and alveolization, although more severe in the ipsilateral side.

When the hernia is small presentation may be delayed. These are often anterior and may mimic a cystic CTM on the CXR. The possibility of this diagnosis should be considered in any child presenting with an air fluid level on a chest radiograph, cystic lesion or where the diaphragm is ill defined. A coexisting pneumonia may further confuse the issue. A barium meal will confirm the diagnosis and operation should proceed immediately diagnosis is made as there is a very real risk of strangulation.

Long-term follow-up of successful neonatal surgical repair shows that although lung volumes may be normal, morphologically the lungs probably remain small (with reduced alveolization). Pulmonary perfusion to the ipsilateral lung remains reduced even in adolescence. Long-term, most survivors do well, although a few have recurrent respiratory infections and a small minority have severe respiratory disability.[371]

Although most diaphragmatic hernias present antenatally or immediately after birth, a few present in mid-childhood. Whether this is truly a congenital defect, or is in fact an acquired diaphragm rupture is disputed. In most cases, pulmonary hypoplasia is minimal if present at all, and this suggests that these children in practice have a very different disease.

If the substance of the diaphragm is deficient, usually on one side, the abdominal viscera are elevated (eventration of the diaphragm). Eventration is believed to result from failure of all or a portion of the normal muscularization of the developing diaphragm which remains thin and translucent. It is usually unilateral and isolated, but occasionally other abnormalities are associated. Isolated unilateral eventration rarely needs treatment; occasionally plication of the diaphragm may be indicated if there are recurrent infections in the associated lung. Fluoroscopy will help to distinguish phrenic nerve palsy where there is paradoxical movement of the diaphragm. In eventration there is little or no movement. Duplication of the diaphragm results in a fibromuscular septum dividing one pleural cavity in two, usually between the right upper and middle lobes.

Asphyxiating thoracic dystrophy (Jeune's syndrome)

This is a rare disorder of the costal cartilages in which the ribs are shortened and the rib cage narrowed so that lung development is retarded and the lungs are small.

ABDOMINAL DISEASE

Any large abdominal mass or fluid may compress the lungs, thus impairing development. Congenital absence of the kidneys causes oligohydramnios and small lungs (above). Rare CTMs may connect with the stomach, and be associated with abdominal visceral malrotation.

MULTISYSTEM DISEASE

Most congenital lung abnormalities are isolated, but a few are part of a more generalized disorder, for example tuberose sclerosis may affect the lung as well as kidneys, heart and brain. Complex abnormalities of lung development may be associated with chromosomal abnormalities.

CHRONIC LUNG DISEASE OF PREMATURITY

INTRODUCTION

Although chronic lung disease (CLD) is usually ascribed to preterm infants, hence CLD of prematurity, it may also affect older more mature infants (Table 18.16). The early course of CLD whilst the infant is in the neonatal intensive care unit is described in Chapter 10. Discussed in this section are the features associated with CLD after the child is discharged. Since CLD predominantly affects the preterm child, most definitions have focused on this group of infants. The earliest definitions described the different stages through which

Table 18.16 Diseases which may lead to a prolonged requirement for oxygen. By far the commonest is oxygen dependency due to prematurity

Preterm	Chronic lung disease of prematurity Wilson–Mikity syndrome Chronic pulmonary insufficiency of prematurity
Term	Meconium aspiration Respiratory infections Pulmonary hypoplasia Muscular disorders
Surgical	Tracheoesophageal fistula Congenital diaphragmatic hernia
Congenital abnormalities	Cystic adenomatoid malformations Congenital lobar emphysema Sequestration of the lung Chylothorax

the infant progressed during development of their disease and the extreme stage (IV on Northway's original classification)[394] with large cystic changes interspersed with areas of collapse was termed bronchopulmonary dysplasia (BPD). Although the term BPD or New-BPD is widely used, the preferred term remains chronic lung disease of prematurity or CLD, since it embraces a wide range of diseases which may lead to the development of oxygen dependency. Many definitions have been proposed but the most commonly used are oxygen dependency beyond 28 days of age with chest radiological changes or oxygen dependency at 36 weeks' postconceptional age.[395] A more recent report from the American Thoracic Society has proposed yet another definition in the face of increasingly preterm infants surviving the early neonatal period.[396] This definition is based on whether the infant is greater than or less than 32 weeks' gestation at birth and also attempts to classify the severity based on respiratory support including oxygen and ventilation requirements. Regardless of the definitions of CLD, it is clearly important to determine why the definition is required in the first instance.[397] For mechanistic studies, the definition is likely to be oxygen dependency at 28 days but for epidemiological studies oxygen dependency at 36 weeks corrected gestation is likely to be more relevant.

INCIDENCE

Estimating the incidence of CLD is problematic because of inconsistencies in case definition between different studies. Furthermore, incidence is often quoted for individual units, which is subject to referral bias and to local practices. Varying approaches between individual units, for instance the approach to extremely preterm infants, will markedly influence the local incidence. There are few comprehensive population studies, which are essential to accurately report the incidence of CLD. In the Trent region of the UK, systematic data have been collected for infants born at less than 32 weeks since 1987. Recent analysis of these data suggested that, despite falling birth rates, the number of babies of < 32 weeks' gestation admitted to neonatal units increased significantly.[398] For the two consecutive 5-year periods 1987–1992 and 1992–1997, during which a number of therapeutic modalities, including regular use of antenatal corticosteroids, exogenous surfactant therapy, high frequency ventilation and postnatal corticosteroids, were introduced, the survival improved for both time periods (Fig. 18.32) (odds ratios adjusted for gestation and birth weight for survival at 28 days of age 1.69 [1.23–2.33] between 1987 and 1992 and 1.90 [1.36–2.64] between 1992 and 1997). During the first of these periods, the odds ratio for CLD, defined as oxygen dependency at 28 days of age, increased (2.20 [1.47–3.30] adjusted for gestation and birth weight). However, during the second period the odds ratio was 0.72 [0.5–1.03] suggesting no further increase despite a further improvement in survival. Taken together these data suggest that the survival of ever increasing preterm infants, in recent years, has not resulted in an increased incidence of CLD.

The reported incidence of CLD (whether defined as oxygen dependency at 28 days or 36 weeks postconceptional age) varies from 18% to 36% between centers.[399–401] In Trent, the unadjusted incidence has remained remarkably stable at 40–45% for infants born < 32 weeks' gestation and who required mechanical ventilation.[402] This is despite interunit differences in practices and approaches to care of extremely preterm infants. Factors which may affect the reporting of the prevalence and incidence of CLD from different units are given in Table 18.17.

PATHOPHYSIOLOGY

The risk factors which lead to the development of CLD are described in Chapter 10. However, it is worth reiterating that although the risk factors for the development of CLD have been accurately described, the mechanisms which lead to the development of CLD are largely unknown. Both antenatal and postnatal factors contribute to the development of lung injury in infants destined to develop CLD.[403] With the survival of extremely preterm infants, the pathological changes observed in infants who do not survive the neonatal course have altered over the years. When CLD affected more mature infants, both lung fibrosis and atelectatic areas were regularly seen.[404] With CLD being largely confined to the smallest immature infants, the picture has changed to one of decreased alveolization rather than of lung fibrosis. The final number of alveoli is decreased markedly and associated with rudimentary air sacs of increased diameter and decreased gas exchanging surface area.[405,406] Whether dysregulated lung growth is due to an arrest of normal lung growth[407] or due to accelerated lung growth resulting in reduced final numbers of alveoli[403] is unknown. The decrease in final numbers of alveoli is also associated with abnormal deposition of components of the extracellular matrix including elastin.[408] Abnormalities are also seen in the larger airways with smooth muscle extending more distally in infants with CLD than is observed in normal lung development.[409] It is likely that this last observation

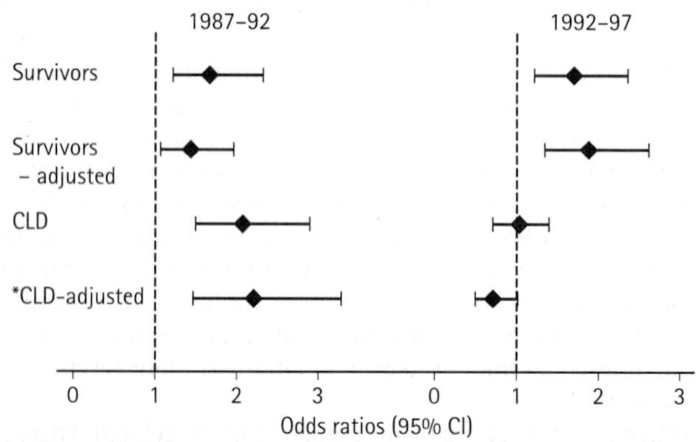

Fig. 18.32 Odds ratios for survival and chronic lung disease (CLD) at 28 days of age between 1987-1992 and 1992-1997. Note improvement in survival between both time periods but with increased incidence of CLD during the first period. * Odds ratios corrected for gestation and birth weight. (Adapted from Manktelow et al 2001[398])

Table 18.17 Factors that may affect the reported incidence and prevalence of chronic lung disease

Population base of community
Social factors
Environmental factors
Age and health structure of community
Ethnic mix of population
Referral patterns of neonatal unit
Obstetric population (high/low risk)
Obstetric practices
Postnatal referrals from less expert units
Morbidity of patients
Early morbidity
Maturity of population
Complication rate
Early mortality rate
Quality of care
Quality and quantity of medical and nursing staff
Quality of equipment
Use of protocols based on scientific data

From Kotecha and Silverman 1999[397]

is responsible for the airway obstruction that is described in infants with CLD. Initially the airways may respond to bronchodilators but with subsequent remodelling and fixed airway obstruction, the response to such treatment becomes less predictable.

CLINICAL FEATURES

The clinical features of infants developing CLD whilst in the neonatal intensive care unit are discussed in detail in Chapter 10. The typical infant with CLD will have been born prematurely and may have received mechanical ventilation and oxygen therapy either from birth or at some stage of the neonatal course.[397] A prolonged oxygen requirement is the most common feature and clinical signs of respiratory distress, including an increased respiratory rate, inter- and subcostal recession, may still be evident even at rest. At the more severe end of the spectrum, the infant may have developed chest abnormalities including a barrel chest reflecting air trapping and Harrison's sulci suggesting increased work of the diaphragm during breathing. Some of these infants may have been discharged home on oxygen. Their appetite and weight gain are likely to be poor despite increased energy intake. Vomiting and feeding difficulties may be present due to gastroesophageal reflux. Other features of being born too early may also be present including poor sucking, retinopathy of prematurity and early evidence of neurodevelopmental delay.

On examination, besides an increased respiratory rate and the features mentioned above, widespread wheezing and/or crackles may be present throughout the lung fields on auscultation. Pulmonary hypertension when present may manifest itself clinically with right ventricular hypertrophy and tricuspid regurgitation. If prolonged endotracheal intubation has been necessary, signs of upper airway obstruction due to subglottic stenosis may also be present.

Chest radiographs are likely to show abnormalities ranging from mild haziness of type I disease (Fig. 18.33a)[410] to large cystic areas interspersed with areas of atelectasis of type II or Northway Stage IV BPD (Fig. 18.33b). Lung function testing in infancy (which remains largely a research tool) may demonstrate evidence of gas trapping. In addition, decreased dynamic and static lung compliance and increased airway resistance are commonly observed. Response to bronchodilators may be variable but may provide a guide to future treatment for the child. Electrocardiography and echocardiography (discussed below) are necessary, especially when pulmonary hypertension is suspected.

Other causes of oxygen dependency other than prematurity are likely to have been excluded by the time the child is discharged from the neonatal unit. Nevertheless, there are a number of associated differential diagnoses which need to be sought and treated as appropriate (Table 18.18). Obstructive disorders are discussed in the section on asthma but other disorders including laryngomalacia, tracheobronchomalacia, subglottic stenosis, laryngeal webs and granulomas, vascular rings and enlarged tonsils should be sought and treated. In one study, 30% of low birth weight infants underwent surgery for upper airway abnormalities.[411]

(a)
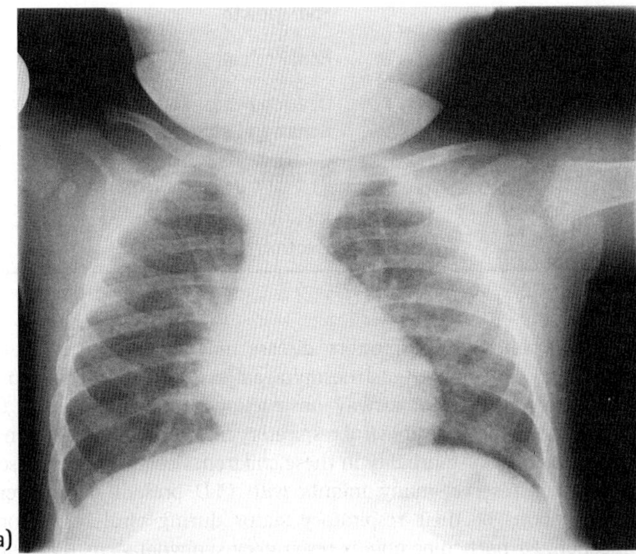

(b)
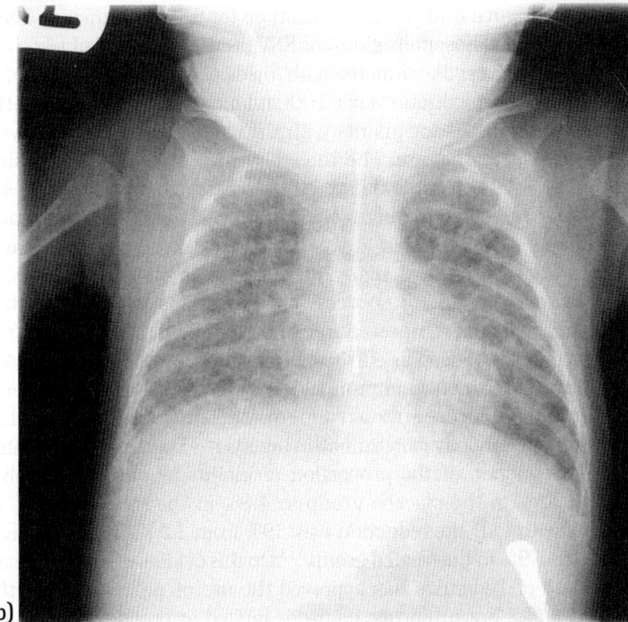

Fig. 18.33 Chest radiograph showing (a) haziness of both lung fields with oxygen dependency typical of type I chronic lung disease (CLD) (Hyde et al 1989[410]), and (b) more cystic changes associated with CLD typical of type II (Hyde et al 1989[410]) or Stage IV CLD (Northway et al 1967[394]). Note also presence of pH probe for assessing presence of gastroesophageal reflux.

Table 18.18 Conditions which may be associated with CLD

System	Clinical manifestation
Respiratory	Oxygen dependency for hypoxia Airway obstructive disease Laryngo-, tracheo- or bronchomalacia Subglottic stenosis Acquired bronchial stenosis Respiratory viral infections Aspiration pneumonitis
Cardiovascular	Pulmonary hypertension Cor pulmonale Arterial hypertension
Gastrointestinal system and growth	Gastroesophageal reflux Malabsorption Poor growth
Renal	Renal calculi
Central nervous system	Developmental abnormalities Behavioral abnormalities
Ophthalmology	Retinopathy of prematurity
Metabolic	Rickets Electrolyte imbalances

Exacerbations of respiratory disease may occur as a result of respiratory infections, gastroesophageal reflux with or without pulmonary aspiration, airway obstruction and heart failure. Of particular importance are viral respiratory infections which remain a common cause of morbidity in these children. Because of decreased respiratory reserve, many infants with CLD present with severe exacerbations of their respiratory status during viral respiratory infection. Of particular note is respiratory syncytial virus (RSV). In one retrospective study of hospitalizations for RSV in Tennessee, USA, there were 40.8 hospitalizations for RSV per 1000 infants of less than 1 year of age.[412] For infants with medical factors the estimated numbers of hospitalizations per 1000 infants of less than 12 months of age were: 388.4 for infants with CLD and 92.2 for infants with congenital heart disease. The rates also increased with decreasing gestation: 57.2 per 1000 children if born between 33 and 36 weeks' gestation, 65.9 if born between 29 and 32 weeks' gestation and increasing to 70.0 if born at less than 28 weeks' gestation. Clearly, respiratory viruses particularly RSV place a great burden on both human and economic resources. Therefore considerable effort has been directed to both prevention and treatment of this infection. Ribavirin has not been as efficacious as initial expectations predicted and intravenous pooled immunoglobulins have had variable success reported. More recently, a randomized controlled trial of the monoclonal antibody palivizumab in infants < 35 weeks demonstrated a 55% reduction of the proportion of infants admitted to hospital from 10.6% in the placebo group to 4.8% in the treated group. In infants with CLD the reduction was 39% from 12.8% in the placebo group to 7.9% in the treated group.[413] On this evidence, the American Academy of Pediatrics has approved the use of palivizumab in the United States but in Europe its use is limited at present by cost and case-mix considerations.[414] Reassuringly, data from the PICNIC study in Canada demonstrated that infants with CLD who acquired RSV and required mechanical ventilation did not fare worse than children with other respiratory disorders (cystic fibrosis, congenital lung malformations, respiratory disease associated with CNS disorders).[415] Respiratory viruses, therefore, remain a common cause of respiratory morbidity in children with CLD and place a great burden both on the parents and on the health services.

EXTRAPULMONARY COMPLICATIONS

Growth and nutrition

Many other systems may be affected in children with CLD either directly as a result of developing CLD or indirectly due to being born prematurely (Table 18.18). Gastroesophageal reflux is common. It may exacerbate the respiratory disease if recurrent aspiration occurs or provoke airway obstruction via reflex neural pathways. Gastroesophageal reflux may present as vomiting, failure to thrive, cough, poor feeding and in the worst cases recurrent lower respiratory tract infections or aspiration pneumonitis. Twenty-four hour esophageal pH monitoring and an upper gastrointestinal tract contrast study are the investigations of choice to confirm gastroesophageal reflux. Medical treatment with a prokinetic agent together with a feed thickener or alginate are the drugs most often used and in the worst cases reduction of gastric acid by H_2 blockers or proton pump inhibitors is useful. Recently erythromycin has been used in low doses for its prokinetic action. Fundoplication is required in some children in whom medical treatment fails, as evidenced by failure to thrive, continuing respiratory exacerbations or rare complications of gastroesophageal reflux including hematemesis, anemia or strictures (see Ch. 17).

Growth failure is common in infants with CLD due to a number of reasons that may include increased work of breathing, hypoxemia, gastroesophageal reflux, neurodevelopmental abnormalities resulting in poor feeding, heart failure and other complications of prematurity including necrotizing enterocolitis. There have been no controlled trials of the benefits of supplemental oxygen treatment on growth in CLD but evidence that oxygen improves growth has been reported.[416] When caregivers abruptly and against medical advice ceased giving oxygen to hypoxic infants with CLD, their growth rates decreased and increased when oxygen was reintroduced although never to previous rates of weight gain. Increased energy intake is necessary in these children to promote growth and high calorie supplements are often essential. In some cases enteral feeds may have to be given or supplemented via a nasogastric or gastrostomy tube.

Cardiovascular system

Cardiac abnormalities are often seen in children with CLD. These include increased pulmonary vascular resistance due to respiratory disease, right-to-left shunting, left ventricular hypertrophy most likely to be due to corticosteroid treatment during the neonatal period, patent ductus arteriosus (which will have been treated in the neonatal period) and fluid overload. One or a combination of these features may result in heart failure manifested as poor feeding and failure to thrive, tachypnea, hypoxemia and worsening respiratory disease, and inappropriate weight gain.

Pulmonary hypertension remains the commonest association with CLD and markedly improves with oxygen treatment.[417,418] Cor pulmonale is now uncommon especially after the introduction of home oxygen programs and with improved neonatal care in general. Electrocardiographs may demonstrate right heart strain or hypertrophy and echocardiograms may be used to estimate the degree of the pulmonary hypertension particularly if tricuspid regurgitation is present. Indirect methods of assessing pulmonary arterial pressures by echocardiography and Doppler have also been used (e.g. the ratio of pulmonary arterial acceleration:right ventricular ejection time).[418] Such measurements may be used to determine the fixed and reversible components of pulmonary hypertension with the child on and off oxygen. The data may be useful in determining when to wean an infant from supplemental oxygen.

Neurodevelopmental complications

It is almost impossible to attribute the risk of developing neurodevelopmental abnormalities exclusively to CLD as sick extremely preterm infants are at risk of developing both conditions. Majnemer et al[419] reported that, when 27 children with CLD were matched with a similar number of controls (preterm controls matched for gestational age, birth weight and year of birth), neurological abnormalities were more prevalent in the CLD group (71%) compared with the controls (19%). A variety of disorders were described including cerebral palsy, subtle neurological disorders, microcephaly and behavioral difficulties. Feeding disorders including dysphagia and sleep disorders are also more prevalent in these children. Retinopathy of prematurity leading to visual impairment, in some cases blindness, and hearing abnormalities are more common in infants with CLD. Respiratory responses to hypoxia may be blunted in infants with CLD when compared with non-oxygen dependent preterm infants, at least in the early stages after weaning from oxygen.

MANAGEMENT

General aspects of management

The management of the oxygen-dependent child with CLD can be divided into pulmonary and non-pulmonary aspects. The latter should focus on maximizing the growth of the child and on treating conditions such as gastroesophageal reflux which may exacerbate existing respiratory disease. Cardiovascular abnormalities should be sought and treated as necessary. Pulmonary hypertension is likely to respond to oxygen therapy and is discussed below. Full immunization of these infants is essential and killed vaccines (e.g. polio) may be required if there has been prolonged corticosteroid treatment. Input from relevant agencies, including community pediatricians, health visitors, dietitians, physiotherapists, speech and occupational therapists and educational psychologists, is usually necessary, especially if neurodevelopmental abnormalities are evident. For established CLD, the mainstay of therapeutic treatment remains:

- Domiciliary oxygen
- Corticosteroids
- Bronchodilators
- Diuretics

Because of the small numbers of infants with established CLD in any one center, there have been very few controlled evaluations of the above treatments in large studies of this group of children. Most studies have been uncontrolled observational studies or have included only small numbers of patients. Almost all studies of these treatments have been confined to the neonatal period and are discussed in Chapter 10. Many such studies have evaluated only short-term outcomes and their relevance to longer term outcomes is unknown. As a result most treatment is empirical and founded on 'best practice' rather than evidence based. Discussed below are current practices drawn from the literature and from the author's personal practice.

Domiciliary oxygen

By definition children with CLD are hypoxemic and their well-being, particularly with regard to growth, development, work of breathing and decreased pulmonary hypertension, may depend on achieving normoxemia using oxygen therapy. The criteria for domiciliary oxygen vary between units but, generally speaking, an infant with an oxygen requirement, i.e. supplemental oxygen is required to achieve arterial PaO_2 of >8 kPa or arterial oxygen saturation (SaO_2) of = 94%, should be considered for domiciliary oxygen if all attempts to wean the child from their oxygen have failed especially if the infant is feeding orally by bottle or breast. Nasogastric feeding may not preclude the child from going home on oxygen but may place a greater burden and stress on the family. Clearly the family should be willing and capable of looking after the child on oxygen. A stable oxygen requirement and a thriving child are ideal but changes to respiratory treatment, particularly the recent cessation of corticosteroids, may result in a rebound increase in oxygen requirements.

Oxygen is most often given by nasal cannulae and is most commonly delivered by an oxygen concentrator.[420] Portable cylinders allow greater mobility and are helpful for emergency use. Liquid oxygen is sometimes necessary if flow rates higher than 1 L/min are required. The general practitioner prescribes the equipment and the local oxygen company provides 24-h backup service. The latter will install and provide initial training for the parents. It is usual to provide two outlets – one in the living room and one for the child's sleeping area.

Monitoring of oxygenation is essential. Oximeters have transformed the monitoring of these children. A small number of units have used *continuous* monitoring with transcutaneous monitors but few have used pulse oximeters in this way partly due to movement artefacts and partly due to the poor quality probes of portable machines for small infants. Therefore, most units have relied on intermittent oxygen saturation measurements on a regular basis. Monitoring should be frequent early after discharge, during intercurrent infections and during weaning of oxygen. Specialist respiratory nurses provide a vital link between the hospital environment (to which the family have 'open' access) and the community. Infants should also be evaluated regularly within the hospital environment in the presence of all relevant agencies. Weaning from oxygen can commence once the child has been stable and thriving.[420] Usually the oxygen saturation is 95% and only insignificant drops occur during feeding and sleep (≤ 4%). Where available, echocardiography can be used to determine the reversible component of pulmonary hypertension by assessing the pulmonary arterial pressures on and off oxygen. Rates of weaning vary greatly from increasing time off oxygen gradually, e.g. 15–30 min every week to completely stopping the oxygen abruptly. Regardless of rates of weaning, it is essential to monitor the child's oxygen saturations once off their oxygen and at times of intercurrent infections. The duration of oxygen dependency varies widely but in one study of infants with CLD discharged at a mean age of 3.7 months, mean duration of oxygen therapy was 97 days (range 15–320 days), and the mean age of discontinuation of oxygen was 6.9 months (range 3–14.7 months).[421] It is necessary to continue to monitor after weaning especially at times of viral upper respiratory tract infections.

Corticosteroids

Corticosteroids remain the main treatment for CLD in newborn infants, especially those who require mechanical ventilation. However, recent data suggest that the administration of corticosteroids to infants, particularly early after birth, is associated with adverse neurodevelopment.[422,423] In contrast to ventilated preterm infants, studies of the use of both systemic and inhaled corticosteroids in established CLD are severely lacking. Caution with the use of dexamethasone, the most frequently used corticosteroid for CLD, was reported by Noble-Jamieson and colleagues in 1989.

They treated 18 non-ventilated infants with CLD with either dexamethasone or placebo[424] and reported that, although there was an initial decrease in oxygenation requirements with steroid treatment, the overall duration of oxygen dependency was similar in both groups. Of particular note was the observation that the treated group had an apparent increase in periventricular abnormalities. In the Cochrane review of the use of inhaled corticosteroids in established CLD,[425] only one study published as an abstract was included.[426] In that single study non-ventilated infants of at least 36 weeks corrected gestation and who were oxygen dependent were included. Budesonide (1 mg) was administered by an Airlife Misty-Neb jet nebulizer three times a day for 7 days. A significant reduction in oxygen requirements was observed by the authors. In another study of 18 preterm infants at a mean postnatal age of 10.5 months, the use of inhaled beclometasone for 6weeks was associated with an improvement in respiratory tract symptoms and functional residual capacity.[427] Since this study did not specify the number of infants with oxygen dependency, it is difficult to extrapolate the results to infants with established CLD. As this set of children forms a large group in the community, there is a clear need to examine the role of both systemic and inhaled corticosteroids in infants with CLD.

Bronchodilators

Several studies have shown that preterm infants who are mechanically ventilated have an improvement in lung compliance and resistance following the administration of bronchodilators.[428] Whether these agents have a beneficial effect on longer term outcomes including symptoms or oxygen dependency is unknown. In established CLD, marked airway smooth muscle hypertrophy is seen.[409,429] It is likely that this increased smooth muscle stabilizes the compliant infant airway but whether relaxation of airway smooth muscle by bronchodilators leads to increased airway resistance by increasing dynamic airway compression is speculative. Few studies have investigated bronchodilators in infants with CLD beyond the neonatal period. Most have examined a small number of children in short-term, observational studies. In one study of 1-year old infants, decreased resistance was noted in half the infants with CLD but half showed no improvement following inhaled salbutamol.[430] Similarly in older children, functional small airway abnormalities remain and a favorable response to salbutamol is seen in some but not all children.[431] Taken together, these data suggest that there is a subgroup of children who had CLD in infancy who have reversible airway obstruction. However, routine use of salbutamol in all children with CLD is not recommended but should be assessed clinically. If no response is observed, the treatment should be stopped.[431]

Similarly, there have been few studies evaluating the benefits of inhaled ipratropium bromide in infants with CLD, especially beyond the neonatal period. Benefit from this treatment has been noted in small studies of ventilated neonates and during early infancy with improvement observed in some children.[432] As with salbutamol, not all children with CLD respond to ipratropium. Another poorly studied area is the optimal method of administering bronchodilators. A metered-dosed inhaler is most frequently used with a spacer device such as the Aerochamber. Questions remain regarding the optimal dose, timing and assessment of clinical response when bronchodilators are used in children with established CLD.

Diuretics

There have been few studies investigating the role of diuretics in CLD beyond the neonatal period. Even those in the neonatal unit have only investigated short-term pulmonary outcomes such as falls in pulmonary resistance, improvements in compliance and oxygen requirements. Recent Cochrane reviews of the use of diuretics have concluded that studies of longer term outcomes are necessary.[433–435] Clearly diuretics are indicated for cardiac failure diagnosed by abnormal weight gain, tachypnea, tachycardia, hepatomegaly and peripheral edema. The short-term benefits on respiratory mechanics from diuretics are likely to result from a direct action on pulmonary vascular resistance and on extracellular pulmonary water. Whether these benefits are associated with improved longer term outcomes, e.g. decreased numbers of days of oxygen dependency, is currently unknown. In addition, adverse effects of long-term diuretic treatment may be clinically significant. The use of diuretics, especially loop diuretics such as furosemide (frusemide), may result in renal calcification and calculi which often but not always resolve on cessation of therapy. It is usual practice to use loop diuretics in the short term and to change over to a combination of a thiazide and spironolactone to decrease the risks of adverse effects, although electrolyte imbalance with hyponatremia and hypokalemia may still be troublesome.

PROGNOSIS

There has been a great improvement in survival of preterm infants and, with home oxygen programs, the outlook for children with CLD has also improved vastly. However, although there is improvement in the respiratory status of preschool children following CLD as infants, as they reach adolescence there remains a degree of respiratory morbidity as evidenced by increased cough, wheezing and decreased exercise tolerance. Lung function improves with time but, compared with healthy controls or preterm controls without CLD, persisting abnormalities, particularly of FEV_1 and more peripheral airway function ($FEF_{25-75\%}$) have been reported.[436,437] The decreased alveolar numbers described in infants with CLD is clearly worrying,[405] but whether these children are candidates for chronic pulmonary dysfunction in later life remains to be seen.

FUTURE

The outlook for children with CLD has improved markedly but there are a number of areas which will require refining over the next few years. These include the role of therapeutic agents such as systemic and inhaled corticosteroids, bronchodilators and diuretics in children with established CLD. Further information regarding efficacy, doses and their timing and routes of administration is required urgently. The roles of antiviral drugs, such as palivizumab, and supportive therapies, such as the effects of nutrition on lung growth, need to be clarified further. Since candidates for developing CLD are preterm and at an early stage of lung development, we need a better understanding of both normal lung development in the fetus and also after the infant is delivered. Only by understanding the underlying mechanisms are we likely to develop therapies which do not have adverse effects including poor neurodevelopment. Ideally, CLD can be 'cured' by preventing preterm labor (a forlorn hope at present!) but alternatively, treatments to abrogate acute lung injury are likely to at least decrease the severity of CLD.

LONG TERM VENTILATION

There is evidence of growing numbers of children who are dependent on long term ventilation, defined as the need for a mechanical aid to breathing after failure to wean 3 months after the initiation of ventilation in children who are otherwise medically stable.[438] Conditions which are associated with chronic respiratory failure and the need for long term ventilation fall into 3 broad categories of increased respiratory load, respiratory muscle weakness and inadequate respiratory drive. Examples of these are shown in Table 18.19.

INCREASED RESPIRATORY LOAD

Upper airway obstruction can often be managed with continuous positive pressure (CPAP) by nasal or face mask alone. This splints the airway and decreases inspiratory resistive load thus reducing work of breathing. CPAP may also have a role in intrinsic lung diseases in which intrinsic positive end expiratory pressure ($PEEP_i$) may also contribute to increased work of breathing. However, upper airway loading and $PEEP_i$ are not the sole mechanisms of hypoventilation in the majority of these cases and intermittent positive pressure or bilevel pressure support is usually required. In patients with cystic fibrosis, positive pressure ventilation was initially introduced as a bridge to transplantation in end-stage lung disease but non-invasive ventilation has evolved as a strategy to treat respiratory failure associated with exacerbations of lung disease and as long term support of nocturnal hypoventilation in this condition.

RESPIRATORY MUSCLE WEAKNESS

Duchenne muscular dystrophy is the single most common indication for long term ventilation of children in the United Kingdom. Progression of respiratory muscle weakness in Duchenne muscular dystrophy inevitably leads to hypercapnic respiratory failure at some point but the rate of progression is variable between individual patients. Respiratory failure is the commonest cause of death in Duchenne muscular dystrophy and may also complicate the cardiomyopthy associated with the condition. Despite initial ethical and practical concerns about long term ventilation of patients with Duchenne muscular dystrophy, there is now good evidence of patient acceptability, improved survival and enhanced health-related quality of life associated with non-invasive ventilation of patients with this disease who have developed hypercapnic respiratory failure.[439] Respiratory support is less commonly required for other types of muscular dystrophy.

Table 18.19 Conditions causing chronic respiratory failure and the need for long term ventilation in children

Increased respiratory load
Upper airway obstruction
Craniofacial abnormalities
Severe tracheobronchomalacia
Intrinsic pulmonary disease
Chronic lung disease of prematurity
Cystic fibrosis
Chest wall abnormalities
Severe kyphoscoliosis
Thoracic dystrophies
Respiratory muscle weakness
Spinal muscular atrophy (SMA)
Congenital myopathies
Duchenne muscular dystrophy
Spinal cord injury
Abnormal control of respiration
Congenital central hypoventilation syndrome (CCHS)

Although respiratory failure is seen as an inevitable consequence of some progressive neuromuscular conditions, non-progressive diseases, such as congenital myopathies, may also result in chronic respiratory failure requiring ventilatory support. This usually occurs at or around the time of puberty when increased functional demands of increasing body mass exceed the capabilities of respiratory muscle strength to meet associated increased ventilatory requirements.

The respiratory consequences of spinal cord injury are largely dependent on the level of the lesion. High spinal cord injury above the level of C3 leads to diaphragmatic paralysis and respiratory failure. Lower cervical or thoracic spinal cord injury may compromise expiratory muscle function leading to a defective cough, atelectasis and frequent respiratory infections and such patients may need respiratory support during exacerbations.

DISORDERS OF CONTROL OF RESPIRATION

The commonest example of respiratory control disorders requiring long term ventilation is congenital central hypoventilation syndrome (see p. 746 Apnea and breathing disorders during sleep).

HOME VENTILATION

There are many potential benefits of home care compared with hospital care, particularly in intensive care settings, for children with long term ventilation needs who are otherwise medically stable. Advances in ventilator technology and increased experience and acceptance of home ventilation have made home care possible for an increasing number of children with chronic respiratory failure. In a postal survey in the United Kingdom in 1997, 68% of 136 children who were receiving long term ventilation were cared for at home.[438] The degree of respiratory support that these patients required ranged from intermittent CPAP via nasal or face mask to 24 h/day controlled positive pressure ventilation through a tracheostomy tube. The duration and mode of ventilation, associated medical conditions, level of support available and ability of the child's family to cope with home ventilation are all factors that may determine the feasibililty and success of long term ventilation in the home. The United Kingdom Working Party on Pediatric Long Term Ventilation has produced core guidelines for home ventilation of children with chronic respiratory failure.[440] These include a stable medical condition, comprising a stable airway, stable oxygen requirements of usually no more than 40% inspired oxygen concentration, the ability to maintain $PaCO_2$ within safe boundaries and adequate nutrition to meet the child's needs for growth and development. In addition, the child's family must have a clear understanding of the prognosis and be willing and able to meet the needs of the child in the home environment and there must be the capability to provide an adequate level of support, intervention and monitoring of the child's condition. Monitoring should usually consist of evaluation of gas exchange before and after the institution of ventilation and during follow up, ideally with the addition of polygraphic recordings of respiration during different behavioral states, including night-time sleep (polysomnography), but the optimal frequency of such assessments has yet to be determined.

The amount of home care support that families will require is determined by a large number of local factors, including the child's ventilator dependency, the means of ventilation, the need for other medical interventions such as overnight enteral tube feeding, whether the child is ambulant or paralyzed, and what other commitments the family have in terms of work and other children. It is important that home carers receive adequate training and supervision and it is recommended that each home care team is led by a nurse with pediatric training.

Many children on long term ventilation can return to mainstream schooling but provision is likely to be needed for their special needs, including trained assistants to supervise ventilation and tracheostomy care where indicated.

Problems that may be encountered in the long term management of children with chronic respiratory failure include equipment considerations, changing ventilation requirements with growth or progression of the underlying disease, associated medical conditions, and possible adverse effects of treatment. Equipment will be selected on the basis of size, robustness, reliability and ease of use and it is essential to ensure that adequate maintenance and service contracts are in place to replace ventilators during routine service and in the event of breakdown. Children who are unable to cope without ventilator assistance for more than 6 h should have a second ventilator available for immediate use. Ventilation requirements should be assessed frequently, particularly in young children, as changes in lung and chest wall mechanics occur with normal growth and development. In some neuromuscular conditions, it may be necessary to consider switching from non-invasive ventilation to tracheostomy ventilation as the disease progresses.

It is important to ensure adequate nutritional support, particularly as many children are undernourished at the time long term ventilator support is initiated. Associated problems such as bulbar dysfunction and gastroesophageal reflux may limit the ability of some children to feed orally and surgical interventions, including fundoplication and gastrostomy, may be indicated for some. Abdominal distension occasionally complicates non-invasive ventilation by face mask but can usually be dealt with by altering ventilator settings. The use of tightly fitting face masks for non-invasive ventilation has been reported to cause mid-face hypoplasia in children so careful monitoring of maxillo-mandibular growth and inspection for signs of pressure to the nose and maxillae should be carried out regularly.

OUTCOMES

The outcome of long term ventilation is dependent on the underlying condition for which ventilation was initiated. Some conditions may be predicted to remain static but ventilation requirements may change as a result of growth and development. Others, such as the muscular dystrophies, may worsen with time whereas some conditions may be expected to improve, such as chronic lung disease of prematurity or tracheobronchomalacia. The initiation of long term ventilation should be based not only on its potential for prolonging life but on the quality of life during the extension that ventilation affords. In addition to correcting gas exchange abnormalities associated with chronic respiratory failure, ventilatory support may retard progression of morbidity associated with suboptimal respiratory and chest wall function including cor pulmonale, recurrent pneumonia and thoracic deformity. There is now good evidence for improved survival with acceptable quality of life for children with neuromuscular and skeletal diseases treated with non-invasive ventilation at home[439] and it is likely that demand for this intervention will continue to increase.

ACUTE RESPIRATORY DISTRESS SYNDROME (ARDS)

Acute respiratory distress syndrome (ARDS), previously termed *adult respiratory distress syndrome*, refers to a combination of severe respiratory failure with refractory hypoxemia and widespread pulmonary infiltrates on chest X-ray. The precise incidence of ARDS has been difficult to establish because of differences in definitions that have been applied in epidemiological studies. However, in 1994, an American–European consensus conference attempted to clarify the definitions and approaches to management of ARDS. In this, it was recognized that ARDS represents part of a continuum of lung injury. An operational definition of *acute lung injury* (ALI) was proposed that included diffuse parenchymal infiltrates (in three or four quadrants on chest X-ray); hypoxemia ($PaO_2/FiO_2 < 300$ mmHg) and pulmonary capillary wedge pressure < 18 mmHg or absence of clinical evidence of increased left heart filling pressure. In clinical practice in the United Kingdom, few children have pulmonary artery catheters (Swan–Ganz) inserted for measurement of pulmonary capillary wedge pressure and clinical/ultrasonographic measurements are used instead. The definition of *acute respiratory distress syndrome* uses similar criteria but with more severe oxygenation deficit ($PaO_2/FiO_2 < 200$ mmHg). Using post-1994 definitions, the incidence has been calculated to be approximately 12.5–13.5/100 000 per annum in separate studies in Scandinavia and the USA.

Although a variety of clinical insults, both direct (pulmonary) and non-direct (non-pulmonary) are associated with ARDS (Table 18.20), it is likely that the final pathophysiological response of the lungs is similar. However, the clinical course and mortality varies according to the initiating process and the presence of other complications of systemic disease, particularly multiorgan system failure. In practice, sepsis is the single most common clinical risk factor for ARDS, which frequently complicates an overwhelming systemic inflammatory response (systemic inflammatory response syndrome or SIRS).

The pathology of the lungs during the development and resolution of ARDS has three distinct stages, although not every patient with ARDS will necessarily progress through all three. The first phase represents *diffuse alveolar damage* (DAD) manifest by extensive epithelial and capillary endothelial cell damage with leakage of protein-rich fluid into the alveolar spaces. Damage to type II pneumocytes results in altered surfactant composition and surfactants are inactivated by alveolar protein content, leading to increased surface tension and atelectasis. There is usually an intense neutrophil response initiated by cellular adhesion molecules, including selectins and beta 2-integrins, and activated by a variety of cytokines, including tumor necrosis factor alpha (TNF-alpha) and interleukins 1, 6, 8 and 10. However, although neutrophils are central to the inflammatory process, it is still possible for neutropenic patients to develop ARDS. Platelet aggregation leads to microthrombi forming in the pulmonary microvasculature resulting in raised pulmonary vascular resistance and pulmonary hypertension. The second phase occurs after 3 to

Table 18.20 Clinical risk factors for acute respiratory distress syndrome

Direct pulmonary injury	Indirect pulmonary response
Aspiration	Sepsis
Pneumonia	Shock
Pulmonary contusion	Trauma
Toxic inhalation	Multiple fractures
Near drowning	Drug overdose
	Multiple transfusions
	Cardiopulmonary bypass
	Burns
	Disseminated intravascular coagulation

10 days and is characterized by fibroproliferation and organization. Type II pneumocytes proliferate and replace type I cells on the denuded basement membrane, collagen is deposited in the alveolar walls and macrophages phagocytose hyaline membranes and cellular debris. This is followed by the final stage of fibrosis, scarring and cyst formation.

The clinical features of ARDS follow these pathological changes. There is an initial period at the initiation of acute lung injury during which the only manifestation may be respiratory alkalosis. This is followed, over a period of several hours to 2 days, by a latent phase during which there is gradual development of widespread patchy infiltrates which correspond to the leakage of fluid into the airspaces (non-cardiogenic pulmonary edema). Acute respiratory failure ensues (ALI) and may progress to a final stage of severe physiological abnormalities with intrapulmonary shunting and severe, refractory hypoxemia with concomitant respiratory and metabolic acidosis.

MANAGEMENT OF ARDS

The key to optimal management of ARDS is supporting adequate tissue oxygen delivery and mechanical ventilation remains the most important component of management strategy. There are few studies of management of ARDS in children alone and much of the available evidence comes from adult studies. The recognition that conventional ventilation of hypoxemic respiratory failure with relatively high tidal volumes can contribute to lung injury by epithelial disruption and release of inflammatory mediators at local and systemic level has led to the development of a lung-protective ventilation strategy. This relies on maintaining the patency of small peripheral airways by keeping PEEP above the point at which airway closure occurs, and using low tidal volumes with resultant 'permissive' hypercapnia (see pp. 724 – Postnatal development). Two controlled trials of protective lung strategy compared with conventional ventilation have demonstrated improved outcomes with the former and this is now recommended as the strategy of choice for ventilating patients with ARDS.[441] Many of the large number of other proposed treatments for ARDS (Table 18.21) have not been subjected to sufficiently large, prospective controlled trials to recommend their use at the present time. A systematic review of inhaled nitric oxide (iNO) treatment in hypoxemic respiratory failure in adults and children concluded that iNO had no effect on mortality and produced only transient improvements in oxygenation.[442] Extracorporeal membrane oxygenation (ECMO) has been evaluated in adults with ARDS in two large randomized controled trials which did not show an advantage over conventional ventilation. However, recent advances in both ECMO and ventilation methods suggest that this intervention should be formally re-evaluated. Exogenous surfactant treatment has been demonstrated to be safe in ARDS but it has not been demonstrated to be efficacious in a large clinical trial. Corticosteroids and other anti-inflammatory/ immune-modulating treatments have been investigated on the basis that ARDS has an inflammatory pathogenesis. However, short courses of steroids during the development of ARDS are ineffective in preventing progression of the disease and the early administration of steroids has not been demonstrated to reduce mortality in ARDS. Recent small studies of corticosteroids in the later, fibroproliferative stage of ARDS have suggested potential benefits in this context but there is still no convincing evidence of their safety and efficacy and there is a need for a large, prospective randomized controlled trial.

Table 18.21 Management strategies for the treatment of acute respiratory distress syndrome

Ventilation	Others
Lung-protective ventilation	Corticosteroids
Non-invasive ventilation (NIPPV)	Non-steroidal anti-inflammatories
Inverse I:E ratio	Epoprostenol (PGI_2)
Partial liquid ventilation (PLV)	Exogenous surfactant
Inhaled nitric oxide (iNO)	Antioxidants
Extracorporeal membrane oxygenation	Anticytokine/antiendotoxin therapies
Positional changes (prone positioning)	Ketoconazole
	Almitrine

OUTCOME

Despite advances in the understanding of the pathophysiology of ARDS, the mortality has remained high at around 40% or more. The highest mortality is observed in ARDS associated with sepsis and multiorgan system failure. In those patients that do survive the acute lung injury, the majority will have persistent decrements in pulmonary function with reduced lung volumes and impaired gas transfer being the most frequently documented abnormalities. Many patients report cough and dyspnea and there is evidence that ARDS survivors have impaired health-related quality of life and a high proportion have impaired cognitive function 1–2 years after hospital discharge.

RARE LUNG DISEASES

The majority of these conditions are so rare that they will be encountered but once in a lifetime by the general pediatrician. Thus early referral for specialist review is recommended in suspected cases.

THE TRUE INTERSTITIAL PNEUMONITIDES

About 50% of children with these conditions present at less than 1 year of age. The spectrum includes chronic pneumonitis of infancy (CPI), desquamative interstitial pneumonitis (DIP, the 'usual' pattern of adults rarely if ever occurs in children), and non-specific interstitial pneumonitis (NSIP), which last may be subclassified by the presence or absence of a fibrotic component.[443] The cause of all these conditions is unknown; some have speculated that CPI, which is characterized by Type 2 cell hyperplasia and intraalveolar lipoproteinaceous material,[444] is a complication of gastro-esophageal reflux and aspiration. Presentation of all these conditions is similar and non-specific, with cough, tachypnea, respiratory distress, failure to thrive and sometimes cyanosis. The physical signs may include digital clubbing and fine crackles. The CXR appearances are non-specific, and include generalized ground glass shadowing, reticular nodular infiltrates and honeycombing. HRCT is performed to confirm that an interstitial disease is present; but unlike in adults, it is relatively rare for a specific diagnosis to be made on the scan alone.[445] Diagnosis requires a lung biopsy; transbronchial biopsy gives only small samples, which may be sufficient for the rare diseases with highly specific histological features such as pulmonary alveolar microlithiasis, and is the investigation of choice in the transplant recipient with possible rejection.[446] Some advocate CT guided, percutaneous needle biopsy, but the complication rate is thought by many to be unacceptable.[446]

Open lung biopsy (OLB) through a mini-thoracotomy, is safe in experienced hands and has a high diagnostic yield.[447] In older children, a video-assisted, thoracoscopic (VATS) procedure may be preferred. It has to be said that there seems to be little relationship between biopsy appearances and response to treatment or prognosis. These conditions are so rare that treatment recommendations are scanty. Most pediatricians would treat with hydroxychloroquine alone, or in combination with prednisolone.[448] If there is no response, recommendations are even more anecdotal; pulse methylprednisolone, azathioprine and ciclosporin have all been tried. Prognosis is variable and unpredictable from either radiology or histological features; in general, the younger the age of onset the poorer the prognosis, but spontaneous and complete resolution of even severe disease is well described. There is a rare familial form of DIP which is an autosomal dominant, for which the gene is currently not identified.

RARE SINGLE SYSTEM DISORDERS

Interested readers are referred to a recent narrative review.[449]

Extrinsic allergic alveolitis. The allergen is usually pigeon or budgerigar excreta or moldy hay. Exposure to bird allergen may be indirect via the clothes of a parent. Presentation is with chronic respiratory distress (birds) or acute symptoms within hours of exposure (moldy hay), confirmed by positive serology. Treatment is allergen avoidance; oral steroids are given for severe acute or chronic progressive disease.

Pulmonary lymphangiectasia. This typically presents with relentlessly progressive respiratory distress in a term baby. CXR may show dilatation of lymphatics and pleural effusions. Treatment is generally hopeless, but octreotide has been used in some cases. Rarely, this condition may present in adolescence, localized to a single lobe.

Pulmonary alveolar microlithiasis. This condition, which may be inherited, has a non-specific presentation but a classical sandstorm appearance on CXR. Calcium carbonate stones are formed within the alveoli; the differential diagnosis is other forms of pulmonary calcification. Pulmonary fibrosis may develop many years later when the patient becomes symptomatic. A recent narrative review discusses these unusual problems in greater depth.[449]

THE LUNG AS PART OF A MULTISYSTEM DISORDER

Causes include conditions thought to be autoimmune (scleroderma, systemic lupus erythematosus, rheumatoid disease); inherited conditions (sickle cell disease, Riley–Day syndrome, mucopolysaccharidoses); and those of unknown cause (sarcoidosis, Langerhans' cell histiocytosis, and the disorders of the pulmonary lymphatics).[450]

The lung in connective tissue diseases. The lung may be affected as part of a systemic vasculitis, such as Wegener's granulomatosis or Churg–Strauss syndrome. Systemic lupus erythematosus may cause a variety of manifestations, including interstitial pneumonitis, obliterative bronchiolitis, respiratory muscle weakness, pulmonary hemorrhage and pleural effusion. Scleroderma is associated with pulmonary fibrosis, and pulmonary hypertension. All these conditions are so rare that referral to a tertiary center is advisable if they are suspected.

Histiocytosis. Lung involvement is usually part of a multisystem disease in children, but in young adults who smoke it may be confined to the lungs. Presentation is with respiratory distress, or sometimes with acute and non-resolving pneumothorax. CXR shows interstitial changes, and HRCT shows characteristic nodules which cavitate, allowing the diagnosis to be made without recourse to further tests. If in doubt, BAL shows increased numbers of Langerhans' cells, and biopsy is definitive. Treatment is smoking cessation, and sometimes prednisolone or a cytotoxic. The disease may progress to respiratory failure, and recur in the transplanted lung.

Sarcoidosis. Pulmonary disease is very rare in children; presentation is more usually with bilateral anterior uveitis, skin rashes and tendon sheath effusions. Diagnosis is on biopsy and is suggested by a high serum level of angiotensin-converting enzyme. Treatment is with steroids, to which may be added hydroxychloroquine and other steroid sparing agents.

Pulmonary lymphangiomatosis

Pulmonary lymphangiomatosis is a manifestation of a systemic lymphatic malformation which may also affect the spleen, heart and bone. It is usually fatal over 5–7 years, whatever treatment is tried.[451]

Alpha-1 antitrypsin deficiency. This is an autosomal recessive disorder which usually presents in adult life with emphysema or sometimes bronchiectasis. In childhood, however, it presents as a neonatal hepatitis. Pulmonary disease is usually not evident until late in adolescence. Children who are known to have this disorder should be advised never to smoke. Many non-smokers with this condition remain asymptomatic for many years, but prognosis for pulmonary function is poor in smokers. Replacement therapy with alpha-1 antitrypsin is now available.

RARE DISORDERS OF THE BRONCHIOLES

The most distal airways are the physiologically silent areas of the lungs, and notoriously difficult to investigate. Currently, patchy air trapping in the absence of overt large airway bronchiectasis, best demonstrated with inspiratory and expiratory HRCT, is the best diagnostic pointer.

Obliterative bronchiolitis

Obliterative bronchiolitis (OB) has been described in association with infections caused by adenovirus types 3, 7 and 21; measles, pertussis, influenza A, mycoplasma; after lung transplantation; and secondary to chronic aspiration.[452] Often the cause remains conjectural. The clinical course is one of cough, wheeze and tachypnea in an infant or young child which may be static if the cause is an infection, or progress at a variable rate to respiratory failure and failure to thrive if there is ongoing aspiration. Chest radiography initially shows generalized hyperinflation. HRCT demonstrates patchy air trapping, particularly if the scan is expiratory. Focal hyperlucency involving a lobe or a whole lung represents the radiological appearance of Macleod's syndrome, in which the affected lung appears small and hyperlucent. This represents long-term damage to lung development, both parenchymal and vascular. HRCT will usually show ipsilateral bronchiectasis, and contralateral, albeit less severe, areas of air trapping. This radiographic appearance should not be confused with other causes of hyperlucency such as hypoplastic pulmonary artery, congenital large hyperlucent lobe (CLHL, congenital lobar emphysema) or ball valve obstruction to a large airway. Radioisotope split lung function studies examining both ventilation and perfusion may help to clarify equivocal radiographic features. In Macleod's syndrome the affected lung is small and both poorly perfused and ventilated.

Lung function studies show severe airway obstruction, and, in pure OB, large lung volumes. Underlying diseases such as cystic fibrosis, immunodeficiency, ciliary dyskinesia and chronic aspiration may need to be ruled out. The main differential diagnosis is fibrosing alveolitis, which should easily be distinguished by HRCT. Management is supportive. Steroids have no proven value. Individuals may find bronchodilators helpful.

The prognosis for OB is most serious after adenoviral disease. Long term oxygen dependency is common.[453] Improvement after 2–3 years may be seen. The condition is usually stable once the initial effects of the devastating infection have burnt out, but some may go on to require lung transplantation. OB developing after lung transplant is eventually fatal, and the results of a second transplantation are very poor.

Follicular bronchiolitis

Follicular bronchiolitis (FB) is part of the spectrum of lymphoid disorders of the lung, which includes lymphoid interstitial pneumonia (LIP). There is a polyclonal expansion of lymphoid tissue, probably part of the bronchus associated lymphoid tissue (BALT), which causes small airway obstruction. Presentation is with chronic respiratory distress, and HRCT demonstrates air trapping, sometimes with associated infiltrates. Such a finding should prompt a full immune workup, including HIV testing (see Ch. 25). If no immune defect is found, anecdotal evidence suggests that treatment with inhaled steroids and long term macrolide antibiotics (clarithromycin, azithromycin) for their anti-inflammatory effects may be worthwhile.

SPONTANEOUS AIR LEAKS

Air leaks such as pneumothoraces, subcutaneous emphysema and pericardial and mediastinal air are very unusual outside the neonatal period, and are usually seen as a complication of positive pressure ventilation. Children with airway obstruction such as asthma or cystic fibrosis are at relatively higher risk. A spontaneous pneumothorax in a previously healthy child is extremely rare, and more often is a sign of an underlying lung disease than in adults.[454] Apical bullae or an isolated lung cyst are sometimes identified on a chest radiograph or CT scan. Rare causes include pulmonary Langerhans' cell histiocytosis and lung metastases from a primary sarcoma. Presenting features include sudden chest pain and breathlessness. There are reduced breath sounds over the affected side. In the management of a first episode the options are observation alone, simple aspiration or tube drainage with pleurodesis, depending on the size of the pneumothorax and on risk factors such as distance from hospital or future air travel, as well as any underlying disease. In spontaneously breathing children with acute asthma, an air leak may be identified on a chest radiograph quite unexpectedly; the majority resolve without intervention. Pneumothorax in a patient with cystic fibrosis is usually a sign of severe underlying disease and carries a poor prognosis. Treatment should be discussed with the local transplant center, to avoid contraindicating lung transplant by too aggressive a pleurodesis.

PULMONARY HEMORRHAGIC DISORDERS

The spectrum of these disorders has been reviewed recently.[455] Idiopathic pulmonary hemosiderosis is characterized pathologically by recurrent alveolar bleeding. Presentation is either as an iron deficiency anemia or with respiratory distress. The anemia may respond to oral iron, and the child has frequently been subjected to numerous invasive gastrointestinal investigations before a CXR is inspected. The respiratory presentation is with tachypnea, cough and sometimes but not invariably, hemoptysis. There may be digital clubbing and crackles, and hepatosplenomegaly in up to 20% of children. Gastric aspirates may be positive for hemosiderin laden macrophages, and the stools positive for occult blood. CXR may show ground glass opacification, or blotchy shadowing. HRCT may strongly suggest the diagnosis, which may also be confirmed by finding hemosiderin laden macrophages in BAL fluid; open lung biopsy is rarely necessary. An association with IgD milk antibodies (Heiner's syndrome) is in fact rarely if ever seen today. Secondary causes of pulmonary hemorrhage, for example pulmonary venous hypertension, must be excluded. Treatment is with hydroxychloroquine,[456] to which prednisolone may need to be added. Relapse is common, and death may be from acute massive bleeding or chronic respiratory failure. Treatment should probably be continued for at least 2 years after the last relapse. Cases apparently resistant to therapy should be referred for OLB, which may show not the expected normal lung architecture with intra-alveolar blood and hemosiderin laden macrophages, but a neutrophilic vasculitis. This picture, which is very rare, responds to cyclophosphamide.

PULMONARY VASCULAR DISEASES CHARACTERIZED BY PULMONARY HYPERTENSION

Primary pulmonary hypertension

Primary pulmonary hypertension (PPH) is a diagnosis of exclusion. Presentation is with non-specific symptoms such as breathlessness and syncope, and the physical signs of pulmonary hypertension (loud pulmonary component of the second heart sound, parasternal heave) may be elicited. Secondary causes such as congenital heart disease are excluded by echocardiography and are discussed in Chapter 19. PPH may be isolated, or inherited as an autosomal dominant, or associated with liver or autoimmune disease, or HIV infection. The gene accounting for some cases of familial PPH has recently been localized to chromosome 2.457 Treatment advice is largely based on adult guidelines,458 which make the assumption that the adult and pediatric diseases are the same. Possible lines of treatment include oxygen at least overnight, to maintain normal arterial saturation; anticoagulation; oral pulmonary vasodilators such as the calcium channel antagonists; and, for those rare children who can tolerate it, a continuous intravenous infusion of epoprostenol (prostacyclin, PGI_2). Recently, there has been interest in orally active PGI_2 analog such as iloprost, and the selective phosphodiesterase 5 inhibitor, sildenafil; currently, such treatment must be considered experimental. If these fail, lung transplantation is the only other option.

Embolic pulmonary hypertension

This presents in a similar manner to primary pulmonary hypertension. Spiral CT with contrast or angiography may lead to suspicion of the diagnosis by the demonstration of large pulmonary artery filling defects. OLB may be needed to confirm the presence of microemboli. Thromboembolic disease is the commonest cause. It may be a manifestation of an underlying congenital or acquired coagulopathy. Other predisposing factors include immobility, and a sluggish circulation, as for example after a Fontan procedure or secondary to right atrial stasis in dilated cardiomyopathy. Tumor emboli are another cause, with Wilms tumor or hepatoblastoma the commonest primary sources. Talc microemboli should be considered in adolescents who abuse substances intravenously; crushed up injected tablets result in talc microemboli. Worldwide, schistosomal disease must be the commonest cause of non-thrombotic embolic disease.

Pulmonary veno-occlusive disease

This condition presents as chronic pulmonary venous hypertension, with pulmonary edema resistant to diuretics.

Cases are usually isolated, but may rarely be familial, or a complication of cytotoxic chemotherapy. Diagnosis may be confirmed at cardiac catheterization or open lung biopsy. There is no known effective treatment, and most die of severe pulmonary hypertension unless transplanted.

Invasive pulmonary capillary hemangiomatosis

This is due to proliferating sheets of thin walled capillary channels infiltrating blood vessels and causing secondary vascular occlusion. Familial cases have been described. Diagnosis is by open lung biopsy, and the condition is usually fatal.

PULMONARY VASCULAR DISEASES CHARACTERIZED BY CYANOSIS WITHOUT PULMONARY HYPERTENSION

Macroscopic pulmonary arteriovenous malformations (PAVM)

PAVM are large malformations which typically present with cyanosis, and sometimes a bruit may be heard over the lung field. There may be an associated cerebral AVM with a bruit heard over the cranium. There is an obvious mass on CXR, and contrast echocardiography or peripheral injection of technetium labeled albumin microspheres confirms a large intrapulmonary right-to-left shunt. Most such PAVMs consist of a direct connection between the pulmonary arterial and venous circulations, but some also have a systemic arterial supply. Treatment is with transcatheter embolization using a balloon or coil. Untreated, complications include polycythemia, and systemic embolization and abscess formation, these last as a result of the systemic venous return bypassing the filtration function of the pulmonary capillary bed. Cerebral abscess or embolic stroke are the most feared complications of PAVM.

Microscopic pulmonary arteriovenous malformations

These may be an isolated finding, or a manifestation of Osler–Weber–Rendu disease. Presentation is with cyanosis without respiratory distress, and a clear CXR. There is no treatment other than lung transplantation.

INHERITED DISORDERS OF SURFACTANT PROTEINS

There are four surfactant proteins, lettered A to D. Surfactant proteins A and D are more properly considered as members of the collectin family, with important functions in host defense, but not much surface active function. Inherited disorders of proteins B and C, with a respiratory presentation, have been described.

Congenital surfactant protein B (SpB) deficiency

This condition presents as relentlessly progressive respiratory distress, usually in a term baby.[459] It is inherited as an autosomal recessive. CXR shows a ground glass appearance. OLB shows alveoli filled with lipoproteinaceous material, and special stains confirm the absence of SpB. Successful treatment with granulocyte-colony stimulating factor has been reported. If this fails, lung transplantation is the only other option.

Congenital surfactant protein C (SpC) deficiency

SpC deficiency has recently been described.[460] The index case was a woman with an interstitial lung disease, who gave birth to an infant with respiratory distress. The mother subsequently died. Molecular studies established the diagnosis. It seems likely that children previously given the diagnosis of CPI will turn out to have subtle inherited defects of surfactant proteins.

Pulmonary alveolar proteinosis (PAP)

Although not apparently related to an inherited surfactant protein deficiency, PAP presents in infancy with progressive respiratory distress. In some children it may be related to a form of immune deficiency such as thymic atrophy, lymphopenia and immunoglobulin deficiency. CXR shows a ground glass appearance, and HRCT a typical cobblestone appearance. Unlike adult PAP, whole lung, large volume lavage is usually only of transient benefit, and the prognosis is very poor. As knowledge of surfactant physiology and genetics increases, it is likely that many of these children will be found to have inherited surfactant protein disorders.

THORACIC TUMORS

Primary and secondary tumors within the thorax are very rare;[461] even within a tertiary practice, thoracic malignancy is usually diagnosed only once or twice a year. Possible presentations include airway compression and stridor; chest wall invasion with either or both of pleuritic chest pain and pleural effusion; systemic symptoms such as fever, malaise and weight loss; or, in the case of a primary tumor, with the effects of secondary systemic disease. The rarity of tumors leads to the very great danger that the possibility is not even considered. Although measurement of catecholamine metabolites, alpha-fetoprotein or beta human gonadotrophin in serum may reveal the diagnosis, surgical biopsy is usually needed. Treatment of all such lesions is the province of the pediatric oncologist.

Benign tumors

These include true benign lesions such as pulmonary hamartomas, and pseudotumors, for example plasma cell granuloma. Carcinoid tumors present as an endobronchial mass which may bleed profusely if biopsied. Some behave as true malignancies.

Primary malignant lung tumors

Less than 2% of childhood cancers are lung primaries. Endobronchial cancer should at least be considered as a possibility in an otherwise unexplained bronchial obstruction. The intrathoracic sarcomas enter the differential diagnosis of large mass lesions within the chest. Whether intrathoracic lymphoma is a true primary pulmonary malignancy is a matter of semantics; suffice it to say that T-cell lymphoma may present as a rapidly progressive upper airway obstruction. Emergency control of the airway may be necessary to prevent asphyxia.

Metastatic tumors

These usually present in the context of a known primary tumor, most commonly osteo- or other sarcoma, Wilms tumor, germ cell tumors, neuroblastoma or hepatoblastoma. Presentation as pulmonary vascular disease is discussed above. Occasionally metastatic disease is found de novo as multiple round lesions on CXR; the differential diagnosis includes multiple lung abscesses and hydatid disease. Occasionally, pulmonary metastases may be cured surgically; specialist advice should always be sought before recommending such a course.

Mediastinal tumors.

These may be benign or malignant, and there is an extensive differential diagnosis. Presentation is with compression of the central airways leading to stridor; compression of the superior caval vein; and as the chance finding of mediastinal widening on the CXR. Although clues as to the likely histology may be obtained from CT and MRI, most lesions will need a surgical biopsy to establish the exact diagnosis.

REFERENCES (* Level 1 evidence)

1 Strachan DP. Hay fever, hygiene and household size. BMJ 1989; 299:1259–1260.

2 Seaton A, Godden DJ, Brown K. Increase in asthma: a more toxic environment or a more susceptible population? Thorax 1994; 49: 171–174.

3 Fogarty A, Britton J. The role of diet in the etiology of asthma. Clin Exp Allergy 2000; 30:615–627.

4 Helms PJ. Corticosteroid-sparing options in the treatment of childhood asthma. Drugs 2000; 59(suppl 1):15–22.

5 Custovic A, Simpson A, Chapman MD, Woodcock A. Allergen avoidance in the treatment of asthma and atopic disorders. Thorax 1998; 53:63–72.

*6 Gotzsche PC, Hammarquist C, Burr M. House dust mite control measures in the management of asthma: meta-analysis. BMJ 1998; 317:1105–1110.

7 Lau S, Illi S, Sommerfeld C, et al. Early exposure to house-dust mite and cat allergens and development of childhood asthma: a cohort study. Multicentre Allergy Study Group. Lancet 2000; 356:1392–1397.

8 Burrows B, Martinez FD, Cline MG, Lebowitz MD. The relationship between parental and children's serum IgE and asthma. Am J Respir Crit Care Med 1995; 152:1497–1500.

9 Britton JR. Effect of social class, sex and region of residence on age at death from cystic fibrosis. BMJ 1989; 298:483–487.

10 Eiser C, Morse RA. Review of measures of quality of life for children with chronic illness. Arch Dis Child 2001; 84:205–211.

11 Reichenber K, Broberg AG. The Pediatric Asthma Caregiver's Quality of Life Questionnaire in Swedish parents. Acta Pediatr 2001; 90:45–50.

12 Harding R, Cock ML, Louey S, et al. The compromised intrauterine environment: implications for future lung health. Clin Exp Pharmacol Physiol 2000; 27:965–974.

13 Barker D, Godfrey K, Fall C, et al. Relation of birth weight and childhood respiratory infection to adult lung function and death from chronic obstructive airways disease. BMJ 1991; 303:671–676.

14 Castro-Rodriguez J, Holberg C, Wright A, et al. Association of radiologically ascertained pneumonia before age 3 years with asthma like symptoms and pulmonary function during childhood: a prospective study. Am J Respir Crit Care Med 1999; 159:1891–1897.

15 Shaheen SO, Barker DJ, Holgate ST. Do lower respiratory tract infections in early childhood cause chronic obstructive pulmonary disease? Am J Respir Crit Care Med 1995; 151:1649–1651.

16 Anderson GG, Morrison JFJ. Molecular biology and genetics of allergy and asthma. Arch Dis Child 1998; 78:488–496.

17 Blouin JL, Meeks M, Radhakrishna U, et al. Primary ciliary dyskinesia: a genome-wide linkage analysis reveals extensive locus heterogeneity. Eur J Hum Genet 2000; 8:109–118.

18 Pasteur MC, Helliwell SM, Houghton SJ, et al. An investigation into causative factors in patients with bronchiectasis. Am J Resp Crit Care Med 2000; 162:1277–1284.

19 Cook DG, Strachan DP. Summary of effects of parental smoking on the respiratory health of children and implications for research. Thorax 1999; 54:357–366.

20 Martinez FD, Morgan WJ, Wright AL, et al. Diminished lung function as a predisposing factor for wheezing respiratory illness in infants. N Engl J Med 1988; 319:1112–1117.

21 Stick SM, Burton PR, Gurrin L, et al. Effects of maternal smoking during pregnancy and a family history of asthma on respiratory function in newborn infants. Lancet 1996; 348:1060–1064.

22 Dezateux C, Stocks J, Dundas I, Fletcher ME. Impaired airway function and wheezing in infancy: the influence of maternal smoking and a genetic predisposition to asthma Am J Respir Crit Care Med 1999; 159:403–410.

23 Gilliland FD, Li Y-F, Peters JM. Effects of maternal smoking during pregnancy and environmental tobacco smoke on asthma and wheezing in children. Am J Respir Crit Care Med 2001; 163:429–436.

24 Mitchell EA. Smoking: the next major and modifiable risk factor. In: Rognum TO, ed. Sudden infant death syndrome: new trends in the nineties. Oslo: Scandinavian University Press, 1995;114–118.

25 Fleming PJ, Blair P, Bacon C, et al. Environment of infants during sleep and risk of the sudden infant death syndrome: results of the 1993–95 case-control study for confidential enquiry into stillbirths and deaths in infancy. BMJ 1996; 313:191–198.

26 Withers NJ, Low JL, Holgate ST, Clough JB. Smoking habits of a cohort of UK adolescents. Resp Med 2000; 94:391–396.

27 World Health Organization. Integrated management of childhood illness. Bull World Health Organ 1997; v75:S1.

28 UNICEF. State of the world's children. Oxford: Oxford University Press; 2002.

29 Cohen S. Social status and susceptibility to respiratory infections. Ann N Y Acad Sci 1999; 896:246–253.

30 Mann SL, Wadsworth ME, Colley JR. Accumulation of factors influencing respiratory illness in members of a national birth cohort and their offspring. J Epidemiol Comm Health 1992; 46:286–292.

31 Rose AMC, Watson JM, Graham C, et al. Tuberculosis at the end of the 20th century in England and Wales: results of a national survey in 1998. Thorax 2001; 56:173–179.

32 Beckhurst C, Evans S, MacFarlane AF, Packe GE. Factors influencing the distribution of tuberculosis cases in an inner London borough. Commun Dis Public Health 2000; 3:28–31.

33 Bennett J, Pitman R, Jarman B, et al. A study of the variation in tuberculosis incidence and possible influential variables in Manchester, Liverpool, Birmingham and Cardiff in 1991–1995. Int J Tuberc Lung Dis 2001; 5:158–163.

34 von Ehrenstein OS, von Mutius E, Illi S, et al. Reduced risk of hay fever and asthma among children of farmers. Clin Exp Allergy 2000; 30:187–193.

35 Prescott SL, Macaubas C, Smallacombe T, et al. Development of allergen-specific T-cell memory in atopic and normal children. Lancet 1999; 353:196–200.

36 Shaheen SO, Aaby P, Hall AJ, et al. Measles and atopy in Guinea-Bissau. Lancet 1996; 347:1792–1796.

37 von Hertzen L, Klaukka T, Mattila H, et al. Mycobacterium tuberculosis infection and the subsequent development of asthma and allergic conditions. J Allergy Clin Immunol 1999; 104:1211–1214.

38 Jones CA, Kilburn SA, Warner JA, Warner JO. Intrauterine environment and fetal allergic sensitisation. Clin Exp Allergy 1998; 28:655–659.

39 Sigurs N. Epidemiologic and clinical evidence of a respiratory syncytial virus–reactive airway disease link. Am J Respir Crit Care Med 2001; 163:S2–S6.

40 Schwartz J. Role of polyunsaturated fats in lung disease Am J Clin Nutrition 2000; 71(suppl 1):393S–396S.

41 Cook D, Carey I, Whincup P, et al. Effect of fresh fruit consumption on lung function and wheeze in children. Thorax 1997; 52:628–633.

42 Moreno-Reyes R, Suetens C, Mathieu F, et al. Kashin-Beck osteoarthropathy in rural Tibet in relation to selenium and iodine status. N Engl J Med 1998; 339:1112–1120.

43 Sempertegui F, Estrella B, Camaniero V, et al. The beneficial effects of weekly low-dose vitamin A supplementation on acute lower respiratory infections and diarrhea in Ecuadorian children. Pediatrics 1999; 104:E1.

44 Fawzi WW, Mbise R, Spiegelman D, et al. Vitamin A supplements and diarrheal and respiratory tract infections among children in Dar es Salaam, Tanzania. J Pediatr 2000; 137:660–667.

45 Demissie K, Ernst P, Donald K, Joseph L. Usual dietary salt intake and asthma in children: a case-control study. Thorax 1996; 51:59–63.

46 Gouveia N, Fletcher T. Respiratory diseases in children and outdoor air pollution in Sao Paulo, Brazil: a time series analysis. Occup Environ Med 2000; 57:477–483.

47 Hajat S, Haines A, Goubet SA, et al. Association of air pollution with daily GP consultations for asthma and other lower respiratory conditions in London. Thorax 1999; 54:597–605.

48 von Mutius E, Fritzsch C, Weiland SK, et al. Prevalence of asthma and allergic disorders among children in united Germany: a descriptive comparison. BMJ 1992; 305: 1395–1399.

49 Wjst M, Reitmeir P, Dold S, et al. Road traffic and adverse effects on respiratory health in children. BMJ 1993; 307:596–600.

50 Bruce N, Perez-Padilla R, Albalak R. Indoor air pollution in developing countries: a major environmental and public health challenge. Bull World Health Organ 2000; 78:1078–1092.

51 Dekker C, Dales R, Bartlett S, et al. Childhood asthma and the indoor environment. Chest 1991; 100:922–926.

52 Burr ML, Anderson HR, Austin JB, et al. Respiratory symptoms and home environment in children: a national survey. Thorax 1999; 54:27–32.

53 Burrows B, Taussig LM. 'As the twig is bent, the tree inclines' (perhaps). Am Rev Respir Dis 1980; 122:813–816.

54 Cooney TP, Thurlbeck WM. The radial alveolar count method of Emery and Mithal: a

reappraisal. 1 – Postnatal lung growth. Thorax 1982; 37:572–579.
55 Hislop A, Muir DC, Jacobsen M, et al. Postnatal growth and function of the pre-acinar airways. Thorax 1972; 27:265–274.
56 Thurlbeck WM, Kida K, Langston C, et al. Postnatal lung growth after repair of diaphragmatic hernia. Thorax 1979; 34: 338–343.
57 Wigglesworth JS, Desai R, Guerrini P. Fetal lung hypoplasia: biochemical and structural variations and their possible significance. Arch Dis Child 1981; 56:606–615.
58 Helms P, Stocks J. Lung function in infants with congential pulmonary hypoplasia. J Pediatr 1982; 101:918–922.
59 Wigglesworth JS, Winston RML, Bartlett K. Influence of the central nervous system on fetal lung development. Arch Dis Child 1977; 52:965–967.
60 Falconer AR, Brown RA, Helms P, et al. Pulmonary sequelae in survivors of congenital diaphragmatic hernia. Thorax 1990; 45:126–129.
61 Taylor B, Wadsworth J. Maternal smoking during pregnancy and lower respiratory tract illness in early life. Arch Dis Child 1987; 62:786–791.
62 Hanrahan JP, Tager IB, Segal MR, et al. The effect of maternal smoking during pregnancy on early infant lung function. Am Rev Respir Dis 1992; 145:1129–1135.
63 Young S, Le Souef PN, Geelhoed GC, et al. The influence of a family history of asthma and parental smoking on airway responsiveness in early infancy, N Engl J Med 1991; [325:747]. 324:1168–1173.
64 Collins MH, Moessinger AC, Kleinerman J, et al. Fetal lung hypoplasia associated with maternal smoking: a morphometric analysis. Pediatr Res 1985; 19:408–412.
65 Vidic B, Ujevic N, Shabahang MM, van de Zande F. Differentiation of interstitial cells and stromal proteins in the secondary septum of early postnatal rat: effect of maternal chronic exposure to whole cigarette smoke. Anat Rec 1989; 223:165–173.
66 Thurlbeck WM. Postnatal lung growth. Thorax 1982; 37:564–571.
67 Polgar G, Weng TR. The functional development of the respiratory system. Am Rev Respir Dis 1979; 120:625–695.
68 Quanjer PH, Helms P, Bjure J, Gaultier C. Standardization of lung function tests in pediatrics. Eur Respir J 1989; 2.
69 Openshaw P, Edwards S, Helms P. Changes in rib cage geometry during childhood. Thorax 1984; 39:624–627.
70 Proctor DF. Physiology of the upper airway. In: Fenn WO, Rahn H, eds. Respiration. Am Physiol Soc. Distributed by Williams & Wilkins, Baltimore; 1964.
71 Davies H, Kitchman R, Gordon I, Helms P. Regional ventilation in infancy. N Engl J Med 1985; 313:1626–1628.
72 West JB. Respiratory physiology – the essentials, 5th edn. Baltimore: Williams & Wilkins; 1995.
73 Stocks J, Sly PD, Tepper RS, Morgan WJ. Infant respiratory function listing. New York: Wiley Liss; 1996.
74 Nielsen KG, Bisgaard H. Discriminative capacity of bronchodilator response measured with three different lung function techniques in asthmatic and healthy children aged 2 to 5 years. Am J Respir Crit Care Med 2001; 164:554–559.
75 Wang XB, Dockery DW, Wypij D, et al. Pulmonary-function between 6 and 18 years of age. Pediatr Pulmonol 1993; 15:75–88.
76 Tsanakas JN, Primhak RA, Milner RD, et al. Unexpectedly high peak expiratory flow rates in normal Greek children. Eur J Pediatr 1983; 141:46–49.
77 Kovatch AL, Wald ER, Ledesma-Medina J, et al. Maxillary sinus radiographs in children with nonrespiratory complaints. Pediatrics 1984; 73:306–308.
78 Deanfield JE, Chrispin AR. The investigation of chest disease in children by high kilovoltage filtered beam radiography. Br J Radiol 1981; 54:856–860.
79 Cave APD, Adam E. Cystic adenomatoid malformation of the lung (Stocker type 111) found on antenatal ultrasound examination. Br J Radiol 1984; 57:176–178.
80 Cartier Y, Kavanagh PV, Johkoh T, et al. Bronchiectasis: accuracy of high-resolution CT in the differentiation of specific diseases. AJR 1999; 173(1):47–52.
81 Siegel MJ, Bhalla S, Gutierrez FR, et al. Post-lung transplantation bronchiolitis obliterans syndrome: usefulness of expiratory thin-section CT for diagnosis. Radiology 2001; 220:455–462.
82 Wood RE, Fink RJ. Applications of flexible fiberoptic bronchoscopes in infants and children. Chest 1978; 73(5 suppl):737–740.
83 Nussbaum E, Zagnoev M. Pediatric fiberoptic bronchoscopy with a laryngeal mask airway. Chest 2001; 120:614–616.
84 Green CG, Eisenberg J, Leong A, et al. Flexible endoscopy of the pediatric airway. Am Rev Respir Dis 1992; 45:233–235.
85 Whitehead B, Scott JP, Helms P, et al. Technique and use of transbronchial biopsy in children and adolescents. Pediatr Pulmonol 1992; 12:240–246.
86 British Thoracic Society. Guidelines on diagnostic flexible bronchoscopy. Thorax 2001; 56(suppl 1):11–21.
87 Barbato A, Magarotto M, Crivellaro M, et al. Use of the pediatric bronchoscope, flexible and rigid, in 51 European centres. Eur Respir J 1997; 10(8):1761–1766.
88 de Blic J, Azevedo I, Burren CP, et al. The value of flexible bronchoscopy in childhood pulmonary tuberculosis. Chest 1991; 100:688–692.
89 European Respiratory Society Task Force on bronchoalveolar lavage in children. Bronchoalveolar lavage in children. Eur Respir J 2000; 15:217–231.
90 Filler RM, Forte V, Chait P. Tracheobronchial stenting for the treatment of airway obstruction. J Pediatr Surg 1998; 33:304–311.
91 Nicolai T, Huber RM, Reiter K, et al. Metal airway stent implantation in children: follow-up of seven children. Pediatr Pulmonol 2001; 31:289–296.
92 Wood RE, Postma D. Endoscopy of the airway in infants and children. J Pediatr 1988; 112:1–6.
93 Barbato A, Novello A Jr, Tormena F, et al. Use of fiberoptic bronchoscopy in asthmatic children with lung collapse. Pediatr Med Chir 1995; 17(3):253–255.
94 Brownlee KG, Crabbe DC. Pediatric bronchoscopy. Arch Dis Child 1997; 77(3): 272–275.
95 Zalzal GH. Stridor and airway compromise. Pediatr Clin North Am 1989; 36:1389–1402.
96 Orlow SJ, Isakoff MS, Blei F. Increased risk of symptomatic hemangiomas of the airway in association with cutaneous hemangiomas in a 'beard' distribution. J Pediatr 1997; 131:643–646.
97 Wood RE. Spelunking in the pediatric airway: explorations with the flexible fiberoptic bronchoscope. Pediatr Clin North Am 1984; 31:785–799.
98 Mahut B, Delacourt C, Scheinmann P, et al. Pulmonary alveolar proteinosis: experience with eight pediatric cases and a review. Pediatrics 1996; 97:117–122.
99 Kurland G, Noyes BE, Jaffe R, et al. Bronchoalveolar lavage and transbronchial biopsy in children following heart–lung and lung transplantation. Chest 1993; 104:1043–1048.
100 Colombo JL, Hallberg TK. Pulmonary aspiration and lipid-laden macrophages: in search of gold (standards). Pediatr Pulmonol 1999; 28:79–82.
101 de Blic J, Delacourt C, Scheinmann P. Ultrathin flexible bronchoscopy in neonatal intensive care units. Arch Dis Child 1991; 66:1383–1385.
102 Fleming P, Bacon C, Blair P, Berry J, eds. Sudden unexpected deaths in infancy. The CESDI SUDI studies. London: The Stationery Office; 2000.
103 Mitchell EA, Thompson JM. Parental reported apnea, admissions to hospital and sudden infant death syndrome. Acta Pediatr 2001; 90:417–422.
104 Guilleminault C, Pelayo R, Leger D, et al. Sleep-disordered breathing and upper airway abnormalities in first degree relatives of ALTE children. Pediatr Res 2001; 50:14–22.
105 Jeffrey HE, Pag M, Post EJ, Wood AKW. Physiological studies of gastroesophageal reflux and airway protective responses in the young animal and human infant. Clin Exp Pharmacol Physiol 1995; 22:544–549.
106 Arad-Cohen N, Cohen A, Tirosh E. The relationship between gastroesophageal reflux and apnea in infants. J Pediatr 2000; 137:321–326.
107 Hewertson J, Poets CF, Samuels MP, et al. Epileptic seizure-induced hypoxemia in infants with apparent life-threatening events. Pediatrics 1994; 94:148–156.
108 Southall DP, Samuels MP, Talbert DG. Recurrent cyanotic episodes with severe arterial hypoxemia and intrapulmonary shunting: a mechanism for sudden infant death. Arch Dis Child 1990; 65:953–961.
109 Fleming PJ, Levine MR, Azaz Y, Wigfield R. The development of thermoregulation and interactions with the control of respiration in infants: possible relationship to sudden infant death. Acta Pediatr Scand 1993; 389(suppl): 57–59.

110 Wigfield RE, Fleming PJ, Azaz Y, et al. How much wrapping do babies need at night? Arch Dis Child 1993; 69:181–186.
111 Kahn A, Groswasser J, Kelmanson I. Risk factors for SIDS: risk factors for ALTE? From epidemiology to physiology. In: Rognum TO, ed. Sudden infant death syndrome. New trends in the nineties. Oslo: Scandinavian University Press, 1995:132–137.
112 Southall DP, Plunket MCB, Banks MW, et al. Covert video recordings of life-threatening child abuse: lessons for child protection. Pediatrics 1997; 100:735–760.
113 Meadow R. Unnatural sudden infant death. Arch Dis Child 1999; 80:7–14.
114 Royal College of Paediatrics and Child Health. The fabricated or induced illness report. London: RCPCH; 2001.
115 Department of Health. Safeguarding children in whom illness is induced or fabricated by carers with parenting responsibilities. www.doh.gov.uk/qualityprotects/info/publications/childprot.htm; 2001.
116 Gray C, Davies F, Molyneux E. Apparent life-threatening events presenting to a pediatric emergency department. Pediatr Emerg Care 1999; 15:195–199.
117 Kahn A, Rhuffat E, Franco P, et al. Apparent life-threatening events and apnea of infancy In: Beckerman RC, Brouillette RT, Hunt CE, eds. Respiratory control disorders in infants and children. Baltimore: Williams & Wilkins, 1992:178–189.
118 Oren J, Kelly DH, Shannon DC. Identification of a high-risk group for sudden infant death syndrome among infants who were resuscitated for sleep apnea. Pediatrics 1986; 77:495–499.
119 Keens TG, Ward SL. Apnea spells, sudden deaths and the role of the apnea monitor. Pediatr Clin North Am 1993; 40:897–911.
120 Gaultier C, Praud JP, Canet E, et al. Paradoxical inward rib cage motion during rapid eye movement sleep in infants and young children. J Dev Physiol 1987; 9:391–397.
121 Marcus CL, Glomb WB, Basinski DJ, et al. Developmental patterns of hypercapnic and hypoxic ventilatory drive from childhood to adulthood. J Appl Physiol 1994; 76:314–320.
122 Hunt CE, Hufford DR, Bourguignon C, Oess MA. Home documented monitoring of cardiorespiratory patterns and oxygen saturation in healthy infants. Pediatr Res 1996; 39:216–222.
123 Keens TG, Hoppenbrouwers T. Congenital hypoventilation syndrome. In: Diagnostic Steering Committee of the American Sleep Disorders Association. The international classification of sleep disorders: diagnostic and coding manual. Lawrence, Kansas: Allen Press; 1990:205–209.
124 Marcus CL, Bautista DB, Amihyia A, et al. Hypercapneic arousal responses in children with congenital central hypoventilation syndrome. Pediatrics 1991; 88:993–998.
125 Paton JY, Swaminathan S, Sargent CW, Keens TG. Hypoxic and hypercapnic ventilatory responses in awake children with congenital central hypoventilation syndrome. Am Rev Respir Dis 1989; 140:368–372.
126 Harper RM, Kinney HC, Fleming PJ, Thach B. Sleep influences on homeostatic functions: implications for sudden infant death syndrome. Respir Physiol 2000; 119:123–132.
127 Weese Mayer DE, Silvestri JM, Huffman AD, et al. Case-control family study of autonomic nervous system dysfunction in idiopathic congenital central hypoventilation syndrome. Am J Med Genet 2001; 100:237–245.
128 Keens TG, Ward SL. Syndromes affecting respiratory control during sleep. In: Loughlin GM, Carroll JL, Marcus CL (eds). Sleep and breathing in children: a developmental approach. New York: Marcel Dekker; 2000.
129 Sakai T, Wakizaka A, Matsuda H, et al. Point mutation in exon 12 of the receptor tyrosine kinase proto-oncogene RET in Ondine-Hirschsprung syndrome. Pediatrics 1998; 101:924–926.
130 American Thoracic Society. Idiopathic congenital central hypoventilation syndrome: diagnosis and management. Am J Respir Crit Care Med 1999; 160:368–373.
131 Weese Mayer DE, Silvestri JM, Kenny AS, et al. Diaphragm pacing with a quadripolar phrenic nerve electrode: an international study. Pacing Clin Electrophysiol 1996; 19:1311–1319.
132 Fodstad H. Phrenicodiaphragmatic pacing. In: Roussos C (ed). The thorax. New York: Marcel Dekker; 1995.
133 Weese Mayer DE, Silvestri JM, Menzies LJ, et al. Congenital central hypoventilation syndrome: diagnosis, management and long-term outcome in thirty-two children. J Pediatr 1992; 120:381–387.
134 Bar A, Taraisuk A, Segev Y, et al. The effect of adenotonsillectomy on serum insulin-like growth factor-I and growth in children with obstructive sleep apnea syndrome. J Pediatr 1999; 135:76–80.
135 Tal A, Leiberman A, Margulis G, Sofer S. Ventricular dysfunction in children with obstructive sleep apnea: radionuclide assessment. Pediatr Pulmonol 1988; 4:139–143.
136 American Thoracic Society. Standards and indications for cardiopulmonary sleep studies in children. Am J Respir Crit Care Medir 1996; 153:866–878.
137 Marcus CL. Sleep-disordered breathing in children. State of the art. Am J Respir Crit Care Med 2001; 164:16–30.
138 Marcus CL, Ward SL, Mallory GB, et al. Use of nasal continuous positive airway pressure as treatment of childhood obstructive sleep apnea. J Pediatr 1995; 127:88–94.
139 Guilleminault C, Partinen M, Praud JP, et al. Morphometric facial changes and obstructive sleep apnea in adolescents. J Pediatr 1989; 11:997–999.
140 Silverman M, Wilson N. Asthma – time for a change in name? Arch Dis Child 1997; 77:62–64.
141 Martinez FD, Morgan WJ, Wright AL, et al. Initial airway function is a risk factor for recurrent wheezing respiratory illnesses during the first three years of life. Group Health Medical Associates. Am Rev Respir Dis 1991; 143:312–316.
142 Bisgaard H. Persistent wheezing in very young preschool children reflects lower respiratory inflammation. Am J Respir Crit Care Med 2001; 163:1290–1291.
143 Stevenson EC, Turner G, Heaney LG, et al. Bronchoalveolar lavage findings suggest two different forms of childhood asthma. Clin Exp Allergy 1997; 27:1027–1035.
144 Dold S, Wjst M, von Mutius E, et al. Genetic risk for asthma, allergic rhinitis, and atopic dermatitis. Arch Dis Child 1992; 67:1018–1022.
145 Wjst M, Immervoll T. An Internet linkage and mutation database for the complex phenotype asthma. Bioinformatics 1998; 14:827–828.
146 Immervoll T, Loesgen S, Dutsch G, et al. Fine mapping and single nucleotide polymorphism association results of candidate genes for asthma and related phenotypes. Hum Mutat 2001; 18:327–336.
147 Postma DS, Bleecker ER, Amelung PJ, et al. Genetic susceptibility to asthma. Bronchial hyperresponsiveness coinherited with a major gene for atopy. N Engl J Med 1995; 333:894–900.
148 Doull IJM, Lawrence S, Watson M, et al. Allelic association of gene markers on chromosomes 5q and 11q with atopy and bronchial hyperresponsiveness. Am J Respir Crit Care Med 1996; 153:1280–1284.
149 Weiss ST. Association studies in asthma genetics. Am J Respir Crit Care Med 2001; 164:2014–2015.
150 Drazen JM, Silverman EK, Lee TH. Heterogeneity of therapeutic responses in asthma. Br Med Bull 2000; 56:1054–1070.
151 Szepfalusi Z, Loibichler C, Pichler J, et al. Direct evidence for transplacental allergen transfer. Pediatr Res 2000; 48:404–407.
152 Zeiger RS, Heller S. The development and prediction of atopy in high-risk children: follow-up at age seven years in a prospective randomized study of combined maternal and infant food allergen avoidance. J Allergy Clin Immunol 1995; 95:1179–1190.
153 Rusconi F, Galassi C, Corbo GM, et al. Risk factors for early, persistent, and late-onset wheezing in young children. SIDRIA Collaborative Group. Am J Respir Crit Care Med 1999; 160:1617–1622.
154 Prescott SL, Macaubas C, Holt BJ, et al. Transplacental priming of the human immune system to environmental allergens: universal skewing of initial T cell responses toward the Th2 cytokine profile. J Immunol 1998; 160:4730–4737.
155 Strachan DP. Family size, infection and atopy: the first decade of the 'hygiene hypothesis'. Thorax 2000; 55(suppl 1):S2–10.
156 Stein RT, Sherrill D, Morgan WJ, et al. Respiratory syncytial virus in early life and risk of wheeze and allergy by age 13 years. Lancet 1999; 354:541–545.
157 Sporik R, Chapman MD, Platts-Mills TA. House dust mite exposure as a cause of asthma. Clin Exp Allergy 1992; 22:897–906.
158 Woodcock A, Custovic A. Allergen avoidance: does it work? Br Med Bull 2000; 56:1071–1086.
159 Hesselmar B, Aberg N, Aberg B, et al. Does early exposure to cat or dog protect against later allergy development? Clin Exp Allergy 1999; 29:611–617.
160 Lewis SA. Animals and allergy. Clin Exp Allergy 2000; 30:153–157.
161 Wickens K, Pearce N, Crane J, Beasley R. Antibiotic use in early childhood and the

development of asthma. Clin Exp Allergy 1999; 29:766–771.
162 Anderson HR, Butland BK, Strachan DP. Trends in prevalence and severity of childhood asthma. BMJ 1994; 308:1600–1604.
163 Ng MK, Proctor A, Billings C, et al. Increasing prevalence of asthma diagnosis and symptoms in children is confined to mild symptoms. Thorax 2001; 56:312–314.
164 Downs SH, Marks GB, Sporik R, et al. Continued increase in the prevalence of asthma and atopy. Arch Dis Child 2001; 84:20–23.
165 Asher MI, Keil U, Anderson HR, et al. International Study of Asthma and Allergies in Childhood (ISAAC): rationale and methods. Eur Respir J 1995; 8:483–491.
166 Peat JK, Toelle BG, Marks GB, Mellis CM. Continuing the debate about measuring asthma in population studies. Thorax 2001; 56:406–411.
167 Santanello NC, Davies G, Galant SP, et al. Validation of an asthma symptom diary for interventional studies. Arch Dis Child 1999; 80:414–420.
168 Cane RS, Ranganathan SC, McKenzie SA. What do parents of wheezy children understand by 'wheeze'? Arch Dis Child 2000; 82:327–332.
169 Christie GL, Helms PJ, Godden DJ, et al. Asthma, wheezy bronchitis, and atopy across two generations. Am J Respir Crit Care Med 1999; 159:125–129.
170 Godfrey S. Bronchial hyperresponsiveness in children. Pediatr Respir Rev 2000; 1:148–155.
171 Godfrey S, Springer C, Bar-Yishay E, Avital A. Cut-off points defining normal and asthmatic bronchial reactivity to exercise and inhalation challenges in children and young adults. Eur Respir J 1999; 14:659–668.
172 National Asthma Education and Prevention Program. National Institutes of Health clinical practice guidelines for the diagnosis and management of asthma 2, 15–17. Bethesda: NIH; 1997.
173 Dales RE, Spitzer WO, Tousignant P, et al. Clinical interpretation of airway response to a bronchodilator. Epidemiologic considerations. Am Rev Respir Dis 1988; 138: 317–320.
174 Ranganathan SC, Payne DN, Jaffe A, McKenzie SA. Difficult asthma: defining the problems. Pediatr Pulmonol 2001; 31:114–120.
175 American Thoracic Society. Guidelines for standardized procedures for the online and offline measurement of exhaled lower respiratory nitric oxide in adults and children. Am J Respir Crit Care Med 1999; 160:2117.
176 Martinez FD. Viruses and atopic sensitization in the first years of life. Am J Respir Crit Care Med 2000; 162: S95–S99.
177 Fuller P, Picciotto A, Davies M, McKenzie SA. Cough and sleep in inner-city children. Eur Respir J 1998; 12:426–431.
178 Wright AL, Holberg CJ, Morgan WJ, et al. Recurrent cough in childhood and its relation to asthma. Am J Respir Crit Care Med 1996; 153:1259–1265.
179* Davies MJ, Fuller P, Picciotto A, McKenzie SA. Persistent nocturnal cough: randomized controlled trial of high dose inhaled corticosteroid. Arch Dis Child 1999; 81:38–44.
180 Chang AB, Phelan PD, Carlin JB, et al. A randomized, placebo controlled trial of inhaled salbutamol and beclomethasone for recurrent cough. Arch Dis Child 1998; 79:6–11.
181 von Mutius E, Schwartz J, Neas LM, et al. Relation of body mass index to asthma and atopy in children: the National Health and Nutrition Examination Study III. Thorax 2001; 56:835–838.
182 Martinez FD, Wright AL, Taussig LM, et al. Asthma and wheezing in the first six years of life. The Group Health Medical Associates. N Engl J Med 1995; 332:133–138.
183 Elphick HE, Sherlock P, Foxall G, et al. Survey of respiratory sounds in infants. Arch Dis Child 2001; 84:35–39.
184 McKenzie SA, Bridge PD, Pao CS. Lung function tests for preschool children. Pediatr Respir Rev 2001; 2:37–45.
185 Sly PD, Flack F. Is home monitoring of lung function worthwhile for children with asthma? Thorax 2001; 56:164–165.
186 Strachan DP. Repeatability of ventilatory function measurements in a population survey of 7 year old children. Thorax 1989; 44:474–479.
187 Eaton T, Withy S, Garrett JE, et al. Spirometry in primary care practice: the importance of quality assurance and the impact of spirometry workshops. Chest 1999; 116:416–423.
188 Gibson NA, Ferguson E, Aitchison TC, Paton JY. Compliance with inhaled asthma medication in preschool children. Thorax 1995; 50:1274–1279.
189 Jonasson G, Carlsen KH, Mowinckel P. Asthma drug adherence in a long term clinical trial. Arch Dis Child 2000; 83:330–333.
190 Crim C. Clinical practice guidelines vs actual clinical practice : the asthma paradigm. Chest 2000; 118:62S–64S.
*191 McKean M, Ducharme F. Inhaled steroids for episodic viral wheeze of childhood. Cochrane Database Syst Rev 2000; CD001107.
192 Majeed A, Moser K. Prescribing for patients with asthma by general practitioners in England and Wales 1994–96. Health Stat Q 1999; 1:16–20.
*193 British Thoracic Society, Scottish Intercollegiate Guideline Network (SIGN). British guideline on the management of asthma. Thorax 2003; 58(suppl 1):1–94.
*194 Haby MM, Waters E, Robertson CF, et al. Interventions for educating children who have attended the emergency room for asthma. Cochrane Database Syst Rev 2001; 1:CD001290.
195 Peat JK, Dickerson J, Li J. Effects of damp and mould in the home on respiratory health: a review of the literature. Allergy 1998; 53:120–128.
*196 Shrewsbury S, Pyke S, Britton M. Meta-analysis of increased dose of inhaled steroid or addition of salmeterol in symptomatic asthma (MIASMA). BMJ 2000; 320:1368–1373.
*197 Tasche MJ, Uijen JH, Bernsen RM, et al. Inhaled disodium cromoglycate (DSCG) as maintenance therapy in children with asthma: a systematic review. Thorax 2000; 55:913–920.
198 Childhood Asthma Management Program Research Group. Long-term effects of budesonide or nedocromil in children with asthma. N Engl J Med 2000; 343:1054–1063.
*199 Qureshi F, Pestian J, Davis P, Zaritsky A. Effect of nebulized ipratropium on the hospitalization rates of children with asthma. N Engl J Med 1998; 339:1030–1035.
200 Nielsen KG, Bisgaard H. The effect of inhaled budesonide on symptoms, lung function, and cold air and methacholine responsiveness in 2 to 5 year old asthmatic children. Am J Respir Crit Care Med 2000; 162:1500–1506.
201 Pao CS, McKenzie SA. Randomized controlled trial of fluticasone in preschool children with intermittent wheeze. Am J Respir Crit Care Med 2002; 166(7):945–949.
*202 Sharek PJ, Bergman DA. Beclomethasone for asthma in children: effects on linear growth. Cochrane Database Syst Rev 2000; CD001282.
*203 Holt S, Suder A, Weatherall M, et al. Dose-response relation of inhaled fluticasone propionate in adolescents and adults with asthma: meta-analysis. BMJ 2001; 323:253.
204 Harrison TW, Wisniewski A, Honour J, Tattersfield E. Comparison of the systemic effects of fluticasone propionate and budesonide given by dry powder inhaler in healthy and asthmatic subjects. Thorax 2001; 56:186–191.
205 Warner JO. The role of leukotriene receptor antagonists in the treatment of chronic asthma in childhood. Allergy 2001; 56:22–29.
206 Milgrom H, Berger W, Nayak A, et al. Treatment of childhood asthma with anti-immunoglobulin E antibody (omalizumab). Pediatrics 2001; 108:E36.
207 Payne N, Beard S, Brocklebank D, et al. Clinical and cost effectiveness of inhaler devices for children with chronic asthma. The National Institute for Clinical Excellence, editor 1–49 NHS R&D HTA Program. London: NICE; 2000.
*208 Cates CJ. Comparison of holding chambers and nebulisers for beta-agonists in acute asthma. 1. Oxford. Airways Module of The Cochrane Database of Systematic Reviews; 2000.
209 McKenzie SA. Sudden death in asthma. Arch Dis Child 1989; 64:1450–1451.
210 Keeley D, Osman L. Dysfunctional breathing and asthma. It is important to tell the difference. BMJ 2001; 322:1075–1076.
211 Balfour-Lynn I. Difficult asthma: beyond the guidelines. Arch Dis Child 1999; 80:201–206.
212 Coren ME, Rosenthal M, Bush A. The use of cyclosporin in corticosteroid dependent asthma. Arch Dis Child 1997; 77:522–523.
213 Hampton FJ, McFadyen UM, Beardsmore CS, Simpson H. Gastroesophageal reflux and respiratory function in infants with respiratory disease. Arch Dis Child 1991; 66:848–853.
*214 Gibson PG, Henry RL, Coughlan JL. Gastro-esophageal reflux treatment for asthma in adults and children (Cochrane Review). In: The Cochrane Library, Issue 4, 2001. Oxford: Update Software.
215 Hilliard TN, Witten H, Male IA, et al. Management of acute childhood asthma: a prospective multicentre study. Eur Respir J 2000; 15:1102–1105.
216 Leone FT, Mauger EA, Peters SP, et al. The utility of peak flow, symptom scores, and beta agonist use as outcome measures in asthma clinical research. Chest 2001; 119:1027–1033.

217 Madge P, McColl J, Paton J. Impact of a nurse-led home management training program in children admitted to hospital with acute asthma: a randomized controlled study. Thorax 1997; 52:223–228.
218 Deshpande A, McKenzie SA. Short course of steroids in home treatment of children with acute asthma. Br Med J 1986; 293:169–171.
219 Male I, Richter H, Seddon P. Children's perception of breathlessness in acute asthma. Arch Dis Child 2000; 83:325–329.
220 Kerem E, Canny G, Tibshirani R, et al. Clinical–physiologic correlations in acute asthma of childhood. Pediatrics 1991; 87:481–486.
221 McKenzie SA, Edmunds AT, Godfrey S. Status asthmaticus: a one year study. Arch Dis Child 1979; 54:486.
222 Inwald D, Roland M, Kuitert L, et al. Oxygen treatment for acute severe asthma. BMJ 2001; 323:98–100.
*223 Cates CJ, Adams N, Bestall J. 2002; Holding chambers versus nebulisers for inhaled steroids in chronic asthma. Cochrane Database Syst Rev 2001; 2:CD001491.
224 British Thoracic Society. British guidelines on asthma management. 1995 Review and Position Statement. Thorax 1997; 52: S21.
225 Rubilar L, Castro-Rodriguez JA, Girardi G. Randomized trial of salbutamol via metered-dose inhaler with spacer versus nebulizer for acute wheezing in children less than 2 years of age. Pediatr Pulmonol 2000; 29:264–269.
226 Plotnick LH, Ducharme FM. Should inhaled anticholinergics be added to beta2 agonists for treating acute childhood and adolescent asthma? A systematic review. BMJ 1998; 317:971–977.
227 Yung M, South M. Randomized controlled trial of aminophylline for severe acute asthma. Arch Dis Child 1998; 79:405–410.
228 Browne GJ, Penna AS, Phung X, Soo M. Randomized trial of intravenous salbutamol in early management of acute severe asthma in children. Lancet 1997; 349:301–305.
229* Rowe BH, Bretzlaff JA, Bourdon C, et al. Intravenous magnesium sulfate treatment for acute asthma in the emergency department: a systematic review of the literature. Ann Emerg Med 2000; 36:181–190.
230 Stack AM, Caputo GL. Pneumomediastinum in childhood asthma. Pediatr Emerg Care 1996; 12:98–101.
231 Fitz Simmons SC. The changing epidemiology of cystic fibrosis. J Pediatr 1993; 122:1–9.
232 Elborn JS, Shale DJ, Britton JR. Cystic fibrosis: current survival and population estimates to the year 2000. Thorax 1991; 46:881–885.
233 Lewis P, Morison S, Dodge J, et al. Survival estimates for adults with cystic fibrosis born in the United Kingdom between 1947 and 1967. Thorax 1999; 54:420–422.
234 Pilewski J, Frizzell R. Role of CFTR in airway disease. Physiol Rev 1999; 79: S215–S255.
235 Welsh M, Smith A. Molecular mechanisms of CFTR chloride channel dysfunction in cystic fibrosis. Cell 1993; 73:1251–1254.
236 Hubert D, Bienvenu T, Desmazes-Dufeu N, et al. Genotype phenotype relationships in a cohort of adult cystic fibrosis patients. Eur Respir J 1996; 9:2207.
237 Stern R, Doershuk C, Drumm M. 3849+10 kb C to T mutation and disease severity in cystic fibrosis. Lancet 1995; 346:274–276.
238 Cystic Fibrosis Genotypesolidus Phenotype Consortium. Correlation between genotype and phenotype in patients with cystic fibrosis. N Engl J Med 1993; 329:1308–1313.
239 Corey M, Edwards L, Levison H, Knowles M. Longitudinal analysis of pulmonary function decline in patients with cystic fibrosis. J Pediatr 1997; 131:809–814.
240 Garred P, Pressler T, Madsen H, et al. Association of mannose-binding lectin gene heterogeneity with severity of lung disease and survival in cystic fibrosis. J Clin Invest 1999; 104:431–437.
241 Di Sant'Agnese P, Darling R, Perera G, Shea E. Abnormal electrolyte composition of sweat in cystic fibrosis of the pancreas. Pediatrics 1953; 12:549–563.
242 Quinton P. The neglected ion: HCO_3^-. Nat Med 2001; 7:292–293.
243 Smith J, Travis S, Greenberg E, Welsh M. Cystic fibrosis airway epithelia fail to kill bacteria because of abnormal airway surface fluid. Cell 1996; 85:229–236.
244 Armstrong DS, Grimwood K, Carzino R, et al. Lower respiratory infection and inflammation in infants with newly diagnosed cystic fibrosis. BMJ 1995; 310:1571–1572.
245 Khan TZ, Wagener JS, Bost T, et al. Early pulmonary inflammation in infants with cystic fibrosis. Am J Respir Crit Care Med 1995; 151:1075–1082.
246 Balough K, McCubbin M, Weinberger M, et al. The relationship between infection and inflammation in the early stages of lung disease from cystic fibrosis. Pediatr Pulmonol 1995; 20:63–70.
247 Smyth RL, Croft N, O'Hea U, et al. Intestinal inflammation in cystic fibrosis. Arch Dis Child 2000; 82:394–399.
248 Bonfield T, Konstan MW, Burfeind J, et al. Normal bronchial epithelial cells constitutively produce the anti-inflammatory cytokine interleukin 10, which is downregulated in cystic fibrosis. Am J Respir Cell Mol Biol 1995; 13:257–261.
249 Kirk J, Keston M, McIntosh I, Al Esia S. Variation of sweat sodium and chloride with age in cystic fibrosis and normal populations: further investigations in equivocal cases. Ann Clin Biochem 1992; 29:145–152.
250 Super M, Schwarz M, Malone G, et al. Active cascade testing for carriers of cystic fibrosis gene. BMJ 1994; 308:1462–1468.
251 Pollitt R. Screening for cystic fibrosis. Semin Neonatol 1998; 3:9–15.
252 Wald N, Morris J. Neonatal screening for cystic fibrosis. BMJ 1998; 316:404–405.
253 Anon. Neonatal screening for cystic fibrosis: position paper. Pediatrics 1983; 72:741.
254 Dankert-Roelse J, te Meerman G. Long term prognosis of patients with cystic fibrosis in relation to early detection by neonatal screening and treatment in a cystic fibrosis centre. Thorax 1995; 50:712–718.
255 Farrell P, Kosorok M, Laxova A, et al. Nutritional benefits of neonatal screening for cystic fibrosis. N Engl J Med 1997; 337:963–969.
*256 Merelle ME, Nagelkerke AF, Lees CM, Dezateux C. Newborn screening for cystic fibrosis (Cochrane Review). In: The Cochrane Library, Issue 3, 2001. Oxford: Update Software.
257 Miedzybrodzka Z, Hall M, Mollison J, et al. Antenatal screening for carriers of cystic fibrosis: randomized trial of stepwise v couple screening. BMJ 1995; 310:353–357.
258 NIH Consensus Development Statement. Genetic testing for cystic fibrosis. Bethesda: NIH; 1997.
259 Smyth RL, van Velzen D, Smyth AR, et al. Strictures of ascending colon in cystic fibrosis and high-strength pancreatic enzymes. Lancet 1994; 343:85–86.
260 Smyth RL, Ashby D, O'Hea U, et al. Fibrosing colonopathy in cystic fibrosis: results of a case-control study. Lancet 1995; 346:1247–1251.
261 Committee on Safety of Medicines MCA. Fibrosing colonpathy associated with pancreatic enzymes: dose-related strictures in children with cystic fibrosis. Curr Probl Pharmacovig 1995; 21:11.
262 Chrispin A, Norman A. The systematic evaluation of the chest radiograph in cystic fibrosis. Pediatr Radiol 1974; 2:101–106.
263 Brasfield D, Hicks G, Soong S, Tiller R. The chest roentgenogram in cystic fibrosis: a new scoring system. Pediatrics 1979; 63:24–29.
264 Conway S, Pond M, Bowler I, et al. The chest radiograph in cystic fibrosis: a new scoring system compared with the Chrispin-Norman and Brasfield scores. Thorax 1994; 49:860–862.
265 Kerem E, Reisman J, Corey M, et al. Prediction of mortality in patients with cystic fibrosis. N Engl J Med 1992; 326:1187–1191.
266 Scott-Jupp R, Lama M, Tanner M. Prevalence of liver disease in cystic fibrosis. Arch Dis Child 1991; 66:698–701.
267 Tanner M. Liver and biliary problems in cystic fibrosis. J R Soc Med 1992; 85:20–24.
268 Carty H. Abdominal radiology in cystic fibrosis. J R Soc Med 1995; 88:18–23.
269 O'Connor P, Southern K, Bowler I, et al. The role of hepatic scintigraphy in cystic fibrosis. Hepatology 1996; 23:281–287.
270 Lanng S, Hansen A, Thorsteinsson B, et al. Glucose tolerance in patients with cystic fibrosis: five year prospective study. BMJ 1995; 311:655–659.
271 Shwachmann H, Kulczycki L. Long-term study of one hundred and five patients with cystic fibrosis. Studies made over a five to fourteen year period. Am Med Assoc J Dis Child 1958; 96:6–15.
272 McCallum S, Corkhill J, Gallagher M, et al. Superinfection with a transmissible strain of Pseudomonas aeruginosa in adults with cystic fibrosis chronically colonized by P. aeruginosa. Lancet 2001; 358:558–560.
273 Geddes D. Of isolates and isolation: Pseudomonas aeruginosa in adults with cystic fibrosis. Lancet 2001; 358:522.
*274 Smyth A, Walters S. Prophylactic antibiotics for cystic fibrosis (Cochrane Review). In: The Cochrane Library, Issue 3, 2001. Oxford: Update Software.

275 Valerius N, Koch C, Hoiby N. Prevention of chronic Pseudomonas aeruginosa colonization in cystic fibrosis by early treatment. Lancet 1991; 338:725–726.
*276 Ryan G, Mukhopadhyay S, Singh M. Nebulized anti-pseudomonal antibiotics for cystic fibrosis (Cochrane Review). In: The Cochrane Library, Issue 3, 2001. Oxford: Update Software.
277 Whiteford M, Wilkinson J, McColl J, et al. Outcome of Burkholderia (Pseudomonas) cepacia colonization in children with cystic fibrosis following a hospital outbreak. Thorax 1995; 59:1194–1198.
278 Ledson M, Gallagher M, Corkhill J, et al. Cross infection between cystic fibrosis patients colonized with Burkholderia cepacia. Thorax 1998; 53:432–436.
279 Cheng K, Smyth RL, Govan JR, et al. Spread of beta lactam-resistant Pseudomonas aeruginosa in a cystic fibrosis clinic. Lancet 1996; 348:639–642.
*280 Elphick HE, Tan A. Single versus combination intravenous antibiotic therapy for people with cystic fibrosis (Cochrane Review). In: The Cochrane Library, Issue 3, 2001. Oxford: Update Software.
*281 Tan K, Bunn H. Once daily versus multiple daily dosing with intravenous aminoglycosides for cystic fibrosis (Cochrane Review). In: The Cochrane Library, Issue 3, 2001. Oxford: Update Software.
*282 Elphick HE, Southern KW. Antifungal therapies for allergic bronchopulmonary aspergillosis in people with cystic fibrosis (Cochrane Review). In: The Cochrane Library, Issue 3, 2001. Oxford: Update Software.
*283 van de Schans C, Prasad A, Main E. Chest physiotherapy compared to no chest physiotherapy for cystic fibrosis (Cochrane Review). In: The Cochrane Library, Issue 3, 2001. Oxford: Update Software.
*284 Thomas J, Cook D, Brooks D. Chest physical therapy management of patients with cystic fibrosis: a meta-analysis. Am J Respir Crit Care Med 1995; 151:846–850.
*285 Cheng K, Ashby D, Smyth RL. Oral steroids for cystic fibrosis (Cochrane Review). In: The Cochrane Library, Issue 3, 2001. Oxford: Update Software.
*286 Dezateux C, Walters S, Balfour-Lynn I. Inhaled corticosteroids for cystic fibrosis (Cochrane Review). In: The Cochrane Library, Issue 3, 2001. Oxford: Update Software.
*287 Dezateux C, Crighton A. Oral non-steroidal anti-inflammatory drug therapy for cystic fibrosis (Cochrane Review). In: The Cochrane Library, Issue 3, 2001. Oxford: Update Software.
*288 Fuchs H, Borowitz D, Christiansen D, et al. Effect of aerosolized recombinant human DNase on exacerbations of respiratory symptoms and on pulmonary function in patients with cystic fibrosis. N Engl J Med 1994; 331:637–642.
*289 Kearney CE, Wallis CE. Deoxyribonuclease for cystic fibrosis (Cochrane Review). In: The Cochrane Library, Issue 3, 2001. Oxford: Update Software.
*290 Wark PAB, McDonald V. Nebulized hypertonic saline for cystic fibrosis (Cochrane Review). In: The Cochrane Library, Issue 3, 2001. Oxford: Update Software.
291 Suri R, Metcalfe C, Lees B, et al. Comparison of hypertonic saline and alternative-day or daily recombinant human deoxyribonuclease in children with cystic fibrosis: a randomized trial. Lancet 2001; 358:1316–1321.
*292 Smyth RL, Walters S. Oral calorie supplements for cystic fibrosis (Cochrane Review). In: The Cochrane Library, Issue 3, 2001. Oxford: Update Software.
293 Boland M, Stocki D, McDonald N, et al. Chronic jejunostomy feeding with a non-elemental formula in undernourished cystic fibrosis patients. Lancet 1986; ii:232–234.
294 Rayner R, Tyrrell J, Hiller E, et al. Night blindness and conjunctival xerosis caused by vitamin A deficiency in patients with cystic fibrosis. Arch Dis Child 1989; 64:1151–1156.
295 Bennett M, Medwadowski B. Vitamin A, vitamin E and lipids in serum of children with cystic fibrosis or congenital heart defects compared with normal children. Am J Clin Nutr 1967; 20:415.
*296 Cheng K, Ashby D, Smyth RL. Ursodeoxycholic acid for cystic fibrosis-related liver disease (Cochrane Review) In: The Cochrane Library, Issue 3, 2001. Oxford: Update Software.
297 Madden B, Hodson M, Tsang V, et al. Intermediate results of heart lung transplantation for cystic fibrosis. Lancet 1992; 339:1583–1587.
298 Balfour-Lynn I, Martin I, Whitehead B, et al. Heart–lung transplantation for patients under 10 with cystic fibrosis. Arch Dis Child 1997; 76:38–40.
*299 Arroll B, Kenealy T. Antibiotics for the common cold (Cochrane Review). In: The Cochrane Library, Issue 3, 2001. Oxford: Update Software.
*300 Jefferson T, Tyrrell D. Antivirals for the common cold (Cochrane Review). In: The Cochrane Library, Issue 3, 2001. Oxford: Update Software.
301 Rudberg R. Acute otitis media: comparative therapeutic results of sulphonamide and penicillin administered in various forms. Acta Otolaryngol 1954; 113:71–79.
302 Burke P, Bain J, Robinson D. Acute red ear in children: controlled trial of non-antibiotic treatment in general practice. BMJ 1991; 303:558–562.
*303 Glasziou P, Del Mar C, Sanders S. Antibiotics for acute otitis media in children (Cochrane Review). In: The Cochrane Library, Issue 3, 2001. Oxford: Update Software.
*304 Kozyrskyj A, Hildes-Ripstein G, Longstaffe S, et al. Short course antibiotics for acute otitis media (Cochrane Review). In: The Cochrane Library, Issue 3, 2001. Oxford: Update Software.
*305 Flynn C, Griffin G, Tudiver F. Decongestants and antihistamines for acute otitis media in children (Cochrane Review). In: The Cochrane Library, Issue 3, 2001. Oxford: Update Software.
306 Burke P, Bain J, Lowes A, Athersuch R. Rational decisions in managing sore throat: evaluation of a rapid test. BMJ 1998; 296:1646–1649.
307 Del Mar C, Glasziou P, Spinks A. Antibiotics for sore throat (Cochrane Review). In: The Cochrane Library, Issue 3, 2001. Oxford: Update Software.
308 Royal College of Paediatrics and Child Health. Guidelines for good practice: management of acute and recurring sore throat and indications for tonsillectomy. London: RCPCH; 2000.
*309 Burton M, Towler B, Glasziou P. Tonsillectomy versus non-surgical treatment for chronic/recurrent acute tonsillitis (Cochrane Review). In: The Cochrane Library, Issue 3, 2001. Oxford: Update software.
*310 Tinnion O, Hanlon M. Acellular vaccines for preventing whooping cough in children (Cochrane Review). In: The Cochrane Library, Issue 3, 2001. Oxford: Update Software.
311 Ranganathan S, Tasker R, Booy R, et al. Pertussis is increasing in unimmunized infants: is a change in policy needed? Arch Dis Child 1999; 80:297–299.
312 Bruss J, Malley R, Halperin S, et al. Treatment of severe pertussis: a study of the safety and pharmacology of intravenous pertussis immunoglobulin. Pediatr Infect Dis 1999; 18:505–511.
313 Mertsola J, Viljanen M, Ruuskanen O. Salbutamol in the treatment of whooping cough. Scand J Infect Dis 1986; 18:593–594.
314 Dodhia H, Miller E. Review of the evidence for the use of erythromycin in the management of persons exposed to pertussis. Epidemiol Infect 1998; 120:143–149.
*315 Ausejo M, Senz A, Pham B, et al. Glucocorticoids for croup (Cochrane Review). In: The Cochrane Library, Issue 3, 2001. Oxford: Update Software.
316 Waisman Y, Klein B, Boenning D, et al. Prospective randomized double-blind study comparing L-epinephrine and racemic epinephrine aerosols in the treatment of laryngotracheitis (croup). Pediatrics 1992; 89:302–306.
317 Prendergast M, Jones J, Hartman D. Racemic epinephrine in the treatment of laryngotracheitis. Can we identify children for outpatient therapy? Am J Emerg Med 1994; 12:613–616.
318 Kessler A, Wetmore R, Marsh R. Childhood epiglottitis in recent years. Int J Pediatr Otorhinolaryngol 1993; 25:155–162.
319 Booy R, Hodgson L, Carpenter L, et al. Efficacy of Haemophilus influenzae type b conjugate vaccine PRP-T. Lancet 1994; 344:362–366.
320 Murrage K, Janzen V, Ruby R. Epiglottitis: adult and pediatric complications. Otolaryngol 1988; 17:194–198.
321 Sobolev I, Plunkett N, Barker I. Acute epiglottitis, sevofluorane and Hib vaccination. Anesthesia 2001; 56:799–820.
322 Bernstein T, Brilli R, Jacobs B. Is bacterial tracheitis changing? A 14 month experience in a pediatric intensive care unit. Clin Infect Dis 1998; 27(3):458–462.
323 Noble V, Murray M, Webb MS, et al. Respiratory status and allergy nine to 10 years after acute bronchiolitis. Arch Dis Child 1997; 76:315–319.
*324 Kellner J, Ohlsson A, Gadomski A, Wang E. Bronchodilators for bronchiolitis (Cochrane Review). In: The Cochrane Library, Issue 3, 2001. Oxford: Update Software.
325 Ho L, Collins G, Landau L, LeSouef P. Effect of salbutamol on oxygen saturation in bronchiolitis. Arch Dis Child 1991; 66:1061–1064.

326 Cade A, Brownlee K, Conway S, et al. Randomized placebo controlled trial of nebulized corticosteroids in acute respiratory syncytial viral bronchiolitis. Arch Dis Child 2000; 82:126–130.
327 Richter H, Seddon P. Early nebulized budesonide in the treatment of bronchiolitis and the prevention of postbronchiolitis wheezing. J Pediatr 1998; 132:849–853.
*328 Randolph A, Wang E. Ribavirin for respiratory syncytial virus infection of the lower respiratory tract (Cochrane Review). In: The Cochrane Library, Issue 3, 2001. Oxford: Update Software.
329 Giffin F, Greenough A, Yuksel B. Antiviral therapy in neonatal chronic lung disease. Early Hum Dev 1995; 42:97–109.
330 Steinhorn R, Green T. Use of extracorporeal membrane oxygenation in the treatment of respiratory syncytial virus bronchiolitis: the national experience, 1983 to 1998. J Pediatr 1990; 116:338–342.
331 Luchetti M, Casiraghi G, Valsecchi R, et al. Porcine-derived surfactant treatment of severe bronchiolitis. Acta Anaesthesiol Scand 1998; 42:805–810.
*332 Wang E, Tang N. Immunoglobulin for preventing respiratory syncytial virus infection. Cochrane Database Syst Rev 2001; (2):CD001725, 2000.
333 Simoes E, Sondheimer H, Top F, et al. Respiratory syncytial virus immune globulin for prophylaxis against respiratory syncytial virus disease in infants and children with congenital heart disease. J Pediatr 1998; 133:492–499.
*334 IMpact-RSV Study group. Palivizumab, a humanised respiratory syncytial virus monoclonal antibody, reduces hospitalisation from respiratory syncytial virus infection in high risk infants. Pediatrics 1998; 102:531–537.
*335 British Thoracic Society standards of care committee. BTS guidelines for the management of community acquired pneumonia in childhood. Thorax 2002; 57:S1.
336 Block S, Hedrick J, Hammerschlag M, et al. Mycoplasma pneumoniae and Chlamydia pneumoniae in pediatric community-acquired pneumonia: comparative efficacy and safety of clarithromycin vs. erythromycin ethylsuccinate. Pediatr Infect Dis J 1995; 14(6):471–477.
337 Harris J, Kolokathis A, Campbell M, et al. Safety and efficacy of azithromycin in the treatment of community-acquired pneumonia in children. Pediatr Infect Dis 1998; 17:865–871.
338 Omidvari K, de Boisblanc B, Karam G, et al. Early transition to oral antibiotic therapy for community-acquired pneumonia: duration of therapy, clinical outcomes and cost analysis. Respir Med 1998; 92:1032–1039.
339 Wilmott RW, Khurana-Hershey G, Stark JM. Current concepts on pulmonary host defense mechanisms in children. Curr Opin Pediatr 2000; 12:187–193.
340 Larsen GL. Host defense systems of the lung. In: Taussig LM, Landau LI, eds. Pediatric respiratory medicine. St Louis: Mosby; 1999:57–75.
341 Houtmeyers E, Gosselink R, Gayan-Ramirez G, et al. Regulation of mucociliary clearance in health and disease. Eur Respir J 1999; 13:1177–1188.
342 Diamond G, Legarda D, Ryan LK. The innate immune response of the respiratory epithelium. Immunol Rev 2000; 173:27–38.
343 Parkin J, Cohen B. An overview of the immune system. Lancet 2001; 357:1777–1789.
344 Meeks M, Bush A. Primary ciliary dyskinesia (PCD). Pediatr Pulmonol 2000; 29:307–316.
345 Bush A, Cole P, Hariri M, et al. Primary ciliary dyskinesia: diagnosis and standards of care. Eur Respir J 1998; 12:982–988.
346 Cowan MJ, Gladwin MT, Shelhamer JH. Disorders of ciliary motility. Am J Med Sci 2001; 321:3–10.
347 Karadag B, James AJ, Gültekin E, et al. Nasal and lower airway level of nitric oxide in children with primary ciliary dyskinesia. Eur Respir J 1999; 13:1402–1405.
348 Ferkol TW, Davis PB. Bronchiectasis and bronchiolitis obliterans. In: Taussig LM, Landau LI, eds. Pediatric respiratory medicine. St Louis: Mosby: 1999:784–792.
349 Coleman LT, Kramer SS, Markowitz RI, Kravitz RM. Bronchiectasis in children. Thorac Imaging 1995; 10:268–279.
350 Nikolaizik WH, Warner JO. Etiology of chronic suppurative lung disease. Arch Dis Child 1994; 70:141–142.
351 Agasthian T, Deschamps C, Trastek VF, et al. Surgical management of bronchiectasis. Ann Thorac Surg 1996; 62:976–978.
352 Peake J, Roberton D. Advances in the diagnosis of primary immunodeficiency disorders in childhood. Curr Pediatr 2001; 11:149–157.
353 Anon. Primary immunodeficiency diseases. Report of an IUIS Scientific Committee. International Union of Immunological Societies. Clin Exp Immunol 1999; 118(S1):1–28.
354 Gennery AR, Cant AJ. Diagnosis of severe combined immunodeficiency. J Clin Pathol 2001; 54:191–195.
355 Goldblatt D, Thrasher AJ. Chronic granulomatous disease. Clin Exp Immunol 2000; 122:1–9.
356 Williams AJ, Duong T, McNally LM, et al. Pneumocystis carinii pneumonia and cytomegalovirus infection in children with vertically acquired HIV infection. AIDS 2001; 15:335–339.
357 Hargreave DR, Hann IM, Richards SM, et al. Progressive reduction in treatment-related deaths in Medical Research Council childhood lymphoblastic leukemia trials from 1980 to 1997 (UKALL VIII, X and XI). Br J Haematol 2001; 112:293–299.
358 Abadco DL, Amaro-Galvez R, Rao M, et al. Experience with flexible fiberoptic bronchoscopy with bronchoalveolar lavage as a diagnostic tool in children with AIDS. Am J Dis Child 1992; 146:1056–1059.
359 Stefanutti D, Morais L, Fournet JC, et al. Value of open lung biopsy in immunocompromised children. J Pediatr 2000; 137:165–171.
360 Schliep TC, Yarrish RL. Pneumocystis carinii pneumonia. Semin Respir Infect 1999; 14:333–343.
361 Bye MR, Cairns-Bazarian AM, Ewig JM. Markedly reduced mortality associated with corticosteroid therapy of Pneumocystis carinii pneumonia in children with acquired immunodeficiency syndrome. Arch Pediatr Adolesc Med 1994; 148:638–641.
362 Salomon N, Perlman DC. Cytomegalovirus pneumonia. Semin Respir Infect 1999; 14: 353–358.
363 Snoeck R, Andrei G, De Clercq E. Current pharmacological approaches to the therapy of varicella zoster virus infections. Drugs 1999; 57:187–206.
*364 Shann F, D'Souza RM, D'Souza R. Antibiotics for preventing pneumonia in children with measles (Cochrane Review). In: The Cochrane Library, Issue 3, 2001. Oxford: Update Software.
365 Muller FMC, Groll AH, Walsh TJ. Current approaches to diagnosis and treatment of fungal infections in children infected with human immunodeficiency virus. Eur J Pediatr 1999; 158:187–199.
366 Kroegel C, Antony VB. Immunobiology of pleural inflammation: potential implications for pathogenesis, diagnosis and therapy. Eur Respir J 1997; 10:2411–2418.
367 Chan PWK, Crawford O, Wallis C, et al. Treatment of pleural empyema. J Pediatr Child Health 2000; 36:375–377.
368 Thomson AH, Hull J, Kumar MR, et al. Randomized trial of intrapleural urokinase in the treatment of childhood empyema. Thorax 2002; 57:343–347.
369 Carey JA, Hamilton JRL, Spencer DA, et al. Empyema thoracis: a role for open thoracotomy and decortication. Arch Dis Child 1998; 79:510–513.
370 Doski JJ, Lou D, Hicks BA, et al. Management of parapneumonic collections in infants and children. J Pediatr Surg 2000; 35:265–270.
371 Zach MS, Eber E. Adult outcome of congenital lower respiratory tract malformations. Thorax 2001; 56:65–72.
372 Bush A. Congenital lung disease: a plea for clear thinking and clear nomenclature. Pediatr Pulmonol 2001; 32:328–337.
373 Durning RP, Scoles PV, Fox OD. Scoliosis after thoracotomy in tracheoesophageal fistula patients. J Bone Joint Surg 1980; 62:1156–1159.
374 Landing BH, Lawrence TK, Payne CV, Wells TR. Bronchial anatomy in syndromes with abnormal visceral situs, abnormal spleen and congenital heart disease. Am J Cardiol 1971; 28:456–462.
375 McCartney FJ, Zuberbuhler JR, Anderson RH. Morphological considerations pertaining to recognition of atrial isomerism. Consequences for chamber localisation. Br Heart J 1980; 44:657–667.
376 Bush A. Left bronchial isomerism, normal atrial arrangement and bronchomalacia mimicking asthma: a new syndrome? Eur Respir J 1999; 14:475–477.
377 Kramer MS. 'Horseshoe' lung: report of five new cases. Am J Roentgenol 1986; 146:211–215.
378 Reale FR, Esterly JR. Pulmonary hypoplasia: a morphometric study of the lungs of infants with diaphragmatic hernia, anencephaly, and renal malformations. Pediatrics 1972; 51:91–96.
379 Johnston RF, Green RA. Tracheobronchiomegaly: report of five cases and demonstration of familial occurrence. Am Rev Respir Dis 1965; 91:35–50.

380 Williams AJ, Schuster SR. Bronchial atresia associated with a bronchogenic cyst. Evidence of early appearance of atretic segments. Chest 1985; 87:396–398.
381 Hislop A, Reid L. New pathological findings in emphysema in childhood: 2. Overinflation of a normal lobe. Thorax 1971; 26:190–194.
382 Aktogu S, Yuncu G, Halilcolar H, et al. Bronchogenic cysts: clinicopathological presentation and treatment. Eur Respir J 1996; 9:2017–2021.
383 Samuel M, Burge DM. Management of antenatally diagnosed pulmonary sequestration associated with congenital cystic adenomatoid malformation. Thorax 1999; 54:701–706.
384 Aulicino MR, Reis ED, Dolgin SE, et al. Intra-abdominal pulmonary sequestration exhibiting congenital cystic adenomatoid malformation – report of a case and review of the literature. Arch Pathol Lab Med 1994; 118:1034–1037.
385 Fraggetta F, Cacciaguerra S, Nash R, Davenport M. Intra-abdominal pulmonary sequestration associated with congenital cystic adenomatoid malformation of the lung: just an unusual combination of rare pathologies? Pathol Res Pract 1998; 194:209–211.
386 Heithoff KB, Sane SM, Williams HJ, et al. Bronchopulmonary foregut malformations: a unifying etiological concept. AJR Am J Roentgenol 1976; 126:46–55.
387 Sade RM, Clouse M, Ellis FH Jr. The spectrum of pulmonary sequestration. Ann Thorac Surg 1974; 18:644–655.
388 dell'Agnola C, Tadini B, Mosca F, et al. Advantages of prenatal diagnosis and early surgery for congenital cystic disease of the lung. J Perinat Med 1996; 24:621–631.
389 Yamanaka A, Hirai T, Fujimoto T, et al. Anomalous systemic supply to normal basal segments of the left lower lobe. Ann Thorac Surg 1999; 68:332–338.
390 Schramel FM, Westermann CJ, Knepen PJ, van den Bosch JM. The scimitar syndrome: clinical spectrum and surgical treatment. Eur Respir J 1995; 8:196–201.
391 Najm HK, Williams WG, Coles JG, et al. Scimitar syndrome: twenty years' experience and results of repair. J Thorac Cardiovasc Surg 1996; 112:1161–1168.
392 Saluja S, Sitko I, Lee DW, et al. Embolotherapy of pulmonary arteriovenous malformations with detachable balloons: long-term durability and efficacy. J Vasc Interv Radiol 1999; 10:883–889.
393 White JES, Veale D, Fishwick D, et al. Generalised lymphangiectasia: pulmonary presentation in an adult. Thorax 1996; 51:767–768.
394 Northway W Jr, Rosan R, Porter D. Pulmonary disease following respiratory therapy of hyaline-membrane disease: bronchopulmonary dysplasia. N Engl J Med 1967; 276:357–368.
395 Shennan AT, Dunn MS, Ohlsson A, et al. Abnormal pulmonary outcomes in premature infants: prediction from oxygen requirement in the neonatal period. Pediatrics 1988; 82:527–532.
396 Jobe AH, Bancalari E. NICHD, NHLBI, ORD Workshop Summary: bronchopulmonary dysplasia. Am J Respir Crit Care Med 2001; 163:1723–1729.
397 Kotecha S, Silverman M. Chronic respiratory complications of neonatal disorders. In: Landau LI, Taussig LM, eds. Textbook of pediatric respiratory medicine. St Louis: Mosby; 1999:488p521.
398 Manktelow BN, Draper ES, Annamalai S, Field D. Factors affecting the incidence of chronic lung disease of prematurity between 1987, 1992 and 1997. Arch Dis Child 2001; 85:F33–F35.
399 Fenton AC, Mason E, Clarke M, Field DJ. Chronic lung disease following neonatal ventilation. II. Changing incidence in a geographically defined population. Pediatr Pulmonol 1996; 21:24–27.
400 Farstad T, Bratlid D. Incidence and prediction of bronchopulmonary dysplasia in a cohort of premature infants. Acta Pediatr 1994; 83:19–24.
401 Fanaroff AA, Wright LL, Stevenson DK, et al. Very low birthweight outcomes of the National Institute of Child Health and Human Development Neonatal Research Network, May 1991 through December 1992. Am J Obstet Gynecol 1995; 173:1423–1431.
402 Field D. Trent Neonatal Survey Department of Epidemiology and Public Health, University of Leicester; 2000.
403 Kotecha S. Lung growth: implications for the newborn infants. Arch Dis Child Fetal Neonatal Ed 2000; 82:F69–F74.
404 Stocker JT. The respiratory tract. In: Stocker JT, Dehner LP, eds. Pediatric pathology. Philadelphia: JB Lippincott; 1992; 533–541.
405 Margraf LR, Tomashefski JF, Bruce MC, Dahms BB. Morphometric analysis of the lung in bronchopulmonary dysplasia. Am Rev Respir Dis 1991; 143:391–400.
406 Husain AN, Siddiqui NH, Stocker JT. Pathology of arrested acinar development in postsurfactant bronchopulmonary dysplasia. Hum Pathol 1998; 29:710–717.
407 Jobe AJ. The new BPD: an arrest of lung development. Pediatr Res 1999; 46:641–643.
408 Thibeault DW, Mabry SM, Ekekezie II, Truog WE. Lung elastic tissue maturation and perturbations during the evolution of chronic lung disease. Pediatrics 2000; 106:1452–1459.
409 Pandya HC, Kotecha S. Chronic lung disease of prematurity: clinical and pathophysiological correlates. Monaldi Arch Chest Dis 2001; 56:270–275.
410 Hyde I, English RE, Williams JD. The changing pattern of chronic lung disease of prematurity. Arch Dis Child 1989; 64:448–451.
411 Fan LL, Flynn JW, Pathak DR. Risk factors predicting laryngeal injury in intubated neonates. Crit Care Med 1983; 11:431–433.
412 Boyce TG, Mellen BG, Mitchel EF, et al. Rates of hospitalisation for respiratory syncyticial virus infection among children in Medicaid. J Pediatr 2000; 137:865–870.
413 Anon. Palivizumab, a humanized respiratory syncyticial virus antibody, reduces hospitalisation from respiratory syncyticial virus infection in high-risk infants. The Impact-RSV Study Group. Pediatrics 1998; 102:531–537.
414 Anon. Prevention of respiratory syncyticial virus infections: indications on the use of RSV-IGIV. American Academy of Pediatrics Committee on infectious diseases and Committee of Fetus and Newborn. Pediatrics 1999; 104:994–995.
415 Arnold SR, Wang EE, Law BJ, et al. Variable morbidity of respiratory syncytial virus infection in patients with underlying lung disease: a review of the PICNIC RSV database. Pediatric Investigators Collaborative Network on Infections in Canada. Pediatr Infect Dis J 1999; 18:866–869.
416 Groothuis JR, Rosenberg AA. Home oxygen promotes weight gain in infants with bronchopulmonary dysplasia. Am J Dis Child 1987; 141:992–995.
417 Abman SH, Wolfe RR, Accurso FJ, et al. Pulmonary vascular response to oxygen in infants with severe bronchopulmonary dysplasia. Pediatrics 1985; 75:80–84.
418 Benatar A, Clarke J, Silverman M. Echocardiographic studies in chronic lung disease of prematurity. Arch Dis Child 1995; 72: F14–19.
419 Majnemer A, Riley P, Shevell M, et al. Severe bronchopulmonary dysplasia increases risk of later neurological and motor sequelae in preterm survivors. Develop Med Child Neurol 2000; 42:53–60.
420 Dunbar H, Kotecha S. Domiciliary oxygen for infants with chronic lung disease of prematurity. Care Crit Ill 2000; 16:90–93.
421 Baraldi E, Carra S, Vencato F, et al. Home oxygen therapy in infants with bronchopulmonary dysplasia: a prospective study. Eur J Pediatr 1997; 156:878–882.
422 Yeh TF, Lin YJ, Huang CC, et al. Early dexamethasone therapy in preterm infants: a follow-up study. Pediatrics 1998; 101:E7.
423 Shinwell ES, Karplus M, Reich D, et al. Early postnatal dexamethasone treatment and increased incidence of cerebral palsy. Arch Dis Child 2000; 83:F177–181.
424 Noble-Jamieson CM, Regev R, Silverman M. Dexamethasone in neonatal lung disease: pulmonary effects and intracranial complications. Eur J Pediatr 1989; 148:365–367.
*425 Lister P, Iles R, Shaw B, Ducharme F. Inhaled steroids for neonatal chronic lung disease (Cochrane Review). In: The Cochrane Library, Issue 1, 2001. Oxford: Update Software.
*426 Dunn M, Pandit P, Magnani L. Inhaled corticosteroids for neonatal chronic lung disease: a randomized, double-blind cross-over study. Pediatr Res 1992; 31:201A.
427 Yuksel B, Greenough A. Randomized trial of inhaled steroids in preterm infants with respiratory symptoms at follow up. Thorax 1992; 47:910–913.
428 Wilkie RA, Bryan MH. Effect of bronchodilators on airway resistance in ventilator-dependent neonates with chronic lung disease. J Pediatr 1987; 111:278–282.
429 Hislop AA, Haworth SG. Airway size and structure in the normal fetal and infant lung and the effect of premature delivery and artificial ventilation. Am Rev Respir Dis 1989; 140:1717–1726.
430 De Boeck K, Smith J, Van Lierde S, Devlieger H. Response to bronchodilators in clinically stable 1-year old patients with bronchopulmonary dysplasia. Eur J Pediatr 1998; 157:75–79.
431 Koumbourlis AC, Motoyama EK, Mutich RL. Longitudinal follow-up of lung function from childhood to adolescence in prematurely born patients with neonatal chronic lung disease. Pediatr Pulmonol 1996; 21:28–34.

432 Yuksel B, Greenough A. Ipratropium bromide for symptomatic preterm infants. Eur J Pediatr 1991; 150:854–857.

***433** Brion LP, Primhak RA. Intravenous or enteral loop diuretics for preterm infants with (or developing) chronic lung disease. Cochrane Database of Systematic Reviews 2000; (2):CD001453.

***434** Brion LP, Primhak RA, Ambrosio-Perez I. Diuretics acting on the distal renal tubule for preterm infants with (or developing) chronic lung disease. Cochrane Database of Systematic Reviews 2000; (2):CD001817.

***435** Brion LP, Primhak RA,Yong W. Aerosolized diuretics for preterm infants with (or developing) chronic lung disease. Cochrane Database of Systematic Reviews 2000; (2):CD001694.

436 Doyle LW, Cheung MMH, Ford GW, et al. Birth weight 1501 g and respiratory health at 14. Arch Dis Child 2001; 84:40–44.

437 Gross SJ, Iannuzzi DM, Kveselis DA, Anbar RD. Effect of preterm birth on pulmonary function at school age: a prospective controlled study. J Pediatr 1998; 133:188–192.

438 Jardine E, O'Toole M, Paton JY, Wallis C. Current status of long term ventilation of children in the United Kingdom: questionnaire survey. BMJ 1999; 318:295–299.

439 Simonds AK, Ward S, Heather S, et al. Outcome of pediatric domiciliary mask ventilation in neuromuscular and skeletal disease. Eur Resp J 2000; 16:476–481.

440 Jardine E, Wallis C. Core guidelines for he discharge home of the child on long term assisted ventilation in the United Kingdom. Thorax 1998; 53:762–767.

***441** McIntyre RC, Pulido EJ, Bensard DD, et al. Thirty years of clinical trials in acute respiratory distress syndrome. Crit Care Med 2000; 28:3314–3331.

***442** Sokol J, Jacobs SE, Bohn D. Inhaled nitric oxide for acute hypoxemic respiratory failure in children and adults. Cochrane Database of Systematic Reviews 2000; CD002787.

443 Nicholson AG, Kim H, Corrin B, et al. The value of classifying interstitial pneumonitis in childhood according to defined histological patterns. Histopathology 1998; 33:203–211.

444 Katzenstein A-L, Gordon LP, Oliphant M, Swender PT. Chronic pneumonitis of infancy. Am J Surg Pathol 1995; 19:439–447.

445 Copley SJ, Coren M, Nicholson AG, et al. Diagnostic accuracy of thin-section CT and chest radiography of pediatric interstitial lung disease. AJR Am J Roentgenol 2000; 174:549–554.

446 Bush A. Diagnosis of interstitial lung disease. Pediatr Pulmonol 1996; 22:81–82.

447 Coren ME, Nicholson AG, Goldstraw P, et al. Open lung biopsy for diffuse interstitial lung disease in children. Eur Respir Dis 1999; 14:817–821.

448 Sharief N, Crawford OF, Dinwiddie R. Fibrosing alveolitis and desquamative interstitial pneumonia. Pediatr Pulmonol 1994; 17:359–365.

449 Spencer D. Rare single system diseases. Pediatr Respir Rev 2001; 2:63–69.

450 Dinwiddie R. The lung in multisystem disease. Pediatr Respir Rev 2000; 1:58–63.

451 Shah AF, Dinwiddie R, Woolf D, et al. Generalised lymphangiomatosis and chylothorax in the pediatric age group. Pediatr Pulmonol 1992; 14:126–130.

452 Chan PW, Muridan R, Debruyne JA. Bronchiolitis obliterans in children: clinical profile and diagnosis. Respirology 2000; 5:369–375.

453 Becroft DM. Bronchiolitis obliterans, bronchiectasis, and other sequelae of adenovirus type 21 infection in young children. J Clin Pathol 1971; 24:72–82.

454 Davis AM, Wensley DF, Phelan PD. Spontaneous pneumothorax in pediatric patients. Respir Med 1993; 87:531–534.

455 Avital A, Springer C, Godfrey S. Pulmonary hemorrhagic syndromes in children. Pediatr Resp Rev 2000; 3:266–273.

456 Bush A. Pulmonary hypertensive disorders. Pediat Respir Rev 2000; 1:361–367.

457 Deng Z, Haghighi F, Helleby L, et al. Fine mapping of PPH1, a gene for familial primary pulmonary hypertension, to a 3-cM region on chromosome 2q33. Am J Respir Crit Care Med 2000; 161:1055–1059.

***458** Paramothayan S, Wells A, Lasserson T, Walters H. Prostacyclin for pulmonary hypertension. [Protocol] Cochrane Airways Group. Cochrane database of systematic reviews Issue 1; 2002.

459 Nogee LM, deMello DE, Dehner LP, Clements JA. Deficiency of surfactant protein B in congenital alveolar proteinosis. N Engl J Med 1993; 328:406–410.

460 Nogee LM, Dunbar E 3rd, Wert SE, et al. A mutation in the surfactant protein C gene associated with familial interstitial lung disease. N Engl J Med 2001; 344:573–579.

461 Hartman GF, Shochat SJ. Primary pulmonary neoplasms of childhood: a review. Ann Thorac Surg 1983; 36:108–119.

19

Cardiovascular disease

Edited by Denise J Kitchiner

PRINCIPLES OF ASSESSMENT OF HEART DISEASE

Detailed clinical evaluation is essential in the assessment of a child suspected of having a cardiac lesion. A comprehensive history provides information on the nature and severity of the condition. It also helps to establish a rapport with the child and family. A thorough physical examination is also necessary. If suspicion of a cardiac lesion exists, an electrocardiogram may give additional information. Chest radiography is seldom helpful in the diagnosis of a specific cardiac lesion. It remains useful in differentiating heart disease from other conditions and in assessing the severity of some lesions. Echocardiography has revolutionized the diagnosis and management of children with heart disease. It must be carried out and interpreted in conjunction with the clinical findings, if errors in diagnosis are to be avoided.[1] Cardiac catheterization is now less frequently used in diagnosis, but transcatheter intervention is performed for a range of conditions. Other investigations are helpful in evaluating some children.

HISTORY

Symptoms can give important clues to the diagnosis and severity of heart disease. The history can also help to differentiate cardiac lesions from other conditions. *Infants* with heart failure present with feeding difficulties and symptoms of respiratory distress. The infant takes frequent small feeds, rapidly becoming exhausted. This results in poor weight gain, which in some children is also due to increased energy expenditure.[2] It is important to assess the volume of feed, or the time taken, if breastfeeding. In warm climates infants may perspire profusely, particularly with feeds. Parents may notice that their baby is breathing rapidly, and suffers from recurrent chest infections. Cyanosis may not be recognized until it is quite severe. Peripheral cyanosis, which does not indicate a cardiac lesion, may cause concern. *Children* often present with an asymptomatic murmur. Heart failure manifests as breathlessness and exercise intolerance. This can be assessed by comparison with peers or by formal exercise testing. Orthopnea and nocturnal dyspnea indicate severe failure. Cyanosis rarely presents in children over a year of age and a history of 'blueness around the lips' is most likely to be due to cold, crying or breath-holding episodes.

A detailed history is also essential when assessing a child with palpitations, dizziness or syncope. In childhood chest pain is rarely cardiac in origin and is more likely to be musculoskeletal, pulmonary or due to anxiety. Angina occurs during activity and is relieved by rest. It is a crushing central chest pain, not related to breathing. It lasts some minutes, unlike muscular pain that is often fleeting and sharp. Symptoms of acquired heart disease such as rheumatic fever, Kawasaki disease and myocarditis are discussed later.

Children may also have symptoms that are unrelated to a cardiac lesion. Non-specific symptoms such as tiredness can also cause concern in a child with a cardiac lesion and reassurance may be necessary if this is not due to the heart condition. A history of prematurity, fetal distress or other congenital lesions may have a bearing on diagnosis. A maternal history of diabetes, systemic lupus erythematosus, phenylketonuria or drug ingestion (e.g. anti-epileptic drugs or alcohol) results in a higher incidence of congenital heart disease. A family history of heart disease, arrhythmias or sudden death, particularly in first-degree relatives[3] or parental consanguinity results in an increased risk.[4]

CLINICAL EXAMINATION

A detailed examination provides essential information for diagnosis, assessment of severity and monitoring of children with heart disease. Systematic examination is preferable, but may be adjusted to obtain the maximum information in young children. It is sensible to listen to the heart with a toddler seated on the parent's lap before attempting to feel the femoral pulses or measuring the blood pressure.

GENERAL EXAMINATION

Children with other congenital abnormalities have a 20–40% incidence of heart disease. Chromosomal abnormalities are found in 10% of children with congenital heart disease and this will increase as more are identified. Down, DiGeorge, Williams, Noonan's and Turner's syndromes are most commonly associated with congenital heart disease, but many other associations have been reported.[1]

Growth and nutrition

Weight and height should be plotted on a growth chart together with birth weight to assess growth. Poor growth is associated with heart failure, cyanosis and some syndromes. It may also be unrelated to a cardiac lesion, particularly in children with dysmorphic features.

Cyanosis and clubbing

Mild central cyanosis may be difficult to detect and must be distinguished from peripheral cyanosis (acrocyanosis) that does not involve well-perfused areas such as the tongue and mucous membranes. Central cyanosis requires the presence of reduced hemoglobin in the arterial circulation so anemia and polycythemia will affect the recognition of cyanosis. Traditionally, detection of cyanosis required the presence of > 5g/dl of reduced hemoglobin in the arterial blood (saturations of 66% with a hemoglobin of 15 g/dl). With the advent of pulse oximetry it has become clear that much milder cyanosis (around 85%) can be detected clinically in children in good light.

Rarely, differential cyanosis involving the lower limbs with pink upper extremities occurs with right-to-left shunt across the arterial duct, together with coarctation. Clubbing of the digits takes months to develop and is not seen in young infants.

Respiratory system

The respiratory rate should be recorded. Normal values are shown in Table 19.1. Upper airway obstruction with stridor can occur in association with a vascular ring. Chronic upper airway obstruction can cause pulmonary hypertension.

Heart failure

Signs of heart failure should be sought in any child suspected of having a cardiac lesion (p. 833). Particular attention should be paid to peripheral perfusion, edema, and respiratory distress. Estimation of the jugular venous pressure is difficult in young children and hepatomegaly is a more reliable indicator of systemic venous congestion.

Pulses

Pulses should be evaluated for rate, rhythm, volume and character. Rate varies with age and ranges are shown in Table 19.1. Faster rates are normal during crying or activity, but persistent tachycardia (> 200 beats/min in neonates, 150/min in infants or 120/min in older children), bradycardia and irregular rhythms should be evaluated with an electrocardiogram. The volume of both arms and femoral pulses should be assessed to exclude coarctation and other arterial anomalies. Radiofemoral delay is difficult to appreciate in children with a rapid pulse, but a difference between the volume of the right axillary and femoral pulse is significant. The femoral pulses should be checked at the postnatal examination, but if the arterial duct is still patent, the pulse may be palpable in the presence of coarctation. The femoral pulses should be checked again, at routine assessments, and if there is a suspicion of heart disease. Poor volume of all pulses reflects a reduced cardiac output indicating hypoplastic left heart syndrome, critical aortic stenosis, severe heart failure or cardiac tamponade. A wide pulse pressure (the difference between systolic and diastolic pressure) produces a collapsing (bounding) pulse in children with a large arterial duct, arteriovenous malformation, severe anemia and severe aortic regurgitation. A slow rising (plateau) pulse is found in severe aortic stenosis.

Blood pressure

Blood pressure should be recorded in *the right arm*, as the measurement in the left may be lower if coarctation is present. Blood pressure should be measured with the child lying or sitting comfortably with the sphygmomanometer at heart level. The inflatable cuff should cover two-thirds of the upper arm from shoulder tip to elbow and completely encircle the arm. A smaller cuff will give a falsely high reading. If there is any suspicion of aortic coarctation, both upper and lower limb pressures should be measured. The blood pressure in the leg is normally higher than the arm. A measurement in the leg that is 10 mmHg or more lower than in the arms is abnormal. Automated oscillometric methods with digital readout of systolic, diastolic and mean pressure are increasingly used. These are reasonably reliable, but inaccuracies occur with movement. Blood pressure in children is labile and a single reading cannot be considered to indicate hypertension unless it is very high. The reading should be repeated and only if the level is elevated on at least three different occasions, can the child be considered to have hypertension. Charts of the 90th and 95th percentile for blood pressure for age, weight and height from birth to 18 years have been published and are shown in the section on Hypertension (p. 881).

Precordial examination

This may reveal a bulge indicating chronic cardiac enlargement. Scars from previous surgery should also be noted. The apex beat is felt at the fourth left intercostal space within the midclavicular line. It is produced by the left ventricle, and is displaced laterally and inferiorly with cardiomegaly. It is palpable on the right in dextrocardia. Left ventricular hypertrophy produces a forceful impulse that is usually not displaced. Right ventricular enlargement

Table 19.1 Normal values of respiratory and heart rates in infants and children (Pelech 1999[1])

	Birth–6 weeks	6 weeks–2 years	2–6 years	6–10 years	Over 10 years
Respiratory rate/min	45–60	40	30	25	20
Heart rate/min	125 ± 30	115 ± 25	100 ± 20	90 ± 15	85 ± 15

produces a diffuse impulse at the lower half of the sternum and in the epigastrium. A poorly felt apex beat suggests a pericardial effusion or severe heart failure. Thrills are palpable over the site of maximum intensity of loud murmurs, but the thrill of aortic stenosis is felt in the suprasternal notch. Thrills are usually systolic; rarely diastolic thrills occur in severe mitral or tricuspid stenosis. The loud second heart sound of severe pulmonary hypertension is sometimes palpable.

Auscultation

Auscultation of all phases of the cardiac cycle should be systematic and include the whole precordium, the axilla and the back. Note changes during inspiration and expiration, and with the child sitting and lying. The heart sounds and high-pitched murmurs are best heard with the diaphragm of the stethoscope, and low-pitched ones with the bell.

The *first heart sound* is caused by mitral and tricuspid valve closure and is best heard at the apex. It is louder with tachycardia as the valve leaflets are further apart in early systole. It is usually single, reflecting mitral closure but split if tricuspid closure is delayed. The *second heart sound* is caused by aortic and pulmonary valve closure and is best heard at the upper left and right sternal borders. During inspiration, pulmonary valve closure is delayed because of the increased volume of blood returning to the right heart, causing audible splitting. On expiration the valves close simultaneously and the sound is normally single. Delayed closure of the pulmonary valve in expiration results in 'fixed' splitting. A single second heart sound occurs when one of the components is inaudible. The pulmonary component of the second heart sound is loud in pulmonary hypertension. A *third heart sound* occurs early in diastole and is caused by rapid ventricular filling. It is low-pitched and heard at the apex in normal children. A *fourth heart sound* occurs late in diastole and is due to atrial contraction. A *gallop rhythm* is caused by rapid diastolic filling of a poorly compliant ventricle and occurs in heart failure. *Ejection clicks* are heard just after the first heart sound. They are due to abnormal but mobile valves or proximal arterial dilatation. Pulmonary ejection clicks are maximal over the pulmonary area, but aortic ejection clicks are best heard at the lower left sternal edge. *Mid-systolic clicks* are due to mitral valve prolapse (at the apex) or Ebstein's anomaly of the tricuspid valve (at the fourth left intercostal space).

Murmurs are described in terms of loudness, quality, timing, site of maximum intensity and radiation. Murmurs are graded from 1 to 6: 1 barely audible, 2 easily audible, 3 loud but no thrill, 4 loud with a thrill, 5 very loud, 6 heard without stethoscope. There is no relationship between loudness and severity of a lesion. The *quality* of a murmur can be distinctive. Innocent murmurs are often vibratory. A high pitched blowing murmur is heard with aortic or mitral regurgitation or a small ventricular septal defect. A lower pitched harsh murmur occurs with outflow stenosis or a perimembranous ventricular septal defect, and a very low-pitched rumble with mitral stenosis. Timing of murmurs is crucial in diagnosis.

Systolic murmurs:

- Early systolic murmur is due to a small muscular ventricular septal defect.
- Ejection (crescendo–decrescendo) murmur is usually due to aortic or pulmonary stenosis, an atrial septal defect or an innocent murmur.
- Pansystolic murmur is due to a ventricular septal defect, mitral or tricuspid regurgitation.
- Late systolic murmur is due to mitral valve prolapse.

In infants with fast heart rates, it can be difficult to distinguish between ejection and pansystolic murmurs. If a distinct first heart sound is audible, it is more likely to be ejection.

Diastolic murmurs are almost always pathological, and rarely occur without a systolic murmur. Early diastolic (decrescendo) murmur is best heard with the diaphragm and the mid-diastolic with the bell of the stethoscope.

- Early diastolic murmurs are due to aortic or pulmonary regurgitation.
- Mid-diastolic murmurs are due to increased flow or stenosis of the mitral or tricuspid valve. Presystolic accentuation indicates significant narrowing.

Continuous murmurs are heard during systole and through the second heart sound into diastole. They occur when an artery communicates with a vessel at lower pressure in systole and diastole such as an arterial duct, systemic to pulmonary (Blalock–Taussig) shunt or an arteriovenous fistula. They may be confused with ejection systolic murmurs closely followed by an early diastolic murmur, or a venous hum.

The *site of maximal intensity and radiation* of a murmur is very helpful in diagnosis. A murmur results from turbulent blood flow and is usually loudest at this site. The typical sites of maximal intensity of the common systolic murmurs are summarized in Figure 19.1. A loud murmur will be conducted widely over the precordium, but most radiate to specific areas. The typical features of individual lesions are discussed separately. Table 19.2 summarizes the typical findings in common types of congenital heart disease.

ELECTROCARDIOGRAPHY

Cardiac muscle, like all muscle, requires an electrical impulse to initiate depolarization. The heart generates and conducts its own electricity and electrocardiography records the cardiac electrical activity, usually from the body's surface. Electrocardiography is a fundamental part of assessment of children with known or suspected congenital or acquired cardiac disease. It provides the main method of evaluation of children with cardiac arrhythmias (p. 866).

Interpretation of the electrocardiogram is a skill acquired only with practice. Whilst the expert can evaluate an electrocardiogram (ECG) almost at a glance, the newcomer should adopt a systematic approach.[5] Knowledge of the patient's age, cardiac (or other) diagnosis, and medications will enhance the interpretation of the ECG. One of the most important influences on interpretation of pediatric ECGs is the change in the normal ECG that occurs with growth and age. Familiarity with the variation in the normal pattern is required before distinction between normality and abnormality can be made with confidence.[6,7]

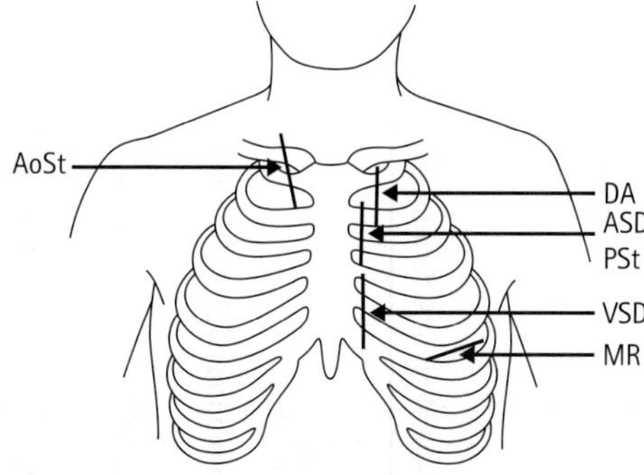

Fig. 19.1 Diagrammatic representation of the precordium showing the usual sites at which the murmur of the most common acyanotic lesions are heard. AoSt, aortic stenosis; ASD, atrial septal defect; DA, ductus arteriosus; MR, mitral regurgitation; PSt, pulmonary stenosis; VSD, ventricular septal defect.

Table 19.2 Typical clinical findings in the most common forms of congenital heart disease

Lesion	Pulses	Ventricular activity	Heart sounds	Systolic murmur	Diastolic murmur	Radiation of murmur
Large ventricular septal defect (VSD)	Normal	Biventricular	Increased P2 if pulmonary hypertension	Pansystolic Lower left sternal edge	Mid-diastolic at apex	Apex and back
Small perimembranous VSD	Normal	Normal	Normal	Loud pansystolic Lower left sternal edge	Nil	Apex and back
Small muscular VSD	Normal	Normal	Normal	Soft early systolic Lower left sternal edge	Nil	Nil
Atrial septal defect	Normal	Right ventricle	Second sound widely spilt and 'fixed'	Ejection Upper left sternal edge	Mid-diastolic at left sternal edge	Back
Large arterial duct	Collapsing	Biventricular	Increased P2 if pulmonary hypertension	Continuous Upper left sternal edge	Mid-diastolic at apex	Back
Small arterial duct	Normal	Normal	Normal	Continuous Upper left sternal edge	Continuous	Nil
Pulmonary stenosis	Normal	Right ventricle (if severe)	Ejection click at pulmonary area	Ejection Upper left sternal edge	Nil	Back
Aortic stenosis	Normal	Left ventricle (if severe)	Ejection click at left sternal edge	Ejection Upper right sternal edge	Nil	Neck
Coarctation of the aorta	Reduced or delayed femoral pulse	Left ventricle (if severe)	Ejection click at left sternal edge (if bicuspid aortic valve)	Ejection Upper left sternal edge	Continuous if collaterals present	Back
Tetralogy of Fallot	Normal	Right ventricle	Single second heart sound ± ejection click	Long ejection Upper left sternal edge	Nil	Back
Transposition of the great arteries	Normal	Right ventricle	Single second heart sound	Nil	Nil	Nil

The ECG is conventionally recorded at a speed of 25 mm/s and at a calibration of 1 cm = 1 mV. Accurate positioning of the leads on the surface of the skin (especially the chest leads) is important. A standard twelve lead ECG includes three standard (bipolar) limb leads I, II, and III, three augmented unipolar limb leads aVR, aVL, and aVF, and six unipolar chest leads, V1–V6. Recordings from children sometimes include additional right chest leads V4R and/or V3R but these are generally less helpful now that echocardiography is widely available.

Routine evaluation of an ECG involves assessment of the heart rate, heart rhythm, QRS axis, then the P waves, QRS complexes, T waves and measurement of the PR, QRS, and QT intervals. Many modern ECG machines automatically measure and display many of these variables. The measurements are usually accurate and reliable but a machine-derived interpretation of the ECG should always be treated with caution, even if it is produced by a pediatric algorithm. The machine often distinguishes between normality and abnormality fairly accurately (assuming the age of the patient is entered into the algorithm) but analysis of the type of abnormality may be less reliable.

THE NORMAL ELECTROCARDIOGRAM

Normal sinus rhythm produces a P wave with a normal axis originating from the high right atrium, normal 1:1 atrioventricular conduction with a normal PR interval, a QRS of normal duration, axis and morphology, and a T wave of normal axis and duration. The rapid evolution in the normal ECG in early infancy mainly reflects the change in ventricular dominance resulting from adaptation to postnatal hemodynamic changes. The changes in the normal pattern with age[8] and many normal values for ECG measurements at different ages[6,7] have been well described.

U waves are commonly seen in children and may be prominent in chest leads. Peaked U waves (especially in lead V2) may occasionally give a notched appearance to the T wave and may simulate atrial tachycardia with 2:1 atrioventricular conduction. Check by examining other leads to confirm the presence of sinus rhythm with 1:1 conduction. One common normal variation is the presence of an RSR′ pattern in lead V1. This does not amount to right bundle branch block, as the QRS duration is normal. T waves in lead V1 also vary considerably with age. They should be inverted between the ages of 7 days and 7 years and precordial T wave inversion may persist into adolescence. A rhythmic variation in sinus rate, related to respiration (respiratory sinus arrhythmia), is very common at all ages and should be regarded as normal. Minor variations in heart rhythm are also common at all ages and should be borne in mind when interpreting 24-h ECG recordings.[9]

In addition to the standard surface electrocardiogram, the exercise ECG may be used for dynamic assessment of children with structural heart disease. Signal averaging of the ECG is occasionally used for detection of underlying abnormalities not visible on a standard 12 lead ECG.[10] Heart rate variability analysis is a subtle form of autonomic evaluation that is still mostly used as a research tool.[11] Ambulatory recording of the ECG, patient-activated event recorders, and implantable loop ECG recorders are available for evaluation of patients with known or suspected cardiac arrhythmias.

THE ABNORMAL ELECTROCARDIOGRAM

The sensitivity and specificity of the ECG in differentiation of normality from abnormality is very variable. The ECG is almost always abnormal in cardiac abnormalities such as atrioventricular septal defect, tricuspid atresia, anomalous origin of the left coronary artery from the pulmonary artery, Wolff–Parkinson–White syndrome, and long QT syndrome but these are relatively rare conditions. However, other than in diagnosis of arrhythmias, there are few situations in which the ECG is diagnostic without being considered alongside the results of other investigations.

The PR interval

The PR interval increases with age and decreases with heart rate. It is shortened in Pompe's disease and in Wolff–Parkinson–White syndrome and is prolonged in conditions such as atrioventricular septal defect or Ebstein's anomaly of the tricuspid valve, by some drugs and in rheumatic fever.

Ventricular hypertrophy

Unfortunately, the ECG performs poorly in evaluation of ventricular hypertrophy, particularly when this is mild, and echocardiography is often a more appropriate investigation.[12] Right ventricular hypertrophy is suspected when there is an upright T wave in lead V1 between the age of 1 week and 7 years or when the height of the R wave in lead V1 is above the 98th centile for age. Other signs include a QR pattern in right chest leads, a deep S wave in lead V6, an RSR′ pattern in V1 (as in atrial septal defect), and right axis deviation. Left ventricular hypertrophy is suspected when the R wave in V5 or V6 or the S wave in V1 exceeds the 98th centile, especially if there is associated lateral T wave inversion. Simply adding the R wave in V5 to the S wave in V2 or the R and S waves in V2 in the hope of detecting significant left ventricular hypertrophy has disappointing sensitivity and specificity.[12] Biventricular hypertrophy may be difficult to recognize. It is suggested when criteria for left and right ventricular hypertrophy are both satisfied, or by a combined R wave and S wave in lead V4 exceeding the 98th centile for age.

Bundle branch block

Right bundle branch block (RBBB) results from a delay in activation of the right ventricle. Early activation of the left ventricle (as in Wolff–Parkinson–White syndrome with a left-sided pathway) gives a similar appearance. RBBB is recognized when the QRS duration is prolonged in association with a broad secondary R wave in V1 and a wide S wave in V6 (Fig. 19.2). It is a common finding after surgery for repair of a variety of congenital heart defects. 'Incomplete' RBBB (with a similar QRS morphology but a normal QRS duration) is a fairly common normal variant and is a characteristic, but not universal, feature of atrial septal defect.

Left bundle branch block (LBBB) is caused by delay in left ventricular activation. It produces a deep S wave or QS complex in lead V1 and a notched R wave in lead V6 (Fig. 19.3). The QRS duration is prolonged. A similar appearance is produced by early right ventricular activation (as in Wolff–Parkinson–White syndrome with a right-sided pathway or in right ventricular paced rhythm). LBBB is rare in children and is always abnormal. It may be seen in advanced aortic valve disease, cardiomyopathy, myocarditis, or after endocarditis.

Other abnormalities of the QRS complex and ST segment

Wolff–Parkinson–White syndrome is the association of an accessory atrioventricular conduction bundle with the propensity to cardiac arrhythmias. It produces a short PR interval and a slurred upstroke to the QRS – the delta wave (Figs 19.2 and 19.3). There is often an abnormal mean frontal QRS axis and T wave inversion but the exact pattern depends on the position of the accessory pathway.

Signs of ventricular ischemia or infarction are rare in children but they may be present in congenital abnormalities of the coronary arteries, Kawasaki disease, cardiomyopathy, and myocarditis. They

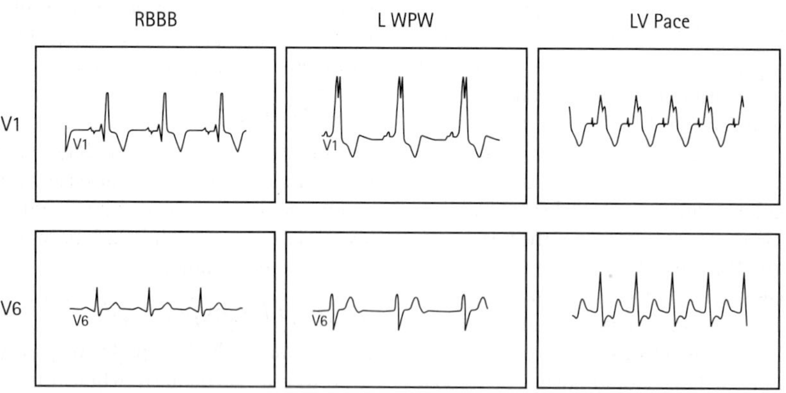

Fig. 19.2 A comparison of the ECG appearances of right bundle branch block (RBBB), Wolff-Parkinson-White syndrome with a left sided accessory pathway (L WPW), and pacing from the left ventricle (LV Pace) in leads V1 and V6. The similarities are due to the fact that in each case the left ventricle is activated before the right ventricle.

include reduction in the height of R waves, abnormal Q waves, abnormalities of the ST segment and T wave inversion. Pericarditis characteristically produces ST segment elevation without T wave inversion. ST shift is also seen in ischemia, metabolic disturbances, and head injury and is sometimes a normal variant in right precordial leads.

Abnormalities of the QT interval

The QT interval is measured from the onset of the QRS complex to the end of the T wave (which is sometimes difficult to define) and is conventionally measured in lead II. It is shortened by hypercalcemia, hypoxia, and digoxin and is prolonged by many factors including hypocalcemia, head injury, antiarrhythmic drugs such as amiodarone and sotalol, and sometimes by other drugs. Perhaps the most important cause of QT prolongation is the long QT syndrome. The QT interval, in common with all other intervals measured on the ECG, varies with the heart rate. It is usually normalized to a heart rate of 60 per minute to produce a corrected value (QTc) by dividing the measured QT interval (in seconds or milliseconds) by the square root of the RR interval (measured in seconds). Thus $QTc = QT/\sqrt{RR}$. The upper limit of QTc is around 440 ms or 0.44 s.

CHEST RADIOGRAPHY

This provides some diagnostic information regarding significant cardiac lesions but is of no value in trivial defects or in distinguishing these from innocent murmurs. Its role in diagnosis has largely been superseded by echocardiography. Chest radiography should be examined for the cardiac size and configuration, pulmonary vascularity and lung disease. Skeletal abnormalities, the thoracic and abdominal situs, and other abnormalities should also be identified. Repeated chest radiographs are of little value in assessing progress of a cardiac lesion.

Cardiac size

A semi-quantitative assessment of the heart size can be calculated from the cardiothoracic ratio. This is the ratio of the cardiac diameter (measured as the sum of the distance from the midline to the right and left margins of the cardiac shadow) to the maximal internal thoracic diameter (Fig. 19.4). In normal children the ratio is less than 0.5 but can be up to 0.55 in the first 2 years of life. It is not possible to detect individual chamber enlargement without an additional lateral film, which is seldom justified. Cardiomegaly is almost always present with a significant cardiac defect, apart from obstructive lesions such as pulmonary or aortic stenosis. It is caused by:

- Ventricular enlargement due to volume overload associated with a left-to-right shunt, valve regurgitation or ventricular dysfunction.
- Atrial enlargement due to tricuspid or mitral regurgitation, or rarely stenosis.
- Pericardial effusion.

Isolated cardiomegaly found when a chest radiograph is taken for another reason is usually spurious. Reasons include a film that

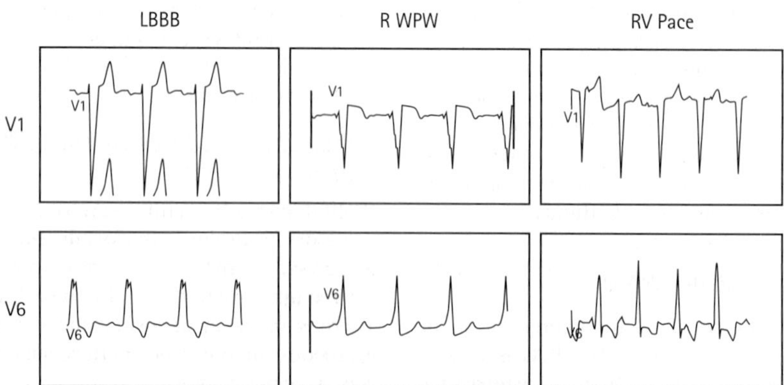

Fig. 19.3 A comparison of the ECG appearances of left bundle branch block (LBBB), Wolff-Parkinson-White syndrome with a right sided accessory pathway (R WPW), and pacing from the right ventricle (RV Pace) in leads V1 and V6. The similarities are due to the fact that in each case the right ventricle is activated before the left ventricle.

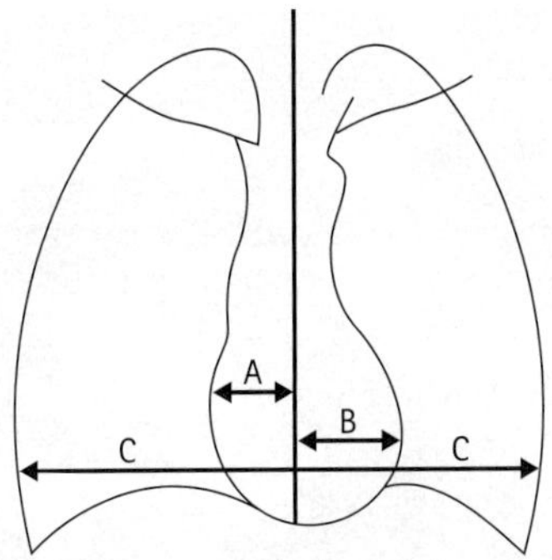

Fig. 19.4 Diagrammatic representation of the measurement of the cardiothoracic ratio:

$$CTR = \frac{A + B}{C} \times 100 \text{ where}$$

A + B = maximum transverse diameter of the heart
C = maximum transverse diameter of the chest.

is not taken in full inspiration or one taken from the front (antero-posterior). Pectus excavatum and other skeletal abnormalities will also give the appearance of cardiomegaly. The thymic shadow in infants overlies the upper mediastinum and can suggest cardiomegaly.

Configuration of the heart

A characteristic appearance may be found with certain congenital cyanotic lesions but these are variable and are only suggestive of the diagnosis. The upper right cardiac border may have a bulge from an anomalous pulmonary venous connection, or an azygous continuation of the inferior caval vein. A dilated ascending aorta or right aortic arch will give a similar appearance. A left superior caval vein or other abnormal systemic or pulmonary venous connection can cause an abnormal appearance of the upper left heart border. Post-stenotic dilatation of the pulmonary artery also causes a prominent shadow at the upper left heart border.

Pulmonary vascularity

Increased pulmonary blood flow from a left-to-right shunt is manifest as large vessels passing outwards from the hilum. With pulmonary edema the hilar vessels are less well defined but the bronchi become more easily seen and, if severe, linear septal shadows appear in the lower lateral aspects of the lung fields. Pulmonary hypertension produces large proximal and small distal vessels. Underperfused (oligemic) lung fields are seen in cyanotic heart disease with reduced pulmonary blood flow.

Pulmonary disease

Chest radiology is important in distinguishing cardiac from respiratory disease in a symptomatic child.

Other abnormalities

A penetrated film demonstrating the bronchi can help to establish the thoracic situs. The left main bronchus arises from the trachea at a less acute angle and its first branch arises more distally. Congenital skeletal abnormalities occurring with certain syndromes such as VACTERL will be apparent. Rib notching may be seen with coarctation of the aorta in older children.

ECHOCARDIOGRAPHY

Echocardiography (the use of ultrasound to examine the heart) is the most important diagnostic technique in congenital heart disease.[13] Pediatric cardiologists rely on it to diagnose structural heart disease by creating moving images of the heart with cross-sectional (or '2D') echocardiography. Cardiac hemodynamics including assessment of pressure gradients across stenoses and septal defects are assessed with Doppler echocardiography. Precise timing of cardiac events and assessment of left ventricular function can be done with the older technique of single beam ultrasound ('M-mode' or movement-mode echocardiography).

Since it is now such a crucial aspect of pediatric cardiology, it is important to know of its indications, strengths and limitations. Some knowledge of cardiac anatomy is also necessary.

Further reading on topics discussed here can be obtained from *Echocardiography for the Neonatologist* (Skinner et al[211]) and *Echocardiography in Pediatric Heart Disease* (Snider & Serwer[212]).

CROSS-SECTIONAL (2D) ECHOCARDIOGRAPHY

Echocardiographers usually use a sector scan; the image that results is shaped like a section of a pie. This sector is built up of many individual lines of ultrasound, which sweep across the sector. Since the heart rate is high in pediatrics, the frame rate (the number of completed sectors per minute) needs to be high to avoid a jerky appearance to the heart movement. The best definition is achieved by using ultrasound with higher frequencies, but the higher the frequency, the poorer the tissue penetration. The best compromise between these two factors means a frequency of 8–12 MHz can be used for preterm infants with often extremely good image quality, but a frequency of 2–3 MHz is needed for the largest children and adults.

Echocardiographic windows

Since ultrasound cannot pass through the air within the lungs, the ultrasonic approach to the heart is through echocardiographic 'windows' where there is little or no air between the transducer and heart. These are subcostal, apical, parasternal and suprasternal, (see Figs 19.5 to 19.8). In the newborn there are large echo windows making imaging easier than in older children and adults, and it is often possible to do most of the scan subcostally.

Imaging axes

Since the heart lies at an angle within the chest, the apex pointing caudal and leftward, the 'standard' anatomical cuts (coronal, sagittal, etc.) are not used. Instead the scanning planes are related to the axis of the heart. There are three axes that form the majority of standard views. They correspond to the mathematical x, y and z axes and are at right angles to each other. They create the long axis, short axis and four chamber views. Examples from the normal infant's heart are shown in Figures 19.5 to 19.8.

Relating normal cardiac anatomy to the standard echocardiographic views

The four chamber views

The plane of this cut through the heart is parallel to the bed upon which the patient is lying. These views, from the apex or subcostal regions (Figs 19.5b and 19.6b), show that the ventricles are caudal and leftward of their corresponding atria. The most caudal valve in the heart is the tricuspid, which is attached to the septum closer to the cardiac apex than the mitral valve. This offsetting of the tricuspid valve (Fig. 19.6b) means that there is an atrioventricular septum dividing the left ventricle from the right atrium; this part of the septum is absent in atrioventricular septal defects. Since a tricuspid valve is always associated with a right ventricle, and a mitral valve with the left, this offsetting can be used to identify which ventricle is which in complex cases.

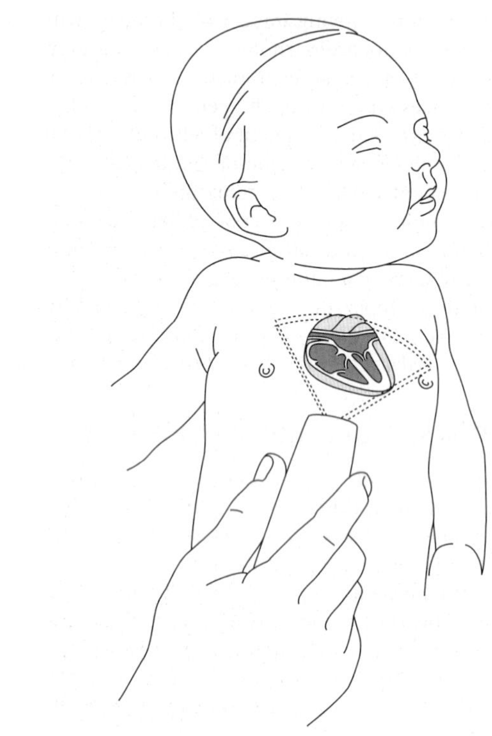

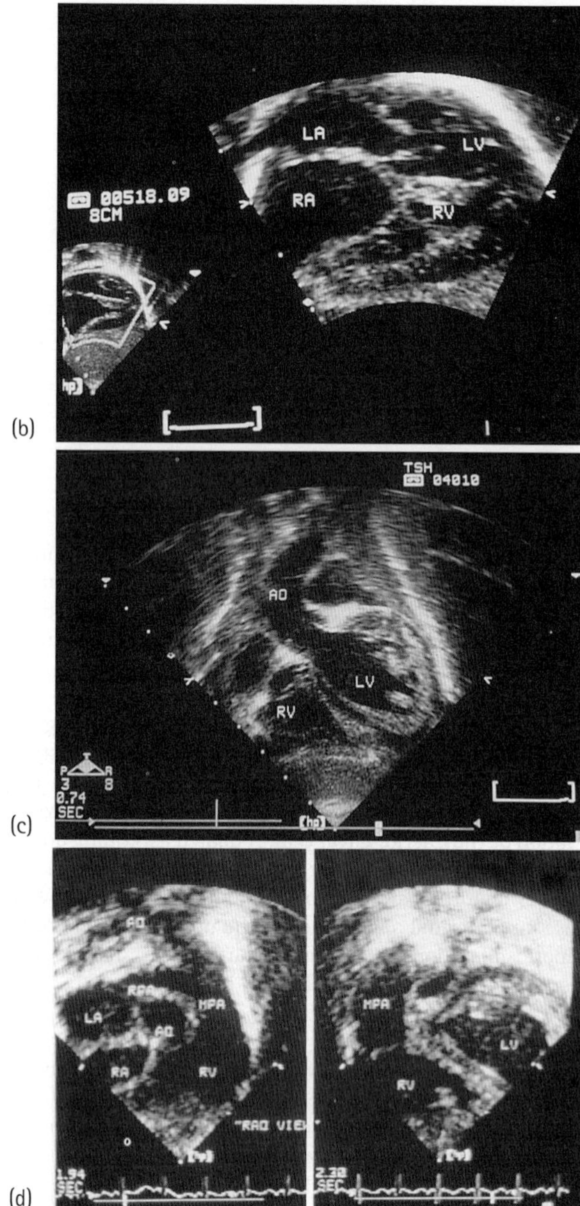

Fig. 19.5 (a) Diagram showing the position of the transducer and orientation of the scanning plane to provide a subcostal four-chamber image of the heart. (b) Subcostal four-chamber image demonstrating the four chambers. This is an ideal view to see atrial septal defects. (c) Tilting the probe anteriorly brings the ascending aorta into view. (d) Left: rotating anticlockwise brings the right ventricular outflow tract and pulmonary arteries into view (subcostal short-axis or 'RAO' (right anterior oblique) view). MPA, main pulmonary artery; RPA, right pulmonary artery. Right: rotating clockwise shows the interventricular septum and another view of the right ventricular outflow tract. These views are especially useful in tetralogy of Fallot to assess obstruction of the right ventricular outflow tract. (From Skinner et al 2000[212])

The atrial septum lies obliquely at 45° to the sagittal plane of the body and is best examined from the subcostal approach (Fig. 19.5b). On the other hand the ventricular septum curves in a complex way from a plane which is nearly sagittal, to one which is nearly coronal, separating respectively the inlet and outlet portions of the two ventricles. Because of this complex shape, the search for ventricular septal defects needs to include all the available views. There is also a tiny component of the septal wall which is not muscular and is known as the membranous septum, closely related to the tricuspid and aortic valves. It has atrioventricular and interventricular portions separated by the attachment of the septal leaflet of the tricuspid valve.

With posterior tilt of the probe in the four chamber planes, the entry of the pulmonary veins into the back of the left atrium can be seen, as can the coronary sinus running in the atrioventricular groove behind the left atrium and opening into the right atrium.

Short axis views

These cut through the heart like transverse slices through a green pepper, and can be obtained from the left parasternum (Fig. 19.7) or subcostally (Fig. 19.5d – left). They show that the right heart 'wraps' around the left heart. The right heart chambers are anterior to the left heart chambers. The left atrium is the most posterior cardiac chamber directly anterior to the esophagus at the bifurcation of the trachea, and has the pulmonary veins draining into the back of it. The right atrium is rightward and anterior, and the tricuspid valve is in a nearly vertical plane.

The aortic valve is seen to lie in a central position (Fig. 19.7d). The pulmonary valve lies anterior and cranially and the atrioventricular valves flank the posterior and caudal margins of the aortic valve. The pulmonary trunk comes from the anterior aspect of the heart, swings to the left side of the ascending aorta, heading posteriorly, bifurcating into the left and right pulmonary arteries. This posterior course of the main pulmonary artery explains why pulmonary valve stenotic murmurs are transmitted to the back.

Angling the short axis cut down towards the apex of the left ventricle brings first the mitral valve structures into view, gaping like a 'fish mouth' as the leaflets open and close (Fig. 19.7c). The cut nearer the apex shows that the mitral valve is tethered and

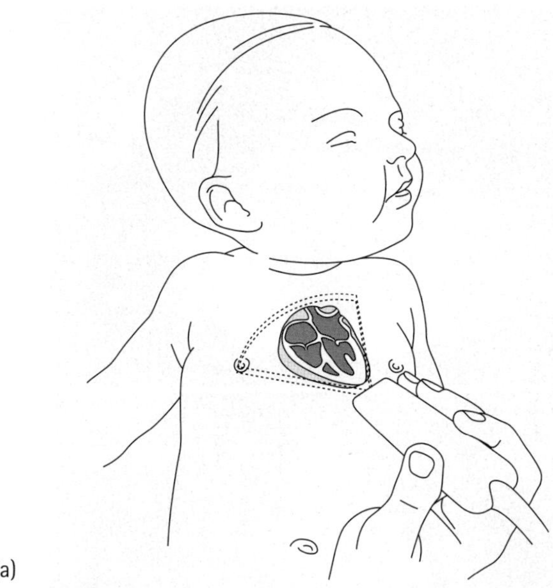

(a)

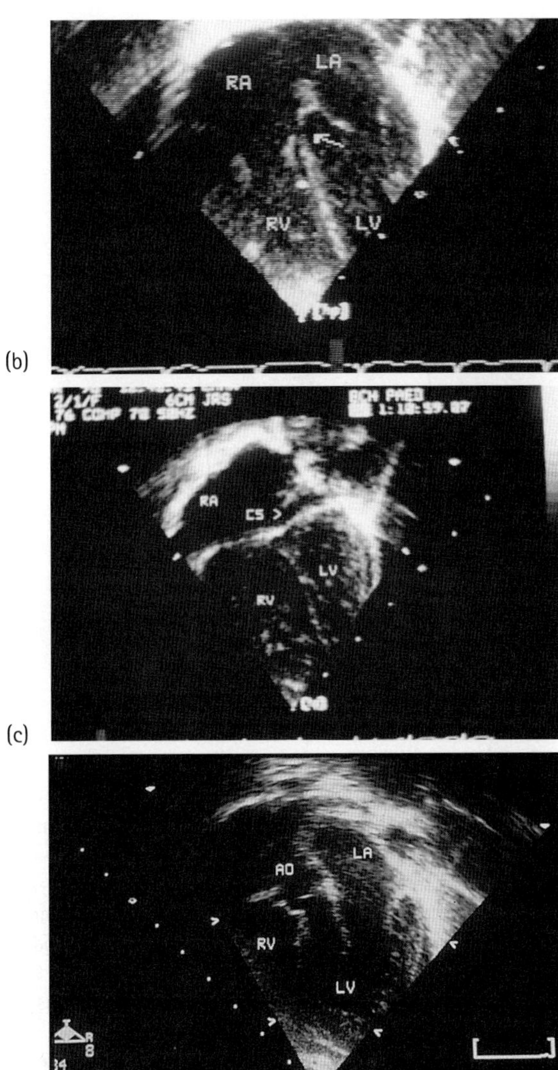

(b)

(c)

(d)

Fig. 19.6 (a) Diagram showing the position of the transducer and orientation of scanning plane to provide an apical four-chamber view of the heart. (b) Apical four-chamber echocardiogram. Note that the screen has been inverted. The arrow indicates the lower position of the tricuspid valve as it arises from the septum. This region between the two atrioventricular valves is known as the atrioventricular septum, dividing the left ventricle from the right atrium. (c) Apical view of the heart with the probe angled posteriorly to bring the coronary sinus (CS) into view (not to be confused with a low atrial septal defect!). (d) Apical view of the heart with the probe angled anteriorly and rotated to the right bringing the left ventricular outflow tract and aortic valve into view - this is an apical long-axis image. (From Skinner et al 2000[211])

supported by two groups of papillary muscles: the anterolateral and posteromedial groups (Fig. 19.7b).

Long axis views

These views (imagine a cut through the stalk and extending into a green pepper) can be obtained from the left parasternum (Fig. 19.8) or the apex (Fig. 19.6c). They show the relatively straight outflow from the left ventricle to the aorta (compare this to the angled outflow of the right ventricle seen in the short axis view). The anterior leaflet of the mitral valve is in fibrous continuity with the aortic valve, whereas there is a muscular infundulum between the tricuspid valve and the pulmonary valve. The ascending aorta passes superiorly, obliquely to the right and slightly forwards towards the sternum.

Suprasternal views

These views (Fig. 19.9) demonstrate the arch of the aorta which supplies origins to the brachiocephalic (innominate) artery and the left common carotid artery as it runs superiorly for a short distance before passing backwards and to the left. The arch finishes on the lateral aspect of the vertebral column after the origin of the left subclavian artery. Aortic coarctation most commonly appears just after this point.

NOMENCLATURE IN CONGENITAL HEART DISEASE

There is a trend to avoid eponyms and Latin terms in congenital heart disease because they may mislead and are confusing to non-specialists; 'solitus' doesn't mean solitary for instance, but 'usual'. 'Inversus' doesn't mean mirror imaged, it actually means 'upside down'. Another essential and helpful part of new cardiac anatomical nomenclature is 'sequential chamber localization' or 'sequential segmental analysis'[14] where congenital heart disease is characterized descriptively using anatomical and physiological terms in a sequential fashion.

SEQUENTIAL CHAMBER LOCALIZATION

If you wish to build a safe house, you first consolidate the foundation before proceeding to the subsequent floors. Taking the same approach to help understand and describe complex heart diseases, the floors, or segments, of the heart are the atria, the ventricular mass and the great arteries. The type of connection between each segment is also described. The possibilities for each segment are shown in Table 19.3.

Thus a normal heart has the usual atrial arrangement, atrioventricular concordance and ventriculo-arterial concordance.

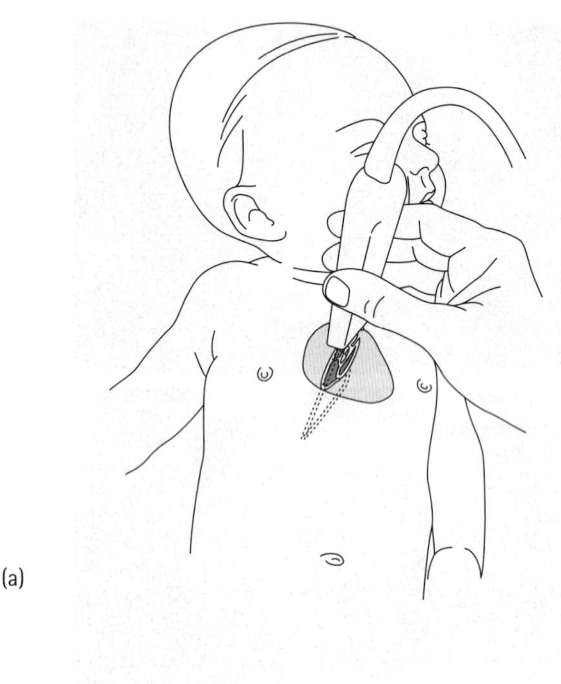

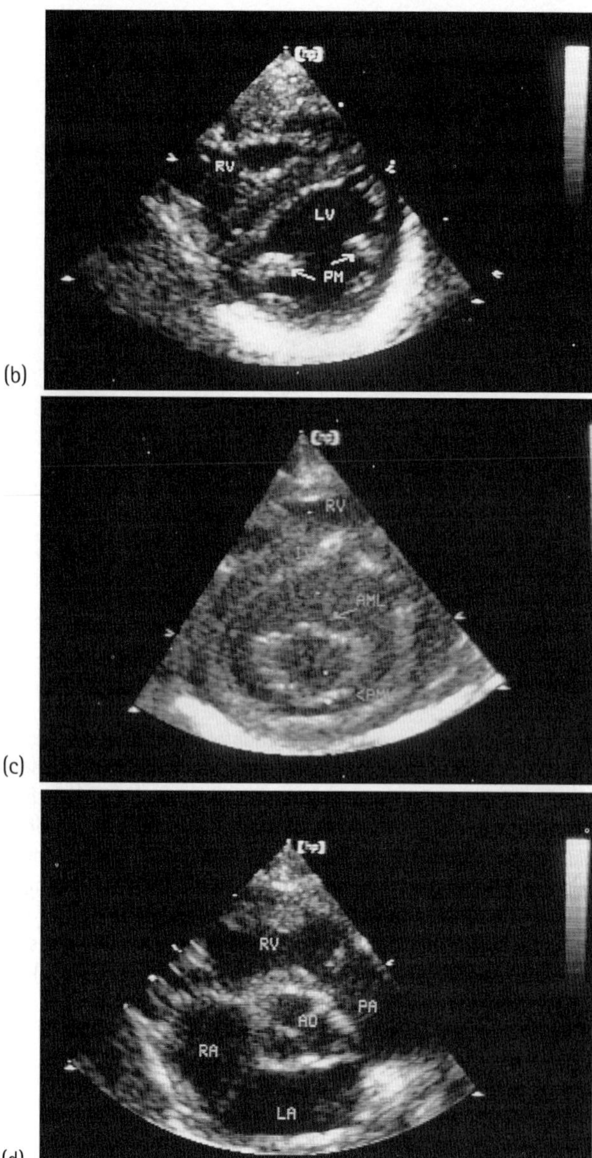

(a) (b) (c) (d)

Fig. 19.7 (a) Diagram showing the position of the transducer and orientation of the scanning plane to provide a parasternal short-axis image of the heart at the aortic valve level. (b) Parasternal short-axis echocardiograph at the level of the papillary muscles (towards the apex of the left ventricle). This image is used to obtain an M-mode cut through the left ventricle to assess left ventricular function (see text). (c) Tilting away from the apex (towards the right shoulder) brings this view of the mitral valve. AML, anterior mitral valve leaflet; PML, posterior mitral valve leaflet. (d) Further tilt shows this cut at the aortic valve (as in (a)). Note here how three aortic valve leaflets are seen, and how the right heart wraps around the aorta. Tilting the probe further still away from the apex demonstrates the pulmonary artery bifurcation. (From Skinner et al 2000[212])

A cyanosed newborn with transposed great arteries has isolated ventriculo-arterial discordance. The condition formally known as 'congenital corrected transposition' is now described as atrioventricular discordance with ventriculo-arterial discordance. The infant is not cyanosed, but the morphological right ventricle is the systemic ventricle. Most pediatric cardiologists start scanning from venous inflow and end with arterial outflow noting abnormalities along the way. In general this means starting with subcostal views and ending with the suprasternal views.

Venous inflow and the atria

In the transverse abdominal cut, the inferior caval vein is normally to the right and the aorta to the left. This is reversed when there is abdominal situs inversus (mirror image position). If the thoracic contents are also mirror imaged, the apex of the heart is seen pointing to the right. The incidence of congenital heart disease is not increased in such cases. It is, though, if only thoracic contents are mirror imaged. Totally anomalous pulmonary venous drainage is seen as failure of the pulmonary veins to connect to the back of the left atrium (Fig. 19.10).

The echocardiogram is not reliable in deciding on the atrial arrangement, since the appearances of the atrial appendages are the only totally reliable way of differentiating the atria and they are often not well seen. Fortunately the plain chest X-ray can help. The atria and lung always go together, thus a short bronchus on the right, on chest radiography, suggests a three-lobed right lung on that side with early branching, and a right atrium on the right. On the left, the bronchus is normally longer and bifurcates to supply a two-lobed lung indicating that the morphological left atrium lies in the left. Mirror imaging of the lungs will give a long bronchus on the right and a short one on the left. Two long bronchi means two left lungs and two short bronchi means two right lungs – left atrial isomerism and right atrial isomerism respectively. Atrial septal defects are best defined from the subcostal position.

Atrioventricular (AV) connection

The connection may be 'concordant' when right atrium leads to right ventricle and left atrium to left ventricle (Fig. 19.6b) or 'discordant' connection when right atrium leads to left ventricle and left atrium to right ventricle. A 'univentricular connection' occurs

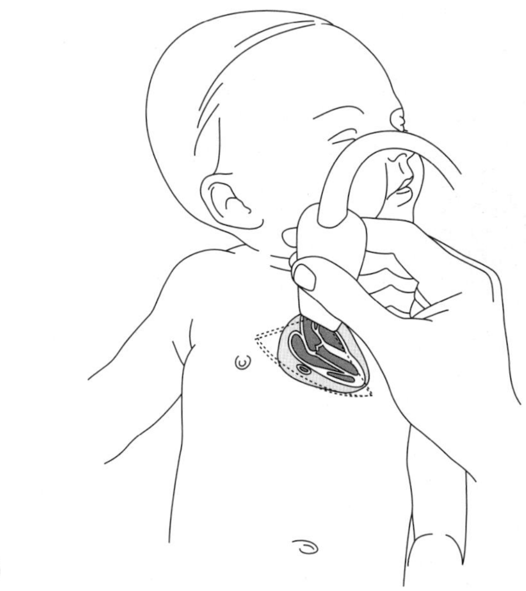

(a)

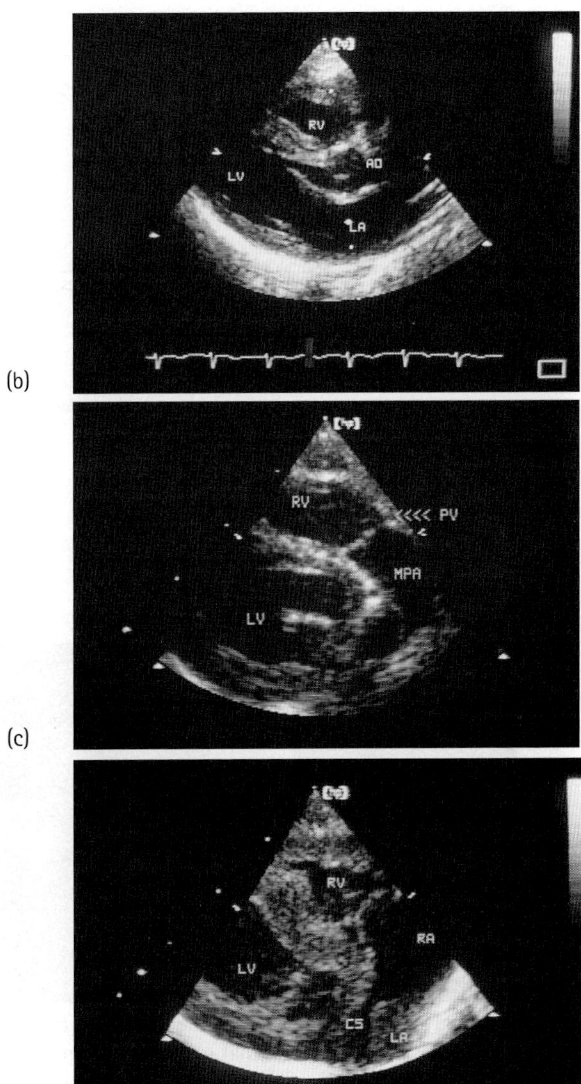

(b)

(c)

(d)

Fig 19.8 (a) Diagram showing the position of the transducer and orientation of scanning plane to provide a parasternal long-axis image of the heart. (b) Echocardiogram showing a standard parasternal long-axis image of the heart, ideal for demonstrating the left heart. The mitral valve is widely open in this diastolic frame. Ao, aorta; LV, left ventricle; RV, right ventricle. (c) Tilting towards the left shoulder reveals a long-axis view of the main pulmonary artery (MPA) and pulmonary valve (PV). (d) Tilting to the right, away from the left shoulder, reveals the tricuspid valve between the right atrium (RA) and right ventricle (RV). The coronary sinus (CS) is seen draining into the right atrium. LA, left atrium. (From Skinner et al 2000[212])

when both atria drain into one ventricle, either a double inlet left or right ventricle (Fig. 19.10). There is another form of univentricular connection where either the right or left connection is absent, either mitral or tricuspid atresia (Fig. 19.10) ('absent left' or 'absent right AV connection' respectively). In the presence of atrial isomerism, the atrioventricular connection is of necessity 'ambiguous' as it cannot be either truly concordant or discordant.

Ventricles

To define atrioventricular concordance the ventricles need to be positively identified, not by position (since a morphological right ventricle can be on the left for example), but by morphology. If there are two ventricles in the heart, the tricuspid valve is always in the right ventricle and the mitral always in the left ventricle. The atrioventricular valve anatomy is, therefore, the most reliable way of identifying the ventricle.

The right ventricle is identified by its heavy trabeculation, a muscular 'moderator band' across its apex, an infundibulum (muscular section dividing inlet from outlet) and a tricuspid valve which attaches directly to the septum and inserts more apically than the mitral valve. The left ventricle in contrast has finer trabeculations, no infundibulum and the mitral valve attached to (usually) two papillary muscles but never attached to the septum.

One or other of the ventricles may be small or even absent. Patients with double inlet left ventricle usually have a small anterior right ventricle connected to the main chamber by a ventricular septal defect and leading to a great artery, frequently the aorta. Very occasionally there are truly single ventricle hearts. Double inlet right ventricles with smaller posterior left ventricles are excessively rare.

Practical points:

- *Characteristic morphological features, identifiable on echocardiography, help to differentiate the right from the left ventricle in complex congenital heart disease.*
- *The tricuspid valve is always associated with the morphological right ventricle, is supported in part from the septum, is not in fibrous continuity with the outlet valve and arises from further down the septum than the mitral valve.*
- *The mitral valve is in fibrous continuity with the outlet valve, has no support from the septum and is always associated with the morphological left ventricle.*

Ventriculo-arterial connections

The aorta is identified by not branching early and having the coronary arteries arising from it. The pulmonary artery bifurcates

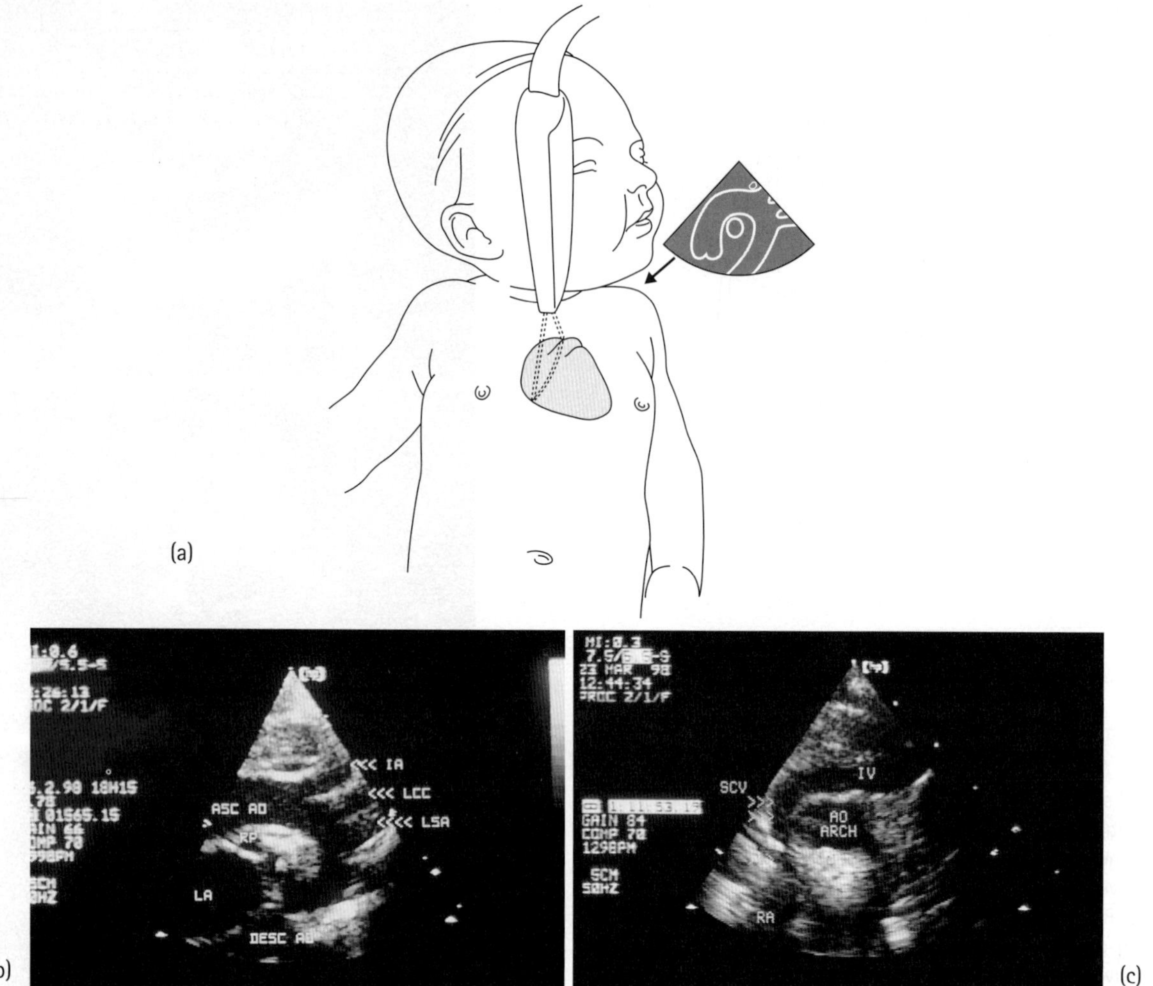

Fig. 19.9 (a) Diagram showing the position of the transducer and orientation of the scanning plane required to obtain views of the aortic arch with a conventional left-sided aorta. Note that a roll has been placed behind the shoulders to extend the neck. (b) Image of the aortic arch and branches obtained from the suprasternal window. IA, innominate artery (or right brachiocephalic artery); LCC, left common carotid artery; LSA, left subclavian artery. Arch interruptions and coarctations are best viewed like this. (c) With a transverse scanning plane, the innominate vein (IV) drains to the superior caval vein (SCV). (From Skinner et al 2000[212])

early into two branches. The connection can be 'concordant' when the right ventricle leads to the pulmonary artery and left ventricle to the aorta or 'discordant' when the right ventricle leads to aorta and left ventricle to pulmonary artery (also known as complete transposition) (Fig. 19.10). 'Double outlet' can be present from either right or left ventricle and 'single outlets' of the heart describe pulmonary atresia, aortic atresia and common arterial trunk.

Having completed the diagnostic process thus far, it remains to identify the associated lesions such as ventricular septal defects and atrial septal defects, arterial valve stenosis, and abnormalities of the great arteries such as a patent arterial duct or aortic coarctation.

DOPPLER ECHOCARDIOGRAPHY

The speed of blood flow can be determined by the Doppler shift created by moving red cells reflecting back ultrasound waves at a different frequency from that which was transmitted by the transducer/receiver. If our brains were programmed like an echocardiography machine, we would be able to determine the speed of an ambulance, with siren blazing, by the increase in pitch as it raced towards us.

The speed of blood flow calculated is, of course, relative to the transducer/receiver and blood flowing at 90° will cause no frequency shift. It is therefore essential to align with flow to determine the true speed. From blood flow velocity it is possible to derive volume of blood flow (cardiac output), and pressure gradients (see below). There are three modes of Doppler ultrasound, pulsed-wave, continuous wave and color Doppler.

Pulsed-wave Doppler ultrasound

Low velocities can be sampled in discrete positions around the heart using pulsed-wave Doppler ultrasound – a small sampling gate can be superimposed on the imaging screen. The receiver only listens for its transmitted pulse when it expects the sound waves to have returned (according to the speed of sound and the distance away).

High velocities cannot be measured reliably with pulsed-wave Doppler due to a problem relating to the sampling frequency needing to be at least half the wavelength of the frequency shift (the Nyquist limit). Instead, high velocities are measured with continuous wave Doppler ultrasound.

Continuous wave Doppler ultrasound

This form of Doppler ultrasound continuously sends and receives its signals. It is not subject to the Nyquist limit and can measure very high velocities accurately. However, since it receives signals

Table 19.3 Possible sequential segmental arrangements in congenital heart disease

Segment	Possibilities	Examples/comments
Great veins	Describe abnormalities of position and connection	e.g. anomalous pulmonary venous drainage, left superior caval vein connecting to coronary sinus
Atria	Usual arrangement	
	Mirror image (left atrium on the right side)	'Situs inversus'
	Two right atria (right atrial isomerism); asplenia is common, pulmonary veins connect abnormally	
	Two left atria (left atrial isomerism), often no inferior caval vein present	
Atrioventricular connection	Concordant (RA-RV, LA-LV)	
	Discordant (RA-LV, LA-RV)	
	Ambiguous (if the two atria are the same morphology)	
	Absent right connection	e.g. tricuspid atresia
	Absent left connection	e.g. mitral atresia
	Double inlet	
Ventricular mass	Two ventricles (biventricular connection)	
	'Single' ventricle (univentricular connection):	
	LV with a rudimentary RV,	This is the most common form
	RV with rudimentary LV,	Very rare
	solitary indeterminate ventricle	
Ventriculo-arterial connection	Concordant (RV-PA, LV-Aorta)	
	Discordant (RV-Aorta, LV-PA)	
	Double outlet	Most common is double outlet RV,
	Single outlet	e.g. common arterial trunk, pulmonary atresia
Great arteries	Describe abnormalities	e.g. patent arterial duct, aortic coarctation, branch pulmonary artery stenosis

LA, left atrium; LV, left ventricle; PA, pulmonary artery; RA, right atrium; RV, right ventricle

back from all along its course, and not at one particular depth, care has to be taken not to be confused by high velocities coming from a valve or vessel further away or closer than that being imaged. An example of a high velocity is shown in Figure 19.11.

Color Doppler ultrasound

This is created by the computerized ultrasound machine placing hundreds of pulsed-wave Doppler sample gates all over the cardiac chamber, and color coding the speed and direction at that point. For example, red and yellow are slow and fast towards the probe respectively, and blue and green are slow and fast away from the probe. Areas of turbulence and high velocity are shown by a mosaic pattern with the colours all jumbled up together. This technique is especially useful in detecting ventricular septal defects, valvar or arterial stenosis, or regurgitation (Fig. 19.11).

Determination of pressure gradient

The simplified Bernoulli equation can be used to estimate pressure drop across a stenosis, across a shunt lesion such as a ventricular septal defect, or across a regurgitant valve, from the peak velocity measured with continuous wave Doppler:

$$P_1 - P_2 = 4V^2$$

Where $(P_1 - P_2)$ is the pressure drop across the obstruction (mmHg) and V is the peak velocity (m/sec). It is imperative that the Doppler beam is in line with flow, to avoid underestimation of the peak velocity.

Valvar stenosis

This technique means that cardiac catheterization is no longer needed to determine pressure gradients across valves. However it has been found that the Doppler gradient is consistently higher than that measured at catheterization. This is because the Doppler gradient is the maximal instantaneous pressure gradient (the largest difference before and after the stenosis at any time in the cardiac cycle), whereas catheter gradients are expressed as the peak to peak gradient (the difference between the highest pressure before and the highest pressure after the stenosis).

Pulmonary arterial (PA) pressure

Pulmonary arterial pressure can be estimated by determining the pressure drop between the right ventricle (RV) and the right atrium (RA) by measuring peak velocity of tricuspid regurgitation (TR).

$$\text{Thus RV systolic pressure} = 4 \times \text{TR jet velocity}^2 + \text{RA pressure}$$

Right ventricular systolic pressure approximates to pulmonary arterial systolic pressure (if the pulmonary valve is not stenotic); right atrial pressure varies little and can in most circumstances be assumed to be 5 or 10 mmHg. The technique is remarkably accurate at all ages and is valuable, because of the high incidence of trivial or mild tricuspid regurgitation in many congenital heart diseases and in the normal population. Pulmonary artery pressure can also be estimated by measuring the peak velocity across a ventricular septal defect, or an arterial duct.

Determination of cardiac output

It is possible to determine left and right ventricular output reasonably reliably in the absence of turbulence in either outflow tract. Cardiac output is equal to stroke volume × heart rate. Left ventricular stroke volume (LVO) is determined by multiplying the flow velocity integral at the aortic valve (measured with Doppler) and the cross-sectional area of the aortic valve (AoCSA) (determined from the valve diameter measured with cross-sectional

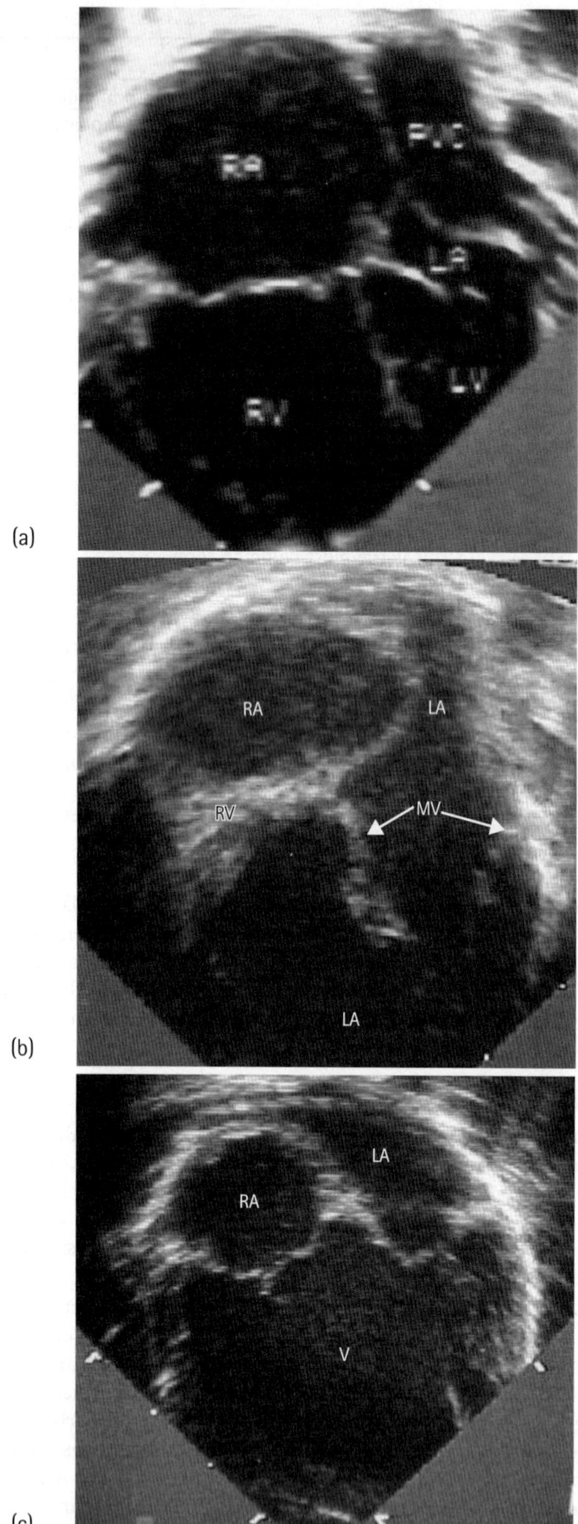

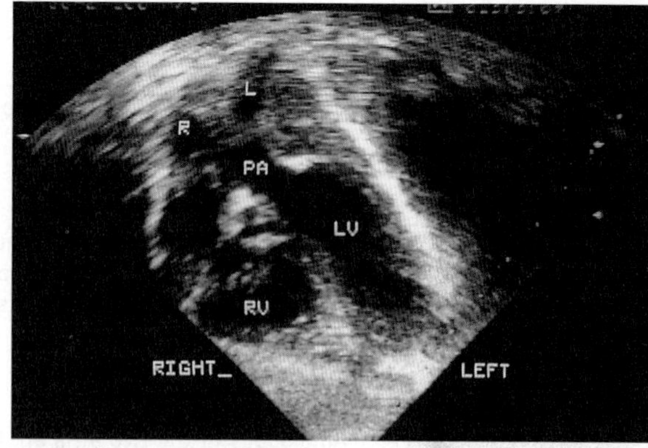

Fig. 19.10 Echocardiographic images in children with abnormal connections. LA, left atrium, RA right atrium. (a) Totally anomalous pulmonary venous drainage. The pulmonary veins drain into a pulmonary venous chamber (PVC) which does not communicate with the left atrium. (b) Absent right atrioventricular connection (tricuspid atresia). The diminutive right ventricle is hardly visible. The interatrial septum bows across to the left, since in this case, the atrial septal defect was restrictive. MV, mitral valve. (c) Double inlet ventricle. Both atrioventricular valves enter into a single large ventricle (V). (d) Ventriculo-arterial discordance. The left ventricle connects with an artery that bifurcates early and is hence the pulmonary artery (PA). This infant was cyanosed due to transposition of the great arteries. (From Skinner et al 2000[212])

echocardiography). The flow velocity integral is the area under the velocity curve, and is often known as the 'stroke distance' (AoSD), since it represents the distance the column of blood ascends the aorta in systole.

$$\text{LV stroke volume (cc)} = \text{AoSD (cm)} \times \text{AoCSA (cm}^2\text{)}$$
$$\text{LV cardiac output (cc/min)} = \text{AoSD (cm)} \times \text{AoCSA (cm}^2\text{)} \times \text{heart rate}$$

It is usual in cardiology to represent ventricular output as an index in relation to body surface area (liters/min/m^2). The technique is of major research interest, especially in intensive care, but is not widely used in pediatric cardiology, largely due to concerns of repeatability error in measurements.

Assessment of valvular regurgitation

Color Doppler is of immense value in assessing regurgitation at all of the valves, but the assessment is subjective and not precisely quantifiable. Other semi-quantitative measurements are added to a visual assessment of the color jet. The more severe the regurgitation, the wider the color jet at the valve. The method is much more sensitive than auscultation. Trivial valvar regurgitation can be seen at all of the valves, except the aortic valve, very commonly, in normal subjects. Severe atrioventricular valve regurgitation is associated with the respective atrium being dilated and reverse flow being detected in the caval veins or pulmonary veins. Severe aortic or pulmonary valve regurgitation leads to dilatation of the right or left ventricle, and reverse flow in the distal pulmonary arteries, or the descending aorta, respectively.

Assessment of ventricular function

Right ventricle

Surprising though it may seem, subjective visual assessment of ventricular function from cross-sectional images (normal, hyperdynamic, mild, moderate or severely depressed), is still the best that can be done when assessing right ventricular function. This is because of the complex shape of the right ventricle, and the difficulty in obtaining repeatable measurements and useful mathematical algorithms.

Left ventricle

The left ventricle is shaped rather like a French rugby football, and is more amenable to mathematical algorithms to determine ejection fraction. However, the single most useful and repeatable technique

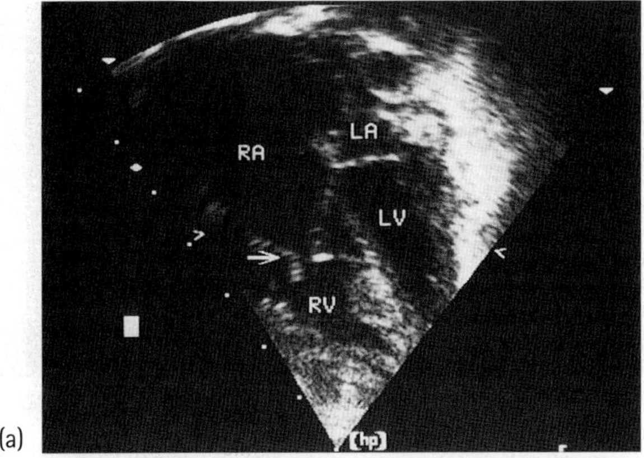

(a)

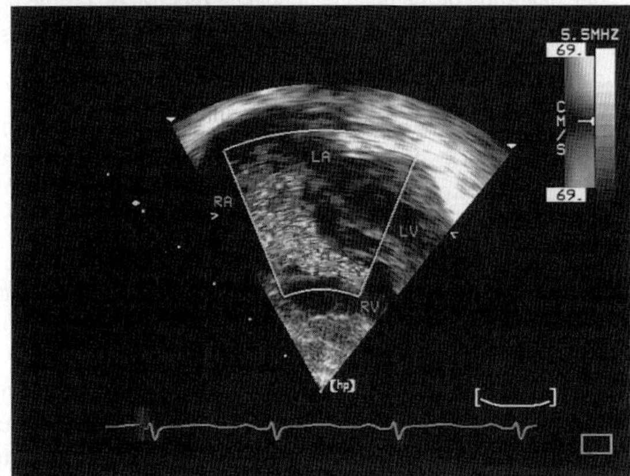

(b)

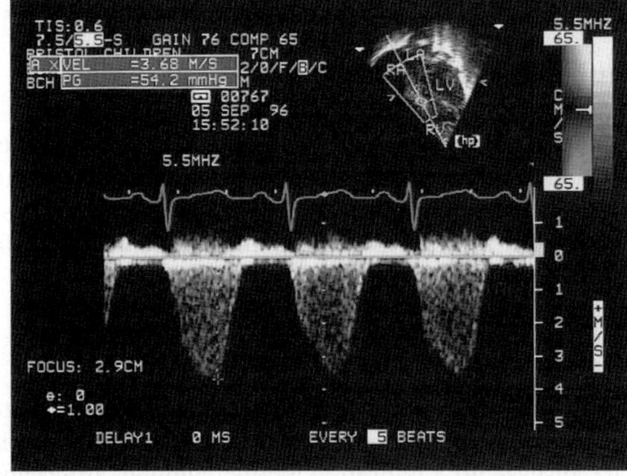

(c)

Fig. 19.11 This example of severe tricuspid regurgitation in a newborn infant demonstrates how several features of echocardiography can be put together in assessing a lesion. (a) The cross-sectional image shows that the tips of the tricuspid valve leaflets do not touch ('coapt') in systole, leaving a large hole for regurgitation. The right atrium (RA) is very dilated. (b) The colour Doppler jet (reproduced here in black and white) shows that the regurgitant jet is wide – the width of the jet helps differentiate grades of severity. (c) The velocity of the jet (3.68 m/sec) is high. When the simplified Bernoulli equation (P = 4V2) is applied to this velocity, the systolic RV-RA pressure drop is 54.2 mmHg. To obtain systolic pulmonary arterial pressure a RA estimate of 10 mmHg is added to the RV-RA pressure drop, so that PA systolic pressure is approximately 64 mmHg. There was significant pulmonary arterial hypertension – near to the aortic pressure in this infant of 80 mmHg at the time. As the pulmonary hypertension resolved the regurgitant jet velocity decreased; it was 2.4 m/sec the next day, though the degree of regurgitation remained severe. (From Skinner et al 2000[212])

avoids such complex formulae and employs M-mode echocardiography to measure the *fractional shortening* (FS) or percentage reduction of the left ventricular diameter in systole. Thus:

$$\text{FS (\%)} = \frac{\text{LV diastolic dimension} - \text{LV systolic dimension} \times 100}{\text{LV diastolic dimension}}$$

The normal value lies between 28 and 44%, is reduced with poor myocardial function, and increased with volume overload, such as with a left-to-right shunt through a ventricular septal defect or arterial duct. The measurements are made just beyond the tips of the mitral valve, from the parasternal position, and accurate measurements of septal and posterior wall thickness can be made in assessing ventricular hypertrophy (Fig. 19.12).

CARDIAC CATHETERIZATION

Diagnostic cardiac catheterization and angiocardiography are undertaken to obtain detailed information on the anatomical abnormality and its hemodynamic effects. The indications for diagnostic catheterization have changed with the widespread availability of high-resolution echocardiography. With hemodynamic information from spectral Doppler studies and color Doppler mapping to assist in shunt detection, most congenital heart disease can be diagnosed and managed using echocardiography alone.[15] Angiography remains useful for coronary and distal pulmonary artery imaging, and clarification of more complex arterial or venous abnormalities. Additional hemodynamic information may be obtained in the assessment of pulmonary vascular disease, measurement of left ventricular end diastolic pressure, and for accurate shunt calculations.[16] The arterial oxygen saturation gives an estimate of the severity of cyanotic congenital heart disease. Catheterization should be undertaken with a clear knowledge of echocardiographic and previous catheterization studies. It is usually performed under general anesthesia, although occasionally procedures in infants and adolescents may be undertaken with local anesthesia and sedation. The approach is generally percutaneous through the femoral vessels, although the brachial, axillary or internal jugular routes are occasionally used. Arterial catheterization can frequently be avoided since the venous catheter may be passed into the left side of the heart through an atrial or ventricular septal defect. An atrial septostomy can be performed through the umbilical vein in the first few days of life, but thereafter it becomes difficult to pass the catheter through the ductus venosus.[17] The catheter course is of limited diagnostic value but, with angiography, may be important in establishing abnormal venous connections.

Calculating the left-to-right shunt

The oxygen saturation is measured in the large veins, atria, ventricles and great arteries. A significant left-to-right shunt is suggested by a rise in oxygen saturation of 5% or more in the right atrium (atrial septal defect), right ventricle (ventricular septal defect) or pulmonary artery (persistent arterial duct). Systemic and pulmonary output can be calculated from the Fick principle[16] and the pulmonary to systemic flow ratio (Qp:Qs) is calculated from the oxygen saturation values in the aorta (Ao), pulmonary artery (PA), left atrium (LA) and the mixed venous saturation (MV) from the formula:

$$\text{Qp}:\text{Qs} = \frac{\text{Ao} - \text{MV}}{\text{LA} - \text{PA}}$$

While these figures give results sufficiently accurate for clinical management, they are not absolute values and will vary with

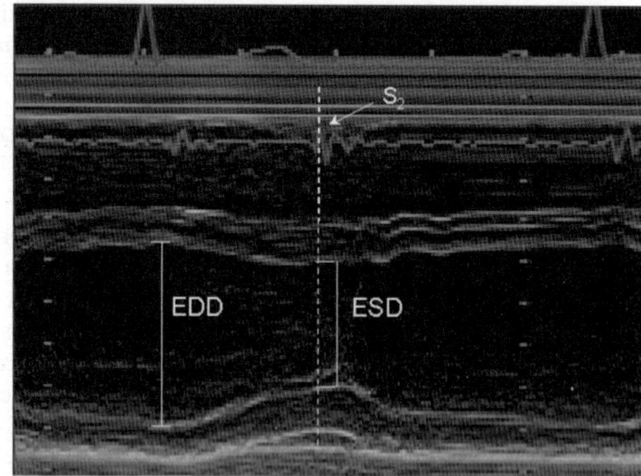

(a)

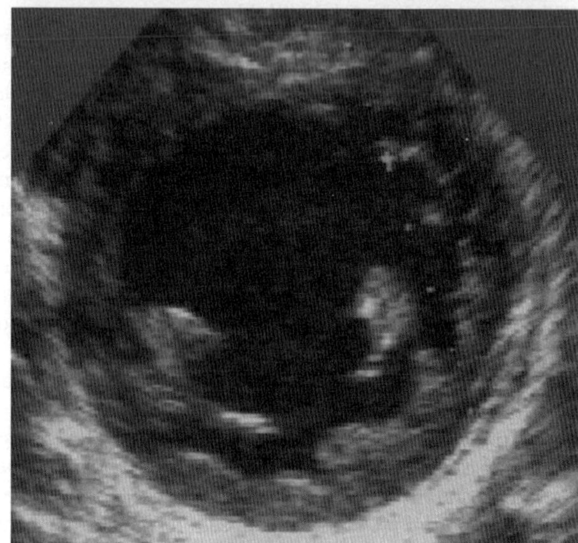

(b)

Fig. 19.12 The M-mode images across the short axis of the left ventricle (a) with the cross-sectional image (b) showing the position from which the M-mode image is derived. Fractional shortening is calculated as end diastolic diameter (EDD) – end systolic diameter (ESD) divided by end diastolic diameter × 100.

time and hemodynamic status. A shunt ratio of more than 1.8:1 is likely to require intervention, whereas one of less than 1.5:1 is insignificant.

Pressure gradients

Pressures are measured in the atria, ventricles and great arteries. Peak pressures in the ventricles and arteries measure transvalvar or arterial gradients. In children, the valve gradient rather than valve area is generally used in deciding on the need for intervention. Pressure gradients show considerable variation with time or sedation. Consideration must be given to whether the need for intervention should be based on a Doppler measurement with the patient awake rather than a lower one obtained at catheterization with the child sedated or anesthetized.

Pulmonary vascular resistance

The mean pressure in the atria and great arteries is required for estimation of pulmonary and systemic vascular resistance, which are indexed for body surface area.[16] The pulmonary vascular resistance, rather than the pulmonary artery pressure, is the main determinant of the prognosis and the operability of a child with a lef-to-right shunt. When it is elevated, it is appropriate to assess whether it is fixed, or can be reduced by the administration of a pulmonary vasodilator such as 100% oxygen or nitric oxide,[16] at the time of the catheter procedure.

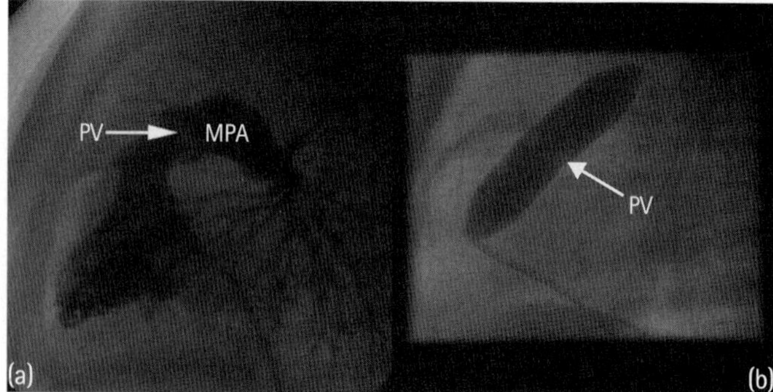

Fig 19.13 (a) Right ventricular (RV) angiogram of a child with pulmonary valve stenosis showing a thickened pulmonary valve (PV) and post-stenotic dilatation of the main pulmonary artery (MPA). (b) The balloon catheter is inflated across the valve resulting in relief of the stenosis.

Angiography

Angiography is performed by the injection of radiological contrast into the chamber or vessel immediately proximal to the abnormality, e.g. left ventricle for ventricular septal defect, right ventricle for pulmonary stenosis (Fig. 19.13), ascending aorta for coarctation. Angiography is now less important for the definition of intracardiac defects, but remains necessary for abnormalities of the great arteries or veins, in particular the anatomy of the pulmonary arteries, when they are reduced in size.

Complications

Although cardiac catheterization is a relatively safe procedure, death can occur, most commonly in patients with severe pulmonary hypertension. Complications include femoral artery occlusion, hemorrhage (from cardiac structures or traversed vessels), arrhythmias, intramyocardial injection with pericardial effusion and cerebral embolism.

INTERVENTIONAL CATHETERIZATION

More than half of all pediatric catheterization is now related to interventional procedures and is a crucial part of the management of heart disease in children.[18] Many complex interventions require imaging, using both radiographic and ultrasound (usually transesophageal) imaging and are performed by trained interventional cardiologists. Balloon atrial septostomy (Fig. 19.14) was the first reported pediatric interventional catheter procedure.[19] It remains life saving for infants with inadequate cardiac mixing, as in transposition of the great arteries, and can be performed using either ultrasound or radiographic imaging.

Balloon valvuloplasty is now the accepted treatment for pulmonary valve stenosis.[20] It is safe and effective (except where there is severe valve dysplasia) and can be performed at any age (Fig. 19.13). Aortic balloon valvuloplasty is an alternative to surgery,[21] in the absence of significant regurgitation. The results are comparable,[18] but both are palliative, and progression occurs. Balloon dilatation does not appear to be effective in the treatment of coarctation in neonates[22] and there is a debate regarding its use in infants and young children who have not had previous surgery.[23] In older children and young adults the risks of surgery for coarctation are greater, and transcatheter treatment may be preferable and

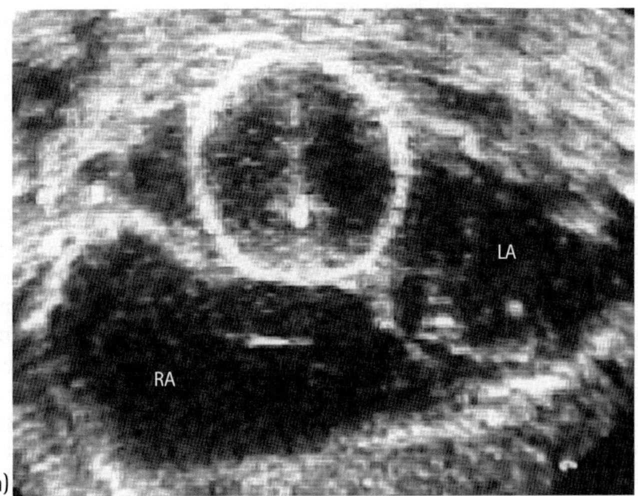

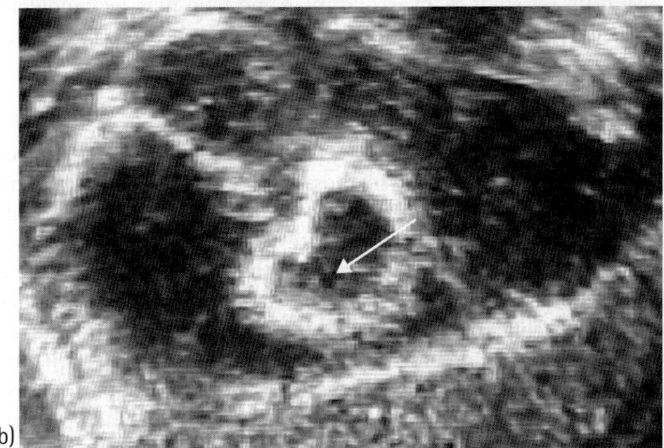

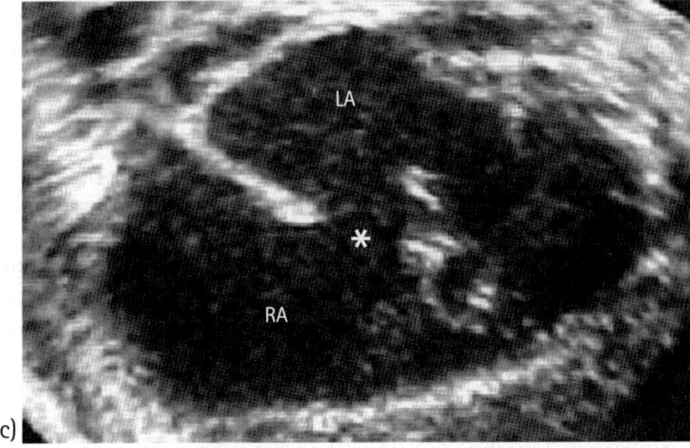

Fig. 19.14 Balloon atrial septostomy using echocardiographic imaging. A balloon septostomy catheter is advanced from the umbilical or femoral vein into the right atrium and across into the left atrium (a). The balloon is inflated in the left atrium and pulled across the atrial septum (b). (c) The atrial septal defect created is identified with the asterisk. LA, left atrium; RA, right atrium.

equally effective.[22] Balloon dilatation is the treatment of choice for most residual or recurrent coarctation following surgery.[24] Balloon expandable metallic stents are used for treatment of both recurrent and native coarctation, in older adolescents and adults, in an attempt to produce more 'permanent' results and reduce the risk of aortic rupture or aneurysm formation.[25] Objective evidence for this is limited and there are concerns regarding the use of stents in young children, because growth will not occur.[24]

Interventional cardiology can be of value for patients with a wide variety of vessel narrowing. In smaller children, balloon dilatation alone is usually performed, but in older children and adolescents, stent placement, although technically challenging, may provide more effective and longer lasting relief of stenoses.[26] These are usually placed percutaneously, but in smaller children, they can be positioned intraoperatively.[27] Radiofrequency energy can be applied to intravascular tissues, using specially designed catheters to ablate arrhythmic substrates and to perforate occluded valves or vessels to allow subsequent balloon dilatation. This is now frequently performed for relief of valvar pulmonary atresia.

Closure of the persistent arterial duct with a coil or device is now the procedure of choice for patients weighing over 5 kg.[18,28] Closure of more than 50% of atrial septal defects[29] is possible with one of a variety of devices. The surgical approach is still required for some anatomical variants, for very large defects or from parental and patient choice. Although the vast majority of hemodynamically significant ventricular septal defects still require surgical closure, transcatheter devices are available for muscular defects that are difficult to close surgically.[18] A wide variety of devices are used to occlude venous collaterals, residual surgical shunts, coronary artery and arteriovenous fistulae. Close collaboration is required between cardiologists and surgeons, with detailed knowledge of anatomy and high quality imaging a prerequisite. Multiple procedures are sometimes required, which raises the issue of radiation dosage.

OTHER CARDIAC INVESTIGATIONS

MAGNETIC RESONANCE IMAGING

Magnetic resonance imaging has become more widely available in recent years. With improvements in imaging quality and acquisition times it is increasingly used for the imaging and assessment of congenital heart disease particularly in complex cases and in older children.[30] It is particularly suitable for imaging the aortic arch (Fig. 19.15), peripheral pulmonary vasculature, and the atrioventricular junction. All images must be gated to the cardiac cycle and preferably also performed during 'breath-holding' to minimize respiratory artifact. To obtain optimal image quality, the child must either be old enough to cooperate fully with the examination or ventilated under general anesthesia. This requires non-ferromagnetically active equipment and adds substantially to costs.[30] Children with pacemakers and some intravascular devices should not undergo magnetic resonance imaging.

RADIONUCLIDE ANGIOGRAPHY

Lung perfusion scanning is particularly helpful in the assessment of children with complex pulmonary vascular abnormalities especially after surgical or catheter interventions. Although used in adult cardiac practice for the assessment of left ventricular function and regional myocardial perfusion, radionuclide scanning is less frequently performed in children. This is partly because echocardiographic imaging is generally of such high quality in children, and also because of the reluctance to expose children to ionizing radiation. However, there are occasions when it may be required (e.g. following Kawasaki coronary arteritis) and it is performed in the same way as in adults.

AMBULATORY ELECTROCARDIOGRAPHIC MONITORING

Continuous ambulatory 24-h electrocardiographic (Holter) monitoring is a well-established technique and assists in the

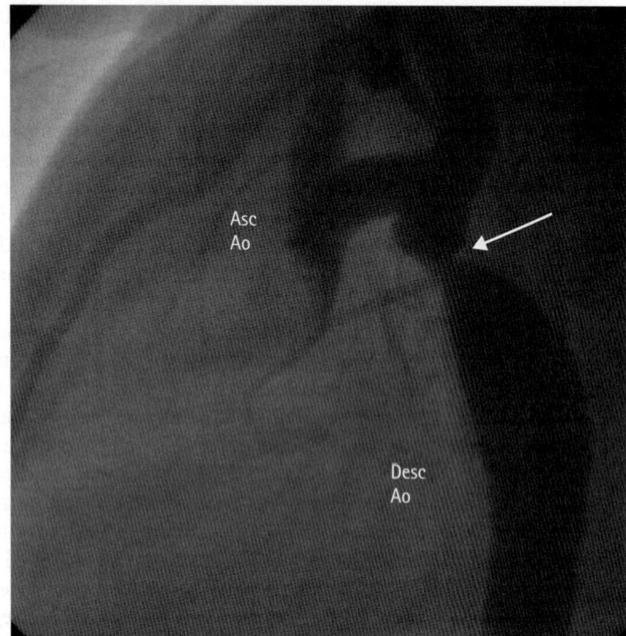

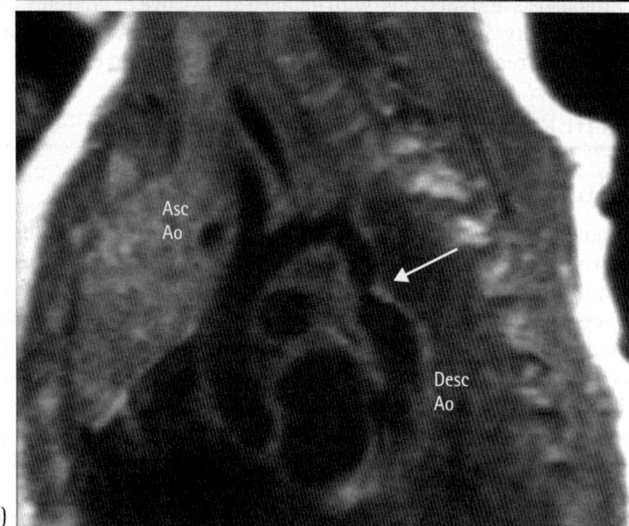

Fig. 19.15 Lateral projection of an aortogram (a) and magnetic resonance image (b) of coarctation of the aorta. The arrow indicates the coarctation. Asc Ao, ascending aorta; Desc Ao, descending aorta.

evaluation of transient events, bradycardia, certain incessant or paroxysmal tachycardia and those associated with symptoms such as syncope. The electrocardiogram is usually recorded continuously for 24 or 48 h and then scanned at high speed, either visually (60 times normal speed), or by computer, with a print-out of any irregularity. Two channel recordings are better than one and an event marker can be used to correlate symptoms with electrocardiographic events. This technique has clarified the variations in heart rate and rhythm that occur in normal healthy children. The heart rate may vary from 45 to 180/min and during sleep, may be as low as 30–70 beats/min.

Many rhythm disturbances occur very infrequently and the chance of detection from a single 24-h electrocardiographic recording may be small. An alternative is to provide the family with an event recorder. These are activated by the child or parent, when a symptom occurs. There are many different types, but most record a short strip in solid state memory. The record can then be played back and analyzed by transmitting it by telephone or returning it to the cardiac center. Another method of detecting infrequent but potentially serous arrhythmias is with an event or loop recorder that is implanted under the skin in the left upper chest.[31] This can be programmed to record significant pauses, bradycardia and tachycardia automatically.

ELECTROPHYSIOLOGICAL STUDIES

Symptomatic tachycardia may be further evaluated by intracardiac electrophysiological studies in which several electrode catheters are passed transvenously to the right side of the heart and intracardiac potentials are recorded from multiple sites, including the bundle of His. Simultaneous recordings of surface and intracardiac electrocardiograms help to determine more precisely the exact site of origin, delay, and direction of impulse conduction in complex arrhythmias. These techniques have their greatest value in defining the exact mechanism of tachycardia and may result in more appropriate therapy, particularly in children who have drug resistant tachyarrhythmias and who may be candidates for radiofrequency catheter ablation therapy of their arrhythmias.

EXERCISE TESTING

Exercise testing is increasingly used in pediatric cardiac practice. The techniques are similar to those used in adults, although end-points and levels of exercise achieved must be adjusted for age. Documentation of peak heart rate, level of exercise achieved and electrocardiographic changes can influence the timing of intervention or evaluate the efficacy of a procedure on effort tolerance. In cyanosed children, saturation monitoring during exercise provides additional information in these situations. Exercise testing can identify and evaluate exercise-related arrhythmias, clarify symptoms in more complex situations and is helpful in long QT syndrome. Measurement of blood pressure response to exercise is important in children following repair of coarctation.[32] Even quite small children can exercise on either the treadmill or a bicycle ergometer, but exercise telemetry or Holter monitoring can also obtain useful information.

HEAD-UP TILT TESTING

Syncope is a common problem in childhood, occurring in one in five adolescents.[31] Most have 'neurally mediated' syncope related to a disturbance of autonomic control of blood pressure and heart rate. This can sometimes usefully be differentiated from other causes of syncope by head-up tilt testing. Protocols vary but generally involve head-up tilting on a table with foot support to an angle of 60° for up to 45 min after an initial horizontal stabilization period. Continuous electrocardiogram and blood pressure monitoring (usually non-invasive) is performed. A positive response usually consists of hypotension and bradycardia before syncope. This provides an explanation for a child's symptoms and paves the way for more successful management.[31]

THE ASYMPTOMATIC CHILD WITH A MURMUR

The incidental finding of a murmur in an asymptomatic child is very common. The physician must decide whether the murmur is innocent, or if further investigation is required. If the murmur is pathological, it is likely that the child will need regular follow-up, antibiotic prophylaxis for dental and other surgical procedures, and possibly treatment for the condition in a specialized center. A careful history is essential but children with an innocent murmur may have unrelated symptoms. Innocent murmurs can be diagnosed accurately by their distinctive features. A thorough examination will identify clinical features that are likely to be associated with heart disease. It is much more common to diagnose an innocent murmur as pathological than to call a cardiac lesion innocent.[33]

INNOCENT MURMURS

Innocent murmurs are the most common murmurs in pediatric practice, occurring in over 30% of children.[34] They are usually heard between 6 weeks and 7 years of age but occur throughout childhood and adolescence. There are a variety of innocent murmurs. A small number of children have more than one – for example a vibratory systolic murmur and venous hum.

Vibratory (Still's) murmur

This accounts for the majority of innocent murmurs.[34] It is characterized by a short vibratory ejection systolic murmur maximal at the lower left sternal edge and radiating towards the base. It changes in intensity on sitting, and on extending the neck. The exact cause is unknown, but is likely to be due to vibration of structures within the ventricles. The differential diagnosis includes small muscular ventricular septal defect and mitral valve prolapse, but if the site of maximal intensity is not accurately defined, it may be confused with mild pulmonary or aortic stenosis or an atrial septal defect.

Pulmonary and aortic flow murmurs

These are soft ejection systolic murmurs maximal in the pulmonary or aortic areas, produced by increased flow across the outlet valves. The common causes are pyrexia, anemia and pregnancy. Review after the fever has subsided prevents referral of a child who no longer has a murmur. The differential diagnosis includes mild aortic or pulmonary stenosis or an atrial septal defect.

Venous hum

This is a continuous murmur maximal in the lower part of the neck and subclavicular area usually on the right. It is due to turbulence in large veins. It is loudest on sitting up and disappears on lying down, turning or lightly compressing the jugular vein in the neck. The differential diagnosis is a persistent arterial duct or arterio-venous fistula.

Features associated with heart disease in the asymptomatic child

McCrindle et al[35] identified a number of specific clinical features that are associated with heart disease. These included a murmur that is

- pansystolic
- grade 3 or more in intensity
- harsh in quality
- maximal at the left upper sternal border.

The presence of an abnormal second heart sound or a click is also an indication that the murmur is not innocent. Outside the neonatal period, a murmur heard in the back is usually pathological and diastolic murmurs are always abnormal. Palpation of the femoral pulses is essential. Other important clinical features that are more likely to indicate a cardiac lesion are feeding difficulties or failure to thrive in infants, dysmorphic features and non-cardiac lesions.

Investigation and management

A complete examination with careful auscultation by a trained clinician is the most useful method of diagnosing an innocent murmur. Chest radiography is likely to be misleading, invasive and unhelpful. An electrocardiogram may be useful in alerting the doctor to the possibility of an atrial septal defect, but may also be misleading. If the murmur is innocent, firm reassurance should be given and the child discharged. Parents should be told that the murmur might be heard intermittently for many years. They should also be reassured that the heart is normal.

If the murmur is not typical of an innocent murmur, or if other features suggest a cardiac lesion, the child should be referred to a pediatric cardiologist. Echocardiographic examination without assessment by a cardiologist is not appropriate as it can be misleading.[1] When a child is referred to a pediatric cardiologist, there is often an expectation that an echocardiogram will be carried out. Although it has been shown that this is usually unnecessary,[34] it may be done to allay fears and prevent the need for further review.

HEART FAILURE

Heart failure occurs when an inadequate amount of oxygen is delivered to the body's tissues, resulting in a series of physiological compensatory mechanisms. These include salt and water retention by the kidneys to increase preload, vasoconstriction through the renin/angiotensin axis to increase afterload and increased circulating catecholamines to increase cardiac output. These compensatory mechanisms will initially result in increased oxygen delivery to tissues, but if the underlying insult continues, these mechanisms overcompensate and heart failure develops.[36]

CLINICAL FEATURES

Heart failure is most frequently associated with congenital heart disease and usually occurs in the first few months of life. The commonest signs are tachycardia, tachypnea and hepatomegaly, the liver size providing an indication of its severity. An ill child will appear upset, fretful, restless and pale. Peripheral perfusion may be poor with a capillary refill time of greater than 3 seconds.

In infants, combined ventricular failure occurs, with the first manifestations usually resulting from pulmonary venous congestion. This produces tachypnea or dyspnea that is more marked on feeding. The association of stiff lung parenchyma with soft, flexible ribs may cause chest deformity with a deep anteroposterior diameter and flaring of the lower part of the rib cage. This combination produces the 'Harrison's sulcus': the name given to the trough which is created just above the lower ribs anteriorly. There may also be intercostal or subcostal indrawing during inspiration (recession). With marked respiratory distress there is an audible grunt and flaring of the alar nasi. Pulmonary edema must be differentiated from respiratory infection. Crepitations are not often heard in the chest and marked edema is rare although some facial puffiness or pitting of the dorsal surfaces of the hands or feet may develop. Pedal edema in the newborn is usually lymphedema associated with Turner's or Noonan syndrome. Sweating at rest and during feeding or exertion may develop, and chronic cardiac failure causes feeding difficulties. Initially, there may be weight gain as fluid is retained, but failure to thrive is seen later. Gallop rhythm and specific auscultatory signs of the cardiac abnormality causing failure may be detected.

Heart failure in older children is relatively uncommon. It usually results from acquired heart disease, and exhibits the clinical features of left or right heart failure as in the adult.

INVESTIGATIONS

Investigation of the child with cardiac failure should be directed at determining its cause. Electrocardiographic changes reflect the underlying diagnosis. Chest radiography usually shows cardiomegaly and plethoric lung fields due to increased flow or venous obstruction. Echocardiography provides information regarding the cardiac lesion and allows assessment of ventricular function.

MANAGEMENT

The treatment of heart failure is directed at maximizing oxygen delivery to tissues by improving myocardial function, reducing afterload and producing a diuresis.[37] Diuretics are the mainstay of treatment, the most widely used being the loop diuretic furosemide (frusemide), in a dose of 2–4 mg/kg/24 h. Potassium depletion may occur and either potassium supplementation or the concomitant administration of a potassium sparing diuretic (spironolactone or amiloride) should be given. Thiazide diuretics may also be used. Supplementary oxygen may be required and anemia should be treated. Digoxin is used principally for its positive inotropic effect, but it also reduces vascular tone. It can be of benefit where there is poor ventricular function, but it is of doubtful value in situations with volume overload, such as a ventricular septal defect.[38] A loading dose of digoxin (20–30 mcg/kg in premature neonates rising to 60–80 mcg/kg in infants) may be given over 24 h as four divided doses, followed by a daily maintenance dose (8–10 mcg/kg/day). Serum levels are of doubtful use, except to check compliance, or when toxicity is suspected.

Angiotensin converting enzyme (ACE) inhibitors (captopril or enalapril) are widely used in heart failure.[39] They prevent the conversion of angiotensin I to angiotensin II, and thus decrease vascular resistance and sodium and water retention. The reduction in vascular tone facilitates left ventricular function in cardiomyopathy and, in ventricular septal defect, reduces the left-to-right shunt by reducing the systemic, and thus left ventricular, pressure. It is recommended that the starting dose of captopril should be 0.1 mg/kg three times daily and this should be increased stepwise to a maximum of 1 mg/kg three times daily. Observation is required for possible hypotension immediately after the initial dose and after any increments.

In an intensive care setting, drug therapy with a number of other agents may be beneficial. Inotropic agents such as dopamine and dobutamine will increase cardiac function. Afterload can be reduced with vasodilators like nitroprusside. Phosphodiesterase inhibitors like milrinone not only have a potent vasodilator effect, but are also positive inotropes. Mechanical ventricular assist devices are now being developed that are small enough to be used in children.

The infant with chronic heart failure will often fail to thrive, so high calorie supplements should be added to the feeds and nasogastric tube feeding is often required. Cardiac failure is often the result of an anatomical abnormality and if the infant does not improve and surgery is available, it is not usually appropriate to persist with medical treatment. Surgical repair or palliation should be undertaken early rather than delay and risk deterioration in the infant's condition. If repair or palliation is not an option the child should be assessed for cardiac transplantation.

INFECTIVE ENDOCARDITIS

Infective endocarditis is rare with an incidence of approximately 4 per 100 000 person-years.[40] It is usually superimposed on underlying congenital or rheumatic heart disease, particularly when a lesion is associated with a high velocity turbulent jet of blood or cardiovascular prosthetic material. A child with a normal heart can also be affected. In the pre-antibiotic era it was universally fatal, but still has a mortality of approximately 20%. Primary prevention of endocarditis whenever possible is therefore very important.

PROPHYLAXIS AGAINST INFECTIVE ENDOCARDITIS

Bacteremia may occur spontaneously or complicate a focal infection. Surgical and dental procedures cause transient bacteremia. Children with a cardiac lesion should be encouraged to keep their teeth and gums in good condition. Poor dental hygiene and inflamed gums that are susceptible to bleeding predispose to endocarditis.[40] The precise risk of endocarditis after dental procedures has never been determined and there is no information on the efficacy of prophylaxis for non-dental procedures.[40,41] In addition the risk of a hypersensivity to antibiotics together with emergence of resistant organisms remains a concern. Nevertheless, antimicrobial prophylaxis is recommended for any procedure likely to cause bacteremia. This includes any dental treatment causing bleeding of the gums, abdominal surgery, surgery or instrumentation of the upper respiratory or genitourinary tract and following burns. It is not considered necessary for gastrointestinal endoscopy without biopsy except in those with intracardiac prostheses. There are some differences in the antimicrobial regimens recommended by the American Heart Association and the British Society for Antimicrobial Chemotherapy.[41,42] Table 19.4 details suitable antibiotic prophylaxis regimens taken from the latter recommendations. Particular care is required in children with an intracardiac prosthesis and parenteral antimicrobial prophylaxis is essential in this situation.

BACTERIOLOGY OF INFECTIVE ENDOCARDITIS

Streptococcus viridans (alpha-hemolytic streptococcus), *Staphylococcus aureus* and *coagulase-negative staphylococci* are the most common bacteria isolated in children.[43] A wide variety of other organisms cause infection on rare occasions. Gram negative and fungal endocarditis occurs in children with an intracardiac prosthesis or following cardiac surgery. In neonates, staphylococcal or candidal infections occur in association with central lines and the prognosis is poor.[44]

CLINICAL FEATURES OF INFECTIVE ENDOCARDITIS

The clinical features and course of the illness vary depending upon the infecting organism and the stage at which the child is seen.[45,46] *Streptococcus viridans* endocarditis presents insidiously and most cases of fulminant endocarditis are caused by *Staphylococcus aureus.* Acute fulminant infection is also more common in children under 2 years of age as part of an overwhelming septicemia, in the setting of an otherwise normal heart.

Unexplained fever in a child with organic heart disease may be the only finding. Non-specific manifestations such as malaise, anorexia, weight loss, arthralgia, backache and hematuria frequently occur. As vegetations increase in size, a murmur may appear or change in character. Splenomegaly may be found and petechiae occur, particularly on the oral mucosa, eyelids or optic fundi (Roth spot). Splinter hemorrhages of the nail bed are also significant. Osler's nodes are red, indurated, tender lesions on the pulps of fingers and toes and also occasionally the palm. These skin lesions, arthralgia and hematuria are immune complex phenomena and not due to emboli. Embolic phenomena have become less common since antimicrobial therapy has been introduced, but occur particularly with fungal endocarditis. Janeway lesions are thought to be due to septic embolization and are transient, non-tender, macular lesions of the palms or soles of the feet. Anemia and leukocytosis are usually present and the erythrocyte sedimentation rate and C-reactive protein are almost always elevated.

Table 19.4 Antibiotic prophylaxis against infective endocarditis

A Dental extractions, scaling or periodontal surgery; surgery or instrumentation of the upper respiratory tract

1. *Under local anesthesia*

Patients not allergic to penicillin and not prescribed penicillin more than once in the last month:

– Amoxicillin as single oral dose taken under supervision 1 h before procedure

Over 10 years	3 g
5–10 years	1.5 g
Less than 5 years	750 mg

Patients allergic to penicillin or prescribed penicillin more than once in the last month:

– Clindamycin or azithromycin as single oral dose taken under supervision 1 h before procedure

Over 10 years	600 mg clindamycin
5–10 years	300 mg clindamycin or 300 mg azithromycin
Less than 5 years	150 mg clindamycin or 200 mg azithromycin

2. *Under general anesthesia*

Patients not allergic to penicillin and not prescribed penicillin more than once in the last month:

– Amoxicillin orally 4 h before and the same dose as soon as possible after the procedure

Over 10 years	3 g	followed by 3 g
5–10 years	1.5 g	followed by 1.5 g
Less than 5 years	750 mg	followed by 750 mg

Or

– Amoxicillin i.v. just before induction then oral dose 6 h later

Over 10 years	1 g i.m./i.v.	then 500 mg orally
5–10 years	500 mg i.m./i.v.	then 250 mg orally
Less than 5 years	250 mg i.m./i.v.	then 125 mg orally

Patients allergic to penicillin or prescribed penicillin more than once in the last month:

Either

Over 10 years	i.v. vancomycin 1 g over at least 100 min then gentamicin 120 mg at induction or 15 min before procedure
Under 10 years	i.v. vancomycin 20 mg/kg over at least 100 min then gentamicin 2 mg/kg at induction or 15 min before procedure

Or

Over 14 years	i.v. teicoplanin 400 mg + gentamicin 120 mg at induction or 15 min before procedure
Less than 14 years	i.v. teicoplanin 6 mg/kg + gentamicin 2 mg/kg at induction or 15 min before procedure

Or

Over 10 years	i.v. clindamycin 300 mg over at least 10 mins at induction or 15 min before procedure then oral or i.v. clindamycin 150 mg 6 h later
5–10 years	i.v. clindamycin 150 mg over at least 10 mins at induction or 15 min before procedure then oral or i.v. clindamycin 75 mg 6 h later
Less than 5 years	i.v. clindamycin 75 mg over at least 10 mins at induction or 15 min before procedure then oral or i.v. clindamycin 37.5 mg 6 h later

3. *Special risk patients (i.e. those who have had a previous attack of endocarditis or have prosthetic valves/intravascular prosthetic material)*

Patients not allergic to penicillin and not prescribed penicillin more than once in the last month:

– Amoxicillin i.v. just before induction then oral dose 6 h later

Over 10 years	1 g i.m./i.v.	then 500 mg orally
5–10 years	500 mg i.m./i.v.	then 250 mg orally
Less than 5 years	250 mg i.m./i.v.	then 125 mg orally

PLUS

– Gentamicin 2 mg/kg body weight to maximum of 120 mg

Patients allergic to penicillin or prescribed penicillin more than once in the last month:

– Same as under general anesthesia

B Genitourinary or gastrointestinal surgery or instrumentation

Cover is directed against fecal streptococci and should be as for special risk above except that clindamycin is not used.
For patients with infected urine, prophylaxis should ensure coverage of the infecting organisms.

C Upper respiratory tract procedures

Cover as for dental procedures. Postoperative dose may be given parenterally if swallowing is painful.

D Obstetric, gynecological and gastrointestinal procedures

Cover only required for those with prosthetic valves or who have had endocarditis. Cover as for genitourinary procedures.

DIAGNOSIS OF INFECTIVE ENDOCARDITIS

Early diagnosis depends on consideration of its possible presence in any child with heart disease and unexplained fever, even when there are no other features of endocarditis. The diagnosis usually depends upon a positive blood culture for an organism known to cause endocarditis. It is therefore vital to take a number of blood cultures *before* starting antibiotics in pyrexial children with heart disease and no obvious source of infection. Three cultures should be performed over a 24-h period and a further three after 24 h if the initial ones are still negative.[47] Bacteremia is a constant feature in infective endocarditis, making timing in relation to spikes of fever unimportant. Culture media should include those for aerobes, anaerobes and fungi and the media should be at a suitable temperature before use (25–35°C).

Repeated sterile blood cultures are strong evidence against infective endocarditis, but do not preclude it, since about 10% of cases are negative on culture. Recent antimicrobial treatment is the most common reason for this, but a right-sided cardiac lesion or infection with non-bacterial agents such as fungi, coxiella, *Chlamydia* or rickettsia should be considered. Echocardiography plays an important role in the diagnosis of infective endocarditis, as identification of vegetations, abscesses, prosthetic valve dehiscence or new valve regurgitation are all highly suggestive of endocarditis. Transesophageal echocardiography is a more sensitive technique and is necessary if inadequate transthoracic views are obtained. The absence of echocardiographic findings does not rule out the diagnosis.

TREATMENT OF INFECTIVE ENDOCARDITIS

Where there is a strong suspicion of infective endocarditis and it appears to be following a fulminant course, antibiotic treatment should be started as soon as a minimum of three blood cultures have been obtained. More commonly antimicrobials should be withheld until the results of blood cultures and sensitivity are available. Bactericidal drugs should be administered parenterally by bolus injection in a dose sufficient to reach therapeutic blood levels and provide a satisfactory minimum inhibitory concentration.[43] However, the clinical response to treatment is more important than the results of in vitro testing. The choice of antimicrobial, dosage schedule, and duration of therapy will depend on the organism and its sensitivity. There is no agreement on specific antimicrobial therapy, but the Working Party of the British Society for Antimicrobial Chemotherapy have produced guidelines for the treatment of endocarditis.[43] Suggested doses of some commonly used antimicrobial drugs are given in Chapter 41. The dosage should be adjusted according to the sensitivity of the organism and blood level of the antimicrobial.

For infections with a highly sensitive *Streptococcus viridans* benzylpenicillin (penicillin G) alone for 4 weeks is probably effective, although low dose gentamicin is usually added, as this has a synergistic effect. Shorter courses for just 2 weeks have been suggested.[43] If the organism is relatively insensitive, penicillin and gentamicin are given for 4 weeks. For staphylococcal infections flucloxacillin is recommended for 4 weeks together with gentamicin for the first week. *Coagulase-negative Staphylococcus* and methicillin-resistant *Staphylococcus* should be treated with vancomycin for 4–6 weeks. Gentamicin may be added for the first week. Rarely longer courses are recommended for certain bacteria such as *Staphylococcus aureus* and enterococci and in children with prosthetic valves. Where the infective agent is unknown, a combination of vancomycin and gentamicin is recommended for 6 weeks and the response assessed.

Penicillin is fundamental to the antibiotic treatment of endocarditis, and hypersensitivity seriously compromises the range of antibiotics that can be used. Parents should be closely questioned about the nature of any suspected penicillin hypersensitivity reaction. Those children who have a clear history of penicillin allergy should receive vancomycin or teicoplanin.

When endocarditis occurs following cardiac surgery in a child with a cardiovascular prosthetic material, surgical removal of the foreign material is often necessary. Active infective endocarditis is not necessarily a contraindication to cardiac surgery. Valve replacement is indicated when valve damage causes moderate or severe heart failure or when recurrent emboli occur. Fungal or coxiella infections respond poorly to medical therapy and surgery may be the only way to eradicate infection.[48]

CONGENITAL HEART DISEASE

INCIDENCE

The incidence of congenital heart disease is between 6 and 8 per 1000 live births with a higher rate in spontaneous abortions and stillbirths (approximately 1/10).[49] Differences in reported frequencies between studies are likely to be due to the method of ascertainment and precise definition of the less severe cardiac malformations. The use of high-resolution echocardiography may increase the detection rate[50] but increased antenatal detection and termination rates could reduce the incidence of the more severe lesions. There is no evidence of racial differences in the incidence of congenital cardiac defects, although there are some differences in the type of lesion.[51] The incidence of recessively inherited lesions such as isomerism (heterotaxy) sequences is increased in consanguineous communities.[4,52] The relative frequency of the most common lesions varies with different reports but nine common lesions form 80% of congenital heart disease. They can be divided into three hemodynamic groups (Table 19.5) and more than one of these lesions may coexist. The other 20% of congenital heart disease consist of many rare or complex lesions.[49,53]

The outlook for a child born with congenital heart disease in the modern era is mainly influenced by the severity of the cardiac disease. Early deaths are uncommon in acyanotic lesions with the exception of coarctation of the aorta and atrioventricular septal defect, and more common in cyanotic lesions, although the outlook is much improved. Between 30 and 40% of early deaths are due to extracardiac malformations, which are frequently associated with congenital heart disease. Prematurity and perinatal complications also contribute to outcome. The mortality rate for untreated congenital heart disease is high. Prior to the introduction of modern surgery, up to one-third of babies born alive with heart disease died from cardiac causes within the first month of life and 60% before the end of the first year.[54] With modern surgery both

Table 19.5 Incidence of common congenital cardiac lesions (Jackson et al 1996[53])

	Condition	Incidence (%)
Left-to-right shunt	Ventricular septal defect	36
	Atrial septal defect	5
	Patent arterial duct	9
	Atrioventricular septal defect	4
Obstructive lesions	Pulmonary stenosis	9
	Aortic stenosis	5
	Coarctation	5
Cyanotic lesions	Transposition of the great arteries	4
	Tetralogy of Fallot	4

'corrective' and palliative, 85–90% of infants born with congenital heart disease are now likely to reach adulthood.[50] The majority enjoy good health but many require lifelong expert follow-up and have special care, counseling and treatment. The incidence of congenital heart disease in adults is now 5/1000 and is rising steadily. As the numbers of survivors with more complex lesions grows,[55] the requirement for further catheter and surgical interventions, including transplantation, will increase further.

ETIOLOGY

Environmental factors and genetic defects can be the cause of congenital heart disease, but in most children no specific cause is found.

Teratogens

In early pregnancy maternal infection, illness or ingestion of certain drugs can result in cardiovascular abnormality. More than a third of children with the congenital rubella syndrome have a cardiovascular malformation, most frequently peripheral pulmonary stenosis or an arterial duct. There is also an increased incidence (4%) of a variety of lesions in the infants of diabetic mothers, with the risk being minimized by good control of the diabetes in early pregnancy. These infants may also have gross cardiac muscle hypertrophy, behaving like hypertrophic cardiomyopathy. Uncontrolled maternal phenylketonuria is associated with heart defects and a low phenylalanine diet should be introduced early, ideally before conception.

Maternal ingestion of some therapeutic drugs has been implicated as the cause of congenital heart disease. This is most frequently reported with lithium (Ebstein's anomaly), phenytoin (semilunar valve stenosis, coarctation, arterial duct), trimethadione, and isotretinoin used for acne (conotruncal malformations).[56,57] Cardiac defects are recognized as a feature of the fetal alcohol syndrome.[58]

Chromosomal and genetic abnormalities

Cardiac defects are associated with a wide range of chromosomal or genetic abnormalities, other syndromes and associations (Table 19.6). It is thus appropriate to perform chromosomal analysis on infants and children with congenital heart disease who have dysmorphic features, low birth weight, other malformations, developmental delay, failure to thrive or short stature. Single gene defects are increasingly being identified and some are associated with congenital heart disease.[59,60]

Five per cent of children with congenital heart disease have trisomy 21[61] and 40% of infants with trisomy 21 have a cardiac

Table 19.6 Congenital disorders associated with cardiac disease in the newborn

Abnormality	Features in the newborn	Chromosome location or abnormality	Percentage with heart disease (%)	Commonest cardiovascular abnormalities associated (not all-inclusive)
Chromosome disorders				
Down	Dysmorphism	Trisomy 21	40–50	AVSDs, VSD, ASD, ToF
Edwards	Dysmorphism	Trisomy 18	90–100	VSD, polyvalve disease, ASD, PDA
Patau	Dysmorphism	Trisomy 13	80	PDA, VSD, ASD
Turner	Puffy feet and hands	XO	15	Coarct, AS, PS
Non-random associations				
Cleft lip and palate	Feeding difficulties		25	VSD, PDA, TGA, ToF
Diaphragmatic hernia	Severe respiratory distress		25	ToF
Lung agenesis	Severe respiratory distress		20	PDA, VSD, ToF, Total or partial TAPVD
Omphalocele			20	ToF, ASD
Intestinal atresia	Bowel obstruction		10	VSD
Unilateral renal agenesis			17	VSD
Tracheoesophageal fistula	Feeding/respiratory difficulties		10	VSD, ToF
Autosomal dominant				
Beckwith–Wiedemann	Hypoglycemia, dysmorphism	11	15+	HCM, ASD, VSD, ToF, PDA
DiGeorge	Hypocalcemia, dysmorphism	22q11	75	Int Ao Arch, ToF, Art Trunk
Goldenhar	Dysmorphism		15	ToF, VSD
Holt–Oram	Bilateral upper limb defects	12q24.1	100	ASD, VSD, PDA
Tuberous sclerosis	Family history	9q34	30+	Rhabdomyomas
Noonan	Dysmorphism, puffy feet	12q22		PS with dysplastic PV, PDA, HCM
Williams	Dysmorphism, hypercalcemia	7q11.2	50-80	Supravalvar AS, stenosis affecting Ao, Cerebral and renal arteries
Autosomal recessive				
Smith-Lemli-Opitz	Dysmorphism	7q32.1	20-100	VSD, PDA, ASD, ToF
Thrombocytopenia absent radius	Thrombocytopenia absent radius		33	ASD, ToF
Syndromes with unknown etiology				
Asymmetric crying facies	Facial nerve palsy		44	VSD
CHARGE association	Multiple features		65–75	ToF, DORV, ASD, VSD, PDA, Coarct, AVSD
VACTERL association	Multiple features		10	VSD, ASD, ToF

Note this list is not inclusive, nor are the cardiac lesions always as most commonly seen!

Art Trunk, common arterial trunk; AS, aortic stenosis; ASD, atrial septal defect; AVSDs, atrioventricular septal defects; Coarct, aortic coarctation; DORV, double outlet right ventricle; HCM, hypertrophic cardiomyopathy; Int Ao Arch, interrupted aortic arch; PDA, patent arterial duct; PS, pulmonary stenosis; PV, pulmonary valve; TAPVD, totally anomalous pulmonary venous drainage; TGA, transposition of the great arteries; ToF, tetralogy of Fallot; VSD, ventricular septal defect.

defect. This is usually an atrioventricular or ventricular septal defect and it is essential to undertake echocardiographic examination in all newborn infants with Down syndrome, even when the clinical examination and electrocardiogram are normal. This information helps parents and health professionals to plan the child's management. There is also a high incidence of cardiac defects in children with trisomy 13 (Patau's syndrome) or 18 (Edwards' syndrome). Most infants die early and since the few longer-term survivors are severely mentally retarded, surgical treatment is indicated only in exceptional circumstances. Turner's syndrome (45 XO) has an association with left heart lesions,[62] and coarctation of the aorta occurs in approximately 15% of these girls.

Autosomal dominant inheritance

DiGeorge syndrome results from a microdeletion within chromosome 22 and arises sporadically in over 70% of children.[63] Seventy five per cent have cardiac (conotruncal) defects[64] and other abnormalities include dysmorphic facial features, thymic aplasia or hypoplasia, cleft palate or velopharyngeal insufficiency, hypocalcemia and renal abnormalities. Noonan's syndrome, which is associated with pulmonary stenosis, has an autosomal dominant inheritance but most cases are due to new mutations. Holt–Oram also has a dominant inheritance. Williams' syndrome is caused by a microdeletion of chromosome 7 and is very occasionally inherited from an affected parent but most cases arise sporadically. Hypertrophic cardiomyopathy has an estimated prevalence of 1:500 persons.[60] Most patients have a positive family history but sporadic cases occasionally occur. Long QT syndrome has a prevalence of 1:5000 persons and sporadic cases are uncommon.[60] Marfan's syndrome is also inherited as an autosomal dominant.

Autosomal recessive inheritance

Pompe's disease and Friedreich's ataxia, which of both cause hypertrophic cardiomyopathy, have an autosomal recessive inheritance. Jervell and Lange-Nielsen syndrome with prolonged QT on the electrocardiogram and deafness is also a recessive condition.

Other relatively common conditions with a usually sporadic occurrence are VACTERL and CHARGE associations.

Polygenic inheritance

It is often considered that congenital heart disease is due to polygenic or multifactorial inheritance, in which, as yet unknown, inherited and environmental factors combine to cause the malformation. The polygenic model for inheritance of congenital heart disease has been supported by the correspondence between the theoretical predicted and reported recurrence risk for first-degree relatives. However, the relatively high incidence in the offspring of those with significant congenital heart disease, who now survive into adult life, may indicate a greater importance for a single gene defect.

RECURRENCE RISK

Recurrence risk for a cardiac defect depends on the nature of the lesion and relationship of the affected person. The risk for another pregnancy rises to about 2% if one previous child is affected; this tends to be highest (3%) for ventricular septal defect, arterial duct, and atrioventricular septal defect.[65] There is a tendency for a related anomaly to recur but this is not necessarily the case. If two previous children are affected the risk rises to 6–8% and recent studies of the offspring of parents with congenital heart disease have indicated a similar risk if the father has congenital heart disease. However, if the mother is affected there is an even higher risk (5–15%) depending on the lesion.[3]

When counseling parents, consideration must be given to known recurrence risks and exposure to possible teratogens, particularly medication. Fetal echocardiography provides an accurate means of diagnosing fetal cardiac abnormalities from about 18 weeks' gestation.[66] In the majority there will be no defect and the family can be reassured. However, the implications for finding a defect, with the possibility of offering termination for severe defects, are major and should be discussed with the parents before the examination is carried out.

FETAL DIAGNOSIS OF HEART DISEASE

RATIONALE

Antenatal ultrasonographic diagnosis of significant congenital heart disease is now possible in around 50% of cases although in the United Kingdom this figure is rarely achieved.[67] Ascertainment of a normal four chamber view with the cardiac apex to the left of the fetus, cardiothoracic ratio < 50%, two atria, two ventricles, normal tricuspid to mitral valve offsetting is a routine part of the standard 18–22 week 'detailed scan'. This should exclude most variations of 'single ventricle' such as hypoplastic left or right heart and common ventricle, as well as most major atrioventricular septal defects (Fig. 19.16) and inlet ventricular septal defects.[66] However, abnormalities of the cardiac outlets such as tetralogy of Fallot, truncus arteriosus, transposition of the great arteries and some ventricular septal defects will be missed in the four chamber view. They can be detected on more detailed 'five chamber or outlet screening' where the integrity of the outlet septum and the ventriculo-arterial connections are also checked. In addition, there are a number of conditions, such as aortic or pulmonary stenosis and coarctation, where any discrepancy in chamber size increases with advancing gestation. Others may only become apparent postnatally when the normal perinatal adaptations fail to

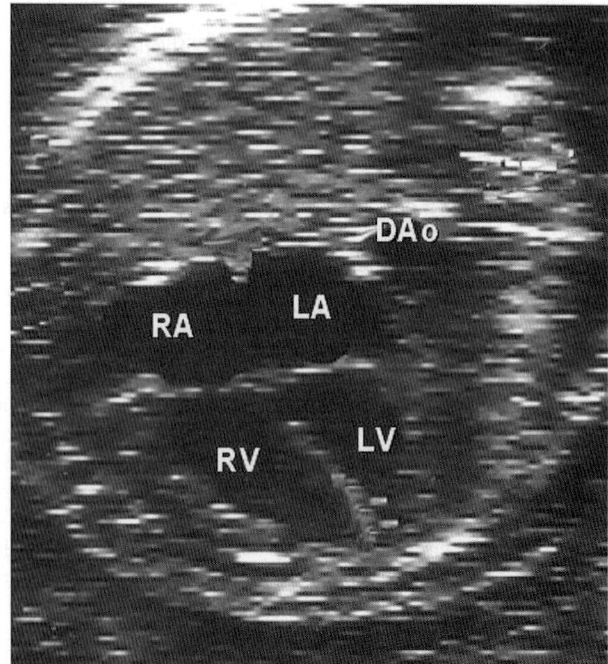

Fig. 19.16 Four chamber view of a fetal heart showing complete atrioventricular septal defect. The left and right components of the atrioventricular valves are at the same level. There is a ventricular septal defect and a primum atrial septal defect. DAo, descending aorta; LA, left atrium; LV, left ventricle; RA, right atrium; RV, right ventricle.

occur, or develop abnormally as in coarctation of the aorta, atrial septal defect and patent ductus arteriosus. Even with detailed cardiac screening performed by an experienced fetal echocardiographer, small septal defects and minor valve abnormalities are frequently outside the resolution and limits of detection of even the most sophisticated ultrasound equipment.

The rationale for antenatal detection of congenital heart disease remains complex and somewhat controversial. There is an increased incidence of congenital heart disease in infants of diabetic mothers, or where there is congenital heart disease in either parent or a first degree relative. Maternal lithium or anticonvulsant therapy and phenylketonuria, as well as twin pregnancies, are associated with an increased risk of congenital heart disease and merit detailed cardiac scanning at around 20 weeks' gestation. The vast majority of these studies will be normal and the main benefit is parental reassurance, although repeated scanning may be required for some progressive conditions to avoid false optimism. Most fetal cardiac abnormalities occur in 'low risk' pregnancies, and in these fetuses, there is a clear indication for further detailed examination of the rest of the fetus. Extracardiac malformations[57] and chromosomal abnormalities[68] are commonly associated with structural heart disease and may adversely affect the cardiac outlook. Cardiac abnormalities are commonly associated with some visceral abnormalities such as exomphalos and diaphragmatic hernia, and this also has prognostic implications. Fetal karyotype can be obtained from placental tissue, amniocytes or fetal blood, and in particular, aneuploidy (trisomy 13, 18 or 21) can be readily excluded. Deletions of chromosome 22 can also be detected by fluorescence in situ hybridization (FISH) analysis and should always be requested in the presence of significant fetal heart disease. When fetal heart block is detected, measurement of maternal autoantibodies (anti-Ro antibodies) will guide towards likelihood of associated structural heart disease and also indicate recurrence risks.

Although some fetal interventions are possible, the main reason for detecting cardiac disease antenatally remains in facilitating parental choice. Fetal diagnosis permits informed consent for termination or continuation of an affected pregnancy and also has implications for perinatal management. Most fetuses with congenital heart disease can be delivered according to normal obstetric parameters, the exceptions being some fetal arrhythmias where intrapartum monitoring may be compromised. Fetuses with known transposition of the great arteries should be delivered in close proximity to a pediatric cardiac center to allow urgent atrial septostomy if the atrial septum is very restrictive. Most other fetuses can be delivered locally provided adequate transport facilities are available for duct dependent neonates. Such infants should be discussed in advance with both obstetricians and neonatologists. There is conflicting evidence available as to whether antenatal detection of congenital heart disease directly influences fetal outcome.[69,70] Antenatal diagnosis of congenital heart disease should permit timely, and appropriate, postnatal management and avoid hemodynamic deterioration and acidosis in duct dependent lesions. However analysis is complicated by the differing severity of the spectrum of congenital heart disease diagnosed prenatally,[71] and prognostication based on postnatally diagnosed series should be offered with some caution.

THE NEONATE WITH A CONGENITAL HEART DISEASE

This section describes the timing and mode of presentation of heart disease in the newborn focusing on the commonest conditions and those that are frequently missed or misdiagnosed. The emphasis is on structural heart disease and the anatomy and physiology of each is described. It discusses the clues and common pitfalls in making the diagnoses and outlines the initial management, followed by a description of the management in the pediatric cardiac center. Arrhythmias are dealt with elsewhere and are mentioned in differential diagnosis only.

DIAGNOSIS

Making the diagnosis

A study of infants with congenital heart disease who died, found that in 30% of cases the diagnosis of a cardiac lesion was not made during life.[72] Some had complex cardiac lesions or severe non-cardiac abnormalities, but if the cardiac diagnosis had been made during life, many were likely to have had a good outcome when treated surgically or with interventional cardiac catheterization.[73] Early detection of these conditions is therefore critical, and health professionals caring for newborns must be constantly alert for the early signs and be prepared to refer to the specialist centers quickly. A delay in referral is as important as a delay in diagnosis, since deterioration can be extremely rapid.

Why is diagnosis delayed?

Most infants appear outwardly normal

Delays in diagnosis occur partly due to false preconceptions that the majority of infants with serious heart disease will have a syndrome such as Down syndrome, or appear unwell immediately after birth. In fact most infants with serious heart disease have no associated syndromes or dysmorphic features. They are often well initially and do not have obvious physical signs until the arterial duct begins to close.

Failure to detect cyanosis

Another frequent cause for delay in diagnosis is the failure to recognize central cyanosis. The most common cyanotic heart diseases in the newborn, transposition of the great arteries and pulmonary atresia, have no associated respiratory distress or other clues to the diagnosis. Central cyanosis must be looked for deliberately on every neonatal check by examining the lips and tongue.[74] Diagnosis is more difficult with dark skinned races, but the tongue and buccal mucosa are reliable in a well-lit room or with a torch. As a rule of thumb, if you think the infant may be cyanosed, she probably is and pulse oximetry should be obtained quickly. Normal values for the neonatal period have been established.[75]

Too much reliance on auscultation alone

Shortly after birth murmurs are common in minor lesions such as small ventricular septal defects, and less common in the most severe conditions such as underdevelopment of the left heart or transposition of the great arteries. More important than auscultation, is careful observation of the infant's color and respiratory pattern, assessment of peripheral perfusion, palpation of brachial and femoral pulses and of the precordium for a prominent pulsation. A normal neonatal examination does not rule out serious heart disease that may present later, usually when the arterial duct closes.[73,76] Equally important is to listen to the parents when they express concern. They often know instinctively that something is wrong!

Practical points:

- *Most infants with life-threatening heart disease have no associated syndrome, a normal outward appearance, are perfectly well and have a normal physical examination for the first day or two after birth.*
- *Look carefully inside the mouth for central cyanosis.*
- *Rely more on observation and palpation than on the stethoscope.*

Hyperoxia test

The normal newborn should have a PaO_2 greater than 70 mmHg (9 kPa). If cyanosis is detected clinically it is usually less than 40 mmHg (5 kPa). In a cyanosed infant, if the arterial PaO_2 rises above 150 mmHg (20 kPa) in 90–100% oxygen, a major right-to-left shunt is unlikely. The test is not completely reliable, but a failure of the PaO_2 to rise strongly suggests a cardiac defect. The PaO_2 can fail to rise for two other reasons:

1. Intrapulmonary shunting in lung disease. Areas of collapsed lung tend to be perfused with blood as well as the well-aerated sections, so some blood returning to the heart is not oxygenated.
2. Failure of the transitional circulation (persistent fetal circulation or persistent pulmonary hypertension of the newborn (Ch. 10). In this condition, the pulmonary vascular resistance fails to fall normally, and right-to-left shunting occurs across the fetal channels, the patent oval foramen and arterial duct. It often coexists with severe neonatal lung disease, causing diagnostic and management dilemmas. Once congenital heart disease is excluded, management is aimed at reducing pulmonary vascular resistance by the treatment of acidosis, and the use of pulmonary vasodilators, in particular inhaled nitric oxide.

THE IMPORTANCE OF THE OVAL FORAMEN IN NEONATAL HEART DISEASE

Patency of the oval foramen is critical for survival where the mitral or tricuspid flow is absent or inadequate, and when mixing at atrial level is essential, as in transposition of the great vessels. In mitral atresia (or hypoplastic left heart), postnatal survival depends on a patent foramen to allow the pulmonary venous blood to enter the right atrium and thence the right ventricle. Blood then reaches the main pulmonary artery and divides between the lungs and the aorta (via the arterial duct). Closure of either the foramen or duct, leads to death. Similarly, in tricuspid atresia, a widely patent foramen is essential for venous return to reach the ventricles via the left atrium. In transposition, the most effective mixing between the systemic and pulmonary circulations is at atrial level and an inadequate or severely restrictive foramen can be life threatening even when the arterial duct is patent.[73] If the oval foramen is inadequate it must be enlarged by cardiac catheter intervention or surgery.

THE IMPORTANCE OF THE ARTERIAL DUCT IN NEONATAL HEART DISEASE

Prostaglandin E2 (dinoprostone) is a physiological compound derived from arachidonic acid and is critical in maintaining duct patency during fetal life. It can be used intravenously in duct-dependent cyanotic and left heart obstructive lesions. The starting dose is 5–10 ng/kg/min and this can be increased to achieve duct patency. Although the arterial duct is functionally closed in most healthy term infants by the second day of life and usually completely closed by day five,[77] persistent or episodic hypoxemia tends to slow down the speed at which the duct closes. Prostaglandin E2 can therefore often be an effective therapy even into the second or third week of life, provided the duct has not completely closed.

Side-effects of prostaglandin therapy

Apnea is a serious side-effect and resuscitation equipment should be available. If doses higher than 10 ng/kg/min are necessary to maintain duct patency, apnea is more frequent. Lower doses can cause apnea in premature infants. If transport to the tertiary center is required, many centers will electively intubate and ventilate such infants.[73] Other common side-effects are jitteriness, fever, hypotension due to systemic vasodilatation, and occasionally hypoglycemia.

PRESENTATION OF HEART DISEASE IN THE NEWBORN

Mode of presentation

As fetal ultrasonographers become increasingly skilled in the detection of heart disease, more infants are born with their diagnosis already made.[67] However, even in the most sophisticated health care systems, the majority of infants with heart disease still present after birth and rely on the vigilance of the clinicians, parents and midwives to be detected.

Symptoms and signs after birth

Neonates almost always present with one of the following:

- cyanosis, with or without respiratory distress;
- heart failure, with or without cyanosis;
- collapse;
- an associated lesion or syndrome;
- an abnormal clinical sign detected on routine examination such as absent femoral pulses or a heart murmur.

Timing of presentation

The age of presentation depends on the effect that the transition from fetal to postnatal circulation has upon the specific lesion. This relates to how the abnormal heart responds to the high pulmonary vascular resistance at birth, the gradual fall of this resistance, and the closure of the arterial duct. Here are three examples:

1. An infant born with a poorly functioning right ventricle and severe tricuspid regurgitation (as with Ebstein's anomaly of the tricuspid valve) will present at birth. This is because the high pulmonary vascular resistance prevents the impaired right ventricle from delivering blood effectively into the pulmonary arteries.
2. An infant with pulmonary atresia, despite having no forward flow from the right ventricle into the pulmonary artery, does not present at birth because the arterial duct is open and blood fills the pulmonary arteries from the aorta. Clinical presentation with severe cyanosis occurs when the duct starts to close a few hours to days after birth.
3. An infant with a large ventricular septal defect has no difficulties at birth, because the high pulmonary vascular resistance prevents excessive pulmonary blood flow. There is hence little flow across the defect from the left to right ventricle. Pulmonary vascular resistance gradually falls after a few weeks and presentation with cardiac failure due to the large left-to-right shunt through the defect typically occurs at 4–6 weeks of age.

When making a diagnosis in a newborn, it is therefore helpful to consider not only the **type** of presentation (cyanosis with or without respiratory distress, cardiac failure, collapse) but also the usual **timing** of presentation (Table 19.7) and the clinical, electrocardiographic and X-ray findings (Table 19.8).

PRESENTATION WITH CYANOSIS WITHOUT RESPIRATORY DISTRESS

The commonest causes of isolated cyanosis are transposition of the great arteries and pulmonary atresia or severe (critical) pulmonary stenosis. Pulmonary atresia can occur with a ventricular septal defect (a variant of tetralogy of Fallot), or without when the right ventricle may be underdeveloped or hypoplastic. Other causes include tricuspid atresia and other complex lesions that have restricted pulmonary blood flow.

Transposition of the great arteries

This is the commonest cyanotic lesion to present in the neonate, accounting for 4–5% of congenital heart disease,[49,53] and occurring more commonly in males.

Table 19.7 Typical timing and mode of presentation of congenital heart disease in the neonate

	EARLY 0–24 hours High pulmonary vascular resistance, arterial duct open	INTERMEDIATE 4 hours–2 weeks Duct closing – 'duct dependent' lesions present	LATE After 2 weeks Duct closed. Pulmonary vascular resistance continues to fall and lesions with left-to-right shunts present
Cyanosis (without congestive failure or respiratory distress)	TGA	Duct dependent for pulmonary blood flow, e.g. Pulmonary atresia with or without VSD Critical pulmonary stenosis (with right-to-left interatrial flow), Tricuspid atresia with small VSD, ^Complex lesions with severe pulmonary stenosis Duct dependent for mixing, TGA (simple and complex)	Tetralogy of Fallot with severe pulmonary stenosis§ ^Complex lesions with pulmonary stenosis
Cyanosis with congestive failure or respiratory distress	Obstructed TAPVD (usually infradiaphragmatic) Severe Ebstein's anomaly	Pulmonary arteriovenous fistulae (rare) Partially obstructed TAPVD	Mixed circulations with unobstructed pulmonary blood flow, e.g. Unobstructed TAPVD (cardiac or supracardiac), Common arterial trunk, Tricuspid atresia with a large VSD. Some complex lesions with high pulmonary blood flow.*
Collapse/shock		Left heart obstruction, e.g. Aortic coarctation or interruption, HLHS, Aortic stenosis	
Congestive cardiac failure (without cyanosis)		Left heart obstruction with a left-to-right shunt, e.g. Aortic coarctation ± VSD Systemic arteriovenous fistulae, e.g. cerebral	Left-to-right shunts, e.g. Large VSD, complete AV septal defect, PDA, aortopulmonary window Complex lesions**

NB. It is important to use this table as a guideline only – each condition can present unusually late or early! Tachyarrhythmias – usually supraventricular tachycardia can present with heart failure or collapse at any of these age groups, as can myocardial failure due to heart muscle disease such as hypertrophic cardiomyopathy or myocardial ischemia secondary to perinatal distress. Cardiovascular collapse in the first few hours is usually related to such myocardial dysfunction; sepsis and metabolic disease should be considered.

HLHS, hypoplastic left heart syndrome; TAPVD, totally anomalous pulmonary venous drainage; TGA, transposition of the great arteries, those without a ventricular septal defect (VSD) and a small oval foramen present earlier.

§In tetralogy of Fallot, only the most severe present as a cyanotic neonate. The less severe forms present typically with cyanotic spells, or with a loud murmur on routine check.

^Examples of complex lesions with low pulmonary blood flow include

1. Any single ventricle with severe pulmonary or subpulmonary stenosis
2. Double outlet right ventricle with severe pulmonary stenosis.

*Examples of complex lesions with high pulmonary blood flow and cyanosis include

1. Double outlet right ventricle with transposed great arteries
2. Pulmonary atresia with large aortopulmonary collateral arteries or large arterial duct.

**Examples of complex lesions with high pulmonary blood flow without cyanosis include

1. Single ventricle without pulmonary stenosis
2. Double outlet right ventricle with normally related great arteries and without pulmonary stenosis.

Anatomy and physiology

In this condition, the aorta and pulmonary arteries are transposed. The right ventricle receiving deoxygenated blood as usual from the right atrium delivers this blood into the aorta (Fig. 19.17). The oxygenated blood returning from the pulmonary veins drains into the left atrium and left ventricle but is pumped directly back into the pulmonary arteries. These two circulations do not mix and this is clearly not compatible with life. Survival in the first few hours is due to mixing at atrial level via a patent oval foramen, and at arterial level via the patent arterial duct. Some infants have a ventricular septal defect, pulmonary stenosis or aortic coarctation.

Clinical features

Cyanosis is sometimes detected at birth. More commonly presentation is over the next 1–3 days, the cyanosis becoming more obvious as the arterial duct closes (Table 19.7). If the atrial communication is small, the infant declines rapidly and will die if the duct is not re-opened with intravenous prostaglandin therapy, or the foramen enlarged by atrial septostomy. No murmurs or physical signs other than cyanosis are present unless there are additional lesions. When a large ventricular septal defect occurs with pulmonary stenosis, the severity of stenosis determines the degree of cyanosis and timing of presentation.

Investigations

The neonate will fail the hyperoxia test and a metabolic acidosis may be present. Right ventricular hypertrophy on the electrocardiogram becomes more obvious with time. Chest radiography shows increased pulmonary vascularity (Table 19.8). In this respect, transposition of the great arteries is unlike most other cyanotic conditions that present early, which have reduced pulmonary blood flow. This is because there are both left-to-right and right-to-left shunting at atrial and ductal levels, combined with hypoxia that causes myocardial dysfunction. The upper mediastinum appears narrow because the aorta lies in front, and slightly to the right, of the pulmonary artery. The 'egg on side' appearance to the heart is not usually seen in the neonatal period. Echocardiography shows the pulmonary artery arising from the left ventricle and the aorta from the right ventricle (Fig 19.10d). A characteristic finding is the parallel relationship of the great vessels.[78] Additional lesions such as a ventricular septal defect, pulmonary stenosis or aortic coarctation can be identified.

Management

Prostaglandin infusion should be commenced immediately, without waiting for the diagnosis to be confirmed. Any metabolic acidosis should be corrected.

Balloon atrial septostomy: This is usually performed to enlarge the oval foramen and promote mixing at this level.[19] This can be done with echocardiographic guidance, on the intensive care unit, or in the cardiac catheterization theater. A catheter with a balloon mounted on the end is advanced from the umbilical,[17] or femoral, vein into the right atrium and across into the left atrium. The balloon is inflated and pulled back to tear the septum (Fig. 19.14).

Surgical management: The arterial switch operation (Fig. 19.18) is performed within the next few days, using cardiopulmonary bypass. The arterial trunks are transected, the main pulmonary artery pulled forward, and the ascending aorta moved posteriorly such that the branch pulmonary arteries straddle the ascending aorta. The coronary arteries are removed with a small button of surrounding arterial wall, and resutured into the new ascending aorta. This operation is usually done in the neonatal period, before the left ventricle becomes adapted to pumping against a low pulmonary vascular resistance and develops thin walls, which are unable to cope with transition to becoming the systemic ventricle. In older infants, a band can be placed around the pulmonary artery to increase left ventricular pressure and 're-train' it to cope with the systemic circulation. Early mortality from the arterial switch operation is now less than 2%, and 10 year survival is 94%.[80] The commonest complication is narrowing of the branch pulmonary arteries as they stretch over the aorta. Myocardial infarction is surprisingly rare.

Previous surgical procedures: Because of the difficult technical problems related to the arterial switch operation, surgery until the mid-1980s consisted of an atrial rerouting operation (Fig. 19.19), the Senning or Mustard procedure. Systemic venous blood is directed from the right atrium by means of a baffle across the atrial septum to the mitral valve, leading into the left ventricle and out to the pulmonary arteries. Pulmonary venous blood is routed via the right ventricle to the aorta. The morphological right ventricle, designed for pumping through a low-pressure circuit to the lungs, pumped blood around the body under high pressure. Although patients do well for the first two decades of life, the right ventricle gradually fails, typically in the third and fourth decade of life, and there is a risk of sudden death from atrial and ventricular arrhythmias.[81,82]

Surgical options for transposition with pulmonary stenosis: After the arterial switch, the stenosed pulmonary valve would become the new aortic valve. Aortic stenosis or regurgitation carries significant lifetime morbidity, so it is inappropriate to perform the switch operation when there is significant pulmonary stenosis as this problem will be transferred to the new aorta. If there is an associated large outlet ventricular septal defect, it is sometimes possible to patch the ventricular septal defect so that the left ventricle leads into the aorta anteriorly, and then place a tube graft (conduit) from the right ventricle to the pulmonary artery (Fig. 19.20). This is known as the Rastelli procedure.[83] The conduit needs to be replaced as the child grows, increasing the cumulative mortality risk.

Tetralogy of Fallot with pulmonary atresia

This condition represents the severe end of the spectrum of this condition. Most children with tetralogy of Fallot have stenosis rather than atresia of the right ventricular outflow tract and present outside the neonatal period, are therefore described later (p. 861).

Anatomy and physiology

Pulmonary atresia is a complete obstruction between the right ventricle and pulmonary arteries. The intracardiac anatomy

Table 19.8 Flow chart for the differential diagnosis of central cyanosis. Assessment of whether pulmonary blood flow is increased or diminished combined with the electrocardiographic findings helps to narrow the diagnostic possibilities

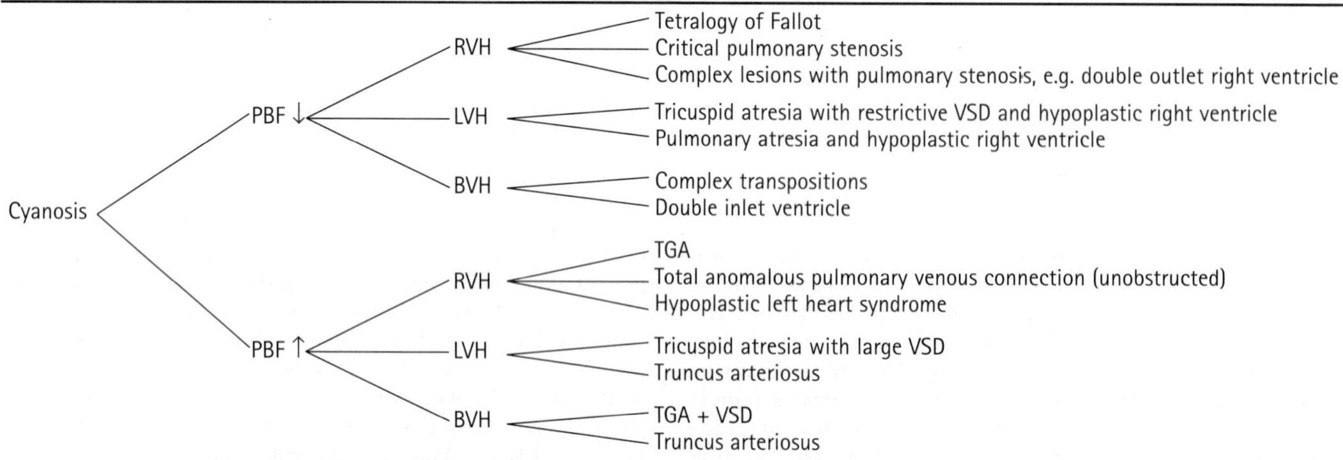

BVH, biventricular hypertrophy; LVH, left ventricular hypertrophy; PBF, pulmonary blood flow; RVH, right ventricular hypertrophy; TGA, transposition of great arteries; VSD, ventricular septal defect

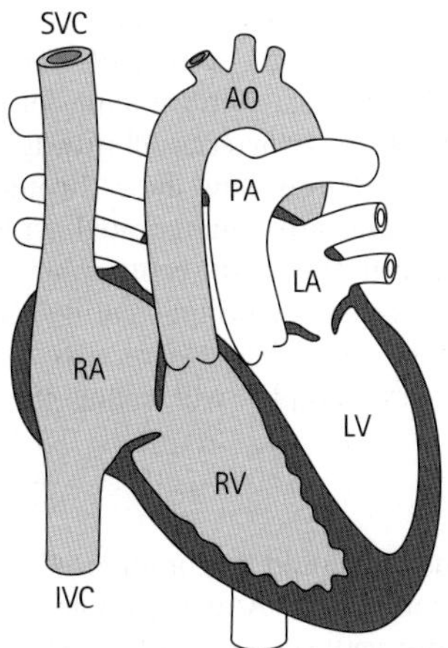

Fig. 19.17 Transposition of the great arteries (atrioventricular concordance, arterioventricular discordance). Shading indicates desaturated/unoxygenated blood. AO, aorta; IVC, inferior vena cava; LA, left atrium; LV, left ventricle; PA, pulmonary artery; RA, right atrium; RV, right ventricle; SVC, superior vena cava.

resembles that of tetralogy of Fallot with a large ventricular septal defect, but the pulmonary arteries are frequently abnormal. The central pulmonary arteries may be confluent and supplied by the arterial duct. Alternatively, or in addition, collateral arteries from the aorta, major aortopulmonary collateral arteries (MAPCAs), supply the lungs and connect with the pulmonary arteries.

Clinical features

When the infant is dependent on the arterial duct, cyanosis develops when it closes in the first days of life (Table 19.7). Major aortopulmonary collateral arteries provide a more stable source of pulmonary blood flow and cyanosis may be mild. A few infants have excessive pulmonary blood flow from these collateral vessels and present in heart failure with minimal cyanosis. The pulses are normal and the right ventricle is prominent on palpation. The first sound is frequently followed by an aortic ejection click, related to the dilated ascending aorta and the second heart sound is single. Continuous murmurs from the collateral vessels are heard widely over the precordium. Almost 50% of children have DiGeorge syndrome.[84]

Investigations

The electrocardiogram shows right ventricular hypertrophy, with persistence of the upright T wave in lead V1. Chest radiography shows pulmonary oligemia (Table 19.8). Right ventricular hypertrophy may produce a 'boot-shaped' appearance to the heart and 25–30% of infants have a right aortic arch. Echocardiography shows the subaortic ventricular septal defect and identifies the central pulmonary arteries. Additional muscular ventricular septal defects and other abnormalities can be identified. Cardiac catheterization is needed, prior to definitive surgery, to accurately define the pulmonary arterial anatomy and aortopulmonary collateral arteries.

Management

Prostaglandin infusion maintains duct patency until the anatomy of the pulmonary arteries is delineated and metabolic acidosis should be corrected.

Infants with duct-dependent pulmonary circulation: Stability is usually achieved by creating a shunt, usually a Gortex tube, from the right innominate or subclavian artery to the right pulmonary artery (modified Blalock–Taussig shunt). This encourages pulmonary arterial growth in preparation for definitive surgery, which consists of closing the ventricular septal defect and placing a conduit from right ventricle to pulmonary artery. It is preferable to defer definitive surgery until the child is older to reduce the number of conduit replacements needed during growth.

Infants with major aortopulmonary collateral arteries: Surgery varies depending on the anatomy of the pulmonary arteries and MAPCAs. The aim is to connect important MAPCAs to the central pulmonary arteries and to place a conduit between the right ventricle and pulmonary artery. The ventricular septal defect is closed.[85] Several staged operations are often needed.

Pulmonary atresia with intact ventricular septum/critical pulmonary valve stenosis

This accounts for about 2.5% of all congenital heart defects.

Anatomy and physiology

The pulmonary valve is imperforate or has a tiny orifice. The ventricular septum is intact and the right ventricle is always abnormal, varying in size from slightly small to severely hypoplastic. The tricuspid valve is usually abnormal, small and regurgitant. Pulmonary blood flow depends on the arterial duct. Cyanosis is caused by right-to-left shunting at atrial level, through a stretched oval foramen. In some

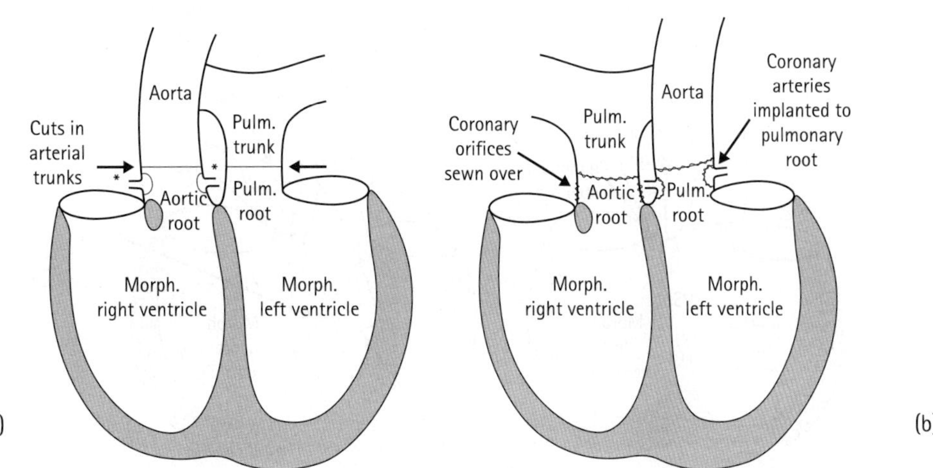

Fig. 19.18 Diagrammatic representations of the arterial switch (a) before and (b) after the procedure. Morph., morphological; Pulm., pulmonary. (From Anderson et al 2002[79])

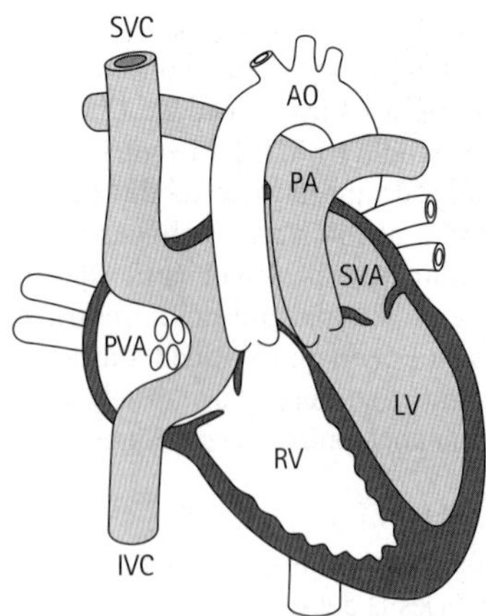

Fig. 19.19 Mustard procedure for transposition of the great arteries. Intra-atrial baffle of pericardium redirects pulmonary and system venous return so that superior vena cava (SVC) and inferior vena cava (IVC) unoxygenated venous blood (shaded) is directed to the left ventricle (LV) and pulmonary venous blood to the right ventricle (RV). PVA, new pulmonary venous atrium; SVA, new systemic venous atrium.

infants with an atretic valve, the small, hypertensive, muscle-bound right ventricle has fistulous connections to the coronary arteries. The coronary arteries may be stenosed, so that the distal part of the coronary circulation depends entirely on flow from the right ventricle. Relief of the pulmonary valve obstruction is dangerous, because the right ventricular pressure falls, reducing coronary arterial flow and causing myocardial infarction.

Clinical features

Neonates present with cyanosis when the arterial duct closes (Table 19.7). There is a single second sound and there may be a soft ductal murmur and a systolic murmur of tricuspid regurgitation. Infants with critical pulmonary stenosis have an ejection systolic murmur audible in the pulmonary area.

Investigations

The electrocardiogram shows right atrial enlargement with tall P waves, and occasionally ST segment changes if there is coronary ischemia. When the right ventricle is hypoplastic, the R wave in V1 is small. Chest radiography shows pulmonary oligemia, with cardiomegaly if tricuspid regurgitation is severe (Table 19.8). Echocardiography shows right ventricular hypertrophy with a varying degree of hypoplasia. Abnormalities of the tricuspid valve can be seen, and pulmonary arteries fill through the arterial duct. Infants with critical stenosis have flow through the pulmonary valve. If coronary fistulae are demonstrated, with continuous color Doppler signals within the right ventricular wall, or suspected because of enlarged coronary origins, cardiac catheterization will delineate them more clearly, and demonstrate coronary supply. Right ventricular angiography will define the right ventricular cavity.

Management

Prostaglandin infusion should be commenced without waiting for diagnosis to be confirmed. Any metabolic acidosis should be corrected. Initial intervention consists of transcatheter perforation and balloon dilatation of the stenosed or atretic valve (Fig. 19.21), surgical valvotomy or a systemic-to-pulmonary shunt. The ultimate clinical course depends on the size of the right ventricle.

Infant with an adequate right ventricle: Infants with critical pulmonary valve stenosis and some patients with atresia will have a right ventricle of good size and, with relief of the obstruction, it will eventually function well.[86]

Infant with a severely hypoplastic right ventricle: If the right ventricle is hypoplastic, the heart has functionally only a left ventricle. Palliation for all children with a single ventricle circulation is outlined later (p. 863).

Tricuspid atresia

This spectrum of conditions, accounting for 1% of congenital heart defects, has in common an absent right atrioventricular connection. Survival requires a large oval foramen, allowing systemic and pulmonary venous return to mix in the left atrium. There are many anatomic and hemodynamic variations, producing widely different clinical features. These depend on the atrial and ventricular septal defects, the size of the right ventricle and the ventriculo-arterial connections (Fig. 19.22). If the ventricular septal defect is small, there will be reduced pulmonary blood flow (discussed below). If the ventricular septal defect is large, excessive pulmonary blood flow will result in cyanosis and heart failure (p. 847). When the pulmonary artery arises from the left ventricle and the aorta from the hypoplastic right ventricle, this constitutes a form of hypoplastic 'left' heart syndrome (p. 850).

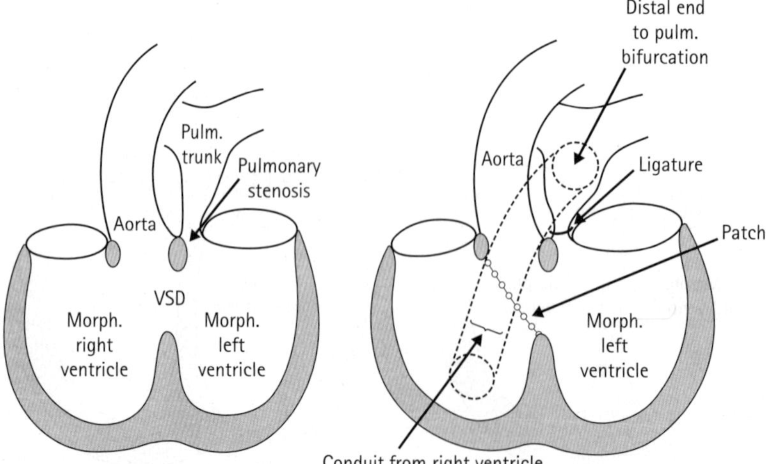

Fig. 19.20 A diagrammatic representation of the steps involved in the Rastelli procedure. Morph., morphological; Pulm., pulmonary; VSD, ventricular septal defect. (From Anderson et al 2002[79])

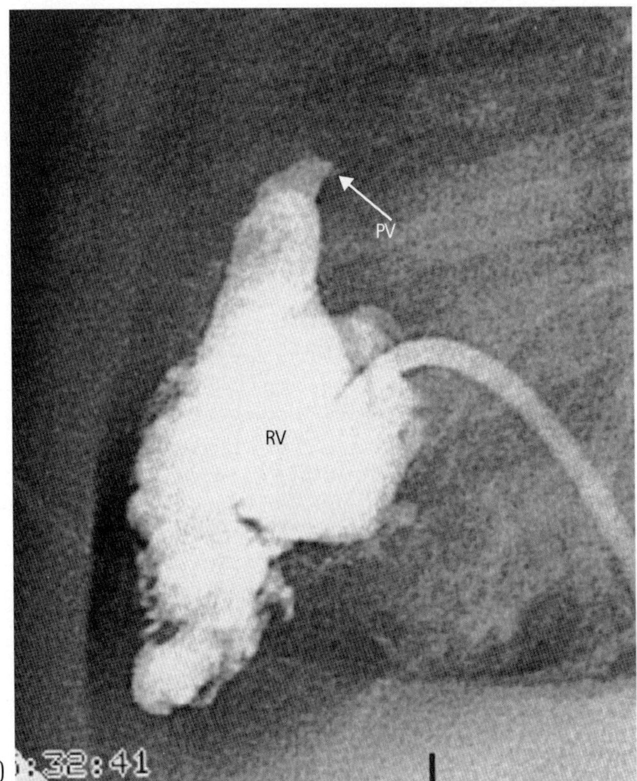

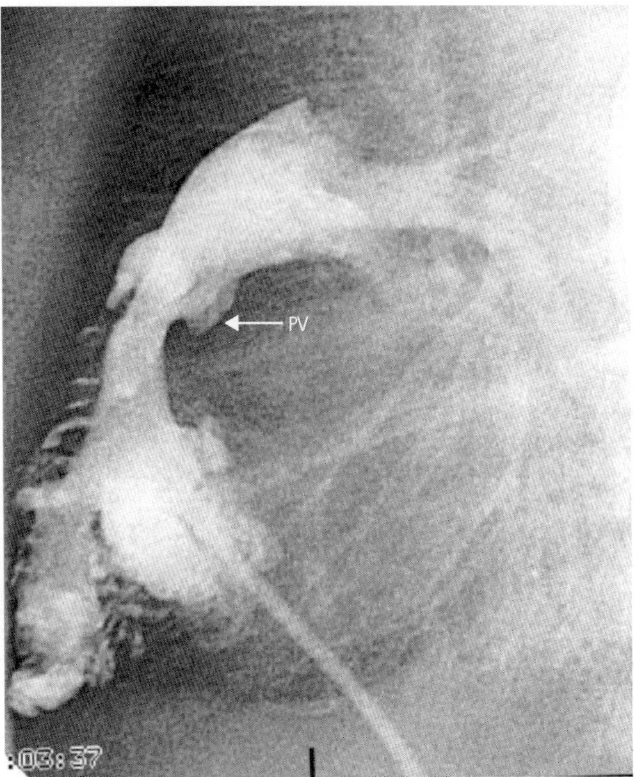

(a) (b)

Fig. 19.21 Right ventricular (RV) angiogram showing pulmonary atresia with an obstruction of the right ventricular outflow tract (a). Following radiofrequency perforation and balloon dilatation, there is flow through the pulmonary valve and into the pulmonary arteries (b). PV, pulmonary valve.

Tricuspid atresia with reduced pulmonary blood flow

Anatomy and physiology

Flow to the pulmonary arteries is via the left ventricle, either through a restrictive ventricular septal defect to the right ventricle and pulmonary artery or through an arterial duct if the pulmonary valve is atretic (Fig. 19.22).

Clinical features

Infants present, in the first few days, with cyanosis (Table 19.7). There is usually a systolic murmur and the second heart sound is single.

Investigations

The electrocardiogram shows a superior (left) axis, left ventricular dominant forces and prominent P waves if the right atrium is enlarged. The lung fields are oligemic on chest radiography (Table 19.8). Echocardiography demonstrates the absent tricuspid valve and other relevant anatomy.[78]

Management

The neonate usually requires prostaglandin to maintain duct patency and a systemic-to-pulmonary shunt to provide a reliable source of pulmonary blood flow. The absent tricuspid valve means that the heart has functionally only a left ventricle. The child will have a single ventricle circulation and palliation is outlined under this condition (p. 863).

PRESENTATION WITH CYANOSIS AND RESPIRATORY DISTRESS

The combination of cyanosis with respiratory distress at birth usually indicates a lung rather than a heart problem. Examples are meconium aspiration syndrome, neonatal pneumonia, or surfactant deficiency in the preterm infant. There is often a history suggesting a respiratory problem such as meconium aspiration. Chest radiography may indicate pneumonia or aspiration with areas of focal lung collapse (atelectasis), hyperexpanded or underdeveloped lungs, a pneumothorax or diaphragmatic hernia. However, it is vital not to miss cyanotic heart disease since the management is so different. Persistent cyanosis in a newborn with respiratory distress is a clear indication for echocardiography. A *hyperoxia test* is useful when this is not immediately available.

Two uncommon congenital heart lesions that present in this way are Ebstein's anomaly and obstructed total anomalous pulmonary venous connection. Ebstein's anomaly is not easily missed. There is typically a huge ('wall-to-wall') heart on chest radiography. Total anomalous pulmonary venous connection is, however, often missed or diagnosed late. Differentiation from persistent fetal circulation or primary lung pathology can be difficult,[73] and since the only effective therapy is urgent surgery, late diagnosis often results in death. Delayed diagnosis also occurs when an infant with a lung problem has a coincident cyanotic heart disease.

Ebstein's anomaly

Anatomy and physiology

The tricuspid valve is displaced down the interventricular septum (Fig. 19.23), towards the apex of the right ventricle, resulting in 'atrialization' of this chamber. This displacement, together with dysplasia of the valve dictates the clinical spectrum, which varies from minimal to severe tricuspid regurgitation. Antenatally, a hugely dilated right heart occupies much of the thorax and the lungs cannot develop normally. Right-to-left shunting at atrial level and little forward flow across the pulmonary valve, which may be stenotic, causes cyanosis at birth. It is uncommon,

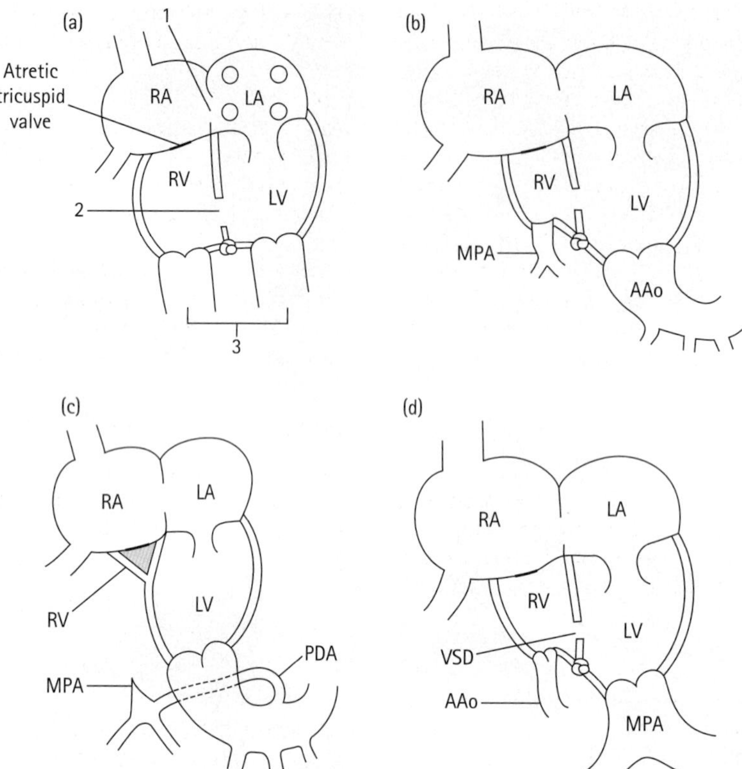

Fig. 19.22 Tricuspid atresia: anatomical variations and physiological implications. (a) The basic structural elements are identified with an atretic tricuspid valve and the three key anatomical-pathophysiological factors: (1) status of the atrial septal defect (ASD), (2) size of the ventricular septal defect (VSD), and (3) great artery connections (normal or transposed). (b) A common form of tricuspid atresia with a large ASD, small-to-moderate VSD resulting in a small right ventricle (RV) and, with normally related great arteries, a small (stenotic) main pulmonary artery (MPA). This patient is likely to have inadequate pulmonary blood flow and need a neonatal shunt. (c) When there is no VSD and normally related great arteries, the RV is absent and MPA is atretic; pulmonary blood flow is dependent on ductal patency. Such patients always need a systemic-to-pulmonary shunt. (d) A small VSD and transposition results in hypoplasia of the RV and aorta; effectively, this is hypoplastic left heart syndrome. (From Skinner et al 2000[212])

comprising less than 1% of congenital heart disease, and is occasionally familial.[87]

Clinical features

The most severe form results in marked tricuspid valve regurgitation and a poorly functioning thin-walled right ventricle, causing fetal or neonatal death. At birth, the infant is deeply cyanosed, with a severe respiratory distress due to the hypoplastic lungs (resulting from intrauterine compression by the large heart) and reduced pulmonary blood flow (Table 19.7). The pansystolic murmur of tricuspid regurgitation together with tricuspid valve clicks may be audible. The liver is markedly enlarged. Mild forms are asymptomatic, presenting with cyanosis, a murmur or supraventricular tachycardia due to the commonly associated Wolff–Parkinson–White syndrome.[88]

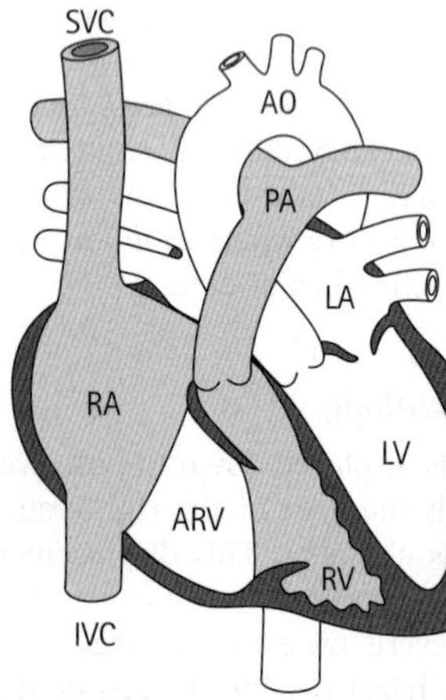

Fig. 19.23 Ebstein's anomaly. The hatched area represents the atrialized portion of the right ventricle (ARV) resulting from the displacement of the septal and posterior leaflets.

Investigations

The electrocardiogram shows right atrial enlargement with large P waves and an incomplete right bundle branch block pattern. Chest radiography shows a markedly enlarged heart and vascularity may be reduced. Echocardiography defines the severity of the lesion.[78]

Management

Successful management of severely affected infants is extremely difficult. Surgical repair of such grossly abnormal valves is impossible. Early therapy includes intensive ventilatory support and treatment with nitric oxide and drugs to encourage a fall in pulmonary vascular resistance. Early mortality is high[88] and long-term outlook poor. Infants with a small right ventricle require management similar to others with a single ventricle circulation (p. 863). Children with a milder form of the condition have a better outlook, but some require surgery to the tricuspid valve in later life.[89]

Total anomalous pulmonary venous connection

This is uncommon, accounting for less than 1% of congenital heart disease. The pulmonary veins join to form a confluence or channel behind the left atrium and eventually drain into the right atrium to mix with the deoxygenated blood returning from the body. The route from the pulmonary venous confluence can be of three types (Fig. 19.24), the commonest being the supracardiac.[90,91] The mode and timing of the clinical presentation depends on whether an obstruction prevents free drainage of the pulmonary venous blood into the right heart (Table 19.7). Infants, with obstruction, present shortly after birth with respiratory distress, cyanosis and cardiac failure. Those without obstruction, present at 2–8 weeks of age, with mild cyanosis and progressive cardiac failure.

Obstructed total anomalous pulmonary venous connection

Anatomy

The infracardiac type is almost always severely obstructed (Fig. 19.24c). The cardiac and supracardiac types are rarely obstructed but this can occur when narrowing is present in other parts of the channel or when a small foramen prevents right-to-left flow at atrial level.

Clinical features

The infant becomes unwell shortly after birth as the pulmonary venous obstruction results in severe pulmonary venous hypertension, cyanosis, cardiac failure and respiratory distress, similar to the picture of persistent fetal circulation.

Investigations

Chest radiography shows pulmonary venous hypertension, but the heart is often not greatly enlarged. The streaky appearance due to the prominent pulmonary veins can easily be mistaken for lung disease, particularly meconium aspiration syndrome. Once the diagnosis is suspected, echocardiography is extremely urgent. Differentiation from persistent pulmonary hypertension of the newborn can be difficult since the left atrium and ventricle are underfilled in both conditions, and compressed by the enlarged right ventricle. There is right-to-left flow across the atrial septum. Diagnosis depends on recognizing the pulmonary venous chamber behind the left atrium but not connecting with it.[78]

Management

Maintaining arterial duct patency with prostaglandin will not help. Ventilatory and circulatory support is necessary and the child transferred urgently for surgery, which is performed without delay. The pulmonary venous chamber is opened into the back of the left atrium, and the abnormal connecting vein ligated. Surgical mortality is high if the infant is extremely acidotic prior to surgery, but overall mortality as low as 7% has been reported.[90] There is a risk of later pulmonary vein stenosis (11%) which can be extremely difficult to manage successfully.

PRESENTATION WITH CYANOSIS AND CARDIAC FAILURE

This is rare presentation, and is usually caused by unobstructed total anomalous pulmonary venous connection, tricuspid atresia with a large ventricular septal defect or common arterial trunk.

Unobstructed total anomalous pulmonary venous connection

Anatomy and physiology

The majority of supracardiac and intracardiac types (Fig. 19.24) are unobstructed. There is a bi-directional shunting at atrial level since the deoxygenated blood from the caval veins mixes with the oxygenated blood from the pulmonary veins in the right atrium. However, the moderate cyanosis is often not detected clinically. As pulmonary vascular resistance falls, the path of least resistance for the blood is now through the tricuspid valve rather than through the oval foramen and the mitral valve. The left-to-right shunting increases and congestive cardiac failure develops due to excessive pulmonary blood flow.

Clinical features

The infant presents, typically after 2 weeks, and sometimes at several months, of age with congestive cardiac failure and moderate cyanosis (Table 19.7). There is a right ventricular heave palpable

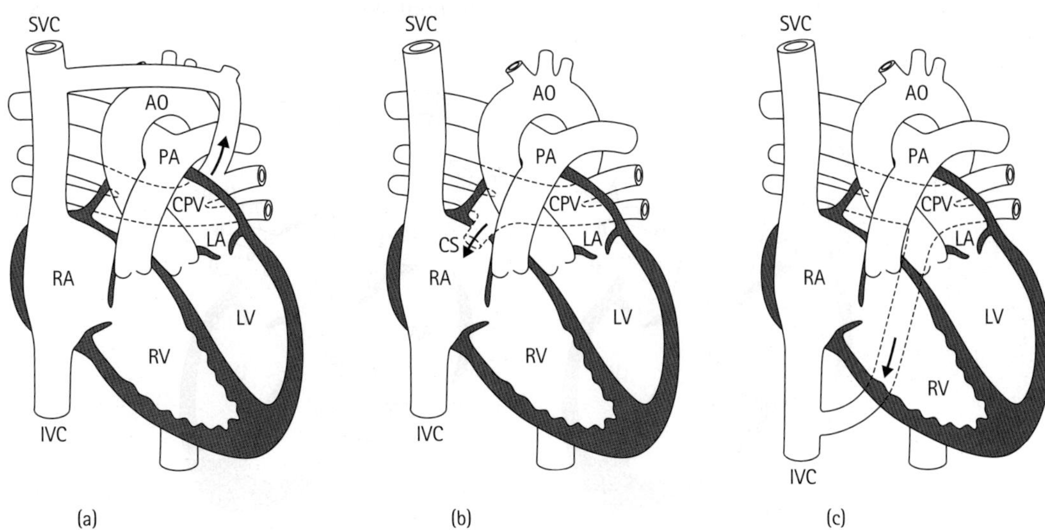

Fig. 19.24 Total anomalous pulmonary venous connection. The three common varieties are shown: (a) supracardiac with the four pulmonary veins draining into a common pulmonary venous channel (CPV) and then via a vertical (ascending) vein to the innominate vein and the right heart; (b) cardiac with the pulmonary veins draining directly to the coronary sinus (CS) as shown or directly to the right atrium (not shown); (c) infracardiac draining into the inferior vena caval or portal vein.

and the second sound is loud and split. There may be a soft ejection systolic murmur caused by increased pulmonary blood flow.

Investigations

The electrocardiogram shows prominent P waves due to right atrial enlargement and right ventricular hypertrophy develops. Chest radiography shows cardiomegaly with right atrial dilatation and pulmonary plethora. The supracardiac type frequently has a broad mediastinum due to the ascending vein, the 'snowman' appearance.

Management

Initial management includes treatment of the cardiac failure with diuretics. Early, but not urgent surgical correction is performed. The pulmonary venous chamber is opened into the back of the left atrium, and the connecting vein is ligated. The results of surgery are good with few long-term complications although early postoperative pulmonary venous obstruction rarely occurs.

Tricuspid atresia with excessive pulmonary blood flow

Anatomy and physiology

There is absence of the right atrioventricular connection and the great vessels are normally related. Systemic venous return passes across the atrial septum to mix with pulmonary venous blood in the left atrium. Flow to the lungs is via the left ventricle, across a large ventricular septal defect to the right ventricle and pulmonary arteries (Fig. 19.22). As the ventricular septal defect is large, pulmonary blood flow is excessive when pulmonary vascular resistance falls.

Clinical features

These infants present with mild cyanosis and congestive cardiac failure after 2 weeks of age (Table 19.7). There may be a soft pulmonary ejection murmur caused by increased blood flow across the pulmonary valve.

Investigations

The electrocardiogram shows a superior axis and the P waves are prominent if the right atrium is enlarged. Chest radiography shows plethoric lung fields (Table 19.8). Echocardiography shows the anatomical features necessary to make the diagnosis.[78]

Management

As the tricuspid valve is atretic, the right ventricle can never function as a normal ventricle and the management will be that of a child with a single ventricle circulation (p. 863). Initially a pulmonary artery band will be needed to limit pulmonaryblood flow.

Common arterial trunk (truncus arteriosus)

This comprises about 1% of congenital heart defects.

Anatomy and physiology

The common arterial trunk fails to divide into aortic and pulmonary components. There is a large ventricular septal defect below the common outlet (truncal) valve, which overrides the ventricular septum. This valve is commonly abnormal, and may have more than three leaflets. It may be stenotic or regurgitant. The condition is subdivided according to the origin of the pulmonary arteries from the arterial trunk (Fig. 19.25). In type 1 they have a common origin; in type 2 they arise separately, but close together, from the back of the trunk, and type 3 separately from the lateral walls of the trunk. Aortic coarctation or interruption is occasionally present.

Clinical features

The mild cyanosis is usually not obvious, and congestive cardiac failure occurs after 2–3 weeks of age due to the high pulmonary blood flow. Clinical signs include brisk pulses, an ejection click from the abnormal valve and cardiac failure. Systolic or early diastolic murmurs occur with truncal valve stenosis or regurgitation. Approximately 35–40% of children have DiGeorge syndrome.[64,84]

Investigations

The electrocardiogram shows biventricular hypertrophy. Chest radiography shows cardiomegaly and plethora, and over 30% have a right aortic arch. Echocardiography shows the ventricular septal defect with overriding truncal valve similar to that in tetralogy of Fallot, but the pulmonary arteries arise from the arterial trunk.[78] Cardiac catheterization is unnecessary unless there is a suspicion of irreversible pulmonary hypertension.

Management

Cardiac failure is managed medically initially, but the large left-to-right shunt and rapid development of pulmonary vascular disease,

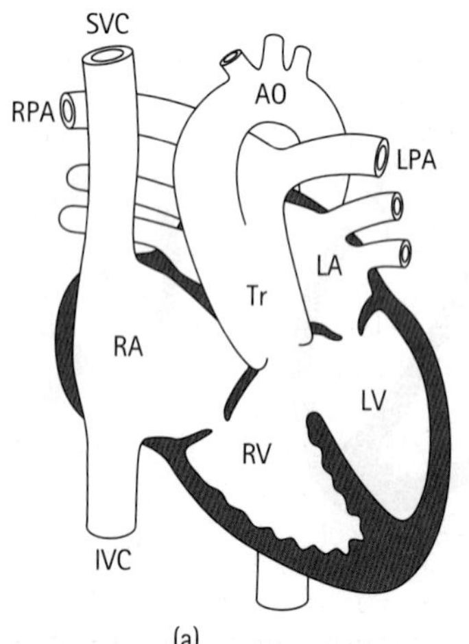

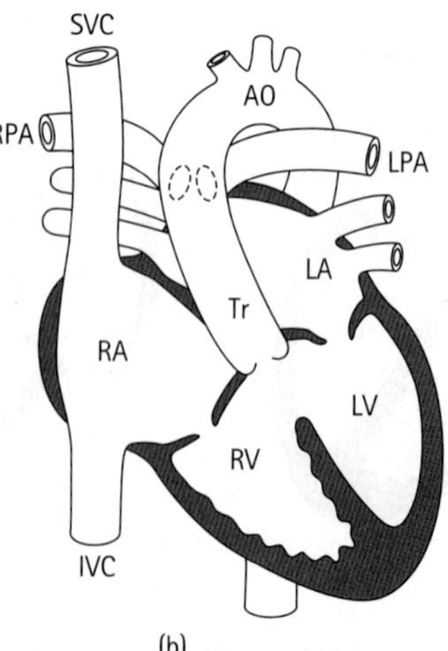

Fig. 19.25 Common arterial trunk: (a) in type 1 the pulmonary arteries arise from the truncus (Tr) with a common origin; (b) in type 2 the pulmonary arteries arise separately from the back. In type 3 (not shown) the pulmonary arteries are more widely reported at origins and arise posteriorly/laterally from the trunk.

makes early surgery necessary. The ventricular septal defect is closed and a valved conduit (usually an aortic homograft) is placed from the right ventricle to the pulmonary artery branches after they are detached from the trunk. Mortality is in the region of 8% and prognosis is largely determined by the function of the truncal valve. A stenotic or regurgitant valve predicts a poor prognosis. The right ventricle to pulmonary artery conduit will need to be replaced as the child grows and the 15 year survival is 83%.[92]

PRESENTATION WITH CARDIOVASCULAR COLLAPSE

Heart disease, especially left heart obstruction, should always be considered in a shocked infant. It is important to feel all the pulses carefully and examine the heart size on chest radiography. Cardiomegaly is usually present with cardiac causes and rare in other conditions.[93] If there is any suspicion of a cardiac lesion, echocardiography is indicated. Other causes of collapse in the neonate include sepsis,[93] respiratory and metabolic disease.

The most common cardiac causes are the left heart obstructive lesions. Supraventricular tachycardia should be considered if the heart rate is over 250 beats per minute.[73] Myocardial disease such as cardiomyopathy (p. 878), either dilated or hypertrophic as seen in infants of diabetic mothers, myocardial ischemia following perinatal distress or anomalous origin of the left coronary artery (p. 865) are rare causes. Pericardial effusion with tamponade occasionally occurs.

Left heart obstructive lesions

Most commonly these are due to severe aortic coarctation or arch interruption, hypoplastic left heart or critical aortic stenosis. Mitral stenosis and pulmonary vein stenosis are rare in isolation. Obstructed total anomalous pulmonary venous connection can present with precipitous cardiovascular collapse, but severe cyanosis and respiratory distress due to pulmonary venous hypertension is usually a more dominant feature. Pulmonary venous hypertension does not occur to the same degree in left heart obstructive lesions, since the left atrium usually decompresses via the oval foramen into the right atrium.

The importance of the arterial duct with critical left heart obstructive lesions

At birth the arterial duct is widely patent and as large as the descending aorta. Thus, when little blood is reaching the distal end of the aortic arch due to an obstruction within the left heart or aorta, the right ventricle is able to supply blood (albeit deoxygenated) to the descending aorta, and the femoral pulses will be palpable. Infants with coarctation have a lower saturation in the legs than in the right arm. In severe aortic stenosis or left heart hypoplasia, the deoxygenated blood from the duct travels retrogradely around the arch and into the head, arms and down the ascending aorta to the coronary arteries. Oximetry in all limbs will reveal deoxygenation. Thus the infant with an obstruction within the left heart will be generally cyanosed, and an infant with isolated coarctation or arch interruption will be cyanosed in the lower body only.

Another interesting presentation is that of cyanosis in the upper body, but normal oxygenation in the lower body. If you can figure out the diagnosis you are beginning to grasp the physiology! It occurs with the combination of transposition of the great arteries and aortic arch interruption or coarctation.

When the arterial duct closes

Since neonates are used to lower blood oxygen levels before birth, they remain well until the duct closes. Flow in the aorta falls with decreased perfusion of vital organs and the deterioration is often dramatic. This effect is made worse in infants with coarctation as ductal tissue around the coarctation site in the aorta produces further narrowing.

Clinical features

All the left heart obstructions share common clinical features related to duct closure. Presentation is usually within 48 h of birth and symptoms include poor feeding, lethargy and pallor. Deterioration is extremely rapid with poor peripheral perfusion resulting in delayed capillary refill time and mottled skin. The pulses are poor and the blood pressure is low. The right ventricle is forceful and murmurs are unremarkable. The infant is usually tachypneic with grunting respiration, the liver is markedly enlarged and urine output is poor.

Investigations

There is a marked metabolic acidosis with abnormal renal and hepatic function, which may result in an abnormal coagulation profile. The electrocardiogram shows right ventricular hypertrophy, and there may be ST depression in the left precordial leads from myocardial ischemia. Chest radiography shows cardiomegaly with a combination of pulmonary plethora and edema. The echocardiographic findings are described under the individual lesions.

Management

Intravenous prostaglandin causes the arterial duct to dilate but the precipitous collapse means that these infants often require endotracheal intubation, inotropic and intensive support. Death can occur if acidosis and renal dysfunction are not corrected. The specific management of individual conditions is discussed below.

Aortic coarctation and interruption of the aortic arch

Anatomy and physiology

Narrowing of the aortic arch commonly occurs at its isthmus between the left subclavian artery and the origin of the arterial duct. This is usually due to a shelf-like obstruction but it can be tubular (Fig. 19.26) and is sometimes associated with hypoplasia of the transverse aorta. About 70% of infants with a coarctation have at least one other associated lesion.[94] The most common are a bicuspid aortic valve, ventricular septal defect and mitral valve anomalies.

Interruption of the aortic arch describes a complete occlusion, which can be classified according to the position. Type A is beyond the left subclavian, type B between the left common carotid and the left subclavian arteries and type C between the carotid arteries.[95]

Clinical features

Most infants present in the first 2 weeks with rapid onset of cardiac failure progressing to cardiovascular collapse as described above. In milder forms the presentation is more insidious, with failure to thrive and cardiac failure. The right arm pulse is strong unless the cardiac function has deteriorated significantly, there is coincident aortic stenosis, or the right subclavian artery has an abnormal origin below the coarctation (an aberrant right subclavian artery). The left arm pulse may be weak if the left subclavian artery arises after the coarctation. The femoral pulses are absent. The right arm blood pressure is high and the blood pressure in the leg is more than 15 mmHg lower. Oscillometric techniques (Dynamap) are not reliable in this setting to record blood pressure in the legs and Doppler sphygnomanometry is more accurate. The right ventricular impulse is prominent and there may be a murmur of mitral regurgitation if the left ventricle is dilated. Murmurs can also be due to associated lesions. Turner's syndrome should be considered in girls with coarctation. Over 50% of infants with type B interruption of the aortic arch have DiGeorge syndrome.[64,84]

Investigations

In addition to the investigations described, echocardiography defines the lesion. The right ventricle and pulmonary artery are enlarged. In infants with coarctation there is an area of narrowing with turbulent flow seen on color Doppler. The Doppler flow pattern through the coarctation has a characteristic 'saw-tooth' appearance with flow continuing into diastole (diastolic tail) (Fig. 19.26). Left ventricular dysfunction may be present. Associated lesions must be assessed together with the size of the arterial duct. Interruption of the aortic arch will be visible on echocardiography.

Management

Surgery is performed when the infant has been stabilized and the acidosis corrected. Infants with coarctation usually have repair through a lateral thoracotomy, and cardiopulmonary bypass is not used unless there is severe hypoplasia of the transverse aortic arch. Repair usually consists of excision of the coarctation and end-to-end anastomosis of the aorta. Infants with an interrupted aortic arch require repair on cardiopulmonary bypass, usually with closure of the associated ventricular septal defect.

Hypoplastic left heart

Anatomy

This is a group of conditions characterized by underdevelopment of the left ventricle, with mitral and aortic atresia or stenosis to a degree that the left ventricle cannot sustain a systemic cardiac output. The ascending aorta is small and most infants (70%) also have coarctation. The milder forms overlap with the severest forms of critical aortic stenosis. Pulmonary venous return is diverted across the oval foramen to the right atrium and ventricle and flow in the aorta is dependent on the arterial duct. As the duct supplies both the systemic and pulmonary circulations, the balance between flow to the body and lungs is critical.[96]

Clinical features

The infant presents acutely with profound collapse (Table 19.7) when the duct closes as described above.

Investigations

The electrocardiogram shows right axis deviation and low left ventricular forces with small R waves in V6. Echocardiography reveals a small left ventricle with stenotic or atretic mitral and aortic

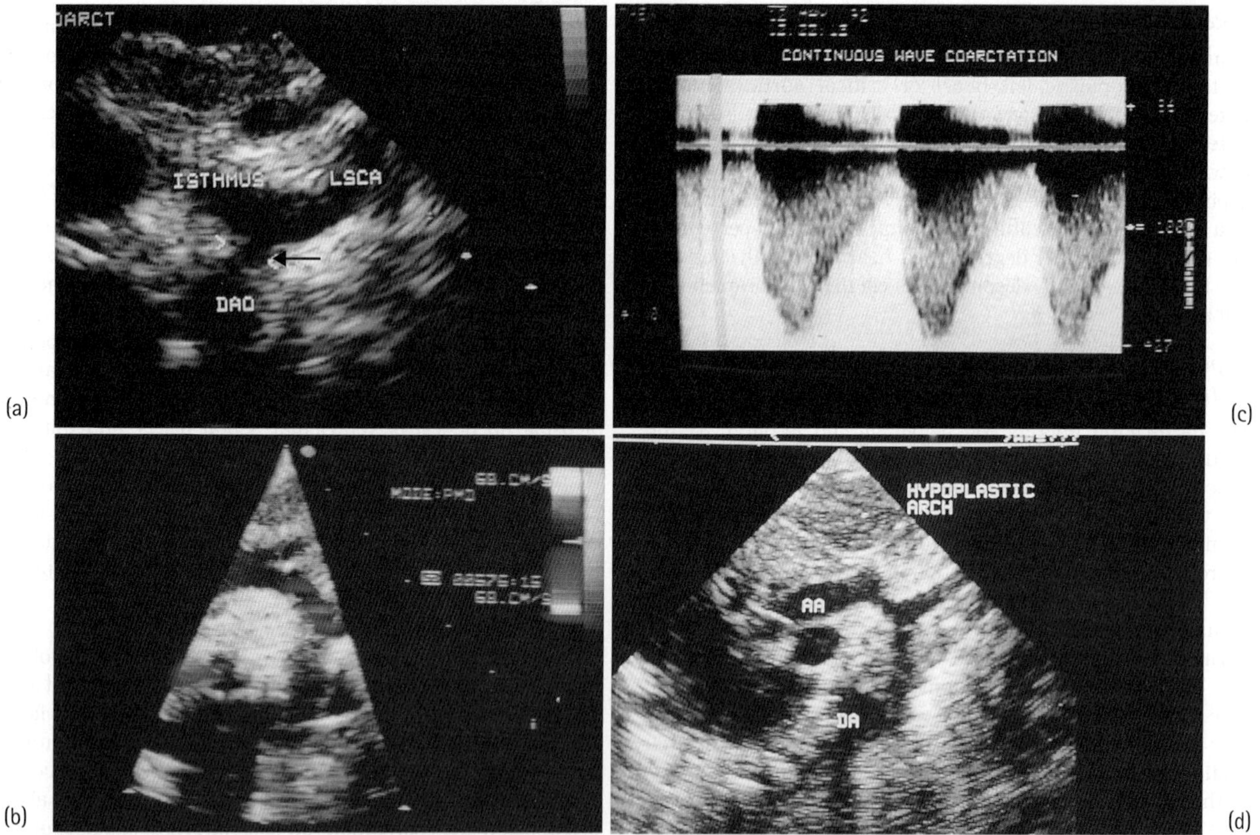

Fig. 19.26 (a) High parasternal greatly magnified view of the isthmus of the aorta, the origin of the left subclavian artery (LSCA) and the descending aorta (DAO). Narrowed area of coarctation is arrowed. (b) Suprasternal view of a baby with coarctation of the aorta. The arch is of reasonable size and the area of coarctation is only clearly identified by the presence of turbulence on the color flow map. (c) Continuous wave Doppler from descending aorta via the suprasternal approach. The classical continuous flow which is seen in coarctation is present. The peak velocity is high and the diastolic velocity never returns to the baseline. (d) Hypoplastic aorta arch in a child who also had coarctation of the aorta. Coarctectomy has been carried out, but there is still isthmal narrowing. AA, ascending aorta; DA, descending aorta. (From Skinner et al 2000[212])

valves. The aortic arch is hypoplastic. The right atrium and ventricle are enlarged, as is the pulmonary artery.

Management

An increasing number of infants, often with an antenatal diagnosis of this condition,[97] are started on prostaglandin infusion soon after birth and are stable enough to undergo the high risk, palliative Norwood operation (Fig. 19.27) in the first days. The aorta is enlarged using part of the pulmonary artery and the distal pulmonary artery is detached and supplied by an aortopulmonary shunt.[98] Further surgery is similar to that for other children with a single ventricle circulation (p. 863). Survival through infancy can now be expected in 30–50%.[97,99]

Critical aortic stenosis

Anatomy and physiology

The aortic valve is thickened, dysplastic and often unicuspid. The right heart is enlarged as it supplies both the pulmonary and systemic circulations through the arterial duct.

Clinical features

These are similar to infants presenting with a hypoplastic left heart. A soft ejection murmur may be audible in the aortic area. An aortic ejection click is seldom audible, as the valve is usually thickened and immobile.

Investigations

These are the same as those described for other infants with left heart obstructive lesions, but there may be left ventricular hypertrophy with a strain pattern on the electrocardiogram. Echocardiography distinguishes it from the other conditions, demonstrating an adequate sized left ventricle, which is either hypertrophied or dilated. The function is usually reduced. The aortic valve is thickened with restricted opening and turbulence is seen on color Doppler. The Doppler velocity across the valve may be increased, or reduced because of poor ventricular function.

Management

Once the infant has been resuscitated and stabilized, transcatheter balloon aortic valvuloplasty or open surgical valvotomy is performed. The results are similar from the two procedures[100,101] but recurrence of the stenosis occurs which requires further intervention later in life.[102]

PRESENTATION WITH CARDIAC FAILURE WITHOUT CYANOSIS

A number of conditions present in early infancy with cardiac failure. These children usually present outside the neonatal period and are discussed later. These include ventricular septal defect (p. 853), atrioventricular septal defect (p. 856), aorticopulmonary window (p. 857), anomalous origin of the left coronary artery (p. 865) and persistent arterial duct (p. 856), which is also covered in the neonatal section. Occasionally infants with cardiomyopathy (p. 878) present in the neonatal period and failure can also be caused by supraventricular tachycardia (p. 868).

PRESENTATION WITH AN ASSOCIATED LESION OR SYNDROME

The most common syndromes likely to be associated with congenital heart disease are shown in Table 19.6. Congenital heart disease should always be considered in infants with a syndrome or dysmorphology. These are discussed in the section on the etiology of congenital heart disease (p. 836).

PRESENTATION WITH AN ASYMPTOMATIC MURMUR

Innocent murmurs are common in the first few days, and are usually related to pulmonary or ductal flow. They are of lower pitch than pathological murmurs, varying with time and heart rate. The murmur of the closing duct may be transient, lasting only one or two days. Physiological branch pulmonary artery stenosis, occurring after duct closure between days one and four, also produces a pulmonary systolic murmur audible in the back. Though more common in the preterm, it can occur in term infants and is almost invariably benign, resolving in a few months.[103]

Since the average heart rate in a newborn is 120 beats per minute, defining niceties of cardiac murmurs is difficult at this age. Even with a calm subject, a lot of practice is required and less than 5% of neonates with a significant murmur will have life-threatening heart disease.[104] Congenital heart lesions that cause a systolic murmur audible from birth are aortic and pulmonary stenosis and tetralogy of Fallot. Small ventricular septal defects are the most common single lesion causing an asymptomatic murmur at this age. This is heard as the right ventricular pressure falls with the postnatal reduction in pulmonary arterial pressure. A patent arterial duct generates a murmur if there is some constriction,

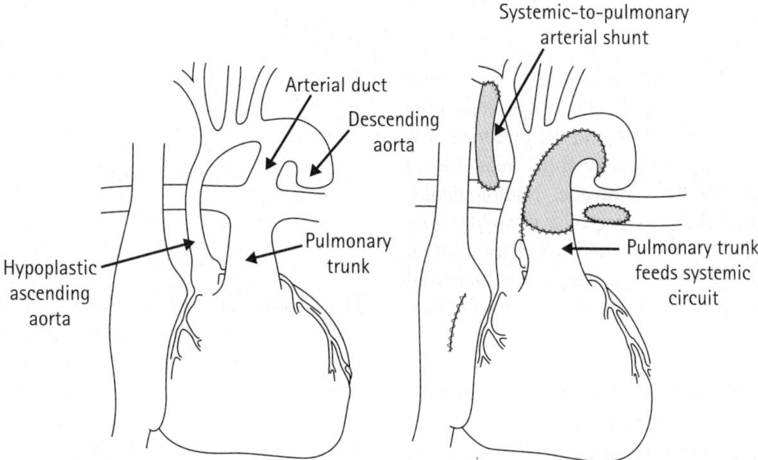

Fig. 19.27 These diagrams show the arrangement of the circulations before and after the classical Norwood procedure, which is the first stage of palliative surgery. (From Anderson et al 2002[79])

allowing the aortic pressure to be higher than pulmonary arterial pressure, but still enough flow through it to generate a noise. In the preterm infant a large left-to-right ductal shunt typically has a systolic rather than a continuous murmur because the aortic and pulmonary arterial pressures are similar in diastole. Tricuspid or mitral regurgitation causes a pansystolic murmur, most commonly in myocardial ischemia following perinatal distress but can represent an isolated valve lesion, or be part of a more complex condition such as an atrioventricular septal defect. A diastolic murmur is always pathological, most commonly due to a large left-to-right shunt later in the first month of life.

MISCELLANEOUS COMPLEX LESIONS

Congenitally corrected transposition of the great arteries

This rare lesion accounts for less than 1% of congenital heart disease.

Anatomy and pathophysiology

This condition has a variety of eponyms including L-transposition and ventricular inversion. It is characterized by discordance of both the atrioventricular and the ventriculo-arterial connection (Fig. 19.28a). The deoxygenated right atrial blood passes through the mitral valve into a morphological left ventricle from which the pulmonary artery arises. The oxygenated pulmonary venous blood passes from the left atrium, through the tricuspid valve, into the morphological right ventricle and thence into the aorta. Thus although there is transposition, the anatomical fault is functionally corrected by the presence of atrioventricular discordance. The aorta is usually located anterior and to the left of the pulmonary artery. Ventricular septal defect is the most frequently associated lesion and commonly occurs with pulmonary stenosis, which may result in cyanosis from shunting of deoxygenated blood into the aorta. A few patients have no other lesions and remain pink. The condition is commonly associated with dextrocardia.

Clinical presentation and course

Associated cardiac lesions usually dictate the clinical presentation and course. If a large ventricular septal defect is present heart failure develops early. Those patients with a ventricular septal defect and pulmonary stenosis present with cyanosis and clinically resemble tetralogy of Fallot. In the absence of associated defects the condition may not be recognized for many years, but left sided atrioventricular valve (tricuspid) regurgitation may develop progressively. Arrhythmias and complete heart block are common.

Investigations

Inversion of the ventricles alters the direction of ventricular septal depolarization and produces the characteristic electrocardiographic finding of the absence of Q waves in V5 and V6 and the presence of Q waves in V4R or V1. The electrocardiogram may show heart block, arrhythmias or Wolff–Parkinson–White syndrome. Radiologically, the condition may be suspected by the presence of a straight upper left heart border produced by the left-sided anterior aorta. Echocardiography will determine the abnormal atrioventricular and ventriculo-arterial connections and define any associated abnormality.

Management

The management is usually that of the associated lesion. Severely cyanosed infants require a systemic-to-pulmonary shunt. For those with heart failure secondary to a large ventricular septal defect, pulmonary artery banding may be indicated. Closure of the ventricular septal defect is associated with a high incidence of complete heart block (30%) and significant mortality. Because of gradual deterioration of the systemic right ventricle and progressive tricuspid regurgitation, surgery, to restore the left ventricle to pump to the systemic circulation, has been performed. This can be achieved by means of the double switch operation (Fig. 19.28).

Double inlet (single) ventricle

This condition is more common than has been previously recognized and may account for up to 2–3% of congenital heart disease. Both atria are connected with a dominant ventricle, usually the left ventricle, the other ventricle being rudimentary (Fig. 19.29).

The main ventricle usually has the morphology of a left ventricle with two inlet valves and the right ventricle is a small outflow chamber. The ventriculo-arterial connection can vary, but most commonly the aorta arises from the rudimentary chamber, and the pulmonary artery from the main ventricular chamber. The outlet chamber communicates with the main ventricular chamber via a ventricular septal defect. The severity of any associated pulmonary stenosis determines the presentation and the management is the same as for other children with a single ventricle circulation (p. 863).

Double outlet right ventricle

Anatomy and physiology

The aorta and pulmonary artery both arise from the right ventricle. There are two common types. In one variation there is a large ventricular septal defect, with no pulmonary stenosis. This is commonly associated with a posterior pulmonary artery and an anterior aorta. The ventricular septal defect is related to the large pulmonary valve and has obvious similarities to transposition with a large ventricular septal defect (known as the Taussig–Bing malformation). In the other variation there is a large ventricular septal defect with pulmonary stenosis and the features mimic tetralogy of Fallot.

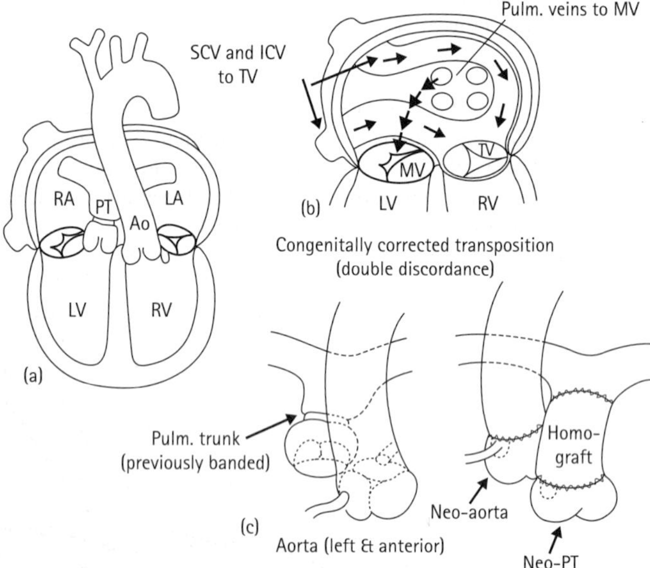

Fig. 19.28 The steps involved in the so-called double switch procedure involve, first, banding of the pulmonary trunk (PT) unless associated lesions have already 'prepared' the left ventricle (a). An atrial redirection procedure (b) is then combined with an arterial switch (c). This then produces both physiological and anatomical correction. Ao, aorta; LA, left atrium; LV, left ventricle; MV, mitral valve; Pulm., pulmonary; RA, right atrium; RV, right ventricle; SCV and ICV, superior and inferior caval veins; TV, tricuspid valve. (From Anderson et al 2002[79])

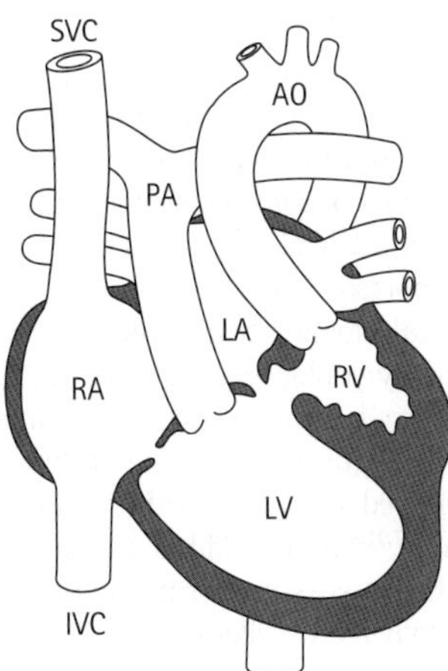

Fig. 19.29 Double inlet ventricle or single ventricle. In the most common variety as here both atrioventricular valves connect to a morphologically normal left ventricle (LV) and the right ventricle is represented by a small rudimentary outflow chamber from which the aorta arises. There is usually arterioventricular discordance.

Clinical features

Depending upon the associated lesions, the clinical features mimic other lesions such as transposition, ventricular septal defect, or tetralogy of Fallot. Echocardiography defines the anatomy and excludes other conditions.

Management

Infants with high pulmonary blood flow require pulmonary artery banding whereas those with severe cyanosis, because of restrictive pulmonary blood flow, may require a Blalock–Taussig shunt. Definitive repair depends upon the site of the ventricular septal defect. Occasionally, only an intracardiac patch may be required, but in other children, arterial switch and closure of a ventricular septal defect, or major reconstruction with the use of a conduit, may be necessary.

Abnormal cardiac positions

Dextrocardia refers only to the situation in which more than half the heart is situated in the right side of the chest. It does not necessarily have implications for the anatomy of the heart itself. Dextrocardia may thus be a primary abnormality of the heart or secondary to other thoracic pathology. Primary dextrocardia is often associated with abnormal positions of the abdominal organs. Complete situs inversus refers to the mirror image arrangement of the organs. It occurs with an incidence of 1 per 7000 to 1 per 10 000 and 90–95% of these individuals have a normal heart. When dextrocardia is associated with abnormal or ambiguous visceral arrangements the heart is usually abnormal; malformations include atrioventricular discordance, univentricular heart, anomalous pulmonary venous drainage and pulmonary atresia. About one-third of patients with asplenia or polysplenia have dextrocardia. The combination of situs inversus, bronchiectasis and paranasal sinusitis, known as Kartagener's syndrome, occurs in 10–15% of patients with mirror-image dextrocardia.

Mesocardia indicates the position of the heart in the center of the thorax, prominent neither to the right, nor to the left. It is usually not recognized clinically and is apparent only from chest radiography. The term *levocardia* need be used only when the left-sided heart is associated with abnormal visceral situs.

The possibility of abnormal cardiac position should always be remembered. The cardiac apex and impulse should be palpated over the right chest if it is not apparent on the left side, and heart sounds should be auscultated on both sides. Abnormal location of the liver edge in the midline or the left side, or the stomach resonance on the right side of the abdomen suggests abnormal abdominal situs, often associated with cardiac malposition.

Chest radiography confirms the position of the heart. The morphology of the bronchi will suggest the thoracic situs, and the position of the stomach and liver, the abdominal situs. Abnormal cardiac or visceral situs is an indication for cardiac review. The electrocardiogram should be performed with the addition of right-sided chest leads (V3R to V7R). In dextrocardia, the QRS complexes are characteristically taller in the right chest leads and become progressively smaller from V3 to V7 in the left-sided chest leads. A negative P wave in lead I indicates reversed atrial arrangement (atrial situs inversus), but does not specify the position of the heart in the chest. Echocardiography provides the best, non-invasive means of identifying the arrangements and anatomy of the atria, ventricles and great vessels and any associated malformations.

Mesocardia and levocardia, with abnormal visceral situs, are commonly associated with asplenia or polysplenia.[105] When asplenia or polysplenia is suspected, splenic ultrasound and examination of the peripheral blood for Howell–Jolly bodies are appropriate. Patients with asplenia should receive pneumococcal vaccine, and prophylactic antibiotic therapy.

THE INFANT AND CHILD WITH CONGENITAL HEART DISEASE

The range of cardiac lesions, together with their presentation and management, is somewhat different from that of neonates. However, there is overlap with a number of cyanotic and acyanotic lesions presenting at any age. Acyanotic lesions fall broadly into two groups; those with heart disease which causes an increased volume load, and those with a lesion which results in pressure loading of the heart.

ACYANOTIC HEART DISEASE WITH INCREASED VOLUME LOAD

Increased volume load is usually caused by a left-to-right shunt, such as an atrial or ventricular septal defect, persistent arterial duct or atrioventricular septal defects. Rare causes include aortico-pulmonary window and large arteriovenous fistula. Valvular regurgitation also produces an increased volume load to the heart.

Ventricular septal defect

Anatomy

Ventricular septal defects occur alone or in association with a range of other cardiac lesions. They are usually small and occur in any part of the membranous or muscular interventricular septum (Fig. 19.30). Those in the membranous septum are called perimembranous, as they extend into the adjacent muscle. They are the most common variant and are usually single. They can extend;

- posteriorly into the muscular inlet between the atrioventricular valves;
- inferiorly into the trabecular portion of the interventricular septum;
- anteriorly into the muscular outlet between the right and left ventricular outflow tracts (as in tetralogy of Fallot). Rarely outlet defects are associated with prolapse of the aortic valve into the defect causing regurgitation.

Muscular defects are completely surrounded by muscle. They also occur in the inlet, outlet or trabecular portions of the muscular septum where they are frequently multiple.

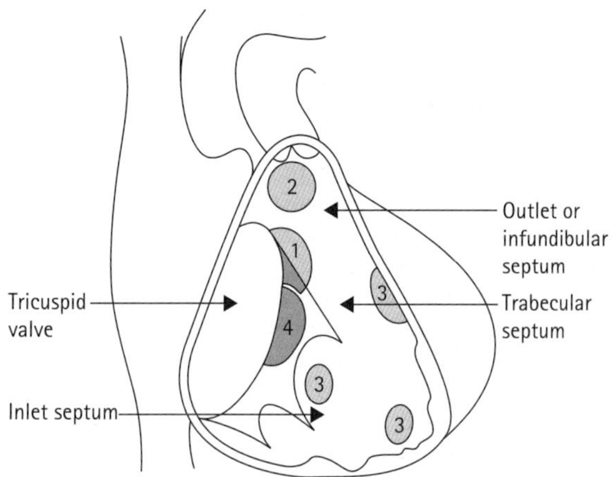

Fig. 19.30 Types of ventricular septal defect: (1) perimembranous; (2) outlet or subarterial; (3) trabecular; (4) inlet.

Physiology

The clinical features and prognosis depend on the size and number of defects, and the volume of blood passing into the right ventricle. Small defects limit the shunt, so pulmonary artery pressure and blood flow are close to normal (restrictive defect). If the defect is large, left and right ventricular pressures are equal (non-restrictive defect) and the volume of shunt depends on the systemic and pulmonary vascular resistances. The fall in pulmonary vascular resistance after birth is delayed and if the pulmonary blood flow remains excessive, irreversible pulmonary hypertension develops (p. 884).

Small ventricular septal defect

Clinical features

Infants present with an asymptomatic murmur, audible in the first few weeks of life, as the pulmonary vascular resistance falls. A perimembranous defect produces a loud, harsh pansystolic murmur at the fourth left intercostal space, usually associated with a thrill. It radiates to the apex and back. A muscular defect gives a short early systolic murmur localized to the fourth left intercostal space that disappears late in systole as the defect closes with ventricular contraction. The rest of the cardiovascular examination is normal unless there are other cardiac lesions.

Differential diagnosis of small perimembranous ventricular septal defect: mitral regurgitation, where the murmur radiates to the axilla, tricuspid regurgitation, where the murmur varies in intensity with respiration. The long ejection systolic murmur of tetralogy of Fallot, or severe subaortic stenosis, can mimic a pansystolic murmur and the site of maximum intensity is similar. In severe aortic and pulmonary valve stenosis, the site of maximum intensity is in the second intercostal space.

Differential diagnosis of small muscular ventricular septal defect: innocent vibratory murmur, mitral valve prolapse, bicuspid aortic valve, mild aortic or pulmonary stenosis, atrial septal defect.

Investigations

The electrocardiogram is normal and chest radiography is not indicated. Echocardiogram confirms the diagnosis. Perimembranous defects often have a small aneurysm of the membranous septum. Color Doppler flow identifies small muscular defects. The velocity across the defect will be over 4 m/sec indicating that the right ventricular pressure is normal. Echocardiography will also identify other cardiac lesions.

Management and prognosis

Over two-thirds of muscular defects, and almost one-third of perimembranous defects, close spontaneously within 6 years.[106] Initially it is necessary to confirm that the pulmonary artery pressure is normal. Thereafter the child is reviewed at infrequent intervals until it has closed. This is most likely in early childhood, but closure into adult life has been reported.[107] Children should be encouraged to lead a normal life. Surgical closure is indicated for patients with aortic regurgitation caused by prolapse of a leaflet into the defect[108] and following endocarditis. A small number of patients (5%) develop subaortic stenosis or right ventricular outflow obstruction (8%). Surgery may be indicated for these or other lesions. Late arrhythmias have been reported[107,109] and sudden death has been described. Antibiotic prophylaxis is necessary for procedures until the defect has closed. Long-term survival is excellent with a 96% 25-year survival.[109]

Large ventricular septal defects

Clinical features

Infants present at 2–8 weeks of age as pulmonary vascular resistance falls and pulmonary blood flow increases. They develop symptoms of heart failure and recurrent respiratory infections. As pulmonary hypertension develops, symptoms disappear and reversal of the shunt causes cyanosis (Eisenmenger syndrome). Some infants, particularly those with Down syndrome, have minimal symptoms because persistently high pulmonary vascular resistance prevents excessive blood flow. The infant is tachypneic with intercostal and subcostal recession. The left precordium is prominent with a right ventricular lift and displaced apex indicating biventricular enlargement. A thrill may be associated with the pansystolic murmur that is maximal at the fourth left intercostal space and radiates to the apex and the back. A mid-diastolic murmur is caused by excessive pulmonary blood flow returning to the left atrium, causing turbulent flow across the mitral valve. It is present at the apex but may be inaudible because of tachypnea and tachycardia. A gallop rhythm may be heard and the liver is enlarged. As pulmonary vascular resistance increases, the murmur becomes softer and the pulmonary component of the second heart sound louder. Older infants and children have signs of pulmonary hypertension (p. 884).

Differential diagnosis: large persistent arterial duct or complete atrioventricular septal defect. Rare conditions include aortico-pulmonary window, cardiomyopathy, severe mitral regurgitation, anomalous origin of the left coronary artery, total anomalous pulmonary venous drainage and complex lesions with unrestricted pulmonary blood flow.

Investigations

The electrocardiogram shows biventricular hypertrophy.[6,7] The QRS axis is usually normal, but children with inlet or multiple muscular defects may have left axis deviation. When pulmonary hypertension develops, right ventricular hypertrophy is dominant. The presence of other cardiac lesions may modify the electrocardiogram. Chest radiography shows cardiomegaly with biventricular and left atrial enlargement with plethora. As pulmonary hypertension develops, the cardiac shadow becomes smaller, the proximal pulmonary arteries larger and the peripheral vessels less prominent ('peripheral pruning').

Echocardiography indicates the site, size and number of defects[110] and other cardiac lesions. Enlargement of the left atrium, left ventricle and pulmonary artery indicates a large shunt. The Doppler velocity across the defect is low, reflecting an elevated right ventricular pressure. Cardiac catheterization is rarely performed, as the information necessary for monitoring and surgical closure can be obtained from echocardiography.[111] It is indicated if there is concern about irreversible pulmonary hypertension, especially in a child who presents late, or to obtain information about other lesions. The increase in oxygen saturation between the systemic veins and pulmonary artery allows calculation of pulmonary blood flow, which is more than twice systemic. Measurement of the pulmonary artery pressure allows assessment of pulmonary hypertension. A high concentration of inspired oxygen will indicate whether pulmonary hypertension is reversible. Angiography in the left ventricle demonstrates the site, size and number of defects. Further angiography may be performed to evaluate other lesions.

Management and prognosis

Treatment is initially for heart failure (p. 833). Nasogastric feeding may help to achieve adequate intake. Added calories are beneficial, but poor weight gain may also be due to increased energy expenditure. Limiting the volume of feeds is only done to control intractable heart failure. Patients with large defects can develop pulmonary hypertension in infancy. Surgery is indicated between 2 and 5 months of age to prevent this and to promote growth. The operative mortality is less than 5% with a similar risk of re-operation. Children with more complex lesions such as multiple muscular defects or chronic lung disease may be unsuitable for primary repair. This may also not be possible if facilities for infant surgery are unavailable. Pulmonary artery banding is palliative, limiting pulmonary blood flow and preventing irreversible pulmonary hypertension until the defects become smaller or the other problems improve. Transcatheter device closure is limited to defects, usually muscular, that are difficult to close surgically.[18] Rarely a large defect will close spontaneously by apposition of part of the tricuspid valve or prolapse of an aortic leaflet into the defect. Muscular defects are more likely, and outlet defects less likely, to close spontaneously. Antibiotic prophylaxis is essential for procedures until the defect is closed. The long-term survival after repair of a ventricular septal defect is excellent, with few late complications.[109]

Some patients have moderate-sized defects without pulmonary hypertension. Surgery can be delayed if the child is asymptomatic, weight gain is satisfactory and there are signs of closure on the echocardiogram. If the pulmonary blood flow remains more than twice systemic, the defect should be closed because of the late development of pulmonary hypertension or chronic volume loading of the heart.

Atrial septal defect

Anatomy

Atrial septal defects are classified according to their position in the atrial septum. (Fig. 19.31) The most common type is the ostium secundum defect, situated in the region of the fossa ovalis. It is usually single, but may consist of multiple small defects (fenestrated). Sinus venosus defects occur in the superior part of the atrial septum and are associated with partial anomalous venous drainage of the right upper pulmonary vein to the superior vena cava or right atrium. Ostium primum defects, at the lower margin of the interatrial septum, are partial atrioventricular septal defects (p. 856). Rarely defects are related to the inferior vena cava or coronary sinus. Occasionally there can be an almost complete absence of the atrial septum (common atrium). A patent oval foramen is normal in infancy and occasionally persists into adult life.

Physiology

The volume of left-to-right shunt depends on the size of the defect and the relative compliance of the ventricles. This determines the size of the right atrium, right ventricle, pulmonary artery and left atrium that receive the excessive blood flow. Pulmonary hypertension does not develop until adult life. A patent oval foramen is not usually hemodynamically significant, but if the right atrial pressure is increased due to another cardiac abnormality, right-to-left shunting can occur with systemic desaturation. It may also be a cause of paradoxical systemic emboli.

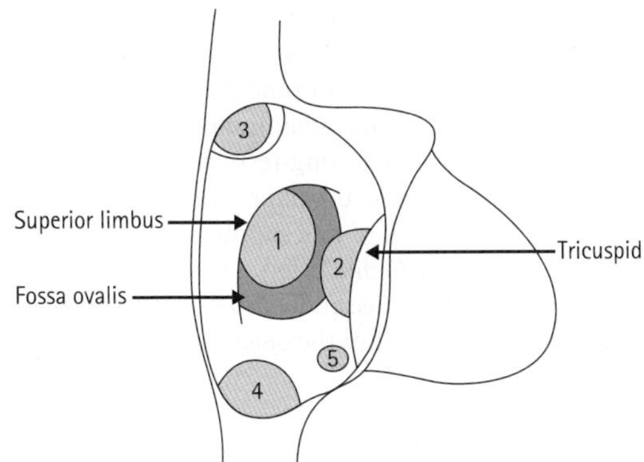

Fig. 19.31 Types of atrial septal defect: (1) ostium secundum; (2) ostium primum; (3) superior sinus venosus; (4) inferior sinus venosus; (5) coronary sinus.

Clinical features

Most children present between 1 and 5 years of age with an asymptomatic murmur. Rarely this condition is familial. Few have failure to thrive or symptoms of heart failure. The right ventricular enlargement results in a slight precordial bulge and diffuse impulse on palpation. Because of excessive pulmonary blood flow, the pulmonary component of the second heart sound is delayed and does not become single during expiration (fixed splitting). This excessive blood flow also accounts for the murmurs, as flow across the actual defect is silent. The ejection systolic murmur in the pulmonary area is due to flow across the pulmonary valve and may be audible in the back. The mid-diastolic murmur at the fourth left intercostal space is caused by increased flow across the tricuspid valve.

Differential diagnosis: innocent murmur, mild pulmonary or aortic stenosis, aortic coarctation and persistent arterial duct with pulmonary hypertension.

Investigations

The electrocardiogram shows incomplete right bundle branch block in over 90% of patients, but this can also be seen in up to 10% of normal children. Chest radiography shows a right atrial, right ventricular, and pulmonary artery enlargement with plethora. Echocardiography confirms the size and type of defect together with a large right atrium, right ventricle and pulmonary artery. The velocity across the pulmonary valve is usually normal, but may be increased due to flow. Cardiac catheterization is seldom necessary for diagnosis, except for sinus venosus defects when the pulmonary venous drainage is unclear. Pulmonary artery pressures are normal or slightly elevated and the increase in oxygen content between systemic veins and pulmonary artery allows the left-to-right shunt ratio to be calculated. Angiography can identify the site of pulmonary venous drainage. Transoesophageal echocardiography also defines the defect and pulmonary veins.

Management and prognosis

The majority of secundum defects seen in the neonatal period will close,[112] as will those smaller than 6 mm in diameter.[113] Defects more than 8 mm are unlikely to close. It is now possible to close central defects by transcatheter route with various devices.[18,114] This technique carries a low risk in selected patients and results in a high closure rate that is comparable with surgery.[29] Surgical closure is either by direct suture or patch. Mortality is less than 1%, with a 10% chance of postcardiotomy syndrome with pericardial effusion, which usually resolves with anti-inflammatory treatment. Closure during early childhood results in long-term survival that is similar to the general population.[115] Closure after 7 years of age results in a progressive increase in the risk of late supraventricular tachycardia because of chronic right atrial dilatation. Pulmonary hypertension may develop in adult life. Infective endocarditis is rare, but antibiotic prophylaxis is recommended until the defect is closed.

Patent arterial duct

Anatomy

The arterial duct connects the pulmonary artery and descending aorta. It usually closes in the first few days of life by contraction of smooth muscle. This is delayed in premature infants (Ch. 10), those born at high altitudes and if there is an abnormality of the duct wall. It may coexist with other congenital heart defects. In the presence of inadequate systemic or pulmonary blood flow, it provides a temporary conduit to compensate for the lesion.

Physiology

Flow across an arterial duct depends on its size and the difference between the systemic and pulmonary vascular resistance. The duct is usually constricted and the pulmonary arterial pressure is lower than systemic, producing continuous systolic and diastolic flow. If it remains large, pulmonary arterial and aortic pressures equalize, and flow depends on the relative resistances. The increased pulmonary blood flow results in enlargement of the left atrium and ventricle. A large shunt causes pulmonary hypertension and flow becomes limited to systole or even reversed (Eisenmenger syndrome).

Small patent arterial duct

Clinical features

The child usually presents with an asymptomatic murmur. A history of prematurity or maternal rubella should arouse suspicion of an arterial duct. Rarely it is familial. Pulses and precordial palpation are normal. A continuous murmur is best heard at the left infraclavicular area.

Differential diagnosis: venous hum (varies with posture and is best heard on the right), arteriovenous connection (e.g. coronary, cerebral, chest wall or pulmonary), ventricular septal defect with aortic regurgitation, ruptured sinus of Valsalva aneurysm.

Investigations

Electrocardiogram and chest radiography are normal. Echocardiography confirms the presence and size of the duct. There is no chamber enlargement and a high velocity flow across the duct confirms that the pulmonary artery pressure is normal. Cardiac catheterization is not necessary for diagnosis, but transcatheter closure with a device is possible.

Management and prognosis

Arterial ducts are unlikely to close spontaneously in an infant more than a few months after term. Although the risk of endocarditis is small, closure is usually recommended as this, together with mild left ventricular volume overload, may cause long-term problems.[116] Transcatheter closure, by a variety of coils or devices, is the method of choice if this is available, with successful occlusion rate of over 98%.[18,28] Significant complications are rare and embolized coils or devices are usually retrieved by catheter. Alternatively, surgical ligation is performed through a lateral thorocotomy. Echocardiography has allowed visualization of ducts that are so tiny that they do not produce an audible murmur. The consensus is that they should not be occluded as this is technically difficult and the risk of endocarditis is remote.[116,117]

Large patent arterial duct

Clinical features

Large arterial ducts are rare and symptoms are similar to those found in infants with a large ventricular septal defect. The pulse is rapid and bounding with a wide pulse pressure, and there are signs of heart failure. The heart sounds are loud and there may be a third sound at the apex. The murmur is best heard in the pulmonary area but radiates down the left sternal border. It peaks late in systole with a soft, short diastolic component. A mid-diastolic murmur at the apex is caused by increased blood flow returning from the lungs to the left atrium and causing turbulence across the mitral valve. If pulmonary hypertension is present, there will be a right ventricular lift, a short systolic murmur and a loud second heart sound. No mid-diastolic murmur will be heard because pulmonary blood flow is reduced.

Differential diagnosis: other conditions presenting with heart failure and a continuous murmur include aorticopulmonary window, pulmonary atresia with major aorticopulmonary collateral arteries, absent pulmonary valve syndrome. Other conditions presenting with heart failure and a systolic murmur are as for a large ventricular septal defect.

Investigations

The electrocardiogram shows biventricular hypertrophy.[6,7] Chest radiography shows left atrial, left ventricular and pulmonary artery enlargement with plethora. As pulmonary hypertension develops, the cardiac shadow becomes smaller, the proximal pulmonary arteries larger and peripheral vessels less prominent ('peripheral pruning'). Echocardiography shows left atrial, left ventricular and pulmonary artery enlargement. The right ventricle is hypertrophied if there is pulmonary hypertension. The duct can be imaged and Doppler evaluation allows an estimation of pulmonary artery pressure.

Management and prognosis

Initial management includes the treatment of heart failure (p. 833). Surgical ligation is necessary if the duct is too large for transcatheter closure. Risks include recurrent laryngeal nerve damage, recanalization and inadvertent ligation of the left pulmonary artery. The operative mortality is less than 0.5%.[116] Recently devices have become available that can occlude large ducts in infants over 5 kg. If the duct is closed before the development of irreversible pulmonary hypertension, the outcome is excellent.

Atrioventricular septal defect

Anatomy

Atrioventricular septal defects represent a spectrum of conditions that have in common a deficiency of the atrioventricular septum and adjacent valves (Fig. 19.32). A partial atrioventricular septal defect is an ostium primum atrial septal defect. A complete atrioventricular septal defect has both atrial and ventricular components (Fig. 19.16). The atrioventricular valves are always abnormal. Partial defects usually have two separate atrioventricular valves at the same level. In the complete atrioventricular septal defect there is a single (common) atrioventricular valve. Occasionally left ventricular outflow tract obstruction[118] or a hypoplastic ventricle can complicate the clinical picture. Tetralogy of Fallot, coarctation or atrial isomerism with asplenia may coexist. Down syndrome occurs in over 65% of children with a complete atrioventricular septal defect[119] and 25% of those with a partial

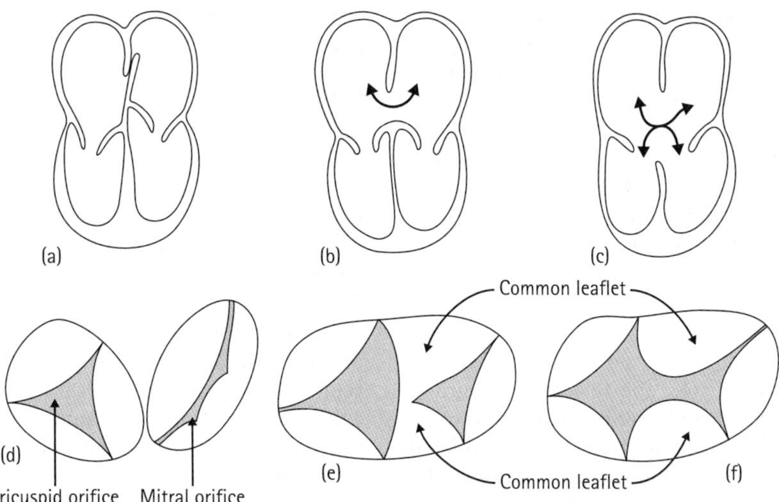

Fig. 19.32 Anatomy of the atrioventricular junction: (a and d) normal septation with no septal communication and separate valve orifices at different levels; (b and e) partial atrioventricular septal defect with atrial shunting, two valve orifices at the same level and a 'cleft' anterior mitral leaflet; (c and f) complete atrioventricular septal defect with interatrial and interventricular communications and a common atrioventricular valve.

defect. This lesion was previously called an endocardial cushion defect or atrioventricular canal.

Physiology

Children with partial atrioventricular septal defects have hemodynamics similar to an atrial septal defect and those with a complete atrioventricular septal defect have features of a ventricular septal defect. The atrioventricular valves are always regurgitant. If this is severe, the hemodynamic effect adds to that of the septal defect. Infants with a complete atrioventricular septal defect may have mild desaturation because of common mixing and pulmonary hypertension. Those with Down syndrome develop pulmonary vascular obstructive disease at a younger age.[120]

Clinical features

Infants may present because of the diagnosis of Down syndrome. The other clinical features are those of an atrial or ventricular septal defect. There is also a pansystolic murmur of left atrioventricular valve regurgitation. If this is severe it will contribute to the clinical features of pulmonary congestion and heart failure.

Investigations

Chest radiography and electrocardiogram correspond to the type of septal defect. There is also left axis deviation on the electrocardiogram. Echocardiography identifies the anatomical type of atrioventricular septal defect and the size of the atrial and ventricular components. It allows evaluation of ventricular size, atrioventricular valve regurgitation and other cardiac lesions. It also provides information on the degree of pulmonary hypertension. Cardiac catheterization may be required to assess pulmonary vascular resistance in older infants and children. Angiography defines the atrial and ventricular septal defects and atrioventricular valve regurgitation.

Management and prognosis

Partial atrioventricular septal defects should be closed surgically between 2 and 5 years of age. Complete atrioventricular septal defects require surgery at 3–6 months of age,[74] to prevent the development of irreversible pulmonary hypertension. Pulmonary artery banding may be performed to defer definitive surgery in infants with other lesions or when surgery carries a high risk. At the time of definitive surgery the left atrioventricular valve is repaired to reduce regurgitation and improve outcome.[118] Re-operation is occasionally necessary for left atrioventricular valve regurgitation or stenosis, or left ventricular outflow tract obstruction. A few patients require a pacemaker for complete heart block after surgery, or develop late supraventricular tachyarrhythmias.

Survival after repair of partial atrioventricular septal defect is excellent with less than 3% early mortality and a 20-year survival of 87%.[118] Early mortality following repair of complete atrioventricular septal defect is about 10% with a 10-year survival of 83%.[119]

Aorticopulmonary window

This is a direct communication between the ascending aorta and the pulmonary trunk, usually between the left side of the ascending aorta and the right side of the pulmonary artery. Most defects are large and increased pulmonary blood flow and pulmonary hypertension occur early in life. Dyspnea, failure to thrive, and congestive heart failure are common in infancy. The pulse is collapsing and there is cardiomegaly on palpation. The pulmonary second heart sound is loud and a systolic rather than continuous murmur is heard over the left sternal border. A mid-diastolic flow murmur may be present at the apex. The findings mimic a large ventricular septal defect or ductus arteriosus with pulmonary hypertension.

Chest radiography shows cardiomegaly with prominent pulmonary trunk and plethoric lungs. The electrocardiogram shows biventricular hypertrophy or left ventricular hypertrophy alone if pulmonary hypertension is mild. The defect is visible on cross-sectional echocardiography and color Doppler imaging. The precise site and size of the defect can be defined with aortic root angiography and surgical closure of the defect should be performed early because of the high risk of pulmonary vascular disease.

Arteriovenous fistulas

Fistulas between a systemic artery and vein can be present anywhere in the body. The common sites are between a cerebral artery and the vein of Galen,[121] the subclavian artery and vein, the hepatic artery and portal vein, the internal mammary artery and the internal mammary vein or the ductus venosus. Cavernous hemangiomas can involve the skin, pelvis or the liver. Acquired fistulas are usually the result of trauma.

The arteriovenous fistula allows run-off of blood from the aorta and increases systemic venous return, the magnitude depending on the size of the vascular communication. Small communications cause no symptoms. Large communications produce increased arterial flow resulting in high output heart failure. A continuous murmur is audible over the involved area, sometimes accompanied by a palpable thrill. Other signs include bounding pulses, systemic venous congestion, cardiomegaly and hepatomegaly. Hepatic artery fistulas may produce liver enlargement. In any infant with heart failure and no obvious precordial or echocardiographic findings, a bruit suggestive of an arteriovenous fistula should be sought over the skull, chest wall and abdomen.

Large fistulas produce cardiomegaly on chest radiography and biventricular hypertrophy on the electrocardiogram. Echocardiography is useful in excluding cardiac pathology while ultrasound of the skull and abdomen may reveal dilated arteriovenous channels. Definitive diagnosis is obtained by catheterization showing increased oxygen saturation in the venous blood draining from the fistulous communication and angiogram on the arterial side showing the number and extent of fistulas. Treatment traditionally required excision of the fistula or ligation of the feeding artery, but recurrence is frequent. The use of transcatheter embolization has recently improved the prognosis,[122] although some infants with symptomatic intracranial or hepatic fistulas still die and others survive with brain damage.

Coronary artery fistula

A coronary artery fistula usually occurs as an isolated malformation. The right coronary artery is more often involved and more than 90% of the fistulas drain into the right heart. The pulmonary-to-systemic flow ratio is seldom more than 2:1. Small fistulas are hemodynamically insignificant. Large fistulas may produce exercise intolerance, dyspnea or angina because of the 'stealing' of blood from the normal coronary circulation. Heart failure is rare. The characteristic finding is a continuous murmur heard over the site of drainage into the heart. It is therefore maximal over the lower right or left sternal border when the fistula drains into the right atrium or right ventricle, and over the upper left sternal border when the fistula drains into the pulmonary artery or left atrium.

Sinus of Valsalva aneurysm

Congenital aneurysm of the aortic sinus (of Valsalva) may rupture into the right ventricle or atrium producing a left-to-right shunt. Symptoms of heart failure develop acutely and a continuous murmur is audible over the mid-left sternal area. Diagnosis is made by echocardiography and treatment is surgical.

Mitral regurgitation

Anatomy

Mitral valve prolapse, cleft mitral valve leaflet and atrioventricular septal defect produce mitral regurgitation. A parachute mitral valve with abnormal papillary muscles that restrict openin may also cause regurgitation. Left ventricular dilatation, due to cardiomyopathy or certain congenital lesions, may result in stretching of the mitral valve and produce regurgitation. Infants with anomalous origin of the left coronary artery have myocardial ischemia that results in left ventricular dilatation. In addition infarction of the papillary muscles of the mitral valve causes regurgitation.

Physiology

Mild regurgitation has little hemodynamic effect. Increasing severity results in volume loading of the left atrium. Excessive flow returning through the mitral valve into the left ventricle causes dilatation.

Clinical features

Mild regurgitation will be asymptomatic, but symptoms of heart failure develop with increasing severity. A blowing pansystolic murmur is maximal at the apex, radiating to the axilla. Severe regurgitation will be associated with left ventricular enlargement, a third heart sound and a mid-diastolic murmur caused by increased blood flow across the mitral valve. Pulmonary hypertension may develop with right ventricular hypertrophy and a loud pulmonary component of the second heart sound. If the regurgitation is severe, the electrocardiogram will show left atrial enlargement and left ventricular hypertrophy. Chest radiography will also show left atrial enlargement. Echocardiography demonstrates the severity of the regurgitation and the anatomy of the valve. Cardiac catheterization is seldom necessary for diagnosis or management.

Management and prognosis

Mild regurgitation requires only observation for increasing severity and antibiotic prophylaxis for surgical procedures. Moderate regurgitation is treated medically with afterload-reducing drugs such as angiotensin converting enzyme inhibitors and diuretics. Severe regurgitation with symptoms is an indication for surgery. This consists of mitral valve repair or replacement.

Aortic regurgitation

Aortic regurgitation rarely occurs in isolation in children although it can occur with a bicuspid aortic valve or ventricular septal defect. It is sometimes the only lesion in children with rheumatic heart disease (p. 876).

Tricuspid regurgitation

Tricuspid regurgitation is usually associated with Ebstein's anomaly of the tricuspid valve (p. 845). Occasionally a dysplastic but not displaced tricuspid valve will cause similar hemodynamic and clinical features.

Pulmonary regurgitation

Isolated pulmonary regurgitation is rare. Trivial regurgitation detected on color Doppler echocardiography is a normal finding. Pulmonary regurgitation is usually well tolerated. Severe regurgitation results in right ventricular volume overload with dilatation.

ACYANOTIC HEART DISEASE WITH INCREASED PRESSURE LOAD

Pulmonary stenosis

Anatomy

Valve stenosis is the most common level of obstruction, but subvalvular or supravalvular stenosis can occur. Thickened and fused valve leaflets open incompletely during systole producing a jet, which causes post-stenotic dilatation of the pulmonary artery. Muscular obstruction develops below a severely narrowed valve. Associated lesions include atrial and ventricular septal defects.

Physiology

Obstruction to outflow increases right ventricular systolic pressure causing hypertrophy. Severe obstruction can raise the right ventricular pressure such that it is greater than left ventricular pressure. The non-compliant right ventricle causes elevated right atrial pressures, stretching of the oval foramen, and right-to-left shunting with cyanosis.

Clinical features

Most children present, with an asymptomatic murmur, before 4 years of age.[123] Supravalvular pulmonary stenosis occurs with Williams, Alagille (dysmorphic facial features, intrahepatic cholestasis and skeletal abnormalities) and congenital rubella syndromes. Noonan's syndrome is associated with valve stenosis, often with a very thickened dysplastic valve.

***Mild stenosis*:** The pulses, precordial pulsation and second heart sound are normal. A short, soft ejection systolic murmur maximal at the second left intercostal space usually radiates to the back. If the valve is mobile, a pulmonary ejection click is heard at the second left intercostal space. It varies with respiration and is not related to the severity of stenosis.

Differential diagnosis: innocent murmur, atrial septal defect, aortic coarctation, mild aortic stenosis, small muscular ventricular septal defect.[124]

***Severe stenosis*:** Infants may be cyanosed because of right-to-left shunting at atrial level. Rarely there is a history of dyspnea, exercise intolerance or syncope. In older children, a prominent 'a' wave is seen in the jugular venous pulse. There is a right ventricular lift, and a systolic thrill may be palpable at the second left intercostal space where the murmur is maximal. The long, harsh, ejection systolic murmur increases in intensity late in systole, radiating to the back and neck. The pulmonary component of the second heart sound is soft and late, as right ventricular ejection is prolonged. A pulmonary ejection click may be heard.

Differential diagnosis: tetralogy of Fallot, severe aortic stenosis, coarctation, perimembranous ventricular septal defect.

Investigations

Severe obstruction causes ventricular hypertrophy on the electrocardiogram. Chest radiography may show post-stenotic dilatation of the pulmonary artery. The vascular markings are usually normal, as blood returning to the right heart must pass through the lungs. However, substantial right-to-left shunting at atrial level results in pulmonary oligemia. Echocardiography usually shows a thickened pulmonary valve and pulmonary artery dilatation. Color Doppler shows turbulence distal to the site of obstruction and the measured velocity indicates the severity. Severe stenosis is associated with right ventricular hypertrophy, muscular subvalve obstruction, tricuspid regurgitation and right atrial enlargement. Cardiac catheterization is not necessary for diagnosis, but transcatheter balloon dilatation is usually the treatment of choice (Fig. 19.13). There is a pressure gradient at the site of the obstruction and systemic desaturation occurs when there is right-to-left shunting. Right ventricular angiography identifies the levels of obstruction, and usually shows a thickened, doming pulmonary valve.

Management and prognosis

Pulmonary stenosis often decreases spontaneously over time, but 27% of children have increasing obstruction.[123] This is frequently gradual but rapid progression occurs in neonates[125] and those with a thickened valve. The electrocardiogram and Doppler echocardiography allow accurate assessment of increasing stenosis. Approximately 17% of children require intervention.[123] This is usually performed when the pressure gradient across the valve exceeds 50 mmHg. Balloon dilatation is the treatment of choice, unless the valve is dysplastic or other lesions require surgery. The gradient is usually markedly reduced or abolished.[18] Pulmonary regurgitation occurs but is well tolerated. The long-term results are excellent,[20] but repeat balloon dilatation is occasionally necessary. Infective endocarditis is rare but antibiotic prophylaxis is recommended irrespective of the site or severity of stenosis.

Aortic stenosis

Anatomy

Aortic valve stenosis is the most common level of obstruction. Subaortic or supravalve stenosis occurs less frequently, and occasionally children have more than one level of obstruction.[126] *Aortic valve stenosis* is due to a thickened valve that is often bicuspid. Post-stenotic dilatation of the ascending aorta may occur. A bicuspid aortic valve without stenosis occurs in 2% of the population. *Subaortic stenosis* is usually due to fibromuscular tissue below the aortic valve, which may be thickened or distorted by the high velocity jet through the narrowed subaortic area. Muscular subaortic obstruction occasionally occurs. *Supravalve stenosis* is due to localized or diffuse thickening and narrowing of the ascending aorta. It is commonly associated with Williams syndrome or a positive family history (autosomal dominant inheritance), but 25% of cases are sporadic.[127] Coronary artery abnormalities can occur.

Clinical features

Children usually present at about 2 years of age with an asymptomatic murmur and features of mild stenosis. The pulses and apex beat are normal. A systolic thrill may be palpable in the suprasternal notch. An ejection systolic murmur is maximal in the aortic area with radiation to the neck and down the left sternal border. If the stenosed valve remains mobile, an ejection systolic click may be audible at the lower left sternal border. It does not vary with respiration. The murmur of subaortic stenosis may be loudest at the lower left sternal edge. A soft, early diastolic murmur of aortic regurgitation is more common with subaortic stenosis, but does occur in valve stenosis.

***Severe aortic stenosis*:** The severity correlates reasonably well with the clinical features, but severe stenosis may occur without these features. Symptoms include dyspnea, syncope or angina on exertion. The pulse is weak and slow rising (plateau) with reduced pulse pressure. The aortic component of the second heart is soft and delayed, resulting in a single second heart sound or paradoxical (expiratory) splitting. The more severe the stenosis, the longer and later the accentuation of the systolic murmur. A long ejection systolic murmur can be difficult to distinguish from the pansystolic murmur of a ventricular septal defect. Most infants with severe (critical) stenosis present in the neonatal period (p. 843), but some develop heart failure in early infancy. The pulses are weak and cardiomegaly is present. A gallop rhythm is heard and the ejection systolic murmur may be soft if left ventricle function is poor. An ejection click is rare, as the valve is thick and immobile.

Investigations

The electrocardiogram is usually normal, but left ventricular strain pattern, with inverted T waves in the left precordial leads, indicates severe stenosis. Chest radiography does not show cardiomegaly in the absence of heart failure. Post-stenotic dilatation of the ascending aorta produces a prominent ascending aorta. Echocardiography shows the site of obstruction and whether left ventricular hypertrophy is present. The Doppler velocity across the outflow tract provides a reliable indication of the severity of stenosis. Turbulence occurs on color Doppler at the level of obstruction. Cardiac catheterization is not necessary for diagnosis, but is undertaken as part of therapeutic balloon dilatation of the aortic valve.

Management and prognosis

Aortic valve stenosis progresses with time. Less than 20% of patients will have mild stenosis after 30 years.[102] Rapid progression may occur in the first 5 years of life and during the adolescent growth spurt. Surgical valvotomy is undertaken when the pressure gradient across the valve exceeds 50 mmHg, or if the child has clinical features of severe stenosis. Transcatheter balloon dilatation is an alternative to surgery.[18] Reduction of valve gradient and the incidence of valve regurgitation are comparable to surgery.[128] Treatment is palliative as re-stenosis and progressive aortic regurgitation do occur. Once severe aortic regurgitation develops, or if obstruction cannot be relieved, valve replacement is necessary. Both aortic homograft and prosthetic valve replacements have potential problems. The Ross procedure has become the operation of choice in children.[129] The aortic valve is replaced by the patient's own pulmonary valve, and a homograft replaces the pulmonary valve. *Subaortic stenosis* is rarely significant during infancy but subsequent progression may be rapid, and the majority of children require surgery. This is recommended when the subaortic gradient reaches 40 mmHg in order to reduce the risk of progressive aortic regurgitation. Subaortic obstruction is not usually relieved by balloon dilatation. Localized *supravalve aortic stenosis* responds well to surgery and re-operation is rarely necessary.[130] Surgery for diffuse narrowing of the ascending aorta produces less favorable results. Balloon dilatation is not recommended, because of the nature of the narrowing and the proximity of the coronary arteries.[18] *Multilevel obstruction* is more severe at presentation and has a worse prognosis than a single level of stenosis. Children are more likely to undergo operation, and have a higher incidence of re-operation.[126] Mortality is higher, emphasizing the difficult surgical problems that these children present.

Sudden death of patients with aortic stenosis is rare, accounting for only 2% of sudden cardiac deaths under 35 years of age.[131] It occurs in less than 2% of patients with aortic stenosis and only in those with severe aortic stenosis.[126] It is unnecessary to restrict activities of children with mild aortic stenosis[126] but regular review and antibiotic prophylaxis for procedures is essential throughout life.

Coarctation of the aorta

Coarctation most commonly presents acutely in the neonatal period when the arterial duct closes (p. 849). In older infants and children the signs are usually more subtle.

Anatomy

The aorta is narrowed at the isthmus between the left subclavian artery and the insertion of the arterial duct. Ductal tissue extending into the aortic wall constricts after birth, producing or increasing an obstruction that is usually discrete. Diffuse hypoplasia of the isthmus or transverse aortic arch may be due to abnormal development caused by decreased flow into the aorta during fetal life. Rarely constriction occurs in the lower thoracic or abdominal aorta. Intercostal, mammary and subclavian arteries gradually produce collateral vessels. Associated cardiac lesions are common, including a bicuspid or stenotic aortic valve, ventricular septal defect and mitral stenosis. Shone's syndrome consists of a number of left sided obstructive lesions including supramitral membrane, mitral valve abnormalities, subaortic stenosis and coarctation. Over 15% of girls with Turner's syndrome have coarctation.

Physiology

Obstruction of the aorta results in pressure overload of the left ventricle. Systemic hypertension is due to mechanical obstruction and neurohumoral mechanisms related to reduced renal perfusion.

Clinical features

Children present with an asymptomatic murmur, weak femoral pulses or systemic hypertension, detected on routine examination. Infants may have features of heart failure. The femoral pulses are less easily felt than the right axillary pulse. The blood pressure in the right arm is greater than the 95th percentile for age, and more than 10 mmHg higher than in the legs. The blood pressure in the left arm depends on the site of the coarctation. Techniques of measuring blood pressure and normal values have been discussed previously (p. 816). The left ventricular impulse is prominent, and there is a short ejection systolic murmur maximal at the second left intercostal space and below the left scapula posteriorly. A continuous murmur of collateral arteries may be heard in older children. Murmurs of other cardiac lesions are frequently audible.

Investigations

The electrocardiogram is usually normal, but left ventricular hypertrophy may be present in older children. Chest radiography may show an abnormal aortic contour ('3 sign') caused by a localized constriction of the aorta at the site of the coarctation. Dilated intercostal arteries cause rib notching in older children. Echocardiography demonstrates the site of the coarctation and whether there is hypoplasia of the aortic arch and isthmus. There is turbulence on color Doppler at the site of obstruction with increased velocity and continuous flow into diastole (Fig. 19.26). Magnetic resonance imaging or cardiac catheterization and angiography demonstrate the gradient and anatomy of the coarctation (Fig. 19.15).

Management and prognosis

Early treatment improves life expectancy.[132] It is undertaken soon after diagnosis, as the incidence of residual systemic hypertension is related to the age at intervention. Severe hypertension results in premature cardiovascular disease, aortic dissection or cerebrovascular accident. There are no clinical trials of appropriate size or design to determine the optimum form of treatment.[24] The surgical repair consists of excision of the narrowed segment and end-to-end anastomosis of the aorta, or left subclavian flap repair. Rarely a patch or tube graft is necessary to relieve the obstruction. The risks of surgery include paraplegia, because of spinal cord ischemia (1%), recurrent laryngeal or phrenic nerve injury and recoarctation (< 4%). Transcatheter balloon angioplasty has been used as the initial treatment for coarctation[22,23] and is the treatment of choice for recoarctation following surgical repair. Complications include femoral artery damage and aortic aneurysm formation. Recoarctation, is more common than following surgical repair, particularly in younger children. The risks of both surgery and angioplasty are similar and mortality is rare in the absence of other lesions. Balloon-expandable stents have been used to prevent recoarctation and reduce the risk of aneurysm formation but there are concerns about their use in children.[24] Other lesions such as left ventricular outflow tract obstruction may require treatment. Follow-up is essential and the risk of infective endocarditis remains.

Left ventricular inflow obstructions

Anatomy

Obstruction between the pulmonary veins or left atrium and the left ventricle is rare. It may be caused by congenital mitral valve stenosis, a supramitral stenotic ring, or cor triatriatum. The supramitral stenotic ring comprises a circumferential ridge of tissue in the left atrium immediately above the mitral valve. Cor triatriatum consists of a fibrous diaphragm dividing the left atrium into two chambers, with a restrictive communication between them.

Physiology

Obstruction from any of these lesions produces elevation of the pressure proximal to the site of obstruction and pulmonary venous congestion. Pulmonary hypertension develops, causing right heart failure.

Clinical features

Children frequently present with associated malformations such as aortic coarctation or ventricular septal defect and the mitral lesion may not be recognized initially. Isolated mitral valve stenosis, supramitral ring or cor triatriatum produce similar manifestations when the obstruction is severe. Symptoms begin in early infancy with dyspnea, cough and poor weight gain. There is right ventricular hypertrophy on palpation. The pulmonary component of the second heart sound is accentuated and there are other auscultatory findings of pulmonary hypertension. An apical mid-diastolic murmur is more often audible in mitral valve stenosis or supramitral ring than in cor triatriatum. Tachypnea and hepatomegaly are present.

Investigations

The electrocardiogram shows right atrial and right ventricular hypertrophy. Left atrial enlargement is seen in mitral valve stenosis or supramitral ring but not in cor triatriatum. Chest radiography shows cardiomegaly with left atrial enlargement, producing a double density shadow at the right heart border. There is a prominent pulmonary artery and pulmonary venous congestion with 'butterfly wing' distribution of vascular markings or ground glass appearance if pulmonary edema is present. Echocardiography provides definitive diagnosis of the lesion and Doppler velocity across the obstruction indicates its severity. The tricuspid regurgitant velocity indicates the severity of pulmonary hypertension. Cardiac catheterization is not usually required, but an end-diastolic pressure difference of more than 5 mmHg across the site of obstruction is significant. Angiography confirms the site of obstruction, but this is better seen on transthoracic or transesophageal echocardiography.

Management and prognosis

Surgical excision of the obstructive membrane is the definitive treatment for cor triatriatum and supramitral ring. For congenital mitral stenosis, the deformity of the valve dictates the surgical approach. Valvotomy with attempts to conserve the native valve is preferred to mitral valve replacement.

Double chambered right ventricle

This is a rare condition resulting from a hypertrophied muscular band in the mid-portion of the right ventricle. It may be associated with a ventricular septal defect and is usually not severe at birth, the obstruction developing with time. The clinical features are similar to pulmonary valve stenosis, but there is no ejection click and the murmur is maximal lower down the left sternal border. Diagnosis is confirmed by echocardiography or cardiac catheterization with right ventricular angiography. Surgery is indicated for significant obstruction and the long-term outlook is excellent.

Peripheral pulmonary artery stenosis

Single or multiple stenoses of the pulmonary arteries occur in isolation or associated with tetralogy of Fallot, pulmonary valve stenosis, supravalve aortic stenosis or septal defects. It also occurs in children with Williams, Alagille and rubella syndromes. The clinical features depend on the severity of obstruction and associated abnormalities. The ejection systolic murmur is prominent in the back and both axillae. Right ventricular hypertrophy on electrocardiography indicates severe obstruction. Proximal stenoses are seen on echocardiography. Cardiac catheterization and pulmonary angiography are more useful in evaluating distal or diffuse obstructions. There is often spontaneous improvement with time. Surgery is most effective for severe proximal stenosis. Distal obstruction may be relieved by balloon dilatation or stent implantation.[18]

CYANOTIC CONGENITAL HEART DISEASE

The majority of children with cyanotic heart disease present in the neonatal period (p. 840). Tetralogy of Fallot is the commonest cyanotic cardiac defect but seldom presents with cyanosis in the newborn period.

Tetralogy of Fallot

Anatomy

This condition consists of subvalvar right ventricular outflow obstruction (often accompanied by valvar and supravalvar stenosis), right ventricular hypertrophy, a large perimembranous outlet ventricular septal defect and an aorta that overrides the ventricular septal defect (Fig. 19.33). The hilar pulmonary arteries are usually small. When more than 50% of the aorta arises from the right ventricle, it is termed 'double outlet right ventricle'. Other lesions include a right-sided aortic arch (20% of children), atrial septal defect or persistent arterial duct. Tetralogy of Fallot with an atrioventricular septal defect occurs with Down syndrome. DiGeorge syndrome is found in 16% of infants.[64]

Physiology

Because the ventricular septal defect is large and non-restrictive, pressures in both ventricles are similar. The hemodynamic effect is labile depending on the degree of right ventricular outflow obstruction and systemic vascular resistance. The obstruction varies in severity, but is always sufficient to result in normal or low pulmonary artery pressure. If it is mild, flow across the ventricular septal defect will be from left to right. Increasing obstruction results in right-to-left shunting and cyanosis.

Clinical features

Neonates with severe outflow obstruction present with marked cyanosis and duct-dependent pulmonary circulation (p. 843). More commonly, infants present with an asymptomatic murmur, minimal cyanosis or heart failure caused by a left-to-right shunt. As right ventricular outflow obstruction increases, cyanosis becomes more noticeable and clubbing develops. Right ventricular hypertrophy is palpable. The second heart sound is single because the pulmonary component is inaudible. An aortic ejection click is occasionally heard. The long loud ejection systolic murmur caused by subpulmonary obstruction is maximal at the third left intercostal space, radiating to the back. With increasing obstruction the murmur becomes shorter and the child develops effort intolerance. The characteristic 'squatting' is not seen if children undergo palliative or definitive surgery in infancy. This maneuver increases systemic vascular resistance thus promoting pulmonary blood flow, and decreases the return of reduced venous blood from the legs.

Differential diagnosis: mild right ventricular outflow obstruction: ventricular septal defect, severe pulmonary or aortic stenosis; severe right ventricular outflow obstruction: other complex cyanotic lesions with pulmonary stenosis.

Investigations

The electrocardiogram shows right ventricular hypertrophy. Chest radiography shows a normal sized heart with an uptilted apex. Concavity of the left heart border (pulmonary bay) indicates a small pulmonary artery. Oligemic lung fields reflect reduced pulmonary blood flow. A right-sided aortic arch will cause deviation of the trachea to the left and a bulge in the right upper mediastinum (Fig. 19.33d). Echocardiography establishes the diagnosis showing the ventricular septal defect, overriding aorta and right ventricular hypertrophy with outflow obstruction. The pulmonary arteries can

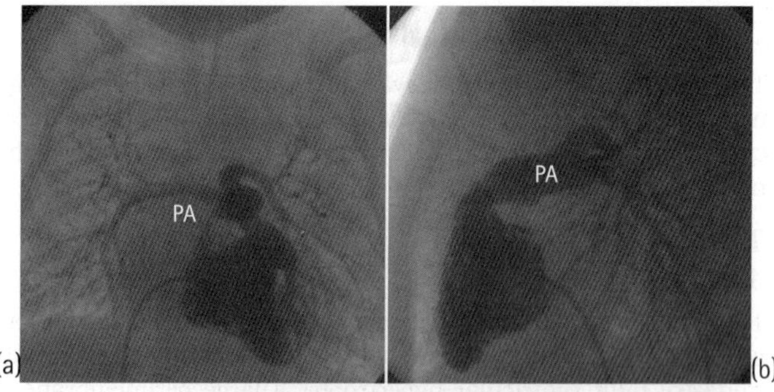

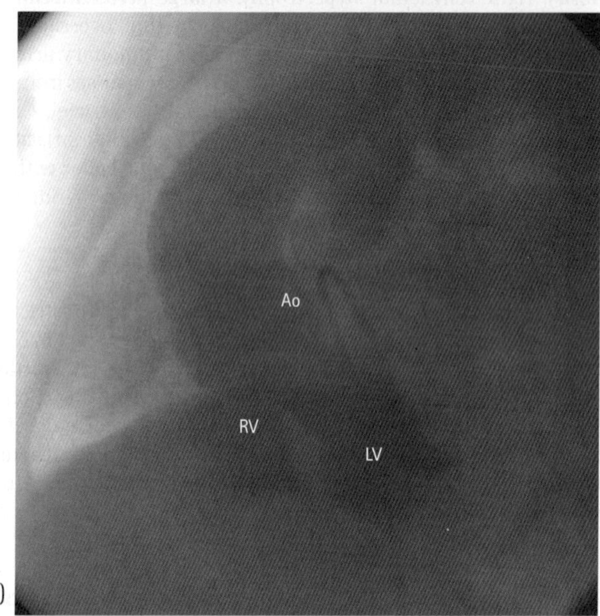

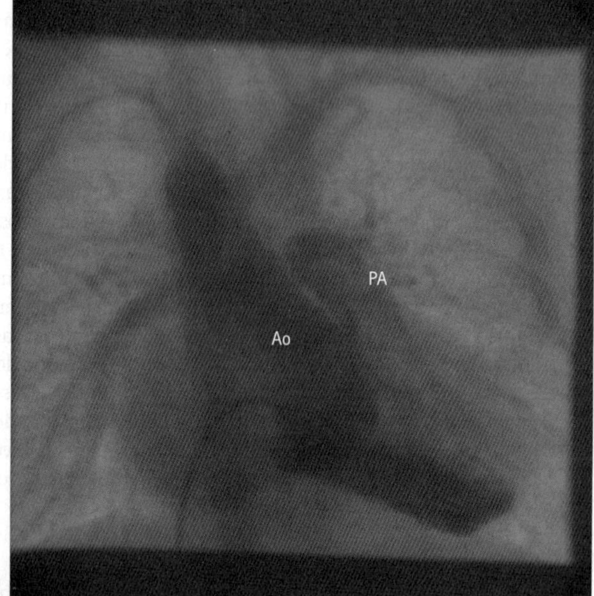

Fig. 19.33 Tetralogy of Fallot: This demonstrates the anteroposterior (a) and lateral (b) view of the right ventricular angiogram. There is infundibular narrowing below the pulmonary valve and small pulmonary arteries. A left ventricular angiogram (c) demonstrates the ventricular septal defect with aortic override. Opacification of the right sided aortic arch (d) to the right of the trachea shows the reason for the characteristic picture on chest radiography. Ao, aorta; LV, left ventricle; PA, pulmonary artery; RV, right ventricle.

be measured and a right aortic arch identified. The Doppler velocity will indicate the pressure difference between the right ventricle and pulmonary artery. Color Doppler shows turbulence below the pulmonary valve, extending into the pulmonary arteries. Chromosome analysis for DiGeorge syndrome should be considered. Cardiac catheterization and angiography are usually performed to provide further information on the anatomy of the coronary and pulmonary arteries.

Management and prognosis

With a move to earlier definitive surgery, complications are less common.

Hypercyanotic attacks (*hypoxic spells*) occur in young children, particularly those with minimal cyanosis. A sudden decrease in pulmonary blood flow causes severe cyanosis and distress. Spells occur in the early morning or after a warm bath and may be initiated by crying, exertion and feeding. The precise cause is unknown but decreased systemic vascular resistance with increased right-to-left shunting may contribute. The murmur becomes short and soft. The child can lose consciousness and spells are life threatening.

Treatment

Flexing the legs onto the abdomen (knee–chest position) increases systemic vascular resistance. Administration of oxygen maximizes inspired oxygen. Morphine appears to have a specific effect in addition to sedation. If there is no immediate venous access, intramuscular morphine injection (0.1 mg/kg) allows valuable time to site a cannula. Severe metabolic acidosis is common and should be corrected with sodium bicarbonate to prevent further episodes. Intravenous propranolol 0.1 mg/kg is effective but should be used with caution in children on beta-blockers. Intravenous phenylephrine is effective in increasing systemic vascular resistance and promoting pulmonary blood flow, but should be used with direct arterial pressure monitoring. A hypoxic spell is an indication for urgent surgical intervention to increase pulmonary blood flow. Prevention of spells with regular beta-adrenergic blockade is beneficial prior to surgery.

- Cerebral thrombosis can result from polycythemia particularly in association with dehydration. The incidence of brain abscess is also increased in children with cyanotic heart disease. Iron deficiency anemia with microcytosis increases the risk of cerebrovascular complications[133] and should be prevented with iron supplements.
- Infective endocarditis is most likely in children with a systemic to pulmonary artery shunt.

Balloon dilatation of the right ventricular outflow tract. This is a palliative procedure used to defer surgery, particularly in small infants. With the move to earlier definitive surgery, this will be performed less frequently.

Palliative surgery. Palliative surgery may be necessary in symptomatic infants with hypoplastic right ventricular outflow tracts and small pulmonary arteries. This may also be preferred in neonates with a duct-dependent pulmonary circulation. It involves insertion of a conduit between the pulmonary and subclavian arteries (modified Blalock–Taussig shunt) (Fig. 19.34). Complications include chylothorax, diaphragmatic paralysis and Horner's syndrome. Definitive repair can be delayed until the child is older and growth of the pulmonary arteries has occurred. Clinical findings include cyanosis and a continuous murmur loudest over the site of the shunt.

Definitive surgery. Primary repair is now commonly performed in the first year of life.[134] The ventricular septal defect is closed with a patch and the right ventricular outflow tract is enlarged by muscle resection, pulmonary valvotomy and sometimes by patch augmentation. Early mortality is less than 5% and complications

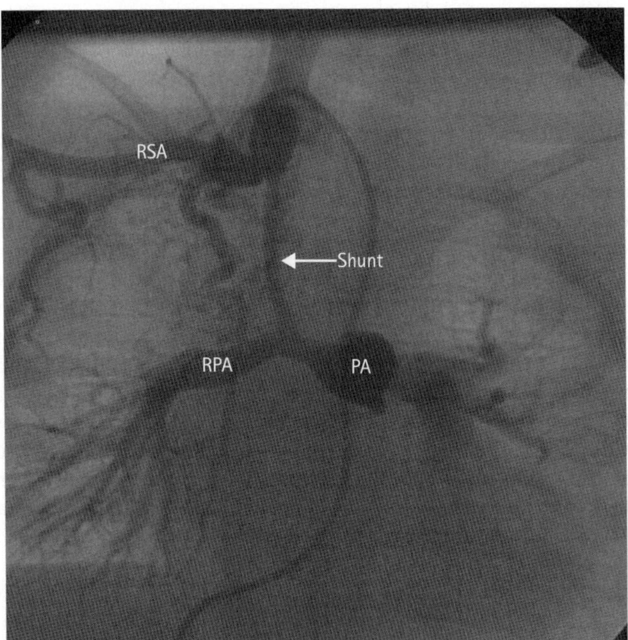

Fig. 19.34 Blalock–Taussig shunt: An angiogram into the right subclavian artery (RSA) at the site of the shunt showing contrast filling the shunt and the pulmonary arteries. The pulmonary valve is atretic. PA, pulmonary artery; RPA, right pulmonary artery.

include right ventricular dysfunction, pleural effusion, and complete heart block. The residual systolic murmur reflects turbulence in the right ventricular outflow tract and the diastolic murmur is due to pulmonary regurgitation. Right bundle branch block may present on the electrocardiogram. Most patients lead normal lives with good effort tolerance. There is a small risk of re-operation for residual ventricular septal defect, pulmonary stenosis or regurgitation.[134] The 20-year survival is over 90%.[135] Patients require follow-up because of a late incidence of ventricular arrhythmias, complete heart block[136,137] and sudden death. Endocarditis prophylaxis must continue.

Pulmonary atresia and ventricular septal defect

Pulmonary atresia with ventricular septal defect is the extreme form of tetralogy of Fallot. Pulmonary blood flow then depends on a persistent arterial duct or major aortopulmonary collateral arteries (MAPCAs). Most present in the neonatal period (p. 843), but diagnosis may be delayed when the collateral vessels provide adequate pulmonary blood flow. Clinical features may include heart failure, mild cyanosis and a continuous murmur in the lung fields.

Tetralogy of Fallot with absent pulmonary valve

This condition is characterized by severe pulmonary regurgitation and aneurysmal dilatation of the pulmonary arteries. This may produce severe upper airways obstruction in infancy with wheeze and recurrent pneumonia. There is mild cyanosis and an ejection systolic murmur is followed by a long diastolic murmur in the pulmonary area.

THE SINGLE VENTRICLE CIRCULATION

This is a complex and diverse group of conditions that have in common the fact that only one ventricle provides the majority of both the systemic and pulmonary blood flow. Surgical correction is not possible and effective palliation is directed towards optimizing the circulation. The aim is to allow the functional ventricle to supply the systemic circulation. Blood returning from the superior and inferior caval veins is directed into the pulmonary arteries driven by the central venous pressure and the negative forces generated by inspiration and ventricular diastole. This separates the pulmonary and systemic venous returns.

Anatomy

The range of conditions is diverse and the specific abnormality is less important than early identification that the anatomy is unsuitable for two-ventricle repair. It includes conditions with hypoplasia or atresia of the mitral or tricuspid valve, or significant hypoplasia of either ventricle.

Physiology

Infants may have:

- inadequate pulmonary blood flow (tricuspid atresia or double inlet left ventricle with pulmonary stenosis, pulmonary atresia with intact ventricular septum and hypoplastic right ventricle, severe Ebstein's anomaly);
- inadequate systemic blood flow (hypoplastic left heart, tricuspid atresia with transposition);
- unrestricted pulmonary blood flow (double outlet right ventricle with hypoplastic left ventricle).

Clinical features

At birth the arterial duct compensates for inadequate pulmonary or systemic circulation and symptoms only develop when the duct closes. Infants with unrestricted pulmonary blood flow develop symptoms when the pulmonary vascular resistance falls and pulmonary blood flow becomes excessive. The clinical features depend on the physiology. Infants with inadequate pulmonary blood flow present with cyanosis. Those with inadequate systemic blood flow present with cardiovascular collapse. Those with unrestricted pulmonary blood flow present with signs of heart failure. Some infants will be diagnosed antenatally, and others will present with a murmur or poor femoral pulses.

Investigations

Findings on electrocardiogram and chest radiography will depend on the underlying condition. Echocardiography will identify the details of the specific cardiac lesion.

Management and prognosis

Initial management is critical to achieve a satisfactory long-term outcome. It involves at least three staged procedures.[138]

Stage 1: Optimizing systemic and pulmonary blood flow. Effective early palliation is critical. From infancy the blood flow into the lungs must be adequate but at low pressure. Neonates with inadequate pulmonary blood flow require a systemic-to-pulmonary (modified Blalock–Taussig) (Fig. 19.34) shunt. Those with inadequate systemic blood flow require a Norwood or Damus Kaye Stansel operation. Those with excessive pulmonary blood flow require a pulmonary artery band placed around the main pulmonary artery and tightened to reduce pulmonary blood flow (Fig. 19.35). A few infants have a cardiac lesion that results in optimal systemic and pulmonary blood flow in that they have pulmonary stenosis and unobstructed systemic blood flow.

The definitive palliative procedure is the Fontan operation. This is usually carried out in two further stages. The first consists of anastomosis of the superior caval vein to the pulmonary artery (superior cavopulmonary anastomosis) (Fig. 19.36). This is followed a few years later by connection of the inferior caval vein to the pulmonary circulation (completion of the modified Fontan operation) (Fig. 19.37). Successful surgery depends on a low pulmonary vascular resistance as blood returning from the body flows directly into the pulmonary arteries, driven by the systemic venous pressure. Any anatomical or physiological abnormality that impedes this must be corrected and other transcatheter and surgical interventions may be necessary to achieve the optimal hemodynamics. The pulmonary artery pressure must be low and the pulmonary arteries of adequate size without localized narrowing. There must also be unobstructed pulmonary venous return, a normal left atrial pressure, good systemic ventricular function and unobstructed systemic outflow.

Stage 2: Superior (bidirectional) cavo-pulmonary anastomosis. This relieves the systemic ventricle of chronic volume and pressure loads that occur regardless of the type of neonatal palliation. It usually decreases the cyanosis and reduces the risks at subsequent surgery. It is performed at 6–12 months of age. The superior caval vein is anastomosed to the proximal right pulmonary artery (Fig. 19.36). If a left superior vena cava is present, this is anastomosed to the left pulmonary artery at the same procedure. If a Blalock–Taussig shunt is present it is ligated. Forward flow through the main pulmonary artery may also be occluded. Residual lesions that may increase the risk of subsequent surgery, such as pulmonary artery narrowing or recoarctation, are corrected. The superior cavo-pulmonary anastomosis is well tolerated, even when combined with other procedures. A superior vena caval syndrome with upper body swelling may occur postoperatively if the pulmonary artery pressure is elevated. During early childhood the relative size of the lower body increases, and the ratio of blood returning from the inferior and superior caval veins alters. This results in increasing cyanosis which may also occur due to venous collaterals that develop between the upper and lower body.

Stage 3: Completion of modified Fontan operation. This is usually performed at 2–5 years of age. Some children will not be suitable for the procedure because of adverse risk factors such as poor systemic ventricular function or elevated pulmonary artery pressure. The inferior vena cava is anastomosed to the pulmonary arteries, either by a baffle that is created inside the lateral wall of the right atrium, or an extracardiac conduit (Fig. 19.37). Creation of a small hole or fenestration between this tunnel or conduit and the left-sided (systemic) circulation produces a small right-to-left shunt. This lowers the central venous pressure, preventing severe venous congestion in the postoperative period but producing systemic desaturation. The fenestration can be closed at a later time if the hemodynamics are suitable.

Prognosis depends on the underlying condition, the success of the various interventions and the long-term function of the systemic ventricle. The 30-day mortality is less than 5%, but the postoperative period may be protracted with high central venous pressure, ascites, pleural effusions and poor cardiac output. Atrial arrhythmias can further destabilize the hemodynamics. The highest death rate is in the first year after operation.[139] Recent figures suggest a 5-year survival of more than 70% but deaths are likely to continue to occur with longer follow-up and the 20-year survival is just under 60%.[139] The quality of life in survivors is satisfactory,[140] but a number of late complications account for a continuing mortality. They include cardiac failure, systemic venous obstruction, persistent fluid accumulation and protein-losing enteropathy. Reports of thromboembolism, both pulmonary and systemic (if a fenestration is present), have resulted in the common practice of long-term anticoagulation. Arrhythmias can produce significant hemodynamic deterioration and need urgent treatment. The only option for a child with a failing 'Fontan' circulation is heart transplant.

MISCELLANEOUS CARDIOVASCULAR LESIONS

Vascular ring

Anatomy

A vascular ring is a malformation of the aortic arch or its brachiocephalic branches encircling and compressing the trachea and esophagus. Double aortic arch is the most common

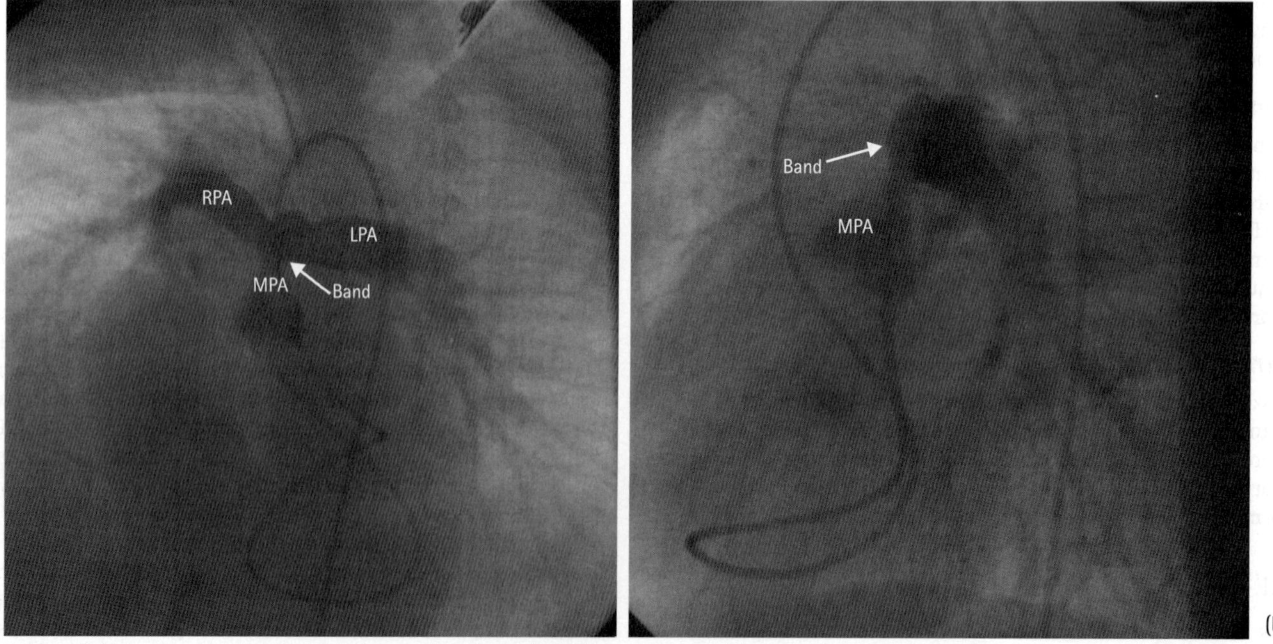

Fig. 19.35 Pulmonary artery band: An angiogram into main the pulmonary artery (a) shows the constriction from the pulmonary artery band distal to the pulmonary valve, before the bifurcation into right and left pulmonary arteries. (b) A lateral projection of the same angiogram. LPA, left pulmonary artery; MPA, main pulmonary artery; RPA, right pulmonary artery.

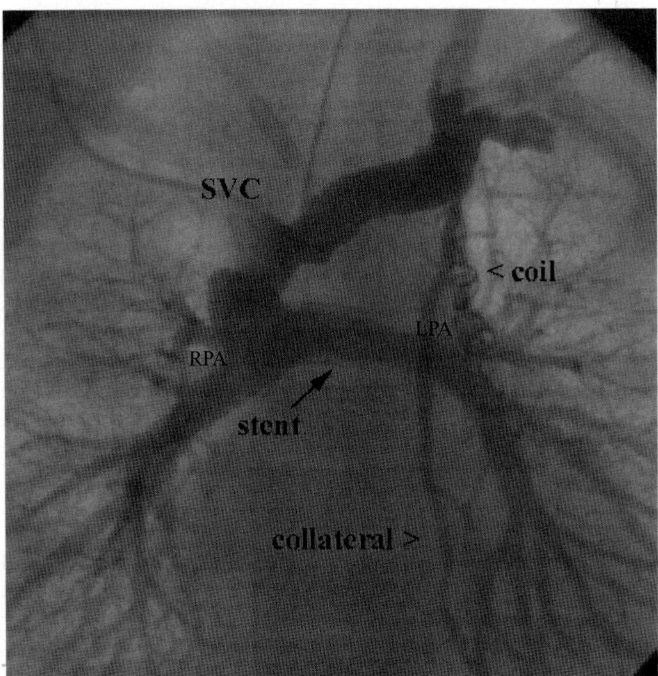

Fig. 19.36 The superior cavopulmonary anastomosis: The angiogram in the superior caval vein shows the connection to the proximal right pulmonary artery. Contrast also fills the innominate vein on the left. Coils have been used to occlude some of the collateral veins from the innominate vein. An intravascular stent was expanded in the proximal left pulmonary artery at the time of surgery. LPA, left pulmonary artery; RPA, right pulmonary artery; SVC, superior caval vein.

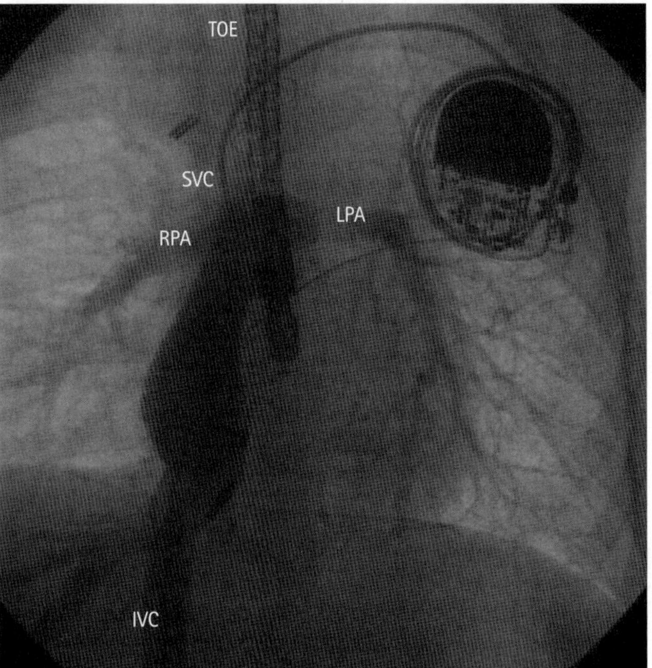

Fig. 19.37 The Fontan operation: The angiogram shows the lateral tunnel connecting the inferior caval vein to the pulmonary arteries. The position of the connection between the superior caval vein and the pulmonary arteries is shown by the pacemaker lead, which passes from the subclavian vein, via the superior caval vein to the atrial wall. The transesophageal probe is visible in the esophagus. IVC, inferior calval vein; LPA, left pulmonary artery; RPA, right pulmonary artery; SVC, superior caval vein; TOE, transesophageal echocardiographic probe.

type. The ascending aorta divides into two vessels that reunite to form the descending aorta. A pulmonary artery sling is anomalous origin of the left pulmonary artery from the right pulmonary artery crossing the midline between the trachea and esophagus and producing severe tracheal compression. Intrinsic narrowing of the trachea often coexists.

Clinical features

Airway obstruction resulting from tracheal compression is progressive and is the most important clinical problem and causes inspiratory stridor, which is usually present soon after birth. Wheezing, cough and recurrent respiratory tract infections are common. Dysphagia due to esophageal compression is rare. The diagnosis is often delayed because of the failure to consider it in the child with respiratory difficulties.

Investigations

A barium swallow is the most useful investigation and demonstrates an indentation of the posterior aspect of the esophagus by a vascular ring. A double aortic arch is suggested by bilateral indentations, usually at different levels, in addition to the posterior indentation. A pulmonary artery sling characteristically produces an anterior indentation, sometimes accompanied by a posterior impression on the air column in the trachea at the same level. A more complete diagnosis of the vascular anatomy requires angiography but lesions are also well demonstrated by magnetic resonance imaging. Echocardiography may show a double arch or pulmonary sling, but in most cases does not completely demonstrate the abnormality.

Treatment

Although spontaneous improvement of respiratory symptoms in patients with a vascular ring have been described, surgery is always indicated. Outcome is generally good although persistent respiratory symptoms may result from tracheal distortion and associated tracheomalacia.

Anomalous origin of the left coronary artery from the pulmonary artery

Anomalous origin of a coronary artery from the pulmonary artery is rare, the left coronary usually being involved. Perfusion of the left ventricle depends on the pressure in the pulmonary artery and the collateral circulation from the right coronary artery. At birth, when the pulmonary pressure is still high, the left ventricular myocardium remains well perfused. Ischemia occurs with the postnatal fall in the pulmonary pressure, its severity depending on the amount of collateral circulation which develops. The manifestations can thus vary from minimal to severe congestive heart failure in early infancy.

The infant with inadequate left ventricular perfusion usually presents in the second month of life with 'anginal attacks', manifested as acute distress with crying, sweating, pallor or gray coloration, often during feeding or defecation. Heart failure develops, the heart is enlarged and gallop rhythm is common. There is often a murmur of mitral regurgitation secondary to left ventricular dilatation. There is marked cardiomegaly and pulmonary venous congestion on chest X-ray. The electrocardiogram characteristically shows an anterior infarction pattern with T wave inversion and deep Q waves in the left chest leads, lead I and aVL. Echocardiography reveals a dilated and poorly contractile left ventricle with an enlarged right coronary artery. The abnormal origin of the left coronary artery may be visualized. Angiography is necessary if ultrasound studies are inconclusive. An aortogram shows a large right coronary artery and its distal anastomosis with the left coronary artery, which then drains into the pulmonary artery.

Children who establish adequate collateral circulation early in life have few symptoms and may have evidence of mitral regurgitation or no cardiac findings. Ischemic symptoms on exertion may occur in adult life and sudden death has been described. Treatment consists of surgical anastomosis of the left anomalous coronary artery to the aorta.

Marfan's syndrome

This is a autosomal dominant inherited disorder of connective tissue. It is characterized by musculoskeletal, cardiovascular and ocular abnormalities, two of which should be present to make the diagnosis. It is caused by various mutations in the FBN1 gene on chromosome 15q and is inherited in about 75% of children, the rest arising because of a new mutation.[60]

Clinical features

The musculoskeletal features include tall stature, long arms and digits, a high arched palate, pectus excavatum and kyphoscoliosis. The cardiovascular manifestations include dilatation of the ascending aorta (and occasionally the descending) due to cystic medial necrosis, aortic regurgitation, and mitral valve prolapse and regurgitation. Disturbances in cardiac rhythm can occur. The ocular abnormalities consist of lens dislocation, myopia, and detachment of the retina. A family history should always be sought.

Investigations

Children should be reviewed regularly with echocardiography to measure the aortic root dimensions and these should be plotted against normal values.[141] Transesophageal echocardiography or magnetic resonance imaging may give additional information, and are valuable when dissection is suspected.

Management

Beta-blockers have been shown to slow the aortic root dilatation.[142] Children should be advised against competitive and contact sports. Surgical replacement of the aortic root should be considered when the aortic root diameter reaches 5.5 cm, with earlier surgery if there is a rapid increase in diameter, in high risk families (with history of aortic dissection) or in young women planning pregnancy.[143]

CARDIAC ARRHYTHMIAS

Over the past few years there have been significant advances in our understanding and treatment of cardiac arrhythmias in children. There is now widespread recognition amongst pediatricians that most arrhythmias result from primary electrical abnormalities of the heart. We also have a greater understanding of the anatomical substrates and electrophysiological mechanisms of arrhythmia. There are now available better non-invasive diagnostic techniques, safer and more effective drugs for acute and long term control and the possibility of cure by catheter ablation.

IDENTIFICATION OF THE ARRHYTHMIA

Cardiac arrhythmias usually affect children with structurally normal hearts but they may also develop in those with congenital heart disease. They make up a significant proportion of the work of pediatric cardiologists and are one of the more common ways in which babies and children with cardiac problems present to the general pediatrician. For this reason it is important for pediatricians to have some understanding of the types of arrhythmia, and familiarity with non-invasive diagnostic techniques and treatment strategies.

If we know the age at onset of an arrhythmia and have good quality recordings of the electrocardiogram (ECG) in sinus rhythm, during arrhythmia, and during adenosine administration we can often make a precise identification of the mechanism of the arrhythmia. This will help to define the prognosis and will guide the choice of treatment. Available diagnostic techniques include standard surface electrocardiography, ambulatory 24-h electrocardiography (Holter monitoring), patient-activated event recorders, invasive electrophysiology studies and implantable loop recorders. The first three are widely available whilst the last two are reserved for specialist assessment.

CLINICAL PRESENTATION OF ARRHYTHMIAS

Cardiac arrhythmias may occur at any age and their differential diagnosis depends upon the age of onset. They may be noticed incidentally in the neonate because of bradycardia, tachycardia or an irregular rhythm but the commonest presentation in infancy is with heart failure, usually as a result of sustained tachycardia. In childhood, by far the most common presentation is with palpitations, usually as a result of paroxysmal tachycardia. Some less common incessant tachycardias may present with heart failure due to secondary myocardial dysfunction. Arrhythmias that present with syncope are rare but are very important to recognize. A few rare but dangerous arrhythmias may result in (and may even present with) sudden death.[144] Some arrhythmic causes of sudden death are familial, so making a diagnosis, although often difficult, is very important. Children who develop arrhythmias after surgery for congenital heart disease should already be under the care of a pediatric cardiologist but may present acutely to a pediatrician.

CLASSIFICATION OF ARRHYTHMIAS

There are several ways of classifying arrhythmias. Tachycardias have conventionally been considered as either 'supraventricular' or ventricular but, as there are many mechanisms of each, this broad classification is relatively unhelpful. The ECG in tachycardia will show QRS complexes that are either normal or broad so these are two clinically useful groups. Arrhythmias in infancy differ in important aspects from those seen in children and so it is helpful to consider them separately.

MECHANISMS OF TACHYCARDIAS

Most of the tachycardias we encounter in clinical practice are due to re-entry by which we mean that there is recirculating electrical activation travelling around an anatomical circuit. Such arrhythmias are usually (but not always) paroxysmal. Re-entry tachycardias usually have fairly constant rates and can be started by pacing and stopped by drugs, pacing and electrical cardioversion. The circuit commonly involves an anatomically abnormal structure – the best example is the accessory atrioventricular connection in Wolff–Parkinson–White syndrome, which is really a form of congenital structural heart disease.[145] In other cases, the circuit probably develops during growth – as in atrioventricular (AV) nodal re-entry tachycardia. Other examples of re-entry tachycardias include atrial flutter, permanent junctional re-entry tachycardia, and late postoperative ventricular tachycardia.

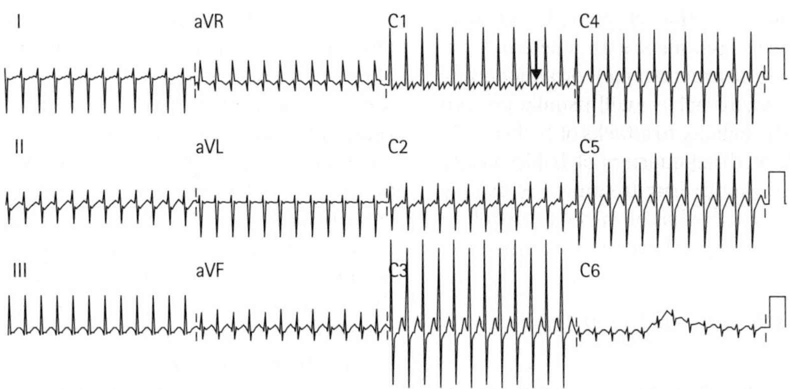

Fig. 19.38 Typical atrioventricular (AV) re-entry tachycardia in a neonate. The ventricular rate is 290 per minute and the QRS is normal. A retrograde P wave is clearly seen in lead C1 (arrow). The timing of the P wave and the age of patient make orthodromic AV re-entry tachycardia via an accessory pathway an almost certain diagnosis.

A less common arrhythmia mechanism is automaticity. Automatic arrhythmias arise from an ectopic focus and overdrive pacing or cardioversion are ineffective. They are usually incessant and often show significant variation in rate. Those most commonly encountered in children are atrial ectopic tachycardia and junctional ectopic tachycardia (His bundle tachycardia).

TACHYCARDIA IN INFANCY

Atrioventricular re-entry tachycardia

The commonest type of 'supraventricular tachycardia' (SVT) presenting in infancy is orthodromic AV re-entry via an accessory pathway (Fig. 19.38). The term orthodromic implies that there is normal (anterograde) conduction over the AV node and retrograde conduction over an accessory muscular atrioventricular connection (accessory pathway). About a third of these connections encountered in infants are capable of anterograde conduction in sinus rhythm, producing ventricular pre-excitation that is recognized as Wolff–Parkinson–White syndrome. More commonly the pathway can only conduct retrogradely so the ECG is normal in sinus rhythm. In tachycardia the QRS is usually normal in infancy although transient rate-related bundle branch block at the onset of tachycardia is not unusual (Fig. 19.39). Tachycardia usually presents with heart failure, more often causing pallor, breathlessness and poor feeding but sometimes severe enough to cause cardiogenic shock. The symptoms are often non-specific and there may be few clinical signs to indicate that there is a cardiac problem. The differential diagnosis includes infection and metabolic problems. The rate of sinus tachycardia in an ill baby may exceed 200 beats/min but AV re-entry tachycardia in infancy is rarely slower than 270 beats/min. It is difficult or impossible to distinguish between these heart rates clinically and some ECG monitors are unreliable in measuring high heart rates. Recording a 12 lead ECG on paper will allow accurate measurement of the heart rate and confirmation of the diagnosis.

The treatment of choice for acute termination of AV re-entry tachycardia is intravenous administration of adenosine. The dose is 150–300 μg/kg (occasionally higher) given by rapid bolus injection (Fig. 19.39).[146] The drug is metabolized very quickly and the dose can be repeated or increased if necessary. Facial immersion in iced water or facial application of an ice pack is also usually effective but is only appropriate in early infancy. Other drugs are not often required for termination of tachycardia in infancy. Verapamil is contraindicated in early infancy because it may accelerate the tachycardia. Synchronized electrical cardioversion is effective but is not usually necessary and, because it requires general anesthetic, is not easily repeated.

The baby's condition will improve once sinus rhythm has been restored. Recurrence of tachycardia in the short term is quite likely so prophylactic drug treatment is usually advised. There are no

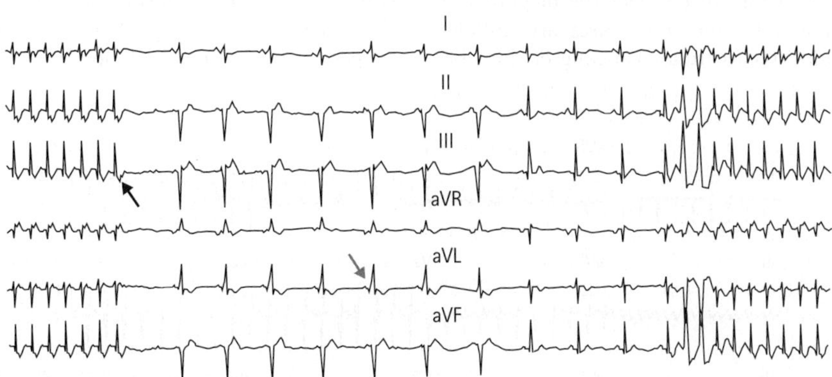

Fig. 19.39 Administration of intravenous adenosine during atrioventricular (AV) re-entry tachycardia in a neonate. Adenosine produces transient AV block and the tachycardia terminates with a non-conducted P wave (black arrow). This is followed by sinus rhythm which for seven beats shows clear evidence of ventricular pre-excitation (gray arrow). As the sinus rhythm speeds up slightly the pre-excitation disappears and there is no delta wave for the next four sinus beats. AV re-entry tachycardia then reinitiates with rate-related bundle branch block during the first two beats of tachycardia.

controlled trials of drug treatment in this situation but digoxin seems to have relatively little effect. Treatment with a beta-blocker, a class IC drug (such as flecainide or propafenone), or amiodarone (or a combination of these in difficult babies) will usually prevent recurrence of the arrhythmia. The liability to attacks of tachycardia will resolve in about two-thirds or three-quarters of babies before the end of infancy so that prophylactic drug treatment is usually withdrawn after 6 or 12 months if there has been good control. In some cases, in which the problem seems to have resolved, there will be a recurrence later in childhood.

Other types of 'supraventricular' tachycardia in infancy

Several less common types of tachycardia may be encountered in infancy. *Atrial flutter* is usually easy to recognize on the ECG at this age as there are often prominent flutter waves with 2:1 AV conduction (Fig. 19.40). Atrial flutter can be terminated by direct current cardioversion or transesophageal overdrive pacing. Recurrence is rare and prophylactic treatment is not usually required. Occasionally the more common type of AV re-entry tachycardia, that can then be treated as discussed above, follows restoration of sinus rhythm. *Chaotic* or *multifocal atrial tachycardia* causes an irregular rhythm with multiple non-conducted P waves of varying morphology (Fig. 19.41). There is usually sufficient AV block to give a more or less normal ventricular rate so treatment is usually unnecessary. Resolution during infancy is likely. *Atrial ectopic tachycardia* may present as a sustained arrhythmia in early infancy (Fig. 19.42). Drug treatment (beta-blocker, flecainide or amiodarone) may be required in the short term, but at this age the problem usually resolves within a few months.[147]

One unusual but important variety of AV re-entry tachycardia presents with an incessant tachycardia and is known as *permanent junctional reciprocating tachycardia* or PJRT.[148] It is recognized on the ECG from the long RP interval and the inverted P waves in inferior leads (Fig. 19.43). Treatment with a beta-blocker, flecainide, or amiodarone will suppress the arrhythmia or control the rate. Spontaneous resolution of PJRT is unusual and radiofrequency ablation will usually be required later in childhood (see below). Congenital *His bundle tachycardia* (*junctional ectopic tachycardia*) is rare and is recognized by the presence of slower dissociated P waves. Long term drug treatment is required. This arrhythmia is more commonly encountered early after infant open heart surgery.

Ventricular tachycardia in infancy

Pediatricians usually seem reluctant to consider the diagnosis of ventricular tachycardia in infants, and most cases are initially mistaken for 'supraventricular' tachycardia. Widening of the QRS can be very subtle in infancy but if the QRS is abnormal the diagnosis of ventricular tachycardia should be considered. The tachycardia is often relatively slow and well tolerated, in which case treatment may not be required and resolution is likely.[149] The most significant type of ventricular tachycardia encountered is incessant infant ventricular tachycardia (VT). It usually presents between 3 months and 2 years of age. The QRS most often shows a right bundle branch block pattern with a superior axis indicating a posterior left ventricular origin for the tachycardia (Fig. 19.44). The underlying problem in most cases is probably a tiny myocardial hamartoma that is beyond the resolution of imaging techniques. The most effective drug for suppression of incessant VT is amiodarone or flecainide, often used in combination with a beta-blocker. This arrhythmia usually resolves before school age and treatment can be withdrawn without recurrence. Other ventricular tachycardias in infancy are rare and require specialist evaluation.[149]

TACHYCARDIA IN CHILDHOOD WITH NARROW QRS COMPLEXES

Atrioventricular re-entry tachycardia

As in infancy, the commonest type of tachycardia encountered in childhood is orthodromic atrioventricular re-entry tachycardia (Fig. 19.38). Relatively few new cases present between 1 and 4 years of age and at this age they are often triggered by fevers. New presentation after early childhood (usually with palpitation) implies only a small chance of long term natural resolution. As in infancy, the ECG may show ventricular pre-excitation in sinus rhythm (Fig. 19.45) but it is more common for the pathway to be 'concealed', that is to be capable of only retrograde conduction. Most episodes of tachycardia during childhood revert to sinus rhythm spontaneously. In some children vagal stimulation slows AV nodal conduction sufficiently to break tachycardia.[150] The most effective techniques include a Valsalva maneuver (such as trying to blow up a balloon) and other methods of breath-holding, facial application of an ice-pack and occasionally inversion into a headstand. Carotid sinus massage and eyeball pressure is relatively ineffective. If the tachycardia is sustained, sinus rhythm can be restored with a rapid intravenous bolus of adenosine 100–300 μg/kg, or with intravenous verapamil. AV re-entry tachycardia in childhood is not an intrinsically dangerous arrhythmia so decisions about long term treatment depend on the frequency, severity and duration of episodes. If attacks are mild and infrequent, treatment may not be required. Long term treatment involves a choice between prophylactic medication and radiofrequency ablation of the accessory pathway. A recent cost effectiveness analysis suggested that catheter ablation had a lower long term morbidity,

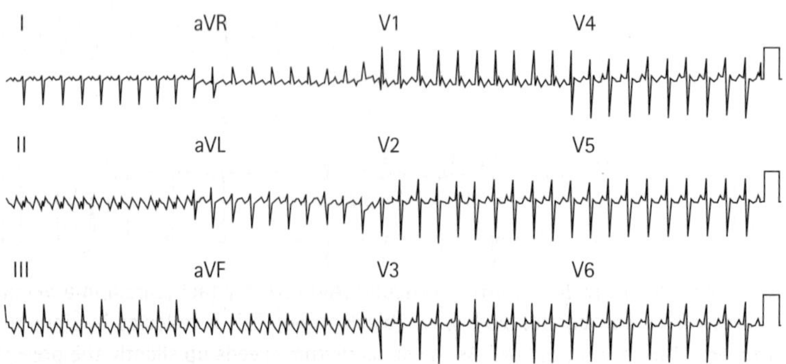

Fig. 19.40 Neonatal atrial flutter. The atrial rate is 460 per minute which, with 2:1 AV conduction, gives a ventricular rate of 230 per minute. Saw-tooth flutter waves are clearly seen in leads II, III, aVF, and V1.

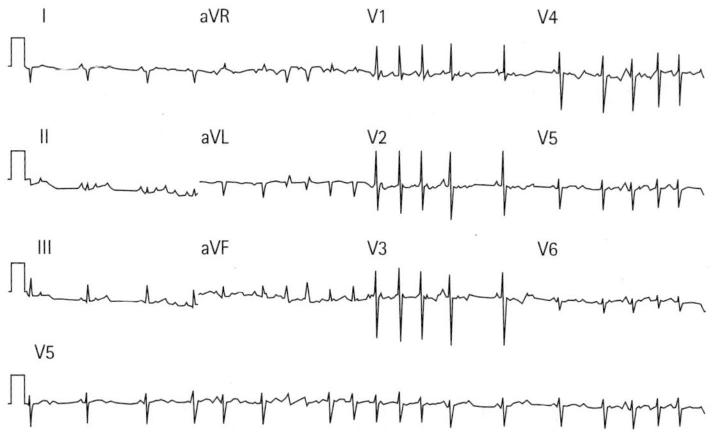

Fig. 19.41 Chaotic atrial tachycardia in infancy. This is also known as multifocal atrial tachycardia. There are several different P wave morphologies and many more P waves than QRS complexes. Many of the P waves are not conducted so the ventricular rate is in fact slightly slow. The extra or early P waves differ in morphology from the sinus beats.

mortality and cost than long term drug treatment.[151] Many children and their parents prefer the prospect of a cure with catheter ablation to the alternative of long term drug treatment.

Many drugs can be used to suppress AV re-entry tachycardia. The literature relating to their use is mainly a series of retrospective reports of clinical experience.[146] There are no blinded or placebo-controlled trials and very few comparisons between drugs. Most anti-arrhythmic drugs have been used for control of this common arrhythmia. Those most likely to be effective include beta-blockers, flecainide, amiodarone and sotalol. Drug treatment may occasionally produce new arrhythmias, a so-called 'pro-arrhythmic' effect. The risk of this is small but difficult to assess.

Radiofrequency catheter ablation was introduced to clinical practice about 10 years ago and it is already regarded as the standard treatment for many arrhythmias. In experienced hands, success rates are high and serious complications are rare.[152] The procedure involves the use of a high frequency electric current to induce a small burn at the point of contact between the catheter and the heart. If the catheter is accurately positioned the arrhythmia substrate will be destroyed. Catheter ablation of accessory pathways involves delivery of a burn to the endocardial surface of the atrioventricular ring and there are some concerns about possible late complications because of the proximity of the main coronary arteries.

Atrioventricular nodal re-entry tachycardia

This arrhythmia is rare before school age but becomes an increasingly important mechanism of SVT during later childhood. It is sometimes difficult to differentiate with confidence from atrioventricular re-entry (Fig. 19.46) but the difference is really only important if catheter ablation is being considered and can easily be established at electrophysiology study. Both arrhythmias can be stopped with vagal maneuvers or intravenous adenosine. AV nodal re-entry has become much better understood and is now known to include the AV node and adjacent low right atrium[153] (it would perhaps be more accurately termed atrionodal re-entry tachycardia). Drug treatment is often relatively ineffective or poorly tolerated. Radiofrequency modification of the AV node is often effective and offers the prospect of a cure but is associated with a small risk of atrioventricular block.[152,153]

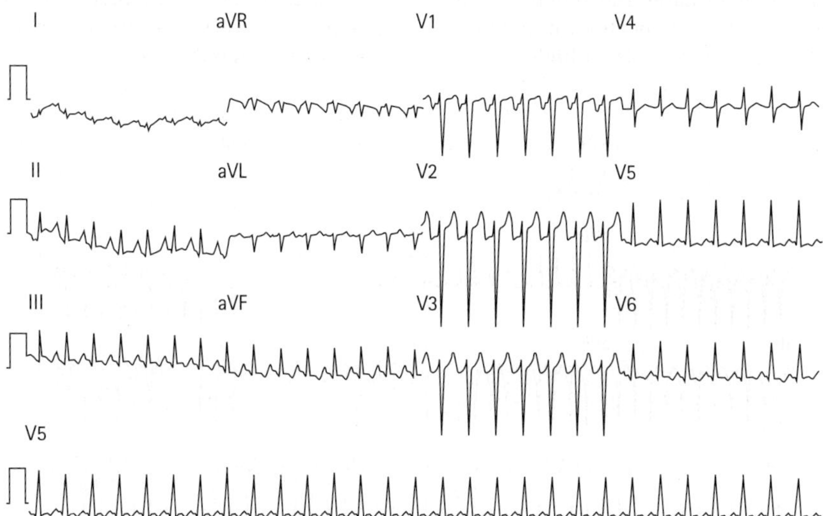

Fig. 19.42 Atrial ectopic tachycardia in a 5-year-old boy. At first glance this looks like a sinus tachycardia but the rate is inappropriately high for the age and clinical situation. The P waves are abnormal and their morphology suggests an ectopic focus in the right atrium. In this example there is 1:1 conduction throughout but transient AV block is not unusual.

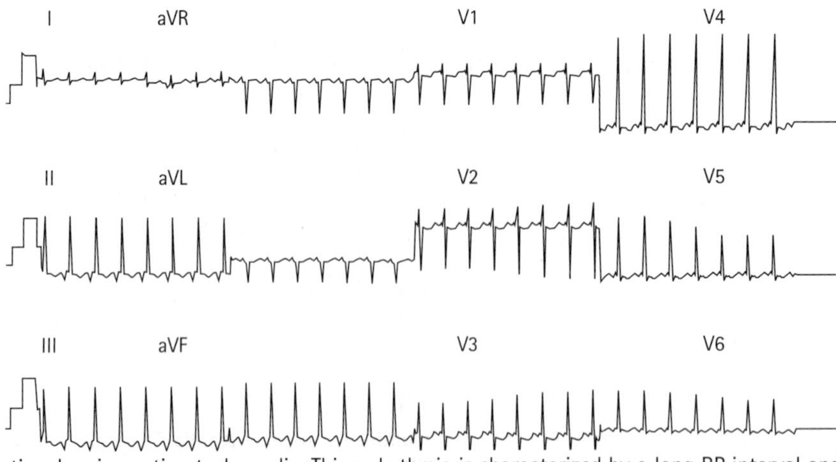

Fig. 19.43 Permanent junctional reciprocating tachycardia. This arrhythmia is characterized by a long RP interval and an abnormal P wave axis with inverted P waves in leads II, III, and aVF. It is usually incessant but will stop transiently with adenosine.

Other tachycardias

Other tachycardias with a normal QRS are unusual in childhood. They include *atrial ectopic tachycardia*, which often presents with heart failure rather than palpitations and may be mistaken for dilated cardiomyopathy (Fig. 19.42). Improvement or normalization of ventricular function usually follows if suppression of the tachycardia is effective. Some cases may resolve spontaneously in the long term but this arrhythmia is also amenable to radiofrequency ablation. *Permanent junctional reciprocating tachycardia* may also present during childhood and is often incessant (Fig. 19.43). Long term resolution is unusual but radiofrequency ablation has a high chance of cure.[148]

TACHYCARDIA IN CHILDHOOD WITH WIDE QRS COMPLEXES

'Supraventricular' tachycardias

Almost any of the tachycardias with normal QRS morphology discussed above may also occur with a wide QRS. This may be due to an underlying permanent right or left bundle branch block, or, more commonly, to rate-related bundle branch block or aberration (Fig. 19.32). In these cases the bundle branch block has no influence on the natural history or choice of treatment but does affect the differential diagnosis. Children with Wolff–Parkinson–White syndrome may occasionally have antidromic AV re-entry in which the re-entry is in the opposite direction to the orthodromic or more common re-entry circuit. There is retrograde conduction through the normal conduction axis and anterograde conduction over the accessory pathway producing maximal pre-excitation and a slow slurred upstroke to the QRS. This is more commonly encountered in the presence of multiple pathways, right sided pathways and Ebstein's malformation of the tricuspid valve. An irregular tachycardia with a similar appearance is due to atrial fibrillation in the Wolff–Parkinson–White syndrome (Fig. 19.47). This is rare in childhood but more often seen in teenage or young adult life. It is potentially dangerous, particularly if the pathway will permit rapid conduction to the ventricle (that is it has a short refractory period). This arrhythmia may present with syncope and is potentially life threatening so it requires urgent specialist evaluation. Radiofrequency ablation of the pathway offers a cure.

Ventricular tachycardia

Ventricular tachycardia is an uncommon but important diagnosis in childhood. It can be conveniently divided into monomorphic and polymorphic forms, based on the ECG appearance. Many subtypes of each of these are recognized, but in some cases precise subclassification is difficult.

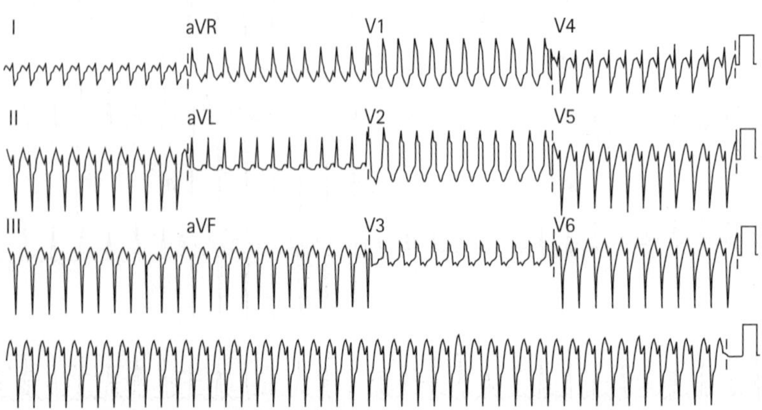

Fig. 19.44 Ventricular tachycardia in an 11-month-old boy. The QRS complexes have an appearance similar to right bundle branch block but the initial R wave in V1 is taller than the secondary R. There is very subtle evidence of ventriculo-atrial dissociation, perhaps best shown by the variable height of the T waves in the rhythm strip at the bottom caused by intermittent superimposition of P waves.

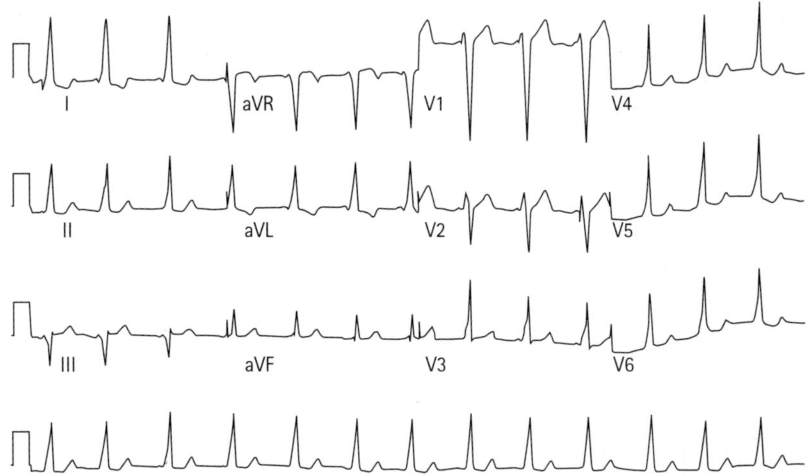

Fig. 19.45 Ventricular pre-excitation in sinus rhythm. In this case pre-excitation produces a pseudo left bundle branch block pattern and the QRS morphology predicts a right sided accessory pathway.

In most types of ventricular tachycardia the QRS complexes are regular and the obvious differential diagnosis is with the various types of 'supraventricular' tachycardia with wide QRS described above. The presence or absence of symptoms is no real guide in differential diagnosis, nor is the ventricular rate. The diagnosis of ventricular tachycardia is proven in the presence of ventriculoatrial block (slower dissociated P waves) and can be strongly suspected from the QRS morphology (Fig. 19.48).

Once the diagnosis of ventricular tachycardia is established, the clinical situation and the electrocardiographic appearance should be compared with the many types of ventricular tachycardia which are recognized in childhood. This will enable the prognosis and the response to treatment to be predicted. There is more variation between individual cases of ventricular tachycardia than is seen with supraventricular tachycardia.

Monomorphic ventricular tachycardia

Idiopathic left ventricular tachycardia has become better recognized in recent years. The commonest type is left posterior fascicular tachycardia that is often precipitated by exercise or emotion. The ECG has a RBBB pattern with a superior axis reflecting the origin of the arrhythmia in the left side of the ventricular septum. It is thought to be due to localized re-entry and may respond to drug treatment or catheter ablation.

Idiopathic right ventricular tachycardia is also described. The commonest type is right ventricular outflow tachycardia that is most frequently seen in older children or teenagers. It often produces no symptoms and seems to be benign. In this case the ECG in tachycardia shows a LBBB pattern with an inferior axis. The tachycardia usually originates just below the pulmonary valve and can be treated by catheter ablation although the need for and wisdom of such treatment has been questioned. Monomorphic ventricular tachycardia may also occur in association with underlying myocardial disease such as myocarditis, dilated cardiomyopathy or arrhythmogenic right ventricular cardiomyopathy.

Polymorphic ventricular tachycardia

Irregular ventricular tachycardia with varying QRS morphology is described as 'polymorphic'. It is a rare, but potentially very dangerous, arrhythmia. It may indicate an intrinsic problem or can be acquired, most often as a pro-arrhythmic effect of drugs. The clinical situation with which it is usually associated is the congenital long QT syndrome, in which life-threatening polymorphic ventricular tachycardia (torsade de pointes) is associated with an

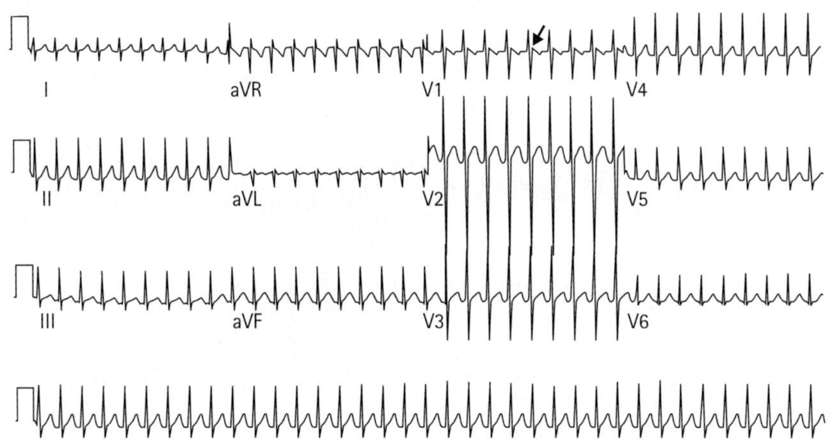

Fig. 19.46 AV nodal re-entry tachycardia in a 14-year-old girl. The ventricular rate is 220 per minute and the QRS is normal. P waves are not easily seen. However, the 'pseudo-R' appearance in lead V1 (arrow) strongly suggests that the P wave is within the terminal portion of the QRS. Comparison with the ECG in sinus rhythm showed this appearance was not present in sinus rhythm, making it probable that this is indeed the P wave.

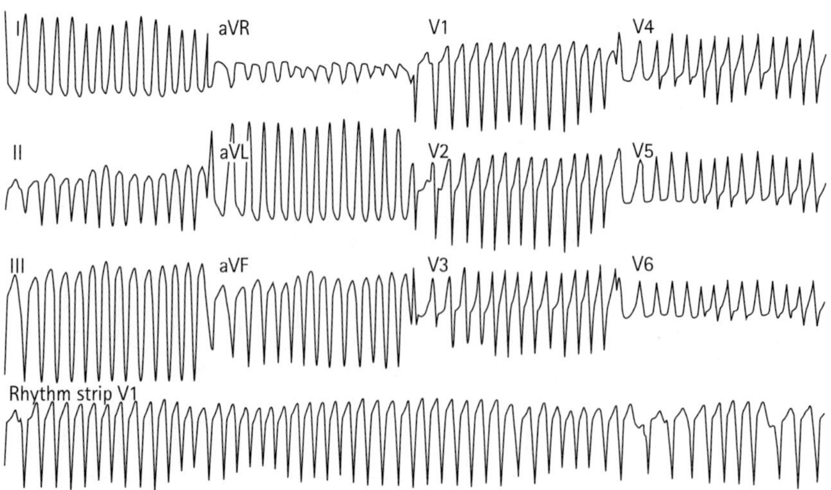

Fig. 19.47 Atrial fibrillation in Wolff-Parkinson-White syndrome. A recording from a 10-year-old girl who presented with syncope. The QRS is very abnormal, being broad with a slurred upstroke. The rhythm is irregularly irregular and the QRS axis is constant. The ECG in sinus rhythm in the same girl showed ventricular pre-excitation with the same activation pattern.

underlying prolongation of the QT interval (Fig. 19.49).[154] Syncope or sudden death occurs during emotional or physical stress. Revised diagnostic criteria were published in 1993.[155] The more common type has a dominant inheritance (Romano–Ward syndrome) and there is a rarer autosomal recessive variety with deafness (Jervell and Lange-Nielsen syndrome). The underlying abnormality is a defective sodium or potassium channel in the myocardial cell wall and many genetic mutations have been identified.[156] Several distinct genetic and clinical varieties have been identified with varying mortality rates and these can sometimes be predicted from the appearance of the ECG. Because of the high risk of sudden death treatment is required even in the absence of symptoms during childhood.[154] Treatment with a beta-blocker, most often nadolol, produces a dramatic reduction in mortality. Patients who remain symptomatic despite treatment with beta-blocking drugs may require pacemaker or defibrillator implantation. Coumel[157] and Brugada[158] have described other rare varieties of polymorphic ventricular tachycardia.

BRADYCARDIA

Bradycardia may result from defective impulse formation or from conduction block. The latter is more common and more significant in pediatric practice.

Complete Atrioventricular Block

Complete atrioventricular block usually presents in infancy, often as a result of detection during labor. The ECG shows a normal atrial rate and a ventricular bradycardia with atrioventricular dissociation (Fig. 19.50). In most cases the heart is structurally normal and the commonest underlying cause is maternal connective tissue disease, which may be subclinical. The AV block in the newborn is caused by transplacental passage of Sjörgren's syndrome antibodies. The risk of recurrence in subsequent pregnancies for antibody positive mothers is around one in six. The main decision to be made in the newborn is whether to implant a permanent pacemaker. The presence of symptoms, or a ventricular rate consistently below 55 per minute will usually be taken as an indication for pacemaker implantation.[159]

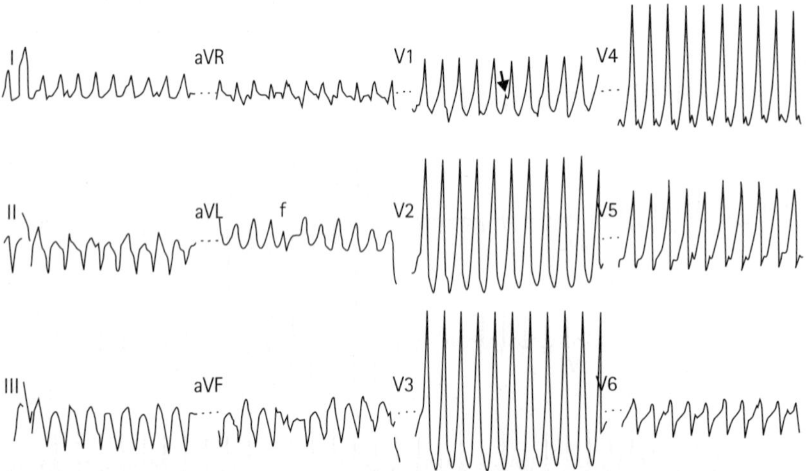

Fig. 19.48 Ventricular tachycardia. The QRS is broad and mostly regular. There is clear evidence of ventriculoatrial dissociation (dissociated P waves – solid arrow). The rhythm is occasionally disturbed by fusion beats (f). The QRS shows a right bundle branch block pattern with a superior axis predicting a left posterior origin for the ventricular tachycardia.

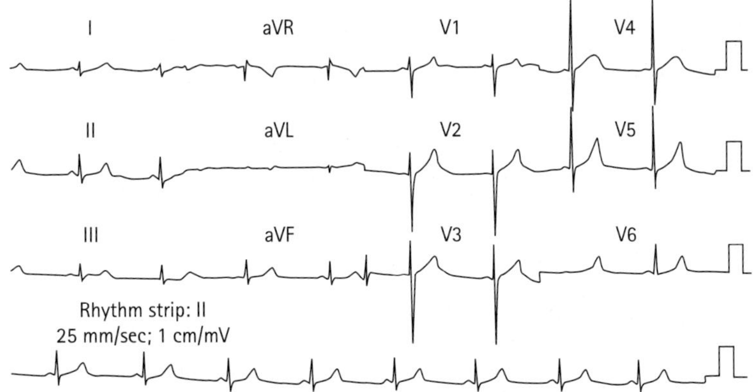

Fig. 19.49 Congenital long QT syndrome. A recording from a 14-year-old boy who presented with syncope. The QT interval is markedly prolonged.

A few infants with complete atrioventricular block have underlying structural heart disease, most commonly left atrial isomerism or congenitally corrected transposition (atrioventricular and ventricular arterial discordance). Complete AV block also occurs after surgical repair of heart disease, in which case pacemaker implantation is almost always required.

While AV block in infancy is rare (with a prevalence at live birth of 1:22 000),[147] a much more common arrhythmia, which may be mistaken for AV block, is produced by atrial premature beats or atrial ectopic beats. These are benign, asymptomatic and usually disappear during infancy. Depending on their prematurity they may be conducted normally, or with a bundle branch block pattern or may be blocked (Fig. 19.51).

Complete atrioventricular block may be detected for the first time in childhood but it is probably most often congenital in origin. An average daytime ventricular rate below 50 per minute may be an indication for pacemaker implantation, even in the absence of symptoms.[159] The presence of symptoms such as syncope, breathlessness or tiredness implies a significant risk and is an absolute indication for a pacemaker.

Other primary bradycardias

Bradycardia may also result from primary failure of impulse formation, known as sinoatrial disease. This is rare in childhood and pacemaker implantation is required only if there are symptoms. It is most often encountered late after cardiac surgery.

CARDIAC ARRHYTHMIAS IN OTHER SITUATIONS

Arrhythmias occurring late after surgery for congenital heart disease

Several cardiac operations are associated with late postoperative arrhythmias that have a significant impact on late morbidity and mortality.[136] Atrial flutter most often complicates atrial repair of transposition of the great arteries (Mustard or Senning operations) or right heart bypass operations for complex malformations (Fontan operation). It may also be a late complication of simpler operations such as repair of atrial septal defect or repair of tetralogy of Fallot. Atrial flutter may be associated with syncope or sudden death and demands expert evaluation and treatment. Postoperative ventricular tachycardia usually complicates operations that involve surgery on the ventricles such as repair of tetralogy of Fallot or Rastelli operation. Again the arrhythmia is potentially dangerous and requires expert assessment.

Asymptomatic Wolff–Parkinson–White syndrome

Ventricular pre-excitation may be found unexpectedly on an ECG. Population studies have shown that two-thirds of children with ventricular pre-excitation have no symptoms. It is likely that the majority of them will never develop an arrhythmia and the risk associated with ventricular pre-excitation in the absence of symptoms is very small. The consensus at present is that treatment is not required although expert assessment and discussion is appropriate.[160]

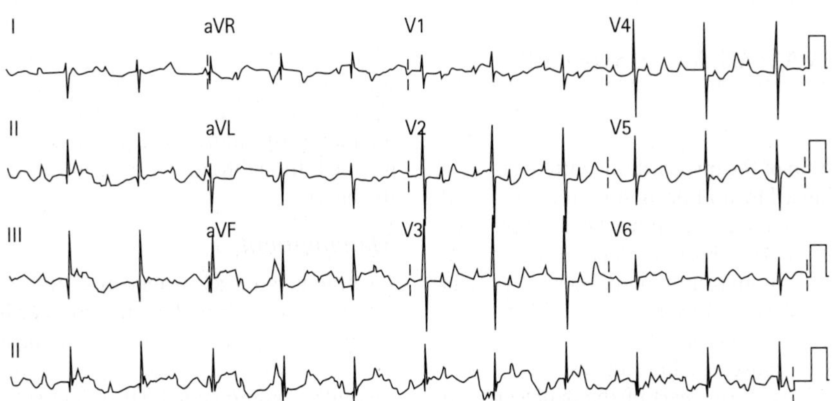

Fig. 19.50 Complete atrioventricular block in a neonate. The atrial rate is 140 per minute. The QRS complexes are regular with a normal morphology at a rate of 67 per minute. The baby's mother has Sjögren's syndrome. Pacing was not required during infancy.

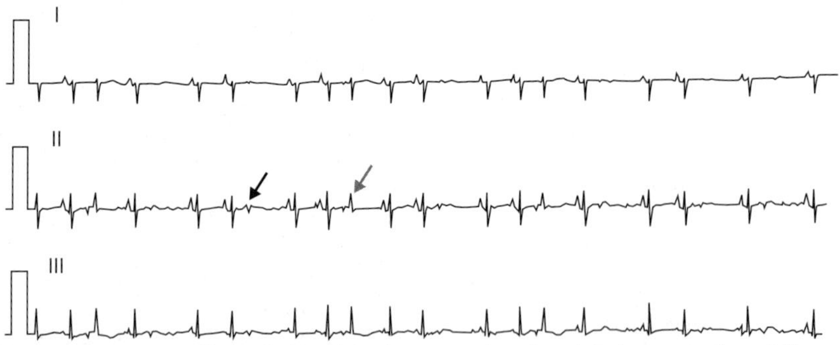

Fig. 19.51 Atrial premature beats in a neonate. The majority of the beats are sinus in origin but several are followed by premature P waves. Some of these are not conducted to the ventricles (black arrow) while others are conducted with a slightly different QRS morphology (gray arrow).

SYNCOPE

Syncope is a common symptom in childhood and in most cases is benign.[31] The commonest mechanism is vasovagal syncope (so-called simple faint) in which there is a transient vagally-mediated bradycardia. Other causes of syncope may be associated with transient bradycardia – such as in reflex anoxic seizures (pallid syncope) in preschool children and in neurocardiogenic syncope in older children. Documentation of bradycardia during syncope in this situation does not necessarily mean that there is a primary cardiac arrhythmia. In most cases the significance of the syncope and the likely underlying cause will be evident from the history.

A few rare but potentially dangerous arrhythmias may present with syncope. They include polymorphic ventricular tachycardia, other types of ventricular tachycardia, and atrial fibrillation in the Wolff–Parkinson–White syndrome (all discussed above). An electrocardiogram should be part of routine assessment of children with syncope but clinical evaluation is necessary before embarking on further investigation. Children with syncope on exertion, or physical signs of possible cardiovascular abnormality, or a family history of syncope or sudden death, or an abnormal ECG should be referred for expert evaluation.[31]

CONCLUSION

Recent years have seen an increased awareness of cardiac arrhythmias amongst pediatricians and pediatric cardiologists and a rapid advance in our understanding of the mechanisms. Non-invasive evaluation will usually identify precisely the type of arrhythmia and will help to define the prognosis and guide treatment. The outlook for most children with arrhythmias is good, especially in the present era of improved acute and long term treatment.

ACQUIRED CARDIOVASCULAR DISORDERS

MYOCARDITIS

Myocarditis is an inflammation of the myocardium with necrosis of myocytes.[161] It is usually caused by an infection with Coxsackie B or adenovirus.[161] Other viral infections have been implicated including cytomegalovirus, ECHO, Ebstein–Barr, influenza A, respiratory syncytial, mumps, human immunodeficiency, rubella and measles. Less frequently infections such as tuberculosis, meningococcus, diphtheria, rickettsia, protozoa, fungi and yeasts have been implicated. Other causes include drugs, toxins and autoimmune disease. Myocarditis forms part of the pancarditis in rheumatic fever and Kawasaki disease. Although viral infection appears to be the most frequent trigger for myocarditis, a subsequent autoimmune response may be responsible for the inflammation and necrosis. The true incidence is difficult to determine, as many cases are subclinical. Not all children infected with Coxsackie or adenovirus develop myocarditis, and genetic predisposition may play a role. Myocarditis has been implicated in sudden infant death syndrome.

Clinical features

The clinical presentation varies widely. At one end of the spectrum it can run a fulminant and rapidly fatal course, particularly in infancy, while at the other end the majority probably go unnoticed. There is frequently a recent history of a flu-like illness or gastroenteritis. Myocarditis should be suspected if there is a persistent, unexplained tachycardia, cardiac arrhythmia, tachypnea or signs of heart failure (p. 833). Survivors may recover completely, often after an illness of many weeks or months, or be left with a dilated cardiomyopathy.[163,164]

Investigations

Chest radiography usually shows cardiomegaly. Electrocardiographic changes are non-specific, but a sinus tachycardia is usually present and conduction disturbances occur. There may be premature atrial and ventricular contractions or occasionally ventricular tachycardia. Decreased QRS voltage with T wave flattening and inversion is commonly found. Echocardiography demonstrates a dilated and poorly contracting left ventricle with a reduced ejection fraction and fractional shortening. Mitral regurgitation is frequently seen and a pericardial effusion may be present. The erythrocyte sedimentation rate, C-reactive protein and cardiac muscle enzyme levels are usually elevated. Evidence of viral infection should be sought. Throat swab and feces should be sent for virology. Serology with rising or falling titers may help to confirm a viral infection, but results are inconclusive in many children. Myocardial biopsy is the gold standard for diagnosis, but is rarely performed in children as inflammatory changes are patchy and normal myocardium may be biopsied. In addition, the procedure carries a risk of perforation of the heart.

Management

Treatment is largely supportive and will depend on the severity of the myocarditis.[164] Initially, cardiac monitoring and rest are advisable. Heart failure is managed as described previously (p. 833). No specific therapy to reverse myocardial damage is currently recommended. The use of steroids or immunosuppressive therapy is controversial.[162] Arrhythmias should be treated aggressively.

PERICARDITIS AND PERICARDIAL EFFUSION

Etiology

Infective and non-infective inflammatory diseases can produce a pericardial exudate, which can be serous, fibrinous, hemorrhagic or purulent.[162] Viral pericarditis is often associated with a myocarditis and is caused by a similar range of viruses. Purulent or tuberculous pericarditis is rare in developed countries but not uncommon in the developing ones. Pericarditis occurs as part of the pancarditis of rheumatic fever and Kawasaki disease. Pericarditis and pericardial effusions are found in children with chronic renal failure, collagen diseases (particularly systemic lupus erythematosus and rheumatoid arthritis) and after cardiac surgery (postcardiotomy syndrome). In children with leukemia or other malignancies pericardial effusion may occur early due to pericardial infiltration, or later as a result of mediastinal irradiation. Sometimes no cause is found. A hemorrhagic pericardial effusion may be caused by chest trauma.

Moderate to large effusions are most common in neoplastic, viral, idiopathic, uremic and collagen disorders,[165,166] and are rare with rheumatic pericarditis and Kawasaki disease.

Clinical features

Signs of pericarditis vary with the primary illness, and with the volume and rate of accumulation of pericardial fluid. A smaller volume is relatively more significant in a younger child, and rapid accumulation is more likely to produce cardiac tamponade. Pain is an uncommon feature in children. Fever is prominent with bacterial infection. Dyspnea and a non-productive cough may develop as the effusion enlarges and a pericardial friction rub may be audible. If the effusion produces tamponade neck vein distension, hepatomegaly, low pulse pressure, pulsus paradoxus and cardiac failure become apparent. Pulsus paradoxus is significant when there is a fall in systolic pressure, on inspiration, of more than 10 mmHg. Since signs and symptoms of purulent pericarditis may be minimal and non-specific in the early stages, or may be missed in the presence of a severe generalized illness, a high index of suspicion is necessary. The onset of cardiac failure in a child with bronchopneumonia, empyema or lung abscess may be the first sign of purulent pericarditis.

Investigations

Electrocardiogram may show diffuse ST segment elevation with diminished QRS voltage if there is a significant effusion and chest radiography may demonstrate an enlarged globular cardiac shadow. Echocardiography is the most sensitive technique to assess the presence and size of a pericardial effusion (Fig. 19.52). Collapse of the right sided heart chambers indicates increased intra-pericardial pressure and, in the absence of clinical features, may be an early sign of tamponade.[166]

Where infective pericarditis is suspected, blood cultures should be performed and pericardiocentesis is mandatory. The fluid should be examined for cells and organisms and cultured for bacteria, viruses, mycobacteria and fungi. When appropriate, serological evidence of a viral infection or autoimmune disease should be sought.

Treatment

Treatment of pericarditis with a small effusion is symptomatic and the disease is often self-limiting. Diuretics and anti-inflammatory doses of aspirin are usually sufficient to treat postcardiotomy syndrome. Suspected purulent or tuberculous pericarditis requires pericardiocentesis to establish the causal agent. High doses of appropriate antibiotics should be given intravenously and surgical drainage may be necessary. Pericardial effusions due to leukemia are likely to resolve with appropriate chemotherapy.

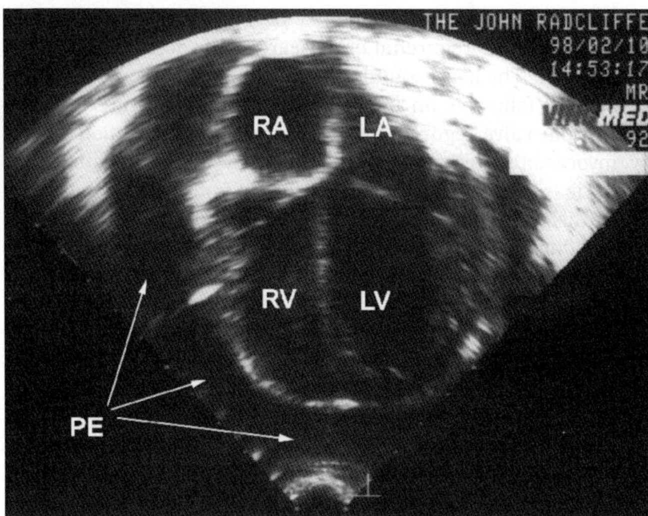

Fig. 19.52 Four chamber echocardiogram view of a pericardial effusion. PE, pericardial effusion; RV, right ventricle; LV, left ventricle; RA, right atrium; LA, left atrium.

Pericardiocentesis is essential and urgent in children with overt tamponade and should be considered if echocardiography shows cardiac compression. Except in an emergency, this is usually carried out in the cardiac catheterization theater, under ultrasound and fluoroscopic guidance, with electrocardiographic monitoring. A sub-xiphoid approach is usually used. It is advisable to leave a drain in situ until the effusion has resolved. Constriction is rare in children and is usually due to tuberculous pericarditis.

RHEUMATIC FEVER AND RHEUMATIC HEART DISEASE

Rheumatic fever is an endemic disease in developing countries with an annual incidence of 100 to 200 per 100 000 school-age children. Despite a dramatic fall in the incidence, it remains the major cause of morbidity and mortality from acquired heart disease in developing countries.[167] Acute carditis with the subsequent development of rheumatic heart disease is the most serious consequence of rheumatic fever,[168] as it is the only one that can cause death or serious disability. The pathogenesis and non-cardiac manifestations of rheumatic fever are discussed in Chapter 27.

Acute carditis

This is a pancarditis, affecting the endocardium with valve involvement, myocardium and pericardium. It occurs in over 50% of children, early in the course of rheumatic fever, usually within the first 3 weeks. It is extremely common in recurrences where carditis has occurred in the initial attack. It is more common in younger children ranging from 90% in those under 3 years, to 30% in adolescents. The development of a significant murmur is the prime clinical indicator of carditis. However, innocent murmurs are common in association with a febrile illness, and an organic murmur may be due to pre-existing congenital or rheumatic heart disease. The demonstration that a murmur has developed recently, or changed in character, is more definite evidence of rheumatic carditis. The most common murmur is an apical pansystolic murmur of mitral regurgitation. This may be due to endocarditis with edema and cellular infiltration of the mitral valve or myocarditis with dilatation of the left ventricle and stretching of the mitral valve. A short apical mid-diastolic flow murmur may be heard. This frequently resolves when the child recovers.

Less commonly the high-pitched decrescendo early diastolic murmur of aortic regurgitation is heard in the aortic area and left sternal edge. The heart sounds are soft.

Cardiac failure is an uncommon presenting feature but may result from valve regurgitation or ventricular dysfunction caused by myocarditis. Pericarditis, recognized by a friction rub, never occurs in isolation and provides evidence of underlying myocarditis. Sinus tachycardia is suggestive of carditis, particularly when it occurs during sleep in the afebrile child. Occasionally a sinus bradycardia occurs.

Investigations

An electrocardiogram and echocardiogram should be performed in all children suspected of having rheumatic fever. Other investigations are discussed in Chapter 27. A variety of electrocardiographic changes have been reported. Prolongation of the PR interval (first degree heart block) is frequently found but does not necessarily indicate carditis. Second degree or complete heart block also occurs. Flattened or inverted T waves over the left precordial leads (V4–V6) are a characteristic finding of myopericarditis. Echocardiography may demonstrate a small pericardial effusion and allows assessment of cardiac chamber sizes and function. A dilated left ventricle occurs with significant myocardial disease or valve regurgitation. Contractility is decreased with myocarditis, but normal or increased with mitral or aortic regurgitation. Approximately 50% of children with rheumatic fever have clinical evidence of carditis, but Doppler and color flow mapping demonstrates valve regurgitation in up to 70%. In a significant number of children the only manifestation of carditis will be echocardiographic, and increasingly this is being accepted as diagnostic of carditis.[169,170] Strict criteria must be applied,[171] however, as minimal mitral regurgitation is a physiological condition.

Prognosis

There has been a marked decrease in mortality and morbidity in the past century as a result of improved socioeconomic standards and treatment with penicillin, particularly as prophylaxis to prevent recurrences. The prognosis is still much worse in less developed countries where severe rheumatic heart disease develops during childhood. The prognosis is also worse in children who have severe cardiac involvement in the initial attack and in those who have recurrences with carditis. Mitral regurgitation can improve with time,[172] but aortic regurgitation is more likely to be permanent.

The prognosis is excellent for patients who escape carditis during an initial attack of rheumatic fever, but this does not preclude carditis in a subsequent attack, so prophylaxis is indicated.

Treatment

Penicillin therapy is given orally for 10 days to eradicate the streptococcal infection. Alternatively a single dose of benzathine penicillin 0.6–1.2 million units is given intramuscularly. Erythromycin is used in children allergic to penicillin. Anti-inflammatory drugs provide dramatic clinical improvement, but there is no evidence that they prevent the development of rheumatic heart disease. Aspirin (75 mg/kg/24 h) is given in four divided doses for 2 weeks with gradual reduction thereafter. Steroids shorten the course of the acute illness but symptoms are likely to return when they are discontinued, and some advocate the use of aspirin as the steroids are reduced. Controlled studies have failed to demonstrate improved long-term prognosis.[173,174] Heart failure is treated as described previously (p. 833).

Rheumatic fever is a recurring disease with relapses most common in young children and in the first 5 years following an episode. Each attack carries an increasing risk of carditis with permanent valve damage and death. It is therefore essential that *continuous* antimicrobial prophylaxis against further streptococcal infection be started as soon as the initial therapeutic course of penicillin has been completed. The most effective form of prophylaxis is an intramuscular injection of 0.6–1.2 million units of benzathine penicillin every 3–4 weeks. It eliminates recurrences and is the treatment of choice.[175] Alternatively oral phenoxymethylpenicillin (penicillin V) 250 mg is given twice daily. Sulfadiazine is recommended for children allergic to penicillin. Prophylactic therapy must be continued throughout childhood and into early adult life. The decision whether to discontinue prophylaxis thereafter depends on the severity of cardiac involvement, time since the last attack, social circumstances and the increased risk of exposure to further streptococcal infections.

Rheumatic heart disease

Rheumatic heart disease occurs in childhood in the many countries where the incidence of rheumatic fever remains relatively high. The prevalence is in the region of 6 per 1000 school-age children.[176,177] The risk of rheumatic heart disease increases with increasing severity of initial cardiac involvement and younger age at the time of the initial attack. The mitral valve is affected in 85% of cases, the aortic valve in 55%, and the tricuspid and pulmonary valves in less than 5%.[178] Isolated aortic valve disease is rare.

Mitral regurgitation is the commonest lesion in children with rheumatic heart disease. In older children and adults it may be associated with mitral stenosis. Where regurgitation is mild, the child is asymptomatic with an apical pansystolic murmur radiating to the axilla. When regurgitation is severe, the child may experience effort dyspnea or palpitations. The apex beat is forceful and displaced and a third heart sound may be prominent, its presence excluding coexisting tight mitral stenosis. The pulmonary second sound is accentuated in the presence of pulmonary hypertension. A mid-diastolic flow murmur is heard with severe mitral regurgitation, because of increased diastolic flow through the mitral valve. Chest radiography shows cardiomegaly and the enlarged left atrium may be seen. Electrocardiography demonstrates left atrial and left ventricular hypertrophy. Echocardiography shows enlargement of the left atrium and left ventricle and color Doppler confirms the presence of regurgitation and gives an estimate of its severity. The mitral valve leaflets are thickened and tethered, with cordal rupture. Cardiac catheterization adds little further information, apart from measurement of pulmonary arterial resistance.

Mitral stenosis may be asymptomatic initially, but effort intolerance and dyspnea progress to orthopnea, paroxysmal nocturnal dyspnea, cardiac failure and hemoptysis. The apex beat is not displaced unless there is also significant mitral regurgitation. The pulse volume may be reduced and the first heart sound is loud. An opening snap early in diastole is followed by a low-pitched rumbling mitral mid-diastolic murmur. Increasing mitral stenosis causes progressive lengthening of the murmur resulting in presystolic accentuation. Atrial fibrillation is rare in children but if it occurs, the presystolic component (related to atrial systole) disappears. A right ventricular parasternal impulse is palpable and the pulmonary second sound is accentuated when pulmonary hypertension occurs.

On chest radiography the heart size is usually normal with left atrial enlargement. Increased left atrial pressure causes dilatation of the upper lobe pulmonary veins and edema of the interlobular septa (Kerley B lines). The electrocardiogram demonstrates the broad, notched P waves of left atrial hypertrophy, if there is moderate or severe mitral obstruction, and right ventricular hypertrophy when pulmonary hypertension develops. Echocardiography shows a large left atrium with thickened and tethered mitral valve leaflets. Fibrosis and calcification of the valve and subvalvar apparatus reduce mobility of the leaflets. M-mode echocardiography demonstrates a reduced closure rate of the anterior mitral valve leaflet, with the posterior leaflet moving anteriorly with it in diastole. The Doppler signal shows an increased velocity and reduced rate of pressure fall across the valve throughout diastole, a quantitative assessment of which is given by the pressure half-time, that is, the time taken for the pressure across the valve to reach half the initial maximum value. This provides some assessment of the severity of the obstruction. In normal adults it is 60 ms and in those with mitral stenosis it is above 100 ms. Cardiac catheterization adds little information to that obtained from echocardiography. It may be performed to assess pulmonary vascular resistance or as part of therapeutic balloon dilatation of the mitral valve.

Aortic regurgitation is not associated with symptoms unless there is severe regurgitation with left ventricular dysfunction, when palpitations, sweating and effort dyspnea occur. The pulse pressure is wide, the pulse collapsing and the apical impulse of left ventricular type. The murmur is a high pitched blowing early diastole murmur, best heard at the upper and middle left sternal edge with the child leaning forward and holding their breath in expiration. An aortic ejection systolic murmur is usually audible when there is marked regurgitation, which in children represents increased flow across the valve, not stenosis. An apical mid and late diastolic murmur (Austin Flint) can be heard if there is severe aortic regurgitation without mitral valve disease. It is due to forward flow through the mitral valve, which is partially closed by the aortic regurgitant jet. It may be indistinguishable from organic mitral stenosis. In severe cases left ventricular failure may produce signs of pulmonary edema.

With moderate or severe regurgitation there will be left ventricular hypertrophy on the electrocardiogram and enlargement on the chest radiograph. Echocardiography will demonstrate a dilated and hypercontractile left ventricle and possibly flutter of the anterior leaflet of the mitral valve. Color Doppler will show the regurgitant flow. Cardiac catheterization adds little information to that obtained from echocardiography.

Management

Children with mild valve disease simply require follow-up and antimicrobial prophylaxis. In addition, life-long prophylaxis against bacterial endocarditis is necessary for dental and other surgical procedures.[41,42] If the lesion is moderate or severe, competitive sport should be avoided.[179]

Indications and timing of mitral and aortic valve surgery remain controversial. If the child is asymptomatic and echocardiography shows normal left ventricular function, surgery is not required. Children who are asymptomatic with significant regurgitation and normal left ventricular function on echocardiography need to be observed closely. Because of the possibility of valve replacement, it is desirable to defer surgery, if possible, until the child is fully grown. However, deterioration in left ventricular dysfunction is an indication for surgery. If this is not done promptly they will have a higher operative mortality, and unrecoverable left ventricular damage may occur. A good result may sometimes be achieved with annuloplasty for mitral regurgitation, or surgical or balloon valvotomy for mitral stenosis. Valve replacement is required for severe aortic regurgitation.

KAWASAKI DISEASE

Kawasaki disease is a generalized vasculitis, of unknown etiology, first reported in Japan in 1967. Since that time, Kawasaki disease has been recognized around the world. The annual incidence varies from 4–5 cases per 100 000 children under 5 years old in the United States, rising to an incidence of 120–150 cases per 100 000 children under 5 years old in Asian populations.[180] While normally self-limiting it is associated with a number of complications, the most important of which is the development of life-threatening coronary artery abnormalities. In the acute phase Kawasaki disease may cause medium and large vessel arteritis, myocarditis and arterial aneurysms, particularly of the coronary arteries. These may thrombose or develop segmental stenosis in the chronic phase of the disease. It is now the most common cause of acquired heart disease in children in the developed world. It remains unclear whether this newly recognized disease has always existed, but has not been diagnosed, or if it is truly a new disease.

The causative agent remains elusive, although an infectious etiology is most likely.[181] The peak incidence is in toddlers, with 85% of cases occurring in children under 5 years of age, and only rare cases in infants under 3 months of age or adults. The disease is 1.5 times more common in males and recurrence rates are low (3%).[182] Diagnosis is based on the presence of characteristic features outlined in Table 19.9 and the exclusion of other diagnoses.[183] Cardiac involvement usually occurs within 2 weeks of the onset of Kawasaki disease. If severe, a friction rub of pericarditis or gallop rhythm of cardiac failure from myocarditis may be apparent. Myocardial ischemia may cause papillary muscle dysfunction and mitral regurgitation.

Investigations

Electrocardiographic abnormalities include sinus tachycardia, reduction in QRS amplitude, flattening of T waves, prolongation of rate, adjusted PR and QT intervals and occasional dysrhythmias. Evidence of ischemia or infarction may be seen during long-term follow-up. Serial echocardiograms are required to evaluate and follow-up coronary artery abnormalities.[184] The initial echocardiogram should be performed at the time of diagnosis, although aneurysms are rarely seen before the tenth day of illness. It should be noted that, while coronary artery aneurysms in a febrile child are almost pathognomonic of Kawasaki disease, their absence does not rule out the diagnosis.

If there is no coronary artery involvement or only mild ectasia, echocardiograms should be repeated at 10–14 days into the illness (if this was not the timing of the first study), at 6–8 weeks and at 6–12 months. If the coronary arteries remain normal, no further follow-up is indicated. If coronary artery aneurysms occur, then follow-up must be modified based on the severity of the lesions and the clinical course.

Management and prognosis

High dose intravenous immunoglobulin (2 g/kg) in conjunction with aspirin lowers the rate of coronary artery aneurysms from

Table 19.9 Diagnostic criteria for Kawasaki disease

Fever persisting at least 5 days and the presence of at least four of the following five principal features:
Changes in extremities:
Acute: erythema and edema of hands and feet
Convalescent: membranous desquamation of fingertips
Polymorphous exanthema
Bilateral, painless bulbar conjunctival injection without exudates
Changes in lips and oral cavity: erythema and cracking of lips, strawberry tongue, diffuse injection of oral and pharyngeal mucosae
Cervical lymphadenopathy (≥ 1.5 cm in diameter), usually unilateral

between 20 and 25% to less than 5%.[185–187] An anti-inflammatory dose of aspirin (30 mg/kg/day in four divided doses) should be continued until clinical and hematological markers of inflammation have settled. Aspirin should then be continued at an antiplatelet dose (3–5 mg/kg/day) until follow-up at 6–8 weeks. If there is no evidence of coronary artery involvement at that stage aspirin can be discontinued. It remains unclear how patients who fail to respond to the initial treatment with intravenous immunoglobulin and aspirin should be managed. There may yet be a role for steroids and other anti-inflammatory agents in this subset of patients.

No restrictions need be applied to children after 6–8 weeks if they do not develop coronary artery abnormalities. In those patients who do go on to develop coronary ectasia or small, single aneurysms the majority regress within 1–2 years. Approximately 1% of patients who recover from Kawasaki disease will develop significant coronary artery aneurysms (Fig. 19.53) or obstruction. This is more likely in children with multiple or large aneurysms. These patients should remain on the antiplatelet dose of aspirin and have annual clinical review with electrocardiography, echocardiography and exercise testing. Those with a suggestion of coronary obstruction should have coronary angiography. In some patients with very large aneurysms, warfarin is indicated in addition to aspirin to prevent clot from embolizing to distal coronary arteries.[188] The results of surgery for coronary artery stenosis are poor, particularly in younger children.

CONNECTIVE TISSUE DISEASE

Cardiac involvement can occur in all connective tissue diseases but is most common in systemic lupus erythematosus. Pericarditis without tamponade is the usual presenting feature. The characteristic atypical verrucose endocarditis (Libman–Sacks) can cause valve regurgitation. Congenital complete heart block can occur in infants of mothers suffering from connective tissue disease who are seropositive for anti-Ro.[189]

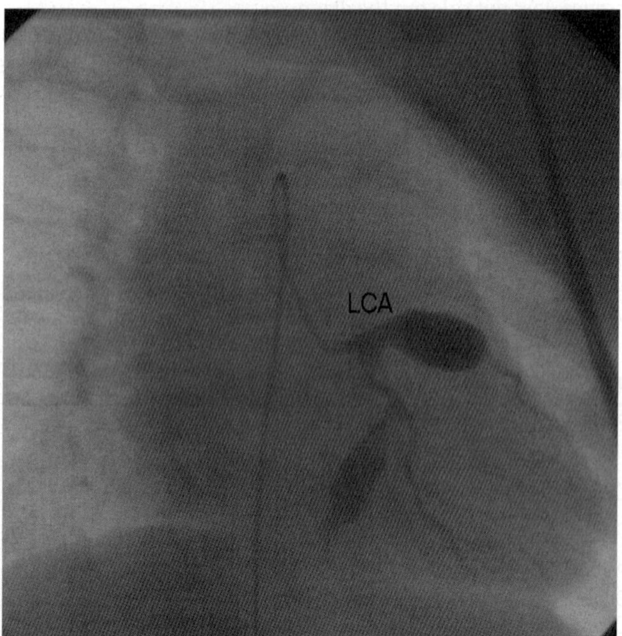

Fig. 19.53 Left coronary arteriogram showing an aneurysm of the main left and anterior descending coronary arteries in a child with Kawasaki disease. LCA, Left coronary artery.

In juvenile rheumatoid arthritis cardiac abnormalities usually occur in the acute systemic form of the disease with pericarditis, myocarditis and occasionally mitral regurgitation. Echocardiography may demonstrate a pericardial effusion in children with no clinical signs of heart disease. Cardiac failure is an uncommon complication but can be fatal. Scleroderma can be associated with diffuse focal fibrosis within the myocardium producing ventricular dysfunction, which may lead to left ventricular failure and death. Polyarteritis nodosa is rare in infants and children, but it follows a more fulminant course. Infantile polyarteritis is usually associated with coronary artery lesions, which can result in myocardial ischemia, cardiac failure and death.

CARDIOMYOPATHIES

Traditionally, the term cardiomyopathy refers only to heart muscle disease of unknown cause. However, with better understanding of the metabolic, genetic and molecular mechanism of cardiomyopathies, many are now known to be secondary, and an extensive search must always be made in children for possible causes. Familial cardiomyopathy is more common than was previously thought, accounting for up to 30% of dilated cardiomyopathy.[190] Cardiomyopathies are broadly divided into dilated, hypertrophic and restrictive, although not all cardiomyopathies fit neatly into this classification.[191]

Dilated cardiomyopathy

Dilated cardiomyopathy is characterized by dilatation and impaired systolic function of the left or both ventricles. Possible causes are outlined in Table 19.10. Dilatation of the mitral valve ring may occur producing mitral regurgitation. Heart failure frequently develops.

Table 19.10 Conditions producing features of dilated cardiomyopathy

Conditions
Other cardiac conditions
Anomalous origin of left coronary artery
Coarctation of the aorta
Arrhythmias (SVT/VT)
Systemic arteriovenous fistula
Infections (myocarditis)
Drug therapy
Anthracyclines
Infection
Viral myocarditis
Fungal/protozoal/metazoal myocarditis
Metabolic causes/storage
Mucopolysaccharidoses
Lipidoses (GM1 gangliosidosis)
Sialic acid storage disorder
Fucosidosis
Metabolic causes/energy production
Carnitine deficiency
Fatty acid oxidation defects (usually thick walls)
'Mitochondrial' abnormalities (usually thick walls)
Aminoacidemias (sick neonate/infant)
Neuromuscular disorders
Muscular dystrophies (late, thin walls)
Rare congenital myopathies ('floppy')
(Friedreich's ataxia: mostly hypertrophic)
Familial – usually autosomal dominant
Chromosomal abnormalities (dysmorphic features)

It is the commonest cardiomyopathy in childhood and the most frequent indication for cardiac transplantation in the pediatric population.

Clinical features

Symptoms vary with the severity of dysfunction and the level of activity of the child. In the acute state there will be marked dyspnea and cardiac failure while less severe states will produce easy fatigue and decreased exercise tolerance. Less commonly the patient may present with a cardiac arrhythmia or conduction defect. Clinical examination will show signs of heart failure (p. 833).

Investigations

A secondary cause should always be sought and Table 19.11 contains a list of appropriate investigations.[192] Chest radiography shows cardiomegaly and pulmonary edema is sometimes present. The electrocardiogram will usually show evidence of hypertrophy and strain. If there are ischemic changes, an anomalous left coronary artery from the pulmonary artery should be ruled out (p. 865). A 24-h electrocardiogram should be performed to rule out an incessant tachycardia as the cause, as well as to document any arrhythmias secondary to the cardiomyopathy. Echocardiography is the most important investigation and will demonstrate a dilated, poorly contracting left ventricle (Fig. 19.54) and mitral regurgitation.

Treatment and prognosis

Initial treatment is symptomatic and non-specific.[193] It takes the form of heart failure therapy, with diuretics, angiotensin converting enzyme (ACE) inhibitors and digoxin. Beta-blockers are increasingly being recognized as playing an important role in the management. Anticoagulation may be necessary to avoid embolization of intracavity thrombus. Intravenous inotropes or vasodilators may be required in severe cases. Arrhythmias should be treated, but can be problematic, as most anti-arrhythmic agents are negative inotropes. Incessant supraventricular tachycardia has been treated with radiofrequency ablation, with improvement in ventricular function.[194] If there is no improvement referral for cardiac transplantation should be considered.[195] Left ventricular assist devices ('artificial hearts') are being developed that may help the recovery phase or act as a bridge to transplant.

The outcome is related to the severity of the dysfunction and whether a secondary cause can be found which is amenable to treatment. Treatment with carnitine in children with carnitine deficiency results in resolution of the cardiomyopathy.[196] As a general rule, one-third of dilated cardiomyopathies get better, one-third stay the same and one-third get worse. Older age at presentation and lack of improvement in systolic function are associated with adverse outcome.[197]

Hypertrophic cardiomyopathy

Hypertrophic cardiomyopathy is the appearance of unexplained ventricular hypertrophy and is usually inherited in an autosomal dominant manner with incomplete penetrance. There are a number of secondary causes of thickening of the ventricle, which are outlined in Table 19.12. It is seen in up to 20% of children with Noonan's syndrome. Neonatal hypertrophic cardiomyopathy is commonly due to maternal diabetes and is caused by the increased fetal insulin acting as a growth factor. It usually resolves spontaneously. By a similar mechanism it is seen in infants with Beckwith–Wiedemann syndrome. The hypertrophy may involve the septum more than the free wall, which can result in a gradient low in the left ventricular outflow tract either at rest or on exercise. There is also left ventricular diastolic dysfunction with reduced distensibility and impaired

Table 19.11 Screening investigations for secondary heart muscle disease

Blood
Autoimmune/connective tissue screen (creatine kinase)
Carnitine (free and acyl carnitine)
Fasting sugar and lactate
Thyroid function
Calcium/phosphate
Full blood count and film (eosinophilia or neutropenia)
Amino acids
Vacuolated lymphocytes
Selenium (if geographical risk)
Iron and iron binding
Viral serology (Coxsackie, ECHO, influenza, parainfluenza, mumps, rubella, rubeola and possibly HIV) – acute and convalescent
Urine
Amino acids

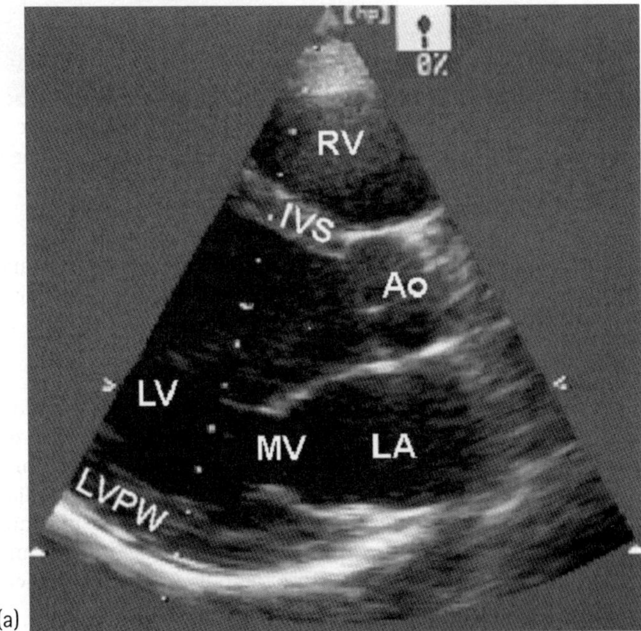

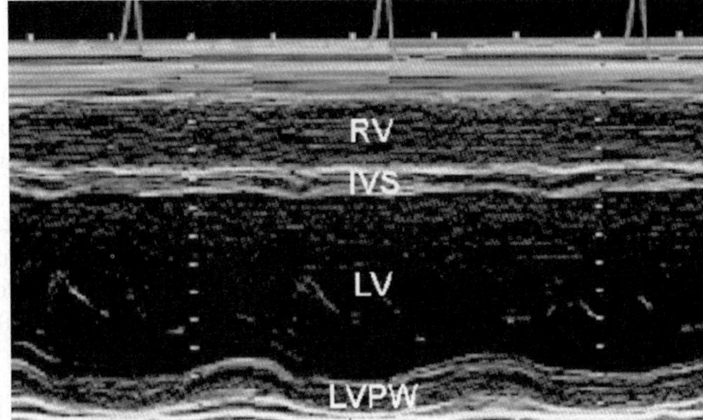

Fig. 19.54 (a) Parasternal long axis view of a child with dilated cardiomyopathy demonstrating a dilated left ventricle. The dashed line marks the line through which the (b) M-mode recording was made and demonstrates poor contractility. Ao, aortic root; IVS, intraventricular septum; LA, left atrium; LV, left ventricle; LVPW, posterior wall of the left ventricle; MV, mitral valve; RV, right ventricle.

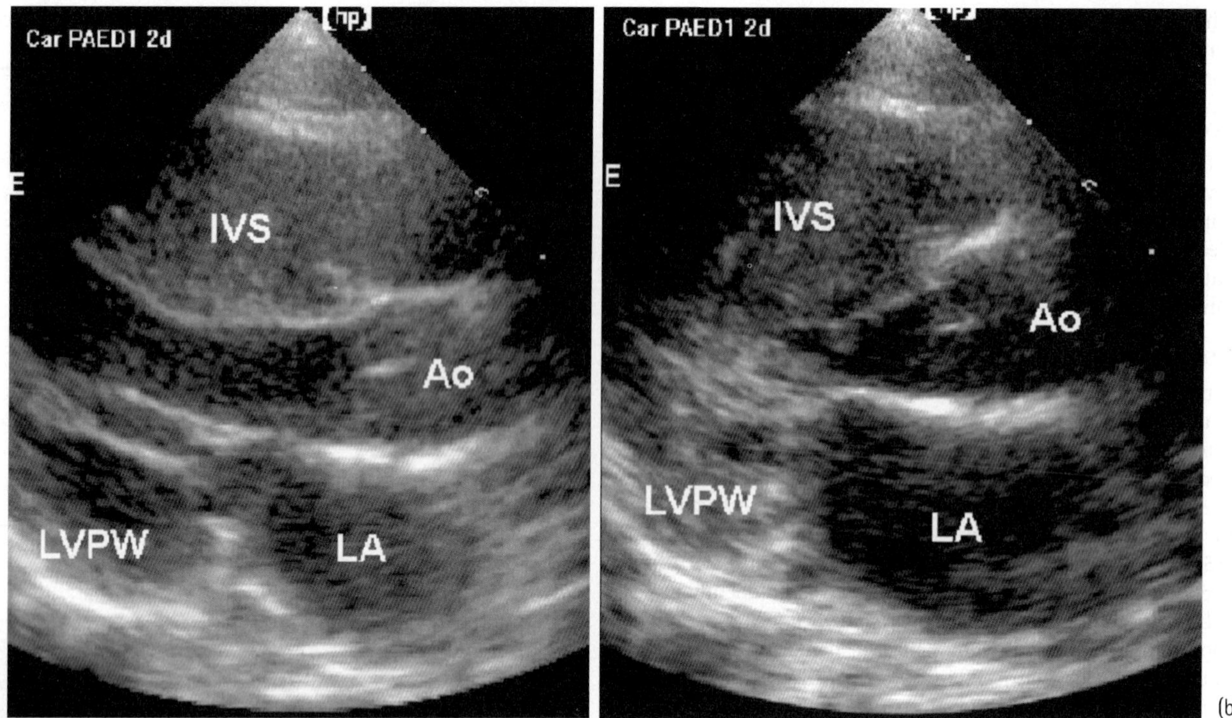

Fig. 19.55 Parasternal long axis views of a child with hypertrophic cardiomyopathy at (a) end-diastole and (b) end-systole. Note the marked hypertrophy of the posterior wall of the left ventricle (LVPW) and the intra-ventricular septum (IVS), which results in significant sub-aortic obstruction at end-systole. Ao, aortic root; LA, left atrium.

relaxation. The condition is often not recognized until adult life and the diagnosis may only be made in a child because they are referred for family screening.

Clinical features

Symptoms are most often associated with a left ventricular outflow tract gradient. In older children, dyspnea or excessive fatigue on exertion are most common but angina, dizziness, syncope and palpitations also occur. Infants may present with congestive cardiac failure, cardiomegaly or cyanosis. An ejection systolic murmur may be audible, maximal at the lower left sternal edge or apex and it may be possible to feel a 'jerky' arterial pulse or a double apical impulse.

Investigations

There is no characteristic electrocardiographic abnormality. There may be left ventricular hypertrophy, ST and T wave abnormalities, deep Q waves, and prolongation of the QT interval. Echocardiography characteristically shows thickening of the septum and posterior left ventricular wall, often with asymmetric septal hypertrophy (ratio of thickness of ventricular septum to left ventricular wall 1.3 or greater) and systolic anterior motion of the mitral valve. Doppler ultrasound may demonstrate increased velocity low in the left ventricular outflow tract with a characteristic signal and an abnormal left ventricular filling pattern.

Treatment and prognosis

The course of the disease is variable. Sudden death occurs in 2–6% of patients per year, probably from ventricular tachycardia, and may be the presenting feature. Attempts have been made to stratify risk,[198] but no single test can reliably predict risk. A family history of cardiac arrest or sudden death is of prognostic importance. Non-sustained ventricular tachycardia, early onset of symptoms in childhood, severe ventricular hypertrophy and exercise-induced hypotension all suggest increased risk of sudden death.

Drug therapy with beta-blockers and verapamil may help with symptoms of obstruction and abnormal filling. These drugs have little influence on the incidence of sudden death but amiodarone may be valuable in this context.[198] Cardiac pacing can be of symptomatic

Table 19.12 Specific heart diseases causing wall thickening

Other cardiac conditions
Coarctation of the aorta
Systemic hypertension
Tumors
Metabolic causes/storage
Glycogenoses (Pompe, GSDIII)
Mucopolysaccharidoses (ASH in older children)
Metabolic causes/energy production
Fatty acid oxidation defects
'Mitochondrial' cardiomyopathies
Organic acidurias
Endocrine
Infant of diabetic mother
Beckwith–Wiedemann syndrome
Pancreatic tumors (severe neonatal hypoglycemia)
Hypothyroidism (ASH)
Neuromuscular disorders
Friedreich's ataxia
Rare congenital myopathies ('floppy')
Syndromes
Noonan
Leopard/neurofibromatosis/Williams
Chromosomal abnormalities

ASH, asymmetric septal hypertrophy.

benefit and implantable defibrillators are now small enough to implant in children and may abort sudden death. Patients with severe left ventricular outflow gradients may also benefit from a septal myomyectomy. Children who are symptomatic, or have signs of significant disease, should have their activities restricted. It is worth noting that although severe exertion is considered a risk factor, in most cases sudden death is unrelated to exertion. Great advances have been made in the genetics of hypertrophic cardiomyopathy, which may help in identifying those most at risk and guiding treatment.

Other cardiomyopathies

Restrictive cardiomyopathies are rare in children. Radiation therapy for malignancies, pseudoxanthoma elasticum and hypereosinophilic syndromes are rare causes in children. Adult causes (amyloid, sarcoid and Fabry's disease) are virtually never seen in children.

Endomyocardial fibrosis is a progressive and usually fatal disease of unknown etiology occurring mainly in children and young adults living in specific regions of the tropics and subtropics, most frequently in Africa. The main pathological finding is an endocardial layer of dense fibrous tissue originating at the apex of one or both ventricles and spreading upwards.

Endocardial fibroelastosis has similar clinical features and evolution to dilated cardiomyopathy, and may be present as part of that disease. It is also seen secondary to left ventricular outflow tract obstruction or coarctation of the aorta and can be primary (congenital).

Arrhythmogenic right ventricular dysplasia is characterized by fatty infiltration and fibrosis of the free wall of the right ventricle. The disease may be familial and symptoms and risk of sudden death due to ventricular tachycardias increase with age.[199]

CARDIAC TUMORS

Primary cardiac tumors are rare in children.[200] The majority are benign, in the histological sense, but, by compressing the conducting tissue or encroaching on the cardiac cavities, they may cause death from arrhythmia or from ventricular or valve dysfunction. Rhabdomyomas are by far the most common tumor in the pediatric age group and if multiple, almost certainly mean the child has tuberous sclerosis. Fibromas and teratomas can occur in infants and young children, including the newborn, and hemangiomas and myxomas only rarely in older children.

Clinical features depend on the site and size of the tumor. Intramural tumors may be asymptomatic or cause an arrhythmia. Tumors within a cavity can cause ventricular outflow obstruction, or obstruction or regurgitation of the atrioventricular valves. Cardiac failure and embolic phenomena can also occur.

Echocardiography and magnetic resonance imaging are both useful techniques to demonstrate intracardiac tumors.[201] Surgical therapy is indicated if there is an intractable arrhythmia or obstruction to the outflow or inflow tracts. Rhabdomyomas may regress spontaneously during infancy.

SYSTEMIC HYPERTENSION

Hypertension in children and adolescents is underdiagnosed, and although in younger patients is often secondary to other diseases, in the older child and adolescent it is at least as frequently of the primary or essential type.[202] Furthermore, evidence suggests that primary hypertension has its origins in early life and those at risk may be identifiable in childhood or adolescence, allowing surveillance and management with the aim of preventing the later development of cardiovascular disease. Measurement of blood pressure should be a part of the clinical examination by pediatricians of all children over 3 years old, and in younger children where appropriate.[203]

There are difficulties in defining hypertension in children since blood pressure rises with age and exhibits considerable variability in an individual. The National High Blood Pressure Education Program Working Group on Hypertension Control in Children and Adolescents[204] has suggested that consistent diastolic values above the 95th centile (p. 883) should be considered to indicate hypertension. On this basis the prevalence of systemic hypertension in children is 5%, but a smaller number will have persistent hypertension.

Etiology

The causes are outlined in Table 19.13. Essential hypertension is most common in adolescents, particularly in those who have a hypertensive first-degree relative or who are overweight. Renal disease accounts for about 95% of cases of secondary hypertension.

Clinical features

Hypertension is frequently discovered on routine examination of a child who has no symptoms directly attributable to it. In a few children with severe hypertension, the diagnosis of hypertension is beyond doubt, but frequently identification is dependent upon an arbitrary definition of the upper limits of normal blood pressure. Techniques of blood pressure measurement are discussed on page 816. 24-hour ambulatory blood pressure monitoring can be performed on older children, and is especially useful in those whose readings might be affected by increased levels of anxiety.[205] Larger children (heavier and taller) have higher blood pressures than smaller ones and if levels between the 90th (Tables 19.14 and 19.15) and 95th percentiles

Table 19.13 Causes of secondary hypertension

Renal
Chronic glomerulonephritis
Reflux nephropathy
Obstructive uropathy
Hemolytic uremic syndrome
Polycystic disease
Dysplastic disease
Cystinosis
Hypoplastic kidneys
Renal tumors
Collagen disease
Vascular
Coarctation of the aorta
Renal artery stenosis
Renal venous thrombosis
Takayashu's disease
Endocrine
Pheochromocytoma
Neuroblastoma
Cushing's syndrome
Primary aldosteronism
Congenital adrenal hyperplasia (17α-hydroxylase or 11-hydroxylase deficiency)
Miscellaneous
Obesity
Increased intracranial pressure
Drugs (corticosteroids, oral contraceptives)
Neurofibromatosis
Lead poisoning
Familial dysautonomia
Porphyria
Turner's syndrome

Table 19.14 The 90th percentile for blood pressure for girls (From the second Report of the Task Force on Blood Pressure control in Children 1987[203] with permission)

	Systolic	Diastolic	Height (cm)	Weight (kg)
Birth	76	68	54	4
1 month	98	65	55	4
6 months	106	66	66	7
1 year	105	67	77	11
2 years	105	69	89	13
3 years	106	69	98	15
4 years	107	69	107	18
5 years	109	69	115	22
6 years	111	70	122	25
7 years	112	71	129	30
8 years	114	72	135	35
9 years	115	74	142	40
10 years	117	75	148	45
11 years	119	77	154	51
12 years	122	78	160	58
13 years	124	80	165	63
14 years	125	81	168	67
15 years	126	82	169	70
16 years	127	81	170	72
17 years	127	80	170	73
18 years	127	80	170	74

Table 19.15 The 90th percentile for blood pressure for boys (From the second Report of the Task Force on Blood Pressure control in Children 1987[203] with permission)

	Systolic	Diastolic	Height (cm)	Weight (kg)
Birth	87	68	51	4
1 month	101	65	59	4
6 months	105	66	72	8
1 year	105	69	80	11
2 years	106	68	91	14
3 years	107	68	100	16
4 years	108	69	108	18
5 years	109	69	115	22
6 years	111	70	122	25
7 years	112	71	129	29
8 years	114	73	135	34
9 years	115	74	141	39
10 years	117	75	147	44
11 years	119	76	153	50
12 years	121	77	159	55
13 years	124	79	165	62
14 years	126	78	172	68
15 years	129	79	178	74
16 years	131	81	182	80
17 years	134	83	184	84
18 years	136	84	184	86

are found, height should be considered.[203] In general, the younger the child and the higher the blood pressure, the more likely it is that the hypertension will be secondary and the more intense should be the search for an underlying cause. Children whose blood pressure is consistently above the 95th percentile should be investigated and treatment should aim to achieve a reduction to below the 95th percentile (Table 19.16). Ideally, an obese child with moderate hypertension should be encouraged to lose weight and the blood pressure subsequently repeated before undergoing investigation and possible treatment.

Symptoms, when they occur, result from the cause or the complications of hypertension.

Symptoms of the cause: the history may suggest a renal cause (past or present kidney disease), pheochromocytoma (episodes of palpitations, excessive sweating, headache), aldosteronism (weakness, polyuria, muscle cramps) or drug ingestion (corticosteroid, oral contraceptive). Inquiry should be made for a family history of eclampsia, essential hypertension, premature coronary artery or cerebrovascular disease, diabetes mellitus, inherited renal conditions and neurofibromatosis.

Symptoms of the complications: hypertension may cause raised intracranial pressure resulting in headache or vomiting, and eventually result in seizures or other neurological disturbances. Visual problems, tiredness, irritability and epistaxis have been described. Left ventricular failure may cause dyspnea or cough. Cardiac failure, respiratory distress, vomiting, irritability or convulsions may be the presenting feature in infants.

Signs of hypertension: physical examination may be normal initially but with established hypertension changes occur in the optic fundi and evidence of left ventricular hypertrophy becomes apparent. Signs of heart failure may be present.

Signs of the cause of hypertension: physical examination must include palpation of the femoral pulses and kidneys, and auscultation of the abdomen and flanks for a bruit suggesting renal artery stenosis. The clinical features of Williams and Turner's syndromes must be considered.

Investigation

This will depend on the child's age, blood pressure level, and the clinical findings. Those with severe hypertension, symptoms, or advanced retinopathy require urgent investigation and treatment. Hypertensive children should have a full blood count, urinalysis and urine culture, and serum electrolytes, urea, creatinine and uric acid concentrations performed. The presence of associated hyperlipidemia, a further risk factor in coronary artery disease, should be excluded.

Other studies may be warranted on the basis of the history, or physical or laboratory findings with the aim of excluding renal and endocrine disease, as detailed in Chapters 16 and 13 respectively. Echocardiography can identify aortic coarctation. The search for a renal cause of hypertension requires additional renal imaging with ultrasound, radioisotope scanning or micturating cystourethrography and measurement of peripheral plasma renin activity. Abdominal angiography is essential for identifying vascular lesions of the renal arteries and may demonstrate tumors such as pheochromocytoma. When a renal lesion contributing to hypertension may benefit from surgery, samples for plasma renin activity should be taken from the inferior vena cava and both renal veins. Increased secretion by an affected kidney with suppression of secretion by the contralateral one suggests that surgery will result in a reduction of blood pressure.

Endocrine causes of hypertension are rare in children and their diagnosis requires specific biochemical tests. Screening tests should include measurement of hydroxymethoxymandelic acid (HMMA) (pheochromocytoma or neuroblastoma), metadrenaline (pheochromocytoma) and homovanillic acid (HVA) (neuroblastoma) and urinary free cortisol and diurnal plasma cortisols (Cushing's syndrome). Hyperaldosteronism is suggested by hypokalemia but this is not a reliable screening test for aldosteronism in children, and plasma aldosterone and plasma renin activity should be measured.

Management and prognosis

Borderline hypertension (below the 95th percentile) does not require drug therapy. Obese children should be encouraged to lose weight. All should be advised not to smoke and to avoid excessive salt intake.

Table 19.16 Classification of hypertension by age group (From the second Report of the Task Force on Blood Pressure control in Children 1987[203] with permission)

Age group	Significant hypertension (mmHg) average systolic and/or diastolic blood pressure ≥ 95th percentile for age with measurements obtained on at least three occasions	Severe hypertension
Newborn		
7 days	Systolic BP ≥ 112	Systolic BP ≥ 106
8–30 days	Diastolic BP ≥ 74	Systolic BP ≥ 110
Infant < 2 years	Systolic BP ≥ 112 Diastolic BP ≥ 74	Systolic BP ≥ 118 Diastolic BP ≥ 82
Children (3–5 years)	Systolic BP ≥ 116 Diastolic BP ≥ 76	Systolic BP ≥ 124 Diastolic BP ≥ 84
Children (6–9 years)	Systolic BP ≥ 122 Diastolic BP ≥ 78	Systolic BP ≥ 130 Diastolic BP ≥ 86
Children (10–12 years)	Systolic BP ≥ 126 Diastolic BP ≥ 82	Systolic BP ≥ 134 Diastolic BP ≥ 90
Adolescents (13–15 years)	Systolic BP ≥ 136 Diastolic BP ≥ 86	Systolic BP ≥ 144 Diastolic BP ≥ 92
Adolescents (16–18 years)	Systolic BP ≥ 142 Diastolic BP ≥ 92	Systolic BP ≥ 150 Diastolic BP ≥ 98

Table 19.17 Antihypertensive drugs for oral use (From Anderson et al 2002[79])

Drug	Major side-effects	Precautions	Dose
Angiotensin-2 converting enzyme inhibitors			
Captopril	Hypotension, rash, cough, agranulocytosis	Avoid in renal artery stenosis	Children 0.1–0.5 mg/kg (maximum 2 mg/kg) three times a day Neonates: 0.01–0.05 mg/kg three times a day
Enalapril	Hypotension, cough	Avoid in renal artery stenosis	0.1 mg/kg (maximum 1.0 mg/kg) once daily (enalapril has been substituted for captopril as 1 mg enalapril per 7.5 mg captopril)
Calcium channel blocker			
Nifedipine	Flushing, tachycardia, headache	–	Capsule: 5–10 mg, three times a day Modified release tablets: 10–20 mg twice a day Slow release tablets: 30–60 mg once a day
Diuretics			
Chlorothiazide	Hypokalemia, hyperuricemia	Renal insufficiency	10 mg/kg (maximum 40 mg/kg) per day
Furosemide (frusemide)	Hypokalemia		1–4 mg/kg once or twice a day
Spironolactone	Hyperkalemia, gynecomastia	Renal insufficiency	1 mg/kg, twice or three times a day
β-Adrenoceptor blockers			
Propranolol	Reduced cardiac output, bradycardia	Cardiac failure, asthma	0.2–2.0 mg/kg three times a day
Atenolol	As propranolol	As propranolol	1–2 mg/kg (maximum 8 mg/kg) once a day
α-Adrenoceptor blocker			
Prazosin	Hypotension after first dose, dizziness	First dose reaction	0.01 mg/kg three times a day; increase to a maximum of 0.5 mg/kg three times a day
Mixed α and β-adrenoceptor blocker			
Labetolol	Rash, dry eyes, dizziness	Cardiac failure, asthma	1–2 mg/kg three or four times a day
Vasodilators			
Minoxidil	Fluid retention, tachycardia, hirsutism	–	0.1 mg/kg twice daily; increase by 0.1 mg/kg per dose every 3 days to a maximum of 0.5 mg/kg twice a day
Hydralazine	Flushing, tachycardia, lupus syndrome	–	0.2–1.0 mg/kg

Girls must be warned of the hypertensive effects of oral contraceptives. Blood pressure should be measured annually. Children with undoubtedly high levels (persistently above the 95th percentile) or symptoms and signs caused by the hypertension must be treated.[206] Emergency treatment for severe hypertension should be sublingual nifedipine or intravenous labetalol or sodium nitroprusside. For less severe hypertension initial therapy is generally with a diuretic or a beta-blocker. In refractory cases the further addition of a vasodilator such as hydralazine, an ACE inhibitor (e.g. captopril) or a calcium channel antagonist (e.g. nifedipine) should be used. Hypotensive drugs have a variety of side-effects and each should be introduced in a low dose that is then increased slowly, up to therapeutic levels (Table 19.17). It is important to monitor renal function as this can deteriorate with the use of some drugs, particularly ACE inhibitors.

PULMONARY HYPERTENSION

Pulmonary hypertension is defined as a mean pulmonary artery pressure > 25 mmHg at rest or 30 mmHg with exercise.[207] The main causes of pulmonary hypertension are listed in Table 19.18. Pulmonary hypertension secondary to congenital heart disease has become less prevalent as surgery is now usually performed before irreversible pulmonary vascular disease develops.[208] Primary pulmonary hypertension, which can be familial, is rare.[209]

Clinical findings usually relate to the cause of the pulmonary hypertension. They can be unremarkable but breathlessness is the most common feature. The cardiac impulse is usually hyperdynamic, and the pulmonary component of the second heart is loud. Once the right-sided pressure in the heart rises higher than systemic, right-to-left shunting can occur and the child may become cyanosed (a phenomenon known as Eisenmenger's syndrome.

Table 19.18 Causes of pulmonary hypertension

1. Congenital heart diseases
   - With increased pulmonary blood flow
     - left-to-right shunts, e.g. VSD, PDA, truncus arteriosus
     - disconnected pulmonary artery
     - total anomalous pulmonary venous drainage
     - transposition of great arteries
   - With pulmonary venous obstruction
     - left ventricular inflow or outflow obstruction
     - obstructed total anomalous pulmonary venous drainage
     - pulmonary vein stenosis or veno-occlusive disease
2. Chronic lung diseases producing hypoxemia
   - airway obstructions, e.g. upper airways obstruction, chronic asthma
   - parenchymal disorders, e.g. cystic fibrosis, neonatal lung disease
   - restrictive disorders, e.g. kyphoscoliosis
3. Pulmonary vascular diseases
   - primary (idiopathic) pulmonary hypertension
   - persistent pulmonary hypertension of the newborn
   - collagen vascular diseases, e.g. systemic lupus erythematosus
   - thromboembolism, e.g. ventriculoatrial shunts for hydrocephalus
   - sickle cell disease
4. Others
   - high altitude
   - drugs and toxins
   - neuromuscular disorders producing hypoventilation
   - familial

PDA, persistent arterial duct; VSD, ventricular septal defect.

Investigation

The electrocardiogram demonstrates right ventricular hypertrophy. Chest radiography shows large proximal pulmonary vessels with small distal branches – peripheral pruning of the pulmonary arterial tree. Echocardiography demonstrates the congenital cardiac lesion if present. Doppler can be used to measure the velocity of tricuspid regurgitation which can accurately reflect right ventricular pressure. Pulse oximetry performed at rest and during a graded exercise test demonstrates the degree of desaturation and exercise capacity. Pulmonary function tests, ventilation perfusion scan, computerized tomography (CT) scan of the lungs and thrombophilia screen may be indicated.

Cardiac catheterization confirms the diagnosis and measures the response of the pulmonary vascular bed (pulmonary vascular resistance) to vasodilators such as oxygen, prostacylin and nitric oxide. The positive response to acute vasodilator testing, with more than 20% reduction in mean pulmonary artery pressure or pulmonary vascular resistance, accurately identifies patients who may respond to long term oral vasodilator treatment such as nifedipine.[207] Lung biopsy may be indicated.

Management and prognosis

Children with a large left-to-right shunt, who have a fall in pulmonary vascular resistance in response to an acute vasodilatation, are suitable for correction of the underlying lesion. Up to 40% of children without a cardiac lesion will respond to acute pulmonary vasodilatation, the youngest having the greatest likelihood of a positive response. These children should be treated with a calcium antagonist. If, however, the pulmonary hypertension is irreversible the prognosis is extremely poor. Prostacyclin and nitric oxide have both been shown to improve survival.[210] Most recently, sildenafil has been used with apparent success, but long-term studies are awaited. Other therapy is directed primarily at ameliorating symptoms and improving survival.[211] Oxygen therapy may provide symptomatic improvement especially in children with pulmonary disease. Anticoagulation with warfarin and antiplatelet agents is recommended as patients are at risk of thrombotic events. Antifailure therapy may provide symptomatic relief. Children with right heart failure or syncope should be palliated with an atrial septostomy. Patients should receive pneumococcal immunization and annual immunization against influenza. Ultimately these patients may require heart–lung transplantation, although results are poor in children.

REFERENCES (* Level 1 evidence)

1 Pelech AN. Evaluation of the pediatric patient with a cardiac murmur. Pediatr Clin North Am 1999; 46:167–188.

2 Mitchell IM, Logan RW, Pollock JCS, Jamieson MPG. Nutritional status of children with congenital heart disease. Br Heart J 1995; 73:277–283.

3 Burn J, Brennan P, Little J, et al. Recurrence risks in offspring of adults with major heart defects: results from first cohort of British collaborative study. Lancet 1998; 351:311–316.

4 Becker SM, Al Halees Z, Molina C, Paterson RM. Consanguinity and congenital heart disease in Saudi Arabia. Am J Med Genet 2001; 99:8–13.

5 Garson A Jr. The electrocardiogram in infants and children: a systematic approach. Philadelphia: Lea & Febiger; 1983.

6 Davignon A, Rautaharju P, Boisselle E, et al. Normal ECG standards for infants and children. Pediatr Cardiol 1979/80; 1:123–152.

7 Rijnbeek PR, Witsenburg M, Schrama E, et al. New normal limits for the paediatric electrocardiogram. Eur Heart J 2001; 22:702–711.

8 Tipple M. Interpretation of electrocardiograms in infants and children. Images Paediatr Cardiol 1999; 1:3–13.
9 Wren C. The presentation of arrhythmias. In: Wren C, Campbell RWF (eds). Paediatric cardiac arrhythmias. Oxford: Oxford University Press; 1996.
10 Fallah-Najmabadi H, Dahdah NS, Palcko M, et al. Normal values and methodologic recommendations for signal-averaged electrocardiography in children and adolescents. Am J Cardio 1996; 77: 408–412.
11 Rosenstock EG, Cassuto Y, Zmora E. Heart rate variability in the neonate and infant: analytical methods, physiological and clinical observations. Acta Paediatr 1999; 88:477–482.
12 Fogel MA, Lieb DR, Seliem MA. Validity of electrocardiographic criteria for left ventricular hypertrophy in children with pressure or volume loaded ventricles: comparison with echocardiographic left ventricular muscle mass. Pediatr Cardiol 1995; 16:261–269.
13 Silverman NH, Hunter S, Anderson RH, et al. Anatomical basis of cross sectional echocardiography. Br Heart J 1983; 50:421–431.
14 Anderson RH, Ho SY. Sequential segmental analysis – description and categorisation for the millennium. Cardiol Young 1997; 7:98–116.
15 Tworetzky W, McElhinney DB, Brook MM, et al. Echocardiographic diagnosis alone for the complete repair of major congenital heart defects. J Am Coll Cardiol 1999; 33:228–233.
16 Wilkinson JL. Haemodynamic calculations in the catheter laboratory. Heart 2001; 85: 113–120.
17 Ashfaq M, Houston AB, Gnanapragasam JP, et al. Balloon atrial septostomy under echocardiographic control: six years' experience and evaluation of the practicability of the umbilical vein route. Br Heart J 1991; 65:148–151.
18 Pihkala J, Nykanen D, Freedom RM, Benson LN. Interventional cardiac catheterisation. Pediatr Clin North Am 1999; 46: 441–464.
19 Rashkind WJ, Miller WW. Creation of an atrial septal defect without thoracotomy. A palliative approach to transposition of the great arteries. JAMA 1966; 196:991–992.
20 Rao PS, Galal O, Patnana M, et al. Results of three to 10 year follow up of balloon dilatation of the pulmonary valve. Heart 1998; 80: 591–595.
21 Bu'Lock FA, Joffe HS, Jordan SC, Martin RP. Balloon dilatation (valvoplasty) as first line treatment for severe stenosis of the aortic valve in early infancy: medium term results and determinants of survival. Br Heart J 1993; 70:546–553.
22 Rao PS. Should balloon angioplasty be used instead of surgery for native aortic coarctation? Br Heart J 1995; 74: 578–579.
23 Shaddy RE, Boucek MM, Sturtevant JE, et al. Comparison of angioplasty and surgery for unoperated coarctation of the aorta. Circulation 1993; 87:793–799.
24 Gibbs J. Treatment options for coarctation of the aorta. Heart 2000; 84:1–13.
25 Harrison DA, McLaughlin PR, Lazzam C, et al. Endovascular stents in the management of coarctation of the aorta in the adolescent and adult: one year follow up. Heart 2001; 85: 561–566.
26 Bu'Lock FA, Tometzki AJP, Kitchiner DJ, et al. Balloon expandable stents for systemic venous pathway stenosis late after Mustard's operation: comparison with balloon angioplasty alone. Heart 1998; 79:225–229.
27 Mendelsohn AM, Bove EL, Lupinetti FM, et al. Intraoperative and percutaneous stenting of congenital pulmonary artery and vein stenosis. Circulation 1993; 88:210–217.
28 Bilkis AA, Alwi M, Hasri S, et al. The Amplatzer duct occluder: experience in 209 patients. J Am Coll Cardiol 2001; 37:258–261.
29 Berger F, Vogel M, Alexi-Meskishvili V, et al. Comparison of results and complications of surgical and Amplatzer device closure of atrial septal defects. J Thorac Cardiovasc Surg 1999; 118:674–678.
30 Baker E. What's new in magnetic resonance imaging? Cardiol Young 2001; 11:445–452.
31 McLeod KA. Dizziness and syncope in adolescence. Heart 2001; 86:350–354.
32 Guenthard J, Wyler F. Exercise-induced hypertension in the arms due to impaired arterial reactivity after successful coarctation resection. Am J Cardiol 1995; 75:814–817.
33 Rajakumar K, Weisse M, Rosas A, et al. Comparative study of clinical evaluation of heart murmurs by general pediatrians and pediatric cardiologists. Clin Pediatrs 1999; 38:511–518.
34 Advani N, Menahem S, Wilkinson JL. The diagnosis of innocent murmurs in childhood. Cardiol Young 2000; 10:340–342.
35 McCrindle BW, Shaffer KM, Kan JS. Cardinal clinical signs in the differentiation of heart murmurs in children. Arch Pediatr Adolesc Med 1996; 150:169–74.
36 O'Laughlin MP. Congestive heart failure in children. Pediatr Clin North Am 1999; 46:263–273.
37 Kay JD, Sinaiko AR, Daniels SR. Pediatric hypertension. Am Heart J 2001; 142:422–432.
38 Salmon AP, Holder R, DeGiovanni JV et al. Effects of digoxin in infants with ventricular septal defects and cardiac failure. Br Heart J 1989; 61:115.
39 Kay JD, Colan SD, Graham TP. Congestive heart failure in pediatr patients. Am Heart J 2001; 142:923–928.
40 Morris AM, Webb GD. Antibiotics before dental procedures for endocarditis prophylaxis: back to the future. Heart 2001; 86:3–4.
41 Dajani AS, Taubert KA, Wilson W, et al. Prevention of bacterial endocarditis. Recommendations by the American Heart Association. Circulation 1997; 96:358–366.
42 Working Party of the British Society for Antimicrobial Chemotherapy. Antibiotic prophylaxis of infective endocarditis. Lancet 1990; 335:88–89 & Lancet 1997; 350:1100.
43 Simmons NA, Ball AP, Eykyn SJ, et al. Antibiotic treatment of streptococcal, enterococcal, and staphylococcal endocarditis. Working Party of the British Society for Antimicrobial Chemotherapy. Heart 1998; 79:207–210.
44 O'Callaghan C, McDougall P. Infective endocarditis in neonates. Arch Dis Child 1988; 63:53–57.
45 Bayer AS, Bolger AF, Taubert KA, et al. Diagnosis and management of infective endocarditis and its complications. Circulation 1998; 98:2936–2948.
46 Brook MM. Pediatric bacterial endocarditis treatment and prophylaxis. Pediatr Clin North Am 1999; 46: 275–287.
47 Washington JA. The microbial diagnosis of infective endocarditis. J Antimicrob Ther 1987; 20 (suppl A):29–39.
48 Donal E, Abgueguen P, Coisne D, et al. Echocardiographic features of *Candida* species endocarditis: 12 cases and a review of published literature. Heart 2001; 86:179–182.
49 Hoffman JIE. Incidence, mortality and natural history. In: Anderson RH, Baker EJ, Macartney FJ, et al (eds) Pediatric cardiology, 2nd edn. Edinburgh; Churchill Livingstone; 2002; 111–139.
50 Samanek M, Voriskova M. Congenital heart disease among 815 569 children born between 1980 and 1990 and their 15 year survival: a prospective Bohemia survival study. Pediatr Cardiol 1999; 20:411–417.
51 Fixler DE, Pastor P, Sigman E, Eifler CW. Ethnicity and socioeconomic status: impact on the diagnosis of congenital heart disease. J Am Coll Cardiol 1993; 21: 1722–1726.
52 Sadiq M, Stumper O, Wright JG, et al. Influence of ethnic origin on the incidence of congenital heart defects in the first year of life. Br Heart J1995; 73:173–176.
53 Jackson M, Walsh KP, Peart I, Arnold R. Epidemiology of congenital heart disease in Merseyside – 1979 to 1988. Cardiol Young 1996; 6:272–280.
54 Macmahon B, McKeown T, Record RG. The incidence and life expectation of children with congenital heart disease. Br Heart J 1953; 15:121–129.
55 Wren C, O'Sullivan JJ. Survival with congenital heart disease and need for follow-up in adult life. Heart 2001; 85:438–443.
56 Lammer EJ, Chen DT, Hoar RM, et al. Retinoic acid embryopathy. N Engl J Med 1985; 313:837–841.
57 Copel JA, Pilu G, Kleinman CS. Congenital heart disease and extracardiac anomalies; associations and indications for fetal echocardiography. Am J Obstet Gynecol 1986; 154: 1121–1132.
58 Beattie JO, Day RE, Cockburn F, et al. Alcohol and the fetus in the west of Scotland. BMJ 1983; 287:17–20.
59 Johnson MC, Payne RM, Grant JW, Strauss AW. The genetic basis of paediatric heart disease. Ann Med 1995; 27:289–300.
60 Vincent GM. Role of DNA testing for diagnosis, management, and genetic screening in long QT syndrome, hypertrophic cardiomyopathy and Marfan syndrome. Heart 2001; 86:12–14.
61 Kenna AP, Smithells RW, Fielding DW. Congenital heart disease in Liverpool: 1960–69. QJM 1975; 44:17–44.
62 Mazzanti L, Cacciari E. Congenital heart disease in patients with Turner's syndrome. Italian Study Group for Turner Syndrome (ISGTS). J Pediatr 1998; 133:688–692.
63 Ryan AK, Goodship JA, Wilson DI, et al. Spectrum of clinical features associated with interstitial chromosome 22q11 deletions: a

European collaborative study. J Med Genet 1997; 34:798–804.

64 Goldmuntz E, Clark BJ, Mitchell LE, et al. Frequency of 22q11 deletions in patients with conotruncal defects. J Am Coll Cardiol 1998; 32:492–498.

65 Nora JJ, Nora AH. Update on counseling the family with a first-degree relative with a congenital heart defect. Am J Med Genet 1988; 29:137–142.

66 Sharland G. Changing impact of fetal diagnosis of congenital heart disease. Arc Dis Child 1997; 77:F1–F3.

67 Bull C. Current and potential future impact of fetal diagnosis on prevalence and spectrum of serious congenital heart disease at term in the UK. Lancet 1999; 354:1242–1247.

68 Allen LD, Sharland GK, Chita SK, et al. Chromosomal anomalies in fetal congenital heart disease. Ultrasound Obstet Gynecol 1991; 1:8–11.

69 Brackley KJ, Kilby MD, Wright JG, et al. Outcome after prenatal diagnosis of hypoplastic left-heart syndrome: a case series. Lancet 2000; 356:1143–1147.

70 Tworetzky W, McElhinney DB, Reddy VM, et al. Improved outcome after fetal diagnosis of hypoplastic left heart syndrome. Circulation 2001; 103:1269–1273.

71 Marek J, Oekovranek J, Povy Ueilova, et al. Effectiveness of fetal heart screening in the Czech Republic. Proceedings of the 2nd world Congress on Pediatric Cardiology and Cardiac Surgery. Hawaii: 1997.

72 Abu-Harb M, Hey E, Wren C. Death in infancy from unrecognised congenital heart disease. Arch Dis Child 1994; 71:3–7.

73 Penny DJ, Shekerdemian LS. Management of the neonate with symptomatic congenital heart disease. Arch Dis Child 2001; 84:F141–F145.

74 Pfammatter J-P, Stocker FP. Delayed recognition of haemodynamically relevant congenital heart disease. Eur J Pediatr 2001; 160:231–234.

75 O'Brien LM, Stebbens VA, Poets CF, et al. Oxygen saturation during the first 24 hours of life. Arch Dis Child Fetal Neonatal Edn 2000; 83:F35–F38.

76 Wren C, Richmond D, Donaldson L. Presentation of congenital heart disease in infancy: implications for routine examination. Arch Dis Child Fetal Neonatal Edn 1999; 80: F49–F53.

77 Skinner JR, Boys RJ, Hunter S, Hey EN. Non-invasive determination of pulmonary arterial pressure in healthy neonates. Arch Dis Childhood 1991; 66:386–390.

78 Waldman JD, Holmes G. The cyanosed newborn: excluding structural heart disease In: Skinner J, Alverson D, Hunter S (eds) Echocardiography for the neonatologist. Edinburgh: Churhill Livingstone; 2000:181–195.

79 Anderson RH, Baker EJ, Macartney FJ, et al (eds). Pediatric cardiology, 2nd edn. Edinburgh: Churchill Livingstone; 2002.

80 Prêtre R, Tamisier D, Bonhoeffer P, et al. Results of the arterial switch operation in neonates with transposed great arteries. Lancet 2001; 357:1826–1830.

81 Gelatt M, Hamilton RM, McCrindle BW, et al. Arrhythmia and mortality after the Mustard procedure: a 30-year single-center experience. J Am Coll Cardiol 1997; 29:194–201.

82 Wilson NJ, Clarkson PM, Barratt-Boyes BG, et al. Long-term outcome after the Mustard repair for simple transposition of the great arteries. 28 year follow-up. J Am Coll Cardiol 1998; 32:758–765.

83 Rastelli GC, McGoon DC, Wallace RB. Anatomic correction of transposition of the great arteries with ventricular septal defect and subpulmonary stenosis. J Thorac Cardiovasc Surg 1969; 58:545–552.

84 Iserin L, de Lonlay P, Viot G, et al. Prevalence of the microdeletion 22q11 in newborn infants with congenital conotruncal cardiac abnormalities. Eur J Pediatr 1998; 157:881–884.

85 Reddy VM, Petrossian E, McElhinney DB, et al. One-stage complete unifocalization in infants: when should the ventricular septal defect be closed? J Thorac Cardiovasc Surg 1997; 113:858–866.

86 Cheung YF, Leung MP, Lee JW, et al. Evolving management for critical pulmonary stenosis in neonates and young infants. Cardiol Young 2000; 10:186–192.

87 Balaji S, Dennis NR, Keeton BR. Familial Ebstein's anomaly: a report of six cases in two generations associated with mild skeletal abnormalities. Br Heart J 1991; 66:26–28.

88 Celermajer DS, Bull C, Till J, et al. Ebstein's anomaly: presentation and outcome from fetal to adult. J Am Coll Cardiol 1994; 23:170–176.

89 Chauvaud S. Ebstein's malformation. Surgical treatment and results. Thorac Cardiovasc Surg 2000; 48:220–223.

90 Hyde JA, Stumper O, Barth MJ, et al. Total anomalous pulmonary venous connection and management of recurrent venous obstruction. Eur J Cardiothorac Surg 1999; 15:735–740.

91 Anderson RH, Macartney FJ. Pulmonary venous abnormalities In: Anderson RH, Baker EJ, Macartney FJ, et al (eds) Pediatric cardiology, 2nd edn. Edinburgh: Churchill Livingstone; 2002:867–899.

92 Rajasinghe HA, McElhinney DB, Reddy VM, et al. Long-term follow-up of truncus arteriosus repaired in infancy: a twenty-year experience. J Thorac Cardiovasc Surg 1997; 113:869–878.

93 Pickert CB, Moss MM, Fiser DH. Differentiation of systemic infection and congenital obstructive left heart disease in the very young infant. Pediatr Emerg Care 1998; 14:263–267.

94 Sinha SN, Kardatzke ML, Cole RB, et al. Coarctation of the aorta in the newborn. Circulation 1969; 40:385–398.

95 Celoria GC, Pattern RB. Congenital absence of the aortic arch. Am Heart J 1959; 56:400–426.

96 Salmon AP. Hypoplastic left heart syndrome outcome and management. Arch Dis Child 2001; 85:450–451.

97 Andrews R, Tulloh R, Sharland G, et al. Outcome of staged reconstructive surgery for hypoplastic left heart syndrome following antenatal diagnosis. Heart 2001; 85:474–477.

98 Norwood WI, Lang P, Hansen DD. Physiologic repair of aortic atresia-hypoplasic left heart syndrome. N Engl J Med 1983; 308:23–26.

99 Mahle WT, Spray TL, Wernovsky G, et al. Survival after reconstructive surgery for hypoplastic left heart syndrome: a 15-year experience from a single institution. Circulation 2000; 102(suppl 3):136–141.

100 Sullivan ID, Wren C, Bain HH, et al. Balloon aortic valvotomy for congenital aortic stenosis in childhood. Br Heart J 1989; 61:186–191.

101 Mosca RS, Iannettoni MD, Schwartz SM, et al. Critical aortic stenosis in neonates. J Thorac Cardiovasc Surg 1995; 109:147–154.

102 Kitchiner D, Jackson, Walsh K, et al. The incidence and prognosis of congenital aortic valve stenosis in Liverpool (1960–1990). Br Heart J 1993; 69:71–79.

103 Arlettaz R, Archer N, Wilkinson AR. Natural history of innocent heart murmurs in newborn babies: controlled echocardiographic study. Arch Dis Child Fetal Neonatal Edn 1998; 78:F166–F170.

104 Rein AJT, Omokhodion SI. Significance of a cardiac murmur as the sole clinical sign in the newborn. Clin Pediatr 2000; 39:511–520.

105 Phoon CKL. Where's the spleen. Looking for the spleen and assessing its function in the syndromes of isomerism. Cardiol Young 1997; 7:347–357.

106 Turner SW, Hunter S, Wyllie JP. The natural history of ventricular septal defects. Arch Dis Child 1999; 81: 413–416.

107 Neumayer U, Stone S, Somerville J. Small ventricular septal defects in adults. Eur Heart J 1998; 19:1573–1582.

108 Leung MP, Beerman LB, Siewers RD, et al. Longterm follow up after aortic valvuloplasty and defect closure in ventricular septal defects with aortic regurgitation. Am J Cardiol 1987; 60:890–894.

109 Kidd L, Driscoll D, Gersony W, et al. Second natural history study of congenital heart defects: results of treatment in patients with ventricular septal defects. Circulation 1993; 87 (suppl I): I38–I51.

110 Sutherland GS, Godman MJ, Smallhorn J F. Ventricular septal defects. Two dimentional echocardiographic and morphological correlations. Br Heart J 1982; 47:316–328.

111 Carotti A, Marino B, Bevilacqua M, et al. Primary repair of isolated ventricular septal defect in infancy guided by echocardiography. Am J Cardiol 1997; 79:1498–1501.

112 Riggs T, Sharp SE, Batton D, et al. Spontaneous closure of atrial septal defects in premature vs. full-term neonates. Pediatr Cardiol 2000; 21:129–134.

113 Helgason H, Jonsdottir G. Spontaneous closure of atrial septal defects. Pediatr Cardiol 1999; 20:195–199.

114 Carminati M, Giusti S, Hausdorf G, et al. A European multicentric experience using the CardioSeal and Starflex double umbrella devices to close interatrial communications holes within the oval fossa. Cardiol Young 2000; 10: 519–526.

115 Murphy JG, Gersh BJ, McGoon MD, et al. Longterm outcome after surgical repair of isolated atrial septal defect: follow-up at 27–32 years. N Engl J Med 1990; 323: 1643–1650.

116 Sullivan I. Patent arterial duct: when should it be closed? Arch Dis Child 1998; 78:285–287.

117 Rao PS. Transcatheter occlusion of patent ductus arteriosus: which method to use and which ductus to close. Am Heart J 1996; 132:905–909.
118 El-Najdawi EK, Driscoll DJ, Puga FJ, et al. Operation for partial atrioventricular septal defect: a forty-year review. J Thorac Cardiovasc Surg 2000; 119:880–889.
119 Najm HK, Coles JG, Endo M, et al. Complete atrioventricular septal defects: results of repair, risk factors, and freedom from reoperation. Circulation 1997; 96(suppl):II-311–315.
120 Clapp S, Perry BL, Farooki ZQ, et al. Down's syndrome, complete atrioventricular canal, and pulmonary vascular obstructive disease. J Thorac Cardiovasc Surg 1990; 100:115–121.
121 McElhinney DB, Halbach VV, Silverman NH, et al. Congenital cardiac anomalies with vein of Galen malformations in infants. Arch Dis Child 1998; 78:548–551.
122 Friedman DM, Verma R, Madrid M, et al. Recent improvement in outcome using transcatheter embolization techniques for neonatal aneurysmal malformations of the vein of Galen. Pediatrics 1993; 91:583–586.
123 Gielen H, Daniëls O, van Lier H. Natural history of congenital pulmonary valvar stenosis: an echo and Doppler cardiographic study. Cardiol Young 1999; 9:129–135.
124 Danford DA, Salaymeh KJ, Martin AB, et al. Pulmonary stenosis: defect-specific diagnostic accuracy of heart murmurs in children. J Pediatr 1999; 134:76–81.
125 Rowland DG, Hammill WW, Allen HD, Gutgesell HP. Natural course of isolated pulmonary valve stenosis in infants and children utilizing Doppler echocardiography. Am J Cardiol 1997; 79:344–349.
126 Kitchiner DJ, Jackson M, Malaiya N, et al. The incidence and prognosis of left ventricular outflow obstruction in Liverpool (1960–1991). Br Heart J 1994; 71:588–595.
127 Kitchiner D, Jackson M, Walsh K, et al. The long-term prognosis of 81 patients with supravalve aortic stenosis (1960–1992). Heart 1996; 76:395–402.
128 Justo RN, McCrindle BW, Benson LN, et al. Aortic valve regurgitation after surgical versus percutaneous balloon valvotomy for congenital aortic valve stenosis. Am J Cardiol 1996; 77:1332–1338.
129 Laudito A, Brook MM, Suleman S, et al. The Ross procedure in children and young adults: word of caution. J Thorac Cardiovasc Surg 2001; 122:147–153.
130 McElhinney DB, Petrossian E, Tworetzky W, et al. Issues and outcomes in the management of supravalve aortic stenosis. Ann Thorac Surg 2000; 69:562–567.
131 Basso C, Corrado D, Thiene G. Cardiovascular causes of sudden death in young individuals including athletes. Cardiovasc Rev 1999; 7:127–135.
132 Cohen M, Fuster V, Steele PM, et al. Coarctation of the aorta. Long-term follow-up and prediction of outcome after surgical correction. Circulation 1989; 80:840–845.
133 Linderkamp O, Klose HJ, Betke K, et al. Increased blood viscosity in patients with cyanotic congenital heart disease and iron deficiency. J Pediatr 1979; 95:567–568.
134 Van Arsdell GS, Maharaj GS, Tom J, et al. What is the optimal age for repair of tetralogy of Fallot? Circulation 2000; 102(suppl 3): III123–129.
135 Nollert G, Fischlein T, Bouterwek S, et al. Long-term survival in patients with repair of tetralogy of Fallot: 36-year follow-up of 490 survivors of the first year after surgical repair. J Am Coll Cardiol 1997; 30:1374–1383.
136 Silka MJ, Hardy BG, Menashe VD, et al. A population-based prospective evaluation of risk of sudden cardiac death after operation for common congenital heart defects. J Am Coll Cardiol 1998; 32: 245–251.
137 Gatzoulis MA, Balaji S, Webber SA, et al. Risk factors for arrhythmia and sudden cardiac death late after repair of tetralogy of Fallot: a multicentre study. Lancet 2000; 356: 975–981.
138 Tweddell JS, Litwin SB, Thomas JP, Mussatto K. Recent advances in the surgical management of the single ventricle patient. Pediatr Clin North Am 1999; 46: 465–480.
139 Freedom RM, Hamilton R, Yoo SJ, et al. The Fontan procedure: analysis of cohorts and late complications. Cardiol Young 2000; 10:307–325.
140 Saliba Z, Butera G, Bonnet D, et al. Quality of life and perceived health status in surviving adults with univentricular heart. Heart 2001; 86:69–73.
141 Groenink M, Rozendaal L, Naeff MS, et al. Marfan syndrome in children and adolescents: predictive and prognostic value of aortic root growth for screening for aortic complications. Heart 1998; 80:163–169.
142 Shores J, Berger KR, Murphy EA, Pyeritz RE. Progression of aortic dilatation and the benefit of long-term adrenergic blockade in Marfan's syndrome. N Engl J Med 1994; 330:1384–1385.
143 Treasure T. Cardiovascular surgery for Marfan syndrome. Heart 2000; 84:674–678.
144 Liberthson RR. Sudden death from cardiac causes in children and young adults. N Engl J Med 1996; 334: 1039–1044.
145 Mazgalev TN, Ho SY, Anderson RH. Anatomic-electrophysiological correlations concerning the pathways for atrioventricular conduction. Circulation 2001; 103: 2660–2667.
146 Wren C. Practical use of antiarrhythmic drugs. In: Wren C, Campbell RWF (eds) Paediatric cardiac arrhythmias. Oxford: Oxford University Press; 1996:279–289.
147 Baursfeld U, Gow RM, Hamilton RM, et al. Treatment of atrial ectopic tachycardia in infants <6 months old. Am Heart J 1995; 129:1145–1148.
148 Dorostkar PC, Silka MJ, Morady F, et al. Clinical course of persistent junctional reciprocating tachycardia. J Am Coll Cardiol 1999; 33: 366–375.
149 Perry JC. Ventricular tachycardia in neonates. PACE 1997; 20:2061–2064.
150 Muller G, Deal BJ, Benson DW. 'Vagal maneuvers' and adenosine for termination of atrioventricular reentrant tachycardia. Am J Cardiol 1994; 74:500–503.
151 Garson A, Kanter R J. Management of the child with Wolff–Parkinson–White syndrome and supraventricular tachycardia. J Cardiovasc Electrophysiol 1997; 8: 1320–1326.
152 Kugler JD, Danford DA, Houston K, et al. Radiofrequency catheter ablation for paroxysmal supraventricular tachycardia in children and adolescents without structural heart disease. Am J Cardiol 1997; 80: 1438–1443.
153 Prystowsky EN. Atrioventricular node re-entry: physiology and radiofrequency ablation. Pacing Clin Electrophysiol 1997; 20:552–571.
154 Garson A Jr, Dick M, Fournier A, et al. The long QT syndrome children. An international study of 287 patients. Circulation 1993; 87:1866–1872.
155 Schwartz PJ, Moss AJ, Vincent GM, et al. Diagnostic criteria for the long QT syndrome: an update. Circulation 1993; 88:782–784.
156 Geelen JLMC, Doevendans PA, Jongbloed RJ, et al. Molecular genetics of inherited long QT syndromes. Eur Heart J 1998; 19: 1427–1433.
157 Leenhardt A, Lucet V, Denjoy I, et al. Catecholaminergic polymorphic ventricular tachycardia in children. Circulation 1995; 91: 1512–1519.
158 Naccarelli GV, Antzelevitch C. The Brugada syndrome: clinical, genetic, cellular, and molecular abnormalities. Am J Med 2001; 110:573–581.
159 Ross BA. Congenital complete atrioventricular block. Pediatr Clin North Am 1990; 37:67–78.
160 Miller JM. Therapy of Wolff–Parkinson–White syndrome and concealed bypass tracts: Part II. J Cardiovasc Electrophysiol 1996; 7:178–187.
161 Batra AS, Lewis AB. Acute myocarditis. Curr Opin Pediatr 2001; 13: 234–239.
162 Oakley CM. Myocarditis, pericarditis and other pericardial diseases. Heart 2000; 84: 449–454.
163 Weinhouse E, Wanderman KL, Sofer S, et al. Viral myocarditis simulating dilated cardiomyopathy in early childhood: evaluation by serial echocardiography. Br Heart J 1986; 56:94–97.
164 Levi G, Scalvini S, Volterrani M, et al. Coxsackie virus heart disease: 15 years after. Eur Heart J 1988; 9:1303–1307.
165 Corey GR, Campbell PT, Van Trigt P, et al. Etiology of large pericardial effusions. Am J Med 1993; 95:209–213.
166 Soler-Soler J, Sagristà-Sauleda J, Permanyer-Miralda G. Management of pericardial effusion. Heart 2001; 86:235–240.
167 Olivier C. Rheumatic fever – is it still a problem? J Antimicrob Chemother 2000; 45:13–21.
168 Groves AM. Rheumatic fever and rheumatic heart disease: an overview. Trop Doct 1999; 29:129–132.
169 Narula J, Chandrasekhar Y, Rahimtoola S. Diagnosis of active rheumatic carditis: the echoes of change. Circulation 1999; 100: 1576–1581.
170 Saxena A. Diagnosis of rheumatic fever: current status of Jones Criteria and role of echocardiography. Indian J Pediatr 2000; 67:283–286.
171 Veasy LG. Rheumatic fever – T Duckett Jones and the rest of the story. Cardiol Young 1995; 5:293–301.
172 Tomkins DG, Boxerbaum B, Lichman J. Longterm prognosis of rheumatic fever patients receiving regular intramuscular benzathine penicillin. Circulation 1997; 45:543–551.
*173 Albert DA, Harel L, Karrison T. The treatment of rheumatic carditis: a review and meta-analysis. Medicine 1995; 74:1–12.

174 Thatai D, Turi Z G. Current guidelines for the treatment of patients with rheumatic fever. Drugs 1999; 57:545–555.

175 Dajani A, Taubert K, Ferrieri P, et al. Treatment of acute streptococcal pharyngitis and prevention of rheumatic fever: a statement for health professionals. Pediatrics 1995; 96: 758–764.

176 McLaren MJ, Hawkins DM, Koornhof HJ, et al. Epidemiology of rheumatic heart disease in black schoolchildren of Soweto, Johannesburg. BMJ 1975; 3(5981): 474–478.

177 Padmavati S. Rheumatic heart disease: prevalence and preventive measures in the Indian subcontinent. Heart 2001; 86:127.

178 Kaplan S. Chronic rheumatic heart disease. In: Moss AJ, Adams FH, Emmanouilides GC (eds) Heart disease in infants, children and adolescents. Baltimore: Williams & Wilkins; 1977:533–547.

179 Kitchiner D. Physical exertion in patients with congenital heart disease. Heart 1996; 76: 6–7.

180 Burns JC, Kushner HI, Bastian JF, et al. Kawasaki disease: a brief history. Pediatrics 2000; 106: e27.

181 Lloyd AJ, Walker C, Wilkinson M. Kawasaki disease: is it caused by an infectious agent? Br J Biomed Sci 2001; 58:122–128.

182 Nakamura Y, Yanagawa H, Ojima T, et al. Cardiac sequelae of Kawasaki disease among recurrent cases. Arch Dis Child 1998; 78: 163–165.

183 Council on Cardiovascular Disease in the Young, Committee on Rheumatic Fever, Endocarditis, and Kawasaki Disease, American Heart Association. Diagnostic guidelines for Kawasaki disease. Circulation 2001; 103: 335–336.

184 McMarrow Tuohy AM, Tani LY, Cetta F, et al. How many echocardiograms are necessary for follow-up evaluation of patients with Kawasaki disease? Am J Cardiol 2001; 88:328–330.

***185** Newburger JW, Takahashi M, Burns JC et al. The treatment of Kawasaki syndrome with intravenous gamma globulin. N Engl J Med 1986; 315:341–347.

***186** Newburger JW, Takahashi M, Beiser AS et al. Single infusion of intravenous gamma globulin compared to four daily doses in the treatment of acute Kawasaki syndrome. N Engl J Med 1991; 324: 1633–1639.

***187** Durongpisitkul K, Gururaj VJ, Park JM, Martin CF. The prevention of coronary artery aneurysm in Kawasaki disease: a meta-analysis on the efficacy of aspirin and immunoglobulin treatment. Pediatrics 1995; 96:1057–1061.

188 Dajani AS, Taubert KA, Takahashi M, et al. Guidelines for long-term management of patients with Kawasaki disease. Report From the Committee on Rheumatic Fever, Endocarditis, and Kawasaki Disease, Council on Cardiovascular Disease in the Young, American Heart Association. Circulation 1994; 89:916–922.

189 Behan WMH, Behan PO, Reid JM, et al. Family studies of congenital heart disease associated with Ro antibody. Br Heart J 1989; 62:320–324.

190 Komajda M. Genetics of dilated cardiomyopathy: a molecular maze? Heart 2000; 84:463–464.

191 Denfield SW, Gajarski RJ, Towbin JA. Cardiomyopathies. In: Garson Jr A, Bricker TJ, Fisher DJ, Neish SR (eds) The science and practice of pediatric cardiology, 2nd edn. Baltimore: Williams & Wilkins; 1998:1851–1884.

192 Burch M. Cardiomyopathy. In: Archer N, Burch M (eds). Paediatric cardiology: an introduction. London; Chapman & Hall; 1998:99–112.

193 Elliot P. Diagnosis and management of dilated cardiomyopathy. Heart 2000; 84: 106–112.

194 De Giovanni JV, Dindar A, Griffith MJ, et al. Recovery pattern of left ventricular dysfunction following radiofrequency ablation of incessant supraventricular tachycardia in infants and children. Heart 1998; 79:588–592.

195 Morrow WR. Cardiomyopathy and heart transplantation in children. Curr Opin Cardiol 2000; 15:216–223.

196 Walter JH. L-Carnitine. Arch Dis Child 1996; 74:475–478.

197 Burch M, Saddiqi AS, Celermajer DS, et al. Dilated cardiomyopathy in children: determinants of outcome. Br Heart J 1994; 72:246–250.

198 Spirito O, Seidman CE, McKenna WJ, Maron BJ. The management of hypertrophic cardiomyopathy. N Engl J Med 1997; 336:775–785.

199 Pinamonti B, Sinagra G, Camerini F. Clinical relevance of right ventricular dysplasia/cardiomyopathy. Heart 2000; 83: 9–11.

200 Becker AE. Primary heart tumors in the pediatr age group: a review of salient pathologic features relevant for clinicians. Pediatr Cardiol 2000; 21:317–323.

201 Shapiro LM. Cardiac tumours: diagnosis and management. Heart 2001; 85:218–222.

202 Kay JD, Smaiko AR, Daniels SR. Pediatric hypertension Am Heart J 2001; 142:422–432.

203 Report of the Second Task Force on Blood Pressure Control in Children. Pediatrics 1987; 79:1–25.

204 National High Blood Pressure Education Program (NHBPEP) Working Group on Hypertension Control in Children and Adolescents. Update on the 1987 Task Force Report in Children and Adolescents: a working group report from the National High Blood Pressure Education Program. Pediatrics 1996; 98:649–658.

205 Gibbs CR, Murray S, Beevers DG. The clinical value of ambulatory blood pressure monitoring. Heart 1998; 79:115–117.

206 Bartosh SM, Aronson AJ. Childhood hypertension. Pediatr Clin North Am 1999; 46:235–252.

207 Gibbs JSR, Higgenbottam TW. Recommendations on the management of pulmonary hypertension in clinical practice. Heart 2001; 86(suppl):i1–i13.

208 Barst RJ. Recent advances in the treatment of pediatric pulmonary artery hypertension. Pediatr Clin North Am 1999; 46:331–345.

209 Rubin LJ. Primary pulmonary hypertension. N Engl J Med 1997; 336:111–117.

210 Wilkins MR, Wharton J. Progress in, and future prospects for, the treatment of primary pulmonary hypertension. Heart 2001; 86: 603–604.

211 Klings ES, Farber HW. Current management of primary pulmonary hypertension. Drugs 2001; 61:1945–1956.

212 Skinner J, Alverson D, Hunter S (eds). Echocardiography for the neonatologist. London: Churchill Livingstone; 2000.

213 Snider AR, Serwer GA. Echocardiography in pediatric heart disease. Chicago: Year Book Medical; 1990.

20

Neurology

Edited by Colin Ferrie, Tim Martland, Richard Newton

THE NEUROLOGICAL CONSULTATION

THE SETTING

To be successful neurological consultations require time. The role of the pediatrician is to help understand the issue of causation, inform the parents of future outlook, deal with any attendant medical problems, give specific treatment where available, and arrange genetic counseling and supportive services. Special investigation is only part of this process: clinical skills are equally important. A child's appearance, pattern of movement, or mode of presentation all give important diagnostic clues and help shape the approach to investigation.

THE HISTORY

Histories are often complex; physical examination requires care; and there are often attendant psychological and educational issues which need definition and planned intervention. Consultations need space; gait assessment is an essential feature as well as observation of patterns of play. Correct choice of room and a correct scheduling for families therefore demands adequate attention.

First impressions are very important and it is helpful to families to be greeted in a friendly way and for those in the room to be introduced to them. Cunningham & Newton[1] showed that parents and children attending hospital still had difficulty in asking about things that worried them most, during consultations, despite a welcoming environment. These questions are often centered on fears and misunderstandings that would not necessarily be on the doctor's standard consultation agenda. An attractive, clear question sheet proved to be a simple but effective intervention. Parents felt empowered to take control. Its use often led to the adoption of a new consultation format that ensured that all parents' questions were addressed and limited time was used to its best advantage.

In history taking it is important to listen to what the child has to say. In their 1998 study Viswanathan et al[2] showed that children's descriptions of their headaches cannot be tidily 'pigeonholed' into traditionally held views on headache classification. It is important to use language appropriate for the particular age of the child and to acknowledge that some things are difficult to describe. It is therefore perhaps better to note an 'indescribable feeling in the head' than trying to persuade them to accede to a proffered descriptive checklist.

Common clinical scenarios demand individual consideration:

Paroxysmal disorders: including seizure disorders, headaches and paroxysmal movement disorders

In the histories related to paroxysmal disorders an accurate description of the episodes, prodromal features, auras, and situations or activities that trigger the bouts should be taken. The child's views and experiences ought to be sought as well as those of witnesses.

Gait disturbance

For gait disturbance a description of the pattern of early ambulation is necessary along with the evolution of the disorder. For subtle difficulties it is good to ask about when the motor system is put to its greatest test; how is the child able to ascend stairs? How does the child fare in school races? Are they picked for the cricket or rounders teams? Is the disorder intermittent? Is there a hint of fatiguability?

Developmental or speech delay

Where communication skills are concerned, if there is difficulty with expressive language it is useful to determine whether the child has a good understanding of imitative gesture. This will signify that some fundamental language concept is present. Listening to sentence construction will indicate if there is a syntax problem and insight into their sense of humour at a later stage will indicate whether there is a semantic/pragmatic language problem. Speech and language disorders are common in childhood, boys being affected twice as often as girls.[3,4] The history highlights whether the language problem is isolated or associated with global developmental delay. An assessment should be made of language opportunity for the child and whether there is any social disadvantage. Children brought up in a bilingual environment tend to develop speech later, but then catch up. Left handedness or ambidexterity is associated with speech disorder in half the children involved. Elective mutism, commoner in boys, can usually be recognized in the context of unresolved predicament. Children with elective mutism often talk freely in certain situations and continue to communicate with gesture.

For children with suspected global learning difficulties, the neurological consultation enables one to determine whether the problems are indeed global or confined to verbal skills, non-verbal skills and/or social issues. Children with learning difficulties present in relatively few, well circumscribed ways: hypotonia in the newborn period, recognized developmental delay later in infancy or in the early toddler age group, language delay, arrest of development, or difficulties at school (see below). In each of these groups the history should detail the pregnancy, including any drug ingestion or early threatened abortion. A history of fetal distress should lead to careful scrutiny of the obstetric notes, though it is now generally accepted that in order to attribute causation to birth asphyxia the presence of neonatal hypoxic–ischemic encephalopathy must be established and there must be an associated motor difficulty compatible with the type of injury sustained. (See cerebral palsy section.) A record of cord, or early, pH measurements, as well as neonatal behavior are important in this respect as not all early neonatal encephalopathy is due to hypoxic–ischemic insult.[5] Parents, in their own minds, often attribute their child's difficulties to the events of labor and it can be helpful for them to be taken through details of the birth.

A detailed family history is clearly of value especially if supplemented by perusal of the family photograph album. These, together with home video recordings, can give a surprisingly clear idea of the evolution of a disorder. Many motor disorders such as the spasticity in cerebral palsy or the extrapyramidal involvement in Rett's syndrome may evolve over a period of time, raising the possibility of a neurodegenerative disorder. Careful scrutiny of the history often reveals that whereas things have changed, skills may not actually have been lost.

All these issues will be dealt with in more detail under separate headings in this chapter, but it is important to say at this early stage that the consultation should deliver the doctor a clear idea of the pattern of developmental delay, conveniently considered under the headings which follow.

Abnormal behavior in the neonatal period

Dysmorphic features, disordered tone, feeding difficulties, irritability and seizures may all signify continuing neurological abnormality. Hypotonia in the limbs and axes raise the possibility of a neuromuscular disorder, the Prader–Willi syndrome and other causes of learning disability. Where hypotonia is confined to the axis, there is usually a central nervous system abnormality such as a neuronal migration disorder, or hypoxic–ischemic encephalopathy. In the latter cases there may be associated full fontanel (due to cerebral edema), irritability, feeding difficulties, and seizures.

The commonest cause of persisting hypotonia or feeding difficulty is the presence of one of the recognizable forms of learning difficulty, of which Down syndrome is the commonest. Of the metabolic disorders, it should be remembered that the cerebrohepatorenal syndrome of Zellweger (one of the peroxisomal disorders) can mimic Down syndrome. It is associated with profound hypotonia as well as a craniofacial dysmorphism, similar to trisomy 21. The use of one of the computer based databases of dysmorphology can be helpful when attempting to establish a dysmorphic diagnosis.

Arthrogryposis should make one think of a neuromuscular problem or a neuronal migration defect particularly if the hands and arms are held in a 'decorticate' posture. Half of the children with arthrogryposis who are ventilator dependent will have a developmental brain abnormality. The presence of scoliosis and pooling of secretions with aspiration makes a congenital myopathy, and particularly nemaline rod myopathy, likely.

Abnormal head size

This common cause of referrals to pediatricians is dealt with below under 'investigation'.

Syndromes of developmental arrest

A number of conditions lead to similar developmental profiles. For example, for a while children seem capable of learning; learning then slows, arrests, some skills may actually be lost, and then learning continues at a slower rate. The child with hydranencephaly (e.g. due to pyruvate dehydrogenase deficiency) may well return the mother's smile before this smile is lost. Deaf children may babble but then, lacking input, their language development will subsequently become deviant if the problem is not identified and treated.

Children with autism often make reasonable developmental progress in the first year or so, their problems only becoming evident when there is a greater demand on social contact and language function. Words originally attained may be lost before the depth of communication difficulty is revealed. A very similar profile is seen in the age related epileptic encephalopathies. West's syndrome often begins too early in infancy for much difference with other children to be noticed, but in the Lennox–Gastaut syndrome, which often presents in the third or fourth year, there is very often an arrest of developmental progress at the time of onset of the seizure disorder. In Rett's syndrome, although in retrospect movements may have had a 'jerky' quality throughout infancy, there is often reasonable early developmental attainment before the process slows and the extrapyramidal features and loss of useful hand function become evident.

GENERAL POINTS ON EXAMINATION

This will be dealt with in detail in Chapter 3. Additionally, points on clinical examination specifically relevant to sections in this chapter will be revisited. Here, an approach to a shortened neurological examination that can be used in everyday clinical practice will be outlined. Hopefully this will avoid the practice seen in some clinical records of simply noting, CNS ✓

In terms of general examination it is always good to look for features of dysmorphism, signs of a neurocutaneous syndrome or the visceromegaly, heart murmur or skeletal abnormality one might associate with a storage disorder. Examination of the eyes should include not only a search for papilledema (which is rare even in the presence of raised intracranial pressure in pediatric practice) but also a careful look at the retina to look for degenerative features or pigmentation that one might associate with a mitochondrial cytopathy, or peroxisomal disorder.

From the age of 5 onwards children will usually cooperate with a formal examination of cranial nerves, coordination and power where required. For the younger child eye movements can be tested through distraction through the various fields of movement. Close inspection of facial expression will reveal any facial weakness. If there is any doubt about hearing, it should be tested formally. Observation of speech and questions about the child's pattern of chewing and swallowing and the ability to handle liquids and solids avoid the need for tongue depressors and more intrusive aspects of physical examination. They will give a good indication of the function of muscles of mastication and the lower brainstem.

Observation of the pattern of movement is more useful than the traditional 'hands-on' approach. Cerebellar function can be tested by holding the arms outstretched and looking for 'drift'. Up to 6% of boys will show choreiform movement of the outstretched hands until the age of about 10. Carrying out the finger/nose test, assessing alternating movements and touching each finger in turn can then further test cerebellar function. (Musical instrument skills are a good reflection of coordination.)

The gait should be observed with particular features in mind. The first question always is whether this is a heel–toe gait, or a toe–heel gait. If there is any doubt the shoes can be inspected for uneven wear. A toe–heel gait may be due to pyramidal or extrapyramidal motor dysfunction, a foot drop due to a lateral popliteal nerve palsy or tight tendo-Achilles due to a neuromuscular problem. Corticospinal posturing in the upper limb leads to adduction, elbow and wrist flexion and pronation; in the lower limb, adduction, internal rotation and flexion at the hip, knee and plantar flexion at the ankle.

Fogg's test may reveal these patterns when subtle. Fogg's test involves walking on the heels, then walking on the outside of the feet and then walking on the inside of the feet. At each stage, children are observed for the degree of associated movement in the upper limb. An undue degree of associated movement is often related to poor sequencing and balance and coordination seen in children with a developmental dyspraxia (see below). Asymmetry over and above what one would see in the dominant hand, as opposed to the non-dominant hand, often reflects contralateral hemisphere dysfunction, which can reflect the presence of a dysgenesis, a space occupying lesion or the site of an epileptogenic focus.

Children with a cerebellar problem have a wide based gait for additional stability and this is often accompanied by a moderate amplitude truncal tremor, deviations off the path, overcorrection and then restitution. Extrapyramidal disorders will give a paucity of movement with a stiff-legged gait or too much movement, as in a dyskinesia.

A wide base, seen continuing for some months after children first begin to walk, may suggest a cerebellar problem, the general hypotonia of the recognizable forms of learning difficulty or a carbohydrate deficient glycoprotein syndrome.

If learning difficulties are present then think of Duchenne muscular dystrophy. The average age at which boys with this disorder are taken to doctors with developmental concerns is 2.5 years, whereas the average age of diagnosis is 5.5 years. A large contribution to this delay is a misunderstanding of Gowers' sign.[6] Most people remember the sign as the need to climb up the legs using the hands when rising from a supine to standing position. The most important component, however, is the need to turn prone and in so doing adopting a 'prayer position' before rising. This overcomes difficulties sustained in attaining a sitting position if the rectus abdominus is weak and furthermore allows the hips to be extended before rising relative to the position of full hip flexion found in the normal squatting position. Most children show a Gowers' or modified Gowers' maneuver before the age of 3 years. If it is seen after the age of 3 then it is highly likely that there is a neuromuscular problem, or a central nervous system disorder with hypotonia.

Neuromuscular problems leading to proximal weakness often lead to a waddling pattern. The weak gluteal muscles lead the body weight to be transferred outside the weight bearing leg; the resulting mechanical advantage avoids dropping of the pelvis away from the weight bearing side.

The presence of choreoathetosis naturally would lead to investigations for basal ganglia dysfunction, but the erratic movements of Angelman syndrome may certainly imitate this, particularly in infancy and it may also be an early feature of Friedreich's ataxia.

If one side of the body 'mirrors' movement seen on the other then agenesis of the corpus callosum should be considered.

Whenever the motor system is examined the examiner should have on their mind, is this normal or abnormal? If it is abnormal is it central nervous or peripheral nervous system, and if it is central nervous system is it corticospinal (voluntary movement), extrapyramidal (where patterns of movement are stored) or cerebellar (the 'air traffic controller')? This in turn will help guide investigation.

Sensory testing is only indicated when the history indicates it should be done (that is sensory symptoms or perhaps features of a peripheral neuropathy or spinal cord lesion). In this eventuality all modalities should be tested working from the point of perceived maximum sensory loss towards more normal areas.

THE INVESTIGATION OF NEUROLOGICAL DISORDERS

This section will give a guide to the general approach to special investigations in common clinical scenarios. Specific approaches are of course given in individual sections.

ABNORMAL BEHAVIOR IN THE NEONATAL PERIOD

The presence of limb and axial hypotonia or arthrogryposis should lead to measurement of serum creatine kinase, electromyography, needle muscle biopsy, and nerve conduction velocity measurement.

Electron microscopy of muscle with membrane protein histochemistry should be performed particularly when congenital myopathy is suspected. It must be remembered that the Prader–Willi syndrome may lead to persisting hypotonia and a karyotype should always be requested in this group with a particular search being made on chromosome 15q. The presence of dysmorphism should also lead to chromosome analysis.

If a neuronal migration problem is suspected magnetic resonance imaging offers exciting detail of underlying structural abnormalities that in turn will lead to growing understanding of the mechanisms and genetics involved. Our experience is that computed tomography carried out in district general hospitals in this respect often misses important detail either through poor quality of the scans or lack of neuroradiological opinion. Neuronal migration problems should be suspected when early ultrasound, either antenatally or postnatally, suggests underlying structural abnormality, or when there is a suggestive pattern of arthrogryposis or seizures.

When hypoxic–ischemic encephalopathy has been ruled out and after excluding more common derangements of glucose homeostasis, urea and electrolytes, calcium and magnesium, the persistence of encephalopathy should lead to a full metabolic workup, looking for the amino or organic acidopathies and urea cycle defects.

DEVELOPMENTAL DELAY

Investigation of children with mild to moderate learning difficulty alone is rarely rewarding. Very occasionally patients with amino or organic acid abnormalities will be detected, but in retrospect there are often clues to their presence in the past medical history. Some disorders, such as homocystinuria, may present with developmental delay before the onset of more classic features of the disease make the diagnosis obvious. Mucopolysaccharidosis type III (Sanfilippo's syndrome) is associated with only mild somatic abnormalities and the earliest clinical presentation is usually with developmental delay alone, particularly speech delay. Later the characteristic behavioral abnormality with progressive loss of skills makes the diagnosis easier. Urine screening for amino acids and organic acids as well as glycosaminoglycans is therefore justified in these children along with a urate and creatine kinase in boys. Detailed lysosomal enzyme studies are not indicated. Children with severe learning difficulties should have chromosome analysis and neuroimaging, preferably with magnetic resonance imaging looking for neuronal migration problems as well as the metabolic investigations detailed above. A search of the skin for depigmented patches and other signs of tuberous sclerosis is always indicated.

GAIT DISTURBANCE

A clinical suspicion of weakness should lead to the estimation of serum creatine kinase, needle muscle biopsy and, where indicated, electromyography and nerve conduction velocity measurement. Pyramidal gait disturbance should lead to neuroimaging, looking for abnormalities of white matter for underlying structural abnormality, blood pH and lactate looking for mitochondrial cytopathies, and arylsulphatase A to exclude metachromatic leukodystrophy. If clinical suspicion of a mitochondrial disorder persists despite a normal or near normal blood lactate, the concentration in the cerebrospinal fluid should be checked and a glucose load with serial estimation of lactates is indicated. Confirmed raised concentrations of lactate should be followed by formal measurement of respiratory chain enzyme activity in muscle and a screen for mitochondrial DNA mutations should also be performed on this tissue.

Extrapyramidal signs should lead to a search for a family history of Huntington's disease (spontaneous mutations are exceptionally rare), a carnitine profile and organic acid to exclude glutaric aciduria and copper and ceruloplasmin estimation for Wilson's disease. Mitochondrial cytopathies should be excluded (above) and neuroradiological investigation should search for caudate atrophy reflecting one of the named striatonigral degenerations. Nerve conduction studies, somatosensory evoked responses and echocardiography may reveal evidence of Friedreich's ataxia, for which a definitive DNA test is now available. Cerebellar signs should lead to a neuroradiological search for a structural abnormality of the cerebellum and the rare abetalipoproteinemia. When seen in the presence of an oculomotor dyspraxia, ataxia telangiectasia, a DNA repair disorder should be considered and investigated with an estimation of alpha-fetoprotein (raised in that condition), immunoglobulins (an immune paresis is common) and, if clinical suspicion is sustained, a gene test for AT mutant protein is available and has superseded chromosome fragility studies. Vitamin E deficiency, as a treatable cause should be excluded.

ABNORMAL LANGUAGE DEVELOPMENT

Investigation of this group of children is rarely rewarding. DNA analysis for fragile X syndrome is justified particularly when the child shows autistic features. Where the language disorder is recently acquired then the Landau–Kleffner syndrome should be suspected.

ABNORMAL HEAD SIZE

The commonest cause of either a small or large head is to have one or both parents with a similar head size. Familial large heads may actually accelerate in growth and cross centiles in the early months of life but growth usually parallels normal centiles after the age of 6 months or so. The serial plotting of the occipitofrontal circumference, beyond infancy if doubt exists, is clearly important for a judgment to be made. A large head requires no investigation where there are no neurological signs and at least one parent also has a large head. It must be remembered that children with familial macrocephaly have the appearance of communicating hydrocephalus on neuroimaging for the first year or so.[7] This observation has led, in the past, to some parents being given inappropriately gloomy information, where scans have been performed (inappropriately!) in this condition.

In the presence of neurological abnormality the large head may reflect hydrocephalus, storage disorder, Canavan's or Alexander's leukodystrophy, congenital tumors or neurofibromatosis.

In early infancy an ultrasound scan will rule out hydrocephalus and, in the absence of other signs, it may be worthwhile adopting a 'wait and see' policy and monitoring head growth. MRI may reveal a leukodystrophy, which in turn will lead to specific neurometabolic investigation. The phenotype in fragile X syndrome is broad. The investigation should be ordered particularly when there is a relatively large head in a child with below average height who has specific difficulties with language and communication. Macro-orchidism in this condition only occurs after puberty. Microcephaly can be the end result of many neurometabolic disorders and it is important to remember maternal phenylketonuria as a potential cause. A congenital infection screen and review of the obstetric notes is indicated.

A small head may reflect an underlying metabolic disorder, neurodegenerative condition, or congenital infection. The retina should be examined for signs of chorioretinitis or pigmentation to reflect a mitochondrial cytopathy or peroxisomal disorder and bone structure and viscera should be examined for signs of abnormal storage.

SYNDROMES OF DEVELOPMENTAL ARREST

Autism, Rett's syndrome, and the epileptic encephalopathies of childhood may all carry their own distinctive patterns on electroencephalography. When the clinical picture and electroencephalographic findings are typical of one of these syndromes no further metabolic investigation is warranted. Where neurodegeneration is suspected children need a full neurometabolic workup including urine for oligosaccharide and glycosaminoglycans excretion, amino and organic acid analyses, very long chain fatty acids and a white cell lysosomal enzyme screen. If these are normal, and degeneration persists, signs of abnormal storage should be sought on a tissue biopsy specimen. Skin, rectum, conjunctiva, and bone marrow have all been used successfully to demonstrate the pathological abnormality.

TROUBLE AT SCHOOL

It is rarely worthwhile carrying out any specific investigation in the 'clumsy child syndrome', as long as there is no suspicion of clinical deterioration. It is more appropriate to ask the remedial therapists and clinical psychology team for their appraisal of the child's educational strengths and weaknesses as a basis for further remediation. The clinician must be aware of other possibilities, however. The authors have known children with Duchenne muscular dystrophy and ataxia telangiectasia referred at the age of 5 with 'clumsiness' as the main feature.

GIVING THE NEWS OF DISABLITY

Much attention has been paid in recent years to how best to impart the news of disability to parents when this first becomes evident. Guidelines have been drawn up expanding on work originally carried out by Cunningham et al[8] and formulated in a British Paediatric Association guideline.[9] The key points are as follows:

1. Parents like to be given the news of disability by someone they are familiar with.
2. They like to be given the news together and if a single parent is involved then a partner, close friend or relative should be encouraged to attend also.
3. They like to be given the truth as early as it becomes known. If there is initial doubt, they respect doctors for sharing doubt, but nonetheless to be included in what is a truthful process.
4. The surroundings need to be quiet, private and adequate time given to the process.
5. If possible, the child should be present also as an indication of inclusion (or lack of rejection).
6. They value time spent alone after the event while they muster their thoughts and begin the adaptation process.
7. They value the opportunity of another meeting at an early stage to go over things they have not fully understood. In the interim it is good for them to have access to another health worker perhaps more familiar to them, such as a health visitor, who can also act as a useful resource for knowledge.
8. They should be directed to useful written material to complement what they have been told as well as to support groups.

Parents will often go through a bereavement-like process with its attendant initial shock and disbelief, anger and resolution. Part of the process ought to be to talk to them about how they are feeling about things, how the two of them may feel different at different times with due emphasis on the need for them to support each other during the process of readaptation. They ought to be taught to recognize how they are feeling about things as being quite separate from the problem the child has. It must be emphasized that they will not always feel this way and that the family will learn to adjust, accommodate to the child's disability and grow strong together once more.

For many conditions there is a clear-cut diagnosis and this model for giving the news becomes a relatively straightforward event. The original research was carried out around the paradigm of Down syndrome. With an evolving condition, such as cerebral palsy, the approach needs modification. Here the situation is that at a fairly early stage a doctor may share the concern raised by a parent that motor development is not proceeding satisfactorily. However, in one longitudinal study,[10] which followed 229 children with cerebral palsy, 118 were free from motor disability at the age of 7 (although up to 25% retained a learning disability). The best approach would seem to be to acknowledge what is seen and what the observation might represent, to lay out a plan of investigation and observation and explain that at that stage it is just too early to tell. Later if the fears come to fruition and a diagnosis of cerebral palsy is established then the process of news giving can be followed in the usual way, but with the family much better prepared.

A third scenario arises where risk factors for cerebral palsy are identified, for example, grade IV intraventricular hemorrhage will lead to 40% of the children affected having a motor deficit. Here again a process of openness and truth is required. The reason for continuing observation in clinics is explained and in the end often turns out to be a more solid foundation for a continuing professional relationship, rather than the alternative 'conspiracy of silence'.

Other conditions bring different challenges where the issue of giving the news is concerned. In a recent study of how 32 UK pediatric neurologists gave the news of epilepsy three approaches were identified (personal communication): i) a proactive approach where many issues surrounding the diagnosis were discussed, including the type of epilepsy, prognosis, stigma, treatment, investigation plan, how to contact and tell others, sources of information, help and reactions and feelings. This approach runs to the risk of overload but recognizes the right of parents to information; ii) a reactive approach which was more individually tailored but assumes that the doctors involved can intuitively judge parental reactions; and iii) a drip feed approach being rather more protective in preselecting topics to meet any given particular situation.

There was little consensus in relation to the use of analogy in explanation and there is often no good knowledge on the usefulness and awareness of available unevaluated literature. All acknowledged the value of a specialist epilepsy nurse, in this context, who is able to visit the family and answer any continuing questions. The doctors involved largely determined consultation content intuitively, rather than on a shared knowledge of the process involved. It is clear that, in this, and in other situations, a more detailed model of the disclosure process needs studying and epilepsy explanations that can be consumer tested need identifying.

Houston et al[11] studied the information needs and understanding of 5–10 year-old-children with epilepsy, asthma or diabetes. They were asked about their knowledge of their condition, psychological effects, medication, restrictions on lifestyle and where they obtained their information if they had unanswered questions. The children with epilepsy had far more unanswered questions and felt excluded from discussions with doctors. They felt reluctant to tell their friends about their diagnosis and often felt stigmatized. The study highlighted a contrast in the understanding of children with epilepsy compared to those with asthma and diabetes. The authors proposed that a simple biological model used to explain epilepsy could aid a child's understanding and reduce their reluctance to disclose the diagnosis.

The subject of written information is important. It is often written using analogy or paradigms that do not specifically relate to biology. It is almost always written without due attention to the reading age of the material involved, and the fact that children at different ages respond to different approaches in this respect. This is an area of research that needs pursuing and with the advent of information technology it should be possible for core information documents to be identified and developed to suit this information need on a national, if not international, basis.

DEVELOPMENT OF THE HUMAN BRAIN

An understanding of normal embryogenesis is the key to understanding the myriad of conditions that may present with motor and/or intellectual impairment. It also helps us to explain the biological processes leading to a particular child's disability even when the definitive cause (such as a particular gene) is unknown. There are a number of well-defined phases:

1. Isolation of the neural groove
2. Germinal zone cellular proliferation
3. Neuronal migration
4. Ventral and horizontal organization
5. Synaptogenesis
6. Myelination.

ISOLATION OF THE NEURAL GROOVE

The neural plate begins to form between 18 and 19 days postfertilization. It develops cranial to the primitive streak along the mid sagittal line. Two neural folds emerge which then fuse at the level of the first pair of somites at 20/21 days, giving the embryonic disc a tubular shape. The neural tube then closes from day 20 through to day 25, with the closing of the anterior neuropore. On day 27 the caudal neuropore closes at the level of somite 31, which will ultimately become the second sacral segment (Figs 20.1 and 20.2).

A stage of rapid differential growth then follows leading to the emergence of flexures. The cervical flexure is prominent at 35 days, by which time a midbrain and pontine flexure can also be seen. The appearance of flexures is associated with segmentation of the central nervous system. At 29 days three brain vesicles or neuromeres are evident for the first time, namely the prosencephalon, the mesencephalon and the rhombencephalon (Fig. 20.3).

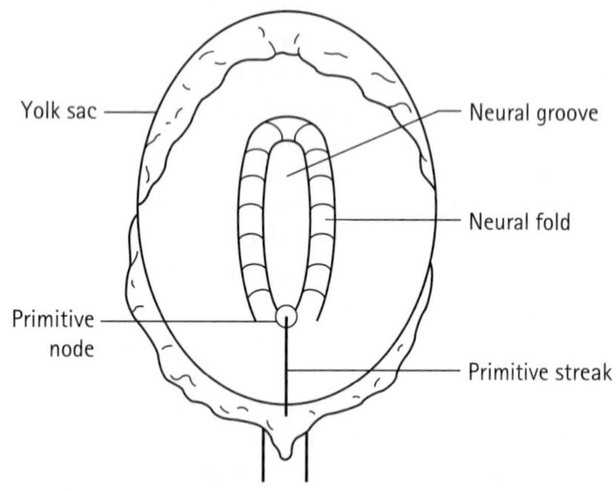

Fig. 20.1 The amnioembryonic vesicle.

At about 29 days postfertilization two telencephalic vesicles appear on the prosencephalon or forebrain. By the end of the embryonic period (8 weeks' gestation) these telencephalic vesicles can be recognized as developing the cerebral hemispheres. They remain smooth initially but after 12 weeks' gestation gyri emerge on the medial aspect.

The mesencephalon changes less than the prosencephalon (forebrain) and the rhombencephalon. It will later contribute the cerebral aqueduct, the cerebral peduncles, and the tegmentum and substantia nigra, which are derived from the basal plate.

Growth in the rhombencephalon shows increasing complexity. At 34 days the pontine flexure is a prominent feature made up by the rhombic lips at the cephalic end and by the developing floor of the fourth ventricle at its caudal end. The rhombic lips contribute significantly to the formation of the cerebellum. At the end of the first trimester the cerebellar hemispheres show a smooth outer surface and the vermis is developing as a medial raphe. Cerebellar foliation follows from 14 weeks' gestation.

GERMINAL ZONE CELLULAR PROLIFERATION OF NEURONES

Following the formation of the neural tube and the prosencephalon, proliferation of new neurones takes place. They originate from the

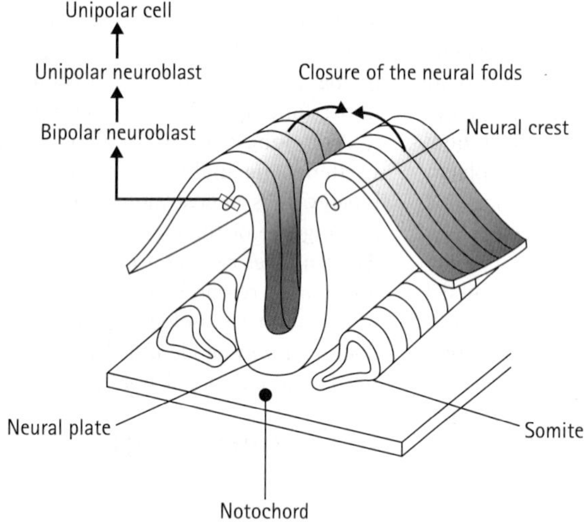

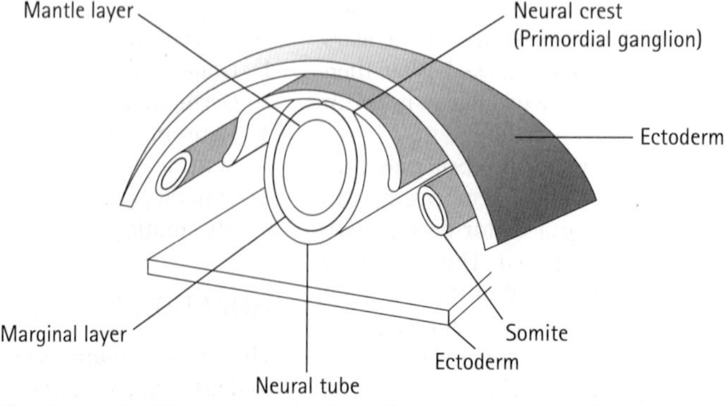

Fig. 20.2 Development of the neural tube from the neural plate 22 days onwards.

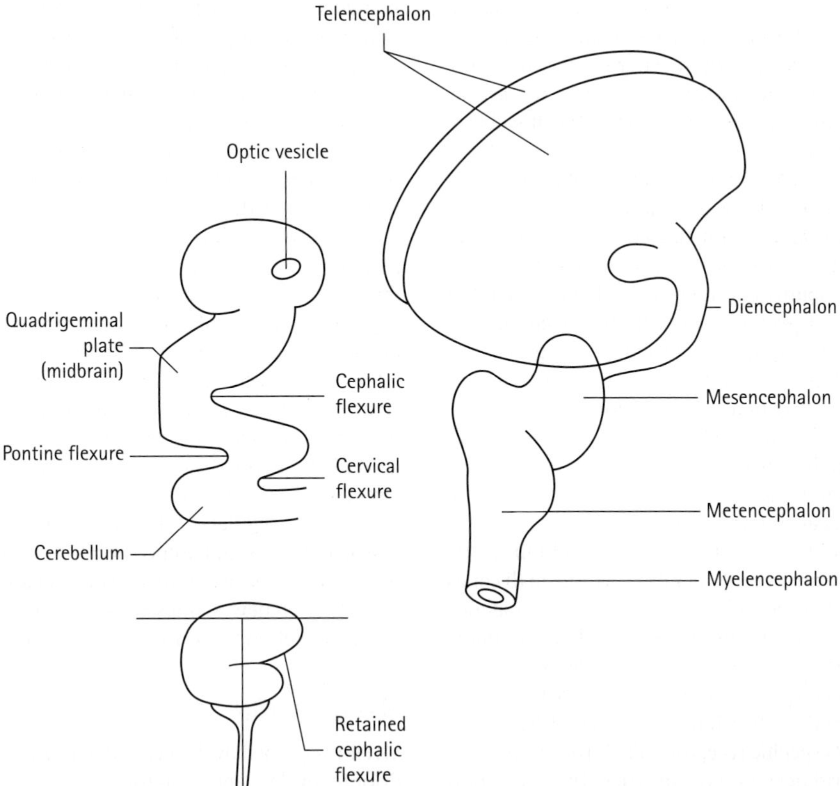

Fig. 20.3 Embryonic flexures of the brain 6 weeks onwards.

pseudostratified ventricular epithelium (PVE). They proliferate in cycles. One cell migrates, and then ceases to proliferate while another returns to the PVE to undergo a new cell cycle. The pace of neurone production is dependent on the exit rate of cells from the PVE. Most nerve cells are formed between the 8th and 18th week of gestation and there is probably no significant neurogenesis after birth, in the human. Neuronal and glial lineaging occurs at this stage, with the emergence of protomap layers so that specific neurones and glial cells are lined up for a particular destination. Cell precursors predestined for the prospective neocortical units appear. Vasoactive intestinal peptide (VIP) appears to be a crucial determinant of central nervous system growth. It is clear that maternal and/or placental environment and the influence of VIP and other circulatory factors are very important at this stage of neuronal proliferation.

The primitive neuroepithelial cells of the embryonic neural tube are the precursors of neurones and glia within the central nervous system. These cells undergo many proliferation cycles in the ventricular zone and then exit from the cell cycle, leave the ventricular zone and migrate centrifugally in a series of waves. They pass through the intermediate zone to form the layer structure of the cerebral cortex between the 8th and 14th week of post-fertilization development (Fig. 20.4).

The earliest migrating neuroblasts form a transient structure, the preplate between the pial surface and the intermediate zone which becomes spilt into deep and superficial layers by later migrating neuroblasts which form the cortical plate. Most preplate neurones are lost by programmed cell death (apoptosis). The deep component of the preplate, called the subplate, plays a role in axonal guidance by serving as an intermediate target for the axons of thalamic neurones during their ascent to synapse with cortical plate neurones. The superficial layer of the preplate forms the cells' sparse marginal zone where the Cajal-Retzius neurones lie (see below).

NEURONAL MIGRATION

The migration of neurones follows to form the primitive plexiform zone (the preplate). Later cells migrate into the preplate and split it into an outer marginal zone (or future layer I) and an inner subplate. Later formed cells migrate past those cells that arrived earlier. The cells in layer II are formed after those in layer VI. Migration mainly occurs between the 12th and 24th weeks of gestational age.

Migrating neurones advance along radial glial cells, which form columns between the PVE and the pia. These radial glial cells

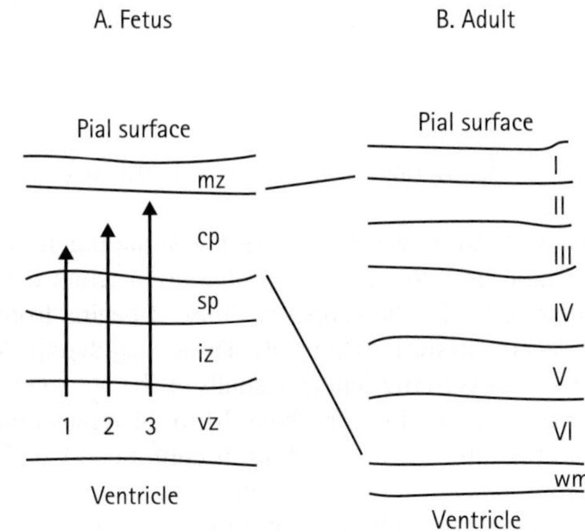

Fig. 20.4 Neuroblasts exit cell cycles and migrate centrifugally along radial glia. Those migrating later pass those migrated earlier to take up more superficial positions. mz, marginal zone; cp, cortical plate; sp, superficial plate; iz, intermediate zone; vz, ventricular zone; wm, white matter.

contain rich amounts of particulate glycogen, which acts as an energy source for migrating neurones which depend on anaerobic glycolysis. Having passed through these energy corridors the migrating neurones then transform from anaerobic to aerobic metabolism in the postmigratory settlement areas then being able to rely on a vascularized cortical plate.

Some of the neurones formed early in the marginal zone secrete a substance known as Reelin. These are the Cajal-Retzius cells. Correct cortical lamination depends on Reelin, which appears to instruct neurones on when to cease their migratory activity.

It was in 1892 that the Spanish anatomist Cajal discovered that neurones have differentiated growth cones at their leading end. These growth cones respond to signals, which can be categorized as: chemo-attractive, chemo-repellent, contact-attractive or contact-repellent. This allows a migrating neurone to respond to substances within its immediate environment. The chemical signals are diffusable molecules, which create gradients over a distance, whereas contact modulating molecules are cell membrane bound, or are to be found in the extracellular matrix.

Many ligand receptor families are known including the semaphorins, of which there are over 30 members. The growth cones probably carry receptors for several classes of these axon guidance molecules. One possible mechanism for guidance is that the inputs from the various molecules integrate and differentially alter cross-membrane calcium levels on one side of the tip or the other.

A number of nerve growth factors have been defined. These are diffusable peptides acting on specific receptors. Their role is probably best defined in the peripheral nervous system where their secretion defines a target for migrating neurones. In the central nervous system nonetheless they appear to act as yet another intrinsic determinant of cortical maturation.

Programmed cell death (apoptosis). Most of the subplate neurones are transient and are eliminated by programmed cell death.

Anomalies of programmed cell death have been implicated in the pathogenesis of certain types of neuronal migration disorder, particularly the heterotopias. It seems that 'pro-death' genes (e.g. Bax, Bad) and 'anti-death' genes (e.g. Dcl) are expressed in cells in varying combinations and amounts under exogenous influences such as survival factors, for instance neurotrophins and apoptosis inducing factors including proteolytic fragments of the laminin. It is the balance between pro- and anti-death genes that determines whether a cell will survive or die. A disruption in this process or an alteration in local environment could well lead to the persistence of cells normally destined to die yielding a neuronal heterotopia.

SYNAPTOGENESIS

In monkey experiments, distinct phases have been identified for this process.

In phase 1 (from 6 to 8 weeks' gestation) synaptogenesis commences at the same time as neuronal proliferation when it is limited to lower structures like the subplate. Phase 2 begins from 12 to 17 weeks, and occurs in the cortical plate. These early synapses are sparse and form contacts in the dendritic shafts of the neurones. Phase 3 is much more rapid and occurs from 20 to 24 weeks and persists up to 8 months after birth. It occurs in conjunction with arborization of axons and dendrites. Phase 4 then proceeds at a very high rate and lasts until puberty. Phase 5 continues up to the age of 70 years, during which time there is also considerable loss. Stage 3 is partially dependent on sensory input, phase 4 much more so.

Excitatory amino acids are the primary neurotransmitter in approximately 50% of mammalian synapses and have an important function in the development of the CNS. They participate in neuronal signal transduction and exert trophic influences on neuronal development. They affect differentiation, growth and survival as well as neuronal circuitry.

Huttenlocher & Dabholkar[12] indicate that although synapse formation begins in the human fetus before 27 weeks' gestation, maximum synaptic density is not seen until after 15 months of age. It occurs concurrently with dendritic and axonal growth and with myelination of the subcortical white matter. Net synapse elimination occurs late in childhood, often extending to mid-adolescence. Synaptogenesis and synapse elimination in humans occur at different times in different cortical regions. Synapse formation appears to be triggered by the contact of two neurites and may occur within minutes of such contact. Initially this appears to be random but then becomes refined selectively through retrograde and anterograde signaling. Neurotransmitter release before synapse formation appears to be an important signaling mechanism. Stabilization appears to be activity dependent. Synaptic contacts that are not included in neuronal circuits are then gradually eliminated. Early synaptogenesis is intrinsically regulated and not under environmental control. For example there is an absence of effects of age of first exposure to light on synaptogenesis in the visual cortex. This contrasts with the formation of new synapses later in life, which have been shown to occur in relation to learning and memory.

MYELINATION

Myelin is formed in the central nervous system by oligodendrocytes. Prior to myelin deposition these cells proliferate and there is a marked increase in vascularization. The myelin is laid down first on the fiber close to the nerve cell body, then deposition proceeds along the axon, the oligodendrocyte wrapping its lipoprotein plasma membranes repeatedly around the axon to produce the myelin sheath.

Cycles of myelination progress at different rates and may not be complete for some structures until several years after birth.

There are probably no myelinated fibers in the CNS before the end of the fifth fetal month. There is no myelination of the forebrain until the seventh fetal month. Most myelination in the telencephalon occurs in the third trimester and postnatally. The first neurones to acquire myelin sheaths are the olfactory, optic and acoustic cortical areas and the motor cortex (pyramidal cells). The last to be myelinated are the projection commissure and association neurones of the cerebral hemispheres (Table 20.1).

Myelination is a critical process for the development of the brain because it enhances the speed of neural communication. It occurs most rapidly during the first 2 years of life, but probably continues until early adulthood. Klingberg et al[14] studied the degree of myelination of young people's brains with magnetic resonance imaging and showed that the maturation of frontal white matter probably continues into the second decade of life.

THE DEVELOPMENT OF SPECIFIC BRAIN STRUCTURES

Forebrain (telencephalon): Initially the cerebral hemispheres are smooth but with growth the sulci and gyri develop. Many gyri are well defined between 26 and 28 weeks' gestation with secondary and tertiary gyri appearing between 40 and 44 weeks' gestation, initially in the frontotemporal areas and later in the orbital and occipital gyri.

The lateral (sylvian) and central (rolandic) fissures appear in month four. The callosal sulcus appears around week 14 together with the corpus callosum. At birth the sulci and gyri are similar in arrangement to that of the adult.

The pyramidal tract is the only tract to span the entire length of the central nervous system without synaptic relay. Association

Table 20.1 Age (in months) at which myelination becomes apparent.

MR Imaging sequence	T1	T2	STIR
Peripheral parts of midcerebellar peduncles	2–3[a]	4	2–3[a]
Folia cerebelli	7[b]	6–7	6–7
Capsula interior (posterior limb)	0	0	0
(anterior limb)	4–5	9–10	5
Corona radiata	0	0–1	0–1
Corpus callosum (splenium)	4–5	6	5–6
(genu)	5–7	7–9	5–9
Optic radiation	0–1	0–1	0–1
Lobar cerebral white matter (central portion)			
paracentral	2	5–7	5–6
occipital	4–6	10–12	7–9
frontal	5–6	11–14	8–12
Completed cerebral white matter arborization			
paracentral	3–6[a]	10–12	7–9[a]
occipital	7–9[a]	18–20	14–16[a]
frontal	8–10[a]	18–22	14–16[a]

From Hittmair et al 1994[13] T1/T2, T1 or T2 weighted images; STIR, Short-inversion-time-inversion recovery images.

fibers connect adjacent areas of the brain whilst comissures connect equivalent areas on opposite sides (Fig. 20.5).

Diencephalon: This is the posterior part of the forebrain. Three swellings emerge to form:

The thalamus – this is located in the superior portion of the diencephalon and is the site of the main relay nuclei receiving sensory input and projecting on to the cerebral cortex.

The epithalamus – this gives rise to the pineal body, the posterior commissure and the nucleus habenulae (an important relay to the thalamus).

The hypothalamus arises in the floor of the diencephalon and from here the mamillary bodies, the tuber cinereum and part of the hypophysial stalk of the pituitary arise.

The medial and lateral geniculate bodies appear later to act as important nuclei for auditory, visual and motor activity caudally to the thalami. The optic vesicles and second cranial nerve grow forward from the diencephalon.

Midbrain (mesencephalon): The lumen of the midbrain is eventually reduced to the narrow cerebral aqueduct of Sylvius connecting the third and fourth ventricles. The dorsal midbrain roof (the tectum) enlarges as two pairs of protuberances, the rostral superior colliculi and the inferior colliculi. The superior colliculi act as relays for visual reflexes and the inferior for auditory reflexes. Several nuclear groups develop from the basal plate in the midbrain floor (the tegmentum): the reticular formation, the red nucleus, the substantia nigra and the nuclei for the third and fourth cranial nerves. The cerebral peduncles develop as small thickenings from the ventral laminae. In the fourth month they increase rapidly in size as the corticopontine, corticobulbar and corticospinal tracts expand and pass through the midbrain area.

Hindbrain (metencephalon): This comprises the cerebellum, the pons and the fourth ventricle lying between the two.

Hindbrain (myelencephalon): This forms the medulla oblongata and is continuous caudally with the spinal cord.

GENES ASSOCIATED WITH BRAIN DEVELOPMENT

A number of genes involved in the formation of the brain have been retained phylogenetically and are to be found in insects and lower vertebrates. They are known as homeotic genes and control the orientation of the embryo, segmentation of the body and segment identity. Clustered homeobox containing genes (the HOX genes) are important. They differentiate the segments of the early embryonic brain. Those expressing many HOX proteins develop as posterior structures, those with lower levels form the anterior part of the axis. EMX and OTX are expressed in the fore- and midbrain region. Mutation of the EMX gene leads to one form of schizencephaly (see below).

Krox-20 is necessary for the development of the cranial nerves in the hindbrain. The Sonic Hedgehog genes determine timing and spacing, for example, which neurones should develop into motor neurones in the spinal cord. If this gene is knocked out all neurones become sensory neurones by default.

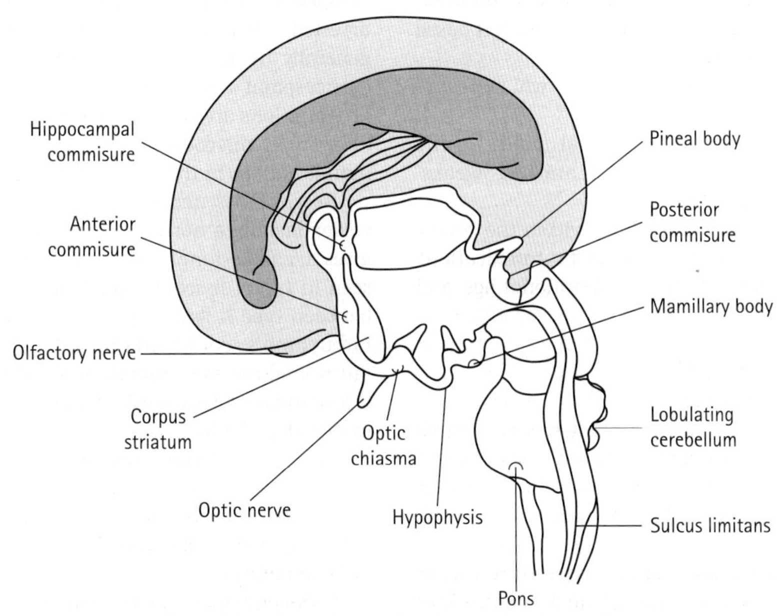

Fig. 20.5 Commissure development at 4 months.

Early specification of the forebrain depends on appropriate expression of a number of homeobox containing and winged helix-containing genes including members of the Otx, Emx, Dlx, BF, Mf, Lhx and Gsh family.

The genes Reelin and Mdab1 are important early in the process of neuronal migration as the preplate does not split into deep and superficial layers in mice mutant for these genes. The cortical plate subsequently in this case develops within an inverted structure. It would seem that Reelin and Mdab1 are needed by neuroblasts to pass one another as they migrate centrifugally.

With Cdk5 and p35 mutant genes later migrating, neuroblasts do not appear to be able to pass early migrating neurones with the resulting disruption to the cortical plate. The LIS1 and doublecortin gene are both implicated in the etiology of lissencephaly in humans. Subcortical band heterotopia arises from cortical plate cells that express the mutant doublecortin gene. The protein kinase C substrate MARCKS appears to be needed to define the pial basement membrane that serves as the external anchoring point for radial glial end feet. Without correct functioning of extracellular matrix models including laminin and collagens at pial limiting membranes, determined by MARCKS, layer II neurones are found heterotopically in the marginal zone or in the subarachnoid space.

The interaction between neuroblasts and radial glia is mediated by a number of molecules including astrotactin and neuroregulin (glial growth factor). erbB receptors are known to transduce signals from neuroregulin. Recent studies demonstrate a neural migration disorder in mice when a knockout mutation of erbB2 gene occurs.

It could well be that normally differentiated cortical cells undergo the genetic change which could trigger the development of a dysplastic lesion. The mutation could lead to cells within the lesion beginning to re-express genes normally only expressed by cells at an earlier stage of differentiation, or genes that characterize a different cell lineage. Somatic mutation is commonly observed in the germinal tumors of many types and has also been inferred from the finding of 'loss of heterozygosity' for polymorphic DNA markers in the lesions of tuberous sclerosis (see below).

UNDERSTANDING ABNORMALITIES OF CEREBRAL CORTEX DEVELOPMENT

Barkovich and colleagues[15] proposed a rational classification system for malformations of the cerebral cortex in 1996. It is based on three embryological stages of cortical formation:

1. Cellular proliferation within the germinal zone, which occurs between 7 and 16 weeks' gestational age.
2. Migration of neuroblast cells from the general matrix to the developing cortex occurring between 12 and 24 weeks' gestational age.
3. Vertical and horizontal organization of cells within the cortex with the establishment of axonal and dendritic ramifications which begins at approximately 22 weeks' gestational age and continues until after birth.

Problems of cellular proliferation

Entities in this category include the following.

Radial micro-brain (also known as lissencephaly type IV) results in a brain of dramatically reduced size but with a normal gyral configuration and cortical thickness. Children with this condition have severe microcephaly and often multiple non-central nervous system abnormalities.

Microcephalia vera (also called lissencephaly type III) results in severe depletion of neurones in cortical layers 2 and 3. A number of genetic and sporadic abnormalities may lead to this condition, which involves a reduced number of neurones in the germinal zones but no evidence of a migratory disorder. Children with this condition often have moderate developmental delay.

Tuberous sclerosis is a disorder of cellular proliferation that results in hamartomatous growths and, at times, neoplasms. The cortical tuber is composed of bizarre giant cells, heterotopic neurones and glial tissue. Defective stem cells in all germ cell layers may underlie the central nervous system manifestations of tuberous sclerosis. The stem cells differentiate into astrocytes and neurones, which lack the ability to integrate themselves further into the brain structure. Some remain in the germinal zone, resulting in the subependymal hamartomas, whereas others migrate along glial fibers in the white matter to the cortex, where they form the disorganized cellular clusters known as tubers.

van der Knaap & Valk[16] in their categorization included the other phakomatoses, such as neurofibromatosis, Sturge–Weber disease, von Hippel–Landau disease and ataxia telangiectasia, in the category of abnormalities of neuronal proliferation, differentiation and histogenesis.

Focal cortical dysplasia of Taylor, although showing a similar histology to tuberous sclerosis, presents as a solitary cerebral lesion with no associated cutaneous manifestations. Balloon cell focal cortical dysplasia of Taylor is associated with focal gray matter thickening contiguous with the linear hyperintense signal, extending through the subcortical white matter on T2 weighted images on MRI. The balloon cells have components of both neurones and astrocytes.

Hemimegalencephaly consists of unilateral cerebral enlargement with associated hamartomatous parenchymal overgrowth. Children present with developmental delay and intractable seizures. There may be an association with linear sebaceous nevus syndrome and unilateral hypomelanosis of Ito.

Focal transmantle dysplasia is characterized by abnormal cortical lamination, white matter astrogliosis and balloon cells. It arises from the maldifferentiation of germinal zone stem cells. Children present with a localization related epilepsy and the focal dysplasia is demonstrable with magnetic resonance imaging.

Disorders resulting from a disorder of migration include: classical (type I) lissencephaly, which is also called agyria-pachygyria. There is absent or marked underdevelopment of the gyri and sulci. The cortex comprises only four layers and migration appears to have been arrested sometime between 12 and 16 weeks' gestation. Children are generally hypotonic at birth with the subsequent development of corticospinal tract signs and seizures. The most striking clinical presentations are seen in children with the Miller–Dieker syndrome (17p13.3 microdeletion) and there are relatively milder manifestations in those with isolated lissencephaly.

In type II lissencephaly there is a severely disorganized thickened cortex lacking a normal layered pattern. MRI scanning sometimes gives a 'cobblestone' appearance though the cortex is thinner than seen in type I lissencephaly. There is considerable clinical overlap between type II lissencephaly, the Walker–Warberg syndrome and Fukuyama's congenital muscular dystrophy which all have autosomal recessive inheritance. MRI imaging reveals a thickened disorganized cortex with shallow sulci and hypomyelinated white matter (Fig. 20.6).

Gray matter heterotopia are foci of normal neurones situated in abnormal locations due to an arrest in the migration process. The heterotopia may be localized or diffuse. Subependymal and band heterotopia are examples of neuronal migration anomalies, which are often diffuse.

Subependymal heterotopia has small ovoid masses of gray matter located along the lateral ventricular walls. Young people with

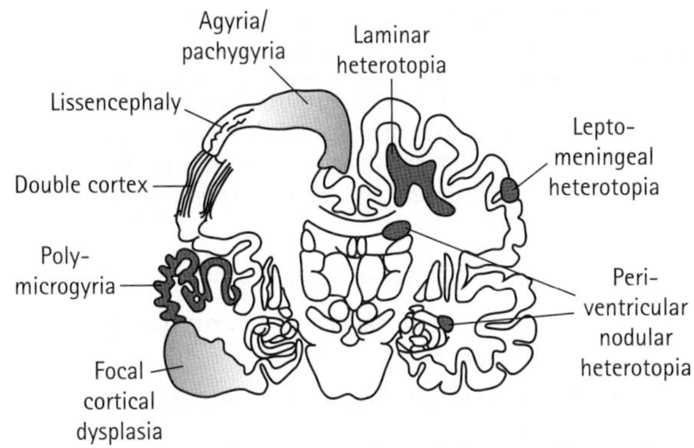

Fig. 20.6 Diagrammatic representation of the more frequent neuronal migration disorders.

this disorder often have normal development and a seizure onset after the first decade of life. The abnormality is readily identifiable with MRI. The nodules do not enhance with gadolinium, in direct contrast to the subependymal nodules seen in tuberous sclerosis.

Band heterotopia, also known as 'double cortex' heterotopia, consists of large circumferential layers of heterotopic neurones that have failed to reach the cortex. The resulting gray matter band is uniform, diffuse and bilateral. Those affected often have moderate to severe learning difficulties and intractable seizures. It must be noted that any of the above neuronal migration anomalies may be very localized as well as diffuse. They have all arisen between 12 and 16 weeks' gestational age. Subcortical heterotopia may exist as an irregular lobulated mass of gray matter situated in the subcortical white matter. These heterotopia tend to be large, extending between lobes. The overlying cortex is thin, with shallow sulci, and there are often associated dysplastic basal ganglia. Those affected often present with learning difficulties, a hemiplegia, or hemi-hypo-esthesia and localization related epilepsy.

Cortical organization follows 24 weeks of fetal development. Abnormalities occurring in this process include focal or diffuse polymicrogyria and schizencephaly. Polymicrogyria results when neurones reach the cortex but distribute in an abnormal fashion creating multiple small gyri with a deranged sixth layer cortex. It may be diffuse, symmetrical and bilateral, as in the bilateral opercular syndrome, or focal and unilateral. The clinical presentation depends on the location and extent of involvement but seizures are seen in up to 80% of those affected.

Schizencephaly consists of gray matter lined clefts that extend through the full thickness of the hemisphere from the cortex to the ependymal lining of the ventricles. The gray matter lining the clefts is often polymicrogyric. If the walls of the cleft are fused it is termed 'closed lip' schizencephaly. If not, it is known as 'open lip'. The clinical course often includes seizures, hemiparesis, with the closed lip varieties tending to be associated with the milder clinical course.

It must be noted that Van der Knaap & Valk[16] placed schizencephaly earlier in the migration sequence than polymicrogyria, proposing a time of onset of 2 months' gestational age for schizencephaly and 5 months for polymicrogyria. As already indicated mutations of the EMX2 gene have been found in humans with schizencephaly.

Agenesis of the corpus callosum involves failure of growth of the main forebrain commissure. It is associated with a number of chromosomal abnormalities, drug ingestion, including valproate, and a number of syndromes. Aicardi syndrome is an X-linked dominant condition in which agenesis of the corpus callosum is associated with infantile spasms, intellectual impairment, vertebral anomalies and retinal lacunae.

EARLIER DEVELOPMENTAL BRAIN ABNORMALITIES

Abnormalities of dorsal induction

The neural plate folds over on itself and fuses to form the neural tube, which will eventually give rise to the brain and spinal cord. This is known as dorsal induction and occurs between the third and fourth weeks of gestation. An insult in this period will lead to defective neural tube closure at either the rostral or caudal end and can result in encephalocele, a Chiari II malformation or myelomeningocele.

Encephaloceles consist of a bony skull defect through which dura and brain parenchyma protrude. They are identified according to the location of the bony defect, e.g. occipital. The brain parenchyma abnormality reflects many disorders of embryogenesis.

The Chiari II malformation is almost always associated with a spinal myelomeningocele and is a complex hindbrain deformity with caudal displacement of the medulla, pons and portions of the cerebellum through an enlarged foramen magnum. There is often associated callosal dysgenesis and cervicomedullary kinking, which may predispose to hydrocephalus.

Disorders of ventral induction

Once dorsal induction is complete, ventral induction follows. This involves the further growth and development of the three vesicles, the prosencephalon to form the forebrain, the mesencephalon to form the midbrain and the rhombencephalon to form the hindbrain, between the fifth and tenth weeks of gestational age. The detail of this has already been described. Congenital abnormalities arising from disorders of ventral induction include holoprosencephaly, the Dandy–Walker syndrome and callosal dysgenesis/agenesis.

Holoprosencephaly results when the prosencephalon fails to cleave laterally and transversely. The result is varying degrees of hemisphere and ventricular fusion bearing the names, alobar, semi-lobar or lobar holoprosencephaly. In alobar holoprosencephaly there is a complete lack of cleavage leading to a horseshoe-shaped monoventricle and absence of the corpus callosum. In semi-lobar holoprosencephaly there are rudimentary temporal occipital lobes with some differentiation of the ventricular system. In lobar holoprosencephaly there may be very mild appearances on MRI including hypoplasia of the frontal horns or underdevelopment of the anterior aspect of the falx.

The Dandy–Walker complex is a spectrum of hindbrain abnormalities incorporating varying degrees of hypoplasia of the cerebellar vermis and/or enlargement of cisterna magna. There is often associated hydrocephalus.

Callosal development occurs between 8 and 20 weeks of fetal life and proceeds in an anterior to posterior direction. Abnormalities result in complete absence of the corpus callosum or simply underdevelopment.

FUTURE CLASSIFICATION SYSTEM

Traditionally, morphological classification schemes have focused on anatomical or histological abnormalities identified at postmortem, complemented over the last decade or so with the findings of more refined imaging systems, especially magnetic resonance imaging. The timing of the interruption of the normal developmental process has then been estimated and the disorder classified (as delineated above) according to whether this was a problem with neurulation, cell migration, axonal projection, synaptogenesis or myelination. As our knowledge of gene receptors and chemotactic agents grows, this system requires refining. Recently, a new system for classification of the malformations of the nervous system has been proposed by Sarnat & Flores-Sarnat.[17] They make the point that, whereas traditionally, a disorder such as holoprosencephaly was subdivided into alobar, semi-lobar and lobar forms (see above), this classification does not accommodate the recent identification of four distinct human genes responsible for various cases of holoprosencephaly. Some of these genes have a ventralizing effect in the vertical gradient (for example, the Sonic Hedgehog gene, SHH at 7q36) whereas others have a dorsalizing influence (for example, Z1C2 at 13q32). At least seven other defective chromosomal loci have been associated with holoprosencephaly. Thus, holoprosencephaly is a common end stage of several different disturbances in cerebral development. Severity does not always correlate well with the associated mid-facial hypoplasia, which may range from mild hypotelorism to extreme forms of cyclopia, or the correlation with diabetes insipidus, in about one-third of affected infants. These correlations most likely relate to the rostrocaudal gradient of the genetic expression, bearing in mind that most rostral neural crest tissue arises in the midbrain and forms not only neural structures but also the membranous bones of the face, orbits and much of the eyeball except the retina, lens and cornea. It must be acknowledged that a scheme purely based on genetic analysis would be very difficult to use for radiologists, pathologists and clinicians. Furthermore, disruption in one gene, particularly one involved in a cascade, may lead to disruption of further genes lying later on in the sequence. For example, defective DAB1 causes under-expression of the downstream genes LIS1, Reelin and EMX2, all of which are important for various stages of neuroblast migration. It must be remembered also that non-genetic malformations secondary to acquired lesions in fetal life (for example infarction to interrupt radial glial fibers and their guidance of migrating neurones) would not be accommodated within a genetic scheme.

Sarnat & Flores-Sarnat, in their paper, took these principles and applied them to known patterns of malformation. It must be noted that a single condition may appear in at least one position in the table, implying that a particular abnormality is a common end point for a number of different mechanisms. There is no doubt that this proposed classification is likely to change in time with the advent of new knowledge (Table 20.2). It nonetheless does offer clinicians, radiologists and pathologists alike an understanding of some of the complex biological processes involved. It also provides the opportunity to give affected families important understanding and appropriate genetic counseling.

Table 20.2 Twelve principles cited by Sarnat & Sarnat[17] involved in genetic programming of the neural tube

Principle 1:	Development genes are re-used repeatedly. For example, an organizer gene establishing axis of growth may appear later in development as a regulator gene for differentiation and maintenance of specific cellular types.
Principle 2:	Domains of organizer genes change in successive stages.
Principle 3:	Relative gene domains may differ in various neuromeres.
Principle 4:	Some genes activate, regulate, activate, regulate or suppress the expression of others.
Principle 5:	Defective homeoboxes usually have reduced domains or result in deletions of entire neuromeres.
Principle 6:	Some genes may compensate for the loss of others if their domains overlap: redundancy and synergy.
Principle 7:	An organizer gene may be upregulated to be expressed in ectopic domains. For example, epithelial growth regulator-2 may be ectopically expressed with the loss of unique identity of those rhabdomeres in which specific cranial nerve nuclei and other structures are generated.
Principle 8:	Developmental genes regulate cell proliferation to conserve constant ratios of synaptically related neurones. For example the regulation of the ratio of Purkinje cells to granule cells is regulated through Sonic Hedgehog (SHH) and the granule cell receptor product of the gene Patched (PTC) and a related additional receptor gene Smoothened. Hemizygous mutations of the PTC gene in mice result in meduloblastoma. Cellular proliferation may be regulated by mitogenic stimulation or by the rate of apoptosis.
Principle 9:	Overexpression of genes programming the ventro-dorsal or dorsoventral gradients, manifest as hypoplasia or duplication of paramedian structures of the neuroaxis.
Principle 10:	Underexpression of genes programming the ventro-dorsal or dorsoventral gradients manifests as aplasia, hypoplasia, or midline fusion of paramedian structures of the neuroaxis.
Principle 11:	Minor genetic mutations may change cell lineage within or between traditional embryonic germ layers.
Principle 12:	Organizer and regulator genes are conserved in a phylogenetic evolution but may form several distinct varieties with related but distinctive functions in more advanced species.

PRENATAL PRESENTATION OF DEVELOPMENTAL BRAIN ABNORMALITIES

As mentioned already, many of the described abnormalities result in motor and/or intellectual impairment and/or epilepsy. Their postnatal presentations will be dealt with in the relevant sections of this chapter. The general pediatrician, or pediatric neurologist, may well be called upon, however, to advise colleagues in radiology and families, at least preliminarily, on brain abnormalities detected antenatally. This is usually following a routine or follow-up ultrasound scan. The more common disorders will be dealt with in this section.

Agenesis of the corpus callosum

Up to 0.7% of the general population may have complete or partial agenesis of the corpus callosum and 85% of these individuals are asymptomatic. The problem may, however, be associated with seizures or learning difficulties. The agenesis here is a marker of other central nervous system abnormality. Many cases are sporadic, but autosomal recessive or X-linked varieties are also described and there is a 1 in 10 risk of an associated chromosomal abnormality, a trisomy being the most common.

Three per cent of all fetuses with ventriculomegaly and 10% of all fetuses with mild ventriculomegaly also have agenesis of the corpus callosum. Those features most commonly associated with a poor prognosis include upward displacement of the third ventricle, widened interhemispheric and atrial diameters, absence of the cavum septum pellucidum, the radial array of the medial gyri and dilated occipital horns.

Approximately 80% of children with partial or complete agenesis of the corpus callosum have associated central nervous system anomalies including ventriculomegaly, porencephaly, microcephaly, encephalocele, holoprosencephaly, lissencephaly, Dandy–Walker malformation and spina bifida. Non-CNS abnormality is also common. Eighty sporadic genetic and chromosomal syndromes have been described with agenesis of the corpus callosum.

Fetal ventriculomegaly

Isolated ventriculomegaly has a prevalence of 1 in 1000 births in the United States. Thirty per cent of fetuses with ventriculomegaly have associated neural tube defects so careful evaluation of the spine should be performed.

Hudgins et al[18] reported that approximately 86% of ventriculomegaly is stable throughout the gestation, 9% progressive and approximately 4–5% resolve. Ventriculomegaly is defined as atrial diameters greater than 10 mm, or above four standard deviations. Measurements are taken at the level of the choroid plexus from the inner border of the medial wall to the inner border of the lateral wall.

Mild idiopathic lateral ventricular dilation defined as atrial dimensions of 10–15 mm encompass approximately 20% of the fetuses with ventriculomegaly and resolution may be seen with ventricular diameters as large as 12 mm. Mild isolated ventriculomegaly during the second trimester has been estimated to occur in 1 in 675 pregnancies. Follow-up shows 80–90% of the fetuses with isolated mild ventriculomegaly develop normally[19,20] whilst 50% of fetuses with mild ventriculomegaly and associated congenital defects are developmentally impaired and there is 36% of developmental delay at 2 years of age in children with mild fetal ventriculomegaly. Fetal hydrocephalus with marked ventriculomegaly is associated with a 55–75% mortality (including elective abortions, intrapartum and postnatal deaths). The prognosis is better where there is no associated abnormality but still 40% survive with severe disability.[21,22] Intrauterine shunting has been shown not to improve outcome.[23] Where the ventriculomegaly is due to hydrocephalus infants do best when the shunt is placed postnatally.

Dandy–Walker malformation

This incorporates cystic dilation of the fourth ventricle, an enlarged posterior fossa with upward displacement of the tentorium and cerebellar vermian hypoplasia. A definitive diagnosis cannot be made until after 18 weeks' gestation as normal cerebellar hemisphere fusion is not complete until 17 weeks' gestation. There is an association between Dandy–Walker malformations and chromosomal abnormality in up to 45%. It must be borne in mind that an enlarged cisterna magna when noted in association with a vermian defect or other cerebellar anomaly may be a benign condition. The outcome for Dandy–Walker malformations and its variants ranges from normal to severe disability. All the clinician can offer is detailed screening for associated abnormality and the assessment of the presence of any chromosomal abnormality, along with the presentation of this information.

Cerebellar hypoplasia

Spinal dysraphism may be associated with cerebellar hypoplasia. Other forms are genetically determined, the most prominent of which is probably Joubert's syndrome, whose postnatal clinical features include episodes of overbreathing, ataxia, abnormal eye movements and severe learning difficulties. Cerebellar hypoplasia may be associated with abnormality of gait, eye movement, epilepsy and learning difficulties, but is compatible with normal neurodevelopmental outcome.

Cranial cystic lesions: developmental or destructive in origin

Midline lesions may include holoprosencephaly, a Dandy–Walker malformation or cerebral hypoplasia. An arachnoid cyst may also be considered. An arachnoid cyst is often associated with underdevelopment of adjacent brain parenchyma. If a cyst is within the third ventricular region an aneurysm of the great vein of Galen should be considered.

If the cyst is asymmetrical or lateralized this is most often associated with destructive causes, which in turn may result from systemic disease of the fetus, mother or placenta. Prognosis will depend on the site and extent of the lesion.

DEVELOPMENT OF THE SPINAL CORD

The spinal cord extends into the tail of the embryo until day 44 to 51. Once the philum terminale and conus medullaris have formed the conus assumes a higher and higher position within the vertebral canal. This is thought to be due to differential growth of the vertebrae, which are growing more rapidly than the spinal cord. By week 31 the spinal cord has reached its adult level of L1.

As the neural folds first fuse to form a tube the walls are composed of a single layer of columnar epithelium. These cells proliferate and the neural tube walls become thickened. The central canal is initially relatively large but as the volume of gray and white matter increases they become smaller. The epithelial layer around the central canal is known as the ventricular zone. A cycle of growth is followed. During week 4 the cells successively retract to the lumen margin of the neural tube and divide. The daughter cell nuclei then migrate back into the layer and reconnect to the outer margin of the neural tube. This process is repeated so that cells eventually give rise to all the neural and macroglial cells in the central nervous system.

Once the neural tube has closed the ventricular layer gives rise to neuroblasts and glioblasts. Radial glial cells are present from the earliest stages and form the glia limitans, along with guiding neurones. Neuroepithelial cells produce ependymal cells, which will intimately line the ventricular system of the brain, choroid plexuses and the central canal of the spinal cord.

At 33–43 days a second layer, the marginal zone (subpial or molecular layer) appears outside the ventricular zone. This eventually forms the white matter.

The neuroepithelial cells proliferate and the lateral walls of the spinal cord thicken but the roof and floor plates remain thin. A shallow grove (sulcus limitans) appears between the dorsum and ventral parts of the spinal cord with the dorsal cord becoming the alar plate (lamina), the ventral part the basal plate (lamina). The alar plate forms the dorsal gray columns, the basal plates the ventral and lateral gray columns. Axons from unipolar neurones in the spinal ganglia enter the spinal cord and form the dorsal root ganglia, as axons from the ventral horns grow out of the spinal cord and form the ventral roots of the spinal cord.

From the beginning of week 12 ascending, descending and propriospinal fibers invade the marginal zone.

The third layer of the neural tube, the intermediate layer (middle or mantle layer) is present by 38–40 days and is located between the ventricular and marginal zones. This layer forms from neuroblasts, which have moved outwards from the ventricular zone. It is destined to form the gray matter.

Three periods of synaptogenesis have been described. These include the spinal reflex activities at 8 weeks when the fibrous connections to the spinal reflex arch are complete, the onset of local activities with a rapid increase in axodendritic synapses (9.5 weeks) and multiple responses at 13–15 weeks with a rapid increase in axosomatic synapses. The first observable movements are seen at 7.5 weeks.

NEURAL TUBE DEFECTS

The term includes anencephaly, encephaloceles, cranial meningoceles and the various forms of spinal bifida.

Primary non-closure of the neural tube is the most likely mechanism in the formation of neural tube defects. The process should be complete by 23–26 days. van Allen et al[24] suggested five separate sites of closure along the length of the neural tube. At the lower sacral end a process of neurulation is followed. There is a condensation of mesenchymal cells arriving from the primitive streak followed by canalization.

Mesodermal defects

There may be bony defects ranging from failure of fusion of the complete spine (total rachischisis) to simple deficiencies of the lower lumbar spinous processes as part of a spina bifida occulta. Hemivertebrae may give a scoliosis and the associated ribs may be absent or fused. Bony spurs occur in diastematomyelia. There may be absence of the sacrum or sacralization of the lower spine. Klippel–Feil anomaly involves fusion of cervical vertebrae, with severe disruption of the cervical spine. This causes marked retroflexion of the head in iniencephalus where there is also complete lack of fusion of the neural tube.

Other mesodermal defects such as angiomas, lipomas, dermoids, renal abnormalities with pelvic kidney or horseshoe kidney may be added to the bony spectrum.

Ectodermal defects

A defect in the neuroectoderm is known as myelodysplasia. This may manifest as disruption of the histological architecture of the spinal cord (multiple anterior horns, several central canals, abnormal neurones), syringomyelia, failure of fusion of the cord so that there is a flat neural plaque rather than a fused tube (myelocele), double neural tube (diplomyelia), tethering of the cord or herniation through the bony defect as a meningocele or meningomyelocele.

Other ectodermal defects include dimples, sinuses, skin defects, hairy patches, tails and cutaneous capillary hemangiomas that can occur in any combination.

INCIDENCE

Cuckle & Wald[25] showed that the birth prevalence of anencephaly and spinal bifida declined by 80% from 3.15 to 0.6 per 1000 births between 1964 to 1972 and 1985. Prenatal diagnosis followed by termination (achieved by measurement of the serum alpha-fetoprotein and by ultrasound) accounted for 31% of the decline. The increased risk in monozygotic twin pairs and in the siblings and half-siblings of affected children indicate a genetic component to the risk. The 1983 UK Medical Research Council trial looking at folic acid, mineral and vitamin supplementation indicated that folic acid had a protective effect of 72% with a recommended daily dose of 5 mg. The first genetic risk factor for neural tube defects identified at a molecular level is C677T (alanine to valine), polymorphism in the gene encoding for the folate dependent enzyme 5,10-methylene tetrahydrofolate reductase (MTHFR). Following the work of the MRC Vitamin Study Group[26] it is now recommended that folic acid, 0.4 mg, should be given to all women planning a pregnancy.

SPINA BIFIDA OCCULTA

Spina bifida occulta may present in several ways.

An incidental radiological finding of a narrow split in the fifth lumbar or first sacral spinous process is of no clinical significance. It is very common in young children and the incidence lessens with age.

A cutaneous lesion in the form of a small nevus, hemangioma, tuft of hair, sacral pit or soft lipomatous swelling should be taken as a warning signal that there may be an underlying abnormality. This may consist of a bony abnormality with bifid spinous processes but can also signify an underlying abnormality of the spinal cord with an associated myelodysplasia, lipoma, diastematomyelia or neuroenteric cyst. These cutaneous lesions should be taken as an indication for imaging of the whole neuraxis, using ultrasonography in babies or magnetic resonance imaging of the spine in older children, even when there is no neurological deficit.

Myelodysplasia

This term is used to indicate that there is an abnormality in the development of the spinal cord. There may be several central canals, several anterior horns or disorganization of the 'muscle nuclei' so that specific muscles do not form properly. The characteristic clinical findings are often referred to as myelodysplasia. There is usually a cavovarus deformity of the foot, which may be small so that shoe sizes are different. The leg on the affected side is shorter and appears to be the leg of a younger child. It is cold and often shows erythrocyanosis. It may be difficult to demonstrate definite weakness.

Tethering

Tethering of the cord refers to persistent caudal attachment through the filum terminale. It may lead to damage from traction, associated with repeated movement of the spine. The child may present with weakness in one leg or with bladder problems and progressive neurological deterioration is a definite indication for surgery. Whether tethering without neurological deterioration in the legs should be operated upon remains an unanswered question. If operation is not undertaken then careful neurological follow-up is mandatory, especially at peak growth periods. With MRI scanning, it is now possible to diagnose the condition more easily and criteria for operation should become clearer. Serial somatosensory potentials may also assist in diagnosis of progression.

Diastematomyelia

A different cause of tethering is a bony or fibrocartilagenous spur, which arises from a vertebral body and passes between the halves of a bifid cord – diastematomyelia. In some cases this fixes the cord and results in increasing traction with growth. In other cases the cord divides well above the spur and passes around the diastematomyelia in two separate dural canals, i.e. a diplomyelia.

Damage from tethering or compression may cause spastic paraplegia. More frequently, however, the child presents with distal weakness of the foot, with clawing of the toes and equinovarus posture and weakness of the peronei. Dribbling incontinence of urine may be an early feature and there may be sensory loss in the sacral territory, loss of ankle jerk and anal reflexes and trophic changes in the feet. Neurological deterioration in the presence of bony spur is an indication for removal, but removal of any bony spur demonstrated to put the cord at risk during growth, should be considered before the development of neurological signs.

Intraspinal lipoma

A cutaneous lipoma or lipomeningocele may penetrate in dumb-bell fashion into the spinal canal. It may cause increase in pressure within the canal. Treatment of a lipoma can be difficult as the cord itself as well as nerve roots may be enmeshed in fatty tissue.

Infection

Infection may be the presenting feature of dermal sinuses. Blind pits over the coccygeal region are rarely associated with communication to the theca but focal infection with abscess formation may be a nuisance. Pits over the sacrum itself, especially at the site of the caudal neuropore, are much more of a concern, as there may be a direct communication with the theca and therefore a risk of recurrent meningitis. These should be electively excised in the neonatal period.

SPINA BIFIDA CYSTICA

Meningocele

In this condition there is a defect in the spinous processes (spina bifida), together with herniation of the meninges through the defect to form a cystic mass on the back (Fig. 20.7).

There may be cover by thick skin with little risk of rupture or infection or by a thin transparent membrane; there may be skin at the sides and a thin blue membrane over the top. There is no myelodysplasia or cord within the sac in the pure cases and the child is neurologically completely normal. Hydrocephalus is usually absent and simple repair of the defect can be carried out as a cold elective procedure. The result should be a normal child. Ultrasound of the head should be performed to be sure that there is no associated hydrocephalus and ultrasound of the abdomen to be sure there is no associated renal abnormality.

Myelomeningocele

Spinal lesion

The spinal cord is an open flat plate on the surface of the bulging meninges. It is not known whether the developmental abnormality itself, intrauterine damage, secondary ischemia, trauma to neural tissue during delivery or postnatal infection is the principal cause of the neurological deficit. Exposure of neural tissue, in normal fetal lambs, to amniotic fluid results in neurological dysfunction of legs and bladder.[27] Stimulation of the exposed neural plate shows that all the muscles of the legs have intact innervation to the exposed plaque. The lower motor neurones are intact but these are not connected to higher centers at the upper end of the plaque. These connections are lost as the plaque dries out or is infected. The fetus at 12 weeks of gestation can be shown to have talipes and evidence of neuromuscular imbalance in utero. There is no doubt that secondary postnatal injury may occur, but the initial claim, that immediate operation at birth reverses all neurological deficit, has been shown not to be the case. A myelomeningocele is an open wound and therefore liable to infection (Fig. 20.8). Surface infection leads to meningitis or ventriculitis, which is the usual cause of death in untreated patients. If the open lesion is not operatively closed and death from infection does not occur, there is gradual epithelialization of the lesion over a period of weeks or months. The end result is inferior to elective surgical closure, as low-grade infection results in further loss of spinal cord function and more impairment and there is an ugly tender scar on the infant's back. Epithelialization may also result in tethering of nerve roots, which can be very difficult to treat at a later date.

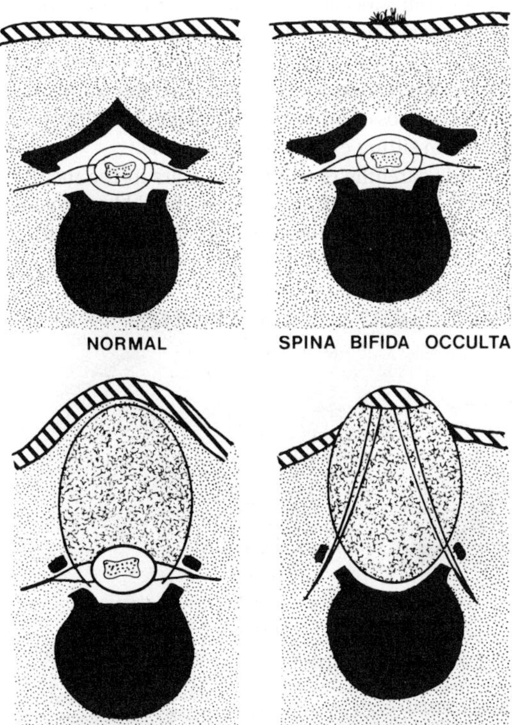

Fig. 20.7 Classification of spina bifida.

Patterns of spinal cord involvement

It is convenient to divide the type of cord lesion into types 1 and 2.

Type 1 cord lesion. In the type 1 lesion there is complete absence of function below a certain segmental level, which results in a flaccid paralysis, loss of sensation and loss of all reflex movement and tendon reflexes below that level. Knowledge of the segmental innervation of the lower limb muscles allows the segmental level to be determined from examination of the lower limbs.

Type 2 cord lesion. In this type there is voluntary control of muscles, which have normal innervation and are in direct communication with the long tracts of the brain above the level of the lesion. At the level of the lesion there may be a complete loss of all function, voluntary and reflex, and of sensation. This may extend over a very short area, i.e. one segment, or over several segments of the spinal cord. The cord then resumes reflex function, as an isolated cord segment. There will be no sensation and no voluntary movement of the muscles in this isolated cord segment. Muscles will, however, respond to dermatome stimulation tapping of the muscle, tapping of the tendon and pinprick.

Examination of the lower limbs is essential in determining the neurological level of paraplegia and also the prognosis for walking, type of deformity and degree of future handicap. The level of the lesion, level of vertebral abnormality and neurological level are not identical and one should not look at the back lesion and guess the neurology is the same.

Direct stimulation of the muscles which do not move is possible by dermatome-to-myotome stimulation, i.e. as the corresponding dermatome is stroked, if there is reflex activity the muscle supplied by that segment will contract. In addition to testing the cremasteric reflex (L1), knee jerk (L3–4), ankle (S1–2), anal and bulbocavernosus reflexes (S4–5), one looks for exaggerated flexor withdrawal reflexes, contraction of the muscles of the perineum on stimulating the perianal region and contraction of the short toe flexors by flicking the toes. Reflexes not normally easily elicited, such as tendon jerks of the hamstring muscles, adductors and tibialis anterior, may be elicited, and in very high lesions, one may see adductor clonus and patella clonus.

If the isolated cord segment is long, then complex reflexes such as flexor withdrawal responses may occur, making one think that the child is actually voluntarily moving the leg. This has led to

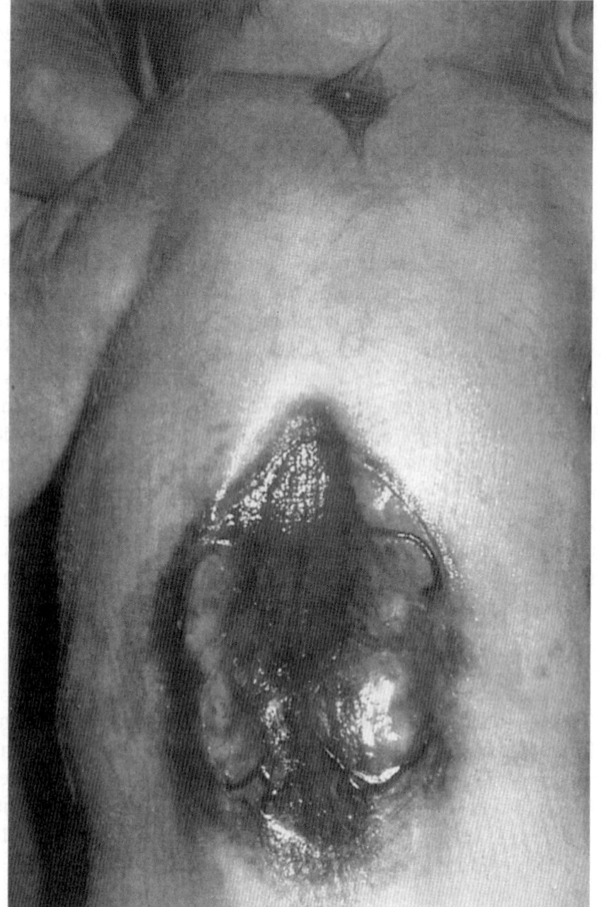

(a)

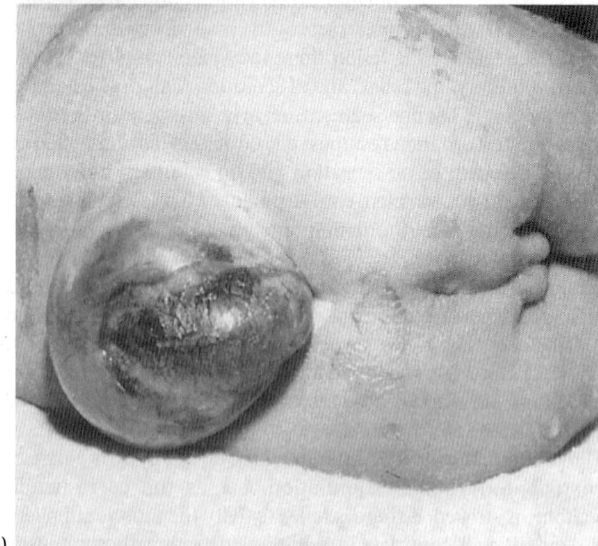

(b)

Fig. 20.8 (a) Meningomyelocele at birth. (b) Bulging meningomyelocele at a few hours of life.

confusion in the past as to the degree of paralysis and the tendency to give a misleadingly good prognosis in the neonatal period.

If the area of isolated cord is limited to the sacral segments, then ankle clonus with a brisk ankle jerk and exaggerated anal reflex will be seen together with a spread of the response when stimulating the perianal region to cause toe flexion and flexion of the lateral hamstrings. Equally, tapping the toes in order to elicit the toe jerk will produce flexion of the knee and a contraction of the anus. The segment of cord showing a lower motor neurone loss of activity is more often in the region of the abdominal muscles, which may be completely paralysed, causing a lumbar hernia and a pot belly.

Mechanism of deformity

The level of deformity often determines the neurological level, e.g. involvement below T8 is associated with paralysis of the abdominal walls and all the lower limb muscles. The lower limb deformities arise from two mechanisms. The first is due to muscle imbalance, e.g. dislocation of the hip when the flexors and adductors (L1–3) overcome the weak gluteal extensors and abductors (S1–2). Hip adduction is a potent cause of posterior hip dislocation. Involvement below L4 causes the lower limb muscles innervated from above this level (hip flexors, hip adductors, quadriceps and tibialis anterior) to be strong and under voluntary control whilst their antagonists are paralysed. This causes the characteristic flexed hip, extended knee (genu recurvatum) and equinovarus foot. If the tibialis anterior is active as a dorsiflexor (L4) whilst the calf muscles as plantar flexors (S1–2) are paralysed, then dorsiflexion and inversion of the foot will occur.

The second cause of deformity results from immobility in utero. The fetus may present as a breech and the immobility results in secondary positional deformities adding to the neurogenic deformity (Fig. 20.9).

In 5% of cases the spinal cord is split with only one half of the cord exposed to the surface; the other half remains in the spinal canal and functions normally. In this case only one leg will have a neurological deficit.

NEONATAL MANAGEMENT OF THE CHILD WITH A NEURAL TUBE DEFECT

The general condition of the infant is assessed to ensure that there are no associated abnormalities, such as chromosome disorder or other malformations of the heart and kidney. The face of a child with a meningomyelocele often has a suggestion of a Down syndrome appearance. The head circumference, sutures and fontanel should be measured and cerebral and renal ultrasound should be routinely performed. X-ray of the spine will show hemivertebrae or gross disruption of the spinal architecture, which would make even sitting eventually impossible.

The lesion is carefully examined for tears in the membranes or leakage of CSF suggesting that operation should be early because of the risk of meningitis. The hips are examined for dislocation.

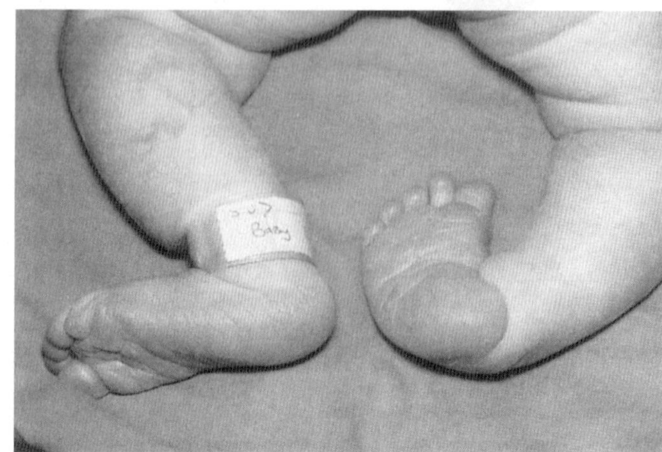

Fig. 20.9 Talipes due to muscle imbalance.

Detailed neurological examination is carried out with the child warm and recovered from the immediate 'birth shock'. Sensory testing is carried out first with the child quiet; the skin is stimulated with the end of a straightened paper clip, starting in the saddle area and progressing through the sacral and lumbar territory. One observes facial grimace or a cry.

Following sensory testing, and with the baby active and crying so that there is spontaneous movement of the upper limbs, one can determine the amount of spontaneous movement in the lower limbs as part of the baby's doggy paddling and cycling movements. It should be possible to give each muscle group an MRC grading of 1–5 and a voluntary motor level down to which the child can move in response to cerebral motor drive can be defined.

Of the factors identifiable at birth, which are predictive of severe disability, one of the most important is gross hydrocephalus, with an occipitofrontal circumference (OFC) more than 20 cm above the 90th centile or a cortical mantle less than 150 mm. Serious spinal deformity, absence of voluntary movement below L2 and the presence of other major defects are the factors which help in deciding whether early immediate operation should be performed or whether one should delay surgery to see how the child progresses over the first week or so. There is no good evidence that early repair of the back lesion will lessen the degree of paralysis in the lower limbs so that one is not jeopardizing the child's future by waiting to see what spontaneous progress occurs. Later plastic repair of the back that has granulated is still feasible.

If immediate closure is not undertaken and the spinal lesion granulates without meningitis developing, hydrocephalus may progress. This may lead to impairment of intelligence, which can be prevented by insertion of a ventriculoperitoneal shunt, so this is the ethical and appropriate intervention in this situation. While the infant is in hospital the parents should be encouraged to visit frequently and be given every opportunity to feed and handle their baby. During this period many questions can be answered, anxieties are allayed and genetic counseling undertaken. The support of a medical social worker is invaluable and the parents can be put in touch with one of the local parent support groups.

Bruner et al[28] reported a 35% reduction following intrauterine repair of myelomeningoceles suggested by a 60% reduction in hindbrain herniation. However the risk of oligohydramnios and preterm labor were significantly increased. Their study compared 29 fetuses operated on between 24 and 30 weeks' gestation with 23 historical controls. Further careful assessment of prenatal intervention is required.

THE LATER MANAGEMENT OF THE CHILD WITH A NEURAL TUBE DEFECT

Motor problems

It should be possible to make a reasonably accurate prediction of the child's future mobility even in the neonatal period if an accurate clinical neurological assessment is made (Table 20.3).

Orthosis refers to light weight plastic splints which are malleable when hot, but firm when cool and can be molded to any required position. Reciprocal gait orthoses are hinged splints, which invoke forward momentum when the weight of the wearer is swung from side to side at the hip. They follow the same principle of the toy animals that will 'walk' down a slope, each limb rocking from side to side.

The child with a purely sacral lesion, as for example with sacral agenesis, or a very low meningomyelocele, will have problems with the feet due to paralysis of the intrinsic muscles of the feet, weak calf muscles and weak hip extensors. He will walk with a waddle and will need boots to support the ankles. He will also have a neurogenic bladder and will require a bladder regime.

Table 20.3 Prediction of walking ability in myelomeningocele

Voluntary motor level	*Probable walking ability*
T6–L2	Chair Crutches – swing through Parapodium Swivel walker RGO, HGO
L3	HKAFO RGO, HGO with sticks or tripods
L4	KAFO, HKAFO AFO
L5	AFO KAFO
Sacral	nil or AFO

RGO, reciprocating gait orthosis; HGO, hip guidance orthosis; HKAFO, hip/knee/ankle/foot orthosis; KAFO, knee/ankle/foot orthosis.

Paralysis below L3–4 is compatible with walking unaided with sticks and below-knee calipers. The spinal lesion may always be complicated by the effects of ataxia from the hydrocephalus or hemiplegia as a result of shunt malfunction, ventriculitis or puncture porencephaly. The child with a high lumbar lesion was in the past sentenced to immobility in a wheelchair but the use of reciprocating gait orthoses or hip guidance orthoses means that these children can now be mobile in the erect posture.

It may be necessary for an orthopedic surgeon to perform tenotomies in the neonatal period or later to correct muscle imbalance, e.g. the very tight tibialis anterior that may occur in an L4 lesion. Talipes will need correcting and hips will need to be released and put back into joint. Scoliosis may require surgery in adolescence.

Non-motor neurological problems

Sensation

The sensory level in myelomeningocele, i.e. the lowest level of normal sensation, is usually within one or two segments of the motor level. As a result of cutaneous anesthesia there is a constant danger of painless ulceration. Pressure sores may develop over the sacral tuberosity, especially if incontinence has led to maceration of the skin. Sensory loss may become more of a problem in the future with the use of reciprocating gait orthoses when the risk of Charcot joints (i.e. neurogenic arthropathy and painless fractures) is added to the list of problems. The feet are often cold, blue and erythrocyanotic due to poor peripheral perfusion.

Burns may occur from hot-water bottles or sitting on radiators. Shoes which are too tight or failure to recognize the effects of intense cold in the winter can both result in gangrene of the toes.

The neurogenic bladder

The bladder receives its nerve supply from three sources. First, the parasympathetic via the nervi erigentes from the sacral roots S2–4 which control detrusor contraction. Second, a sympathetic component supplies the trigone and internal sphincter and allows opening of the bladder neck during micturition. It is also important in sexual function when the internal sphincter is closed without any contraction of the detrusor. The third supply is via the pudendal nerve, which carries the voluntary control of the striated external sphincter.

The bladder and bowel will be involved in most cases, but the type of bladder involvement depends upon the type of lesion.[29]

If the lower limbs show signs of lower motor neurone denervation in the muscles innervated from S2–4 (type 1 lesion), e.g. calf, intrinsic muscles of the foot, anal sphincter and pelvic floor, then a weak or totally paralysed bladder (acontractile) is to be expected. Lack of tone in the anal sphincter shows as a patulous anus, dribbling of urine and loss of the normal gluteal fold so that the anus appears wide open on top of a mountain rather than in a valley.

Depending on the degree of resistance of the bladder outlet, such infants may have constant dribbling of urine with an empty bladder or overflow incontinence from a distended bladder. Ureteric reflux may occur at low pressures from such inert bladders in which the valvular effect of the intramural ureter is lacking.

In infants with an isolated cord lesion (type 2 lesion), where examination of the limb shows purely reflex activity in S2–4 (i.e. spastic calves, toe flexors with exaggerated reflexes, a very brisk anal reflex), a reflex type of bladder (contractile) is to be expected. The ideal automatic bladder, i.e. one with periodic complete reflex emptying, is rare in myelomeningocele. At best an intermittent detrusor contraction results in voiding of up to 100 ml of urine; at worst persistent dribbling may result from constant poorly coordinated detrusor contractions. Despite an active detrusor, which may generate pressures of over 100 mmHg in a small infant, the bladder emptying may be poor because of a high urethral resistance. This outlet obstruction is probably due to failure of relaxation of the striated external sphincter, which is normally under voluntary control via the pudendal nerve. This type of spastic bladder neck responds to stretching by further contraction and very high pressures result in back pressure with acute and severe hydroureter and hydronephrosis. Bladder rupture and urinary ascites can occur in utero. True bladder neck obstruction is relatively uncommon. Dilation of the upper urinary tract may occur in both the flaccid and the high pressure bladder. Stagnation with incomplete bladder emptying and dilation of the upper urinary tract inevitably leads to the risk of infection. Chronic pyelonephritis may lead to renal failure and hypertension before adult life is reached.

Assessment of the upper renal tract

The presence of hydronephrosis is detected using ultrasound. The presence of ureteric reflux and the adequacy of the bladder neck and urethra can all be assessed using cystourethrography. Renal function is assessed using biochemical estimations such as urea, electrolytes and creatinine together with a chromium or DMSA scan.

Assessment of the neurogenic bladder

Clinically the most important part of the assessment is to watch a child actually pass urine. If the urine can be passed in a stream one knows that there must be a coordinated detrusor contraction. If the stream is a good one, i.e. the child can 'pee in a parabola', there can be no serious bladder neck obstruction. In the older child, the rate of passing urine can be measured as ml/unit time by getting the child to pass urine into a container with an electronic measuring device which draws out a graph of the rate of urination. This is a measure of detrusor contraction and bladder neck obstruction. The infant should be held up to see if there is any dribbling dependent on position and light suprapubic pressure applied to assess effective bladder neck contraction to allow continence and bladder filling.

Investigation of the bladder in the neonatal period is undertaken to decide whether the infant has a safe or dangerous bladder, i.e. whether early intervention is necessary or not. If the upper renal tract is normal on ultrasound and the baby passes urine or it can be easily expressed, one can wait until 4 months of age for detailed urinary investigations. If, however, there appears to be bladder outlet obstruction, high pressure bladder and dilation of the upper renal tract then catheterization from birth may be necessary in order to preserve renal function.

Cystometrogram

This is performed either by a urethral catheter into the bladder when the effects of adding small aliquots of saline upon the pressure is monitored or, more physiological but more invasive, a suprapubic cystometrogram is performed using two catheters inserted into the bladder by suprapubic puncture. One of these is used to fill the bladder at the physiological rate of 2 ml/min and the second to measure pressure. The bladder volume, sensation and pressures at which urethral sphincters open can then be measured and it is possible to look at micturition and urethral resistance in a way that is not possible with a catheter per urethra.

Management of the neurogenic bladder

The infants are divided into those with a safe bladder and those with an unsafe bladder. For safer definition all children with known or suspected spina bifida should have videourodynamic assessment.[30]

The safe bladder. By safe it is meant that there is a normal upper renal tract with normal renal function and no secondary pressure transmitted to the ureter or renal pelvis. There is a residual urine of less than 20 ml with normal pressures and no outlet obstruction. This may be due to the fact that the bladder is in fact completely normal and a toilet-training program is all that is required, or it may be due to the fact that the child can safely empty the bladder by suprapubic manual pressure. This requires careful monitoring for urinary tract infection as well as regular monitoring of the upper renal tract to be sure that secondary damage is not occurring.

The unsafe bladder. In this situation there is already hydronephrosis and hydroureter, a high residual urine, a high intravesical pressure and/or the presence of outlet obstruction. There is a need for adequate bladder drainage to avoid progressive damage to the kidneys, with resultant renal failure. The unsafe bladder may require catheterization in the immediate neonatal period. A silicone catheter may be changed every 4–6 weeks in the first few years of life after which intermittent self-catheterization can be taught once the child is old enough. Urinary diversions such as ureterostomy or a colonic loop are now only rarely indicated. Bladder neck obstruction can be treated by per urethral resection or pudendal neurectomy or bladder neck Y-V plasty may be required later to try and achieve relief of bladder neck obstruction without producing incontinence.

Toilet training is important in these children, as one will occasionally achieve continence in the presence of a neurogenic bladder that was not thought to be under voluntary control. There is a need to regulate fluid intake, e.g. at night, and to go to the toilet regularly, utilizing suprapubic pressure to induce voiding, at first hourly. Constipation should be avoided, urinary tract infections carefully monitored and when there is voluntary control, double micturition should be practiced as a routine. Pelvic floor stimulators are not of proven benefit. They can be useful in selected cases in the short term, but have many complications.

Most children are managed nowadays either by a simple toilet-training regime or with indwelling and then intermittent catheterization. One of the problems associated with intermittent catheterization is how to keep the child dry between catheterizations. Drugs may be used to increase or decrease bladder tone and capacity.

Cholinergic drugs such as carbachol, bethanechol chloride or distigmine bromide will increase detrusor contraction whilst anticholinergic drugs such as propantheline, imipramine and oxybutynin will decrease detrusor contractions. Beta-adrenergic agonists such as ephedrine will increase the tone in the bladder neck whilst alpha-adrenergic blockers such as phenoxybenzamine will decrease the tone in the bladder neck. These have a useful but limited place in a small percentage of children.

Urinary tract infection is a constant hazard with the risk of pyelonephritis and this, together with the effects of back pressure on the kidney, may result in renal failure by the teenage years.

Sexual function

Motor problems are likely to lead to physical difficulty and result in problems with sexual intercourse. Only small numbers of young adults with spina bifida have any sexual experience and very few females have children even though there is no reason why they should not become pregnant and have a normal delivery. In the male, impotence will depend upon a sympathetic and parasympathetic involvement. Failure of closure of the bladder neck during ejaculation means that sperm enters the bladder and not the posterior urethra.

Bowel

Chronic constipation, with gross dilation of the descending colon and overflow incontinence, is common. Prolapse of the rectum may occur in infancy, but rarely remains into school age. Chronic fecal retention may further impede bladder drainage. The anal sphincter, like the bladder neck, may be either patulous and incompetent or tight and spastic. Sensation may be absent so that severe constipation, with retention of feces or fecal incontinence, may occur. In spite of the neurogenic problems, the bowel appears to be more amenable to training in the long run than the bladder. The child should take a high-fiber diet and it may be necessary to use stimulative laxatives such as Senokot or fecal softeners such as Dioctyl. The time of day when the bowel would naturally empty should be sought. This need not necessarily be the morning and toilet training with abdominal pressure will be successful in at least half of the cases. Fecal impaction should be avoided as this presses on the bladder neck and may result in both urinary incontinence and secondary spurious diarrhea, which can be cured by emptying the bowel. In occasional patients regular manual evacuation is necessary to maintain continence.

Teenage problems

As the pubertal growth spurt occurs, several problems result. Sexual problems have already been discussed. The realization of the degree of handicap may cause profound reactive depression. The renal tract problems cause most anxiety, especially if renal damage has progressed to the point of considering the ethics of chronic dialysis or transplant. Scoliosis may be greatly aggravated by growth and pain at the site of the healed lesion may cause a lot of discomfort. Traction on the nerve roots due to tethering may cause downward pull at the foramen magnum. It is the medullary cervical junction which causes most problems and is the most difficult to deal with. Stretching of the medulla with obstruction at the aqueduct and the fourth ventricular foramina from the Arnold–Chiari formation may cause an isolated fourth ventricular hydrocephalus. This may require separate shunting. The pressure may be projected down the central canal of the spinal cord so that a hydromyelia results with gross distension of the cord, producing a string-of-sausages appearance. A localized dilation may occur as a syringomyelia. These brainstem and cervical spinal abnormalities present as drooling, swallowing difficulties, bilateral sixth and seventh paresis, Erb palsy posture, weakness of shoulder elevation or wasting, weakness and loss of use of the hands. Removal of tethering, shunting fourth ventricles, cerebellar tonsillectomy and removal of the arch of the atlas and part of the foramen magnum-impacted tissue may be attempted to try and prevent progressive loss of function.

HYDROCEPHALUS

DEFINITION

Hydrocephalus denotes an increase in size of the CSF spaces associated with an increase in intracranial pressure (ICP), secondary to a pathophysiological process.

INCIDENCE

The incidence of hydrocephalus per 10 000 births around the world is particularly high in Alexandria (20.8), Belfast (12.5) and Dublin (35). A collaborative perinatal survey[31] found an incidence of 15 per 10 000 births, only half of whom were evident at birth. These figures are, however, now too high for the UK, as hydrocephalus associated with spina bifida, secondary to intraventricular hemorrhage in the premature infant and secondary to haemophilus meningitis and tuberculous meningitis have all declined. The current prevalence[32,33] of congenital and infantile hydrocephalus is between 0.48 and 0.81 per 1000 births (live and still). The ability to diagnose severe hydrocephalus antenatally by ultrasound means that some cases are prevented by termination.

PATHOPHYSIOLOGY

Factors that cause ventricular dilation

The normal intracranial pressure in the human represents a balance between the intracranial contents, i.e. blood, brain and CSF. For the CSF compartment, any increase in production or obstruction of flow or absorption will result in ventricular dilation.

Production of CSF

In normal subjects, CSF is formed at a rate of 0.3–0.5 ml/min. In hydrocephalic patients on external drainage the CSF production rate is similar. CSF production occurs by two mechanisms.

1. That dependent on choroidal capillary blood flow. This is a two-step process with, first, an ultrafiltrate of plasma produced hydrostatically through the lax choroidal capillary endothelium (blood–CSF barrier) and, second, an active process involving secretion of sodium into and out of the apical choroidal villi. The raised osmotic pressure causes water to follow passively.
2. That due to a direct neurogenic stimulation of choroidal villi (which have beta2-adrenergic receptors, cholinergic receptors, GABA receptors), which is independent of choroidal blood flow. Stimulation of adrenergic fibers may reduce CSF flow by approximately one-third.

The production rate is similar in newborn and older children, despite the obvious difference in size of the choroid plexus. It is postulated that early maturation of enzyme systems may be responsible for the similar production rates.

A number of factors influence the CSF formation rate. Increased secretion may occur with a choroid plexus papilloma. Furosemide (frusemide) and acetazolamide reduce CSF production. Hypothermia will also reduce the rate of production and although the CSF formation rate is usually independent of the intracranial pressure, when high intraventricular pressures exist the production rate falls, due to decreased choroidal perfusion. Ventricular outflow rates appear to be pulsatile so that peaks and troughs of CSF evacuation occur from the ventricles when measured objectively in children undergoing closed ventricular drainage.[34]

Obstruction

A choroid plexus tumor may not only induce excessive CSF production, but may also block the outlet of the ventricle. Intracranial hemorrhage or meningitis may cause leptomeningeal adhesions and obstruction to the CSF flow as well as impairing absorption by blocking arachnoid granulations. A common site for obstruction is the aqueduct of Sylvius. Congenital atresia may result in an inadequate lumen or a total blind-ending channel with forking of the upper and lower components of the aqueduct. Occasionally there is a filamentous or membranous obstruction, which may be broken down either by an increase in the intraventricular pressure or by surgical bouginage from the fourth ventricle. This rarely results in an effective reduction of the hydrocephalus because inadequate development of the peripheral subarachnoid pathways, which has resulted from the non-communicating hydrocephalus, means the dynamics are only changed from a non-communicating to a communicating hydrocephalus. The aqueduct of Sylvius may also be occluded by organized blood clot after intracranial hemorrhage, inflammatory exudate following ventriculitis or from an aqueductitis resulting from mumps.

Obstruction to CSF flow at the outlet foramina of the fourth ventricle may be secondary to intracranial hemorrhage or infection or may be due to congenital failure of the foramina of Magendie and Luschka to open during development. Occlusion of the fourth ventricle foramina results in a fourth ventricular cystic dilation with atrophy of the cerebellum (the Dandy–Walker cyst). Tumors or clots, cysts or abscesses within or adjacent to the ventricular system may result in hydrocephalus. Thalamic tumors, and giant cell astrogliomas in tuberous sclerosis may obstruct the foramen of Monro and third ventricle and pontine or brainstem gliomas may distort the aqueduct of Sylvius, although frequently such pontine gliomas are invasive throughout the brainstem and do not usually cause a gross hydrocephalus. Cerebellar tumors will affect the CSF flow from the fourth ventricle. A choroid cyst of the third ventricle may give rise to intermittent high pressure and hydrocephalus, by obstructing the foramen of Monro in a 'ballcock' fashion. During distention of the cyst or venous distention about it there is obstruction of CSF flow through the foramen of Monro. With a possible change of posture, the obstruction may be rapidly released and the pressure decline. Children with cysts of the third ventricle frequently present with a 'bobble-headed doll' syndrome and progressive loss of intellect with frontal horn dilation.

Decreased absorption

Decreased absorption may result from obstruction of the arachnoid villi or other peripheral subarachnoid pathways. Absorption (unlike formation) of CSF is a pressure-dependent phenomenon and increases linearly with CSF pressure. Normally CSF absorption begins at a mean pressure of 5 mmHg.

Factors causing progression of hydrocephalus

Observations in experimental hydrocephalus suggest that after CSF obstruction the ICP rises acutely. This is followed by a stage of periventricular edema with expanded ventricles and subsequently by an increase in CSF absorption. Ventricular dilation and its eventual size depend on the external support of the brain. In infants up to 16 months of age the support of the brain is weak from the poorly myelinated soft parenchyma and there are unfused sutures. Clearly the level of pressure is important at first in the pathogenesis of ventricular dilation, together with the known increase in the outflow resistance and a higher 'pressure volume index' (PVI) than could be predicted from the volume of the cranial and spinal axis.

In term and preterm infants we frequently see levels of intraventricular pressure of 5 mmHg (above normal for age) which are sufficient to interfere with the cerebral blood flow velocity and have the potential to cause ischemia.

A number of physiological buffers come into play in response to the hydrocephalus. There is collapse of cerebral veins, a shunting of CSF from the ventricular to the spinal CSF compartment, expansion of the skull and an increase in the CSF absorption from the raised pressure. There may also be increased CSF absorption about the spinal nerve roots and paranasal sinuses. Once these compensatory mechanisms have been exhausted, then further progression of the hydrocephalus will occur.

The sequence of events is that at first the pressure will increase. The dilation of the ventricles in response to this high pressure is termed 'active or progressive hydrocephalus'. Finally the pressure returns to the normal levels with severely dilated ventricles, a state of arrest (*compensated or arrested hydrocephalus*). Sometimes the active process may be followed by an intermittent pressure pattern with ventricular dilation until the arrested state is reached. This intermittent pattern may be reversible. However, significant elevation of the pressure with increasing ventricular dimensions to the point where brain perfusion is compromised necessitates CSF diversion procedures before shunt-dependent or compensated arrest occurs.

The effects of raised ventricular pressure

Raised intracranial pressure results in either ischemia or brain shift. The ischemia results from a reduced cerebral perfusion pressure (CPP) (mean arterial blood pressure minus intracranial pressure). At levels of CPP below 60 mmHg, in the older child, there is a progressive reduction in brain perfusion. At 40–50 mmHg, profound ischemia results. In the newborn, cerebral perfusion pressures of 30 mmHg may be associated with a normal neurodevelopmental outcome.

The subarachnoid space and the aqueduct are obliterated after shunting, presumably because they are used less, and the patient becomes totally shunt dependent.

Fourth ventricular entrapment, with ataxia, vomiting, cranial nerve disturbances and headache, is a result of outlet obstruction. Treatment is shunting of the ventricle itself. Fistulous communications and diverticulae of the ventricles are usually an accompaniment of severe ventricular dilation. This produces a complex CT scan appearance and intraventricular contrast studies are needed to distinguish these from primary subarachnoid cysts.

CLASSIFICATION AND ETIOLOGY

Terminology

Internal or non-communicating hydrocephalus: excess of CSF within the ventricular system up to the level of the outlet foramina of the fourth ventricle. The common sites of obstruction are at the outlet foramina of the fourth ventricle, the aqueduct of Sylvius or at the foramen of Monro.

External or communicating hydrocephalus: an increase in the ventricular volume and the subarachnoid spaces of the cranium and spine. The sites of obstruction are at the arachnoid villi or in the basal cisterns.

Panventricular hydrocephalus: dilation of the lateral, third and fourth ventricles (in aqueduct stenosis the fourth ventricle is small

Table 20.4 Etiology of hydrocephalus

Causes of prenatally determined hydrocephalus
Congenital (chromosomal) malformations
Maternal diabetes resulting in holoprosencephaly
Neural tube defects
Occipital meningocele and encephalocele
The Cleland–Chiari II malformation
Dandy–Walker syndrome
Hydranencephaly
Multicystic encephalomalacia
Schizencephaly
Achondroplasia
Arachnoid cysts
Quadrigeminal plate cysts, retrocerebellar cysts, cysts of the cerebellopontine angle and supracellar cysts
Congenital craniosynostosis (e.g. Apert's syndrome)
Agenesis of the corpus callosum and cysts of the cavum septum pellucidum and cavum vergae
Encephalocraniocutaneous lipomatosis
Isolated stenosis of the aqueduct of Sylvius
Sex-linked stenosis of the aqueduct of Sylvius
Hydrocephalus associated with giant hairy nevus (melanosis of the leptomeninges)
Aneurysm of the great vein of Galen
Hurler's disease
Basilar impression
Osteogenesis imperfecta (rarely)
Paget's disease
Colpocephaly
Lissencephaly
Say–Gerald syndrome
Causes of acquired hydrocephalus
Posthemorrhagic causes
Neonatal intraventricular hemorrhage
Subarachnoid hemorrhage
Subdural hemorrhage
Postmeningitic
Toxoplasmosis
Mumps (aqueductitis, ependymitis)
Pyogenic organisms (pneumococcus, haemophilus, etc.)
Cytomegalovirus
Other viral meningitides
Rubella
Tuberculous meningitis and tuberculoma
Space-occupying lesions
Tumor
Clot
Cyst
Abscess
Postasphyxial
Injury
Other causes
Stenosis of the aqueduct of Sylvius
1. Due to raised intracranial pressure with secondary kinking of the aqueduct
2. Due to aqueductitis and ependymitis associated with mumps, toxoplasma, tuberculomas, pyogenic meningitis, rarely cytomegalovirus, rubella and tumors
Dystrophia myotonia
Otitic hydrocephalus
Choroid plexus papilloma
Intrathecal contrast agents
Fungal infection (cryptococcus and blastomyces)
Cysticercosis
Sarcoidosis
Spinal tumor
Dural venous thrombosis
Isolated Chiari type I deformity

or of normal size – 'triventricular hydrocephalus'). An *isolated fourth ventricle* ('double compartment hydrocephalus' or 'trapped fourth ventricle') occurs when there is outlet obstruction from that ventricle and stricture of the aqueduct.

Unilateral hydrocephalus: abnormal dilation of the body, frontal and/or posterior horn of the lateral ventricle on one side. This may be due to compression of the ventricular system on the opposite side, obstruction to one foramen of Monro, slit ventricle syndrome or a hemiparenchymal atrophy.

Slit ventricles: a reduction in the size of the ventricular system seen on CT scan, usually in response to excessive CSF drainage. The slit ventricle *syndrome* is distinguished from radiological slit ventricles by the presence of symptoms and clinical signs attributable to this overdrainage. The etiology of hydrocephalus is given in Table 20.4.

DIAGNOSIS AND ASSESSMENT

Clinical features of progressive hydrocephalus

The symptoms and signs of progressive hydrocephalus in infants are shown in Table 20.5.[35] The symptoms of infantile progressive hydrocephalus are vague and consist of irritability and vomiting but about half are without symptoms. The most common clinical sign is an inappropriately increasing head circumference, followed by a tense non-pulsatile fontanel, then clinical and radiological separation of the sutures, scalp vein distension with taut skin over the scalp. It is important to realize that the classic adult presentation of raised intracranial pressure is rare in children (headache, vomiting, papilledema). Vomiting is a non-specific symptom in childhood, as are behavioral changes (irritability).

The most common sign of hydrocephalus is really a sign of compensation for the raised ventricular pressure. 'Sunsetting' – the inability to look upwards, with depression of both eyes – may initially be intermittent and later continuous (Fig. 20.10). It is due to pressure on the superior quadrigeminal plate against the free edge of the tentorium causing a supranuclear paresis, which may be accompanied by paralysis of the fourth nerve.

Neurogenic stridor is a result of deranged lower brainstem function caused by bilateral corticobulbar disruption and is a feature of pseudobulbar paresis. Abnormalities of sucking and feeding may also occur with seriously raised intracranial pressure. Papilledema is rare, but distended retinal veins are common.

The symptoms of *chronic hydrocephalus* are an insidious deterioration in school performance, intermittent headaches over

Table 20.5 Most common clinical features of progressive infantile hydrocephalus (50% of cases are asymptomatic)

Symptoms
Headache or irritability
Vomiting
Anorexia
Drowsiness or lethargy
Signs
Inappropriately increasing occipitofrontal circumference (approx 75%)
Tense anterior fontanel
Splayed sutures
Scalp vein distention
Sunsetting (loss of upward gaze)
Neck retraction or rigidity
Pupillary changes
Neurogenic stridor
Decerebration

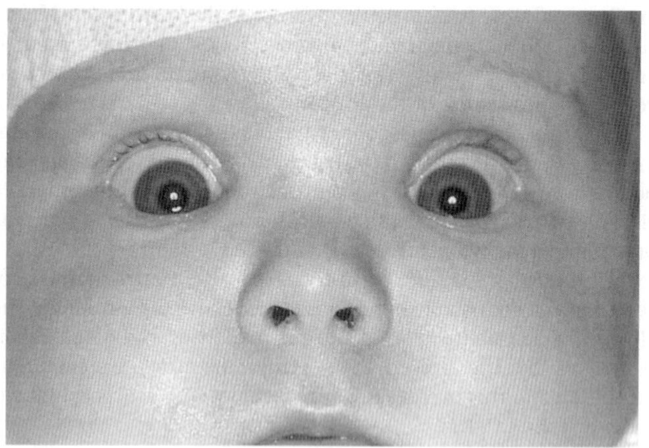

Fig. 20.10 'Sunsetting' due to loss of upward conjugate gaze.

many months, behavioral and personality changes, failure to thrive and dizziness. These are distinct from the signs and symptoms of *arrested hydrocephalus* of long standing which include features of ataxic and spastic cerebral palsy, precocious puberty, mental retardation and specific learning problems. The clinical features of hydrocephalus with raised intracranial pressure may be extremely variable and any infant with a rapidly increasing head circumference should have a cranial imaging.

It should be considered in the older infant who presents with an enlarged head circumference and developmental delay (considering also other syndromes of macrocephaly including fragile X and neurofibromatosis).

Clinical features of decompensated hydrocephalus

Additional signs of raised pressure (Table 20.6) suggest the possibility of a shunt blockage. The median survival time for a ventriculoperitoneal shunt was 4.31 years in the Edinburgh study.[36]

Unusual features of raised ventricular pressure include neurogenic pulmonary edema, profuse sweating, ptosis, neurogenic stridor, pseudobulbar paresis and skin rashes.[35]

Imaging

X-ray examinations of the skull, although not routinely indicated, may show a 'copper-beaten' appearance, shallow orbits and splayed sutures. Computed axial tomography, ultrasound or magnetic resonance image scans will all define ventricular size. Although repeated ultrasound examinations may show progressive hydrocephalus, it is advisable to have a definitive CT or MRI investigation prior to any surgical intervention. The CT scan requires sedation or anesthetic for small children and provides information about the size and symmetry of the ventricles and whether there is any underlying pathology. A single CT scan, like a single ultrasound or MRI scan, may not reveal whether there is a progressive or an arrested hydrocephalus. When there is significantly elevated intraventricular pressure from progressive hydrocephalus, periventricular lucencies, rounding of ventricles, absence of a cortical subarachnoid space and a spherical appearance of the third ventricle (instead of the usual barrel appearance) is seen on CT scan. It is not sufficient to rely on the skull circumference measurements alone and repeated ultrasound scans are the most useful arbiter.

The most commonly used index of ventricular dilation is the V/P ratio, that is, the ventricular diameter at the mid-portion of the lateral ventricles divided by the biparietal diameter from inner table to inner table. Hydrocephalus is defined as a ratio higher than 0.26.

Antenatal ultrasound for assessment of fetal hydrocephalus is indexed slightly differently. The commonly used parameters are biparietal diameter and the ratio of the lateral ventricular width divided by the width of the head. The latter is approximately 0.61 at 14 weeks, 0.29 at 27 weeks and 0.29 at term. Absolute measurements of ventricular width are done using the atrium as reference point. Ultrasound estimates of ventriculomegaly in utero may be exaggerated by a factor of about 10%, due to the distortion of sound signals passing through two fluids (amniotic and CSF). If hydrocephalus is suspected, ultrasound is done weekly until elective cesarean section at 36 weeks (intraventricular hemorrhage is maximal before 34 weeks). Intracranial Doppler blood flow velocities should be measured in addition to the biparietal diameter.

Table 20.6 Clinical features of decompensated hydrocephalus (children with shunts)

Symptoms
Vomiting
Drowsiness or lethargy
Headache
Behavioral change
Anorexia
Valve malfunction
Sleep disturbance
Seizures
Signs
No clinical signs (approx 25%)
Decreased conscious level
Acute squint
Neck retraction
Distended retinal veins
Sluggish palpable valve mechanism

Intracranial pressure

Ventricular CSF pressure monitoring is the only accurate way of assessing the activity of the hydrocephalus. This can be achieved by direct puncture of the ventricle via the anterior fontanel until it is closed at 18 months. Should repeated ventricular punctures be required then a frontal ventricular access device (Rickham or Ommaya reservoir) should be inserted into the frontal horn of the right lateral ventricle to allow sequential pressure measurements. Repeated brain puncture may cause a puncture porencephaly. A single measurement of intracranial pressure is of limited value. The cerebral perfusion pressure (CPP) should be calculated by subtracting the intracranial pressure (mean ICP) from the mean systemic arterial pressure. For neonates the mean upper normal limit of intracranial pressure is 3.5 mmHg compared to 5.8 mmHg for infants up to 12 months, 6.4 mmHg from 1 to 3 years and 15 mmHg in adults.[37]

For children who present with symptoms of shunt malfunction, due to blockage or infection, and who already have CSF shunting devices in situ, pressure measurements via a 'CSF access device' may be done continuously or overnight. This can indicate when raised pressure should be treated at the bedside and overnight measurements are a way of assessing whether the hydrocephalus is arrested or whether there is an intermittently active component. The rapid eye movement phase of sleep is associated with an increase of cerebral blood flow of about 40% in certain areas of the brain. This increase in intracranial volume has to be buffered if raised pressure is not to occur. In children with abnormal intracranial dynamics, raised pressure is seen particularly during rapid eye movement (REM) sleep and, to a lesser extent, during stage 2 non-REM sleep.

Cerebral blood flow

The cerebral perfusion pressure gives an indication of the potential for anoxic, ischemic damage to the brain. There are a number of methods available for measuring the blood flow velocity or perfusion to the brain, including flow meters, electrical impedance, autoradiography, wash-out and wash-in techniques, microspheres, ultrasound, MRI, Single photon emission tomography (SPECT), positron emission tomography (PET) and first pass (mean transit time). Our own studies of the first pass method measuring the net mean cerebral transit time use an isotope (sodium pertechnetate or technetium albumin) and were performed on 11 hydrocephalic children. The transit time values correlated with cerebral perfusion pressure values.[38] Children with arrested hydrocephalus had transit times within the normal range, while those with progressive hydrocephalus had up to 15% of their sleep time with a cerebral perfusion pressure of less than 50 mmHg.

It is possible also to use a resistance index (systolic minus diastolic over systolic pressure (S – D)/S) or the area under the curve obtained by pulsed Doppler measurements of the major cerebral arteries as a measure of the cerebral blood flow velocity. The most useful vessel is the middle cerebral artery and an estimate of the velocity is best obtained through the squamous window of the temporal bone, rather than via the open anterior fontanel (Fig. 20.11).

The resistance index correlates significantly with the intracranial pressure[34] MINNS ET AL 1990 and the mean cerebral blood flow velocities fall with elevated ICP measurements. Doppler measurements can be performed intermittently or even continuously in hydrocephalic infants. Since the main effects of raised intracranial pressure are to produce ischemia and brain shifts, an increase in the ventricular pressure sufficient to impair blood flow is an indication for insertion of a CSF shunt or third ventricular ventriculostomy. Despite the low values of ICP in normal newborn infants and the relatively low values in infantile and neonatal hydrocephalus, small rises may be sufficient to impair cerebral blood flow. It is our practice to measure both the pressure and the cerebral blood flow velocity sequentially on these infants and the volume of CSF which needs to be removed in order to produce and maintain a normal resistance index (normal equals 0.68); this will indicate whether the hydrocephalic process is arresting spontaneously or whether it is progressing.[39]

TREATMENTS

Shunts

The usual treatment of progressive hydrocephalus is to divert CSF from the ventricular system to another site. There are numerous valves and shunt systems available, which take CSF out of the head

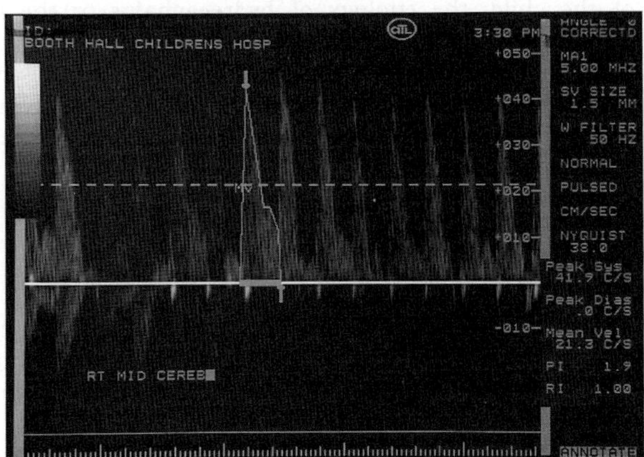

Fig. 20.11 Ultrasound demonstrating flow pattern in left middle cerebral artery with resistance index of 1.22.

for it to be absorbed elsewhere (Spitz–Holter valve, Pudenz–Hakim, Raimondi, the Indian valve, the Denver, etc.). The author favors the unitised Pudenz with a proximal valve. There are now more sophisticated types (the Sophy programmable and multiprogrammable and the Cosman ICP telesensor) with various types of opening pressure device incorporated into the shunt system.

There are many variations on the basic shunt system, which include a ventricular catheter with a flanged end to cause the choroid plexus to waft away from the drainage holes and so lessen proximal blockage. Some shunt systems have a twin valve, one arranged proximally and another distally, and some include a pump or flushing device. The valve usually has a distinct opening pressure, either 2–4, 4–6 or 6–8 cmH_2O, the CSF draining when this pressure is exceeded. In the newborn, a device that opens at low pressure is advisable, but as the child grows, it may be necessary to replace this with one opening at a higher pressure to avoid the development of overdrainage and craniocerebral disproportion. A valve may be incorporated in the pump (Spitz–Holter system) or it may be a distal 'slit valve' at the peritoneal end. It may be a single continuous stiff tube with radiopaque gradations to avoid kinking, such as the Raimondi system. Many different valves and shunt system combinations therefore exist. Our reason for choosing the unitised system with a proximal valve is to avoid the overdrainage, which frequently results by a siphon effect from a long distal catheter.

Various routes of drainage have been used. The earliest was the ventricular atrial route in which the distal tube was passed by the common facial vein into the right atrium. On occasions a ventriculoazygous route was employed. The potential complications from ventriculoatrial shunts were serious, with infection occurring in between 10 and 30% (Table 20.7). Acute infection with these shunts is automatically accompanied by septicemia and chronic infection may result in shunt nephritis or unexplained rashes of a vasculitic nature due to complement activation from chronic septic emboli. The other chronic effects are right heart failure from pulmonary hypertension (the end result of chronic embolic phenomena from the catheter tip lying in the right atrium) and bacterial endocarditis, thrombosis of the superior vena cava with superior vena caval syndrome arrhythmias and possible perforation of the myocardium. Most centers have now turned to the peritoneal route for drainage.

Ventriculoperitoneal shunts may also have complications, and on at least one occasion, shunt nephritis has been recorded (Table 20.7). More common is distal blockage due to pocketing of CSF from adhesions, preventing CSF spreading through the peritoneum. This may result eventually in pseudocyst formation. Other complications include penetration of the distal end into a viscus or through the gut wall and it has been known for ventriculoperitoneal (VP) shunts to appear per rectum. When infection of the shunt spreads distally, peritonitis may result.

Thecoperitoneal shunts or lumboperitoneal shunts have been largely replaced. They were useful in cases of communicating hydrocephalus following hemorrhage or infection but now are reserved for benign intracranial hypertension and occasionally posthemorrhagic hydrocephalus. Insertion of this shunt requires a laminectomy and hyperlordosis of the spine above the level of shunt insertion may develop. Recent studies also show there is a chronic distortion of the brainstem at the level of the foramen magnum. It is not nowadays considered a long-term option. It is advisable when these operations are used that additional supratentorial access is maintained by means of a reservoir into the frontal horn of the right lateral ventricle. On the positive side, shunting from the peripheries of the CSF fluid circulation encourages reopening of the subarachnoid pathways, which does not happen with VP anastomoses, and the risk of infection from thecoperitoneal shunts

Table 20.7 Complications of CSF shunting

Blockage by choroid plexus, fibrin, neuroglia, blood clot and brain fragments causing raised intracranial pressure
Fractured tubing: fracture of the distal tubing may occur in the neck as a result of direct trauma or kinking of the tubing with repeated movements (fracture can also occur over the surface of the chest and exaggerated flexion/extension movements may result in a crack in the distal tube)
Infection (colonization and ventriculitis) with raised intracranial pressure
Shunt dependence
Slit ventricle syndrome
Other decompressive effects (e.g. subdural hematoma)
Migration of the tubing proximally or distally: cases have been reported of migration of the distal tubing through the gut wall or penetration of other organs. (Cases are known where the tubing has dramatically retracted from the abdominal cavity to the intracranial space. Migration of the distal tubing may cause a volvulus. Commonly if insufficient length is implanted initially, the tubing may retract subcutaneously over the chest wall with growth. Migration of the proximal tubing may result in the proximal catheter extending into a different ventricle or into subcortical structures)
Intestinal obstruction (volvulus)
Peritonitis and peritoneal fibrosis
Endocarditis (VA shunts)
Chronic pulmonary hypertension (VA shunts)
Superior vena caval syndrome (VA shunts)
Arrhythmias (VA shunts)
Shunt nephritis (VA shunts): a case has been reported of shunt nephritis following a VP shunt
Hyperlordosis (TP shunts)
Acute non-communication (with TP shunts)
Product failure due to mechanical deficiency and a faulty valve
Surgical technique (malplacement or displacement)
Ventricular collapse from excessive drainage causing the tip of the catheter to impinge through the ependyma or brain substance
Pseudocyst formation with defective drainage

VA, ventriculoatrial; VP, ventriculoperitoneal; TP, thecoperitoneal.

is about the same as for ventriculoperitoneal shunts but the technique avoids the need for cortical puncture. The opposite may occur with VP shunts, the aqueduct may close and the patient become totally shunt dependent. More recent lumboperitoneal shunt operations can be performed without a laminectomy.

Various other routes, such as ventriculopleural, ventriculo-thoracic duct, etc., have been used but are not a modern practical alternative.

Shunt and separate reservoir

Separate reservoirs have been used for acute surgical decompression since the early 1960s. They have been used to instil chemotherapeutic agents into the CNS in malignant disease and in the management of preterm intraventricular hemorrhage.

In Edinburgh the management of children with hydrocephalus has involved both the use of a shunt and a separate CSF access device (reservoir), which is inserted into the frontal horn of the right lateral ventricle at the same time as the primary shunt surgery. A study to assess the risks attendant on this policy showed no extra mortality or morbidity.[36] There was less chance of the initial shunt blocking and a lesser incidence of visual and schooling handicap. The double cortical puncture did not result in an increased incidence of hemiplegia or epilepsy. The separate reservoir greatly eased the detection and management of raised intracranial pressure, shunt infection and ventriculitis. Children who only have shunts in situ may have optic discs that become scarred and unreliable as indicators of raised intracranial pressure and frequently the presentation may be subtle with, for example, a decline in school performance. Since there are no absolutely reliable signs or symptoms of raised pressure, the only means of detection is by direct measurement of the intraventricular pressure, which is easy when the reservoir is present.

Many children with shunted hydrocephalus will still present with the usual childhood illnesses and infections and symptoms of these are often impossible to differentiate from those due to shunt malfunction. With the facility for intracranial monitoring via a reservoir, the presence of raised pressure or infection can be detected in a matter of minutes rather than with prolonged inpatient observation and repeated CT scanning, etc. In the Edinburgh study,[36] in 58% of admissions where a tap was thought necessary to exclude raised pressure or infection, normal values for both pressure and cell counts were obtained, thus avoiding the need for unnecessary emergency shunt surgery. If raised pressure is found, it can be lowered by CSF removal via the reservoir. If repeated taps do not effectively normalize the pressure, closed external ventricular drainage can be easily instituted via the reservoir, allowing replacement of the shunt by elective rather than emergency surgery. This was the case in 60 admissions, in the above series, where the intracranial pressure was controlled by intermittent or continuous ventricular drainage.

The presence of a reservoir also has the advantage of an immediate diagnosis or exclusion of ventriculitis and therapy can be immediately instituted by direct instillation of the appropriate antibiotic into the ventricles, with monitoring of the CSF cell counts and antibiotic levels. In the Edinburgh series,[36] in 28 admissions, the reservoir was used to treat the infection while simultaneously controlling the raised intracranial pressure. With this method of management there is virtually no mortality from ventriculitis and one also expects a near zero infection rate from shunt and reservoir replacement (Table 20.7).

Shunt blockage

The Edinburgh series is shown in Table 20.8.[36] Survival analyses showed no significant relationship between the onset of mechanical blockage and the type of shunt, the age at reservoir insertion, the sex of the child, the etiology of hydrocephalus or the time relationship of the shunt insertion to reservoir insertion. The reduction in complications with the introduction of the reservoir may be due to the ability to measure directly the intracranial pressure and so reduce the number of unnecessary shunt revisions (Table 20.8).

Ventriculitis

Ventriculitis is diagnosed on the basis of a positive ventricular CSF culture with or without pleocytosis.

Many factors influence the incidence of shunt infection, such as the length of operation, the skin preparation and the type of shunt, but infection remains a problem in a significant number of children with shunts. It can be difficult to diagnose and there is still controversy about the optimum management. Several different treatment regimes have been suggested, including vancomycin into the shunt and systemic therapy with oral trimethoprim and

Table 20.8 Incidence of shunt problems before and after reservoir insertion

Period	Number of episodes (episodes per child shunt year)			
	Serious shunt failure	Blockage	Infection	Ventriculitis
Prereservoir period 219 child shunt years	99 (0.45)	75 (0.29)	24 (0.11)	37 (0.17)
Postreservoir period 269 child shunt years	77 (0.29)*	55 (0.20)*	22 (0.08) ns	28 (0.10) ns

Figures in brackets = per child shunt year.
* = *P* 0.01 cf. pre- and postreservoir periods.

rifampicin. Others have advocated that infection can only be eradicated successfully by removal of the shunt.

It is our practice to subject the CSF to cytological techniques of cytocentrifugation and millipore filter collection. This improves the identification of cell types in the CSF. It is especially useful in cases of mild CSF pleocytosis. Routine biochemistry is also performed on the separated CSF specimen. The vast majority of episodes of ventriculitis are due to *Staphylococcus albus* with occasional cases of *Escherichia coli*. Neurosurgical intervention increases the number of cells in the CSF transiently but infection may occur in the early postoperative period so the need for accurate cell type identification is clear. Macrophages can persist in the CSF for a long time and these need to be distinguished from the mild persisting pleocytosis of active infection when there are equal numbers of neutrophils, lymphocytes and macrophages. Macrophages indicate that there is an active repair process going on. Intrathecal penicillin and cephalosporins can also produce a CSF pleocytosis, i.e. a chemical ventriculitis.

It is imperative that treatment is begun immediately. Intrathecal and intravenous vancomycin is now preferred to gentamicin, complemented by intravenous rifampicin. Where hypersensitivity or resistance is a problem teicoplanin or meropenem offer useful alternatives. Raised ventricular pressure is controlled. Occasionally there may be organisms present in the CSF which have not yet excited a cellular response, and very few cells are found. In only three episodes of ventriculitis, in our series, were there less than 100 cells/ml. Shunt infections may also be associated with a negative organism culture. Because many of these children are highly shunt dependent, once the shunt is removed (which is necessary in ventriculitis because the organisms hide within mucoprotein colonies within the shunt tubing) it is imperative that their pressure is managed by tapping or draining CSF from the reservoir. It is also critical that shunt reinsertion is not done before the CSF is sterilized.

There is a significant discordance between lymphocytes and macrophages in the CSF. Neurosurgery may lead to a 20% increase in neutrophils on the first postoperative day with a progressive decline to a mean of 10 cells (range 7–12) on the fourth postoperative day. There is also a small decrease in the number of lymphocytes on the first postoperative day followed by an increase on the second day. Macrophages are reduced by 12% on the first postoperative day and then steadily increase from the second to the fourth day.

Slit ventricle syndrome

Effects of acute CSF decompression. This results in a low-pressure headache, delayed valve pump refilling, a depressed fontanel and possibly an upward brainstem cone (apnea, bradycardia, syncope, hypotension, stridor and hemiparesis).

Effects of chronic CSF decompression. These include acquired craniosynostosis, skull deformity, a thickened skull vault, microcephaly, hyperpneumatization of the sinuses, pneumocranium (tension), subdural hematoma, hygroma, cephalocranial disproportion, slit ventricle syndrome (total or partial ventricular collapse), enlarged cortical vascular bed, partial stripped ependymal lining, gliotic scar tissue (subependymal and white matter), wide open Virchow–Robin spaces and decreased intracranial compliance.

In patients with normotensive hydrocephalus the normal ICP in the sitting position is negative and approximately −5 mmHg. Following a shunt insertion in the erect position, the pressures are approximately −18 mmHg. Therefore, in most situations, with the patient upright and mobile during the day, the pressures will be negative, but when supine and during REM sleep, there may be significant elevation of pressure. This has given rise to the concept of slit ventricles and the 'slit ventricle syndrome'. Our own studies suggest 10% have radiological slit ventricles, but only 1% were symptomatic.

The slit ventricle syndrome incorporates three components: intermittent or chronic headache secondary to episodic ventricular catheter obstruction; slit-like (Y shaped) ventricles on CT scan; and a slowed refill of the palpable valve mechanism.

The pathogenesis of the slit ventricle syndrome involves a siphon effect of continuing CSF flow down a shunt tubing (particularly with the ventriculoperitoneal route), excessive drainage from thecoperitoneal shunts in patients who are predominantly in the upright posture and the possibility that, with ventriculoatrial shunts, the diastolic phase of blood flow may encourage CSF withdrawal from the distal end of the shunt.

The management of slit ventricle syndrome has involved several procedures such as the use of high-pressure valves, an antisiphon device, a valve upgrade together with an antisiphon device, a subtemporal decompression, a volume-regulated shunt system, an antisiphon ventricular catheter (that is incorporated into the shunt) and lastly the use of steroids and the head-down position.

OTHER TREATMENTS

Choroid plexectomy

This operation has been used to treat hydrocephalus, but in most cases hydrocephalus is due to an increased resistance to drainage rather than an oversecretion of CSF and a reduction of over 50% of CSF production may not produce any substantial effect on the degree of hydrocephalus or pressure. Even patients showing relief of symptoms may relapse after a period of months. Animal experiments have shown that, in those plexectomized, the CSF production rate falls by about one-third.

Drug effects on CSF production

A number of drugs have been shown to have an effect on the rate of production of CSF, but it is unlikely that even with a substantial reduction in CSF this could be a definitive management for progressive hydrocephalus. However, there may be additional measures to help control CSF pressure in different situations, e.g. with the patient on external ventricular drainage due to ventriculitis. Furosemide (Frusemide) and acetazolamide reduce CSF production by virtue of their carbonic anhydrase inhibitory effect. Acetazolamide, while it reduces CSF production, has only a transitory effect and isosorbide (a sorbitol derivative), which acts as an osmotic diuretic, is unpalatable and may produce hypernatremia and metabolic acidosis. For any acute rise in intracranial pressure associated with hydrocephalus, mannitol may reduce the pressure sufficiently to prevent coning. Other drugs with receptor sites on the choroid plexus may also reduce CSF production without diminishing overall choroidal perfusion.

Other procedures

Additional procedures include third ventriculostomy (the opening of the ventricular CSF system into the subarachnoid space via the lamina terminalis) and ventriculocisternostomy (Torkildsen shunt) between the ventricle and the basal cisterns. These are reliant on a block being present in the CSF outflow from the ventricles with an intact subarachnoid space and surface CSF pathways, with a normal reabsorptive capacity. In purely obstructive hydrocephalus, such as aqueduct stenosis, 70% require no further surgical intervention. Its use in other circumstances, and in particular those under 6 months of age, requires further study and definition.[40]

When there is ventriculitis, meningitis, blood in CSF or other factors making the insertion of a CSF shunt impracticable, then a temporary measure may be necessary, such as ventricular tap through the anterior fontanel. As previously mentioned, a puncture may result in porencephaly and it is preferable to have neurosurgical assistance and have a temporary reservoir implanted.

SPECIFIC TREATMENT REGIMENS

Posthemorrhagic hydrocephalus

This is common in premature infants following periventricular hemorrhage (PVH) but may occur in other age groups as well. Posthemorrhagic ventricular dilation in prematures may be assessed by serial ultrasound to compare the ventricular index (above) to the centiles for age. Approximately one-third of infants with a PVH will develop posthemorrhagic ventricular dilation and one-fifth of these will require a CSF shunt. Only about one in five cases of dilation are due to outlet obstruction at the fourth ventricle.

Distinguishing progressive hydrocephalus with high pressure, i.e. pressure-driven ventricular dilation, from brain atrophy in such circumstances requires ultrasound or imaging scans and pressure measurements. In atrophy the ventricles retain their usual configuration and do not have loss of the normal angles of the lateral ventricles.

There is no ideal or single method for managing posthemorrhagic hydrocephalus. Repeated lumbar punctures may prevent the need for shunting and will certainly ameliorate progressive ventricular dilation but the pressure should be measured at the same time with CSF removal to reduce the pressure level to normal. It is associated with an increased risk of infection[41] and it has been suggested that it be replaced with alternatives[42] such as early ventriculosubgaleal shunting.[43]

Acetazolamide in a dose 100 mg/kg per 24 h, and furosemide (frusemide) in a dose of 1 mg/kg per day have been shown to be ineffective in decreasing the rate of shunt placement.[44] Ventriculoperitoneal shunting is not done until the CSF hemorrhage has cleared sufficiently to avoid blocking the shunt. Brydon et al[45,46] indicate that it is cells that adversely affect shunt performance rather than CSF protein concentration.

The elective insertion of a ventricular reservoir will allow measurement and treatment of raised pressure by sequential taps. The hydrocephalus may arrest or the patient may subsequently need a ventriculoperitoneal shunt.

Tuberculous meningitis

Details of its presentation and management are given in the central nervous system infection section. Here special consideration will be given to its presentation with coma or deterioration with coma once treatment is initiated. Ventricular dilation is present in nearly 80% of these cases though it is uncommon in adult tuberculous meningitis. The immediate management is to have a CT scan done and to attend to the raised ventricular pressure; the child may sustain serious sequelae, or die, as a result of untreated or unrecognized pressure. The emergency insertion of a ventriculostomy reservoir allows measurement of the ventricular pressure and decompression by CSF removal. A diagnostic lumbar puncture may then be carried out. Pressure is measured at the time of lumbar puncture and comparison can be made with the ventricular measurement to see whether there is any spinal block (Froin's syndrome). CSF is then removed for cytocentrifuge cell count, protein, Ziehl–Nielsen, etc. in order to confirm the diagnosis of tuberculous meningitis.

The raised pressure, which may continue for many days, can be treated by intermittent taps of the reservoir, or by closed external ventricular drainage against a pressure head of 10 mmHg. Routine antituberculous chemotherapy is commenced and both the infection and the pressure are monitored and treated carefully over the next 2 weeks. The use of intrathecal steroid preparations may be necessary if there is a spinal block or a basal adhesive arachnoiditis.

Early CSF shunting is an alternative way to control the pressure while treating the infection, but the shunt will need to be replaced if it becomes colonized and shunt dependence continues. Alternatively a temporary shunt may be sufficient to control the pressure while attempting to sterilize the CSF. Although earlier practice was routinely to carry out a lumbar puncture in suspected tuberculous meningitis (in most cases safely), there remains the possibility of coning at the time of diagnosis. These patients, and others who present in coma, must not have a lumbar puncture until a CT scan has been performed and the basal cisterns are seen to be patent.

Fetal hydrocephalus

See above under the Prenatal presentation of developmental brain abnormalities.

Prognosis

Natural history of untreated hydrocephalus

Several studies detail the course of untreated hydrocephalus. An average result from these studies indicates that approximately 50% survive and of the survivors, 25–30% have normal intelligence and 25–30% have severe motor and other handicaps.

Epilepsy

Localized injury to the frontal cortex raises a theoretical risk of precipitating seizures from frontal reservoirs. Also with a reservoir there are two cortical insults. Seizure disorders follow in about one in six children compared with a one in two risk with the siting of a single VP shunt frontally.

Hemiplegia

Hemiplegia is the commonest type of cerebral palsy complicating hydrocephalus associated with spina bifida. This accounts for about 20% of children with congenital hemiplegic cerebral palsy.

The hemiplegia in hydrocephalus may be due to the etiology (e.g. prematurity or meningitis) or may be a complication of the hydrocephalus as a result of parenchymal hemorrhage from brain puncture, traumatic puncture of the internal capsule, siting of the shunt to involve the motor strip, subdural hematomata as a result of overdrainage, cortical thrombophlebitis or basilar arachnoiditis or precipitation of status epilepticus with postconvulsive hemiplegia or puncture porencephaly.

Vision

Blindness is not a problem of untreated hydrocephalus but sudden total blindness may result from raised pressure due to shunt malfunction. Gaston,[47] in studying a group of spina bifida children, found only 27% of 322 had normal visual function. In the Edinburgh study only one child (n = 56 over 12 years) had visual handicap which was of a severity for the child to be registered as blind and 88% had normal visual function. Visual impairment in children with hydrocephalus may result from optic atrophy secondary to chronic papilledema, distension of the third ventricle with chiasmal compression, posterior cerebral artery compression with ischemia of the optic radiation or calcarine cortex or selective posterior horn dilation leading to gross thinning of the calcarine cortex. These are all due to raised pressure with hydrocephalus.

Intelligence

Some 50–60% of shunted hydrocephalic children have normal IQs. In our study group 65% of children were in normal education, 29% were educated in special schools and 6% were in residential care for the severely handicapped. The pathophysiological mechanisms whereby learning is impaired include an associated cortical dysplasia, marked thinning of the cortical mantle (less than 15 mm), ventriculitis, chronically reduced cerebral perfusion pressure and coincidental parenchymatous brain damage (meningitis, asphyxia, etc.).

THE NEUROCUTANEOUS DISEASES

The last decade has seen important advances in the identification of the causes of the neurocutaneous syndromes. Neurofibromatosis 1 (NF1) and NF2 are two diseases caused by separate genes, whilst tuberous sclerosis (TSC) 1 and 2 is one disease caused by separate genes. Increasing involvement by parents and families, advances in neuroimaging and molecular genetics have all led to important advances in our understanding of these disorders.

NEUROFIBROMATOSIS 1 IN CHILDHOOD

NF1 is the most common single gene disorder to affect the human nervous system with an estimated incidence of 1 in 3000.

Diagnostic criteria for NF1: Two or more of the following are required:

1. six or more café-au-lait spots (at least 1.5 cm post-puberty, at least 0.5 cm pre-puberty);
2. two or more neurofibromas or one or more plexiform neurofibromata;
3. axillary or inguinal freckling;
4. optic glioma;
5. two or more Lisch nodules (benign iris hamartomas);
6. osseous dysplasia on the sphenoid bone or cortex of a long bone;
7. a first degree relative with NF1.[48]

About a third of young people with NF1 have short stature and almost 50% have a head circumference at or above the 97th centile. NF1 is a multisystem disorder associated with a wide variety of complications. The most common are plexiform neurofibromas, learning disability, optic gliomas and scoliosis occurring in 15–50% of affected individuals. More than 50% of people with NF1 will be mildly affected and may not even know they carry the gene.

Plexiform neurofibromas occur in about 25% of individuals with NF1. They carry the potential for cosmetic disfigurement and malignant transformation often extending deeply into underlying tissues. Here they may cause compression or distortion of adjacent structures.

Specific learning difficulties are most common in NF1 with a frequency of between 30 and 60%. The frequency of global learning difficulties is only slightly higher than in the general population. There is no specific learning disability profile.

Optic nerve gliomas are the most common central nervous system tumors in NF1 occurring in up to 20% but only 30–50% will become symptomatic. They can involve any part of the visual pathway and take the form of low-grade pilocytic astrocytomas. All symptomatic tumors are diagnosed before 6 years of age. They rarely progress once they have been discovered. Thus whereas formal ophthalmological assessment is indicated up to the age of 10 years, after this age annual routine clinical assessment of acuity and visual fields is sufficient.

A scoliosis occurs in up to 20% of those with NF1 and usually appears before the age of 10 years of age if it is going to appear.

Neuroimaging features

Areas of increased signal intensity on T2 weighted images with magnetic resonance imaging occur in 60–70% of children. They have been referred to as UBOs (unidentified bright objects). They generally disappear during late teenage years or the early 20s.

The genetics of NF1

This is an autosomal dominant disorder although 50% of cases are sporadic. The NF1 gene has been mapped to chromosome 17 and codes the protein Neurofibromin. This has a high sequence homology with GAP (GTPase) activator protein. These proteins have an important role in cell growth and differentiation. The genetics of the disorder will be dealt with in more detail in Chapter 12.

NEUROFIBROMATOSIS 2 (NF2)

The diagnosis is based on the following criteria:[48]

1. Bilateral VIII nerve masses detected on neuroimaging.
2. A first degree relative with NF2 and either unilateral VIII nerve mass or two of the following:
   - Neurofibroma
   - Meningioma
   - Glioma
   - Schwannoma
   - Juvenile posterior subcapsular lenticular opacity.

NF2 usually presents in adult life, though many childhood cases have been described. Presentation is usually with progressive deterioration associated with tumors with loss of hearing, difficulty with walking, loss of sight or chronic pain being the most common features.

NF2 should be suspected in children presenting with any of these tumors but fewer than six café-au-lait patches.[49] It is unusual for children with NF2 to present with features other than those due to a tumor.

The genetics of NF2

NF2 is very rare with a birth incidence of 1 in 40 000. It shows autosomal dominant transmission with nearly full penetrance.

The NF2 gene maps to the long arm of chromosome 22 and codes a member of the protein 4.1 family of cytoskeletal associated elements. For further details see Chapter 12.

Subtle skin tumors often characterized by small well conscribed lesions found on the trunk or face, which after adolescence become roughened with overlying coarse hair, are a clue to the disorder, along with the lenticular opacities. A meningioma or Schwannoma in the child should raise the possibility of NF2.

TUBEROUS SCLEROSIS COMPLEX

There have been recently revised diagnostic criteria for tuberous sclerosis complex (TSC).[50]

Major features:

1. Facial angiofibromas or forehead plaque
2. Non-traumatic ungual or periungual fibroma
3. Hypomelanotic macules (more than three)
4. Shagreen patch (connective tissue nevus)
5. Multiple retinal nodular hamartoma
6. Cortical tuber
7. Subependymal nodule
8. Subependymal giant cell astrocytoma
9. Cardiac rhabdomyoma, single or multiple
10. Lymphangiomyomatosis
11. Renal angiomyolipoma.

Minor features:

1. Multiple randomly distributed pits in dental enamel
2. Hamartomatous rectal polyps
3. Bone cyst
4. Cerebral white matter radial migration lines
5. Gingival fibromas
6. Non-renal hamartoma
7. Retinal achromic patch
8. 'Confetti' skin lesions
9. Multiple renal cysts.

Definite TCS: Either two major features or one major feature plus two minor features.

Probable TCS: One major plus one minor feature.

Possible TCS: Either one major feature or two more minor features.

Clinical presentation

Seizures are by far the most common neurological condition in TSC, occurring at some point in up to 90% of young people with the disorder. Infantile spasms occur in about one-third. The earlier the onset of seizures, the greater the risk of them being intractable and being associated with cognitive and behavioral impairments. If seizures present after the age of 2 years then attendant learning difficulties may be mild or absent.

The antiepileptic drug vigabatrin is noted to be particularly efficacious in tuberous sclerosis. The risk of associated retinopathy always needs to be considered carefully when this drug is used. As in all children where the epilepsy is intractable the question of the use of surgery for epilepsy needs to be considered. Multifocal lesions often make this impracticable.

Learning difficulties are commonly (probably up to 40%) found in TSC. There is also a strong association between TSC and autism, particularly as an outcome of infantile spasms. Early reported associations between autism and temporal lobe lesions or a high number of tubers seem not to have been borne out by more recent study.

It is the skin lesion, hypomelanotic (ash leaves) macules, periungual or gingival fibromas and thickened firm areas of subcutaneous tissue often on the lower back (shagreen patch) or forehead and face (fibrous plaques), which offer the most ready diagnostic clue. Adenoma sebaceum does not occur until late childhood or early adolescence. It is an angiofibroma (cutaneous hamartoma) (Figs 20.12, 20.13a and b) which initially appears as flat reddish macular lesions, which become increasingly erythematous. Papular nodules over the bridge of the nose and higher cheek (in a butterfly distribution), often noted in the presence of examination of a child with epilepsy, bring the disorder to the attention of clinicians. Magnetic resonance imaging usually then confirms the diagnosis by revealing tubers, subependymal nodules or subependymal giant cell astrocytomas. CT scanning is less sensitive and often fails to identify tubers. Subependymal calcification is often not present until the second year of life. In the first year of life ultrasound of the heart will reveal cardiac rhabdomyomas in up to 60% with TCS. Put the other way round any child with a rhabdomyoma in infancy is likely to have TSC. They later regress but occasionally may be the presenting feature where they lead to an obstructive cardiomyopathy.

Angiomyolipomas and renal cysts are noted in 45–50% of people with TCS. Renal disease is uncommon in childhood except in cases of polycystic disease. Pulmonary involvement is seen exclusively in adult women where cysts or lymphangioliomyomatosis may be associated with respiratory symptoms and hypertension.

Managing people with TS

The management of attendant epilepsy and learning difficulties is discussed in the relevant sections. In relation to problems, which are specific for TSC, it has been recommended that neuroimaging be carried out, perhaps two yearly, to check for the growth of subependymal giant cell astrocytomas. The cost effectiveness of the screening examinations is not clearly known. Our own policy is to respond to the assessment of new symptoms if they present.

Renal ultrasound needs to be carried out on presentation and then every 2–3 years to assess changes in angiomyolipomas or cysts, hopefully to allow operative intervention before the development of renal failure. An ECG is useful on presentation to

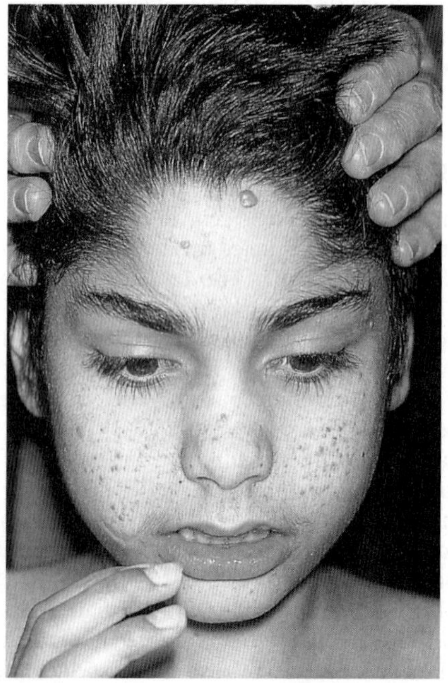

Fig. 20.12 Tuberous sclerosis: adenoma sebaceum.

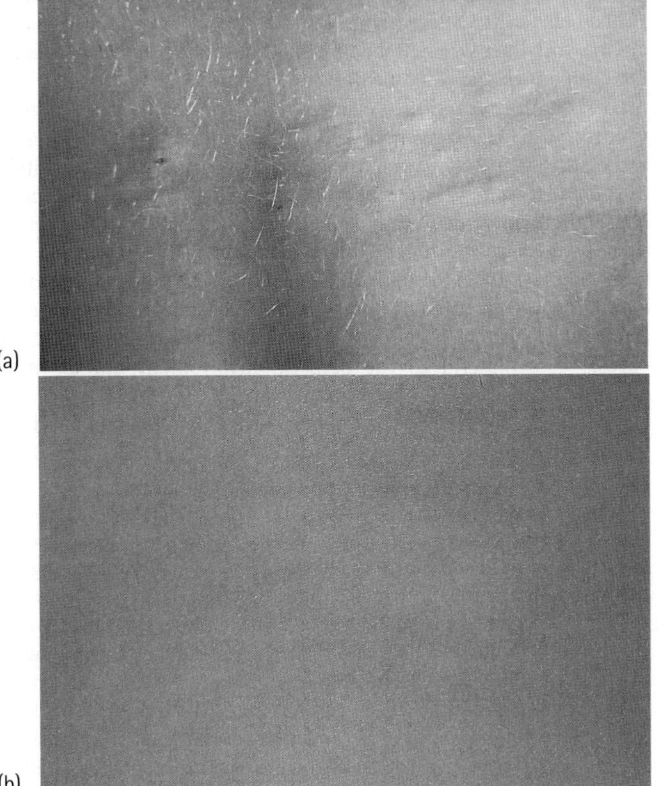

Fig. 20.13 Tuberous sclerosis: (a) Shagreen patch; (b) depigmented patches.

screen for the presence of any potentially life threatening cardiac arrhythmias.

The genetics of TCS

This is an autosomal dominant condition with a high spontaneous mutation rate. Gene loci for TSC have been identified on chromosome 9q34 (TSC1) and on chromosome 16p13 (TSC2). The TSC1 product is Hamartin and may act as a tumor suppressor. TSC2 encodes for Tuberin, which has GTPase activating properties and seems to function as a tumor suppressor. Hamartin and Tuberin cooperate to regulate cellular growth and differentiation. The genetics of TSC will be dealt with in more detail in Chapter 12.

ATAXIA TELANGIECTASIA

This is a rare autosomal recessive disorder with incidence between 1 in 40–300 000.

Presentation

The main neurological feature is the ataxia. Children often learn to walk at a normal age, but throughout the toddler years appear to be clumsy. Then often after entering school the clumsiness becomes more evident and leads to referral. They have a wide based gait but often demonstrate excessive adduction of the leg during the passing phase on foot strike causing a stagger to the outside of the base. They may choose a toe-walking gait and prefer to run everywhere rather than walk. More typical features of cerebellar ataxia then ensue often superimposed by choreiform movement, the latter being a variable feature.

Very often children lose the ability to walk independently between the ages of 8 years and about 12 years. Similarly after the age of 5 there is a deterioration of speech, the pattern of which carries the features of cerebellar dysfunction. Bulbar function then becomes increasingly involved raising the risk of aspiration. This often in due course leads to the requirement for gastrostomy feeding.

Children with the condition also demonstrate an oculomotor dyspraxia. This involves no problem with vertical eye movement, but when trying to follow an object through the horizontal plane the head is moved quickly to follow the object leaving the eyes behind, the latter then restituting on the object once it has stopped moving. This leads to a characteristic flick of the head that is readily perceived.

Around the age of 10 years an axonal polyneuropathy appears with loss of the deep tendon reflexes.

The associated telangiectasia is often evident across the top of the shoulders, on the ears, and on the conjunctiva. This tends to become more obvious as children get older.

Premature aging features often appear in people as they move through the teenage years and early adult life with the appearance of gray hairs and aging of the skin with diminution of subcutaneous tissue. Vitiligo may also appear along with hyperpigmented areas.

Up to 80% of children with the condition will have diminished levels of IgA and IgG 2 (less frequently IgE and IgM). They have a diminished cell-mediated response to intradermal antigens and atrophy of the thymus. Infections of the sinuses and lungs are common with bacterial pneumonia being the major cause of death.

The problem with immunity is also associated with malignancy, tending to be lymphoreticular disorders in childhood and solid tumors in adult life.

Genetics of ataxia telangiectasia (AT)

The gene known as ataxia telangiectasia mutated (ATM gene) is found at chromosome location 11q22–23. ATM deficient cells lack of sensor of double stranded DNA breaks, which would normally suppress the mitotic cycle pending repair. Cell division therefore proceeds and is likely to be directly responsible for the frequent chromosomal rearrangements seen in AT cells.

Diagnostic criteria

The clinical diagnosis is usually straightforward due to the constellation and characteristic features including the oculomotor dyspraxia and deteriorating cerebellar signs. With the identification of the ATM gene a new molecular standard of diagnosis is available. The finding of an elevated alpha-fetoprotein (at least twice the upper limit) along with reduced immunoglobulin levels in the presence of the typical neurological picture, substantiates the case for requesting the genetic study. The gene test has now replaced chromosome fragility studies.

It must be remembered some children present, before neurological signs have appeared, with acute lymphoblastic leukemia. If these children have an oculomotor dyspraxia then a careful search of the skin ought to be made for the telangiectasis and the ATM gene analysis.

OTHER DNA REPAIR DISORDERS

Xeroderma pigmentosum

This is also a DNA repair disorder with autosomal recessive inheritance. Its cardinal feature is acute sun sensitivity, often leading in infancy to erythematous and bullous skin lesions. Freckles and hypopigmentation are common, along with dryness, telangiectasis and, at times, skin atrophy. Ectoderm around the eye also shows light sensitivity and may lead to blepharitis, iritis or conjunctivitis with keratitis and edema of the cornea, occasionally leading to ulceration and opacification. Susceptibility to skin neoplasia is very high, and all affected young people should have their eyes and skin inspected weekly for new lesions.

About 20% have associated neurological problems (a much higher percentage in Japan) and, in its severest form, microcephaly, progessive dementia, choreoathetosis, ataxia and spasticity are seen, along with a progressive peripheral neuropathy. Sensorineural deafness may also be progressive.

Management is by way of reducing exposure to ultraviolet light as much as possible and the aggressive early treatment of skin cancer.

Cockayne syndrome

This autosomal recessive condition leads to small stature, severe sun sensitivity, ocular, skeletal and neurological abnormalities. The most common findings are optic atrophy, pigmentary retinal degeneration, cataracts, sensorineural deafness and an extrapyramidal movement disorder, in addition to spasticity of the lower extremities with flexion contractures.

At birth, babies are of normal size but significant feeding difficulties and subsequent growth failure leads them to become progressively cachetic. At this time they acquire a distinctive facial appearance with a thin prominent nose and zygomatic processes, prognathism, enophthalmos and absent fat. This appearance is usually well developed by the teens, and neurological abnormalities largely resemble those of xeroderma pigmentosum, which may well exist in some young people. Many young people die in their teens in status epilepticus or with malignant hypertension, or renal and pulmonary dysfunction.

Incontinentia pigmenti

As this condition predominantly affects girls, it is thought to be an X-linked dominant condition, probably lethal in males in utero. The central nervous system is involved in 30–50%. A cerebral dysgenesis leads to delayed development with seizures, spastic paralysis and cerebellar signs in some. The degree of learning difficulty varies greatly. Associated with this there may be a retinal dysplasia leading to a retrolental mass and skeletal and teeth abnormalities.

The skin abnormality is seen in three distinct stages. In the first 2 weeks of life erythematous, macular, papular, vesicular, bullous or pustular lesions occur proximally in a linear distribution. This is in association with an eosinophilia. In the following 2–3 weeks pustular, lichenoid, verrucous, keratotic and dyskeratotic lesions occur more distally and as they resolve, often leave areas of atrophied skin. In the third stage, areas of pigmentation appear over a period of some weeks.

OTHER NEUROCUTANEOUS SYNDROMES

Sturge–Weber syndrome

This is a sporadic condition involving a malformation of cephalic-venous microvasculature. There is an abnormality in the growth of the primordial vascular plexus in cephalic mesenchyme as it lies between the epidermis and the telencephalic vesicles in close proximity to the optic cup. This leads in its fullest form to a cavernous angioma of the leptomeninges, a facial angiomatous nevus and a choroidal angioma of the eye. The lesion may be unilateral or bilateral and in individual children may affect one or all of brain, eye or skin tissue. The lack of cerebral or ocular symptoms does not preclude them developing at a later date where the facial nevus is present. Sturge–Weber syndrome is not usually applied when neither cerebral nor ocular symptoms have appeared.

The port wine-colored stain on the face is evident at birth and always involves the first division of the trigeminal nerve. Involvement of the skin on that side may be more widespread and there is an association in some with the Klippel–Trenauney syndrome. This syndrome involves angiomatous skin nevi in association with bony hypertrophy, lymphangiomas or varicosities; the genetics are not defined. A bilateral facial nevus does not mean bilateral cerebral involvement. Seizures are seen in up to 90% of those involved. Abnormal venous return with blood stagnation and hypoxemia coupled with a high metabolic demand of neurones exhibiting seizure activity often lead to a progressive functional problem. Neurological signs emerge, often starting as a postictal paresis contralateral to the cerebral involvement but at times consolidating into a permanent paresis as time goes on. Hemianopias, dysphasias, or quadriparesis may also occur. Where the seizures are intractable and infrequent there are very often associated learning difficulties.

Buphthalmos or glaucoma may accompany a choroidal angiomatous lesion and may be present at birth. Rarely, hydrocephalus has been reported but intracranial hemorrhage is exceptionally rare.

In the presence of a facial nevus full radiological assessment of the brain should be carried out with serial CT scanning with contrast to define the extent of the angiomatous lesion. Magnetic resonance imaging offers an even more sensitive technique for this. Intracerebral angioma may become more obvious with the passing of time. Calcification of the lesion becomes prominent. This should be accompanied by a full electroencephalographic assessment of seizure activity.

Management involves regular assessment of ocular pressure. Seizure control is difficult to attain at times. Where the vascular anomalies and seizure discharge are confined to one hemisphere, an early surgical resection of the lesion may offer benefit where the seizures are intractable. The evidence shows that residual handicap is minimized when lobectomy or hemispherectomy is performed in the early weeks with many children surviving with little sign of a hemiparesis or hemianopia. However, exact criteria for this early intervention have yet to be laid down, as there are some children in whom a seizure disorder presenting at an early stage stabilizes.

Hypomelanosis of Ito

In some families, this is an autosomal dominant disorder, but in most there is no clear family history. Chromosomal abnormalities including balanced translocation have been described in at least two children. The skin lesion is of linear vorticose or irregular areas of hypopigmentation. These may affect one or both sides of the body and be associated with lesions of the iris or hemihypertrophy.

The central nervous system is affected in at least 50%. Those with seizures in the first year of life are most likely to have a static encephalopathy associated with significant learning difficulties.

The pathology of both skin and brain is very reminiscent of that seen in tuberous sclerosis, neurofibromatosis and in incontinentia pigmenti. They are considered the non-specific result of a dysplasia or embryopathy affecting the central nervous system and the skin. At about 15 weeks' gestation the melanoblasts migrate from the neural crest and mature to melanocytes in the skin. In the sixth month, the hair anlage is present, accounting for an association between abnormalities of cerebral cortex and hair. The number, size and pigment content of melanocytes in the basal area of the epidermis is generally reduced and in the brain the signs are of a neuronal migration defect, with microcephaly and a rostral displacement.

Linear sebaceous nevus syndrome

In its complete form, this syndrome includes a cutaneous nevus, with neurological and ocular abnormalities. The skin lesion may be of several types. The typical Jadassohn nevus may be visible at birth or in infancy, or become evident only after a few years. It is a slightly raised, yellow–orange, smooth, linear plaque that abuts the midline of the forehead, nose or lips and often involves the scalp. Over years, the lesion tends to become darker and verrucous. Early in life there is little pigment, and sebaceous glands are often not prominent. Later, sebaceous glands proliferate throughout the thickness of the skin.

Neurological manifestations consist mainly of learning disability, seizures and asymmetrical macrocephaly. Seizures are often partial, but infantile spasms have been reported. Hamartomatous tumors may be present and various other abnormalities have been seen including porencephaly arterial aneurysms, abnormal venous return and arachnoid cysts along with hemihypertrophy.

The most common eye abnormalities are dermoids or epidermoids of the conjunctiva and colobomas of the iris, choroid, retina or optic nerve.

The diagnosis may be difficult in early cases without visible nevus. Imaging reveals hypertrophy of one hemisphere, usually on the same side as the nevus, with enlargement of the ipsilateral ventricle and pachygyria with hypodense white matter.

SEIZURES, EPILEPSY AND OTHER PAROXYSMAL DISORDERS

INTRODUCTION

A seizure is any sudden clinical event. As such it is non-specific in its etiology and could arise as a result of a neurological or non-neurological disturbance. However, the term is often used synonymously with epileptic seizure, which can be defined as any clinical event arising as a result of epileptic activity of neurones in the brain. Epileptic activity involves the excessive and/or hypersynchronous electrical discharge of neurones, which, for practical purposes, are located within the cerebral cortex. Epilepsy is the tendency to have recurrent epileptic seizures. The term 'fit' is a lay term whose meaning is almost synonymous with epileptic seizure. A convulsion is any seizure (not necessarily epileptic) characterized by excessive, abnormal muscle contractions, which are usually bilateral. Epileptology abounds with terms many of which, though still used, are now obsolete. Included are 'grand mal' (big attack) and 'petit mal' (little attack).

The basic mechanisms which underlie the generation of seizures are incompletely understood, but involve abnormalities at the cell membrane level (ion channels and receptors) and in neuronal circuits. The electrical behavior of neurones is determined by ionic channels in the neuronal membrane, which are either voltage-gated or receptor (ligand)-gated. Voltage-gated ion channels determine the excitability of neurones as well as participating in the release of neurotransmitters. They are membrane-spanning proteins with a pore through which the ion can pass. A voltage sensor controls the opening of the pore and a selectivity sensor determines which type of ion can pass through the pore. Three main classes of voltage-gated ion channels have been described: Na^+, Ca^{2+}, and K^+. Sodium currents are involved in the generation of action potentials. Potassium currents cause hyperpolarization and hence stabilize the neuronal membrane. Both calcium and sodium currents are involved in the generation of burst discharges. These are discharges generated by certain classes of neurones when excited. They consist of a burst of action potentials produced as an all-or-nothing phenomenon. It is likely that burst discharges and other similar phenomena are important in the generation of some types of seizures. Ligand-gated ion channels are activated by the binding of a neurotransmitter to the ion channel's receptor. Gamma-aminobutyric acid (GABA) and glycine are inhibitory neurotransmitters whilst glutamate and aspartate are excitatory neurotransmitters. A useful, though simplistic model of epilepsy is that it involves an imbalance of excitatory and inhibitory neurotransmitter systems within the CNS.

It is likely that ion channel abnormalities (channelopathies) cause many epilepsies, particularly idiopathic epilepsies. For example, mutations in a neuronal nicotinic acetylcholine receptor have been shown to be associated with familial nocturnal frontal lobe epilepsy, in a potassium channel with benign familial neonatal seizures and in a sodium channel with generalized epilepsy with febrile seizures and severe myoclonic epilepsy of infancy.[51–55] Many antiepileptic drugs block voltage-gated ion channels. These include carbamazepine and phenytoin, both of which block sodium channels. Other antiepileptic drugs act either at ligand-gated ion channels or else interfere with the production, release, function or catabolism of neurotransmitters. For example, benzodiazepines and barbiturates bind to specific domains on subtypes of the GABA receptor and vigabatrin increases GABA inhibition by preventing the breakdown of GABA at synaptic clefts.[56]

Epileptic seizures involve groups of neurones interacting together abnormally. Neurones within the brain work within physiologically and anatomically defined circuits. Some of these are important in particular types of epilepsy. They include neocortical circuits involved in, for example, frontal and occipital lobe seizures, the limbic system, involved in mesial temporal lobe seizures and thalamocortical circuits involved in generalized epilepsies, particularly absence seizures.

The neocortex comprises six distinct layers. Function occurs within vertically arranged columns. However, there are abundant excitatory horizontal connections. It is thought that it is these columns which allow the rapid seizure propagation, which is a feature of many neocortical epilepsies. Moreover, the neocortex contains intrinsically bursting pyramidal cells, which may be involved in seizure initiation.

At least in adults, mesial temporal lobe epilepsy is the commonest cause of drug-resistant seizures. The mesial temporal lobe structures, including the hippocampus and amygdala are part of the limbic system. Groups of neurones within parts of the limbic system have relatively low thresholds for seizure generation. Again, this may relate in part to neurones with intrinsic bursting activity and may be augmented by loss of particular classes of neurones caused, for example, by prolonged febrile convulsions. Intimate connections within the limbic system allow seizures to propagate and determine the semiology of mesial temporal lobe seizures.

The thalami have rich connections to the cerebral cortex. Intrinsic membrane properties of thalamic neurones arising as a result of so-called low threshold calcium channels, cause it to generate low frequency oscillatory rhythms which appear to underlie both certain physiological phenomena and also pathological ones such as the 3 Hz spike–wave discharge seen in idiopathic generalized epilepsies. These consist of a spike caused by action potentials in both thalami and cortex followed by an after coming slow wave due to prolonged inhibition within the cortex.

EPIDEMIOLOGY AND NATURAL HISTORY

Epilepsy is the commonest serious neurological condition of childhood. However, it is not a single condition, but comprises many

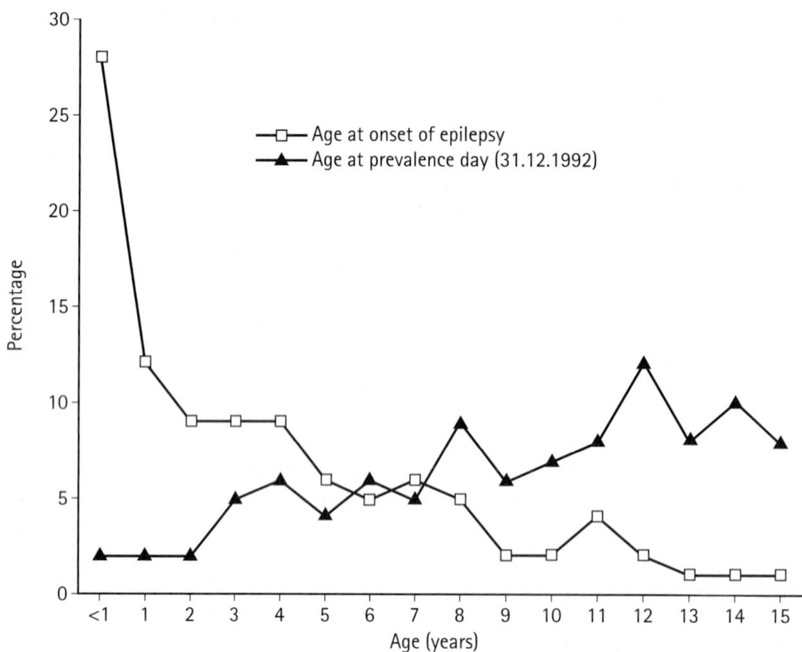

Fig. 20.14 Age specific incidence and prevalence of epilepsy in children. (From Eriksson & Koivikko 1997,[59] reprinted by permission of the journal Epilepsia)

different conditions. Epidemiological studies are bedevilled with problems as to which subjects to include. Rates vary according to whether neonatal, febrile and single seizures are included and according to how 'active epilepsy' is defined.[57]

In developed countries the crude annual incidence of epilepsy in children (excluding neonates) is around 60/100 000 children.[58] Rates are higher in developing countries. The incidence varies markedly with age (Fig. 20.14) and most studies report slightly higher rates in boys. The point prevalence of epilepsy in children is 3–6/1000.[58] Cumulative incidence rates are much higher than annual incidence rates. During childhood, prevalence rates for active epilepsy increase but not as fast as cumulative incidence rates, reflecting the effect of remission (Fig. 20.15).[61] The British National Child Development Study reported cumulative incidence rates for epilepsy of 4, 5, 7 and 8 per 1000 at ages 7, 11, 16 and 23 years

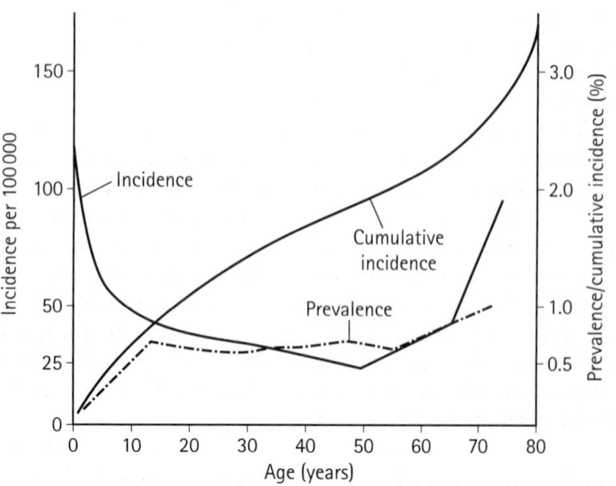

Fig. 20.15 Incidence, prevalence and cumulative incidence rates for epilepsy in an American population. (From Shorvon 1996,[60] reprinted by permission of the journal Epilepsia)

respectively and prevalence rates of 4, 4, 5 and 6 per 1000 at the same ages.[61] The lifetime prevalence of non-febrile seizures is between 1.5 and 5% of the population.[57] In other words, up to 5% of people will have at least one non-febrile seizure at some point in their life.

Recent data suggest that the incidence of epilepsy is falling in children but rising in the elderly. This may relate to improved standards of pre- and postnatal medical care, to better standards of maternal and child health and to the rise in life expectancy in the elderly coupled with more cerebrovascular disease. Although age-specific incidence and prevalence rates for epilepsy are higher in children than in adults (excluding extreme old age), the rates for treated epilepsy may be higher in adults than in children.[54] Epidemiological studies in both adults and children, which have taken particular care to classify seizure type, have suggested that focal epilepsies are more common than generalized epilepsies. In the British National Child Development Study after 23 years follow-up about 70% of those whose seizures were classifiable had focal epilepsies and 30% had generalized epilepsy; around 45% of both were symptomatic or probably symptomatic. The type of epilepsy could not be determined in around a fifth of subjects.[61] A number of recent studies have given information on the epidemiology of specific epilepsy syndromes in children.[59,62,63]

The previous view that epilepsy is a chronic disorder with little prospect of remission was mistaken. The majority of children who have a seizure have a good prognosis both in terms of the likelihood of seizure recurrence and of obtaining remission should recurrent seizures (i.e. epilepsy) develop. The risk of a further seizure is greatest immediately after the first and declines thereafter. Forty-five per cent of children who have a single seizure have a recurrence within 5 years, and once there has been one recurrent seizure further seizures become likely. The risk of having a third after a second, and a fourth after a third seizure at 5 years is 71 and 81% respectively.[64] Etiology is the main determinant of the risk of recurrence.[64–68]

Once recurrent epileptic seizures have occurred, an important issue is the probability of early remission. In a large prospective study 57% of children, 2 years after a diagnosis of epilepsy, had a 'good outcome' (a remission which had lasted more than 12 months), 12%

had a 'fair outcome' (a remission which had lasted 6–12 months) and 31% had a 'poor outcome' (a remission which had lasted less than 6 months).[69] Another study reported that at 2 years after diagnosis of epilepsy 53% of children had a 'good outcome' (a remission of more than a year), 8% had a 'bad outcome' (two or more antiepileptic drug failures and at least one seizure per month over an 18-month period) and 38% had an 'intermediate outcome'.[70] In about 80% of children who were followed for 4 or more years the outcome was similar to that at 2 years. However, around half of those with an intermediate outcome at 2 years achieved remission and 8% became intractable. Factors which are associated with the likelihood of a poor outcome include young age at seizure onset, symptomatic etiology, an initial presentation with status epilepticus or infantile spasms and high initial seizure number.[64,65,67]

Information on the long term prognosis of children with epilepsy is provided by the British National General Practice Study of Epilepsy.[71] In this study 86% of children of all ages, with a diagnosis of definite epilepsy, achieved a 3-year remission and 68% a 5-year remission, after 9 years. 'Remission' referred to a remission at any stage in the 3 or 5-year period. The proportions achieving a terminal remission (i.e. seizure free at the end of the follow-up period) of 3 and 5 years were 68% and 54% respectively, indicating that some children with prolonged remission subsequently relapsed. A very long prospective follow up study of childhood-onset epilepsy found that 64% of children had been seizure free for at least 5 years of whom 47% were not taking antiepileptic drug medication.[72] The study showed that the cumulative probabilities of a 5-year remission, at any point, with or without drugs, all increased with increasing years after the onset of epilepsy.

Long-term outcome studies have shown that epilepsy has adverse social outcomes whether or not the epilepsy was symptomatic and whether or not remission was achieved.[72,73] However, the outlook is considerably better in those with idiopathic seizures who achieve remission. Children with idiopathic epilepsies are reported, as adults, to have similar socioeconomic and/or employment status compared to matched controls without epilepsy, but they are less likely to marry.

The standardized mortality ratio of people with epilepsy (children and adults) is 2–3 times that of the general population.[74] Causes of death in children with epilepsy include accidents, status epilepticus and occasionally idiosyncratic reactions to drugs. As they enter teenage and adult years, suicide becomes increasingly important. Finally seizure-related death (death during or shortly after a seizure when there is no evidence of status epilepticus or when no other explanation for death is found at autopsy) and sudden unexpected death in epilepsy (SUDEP) (a non-traumatic, unwitnessed death occurring in a child with epilepsy who had previously been relatively healthy and for whom no cause of death is found even after postmortem examination) have been the subject of recent interest. By definition, the cause of such deaths is unknown. However, at least some may be caused by seizure-related cardiac arrhythmias. A population based study of SUDEP found an incidence of 0.27 per 1000 person-years in those under 14 years of age.[75]

The question as to whether antiepileptic drug treatment affects the prognosis for epilepsy (in terms of eventual remission of seizures) has perplexed clinicians and scientists. Although there are theoretical arguments why it might do, there is no evidence that it does.[65,76,77] Antiepileptic drugs may be used to suppress distressing symptoms, but not in the expectation that they are likely to change the natural history of the condition, at least in the large majority of children. Possible exceptions to this are some of the epileptic encephalopathies.

INVESTIGATIONS

EEG

Introduction

The EEG is the single most useful investigation in children with seizure disorders. However, it is frequently misused, overinterpreted and, because many clinicians are unaware of its full potential, underutilized.

The EEG gives a visual representation of differences in electrical potential between different areas of the brain. These reflect underlying neuronal activity. Most EEGs are recorded from the scalp using an array of 20 electrodes, although smaller numbers are sometimes used, particularly in young children. The EEG does not record the absolute potential at a particular electrode. Rather differences in potential between consecutive pairs of electrodes may be recorded (bipolar recordings) or else differences in potential between each electrode may be compared to a common reference electrode (referential recording). The EEG was traditionally recorded on paper, with the potential at each electrode used to cause a deflection of a marker pen. The sequence of electrodes displayed on the EEG trace is called the montage. In any one paper recording, a number of different montages using both bipolar and referential recordings is used in order to best detect normal and abnormal EEG features originating from different parts of the brain. Today most EEGs are recorded digitally and displayed on VDU screens. Other than storage considerations, the advantage of digital recording is that once the data are recorded, computerized reformating and manipulations enable far more information to be obtained than was possible on paper systems. It is, for example, possible to display the same data in numerous different bipolar and referential montages, filters can be added or taken away to remove artefacts which obscure the underlying EEG and EEG features can be precisely timed.

Interictal EEG

Most EEGs are recorded between seizures (interictal recording). A standard interictal EEG is usually recorded for 10–60 min. The EEG trace can be analyzed in terms of ongoing or background activity and episodic or paroxysmal activity. For both, normal and abnormal patterns occur. The background activity includes various physiological rhythms, including the well-known alpha rhythm. It is dramatically different in the premature neonate compared with the mature adult. In general, the EEG becomes increasingly synchronized and physiological rhythms become faster with maturity. The background EEG also changes with the level of arousal. For example, as an older child passes from alert to drowsy to light and then to deep sleep, a drop out in the alpha rhythm occurs, followed by progressive slowing.

Paroxysmal EEG activity is any activity which stands out from the background. There are numerous physiological paroxysmal EEG features which, like background features, are age and state dependent.

Most EEGs also contain artefact, which is not caused by electrical activity of the brain. Some artefacts relate to physiological functions such as eye, head and breathing movements and the electrical activity of the heart. Muscle artefact, which is in effect an EMG recording, is also common. Extraneous artefacts may be caused by poor electrode contact, by the mains electrical source and by nearby electrical equipment. Some artefacts can be very difficult to distinguish from cerebral activity.

Abnormalities of the EEG background are usually rather non-specific and of limited value when investigating children with seizure disorders. Focal background abnormalities, generally with slowing, reduction in amplitude and loss of physiological rhythms may reflect focal brain abnormalities giving rise to seizures, such as brain tumors, infarcts and abscesses. However, all are better diagnosed by neuroimaging. In children whose epilepsy is part of a static or progressive encephalopathy diffuse slowing and attenuation of the background EEG is expected.

Of most use in the investigation of children with seizure disorders is the detection of abnormal paroxysmal activity. Abnormal paroxysmal activity on interictal EEG can be divided into two broad categories: epileptiform and non-epileptiform abnormalities. Epileptiform abnormalities are those which have an association with the occurrence of epileptic seizures. In addition to being paroxysmal they are also usually abrupt and short-lived giving rise to spikes and sharp waves. Interictal spikes and waves are often followed by slow waves (paroxysmal EEG abnormalities which are of longer duration and blunter), constituting spike–wave complexes.

The non-specialist is often confused by reports of EEG abnormalities. These are often all incorrectly considered to support or even confirm a diagnosis of epilepsy. Common mistakes are:

- The assumption that focal, paroxysmal, slow wave activity supports the diagnosis of epilepsy. This is a non-specific finding, occurring frequently in normal children, especially younger children and if the child is drowsy. It can be a postictal phenomenon but this is a relatively rare cause.
- The assumption that all spikes and sharp waves are epileptiform. Although the spike and to a lesser extent, sharp waves, are considered the paradigm epileptiform abnormality, there are some 'physiological' spike and sharp wave paroxysmal EEG features.
- The assumption that the detection of epileptiform paroxysmal abnormalities necessarily implies that the child has seizures. Some such abnormalities, though more frequent in people with epilepsy than in the general population, are more frequently seen in people with cerebral disease but without seizures. Others have a strong association with epilepsy. They also occur in small numbers of people with other disorders and without seizures. For example, occipital spikes are common in blind people and centrotemporal spikes occur in some children with cerebral palsy and in boys with fragile X syndrome. Finally, a small number of normal children who have never had and never will have a seizure have epileptiform EEG abnormalities.

Certain EEG abnormalities can be activated by physiological maneuvers. These include sleep, hyperventilation and photic stimulation. Sleep (especially light sleep) is a powerful activator of many EEG abnormalities and if an awake recording is unhelpful it is usually worth obtaining a sleep recording. This can be achieved using natural sleep, following partial sleep deprivation or by drug-induced sedation. When sleep is induced by drugs it should be remembered that these may influence the EEG beyond causing sleep. Benzodiazepines and barbiturates often cause excessive fast activity and suppress many EEG abnormalities; they are therefore best avoided. Major tranquilizers such as chlorpromazine can decrease seizure threshold and may activate EEG abnormalities through mechanisms other than by sleep induction. Chloral hydrate and melatonin appear not to have significant effects on the EEG. The recording should be continued whilst the person is awakening as this may also provoke epileptiform abnormalities.

Hyperventilation, which should be included in the protocol for standard EEG recordings, is of particular use in investigating subjects with idiopathic generalized epilepsies in whom it frequently activates generalized spike–wave discharges. Apparently 'subclinical' discharges can often be shown to be associated with transient cognitive impairment if combined with breath counting during hyperventilation. Other epileptiform abnormalities are less reliably activated by hyperventilation. Hyperventilation often causes bilaterally synchronous slow wave activity in normal children. This physiological response must not be misinterpreted as indicating the likelihood of a seizure disorder.

Photic stimulation should also routinely be applied during standard EEG recordings. 'Photic-driving' or 'following' is a normal response and the 'photomyoclonic response' is a non-epileptiform abnormality often seen in anxious subjects. Photoparoxysmal responses are epileptiform abnormalities in which spikes and/or spike–wave discharges are produced by intermittent photic stimulation (Fig. 20.16). They are usually generalized but can be confined to the occipital regions. Generalized photoconvulsive responses are most often seen in subjects with idiopathic generalized epilepsies but occur in a variety of other epilepsies and rarely in normal children. Occipital photoconvulsive responses are occasionally seen in subjects with occipital lobe seizures.

Ictal EEG

During routine EEG recordings it is rare to record a seizure. An exception to this is in children with typical absences, which often occur during recordings, especially during hyperventilation. Ictal records usually require prolonged recording (24 h or more) and even then are only likely to be obtained if seizures are frequent. Two types of prolonged EEG are commonly employed. Ambulatory cassette EEG usually record eight channels of EEG using a cassette recorder. The EEG is later analyzed at high speed on a VDU screen with events electronically marked by the child or witness analyzed in detail. Video-EEG telemetry involves the subject staying in hospital whilst a 20 lead EEG is recorded, usually digitally, with simultaneous time-locked video recording. Again the whole record can be viewed at high speed with events analyzed in detail. Prolonged recordings are useful to:

- Help decide if paroxysmal clinical events are epileptic.
- Localize the onset of focal seizures. This is usually done as part of a presurgical workup in refractory epilepsy and requires video telemetry rather than a cassette recording.
- Establish the frequency of seizures and interictal epileptiform discharges. This may be useful if a child with epilepsy is performing less well at school than expected and it is considered that this might reflect under-recognized seizure activity.

Special techniques

The sensitivity of EEG recordings can be increased by using additional electrodes. Foramen ovale and sphenoidal electrodes are semi-invasive electrodes used to increase the detection of temporal lobe discharges. They are rarely used in children, in whom cheek electrodes have been suggested as an alternative. Invasive EEG recordings, with recording directly from the surface of the brain (subdural recordings) or from within the substance of the brain (intracerebral recordings) are used in a minority of children undergoing presurgical evaluation. They are employed to precisely localize the onset of seizures and are available only in specialized centers.

Polygraphic recordings, in which a number of physiological variables such as ECG, chest and abdominal wall movements, airflow at the nose and esophageal pH are recorded simultaneously with the EEG, and often video, are particularly useful in investigating children with recurrent apnea and life-threatening events, including Munchausen's syndrome by proxy. It should be noted that all EEG recordings should routinely include an ECG lead and if subtle myoclonus is suspected an EMG lead may be useful.

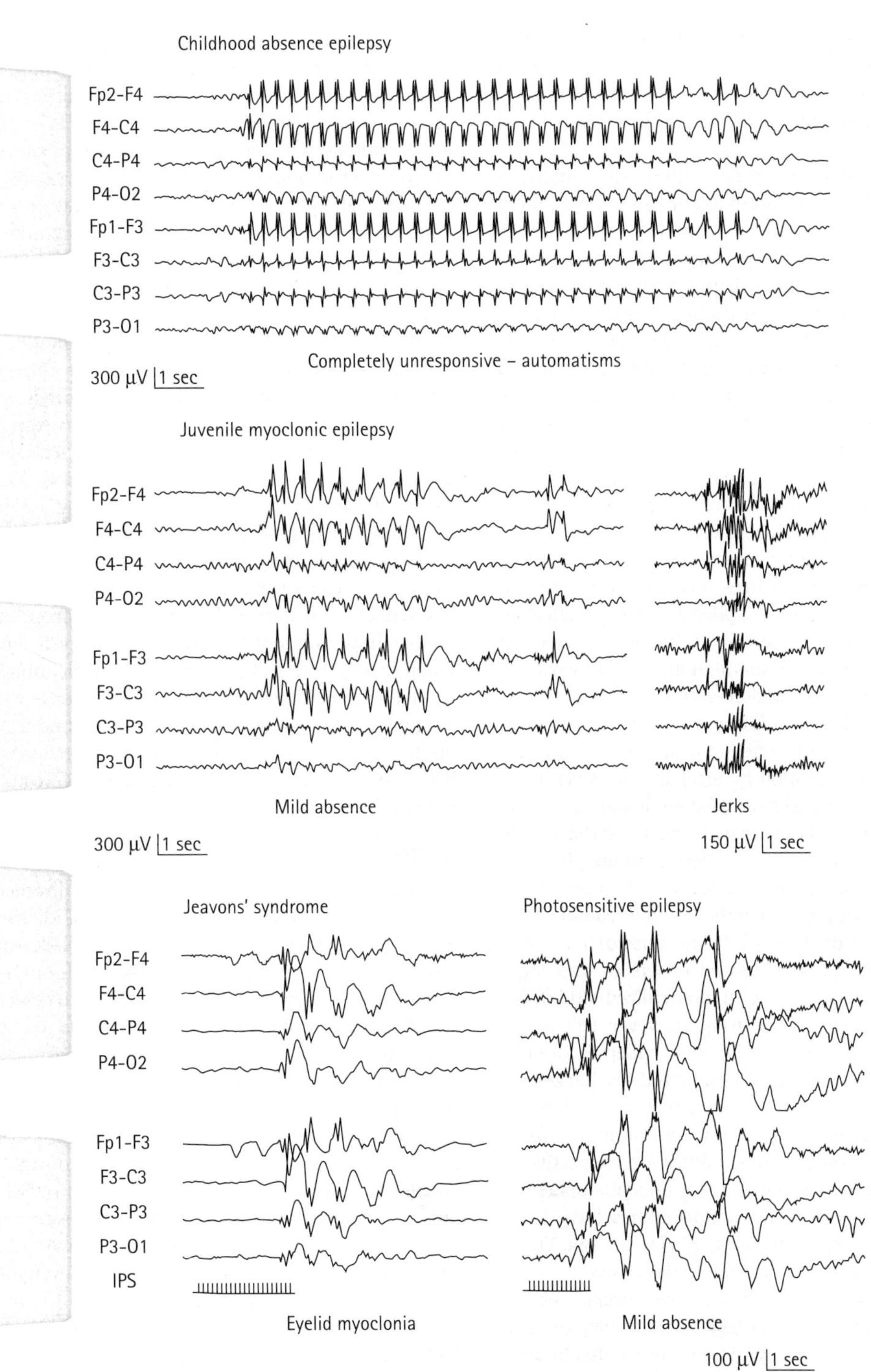

Fig. 20.16 Samples of video-EEG in some idiopathic generalized epilepsies of childhood. **Top:** Childhood absence epilepsy, a regular spike–wave discharge at 3 Hz is associated with complete unresponsiveness and automatisms. **Middle:** Juvenile myoclonic epilepsy. **Left:** an irregular and brief spike and polyspike discharge is associated with mild impairment of cognition. **Right:** A brief multiple spike discharge associates with myoclonic jerks without absence. **Bottom:** Response to intermittent photic stimulation. **Left:** A generalized discharge of irregular spike and wave is associated with marked eyelid myoclonia in eyelid myoclonia with absences (Jeavons' syndrome). **Right:** A similar generalized discharge is associated with a mild absence in another child with idiopathic generalized epilepsy and photosensitivity. With thanks to CP Panayiotopoulos.

Using the EEG in clinical practice

The EEG is used for six principal purposes:

- to help establish the likely diagnosis of epilepsy;
- to help establish the type of epilepsy;
- to help identify possible precipitants to epileptic seizures;
- to investigate the cause of cognitive decline;
- to help localize the onset of focal seizures;
- to monitor treatment, including the timing of drug withdrawal.

The usefulness of any investigation in helping to establish a diagnosis depends on its sensitivity and specificity. 2.2–3.5% of normal children have interictal epileptiform abnormalities whilst, in children with infrequent seizures, the yield of interictal epileptiform

EEG abnormalities on initial EEG is probably under 30%.[78] Over-reliance on interictal EEG for diagnosing epilepsy leads to frequent misdiagnoses. The clinical utility of recording interictal epileptiform discharges is exponentially related to the strength of the clinical suspicion of epilepsy.[79]

Some children with epilepsy have persistently normal interictal EEGs. This is often because the epileptiform discharges are infrequent and likely to be missed during a 30–60 min recording. Increasing the length and/or number of recordings or activating discharges, for example, by obtaining a sleep recording will increase the yield in these children. However, in some children, interictal abnormalities may be highly localized and/or attenuated by the dura, skull and scalp and therefore not detected by the standard array of electrodes used with a surface EEG. Many areas of the cortex, including the basal frontal and medial temporal regions are not directly accessible to scalp recordings and therefore only discharges which propagate will be detected. Obtaining an ictal recording may be the best strategy here. Antiepileptic drug treatment can affect the yield of EEG recordings.[80] Barbiturates and benzodiazepines are reported to reduce the abundance of epileptiform abnormalities and drugs effective in controlling typical absence seizures are likely to reduce epileptiform abnormalities in absence epilepsies. Drugs effective against photosensitive seizures reduce the likelihood of detecting photosensitivity on intermittent photic stimulation. Most antiepileptic drugs have little effect on the EEG of children with focal epilepsies.

It is unusual for an ictal EEG recording not to show epileptiform activity. However, it may fail to clarify whether a paroxysmal attack is epileptic or not because of obscuration by artefact. Moreover, focal seizures in which there is no disturbance of consciousness (simple focal seizures) often show no EEG changes because of the highly localized nature of the discharges. This is less common in focal seizures in which there is impairment of consciousness (complex focal seizures) but may occur, particularly when the origin is frontal.[81]

In routine clinical practice the EEG is at its most useful in helping to classify the type of epilepsy. Generalized epilepsies and focal epilepsies are commonly associated with generalized and focal interictal epileptiform discharges respectively. However, this is not absolute and in young children in particular, focal epilepsies are not infrequently associated with apparently generalized discharges. In idiopathic epilepsies the background is expected to be normal. Focal background abnormalities are frequent in symptomatic focal epilepsies. Generalized background abnormalities are suggestive of symptomatic generalized epilepsies and epileptic encephalopathies. Finally many more-or-less specific EEG abnormalities have been described for specific epilepsy syndromes (Figs 20.16–20.18). These will be described when the relevant syndrome is discussed.

A small minority of people with epilepsy have specific seizure precipitants. This is exemplified by photosensitive epilepsies, the evaluation of which is greatly aided by photic stimulation. In children in whom other precipitants appear important the recording conditions of the EEG can often be modified to investigate a particular precipitant's role.

Occasionally children with epilepsy show a stagnation or decline in their cognitive performance. The EEG can be useful in investigating the possible role of epileptiform activity in causing this. In some children, especially those with idiopathic generalized epilepsies, frequent interictal and subtle ictal discharges are responsible and can be detected on prolonged EEG recordings, preferably with simultaneous video recording. In others, electrical status during slow wave sleep may be responsible for cognitive problems and this possibility should be investigated by a sleep recording. Finally, some children with apparent cognitive decline are in non-convulsive status epilepticus. This is usually obvious on a standard EEG.

The EEG has an important role in the localization of the site of onset of focal seizures. However, it is important to remember its limitations. If ictal or interictal discharges originate from areas of the cortex 'hidden' to the scalp EEG, any associated EEG abnormalities will reflect discharge propagation rather than site of origin. Additionally, some discharges rapidly spread giving rise to bilateral EEG abnormalities. Finally, interictal epileptiform abnormalities may originate from sites remote from those giving rise to habitual seizures. For example, in mesial temporal lobe epilepsy it is common to find independent bilateral interictal discharges in people whose seizures all originate from one side.

Intuitively, it would seem likely that the EEG could help predict the likelihood of recurrence after an initial seizure and the prognosis for seizure recurrence after drug withdrawal. Studies have confirmed that this is the case.[78] However, a lack of sensitivity means that, clinically, its role in this regard is limited. The type of epilepsy, including the syndromic diagnosis, is probably a more useful guide. Illustrative examples may be helpful. In benign childhood epilepsy, with centrotemporal spikes, the abundance of interictal discharges varies markedly between EEGs done in the same child. Moreover, they often persist long after clinical remission of seizures has occurred. It would be inappropriate to use the EEG to predict how frequent seizures were likely to be or to help decide when to withdraw antiepileptic drug medication. On the other hand a child with an idiopathic generalized epilepsy whose EEG continues to show frequent spike–wave discharges and a positive response to photic stimulation, despite clinical remission of seizures, would have a high chance of relapse and the EEG result might reasonably help in the decision to continue antiepileptic drug medication.

Neuroimaging

For the majority of children with seizure disorders, MRI is the only brain imaging method of importance. Skull X-rays are only now indicated if a child presents with a seizure following a head injury in order to detect skull fractures. The main role of CT is also in the acute situation, in which its ability, unlike MRI, to detect skull fractures, its superior ability to detect fresh blood, and its ready availability, makes it the imaging method of choice when an unwell child presents with seizures of obscure origin. CT may also be useful in young children with seizures in whom neuroimaging is indicated to exclude, for example, space-occupying lesions, but in whom MRI would require a general anesthetic. The reassurance of a normal CT may reasonably enable the clinician to delay obtaining an MRI until this can be obtained without anesthetic. Cranial ultrasound is a useful imaging method in the neonatal period. However, its limitations must be appreciated. In particular it will miss many important lesions encountered in children with seizures.

MRI (Fig. 20.19) enables the following conditions associated with epilepsy to be detected:

- Brain malformations and maldevelopments such as agenesis of the corpus callosum, septo-optic dysplasia, holoprosencephaly, hemimegalencephaly, neuronal migration disorders and lesions associated with neurocutaneous disorders including tuberous sclerosis and Sturge–Weber syndrome
- Vascular disorders such as arteriovenous malformations
- Areas of sclerosis and gliosis associated with old infarcts, hypoxic–ischemic insults and infection
- Tumors, including low grade gliomas and dysembryoplastic neuroepithelial tumors.

There is an almost limitless number of potential MRI sequences. Close liaison between the clinician and radiologist is essential in order to ensure the most appropriate ones are obtained in an individual child. There are many excellent reviews on the role of MRI in the

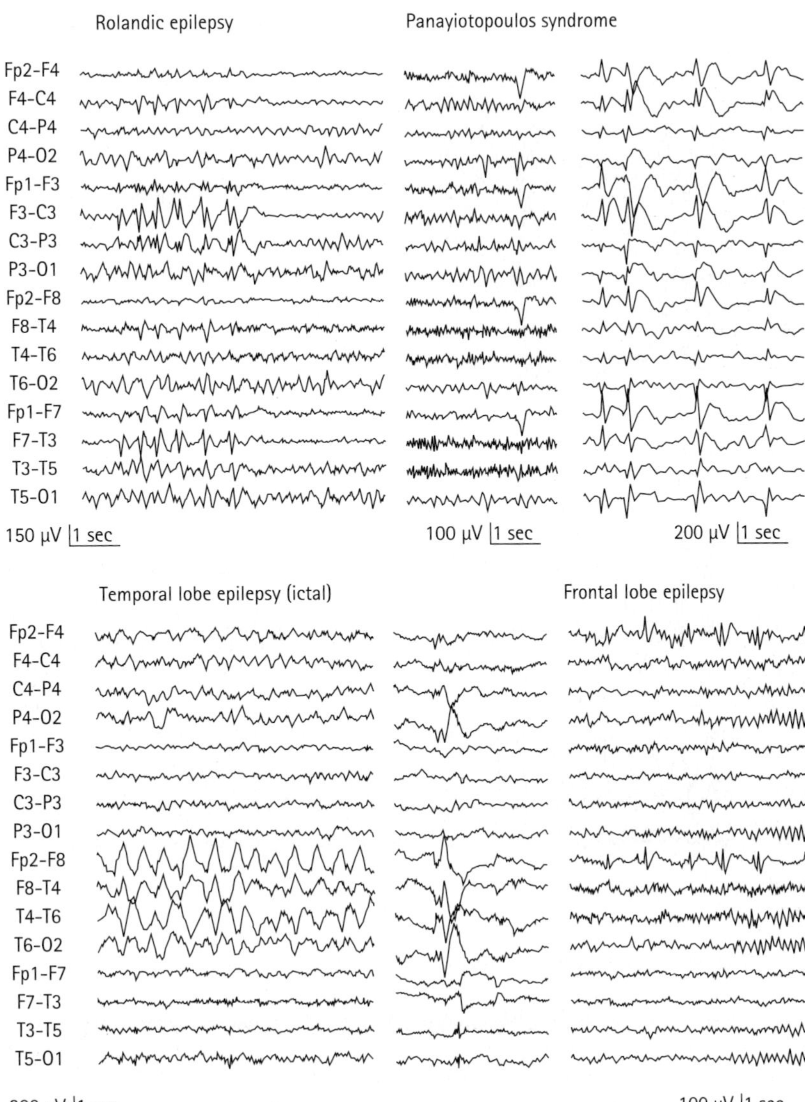

Fig. 20.17 EEGs in some focal epilepsies of childhood. **Top:** Benign childhood epilepsies. **Left:** Benign childhood epilepsy with centrotemporal spikes (Rolandic epilepsy) – focal high amplitude spike-wave discharges occur mainly in the left centrotemporal regions. These are typical of the EEG abnormalities expected in this syndrome. Some independent sharp waves are also seen in the posterior regions. These are less typical of the syndrome but nevertheless common. **Middle and Right:** EEG of two different patients with Panayiotopoulos syndrome. Despite similar lengthy seizure typical of the syndrome, EEG shows occipital spikes in the first (middle) and cloned-like repetitive multifocal spike-wave complexes, which are mainly frontal in the other (left). **Bottom:** Focal symptomatic epilepsies. **Left and middle:** Temporal lobe seizure of a child with right hippocampal sclerosis. High amplitude rhythmic slow wave activity over the right hemisphere occurred during the seizure; the child complained of 'tummy ache and panic' (left). High amplitude sharp and slow waves in the same regions persisted postictally (middle). **Right:** Frontal lobe epilepsy. Frequent spike and slow wave complexes are strictly localized in the right frontal regions. With thanks to CP Panayiotopoulos.

investigation of children with epilepsy.[82–84] Most brain malformations and maldevelopments comprise 'normal' brain tissue arranged abnormally and are best detected with sequences which give good anatomical definition, such as T1 weighted images. On the other hand 'foreign' tissue including tumors and gliotic tissue is usually best detected with T2 weighted images. The contrast agent gadolinium is rarely helpful and is not indicated as a routine. However, it can be helpful in conditions associated with breakdown in the blood–brain barrier, such as some tumors and vascular malformations. Proton density and fluid attenuated inversion recovery (FLAIR) sequences give improved contrast between brain lesions and CSF.

Detection of mesial temporal sclerosis, the pathological substrate underlying mesial temporal lobe epilepsy, deserves special mention (Fig. 20.19). It is usually not detected with 'standard' T1 and T2 weighted axial images. The important features are decreased volume (atrophy) and increased signal on T2 weighted and FLAIR sequences in the hippocampus and/or amygdala often with dilatation of the temporal horn. Its detection requires thin heavily T1 weighted and T2 weighted coronal images taken orthogonal to the long axis of the temporal lobe. More specialist techniques, which may improve detection further but which are not widely available, include T2 relaxometry and volumetric analysis.

An important question for the clinician is which children with epilepsy require neuroimaging. It is easier to say which children do not. One reasonable approach is to image all children with focal epilepsies except those with a pattern of epilepsy which corresponds

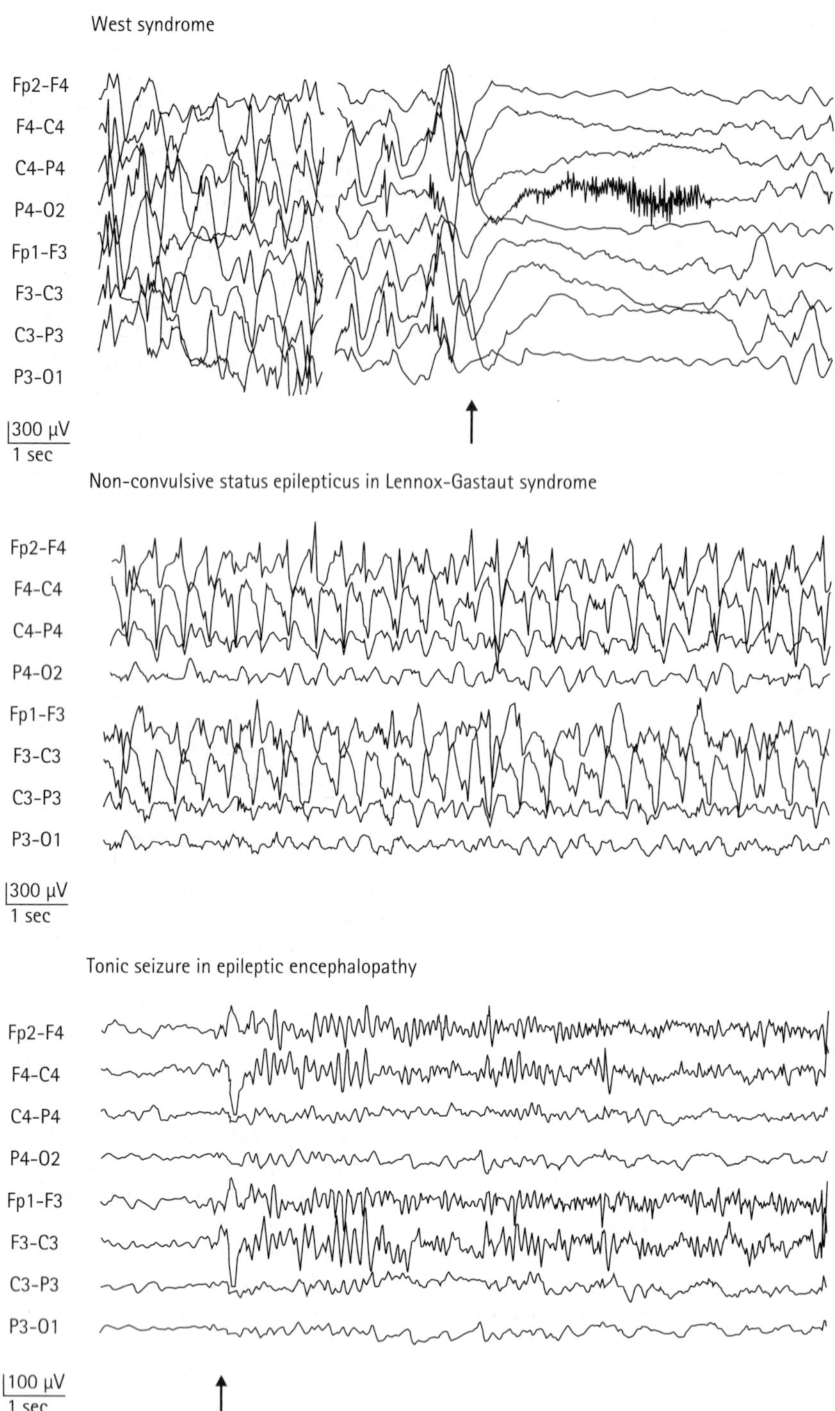

Fig. 20.18 The EEGs in some epileptic encephalopathies of childhood. **Top:** West syndrome showing typical hypsarrhythmia – the arrow indicates the onset of an epileptic spasm. This is accompanied by a high amplitude slow wave followed by flattening of the EEG (an electrodecremental response). **Middle:** Non-convulsive status epilepticus in Lennox-Gastaut syndrome showing continuous slow spike and wave. **Bottom:** A tonic seizure in Lennox–Gastaut syndrome – the onset of the seizure (arrow) is accompanied by a generalized discharge of spikes (fast spike discharge). With thanks to CP Panayiotopoulos.

clinically and on EEG with the syndrome of benign epilepsy of childhood, with centrotemporal spikes. Children with features of one of the idiopathic generalized epilepsies do not require imaging provided they respond as expected to appropriate medication. Another approach is to image children only if there are interictal neurological signs, or if seizures do not come under complete control after the first line antiepileptic drug.

Currently, functional brain imaging's role in the investigation of childhood epilepsy is confined to those in whom epilepsy surgery is being considered. During seizures, seizure foci are metabolically more active and require an increased blood flow. Between seizures, they are often less metabolically active and require less blood. In positron emission tomography (PET) a positron emitting ligand is injected into the subject and is then distributed around the body.

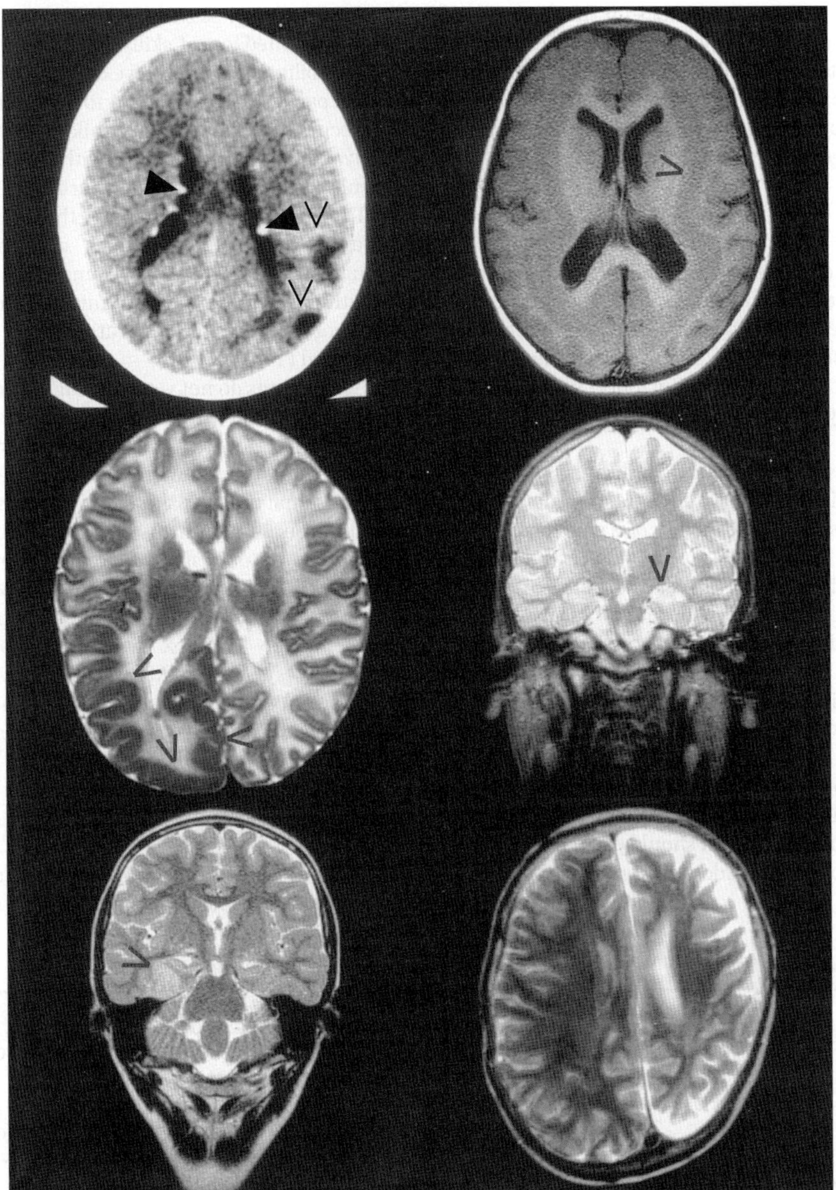

Fig. 20.19 Neuroimaging in some symptomatic childhood epilepsies. **Top left:** Non-enhanced CT showing calcified subependymal nodules (arrowheads) and multiple cortical tubers manifested as low attenuation areas (open arrows). **Top right:** T1 weighted axial MRI image showing subcortical band heterotopia ('double cortex') (arrow). **Middle left:** T2 weighted axial MRI image showing extensive right sided temporoparieto-occipital polymicrogyria (arrows). The child presented with very frequent occipital seizures and episodes of focal status epilepticus. All seizures ceased following a right temporoparieto-occipital resection. **Middle right:** T2 weighted coronal MRI image showing left mesial temporal sclerosis (arrow). The hippocampus is shrunken and of high signal and there is associated dilation of the temporal horn. **Bottom left:** T2 weighted coronal image showing a right sided dysembryoplastic neuroepithelial tumor in the right mesial temporal lobe (arrow). The tumor is cortical and of moderately high signal. **Bottom right:** T2 weighted image of a child with hemiconvulsion-hemiplegia-epilepsy syndrome (HHE syndrome) following haemophilus meningitis. There is left hemiatrophy. With thanks to JH Livingston and S Yeung.

In epilepsy studies, the ligand is usually ^{18}fluorodeoxyglucose (FDG), which is an analog of glucose. FDG enters the glycolytic pathway but cannot proceed beyond the initial steps. It therefore accumulates within tissues, the accumulation being proportional to the metabolic activity of the tissue. The rate of positron emission is detected by the PET scanner. FDG PET is, for a variety of reasons, unsuitable for ictal studies; the vast majority of FDG PET studies are interictal with the aim of detecting focal areas of hypometabolism. Single photon emission tomography (SPECT) is based upon the emission of photons from radioligands. These can be detected using conventional gamma cameras. In epilepsy studies, ^{99m}Tc-hexamethyl-propyleneamine (HMPAO) is the most widely used radioligand. Its distribution around the body reflects blood flow. The main advantage of SPECT over PET is its wide availability, as it utilizes commercially prepared radioligands and conventional gamma cameras which are available in all nuclear medicine departments. In addition, the pharmacokinetics of the distribution of HMPAO make it suitable for injection ictally. Unfortunately interictal SPECT has proved relatively insensitive in the detection of surgical foci and has largely been abandoned. Interictal PET and ictal SPECT appear to have similar sensitivities for the detection of temporal and extra temporal epileptic foci. The reader is referred to recent reviews for more details on these methods.[85–89]

Functional MRI holds great promise for the future, but is currently mainly a research tool. It may be used to map eloquent cortex before epilepsy surgery, lateralize language dominance and localize epileptic foci.

Other investigations

Most children with seizure disorders require no investigations other than EEG and structural brain imaging. However, there are children in whom seizures dominate the clinical picture but who have other features which suggest the possibility of an underlying genetic, metabolic or degenerative condition. These include:

- Early onset of refractory seizures in the neonatal or early postnatal period
- Stormy onset of seizures in the previously well child
- Occurrence of seizures in children with mental retardation of unknown cause (suggesting the possibility of a genetic or chromosomal disorder)
- Occurrence of seizures in children with dysmorphic features (suggesting genetic and chromosomal disorders. Peroxisomal disorders and the carbohydrate-deficient glycoprotein syndrome are also associated with dysmorphism)
- Occurrence of seizures in children with episodes of unexplained drowsiness or confusion (suggesting the possibility of an amino or organic acid disorder, a urea cycle defect or a mitochondrial disorder)
- Occurrence of seizures in children with neurological abnormalities on examination; ataxia should particularly raise suspicion (many degenerative disorders can produce this picture)
- Occurrence of seizures in children in whom there is a documented loss of skills, including visual skills (suggesting the possibility of degenerative disorders; the ceroid lipofuscinoses are particularly important to consider in children)
- Occurrence of seizures in children in whom there is evidence of dysfunction in systems outwith the CNS (suggesting mitochondrial disorders in particular).

The investigation of many of these disorders is best undertaken by a pediatric neurologist in conjunction with a metabolic pediatrician and clinical geneticist. However, the general pediatrician will not wish to miss potentially treatable conditions and should understand the rationale for the various investigations performed (Table 20.9).

Genetic tests do not yet play a significant role in the investigation of most children with seizure disorders. This may soon change dramatically. However, seizures are a prominent feature of the clinical phenotype of many chromosomal disorders and therefore chromosomal analysis should be a routine part of the investigation of children in whom seizures are accompanied by learning difficulties and/or dysmorphic features. In addition, there are many other genetic syndromes in whom seizures are prominent and which can now be diagnosed with molecular DNA techniques. These include fragile X syndrome, Wolf–Hirschhorn syndrome, Angelman syndrome, Miller–Dieker syndrome, Smith–Magenis syndrome, Pallister–Killian syndrome and Rett's syndrome. The clinical geneticist plays an important role in the evaluation of children with intractable seizures.

CLASSIFICATION

Classification profoundly affects our approach to medical disorders. In the past it was common to confuse classification of

Table 20.9 Investigations useful in children with seizure disorders in whom neurometabolic conditions are suspected

Disorder	Available tests	Comment
Biotinidase deficiency	Plasma biotinidase Urine organic acids	Treatable; worth excluding in all refractory childhood epilepsies
Amino acid disorders	Plasma and urine amino acids	Wide range of phenotypes. Worth performing in all children with early onset seizures and in all children in whom seizures are associated with mental retardation or loss of skills
Organic acidurias	Plasma organic acids	Worth performing in all children in whom seizures occur in association with intermittent vomiting and/or lethargy
Peroxisomal disorders	Very long chain fatty acids and phytanic acid	Consider especially in children with 'Zellweger' facies, mental retardation and profound hypotonia
Carbohydrate-deficient glycoprotein syndromes	Transferrin electrophoresis	Wide, incompletely described phenotype. Characteristic dysmorphic features
Menkes' disease	Serum copper and ceruloplasmin levels	Consider in boys with neonatal and early postnatal seizures
Folate and B_{12} disorders	Plasma and urine amino acids, urine organic acids, blood and CSF folate	Extremely rare; present in infancy
Molybdenum cofactor deficiency	Plasma urate level (low) and urinary sulfite excretion on dipstick test	Extremely rare
Purine and pyrimidine disorders	Urine purine and pyrimidine studies	Extremely rare
Creatine deficiency syndrome	Consistently low plasma creatinine levels	Extremely rare
Mitochondrial disorders	Plasma and CSF lactate levels	Huge variation in clinical phenotype. Suspect when there is evidence of multisystem disease
Storage disorders	White cell enzymes Specific enzyme assays for the ceroid lipofuscinoses	The main disorders which can present primarily as an epilepsy are the sialidoses, type 3 Gaucher disease and the ceroid lipofuscinoses
Glucose transporter protein deficiency	Paired CSF and blood glucose levels	Extremely rare
Pyridoxine dependency and deficiency	Trial of oral or intravenous vitamin B_6 (pyridoxine)	Consider in neonates and younger children with intractable seizures

epileptic seizure types (i.e. symptoms) with types of epilepsy (i.e. syndromes and diseases). A major advance in the last few decades has been the widespread acceptance of classification schemes for both epileptic seizures and epilepsy syndromes proposed by the International League Against Epilepsy (ILAE). Until very recently the classifications of seizures and of syndromes used worldwide were those proposed by the ILAE in 1981 and 1989 respectively.[90,91]

The 1981 classification divided seizures according to whether on clinical and EEG grounds they appeared to begin in a localized group of cortical neurones in one cerebral hemisphere (partial, focal or localization-related seizures) or whether both cerebral hemispheres appeared to be involved from the start (generalized seizures). The list of generalized epileptic seizures was similar, though not identical, to that in the new system discussed later. Partial epileptic seizures were divided into simple partial (implying no impairment of consciousness), complex partial (implying impairment of consciousness as assessed by the children's reduced reactivity to external stimuli and amnesia for the event) and partial evolving into generalized tonic–clonic seizures. The occurrence of various symptoms (motor, somatosensory, special-sensory symptoms, autonomic and psychic) was the basis for further subdivision.

The 1989 classification of 'epilepsies and epileptic syndromes' introduced a new concept, which has gained widespread acceptance, namely that of epileptic syndromes. This was in recognition of the fact that the etiology, pathogenesis and clinical features were established for very few epileptic conditions and that it was therefore inappropriate to consider them as diseases. An epileptic syndrome is defined by the non-fortuitous clustering of various features of which the most useful are the type(s) of epileptic seizure, EEG features and age of onset. The two main components of the classification were: (i) the division of epilepsies and epileptic syndromes into those with generalized seizures (generalized epilepsies and syndromes) and those with partial seizures (partial epilepsies and syndromes) and (ii) the division of both generalized and partial epilepsies and syndromes according to whether the cause was unknown and there was no suggestion of an underlying cause other than a possible hereditary predisposition (idiopathic epilepsies), whether the cause was unknown but an underlying cause was suspected (cryptogenic epilepsies) or whether the epilepsy occurred as a consequence of a known disorder of the CNS (symptomatic epilepsy).

In 2001 the ILAE published new classification proposals which are likely to gain wide acceptance.[92,93] They contain radical changes:

Rather than two classifications, one of seizures and the other of epilepsies and syndromes, there is a diagnostic scheme based on five axes. These are:

1. a glossary of terms used in epileptology
2. a list of epileptic seizure types
3. a list of epilepsy syndromes
4. an etiological classification
5. a classification of impairments arising as a consequence of the patient's condition.

- The terms 'partial' and 'localization-related' are abandoned in favor of 'focal'.
- The division of focal seizures into simple and complex is abandoned, partly because of conceptual difficulties with the notion of consciousness and the relative lack of importance of this feature anyhow. A new term 'dyscognitive seizure' has been introduced. This is a seizure in which disturbances of cognition are prominent.
- The term 'cryptogenic', which was considered confusing, is abandoned and is replaced by 'probably symptomatic'.

A number of new terms are introduced. These include:

1. Epileptic disease. This is a pathological condition with a single specific, well-defined etiology, e.g. tuberous sclerosis.
2. Epileptic encephalopathy. This is a condition in which the epileptiform abnormalities themselves are considered to cause a progressive disturbance in cerebral function.
3. Benign epilepsy syndrome. This is a syndrome in which seizures are easily treated, or require no treatment, and remit without sequelae.

Epileptic seizures

Axis 2 of the ILAE proposals classifies seizures into self-limited and continuous seizure types (status epilepticus). Each of these is then subdivided into generalized and focal seizures, whose meaning is unchanged from before.

Generalized, self-limited seizures[92,93]

Generalized tonic–clonic seizures (GTCS) involve an initial, bilaterally symmetrical, sustained contraction of the muscles (tonic phase) followed by bilateral repetitive, rhythmical contractions of the limbs (clonic phase). There is usually a phase of postictal drowsiness, of variable duration. During GTCS, manifestations such as tongue biting, cyanosis of the lips and incontinence are frequent. However, their usefulness in distinguishing between epileptic and non-epileptic seizures has been overemphasized. *Tonic seizures* are characterized by sustained muscle contractions lasting a few seconds to minutes. They may involve the whole, or greater part, of the body or be confined to particular parts of the body. For example, tonic seizures may be manifested by opisthotonos or by a subtle elevation of the eyebrows.

Clonic seizures are manifested by rhythmical contractions of the limbs. An alternative term is rhythmic myoclonus.

Myoclonic seizures are characterized by sudden, brief (<100 msec), involuntary, single or multiple contraction(s) of muscle(s) or muscle groups. They may be massive, involving axial and proximal limb muscles, or subtle and fragmentary involving distal muscles. Facial muscles, such as the eyelids, may be involved. A number of special types of myoclonic seizure are described. These include *myoclonic absence seizures* (characterized by a typical absence seizure with rhythmical myoclonus usually involving the head and proximal muscle of the upper limbs); *eyelid myoclonia* (characterized by rhythmical myoclonia of the eyelids sometimes accompanied by a brief typical absence seizure) and *myoclonic atonic seizures* (consisting of a brief jerk followed by a diffuse loss of tone). *Negative myoclonic seizures* involve an interruption of tonic muscular activity for <500 msec without any preceding myoclonus.

Atonic seizures are characterized by a sudden diminution of muscle tone lasting a second or longer, and involving the head, trunk, jaw or limb musculature.

An astatic seizure, also called a *drop attack*, is one in which there is a loss of erect posture resulting from an atonic, myoclonic or tonic mechanism.

Epileptic spasms (previously called infantile spasms) consist of a sudden flexion, extension or mixed extension–flexion of, predominantly proximal and truncal, muscles which is more sustained than myoclonus but briefer than a tonic seizure (approx. 1 s). They frequently occur in clusters and it is now recognized that their occurrence is not limited to infancy or to West syndrome (see p. 932).

Absence seizures are characterized clinically by a brief impairment of consciousness. In *typical absence seizures* this is of abrupt onset and cessation with no postictal symptoms. In *atypical absence seizures* the onset and cessation may be less clearly defined, with the person appearing to drift into and out of the seizure. Typical absence seizures are accompanied, on the EEG, by generalized 3 Hz spike–wave discharges. Atypical absence seizures are usually accompanied by generalized spike–wave discharges at frequencies under 2.5 Hz. The depth of impairment of consciousness during absences varies. Unless mild, automatisms (defined as more or less coordinated, repetitive, motor activity usually occurring when cognition is impaired and for which the subject is usually amnesic afterwards) are frequent. They are usually relatively simple, for example lip smacking and fumbling with hands. Mild clonic, myoclonic and atonic phenomena may also occur during absences.

Focal, self-limited seizures [92,93]

Focal motor seizures involve muscle activity in any form, with either an increase or decrease in muscle contraction. Subtypes include:

- *Focal motor seizures with elementary clonic motor signs.* The term 'elementary' implies that a single type of contraction of a muscle or group of muscles is involved; 'clonic' implies regular repetitive contractions. Such seizures often imply involvement of the primary motor area of the frontal lobe and may include a Jacksonian march with spread of clonic movements through contiguous body parts.
- *Focal motor seizures with asymmetric tonic motor signs.* These seizures are characterized by an asymmetrical, sustained increase in muscle contractions, causing, for example, the child to adopt a 'fencing' posture. Such seizures are characteristic of those involving the supplementary motor areas of the frontal lobes although they can arise from other frontal lobe regions and from extrafrontal lobe sites.
- *With typical (temporal lobe) automatisms* as occurs in mesial temporal lobe seizures (described later).
- *With hyperkinetic automatisms* (such as pedalling, thrashing and rocking movements). Such seizures usually imply a frontal lobe origin.
- Rarer seizure types include *focal negative myoclonus* and *seizures with inhibitory motor signs* (implying a loss of muscle contraction as in motor arrest).

Focal sensory seizures are characterized by a perceptual experience not caused by appropriate stimuli in the external world. Subtypes include:

- *Focal sensory seizures with elementary sensory symptoms.* Here the term 'elementary' is used to imply a single, unformed phenomenon involving one primary sensory modality, e.g. somatosensory (parietal lobe seizures), visual (occipital lobe seizures), auditory, olfactory, gustatory, epigastric or cephalic.
- *With experiential sensory symptoms.* By this it is meant affective symptoms (fear, depression, anger, etc.), distortions of reality (déjà vu, jamais vu), feelings of depersonalization and formed illusionary or hallucinatory events. These are characteristic of seizures involving the junction of the temporal, parietal and occipital lobes.

Gelastic seizures are characterized by ictal laughter or giggling, usually without an appropriate affective tone. Such seizures often involve the hypothalamus.

Hemiclonic seizures are characterized by rhythmical clonic jerking involving one side of the body.

Secondary, generalized seizures are seizures whose onset is focal (e.g. motor or sensory) and then becomes generalized usually as a tonic–clonic seizure.

The term aura, which had recently fallen from use, has now been defined as a subjective ictal phenomenon that, in a given child, may precede an observable seizure; if it occurs alone, it constitutes a sensory seizure.

Continuous seizure types (status epilepticus)

Status epilepticus is defined by the ILAE as 'a seizure which shows no clinical signs of arresting after a duration encompassing the great majority of seizures of that type in most children or recurrent seizures without resumption of baseline central nervous system function, interictally'.[92] However, operationally it is usually defined as 'recurrent epileptic seizures continuing for more than 30 minutes without full recovery of consciousness before the next seizure begins, or continuous clinical and/or electrical seizure activity lasting for more than 30 minutes whether or not consciousness is impaired'.[94] For each type of epileptic seizure it is possible to define a corresponding type of status epilepticus:

- Generalized status epilepticus
  - Generalized tonic–clonic status epilepticus
  - Clonic status epilepticus
  - Absence status epilepticus
  - Tonic status epilepticus
  - Myoclonic status epilepticus
- Focal status epilepticus
  - Epilepsia partialis continua (of Kozhevnikov)
  - Aura continua
  - Limbic status epilepticus (psychomotor status)
  - Hemiconvulsive status with hemiparesis

Some authorities recognize continuous spike and wave during slow sleep and hypsarrhythmia as special forms of 'electrical status'.[95]

A pragmatic clinical classification defines two main groups, convulsive and non-convulsive status epilepticus. The former includes generalized tonic–clonic, clonic, tonic and myoclonic status epilepticus, epilepsia partialis continua and hemiconvulsive status with hemiparesis as convulsive status epilepticus and the others as non-convulsive status epilepticus. Status epilepticus can also be defined according to etiology:

- Febrile status epilepticus – essentially a febrile convulsion lasting over 30 min. This is the commonest cause in children aged 1–3 years
- Idiopathic status epilepticus – status epilepticus occurring without evidence of any previous CNS dysfunction (except possible previous seizures), and in the absence of an acute CNS or systemic disorder
- Remote symptomatic – status epilepticus occurring in the context of a child with pre-existing static or progressive brain damage or dysfunction
- Acute symptomatic – status epilepticus occurring during the course of an acute brain disorder caused by, for example infection, trauma, hypoxic–ischemic insults, stroke, intoxication, metabolic and electrolyte disturbances, tumor and drugs, including antiepileptic drug withdrawal.

The clinical features of the different types of status epilepticus can generally be deduced from their names. However, it is worth noting that the clinical manifestations of both convulsive and non-convulsive forms often become subtle as the seizure progresses. Hence, late in generalized tonic–clonic status, clonic movements may consist of barely perceptible stiffening of the limbs, whilst long lasting tonic status may mainly be manifested with hypoventilation, salivation and cyanosis. Non-convulsive status may present with a child who is confused or is performing less well than is usual.

The effects and treatment of status epilepticus are considered elsewhere in this book.

Epilepsies and epilepsy syndromes

The following summarizes the principal features of epilepsies and epilepsy syndromes currently recognized by the ILAE. More detailed accounts are given elsewhere.[96,97]

Syndromes with onset in the neonatal period

The incidence of seizures in the neonatal period is higher than at any time. Neonatal seizures can be classified as:

- Focal clonic – repetitive, rhythmic, unifocal or multifocal contractions of muscle groups of the limbs, face or trunk
- Focal tonic – sustained posturing of a single limb or asymmetrical posturing of the trunk or sustained eye deviation
- Myoclonic – generalized, focal or fragmentary arrhythmic shock-like contractions of muscle groups often provoked by stimulation
- Generalized tonic – sustained symmetrical posturing of limbs, trunk and neck
- Subtle seizures (often called motor automatisms) – these include random, roving eye movements, sucking, chewing and tongue protrusions and rowing, swimming and peddling movements of the limbs.

There is considerable debate as to whether all of these seizure types are epileptic in origin.[98] Clonic, focal tonic, generalized myoclonic and some subtle seizures are usually accompanied by ictal EEG discharges, are not usually provoked by stimuli and cannot be terminated by restraint or repositioning. They are probably epileptic in origin. Generalized tonic, focal and fragmentary myoclonic, and some subtle seizures, are usually not accompanied by ictal EEG discharges, can often be provoked by stimulation and terminated by restraint and repositioning. Many are probably not epileptic in origin, but may arise due to loss of cortical inhibition on lower centers.

The interictal EEG is of limited value in the investigation of neonatal seizures. Sharp waves, and even spikes, may be normal features and are not regarded as 'epileptiform abnormalities' as in older children. They are unlikely to be of significance, unless markedly asymmetrical in distribution. Asymmetries and absence of normal elements appropriate for the gestational age are of more help, but are indicators of brain dysfunction rather than specifically of seizure activity. Because neonatal seizures are often very frequent, ictal recordings are often obtained. Ictal discharges take many different forms but generally comprise combinations of repetitive sharp waves or spikes and abnormal paroxysmal rhythms. Discharges are often highly localized or may be confined to one hemisphere. They frequently move during the same recording. Generalized discharges are rare. Neonatal seizures are often unaccompanied by EEG discharges; conversely 'ictal' EEG discharges are frequently unaccompanied by clinical seizures. The clinical significance of such events is unclear.

A majority of neonatal seizures are symptomatic arising as a consequence of pre-, peri- or postnatal insults to the brain, including:

- Hypoxic–ischemic insults (including intrapartum hypoxia)
- Infection – including congenital infections, meningitis and encephalitis
- Hemorrhage – including intraventricular, intracerebral, subdural and subarachnoid
- Infarction
- Malformations and maldevelopments of the brain
- Metabolic problems including hypoglycemia, hypocalcemia, hypomagnesemia and inborn errors of metabolism.

The prognosis for neonatal seizures is heavily dependent on their etiology. It remains controversial as to whether the seizures themselves are damaging. This has lead to uncertainty as to how aggressively they should be treated. Many clinicians only treat clinical seizures accompanied by ictal EEG changes (or if no ictal EEG is available, clinical seizures likely to be accompanied by ictal EEG changes). The treatment of neonatal seizures is considered in detail elsewhere.

Two specific symptomatic or probably symptomatic epilepsy syndromes of the neonatal period are described. These are *early myoclonic encephalopathy and Ohtahara's syndrome.* Both usually have their onset within the neonatal period or first few months of life and are associated with an identical abnormal EEG pattern known as suppression-burst. Early myoclonic encephalopathy is characterized by the occurrence of frequent, refractory generalized, focal or fragmentary myoclonia, focal clonic seizures and epileptic spasms. There is a high frequency of familial cases and the syndrome is often a manifestation of an inborn error of metabolism, especially non-ketotic hyperglycinemia. It is highly resistant to treatment, carries a high mortality and survivors are nearly all severely retarded. Ohtahara's syndrome is characterized by frequent tonic spasms. The etiology is heterogeneous but structural brain abnormalities are common. It often evolves to West syndrome (see below). Seizures are highly resistant to treatment and again, there is an appreciable mortality with survivors nearly always being severely retarded.

Not all seizures in the neonatal period are a manifestation of a severe underlying problem. Two benign syndromes of neonatal seizure have been described. *Benign familial neonatal seizures* is an autosomal dominant epilepsy syndrome caused by mutations on voltage-gated potassium channels coded for on chromosomes 8 and 20.[52,53,99] The seizures occur in babies, who are otherwise well, and who remain well. They usually begin on the second or third day of life, but can be delayed up to the third month. A variety of seizure types have been described, but most appear to involve an initial tonic component followed by autonomic changes (especially apnea and heart rate changes) and clonic components. Seizures are often initially frequent, but usually abate within a few days or weeks. The interictal EEG is usually normal. The ictal EEG usually shows generalized flattening, often followed by localized or generalized spikes or slow waves. There is no consensus regarding treatment, which is probably not necessary. Although the outlook is good, there is a significantly higher incidence of febrile and non-febrile seizures in later childhood. *Benign idiopathic neonatal seizures* ('fifth day fits') is a non-familial condition occurring in otherwise normal babies.[99] Epidemiological data suggest clustering of cases, with at times epidemics, leading to the hypothesis of an infective etiology. Seizures, often frequent and prolonged, begin between days 1 and 7 of life and are mainly focal clonic in type, often with apnea. Drowsiness and hypotonia are common during the evolution of the disorder. A variety of interictal EEG patterns have been described. Ictal EEGs show rhythmic spikes or slow waves localized to various locations, particularly the rolandic regions. Generalized discharges also occur. As for benign familial neonatal seizures, antiepileptic drug treatment may not be required. The duration of active seizures is short, usually under a day. The long-term outlook is generally considered good, although detailed prospective studies are lacking.

Syndromes with onset in infancy and early childhood

This period is marked by a high incidence of symptomatic and probably symptomatic epilepsies. Nevertheless, benign syndromes do occur, including that of febrile seizures (this term is preferred in the new ILAE classification to 'febrile convulsions'), which is the most common of all the benign seizure syndromes. A notable feature of this period is the occurrence of the epileptic encephalopathies. These are conditions in which intense epileptiform activity appears to cause or contribute to neurodevelopmental problems.

Benign epilepsies of infancy are rare. The best known is *benign myoclonic epilepsy of infancy.*[100] This is an idiopathic, generalized epilepsy with onset between 4 months and 3 years. The characteristic seizures (indeed the only seizure type considered compatible with the diagnosis) are myoclonic jerks, which can be single or repeated, subtle, for example causing only head nods, or massive, causing falls. Seizures can occur at any time whilst awake or asleep but often cluster when the infant is tired or on awakening. The seizures are accompanied on the EEG by a generalized discharge of spike or polyspike and waves. The interictal EEG, whilst awake, is usually normal, but sleep leads to a dramatic activation of spike or polyspike and wave discharges. As expected in an idiopathic epilepsy, neurodevelopmental progress prior to seizure onset is normal and there is often a family history of seizure disorders. Benign myoclonic epilepsy of infancy usually responds well to sodium valproate; treatment is generally recommended and is said in uncontrolled studies to improve prognosis. The period of active seizures probably lasts for up to 3 years. Some children later develop other generalized epilepsies. Although considered a benign condition, a relatively high proportion of children are subsequently said to have schooling problems. Children with a condition similar to benign myoclonic epilepsy of infancy, but whose seizures are provoked by acoustic and tactile stimuli, have been described.

Benign partial epilepsies in infancy are rare but a number of syndromes have been described, including *benign infantile seizures (non-familial), and benign familial infantile seizures.* All occur in otherwise normal infants, with no identifiable predisposing factor, other than a positive family history in the latter. Onset is from 3 to 20 months for the non-familial type and from 4 to 7 months in the familial type. Seizures are focal, with rare secondary generalization and often occur in clusters. Interictal EEG is usually normal. The gene responsible for benign familial infantile seizures maps, at least in some families, to chromosome 19. In both syndromes the prognosis appears to be excellent.

West syndrome (with an incidence of 1.6–4.3 per 10 000 live births) is the best known epilepsy syndrome of infancy. It consists of a triad of epileptic spasms (this term is now preferred to infantile spasms and all other synonyms), hypsarrhythmia and psychomotor regression. Its onset is nearly always within the first year of life, and typically between 3 and 7 months of age.

Epileptic spasms involve a contraction of the axial muscles causing flexion, extension or both. They may be symmetrical or asymmetrical. The latter is a feature of focal brain lesions. Spasms may be single, but more typically occur in clusters and may occur at any time. However, they are particularly likely to occur when drowsy and on arousal and are rare in sleep. Spasms, particularly at onset, may be subtle, causing only brief head nods. Others are massive and cause distress. Other seizure types may precede, accompany or follow spasms. Of particular importance are spasms preceded by focal seizures, as this may indicate an operable lesion.

Typical hypsarrhythmia is defined as a more or less continuously abnormal EEG with high amplitude, irregular and asymmetric slow wave activity across all leads with random sharp waves and spikes producing a chaotic pattern (Fig. 20.18). Spasms are often accompanied by electrodecremental responses in which the EEG briefly assumes a more normal appearance. Typical hypsarrhythmia occurs in under half of all cases of West syndrome. Modified forms include cases with some preservation of normal background activity, cases with synchronized bursts of generalized spike and wave activity and cases with significant asymmetries. Other EEG patterns which may occur include constant spike foci and burst-suppression. Hypsarrhythmia may be absent during awake recordings, but present in slow wave sleep.

Psychomotor stagnation and regression is extremely frequent, but not constant, in West syndrome. It often precedes the onset of spasms. Particularly prominent is loss, mostly visual, of interest in the environment.

An underlying cause for West syndrome can be identified in 85–90% of cases. Causes include:

- Neurocutaneous syndromes (tuberous sclerosis is the commonest single cause)
- Brain malformations (such as Aicardi syndrome, agyria-pachygyria, laminar heterotropia, hemimegalencephaly and other migrational disorders)
- Chromosomal abnormalities, including Down syndrome
- Neurometabolic and degenerative diseases, including aminoacidurias, non-ketotic hyperglycinemia, organicacidurias, urea cycle defects, mitochondrial disorders, CDG (carbohydrate-deficient glycoprotein) syndrome, pyridoxine dependency, biotinidase deficiency and PEHO (progressive encephalopathy with edema, hypsarrhythmia and optic atrophy) syndrome
- Pre-, peri- and postnatal destructive lesions of the brain whether due to infection, hypoxic–ischemic insults, hypoglycemia, trauma or hemorrhage
- Brain tumors.

Recently an X-linked form of the disorder has been described.[101]

The use of the terms 'cryptogenic' and 'idiopathic' are somewhat confusing when applied to West syndrome. Traditionally the former was used if no cause could be found, particularly if development prior to onset of spasms was normal. No idiopathic category was recognized. However, some children with West syndrome of unknown cause are normal prior to onset of spasms, have spasms (accompanied by typical hypsarrhythmia) for a short period during which development is relatively unaffected. Most authorities now recognize these as true idiopathic cases.[102]

The treatment of infantile spasms is controversial with the major areas of debate centering around whether vigabatrin or hormonal treatment should be used first line and the type, dosage and duration of hormonal treatment.[103,104] The efficacy of vigabatrin in treating infantile spasms was first reported in the early 1990s.[105] It has been shown to be more efficacious than placebo.[106] Retrospective studies have suggested similar response rates to vigabatrin and hormonal therapy.[104] In an open, randomized, prospective study comparing vigabatrin and adrenocorticotropic hormone (ACTH) no significant difference in the response to the two drugs was shown, although more subjects showed an initial good response to ACTH.[107] Until recently vigabatrin was perceived to lack serious adverse effects. However, it is now known to cause irreversible visual field defects. The clinician must make a choice between drugs of similar efficacy but completely different unwanted effects. The unwanted effects of hormonal treatment are more or less predictable, detectable and reversible but occasionally fatal whilst the visual field defects caused by vigabatrin are currently unpredictable and, in infancy and early childhood, undetectable, but certainly not fatal.

When a response occurs to vigabatrin it is apparent within days. It should be started at relatively modest doses of around 50 mg/kg/day and the dose increased in non-responders every few days to around 180 mg/kg/day before concluding that it has been ineffective. It is usually possible to establish efficacy within a period of 2–3 weeks. Significant drowsiness is likely. Subjects who fail to respond to vigabatrin or who relapse often respond to subsequent hormonal treatment.

There is a multiplicity of studies comparing different hormonal regimens for the treatment of infantile spasms. Unfortunately, these have not yet yielded unequivocal answers and as yet, there are no placebo-controlled trials of either ACTH or corticosteroids. A recent review concluded that:[108]

- Cessation or improvement in spasms occurs in 50–75% of subjects
- The effect is apparent within a couple of weeks
- Studies suggest either that prednisolone and ACTH are equally effective or that ACTH is more effective
- Subjects who fail to respond to ACTH or prednisolone may subsequently respond to the other agent
- There is no clear evidence that larger doses (150 U/m^2/day) of ACTH are more effective than lower doses (20–30 U/day).
- Longer treatment periods do not usually improve remission rates.
- Relapses occur in – 1/12 of subjects although second courses of treatment may be effective.

In the UK, short regimens of 4–6 weeks, using either oral prednisolone at 2 mg/kg/day or intramuscular ACTH (as opposed to tetracosactide which has more unwanted effects) at 20–30 U/day, given as a single morning dose appear to be favored. Before starting hormonal treatment, infection should be excluded. Frequent monitoring of blood pressure, urine (for glycosuria) and serum electrolytes is important. Hypertensive children should be evaluated for cardiomyopathy. Hypertension and glycosuria may respond to a reduction in dose. Some authorities recommend tapering ACTH and prednisolone over a 1-week period, even when used for only short periods. If high dose and/or prolonged treatment regimens are used longer tapering courses are necessary; evaluation of the hypothalamic–pituitary axis at the end of therapy is advocated by some.

Infantile spasms complicating tuberous sclerosis respond much better to vigabatrin than to hormonal treatment.[109] Otherwise, the response rate is better in those in whom no underlying cause can be found. It is not clear whether it is appropriate to use different agents first line in the treatment of cryptogenic and symptomatic spasms.

Many other agents have been suggested for the treatment of spasms, whether as initial treatment or as add-on therapy. These include: benzodiazepines, especially nitrazepam; sodium valproate (used in doses considerably higher than usual); pyridoxine; topiramate; lamotrigine; zonisamide and immunoglobulins.

A small, but important, group of children with focal brain lesions develop West syndrome. These may respond best to drugs like carbamazepine. Non-responders may be candidates for early resective surgery. Suggestive features are: focal neurological signs; focal epileptic seizures, prior to the onset of or concurrent with epileptic spasms; focal onset of spasms or asymmetrical spasms; asymmetrical hypsarrhythmia or fixed EEG foci. All children with West syndrome require early evaluation with structural brain imaging, preferably MRI. Video-EEG may be necessary to detect focal onset of spasms or asymmetrical spasms.

The overall prognosis for West syndrome is poor and it has not been established whether drug treatment has any impact on the ultimate outcome. Spasms usually remit in infancy or early childhood, but may continue. However, 50–75% of children develop other forms of epilepsy, particularly the Lennox–Gastaut syndrome. 70–90% of infants with West syndrome are mentally retarded and a significant minority have cerebral palsy and/or neuropsychiatric disorders, including autism.[108] West syndrome carries an increased mortality of perhaps around 5%. The main determinant of prognosis is the etiology. Those with cryptogenic, and especially idiopathic, spasms, have the best prognosis, both in terms of becoming seizure free and in developing normally. However, symptomatic spasms complicating Down syndrome and neurofibromatosis are said to carry a better prognosis. Other good prognostic factors include normal neurodevelopment prior to onset of spasms, older age at onset and short duration of spasms. Early effective treatment is felt likely to improve outcome but remains to be shown conclusively.

Severe myoclonic epilepsy in infancy (now termed *Dravet syndrome* by the ILAE) has only been recognized for the last two decades but is amongst the most distinctive of the severe epilepsies occurring in infants and young children.[110] The key features for its recognition are the occurrence of febrile, or afebrile, clonic, or tonic–clonic, seizures, often unilateral and sometimes prolonged occurring in the first year of life in an otherwise normal infant. Initial development continues to be normal. However, somewhere between the second and fourth years of life, other seizure types occur, notably myoclonic seizures, atypical absences, absence status, and focal seizures. This is accompanied by psychomotor delay, with nearly all children eventually being severely retarded. This justifies its inclusion within the epileptic encephalopathies. Ataxia, mild pyramidal signs and behavioral problems are also common. The interictal EEG is initially normal, except for early photosensitivity in a significant minority of children. With the onset of the polymorphous seizures in the second year of life, spike, polyspike and spike and wave discharges occur. The background may remain normal or show progressive slowing. There is evidence that the syndrome may be a channelopathy.[55] Otherwise, the etiology is unknown. However, a detailed evaluation with structural neuroimaging and neurometabolic studies is probably indicated. The syndrome is highly resistant to treatment. Sodium valproate is probably the initial drug of choice. Benzodiazepines and ethosuximide may also be useful. Given the focal nature of many of the seizures, carbamazepine may be tried, but may exacerbate the myoclonus. Lamotrigine may also exacerbate seizures.[111]

Rarer and less well-characterized severe epilepsies occurring in infancy and early childhood include *migrating partial seizures of infancy, myoclonic status in non-progressive encephalopathies* and *hemiconvulsion–hemiplegia syndrome*.[112] The first of these is characterized by an onset at around 3 months of age of intractable and escalating focal seizures (usually focal motor), which characteristically involve one area of the body before shifting to another. Myoclonic status in non-progressive encephalopathies is characterized by repeated episodes of myoclonic status epilepticus occurring in children with non-progressive 'static' encephalopathies, including cerebral palsy, Angelman syndrome and Prader–Willi syndrome. Hemiconvulsion–hemiplegia syndrome (HH syndrome) has been long recognized, but appears to be declining in frequency. Its cardinal features are the occurrence, in an otherwise normal child, of a prolonged unilateral, usually clonic, febrile seizure, either in the course of a trivial infection or else symptomatic of a severe acute brain disorder such as meningitis, followed by atrophy of one cerebral hemisphere and hemiplegia. Epilepsy supervenes after a variable period. Both focal and generalized seizures may occur. Prevention with rapid termination of prolonged febrile seizures is important and may help explain its decline in frequency.

Syndromes with onset in mid and late childhood and adolescence

This age group is associated with a decline in the incidence of epilepsy and by a number of relatively common and well-characterized epilepsy syndromes, which are almost certainly genetic in origin and many of which carry an excellent prognosis. These can be conveniently considered under the categories of the idiopathic focal and generalized epilepsies of childhood and adolescence. Symptomatic and probably symptomatic epilepsies are also important in this age group. They include focal epilepsies, most notably mesial temporal lobe epilepsy, and a number of epileptic encephalopathies such as the Lennox–Gastaut syndrome and the Landau–Kleffner syndrome.

The idiopathic generalized epilepsies.[113] These are characterized by:

- Occurrence in otherwise normal children and adolescents
- Strong family history of epilepsy, including, but not restricted to, idiopathic epilepsies
- A preceding history of febrile convulsions in many subjects
- The occurrence in various combinations of three seizure types: generalized tonic–clonic seizures; typical absence seizures; and myoclonic seizures
- EEGs in which the background is generally normal with paroxysmal regular or irregular spike or polyspike and wave abnormalities at 3Hz or greater.

The three best-characterized, idiopathic generalized epilepsies are childhood absence epilepsy, juvenile absence epilepsy and juvenile myoclonic epilepsy. *Childhood and juvenile absence epilepsies* are both characterized by the occurrence of typical absence seizures. In both these are relatively prolonged, typically 10–20 s, with severe impairment of consciousness such that automatisms are common. Other features during the absences such as eyelid blinking, mild clonic movements around the mouth and head nods may occur but are not prominent. In childhood absence epilepsy, absences are very frequent, occurring many times a day – hundreds may be recorded on video-EEG. In juvenile absence epilepsy they are less frequent, occurring at most a few times a day. Except for febrile convulsions, other seizure types occur only very rarely in childhood absence epilepsy. Occasional myoclonic jerks may occur in juvenile absence epilepsy and up to 80% of subjects with juvenile absence epilepsy have, or develop, generalized tonic–clonic seizures, which are usually infrequent. Many authorities consider that photosensitivity is not compatible with the diagnosis of childhood absence epilepsy, whilst it is probably permissible, although relatively rare, in juvenile absence epilepsy. Childhood absence epilepsy usually has its onset between 4 and 8 years and generally remits by about the age of 12. Occasional children (perhaps around 3%) will develop generalized tonic–clonic seizures in their teenage years or adult life. Juvenile absence epilepsy usually has its onset between 7 and 16 years and is usually long lasting with susceptibility to seizures continuing into adult life.

The EEG in childhood and juvenile absence epilepsies is similar and is characterized by regular generalized spike and wave discharges at around 3 Hz (Fig. 20.16). The discharges are increased during sleep and on awakening and are provoked by hyperventilation.

Juvenile myoclonic epilepsy is characterized by a triad of seizure types. Typical absences occur in about one-third of children, usually in late childhood or early adolescence. They are usually brief (a few seconds), mild and unaccompanied by automatisms. However, if they start in younger children they may resemble those of childhood absence epilepsy. Myoclonic seizures occur in all individuals, usually starting in early to mid adolescence. They may be massive (causing falls), or confined to the limbs, or extremities. They may be single or multiple and rhythmic. They usually cluster in the period shortly after awakening with a second cluster towards the end of the day. They are often not reported spontaneously, as the child considers them as a normal feature of everyday life. Enquiries should be made as to whether the child is considered 'clumsy' in the morning or has the 'shakes' with a tendency to spill drinks. Generalized tonic–clonic seizure occurs in nearly all untreated children, usually a few years after the onset of myoclonic jerks. They usually cluster in the morning and may be heralded by a shower of myoclonic jerks or absences, sometimes leading to an erroneous diagnosis of secondary generalized tonic–clonic seizures. Photosensitivity, both clinical and on EEG, is common. The EEG in juvenile myoclonic epilepsy is characterized by irregular discharges of fast spike, or more often polyspike and wave (Fig. 20.16). Myoclonic seizures are usually accompanied by brief polyspike or polyspike and wave discharges. Although the background EEG is usually normal, focal abnormalities occur in a minority. These have the appearance of abortive generalized discharges and vary in location.

Epilepsy with generalized tonic–clonic seizures only is a somewhat controversial syndrome, usually beginning in adolescence or young adult life, in which generalized tonic–clonic seizures occur exclusively, or predominantly, on awakening (hence the old name 'epilepsy with grand mal on awakening'). At least six such seizures are considered necessary to establish the diagnosis. It should be noted that generalized tonic–clonic seizures, occurring predominantly on wakening, occur in a number of epilepsy syndromes, including juvenile myoclonic epilepsy. It is the lack of other seizure types which distinguishes the syndrome.

The new ILAE classification suggests inclusion of two syndromes, *epilepsy with myoclonic astatic seizures and epilepsy with myoclonic absences,* hitherto usually considered amongst the cryptogenic or symptomatic generalized epilepsies, within the idiopathic generalized epilepsies. The former (also known as Doose syndrome) usually has its onset within the first 5 years of life.[114] The defining seizure types are atonic and myoclonic, which are often combined (myoatonic seizure) and are often manifested as drop attacks. Episodes of non-convulsive status epilepticus are common. The characteristic EEG feature is spike or polyspike and wave discharges, often with photosensitivity. The prognosis is variable. Many children continue to develop normally and seizures eventually remit. However, others, especially those with repeated episodes of non-convulsive status epilepticus, show cognitive decline. In epilepsy with myoclonic absences, the characteristic seizures are typical absences, accompanied by marked rhythmical myoclonia, mainly affecting the upper limbs and head.[115] These seizures can occur in otherwise normal children, but many have pre-existing neurodevelopmental problems. In children who do not, such problems often supervene. The EEG is very similar to that seen in childhood absence epilepsy. However, video-EEG or an EMG lead applied over the deltoids will reveals myoclonus accompanying each spike–wave discharge.

There are many children with epilepsy with features suggestive of an idiopathic generalized epilepsy who do not fit within the above syndromes. In recent years a number of other syndromes have been suggested and are more or less well characterized. In *eyelid myoclonia with absences (Jeavons' syndrome)* the characteristic seizure consists of brief episodes of marked jerking of the eyelids usually accompanied by upward deviation of the eyes. These usually start in childhood, are often very frequent, and may be misdiagnosed as ticks. On EEG, the seizures occur on eye closure and are associated with generalized polyspike and wave discharges (Fig. 20.16). All children are photosensitive and there is continued debate about the role of self-induction of the seizures. Despite the name, absences are usually inconspicuous. The condition usually continues into adult life and generalized tonic–clonic seizures commonly develop. *Perioral myoclonia with absences* is a syndrome in which typical absences are accompanied by marked rhythmical myoclonia of the perioral and /or jaw muscles. Episodes of absence status appear to be common as are generalized tonic–clonic seizures. The most recently described epilepsy to be placed by the ILAE with the idiopathic generalized epilepsies is *generalized epilepsy with febrile seizures plus.*[116] This is an autosomal dominant condition in which different family members have variable phenotypes including febrile seizures only, febrile seizures with other, mainly generalized, seizure types, and myoclonic–astatic seizures.

The idiopathic generalized epilepsies usually show an excellent response to sodium valproate, which is the drug of first choice for all of them. Lamotrigine is a useful second line agent and may become preferable to sodium valproate in adolescent girls as it may have fewer teratogenic effects. Ethosuximide is a useful drug for childhood absence epilepsy, but is considered to be ineffective against generalized tonic–clonic seizures. Combined therapy, with two, or even all three, of these agents, is occasionally useful in refractory cases. Benzodiazepines, including clobazam and clonazepam, are also useful, particularly against myoclonic seizures. Sodium valproate and lamotrigine are both active against photosensitive seizures. Carbamazepine, vigabatrin, tiagabine and probably also phenytoin are generally ineffective and may exacerbate existing seizures and precipitate new seizure types: their use is contraindicated except in exceptional circumstances.[117]

The idiopathic focal epilepsies.[118] These are characterized by:

- Normal preceding neurodevelopment
- A strong family history of epilepsy including, but not restricted to, idiopathic epilepsies
- A strong history of preceding febrile seizures
- Stereotyped seizures reflecting the site of ictal onset and spread
- EEGs in which the background is normal but in which highly characteristic interictal focal spike and wave abnormalities are frequent.

Benign childhood epilepsy with centrotemporal spikes (commonly called *rolandic epilepsy* or *BECTS)* is the commonest of these epilepsies, and indeed may account for around 20% of all new onset epilepsies in young school-age children who are otherwise normal. The seizures have their onset in the lower rolandic cortex representing the face and oropharynx. Seizure onset peaks between 7 and 10 years. Seizures occur in sleep in only around 70% of children, in both sleep and awake in 15%, and whilst awake, only in 15%. Seizures during sleep often occur shortly after falling asleep or shortly prior to awakening. The seizures are most characteristically unaccompanied by any impairment of consciousness (simple focal in the old terminology), but those during sleep may evolve (often rapidly) with disturbance of cognition (complex focal) and/or secondary generalized tonic–clonic or hemiconvulsions. BECTS should always be considered in a child, of appropriate age, who presents with nocturnal generalized seizures. The seizures usually begin with somatosensory symptoms in and around the mouth. The child often complains of paresthesiae, numbness, 'heaviness' or 'thickness' of the lips, gums, inner cheek and tongue. This is often followed by clonic jerking of the perioral muscles, lips and tongue. Salivation is often prominent. Speech arrest may be due to either laryngeal involvement, or to involvement of nearby speech areas. Seizures usually last only a few seconds to a few minutes but status epilepticus has been described. Total seizure count is usually low; many children have a single seizure only. However, some children may have numerous seizures, sometimes with more than one in a single night. The EEG is highly characteristic with interictal sharp and slow wave complexes in the left and/or right central and/or mid temporal region (Fig. 20.17). They may be unilateral or bilaterally synchronous or asynchronous. They are strongly activated by sleep. Similar abnormalities occur in a minority of children in other brain regions. BECTS has an excellent prognosis. It usually remits within 1–2 years of onset and certainly before mid adolescence. It is exceptional for seizures to occur in adult life.

The second most common benign partial epilepsy of childhood is *Panayiotopoulos syndrome (early-onset benign childhood occipital epilepsy)*.[118,119] It is encountered two to three times less frequently than BECTS. It predominantly affects younger children aged 3–6 years old. Seizures manifest with autonomic symptoms, particularly nausea, retching and vomiting. Often the seizure onset is inconspicuous with the child simply appearing unwell, pale, quiet or irritable. They may complain of feeling sick. Other autonomic manifestations include pallor, pupillary, cardiorespiratory and probably thermoregulatory changes. As the seizure progresses, there is frequently deviation of the eyes and head and impairment of consciousness. Unresponsiveness may be accompanied by marked loss of postural tone. The term 'ictal syncope' has been suggested for this. Around half of the seizures end in secondary generalization. Two-thirds of seizures start in sleep. An important and unusual feature in Panayiotopoulos syndrome is that around half of all seizures last for more than half an hour (sometimes for many years) constituting (autonomic) status epilepticus. During such episodes the child's conscious level fluctuates and there is often intermittent retching and vomiting and eye and head deviation. The status may terminate with a hemiconvulsion or a generalized tonic–clonic seizure. Status in Panayiotopoulos syndrome is frequently not recognized as being epileptic in nature, but may lead to admission to an intensive care unit, with a suspected grave cerebral insult.

The interictal EEG usually reveals abnormalities similar to those seen in BECTS – sharp and slow waves or spikes – but predominating in the occipital regions (Fig. 20.17). As a consequence, Panayiotopoulos syndrome has been classified as an occipital epilepsy. However, this may not be appropriate given the frequency of extraoccipital EEG abnormalities and the predominantly autonomic seizure manifestations. Panayiotopoulos syndrome is amongst the most benign of all epilepsies. Total seizure count is usually low; many children have only a single seizure and seizures generally remit within 1–2 years of onset.

Late-onset childhood occipital epilepsy (Gastaut type or CEOP) begins predominantly in mid–late childhood with a peak age of onset around the age of 7–9 years. It is characterized by relatively frequent, usually brief, visual seizures occurring whilst awake. These occur in full consciousness and are mainly manifested by elementary visual hallucinations of, for example, colored balls (Fig. 20.20). In contrast, in migraine, visual hallucinations are usually black and white and jagged or sharp in outline.[120] Less commonly, visual hallucinations in CEOP are complex, e.g. of figures. Visual illusions, such as micropsia, visual field defects and episodes of ictal blindness also occur. Headache, often hemicranial, is common either ictally or postictally and misdiagnosis as migraine is common. The EEG is characterized by occipital paroxysms, which are runs of high-amplitude spike–waves or sharp waves, occurring in the posterior regions. Prognosis is less clear than with either BECTS or Panayiotopoulos syndrome – many individuals continue to have seizures in adolescence and adult life and some develop occasional generalized tonic–clonic seizures.

A third idiopathic occipital epilepsy syndrome in children – *idiopathic photosensitive occipital lobe epilepsy* – will be described later (p. 939) when reflex epilepsies are discussed.

A number of other epilepsy syndromes with certain similarities to BECTS and Panayiotopoulos syndrome have been proposed but are less well characterized. These include *benign partial epilepsy with affective symptomatology, benign partial seizures in adolescence, benign epilepsy with 'extreme' somatosensory evoked potentials* and *benign frontal lobe epilepsy*. These demonstrate that there are many children who have features suggestive of benign focal epilepsy, but whose electroclinical features do not fit within existing syndromes.

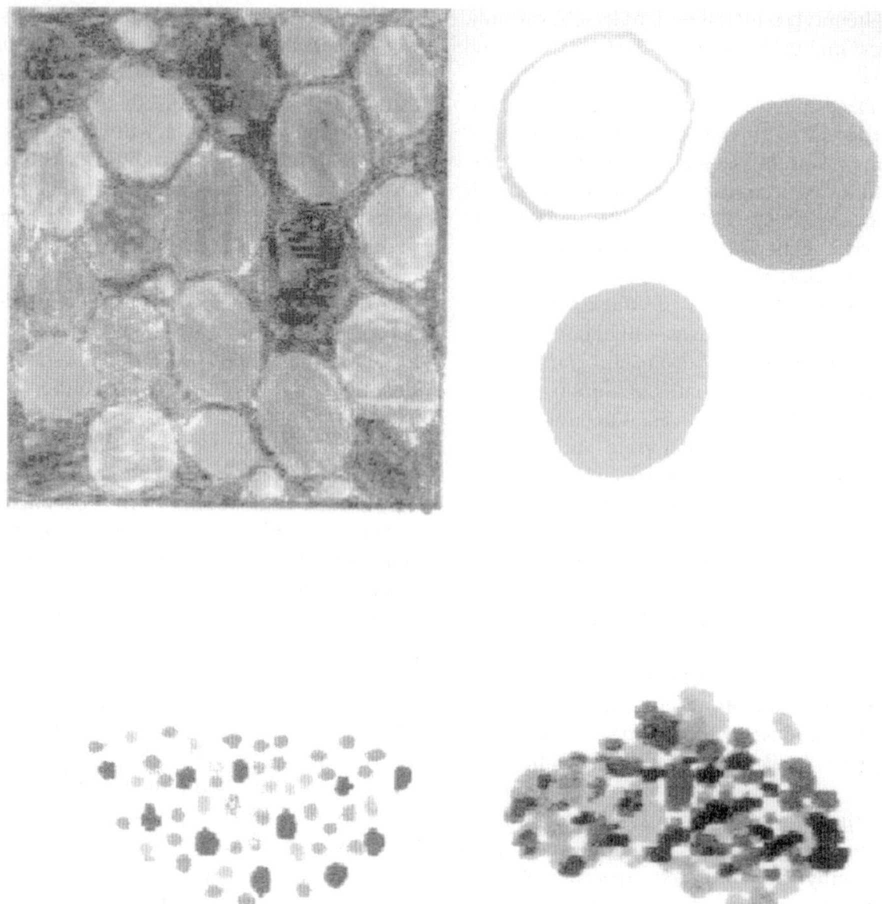

Fig. 20.20 Patient's illustrations of visual hallucinations in childhood occipital epilepsy (Gastaut type). (Modified from Panayiotopoulos 1999[118] with permission of the BMJ Publishing Group)

In recent years, a number of idiopathic focal epilepsies, inherited in an autosomal dominant manner, have been described. The best characterized is *autosomal dominant nocturnal frontal lobe epilepsy*. This usually begins in childhood, but has an exceptionally wide age range of onset. The seizures are characteristically brief and occur during light sleep. They may be repeated many times per night. Motor symptoms predominate. A grunt, groan, or more complex vocalization, often heralds the seizure, followed by hyperkinetic motor behaviors (e.g. thrashing, thrusting and rocking movements) or tonic or dystonic posturing, sometimes with clonic components. The occurrence of dystonic features gave rise to the designation 'nocturnal paroxysmal dystonia', which was previously considered non-epileptic. The EEG is frequently normal, even during attacks. A minority show focal frontal interictal and ictal abnormalities. Neuroimaging is normal. The condition appears to be life long. A good response to carbamazepine is seen in some, but not all, patients. Other autosomal dominant focal epilepsies include *familial temporal lobe epilepsy* and *familial focal epilepsy with variable foci*.[121,122]

In children with benign focal seizures who have few seizures, particularly if seizures cause little distress, and in whom remission is expected (i.e. BECTS and Panayiotopoulos syndrome), it is reasonable not to treat with antiepileptic drugs and to await spontaneous remission. When treatment is given, it is important to ensure that the unwanted effects are not more troublesome than the seizures. Occasionally the idiopathic focal epilepsies can be made more severe with antiepileptic drug treatment. This is particularly described with carbamazepine.[123]

Symptomatic and probably symptomatic focal epilepsies. These epilepsies are mainly defined by their site of origin and, to a lesser extent, by their etiology. A broad distinction is made according to whether the site of origin is in the limbic system or in the neocortex (including the lateral temporal lobes). Of the limbic epilepsies mesial temporal lobe epilepsy is the most important. Neocortical epilepsy syndromes include Rasmussen's syndrome.

Mesial temporal lobe epilepsy with hippocampal sclerosis (often referred to simply as *mesial temporal lobe epilepsy*) is of considerable importance because it is the single largest cause of refractory epilepsy in adults and the commonest reason for undertaking epilepsy surgery. Mesial temporal sclerosis consists of severe loss of specific neurones in the hippocampus along with synaptic reorganizations. This probably results from a previous cerebral injury rather than as a consequence of repeated seizures and, at least in adults undergoing epilepsy surgery, is strongly associated with prolonged febrile convulsions in early childhood. It is not established whether these are the cause of mesial temporal sclerosis, or another manifestation of it. Genetic factors are also important and there is an increased incidence of various seizure disorders in the families of subjects with mesial temporal lobe epilepsy.

The following represents the sequence typical in mesial temporal lobe epilepsy, although there is considerable variation:

- Complicated febrile convulsion(s) in infancy/early childhood
- Later onset of habitual seizures, usually in childhood, which characteristically respond well to initial treatment

- Return of habitual seizures in adolescence/early adult life, which often become refractory to treatment.

The habitual seizures of mesial temporal lobe epilepsy often begin with an aura, manifestations of which may include autonomic features such as a rising sensation in the epigastrium, psychic features such as fear, déjà vu and feelings of depersonalization, visual illusions such as micropsia and macropsia and olfactory hallucinations such as unpleasant smells. Formed visual and auditory hallucinations are said not to occur. Many seizures do not progress beyond the aura. In the old terminology they were classed as simple focal seizures. However, they often progress such that there is impaired cognition, perception, attention and memory (dyscognitive seizure or 'complex partial' in the old terminology). Motor manifestations are often prominent and include motor arrest, oral–alimentary and manual automatisms and lateralized motor manifestations such as forced head and eye deviation and tonic or dystonic posturing. Language disturbances also occur. Secondary generalization is often not a prominent feature. The postictal period is typically characterized by a variable period of confusion, disorientation, language disturbances and either relaxation or automated semipurposeful movements. Contralateral Todd's paresis may occur. More details on the lateralizing features of mesial temporal lobe seizures are to be found elsewhere.[124,125]

The characteristic interictal EEG abnormality is anterior temporal sharp waves, spikes and slow waves (Fig. 20.17). These are quite frequently bilateral, even in children in whom habitual seizures are unilateral. In younger children, bilateral synchronous spike–wave discharges may occur. A repeatedly normal, interictal EEG is common. MRI has revolutionized the detection of hippocampal sclerosis. Thin coronal slices orthogonal to the long axis of the temporal lobes usually reveal hippocampal atrophy, temporal horn dilatation (both best appreciated on T1 weighted sections) and, on T2 weighted images, high signal in the hippocampus (Fig. 20.19).

The drug of choice for mesial temporal lobe epilepsy is carbamazepine. Initial response is usually good, but may not be maintained. There is currently no information about what percentage of children gain permanent seizure remission and how many develop refractory epilepsy. When carbamazepine fails, other drugs active against partial seizures should be tried. However, surgery offers the prospect of 'cure' in around 80% of children and should not be unduly delayed through a desire to exhaust all medical options.

Mesial temporal lobe epilepsy can also be caused by cortical dysplasias, tumors (particularly dysembryoplastic neuroepithelial tumors), hamartomas and chronic encephalitis and other destructive lesions.

The neocortical epilepsies are a heterogeneous group of epilepsies arising from the frontal lobes, lateral temporal lobes, parietal and occipital lobes. *Lateral (neocortical) temporal lobe epilepsy* is uncommon. Compared to mesial temporal lobe epilepsy seizures are more likely to give rise to auditory, vertiginous and complex visual hallucinations and less likely to give rise to motor manifestations.

Frontal lobe epilepsies are relatively common and probably under-recognized. They pose particular diagnostic problems. Three main seizure types have been described:

- Focal clonic seizures. These characteristically occur in clear consciousness and involve localized rhythmical jerking of a limb. A Jacksonian march, consisting of sequential involvement of contiguous areas of the body in a focal motor seizure, may be seen. Such activity implies seizure activity in the primary motor area.
- Focal motor seizures with asymmetric tonic motor seizures (asymmetrical tonic seizures, supplementary motor seizures). These are characterized by the assumption, usually suddenly, of fixed and abnormal postures, the most classical being the so-called 'fencing posture'. Motor manifestations are often preceded by somatosensory sensations of numbness and tingling. Other ictal features are speech arrest or forced vocalizations and secondary generalization. Asymmetrical tonic seizures are characteristic of seizures arising in the supplementary motor area of the frontal lobes.
- Focal motor seizures with hyperkinetic automatisms (frontal lobe complex partial seizures, hypermotor seizures). These seizures occur in association with impaired cognition and are characterized by complex motor automatisms. Frenetic, agitated, and sometimes sexual, behavior is often seen, along with vocalizations, ranging from humming to the shouting of obscenities. Such seizures can originate from many areas of the frontal lobes.

The reader requiring fuller descriptions is referred elsewhere.[126] Frontal lobe epilepsies are often characterized by frequent, mainly nocturnal, seizures, with little if any postictal drowsiness. The interictal and even ictal EEG is often normal, reflecting the fact that large areas of the mesial and inferior frontal lobes are not directly accessible by scalp EEG. They are often confused with psychogenic seizures, which, however, rarely occur whilst the child is asleep and usually last longer.

Occipital lobe epilepsies are relatively uncommon. Characteristic ictal features include elementary and sometimes complex visual hallucinations. The most common are hallucinations of colored spots or geometric forms similar to those described for late-onset childhood occipital epilepsy (Gastaut type). Ictal blindness may also occur. Other features are a variety of abnormal eye movements such as tonic deviation, nystagmoid movements, forced blinking and eyelid flutter. Many different patterns of spread can occur, giving rise to features more typical of temporal or frontal lobe seizures. The interictal and ictal EEG is generally useful in the diagnosis of occipital epilepsies. However, occasionally discharges confined to mesial or inferior aspects of the occipital lobes may be undetected by scalp EEG and the propensity of seizures to spread may impede localization. The range of pathologies causing occipital lobe epilepsy is similar to that of other neocortical epilepsies. However, in addition, a syndrome of *occipital lobe epilepsy with bilateral occipital calcifications and celiac disease* has been described.[127] The relationship between occipital lobe epilepsies and migraine has also aroused much debate. Occipital epilepsy and migraine are often confused because both are characterized by visual hallucinations and by headache, often hemicranial. In addition, it is possible that occipital (and other) epilepsies may occasionally trigger migraine attacks. Whether epileptic seizures are ever caused by migraine remains to be established.[118]

Parietal lobe epilepsy is rare. Ictal manifestations include somatosensory symptoms, particularly unilateral paresthesiae and pain (including abdominal pain), speech problems, dyspraxias and agnosias. Many parietal lobe seizures are 'silent' unless they spread. Interictal and even ictal EEG is often unhelpful.

Rasmussen's syndrome (often called *Rasmussen's encephalitis*) is a symptomatic, neocortical epilepsy syndrome of unknown cause, characterized pathologically by so-called 'chronic encephalitis'. Its onset is usually between 1 and 15 years and may present either with focal seizures, which quickly become more and more frequent, or as status epilepticus, which is usually focal in nature. The most characteristic seizure type is focal motor seizures, often highly localized, for example to an extremity of one limb or around the mouth. However, impaired cognition during seizures is not uncommon, particularly as the condition progresses. Epilepsia partialis continua is seen at some time in the disease in the majority of patients. The disease is nearly always strictly unilateral at onset, but 'spread' to the other hemisphere can occur with time. A hallmark of the disease is progressive cerebral atrophy, usually confined to one hemisphere, at least initially. This is accompanied by a progressive hemiparesis whose onset can occur within weeks of the onset of clinical seizures or be delayed for years. It is accompanied by cognitive decline. Interictal EEG may show progressive background slowing of the involved hemisphere. Ictal EEG is often lateralizing but rarely localizing. Structural imaging early in the disease may show focal high signal on T2 weighted images, particularly in the cerebral cortex. Later atrophic changes are seen.

The management of Rasmussen's syndrome should involve early referral to an epilepsy surgery center, since early hemispherectomy is considered by many to be the treatment of choice. Localized resections are generally ineffective. Medical therapy with conventional antiepileptic drugs is nearly always unsuccessful in the long term although short term control of seizure may be achieved. Immunotherapy with either steroid medication or intravenous immunoglobulin may be of benefit in some children and may avoid the need for hemispherectomy. The condition has recently been reviewed in detail.[128]

Epileptic encephalopathies. The best known epileptic encephalopathy of childhood is *Lennox–Gastaut syndrome*. However, there is considerable variation in how this syndrome is defined. At one extreme it has been used to designate virtually any seizure disorder in childhood characterized by drug resistant seizures and impaired mental abilities. Alternatively, as here, it is used to designate a narrowly defined symptomatic, or probably symptomatic, generalized epilepsy. Its onset is usually between 3 and 5 years of age; onset after 10 years of age is exceptional. The defining features are:

- The occurrence of mixed generalized seizure types of which tonic, atonic and atypical absences are the most prominent
- Interictal EEG patterns with generalized slow spike and wave discharges and, in sleep, bursts of fast rhythms at 10–12 Hz (Fig. 20.18)
- Psychomotor delay.

Lennox–Gastaut syndrome has multiple causes, similar to those of West syndrome, from which it sometimes evolves. Indeed virtually any cortical brain pathology, whether focal or generalized, can cause it. True idiopathic cases are not generally recognized, patients in whom no cause can be found being classified as probably symptomatic.

The characteristic seizures of Lennox–Gastaut syndrome can be present from the start. Alternatively, they may be preceded by other seizure types, including focal seizures. Seizures tend to be frequent, occurring many times a day, and tonic and atonic seizures often cause falls ('drop attacks'). During sleep, tonic seizures are particularly characteristic and are associated with 10–12 Hz fast rhythms. Episodes of non-convulsive status epilepticus are common. Virtually any other seizure type can occur, including (according to many but not all authorities), focal seizures. However, myoclonic seizures are not usually prominent. Their occurrence, especially if associated with EEG patterns other than slow spike and wave, should make one consider other severe epilepsies, such as severe myoclonic epilepsy in infancy. However, a myoclonic variant of the Lennox–Gastaut syndrome is recognized. Occasionally, children and adolescents with apparently idiopathic epilepsies develop features of the Lennox–Gastaut syndrome.[129,130] In some cases this may be drug induced.

Mental retardation is often pre-existing. However, the onset of the syndrome is nearly always accompanied by a slowing in development or even apparent regression. This is not of the relentless nature, which is seen in neurodegenerative conditions. It often appears to mirror seizure control, with improvement occurring during quiescent periods. However, a majority of children eventually become mentally retarded, and this is often severe. Behavioral problems, including autistic behaviors, may coexist. A small number of children with otherwise typical Lennox–Gastaut syndrome develop normally.

Lennox–Gastaut syndrome is highly resistant to therapy. There are many different recommendations but in general it is best to use broad-spectrum agents such as sodium valproate and lamotrigine rather than narrower spectrum agents such as carbamazepine and vigabatrin. However, there is no doubt that the latter have benefited individual children. Other drugs, usually used as concomitant therapy, which may be useful, include the benzodiazepines, ethosuximide and acetazolamide. Controlled trials have demonstrated efficacy of lamotrigine, topiramate and felbamate in the Lennox – Gastaut syndrome.[131–133] Monotherapy should always be attempted, but many children do best on two, or occasionally three, drugs. Polytherapy carries significant risks of making seizures worse, particularly if they induce drowsiness. In children with Lennox–Gastaut syndrome it is important to define a realistic aim for drug therapy. This will involve accepting that complete seizure control is unlikely and that maximizing function and quality of life is of more importance. The natural history of the disorder is marked by fluctuations in the activity of seizures. This must be recognized, when making decisions regarding drug treatment.

Other treatments, which may be helpful in Lennox–Gastaut syndrome, include the ketogenic diet, steroids, intravenous immunoglobulins and surgery. Except in very rare occasions when a focal or strictly hemispheric lesion gives rise to Lennox–Gastaut syndrome, resective surgery is not an option. However, corpus callostomy may be helpful if atonic drop attacks are a major problem. Vagal nerve stimulation may also be useful.[134]

The overall prognosis for Lennox–Gastaut syndrome is poor. A small number of previously normal subjects, particularly those whose condition is of later onset and who have the condition for only a short period of time, have a favorable outlook. The remainder continue to have seizures for many years. These may continue to show the characteristics of the Lennox–Gastaut syndrome or there may be an evolution into other types of epilepsy.

The Landau–Kleffner syndrome and *epilepsy with continuous spike–waves during slow-wave sleep* are closely related epilepsy syndromes. The EEG pattern of continuous spikes and waves during slow sleep (CSWS) consists of bilateral generalized spike and wave discharges present for at least 85% of slow-wave sleep. This pattern is occasionally encountered in the course of a number of epilepsies. For example, it is occasionally described in children with benign childhood epilepsy with centrotemporal spikes in whom it may be associated with a decline in cognitive performance. It has also been described as a separate, and rather poorly defined, syndrome (epilepsy with continuous spike–waves during slow-wave sleep). Finally it is very common in the Landau–Kleffner syndrome. The latter is an epilepsy syndrome occurring in previously normal children, usually between 3 and 8 years of age, but occasionally younger, who develop an aphasia, which initially is mainly receptive, but often becomes global. Deafness is frequently suspected. Many children become totally mute and may fail to understand environmental noises. A notable feature of the syndrome is severe behavioral problems. Epileptic seizures are usually relatively infrequent and may be totally absent. They can be of various types. The awake EEG may be normal or else show focal, hemispheric or generalized spike–wave abnormalities. The sleep EEG often, but not invariably, shows CSWS. Sophisticated EEG techniques often indicate that the EEG abnormality is maximal in one or other posterior temporal electrodes. MRI is nearly always normal but PET and SPECT often show localized or hemispheric metabolic and perfusion abnormalities. All children with suspected Landau–Kleffner syndrome and/or CSWS require detailed neuropsychological evaluation.

Seizure control in these syndromes may not be difficult and may lead to improved language function. However, the syndrome frequently fails to respond to conventional antiepileptic drug medication. Most authorities appear to treat initially with sodium valproate. However, if an inadequate response is obtained, hormonal treatment (steroids or ACTH) is indicated and the response may be dramatic. Unfortunately relapses are common. The technique of multiple subpial transection has been pioneered for the treatment of Landau–Kleffner and appears to improve the outlook.[135] It is based on the functional organization of the cerebral cortex vertically but with the connections involved in the spread of seizures being arranged horizontally. The horizontal connections are disrupted by making multiple cuts perpendicular to the cortical surface whilst preserving the vertically orientated fibers. Eventually Landau–Kleffner syndrome remits. This can occur after only a few weeks or after many years. The long-term outlook in Landau–Kleffner syndrome reflects the duration of the condition;[136] most subjects have permanent language problems unless the stage of active disease was very short.

The widespread recognition of the Landau–Kleffner syndrome has lead to renewed interest in the cognitive effect of seizures in other epilepsies.[137] It is now increasingly accepted that specific cognitive and/or behavioral disturbances may have an epileptic basis even when overt seizures are infrequent or absent. Recognition can be a major problem. Clues include fluctuations, sometimes abrupt, in aspects such as mood, attention, memory and performance. Sophisticated EEG techniques coupled with neuropsychological evaluation are necessary to investigate such 'cognitive seizures'. The role of antiepileptic drug treatment is uncertain, but a trial of therapy is probably justified if there is reasonable evidence that cognitive problems are the result of epileptic activity. However, the possibility of inducing cognitive problems with antiepileptic drugs must constantly be borne in mind.

Reflex epilepsies. Reflex seizures are seizures precipitated by sensory stimuli. The stimulus may be simple such as flashes of light, touch or unexpected loud noises or complex such as colored pictures, eating, etc. Most stimuli inducing reflex seizures are extrinsic. However, intrinsic stimuli such as proprioception can occasionally induce seizures. The 2001 ILAE definition precludes seizures provoked by higher brain functions, such as cognition and specific emotions. However, these have conventionally been considered with reflex seizures. The range of stimuli, which have been linked to seizure provocation, is wide and the clinician should be alert to the possibility of reflex seizures even if the stimulus seems bizarre and novel. Seizures precipitated by fever, alcohol, drugs and trauma are not considered to be reflex seizures. Reflex seizures occur in many epilepsy syndromes.

Light induced seizures (photosensitive seizures) are by far the most common reflex seizures. Photosensitivity appears to be a genetically determined trait. It can be assessed in the EEG laboratory by the response to intermittent photic stimulation (IPS). Normally IPS induces so-called 'photic following responses' which must not be interpreted as indicating photosensitivity. A number of abnormalities, both focal (nearly always occipital) and generalized, can be evoked by IPS in susceptible subjects and these may be associated with clinical photosensitivity. Of most significance is generalized spike and wave activity or multiple spikes, which continue for at least 100 msec after the train of flashes ends (Fig. 20.16). Light induced seizures are most commonly generalized, particularly generalized tonic–clonic seizures, absences and myoclonic jerks. However, partial seizures, often but not exclusively with features suggesting occipital lobe onset, are increasingly recognized. Among the important clinical precipitants of light induced seizures are television, video-games, VDU screens (which nevertheless are much less provocative than TV screens), discotheques (particularly stroboscopic lights), and natural flickering light, for example caused by light shining through trees or fences or reflected off water. Some people with light induced seizures are also sensitive to specific patterns such as striped wallpaper and certain patterns on clothing. Very rarely pattern sensitivity can occur without photosensitivity. Some subjects who are photosensitive can, and habitually do, self-induce seizures. This may be achieved by waving the outstretched hand in front of the eyes, viewing provocative patterns, or watching TV sets extremely close up.

Light induced seizures are particularly common in idiopathic generalized epilepsies. They occur in more than a third of children with juvenile myoclonic epilepsy and are universal in eyelid myoclonia with absences. In addition, many children with idiopathic generalized epilepsies, who have typical absence seizures, and do not fit within the patterns of currently recognized syndromes, have light induced seizures. Their prognosis, in terms of remission of seizures, is much poorer than children with childhood absence epilepsy. Significant numbers of children and adults have focal seizures, all of which have been provoked by photic factors. *Idiopathic photosensitive occipital lobe epilepsy* is an epilepsy syndrome beginning in late childhood and adolescence. It is characterized by focal seizures with symptomatology suggesting occipital lobe onset (elementary visual symptoms, head and eye deviation, headache), often with secondary generalization. Seizures are provoked by visual stimuli and the interictal EEG shows occipital spike and waves and generalized or occipital photoparoxysmal responses on IPS.

Light induced seizures are also characteristic of a number of symptomatic epilepsies and epileptic encephalopathies, including severe myoclonic epilepsy of infancy, epilepsy with myoclonic–astatic seizures, Unverricht–Lundborg disease and Lafora disease.

Some subjects with photosensitive seizures may be able to avoid the provoking factor. Most, however, will require antiepileptic drug treatment. Sodium valproate and lamotrigine are the main drugs effective against photically induced seizures. Other measures depend on the fact that photically induced seizures are more likely, the larger the area of retina stimulated. Hence TV should be watched from the maximum comfortable viewing distance and a remote control should be used to change channels. Fully covering one eye may be advised if the child cannot watch TV safely otherwise and is useful if the subject is caught unawares, for example at a disco if a strobe is suddenly used. TV should also be watched in a well-lit room. Factors such as fatigue and sleep deprivation are likely to also play a role and therefore photosensitive subjects should be advised to avoid watching TV or playing video-games for prolonged periods and if tired.

Primary reading epilepsy is a rare, probably genetically determined, epilepsy, which usually starts in late childhood and adolescence and is characterized mainly by jaw jerks, sometimes with spread, occurring whilst reading. Seizures may also be provoked by speaking. Interictal EEG is usually normal; an ictal recording is often easy to obtain.

Seizures evoked by unexpected auditory or somatosensory stimuli are most often encountered in children with symptomatic generalized epilepsies, who usually also have spontaneous seizures. They are sometimes seen in children with Down syndrome.

Occasionally all seizures may be provoked by startle (*startle epilepsy*). The seizures are usually tonic but may be atonic or myoclonic. Obtaining an ictal EEG can be very helpful. Clonazepam is probably the most effective drug.

Seizures not necessarily requiring a diagnosis of epilepsy. This inelegant term is used to designate conditions in which recurrent epileptic seizures may occur (the usual pragmatic definition of an epilepsy), but in whom the term 'epilepsy' is, for a variety of reasons, inappropriate. The most important example is febrile seizures (the term 'febrile convulsions' is discouraged), which is distinguished from epilepsy principally to remove the stigma associated with epilepsy when describing a generally benign condition. A similar argument could be made for benign childhood epilepsy with centrotemporal spikes and Panayiotopoulos syndrome, which are equally self-limiting.

Febrile seizures are usually defined as epileptic seizures precipitated by fever (usually defined as above 38°C), not due to an intracranial infection or other definable CNS cause and not preceded by afebrile seizures. They are the most common form of epileptic disorder and affect about 3% of children. They generally occur between 6 months and 4 years of age, although younger and older children may be affected.[138] Prevalence in boys is slightly higher than in girls. Most febrile seizures are generalized tonic–clonic (or purely clonic) seizures. Focal and atonic febrile seizures also occur. A simple febrile seizure is generalized, lasts under 15 min and is not repeated during the same illness. Complex febrile seizures are focal and/or last over 15 min and/or recur during the same febrile illness. The focal nature of a febrile seizure may be revealed by a Todd's paresis. Febrile status epilepticus is defined as lasting over 30 min. Approximately 6% of febrile seizures are prolonged, with 80% of these being the initial seizure.

Genetic factors are important in the etiology of febrile seizures.[139] Children of parents who had febrile seizures have a risk four times that of the general population and siblings of probands have a risk 3.5 times that of the general population. There is a high concordance in monozygotic twins. Polygenic inheritance, or autosomal dominant inheritance with reduced penetrance, are considered the most likely modes of inheritance. Although the usual definition of febrile seizures precludes children with known brain disorders, epidemiological studies have shown an increased risk of febrile seizures in children whose developmental milestones are slow (but not necessarily outwith the normal range). All infections which cause fever, may be associated with febrile convulsions, but some infections are more prominent. Roseola infantum and shigella dysentery are said to be associated with a particularly high risk of febrile seizures. Vaccinations, especially diphtheria, tetanus and pertussis (DTP) and against measles, may also be associated.[140] A rapid rise in the temperature is said to be important although data to prove this are lacking. However, it is certainly the case that febrile seizures often arise early in the course of the illness; it is often the first indication that the child is unwell.

The clinical skill in managing a child presenting with a suspected febrile seizure involves confirming that the event was probably epileptic, since a number of non-epileptic disorders (syncopes occurring during febrile illnesses, delirium and rigors) are commonly misdiagnosed as febrile seizures. It is important to exclude serious infections (particularly meningitis and encephalitis) in which both fever and seizures may occur. The evaluation must include a detailed history and examination. It is particularly important to obtain a detailed description of the attack and the circumstances in which it took place. Many children, when first seen, will have recovered and will be fully conscious. Febrile convulsions are rare under 6 months of age and in this age group, examination of the CNS is almost mandatory. Between 6 and 18 months febrile seizures are common but meningitis can present in this age group without meningism. Many authorities advocate lumbar puncture in all children in this age group presenting with a first febrile seizure;[139] meningitis often occurs in children with coexisting respiratory tract infections, including otitis media. However, the value of this approach has recently been questioned.[141] Beyond 18 months of age lumbar puncture can be avoided if there is no meningism and a clear focus of infection is found. Investigations, other than those looking for sources of infection, are generally not required. Children who are unconscious when first seen should be assessed along standard lines. The risk of inducing brain herniation is such that lumbar puncture should be delayed unless the subject is localizing pain, has no focal neurological signs and no papilledema. Most children will recover consciousness within half an hour or so of the seizure. If the child is otherwise well, it is reasonable to wait a short period of time to see if the expected recovery occurs. If it does not, then the child must be managed as a case of coma. Empirical treatment with antibiotics and antiviral agents to cover the risk of bacterial meningitis and encephalitis should be started and lumbar puncture delayed until clinical and radiological assessment suggests that it can be done safely.

Children are often admitted to hospital following their first febrile seizure. However, admission is not always necessary.[141] A reasonable alternative is for the child to be observed for several hours. If the child has fully recovered and a source of infection has been identified, s/he can be discharged, with advice given to the parents. Children with complex febrile seizures probably all warrant admission.

The overall prognosis for febrile seizures is excellent.[142] However, around one-third will have at least one recurrence and 9% of children will have over three febrile seizures. The majority of recurrences occur within the year following the first seizure. Recurrences are more likely if the seizure has been complex, if there is a family history of febrile or non-febrile seizures and if the initiating temperature for the seizure was relatively low. Meta-analyses have failed to show any benefit of continuous antiepileptic drug medication in preventing febrile convulsions and there is now almost universal agreement that it is not indicated.[142,143] The parents of children who have had febrile convulsions are generally given antipyretic advice, although this on its own offers poor protection from recurrences. Removal of excessive clothes and blankets is recommended. Occasionally tepid sponging may be useful, but cold baths and fans played directly onto the child should be avoided as they may increase core temperature. Antipyretic agents such as paracetamol and ibuprofen should be given. Intermittent prophylactic therapy with oral or rectal benzodiazepines has been advocated but is rarely used. Most authorities consider the most appropriate management is for the parents to have clear first aid instructions and advice as to when to call for emergency help. Depending on circumstances, it may be appropriate for the family to have a supply of either rectal diazepam or midazolam to be used nasally or buccally for prolonged seizures.[144,145] An important aspect of management is reassurance of the parents, who almost certainly will have been greatly traumatized by the event.

The risk of developing epilepsy in children who have had febrile seizures is increased compared to that of the general population. The risk is 2% at 5 years, 4.5% at 10 years, 5.5% at 15 years and 7% at 25 years.[146] The risk is greater if the febrile seizures started under the age of 1 year, in the presence of any preceding neurodevelopmental problem, if there is a family history of epilepsy and if the febrile seizures have been complex. Generalized epilepsies tend to follow when there is a family history of non-febrile seizures and a large number of simple febrile seizures. Partial epilepsies are more common if there have been prolonged lateralized seizures. Although it is clear that the overall prognosis for children who have had febrile seizures, even if complex, is excellent, clinicians should avoid overoptimism. They should be particularly wary in cases where prolonged, often asymmetrical, febrile seizures have occurred in association with relatively mild febrile illnesses since this may be the herald of severe myoclonic epilepsy in infancy. In addition, as previously discussed, the majority of children who subsequently develop refractory mesial temporal lobe epilepsy have had prolonged, often lateralized febrile seizures. The intellectual and behavioral outcome of febrile seizures is excellent.[147]

The EEG has very little role to play in the management of febrile seizures. Within a week of the attack a variety of non-specific abnormalities may be seen. In addition, various generalized or focal epileptiform abnormalities occur in the EEG of children who have had febrile seizures but are of poor prognostic significance.

Post-traumatic seizures are classified as early (occurring within a week of the trauma) and late. The former include immediate seizures, which occur within 24 h of the injury. Only recurrent, late, post-traumatic seizures are considered a manifestation of epilepsy. Immediate and early post-traumatic seizures are much more common in children than in adults. They occur in up to 5% of all children and are usually focal, but can be generalized. In up to one-fifth of cases they take the form of status epilepticus. Following severe head injuries the risk may be as high as 35%.[148,149] Late, post-traumatic seizures can occur at any time following the trauma but usually within 2 years. They are less common in children than in adults. In a large population based study they occurred in 7.4% of children following head injury.[148] The risk is determined by the severity and type of head injury. There is no increased risk following mild closed head injuries. The risk is increased by early post-traumatic seizures, intracranial bleeding and depressed skull fracture. Both focal and generalized seizures can occur. Prophylactic antiepileptic drugs probably do not decrease the risk of developing late post-traumatic seizures and are not indicated.[150] Phenytoin is generally used in the acute situation for treatment and prevention of early post-traumatic seizures.

Seizures can occur as a complication of a large number of disturbances in body homeostasis. Generally these only occur whilst the disturbance persists and hence a diagnosis of epilepsy is inappropriate. They include seizures occurring during hyponatremia, hypocalcemia and hypomagnesemia. Seizures may also be a feature of uremia, the treatment of renal failure with dialysis and during renal transplant rejection. Epileptic seizures are a well-known feature of hypoglycemia; they may also occur during hyperglycemic comas in diabetic children. Epileptic seizures are also an occasional occurrence in individuals with a variety of endocrine disorders.

There are many children and adults who have only a single seizure during their lifetime, or else a cluster of seizures over a short period of time with no further seizures, or else very occasional seizures with long periods between seizures. These individuals do not warrant a diagnosis of epilepsy. They probably represent a heterogeneous group, with the milder forms of different types of epilepsy. Seizures are liable to occur during periods of emotional or physical stress such as at exam times, when sleep deprived, or when drinking unaccustomed alcohol.

DISEASES FREQUENTLY ASSOCIATED WITH EPILEPSY

Epileptic seizures occur in children with a huge range of different diseases and the manifestations of the seizures often show disease specific characteristics. The following is a survey of some of the clinically relevant features of epileptic seizures as they manifest in diseases encountered in childhood. Comprehensive descriptions of many of these disorders are given elsewhere in this text.

The progressive myoclonic epilepsies

Most pediatricians find the concept of the progressive myoclonic epilepsies a difficult one. Nevertheless they often undertake extensive neurometabolic investigations. These are to a large extent designed to detect the progressive myoclonic epilepsies. The conditions included are all rare such that most pediatricians might see only one or two cases throughout their career. Their key characteristics are:

- An epilepsy characterized by myoclonic and other seizure types, including generalized tonic–clonic seizures. The seizures are often precipitated by factors such as touch, action or intention
- Neurological problems, usually including cerebellar signs, and often progressive
- Mental deterioration, of varying degrees, but often eventually leading to dementia.

These features typify the 'core group' of progressive myoclonic epilepsies. In other progressive myoclonic epilepsies atypical features are present whilst in some other progressive epilepsies, myoclonic seizures occur but are overshadowed by other manifestations.[151] In the latter group the epilepsy is almost an incidental problem and its characterization is of limited value in recognizing the disorder. Included are: non-ketotic hyperglycinemia; D-glyceric aciduria, biopterin deficiency, Menkes' disease, Krabbe disease; Tay–Sachs disease; Sandhoff disease and Niemann–Pick C disease.

The core conditions included in the progressive myoclonus epilepsies are:

- Lafora disease
- Unverricht–Lundborg disease
- Sialidosis (types I and II)
- Gaucher disease (type III)
- Neuroaxonal dystrophy
- Myoclonic epilepsy with ragged red fibers (MERRF)
- Dentatorubropallidoluysian atrophy.

Lafora disease is an autosomal recessive disorder, common in the Mediterranean, and caused by mutations of the EPM2A gene on chromosome 6.[152] It usually presents between 6 and 19 years of age. Two features of the epilepsy are distinctive: (i) the precipitation of myoclonia by action and intention and (ii) the occurrence of partial seizures with elementary visual phenomena. Mental and neurological decline with pyramidal, extrapyramidal and cerebellar signs appear, leading to early death. Diagnosis is now by molecular genetics, but previously relied on identification of so-called Lafora bodies on biopsy, particularly of apocrine sweat glands. No specific treatment is available.

Unverricht–Lundborg disease (Baltic myoclonus/Mediterranean myoclonus) is an autosomal recessive disorder caused by a disease causing mutation in the cystatin B gene on chromosome 21.[153] The age of onset is similar to that of Lafora disease. The distinctive features of the epilepsy are the precipitation of myoclonic seizures by maintenance of posture or intended movements and photosensitivity. Neurological and mental decline is usually very slow and prolonged survival is expected. Valproate is the treatment of choice; phenytoin is contraindicated as it appears to increase the rate of deterioration.

The ***sialidoses*** and ***Gaucher disease type III*** are lysosomal storage disorders caused by deficiencies of alpha neuraminidase and beta-glucocerebrosidase respectively. They present in childhood or adolescence with features of a myoclonic epilepsy and variable evidence of visceral storage and dysmorphism. Cherry red spots may be seen. Gaucher disease type III is characterized by horizontal ophthalmoplegia.

The extremely rare juvenile form of *neuroaxonal dystrophy* causes a progressive myoclonic epilepsy in late childhood or adolescence often with retinal degeneration. The pathological hallmark is the demonstration of axonal spheroids on rectal or skin biopsy.

Epileptic seizures occur in a number of mitochondrial disorders.[154] However, the most characteristic is *MERRF* in which myoclonic epilepsy is associated with cerebellar signs, myopathy and often with other features seen in mitochondrial disorders. Ragged red fibers may be seen on muscle biopsy, but it can also be diagnosed on the basis of mitochondrial DNA mutations.

Dentatorubropallidoluysian atrophy is an autosomal dominant disorder with anticipation due to a trinucleotide repeat on chromosome 12. It is mainly seen in adults from Japan but does occur in children and in non-Japanese. Features of progressive myoclonus epilepsy are combined with an extrapyramidal movement disorder and dementia.

Diseases in which features of progressive myoclonus epilepsy occur which are atypical or which are associated with other prominent manifestations include:

- The neuronal ceroid lipofuscinoses
- Poliodystrophies (Alper's disease)
- Childhood onset Huntington's chorea (myoclonic variant)
- Hallovorden–Spatz disease
- Biopterin deficiency
- Other mitochondrial disorders including mitochondrial encephalomyopathy, lactic acidosis and stroke-like episodes (MELAS).

Special mention should be made of the *neuronal ceroid lipofuscinoses*.[155] These disorders were previously diagnosed pathologically and are characterized by the accumulation of ceroid lipofuscin in neurones. All the common forms can now be diagnosed enzymatically or by molecular DNA analysis. Epilepsy occurs in all forms of the disorder, but is a particularly prominent and early feature of the late infantile form which may be mistaken for the Lennox–Gastaut syndrome.

The neurocutaneous disorders[156,157]

Many neurocutaneous disorders are associated with seizures (e.g. tuberous sclerosis, neurofibromatosis, Sturge–Weber syndrome, West syndrome, epidermal nevus syndrome, hypomelanosis of Ito and incontinentia pigmenti.

Brain malformations and maldevelopments[157–160]

One of the major impacts of MRI has been the realization that many epilepsies arise as a consequence of malformations and maldevelopments of the brain (Fig. 20.19). Together these causes probably outweigh perinatal problems in the causation of neurodevelopmental problems. Milder disorders may be silent. When overt they present with combinations of mental retardation, cerebral palsy and epilepsy.

A large number of conditions may be associated with neuronal migration disorders. These include: metabolic diseases such as peroxisomal disorders and Menkes' disease; chromosomal disorders including Edwards (trisomy 18), Patau (trisomy 13), Down (trisomy 21), Smith–Magenis (deletion 17p) and Wolf–Hirschhorn (deletion 4p) syndromes; neuromuscular diseases including some forms of congenital muscular dystrophy and myotonic dystrophy; neurocutaneous syndromes; multiple congenital anomaly syndromes and infective and toxic causes. Among the latter prenatal cytomegalovirus infection and fetal alcohol syndrome merit special mention.

Heterotopias, including periventricular, subcortical and laminar (or band) heterotopias; agyria-pachygyria, including lissencephaly types I and II and focal pachygyria; polymicrogyria; schizencephaly and hemimegalencephaly are migrational disorders and are often highly epileptogenic, giving rise to focal or generalized seizure disorders, including epileptic spasms. They are dealt with in detail elsewhere in this chapter. Agenesis of the corpus callosum is also commonly associated with seizures. Aicardi syndrome is an X-linked dominant disorder almost confined to females. The brain abnormality is complex with agenesis of the corpus callosum (in most but not all cases), periventricular heterotopias, variable dysplasias of the cortex and ependymal cysts. Choroidal lacunae, often with coloboma of the optic discs are a characteristic feature. Severe mental retardation and epileptic spasms are characteristic.

Cortical microdysgenesis implies a postmigrational defect in cortical organization. It comprises minor malarrangements and malorientations of cells within the cortex and is postulated to be a substrate for seizures in some children. It is not diagnosable in life.

The epilepsy complicating cerebral maldevelopments and malformations is for the most part treated along standard lines. Vigabatrin is often considered as particularly useful although this has not been confirmed by rigorous trials. Children with focal cortical malformations may be candidates for resective surgery. Hemimegalencephaly, a cause of catastrophic epilepsy in infancy, may be treated by hemispherectomy.

Brain tumors[161]

Brain tumors are an uncommon, but important and potentially curable, cause of epilepsy in children. Slow growing tumors of the cerebral hemispheres, such as low-grade astrocytomas, oligodendrogliomas, gangliogliomas and gangliocytomas are more likely to present with seizures than are malignant tumors. Diagnosis may be delayed for many years. Seizures are mainly focal, but generalized seizures, with generalized EEG abnormalities, are well recognized.[162] Intellectual ability and neurological examination is often normal. Treatment may be expectant if seizures are controlled by antiepileptic drugs and no tumor growth is observed on serial brain scans. However, surgery often offers a good hope of cure. Gelastic seizures, which often begin in infancy or early childhood, are characterized by laughter, usually without an appropriate affect. They are strongly suggestive of tumors of the floor of the third ventricle, especially hypothalamic hamartomas. Unfortunately these tumors are not easily resected, although there have been encouraging recent reports. Intractable epilepsy, mental retardation, behavioral problems and endocrine problems are frequent. Dysembryoplastic neuroepithelial tumors (DNET) are benign supratentorial tumors which are often located deep in the temporal or frontal lobes and are often associated with intractable focal seizures (Fig. 20.19). Treatment is usually by resection.

Although most brain tumors will be apparent on CT, especially if contrast is used, some may be missed. MRI is superior and is the imaging method of choice.

Cavernous angiomas

These are thin walled clusters of dilated blood vessels whose commonest manifestation is focal epilepsy, often intractable. They may be revealed on CT by areas of calcification. MRI is superior. They are often not apparent on angiograms. Minor bleeding is common; major bleeds are uncommon but occur. Some progressively enlarge and act as space occupying lesions. Treatment is surgical if the lesion is accessible. Radiotherapy is an alternative.

Genetic or presumed genetic disorders[156,163]

Numerous chromosomal and other genetic disorders feature seizures as a prominent or occasional manifestation. Some have already been mentioned.

Angelman syndrome is complicated by epilepsy in up to 90% of children. The characteristic jerky movements of the upper limbs and trunk which gave rise to the eponymous name 'happy puppet syndrome' are caused by a unique form of cortical myoclonus which is reported to respond to piracetam. Epileptic seizures can start at any time from childhood to young adult life, but usually begin in infancy and early childhood. Epileptic spasms are rare. Seizure types include generalized tonic–clonic seizures, clonic seizures, myoclonic seizures, atypical absences and focal seizures, possibly with occipital lobe onset. Episodes of non-convulsive status epilepticus or myoclonic status epilepticus are relatively common and may be recurrent. They are particularly troublesome in early to mid childhood. The severity of the epilepsy often appears to subside in later childhood. Most authorities favor treatment with broad-spectrum antiepileptic drugs or drugs useful against generalized seizures such as sodium valproate, lamotrigine and ethosuximide. Benzodiazepines are useful against episodes of status. Carbamazepine may cause myoclonic and absence seizures.

Rett's syndrome is an X-linked dominant mental retardation disorder. Epileptic seizures are particularly associated with the third or 'pseudostationary' period of the disease, from about 2–10 years of age. Atypical absences are particularly prominent but partial and generalized tonic–clonic seizures also occur. Hyperventilation is a particularly striking feature of the condition. It may provoke atypical absences but many of the phenomena associated with the hyperventilation are probably non-epileptic; certainly the response to antiepileptic drugs is poor. Seizures often show spontaneous improvement or even resolution in later childhood or adolescence. Atypical forms of Rett's syndrome may present with epileptic seizures including epileptic spasms.

Fragile X syndrome is associated with epilepsy in about a fifth of affected boys. The epilepsy is usually mild with relatively infrequent seizures and a tendency for remission in the teenage years. Both focal and generalized seizures are described. The EEG often shows paroxysmal abnormalities similar to those seen in benign childhood epilepsy with centrotemporal spikes.

PEHO (progressive encephalopathy with edema, hypsarrhythmia and optic atrophy) syndrome is a rare, probably autosomal recessive, disorder presenting in early life with drug resistant epileptic spasms, retardation, hypotonia, blindness and optic atrophy. The children are generally almost immobile and have characteristic peripheral edema. Progressive microcephaly and marked cerebellar atrophy are other features.

Metabolic disorders[164]

Virtually all the metabolic disorders which occur in childhood are associated with seizures. However, these are rarely the major feature and certainly the characteristics of the epilepsy are rarely of significance in establishing the correct diagnosis. Important exceptions to this are:

- *Non-ketotic hyperglycinemia* in which early myoclonic seizures and Ohtahara's syndrome are characteristic. Diagnosis is made by demonstrating a raised absolute or relative (to blood and urine) CSF glycine level.
- *Pyridoxine (vitamin B_6) dependent seizures.*[165] These typically begin in the neonatal period or infancy, but may begin prenatally (revealed by hiccups) or up to early childhood. Any seizure type, including epileptic spasms, may occur and frequently become intractable. They respond poorly to conventional antiepileptic drugs. Usually a dramatic cessation of seizures occurs on the intravenous administration of pyridoxine (doses of 40–300 mg). However, this may cause profound apnea and some authorities suggest giving a trial of oral pyridoxine. The condition is autosomal recessive. Measurement of the CSF GABA level (reduced) and glutamate level (raised) may be helpful in diagnosis and management.
- *Biotinidase deficiency.* This autosomal recessive disorder can present in the neonatal period, or beyond, with isolated seizures or seizures in association with skin rashes, alopecia, ataxia and various other neurological abnormalities. It can be detected by the production of a characteristic organic aciduria but more reliable and widely available is testing for deficiency of biotinidase in the blood. Seizures respond to biotin replacement.
- *Glucose transporter deficiency* presents with seizures in infancy and is associated with a deficiency in the transport of glucose across the blood–brain barrier. It is detected by an abnormally low CSF : blood glucose ratio (< 0.35) and responds to the ketogenic diet.

Cerebral palsy[166]

Cerebral palsy is not a disease, but a collection of conditions characterized by abnormalities of movement and posture, caused by non-progressive disorders of the developing brain. Epilepsy has been estimated to occur in 10–40% of cases, but its likelihood depends on the type of cerebral palsy. Cerebral palsy involving damage to the cerebral cortex has a high risk for the development of epilepsy. Hence spastic hemiplegic and quadriplegic cerebral palsy are often accompanied by seizures, whilst these are rarer in spastic diplegic, dyskinetic and ataxic forms of cerebral palsy. Various types of seizure may occur. However, in hemiplegic cerebral palsy, focal motor seizures, often with a Jacksonian march, and secondary generalized tonic–clonic seizures are characteristic. In quadriplegic cerebral palsy generalized seizures (both primarily and secondarily generalized) predominate. Some such children develop epileptic encephalopathies, such as the Lennox–Gastaut syndrome. Startle seizures are relatively common in children with severe forms of cerebral palsy.

MANAGEMENT OF CHILDHOOD EPILEPSY

General principles

Education is the cornerstone to the management of children with any form of seizure disorder. Children, and more especially the families of children, who have had a first epileptic seizure, particularly if convulsive, will almost certainly have been extremely frightened. Initial reassurance should allay the fear that seizures are likely to be life threatening and/or cause brain damage. However, it is wrong to trivialize what has occurred. It is also a mistake to suggest that the attack is unlikely to ever happen again. This is a reasonable hope but is an unreasonable expectation. Education should cover the following points:

- An explanation of the terms 'epileptic seizure' and 'epilepsy'. This should stress the multiplicity of conditions covered by the latter and the huge range in their 'seriousness'.
- A specific explanation as to what type of seizure disorder the child has or may have.
- The impact this is likely to have on the child's future. A frank acknowledgment of uncertainties, which are often considerable, is appropriate.
- Treatment options available.
- 'First aid' measures to be taken in the event of further seizures, including detailed advice as to when medical help should be summoned.
- An exploration of the role of possible precipitants and measures which might be taken to reduce the risk of recurrence.

- Sensible restrictions which should be considered to ensure the child's safety and restrictions which are not required.
- What to tell other people, including the school.

The clinician should also explore the family's own beliefs about seizures and epilepsy. Highly prejudicial attitudes are surprisingly common and may require to be challenged directly.

Written and video information is usually greatly appreciated and all clinicians involved in treating a child with epilepsy should have access to a range of suitable material. Charities and self-help societies produce high-quality material, which is usually free or obtainable at nominal expense. Guiding families to useful websites is increasingly important and clinicians increasingly have to be prepared to counteract misleading information obtained from the Internet.

A number of factors are likely to lower the seizure threshold in anyone with a seizure disorder. Knowledge of these is relevant to all children with epilepsies, although they operate most powerfully in the idiopathic generalized epilepsies. They include fatigue, sleep deprivation, emotional stress and anxiety, excitement, hunger and alcohol.

Undue restrictions are often imposed on children with epilepsy.[167] These have the potential to lead to overdependence in later life. The principal dangers are from drowning and falls. A child with continuing seizures (this might reasonably be defined as a daytime seizure within the last year) should be closely supervised during swimming by a responsible adult capable of rescuing the child if a seizure occurs in the water. Similarly baths for younger children should be supervised and showers encouraged for older children. Climbing, unless protected, is ill-advised. Cycling on busy roads should be avoided if seizures are active. Otherwise cycling with a helmet poses few additional dangers. Most other sports and leisure activities should be encouraged unless there is clear evidence in an individual case that it is associated with a substantially increased risk. Detailed advice about individual sports can be obtained from the websites of the British Epilepsy Association (www.epilepsy.org.uk) and the National Society for Epilepsy (www.epilepsynse.org.uk).

Teenagers with epilepsy should be given the opportunity to discuss issues regarding sex, genetic implications, fertility, contraception and teratogenicity.[168] For up to date information regarding driving and employment issues in the UK the reader is again referred to appropriate websites.

Finally the clinician should be aware that most parents who have lost a child with epilepsy report that they would have wished to know about the increased mortality of children with epilepsy.

Non-drug treatment and intermittent drug treatment

Although antiepileptic drugs play an important part in the management of children with seizure disorders, there are many children in whom regular antiepileptic drug treatment is not or may not be required. This includes:

- Children who have had a single seizure or who only have infrequent seizures.
- Children whose seizures have occurred in the context of a temporary state, for example during a period of hyper- or hyponatremia, or immediately after a head injury; acute treatment with antiepileptic drugs may be required but these should be withdrawn quickly.
- Children with febrile seizures.
- Children whose seizures are all provoked by a stimulus which can reasonably be avoided.
- Children with certain benign focal epilepsies characterized by infrequent seizures, often at night, causing minimal disturbance and with a high probability of remission. This includes many children with benign childhood epilepsy with centrotemporal spikes and Panayiotopoulos syndrome.

Consideration should be given as to whether, as part of an overall regime to be followed if seizures occur, an antiepileptic agent should be provided for intermittent use in the event of prolonged convulsive seizures. Diazepam administered rectally is most often used, although midazolam administered bucally, sublingually or nasally is an unlicensed alternative. Convulsive seizures generally last less than 2 min and it is therefore appropriate to recommend administering the drug either if the seizure lasts longer than usual or after 2 min.

Antiepileptic drug treatment

There are a large number of antiepileptic drugs available to treat seizures in children. Before prescribing an antiepileptic drug the prescriber needs to consider:

- Its efficacy in the particular type of epilepsy
- Potential adverse effects
- Possible interactions with other drugs, including other antiepileptic drugs and the contraceptive pill
- Route of elimination (essential knowledge if prescribing to children with renal or hepatic impairment)
- Its ease of use (related to formulations available, dosing frequency and need for monitoring of levels and other parameters).

Much of our knowledge concerning the efficacy of antiepileptic drugs in humans is derived from clinical observation. The older agents were introduced at a time when classification mainly consisted of a division into grand mal and petit mal seizures. All the new drugs were introduced into clinical practice following trials in children, mainly adults, with focal seizures. These were designed to obtain licensing approval for the drugs rather than to help guide clinical practice. Some antiepileptic drugs have a wide spectrum of action across both generalized and focal epilepsies. These include sodium valproate and lamotrigine and, probably also, topiramate and levetiracetam. Phenobarbital is also broad spectrum but may exacerbate absences. Other drugs, notably carbamazepine, vigabatrin, gabapentin, and, probably also, tiagabine and, to a lesser extent, phenytoin are narrow spectrum agents with efficacy principally against focal epilepsies; they may exacerbate generalized epilepsies. However, vigabatrin has unique activity against epileptic spasms and all seizure types in tuberous sclerosis. Ethosuximide is active against absences and to a lesser extent atonic and myoclonic seizures. Piracetam is mainly used for cortical myoclonus, for example in Angelman syndrome. The benzodiazepines and acetazolamide are usually used as adjunctive agents in children with refractory focal and generalized epilepsies. Clonazepam may be particularly useful against myoclonic seizures. Historically, nitrazepam has tended to be used for treating epileptic spasms.

All antiepileptic drugs have potentially serious adverse effects. These are reviewed in detail elsewhere.[169] Here, only those adverse effects seen commonly or which are likely to influence prescribing habits are discussed.

All antiepileptic drugs are psychoactive and all have the potential to cause CNS unwanted effects such as drowsiness, sedation, dizziness and ataxia. However, such effects are more likely, even with standard dose regimens, with carbamazepine, phenytoin, phenobarbital, topiramate and the benzodiazepines than with sodium valproate and lamotrigine. Both phenobarbital and phenytoin are considered to impair cognitive function (impaired concentration, decreased motor speed and memory problems) even at normal dosages. Behavioral side-effects, including hyperactivity and aggression have been particularly reported with phenobarbital and vigabatrin. They are so common with the former as to have caused its use to sharply decline in developed countries. Overall studies on the effects of other agents have been reassuring[170] but the clinician must always be alert to the potential deleterious effect on cognitive function of antiepileptic drugs in individual children. Many antiepileptic drugs, but notably sodium valproate, lamotrigine and ethosuximide, cause gastrointestinal upsets, particularly pain, nausea and vomiting. Hypersensitivity reactions, particularly rash, generally occur within a few weeks of starting the drug, but may occasionally be delayed. They are particularly a problem with lamotrigine, which has been associated with a widespread erythematous rash and Stevens–Johnson syndrome. If this occurs, the drug must be immediately discontinued. The risk of it occurring can be substantially reduced by slow titration, particularly in children also on sodium valproate. Rash is also regularly encountered with carbamazepine, oxcarbazepine, phenytoin and phenobarbital.

A few drugs have unique adverse effects. These include hair thinning and loss, weight gain and tremor with sodium valproate, appetite suppression and weight loss with topiramate, renal calculi with topiramate and acetazolamide and constriction of the visual fields with vigabatrin. The latter appears to be common and sometimes irreversible.[171] Because of it, vigabatrin should only be used to treat epileptic spasms, seizures in tuberous sclerosis and those children in whom other options have been exhausted. In those treated and who have a mental age of over 7 years detailed assessment of visual fields every 6–12 months is recommended.[172] Carbamazepine and oxcarbazepine can both cause hyponatremia, although this is rarely severe.

Of the rare, potentially fatal adverse effects of antiepileptic drugs, particular attention has been paid to blood dyscrasias with phenobarbital, phenytoin, carbamazepine and ethosuximide, and to severe hepatic toxicity with sodium valproate. The origin of the latter is poorly understood. It is especially common in infants with developmental delay treated with multiple antiepileptic drugs. An underlying metabolic disorder may be implicated and the drug should be avoided where such conditions seem likely. It is unrelated to the mild hyperammonemia seen in many subjects treated with the drug and cannot be predicted by blood tests taken prior to or after starting the drug.

Long-term cumulative adverse effects do not occur with the commonly prescribed agents but phenobarbital and phenytoin can cause connective tissue disorders and metabolic bone disease with the latter also being associated with a cerebellar syndrome, intellectual blunting, coarsening of the facies, gum hypertrophy (partially avoidable with good oral hygiene) and hirsutism.

Many of the commonly prescribed antiepileptic drugs interact with other antiepileptic drugs and with non-antiepileptic drugs. Many interactions are rarely of clinical importance. In general, interactions between antiepileptic drugs either lower the effective concentration of one or both of the drugs increasing the risk of seizures or raise the plasma level of one of the drugs (or a metabolite) increasing the risk of toxicity. These effects can occur at the time of drug withdrawal as well as when a new drug is introduced. At such times, the clinician must carefully evaluate whether adjustments to the dosages of concomitantly prescribed antiepileptic drugs are needed. Carbamazepine (and oxcarbazepine), phenytoin and phenobarbital are enzyme inducers and increase the metabolism of other drugs eliminated by the liver. The effect is of significance when one or other of these drugs are administered together and also when they are administered with sodium valproate, lamotrigine and topiramate. Carbamazepine also causes significant autoinduction and hence carbamazepine levels often fall after a few weeks treatment. Enzyme inducers may also cause significant interactions with other prescribed drugs; most notably they decrease the effectiveness of the oral contraceptive pill.

Sodium valproate inhibits the hepatic metabolism of many antiepileptic drugs. In most cases this is of little significance. However, it causes an effective doubling of the half-life of lamotrigine. Clinically significant increases in the plasma levels of phenobarbital may also occur.

Phenytoin is a difficult drug to use for a number of reasons. Besides being an enzyme inducer it has zero order pharmacokinetics, which means that small changes to the dose can lead to marked changes in plasma levels. It is also extensively protein bound. This means that other protein-bound drugs may cause rises in the unbound fraction of the drug by displacing phenytoin.

Unexpected carbamazepine toxicity may arise as a consequence of inhibition of its metabolism by macrolide antibiotics such as erythromycin. It also occasionally occurs due to inhibition of the metabolism of its pharmacologically active epoxide residue by sodium valproate and lamotrigine.

Vigabatrin, gabapentin, tiagabine, piracetam and levetiracetam are relatively free of significant interactions.

Knowledge about the elimination of antiepileptic drugs is useful to the clinician both because it helps predict possible interactions and is essential when treating children with hepatic or renal impairment. Carbamazepine, phenytoin, sodium valproate, lamotrigine, ethosuximide, oxcarbazepine, the benzodiazepines and tiagabine are all exclusively or predominantly eliminated by hepatic metabolism. Vigabatrin, gabapentin, levetiracetam and acetazolamide are excreted unchanged by the kidneys. Phenobarbital and topiramate are eliminated both by hepatic metabolism and by the kidneys.[173]

Although there have been numerous trials, particularly of the newer antiepileptic drugs, many of these were conducted primarily for licensing purposes and have limited relevance to the clinician in helping to choose between available options. To a considerable extent the way in which clinicians use antiepileptic drugs is based upon the results of uncontrolled clinical studies, their own experience and the advice of trusted colleagues. Table 20.10 details the author's practice aided by the published experience of respected experts.[174,175]

Using antiepileptic drugs

The decision to initiate treatment with an antiepileptic drug should not be taken lightly. Treatment is likely to be prolonged and the risk of adverse effects is significant. Treatment should only be started after a definite diagnosis has been made. A therapeutic trial of an antiepileptic drug in children where a definitive diagnosis has not been made should be avoided. The risk of treating a child who does not have epilepsy with multiple antiepileptic drugs is high. Because of their high prevalence, children with seizure disorders are often treated by clinicians whose knowledge and experience of epilepsy is limited. In developed countries, it should be considered unacceptable to treat a child for epilepsy unless the clinician can recognize the common types of seizure disorders, has access to suitable investigational facilities, including EEG and MRI and has a reasonable knowledge of the available treatments. All children with rare, atypical or unclassifiable seizure disorders, seizure disorders which require special investigational facilities (such as video-EEG) or treatments (such as steroids) or whose seizures continue despite initial treatment should be assessed by a clinician with a special expertise in the epilepsies.

All children should initially be started on monotherapy. Use of more than one drug increases the risk of adverse effects. Large studies of children with new-onset seizures have failed to show a convincing

Table 20.10 Suggested dosage regimens for antiepileptic drugs available in the UK. These are likely to vary from the manufacturers' published information. Many of these drugs are unlicensed or have restricted licences for use in children in the UK

Antiepileptic drug	Initial dose (mg/kg/day)	Usual maintenance dose (mg/kg/day)	Dosage interval	Comments
Carbamazepine	5	10–20; may be up to 30	bd	Liquid and chewtab preparations as well as tablets; slow release preparation has significant advantages
Sodium valproate	10	20–30; occasionally up to 40	bd	'Chrono' preparation has limited advantages
Phenytoin	<3 yrs – 8 >3 yrs – 5	As determined by response and levels	od or bd	Liquid, tablets and capsules available. Prescribe by brand to avoid bioavailability problems
Phenobarbital	5	5; occasionally up to 10	od	
Ethosuximide	10	30–40	bd	
Acetazolamide	5	0–1 yr – 10 >1 yr -20–30	bd	
Clobazam	0.25	0.25–1.0; occasionally up to 2.0	bd	
Clonazepam	0.01	0.05; occasionally up to 0.3	bd or tds	
Nitrazepam	0.05	0.25–1.0	bd	
Vigabatrin	40	60–80; up to 180 in epileptic spasms	od or bd	Sachets of dissolvable powder available
Lamotrigine	Monotherapy – 0.5	Monotherapy – 2–10; occasionally up to 15	od or bd	Dispersible tablets available
	With enzyme inducers – 1.0	5–15	bd	
	With sodium valproate – 0.2	1–5	od or bd	
Gabapentin	15	30–90	tds	Only capsules available
Topiramate	1.0	4–10; sometimes up to 18	bd	Sprinkle granules available
Tiagabine	0.1	0.3–1.5	tds	Only tablets available
Oxcarbazepine	20	50–90	bd	
Levetiracetam	10	20-40	bd	Only tablets available

difference in efficacy between the standard antiepileptic drugs.[176,177] A systematic review concluded that there is no evidence to support the choice of sodium valproate compared to carbamazepine in generalized epilepsies.[178] However, this emphasizes the limitations of over-reliance on such studies since there is compelling evidence that carbamazepine may aggravate some generalized epilepsies in which it should be considered contraindicated.[117] Most authorities consider that sodium valproate is the drug of first choice for generalized epilepsies (whether idiopathic or symptomatic). Some authorities recommend lamotrigine in teenage girls because of concerns about weight gain, decreased fertility and the teratogenicity of sodium valproate. However, lamotrigine also has significant adverse effects and has not yet been shown to be safe in pregnancy. Ethosuximide is an alternative for childhood absence epilepsy but is less well tolerated. Carbamazepine is generally considered the drug of first choice for most focal seizure disorders, including secondary generalized epilepsies. Some support for this practice was found in a systematic review comparing carbamazepine and sodium valproate monotherapy.[178] However, sodium valproate is a suitable alternative for the benign focal epilepsies of childhood. Sodium valproate (or lamotrigine) is the drug of choice for all photosensitive seizures. If it has not proved possible to reliably distinguish focal from generalized seizures it is sensible to treat with a broad spectrum agent such as sodium valproate to avoid the possibility of exacerbating generalized seizures.

When initiating treatment, it is generally advisable to start with modest doses and to build the dose up as required. This reduces the risk of adverse CNS and gastrointestinal unwanted effects. Although many clinicians aim to achieve a 'target dose' seizure control may be achieved at remarkably low doses in some children. Although the manufacturers of some drugs recommend measurement of various blood parameters prior to initiating, and during, therapy in order to avoid/detect early adverse effects there is no evidence that this is effective and is rarely necessary.[179] Similarly blood monitoring of antiepileptic drug levels, although widely available, is usually unhelpful. The so-called target ranges for individual drugs are defined according to the levels at which a majority of responders to the drug achieved seizure control. Significant numbers of children will respond at lower or higher levels and unwanted effects may occur at levels within the therapeutic range, or may not occur despite levels being considerably above the range. Most epileptologists rarely perform antiepileptic drug levels, relying instead on careful clinical monitoring of both efficacy and for adverse effects. Exceptions to this are:

- With phenytoin whose complex pharmacokinetics means that levels should be monitored.
- In children in whom detection of unwanted effects may be difficult. This is particularly the case in those with severe learning difficulties.
- As a check on compliance.

The limitations of blood levels should be appreciated. For drugs such as phenytoin, in which there is significant binding to plasma proteins, it is the free drug which is of importance both in terms of efficacy and safety. Measurement of the total plasma concentration may be misleading in circumstances in which there is altered protein binding. Saliva levels, though not widely available, may be more relevant.

A majority of children treated with antiepileptic drugs will become seizure free and most should be subsequently withdrawn from antiepileptic medication. However, the maxim of withdrawing treatment after two seizure-free years is an oversimplification.[180] The best predictor of relapse is the epilepsy syndrome. Relapse is very unlikely in benign childhood epilepsy with centrotemporal spikes and benign childhood occipital epilepsy (Panayiotopoulos type) and almost certain in juvenile myoclonic epilepsy. Relapse rates are intermediate for other commonly encountered syndromes. Other predictors, all imperfect, of the likelihood of relapse are age (greater risk with onset of seizures in infancy or very early childhood), symptomatic etiology, EEG abnormalities (photosensitivity appears to be strongly correlated with relapse) and severity of epilepsy prior to control being achieved.[181] The decision as to whether antiepileptic drugs should be withdrawn needs to be an individual one based on a detailed analysis with the child and family which takes into account the likely consequences should a relapse occur. For all children with epilepsies in whom there is a good prospect for successful withdrawal (benign focal epilepsies, childhood and to a lesser extent juvenile absence epilepsy) withdrawal should be attempted after two seizure-free years, or even earlier.[182] Persisting EEG abnormalities, except possibly photosensitivity, should not unduly influence this decision. For children with epilepsies which have proved difficult to control a longer period free of seizures (perhaps 2–5 years) is advisable. It is probably not justified in recommending drug withdrawal in juvenile myoclonic epilepsy or photosensitive epilepsies in children who remain highly photosensitive on EEG testing.

Children who have been on benzodiazepines and barbiturates for anything other than brief periods should be withdrawn very slowly over many months or even years as the risk of withdrawal seizure is considered high, although this has recently been questioned.[183] Other drugs can usually be safely withdrawn over 1–2 months. Detailed instructions as to what measures to take should a seizure occur during withdrawal should always be given. Some families appreciate being provided with an agent such as diazepam for emergency use. However, they should be reassured that status epilepticus is extremely rare during antiepileptic drug withdrawal.[181] Overall the risk of relapse in children withdrawn from antiepileptic drugs is around 20% at 6 months, rising to 35% at 4 years.[181] Relapses usually occur within a year of withdrawal. If seizures recur during or after withdrawal the drug should generally be restarted and the prospect of regaining control is very good but not assured.[184,185]

If the child fails to respond to an antiepileptic drug it is important to reconsider the diagnosis: misdiagnosis of epilepsy remains a major problem. Sometimes a child will have responded to a drug but intolerable unwanted effects cause it to be stopped. It is usually easy in this situation to choose a suitable alternative. If, however, seizures have not been controlled despite pushing the first drug to the limit of tolerability or to the maximum reasonable dose then a second drug should be tried as monotherapy. A recent study found that 42% of children who failed on initial monotherapy subsequently had a complete remission on other agents.[186] Different clinicians vary in how this is achieved. Some prefer to wean off the first drug as the new drug is being introduced. However, if some response has occurred this may lead to an increase in seizures. The alternative approach is to introduce the second drug whilst maintaining the child on the first drug. The dose of the first drug may need to be adjusted. When seizures have been controlled the first drug can be withdrawn. The difficulty with this approach is that there is often an understandable reluctance to alter things once seizures have been controlled. For generalized epilepsies, assuming that sodium valproate has been tried initially, the second line drug of choice is probably lamotrigine. However, for childhood absence epilepsy ethosuximide would be an alternative. Moreover, in juvenile myoclonic epilepsy if absences and generalized tonic–clonic seizures are completely controlled but myoclonic jerks remain problematic a small dose of a benzodiazepine, such as clonazepam, is a suitable alternative. For focal epilepsies, assuming carbamazepine has been the first line drug, a large number of suitable second line agents, including sodium valproate, are now available and it is not possible to give a blanket recommendation. All the recently introduced drugs have been shown in double-blind, placebo-controlled trials to be efficacious against partial seizures. Moreover systematic reviews have concluded that gabapentin, lamotrigine, topiramate, levetiracetam and oxcarbazepine are effective at least in the short term as add-on treatment in patients with drug-resistant focal epilepsies.[187–192] However, there are very few studies reported comparing them 'head-to head'. When a child has failed to respond to two suitable major antiepileptic drugs pushed to their maximum dose, the chances of achieving complete seizure control rapidly diminishes. Many different strategies exist but a number of principles should be emphasized:[193]

- There is evidence that control is sometimes better with two and occasionally three antiepileptic agents. However, there is no evidence that four antiepileptic drugs are ever appropriate.
- If more than one drug is to be used the approach taken should be rational. Some combinations of drugs are more appropriate than others. For example when treating drug resistant focal seizures it may be wise to use combinations of drugs with different modes of action. Moreover, drugs with similar adverse effects such as benzodiazepines and phenobarbital should be avoided.
- Polypharmacy has many potential problems:
  Increased risk of adverse effects
  Risk of exacerbating seizures, particularly if drowsiness is a problem
  Risk of drug interactions causing all the drugs to be at subtherapeutic levels – drug levels may be helpful.
- The aim of therapy is to improve quality of life not necessarily to render the child totally seizure free.
- The diagnosis should be re-evaluated periodically. Pseudoseizures should be among the considerations.
- Compliance may need to be checked.
- If seizures are only being reported by one party the possibility of 'misreporting' by the carer to gain attention or benefits should be considered.
- A systematic approach should be adopted whereby each agent tried is given an adequate trial before deciding that it is ineffective.

In children with drug resistant epilepsies thought should be given to trying less conventional medication such as short courses of steroids or ACTH and immunoglobulins. Anecdotal evidence suggests that these may be effective in individual children.

The ketogenic diet

Ketogenic diets have been used in the treatment of drug resistant epilepsies for decades. It has not been established if they are particularly indicated for any particular seizure or epilepsy syndrome type and have been advocated for children with drug resistant seizures of any type and from any cause. However, they should be avoided in children with mitochondrial diseases, particularly pyruvate carboxylase deficiency.[194] A recent review concluded that complete seizure control occurs in 20–30% of children, a greater than 50% reduction in seizures in 60–80% of children whilst 20–40% of children gain no benefit.[195] The mechanism of action remains obscure. All ketogenic diets aim to induce ketosis by providing the child's caloric needs predominantly as ketogenic foods (fats). The classic (4 : 1) diet uses 4 g of fat to every 1 g of non-ketogenic foods (protein and carbohydrate). The medium-chain triglyceride and the modified medium-chain triglyceride diets utilize medium-chain triglycerides, which are more ketogenic and hence allow a lower ratio of fats to other foods to be given. The diet is usually initiated by fasting in hospital with the aim of achieving and maintaining 3–4+ ketonuria. Acetazolamide and topiramate should be withdrawn first because severe acidosis may occur. Other antiepileptic drugs are usually continued, at least initially. A skilled dietitian is essential. Unwanted effects include hypoglycemia (usually only a problem when the diet is first initiated), hunger and thirst, weight problems, antiepileptic drug toxicity and renal stones. The diet must be kept to strictly; even sugar containing medicines can reduce its efficacy. Regular monitoring of growth and of blood electrolytes, liver function tests, lipids, proteins and full blood count is generally advocated. If successful, the diet is usually continued for at least 2 years. It should be stopped gradually.

The vagal nerve stimulator

This is a relatively new technique involving intermittent stimulation of the left vagus nerve in the neck. A pulse generator is implanted subcutaneously in the upper chest. Leads convey electrical impulses from it to the vagus nerve and are then transmitted up the nerve to the nucleus solitarius. The antiepileptic action of vagal nerve stimulation is poorly understood, but presumably relies on projections from the nucleus solitarius to cortical and subcortical structures. The generator is programmed using a PC and 'wand' to give chronic intermittent stimulation. A systematic review concluded that vagal nerve stimulation appears to be an effective and well-tolerated treatment for focal seizures.[196] There is currently no clear indication as to which children with refractory epilepsy should be offered this treatment. There is as yet no large randomized study reported from children but a median reduction in seizures of up to 43% has been reported in a small group with epileptic encephalopathies.[197] Very few children become seizure free. Efficacy appears to improve with time.

Epilepsy surgery

A significant minority of children with medically refractory epilepsy can benefit from surgery. All children with ongoing seizures, despite medical treatment, should be evaluated in a center with the facilities and expertise to assess their suitability for surgical treatment. Epilepsy surgery can be resective or functional. The former involves removing epileptogenic tissue, aiming to 'cure' the epilepsy. The latter modifies brain function in order to interrupt the transmission of epileptic discharges. Its aim is to improve seizure control, to modify seizure type or to minimize the deleterious effects seizures can have on cerebral function.

The evaluation and selection of children for any type of epilepsy surgery is multidisciplinary, involving pediatric neurologists, neurophysiologists, neuropsychologists, neuroradiologists, nuclear medicine physicians and child psychiatrists as well as the neurosurgeon. Severe learning difficulties and behavioral problems are relative, but not absolute, contraindications to surgery.

A prerequisite of resective surgery is that seizures are focal in origin or arise from one cerebral hemisphere. Identification of the seizure focus involves integration of multiple sources of data. In all cases this involves:

- A detailed clinical assessment. Seizure sociology along with the findings on neurological examination may give useful information regarding seizure localization.
- Detailed scalp EEG studies. These will include interictal and ictal recordings with recordings during awake and sleep. Video-EEG is essential and it is usual to try to capture a number of the child's habitual seizures.
- High quality structural imaging with MRI; the prospects for surgery are considerably enhanced if a structural lesion can be identified.
- Neuropsychological evaluation. This may provide further useful information on the likely lateralization and even localization of the epileptic focus. In addition it seeks to identify cerebral dominance for speech and to give a baseline of the child's cognitive abilities.

If the data from these studies are congruent it is often possible to proceed to surgery without further investigations. However, if the site of the epileptic focus is still unclear further investigations are carried out. These may include:

- Semi-invasive EEG studies (foramen ovale or sphenoidal electrodes)
- Functional neuroimaging usually with ictal SPECT or interictal PET
- Invasive EEG studies using subdural grids of electrodes or depth electrodes.

In older children and teenagers undergoing resective surgery it is usual to establish the dominant hemisphere for language and memory using the carotid amytal test. Resecting a temporal lobe in which memory resides would result in a dense amnesia.

The majority of resections in both adults and children are of the temporal lobe. However, whereas in adults mesial temporal sclerosis is the predominant pathology, in children, tumors, cortical dysplasias and other focal pathologies are also relatively common.[198] In the Maudsley series of 41 children 15 years or younger 80% became seizure free. There was no mortality and series morbidity occurred in only 1–2%.[198] Extratemporal resections are less commonly performed and the outcome poorer with seizure free rates of well under 50%.[199]

Hemispherectomies and multilobar resections are performed considerably more often in children than in adults. They are indicated for some of the catastrophic epilepsies of infancy such as Sturge–Weber syndrome and hemimegalencephaly. Hemispherectomy is the treatment of choice in Rasmussen's disease and has been used to treat severe epilepsies due to extensive unilateral infarctions. It is generally reserved for people with already established hemiplegias. Depending on the underlying pathology, up to 70–80% of children become seizure free.[200]

Functional procedures include callostomy, stereotactic lesioning (for example with the gamma knife) and multiple subpial resection. The indications for callstomy are still disputed. However, it is generally reserved for children with seizures presumed to be of focal onset but in whom rapid bilateral synchrony occurs. It seems to be most effective against atonic drop attacks. Few children become seizure free, but in many the seizures postoperatively are less disabling. Significant neuropsychological deficits may occur, particularly if the posterior part of the corpus callosum is divided. Multiple subpial transection involves sectioning horizontal cortical fibers thought to be responsible for seizure propagation, leaving vertically orientated fibers, responsible for normal function, intact. It has mainly been used in the Landau–Kleffner syndrome.

NON-EPILEPTIC PAROXYSMAL DISORDERS

The conditions described here are frequently misdiagnosed as epilepsy. Their recognition is important, not only to avoid this, but because they are important conditions in their own right, requiring investigation and explanation. Moreover, for many specific and effective treatments exist. The reader who requires more information is referred to Stephenson's unique text.[201]

Syncopes and anoxic seizures

A syncope or faint is a sudden loss of consciousness and postural tone caused by a cessation in the supply of energy substrates to the cerebral cortex. The latter is usually a result of hypoxia or reduced cerebral perfusion or a combination of both. An anoxic seizure is a non-epileptic seizure caused by syncope. In effect, it is a severe form of syncope. The clinical features consist of an initial loss of consciousness and postural tone (this phase may be brief) followed by tonic stiffening and/or clonic movements. If an EEG is recorded during an anoxic seizure it shows slowing, followed by flattening during the tonic phase, followed by the reappearance of slow waves, often coinciding with clonic jerks. No epileptiform abnormalities are seen. It should be noted that there are no unique features of syncopes and anoxic seizures that reliably distinguish them from epileptic seizures: eye rolling, tongue biting and urinary incontinence occur in both. Moreover, although many syncopes are short, both these and reflex anoxic seizures can be prolonged. Postictal drowsiness can follow epileptic seizures, syncopes and anoxic seizures. It is the circumstances in which syncopes and anoxic seizures occur which often allows them to be distinguished from epileptic seizures. However, in some cases definite distinction requires prolonged polygraphic recording.

The commonest forms of syncope are *simple faints* or *vasovagal syncopes*. The most important distinguishing feature is the circumstance of occurrence, which is often stereotyped for the individual. Common provoking factors are stress, emotion and upright posture, especially in confined spaces. Older children may recount initial symptoms of light-headedness and graying of vision. Abdominal pain is also said to be common. During the attack the child is usually pale, limp and the pulse may be slow. Attacks may occur when supine, clonic limb movements are common and postictal confusion may occur. There is often a family history of similarly affected relatives. Head-up tilt testing may help if the diagnosis remains in doubt. Vasovagal syncopes are considered to arise as a consequence of a vasodepressor mechanism, sometimes combined with vagally mediated cardio-inhibition. *Vagovagal syncopes* in which a reflex bradycardia or asystole follows vagal stimulation by swallowing or vomiting are more rare. Syncopes can also arise due to *orthostatic hypotension*, rare in children but more common in adolescence.

Reflex anoxic seizures are a relatively common form of syncope in young children. The precipitant is usually a minor bump to the head provoking a vagally mediated cardiac asystole, which may last many seconds. Clinically the child simultaneously loses consciousness and becomes floppy and extremely pale (pallid syncope). Subsequent tonic stiffening and clonic movements are common. Although the heart quickly restarts the loss of consciousness may be prolonged. Reflex anoxic seizures should be distinguished from *breath-holding attacks (blue syncopes, prolonged expiratory apnea)*. The pathophysiology of these relatively common attacks is still incompletely understood, but they are not behavioral in origin. They are provoked by fright, pain, anger or frustration. Crying is followed by the breath being held in expiration. Cyanosis and then loss of consciousness and limpness follows. If severe, tonic stiffening may follow.

All the syncopes discussed so far are benign, although attacks similar to breath holding attacks occurring in some neurologically impaired children may not be so. Reassurance and explanation is all that is generally required. Simple faints wax and wane in their frequency, often being particularly troublesome in the teenage years. Most, but not all, infants with reflex anoxic seizures and breath-holding attacks eventually become free of the attacks in mid to late childhood. Specific treatment is not required although some advocate the use of atropine in reflex anoxic seizures. When very severe, these may also be helped by cardiac pacing.[202]

Some forms of syncope are less benign. Retarded children sometimes provoke 'drop-like attacks' by a *Valsalva maneuver*. Occasionally these have been fatal. *Gastroesophageal reflux* occasionally provokes apnea, sometimes followed by an anoxic seizure. The mechanism may be vagally mediated cardiac inhibition or laryngospasm and appears to be a feature of the awake state. Whether this is one cause of apparent life-threatening events and sudden infant death syndrome is controversial. Treatment is of the gastroesophageal reflux.

Cardiac syncopes are important and potentially life threatening.[203] Syncopes and anoxic seizures can be a manifestation of various cardiac arrhythmias and of structural heart disease. Particularly important to recognize are the *prolonged QT syndromes*. These ion channel disorders are characterized by anoxic seizures occurring during exercise and sleep. They are potentially fatal. In most but not all cases the corrected QT interval (QTc) is greater than 440 msec. If the clinical history is suggestive but the QT interval on a standard EEG is normal, prolonged ECG monitoring and exercise ECG is indicated.

Craniocervical junction disorders such as Chiari malformations may be associated with apneas and syncopes occurring during activities which increase intracranial pressure.

Imposed suffocation is a relatively common manifestation of *Munchausen's syndrome by proxy*.[204] Attacks all begin in the presence of the perpetrator, usually the mother. Others may witness the conclusion of the attacks.

Movement disorders and related conditions[205]

A large number of paroxysmal movement disorders occur in children and can be mistaken for epilepsy. The *episodic ataxias* are familial ion channel disorders.[206] Episodic ataxia provoked by factors such as startle or exercise often provides the clue to diagnosis and may be isolated or coexist with a variety of other problems including cerebellar signs. They may respond to acetazolamide. A variety of conditions are described in which paroxysmal dystonia or dyskinesia or choreoathetosis occurs. The two best characterized conditions are *paroxysmal kinesigenic choreoathetosis* and *paroxysmal non-kinesigenic choreoathetosis*, both of which are autosomal dominant. The former is characterized by very frequent short episodes, unilateral or bilateral, of dystonia or choreoathetosis provoked by sudden movement. Although not an epilepsy, it frequently responds to antiepileptic drugs such as carbamazepine and phenytoin. The non-kinesigenic form is characterized by less frequent longer attacks precipitated by stress, coffee or alcohol. It may respond to clonazepam.

Benign myoclonus of infancy may be mistaken for epileptic spasms. It is unrelated to *benign neonatal sleep myoclonus* which is relatively common and frequently mistaken as epileptic. It is characterized by repetitive, usually rhythmic jerks of one or more limbs in sleep. *Shuddering attacks* occur in the same age group or in older children. They may be accompanied by urination and are said sometimes to be a herald of essential tremor.

Various abnormal head movements are described. These include repetitive *head bobbing* and *banging*. The latter sometimes occurs in understimulated children. *Tics* are occasionally confused with seizures.

Paroxysmal vertigo, occurring in children between 1 and 5 years of age, and manifest as the child suddenly appearing distressed, pale and unsteady, sometimes with nystagmus, may be related to *benign paroxysmal torticollis of infancy*. In the latter repeated attacks of distress, vomiting and head tilt occur. In turn both conditions may be related to migraine.

Benign paroxysmal tonic up-gaze of childhood may be responsive to L-dopa.

Sandifer's syndrome refers to dyskinetic neck movements occurring in children with gastroesophageal reflux often in association with hiatus hernia.

Drug induced dystonic reactions, including oculogyric crises are seen with psychotropic drugs, particularly the phenothiazines and metoclopramide. Intravenous benzotropine or a benzodiazepine will abort attacks.

Tetany with carpopedal spasm and laryngospasm is a manifestation of hypocalcemia or hypomagnesemia, both of which can also cause epileptic seizures.

Hyperekplexia

This is usually an autosomal dominant condition; less commonly it is recessive. It is caused by mutations in a subunit of the glycine receptor on chromosome 5. It is conventionally divided into major and minor forms. The latter is manifested by generalized hypertonia (which may lead to an erroneous diagnosis of cerebral palsy) and excessive startles to auditory, visual and somatosensory stimuli. In the major form there are, in addition, attacks of severe tonic stiffening with apnea. These can be life-threatening.

A useful diagnostic test is nose-tapping which causes an excessive and reproducible startle. Clonazepam and valproate are useful. In addition, the forced flexion maneuver consisting of sudden flexion of the head and limbs can be life saving during severe apneic attacks.

Familial rectal pain syndrome

This is a rare, usually autosomal dominant condition, which is probably manifest throughout life. It is characterized by discrete attacks with marked autonomic features. The most prominent of these is the sudden onset of excruciating pain that can be generalized or localized to sites such as the rectum, genitalia and face. Harlequin color changes may be conspicuous. Some attacks may be associated with severe apneas and asystoles. The risk which these pose is unknown. Many attacks are unprovoked but triggers include startles, defecation, wiping of the nappy area, urination, eating and drinking. Carbamazepine is of some benefit.

Sleep disorders

A number of different movement disorders related to sleep are described. These include *benign neonatal sleep myoclonus, periodic movements of sleep, restless leg syndrome, jactatio capitis nocturna* (repetitive head banging), *hypnagogic jactitations* (myoclonic jerks, usually of the legs, on falling asleep) and *nocturnal myoclonus*. These are all benign phenomena requiring reassurance only.

Night terrors are occasionally confused with frontal lobe seizures. They occur in infancy and early childhood and are associated with partial arousal from deep slow sleep. They usually occur early in the night and are manifested with the child screaming as if terrified. Although appearing awake, the child cannot be consoled and appears not to recognize his parents. There is no recollection next morning. *Nightmares* are a phenomenon of rapid eye movement sleep. *Sleepwalking* and *sleep talking* often occur together, usually in older children and adolescents who previously had night terrors. Again reassurance is all that is required along with advice about sensible safety precautions. *Hypnagogic hallucinations and illusions*, usually visual or auditory, occur in the transitions between wakefulness and sleep and are considered normal phenomena.

Narcolepsy is usually an autosomal dominant disorder which in its full form features:[207]

- Excessive daytime sleepiness with frequent daytime naps
- Cataplexy, i.e. attacks of sudden loss of tone causing falls in full consciousness, often precipitated by laughter or excitement
- Hypnagogic hallucinations
- Sleep paralysis manifested by attacks of inability to move or to move a limb occurring as the subject is wakening.

The disorder is probably underdiagnosed in childhood as it is usually manifested only as excessive daytime sleepiness with frequent daytime naps, the other features appearing in adolescence and adult life. However, its recognition is important as it can lead to school failure.

The diagnosis is essentially clinical. However, multiple sleep latency studies can offer confirmatory information. Subjects with narcolepsy have a short latency for entering rapid eye movement sleep and may pass straight into it from the awake state. In addition there is a very strong association with HLA-DQB1 0602, present in up to 98% of subjects. It is important to exclude nocturnal hypoventilation, a much commoner cause of daytime sleepiness than narcolepsy. The most important aspect of management of narcolepsy is ensuring that the family and school understand the nature of the condition and that the child has an appropriate period of night-time sleep (paradoxically night-time insomnia can be a problem), along with daytime naps. It is sensible to present the most important educational material early in the day when the child is likely to be at its brightest. Amfetamines have traditionally been the main pharmacological agent used to treat excessive sleepiness in narcolepsy but modafinil is being increasingly preferred. Imipramine and clomipramine can be useful in cataplexy.

Psychological and psychiatric disorders

Many different psychological and psychiatric disturbances can present as paroxysmal episodes and are important in the differential diagnosis of epilepsy. *Masturbation* occurs at all ages and may be more or less obvious. In young girls it often involves adduction of the thighs and rhythmic hip flexion. The child is characteristically vacant, rigid and flushed. Other gratification phenomena are described and are manifested with stereotyped behaviors during which the child appears withdrawn. *Daydreams* are particularly prone to misinterpretation by school teachers. They occur when bored or fatigued and generally involve the child's attention gradually drifting away.

Hyperventilation is relatively common, especially in teenage girls. It provokes sensations of light-headedness, chest pain and paresthesiae. It may also be manifested with carpopedal spasm as in tetany. Hyperventilation is often a symptom of anxiety and may be helped by psychological intervention. Milder cases may be helped by rebreathing into a paper bag.

Non-epileptic attack disorder (pseudoseizures) occur in mid and late childhood and adolescence. Some are easily distinguished from epileptic seizures whilst in others the distinction may be extremely difficult. Pseudoseizures may mimic any type of epileptic seizure, including status epilepticus. There are no hard and fast rules whereby epileptic and pseudoseizures can be reliably separated. However, movements in the latter are usually thrashing and semipurposeful rather than rhythmic clonic jerks. Induction by suggestion can be very helpful. A major difficulty is in distinguishing frontal lobe seizures from pseudoseizures. Pseudoseizures are probably most common in children who also have epileptic seizures. However, they also occur in children who had epileptic seizures but whose seizures have stopped and in children who have never had an epileptic seizure, although a friend or relative may.

An ictal EEG recording which shows no epileptiform abnormalities is suggestive, but not conclusive, evidence of pseudoseizures; the ictal EEG is often normal during, for example, frontal lobe seizures and elementary focal seizures. Measurement of serum prolactin levels is occasionally useful, levels increasing after generalized tonic–clonic seizures and some focal seizures, but not usually after frontal lobe seizures or elementary focal seizures. It is crucial to have an accurate baseline measurement and to take the sample at the appropriate time after the start of the seizure.[208]

Confidently distinguishing between epileptic seizures and non-epileptic attack disorder may be impossible, even after extensive history taking and detailed investigations. However, if the latter seems more likely it is inappropriate to treat with antiepileptics in the hope that it might be. It must be accepted that even the best clinician will be mistaken from time to time. What is required is the honesty to review the diagnosis if the management offered fails. All children who have or are suspected of having non-epileptic attack disorder require the input of a child psychologist or psychiatrist. Often there is no serious underlying psychological or psychiatric problem and the prognosis is excellent. However, children who are, or have been, abused physically or sexually may present in this way.

Other conditions to consider in the differential diagnosis of paroxysmal disorders include the effects of *substance abuse, early-onset schizophrenia* with hallucinations and attacks of ***rage*** seen in older children and adolescents.

Other neurological conditions

Migraine, which is considered in detail elsewhere (p. 952), may be confused for epilepsy and vice versa. Some epileptic seizures, particularly of occipital lobe origin, superficially resemble migraine attacks.[118] In addition, given that both conditions are relatively common, it is not surprising that some children will be encountered with both conditions. Both migraine and some forms of epilepsy are regularly provoked by endogenous and exogenous factors. Therefore, it is likely that occasionally a migraine will provoke an epileptic seizure and vice versa. Exceptionally a severe migraine may result in an ischemic lesion, which acts as an epileptic focus.

Alternating hemiplegia of childhood is a rare disorder which begins within the first year of life, usually with brief tonic attacks, often unilateral with eye movement abnormalities, accompanied by general misery.[209] Shortly after attacks of alternating hemiplegia begin and are usually frequent. They may be provoked by various triggers. A striking feature is disappearance of the hemiplegia with sleep, often with its reappearance shortly after awakening. Although some response to flunarizine is reported, the condition is progressive with mental retardation and a variety of motor problems. Structural neuroimaging is normal.

HEADACHE AND MIGRAINE

HEADACHE

Headache is one of the most common childhood health complaints reported by adolescents and their parents. It has been reported in children of all ages from infancy to adolescence and from all ethnic groups and socioeconomic backgrounds. Chronic recurrent headaches have long-term health implications on children as they commonly grow up to become adults with chronic headache.[210]

Population-based studies of headache in schoolchildren have shown that 66% of all children between 5 and 15 years had suffered at least one episode of headache during a 1-year period and in 22% the headache was severe enough to interfere with daily activities.[211] The prevalence of headache increases steadily from early age to adolescence. By the age of 12–13 years, the prevalence rate of headache reaches adult levels of around 90%.[212]

Headache during infancy is usually secondary to underlying systemic diseases and viral illnesses. The prevalence rate of headache during the first 2 years of life is difficult to estimate, but it is not unusual for children with migraine to have early attacks dating back to the first year of life. During the preschool years, the prevalence rate of headache increased from 13.5% at age 3 to 25.6% at age 4 years in a population of an urban general practice in the UK.[213] The prevalence rate increases suddenly during the first year at school reaching a peak of 40–50% followed by a slight drop in the following 1–2 years.[214]

In many children, headache is benign and infrequent. At least 40% of schoolchildren, over the age of 11 years, use over-the-counter painkillers to treat their own headache.[215,216] Also it is common for parents to treat their children's headaches, though, on many occasions, inappropriately. A study of 100 caregivers showed that only 30% were able to determine the correct dose of paracetamol for their children and to accurately measure the intended dose.[217] Other children may seek medical advice from general practitioners, general pediatricians, pediatric neurologists, neurosurgeons, child psychiatrists, ENT surgeons and ophthalmologists.

Headaches can be classified according to their clinical presentation, duration of illness and the frequency of attacks as acute, recurrent or chronic in nature (Table 20.11).

Acute headaches

Children present with single or isolated attacks of headache. The headache is commonly associated with other symptoms indicating an underlying local or systemic illness. The causes of acute headache in 150 unselected children attending an accident and emergency department were upper respiratory tract infections (57%), migraine without aura (18%), viral meningitis (9%), brain tumor (2.6%), ventriculoperitoneal shunt dysfunction (2%), intracranial hemorrhage (1.3%), postictal headache (1.3%), post-concussion (1.3%) and undetermined causes (7%).[218] A similar pattern was also seen in 634 children attending general practice,[219] whose acute headache was due to febrile illnesses (56.8%), idiopathic headache (8.8%), tension headache (5.7%), migraine (3.3%) and other causes in 25.3%.

Chronic headaches

Children usually present with at least 3 months' history of constant headache or a headache with a fluctuating intensity, but with no

Table 20.11 Main causes of headache in children and adolescents

Acute headaches
Viral illnesses: respiratory, gastrointestinal and flu-like illnesses
Bacterial infections: tonsillitis, pharyngitis, sinusitis, pneumonia
Intracranial infections: viral or bacterial meningitis, encephalitis
Intracranial bleeding
Head trauma
Migraine headache
Others
Recurrent headache
Migraine: migraine without aura, migraine with aura, complicated migraine
Tension-type headache: episodic tension headache, chronic tension headache
Short-lasting unilateral headaches: cluster headache, neuralgias
Others
Chronic headache
Raised intracranial pressure: brain tumor, hydrocephalus, benign intracranial hypertension
Hypertension
Substance induced: intoxication, medications
Others

periods of complete recovery. Chronic headaches are rare in children, but brain tumors are the main concern to the parents and their pediatricians. Headache is rarely the only complaint and other symptoms may be more prominent in the clinical presentation.

Recurrent headaches

The headache disorder usually runs a chronic course and a history of at least 6 months of recurrent episodes is common. Idiopathic or primary headache is the most common cause and the attacks of headache are clearly separated by periods of complete normality. In a population-based study,[211] migraine (with or without aura) was the most common cause of recurrent headache in schoolchildren accounting for 77.2% of cases. Other causes were tension headache (episodic and chronic tension headache) in 11.7%, non-specific headache in 9.7% and headache associated with specific illnesses such as asthma, hay fever, allergy and constipation in 1.5%. Similar causes, but in different proportions, are reported in children attending specialist clinics: 34% had migraine (of whom 82% without aura and 18% with aura), 32% tension headache (of whom 64% chronic and 36% episodic), 12.6% mixed migraine and tension headaches, 10.4% unclassified headaches and 10.9% had other causes or combination of causes.[220]

Clinical classifications of recurrent headache

The 1988 International Headache Society's (IHS) classification of headache and facial pain[221] is the most widely used and tested criteria for the diagnosis of several types of recurrent headache in children and in particular migraine and tension headache. Several minor modifications for the diagnosis of childhood migraine[211,213,222] and tension headache[220,223] have been suggested.

The classification of recurrent headaches is based mainly on the presence or absence of specific clinical features. Therefore, different types of headache may have different numbers and combinations of symptoms that may make it possible to view the different types of recurrent headache as a disease continuum on a headache spectrum.[224] Clinical features such as the pain quality, site of maximal intensity, severity of the pain and the number and nature of the associated symptoms during headache attacks may determine the clinical headache diagnosis. Tension-type headache is commonly mild to moderate in intensity, dull aching in nature and poorly localized or affects the whole of the head. Also tension headache is rarely associated with other sensory, vasomotor or gastrointestinal symptoms. Episodic tension-type headache with its infrequent number of attacks may represent the mild end of the headache spectrum. On the other end of the spectrum the pain during migraine attacks is more intense (moderate or severe), more localized (unilateral or frontal), throbbing or stabbing in character and is associated with a variable number of sensory, vasomotor or gastrointestinal symptoms. Migraine without aura can bear similarities to episodic tension-type headache with some blurred borders separating the two conditions midway in the headache spectrum. Migraine with aura at the extreme end of the spectrum has a well-defined symptom constellation that may also include complicated attacks of migraine with dysphasia, hemiplegia or prolonged aura. The concept of the headache continuum encompassing all types of headache into one clinical spectrum has gained a wide interest, but is not yet universally accepted.[225]

Evaluation of the child with recurrent headaches

The diagnosis of most types of recurrent headache is dependent on full clinical history and physical examination. A specific diagnosis can be made in the majority of patients on the basis of clinical history, physical examination, appropriate investigations and the recording of headache diaries. Detailed clinical history and diary analysis should allow the distinction between the several coexisting types of headache. Some types of headache may have some overlap in their clinical features and in some patients more than one type of headache may coexist.

Clinical history of headache

Complete clinical history is paramount in the evaluation of the child with headache. Young children may find difficulties in describing pain and its characteristics. Therefore, the child should be encouraged to use his/her own words and be assisted with visual images to describe certain ideas such as the severity of pain. Assessment of the headache should document when the disease started, frequency of attacks, duration of each attack, severity, site of maximal intensity and quality of pain. Possible trigger factors, warning signs and aura symptoms that precede the onset of headache should be recorded. Associated clinical features that may accompany headache attacks such as anorexia, nausea, vomiting, light, noise or smell intolerance, pallor, visual disturbances, dizziness, confusion, abdominal pain and motor or sensory deficits should also be carefully assessed and recorded. Assessment should also be made of aggravating and relieving factors and the patients' own treatment strategies. It should also be determined if there are continuing sensory, motor or gastrointestinal symptoms between attacks of headache or a complete resolution of symptoms and a full return to normality. The complete clinical description of these features is best collected prospectively, for example, by using a diary to record the events as they happen.

Physical examination

All patients should have a complete physical examination including the measurement of blood pressure. Neurological examination should be thorough and complete including the measurement of the head circumference. Of particular importance is the detection of signs and symptoms of raised intracranial pressure (papilledema, squints and pupillary abnormalities), cerebellar dysfunction (nystagmus, ataxia, intention tremor or torticollis), focal neurological deficits and brainstem disease (and cranial nerve palsies).

Investigations

Investigations are only needed in minority of children with chronic or recurrent headache. Neuroimaging, with computerized tomography (CT) or magnetic resonance imaging (MRI) of the brain, is indicated in patients with the following features:

- focal neurological deficits
- recent onset squint
- signs of cerebellar dysfunction and features
- features suggestive of raised intracranial pressure
- children younger than 5 years of age with short duration of illness, difficult to obtain clinical history of headache and/or difficult to carry out a physical examination
- recent change in character or quality of headache
- deterioration in schoolwork or behavior.

Lumbar puncture and measurement of opening pressure is indicated if infection or benign intracranial hypertension is suspected.

CHILDHOOD MIGRAINE

It is estimated that around 1 in 10 schoolchildren suffers from migraine. The prevalence rate is estimated at 1.3% in children between 3 and 5 years of age[213] and 3.4% at age 5 with a steady increase to 19.1% at 12 years of age. After the age of 12 the prevalence rate drops slightly to reach adult prevalence rates.[211] Boys and girls under the age of 12 years are almost equally affected with migraine, but in children older than 12 years migraine is commoner in girls than in boys.

The etiology of migraine is not known, but it has a familial tendency. The risk for first degree relatives of patients with migraine without aura increases by 1.9-fold and that for migraine with aura increases by four-fold as compared to the general population, indicating both genetic and environmental factors are involved in its etiology.[226] The concordance rates of migraine without aura are higher in monozygotic (MZ) at 28% than in dizygotic (DZ) twins at 18%.[227] The concordance rates of migraine with aura are also higher in MZ (34%) than in DZ twins (12%) ($p < 0.05$).[228] Molecular genetic studies have identified so far at least one gene (19p13) in patients with familial hemiplegic migraine establishing a link between migraine and calcium channel disorders.[229]

Pathophysiology of migraine

The pathophysiological changes are triggered by appropriate physical or environmental factors in genetically predisposed individuals. The initiating steps in the pathophysiological cascade of migraine attacks may have neural, vascular, autonomic or biochemical origin. The recent progress in the understanding of the role of the neurotransmitter 5-hydroxytryptamine (5HT) and its several different receptors in the brain have made it possible to understand some mechanisms responsible for the initiation and progression of migraine attacks. Regardless of the exact initiating factors, it seems that the principal pathway in migraine attacks involves the activation of the trigeminovascular system. The interactions between the cranial vascular system and the trigeminal nucleus are complex and inter-related. Stimulation of the trigeminal sensory nerves either naturally by specific trigger factors or experimentally by electrical impulses in laboratory animals may induce the release of vasoactive neuropeptides. The release of vasoactive neuropeptides (substance P, neurokinin A and calcitonin gene-related peptide) initiates a process of microneurogenic inflammation followed by vasodilatation, mast cell degradation and plasma extravasation. Dihydroergotamine and sumatriptan as $5HT_{1B/D}$ receptor agonists can inhibit this process. As a result of the neurogenic inflammation, nociceptive impulses travel inferiorly to the trigeminal nucleus caudalis and superiorly to the thalamus and the cerebral cortex.[230] Diffuse projections from the locus ceruleus to the cerebral cortex may initiate a process of cortical oligemia that is better known as 'spreading depression of Leo' and may account for the aura symptoms. These may occur independently of headache. Interaction of brainstem and afferent impulses from cranial blood vessels may lead to vasomotor changes and the characteristic throbbing headache.

Clinical features and diagnostic criteria

The International Headache Society classified migraine into two major forms: migraine without aura and migraine with aura. Other less common forms were also recognized and defined. The majority of children with migraine (75–85%) suffer from migraine without aura.

Both forms of migraine may be present in the same patient.

Criteria have been established by the IHS for the diagnosis of migraine (Table 20.12). Migraine headache is typically recurrent in nature with complete recovery between attacks. Stress and anxiety are the most commonly identified trigger factors. Only 10–15% of patients can identify a certain type of food as a trigger factor such as cheese, chocolates and caffeine-containing soft drinks. Aura symptoms, if present, precede the onset of headache and are commonly visual in nature (blurred vision, tunnel vision, blind spots [scotomata] or zigzag colored lines in front of the eyes). Rarely the aura symptoms are sensory (tingling or numbness), motor (hemiplegia or speech disturbances), autonomic or non-specific.

The headache starts as a mild pain that does not interfere with normal activities. It increases in intensity over 30–60 min to a moderate intensity that may stop some activities or severe intensity that stops all activities. The pain is commonly described as throbbing, but some children may not be able to describe the pain or may refer to it as 'just sore'. In most patients the site of maximal intensity is either unilateral or frontal in location.

During the attack of migraine the child is described by parents as pale, quiet and wants to be left alone. The child refuses food and drink, feels nauseated and may vomit. Light, noise, smell and physical exercise may aggravate pain. Dizziness (unreal sensation of movement), abdominal pain, visual disturbances and sensory or motor deficits may also be associated, but to a lesser degree. Some patients describe unusual visual hallucination or distortion of images including micropsia, macropsia or a combination of both called *the Alice in Wonderland syndrome*.[231] Sleep, rest and simple analgesics may relieve symptoms. The attack lasts for at least 1 h and is followed by gradual resolution.

The clinical features of migraine can be dominated by transient symptoms of cerebellar and brainstem dysfunction such as vertigo,

Table 20.12 Diagnostic criteria of the International Headache Society (IHS)

IHS criteria for the diagnosis of migraine without aura

A. At least five attacks fulfilling B-D

B. Headache lasting 4–72 h (untreated or unsuccessfully treated)

C. Headache has at least two of the following characteristics:
   1. unilateral location
   2. pulsating quality
   3. moderate or severe intensity (inhibits or prohibits daily activities)
   4. aggravation by walking stairs or similar routine physical activity

D. During headache, at least one of the following:
   1. nausea and/or vomiting
   2. photophobia or phonophobia

E. No evidence of organic disease

IHS criteria for the diagnosis of migraine with aura

A. At least two attacks fulfilling B

B. At least three of the following four characteristics:
   - one or more fully reversible aura symptoms indicating focal cerebral cortical and/or brainstem dysfunction
   - at least one aura symptom develops gradually over more than 4 min, or two or more symptoms occur in succession
   - no aura symptom lasts more than 60 min. If more than one aura is present, accepted duration is proportionally increased
   - headache follows aura with a free interval of less than 60 min (it may also begin before or simultaneously with the aura)

C. No evidence of organic disease

Criteria for the diagnosis of abdominal migraine

1. Pain is severe enough to interfere with normal daily activities
2. Pain is described as dull or sore in nature
3. Pain is periumbilical or poorly localized
4. Pain is associated with any two of the following: anorexia, nausea, vomiting, pallor
5. Each attack lasts for at least 1 h
6. There is complete resolution of symptoms between attacks
7. Attacks occur at least twice a year

Criteria for the diagnosis of cyclical vomiting syndrome

- Recurrent, severe, discrete episodes of vomiting
- Various intervals of normal health between episodes
- Duration of vomiting episodes from hours to days
- No apparent cause of vomiting

ataxia, blurred vision, visual field defects, motor deficits, dysphasia and confusion. These features were attributed to vascular constriction in the territory of the basilar artery and hence described as *basilar migraine*.[232]

Some attacks of migraine are triggered by minor head injury and can be complicated with a disturbed level of consciousness and are commonly called *confusional migraine*. They occur mainly in children and are commoner in boys than in girls. The clinical features include an aura, followed by headache of variable severity and duration. There is an associated state of drowsiness, irritability, agitation, disturbed speech, aggressive behavior and amnesia. Blurred vision, nausea and vomiting are common features. The attacks may last between a few hours to a few days.

Migraine attacks can be complicated in some children with paralysis or paresis of the extraocular muscles, ptosis and pupillary dilatation, but with no associated confusion or loss of consciousness. These attacks are called *ophthalmoplegic migraine* and the eye features may not resolve until days or occasionally weeks after the resolution of headache. Some cases are indistinguishable from Tolosa–Hunt syndrome with MRI evidence of cavernous sinus dilatation and inflammatory process.

Attacks of migraine can be complicated with unilateral weakness, impaired speech or sensory loss. The neurological deficits are transient, fully reversible and may start before, with or after the onset of the headache. The neurological deficit may last longer than the duration of headache. The disease can be familial and is called *familial hemiplegic migraine* with an autosomal dominant inheritance or sporadic occurrence. Inherited cases may demonstrate a deletion of the calcium channel gene CACNA 1A on 19p13.

Treatment

The treatment of migraine includes reassurances to the child and the parents about the benign nature of the disorder and education concerning its natural course of remissions and relapses. Satisfactory management of the child with migraine may require more than one consultation in order to establish a good understanding of the condition and to address the individual concerns. Children should be encouraged to identify their own trigger and relieving factors and explore their own strategies of treatment. The judicial use of analgesics and other medications should be discussed from early on as many children and their parents use over-the-counter medications or have already received advice from their primary care physician.

Management of acute attacks of migraine

In the majority of patients an effective treatment of the acute attacks is the cornerstone of management and prophylaxis is not necessary. The treatment of acute attacks of migraine should start as early as possible after the onset of headache. Children should be allowed to rest and lie down in a quiet environment. Early administration of anaglesics is commonly associated with good results.

Paracetamol and ibuprofen are the first line of treatment. The analgesic effects of paracetamol are probably mediated centrally with possible indirect action on spinal serotonin receptors. Ibuprofen is a non-steroidal anti-inflammatory drug (NSAID) that inhibits the cyclo-oxygenase enzyme and hence prostaglandin synthesis. The analgesic effects of ibuprofen may also be mediated through independent spinal mechanisms.

In children under 15 years of age, paracetamol in single doses of 15 mg/kg body weight and ibuprofen (10 mg/kg) were effective and well tolerated in the treatment of headache and migraine.[233] Paracetamol had a more rapid onset than ibuprofen, but ibuprofen was twice as effective to abort migraine within 2 h. No other non-steroidal anti-inflammatory analgesics have been investigated in the acute treatment of migraine in children. Aspirin is an effective analgesic in migraine, but its association with Reye's syndrome has limited its use in children under the age of 12 years, especially in the presence of symptoms or signs of viral infection. Over-the-counter analgesics may contain any combination of drugs that have not been investigated in children. Occasionally a stronger analgesic such as codeine sulfate may be necessary.

Sumatriptan is a specific antimigraine medication with a good efficacy and safety record in adult patients. Sumatriptan is a selective agonist of $5HT_{1B/D}$ receptors. It causes constriction of cerebral blood vessels and blocks nociceptive impulses. Sumatriptan is available in subcutaneous autoinjection, oral tablets and as a nasal spray. Oral sumatriptan (doses between 50–100 mg) has been shown to be less effective in children than in adults in a placebo-controlled crossover study of 23 children, aged 8–16 years.[234] An open study of subcutaneous injections of sumatriptan (0.06 mg/kg) in 50 children between 6 and 18 years of age showed only a limited benefit.[235] Nasal sumatriptan is more effective than the oral preparation. A large multicenter double-blind placebo-controlled study of 653 adolescents aged 12–17 years has shown beneficial effects of nasal sumatriptan at a dose of 20 mg with bad taste being the most commonly reported side-effect.[236] Other similar triptans are also available, but their efficacy in childhood migraine is not proven yet.

Metoclopramide or prochlorperazine may alleviate nausea and vomiting during migraine attacks, but there are no controlled trials on their use in children. Concerns about possible extrapyramidal symptoms and dystonic reactions may preclude their use.

Prevention of migraine

Non-pharmacological strategies for the prevention of migraine attacks should include avoidance of specific trigger factors if identified. Dietary exclusion is only recommended in children with confirmed food triggers. All children with migraine should be encouraged to assume a good healthy lifestyle with regular pattern of sleep and meals and appropriate balance between rest and exercise. They should avoid spending excessive amounts of time on computer and video games and teenagers should be discouraged from smoking.

Pharmacological prophylactic treatment is not reliable and success is not always predictable. There is no consistent evidence for the efficacy and tolerability of any prophylactic agent. Therefore, treatment is only indicated if acute treatment is unsuccessful and migraine attacks are frequent (more than two attacks per month), prolonged and severe enough to interfere with school attendance and education. Prophylactic treatment should be continued for at least 6 weeks before considered ineffective and polytherapy should be avoided. Prophylactic treatment may be discontinued after 6 months, but could be restarted if necessary. Propranolol was shown to reduce the frequency of migraine attacks in a double-blind placebo-controlled trial,[237] but the results were not confirmed in a similar trial.[238] In children over 7 years of age, propranolol may be given in a dose of 1–2 mg/kg/day in two divided doses. The mechanism of action is not clear, but can involve inhibition of the catecholamine-induced platelet aggregation and release of platelets' serotonin. Side-effects may include hypoglycemia, hypotension, tiredness and mood changes.

The evidence for efficacy of other medications (pizotifen, clonidine and valproate) is either inconsistent or based on studies related to adult patients. Pizotifen was found to be effective in the treatment of abdominal migraine only,[239] but not in migraine.[240] Flunarizine, a cerebral calcium channel antagonist, can be effective in a dose of 5–10 mg per day,[241] but its use is associated with excessive side-effects such as drowsiness, depression and weight gain. Valproic acid is shown to be effective in adults, but has not been studied in children.[242] Amitriptyline was shown to be very effective in prevention of chronic headache in a large open observational study.[243] Amitriptyline, a tricyclic antidepressant, may block the reuptake of both serotonin and noradrenaline and its prophylactic property on migraine is independent of its antidepressant actions. A study of the efficacy of amitriptyline, (1.5 mg/kg/day) in the prevention of migraine in 19 children (6–12 years of age) has shown only a modest benefit.[244] Unlike in adult studies, amitriptyline did not influence the duration of migraine attacks and drowsiness was the most common adverse effect.

Prognosis

The natural course of migraine is of remissions and relapses, but with tendency for permanent remission with increasing age. Remissions of at least 1 year have been recorded in up to 58% of patients during periods of follow-up of at least 5 years.[245] Long-term follow-up studies of 73 children with migraine showed that 34% became headache free after 6 years, 62% after 16 years and 40–47% after 22–40 years.[210,246,247]

Alternating hemiplegia of childhood

Alternating hemiplegia of childhood (AHC) is a progressive disabling disorder of unknown etiology, but has long been considered as a form of 'complicated migraine'.[248] Affected children present in early infancy and may pass through three distinct clinical phases.[249] During the first year of life (phase I) children show signs of delayed development, abnormal eye movement and episodes of dystonia. During the second year of life (phase II) they show the typical hemiplegic spells that alternate between sides and last between a few days to a few weeks. By the age of 5 years (phase III), patients have fixed neurological deficits and variable degrees of disability, developmental delay, spasticity and epilepsy.

The diagnosis is usually based on the typical clinical course. CT and MRI scans of the brain do not show any specific patterns. Long term treatment with flunarizine (a specific calcium channel blocker) results in reduced number and severity of hemiplegic spells, but it is unlikely to change the natural course of the disease. The relationship of AHC to migraine is based on its paroxysmal nature, the occurrence of headache during some attacks and the apparent high prevalence of migraine with aura among the relatives of patients. However, the progressive nature of the disease and the permanent neurological and learning disabilities suggest a pathophysiological process that is unrelated to migraine.

Benign paroxysmal torticollis of infancy (BPTI)

BPTI is a benign disorder of early childhood characterized by self-limiting episodes of head tilt lasting a few hours to a few days. Attacks start during the first year of life and resolve completely by the age of 5. The attacks are sudden in onset and resolution and may alternate between sides.[250] BPTI has been linked to migraine and benign paroxysmal vertigo on clinical and epidemiological bases. The pathophysiology is not clear, but surface electromyography (sEMG) of the sternomastoid muscle during attacks shows dystonic phenomena.[251] The diagnosis is based on the typical episodic clinical features. The attacks start suddenly with the head held to one side. The neck muscles on the side of the tilt, particularly the sternomastoid, are stiff and tense. During attacks the child may also have pallor, nausea, vomiting, ataxia and irritability.

Neuroimaging and electroencephalography (EEG) are indicated in order to exclude intracranial pathology, cerebellar lesions and epilepsy. A definite diagnosis should be followed by reassurance to parents about the benign nature of the condition. The majority of cases resolve by the age of 3 and almost all by the age of 5 years. No treatment is necessary.

Benign paroxysmal vertigo

Benign paroxysmal vertigo (BPV) is a syndrome characterized by recurrent episodes of unreal sensation of movement of the child or his or her surrounding environment. Each episode lasts for a few minutes, but occasionally may continue for hours or up to 2 days.

Early onset BPV is uncommon, but affects children between the ages of 2 and 4 years. It is characterized by sudden episodes of pallor, screaming, unsteadiness, nystagmus, nausea and occasionally vomiting.[252] The child either sits or clings to his or her parent in fear. The attacks terminate spontaneously and the child returns to normal. There is no loss of consciousness and the child is aware and responsive during the event. Episodes of BPV decrease in frequency by age 5 years and may be replaced by episodes of headache typical of migraine.

Late onset BPV is common among schoolchildren[253] with a prevalence rate of 2.6%. Older children are able to describe the unreal sensation of movement. The attacks last for seconds to minutes and average about one attack per month. The only abnormal finding on physical examination during attacks is horizontal nystagmus. Migraine is more common among children with BPV and among their first degree relatives than in matching control children.[253]

The diagnosis of BPV is based on excluding underlying neurological causes, vestibular disorders, epilepsy, medications and toxic substances by appropriate investigations such as neuroimaging and EEG. Treatment is not needed, apart from reassurance about the benign nature of the condition. Some children may benefit from the antihistamine betahistine.[254]

Abdominal migraine

Recurrent abdominal pain (RAP) is a common problem affecting around 8% of schoolchildren. Half the children with RAP (4%) have abdominal migraine[255] as defined by the clinical criteria in Table 20.12. Abdominal migraine is characterized by recurrent episodes of a dull abdominal pain lasting between 1 and 72 h. Between attacks the child is completely well. The clinical pattern of trigger factors, associated symptoms and relieving factors of abdominal migraine is similar to that of migraine headache in children. Attacks of abdominal migraine have been reported to start at any age from early infancy with a mean age of onset at around 7 years. Follow-up studies showed that at least one-third of children continue to suffer attacks of abdominal migraine late into their teenage years and 70% have a current (52%) or past (18%) history of migraine.[256]

The management of affected children starts with the confirmation of the diagnosis, reassurance to parents and identification and avoidance of trigger factors. Acute attacks should be treated with simple analgesics, rest, and fluid replacement and occasionally with antiemetics. There are no published data on the use of specific antimigraine agents such as sumatriptan. Drug prophylaxis has been evaluated in a randomized double-blind placebo-controlled trial of pizotifen. It was shown to be effective in the prevention of abdominal migraine.[239] Evidence for the value of other drugs such as propranolol and cyproheptadine is based on open trials only.[257]

Cyclical vomiting syndrome (CVS)

CVS is a disease mainly of early childhood and closely related to migraine. It presents with sudden episodes of anorexia, nausea, vomiting, lethargy and intolerance to light, noise and exercise. During the attack the child looks unwell, pale and miserable. The attacks can be severe enough to stop activities and may lead to dehydration especially if prolonged. The attacks last from a few hours to a few days and the child is completely well between attacks. It is estimated that around 2% of schoolchildren may have unexplained attacks of vomiting that fulfil the criteria for the diagnosis of CVS (Table 20.12).[258] The disease may begin during infancy and occasionally during the first year of life. As the child grows up typical episodes are associated with headache that fulfils the criteria for the diagnosis of migraine. Children with CVS who were followed up for 7–10 years had a high prevalence rate of migraine (46%) as compared to a matching control group of children (12%). Also 50% of children continued to suffer from attacks of CVS into teenage and early adult life.[259] The treatment of acute attacks aims to stop vomiting and prevent dehydration. Early administration of oral or intravenous antiemetic drugs such as ondansetron may abort attacks. Prophylactic treatment with erythromycin as a prokinetic agent may reduce the number and severity of attacks.

TENSION-TYPE HEADACHE

Tension type headache (TTH) is common among children and adolescents who seek medical advice for their headache. TTH is also known as psychogenic headache, muscle contraction headache or non-vascular headache. Tension-type headache may be episodic or chronic in nature. *Episodic tension-type headache (ETTH)* is defined by the International Headache Society[221] as recurrent episodes of headache lasting 30 min to 7 days with a frequency of less than 15 days per month. The pain is typically felt as pressure or tightening of mild to moderate severity. It is bilateral in location and does not worsen with routine activities. It may be associated with photophobia or phonophobia, but not nausea or vomiting. *Chronic tension-type headache (CTTH)* is defined when headache attacks are present for at least 15 days per month for at least 6 months. The pain is similar to ETTH and can be associated with photophobia, phonophobia or nausea. CTTH commonly evolves from long standing ETTH or migraine.

The prevalence rate of TTH in the general childhood population is not known. In one population-based study of childhood headache, the prevalence rate of CTTH was estimated at 1%.[211] However, TTH is common among children and adolescents attending accident and emergency departments, general practice and hospital clinics for headache as their chief complaint. Both males and females are equally affected and TTH is commoner in older children (over the age of 12 years) and adolescents. TTH is rare in children under the age of 6 years.

The etiology of tension-type headache is not known, but there is evidence of familial tendency, especially in CTTH, and significant environmental influences. CTTH may evolve from ETTH or may start as chronic from the onset. It may be induced by chronic use of analgesics or high daily caffeine intake. It has been noted that children with CTTH have a higher than expected incidence of major life events such as chronic disease, family illnesses and bereavements that may predispose to or complicate the course of headache.[220] The pathophysiology of TTH is not understood. Several initiating mechanisms have been suggested including muscle contraction, physical strain, anxiety and stress. No consistent biochemical or physiological (EMG) changes have been found.

The clinical features of ETTH can sometimes be indistinguishable from those of migraine without aura and the correct diagnosis is best made by the use of headache diaries. In some patients both migraine without aura and episodic tension headache coexist. The distinction between the two conditions is important, as the response to treatment with painkillers is different.

The diagnosis of TTH is made on the basis of the typical clinical history and normal neurological examination and investigations are not needed in the majority of patients. Treatment with analgesics is often unsuccessful and should be discouraged in children with CTTH, as some may develop analgesia-induced headache on long term use. The management of the child with TTH can be complex and multidisciplinary. The treatment should aim at reassuring the child and the parents of the absence of any sinister cause and to offer general advice on healthy lifestyle. Children should be encouraged to adopt predictable patterns of sleep, regular meals, balanced diets, adequate exercise and rest. Successful management will need the full involvement of the children, their parents, schoolteachers or nurses, and occasionally clinical psychologists. Attention should be paid to possible underlying chronic physical, psychological or emotional problems. The expertise of a clinical psychologist may also help in the management of acute headache attacks and in helping the child and the family to develop their own strategies in dealing with pain in general. The prognosis of TTH is variable and patients may run a course of remissions and relapses.

CLUSTER HEADACHE

Cluster headache is uncommon in children, but cases were reported in children as young as 1 year of age.[260] In many adult patients the onset of headache is before the age of 18 years and in some before the age of 10 years.[261] Episodic cluster headache is more common (affecting around 80% of patients) than the chronic form and more males are affected than females.

The cause of cluster headache is not known, but there is a strong familial tendency to suggest genetic predisposition. The changes during attacks are consistent with neuronal, endocrine and vascular mechanisms involving trigeminovascular activation.[262]

The clinical features of cluster headaches during childhood are similar to those which typically occur in adult life with a tendency for the frequency and duration of cluster periods and the frequency of the individual headache episodes to increase with age. Headache attacks are short (up to 90 min) and have a well-defined periodicity. The pain is severe, sharp and reaches its peak intensity within 5–15 min and may provoke intense emotions and violent behavior. The pain is almost always unilateral with maximal intensity around the eye and can be associated with nausea and vomiting. Autonomic symptoms (nasal congestion, forehead sweating, conjunctival injection, miosis, lacrimation and ptosis) are common and are almost always on the same side of the pain and resolve with the resolution of pain.

Atypical attacks (cluster headache-like disorders) have been reported in a small number of children. The headache is bilateral, the pain is not periorbital and children exhibit unusual motor behavior consisting of thrashing of limbs and irritability.[263] Early administration of high flow oxygen (7 L/min via a facial mask), subcutaneous injection or nasal administration of sumatriptan may relieve acute attacks. A short course of steroids (prednisolone or dexamethasone) can induce remission and verapamil, valproate, melatonin or topiramate may be given as prophylactic maintenance therapy.

CHRONIC POST-TRAUMATIC HEADACHE (CPTH)

Episodes of headache start within 2 weeks of head injury including minor trauma. The headache episodes continue for at least 8 weeks.

The prevalence rate of CPTH in children is not known, but a follow-up study, 12–18 months after head injury, has shown that 29% of 138 children (mean age 9.2 years) suffered from recurrent headaches.[264]

The cause of CPTH is not fully understood, but the pathogenesis is likely to be complex and may involve premorbid predisposition to headache and other psychosocial factors.

The clinical features are those of idiopathic recurrent headaches (migraine and tension headache of childhood). Other symptoms of postconcussion syndrome may be present, but physical and neurological examinations are completely normal.[265] In children with typical presentation neuroimaging is not indicated.

Treatment includes reassurance and appropriate use of simple analgesics as necessary.

HEADACHE DUE TO INTRACRANIAL DISORDERS

Brain tumors

Headache is a common symptom of brain tumors and has been reported in 62% of 3291 children with brain tumors.[266] It is almost always associated with at least one other specific feature such as ataxia, nystagmus, intention tremor, effortless vomiting, headache during sleep, focal neurological deficits, acquired squint, papilledema, personality change or deteriorating schoolwork. In 8–10% of children, headache may be the only presenting symptom.[267,268]

When headache is the only presenting symptom of brain tumor or raised intracranial pressure, it may have no specific features or may have features similar to those of migraine or tension-type headache leading to a delay in the diagnosis of the underlying cause. However, a detailed history may elucidate some clues pointing to the cause. In a study of 600 children with migraine and 67 children with brain tumor, the most important headache features in children with brain tumors were nocturnal headache and headache present on arising.[269]

In a retrospective study of 74 children with brain tumors,[270] the mean duration of symptoms before diagnosis was 20 weeks. The most common symptoms were vomiting (65%) and headache (64%). Only 34% of headaches were always associated with vomiting and only 28% occurred 'early morning'.

Benign intracranial hypertension (BIH)

BIH is a rare clinical syndrome of raised intracranial pressure and headache. It occurs in all ages including infancy. No specific causes have been identified in children and the pathogenesis is not clear. Clinical features are those of raised intracranial pressure and headache is the most common symptom occurring in the majority of patients. Headache is often located at the forehead and is worse on lying down or on awakening up in the morning.[271] Other symptoms may include nausea, vomiting, visual disturbances (diplopia, visual loss, blurred vision and visual field defects), lethargy, dizziness and behavioral problems. There is no deterioration in the level of consciousness. On examination, papilledema is the most common sign occurring in the majority of patients followed by sixth cranial nerve palsy and defects of visual acuity.[272]

Ophthalmological examination is an essential part in the assessment of the child with BIH and children often have their first presentation to the opticians or the ophthalmologists.

Neuroimaging with CT or MRI excludes other causes of increased intracranial pressure and demonstrates normal structure of brain and the ventricular system. Lumbar puncture shows increased CSF pressure above 200 mm water and a normal CSF analysis.

The diagnosis of BIH is based on fulfilling the following International Headache Society's clinical criteria:[221]

1. cerebrospinal fluid (CSF) pressure above 200 mm water;
2. normal neurological examination except for papilledema and possible sixth cranial nerve palsy;
3. no mass lesion and no ventricular enlargement on neuroimaging;
4. normal or low protein concentration and normal white cell count in the CSF; and
5. no clinical or neuroimaging evidence of venous sinus thrombosis.

BIH is largely a self-limiting condition, but unfortunately permanent loss of visual field and reduced visual acuity can occur in 13–27% of children.[272] Therefore, early recognition and treatment are necessary to avoid visual complications. Regular ophthalmological reviews are recommended from the time of diagnosis. A number of treatment measures have been shown to be effective in reducing the intracranial pressure. Repeated lumbar punctures with CSF removal may initially be required daily and thereafter at reducing intervals. Steroids have not been properly evaluated for this condition but various single reports suggest that the pressure drops within 24 h. Acetazolamide is often given to patients who have an inadequate steroid response: large doses are required to be effective and sometimes the acetazolamide is combined with a loop diuretic. A lumboperitoneal or ventriculoperitoneal shunt may be necessary for those who have failed medical treatment and symptomatic relief may occasionally be required by optic nerve decompression.

HEADACHE DUE TO SINUSITIS

Sinus diseases are unusual during early childhood, as paranasal sinuses are not fully developed before the age of 8 years. In children with acute sinusitis the headache is usually mild and its site of maximal intensity is related to the affected sinuses. The International Headache Society described the headache of acute frontal sinusitis as 'located directly over the sinus and may radiate to the vertex or behind the eyes'. In maxillary sinusitis 'the headache is located over the antral area and may radiate to upper teeth or to the forehead'. In acute ethmoiditis 'the headache is located between and behind the eyes and may radiate to the temporal area'.[221] The headache of acute sinusitis is almost always associated with other features of upper airway disease, e.g. nasal congestion, discharge, sneeze and cough, making the diagnosis of acute sinusitis relatively easy.

Headache due to chronic sinusitis may be present with or without upper respiratory tract symptoms and the diagnosis, therefore, can be less obvious. Therefore, sinusitis should be suspected as the cause of chronic headache in the presence of clinical features related to upper airway disease such as sleep disturbance, nasal discharge, nasal blockage and decreased sense of smell. In other children, headache can be the only symptom for a 'silent' sinus disease.

The diagnosis of chronic sinusitis should confirmed with appropriate imaging. Medical treatment should include anti-histamine decongestants, antibiotics and simple analgesia. Surgical treatment is rarely needed except in the presence of underlying predisposing factors or nasal polyps causing obstruction.

DISORDERS OF MOVEMENT

EXTRAPYRAMIDAL DISORDERS, BASAL GANGLIA DISORDERS

Extrapyramidal movement disorders (involuntary movements) accompany many diseases thought to originate from the basal ganglia. Some are amongst the most benign of neurological disorders but others are progressive. There are no clear figures concerning the incidence and prevalence of movement disorders. However, movement disorders are not uncommon.

The underlying causes include infections, metabolic disorders and neurotransmitter imbalance. However, the cause of many is unknown. The basal ganglia are particularly susceptible to hypoxia. This is seen in carbon monoxide poisoning, neonatal asphyxia and post cardiopulmonary bypass. Heavy metals also appear to have a special affinity for this part of the brain (e.g. copper deposition with Wilson's disease, iron deposition in Hallervorden–Spatz disease and the dyskinesias of manganese, molybdenum and thallium poisoning). Metabolic diseases such as phenylketonuria, Leigh's encephalopathy and glutaric aciduria may present with a predominant dyskinetic clinical picture.

Anatomy of the basal ganglia

The extrapyramidal system in classic neurology consists of part of the cerebral cortex anterior to the motor strip and several masses of gray matter deep in the hemisphere white matter and the upper brainstem. The nomenclature has been rather confusing as words such as basal ganglia, striatum, corpus striatum, and lenticular nucleus are either synonyms or groupings of nuclei. The corpus striatum is the name given to the lentiform nucleus (i.e. the combined putamen and globus pallidus) and the caudate nucleus. It is more appropriate to think in terms of the caudate, putamen and globus pallidus in the cerebral hemisphere together with the substantia nigra in the upper brainstem and the subthalamic nucleus of Luys as constituting together the basal ganglia.

The basal ganglia can be regarded as a major motor computation center receiving information from the cortex about movements being planned together with information from the parietal cortex about body image and from vision. They receive input regarding the force, speed and direction of movement planned by the cerebellum together with information on the position of the head and eyes from the labyrinth and information about body contact and visual information on the position of the body in space. The basal ganglia and extrapyramidal motor cortex inhibit certain primitive brainstem reflexes such as the asymmetrical tonic neck reflex, primitive walking and swimming reflexes and probably store more sophisticated patterns of movement.

Biochemistry of the basal ganglia

The main interest in biochemistry of the basal ganglia stems from the discovery of the dopaminergic pathways from the substantia nigra, the effects of L-DOPA in parkinsonism and the study of the extrapyramidal side-effects of drugs like the phenothiazines.

Classic parkinsonism has three components – tremor, bradykinesia and rigidity – and although the symptoms and signs of basal ganglia disease will be discussed in more detail later (see below), it is necessary to consider some aspects to understand the role of dopamine and L-DOPA in normal basal ganglia function and in disease. The three components appear independently determined because the tremor may be made worse by L-DOPA but helped by surgery; the bradykinesia is helped by L-DOPA but surgery has no effect; the rigidity is helped by L-DOPA and surgery and is especially helped by anticholinergics. Current evidence suggests that cholinergic, serotonergic and gabanergic pathways are normally balanced (inhibited) by dopamine and that while dopamine is important in inhibiting rigidity, it is involved in the causation of the hyperkinetic dyskinesias. Rather confusingly, however, there are some children with dyskinesias involving too much movement who are helped by L-DOPA. In tardive dyskinesia and chorea there should be inherent dopamine excess or drugs that directly stimulate dopamine receptors could be responsible. Drugs which cause tardive dyskinesias such as the phenothiazines, are known to have anticholinergic, antiserotoninergic and antihistaminergic effects and to leave dopamine unopposed. Drugs which reduce dopamine action such as tetrabenazine, haloperidol and reserpine, will reduce the involuntary movements in chorea, but are more likely to induce a parkinsonian picture as a side-effect. Parkinsonism can be induced either by depleting the brain's production of dopamine, as occurs with reserpine and tetrabenazine when the dopamine receptors remain free, or alternatively it can be caused by blocking the dopamine receptors by such drugs as haloperidol when L-DOPA cannot reverse the parkinsonism so produced.

Some other drug effects are also important. Thus multiple tics may appear as a complication of chronic amfetamine use or chronic overdose by methylphenidate (Ritalin). Both of these drugs increase brain dopamine as well as having a noradrenergic effect. 5-hydroxytryptophan has been given to patients with Lesch–Nyhan syndrome, and in this disorder, it appears to lessen self-mutilation. In the past, it has also been used in children with Down syndrome in the hope that it would improve muscle tone and motor performance, but it was found to produce marked rigidity and myoclonic jerks. Cholinergic drugs such as physostigmine will make parkinsonism worse, but will lessen choreiform movements. Together clinical anatomy, physiology, biochemistry and pharmacology help to explain the diverse clinical signs and symptoms which occur in disorders of the basal ganglia.

Movement disorders: general considerations

Many neurological diseases have movement disorders as the main presentation or part of it. These movements are often misdiagnosed as epilepsy, behavioral disorder or tics.

A good eyewitness description is important. However, where possible, it is essential to observe the movements. Videotapes are an excellent way of achieving this especially when they are infrequent or episodic.

Movement disorders may present as more or less continuous abnormal movements or posture or these may fluctuate with time and in relation to emotional state and anxiety. In addition, they may present as paroxysmal episodes mimicking epileptic attacks. Movement disorders may be benign and transient such as benign myoclonus of infancy and dyskinesia after the withdrawal of benzodiazepines (especially i.v. midazolam), or phenytoin in the pediatric intensive care unit (Table 20.13).

It is necessary to observe the child at rest, whilst sustaining postures, such as outstretching the limbs, during active movement, such as tying shoelaces, and, if possible, under stress. Although involuntary movements often present at rest, they are usually more pronounced with volitional execution of a motor task and may significantly disrupt the motor activities. Children often try to mask abnormal movements by combining them with a normal movement pattern. For example, children with chorea usually mask their abnormal movements by scratching the nose or forehead or by clenching the fingers together. The clinician should not be misled and should notice that these normal movements are not purposeful. Movement disorders are almost always absent during sleep. They are not associated with loss of consciousness and children have full recall of the episodes.

Sometimes, the involuntary movements are a mixture of several types such as choreoathetosis and myoclonic dystonia. The correct classification is often difficult and requires experience and skill. More clinical details will come later regarding specific types of movement disorder and associated conditions.

Investigation of movement disorders

Identification of the movement disorder type should be attempted but is not always possible. Investigations are directed toward the

Table 20.13 Transient movement disorders in childhood

Benign paroxysmal torticollis of infancy
Benign myoclonus of the newborn
Benign myoclonus of infancy
Jitteriness
Transient paroxysmal dystonia of infancy
Spasmus nutans

suspected most likely diagnosis. Many diseases may cause more than one type of movement disorder. This includes tumors of the basal ganglia, which makes it reasonable to perform neuroimaging in all children with acquired movement disorder. On the other hand, a single type of movement disorder can be caused by many different diseases. Treatable conditions, such as Wilson's disease, should be looked for early as more benefit is obtained with early treatment. Specific investigations for each movement disorder and related conditions will be dealt with later.

Classification of movement disorders

Movement disorders (dyskinesias) can be classified in many ways (Table 20.14). An anatomical classification may conclude that lesions of the globus pallidus cause parkinsonism or a lack of movement, lesions of the putamen cause athetosis and lesions of the caudate cause chorea. However this is a gross oversimplification. Alternatively, they can be classified on the basis of clinical presentation, i.e. whether there is an acute dyskinesia, progressive dyskinesia or chronic non-progressive dyskinesia. A third method is according to the predominant type of movement, i.e. chorea and choreoathetosis, dystonia, and tremor. Also, movement disorders can be classified as hyperkinetic or hypokinetic.

Hyperkinetic dyskinesias

These are typified by the choreas, hemiballismus, tics and orofacial dyskinesias. This group is most often associated with a reduction in muscle tone and the movements disappear in sleep, or if the child is totally relaxed and lying down. Symptomatically there is a close link between this group of disorders and cerebellar dysfunction, e.g. myoclonus can occur in both. In the hyperkinetic dyskinesias the child is restless, fidgety, cannot sit still, stamps his feet, grimaces, shakes his head, may get a constant urge to run, may grunt, make clucking noises and show respiratory irregularity. Difficulty keeping still is referred to as akathisia. The hyperkinetic dyskinesias tend to be associated with high levels of dopamine or noradrenergic substances.

Table 20.14 Classification of movement disorders

Dyskinesias
Hyperkinetic
Hypokinetic
Akinetic
Anatomical
Lesion of the putamen
Lesion of the caudate
Lesion of the globus pallidus
Clinical presentation
Acute
Progressive
Chronic
Type of predominant movement
Chorea/athetosis
Dystonia
Tremor
Tics

Hypokinetic dyskinesia

In the most severe cases there is akinesia and the child cannot initiate any movement even though not paralysed. Less severe cases with bradykinesia are associated with difficulty in initiating movements, e.g. difficulty in running is characteristic. The most characteristic hypokinetic state is parkinsonism, which is classically associated with dopamine depletion.

Diseases will be discussed depending on the predominant disorders. Many of these conditions, especially the metabolic, will be discussed in the related chapters.

CHOREA AND ATHETOSIS

Definition and general considerations

Chorea is rapid, repetitive, jerky movements affecting any part of the body. It may be unilateral or bilateral and affect the face and trunk as well as the limbs. The movements are neither rhythmic nor stereotyped and they migrate from side to side and limb to limb. True choreiform movements tend to be jerky, unpredictable and random and differ from tics in that they have no pattern of repetition, but the so-called convulsive tic with repeated wild flinging movements of the arms and lateral jerking of the head may resemble hemiballismus. Chorea may be incorporated into a voluntary movement. The sudden wild flinging of the arm or the head in chorea is made semipurposeful by pretending to scratch the head or straighten the hair. The child may sit on the affected hand, or the tongue is held between the teeth to try to lessen the movements. Walking and feeding may become impossible due to the repeated jerks of the head and limbs together with involvement of the lips, tongue and palate.

True choreiform movements can be appreciated most easily by getting the child to stand still, arms outstretched when the jerks appear as a gross caricature of the milder constant readjusting movements seen in pure cerebellar disease, as if there was a total absence of damping, with wild overswings of correction. The head and upper limbs are affected more than the trunk and lower limbs, and total relaxation in the supine position lessens the movements as maintenance of posture and initiation of voluntary movement seems to be important in triggering them off. The face and bulbar muscles are involved when there are bilateral choreiform movements of the arms (a tic may be unilateral and have bulbar involvement). It must be remembered that low amplitude choreiform movement of the outstretched hands as a normal physiological variant is a frequent finding in boys of early primary school age.[273]

Athetosis literally means without posture, i.e. it is a posture that is constantly changing. It is a slow, writhing movement of the limbs that is frequently associated with chorea (choreoathetosis). Isolated athetosis is almost always due to perinatal asphyxia. Previously, kernicterus was the major cause. The movements in the athetoid child are slower than those in a child with pure chorea and they involve gradual changes in posture secondary to changes in muscle tone. The upper limbs appear to be constantly moving between the primitive extensor posture and the hemiplegic flexor posture. The fingers start in the hemiplegic position with the hand closed across the adducted thumb and flexed at wrist and elbows. The fingers then extend and the arm extends, abducts and internally rotates into the extended (also called avoiding) position. Since the leg is extended in both postures, it remains in equinus and does not show the same movements as occur in the arms. Feeding, especially chewing, is difficult and speech is always affected. Walking may be possible, with a reeling gait and contortions of the trunk, yet surprisingly few falls result.

Athetosis of the hands, dilation of the alae nasae and fanning of the toes is often seen in normal infants at birth and may become very obvious after relatively mild asphyxia. Pathological athetosis rarely appears in the first year of life in brain damage syndromes. Dystonic extension appears at about 4 months of age and athetosis may not occur for a further 2 or 3 years. Grimacing, laughing, crying and inappropriate emotional responses can accompany the fluctuating muscle tone.

Differential diagnosis

The conditions which present with chorea/choreoathetosis may be acute (Table 20.15), chronic and progressive (Table 20.16) or chronic and non-progressive (Table 20.17). Some conditions are genetic (Table 20.18), systemic, metabolic, or secondary to infections and vascular diseases. Chorea might be the initial or most prominent symptom or may be present as an associated symptom. Some of these conditions will be discussed in this chapter. The rest are discussed elsewhere.

Table 20.15 Acute-onset choreiform disease

Sydenham's chorea
Toxic dystonic/chorea
Phenothiazines – chlorpromazine (Largactil), trifluoperazine (Stelazine), fluphenazine (Moditen), thioridazine (Melleril)
Phenytoin
Carbamazepine (tics and dystonia)
Maxolon
Prochlorperazine (Stemetil)
Lithium
Tricyclics – amitriptyline
Manganese poisoning
Thallium poisoning
Hydrogen sulfide
Fentanyl
Propofol
Serotonin reuptake inhibitors – paroxetine
Bethanechol
High estrogen contraceptive pill
Lamotrigine
Chorea gravidarum
Chorea and the contraceptive pill
Chorea and lupus erythematosus
Chorea and Henoch–Schönlein purpura
Hemolytic uremic syndrome
Hypoparathyroidism
Paroxysmal kinesiogenic dystonia
DOPA-sensitive dystonia (Segawa)
Carbon monoxide poisoning
Following cardiac bypass surgery
Postdialysis dyskinesia
After burns – burns shakes
Metabolic diseases – Leigh's disease
Familial paroxysmal choreoathetosis
Infections
Encephalitis lethargica
Toxoplasmic encephalitis
Coxsackie, echo and varicella encephalitis
Haemophilus influenzae B meningitis
AIDS encephalopathy
Neurosyphilis
Epidemic rubeola

Table 20.16 Progressive diseases associated with chorea

Huntington's chorea
Idiopathic torsion dystonia
DOPA-sensitive dystonia of Segawa
Metabolic
Wilson's disease
Glutaric aciduria
Phenylketonuria
Leigh's encephalopathy
Mitochondrial diseases (MELAS, MERRF)
Homocystinuria
Triosephosphate isomerase deficiency
Sulfite oxidase deficiency
Methylmalonic acidemia
Dihydropteridine reductase deficiency
Hexosaminidase A and B deficiency (onset 10 years with dystonia)
Lesch–Nyhan syndrome
Lysosomal enzyme disorders – G_{M1}, G_{M2}, Krabbe and metachromatic leukodystrophy
Fahr's syndrome (basal ganglia calcification)
Hypoparathyroidism
Infectious origin
Subacute sclerosing panencephalitis
AIDS encephalopathy
Infantile bilateral striatal necrosis
Hallervorden–Spatz disease
Ataxia telangiectasia
Ataxia with ocular dyspraxia (Aicardi)
Pelizaeus–Merzbacher disease
Familial dystonic paraplegia
Paroxysmal dystonia with myoclonus
Paroxysmal sleep dystonia
Neuraxonal dystrophy
Parkinson's disease
Hunt's juvenile parkinsonism (striatonigral degeneration)
Hunt's pallidocerebellar degeneration
Pilocytic astrocytomas

MELAS, mitochondrial encephalomyopathy, lactic acidosis, and stroke-like episodes; MERFF, myoclonic epilepsy with ragged red fibers.

Specific syndromes

Genetic diseases

Huntington's chorea. This dominantly inherited condition characteristically appears in adults around 30 years with dementia, rigidity and chorea as well as psychological and behavior changes. Ten per cent of cases start in childhood and inheritance is usually from the father. It is therefore an imprinted disorder with spontaneous mutations being very rare. It is a triple codon repeat disease: 35–90 repeats of trinucleotide CAG are diagnostic on chromosome 4p16.3. Diagnosis of suspected childhood cases is now possible. Presentation can be with seizures in 50% of cases, thus differing from the adult who presents with dementia or dystonia. However, up to 50% will present with dementia, manifested by a fall off in schoolwork before the rigidity, which is often asymmetrical. MRI scan shows selective atrophy of the head of the caudate nucleus.

Benign familial (hereditary) chorea. This is a rare dominantly inherited disorder. The onset is usually in early childhood. It starts

Table 20.17 Chronic non-progressive disease (cerebral palsies)

Bilirubin encephalopathy
Hypoxic–ischemic encephalopathy
Autosomal recessive striatonigral dysplasia
Dystonia of prematurity

Table 20.18 Inherited choreas

Benign familial chorea	AD or AR
Dentatorubropallidoluysian atrophy (DRPL)	AD
Familial paroxysmal choreoathetosis	AD
Huntington's chorea	AD
Neuroacanthocytosis	AD or AR
Pontocerebellar hypoplasia type 2	AR

AD, autosomal dominant; AR, autosomal recessive

with the child's first steps. Intelligence is usually normal. Chorea may associate with athetosis, hypotonia and tremor. The condition becomes less pronounced by adolescence and may disappear in some affected adults.

It is difficult to distinguish between this condition and other causes of chorea, especially familial paroxysmal chorea. The family history and the continuous, non-episodic chorea are important pointers. Treatment with anticonvulsants, chlorpromazine or haloperidol is beneficial in some.

Hallervorden–Spatz syndrome. The basal ganglia are very rich in iron. The reason for this is not known nor is it understood why the basal ganglia are so selectively vulnerable to heavy metal toxicity. Hallervorden–Spatz syndrome, a recessive condition, is associated with an increase of the amount of stainable iron. The globus pallidus and substantia nigra are affected with accumulation of iron pigments, a decrease in myelin and axonal swellings (spheroids). The clinical picture is not of parkinsonism but of spasticity with brisk reflexes, extensor plantar responses and increasing extrapyramidal rigidity of a hemiplegic dystonic type affecting all four limbs. When progression is very slow, the child may be thought to have cerebral palsy. Usually by the age of 10 years there is fixation of posture with varying degrees of choreoathetosis. Death usually occurs in the early 20s. There is no definitive diagnostic test, but as the condition progresses many children on MRI show an appearance of the basal ganglia which is typical and has been likened to a 'tiger's eye'. Genetically the syndrome appears to be heterogeneous.[274] Brain biopsy does not help unless one is fortunate enough to see circular inclusions known as spheroids. Iron metabolism, as judged by the measurement of serum iron, transferrins or iron absorption, is normal. No treatment is of any avail. The disease is rare and differentiation from metachromatic leukodystrophy, Alexander's disease and Pelizaeus–Merzbacher disease can be clinically difficult. All may be misdiagnosed initially as cases of cerebral palsy.

Paroxysmal choreoathetosis. This is an odd condition with grimacing, choreiform movements and abnormal posturing, which occur in episodes. It may be difficult without a continuous 24-h EEG recording to differentiate sporadic cases from epilepsies manifested with similar abnormal movements. The condition does not progress and is not associated with dementia. Onset may be as early as 6 months of age. Examination between episodes is normal, as is the EEG. It is dominantly inherited and no biochemical abnormality has been found. Sudden movement, or a particular movement, may precipitate bouts of choreoathetosis. The episode may be brief or may last several hours. Consciousness is usually maintained, even in paroxysmal choreoathetosis lasting hours or days. Paroxysmal choreoathetosis can also occur as a consequence of lesions to the basal ganglia, such as low grade astrocytomas. Dystonia or athetoid posturing precipitated by movement, i.e. paroxysmal kinesiogenic dystonia, may be very sensitive to carbamazepine.

Initial treatment is with anticonvulsants, particularly carbamazepine and phenytoin. If unsuccessful, prolonged episodes can be treated with anticholinergics such as benzatropine.

Systemic diseases

Sydenham's chorea. This is the most common acquired chorea in children. It is a cardinal feature of rheumatic fever and alone is enough for the diagnosis. The onset is usually 4 months after the initiating streptococcal infection.

The onset is usually insidious and diagnosis is often delayed. Chorea, hypotonia, dysarthria, restlessness and emotional lability are essential features. An early feature is an unexplained deterioration in school work with the affected child being accused of 'messing about'. Obsessive–compulsive behavior may be present.

On examination the child looks fidgety with migratory chorea of limbs and face. This may be unilateral initially but eventually becomes generalized in most. The child tries to mask the chorea with voluntary movements, which gives the appearance of restlessness.

Gradual improvement occurs over several months, and most young people recover completely. Rheumatic valvular heart disease develops in one-third of untreated cases.

The diagnosis is essentially clinical. The differential diagnosis includes drug-induced chorea and systemic lupus erythematosus, making measurement of lupus antinuclear antibody titers worthwhile. Antistreptolysin O titer is usually back to normal or only slightly raised by the time of presentation.

All children with Sydenham's chorea should be treated with high doses of penicillin for 10 days to eradicate active streptococcal infection and should continue with prophylactic penicillin until the age of 21. Pimozide usually controls the neurological symptoms without sedation. Alternatives are tetrabenazine, benzodiazepines, phenothiazines or haloperidol.

Chorea gravidarum. Chorea can complicate pregnancy. The likely explanation is that it may be the initial attack or recurrence of Sydenham's chorea or lupus erythematosus triggered by the pregnancy.[275]

Choreas associated with systemic lupus erythmatosus and hyperthyroidism.

Tumors. Although chorea is a rare presentation of tumors compared with seizures or a slowly evolving paresis, cerebral hemisphere tumors may be associated with any types of movement disorder.

DYSTONIA

Definition

Dystonia is an abnormal posture caused by the simultaneous contraction of agonist and antagonist muscles.

Differential diagnosis

Dystonia may be focal, affecting a single body part, segmental affecting contiguous parts, hemidystonia, affecting one side or generalized, affecting both sides of the body. The differential diagnosis of dystonia is listed in Table 20.19; other conditions associated with abnormal postures are listed in Table 20.20.

Specific syndromes

Focal dystonias

Benign paroxysmal torticollis. This is a self-limiting, benign condition that starts in the first year of life with repeated attacks of sickness, apparent discomfort and tilting of the head to one side and often associated with eye deviation to the same side. This may be repetitive. The affected side may change from one to another. Occasionally the trunk might incline to the same side and this may be associated with a degree of ipsilateral stiffness. Ataxia is not

Table 20.19 Differential diagnosis of dystonia in children

Focal dystonias
Torticollis
Writer's cramp
Blepharospasm
Drug induced dystonia
Generalized dystonia present initially with focal dystonia
Drug reaction
Hemidystonia
Basal ganglia tumors
Cerebral tumors
Antiphospholipid syndrome
Dopa responsive dystonia
Glutaric aciduria type 1
Hallervorden–Spatz disease
Idiopathic generalized dystonia
Infantile bilateral striatal necrosis
Wilson's disease
Ceroid lipofuscinosis
Generalized symptomatic dystonias
Drug reaction
Post encephalitis/meningitis
Post traumatic
Cerebral palsy
Post stroke
Sandifer's syndrome

uncommon, especially later in the course of the disease. Shifting torticollis that occurs in attacks suggests the diagnosis. The combination of head tilt and nystagmus is termed spasmus nutans.

Although the initial presentation may suggest a posterior fossa tumor, the attacks rapidly subside leaving a normal child with no neurological abnormalities.

There is a well-recognized relation between this condition and migraine as with paroxysmal vertigo, and a family history of migraine may be relevant to the diagnosis.

Dystonia associated with hiatus hernia: Sandifer's syndrome. Hiatus hernia may be associated with sudden spastic opisthotonic extension of the head, neck and sometimes of the upper part of the trunk. The head may move from side to side with the upper trunk bent to one side. All manner of bizarre posturing predominantly of the upper torso and arms may be seen. These bouts usually cease during sleep and may increase during, or shortly after, feeding. Vomiting and other symptoms of the hernia may be obvious or occult.

The condition may be underdiagnosed or misdiagnosed as one of the idiopathic movement disorders leading to unnecessary treatment and intervention. The key is to consider the possibility and then treat the hernia and associated reflux as appropriate.

Generalized dystonias

Flexor dystonia is a feature of carbon monoxide poisoning, head injury and encephalitis. The affected child may lie curled up with marked flexor dystonia and complete akinesia. In less severe cases the child may be stooped, flexed at the elbows, knees and hips with the head bent forward. Classically, the arms are flexed and resist passive extension and the legs are flexed on the abdomen with the toes tending to claw. The asymmetrical tonic neck reflexes and progression reflexes are absent. It is not influenced by anxiety and does not disappear in sleep. Chorea and athetosis are not seen. L-DOPA will release the patient from the flexor rigidity.

Table 20.20 Conditions associated with abnormal posture

Dystonia
Myotonia
Spasticity
Neuromuscular conditions
Stiffman syndrome
Hysteria

Extensor dystonia occurs most commonly in children as the dystonic phase of cerebral palsy. It is not caused by a known neurotransmitter imbalance but may be seen as part of some of the very acute dystonic reactions described later as unwanted effects of certain neuroleptic drugs, in which case they are rapidly abolished by anticholinergics. Extensor dystonia corresponds to the physiological second stage of extension seen in normal child development between 6 weeks and 4 months after birth. In the abnormal or diseased state it is an obligatory exaggeration or caricature of this normal physiological developmental state. It is the hallmark of the cerebral palsies which follow kernicterus before choreoathetosis makes its appearance, of dystonia associated with prematurity or due to basal ganglia damage following perinatal asphyxia.

Juvenile parkinsonism. The clinical picture of tremor, bradykinesia and flexor rigidity has already been outlined. Parkinsonism is a form of dyskinesia rarely seen in children (Table 20.21).

Treatment of parkinsonism consists of L-DOPA combined with inhibition of the peripheral tissue breakdown by a specific carboxylase which increases the concentration of L-DOPA in the brain. This is often combined with an anticholinergic such as benzatropine. Surgery does not have a place in most of the cases of childhood parkinsonism.

Dopa-responsive dystonia. Dopa-responsive dystonia (DRD) is also known as hereditary progressive dystonia with diurnal variation (HPD) and Segawar's disease. The onset usually is between 2 to 9 years.

The striking feature of the disease is the fluctuation of dystonia in relation to the sleep-waking cycle. The child may be normal on waking, but after 30–60 min the dystonic movements start and increase with time. The response to low dose L-DOPA is dramatic, with restoration of normal mobility.

The initial presentation is with gait disturbance, difficulties walking and frequent falls. Dystonia usually affects one of the lower limbs and then spreads to others. Rarely it involves the truncal muscles.

Sometimes, the diurnal fluctuation might not be prominent, the family history may be absent and the response to L-DOPA may not be dramatic. It is essential to give the medication a full 3 months' trial. It is also very important to consider the diagnosis of a dopa-responsive dystonia in children with a symmetrical cerebral palsy where the investigations, including neuroimaging, are normal and there have been no antenatal/perinatal risk factors (such as prematurity in a child with a diplegia). It is particularly important to think of this possibility where the signs continue to evolve after the first 2 years or so, into later childhood.

Table 20.21 Causes of parkinsonism in children

1. Familial striatonigral degeneration of Hunt
2. Postencephalitic
3. Drug induced – haloperidol, reserpine, phenothiazine
4. Subacute sclerosing panencephalitis – measles
5. Batten's disease
6. Phenylketonuria – lack of tyrosine
7. Head injury, e.g. boxers
8. Lewy body idiopathic
9. Methyl-4-1,2,3,6-tetrahydropyridine (MPTP) toxicity
10. Manganese toxicity

In many children in this undoubtedly heterogeneous group, DRD is inherited as a dominant trait with low penetrance. The gene is mapped to chromosome 14 and codes for the enzyme GTP cyclohydrolase 1 which is involved in the synthesis of biopterin. Several different mutations are reported.

Treatment is with L-DOPA along with an inhibitor of peripheral catabolism. The required dose is usually small (50–250 mg/day). Considering the existence of atypical responses, higher doses up to (750 mg/day) may need to be tried. Table 20.22 shows other conditions which respond to L-DOPA. Some people have been treated now for 30 years or so with no reports of long term unwanted effects or signs of tolerance.

Dystonia musculorum deformans. Idiopathic torsion dystonia (ITD) is a severe dystonia that occurs in many of the diseases already described. The term is usually restricted, however, to unilateral torticollis extension of the leg, torsion of the trunk, extension and internal rotation of the arm (Fig. 20.21).

Although the condition can be seen in some cases of dyskinetic cerebral palsy and in some children with a relatively pure dyskinetic hemiplegia, there are two genetic forms, autosomal recessive and autosomal dominant. The former is more common in Ashkenazi Jews. A large proportion of the early onset dominant form have a coding sequence deletion in the GAG trinucleotide repeat in the DYT1 gene on chromosome 9q34. This offers a useful diagnostic test.[276] Treatment is with L-DOPA, anticholinergics, and benzodiazepines (Table 20.23).

A group of children with onset of a paroxysmal dystonia, which is better in the mornings and worse as the day wears on, has been described. Rest does not reduce the dystonia but rapid eye movement (REM) sleep results in alleviation for a short time. The condition may be associated with a severe generalized dystonia with brisk reflexes and extensor plantar responses and may progress to the point where the child cannot walk. The importance of this subgroup of dystonia musculorum deformans is that these children are extremely sensitive to L-DOPA and 25 or 50 mg of the drug together with a peripheral carboxylase inhibitor results in very dramatic improvement.

Wilson's disease. This is an important cause of dystonia and is discussed in Chapter 24.

Glutaric aciduria type 1. In this condition, episodes of crying, cyanosis, pallor, lethargy and hypotonia may commence early in the first year of life. From about 5 months onwards an acute onset with tachypnea, acidosis and stiffness following a minor infection is common. There may be associated seizures, suggesting a diagnosis of febrile convulsions, or encephalitis, in the first instance. The episodes tend to be repeated and dystonia and choreoathetosis, if not present initially, gradually appear. The caudate and putamen show a loss of nerve cells and gliosis. Organic acid analysis shows raised glutaric and betahydroxyglutaric acid excretion in most, but not all cases. Serum L-carnitine is usually reduced. Glutaryl CoA dehydrogenase assay in fibroblasts gives the definitive diagnosis. Treatment with a low lysine and tryptophan diet has been tried without dramatic clinical improvement.

Choreoathetosis can also be a symptom of other metabolic disorders such as D-glyceric acidemia and sulfite oxidase deficiency, underlining the importance of a full metabolic screen with appropriate specialist advice in this group of disorders.

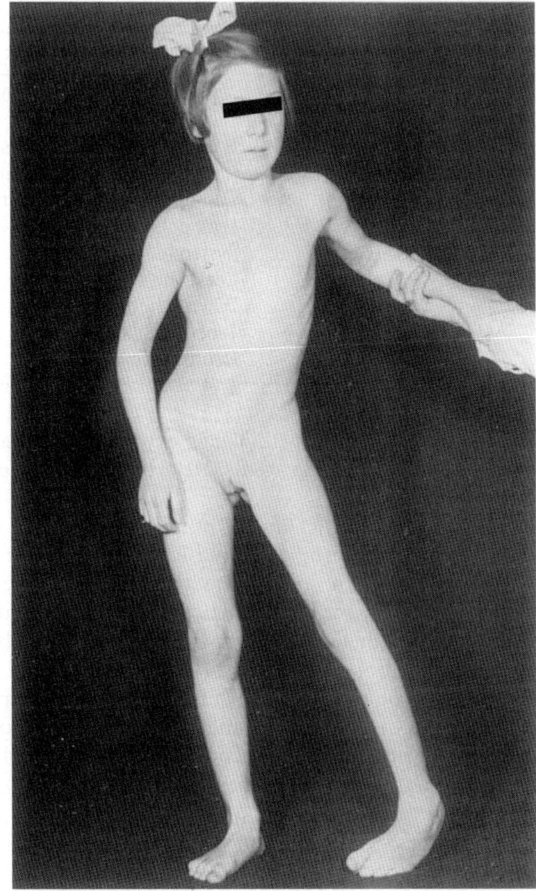

Fig. 20.21 Characteristic posture of the left lower limb in dystonia musculorum deformans. Mother and an uncle also suffered from the condition.

Dystonia with basal ganglia calcification. With the advent of modern imaging, basal ganglia calcification is a relatively common finding. There are many causes (Table 20.24) and the movement disorder may not be the initial or sole presentation.

Symptomatic generalized dystonia. Many diseases and disorders such as brain tumors, the effect of hypoxia, stroke, head injury and encephalitis may cause dystonia. The onset of dystonia may be during the acute illness or several years later.

Drug induced movement disorders

In pediatric practice, drug induced dyskinesias are usually idiosyncratic reactions or the result of toxicity and not related to the principal pharmacological action of the specific causative drug. Drug induced dyskinesias are particularly likely with major tranquilizers (phenothiazines and butyrophenones) and the newer antipsychotic agents, which may cause parkinsonism, tardive dyskinesia and acute dystonic reactions, the latter presenting as opisthotonos and

Table 20.22 Movement disorders which may respond to L-DOPA

Dopa-responsive dystonia
Striatonegral degeneration*
Pallidopyramidal syndrome*
Juvenile idiopathic parkinsonism
Parkinsonism secondary to hydrocephalus*

* Not all the cases, but worth trying.

Table 20.23 Treatment of idiopathic torsion dystonia

Levodopa/cabidopa
Anticholinergics
Benzodiazepines (clonazepam, tetrabenazine)
Others (baclofen, carbamazepine)
Mixed treatments (e.g. anticholinergics + baclofen +/– pimozide and/or tetrabenazine and/or haloperidol)

Table 20.24 Causes of basal ganglia calcification

Endocrine	Congenital and metabolic disease	Infection	Neoplasms
Hypoparathyroidism Pseudo hypoparathyroidism Pseudopseudo hypoparathyroidism Hyperparathyroidism Hypothyroidism	Mitochondrial encephalopathies Leigh's encephalopathy Hallervorden–Spatz disease Chronic methemoglobinemia Carbon monoxide poisoning Lead poisoning Systemic lupus Cockayne's syndrome Down syndrome Tuberous sclerosis Neurofibromatosis	Toxoplasmosis Subacute sclerosing panencephalitis Cytomegalovirus infection Congenital rubella AIDS	Craniopharyngioma Optic nerve glioma Radiotherapy Methotrexate therapy for leukemia

oculogyric crises. Treatment is with diphenylhydramine (2 mg/kg), tetrabenazine or anticholinergic agents. Metaclopramide can cause an identical clinical picture.

Opisthotonos, muscular rigidity and other extrapyramidal signs association with hypothermia, decreased consciousness and autonomic disturbance occur in the neuroleptic malignant syndrome precipitated by certain inhalational anesthetic agents.

Stimulants (e.g. methylphenidate) cause motor tics and chorea and are a cause of Tourette-like disorder (see below).

The selective serotonin reuptake inhibitors (SSRIs), used in pediatric practice for depression and obsessive–compulsive disorder, may produce a hyperkinetic movement disorder with myoclonus and tremor as part of the serotoninenergic toxic syndrome.

MYOCLONUS

Myoclonus is a brief, sudden, involuntary, shock-like muscle contraction arising from the central nervous system. It is usually associated with co-contraction of agonist muscles. A distinction of practical clinical importance is epileptic versus non-epileptic myoclonus. Both types may be focal or generalized and repetitive or non-repetitive. Further division into rhythmic myoclonus (of brainstem or spinal origin) and arrhythmic myoclonus (cortical or subcortical in origin and due to lack of inhibition) is useful clinically.[277]

Epileptic myoclonus occurs in many different epilepsies. It is a prominent feature of some idiopathic generalized epilepsies, e.g. juvenile myoclonic epilepsy, of the symptomatic and probably symptomatic encephalopathies of the infant and preschool child and is a prominent feature of the epilepsies associated with inherited metabolic disorders, e.g. mitochondrial disorders.

Benign myoclonus of early infancy very closely resembles infantile spasms but is non-epileptic. The infant is not encephalopathic and the EEG is normal.[278]

In benign neonatal sleep myoclonus focal or generalized myoclonic jerks occur in slow wave sleep. It is a common condition and myoclonus may be very frequent. Anticonvulsants are often prescribed inappropriately. Myoclonus does not occur in wakefulness and may be present for some months beyond the neonatal period into infancy. There may be a family history of the condition.[279]

Essential myoclonus is an extrapyramidal disorder of dominant inheritance and is non-progressive. Myoclonus is worse on movement. EEG is normal, intellectual impairment absent and the condition is not progressive.

Myoclonus is a feature of a wide range of serious neurological disorders. Metabolic disorders in which myoclonus is a feature include aminoacidopathies (hyperglycinemia, phenylketonuria and maple syrup urine disease), sialidosis – cherry red spot myoclonus, Unverricht–Lundborg disease, mitochondrial cytopathies, the late infantile neuronal ceroid lipofuscinoses, Menkes' disease, sphingolipidoses and Wilson's disease.

A curious form of upper limb myoclonus is seen in slow virus infections, including subacute sclerosing panencephalitis in which the myoclonus is 'hung up', i.e. sudden contraction of muscles followed by delayed relaxation.

Symptomatic myoclonus may occur in conditions characterized by brain malformations, such as Aicardi syndrome, tuberous sclerosis and Sturge–Weber syndrome.

When myoclonus is symptomatic it is never the only neurological symptom, but it may be the only symptom at presentation and for a time thereafter. Symptomatic myoclonus may arise from pathology at any level of the neuroaxis and is the result of hyperexcitability (or lack of suppression) of gray matter in the cortex, basal ganglia, brainstem and spinal cord. Cortical myoclonus, in which there is increased cortical excitability with giant sensory and action potentials results from localized brain lesions, e.g. space-occupying lesions of the sensorimotor cortex, or, more frequently, is of multifocal origin following cerebral hypoxia.[280] In the latter situation, the myoclonus may be generalized or focal.

In celiac disease the syndrome of progressive myoclonic ataxia is seen. This is not responsive to a gluten free diet and an autoimmune etiology has been suggested.

An autoimmune etiology has also been proposed in the opsoclonus–myoclonus (dancing eye) syndrome. This serious disorder presents in the infant or toddler with irritability, loss of skills, generalized myoclonus, ataxia and chaotic eye movements (opsoclonus). The condition has a postinfectious etiology in around 50% of cases but an association with neural crest tumors, particularly neuroblastomas is recognized. The pathophysiology involves binding of specific autoantibodies to the Purkinje cells of the cerebellum. Steroids and intravenous immunoglobulins are effective treatments but the course is often relapsing and half of those affected have persisting neurodevelopmental impairments.[281]

Spinal myoclonus is segmental or involves multiple spinal segments. Segmental myoclonus is usually symptomatic of a structural cord lesion.

Treatment of symptomatic, non-epileptic myoclonus is of the underlying cause. Piracetam, clonazepam and valproate may be helpful but pharmacological treatment of symptomatic myoclonus is often disappointing.

TICS AND TOURETTE SYNDROME

Tics are involuntary, purposeless contractions of functionally related groups of skeletal muscles. They are brief, repetitive, stereotyped, non-rhythmic movements or vocalizations. Motor tics persist in sleep (which is unusual in movement disorders).

Transient tic disorder is common. Estimates vary from 5 to 25% of all children at some time in childhood.[282] Most people have some stereotyped movement that they pursue when tired, bored or stressed. A ride on a bus, a glance around a lecture or committee meeting will reveal an array of hair twiddlers, nail biters or pickers, finger drummers or foot tappers. Most people keep these idiosyncrasies throughout their lives, with periods in which the habit is more or less obvious. The adoption in some diagnostic classifications such as DSM-IV of a fixed time course in some of its definitions (see Table 20.25) is therefore problematic.[283]

Those who have movements above the shoulders often get taken to doctors as they are less likely to be accepted in social settings. It is rare to be presented with a finger tapper, much more commonly a blinker. Many children with tics persisting for more than 1 year have Tourette syndrome, which is increasingly recognized as having great variation in severity. Tourette syndrome is a chronic disorder characterized by multiple motor and at least one vocal tic waxing and waning but present for at least 1 year with onset most commonly between 4 and 11 years of age. It is no longer regarded as rare – the prevalence is 1: 2000 and the male to female ratio 4 : 1.[284]

Simple tics presenting to doctors usually involve the face or shoulders – blinking, stretching facial muscles, head flicking, shoulder shrugging, etc. More complex tics include forced touching, sniffing, or licking and there is a close association with obsessive–compulsive disorder (OCD). Premonitory sensory sensations preceding the tics are common. Tics can be voluntarily suppressed for a short time but this is distressing if continued. 'Sensory tics' can occur alone.

Simple vocal tics include grunting, throat clearing, coughing, barking and complex vocal tics include echolalia phrases. Coprolalia (obscene words), though well known, is rare, occurring in less than 10% of cases.

Although tics are the most common clinical manifestation of Tourette syndrome, it is often the associated psychopathology that produces most impairment. These include obsessive–compulsive disorder, attention-deficit-hyperactivity disorder (ADHD), depression, anxiety and specific learning difficulties, particularly dyscalculia. There is often a strong family history of tic disorder or psychopathology with OCD being particularly common.

As with most tic disorders people with Tourette syndrome have a life-long tendency to the disorder with good spells and bad spells and often an exacerbation during adolescence.

Treatment is multi disciplinary. It is important to support the family and the child in education. Occasionally behavioral treatments for tics and obsessive–compulsive symptoms may be helpful. Neuroleptics, sulpiride and haloperidol are highly effective. Tranidine is useful for treatment of ADHD. Drug holidays are indicated and families must be warned about the rare but serious occurrence of tardive dyskinesia with chronic neuroleptic use.

A Tourette-like disorder with tics, but without the psychopathology of Tourette syndrome, may occur secondary to acquired brain injury, such as following head injuries. Pediatric autoimmune neuropsychiatric disorder associated with streptococcal infection (PANDAS) is of interest in that in a significant number of children with Tourette syndrome group A streptococcal infection is associated with antibodies that crossreact with putaminal neurones. Some children in whom traditional pharmacotherapy treatment has failed have responded to steroids or immunomodifying therapy.[285]

TREMOR

Tremor is a continuous rhythmic and involuntary movement disorder of a body part and results in alternating contractions of agonist and antagonistic muscles.

A clinically useful classification is tremor at rest, tremor on maintenance of a posture (postural tremor) and action tremor, i.e. tremor occurring on performance of a voluntary activity. It must be noted that action tremor is not synonymous with the intention tremor of cerebellar disease. Intention tremor is one type of action tremor and is characterized by accentuation of tremor just before the target is reached on finger/nose testing. At its most extreme the oscillations in terminal intention tremor as seen in Wilson's disease, may be so violent that there is a risk of self-injury. A similar gross intention tremor can be seen after traumatic brain injury.

Resting tremor is not common in pediatric practice. Causes include Wilson's disease, juvenile Parkinson's disease and neuroleptic drugs.

Postural tremor is tested by asking the child to stand with arms outstretched or to hold arms abducted and flexed at the elbows, with the hands brought to the mid line and the fingers of one hand almost, but not quite touching the fingers of the other hand. The commonest cause of postural tremor is physiological tremor.

Familial essential tremor is often of dominant inheritance and both postural and action tremor are present. Whilst there is a danger of overdiagnosis of essential tremor (particular care is necessary if family history is negative), most high frequency low amplitude tremors are physiological. If an essential tremor is widespread, the legs may be involved, and titubation, producing head nodding, may be present. Shuddering attacks in infants are an early manifestation.[286] Essential tremor may worsen during childhood. Treatment should be

Table 20.25 DSM-IV criteria for tic disorders*

Common criteria
The tics occur many times a day (usually in bouts) nearly every day
The disturbance causes marked distress or significant impairment in social, occupational or other important areas of functioning
Onset is before age 18 years
The disturbance is not due to the direct physiological effects of a substance or a general medical condition
Tourette syndrome
Both multiple motor and one or more vocal *tics* have been present at some time during the illness, although not necessarily concurrently, throughout a period of more than 1 year, and during this period there was never a tic-free period of more than 3 consecutive months
Chronic tic disorder
Single or multiple motor or vocal tics, but not both, have been present at some time during the illness throughout a period of more than 1 year, and during this period there was never a tic-free period of more than 3 consecutive months.
Transient tic disorder
Single or multiple motor and/or vocal tics for at least 4 weeks but not longer than 12 consecutive months
Tic disorder not otherwise specified
Cases that do not meet the criteria for a specific tic disorder.

*Adapted from APA.[283]

considered if writing is seriously impaired. Propranolol and primidone may help but unwanted effects limit usefulness.

Symptomatic causes of tremor include traumatic brain injury (tremor may become evident in the first year post injury and subsides spontaneously in 50% of cases), juvenile Parkinson's disease, severe malnutrition with cobalamin deficiency, Wilson's disease, hepatic encepalopathy, as a drug side-effect (e.g. sodium valproate), in juvenile multiple sclerosis, galactosemia, hereditary and acquired ataxias, Hartnup disease, hereditary fructose intolerance, thalamic tumor, vascular accidents involving the thalamus and internal capsule, spinal muscular atrophies and occasionally in hereditary motor and sensory neuropathies. Treatment is of the underlying cause.

NYSTAGMUS

Nystagmus is a tremor of the eyes, which may involve rhythmical conjugate oscillatory movement in any plane. It usually involves an initiating component and a fast correcting component. Clinically, different patterns of movement may be recognized. In pendular nystagmus the oscillations are slow in each direction with the eyes in a neutral position but on lateral gaze they may show a jerky quality. Jerk nystagmus indicates a slow phase in one direction followed by a fast corrective jerk in the other. It is the direction of the fast component that conventionally defines the direction of the nystagmus. When gaze is in the direction of the fast phase the intensity of the nystagmus increases.

Nystagmus should be differentiated from the roving eye movements of a blind child or one with significantly reduced acuity, particularly in the first 2 years of life. Opsoclonus involves very fast saccadic eye movement in all directions occurring in sudden bursts. It is associated with the dancing eye syndrome and its underlying causes, notably neuroblastoma. Ocular bobbing and dipping involve downward movement of the eyes with corrective movement to the mid-position. They indicate brainstem dysfunction often seen in comatose children. Oculomotor dyspraxia, commonly associated with ataxia telangiectasia, involves difficulty with horizontal saccadic eye movement. The eyes are often left behind the position of the head, later to be restituted with a characteristic flick of the head.

The most common cause of jerk nystagmus is gaze-evoked nystagmus reflecting dysfunction of the posterior fossa centers responsible for holding the eyes in an eccentric position. Vestibular nystagmus is also a jerk nystagmus resulting from involvement of the vestibular end-organ or its central pathways and nuclei.

Congenital nystagmus may be sensory, due to low acuity, or motor, due to a defect in the slow eye movement system. It is usually evident from birth and dominant, recessive and X-linked inheritance is described. It is usually horizontal (even on upgaze) but may be vertical or rotary. Pendular nystagmus is almost never acquired. Congenital nystagmus is abolished by sleep and increased by attempts at fixation. Up to 8.0% of children may have associated head bobbing.

ATAXIA

Definition and types

Ataxia is incoordination of movement not due to weakness, involuntary movements or abnormal muscle tone and is the major clinical sign of cerebellar disease. Sensory ataxia results when there is impaired afferent input into the cerebellum via the spinocerebellar pathways.

The three types of ataxia resulting from cerebellar disease are gait, truncal and limb and each has anatomical localizing value. Gait and truncal ataxia are due to lesions of the vermis or brainstem cerebellar connections; limb ataxia results from ipsilateral cerebellar hemisphere lesions. The causes are summarized in Table 20.26.

Examination

An infant is best examined on the parent's knee and encouraged to reach out with each hand. Intention tremor is distinctive, of maximum amplitude at the beginning and end of the range of movement and is irregular. Dysmetria is error in the estimation of the amplitude of movement.

In the older infant a delay in gaining independent walking, having cruised at a normal age, may be the first manifestation of gait ataxia. A child with truncal ataxia will not sit without supporting himself or is easily knocked off balance when sitting.

It is important when using the finger/nose test to ensure maximum range of movement, by ensuring that the child's arm is not held adducted against his trunk and that the child's arm is fully extended during finger/nose testing.

A child with gait ataxia stands and walks with feet widely apart and cannot place one foot directly in front of the other (tandem walking). This is best demonstrated to the child. Most 5-year-old children can tandem walk easily, when shown what to do by the examiner.

Rapid alternating movements (dysdiadochokinesis) are tested by rapid pronation and supination of the forearm.

Every ataxic child should have careful fundal examination for papilledema, plotting of head circumference and, in the infant,

Table 20.26 Selected causes of ataxia in childhood

Progressive/inherited
Friedreich's ataxia
Ataxia telangiectasia
Spinocerebellar degeneration (SCA)/olivopontocerebellar ataxias
Cockayne syndrome
Pelizaeus–Merzbacher disease
Ramsay Hunt syndrome
Metabolic
Any cause of fat malabsorption
Abetalipoproteinemia
Vitamin E deficiency
Mitochondrial cytopathies
Refsum disease
Sialidosis
Neuronal ceroid lipofuscinosis (late infantile)
Biotinidase deficiency
Metachromatic leukodystrophy
Organic acidemias
Urea cycle disorders
Acute/subacute
Acute cerebellar ataxia
Posterior fossa tumor/space occupying lesion
Acute disseminated encephalomyelitis
Miller-Fisher syndrome
Postinfectious polyneuropathy
Acute labyrinthitis
Hydrocephalus
Traumatic brain injury
Toxic/poisoning
Non-convulsive status
Non-progressive
Ataxic cerebral palsy
Congenital cerebellar abnormalities
As part of a complex syndrome
Dandy–Walker
Joubert
Angelman
Chiari malformation
Basilar impression

assessment of fontanel pressure, as posterior fossa space occupying lesions often present with ataxia.

Other signs of cerebellar dysfunction commonly seen in ataxia are jerk nystagmus, hypotonia and diminished reflexes.

Causes of ataxia

Ataxia is always of significance and requires full investigation. It is rare for a definitive diagnosis not to be made.

Tumors

Infratentorial tumors. Infratentorial tumors often involve the cerebellar vermis producing gait ataxia. Any unsteady child with headache or sleepiness must be assumed to have a posterior fossa tumor. There may be no long tract signs. The commonest tumors are medulloblastoma/primitive neuroectodermal tumors, which produce obstructive hydrocephalus with headache, vomiting and ataxia. Cerebellar hemisphere astrocytomas do not usually produce obstructive hydrocephalus, are indolent, of good prognosis and produce ipsilateral ataxia. Diffuse astrocytomas also occur. Ependymomas produce fourth ventricle obstruction.

Intrinsic brainstem tumors. These present with gait and truncal ataxia, with cranial nerve dysfunction and long tract signs. Cranial nerve dysfunction is often evidenced by dysphagia, lower motor neurone facial palsy and gaze palsy or nystagmus. The duration of ataxia before diagnosis may be as short as a few weeks and a mistaken diagnosis of acute cerebellar ataxia may be made if specific signs, particularly lower motor neurone cranial nerve dysfunction, are not sought.

Cranial MRI is almost invariably abnormal though CT may be normal. Cranial MRI shows an intrinsic brainstem lesion, a cystic mass or an exophytic lesion. Histological diagnosis is difficult because of the site of tumor and danger of brainstem swelling with biopsy. Biopsy is now no longer usually performed in typical cases. Prognosis is generally poor, with death within 2 years, but a small number are long-term survivors with only very slow progression.

Acute ataxias

The commonest neurological causes of acute ataxia are infectious or postinfectious.

Acute cerebellar ataxia often follows a viral infection, commonly varicella. It is most common in children under the age of 4 years. It often presents with the child suddenly stopping walking. He may revert to crawling and ataxia may be difficult to demonstrate. The infant is not weak and reflexes are present, although they may be depressed. There is no cranial nerve involvement other than nystagmus (in 50% of cases). However, the child may be dysarthric. Differential diagnosis includes posterior fossa or brainstem tumor and if cranial MRI is available it should be done. CSF is usually normal. It is particularly important to note that CSF protein is normal early in the course of the condition. The importance of this finding is that CSF protein is usually elevated in postinfectious polyneuropathy, which may present as gait ataxia. The child with acute postinfectious cerebellar ataxia is not encephalopathic and not distressed (pain is an important early feature of postinfectious polyneuropathy). Recovery is rapid (weeks) but occasionally takes months and in a very small number of children ataxia persists.

A rare type of postinfectious polyneuropathy is the Miller–Fisher syndrome, which presents with an acute cerebellar ataxia, ophthalmoplegia and areflexia but with no weakness. CSF protein is elevated and serum antibodies against ganglioside CQ1B may be found. Antibodies against this ganglioside recognize epitopes from *Campylobacter jejuni* indicating crossreactivity. Urgent MRI is indicated by the combination of ophthalmoplegia and ataxia. The cause of ataxia in the Miller–Fisher syndrome is unknown. Recovery is over weeks and is usually complete. Intravenous immunoglobulins may help as in postinfectious polyneuropathy.

Many metabolic disorders include ataxia in their clinical phenotype. In females with X-linked ornithine transcarbamylase deficiency, ataxia (which is often of acute onset) and vomiting occur during metabolic decompensation. Ammonia is elevated. Other metabolic disorders presenting with acute ataxia include mitochondrial cytopathies, maple syrup urine disease and Hartnup disease. Ataxia is a feature of Batten's disease and metachromatic leukodystrophy. In these conditions ataxia is of subacute onset.

Distinguishing acute ataxia from acute labyrinthitis is difficult in a young child. The child with labyrinthitis is distressed, vomiting and does not have limb ataxia when encouraged to reach.

Acute ataxia as a result of poisoning or intoxication is caused by anticonvulsants (particularly carbamazepine and benzodiazepines), alcohol and thallium containing insecticides.

In non-convulsive status epilepticus, and the symptomatic and probably symptomatic age dependent epileptic encephalopathies ataxia, initially intermittent, may be the presenting feature with regression of speech and cognition.

Inherited ataxias

The inherited ataxias are of recessive, dominant or X-linked inheritance and many are triplet repeat diseases. The commonest is Friedreich's ataxia; the others are summarized in Table 20.27.

Friedreich's ataxia and other spinocerebellar degenerations

This has a prevalence of 1 : 48 000 and is a progressive disorder with most children having very severe physical disability by adulthood although survival to the fifth or sixth decade is possible.

Friedreich's ataxia is recessively inherited. The gene is mapped to 9q13 and codes for the protein frataxin, an 18 kb soluble mitochondrial protein with 210 amino acids. The GAA triplet repeat expansion produces frataxin deficiency with clinical severity related to the GAA expansion size. The protein function is unknown. Truncal ataxia is the first symptom, with onset as young as 2 years, followed by dysarthria, limb ataxia and evolving kyphoscoliosis. Findings include nystagmus, pes cavus, distal weakness, posterior column dysfunction, areflexia and extensor plantars.

All children require cardiological assessment and review. Hypertrophic cardiomyopathy and ECG abnormalities (T wave abnormalities and heart block) are found. Diabetes and impaired color vision also occur. Friedreich's ataxia is relentlessly progressive and there is no specific medical treatment of proven benefit. However, much can be done to help the child and family by rehabilitative management ensuring access to education, independent mobility (often with a powered chair) and help with activities of daily living.

Diagnosis is by determining the number of GAA repeats in a child with progressive ataxia.

All of the inherited spinocerebellar ataxias have varying degrees of pyramidal and extrapyramidal involvement. There are 10 autosomal dominant hereditary ataxias (spinocerebellar ataxias, SCAs) separated by genotype. Most are triplet repeat diseases.[287]

Ataxia telangiectasia

The second commonest cause of progressive ataxia in childhood is ataxia telangiectasia which is discussed elsewhere in this chapter (pp 917).

Table 20.27 The spinocerebellar ataxias: genotypes and main clinical features

Name	Gene locus	Autosomal inheritance	Triplet repeat	Anticipation	Chorea	Dementia	Sensory loss	Retinal degeneration
SCA-1	6p23	AD	CAG	P			+	
SCA-2	12q23	AD	CAG	P	+	+		
SCA-3/MJD	14q32.1	AD	CAG	P			+	
SCA-4	16q24	AD	?	?			+	
SCA-5	11cent	AD	?	M				
SCA-6	19p13	AD	CAG	P			+	
SCA-7	3p12-13	AD	CAG	P			+	+
DRPLA	12p12	AD	CAG	P	+	+		
SCA-?9	13q21	AD	CTG	M			+	
SCA-10	22q13	AD	?	?		+		
SCA-11	15q14-21	AD	?	?		+		
SCA-12	–	AD	CAG	?				
Friedreich	20 9q13	AR	GAA	–			+	
A VED	8q13	AR		–			+	
ABLP	4q22-24	AR		–			+	+
SCA-8/ IOSCA	10q24	AR	?	–	+			+

All show cerebellar ataxia
P, with paternal transmission; M, with maternal transmission
?: Not yet identified
IOSCA, Infant onset spinocerebellar ataxia; MJD, Machado-Joseph disease
AD, autosomal dominant; AR, autosomal recessive
After Morrison.[287]

Inherited vitamin E deficiency

Any chronic disorder causing intestinal fat malabsorption may result in vitamin E deficiency and hence features of spinocerebellar degeneration. Vitamin E deficiencies, due to abetalipoproteinemia and familial vitamin E deficiency, are recessive ataxias. The importance of the latter is that the phenotype is of Friedreich's ataxia though cardiomyopathy is rare. In hereditary vitamin E deficiency the gene is located on 8q13 and codes for alpha tocopherol transfer protein. Large doses of vitamin E can halt progression and occasionally improve neurological function.

NON-PROGRESSIVE ATAXIAS AND ATAXIC CEREBRAL PALSY

Congenital non-progressive ataxia is synonymous with ataxic cerebral palsy and many non-progressive ataxias of early onset, particularly if associated with learning difficulties, are inherited. Even if there is a history of intrapartum asphyxia, attributing ataxic cerebral palsy to this cause is likely to be wrong and there may be recurrence in future children. Inheritance is usually recessive, occasionally dominant. All such children should undergo MRI scanning, which often shows congenital cerebellar abnormalities, such as vermian or generalized cerebellar hypoplasia.

In ataxic diplegia there are components of both ataxia and spastic cerebral palsy. The causes are similar to spastic diplegia and both are associated with prematurity. In addition it is a characteristic feature of 'neglected' hydrocephalus. Inherited forms of ataxic diplegia occur.

SYNDROMES FEATURING ATAXIA

Children with Angelman syndrome have severe learning difficulties, a jerky ataxia (hence the former derogatory term 'happy puppet') and (usually) a submicroscopic deletion of maternally derived 15q11-q13.

Ataxia is found in Joubert's syndrome, Dandy–Walker cyst and Chiari malformation but in these cases ataxia is but one feature of a complex syndrome. Other causes of ataxia are summarized in Table 20.26.

THE CARBOHYDRATE-DEFICIENT GLYCOPROTEIN SYNDROMES

This group of disorders is dealt with in detail in Chapter 24. The diagnosis should be considered whenever ataxia is accompanied by a learning disability, epilepsy or dysmorphism. Transferrin isoelectric focusing is a useful diagnostic test but will not detect all cases.

CEREBRAL PALSY

INTRODUCTION

Despite immense changes in obstetric and pediatric practice since William Little[292] ascribed cerebral palsy to perinatal causes, and a major decline in neonatal death rate, the incidence of these disorders has remained relatively unchanged at about 2 : 1000 children for the last 40 years.[293,294] The widespread lay belief that cerebral palsy is likely to be the consequence of brain damage (asphyxia) at birth has led to extensive litigation. Yet this is only the case for a small minority (about 10%),[295,296] and most of these have suffered an unforeseen disaster rather than lack of care.[297] In an Oxford study comparing the relationship between quality of intrapartum care for 34 children with cerebral palsy compared with 377 controls[298] only 2.9% of the cerebral palsy cases were considered to have experienced suboptimal care in labor compared with 14.5% of controls. None of the cerebral palsy cases had received suboptimal quality of care in response to fetal distress compared with 1.4% of controls. A change in practice towards no-fault compensation and a care package for children with cerebral palsy has been proposed. This would have the advantage of relative speed and would obviate the need to prove negligence in a protracted medicolegal process. However the diagnosis of cerebral palsy in early childhood is difficult and often changes with time.

Children may go through periods of transient motor abnormalities and may outgrow cerebral palsy in the same way as the motor signs abate after head injuries and acquired brain diseases.[299] Other conditions may resemble cerebral palsy.[300] Brain magnetic resonance imaging is helpful in distinguishing genetic-metabolic from acquired causes of extrapyramidal cerebral palsy.[301] Premature infants may go through a period of stiffness around what would have been term (dystonia of prematurity) but only rarely does this persist. In a very large American cohort most children considered to have definite cerebral palsy at 1 year had outgrown it by 7 years and very few of those considered to have probable or possible cerebral palsy had abnormal motor signs by this age.[299] In a study conducted in 1975 of children considered to show symptomatic asphyxia only a quarter showed continuing motor signs in later childhood,[302] though there was an excess of children with learning difficulties.

Infants withstand 10 min of total intrapartum asphyxia without long-term consequences, but are very unlikely to survive more than 20 min of this. Of those who have suffered an intervening period of total asphyxia, the effects are variable. The typical outcome is one of dyskinetic cerebral palsy, with or without seizures but with relative intellectual sparing or normal intelligence. MRI scans show lesions in the basal ganglia and/or thalamus in most affected children.[303] Only with very prolonged subtotal intrapartum asphyxia is it likely that a child will suffer major learning difficulties[304,305] and only in association with severe cerebral palsy (as with sensorineural hearing loss). Children with known biomedical causes of learning disability can have low Apgar scores at birth without any asphyxia.[306] The combination of low tone and severe learning disability in a child of school age is likely to be the result of a constitutional disorder, not acquired intrapartum damage.

In court, much may be made of cardiotocographic abnormalities but this is an unsatisfactory technique for preventing symptomatic asphyxia.[307,308] The practice, during the last 40 years, of widespread continuous fetal heart monitoring has led to increased cesarean section rates, with associated maternal morbidity and mortality and no significant effect on perinatal morbidity or mortality,[309,310] though conflicting opinions have been expressed.[311] It has been of minimal benefit for low risk patients and its use in high risk patients has yet to be subjected to adequate evaluation. In the current medicolegal climate perhaps it never will be. If midwifery staffing is adequate, as it should be, intermittent fetal heart recording by Pinard stethoscope or hand held ultrasound monitors is competent practice. This would not detect total asphyxia due to placental separation during the second stage in a breech delivery but cesarean section is not an option in such circumstances and attempts at heroic emergency vaginal deliveries are likely to cause more harm than good. When staffing is inadequate there is a temptation to use cardiotocography as an electronic babysitter.

The greater number of premature infants who survive with cerebral palsy reflects a greater survival of such infants, most of whom survive in a healthy condition,[312] rather than an increased risk of cerebral palsy for such children. This justifies the enthusiasm for high quality neonatal care for premature infants. The changes in causes of cerebral palsy indicate a shift from the consequences of traumatic delivery of term infants many years ago to the higher proportion of very low birth weight survivors who would have died in time past. Overall the prevalence of cerebral palsy remains little changed.

The contribution of survivors of < 1500 g birth weight largely accounts for the proportion of children with cerebral palsy who have acquired it postnatally increasing to 18% in the Mersey region between 1966 and 1977.[313] The expected proportion is about 10%.[314,315] In three series from New York, Chicago and Western Australia, quoted by Stanley et al[316] CNS infection accounted for over 60% of 856 cases of postnatal cerebral palsy. It is hoped that the subsequent introduction of immunization against measles, mumps, rubella, *Haemophilus influenzae* and meningococcus C has reduced the risk of postnatal cerebral palsy. Other causes include accidental and non-accidental head injury, anoxia and cerebrovascular accidents.

DEFINITION

Cerebral palsy is a disorder of posture movement and tone due to a static encephalopathy acquired during brain growth in fetal life, infancy or early childhood. Though the brain disorder is unchanging, the effects are dynamic, as the brain matures, and the child's developmental capabilities extend.

CLASSIFICATION AND EPIDEMIOLOGY

Cerebral palsy syndromes are classified according to the type of motor disorder and the topographical distribution of the condition.[317–319] Spasticity was the commonest motor impairment, reported to be present in 85% of a West Swedish series of 328 children,[320] or about 1 : 500 children. Dyskinetic cerebral palsy was found in 8.5% and simple ataxia in 6.5%. This means that dyskinetic cerebral palsy occurs in about 1 : 5000 children and simple ataxia in 1 : 6500 children. An average general practitioner (GP) has 25 babies born into the practice per year and the average health visitor (HV) has a caseload of up to 100 new babies per year. So those providing generic services see newly born children with spastic cerebral palsy quite infrequently – a GP once in 20 years and a HV once in 5 years. Only one GP in six and one HV in two will ever have a child patient with dyskinetic cerebral palsy throughout a whole working life. One GP in eight and one HV in three will ever look after a child with simple ataxic cerebral palsy. An individual child may have both ataxia, affecting the whole body, and spasticity, mainly affecting the legs, for instance, or other combinations of signs. As the diagnosis of cerebral palsy is made by increasing suspicion over time, it is not easy for clinicians who have never seen the condition before.

The other way cerebral palsy is classified is by its taxonomic distribution. Thus hemiplegia describes cerebral palsy affecting one half of the body predominantly, the upper limb more than the lower limb, normally sparing the bulbar muscles. Quadriplegia, or tetraplegia affects all four limbs, upper limbs more than lower limbs. It is sometimes described as a double hemiplegia and is usually associated with a bulbar palsy. When all four limbs are affected, but the upper limbs are affected less than the legs, this is described as a diplegia. If the part of the body affected predominantly is the bulbar muscles, this is described as congenital suprabulbar paresis or Worster-Drought syndrome.[321] When specialists write to primary care colleagues they should not presume expertise in the condition. 'This child with a typical left hemiplegia' is not a helpful way to write. No two children with cerebral palsy are the same.

ETIOLOGY OF CEREBRAL PALSY

Cerebral palsies may arise from genetic causes,[322] developmental brain anomalies, e.g. bilateral perisylvian polymicrogyria in some children with congenital suprabulbar paresis,[323] aqueduct stenosis and Arnold–Chiari malformation of the cerebellum in children with ataxic diplegia, or from a host of acquired causes including intrauterine infection. In a study of 276 term infants with moderate or severe newborn encephalopathy and 564 controls, birth defects were found in 27.5% of the former but only 4.3% of the latter.[324]

Spastic diplegia is the commonest form of cerebral palsy. The children have four limb cerebral palsy, but the legs are more affected than the arms and bulbar involvement is relatively slight. A minority have ataxia also, mainly truncal (ataxic diplegia). Two-thirds of children affected are preterm, but almost always appropriate for gestational age. The characteristic pathology is periventricular leukomalacia (PVL), which occurs when the periventricular structures are particularly vulnerable to hypoperfusion (26–36 weeks' gestation), usually in utero.[325] Birth asphyxia is only recorded for a tenth of these children and is never the single risk factor.[326] Periventricular venous infarction may coexist with intraventricular hemorrhage in these children, sometimes leading to striking asymmetries of neurological findings in later childhood. In term diplegic infants, with no history of asphyxia, it is common to find periventricular myelin defects indicating early prenatal origin from the early third trimester.[327]

Hemiplegia is the commonest form of cerebral palsy in term infants and is second only to diplegia amongst preterms. The proportion of infants with hemiplegia born at term is about 80%.[328] Hemiplegia derives, usually, from prenatal circulatory disturbances during pregnancy, the commonest, affecting over a third, being periventricular leukomalacia (PVL) due to hypoperfusion of the brain early in the third trimester.[329] Cerebral maldevelopments and major cortical/subcortical lesions ('holes' in the brain) each account for about a sixth of cases. Though two-thirds of children with hemiplegia have unilateral lesions (rare in other types of cerebral palsy), one-third have bilateral lesions.[330] Conversely, children with unilateral lesions, even agenesis of a cerebral hemisphere, do not necessarily show a hemiplegia. The relationship between structural lesions demonstrated by imaging, both in infancy and later childhood, and neurological function is complex, reflecting the brain's capacity for plasticity in response to dysgenesis or damage.[331]

Spastic quadriplegia (tetraplegia) is a severe form of four limb cerebral palsy, arms more affected than legs, with bulbar palsy. All have severe or profound learning difficulties; up to 90% have epilepsy; bulbar palsy is often severe and about half have cortical blindness. Currently about a third to 40% were born preterm, including children who would not have survived in the past. Children with acquired spastic diplegia of prematurity almost always show evidence of PVL, whereas those with acquired spastic quadriplegia may show PVL, but more commonly show full-term-type border zone infarcts, bilateral basal ganglia/thalamic lesions, subcortical leukomalacia and multicystic encephalomalacia.[330] Severe PVL is characteristic of children whose gestational age at birth is between 25 and 32 weeks, whereas term babies tend to have mild PVL. Diplegia is of course the ascription when the legs are more affected than the arms. In quadriplegia the arms are more affected. Nonetheless despite this clinical difference and the different causation some studies and some doctors in their clinical notes include severely affected diplegic children in this quadriplegic category.

Dyskinetic cerebral palsy is a form of cerebral palsy where there is four limb involvement and bulbar palsy, with fluctuating tone and involuntary movements. Magnetic resonance imaging has helped our understanding of acquired dyskinetic cerebral palsy. Acute near-total intrapartum asphyxia for 10–20 min causes damage predominantly in the subcortical gray matter.[303]

It is prudent to test the blood of children with cerebral palsy for evidence of congenital rubella, toxoplasmosis or cytomegalovirus and to culture urine for rubella and cytomegalovirus, which may be excreted for 3–5 years. Serological tests for syphilis will have been part of the mother's antenatal care but this should be confirmed from the maternity records. A cause of cerebral palsy, particularly spastic cerebral palsy, which has emerged in recent years, is congenital infection with human immunodeficiency virus (HIV). This causes a low-grade chronic brain infection, which may not be evident on CT scan. The processes of brain development interact with, and partly overcome, the destructive effects of the encephalopathy so that the child appears to be developmentally delayed, but improving over the first 2 years. Signs of apparent cerebral palsy emerge, but the child may appear to progress up to a point – e.g. sitting and crawling – before regression sets in. Such children do not show signs of full AIDS with a sequence of major infections and bowel upsets. The first serious infection may be *Pneumocystis carinii* pneumonia. This is difficult to diagnose clinically though the chest X-ray is characteristic with a 'ground glass' appearance in the lung fields and a hypoplastic thymus. Opportunistic superinfection, with other organisms such as toxoplasma or cytomegalovirus, may occur and may cause an encephalopathy in their own right. The diagnosis is by detection of HIV antibody titers and characteristic CD4 : CD8 lymphocyte counts.

Herpes simplex infection can be picked up from the genital tract during birth, leading to a destructive encephalopathy, one consequence of which is a spastic quadriplegia, usually with cortical blindness and epilepsy. The acronym 'TORCH screen' is an aide-mémoire although toxoplasma, rubella and cytomegalovirus cause intrauterine infection whereas herpes simplex virus causes brain damage in an acute, usually obvious, illness after birth. Perhaps the H should now be for HIV.

One mechanism proposed for causing cerebral palsy is the effect of the vanishing twin.[332,333] The proposal is that twin-to-twin transfusion occurs in the first trimester in monochorionic twins through a vascular anastomosis. Following the death of one twin, thromboplastin-like material passes through the vascular connection into the survivor's circulation resulting in end organ damage (the embolic theory). Alternatively the survivor's blood may be shunted into the low-resistance vascular system of the dead fetus causing acute hypovolemia, ischemia and end-organ damage (the ischemic theory). A 'prevanishing twin' syndrome before sonographic detection of two gestational structures may be supported by chorionic villus sampling (CVS). Cytogenetic evidence for this syndrome has been found in 1 : 2000 singleton pregnancies undergoing CVS.[334] The combination of placental chimerism (rather than mosaicism) and unlike-sexed cell lines, including cells with a chromosome abnormality not found in the surviving fetus is suggestive of twin-to-twin tranfusion early in the first trimester in dichorionic twinning.

PREVENTION OF CEREBRAL PALSY

Stanley et al[335] reviewed causal pathways to the cerebral palsies: a new etiological model and also possibilities for the prevention of the cerebral palsies, i.e. social and medical factors. They quote Hill & Hill's[336] criteria suggesting a causal link should be:

- Strong: high relative risks or odds ratios
- Consistent: cohorts from different geographic populations/time periods show the same patterns of causal associations
- Specific: the disease occurs only following exposure to the putative cause and not to other exposures. The exposure is followed by one specific disease, rather than by many diseases
- Time sequence: the putative cause precedes the outcome
- Dose dependent, or with a biological gradient: the degree of association increases with increasing intensity of exposure
- Biological plausibility: a biologically plausible mechanism for the causal association exists
- Coherence of evidence: the proposed mechanism is consistent with current biological wisdom.

These, often called the Bradford Hill criteria, and the analytical methods to measure the associations, such as multivariate analyses, are largely based on *single and sufficient* or, less often, *multiple independent* causal models. Links between factors on a causal pathway operate in two ways:

1. Independent but their coincidence is necessary for the consequence, e.g. a Rh-ve mother has a Rh+ve partner hence the possibility of a Rh incompatible fetus
2. Cascade: A causes, or predisposes, to B, which causes or predisposes to C, e.g. a multiple pregnancy predisposes to premature delivery and higher risk for intracerebral hemorrhage

There are many interventions which could prevent cerebral palsy. These may be considered as follows:

- Proven: MMR vaccination, iodine supplementation in iodine deficient areas, anti-D for RH-ve women, reducing risk of methylmercury exposure, transfer of the very preterm infant in utero to a tertiary center, reducing embryos transferred in infertility treatments to three or less, fencing swimming pools, home support for socially disadvantaged parents
- Probable: early routine ultrasound, avoiding excessive alcohol intake in pregnancy, phototherapy for neonatal jaundice, vitamin K at birth to prevent brain hemorrhage, infant restraints in cars, child abuse prevention strategies, sudden infant death syndrome prevention strategies
- Possible: mode of delivery for very preterm births including breech presentations, zinc, folate or fish oil to prevent intrauterine growth retardation (IUGR), methods of detecting IUGR, operative delivery for fetal distress, amnioinfusion for umbilical cord compression, rescue therapy for birth asphyxia
- Doubtful: electronic fetal monitoring for fetal distress – addition of fetal scalp sampling or ECG, bedrest for growth restriction, hospitalization for multiple pregnancies, multifetal pregnancy reduction for high order multiples, antenatal indometacin or thyrotropin-releasing hormone.

In spite of the proven or probable interventions available, the rate of cerebral palsy remains steady. Such interventions might not be enough. We may not understand all the steps in a complex causal pathway. There may be social factors, which influence people's decisions, which affect the outcome – access to a telephone, care of other children, independent transport, for instance. The balance between death and cerebral palsy may be irreducible. Even if it were possible to prevent the occurrence of cerebral palsy in children who entered labor as healthy, but who showed signs of intrauterine asphyxia, to reduce by a quarter the 25% of cerebral palsy cases born preterm, and to prevent the 2% of cases secondary to intrauterine infection, the total reduction in cerebral palsy cases would not exceed 20%. The effect of such prevention might not be evident if the program of prevention enabled children who previously would have died before their cerebral palsy was identified, to survive and be diagnosed as having cerebral palsy.

CLINICAL FEATURES

Spastic diplegia

By the time diplegic children reach the age of 5 years or so they show spasticity in their legs more, or far more, than in their arms (Fig. 20.22). If the signs are restricted to the legs, investigation of the spinal cord for a paraplegia should be undertaken, even though there is known to be brain damage from intracerebral bleeding, ischemia, meningitis or other conditions in infancy. Such spinal lesions as diastematomyelia, neurenteric or dermoid cysts, myelodysplasia, neurofibromata or vascular infarction may be found. The signs in the diplegic child's arms vary from mild spasticity to manual dyspraxia or dyskinesia, which may have emerged when the child was 3 or 4 years old.

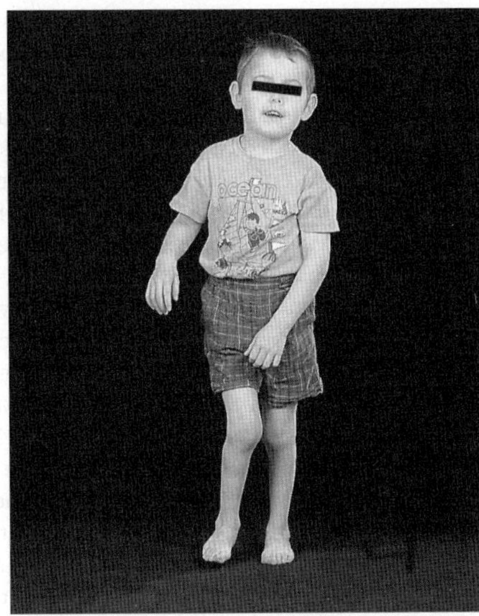

Fig. 20.22 Diplegic gait. Internal rotation with hip adduction.

Premature infants in the special care baby unit commonly show neurological abnormalities or ambiguities, which are hard to assess. They may show increased or decreased tone. Episodes are observed which may be seizures. The need for parenteral or nasojejunal feeding removes oral feeding behavior as an indicator of health. Ultrasound scans may show focal lesions of uncertain significance. Risk of cerebral palsy is known to be high for extremely low birth weight premature babies, though most premature babies grow up to be healthy children, free of neurological deficits. Parents and health professionals are bound to be concerned for each individual baby: 'is he/she going to be all right?' Unless the neonatal scans show advanced and extensive PVL or multicystic lesions or the child has had bacterial meningitis, which carries a high risk of morbidity, the answer is 'probably yes'. When this is, happily, borne out, the children and their families get on with their lives, free of medical or therapy appointments. When the child turns out to have cerebral palsy, the parents often say that they've been asking questions for months and the doctors haven't been giving them a straight answer.

Dystonia of prematurity is a form of extensor hypertonus emerging around 40 weeks' gestational age and reaching its peak by 4 months old. This causes much parental concern and makes affected children difficult to handle in the first 7 or 8 months. It is most marked when the infant is lying supine, with the neck extended, or when the child is suspended under the armpits. The arms become extended rigidly with internal rotation and fisting of the hands. The mouth may open widely, the legs become extended and stiff, the feet adopt an equinus posture with a spontaneous extension of the big toes and fanning of the other toes. Clonus is not seen. The back arches in extension, even opisthotonos, if the feet come in contact with a firm surface. When the head is turned to the side there is an obligatory asymmetrical neck reflex in the first few months. Attempting to position the child in a sitting position is unsuccessful, as the child remains stiff as a board. When the feet touch the floor, with the child suspended, rapid automatic walking is observed, with a degree of scissoring so that the feet tread on each other. The signs are most marked when the child is agitated, hungry, in discomfort or even at the beginning of feeding. However when the child is turned over into a prone position, especially when the neck is flexed, the child adopts a flexed posture. If a child has spastic cerebral palsy by this age, which is rare, posture does affect the degree of spasticity but turning the child into a prone position does not abolish spasticity or increased extensor tone.

Dystonia of prematurity, unless severe, resolves spontaneously in most children, leaving no persistent motor signs. While it is present, however, it is helpful for parents to be advised on handling and activities by a physiotherapist. In a small proportion of children the dystonia persists and may be a life-long condition. It is exceedingly difficult, if not impossible, to examine such children at 4–6 months and predict who is going to show complete resolution and who is going to have cerebral palsy. It is fair to offer physiotherapy advice to parents of all the children, explaining to parents that the problems may or may not resolve. In children who turn out to have spastic cerebral palsy, the dystonia merges into spasticity, after a period of mixed rigidity and spasticity in the legs. The dystonia in the neck, trunk, arms and hands resolves leading to a spurt in development, especially hand function. Sitting is late, but is achieved. Spasticity may first be noted at the ankles where clonus can be elicited. It soon becomes evident in the hip adductors and the hamstrings. In some children the spasticity is not demonstrable at rest and is only observed during exertion.

Spastic quadriplegia

The children with spastic quadriplegia have a high risk of associated learning disability and epilepsy (Fig. 20.23). They may be hypotonic in early infancy but spasticity emerges in the early months of life. There is a continuing need to find suitable positioning and seating. Gastrostomy feeding is often indicated. Standing frames give experience of upright position and promote stronger bone growth. Hydrotherapy is beneficial. However medication for spasticity in cerebral palsy is disappointing. It is rare for baclofen or diazepam to be beneficial in doses which are free of causing unacceptable levels of drowsiness or vomiting. Botulinum toxin, in experienced hands, has a place in prevention of fixed deformities.

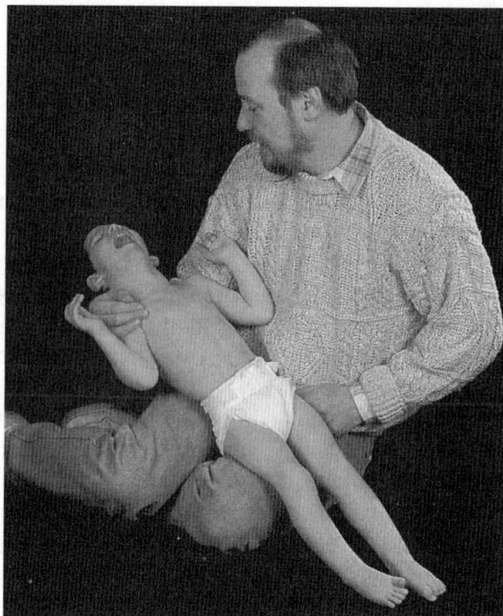

Fig. 20.23 Four limb cerebral palsy.

Ataxic cerebral palsy

In infancy, children who develop ataxic cerebral palsy show hypotonia and very delayed motor development (Fig. 20.24). Sitting is long delayed. Truncal ataxia predominates over limb dysmetria. Eventually they may cruise round furniture or walk with support for many months before walking independently. Even then they may be advised to use a walking aid. Hydrotherapy is much enjoyed by ataxic children.

ATAXIC DIPLEGIA

Children who grow up to demonstrate signs of ataxic diplegia do not go through a dystonic phase. On the contrary, they show very low tone in the trunk and limbs until signs of spasticity evolve, usually distally in their legs. Motor development is markedly delayed, usually more by the ataxia than the spasticity.

Autosomal recessive diplegia

Children who turn out to have genetic diplegias show normal tone in early infancy but begin to show signs of spasticity distally at about a year. It is important to remember that children who have a symmetrical diplegia or quadriplegia involving dystonia may have a dopa-responsive dystonia, especially where investigations are normal (see section on movement disorders).

Differential diagnosis: at first it may be difficult to know whether the tightness at the ankles indicates Duchenne muscular dystrophy, metachromatic leukodystrophy or some other progressive disorder. These conditions have to be distinguished from hereditary spastic paraplegias, some of which are autosomal dominant though autosomal recessive forms also occur associated with loci mapping to chromosome 8 (spg5), 15 (spg11) and 16 (spg7 which encodes for the protein paraplegin, apparently involved in mitochondrial function). In these disorders, which are of unknown pathogenesis, there is a progressive gait disturbance due to lower limb spasticity. They have hyperreflexia in their legs and extensor plantar responses. Ataxia, amyotrophy, neuropathy, extrapyramidal signs or pigmentation may be found also. In the dominant form there is an affected parent. In the recessive form more than one sibling is affected with or without parental consanguinity or there is an isolated patient with parental consanguinity.

Hemiplegia

Children present in the second half of the first year of life when pincer grasp, individual finger movements, bimanual activities and

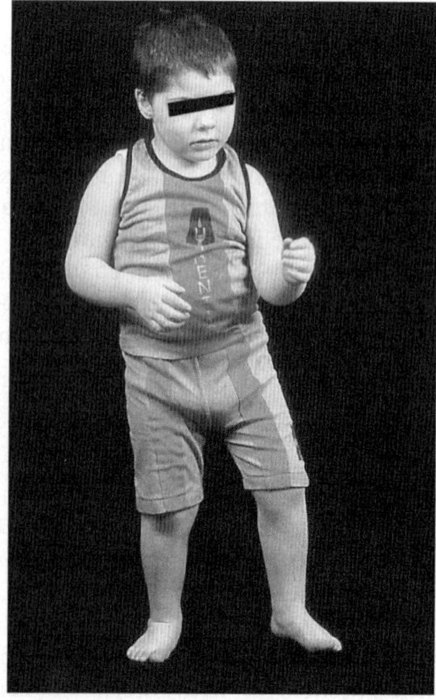

Fig. 20.24 Ataxic 3-year-old child showing broad based gait and elevated arms.

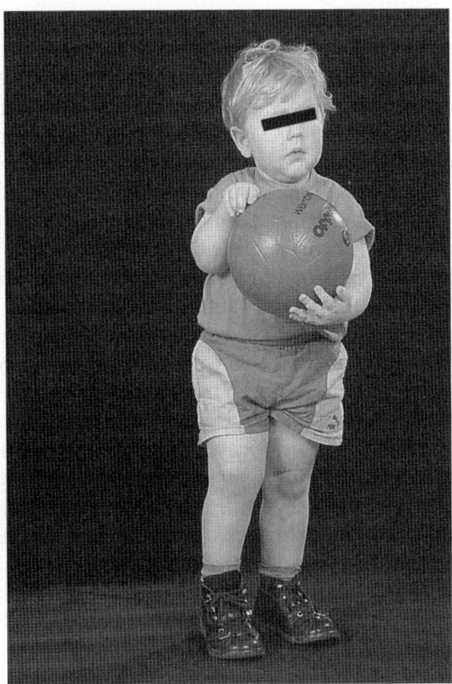

Fig. 20.25 Spastic hemiplegia, right-sided – hyperpronated right arm.

manipulation of objects are seen to be asymmetrical (Fig. 20.25). At first it may be attributed to the unaffected side being unusually dominant, an inappropriate conclusion so early in life. However it is evident that the affected hand tends to be fisted and there is poverty of movement in this arm and hand. If the child is able to sit unsupported, the lateral guarding reaction when the child is pushed to that side is absent or much less than on the unaffected side. The forward parachute reaction is asymmetrical. Hemiplegic children are a little late to pull to stand, to cruise around furniture and to walk independently, but not to a marked degree unless there is a comorbid global learning disability. A striking feature is that the child tends to go up on the toes of the affected foot. When walking begins, the heel tends to remain off the ground. As children grow older it is helpful to examine their outdoor shoes when they have been using them for some weeks. It is evident that there is a marked asymmetry with excessive wear at the toe and little or no wear at the heel compared with the unaffected side. As years pass there comes to be a clear asymmetry of growth between the limbs on the affected and unaffected sides, most evident in the hands and feet, in distinction from the symmetrical findings in children with acquired hemiplegia in later childhood.

Children with hemiplegia may have associated sensory loss on the affected side of the body and may also have a partial or complete hemianopia. As they grow older, some develop dyskinetic movements on the affected side. It may also become clear that there are mild signs of spasticity and increased reflexes on the supposedly unaffected side so that the condition is a markedly asymmetrical form of spastic quadriparesis. About a third of hemiplegic children have seizures and these are the first presentation in some of them. A surprising proportion of hemiplegic children have sufficient associated learning difficulties or other disabilities to attend special schools. In Salford, Manchester, in 1988, of 110 children with cerebral palsy, 27 had a hemiplegia of whom 17 attended special schools.[337]

Dyskinetic/dystonic cerebral palsy

Though pediatric neurologists with a regional practice will have a number of patients with dyskinetic/dystonic cerebral palsy, the condition arises infrequently in any local service, whether as a consequence of acute near-total intrapartum terminal asphyxia or as an autosomal recessive disorder (Fig. 20.26). About 1 : 7000 children is affected. Only one in ten primary care physicians (general practitioners) will ever have such a child born into his or her practice in a working lifetime. Though families may expect their doctors to know about the condition, it is only through close liaison with therapy and specialist neurology services that knowledge and confidence will grow.

In infancy the children seem hypotonic with poor conjugate use of their eyes to follow people or objects. They have impassive facies, do not learn to speak, and have major feeding difficulties. Hand function is of little or no functional benefit. Dystonic posturing may make the child hard to handle. Commonly these children show emotional lability and they are easily distressed. It is very difficult for such children to demonstrate their intelligence. The involuntary choreiform or athetoid movements do not appear till the second year or subsequently. Parents may be convinced of their child's intelligence yet the standardized developmental assessments of ability yield results suggesting very low function.

As these children grow up they need expert advice on seating, feeding and communication particularly.[338] Saddle seating may be more secure and more suitable than conventional seating. Gastrostomy feeding may be required, at least for a time. There are a number of Advisory Centers for Education around Britain to give advice on aids to communication for personal and educational purposes.[339] Expert advice on physiotherapy,[340,341] hydrotherapy, horse riding[342] and other forms of exercise should be sought. Medication may be considered, only to be rejected.[343] It is exceptional for a child to benefit from drug therapy. A conceptual framework for reviewing outcomes in developmental disabilities has been proposed[344] but more research is needed.[345] As school leaving age approaches, there should be a multidisciplinary approach to transition planning and a college with the appropriate expertise should be sought. Expert careers advice is invaluable and suitable recreational opportunities

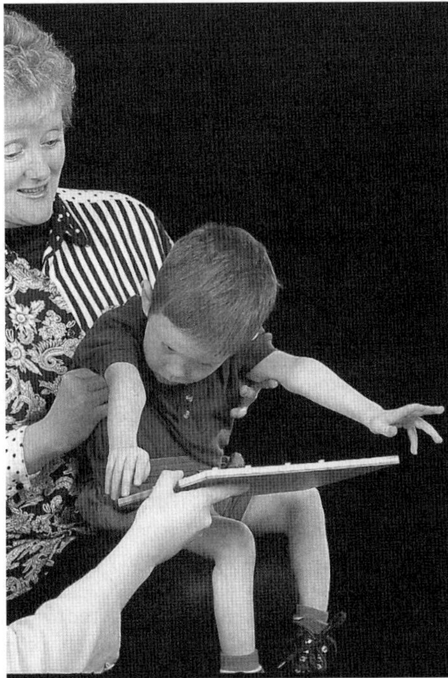

Fig. 20.26 A child with dyskinetic cerebral palsy, showing uncontrolled patterns of movement and flaccid trunk, whilst attempting to reach out.

should be investigated. There is justified concern for the decline in adult rehabilitation services over the past 30 years.[346,347]

Clinical progress

In early childhood the principal parental concern is to promote independent walking in children with diplegia or other forms of cerebral palsy.

MULTIDISCIPLINARY TEAMS AND CHILD DEVELOPMENT CENTERS

For parents of children with cerebral palsy, the discovery of the many associated potential problems can be daunting. There may be a multiplicity of appointments with different medical specialists, including dietitians, therapists, specialist nurses, orthoptists, audiometricians, medical social workers and diverse doctors. Co-ordination of investigation and treatment is best carried out through a child development team[348] based in a child development center[349,350] as recommended in the Court Report.[351] The nature of such teams and the facilities in these centers differ from place to place,[352] not least because of diversity of services from agencies other than health services. Making the services work in cooperation needs continuous attention as personnel and policies change frequently. These are among the keys to successful provision:

- Good coordination of health, education and social services
- Clear lines of communication between primary care and specialist health services
- Shared single set of case notes for hospital and community health services
- Access to necessary expertise including seating, communication aids, orthotics, prosthetics, clinical psychology, dental services, feeding team
- Medical specialist services: vision, hearing, epilepsy service, orthopedics, psychiatry, genetics
- Close links with voluntary organizations
- Parental choice at all times
- Parent-held records
- Children's needs are paramount.

ASSOCIATED HEALTH PROBLEMS IN CEREBRAL PALSY

Feeding problems due to bulbar palsy, handling and seating difficulties, involuntary movements or posture and tone problems are a common first presentation. The children are prone to oral hypersensitivity and to bite on whatever is put in their mouths. Parents can be taught to desensitize the child's mouth before feeds. The reverse may be the case and the child's mouth may need stimulation during feeds. There may be aspiration of food with consequent respiratory symptoms. When this is chronic, the chest develops an increased anteroposterior diameter. Gastroesophageal regurgitation may occur leading to postprandial dyspepsia (heartburn) and vomiting. These symptoms may provoke crying or reflex syncope. Food thickeners and barrier treatment such as Gaviscon can be used as well as an upright position after meals. They may drool saliva. If this is persistent, they may benefit from hyoscine skin patches behind the ear or between the scapulae or from oral glycopyrrolate. Surgery on salivary glands or salivary ducts is not very successful in the long term.

Gastrostomy will be considered for those children with an unsafe swallow or whose intake is insufficient for growth, reflected in a markedly delayed bone age. A multidisciplinary team makes the assessment and simpler management strategies will be tried first. Assessment for gastrostomy includes a videofluoroscopy, by an experienced radiologist, with the child's speech and language therapist in attendance. The procedure is seen as mutilating, so parents need careful preparation and support. However, their subsequent satisfaction is usually good, because they observe less coughing and choking in their children, medication can be given more reliably and feeding time is improved, allowing the parent to spend more time doing other things with the child including play, and with other children.[353] A dietitian will advise on the content of gastrostomy feeds. A common practice is to give a slow overnight infusion of feed by syringe pump, to reduce the volume that has to be given in the day. The cost–benefit of tube feeding has been questioned by Strauss et al[354] who demonstrated an increased mortality risk in tube-fed children (relative risk 2.1, with no increased risk in the most severely disabled children, but a doubled risk in those with less severe disabilities with increased risk of aspiration of vomit), but the lesson may be in the selection process and the appropriate use of fundoplication. There is a need for prospective studies[355] including comparison of the available gastrostomy tubes.

When reflux and vomiting are troublesome and persistent, and this can become more of a problem after gastrostomy, as feeding volume increases, *fundoplication* is considered. This is a major procedure and requires postoperative high dependency backup till breathing is safe. The procedure – wrapping part of the fundus of the stomach round the lower part of the esophagus – is not an exact science. Sometimes it turns out to be too tight and swallowing becomes difficult, as is burping air. Sometimes it turns out to be too slack and makes little difference. So re-operation may be required. When it works well it makes a great difference to reflux and vomiting. There is, however, a significant risk of complications with gastrostomy and fundoplication.[356,357]

Constipation is a risk in all children who are inactive and if this is allowed to persist there is a risk of acquired megacolon, a lot of colicky pain after meals and soiling with overflow. Sometimes constipation can build up when the child is unwell. Pushing frequent fluids is wise.

The mainstays of treatment are:

- Adequate, frequent fluid intake including fresh fruit juice especially during fever
- Varied, stimulating diet
- Communicative mealtimes – social occasions not just 'feeding time'
- Some pureed fruit and fiber in the diet but not too much as it packs the colon
- Exercise including hydrotherapy
- Relaxed but consistent toileting
- Lactulose as a stool softener morning and evening mixed with a cordial
- Senokot syrup in the morning

Prune juice and syrup of figs are effective but are used less than they used to be, probably because children don't like the tastes. There is a range of unstandardized herbal preparations of cascara, frangula, rhubarb, senna, aloes, colycynth and jalap which should be avoided in children because of their unpredictable laxative effects. Osmotic laxatives such as magnesium hydroxide (milk of/cream of magnesia) or magnesium sulfate (Epsom Salts, Andrews Liver Salts) can be used in older children.

Judicious short-term use of sodium picosulfate can help clear the bowel but is not appropriate in very young children.

Incontinence is persistent for children with severe cerebral palsy. It is also a problem, alongside enuresis, for many less severely affected children for longer than is seen in most children. Toileting routines should be attempted when the child is ready developmentally. Extra consideration is needed for time taken to go to the toilet, transfer from a wheelchair in some, unfastening and fastening clothes, for balancing on the toilet, with help from a rail if needed, and for wiping, which may be difficult. While parents and care staff will help young children, this is not appropriate from the onset of puberty when a toilet that washes, then dries, the youngster's bottom is a more dignified solution. For those who are not capable of a continence program there needs to be a regular supply of nappies of appropriate size.

Osteopenia is a risk in immobile children with cerebral palsy, with consequent increased risk of fractures. This is not due to abnormalities of vitamin D or parathyroid hormone.[359] While enabling children to spend part of each day in a standing frame and promoting physical activity, e.g. with hydrotherapy, is likely to promote improved bone density, use of bisphosphonates for 12–18 months has been shown to increase bone density by 20–40%, with no apparent adverse effects.

A third of the children have a *global learning disability*, which may be moderate or severe. It may be thought that this is also true of children with dyskinetic cerebral palsy because there is so little that they can do; their eye movements may be all over the place and communication is extremely difficult. Beware – some of these children are very intelligent but remain 'locked in' until technological means are found to enable them to control speech synthesizers, computers, environmental control systems and other technology. In the past, many such children and adults have languished, completely inappropriately, in provision for people with profound and multiple disabilities. A third of children have patchy or *specific learning difficulty*. The commonest specific difficulties are in language and communication, in visual perception or in mathematical tasks and calculation. There has been little reliable research into the communication difficulties of children with cerebral palsy[359–362] and the subject has been referred to only briefly in standard texts. Yule & Rutter[360] suggest that this is because few therapists work with children with physical disabilities. Careful attention to hearing testing is important, because there is a substantial risk of hearing impairment in children with cerebral palsy, either from associated sensorineural loss or from secretory otitis media, which is very common in children with eustachian tube dysfunction in bulbar palsy. There has been a good deal of attention to communication before speech and to means of augmented communication (signing and symbol systems, information technology, speech synthesizers for instance) among practitioners. Doctors rely on advice from their speech and language therapy colleagues throughout. It is wise to beware early judgments on the communication potential of children with choreoathetoid (dyskinetic) cerebral palsy. So often they turn out to be much more capable than first thought. Perceptual difficulty may make it difficult for children to tell the time from a conventional clock, to understand maps and diagrams or to find their way about, including difficulty in avoiding obstacles with their wheelchairs.

Hearing impairment is very common in children with cerebral palsy, usually from fluctuating loss with secretory otitis media, but sometimes from sensorineural loss, or a combination of the two. Grommets can produce dramatic short-term benefits but hearing aids may be the more effective long-term solution, combined with expert learning support services.

Visual impairment is common in children with cerebral palsy, more than half of whom have visual problems for several reasons.[363] The condition causing the cerebral palsy such as congenital cytomegalovirus, toxoplasmosis or rubella may also have caused a cataract, colobomas or retinal lesions including pigmentary retinopathy. Retinopathy of prematurity is amenable to control by laser therapy or cryotherapy, but skilled ophthalmic examination of preterm infants' eyes has been available in recent years. The eyes may be too small (microphthalmia) or too big (buphthalmos or congenital glaucoma). The child may be shortsighted or longsighted. Cortical visual defects are common.

Epilepsy is common in children with cerebral palsy, affecting about a third over all.[364] Hadjipanayis et al[365] reported a prevalence of epilepsy of 41.8% in 323 patients with cerebral palsy in Athens, Greece. However the rate varies between studies, as the type of cerebral palsy in children in each study is different. The risk of epilepsy varies from rare, in pure ataxic cerebral palsy, to very high (up to 94% in some series but 71% would be more typical) in children with spastic quadriplegia and severe learning disability.[365] The prevalence of epilepsy in spastic or ataxic diplegia is 16–27%, but only 3% in encephalopathy of low birth weight (Little's disease). In dystonic/dyskinetic cerebral palsy the prevalence is about a quarter and in hemiplegia between 30 and 50%.[365] Diagnosis of the condition is difficult enough in general[366,367] in children. This is more difficult in a child with cerebral palsy, who may have difficulty describing symptoms. It depends on careful observation and history taking while detection of side-effects requires constant vigilance. A child considered to have lost her sitting from a progressive undiagnosed degenerative ataxic disorder got better when her phenytoin was stopped. Another child with a cachectic state was considered to have a mysterious malignancy till his carbamazepine was stopped and he regained his weight. Vigabatrin is licensed for infants with infantile spasms, but up to 90% of them turn out to have severe learning difficulties. The finding of visual field defects in such children is difficult, though there is a program to attempt to do this. Sodium valproate can lead to considerable weight gain. As ever in epilepsy, the doctor, family and sometimes the affected child weigh costs versus benefits.

Psychiatric aspects

The commonest psychiatric reactions to having cerebral palsy are anxiety, depression and/or withdrawal. Other features include attention deficit hyperactivity disorder, tantrums, social naivety, passivity and autistic spectrum disorders which Nordin & Gillberg[368] found in 10.5% of children with cerebral palsy. The implications of the differences in neurobiological findings between children with cerebral palsy and those with learning disability or autism are not understood. Concentrations of neuropeptides and neurotrophins are raised in the blood of newborn infants who subsequently go on to develop severe learning disability and/or autism, but not in children with cerebral palsy.[369] Conversely altered secretion of androgens is a feature of children with cerebral palsy, but is not a feature of children with autism or learning disability.

Sleeping difficulties

It is very common for children with cerebral palsy to be difficult to settle at night, or to wake up unduly frequently during the night. For those with four limb involvement or with severe spasticity in the legs the lack of activity in the day does not leave them tired at night. They may benefit from melatonin, 2 mg half an hour before a bedtime routine. Some require a higher dose of 4 mg.[370] If this does not help, it is worth trying 6 mg daily for a month. Of the other night sedatives, among the most reliable is chloral hydrate elixir. Though it tastes strongly and needs to be mixed with a palatable disguise, it does not suppress dreaming sleep and can be omitted without causing withdrawal symptoms. Some children with cerebral palsy cannot turn in bed and become uncomfortable unless supplied with a sheepskin, a ripple mattress, special cushion or need to be turned in bed on a regular basis. Antihistamine analogs such as alimemazine tartrate (Vallergan) can help on a one-off basis, but they may have a paradoxical effect of exciting the child or provoking seizures.

TREATMENTS FOR CEREBRAL PALSY

Treatment of spasticity

Parents and carers may seek treatment for spasticity with expectations that exceed clinical possibilities. The most important starting point is an understanding of the limitations of all forms of treatment, alongside the usually moderate gains that can be made. A spastic diplegic gait will always be recognizable as such but improved function, efficiency and comfort are all worthwhile. A child will be well advised to walk a little, without rushing, in as good a gait as possible, rather than walk as far or as fast as possible. Unrealistic expectations will burden the child, as well as the physician, with a sense of failure.

Dynamic spastic tone can be modified by ankle–foot orthoses, serial casting with progressive dorsiflexion of the ankle, medication or surgical procedures. The balance to be struck is between useful relaxation on the one hand and undesirable weakness or constitutional side-effects on the other. Scoliosis may be contained by wearing bracing or jackets. Children with ataxic or dyskinetic cerebral palsy may feel more secure in Lycra splinting but this has little part to play for spasticity.

Fixed contractures may be released by orthopedic operations, but these must be carefully selected so that the child does not consequently suffer any deterioration in functional level.

The aims for the child are to relieve pain and discomfort, improve function, facilitate care and contain contractures.[371] The authors' approach to therapy is summarized in Table 20.28.

Table 20.28 Schema for the treatment and management of cerebral palsy

Goals[371]	
1. Facilitating care 2. Improving function 3. Containing contractures 4. Relieving pain and discomfort	
Spasticity	
Medication	Baclofen Tizanidine Benzodiazepines, esp. Valium Intramuscular – botulinum toxin
Surgery	Release of contractures, Tendo-Achilles, hamstrings, hip adductors Scoliosis – spinal brace (operative fixation rarely?) Hip dislocation –*prevention:* adductor tenotomy/obturator neurectomy, derotation osteotomy –*correction:* open reduction, resection of head of femur (Girdlestone procedure) Upper limb – hand surgery? Reasons for (hygiene)
Neurosurgery	Intrathecal baclofen Dorsal rhizotomy
Physical and occupational therapy	Stretching, splinting, seating, standing, walking aids Home and school, aids and adaptations Advice on handling and posture
Paediatrician	Attention to associated conditions that will *exacerbate* spasticity: pain (e.g. ear infection, pressure area), reflux esophagitis, constipation, upper airways obstruction Or *compound* it, as with sleep disorder, seizures, failure to thrive
Athetosis and dyskinetic cerebral palsy	Medication most difficult, consider L-Dopa, Valium and possibly oral baclofen for dystonia For children with later acquired disorder consider biotin and pyridoxine Physical/occupational therapy as above (? Lycra suits) Pediatrician as above Orthopedic surgery as above Neurosurgery? stereotactic basal ganglia stimulation
Ataxia	Supportive therapy only – walking frames/Lycra suits?

Oral medication

Baclofen acts at the level of the neurones in the spinal cord, enhancing gamma-aminobutyric acid (GABA) activity as a GABA agonist, inhibiting some of the excess excitatory activity responsible for spastic tone. Dosage is built up gradually, according to effect and tolerance, to 2 mg/kg/day. Its effect will be global, rather than targeted, which may produce undesirable hypotonia of truncal muscles, adversely affecting sitting posture, for instance. It is essential that all treatments should be monitored in conjunction with physiotherapy assessments as well as the observations of the carers. This is very important for the child with four-limb spasticity in whom important side-effects may be overlooked, and who is especially susceptible to increasing polypharmacy. When there is doubt about benefit, then a planned withdrawal gradually (so as to avoid rebound spasticity, fits or hallucinations) will usually clarify its role.

Adverse effects on the child's alertness, diminished appetite, nausea or vomiting, and exacerbation of epilepsy should all be looked for. As for any treatment, there should be a general agreement between doctor and carer that only substantial, trouble free gains from treatment can justify its prolonged prescription.

Dantrolene acts on calcium channels, reducing the power of muscle contraction. Relaxation may be at the cost of reduced function. Side-effects also include nausea, vomiting and diarrhea. Hepatotoxity has been reported.

Tizanidine is an alpha2-adrenergic agent, which modifies excitatory transmitter activity. It has not been fully appraised for spastic cerebral palsy, in spite of manufacturers' claims that it may have a better side-effect profile for some patients compared with baclofen.

Diazepam can be a very effective muscle relaxant, but its use is limited by systemic side-effects of drowsiness. However this is not inevitable, and when spastic tone is distressing, it is worth a trial. It can be very helpful, for instance in seeing a child through a painful episode such as a fracture. Rebound spasticity can be severe following a prolonged period in plaster. Baclofen can also give relief at such times. Botulinum toxin (see below) may have a similar role.

Botulinum toxin

Botulinum toxin A (BTA) is a paralysing agent derived from *Clostridium botulinum*. It causes muscle relaxation by chemically blocking acetylcholine release, with the loss of motor end plates. Its effect reverses over 3–6 months as affected nerve roots sprout forming new junctions. It is given intramuscularly, usually targeting lower limb muscle groups in spastic diplegic children. These include hip adductors, hamstrings, gastrocnemius and soleus, which all contribute to the classical crouched gait and scissoring typical of this group. Multiple site injections, selected after clinical and video assessment by a multidisciplinary team are most effective. The team usually comprises at least a dedicated physiotherapist, an orthopedic surgeon and pediatric neurologist.

Three groups of patients may benefit: 1) ambulant children with a dynamic equinus throughout the gait cycle with knee flexion > 20 degrees or scissoring; 2) children who are losing ability to get to standing or maintain standing; 3) children of any functional category who are in pain or discomfort around the hip, or where adductor spasm seriously hampers care and hygiene.

The treatment is only effective for dynamic spasticity, especially in the young child, where therapeutic gains are greater and realistic aims to delay surgery beyond 8 years of age likely to be achieved by repeated injections. Towards adolescence many patients experience diminishing returns because of the added problems of growth. It is probably best considered as a possible treatment for windows of time in the child's life.[372] It must always be complemented by continuing physiotherapy and conventional containment of contractures, e.g. with orthoses.

The injections are painful, requiring sedation and local anesthetic cream for most children. Dose guidelines must be carefully followed, since it is a paralysing agent. Systemic spread from an injection site can cause bladder incontinence, lethargy and laryngeal weakness temporarily in a few children, though in the main side-effects are not common.

Orthopedic surgery

The consensus in orthopedic intervention is for multilevel surgery delayed until the age of 8–11 years for the release of contractures at tendo-Achilles (TA), hamstrings and hip adductors. The skill is as much in selecting the operation that is right for the child as in performing it. An ill-chosen isolated release of the TAs may bring the foot out of equinus, but put the child into a worsened crouch at the hips and knees, speeding their progression to wheelchair dependence. Hamstring release may weaken hip extension, worsening the crouch position at the hip.

Hip subluxation can be contained by timely release of psoas and adductor muscles. The adducting hip is the one at risk of dislocation, but in the windswept posture the opposite abducting hip can also develop an abduction contracture, hampering seating. Femoral osteotomy can realign the femoral head into the acetabulum, correcting a persisting fetal alignment that lends to dislocation. In more severe cases the acetabulum may be refashioned as well. In extreme cases the femoral head may be resected (the Castle procedure) but sitting balance, if present, is likely to be lost.

Scoliosis is most common in non-ambulant four-limb spasticity. Early attention to seating with scoliosis support inserts is important, as is standing time in a frame, use of bracing or moulded jackets. Spinal fixation is a major operation which may be selected for some patients with a curve of > 40 degrees before the age of 15 years. However the general state of health of the child with respect to risks and likely change in quality of life postoperatively have all to be weighed thoughtfully.

Neurosurgery

Intrathecal baclofen delivered at very low doses through a pump driven by an implanted battery may be very effective for children with four-limb spasticity. The implant is positioned subcutaneously or subfascially in the abdomen or loin. A fine tube leads intrathecally to the mid to lower thoracic level, and there is a reservoir of baclofen that is replenished at intervals by injection. Complications include infection and meningitis, CSF leaks and wound infection. The system itself can become displaced or disconnected.

It has been used less hitherto in the UK for ambulant patients than in the USA. However it does have the advantage of an effective preoperative assessment by injecting a test dose at lumbar puncture. The response is measurable in a few hours.

Selective dorsal rhizotomy is a neurosurgical procedure by which selected lower nerve roots in the lumbar sacral distribution are partially deafferented. This reduces spasticity permanently. It is thought to work by reducing the afferent stimulation of alpha motor neurones, which already lack inhibition from the dysfunctional or damaged corticospinal tracts. There can be bladder dysfunction as a complication and significant muscle weakness that impairs function. Functional improvement has not been demonstrated in all studies and therefore it is a form of treatment that is still being assessed.

DISCLOSURE OF DIAGNOSIS OF CEREBRAL PALSY

As soon as it becomes clear that the child is developing signs of spastic diplegia or any other form of cerebral palsy, arrangements should be made for a senior doctor to discuss the findings with the parents. Guidelines on good practice have been published by the UK based charity Scope[373] based on the recommendations of Cunningham et al[374] in relation to infants with Down syndrome, which is a life-long condition, diagnosable at birth. The reason for including this in the section on spastic diplegia is that there are many reasons for clinical uncertainty on the way to making this diagnosis. Yet there comes a time when it is possible to be reasonably confident. It is a way of describing how a child functions at present. In future it is possible for some children to grow out of this condition or other forms of cerebral palsy[299] so this, and other uncertainties, will be part of the discussion with parents.

- Planned appointment as soon as feasible after diagnosis made
- Both parents present
- With a relative, friend or professional (nurse, social worker, therapist) if parents wish
- Senior doctor with wide experience of developmental disabilities
- Trainee present if parents agree
- Quiet, comfortable room, free of interruption or disturbance
- As much time available for discussion as parents find helpful
- A full account of the condition and possible associated problems
- Details of further investigations or assessments
- Explanation of treatment plans and timetable
- Permission to notify the local education authority that the child may have special educational needs
- Information about help available from the social services department
- Details of local and national voluntary organizations who can help (photocopy the relevant pages of the Contact a Family Directory)
- Write in the parent-held child health record
- Let parents have a copy of the clinic letter to the general practitioner
- Offer a home follow-up visit by a colleague to help the parents understand what they have been told
- Arrange a follow-up clinic visit and encourage parents to make a list of questions
- Assure parents of your willingness and that of your colleagues to help their child to find what he/she can do best and to make the most of that at each stage through childhood and adolescence
- At all times show willingness to seek a second opinion.

LIFE EXPECTANCY

The life expectancy of children and adults with cerebral palsy is reduced but this is explained, almost entirely, by those with four-limb involvement lacking independent movement and self-care abilities. Strauss & Shavelle[375] reported findings on 24 768 individuals aged

15 or over and receiving services in California between January 1980 and December 1995. This work was extended, in a study period from 1986 to 1995, to a Californian population of 45 292 individuals of all ages with cerebral palsy.[376] Detection of other conditions was poorer in people with cerebral palsy, so that mortality from breast cancer was three times that of the general population. The risk of brain tumors was raised dramatically, especially in children (standardized mortality ratio = 24) indicating an increased risk in those diagnosed as having cerebral palsy. There was a range of life expectancy of over 40 years in the adult study, according to the functional level. Some with the least independent function had a life expectancy of only 11 years. Similar findings have been reported in North East and South East Thames Regions in Britain,[377–379] in British Columbia, Canada,[380] and in Western Australia.[381]

In South East Thames, 79% of children with severe learning disability and cerebral palsy survived to a mean age of 16 years. This is higher than in an earlier study in Rochester, Minnesota over the period 1950–1976.[382] In the Australian study, half the children with profound and multiple learning disability, with cerebral palsy (DQ < 20) lived to adult life. Of those with a DQ of 20–34, 76% survived to adult life, while 92% of those with higher ability did so. Those who reached 25 years had good subsequent life expectancy. There was no evidence in this study that advances in medical care and improvement in community awareness had improved the survival of people with cerebral palsy. It is premature to judge the impact on life expectancy of gastrostomy feeding, food supplements and the involvement of speech and language therapists, dietitians and others in feeding teams, tracheostomies for those prone to respiratory failure and the contemporary range of antiepileptic drugs. There is evidence of improved quality of life but, as yet, not of significant change in length of life. Comparison between the survival data from Western Australia and California was made by examination of both databases by Shavelle et al[383] and the differences were found to be slight if severity of learning disability was controlled for. The apparent disparity in survival was not due to differences in care, but because the Australian population included a higher proportion of mildly affected people and a lower proportion of people with severe or profound learning disability. This is the first published controlled comparison of survival in cerebral palsy between countries.

The interaction between cerebral palsy and learning disability in life expectancy has been reported to be an increasing problem (from 0.7 to about 0.9/1000 live births over the decade studied by Nicholson & Alberman[384]) Learning disability is, in itself, a risk factor for early death, especially from respiratory disease, which is three times commoner than in the general population.[385] Whereas 83% of the whole population live to be 65 years old or more, fewer than 50% of 2000 with an IQ < 70 and known to services in two London districts did so in this 8 year study. The risk of death before 50 was 58 times higher than in the population of England and Wales. Early death was associated with cerebral palsy, incontinence, problems of mobility and residence in hospital. Nonetheless, for children and adolescents with cerebral palsy and learning disability we must plan for their survival into adult life and advocate their case for transition into suitable health services when they leave pediatric care.

QUALITY OF LIFE AND COSTS OF CARING

In a review of 1365 published measures of quality of life only 5% were found to be applicable to children.[386] There are few published data on the views of children with disabilities on their quality of life and none of children with cerebral palsy and/or learning disability. Quality of life assessments of and by children with epilepsy have been reported.[387] Sociometric study of fifty-five 9–11-year-old children with hemiplegia in 54 mainstream schools has demonstrated increased risk of peer rejection, lack of friends and victimization.[388] As increasing inclusiveness is promoted for children with disabilities in mainstream schools there is a need to make provision for their social as well as physical and academic development. Fostering the social skills of children with disabilities may reduce the risk of social disadvantage.

The views of children with ADHD concerning behavior disturbance, social competence and familial environment have been found to differ from those of their parents.[389] Children perceived themselves as equally competent and socially accepted as their peers, in contrast to their parents' ratings. Though parenting a preschool child with ADHD was found to be stressful it was not considered by parents or children to affect family functioning adversely. Parents of children with physical and/or learning disabilities have reported lower quality of life in all family members compared with parents of children without disabilities.[390,391] The substantial impact of severe disablement in a child on parental careers, family income and expenditure patterns has been demonstrated clearly in a study of nearly 500 children with disabilites and nearly 700 controls.[392] In that study, 67% of mothers of children with disabilities were unable to enter or keep paid employment after the birth of their child compared with 60–69% of mothers of children without disabilities who are able to do this.[393–395] In a study of time costs of caring for 16 children with severe disabilities, including cerebral palsy, compared with 31 children without disabilities, it was found that personal care time was significantly greater per waking hour throughout the day for the former.[396] Twelve of the 16 mothers of children with disabilities were not in paid employment. Twelve had little or no extended family support. Care needs did not decline with increasing age, preventing mothers working outside the home outwith school hours. (The same would be true of fathers when, as is now increasingly common, they act as main carers.) This is the only published study of time costs of caring for a child with a disability carried out entirely in the family home. Two previous studies were based on observation of institutional care[397,398] while that of Edebol-Tysk[399] was a study partly in an institution and partly at home.

Most parents do not regret the changed way of life consequent upon having a child with a disability but some find it a struggle. In a study of 110 children with cerebral palsy in Salford[337] 39% of the children attended mainstream schools. Of those attending special schools 22% had attended mainstream schools but the placement had broken down. Thirty-nine per cent of those now in mainstream had been in a special school or nursery in the past. Of the children attending mainstream schools 88% were community ambulant compared with 17% in special schools. Two of the mainstream children were partially sighted compared with 11 who were partially sighted and 11 who were blind in special schools. Of the mainstream children 95% could feed themselves compared with 36% in special schools. Only 5% of those in mainstream school had current epilepsy compared with 52% of those in special schools. No mainstream child was bowel or bladder incontinent though help was needed for 17%/9% of the children for these functions. Fifty-three per cent of the special school children were incontinent and an additional 18%/12% needed help for bladder or bowel function. Thus the children in special schools had more severe and complex disabilities than the mainstream children. Of the mainstream children 11% had a single parent compared with 35% of the special school children. Fifteen (14%) of these 110 children with cerebral palsy were on or had been on the child protection register compared with 1 : 500 in Salford children in general at that time. Four per cent of mainstream children and 18% of special school children were in residential or foster care and two children had been adopted. In addition a further child had suffered a skull fracture, one had sustained extensive scalds in the bath, one had asphyxiated as a result of having a large screw in his mouth and another had a sibling on the child protection register.

Knowing of the pressures experienced by families of children with disabilities should prompt services to go out of their way to be helpful, to be pre-emptive and to minimize the risks of dysfunction.

TRANSITION TO ADULT SERVICES

As school leaving age approaches, there should be a multidisciplinary approach to transition planning and a college with the appropriate expertise should be sought. Expert careers advice is invaluable and suitable recreational opportunities should be investigated. An adult specialist resource should be sought as a source of advice in future. Such services have been difficult to find in many places. Many adults with cerebral palsy and other disabling conditions are either not in touch with social services or specialist medical advice or are dissatisfied with the services received.[400] There is justified concern for the decline in adult rehabilitation services over the past 30 years.[346,347]

DEGENERATIVE BRAIN DISORDERS

INTRODUCTION

The neurodegenerative disorders of childhood are a heterogeneous group of diseases that result in the progressive deterioration of neurological function with loss of speech, vision, hearing or locomotion, often associated with seizures, feeding difficulties and intellectual impairment. They are caused by specific genetic and biochemical defects, chronic infections or toxins. A considerable number remain poorly understood. Their recognition and diagnosis, where possible, is important as some of them are treatable, their management and ultimately terminal care needs planning and most of them have specific genetic implications. There has been a huge growth in neurogenetic knowledge in recent years. We are coming to realize that one phenotype may be explained by a number of genotypes and vice versa. A rational approach to specific gene testing will emerge in time. Meanwhile the focus of this section will stay on clinical diagnosis and management.

CLINICAL APPROACH

A history of loss of skills helps distinguish the neurodegenerative from static, non-progressive conditions. Usually, initial development is either normal or slightly delayed. Development then plateaus over a period of time with no acquisition of new skills followed by loss of previously acquired skills. The onset may be insidious or conversely acute sometimes in association with viral infections. Both may cause diagnostic difficulty. Regression may progress steadily at varying speeds or else spasmodically, with periods of progression followed by a plateauing of abilities prior to the next period of deterioration. Again, periods of deterioration may be triggered by intercurrent viral infections. Sometimes the presentation is with behavioral or psychiatric disturbances, or educational difficulties. Neurodegenerative conditions in early childhood often present with or include myoclonic or pleomorphic seizures so that an epileptic encephalopathy, such as the Lennox–Gastaut syndrome may be suspected.

Some neurodegenerative conditions are localized to white matter or else gray matter. White matter involvement leads to upper motor neurone signs, episodic hypertonia and difficulties in mobility. Gray matter involvement is associated with intellectual and visual impairment and seizures.

The involvement of other organs is common. Physical examination should include a search for visceromegaly and skeletal deformity. The retina should be examined carefully for pigmentation which might, for example, suggest a peroxisomal disorder or a mitochondrial cytopathy and for cherry-red spots reflecting macular degeneration seen in a number of lysosomal storage disorders.

Family history, including a history of consanguinity, may be important as most of these conditions, especially the neurometabolic, are autosomal recessive.

AGE-RELATED PRESENTATIONS

Infancy

A loss of motor skills may not be appreciated in infancy. Regression at this age often presents with a loss of interest which may be visual or in non-verbal communication.[408] Hypothyroidism, the aminoacidopathies, and metabolic (organic) acidosis are the main conditions associated with regression without obvious clinical clues. Non-ketotic hyperglycinemia and Menkes' kinky hair disease often present with seizures. A number of conditions presenting in this age group feature prominent irritability with arching with or without organomegaly (Table 20.29).

The toddler age group

In the toddler, changes are seen in speech and behavior as well as in motor difficulties.[408] In some conditions, there are specific, but often subtle features suggesting a specific diagnosis, such as Sanfilippo disease (soft dysmorphic features, very small spleen or might be not palpable), Moya Moya (dementia and regression) disease and HIV dementia (failure to thrive, brain atrophy on the CT scan). In others, specific neurological signs at presentation may suggests the diagnosis such as peripheral neuropathy with ataxia and bulbar signs suggests metachromatic leukodystrophy, ataxia with ocular apraxia and conjunctival capillary dilatation suggests ataxia telangiectasia, progressive cerbellar ataxia with mild dementia in juvenile Sandhoff disease, impairment of eye movement control and respiration and ataxia in Leigh's disease and splenomegaly with impaired saccadic eye movements suggest Niemann–Pick disease type C. The clinical manifestations of some conditions with autistic features such as Rett's and Angelman syndromes and a number of psychoses also start in this age group. Again, epilepsy can be the presenting feature (Table 20.30).

Table 20.29 Regression in infancy

With no obvious clue:
Hypothyroidism
Aminoacidopathies
Metabolic (organic) acidosis
With seizures:
Tuberous sclerosis
Angelman syndrome
Menkes' kinky syndrome
Non-ketotic hyperglycinemia
With irritability:
Krabbe's
Infantile Gaucher
Tay–Sachs
Niemann–Pick
Glutaric aciduria type 1
Pelizaeus–Merzbacher

Table 20.30 Regression in toddlers

With neurological signs:
Metachromatic leukodystrophy
Juvenile Sandhoff
Ataxia telangiectasia
Leigh's disease
Niemann–Pick type C
With autistic features:
Rett's syndrome
Angelman syndrome
Infantile Batten's disease
Missed phenylketonuria
With seizures:
Late infantile Batten's disease
Alper's disease

The school-age child

In the school-age child regression is often manifested with a decline in school performance, including concentration and pencil skills. New learning is hindered because of poor memory and coordination is impaired.[408] A wide range of conditions are present with or without epilepsy in this age-group (Table 20.31).

CLASSIFICATION OF DEGENERATIVE BRAIN DISEASES

Neurometabolic disorders

These conditions have recognized biochemical markers. The neurological deterioration and dementia are the direct result of enzymatic defects, which lead either to the storage of abnormal metabolites, or to a lack of an intermediate or the essential end product of the biochemical pathway. They are grouped according to the enzymatic defect or the abnormal stored material and are summarized in Tables 20.32–20.37. Other different conditions with biochemical defects including carbohydrate-deficient glycoprotein syndrome (CDG) are summarized in Table 20.38.

The leukodystrophies

The leukodystrophies are disorders of cerebral white matter, either alone or combined with other CNS or peripheral nervous system problems. Some, such as metachromatic leukodystrophy, have known metabolic defects (Table 20.32) while there is an expanding group whose underlying cause remains unknown. Some of these, such as Pelizaeus–Merzbacher disease, are clinically well defined (Table 20.41); others are grouped as unclassified leukodystrophies. Each disorder represent a phenotype which can be distinguished on the clinical and/or neuroimaging characteristics such as the age of onset, predominant features and distributions of the changes in the MRI.

Table 20.31 Regression in school age

With seizures as a prominent feature:
Juvenile Batten's disease
Lafora body disease
Sialidosis type 1
Myoclonic epilepsy with ragged red fibers
Juvenile Gaucher's disease
Juvenile GM2 gangliosidosis
With epilepsy is *not* a presenting picture:
Juvenile metachromatic leukodystrophy
Adrenoleukodystrophy
Subacute sclerosing panencephalitis
Wilson's disease
Juvenile Huntington's disease
Hallervorden–Spatz disease

Rare leukodystrophies

Leukodystrophies with vanishing white matter is a group of conditions with extensive MRI changes restricted to white matter. They present with progressive spasticity and ataxia. They often show step-wise progression with a sudden onset of symptoms, followed by a period of stability and then further deterioration. They vary in age of onset, are thought to be familial and no underlying cause is yet known.

van der Knaap et al[409] described families with MRI scan changes restricted to the white matter with cavitation in the frontal and/or temporal lobes. Affected patients had a relatively mild clinical course presenting with late spasticity, cerebellar signs and macrocephaly. A more rapid course was reported in three siblings without cystic changes.[410] They presented with progressive diplegia and ataxia.

Yet other cases, reported from the Netherlands[411] with early onset in infancy or early childhood, presented with steadily progressive ataxia and spasticity with exacerbations with infections and mild head trauma. Extensive cavitation of the white matter was found in one autopsy.

Spinocerebellar and peripheral nerve degenerations

(Table 20.39)

These are primary neuronal degenerations, without metabolic markers. Their common features are their selective nature affecting one or only a few parts of the central or peripheral nervous system, their progressive nature though not necessarily fatal, and the likelihood of symmetrical involvement. With the rapid advances in neurogenetics, many of them now have a specific test related to a gene or gene locus. As knowledge of the different genotypes grows, it is evident that the same gene defect can lead to heterogeneous clinical features. This variable clinical picture with overlapping symptom and sign complexes has made classification difficult. The recognized conditions included in the group are summarized in Table 20.39. Particularly rapid advances have been made in the genetics of the spinocerebellar degenerations (see section on spinocerebellar ataxias) and in ataxia telangiectasia (see above).

Neuroaxonal dystrophy

This is an autosomal recessive condition or conditions. The histopathological hallmark is the spheroid which is an axonal swelling formed by branched tubular structure and bundles of filament with mitochondria. Spheroids are present in peripheral nerves, especially presynaptically, but are also widespread throughout the CNS.[412]

The infantile form starts between 6 months and 2 years of age with motor difficulties. The child is hypotonic but with pyramidal signs differentiating it from a neuromuscular condition. The condition progresses to severe dementia with spasticity and eventually decorticate rigidity. Nystagmus and optic atrophy commonly occur by the age of 3 years while seizures are a late feature. Death occurs by 5–10 years. Neuroimaging reveals cerebellar atrophy with, on MRI, increased signal on T2 in the cerebrum and cerebellum and sometimes basal ganglia calcification. EMG shows denervation with nerve conduction studies being normal. Visual evoked potentials disappear after a few months. The diagnosis is confirmed by the finding of spheroids on peripheral biopsy of skin, conjunctiva, nerves and/or muscle.

Table 20.32 Lysosomal storage disorders – lipidoses and sphingolipidoses

Disorder	Age of onset	Clinical features
GM1 gangliosidosis	Infantile (type I) (0–6 months)	Mental and motor retardation Hepatosplenomegaly, fits, skeletal changes, hypotonia, blindness, cherry red spot (~50%), startle response, vacuolated lymphocytes, foam cells
	Juvenile (type II) (6–20 months)	Mental and motor retardation, fits, startle, response, ataxia, vacuolated lymphocytes, mild skeletal changes, foam cells
	Adult (type III) (teens)	Mental and motor retardation, progressive spasticity and ataxia, dysarthria, mild skeletal changes
Sandhoff disease (GM2 gangliosidosis)	Infantile (3–6 months)	Mental and motor retardation, fits, hypotonia No hepatosplenomegaly, cherry red spot, early blindness, doll-like face, foamy histiocytes in kidney, lung, spleen, etc., startle response
Tay–Sachs (GM2 gangliosidosis, B variant)	Classically infantile (3–6 months)	Common in Ashkenazi Jews where carrier frequency is 1/30 Doll-like face, mental and motor retardation, fits, early blindness, hypotonia and hyperekplexia, startle response, cherry red spot at macula
	Juvenile and adult variants, adult forms reported	Spinocerebellar degeneration, spinal muscular atrophy
Fabry (angiokeratoma corporis diffusum)	Usually in childhood or early adulthood	Cerebrovascular disease Cardiac and renal complications Progressive accumulation of lipid in vascular epithelium leads to increasing morbidity; excruciating pain especially at extremities, angiokeratomas particularly distributed around umbilicus, knees, flanks and scrotum; corneal opacity seen on slit lamp; mild disease may be expressed in heterozygous females
Wolman	Infancy	Non-specific progressive mental deterioration, hepatosplenomegaly, diarrhea, vomiting, and marked failure to thrive, anemia, vacuolated lymphocytes and foamy histiocytes in marrow, adrenal calcification a pathognomonic feature not present in the milder variant, cholesterol ester storage disease
Metachromatic leukodystrophy	Late infantile form 2 years	Unsteady gait and slow learning, blindness, bulbar palsy, quadriparesis No hepatosplenomegaly, loss of speech, loss of white matter may be seen on CT scan of brain as diffuse symmetrical loss in density; peripheral neuropathy, ataxia, dementia
	Juvenile type 6–14 years	Difficulties with mental ability, no hepatosplenomegaly, ataxia, spasticity; extrapyramidal dysfunction, pseudobulbar palsy, seizures features as for late infantile type
	Adult type 16 years–adulthood	Behavioral changes – psychosis, no hepatosplenomegaly, dementia, ataxia, spasticity
Krabbe	3–6 months but late onset (2–6 years) and adult forms are reported	Irritability, hypertonia with psychomotor neuropathy, fits and optic atrophy; deaf and blind; no hepatosplenomegaly, pathology confined to the nervous system Loss of deep tendon reflexs due to demyelinating neuropathy
Gaucher	Adult type I Childhood/adulthood	Normally no neurological involvement, hepatosplenomegaly, bone infiltration, pain/osteomyelitis/collapse of femoral head; hematological characteristic foamy macrophages (Gaucher cells) in bone marrow
	Infantile type II Infancy	Fits and psychomotor retardation, pyramidal tract dysfunction, hypertonic brisk reflexes; bulbar signs, strabismus, loss of saccadic eye movements, progressive hepatosplenomegaly, hematological complications, Gaucher cells in bone marrow
	Juvenile type III Childhood	Subacute neuropathy, hepatosplenomegaly, bleeding tendency, psychomotor development retardation, ataxia, strabismus; defective horizontal saccadic eye movement, skeletal involvement
Niemann–Pick	Type A Infancy	Neurological deterioration, hypotonia, blindness; massive hepatosplenomegaly Rapidly progressive with marked failure to thrive, areflexia, slow motor nerve conduction velocity suggests demyelinating neuropathy, cherry red spot in eye with corneal opacification; characteristic foamy histiocytes (may be sea-blue) especially in bone marrow
	Type B Childhood	No neurological involvement, marked hepatosplenomegaly, hematological complications, lung infiltration and histiocytes in bone marrow
	Type C, variable from infancy to adulthood	Neurological deterioration with variable time course; hypotonia Moderate splenomegaly, mental and motor regression, pyramidal tract involvement; in others unsteady gait and cerebellar ataxia, lack of coordination, dysarthria, cataplexy, fits, dystonia, supranuclear ophthalmoplegia, 'sea-blue' histiocytes in bone marrow
	Type D, similar to type C (above)	Similar to type C (above)
Farber	Infants generally	Progressive psychomotor impairment, no marked hepatosplenomegaly, striking clinical features include numerous subcutaneous nodules, arthritis with painful and deformed joints, hoarseness due to laryngeal involvement which may lead to breathing and swallowing difficulties

Table 20.33 Disorders of glycoprotein and oligosaccharide metabolism including mucolipidoses

Disorder	Age of onset	Neurology	Visceral involvement	Other clinical features
Aspartyl-glucosaminuria	About 6 months onwards	Mental retardation from almost 5 years of age, behavioral problems	Generally no hepatosplenomegaly	Coarse featured with loose skin, mild dysostosis multiplex, short stature, lens opacity, acne vacuolated lymphocytes
Fucosidosis	Two phenotypes: type I 3–18 months, type II 1-2 years	Psychomotor retardation, more marked deterioration in type I	Hepatosplenomegaly may be present	Mildly coarse featured, short stature, dysostosis multiplex but less marked in type II; increased sweat NaCl in type I and angiokeratoma in the longer surviving type II; vacuolated lymphocytes in both types
Mannosidosis	Two phenotypes Type I 3–12 months, type II 1–4 years	Psychomotor retardation, deafness	Hepatosplenomegaly	Coarse featured, dysostosis multiplex and characteristic corneal and lens opacities, especially in type I; vacuolated lymphocytes in types I and II
β-Mannosidosis	Variable	Mental retardation, deafness	No hepatosplenomegaly	Only three families so far, all with different phenotypes
α-N-acetyl galactosaminidase deficiency	~9 months	Severe psychomotor retardation, cortical blindness, myoclonic seizures, neuroaxonal dystrophy	No hepatosplenomegaly	Recently described disease, only in one family so far
Sialic acid storage disease	1-2 months	Mental retardation, slow regression	Hepatosplenomegaly	Coarse facies and short stature, dysostosis multiplex but clear corneas: hypopigmentation (fine wispy hair); vacuolated lymphocytes and punctuate calcification; beware, some features like Zellweger syndrome; may present as hydrops fetalis: a milder variant known as Salla disease is common in Finland
Mucolipidosis I (sialidosis)	Type 1 18–20 years, type 2 variable, infancy–late childhood	Type 1 myoclonic seizures, cherry red spot in eye, psychomotor retardation in some Type 2, cherry red spot, seizures	Type 1 no hepatosplenomegaly Type 2 hepatosplenomegaly	Considerable variation in phenotype, type 1 patients not dysmorphic, but type 2 patients dysmorphic and coarse featured, short stature with dysostosis multiplex; vacuolated lymphocytes in both types
Galactosialidosis	Variable	Similar to mucolipidosis I (type 2)	No hepatosplenomagaly	Similar to mucolipidosis (type 2) but with angiokeratoma in some patients; primary defect in combined enzyme protective protein. May lead to hydrops fetalis
Mucolipidosis II (I-cell disease)	Neonates and infants	Psychomotor retardation	Usually hepatosplenomegaly and cardiomegaly	Coarse facies, marked skeletal deformities including gibbus and kyphoscoliosis, short stature; joint contractures, 'puffy' eyes and gingival hyperplasia; little or no corneal clouding; characteristic intracellular inclusions (hence I-cell) in certain cell types, especially cultured fibroblasts; primary defect in Golgi enzyme responsible for phosphorylation of lysosomal glycoproteins including most lysosomal hydrolases; defect results in failure of receptor mediated uptake into lysosomes
Mucolipidosis III (pseudo-Hurler polydystrophy)	About 4-5 years	Slow psychomotor retardation	Possibly mild hepatosplenomegaly	Mild phenotype of mucolipidosis II; usually presenting features include stiff joints
Mucolipidosis IV	In the first year	Marked psychomotor retardation, visual impairment	No hepatosplenomegaly	Corneal opacities with retinal degeneration; short stature, foamy histiocytes in bone marrow

Table 20.34 Mucopolysaccharidoses – MPS disorders

Disorder	Age of onset	Neurology	Visceral involvement	Other clinical features
MPS I Hurler-Scheie	2/3 phenotypes (i) Hurler - onset in first year and death usually by 10 years	Marked psychomotor retardation, hydrocephalus	Hepatosplenomegaly and cardiomegaly	Coarse features, stunted growth, dysostosis multiplex, lumbar lordosis, stiff joints and claw hand; characteristic radiological changes (skull, vertebrae, ribs and clavicle); umbilical hernia and progressive corneal clouding
	(ii) Scheie - onset during childhood or adulthood (formerly designated MPS V)	No neurological deficit	No visceromegaly normally seen	Milder clinical phenotype than in Hurler; mildly coarse facies and skeletal deformities but normal stature; corneal opacities; note: an intermediate phenotype, Hurler-Scheie may result from a genetic compound
	(iii) Hurler–Scheie (intermediate type)			
MPS II Hunter	Usually between 2 and 5 years, but milder types survive to late adulthood	Slowly deteriorating, mental retardation	Hepatosplenomegaly Cardiac defects due to infiltration into valves and arterial walls	Normally no clouding but papilledema may lead to blindness, also differs from Hurler in absence of gibbus; pale nodular skin lesions, especially over scapulae; recurrent respiratory infections, cardiac abnormalities (murmurs), stunted growth, dysostosis multiplex, claw hands, coarse featured, hernias, progressive deafness, not: milder variant surviving into late adulthood – carpal tunnel syndrome
MPS III Sanfilippo	All types similar, usually between 2 and 6 years	Severe and progressive mental deterioration, usually impairment of complete extension of the fingers	Mild or no hepatosplenomegaly	All four types are clinically indistinguishable. In UK, the most common appears to be MPS IIIA and MPS IIID the least frequent; relatively mild skeletal and somatic involvement and generally no corneal clouding; often main feature is behavioral disturbance with hyperactivity and sleep problems; many become institutionalized
MPS IV Morquio	Usually first years of life	No primary neurological involvement in either type but quadriplegia and myelopathy may result from compression of the cervical cord	Mild, no hepatosplenomegaly	Characteristic skeletal dwarfism, corneal clouding, thin dental enamel
MPS VI Maroteaux-Lamy	Usually first years of life	No primary neurological involvement but secondary problems as in MPS IV	Hepatosplenomegaly	Marked skeletal abnormalities with corneal clouding, characteristic leukocyte inclusions
MPS VII Sly	Variable (only few patients)	Variable but may have mental retardation	Hepatosplenomegaly	Few patients described; spectrum of severe (hydops fetalis) to adult forms
Multiple sulfatase	1-2 years usually	Marked psychomotor deterioration, deafness and abnormal gait	Hepatosplenomegaly	Combines features of mucopolysaccharidosis with those of metachromatic leukodystrophy; mildly dysmorphic, high CSF protein and ichthyosis present; no corneal clouding, enzyme deficiency may be variable in expression and both leukocytes and fibroblasts should be studied for several sulfatase activities

Table 20.35 Peroxisomal disorders

Disorder	Age of onset	Neurology	Visceral involvement	Other clinical features
Zellweger (cerebro-hepatorenal syndrome)	At birth/neonate, most succumb by 6 months	Severe hypotonia, seizures, psychomotor retardation, areflexia, deaf and blind, flat electroretinogram	Hepatomegaly renal cysts, adrenal atrophy, no peroxisomes seen on liver microscopy	Multiple abnormalities; characteristic facies, high forehead, epicanthus, low set ears and high arched palate; large fontanel; cataract/retinal pigmentation and/or pale optic disc; failure to thrive, jaudice, raised LFT and diminished response to ACTH; punctate calcification especially in neonate, simian crease, cryptorchidism; these patients appear to lack peroxisomes in all cells
Neonatal adreno-leukodystrophy	At birth/neonates, most succumb by 6 years	Similar to Zellweger but less marked, severe neuro-degeneration	Similar to Zellweger (above)	Similar to Zellweger but less marked craniofacial abnormality, but generally blind and deaf. More marked adrenal atrophy but less marked renal cysts. Punctate calcifications not usually found. Numerous foamy macrophages esp. in adrenal, with characteristic lamellar inclusions. Patients appear to lack peroxisomes
Infantile Refsum	Usually in the first months, but generally not in neonatal period; may survive into teens	Neurological symptoms become more evident after 6 months when regression develops, with psychomotor delay and hypotonia; autistic behavior with impaired vision and hearing	Only mild hepatomegaly	Only mildly dysmorphic like Zellweger
Zellweger-like syndrome	Neonate	As for Zellweger	As for Zellweger	Apart from the presence of peroxisomes, this condition appears to be similar to Zellweger
Peroxisomal β-oxidation defects (a) Pseudo-Zellweger	Neonate	Severe hypotonia similar to Zellweger	Mild hepatomegaly, renal cysts present	Presents like Zellweger but peroxisomes present and dihydroxyacetone phosphate acyltransferase activity normal; no punctate calcification and no simian crease
(b) Pseudo-neonatal adrenoleukodystrophy	Neonate	Similar to neonatal adrenoleukodystrophy	No, or mild hepatomegaly	Similar to neonatal adrenoleuko-dystrophy but peroxisomes present as above, not markedly dysmorphic
(c) Bifunctional enzyme deficiency	Neonate	Similar to neonatal adrenoleukodystrophy	See (b)	Similar to (b)
Rhizomelic chondrodysplasia punctata (type of Conradi syndrome)	At birth but usually succumb in first year	Marked psychomotor retardation and failure to thrive	No hepatosplenomegaly reported	Severe and symmetric dysmorphology, microcephaly, prominent forehead and flattened nasal bridge; proximal limb shortening and joint contractures; punctate calcifications, especially of epiphyses; cataracts and ichthyosis; several peroxisomes present. Normal levels of very long chain fatty acids and bile acid intermediates
Adrenoleukodystrophy (Addison's disease with cerebral sclerosis, Schilder disease)	Usually 4-8 years but milder adrenomyelo-neuropathy at 20-30 years	Progressive psychomotor deterioration, ataxia, dementia, loss of vision and hearing	No hepatosplenomegaly	CT-symmetrical white hypo-densities especially in occipital poles; CSF protein increased; oligoclonal bands commonly present; affected males have neurological symptoms with loss of adrenal function; bronzing of skin, characteristic curvilinear storage bodies especially

(Continued)

Table 20.35 Peroxisomal disorders (*Continued*)

Disorder	Age of onset	Neurology	Visceral involvement	Other clinical features
				in adrenal cortex, peripheral nerve and CNS; the milder adrenomyeloneuropathy may present with leg stiffness and peripheral neuropathy
Refsum (heredopathia atactica polyneuritiformis)	1-20 years	Polyneuropathy, ataxia, loss of vision (retinitis pigmentosa), loss of hearing and smell	No hepatosplenomegaly	Skeletal changes, e.g. shortened metatarses, cardiac arrhythmias and ichthyosis (which may respond to dietary restriction of phytanate); anosmia is one of the first and most consistently presenting features

Rare cases of late onset (juvenile type) neuroaxonal dystrophy are reported. Onset is in late childhood with progressive myoclonic epilepsy and retinal degeneration. The diagnosis is by rectal or skin biopsies.[413]

No treatment or antenatal diagnosis is available for neuroaxonal dystrophy.

Neurodegenerative disorders with involvement of the basal ganglia

Most of these conditions have a metabolic or genetic basis. They commonly present as a movement disorder and are discussed elsewhere in this book.

Infectious and progressive encephalitides

Some neurodegenerative conditions result from some slow viral infections. The main examples are: subacute sclerosing panencephalitis (SSPE), progressive rubella panencephalitis, Lyme disease and HIV dementia. The latter two conditions are discussed in the section on aseptic meningitis in this chapter and in Chapters 27 and 25 respectively.

Subacute sclerosing panencephalitis (SSPE)

SSPE is by far the most common of the chronic encephalitides. It most frequently follows measles infection in the first 2 years of life with an incidence of 1 : 1 000 000. It represents an altered host response to the virus. The interval between measles and the onset of SSPE is usually 5–7 years. The onset is often insidious with slow intellectual and bizarre behavior followed by the onset of intractable myoclonus. Occasionally unilateral symptoms and signs make early diagnosis difficult. Extrapyramidal and pyramidal features follow and the condition progresses to dementia. The speed of progression

Table 20.36 Mitochondrial disorders and Leigh's encephalopathies

Disorder	Age of onset	Neurology	Visceral Involvement	Other clinical features
Kearns–Sayre	Before 15 years	Cerebellar involvement, ophthalmoplegia and retinal degeneration, ataxia	Cardiomyopathy with arrhythmias	High CSF protein; myopathy of skeletal muscle including oculomotor and cardiac muscle; ragged red muscle fibers, weakness of facial muscles, short stature, possibly a heterogeneous group of disorders, including some with mitochondrial respiratory chain defects
Mitochondrial encephalomyopathy, lactic acidosis and stroke-like episodes (MELAS)	Childhood	Cortical blindness, hemiparesis and deafness, seizures	None reported	Stunted growth, episodic vomiting, ragged red muscle fibers and spongy degeneration of brain at postmortem, probably a heterogeneous group of disorders including patients with respiratory chain defects
Myoclonic epilepsy with ragged red fibers (MERRF)	Before 20 years	Myoclonus, ataxia, weakness and seizures	None reported	Some patients may present as Friedreich's ataxia but this is probably a heterogeneous group of disorders; ragged red muscle fibers found but no specific enzyme deficiencies yet identified
Leigh's subacute necrotizing encephalopathy	Early childhood	Marked neurodegeneration, deafness, blind and progressive spasticity, eye movement control, control of respiration, ataxia possible, peripheral neuropathy	None	Appears to be a heterogeneous group of conditions often associated with specific enzyme deficiencies; deficiencies are not specific to Leigh's and many patients have no known enzyme deficit; deficiencies may be tissue/cell specific; CT: low densities in putamen, cerebellum and brainstem
Fumarase deficiency	Infancy	Developmental delay, hypotonia and cerebral atrophy	None	Progressive neurological disorder which present as 'mitochondrial myopathy', with lethargy and failure to thrive

Table 20.37 Disorders of carbohydrate metabolism

Disorder	Age of onset	Neurology	Visceral involvement	Other clinical features
Glycogenosis type I (Von Gierke)	Unusually in infancy	Secondary to hypoglycemia as convulsions, coma	Massive hepatomegaly and enlarged kidneys	Primary liver and kidney involvement with short stature, usually marked hypoglycemia, with raised lactate, blood lipids and uric acid; three variants; type 1a: glucose-6-phosphatase deficiency; type 1b: microsomal glucose-6-phosphate transporter, more severe disorder with neutropenia; type 1c: microsomal phosphate translocase
Glycogenosis type II (Pompe)	Two types: generalized infantile form and adult myopathic form (infant-adult onset)	Marked hypotonia in infantile form	Marked cardiomegaly with hepatomegaly	Severe and generalized condition with cardiorespiratory involvement and failure to thrive; patients are grayish, pale and listless, and tongue may be enlarged, vacuolated lymphocytes present, most patients succumb in first year
		Progressive muscle weakness in adults		Variable presentation in children and adults; skeletal and respiratory muscle involvement especially in trunk and proximal limbs
Glycogenosis type III (Cori)	Usually in infancy	Muscle wasting and myopathy in some patients	Massive hepatomegaly and moderate splenomegaly	Infants may appear to be obese with rosy cheeks; muscle involvement may extend to heart and lead to hypertrophy and sudden death; hypoglycemic generally only after fasting; different variants without muscle involvement known
Glycogenosis type IV (Anderson)	Infancy	Poor development, hypotonia, muscular atrophy	Hepatosplenomegaly	Marked failure to thrive with ascites and progressive cirrhosis; abnormal storage bodies in CNS and peripheral nerves
Glycogenosis Type V (McArdle)	Childhood and young adults	Muscle weakness, cramps on exercise	No visceromegaly	No increase in venous lactate after ischemic exercise, myoglobinuria; a severe infantile type has been reported, muscle phosphofructokinase deficiency (Tarui disease) is clinically similar
Glycogenosis type VI	Infants	No neurological symptoms usually	Hepatomegaly	This type should not present as a neurological problem

is variable, but more than half of the patients have a rapid course. Most survive for 1–3 years after. An apparent remission is reported in less than 10% of cases.[414]

The EEG shows a characteristic pattern with periodic complexes. The CSF shows evidence of intrathecal antimeasles antibody production. CT scan and MRI may be normal especially early in the disease. Later, they may show variable cortical atrophy and ventricular dilatation. Focal or multifocal white matter abnormalities may also be seen.

No effective treatment is available. Antiviral agents (inosiplex) were claimed to slow the progression of the condition and to prolong the survival[414] but SSPE invariably results in profound disability or death.

Prion diseases

Prions are infectious agents which affects only the CNS, are distinct from viruses and have very long incubation periods. The diseases caused by these agents were previously called the transmissible spongiform encephalitides and include scrapie in sheep, the human disease Kuru and Creutzfeldt–Jakob disease (CJD). Attempts to identify specific nucleic acid within highly purified preparations of prion were not successful.[419]

The major infectious component of prions is composed of a protein designated PrPSc. Cloning the prion protein gene resulted in the discovery of a point mutation for humans with familial CJD and established that prion diseases are genetic and infectious in humans.

Creutzfeldt–Jakob disease

Progressive dementia, loss of intellectual functions, sometimes with cerebellar and visual defects are the main characteristics of CJD. The onset is usually in adults though there is a reported case in a 10 year old. CJD is transmissible through growth hormone derived from human pituitary glands, through corneal transplants and by contaminated surgical instruments. The infectious agent is highly resistant to sterilization.[415]

New CJD variant

Recently in the United Kingdom, there have been reports of a new variant of CJD occurring in adolescents and young adults.

Table 20.38 Other conditions with biochemical defects

Disorder	Age of onset	Neurology	Visceral involvement	Other clinical features
Carbohydrate-deficient glycoprotein syndromes (CDG)	CDG1 Infantile from neonatal period through late infancy	Floppiness, psychomotor retardation, severe gross motor delay, axial hypotonia, muscular weakness, acquired microcephaly, roving eye movement Neuroimaging: rapidly progressive brainstem and cerebellar hypoplasia with usually normal supratentorial structures	Mild hepatomegaly Enlarged kidneys	Failure to thrive, congenital cataracts, some facial dysmorphism, limb joint restriction, unusual lipodystrophy, multiple organ failure
	CDG 1 Childhood	Non-progressive mental deficiency, IQ around 50, cerebellar ataxia, peripheral neuropathy, stroke-like episodes (in 50%), epilepsy (in 50%)		
	CDG 1 Adolescence and adulthood	Static condition, most patients remain independent and achieve some social functioning		
	CDG 2	Severe developmental delay No peripheral neuropathy, and normal cerebellum in the MRI	Two cases reported, more pronounced dysmorphic features	
	CDG 3	Neonatal floppiness, motor, mental and visual impairment; infantile spasm	Dysmorphic features Later, areas of patchy skin depigmentation, two cases reported	
	CDG4	Neonatal onset of severe epilepsy	Two cases reported	
Abeta-lipo-proteinemia	Childhood onwards; common in Jews	Progressive spinocerebellar ataxia; peripheral neuropathy; pigmentary retinopaphy	Not usually involved	Acanthocytosis of erythrocytes; hematological complications; fat malabsorption with gastro-intestinal manifestations of celiac disease
Acute intermittent porphyria	Latent condition, with attacks after puberty	Acute neuropathic episodes; muscle weakness; mental disturbance	None	Acute abdominal pain; vomiting; tachycardia, attacks precipitated by drugs
Lesch–Nyhan	3–6 months	Choreoathetosis: spasticity, mental retardation; self-mutilation	None	Renal stones and obstructive neuropathy; gouty arthritis
Non-ketotic hyperglycinemia	Neonate	Muscular hypotonia; marked seizures; apneic attacks; lethargy and coma	None	Generally fatal condition but some milder phenotypes have been reported
Homocystinuria	Early childhood	Mental retardation and convulsions; cerebrovascular accidents	None	Lens dislocation is common; osteoporosis and marfanoid features with elongated long bones; thromboemolism a major cause of morbidity
Phenylketonuria	If missed in neonatal screen Onset ~6–12 months	Seizures and increased muscle tone, agitated behavior	None	Fair hair, blue eyes and eczema
Biotinadase deficiency	3–6 months	Seizures; hypotonia, ataxia; developmental delay	None	Skin rash, alopecia

(*Continued*)

Table 20.38 Other conditions with biochemical defects (*Continued*)

Disorder	Age of onset	Neurology	Visceral involvement	Other clinical features
Menkes' disease (kinky or steely hair disease)	2–4 months	Neurological degeneration, fits, hypothermia	No hepato-splenomegaly	Abnormal hair (pili torti) hence kinky/steely hair syndrome; unusual face, bony changes and fractures, tortuosity of blood vessels and aneurysms
Wilson's disease (hepatolenticular degeneration)	8 years–adulthood	Neurological involvement often later in onset, as dysarthria, uncoordinated movement; pseudobulbar palsy	Liver disease, often acute, renal stones	Characteristic Kayser–Fleischer rings in cornea of eye, esp. in neurologically affected patients; bone and joint disorders; low serum copper and ceruloplasmin common but not diagnostic
Combined sulfite oxidase and xanthine oxidase deficiency	Neonate	Severe psychomotor retardation and regression, tonic seizures; lens dislocation and dysmorphism	None	A rapidly degenerating leukodystrophy. Most patients die by 18 months; biochemical defect recently described
Canavan (spongy degeneration of CNS)	Early infancy	Megalencephaly, visual loss, marked degeneration of white matter; severe mental deficit, blind, atonic neck muscles and hyperextension of legs	None	A rapidly degenerating leukodystrophy, most patients die by 18 months; biochemical defect recently described (N-acetylaspartic aciduria)
Sjögren–Larrson syndrome	Skin lesions at birth, neuro-	Mental retardation, spasticity, neurological deficit around 3 years	None	Ichthyosis of skin and glistening spots in ocular fundus

The characteristic features are personality changes, mental disturbance, dysesthesia and progressive dementia and ataxia. Affected young people often present with severe depression. A period of dysphoria follows accompanied by the onset of a florid, worsening ataxia. Dementia and an evolving spastic quadriparesis then follow with death occurring in 2 years or so. MRI shows high signal in the posterior thalamus. The place of tonsillar biopsy and specific CSF proteins in diagnosis is being defined. The histopathology is different from that of classical CJD.

Miscellaneous

Batten's disease (neuronal ceroid lipofuscinosis, NCL)

The ceroid lipofuscinoses are characterized by the storage of certain lipo-pigments that present morphological and tinctorial similarities with ceroid and lipofuscin. The chemical nature of these pigments is unknown. They normally accumulate in neurones with age and present in external tissues outwith the CNS.

The molecular genetic basis of all the common forms and most of the rare forms of the neuronal ceroid lipofuscinoses have been characterized in recent years.[416] The responsible genes are located on 1p32 (infantile, variant infantile with granular osmophilic deposits – GROD - typical of infantile NCL, and variant juvenile with GROD), 11p15 (Late infantile), 13q22 (Finnish variant late infantile), 15q21-q23 (Variant late infantile), 16p12 (variant late infantile) and 8p23 (Progressive epilepsy with mental retardation). The genes code for enzymes essential in nerve membrane lipid metabolism.

The three common phenotypes are summarized in Table 20.40. They overlap considerably. Early onset cases present with intractable myoclonic epilepsy, ataxia and dementia; visual failure occurs late. Later presentation is usually with visual failure, the other features following later.

Other conditions

Alper's disease, Alexander's disease, Alzheimer's disease, central pontine myelinolysis and Pelizaeus–Merzbacher disease are neurodegenerative conditions without biochemical markers and unclear pathophysiology. However, defective biosynthesis of proteolipid protein (PLP) was shown in a patient with Pelizaeus–Merzbacher and recent genetic studies have indicated point mutations[417] and duplications[418] in PLP gene. These are summarized in Table 20.41.

INVESTIGATION OF DEGENERATIVE DISEASES

The clinical history, including the age of onset of the condition, together with specific clinical features referable to the nervous and other systems, may suggest a differential diagnosis. However, frequently specific features are lacking and in such cases 'screening' in relation to the age of onset can be useful. In all cases MRI is required.

In infancy, screening should include thyroid function tests (for hypothyroidism), urine and plasma amino acids (for aminoacidopathies), urine organic acids (for organic acidosis) and white cell enzymes (WCE) (for the neurolipidoses such as Niemann–Pick and Tay–Sachs diseases). EEG can sometimes be useful, for example revealing hypsarrhythmia, suggesting infantile spasms as a cause of apparent regression or a burst suppression pattern in non-ketotic hyperglycinemia. Other investigations which may be useful include plasma copper (low in Menkes' kinky hair syndrome), CSF with simultaneous blood and urine glycine (raised in non-ketotic hyperglycinemia), and DNA studies such as for Pelizaeus–Merzbacher disease mitochondrial cytopathies.

Table 20.39 Spinocerebellar and peripheral nerve degenerations

Disorders	Genetics	Age at onset	Neurology and other clinical features
Dentatorubral atrophy (Ramsay Hunt syndrome)	Familial	Late childhood to adolescence	Myoclonic epilepsy; cerebellar ataxia
Friedreich's ataxia	AR (chromosome 9)	Mean 10.5 years (range 2–16 years)	Presenting: ataxia (limbs and trunk), scoliosis, tremor, cardiomyopathy (T inversion and LVH). Later: dysarthria, pyramidal signs with extensor plantars and diminished reflexes, proprioceptive loss, pes cavus, distal amyotrophy (distal wasting and weakness), optic atrophy and nystagmus, deafness, CCF or arrhythmias, gradually progressive diabetes mellitus; sudden cardiac death in the 30s
Familial spastic paraplegia	AR AD	11.5 years 18.5 years	Slow learning to walk; mild spastic paraplegia; stiff gait; scissoring of legs; slowly progressive (variable)
Progressive cerebellar ataxia	AR	Mean 9.4 years	Dysarthria, pyramidal signs, absent ankle jerks (others normal); sensory loss. Better prognosis than Friedreich's ataxia
Familial spastic-ataxic syndrome	AR		Progressive insidious involvement with signs relative to cerebellum, corticospinal tract and occular signs Death over 5–20 years
Olivopontocerebellar atrophy (OPCA) (Types I–V)	AD–OPCA (Types I, III, IV, V) AR–OPCA (Type II)		With retinal degeneration, progressive cerebellar ataxia; parkinsonian rigidity; resting tremor; impairment of speech
Ataxia telangiectasia (Louis–Barr syndrome)	AR (chromosome 11)		Progressive neurological deterioration with ocular and cutaneous telangiectasia. Early: cerebellar ataxia (often less than developmental progress). Later: decreased IgA, dysarthria; choreoathetosis; titubation. Sometimes progressive dementia. Telangiectasia of conjunctiva, pinnae, face, V of the neck, and flexures begins after 3 years; oculomotor dyspraxia, growth retardation; with wheelchair by 10–12 years; survivors show distal weakness, wasting, posterior column signs after 10 years; death before adulthood. Immunological: tonsils hypoplastic, abnormal IgM, thymic hypoplasia. Neoplasia: lymphomas, sarcomas, leukemia, Hodgkin's, lymphosarcomas, ovarian and gastric tumors. Blood: lymphocytopenia. Endocrine: abnormal carbohydrate metabolism
Infantile neuroaxonal dystrophy	AR	6 months–2 years	Loss of motor and mental milestones with regression; early visual involvement (ocular wobble); symmetrical pyramidal tract signs; marked hypotonia; anterior horn cell involvement (peripheral motor and sensory defect); dementia and decerebration
Multiple sclerosis in childhood		12–13 years	Death less than 10 years. Remitting course (1–2 episodes in childhood); optic/retrobulbar neuritis bilaterally (a quarter of childhood cases subsequently develop MS); gait disorder (with spasticity or ataxia)
Giant axonal neuropathy	AR	Early school years	Chronic peripheral mixed neuropathy; regression of gait, movement and IQ; fits; nystagmus; precocious puberty; pale, slightly reddish tightly curly hair

Screening in toddlers should include urine and plasma amino acids and urine organic acids. Metachromatic leukodystrophy (MLD) and the neurolipidoses can be detected from WCE. The diagnosis of Batten's disease is undergoing a transformation. Previously neurophysiological studies along with skin and rectal biopsies (to detect neuronal inclusions) were required. However, nearly all cases can now be diagnosed using a combination of enzyme assays done on blood combined with molecular DNA studies. DNA studies now also assist in the diagnosis of Rett's syndrome. Liver function tests and CSF and blood lactate levels can be helpful in Alper's disease due to mitochondrial cytopathies.

In school-age children (Table 20.42) investigations should include WCE for juvenile metachromatic leukodystrophy, juvenile Gaucher's disease and juvenile GM2 gangliosidosis; investigations (as above)

Table 20.40 Batten's disease (neuronal ceroid lipofuscinosis)

Type	Genetics	Age of onset	Neurology	Other clinical features
Late infantile form (Bielschowsky and Jansky) 11p15 pepstatin-insensitive lysosomal peptidase	AR	22 months	Slowing of development (may be masked by seizures), seizures (especially myoclonic); cerebellar ataxia; increasing spasticity; pigmentary maculae and retina; optic atrophy	Death 6–7 years
Juvenile form (Speilmeyer-Vogt) 16p12 438 amino acid membrane protein	AR	5–7 years	Progressive visual failure (pigmentary retinopathy and later optic atrophy); seizures (later); dementia; extrapyramidal and cerebellar signs (later)	Death 13–20 years +
Infantile form 1p32 palmitoyl protein thioesterase	AR	8–18 months	Progressive mental deterioration with microcephaly; ataxia; visual failure (optic) atrophy and brown discoloration of maculae; myoclonic jerks; pyramidal signs and contractures (later); 'hand knitting' behavior; autistic appearance	Rapid course, especially Finland. Death 8–9 years

Table 20.41 Miscellaneous regression

Disorders	Genetics	Age of onset	Neurology	Other clinical features
Alper's disease (Huttenlocher's disease)	AR	1–3 years	Probable group of disorders with degeneration of gray matter; convulsions (myoclonic); dementia; spasticity; opisthotonos	Sclerosis and coagulation defects; death in 10 months
Alexander's leukodystrophy and spongiform degeneration	Sporadic childhood	Infancy	Insidious, slowly progressive dementia; seizures; spasticity; megalencephaly	Persistent hiccup Emaciation (late)
Alzheimer's disease		Rarely less than 10 or 20 years, females predominate	Onset dysmnesia; seizures	
Central pontine myelinosis			Palatal palsy; dysarthria; ophthalmoplegia; ataxia; decerebrate postures; return of primitive reflexes; tetraplegia; respiratory difficulty	
Pelizaeus–Merzbacher disease	Sex-linked recessive (more common); autosomal dominant later onset	Infancy	Slowly progressive in a previously normal infant; nystagmus and roving eye movements; dystonia; rotatory head movements and ataxia with arrhythmic trembling and poor head control; tetraplegic spasticity (later)	

for Batten's disease; DNA for juvenile Huntington's and in some cases of Hallervorden–Spatz diseases; muscle biopsy, EEG and DNA for mitochondrial cytopathies; very long chain fatty acids for adrenoleukodystrophy; EEG and CSF measles antibodies for SSPE; plasma ceruloplasmin and copper and urine copper for Wilson's disease. Depending on the clinical picture, other investigations may need to be considered but the temptation to undertake all known tests should be resisted.

Table 20.42 Investigation for neurodegenerative conditions in school-age children

Plasma
Liver function tests
Copper, ceruloplasmin
Lactate
Amino acids
Very long chain fatty acids
Uric acid
Immunoglobulins
Urine
Amino acids
Renal epithelial metachromatic granules
CSF
Immunoglobulins
Cells (cytospin)
Measles IgG
Lactate
Neurotransmitters
White cell enzymes
Neurophysiology
EEG
Electroretinogram
Visual evoked potentials
Neuroimaging
CT scan
MRI

NEUROMUSCULAR DISEASE

MODES OF PRESENTATION

Neuromuscular diseases are disorders in which the principal problem lies at the anterior horn cell (the spinal muscular atrophies), the peripheral nerve (the peripheral neuropathies), the neuromuscular junction (the myasthenic syndromes) or the skeletal muscle (the myopathies and muscular dystrophies). Classically the central nervous system was considered not to be involved. However, it often is. For example in Duchenne muscular dystrophy learning difficulties are common whilst the congenital muscular dystrophies are associated with a variety of structural brain disorders. Mitochondrial cytopathies often feature prominent muscle involvement but are of course multisytem disorders. Clinical evaluation can often be helpful in defining the likely site of involvement in neuromuscular disorders. Hence fasciculation, muscle atrophy and severely decreased or absent tendon reflexes are characteristic of anterior horn cell disease. In peripheral neuropathies absent tendon reflexes and muscle atrophy, but not fasciculation are characteristic. Myasthenia is characterized by fatiguability. Tendon reflexes are usually normal or only slightly depressed. In the myopathies and muscular dystrophies the main finding is of weakness; tendon reflexes are usually preserved. Beyond such broad generalizations, the presentation of neuromuscular disorders shows considerable variation according to the age of the child.

Neonatal period

Pregnancy with a fetus with a neuromuscular condition may be complicated by polyhydramnios and reduced fetal movement.

Neuromuscular conditions must be suspected in infants who have arthrogryposis, are hypotonic, have feeding difficulties, respiratory problems or a need for respiratory support in the absence of any significant pulmonary pathology.

As any examination candidate knows conditions which may lead to a 'floppy infant' are legion. How does one distinguish infants who may have a neuromuscular condition? The traditional teaching, that these infants are weak in addition to being hypotonic, holds true. However, even if an infant is profoundly weak, without any antigravity limb movement, there are pitfalls to recognizing that the infant has a neuromuscular condition. An infant who unexpectedly fails to breathe after birth may be thought to have a hypoxic–ischemic encephalopathy and subsequent lack of movement may be attributed to the sequelae of this. Indeed, to confuse matters further, the infant may have had a degree of hypoxic–ischemic encephalopathy secondary to profound respiratory muscle weakness. Assessment of level of consciousness is difficult in neonates and is particularly difficult in an infant with ptosis and facial weakness.

Arthrogryposis may be caused by any condition resulting in restricted fetal movement. Neuromuscular disorders reported in patients with arthrogryposis include distal spinal muscular atrophy, neuropathy, congenital myopathy and congenital muscular dystrophy.

Feeding difficulties may be profound, with inability to suck and swallow and respiratory embarrassment on attempted feeding, or may mean feeds take longer than expected with weight gain less than ideal.

Conditions presenting in the neonatal period with limb weakness and respiratory and feeding difficulty include myotonic dystrophy and the congenital myopathies. The birth of an infant with congenital myotonic dystrophy is often the first presentation of this condition in the family. It is always useful to examine the mother of a weak neonate for ptosis, facial weakness and myotonia. The congenital myopathies, which are most likely to present with a need for respiratory support, are nemaline myopathy and myotubular myopathy. Ophthalmoplegia in a male infant is particularly suggestive of myotubular myopathy and there may be a history of neonatal death in other males in the family. Antenatal onset of spinal muscular atrophy is rare but severely affected neonates with deletions in the SMN1 gene are described.[420]

Congenital myasthenic syndromes must always be considered in neonates with feeding difficulty and episodes of respiratory distress or apnea.

Infancy and early childhood

Delayed motor development with age appropriate cognitive abilities should prompt consideration of a neuromuscular condition. Global developmental delay may be the presenting feature in dystrophinopathies[421] and, in a boy with developmental delay, investigation should always include creatine kinase estimation. Episodic weakness or exacerbations of weakness during intercurrent illnesses suggest metabolic myopathy or congenital myasthenic syndrome.

Later childhood

The manifestations of limb muscle weakness include difficulty with or inability to run, abnormal gait, difficulty climbing stairs and rising from the floor (Fig. 20.27). Fatiguability should suggest a myasthenic disorder. Muscle pain or cramp on exertion and episodes of rhabdomyolysis are suggestive of metabolic myopathy.

Occasionally neuromuscular disease presents with 'abnormal liver function tests'. When creatine kinase is very elevated, other enzymes such as alanine transferase (ALT) may also be elevated, leading to the suspicion of liver disease. When ALT is elevated but other measures of liver function such as bilirubin and coagulation studies are normal, checking the creatine kinase level may reveal the true source of this enzyme and lead to appropriate investigations.

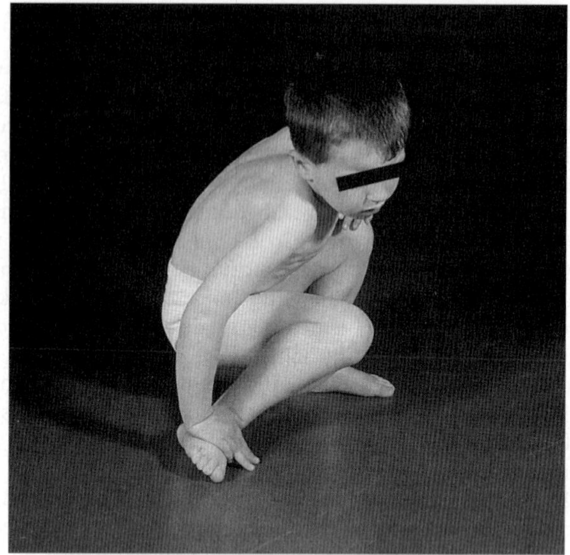

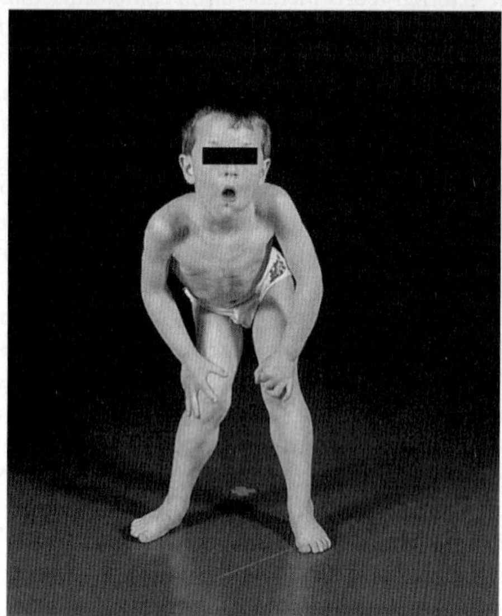

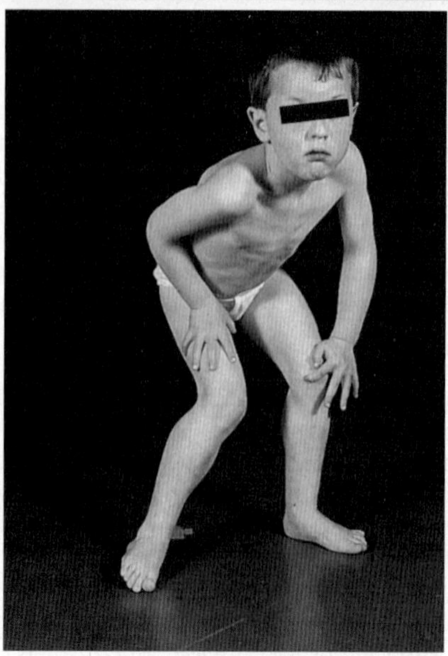

Fig. 20.27 A child with hip girdle weakness demonstrates a Gowers' maneuver: on rising from supine he turns prone then pushes himself up with his hands on his legs to the standing position.

Table 20.43 DNA analysis in investigation of neuromuscular disease

DNA analysis for diagnosis	DNA helpful following diagnosis
Myotonic dystrophy	Charcot–Marie–Tooth 1
Spinal muscular atrophy	Limb girdle dystrophy
Facioscapulohumeral MD	Congenital muscular dystrophy
+/- dystrophinopathy	Nemaline myopathy
	Myotubular myopathy
	Emery–Dreifuss MD
	Myotonia/paramyotonia congenita

Toe walking may be a manifestation of many conditions in childhood. Neuromuscular conditions, particularly dystrophinopathy, Emery–Dreifuss muscular dystrophy and Charcot–Marie–Tooth disease (CMT), must be considered in the differential diagnosis. Foot deformity is a frequent presenting feature of CMT and is also seen in distal spinal muscular dystrophy.

INVESTIGATION

Appropriate investigation is only possible when preceded by comprehensive clinical assessment with particular attention to pattern of muscle weakness.

There are a few neuromuscular conditions in which specific and highly sensitive DNA tests are available (Table 20.43). These are myotonic dystrophy, spinal muscular atrophy and fascioscapulohumeral muscular dystrophy. DNA analysis is an appropriate first line investigation for such conditions. Around 65% of boys with dystrophinopathy have a deletion in the dystrophin gene. DNA analysis for such a deletion is an appropriate early investigation to confirm the clinical diagnosis. If such a deletion is found opinion is divided as to whether muscle biopsy is indicated in order to determine with certainty whether the boy has Duchenne or Becker muscular dystrophy. In boys in which initial DNA analysis is negative but a dystrophinopathy is confirmed on muscle biopsy further more detailed DNA analysis may detect other defects, such as point mutations. In a large number of other neuromuscular conditions DNA analysis can be helpful in confirming or further defining the diagnosis. However, in such conditions it is not sufficiently sensitive to enable it to reliably refute the clinical diagnosis and should only be performed when indicated by other investigations.

Muscle biopsy

Muscle biopsy may be by needle or with an open technique. Needle muscle biopsy is usually sufficient but may not yield enough muscle for biochemical enzyme analysis or comprehensive immunoblotting in limb girdle dystrophy.

Analysis of muscle biopsy may include:

Hematoxylin and eosin
Fiber typing
Immunohistochemistry
Oxidative enzyme staining
Immunoblotting
Enzyme analysis
Mitochondrial DNA analysis
Electronmicroscopy

Neurophysiology

Nerve conduction studies will usually confirm the presence of neuropathy and define whether this is of the demyelinating or axonal type. DNA studies are only appropriate in inherited demyelinating neuropathy (CMT 1).

EMG may show a clear myopathic or denervating pattern, however the picture is often mixed. Moreover, it is often normal even in confirmed myopathies.

Repetitive stimulation and single fiber EMG may be helpful in confirming a defect of neuromuscular transmission.

Biochemistry

The following biochemical tests may be useful in the investigation of neuromuscular disorders (Table 20.44).

Muscle imaging

Muscle ultrasound can be valuable in detecting myopathies and muscular dystrophies, both of which are associated with increased echogenicity of involved muscles. MRI can identify the pattern of muscle groups involved. Currently information is being gathered, largely in relation to the congenital myopathies, which may ultimately become a useful clinical tool. The place of MR spectroscopy in helping to define the metabolic myopathies is still at the research stage.

MANAGEMENT

Accurate diagnosis is the first step in management and allows some estimation of the future course of the child's condition. Accurate diagnosis can also predict the need to be watchful for the development of particular complications such as respiratory insufficiency in minicore myopathy (see below). If a molecular genetic diagnosis can be made this allows accurate genetic counseling and antenatal testing.

To date, with the exception of some of the congenital myasthenic syndromes, there is no specific treatment for inherited neuromuscular conditions.

The aims of management are therefore:

(i) family support and education
(ii) prevention and management of complications
(iii) enhancing function
(iv) palliation of symptoms.

Family support and education

Family support is vitally important, not only following diagnosis, but also in negotiating the various hurdles encountered by the family of a child with physical disability. Families now have access to a vast array of information about their child's condition but making sense of what all this means for an individual child can be challenging. Although there are principles for good practice, for example in disclosing a diagnosis, families vary and no single approach fits all so it is important support is tailored to an individual family's need with the aim of enabling them to achieve the best for their child.

Table 20.44 Biochemical investigations

Creatine kinase	Marked ↑ in most muscular dystrophies, may be mildly ↑ in neuropathic conditions. Often normal in myopathies
Lactate	↑ may occur in mitochondrial myopathy
Carnitine/acylcarnitine profile	May be helpful in fatty acid oxidation defects
Glycolytic enzyme analysis	Useful in metabolic myopathy
Forearm ischemic exercise test	<fivefold rise in lactate in glycogen storage defect <fivefold rise in ammonia in adenylate deaminase deficiency

Prevention and management of complications

Contractures

Contractures are inevitable in neuromuscular conditions when there is marked weakness. In some conditions there is a propensity to early contractures, for example in Emery–Dreifuss muscular dystrophy flexion contractures at the elbows and Achilles tendon contractures develop in the presence of only mild weakness.

Passive stretching of joints and splinting are the mainstays of contracture prevention. Physiotherapy entailing extensive exercises may be recommended, but there is no evidence that it is helpful and it is very difficult to comply with. Brief passive joint stretching is more likely to be tolerated by child and parents. Achilles tendon stretching can be carried out for a few minutes twice a day without major interruption of daily routine. A period of prone lying will stretch the hip flexors.

When there is useful muscle strength around a joint, splints which interfere with function are unlikely to be worn. In the prevention and management of Achilles tendon contractures, daytime ankle–foot orthoses (AFOs) will be helpful if there is marked ankle dorsiflexion weakness. If ankle dorsiflexion is not weak or there is a dynamic advantage from toe walking, daytime AFOs will not be tolerated and night splints can be used. For example, in ambulant boys with dystrophinopathy daytime AFOs are unlikely to be tolerated so night splints are used; once ambulation is lost AFOs can also be used.

Surgery for release of contractures is of benefit in ambulant patients or may be needed prior to rehabilitation in knee–ankle–foot orthoses. Particular care is required in assessing the role of surgery in children with Achilles tendon contractures and weak hip flexors as tendon lengthening may cause a loss in ambulation.

Scoliosis

Bracing probably does not prevent progression of scoliosis in neuromuscular conditions; however it may facilitate seating in a child with marked truncal weakness.

Surgery is well established in the management of neuromuscular scoliosis. Posterior fusion is the procedure usually performed as respiratory compromise usually precludes an anterior approach.[422,423] More recently, rods which may be repeatedly extended have been useful in children who require surgery at a younger age and risk the development of secondary crankshaft deformity during the adolescent growth spurt. Careful attention must be paid to respiratory function in this group, so that completion of lengthening is performed while the child is still fit for surgery.

Respiratory management

Respiratory insufficiency is inevitable in the late stages of progressive neuromuscular conditions. In some conditions, however, respiratory muscles are selectively involved so respiratory insufficiency may occur when limb weakness is mild.

Weakness of inspiratory muscles restricts lung capacity, weakness of inspiratory and expiratory muscles reduces the effectiveness of the cough. Bulbar dysfunction and aspiration will also contribute to respiratory compromise. The presence of a scoliosis or spinal rigidity will also complicate the picture.

Regular monitoring of forced vital capacity (FVC) is important in predicting the development of symptoms and should be performed at each clinic visit and before surgery is contemplated. When FVC is 50% of predicted for height (arm span equates well with height in those unable to stand) there is a high risk of respiratory complications.

Table 20.45 Assessment of bulbar function

Questions in clinic	Any coughing or choking on eating or drinking? How long does it take to complete meals? What consistency of food can be managed?
Specialist assessment	Speech and language therapy assessment Videofluoroscopy of swallowing

Assessment of bulbar function is important (see Table 20.45) and the possibility of gastroesophageal reflux with aspiration also needs to be considered. If there is significant risk of aspiration because of bulbar weakness it may be necessary to limit oral intake giving most of the nutritional requirements by nasogastric tube or gastrostomy.

Haemophilus influenzae vaccination is included in routine childhood immunizations. Pneumococcal vaccine and an annual flu vaccine should be offered to those at risk of respiratory problems. Chest physiotherapy is helpful during respiratory infections and when there are retained secretions. There is conflicting evidence about the relative efficacy of the various methods available. Cough assist devices may also be helpful in removing secretions. There is no strong evidence that respiratory muscle training is of benefit.

Respiratory tract infections should be treated early and aggressively.

The first stage of respiratory failure is the development of nocturnal hypoventilation with oxygen desaturation during rapid eye movement (REM) sleep. Sleep is disturbed so the affected child wakes more frequently (this may be attributed to a need for turning), is not refreshed after the night's sleep and is tired during the day. Nocturnal hypoxemia with hypercapnia causes morning headache and a loss of appetite for breakfast. Left untreated, daytime hypoxemia and hypercapnia will ensue, with eventual cor pulmonale.

Nocturnal hypoventilation can be effectively managed with nocturnal non-invasive positive pressure ventilation (NIPPV). In boys with dystrophinopathy this has been shown to prolong life and provide a quality of life equivalent to that of individuals with non-progressive conditions receiving ventilatory support.[424,425]

Respiratory complications vary in different conditions. For example, in the dystrophinopathies and limb girdle dystrophies, respiratory muscle weakness will usually lead to nocturnal hypoventilation before there are significant bulbar problems. In spinal muscular atrophy, bulbar weakness often, but not invariably, contributes to recurrent respiratory tract infections before nocturnal hypoventilation occurs.

Cardiac complications

Ventricular dysfunction may be seen in many of the muscular dystrophies, in female dystrophinopathy carriers and in metabolic and congenital myopathies. Treatment for cardiac failure will relieve symptoms. Some children with dystrophinopathy with mild or even no skeletal muscle involvement may develop severe cardiomyopathy necessitating cardiac transplant.

Young people with some neuromuscular conditions have a propensity to develop cardiac dysrhythmias. Those with Emery–Dreifuss muscular dystrophy should have annual 24 h ECG monitoring. Individuals with myotonic dystrophy are also predisposed to cardiac dysrhythmias.

Malnutrition

Malnutrition at both ends of the scale is seen. Children who have restricted mobility can easily gain weight excessively and the encouragement of healthy eating habits from the time of diagnosis is recommended. Bulbar weakness and secondary orthodontic problems may cause failure to thrive. Assessment of swallowing and dietary intake will indicate appropriate lines of management, which may be nutritional supplements, advice on consistency of food, or need for supplementary feeds via nasogastric tube or gastrostomy (Table 20.45).

Enhancing function

Prolonging mobility and standing. Prolongation of mobility and standing has been shown to delay the onset of scoliosis. Mobility may be prolonged with the use of ischial weight bearing long leg splints, knee–ankle–foot orthoses (KAFOs). These may be used in any neuromuscular condition. The use of a standing frame is of particular benefit in children with spinal muscular atrophy type II and in children with congenital myopathies and congenital muscular dystrophy.

Independent mobility. It is important that children are sufficiently independently mobile to partake safely in activities with their peers. Electrically powered indoor–outdoor chairs (EPIOCs) allow children who are not ambulant or who have only very limited mobility to join others safely in the playground or elsewhere.

Education. Physical disability should not preclude education in mainstream school with access to the full curriculum. Adaptations may be needed. Use of information technology may be helpful, for example many children find the use of a keyboard allows them to be more productive than they can be when writing. Many children with neuromuscular conditions will also have learning needs which will also need to be addressed.

Adaptations and aids. Adaptations to the home and the use of environmental controls increase the independence of young people with neuromuscular conditions. Accessibility to public buildings and transport also allow a degree of independence.

Allowances

Individuals with physical disability and care needs may be entitled to financial help.

Palliative care

Most care in neuromuscular disease is palliative rather than curative. It is important that not only the physical but also the psychosocial and spiritual needs of the individual are met. Affected young people and their families should have an understanding of the benefits and burdens of treatment, be given an opportunity to express their views on those benefits and burdens and an assurance that there will be appropriate action in the light of those views.

In the progressive conditions, however, there comes a time when despite active management a terminal stage is reached, at which time alleviation of symptoms should be a priority.

MUSCULAR DYSTROPHIES

This group of conditions is characterized by the finding of dystrophic change on muscle biopsy: variation in fiber size, fiber splitting, necrotic fibers, excess of fatty and fibrous tissue. Classification was originally according to clinical phenotype but now these conditions can frequently be defined at the level of the specific protein deficiency by immunohistochemistry and immunoblotting and at DNA level by mutation analysis.

Duchenne and Becker muscular dystrophy – dystrophinopathy

The dystrophinopathies are the most common form of muscular dystrophy seen in pediatric practice and have X-linked recessive inheritance. There is a wide spectrum of severity, boys with loss of ambulation before 13 years of age are considered to have Duchenne muscular dystrophy (DMD), those with preservation of ambulation beyond 16 years are considered to have the Becker variant. Boys losing ambulation between 13 and 16 years of age are said to have an intermediate type.

Dystrophin is a 427 kDa protein, which forms part of the cytoskeleton of the muscle cell plasma membrane. It consists of an N-terminal domain, which binds actin, a central rod domain, a cysteine rich domain, and a C-terminal globular domain. The N-terminal and rod domains bind to actin filaments with the greatest affinity at the N-terminal; the C-terminal domains bind to the transmembrane dystroglycan complex. The cysteine rich domain, the beginning of the C-terminal globular domain and the N-terminal actin binding domain are very important for dystrophin function, with those deleted for this region having more severe phenotypes. The central rod domain is less important with deletions for much of this region resulting in mild phenotypes.

The dystrophin gene is located on the X chromosome and at 14 kb is the largest human gene cloned so far. Around 65% of males with dystrophinopathy are found to have a deletion mutation of one or more exons of the gene, 5% have a duplication, the remainder have point mutations. Approximately one-third of the mutations are new mutations. The clinical phenotype depends on the amount of functional dystrophin. Boys with the more severe Duchenne phenotype have absence of dystrophin, males with the milder Becker phenotype have partial dystrophin deficiency.[426–428] Clinical severity cannot be predicted by the size of the deletion or the region of the gene deleted.[429] The main factor that appears to determine clinical severity is whether there is disruption of the reading frame.[430] If the exons flanking the deletion share the same reading frame, protein translation can continue to produce a protein which, although it is missing amino acids, retains some biochemical function. If there is disruption to the reading frame no functional protein is produced.

With the identification of the gene and its protein product has come the realization that the clinical phenotype of dystrophinopathy is very wide indeed and includes asymptomatic cases with elevated creatine kinase (CK) only, cases with dilated cardiomyopathy and no skeletal muscle involvement and cases with elevated CK, cramps and myalgia.

Occasional female cases are seen, with a translocation involving the X chromosome.[431,432] Female carriers, heterozygous for a dystrophin gene mutation, occasionally exhibit overt muscle weakness, which can often be asymmetric. Approximately 10% of isolated females, with a muscular dystrophy with high Creative kinase (CK) and proximal muscle weakness, can be shown to be manifesting carriers.[433,434] About 17% of female carriers have some demonstrable muscle weakness. Female carriers without muscle weakness may have cardiac involvement, with approximately 8% showing evidence of dilated cardiomyopathy.[435]

In a study of a cohort of 33 males born between 1953 and 1983, the mean age of diagnosis of DMD was 4.6 years, the median age of wheelchair dependency was 10 years and the median age of death 15 years.[436] Non-invasive ventilatory support can extend the length and quality of life considerably. The rate of learning disability is higher in the population with DMD than in the normal population. A meta-analysis of 1224 cases of DMD found a mean full scale IQ (FIQ) of 80.2. Of these children, 34.8% had a FIQ less than 70, of these 79.3% had mild (FIQ 50–70) learning difficulty, 19.3% moderate (FIQ 35–50), and 1.1% profound learning difficulty. In this study 6% of the children had FIQ >110.[437]

Fatal rhabdomyolysis during anesthesia has been reported in a patient with BMD.[438] Smooth muscle involvement also occurs with acute gastric dilatation and intestinal pseudo-obstruction.[439] Boland et al[436] found cardiac failure in 21% of males with DMD at a median age of 21.5 years.

Limb girdle dystrophy (LGMD)

This is a group of genetically heterogeneous conditions which have in common a syndrome of proximal limb weakness. Each condition can vary in severity from a severe Duchenne type phenotype to a mild phenotype. Even within a family there may be variation in severity between affected family members.

Classification of limb girdle dystrophies is now by mode of inheritance (1 autosomal dominant, 2 autosomal recessive), protein deficiency and gene mutation. To date, the protein deficiency in three autosomal dominant and eight autosomal recessive LGMD have been identified (Table 20.46). In addition, the gene loci for two more autosomal dominant and two autosomal recessive LGMD have been identified.

Facioscapulohumeral dystrophy

Facioscapulohumeral muscular dystrophy (FSHMD) is an autosomal dominant condition. The characteristic pattern is of facial weakness and weakness of scapular fixation, with winging of the scapulae and difficulty raising the arms. Weakness is frequently asymmetrical. Later there is weakness of biceps and triceps, truncal weakness and lower limb weakness, which usually starts distally, but proximal lower limb weakness is frequently present.

In the severe infantile onset FSHMD there is marked facial weakness and a severe lumbar lordosis.

High frequency hearing loss is detected in most affected individuals. This is most likely to be clinically significant in the infantile onset FSHMD. The majority of affected individuals also have retinal telangiectasia on fluorescein angiography; only rarely does Coats' syndrome, an exudative retinopathy with retinal detachment, occur.

Cardiac involvement is rare and is most commonly manifest as dysrhythmia.

FSHMD is linked to 4q35. There is a deletion of an integral number of copies of a 3.3 kb DNA repeat. Affected individuals have 10 or fewer repeats, normal individuals 15 or more repeats.[440] No transcribed gene sequences are contained within this area. The proposed mechanism by which the deletion produces the condition is by position effect variegation, where the deletion may influence expression of distant genes.[441]

Emery–Dreifuss muscular dystrophy

Emery–Dreifuss muscular dystrophy (EDMD) is characterized by early contractures, particularly involving Achilles tendons, elbows and paraspinal muscles causing spinal rigidity, slowly progressive muscle weakness in a humeroperoneal distribution and cardiomyopathy with a propensity to conduction block and a risk of sudden death.

Table 20.46 Limb girdle muscular dystrophy

Inheritance	Classification	Gene product
Autosomal dominant	LGMD1A	myotilin
	LGMD1B	laminA/C
	LGMD1C	caveolin-3
Autosomal recessive	LGMD2A	calpain 3
	LGMD2B	dysferlin
	LGMD2C	γ-sarcoglycan
	LGMD2D	α-sarcoglycan
	LGMD2E	β-sarcoglycan
	LGMD2F	δ-sarcoglycan
	LGMD2G	telethonin
	LGMD2I	fukutin related protein

EDMD is genetically heterogeneous. Two genes have been identified so far, the emerin gene on Xq28 and the laminA/C gene on 1q11-q13. The products of both these genes form part of the inner nuclear membrane. Emerin deficient EDMD is inherited in an X-linked recessive fashion. Female carriers may occasionally have cardiac conduction abnormalities and so warrant cardiology assessment. EDMD due to laminA/C deficiency may be inherited in an autosomal dominant or recessive fashion.

CONGENITAL MYOPATHIES

The congenital myopathies are a group of conditions that frequently, but not always, manifest in infancy with hypotonia and motor delay. Classification has traditionally been on a morphological basis. It has long been recognized that the morphological appearances may not be specific and some changes may be seen in other conditions. With the elucidation of the genetic basis of some of these conditions it appears that the same morphological changes and clinical features may be seen in genetically heterogeneous conditions; most notably to date, nemaline myopathy may be caused by defects in six different genes (Table 20.47). Determination of the genotype in a child with a congenital myopathy allows more informative genetic counseling and the possibility of antenatal diagnosis.

Most of these conditions are apparently non-progressive, or only very slowly progressive, but important specific clinical features may occur, for example respiratory failure and paraspinal muscle contractures in minicore myopathy.

Myotubular myopathy and centronuclear myopathy

These terms may be used interchangeably or myotubular myopathy may be used for the severe X-linked early onset form and centronuclear myopathy used for sporadic, dominant or recessive cases. Muscle fibers, with centrally located nuclei with a surrounding halo devoid of myofilaments, resemble myotubes. In all types, ptosis and ophthalmoplegia are frequent features. Calf hypertrophy is described in late onset cases.

The X-linked form is due to mutation in the myotubularin (MTM1) gene. The gene product is a protein tyrosine phosphatase, which is required for muscle cell differentiation.[442]

The severe X-linked early onset form is frequently associated with respiratory insufficiency and ventilator dependency. In a study of 55 males with confirmed MTM1 mutations Herman et al[443] found a survival rate at 1 year of age of 74%; 80% of these remained ventilator dependent. Care must be taken to distinguish this condition from congenital myotonic dystrophy. In the latter condition, examination of the mother may be helpful and DNA analysis will identify the CTG triplet repeat (see below).

Spherocytosis, gallstones, renal stones and a vitamin K-responsive coagulopathy are described[443] and it is prudent to assess coagulation prior to any operative procedures.

Table 20.47 The congenital myopathies

Congenital myopathy	Pathology	Important clinical features	Inheritance	Gene locus	Gene product
Myotubular	Central nuclei surrounded by clear area without myofibrils	Ophthalmoplegia, respiratory insufficiency in neonatal period, coagulopathy and hepatic dysfunction with subcapsular hemorrhages	XR	Xq28	MTM1 Myotubularin
Nemaline	Rod bodies derived from Z-band material	Respiratory insufficiency in neonatal period, occasional cardiomyopathy, selective diaphragmatic involvement with early respiratory insufficiency in milder cases	AD	1q21-q23	NEM1 α-tropomyosin
			AR	2q21.2-q22	NEM2 nebulin
			AD/AR	1q42.1	ACTA1 Alpha actin, skeletal muscle
			AD	9p13.2-p13.1	TPM2 β-tropomyosin
			AR	19q13.4	TNNT1 troponin T1
			AD	15q21-q24	?
Central core	Central areas of derangement of sarcomeres with absence of oxidative enzyme activity	Congenital hip dysplasia may occur, cardiomyopathy and respiratory insufficiency rare	AD	19q13.1	CCD Skeletal muscle ryanodine receptor
Minicore	Multiple small areas devoid of oxidative enzyme, type 1 fiber predominance	Contracture of paraspinal muscles with complicated scoliosis, early diaphragmatic involvement and respiratory insufficiency	?AR	?	

Later onset disease is usually only very slowly progressive. Cardiomyopathy is rare but has been reported as the presenting feature. No gene loci have yet been identified for autosomal dominant or recessive varieties. In females, care must be taken to exclude manifesting carrier status for the X-linked variety.

Nemaline myopathy

Nemaline myopathy is defined by the presence of nemaline rods in muscle fibers. These rods contain Z disc material. Intranuclear rods, which are identical to cytoplasmic rods, may be seen and may indicate an unfavorable prognosis.[444]

Various clinical phenotypes are seen. In the severe congenital form, there are no spontaneous movements or respiration. In the typical congenital type, onset is in infancy or early childhood with weakness predominantly affecting neck flexors, facial, bulbar and respiratory muscles. The course is slowly progressive but respiratory insufficiency may occur. Onset in later childhood or adult life may also occur. Nemaline myopathy has also been reported in the fetal akinesia sequence.[445]

Mutations in five genes: alpha-tropomyosin (TPM3)[446] nebulin (NEB), alpha-actin (ACTA1),[447] beta-tropomyosin (TPM2)[448] and troponin T1 (TNNT1)[449] have been found in nemaline myopathy. A further gene locus (15q21-q24) has been identified. Autosomal dominant and autosomal recessive inheritance has been found in families with TPM3 and ACTA1 mutations. All TPM2 mutations have been autosomal dominant and all NEB and TNNT1 mutations autosomal recessive.

Genotype and mode of inheritance cannot be predicted from the clinical severity. Neonatal presentation has been seen with recessive mutations in NEB and TPM3 and dominant mutations in ACTA1. In the group with adult onset only dominant mutations have been found.

Central core disease (CCD)

The characteristic histological feature of CCD is the presence of central cores devoid of oxidative enzyme activity in type 1 muscle fibers (Fig. 20.28). In addition there is type 1 fiber predominance.

Inheritance is autosomal dominant but a description of two severely affected cases suggests possible autosomal recessive inheritance.[450] Linkage to chromosome 19q13.1 has been found in a few families with CCD. Mutations in the ryanodine receptor gene (RYR1) have been identified in a few patients with CCD.[451] Mutations in this gene have also been found in families with susceptibility to malignant hyperthermia and these two conditions may coexist within a few patients and families.

CCD is usually non-progressive or only very slowly progressive even in the severe cases described.[450] Presentation is usually with hypotonia and delayed motor development in infancy. Congenital hip dislocation, contractures, scoliosis or foot deformity may occur.[452] Cardiac involvement and respiratory insufficiency do not usually occur.

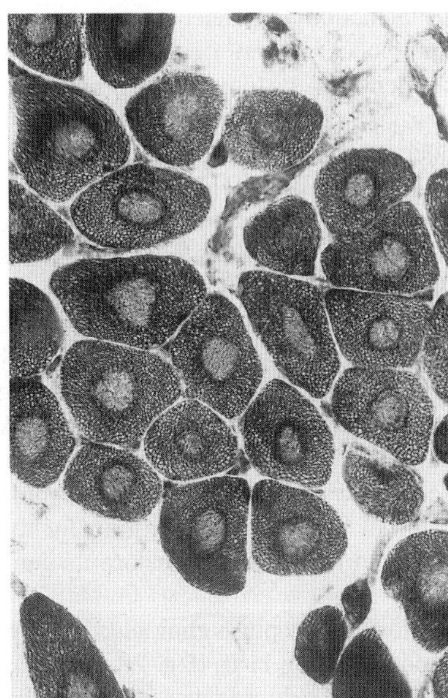

Fig. 20.28 Central core disease: the cores show absence of staining with NADH.

Minicore myopathy

Minicore myopathy is defined by the presence of small cores, which do not extend through the full fiber length but are histochemically and ultrastructurally similar to central cores. They are not confined to type 1 fibers.

Sporadic cases, autosomal recessive inheritance and, in a few families, autosomal dominant inheritance have been described. No gene loci have been identified yet.

Presentation is most frequently with hypotonia and delayed motor development. Muscle weakness is most marked in axial muscles and proximal limbs. Ophthalmoplegia is described. The weakness is static or very slowly progressive. Scoliosis, cardiomyopathy and respiratory insufficiency may occur in ambulatory patients.[453,454]

Other congenital myopathies

Other congenital myopathies occur more rarely. Desmin-related myopathies are clinically and genetically heterogeneous. Some types are associated with cardiomyopathy, others with respiratory insufficiency. Actin-related myopathy, a congenital myopathy with an excess of thin myofilaments, has been described in a small number of severely affected infants and has been associated with mutations in the ACTA1 gene.

CONGENITAL MUSCULAR DYSTROPHY

The congenital muscular dystrophies are a group of genetically heterogeneous conditions. The clinical features which they have in common are muscle weakness and hypotonia, which is present from birth or the first few months of life, contractures, which occur early or may be congenital, raised or normal CK levels and dystrophic changes on muscle biopsy. All are autosomal recessive and a number of gene defects have been identified to date. Most of the defective proteins responsible for congenital muscular dystrophy (CMD) interact with components of the extracellular matrix.

Important clinical features, which may help define a specific diagnosis, include whether intellect is normal or there is associated learning difficulty, the presence of muscle hypertrophy or distal joint laxity. Brain MRI may be normal or may show the presence of abnormalities such as white matter changes, neuronal migration disorder, cerebellar or brainstem abnormalities. There may also be associated eye abnormalities such as myopia, glaucoma, cataract and retinal dysplasia.

Congenital muscular dystrophy without mental retardation

Primary laminin-α2 (merosin) deficiency

This is the most common form of CMD and accounts for 50% of CMD cases in the Caucasian population.[455] Severe muscle weakness involves the face, trunk and limbs symmetrically and is present from birth. CK is markedly elevated. Feeding and respiratory difficulties are common. Some improvement in muscle strength is usually seen so that independent sitting is achieved. Only very few children with complete laminin-α2 deficiency are able to stand or walk a few steps. Muscle strength tends to remain fairly stable through childhood.

All patients have white matter changes on brain imaging[456] (Fig. 20.29). Structural abnormalities such as occipital agyria and cerebellar hypoplasia have also been reported.[457] Most children are of normal intelligence unless there is gross occipital agyria. Epilepsy occurs in up to 30% of affected children.[457] A demyelinating neuropathy also occurs in this condition.[458]

Patients with partial laminin-α2 deficiency may have a clinical phenotype ranging from early onset of weakness and hypotonia to adult onset of limb girdle weakness.

Laminin-α2 is expressed in skin basement membrane and in the trophoblast. Immunofluorescence of fetal trophoblast may be used along with haplotype analysis or mutation analysis for antenatal diagnosis.

Secondary laminin-α2 (merosin) deficiency

Several families with an abnormality of laminin-α2 staining, but not linked to the LAMA-2 gene on chromosome 6q2, have been described. Mutations in a fukutin-related protein gene (FKRP) on chromosome 19q13.3 have been found in a number of families.[459] The clinical features are onset in the first weeks of life, severe weakness and wasting of the shoulder girdle muscles, hypertrophy and weakness of leg muscles with inability to walk and respiratory failure in the second decade. Mutations in this gene are also described in children with limb girdle dystrophies of varying severity.

Ullrich syndrome

Recently mutations in the collagen VI genes COL6A1, COL6A2 and COL6A3 have been demonstrated in this condition.[460] The characteristic clinical features are proximal contractures and marked distal joint laxity. Intelligence is normal.

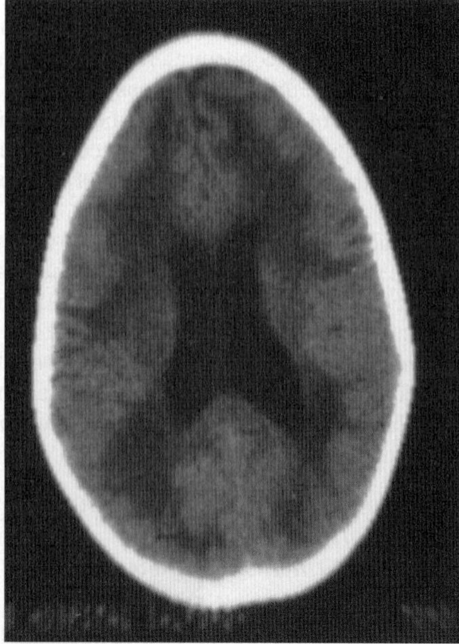

Fig. 20.29 CT scan in laminin-α2 deficiency showing extensive white matter changes.

Congenital muscular dystrophy with mental retardation

Fukuyama congenital muscular dystrophy (FCMD)

This condition is essentially only seen in the Japanese population or patients of Japanese descent. Muscle weakness and learning difficulty are usually severe. Seizures occur in around 60%. Over 80% have high myopia, 60% glaucoma and 90% retinal dysplasia. The MRI brain scan shows abnormal signal in periventricular white matter in addition to neuronal migration defects.

Mutations in the fukutin gene on chromosome 9q3 are responsible for the condition.

Muscle eye brain disease (MEB)

Most children with MEB are severely affected. Brain MRI shows neuronal migration defects in addition to partial absence of the septum pellucidum, corpus callosum dysplasia, hydrocephalus, pontine and cerebellar hypoplasia and periventricular white matter changes. Eye abnormalities are severe with severe myopia and glaucoma. Most patients have severe visual handicap.

Mutations in a glycosyl-transferase gene (OMGnT) on chromosome 1p3 have been found in this condition.[461]

Walker–Warburg syndrome

In this condition there is almost complete lissencephaly (absence of cortical sulcation), microphthalmia with persistence of hyaloid vasculature and retinal detachment in combination with a muscular dystrophy. Other features may include encephalocele, ocular colobomas, cataract, genital abnormality and cleft lip and palate.[462]

No gene locus has yet been identified.

MYOTONIC DYSTROPHY

Myotonic dystrophy is a condition with effects on other systems in addition to muscle. Muscle weakness predominantly affects facial muscles, levator palpebrae, neck flexion and distal limb muscles. Muscle weakness is commonly more extensive and the diaphragm and intercostal muscles are commonly involved. Myotonia is unusual before the age of 6 years. Smooth muscle involvement causes dysphagia, which may be life threatening, and bowel dysfunction. Cardiac conduction defects and tachyarrhythmias are common and may occur when neuromuscular involvement is mild.[463] Central nervous system involvement causes learning difficulty in children and the somnolence and lethargy of older individuals. Endocrine disturbances occur, subfertility occurs and in females there is a high rate of fetal loss.[464]

The genetic defect in myotonic dystrophy is a trinucleotide repeat disorder with an expansion of CTG repeats. There is a relationship between the size of DNA expansion and clinical severity.[465] Thus those presenting with the condition in adult life will have a DNA expansion band size between 0.25 and 3.5 kb, whereas about one in three children presenting in the newborn period will have DNA band expanded above 5 kb. Germline instability accounts for the tendency of the mutation to expand in subsequent generations, diminution may occur but is much less frequent. Expansion of the mutation accounts for the anticipation recognized clinically in this condition before its genetic basis was elucidated.

Congenital myotonic dystrophy is characterized by marked muscle weakness and hypotonia from birth (Fig. 20.30). Affected neonates have feeding difficulty with reduced reflexes and may have respiratory insufficiency. Mechanical ventilation may be required and the need for this is associated with a high mortality. Affected babies have a

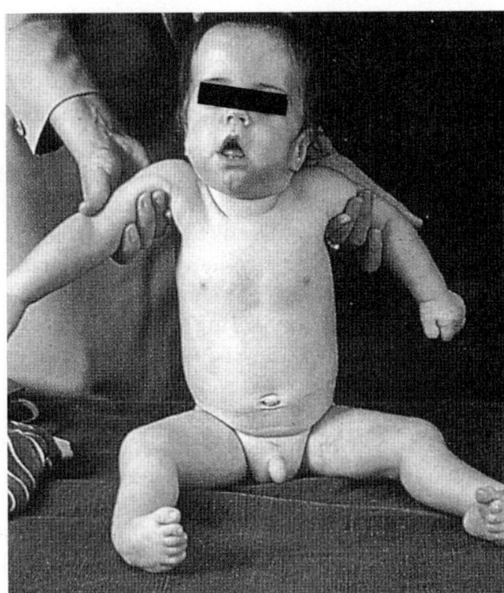

Fig. 20.30 Congenital myotonic dystrophy in a year old child with facial weakness, foot deformity and developmental delay.

characteristic facial muscle posture with an open mouth and a tent shaped or inverted V shaped upper lip. Talipes and hip joint dislocation are occasionally seen. The finding of a large head with ventricular dilatation in association with talipes on an antenatal ultrasound scan should prompt consideration of this diagnosis. All have learning difficulties with a wide spread of ability, some mild, some severe though few are able to obtain employment in adult life.[466]

With few exceptions congenital myotonic dystrophy is maternally transmitted.[467,468] Two-thirds of the affected mothers have minimal or no symptoms of their own disease at the time of delivery.

Children with congenital myotonic dystrophy have a 25% chance of death before 18 months and a 50% chance of survival into the mid-30s.[466] Life expectancy for adults is shortened, with a mean of about 60 years for men and women. Death usually results from respiratory insufficiency or cardiac arrhythmias (a cardiomyopathy is relatively rare). About half those with adult onset disease become wheelchair users. A higher proportion of those with childhood onset disease will use a wheelchair for mobility.

As childhood progresses, and particularly through adolescence, treatment for myotonia can be considered. Phenytoin and procainamide have been used successfully.

CHANNELOPATHIES: THE NON-DYSTROPHIC MYOTONIAS AND PERIODIC PARALYSES

This group of disorders is caused by abnormalities of membrane excitation caused by specific mutations in genes coding for various ion channels in the muscle fiber membrane.

Point mutations or deletions in the gene encoding the skeletal muscle chloride channel, CLCN1 on chromosome 7q35 cause myotonia congenita. Mutations in the gene coding for the skeletal muscle sodium channel, SCN4A on chromosome 17q23.1-q25.3, lead to a variety of conditions including paramyotonia congenita, potassium aggravated myotonia, hypo- and hyperkalemic periodic paralysis. Some families with SCN4A mutations may manifest both paramyotonia and periodic paralyses. Point mutations in the gene encoding the muscle L-type calcium channel, CACNL1A3 on chromosome 1q31-q32 lead to hypokalemic periodic paralysis.

In this group of conditions symptoms are caused by long lasting depolarizations of the muscle fiber membranes. Myotonia may be present at birth, whereas spontaneously occurring episodes of weakness usually start in the first or second decade of life.

MYOTONIA CONGENITA

This is a disorder of the major chloride channel of adult skeletal muscle. The recessive form is more common with an incidence of about 1 in 50 000. Females are affected to a much lesser degree. A dominant form of the same clinical condition is much rarer.

Clinical signs of dominant myotonia congenita (Thomsen disease)

This is usually present from early childhood with generalized myotonia, the legs being affected more than the arms. Chewing may be affected. Myotonic stiffness is more pronounced when a forceful movement is abruptly initiated after a period of rest. Repeating a movement will ablate the myotonia, but it always recurs following rest. A sudden fright may cause instantaneous generalized stiffness, the child falling to the ground, remaining rigid and helpless for some seconds or even minutes. Muscle hypertrophy is a feature and strength may be increased. Tightness of the tendo-Achilles is often seen. Tapping a muscle produces an indentation for a few seconds (percussion myotonia). Lid lag and/or blephrospasm may be present.

Clinical signs of recessive myotonia (Becker type)

The clinical features are very similar to the dominant type, but they often appear after the age of 10 years and it is generally more severe than seen in the dominant type. There is usually generalized muscle hypertrophy, on initiating movement there is muscle weakness but after a few contractions muscle strength becomes normal.

DNA testing is now available to confirm the diagnosis.

Should treatment be necessary, the myotonic stiffness responds well to drugs that reduce the increased excitability of the cell membrane by interfering with the sodium channel and these include local anesthetics, antifibrillar and antiarrhythmic drugs with mexiletine being the drug of choice.

Paramyotonia congenita

The cardinal feature of this condition is mytonia that appears with exercise and increases with continued exercise. It is made worse by the cold and is most obvious in the muscles of the face, neck and distal upper extremities. Weakness after prolonged exercise and exposure to cold is seen in most cases. Spontaneous bouts may occur in some families, much as those seen in hyperkalemic periodic paralysis (see below). It is a dominant condition with complete penetrance.

Symptoms are usually present from birth, though bouts of weakness, with hyperkalemia may not appear until after adolescence if at all. Sensitivity to hot and cold environments varies tremendously. Ingestion of potassium can induce bouts of paramyotonic hyperkalemic periodic paralysis. EMG always shows myotonic discharges and the CK is often elevated. Both the stiffness and weakness are caused by long lasting depolarization of the muscle fiber membrane.

Antiarrhythmic drugs such as mexiletine are effective in preventing muscle stiffness and weakness induced by physical activity or a cold environment. The majority require no treatment.

In paramyotonic hyperkalemic periodic paralysis the combined use of mexiletine and hydrochlorothiazide can prevent stiffness and weakness induced by the cold and spontaneous bouts of paralysis.

OTHER FORMS OF MYOTONIA

There can be considerable clinical heterogeneity between families with SCN4A mutations.[469] Individuals with paramyotonia, showing cold and exercise induced stiffness but no cold induced weakness are described. Another group of children show fluctuating stiffness throughout the day (myotonia fluctuans) but never show weakness and are not cold sensitive. Their symptoms are exercise provoked (they are often acetazolamide responsive). A further form leads to severe and permanent myotonia (myotonia permanens) that shows continuous myotonia, particularly affecting muscles of the neck, shoulder and chest. At times this leads to impairment of ventilation, hypoventilation with cyanosis and loss of consciousness with the possibility of a misdiagnosis of epilepsy. Treatment with carbamazepine can be successful.

In all these children careful assessment of the history, clinical examination, neurophysiology and DNA testing should lead to the correct diagnosis and approach to therapy.

Hyperkalemic periodic paralysis

This is a dominantly inherited condition with complete penetrance in both sexes. It may present with or without myotonia or with paramyotonia. Attacks usually begin before the age of 10 and slowly increase in frequency. A common time of presentation is before breakfast and episodes may last from 15 min up to an hour and then spontaneously disappear. The episodes are triggered by rest and they are often provoked by previous exercise. Potassium loading often precipitates an episode, and these are worsened by the cold, stress, glucocorticoids or pregnancy. Some episodes are heralded by paresthesia or a sensation of muscle tension.

The generalized weakness is usually accompanied by a significant increase in serum potassium (up to 5 to 6 mmol/L). Just occasionally the potassium can reach cardiotoxic levels. Cooling can induce weakness but not stiffness and reheating restores power.

Although probably caused by the common Val-704-MET mutation in the SCN4A gene, normokalemic period paralysis differs from the hyperkalemic form by showing urinary potassium retention, a lack of a beneficial effect of glucose and failure of the serum potassium to increase during episodes.

Diagnosis of hyperkalemic periodic paralysis is based on the presence of a history of typical bouts of weakness, paralysis, myotonia or paramyotonia and a family history. The muscles are often well developed, the CK mildly elevated. Where diagnostic doubt exists, a potassium load may induce an episode.

During an episode the sodium channels open and the sodium moves into muscle cells causing a fall in serum sodium of between 3 and 9 mmol/L. Water follows the sodium causing hemo-concentration and an increase in the serum potassium. This in turn leads to potassium excretion in the urine, which may itself curtail the attack. Five mutations in the SCN4A gene are associated with the clinical syndrome of hyperkalemic periodic paralysis.

Preventative therapy consists of frequent meals, rich in carbohydrate, a low potassium diet and the avoidance of fast and strenuous work and exposure to cold. The prompt intake of a thiazide diuretic or acetazolamide or the inhalation of a beta-adrenergic agent can curtail episodes in some people. Continuous use of these diuretics is not recommended.

Familial hypokalemic period paralysis

The incidence of this disease is estimated to be about 1 in 100 000, making it the most common of the familial periodic paralyses. It is an autosomal dominant trait with reduced penetrance in women (the male to female ratio is 3–4 : 1). It is linked to 1q31-q32 and co-segregates with the gene encoding the alpha-one subunit of the L-type calcium channel skeletal muscle.

Most people with the condition present in childhood. Initially episodes are infrequent and gradually become more frequent and ultimately daily.

Episodes vary in severity from slight temporary weakness of an isolated muscle group to generalized paralysis. Episodes usually occur in the second half of the night and on awakening the arms, legs or trunk cannot be moved. Occasionally respiratory failure can occur. Strength gradually increases as the day goes on.

Episodes are triggered by strenuous physical activity or a carbohydrate rich meal on the preceding day. There may be an associated bradyarrhythmia. During episodes the potassium decreases (not always below normal) and there is urinary retention of sodium, potassium, chloride and water.

If the serum potassium cannot be investigated during a spontaneous attack, a provocation test in a specialized unit can be pursued using glucose load or glucose plus insulin to cause hypokalemia.

Mild episodes need no treatment. Generalized paralysis should be treated with potassium. General advice includes the avoidance of heavy exercise and the ingestion of carbohydrate rich meals. The medication of choice is acetazolamide.

THE INFLAMMATORY MYOPATHIES

Juvenile dermatomyositis (See also Ch. 27)

The estimated incidence of juvenile dermatomyositis in the UK and Ireland is 1.9 per million aged under 16 years.[470] The median age of onset in this study was 6.8 years with five girls affected to each boy. The cause remains unknown. There is an association with HLA-B8/DR3 but the adult association with malignancy is not seen in children. It is a systemic vasculopathy associated primarily with inflammation of skin and muscle. About 10% of children with dermatomyositis test positive for myositis-associated antibody (MSA) (compared to about 50% of adults), and 60% are positive for antinuclear antibodies. The MSA is directed against Mi-2 most commonly (in adults it is most often toward one of the tRNA synthetases). About 50% of children have circulating evidence of endothelial damage, whilst others have different indicators of disease activity such as elevated neopterin, or increased circulating B cells with peripheral lymphopenia.[471] Heterogeneity of this sort may well be associated with differing outcomes and in time define more specific approaches to therapy.

Presentation

The onset is usually insidious with slowly increasing proximal muscle weakness. Affected muscles are stiff, sore and tender and occasionally indurated. Non-pitting edema or thickening of the overlying skin may be seen. Bulbar muscles may be involved and occasionally weakness is so severe that respiratory failure ensues.

The skin lesions often have a characteristic violaceous (heliotrope) hue best seen on the eyelids (Fig. 20.31). The skin over the extensor surfaces of joints often becomes erythematous, atrophic and scaly, capillary loops may be prominent in the nail beds. Pigmentation may appear in these areas in time. A papular or pustular eruption may appear in the same position in oriental children.[472] A malar butterfly rash may appear similar to that seen in systemic lupus erythematosus. Calcification of subcutaneous tissues may occur.

There may be gastrointestinal involvement with functional large or small bowel symptoms or bleeding, arthropathy, fever, pulmonary disease, iritis and very occasionally seizures.

Diagnosis

High levels of muscle enzymes usually mirror muscle inflammation. Biopsy shows an inflammatory infiltration with

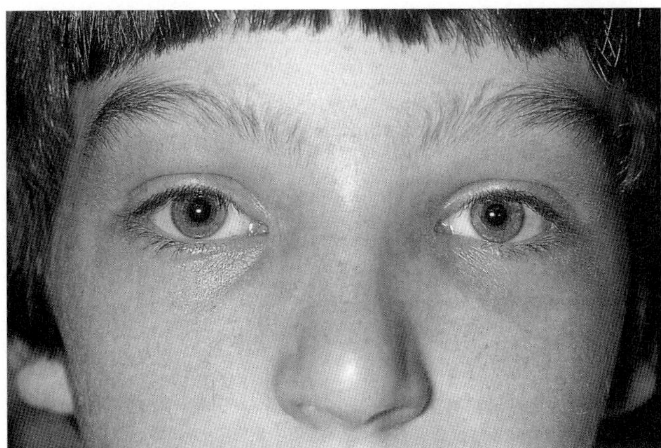

Fig. 20.31 Dermatomyositis: heliotrope rash around eyes.

muscle fiber necrosis and macrophage activity. Real diagnostic difficulty only arises when the rash is not evident. The differential diagnosis then includes conditions that may give insidious weakness including postinfectious polyneuropathy, metabolic and endocrine myopathies, myasthenia gravis or acute infectious myopathies.

Treatment

Many children will respond well to corticosteroid treatment. A starting dose of prednisolone 1 mg/kg/day is used, tapering off over 6–12 months. Further immunosuppression may be required and azathioprine is a valuable agent in a dose of 2.5 mg/kg/day. Low dose ciclosporin may also be used starting at 4 mg/kg/day.

A number of centers have reported that intravenous immunoglobulin therapy has allowed the dose of steroid to be reduced in resistant cases.[473] Intravenous methylprednisolone and methotrexate may prove to be effective in children with severe dermatomyositis – defined as those with associated dysphagia and severe vasculitis.[474] Great care must be taken with the supportive care of those children with bulbar involvement. Oral feeding should be suspended when dysphagia is present and serial measurements of forced expiratory volume made. Ventilatory support may be required.

Outcome

The outlook with modern immunosuppressant therapy is generally good. Before steroids up to 40% died, usually from bulbar and respiratory involvement. Tabarki et al[475] followed 36 children for a mean of 4.9 years. Twenty-eight of the children (78%) were well without functional impairment; five had inactive disease but with functional impairment and three had retained their active disease. Fifteen children developed dystrophic calcifications, which in five affected function. There is no satisfactory treatment for calcinosis though aluminum hydroxide[476] and alendronate[477] have both been reported to bring benefit. Excision might be considered where functional impairment is significant. The best indicators of a good outcome were early treatment and a low creatine kinase level at diagnosis.

Acute infectious myositis

Viral myositis

This may occur in association with Coxsackie, echo and influenza viral infections. The presentation is of acute, distressing muscle aches, which are often symmetrical, and most commonly affects the thighs. There may be associated weakness. Occasionally it is very focal, affecting only one group of muscles. Viral invasion of muscle has not been demonstrated, but biopsy does show muscle cell necrosis and an inflammatory cell infiltrate. The creatine kinase may not be raised, although it usually is. Treatment is symptomatic and the condition is self-limiting and benign.

Pyogenic myositis

The commonest cause is *Staphylococcus aureus*. It is usually secondary to a penetrating injury, although in the tropics it may result from spreading infection from a superficial wound. There is intense local pain, swelling and loss of function. Treatment is with antibiotics and drainage as appropriate.

Parasitic myositis

Infestation with *Trichinella spiralis* results from the ingestion of undercooked, infested pork. Fever and myalgia are the commonest presentations. There may be periorbital edema, if periorbital muscles are involved or even dysphagia where bulbar muscles are involved. The calves, forearms or paraspinal muscles may be painful. Treatment is with thiabendazole 25–50 mg/kg/day or with mebendazole 100–200 mg twice daily and steroids. Mebendazole may have fewer unwanted effects.[478] Recovery is usually complete.

In cysticercosis, if infection is heavy, then muscle may be affected.

Rarer forms of myositis

Congenital or infantile myositis

This was described by Shevell et al[479] and more recently by Vajsar et al.[480] Hypotonia and weakness are marked. Ventilatory support has often been required. The diagnosis is by muscle biopsy. Some cases are steroid responsive but the pathophysiology is poorly understood.

Inclusion body myositis

This is exceptional in childhood and presents as a chronic myositis simulating a dystrophy. The biopsy shows sarcoplasmic vacuoles containing basophilic and eosinophilic inclusions. The cause is unknown and treatment is usually ineffective.

METABOLIC MYOPATHY (see also Ch. 24)

Metabolic myopathies are the result of genetic defects of energy production, which may affect muscle alone or may also affect other high energy dependent tissues. The defect may be in glycogen or fatty acid metabolism or in mitochondrial oxidative phosphorylation.

Presentation may be with progressive weakness, recurrent symptoms of exercise intolerance, reversible weakness and myoglobinuria or both. Neonates and infants frequently present with severe multisystem disorders. In recent years advances in the understanding of the biochemical and genetic basis for many of these disorders has lead to new diagnostic tests. Nonetheless a specific enzyme abnormality could be detected in only 24% in a series of children with recurrent myoglobinuria.[481]

The glycogenoses

These defects of glycogen metabolism are rare and only those with prominent muscle involvement are included in Table 20.48.

Defects of mitochondrial fatty acid oxidation

Beta-oxidation results in the sequential cleavage of two carbon atoms from fatty acids and provides an important energy source during times of fasting and metabolic stress. Clinical features of muscle involvement include recurrent rhabdomyolysis and/or weakness and muscle pain provoked by prolonged exercise, which may occur some time after the

Table 20.48 Glycogen storage diseases with muscle involvement

Enzyme defect	Clinical features		Inheritance
Acid maltase (Pompe's disease)	Infantile	Hypotonia, weakness, cardiomegaly, hepatomegaly, respiratory and feeding difficulty, death usually before 2 years	AR
	Juvenile	Muscle weakness proximal > distal, selective respiratory muscle involvement	
	Adult	Slowly progressive myopathy, one-third present with respiratory failure	
Myophosphorylase (McArdle's disease)	Muscle pain, weakness, stiffness during slight-moderate exertion, 'second wind' phenomenon, ↑ CK		AR
Phosphofructokinase (Tarui's disease)	Exercise intolerance, hemolysis		AR
Phosphoglycerate kinase	Exercise intolerance, muscle cramps, myoglobinuria, CNS involvement-learning difficulty epilepsy		XR
Debranching enzyme deficiency	Protuberant abdomen, muscle aching, progressive weakness		AR

exercise. Rhabdomyolosis may also occur during intercurrent infection. Proximal weakness without pain or rhabdomyolysis may also occur. Cardiomyopathy frequently occurs with dysrhythmia and/or progressive cardiac failure. Pigmentary retinopathy and peripheral neuropathy may also be seen. The most common presentation of this group of conditions in childhood is with hypoketotic hypoglycemia. These are all autosomal recessive conditions.

Diagnosis of these conditions requires a high level of suspicion. It is essential to obtain urine and blood samples during the acute episode and biochemical abnormalities may not be present when the patient is well. Initial investigations should include urine organic acids, CK, lactate, carnitine and acylcarnitine profile. Mutational analysis is available for the common mutations found in medium chain acyl-CoA dehydrogenase (MCAD) and long chain 3-hydroxyacyl-CoA dehydrogenase (LHCAD) deficiency. Specific enzyme analysis can be performed for many of these conditions on cultured fibroblasts. Table 20.49 lists the features of muscle involvement in some defects of beta-oxidation.

Defects of oxidative phosphorylation (OXPHOS)

Oxidative phosphorylation occurs in the mitochondria. Mitochondrial DNA encodes for only 13 subunits of the OXPHOS enzymes with more than 70 nuclear encoded subunits.

Isolated muscle involvement is unusual in this group of conditions in childhood. In a population based study of OXPHOS disorders in childhood in Sweden 8 out of 32 patients had myopathy, 6 infantile mitochondrial myopathy with cytochrome oxidase (COX) deficiency and 2 myopathy.[482]

A defect of OXPHOS is suggested by high plasma lactate, the finding of ragged red fibers or COX-deficient fibers on muscle biopsy. Electron microscopy of muscle biopsy may show structurally abnormal mitochondria with paracrystalline inclusions. OXPHOS enzyme analysis can be performed on muscle.

THE MYASTHENIC SYNDROMES

Myasthenia gravis

This is an autoimmune disorder, which is heterogeneous with respect to age at onset, ophthalmic changes and distribution of muscle weakness. Our knowledge of immunogenetic factors and thymic abnormalities in the causes of the different forms is still emerging.

The annual incidence is between 0.25 and 2 people per 100 000. Although there has been an increase in the incidence for the over 40s, in the childhood age range, incidence appears to be static. Boys and girls are equally affected in the first decade although the incidence in adolescence rises in girls with a ratio of three girls to two boys.

In most young people, myasthenia gravis is caused by autoantibodies specific for the human nicotinic acetylcholine receptor (AChR), which is concentrated at the postsynaptic region

Table 20.49 Defects of beta-oxidation of fatty acids

	Clinical features
Primary carnitine deficiency	Progressive muscle weakness, cardiomyopathy, hypoglycemia in some
Carnitine palmitoyl transferase II deficiency	Recurrent myalgia, rhabdomyolysis induced by fasting or prolonged exercise
Very long chain acyl-CoA dehydrogenase deficiency	Exercise induced myalgia and rhabdomyolysis (presentation most often with hypoglycemia)
Medium chain acyl-CoA dehydrogenase deficiency	Rarely muscle pain, lipid storage myopathy, rhabdomyolysis
Short chain acyl-CoA dehydrogenase deficiency	Slowly progressive proximal lipid storage myopathy, secondary carnitine deficiency
Riboflavin responsive multiple acyl-CoA dehydrogenase deficiency	Muscle pain, proximal weakness, improvement with riboflavin
Long chain 3-hydroxyacyl-CoA dehydrogenase deficiency and mitochondrial trifunctional protein deficiency	Proximal myopathy, rhabdomyolysis, peripheral neuropathy, pigmentary neuropathy

of the neuromuscular junction. These antibodies cause impaired neuromuscular transmission and muscle weakness.

There appears to be an immunogenetic predisposition to the development of idiopathic myasthenia gravis. Those with early onset myasthenia gravis have different HLA associations from those with late onset myasthenia gravis. Those with onset in childhood and adolescence also have an increased frequency of other autoimmune diseases. Monozygotic twins are at increased frequency of concordance and some families have more than one member affected. In Chinese and Japanese populations up to 30% present in early childhood, many with ocular myasthenia only. They show an association with HLA-BW46. This suggests that a particular environmental agent could be important. In Caucasians, about 60% of those with early onset myasthenia gravis are HLAB8 and DR3 positive.

Myasthenia gravis is associated with 30–60% of thymomas and about 10% of affected people of all ages have a thymoma.

Clinical features

The onset may be insidious or sudden. A common presentation is with ptosis and diplopia due to weakness of the extraocular levator palpebrae muscles. This may or may not then spread to involve proximal limb and bulbar muscles. Respiratory muscles may also be involved. Lower limb muscle involvement is relatively rare. The weakness is variable and commonly progresses as the day goes on. This may lead a child to have difficulty with chewing and swallowing at the time of the evening meal. The weakness can remain localized to one group of muscles for many years, commonly the eye muscles. In some the weakness may only be obvious with tests of fatigue, for example, sustained upward gaze or repetitive shoulder abduction. Tendon reflexes are normal and there is no sensory impairment.

If symptoms and signs remain confined to the eyes (ocular myasthenia) for longer than 2 years the risk of subsequent development of generalized myasthenia gravis is low. Titers of antibodies to AChR are lowest in ocular myasthenia, although if the disease does become generalized the antibody titers tend to become positive.

Hoch and colleagues[483] showed that a high proportion of people without antibodies to AChR have antibodies to a muscle specific receptor tyrosine kinase, MuSK.

Antibodies in myasthenia gravis lead to a functional loss of acetylcholine receptors at the neuromuscular junction by complement-dependent lysis of the postsynaptic membrane; cross-linking AChRs on the surface of the membrane lead to an increase in the rate of internalization and degradation of AChR and also direct inhibition of AChR function.

The importance of the recently discovered presence of MuSK antibodies in AChR negative myasthenia gravis has yet to be defined. MuSK is an essential component of the developing neuromuscular junction and MuSK antibodies might cause complement-mediated damage to the neuromuscular junction.

The thymus gland is probably necessary for the deletion of auto-reactive T cells and has an important role in the pathogenesis of myasthenia gravis, even without the presence of a thymoma. In most children and adolescents the thymus is typically enlarged and contains many germinal centers with T and B cell areas very similar to those seen in lymph nodes. B cells obtained from the thymus spontaneously synthesize anti-AChR and thymic T cells are clonally restricted. A few T cells cloned from the thymus have proved specific for AChR epitopes. It seems probable that thymoma epithelium sensitizes T cells to these AChR epitopes and that T cells leave the thymus and initiate antibodies against AChR and other muscle antigens.

Investigations

AChR antibodies are positive in 85% of young people with generalized disease. When present this finding is diagnostic. Peripheral neurophysiology shows an increased decrement (greater than 10%) of the evoked compound muscle action potential in response to repetitive supramaximal stimulation.

Edrophonium (Tensilon) is a short acting anticholinesterase. When this is given intravenously there is a rapid (usually within 2 min), but often short lived (less than 5 min) improvement in strength (Fig. 20.32). Interpretation can be difficult, however. It must be remembered there is a small risk of inducing a cholinergic crisis with respiratory arrest.

Once the diagnosis is made, computed tomography or magnetic resonance imaging of the mediastinum should be carried out to exclude an associated thymoma. Thyroid function and thyroid antibodies should be measured because of the association with other autoimmune disease.

In childhood and adolescence, where ocular myasthenia is relatively common, the main diagnostic dilemma is distinguishing it from mitochondrial cytopathy. It must be remembered that 50% of those with ocular myasthenia are AChR antibody negative. For those with generalized myasthenia who are also antibody negative the difficulty is differentiating their problem from other neuromuscular disorders and other disorders of the neuromuscular junction. If the onset of bulbar myasthenia is sudden, a brainstem stroke also enters the differential diagnosis.

Treatment

The first line management is with oral anticholinesterase drugs such as pyridostigmine. The dose should be titrated carefully with the response, remembering that too high a dosage can lead to a cholinergic crisis. Children under 20 kg should receive a dose of 30 mg initially. Those over about 20 kg should have 60 mg initially. The dosage can then slowly be increased in increments of 15–30 mg daily until maximum improvement is obtained. Total daily requirements are usually in the range of 30–360 mg. The effect of the drug usually wears off within 3–4 h and the timing of the doses needs to be made accordingly. Unwanted gastrointestinal effects may occur, in particular abdominal pain and diarrhea. These may be countered with the use of propantheline.

Thymectomy is usually performed in children or adolescents who are AChR antibody positive with generalized myasthenia. Evidence from retrospective uncontrolled studies suggests benefit.[484] Thymectomy is rarely carried out for ocular myasthenia and for those who are AChR antibody negative. It nonetheless demands careful consideration where the symptoms prove to be anticholinesterase resistant.

Where symptoms are not well controlled, immunosuppression is indicated. Alternate day prednisolone is generally used, starting with a low dose, which is gradually increased (high doses may exacerbate myasthenia). On remission, the dose is gradually reduced. Azathioprine may have a steroid sparing effect. In severely affected young people, plasma exchange or intravenous immunoglobulins can bring temporary improvement. These are useful strategies if the person involved poses an anesthetic risk prior to thymectomy.

Other neuromuscular junction disorders

The Lambert–Eaton syndrome

This is caused by antibodies to voltage gated calcium channels on the presynaptic nerve terminals of the motor nerve. Peripheral neurophysiology reveals a small compound muscle action potential at rest and an increase in the amplitude of the action potential after maximal voluntary contraction. Antibodies to voltage gated

(a)
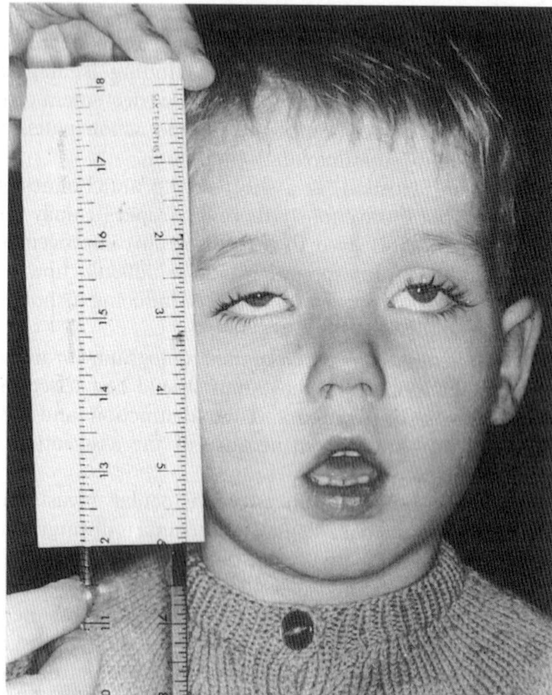

(b)
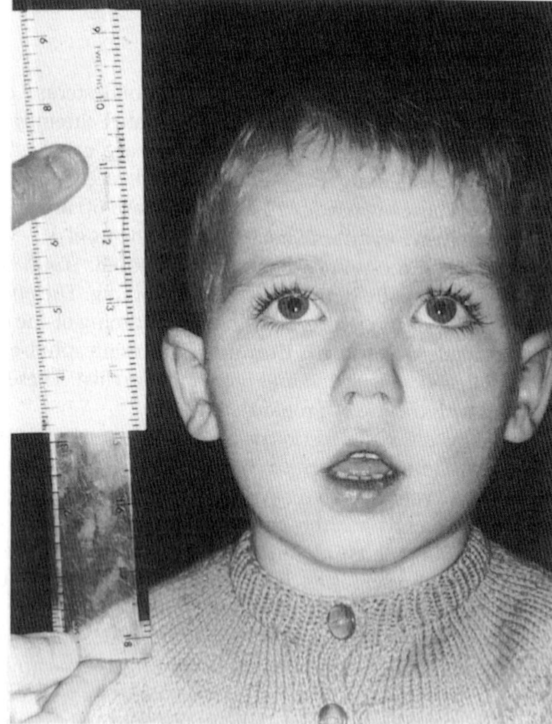

Fig. 20.32 Myasthenia gravis (a) before and (b) after intravenous edrophonium.

calcium channels can be detected in most. 3,4-Diaminopyridine prolongs the motor nerve action potential thus increasing neurotransmitter release. It can be effective when used in combination with the anticholinesterases.

Acquired neuromyotonia

This is caused by antibodies to the voltage gated potassium channels present on motor nerve terminals. Most patients present with muscle twitches (fasciculations and myokymia) and cramps. The condition may be present alongside neuropathies or those with myasthenia gravis (particularly in the presence of a thymoma). Muscle weakness is often the major complaint. Membrane stabilizers such as carbamazepine may improve symptoms.

Congenital myasthenic syndromes

The congenital myasthenic syndromes are a group of genetic disorders of neuromuscular transmission. Fatiguable muscle weakness occurs and in some, progressive weakness and wasting may occur. They are very rare conditions but notable because respiratory crises may occur, especially in childhood, and some will benefit from treatment with anticholinesterases. The defect may be presynaptic, synaptic or postsynaptic. Gene mutations responsible for a number of these conditions have now been identified.

In childhood, presentation is usually with feeding difficulty, episodic respiratory difficulty, motor delay, facial weakness, impaired eye movements and fatiguable ptosis. With the exception of slow-channel syndrome, inheritance of these conditions is autosomal recessive.

Confirmation of the diagnosis may be difficult. Brief improvement in muscle strength following i.v. injection of edrophonium may help confirm clinical suspicion but some conditions will not respond to anticholinesterases or may even be worsened. Neurophysiology may be helpful especially if a decrement of more than 10% in compound muscle action potential occurs on repetitive stimulation or increased jitter on single fiber EMG. Cytochemical and morphological analysis of the neuromuscular junction is confined to centers with a research interest in this group of conditions. Increasingly the underlying genetic defect will be used in diagnosis and classification of these conditions (Table 20.50).

SPINAL MUSCULAR ATROPHY

Spinal muscular atrophy (SMA) is the result of anterior horn cell disease. The spinal muscular atropies are clinically and genetically heterogeneous. By far the most common type of SMA is proximal SMA caused by deletions in the SMN1 gene. Other types of SMA are very much rarer.

Proximal SMA

Spinal muscular atrophy (SMA) is the second most frequent lethal gene disorder in Caucasians after cystic fibrosis. Prevalence is 1/10 000. SMA is inherited in an autosomal recessive fashion; carrier frequency is estimated to be 1/40–1/60. The majority of cases are due to deletions within the SMN1 gene, the telomeric copy of the Survival of Motor Neurone gene on chromosome 5q12.2-q13.3. This area on the short arm of chromosome 5 is complicated with an inverted duplication containing the SMN, Neuronal Apoptosis Inhibitor Protein (NAIP) and P44 genes.[485] The SMN1 gene is the causative gene in SMA but the NAIP gene may influence severity with 67% of type I patients having deletions in the first two exons. The telomeric copy (SMN1) and the centromeric copy (SMN2) of the SMN gene differ by 7 base pairs, which results in a splicing difference. There is evidence in transgenic mice that increasing the number of copies of the SMN2 gene ameliorates the severity of the disease. In humans some mutations in SMAII and SMAIII patients may be gene conversions with SMN1 being replaced by SMN2.[486] There is some correlation between SMN protein levels and disease severity.

In proximal SMA, weakness is more severe in the legs than the arms and is more marked proximally than distally. Intercostal muscles are affected with diaphragmatic sparing. Clinically there is

Table 20.50 The classification of the congenital myasthenic syndromes

		Clinical features	Response to anticholinesterase	Inheritance	Gene defect
Presynaptic	Familial infantile myasthenia	Onset in neonatal period Severe episodic respiratory and bulbar weakness Facial weakness Fatiguable ptosis No eye movement impairment	+	AR	Unknown
Synaptic	End plate acetylcholinesterase (AChE) deficiency	Early onset Fatiguable generalized weakness Slowly progressive	–	AR	ColQ mutations (ColQ polypeptide binds AChE tetramers)
Postsynaptic	Acetylcholine receptor (AChR) deficiency	Early onset Feeding difficulty Ptosis Impaired eye movements Motor delay	+ 3,4-Diaminopyridine may also be useful	AR	AChR ε subunit mutations
	Fast channel syndrome	Similar to AChR deficiency	–	AR	AChR ε subunit AChR α subunit mutations
	Slow channel syndrome	Onset variable Weakness of scapular muscles and finger extensors Slowly progressive	– Quinidine sulfate is beneficial	AD	Mutations described in AChR α, β, δ, ε subunits

a wide spectrum in the severity of SMA. Classification is clinical and based on age of onset and motor function. Life span however depends on respiratory and bulbar function. Within a type there is also a range of severity such that Dubowitz suggested classification should be on a decimal scale, type 1.0 to 1.9 and so on.[487]

Onset may be prenatal, with profound weakness, including facial weakness, contractures and respiratory failure in the neonatal period. Onset within the first 2 months of life is associated with early death. A few infants with SMA type I will have more prolonged survival. Infants with SMA type I are alert with normal facial expression; there is tongue fasciculation, and the limbs are profoundly weak (Fig. 20.33). Often the forearms are contracted in pronation leading to the classic 'jug handle' posture. Bulbar problems with aspiration and the need for tube feeding are invariable. Death is from respiratory causes.

Children at the more severe end of SMA type II may develop respiratory compromise early and will benefit from aggressive management of respiratory complications including the use of NIPPV. The majority of children with type II SMA can be expected to survive beyond childhood. Children with SMA have a hand tremor, polyminimyoclonus, which is very characteristic.

Individuals with SMA type III walk with a waddling gait and increased lumbar lordosis. Life expectancy is not affected (Table 20.51).

Spinal muscular atrophy with respiratory distress (SMARD)

The presentation of this condition is usually with respiratory distress due to diaphragmatic paralysis; often there is eventration of the diaphragm. Limb weakness is more marked in the upper limbs and distally.

SMARD is genetically heterogeneous. Inheritance is autosomal recessive and recently mutations in the immunoglobulin mu-binding protein2 have been found in patients with the condition.[488]

Pontocerebellar hypoplasia type 1 (PCH 1)

This condition is characterized by neonatal onset, congenital contractures, ventilatory insufficiency and early death.[489] There is neurophysiological and histopathological evidence of anterior horn cell disease. Hypoplasia of the brainstem and cerebellum is seen on brain imaging. Linkage to the SMN1 gene has been excluded.[490] No gene locus has yet been identified.

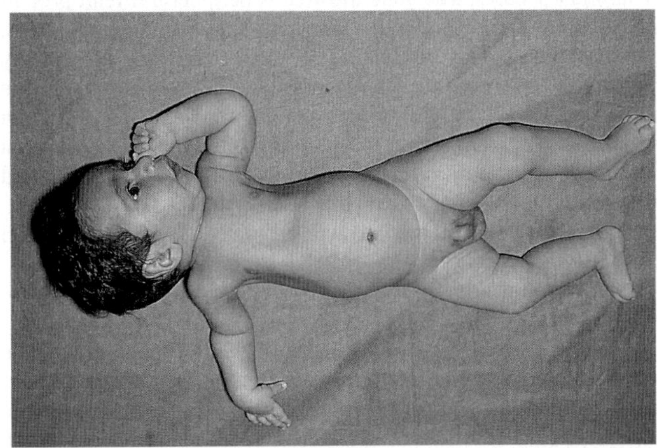

Fig. 20.33 SMA type I: alert infant with severe limb and intercostals muscle weakness.

Table 20.51 SMA; clinical spectrum

Type	Age of onset	Motor skills	Life expectancy
I Werdnig–Hoffmann	<6 months	Never sits alone	80% die by 1 year
II Intermediate	6–18 months	Sits alone, unable to walk	Variable
III Kugelberg–Welander	>18 months	Walks more than 4 steps alone	Normal

Spinal muscular atrophy, congenital benign with contractures

A number of families have been described with lower limb deformity present at birth and complete sparing of the upper limbs.[491] Motor and sensory nerve conduction is normal with giant motor units present on EMG. The condition is non-progressive and inheritance is autosomal dominant. The gene locus is on chromosome 12q23-q24.[492]

THE INHERITED NEUROPATHIES

Introduction

Tooth, in 1886, described five cases with predominantly distal limb weakness and wasting, later referred to as peroneal muscular atrophy, suggesting that the primary pathology was in nerve.[493] In the same year Charcot and Marie described five further cases of peroneal muscular atrophy.[494] Despite their conclusion that the primary pathology was probably in the spinal cord, their names along with that of Tooth became eponymously associated with inherited neuropathies. Over the past decade, rapid progress has been made in defining the mutant genes causing this heterogeneous group of conditions. The nomenclature used has therefore also been in a state of flux with neurologists tending to use the term hereditary motor sensory neuropathy (HMSN) and in the genetic literature the term Charcot–Marie–Tooth is more commonly found. The CMT nomenclature is now in more widespread use and applies to a wide range of hereditary peripheral neuropathies with a population prevalence of approximately 1 in 2500.

The basic division of CMT is into type 1, representing demyelinating neuropathies, and type 2 representing axonal neuropathies. The division is based on electrophysiological criteria, the demyelinating group demonstrating a median nerve motor conduction velocity of less than 38 msec and the axonal group a velocity of greater than 38 msec.

The genes and proteins involved

CMT 1A is the most common form of CMT 1 and is caused by a 1.5 Mb duplication of chromosome 17p11.2.[495] This accounts for 70% of all CMT 1 cases. The gene involved is peripheral myelin protein 22 gene (PMP22). Deletions in this gene, rather than duplications, can also occasionally cause CMT 1A, although they are usually responsible for hereditary neuropathy with liability to pressure palsies (HNPP).[496] HNPP presents in adult life. Human myelin protein 0 (P_0) gene is on chromosome 1q22-q23. Autosomal dominant point mutations in this gene lead to CMT 1B and occasionally the axonal neuropathy CMT 2 phenotype.[497]

Mutations in the early growth response 2 gene (EGR2) on chromosome 10 cause the rare CMT 4.[498]

Point mutations in the Connexin 32 gene (CX32) cause X-linked CMT.[499]

The myelin proteins PMP22, P_0 and CX32 all play a part in the maintenance of myelin integrity. P_0 is an abundant myelin protein accounting for 50% of peripheral myelin protein. It transverses the Schwann cell membrane once and contributes the homophilic linkages between adjacent myelin lamellae thus bonding together the concentric myelin wraps.

PMP22 accounts for only 2–5% of peripheral myelin protein. Its role is unknown, though it is thought to play a part in cellular growth.

Connexin 32 is a gap junction protein. It mediates the formation of intracellular gap junctions between the folds of Schwann cell cytoplasm, particularly in the paranodal regions. These act as a channel for the transport of electrolyes and metabolites between the myelin wraps of an individual cell, the flow extending to the axon.

Phenotypes

CMT 1 refers to autosomal dominant demyelinating CMT. Most affected people present in childhood or adolescence with a slowly progressive distal wasting and weakness, associated with evolving areflexia, distal sensory loss and pes cavus. Affected people show evidence of demyelination and remyelination with onion bulb formation and Schwann cell proliferation on nerve biopsy.

Affected males with the disease arising from point mutations in the CX32 gene present in a way indistinguishable from those with CMT 1. Carrier females are mildly affected.

Dejerine–Sottas disease and congenital hypomyelinating neuropathy (CHN) represent a more severe phenotype. They present in the first 10 years of life with extremely slow motor conduction velocities. Point mutations in PMP22, P_0 and EGR2 can exist in either the heterozygous or the homozygous state, meaning these conditions may be either dominant or recessive.

A number of gene loci have been identified in families with autosomal recessive demyelinating neuropathies (referred to as HMSN type 1 autosomal recessive or CMT 4). To date eight loci have been identified and three genes discovered on chromosomes 11, 8 and 19.

Autosomal dominant CMT 2 carries the same phenotype as CMT 1 though symptoms tend to develop later, in less severe form with preserved reflexes. Six loci and two genes are described. One gene is on chromosome 8p21 and is involved in neurofilament organization and regulation.[500] A further gene on chromosome 1p35-p36 is a member of the kinesin family of proteins, which are important in the transportation of mitochondria.[501] An X-lined form of CMT 2 has been described in association with deafness and mental retardation.[502]

No causation genes have been identified for the recessive forms of CMT 2.

The clinical approach

Most children presenting with CMT present with motor difficulties of some sort. There may be an earlier history of motor developmental delay and hypotonia, or the story may be of slowly increasing unsteadiness, falling off in performance in games at school, or increasing tightness in the tendo-Achilles with the emergence of pes cavus making shoe fitting ever more difficult. Sensory symptoms tend to be mild and late.

More severe forms, the recessive variety of CMT 1 and CMT 2 in particular, may present with what appears to be a cerebellar ataxia with a scanning dysarthria. This means when children are investigated for ataxia the possibility of CMT should be considered.

The common clinical picture is that of a pattern of wasting and weakness of the calves and small muscles of the feet, pes cavus, hammer toes and broadening of the forefoot appearing later (Fig. 20.34). Weakness and wasting of intrinsic hand muscles is also frequently present (Fig. 20.35). The tendo-Achilles tend to be tight. In the forms of CMT with a faster rate of progression, bilateral foot drop may emerge. These forms tend to have an earlier loss of tendon reflexes with the emergence of sensory symptoms and signs.

The first investigation is peripheral neurophysiology. In most children, assessment of the motor nerve conduction velocities will help define whether this is a demyelinating or axonal neuropathy. Where the neuropathy is demyelinating a common duplication in the PMP22 gene can be sought. This will account for almost 70% of children in the CMT 1 group.

When interpreting the nerve conduction velocity results it must be remembered that when the nerves are inexcitable, this may not necessarily be due to severe demyelination. Not infrequently nerves undergoing severe axonal degeneration become inexcitable also.

Clearly the family history is a useful adjunct in reaching a diagnosis and in this way the CMT may be classified as dominant, recessive or in the absence of male to male transmission probably X-linked. In a typical small family, however, this is often impossible.

Many laboratories also offer screening for PMP22, P_0 and CX32 point mutations though the other rarer genes mentioned have only been identified in interested research laboratories.

In a child or adolescent with clinical and neurophysiological CMT 1, where there is no evidence of male to male transmission, no chromosome 17 duplication and nothing to suggest Dejerine–Sottas disease or congenital hypomyelinating neuropathy, screening should be carried for CX32 mutations. If negative, mutations in P_0 and PMP22 should then be screened, followed lastly by ERG2, if available. In the very small number of remaining demyelinating cases, especially the more severe ones with a suggestion of recessive transmission, MTMR2 and perixin should be screened where possible.

In the axonal form of CMT most genes are not yet known. If there is no male to male transmission, and especially if the index case is female, CX32 should be screened first. If this is negative, P_0 should be screened next as in all other cases. If these are both negative the rarer genes might then be sought.

In the intermediate cases, as always the first check should be for the duplication on chromosome 17. If this is negative and there is no male to male transmission it is advisable to check CX32 next and then P_0 in all remaining negative cases. Finally if this is negative it is worth checking PMP22 and ERG2 for point mutations.

Hereditary sensory and autonomic neuropathies (HSAN)

Hereditary sensory neuropathies are rare, accounting for 3% of hereditary neuropathies in the European population.[503] In this group of disorders there is loss of one or several modalities of sensation with less prominent clinical involvement of motor and autonomic function. Prominent features in presentation therefore are a conspicuous alteration of pain sensation related to the preferential progressive atrophy of small myelinated (delta) and usually the unmyelinated (C) nerve fibers.

Affected children may well therefore cause concern with painless burns, fractures, indolent ulcers and self-mutilation in infancy. Repeated injury may lead to an incorrect diagnosis of non-accidental injury.[504]

The HSANs are clinically and genetically heterogeneous; Table 20.52 gives the characteristics of the main types.

ACUTE NEUROLOGICAL CONDITIONS

The approach to the child with decreased conscious level should be systematic. There are many potential causes and many specific treatments need to be considered. Reduced conscious level may be difficult to detect in infants and in all children may be obscured by the other features at presentation.

Initially it may not be apparent that the child has a primary neurological problem. For example, a high fever or abnormal cardiac or respiratory signs may distract the clinician. Conversely, reduced conscious level is most commonly caused by problems outside the CNS, e.g. hypoxia of primary respiratory or cardiac origin. Treatment of these will often improve CNS function and conscious level. In the emergency situation, the approach recommended in the APLS (Advanced pediatric life support) manual[505] should be followed. These follow the ABC (Airway, Breathing, Circulation) principles of resuscitation. This systematic approach will address problems in other organ systems that are affecting the CNS. For example, in a child with meningococcal septicemia, reduced conscious level may be prominent at presentation but securing an adequate airway, optimizing oxygenation and treating shock will improve CNS function.

CLINICAL ASSESSMENT

The main causes of decreased conscious level are shown in Table 20.53. The initial history should concentrate on detecting these and, for example, a history of recent trauma, previous seizures or potential drug ingestion will guide appropriate investigations and may suggest specific treatments.

Symptoms of raised intracranial pressure (ICP) include poor feeding, vomiting, irritability, lethargy and seizures. Signs include a full fontanel (in babies), scalp vein distension, macrocephaly,

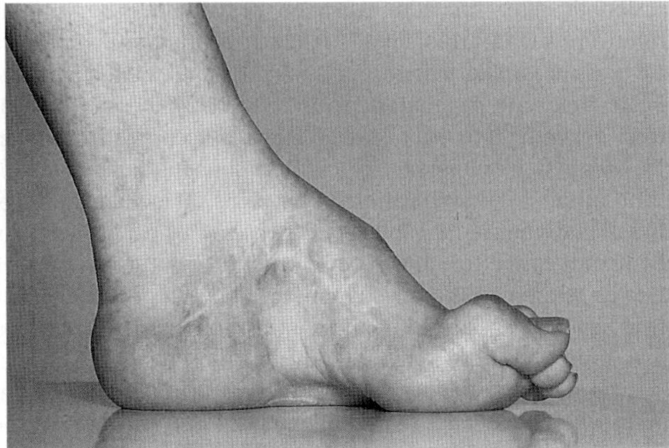

Fig. 20.34 CMT: pes cavus and clawing of toes.

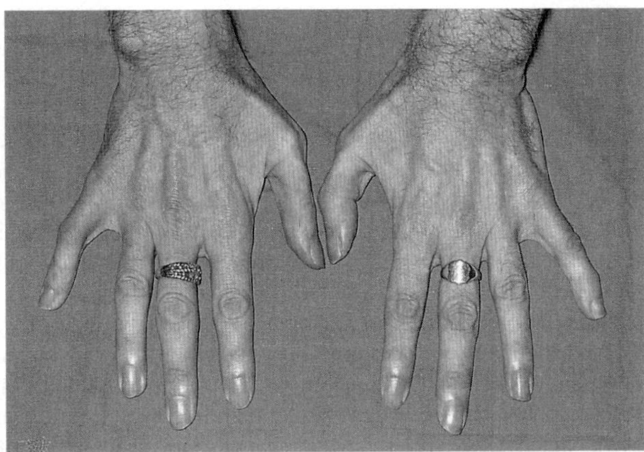

Fig. 20.35 CMT: wasting of intrinsic hand muscles.

Table 20.52 The current classification of HSAN

Type	Clinical features	Inheritance	Gene
I	Onset after first decade Lack of pain sensation, reduced sweating especially over distal lower limbs Mild-moderate lower limb weakness Hyporeflexia Abnormal sensory conduction, motor conduction normal	AD	SPTLC1 (Serine palmitoyl transferase long chain base subunit 1)
II	Early onset Fungiform papillae absent from tongue Repeated trauma, ulcers, infected sores on hands and feet Diminished pain, temperature and touch sensation No weakness Reflexes absent or decreased Absent sensory nerve action potentials, normal motor nerve conduction velocities	AR	Unknown
III Riley-Day	Feeding difficulty from birth Absence of tears Abnormal temperature control Postural hypotension Emotional lability Absent fungiform papillae from tongue Absent corneal reflexes Relative indifference to pain Absent flare to intradermal histamine Reflexes decreased or absent Motor nerve conduction velocities slightly slow Sensory conduction normal	AR	IKBKAP (Inhibitor of kappa light polypeptide gene enhancer in B cell, kinase complex-associated protein)
IV	Anhydrosis with recurrent fevers Painless injury and self-mutilation Learning difficulty frequent Reflexes preserved	AR	Receptor tyrosine kinase for nerve growth factor TRKA
V	Early onset Painless injuries of extremities No weakness Normal reflexes Normal motor and sensory conduction	Uncertain, presumed AR	Unknown

bradycardia, hypertension, abnormal respiratory patterns, and focal neurological deficits including false localizing signs, particularly sixth nerve palsies.

Clinical examination should be thorough. General examination should seek signs suggestive of the causes in Table 20.53, e.g. the rash of meningococcal disease. In school-age children the conscious level should be assessed using the Glasgow Coma Score (GCS) (Table 20.54). In the preschool child the verbal response component of the GCS is unreliable and modified coma scores have been proposed (Table 20.54). In the intubated child modifications to the GCS use grimace rather than vocalization. Whilst in adults the GCS is well validated and scores have been shown to have prognostic significance, this is not yet the case in children. However, a coma score of 8 or less should generally prompt intubation, as the child is unlikely to be able to protect the airway adequately. The coma score is a useful tool for the ongoing assessment of the encephalopathic child, in order to detect improvement or deterioration in the child's condition.

It is important to complete and document a neurological examination early in the assessment of the unconscious child. Management of the child may include ventilation, sedation and muscle paralysis, which are likely to interfere with later assessments. Particular attention should be paid to pupil size and reactivity. Pinpoint pupils may be a sign of poisoning, particularly with opiates and barbiturates. Small reactive pupils are a feature of medullary lesions and mid-size, non-reactive pupils of mid-brain lesions. Fixed dilated pupils are an ominous sign, often indicating terminal coning, but can also occur temporarily, after severe hypoxia and as a consequence of hypothermia, seizure activity and occasionally after the administration of certain drugs, notably barbiturates such as thiopental. Metabolic conditions can cause all these types of pupillary abnormality. A unilateral dilated pupil may indicate incipient herniation, causing dysfunction of the third cranial nerve. This is particularly likely to occur with ipsilateral space occupying lesions, such as extradural hematomas.

The fundi should be examined for signs of metabolic disease, retinal hemorrhage and papilledema. Absence of papilledema does not rule out raised ICP and does not indicate that it is necessarily safe to do a lumbar puncture. Voluntary and reflex eye movements should be assessed, facial weakness and asymmetry looked for and bulbar muscle functions tested. When oculocephalic reflexes are preserved (doll's eye movements) the eyes are able to maintain fixation when the head is moved side to side or up and down. When these are lost the eyes move with the head. Oculovestibular reflexes (caloric responses) are usually tested as part of brainstem death

Table 20.53 Important causes of acute encephalopathy

Infectious and parainfectious encephalopathies
Meningitis (mainly bacterial, rarely fungal, protozoal and viral)
Cortical thrombophlebitis
Cerebral abscess and empyema
Primary viral encephalitis
Postinfectious encephalitis
Acute disseminated encephalomyelitis
Cerebral malaria
Severe systemic infections, including septicemia
Hypoxic ischemic encephalopathies
Perinatal asphyxia
Severe pulmonary disease
Carbon monoxide poisoning
Methemoglobinemia
Severe anemia
Status epilepticus
Near miss sudden infant death syndrome
Post cardiac arrest
Cardiac bypass surgery
Near drowning
Cardiac arrhythmias
Congestive cardiac failure
Hypotension
Disseminated intravascular coagulation
Hypoglycemia
Anesthetic accidents
Vitamin or cofactor deficiencies (B_{12}, B_6, folate, etc.)
Trauma
Accidental
Non-accidental
Exogenous toxins
Drugs:
Antihistamines, anticholinergics, antidepressants, hypnotics & sedatives, analgesics, antiepileptics, anti-inflammatory, antimetabolites, antibiotics, etc.
Illicit substances:
Alcohol, solvents, cannabis, cocaine, amfetamines, opiates
Environmental toxins:
Carbon monoxide, phosphates, DDT, iron, lead, pesticides, heavy metals, insect & snake venoms, plants, etc.
Hypothermia
Heat stroke
Endogenous agents
Water intoxication
Electrolyte imbalances, esp. hypo & hypernatremia
Acidosis & alkalosis
Scalds
Endocrine disorders:
Diabetes mellitus, hypoglycemia, hypo & hyperthyroidism, hypo & hyperparathyroidism, hypopituitarism, hypoadrenalism
Organ failure:
Hepatic, renal, pancreas
Hypertension
Inborn errors of metabolism:
Aminoacidopathies, organicacidurias, urea cycle defects, fatty acid oxidation defects, mitochondrial disorders, carnitine deficiency, porphyria
Cerebrovascular disease
Hemorrhagic stroke
Ischemic stroke
Epileptic seizure related
Postictal
Nonconvulsive status epilepticus
Postconvulsive status epilepticus

tests and require the eardrum to be intact. Deviation of the eyes towards a cold water stimulus and away from a warm water stimulus occurs.

The child's body posture and any abnormal movements should be noted. The presence of decorticate (arms flexed, legs extended) or decerebrate (arms and legs extended) postures are particularly significant. Tone, power, reflexes and plantar responses in the limbs should be documented and interpreted in the light of recently administered drugs such as neuromuscular blockers.

INVESTIGATIONS

During the primary assessment and resuscitation blood should be taken for FBC, U&E, calcium, blood cultures and blood glucose. Specific treatments such as glucose for hypoglycemia, antibiotics for meningococcal septicemia and calcium for seizures caused by hypocalcemia may be indicated. Further investigations which will aid the supportive care of the child include arterial blood gases, coagulation screen and urine and plasma osmolality (Table 20.55).

Subsequently, further investigations may be indicated for specific conditions. These may include a toxicology screen, blood alcohol level, specific drug levels (such as anticonvulsants), plasma ammonia and lactate levels and liver function tests. Urine for amino and organic acids and porphyrins should be collected. An early CT scan is usually indicated unless a cause for the child's condition is apparent. Lumbar puncture should usually be deferred at least until the results of this are known.[506,507] An X-ray skeletal survey may be useful at this point if non-accidental injury is suspected. Children who are hypoglycemic should have blood and urine collected whilst hypoglycemic or immediately thereafter for later metabolic investigations. Laboratory advice should be sought on the samples required and their subsequent handling and storage.

CONTINUING MANAGEMENT

The continuing management of the child with reduced conscious level is directed at maintaining homeostasis and at detecting and treating the underlying cause. Maintenance of cerebral perfusion pressure (CPP), cerebral blood flow (CBF) and normal cerebral metabolism are important. Raised ICP should be detected and treated. However, CPP is also affected by systemic factors such as hypotension. Children in coma require repeated reassessment and skilled neurological nursing usually on an intensive care or high dependency unit. Specific therapy for certain causes of encephalopathy, such as hemodialysis for removal of drugs after overdose, may be required.

The physiology of intracranial pressure, cerebral perfusion pressure and cerebral blood flow

Intracranial pressure

Raised ICP can arise by a number of different mechanisms. The commonest causes are intracranial space occupying lesions, CNS infections, hydrocephalus, intracranial hemorrhage, metabolic disease (with cerebral edema), meningeal inflammation (reducing CSF resorption) and dural sinus thrombosis (raising

Table 20.54 Glasgow Coma Scale and Children's Coma Scale (modified Glasgow Coma Scale)

Eyes	Score	Best motor response	Score	Best verbal response		Score
Glasgow Coma Scale						
Open		*To verbal command*				
Spontaneously	4	Obeys	6	Orientated and converses		5
To verbal command	3	*To painful stimulus*		Disoriented and converses		4
To pain	2	Localizes pain	5	Inappropriate words		3
No response	1	Flexion – withdrawal	4	Incomprehensible sounds		2
		Flexion abnormal	3	No response		1
		Extension	2			
		No response	1			
Children's Coma Scale						
Spontaneous	4	Spontaneous (obeys verbal command)	6	Smiles, orientated to sound, follows objects, interacts		5
Reaction to speech	3	Localizes pain	5	*Crying*	*Interacts*	
Reaction to pain	2	Withdraws in response to pain	4	Consolable	Inappropriate	4
No response	1	Abnormal flexion in response to pain (decorticate posture)	3	Inconsistently consolable	Moaning	3
		Abnormal extension in response to pain (decerebrate posture)	2	Inconsolable	Irritable restless	2
		No response	1	No response	No response	1

GCS total 3–15; CCS total 3–15

venous pressure) are the commonest. A rise in ICP may lead to secondary brain shifts with herniation of brain contents. A critical reduction in perfusion to the brain may result leading to disability or death.

Cerebral edema has several pathological types. Both focal and generalized cerebral edema can cause raised ICP and decreased consciousness. Focal cerebral edema may be associated with localized brain dysfunction and focal neurological signs. Generalized cerebral edema may be associated with false localizing signs. Vasogenic edema results from changes in capillary permeability and occurs with CNS infections, head trauma and in encephalopathies due to toxins, hypertension and seizures. Osmotic edema is seen in hyponatremia, diabetic ketoacidosis and excessive fluid resuscitation. Cytotoxic edema is secondary to intracellular energy failure and occurs with hypoxic–ischemic insults, status epilepticus and severe infection. Hydrocephalus may result in transependymal resorption of CSF and periventricular interstitial edema. Finally, loss of cerebral autoregulation as occurs with systemic hypertension and in hypercapnia results in hydrostatic edema.

Table 20.55 Useful investigations in coma

Basic hematological & biochemical investigations, including glucose, Ca, Po_4, Alk P & LFTs
Markers of inflammation, including ESR & CRP
Blood & urine osmolality
Blood clotting studies
Bacteriological & virological studies including cultures, serology, PCRs, Mantoux, etc.
Neuroimaging:
Ultrasound, CT, MRI
Blood gases
Plasma ammonia
Plasma lactate
Urine toxicology
Blood toxicology – alcohol, lead & specific toxins where indicated
Blood anticonvulsant levels
Urine metabolic screen
Urine amino and organic acids
CSF examination including lactate and glycine if indicated
TFTs & other endocrine investigations if indicated
Blood & urinary porphyrins
Skeletal survey
EEG

In children under 12–18 months the open sutures enable the skull volume to increase and large intracranial masses may accumulate without rapid or large rises in ICP. After 2 years of age the cranial cavity behaves more like the adult with a fixed volume. The development of cerebral edema as a normal response of the central nervous system to injury causes an increase in the volume of the brain. With the volume of the skull cavity fixed there will inevitably be either diminution in the total volume of CSF spaces and/or diminution of the pool of venous blood within the skull. As ICP increases there will be an increased resistance to inflow of arterial blood and thus a fall in the cerebral perfusion pressure. Cerebral perfusion pressure (CPP) = the mean systemic blood pressure (SBP) – the mean ICP. A fall in CPP leads to a fall in the CBF and if this is below 20 ml/100 g of tissue per min, brain ischemia will develop. Brain ischemia further increases the formation of cerebral edema leading to a further rise in ICP. If CBF falls below 10 mL/100 g per min electrical dysfunction of the neurones and loss of intracellular ion homeostasis occurs.

Generalized rises of ICP will first cause transtentorial and eventually transforaminal herniation. Unilateral increases in ICP, for example secondary to hematoma, will cause ipsilateral uncal herniation and compression of the third nerve against the free border of the tentorium with ipsilateral pupillary dilation secondary to loss of parasympathetic constrictor tone to the ciliary muscles. Uncontrolled further herniation will cause, in addition, contralateral third nerve palsy. At the same time the brainstem is shifted downward to the foramen magnum, which impairs the blood supply to the brainstem from the perforating branches of the basilar artery and results in brainstem ischemia. The signs of cingulate gyrus herniation, tentorial herniation and foramen magnum coning are given in Table 20.56.

Monitoring ICP can be useful in head trauma, certain metabolic encephalopathies and in intracranial infection. There is little evidence

Table 20.56 Clinical features of brain herniation

Tentorial
Sunsetting
Dilated pupils
VI nerve palsy
Cortical blindness
Hemiplegia
Extensor motor pattern (decerebrate)
Coma
Respiratory irregularity
Systemic hypertension
Tonic seizures
Cingulate gyrus herniation
Diplegia or hemiplegia
Visual symptoms
Foramen magnum cone
Cardiorespiratory arrest
Bulbar palsy
Neck stiffness
Hypotonia
Stridor
Spinal flexion
Hypotension
Hyperthermia

of benefit in Reye's syndrome, hepatic encephalopathy or hypoxic–ischemic injury (such as post cardiac arrest). A number of techniques have been described for monitoring ICP.[508] All depend on the principle, which is generally but not invariably correct, that the pressure within the cranium is the same in all departments. The preferred technique will depend on whether ventricular dilation is present or whether the ventricles are small and shifted as a result of the brain swelling. In the child with cerebral edema it is possible to monitor the ICP continuously by the use of a subdural or subarachnoid Teflon catheter. In infants this can be placed percutaneously through the anterior fontanel. Ventricular transducers record either the ventricular pressure, or if not in the ventricle, the brain parenchymal pressure. Cerebral intraparenchymal devices are also available. The normal ICP in adults is 0–15 mmHg (0–2 kPa). In the newborn, older infants and toddlers the upper limits are 3.5 mmHg, 5.5 mmHg and 6.5 mmHg respectively.[509]

Brief rises in ICP may occur during coughing, straining and crying, as well as other physiological activities that increase the central venous pressure. Sustained elevations or intermittent rises in pressure in the form of pressure waves may also occur and may require treatment. An increase in the ICP may come about as a result of increasing the brain, blood or CSF contents of the skull. The increase in ICP that results from a given increment in volume depends on the ICP–volume status. As the ICP increases small changes in volume may result in significant changes in pressure.

Cerebral perfusion pressure

With increasing ICP there is an increase in the cerebral venous pressure. This remains about 3 mmHg below the ICP so that cerebral circulation continues. The cerebral perfusion pressure is the difference between the mean systemic arterial pressure (MAP) and the ICP, i.e. CPP = MAP – ICP.

The relationship between ICP and cerebral perfusion pressure is complex. Raised ICP may be caused by an increase in CBF or it may be the limiting factor producing a reduction in CBF. In encephalopathies the brain is frequently pale and devoid of blood flow as a result of raised ICP producing ischemia. The normal cerebral perfusion pressure is 60–70 mmHg. There is a progressive fall in brain perfusion with decreasing CPP down to a CPP of 40 mmHg. Below this ischemic infarction may result.

Cerebral blood flow

During acute encephalopathy there are changes in general and regional cerebral blood flow (CBF). Cerebral autoregulation is the maintenance of cerebral blood flow by alteration of the cerebral blood volume in response to large changes (increases or decreases) in the systemic perfusion pressure. Cerebral autoregulation is often impaired (globally or regionally) with encephalopathy so that CBF is related directly to systemic arterial pressure. Excessive blood flow (luxury perfusion) is sometimes seen after hypoxic–ischemic injury. It is possible using the Fick principle to measure changes in CBF but this is rarely used in clinical practice. Ordinarily there is coupling between CBF and brain metabolism but in coma the cerebral metabolic rate for oxygen falls as well as the CBF.

The main determinant of CBF is the arterial $PaCO_2$. Increases in the arterial $PaCO_2$ increase CBF due to cerebral vasodilatation whilst decreases in arterial $PaCO_2$ reduce CBF due to cerebral vasoconstriction. Changes in CBF cause changes in the cerebral blood volume and this influences the ICP. Inducing hypocapnia by hyperventilation can reduce ICP (if the raised ICP had been due to cerebral vasodilatation). If, however, the CBF is already low from cerebral edema then hyperventilation will result in worsening ischemia. The cerebral circulation will readjust vascular tone to lowered $PaCO_2$ levels over time. The effect of hyperventilation can be used for controlling acute rises in ICP. In the intensive care setting $PaCO_2$ is generally kept at 4.0–4.5 kPa. Levels below this risk causing infarction in areas of relative ischemia.

Treatment of raised ICP

Major principles involved in the treatment of raised ICP are summarized in Table 20.57. The child's airway should be secured. Intubation is usually indicated if the GCS is 8 or less. As previously discussed, the arterial concentration of CO_2 has a significant effect on CBF and hence cerebral perfusion. Maintenance of a normal or high normal blood pressure is beneficial and inotropic support is

Table 20.57 Management of raised intracranial pressure

1. Optimize metabolic state	Maintain normal blood glucose Avoid hyponatremia and hypocalcemia Maintain normal temperature
2. Maintain cerebral perfusion	Maintain cerebral perfusion pressure above 60 mmHg Maintain BP at normal levels or above Ventilate to achieve low normal $PaCO_2$ (4.0–4.5 kPa) Maintain high-normal oxygenation PaO_2 (12–14 kPa)
3. Improve cerebral venous return	Head-up tilt (15–20 degrees)
4. Reduce effect of cytotoxic edema	Fluid restriction to 75% of maintenance Once hemodynamically stable give intravenous mannitol (0.2–0.5 g/kg)
5. Avoid secondary insults	Prompt treatment of seizures (anticonvulsants) Minimize external stimuli (appropriate sedation and paralysis)

often beneficial. Adequate pain relief and sedation are important to reduce changes in ICP from arousal, coughing, etc. Reducing fever will reduce whole body and cerebral metabolism.

Specific treatment may be aimed at reducing the volume of CSF, blood or brain (including brain edema). Removal of CSF is possible through a ventricular cannula but this may not be possible if the ventricles are compressed. The technique has been particularly advocated in tuberculous meningitis. Hyperventilation should not be used prophylactically, as prolonged hyperventilation is associated with a significant risk of brain ischemia. However, it can be useful to treat episodic increases in ICP. The $PaCO_2$ level should be reduced to no lower than 3.5–4.0 kPa. At other times it should be kept at 4.0–4.5 kPa.[510]

Seizure activity should be promptly controlled. Clinical detection of seizures may be difficult or impossible, particularly when neuromuscular blocking agents are being used. Continuous EEG monitoring has an important role. Phenytoin and phenobarbital are the antiepileptic drugs most commonly used in the ICU setting. Both have important cardiorespiratory depressant effects and these should be looked for carefully.

There is no role for the routine use of steroids to control raised ICP.[511,512] However, they are useful in reducing the focal edema around mass lesions and postoperatively. In haemophilus meningitis, steroids reduce the incidence of subsequent sensorineural deafness.[513]

Mannitol increases serum osmolality and reduces brain water by controlled hyperosmolar dehydration. If mannitol and furosemide (frusemide) (dose 0.5–1 mg/kg) are used together, the circulating volume is decreased and, depending on the central venous pressure, volume expansion may be necessary. Mannitol is given in a dose of 0.25 to 0.5 g/kg per dose. The effect may last only 6 h and rebound rises in ICP may be seen. Mannitol is used to treat acute rises in ICP rather than as a regular or prophylactic agent. It should be used with caution in the presence of impaired renal function as hyperosmolality and renal failure may ensue.[514]

Barbiturates produce a reduction in cerebral metabolic rate and CBF. Their use is restricted to those patients with unrelieved raised ICP despite appropriate use of other therapies such as inotropes, ventilation, mannitol and, if appropriate, steroids. It is important to monitor the systemic blood pressure carefully during their use since hypotension, causing a reduction in the cerebral perfusion pressure often occurs. Inotropes are usually needed.

The role of controlled hypothermia in the treatment of raised ICP is controversial. There are theoretical benefits from reduction of cerebral metabolism. Complications of hypothermia include respiratory infection and cardiovascular compromise that impair optimal oxygenation and could have a deleterious effect. Current published studies are inconclusive. Reports of the benefits of decompression craniotomy are anecdotal.

Once the ICP has remained normal for 48 h the measures instituted can be gradually reversed, one at a time whilst monitoring continues.

OUTCOME

The underlying cause of the coma determines the outcome. In non-traumatic encephalopathy, overall mortality is around 30%. In those children who survive, 25% will have a degree of neurological impairment. Children whose encephalopathy has an infectious or hypoxic–ischemic cause do worst whilst children with metabolic causes for their coma generally do better. The factors affecting outcome in traumatic head injury are dealt with in the relevant sections below. As children recover from their encephalopathy regular neurological and developmental assessment is required in order to detect impairments. Physical problems such as hemiparesis or quadraparesis are often detectable within the first few weeks. Cognitive, psychological and behavioral impairments may take months to become apparent. This is particularly recognized after traumatic brain injury. Tests of hearing and vision should be routinely undertaken. Involvement of a clinical or neuropsychologist in the rehabilitation period to assess deficits and advise on behavioral and educational support is useful. The establishment of dedicated rehabilitation teams, often nurse led, will facilitate optimal recovery[515] and give expert advice to hospital and community services with regard to long term management.

The persistent vegetative state

There has been considerable interest in the diagnosis of the persistent vegetative state. This is characterized by the patient being awake, but without being aware, and occurs in those who have suffered severe and irreversible damage to their cerebral cortex, but whose brainstem function remains to some degree intact. Those affected may open their eyes, have sleep–wake cycles and chew and swallow. Such skills may be misinterpreted as signs of awareness. The diagnosis is particularly difficult in children and it is extremely hard for the family not to hope for improvement. There is a continuum of awareness and responsiveness and it may not be possible to draw a line beyond which a child is said to be in the persistent vegetative state, even for legal purposes. In children who have very low levels of functioning, good nursing care and support for the family is important. Decisions around resuscitation, should deterioration or cardiac arrest occur, should only be made after full discussion with the family and should be regularly reviewed to ensure they are still appropriate. Cultural and religious views must be taken into account. With the recent adoption of the Human Rights Act, ethical issues in this area may change.

Brain death

In the UK it is accepted that permanent functional death of the brainstem is equivalent to brain death. In patients where brainstem death is established actual death always follows, although this may be delayed if mechanical ventilation is continued. Its diagnosis depends on the absence of brainstem function for at least 24 h, once hypothermia and drug intoxication have been excluded. At least in the UK, EEG evidence is not needed and the diagnosis remains clinical. The use of organs of brain dead individuals for transplantation has led to standardized methods for diagnosis of brain death.

Two senior doctors working independently perform tests of brainstem function. The core temperature should be above 35°C and there should be no hypovolemia or biochemical abnormalities. No drugs that can affect the level of consciousness or respiratory function should be still acting. It may be difficult to establish if this criterion is satisfied in children who have been given anticonvulsants, especially barbiturates, during their illness. Drug levels may be helpful. There should be no treatable metabolic or endocrine cause for the coma. The mechanism of injury or underlying cause for the irreversible coma should be known. The child must be unconscious with no change in state and no sleep–wake cycles. There should be no response, including heart rate, to a central painful stimulus, e.g. supraorbital pressure. There must be ophthalmoplegia with fixed dilated pupils and no gag, cough, oculocephalic or oculovestibular reflexes. An apnea test is carried out (5–8 min of apnea without any ventilation at the end of which the $PaCO_2$ should be equal to or greater than 6.7 kPa or 56 mmHg). Adequate oxygenation is provided throughout the test by oxygen introduced at 6–10 L/min via a tracheal cannula.

If the brain death criteria are satisfied, then ventilation may be terminated or, where indicated by the relatives and where there is no objection from the legal authorities (coroner in England and Wales, Procurator Fiscal in Scotland), organ donation may take place.

It has been debated whether adult criteria for brainstem death apply to children, particularly infants. The President's Commission in the USA, that developed brain death criteria there, believed that they did. In the USA, evidence of the cessation of higher mental function, in addition to that obtained from clinical evaluation, is required. This may involve the use of EEG and brainstem evoked potentials along with techniques to demonstrate absence of CBF. These include radionuclide cerebral angiography, cerebral Doppler ultrasound and xenon CT. Such techniques may be particularly useful if the administration of drugs makes clinical assessment difficult. There are no published reports of children who have survived after fulfilling adult brain death criteria.

SPECIFIC CAUSES OF ACUTE ENCEPHALOPATHY

Traumatic brain injury

Accidental head injuries are common in children and the majority will have a straightforward course with a good outcome. However, head injury causes one-third of accidental deaths in children. Boys outnumber girls at all ages and there is a preponderance of children from lower socioeconomic groups and children with previous learning and behavioral difficulties. The population incidence is 2–3 per 1000 per year. Around 5% of these are severe injuries (GCS 8 or less) and 5–10% are moderate (GCS 9–12) (Table 20.54).

Most reports on the epidemiology of head injuries in children obtain data from recordings of hospital admissions, attendances at accident and emergency departments or from returns on death certificates, giving mortality rates. However, many factors will affect these figures such as the degree of access to local hospitals, the provision of local health care facilities, medical admission policy, socioeconomic status of the patients, the local environment (city or rural) and the amount of preventive legislation.[516] It is probable that published figures for both incidence and mortality of head injury are an underestimate of the true figures. Though mortality is reducing with modern assessment and management (Fig. 20.36) there is still a major role for preventative measures. These include compulsory seat belts, back-facing baby car seats, speed control by cameras and traffic calming measures, cycle helmets and modification of children's playgrounds with a forgiving surface such as forest bark and rails on slides. Most injuries result from falls or road traffic accidents, with the child as pedestrian, although the causes of head injury vary with the age of the child (Fig. 20.37).

The Royal College of Paediatrics and Child Health have recently published guidelines on the acute management of head injury in children.[517]

Mechanisms of brain injury

Trauma can cause brain primary (or immediate) brain injury and secondary (or delayed) head injury.

Primary brain injury

A high velocity, high energy impact over a small area will cause a depressed or complex skull fractures and penetrating trauma. Knives, scissor blades and screwdrivers can penetrate the vault of the skull. Gunshot wounds are rare in the UK. Accidental penetrating injuries through the orbit or nose with sticks, pencils and toys occur. Objects in the mouth may penetrate the tonsillar fossa and cause carotid artery injury. There may be a delay of a day or more before the onset of neurological signs, as a dissecting aneurysm forms. Cavernous sinus thrombosis or caroticocavernous fistulae can result from intracranial injuries to the carotid artery. Blows, car accidents and falls commonly cause low velocity impacts and often lead to linear skull fractures. At the time of injury, linear or rotational forces of acceleration or deceleration cause deformation of the skull and its contents. The commonest primary brain injuries seen are due to shearing or contusion.

Shearing injury occurs when the brain moves, often with a rotational component, at the time of impact. There is disruption of axons in the subcortical or deep white matter with associated hemorrhage. Lesions may also be seen in the corpus callosum particularly on MRI. In children with significant diffuse axonal injury, early CT scans may appear normal. Some axonal disruption can be shown pathologically even following minor head injury associated with loss of consciousness. Contusion of the brain is often seen on the side opposite to the site of impact (contra coup injury). This most usually affects the frontal or temporal lobes. It is thought to be secondary to the brain abutting the bony prominences in these areas. Areas of edema, with small hemorrhages, represent localized nerve damage and disruption. Compression injuries and lacerations of the brain are occasionally seen.

Secondary brain injury

Much of the focus in the management of head injury has been on the prevention of secondary brain injury. It is assumed that primary

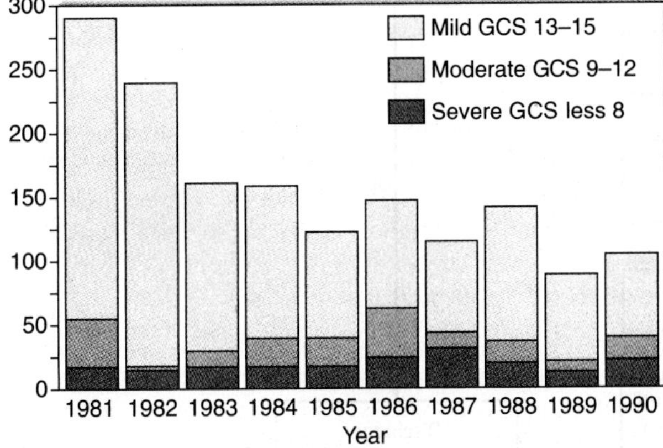

Fig. 20.36 Head injury in children under 16 years over a 10-year period. GCS, Glasgow Coma Score.

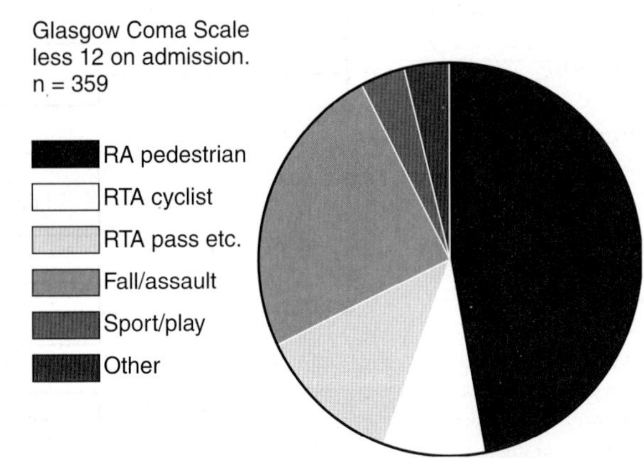

Fig. 20.37 Causes of accidental head injury in children under 16 years.

brain injury is established by the time the child is seen at hospital. The clinical scenario of the child who 'talks and dies' is well known and although not all of these deaths are preventable, a number are.[516]

Associated thoracic, abdominal and pelvic injuries have the potential to cause additional brain injury. Skilled resuscitation will minimize the impact of these on the brain. Hypoxic–ischemic injury may be secondary to airway or chest trauma, blood loss or direct injury to cerebral vessels. Raised ICP and status epilepticus need to be recognized and promptly treated. Cerebral autoregulation may be impaired. Diffuse brain swelling is common following severe head injury in children and may have a number of causes. It may take 24 h or more to reach its peak. Monitoring of ICP and treatment of raised ICP and/or CPP following traumatic brain injury is widely advocated. The use of controlled hypothermia is routine in some neurosurgical units.

Intracranial hemorrhage (extradural hematoma, acute subdural hematoma, subarachnoid and intracerebral hemorrhage) may occur soon after injury or be delayed by several weeks (chronic subdural hematoma). It is unusual, even in infants, for the amount of blood loss intracranially to, by itself, cause shock and other sources of blood loss should be sought. Intracranial hemorrhages are usually seen in moderate or severe head injuries and rarely occur as an isolated injury.

Neuroimaging

The use of CT scanning has revolutionized the management of head injuries. CT scans are excellent for visualizing blood, bone and CSF. The main advantages are precise anatomical location of intracranial hematomas and accuracy in the diagnosis and differentiation of intracerebral, subdural and extradural hematomas.

Ultrasound may be useful in young children with an open anterior fontanel both for imaging and by utilizing Doppler for monitoring possible raised ICP and its subsequent response to treatment. There are great advantages in a portable, bedside and easily repeatable investigation with no radiation risk. The main disadvantages are the need for a 'window' through the skull through which to operate. Magnetic resonance imaging is mainly used to correlate neuroradiological abnormalities with functional disability in those children with residual neurological or neuropsychological deficits.[518]

Guidelines published on neuroimaging following head injury by the Royal College of Paediatrics and Child Health are shown in Figure 20.38.

Early complications of traumatic brain injury

Skull fractures

Forty per cent of infants hospitalized with cranial trauma have skull fractures, but sequelae in the form of intracranial hematoma occur in only 8–22%. Leggate et al[519] showed that all infants, under 6 months of age, operated on for an extradural hematoma, had either a skull fracture or suture separation seen on X-ray. In a group of 40 infants with extradural hematomas, 90% had an abnormal X-ray. Most skull fractures are linear.

The skull in the neonate consists of poorly mineralized membranous bone. Linear fractures due to birth trauma occur but are rare in the compressive head injuries associated with traumatic

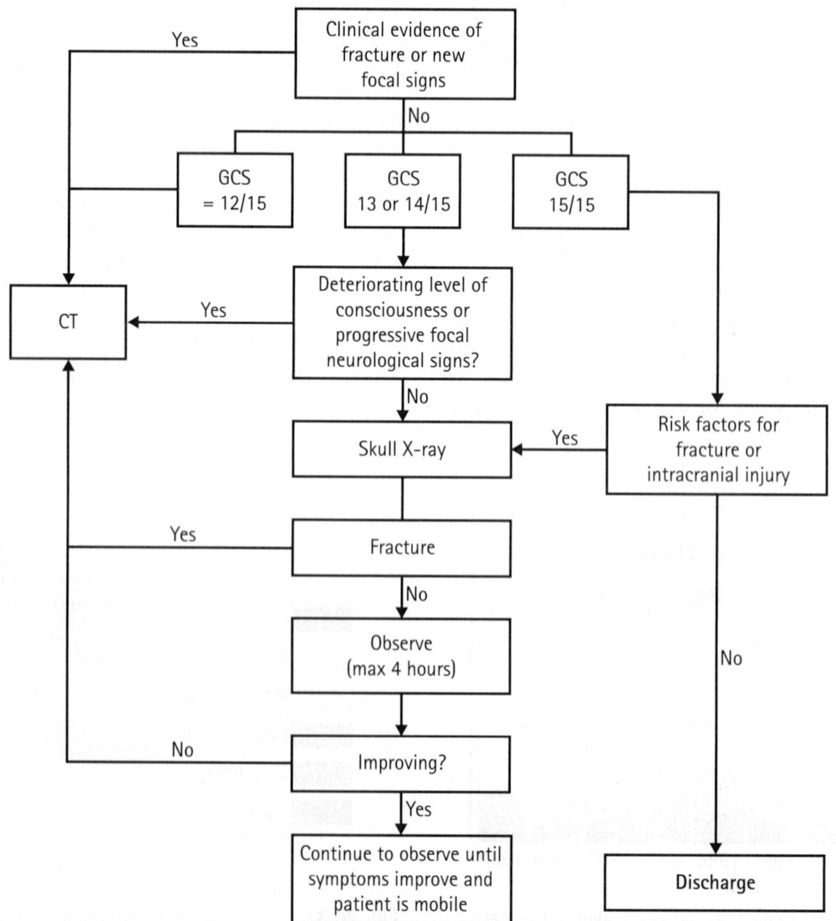

Fig. 20.38 Use of radiographic investigations in patients (> 5 years of age) with a head injury.

deliveries, unless the baby is postmature. Under these circumstances, it offers little protection to the underlying brain, which is easily compressed in a ping-pong ball or Pond fracture. These may be associated with severe localized bruising and hemorrhage into the brain with minimal fracture.

Skull fractures do not heal by callus formation and so dating of the time of injury is difficult. If the edges are rounded and smooth, it is more than 2 weeks old. At autopsy, the margins are heaped, smooth and discolored with hemosiderin. A skull fracture normally heals in 2–3 months and has disappeared on X-ray by 6 months. In small infants the fracture site may not heal but form a growing skull fracture. This may present as a palpable, pulsating lump. Diagnosis is by X-ray. Management consists of closure of the underlying dural defect with natural or artificial membrane and closure of the bony defect either with an acrylic graft or a graft from the patient's own bone.

Most skull fractures are only medically significant if they:

- are depressed
- go through the anterior fossa and cribriform plate, allowing CSF rhinorrhea and a risk of meningitis
- go through the petrous temporal bone into the ear, allowing CSF otorrhea and a risk of meningitis
- enter the sinuses or is across the skull base with brainstem injury.

Compound fractures, secondary to penetration injuries, may be obvious, or subtle (e.g. orbital trauma from an object such as a pencil or sharp pointed stick penetrating the medial aspect of the orbit, passing into the ethmoid sinus and through the cribriform plate into the intracranial cavity in its subfrontal compartment). Another common site for a penetrating injury is the temporal region. In all such cases, extensive preoperative investigation is required, including CT scanning and MRI angiography, prior to a thorough exploration of the penetrating tract with debridement of damaged brain and formal closure of the dura. The use of prophylactic antibiotics is controversial, but intravenous cefotaxime is often used.

Basal skull fractures are uncommon in pediatric trauma but, when present, manifest with bilateral 'black eyes', CSF leaks, otorrhea, or rhinorrhea. In the case of fractures of the petrous temporal bone there may be an ipsilateral facial nerve palsy. Management is conservative, the main complication being meningitis. Again, the use of prophylactic antibiotics is controversial, but careful observation is always required. CT scan will help in assessing the safety of performing lumbar puncture. In a large proportion of cases, there will be traumatic subarachnoid hemorrhage and the signs of meningitis (neck stiffness, pyrexia, headache, nausea, vomiting and photophobia) may all be the result of blood in the CSF rather than bacterial meningitis.

Extradural hematomas

An extradural hematoma consists of a collection of blood lying between the skull and the dura. It results either from torn dural veins or bleeding from meningeal arteries. Half of all cases occur in children under 2 years. The development of symptoms and signs may be rapid but, often in children, occur over several hours or days. Following a significant head injury, the child will become progressively drowsy with a deterioration in the GCS. Vomiting, focal weakness and ipsilateral third nerve palsy may be seen. A skull fracture is seen in only half of children. CT scan will show the hematoma. Neurosurgical evacuation is usually necessary although a few cases may be managed conservatively.

Subdural hematomas

These result from tearing of the bridging veins as they cross the subdural space. The hematoma lies between the dural and the arachnoid membranes. Subdural hematomas are conventionally classified as acute or chronic although there is significant overlap. Subdural hematomas are nearly always caused as a result of trauma, with rotation between brain and dura. This causes shearing of bridging veins and is the likely mechanism in non-accidental injuries caused by shaking, with or without impact. Subdural hematomas are occasionally seen as a consequence of bleeding from penetrated vessels in depressed skull fractures[520] or in primary penetrating injuries, or in association with brain contusions with oozing from surface veins.

Acute subdural hematomas may be isolated or can be associated with brain contusion and/or skull fracture. The symptoms are those of raised ICP. Seizures are common. If there is no clear history of significant accidental trauma then the possibility of non-accidental injury should be considered. The management is that of raised ICP, with possible evacuation of the hematoma. Some thin hematomas with no evidence of midline brain shift or significantly raised ICP can be managed non-operatively. All should be discussed with a neurosurgical team. CT scan will show a high density, often unilateral, collection. If the scan is done some days after the injury, the collection may be isointense to brain and can be missed. After 2–4 weeks it becomes hypodense in comparison with brain tissue.[521] The collection usually lies over the convexity of the cerebral hemispheres, but may involve the posterior fossa, particularly in babies and infants. Underlying brain injuries may best be visualized with ultrasound and MRI.

Chronic subdural hematomas occur mainly in children under 1 year of age and may follow known trauma or may be apparently idiopathic. They may arise following instrumental delivery. Non-accidental injury must always be considered. The presentation may be with signs and symptoms of raised ICP, isolated macrocephaly, vomiting, failure to thrive or seizures. Chronic subdurals are usually bilateral lying over the frontoparietal regions. Though bleeding is probably responsible for initiating the process, why the hematoma organizes and becomes chronic is incompletely understood. A membrane surrounds the clot and fluid is probably absorbed across it by osmosis. The collection acts as a space-occupying lesion. There may be associated hydrocephalus, although the role of subarachnoid blood should then be considered.

The most appropriate management of chronic subdural hematomas is not straightforward. If the collection is evacuated, it will often reform within 24 h or so, since a gap between brain and skull is formed by the chronic nature of the lesion allowing fluid to collect again. Tapping is usually reserved for treatment of symptoms of raised ICP rather than done routinely. In some children, placement of a subdural-peritoneal shunt may be required if accumulation of fluid continues.

Chronic subdural hematomas on CT scan appear as extra-axial collections of fluid iso- or hypointense to brain tissue. Depending on whether there has been associated damage to the brain, brain atrophy may be seen. MRI scanning may be helpful in determining the age of the collections.

The prognosis for subdural hematomas depends on the underlying cause and any associated brain injury from raised ICP or direct trauma. There is a mortality (mainly from acute subdural hematomas) of up to 3%. At follow-up 57–80% of survivors have normal development.

Intraparenchymal hemorrhage

Most intraparenchymal hemorrhages are associated with edema or contusion and are small in size, although often multiple. They are usually seen in the white matter, brainstem, cortex and corpus callosum. Operative treatment is rarely needed. Management is of the raised ICP, which almost always accompanies intraparenchymal hemorrhages. Intracerebellar hemorrhage is rare but may present with acute cerebellar signs, raised ICP, bilateral sixth nerve palsies or acute hydrocephalus.

Hydrocephalus

This may occur early in the period after head injury, in association with subarachnoid or intraventricular hemorrhage or localized brain edema. It may also be seen in the weeks or months following injury resulting in prolonged coma. It can be difficult, in some cases, to distinguish between hydrocephalus and post injury cerebral atrophy with ventricular dilatation. Pressure monitoring may be required. Treatment is by ventriculoperitoneal shunt or third ventriculostomy.

Seizures

In the conscious or non-paralysed child, seizures will usually be clinically obvious. In an unconscious or paralysed, ventilated child there may be clinical signs of seizures such as changes in systemic blood pressure or ICP, accompanied by tachycardia with or without pupillary dilation. Similar signs can also be seen during the recovery period after head injury as a non-epileptic phenomenon and are termed brainstem release symptoms. Immediate control of the seizure may be effectively obtained with lorazepam (0.1 mg/kg) given intravenously or diazepam (0.5 mg/kg) given rectally. Continuing treatment consists of intravenous phenytoin (18 mg/kg) or phenobarbital (15–20 mg/kg) and thereafter by maintaining blood levels in the therapeutic range. Resistant seizures may require control with a thiopental or midazolam infusion.

Infection

A high index of suspicion must always be maintained for the development of meningitis in an unconscious child with an open head injury, such as a basal skull fracture. A persistently raised core temperature with evidence of infection from the peripheral white count and persistent tachycardia are important signs of possible meningitis. The possibility can only be eliminated confidently by lumbar puncture, but this should only be carried out after CT examination has confirmed the presence of open CSF cisterns and free communication between the supra- and infratentorial compartments. If there is any doubt about the safety of a lumbar puncture, it should not be carried out. CSF can be obtained either from a ventricular tap or by swabbing the cerebral cortex after making a small burr hole (note that a clear ventricular tap does not exclude the diagnosis of meningitis in the subarachnoid spaces). Where a high index of suspicion for meningitis exists and CSF cannot be safely obtained, then antibiotics should be given. A third-generation cephalosporin (with metronidazole if anaerobic infection is possible as with penetrating wounds), given intravenously, is the preferred choice.

Diabetes insipidus

Diabetes insipidus may be seen following basal skull fractures and following any brain injury. Most cases are transient. Management consists of maintenance of the systemic blood pressure by adequate fluid replacement and DDAVP to reduce the continuing urine output. In other cases, diabetes insipidus develops following profound and prolonged raised ICP. This is a poor prognostic indicator and is often accompanied by incipient brain death.

Outcome

The prognosis for a head-injured child is related to the severity of the initial impairment of consciousness. Modern imaging techniques and easy access to neurosurgical units have diminished the mortality of treatable lesions such as acute extradural hematomas. The mortality of extradural hematoma in the pre-CT scan era was between 10 and 30% but is now reduced to almost zero. Overall most series of severely head-injured patients show a combined mortality and morbidity of approximately 30%. About 10% will die, 5% at the accident scene and 5% in the first few days. Details concerning the long-term morbidity of head injuries is given in the section, in this chapter, on rehabilitation.

NON-ACCIDENTAL HEAD INJURY (see also Ch. 5)

Child abuse has an incidence of 6/1000 of the childhood population.[522] However, less than 10% of all physically abused children will have a significant head injury, with brain involvement. In these children, approximately 75% also have bruises, 20% have burns, 40% have fractures and intracranial damage is seen in 40%. All socioeconomic groups are involved and 60–90% of abusers were themselves abused as children. Children born prematurely, children with learning difficulties and those with cerebral palsy are especially vulnerable. The outlook for children who survive non-accidental head injury is worse than following accidental injury. Neurological sequelae were reported in 30% of survivors with 57% having an IQ below 80.[523]

Neurological presentation of child abuse

The neurological presentation is not specific and may not immediately suggest abuse. The history may be vague. The child may present as an acute encephalopathy. Meningitis, encephalitis or metabolic disease may be suspected, rather than poisoning or shaking. Some children may present with repeated episodes of encephalopathy. Fabrication of symptoms, especially seizures (fictitious epilepsy), is a form of child abuse in Munchausen by proxy (Meadows syndrome). Seizure or status epilepticus is a possible presentation of non-accidental head injury; they are usually accompanied by encephalopathy. Attempts at suffocation may present as odd turns, seizures, apneic attacks, cyanotic attacks, rigidity or coma. It may be perpetrated in hospital as well as at home.[524]

The abused child may present with a traumatic head injury with scalp bruising, swelling, lacerations, skull fracture and neurological signs and symptoms. Injuries remote from the head may cause seizures and coma (e.g. burns, encephalopathy). In shaking injury, there may be no evidence of trauma to the head unless there has been an associated impact. The commonest presentation is as an unwell child who is irritable or excessively quiet, refusing feeds and vomiting. The infant is often hypothermic, pale and shocked with low blood pressure and tachycardia suggesting sepsis, hypoglycemia or intussusception. There may be seizures, tonic extensor spasms, breathing difficulties and cyanotic attacks.[525] A history of an attempted resuscitation is often given. It may be contended that the child was shaken because they were found gravely ill rather than this being the cause of the illness. Studies have shown that the force required to produce shaking injury in an infant is such that 'no reasonable parent would apply such force' (American Academy of Pediatrics). Rib fractures and retinal hemorrhages are commonly associated and are extremely rare after cardiopulmonary resuscitation.[526,527]

Skull fractures

Most accidental fractures are simple linear fractures, usually parietal and over the vertex or coming from the coronal suture. If the fracture line branches, crosses suture lines, is bilateral, stellate, multiple with separate fractures, more than 50 mm wide at presentation or expands as a growing fracture, then non-accidental fracture is more likely. A depressed fracture, especially of the occipital bone in a child under 3 years, is suggestive of abuse. Any of these features merits a full skeletal survey.[528]

A history that the infant fell from a couch or suffered some similar trauma is often obtained. Of 330 children under 2 years of age who were witnessed falling from couches, cots, etc., skull fractures occurred in only three and a subdural hematoma in only one. Fewer than 10% had evidence of concussion.[529]

Shaking whiplash injuries

The injury most characteristic of non-accidental head injury is the whiplash shaking injury. The full picture, originally described by Caffey,[530] consists of a subdural hematoma, massive cerebral edema, hemorrhagic retinopathy, fractured ribs and metaphyseal injury. These may occur in any combination. Often there is no skull fracture, bruising of the scalp, scalp edema or other evidence of direct head trauma. However, when present, these features suggest direct impact. This may be due to the head banging against a hard surface during the shaking, or the child may be thrown or dropped on the floor after the shaking or may be hit against a wall. The manner in which shaking injuries are caused have been admitted to by a number of perpetrators.[525,531,532]

The commonest age for shaking injury is 5 months. In children under 2 years of age 64% of head injuries and 95% of severe head injuries are due to abuse.[533] Of 100 children studied in a carefully controlled prospective study,[534] 24% of head injuries were presumed inflicted and these carried a higher mortality and risk of permanent brain damage than true accidental injuries. Many children die from their injuries.

The child may be shaken by the shoulders and upper arms, causing spiral humeral fractures or periosteal avulsion. Humeral fractures in very young children, excluding supracondylar fractures, were all found to be due to child abuse.[535] Alternatively the smaller child may be held by the rib cage, which is often severely squeezed, leaving finger-mark bruising and fractured ribs and causing a high central venous pressure which may contribute to the retinopathy. Rib fractures are very rarely caused in young infants by falls, coughing or birth injury; even very vigorous cardiac massage and resuscitation do not normally fracture ribs.[526] Concurrent injuries to the cervical spine with spinal epidural hemorrhage and bruising of the cervicomedullary junction are probably underestimated; they were found in five of six fatal cases of whiplash shaking injury by Hadley et al.[536]

Pathophysiology of brain injury from shaking

Shaking causes the brain to swirl first in one direction and then the reverse. The brain and skull start and stop rotating at different times causing tearing of bridging veins. Gray matter is firmer than white matter and they move at different velocities causing small tears that can best be demonstrated on ultrasound imaging.[537] The tentorium anchors the brainstem and the mid-brain acts as a pivot upon which the cerebral hemispheres can rotate. This may cause a primary brainstem injury with concussion.

In child abuse, tears in the white matter of the orbital, first and second frontal convolutions and temporal lobe are common. Shaking may cause slit-like cavities in white matter and the ependyma may be torn so that necrotic brain extrudes into the ventricles.[538] Shearing injuries occur in the white matter of the hemispheres, particularly the corpus callosum, superior cerebellar peduncle and in the mid-brain. Lesions in the latter may be unilateral or bilateral but are usually asymmetrical and often multiple. Although CT is the initial imaging method of choice, in cases of suspected non-accidental injury, MRI should also be obtained and serial imaging performed. This greatly helps in dating injuries, particularly subdural hematomas.[539]

In shaking injuries combined with impact, cerebral edema is often very severe but may take some hours to appear after the injury. The cause of the edema is probably multifactorial.[540]

Retinal hemorrhages are most characteristic of non-accidental shaking injuries with chest compression. In Duhaime's series nine out of 10 children with retinal hemorrhage had been subjected to physical abuse; the one other case was a fatal high speed impact injury in a car.[534] Retinopathy can occur without subdural hemorrhage or cerebral edema but is seen in 50–70% of subdural hematomas. The bleeding involves all retinal layers and is also preretinal, extending into the vitreous or backwards, i.e. subretinal, to cause retinal detachment. Severe visual defects are common in survivors.

Subdural hematomas in the first 2 years of life are more commonly acute and due to child abuse than birth injury or accidental injury. Interhemispheric hematomas are particularly likely to be the result of being shaken. Most fatal non-accidental head injuries and many of those with persisting handicap have subdural hematomas (Fig. 20.39). Seventy-five per cent of subdural hematomas are bilateral, 90% are supratentorial and 10% infratentorial. Eighty per cent of interhemispheric subdural hematomas, caused by non-accidental injury, have an associated retinopathy.

Arteriovenous malformations can bleed into the subdural space and hemorrhagic diatheses can cause spontaneous subdural bleeding, but this is rare without trauma. Scurvy, Menkes' disease, osteogenesis imperfecta, coagulopathies, thrombocytopenia and glutaric aciduria must also be included in the differential diagnosis.

The majority of small acute subdural hematomas, without mass effect, will resolve spontaneously. Larger or persisting hematomas can be treated by aspiration through the fontanel or drained via burr hole. This may, in addition to relieving symptoms, also be of medicolegal significance. The hematoma may re-accumulate. If it becomes chronic, a subduroperitoneal shunt may be required.

HYPOXIC–ISCHEMIC ENCEPHALOPATHY

Children who are successfully resuscitated from cardiac arrest may have experienced a critical period of hypoxia and/or ischemia.

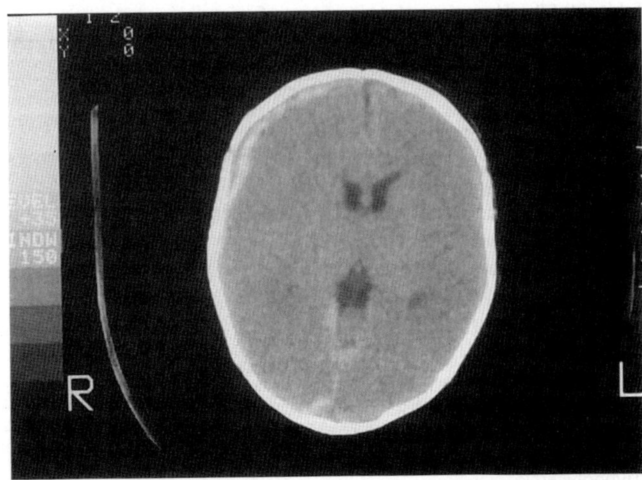

Fig. 20.39 Acute subdural hemorrhage over right hemisphere with hemispheric swelling and poor gray–white differentiation and some shift of midline.

If this has been severe, the child may not recover consciousness and criteria for brain death may be fulfilled. Unlike adults, in whom primary cardiac arrest is common, most children who suffer cardiac arrest have had a period of respiratory and/or cardiovascular failure prior to the arrest.

Initial hypoxia is followed by a build-up of carbon dioxide and lactic acid leading to acidosis. There then follow two major mechanisms:

1. Ion pumps on the brain cell membranes are inhibited resulting in accumulation of extracellular K^+ and intracellular Na^+ and Ca^{2+} and in depletion of ATP and phosphocreatine. The result is cytotoxic edema, which contributes to raised ICP and infarction. The release of glutamate causes a rise in intracellular calcium and this activates proteases resulting in secondary cell death.
2. Cardiac muscle dysfunction results in a fall in systemic blood pressure below that necessary to maintain cerebrovascular autoregulation. This results in a failure of cerebral perfusion and ischemic infarction is added to the hypoxia. The low systemic pressure also causes a degree of vasogenic brain edema.

The brain is able to withstand hypoxia without ischemia by anaerobic metabolism but is especially vulnerable to ischemia, which is associated with a failure in the delivery of metabolic substrates and an accumulation of lactic acid causing severe intracellular acidosis. This inhibits the activity of enzymes causing lysosomes to rupture.

The hypoxic–ischemic causes of encephalopathy and coma are listed in Table 20.58.

CT scan done within hours of resuscitation from an hypoxic–ischemic insult may be normal. Progressive edema may then be seen over the following 24–48 h. Changes indicating severe brain injury include generalized hypodensity of cerebral cortex, marked brain swelling and loss of gray–white differentiation. Low density areas indicating infarction in the cortex or basal ganglia may take 1–2 weeks to become apparent.

Decisions on whether active treatment is appropriate following hypoxic–ischemic insults are heavily influenced by the likely severity of subsequent neurological sequelae. However, early on, the extent of long-term damage may be very difficult to predict. The presence of a burst suppression pattern on EEG is associated with a poor outcome, but lesser abnormalities are not very helpful in predicting outcome. Children with encephalopathy due to hypoxic–ischemic injury generally have a worse outcome than other causes of acute encephalopathy. No specific interventions have been shown to be effective. The use of calcium channel blockers and glutamate antagonists is not supported by clinical trial data.

Table 20.58 Hypoxic–ischemic causes of acute encephalopathy

Perinatal asphyxia
Pulmonary disease (upper airways obstruction, laryngeal TB, epiglottis)
Alveolar hypoventilation
CO poisoning
Methemoglobinemia
Anemia
Status epilepticus
Near miss sudden infant death syndrome
Postcardiac arrest (any cause)
Cardiac bypass surgery
Near drowning
Cardiac dysrhythmia
Congestive cardiac failure
Hypotension
Disseminated intravascular coagulation
Hypoglycemia
Vitamin or cofactor deficiency (B_{12}, B_6, folate, etc.)
Anesthetic accidents

It is important, when cardiac arrest follows near drowning, that resuscitation is continued until the child is no longer hypothermic.[541] However, in a study[542] all patients submerged for more than 9 min and requiring more than 25 min of cardiopulmonary resuscitation either died or were severely impaired.

ACUTE INFECTIOUS, INFLAMMATORY ENCEPHALOPATHIES AND ASSOCIATED CONDITIONS

(see also Ch. 26)

Most organisms are capable of invading the nervous system. Direct effects can include cerebral edema, cerebritis, encephalitis, cerebral congestion, hydrocephalus, subdural effusion, empyema, ventriculitis, thrombophlebitis and abscess. Encephalopathy may also result from the effects of extracranial infection by inappropriate antidiuretic hormone secretion, inflammatory brain edema, thrombophlebitis, status epilepticus, severe endotoxemic shock and disseminated intravascular coagulation. *Escherichia coli* O157, *Shigella* and *Campylobacter* secrete neurotoxins that can cause coma and/or seizures.

Viruses may cause an acute encephalopathy by direct invasion of the brain or may attack specific parts of the central or peripheral nervous systems, e.g. polio and the anterior horn cells, causing limb paresis, chickenpox and the cerebellum, causing ataxia and mumps and the aqueduct of Sylvius, leading to hydrocephalus. Viruses may also produce an acute postinfectious encephalitis that is characterized by demyelination.

Bacterial meningitis

Bacterial meningitis remains a significant cause of acute encephalopathy in childhood despite the introduction of vaccination for *Haemophilus influenzae* and *meningococcus* group C. Children usually present with the classical symptoms of headache, photophobia, vomiting, neck stiffness with fever and encephalopathy. The characteristic rash may be present in meningococcal disease. In infancy, the classical symptoms and signs are often absent. The child is often non-specifically unwell with vomiting, fever, pallor and lethargy. A bulging fontanel may be present where the ICP is raised. Seizures, either focal or generalized, or tonic extensor spasms caused by raised ICP are a common accompaniment.

In acutely unwell children broad-spectrum antibiotics such as cefotaxime or ceftriaxone should be given immediately after taking blood cultures. Antibiotics vary in their ability to penetrate the CSF but third generation cephalosporins are broad spectrum and penetrate CSF quite well. Papilledema is usually absent initially. Lumbar puncture should be deferred in any child with a GCS of less than 13, focal symptoms or signs, papilledema or radiological evidence of raised ICP. A normal CT scan does not exclude raised ICP. Characteristically the CSF shows a raised white cell count (predominantly neutrophils), a raised protein level and a low glucose level compared to the blood glucose level. More details of the CSF features of bacterial meningitis are discussed elsewhere along with details on the responsible organisms and drug treatment.

Seizures occur in 30–40% of children with meningitis and are managed as in any child with acute encephalopathy. A vasculitis often complicates bacterial meningitis with both arterial and venous occlusion and infarction causing focal deficits, including spinal cord infarction. Subdural effusions are commonly seen but rarely require intervention. Subdural empyema is rare. Raised ICP in meningitis may be secondary to cerebral edema, acute hydrocephalus, venous sinus thrombosis or cerebral abscess. Fever is prolonged for more than 10 days in 13% of patients and usually no cause is found.

The outcome from bacterial meningitis in childhood varies according to the organism involved, the delay in starting treatment and the development of complications. In a review of outcome data from 45 published reports Baraff et al[543] found a mortality rate of 5–8%, but no major sequelae in 74–83%. Deafness was seen in 10% and was profound in 5%. The use of steroids in *H. influenzae* meningitis may reduce this figure.[513] Severe learning difficulties are unusual, but in prospective studies, up to 40% of children were found to have subtle learning deficits. Major motor deficits occurred in 4%.

Bacterial meningitis in the first month of life differs from that seen later. The signs and symptoms at presentation are less specific. Common presentations are with irritability, drowsiness, poor feeding, prolonged jaundice and focal seizures. Some babies look clearly septic. Interpretation of CSF results may be difficult. Many healthy newborns have up to 10 white cells/mm^3 and a raised protein level. The most common causative organisms are *E. coli* and the beta hemolytic streptococcus. However, many other organisms have been reported. Initial antibiotic treatment is often with ampicillin and gentamicin or a cephalosporin. The outcome is poorer than in older children. Mortality is 25% and up to 50% of survivors have cognitive and/or neurological deficits.[543] Hydrocephalus and epilepsy are frequent.

Viral encephalitis

Viruses can cause encephalitis either by direct infection of the CNS (primary viral encephalitis) or by indirect immune mediated mechanisms (postinfectious viral encephalitis). Viral encephalitis, especially if postinfectious, often has a rather insidious onset compared to meningitis. There may be a history of headache, lethargy, vomiting and behavioral change in the few days prior to more definite encephalopathic features. The depth of the impairment of consciousness is variable and focal neurological signs, referable to any part of the brain may occur. Seizures, particularly focal, are common. They may be difficult to control with status epilepticus. In a series from the USA, examining status epilepticus in pediatric intensive care 50% of cases were associated with viral encephalitis.[544] In the UK it has become accepted practice to treat children presenting with encephalopathy and seizures with intravenous aciclovir, to cover herpes simplex virus infection, a third generation cephalosporin, to cover meningitis and erythromycin, to cover mycoplasma infection, whilst further investigations are undertaken.

Enteroviruses such as Coxsackie virus, herpesviruses (simplex, zoster and HHV6), measles virus and mumps virus are amongst the more frequent causes of viral encephalitis in the UK. Many of these can cause both primary and postinfectious viral encephalitis. The specific cause of encephalitis is often not found despite appropriate investigations having been undertaken. These include blood serology, viral cultures (throat, stool and CSF) and polymerase chain reaction (PCR) for specific pathogens. Although false positive and false negative results occur, PCR offers an extremely useful test for the rapid diagnosis of, in particular, herpes simplex encephalitis.

Herpes simplex virus is the commonest single identified cause of viral encephalitis in the UK. It has a predilection for the temporal lobes, but other parts of the brain may be involved, particularly in younger children. The 'typical' EEG pattern of triphasic waves over the temporal lobes is neither particularly sensitive nor specific for herpes simplex encephalitis. Brain biopsy is no longer recommended.

The CSF in viral encephalitis may be acellular or show an increased white cell count usually lymphocytes. The protein level is normal or slightly raised and the glucose level is normal. In some patients, initial CSF examination is normal and a repeat may be necessary after an interval of 5–7 days. CT scans are often normal, particularly in the early stages of the illness. MRI scanning, particularly if contrast and techniques such as diffusion weighted imaging are used, is more sensitive and may show localized areas of inflammation, particularly in herpes simplex encephalitis. In many cases, brain imaging shows evidence of diffuse brain swelling, which if severe, may be associated with herniation.

Specific antiviral treatment with aciclovir is available for herpes simplex encephalitis. It must be given intravenously and for at least 10 days and possibly longer.[545] Other agents are active against certain other causes of viral encephalitis and can be especially useful in immunocompromised children. Advice from a virologist should be sought.

Neurological sequelae are common following viral encephalitis. Cognitive and motor deficits, epilepsy and behavioral change are present in up to 50% of survivors.[546] The immunocompromised child is especially vulnerable.

Tuberculous meningitis, causing acute encephalopathy

Though this is not often seen in the UK now it remains an important cause of death and neurological disability worldwide. Tuberculous meningitis can occur despite BCG immunization. The clinical manifestations are extremely variable and virtually any combination of neurological symptoms and signs can occur. A prodromal phase of irritability, vomiting and apathy is often followed by fever, headache, focal neurological signs and meningism. Signs of raised ICP and coma will occur if treatment is not started. Ventricular dilation is present in nearly 80% of cases and urgent ventricular drainage may be needed.

There is often no history of exposure to TB and skin testing is unreliable. CT scanning is often done in the initial assessment and may show tuberculomas, hydrocephalus or meningeal enhancement. Lumbar puncture should be deferred until after CT scan. CSF usually contains a high lymphocyte count, a raised protein (often > 1g/L) and a low CSF glucose. Acid fast bacilli are rarely seen but culture may be positive in up to 50%. The use of PCR for mycobacterium DNA on blood and CSF has aided rapid diagnosis but false positives are seen. Further consideration is given to this illness under aseptic meningitis below.

Cerebral abscess and subdural empyema

Cerebral abscesses can result from hematogenous spread of infection, often in association with congenital heart disease, local spread of infection from sinusitis or mastoiditis or arise as a complication of meningitis. Streptococcus, Staphylococcus and anaerobic organisms are the most common causes, but many other organisms have been reported. Abscesses are usually located in the cerebral hemispheres and present with encephalopathy, seizures and sepsis. CT with contrast is usually diagnostic often showing enhancement of the abscess cavity with intense surrounding edema.

Intravenous antibiotics are the main treatment although surgical drainage may be needed. A prolonged course of 4–6 weeks is often needed with progress monitored by serial scans. Mortality is around 10% with 30% of survivors developing epilepsy.

Subdural empyemas are essentially abscesses lying in the subdural space. Their presentation is similar to that of cerebral abscesses in general. Surgical evacuation is usually necessary combined with prolonged antibiotic treatment.

Acute disseminated encephalomyelitis (ADEM)

This acute patchy demyelination, occurring in the central nervous system, is thought to be an abnormal immunological response to infection. It may be considered a special form of postinfectious encephalitis. After an interval, following the precipitating viral infection, the child develops focal neurological signs, headache, mild encephalopathy and occasionally seizures. The focal neurological deficits depend on the sites of demyelination and may follow any pattern. There may be fluctuation or progression of signs in the days after presentation. CT scanning in the acute phase may be normal. MR scanning is usually diagnostic. The spinal cord may be involved. CSF examination characteristically shows a mild pleocytosis, usually lymphocytic, a normal or mildly raised CSF protein level and a normal glucose level. Oligoclonal bands may be present in some patients. Investigations looking for evidence of the precipitating infection often prove negative.

A good response is usually seen to steroids although it is unclear if the final outcome is influenced by such treatment. A 3–5 day course of intravenous methyl prednisolone is often given. More than 90% of children with ADEM make a full recovery from the initial episode, although this may take many months. Relapses are occasionally described.

Multiple sclerosis

Clinically it is not possible to distinguish between ADEM and the first attack of demyelination due to multiple sclerosis. Long term follow-up studies have suggested that as many as 10% of patients with ADEM later develop multiple sclerosis. 2.7% of adults with MS had onset before 16 years of age, but it is rare under the age of 10 years. Clinical features include the relapsing remitting course. Visual and sensory symptoms are prominent as in adults. Seizures occur more commonly than in adults. Optic neuritis is characterized by a sudden reduction in monocular or binocular vision. A large central scotoma and papillitis are usually found on ocular examination. Though often considered a principal feature of multiple sclerosis in adults, few children with optic neuritis go on to develop multiple sclerosis.

Diagnosis of multiple sclerosis depends principally on the clinical picture combined with the results of MRI. CSF examination and visually evoked responses remain useful adjuvant investigations. High dose steroid treatment is effective for acute relapses but the use of beta-interferon remains controversial.

CHRONIC INFLAMMATORY AND INFECTIOUS MENINGOENCEPHALOPATHIES

Aseptic meningitis

Not all children with CNS sepsis present with acute encephalopathy. The onset may be insidious, diagnostically confusing, and if appropriate therapy is not initiated significant disability may result. Thus, the child with subacute or chronic meningitis who fails to respond to adequate antibiotic therapy presents the pediatrician with a worrying and perplexing problem. Most of these children will present with fever, nuchal rigidity and headache, probably after an insidious prodromal illness of general malaise and anorexia. The CSF initially may show pleocytosis changing to lymphocytosis within a few hours or a day or two. Antibiotic therapy for at least 48 h is appropriate until cultures are shown to be negative, along with supportive therapy with fluids, analgesia and antipyretics.

As for acute encephalopathy a variety of viruses are potentially implicated. The enteroviruses account for 80% of all cases of aseptic meningitis in American studies. The UK picture is similar in infancy, but the mumps virus is a more common pathogen in the 1–9-year-old age group. This may change with the advent of mumps, measles, and rubella vaccination. Other common causes of aseptic meningitis include herpes simplex, adenovirus, measles, cytomegalovirus, rubella, varicella, Epstein–Barr, influenza, parainfluenza and rotavirus. The Epstein–Barr and Coxsackie virus in particular may run a subacute or chronic course. A rash may accompany the illness, which can be specific. Febrile convulsions may occur. Generally, younger children are irritable and resent handling, whilst older children complain of myalgia, photophobia and retrobulbar pain with evidence of nuchal rigidity in only about 50%.

It is generally accepted that after 12 h of illness, almost all (97%) of the cellular response in CSF will be lymphocytic and that antibiotics can be withheld if the child seems otherwise well. CSF glucose may be low in up to 20% and CSF protein may be increased in up to 50%. Laboratory tests for bacteria will be negative but should be complemented by specific viral culture of CSF and other sites, including throat, feces and urine, as well as the measurement of serum viral-antibody titers. Raised alpha-interferon levels usually indicate a viral meningoencephalitic illness, but slightly raised levels may also occur in bacterial infection. Viral identification can shorten antibiotic courses and reduce time spent in hospital.

After 48 h of treatment the main alternative diagnoses to consider with a sterile polymorphic or pleocytic CSF are partially treated bacterial or tuberculous meningitis (TBM). Partially treated meningitis is particularly likely if there is a history of a course of oral antibiotics given for an intercurrent infection. This treatment may render microbacterial techniques unreliable, and it is reasonable at this stage to stop all antibiotics in order to clarify the situation. If deterioration ensues, antibiotic therapy may be reinstituted.

Tuberculous meningitis

Tuberculosis (TB) of the CNS occurs in all ethnic groups; diagnosis and treatment are difficult. Late diagnosis carries an associated high morbidity and mortality. The incidence of TB of the CNS is increasing in part as a result of the acquired immunodeficiency syndrome becoming more common. In children, TB of the CNS is often a complication of primary infection with or without miliary spread. TB of the CNS should be considered in any child with a subacute history of fever, headache, seizures, vomiting, behavioral change or impairment of consciousness. Respiratory symptoms may or may not be present. It is important to note that tuberculous meningitis (TBM) results from Rich's focus produced in an intensive inflammatory response, particularly at the base of the brain. There is an associated vasculitis, which may result in convulsions, cranial nerve palsies, dyskinesia, hemiparesis, or signs of a mild radiculopathy.

The CSF sugar is typically low, but may be normal in up to 10% of patients. When the ratio of blood to CSF sugar is greater than 2 : 1 in the presence of a lymphocytic meningitis, TBM must be given very serious consideration. The Mantoux test may remain negative for some weeks due to anergy following primary exposure; the combination of lobar consolidation on a chest X-ray and aseptic meningitis is a particularly strong indication for antituberculous therapy. The decision to treat is rather easier when the X-ray shows classical miliary mottling, or examination of the fundi reveals choroidal tubercles.

Neuroimaging with MRI or CT with contrast may be helpful in diagnosis; tuberculomas may not be evident on an unenhanced scan. Lumbar puncture may be negative for culture of acid-fast bacilli, this diagnosis being made only on ventricular drainage. Acid-fast bacilli have to be searched for carefully in CSF specimens. The use of the polymerase chain reaction to detect antigen or metabolic products of tubercle bacilli can be misleading, with a one in ten false positive rate.

Treatment of tuberculous meningitis involves administration for at least a year of two antituberculous therapeutic agents that penetrate the blood–brain barrier and tuberculomas. Isoniazid and rifampicin are the mainstay of continued treatment during this period. Initially, four drugs are required, usually rifampicin, isoniazid, pyrazinamide and ethambutol. Steroids are of value when there is progressive neurological disorder or deteriorating consciousness, once appropriate antituberculous chemotherapy is begun. Further detail on treatment is given in Chapter 26.

Other causes

When a child with lymphocytic CSF does not improve as expected, a full reappraisal of the history and findings is appropriate, and thoughts on differential diagnosis should be broadened. Possibilities are rarer bacteria (see below), an immune paresis with opportunistic infection, a fistula, autoimmune disease or toxins.

Five per cent of all children with acute lymphoblastic leukemia have CNS disease at presentation. The CNS is the most common site for relapse. Usually, associated signs of bone marrow failure (anemia, thrombocytopenia, recurrent infection) will aid diagnosis. Rarely, primary CNS lymphoma may present in this way. It is essential that bone marrow investigation is performed before the use of steroids.

In an immunocompromised or severely debilitated child, fungal infection, including candida and cryptococcus may spread to the CNS from specific skin or oral lesions. Stains for fungi, swabs, cultures, antibody titers and urine microscopy should identify the cause. When the degree of debility is severe, and particularly when there is marked and rapid wasting of muscles, it may be justified to administer a course of amphotericin. In immunocompromised children, in addition to severe illnesses caused by the common agents, opportunistic pathogens may cause an encephalopathy.

Neurological manifestations of nervous system infection with *Borrelia burgdorferi* (a spirochete) are protean. It is a multisystem disorder, known also as Lyme disease, affecting the skin, joints, nervous system and cardiovascular system. Borrelia inhabits the gut of the *Ixodes* tic. The tic is widespread throughout the UK but found in greater numbers in woodland.

Man is infected by the bite of a tic producing (in most cases) a slowly enlarging patch of erythema (erythema chronicum migrans). A non-specific flu-like illness may occur at this stage. These symptoms may be followed by cranial poly- or mononeuropathies, aseptic meningitis, transverse myelitis, postinfectious polyneuritis and encephalitis. A history of skin lesion or a tic bite is not always obtained.[547] Diagnosis is difficult, and serological studies may not be positive at the time of neurological presentation. Specific IgM is the most valuable serological test and intrathecal synthesis of specific antibodies which immunoblot the spirochetal antigen may also (in due course) be helpful diagnostically. Treatment in childhood is usually with penicillin or erythromycin. Nervous system disease must be treated aggressively as chronic encephalopathy may ensue. There is increasing evidence[548,549] in neuroborreliosis that intravenous cephalosporins are superior to penicillin, because of the latter's relatively poor CNS penetration.

The protozoon *Toxoplasma gondii* may cause meningitis in immunosuppressed children. It is usually accompanied by lymphadenopathy. The histology of an affected node may give the diagnosis, as may the presence in the serum of specific IgM. Treatment with sulphonamides, pyrimethamine or spiramycin is effective.

Leptospirosis results from contact with infected animal urine (mainly rats), usually in contaminated water or from farm machinery. After an incubation period of 10 days, the illness typically produces a high fever, sweating, headaches, conjunctival suffusion, muscle tenderness and pain with meningitis. Cardiac or renal failure may occur, with spontaneous improvement after 3 weeks. Diagnosis is based on cultured blood and urine and rising antibody titers after the first week. Penicillin, erythromycin and tetracycline are the treatment options, along with supportive therapy, though the immune-mediated effects of the illness may not be affected. Tetracyclines are contraindicated in renal failure and, depending on the severity of the illness, are contraindicated in children. Usually high doses are given for 10 days. Cerebral malaria may need to be considered in those who have recently traveled abroad.

Mycoplasma pneumoniae is reported to cause CNS disease in 7% of those admitted to hospital with associated upper or lower respiratory tract illness. A meningoencephalitis, which may be severe, is the commonest result, but polyneuropathy or transverse myelitis may also occur.

Neurobrucellosis may also cause meningoencephalitis. It is usually contracted from animals known to harbor the organism, or from the ingestion of unpasteurized milk products. Sweating, abdominal pain, fever, hepatosplenomegaly and arthritis commonly accompany the illness. Axonal polyneuropathy has been reported. *Brucella melitensis* may be isolated from CSF and there may be rising antibody titers. Regimens advocated include (either alone or in combination) co-trimoxazole, rifampicin or streptomycin. In chronic brucellosis suppression of intracellular infection may be attempted in the hope that the host's immunity will eventually eliminate or contain infection. Regimens advocated include protracted courses of the antibiotics used in acute brucellosis. Tetracyclines are useful but obviously cannot be used in children unless there is no alternative. Most children make a full recovery.

Kawasaki disease or mucocutaneous lymph node syndrome is a relatively uncommon disorder. It predominates in the under-fives and, although the etiology is uncertain, infective agents have been implicated in its etiology. Presentation is with persistent fever, characteristic skin rashes, with desquamation of the extremities, mucosal and buccal involvement and lymphadenopathy. It may be associated with aseptic meningitis though rarely as an isolated feature. The association of aseptic meningitis with an autoimmune vasculitis is dealt with in Chapter 27.

Aseptic meningitis may follow the administration of certain drugs. These include OKT3 (in renal transplantation), immunoglobulin (in idiopathic thrombocytopenic purpura and Kawasaki disease), isoniazid, sulfamethiazole, co-trimoxazole and azathioprine. A cellular response has also been reported in lead poisoning, although meningism is rare and reduced conscious level common.

It must also be remembered that migraine at times leads to a cellular response in the CSF, particularly in complicated migraine. If the hemiplegia is fleeting, the child's presentation at hospital may be with headache and the picture of an aseptic meningitis. Migraine may also present with fever, neck stiffness and aseptic meningitis. Although uncommon, recognition of this syndrome should help to avoid unnecessary invasive investigations.

The clinician needs to be aware that aseptic meningitis may well be the presenting feature of a number of less common, but important conditions specified here. While the diagnosis is being investigated, due attention should be paid to the child's parents, who will also be feeling worried and perplexed. Adequate time needs to be allocated to inform them of investigation and treatment strategy at each stage, in order to maintain their confidence at a time when the medical team themselves may be feeling unsure.

Recurrent or chronic meningitis

Recurrent meningitis may result from anatomical abnormalities of the inner ear or craniovertebral axis. The causes are acquired (following trauma) or congenital, immunodeficiency or distant untreated foci of infection.

In any child with recurrent meningitis, a communication between the CNS and the exterior must be assiduously sought. Congenital abnormalities of the inner ear leading to fistulae may present with recurrent meningitis. Otoscopy is usually normal, and diagnosis requires expert neuroradiological and possibly radioisotope investigation. CSF fistulae may also result from trauma or infection. Recurrent meningitis (often with unusual organisms for age) may result from infection via a midline dermal fistula (often referred to as a sinus), usually associated with spina bifida occulta. The fistula can occur at any point in the midline, though the natal cleft is the commonest site. There may be associated cord tethering, intraspinal dermoid, lipoma or cyst or diastematomyelia.

The second commonest site for a fistula is the occiput, and there may be associated cerebellar or brainstem signs of hydrocephalus. Infection of a dermoid cyst and proximal end of a neurodermal sinus may result in intraspinal abscess rather than meningitis.

Any neurodermal sinus that ends above the sacrum should be dealt with neurosurgically. Surgical results are poorer when definitive treatment is delayed until after the occurrence of meningitis.

Other infectious encephalopathies

Chronic encephalitides include subacute sclerosing panencephalitis (SSPE), progressive rubella panencephalitis and HIV encephalopathy. SSPE is an exceptionally rare disease caused by direct invasion by the measles virus of the CNS and usually first manifests some years after the initial measles illness, which has often occurred within the first 2 years of life. It has been described after measles immunization. An initial stage marked by intellectual and behavioral changes is followed by repetitive involuntary movements, resembling myoclonus. Dementia and early death follow inexorably. Diagnosis is by the detection of an oligoclonal CSF pattern and raised measles antibody titers in the CSF. SSPE is covered in detail in the section on neurodegenerative conditions. There is no specific treatment. HIV encephalopathy is dealt with in detail elsewhere.

HYDROCEPHALUS

The main features of hydrocephalus are dealt with elsewhere in this chapter. The child with acute hydrocephalus may present with vomiting, drowsiness, headache and seizures. The cause of the acute encephalopathy is usually apparent on neuroimaging. A subacute presentation with intermittent drowsiness, headache, occasional vomiting and false localizing signs is also common. The presentation of hydrocephalus secondary to congenital brain malformations, such as aqueduct stenosis, can be delayed until later in childhood.

Hydrocephalus is often a complication of other brain disorders causing encephalopathy, e.g. hemorrhage, tumors and meningitis.

CEREBRAL TUMORS

Impairment of consciousness is often present at the time of initial diagnosis of brain tumors but is often not the most prominent feature. Cerebral hemisphere lesions usually present with focal deficits related to the site of tumor, seizures, headache, vomiting and drowsiness. It is unusual for cerebral hemisphere tumors to present with coma prior to diagnosis. Thalamic tumors may obstruct the foramen of Monro and third ventricle and brainstem gliomas may distort the aqueduct of Sylvius causing raised ICP due to hydrocephalus. Choroid cysts of the third ventricle may give rise to intermittent hydrocephalus by obstructing the foramen of Monro in a 'ballcock' fashion. Changes of posture may lead to rapid release of the pressure. Children with cysts of the third ventricle may present with a 'bobble-headed doll' syndrome and progressive loss of intellect with frontal horn dilatation.

Tumors in the posterior fossa often present with weakness, truncal and limb ataxia, headache, vomiting and drowsiness. These tumors may present acutely with features of raised ICP because they frequently lead to acute hydrocephalus due to obstruction at the aqueduct or fourth ventricle. High dose steroid treatment may relieve the pressure but many children require urgent decompression.

In tuberous sclerosis subependymal giant cell astrocytomas can cause acute hydrocephalus as a consequence of blockage at the foramen of Monro. This can be difficult to recognize as a consequence of the motor, cognitive and behavioral impairments characteristic of tuberous sclerosis. Symptoms may include a change in behavior, altered seizure pattern or periods of decreased awareness.

STATUS EPILEPTICUS AND RELATED ISSUES

This is conventionally defined as an epileptic seizure lasting for more than 30 min or frequent seizures for the same period without recovery of consciousness between seizures. Convulsive status epilepticus (CSE) in childhood is a life-threatening condition with serious risk of neurological sequelae[550–552] and constitutes a medical emergency. Although the outcome from an episode of CSE is mainly determined by its cause, the duration of CSE is also important. In addition, the longer the duration of the status, the more difficult it is to terminate.[552,553] Treatment of convulsive seizures lasting more than 5 min is recommended in order to prevent the development of CSE.

Data from epidemiological studies suggest that 4–8 children per 1000 have an episode of CSE before the age of 15 years[554] and 17% of children with seizures present with CSE as their first unprovoked seizure.[555] CSE in children has a mortality of approximately 4%.[556] Neurological sequelae of CSE (epilepsy, motor deficits, learning difficulties and behavior problems) are age dependent, occurring in 6% of those over 3 years but in 29% of those under 1 year.[556] Important causes of CSE are febrile seizures and those with epilepsy in whom antiepileptic drug treatment is being modified. Idiopathic CSE is also relatively common.

An evidence-based approach to the prevention/treatment of CSE is shown in Figure 20.40.[557] Initial management should follow the ABC principle of resuscitation. High flow oxygen should be given and the blood glucose measured by stick testing. It is important to emphasize that not all episodes of apparent status epilepticus are in fact epileptic. A brief history and clinical examination should therefore be undertaken to confirm that the seizure activity is likely to be epileptic and not, for example, a drug-induced dystonic reaction, a tonic spasm due to raised ICP or a psychogenic (pseudo-epileptic) attack.

If the seizure does not rapidly respond to initial treatments, or if there is significant respiratory, cardiovascular or neurological compromise the child should be intubated, artificially ventilated and treated in an intensive care setting. Monitoring of vital signs, including pulse, blood pressure and blood gases is essential to ensure that a hypoxic–ischemic insult is not added to the direct effects of the status epilepticus. A small number of children will continue to convulse despite treatment with thiopental (refractory CSE). The most appropriate subsequent anticonvulsant management is unclear. Regimens using continuous intravenous agents such as midazolam[558] and inhalational anesthetic agents such as isoflurane[559] have been reported but are not fully evaluated.[560] During CSE, depletion of intracellular energy stores in

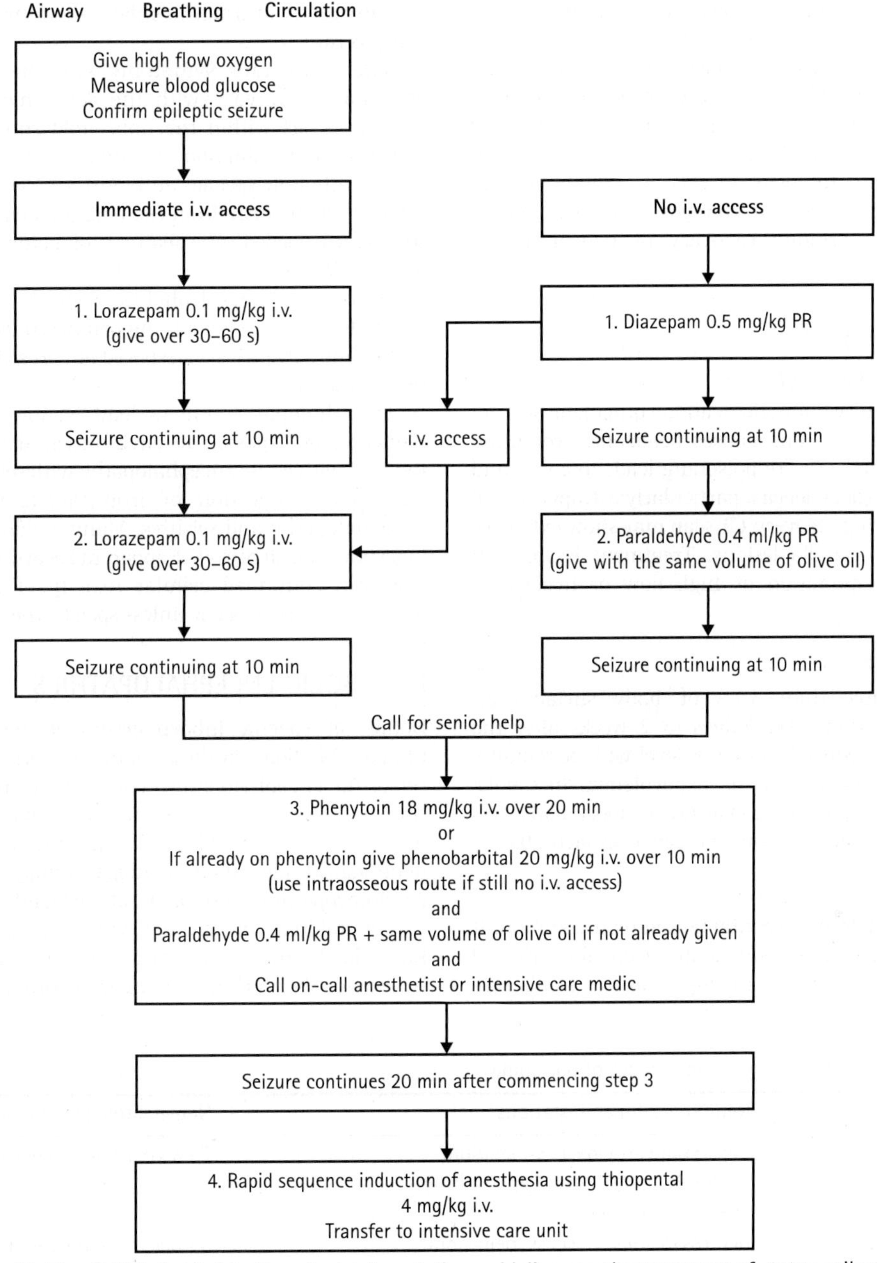
Airway Breathing Circulation
Give high flow oxygen
Measure blood glucose
Confirm epileptic seizure
Immediate i.v. access
No i.v. access
1. Lorazepam 0.1 mg/kg i.v.
(give over 30–60 s)
1. Diazepam 0.5 mg/kg PR
Seizure continuing at 10 min
i.v. access
Seizure continuing at 10 min
2. Lorazepam 0.1 mg/kg i.v.
(give over 30–60 s)
2. Paraldehyde 0.4 ml/kg PR
(give with the same volume of olive oil)
Seizure continuing at 10 min
Seizure continuing at 10 min
Call for senior help
3. Phenytoin 18 mg/kg i.v. over 20 min
or
If already on phenytoin give phenobarbital 20 mg/kg i.v. over 10 min
(use intraosseous route if still no i.v. access)
and
Paraldehyde 0.4 ml/kg PR + same volume of olive oil if not already given
and
Call on-call anesthetist or intensive care medic
Seizure continues 20 min after commencing step 3
4. Rapid sequence induction of anesthesia using thiopental
4 mg/kg i.v.
Transfer to intensive care unit

Fig. 20.40 British Paediatric Neurologist Association guidelines on the treatment of status epilepticus.

muscle may lead to reduction in muscle activity. This may be misinterpreted as 'the seizure settling down', whereas the cerebral activity and damaging metabolic derangements are continuing. Careful examination, and EEG, if available, will help determine if there is ongoing seizure activity.

Impairment of consciousness following a seizure is common. This postictal impairment is easy to diagnose if the seizure has been witnessed, but may present difficulties if it has not. Although the coma score may be very low, supportive care is usually all that is required, provided steady improvement is documented. A cause for the seizure such as hypoglycemia or infection should be sought. Drug treatment with agents such as lorazepam and diazepam will greatly prolong the recovery period.

Non-convulsive status epilepticus (NCSE) may present as a child with reduced conscious level. The child has continuous, or very frequent absence, atypical absence or complex partial seizures so that an enduring epileptic state is present. The child is unaware, or has severely impaired awareness, is ataxic, drooling and uncommunicative and may manifest minor jerks and myoclonus. This seizure state rarely happens as the first manifestation of epilepsy. It is usually seen as part of an epileptic encephalopathy such as the Lennox–Gastaut syndrome, but can occur in idiopathic epilepsies and may be provoked by inappropriate antiepileptic drug treatment, such as giving carbamazepine to children with absences. The parents or carers will often be aware of the cause of the impaired consciousness. An EEG will usually show continuous spike and wave activity. There is not the same degree of urgency in treating non-convulsive as compared to convulsive status epilepticus. However, prolonged episodes of non-convulsive status epilepticus have been linked to intellectual decline. Oral, rectal and intravenous benzodiazepines or steroids are often used. Occasionally benzodiazepines may provoke tonic status epilepticus.

In a child who has had seizures as part of their encephalopathy the possibility that subclinical or subtle seizures are continuing to impair consciousness should be considered. Such seizures may be difficult to detect and an EEG or continuous EEG monitoring may be required. The decision as to whether to treat an abnormal EEG without clear clinical seizure activity is a difficult one. In practice it is often possible to correlate EEG abnormalities with subtle seizure signs or physiological changes. Overtreatment of EEG abnormalities may prolong recovery of consciousness unnecessarily.

TOXIC ENCEPHALOPATHIES

Carbon monoxide poisoning

This may be caused by faulty domestic heating equipment or from car exhaust fumes. Mild poisoning causes headaches, vomiting, sweating and breathlessness. Severe poisoning leads to coma and seizures. Residual neurological deficits, particularly extrapyramidal signs, are common following recovery. CT scan may show extensive white matter and basal ganglia lesions. Treatment is through supportive care and the provision of high flow or hyperbaric oxygen.[561]

Burn encephalopathy

In severe burns (greater than 30% of body surface) an encephalopathy may be seen several days to 2 weeks after the injury. Seizures, lethargy, reduced conscious level with personality change are common.[562] Correction of hypovolemia, metabolic abnormalities and treatment of infection are also important aspects of management in this setting. The course is generally favorable.

Drug poisoning

In toddlers and young children accidental poisoning is common. It should be considered in all children with acute encephalopathy and samples for urine and blood toxicology taken. Deliberate administration of drugs to children in Munchausen's syndrome by proxy is rare.

The signs and symptoms seen in association with the encephalopathy vary with the drug ingested. A history of all possible drugs within the household should be elicited. Specific features on examination or initial investigations may give further clues. Although specific antidotes are rarely available, enhanced removal of the drug from the body by hemofiltration or dialysis is sometimes needed. The features of common poisons are shown in Table 20.59.

In older children alcohol intoxication is common. Detection of associated hypoglycemia is important. Abuse of cannabis, cocaine, heroin and solvents is widespread but presents infrequently to acute medical services.

Encephalopathy due to lead is now rarely seen since the reduction of exposure to environmental lead. It may present in toddlers with acute encephalopathy with seizures, ataxia and visual loss. Acute ingestion of iron tablets may also lead to an encephalopathy and seizures. Many children with accidental iron ingestion show a period of apparent recovery after the initial illness. However, continued cellular toxicity of iron is occurring and deterioration may occur unless specific therapy is given.

METABOLIC ENCEPHALOPATHIES

Details of specific inborn errors of metabolism are given in Chapter 24. Some of these conditions can present with an acute or relapsing encephalopathy. The history may highlight previous similar episodes or features of chronic illness such as poor growth or intermittent vomiting. Examination, in addition to the neurological signs of encephalopathy, may show liver enlargement, cardiomyopathy or respiratory abnormalities.

All children who present with acute encephalopathies should have blood glucose, urea and electrolytes checked. If the glucose is low or borderline on stick testing, a laboratory glucose

Table 20.59 Clinical features following common types of poisoning

Drug	Neurological manifestations	Non-neurological manifestations
Amfetamines	Depressed consciousness, delirium, agitation, mydriasis, hyperreflexia, choreiform movements	Cardiac arrhythmias, hyperpyrexia, hypertension, sweating, tachycardia
Anticonvulsants	Depressed consciousness, behavioral disturbances, ataxia, diplopia, seizures	Cardiac arrhythmias & hypotension (phenytoin), hyponatremia (carbamazepine), blood dyscrasias
Antidepressants (tricyclics)	Agitation, muscle rigidity, seizures, coma, mydriasis	Sweating, tachycardia, hyperpyrexia, vomiting
Antihistamines	Depressed consciousness, hallucinations, tremulousness, mydriasis, convulsions	Dry mouth, urinary retention, hypotension
Barbiturates	Ataxia, coma, absent tendon reflexes, miosis, respiratory depression	Hypothermia, hypotension
Lithium	Nausea, drowsiness, dysarthyria, tremor, ataxia	Vomiting, cardiac arrhythmias
Methadone	Depressed consciousness, respiratory depression, miosis	Fecal & urinary retention, hypotension
Phenothiazines	Dystonia, extrapyramidal signs, lethargy	Hypotension
Piperazine	Ataxia, hypotonia	Vomiting, diarrhea
Salicylates	Depressed consciousness, convulsions, tinnitus	Hyperventilation, hyperpyrexia, hypoglycemia, metabolic acidosis
Theophylline	Seizures, depressed consciousness	

measurement should be taken before dextrose therapy is given. If hypoglycemia is the cause of the encephalopathy then further specialist advice should be sought and investigations undertaken to determine the cause of hypoglycemia. Although it is common for children who are acutely unwell to become hypoglycemic, this should not be assumed.

Encephalopathy from hyperammonemia, secondary to urea cycle disorders, is an important consideration. Measurement of the ammonia should be undertaken. The incidence of Reye's syndrome, in the UK, has decreased significantly since the reduced use of aspirin in children. The clinical picture of vomiting and deteriorating level of consciousness, hypoglycemia, abnormal liver function tests and hyperammonemia is characteristic. Some inborn errors of metabolism such as mitochondrial beta-oxidation defects and organic acidemias can present with a Reye-like illness. Specialist advice and specific investigations will determine the cause of hyperammonemia. In addition to the general care of any child with encephalopathy, specific treatment with sodium benzoate and sodium phenylbutyrate can help to reduce the blood ammonia and subsequent cellular damage.

Lactic acidosis in association with encephalopathy may be caused by a mitochondrial disorder. Many children who are critically ill, particularly with septicemia, will have a lactic acidosis and differentiating these in the acute phase may not be possible. Other signs of mitochondrial disorders such as poor growth, intermittent vomiting, retinopathy, seizures or nerve deafness should be sought. Mitochondrial disorders can mimic many neurological conditions and are often considered in the differential diagnosis. Investigations including blood and CSF lactate, skin and muscle biopsies with assay of respiratory chain enzymes are often necessary to pinpoint the metabolic defect. Although mitochondrial DNA sequencing is now widely available, many mitochondrial disorders are nuclear in origin and diagnostic testing is difficult.

THE CHILD WITH ACUTE WEAKNESS

It may be difficult to determine if an unwell child has actual muscle weakness. Many children present with non-specific symptoms of irritability, lethargy and pallor. Some conditions with acute weakness are commonly associated with encephalopathy and this may be the predominant feature at presentation. Children with abnormal gait, limp or refusing to walk may present to orthopedic or trauma clinics, or be suspected of 'putting it on'. Failure to consider a neurological cause for non-specific presentations is a common reason for delay in diagnosis of treatable conditions such as Guillain–Barré syndrome and acute myelopathy.

Initial assessment of any acutely ill child should concentrate on the ABC principles of resuscitation especially where there is co-existing encephalopathy. Neurological assessment should determine the pattern of weakness so that it can be classified according to the likely site of the lesion. The pattern of weakness will generally be that of hemiplegia, quadriplegia, paraplegia or asymmetrical variants of these. Further information from the pattern of tendon reflexes, sensory signs and symptoms of bladder and/or bowel involvement are important. Although not always clear after the initial neurological examination, it should be possible to determine whether the weakness is due to a lesion in the brain, spinal cord, anterior horn cell, peripheral nerve, neuromuscular junction or muscle. Points on history taking which aid the diagnosis are dealt with in the relative sections below.

Children with weakness due to upper motor neurone lesions present initially with a flaccid limb weakness and loss of reflexes. Typical upper motor neurone signs of increased tone and brisk reflexes may not be present for several days or weeks.

There are a number of conditions that present with acute weakness where specific treatment is available and improves long-term outcome. Diagnosis of these and early referral to specialist advice is important. Guillain–Barré syndrome, acute myelopathy due to cord compression and myasthenia gravis are important examples. In the child with an acute hemorrhagic or ischemic stroke, neurological and neurosurgical advice should be sought immediately. Children with acute stroke often have associated cerebral edema and raised ICP.

In children who present with an acute hemiparesis the differential diagnosis includes hemorrhagic and ischemic stroke, brain tumor, extradural or subdural hematoma, focal central nervous system infection (encephalitis or abscess), hemiplegic migraine, Mitochondrial encephalomyopathy, lactic acidosis and stroke-like episodes (MELAS), acute demyelination and Todd's paresis secondary to an epileptic seizure.

The differential diagnosis in children with paraplegia or quadriplegia includes Guillain–Barré syndrome, acute dermatomyositis, myasthenia gravis, acute peripheral neuropathy other than Guillain–Barré syndrome, CNS infection such as poliomyelitis or spinal cord abscess, acute transverse myelitis, spinal cord compression from tumor, abscess or hematoma and multifocal cerebral cortical dysfunction (although in the latter an encephalopathy is often prominent).

ACUTE PARAPARESIS AND QUADRIPARESIS

In paraparesis the weakness is confined to the lower limbs. A quadriparesis affects all four limbs. In the acute situation these are usually caused by lesions of the spinal cord, although anterior horn cell disease such as poliomyelitis and polio-like illnesses due to enteroviruses, lesions of the cauda equina or peripheral nerves, such as in Guillain–Barré syndrome, also need to be considered. Vascular lesions of the cord such as anterior spinal artery infarction and spinal arteriovenous malformations may need excluding. A very acute onset of dermatomyositis may present in a similar way. A raised CPK, heliotrope rash, muscle tenderness and irritability are useful diagnostic clues. Acute periodic paralysis should also be considered in the differential diagnosis. Vertebral osteomyelitis or discitis can present with lower limb weakness.

The main clinical distinction to be made is usually between spinal cord compression and Guillain–Barré syndrome. The onset of spinal cord dysfunction may be very acute, such as in transverse myelitis, or

Table 20.60 Metabolic causes of cerebral edema

Inherited metabolic
Aminoacidopathies
Organic acidopathies
Hyperammonemia
Porphyria
Non-ketotic hyperglycinemia
Organ failure
Uremia
Hepatic failure
Electrolyes, minerals and vitamins
Hypercalcemia
Hypernatremia
Water intoxication
Lead poisoning
Vitamin A toxicity
Other
Hypoglycemia
Hypoxia-ischemia

slowly progressive. A history of bony dysplasias or storage disorders such as a mucopolysaccharidosis suggest spinal cord compression. Guillain–Barré syndrome can have a very acute onset and differentiating it in the early phase of the illness can be difficult. Both disorders will show a flaccid, relatively symmetrical weakness of the lower limbs and trunk (depending on the site and extent and of the lesion). Autonomic dysfunction may be seen in both with skin changes, sweating and pulse and blood pressure instability. Cardiovascular instability can be life threatening. There may be dysfunction of bladder and bowel in both disorders although it is more consistently present in spinal cord lesions. Sensory signs with loss of pain, light touch, temperature discrimination and proprioceptive loss are commonly seen in spinal cord lesions. A sensory level may be apparent. Although sensory symptoms are present in Guillain–Barré syndrome, sensory signs are usually absent.

Spinal cord compression

In children in whom spinal cord compression is slow in onset a history of progressive weakness and spasticity on examination may be seen. If the posterior columns are involved a loss of proprioception is expected. More extensive compression involving spinothalamic tracts will impair pain and temperature sensation. Corticospinal tract involvement leads to weakness, spasticity, hyperreflexia and extensor plantar response. Symptoms related to spinal route compression are unusual in childhood but may be seen in children with bony abnormalities or neurofibromatosis. Voluntary control over the bladder may be affected with difficulty in initiating micturition. Constipation may be seen.

Acute and severe spinal cord compression may cause spinal shock. There is complete flaccid paralysis, loss of reflexes and retention of urine and feces. Autonomic involvement may be severe and life threatening. In spinal shock there is both a direct effect on nerve conduction by the compressing lesion and also an indirect effect due to compromise of the vascular supply to the cord leading to ischemia and edema below the site of compression.

The commonest cause of acute spinal cord injury is trauma. In children with pre-existing spinal cord or vertebral column malformations this may be minor. Compression of the cord from a tumor, spinal abscess or intraspinal hematoma can be diagnosed on MRI. Acute transverse myelitis may show little change on MRI in the acute phase and imaging may need to be repeated.

When a child presents with acute spinal cord injury the ABC principles of resuscitation are paramount. Cervical cord lesions in particular may lead to respiratory, muscle and diaphragmatic weakness and require immediate intubation and ventilation. In trauma situations, the use of an appropriate sized hard cervical collar with cervical immobilization is vital. This should continue until the spine is deemed to be stable by an experienced neurosurgeon. Urgent MRI imaging is necessary. Immediate decompression of the cord may be possible. The use of intravenous dexamethasone is of proven benefit. Bladder catheterization is usually necessary.

The continuing approach to management will depend on the site and extent of the lesion. In all cases a multidisciplinary rehabilitation approach is best. Involvement of a regional spinal injuries unit early in management is helpful. Major difficulties in the long-term management often concern problems due to spasticity, pressure areas, bladder and bowel function and in cervical cord lesions, respiratory function. Techniques for long-term home ventilation are well established.

Transverse myelitis

This is an inflammatory lesion of the spinal cord thought to be immune-mediated. Pathologically changes are similar to acute disseminated encephalomyelitis (ADEM) and similar preceding illnesses have been implicated. Direct viral infection of the spinal cord is unusual, but needs to be considered, and treatment with aciclovir may be necessary until herpes simplex virus infection is excluded. Borrelia infection may present in this way.

Transverse myelitis often presents over a matter of hours or days with symptoms and signs of acute spinal cord dysfunction, both sensory and motor. In 80%, the level is thoracic. Segmental edema of the spinal cord is seen on MRI imaging, although this may not be clear in the acute phase. An intraspinal tumor may be difficult to exclude on initial imaging.

There is no treatment that is of proven benefit. Steroids and intravenous immunoglobulin have been given to patients, but no systematic trials support their use. Investigation of blood and CSF for evidence of viral infection is often undertaken but rarely reveals a specific cause.

Clinical management follows the same lines as acute cord compression. Recovery from transverse myelitis may continue for 2 or 3 years. Return of sensation, motor function and finally bladder function often occurs sequentially. The prognosis, however, is difficult to predict. Approximately 20% of children have little or no recovery of function. Others recover fully.

Progressive myelopathy

Children who develop slowly progressive compression of the spinal cord may present diagnostic difficulties. Initial symptoms are usually a subtle stiffening of the legs followed by increasing difficulty caused by weakness of hip flexion and ankle dorsiflexion. Pyramidal weakness with hyperreflexia may then become apparent. Initial sensory involvement may cause paresthesiae below the level of the lesion, or if spinal thalamic pathways are involved, unpleasant and painful limb sensations.

Conditions that predispose to progressive myelopathy, particularly cervical myelopathy, include Down syndrome, the mucopolysaccharidoses and other storage disorders, bony dysplasias such as spondylometaphyseal dysplasia and, in children with CNS malformations, particularly, hindbrain malformations. It is important in boys to consider the peroxisomal disorder adrenomyelopathy, which is a form of adrenoleukodystrophy.

Children with spinal cord developmental disorders may develop progressive myelopathy due to lesions in the lumbar spinal cord or cauda equina. A small number of these may be due to the effect of tethering of the spinal cord and neurosurgical release of this may be useful. Tethering of the cord may lead to damage from traction as the cord cannot ascend with growth of the spinal column. The child may present with weakness in one leg or with bladder or bowel problems. Progressive neurological deterioration is an indication for surgery. If prophylactic untethering is not undertaken then careful neurological follow-up is mandatory, especially at peak growth periods. With modern MRI scanning it is now possible to diagnose the condition with more accuracy and criteria for operation should become clearer.

An important cause of tethering is a bony or fibrocartilaginous spur, which arises from a vertebral body and passes between the halves of a bifid cord – diastematomyelia. In some cases this fixes the cord and results in increasing traction with growth. In other cases the cord divides well above the spur and passes around the diastematomyelia in two separate dural canals – diplomyelia.

Damage from tethering or compression may cause spastic paraplegia. More frequently, however, the child presents with distal weakness of the foot with clawing of the toes and equinovarus posture and weakness of the peronei. Dribbling incontinence of urine may be an early feature and there may be sensory loss in the sacral territory, loss of ankle jerk and anal reflexes and trophic changes in the feet.

The presence of a cutaneous lipoma or lipomeningocele may penetrate in dumb-bell fashion into the spinal canal. It may cause an increase in pressure within the canal. Treatment of the lipoma can be difficult, as the cord itself, as well as nerve roots, may be enmeshed in fatty tissue.

Guillain–Barré syndrome

This is a form of acute or subacute polyneuropathy seen at all ages. Several variants are described including acute inflammatory demyelinating polyneuropathy, acute motor axonal neuropathy and Miller–Fisher syndrome. All have an immunological basis.

The clinical presentation in Guillain–Barré syndrome is with progressive motor weakness of more than one limb, and areflexia, of varying degree. The weakness should not be still progressing 4 weeks into the illness and should be relatively symmetrical. Most patients report a prodromal upper respiratory or gastrointestinal illness in the 4 weeks prior to the onset of weakness. Pain and paresthesia, without sensory signs, is a common feature at presentation. Autonomic symptoms, such as constipation, urinary retention and vasomotor disturbances, may occur. Although lower limb weakness is the usual presentation, it may be generalized and proximal or distal. Facial and bulbar weakness occurs in around a quarter of children. Abnormal eye movements, meningeal irritation and papilledema (rarely) may be present, making distinction from a primary cerebral problem difficult. Deep tendon reflexes are lost in most children early in the illness, but this is variable.

The most serious complication of Guillain–Barré syndrome is respiratory failure and ventilation is required in around 10% of cases. A rapid onset, cranial nerve involvement and high CSF protein are associated with the need for ventilation.[563] Monitoring of respiratory function through peak flow or formal forced vital capacity measurements (which may be difficult in the preschool child) is essential.

The maximum weakness is often present for several days before improvement starts. Recovery may take several months, but is complete in the majority of children. In 25% or so of children mild long-term problems such as foot drop or hand weakness is found. Mortality is 2–5%, usually related to respiratory failure. Features influencing prognosis include severity of distal weakness and length of time from maximal weakness to onset of recovery.

The CSF protein level is raised in almost all children with Guillain–Barré syndrome. The cell count should be >10 cells/mm^3. However, the protein may be normal during the first week of the illness. Nerve conduction studies characteristically show a patchy conduction block consistent with demyelination. They also may be normal in the first week of the illness. Investigation for the preceding infection may be useful. Many cases are associated with *Campylobacter jejuni* infection. This in turn may be associated with antiganglioside antibodies.

Treatment in Guillain–Barré syndrome is mainly symptomatic and supportive. Particular attention must be paid to symptoms and signs suggesting respiratory failure and autonomic instability. Regular measurement of respiratory function and consideration of elective ventilation are vital. Bulbar dysfunction may require nasogastric feeding. Chest and limb physiotherapy are helpful.

Specific treatment is now by the use of intravenous immunoglobulin (IVIG) or plasmapheresis. Studies have shown these to be equally effective.[564] The former is considerably easier to administer. IVIG in a dose of 2 g/kg split over 5 days is the conventional regimen although single dose regimens and regimens given over 3 days are also described. Treatment is usually given when the patient is non-ambulant or appears to be losing the ability to walk. Steroids are not beneficial. Symptomatic treatment for pain and paresthesia may be needed.

ACUTE HEMIPARESIS

The commonest cause of acute hemiparesis is a Todd's paresis secondary to a prolonged partial seizure. This is usually obvious in a child with an established history of epilepsy, but diagnostic difficulties may arise if the child is not known to have epilepsy. Unrecognized nocturnal partial seizures may also cause diagnostic difficulty. Investigation for stroke or transient ischemic episodes may be necessary in this situation.

Hemiplegic migraine is also a common cause of acute hemiparesis. There is often a family history of hemiplegic migraine. Hemiplegic migraine is an ion channel disorder and in some families a gene has been identified linked to chromosome 19q12. In the absence of a family history, or previous attacks of migraine, the diagnosis may be difficult. The hemiparesis usually resolves within 24 h.

Other conditions that present with acute hemiparesis such as central nervous system infection (encephalitis, meningitis or cerebral abscess), demyelination, extradural, subdural hematoma are usually readily apparent on initial imaging. Where the area of radiological abnormality does not fit with a vascular distribution then the possibility of metabolic stroke as in MELAS and other mitochondrial disorders should be considered. In up to 20% of children who are fully investigated after an apparent ischemic cerebrovascular event no cause will be found.[565]

Cerebrovascular disease

Stroke in childhood has an incidence of three per million. Approximately half of all strokes are hemorrhagic and half are ischemic. Both require urgent neurological/neurosurgical assessment. In the postneonatal period the commonest cause of intracranial hemorrhage is head trauma. Spontaneous intracranial hemorrhage is usually either subarachnoid or intracerebral with subdural bleeding being extremely rare. Infarction of the brain may result from many causes including vascular thrombosis, cerebral embolism, watershed zone infarction, vascular compression or vascular injury. Most children present with an acute hemiparesis. This may be associated with a visual field defect, sensory symptoms, headache and focal seizures.

Some children will present with a stroke-like episode, which resolves within 24 h. Although this is more likely to be due to a Todd's paresis or hemiplegic migraine, cerebrovascular disease should be considered and investigations may be necessary. Most children who present with acute stroke are previously healthy but some conditions such as congenital heart disease and sickle cell disease are associated with a high incidence of stroke. In previously well children it is important to determine if there has been any preceding trauma that may suggest acute carotid dissection. Strokes are also associated with certain infections particularly varicella zoster and acute meningoencephalitis. Treatment with cefotaxime and aciclovir may be required in the acute phase until the cause of the stroke is known.

Initial management of stroke

Initial management following presentation with an acute stroke is along the ABC principles of resuscitation. However, intubation is rarely required. There is often an associated encephalopathy. Cerebral edema secondary to a hemorrhage or infarction is common and may persist for several days. With large infarcts, conscious level may deteriorate over the first 24 h and vigilance is required. Correction of any associated metabolic disturbance and control of seizures are important. In the acute phase, CT scanning is the imaging method of choice as it readily shows fresh hemorrhage. In ischemic stroke, particularly early on, CT may be normal. All children with non-hemorrhagic stroke should have an MRI scan with MR angiography as soon as practically possible. The role of acute thrombolysis in the management of childhood stroke has yet to be investigated and is not generally recommended. In children with sickle cell disease exchange transfusion is beneficial. Most authorities do not recommend use of anticoagulants and antiplatelet drugs in the acute phase of management. An exception is if a dissection has been demonstrated, when acute anticoagulation may be indicated. Likewise, some authorities suggest the use of anticoagulation following ischemic stroke associated with cerebral venous thrombosis. However, there is a significant risk of causing hemorrhagic transformation. Occasionally, children with large middle cerebral artery infarctions with massive cerebral edema benefit from surgical decompression.

Investigation of stroke

In children with hemorrhagic strokes, coagulopathies should be excluded. When the site of bleeding is not obvious on initial imaging, early cerebral angiography should be considered. However, this is not without risk and is often deferred.

Causes of ischemic stroke are numerous. A list of useful investigations is given in Table 20.61. Cardiac disease is strongly associated with cerebrovascular accident and ECG and echocardiogram should be done in all children. Transesophageal echocardiography may be necessary to fully exclude cardiac causes of ischemic stroke. Detailed hematological investigations for hemoglobinopathies and procoagulable states are necessary in all cases and, since the range of such disorders known to be associated with childhood stroke is increasing rapidly, a hematologist should be consulted. Biochemical investigations should include serum lipids and cholesterol, urine amino and organic acids and plasma, and in selected cases CSF, lactate levels. Inflammatory vasculitides should be screened for with measurement of the ESR and CRP, rheumatoid and antinuclear factors. If there is a history of recent chickenpox infection chickenpox antibodies in the CSF can be measured.

Brain imaging with MRI and MR angiography will determine the extent of the infarction and will show the nature of the large vessels in the neck and the circle of Willis. Carotid Doppler ultrasound is often helpful in looking for acute carotid dissection. In those children in whom the cause of ischemic stroke remains undetermined, formal cerebral angiography, after an interval of several weeks, is usually recommended, as potentially treatable conditions such as Moya Moya disease may otherwise be missed.

Table 20.61 Investigations in childhood stroke

Investigations in hemorrhagic stroke
FBC, U&Es, glucose
Clotting studies
CT, MRI, magnetic resonance angiography
Formal angiography
Investigations in ischemic stroke
FBC, U&Es, glucose
ESR/CRP
Clotting screen
Sickle cell screen
Studies for procoagulable states:
protein C, protein S, protein C resistance factor, factor V Leiden mutation, antithrombin III, lupus anticoagulant, anticardiolipin antibodies
Blood & CSF lactate – more detailed mitochondrial studies in selected cases
Urine amino acids (for homocystinuria)
Plasma lipids & cholesterol
Rheumatoid factor & antinuclear factor
CT, MRI, magnetic resonance angiography
Formal angiography in selected cases
Doppler studies
Cardiological investigations, including echocardiogram/ transesophageal echocardiogram
Investigations in venous sinus thrombosis
FBC, U&Es, glucose
ESR/CRP
Plasma viscosity
Detailed investigations for sepsis, including infections of the sinuses
Sickle cell screen
Clotting studies
Studies for procoagulable states (as above)
Urine amino acids
CT, MRI, magnetic resonance venography
Cardiological investigations (mainly associated with cyanotic heart disease & congestive cardiac failure)

Continuing management

A multidisciplinary team approach is important in the rehabilitation of children following strokes. The prognosis is variable depending on whether an underlying cause for the stroke can be found. In many children full investigation fails to reveal a specific cause; this is often regarded as a good prognostic feature.

In adults, large studies have shown clinical benefit in terms of prevention of recurrence of ischemic stroke from low dose aspirin therapy. Benefits of long-term anticoagulation with warfarin are not proven and this is now generally discouraged. In children, the role of low dose aspirin is unproven but the drug is widely given. Some authorities recommend doses as low as 1 mg/kg/day whilst others use up to 3 mg/kg/day.[566] The duration of therapy is uncertain but most neurologists recommend treatment for a minimum of 2 years. If MR, or conventional angiography, has revealed abnormalities of the cerebral vessels, repeat imaging may be used to guide the duration of treatment with aspirin. In children with hemoglobinopathies and coagulopathies specific treatment can help to reduce the risk of recurrent stroke.

Children who have bled from arteriovenous malformations, cavernous hemangiomas, and aneurysms or in association with Moya Moya disease have a significant risk of further strokes.

Arteriovenous malformations (AVM) have a life-long risk of re-bleeding of 2–3% per year. They are most commonly located supratentorially but may occur anywhere in the brain. Hemorrhagic stroke is the commonest presenting feature but they may also present with seizures or progressive neurological deficits including hemiplegia, visual field and eye movement disorders. They may give rise to a bruit on auscultation of the skull. Hemorrhagic stroke from AVM currently has a mortality of 15%. The risk of re-bleeding has persuaded most authorities that active treatment of AVM is necessary. Options include resection, interventional neuroradiology with occlusion by coils or glue and stereotactic radiosurgery. *Cavernous hemangiomas* consist of vascular spaces within endothelium and collagen. They are often calcified and are rare in childhood. Children usually present with epilepsy, but in those who present with bleeding, there is a high risk of re-bleeding. Management is along similar lines to that for AVM.

Intracranial aneurysms are much less common in children than adults. Most occur supratentorially and are only rarely multiple. The usual presentation is with acute hemorrhage. There is an association with coarctation of the aorta, congenital bilateral polycystic kidneys and Ehlers–Danlos syndrome. Mortality rate from bleeding is 30% and in the first month there is a re-bleed rate of 50%. Diagnosis is by CT scanning initially, followed by cerebral angiography. MR angiography does not have sufficient resolution to detect small aneurysms. Definitive treatment is either by resective surgery or by interventional radiology with occlusion.

Aneurysms of the vein of Galen may present with congestive heart failure or obstructive hydrocephalus or later in childhood with progressive pyramidal and cerebellar signs. A few children present with transient or permanent hemiplegia. Subarachnoid hemorrhage is rare. Treatment is often very difficult but embolization may be possible.

Moya Moya disease, although initially reported in Japan, affects all races and is increasingly recognized as a treatable cause of both ischemic and hemorrhagic stroke. Pathologically there is progressive arterial occlusion of the internal carotid and circle of Willis resulting in the development of fragile collateral vessels. Moya Moya disease may present with transient ischemic episodes, seizures, chorea or progressive intellectual deterioration as well as stroke. There is an association with neurofibromatosis, Down syndrome, sickle cell disease and previous cranial irradiation. Initial neuroimaging may show the clinical effects of stroke. MRI may show multiple flow voids around and in the basal ganglia. The collateral vessels may be seen on MR angiography with occlusion of the internal carotids. Formal cerebral angiography is usually necessary to confirm the diagnosis.

Around 50% of children with Moya Moya disease will have no long-term sequelae if left untreated. However, a proportion develop intellectual and motor impairment and early death and treatment is usually indicated. Anticoagulation and antiplatelet agents are of no proven benefit. The surgical creation of an anastamosis between the external and internal carotid circulation appears to be the most effective treatment.

DEVELOPMENTAL MEDICINE

INTRODUCTION

The development of the fetus, through infancy to adolescence, covers a period of evolution of the nervous system. This was first studied at an anatomical and microscopic level, and now genetic mechanisms of control begin to be understood in terms of molecular biology. The molecular mechanisms offer hypotheses for the influence of the environment and nurture on child development and this has been studied in detail in the opening section of this chapter.

The interaction of these factors is of importance to the parents and carers of children with disability, and often their concerns and questions on these aspects exceed the doctors' ability to provide answers. It is important for everyone practicing in this field to remain aware of advances in genetics.

Neuroimaging has identified structural changes, which are associated with developmental syndromes and cerebral palsy, such as hydrocephalus, neuronal migration disorders, callosal agenesis, or periventricular white matter change. Metabolic abnormalities may also lead to imaging changes, e.g. mitochondrial disorders with basal ganglia signal change and leukodystrophies. Cortical dysplasia is most likely to occur during neuroblast proliferation and migration. However there may be other ontogenic stages where this can occur, implicating environmental factors, including intrauterine infection, alcohol and drugs.

Behavioral development, up to 2 years, has been considered in its temporal relationship to maturational changes in the prefrontal cortex, language related cortical areas, the hippocampus, cerebellum and basal ganglia.[571,572] Environmental disadvantages, such as severe malnutrition during early postnatal life, produce neuro-integrative disorders and mental retardation. Dendritic abnormalities have been demonstrated which may be related.[573] Further advances in such research promises to integrate biological, social and environmental factors in child development. Biological factors correlate strongly with poor developmental attainment. Social and environmental factors continue to play a role in older children.[574]

Development and neurological disorders

Neurological disorders interact with developmental processes in ways which may be characteristic of different categories of disease. Rett's syndrome, for instance, has a disintegrative effect on normal development, usually during the first year of life, leading to regression in hand function, gross motor ability and communication. Hemiplegic cerebral palsy emerges at stages of hand function like reaching. Metabolic abnormalities, such as mitochondrial disorder, can set back development after an encephalopathic presentation. Other neurodegenerative disorders can have a more insidious course, like the ceroid lipofuscinoses (Batten's disease) causing loss of vision, loss of motor skills accompanied by dementia and epilepsy at ages varying according to the genetic abnormality.

Therefore it is essential to document development in a way that profiles the individual child being assessed. The neurological history can be expected to take longer than the clinical examination, to gain a thorough understanding of the problem. Neurodegenerative disorders may present with a stagnation of development in some, or regression in others. Growth is an important aspect, including weight, height, head circumference and pubertal staging. Dysplastic cerebral conditions, such as septo-optic dysplasia, may present with deficiences of the pituitary–hypothalamic axis as well as developmental delay.

Structured developmental assessment may be important to the neurological diagnosis, prognosis and support strategies in education and the community for the child and family. Table 20.62 lists psychometric tests most often used.

These tests are standardized examinations performed by educational or clinical child psychologists. The Griffiths' assessment is carried out by appropriately trained doctors in child development centers and in community child health settings. Each test has a formal scored structure with normative reference values. They may be used for one off assessments, or can be repeated over time as long as a minimum interval of 6 months separates longitudinal tests to avoid bias due to learnt responses.

Family functioning and developmental delay

The parents' ability to cope with their child's disability will be influenced by the information they receive, the way it is presented and the support they receive. They need to know what will be done for them, their family and for their child and to be guided in the spectrum of prognosis. Early liaison between neonatal and community, or acute pediatric and community services is essential.[575] Early intervention can do something to alleviate distress, anxiety and depression, with a positive influence on parents' perceptions of their child and their own parenting role.[576] The child's self-esteem is likely to be enhanced by positive perceptions.[577]

Table 20.62 Developmental measures

	Age range
Bayley Infant Neurodevelopmental Scales II	1–42 months (Bayley[609])
Denver – II	0–72 months (Frankenburg[610])
Griffiths Scales of Mental Development	Infants–6 years (Griffiths[612,613])
WISC – III (Wechsler intelligence scale for children)	16 years 11 months (Wechsler[611])

PATTERNS OF DEVELOPMENT

Motor

General introduction

Table 20.63 sets out a framework upon which to judge a child's development at different ages. However, there is individual variation for every child. It is not helpful to list only negative factors, but to find out what the child can do and how he/she performs. Some of this will emerge from the history, but other features come from informal observation of the child's activities. Parents enjoy describing their child's successes and children enjoy showing what they can do. The clinical setting should be comfortable, relaxed and attractive. Whilst the history is taken, if the child is able to be left to explore or play, he should be allowed to do so and should remain within the clinician's view. The floor is the safest place for a collection of interesting toys to motivate play and movement. Degrees of motivation, hand skills, and mobility may be demonstrated, whereas formal examination, essential as it is, may cause the child to withdraw.

The history should be left as much as possible to the parents to present in their own words and with as little interruption as possible. For instance the parents will recall when they first had concerns about the child, and this may pre-date the time of concern expressed in the referral letter. This approach helps to promote trust and minimize misunderstanding in the therapeutic relationship.

Children's development has to be understood as a whole. There is a vast difference between a child aged 1 year who can only sit without progressing and is content so to be, compared with a child who is normally motivated but frustrated by their plight. The former prompts concern about intellectual development. Motor development must be appraised alongside the way the child is developing altogether.

Key historical aspects

In taking a history the aim is to clarify the specific nature of the problem in the context of the child's overall development, social/family circumstances and general health. It is essential to understand who is concerned about the child (e.g. parent or professional or both) and the reason for the concern. Parents are encouraged to write down questions for which they want answers and some clinics offer a pre-clinic visit by a specialist nurse or social worker to help parents prepare for the consultation. On the day, time passes quickly and much information may be difficult to take in. If parents wish, there is much to be said for them bringing an experienced professional or a relative to listen with them, maybe to take notes and to visit them at home later. In a familiar setting the supporter can find out whether the parents asked the questions they wanted to ask, understood the answers and want to know more. It is often helpful to arrange a second appointment soon after the first to deal with anxieties, further questions and plans for help in the future.

Pregnancy. Threatened abortion, antepartum hemorrhage, hypertension, pre-eclampsia, the continuity of fetal movements and the outcome of antenatal scanning are all relevant. The loss of fetal movements for more than 12 h may signal a stroke-like event in the fetus. Maternal illness and the need for medication, such as anticonvulsants in pregnancy, can be associated with an adverse fetal outcome. Past obstetric history, such as fetal loss, may be of genetic significance.

Birth and neonatal period. The reasons for induction of labor should be explored. The mode of delivery and immediate health of the infant are usually recalled clearly by the mother. Comments on the need for resuscitation will require clarification by reference to the neonatal notes. The baby's weight and maturity, and degree of vigor in feeding are markers for later development. Need for tube feeding may signal early cerebral palsy, syndromal diagnoses such as Prader–Willi syndrome, neuromuscular disorder including dystrophia myotonica, hypoxic–ischemic encephalopathy or anatomical palatal problems. Hypoglycemia can lead to occipital ischemic change, and may be associated with pituitary–hypothalamic insufficiency as in septo-optic dysplasia. Seizures are likely to be symptomatic, possibly underlining the significance of hypoxic–ischemic injury, neonatal sepsis, a metabolic disorder, or the onset of epilepsy related to antenatal cerebral dysgenesis.

Table 20.63 Framework for developmental appraisal

Newborn period	Well-being of infant at birth Feeding ability – duration of feeds – ability to thrive
Infancy	Early watching and smiling Manipulative skills – ensure bimanual in infancy Independent sitting Age at independent walking Means of mobility before walking – crawling, bottom-shuffling, etc. Motivation to move – goal-directed
Toddler and preschool	Speech – vocabulary, clarity, grammar, context. Ability to talk about pictures that tell a story. Play – interactive, imaginative, imitative, flexible Social awareness – aware of strangers, biddable, able to share, no excessively rigid fixations, appropriate perception of sadness and humour Motor ability to run, jump, climb stairs, get up from falls Drawing skills, shape recognition, colours Self-care – feeding, dressing, and toilet training
School entry	Emotional adjustment Academic progress Behavior in class, and at home Friendships with peers Evidence of clumsiness Attention span
General health	Appetite and growth, monitoring height, weight, and head circumference Quality of sleep Significant intercurrent illness, especially evidence of encephalopathic episodes, e.g. vomiting and drowsiness

Milestones. Details of developmental milestones may tax the memory of parents and it may be helpful to refer to contemporary records, including baby books, parent-held child health records, photographs and videos. However, if the child is walking, age of first walking independently is usually recalled accurately and is a good starting point. It is then helpful to ask how the child moved before walking, or moves now if they are not walking. This may reveal alternative patterns of movement which may be a normal, familial variant associated with low tone and hypermobile joints, like creeping, rolling or bottom shuffling.[578] In such children, the median age of walking independently is 19 months and some are not walking independently until 30 months. Often a parent/sibling will have had a similar developmental history though there may also be a family history of children who 'just stand and walk' before a year old. Crawling beyond 2 years, however, is likely to signal an ataxic pattern of development.

Speech and language difficulties may be associated with motor developmental problems in a spectrum from habitual toe-walking,[579] developmental dyspraxia to a neuromuscular disorder like the Xp21 dystrophinopathies[580] and cerebral palsy.

Table 20.64 The floppy infant: investigations and related etiologies

Chromosomes	Down syndrome and other genetic diagnoses
DNA analysis	Prader–Willi syndrome Congenital myotonic dystrophy Spinal muscular atrophy
Creatine phosphokinase	Congenital muscular dystrophy
Tensilon test	Maternal myasthenia gravis Congenital myasthenia
Urinary amino acids organic acids mucopolysaccharides oligosaccharides	Inborn errors of metabolism, e.g. methyl malonic aciduria, propionic aciduria
Biotinidase	Biotinidase deficiency
Calcium FISH analysis chromosome 22	DiGeorge spectrum/ 22q11 deletions
Glucose Thyroid function (TSH & FT4) Electrolytes	Optic nerve hypoplasia/septo-optic dysplasia spectrum and hypopituitarism
White cell enzymes	Pompe's disease/glycogenosis type II
Transferrin isoelectric focusing	Congenital glycoprotein disorders especially Type Ia and Ic
Serum lactate CSF lactate and protein Mitochondrial DNA analysis	Mitochondrial cytopathies
Very long chain fatty acids	Peroxisomal disorders (Zellweger's disease)
Magnetic resonance imaging of brain	Lissencephaly and other cerebral dysplasias and cell migration disorders Cerebral hypoxia/ischemia of intrauterine origin (e.g. spastic or athetoid cerebral palsy)
Muscle biopsy (respiratory chain enzyme analysis)	Discussed in section on neuromuscular disorders

Hand preference acquired in the first year often indicates a hemiplegia on the opposite side. Neglect of reaching with one hand may be interpreted as early dominance in the other. Observation of the child will indicate neglect of the affected arm and hand with poverty of movement, failure to use the limb to maintain balance and persistent fisting. When standing with support, the child may be up on the toes of the affected side. All infants should be bimanual.

Early school progress is worth documenting in all relevant age groups, including older children and adolescents. By junior and senior years, school progress may be difficult for parents to comment on. Emotional difficulties settling into early school and the need for early help with reading, writing and maths recalled by parents may still have relevance to the child later on. An assessment of the child's social and peer group skills is important. These aspects inform the clinician as to the impact of the child's condition on daily living, including happiness and confidence.

General health. Frequent chest infections may be relevant to the feeding and swallowing difficulties of infants with cerebral palsy. The immune system can be affected in the DiGeorge spectrum of chromosome 22q11 disorders, and in ataxia telangiectasia. Growth retardation or failure to thrive may indicate underlying metabolic disease or pituitary–hypothalamic involvement, oropharyngeal feeding difficulties, malabsorption or neglect. Seizures may weigh more towards central nervous system diagnoses but need to distinguished from syncope, breath-holding attacks, night terrors, vertigo, daydreaming and other non-epileptic phenomena. Myoclonic seizures may have to be demonstrated to parents who otherwise regard them as 'normal' startles. Tics are common in later childhood. They may be familial. Though doctors regard these and other phenomena as of no importance clinically, they often cause concern in families.

Family history. A family tree provides the clearest documentation of the family. It helps to highlight possible dominant, recessive or X-linked mechanisms of inheritance. A family history may also give insight into concerns and preoccupations. Aunt Helen may be understood to have drowned in an epileptic seizure. Mother's sister Judith may have been cared for in a home. Uncle Tom has a long psychiatric history. Father's uncle Ron committed suicide. The stories explain the family's reaction to possible diagnoses in their children even though there is no genetic link between the affected relative and their child. Some assessment of parental educational achievement, employment and hobbies can be relevant to children with dyspraxic, speech and language, learning and social developmental difficulties.

FAILURE TO PROGRESS IN THE FIRST 18 MONTHS

The floppy infant (Table 20.64)

Diminished muscle tone may herald cerebral palsy in any of its categories of spasticity, athetosis or ataxia. Neuromuscular presentations are described elsewhere, and it is possible for central and peripheral pathology to coexist. Hence the latter category should not be ruled out too readily. Genetic syndromes, including Down syndrome and Prader–Willi syndrome, cerebral dysplasia, hydrocephalus, inborn errors of metabolism and endocrine disorders are other possible etiologies for floppiness in infancy. The former term 'benign central hypotonia' refers to children with a familial variant of normal development who do not crawl and who show joint hypermobility. (Though the outcome is benign for most there is an increased risk of panic attacks and phobic disorders when this is associated with an interstitial duplication of chromosome 15q24-q26 (named DUP25).[581])

Examination

Observation of movements against gravity needs to be opportunistic. Patterns of movement and posture should be observed with changes of state in the infant; a very hypotonic state in a sleepy infant may change to stiff extensor posturing and arching in an alert state in dyskinetic–athetoid presentations. Reflexes are important to document. Facial expression and eye movements may be induced by the examiner's social interaction with the baby. The degree of success of this may reflect upon the infant's use of vision or cognitive development. A restricted range of horizontal or vertical eye movements may be a sign of mid-brain abnormalities or an active hydrocephalus. Expert assessment of the optic fundi is essential when considering intrauterine infection, optic nerve hypoplasia and pigmentary retinal abnormalities, in mitochondrial cytopathy for instance. A search for dysmorphic features and general systems examination including inspection of the anatomy of the genitalia are also important to neuro-metabolic/genetic diagnoses.

Growth must be assessed in the parameters of weight, length and head circumference with attention to trends over time. Failure to thrive may be a consequence of feeding difficulties, metabolic disorder, or endocrine deficiency, including hypothyroidism.

A growth chart which shows head circumference crossing the percentiles in either direction is a reason for further investigation including brain imaging and, in the case of microcephaly or marked skull asymmetry, skull X-ray for synostosis.

Delayed walking

Physiological alternative patterns of movement, such as bottom shuffling or bunny hopping are often associated with delayed walking. The mean age of walking for bottom shufflers is 19 months. Bottom shuffling is largely benign, but only if it is dissociated, i.e. all other developmental parameters are normal. Abdominal crawling in a commando style raises the possibility of spastic diplegia, where it is goal directed. However a dyspraxic pattern of abdominal crawling, lacking goal directed achievement without frustration usually signals associated learning difficulties, walking coming late. Prolonged crawling and continuing crawling after walking has been achieved with delay, is a strong pointer to ataxia. Regression to crawling with loss of pulling to stand should alert to hip girdle weakness or a progressive cerebellar lesion.

Examination

Observation of natural movement and reaching will be most informative. A specific search for lower limb signs can be achieved first with the child more happily seated on the edge of the parent's knees. Hip adductor spasm, ankle clonus, tightness of the tendo-Achilles and hyperreflexia are long tract signs of spasticity. Signs of hypotonia also may be demonstrated in this situation. In the upper limbs, proximal shoulder girdle power may be estimated by lifting the child under the axillae, when the child should easily hold on by the strength of shoulder adduction. This maneuver will also demonstrate 'sitting on air' in bottom shufflers. The spine must be fully examined in the undressed child for scoliosis and midline defects. Examination in the supine position allows assessment of hip flexor contracture and politeal angle as well as hip symmetry and stability.

INVESTIGATION IN THE UNDER 18-MONTH-OLD CHILD

It is important to gain a mutual perspective with the parents on the child's presentation before discussing investigations. This is an anxious time for the family, and that anxiety may be heightened if the parents consider that the doctor either over- or underestimates their child's problem. Often parents expect that investigations will lead to diagnosis, treatment and cure. It is important to discuss the aspects of investigations that may well not lead to treatment. The priorities in investigation, though, are to seek treatable conditions, or those with genetic implications. A positive diagnosis will help towards awareness of the health care that the child needs now and in the future; it can have genetic implications for the reproductive prospects of the couple, their siblings and possibly the siblings of the child. Iron deficiency, sometimes with anemia, is common and should not be forgotten as a treatable cause of delayed development.[582] Excluding neurometabolic and genetic syndromes will also assist in that process.

The range of investigations relevant to these presentations is very extensive[583] and good practice demands a selective approach. That may mean that the investigation process is in stages, if first line tests prove negative. Parents need preparation for this, and planning should include, where possible, arranging for tests, such as imaging, which require sedation or anesthesia, to be done together as part of the same procedure, for the child's comfort. A considerable proportion of children will remain without a definitive diagnosis. It is important that such children are kept under occasional review to reconsider a diagnosis over time. In time, the child may reveal more informative clinical signs, or diagnostic advances may be made.

Table 20.65 lists tests relevant to the child with delayed walking, who usually presents around 18 months but who can present later. Metabolic tests are relevant to conditions associated with encephalopathic episodes, often precipitated by intercurrent infection such as mitochondrial cytopathy or beta-oxidation defects. Magnetic resonance brain imaging is more informative to developmental disorders than computed tomography. Where neurometabolic and genetic tests are negative, the MR scan is likely to reveal some anatomical abnormality in about one-third of children, but this may not constitute a specific diagnosis.

Tissue biopsy, such as skin conjunctival biopsy, is still important to the diagnosis of the ceroid lipofuscinoses by electron microscopy. It is also relevant to genetic studies on skin fibroblast culture. Muscle biopsy will normally be reserved for the diagnosis of neuromuscular disorders in children with muscle weakness, by needle biopsy, or in the search for a mitochondrial disorder where sufficient sample for respiratory enzyme analysis is usually obtained by open biopsy.

Management

Apart from benign presentations of dissociated motor development, infants and children with motor developmental delay should be referred early to their community pediatrician and child development center (CDC). This does not need to wait until the search for a diagnosis is complete. Much is to be gained from an early referral. Parents need the support of experienced CDC staff, including therapists, health visitor, play therapist and social worker. The team supports both the parents and the investigating pediatrician, helping to review the child's progress and recognizing

Table 20.65 Delayed walking and abnormal gait: investigations and associated etiologies

Consider all investigations for the floppy infant (Table 20.64) and the following:	
Creatine phosphokinase	Xp21 and other dystrophies
Magnetic resonance imaging brain/spinal cord:	
Cerebellar vermis	Congenital glycoprotein disorders Joubert's syndrome Cerebellar hypoplasia
Ventriculomegaly	Hydrocephalus and associated cerebral dysplasias
Craniocervical junction	Arnold–Chiari malformation
Spinal cord	Syringomyelia
Cortex and subcortex	Dysplasia and hypoxic-ischemic injury, e.g. spastic cerebral palsy
White matter	Leukodystrophic conditions: Van der Knaap's leukodystrophy, Pelizaeus–Merzbacher disease
Basal ganglia	Hypoxic-ischemic injury Mitochondrial cytopathy Glutaric aciduria Wilson's disease Hallervorden–Spatz disease
Alpha-fetoprotein Immunoglobulins Chromosome fragility test	Ataxia telangiectasia
Nerve conduction studies DNA analysis	Hereditary motor sensory neuropathies, hereditary peripheral neuropathies
Vitamin E level	Ataxia and peripheral neuropathy
Frataxin DNA analysis	Friedreich's ataxia

new problems such as social/language delay or seizures. It is essential that preschool assessments allow time for setting up supported school entry, such as the need for formal assessment ('statementing').

The CDC team will also be a focal point for the family who may need to see a range of specialists before their child's medical assessment is complete. It is a resource for information about the child's condition, such as the Contact a Family Directory[584] (a collection of parent support organizations renewed annually), plus local support groups and liaison with local education and social services, including housing departments. Children with motor delay may be seen, in turn, by a hospital pediatrician, a pediatric neurologist, a geneticist and an orthopedic surgeon. If there is global delay, in addition, they may have appointments also with ophthalmology and audiology, which are often organized within the community sphere.

Specific physical management will be discussed in the section on cerebral palsy.

ABNORMAL GAIT

Etiology

Presentations with this complaint usually begin around the age of 3 years onwards. Parents may present their child as constantly tripping, falling over, fatiguing or simply as 'not walking properly'. In the young child especially these features may be difficult to distinguish from the normal spectrum of development. If there is a regression of abilities then pathology is expected.

An acute deterioration over days or a few weeks may indicate a peripheral demyelinating condition such as Guillain–Barré syndrome or acute demyelinating encephalomyelitis (ADEM). Infective causes like discitis, osteomyelitis, tuberculosis of the spine and possibly polio should be considered. On a similar time-scale, loss of balance or focal weakness may indicate an intracranial space-occupying lesion. Spinal lesions tend to have a more insidious onset and can present for some time as an abnormal gait, without formal neurological deficit, or simply as back pain.

Non-progressive, or slowly progressive presentations are historically bound with the child's development, emerging with growth and time. Conditions associated predominantly with muscle weakness are discussed in detail in the section on neuromuscular disorders. The static encephalopathies are discussed under cerebral palsy.

Spasticity does not always signify cerebral palsy. Progressive spasticity may be genetic, as in hereditary spastic paraplegia, or metabolic, as in the leukodystrophies, or structural, in the spinal cord, such as Arnold–Chiari malformation with a syrinx. If the upper limbs show no deficit at all, then caution should apply before diagnosing spastic diplegia, as a spinal abnormality must be eliminated.

Discrepancies of growth of a limb often accompany congenital spastic cerebral palsy, as in hemiplegia or monoplegia. Lower limb shortening may be real, in hip subluxation, or apparent in pelvic tilt, which may be associated with a scoliosis. Scoliosis demands spinal imaging apart from the long C-curve, which develops in most children with four-limb cerebral palsy. Dwarfing of one lower limb that is noted at birth raises the possibility of a low cord anomaly like spinal dysraphism, or a tethered cord with an intrathecal lipoma.

Examination

Features of a normal gait

There are fundamental elements of a normal gait that can be helpful to look for in the analysis of an abnormal gait. The first is the normal pattern of heel strike and toe lift off. A tempo or cadence accompanies this, which is regular. The distance between the fe during walking is the base of the gait, which is normally narrow and constant, following a straight line. There are degrees of hip and knee flexion, which may be exaggerated in abnormal gait. In the upper limbs, reciprocal swinging of the arms should be observed, which becomes more emphasized in running, with increased flexion at the elbows. Finally the trunk should remain relatively still as judged by the pattern of movement at the shoulders.

Patterns of abnormal gait

When judging an abnormal gait, the examiner should strive to discern weakness, spasticity, ataxia, dyskinesia and dystonia. If no such signs can be found, the gait may be dyspraxic, or, after careful elimination of pathology including spinal pathology, it may betray an illness pattern of behavior in older children.

Side to side swinging of the shoulders suggests a waddling gait and the possibility of hip girdle weakness. This must be explored more formally, with attention to the presence of a full Gowers' maneuver or modified Gowers' sign.[585] A modified Gowers' sign may also be exhibited by the child with ataxia as they rise from the floor. Formal examination for neuromuscular disorder must follow.

Toe strike may indicate tendo-Achilles tightness, which may be fixed in a contracture, and/or dynamic as in spasticity, dystonia or habitual toe walking. Any condition affecting the gastrocnemius or soleus muscles can lead to this, ranging from spasticity, through peripheral neuropathy to dystrophic change or spinal muscular atrophy. Children with distal arthrogryposis will have more complex distal joint deformities with wasting below the knee. A high stepping flexion at the hips and knees suggests peripheral weakness. Hyperextension at the knee may be a feature of hypotonia as in peripheral neuropathy, or a compensatory mechanism to achieve toe strike in spastic or dystonic tightness of the tendo-Achilles.

A generally flexed pattern at the hips and knees throughout walking describes a crouched gait. This is typical of spastic diplegia, when scissoring of the legs is often seen. Most of these children, but not all, also demonstrate toe strike. Their walking can appear superficially quick with a short stride, but in terms of velocity and energy demands, it is inefficient.

The child with ataxia loses practically all of the normal features of gait. There is lack of heel strike with a flat-footed strike instead. The rhythm and base of the gait are irregular with a tendency to stagger on turning. Reciprocal arm swing is lost, being replaced by an elevated, balancing position of the upper limbs as in early toddler walking. These children usually cannot run, and if they attempt to, they are very likely to fall.

Dyskinetic and dystonic patterns of walking are often misjudged as hysterical, partly because the limb movements and postures can appear bizarre, and because they fluctuate according to the emotional state of the child. A fearful or excited child with these difficulties will exhibit obvious signs that may be harder to recognize when they are relaxed, leading to the misconception that they are 'put on'.

Dystonic patterns often reveal themselves in an exaggerated extension of the trunk and lower limbs, placing the child on their toes with tight plantar flexion and internal rotation at the hips with extension at the knees and/or scissoring. The upper limbs may take up bizarre, uncomfortable positions, such as flexing behind the back. Dyskinetic movements are transient involuntary movements, which can interrupt the fluency of walking. When they occur in the upper limb the child often tries to hide them by holding the limb with the other arm, or pretending that they intended to move it, for instance to stroke their neck or touch their clothes.

If none of the above features of abnormal gait can be discerned, and yet the child's walking and running do look awkward, they may well have developmental dyspraxia. Fogg's test can be helpful, showing symmetrical exaggeration of associated movements for the child's age. The child often has difficulty reproducing the patterns of movement that they are asked to perform. For instance serial finger to thumb sequencing or rapidly alternating hand movements may prove impossible even though they clearly understand the task. This is often solved by the child, who employs the other hand to make the fingers under examination 'work'. Some of these children will exhibit tongue dyspraxia, being unable to 'paint' their upper lip with the tip of their tongue.

Formal neurological examination must be incorporated into the final analysis of observations on gait. Consideration of the presence or absence of weakness or wasting, its distribution and associated deep tendon reflexes will help to clarify the motor categories above.

Investigations

Investigations, according to diagnostic categories, are covered in Tables 20.64 and 20.65.

Management

The care of the child after diagnosis is discussed in the relevant section on neuromuscular disease for children with weakness, and in the relevant section for children with cerebral palsy. Children with developmental motor dyspraxia should be considered in a broader perspective than motor deficits alone. There may be overlapping diagnostic circles with attention deficit and hyperactivity disorder, speech and language delay, specific learning difficulty, habit spasms and the Tourette's syndrome spectrum, social developmental difficulties, as well as behavior disorder. Successful management relies on an integrated approach between health, education and social services, which includes the community pediatric services.

For children with dyspraxic motor deficits there is a risk that their problem falls between the perceived remit of each agency. There is a good case for interagency in-service training and development of local policies. Occupational therapy and pediatric physiotherapy assessments are a scarce resource and dyspraxic children are given low priority. Many therapists believe that the children's problems are of an educational special need rather than a health issue, whether or not there is any educational provision for dyspraxic children. There is little point in referring to a service with a 2-year waiting list. For carefully selected children, therapy review in school can help the child and teacher resolve problems of visual perception and handwriting. Keyboard and computer skills or audiotaped lessons may be needed.

Enhancement of the child's age-appropriate independence in self-help skills is a key aim. There is no research evidence that gross motor physical exercises improve coordination in the long term. Self-esteem and happiness factors may not be improved by a demand to 'practice' that which the child finds intrinsically difficult. An aim is to find activities at which the child can be successful and which promote satisfaction and self-confidence. Group physiotherapy or drama groups for such children may improve confidence for the child and assist the parents' perceptions of the problem. They require a high adult to child ratio. Having dyspraxia in common is no barrier to remorseless mutual criticism.

CLINICAL PRESENTATIONS OF LEARNING DIFFICULTY

Infancy

When an infant presents with developmental delay it is usually with poor motor progress. Sometimes patterns of movement and posture are seen which improve over time such as hypotonia, mild dystonic posturing and elements of disorganized patterns of movement (developmental dyspraxia). Such children are best followed up by community assessment teams. The early parental concern about motor development may be replaced by concerns over language and communication, social awareness and behavior, and ultimately school performance and learning difficulty.

Associated features of concern are lack of sustained visual attention and/or auditory attention to age 6 months or more, as well as the 'too contented' 12-month-old who lacks frustration at their immobility and lacks motivation to move. The absence of goal directed behavior comes into the same category.

There may be a number of recognizable etiologies in this group, including chromosome abnormalities including sex chromosome abnormalities, cerebral palsy, especially the ataxic category; a number of genetic syndromes, such as Prader–Willi and Williams syndromes; inborn errors of metabolism, such as congenital disorders of glycosylation; and structural cerebral abnormalities such as hydrocephalus or degrees of migration disorder such as lissencephaly. Early diagnosis is often difficult and it is these children who will benefit from occasional follow-up in the longer term when further diagnostic features may develop.

The preschool child

Beyond the first 2 years of life presentations possibly associated with learning difficulty are likely to be in the areas of language delay, social awareness, behavior problems and hyperactivity. Gillberg[585a] and Kadesjo & Gillberg[585b,585c] emphasize the importance of overlapping developmental domains in these disorders with a child rarely fitting neatly into one particular category.

Clumsiness, developmental coordination disorder or developmental dyspraxia may be associated with any of the above or may stand on its own. Early school progress for some of the dyspraxic children gives clues to associated specific learning difficulty, e.g. in language. Observation by staff in nursery and infant classes complements parental observations. Dyspraxia is commonly associated with anxiety, depression and withdrawal. Behavior problems, including clinging and attention seeking, are commoner in boys and often reflect anxiety. Depression is commoner in girls who are less likely to be referred to specialists.

Diagnoses which are important to consider at this age include Xp21 muscular dystrophy; neurofibromatosis; the autistic spectrum, especially Asperger's syndrome; and an underlying hydrocephalus. Children with focal epilepsy may present at this age. Those with frontal or temporal foci are likely to have difficulty in all domains of learning compared with their unaffected siblings.[585d] Language-based learning and memory are particularly vulnerable. The effect is less in the early years of schooling when the children are taught by one teacher than when they face the complex demands of secondary school after the age of 11 years.

The mainstream school child

Children with learning difficulties in mainstream school may be assessed to require transfer to special schools, but more often they will be found to be within the normal range in their general intelligence quotient. It will be the uneven profile of individual scores in different domains of learning that underlies their difficulties, i.e. specific learning difficulty (SpLD). This may not be clear until psychometric assessment is performed, school reports alone sometimes being misleading. At the extremes, children who are well behaved with their SpLD may not come to teachers' attention as any more than slow learners, while children with behavior problems may be regularly excluded. Unrecognized SpLD can be expected to cause individuals stress as they struggle to achieve, often experiencing criticism from teachers and reflected anxiety and criticism from their parents. The child with a high verbal score and low performance (visual–perceptual–motor) score may engage well in class discussions but fail to meet the same standard on paper. Children with low verbal scores and low reading age will struggle to gather and order their ideas. They may spend a long time writing very little on a given topic.

Clinically these issues should be considered in a number of common pediatric presentations. These include: headaches; abdominal pain; leg pains; emotional and behavior problems, the recovery phase post brain injury, medical or traumatic; focal epilepsy; and the broad canvas of illness behavior. Commonly, though not invariably, the child has excessive absence from school, bordering on school refusal, but often attributed to minor intercurrent ailments. It is remarkable how other children with notably debilitating episodes of migraine, or treatment resistant epilepsy still maintain a good school attendance record.

Children with Asperger's syndrome deserve a special place in this group. Their rigidities, lack of social and academic flexibility, concrete and literal use of language, developmental coordination difficulties, disinhibition and low threshold to frustrated behavior, alongside their selectively high abilities in particular idiosyncratic fields throw up perplexing school challenges. Peer relationships are scanty and unhappy and such children are vulnerable to bullying. Yet they may converse confidently, albeit pedantically, and at length, with adults. Teachers see areas of ability but struggle to help the children apply them successfully. Often teachers find it difficult to express and identify their concerns for these children.

Management

Infants and preschool children need a multidisciplinary approach involving the community pediatric team when problems are identified by parents, health visitors or preschool teachers. The diagnostic phase requires input from pediatric neurology and clinical genetics services, if there are abnormal neurological signs or dysmorphic features.

It is important that there is a multidisciplinary approach to mainstream school children with learning difficulties from the start – medical investigations, educational assessment and, if indicated, clinical psychology support should run together. This helps to avoid the impasse that follows in illness behavior when no 'medical cause' can be found. It is also essential for the child with Asperger's syndrome, who may well need a diminished and adjusted timetable in the years of GCSE school examinations to take the pressure off them and their families.

Rather than concentrating on the children's weaknesses and making them practice these, a more successful educational and parenting style is to seek the activities in which the child can experience success and help the child develop these. Recognizing that a child has a difficulty in language comprehension or coordination and making appropriate allowances can lead to a marked improvement in behavior and self-esteem. Children with coordination problems may enjoy physical activities nonetheless, provided the demands made on them are realistic. Children with language comprehension and expressive difficulties calm down and thrive when dealt with appropriately.

Global learning disability (mental retardation)

About 3% of children have moderate learning disability (MLD) and four per thousand have severe learning disability (SLD). Only a minority of children with MLD have a known medical diagnosis. Between 33 and 40% of children with SLD have no medical diagnosis. Presentation is usually by delayed motor development and delayed language development. Children with MLD/SLD may be thought to be unusually quiet and inactive when young, but some are hyperkinetic, aggressive and irritable or prone to self-injury. MLD is the commonest reason for children not walking at 18 months, other than normal variants associated with familial joint hypermobility – bottom shufflers, rollers and creepers for instance. Only one in six children with SLD will be walking by 18 months. A third of boys with Duchenne muscular dystrophy are not walking by 18 months and some of them also have delayed language development, MLD or even SLD and autism. In assessing the significance of late walking it is important to assess development as a whole – especially language comprehension. Parents of children with MLD may say 'he understands everything I say' without realizing how many non-verbal cues and contextual prompts they are using.

Investigation

There are numerous reasons for children having MLD or SLD. Some are constitutional such as chromosome disorders, dominant, recessive or X-linked genetic disorders, polygenic conditions and dysmorphic or disorders of brain development. Some are constitutional and amenable to treatment – such as inborn errors of metabolism. Others have environmental causes – intrauterine infection, fetal alcohol syndrome, lead poisoning or brain damage from trauma for instance. Neglect is a reason for developmental delay or apparent MLD so enquiry into home circumstances is appropriate. A more detailed guideline to investigation is given in the introductory section to this chapter.

Management

Whether or not investigation of the medical cause of learning disability is successful, it is always appropriate to offer genetic counseling. The local education authority should be notified, with parental consent, of the child's likely future special educational needs in preschool and school years. The social services department should be informed, also with parental consent, so that families may benefit from their support and information. Parents should be informed of relevant voluntary agencies. The multidisciplinary child development team will be mobilized to explore possible ways of helping the child to achieve his/her potential. The emphasis is of finding remediable aspects – vision, hearing, epilepsy, diet, bowel function for instance – and coordinating such help as the parents think appropriate. This is the guiding principle of management throughout childhood.

ACQUIRED BRAIN INJURY

SCIENTIFIC BACKGROUND

Etiology

Acquired brain injury may be traumatic (TBI) or medical in origin. Admissions to hospital in the UK are about 4 per 1000 children per year aged 15 or under due to TBI. The majority are minor head injuries and about 8% are moderate or severe according to definitions based on the depth and/or duration of coma. Definitions of severe head injury vary between publications, though the consensus favors a Glasgow Coma Score (GCS) of 8 or less at presentation. The brain injury may be multifactorial in origin, especially when significant extracranial injuries exist, such as chest or abdominal injuries with consequences for cerebral oxygenation and perfusion. The incidence increases with increasing age and relaxation of supervision. In the first year of life the majority are due to non-accidental injury. Overall there is a male to female ratio of 2.75 : 1 in severe brain injury.

Non-traumatic, or medical brain injury arises from a variety of causes including CNS infection, e.g. meningoencephalitis, hypoxic–ischemia, as in post cardiac arrest or near drowning, stroke or metabolic encephalopathy. As these are covered in the section on acute encephalopathy, the discussion here will focus on TBI. However, the principles of rehabilitation are the same for all categories of acquired brain injury.

PATHOPHYSIOLOGY

In severe traumatic brain injury the brain is subjected to direct contusional injury, as well as forces that diffusely shear neuronal axons, and subsequently there is cerebral edema and compromise of cerebral perfusion. Lesions are best demonstrated on magnetic resonance imaging (MRI). Deeper lesions correlate with poorer functional outcome at discharge from rehabilitation, whereas initial GCS is more predictive of outcome at 12 months.[586] The brainstem is susceptible to shearing injury because of the differential density between it and the cerebrum. The frontal lobes are commonly affected, even in the absence of focal lesions on MRI.[587]

Collections of blood intraparenchymally, in the subarachnoid space, subdural or extradural spaces will add to cerebral irritation and increase intracranial pressure, diminishing cerebral blood flow.

Regional cerebral blood flow varies within a contused area compared with the surrounding brain, being reduced in the contusion.[588] Also cerebral vascular reactivity varies over time.[589] Such findings have consequences for targeting therapy. Ischemic change occurs in three phases.[590] The first is one of depressed metabolism with increased extracellular K^+ and intracellular Ca^+. The second phase is one of energy failure and anoxic depolarization with loss of normal electrochemical gradients across the neuronal cell wall for different ions and concomitant release of neurotransmitters.[591] The third phase is neurodegenerative, which may take hours or days. The effectiveness of reperfusion and recovery processes will influence the final outcome.

CONSEQUENCES

Physical

Physical neurological deficits often appear the most serious initially. Occasionally a severe physical deficit may remain with long term dependency. More often, sometimes several weeks or days from the injury, an accelerated phase of recovery is seen, leading to independent walking and restoration of fine motor skills for self-care. Fine motor deficits tend to be more prevalent than gross motor 12 months into recovery.[515] Where there has been basal ganglia injury there can be a delayed onset of choreoathetosis, which is difficult to treat. Early onset visual impairment and extrapyramidal signs often settle over the early weeks though visual perceptual difficulties may persist for longer. Otherwise measurable improvement in physical recovery may be detectable over 2 years or more.

Problems with feeding and swallowing, and protection of the airways may be pseudobulbar or dyspraxic in origin. Delayed return of language and articulation difficulties can be expected in this situation. A tracheostomy may be required to enable the child to be weaned from the ventilator, but was required in the long term in only 1 out of 82 children in the North West brain injury rehabilitation study.[515]

Seizures

Seizures following TBI are classified as early in the first week, and thereafter they are classified as late. A Finnish study[592] showed that children of 7 years or under were more likely to have early seizures than adolescents or adults. Overall early fits with depressed skull fracture related to the origin of late post-traumatic seizures. Risk factors for late seizures include persisting neurological deficit, linear skull fracture and a persisting lesion on imaging. Late seizures did relate to a worse functional outcome in this study, and in the North West brain injury rehabilitation study[515] the need for anticonvulsants at 12 months from discharge correlated with a worse cognitive and behavioral outcome. In the Finnish study there was no correlation between late seizures and severity of brain injury scores without focal lesions. Barlow et al in Edinburgh concluded that the severity of early post-traumatic seizures related to the severity of the primary brain injury and the neurodevelopmental outcome.[593]

A large study of 4541 children and adults with TBI of varying severity showed an overall standardized incidence ratio for late epilepsy of 3.1. This ranged from 1.5 for mild head injury, 2.9 for moderate head injury to 17.0 for severe brain injury. Significant risk factors for late seizures in this study included cerebral contusion with subdural hematoma, skull fracture, loss of consciousness or amnesia for > 24 h and an age > 65 years.[594]

In the acute phase of injury antiepileptic drugs can be used to treat observed seizures. However EEG monitoring has shown that electrical seizures may still be recorded in spite of apparently protective levels of medication.[595] There is no evidence that continuation of treatment after the acute phase is protective against late seizures. With increasing awareness of potentially adverse effects of anticonvulsants on neurodevelopmental pathways such as the promotion of apoptosis, prophylactic treatment is not recommended.

LANGUAGE, BEHAVIOR AND COGNITION

These have overlapping consequences for return to the family environment, to education and to society at large. Long-term disorders are common, having far reaching effects beyond childhood into adult prospects for family life and success in the workplace. Behavioral change has been reported by mothers of brain injured children and young men 13 years after injury. Significantly those mothers were more likely to suffer from depression.[596]

Language

Language involvement is obvious in a mute or grossly dysphasic child but lesser degrees will be missed unless a planned assessment approach is adhered to. This is important because impairments of more complex higher language processing will disable information processing. This has consequences for education and social integration, compounding behavioral disorder. Language deficits detected by speech therapy assessment into the second year of recovery are associated with long-term problems in written expressive language.

Early speech difficulties range from mutism, through dyspraxia to dysarthria and related swallowing difficulties.[597] Word finding problems are common, as is lack of organization of thoughts, leading to expressive limitations that can be frustrating for the child with consequent behavioral reactions. The use of language can become concrete, alongside inappropriate social interactions such as impulsiveness, a tendency to tactless outspokenness and untimely interruption.

Behavior

The emotional and behavioral characteristics of frontal lobe dysfunction are most frequently associated with TBI. Executive functioning is usually affected, influencing cognitive as well as social performance. Normal executive function allows individuals to recognize when a problem-solving strategy is failing, moving them on to another logical approach. In executive dysfunction the individual is distractable/haphazard in the approach to problem solving and may return to failed strategies.

Prefrontal and frontotemporal damage may lead to typical psychiatric symptoms of mood swings, impulsiveness, attention deficit, disinhibition, aggressive reactions and agitation. Other features may include over-talkativeness, repetition and obsession with ideas that, in extreme cases, may lose touch with reality. This can be associated with extreme restlessness, making the child difficult to contain. Over-familiarity and lack of normal social inhibition frequently disenchants friends and teachers who regard the child as rude and disruptive. The child's social set of friends may change on return to school as they may attract more dysfunctional children, leading them into trouble or delinquency. Frontal lobe dysfunction is found in about two-thirds of severely brain injured children.[515]

Family functioning is affected.[598] In the home environment, parents experience the effects of the cognitive and emotional changes in terms of the child's impulsivity, flaring tempers, lack of motivation and poor judgment. The stress is multifactorial for a parent trying to steer between safe containment on the one hand, and encouragement towards independence on the other. Siblings are affected and family happiness may be seriously diminished.

Though the concept of plasticity of the immature brain may apply to aspects of severe brain injury recovery, there is a lack of evidence for the popular concept that the young recover better. In one study of 118 head injured children under 12 years, children injured under the age of 5 years with left hemisphere injury had the poorest cognitive scores.[599] Frontal lobe damage at such an age may not become fully apparent in its social consequences until adolescence when frontal lobe development accelerates.

Cognition

Recent learning may be lost in severe head injury and the processes of new learning affected. Problems reside with attention, encoding information into memory, and retrieval of information when needed. Classroom learning will be hindered also by the distractions in that environment. Studying or revising for examinations becomes difficult and stressful, increasing the cycle of behavioral dysfunction with anxiety, poor self-esteem and possibly depression. Protracted post injury headache patterns and fatigue are likely to worsen in an unsupported school situation.

It usually takes between 6 and 9 months for behavioral and cognitive consequences to be recognized. By this time, the child may seem to his/her teachers to be the same person physically as before the injury. The outcome, without planned re-entry to education, is usually criticism of behavior and 'lack of effort', leading to failure or even exclusion from school. In secondary years, leading to important exam years, the timetable may be overwhelming for the severely or moderately head-injured teenager. A reduction in timetable can allow achievement to progress in time to consolidate that aspect of recovery, especially into the second year. Otherwise the child may 'drop out' of educational opportunities altogether, with all the associated adverse consequences for adult life.

The effects of language deficits on learning have been discussed above. Dominant hemisphere injury may hinder sequencing abilities important to spelling and mathematical concepts. Additionally, frontal lobe deficits in executive functioning interfere with the logistical approach to problem solving. Visual–perceptual deficits as well as fine motor problems will impair the accurate and speedy recording of work. It is easy to conceive how such deficits will be compounded by frontal lobe dysfunction.

Detailed psychometric testing, as well as clinical psychological support for the child and family is essential but the timing is crucial, as tests done too soon will be too pessimistic in an evolving recovery.

PREDICTION OF OUTCOME

The GCS 72 h after injury was found to correlate with survival and degree of disability of the child at discharge in a study by Michaud et al.[600] The quality of eye movements has also been shown to relate to outcome. Children may recover from ventilation and sedation initially with purposive movements, which are then lost in a phase of brainstem release mechanisms of extensor posturing, sweating and sympathetic instability. This may take a number of weeks to subside before more encouraging physical signs emerge. It is important to be alongside the child to assess the early examination in the recovery phase. Jaffe et al[601] found a correlation between the GCS in the emergency admission room and later cognitive impairment. Post-traumatic amnesia (PTA) lasting for more than 7 days is also associated with greater cognitive and psychiatric deficits. PTA parallels neurosurgical severity of injury scores in this way.

Intracranial pressure measurements above 20 mmHg appear to correlate adversely with survival rather than quality of outcome in Michaud's study of TBI. In Minns' study of medical brain injury, cerebral perfusion maintained above 40 mmHg predicted a better quality of survival.[602]

Mention has already been made of the relationship between the depth of MR scan lesions and the severity of head injury.[586] Single photon emission tomography (SPECT) has a stronger relationship with neuropsychological outcome than MR findings.[603] Functional MR is likely to be more informative still, but limited in its availability at this time.

REHABILITATION

In ITU

In a severe brain injury this is a time of invasive procedures and intensive monitoring, such as the evacuation of extradural collections, exploration of depressed fractures and insertion of intracranial pressure monitoring systems. Many disciplines may be involved in the circumstances of multiple injury. The records quickly bear witness to important multidisciplinary interventions. However it is very important to find time to document a full pediatric history and examination. It is very occasionally the case that the 'head injury' may not be the cause of the child's loss of consciousness. The history also allows the pediatric neurologist to get to know the child and family, which may be important to the clinical care of the child in ITU, and will most certainly be of prime importance in supporting and providing for the child and family in the recovery phase. For those children who do not survive, this getting to know stage is of no less importance for later counseling.

The neurological examination is important in interpreting possible seizures and abnormal patterns of posture and movement. Purposeful movements recorded when sedation is first lifted may be overwhelmed by a phase of brainstem reflexes with increased extensor tone and excessive sympathetic drive. This is reflected in periods of hypertension, excessive sweating with notable sodium losses and blotchy flushing of the skin. Most often the original picture of purposeful patterns of movement will reappear with a resumed recovery, though uncertainties may reign over a period of weeks.

The family needs preparation and explanation of the stages ahead. These stages will entail adjustments to new environments such as a high dependency ward, a children's ward, and eventually the care of the pediatric teams in the child's district of residence.

It is advantageous to the child and family to coordinate the continuing care of various surgical specialties in a neuro-rehabilitation setting.

The rehabilitation ward

After ITU, multidisciplinary care is essential. Crucial to the effectiveness of this time is a coordinated approach, allowing all participants to meet on a regular basis to share information and observations. This needs to be facilitated by a nominated member of that team to whom the family and various specialties can refer. Such meetings can be kept concise and useful on a weekly basis. When the child is well enough it is important to include them according to age and awareness, and sometimes siblings can join in to the mutual benefit of the child and his/her sibling. The consultant community pediatrician (CCP) for the child's district should be informed at an early stage. A visit by the CCP and relevant district therapy representative enhances the early provision of services, and some will be assisted by a period of stay in their district hospital to allow all members of the CDC team to plan continuation of rehabilitation.

Those involved will include a combination or all of the following.

The child and family

The family supply information about the child before the injury. This is important on a clinical and developmental level, and is important to the understanding of the child's personality, likes and dislikes. Parents need to express their concerns and receive support and understanding at a time which is inevitably fraught. They will be most aware of subtle changes in their child and provide one of the few constant factors in this situation. Parents need to have their confidence restored by being involved in their child's care, after the experience of ITU, when they handed over that role to others. They need to learn about the likely recovery pattern clinically, and the recovery pathway practically and temporally. There will be many items important to them and the child, like returning to favorite activities, advice on degrees of freedom and supervision, and how they will get back to their school and friendships. There must be a point of contact made clear before discharge.

The child and family will need to be encouraged to engage with changing teams of carers in the moves from ITU to the ward, on to district level and finally home. Teams in these different situations need to be mutually supportive and share information. However, no matter how much information is handed over, each service has to be allowed space and opportunity to get to know the child and create their own relationship with the child and family. Each team must use their own skills and initiative to assess changing needs in an evolving recovery. The need for team meetings carries on through all stages of recovery, including predischarge planning meetings with community services and in the early months/years of return to education. Specialist head injury liaison nurses play a valuable role.

Pediatrician/pediatric neurologist

Regular examination, integration of advice from other specialties and facilitation of team meetings constitute the main elements of care. The importance of pediatric input at every stage has been discussed above, especially to communicate with the child and family.

Nursing staff

Nurses spend most time with the child and family. They will be next to the parents in their perception of the child's recovery, physically and psychologically. Parents tend to share their anxiety or frustration first with them, and in this way the nurses can alert appropriate team members to address those problems. They are in a position of advocacy for the child and family, and are able to look ahead at the practical challenges of living at home.

Physical therapists

Physiotherapy and occupational therapy need a distraction free working area and access to equipment. Therapy may be passive in the bed bound patient, to limit contractures and provide chest care. As awareness improves they will work through elements of postural control. Early therapy may be limited by a confused pattern of recovery in the child who resists interaction. Such a pattern is often followed by fluctuating lucidity interspersed with intense tiredness and the need to sleep. All the team then need to plan their interventions so as to take advantage of the more wakeful times without overwhelming the child.

Equipment that can be important at this time includes tilt tables enabling a gradual readjustment to the upright posture as well as stretching tight Achilles tendons; wheelchair; walking aids; orthoses to help contain positional deformities; access to pool therapy and gymnasium areas.

Therapists work to restore independence to the child for personal and everyday needs. Occupational therapists contribute to the assessment of the child in the preparation for return to school, including implications of fine motor and perceptual deficits. Keyboard skills may need to be introduced to enhance the recording of work. Fine motor control and sitting position may also be crucial to an appraisal of feeding, which overlaps with the speech therapist's and nurses' roles.

In the community, the therapists need to plan ahead with colleagues for the return home, including housing implications and school placement. They will visit and assess those environments to give advice for adaptations and supervision. Initial school timetables can depend to some extent on the outcome of these assessments.

Speech therapy

Where there is bulbar and brainstem dysfunction affecting mouth opening and safe swallowing, the speech therapist may first have a role in desensitization programs to overcome reflex patterns before tastes or feeds are offered. They may contribute to assessments of tongue, lip and palate movements when airway protection is uncertain. Augmentive communication (the use of communication aids) is very important to children who have lost speech centrally with aphasia or dyspraxia, or peripherally with bulbar weakness. Awareness and degrees of understanding return in advance of expressive language, leading to frustration for the child who cannot speak. Where there has been base of skull fracture, the possibility of deafness must be examined.

Examination of higher functioning complex language performance is extremely important as a more likely long-lasting disability, especially when detected into the second year of recovery. Deficits have consequences for cognitive performance in the long term. Social language tends to return to a degree that may mask higher deficits. Semantic-pragmatic difficulties may be perceived alongside frontal lobe dysfunction as subtle personality change by family and friends.

Teaching

A hospital based teaching facility is an essential component of rehabilitation, concerned with assessing and facilitating remediation of learning difficulties consequent upon brain injury. The teacher needs to be involved at an early stage of ward recovery, even when the patient is still drowsy or confused. This assists in planning assessments according to the pattern of recovery. Fundamental elements of learning are worked through so as not to take anything for granted in terms of basic perceptual skills. Dedicated teaching areas with mainstream curriculum facilities are essential, and it is important to be aware that the availability of teaching in hospital for children with acquired disability such as traumatic brain injury is a statutory right of the child under the amendment to the Education Act 1994 and the Special Educational Needs Code of Practice.[604]

Parental permission should be obtained early to allow the hospital teacher to contact the child's mainstream school to obtain background information on pre-injury ability and attainment, and to inform the child's school about the likely degree of recovery and persisting difficulties when the child returns to education. The school's special educational needs coordinator should be encouraged to visit and should be involved in discharge planning meetings.

The school health service, including community pediatric nurses, will support teachers as they get to know the child during home teaching and as reintegration into school takes place. The community pediatrician will liase with the Educational Psychology Service, which will be notified well before discharge.

Educational psychology involvement needs to be more flexible than the standard approach in the UK of a statement of special educational needs. In the 6 months that assessment and provision usually takes, the child with brain injury is likely to have changed, usually improved, in their abilities. A modification of the child's school timetable or a reduction in the proposed number of state examination subjects, including a reassessment of aims for post 16 years is essential for children entering years 10 and 11 of mainstream school.

Clinical psychology and psychiatry

The clinical psychologist provides an essential understanding of the emotional, behavioral and psychometric consequences of the injury. This involves an inclusive approach to the family, including siblings. The consequences of frontal lobe dysfunction can be modified by a behavioral approach, and the clinical psychologist can engage directly with education in the formulation of a return to school. The psychologist's input into team meetings very often provides support to the team as well.

Psychiatry and psychology roles overlap, since social disinhibition is a specific psychiatric feature characteristic of traumatic brain injury. Occasionally the marked restlessness and aggressive mood swings that accompany the early confused phase of recovery merit treatment with medication such as methylphenidate or risperidone.

Social services

The learning support limb of the social services team can provide important practical support to families on discharge where safe containment of the child is an issue. They also have a role, with community occupational therapy advice, in assessing housing needs, including access (steps and stairs, corridors and doorways, toilet and bathing facilities, seating) and financial budgeting for adaptations in the home in the event of persisting physical deficits.

Discharge planning

The success of this depends on early involvement of the district community team of CCP and therapists. In fact it is likely that the severely injured child will need a period of time in their district hospital under the care of the CCP to enable all of this team to get to know the child and embark on their own problem solving approach. The North West rehabilitation study[515] showed that this enhances discharge provision of need compared to those children who have no CCP visit or district stay.

Whilst the child is an inpatient, it is essential that the family, including the child whenever possible, should participate in weekly rehabilitation meetings where progress reports can be shared and plans adjusted accordingly. Caregivers need to understand the program that will take over well before discharge. Restrictions on activities need to be considered in a practical way that does not stifle the child's independence nor expose them to physical risk. This situation must be revisited and the family helped to adjust as recovery continues.

Children injured in their early years may not reveal the full consequences of frontal lobe dysfunction until adolescence, when frontal lobe development occurs. It is advisable therefore to follow all these children throughout their school years, with good liaison between Community Child Health, Social Services and Education. A proportion will need support into adulthood. There can be long-term effects on employment prospects, social integration and prospects for a family life.

Outcome measures and standards of service provision

Outcome and standards of care are linked, one influencing the other. Standards of care should be part of the clinical process, and the outcomes should allow comparison. Disability outcome scores may attempt to incorporate the adequacy of provision of need, but generally this is confounded by the influence of medical factors that may not lend themselves to therapeutic correction. It is difficult to show the outcome benefit of, for instance, physiotherapy, occupational therapy, speech therapy, or even surgical intervention such as intracranial pressure monitoring on the basis of disability scores. This is the problem when considering impairments consequent upon irreversible aspects of neurological injury. The King's Outcome Scale for Childhood Head Injury (KOSCHI) is a modification of the Glasgow Coma Scale for children.[605] Outcome is expanded descriptively under categories 1 to 5 as follows:

1. Death
2. Vegetative
3a and b. Severe disability
4a and b. Moderate disability
5a and b. Good recovery.

Interobserver reliability is less good for categories 3, 4, and 5, than 1 and 2. More studies are needed on the ways that effective help can be delivered to children with deficits and to their carers.[606]

This demands an agreed assessment of need, provision of care, assessment of progress, and quality of life scores that take account

Table 20.67 The causes of pathological speech and language delay/disorder

Neurological
Global learning disability (mental retardation)
Cerebral palsy
Autism
Developmental dysphasia
Selective mutism
Congenital suprabulbar palsy
Acquired epileptic aphasia
Acquired brain injury
Neuromuscular
Duchenne muscular dystrophy
Dystrophia myotonica
Congenital bulbar palsy (nuclear agenesis)
Local structural
Malformations: tongue, lips, palate, teeth
Sensory
Bilateral sensorineural hearing loss
Deafblindness
Severe visual impairment
Mixed

of the adaptive competence of the child and their environment. Adult studies have shown that patients self-report a greater recovery than do their relatives or clinicians. Patients focus on residual physical deficits, whereas carers are more aware of cognitive and behavioral change.[607] This may partly reflect the lack of insight accompanying frontal lobe dysfunction. Relatives' questionnaires show a large degree of consistency over time.[608] Such a comparative study would be difficult in children.

Setting standards according to unmet needs requires an approach to care that serves a spectrum of disorders needing rehabilitation and identifies environmental and personal factors, which may act as barriers or facilitators towards a successful outcome. It allows monitoring according to met and unmet needs. Key outcomes such as family adjustment, psychosocial adjustment, re-entry to education, the attainment of life skills progressing to employment and later family life all identify the essential members of a rehabilitation team. Standards of care start with the resourcing of these services, according to the phase of recovery, not only in pediatric hospitals but also locally with community pediatric services, educational services and transitionally into adult services as well.

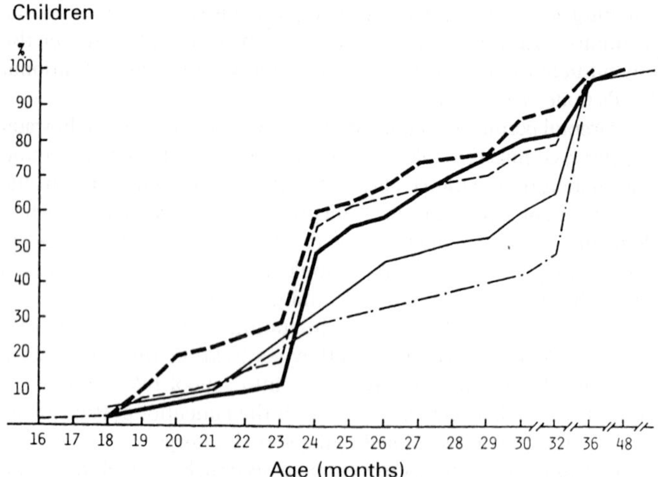

Fig. 20.41 Onset of four-word sentences. Term boys –, term girls - -, preterm boys – and girls - - wihtout cerebral palsy; boys and girls with cerebral palsy –· –·. (From Largo et al 1986[620])

SPEECH AND LANGUAGE DELAY AND DISORDERS

INTRODUCTION

Children have inbuilt capacities to communicate by words, sounds, gestures and music.[615] Even neonates when awake and not hungry will show interest in a face and will mimic a facial expression. From early infancy, children will enjoy making reciprocal noises when alert and comfortable. Babble, which is the same throughout the world, emerges any time after 6 months and subsides by about 15 months. Children with severe hearing impairment babble normally, but fall silent thereafter. The function of babble is to engage adults in conversation. The nature of the words the child learns to speak depends on the adult language they hear. Later, the accent they use depends on that of their peers. There are inbuilt capacities to infer language rules to save time in learning. Sometimes these will lead a child to say words they have never heard from anyone else–'I goed to my gran's', 'I got some chocolate mices' – for instance. The alternative – learning all language by listening and copying would take far too long.

Delay refers to a normal pattern of speech and language acquisition but at a later age than most children. It may be specific in a child whose development is otherwise age appropriate. It may be associated with other specific delays, e.g. in motor development.[616] In children with global moderate learning disability the usual pattern of speech and language development is one of delay. Disorder refers to a pattern of development that is not seen in general. Speech examples include dysarthria or dyspraxia. Language disorders include word finding difficulty, receptive or expressive dysphasia or the excessively literal 'concrete thinking' of autistic children.

The age of uttering first words is variable, from well before the first birthday, to long after the second, in children who turn out to be university graduates, never mind mainstream schoolchildren. It is not related to social class, but there may be a family history of late talking and a higher proportion of boys are late to talk. By the age of 2 years, all but 6% of children have uttered their first words.[617] By the age of 3 years all but 4% can utter appropriate three-word phrases (Fig. 20.41).[618] Extension of language into phrases and sentences is related to social class and is predictive of subsequent academic progress. Of children not yet talking in phrases at 3 years, 30% have walked before one year and 40% walked between 12 and 16 months but 30% walked after 16 months. Early talking in phrases and sentences predicts a good academic performance. Late talking in sentences, but early walking (before 12 months) predicts a good outcome, but with an increased risk of literacy difficulties (dyslexia). Late talking in sentences and walking after 16 months predicts limited academic performance and an increased likelihood of a need for learning support or special education.

Two thirds of children[619] have:

- first words between 9 months and 1 year
- first phrases between 17 months and 2 years
- and are intelligible to strangers at 2 years.

Children seem much more intelligible to those who hear them speak regularly – siblings and mothers particularly – than to professionals or strangers. By 3 years 9 months Morley reported that only 6% had incomplete sentences, but that 11% were unintelligible to strangers and 10% to health visitors, who reported 5% as unintelligible at 4 years 9 months and 0.7% as unintelligible at 6 years 6 months. The improvements were the consequence of maturation rather than treatment. In the National Child Development Study,[617] reduced intelligibility at 7 years was reported for 14% of children by doctors (but only for 1.4% was the problem marked). Teachers reported reduced intelligibility in 11% of the same children (marked in 2.6%). Phonological difficulties such as omissions, substitutions and reversals are common and are seen in early written work also.

PRESENTATION OF SPEECH AND LANGUAGE DISORDERS

When children have difficulty understanding speech they may be thought to be disobedient or deaf. When they have difficulty expressing themselves in speech they may become aggressive or frustrated and may have tantrums or behave destructively. Attempts to attract the attention of others by tapping them or pulling on their sleeves may be interpreted as aggressive behavior. In children who are late to talk, evidence of good comprehension is reassuring. Pure expressive dysphasia is rare and it is more likely that the child is simply showing a variant of normal development and will be fine shortly. Autistic children usually show signs of being remote from the first weeks of life, but a fifth show promising early development then regress. In girls, this should prompt consideration of Rett's syndrome.[621] However Rett's syndrome only affects 1 girl in 20 000 and the usual diagnosis is idiopathic autism or acquired aphasia. In boys, it is likely to be diagnosed as idiopathic autism. Some consideration may be given to fragile X, in that some children who appear odd, very withdrawn and uncommunicative in groups may have this condition, even though in individual consultation the child's communication is not autistic. Children who have communication problems, including those who are deaf, may be thought to be hyperactive until the problem is diagnosed.

PATHOLOGICAL SPEECH AND LANGUAGE DELAY AND DISORDER

There may be a known pathological cause for speech and/or language difficulties (Table 20.66). The child may have a *global learning disability*, due to a chromosomal abnormality, or other demonstrable medical cause. The child may have a suprabulbar palsy, due to *cerebral palsy*. There may be a bulbar palsy, due to a *neuromuscular disorder*. The mean verbal quotient of boys with Duchenne muscular dystrophy is 80 with a distribution from profound communication difficulty and autism to superior intelligence, compatible with university education. In the mouth there may be structural malformations such as *cleft palate* or *micrognathia* (moderate in Down syndrome and severe in Pierre Robin syndrome). One child in 500 has bilateral severe *sensorineural hearing loss*, which explains lack of early speech and language. *Central auditory inattention*[622] describes a condition in which the child behaves as if deaf although the ears can be demonstrated to hear normally by physiological tests. It is analogous to developmental visual inattention and, as with that condition, may resolve spontaneously.

Semantic and pragmatic language disorders are seen in children with *autism/autistic spectrum disorders*, which it is considered result from a developmental brain disorder. The condition known as *selective mutism* is a very persistent condition, often continuing into adult life, with a probable biological cause. Congenital suprabulbar palsy[623–625] may be associated with bilateral parasagittal areas of cortical dysplasia or with an abnormality of chromosome 22. Around the age of 3–9 years some children who have seizures, not necessarily severe ones, may lose their receptive language skills, either acutely or progressively over time, with acquired epileptic aphasia.[626–629] This condition has no known cause and can occur in children. About a third of all cases have not had seizures, but show left hemisphere seizure discharge on EEG.[630] The type with acute onset has a better prognosis for recovery. Cerebrovascular accidents, head injury, accidental or abusive, meningoencephalitis and encephalitis are causes of acquired pathological speech and language disorders (Table 20.67).

AUTISM AND AUTISTIC SPECTRUM DISORDERS

Autism, Asperger's syndrome, high functioning autism, autistic spectrum disorders, atypical autism and pervasive developmental disorders are discussed elsewhere from a child psychiatric perspective (Ch. 33). Here they are considered within the context of speech, language and communication disorder, which is a core feature of the autistic syndrome. Autistic behavior has long been regarded by pediatricians and pediatric neurologists as a familiar feature of children who have had infantile spasms which were idiopathic or associated with tuberous sclerosis.[631] It is also seen as a symptom in some children with idiopathic learning disability and/or in some children with epilepsy. This triad causes confusion for parents in the sense that they ask 'what is wrong with my child – is it learning disability, autism or epilepsy?'

For the pediatrician, all of these are symptoms of an underlying biological disorder of brain development, to be diagnosed medically if possible as the cause of the child's condition. To give autism, learning disability or epilepsy as 'the diagnosis' risks closing minds to the need to continue to search for the cause. However, in spite of much excellent work on the subject[632–637] it remains the case that an underlying medical cause is still unknown for most autistic children. There is an excess in males, which is still present when boys with fragile X are excluded. The concordance for autism in monozygotic twins is 36–89% in published studies. Concordance in dizygotic twins is up to 30% and there is a substantial excess of autism (about 3%) and heterogeneous developmental language disorders in non-autistic twins and siblings of autistic children.

There has been a growing acknowledgment amongst pediatricians that children with autistic behavior present particular challenges to their families, their teachers and all who come in contact with them. It has implications for teaching methods, for speech and language therapy and for behavioral management. The voluntary organizations for families of autistic children have published very helpful and informative literature for parents and professionals. They put parents in touch with each other and provide innovative, appropriate local and national services for autistic people. For such reasons, pediatricians have become increasingly willing to diagnose children as having an autistic disorder, to discuss this with families and colleagues and to seek help from child mental health services. Many children who would have been considered to be 'loners', dyspraxic, eccentric or to have a schizoid personality disorder, in the past, are now being recognized as having autistic features. This increasing identification has contributed to the apparent increase in the prevalence of autistic children in recent years. The Medical Research Council in Britain has published an extensive Autism Review[638] on the Internet.

Childhood autism is characterized by the following developmental features:

- communication difficulties
- problems with social interaction
- behavioral problems including stereotopies and obsessional interests and
- onset in the first 3 years.

The communication difficulties in higher functioning autistic children, or children with Asperger's syndrome, are described as a semantic/pragmatic disorder.[639] By this is meant that children use words without understanding their meaning and in an inappropriate context. It is a sophisticated form of echolalia. Some such children can pick up and repeat long passages of filmscore in appropriate accents. They may come out with apparently grown-up language, in a variety of settings, throughout the day but, if pressed, cannot explain their utterances. Their speech is monotonous in tone (a disorder of prosody). They do not understand similes or metaphors, and have a very concrete, literal understanding of words and objects. They do not understand or engage in symbolic play where one object can represent something

Table 20.66 Investigation of children with speech and language delay/disorder

Hearing
Chromosomes especially for sex chromosome abnormalities, e.g. XXX, XXY, fragile X
Amino acid chromatogram, e.g. phenylketonuria
Creatine kinase in boys
EEG, e.g. in acquired aphasia
CT scan, e.g. in tuberous sclerosis or with partial complex seizures
MRI scan in congenital suprabulbar palsy

else, e.g. a box representing a boat or a pencil representing a rocket. Their visual learning may be well be ahead of their auditory learning and they may be hyperlexic (much better at the mechanics of reading than at reading comprehension). The use of visual prompts may be helpful in structuring their learning and other activities.

A key component of their problems with social interaction is a lack of empathy, analogous to color blindness, in that it cannot be taught. This inability to know how others are feeling or to predict how others would be likely to feel in response to the autistic child's remarks or behavior leads to much conflict and confusion. Autistic children will regard the responses of others as bullying, persecution and utterly unjust. The children will involve themselves in activities along with other children, but not in a collaborative manner. Their highly developed sense of rules may lead them to remonstrate with other children, who may be up to mischief, or to report such children to their teachers, which is not the best way to make friends. The ability to ignore social constraints in able autistic people can lead to unconventional inventions and solutions to problems so there may be a biological advantage to society in having some autistic people amongst us.

The behavioral problems of autistic children are often misconstrued. Their communication and social disabilities can lead to considerable anxiety and a difficulty in coping. This may boil over into tantrums and screaming, e.g. in response to the request from a teacher to 'give me your hand' prior to crossing a road. They are prone to obsessional interests and may break into a rage if their routines are not followed. Reorganization of furniture, redecoration, tidying up toys without discussion, a clock telling the wrong time, taking a different route for a walk, a different vehicle being supplied for transport home from school, interruption of a wheelspinning ritual, siblings or friends playing football in the garden are factors which may provoke tantrums in autistic children. These become much less frequent when all those dealing with and caring for the child work out how his/her mind works.

An autistic 12-year-old boy began to try to kiss other boys and girls at his school. There was concern that he might have been the recipient of inappropriate sexual behavior. It transpired that he had been watching a repeat television transmission of the Morecambe and Wise show. At the end of the program, Ernie Wise berated Eric Morecambe at length for behaving so badly throughout the show. In response, Morecambe leant forward and said to Wise 'Give us a kiss'. This 'brought the house down' (an expression the boy would not have understood but he did realize that the offer of a kiss could have sensational results – as he found out for a while). He was told he must not kiss other pupils or staff at school and stopped trying to do this immediately.

Obsessional interests may be harmless, e.g. stick insects. Young people need to be told before they leave school how to conduct themselves at interview and to refrain from telling the panel, for example, about the life story of Bruce Lee. Occasionally an autistic pupil will reveal an alarming preoccupation in a clinic, having said nothing about this to parents or teachers, e.g. ways of killing people without weapons. Sometimes there are reinforcements for such interests within the home and a residential school may be considered.

Early behavioral intervention by families for children with autism has become popular, e.g. by the Lovaas method,[640] although there is a dearth of published research evidence for benefit of this therapy. UK parents, prompted by American experience, set up their own support group, in 1996: Parents for the Early Intervention of Autism in Children (PEACh UK). By the summer of 1999, 250 Lovaas-style programs had been established for autistic children in Britain. Of these, 109 had taken their local authorities to court to fund the program and 100 of these cases had succeeded. Families from PEACh UK took part in an audit of their experience of this method. They report that it is helpful to have the support of a therapy team, especially if staffing is stable, but find the limiting factors include their own time availability and their energy.

All sorts of anecdotal reports of remedies for autism are picked up by newspapers and from the Internet. Some are inherently improbable (e.g. brushing the skin with paint brushes, serotonin therapy, gluten and milk-free diets, swimming with dolphins or trace element and multivitamin therapy based on analysis of hair samples). None has been shown to be beneficial in any published scientific study. A randomized, double-blind, placebo-controlled trial of the effectiveness of intravenous porcine secretin on autistic behavior in 95 children aged 2–7 years showed no benefit in language development or autistic behavior 3 weeks after treatment. Yet many parents have spent a lot of money pursuing secretin and other treatment. When a condition has no medical cure it is understandable that parents choose to try alternative remedies. A British Paediatric Association working party[641] proposed criteria for health service purchasers considering requests for funding for alternative treatment:

- The scientific plausibility of the program proposed
- The evidence for its effectiveness (if available)
- The extent to which parents may benefit from the opportunity to try the method they prefer
- The right of parents to choose
- The potential difference in benefit between orthodox programs and the one favored by the parents
- Whether the magnitude of the difference could justify the difference in cost between the management available in the local statutory services and that desired by the parents.

There are professional responsibilities to protect parents from exploitation, to ensure regular pediatric review of the children and to understand that rejection of statutory services may be an expression of anger within the grief process. When there is anxiety from parents or professionals that treatment is harmful or causing distress, it is necessary to weigh this against observed benefits to the child and family and to come to an individual decision for counseling.

MMR VACCINE AND REGRESSION IN COMMUNICATION INCLUDING AUTISM

Some newspapers and anti-vaccine parent lobbies exploited the publication of small studies by Thompson et al[642] and Wakefield et al[643] to whip up panic about MMR vaccine which had replaced single vaccines in 1988. Wakefield et al did not claim to show evidence that MMR vaccine had caused either autism or inflammatory bowel disease. They have not replicated their initial research and nor has any other research team in the world. The accumulation of scientific evidence to support the use of the vaccine in 94 countries worldwide became a misplaced argument about families' rights to choose vaccination methods with an implication that there was an official cover-up of 'vaccine damage' caused by MMR in the British government's attempt to induce doctors to hit immunization targets. A factor in this was the lack of preparation of professionals for the introduction of the MMR booster.[644] However a review of the data on 473 children with classical or atypical autism in five health districts in north east London from 1979 to 1998[645] has shown no significant change in the proportion of autistic children with a regressive history (25%), or bowel symptoms (17%) throughout the study, before or after the introduction of MMR vaccine in the middle of the assessment period of the register. Their data showed a possible association between the regressive form of autism and bowel symptoms, but no evidence of a new variant form of autism.

Treatment and management of autistic children

The principal elements in helping autistic children are consistent, appropriate management at home and suitable educational provision. Health input comes, mainly, from speech and language therapists and clinical psychologists after the initial diagnostic work by pediatricians and child psychiatrists. Teachers work closely with health colleagues, parents, social services and voluntary agencies in working out the best means of helping the children to learn academically and socially. Whether the children are educated in mainstream schools with support, in language units within mainstream schools, in special schools for children with learning disability or in schools for autistic pupils depends in part on local availability and in part on associated cognitive and social capabilities of the child. The presumption is that the most inclusive provision is the first priority. Some children's needs are so complex and their capacity to cope with the hurly-burly of mainstream education is so problematic, in spite of good support, that special provision is required.

Medical help may be needed in the management of behavior problems. Pediatricians are wise to liaise with psychiatric colleagues before using medication in these children, some of whom benefit from methylphenidate, carbamazepine or lamotrigine, used for their psychotropic properties. A third of the children experience epilepsy at some stage in childhood or adolescence and require antiepileptic drug therapy, puberty being a time of higher risk. Melatonin has a place in helping autistic children to get to sleep. When the problem is night waking, chloral hydrate may be used though it leaves some hangover effects next day. Administration may be a problem as autistic children can be adamant as to what they are or are not prepared to eat and drink.[646]

SPEECH AND LANGUAGE DELAY AND DISORDER IN CHILDREN WITH GENERAL LEARNING DISABILITY

Speech and language delay/disorder may be a feature of general learning disability (moderate or severe mental retardation). The communication ability may be similar, developmentally, to the rest of the child's age-equivalent progress. It is quite common for children with learning disability to have greater difficulty with communication than with practical and social development. It may be thought by parents that the only problem faced by such children is their speech ('he understands everything'). It requires careful observation by professionals alongside the parents and detailed developmental assessment by a clinical psychologist, as well as full assessment by a speech and language therapist, to understand the child's condition accurately. Such children's communication needs deserve full attention, including consideration of augmented communication when appropriate, within a context which understands their learning disability.

SPECIFIC DEVELOPMENTAL SPEECH AND LANGUAGE DELAY AND DISORDER

When no underlying cause has been discovered for the child's communication difficulties, the child is described as having a specific developmental speech and language delay or disorder. This is frustrating and unsatisfactory for parents and professionals who would like a medical explanation. Nonetheless this is how it is for about 85% of children who present.[618] There are some known risk factors and associated features:

- Social class 4 and 5
- Males/females 2 : 1
- Unremarkable home background (not abusive or disturbed)
- Later children
- Large families
- Family history of language, literacy or autistic problems
- Average or near to average general intelligence
- Higher chance of left-handedness
- Hearing normal or fluctuating hearing loss
- Often a mixed receptive/expressive language and articulatory problem
- May have general developmental coordination difficulties
- May have features of autistic spectrum disorder in early years
- Problems with reading and spelling in school

Examples of developmental speech and language delay/disorder
- *Mild to moderate phonological*
  - *lisping – a form of dyslalia*
  - *stammering – dysfluency (Gordon[647])*
  - *sound substitutions, omissions and reversals*
- *Moderate articulatory*
  - *developmental verbal dyspraxia*
- *Moderate to severe language difficulty*
  - *word finding difficulty*
  - *expressive dysphasia*
- *Severe language difficulty*
  - *receptive dysphasia*
  - *mixed receptive/expressive dysphasia*
- *Profound communication difficulty*
  - *central auditory processing difficulty (auditory imperception)*

The part played by fluctuating hearing loss with secretory otitis media with effusion (OME) has been investigated extensively but inconclusively.[648–651] The nasopharynx increases in size with age but, between the ages of 3 and 5 years, the adenoids grow more rapidly and decrease the size of the palatal airway, particularly in those children who develop OME. Children with Down syndrome have a smaller nasopharynx than most children and are at particular risk from adenoidal encroachment. Subsequently the adenoids remain relatively constant while the nasopharynx increases, so the airway enlarges. Surgical procedures produce good short-term gains but less predictable long-term benefits. Maw[651] reviews the findings of numerous prospective studies over 15 years and proposes recommendations based on factual evidence rather than anecdotal practice. Only 1 : 40 children with developmental speech and language problems will be found to have moderate or severe bilateral sensorineural hearing loss. However high quality hearing testing is essential for all.

COMMUNICATION BEFORE SPEECH

From birth onwards an alert infant interacts with carers by attending to their faces, by phonating and by movements such as wriggling when held. Fixation on faces and smiling emerge in the early weeks after birth, often long before the frequently quoted 6 weeks milestone. Facial expressions can be imitated from the first days of life. Attention to movement of other people, to patterns, preferably complex ones, and to handling begins in the early weeks. Reciprocal phonation with others begins then too. Parents of no experience may say that there is no point talking to babies because they cannot talk back. The reverse is the case. Infants have a repertoire of types of cry – tired, hungry, uncomfortable, experimental – to which parents become attuned and to which they become responsive. The biological purpose of incessant crying at 3 months ('colic') is hard to fathom – it is certainly a test of parental commitment and resourcefulness. When parents are intolerant of this, their children are in grave danger.

Reaching for objects and for the faces of carers becomes increasingly rewarding for the infant as control improves and the child finds that actions can have gratifying and predictable results. This progresses to pointing and imitation of gestures later in the first year. Phonation gives way to babble, which is international and uttered by children with severe hearing impairment. Adults babble back with variations of inflection, which amuses the child. They also talk to the child, who begins to show signs of comprehension. At the end of the first year or early in the second year the child will begin to indicate body parts on request and will be pleased by adult approval. Requests will be indicated by pointing, gestures and phonation. When adults 'misunderstand' as part of a game it amuses the child up to a point. Then it is 'game over'. In the child with severe hearing impairment, babble gives way to silence, but in the hearing child it develops into jargon – word-like noises which are incomprehensible. Even when understandable words emerge, such as doggie, names of family members, juice, no, more, ta, there are other 'words' which are consistent but jargon, e.g. loadalah (motor car) or brewstie (what are you doing? I'm doing a brewstie – the child was pinching the thumb and forefinger and never explained the term). In children with learning disability, the era of communication before speech is much extended. Interpretation is rewarding and development of gestures into signing or of pointing into pointing at symbols can develop into a method of communication, which takes the pressure off the dearth of expressive language. Far from delaying speech it seems to accelerate it.

TREATMENT AND MANAGEMENT OF CHILDREN WITH SPEECH AND LANGUAGE DELAY OR DISORDER

- Identify the problem
- Investigate possible causes which can be treated, or which have genetic implications
- Assess the child's general development including a clinical psychology assessment and motor coordination assessment
- Assess speech and language function: expert help from a speech and language therapist
- Discuss the findings with the parents who may bring a grandparent, friend or professional
- Inform the local education authority
- Contribute to the interdisciplinary process of considering the appropriate form of education
- Review progress at regular intervals – discuss findings with teachers, therapists and parents

Speech and language therapists have a key role as consultants and advisers of parents, teachers, doctors and others in regular contact with children affected by speech and language delay and disorder. They are the experts, in collaboration with clinical psychologists, teachers and parents in working out the way children's minds are working, in the way they are understanding and using language, including context and syntax and in the state of their phonological development. However the 'treatment' is not in the therapy sessions but in the day to day communication between adults and children, the anticipation and avoidance of frustration and the way the children are encouraged to succeed. Progress reassessment and revision of goals by therapists guide those who are in daily contact in helping the children. Sometimes parents complain that it seems they are being expected to adopt a treatment role but they should not be expected to spend too much time grappling with the limits of the child's ability. Rather they will be helping their children to consolidate on their abilities, finding out what their children do best and helping them to make the most of these.

AUGMENTED COMMUNICATION

There are many ways of augmenting spoken language in everyday life. Gestures and other forms of body language are part of our repertoire. Actors develop these to a subtle and remarkable extent. For children whose speech is lacking or incomprehensible, systems involving gestures or symbols can be beneficial. Instead of being reactive, the child can become proactive for the first time. There are specialist centers for augmentative communication, with expertise in signing, symbol and switching methods. The local speech and language therapy service will have a specialist expert who can advise on the best source of help (Fig. 20.42).

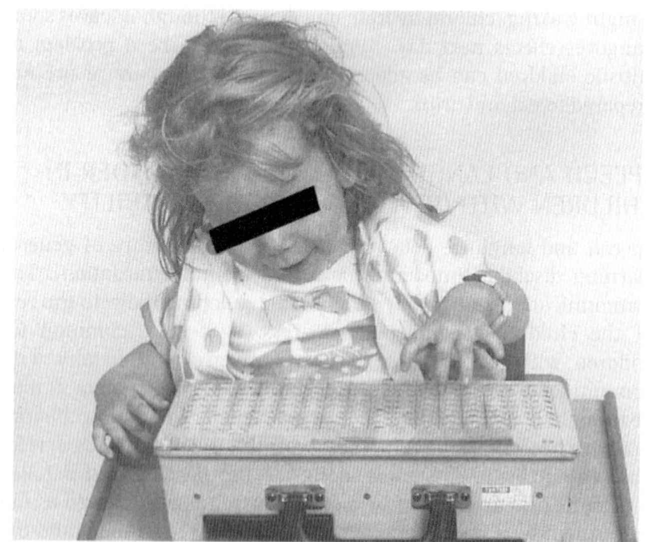

Fig. 20.42 Augmentative communication with Reybus Introtalker (pictograms) being used by an anarthric child with severe mixed cerebral palsy.

REFERENCES (* Level 1 evidence)

THE NEUROLOGICAL CONSULTATION

1 Cunningham C, Newton R. A question sheet to encourage written consultation question. Qual Health Care 2000; 9:42–46.

2 Viswanathan V, Bridges SJ, Whitehouse W, Newton RW. Childhood headaches: discrete entities or continuum? Dev Med Child Neurol 1998; 40:544–550.

3 Silva PA. Epidemiology, longitudinal course and some associated factors: an update in language developments and disorders. In: Yule W, Rutter M (eds). Clinics in Developmental Medicine. 101/102. Oxford: Mac Keith Press; 1987:12–15.

4 Lees J, Urwin S. Children with language disorders. London: Whurr Publishers; 1997.

5 Levene MI. The asphyxiated new born infant. In: Levene MI, Chervenak FA, Whittle M (eds). Fetal neonatal neurology and neurosurgery. London: Churchill Livingstone; 2001:487–498.
6 Wallace GB, Newton RW. Gowers' sign revisited. Arch Dis Child 1989; 64: 1317–1319.
7 Alvarez LA, Maytal J, Shinnar S. Idiopathic external hydrocephalus: natural history and relationship to benign familial macrocephaly. Pediatrics 1986; 77:901–907.
8 Cunningham CC, Morgan PA, McGucken RB. Down's syndrome: is dissatisfaction with disclosure of diagnosis inevitable? Dev Med Child Neurol 1984; 26:33–39.
9 Lingham S, Newton RW. Giving the news of disability – paediatric practice guideline. London: Royal College of Paediatrics and Child Health; 1996.
10 Nelson KB, Ellenberg JH. Children who outgrew cerebral palsy. Paediatrics 1982; 69:529–536.
11 Houston EC, Cunningham CC, Metcalfe E, Newton R. The information needs and understanding of 5 to 10 year old children with epilepsy, asthma or diabetes. Seizure 2000; 9:340–343.

DEVELOPMENT OF THE HUMAN BRAIN
12 Huttenlocher PR, Dabholkar AS. Regional differences in synaptogenesis in human cerebral cortex. J Comp Neurol 1997; 387:167–178.
13 Hittmair K, Wimberger D, Rand T, et al. MR assessment of brain maturation: comparison of sequences. Am J Neuroradiol 1994; 15:425–433. © American Society of Neuroradiology (www.ajnr.org).
14 Klingberg T, Vadya CJ, Gabrieli JDE, et al. Myelination and organisation of the frontal white matter in children: a diffusion tensor MRI study. Neuro Report 1999; 10:2817–2821.
15 Barkovich AJ, Kuzniecky RI, Dobyns WB, et al. A classification scheme for malformations of cortical development. Neuropediatrics 1996; 27:59–63.
16 van der Knapp MS, Valk J. Classification of congenital abnormalities of the CNS. Am J Neuroradiol 1988; 9:315–326.
17 Sarnat HB, Flores-Sarnat L. A new classification of malformations of the nervous system: an integration of morphological and molecular genetic criteria as patterns of genetic expression. Eur J Paediatr Neurol 2001; 5:57–64.
18 Hudgins RJ, Edwards MSB, Goldstein R, et al. Natural history of foetal ventriculomegaly. Pediatrics 1988; 82:692–697.
19 Gupta JK, Bryce FC, Lilford RJ. Management of apparently isolated foetal ventriculomegaly. Obstet Gynecol Surv 1994; 49:716–721.
20 Pilu G, Falco P, Gabrielli S, et al. The clinical significance of foetal isolated cerebral borderline ventriculomegaly: report of 31 cases and review of the literature. Ultrasound. Obstet Gynecol 1999; 14:320–326.
21 Serlo W, Kirkinen P, Jouppila P, Herve R. Prognostic signs in foetal hydrocephalus. Childs Nerv Syst 1986; 2:93–97.
22 Chervenak FA, Duncan C, Ment LR, et al. Outcome of foetal ventriculomegaly. Lancet 1984; 2:179–181.
23 Adzick NS, Harrison MR. Foetal surgical therapy. Lancet 1994; 343:897–902.

NEURAL TUBE DEFECTS
24 van Allen MI, Kalousek DK, Chernoff GF, et al. Evidence of multi-site closure of the neural tube in humans. Am J Med Genet 1993; 47:723–743.
25 Cuckle H, Wald N. The impact of screening for neural tube defects in England and Wales. Prenat Diagn 1987; 7:91–99.
*26 Medical Research Council Vitamin Study Group. Prevention of neural tube defects: results of the Medical Research Council vitamin study. Lancet 1991; 238:131–133.
27 Meuli M, Meuli-Sommen C, Hutchins GM, et al. In utero surgery rescues neurological function at birth in sheep with spina bifida. Nat Med 1995; 1:342–347.
28 Bruner JP, Tulipan N, Paschall RL, et al. Foetal surgery for myelomeningocele and the incidence of shunt dependent hydrocephalus. JAMA 1999; 282:1819–1825.
29 Minns RA. The management of children with spina bifida. In: Gordon N, McKinlay I (eds). Neurologically handicapped children. Oxford: Blackwell; 1986.
30 Johnston LB, Borzyskowski M. Bladder dysfunction and neurological disability at presentation in closed spinal bifida. Arch Dis Child 1998; 79:33–38.

HYDROCEPHALUS
31 Cheung CS, Myrinthopolous NC. Factors affecting risks of congenital malformations. Report from the Collaborative Perinatal Project. Birth Defects 1975; 11:1–22.
32 Blackburn BL, Fineman RM. Epidemiology of congenital hydrocephalus in Utah, 1940 to 1979: report of an aetrogenically related epidemic. Am J Med Genet 1994; 52:123–129.
33 Fernell E, Hagberg G, Hagberg B. Infantile hydrocephalus epidemiology. An indicator of enhanced survival. Arch Dis Child. Fetal Neonatal Ed 1994; 70:F123–F128.
34 Minns RA, Brown JK, Engelman HM. CSF production rate: real time estimation. Z Kinderchir 1987; 42 (suppl I):36–40.
35 Kirkpatrick M, Engelman HA, Minns RA. Symptoms and signs of progressive hydrocephalus. Arch Dis Child 1989; 64:124–128.
36 Leggate JRS, Baxter P, Minns RA. Role of a separate subcutaneous cerebrospinal fluid reservoir in the management of hydrocephalus. Br J Neurosurg 1988; 2:327–337.
37 Minns RA, Engelman HM, Sterling H. A cerebrospinal fluid pressure in pyogenic meningitis. Arch Dis Child 1989; 64:814–820.
38 Minns RA, Merrick MV. Cerebral perfusion pressure and net cerebral mean transit time in childhood hydrocephalus. J Paediatr Neurosci 1989; 5(2):69–77.
39 Minns RA, Goh D, Pye S, Steers J. A volume–blood flow relationship derived from CSF compartment challenge as an index of progression of infantile hydrocephalus. Proc International Symposium on Hydrocephalus, Japan, November 1990.
40 Chumas Tyagia, Livingston J. Hydrocephalus – what's new? Arch Dis Child Fetal Neonatal Ed 2001; 85: F149–F154.
*41 Anonymous. Randomised trial of early tapping in neonatal haemorrhagic ventricular dilatation. Ventriculomegaly Trial Group. Arch Dis Child 1990; 65:3–10.
42 Tortorolo G, Luciano R, Papacci P, Tonelli T. Intraventricular hemorrhage: past, present and future, focusing on classification, pathogenesis and prevention Childs Nerv Syst 1999; 15:652–661.
43 Fulmer BB, Grabb PA, Oakes WJ, Mapstone TB. Neonatal ventriculo subgaleal shunts. Neurosurgery 2000; 47:80–83.
*44 Kennedy CR, Ayers S, Campbell MJ, et al. Randomised, controlled trial of acetazolamide and furosemide. In: posthemorrhagic ventricular dilation in infancy: follow–up at 1 year. Pediatrics 2001; 108:597–607.
45 Brydon HL, Bayston R, Hayward R, Harkness W. The effect of protein and blood cells on the flow pressure characteristics of shunts. Neurosurgery 1996; 38:498–504.
46 Brydon HL, Hayward R, Harkness W, Bayston R. Does the cerebrospinal fluid protein concentration increase the risk of shunt complications? Br J Neurosurg 1996; 10:267–273.
47 Gaston H. Does the spina bifida clinic need an ophthalmologist? Z Kinderchir 1985; 40 (suppl 11):45–50.

THE NEUROCUTANEOUS DISEASES
48 Gutmann DH, Aylsworth A, Carey JC, et al. The diagnostic evaluation and multidisciplinary management of neurofibromatosis I and neurofibromatosis II. JAMA 1997; 278:51–57.
49 Evans DJR, Birch JM, Ramsden RT. Paediatric presentation of type 2 neurofibromatosis. Arch Dis Child 1999; 81:496–499.
50 Roach ES, DiMario FJ, Candt RS, Northrup H. Tuberose Sclerosis Consensus Conference: Recommendations for diagnostic evaluation. National Tuberose Sclerosis Association. J Child Neurol 1999; 14:401–407.

SEIZURES, EPILEPSY AND OTHER PAROXYSMAL DISORDERS
51 Steinlein OK, Mulley JC, et al. A missense mutation in the neuronal nicotinic acetylcholine receptor alpha 4 subunit is associated with autosomal dominant nocturnal frontal lobe epilepsy. Nat Genet 1995; 11(2):201–203.
52 Biervert C, Schroeder BC, et al. A potassium channel mutation in neonatal human epilepsy. Science 1998; 279(5349):403–406.
53 Singh NA, Charlier C, et al. A novel potassium channel gene, KCNQ2, is mutated in an inherited epilepsy of newborns. Nat Genet 1998; 18(1):25–29.
*54 Wallace H, Shorvon S, et al. Age-specific incidence and prevalence rates of treated epilepsy in an unselected population of 2,052,922 and age-specific fertility rates of women with epilepsy [see comments]. Lancet 1998; 352(9145):1970–1973.
55 Claes L, Del-Favero J, et al. De novo mutations in the sodium-channel gene SCN1A cause severe myoclonic epilepsy of infancy. Am J Hum Genet 2001; 68(6):1327–1332.

56 Macdonald RL. Cellular effects of antiepileptic drugs. In: Pedley TA (ed.) Epilepsy: a comprehensive textbook. Philadelphia: Lippincott-Raven; 1997:1383–1391.

57 Sander JW, Shorvon SD. Epidemiology of the epilepsies [erratum appears in J Neurol Neurosurg Psychiatry 1997 Jun62(6):679]. J Neurol Neurosurg Psychiatry 1996; 61(5):433–443.

58 Forsgren L. Epidemiology: incidence and prevalence. In: Wallace S (ed.) Epilepsy in children. London: Chapman & Hall; 1996:27–37.

*59 Eriksson KJ, Koivikko MJ. Prevalence, classification, and severity of epilepsy and epileptic syndromes in children. Epilepsia 1997; 38(12):1275–1282.

60 Shorvon SD. The epidemiology and treatment of chronic and refractory epilepsy. Epilepsia 1996; 37 (suppl 2): S1–S3.

*61 Kurtz Z, Tookey P, et al. Epilepsy in young people: 23 year follow up of the British National Child Development Study. BMJ 1998; 316(7128):339–342.

62 Berg AT, Shinnar S, et al. Newly diagnosed epilepsy in children: presentation at diagnosis. Epilepsia 1999; 40(4):445–452.

*63 Shinnar S, O'Dell C, et al. Distribution of epilepsy syndromes in a cohort of children prospectively monitored from the time of their first unprovoked seizure. Epilepsia 1999; 40(10):1378–1383.

*64 Shinnar S, Berg AT, et al. Predictors of multiple seizures in a cohort of children prospectively followed from the time of their first unprovoked seizure [see comments]. Ann Neurol 2000; 48(2):140–147.

*65 Berg AT, Levy SR, et al. Predictors of intractable epilepsy in childhood: a case-control study. Epilepsia 1996; 37(1):24–30.

*66 Hauser E, Freilinger M, et al. Prognosis of childhood epilepsy in newly referred patients. J Child Neurol 1996; 11(3):201–204.

*67 Casetta I, Granieri E, et al. Early predictors of intractability in childhood epilepsy: a community-based case-control study in Copparo, Italy. Acta Neurol Scand 1999; 99(6):329–333.

68 Duchowny M. Seizure recurrence in childhood epilepsy: the future ain't what it used to be [letter comment]. Ann Neurol 2000; 48(2):137–139.

*69 Arts WF, Geerts AT, et al. The early prognosis of epilepsy in childhood: the prediction of a poor outcome. The Dutch study of epilepsy in childhood. Epilepsia 1999; 40(6):726–734.

70 Berg AT, Shinnar S, et al. Defining early seizure outcomes in pediatric epilepsy: the good, the bad and the in-between. Epilepsy Res 2001; 43(1):75–84.

*71 Cockerell OC, Johnson AL, et al. Prognosis of epilepsy: a review and further analysis of the first nine years of the British National General Practice Study of Epilepsy, a prospective population-based study. Epilepsia 1997; 38(1):31–46.

*72 Sillanpaa M, Jalava M, et al. Long-term prognosis of seizures with onset in childhood. N Engl J Med 1998; 338(24):1715–1722.

*73 Wakamoto H, Nagao H, et al. Long-term medical, educational, and social prognoses of childhood-onset epilepsy: a population-based study in a rural district of Japan. Brain Dev 2000; 22(4):246–255.

74 Ficker DM. Sudden unexplained death and injury in epilepsy. Epilepsia 2000; 41 (suppl 2):S7–S12.

*75 Ficker DM, So EL, et al. Population-based study of the incidence of sudden unexplained death in epilepsy. Neurology 1998; 51(5):1270–1274.

76 O'Donoghue M, Sander JW. Does early anti-epileptic drug treatment alter the prognosis for remission of the epilepsies? J R Soc Med 1996; 89(5):245–248.

77 Shinnar S, Berg AT. Does antiepileptic drug therapy prevent the development of chronic epilepsy? Epilepsia 1996; 37(8):701–708.

78 Walczak TS, Jayakar P. Interictal EEG. In: Pedley TA (ed.) Epilepsy: a comprehensive textbook. Philadelphia: Lippincott-Raven; 1997:831–848.

79 Goodin DS, Aminoff MJ. Does the interictal EEG have a role in the diagnosis of epilepsy? Lancet 1984; 1(8381):837–839.

80 Schmidt D. The influence of antiepileptic drugs on the electroencephalogram: a review of controlled clinical studies. Electroencephalogr Clin Neurophysiol Suppl 1982; 36:453–466.

81 Sperling MR, Clancy RR. Ictal EEG. In: Pedley TA (ed.) Epilepsy: a comprehensive textbook. Philadelphia: Lippincott-Raven; 1997:849–885.

82 Cascino G. Structural brain imaging. In: Pedley TA (ed.) Epilepsy: a comprehensive textbook. Philadelphia: Lippincott-Raven; 1997:937–946.

83 Raybaud C, Guye M. et al. Neuroimaging of epilepsy in children. Magn Reson Imaging Clin N Am 2001; 9(1):121–147, viii.

84 Ruggieri PM, Najm IM. MR imaging in epilepsy. Neurol Clin 2001; 19(2):477–489.

85 Berkovic SF, Newton MR. Single photon emission computed tomography. In: Pedley TA (ed.) Epilepsy: a comprehensive textbook. Philadelphia: Lippincott-Raven; 1997:969–975.

86 Henry TR. Positron emission tomography. In: Pedley TA (ed.) Epilepsy: a comprehensive textbook. Philadelphia: Lippincott-Raven; 1997:947–968.

*87 Devous MD Sr, Thisted RA, et al. SPECT brain imaging in epilepsy: a meta-analysis. J Nucl Med 1998; 39(2):285–293.

88 Robinson RO, Ferrie CD, et al. Positron emission tomography and the central nervous system. Arch Dis Child 1999; 81(3):263–270.

89 Lawson JA, O'Brien TJ, et al. Evaluation of SPECT in the assessment and treatment of intractable childhood epilepsy. Neurology 2000; 55(9):1391–1393.

90 Commission. Proposal for revised clinical and electroencephalographic classification of epileptic seizures. From the Commission on Classification and Terminology of the International League Against Epilepsy. Epilepsia 1981; 22(4):489–501.

91 Commission. Proposal for revised classification of epilepsies and epileptic syndromes. Commission on Classification and Terminology of the International League Against Epilepsy. Epilepsia 1989; 30(4):389–399.

92 Blume W, Luders H, et al. Glossary of descriptive terminology for ictal semiology: report of the ILAE task force on classification and terminology. Epilepsia 2001; 42:1212–1218.

93 Engel J Jr. A proposed diagnostic scheme for people with epileptic seizures and with epilepsy: report of the ILAE Task Force on Classification and Terminology. Epilepsia 2001; 42(6):796–803.

94 Treiman DM. Generalized convulsive status epilepticus in the adult. Epilepsia 1993; 34 (suppl 1): S2–S11.

95 Livingston J. Status epilpeticus. In: Wallace S (ed.) Epilepsy in children. London: Chapman & Hall; 1996:429–448.

96 Roger J, Bureau M, et al. Epileptic syndromes in infancy, childhood and adolescence. London: John Libbey; 1992.

97 Engel J, Pedley TA. Epilepsy: a comprehensive textbook. Philadelphia: Lippincott-Raven; 1998.

98 Mizrahi EM, Kellaway P. Characterization and classification of neonatal seizures. Neurology 1987; 37(12):1837–1844.

99 Plouin P. Benign familial neonatal convulsions and benign idiopathic neonatal convulsions. In: Pedley TA (ed.) Epilepsy: a comprehensive textbook. Philadelphia: Lippincott-Raven; 1997:2247–2255.

100 Dravet C, Bureau M, et al. Benign myoclonic epilepsy in infants. In: Wolf P (ed.) Epileptic syndromes in infancy, childhood and adolescence. London: John Libbey; 1992:67–74.

101 Bruyere H, Lewis S, et al. Confirmation of linkage in X-linked infantile spasms (West syndrome) and refinement of the disease locus to Xp213–Xp221. Clin Genet 1999; 55(3):173–181.

102 Vigevano F, Fusco L, et al. The idiopathic form of West syndrome. Epilepsia 1993; 34(4):743–746.

103 Koo B. Vigabatrin in the treatment of infantile spasms. Pediatr Neurol 1999; 20(2):106–110.

104 Riikonen RS. Steroids or vigabatrin in the treatment of infantile spasms? Pediatr Neurol 2000; 23(5):403–408.

105 Chiron C, Dulac O, et al. Therapeutic trial of vigabatrin in refractory infantile spasms. J Child Neurol 1991; Suppl 2: S52–59.

106 Appleton RE, Peters AC, et al. Randomised, placebo-controlled study of vigabatrin as first-line treatment of infantile spasms. Epilepsia 1999; 40(11):1627–1633.

107 Vigevano F, Cilio MR. Vigabatrin versus ACTH as first-line treatment for infantile spasms: a randomized, prospective study. Epilepsia 1997; 38(12):1270–1274.

108 Wong M, Trevathan E. Infantile spasms. Pediatr Neurol 2001; 24(2):89–98.

109 Hancock E, Osborne JP. Vigabatrin in the treatment of infantile spasms in tuberous sclerosis: literature review. J Child Neurol 1999; 14(2):71–74.

110 Dravet C, Bureau M, et al. Severe myoclonic epilepsy in infants. In: Wolf P (ed.) Epileptic syndromes in infancy, childhood and adolescence. London; John Libbey; 1992:75–88.

111 Guerrini R, Dravet C, et al. Lamotrigine and seizure aggravation in severe myoclonic epilepsy. Epilepsia 1998; 39(5):508–512.

112 Guerrini R, Dravet C. Severe epileptic encephalopathies of infancy, other than West

syndrome. In: Pedley TA (ed.) Epilepsy: a comprehensive textbook. Philadelphia: Lippincott-Raven; 1997:2285–2302.

113 Duncan JS, Panayiotopoulos CP. Typical absences and related epileptic syndromes. London: Churchill Communications; 1995.

114 Aicardi J. Myoclonic-astatic epilepsy. In: Wallace S (ed.) Epilepsy in children. London: Chapman & Hall; 1996:263–270.

115 Tassinari, CA, Bureau M, et al. Epilepsy with myoclonic absences. In: Wolf P (ed.) Epileptic syndromes in infancy, childhood and adolescence. London: John Libbey; 1992:151–160.

116 Singh R, Scheffer IE, et al. Generalized epilepsy with febrile seizures plus: a common childhood-onset genetic epilepsy syndrome. Ann Neurol 1999; 45(1):75–81.

117 Parker AP, Agathonikou A, et al. Inappropriate use of carbamazepine and vigabatrin in typical absence seizures. Dev Med Child Neurol 1998; 40(8):517–519.

118 Panayiotopoulos CP. Differentiating occipital epilepsies from migraine with aura, acephalic migraine and basilar migraine. Benign childhood partial seizures and related epileptic syndromes. London: John Libbey; 1999:281–302.

119 Ferrie CD, Grunewald RA. Panayiotopoulos syndrome: a common and benign childhood epilepsy. Lancet 2001; 357(9259):821–823.

120 Panayiotopoulos CP. Elementary visual hallucinations in migraine and epilepsy. J Neurol Neurosurg Psychiatry 1994; 57(11):1371–1374.

121 Berkovic SF, McIntosh A, et al. Familial temporal lobe epilepsy: a common disorder identified in twins. Ann Neurol 1996; 40(2):227–235.

122 Scheffer IE, Phillips HA, et al. Familial partial epilepsy with variable foci: a new partial epilepsy syndrome with suggestion of linkage to chromosome 2. Ann Neurol 1998; 44(6):890–899.

123 Corda D, Gelisse P, et al. Incidence of drug-induced aggravation in benign epilepsy with centrotemporal spikes. Epilepsia 2001; 42(6):754–759.

124 Elger CE. Semeiology of temporal lobe seizures. In: Oxbury JM, Polkey CE, Duchowny M (eds) Intractable focal epilepsy. London: WB Saunders; 2000:63–68.

125 Avanzini G, Beaumanoir A, et al. Limbic seizures in children. London: John Libbey; 2001.

126 Bartolomei F, Chuvel P. Seizure symptoms and cerebral localization: frontal lobe and rolandic seizures. In: Oxbury JM, Polkey CE, Duchowny M (eds) Intractable focal epilepsy. London: WB Saunders; 2000:55–62.

127 Gobbi G, Bouquet F, et al. Coeliac disease, epilepsy, and cerebral calcifications. The Italian Working Group on Coeliac Disease and Epilepsy. Lancet 1992; 340(8817):439–443.

128 Hart Y, Andermann F. Rasmussen syndrome. In: Oxbury JM, Polkey CE, Duchowny M (eds) Intractable focal epilepsy. London: WB Saunders; 2001:233–248.

129 Aicardi J, Chevrie JJ. Atypical benign partial epilepsy of childhood. Dev Med Child Neurol 1982; 24(3):281–292.

130 Doose H, Hahn A, et al. Atypical benign partial epilepsy of childhood or pseudo-Lennox syndrome. Part II: family study. Neuropediatrics 2001; 32(1):9–13.

*131 Anonymous. Efficacy of felbamate in childhood epileptic encephalopathy (Lennox–Gastaut syndrome). The felbamate study group in Lennox–Gastaut syndrome. N Engl J Med 1993; 328:29–33.

*132 Motte J, Trevathan E, et al. Lamotrigine for generalized seizures associated with the Lennox–Gastaut syndrome. Lamictal Lennox–Gastaut Study Group. N Engl J Med 1997; 337(25):1807–1812.

*133 Sachdeo RC, Glauser TA, et al. A double-blind, randomized trial of topiramate in Lennox–Gastaut syndrome. Topiramate YL Study Group. Neurology 1999; 52(9):1882–1887.

134 Ben-Menachem, E, Hellstrom K, et al. Evaluation of refractory epilepsy treated with vagus nerve stimulation for up to 5 years [see comments]. Neurology 1999; 52(6):1265–1267.

135 Irwin K, Birch V, et al. Multiple subpial transection in Landau–Kleffner syndrome. Dev Med Child Neurol 2001; 43(4):248–252.

136 Robinson RO, Baird G, et al. Landau–Kleffner syndrome: course and correlates with outcome. Dev Med Child Neurol 2001; 43(4):243–247.

137 Deonna, T. Epilepsies with cognitive symptomatology. In: Wallace S (ed.) Epilepsy in children. London: Chapman & Hall; 1996:315–322.

*138 Verity CM, Butler NR, et al. Febrile convulsions in a national cohort followed up from birth. II – Medical history and intellectual ability at 5 years of age. (Clin Res Ed) 1985; 290(6478):1311–1315.

139 Wallace SJ. Febrile seizures. In: Wallace S (ed.) Epilepsy in children. London: Chapman & Hall; 1996:185–198.

140 Barlow WE, Davis RL, et al. The risk of seizures after receipt of whole-cell pertussis or measles, mumps, and rubella vaccine. N Engl J Med 2001; 345(9):656–661.

*141 Offringa M, Moyer VA. Evidence based paediatrics: evidence based management of seizures associated with fever. BMJ 2001; 323:1111–1114.

142 Knudsen FU. Febrile seizures: treatment and prognosis. Epilepsia 2000; 41(1):2–9.

143 Baumann RJ, Duffner PK. Treatment of children with simple febrile seizures: the AAP practice parameter. American Academy of Pediatrics. Pediatr Neurol 2000; 23(1):11–17.

*144 Scott RC, Besag FM, et al. Buccal midazolam and rectal diazepam for treatment of prolonged seizures in childhood and adolescence: a randomised trial [see comments]. Lancet 1999; 353(9153):623–626.

*145 Lahat E, Goldman M, et al. Comparison of intranasal midazolam with intravenous diazepam for treating febrile seizures in children: prospective randomised study. BMJ 2000; 321(7253):83–86.

*146 Annegers JF, Hauser WA, et al. Factors prognostic of unprovoked seizures after febrile convulsions. N Engl J Med 1987; 316(9): 493–498.

*147 Verity CM, Greenwood R, et al. Long-term intellectual and behavioral outcomes of children with febrile convulsions. N Engl J Med 1998; 338(24):1723–1728.

*148 Annegers JF, Grabow JD, et al. Seizures after head trauma: a population study. Neurology 1980; 30(7 Pt 1):683–689.

149 Hahn YS, Fuchs S, et al. Factors influencing posttraumatic seizures in children. Neurosurgery 1988; 22(5):864–867.

150 Chandler C. Posttraumatic seizures and posttraumatic epilepsy. In: Oxbury JM, Polkey CE, Duchowny M (eds) Intractable focal epilepsy. M Duchowny. London: WB Saunders; 2000: 185–193.

151 Aicardi J. Atypical semiology of rolandic epilepsy in some related syndromes. Epileptic Disord 2000; 2(suppl 1): S5–S9.

152 Minassian BA, Ianzano L, et al. Identification of new and common mutations in the EPM2A gene in Lafora disease. Neurology 2000; 54(2):488–490.

153 Lehesjoki AE, Koskiniemi M. Progressive myoclonus epilepsy of Unverricht–Lundborg type. Epilepsia 1999; 40 (suppl 3):23–28.

154 Cock H, Schapira AH. Mitochondrial DNA mutations and mitochondrial dysfunction in epilepsy. Epilepsia 1999; 40 (suppl 3):33–40.

155 Mole S, Gardiner M. Molecular genetics of the neuronal ceroid lipofuscinoses. Epilepsia 1999; 40 (suppl 3):29–32.

156 Cassidy G, Corbett J. Learning disorders. In: Pedley TA (ed.) Epilepsy: a comprehensive textbook. Philadelphia: Lippincott-Raven; 1997:2053–2063.

157 Kuzniecky RI, Jackson GD. Developmental disorders. In: Pedley TA (ed.) Epilepsy: a comprehensive textbook. Philadelphia: Lippincott-Raven; 1997:2517–2532.

158 Menkes JH, Sarnat HB. Malformations of the central nervous system. In: Menkes JH, Sarnat HB (eds) Child neurology, 6th edn. Philadelphia: Lippincott Williams & Wilkins; 2000.

159 Sarnat HB, Menkes JH. The new neuroembryology. In: Menkes JH, Sarnat HB (eds) Child neurology, 6th edn. Philadelphia: Lippincott Williams & Wilkins; 2000:277–304.

160 Sisodiya SM, Squier MV, et al. Malformations of cortical development. In: Oxbury JM, Polkey CE, Duchowny M (eds). Intractable focal epilepsy. London: WB Saunders; 2000:99–130.

161 Riviello JJ, Honavar M, et al. Tumors and partial seizures. In: Oxbury JM, Polkey CE, Duchowny M (eds) Intractable focal epilepsy. London: WB Saunders; 2000: 195–212.

162 Ferrie CD, Giannakodimos S, et al. Symptomatic typical absence seizures. In: Panayiotopoulos CP (ed.) Typical absences and related epileptic syndromes. London: Churchill Communications; 1995:241–252.

163 Guerrini RG, Gobbi, et al. Chromosomal abnormalities. In: Pedley TA (ed.) Epilepsy: a comprehensive textbook. Philadelphia: Lippincott-Raven; 1997:2533–2546.

164 Garcia-Alvarez M, Nordli DR, et al. Inherited metabolic disorders. In: Pedley TA (ed.) Epilepsy: a comprehensive textbook. Philadelphia: Lippincott-Raven; 1997: 2547–2562.

165 Baxter P. Pyridoxine-dependent and pyridoxine-responsive seizures. Dev Med Child Neurol 2001; 43(6):416–420.

166 Curatolo P. Epilepsies symptomatic of structural lesions. In: Wallace S (ed.) Epilepsy in children. London: Chapman & Hall; 1996: 399–415.

167 Austin JK, de Boer HM. Disruptions in social functioning and services facilitating adjustment for the child and adult. In: Pedley TA (ed.) Epilepsy: a comprehensive textbook. Philadelphia: Lippincott-Raven; 1997: 2191–2201.

168 Yerby MS, Collins SD. Teratogenicity of antiepileptic drugs. In: Pedley TA (ed.) Epilepsy: a comprehensive textbook. Philadelphia: Lippincott-Raven; 1997: 1195–1203.

169 Timmings P. Toxicity of antiepileptic drugs. In: Pedley TA (ed.) Epilepsy: a comprehensive textbook. Philadelphia: Lippincott-Raven; 1997: 1165–1173.

170 Kasteleijn-Nolst Trenite D. Cognitive aspects. In: Wallace S (ed.) Epilepsy in children. London: Chapman & Hall; 1996:581–599.

171 Kalviainen R, Nousiainen I. Visual field defects with vigabatrin: epidemiology and therapeutic implications. CNS Drugs 2001; 15(3):217–230.

172 Appleton RE. Guideline may help in prescribing vigabatrin. BMJ 1998; 317(7168): 1322.

173 Perucca E. Pharmacokinetics. In: Pedley TA (ed.) Epilepsy: a comprehensive textbook. Philadelphia: Lippincott-Raven; 1997: 1131–1153.

174 Aicardi J. Epilepsy and other seizure disorders. Diseases of the nervous system in childhood. London: Mac Keith Press; 1998: 575–637.

175 Gilman JT. Drug treatment: children. In: Oxbury JM, Polkey CE, Duchowny M (eds) Intractable focal epilepsy. London: WB Saunders; 2000: 491–504.

*176 Mattson RH, Cramer JA, et al. A comparison of valproate with carbamazepine for the treatment of complex partial seizures and secondarily generalized tonic–clonic seizures in adults. The Department of Veterans Affairs Epilepsy Cooperative Study No 264 Group. N Engl J Med 1992; 327(11): 765–771.

*177 Verity CM, Hosking G, et al. A multicentre comparative trial of sodium valproate and carbamazepine in paediatric epilepsy. The Paediatric EPITEG Collaborative Group. Dev Med Child Neurol 1995; 37(2):97–108.

*178 Marson AG, Williamson PR, et al. Carbamazepine versus valproate monotherapy for epilepsy. Cochrane Database Syst Rev 2002.

179 Camfield C, Camfield P, et al. Asymptomatic children with epilepsy: little benefit from screening for anticonvulsant-induced liver, blood, or renal damage. Neurology 1986; 36(6):838–841.

*180 Sirven JL, Sperling M, et al. Early versus late antiepileptic drug withdrawal for people with epilepsy in remission. Cochrane Database Syst Rev 2002; 1.

*181 Berg AT, Shinnar S. Relapse following discontinuation of antiepileptic drugs: a meta-analysis. Neurology 1994; 44(4):601–608.

*182 Verrotti A, Morresi S, et al. Discontinuation of anticonvulsant therapy in children with partial epilepsy. Neurology 2000; 55(9):1393–1395.

*183 Chadwick D. Does withdrawal of different antiepileptic drugs have different effects on seizure recurrence? Further results from the MRC Antiepileptic Drug Withdrawal Study. Brain 1999; 122(Pt 3):441–448.

*184 Todt H. The late prognosis of epilepsy in childhood: results of a prospective follow-up study. Epilepsia 1984; 25(2):137–144.

185 Matricardi M, Brinciotti M, et al. Outcome after discontinuation of antiepileptic drug therapy in children with epilepsy. Epilepsia 1989; 30(5):582–589.

186 Camfield PR, Camfield CS, et al. If a first antiepileptic drug fails to control a child's epilepsy, what are the chances of success with the next drug? J Pediatr 1997; 131(6):821–824.

*187 Castillo S, Schmidt DB, et al. Oxcarbazepine add-on for drug-resistant partial epilepsy. Cochrane Database Syst Rev 2002; 1.

*188 Chaisewikul R, Privitera MD, et al. Levetiracetam add-on for drug-resistant localization related (partial) epilepsy. Cochrane Database Syst Rev 2002; 1.

*189 Jette NE, Marson AG, et al. Topiramate add-on for drug-resistant partial epilepsy. Cochrane Database Syst Rev 2002; 1.

*190 Levy R. Lamotrigine add-on for drug-resistant partial epilepsy. Cochrane Database Syst Rev 2002; 1.

*191 Marson AG, Kadir ZA, et al. Gabapentin add-on for drug resistant partial epilepsy. Cochrane Database Syst Rev 2002; 1.

*192 Ramaratnam S, Marson AG, et al. Lamotrigine add-on for drug-resistant partial epilepsy. Cochrane Database Syst Rev 2002; 1.

193 Aicardi J, Shorvon S. Intractable epilepsy. In: Pedley TA (ed.) Epilepsy: a comprehensive textbook. Philadelphia: Lippincott-Raven; 1997:1325–1331.

194 Nordli DR, De Vivo DC. Dietary measures. In: Oxbury JM, Polkey CE, Duchowny M (eds) Intractable focal epilepsy. London: WB Saunders; 2000:530–536.

195 Vining EPG. Ketogenic diet. In: Pedley TA (ed.) Epilepsy: a comprehensive textbook. Philadelphia: Lippincott-Raven; 1997:1339–1344.

*196 Privitera MD, Wely TE, et al. Vagus nerve stimulation for partial seizures. Cochrane Database Syst Rev2002; 1.

197 Parker AP, Polkey CE, et al. Vagal nerve stimulation in epileptic encephalopathies. Pediatrics 1999; 103(4 Pt 1):778–782.

198 Polkey CE. Temporal lobe resections. In: Oxbury JM, Polkey CE, Duchowny M (eds) Intractable focal epilepsy. London: WB Saunders; 2000:667–695.

199 Silfvenius H. Extratemporal cortical excisions for epilepsy. In: Oxbury JM, Polkey CE, Duchowny M (eds) Intractable focal epilepsy. London: WB Saunders; 2000:697–714.

200 Tuite GF, Polkey CE, et al. Hemispherectomy. In: Oxbury JM, Polkey CE, Duchowny M (eds) Intractable focal epilepsy London: WB Saunders; 2000:715–733.

201 Stephenson JBP. Fits and faints. Oxford: Mac Keith Press; 1990.

202 McLeod KA, Wilson N, et al. Cardiac pacing for severe childhood neurally mediated syncope with reflex anoxic seizures. Heart 1999; 82(6):721–725.

203 Zaidi A, Clough P, et al. Misdiagnosis of epilepsy: many seizure-like attacks have a cardiovascular cause. J Am Coll Cardiol 2000; 36(1):181–184.

204 McClure RJ, Davis PM, et al. Epidemiology of Munchausen syndrome by proxy, non-accidental poisoning, and non-accidental suffocation. Arch Dis Child 1996; 75(1):57–61.

205 Fernandez-Alvarez E, Aicardi J. Movement disorders in children. London: Mac Keith Press; 2001.

206 Surtees R. Inherited ion channel disorders. Eur J Pediatr 2000; 159 (suppl 3): S199–203.

207 Stores G. Recognition and management of narcolepsy. Arch Dis Child 1999; 81(6):519–524.

208 Betts T. Psychiatric aspects of nonepileptic seizures. In: Pedley TA (ed.) Epilepsy: a comprehensive textbook. Philadelphia: Lippincott-Raven; 1997:2101–2116.

209 Mikati MA, Kramer U, et al. Alternating hemiplegia of childhood: clinical manifestations and long-term outcome. Pediatr Neurol 2000; 23(2):134–141.

HEADACHE AND MIGRAINE

*210 Bille BA. 40-year follow-up of school children with migraine. Cephalalgia 1995; 17:488–491.

*211 Abu-Arafeh I, Russell G. Prevalence and causes of headache in schoolchildren. BMJ 1994; 309:765–769.

212 Pothmann R, v. Frankenberg SV, Mueller B, et al. Epidemiology of headache in children and adolescents: evidence of high prevalence of migraine among girls under 10. Int J Behavior Med 1994; 1:76–89.

*213 Mortimer MJ, Kay J, Jaron A. Childhood migraine in general practice: clinical features and characteristics. Cephalalgia 1992; 12:238–243.

*214 Sillanpää M, Anttila P. Increasing prevalence of headache in 7-year-old schoolchildren. Headache 1996; 36:466–470.

*215 Chambers CT, Reid GJ, McGrath PJ, et al. Self-administration of over-the-counter medication for pain among adolescents. Arch Pediatr Adolescent Med 1997; 151(5):449–455.

216 Dengler R, Roberts H. Adolescents' use of prescribed drugs and over-the-counter preparations. J Public Health Med 1996; 18(4):437–442.

217 Simon HK, Weinkle DA. Over-the-counter medications. Do parents give what they intend to give? Arch Pediatr Adolescent Med 1977; 151(7):654–656.

218 Lewis DW, Qureshi FA. Acute headache in the pediatric emergency department. Headache 2000; 40:200–203.

219 van der Wouden JC, van der Pas P, Bruijnzeels MA, et al. Headache in children in Dutch general practice. Cephalalgia 1999; 19(3):147–150.

220 Abu-Arafeh I. Chronic tension type headache in children and adolescents, Cephalalgia 2001; 21:830–836.

221 Headache Classification Committee of the International Headache Society. Proposed classification and diagnostic criteria for headache disorders, cranial neuralgias, and facial pain. Cephalalgia 1988; 8(7):9–96.

222 Seshia SS, Wolstein JR, Adams C, et al. International Headache Society criteria and childhood headache. Dev Med Child Neurol 1994; 36:419–428.

*223 Wöber-Bingöl C, Wöber C, Karwautz A, et al. Diagnosis of headache in childhood and adolescence: a study in 437 patients. Cephalalgia 1995; 15:13–21.

224 Viswanathen V, Bridges S, Whitehouse W, et al. Childhood headaches: discrete entities or continuum? Dev Med Child Neurol 1998; 40:544–550.

225 Blumenthal HJ, Rapoport AM. The clinical spectrum of migraine. Med Clin North Am 2001; 85(4):897–909.

226 Russell MB, Iselius L, Olesen J. Migraine without aura and migraine with aura are inherited disorders. Cephalalgia 1996; 16:305–309.

*227 Gervil M, Ulrich V, Kyvik KO, et al. Migraine without aura: a population-based twin study. Ann Neurol 1999; 46:606–611.

*228 Ulrich V, Gervil M, Kyvik KO, et al Evidence of a genetic factor in migraine with aura: a population-based Danish twin study. Ann Neurol 1999; 45(2):242–246.

*229 Ophoff RA, Terwindt GM, Vergouwe MN. Familial hemiplegic migraine and episodic ataxia type-2 are caused by mutation in Ca++ channel gene CACNLA4. Cell Tissue Res 1996; 87:543–552.

230 Sanchez del Rio M, Moskowitz M. The trigeminal system. In: Olesen J, Tfelt-Hansen P, Welch KMA (eds) The headaches. Philadelphia: Lippincott Williams and Wilkins; 2000: 141–149.

231 Golden GS. The Alice-In-Wonderland syndrome in juvenile migraine. Pediatrics 1979; 65:517–519.

232 Bickerstaff ER. Basilar artery migraine. Lancet 1961; 1:15–17.

*233 Hämäläinen ML, Hoppu K, Valkeila E, et al. Ibuprofen or acetaminophen for the acute treatment of migraine in children – a double-blind, randomized, placebo-controlled, crossover study. Neurology 1997; 48:103–107.

*234 Hämäläinen ML, Hoppu K, Santavuori P. Sumatriptan for migraine attacks in children: a randomized placebo-controlled study – Do children with migraine respond to oral sumatriptan differently from adults? Neurology 1997; 48:1100–1103.

235 Linder SL. Subcutaneous sumatriptan in the clinical setting – the first 50 consecutive patients with acute migraine in a pediatric neurology office practice. Headache 1996; 36:419–422.

*236 Winner P, Rothner AD, Saper J, et al. A randomized, double-blind, placebo-controlled study of sumatriptan nasal spray in the treatment of acute migraine in adolescents. Pediatrics 2000; 106:989–997.

237 Ludvigsson J. Propranolol used in prophylaxis of migraine in children. Acta Neurol Scand 1974; 50:109–115.

238 Forsythe WI, Gillies D, Sills MA. Propranolol ('Inderal') in the treatment of childhood migraine. Dev Med Child Neurol 1984; 26:737–741.

*239 Symon DN, Russell G. Double blind placebo controlled trial of pizotifen syrup in the treatment of abdominal migraine. Arch Dis Child 1995; 7(21):48–50.

*240 Gillies D, Sills M, Forsythe I. Pizotifen (Sanomigran) in childhood migraine. A double-blind controlled trial. Eur Neurol 1986; 25:32–35.

*241 Sorge F, De Simone R, Marano E, et al. Flunarizine in prophylaxis of childhood migraine. A double-blind, placebo-controlled, crossover study. Cephalalgia 1988; 8:1–6.

242 Caruso JM, Brown WD, Exil G, et al. The efficacy of divalproex sodium in the prophylactic treatment of children with migraine. Headache 2000; 40:672–676.

243 Hershey AD, Powers SW, Bentti AL, et al. Effectiveness of amitriptyline in the prophylactic management of childhood headaches. Headache 2000; 40:539–549.

244 Sorge F, Barone P, Steardo L, et al. Amitriptyline as a prophylactic for migraine in children. Acta Neurol Napoli 1982; 4: 362–367.

245 Sillanpää M. Changes in the prevalence of migraine and other headaches during the first seven school years. Headache 1983; 23:15–19.

246 Bille B. Migraine in childhood and its prognosis. Cephalalgia 1981; 1:71–75.

247 Bille B. Migraine in childhood: a 30 year follow-up. In: Lanzi G, Balottin U, Cernibori A, (eds) Headache in children and adolescents. Amsterdam: Elsevier Science; 1989:19–26.

248 Verret S, Steele JC. Alternating hemiplegia in childhood: a report of eight patients with complicated migraine beginning in infancy. Pediatrics 1971; 47:675–680.

249 Mikati MA, Kramer U, Zupane ML, et al. Alternating hemiplegia of childhood: clinical manifestation and long-term outcome. Pediatr Neurol 2000; 23:134–141.

250 Deonna T, Martin D. Benign paroxysmal torticollis in infancy. Arch Dis Child 1981; 56:956–959.

251 Kimura S, Nezu A. Electromyographic study in an infant with benign paroxysmal torticollis. Pediatr Neurol 1998; 19:236–238.

252 Watson P, Steele JC. Paroxysmal dysequilibrium in the migraine syndrome of childhood. Arch Otolaryngol 1974; 99(3):177–179.

*253 Abu-Arafeh I, Russell G. Paroxysmal vertigo as a migraine equivalent in children: a population-based study. Cephalalgia 1995; 15(1):22–25.

254 Fischer AJ. Histamine in the treatment of vertigo. Acta Otolaryngol Suppl 1991; 47(9):24–28.

*255 Abu-Arafeh I, Russell G. Prevalence and clinical features of abdominal migraine compared with those of migraine headache. Arch Dis Child 1995; 72:413–417.

*256 Dignan F, Abu-Arafeh I, Russell G. The prognosis of childhood abdominal migraine. Arch Dis Child 2001; 84:415–418.

257 Worawattanakul M, Rhoads JM, Lichtman SN, et al. Abdominal migraine: prophylactic treatment and follow-up. J Pediatr Gastroenterol Nutr 1999; 28:37–40.

*258 Abu-Arafeh I, Russell G. Cyclical vomiting syndrome in children: a population-based study. J Pediatr Gastroenterol Nutr 1995; 21(4):454–458.

*259 Dignan F, Symon DN, Abu-Arafeh I, et al. The prognosis of cyclical vomiting syndrome. Arch Dis Child 2001; 84(1):55–57.

260 Terzano MG, Manzoni GC, Maione R. Cluster headache in one year old infant? Headache 1981; 21(6):255–256.

261 Maytal J, Lipton RB, Solomon S, et al. Childhood onset cluster headaches. Headache 1992; 32(6):275–279.

*262 Goadsby PJ, Edvinsson L. Human in vivo evidence for trigeminovascular activation in cluster headache. Brain 1994; 117:427–434.

263 McNabb S, Whitehouse W. Cluster headache-like disorder in childhood. Arch Dis Child 1999; 81(6):511–512.

264 Lanzi G, Balottin U, Borgatti R, et al. Late post-traumatic headache in pediatric age. Cephalalgia 1985; 5:211–215.

265 Callaghan M, Abu-Arafeh I. Chronic posttraumatic headache in children and adolescents. Dev Med Child Neurol 2001; 43:819–822.

266 The Childhood Brain Tumor Consortium. The epidemiology of headache among children with brain tumor. Headache in children with brain tumors. J Neuroncol 1991; 10:31–46.

267 Vazquez-Barquero A, Ibanez FJ, Herrera S, et al. Isolated headache as the presenting clinical manifestation of intracranial tumors: a prospective study. Cephalalgia 1994; 14(4):270–272.

268 Battistella PA, Naccarella C, Soriani S, et al. Headache and brain tumours: different features versus primary forms in juvenile patients. Headache 1998; 9:245–248.

269 Rossi LN, Vassella F. Headache in children with brain tumors. Childs Nerv Syst 1989; 5:307–309.

270 Edgeworth J, Bullock P, Bailey A, et al. Why are brain tumours still being missed? Arch Dis Child 1996; 74(2):148–151.

271 Soler D, Cox T, Bullock P, et al. Diagnosis and management of benign intracranial hypertension. Arch Dis Child 1998; 78:89–94.

272 Salman MS, Kirkham FJ, MacGregor DL. Idiopathic benign intracranial hypertension: case series and review. J Child Neurol 2001; 16(7):465–470.

DISORDERS OF MOVEMENT

273 Towen BC, Sporrel T. Soft signs and MBD. Dev Med Child Neurol 1979; 21:528–530.

274 Zhou B, Bae SK, Malone AC, et al. hGFRalpha-4: a new member of the GDNF receptor family and a candidate for NBIA. Pediatr Neurol 2001; 25:156–161.

275 Fenichel GM. Movement disorders. In: Fenichel GM (ed.) Clinical pediatric neurology, 4th edn, Philadelphia: WB Saunders; 2001:281–299.

*276 Bressman SB, Sabatti C, Raymond D, et al. The DYT1 phenotype and guidelines for diagnostic testing. Neurology 2000; 54:1746–1753.

277 Swaiman KF Movement disorders and disorders of the basal ganglia. In: Swaiman KF, Ashwall S (eds) Pediatric neurology, 3rd edn, St Louis: Mosby; 1999:801–809.

278 Darvet C, Griaud N, Burean M. Benign myoclonus of early infancy. Neuropediatrics 1986; 17:33–38.

279 Di Capua M, Furio L, Ricci S, Vigevano F. Benign neonatal sleep myoclonus. Mov Disord 1993; 8:191–194.

280 Brown P. Cortical myoclonus. Curr Opin Neurol 1996; 9:314–316.
281 Kinsbourne M. Myoclonic encephalopathy of infancy. J Neurol Neurosurg Psychiatry 1962; 25:271–276.
282 Comings DE. Tourette syndrome and human behavior. Duarte CA: Hope Press; 1990.
283 APA diagnostic and statistical manual of mental disorders, 4th edn. Washington DC: American Psychiatric Association; 1994. In: Fernandez-Alvarez E, Aicardi J (eds) Tic disorders in movement disorders in children. London: Mac Keith Press for the International Child Neurology Association; 2001.
284 Robertson MM. Tourette syndrome, associated conditions and the complexities of treatment. Brain 2000; 123:425–462.
285 Swedo SE. Paediatric autoimmune neuropsychiatric disorders associated with streptococcal infections, Clinical description of the first fifty cases. Am J Psychiatry 1998; 155:264–271.
286 Vanasse M, Bedard P, Andermann F. Shuddering attacks in children and early manifestation of essential tremor. Neurology 1976; 6:1027–1030.
287 Morrison PJ. The spinocerebellar ataxias: molecular progress and newly recognized paediatric phenotypes. Eur J Paediatr Neurol 2000; 4:9–15.
288 Brett EM. Some syndromes of involuntary movements. In: Brett EM (ed.) Paediatric neurology, 3rd edn. Edinburgh: Churchill Livingstone; 1997:275–290.
289 Fernandez-Alvarez E, Aicardi J. Movement disorders in children. London: Mac Keith Press; 2001.
290 Haslam RH. Movement disorders: the nervous system. In: Behrman RE, Kliegman R, Nelson WE, Vaughan VC III (eds) Nelson textbook of pediatrics, 14th edn, Philadelphia: Saunders; 1992:1723–1728.
291 Tucker DM, Leckman JF, Scahill JF, et al. A putative post-streptococcal case of OCD with chronic tic disorder, not otherwise specified. J Am Acad Child Adolesc Psychiatry 1996; 35:1684–1691.

CEREBRAL PALSY

292 Little WJ. On the influence of abnormal parturition, labour, premature birth and asphyxia neonatorum on the mental and physical condition of the child especially in relation to deformities. Transactions of the Obstetric Society of London 1862; 3, 293–344 (reprinted Cerebral Palsy Bulletin 1958; 1, 5–36).
293 Stanley FJ, Blair E, Alberman E. How common are the cerebral palsies? In: Stanley F, Blair E, Alberman E, (eds) Cerebral palsies: epidemiology and causal pathways. London: Mac Keith Press/Cambridge University Press; 2000: pp 22–39.
294 Hagberg B, Hagberg GF, von Wendt L. The changing panorama of cerebral palsy in Sweden. 7. Prevalence and origin in the birth year period 1987 to 90. Acta Paediatr 1996; 85:954–960.
295 Pschirrer ER, Yeomans ER. Does asphyxia cause cerebral palsy? Semin Perinatol 2000; 24(3):215–220.
296 Blair EM, Stanley FJ. Intra-partum asphyxia: a rare cause of cerebral palsy. Paediatrics 1988; 133:955.
297 Bakketeig LS. Only a minor part of cerebral palsies cases begin in labour: but still room for controversial child birth issues in court. BMJ 1999; 319:1016–1017.
298 Niswander KR. In: Stanley FJ, Chalmers I. Cerebral palsy, intrapartum care and a shot in the foot. Lancet 1989; 2:1251–1252.
299 Nelson KB, Ellenberg JH. Children who outgrew cerebral palsy. Paediatrics 1982; 69:529–536.
300 Gupta R, Appleton RE. Cerebral palsy: not always what it seems. Arch Dis Child 2001; 85:3556–3560.
301 Hoon AH, Reinhardt EM, Kelley RI, et al. Brain magnetic resonance imaging and suspected extrapyramidal cerebral palsy: observations in distinguishing genetic–metabolic from acquired causes. J Pediatr 1997; 131:240–245.
302 Brown JK. Infants damaged during birth: perinatal asphyxia In: Hull D (ed) Recent advances in paediatrics. Edinburgh: Churchill Livingston; 1976:57–88.
303 Pasternak JF, Gorey MT. The syndrome of acute near-total intrauterine asphyxia in the term infant. Paediatr Neurol 1998; 18:391–398.
304 Nelson KB, Ellenberg JH. Antecedents of cerebral palsy. Multivariate analysis of risk. N Engl J Med 1986; 315:81–86.
305 Yeargin-Allsopp M, Murphy CC, Cordero JF. Reported biomedical causes and associated medical conditions for mental retardation among 10 year old children: Metropolitan Atlanta, 1985–1987. Dev Med Child Neurol 1997; 39:142–149.
306 Low JA, Muir DW, Pater EA, Karchmar EJ. The association of intrapartum asphyxia in the mature fetus with newborn behaviour. Am J Obstet Gynecol 1990; 163:1131–1135.
*307 Neilson JP, Levene MI. The Cochrane Collaboration: Progress in perinatal medicine. Arch Dis Child 1997; 77F:176–177.
308 Umstad MP, Permezel M, Pepperell RJ. Litigation and intra-partum cardiotocograph. Br J Obstet Gynaecol 1995; 102:89–91.
309 Savage LW. The rise in caesarean section: anxiety or science? In: Chard T, Richards MPM (eds) Obstetrics in the 1990s: current controversies. London: Mac Keith Press; 1992; 167–191.
310 Smith JH. Is continuous intra-partum foetal monitoring necessary? In: Chard T, Richards MPM (eds) Obstetrics in the 1990s: current controversies. London: Mac Keith Press; 1992; 192–201.
311 Edington PT, Sibanda J, Beard RW. Influence on clinical practice of routine intra-partum foetal monitoring. BMJ 1975; 3:341–343.
312 Forfar JO, Hume R, McPhial FM, et al. Low birth weight: a 10 year outcome study of the continuum of reproductive casualty. Dev Med Child Neurol 1994; 36:1037–1048.
313 Pharoah POD, Cooke T, Cooke RWI, Rosenbloom L. Birth weight specific trends in cerebral palsy. Arch Dis Child 1990; 65:602–606.
314 Stanley FJ, Alberman E. Birth weight, gestational age and the cerebral palsies In: Stanley FJ, Alberman E (eds) The epidemiology of the cerebral palsies. Spastics International Medical Publications. Oxford: Blackwell; 1984: 57–68.
315 Pharoah POD, Cooke T, Rosenbloom I, Cooke RWI. Trends in birth prevalence of cerebral palsy. Arch Dis Child 1987; 62:379–383.
316 Stanley FJ, Blair E, Alberman E. Postneonatally acquired cerebral palsy: incidence and antecedents. In: Stanley FJ, Blair E, Alberman E (eds) Cerebral palsies: epidemiology and causal pathways. London: Mac Keith Press, Cambridge University Press; 2000: 124–137.
317 Rosenbloom L. Diagnosis and management of cerebral palsy. Arch Dis Child 1995; 72:350–354.
318 Surveillance of Cerebral Palsy in Europe (SCPE). Surveillance of cerebral palsy in Europe: a collaboration of cerebral palsy surveys and registers. Dev Med Child Neurol 2000; 42:816–824.
319 Wood E, Rosenbaum P. The gross motor function classification system for cerebral palsy: A study of reliability and stability over time. Dev Med Child Neurol 2000; 42:292–296.
320 Hagberg B, Hagberg G. Dyskinetic and dystonic cerebral palsy and birth. Acta Paediatr 1992; 81:93–94.
321 Neville B. The Worster-Drought syndrome: a severe test of paediatric neurodisability services? Dev Med Child Neurol 1997; 39:982–984.
322 Hughes I, Newton R. Genetic aspects of cerebral palsy. Dev Med Child Neurol 1992; 34:80–86.
323 Kuzniecky R, Andermann F, Guerrini R. Congenital bilateral peri-Sylvian syndrome: study of 31 patients. The CBPS Multicentre Collaborative Study. Lancet 1993; 341:608–612.
324 Felix JF, Badawi N, Kurinczuk JJ, et al. Birth defects in children with newborn encephalopathy. Dev Med Child Neurol 2000; 42:803–808.
325 Volpe JJ. Brain injury in the premature infant: Is it preventable? Paediatr Res 1990; 27(suppl):S28–S33.
326 Veelken N, Hagberg B, Hagberg G, Olow I. Diplegic cerebral palsy in Swedish term and preterm children – differences in reduced optimality, relations to neurology and pathogenetic factors. Neuropediatrics 1983; 14:20–28.
327 Krägeloh-Mann I, Hagberg B, Petersen D, et al. Bilateral spastic cerebral palsy. Pathogenetic aspects from MRI. Neuropediatrics 1992; 23:46–48.
328 Brown JK, Lin JP, Minns RA. Causes of congenital hemiplegic cerebral palsy. In: Campbell AJM, MacIntosh N (eds) Forfar & Arneil's Textbook of Pediatrics, 5th edn. Edinburgh: Churchill Livingstone; 1998:741.
329 Wiklund LM, Uverbrandt P, Flodmark O. Computed tomography as an adjunct to aetiology analysis of hemiplegic cerebral palsy. 1. Children born pre-term. 2. Children born at term. Neuropediatrics 1991; 22:50–56, 121–128.
330 Okumura A, Hayakawa F, Kato T, et al. MRI findings in patients with spastic cerebral

palsy. 1. Correlation with gestational age at birth. 2. Correlation with type of cerebral palsy. Dev Med Child Neurol 1997; 39:363–368, 369–372.
331 Lebeer J. How much brain does a mind need? Scientific, clinical, and educational implications of ecological plasticity. Dev Med Child Neurol 1998; 40:352–357.
332 Pharoah POD, Cooke T, Cooke, RWI. Hypothesis for the aetiology of spastic cerebral palsy—the vanishing twin. Dev Med Child Neurol 1997; 39:292–296.
333 Blickstein I. Reflections on the hypothesis for the aetiology of spastic cerebral palsy caused by the vanishing twin syndrome. Dev Med Child Neurol 1998; 40:358.
334 Association of Clinical Cytogenetists Working Party on Chorionic Villi in Prenatal Diagnosis. Cytogenetic analysis of chorionic villi for prenatal diagnosis: an ACC collaborative study of UK data. Prenat Diagn 1994; 14:363–379.
335 Stanley FJ, Blair E, Alberman E. Causal pathways to the cerebral palsies: a new aetiological model. In: Stanley F, Blair E, Alberman E (eds) Cerebral palsies: epidemiology and causal pathways. London: Mac Keith Press, Cambridge University Press; 2000.
336 Hill AB, Hill ID. Statistical evidence and indifference. In: Hill AB, Hill ID (eds) Bradford Hill's principles of medical statistics, 12th edn. London: Edward Arnold; 1991:272–276.
337 McKinlay IA, Ismail H. Health services for children with neurodevelopmental disabilities. In: Petridou E, Nakou S. Children and families with special needs: the right to hope. Athens: European Society for Social Pediatrics; 1991.
338 Almost D, Rosenbaum P. The effectiveness of speech intervention for phonological disorders: a randomised controlled trial. Dev Med Child Neurol 1998; 40:319–325.
339 Ko MLB, McConachie H, Jolleff N. Outcome of recommendations for augmentative communication in children. Child Care Health Dev 1998; 24:195–205.
340 McKinlay IA. Physical therapies for cerebral palsies In: Jukes AM (ed.) Baclofen: spasticity and cerebral pathology. Northampton: Cambridge Medical Publications; 1978:4–6.
341 McKinlay I. Autism: the paediatric neurologist's tale. Br J Disord Commun 1989; 24:201–207.
342 Sterba JA, Rogers BT, France AP, Vokes DA. Horseback riding in children with cerebral palsy: effect on gross motor function. Dev Med Child Neurol 2002; 44:302–308.
343 McKinlay I, Hyde E, Gordon N. Baclofen: a team approach to drug evaluation of spasticity in childhood In: Boyle IT, Johnston RV, Forbes CD (eds) Baclofen: a broader spectrum of activity. Scott Med J 1979; S26–S28.
344 Butler C, Chambers H, Goldstein M, et al. Evaluating research and developmental disabilities: A conceptual framework for reviewing treatment outcomes. Dev Med Child Neurol 1999; 41:55–59.
345 Sussman M. Why don't we know more about what we are doing? Dev Med Child Neurol 2001; 43:507.
346 Dyson R. Shortage of therapists: radical solutions will be needed. BMJ 1990; 300:4.
347 Grahame R. Decline of rehabilitation services and its impact on disability benefits. J R Soc Med. 2002; 95:114–117.
348 Robards MF. Running a team for disabled children and their families. London: Mac Keith Press, Cambridge University Press; 1995.
349 Bax MCO, Whitmore K. District handicapped teams in England, 1983–8. Arch Dis Child 1991; 66:656–664.
350 Bax MCO, Whitmore K. District handicapped teams in England 1983–8 Arch Dis Child 1991; 66:1103 (letter).
351 Court Report: Fit for the future. Report of a Committee on Child Health Services. Vol 1. C mnd.6684. London: HMSO; 1976.
352 Bax MCO, Whitmore K. District handicapped teams: structure, function and relationships. Report to DHSS London, Community Paediatric Research Unit, Westminster Children's Hospital; 1985.
353 Tawfik R, Dickson A, Clarke M, Thomas AG. Care givers perceptions following gastrostomy in severely disabled children with feeding problems. Dev Med Child Neurol 1997; 39:746–751.
354 Strauss D, Kastner T, Ashwal S, White I. Tube feeding and mortality in children with severe disabilities and mental retardation. Pediatrics 1997; 99:358–362.
355 Sullivan PB. Is tube feeding in disabled children associated with excess mortality? J Pediatr Gastroenterol Nutr 1998; 27(2):240–241.
356 Kuttiyanawala MA. Gastrostomy complications in infants and children. Ann R Coll Surg Engl 1998; 80:240–243.
357 Khattak IU. Percutaneous endoscopic gastrostomy in paediatric practice. Complications and outcome. J Pediatr Surg 1998; 33:67–72.
358 Shaw NJ, White CP, Fraser WD, Rosenbloom L. Osteopenia in cerebral palsy. Arch Dis Child 1994; 71:235–238.
359 Lassman FM, Fisch RO, Vetter DK, La Bens ES. Early correlates of speech, language and hearing; the collaborative perinatal project of the National Institute of Neurological and Communicative Disorders and Stroke. Littleton, Massachusetts: PSG Publishing; 1980:140–144, 220–225.
360 Yule W, Rutter M. Language development and disorders. Oxford: Mac Keith Press; 1987:20–21, 357–358.
361 Haynes C, Nidoo S. Children with specific speech and language impairment. Oxford: Mac Keith Press; 1991: 202–203.
362 Lees J.Urwin S. Children with language disorders. London: Whurr Publishers; 1991:197–202, 211–212.
363 Fielder AR, Best AB, Bax MCO. The management of visual impairment in childhood. London: Mac Keith Press, Cambridge University Press; 1993:32–33.
364 Wallace SJ. Epilepsy in cerebral palsy. Dev Med Child Neurol 2001;43:713–717.
365 Hadjipanayis A, Hadjichristodoulou C, Youroukos S. Epilepsy in patients with cerebral palsy. Dev Med Child Neurol 1997; 39:659–663.
366 Clinical Standards Advisory Group. Services for people who have epilepsy. London: Department of Health; 2000.
367 Chadwick C, Smith D. The mis-diagnosis of epilepsy. BMJ 2002; 324:495–496.
368 Nordin V, Gillberg C. Autism spectrum disorders in children with physical or mental disability or both. 1: Clinical and epidemiological aspects. Dev Med Child Neurol 1996; 38:297–313.
369 Nelson KB, Jarether JK, Croen LA, et al. Neuropeptides and neurotrophins in neonatal blood of children with autism or mental retardation. Ann Neurol 2001; 49:597–606.
370 Jan JE, Espezel H, Appleton RE. The treatment of sleep disorders with melatonin. Dev Med Child Neurol 1994; 36:97–107.
371 Neville B, Albright AL. The management of spasticity associated with the cerebral palsies in children and adolscents. Secaucus, NJ: Churchill Communications; 2000.
372 Carr LJ, Cosgrove AP, Gringras P, Neville BG. Position paper on the use of botulinum toxin in cerebral palsy. UK Botulinum Toxin and Cerebral Palsy Working Party. Arch Dis Child 1998; 79:271–273.
373 Scope. Right from the start. London: Scope; 1994.
374 Cunningham CC, Morgan PA, McGucken RB. Down's syndrome: is dissatisfaction with disclosure of diagnosis inevitable? Dev Med Child Neurol 1984; 26:33–39.
375 Strauss D, Shavelle R. Life expectancy of adults with cerebral palsy. Dev Med Child Neurol 1998; 40:369–375.
376 Strauss D, Cable W, Shavelle R. Causes of excess mortality in cerebral palsy. Dev Med Child Neurol 1999; 41:580–585.
377 Williams K, Alberman E. Survival in cerebral palsy: the role of severity and diagnostic labels. Dev Med Child Neurol 1998; 40:376–379.
378 Evans PM, Alberman E. Certified cause of death in children and young adults with cerebral palsy. Arch Dis Child 1990; 65:325–329.
379 Evans PM, Evans SJW, Alberman E. Cerebral palsy: why we must plan for survival. Arch Dis Child 1990; 65:1329–1333.
380 Crichton JU, Mackinnon M, White CP. The life expectancy of persons with cerebral palsy. Dev Med Child Neurol 1995; 37:567–576, 1032–1033 (letters).
381 Blair E, Watson L, Badawi N, Stanley FJ. Life expectancy among people wih cerebral palsy in Western Australia. Dev Med Child Neurol 2001; 43(8):508–515.
382 Kudrjavcev T, Schoemberg BS, Kurland LT, Grover RV. Cerebral palsy: survival rates, associated handicaps and distribution by clinical sub-type (Rochester MN, 1950–1976). Neurology 1985; 35:900–903.
383 Shavelle RM, Strauss VJ, Day SM. Comparison of survival in cerebral palsy between countries. Dev Med Child Neurol 2001; 43:574.
384 Nicholson A, Alberman E. Cerebral palsy—an increasing contributor to severe mental retardation? Arch Dis Child 1992; 67:150–155.
385 Hollins S, Attard MT, Fraunhofer N, et al. Mortality in people with learning disability: risk causes, and death certification findings in London. Dev Med Child Neurol 1998; 40:50–56.

386 McLaughlin JF, Bjornson KF. Quality of life and developmental disabilities. Dev Med Child Neurol 1998;40:435.

387 Ronen GM, Rosenbaum P, Law M, Streiner DL. Health-related quality of life in childhood epilepsy: the results of children's participation in identifying the components. Dev Med Child Neurol 1999; 41:554–559.

388 Yude C, Goodman R. Peer problems of 9–11 year old children with hemiplegia in mainstream schools Can these be predicted? Dev Med Child Neurol 1999; 41:4–8.

389 De Wolfe NA, Byrne JM, Bawden HN. ADHD in pre-school children: parent rated psycho-social correlates. Dev Med Child Neurol 2000; 42:825–830.

390 Andrew FW, Withey SB. Social indicators of well-being. London: Plenum Press; 1976.

391 Bode H, Weidner K, Stork M. Quality of life in families with children with disabilities. Dev Med Child Neurol 2000; 42:354.

392 Baldwin S. The costs of caring families with disabled children. London: Routledge & Keegan Paul; 1985.

393 Kew S. The cost of handicap. Health Social Serv J 1973; 14:860-861.

394 Baldwin S. Disabled children. Counting the costs. London: The Disability Alliance; 1977.

395 Lawton D. The family fund database. York UK: University of York; 1996.

396 Curran AL, Sharples PM, White C, Knapp M. Time costs of caring for children with severe disabilities compared with caring for children without disabilities. Dev Med Child Neurol 2001; 43:529–533.

397 Hagberg B, Edebol-Tysk K, Edstrom B. The basic care needs of profoundly mentally retarded children with multiple handicaps. Dev Med Child Neurol 1988; 30:287–293.

398 Barabas G, Matthews W, Zumoff P. Care-load for children and young adults with severe cerebral palsy. Dev Med Child Neurol 1992; 34:979-984.

399 Edebol-Tysk K. Evaluation of care-load for individuals with spastic tetraplegia. Dev Med Child Neurol 1989; 31:737–745.

400 Thomas A, Bax M, Coombes K, et al. The health and social needs of physically handicapped young adults: are they being met by the statutory services? Dev Med Child Neurol 1985; 27: supplement no 50.

401 Thomas AP, Bax MCO, Smyth DPL. The health and social needs of young adults with physical disabilities. Oxford: Blackwell; 1989.

402 Abercrombie MLJ. Perceptual and visuo-motor disorders in cerebral palsy. A survey of the literature. Little Club Clinics in Developmental Medicine No. 11. London: William Heinemann; 1964.

403 Charman T, Baird G. Practitioner review: diagnosis of autism spectrum disorder in 2- and 3-year-old children. J Child Psychol Psychiatry 2002; 43:289–305.

404 Jacobson LK, Dutton GN. Periventricular leucomalacia: an important cause of visual and ocular motility dysfunction in children. Surv Ophthalmol 2000; 45:1–12.

405 Law M, Russell D, Pollock N, et al. A comparison of neurodevelopmental therapy plus casting and a regular occupational therapy programme for children with cerebral palsy. Dev Med Child Neurol 1997; 39:664–670.

406 Lowe JA. Intra-partum foetal asphyxia: Definition, diagnosis and classification. Am J Obstet Gynecol 1997; 176:957–959.

407 Smith VH (ed.) Visual disorders in cerebral palsy. Little Club Clinics in Developmental Medicine No 9. London: William Heinemann; 1963.

DEGENERATIVE BRAIN DISORDERS

408 Stephenson JBP, King MD (eds). Regression. In: Handbook of neurological investigations in children. London: Wright; 1989:209–222.

409 van der Knapp MS, Lyter PR, et al. Leukoencephalopathy with swelling and a discrepantly mild clinical course in eight children. Ann Neurol 1995; 37:324–334.

410 Hanefeld F, Holzbach U, Kruse B, et al. Diffuse white matter disease in children: an encephalopathy with unique features on magnetic resonance imaging and proton magnetic resonance spectroscopy. Neuropediatrics 1993; 24:244–248.

411 van der Knapp MS, Gabreels FJM, et al. A new leukoencephalopathy with vanishing white matter. Neurology 1997; 48:845–855.

412 Aicardi J. Heredodegenerative disorders of the CNS. In: Diseases of the nervous system in childhood 2nd edn. London: Mac Keith Press; 1998:241–322.

413 Dorfman LJ, Pedley TA, et al. Juvenile neuroaxonal dystrophy: clinical, electro-physiological and pathological features. Ann Neurol 1978;3:419– 428.

414 Asber DM. Slow viral infections. In: Behrman RE, Kliegman R, Nelson WE, Vaughan VC III (eds) Nelson textbook of pediatrics 15th edn. Philadelphia: WB Saunders; 1996:1723–1728.

415 Levin M, Walter S. Infections of the nervous system. In: Brett E (ed.) Paediatric neurology, 3rd edn. London: Churchill Livingstone; 1998: 621–690.

416 Mole S. Neuronal ceroid lipofuscinoses. Eur J Pediatr Neurol 1999; 3:43–44.

417 Hudson LD, Pucket C, Berndt J, et al. Mutation of the proteolipid protein gene PLP in human X chromosome-linked myelin disorder. Proc Natl Acad Sci USA 1989; 86:8128–8131.

418 Ellis D, Malcolm S. Proteolipid protein gene dosage effect in Pelizaeus-Merzbacher disease. Nat Genet 1994; 6:333–334.

419 Meyer N, Rosenbaum V, et al. Search for putative scrapie genome in purified prion fraction reveals a paucity of nucleic acids. J Gen Virol 1991; 72:37– 49.

NEUROMUSCULAR DISEASE

420 MacLeod MJ, Taylor JE, Lunt PW, et al. Prenatal onset of spinal muscular atrophy. Eur J Paediatr Neurol 1999; 2:65–72.

421 Essex C, Roper H. Lesson of the week: late presentation of Duchenne's muscular dystrophy as global developmental delay. BMJ 2001; 323:37–38.

422 Westerlund LE, Gill SS, Jarasz TS, et al. Posterior only unit rod instrumentation for neuro-muscular scoliosis. Spine 2001; 26:1984–1989.

423 Hopf CG, Eysel P. One stage versus two-stage spinal fusion in neuromuscular scoliosis. J Pediatr Orthop B. 2000; 9:234–243.

424 Simonds AK. Nasal ventilation in progressive neuromuscular disease: experience in adults and adolescents. Monaldi Arch Chest Dis 2000; 55:237–241.

425 Simonds AK, Ward S, Heather S, et al. Outcome of paediatric domiciliary mask ventilation in neuromuscular and skeletal disease. Eur Respir J 2000; 16:476–481.

*426 Arahata H, Ishiura S, Ishiguro T, et al. Immunostaining of skeletal and cardiac muscle surface membrane with antibody against Duchenne muscular dystrophy peptide. Nature 1988; 333:861–863.

*427 Bonilla E, Samitt C, Miranda A, et al. Duchenne muscular dystrophy: deficiency of dystrophin at the muscle cell surface. Cell 1988; 54:447–452.

428 Hoffmann EP, Fischbeck KH, Brown RH, et al. Characterisation of dystrophin in muscle biopsy specimens from patients with Duchenne's or Becker's muscular dystrophy. N Engl J Med 1988; 318:1363–1368.

429 Koenig M, Beggs AH, Moyer M, et el. The molecular basis for Duchenne versus Becker muscular dystrophy: correlation of severity with type of deletion. Am J Hum Genet 1998; 45:498–506.

430 Monaco AP, Bertelson CJ, Leichti-Gallati S, et al. An explanation for the phenotypic differences between patients bearing partial deletions of the DMD locus. Genomics 1988; 2:90–95.

431 Greenstein RM, Reardon MP, Chan TS. An X-autosome translocation in a girl with Duchenne muscular dystrophy – evidence for DMD gene localisation. Pediatr Res 1977; 11:457. (abstract)

432 Verellen-Doumoulin C, Freund M, De Mayer R, et al. Expression of an X-linked muscular dystrophy in a female due to translocation involving Xq21 and non-random inactivation of the normal X chromosome. Hum Genet 1984; 67:115–119.

433 Arikawa E, Hoffmann EP, Kairdo M, et al. The frequency of patients having dystrophin abnormalities in a limb girdle patient population. Neurology 1991; 41:1491–1496.

434 Hoffmann EP, Arahata K, Minetti C, et al. Dystrophinopathy in isolated cases of myopathy in females. Neurology 1992; 42:967–975.

435 Hoogerwaard EM, Bakker E, Ippel PF, et al. Signs and symptoms of Duchenne muscular dystrophy and Becker muscular dystrophy among carriers in the Netherlands: a cohort study. Lancet 1999; 353:2116–2119.

436 Boland BJ, Silbert PL, Groove RV, et al. Skeletal, cardiac and smooth muscle failure in DMD. Pediatr Neurol 1996; 14:7–12.

*437 Cotton S, Voudoria NJ, Greenwood KM. Intelligence and Duchenne muscular dystrophy: full-scale, verbal and performance intelligence quotients. Dev Med Child Neurol 2001; 43:497–501.

438 Bush A, Dubowitz V. Fatal rhabdomyo-lysis complicating general anaesthesia in a child with BMD. Neuromuscul Disord 1991; 1:201–204.

439 Barohn RJ, Levine EJ, Olson JO, Mendell JR. Gastric hypomotility in Duchenne muscular dystrophy. N Engl J Med 1988; 319:15–18.

*440 van Deutekom JCT, Wijmenga C, van Tienhoven EA, et al. FSHD associated DNA rearrangements are due to large deletions of integral copies of a 32kb tandemly repeated unit. Hum Mol Genet 1993; 2:2037–2042.

441 Winokur ST, Bengtsson U, Feddersen J, et al. DNA rearrangement associated with facioscapulohumeral muscular dystrophy involves a heterochromatin-associated repetitive element: implications for a role of chromatin structure in the pathogenesis of the disease. Chromosome Res 1994; 2:225–234.

442 Taylor GS, Maehama T, Dixon JE. Myotubularin, a protein tyrosine phosphatase mutated in myotubular myopathy, dephosphorylases the lipid second messenger phosphatidylinositol 3-phosphate. Proc Natl Acad Sci USA 2000; 97:8910–8915.

443 Herman G, Finegold M, Zhao W, et al. Medical complications in long-term survivors with X-linked myotubular myopathy. J Pediatr 1999; 134:206–214.

444 Goebel HH, Warlo I. Nemaline myopathy with intranuclear rods – intranuclear rod myopathy. Neuromuscul Disord 1997; 7:13–19.

445 Lammens M, Moerman P, Fryns JP, et al. Fetal akinesis sequence caused by nemaline myopathy. Neuropediatrics 1997; 2:116–119.

*446 Laing NG, Wilton SD, Akkari PA, et al. A mutation in the alpha-tropomyosin gene TPM3 associated with autosomal dominant nemaline myopathy NEM1. Nat Genet 1995; 9:75–79.

*447 Nowak KJ, Wattanasirichaigoon D, Goebel HH. Mutations in the skeletal muscle alpha-actin gene in patients with actin myopathy and nemaline myopathy. Nat Genet 1999; 23:208–212.

448 Donner K, Ollikainen M, Ridanpää M, et al. Mutations in the β-tropomyosin (TPM2) gene – a rare cause of nemaline myopathy. Neuromuscul Disord 2002; 12:151–158.

449 Johnston JJ, Kelley RI, Crawford TO, et al. A novel nemaline myopathy in the Amish caused by a mutation in troponin T1. Am J Hum Genet 2000; 67:814–821.

450 Manzur AY, Sewry CA, Ziprin J, et al. A severe clinical and pathological variant of central core disease with possible autosomal recessive inheritance. Neuromuscul Disord 1998; 8:467–473.

451 Quane KA, Healy JM, Keating KE, et al. Mutations in the ryanodine receptor gene in central core disease and malignant hyperthermia. Nat Genet 1993; 5:51–55.

452 Nagai T, Tsuchiya Y, Maruyama A, et al. Scoliosis associated with central core disease. Brain Dev 1994; 16:150–152.

453 Jungbluth H, Sewry C, Brown SC, et al. Minicore myopathy in children: a clinical and histopathological study of 19 cases. Neuromuscul Disord 2000; 10:262–273.

454 Rowe PW, Eagle M, Pollitt C, et al. Multicore myopathy: respiratory failure and paraspinal muscle contractures are important complications. Dev Med Child Neurol 2000; 42:340–343.

455 Dubowitz V. Workshop report: the 41st ENMC sponsored workshop on congenital muscular dystrophy. Neuromuscul Disord 1996; 6:295–306.

456 van der Knaap M, Smit LM, et al. Magnetic resonance imaging in classification of congenital muscular dystrophies with brain abnormalities. Ann Neurol 1997; 42:50–59.

457 Philpot J, Cowan F, Pennock J, et al. Merosin deficient congenital muscular dystrophy: the spectrum of brain involvement on magnetic resonance imaging. Neuromuscul Disord 1999; 9:81–85.

458 Shorer Z, Philpot J, Muntoni F, et al. Demyelinating peripheral neuropathy in merosin-deficient congenital muscular dystrophy. J Child Neurol 1995; 10:472–475.

*459 Brockington M, Blake DJ, Prandini P. Mutations in the fukutin related protein gene (FKRP) cause a form of congenital muscular dystrophy with secondary laminin-α2 deficiency and abnormal glycosylation of α-dystroglycan. Am J Hum Genet 2001; 69:1198–1209.

*460 Camacho Vanegas O, Bertini E, Zhang RZ, et al. Ullrich scleroatonic muscular dystrophy is caused by recessive mutations on collagen type VI. Proc Natl Acad Sci USA 2001; 98:7516–7521.

461 Kobayashi K, Yoshida A, Manya H, et al. Muscular dystrophy and neuronal migration disorder caused by mutations in a novel glycosyltransferase. 51st ASHG Conference, San Diego, California, 12–16 October 2000, abstract 267.

462 Dobyns WB, Pagon RA, Armstrong D, et al. Diagnostic criteria for Walker Warburg syndrome. Am J Med Genet 1998; 32:195–210.

463 Phillips MF, Harper PS. Cardiac disease in myotonic dystrophy. Cardiovasc Res 1997; 33:13–22.

464 O'Brien T, Harper PS. Reproductive problems and neonatal loss in women with myotonic dystrophy. Clin Genet 1984; 23:366–369.

465 Harley HG, Brook JD, Rundle SA, et al. Expansion of an unstable DNA region and phenotypic variation in myotonic dystrophy. Nature 1992; 6:545–546.

466 Reardon W, Newcombe R, Fenton I, et al. The natural history of congenital myotonic dystrophy: mortality and long term clinical aspects. Arch Dis Child 1993; 68:177–181.

467 Bergoffen J, Kant J, Sladky J, et al. Paternal transmission of congenital myotonic dystrophy. J Med Genet 1994; 31:518–520.

468 Ohya K, Tachi N, Chiba S, et al. Congenital myotonic dystrophy transmitted from an asymptomic father. Neurology 1994; 44:1958–1960.

469 Plassart E, Reboul J, Rime CS, et al. Mutations in the muscle sodium channel gene (SCN4A) in 13 French families with hyperkalaemic periodic paralysis and paramyotonia: phenotype to genotype correlation and demonstration of the predominance of two mutations. Eur J Hum Genet 1994; 2:110–124.

470 Symmons DPM, Sills JA, Davis SM. The incidence of juvenile dermatomyositis: results from a nationwide study. Br J Rheumatol 1995; 34:732–736.

471 Pachman LM. An update on juvenile dermatomyositis. Curr Opin Rheumatol 1995; 7:437–441.

472 Lister RK, Cooper ES, Paige DG. Papules and pustules of the elbows and knees: an uncommon clinical sign of dermatomyositis in oriental children. Pediatr Dermatol 2000; 17:37–40.

473 Al-Mayouf SM, Laxer RM, Schneider R, et al. Intravenous immunoglobulin therapy for juvenile dermatomyositis: efficacy and safety. J Rheumatol 2000; 27:2498–2503.

474 Al-Mayouf S, Al-Mazyed AA, Bahbri S. Efficacy of early treatment of severe juvenile dermatomyositis with intravenous methylprednisolone and methotrexate. Clin Rheumatol 2000; 19:138–141.

475 Tabarki B, Ponsot G, Prieur A-M, Tardieu M. Childhood dermatomyositis: clinical course of 36 patients treated with low doses of corticosteroids. Eur J Paediatr Neurol 1998; 2:205–211.

476 Aihara Y, Mori M, Ibe M, et al. A case of juvenile dermatomyositis with calcinosis universalis – remarkable improvement with aluminium hydroxide therapy. Ryumachi 1994; 34:879–884.

477 Mukamel M, Horev G, Mimouni M. New insight into calcinosis of juvenile dermatomyositis. J Pediatr 2001; 138:763–766.

478 Watt G, Saisorn S, Jongsakul K, et al. Blinded, placebo-controlled trial of antiparasitic drugs for trichinosis myositis. J Infect Dis 2000; 182:371–374.

479 Shevell M, Rosenblatt B, Silver K, et al. Congenital inflammatory myopathy. Neurology 1990; 40:1111–1114.

480 Vajsar J, Jay V, Babyn P. Infantile myositis in the newborn period. Brain Dev 1996; 18:415–419.

481 Tein I, DiMauro S, DeVivo D. Recurrent childhood myoglobinuria. Adv Pediatr 1990; 37:77–117.

482 Darin N, Oldfors A, Moslemi A-R, et al. The incidence of mitochondrial encephalomyopathies in childhood: clinical features and morphological, biochemical and DNA studies. Ann Neurol 2001; 49:377–383.

483 Hoch W, McConvill J, Melms A, et al. Autoantibodies to the receptor tyrosine kinase MuSK in patients with myasthenia gravis without acetylcholine receptor antibodies. Nat Med 2001; 7:365–368.

484 Gronseth GS, Barohn RJ. Practice parameter: thymectomy for autoimmune myasthenia gravis (an evidenced based review): Report of the Quality Standards Subcommittee of the American Academy of Neurology. Neurology 2000; 55:7–15.

485 Lefebvre S, Burglen L, Reboullet S. Identification and characterisation of a spinal muscular atrophy determining gene. Cell 1995; 80:155–165.

486 Campbell L, Potter A, Ignatius J, et al. Genomic variation and gene conversion in spinal muscular atrophy: implications for disease process and clinical phenotype. Am J Hum Genet 1997; 61:40–50.

487 Dubowitz V. Chaos in the classification of SMA: a possible resolution. Neuromuscul Disord 1995; 5:3–5.

*488 Grohmann K, Scheulke M, Diers A, et al. Mutations in the gene encoding the immunoglobulin mu-binding protein 2 cause spinal muscular atrophy with respiratory distress type 1. Nat Genet 2001; 29:75–77.

489 Goutières F, Aicardi J, Farkas E. Anterior horn cell disease associated with pontocerebellar hypoplasia in infants. J Neurol Neurosurg Psychiatry 1977; 40:370–378.

490 Muntoni F, Goodwin F, Sewry C. Clinical spectrum and diagnostic difficulties of infantile pontocerebellar hypoplasia type 1. Neuropediatrics 1999; 30:243–248.
491 Frijns CJM, Van Deutekom J, Frants RR, et al. Dominant congenital benign spinal muscular atrophy. Muscle Nerve 1994; 17:192–197.
492 van der Vleuten AJW, van Ravenswaaij-Arts CMA, Frijns CJM. Localisation of the gene for a dominant congenital spinal muscular atrophy predominantly affecting the lower limbs to chromosome 12q23–q24. Eur J Hum Genet 1998; 6:376–387.
493 Tooth HH. The peroneal type of muscular atrophy. London: HK Lewis;1886.
494 Charcot JM, Marie P. Su rune forme particuliére d'atrophie musculaire progressive souvent familiale, debutante par les pieds et les jambes, et atteignant plus tard les mains. Rev Med Fr 1886; 6:97–138.
495 Timmerman V, Nelis E, Van Hul K, et al. The peripheral myelin protein gene PMP–22 is contained within the Charcot–Marie–Tooth disease 1A duplication. Nat Genet 1992; 1:171–175.
496 Nicholson GA, Valentijn LJ, Cherryson AK, et al. A frame shift in the PMP 22 gene in hereditary neuropathy with liability to pressure palsy. Nat Genet 1994; 6:263–266.
497 Hayasaka K, Himoro M, Sato W, et al. CMT neuropathy type 1B is associated with mutations of myelin P0 gene. Nat Genet 1993; 5:31–34.
498 Warner LE, Mancias P, Butler IJ, et al. Mutations in the early growth response 2 (EGR2) gene are associated with hereditary myelinopathies. Nat Genet 1998; 18:382–384.
499 Bergoffen J, Scherer SS, Wang S, et al. Connexin mutations in X-linked Charcot–Marie–Tooth disease. Science 1993; 262:2039–2042.
500 Mersiyanova IV, Perepelov AV, Polyakov AV, et al. A new variant of Charcot–Marie–Tooth disease type 2 is probably the result of a mutation in the neurofilament-light gene. Am J Hum Genet 2000; 67:37–46.
501 Zhao C, Takita J, Tanaka Y, et al. Charcot–Marie–Tooth disease type 2A caused by mutations in a microtubule motor K1F1B-beta. Cell 2001; 105:587–597.
502 Priest JM, Fischbeck KH, Nouri N, et al. A locus for axonal motor-sensory neuropathy with deafness and mental retardation maps to Xq24–26. Genomics 1995; 29:406–412.
503 Hagberg B, Lyan G. Pooled European series of hereditary peripheral neuropathies in infancy and childhood. Neuropediatrics 1981; 12:9–17.
504 Makari GS, Carroll JE, Burton EM. Hereditary sensory neuropathy manifesting as possible child abuse. Pediatrics 1994; 93:842–844.

ACUTE NEUROLOGICAL CONDITIONS
505 Advanced Life Support Group. Advanced paediatric life support. The practical approach. 3rd edn. London: BMJ Books; 2001.
506 Addy DP. When not to do a lumbar puncture. Arch Dis Child 1987; 62:873.
507 Archer BD. Computed tomography before lumbar puncture in acute meningitis: a review of the risks and benefits. CMAJ 1993; 148:961–965.
508 Leggate JRS, Minns RA. Intracranial pressure monitoring – current methods. In: Minns RA (ed) Problems of intracranial pressure in childhood. Clinics in developmental medicine Nos 113–114. London: Mac Keith Press; 1991:123–140.
509 Minns RA, Merrick MV. Cerebral perfusion pressure and net cerebral mean transit time in childhood hydrocephalus. J Pediatr Neurosci 1989; 5(2):69–77.
*510 Schierhout G, Roberts I. Anti epileptic drugs for preventing seizures following acute traumatic brain injury (Cochrane Review). In: The Cochrane Library, Issue 2, 2002. Oxford: Update Software.
*511 Alderson P, Roberts I. Corticosteroids for acute traumatic brain injury. Cochrane Database Syst Rev 2000; 2:CD000196.
*512 Roberts I, Schierhout G, Alderson P. Absence of evidence for the effectiveness of five interventions routinely used in the intensive care management of severe head injury: a systematic review. J Neurol Neurosurg Psychiatry 1998; 55:729–733 (Review).
513 Schaad UB, Lips U, Grehm HM, et al. Dexamethasone treatment for bacterial meningitis in children. Lancet 1993; 342:457–461.
*514 Schierhout G, Roberts I. Mannitol for acute traumatic brain injury (Cochrane Review). In: The Cochrane Library, Issue 2, 2002. Oxford: Update Software.
515 Tomlin PI, Clarke MA, et al. Rehabilitation in severe head injury in children: outcome and provision of care. Dev Med Child Neurol 2002; 44 (12):828–837.
516 Sharples PM, Storey A, Aynsley-Green A, Eyre JA. Avoidable factors contributing to death of children with head injury. BMJ 1990; 300:87–91.
517 Royal College of Paediatrics and Child Health. Guidelines for good practice: early management of patients with a head injury. London: RCPCH; 2001.
518 Levin HS, Eugenio GA, Eisenberg HM, et al. Magnetic resonance imaging after closed head injury in children. Neurosurgery 1989; 24(2):223–227.
519 Leggate JRS, Lopez-Ramos N, Genitori L, et al. Extradural haematoma in infants. Br J Neurosurg 1989; 3:533–540.
520 Choux M, Lena G, Genitori L. Intracranial haematomas. In: Raimondi AJ, Choux M, di Rocco C (eds) Head injuries in the newborn and infant. Heidelberg: Springer-Verlag; 1986: 203–216.
521 Faerber EN. Intracranial tumours. In: Faerber EN (ed) CNS magnetic resonance imaging in infants and children. Clinics in developmental medicine, no 134. London: Mac Keith Press; 1995:165–172.
522 Barlow KM, Minns RA. Annual incidence of shaken impact syndrome in young children. Lancet 2000; 356(9241):1571–1572.
523 Elmer and Gregg 1967.
524 Southall DP, Stebbens VA, Rees SV. Apnoeic episodes induced by smothering: two cases identified by covert video surveillance. BMJ 1987; 294:1637–1641.
525 Duhaime AC, Gennarelli TA, Thibault LE, et al. The shaken baby syndrome. Journal of Neurosurgery 1987; 66:409–415.
526 Feldman KW, Brewer DK. Child abuse, cardiopulmonary resuscitation and rib fractures. Pediatrics 1984; 73:339–342.
527 Odom A, Christ E, Kerr N, et al. Prevalence of retinal hemorrhages in pediatric patients after in-hospital cardiopulmonary resuscitation: a prospective study. Pediatrics 1997; 99:E3.
528 Carty H. Skeletal manifestations of child abuse. Bone 1989; 6:3–7.
529 Kravitz H, Driesen G, Gomberg R, Konch A. Accidental falls from elevated surfaces in infants from birth to 1 year of age. Pediatrics 1969; 44:869–876.
530 Caffey J. The whiplash shaken infant syndrome. Pediatrics 1974; 54:396–403.
531 Kleinman PK, Blackbourne BD, Marks SC, et al. Radiological contributions to the investigation and prosecution of cases of fatal infant abuse. N Engl J Med 1989; 320:507–511.
532 Aoki N, Masuzawa H. Subdural haematomas in abused children: report of six cases from Japan. Neurosurgery 1986; 18:475–477.
533 Billmire ME, Myers PA. Serious head injury in infants: accident or abuse? Pediatrics 1985; 75:340–342.
534 Duhaime AC, Alario AJ, Lewander WJ, et al. Head injury in very young children: mechanisms, injury types and ophthalmological findings in 100 hospitalized patients younger than 2 years of age. Pediatrics 1992; 90:179–185.
535 Thomas SA, Rosenfield NS, Leventhal JM, Markowitz RI. Long bone fractures in young children: distinguishing accidental injuries from child abuse. Pediatrics 1991; 88:471–476.
536 Hadley MN, Sonntag VKH, Rekate HL, Murphy A. The infant whiplash-shake injury syndrome: a clinical and pathological study. Neurosurgery 1989; 24:536–540.
537 Jaspan T, Narborough G, Punt JAG, Lowe J. Cerebral contusional tears as a marker of child abuse – detection by cranial sonography. Pediatr Radiol 1992; 22:237–245.
538 Rorke LB. Neuropathology of homicidal head injury in infants. Childs Nerv Syst 1990; 6:295 (abstract).
539 Barlow KM, Gibson RJ, McPhillips M, Minns RA. Magnetic resonance imaging in acute non-accidental head injury. Acta Paediatr 1999; 88(7):734–740.
540 Barlow KM, Minns RA. The relation between intracranial pressure and outcome in non-accidental head injury. Dev Med Child Neurol 1999; 41(4):220–225.
541 Shaw KN, Briede CA. Submersion injuries: drowning and near drowning. Emerg Med Clin North Am 1989; 7:355–370.
542 Ashwal S, Schneider S, Tomasi L, Thompson J. Prognostic implications of hyperglycaemia and reduced cerebral blood flow in children with near drowning. Neurology 1990; 40:820–823.
543 Baraff LJ, Lee SI, Schiger DL. Outcome of bacterial meningitis in children: a meta analysis. Pediatr Infect Dis J 1993; 12:389–394.

544 Trinka E, Dubeau F, Andermann F, et al. Clinical findings, imaging characteristics and outcome in catastrophic post-encephalitic epilepsy. Epileptic Disord 2000; 2(3):153–162.

545 Ito Y, Kimura H, Yabuta Y, et al. Exacerbation of herpes simplex encephalitis after successful treatment with acyclovir. Clin Infect Dis 2000; 30(1):185–187.

546 Schmutzhard E. Viral infections of the CNS with special emphasis on herpes simplex infections. J Neurol 2001; 248(6):469–477 (Review).

547 Bingham PM, Galetta SL, Arhreya B, Sladky J. Neurologic manifestations in children with Lyme disease. Pediatrics 1995; 96:1053–1056.

548 Li M, Masuzawa T, Wang J, et al. In-vitro and in-vivo antibiotic susceptibilities of Lyme disease Borrelia isolated in China. J Infect Chemother 2000; 6(1):65–67.

549 Klempner MS, Hu LT, Evans J, et al. Two controlled trials of antibiotic treatment in patients with persistent symptoms and a history of Lyme disease. N Engl J Med 2001; 345(2):85–92.

550 Anonymous. Stopping status epilepticus. Drug Ther Bull 1996; 34:73–75.

551 Scott RC, Surtees RAH, Neville BGR. Status epilepticus: pathophysiology, epidemiology, and outcomes. Arch Dis Child 1998; 79:73–77.

552 Shorvon S. Status epilepticus: its clinical features and treatment in adults and children. Cambridge: Cambridge University Press; 1994.

553 Knudsen FU. Rectal administration of diazepam in solution in the acute treatment of convulsions in infants and children. Arch Dis Child 1979; 54:855–857.

554 DeLorenzo RJ, Pellock JM, Towne AR, Boggs JG. Epidemiology of status epilepticus. J Clin Neurophysiol 1995; 12:316–325.

555 Shinnar S, Berg AT, Moshe SL, et al. The risk of seizure recurrence after a first unprovoked afebrile seizure in childhood: an extended follow-up. Pediatrics 1996; 98:216–225.

556 Maytal J, Shinnar S, Moshe SL, Alvarez LA. Low morbidity and mortality of status epilepticus in children. Pediatrics 1989; 83:323–331.

557 The Status Epilepticus Working Party. The treatment of convulsive status epilepticus in children. Arch Dis Child 2000; 83:415–419.

558 Lal Koul R, Aithala GR, Chacko A, et al. Continuous midazolam infusion as treatment of status epilepticus. Arch Dis Child 1997; 76:445–448.

559 Kofke WA, Young RSK, Davis P, et al. Isoflurane for refractory status epilepticus: a clinical series. Anesthesiology 1989; 71:653–659.

560 Tasker RC. Emergency treatment of acute seizures and status epilepticus. Arch Dis Child 1998; 79:78–83.

561 Hawkins M, Harrison J, Charters P. Severe carbon monoxide poisoning: outcome after hyperbaric oxygen therapy. Br J Anaesth 2000; 84:584–586.

562 Antoon AY, Volpe JJ, Crawford JD. Burn encephalopathy in children Pediatrics 1972; 50:609–616.

563 Rantala H, Uhari M, Cherry JD, Shields WD. Risk factors for respiratory failure in children with Guillain–Barré syndrome. Pediatr Neurol 1995; 13:289–292.

564 van Der Meche FGA, Schmitz PIM and the Dutch Guillain–Barré N Engl J Med 1992; 326(17): 1123–1129.

565 Kirkham FJ. Stroke in childhood. Arch Dis Child 1999; 81:85–89.

*566 CAST (Chinese acute stroke trial) collaborative group. CAST: randomised placebo-controlled trial of early aspirin use in 20,000 patients with acute ischaemic stroke. Lancet 1997; 349:1641–1649.

567 International stroke trial collaborative group. The international stroke trial (IST): a randomised trial of aspirin, subcutaneous heparin, both, or neither among 19,435 patients with acute ischaemic stroke. Lancet 1997; 349:1569–1581.

568 Barlow KM, Spowart JJ, Minns RA. Early posttraumatic seizures in non-accidental head injury: relation to outcome. Dev Med Child Neurol 2000; 429:591–594.

*569 Gadkary CS, Alderson P, Signorin DF. Therapeutic hypothermia for head injury (Cochrane Review). In: The Cochrane Library, Issue 2, 2002. Oxford: Update Software.

570 Kempe CH. Paediatric implications of the battered baby syndrome. Arch Dis Child 1971; 46:28–37.

DEVELOPMENTAL MEDICINE

571 Herschkovitz N, Kagen J, et al. Neurobiological basis of behavioural development in the second year. Neuropediatrics 1999; 30:221–230.

572 Herschkovitz N. Neurological basis of behavioural development in infancy. Brain Dev 2000; 22:411–416.

573 Benitez-Brbiesia L, De la Rosa-Alvarez I, et al. Dendritic spine pathology in infants with severe protein-calorie malnutrition. Pediatrics 1999; 104(2): http://www. pediatrics.org/cgi/content/full/104/2/e21.

574 To T, Caderette SM, Liu Y. Biologic, social, and environmental correlates of preschool development. Child Care Health Dev 2001; 27(2):187–200.

575 Baird G, McConachie H, Scrutton D. Parents' perceptions of disclosure of the diagnosis of cerebral palsy. Arch Dis Child 2000; 83(6):475–480.

576 Pelchat D, Bisson J, et al. Longitudinal effects of an early family intervention programme on the adaptation of parents with a child with a disability. Int J Nurs Stud 1999; 36(6):465–477.

577 Wolman C, Resnick MD, et al. Emotional well-being among adolescents with and without chronic conditions. J Adolesc Health 1994; 15(3):199–204.

578 Robson P. Shuffling, hitching, scooting or sliding: some observations in 30 otherwise normal children. Dev Med Child Neurol 1970; 12:608–617.

579 Mohamed K, Appleton R, Nicolaides P. Delayed diagnosis of Duchenne muscular dystrophy. Eur J Paediatr Neurol 2000; 4(5):219–223.

580 Shulman LH, Sala DA, et al. Developmental implications of idiopathic toe-walking. J Pediatr 1997; 130(4):541–546.

581 Gratacos M, Nadal M, Martin-Santos R, et al. A polymorphic genomic duplication on human chromosome 15 is a susceptibility factor for panic and phobic disorders. Cell 2001; 106:367–379.

582 Saloojee H, Pettifor JM. Iron deficiency and impaired child development. BMJ 2001; 323:1377–1378.

583 Newton RW, Wraith JE. Investigation of developmental delay. Arch Dis Child 1995; 72:460–465.

584 Contact a Family, 170 Tottenham Court Road, London W1P 0HA.

585 Wallace GB, Newton RW. Gower's sign revisited. Arch Dis Child 1989; 64(9):1317–1319.

585a Gillberg C, Billstedt E. Autism and Asperger syndrome: coexistence with other clinical disorders. Acta Psychiatr Scand 2000; 102(5):321–330.

585b Kadesjo B. Gillberg C. Tourette's disorder: epidemiology and comorbidity in primary school children. J Am Acad Child Adolesc Psychiatry 2000; 39(5):548–555.

585c Kadesjo B. Gillberg C. The comorbidity of ADHD in the general population of Swedish school-age children. J Child Psychol Psychiatry 2001; 42(4):487–492.

585d Schoenfeld J, Seidenberg M, Woodward A, et al. Neuropsychological and behavioral status of children with complex partial seizures. Dev Med Child Neurol 1999; 41:724–731.

586 Grados MA, Slomine BS, et al. Depth of lesion model in children and adolescents with moderate to severe traumatic brain injury: use of SPGR MRI to predict severity and outcome. J Neurol Neurosurg Psychiatry 2001; 70(3):350–358.

587 Berryhill P, Lilly MA, et al. Frontal lobe changes after severe diffuse closed head injury in children: a volumetric study of magnetic resonance imaging. Neurosurgery 1995; 37(3):392–399.

588 Hoelper BM, Reinhert MM, et al. RCBF in haemorrhagic, non-haemorrhagic and mixed contusions after severe head injury and its effect on perilesional cerebralblood flow. Acta Neurochir Suppl 2000; 76:21–25.

589 Jackson SA, Piper I, et al. Assessment of the variation in cerebrovascular reactivity in head injured patients. Acta Neurochir Suppl 2000; 76:445–449.

590 Tasker RC. Pharmacological advance in the treatment of acu11te brain injury. Arch Dis Child 1999; 81:90–95.

591 Gopinath SP, Valadka AB, et al. Extracellular glutamate and aspartate in head injured patients. Acta Neurochir Suppl 2000; 76:437–438.

592 Asikainen I, Kaste M, Sara S. Early and late post-traumatic seizures in traumatic brain injury rehabilitation patients: brain injury factors causing late seizures and influence of seizures on long-term outcome. Epilepsia 1999; 40(5):584–589.

593 Barlow KM, Spowart JJ, Minns RA. Early posttraumatic seizures in non-accidental head injury: relation to outcome. Dev Med Child Neurol 2000; 42(9):591–594.

594 Annegers JF, Hauser WA, et al. A population based study of seizures after traumatic brain injuries. N Engl J Med 1998; 338(1):20–24.

595 Vespa PM, Nuwer MR, et al. Increased incidence and impact of non-convulsive and convulsive seizures after traumatic brain injury as detected by continuous electro-encephalographic monitoring. J Neurosurg 1999; 91(5):750–760.

596 Kinsella G, Packer S, Olver J. Maternal reporting of behaviour following very severe blunt head injury. J Neurol Neurosurg Psychiatry 1991; 54(5):422–426.

597 Massagli TL, Jaffe KM. Pediatric traumatic brain injury: prognosis and rehabilitation. Pediatr Ann 1994; 23(1):29–36.

598 Rivara J-MB. Family functioning following pediatric traumatic brain injury. Pediatr Ann. 1994; 23(1):38–44.

599 Chadwick O, Rutter M, et al. Intellectual performance and reading skills after localised head injury in childhood. J Child Psychol Psychiatry 1981; 22(2):117–139.

600 Michaud LJ, Rivara GP, et al. Predictors of survival and severity of disability after severe brain injury in children. Neurosurgery 1992; 31:254–264.

601 Jaffe KM, Fay GC, et al. Severity of pediatric traumatic brain injury and early neurobehavioural outcome. Arch Phys Med Rehabil 1992; 73:540–547.

602 Minns RA. Intracranial pressure monitoring. Arch Dis Child 1984; 59(5): 486–488.

603 Goldenberg G, Oder W, et al. Cerebral correlates of disturbed executive function and memory in survivors of severe closed head injury. J Neurol Neurosurg Psychiatry 1992; 55:362–368.

604 Department for Education and Skills. Special Educational Needs Code of Practice: SEN Toolkit, Section 7: Writing a Statement of Special Educational Needs, Section 12: The role of Health Professionals. DfES Publications. Available from DfES Publications, PO Box 5050, Sherwood Park, Annesley, Nottinghamshire NG15 0DJ 2001.

605 Couchman M, Rossiter L, et al. A practical outcome scale for paediatric head injury. Arch Dis Child 2001; 84(2):120–124.

606 Helders PJ, Engelbert RH, et al. Paediatric rehabilitation. Disabil Rehabil 2001; 23:497–500.

607 Powell JM, Machamer JE, et al. Self-report of extent of recovery and barriers to recovery after traumatic brain injury: a longitudinal study. Arch Phys Med Rehabil 2001; 82(8):1025–1030.

608 Hellawell DJ, Signorini DF, Pentland B. Reliability of the relative's questionnaire for assessment of outcome after brain injury. Disabil Rehabil 2000; 22:446–450.

609 Bayley N. Bayley scales of infant development. San Antonio,Tx: The Psychological Corporation; 1993.

610 Frankenburg WK, et al. The Denver II: a major revision and restandardisation of the Denver Developmental Screening Test. Pediatrics 1992; 89:91–97.

611 Wechsler D. Wechsler intelligence scale for children – III. New York: The Psychological Corporation; 1991.

612 Griffiths R. The abilities of young children. London: Child Development Research Centre; 1970.

613 Griffiths R. The abilities of young children. Amersham: ARICD; 1984.

614 McCarthy DA. Manual of the McCarthy scales of children's abilities. New York: The Psychological Corporation; 1972.

SPEECH AND LANGUAGE DELAY AND DISORDERS

615 Bishop DBM. How does the brain learn language? Insights from a study of children with and without language impairment. Dev Med Child Neurol 2000; 42(2):133–142.

616 Owen SE, McKinlay IA. Motor difficulties in children with developmental disorders and speech and language. Child Care Health Dev 1997; 23(4):315–325.

617 Davie R, Butler N, Goldstein H. From birth to 7: A report of a National Child Development Study. London: Longman; 1972.

618 Fundudis TI, Kolvin I, Garside RF. Speech retarded and deaf children, their psychological development. London: Academic Press; 1979.

619 Morley ME. The development and disorders of speech in childhood 2nd edn. Edinburgh: E & S Livingstone; 1965.

620 Largo RH, Molinari L, Comenale Pinto L, et al. Language development of term and preterm children during the first five years of life. Dev Med Child Neurol 1986; 28:33–35.

621 Hagberg B. Rett syndrome – clinical and biological aspects. London: Mac Keith Press, Cambridge University Press; 1993.

622 Gordon N. The concept of central deafness. In: Renfrew C, Murphy K (eds) The child who does not talk. Clinics in Developmental Medicine 13. London: William Heinemann; 1964.

623 Worster-Drought C. Congenital suprabulbar paresis. J Laryngol Otol 1956; 70:453–463.

624 Kuzniecky R, Andermann F, Gurerrini R. Congenital bilateral peri-sylvian syndrome: study of 31 patients. The CBPS Multicentre Collaborative Study. Lancet 1993; 341:608–612.

625 Gordon NS. Worster-Drought and congenital bilateral peri-sylvian syndromes. Dev Med Child Neurol 2002; 44:201–204.

626 Landau WM, Kleffner FR. A syndrome of acquired aphasia with convulsive disorder in children. Neurology 1957; 7:523–530.

627 Lees J, Urwin S. Acquired childhood aphasia. In: Children with language disorders. London: Whurr Publishers;1991:179–210.

628 Mantovani JF. Autistic regression and Landau–Kleffner syndrome: progress or confusion? Dev Med Child Neurol 2000; 42:349–353.

629 van Slyke PA. Classroom instruction for children with Llandau–Kleffner syndrome. Child Lang Teaching Ther 2002; 18:23–42.

630 Deonna T, Beaumanoir A, Gaillard P, Assal G. Acquired asphyxia in childhood with seizure disorder. A heterogeneous syndrome. Neuropediatriä 1977; 8:263–273.

631 Ferguson AP, McKinlay IA, Hunt A. Care of adolescents with severe learning disability from tuberose sclerosis. Dev Med Child Neurol 2002; 44:256–262.

632 McKinlay IA. Autism: the paediatric neurologists tale. Br J Disord Commun 1989; 24:201–207.

633 Gillberg C, Coleman M. The biology of the autistic syndromes. Oxford: Mac Keith Press; 1992.

634 O'Brien G, Yule W. Why behavioural phenotypes/methodological issues in behavioural phenotypes research. In: O'Brien G, Yule W (eds) Behavioural phenotypes. London: Mac Keith Press, Cambridge University Press; 1995: 1–23, 35–44.

635 Gillberg C, Coleman M. Autism and medical disorders: a review of the literature. Dev Med Child Neurol 1996; 38:191–202.

636 Rutter M. Autism: two-way interplay between research and clinical work. J Child Psychol Psychiatry 1999; 40:169–188.

637 Lauritsen M, Mors O, Mortensen PV, Ewald H. Infantile autism and associated autosomal chromosomal abnormalities. A registered based study and a literature survey. J Child Psychol Psychiatry 1999; 40:335–345.

638 Medical Research Council. Review of autism research: epidemiology and causes. www.mrcac.uk 2001.

639 Bishop DBM. Autism, Asperger's syndrome, and semantic-pragmatic disorders. Where are the boundaries? Br J Disord Commun 1989; 24:107–121.

640 Johnson E, Hastings RP. Facilitating factors and barriers to the implementation of intensive home based behavioural intervention for young children with autism. Child Care Health Dev 2002; 28:123–129.

641 British Paediatric Association. Services for children and adolescents with learning disability (mental handicap): report of a BPA Working Party. 1994. Available from Royal College of Paediatrics & Child Health, 50 Hallam Street, London W1W 6DE.

642 Thompson NP, Montgomery SM, Wakefield AJ, Pounder RE. Is measles vaccination a risk factor for inflammatory bowel disease? Lancet 1995; 345:1071–1074.

643 Wakefield AJ, Murch SH, Linnel AAJ, et al. Ileal-lymphoid-nodular hyperplasia, non-specific colitis and pervasive developmental disorder in children. Lancet 1998; 351:637–641.

644 Smith A, McCann R, McKinlay I. Second dose of MMR vaccine: health professionals level of confidence in the vaccine and attitudes towards the second dose. Commun Dis Public Health 2001; 4:273–277.

645 Taylor B, Miller E, Lingam R, et al. Measles, mumps and rubella vaccination and bowel problems or developmental regression in children with autism: population study. BMJ 2002; 324:393–396.

646 Legge B. Can't eat, won't eat. London: Jessica Kingsley; 2002.

647 Gordon NS. Stuttering: incidence and causes. Dev Med Child Neurol 2002; 44:278–281.

648 Martin JAM. Hearing loss and hearing behaviour. In: Rutter M, Martin JAM (eds) The child with delayed speech. Clinics in Developmental Medicine 43: Spastic International Medical Publications. London: William Heinemann; 1972:83–94.

649 Lassman FM, Fisch RO, Vetter DK, La Benz ES. Early correlates of speech, language, and hearing loss. Littleton, MA:PSG Publishing; 1980.

650 Chalmers D, Stewart I, Silver P, Mulvena A. Otitis media with effusion in children – the Duneden study. Oxford: Mac Keith Press; 1989.

651 Maw AR. Glue ear in childhood: a prospective study of otitis media with effusion. London: Mac Keith Press, Cambridge University Press;1995.

652 Dunn-Gaier J, Hoe HH, Auersperg E, et al. The effect of secretin on children with autism: a randomised controlled trial. Dev Med Child Neurol 2000; 42:796–802.

653 Patja A, Davidkin I, Kurki T, et al. Serious outburst events after measles, mumps, rubella vaccination during a 14-year prospective follow-up. Pediatric Infect Dis J 2000; 19:1127–1135.

654 Peltola H, Patja A, Leinkki P, Valle M. No evidence for measles, mumps and rubella vaccine-associated inflammatory bowel disease or autism in a 14-year prospective study. Lancet 1998; 351:1327–1328.

(a)

(b)

(c)

(d)

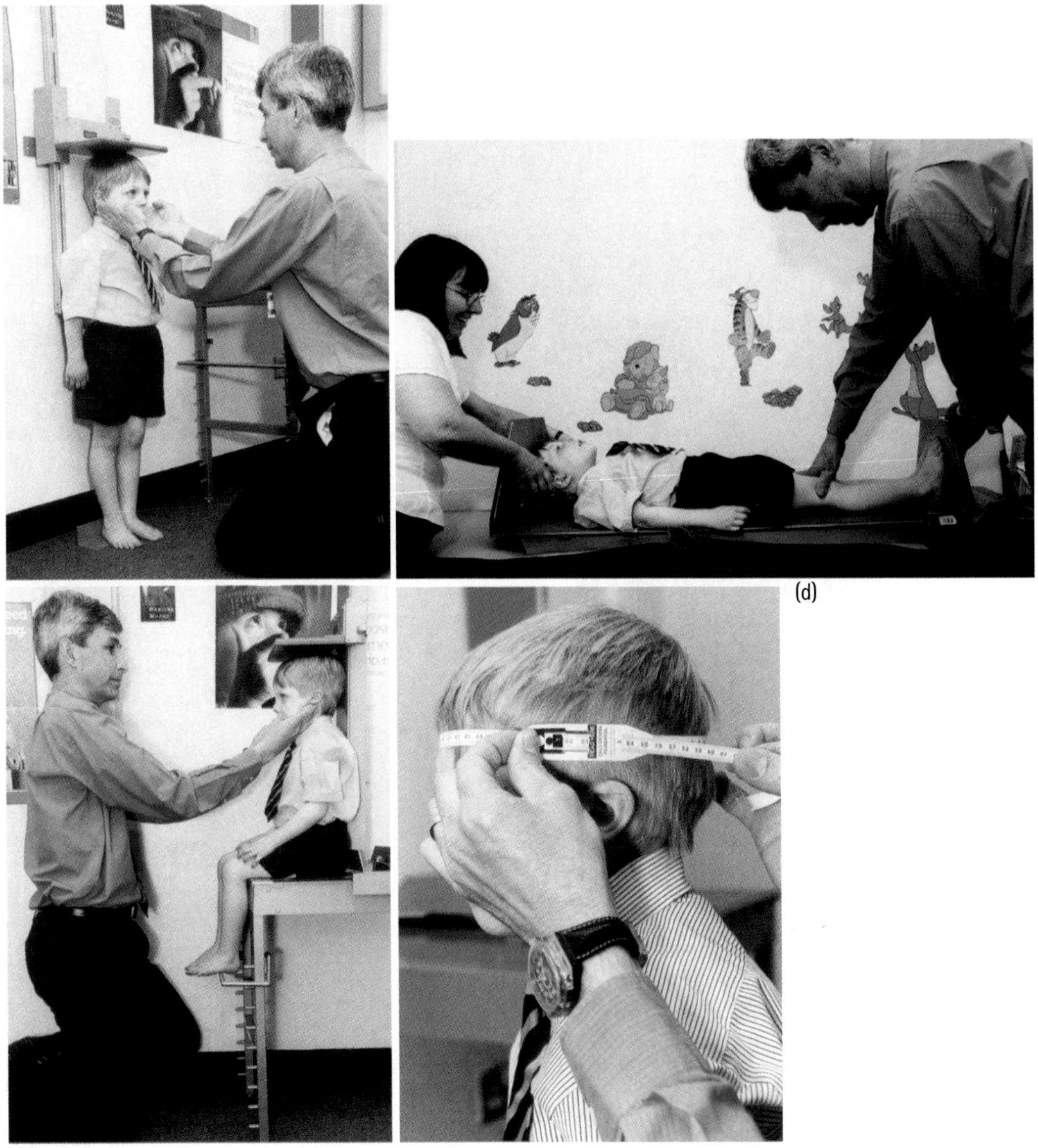

Plate 13.15 Correct positioning and technique for accurate measurement of (a) height, (b) supine length, (c) sitting height, (d) head circumference. For description see text (see p. 466, 467).

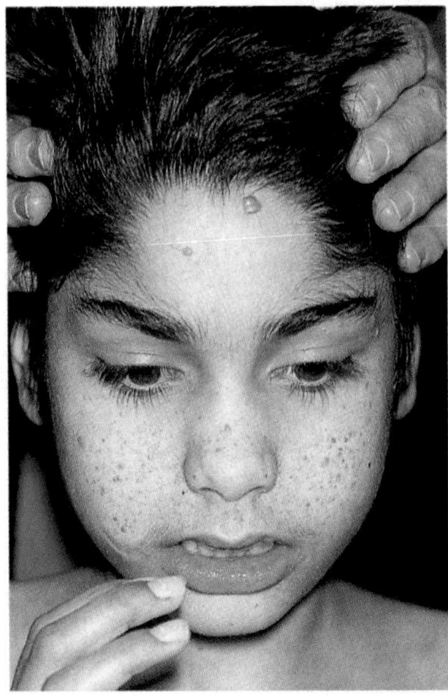

Plate 20.12 Tuberous sclerosis: adenoma sebaceum (see p. 916).

(a)

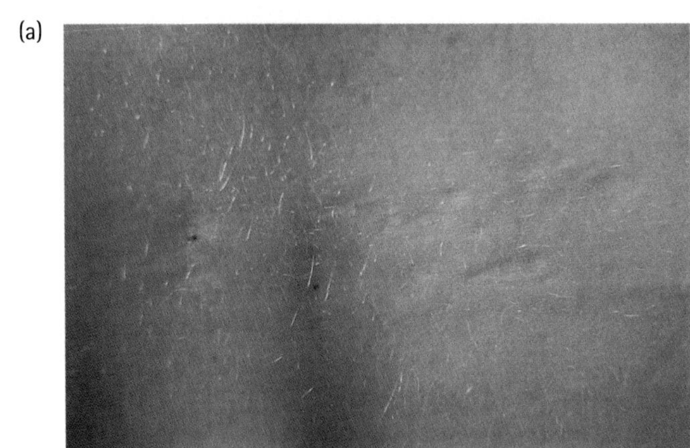

Plate 20.13 Tuberous sclerosis: (a) Shagreen patch; (b) depigmented patches (see p. 917).

(b)

Plate 20.13 (b) Cont'd

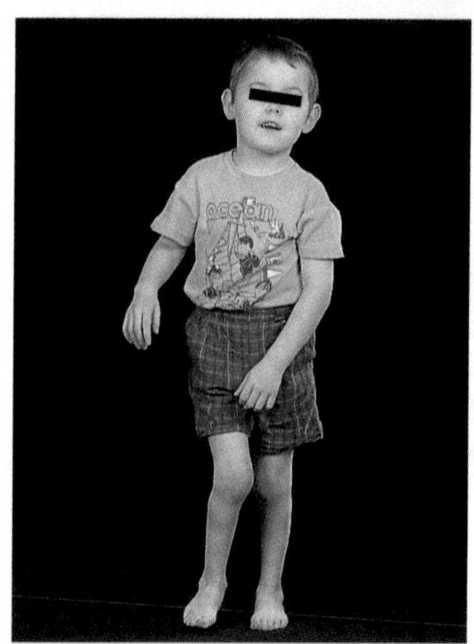

Plate 20.22 Diplegic gait. Internal rotation with hip adduction (see p. 971).

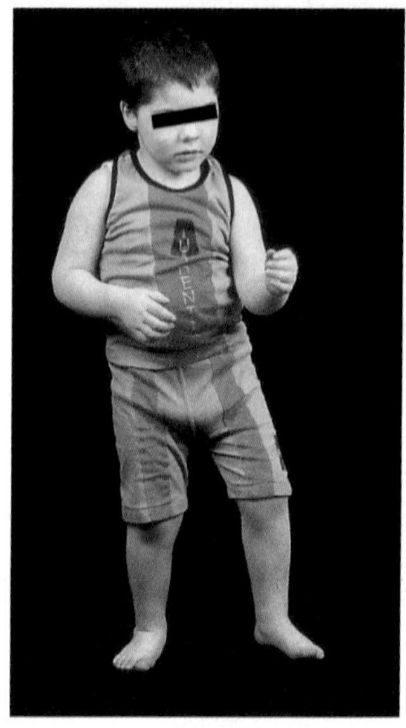

Plate 20.24 Ataxic 3-year-old child showing broad based gait and elevated arms (see p. 972).

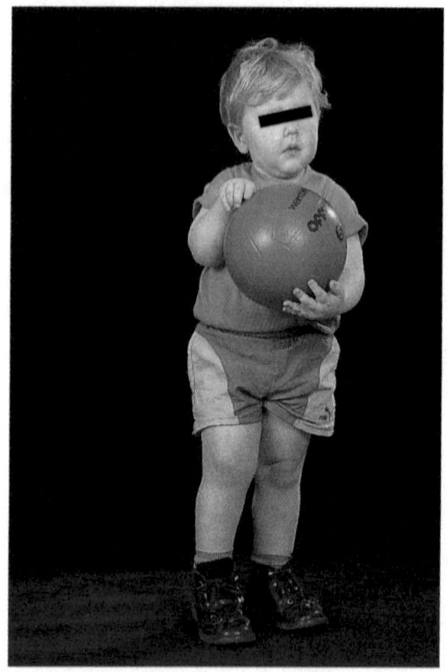

Plate 20.25 Spastic hemiplegia, right-sided – hyperpronated right arm (see p. 973).

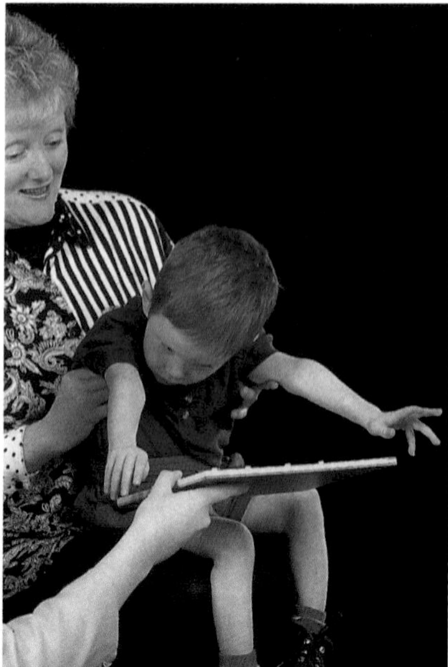

Plate 20.26 A child with dyskinetic cerebral palsy, showing uncontrolled patterns of movement and flaccid trunk, whilst attempting to reach out (see p. 973).

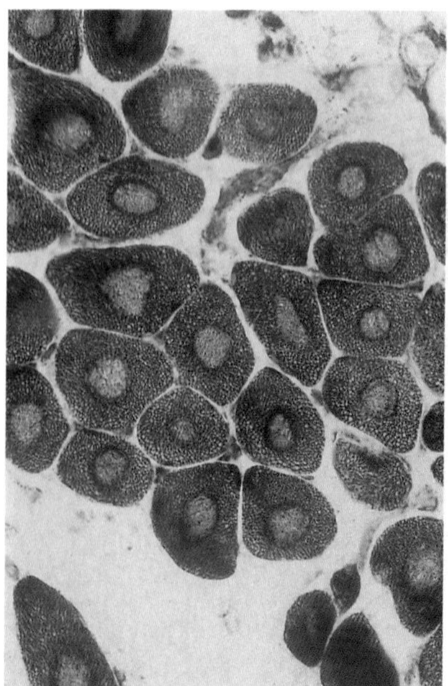

Plate 20.28 Central core disease: the cores show absence of staining with NADH (see p. 997).

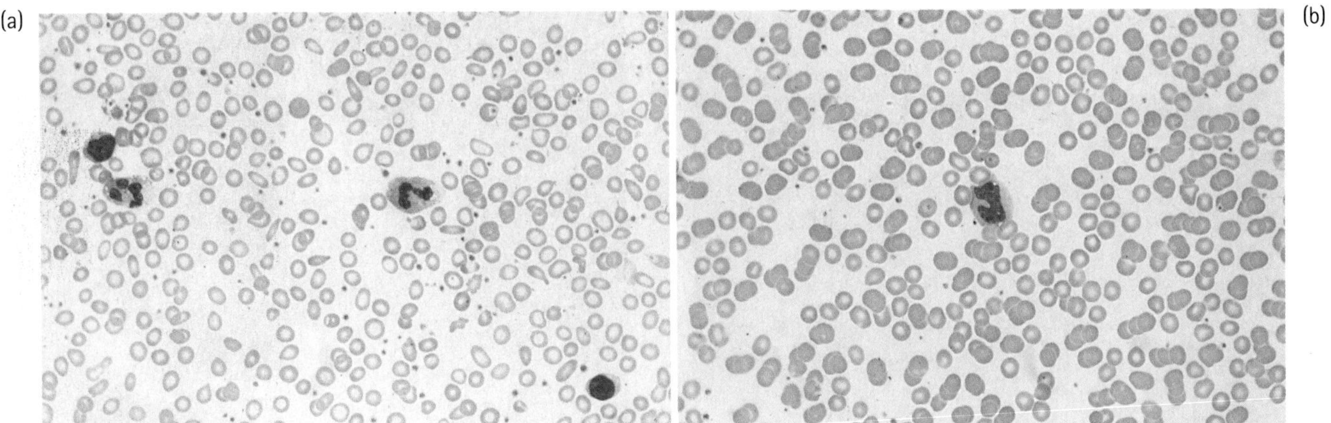

Plate 21.5 Peripheral blood appearances in severe hypochromic iron deficiency with microcytic red cells (a) compared with a normal film (b) (same magnification) (see p. 1063).

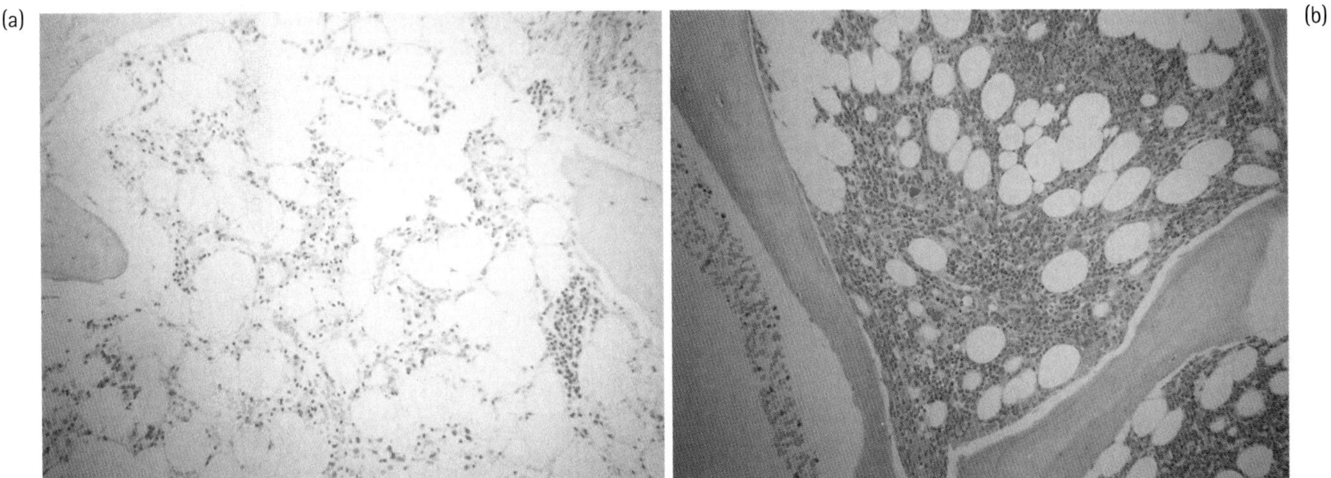

Plate 21.7 The appearances of aplastic bone marrow (a) with a normal marrow (b) for comparison (trephine biopsy) (see p. 1065).

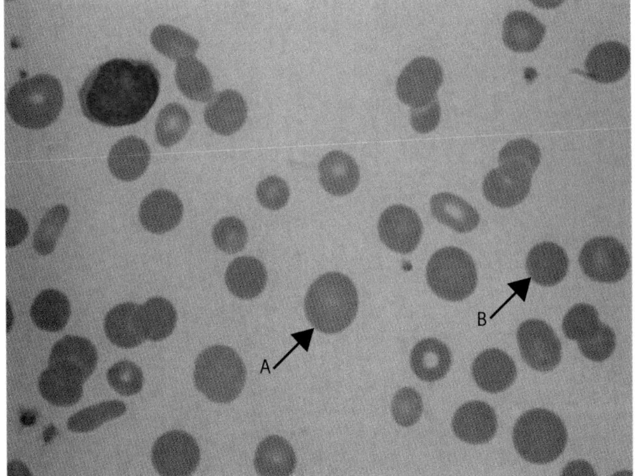

Plate 21.10 Peripheral blood appearance in spherocytosis with spherocytes and polychromasia. A, polychromatic cell; B, microspherocyte (see p. 1068).

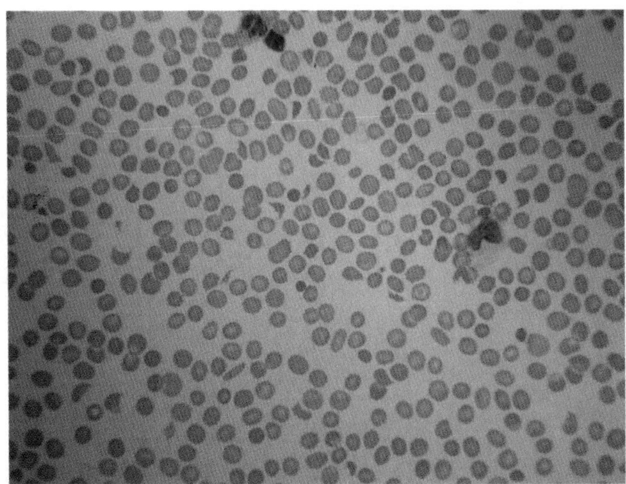

Plate 21.12 Red cell appearances in red cell fragmentation syndromes (see p. 1070).

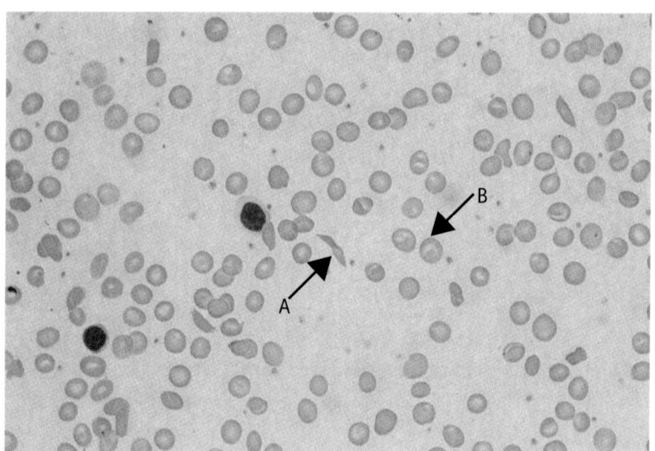

Plate 21.15 Peripheral blood appearance in homozygous sickle cell disease with target cells, polychromasia and distorted red cells (A, sickle cell; B target cell). (From Lissauer & Clayden 2001[37] with permission) (see p. 1072).

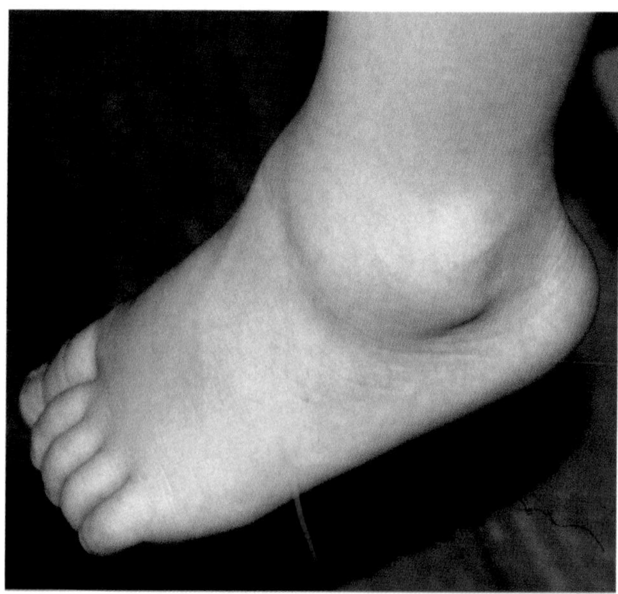

Plate 21.20 Acute ankle hemarthrosis in a child with severe hemophilia A (see p. 1081).

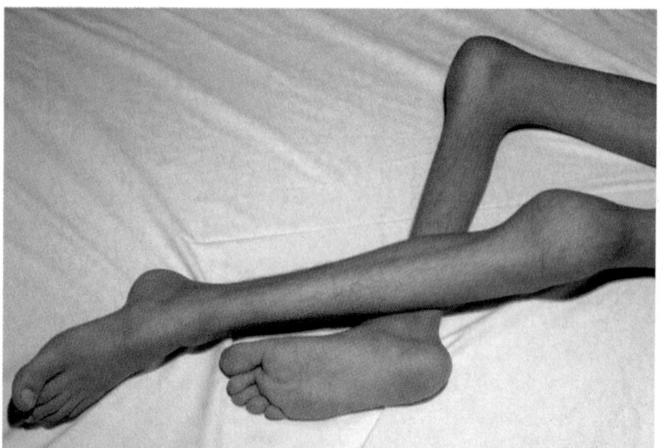

Plate 21.21 (a) Severe hemophilia in an adolescent showing fixed flexion of R knee, marked arthropathy of L knee and muscle wasting (see p. 1082).

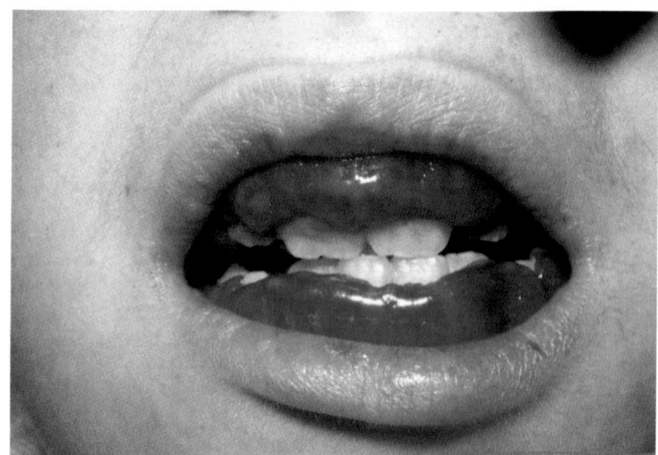

Plate 21.26 Acute monocytic leukemia causing gum infiltration (see p. 1088).

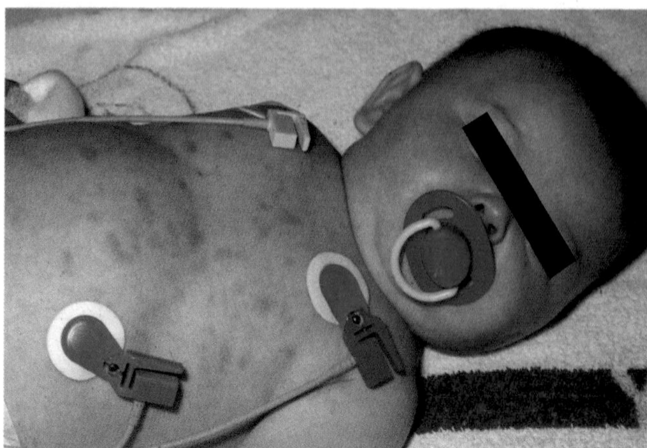

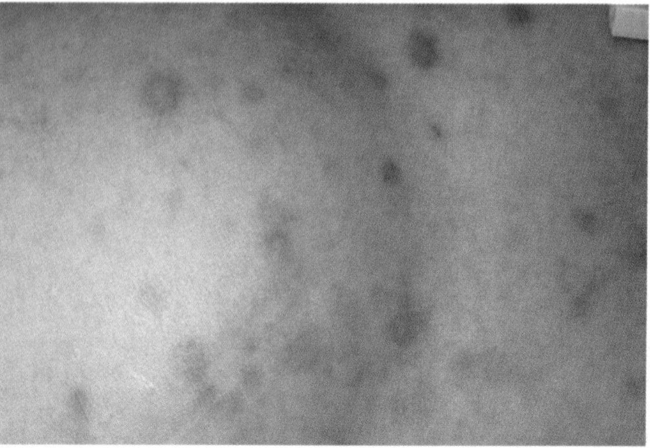

Plate 21.27 Skin infiltration in an infant with acute monocytic leukemia (see p. 1088).

21

Disorders of the blood and bone marrow

Paula Bolton-Maggs, Angela Thomas

Many different factors, including environment, diet and illness can affect the blood picture, so that 'abnormalities' of the blood count are relatively common in childhood. Children tend to have more reactive bone marrow than adults resulting in more impressive changes with relatively smaller stimuli. It is common to see a mild or moderate degree of anemia with infection; it is particularly common to see elevations of the platelet count. The more serious hematological disorders will form the focus of this chapter. It is important to assess hematological laboratory parameters in children against normal ranges for age as these may be significantly different from adults. A table of normal ranges is given in Chapter 40. Developmental hemopoiesis is covered in Chapter 10. Normal ranges for hematological values in the neonatal period, including coagulation factors are given in Chapter 10.

HEMATOLOGICAL ASSESSMENT IN CHILDHOOD

Children with hematological disorders present clinically with very non-specific symptoms. Anemia may be profound before a child has any significant symptoms – pallor is eventually noted in an otherwise well child. Children with severe anemia may also present with respiratory distress and be misdiagnosed.[1] Children with problems in the white cell series may present with infection; thrombocytopenia is often silent until the count is profoundly low (less than 10×10^9/L) when purpura and/or mucosal bleeding bring the child to attention. Demonstration of anemia, or a reduction of any one of the cell lines is not a diagnosis in itself. Once an abnormality has been identified the next step is to establish the diagnosis. The cause will determine the course of action to be taken.

The quality of the blood sample from a child is important. Traumatic or lengthy venepuncture or a difficult capillary collection often results in activation and partial coagulation of the sample. While this may be visible it is possible to miss small clots in a sample. The most common cause of a low platelet count is a poorly collected sample; this can also result in a falsely low white cell count or low hemoglobin. Fortunately modern instruments can handle very small samples of 0.5 ml or less for many tests making collection easier, even from neonates.

ANEMIA

APPROACH TO ANEMIA

Anemia is a sign, not a diagnosis in itself. The diagnosis may be clear from the history and examination together with the result of the blood count.

1. Is the child anemic? The blood count results must be assessed against the normal ranges for age. It should be noted that many hospitals only quote the adult normal ranges; this may lead to a mistaken diagnosis of anemia in a child, as the normal range is lower.
2. What are the characteristics of the red cells? The red cell indices and morphology described by the laboratory staff will suggest potential diagnoses and initial investigations (Fig. 21.1[2] and Table 21.1).
3. What is the pathophysiological mechanism of the anemia? This requires synthesis of the clinical and laboratory findings, and consideration of the mechanisms shown in Figure 21.2.

DEFICIENCY ANEMIAS

Iron deficiency anemia is very common in childhood. Iron deficiency without anemia is significant because iron is also required for the normal development of the central nervous system (CNS). Although deficiencies of other hematinics can occur, by contrast with iron deficiency they are extremely rare.

IRON DEFICIENCY

Etiology

In contrast to adults where the diagnosis of iron deficiency prompts a search for a source of blood loss, the commonest cause of iron deficiency in children is an inappropriate diet; blood loss is uncommon. Iron deficiency occurs from 6 months of age onwards when the child's total body mass is expanding in the face of an inadequate iron intake (Fig. 21.3).[3]

Studies show that 10–18% of Caucasian children, and 17–31% of children of ethnic minorities, have iron deficiency with hemoglobin levels of less than 11 g/dl. Many other infants will be iron deficient (serum ferritin < 12 µg/L) without anemia. Iron is required for the developing brain (see below) as well as for red cell production, so that it is important that iron deficiency, even without anemia, is corrected. Iron deficiency is a significant public health problem. Many infants and young children admitted to hospital for other reasons have blood tests which indicate iron deficiency as an incidental finding. It is important not to miss this opportunity to correct iron deficiency in these children by a combination of therapy and dietary re-education.

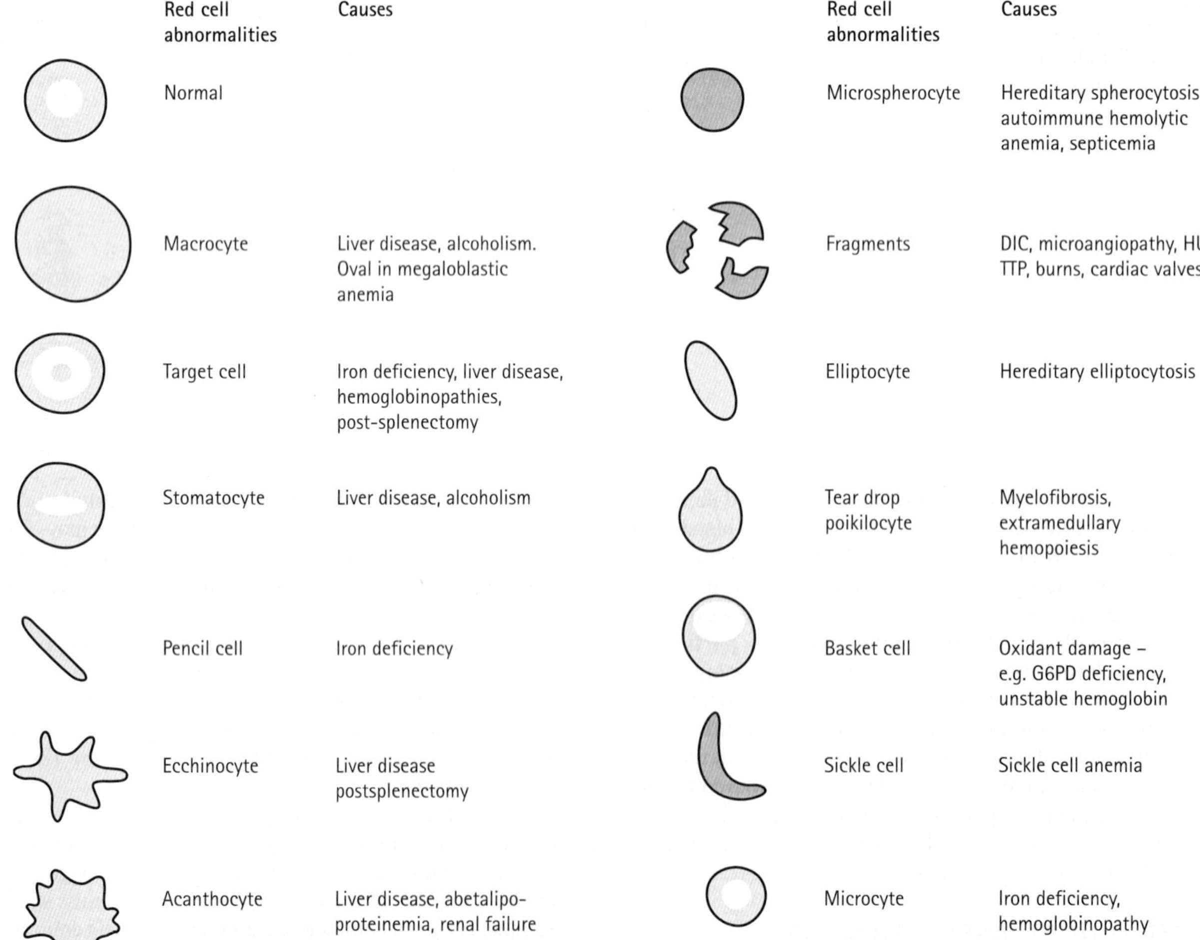

Red cell abnormalities
Causes
Normal
Macrocyte
Liver disease, alcoholism. Oval in megaloblastic anemia
Target cell
Iron deficiency, liver disease, hemoglobinopathies, post-splenectomy
Stomatocyte
Liver disease, alcoholism
Pencil cell
Iron deficiency
Ecchinocyte
Liver disease postsplenectomy
Acanthocyte
Liver disease, abetalipo-proteinemia, renal failure
Red cell abnormalities
Causes
Microspherocyte
Hereditary spherocytosis, autoimmune hemolytic anemia, septicemia
Fragments
DIC, microangiopathy, HUS, TTP, burns, cardiac valves
Elliptocyte
Hereditary elliptocytosis
Tear drop poikilocyte
Myelofibrosis, extramedullary hemopoiesis
Basket cell
Oxidant damage – e.g. G6PD deficiency, unstable hemoglobin
Sickle cell
Sickle cell anemia
Microcyte
Iron deficiency, hemoglobinopathy

Fig. 21.1 Morphological appearance of red blood cells in different anemias. DIC, disseminated intravascular coagulation; G6PD, glucose-6-phosphate dehydrogenase; HUS, hemolytic uremic syndrome; TTP, thrombotic thrombocytopenic purpura. (From Hoffbrand et al 2001[2] with permission)

Table 21.1 Morphological diagnosis of anemia

Red cell appearances	Hypochromic microcytic		Normochromic normocytic		Macrocytic	
Discriminatory test	Serum ferritin		Reticulocyte count		B_{12}/ Folate assay Bone marrow examination	
Result	Reduced	Normal or increased	Reduced	Normal or increased	Megaloblastic	Non-megaloblastic
Possible diagnoses	Iron deficiency	Thalassemia Hemoglobinopathy Sideroblastic anemia	Bone marrow hypoplasia Red cell aplasia	Hemolysis Blood loss Secondary anemia	Deficiency of B_{12}/folate Abnormality of B_{12}/folate metabolism	Liver disease Thyroid disease Congenital dyserythropoietic anemia

Diagnosis

Iron deficiency may present with pallor – it is not uncommon for the hemoglobin level to be extremely low (3–5 g/dl) with no symptoms. Pica (the persistent compulsive ingestion of food or non-food substances) is an insufficiently well known, important and often overlooked clue. The choice foods are soil, stones, chalk, sand, foam rubber and carpet. Usually, but not invariably, these cravings cease with correction of the iron deficiency, and the parents are often extremely grateful. Other signs (such as koilonychia or angular cheilitis) are very rare indeed. Iron deficiency causes serial changes in the blood that can be detected before anemia develops (Fig. 21.3).[3] Serum ferritin is reduced before there are any abnormalities in the red blood cells. Eventually a microcytic, hypochromic anemia results. Usually the mean cell volume (MCV) and mean cell hemoglobin (MCH) fall before the hemoglobin, but the changes can occur together. The mean cell hemoglobin concentration (MCHC) is less useful because it is often normal in the face of hypochromia. [The value is calculated from the packed cell volume (PCV) and hemoglobin and may be falsely elevated due to trapped plasma in the hematocrit where there are abnormal red cells.]

Iron deficiency is suspected when:

1. the hemoglobin is normal but the MCV and MCH are slightly reduced (the most important differential diagnosis is from thalassemia traits);
2. the hemoglobin is reduced with low MCV and MCH (Fig. 21.5) (the reductions in MCV and MCH are usually proportional to the reduced hemoglobin level, for example, with hemoglobin of 3–4 g/dl, the MCV and MCH will be markedly low, e.g. 50 and 18 respectively).

When the diagnosis is not clear it should be confirmed by measurement of serum ferritin (reduced) or zinc protoporphyrin (raised). A low ferritin is diagnostic of iron deficiency. (Note that serum ferritin is an acute phase reactant and will be elevated in acute inflammatory states and in the presence of liver disease. A normal ferritin therefore does not absolutely rule out iron deficiency.) Measurement of the serum iron and iron binding capacity (transferrin saturation) adds little to the diagnosis in straightforward cases. The serum iron level on its own is very unreliable having significant diurnal variation. It may be helpful to request these additional tests in children with chronic disease and in those with suspected iron overload.

Differential diagnosis: Other causes of a hypochromic microcytic blood picture, which should be considered (see later), are:

1. anemia of chronic disease (malutilization of iron);
2. thalassemia traits – these require quantitation of hemoglobins A2 and F, and not simply hemoglobin electrophoresis [thalassemias may not be excluded by normal results and further tests (genetic analysis) may be required – the advice of a hematologist should be sought];
3. sideroblastic anemias (see below).

Iron deficiency and neuropsychological effects

Animal experiments have clearly shown that early iron deficiency irreversibly affects brain iron content and distribution, leading to neurotransmitter and behavioral alterations. Anemia due to iron deficiency has been shown to be significantly associated with poorer scores in developmental testing when compared with controls, particularly in coordination and spatial orientation skills. Some trials have shown a definite benefit in treating the iron deficiency, but have suggested that not all the neurological deficit is reversed. Treating the hemoglobin level without replenishing iron stores is probably insufficient. Children should be treated until the ferritin is normal. Further trials are needed looking at long term school performance, academic achievements and career patterns in relation to iron deficiency in infancy but would be very difficult to do. Prevention of iron deficiency is much better than attempts to reverse damage done. This topic is reviewed by various authors,[4,5]

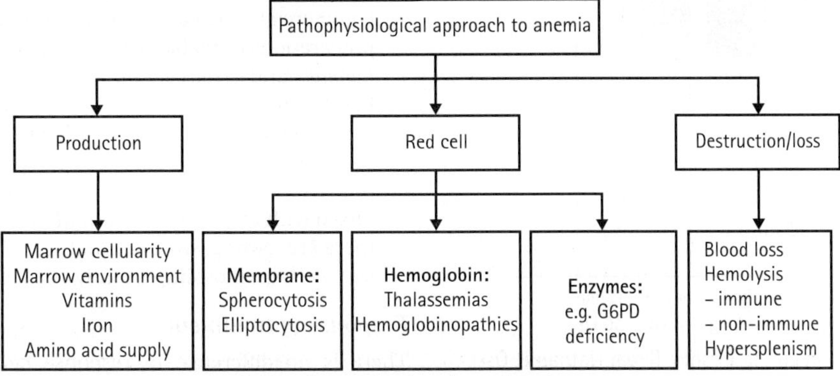

Fig. 21.2 Pathophysiological approach to anemia. G6PD, glucose-6-phosphate dehydrogenase.

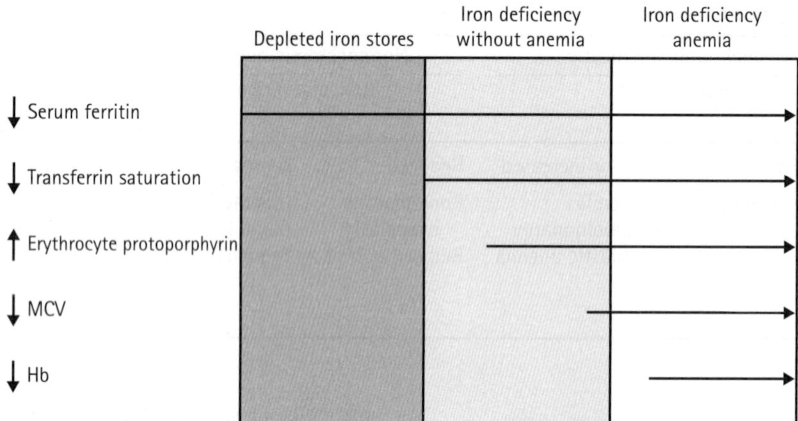

Fig. 21.3 Three stages of iron depletion based on results of laboratory tests. Hb, hemoglobin; MCV, mean cell volume. (From Nathan & Oski 1992[3] with permission)

and the impact of iron therapy on psychomotor development and cognitive function in children under the age of 3 years has been considered in a recent Cochrane review.[6]

Nutritional aspects and diet

Iron requirements are relatively high in infancy and early childhood because these are periods of rapid growth (Fig. 21.4). Stores laid down in pregnancy are depleted after 6 months of age so it is important to establish a good intake of dietary iron early in weaning. Preterm infants have lower iron stores at birth and may become iron deficient as early as 3 months of age.

Dietary iron occurs in two forms – heme and non-heme. Heme iron is well absorbed and its bioavailability is not affected by other dietary factors. It is present in meat, fish and poultry. Non-heme iron is less well absorbed and its bioavailability is affected by dietary factors because of the way it is bound in foods. It is present in beans, pulses, peanut butter, green leafy vegetables, dried fruit and fortified breakfast cereals. Absorption is enhanced by vitamin C and protein food. Absorption is inhibited by a number of different constituents of food and drink, for example tannins (found in tea and legumes), phytates (found in unrefined cereals), phosphates (in eggs), oxalates (in rhubarb, spinach) and polyphenols (in spinach, coffee). The main causes of iron deficiency are delayed weaning, use of cows' milk before 1 year as a main drink, excessive intake of milk and other drinks in older children, a diet low in iron-rich foods, poor intake of vitamin C and an increased intake of food which inhibits iron absorption, e.g. tannins in tea, high fiber food. Education about iron and its absorption should be started early. Primary care support and education should be aimed towards establishing good weaning practices and continued good eating patterns in later childhood.

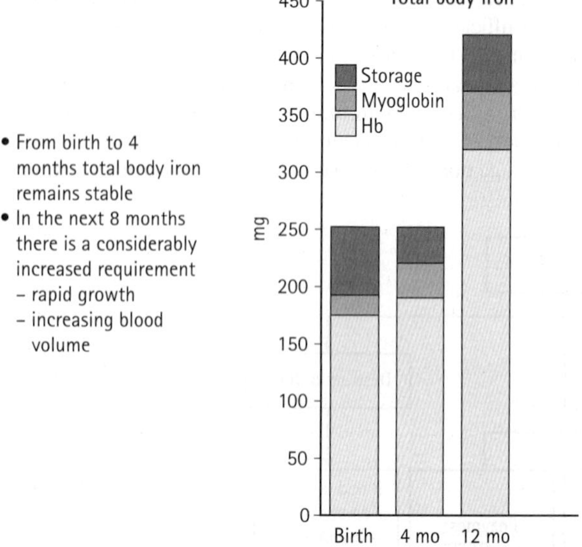

Fig. 21.4 Changes in body iron during infancy. (From Nathan & Oski 1992[3] with permission)

Therapy

Choice of preparation

The daily iron requirement for full-term infants is 1 mg/kg/day (maximum total daily dose 15 mg) starting no later than 4 months of age until 3 years of age. Between 4 and 10 years, the requirement is 10 mg/day and above 11 years and through adolescence, 18 mg/day. The treatment dose for iron deficiency is 3 mg iron/kg body weight/day up to a maximum of 180 mg daily.

When a child fails to respond to iron therapy, the commonest reason is failure of compliance. Although many preparations may be prescribed three times a day, better compliance may be achieved with a single daily dose or twice daily dosing. Iron is available as iron salts and iron chelates.

1. Iron salts (e.g. sulfate, fumarate, gluconate and glycine sulfate). Although ferrous sulfate is a good iron preparation for adults, the mixture (liquid) is no longer recommended. It is not commercially available, and tastes unpleasant. There are other preparations available either as tablets, or liquids such as *ferrous fumarate* and *ferrous glycine sulfate* 141 mg (equivalent to 25 mg Fe) in 5 ml.
2. Iron chelates (sodium iron edetate, and polysaccharide iron complex) have major advantages over standard salts in pediatric practice – they do not stain the teeth, sodium iron edetate can be mixed with milk or juice without altering absorption, in general there are fewer gastrointestinal side-effects, and they are sugar-free. Perhaps most importantly, the child usually likes them.

Response to treatment

There is no difference in response between the types of iron medication used, providing sufficient iron is given. Importantly,

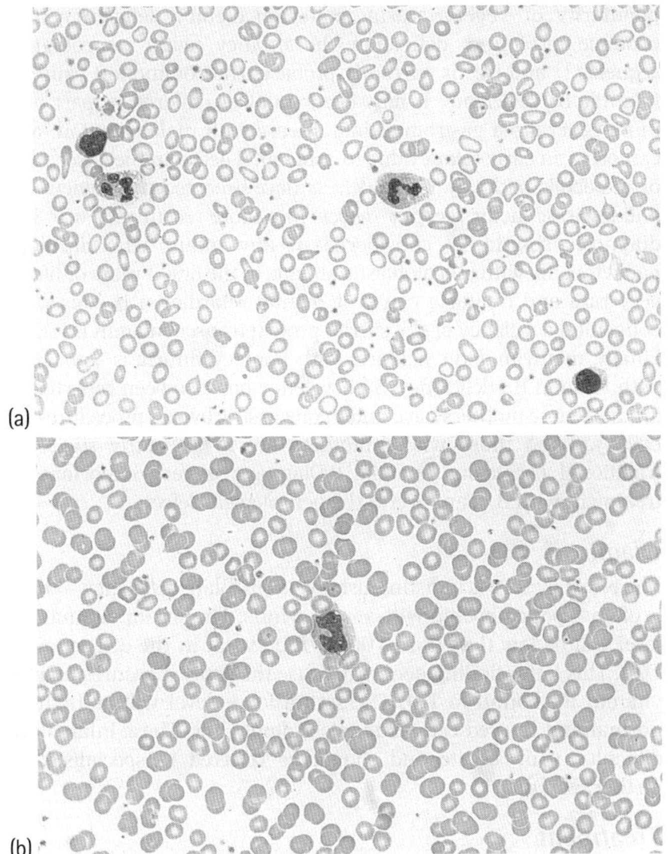

Fig. 21.5 Peripheral blood appearances in severe hypochromic iron deficiency with microcytic red cells (a) compared with a normal film (b) (same magnification).

however severe the anemia, there is no advantage in giving iron parenterally. The hemoglobin can increase by about 1 g/dl per week if compliance is good. If the hemoglobin is repeatedly less than 6 g/dl admission to hospital may be considered for a short period in order to monitor compliance and enhance dietary education of parents. In severe iron deficiency anemia (hemoglobin < 6.0 g/dl) the hemoglobin should be checked within 2 weeks to ensure that the child is responding (complying). If a child has very severe iron deficiency (e.g. hemoglobin of 3 g/dl) leading to a need for early monitoring (e.g. within 3–4 days), the first sign will be an increase in the red cell distribution width (RDW) on the automated count, and of the appearance of some polychromasia on the film. If responding, the interval can then be extended to 1 month, and then to 3 months. Children with severe iron deficiency will need a minimum of 3 months iron therapy, often considerably more. The ferritin can be used to monitor treatment once the anemia and abnormal indices (hypochromia and microcytosis) have been corrected. There is no point in checking the ferritin while these are still abnormal. In older children, the question of occult intestinal blood loss should be more formally investigated.

Conditions that may be associated with iron deficiency – lead poisoning

Although lead toxicity is thought to lead to anemia, severe lead toxicity manifested by the serious neurological effects, can occur without anemia. Coincidental iron deficiency is probably the cause of anemia; lead poisoning and iron deficiency are likely to occur in the same population. Lead poisoning and its management has been reviewed in detail.[7] Typically there is punctate basophilia on the blood film.

Anemias that can be confused with iron deficiency – the sideroblastic anemias and thalassemia traits (see later)

Sideroblastic anemias are rare, and in childhood usually congenital, and may exhibit X-linked inheritance. The red cells are usually hypochromic and microcytic. The ferritin is normal or raised, and the anemia is characterized by erythroid hyperplasia and the presence of abnormal iron staining (ringed sideroblasts) in the bone marrow. Some drugs can also induce sideroblastic change, but this is rare in children.

Sideroblastic anemia (sometimes transient) may be the presenting feature of Pearson's syndrome, a serious multisystem disease due to mitochondrial DNA deletions usually with pancreatic insufficiency, neurological involvement and a tendency to episodes of lactic acidosis and liver failure.

FOLATE DEFICIENCY

Etiology

All causes of megaloblastic anemia in children are very rare indeed but when this does occur it is most commonly due to folate deficiency. Unlike iron, folate stores are relatively labile and in constant need of replenishment. Folates are required for nucleic acid synthesis and 1-carbon unit transfer in all cells of the body, particularly growing tissues (Fig. 21.6).[8] Breast milk from a folate-replete mother contains about 25 μg/L of folate and provides enough for the normally developing child. However, if preterm babies are not supplemented with oral folate about a third will develop low serum folate levels by 6 weeks of age and 10% develop megaloblastic anemia by 8 weeks of age when the hepatic stores have been depleted. Heating of milk results in a 40% loss of folate and reheating of pasteurized milk causes an 80% loss. All babies are in a precarious state of folate balance during the first weeks of life. Rapid growth, fever, infection, diarrhea or hemolysis all increase folate requirements and may lead to clinical deficiency.

Folate is absorbed in the upper jejunum by an active transport mechanism that is impaired in malabsorption states, particularly celiac disease. In these disorders the deficiency does not usually produce a frank megaloblastic anemia. Other malabsorptive disorders such as tropical sprue, Crohn's disease, multiple diverticulae of the small intestine and blind loop syndrome will frequently produce folate deficiency.

Increased requirements for folate and subsequent deficiency occur in chronic hemolytic anemias, but because most children consume in excess of the necessary recommended daily intake, folate deficiency is very rare. Although regular folate therapy is recommended in chronic hemolytic states such as sickle cell disease and hereditary spherocytosis there is little evidence that this is always needed, and a double blind controlled trial of folate therapy in sickle cell disease led the authors to conclude that this policy needs critical review.[9] Various drugs are associated with deficiency of folate, e.g. phenytoin, barbiturates, methotrexate, pentamidine and trimethoprim. Congenital deficiency of several enzymes in the folate pathway has been reported; details can be found in a review.[10]

Clinical features and diagnosis

The presentation, like many hematological disorders, is very non-specific. Folate deficiency will produce macrocytosis (which can be masked by associated iron deficiency in conditions with

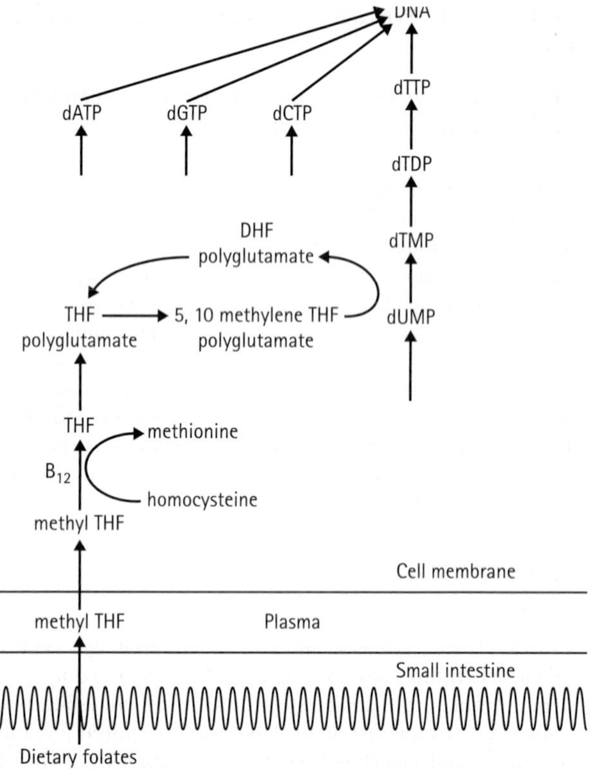

Fig. 21.6 Role of vitamin B_{12} and folate in DNA synthesis. Dietary folates are converted to methyltetrahydrofolate (methyl THF) by the small intestine. Inside marrow and other cells, methyl THF transfers a methyl group to homocysteine to form methionine. Vitamin B_{12} (B_{12}) is needed for this reaction. The THF formed is conjugated to the polyglutamate form possibly after formulation. 5,10-methylene THF polyglutamate is coenzyme for thymidylate synthetase, responsible for the methylation of the pyrimidine deoxyuridine monophosphate (dUMP). The folate coenzyme is oxidized to dihydrofolate (DHF) polyglutamate which is recycled to the fully reduced (THF) form by the enzyme dihydrofolate reductase (DHFR). dTMP is phosphorylated to thymidine triphosphate (dTTP). This is polymerized with the other three deoxyribonucleoside triphosphates, dA (deoxyadenosine) TP, dG (deoxyguanosine) TP, and dC (deoxycytidine) TP to form DNA. (From Hoffbrand 1983[8] with permission)

malabsorption); more severe forms will be associated with leucopenia and thrombocytopenia. Hypersegmented neutrophils seen on the blood film are an important clue. Serum and red cell folate levels should be requested to confirm the diagnosis.

Treatment

Treatment is straightforward with oral folic acid in a dose of 1 to 5 mg daily, and should be continued for several months. Where demand for the folate remains high (e.g. in chronic hemolytic anemias) life-long supplementation may sometimes be required. There is often a dramatic clinical response within a few days and a reticulocytosis can be demonstrated by the end of a week.

VITAMIN B_{12} DEFICIENCY

Vitamin B_{12} deficiency is very rare indeed in childhood. The infant usually has an insidious onset of pallor, lethargy and anorexia. In some cases neurological defects may predominate. With the popularity of vegetarianism, maternal dietary deficiency may produce profound deficiency in infancy with neurological sequelae,[11] and this is currently probably the commonest cause of infantile B_{12} deficiency. It may occur in older children as part of a more generalized gastrointestinal disease with malabsorption, and can occur in early infancy due to congenital defect in the absorption or metabolic pathway. These defects have been recently reviewed[12] and intrinsic factor receptor defects in a more recent review.[13] The diagnosis should be considered in any infant who develops pancytopenia with megaloblastic anemia in the first 3 years of life. A very rare and treatable cause of mental retardation is caused by congenital deficiency of the carrier protein transcobalamin II (TCII). Finally, methylmalonic aciduria with homocystinuria is associated with vitamin B_{12} deficiency. B_{12} deficiency has also been reported in infants whose mothers have undergone gastric bypass procedures for obesity,[14] and those whose mothers are in the early stages of traditional pernicious anemia.[15] Diagnosis is very important as treatment with B_{12} can reverse the neurological defects.[16]

Diagnosis

The blood picture is indistinguishable from folate deficiency – there is often a pancytopenia with macrocytosis. The serum vitamin B_{12} level will be low (less than 100 μg/ml) except in the deficiency of TCII. This latter finding occurs because the assay measures mainly vitamin B_{12} bound to TCI. The serum folate level will be high or normal and the red cell folate misleadingly low. These infants are difficult to investigate and should be referred to specialists for further workup.

Treatment

The usual dose of vitamin B_{12} (as hydroxycobalamin) for children is 100 μg given intramuscularly, three times a week until the hemoglobin is normal, followed by 100 μg monthly thereafter. Some disorders may be successfully treated with oral B_{12} therapy.[17] The neurological defects may take longer to recover. In TCII deficiency very large doses are required.

OTHER CAUSES OF MEGALOBLASTIC ANEMIA

There are other metabolic disorders which are associated with megaloblastic anemia such as orotic aciduria, Lesch–Nyhan syndrome, and thiamine responsive congenital dyserythropoietic anemia type I.

APLASTIC ANEMIAS

Bone marrow failure usually presents with pancytopenia that may be moderate or severe, or initially there may only be a single lineage affected with evolution to full aplasia over months or years. Aplastic anemia may be idiopathic (70–80%) or secondary to a constitutional abnormality. Table 21.2[18] lists those agents that may be associated with aplastic anemia. In many cases it is not possible to be certain about their etiological role. Withdrawal of these agents may lead to improvement in the pancytopenia. Marrow aplasia is diagnosed by bone marrow examination, including trephine biopsy (Fig. 21.7). Whatever the underlying cause, severe disease (70%), defined as pancytopenia with neutrophils $< 0.5 \times 10^9/L$, platelets $< 10 \times 10^9/L$ and reticulocytes < 1%, with documented bone marrow hypocellularity, is associated with a high mortality from infection or bleeding. Good supportive care is essential, and early bone marrow transplantation (BMT) from a human leukocyte antigen (HLA)-matched sibling donor is the optimal definitive treatment. These children should be referred to a specialist service early. If a sibling

Table 21.2 Agents associated with aplastic anemia

Drugs	
Acetazolamide	Phenylbutazone
Amodiaquine	Pyrimethamine
Arsenicals	Quinacrine
Barbiturates	Quinidine, quinine
Chloramphenicol	Streptomycin
Chlordiazepoxide	Sulfonamides
Cimetidine	Thiazides
Colchicine	Thiocyanate
Hydantoins	Thiouracils
Meprobamate	
Phenothiazines	
Insecticides	*Solvents*
Chlordane	Benzene
DDT	Carbon tetrachloride
Gamma benzene hexachloride	Stoddarts solvent
Parathione	Glues
	Toluene
Radiation	
Trinitrotoluene	

(After Alter et al 1978[18])

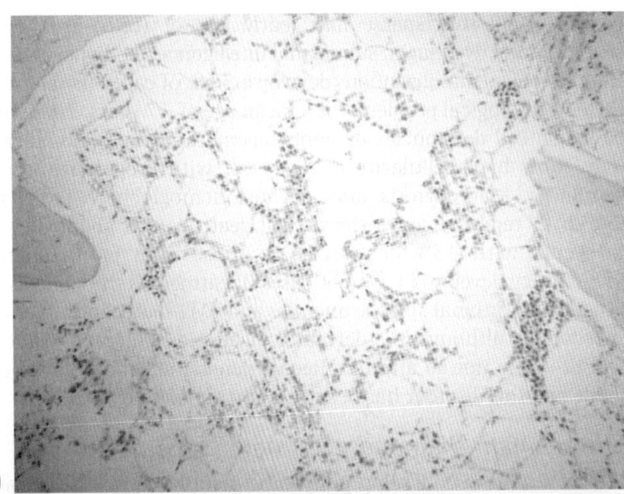
(a)

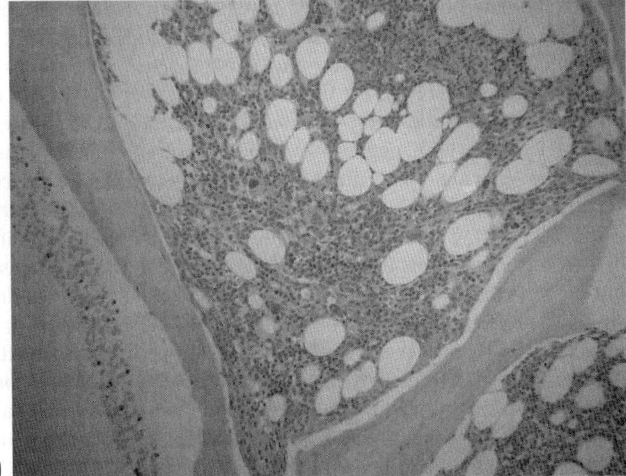
(b)

Fig. 21.7 The appearances of aplastic bone marrow (a) with a normal marrow (b) for comparison (trephine biopsy).

donor is not available the most appropriate treatment is intensive immunosuppression using antilymphocyte globulin combined with ciclosporin. Immunosuppression produces a response in over two-thirds of patients but over a long period of follow-up many patients develop myelodysplasia or leukemia suggesting ongoing clonal stem cell disorder.[19] An international group have published guidelines on the management of aplastic anemia.[20]

CONSTITUTIONAL APLASTIC ANEMIAS

These inherited bone marrow failure syndromes are important and are responsible for about 25% of children with aplastic anemia. Patients with these disorders have a genetic propensity for bone marrow failure presenting at birth or developing later.[21]

Fanconi's anemia (FA)

This rare and heterogeneous disorder can present from birth to 35 years of age although 75% present between 3 and 14 years of age. More than 1000 cases are now described.[21] The most common presentation is with pancytopenia, single lineage defects (particularly thrombocytopenia) or malignancy (particularly leukemia). Half have typical physical findings especially hyperpigmentation, café-au-lait spots, microsomy, microcephaly, thumb, ear, genital and renal anomalies, other skeletal abnormalities, microphthalmia and mental retardation. FA is inherited as an autosomal recessive with a heterozygote frequency of about 1 in 200.[22]

Children may present with single lineage failure, particularly thrombocytopenia. Other clues are macrocytosis and fetal characteristics of red cells [raised fetal hemoglobin (HbF) and an increased expression of i antigen]. Chromosome fragility is the hallmark of this disorder, readily seen in metaphase spreads from blood lymphocytes stimulated with suitable agents. These abnormalities occur either because DNA repair is defective or the cells are unable to remove cell-damaging oxygen free radicals.

Treatment of FA is difficult – the median survival reported in 1989 was 25 years.[22] Allogeneic BMT may be curative but is associated with significant problems of graft-versus-host disease – transplant experience in 69 patients in Europe has been reported with a 33% 3-year survival, illustrating the adverse effects of the additional abnormalities on outcome in this group of patients.[23] Patients with FA do not tolerate irradiation therapy well and thus highly modified conditioning is required. As with all cases of pancytopenia, good supportive care with red cell and platelet transfusion and antibiotics is essential until more specific therapy can be instituted. Androgen therapy has been used for many years with some success in FA.

More than 20% of FA patients develop a malignancy, the risk increasing with age. Half will be leukemias, usually myeloid. Androgens may well exacerbate a genetic risk for liver tumors. Whether or not the risk of malignancy persists after 'curative' bone marrow transplantation remains to be seen. Recent significant advances in genetics, pathology and management are reviewed by Dokal.[24,25] At least eight separate genes can be implicated in FA. Some individuals with FA have given birth to children, genetic in utero testing is possible for some cases, and gene therapy may become a reality in the future.[22]

Dyskeratosis congenita

Ectodermal dysplasia and X-linked recessive inheritance characterize this disorder. Skin manifestations begin during the first decade and progress. Features include reticulated hyperpigmentation of the face, neck and shoulders; dystrophic nails; mucous membrane leukoplakia; epiphora; hyperhidrotic palms and soles;

poikiloderma; thin sparse hair; early loss of teeth; esophageal strictures and dysphagia; subnormal intelligence and hypogenitalia. Hematological manifestations develop in 56% of cases, usually after the dermatological problems, at a mean age of 17 years. There may be single cell deficiencies or pancytopenia and the bone marrow may show hypercellularity at the onset with progressive loss of cellularity. Macrocytosis and elevated hemoglobin F levels are found. In reported series the overall death rate is about 33% at 20 years with 45% death rate in those with pancytopenia. Malignancy develops in 13% of cases. Treatment is the same as for other constitutional aplastic anemias and BMT has been carried out successfully although the dermatological and malignant sequelae will probably not be affected. Recent genetic advances have been made and this disorder has been recently reviewed by Dokal.[26]

Shwachman–Diamond syndrome (SDS)

Children with SDS develop pancreatic insufficiency with variable blood abnormalities (commonly neutropenia) usually detected in infancy, often with skeletal abnormalities. Anemia or thrombocytopenia can occur, and pancytopenia supervenes in many.[27] The genetic basis for this disorder is not yet known but the marrow abnormalities may be caused by increased apoptosis.[28] Supportive care with aggressive management of infections, and pancreatic enzyme replacement are the key therapies. The marrow stroma is abnormal in addition to stem cells and there is a high risk of transformation to myeloid leukemia,[29] often with abnormalities of chromosome 7.[30] The median survival is greater than 20 years but patients die of infection, bleeding and leukemia. Such children should be referred for early consideration of BMT but this may be associated with higher mortality than in other indications. It is important to distinguish this disorder from Pearson's syndrome where affected children have pancreatic insufficiency and vacuolation of marrow precursors in association with congenital sideroblastic anemia (which may show spontaneous recovery). This disorder is caused by mitochondrial DNA deletions, is associated with other features of mitochondrial disruption (neurological deterioration, retinitis pigmentosa and a tendency to liver failure and lactic acidosis) and is usually lethal early in life.

Congenital amegakaryocytic thrombocytopenia (CAT)

Thrombocytopenia in infancy can be caused by this disorder and usually presents with purpura and bleeding within a few months. About half the children have additional congenital abnormalities, particularly cardiac or neurological. Treatment is difficult, and these children need urgent referral for consideration of BMT. The mechanism for disease in some of these patients is caused by mutations in the thrombopoetin receptor.[31] Other children have upper limb abnormalities showing some overlap with other congenital disorders (thrombocytopenia with absent radii, and FA).[32]

PURE RED CELL APLASIA (PRCA)

PRCA in childhood is caused by transient erythroblastopenia or constitutional red cell aplasia.

Transient erythroblastopenia of childhood (TEC) is an important cause of transient red cell aplasia, causing unexplained, sometimes severe, anemia in young children and toddlers.[33] The cause is unknown and may be related to infection, but parvovirus B19, implicated in aplastic crises in hemolytic states, is not the cause. Diamond–Blackfan syndrome – constitutional and congenital red cell aplasia – presents usually at an earlier age, in the first year of life; 95% of cases occur by 2 years of age with occasional cases occurring up to 6 years. Diagnosis of either of these is made by the presence of anemia with reticulocytopenia and very few marrow erythroid precursors. TEC recovers within days or weeks, Diamond–Blackfan anemia (DBA) does not. Children with TEC may need transfusion to tide them over, but usually do not.

DBA is a heterogeneous disorder which occurs with an incidence of 4–7 per million live births. There is a familial incidence of 10–20%. About 50% children have other physical abnormalities, particularly craniofacial or thumb. Some children with DBA respond to steroids (70%) but many remain steroid dependent (45%) and others require life-long regular transfusion therapy (39%) with iron chelation with subcutaneous desferrioxamine. This disorder has recently been reviewed.[34–36]

HEMOLYTIC ANEMIAS

GENERAL FEATURES

Hemolysis is defined by an increased rate of red cell destruction with a shortening of the normal life span of the cell from the normal 120 days to as little as a few days in severe hemolysis. The marrow can increase erythrocyte production six- to eightfold so mild degrees of hemolysis are not associated with anemia. Mild hemolysis may be almost undetectable with no clinical clues; severe hemolysis can lead to a rapid and profound fall in hemoglobin, and be life threatening. The hemoglobin level is a balance between the increased red cell destruction and the ability of the bone marrow to compensate. Hemolysis is suspected when there are polychromatic cells on the blood film (reticulocytes); further diagnostic and confirmatory tests are then indicated. A simplified diagnostic classification of causes is shown in Figure 21.8.[37] Hemolysis is usually associated with raised blood unconjugated bilirubin. Generally hemolytic states are divided into those with spherocytes and those without where the morphology may be normal, or characteristic of the underlying disorder. Hemolysis can be caused by inherited or acquired disorders. Diagnosis of the cause of the hemolysis is made by consideration of the family history, together with clinical features and red cell morphology that will indicate what further laboratory tests are required. Marrow examination is generally unnecessary.

The child with hemolysis may be pale with fluctuating jaundice (usually mild) and splenomegaly. Pigment gallstones may complicate the disorder – hemolytic anemia should always be excluded in a child with gallstones. Aplastic crises may occur, usually precipitated by parvovirus infection or rarely by folate deficiency, both of which are characterized by 'switching off' of erythropoiesis. This leads to reticulocytopenia and anemia. Parvovirus infection typically produces severe anemia sometimes requiring transfusion, and a modest thrombocytopenia and leucopenia. Folate deficiency is uncommon.

HEREDITARY HEMOLYTIC ANEMIAS

Membrane defects

Hereditary spherocytosis (HS)

HS is the commonest hereditary hemolytic anemia in north Europeans, caused by a variety of different genetic defects in the red cell skeletal proteins, ankyrin, spectrin, band 3 or protein 4.2 (Fig. 21.9).[2] It is dominantly inherited in 75% of families. There may be variable expression – investigation of other family members may identify asymptomatic individuals with a milder phenotype. The blood film shows the typical features – multiple small dense cells termed microspherocytes. The marrow produces normally shaped biconcave cells and progressive loss of membrane results in the spherical shape (Fig. 21.10). In an individual with spherocytes and

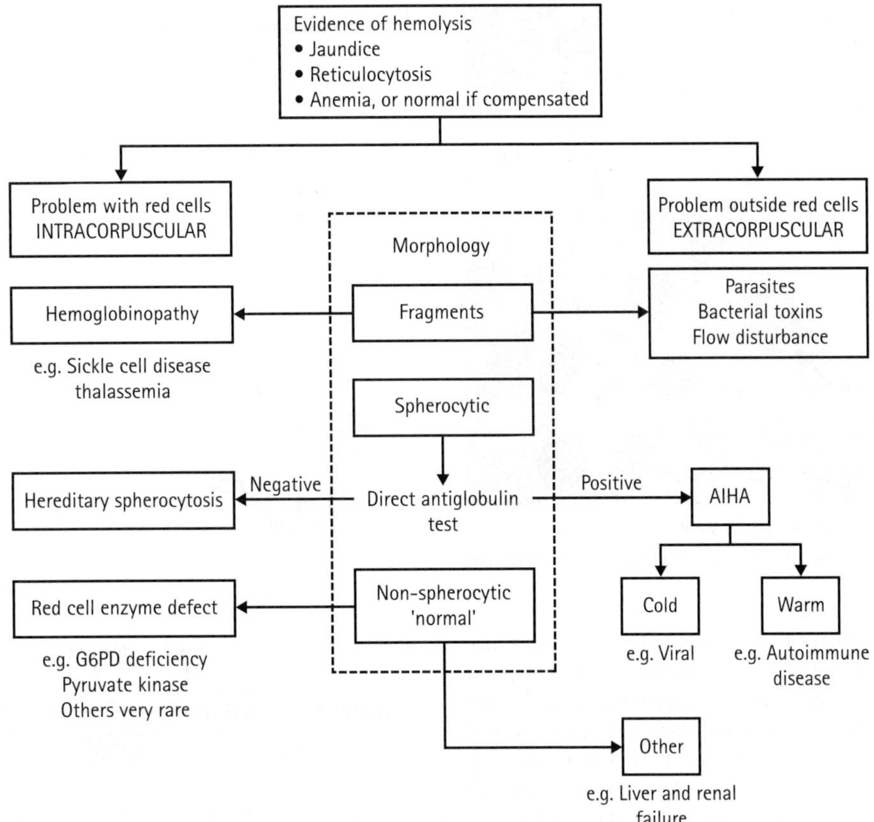

Fig. 21.8 A diagnostic approach to hemolytic anemia. AIHA, autoimmune hemolytic anemia; G6PD, glucose-6-dehydrogenase. (From Lissauer & Clayden 2001[37] with permission)

no other affected family members autoimmune hemolysis must be excluded by a negative direct antiglobulin test. The child may or may not have jaundice and anemia, but splenomegaly is usual. (This is not associated with an increased risk of rupture, and these children should lead a normal active life.) Laboratory diagnosis is usually straightforward and the osmotic fragility test is not necessary for confirmation. For difficult cases there are additional investigations (membrane protein analysis).

Individuals with HS are usefully classified as mild, moderate or severe by their baseline hemoglobin, reticulocyte count and bilirubin level. This classification, which should be made when the individual is well, helps to indicate those in whom splenectomy is beneficial – generally those with severe and moderate disease.[38] Individuals with severe disease should probably receive folate supplements although the evidence for this is scarce.[39]

Splenectomy cures all the clinical manifestations of HS by removing the site of destruction of the abnormal red cells, but is associated with a life-long risk of overwhelming sepsis particularly with encapsulated organisms (*Pneumococcus*) and so should be avoided in all but the most severe cases during the first 10 years of

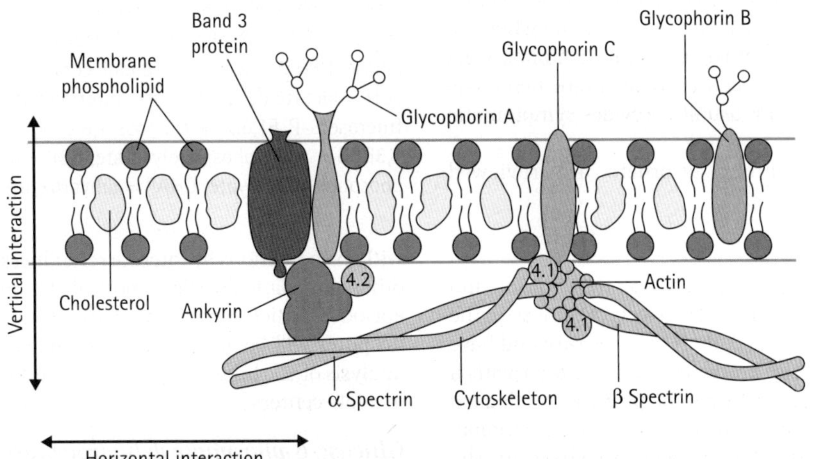

Fig. 21.9 Schematic structure of the red cell membrane. Some of the penetrating and integral proteins carry carbohydrate antigens; other antigens are attached directly to the lipid layer. (From Hoffbrand et al 2001[2] with permission)

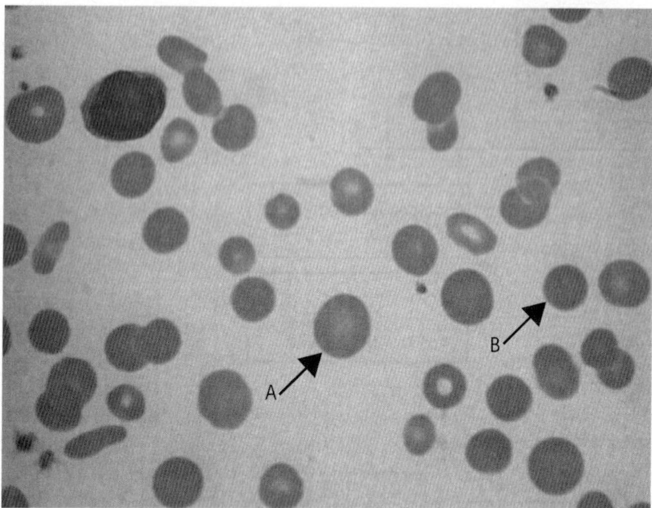

Fig. 21.10 Peripheral blood appearance in spherocytosis with spherocytes and polychromasia. A, polychromatic cell; B, microspherocyte.

life when the risk of postsplenectomy sepsis is highest. There are guidelines for the management of splenectomized individuals, and in families with HS there may be others who have had splenectomy in the past who need information about their increased risks of infection.[40] Patients should be immunized with pneumococcal, hemophilus and meningococcal vaccines before splenectomy and warned of their increased risk of infection with malaria. Antibiotic prophylaxis should be given on a long term basis but compliance may be poor. Patients should be issued with a medical card indicating they have had a splenectomy and warned about the importance of early reporting of symptoms of infection. Children with HS may develop gallstones in the first decade of life. This is an indication for both cholecystectomy and splenectomy at the same time. Following splenectomy the individual usually has a normal hemoglobin and near-normal red cell life span. Annual follow-up may serve to remind the individual about the postsplenectomy risks. Immunity to pneumococcus and hemophilus may wane with time, and survey of antibody levels to these agents may provide a more evidence-based foundation for repeat immunizations. There is currently no consensus in this area.[39]

Hereditary elliptocytosis (HE)

This common disorder is usually inherited as an autosomal dominant trait, usually diagnosed as an incidental finding when the blood count is performed for some other reason. Rare homozygous variants have been described in which chronic severe hemolysis occurs; in these cases splenectomy usually provides symptomatic improvement.

Other less common membrane disorders are reviewed elsewhere.[41]

Red cell enzyme defects

Figure 21.11 shows the pathways of glucose metabolism and energy production in the red cell. Although defects of almost all the separate enzymes have been described, most are very rare and have recently been reviewed.[42,43] They are generally associated with a non-spherocytic blood picture, with no helpful morphological features of the red cells (apart from one or two exceptions). Deficiencies of almost all of the enzymes involved in the Embden–Meyerhof pathway and hexose monophosphate shunt can be associated with significant hemolysis. Some of these are chronic

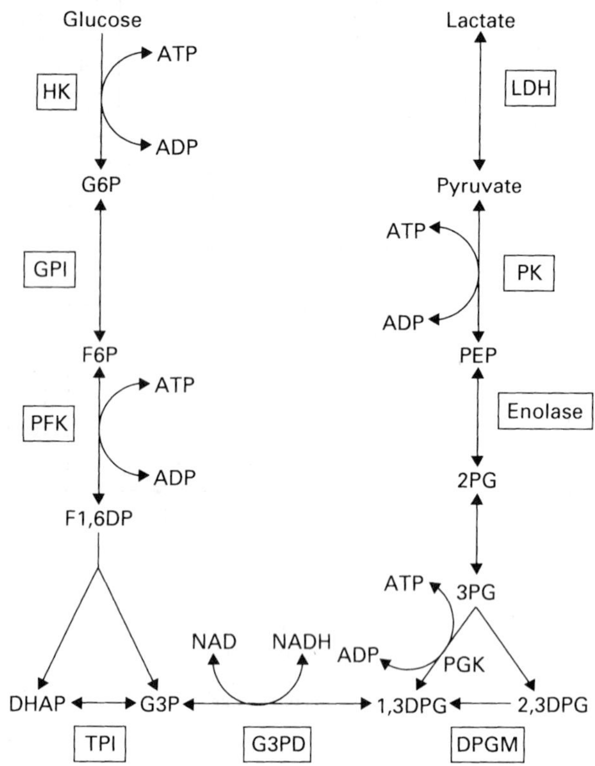

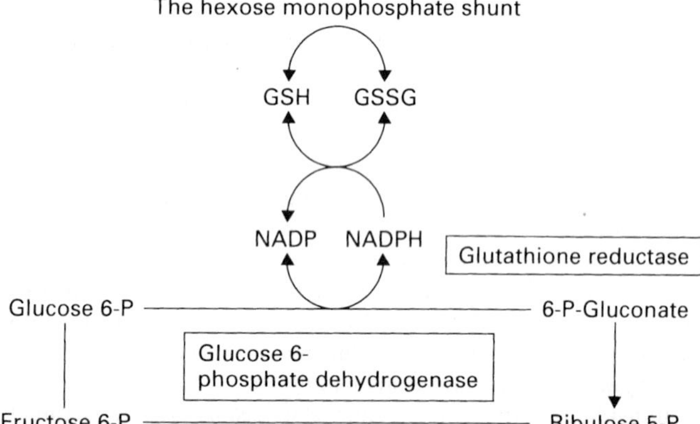

Fig. 21.11 The Embden–Meyerhof pathway and hexose monophosphate shunt. Enzymes: HK = hexokinase, GPI = glucose phosphate isomerase, PFK = phosphofructokinase, TPI = triose phosphate isomerase, G3PD = glucose 3-phosphate dehydrogenase, PGK = phosphoglycerate kinase, DPGM = 2,3-diphosphoglycerate mutase, PK = pyruvate kinase, LDH = lactate dehydrogenase. Intermediates: G6P = glucose 6-P, F6P = fructose 6-P, F1,6DP = fructose 1,6 di-P, 3PG = 3-P glycerate, 1,3DPG = 1,3-diphosphoglycerate, G3P = glyceraldehyde 3-P, PEP = phosphoenolpyruvate, DHAP = dihydroxyacetone P.

with exacerbations by intercurrent illnesses such as viral infections, others are clinically silent most of the time with sudden hemolytic episodes which bring the patient to medical attention. Most hospitals will be able to diagnose the two commonest deficiencies; analysis of the others requires specialist investigation only available in a few centers.

Glucose-6-phosphate dehydrogenase (G6PD) deficiency

This is the commonest cause of hemolysis worldwide, and is caused by a number of different mutations in the gene, which is on the

Table 21.3 Drugs and chemicals associated with hemolysis in G6PD deficient subjects

Group	Drugs
Antimalarials	Primaquine, pamaquine, quinacrine, quinine
Sulfonamides	Sulfapyridine, sulfisoxazole, salicylazosulfapyridine
Nitrofurans	Nitrofuranatoin, furaltadone
Analgesics and related compounds	Acetylsalicylic acid, para-aminosalicylic acid
Miscellaneous	Synthetic water-soluble vitamin K analogs, chloramphenicol, phenylhydrazine, naphthalene, aniline dyes, nalidixic acid

X chromosome. These produce different phenotypes; most are associated with episodic hemolysis, the blood picture being normal at other times. A few variants are associated with chronic hemolysis. G6PD maintains glutathione in its reduced state and so is one of the vital mechanisms for protecting red cell membranes from oxidant stress. Oxidative stress induced by drugs, chemicals (Table 21.3) or an intercurrent infection can produce hemolysis. The different mutants of G6PD occur in different racial groups with differences in clinical severity. The racial incidence varies greatly from extreme rarity in northern Europeans through 1–35% in different Mediterranean races, up to 10% in African Negroes. Neonatal jaundice is more common in oriental male babies especially in the presence of infections or acidosis or if oxidant drugs are given to the mother in late pregnancy or to the neonate. Infections and diabetic ketoacidosis can precipitate hemolysis at all ages. Favism (eating broad beans) produces severe hemolysis, and is commonest in Mediterraneans and in the Middle East although it does occur in Orientals and Europeans. Rare cases of chronic hemolysis in northern European races have also been described.

Hemolytic crises vary in severity and degree. Favism is associated with the most explosive course and intravascular hemolysis. A typical sign is the dramatic darkening of the urine with hemoglobin and urobilinogen to produce so-called 'Coca-Cola' urine. This may lead to renal dysfunction (sometimes severe). Diagnosis depends on an enzyme assay but reticulocytes nearly always have higher levels of all red cell enzymes so the test is best done when the child (usually male) has recovered from the acute episode.

Neonatal jaundice may require exchange transfusion. At other times all that is necessary is to be aware of the problem in appropriate ethnic groups and to avoid the precipitating factors. Patients should be informed of the hazards and supplied with written information about which foods and drugs to avoid (Table 21.3).

Pyruvate kinase (PK) deficiency

PK deficiency is the commonest cause of non-spherocytic hemolysis in northern Europe. It is autosomal recessively inherited and produces chronic hemolysis with varying grades of severity in different individuals. Neonatal jaundice occurs and infection can also precipitate more severe hemolysis. Parvovirus infection can, as in other hemolytic states, produce a dramatic aplastic crisis. Splenomegaly is usually present. Drugs do not precipitate crises.

The blood film in PK deficiency does not have any specific diagnostic features although irregularly contracted cells are seen especially after splenectomy. Diagnosis depends on measurement of the enzyme level, which must be carefully corrected for the high reticulocyte count. Unfortunately some poorly functioning variants of PK can produce normal assay results; this can be sorted out by specialist measurement of the intermediate products of the Embden–Meyerhof pathway in order to demonstrate a block at the appropriate point.

Because of its position in the energy pathway, PK deficiency causes a rise in 2,3 diphosphoglycerate (2,3-DPG) levels and thus a shift to the right in the oxygen dissociation curve and a consequent improvement in oxygen availability. For this reason, patients with PK deficiency can tolerate very low hemoglobin levels (and conversely hexokinase-deficient patients may require blood transfusion at relatively high hemoglobin levels). Thus, it is very important not to transfuse PK-deficient patients unless they are clinically unwell, failing to thrive or are otherwise genuinely symptomatic. Many patients are transfused unnecessarily on the basis of a perfectly acceptable hemoglobin level of about 5–6 g/dl. Severely affected patients may require intermittent transfusions when decompensated by infections, and occasional patients require regular transfusions with iron chelation. In these children, splenectomy usually produces a beneficial reduction or abolition of the need for blood transfusion and should be considered in severe cases.

ACQUIRED HEMOLYTIC ANEMIAS

Acquired hemolysis in childhood is relatively uncommon but can be severe; it is important to make the correct diagnosis.

Autoimmune hemolytic anemias (AIHA)

The development of hemolysis caused by autoantibodies to red cell antigens is uncommon and can occur as a complication of some viral infections, as part of a larger dysregulation of immune function, either in autoimmune diseases such as systemic lupus erythematosus, or in some forms of immune deficiency. Autoimmune hemolysis is suspected when the child has anemia with a reticulocytosis sometimes with jaundice, and splenomegaly. The blood film usually shows spherocytes, and the condition is differentiated from HS by a positive direct antiglobulin test due to antibodies (IgG) or complement (in IgM associated AIHA) attached to the red cells. After viral infections the antibody is usually IgM, and reactive in tests at room temperature ('cold') rather than at 37°C which is typical of IgG ('warm') antibodies. Infectious mononucleosis, cytomegalovirus (CMV) and mycoplasma are infections most commonly implicated in 'cold' autoimmune hemolysis (caused by antibodies to the i/I red cell antigens). These antibodies cause intravascular red cell destruction and may present with brown urine (hemoglobinuria) which is not usually seen in IgG-induced hemolysis where the red cells are destroyed predominantly in the spleen. Another type causing sudden onset of hemoglobinuria is paroxysmal cold hemoglobinuria caused by an unusual type of red cell antibody, a complement-fixing IgG which attaches to the red cells in the cold and lyses the cells in the warm – the Donath–Landsteiner antibody. Treatment is rarely required, the hemolysis being short lived and resolving with the infection. It is prudent to keep the child warm; occasionally transfusion and steroids may be required. Hemolysis occurring as part of a wider autoimmune process can be chronic and difficult to manage; steroid therapy may be beneficial, transfusion is often difficult and best avoided because the antibodies react with all donor blood. Warm AIHA (rare in childhood) can also be caused by drugs.

Immune hemolysis caused by maternal antibodies is discussed in detail elsewhere (Ch. 10). AIHA may occur with immune thrombocytopenic purpura when it is known as Evans syndrome.

Microangiopathic hemolytic anemia (MAHA)

Red cell fragmentation on the blood film (schistocytes – Fig. 21.12) is the pathognomonic feature, associated with reticulocytosis. This may be associated with thrombocytopenia, depending upon the underlying cause (Table 21.4). The red cells are damaged by fibrin strands deposited in small blood vessels and consumption of platelets within the resultant microthrombi, or by trauma passing through a damaged heart valve or other cardiac abnormality. A variety of causes are recognized, particularly hemolytic uremic syndrome (HUS) described more fully elsewhere (Ch. 16). MAHA may be the first signal of a problem with a replaced heart valve or other cardiac lesion. Disseminated intravascular coagulation from any cause may be associated with MAHA.

Table 21.4 Causes of red cell fragmentation syndromes

Microangiopathic
Hemolytic uremic syndrome
Thrombotic thrombocytopenic purpura
Meningococcal sepsis
Disseminated intravascular coagulation
Cardiac valves or arterial grafts
March hemoglobinuria
Infections – malaria, clostridia
Chemical and physical – burns
Liver and renal disease

Other causes of hemolysis

Hypersplenism

Splenic enlargement, from any cause, such as portal hypertension, leishmaniasis and storage disorders, may produce a shortening of red cell survival due to excessive sequestration in the expanded reticuloendothelial system. The anemia is mild and usually associated with mild leucopenia and thrombocytopenia.

Infections

Malaria is an infection in which microorganisms are present within red cells at the time of hemolysis. Mild hemolysis may occur with many other infectious processes. Septicemia, particularly due to clostridial organisms, may produce an acute hemolytic process usually as part of a consumptive coagulopathy. *Bartonella* infection is another documented cause of hemolysis (Ch. 26).

DISORDERS OF HEMOGLOBIN SYNTHESIS

HEMOGLOBINOPATHIES AND THALASSEMIA

Etiology

Hemoglobin is the essential pigment that makes blood red, and carries oxygen to the tissues. There are several different normal hemoglobins suited to different ages; the basic structure is two pairs of globin chains, each containing a heme group which can bind oxygen (Fig. 21.13).[44] Some hemoglobins are only evident during early stages of gestation; later in fetal life the predominant hemoglobin is hemoglobin F (alpha2 gamma2). After birth, when the oxygen affinity does not need to be so high, hemoglobin A (alpha2 beta2) gradually replaces hemoglobin F, the switch starting at about 32 weeks' gestation. Normal blood also contains a small amount of hemoglobin A2 (alpha2 delta2) (Table 21.5). Various hemoglobin abnormalities result in clinically significant effects. There may be a qualitative or quantitative defect. The most common are discussed here, but there are many others that are described in more specialist texts.

The sickling disorders

The most important structural hemoglobin disorder is due to a single amino acid change affecting the ability of hemoglobin to remain in solution. Sickle hemoglobin is produced by a point mutation at beta6 (adenine to thymine) resulting in an amino acid change of glutamic acid to valine. Sickle hemoglobin forms crystals at low oxygen tension; these polymerise into long strands. The sickle gene has occurred from at least four separate mutation events, and is most common across the tropical zones, as shown in Figure 21.14.[45] The high frequency of the gene in these areas relates to protection against infection by malaria parasites conferred by heterozygosity for the sickle cell gene.

The clinical outcome depends upon whether the sickle gene is inherited from one or both parents, (sickle cell trait, AS or sickle cell disease, SS) and whether it is inherited with another hemoglobin disorder that modifies the effects (hemoglobin C, beta thalassemia, alpha thalassemia). It is therefore very important to make the precise diagnosis. Screening tests alone only detect the presence of sickle hemoglobin without any indication of the quantity, and give no information about other possible abnormalities. Full diagnosis requires analysis of the full blood count, blood film, analysis of red

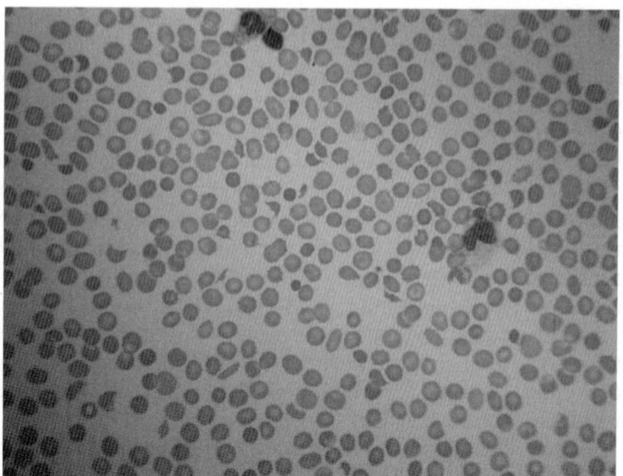

Fig. 21.12 Red cell appearances in red cell fragmentation syndromes.

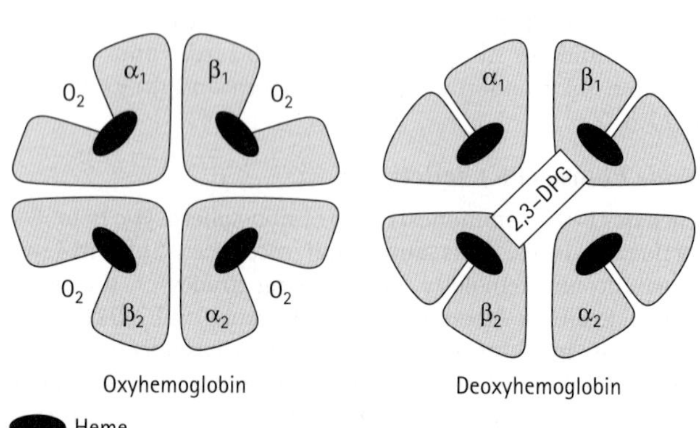

Fig. 21.13 The oxygenated and deoxygenated hemoglobin molecule. Alpha, beta globin chains of normal adult hemoglobin (hemoglobin A); 2,3-DPG, 2,3 diphosphoglycerate. (From Hoffbrand & Lewis 1993[45] with permission)

Table 21.5 The types and quantities of different hemoglobins in infancy and adulthood

Type of Hb	HbA	HbF	HbA_2
Notation	$\alpha2\beta2$	$\alpha2\gamma2$	$\alpha2\delta2$
Normal % at birth	20	80	<1
Normal % in older children	98	<1	2

cell indices, hemoglobin electrophoresis with quantification of S and other hemoglobins. The affected individual then requires adequate information and counseling about the genetic implications, even if clinically mild or insignificant.

Sickle cell trait (AS)

Sickle cell trait (AS) is not a disease; affected individuals have less than 50% hemoglobin S, normal red cell indices and no adverse clinical sequelae unless exposed to severe hypoxic conditions. They should be treated as normal and reassured, but given appropriate genetic advice about the risk of passing on the abnormality. No special precautions are required for anaesthesia or other medical interventions in these individuals.

Sickle cell disease (SS)

Sickle cell disease, i.e. homozygous SS, is a very variable disorder, but affected individuals are prone to a number of serious complications which need careful management. The red cells have reduced survival, and chronic hemolytic anemia (hemoglobin 6–9 g/dl) leads to marrow expansion with typical bossing of the skull. Growth is often less than anticipated. Some individuals have a relatively trouble-free life; others have many vaso-occlusive crises. The relatively insoluble hemoglobin S precipitates into crystals distorting the red cell shape (sickle cells) (Fig. 21.15a);[37] there is microvascular sludging and infarction of surrounding tissues producing ischemic pain. In the infant the first sign may be dactylitis (Fig. 21.15b),[37] in older children the long bones are more commonly affected. These attacks may be precipitated by a variety of external events of which the most important is probably intercurrent infection. Sickling episodes can be life threatening, particularly if the lungs are involved, and are usually very painful. Early and adequate pain relief is an important component of the management, which also includes a diligent search for infection, and good hydration; sickle cell disease usually produces a urinary concentrating defect. Sickling causes necrosis in bones – while the changes may be reversible, avascular necrosis of the femoral or humoral heads leads to early and severe disability. In early life the child typically has an enlarged spleen but with time this gradually infarcts (autosplenectomy) leading to the risk of overwhelming sepsis as with other asplenic individuals.[46] There is evidence that in this group prophylactic penicillin is protective; other postsplenectomy guidance should be followed, in particular appropriate immunization with pneumococcal vaccine (guidelines published in 1996). Such children need open access to an experienced team. Hospitals with few such patients should ensure that appropriate management protocols are available. Other serious complications of sickle cell disease are aplastic crises, most commonly associated with parvovirus B19 (as with all types of hemolysis), and the rare sequestration crises in which there is sudden and dramatic pooling of blood in the spleen or liver; the child presents with very rapidly falling hemoglobin. Splenic sequestration

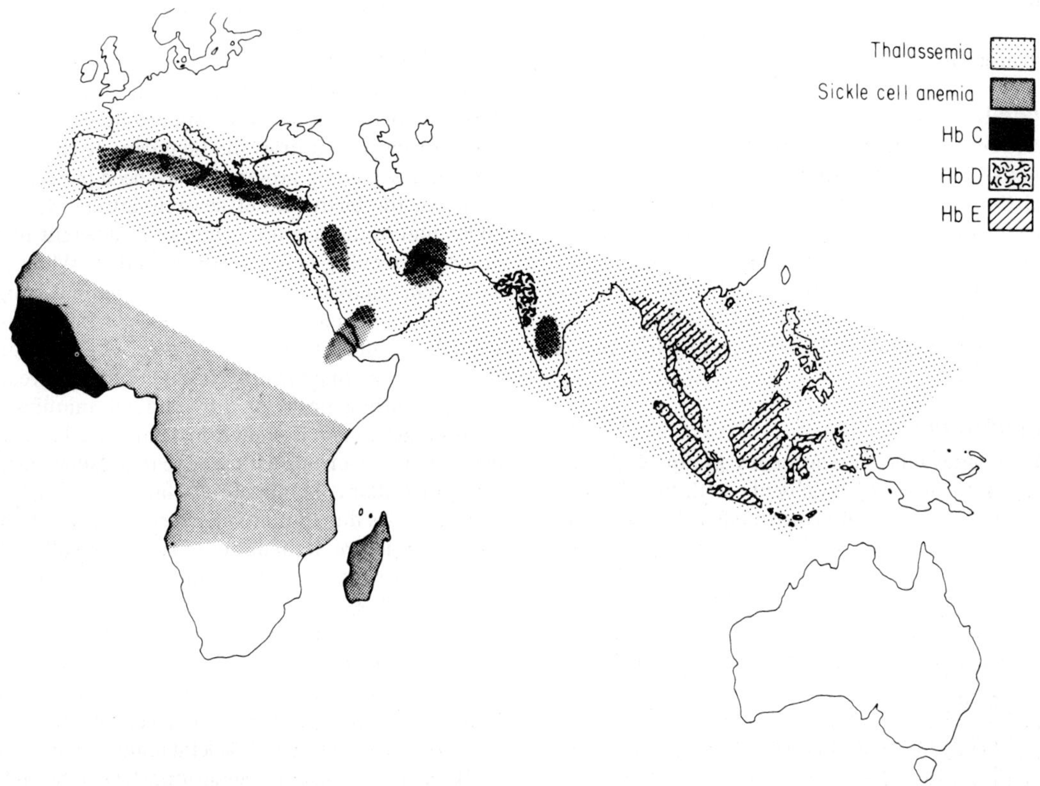

Fig. 21.14 The geographical distribution of the thalassemias and more common inherited structural hemoglobin abnormalities. (From Hoffbrand & Pettit 1993[45] with permission)

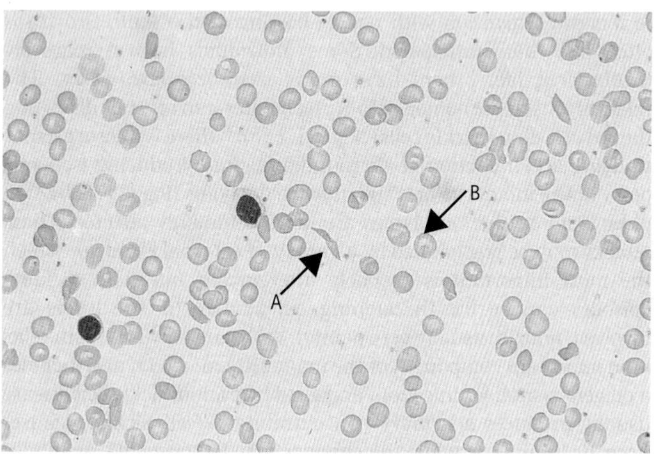

Fig. 21.15 (a) Peripheral blood appearance in homozygous sickle cell disease with target cells, polychromasia and distorted red cells (A, sickle cell; B target cell). (b) Swelling of the fingers from dactylitis, a common mode of presentation of sickle cell disease in late infancy. (From Lissauer & Clayden 2001[37] with permission)

is an indication for splenectomy. Other important complications occur – chronic hemolysis predisposes to the development of gallstones; vascular occlusion can result in stroke, priapism, and leg ulcers and retinal vaso-occlusion leads to proliferative retinopathy.

Management in sickle cell disease is supportive; blood transfusion is required only under some circumstances – occasionally exchange transfusion is required for serious complications, or as prophylaxis following a stroke, but not simply to raise the hemoglobin level. Recent trials have demonstrated that it is feasible to reduce clinical severity by increasing the proportion of hemoglobin F using hydroxyurea.[47] Bone marrow or stem cell transplantation may be curative but selection of suitable patients is difficult and controversial.[48–50]

Sickle cell variants

Hemoglobin S can be inherited with hemoglobin C, each parent being heterozygous. The child with SC disease has a higher hemoglobin level than SS individuals, usually has fewer painful crises, but is nevertheless more prone to avascular necrosis, and to neovascularization of the eyes; these children should have regular ophthalmic review. When hemoglobin S is inherited with beta thalassemia the disorder may be less severe, but this depends upon the type of beta thalassemia (Table 21.6). For further information the reader is referred to Serjeant.[51]

Thalassemia syndromes

Thalassemias are a large and heterogeneous group of red cell disorders resulting from impaired or absent synthesis of globin chains. The different globin chains are coded for on either chromosome 16 (alpha-like) or 11 (beta, delta and gamma chains) shown in Figure 21.16a.[44] If alpha chains are affected alpha-thalassemia results, if beta chains, beta-thalassemia results. The clinical effects depend upon both the type and extent of gene mutations and upon whether inherited from one or both parents (thalassemia trait or a more serious disorder). Large gene deletions on chromosome 11 may affect more than one globin gene producing more complex gamma delta thalassemia. Some disorders which affect only hemoglobin F (gamma chain mutations) may produce only transient disorders (e.g. hemolytic anemia due to unstable gamma chains) in the neonatal period that disappear as the hemoglobin F is replaced by hemoglobin A. The racial and geographic origin of the patient will help point towards which type of hemoglobinopathy is likely and will help guide investigations. The pathology of the thalassemias is related to globin chain imbalance; a reduction of one chain leads to an excess of the other; this disturbs red cell production leading to anemia and other consequences of ineffective erythropoiesis.

Table 21.6 The sickle syndromes – variable clinical severity

Most severe	Homozygous SS, HbS/β^0 thalassemia (β globin mutation with no β globin chain produced)
Intermediate	Hb SC disease
Least severe	HbS/β^+ thalassemia (some β chains produced)
Severity also reduced by:	High HbF level Coincidental inheritance of α thalassemia genes

Alpha thalassemias

Because alpha globin chains are a normal part of fetal hemoglobin, disorders affecting alpha chains may be evident at or before birth, depending upon the severity. There are four alpha globin genes; the clinical phenotype depends upon the number of genes affected (Fig. 21.16b).[44] The most severe form, where all four alpha genes are deleted, is incompatible with life and leads to hydrops fetalis (Fig. 21.16c).[44] The milder forms may lead to a mild hemolytic anemia due to globin chain imbalance. The red cells contain tetramers of beta globin, hemoglobin H, which tends to precipitate out and may be visualized on the blood film with special stains. The mildest forms of alpha thalassemia manifest red cells with reduced MCV and MCH. The alpha thalassemia genes are particularly common in Asia, but mild genotypes are also common in Africa, where they may modify the clinical severity of sickle cell disease.

Beta thalassemias

The beta thalassemias occur mainly in countries bordering the Mediterranean but are also important in Asia. In some of the Mediterranean countries the heterozygote rate is as high as 20%; antenatal screening programs have been particularly important in reducing the birth rate of severely affected homozygous infants. Individual mutations are common in different populations which enables screening by mutation detection. While the heterozygote state, beta thalassemia trait, is usually without symptoms or serious sequelae, the homozygous state results in beta thalassemia major – the child is unable to make hemoglobin A and usually presents with progressive anemia towards the end of the first year of life.

The pathogenesis of the clinical manifestations of beta thalassemia major is shown in Figure 21.17. Untreated, a child develops severe anemia with growth retardation, hepatosplenomegaly (extramedullary hemopoiesis) failure to thrive, and skeletal abnormalities due to marrow hyperplasia. The bones are thin and prone to fracture. In addition to typical maxillary bone expansion which gives rise to the thalassemic facies, the skull X-ray has typical 'hair-on-end' appearance due to medullary expansion as shown in Figure 21.18a, and there is a characteristic peripheral blood picture (Fig. 21.18b). Children with beta thalassemia major require regular transfusions of red cells to maintain adequate hemoglobin levels, promote normal growth and development, and suppress the erythroid hyperplasia and skeletal manifestations.

Before embarking on regular transfusion the child should receive hepatitis B vaccine, and the red cells should be more fully phenotyped, so that blood additionally matched for some of the other

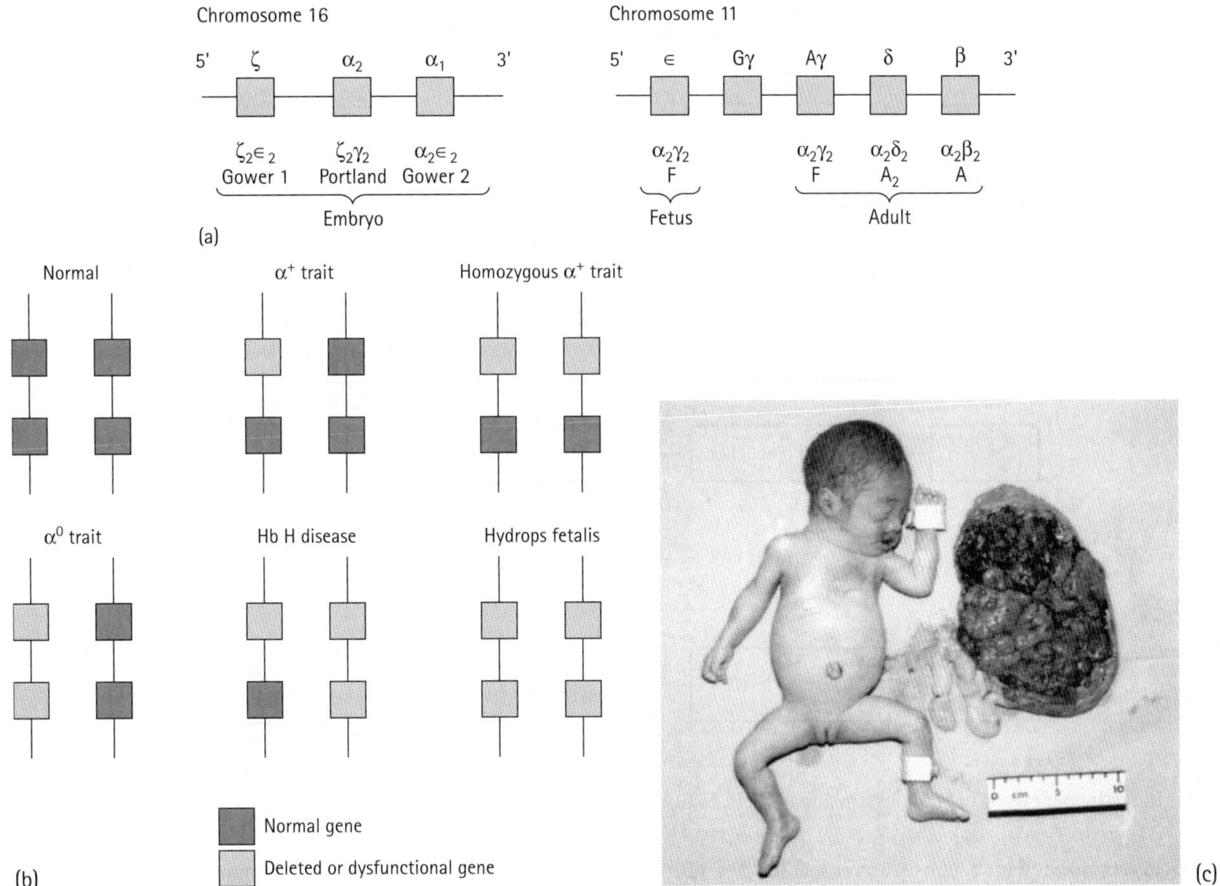

Fig. 21.16 (a) Globin gene clusters on chromosomes 11 and 16. (b) The genetics of alpha thalassemia. (c) Alpha thalassemia hydrops fetalis, the result of deletions of all four alpha globin genes (From Hoffbrand & Lewis 1993[44] with permission)

antigenic red cell groups can be regularly obtained. This is particularly important where the child is of a different ethnic group (and therefore likely to have a different frequency of some of the other red cell antigens) compared to the local blood donor population. The principal adverse outcome of transfusion is iron loading, which is inevitable and must be treated with an iron chelator to remove the excess. Currently the standard iron chelator is desferrioxamine usually given by subcutaneous infusion over several hours daily for maximal effect. Iron loading results in tissue damage to endocrine glands (parathyroids, pancreas), failure to progress through puberty, skin discoloration, but most seriously can lead to heart failure and dysrythmias. Cardiac iron loading causes death in inadequately chelated patients, often before the end of the second decade. Compliance is a major issue for many children, especially in teenage years. Desferrioxamine itself has side-effects and the dose regimen must be carefully calculated. Children should be monitored regularly for ear and eye toxicity. There is good evidence that iron overload, as measured by high ferritin levels and liver biopsy, is clearly related to mortality. Oral iron chelation has been tried but is not as effective and possibly more toxic.[52–54] The transfusion requirements (transfusion of packed red cells exceeding 180–200 ml/kg/year) will often indicate when removal of the enlarged spleen, which acts as a reservoir, may be of benefit. Patients often benefit from contact with other affected individuals and patient support groups.

Some individuals who are homozygous for beta thalassemia show a clinically less severe course (thalassemia intermedia). These individuals may not be transfusion dependent but can show other complications, such as the skeletal manifestations, of beta thalassemia major to a varying degree. Management may be difficult and such children should be referred to thalassemia specialists.

BMT is potentially curative in beta thalassemia major.[55] Initially pioneered in Italy, three risk factors – hepatomegaly, liver fibrosis and quality of iron chelation treatment – were found to predict transplant-related morbidity and mortality. Increased evidence of liver disease, and poor chelation predicted a worse outcome. In patients lacking any risk factors the overall survival was 96% at 10–11 years with an event-free survival of 92%, whereas patients with all three risk factors had an overall survival of 76% with an event-free survival of 53% at 10–11 years. These results suggest that if BMT is undertaken it should be in young children before there has been significant transfusion iron overload.[56–58] Cord blood from a sibling can also be used for transplant into these children.[59]

Rare hemoglobin disorders

A variety of mutations have been recognized which lead to destabilization of the structure of the globin complex. Some produce congenital Heinz body hemolytic anemia. (Heinz bodies are red cell inclusions seen best by staining with methyl violet.) These vary from those with severe clinical manifestations to those which are found incidentally; those affecting the beta chains tend to be worse than the alpha chain variants. Children may present with chronic hemolytic anemia or with a more sudden event such as aplastic crisis with parvovirus or an exacerbation of hemolysis with an infection. Others can produce a picture very similar to thalassemia. Other hemoglobin

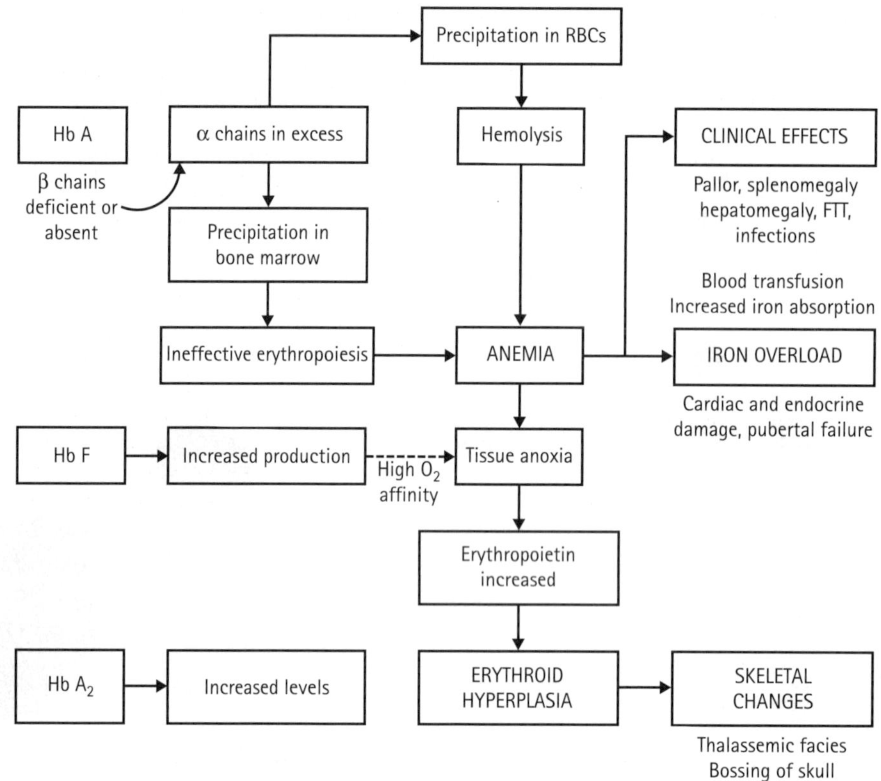

Fig. 21.17 The pathogenesis of beta thalassemia major. FTT, failure to thrive; RBCs, red blood cells.

variants are recognized which cause increased oxygen affinity (leading to polycythemia), decreased oxygen affinity, or those which have oxidized heme iron to the ferric state (resulting in methemoglobinemia). These are reviewed by Kulozik.[60]

SECONDARY ANEMIAS

The normal bone marrow produces 10^{11} red cells daily – disease processes readily affect this activity. Children often develop anemia as a consequence of some other illness. Even a transient infection may cause a significant fall in hemoglobin, but this will recover rapidly when the infection clears. More chronic illness is often complicated by anemia – 'the anemia of chronic disease' – which is at least partly caused by inflammatory cytokines leading to reduced erythropoietin production and a reduced response.[61] The anemia may be mild and normochromic or severe and microcytic. Chronic inflammatory disorders such as rheumatoid arthritis and other connective tissue disorders are commonly associated with this. There may be a low serum iron and transferrin and normal ferritin, as iron is not properly utilized. Patients may become genuinely iron deficient because of poor diet or blood loss from the gut (possibly due to non-steroidal anti-inflammatory drugs). Rheumatoid arthritis is particularly complex because the patients may also develop marrow hypoplasia due to drugs, e.g. gold therapy. Patients with connective

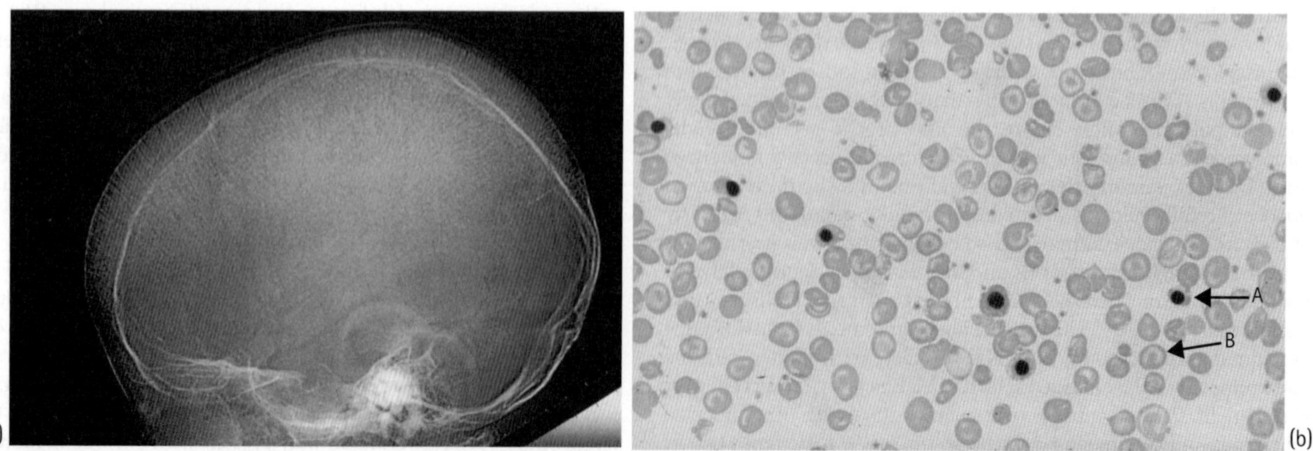

Fig. 21.18 Beta thalassemia major. (a) Skull X-ray showing 'hair on end' appearance caused by marrow hyperplasia and expansion. (b) Peripheral blood (postsplenectomy) showing target cells, nucleated red cells, red cell fragments and hypochromia. A, nucleated red cell; B, target cell.

tissue disorders such as systemic lupus erythematosus (SLE) can develop autoimmune hemolysis. Other important diseases associated with anemia are acute and chronic renal failure, and some endocrine disorders, particularly hypothyroidism.

DRUGS

Drugs must always be considered as a cause of blood dyscrasias; there are several different potential mechanisms such as blood loss (aspirin and other non-steroidal anti-inflammatory agents), development of immune phenomena or marrow suppression.

NEUTROPENIA

The time taken to develop from a stem cell to a mature neutrophil is only 24 h; the mature neutrophil may then spend up to 10 days in a marrow storage site before release when it then only circulates in the peripheral blood for 6–10 h. A proportion is 'marginated' along the endothelium and are not counted in the full blood count, so use of the peripheral blood neutrophil count alone to determine risk of bacterial sepsis can be misleading. The neutrophil reserve (marrow storage pool) is about 13 times the number in the blood. The most important functions of the neutrophils are to phagocytose and kill bacteria. Disorders of neutrophil function are considered in Chapter 25.

The neutrophil count tends to be lower in children, particularly infants, than in adults, and there are racial variations – black races have absolute neutrophil counts that are 0.2 to 0.6 × 10^9/L lower than Caucasians. If blood is left to stand for several hours before being analyzed, the neutrophil count will be falsely low. Neutropenia is defined as a reduction of the absolute neutrophil count below the normal for age, and is divided according to severity, giving some indication of the likely clinical consequences, although this is heavily dependent upon the cause.

- Mild: 1.0– 1.5 × 10^9/L (adjust for the first 6 months of life) – usually no clinical problems;
- Moderate: 0.5– 1.0 × 10^9/L – clinical problems more common;
- Severe: less than 0.5 × 10^9L – risk of life-threatening sepsis, especially if neutropenia is prolonged beyond a few days.

Fortunately severe neutropenia in childhood is rare. Intercurrent viral infection is the commonest reason for mild neutropenia (neutropenia occurring during the first 24–48 h and persisting for up to 6 days). If this is the likely cause, then there is no need to repeat the blood count when the child recovers just to see if the count is back to normal. It is more important to be guided by the clinical picture.

NEUTROPENIAS SECONDARY TO MARROW FAILURE OR INFILTRATION

In children with marrow failure or infiltration the risk of serious sepsis is logarithmically increased at neutrophil counts of less than 0.1 × 10^9/L. In this group a responsible organism is identified in infections in all cases with persistent neutropenia for more than 12 weeks.[62] Endogenous organisms (i.e. part of the resident flora) result in the high risk of serious septicemia. Pathogenic organisms (such as *Pseudomonas*, *Klebsiella* and *Proteus* species) often replace normal less pathogenic flora in many patients with serious underlying disorders such as malignancy. *Staphylococcus aureus* and Gram negative bacilli translocate from the gastrointestinal tract when mucosal defences are breached, for example by the disease or chemotherapy. Neutrophils are normally responsible for some of the clinical features of acute inflammation such as redness, pus and swelling. Such features are therefore often minimal or absent in severe neutropenia. Because of this, and the speed with which sepsis can be fatal, any child with severe neutropenia who develops a significant fever (for example, one reading over 39°C or two over 38°C half an hour apart) should be admitted to hospital, have blood and other relevant cultures sent, and be started on broad spectrum parenteral antibiotics while the culture results are awaited. Patients with chronic severe neutropenia should either have open access to a familiar ward, or carry a letter detailing the importance of blood culture as an initial investigation followed by admission for parenteral antibiotics if they attend the general practitioner or hospital emergency room with a fever. As most infections are caused by the child's own resident flora, the addition of protective isolation is not of any proven benefit. It is more important to screen regularly (surveillance throat and rectal swabs) for colonization by the more pathogenic Gram negative organisms (*Klebsiella* and *Pseudomonas* species which confer a higher risk of serious septicemia) and to use selective non-absorbable antibiotics for gut decontamination. Good hygiene (including mouth and dental care) and prophylaxis against *Candida* are also beneficial. Salads may be significantly contaminated with *Pseudomonas* and other Gram negative organisms and are best avoided.

In other children with neutropenia where there is normal marrow reserve (see below) there is a reduced risk of serious sepsis despite the low count.

AUTOIMMUNE NEUTROPENIA

Autoimmune neutropenia is probably the commonest cause of persistent neutropenia in childhood occurring in perhaps 1 in 100 000 children per annum. It is rarely associated with severe sepsis and usually resolves spontaneously after a variable period of time. Typically the child, who may be of either sex, is aged between 5 and 24 months at presentation. A useful review[63] described 240 children with autoimmune neutropenia aged 5–15 months at diagnosis. Of these 90% had benign infections and 95% recovered spontaneously within 7 to 24 months. Bone marrow examination may show maturation arrest, with lack of the more mature precursors, or some myeloid hyperplasia, or can be normal. Antineutrophil antibodies can usually be demonstrated in the serum, which is helpful in confirming the diagnosis. Until the clinical pattern is clear, fever should be managed carefully with appropriate cultures and parenteral antibiotics, while excluding significant infection. When the diagnosis is clear, these children can be managed conservatively and the parents should be encouraged to continue with normal living. Fevers and other infections can be managed in the same way as any other non-neutropenic child. In the rare case with severe infection (usually the younger child) neutrophils have been temporarily increased by steroids or intravenous immunoglobulin. Both these treatments have disadvantages, and the commercially available cytokine, granulocyte colony stimulating factor (G-CSF) is now the treatment of choice for severe infection or to cover surgery. This usually increases the absolute neutrophil count within 24–48 h and has an additional beneficial effect upon neutrophil function.

SEVERE CONGENITAL NEUTROPENIAS

These disorders are fortunately rare, but very important to recognize because of their potential seriousness and the need for aggressive management of infection. The important difference from autoimmune neutropenia is that these children are likely to present with septicemia or other severe bacterial infections that can lead to early death if not appropriately managed. As neutropenia can occur as a secondary feature in the course of severe sepsis (particularly in neonates and in the presence of endotoxemia), the nature of such a disorder is often not clear at initial presentation. Any child with severe sepsis in whom neutropenia persists should be investigated with bone marrow examination.

Kostmann described 24 cases of severe neutropenia (neutrophils $< 0.2 \times 10^9$/L) in a consanguineous Swedish family in 1956. About 200 similar cases have been described in the literature, but this is now recognized to be a heterogeneous group – some children have been shown to have mutations in the G-CSF receptor gene. Presentation is usually before 6 months of age with severe pyogenic infections – half present in the first month of life, and the outlook was poor before the advent of BMT and the use of G-CSF. The bone marrow shows maturation arrest. Such children should be referred to a pediatric hematologist and usually do well on daily injections of G-CSF. In addition, they should receive mouth care and antibiotic prophylaxis. There is now an international registry so hopefully sharing knowledge will expand our understanding of these rare conditions. There is an increased risk of developing acute leukemia, but it is not clear whether this is related to the underlying disorder or to the therapy with G-CSF. Because of this concern, these children should have regular bone marrow examinations with cytogenetic analysis.

Reticular dysgenesis is another form of severe neutropenia described in Chapter 25.

Cyclical neutropenia

This is a very rare disorder in which there is a nadir of the neutrophil count, usually every 21 days, with a count below 0.2×10^9/L. During the neutropenia the child may have mouth ulcers, gingivitis, malaise and fever, and other evidence of bacterial sepsis. There is often some asymptomatic cycling of other blood parameters. Diagnosis requires twice weekly blood counts for 6 weeks in order to document clear cycling of the absolute neutrophil count. The bone marrow can show either hypoplasia or maturation arrest of the myeloid series. The condition may improve with age. G-CSF therapy, timed to prevent the neutropenic phase, can give good relief. There is no clear evidence that these patients have an increased risk of hematological malignancy.

It is important to establish whether the neutropenia is associated with any other congenital abnormalities. Neutropenia is a well-recognized feature in about two thirds of cases of Shwachman–Diamond syndrome (see above), and may also be seen in other congenital immune deficiency states, such as antibody deficiency.

ACQUIRED NEUTROPENIA

This is most commonly due to intercurrent viral infection or can occur secondary to drug ingestion. The neutrophil count may fall to less than 0.2×10^9/L in an idiosyncratic and unpredictable way; any drug associated with the onset of neutropenia must be considered suspect and evidence sought from the literature. In the face of unexplained neutropenia it is advisable to stop the drug. Many different mechanisms have been implicated and there is no convenient diagnostic test.

EOSINOPHILIA

Eosinophilia is arbitrarily defined at a level of greater than 0.5×10^9/L. The commonest cause is the presence of allergic disease, especially atopy – asthma or eczema. Parasitic diseases such as hookworm, ascariasis, tapeworm and schistosomiasis should be sought when eosinophilia persists. Inquiry concerning overseas travel is an essential part of the clinical history taking. There are other causes that are listed elsewhere.[64]

DISORDERS OF HEMOSTASIS

The normal hemostatic mechanism depends upon the integrity of the vessel wall, and in particular the endothelial cells, the presence of normal numbers and function of platelets, and a normal coagulation mechanism. When an injury occurs, these components act in concert to prevent excessive bleeding. The blood vessel wall contracts, the endothelial cells become procoagulant, platelets and the coagulation factors are activated, resulting in a platelet plug stabilized by fibrin. Several other homeostatic mechanisms come into play – activation of the natural anticoagulant systems and fibrinolytic pathway limit the extent of fibrin formation and maintains the patency of the vessels. Clinical problems with bruising or bleeding can be caused by abnormalities of any part of the hemostatic mechanism.

Differentiation of bleeding disorders from non-accidental injury may be difficult. Investigation of a bruised child is mandatory in all cases where the bruising is unexplained or implausible. The history (particularly a detailed family history of any other bleeding tendency – menorrhagia, bleeding after surgery and dental extractions) and examination play an important part in their differentiation. Screening investigations should aim to identify the commonest disorders and those associated with significant bleeding. A full blood count including a platelet count, and a coagulation screen prothrombin time (PT), activated partial thromboplastin time (APTT) and fibrinogen level should be performed. Measurement of plasma factor VIII and factor IX level is recommended, as significant deficiencies can occur with a near normal coagulation screen. Von Willebrand factor (vWf) antigen and activity should be measured, because von Willebrand disease (vWd) is the commonest inherited bleeding disorder and often gives normal results in a coagulation screen. Interpretation of these investigations, if abnormal, may need the advice of a hematologist. It must be remembered however, that demonstration of a bleeding diathesis does not rule out the diagnosis of non-accidental injury and these children may be at greater risk of harm from such injury due to their bleeding disorder.

PLATELET DISORDERS

Thrombocytopenic purpuras

Thrombocytopenia is common in pediatrics. It is very important to be aware that a poorly taken blood sample is often responsible – if the low platelet count is unexpected it may need repeating to ensure that it was not a spurious result. Thrombocytopenia is often secondary to infection; sick neonates usually have low platelet counts, and the count may drop in a variety of viral infections, either due to mild and temporary marrow suppression, or occasionally by an autoimmune mechanism.

Symptoms are related to the degree of thrombocytopenia, and if the function is normal, there may be very few symptoms until the count is less than 10×10^9/L (Table 21.7a). A raised platelet count is common in pediatrics and is nearly always 'reactive' (Table 21.7b); in most cases it does not require any specific investigation or treatment. The causes of thrombocytopenia are usefully divided into those with normal or increased numbers of megakaryocytes in the marrow (thrombocytopenia caused by increased peripheral destruction) and those with reduced or absent megakaryocytes (failure of production) (Table 21.8a). Thrombocytopenias in children are most commonly caused by increased destruction. The hemostatic defect is mainly due to failure of formation of an adequate platelet 'plug' at the site of damaged capillaries, small arterioles and venules. Coagulation

Table 21.7a Clinical presentation of thrombocytopenia (normal range = 150–450 × 10^9/L)

Platelet count × 10^9/L	Symptoms
50–100	Bleeding only produced by trauma or surgery. Often no symptoms at all.
30–50	Bruising with minor trauma
10–30	Spontaneous bruising and dependant purpura. Menorrhagia, epistaxis
Less than 10	Spontaneous bruising and purpura. Mucosal bleeding. At risk for more serious bleeding, e.g. from the gastrointestinal tract or in the central nervous system, depending upon cause of thromobocytopenia (much more likely in circumstances with reduced production than increased destruction)

Table 21.7b Causes of a raised platelet count (thrombocytosis)

In children nearly always reactive or secondary
Infection
Iron deficiency
Postoperative
Inflammation
Malignancy
Hemorrhage
Primary disease of the marrow is very rare

screening tests such as the PT, thrombin time and partial thromboplastin time will be normal.

Differential diagnosis

A careful clinical history and examination will point to the cause, bearing in mind the likelihood of the different disorders.

Congenital thrombocytopenias are very rare and so may be missed. The time of onset of symptoms should be carefully defined, as patients with congenital disorders will have a life-long history. There may be a family history but many of these disorders are inherited recessively. Consanguinity of parents will increase the risk, so that autosomal recessive disorders such as Bernard–Soulier syndrome are commoner in populations where first cousin marriage is common.

Bernard–Soulier syndrome is caused by a lack of platelet glycoprotein 1b, resulting in thrombocytopenia (typically 30–40 × 10^9/L) and defective function so that the bleeding manifestations (bruising, mucous membrane bleeding) occur at a higher platelet count than expected. The blood film shows giant platelets.

Wiskott–Aldrich syndrome is an X-linked disorder that in classical form leads to severe thrombocytopenia with small platelets. It is associated with eczema, immune defects and a significant risk of transformation to malignancy. Not all patients have eczema at the time of presentation with bleeding. In some the bleeding symptoms may be very severe and life threatening. In these patients BMT has been curative.

Clearly the implications of a diagnosis of one of these disorders are quite different from immune thrombocytopenias (see below). There are several other forms of inherited thrombocytopenias, some of which are associated with other physical abnormalities. In many of these disorders the children have a life-long bleeding tendency that can be very difficult to manage, and need expert management in a specialist center. These disorders are reviewed by Warrier T & Lusher.[65]

Thrombocytopenia may be the presenting feature of a more sinister disorder, such as idiopathic aplastic anemia, or one of the constitutional marrow failure syndromes (see above), e.g. Fanconi syndrome. Limping or bone pain, with lymphadenopathy or splenomegaly, suggest leukemia, but it is rare for this to present without other abnormalities in the blood count. Consideration of these diagnoses will determine whether a bone marrow examination will help (to rule out aplasia or malignancy) or whether other tests of platelet function and surface molecules are required to exclude the congenital disorders. Careful examination of a peripheral smear by an experienced hematologist in possession of the full clinical history is essential.

Coagulation screening tests are not usually indicated unless there is a possibility of consumptive coagulopathy (e.g. in association with suspected sepsis) or hypersplenism that may be associated with hepatic dysfunction. Generally in a well child with purpura alone the coagulation screen is normal and unnecessary. Purpura is not a symptom of a coagulation factor defect. In a child with thrombocytopenia and a hemangioma, even if very small, a coagulation profile is essential as this may indicate Kasabach–Merritt syndrome with a potentially serious consumption coagulopathy. This combination is fortunately rare, but may be very difficult to manage, with life-threatening bleeding. The pathogenesis and management of this disorder has been reviewed by Hall.[66]

Idiopathic thrombocytopenic purpura (ITP)

Immune thrombocytopenia can be caused by a number of different mechanisms (Table 21.8b) but ITP is the most common. Despite this, it is not a common condition; the incidence is about the same as acute leukemia, 1 in 25 000. Many pediatricians will therefore see this infrequently. The disorder is caused by antibody production against platelet antigens, perhaps switched on as an inappropriate immune response to a trivial viral infection or immunization. There are well-recognized associations with varicella, measles, mumps and rubella (MMR) vaccine and with infectious mononucleosis.

The clinical onset is usually abrupt with presentation to medical attention within 24–48 h. Although the platelet count is dramatically decreased (80% have a platelet count less than 20 × 10^9/L), the typical child, a boy or girl aged 1 to 10 years, will have predominantly or exclusively cutaneous symptoms and signs often with florid purpura and easy bruising. Mucosal bleeding is less common, with epistaxis occurring in 20%, and usually not severe. Severe bleeding symptoms such as torrential nose bleeds, hematemesis, melena, menorrhagia or frank hematuria are much less common, occurring in about 4%.[67] Intracranial hemorrhage is rare and not as high as the 1–3% often quoted. The incidence is much closer to 1 in 500 or 1 in 1000, is not confined to early in the course of the disorder, is not necessarily fatal and may be caused by an additional underlying abnormality or provoked by an injury.[68] The outlook in childhood ITP is very good; most children will fully recover within a short time, sometimes even within a few days, and mostly within 6 weeks.

There is no diagnostic test; other disorders have to be considered and excluded as appropriate. No additional tests will confirm the diagnosis. Bone marrow aspiration is not required unless there is

Table 21.8a Causes of thrombocytopenia

Decreased production - Congenital – rare - Acquired
Increased destruction - Immune (common) - Non-immune Disseminated intravascular coagulation Hemolytic uremic syndrome and its variants Hypersplenism

Table 21.8b Causes of immune thrombocytopenia

Idiopathic autoimmune (ITP or AITP) acute (80–90% in children) chronic (i.e. > 6 months duration)
Alloantibodies neonatal (NAIT) post-transfusion purpura
Drug-induced Disease-associated (e.g. systemic lupus erythematosus, immunodeficiency and some infections)

doubt about the diagnosis, as it can only exclude other disorders and show a picture that is consistent with increased peripheral destruction (an increase of megakaryocytes in an otherwise normal marrow).

The management of this disorder is controversial because many doctors fear that a very low platelet count carries a high risk of serious or life-threatening bleeding. The evidence does not support this. Guidelines published in the UK in 1992[69] indicated that 'no treatment' is an acceptable policy in children with clinically mild disease; more recent surveys from Germany[70] and the UK illustrate the safety of a 'no treatment' policy based on mild clinical presentation rather than the platelet count.[71] New standardized parameters are required for the assessment of these children which take into account symptoms as well as the platelet count.[72] A useful clinical classification is shown in Table 21.9. When treatment is required for bleeding symptoms the choice is between oral steroids in high doses (e.g. 1–2 mg/kg/day for 2 weeks; 4 mg/kg/day for 4 days), or intravenous immunoglobulin (IVIG). If a child is treated for a low platelet count alone, it becomes difficult to withdraw steroids, as the count drops when the steroid dose is lowered. Steroids given at high dose over a long period of time have unacceptable side-effects. IVIG is a blood product (from pooled plasma donations), so may carry a risk of infection (hepatitis C has been transmitted in the past); it has a high frequency of side-effects (fever, headache, malaise) and has to be given by intravenous infusion. The original dose regimen was 400 mg/kg daily for 5 days, but many clinicians use 1 g/kg daily for one or two doses and 800 mg/kg as a single dose may be sufficient. It is valuable in the child with a significant bleed (less than 4% of children) as it raises the platelet count faster than oral steroids. Many other agents have been used for the very rare child with serious hemorrhage who is refractory to steroids and IVIG. These complex cases should be referred to a specialist.

About 15% children do not remit within 6 months and this is the accepted cut-off for defining 'chronic'. These children still have a good chance of remitting (60% over 10 years) so that the management can continue to be expectant.[73] Chronic ITP is generally thought to be more common in children over 10 years of age, and females. These children may develop other features of autoimmune diseases and may be screened for these on an annual basis (antinuclear factor, antidouble stranded DNA, lupus anticoagulants, anticardiolipin antibodies). In the absence of symptoms, the finding of other autoantibodies may not alter the management, but will be a useful forewarning of possible trouble to come.

Splenectomy may be considered for children with severe bleeding problems, preferably more than 6 months from diagnosis; again it is important not to take this step on the basis of the platelet count alone. The child's lifestyle may be taken into consideration, but it must be remembered that about 25% will not remit despite splenectomy and evidence suggests that the longer the splenectomized individuals are followed, the higher the relapse rate, with no evidence of a plateau. Splenectomy is associated with a small but life-long increased risk of infection (see above).

Thrombocytopenia secondary to infection

Mild thrombocytopenia of the order of 50–100 × 10^9/L is common following recent infection in young children. Sometimes there is accompanying splenomegaly and both resolve within a week or two. The infection is often a simple upper respiratory tract infection but is sometimes due to specific causes such as glandular fever, CMV or toxoplasmosis. Many of the more serious infections (particularly meningococcal disease) produce consumptive coagulopathy. Thrombocytopenia is common in human immunodeficiency virus (HIV) infection, and may be the presenting feature in adults.

Drug-induced thrombocytopenia

Drugs such as alkylating agents and antimetabolites used in leukemia treatment regularly produce a dose-dependent general marrow suppression. The other main type of drug-induced thrombocytopenia is that produced by immunological mechanisms,

Table 21.9 Clinical bleeding assessment in children with immune thrombocytopenic purpura – irrespective of platelet count

Bleeding category	Clinical description
Asymptomatic	No symptoms. Low platelet count found incidentally
Mild	Cutaneous features only; purpura and bruising; occasional mucosal lesion; trivial nosebleeds. No interference with normal living
Moderate	More troublesome bleeding including menorrhagia, more severe nosebleeds, moderate interference with daily living
Severe	Bleeding requiring hospital admission and/or blood transfusion. Gastrointestinal bleeding; torrential nosebleeds. Serious life threatening bleeding such as intracranial hemorrhage

usually of the drug–hapten variety. This has been shown in adults to occur with Sedormid, quinidine, quinine, sulfamethazine, antazoline and other drugs. Antiepileptic medication can rarely produce marrow toxicity with both thrombocytopenia and leucopenia. Heparin-induced thrombocytopenia (type 2) is a rare but important side-effect of heparin (mainly unfractionated) where a previously exposed individual produces antibodies which complex with heparin-platelet factor 4 to activate platelets, induce thrombocytopenia associated with serious thrombotic events. Heparin must be stopped immediately and an alternative anticoagulant used. This diagnosis must always be considered in the appropriate clinical setting as prompt appropriate management may be life saving.

Disorders of platelet function

Inherited disorders of platelet function are rare; there are many more common acquired conditions in which moderate platelet dysfunction can play a role. Platelet disorders typically lead to mucosal bleeding, prolonged bleeding from superficial cuts, bruising and purpura. The extent of bleeding is related to the severity of the disorder.

Acquired

The main causes of acquired platelet dysfunction are indicated in Table 21.10. Many drugs cause some platelet dysfunction. Aspirin is the most well known, and causes inhibition of prostaglandin synthetase and impaired thromboxane A2 synthesis. There is a failure of the release reaction and aggregation with adrenalin and adenosine diphosphate (ADP). A single small dose can have an effect for the life span of the platelet, 7–10 days. Other non-steroidal anti-inflammatory drugs cause variable interference with platelet function. Heparin and intravenous antibiotics may become important in the seriously ill patient with multiorgan failure in intensive care. Uremia and liver dysfunction may be contributory. Myeloproliferative disorders are extremely rare in childhood. Although in adults a high platelet count may indicate a marrow disorder, in children a raised platelet count is common, and it is nearly always reactive. It is a marker of inflammation and challenge in a non-specific manner similar to the erythrocyte sedimentation rate, and does not need further investigation or repeated measurement.

Hereditary

Glanzmann's disease or thrombasthenia, is a serious bleeding disorder that usually presents early in life with bruising and mucous membrane bleeding. As with other autosomal recessive disorders, cases are commonest in families with consanguineous marriages. The platelet membrane lacks the IIb/IIIa receptor complex that is critical for normal platelet function. The platelet count is normal, laboratory testing shows that the platelets fail to aggregate with any of the usual agonists. Serious bleeding episodes require treatment with platelet transfusions, but these carry a risk of alloantibody stimulation, and so should be used very judiciously. Patients may need bone marrow transplant. Recent experience suggests that a concentrate of recombinant activated factor VII may be a useful agent for hemostasis, but the high cost precludes use except in severe bleeding episodes.

Platelets are complex organelles with several types of granule that are important for function. There are a number of inherited platelet storage pool diseases resulting in defective platelet function that usually produce only a mild bleeding tendency. The investigation of these in children is unsatisfactory, and specialist advice should be sought. The association with tyrosinase-positive albinism is called Hermansky–Pudlak syndrome and the bleeding problems are usually mild.

Table 21.10 Causes of acquired platelet dysfunction

1. Drugs
   - Inhibition of cyclo-oxygenase – e.g. aspirin and other non-steroidal anti-inflammatory agents
   - Elevation of cyclic AMP levels –
     - Inhibitors of phosphodiesterase – dipyridamole
     - Activators of adenyl cyclase
   - Antibiotics – penicillins and cephalosporins
   - Heparin
   - Alcohol
2. Uremia
3. Disseminated intravascular coagulation
4. Primary marrow disorders
   - Acute leukemias
   - Myeloproliferative disorders (very rare in children)
5. Cardiac bypass surgery

COAGULATION DISORDERS

Normal blood coagulation has been described as a 'cascade' where a series of enzymes are activated sequentially, each step adding magnification to the process, leading to the formation of a fibrin clot. In recent years this theory has been revised, and it is now more helpful to visualize the relevant factors being brought into proximity with one another on cell surfaces, which are crucial to normal coagulation (Fig. 21.19a).[74] Coagulation screening tests give important indications of where a coagulation problem lies, but do not take into account many other important physiological systems which add to the balance of hemostasis and thrombosis. In addition to the coagulation factors that contribute to the formation of the fibrin clot, the naturally occurring anticoagulants, antithrombin, protein C and its cofactor protein S, and tissue factor pathway inhibitor are important in preventing excessive coagulation activation. Other so-called coagulation factors, such as factor XII, whose deficiency may produce an abnormal screening test, have no physiological role in coagulation; a defect is not associated with a bleeding disorder. Some of these interactions are shown in Figure 21.19b.

Although the hemophilias are the best characterized of the inherited coagulation disorders, the rare ones have taught us much about normal hemostasis. The physiological pathway for a fibrin clot is the stimulation of tissue factor – factor VII. Infants with complete deficiency of either factor VII or factor X are particularly at risk of intracranial hemorrhage in the first week of life (also a major risk for the same reason in vitamin K deficiency), in contrast to severe factor VIII or IX deficiency where this complication is much less common.

Coagulation tests do not give any information about the fibrinolytic system, complement activation, the activity of the endothelial cell (a very important regulator of hemostasis) or of the other cell systems which may be implicated, such as monocytes and neutrophils where tissue factor expression can vary; upregulation can produce a thrombotic milieu. At present there are no satisfactory routine ways of examining these other homeostatic mechanisms.

HEREDITARY COAGULATION DEFECTS

The three most common serious defects are due to deficiency of factors VIIIC and IXC and vWf. The other disorders are autosomally

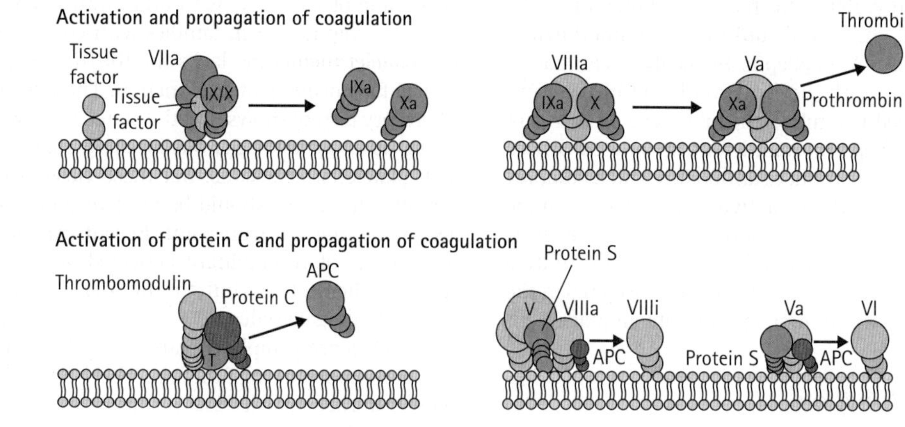

(a)

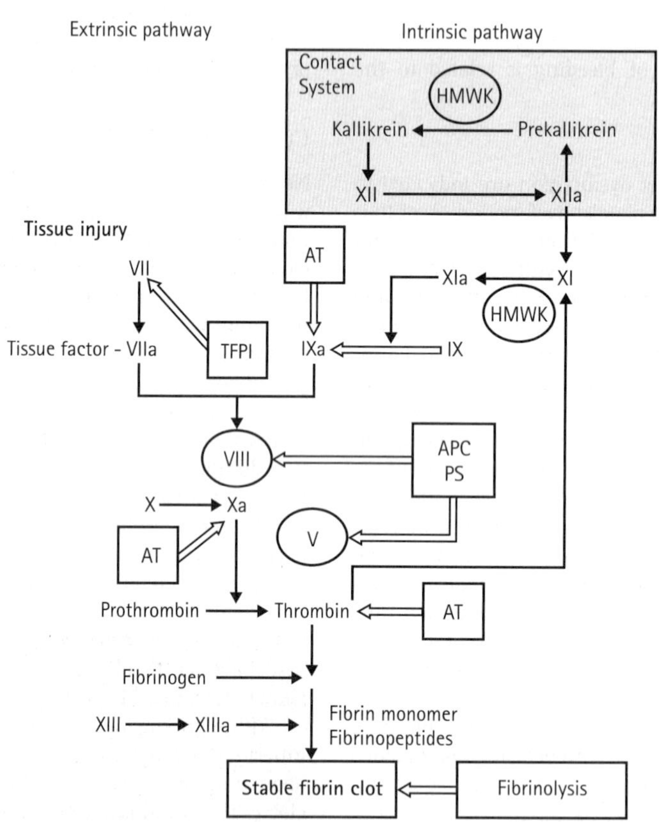

(b)

Fig. 21.19 Coagulation pathways. (a) Schematic models illustrating some of the phospholipid-bound reactions that are involved in the activation and regulation of coagulation. Factor VIIa binds to tissue factor and activates factors IX and X. Factors IXa and Xa together with factors VIIIa and Va, respectively, from the tenase and prothrombinase complexes that activate factor X and prothrombin, respectively. Thrombin-mediated activation of factor XI, factor V, and factor VIII, which gives positive feedback amplification of the system, is not shown. Thrombomodulin is present on endothelial cells. Thrombin generated in the vicinity of intact endothelial cells binds to thrombomodulin and efficiently activates protein C. Activated protein C (APC) and protein S form a complex to the plasma membrane of endothelial cells and possibly also on other cells. This complex inactivates factors Va and VIIIa, which results in down-regulation of the coagulation system. The degradation of factor VIIIa by APC is stimulated by protein S and by factor V, which in this context functions as an anticoagulant protein. (From Dahlback 2000[74] with permission). (b) Schematic representation of the coagulation pathways. The physiological activation of coagulation occurs via the extrinsic system, after activation of tissue factor VII. The end result of activation is the production of a stable fibrin clot. Open shafted arrow, inhibitory action. Inhibitors: APC, activated protein C; AT, antithrombin; PS, protein S; TFPI, tissue factor pathway inhibitor. Tint box outlines the contact system; factors in this box affect the laboratory tests but do not play a significant role in hemostasis. Ovals indicate cofactors; HMWK, high molecular weight kininogen. (From Lissauer & Clayden 2001[37] with permission)

Table 21.11 Hemorrhagic disorders

Deficient factor	Site of production	Synonym	Inheritance	Approximate incidence
VIIIC	Liver	Hemophilia A	X-linked	1:10 000 males
IXC	Liver	Hemophilia B, Christmas	X-linked	1:150 000
VWF	Endothelial cell and platelets	von Willebrand's	Autosomal	1:30 000
XIC	Liver	PTA	Autosomal	Approximately 8% Ashkenazi Jews are heterozygous
XC	Liver	Stuart Prower	Autosomal recessive	1:100 000
VIIC	Liver	Proconvertin	Autosomal recessive	1:500 000
I	Liver	Fibrinogen	Autosomal recessive	1:1 000 000
IIC	Liver	Prothrombin	Autosomal recessive	1:2 000 000
XIII	Liver or platelets	Fibrin stabilizer	Autosomal recessive	1:2 000 000

C, coagulant activity; PTA, plasma thromboplastin antecedent; vWF, von Willebrand factor.

inherited and either very rare (e.g. factor VII and X deficiencies, afibrinogenemia) or they produce less severe bleeding problems (factor XI deficiency). Inheritance patterns and incidence are detailed in Table 21.11.

Hemophilia A and B

Hemophilia A occurs with an incidence of 1 in 10 000 male births, and is thought to be of similar incidence in all the populations of the world. Factor IX deficiency, hemophilia B, is about five times less common, but all the clinical manifestations are as for hemophilia A, and both are inherited as X-linked disorders. The degree of factor VIII or IX deficiency varies in different families, but remains constant within a kindred. They are divided clinically into mild, moderate and severe on the basis of the factor level, which predicts bleeding (Table 21.12). Boys with severe hemophilia often present at 12–18 months of age with joint bleeds when they begin to walk, or with mucosal bleeding from the mouth as a result of a fall. Bleeding is typically not severe but rather a constant ooze, or there may be temporary cessation with a friable clot, which is easily dislodged leading to further bleeding. These infants may also show impressive easy bruising leading to the suspicion of non-accidental injury. Children with moderate hemophilia will mostly have been diagnosed by the age of 5 years, but those with mild hemophilia may only be diagnosed much later (even in adulthood) when they present with bleeding after dental extraction or other challenges.

The hallmark of severe hemophilia is recurrent bleeding into joints and muscles starting in infancy (Fig. 21.20). If inadequately treated, these result in progressive joint deformity and a severe destructive arthropathy (Fig. 21.21a and b). Muscle bleeds can result in permanent damage due to fibrosis and contractures.

Table 21.12 Hemophilia A and B – level of clotting factor related to clinical features

Level of clotting factor (% of normal)	Clinical features
< 1%	Severe disease Spontaneous bleeding into joints and muscles
1–5%	Moderate disease Bleeding after trauma Occasional spontaneous bleeding
5–40%	Mild disease Bleeding after trauma

Relatively minor trauma can also lead to life-threatening bleeding. Bleeding initially appears relatively mild, but is persistent and can last for weeks if no treatment is available; for example an undiagnosed child with a bitten tongue may bleed intermittently for 3 weeks resulting in a profound fall in hemoglobin so that not only is the correct replacement therapy required, but also a blood transfusion. Children with all grades of severity are at risk of bleeding after surgery, particularly in areas of increased fibrinolysis such as the mouth (dental extractions) and genitourinary tract (circumcision). Surgery should never be performed in a hemophiliac without appropriate replacement therapy, and should be carried out in a specialist hemophilia center.

Diagnosis

Severe hemophilia can be diagnosed at birth in an infant with a known family history as the factor VIIIC level at birth is already at normal adult levels. The initial screening test will show a markedly prolonged APTT. This will not distinguish between factor VIIIC and IXC deficiency – the appropriate factor assay must be performed. Severe hemophilia B can also be diagnosed at birth, but milder

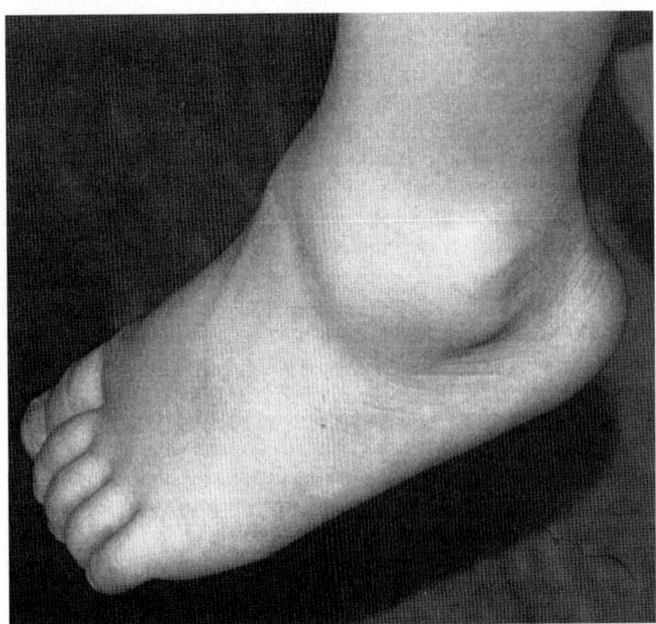

Fig. 21.20 Acute ankle hemarthrosis in a child with severe hemophilia A.

(a)
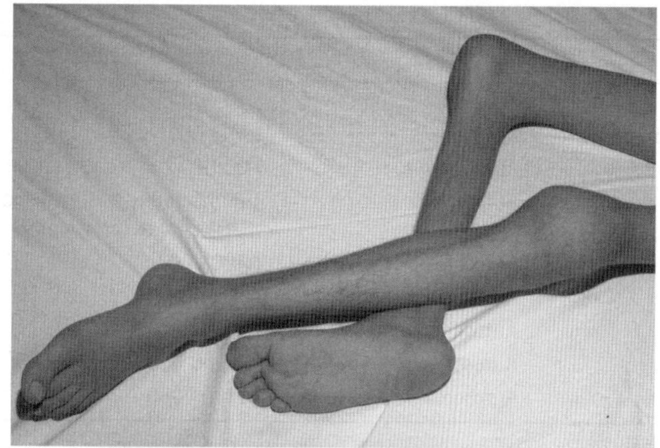

(b)
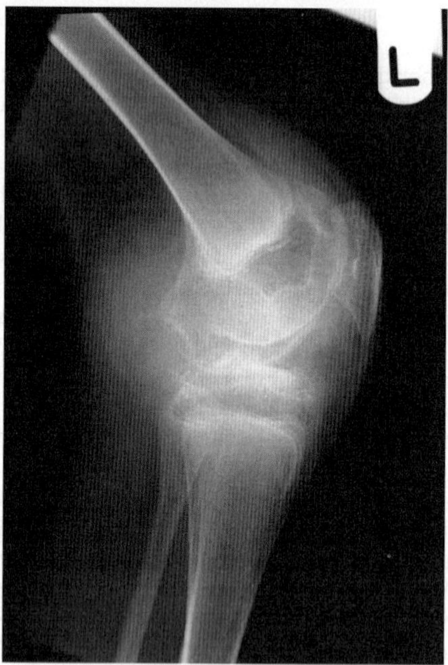

Fig. 21.21 (a) Severe hemophilia in an adolescent showing fixed flexion of R knee, marked arthropathy of L knee and muscle wasting. (b) Radiological appearance of L knee.

forms may not be reliably diagnosed within the first 6 months as the factor IX level only reaches adult levels later. It must be emphasized that the quality of the blood sample for coagulation testing and factor assays is crucial. Traumatic samples may contain tissue factor causing activation of the coagulation pathways and give inaccurate and falsely normal results.

Genetics and counseling

About a third of hemophiliacs have no known family history because either they represent new mutations, or the abnormal gene has been transmitted via asymptomatic women over many generations. It should be noted that about a third of female carriers have low factor VIIIC levels, because in each cell one X chromosome is inactivated (the Lyon hypothesis). On average, the factor VIIIC or IXC in carriers is half of normal, but in some it is low enough to cause bleeding symptoms after trauma or surgery (mild hemophilia). The relevant female relatives of any hemophiliac should therefore have factor VIIIC or IXC assays performed. A normal level will not exclude carrier status, which can generally be detected by mutation analysis of the index patient in the kindred and testing of possible carriers for the known mutation. This should not be performed without consent from the possible carrier and should be delayed until the girl is old enough to understand and consent to the test.

About 500 different mutations have so far been reported for the factor VIIIC gene, and about 700 for the factor IX gene (a complete list of all mutations may be seen at www.hgmd.org, a genetics site maintained at the University of Wales in Cardiff). It is very important to identify which women are at risk of giving birth to a severely affected boy. Parents need the opportunity to consider this, and appropriate management plans need to be in place for delivery. Most hemophiliac babies are born by normal vaginal delivery, but instrumentation should be avoided, and male infants tested at birth. It is possible to undertake antenatal testing in consultation with the appropriate services.

Management

Severe hemophilia is a serious life-long disorder. Families can be taught to manage this very well indeed, but this requires considerable investment of time and support, best provided by specialist centers (hemophilia centers). In addition to information and training, families are often helped by being put in touch with one another, and with support organizations (e.g. the UK Haemophilia Society). Families need to learn how to live with the disorder. Fortunately, with current treatment options there need to be few restrictions on activity. Contact sports should be avoided, but sport is generally beneficial; children should be encouraged to be fit, but regular soccer football is likely to lead to damaged ankle joints in the long term. The important principle is to give replacement therapy for bleeding episodes. Treatment can be given on demand for bleeds in severe and moderate hemophilia. A concentrate of factor VIIIC is used (or factor IXC in factor IX deficiency), either plasma-derived or genetically engineered (recombinant). Fresh frozen plasma contains factor VIIIC and IXC but an unacceptably large volume would be required for an adequate factor increase. Cryoprecipitate is effective in hemophilia, A (but not hemophilia B) but is not virally inactivated and is less convenient because of the volume required. Plasma-derived factor concentrates have been available in developed countries since the 1970s and have changed the lives of severe hemophiliacs, early and adequate treatment of joint bleeds preventing severe joint deformity in many young men. Unfortunately the early products transmitted both hepatitis C and HIV infection, with tragic consequences. More than 1000 of the total of 5000 people with hemophilia A in the UK were infected with HIV between 1979 and 1985, and more than 3000 people have been infected with hepatitis C.[75–77] Viral inactivation steps were introduced in the 1980s and since 1986–1987 these products have not transmitted either of these viruses. In many countries recombinant products are the treatment of choice, but at a high cost. The half-life of factor VIII in the circulation is only 8–12 h, and is less in small children. This means that doses need to be given twice or three times daily for surgery where the aim is to keep the factor VIIIC level above 50 iu/dl. Minor bleeding episodes respond rapidly to a single dose of 20–25 u/kg; more severe bleeds may need higher initial doses and repeat doses over a few days. Factor IXC needs to be given in higher dosage as the recovery is less (40–50 u/kg) but less frequently as the half-life is longer.

Current treatment recommendations aim to prevent joint damage by giving prophylactic therapy. The principle is to give factor VIIIC three times a week or on alternate days at a dose sufficient to prevent the trough level of factor VIII falling below 2 iu/dl, in effect converting severe to moderate hemophilia which is far less likely to be complicated by recurrent joint and muscle bleeds. Experience from Sweden, where this has been normal practice since 1958, has shown convincing benefit in serial cohorts monitored over decades.[78]

Additional suggestive data were produced by the orthopedic outcomes study (data collected from 21 centers worldwide) in which those patients who had more than 45 weeks of regular prophylaxis per year had better joint function at 6-year follow-up than those who were treated 'on demand'. There was also a correlation between the total factor VIII usage per annum and outcomes; in general, more treatment was associated with a better outcome.[79]

These and many other studies have encouraged the adoption of prophylaxis as optimal therapy for young hemophiliacs by the World Health Organization and the World Federation of Hemophilia. This is generally with a regimen of alternate day (or 25 u/kg three times a week) therapy in hemophilia A, and twice weekly (40 u/kg) injections for hemophilia B, starting in the first or second year of life. These regimens are chosen because they are achievable, but more recent data from Sweden suggest that smaller doses given more frequently may be ideal.[78] Prophylaxis has been usefully divided into categories: primary, started before the age of 2 years, or after the first joint bleed; secondary, either as continuous therapy starting after the age of 2, or after two or more joint bleeds. Secondary can also be periodic treatment given to settle a series of repeated bleeds. Confirmation of these findings by controlled trials is desirable, as there are a number of legitimate criticisms of historical studies, and new studies, which may help evaluate which are the best regimens, are underway in the USA, Canada and Italy.

Several questions remain, such as should prophylaxis be started in the first year of life before there are any joint bleeds? (Not all individuals with very low factor levels have repeated joint bleeds.) Venous access is usually very difficult in the young child – perhaps dosing weekly with escalation with age as veins become more accessible may be as effective. Central venous lines have advantages but they have a significant incidence of infection and thrombosis which will necessitate their removal. While the Swedish and other smaller uncontrolled studies of prophylactic therapy demonstrate improvement in quality of life (reduced days off school and greater satisfaction among the families), other families have found it very hard to persist with the regular injections. There is also no doubt that the availability and cost of factor concentrates is a major issue, even in developed countries. Within the European Network of 20 hemophilia centers (16 countries) the proportion of severe hemophiliac children on continuous prophylaxis varies from 15 to 100%.[80] The unforeseen consequences of blood product infusion [HIV and hepatitis C virus (HCV) infection] have made both patients and their physicians more cautious about the repeated injection of a foreign protein; these concerns are most important to families who have personal experience of the consequences of these viral infections, and who watch the debate about prion disease with understandable anxiety.

Mild hemophilia A (but not hemophilia B) can often be treated with a slow intravenous infusion of high dose desmopressin (1-desamino-8-D-arginine vasopressin; DDAVP). This stimulates release of factor VIIIC from storage sites and can increase the level threefold within an hour of the end of the infusion. This is usually appropriate for minor procedures such as tooth extraction. DDAVP, an antidiuretic hormone (ADH) analog, causes fluid retention. Children should be monitored for this complication, because there is a risk of fits due to cerebral edema, particularly in small infants. Because of this DDAVP is not usually given to infants less than 2 years of age. Major procedures can also be managed in this way although the response declines after several days (tachyphylaxis).

Von Willebrand disease (vWd)

This disease is important, as it is the commonest inherited bleeding disorder with a prevalence of 1 in 100 to 1 in 1000. The defect is in the vWf with secondary effects on factor VIIIC. Binding to vWf protects factor VIIIC from degradation in the circulation. VWf itself has an important role in binding platelets to the vessel wall. This activity is mediated through the glycoprotein 1b receptor on the platelets. VWd has many subtypes. VWf is a large molecule and genetic defects may be either quantitative (type I) or qualitative (type II). VWd is most commonly a mild clinical disorder which is inherited autosomally. Expression in different family members is often variable. A good family history is essential and the implications of the diagnosis explained carefully to other members of the family. Symptoms are those of 'platelet-type' bleeding – bruising, mucous membrane bleeding including epistaxis and menorrhagia in women. This latter is an important and often overlooked symptom. Affected individuals are likely to bleed excessively after surgery.

Laboratory diagnosis

Laboratory diagnosis may not be straightforward and generally full workup should be performed in a hemophilia center with adequate diagnostic facilities. Mild vWd is not usually detected by a 'routine coagulation screen' because the factor VIIIC and APTT are often normal. Assays of the vWf (both immunological and functional) are undertaken, often performed three times because both factor VIIIC and vWf are elevated by stress and may be within the normal range on the first occasion. The bleeding time is not usually helpful in small children and difficult to perform reliably. It is the least sensitive diagnostic test in mild vWd. Severe vWd is more easily diagnosed; the factor VIIIC and vWf are markedly reduced. Genetic analysis for vWd is increasingly available from hemophilia centers.

Treatment

No routine treatment is required in mild vWd. Mucous membrane bleeding (including menorrhagia) in mild vWd is often helped by use of antifibrinolytic drugs such as tranexamic acid. Surgery can often be managed with DDAVP infusions. However, there are some subtypes of vWd with platelet hyperaggregability in which DDAVP is contraindicated. Patients with any form of vWd should always be managed with appropriate hematological advice.

Severe vWd is fortunately rare, usually occurring when each parent has a vWf gene defect which may be asymptomatic or expressed as mild vWd. These individuals may experience joint bleeds similar to severe hemophilia. Treatment will require vWf replacement. Some individuals with recurrent joint bleeds may require prophylaxis with regular treatment. This may be with a plasma-derived factor VIIIC concentrate that contains vWf, or a vWf concentrate. Cryoprecipitate should no longer be used as concentrates are safer and usually effective.

Other hereditary bleeding disorders

Congenital deficiencies of all the coagulation factors have been described but are rare. A coagulation screen will indicate where the defect lies, and which further tests and assays are required. Bleeding symptoms should always be investigated. Families with all types of bleeding disorders are often misdiagnosed initially as non-accidental injury as sadly, this is more common. Specific factor concentrates are available for some of the severe homozyogous disorders (factor VII; factor X is contained in plasma-derived factor IX concentrates). Factor XI deficiency is clinically mild even in severe deficiency and more common amongst Jewish people (with a carrier rate of 8%). Factor XIII is the fibrin-stabilizing factor and its deficiency typically produces delayed hemorrhage 24–36 h after injury, with delayed wound healing and sometimes scarring. Bleeding from the umbilical stump and delayed separation of the cord also occur and give a clue to the diagnosis. Specific assays define the diagnosis of all of these disorders.

ACQUIRED COAGULATION DEFECTS

Although the congenital coagulation deficiencies are important, in clinical practice the acquired causes are much more common, and are usual in the sick child.

Deficiency of vitamin K-dependent coagulation factors

Factors II, VII, IX and X, synthesized in the liver, require vitamin K-dependent addition of the gamma-carboxyl group to make a functional protein. Deficiency can cause a very serious bleeding disorder with a risk of intracranial hemorrhage. Vitamin K is fat soluble and obtained from green vegetables and bacterial synthesis in the gut. Vitamin K-dependent factors are low at birth and fall further in breast-fed infants in the first few days of life. Premature and ill babies are prone to deficiency and should always be supplemented. Classical hemorrhagic disease of the newborn is rarely seen in developed countries, partly because of the national prophylaxis strategy (vitamin K is given to all neonates to prevent the development of bleeding due to deficiency) but also due to general good standards of living. Later presentation of vitamin K deficiency can occur in infants with malabsorption and should be screened for in children with celiac disease, cystic fibrosis and other long term gastrointestinal disorders including obstructive jaundice, pancreatic and small bowel disease. Prophylaxis can be achieved with 5 mg vitamin K orally daily. The PT is very sensitive to factor VII deficiency and is a useful screening test; the APTT will also be long.

Parenteral vitamin K produces a shortening of the PT rapidly, within 2–4 h, but serious bleeding must be treated immediately with fresh frozen plasma (preferably pathogen inactivated). Oral supplements can be used where absorption is likely to be normal.

Liver disease

Liver disease can produce a variety of complex alterations in hemostasis. Acute hepatocellular failure produces a rapidly progressive failure of coagulation factor synthesis, detected initially as marked prolongation of the PT (effect on factor VII) and reduction in fibrinogen. Chronic disease produces variable effects often associated with thrombocytopenia. Liver dysfunction can lead to disruption of fibrinogen synthesis with abnormal forms, but these do not predict bleeding. It also affects the fibrinolytic system and can be prothrombotic because of failure of clearance of activated coagulation proteins.

Consumptive coagulopathy – disseminated intravascular coagulation (DIC)

Blood coagulation is kept in a fine balance with other homeostatic pathways: anticoagulant, proinflammatory, fibrinolytic. Under many conditions these are disturbed, resulting in profound clinical derangements. Normal coagulation is triggered by tissue factor activation. Diverse agents and endothelial damage leading to a procoagulant state can increase tissue factor expression. The endothelial cell has a key role as gatekeeper, regulating not only blood flow but also the pro- versus anticoagulant properties.

Any condition which causes endothelial disturbance (shock from any cause) and sepsis can lead to activation of coagulation with consumption of platelets and coagulation factors. This leads to disseminated intravascular coagulation. Microvascular thrombosis leads to end-organ dysfunction; consumption of factors and triggering of fibrinolysis lead to a bleeding diathesis. The condition varies from subclinical, detectable by testing only, to an acute florid hemorrhagic state. There are no diagnostic laboratory tests, rather a constellation of abnormalities associated with the appropriate clinical circumstances lead to the diagnosis.

The commonest triggers in pediatric practice are infections, particularly Gram negative sepsis and meningococcal infection, and vascular injury (trauma, burns). Neonates with shock are particularly vulnerable resulting in profound hypofibrinogenemia, very long coagulation screening tests and thrombocytopenia. The picture may be rapidly evolving, and in the acute situation repeated monitoring is essential. The key principle in management is to treat the underlying cause – remove the trigger. The bleeding child will need replacement therapy with blood products dictated by the laboratory tests (cryoprecipitate for a low fibrinogen, platelet transfusions for severe thrombocytopenia, and possibly plasma as well). Recently appreciated is that the natural anticoagulants, proteins C and S, and antithrombin, is are usually consumed in addition; there may be a role for replacement of these, particularly in severe sepsis with protein C deficiency.[81]

THROMBOSIS IN CHILDREN

Thrombosis has generally been thought rare in children; indeed the incidence of venous thrombosis is 0.6 per 100 000 of the Dutch population under 14 years of age, compared to 20.2 in those aged 15–24 years, 37 in those aged 25–39 years and 74 in those aged 40–54 years. Nevertheless recent Canadian studies have clearly shown that children are at risk, particularly very ill children with central venous lines.[82] There is a high incidence of thrombotic events in neonates again often related to the use of central lines. In addition to such acquired causes, there is increasing interest in a number of inherited risk factors that predispose to thrombosis in adults. A mutation in the factor V gene (factor V Leiden) which makes the activated factor resistant to breakdown is particularly common in northern Europeans (2–7% of the population).

Protein C, protein S and antithrombin deficiency also increase the risk of thrombosis in heterozygotes, but screening for these deficiencies in asymptomatic offspring of an adult with thrombosis is not justified, and the relevance of these heterozygous states for children with thrombosis is not clear. Such genetic screening should only be performed with appropriate consent. Infants with severe protein C deficiency have a severe thrombotic phenotype that usually presents at, or shortly after, birth with intracerebral thrombosis, blindness and microvascular thrombosis of the skin that is typical (Fig. 21.22). Diagnosis in such infants is urgent as treatment is available with protein C concentrate. Severe protein S deficiency may

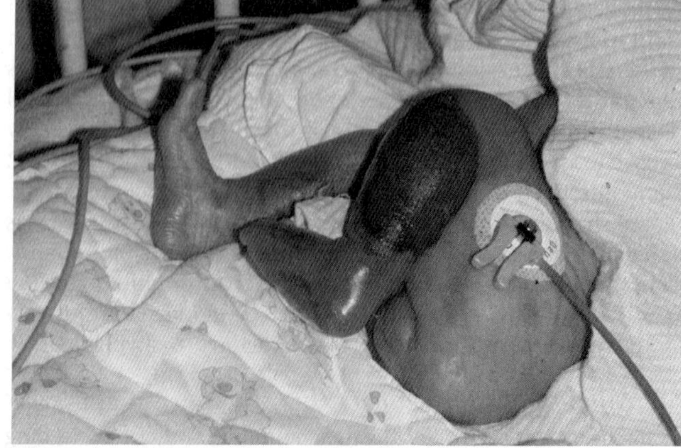

Fig. 21.22 Infant with severe congenital protein C deficiency. Microvascular thrombosis of the skin.

produce a similar picture. Homozygous antithrombin deficiency has not been reported; it is probably incompatible with life. Anticoagulant therapy is appropriate for many of these children, and appropriate protocols are now available, but a hematologist with experience should supervise such children carefully.

LEUKEMIA

INCIDENCE

Leukemia is the commonest malignancy of childhood accounting for approximately 35% of the total. Acute lymphoblastic leukemia (ALL) is much commoner than acute myeloid leukemia (AML) representing 80–85% of all leukemias in this age group. The incidence of leukemia is not constant throughout the world and this can partly be explained by genetic and environmental differences. In Western countries, the incidence is approximately 4/100 000 children up to the age of 15 years,[83] with boys having an incidence 1.2 higher than girls.

CLASSIFICATION OF LEUKEMIA

Distinction between the different types and subtypes of leukemia is essential for optimizing treatment and predicting outcome of disease. Leukemias are classified firstly into acute or chronic forms, indicating the speed of progression of the disease without treatment. Chronic leukemia in children is very rare and is confined to chronic myeloid leukemia (CML). CML accounts for between 2 and 5% of all childhood leukemias and presents as one of two forms: chronic granulocytic leukemia (CGL), which is identical to the adult type CGL or juvenile CML (JCML), recently renamed juvenile myelomonocytic leukemia (JMML),[84] which is a form of myelodysplasia. CGL, JMML and other forms of myelodysplasia carry a risk of progression to acute leukemia.

Cases of acute leukemia can be classified on the basis of morphology, cytochemistry, immunophenotype or cytogenetic abnormality, or by combinations of these characteristics. Ideal classifications of acute leukemias do not yet exist and so information from all these sources must be used together (Table 21.13).[84–87]

Morphologically, the acute leukemias are divided into ALL and AML. The classification most widely used now was first described by the French–American–British (FAB) group in 1976[88] and has subsequently been expanded, modified and clarified over the years. Pediatric myelodysplasia is now recognized as a distinct entity and a prognostic scoring system has been described by Passmore et al.[86] The classification of all these disorders requires both peripheral blood and bone marrow films to be examined and for differential counts to be performed on both. Cytochemical staining can help distinguish lymphoid from myeloid leukemia and also assign the two different leukemias to specific subtypes. This can be important for both informing treatment decisions and predicting outcome. Occasionally acute leukemia cells can show features of both lymphoid and myeloid lines and are described as biphenotypic.

Immunological typing of leukemic cells utilizes immunoenzymatic and immunofluorescent techniques employing a panel of antibodies which recognizes particular cell-surface or cytoplasmic antigens on the blast cells. Immunophenotyping is particularly useful in ALL and in classifying certain types of AML

Table 21.13 The leukemias and myelodysplastic syndromes (After Emanuel 1999,[84] Bennett et al,[85] Passmore et al[86] and Bain[87])

Main group	Subtypes		Chromosomal associations
Acute lymphoblastic leukemia	Early B-precursor	immunophenotype	t(12;21), t(1;19), t(4;11)
	Common		t(12;21), high hyperdiploidy
	Pre-B		
	Null		
	T		t(10;14)
	B		t(8;14); t(8;22), t(2,8)
	L1	morphological	t(12;21), high hyperploidy
	L2		t(12;21), high hyperdiploidy
	L3		t(8;14), t(8;22), t(2;8)
Acute myeloblastic leukemia	M0 undifferentiated		
	M1 without maturation		
	M2 with granulocytic maturation		t(8;21)
	M3 promyelocytic		t(15;17)
	M4 myelomonocytic		
	M4Eo myelomonocytic with eosinophils		inv(16) or t(16;16)
	M5 monocytic/monoblastic		11q23
	M6 erythroleukemia		
	M7 megakaryoblastic		t(1;22)
Myelodysplasia	RA refractory anemia		
	RARS refractory anemia with ringed sideroblasts		
	RAEB refractory anemia with excess blasts (5–20%)		
	RAEBT refractory anemia with excess blasts in transformation (20–30%)		
	JMML juvenile myelomonocytic leukemia		Monosomy 7, never *bcr/abl+*
	Imo 7 infantile monosomy 7		Monosomy 7
	EOS eosinophilia		

(M0 and M7) where the blasts are not easily classifiable morphologically. It will also help identify biphenotypic leukemias where there is expression of the specific markers from both lymphoid and myeloid lines. In ALL, it confirms the diagnosis and separates cases into leukemias of T cell and B cell lineage. Further separation into categories reflecting the stage of maturation at which the abnormal clone expanded is possible. This is so particularly for the B cell leukemias where precursor B cell leukemias (null, pre-B and common) are distinguishable from mature B cell leukemia. These categories show some correlation with cytogenetic subsets and consequently indicate differences in prognosis. It is important to identify mature B cell leukemia which is also identifiable morphologically (FAB L3), and cytogenetically t(8;14) (Table 21.13), since this is treated with chemotherapy designed for B cell non-Hodgkin's lymphoma, not standard ALL therapy.

The mainstay of classification of AML is by morphological characteristics seen on both an ordinary, stained bone marrow aspirate film and those after specific cytochemical staining. Sometimes monoclonal antibody staining is required for precise classification as in megakaryoblastic leukemia (M7). The FAB classification is based on identifying the predominant cell type and the degree of differentiation of the cells. Certain types have characteristic laboratory or clinical features such as disseminated intravascular coagulation with promyelocytic leukemia (M3), gum hyperplasia, skin rash and raised lysozyme levels with monoblastic leukemia (M5) and osteosclerosis and Down syndrome with M7. Certain cytogenetic abnormalities are also associated with specific morphological types and can be important prognostic indicators. These include t(15;17) with M3 and inv(16) with myelomonocytic leukemia with eosinophils (M4Eo), both associated with a good prognosis in children.

Myelodysplasia of the bone marrow was described in the 1930s and 1940s in a variety of ways including primary refractory anemia and preleukemia. The myelodysplastic syndromes (MDS) have been increasingly recognized since then but are rare in childhood and represent between 1 and 9% of all pediatric hematological malignancies.[89] They are often associated with other conditions such as Down syndrome, cardiac abnormalities, neurofibromatosis type 1 and congenital bone marrow disorders. These include Fanconi's anemia and Shwachman–Diamond syndrome which may progress to acute leukemia. Classification by the FAB group[85] is not ideal in childhood as it does not accommodate JMML or infantile monosomy 7, a myelodysplastic condition accurring in young infants which shares many characteristics with JMML. In addition, MDS occurring in association with the congenital bone marrow disorders may not be classifiable, as the bone marrow is often hypoplastic, whereas in adult MDS this occurs in only 10% of cases.

Refractory anemia (RA), where there is anemia with myelodysplastic features, with or without a few ringed sideroblasts, is rare and must be distinguished from the congenital dyserythropoietic anemias (Ch. 10) and megaloblastic anemia (see above). Refractory anemia with ringed sideroblasts (RARS) is exceptionally rare in childhood and must be distinguished from a mitochondrial cytopathy such as Pearson's syndrome (see above). RA and RARS can only be diagnosed with confidence in the presence of clonal cytogenetic abnormalities, but both carry a much better prognosis than other MDS in adults. The distinction between the other types of myelodysplasia, such as refractory anemia with excess blasts (RAEB) or refractory anemia with excess blasts in transformation (RAEBT) and AML depends on the percentage of blasts in the bone marrow. The distinction is potentially important as AML may respond more favorably to chemotherapy. Careful morphological review, to detect multilineage dysplasia seen in true MDS, and cytogenetic analysis, which may be characteristic of one or other condition, may be helpful. The FAB classification has been expanded and a scoring system developed taking into consideration the level of hemoglobin F, platelet count and complexity of karyotype.[86] A favorable score gives a 5-year survival of approximately 60% with all of those with an unfavorable score being dead within 4 years of diagnosis.

CLINICAL TRIALS

It is well recognized that the prognostic significance of nearly all variables depends on the type and intensity of treatment. However, within a particular regimen, it is possible to increase intensity for those at highest risk while decreasing intensity for those with the best prognosis, thus reducing both early and late toxicity. Classification of leukemias morphologically, immunologically and cytogenetically along with certain clinical features has enabled stratification of children into different risk groups within a given type of leukemia, making it possible to give risk-adapted therapy. Many groups have developed different treatment regimens over the past 30 years, building on experience and introducing new drugs or methods of delivery in a controlled way to enable the true effect of any change to be determined. In the UK, > 90% of children with acute leukemia are treated within clinical trials. This enables reliable comparisons between treatments and advances to be made. By standardizing risk categories internationally,[90] it is also possible to compare results from trials conducted in the USA or other parts of Europe, for example.

PRESENTATION

Acute myeloblastic leukemia has a steady incidence throughout childhood although the monoblastic/monocytic types tend to occur relatively more often in infancy. Acute lymphoblastic leukemia is most common between the ages of 2 and 5 years with an increased incidence in boys (ratio M to F is 1.2). Rare cases of congenital leukemia do occur and these are usually but not exclusively malignancies of early B cells. JMML and monosomy 7 tend to occur in infants.

The diagnosis of acute leukemia usually starts from a clinical suspicion. Only very occasionally is it discovered serendipitously when a blood count is done for another reason. The clinical presentation is, for the most part, determined by the degree of bone marrow failure, but other features, secondary to the infiltration of different organs, may give specific signs and symptoms.

General symptoms and signs

The majority of children will give a short history of less than 4 weeks, although a prodrome of a few months is also seen. General symptoms include lethargy, loss of appetite and exhaustion. Bone marrow failure results in anemia, neutropenia and thrombocytopenia.

Anemia

This occurs in most cases but the fall in hemoglobin is gradual and can be very well tolerated initially. The low hemoglobin causes some of the commoner symptoms and signs such as pallor, lethargy, anorexia and breathlessness. Cardiac failure is uncommon even at very low levels of hemoglobin, but tachycardia and flow murmurs are common.

Infection

Susceptibility to infection may be apparent for some time before presentation and some patients may have a serious infection at diagnosis. Pyrexia at presentation may be due to the disease process itself, but since many children are neutropenic, and all are immunosuppressed, the child should be treated for infection with broad-spectrum intravenous antibiotics.

Hemorrhage

This is a frequent presenting feature and can be catastrophic. This is still the commonest cause of the rare deaths, which occur during the first few hours in hospital, and there is a strong association with leukostasis secondary to very high blast counts in the peripheral blood. Most bleeding episodes are milder and secondary to thrombocytopenia. Thrombocytopenia leads to petechiae and other hemorrhagic manifestations, especially mucosal bleeding and easy bruising. Bleeding may also be due to hepatic dysfunction and disseminated intravascular coagulation, the latter particularly with acute promyelocytic leukemia (M3).

Bone and joint involvement

Orthopedic surgeons, rheumatologists and accident and emergency staff frequently see children with bone pain and/or arthralgia and accompanying limp or failure to walk. Up to two-thirds of children with ALL present with bone pain and therefore a full blood count should be checked in children with such symptoms. Examination for hepatosplenomegaly and lymphadenopathy may also help to identify the true diagnosis. Roentgenograms for these children will show changes in at least half, the most frequent of which are transverse radiolucent lines at the metaphyses (Fig. 21.23) and osteopenia sometimes with vertebral collapse. In acute megakaryoblastic leukemia (M7) and other types of leukemia, osteosclerosis can occasionally occur. The bone pain responds rapidly to antileukemic therapy although there may be some exacerbation as treatment starts. Another childhood malignancy, neuroblastoma, may also present with bone pain and anemia with or without thrombocytopenia. However, abnormal cells are rarely seen on the blood film although the bone marrow may be virtually replaced by malignant cells. Immunophenotyping may be helpful and specific tests for neuroblastoma such as urinary catecholamines should be performed.

Hepatosplenomegaly, lymphadenopathy and other organ enlargement

Splenomegaly is present in up to 80% of children with acute leukemia. It is particularly marked in CGL and JMML. The enlargement is smooth, firm and non-tender unless it is chronically enlarged as in CGL when infarction can cause pain and tenderness. Hepatosplenomegaly is present in up to 60% of patients and the kidneys are palpable only occasionally, although abdominal ultrasound will reveal non-palpable renal enlargement quite often in ALL and acute monoblastic leukemia (M5). Ovarian and testicular enlargement are rarely found at diagnosis but regular examination of the testes throughout follow-up, both on and off treatment, is essential as relapse at this site is quite common. Mediastinal enlargement, seen on chest roentgenogram, is almost exclusive to those with T cell ALL and can cause superior vena cava obstruction (Fig. 21.24). Abdominal masses of leukemia/lymphoma tissue not related to the liver and spleen typically occur in B-ALL cases. Infiltration of the sinuses may also occur (Fig. 21.25).

Gum hypertrophy occurs with all types of leukemia but is particularly common with M4 and M5 types (Fig. 21.26). Skin infiltration with leukemia is rare but does occur in the neonatal variety, when it is seen as bluish papules, and can also be seen in M4 and M5 (Fig. 21.27). JMML is associated with a non-specific skin rash, especially on the face.

Meningeal leukemia

Children with ALL virtually all have presymptomatic meningeal leukemia at the time of diagnosis as shown by the inevitability of relapse in those who do not receive CNS-directed therapy. However, a proportion present with blast cells in the CNS, which are often asymptomatic, but can give rise to diffuse or focal neurological signs. The commonest time to present is once treatment has stopped and such a relapse is frequently associated with the symptoms of raised intracranial pressure such as vomiting and severe headaches. Papilledema may be seen and cranial nerve palsies especially of the VIth nerve are common. CNS leukemia rarely presents with hypothalamic involvement, giving rise to hyperphagia and emotional disturbances.

Tumor lysis syndrome

In children with hyperleukocytosis and/or a high leukemia burden secondary to massive organ infiltration, metabolic abnormalities

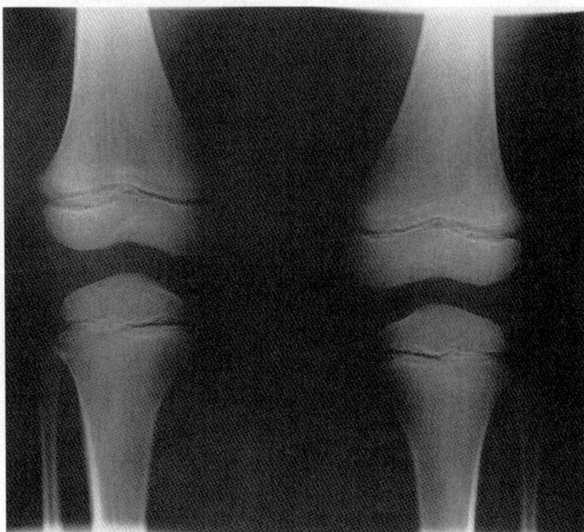

Fig. 21.23 Lymphoblastic leukemia. Knees showing generalized osteoporosis with transverse radiolucent bands across long bone metaphyses adjacent to metaphyseal bone ends, found in malignant infiltration of bone marrow.

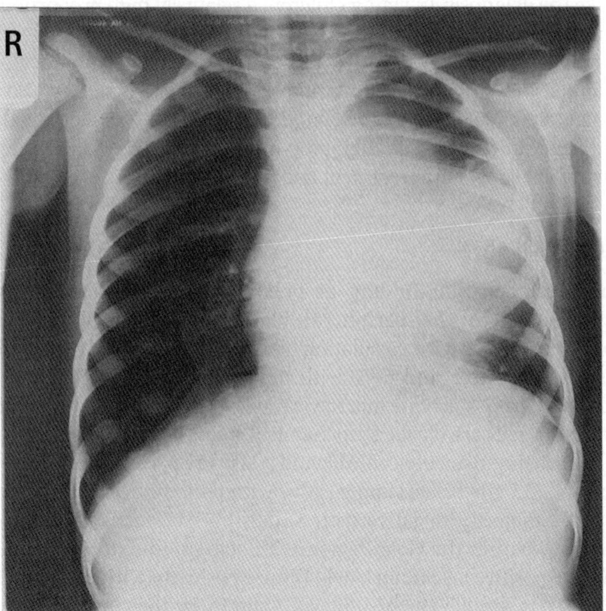

Fig. 21.24 Chest X-ray appearances in acute T cell leukemia with mediastinal widening and hilar lymphadenopathy causing superior vena cava obstruction.

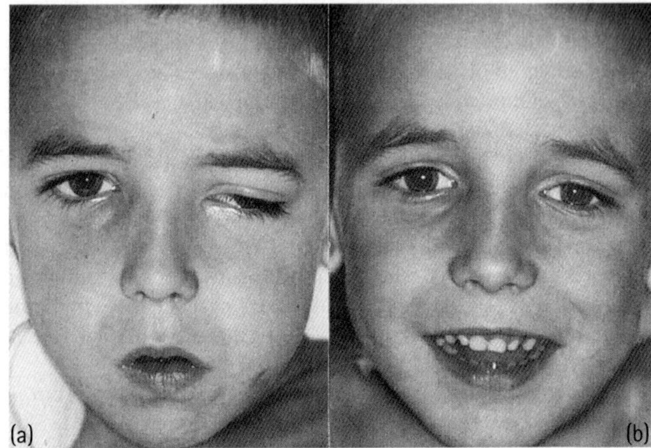

Fig. 21.25 Acute B cell leukemia causing sinus infiltration and 3rd nerve palsy. (a) At presentation. (b) After 3 days of therapy.

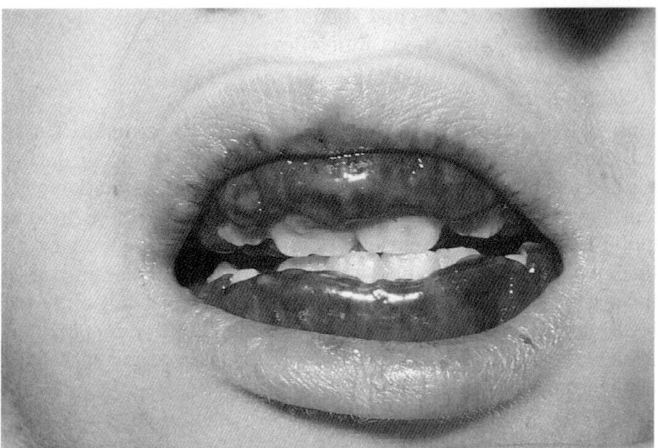
Fig. 21.26 Acute monocytic leukemia causing gum infiltration.

such as hyperkalemia, hyperphosphatemia and hypocalcemia are seen. This is a particular hazard in B-ALL. Hyperuricemia to a varying degree is a common finding at presentation but can be very marked in this syndrome. As treatment is started and there is further lysis of the leukemic cells, the metabolic abnormalities worsen and can lead to renal failure and death. A forced diuresis, a uric acid lowering agent and careful steroid-based cytoreductive treatment may avoid this complication. Renal dialysis may be required in severe cases and leukophoresis or exchange transfusion may be useful.

DIAGNOSIS

It is essential before starting treatment for leukemia that the diagnosis has been made with certainty. Clinical examination and morphological review of well-stained blood and bone marrow films remain the most important parameters for diagnosis. If the bone marrow aspirate is inadequate, a repeat sample with a bone marrow trephine (biopsy) is mandatory. Other diagnostic techniques such as immunophenotyping are complementary but cannot alone be used to make the diagnosis. In young children, a relatively high proportion of lymphocytes both in the blood and bone marrow will express more immature markers, especially if there is a reactive lymphocytosis secondary to an infection for example. Aplastic anemia may also be mistaken for leukemia, as the bone marrow aspirate is often difficult and again may contain a high proportion of early B cells. If there is any doubt, supportive treatment and repeat sampling is essential.

MORPHOLOGY

The most constant finding at presentation of leukemia is an abnormality in the peripheral blood with 99% of children presenting either with circulating blasts and/or thrombocytopenia, 90% with anemia and 67% with neutropenia. Acute leukemia is diagnosed from the bone marrow sample if at least 30% of the total nucleated cells are blasts. Cytochemical stains can then be prepared to help distinguish between ALL and AML. In approximately 80% of cases of ALL the blasts stain positive with periodic acid Schiff (PAS) and the majority negative with Sudan black. T cells show block positivity within the Golgi region with acid phosphatase and AML cells are positive for Sudan black. Diffuse positivity with non-specific esterases is specific for monoblasts. Criteria for the classification of the acute leukemias have been described above.

The presence of CNS disease is assessed from cytospin preparations of cerebrospinal fluid (CSF). The CSF is considered to be positive if > 5 cells/mm^3 with recognizable blast cells are present. Immunophenotyping may be helpful in equivocal cases, as well as cytogenetic analysis, if enough material can be obtained. It is important to determine whether there is involvement with leukemia or not since these patients usually receive more intensive intrathecal chemotherapy and, if over the age of 2 years, cranial irradiation.

In CGL the most consistent finding in the peripheral blood is a leukocytosis, predominantly of mature neutrophils and their precursors (myelocytes and promyelocytes). Eosinophilia and

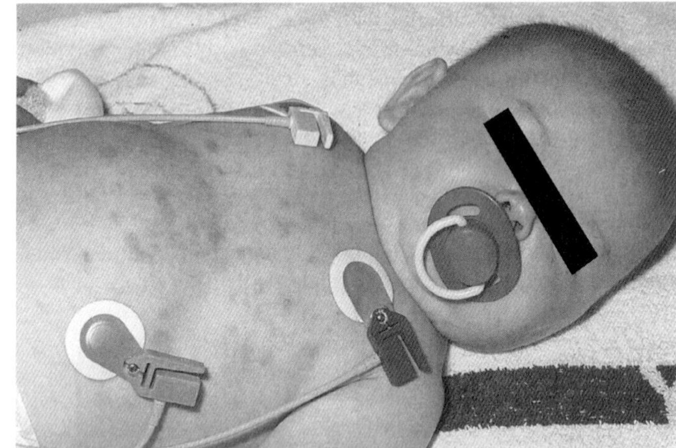
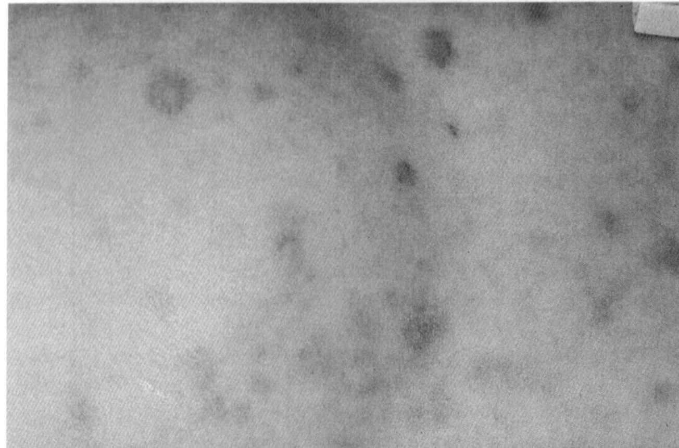
Fig. 21.27 Skin infiltration in an infant with acute monocytic leukemia.

basophilia are commonly present and the white cell count is usually $> 100 \times 10^9$/L at diagnosis. Anemia is usual and platelets are often normal or slightly raised. The bone marrow is markedly hypercellular due to hyperplasia of the granulocyte series. In its chronic phase, blasts constitute < 5% of nucleated cells but increase in the accelerated phase and blast crisis. Cytogenetic analysis shows the Philadelphia chromosome t(9;22) in 90% of patients and the bcr/abl fusion gene can be detected in a proportion of Ph-negative patients.

JMML usually presents with thrombocytopenia and a dysplastic blood film with abnormal monocytes and blast cells. The marrow can be relatively uninformative but associated features include a reversion to a fetal type of hemopoiesis with a high hemoglobin F and the 'i' red cell antigen, and sometimes monosomy 7.

Immunophenotyping

It must be remembered that immunophenotyping is complementary to morphological diagnosis and does not replace it; mistakes in diagnosis can be made if this technique is relied upon in isolation.[91] Immunophenotyping is particularly useful in cases of acute leukemia that are not obviously myeloid, so that a positive diagnosis of ALL can be made and cases of M0 and M7 AML identified. A panel of monoclonal antibodies is used which combines both highly specific and highly sensitive antibodies. Additional antibodies are required for conformation of erythroid leukemia (M6) and M7. Specific antibodies include cytoplasmic (cy) CD22 for B lineage, cy CD3 for T lineage and antimyeloperoxidase (MPO) for myeloid lineage. Sensitive antibodies include CD19, expressed on B cells, CD7 on T cells and CD13/33 on myeloid cells but all may be expressed on cells of other lineage. This aberrant antigen expression is a feature of both ALL and AML and does not mean that the leukemia is biphenotypic. This description is reserved for those leukemias where the more specific antigens (e.g. CD22, CD3, MPO) of more than one lineage are expressed. The prognosis of such leukemias is related to the accompanying cytogenetic abnormalities and many are associated with the Philadelphia chromosome.

Chromosomal analysis

Cytogenetic analysis is carried out by microscopic analysis of cells in metaphase when suitably stained. This technique can be supplemented by fluorescent in situ hybridization (FISH). Molecular cytogenetic analysis, where the DNA from the abnormal cells is analyzed using Southern blotting or polymerase chain reaction (PCR) for example, can be used to establish clonality and also used for detection of minimal residual disease (MRD) to help direct therapy (see later). While some cytogenetic abnormalities identify subtypes of leukemia in a highly specific way, some chromosomal abnormalities occur in both acute and chronic leukemias, ALL and AML and also MDS. Specific cytogenetic abnormalities include t(15;17) in M3, inv(16) in M4Eo and t(8;14) in mature B cell ALL. Other cytogenetic abnormalities such as the Philadelphia chromosome, t(9;22) and monosomy 7 can arise in a variety of leukemias and MDS. In addition to confirming the presence of an abnormal clone in the diagnosis of leukemia or MDS, cytogenetic analysis can also inform both treatment decisions and prediction of outcome.

PROGNOSTIC INDICATORS

The most important prognostic determinants in ALL are the type and intensity of treatment and changes in therapy may alter the significance of other risk factors. Prognostic factors are used to stratify children into different risk groups allowing intensification of therapy in those at highest risk of relapse while decreasing intensity in those in the best prognostic group. In AML, the two parameters of greatest prognostic significance are the karyotype of the malignant cells and response to therapy.

Demographics

In ALL, there is a significant influence of age, sex and presenting white cell count on outcome. The US National Cancer Institute (NCI) set criteria which have been agreed internationally for risk classification based on these parameters.[90] Standard risk patients are aged between 1 and 9 years and have a presenting white cell count of $< 50 \times 10^9$/L, while high risk patients are aged ≥ 10 years or have a white cell count at presentation of $\geq 50 \times 10^9$/L. Approximately 75% of patients with B lineage leukemia are in the standard risk group, while 75% of patients with T lineage leukemia are in the high risk category. Boys have a worse prognosis than girls even after adjusting for age and white cell count. CNS disease at diagnosis is not of prognostic significance.

Morphology

The original morphological classification in ALL is of less prognostic importance than had been supposed[92] but has been of importance in identifying those mature B cell leukemias with a specific morphology (L3). This subtype requires different therapy from the other types of ALL (pre-B and T cell ALL).

In AML, morphology is closely associated with karyotype and this has the most significant influence on outcome.

Chromosomes

For ALL, at the time of the proposed NCI classification, the importance of both cytogenetics and molecular genetics was recognized but were not included in the risk criteria as the tests were not then widely available. Karyotype has now been included in risk stratification, (see above) with those with bcr/abl, hypodiploidy (< 45 chromosomes), or, if 12–24 months old, an MLL gene rearrangement being in the worst prognostic category. The MLL gene rearrangement has a particularly poor prognosis if associated with the translocation t(4;11). By contrast, those with a high hyperdiploid karyotype, that is > 50 chromosomes per cell, do particularly well.[93]

In AML, favorable karyotypes are those with t(8;21), t(15;17) seen with the M3 subtype and inv(16) seen with M4Eo.

Response to treatment

Analysis of the United Kingdom Medical Research Council trials for ALL (UKALL), 1980–1997, has shown that speed of response to treatment is a consistently significant predictor of outcome.[93] The current UKALL trial has included three risk groups taking both response to treatment and karyotype into consideration. The standard risk group (60–65% of children) is as previously defined by NCI criteria; the intermediate risk group (20% of children) has the same parameters as the previous high risk group. A new high risk group (10–12% of children) includes all children irrespective of initial risk group, who have a slow early response to treatment (assessed on bone marrow samples at day 15 for standard risk patients and day 8 for intermediate risk patients) or who have an unfavorable karyotype (see above).

In AML, complete remission (CR), that is < 5% leukaemic cells in the bone marrow after the first course of chemotherapy, confers the best prognosis, while partial remission (PR), that is 5–20% leukaemic cells, is only slightly worse. Patients with resistant disease (RD), defined as > 20% leukaemic cells in the bone marrow after the first course of chemotherapy, have a very poor outlook. There is a correlation between karyotype and bone marrow status such that patients with favorable karyotypes tend to be in CR or PR after one course. Patients with favorable karyotypes who have resistant disease after course 1 appear to have a good prognosis, although the number in this group is very small. Good risk patients are therefore defined as those with a favorable karyotype regardless of their bone marrow status after course 1. Standard risk patients include all those who have no favorable karyotype and do not have RD after course 1. The poor risk group includes all those with RD after course 1 except those with a favorable karyotype.

Minimal residual disease (MRD)

It is hoped that MRD, as a more sensitive measure of response to treatment, will allow a much more accurate stratification of relapse risk than the prognostic indicators described above. MRD detected prior to bone marrow transplant predicts relapse post-transplant and would allow pretransplant intensification.[94] Improved techniques for detection of MRD and long term prospective study of large, comparable cohorts of patients has shown that clearance of MRD is an independent prognostic factor in childhood ALL.[95] This has opened the way for clinical application of MRD measurement in the management of ALL.

In AML, studies on the use of MRD measurement and drug resistance are underway.

TREATMENT

The treatment of acute leukemia requires both the eradication of the leukemic clone, in order that normal bone marrow function may be restored, and supportive care during the period of bone marrow failure, both secondary to the disease itself and to the treatment. AML and ALL are both treated with a combination of chemotherapeutic drugs, with or without radiotherapy, but the pattern of treatment is quite different. In AML, the treatment is concentrated in four or five intensive blocks over a period of 6 months or so whereas in ALL, the treatment begins with an induction block, then intensification blocks followed by a period of maintenance for up to 2 years in girls and 3 years in boys.

Supportive care

Intensive chemotherapy requires expert supportive care and this is best given in a limited number of centers familiar with the treatment of leukemia in children. A multidisciplinary team delivering all aspects of hospital treatment and care of the child at home is necessary and will include nurses, physiotherapists, pharmacists and social workers. In the UK most children are treated within United Kingdom Children's Cancer Study Group (UKCCSG) centers and results from these centers have proved superior to ad hoc therapy elsewhere. Hospitals where pediatricians are able to share care with such centers have been identified so that the majority of therapy can be managed closer to the patients' homes. Supportive care must include easy access to blood products such as platelets and red cell concentrates and the prompt identification and aggressive treatment of infections. Placement of central venous access devices has aided safe delivery of treatment and improved ease of monitoring and delivery of supportive care. Good communication with the parents and patient is essential since understanding the treatment process and its effects will allow families to support their child through the illness more effectively and safely.

Acute lymphoblastic leukemia

The dramatic increase in survival rates from ALL has been achieved by carefully planned progressive randomized trials.[96] Most regimens for ALL are based on the schema in Figure 21.28 and the drugs used are variations of these. With this type of treatment over 97% of patients achieve a remission within the first 4 weeks. Following this period, additional blocks of intensification are required, including drugs not used in the first phase, to eradicate residual resistant leukemic clones. CNS-directed therapy – intrathecal (i.t.) chemotherapy, high-dose intravenous (i.v.) chemotherapy or CNS irradiation – is given during this phase. For those with CNS disease, i.t. methotrexate and cranial irradiation are given, but this is not required if the CSF is negative for leukemic cells. In those with a negative CSF and a peripheral white cell count $< 50 \times 10^9/L$, a long course of i.t. methotrexate achieves the same disease-free survival as those given high-dose i.v. methotrexate with i.t. methotrexate.[93] For those with counts $\geq 50 \times 10^9/L$ no difference was seen in event-free survival at 8 years for those who received high-dose i.v. methotrexate and i.t methotrexate compared to cranial irradiation and i.t. methotrexate.

The overall 10 year event-free survival in the most recent UKALL study, UKALL XI (1990–1997), was 60%.[93] These results are not as good as others such as those from the US Children's Cancer Study Group (USCCSG) during the same time period. However, overall survival, 79% at 9 years, is comparable and is due to a good response to salvage therapy (see below). Although patients may be salvaged with retreatment, it is at the price of greater toxicity. To try to address the lower event-free survival, in the current Medical Research Council (MRC) trial, MRC ALL 97/99, the three different risk categories have varying intensity of induction therapy and intensification blocks. Once completed, maintenance therapy of a daily thiopurine, weekly oral methotrexate and monthly pulses of vincristine with 5 days of steroid continues until the total treatment period is just over 2 years for girls and 3 years for boys.

Patients with high risk factors such as bcr/abl, hypodiploidy or t(4;11) can be considered for allogeneic transplantation during first remission of disease.

Relapsed ALL

Nowadays most relapses occur following cessation of therapy. Most of these occur in the first year after stopping therapy and there is a diminishing risk thereafter. Any type of relapse that occurs whilst treatment is still being given carries a very poor prognosis

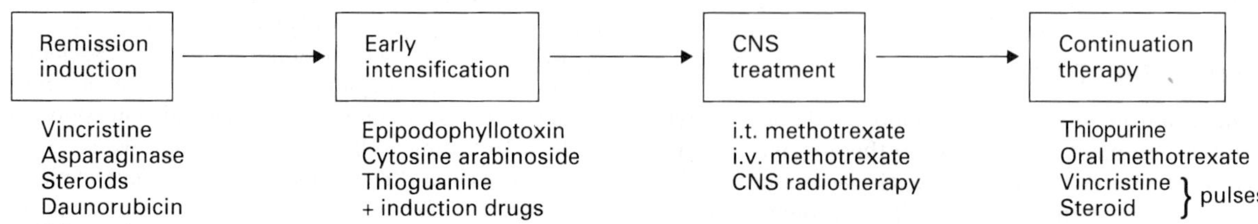

Fig. 21.28 Scheme for treatment of acute lymphoblastic leukemia. Drugs listed are only examples of those which can be used.

and allogeneic transplantation from a histocompatible donor, related or unrelated, should be considered.

The commonest type of relapse is that occurring in the bone marrow following cessation of therapy. In a number of cases, further investigation reveals disease in other sites, either the CNS or testicles or both. Relapse at other sites such as the ovary, eye, tonsils and skin is very rare. All such relapses require intensive chemotherapy with CNS-directed therapy and appropriate local therapy. The intensity of treatment prior to relapse appears to influence the chance of success of retreatment. In the UKALL XI trial, those who relapsed after two intensification modules were more salvageable than those relapsing after three.[93] The usual plan for retreatment includes the standard four-drug induction therapy and then to intensification of treatment with different drugs in high dosage in an attempt to eradicate the residual resistant disease. The results of the most recent UKALL study in relapsed ALL, UKALL R1, show a greater success in retrieving patients within the UK, at least those who relapsed more than 6 months off treatment (5-year event-free survival of 57%), with chemotherapy alone, compared with other published series.[97] Where the relapse has occurred early, fewer than 6 months off treatment, once remission has been achieved, allogeneic bone marrow treatment from a related or unrelated donor is indicated.

CNS relapse is the next most common site after bone marrow relapse. It should be regarded, as in other 'isolated' extramedullary relapses, as a local manifestation of systemic disease and treatment should include intensive systemic therapy as well as local therapy. Local therapy includes extended i.t. therapy and cranial or craniospinal irradiation at a dose dependent on the dose, if any, given during first-line therapy. With this type of therapy, about one-half of patients achieve a long term remission (> 5 years).

Testicular relapse is the third most common site of relapse but can be treated with a good chance of success, especially if isolated. With intensive systemic therapy, CNS-directed therapy and testicular irradiation, there is a > 70% chance of cure.

AML

Therapy in AML includes remission induction, CNS-directed therapy and postremission therapy. However, in contrast to treatment for ALL, the therapy is given in intensive blocks over a shorter duration. This, along with improved supportive care, has resulted in a significant increase in survival over the past 15 years. The current MRC AML trial is based on risk directed therapy, taking account of karyotype and response to treatment (see above). In the good and standard risk groups, chemotherapy alone is recommended, whereas in the poor risk group, transplantation is considered if there is a matched sibling donor.

The results of the MRC AML 10 trial, which included adults and children, show a complete remission rate of 92% in children and an overall 7-year survival from entry of 56%.[98] However, when the pediatric data were analyzed by risk category, the 5-year survival for the good risk group (20% of children) was 77%, for standard risk (67% of children) 63% and for poor risk (10% of children) 15%. Autologous transplantation in this trial did not confer a survival benefit. Specific therapy for different subtypes of leukemia is not given except in the case of M3 which responds to all-trans retinoic acid (ATRA) in conjunction with the standard chemotherapy. CNS-directed therapy is given as three courses of i.t. therapy with three agents, methotrexate, cytosine arabinoside and hydrocortisone, if there is no CNS disease. If CNS disease is present, an extended course of i.t. therapy is given with cranial irradiation at the end of treatment for those > 2 years of age.

BMT

The principle of BMT is the provision of a source of hemopoietic stem cells to repopulate the bone marrow after conditioning therapy has destroyed the patient's own bone marrow cells. The term bone marrow transplant is becoming outdated as alternative sources of hemopoietic stem cells are found, e.g. peripheral blood stem cells and cord blood stem cells.

Allogeneic stem cells may be obtained either from an HLA-identical sibling, partially matched relation or unrelated donor. The most well-evaluated transplants at present are those with matched sibling donors, although increasing experience is being gained with unrelated donor transplantation. Partially matched family donors have mostly been used for transplantation of those with a primary immune deficiency where it is showing some success.

Preparative or conditioning therapy in leukemia is designed to eradicate residual leukemia, immunosuppress sufficiently to prevent graft rejection and to make space for new marrow. Preparative regimens include high dose chemotherapy, with or without total body irradiation (TBI). The morbidity of BMT, both early and late, is considerable and there is a significant mortality associated with the procedure. It is essential that the use and effectiveness of BMT in the treatment of leukemia be carefully monitored in controlled trials to ensure that the benefits outweigh the morbidity and mortality.

Late sequelae of leukemia therapy

About 30 years ago very few children recovered from leukemia, now more than half survive. Currently around one in a thousand adolescents is a survivor of malignant disease in childhood, many of whom will have been treated in an era of less intensive therapy. Recognition of the long term effects of therapy and their impact upon quality of life is therefore gaining increased importance in the management of leukemia. Risk stratification is used to try to identify those who will be cured with less intensive therapy thus reducing toxicity and targeting the more intensive therapy at those at greatest risk of relapse. Both chemotherapy and irradiation have long term effects but those secondary to irradiation can be particularly marked. Sequelae include cardiotoxicity, predominantly from anthracycline use, and growth retardation, cataracts, hypothyroidism, infertility and other endocrine function disturbances, predominantly from TBI and/or cranial irradiation. The neuropsychologic effects of TBI are unknown and likewise, the different modes of CNS-directed therapy. These are being evaluated in a cohort of patients in the UKALL XI trial.

The risk of developing a second malignancy after successful treatment of leukemia is low with an estimated cumulative risk of around 2.5% at 15 years. The majority of tumors develop in the radiation field and exposure to radiotherapy appears to have a continuous risk of a second neoplasm.

It is essential that long-term survivors of childhood malignancy are carefully followed up and late effects recorded so that appropriate modifications to therapy can be made for current and future generations of patients.

REFERENCES (* Level 1 evidence)

1 Hetzel TM, Losek JD. Unrecognized severe anemia in children presenting with respiratory distress. Am J Emerg Med 1998; 16(4):386–389.

2 Hoffbrand AV, Pettit JE, Moss PAH. Essential haematology, 4th edn. Oxford: Blackwell Science: 2001:23.

3 Nathan DG, Oski FA. Hematology of infancy and childhood, 4th edn. London: WB Saunders; 1992.

4 Walter T. Effect of iron-deficiency anaemia on cognitive skills in infancy and childhood. Baillieres Clin Haematol 1994; 7(4):815–827.

*5 Grantham-McGregor S, Ani C. A review of studies on the effect of iron deficiency on cognitive development in children. J Nutr 2001; 131(2S-2):649S-666S, discussion 666S–668S.

*6 Logan S, Martins S, Gilbert R. Iron therapy for improving psychomotor development and cognitive function in children under the age of three with iron deficiency anaemia (Cochrane Review). Cochrane Database Syst Rev 2001; 2:CD001444.

7 Piomelli S. Lead poisoning. In: Nathan DG, Orkin SJ, eds. Hematology of infancy and childhood. Vol 1. Philadelphia: W.B.Saunders; 1998:480–496.

8 Hoffbrand AV. Pernicious anemia. Scot Med J 1983; 28:218–227.

*9 Rabb LM, Grandison Y, Mason K, et al. A trial of folate supplementation in children with homozygous sickle cell disease. Br J Haematol 1983; 54(4):589–594.

10 Zittoun J. Congenital errors of folate metabolism. Baillieres Clin Haematol 1995; 8:603–616.

11 Lovblad K, Ramelli G, Remonda L, et al. Retardation of myelination due to dietary vitamin B12 deficiency: cranial MRI findings. Pediatr Radiol 1997; 27(2):155–158.

12 Linnell JC, Bhatt HR. Inherited errors of cobalamin metabolism and their management. Baillieres Clin Haematol 1995; 8(3):567–601.

13 Grasbeck R. Selective cobalamin malabsorption and the cobalamin-intrinsic factor receptor. Acta Biochim Pol 1997; 44(4):725–733.

14 Grange DK, Finlay JL. Nutritional vitamin B12 deficiency in a breastfed infant following maternal gastric bypass. Pediatr Hematol Oncol 1994; 11(3):311–318.

15 Monagle PT, Tauro GP. Infantile megaloblastosis secondary to maternal vitamin B12 deficiency. Clin Lab Haematol 1997; 19(1):23–25.

16 Salameh MM, Banda RW, Mohdi AA. Reversal of severe neurological abnormalities after vitamin B12 replacement in the Imerslund-Grasbeck syndrome. J Neurol 1991; 238(6): 349–350.

17 Altay C, Cetin M. Oral treatment in selective vitamin B12 malabsorption. J Pediatr Hematol Oncol 1997; 19(3):245–246.

18 Alter BP, Potter NU. Classification and aetiology of the aplastic anemias. Clin Haematol 1978; 7:431–466.

19 Ball SE. The modern management of severe aplastic anaemia. Br J Haematol 2000; 110(1):41–53.

20 Schrezenmeier H, Bacigalupo A, Aglietta M, et al. Guidelines for the treatment of aplastic anemia. Consensus document of a group of international experts. In: Schrezenmeier H, Bacigalupo A, eds. Aplastic anemia. Cambridge: Cambridge University Press; 2000:308.

21 Alter BP. Aplastic anemia, pediatric aspects. Oncologist 1996; 1(6):361–366.

22 Freedman MH, Doyle JJ. Inherited bone marrow failure syndromes. In: Lilleyman JS, Hann IM, Blanchette VS, eds. Pediatric hematology. London: Churchill Livingstone; 1999:23–49.

*23 Guardiola P, Pasquini R, Dokal I, et al. Outcome of 69 allogeneic stem cell transplantations for Fanconi anemia using HLA-matched unrelated donors: a study on behalf of the European Group for Blood and Marrow Transplantation. Blood 2000; 95(2):422–429.

24 Dokal I. Severe aplastic anemia including Fanconi's anemia and dyskeratosis congenita. Curr Opin Hematol 1996; 3(6):453–460.

25 Dokal I. The genetics of Fanconi's anaemia. Baillieres Best Pract Res Clin Haematol 2000; 13(3):407–425.

26 Dokal I. Dyskeratosis congenita in all its forms. Br J Haematol 2000; 110(4):768–779.

27 Smith OP, Hann IM, Chessells JM, et al. Haematological abnormalities in Shwachman–Diamond syndrome. Br J Haematol 1996; 94(2):279–284.

28 Dror Y, Freedman MH. Shwachman–Diamond syndrome marrow cells show abnormally increased apoptosis mediated through the Fas pathway. Blood 2001; 97(10):3011–3016.

29 Dror Y, Freedman MH. Shwachman–Diamond syndrome: an inherited preleukemic bone marrow failure disorder with aberrant hematopoietic progenitors and faulty marrow microenvironment. Blood 1999; 94(9): 3048–3054.

30 Dror Y, Squire J, Durie P, et al. Malignant myeloid transformation with isochromosome 7q in Shwachman–Diamond syndrome. Leukemia 1998; 12(10):1591–1595.

31 van den Oudenrijn S, Bruin M, Folman CC, et al. Mutations in the thrombopoietin receptor, Mpl, in children with congenital amegakaryocytic thrombocytopenia. Br J Haematol 2000; 110(2):441–448.

32 Thompson AA, Woodruff K, Feig SA, et al. Congenital thrombocytopenia and radio–ulnar synostosis: a new familial syndrome. Br J Haematol 2001; 113(4):866–870.

33 Farhi DC, Luebbers EL, Rosenthal NS. Bone marrow biopsy findings in childhood anemia: prevalence of transient erythroblastopenia of childhood. Arch Pathol Lab Med 1998; 122(7):638–641.

34 Ball SE, McGuckin CP, Jenkins G, et al. Diamond–Blackfan anaemia in the UK: analysis of 80 cases from a 20-year birth cohort. Br J Haematol 1996; 94(4):645–653.

35 Willig TN, Ball SE, Tchernia G. Current concepts and issues in Diamond–Blackfan anemia. Curr Opin Hematol 1998; 5(2):109–115.

36 Freedman MH. Diamond–Blackfan anaemia. Baillieres Best Pract Res Clin Haematol 2000; 13(3):391–406.

37 Lissauer T, Clayden G, eds. Illustrated textbook of paediatrics, 2nd edn. Edinburgh: Mosby; 2001:301.

38 Agre P, Asimos A, Casella JF, et al. Inheritance pattern and clinical response to splenectomy as a reflection of erythrocyte spectrin deficiency in hereditary spherocytosis. New Engl J Med 1986; 315(25):1579–1583.

39 Bolton-Maggs PH. The diagnosis and management of hereditary spherocytosis. Baillieres Best Pract Res Clin Haematol 2000; 13(3):327–342.

40 Guidelines for the prevention and treatment of infection in patients with an absent or dysfunctional spleen. Working Party of the British Committee for Standards in Haematology Clinical Haematology Task force. BMJ 1996; 312:430–434.

41 Mentzer WC, Lubin BH. Red cell membrane abnormalities. Pediatric hematology. London: Churchill Livingstone; 1999:257–283.

42 Jacobasch G. Biochemical and genetic basis of red cell enzyme deficiencies. Baillieres Best Pract Res Clin Haematol 2000; 13(1):1–20.

43 Beutler E, Luzzatto L. Hemolytic anemia. Semin Hematol 1999; 36(4 Suppl 7):38–47.

45 Hoffbrand AV, Pettit JE. Essential haematology, 3rd edn. Oxford: Blackwell; 1993.

46 Overturf GD. Infections and immunizations of children with sickle cell disease. Adv Pediatr Infect Dis 1999; 14:191–218.

47 Davies S, Olujohungbe A. Hydroxyurea for sickle cell disease (Cochrane Review). Cochrane Database Syst Rev 2001; 2:CD002202.

48 Walters MC. Bone marrow transplantation for sickle cell disease: where do we go from here? J Pediatr Hematol Oncol 1999; 21(6):467–474.

*49 Walters MC, Storb R, Patience M, et al. Impact of bone marrow transplantation for symptomatic sickle cell disease: an interim report. Multicenter investigation of bone marrow transplantation for sickle cell disease. Blood 2000; 95(6):1918–1924.

50 Hoppe CC, Walters MC. Bone marrow transplantation in sickle cell anemia. Curr Opin Oncol 2001; 13(2):85–90.

51 Serjeant G. Sickle cell disease. In: Lilleyman JS, Hann IM, Blanchette VS, eds. Pediatric hematology. London: Churchill Livingstone; 1999:219–230.

52 Olivieri N. Thalassaemia: clinical management. Baillieres Clin Haematol 1998; 11(1):147–162.

*53 Olivieri NF, Brittenham GM, McLaren CE, et al. Long-term safety and effectiveness of iron-chelation therapy with deferiprone for thalassemia major. New Engl J Med 1998; 339(7):417–423.

54 Olivieri NF. The beta-thalassemias. New Engl J Med 1999; 341(2):99–109.

55 Mentzer WC. Bone marrow transplantation for hemoglobinopathies. Curr Opin Hematol 2000; 7(2):95–100.

56 Lucarelli G. Bone marrow transplantation for thalassaemia. J Intern Med Suppl 1997; 740:49–52.

57 Lucarelli G, Galimberti M, Giardini C, et al. Bone marrow transplantation in thalassemia. The experience of Pesaro. Ann N Y Acad Sci 1998; 850:270–275.

58 Lucarelli G, Clift RA, Galimberti M, et al. Bone marrow transplantation in adult thalassemic patients. Blood 1999; 93(4):1164–1167.

59 Miniero R, Rocha V, Saracco P, et al. Cord blood transplantation (CBT) in hemoglobinopathies. Eurocord. Bone Marrow Transplant 1998; 22(suppl 1):S78–79.

60 Kulozik AE. Hemoglobin variants and the rarer hemoglobin disorders. In: Lilleyman JS, Hann IM, Blanchette VS, eds. Pediatric hematology. London: Churchill Livingstone; 1999:231–256.

61 Spivak JL. The blood in systemic disorders. Lancet 2000; 355(9216): 1707–1712.

62 Bodey GP, Buckley M, Sathe YS, et al. Quantitative relationships between circulating leukocytes and infection in patients with acute leukemia. Ann Intern Med 1966; 64(2):328–340.

63 Bux J, Behrens G, Welte K. Diagnosis and clinical course of autoimmune neutropenia in infancy: analysis of 240 cases. Blood 1998; 91(1):181–186.

64 Dinauer MC. The phagocyte system and disorders of granulopoiesis and granulocyte function. In: Nathan DG, Orkin SH, eds. Hematology of infancy and childhood. Vol. 1. Philadelphia: WB Saunders; 1998:922.

65 Warrier I, Lusher JM. Congenital thrombocytopenias. Curr Opin Hematol 1995; 2(5):395–401.

66 Hall GW. Kasabach–Merritt syndrome: pathogenesis and management. Br J Haematol 2001; 112(4):851–862.

67 Bolton-Maggs PH, Moon I. Assessment of UK practice for management of acute childhood idiopathic thrombocytopenic purpura against published guidelines [see comments]. Lancet 1997; 350(9078):620–623.

68 Lilleyman JS. Intracranial hemorrhage in chronic childhood ITP [editorial]. Pediatr Hematol Oncol 1997; 14(5):iii–v.

69 Eden OB, Lilleyman JS. Guidelines for management of idiopathic thrombocytopenic purpura. The British Paediatric Haematology Group. Arch Dis Child 1992; 67(8):1056–1058.

70 Dickerhoff R, von Ruecker A. The clinical course of immune thrombocytopenic purpura in 55 consecutive children who did not receive intravenous immunoglobulin or sustained prednisone. J Pediatr 2000; 137(5):629–632.

71 Bolton-Maggs PH, Dickerhoff R, Vora AJ. The nontreatment of childhood ITP (or the art of medicine consists of amusing the patient until nature cures the disease). Semin Thromb Hemost 2001; 27(3):269–275.

72 Buchanan GR, Adix L. Outcome measures and treatment endpoints other than platelet count in childhood idiopathic thrombocytopenic purpura. Semin Thromb Hemost 2001; 27(3):277–285.

73 Lilleyman JS. Management of childhood idiopathic thrombocytopenic purpura. Br J Haematol 1999; 105(4):871–875.

74 Dahlback B. Blood coagulation. Lancet 2000; 355(9215):1627–1632.

75 Rizza CR, Spooner RJ, Giangrande PLF on behalf of the UK Haemophilia Centre Directors' Organisation. Treatment of haemophilia in the United Kingdom 1981–1996. Haemophilia 2001; 7:349–359.

76 Darby SC, Ewart DW, et al on behalf of the UK Haemophilia Centre Directors' Organisation. Mortality before and after HIV infection in the complete UK population of haemophiliacs. Nature 1995; 377:79–82.

77 Darby SC, Ewart DW, et al for the UK Haemophilia Centre Directors' Organisation. Mortality from liver cancer and liver disease in haemophilic men and boys in the UK given blood products contaminated with hepatitis C. Lancet 1997; 340:1421–1431.

78 Ljung RC. Prophylactic treatment in Sweden – overtreatment or optimal model? Haemophilia 2000; 4(4):409–412.

79 Aledort LM, Haschmeye RH, Pettersson H. A longitudinal study of orthopaedic outcomes for severe factor-VIII-deficient haemophiliacs. The Orthopaedic Outcome Study Group. J Intern Med 1994; 236(4):391–399.

80 Ljung R, Aronis-Vournas S, Kurnik-Auberger K, et al. Treatment of children with haemophilia in Europe: a survey of 20 centres in 16 countries. Haemophilia 2000; 6(6):619–624.

*81 Bernard GR, Vincent JL, Laterre PF, et al. Efficacy and safety of recombinant human activated protein C for severe sepsis. New Engl J Med 2001; 344(10):699–709.

82 Andrew M, David M, Adams M, et al. Venous thromboembolic complications (VTE) in children: first analyses of the Canadian Registry of VTE. Blood 1994; 83(5):1251–1257.

83 Parkin DM, Stiller CA, Draper GJ, et al. The international incidence of childhood cancer. Int J Cancer 1988; 42(4):511–520.

84 Emanuel PD. Myelodysplasia and myeloproliferative disorders in childhood: an update. Br J Haematol 1999; 105(4):852–863.

*85 Bennett JM, Catovsky D, Daniel MT, et al. Proposals for the classification of the myelodysplastic syndromes. Br J Haematol 1982; 51(2):189–199.

*86 Passmore SJ, Hann IM, Stiller CA, et al. Pediatric myelodysplasia: a study of 68 children and a new prognostic scoring system. Blood 1995; 85(7):1742–1750.

87 Bain BJ. Acute leukemia: immunophenotyping, cytogenetics and molecular genetics – the MIC and MIC-M classifications. In: Bain BJ, ed. Leukemia diagnosis. Blackwell Science; 1999:53–112.

*88 Bennett JM, Catovsky D, Daniel MT, et al. Proposals for the classification of the acute leukemias. French–American–British (FAB) co-operative group. Br J Haematol 1976; 33(4):451–458.

89 Chessells JM. Myelodysplastic syndromes. In: Lilleyman JS, Hann IM, Blanchette VS, eds. Pediatric hematology. London: Churchill Livingstone; 1999:83–101.

90 Smith M, Arthur D, Camitta B, et al. Uniform approach to risk classification and treatment assignment for children with acute lymphoblastic leukemia. J Clin Oncol 1996; 14(1):18–24.

91 Chessells JM. Pitfalls in the diagnosis of childhood leukaemia annotation. Br J Haematol 2001; 114(3):506–511.

*92 Lilleyman JS, Hann IM, Stevens RF, et al. Cytomorphology of childhood lymphoblastic leukaemia: a prospective study of 2000 patients. United Kingdom Medical Research Council's Working Party on Childhood Leukaemia. Br J Haematol 1992; 81(1):52–57.

*93 Eden OB, Harrison G, Richards S, et al. Long-term follow-up of the United Kingdom Medical Research Council protocols for childhood acute lymphoblastic leukaemia, 1980–1997. Medical Research Council Childhood Leukaemia Working Party. Leukemia 2000; 14(12):2307–2320.

94 Goulden N, Oakhill A, Steward C. Practical application of minimal residual disease assessment in childhood acute lymphoblastic leukaemia annotation. Br J Haematol 2001; 112(2):275–281.

*95 Coustan-Smith E, Sancho J, Hancock ML, et al. Clinical importance of minimal residual disease in childhood acute lymphoblastic leukemia. Blood 2000; 96(8):2691–2696.

*96 Schrappe M, Camitta B, Pui CH, et al. Long-term results of large prospective trials in childhood acute lymphoblastic leukemia. Leukemia 2000; 14(12):2193–2194.

*97 Lawson SE, Harrison G, Richards S, et al. The UK experience in treating relapsed childhood acute lymphoblastic leukaemia: a report on the medical research council UKALLR1 study. Br J Haematol 2000; 108(3):531–543.

*98 Stevens RF, Hann IM, Wheatley K, et al. Marked improvements in outcome with chemotherapy alone in paediatric acute myeloid leukemia: results of the United Kingdom Medical Research Council's 10th AML trial. MRC Childhood Leukaemia Working Party. Br J Haematol 1998; 101(1):130–140.

22

Oncology

Tim Eden, Guy Makin

INCIDENCE AND PREVALENCE

Childhood cancer is relatively rare in the United Kingdom with cumulative incidence rates up to age 15 reported for the time period 1981–1990 of 1774 per million with an age standardized rate of 122.1 per million for England and Wales.[1] In Scotland the rates are marginally higher at 1806 and 124.9 per million respectively.[2] These figures mean that of the 10 million children in the United Kingdom approximately 1200 (1 in every 8000) are diagnosed with the disease each year, which amounts to about 1 child in every 600 developing a malignancy before their fifteenth birthday.[3] Relative and absolute incidence figures for individual tumor types are shown in Tables 22.1 and 22.2 (derived from Parkin et al[3]). Compared with adults the total incidence of childhood tumors is relatively constant around the world, with cumulative incidences (0–15 years) in the range of 1–2.5 per 1000 and age standardized rates between 70 and 160 per million.[3] However there are quite marked variations in the incidence of particular types of childhood cancer between countries. These variations can be related to other diseases masking cancer, variable diagnostic and reporting methods, as well as genuine variations in incidence due to differences in a variety of genetic and environmental factors.

It is essential to have population based registration of all cancers in a particular region or country before firm conclusions can be reached about such definite diagnostic variations. Such registration also requires there to be universal agreement on tumor classification which is especially important in childhood where tumor types are histologically very diverse. The standard system used is the international classification of childhood cancer[4] developed in collaboration with the International Society of Pediatric Oncology based on the Birch & Marsden scheme.[5]

Acute leukemia, the commonest individual malignancy in the UK, accounts for 30% of tumors with acute lymphoblastic leukemia predominating (80–85% of cases). A childhood peak (2–6 years) is seen in resource rich countries but is missing in many less privileged communities (see below for etiology). Acute myeloid leukemia (AML) shows rather less variation except for apparently high rates amongst indigenous Pacific Island populations. Genetic variations may alone or in combination with environmental factors explain the high rates of certain tumors, for example retinoblastoma in North East India and sub-Saharan Africa. Environmental factors undoubtedly explain the very high incidence of B cell lymphomas in equatorial Africa and variations in overall and subset types of Hodgkin's disease around the world. Some variations such as the low incidence of Ewing's sarcoma seen in West Africa and amongst American blacks have not yet been fully explained. Similarly the reason for sex differences in incidence and indeed survival seen for many tumors also remain incompletely explained (see Table 22.2).

The incidence of some tumors appears to be increasing, at least in some parts of the United Kingdom. Significant linear increases in acute lymphoblastic leukemia (ALL) of precursor B cell origin (average annual increase 0.7%), most commonly in boys and Hodgkin's disease (1.2% average annual rise) have been reported in the North West of England over the 45 year time period 1954–1998.[6–8] Variations in AML incidence are not reported in that series but have been identified elsewhere. In addition McNally et al.[6–8] also reported a rising incidence of solid tumors, most notably an annual increase of 1% in pilocytic astrocytoma and primitive neuroectodermal tumors and even higher rises in miscellaneous gliomas (2.3%) and of germ cell tumors (2.6%). The increases are not attributable to changes in diagnostic or reporting practice.[8]

Table 22.1 Crude relative incidence figures for childhood cancers and relative percentage for ages 0–15 years

Tumor type	England and Wales		Nigeria Ibadan		India Madras	
	M/F	Rel %	M/F	Rel %	M/F	Rel %
Leukemia	1.2	32.6	2.1	12.0	1.7	29.4
ALL	1.3	26.1	2.8	3.9	1.7	22.1
ANLL	1.0	5.3	3.0	1.0	1.7	5.3
Lymphomas	2.4	10.0	2.3	39.7	2.8	23.0
Hodgkin's	2.2	4.3	8.0	4.7	3.1	10.3
Non-Hodgkin's	2.5	4.9	1.8	2.9	2.6	8.4
Burkitt's	3.2	0.4	2.0	26.6	1.5	0.5
Unspecified	1.9	0.2	2.5	5.5	2.4	3.8
Brain and spinal neoplasms	1.2	22.5	1.3	15.9	1.7	10.4
Neuroblastoma (& other sympathetic nervous system)	1.1	7.0	–	0.3	1.0	2.4
Retinoblastoma	1.2	2.7	1.5	9.7	1.0	9.4
Renal	0.9	5.8	0.7	6.5	1.0	4.5
Wilms'	0.9	5.7	0.6	6.3	1.0	4.5
Hepatic	1.4	0.9	1.0	1.6	2.7	1.0
Hepatoblastoma	1.4	0.7	–	0.8	2.5	0.6
Malignant bone	0.9	4.8	1.8	2.9	1.2	4.8
Osteosarcoma	0.9	2.5	2.0	0.8	1.3	1.9
Ewing's sarcoma	1.0	2.1	–	–	0.6	2.0
Soft tissue sarcoma	1.2	6.8	1.4	7.6	1.5	5.6
Rhabdomyosarcoma	1.2	4.3	1.0	5.2	1.5	3.1
Germ cell and gonadal	0.9	3.5	–	0.5	0.3	3.0
Carcinomas and epithelial	0.8	3.0	3.5	2.3	1.3	3.6

Data derived and modified from Parkin et al 1998[3]
(England and Wales Registry – Stiller et al 1998,[1] pp 365–367; Ibadan Nigeria – Thomas JO, Aghadiuno PU, pp 43–45; India Madras – Shanta V, Gajalakshmi CK, Swaminathan R, pp 169–171.)
M/F ratio, male to female ratio; ALL, Acute lymphoblastic leukemia; ANLL, Acute non-lymphoblastic leukemia.

Table 22.2 Age standardized incidence rates per million children for ages 0–15 by sex

Tumor type	England & Wales		USA, SEER			
			White		Black	
	Male	Female	M	F	M	F
All tumors	130.8	113.1	160.7	139.3	116.3	119.6
Leukemias	43.7	37.7	50.8	42.8	30.9	27.9
Lymphomas	15.3	6.8	19.9	10.2	13.0	8.1
Hodgkin's	6.2	2.9	7.1	5.2	5.4	3.2
Non-Hodgkin's	7.8	3.4	7.6	3.5	5.5	3.7
Burkitt's	0.7	0.2	4.1	0.7	0.9	0.3
Brain & spinal	28.7	25.1	34.0	29.5	27.6	27.1
Neuroblastoma	9.4	9.2	13.3	12.2	8.9	10.4
Retinoblastoma	4.0	3.5	4.8	5.0	5.6	5.1
Renal	7.2	8.1	10.0	10.1	8.3	10.9
Wilms'	7.1	8.1	9.9	10.0	7.4	10.3
Hepatic	1.3	1.0	2.3	2.3	2.2	1.6
Hepatoblastoma	1.0	0.8	1.9	2.1	1.7	1.4
Bone	4.8	5.4	6.6	6.3	2.9	5.0
Osteosarcoma	2.4	2.8	3.4	3.2	2.6	4.1
Ewing's sarcoma	2.2	2.3	2.7	2.6	0.3	0.3
Soft tissue sarcoma	8.9	7.7	10.9	9.1	11.2	11.5
Rhabdomyosarcoma	5.8	4.9	6.4	4.3	5.8	4.7
Germ cell/gonadal	4.1	4.3	3.5	5.1	1.8	7.8
Carcinomas	2.8	3.6	3.5	5.9	3.2	2.6
Other and unspecified	0.5	0.3	0.6	0.5	-	1.3

Data derived from Parkin et al 1998.[3] England and Wales from Stiller et al 1998.[1] USA SEER – The Surveillance, Epidemiology and End Results Program of the National Cancer Institute, Ries et al 1998, all reported in IARC Scientific Publications No 144.

Table 22.3 Five-year actuarial survival percentage of patients treated in United Kingdom Children's Cancer Study Group Centers 1977–1999 by period of diagnosis

Tumor type	77–84	85–89	90–94	95–99	X^2(1df) for trend
ALL	63	72	80	82	246.3***
ANLL	21	42	52	62	132.3***
Hodgkin's disease	90	93	94	91	4.43*
Non-Hodgkin's disease	60	76	76	83	61.5***
Ependymoma	42	45	54	69	14.6***
Low grade astrocytoma	81	84	89	93	19.3***
High grade astrocytoma	38	27	19	20	(7.34)**
PNET (inc medulloblastoma)	52	46	45	56	0.59
Neuroblastoma	37	39	50	58	82.6***
Retinoblastoma					
Bilateral	94	91	91	96	3.65
Unilateral	89	93	97	98	6.72**
Wilms'	81	84	81	89	5.63*
Hepatoblastoma	37	41	68	69	23.9
Osteosarcoma	44	56	55	58	8.81**
Ewing's sarcoma	40	55	65	74	30.5***
Rhabdomyosarcoma	56	60	63	65	12.6***
Germ cell					
CNS	48	59	63	82	8.62**
Non-CNS, non-gonadal	47	82	80	80	15.0***
Gonadal malignant	87	96	97	97	12.3**

+ $p < 0.05$; ** $p < 0.01$; *** $p < 0.001$.
If X^2 in ( ) = negative trend (decreasing survival) which appears to be as a result of increased referral to centers of high risk patients who do not survive long enough to receive adjuvant therapy.
Data derived from United Kingdom Children's Cancer Study Group Scientific Report 2002, compiled by Stiller CA – personal communication.
ALL, acute lymphoblastic leukemia; ANLL, acute non-lymphoblastic leukemia; PNET, primitive neuroectodermal tumor.

The prevalence of childhood cancer patients is clearly rising, largely as a result of improved disease control and supportive care. Table 22.3 shows the survival trends for individual tumor types over the last two decades (data derived from the UKCCSG scientific report compiled by Stiller[9]). Approximately 1 in 900 individuals aged 20 years are now cancer survivors, and as a result any long term effects of their cancer and its treatment present a significant public health concern. Furthermore tumors still constitute the second commonest cause of death after accidents for those aged 5–14 years. After the first month of life cancer deaths make up 1 in 10 of all childhood mortality.[10]

FACTORS INFLUENCING SURVIVAL[11]

Table 22.3 shows 5-year actuarial survival with evidence of significant improvement for the majority of tumors but with some notable exceptions, for example, high grade astrocytomas, and in others a more recent plateau effect in terms of improvement, e.g. acute lymphoblastic leukemia, Hodgkin's disease and primitive neuroectodermal tumors. Prognostic factors for each tumor type will be discussed in subsequent sections but some general factors are relevant. Improvement from 10 to 70% overall event free survival and 60% long term cure for all childhood cancers over the last 30 years has been achieved by the use of multiagent chemotherapy along with appropriate use of radiotherapy and surgery for local tumor control. The acute morbidity of therapy makes it essential that treatment is delivered in specialized centers with a multidisciplinary team approach. Intensive nursing support, a comprehensive blood transfusion service and laboratory backup are all required. Worldwide 'modern era' therapy is only available to approximately 15% of all children. One of the great challenges of this decade is to extend the availability of better care throughout the world.[12]

Pediatric oncology is one of the specialties which has vigorously adopted the approach of randomized controlled trials and more recently the use of overview analyses.[13] Stiller & Eatock[14] reported a rise in treatment for childhood leukemia at specialized centers from 77% in the years 1980–1984 to 89% in the period 1990–1994. Five-year survival rose from 67 to 81% over this time. Entry of patients into therapeutic trials showed an even greater difference with 5-year survival figures of 64% for those treated off protocol in 1980–1984 compared with 70% when treated on a trial whilst for the later time period (1990–1994) the figures were 84% for trial entrants and only 68% for those treated off trial. These figures translate into an increased annual survival of over 50 patients who would have died of their disease in the 1980s. Earlier centralization of care had also been demonstrated to improve survival for acute non-lymphoblastic leukemia, non-Hodgkin's lymphoma, nephroblastoma, osteosarcoma, Ewing's sarcoma and rhabdomyosarcoma.[15] The effect of trial entry includes emphasis on compliance, more consistent supportive care, audit and sharing of toxicity data and international exchange of information. Adoption of the 'best' therapy from other reported trialists has become a feature of modern oncology therapy. Treatment by non-experienced doctors and centers may lead to failure to actually recognize the true extent of disease without appropriate modification of therapy leading to undertreatment or conversely overtreatment with excessive toxicity.[16]

AETIOLOGY

Compared with adults where environmental factors clearly play a significant part, e.g. smoking, relatively little is yet known about the cause of most childhood cancers. Known genetic predisposition syndromes (see Tables 22.4–22.7) are estimated to account for up to 5% of childhood cancers. Increasingly genetic susceptibility or variation leading to either poor or abnormal handling of environmental factors or failure to repair genetic damage leading to a malignant phenotype in target cells is thought to play a crucial role in the development of childhood malignancy. The paradox of childhood cancer is that it should occur at all, since accumulation of genetic damage leading to a fully malignant phenotype takes time, hence the rising incidence of cancer with age. This has led to considerable research into genome–environmental interactions. Indeed a UK wide National Case Control Study was established in 1991 to test five broad hypotheses regarding childhood cancer etiology.17 The hypotheses being investigated were:

1. exposure to ionizing radiation natural or manmade;
2. similar exposure to potentially hazardous chemicals;
3. exposure of parental germ cells to either radiation or hazardous chemicals before conception;
4. extreme low frequency electromagnetic field exposure postnatally particularly in the case of brain cancers and leukemia;
5. abnormal responses to one or more common infectious agents, as potential factors in childhood cancer and leukemia. The infection relationship was thought to be with leukemia although evidence is accumulating that infections may play a part in other tumor etiology. The infection hypothesis includes speculation that there is a paucity of infection exposure in infancy and subsequent late or delayed exposure shortly before the onset of cancer symptoms. In addition the risk might be increased for children in rural areas of marked population mixing. In either of these scenarios there may be an association with genetic factors which influence the host response to infection (see below).

INHERITED PREDISPOSITION TO PEDIATRIC CANCER

Although there is somatic cell DNA damage in all cancers, the percentage of childhood tumors which are truly hereditary is low, estimated not to exceed 5%. Germline mutations may be inherited from parents (e.g. the retinoblastoma gene in familial retinoblastoma or the p53 gene in Li–Fraumeni syndrome and in adrenocortical carcinomas). It may also arise as mutations/rearrangements within the oocyte or sperm prior to fertilization (e.g. in Down syndrome where there is a significantly increased risk of developing leukemia). Some tumors, for example nephroblastoma, are associated with more than one genetic rearrangement and some other cancers do cluster in families (where the predisposing genes are not yet fully defined). Predisposing genes give a high relative risk for the individual but an overall low attributable risk for all cancers. Such inherited predisposition can be subdivided.

Constitutional chromosomal disorders

These disorders (see Table 22.4) are usually characterized by phenotypic features, congenital abnormalities, often failure to thrive and increased risk of malignancy. Altered chromosome number (aneuploidy) or structural rearrangements are easily detectable by routine karyotyping. The most common abnormality is seen in children with constitutional trisomy 21 who have a nearly 20-fold increased risk of developing leukemia (1 in 100 compared with the general population of 1 in 2000 by the age of 10 years).[18,19] Interestingly many childhood ALL patients have leukemic cell trisomy 21 but the crucial genes involved have not yet been fully elucidated. Both ALL (60%) and AML (40%) occur in Down syndrome but with many more AML cases in young children (under 2 years) than seen in the overall childhood leukemic population. A high percentage of such patients have acute megakaryocytic leukemia (M7) which is very responsive to therapy. Provided toxicity can be controlled Down patients fare as well as if not better than non-Down patients. Further studies are now underway to explore why excess chromosome 21 material does so affect progenitor cells leading not only to leukemia but also excess cytotoxicity.

Numerical or structural sex chromosome abnormalities clearly also predispose to malignancy as seen in Table 22.4 but because of the rarity of these disorders it is difficult to define the precise cancer risk for any individual affected child. The extra X chromosome material seen in Klinefelter's syndrome predisposes not only to breast carcinoma but also to acute leukemia, lymphoma and extra gonadal germ cell tumors. Sex chromosome aneuploidy is associated with retinoblastoma in the conditions where there is excess of Y chromosome material.

Studies of the WAGR syndrome[20] (consisting of Wilms' tumor, aniridia, genital abnormalities and mental retardation) led to greater understanding of and indeed the initial identification of the WT1 gene. A number of children with these abnormalities were found to have a deletion of 11p13. Then looking at a large series of Wilms' tumor patients a small percentage (1–3%) were identified as having aniridia often with a degree of developmental delay and genital abnormalities including hypospadias. The WT1 gene was identified at 11p13.[21] Subsequently it has been identified that point mutations (mainly missense but frameshift mutations and aberration RNA splicing also) at this locus are found in the Denys–Drash syndrome (characterized by severe urogenital abnormalities and Wilms' tumor). However the issue is even more complex since there are other families reported with apparent dominant inheritance of Wilms' tumor that do not have mutations at 11p13. There are now thought to be a number of other genes that are involved in the genesis of this tumor. This includes two syndromes involving tissue overgrowth, Beckwith–Wiedemann (intrauterine and postnatal overgrowth, organomegaly, macroglossia and linear ear creases linked with nephroblastoma and hepatoblastoma) and hemihypertrophy (asymmetrical overgrowth of one side of body, or face alone, linked with Wilms' tumor). The risk in both is high enough to warrant regular abdominal ultrasonography in patients recognized to have such overgrowth. The genetics of these syndromes is complex (autosomal inheritance involving 11p15 most frequently of

Table 22.4 Some constitutional chromosomal abnormalities associated with malignancy

Chromosome involved	Defect	Tumor	Estimated risk
21	Trisomy (Down)	Acute leukemia (especially M7 in infancy) Testicular Retinoblastoma*	1 in 100
13	Trisomy	Teratoma Leukemia Neurogenic tumors	?
13	Deletion q14	Sporadic retinoblastoma Osteosarcoma Pinealoblastoma	?
11	Interstitial deletion 11p13 11p15	Wilms' tumor (+ aniridia, genital abnormalities and mental retardation) WAGR	?
	Maternal deletion, uniparental disomy, or disordered imprinting	Hemihypertrophy and Beckwith-Wiedemann syndrome	
X	Monosomy	Post estrogen endometrial carcinoma in Turner's syndrome ?leukemia ?neurogenic tumors	?
X	Extra (Klinefelter's)	Breast carcinoma Acute leukemia + non-Hodgkin's lymphoma Extra gonadal germ cell	?

*Often in trisomy 21 associated with sex chromosome aneuploidy

maternal origin, rearrangements of 11p15 as result of paternal 11p duplications, or loss of normal imprinting). Insulin-like growth factor 2 gene (IGF2) which is a maternally imprinted gene but expressed from the paternal copy, is the gene involved in Beckwith–Wiedemann syndrome.

Single gene disorders

Table 22.5 shows some of the disorders predisposing to childhood tumors, inherited in an autosomal dominant fashion. Because of their inherited nature there is frequently involvement of several family generations but there may be variable expression within any individual family (even with skipped generations) because of incomplete penetrance of the phenotype. Strangely there may be individuals with the same genetic mutation who have no or minimal overt manifestations of the malignant phenotype. The characteristics of these autosomal dominant cancer family syndromes are that

1. inheritance can be from either father or mother;
2. multiple generations are most likely to be involved;
3. onset of the cancer will be at an earlier age compared with sporadic cases;
4. there are more likely to be multiple rather than single tumors;
5. there may be a clustering of increased risk of one or several different types of tumor within the family.

Explanation of all the conditions is beyond the scope of this text but a few examples do clarify the varying genetic mechanisms involved.

Retinoblastoma is the most carefully documented genetically determined tumor of childhood. In 1971 Knudson proposed that bilateral retinoblastoma was the familial form of this condition and patients had already acquired a mutation in the germline. His two-hit hypothesis proposed that such patients only required a further somatic cell hit for the tumor to develop whereas sporadic retinoblastoma which occurs at an older age requires at least two somatic cell mutations in order for the tumor to develop. Mutation in the Rb1 gene was localized to chromosome 13 (q14). The normal function of the Rb gene is to negatively regulate cell division (tumor suppression) and with loss of this function tumors can develop. Since in the inherited form all cells of the body contain the first mutation, tumors can arise not only in the retina but also anywhere else, especially in the pineal gland, bone and soft tissue (particularly in response to irradiation) and skin (melanoma). In the non-hereditary form only retinal tumors develop. We now know that in the inherited form the second event may include loss of the whole chromosome 13, deletions and gene conversion. The retinoblastoma story is slightly complicated by the fact that about 15% of unilateral retinoblastoma is of the inherited type. Again probably due to variable expressivity. There may also be no family history, either because the mutation has started de novo in the affected child or because there may be a mild form of the tumor in parents (known as a retinoma) which has spontaneously regressed and which sometimes can be identified by careful examination of the retina. Life-long follow-up of patients with inherited retinoblastoma shows them to progressively develop other malignancies over their lifetime including osteosarcoma and malignant melanoma as well as, in later life, carcinomas.[22] Knudson's two-hit hypothesis has subsequently been shown to be much more widely applicable in tumorigenesis (see below).

Another tumor suppressor gene involved in pediatric and familial cancers is the TP53 gene located at 17q12–13. Li & Fraumeni[23] identified an increased incidence of breast cancer in mothers of young children with soft tissue sarcoma. On further

Table 22.5 Single gene disorders inherited in an autosomal dominant fashion predisposing to childhood malignancy

Hereditary disorder	Site of genetic defect	Gene mechanism	Tumor type
Familial retinoblastoma	13q14	Rb1 gene tumor suppressor (2 hits required)	Retinoblastoma, pinealoblastoma, melanoma, bone and soft tissue sarcomas, carcinomas (in adult life)
Li-Fraumeni cancer family syndrome	17q12	TP53* (tumor suppressor) (2 hit)	Early onset soft tissue sarcomas Brain tumors Leukemias Adrenocortical carcinoma Breast cancer (early onset) Other carcinomas
Adenomatous polyposis coli (APC)	5q21	APC gene (tumor suppressor) (2 hit)	Colonic polyps (10–20 yrs) + Carcinoma (20–30 yrs) + Extracolonic features Dermoid cysts, mandible cysts, osteomas (Gardner's)
Hereditary non-polyposis colon cancer	2p22–p21 (for hMSH2) 3p21.3 (hMLH1) 7p22 (hPMS2)	HMSH2 (+ other mismatch repair genes) (2 hit)	Right sided colon cancer
Multiple endocrine neoplasia 2A and 2B	10q11.2	RET (receptor tyrosine kinase gene) (oncogene activation)	2A – medullary thyroid carcinoma, pheochromocytoma 2B – similar + ganglioneuromas + skeletal
Neurofibromatosis type I	17q11.2	NF1 gene ↓ Neurofibromin (tumor suppressor) (of Ras gene signalling) (2 hit)	Peripheral neurofibromas, optic tract gliomas, other gliomas, pheochromocytomas, malignant peripheral nerve sheath tumors, sarcomas, leukemias (especially myeloid)

*See Birch et al[27]

exploration they and others have identified in such families considerable clustering of cancers including sarcomas and breast carcinoma but also leukemias, brain tumors and adrenocortical carcinomas.[24,25] Malkin et al[26] reported germline point mutations in the TP53 gene in a large number of such families. Tumor cell p53 mutation is extremely common in a range of malignancies. In some families with such a pattern of increased incidence of malignancy no p53 mutations have been identified and this has led to speculation that other suppressor or key checkpoint genes (e.g. CHK2) may be involved in some cases. There is also some evidence of a relationship between specific breakpoints within the gene and malignant phenotype. It is estimated that about 3% of osteosarcomas, 5% of rhabdomyosarcomas and probably all adrenocortical carcinomas have germline TP53 mutations.[27]

Adenomatous polyposis coli[28] and Gardner's syndrome[29] which are characterized by development of multiple colonic polyps developing in childhood and adolescence with almost universal progression to colonic carcinoma in the second and third decade also have an increased risk of other gastrointestinal and liver malignancies (including childhood hepatoblastoma). The syndrome involves a gene at 5q21 (the APC gene). Molecular diagnostic testing in at risk family childhood members, regular flexible colonoscopy and surgical intervention is of life saving benefit in such young patients. Inheritance appears to be dominant. The precise role of the APC gene in the oncogenic process is being explored.

Another familial condition, hereditary non-polyposis colon cancer syndrome (HNPCC), involves characteristically right sided colon tumors arising as early as the second decade of life. Such tumors have been shown to have microsatellite instability (variations in length and number of intragenic repeat DNA sequences) and mutation of the mismatch repair gene hMSH2.[30] There are now recognized a series of such genes required to provide DNA stability, to repair single mismatch errors and prevent recombination between non-homologous molecules. Mutations of these genes prime cells for mutagenesis. In some HNPCC families other mismatch repair genes have now been identified. The two-hit hypothesis also applies in this syndrome. Turcot syndrome in which familial clustering of brain tumors in childhood and polyposis/colon cancer is found, has been shown to involve mutations of the APC gene in some families and of mismatch repair genes in others (hMLH1 and hPMS2).

There are at least three forms of the multiple endocrine neoplasia (MEN) syndrome, all inherited in an autosomal dominant fashion. MEN2A arises in children (medullary thyroid carcinoma, pheochromocytoma), MEN2B arises in infancy (is related to MEN2A but also includes ganglioneuromas of the gut and skeletal abnormalities). The gene involved in MEN2A is the proto-oncogene RET located on chromosome 10q11.2 (receptor tyrosine kinase gene) and mutations involve replacement of one of four cysteines in the extracellular domain of the protein, encoded by exons 10 and 11.[31] Specific mutations correlate with malignant phenotype (e.g. cysteine 634 mutation and pheochromocytoma). A missense mutation in RET seems to be involved in MEN2B. The two-hit hypothesis does not appear to be relevant here but the single gene mutation activates an oncogene. Screening of sporadic medullary thyroid carcinoma tumors shows a wide range of mutations in the RET gene.

Neurofibromatosis type 1 which affects 1 in 2500 of the population is described elsewhere in greater detail in the text. The NF1 gene (17q11.2) has been identified for over a decade. Its product, neurofibromin, acts as a negative regulator of Ras signalling. Mutations are associated with a range of benign and malignant neoplasms as well as the characteristic stigmata of the syndrome (see Table 22.5). The two-hit hypothesis does apply in NF1. NF2 which is clearly much rarer is related to a separate gene on chromosome 22 and is characterized by café-au-lait spots, bilateral vestibular schwannomas, neurofibromas and meningiomas and rarely presents in adolescence.

Other phakomatoses including tuberous sclerosis (a genetically complex disorder involving at least two genes) and von Hippel–Lindau disease (VHL gene on 3q interacts with transcriptional factors) are associated with a range of benign and malignant neoplasms. In tuberous sclerosis these are retinal hamartomas, giant cell astrocytomas, other brain tumors and rhabdomyosarcomas; in VHL renal cysts and carcinomas, pheochromocytomas, cerebellar hemangioblastomas and retinal angiomas. The nevoid basal cell carcinoma syndrome (Gorlin's) is characterized by an association of early onset basal cell skin lesions and medulloblastomas.

Disorders which are recessively inherited appear to be less frequently associated with cancer (see Table 22.6). Some of that rarity may relate to failure to recognize the recessive disorder, without obvious family history and overt signs of disease at the time of cancer diagnosis. There are however some notable exceptions in childhood which predominantly involve DNA repair or checkpoint genes leading to increased DNA fragility (spontaneous or in response to exogenous DNA damage, e.g. by irradiation or chemicals).

Xeroderma pigmentosa is characterized by eye and skin sensitivity progressing to basal and squamous cell carcinomas, melanomas and tip of tongue carcinomas. These lesions are all in sun exposed areas but internal malignancies may occur. Some children show neurological deterioration. Mutations in at least seven different genes can result in the disorder which is characterized by a defect in nucleotide excision repair.[33] There are related disorders, trichothiodystrophy and Cockayne syndrome. There is considerable overlap in the genes involved between repair and transcription. At least one of the genes involved encodes a DNA helicase.

Ataxia telangiectasia (AT) presents in childhood with progressive truncal and subsequent limb ataxia, choreoathetosis, and ocular motor apraxia.[34] Telangiectasias usually start in the conjunctivae in the first 5 years of life. However many patients are missed until they present with leukemia and/or lymphomas, but also a range of other solid tumors.[35] Thirteen per cent of UK registered cases of AT have leukemia or lymphoma. There is associated deficiency of IgA and IgG_2 levels leading to sinopulmonary infections. It would appear that AT heterozygotes (1–2% of the population) are at risk of developing breast cancer at a much higher rate than the general population, possibly due to increased sensitivity to naturally and man made ionizing irradiation. Certainly the DNA of homozygotes is highly sensitive to damage from radiation and some chemicals. There is loss of checkpoint control so that damaged cells continue through the cell cycle and are not arrested at G1–G2. The AT gene originally localized to chromosome 11q22–33 has now been cloned[36] and appears to encode a kinase with signal transduction function.

Table 22.6 Single gene disorders inherited in an autosomal recessive fashion predisposing to childhood malignancy

Hereditary disorder	Site of genetic defect	Gene deficit	Tumor type
Xeroderma pigmentosa		At least 7 different genes Nucleotide excision repair deficits (sensitivity to ultraviolet light)	Basal and squamous cell carcinoma of skin Melanoma Tongue carcinoma ?internal malignancies
Ataxia telangiectasia	11q22–23	Kinase with signal transduction function (marked radiation and chemical sensitivity)	Leukemia Lymphomas Stomach cancer Other cancers Brain tumors (heterozygote – breast cancer)
Fanconi anemia	Fanc A 16q24.3 Fanc C 9q22.3	8 genes (?all involved) DNA damage repair (chromosomal fragility)	Acute myeloid leukemia Squamous cell carcinoma Hepatic adenomas + carcinomas (?following androgen therapy)
Bloom's syndrome	15q26.1	DNA repair (chromosomal breaks and sister chromatid exchanges)	Myeloid leukemia Lymphoma Squamous cell carcinoma

Modified from Strong 1984[32]

Table 22.7 Some of the immunodeficiency disorders predisposing to childhood tumors

Immunodeficient condition	Inheritance	Tumors
Purtillo syndrome	XR	Burkitt 'like' + other lymphomas
Bruton/ agammaglobulinemia	XR	Lymphoma Leukemia Brain
Severe combined immunodeficiency	XR	Lymphoma Leukemia
Wiskott–Aldrich	XR	Lymphoma Leukemia
Chediak–Higashi	AR	Pseudolymphoma
True IgA deficiency	?AD	Lymphoma Leukemia Gastrointestinal Brain

XR, X-linked recessive; AR, autosomal recessive; AD, autosomal dominant

The rare inherited disease Fanconi anemia (FA) provides the paradigm of a genetically determined disease. FA cells are hypersensitive to damage by bifunctional DNA crosslinkers such as mitomycin C and diepoxybutane. FA patients exhibit complex and variable birth defects, progressive marrow failure but a very significantly increased risk of developing acute myeloid leukemia (a 15 000-fold increase has been claimed). There are now at least eight FA genes demonstrated by cellular complementation studies, with four mapped (Fanc A, C, D and G0) and three (FANCC C, A and G) cloned and sequenced.[37] Approximately two-thirds of Fanconi anemia patients have mutations of the A gene (16q24.3). The FA proteins are clearly involved in DNA damage repair, they appear to be interactive but their exact individual roles remain to be elucidated. Studies are progressing to explore if polymorphic variations within the Fanconi genes may play a role in the etiology of sporadic leukemia.[38]

Genetically determined immunodeficiency

Where immune competence is impaired by inherited defects there is a high risk of leukemia and lymphoma development[39] (see Table 22.7). Similarly acquired immunodeficiency secondary to chemotherapy, intensive immunosuppression and infection (especially HIV infection) also predisposes to malignancy (see below under lymphomas).

GENETIC SUSCEPTIBILITY

The concept that some individuals especially children may be more susceptible to DNA damage leading to malignancy has recently attracted much attention. Even amongst the genetic predisposition syndromes described above abnormal or excessive response/failure to repair adequately is a feature of xeroderma pigmentosa in response to ultraviolet light and in ataxia telangiectasia in response to irradiation and some chemicals. For most childhood tumors we now suspect a combination of environmental factors with an inherent defective or aberrant response, probably genetically determined, to be at the root cause of the malignant phenotype in most tumors.

Most progress has been made in our understanding of infant and childhood peak acute lymphoblastic leukemia. Evidence from identical twins and retrospective scrutiny of neonatal blood spots has identified that, for some, if not all such leukemias initiation of the first genetic damage occurs during early intrauterine life.[40,41] Rearrangements of the MLL gene present in the majority of infant leukemias in hemopoietic stem cells appear adequate for development of overt leukemia, whilst for precursor B cell ALL (peak age 2–6 years) further genetic events are required. Greaves[42] has demonstrated carriage of the commonest leukemia associated gene rearrangement TEL-AML1 (cryptic translocation involving chromosomes 12 and 21) in 1–2% of normal cord bloods. But what causes the first genetic event in utero?

The risk of developing infant MLL associated leukemia is greatly increased in pregnancies where the mother carries a low functioning polymorphic variant of the metabolizing NQ01 gene.[43] This protein is crucial for detoxification of quinone containing substances which include both naturally occurring (widely present in food)[44] and synthetic topoisomerase 2 inhibitors plus other quinone containing chemicals, e.g. pesticides.[45] Topoisomerase inhibitors cause DNA breaks to be inappropriately religated and may lead to genetic rearrangement. Strick et al[46] have shown that dietary bioflavonoids do induce MLL cleavage and may contribute to infant acute leukemia. Conversely low function of the key, 1 carbon pool pathway enzyme, methylene tetrahydrofolate reductase (MTHFR) appears to confer protection against infant leukemia and precursor B cell ALL with hyperdiploidy. Low function MTHFR leads to greater available folate and increased DNA stability.[47] Recently there has been evidence that dietary supplementation with folate early in pregnancy may afford some protection against the development of childhood peak ALL.[48] In all of these instances dietary factors interact with ability to metabolize/detoxify and appear to increase or decrease the risk of DNA damage. Whether other genetically determined factors such as polymorphic variation within the more than 130 DNA repair/surveillance genes now identified, play a part in leukemogenesis is not yet clear.

In precursor B cell ALL abnormal response to infection may play a part in later events or proliferation of the malignant clone. There is evidence that HLA class II alleles do influence risk.[49] Supportive evidence for a role of environmental, possibly infectious, agents in causation of childhood cancer comes from epidemiological evidence of rising incidence,[7,8] onset seasonality[50] and space time clustering[51] in leukemia, some lymphomas and solid tumors.

ENVIRONMENTAL FACTORS

Ionizing radiation

Prenatal exposure

Stewart et al[52] first reported an approximately 1.5-fold increase in childhood cancer for those fetuses exposed to X-rays performed on the maternal abdomen and pelvis during the first trimester of pregnancy. There appeared to be a dose–risk relationship. Some but not all subsequent studies have confirmed the findings. In a series of studies on the 1599 children born to mothers exposed to the Hiroshima and Nagasaki atomic bombs, those who received doses above the threshold of 10–20 cSv showed evidence of small head size, mental retardation and seizures.[53] Yoshimoto et al[54] reported a 38% increase in cancer, with no dose threshold for those exposed in utero to A bomb irradiation, a similar rate to those exposed in the first decade of life in Japan. In recent times there has been an interest in the concept of preconception effects particularly from radiation to the paternal germline.[55] Gardner's findings were controversial and there has been inconclusive evidence with regard to a mechanism whereby relatively low doses of irradiation could cause classical gene mutations but intriguing reports on increased minisatellite mutation rates, whereby the overall DNA is destabilized, require further clarification.[56]

Postnatal exposure

Children who were within 1 kilometer of the epicenter of the Hiroshima bomb experienced an excess of acute and chronic myelogenous leukemia and acute lymphoblastic leukemia 3–10 years after the exposure. Young people surviving the atomic bomb are still developing thyroid and other adult cancers even after 50 years.

Therapeutic (low dose) external irradiation delivered to the scalp for tinea capitis or to the thymus have both been associated with significant increases in leukemia, brain tumors and thyroid carcinoma.[57,58] Dosages to the infant thyroid as low as 0.2 cGy have been reported in association with the development of carcinoma 12–17 years later. Speculation about the effects of radionucleotide ingestion from fallout has mostly centered on military personnel observing nuclear tests, although there has been a reported excess of childhood leukemia in Utah following exposure to fallout from atmospheric nuclear detonations.[59]

An increased risk of childhood malignancy, specifically leukemia (although at Sellafield solid tumors also), has been reported around nuclear reprocessing plants in the United Kingdom, both at Sellafield and Dounreay.[60–63] Studies of known environmental nuclide levels, routes of access and associated exposure to chemicals have failed so far to explain this risk, although Kinlen et al[64] have postulated extreme population mixing, and Greaves[65] abnormal infection response as possible etiological factors in these remote and unusual communities. Speculation behind the 'infective' hypothesis is that children who have a dearth of infection in early life, may respond abnormally later in childhood. Higher birth weight and socioeconomic status have been associated with common ALL and linked to decreased early infection exposure.

Irradiation (and chemotherapy) for a primary malignancy carries with it a definitive risk for development of a second tumor (see Late Effects section). The UK National Case Control Study has failed to show any relationship between household radon or gamma irradiation on the incidence of childhood malignancy.[66,67] (Cartwright R – personal communication).

There may be a life-long risk for children who receive extensive diagnostic X-rays with radiation dosages in excess of 10 cSv, in terms of developing breast and prostate cancer and leukemia in later life. Since such procedures cannot often be avoided clinicians need to be careful in their choice of procedure and avoid repetitive scanning wherever possible (a computerized demographic scan of the head and body gives an effective body radiation dose of 0.1 cSv, whilst for a plain chest X-ray the dose is 0.008 cSv).

It is clearly important to remember that some children (e.g. with germline mutations of the Rb1, ATM or nevoid basal cell carcinoma genes) are particularly sensitive to ionizing irradiation, and that they may not be recognized as carrying the risk at the time of X-ray exposure.

Ultraviolet radiation

The fastest rising cancer incidence in the UK is for skin malignancy secondary to increased sunlight exposure following an increase in sunshine holidays and sunbed usage. The risk begins in childhood with unprotected and excessive sun exposure although the actual incidence of skin cancer in childhood is relatively low.[68] Preventative measures are effective and population education needs to be enhanced (use of hats, clothing, sunscreens and avoidance of prolonged and/or repeated exposure to sun in childhood). The pediatrician has a key role in such education. Patients with xeroderma, Gorlin's syndrome and albinism are clearly at considerable risk. The risk of developing melanoma appears to be increased if the sun exposure is obtained in conjunction with repeated exposure to chlorinated water in open air swimming pools. Some by-products of chlorination are clearly mutagenic.[69]

Electricity and electromagnetic fields

Wertheimer & Leeper[70] reported an excess of childhood cancer in those exposed to excess electromagnetic fields derived from household electricity wiring. Subsequent studies where actual magnetic field measurements have been recorded have not consistently supported that. In the UK as part of the large National Case Control Study no evidence to support such a relationship has been found[71] although the percentage of UK houses found to have high levels of exposure (greater than 0.4 micro-Tessler) was very small. In contrast a Swedish study relating proximity to power lines and generated magnetic fields showed an apparent dose relationship with leukemia but not for all cancers, brain tumors or lymphomas.[70] Overall analysis does suggest the differences in mode of electricity supply, wiring patterns as well as study design differences do explain the conflicting results but for the vast majority of UK homes there appears to be no risk from generated electromagnetic fields nor from adjacency to power lines.

Drugs

Prenatal

Maternal ingestion of diethylstilbestrol is associated with clear cell carcinoma of the vagina and cervix in female offspring as well as genital anomalies in both sexes, maternal phenytoin with neural crest tumors, alcohol with adrenal, neural crest and liver tumors and teratomas and barbiturates possibly with brain tumors. There may be a long latent period, e.g. the vaginal tumors did not occur until the children exposed before 20 weeks of gestation were aged 14–23 years. Other sedatives taken in pregnancy are also under scrutiny.[73] The effect of phenytoin in inducing lymphoproliferation may be related to its immunosuppressive effect.[74]

Postnatal exposure

Intensive immunosuppression as in renal transplantation is associated with a 20–40-fold increased risk of lymphoma development, especially of intracerebral tumors with a short latent period. Modern intensive cancer therapy carries an increased risk of inducing secondary leukemia (mostly acute non-lymphoblastic leukemia) and other neoplasms (e.g. brain). Chronic malnutrition, by inducing immune paralysis, coupled with chronic infective antigenic stimulation may be important in the induction of B cell neoplasias in tropical Africa.

There is an increased risk of developing (acute non-lymphoblastic leukemia ANLL) for those treated with alkylating agents for other tumors (at the rate of 5–10% over the 10 years following exposure). The most common alkylating agent used, cyclophosphamide, can induce hemorrhagic cystitis. This has also been incriminated as causative of bladder cancer.[73] The exact risk for children treated with cyclophosphamide for either cancer or renal problems has not been adequately quantified but the avoidance of combined irradiation and alkylating agents especially when the bladder is involved appears wise. The increasing use of the highly effective cytotoxics, the topoisomerase 2 inhibitors (epipodophyllotoxins and anthracyclines) has been associated with a rise in early onset (median 30 months) therapeutically induced acute myeloid leukemia. The risk appears to be dose and scheduled dependent.[76] For both alkylators and topoisomerase 2 inhibitors concurrent use of other cytotoxics and irradiation may increase the risk.

Long term use of androgens and other anabolic steroids has been associated with the development of hepatomas in patients with Fanconi's anemia.[77] Most tumors are benign, but hepatocellular carcinoma has been described. Such tumors have been reported in other conditions and in athletes taking long courses of anabolic steroids without any known underlying genetic instability. Phenytoin given to children for seizures can induce a benign lymphadenopathy, a self-limiting pseudolymphomatous condition and rarely a true lymphoma. Barbiturates used frequently and in high dosage in early infancy have also been incriminated in brain tumor formation but definitive evidence does not exist.

Golding et al[78] reported that neonates receiving intramuscular vitamin K prophylaxis had a nearly threefold increased risk of developing leukemia. Subsequent studies and a recent pooled analysis of the six major case control studies including that of Golding et al has found no convincing evidence to support the link.[79] The studies however have shown up major variations in clinical practice which need addressing. The risks of hemorrhage in the newborn appear to far outweigh any other risks of vitamin K prophylaxis.

Chemicals

Table 22.8 shows some of the parental occupations or exposures which have been incriminated in childhood tumor formation.[80] The exposure may be maternal or paternal, e.g. solvent exposure in the aircraft industry may act on the male germ cell line which is then transmitted to the fetus. Although close exposure to asbestos mines in childhood was associated with the development in later life of mesotheliomas in the South African population, the rare mesotheliomas of childhood do not appear to be related to asbestos exposure. What has proved very difficult regarding chemicals, unlike with radiation, has been the ability to assess evidence of real exposure and its extent, plus to quantify risks.

There is conflicting evidence regarding parental smoking and alcohol consumption with regard to childhood cancer. Recently some association between smoking and particular subtypes of AML (M_1/M_2) have been suggested for young adults.

Viruses

Although infectious agents have been repeatedly associated with childhood leukemia and cancer no definite evidence has emerged to link any of the common viral agents known to cause intrauterine infection with oncogenesis. To date repeated searches for viral genomic inclusion in ALL patients has proved negative, especially for herpes viruses, simian 40, JC and BK virus sequences.[81–83]

Postnatal exposure to Epstein–Barr virus (EBV) is associated with B cell lymphoid malignancies (Burkitt's lymphoma and leukemia) in malarial areas of Africa where they comprise up to 50% of all childhood tumors. African Burkitt's lymphoma occurs almost exclusively in areas of endemic malaria where early exposure (almost the whole population has been exposed by the age of 3 years) and high titers to EBV are expected. Most of the tumors in endemic areas show evidence of inclusion of viral DNA and the most consistently detectable antigen is the EBV surface capsid antigen. Infection early in life is thought to increase the size of certain pre B and B cell populations and maintains them in a proliferative state making them more likely to genetic change. Alternatively EBV may produce an immortal cell clone with genetic translocation already present. Repeated infection, in particular with malaria (itself a T cell suppressor and B cell mitogen), and malnutrition lead to a major degree of T cell immunosuppression and B cell hyperplasia with tumor formation likely. We do not know whether the initial infection or subsequent events lead to the very characteristic translocation of DNA from chromosome 8 into the immunoglobulin coding sites on chromosomes 14, 2 or 22. The role of other cofactors, such as plant extracts, in promoting proliferation has not yet been fully evaluated. Outside equatorial Africa where exposure to EBV is usually much later, B cell tumors, especially extensive abdominal lymphomas have been shown to contain viral antigen also but in a lower percentage of cases. There are other differences between the endemic and sporadic cases but the same genetic translocation may be found in both forms. EBV has also been associated with nasopharyngeal carcinoma in non-malarial areas and rare familial cases of both Burkitt's lymphoma and nasopharyngeal carcinoma have been observed in tropical Africa.

EBV has also been linked to Hodgkin's disease (HD). In children and young adults it has been postulated that HD represents an abnormal outcome of delayed exposure to a common infectious agent. EBV is found in Hodgkin's–Reed–Sternberg cells in a significant percentage of young cases, especially in boys and those with mixed cellularity subtype. What is not yet clear is whether the EBV is causative, contributory or a bystander in young people with altered immune responses.[84–86] Immune response genes may play a critical role in susceptibility to Hodgkin's disease.[87,88]

Post transplantation and following severe immunosuppression for other conditions on EBV driven lymphoproliferative disorder is increasingly observed (see lymphoma section).

Retroviruses alter the growth and differentiation of cells from various hemopoietic lineages. Abelson murine leukemia virus can induce non-thymic lymphomas in mice while feline leukemia is associated with another retrovirus. There is a clear relationship between infection with the retrovirus HTLV1 and a form of adult T cell leukemia and lymphoma[89] and although there has been recent speculation about in utero transmission no childhood case has yet been reported. HIV infection, presumably as a result of its profound effect on helper T cells, predisposes to the development of a particularly virulent lymphoma in young adults. An increasing incidence of Kaposi's sarcoma has been reported in African children.

Hepatitis B infection has long been associated with hepatocellular carcinoma possibly linked with aflatoxin. The mechanism of oncogenesis and the role of the two agents still requires clarification. Although some viruses may cause tumors by direct genetic transformation, some clearly induce host responses but the majority so far identified appear to function by oncogene activation. This can lead to interference with cell cycle control

Table 22.8 Possible parental occupations associated with childhood malignancy

Occupation	Exposure	Tumor type
Petroleum industry Lead industry	Petroleum Hydrocarbons Lead	CNS Wilms' (lead)
Aircraft manufacturer Painting	Organic solvents	CNS Leukemia ?Hepatoblasoma (paints/pigments)
Paper/pulp mill workers Printing industries	Organic solvents	CNS Leukemia (sawdust)
Farming	Pesticides	CNS Leukemia Wilms'
Metal industries	Heavy metal solvents	Brain Leukemia (metal dust) Lymphoma (foundries)

(e.g. HPV, E6, E7), or immortalization (EBV–EBNAs) or persistent activation of, for example, NFkB pathway with upregulation of the cytotoxic cascade (e.g. HTLV1 and Tax, or EBV and LMP-1) or promotional effects (mitogen exposure leads directly to proliferation, e.g. HTLV1–Tax gene leading to viral replication, HbV and HcV).

EPIDEMIOLOGICAL CONCLUSIONS

Unlike in adults (smoking, alcohol, sun, sex) we have so far failed to identify significant connections between environmental factors and the majority of childhood cancers. Highly penetrant genetic predisposition accounts for only about 5% of cases but increasingly it is recognized that genetic susceptibility may play a significant part in a large number of tumors by altering response to or repair of damage caused by exogenous factors including viruses, chemicals, irradiation, etc. Initiation of the genetic damage, accumulation of a full malignant phenotype and ultimately proliferation of a premalignant clone require an accumulation of contributory factors. Each childhood tumor is likely to have a different combination of such factors in its etiology.

GENERAL PRINCIPLES OF DIAGNOSIS

A complete history and thorough clinical examination will suggest a diagnosis in most childhood malignancies. Investigations are designed to confirm the histology, determine the extent of disease, identify markers by which therapeutic response can be monitored and identify biochemical status as a baseline prior to therapy. Some tumors are very specifically associated with biochemical disturbance (e.g. tumor lysis syndrome in extensive lymphomas) prior to commencement of treatment.

PATHOLOGY

Prior to any biopsy the pathologist should be consulted in order to optimize use of the specimen. Nowadays routine histology is complemented by immunocytochemistry, cytogenetics, and DNA studies for specific rearrangements or oncogene expression. Parental consent should be sought for tumor storage for future study. The collection of constitutional DNA from peripheral blood is increasingly useful in identification of predisposing genetic abnormalities. The pathologist is a key member of the team identifying unfavorable histological features and without whom true incidence and survival figures would not be possible. In these rare tumors central review has enabled audit and consistency of diagnosis. Biopsies are frequently now possible under ultrasound or CT scan guidance but whatever technique is used an adequate sample must be obtained.

RADIOLOGY

Specific radiological investigations will be discussed under each tumor heading but some general principles are important. Plain X-rays may be very suggestive of a specific diagnosis, e.g. suprarenal calcification and neuroblastoma, or onion skin periosteal reaction and Ewing's sarcoma, but are never diagnostic. As far as possible investigations should be rapid, non-invasive and avoid the need for general anesthetic (not always possible in the very young). Ultrasound examination is very useful as a first line, as sedation is rarely needed. Spiral CT scanners and MRI technology enable very precise tumor delineation. MRI is especially helpful for brain, spinal and liver tumors, whilst CT is particularly good for the detection of small chest metastases. Positron emission tomography (PET) scanning is an exciting technique, little used to date in children, which offers an excellent means for monitoring residual disease.[90]

BIOCHEMICAL MARKERS

A few tumors secrete specific markers which can assist in diagnosis and in monitoring the response to treatment. Re-emergence of identifiable markers frequently precedes clinical relapse. Examples are catecholamine excretion in neuroblastoma (total catecholamines, VMA and HVA); serum alpha-fetoprotein (AFP) in hepatoblastoma and teratomas; and human chorionic gonadotrophin in (HCG) some germ cell tumors. Non-specific markers, such as the ESR and serum copper levels in lymphomas are modified by too many factors to be useful.

MOLECULAR AND CYTOGENETICS

Banding techniques and in situ hybridization studies have revolutionized routine karyotyping and tumor cytogenetics respectively. Increasingly, application of probes for specific breakpoints or cloned genes, coupled with polymerase chain reaction amplification of nucleic acid sequences are enabling oncologists to better define tumors. It is essential to combine tumor studies (appropriate specimens required) with analysis of non-tumor DNA to exclude constitutional defects.

BONE MARROW EXAMINATION

Most childhood tumors are highly malignant and likely to be disseminated at presentation, with many (e.g. neuroblastoma, lymphoma, rhabdomyosarcoma, Ewing's sarcoma, retinoblastoma) potentially metastasizing to the bone marrow. To exclude infiltration two aspirates and two trephines from different sites are considered a minimum requirement. The posterior iliac crest is normally more cellular in children. The use of immunophenotyping with a battery of specific monoclonal antibodies has enhanced tumor recognition (especially in lymphomas and neuroblastoma).

PRINCIPLES OF THERAPY

Malignant childhood tumors must always be presumed to be disseminated, and require chemotherapy. Most chemotherapeutic agents are poorly active against resting (G_0) cells but have potentially lethal effects upon normal proliferating cells, especially the gastrointestinal mucosa and hemopoietic cells (especially marrow progenitor cells which can be destroyed by injudicious drug therapy). For most tumors there is some difference in cell cycle duration and this is usually longer than for normal cells even within the same organ. Tumors continue to grow because they appear to overcome normal apoptotic (programmed cell death) mechanisms.[91,92] Some tumor cells will undergo a degree of differentiation, some will go into resting phase while the majority in pediatric tumors will be recruited into the active growth fraction. For any specific tumor a complex interaction of specific gene expression (e.g. Bcl-2, Bax), growth factor activation by oncogene amplification and cytokine stimulation will determine the proliferative rate. Therapy must destroy dividing, resting and maturing cells, and should assist the normal processes of limiting nutrition, vascular supply and oxygenation to the tumor bulk. Normal immune surveillance appears to be overwhelmed by tumor presence. Sometimes within tumors or surrounding nodes, lymphoid hyperplasia, although apparently increasing tumor bulk, is antitumor in effect and caution must be used so as not to completely destroy normal immune responses. Some drugs, for example vincristine, cytosine or hydroxyurea, are phase specific (for the DNA-specific phase) in the cell cycle and should be given at intervals greater than the median duration of the cell cycle in order to kill all the cells passing through the S phase. Other drugs, for example the alkylating agents or external beam irradiation, are cytotoxic at all phases of the cell cycle (cycle specific). Such drugs are best given as a single maximally tolerated dose with a gap between doses to allow for host cell recovery.

One of the major obstacles to the effective kill of all tumor tissue is the presence of hypoxic and nutritionally depleted cells which remain non-proliferative at the time of therapy but retain proliferative capacity and only start to divide when more favorable circumstances prevail. Although the true resting G_0 cell may be as sensitive to radiation as proliferating cells, it is relatively untouched by most antimitotic drugs. Another major reason for failure of therapy in childhood tumors is the use of local therapy without taking into account the fundamentally disseminated nature of all childhood tumors. Tumor cells may metastasize to pharmacological sanctuaries where drugs penetrate poorly, e.g. the brain in leukemia.

Greater understanding of the cellular mechanisms particularly of apoptosis and cellular triggers for proliferation will in the future enable a much more subtle approach to antitumor therapy.[91]

TUMOR CELL RESISTANCE

There are a number of mechanisms that operate to prevent tumors being effectively killed by drugs.[93]

Primary resistance

This may be either extrinsic or intrinsic. Extrinsic means that the drug does not reach the tumor cells in adequate concentration. This can arise from poor bioavailability of a drug, or its metabolism or excretion, or from inbuilt barriers to drug penetration such as the blood–brain barrier. There may be limited drug diffusion into a very large tumor or it may be that the concentration needed to kill the tumor produces excessive host toxicity and therefore cannot be used. In ALL therapy where at least 2 years of continuing oral therapy is utilized, recent studies have shown that poor patient compliance as well as variable drug metabolism do contribute to worsened prognosis.[94] As tumors develop, mutation, deletion, gene amplification, translocation or chromosomal rearrangement can lead to the spontaneous generation of drug-resistant cells which clearly have a survival advantage (e.g. wild type p53 gene appears to inhibit multiple drug-resistant gene expression, see below, but mutant p53 enhances it). Inherent primary resistance of this type is not prominent in pediatric tumors.

Secondary resistance

This is more common in pediatric tumors. Relapse follows a good initial response to treatment and is often after cessation of chemotherapy. The failure of adequate dose therapy to kill leukemic cells, for example within the brain, can lead to secondary resistance. As the cells within pharmacological sanctuaries begin to replicate any mutation which produces resistance, particularly to low levels of cytotoxic agents, will have selective advantage. Resistance may be against a single cytotoxic mechanism or against a battery of cytotoxic agents with different mechanisms. To prevent such resistance developing, pediatric oncologists have developed the strategy of exposing tumor cells to a battery of agents in as short a time as possible with complementary or synergistic combinations delivered in quick succession. A number of mechanisms for the development of tumor cell resistance are now known:

1. *Tumor cell overproduction of the drug target*: For example the enzyme dihydrofolate reductase is the target for methotrexate within the cell. Overamplification of the gene for this enzyme has been demonstrated. In addition an enzyme with low affinity for methotrexate has also been demonstrated. In both circumstances the efficacy of methotrexate will be affected.
2. *Transport resistance*: There may be diminished intracellular transport or enhanced outward transport of a drug from the cell. Methotrexate inhibits folate-specific transmembrane transport, polyglutamation (essential for effective action) and activation of thymidine salvage pathways (used to counteract methotrexate effect). Enhanced outward transport has been demonstrated with many drugs ranging from the vinca-alkaloids to the anthracyclines. Juliano & Ling[95] and Roninson et al[96] demonstrated the activation of a multiple drug resistance gene. Initially identified in Chinese hamster cells, this gene encodes for a membrane transport glycoprotein (p-glycoprotein) which enhances the elimination of drugs from cells. Kartner et al[97] demonstrated activation of this gene in multiple cell lines. This appears to be the principal mechanism of pleiotropic resistance development whereby there is decreased intracellular drug accumulation and an increase in the activity of an energy-dependent efflux pump protein (p-glycoprotein). Other mechanisms and other resistance genes have been identified. Mdr-1 gene (which encodes for p-glycoprotein) expression has been identified in normal liver, kidney, colon, adrenal and blood vessel endothelial cells as well as in the cells of ALL, neuroblastoma, rhabdomyosarcoma, and some bone sarcomas. Although rarely significant at initial presentation, it increases in response to therapy and whenever present confers a worsened prognosis for the patient.
3. *Enhanced biochemical detoxification*: Anthracyclines, alkylators and radiation all produce active antigenic metabolites which the metathione redox system renders harmless. Overproduction of glutathione within cells inactivates these agents.
4. *Activation of DNA repair system*: This occurs with alkylating agents, anthracyclines and radiation. Tumor cells developing resistance to these agents have been shown to have enhanced DNA repair.

To overcome resistance the Goldie–Goldman model[98] can be utilized with rapid alternating drug therapy. High dose chemotherapy potentially toxic to normal cells can be used with peripheral stem cell (with or without growth factor stimulation) or marrow transplantation (autologous or allogeneic) to rescue the normal hemopoietic cells.[99] In vitro partial reversal of mdr-1 expression has been possible with calcium channel blockers such as verapamil. This is cardiotoxic and more success has been obtained using ciclosporin. New in vitro and in vivo studies with non-immunosuppressive ciclosporin analogues are looking promising.

SURGERY AND IRRADIATION

As a general principle surgery can remove large masses of tumor (which may be insensitive to drugs and irradiation) with minimal toxicity. Irradiation can effectively deal with microextensions of malignant cells which have spread to adjacent tissues or nodes. Both surgery and irradiation are effective in sites such as the lung, brain or bone, especially with isolated deposits where drugs may be ineffective. Since most childhood tumors are disseminated at diagnosis the principal place for surgery is in obtaining material for diagnosis though there are notable exceptions which will be mentioned later. The main limitation of irradiation is the ill-effect on normal tissues. The therapeutic ratio depends on the sensitivity of the tumor and the tolerance of neighboring tissues and organs. Megavoltage therapy has a sharper beam edge, better depth of penetration and can give a more even dose distribution avoiding damage to skin and overlying tissues when administered to deep organs. When therapy is planned, careful clinical and radiological assessment of the tumor is undertaken so that radiation fields can be drawn up with plans to shield vital organs such as the kidney or liver if they are not actively involved in disease. New radiation technology is facilitating much more focused therapy with sharp cutoff to minimize damage to surrounding normal tissues. When irradiation is included with chemotherapy in treatment protocols there is a potential for additive toxicity as well as efficacy. The most worrying combination is that of alkylating agents and irradiation, where there is increased risk of the development of secondary neoplasms.

Enhancement of normal cell-mediated immunity using immunotherapy, for example BCG immunization, has proved disappointing for pediatric cancers. Other agents although toxic such as gamma-interferon, and the cytokines (e.g. IL2) may have some place in treatment of resistant disease.

MONITORING TUMOR RESPONSE

Standardization of tumor response criteria is essential to facilitate comparison of treatment protocols. What constitutes each category of response is not always easy in any specific tumor.

1. *Complete regression* (CR): complete macroscopic regression of all apparent tumor.
2. *Partial regression* (PR): more than 50% reduction, but less than 100% of any single measurable lesion without any new lesions appearing or growth of other identifiable lesions. (This category is sometimes split into good partial response and poor partial response.)
3. *Stable disease*: no change in any tumor as defined by less than 50% reduction of any single measurable lesion without any new lesions appearing. In pediatric tumors stable disease represents an unacceptable response.
4. *Progressive disease*: enlargement of at least one measurable lesion and/or the development of new lesions while on therapy.

SPECIFIC EFFECTS OF TREATMENT

Ionizing irradiation

Ionizing irradiation may kill or severely damage a cell. Sublethal cell damage, particularly to normal tissue surrounding a tumor, can cause tissue aging, malformation, growth impairment or induce carcinogenesis. Irradiation is generally given in daily fractions to facilitate normal cell recovery but hopefully not that of tumor cells. As cells in the periphery of the tumor mass are killed, more centrally placed and hypoxic cells will undergo a reoxygenation process and will become susceptible to therapy, particularly if there is an interval between radiation exposures.

Multiple fractions of radiation produce the same effect as a single large dose, but are better tolerated and more efficacious for most tumors. Tolerance curves can be produced for normal and malignant tissues. It is sometimes possible to calculate split course therapy during the intervals of which normal tissues can repair and some tumor cells will be recruited into the proliferative phase where they will be more susceptible to therapy.

Chemotherapy

Table 22.9 shows some adverse drug effects. Most produce alopecia, some gastrointestinal upset and myelosuppression. Patients worry most about the nausea and vomiting, physicians about infection risks and hemorrhage.

Hematological toxicity

The degree and duration of neutropenia increases the risk of sepsis with leukemia patients at greater risk than those with solid tumors.[100] The risks are greater before remission has been achieved. Regular monitoring of counts and careful education of parents as to the risks are essential.[101]

Neutropenia and infection

Neutropenia secondary to marrow infiltration or treatment leads to a significant risk of bacterial and fungal sepsis when the total neutrophil count is less than 1.0×10^9/L and grave risk to life when less than 0.2×10^9/L. The patient's own skin, mucosal surface and gastrointestinal flora may penetrate local defense mechanisms and produce septicemia. In most series the commonest isolated organisms are Gram positive skin flora, including *Staphylococcus albus*, *Staph. aureus* and *Staph. epidermidis*, but the gravest threat to life comes from the Gram negative bowel organisms including *Escherichia coli*, *Proteus*, *Klebsiella* and *Pseudomonas*.[102]

Meticulous hand washing techniques by all staff prior to patient contact can reduce nosocomial infection including colonization with some pathogens. Good oral hygiene reduces secondary infection in drug-induced mucositis, although there is still controversy as to whether oral antiseptic gargling is just as effective as antifungal agents, e.g. nystatin. Absorbed or semi-absorbed antifungals are more effective in preventing oral candida than oral nystatin.[103] The avoidance of vigorous tooth brushing reduces gum trauma.

The increased use of central venous lines has been associated with a rise in Gram positive sepsis, some of which can be avoided by expert placement (tip in right atrium or low superior vena cava) when the patient is not neutropenic, and by meticulous care thereafter. All rectal procedures should be prohibited during neutropenia unless absolutely unavoidable. The only prophylactic antibiotic of proven value in pediatric practice is oral co-trimoxazole to prevent *Pneumocystis carinii* pneumonitis.[104]

The rapid introduction of intravenous antibiotics for any child with less than 1×10^9/L neutrophils and a sustained fever (> 2 h) of 38.5°C has reduced mortality. Clinical signs of infection without fever necessitate a similar response. The antibiotic regimen chosen must take into account hospital and unit infection and sensitivity profiles (require careful monitoring) but must cover both Gram negative and Gram positive organisms (e.g. an aminoglycoside and third generation cephalosporin). In a recent survey of our unit 50% of leukemia patient admissions and 34% of patients with solid tumors were for infections. With more use of broad spectrum antibiotics fungal infection rates have increased. Whether effective oral prophylaxis to reduce gastrointestinal (GI) tract colonization reduces systemic infection is unproven. Failure of resolution of pyrexia after 48–72 h of effective i.v. antibiotics or if there is clinical deterioration, are indications for systemic antifungal therapy with amphotericin (or its liposomal equivalent). Fungal infections are particularly problematic in patients with prolonged neutropenia (> 10 days).

Prior to antibiotic therapy bacterial cultures should be taken from blood, throat, nose, any superficial skin lesion and urine. Stool cultures are useful in the presence of gut dysfunction. Fungal and viral cultures plus serology should be performed if there is poor response. Chest X-ray is indicated in the presence of respiratory symptoms or lack of resolution of fever. An aggressive search for the culpable organism is necessary. However in nearly two-thirds of patients an initial focus of infection is not identified.

Table 22.9 Specific drug toxicity effects of some commonly used chemotherapeutic agents

Drug	Myelo-suppression	Immuno-suppression	Tissue irritant	Nausea + vomiting	Cystitis	Nephrotoxicity	Cardiotoxicity	Neuropathic	Ototoxicity	Pulmonary	Hepatotoxicity
Anthracyclines (adriamycin + daunomycin)	++	+	+++	++	–	–	+++	–	–	–	Radiation recall effect
Actinomycin	++	+	+++	++	–	–	–	–	–	–	Radiation recall effect + VOD
Bleomycin	–	+/-	+	+/-	–	–	–	–	–	++	–
Alkylating agents											
Cyclophosphamide	++	++	+	++	++	+	+ (high dose)	+ (IADH)	–	+	–
Ifosfamide	++	++	+	++	+++	++	?++	++ (> in adults)	–	+	–
(Nitrosoureas, e.g. CCNU)	+++ (cumulative)	++		++	–	++ (cumulative)	–	+ (rare)	–	++	–
Non-classical alkylating											
Cisplatinum	+	+	+/-	+++	–	+++	–	++	+++ (cumulative)	–	–
Dacarbazine DTIC	+	+/-	+ (+ pain)	++	–	–	–	–	–	–	++ (+ VOD)
Antimetabolites											
Methotrexate oral, i.v., i.m., .it.	++	++	–	Mucositis ++ (high dose)	–	++ (high dose)	–	++ (high dose systemic + chronic i.m.)	–	+ + (acute/ chronic)	+ +
6-mercaptopurine oral + i.v.	+	+	–	Rarely	–	–	–	–	–	–	+
Cytosine i.v./i.m.	++	++	–	++ (diarrhea)	–	–	–	Cerebellar (High dose)	–	–	–
Vinca alkaloids									+++		
Vincristine	+/-	++	+++	–	–	–	–	+++ (+ IADH)	–	–	–
Vinblastine	++	++	+++	+/-	–	–	–	+/-	–	–	–
Epipodophyllotoxins											
Etoposide	++	+	+	+/- Mucositis	–	–	± (hypotension)	+ (mild peripheral)	–	–	+ (enzymes)
Steroids	–	+++	High dose pain	–	–	–	–	–	–	–	–
Asparaginase	++	++	–	–	–	–	–	Encephalopathy	–	–	++

In addition epipodophyllotoxins, asparaginases, bleomycin and rarely cytosine + cisplatinum are associated with acute life threatening hypersensitivity reactions
+–+++ denotes varying degree of toxicity
– denotes no recorded toxicity of type
VOD, veno-occlusive disease

Altered vital signs and signs of shock necessitate the addition of plasma expanders and i.v. inotropes starting with dopamine to maintain renal perfusion. Junior medical staff and nurses require expert training to respond to such life-threatening crises.

Immunosuppression

Both chemotherapy (especially leukemia treatment) and radiotherapy can induce lymphopenia and impaired T and B cell function. Viral infections may not be adequately cleared and common viruses may be excreted for months. Chickenpox and measles pose major risks. De novo or reactivated varicella infection formerly carried a 10% mortality but aciclovir therapy given prophylactically on contact history (200–400 mg q.d. for 21 days) or therapeutically 5–10 mg/kg i.v. 8-hourly for at least 5 days followed by at least 2 weeks of oral therapy to prevent recrudescence has dramatically reduced the risk. Immunosuppressed patients contracting measles and developing either immune encephalitis (weeks or months postinfection) or giant cell pneumonitis have a near 100% mortality.[105] Human immunoglobulin in a dose of 1 g/m^2 given i.m. within 72 h of contact may reduce the risk of the patient contracting the infection, although this has never been proved by a controlled trial. Higher titer immunoglobulin and interferon have been used for neurological and pneumonic signs but clear evidence of benefit is not available.[106] Prevention of measles in the patient with malignancy is best achieved by high community uptake of measles vaccination and avoidance of close contact with cases at school or in the community. Although immunization programs have reduced measles prevalence, only uptake rates in excess of 90% will make epidemics a feature of the past. Herpes simplex (HS) and cytomegalovirus (CMV) infections can be very troublesome after bone marrow transplantation. Prophylactic aciclovir may reduce the risk from both organisms. CMV infection can significantly impair marrow engraftment after transplantation.

Pneumocystis carinii pneumonitis may occur during periods of profound lymphopenia. It presents with intractable fever and tachypnea often with no clinically detectable chest signs despite florid radiographic changes. It can be prevented by the use of oral long-term co-trimoxazole. Treatment of the pneumonitis requires a higher dose (trimethoprim 20 mg/kg/day and sulfamethoxazole 100 mg/kg/day given in two divided doses daily). About 80% of patients respond, with some doing so only on the addition of steroids.[104] A small percentage of patients respond only to intramuscular pentamidine which is nephrotoxic and can produce marked hypoglycemia. Aerosol pentamidine can be used for prophylaxis in those hypersensitive to sulfonamides but has had disappointing results in leukemic patients. Cytomegalovirus may coexist with pneumocystis and can alone produce a similar pneumonitis. Ideally bronchoalveolar lavage or lung biopsy should be performed to confirm the diagnosis, certainly if there is poor response to therapy. Disease infiltration, fungi and drug reactions can all mimic *Pneumocystis carinii* pneumonitis.

Live vaccines, including measles and polio, must be avoided during therapy but killed vaccines such as those for diphtheria, pertussis and tetanus are permitted although they may be less effective than in the normal child because of the immunosuppression.

Bleeding

The development of efficient blood transfusion services has facilitated the advances made in the therapy of childhood cancer over the last 20 years. Red cells and platelets for transfusion have reduced morbidity and mortality from bleeding. Children have more efficient platelets and good blood vessel wall support when compared with adults and only tend to bleed overtly at very low platelet counts ($< 10 \times 10^9$/L) except in the presence of severe infection. There is little evidence in favor of prophylactic 'platelets' given at specific levels. Indications for platelet transfusion should be mucosal bleeding and/or florid skin petechiae with counts less than 20×10^9/L or at higher counts if fever is present. If invasive high risk procedures, such as lumbar punctures, are to be carried out, it is advisable to keep counts above 50×10^9/L for 24 h. Extradural hematomata have been reported when counts are not maintained after lumbar punctures. Frequent platelet transfusion leads to antibody development with poor increases in platelet number (children receive blood products from three to six donors for each platelet transfusion). The CMV immune status should be assessed for all patients at diagnosis and only CMV-negative donors used for those with no immunity. There is a significant risk of transfusion related graft versus host disease in patients with profoundly compromised cell mediated immunity. In oncological practice this includes all patients with Hodgkin's disease, bone marrow transplant recipients and any patient who has received fludaribine. To minimize this risk, these patients should receive irradiated blood products at all times.

Local tissue toxicity

Many antimitotics are tissue toxic if they extravasate (e.g. vincristine and anthracyclines). Use of central lines has decreased the risks although these are associated with an increase in infections. For both central and peripheral lines, only experienced fully trained staff should give cytotoxics and correct line placement should always be checked prior to injection (good blood flow back, easy flushing with saline and no pain).

Nausea and vomiting

Many drugs, e.g. the alkylators and platinum analogues, can produce profound nausea and vomiting. Control has been greatly enhanced by use of the 5-HT$_3$ receptor antagonists which avoid the extrapyramidal effects of agents such as the phenothiazines.[107] Seventy to eighty per cent of vomiting can be controlled by regular dosing starting before or just after chemotherapy. The addition of i.v. dexamethasone yields nearly 100% control in children, although hypertension and glycosuria must be checked for. Metoclopramide is an alternative but because of its short half-life really requires frequent (every 3–4 h) administration which can induce 'dystonia'. High dose regimens used in adults are not well tolerated in children. Initial bad experiences with chemotherapy may induce anticipatory vomiting especially in older children, for which oral anxiolytics (e.g. benzodiazepines) 12 h prior to therapy and even added to the ongoing regimen, relaxation and/or abreaction therapy or even hypnosis may be necessary.[108] Late or persistent vomiting can be a problem with the platinum compounds but also should alert the physician to possibilities of infection, hepatotoxicity or ongoing anxiety and psychological problems.[109] Repeated emesis can clearly cause significant fluid and electrolyte imbalance which requires correction.

Mucositis

Methotrexate, the anthracyclines and actinomycin all induce mucositis which is frequently complicated by secondary infection especially candida. Oral herpetic infection and neutropenia can mimic drug-induced ulceration.There is some evidence that ice chips can prevent mucositis but none of the other currently used prophylactic agents is effective. There is evidence that prophylactic absorbed antifungal agents can reduce the clinical signs of oral candidiasis.[103] Mucositis can be extremely painful and opiate analgesia should be used at an early stage.

Bowel dysfunction

High dose chemotherapy (e.g. melphalan, or busulfan and cyclophosphamide pretransplantation) can produce profound watery diarrhea as can continuous infusion or twice-daily cytosine arabinoside. Mucositis and such diarrhea can produce significant (> 10% of body weight) weight loss for which parenteral nutrition is required. In the absence of diarrhea such weight loss is due to tumor cachexia and loss of appetite is an indication for enteric feeding.

The vinca alkaloids produce severe constipation and ileus. This autonomic neuropathy may be complicated by enterocolitis, bowel wall edema and even intussusception. Regular use of bowel softeners (e.g. lactulose) may decrease the risk but when established it may require bowel stimulants, suppositories or enemas which carry infection risks in the neutropenic. Prevention by attention to fluid intake, maximizing activity, avoidance of excess narcotics and stool softeners is preferable.

Renal toxicity

Cisplatin causes progressive tubular and glomerular deterioration with increasing cumulative dosage and occasionally acute tubular necrosis. Vigorous hydration (saline and mannitol) can protect to some degree. Concomitant diuretics and aminoglycoside antibiotics should be avoided. Hydration should be continued for 24 h after cisplatinum. Glomerular function should be monitored regularly and no further cisplatinum should normally be given if the glomerular filtration rate falls below 60 ml/min/1.73m^2. Profound leakage of magnesium and calcium can produce weakness and tetany and require careful replacement. Systemic methotrexate and melphalan if given when renal function is impaired can cause further nephrotoxicity, delaying their own clearance and producing severe myelosuppression.

Cyclophosphamide and ifosfamide cause hemorrhagic cystitis if their metabolites are not voided from the bladder. Regular voiding and hydration for 24 h after administration are essential. The metabolites can be inactivated by concomitant equivalent doses of 2-mercaptoethane sulfonate sodium (Mesna).

The alkylators and vincristine can have an antidiuretic hormone effect with resultant fluid overload and dilutional hyponatremia. Seizures can result especially in the very young. Urinary flow must be maintained, if necessary with diuretics. Ifosfamide also can produce long-lasting renal tubular defects with hypophosphatemia, clinical rickets and reduction in glomerular filtration rate with cumulative dosage.

The nephrotoxicity of the commonly used antifungal agent amphotericin is an additive problem for these patients. Renal tubular damage can render them dependent upon electrolyte supplementation for prolonged periods. These problems can be largely avoided by the use of the liposomal formulations of this drug.

Cardiotoxicity

The anthracyclines produce cardiotoxicity. Acute toxicity with arrhythmias, conduction defects and fall in left ventricular output is relatively rare, transient and does not absolutely prevent future use of the drugs. Late cardiomyopathy is related to cumulative dosage with the incidence of congestive cardiac failure increasing steeply beyond 450 mg/m^2 of doxorubicin. Doppler M mode echocardiography and endomyocardial biopsies have, however, demonstrated functional abnormalities and loss of myofibrils at much lower cumulative dosages.[110] Dose rate and infusion time both affect toxicity.[111] Studies have reported echocardiographic changes in children who have received only 200–250 mg/m^2 of doxorubicin.[112] Up to 5% of patients will develop anthracycline-induced clinical heart failure 15 years after treatment, and those receiving more than 300 mg/m^2 are at highest risk.[113] Careful monitoring of ventricular end diastolic function and cessation of drug when abnormal, concomitant use of cardioprotectants such as ICRF 187 (chelates iron, which is a cofactor in the anthracycline free radical reaction inducing the damage)[114] and altering peak concentrations have all been tried in adults and more recently in children. Weekly scheduling of lower drug dose fractions or continuous infusions may offer a solution, although in adults infusion times beyond 96 h were necessary to provide significant benefit.[115] New analogues (e.g. idarubicin or epirubicin) may be less cardiotoxic especially those where the anthraquinine moiety can be omitted or modified. We do not yet know what the true long-term risk will be.

Neurotoxicity

Vincristine can produce peripheral neuropathy (ranging from loss of ankle jerks during therapy, through foot drop, 5%, wrist drop, 2% to slapping gait and paresthesia of extremities), and rarely convulsions and encephalopathy.[116] The central effects may be complicated by an antidiuretic hormone (ADH) effect with dilutional hyponatremia and seizures. The neuropathy can be very painful and is effectively treated with either amitriptyline or gabapentin. Encephalopathy has most often been recorded with leukemic induction therapy of weekly vincristine. However, such patients receive concomitant l-asparaginase (can produce cerebral hemorrhage, thrombosis, high ammonia levels and asparagine depletion) and intrathecal methotrexate both of which can induce seizures and encephalopathic features.

CNS-directed therapy in leukemia can cause a leukoencephalopathy, most commonly if intrathecal or systemic methotrexate is administered after cranial irradiation. The least toxic modality is continuing intrathecal methotrexate alone (see below); ifosfamide produces an encephalopathy more commonly in adults than in children.[117]

Ototoxicity

Platinum analogues especially cisplatinum cause progressive high tone deafness with increasing cumulative dosage. Tinnitus and, especially if combined with cranial irradiation, rapid deterioration of hearing can occur.[118]

Hepatotoxicity

Oral methotrexate can induce a cirrhotic state and mercaptopurine cholestatic jaundice. High dose i.v. methotrexate can induce florid hepatic disturbance with mucositis and severe myelosuppression (more likely if combined with other drugs cleared by the liver). Actinomycin and anthracyclines should be avoided if possible for the first 4–6 weeks following abdominal (liver encroachment) irradiation. These and busulfan/cyclophosphamide conditioning for transplantation have been associated with veno-occlusive disease (VOD). This condition presents with hepatomegaly, ascites, encephalopathy and thrombocytopenia 5–10 days after actinomycin treatment.[119] An incidence of 1.2% has been reported for this condition in patients treated on the IRS IV protocol,[120] and as high as 8% for children treated for Wilms' tumor.[121] It can be associated with multiorgan failure and death. A strong case can be made for the avoidance of any further actinomycin in patients who have even a mild episode of VOD. The most effective therapy remains in doubt.

Biochemical disturbance

Either spontaneously or following treatment, tumor cell breakdown can result in a lysis syndrome, most commonly in T and B cell lymphoblastic disorders. Hyperkalemia (from cell death), hyperphosphatemia (high content in lymphoblasts) and consequent hypocalcemia, hyperuricemia (and oxypurines from nucleic acid breakdown), renal tubular urate deposition, and azotemia can occur. The risks can be reduced by phased drug introduction, avoidance of citrated blood (exacerbates hypocalcemia), control of any infection, high fluid intake (2.5–3 L/m^2/day), allopurinol (10 mg/kg/day in divided doses, i.v. if necessary) and careful urinary alkalinization with i.v. bicarbonate. In patients at greatest risk of tumor lysis syndrome recombinant urate oxidase is highly effective at preventing its development.[122] The aim is to keep the urine at pH 6.5–7.0 to keep urate and xanthine in solution. At higher pH values phosphate may precipitate in the renal tubules. Blood phosphate levels can be reduced by oral aluminum hydroxide. Intravenous calcium should be avoided (it will be tissue deposited) and careful i.v. injection of magnesium preferred to relieve tetany.

Acute psychological effects

Painful procedures and toxic therapy can become intolerable for the child unless reduced to a minimum by a closely coordinated team of doctors and nurses. The family need to make the child realize the absolute need for such treatment and must tolerate but not overindulge the natural reaction to the treatment and show that they care for their child as a special individual. Displays of personal warmth by the pediatrician can be amazingly effective in defusing emotional crises. The pediatric oncologist must support and help not only the child but the whole family. The parents must know and understand the diagnosis, the nature of cancer and the effect of treatment if the child is to come through emotionally intact. It is essential from the start to explain repeatedly in everyday language what is happening, the likely diagnosis and what it means to the child. The initial shock or numbness at the news precludes 'real' hearing and subsequently, phases of anger at the apparent injustice are often misdirected at the staff.[123] This must be tolerated and emphasis placed on the team approach necessary to help their child through. Excess optimism or pessimism must be avoided but if treatment is offered and accepted, some feeling of hope must be conveyed. Involvement in the simpler aspects of nursing their child often provides a sense of purpose for parents. As they come to terms with the shock of diagnosis, parents frequently ask more searching questions which must be answered truthfully. If more than one member of staff explains matters, it is essential to stress that words used may be different but the meaning is the same. The caring team must be both seen to be and in fact coordinated, and unit meetings are essential for this purpose. There are a few genuine circumstances where the extent of disease or nature of tumor diagnosis precludes cure. For such a child where there is no realistic treatment option and if parents agree, support for the whole family is even more important. Parents must realize that they are always told the truth, 'good' means good and the converse is true about any bad news. Parents may wish their child to be protected from the facts of the disease and diagnosis, but for the majority of children this is a mistake. Children are usually much more resilient than adults and provided appropriate words are used, and they have confidence in the person conveying the problem, they can cope admirably with even the worst of news. Time is necessary to build up confidence for the child and parents, and if such time is not spent at the beginning, management will become fraught with problems. Secrets about the disease within the family, especially keeping facts from siblings, is also unwise. When trust has developed, even if treatment fails and the patient becomes terminal, the team can usually support the patient and family through the final illness more adequately.

For teenagers striving to find themselves and being naturally rebellious against parental and other authority, the news of cancer and its necessary treatment can be particularly hard as it inevitably requires compliance with and dependence upon those from who they are striving to emotionally separate. They require great understanding and sometimes even a little support in their rebellion.

The involvement of a dedicated child psychiatrist in the team who can help staff to understand family interactions and can guide both staff and family through specific crises has proved very useful in many oncology centers. It may be that help is required by specific families where stress has become too great or where previous psychopathology is present. Cancer does not select specific families but affects the spectrum of the population independent of intelligence, insight and behavior.

LONG TERM SEQUELAE

Table 22.10 lists the potential long term sequelae seen in childhood cancer survivors.

Late recurrence

Patients and parents worry most about disease recurrence. Hawkins[124] followed up over 11 000, 3-year cancer survivors, for at least 10 further years (Table 22.11). He found no excess late deaths and consequently cure was possible in non-Hodgkin's lymphoma and non-genetic retinoblastoma. The late excess deaths in ALL were largely confined to boys with recurrent leukemia which has been reported beyond 10 years from diagnosis. Young age was a definite advantage in nephroblastoma and neuroblastoma in reducing the risk of later recurrence; indeed late relapses in both tumors are rare (less than 1 in 200). Over 75% of late deaths were due to primary disease. Second tumors caused the excess deaths in genetic retinoblastoma and Hodgkin's disease, not recurrence of the primary disease. With improving event free survival (EFS) after very intensive treatment for the primary cancer this pattern of late events may well change.

Second tumors

The Late Effects Study Group (USA) studied 9000 childhood tumor patients diagnosed between 1936 and 1979 and reported a second neoplasm incidence of 8% at 20 years from diagnosis which is 15 times higher than the general population at this age range.[125] In the more recent era the risks may be different as a result of increasing survival after the first tumor following more intensive therapy larger population at long term risk but with decreasing use of mixed modality therapy radiotherapy as well as chemotherapy which is known to have

Table 22.10 Potential long term sequelae of childhood cancer

Late recurrence of primary cancer
Second malignancy
Impairment of normal growth
Endocrine dysfunction
Infertility
Educational and psychological dysfunction
Other organ toxicity, e.g. cardiac, pulmonary
Impairment of normal life, e.g. obtaining work, insurance, being allowed to adopt children

Table 22.11 Long term survivors in childhood cancer

Tumor type	% of survivors at 3 years still alive at +10 years	Excess deaths (per n survivors at +10 years)
Acute lymphoblastic leukemia	60%	1 in 100
Hodgkin's disease	74%	< 1 in 100
Non-Hodgkin's lymphoma	85%	None
Neuroblastoma	89%	< 1 in 200
Nephroblastoma	94%	< 1 in 200
Retinoblastoma		
Genetic	93%	1 in 200
Non-genetic	100%	None

Data derived from Hawkins 1989[124]

increased the incidence of soft tissue and bony sarcomas. Meadows et al[125,126] identified in that initial series that 'genetic' retinoblastoma and Hodgkin's disease (HD) were the most frequent primary tumor in patients developing second tumors, identifying the risk factors to be genetic susceptibility (with Rb1 gene mutation up to 30% will develop a second tumor[22]) and a combination of irradiation with alkylators in Hodgkin's disease, respectively. Other genetic disorders predisposing to multiple malignancies in childhood are clearly germline TP53 mutation (Li–Fraumeni syndrome), neurofibromatosis type 1, and nevoid basal cell carcinoma syndrome. Emphasizing the contribution of irradiation, two-thirds of all the second solid tumors occurred within radiation fields (30% being soft tissue or bony sarcomas). Such solid tumors have a long latency (median of 10–15 years). Total dosage (greater than 30 Gy), orthovoltage treatment (largely replaced now by megavoltage) and young age increased the risk.[75,127] In the Late Effects Group series secondary leukemia was most consistently associated with previous receipt of alkylators (dose dependent).[75] Ng et al[76] have reviewed the risks in the more modern era where secondary acute non-lymphoblastic leukemia with a shorter latency period (median 30 months) than seen with alkylators (median 5–7 years) has been increasingly described in patients exposed to topoisomerase 2 inhibitors (epipodophyllotoxins such as etoposide and tenoposide plus anthracyclines). The risk appears to be total dose and schedule dependent (once or twice weekly without allowing for DNA recovery time).[128] However even with low dosage and 'safe' schedules there is a risk which is probably a reflection of genetic susceptibility either to increased DNA damage or failure to repair it adequately following the double DNA strand induced by the drugs.[76,129]

The risk of developing second tumors after treatment for acute lymphoblastic leukemia appears to be relatively low at 2.5–3% at 15 to 20 years from diagnosis.[130,131] The commonest tumors seen are gliomas and meningiomas in cranial irradiation fields. It has been reported that the risk continues to increase with time from treatment well beyond 20 years and may be exacerbated by defective concurrent thiopurine metabolism.[132] Thyroid and tongue carcinomas (both organs at the periphery of cranial irradiation fields) have been described.[133,134]

Growth impairment

The tumor itself, poor nutrition and infection as well as treatment can all impair growth and cause weight loss but there is usually catch up once remission is achieved. Direct radiation damage to the hypothalamic–pituitary axis (from cranial irradiation) impairs growth hormone production or release and in higher total dosage greater than 30 Gy (also dependent on fractions) also gonadotrophic and adrenocorticotrophic hormone secretion.[135] Since the hypothalamus is more sensitive to irradiation than the pituitary the primary event is one of subnormal secretion of growth hormone releasing hormone (GHRH) rather than growth hormone production especially when radiation doses are less than 30 Gy.

Spinal irradiation will significantly impair final height achievement. The younger the child at treatment the greater the height lost (if irradiated at 1 year 9 cm, if at 10 years 5.5 cm). Precocious puberty can occur in children receiving cranial irradiation as part of treatment for leukemia (total dosage in the range 18–24 Gy) or even more so in those with brain tumors (radiation to hypothalamic–pituitary axis greater than 30 Gy). Young age at treatment increases the risk. In girls but possibly not in boys puberty may be both premature and foreshortened, further reducing final height and giving less time during which growth hormone replacement can be delivered. Growth hormone may need to be given in combination with gonadotrophin releasing hormone (GnRH) to attempt to arrest pubertal maturation. Growth hormone replacement may be less effective in gaining height for such patients than it is in idiopathic growth hormone deficiency. This is particularly noted in patients who have received total body irradiation for marrow transplantation. In them spinal irradiation, thyroid deficiency, epiphyseal plate damage, chronic graft versus host disease and malnutrition may all contribute. Growth hormone therapy appears totally safe to administer to patients with previous malignancies provided at least 1 year (but normally 2 years) have elapsed from treatment, and the patient is in full remission. To date there has been no convincing evidence of tumor reactivation or induction of second malignancies by growth hormone.[136]

Progressively more intensive chemotherapy used with cranial irradiation for childhood leukemia appears to increase the risk of growth impairment[137] and Davies et al[138] reported increased body disproportion with short spines in children treated with cranial irradiation and chemotherapy. In vitro there is evidence of a direct effect of cytotoxics on chondrocytes.[139]

Now that cranial irradiation is only used in a small minority of ALL patients, we will obtain a clearer picture of the effect on growth of intensive chemotherapy alone. Other effects of treatment for leukemia during childhood using chemotherapy and cranial irradiation include altered body composition with central obesity, hyperleptinemia[140] and reduced bone mineral density.[141] Such patients in adulthood might require and benefit from some growth hormone replacement. The evidence to date is that with chemotherapy alone bone mineral density is not significantly affected (Brennan 2003 – personal communication).

It is essential that all children with malignancies who receive cranial, craniospinal, abdominal and total body irradiation and those treated with intensive chemotherapy should be regularly assessed for linear growth, pubertal status and weight, not just whilst on therapy but on a long term basis until they have reached maturity.

Thyroid dysfunction

Thyroid radiation damage results in a rise in thyroid stimulating hormone (TSH) and then hypothyroidism. This follows total body, craniospinal and local neck irradiation (e.g. in Hodgkin's disease). Low doses (100 cGy) may be enough to induce damage, even after cranial irradiation (up to 7.5% scatter may impinge on the gland). Thyroid adenomas and carcinomas have been induced.[133] Tumors are thought to result from prolonged overdrive by elevated TSH. Persistent TSH elevation on follow-up requires replacement even in the absence of clinical or biochemical hypothyroidism. It is not clear whether chemotherapy enhances the radiation damage of the thyroid gland.

Gonadal dysfunction and infertility

From spinal irradiation there will be a scatter to the ovaries (90–1000 cGy depending on the field and dosage) and testes (40–1020 cGy) potentially affecting fertility. Direct testicular therapy in leukemia (20–24 Gy) for testicular relapse ablates the germinal epithelium leading to infertility and in addition the younger the patient the more likely it will also damage Leydig cell function – raised basal levels of follicle stimulating hormone (FSH) and luteinizing hormone (LH), low testosterone and impaired response to HCG. If present, androgen replacement will be required from age 12–13 years. Total body irradiation (TBI) will impair spermatogenesis, and have a variable effect on testicular endocrine function depending on the total dose, fraction and whether any gonadal boost has been given. Ovarian function is dependent on the dose delivered, with variable endocrine and oogenic consequences. TBI invariably causes secondary amenorrhea in postpubertal females from which there may be some recovery with time.

Drugs have a variable impact on gonadal function. The nitrosoureas (BCNU and CCNU) and procarbazine produce primary gonadal failure with elevated basal FSH and sometimes LH levels. Girls achieve puberty at a normal age with regular menses but whether these are ovulatory cycles or whether reproductive life may be shortened is unclear. Testicular size is reduced postpubertally with oligospermia and in some total infertility. There is no evidence of recovery for boys. Chemotherapy compounds irradiation effects. Testicular germinal epithelial damage is particularly common with cyclophosphamide and cytosine although some recovery of spermatogenesis may occur with these drugs over time. Leydig cell function is minimally affected by these agents. In standard Hodgkin's disease therapy including alkylating agents, the germinal epithelium of boys may be severely and apparently irreversibly affected while Leydig cell function may be near normal. In adolescents and young adults sperm banking is now recommended before treatment.[142] In young girls ovarian damage is not clinically obvious but for postpubertal women ovarian failure may occur in up to 60% of patients. This demonstrates the complexity of endocrine disorders and an endocrinologist should be involved in the long term follow-up and management of childhood cancer survivors.[143] In the future the current experimental approaches of ovarian and testicular tissue storage with later reimplantation may have a place in therapy.

Educational and psychosocial effects

Time lost from nursery and schooling at critical stages of learning, e.g. during the peak age range of childhood leukemia (2–6 years) may impair educational achievement. This may result from illness, sequelae of treatment and parental anxiety about allowing the child to mix in 'society'. CNS directed radiation therapy for leukemia (in the range 18–25 Gy) and even more so for CNS tumors (whole brain doses in excess of 30 Gy) produces long standing neuropsychological sequelae (cognitive dysfunction, short term memory impairment and difficulties in problem solving). Young age at the time of treatment (especially under 3 years) affords a special risk of damage.[144] These findings occur in patients without necessarily evidence of any structural abnormalities although there are a whole range of more severe neurological sequelae in leukemic patients including subacute leukoencephalopathy, mineralizing angiopathy, subacute necrotizing leukomyelopathy and cortical atrophy.[145] The combined effect of cranial irradiation in leukemia patients on both growth and educational achievement has led to alternative CNS directed strategies being utilized (prolonged course of intrathecal methotrexate injections with or without high dose systemic methotrexate). Such approaches are effective in controlling CNS disease but are not totally without some effect on neuropsychological functioning albeit apparently less than with cranial irradiation.[146,147] Maintenance of verbal proficiency may mask poor overall performance.

The incidence of long term overt psychological and psychiatric problems appears remarkably low amongst cancer survivors. However, many patients, particularly those who have received cranial irradiation, appear to be 'loners' with low self-esteem, working but in jobs requiring less than they are capable of and are much less likely than their peers to be in long term relationships. Child–parent relationships and life-long family coping does seem to influence psychological outcome. Recently reported is a trend for paternal emotional distancing from affected children which may underpin some of the abnormal long term psychosocial adjustment. The impact of 'waiting for a relapse' is too much for some families to cope with.[148] Nevertheless the vast majority of childhood cancer patients complete normal education, have higher rates of employment than their matched peers[149] but some as described above function below their level of competence. Some face outdated prejudice from employers, some insurance and pension schemes (excessive weighting of premiums long term) and have difficulty of being considered as adoptees when rendered infertile by treatment.

Cardiorespiratory

Acute cardiac effects after anthracycline drugs have been described above, but the extent of the long term effects on endocardial muscle remains controversial. There are reports of cardiac failure leading to sudden death after strenuous exercise (e.g. weight lifting) or during pregnancy, and deteriorating cardiac function only rescued by cardiac transplantation in others. Total anthracycline doses in excess of 200 mg/m^2 have been associated with long term echocardiographic changes but how many progress to overt severe cardiac disease in mid life is still not clear.[111,150] Other cytotoxics, for example high dose cyclophosphamide, and irradiation have been implicated in contributing to late cardiac dysfunction.

Sixty-five per cent of 5-year leukemia survivors in one study showed one or more defects of low vital capacity, total lung capacity, residual volume or transfer factor[151] but very few were symptomatic. These features represent impairment of lung growth during the first 5–6 years of life. This may be of significance especially amongst smokers, later in life. Amongst solid tumor survivors chest wall growth impairment, restriction defects and/or fibrosis are more frequently identified, especially where the lungs have been irradiated.[152, 153]

Conclusions on sequelae

Without intensive treatment most children with cancer died 30–40 years ago. Now approximately 60% survive long term and most have good quality of life. Some sequelae such as gonadal failure and infertility may be an acceptable, if regrettable, price for life but second tumors and late cardiac deaths are not. It is essential that all childhood cancer patients are followed for life so that lessons can be learnt and therapy modified where appropriate without any loss of efficacy.

CENTRAL NERVOUS SYSTEM TUMORS

Central nervous system tumors constitute the commonest solid tumors of childhood. The commonest – embryonal medulloblastomas – are quite distinct from the common adult gliomas.[154] Recognized etiologic factors are shown in Table 22.12, and Table 22.13 shows

Table 22.12 Etiological factors for CNS tumors

Heritable syndromes
- Neurofibromatosis (visual pathway tumors + gliomas)
- Tuberous sclerosis (glial ependymomas)
- Von Hippel–Lindau (cerebellar + retinal + pheochromocytomas)

Familial clustering without identifiable genetic factor (various tumors including pinealomas)

Familial with autosomal dominant inheritance: astrocytoma

Retinoblastoma and pinealoblastoma (13q-)

Rhabdoid renal tumors and primitive neuroectodermal tumors of brain

Monosomy 22: meningiomas + acoustic neuromas

Ionizing irradiation: after low dose scalp irradiation and possible dental investigations

Immunodeficiency (intracerebral lymphomas) especially:
- a. postrenal transplantation
- b. Wiskott–Aldrich
- c. ataxia telangiectasia

Parental exposure to organic compounds such a nitrosamines and polycyclic hydrocarbons

the incidence of different childhood brain tumors. Universal agreement about classification is lacking. Most modern schemes divide them into four broad categories:[155] 1) glial, 2) neuronal, 3) primitive neuroectodermal tumor (PNET) and 4) pineal cell tumors. Attempts to grade tumors by the degree of anaplasia have only been partially successful. With modern immunohistochemistry and molecular biological methods it is possible to more accurately identify the cells within CNS tumors.[156] Markers include antibodies detecting glial fibrillary acidic protein, S100 protein, neuron specific enolase and neurofilament protein. These are coupled with non-neuronal markers such as cytokeratin, vimentin, desmin and AFP to enable the pathologist to more accurately determine the cellular nature of the tumors. More than 60% of childhood brain tumors are infratentorial and nearly half are undifferentiated embryonal tumors (Table 22.14). Only modification of the WHO classification takes all these pediatric features into account.[155]

The primitive neuroectodermal tumor (PNET) which occurs almost exclusively in childhood, in or around the cerebellum, is usually identified as a medulloblastoma. Similar tumors may occur in the cerebrum, the pineal region, the brainstem or in the cord

Table 22.13 Relative incidence of CNS neoplasms in childhood (1981–1990) with male/female ratio of each group of tumors

Tumor type	Percentage	M/F ratio
Astrocytoma	38.3	1.1
Primitive neuro-ectodermal tumors	21.2	1.7
Ependymoma	10.8	1.4
Other gliomas	15.2	1.1
Other specified	8.6	1.1
Unspecified	5.9	0.9

Data from Parkin et al 1998[3]

Table 22.14 World Health Organization classification of pediatric brain tumors

A. Glial tumors
1. Astrocytic astrocytoma
2. Oligodendroglial tumors
3 Ependymomal tumors including ependymoma
4. Choroid plexus tumors
5. Mixed gliomas
6. Glioblastoma multiforme

B Neuronal tumors
1. Gangliocytoma } including primary intracranial neuroblastoma
2. Ganglioglioma } including primary intracranial neuroblastoma
3. Anaplastic ganglioglioma

C. Primitive neuroectodermal tumors (PNET)
1. PNET not otherwise specified = medulloblastoma
2. PNET with differentiation
3. Medulloepithelioma

D. Pineal cell tumors
1. Pineocytoma
2. Pineoblastoma (PNET)

where they may be labeled ependymoma, pinealoma, retinoblastoma or even infratentorial–cerebral neuroblastoma. Controversy exists as to whether all these tumors should be called PNET and how the differentiation between them should be made.

SYMPTOMS AND SIGNS

The presenting symptoms and signs of brain tumors in childhood depend more on the site than on type of tumor. Neurological features are due to infiltration, compression of neuronal structures or raised intracranial pressure secondary to obstruction of CSF pathways. Raised intracranial pressure presents early in the majority of the infratentorial tumors with the classic triad of morning headache, vomiting and visual disturbance. There may be more vague symptoms of tiredness, deteriorating school performance, personality change and non-localized headache for a variable period before the classic triad presents.

Headaches in young children should always be taken seriously and investigated. In infants presenting symptoms may be irritability, loss of appetite and developmental delay or even the loss of acquired skills. Even with large tumors full neurological examination may yield few signs. Infants under 2 years may develop an increase in OFC with springing of the sutures as intracranial pressure increases and in babies the 'setting sun' sign may be seen. Fundi are frequently pale with just the early signs of papilledema. Fundal examination can be very difficult and sedation and pupillary dilatation may be appropriate. Developmental assessment should be part of the full examination. Specific signs depend on the site of the tumor.

Infratentorial lesions

Raised intracranial pressure and disturbance of balance (truncal and extremity) and specific cranial nerve dysfunction are the cardinal signs of the well-established tumor. Midline medulloblastomas may present only with raised intracranial pressure and truncal unsteadiness and without localizing features while the cerebellar hemisphere lesions (e.g. astrocytomas) may present with lateralizing features before intracranial pressure is evident. It is, however, usually not possible to distinguish between astrocytoma and medulloblastoma clinically. VI nerve palsy may be a false localizing sign arising from raised intracranial pressure. When present bilaterally and especially when in combination with V, VII or IX nerve palsies, brainstem involvement is likely. Head tilt is frequently seen together with cochlear nerve palsy and vertical or horizontal diplopia when cerebellar tonsillar herniation occurs.

Supratentorial lesions

Both the site and the size of the tumor determine the presenting signs. With these lesions non-specific headaches, seizures of all types and long tract signs may predominate. Raised intracranial pressure may be the first sign of tumors in relatively silent areas of the cortex (frontal, parietal or occipital) and the tumor may be very large. Raised pressure may be an early feature in small 3rd ventricular lesions. Visual field defects may help to localize tumors. In primitive neuroectodermal tumors such as medulloblastoma, dissemination throughout the CNS via the cerebrospinal fluid may lead to symptoms and signs far removed from the primary lesion with consequent diagnostic confusion. Careful documentation of all signs and symptoms in the order that they appear is important and their disappearance with treatment should be monitored for response rates.

DIAGNOSIS

CT and MR scanning have revolutionized the diagnosis of pediatric brain tumors. CT is useful for rapid identification of hydrocephalus and mass effect but MRI is preferred for precise tumor definition in multiple planes prior to surgery (especially for brainstem gliomas and spinal tumors).[157] Positron emission tomography (PET) may prove useful in detecting variations in metabolism between residual tumor and normal brain, and MR spectroscopy may also prove useful in non-invasive diagnosis.[158] For the PNETs, exclusion of spinal deposits by MR scanning is essential.

GENERAL PRINCIPLES OF TREATMENT

Surgery

Preoperative steroids to reduce edema, external decompression of hydrocephalus and new scanning techniques have facilitated more complete surgical removal of visible tumor without increased morbidity. Extent of excision is a determinant of outcome for many tumor types.[159,160] Midline posterior fossa tumors more frequently require long-term ventriculoperitoneal shunting. There is no evidence that this increases the likelihood of extracerebral metastases. Surgeons reduce peripheral damage by use of operative microscopes, ultrasonic aspirators and lasers. Operative mortality for most tumors has been reduced to under 1% although morbidity may be as high as 20%. For some (e.g. cerebellar astrocytomas) excessive attempts to excise all of the tumor initially may be contraindicated (see below).

Radiotherapy[161]

Fields and volumes treated should be limited to minimize normal tissue damage. Astrocytomas of Grade III and IV do require whole brain irradiation and medulloblastomas, ependymomas, PNETs and some germ cell tumors, craniospinal irradiation. Although local areas can tolerate total dosages as high as 50–55 Gy, whole brain dosages over 35 Gy are associated with significant sequelae. Fraction size, number of fractions and duration of treatment all influence toxicity. Hypoxic cell sensitizers have not yet found a place in pediatric practice.

Acute radiation side-effects include headache (hot head), vomiting, skin erythema, alopecia and otitis externa. Lymphopenia is universal and may persist for 6 months. Profound myelosuppression may follow spinal irradiation and make subsequent chemotherapy difficult to deliver. Five to ten weeks after cranial irradiation 'somnolence syndrome' can occur (profound sleepiness, mild pyrexia, and some have GI upset) owing to a temporary disturbance of myelination. A similar effect on the spine produces Lhermitte's sign (shooting arm pains). Long-term effects are described above.

Chemotherapy

The vulnerability of the developing CNS to radiation-induced damage, coupled with the poor survival for many types of tumor has resulted in considerable interest in the role of chemotherapy. The blood–brain barrier limits access to the brain of most drugs. At the margins of tumors, the tight capillary endothelial junctions persist, while neoplastic neovascularity makes the core of tumors more accessible. Lipid solubility, molecular size, protein binding and plasma concentration all determine the ability of a drug to penetrate the CNS. Lipophilic drugs (e.g. nitrosoureas) will penetrate tumor margins and water-soluble agents (e.g. cisplatinum) the core. The initial goal of many of the early studies of chemotherapy for CNS tumors was to delay or avoid radiotherapy especially in the very young. A large number of such 'baby brain' studies have now been reported (reviewed in Kellie[162]) with varying degrees of success, and such a strategy is now routinely adopted for most infants. The use of multiagent chemotherapy with curative intent is variable between tumor types and for most randomized prospective trials are only just beginning to be done to determine the role of chemotherapy in a multimodality treatment plan.

MEDULLOBLASTOMA (PNET OF CEREBELLUM) (20% of CNS tumors)

This is a midline vermis PNET arising adjacent to the roof of the fourth ventricle. The peak age incidence is 5 years (some series show a second peak at 10–12 years). There is a male preponderance.

Presentation

Obstruction of the fourth ventricle leads to raised intracranial pressure, progressive ataxia of the lower limbs, diplopia, and V, VII and other cranial nerve deficits. Long tract signs appear rather later. Nuchal rigidity and/or head tilt suggests cerebellar tonsillar herniation and necessity for rapid relief. The differential diagnosis includes cerebellar astrocytoma, ependymoma, brainstem glioma, and infectious encephalitis (although the last is usually of more acute onset). CT scan shows a solid homogeneous, iso- or hyperdense lesion which is enhanced by contrast but these features are not unique to medulloblastoma. An MR scan may more easily differentiate a medulloblastoma from the other tumors by clearly showing the site of origin.[157] Lumbar CSF examination should *not* be performed before surgery.

Prognostic features

In 1969 Chang devised a staging system based on tumor size, local extension and presence of metastases.[163] Degree of resection rather than size of tumor per se may influence prognosis. Any subarachnoid spread and of course extraneural disease significantly worsens prognosis but isolated positive CSF cytology does not. Young age (under 5 but especially under 2) is adverse with likelihood of large tumor bulk and treatment modification to prevent neuronal damage. A diploid DNA content within tumor cells worsens prognosis (35% at 4 years compared with 85% in hyperdiploidy in one series). c-myc oncogene amplification and differentiation within the tumor may prove to be adverse features.

Pathology

This is a highly cellular soft and friable tumor full of small round undifferentiated cells with hyperchromatic nuclei and abundant mitoses. There can be variable glial or neuroblast differentiation which may be of prognostic significance.

Management

Complete macroscopic resection is achievable in about 50% of cases. One-year disease-free survival figures appear to be 30–50%, better for those with complete resection, but at 5 years the improvement is down to about 10%. Provided there is no evidence of morbidity during the procedure, complete removal should be attempted. These tumors are the most radiosensitive of the primary CNS childhood tumors and radiotherapy is required to the whole neuraxis with at least 50 Gy to the posterior fossa. Attempts to reduce whole craniospinal dosages by use of chemotherapy have resulted in worsened prognosis.

Three-year survival figures of up to 60% have been reported for surgical resection followed by craniospinal irradiation.[160] These patients have high morbidity from whole CNS irradiation (intellectual impairment and growth). Medulloblastoma has been shown to be chemosensitive in relapse schedules and in vitro. Although early multicenter trials (SIOP I, II) were unable to confirm the survival advantage seen with adjuvant chemotherapy in single-center trials, SIOP PNET 3 showed a significant increase in EFS for patients treated with etoposide, vincristine, cyclophosphamide and carboplatin as opposed to those receiving radiotherapy alone (3-year EFS 78% v 65%).[164] Excellent results have also been reported using cisplatin, vincristine and CCNU[165,166] and this combination is now the recommended treatment in most studies.

EPENDYMOMA (5–10% of CNS tumors)

These arise from the lining of the ventricular system and central canal of the spinal cord (75% in the posterior fossa, 25% in the cord). The peak age of onset is in the first 2 years of life. Like the medulloblastomas they may be a heterogeneous group; most are well demarcated but with areas of hemorrhage and cyst formation internally. There is considerable variation in anaplasia, pleomorphism and differentiation. The *subependymoma* is often silent and found coincidentally at autopsy. The ependymomas spread locally and disseminate. Spinal subarachnoid space involvement is much more likely with infratentorial tumors (20–30%) than with the supratentorial tumors (3–8%). High grade ependymomas may disseminate within the CNS through the CSF but systemic spread is rare.

Presentation

Raised intracranial pressure is common in all posterior fossa tumors. There may be some cerebellar dysfunction. Local cranial nerve deficits are more commonly seen than in medulloblastoma because of local infiltration and invasion of the floor of the fourth ventricle and brainstem. Supratentorial ependymomas more commonly present with seizures and long tract signs. The duration of the history depends on the site and the grade of the tumor ranging in high grade tumors to just 3 or 4 weeks and in lower grade ones, up to 1 year. The differential diagnosis will include astrocytomas, medulloblastomas, brainstem gliomas and, where they arise in the lateral or third ventricles, choroid plexus tumors or astrocytomas.

Diagnosis

CT scans will show a hyperdense and contrast-enhancing tumor with hydrocephalus. Internally there will frequently be hemorrhage and cysts; MR scanning will delineate infiltration. CSF examination is needed postoperatively along with myelography or MR scanning.

Prognostic features

Spinal cord and especially myxopapillary cauda equina tumors fare better but otherwise site is not of prognostic significance. It is unclear for ependymomas whether histology (anaplasia) or degree of resection are of significance. Young age (< 5 years) and brainstem invasion do adversely affect outcome.

Management

Attempts at primary total resection are indicated and usually possible for supratentorial tumors, less so in the posterior fossa where brainstem infiltration increases perioperative morbidity (5–10%). With surgery alone 5-year survival is 15–20%. For supratentorial tumors extended local field irradiation to a total dose of 50–55 Gy (tumor + 1- to 2-cm margin) and for posterior fossa lesions a field to extend down to C3–4 are indicated. Most relapses are local but 10–15% have subarachnoid spread. This may be greater in posterior fossa and anaplastic tumors; for them, craniospinal irradiation has been recommended. For low grade tumors, surgery and extended field radiotherapy yield 50% 5-year survival. Intramedullary spinal cord tumors may be cured by complete microsurgical resection. Chemotherapy has not been shown to significantly improve survival[167] although ependymoma has been shown to be chemosensitive especially in infants, and trials of adjuvant chemotherapy are ongoing.

CEREBELLAR ASTROCYTOMAS (10–20% of CNS tumors)

These occur throughout childhood without an obvious age peak but there is a slight male preponderance. Four-fifths are pilocytic with areas of loose cellularity or cyst formation intermixed with more compact cellular areas. The remainder are termed diffuse astrocytomas. These more solid tumors appear to have a poorer prognosis. Most cerebellar astrocytomas are well localized although occasional reports of non-contiguous spread have occurred even in the pilocytic tumors. It is possible that some of these deposits represent multifocal disease. Very rarely high grade astrocytomas do arise in the cerebellum.

Presentation

Because of their usual slow growth, these tumors are often associated with less acute clinical onset and symptoms present for longer than in medulloblastoma. Presentation is usually with the symptoms and signs of raised intracranial pressure, although involvement (pressure or invasion) of the cerebellar peduncles and brainstem may give cranial nerve and long tract signs.

Diagnosis

Distinction from medulloblastoma is often difficult although on CT astrocytomas are usually less dense and often have a cystic component (the wall and nodule of which contrast enhance). MR scans usually show sharper demarcation of tumor margins.

Management

Lateral tumors should be removed as completely as possible. While this may be more difficult for midline or peduncular tumors, between 80 and 90% of all low grade cerebellar astrocytomas can be fully resected with less than 1% mortality. Some patients require preoperative and some long-term CSF shunting. After complete resection about 90% of patients in most series remain alive and well, requiring no further treatment. For tumors that can not be completely resected a period of close observation followed by further surgery, should tumor regrowth occur, is justified. Radiotherapy does not significantly influence survival following surgical resection and should only be used where repeat operation is not possible. With improved surgical techniques, smaller residual loads remain and survival figures for those with incomplete resection are now 60–70%. There would appear to be little or no place for chemotherapy in treatment of low grade tumors.

SUPRATENTORIAL ASTROCYTOMAS (up to 35% of CNS tumors)

There is a peak age incidence of these tumors at 3 years and a second peak in adolescence with twice as many males affected as females. Cystic tumors often occur in the diencephalon and ventricles and have a good prognosis. Fibrillary tumors with more dense cellularity and less cystic change occur particularly in the cerebral hemispheres. They are mostly low grade, grow slowly and have a fair prognosis. Anaplastic tumors including glioblastoma multiforme and anaplastic astrocytoma are rapidly growing aggressive tumors also most frequently found in the hemispheres. Glioblastomas in particular will spread widely within the CNS and even systemically.

Presentation

For all sites the predominant presenting features (75%) are those of raised intracranial pressure. Seizures are seen in 25% of supratentorial tumors especially low grade ones (may precede all other symptoms/signs). Twenty-five to fifty per cent may have visual disturbances, weakness, hemiplegia or cranial nerve deficit. Diencephalic tumors may present with the classic syndrome of emesis, emaciation and even euphoria or with CSF obstruction. Dysmetria and chorea is seen in basal ganglia and optic atrophy with neuroendocrine disturbance in hypothalamic tumors. Neurofibromatosis type 1 (NF1) is associated with 10–20% of diencephalic lesions.

Diagnosis

Low grade astrocytomas on CT scanning are usually of low density with minimal enhancement in contrast to high grade tumors which have more variable density, marked enhancement and greater mass effect. MR scanning always defines more tumor than CT and is better able to distinguish edema from infiltrating neoplasia.

Prognostic features

Low grade (I and II) especially pilocytic varieties fare better than high grade (III and IV) and fibrillary tumors which are more common. Children fare better than adults, except infants where higher grade tumors and greater surgical risks coexist. Degree of resection influences outcome. Site is not a significant independent prognostic variable.

Management

Complete resection should be attempted (40–80% possible in supratentorial, less than 40% in diencephalon). In low grade tumors complete resection may lead to 80% survival at 7 years;[168] with incomplete removal survival is only 14–48% at 10 years even with radiotherapy. Whether there is long-term benefit for radiotherapy is unclear, most studies are retrospective and usually single center.[169] In partially resected low grade tumors it may be reasonable to delay radiotherapy until there is tumor regrowth. In low grade tumors associated with NF1 there is a high risk of multiple tumors and radiotherapy should only be used if there is tumor progression or deteriorating vision for tumors of the optic tract. There is no evidence from prospective randomized trials for the use of chemotherapy; however responses have been seen with a number of agents and a SIOP study evaluating the combination of vincristine and carboplatin is in progress. High grade tumors do require postoperative radiation although 5-year survival in Grade IV tumors is poor (5–25% at 5 years). Extended field irradiation with a tumor bed dosage of 50–55 Gy is used in Grade III and IV lesions (90% of recurrences are local). Because of the poor survival rates for such tumors chemotherapy with vincristine and cyclophosphamide or vincristine, CCNU and prednisolone have been tried. Forty to fifty per cent response rates are reported. The use of this combination in infants with high grade astrocytomas, followed by delayed radiotherapy, produced a 5-year overall survival of 50%.[170] No benefit has been shown from using more intensive chemotherapeutic regimens for these patients.[171] High dose chemotherapy with autologous marrow rescue has been used in several small studies but evidence for improvement in survival is lacking.[172]

BRAINSTEM GLIOMAS (10–20% of CNS tumors)

These have a peak incidence between 5 and 8 years but no sex difference. Seventy-five per cent occur in the pons and the rest in the medulla and midbrain. About 50% are of low grade malignancy, graded I or II mostly with a fibrillary histology, and a few are pilocytic. Thirty-five to forty per cent are high grade anaplastic astrocytomas or glioblastoma multiforme. Ten per cent are ependymomas and primitive neuroectodermal tumors.

Presentation

Raised intracranial pressure and hydrocephalus develop slowly with non-specific, non-localizing features of headache, nausea and vomiting but only with late papilledema. Emesis may be related to infiltration of local nuclei. Cranial nerve palsies (III, V, VI, VII, IX and X) are common and cerebellar and long tract signs may all be found. Pontine tumors may cause behavioral and emotional changes.

Diagnosis

On CT most are hypo- or isodense, and poorly enhancing while MR T1 weighted images show hypodensity and T2 images a hyperdense mass. MR much more accurately defines tumor extent especially exophytic components.

Prognostic features

Low grade tumors have improved survival (50–60% at 2 years for Grade I + II; 0–15% for Grade III and IV). The presence of calcification, Rosenthal fibers and no mitoses are favorable features. Midbrain and medullary sites have improved outcome compared with pontine tumors. Pontine tumors present rapidly, with cranial nerve defects. Patients with diffuse infiltrating tumors fare very badly; 90% will be dead within 18 months.[173] Patients with dorsal exophytic tumors have a gradual onset of symptoms and do well (up to 90% survival at 4–5 years).

Management

Attempts at resection are hazardous. For dorsal exophytic, cervicomedullary junction, and non-enhancing cystic or small tumors subtotal resection should be attempted. For diffuse pontine glioma the clinical and radiological appearances are so characteristic that even stereotactic biopsy is probably unnecessary, and may worsen the patient's neurological condition.[174] With radiation (45–50 Gy to tumor field) in the majority of pontomedullary tumors, the best survival quoted is 30% at 3–5 years. Hyperfractionated therapy (total dose up to 72 Gy) has proved disappointing.[175] To date no clear benefit has been shown from chemotherapy.[176] A UKCCSG trial of tamoxifen as adjuvant therapy is ongoing.

OPTIC GLIOMAS (OPTIC NERVE, CHIASMA AND TRACTS) (5% of CNS tumors)

Three-quarters occur before 10 years but chiasmal tumors tend to occur in older children. There is no sex difference. Neurofibromatosis is seen in up to 75% of patients with optic nerve tumors but is less frequent in those with more central lesions. The tumors tend mostly to be astrocytomas of low grade malignancy with a tendency for local infiltration along the optic tracts but also into the frontal lobes, hypothalamus, thalamus and other midline structures especially from the chiasma. Growth tends to be erratic but slow.

Presentation and diagnosis

Clinical features depend on the site and the age of the patient. The young usually present with squint, nystagmus, mild proptosis or developmental delay rather than loss of vision. The discs may be pale and atrophied but signs of raised intracranial pressure may occur in large chiasmal or hypothalamic tumors. Visual loss can be very profound; intraorbital lesions leading to central vision loss; chiasmal lesions to temporal hemianopia. In addition there is often a very fine and rapid unilateral or bilateral nystagmus. Lesions that spread to the hypothalamus may be associated with endocrine disorders or growth failure and even the diencephalic syndrome. Differential diagnosis will include rhabdomyosarcoma and neuroblastoma in the orbit; angiomas, lymphangiomas and meningiomas of the optic sheath; and in infants spasmus mutans (for chiasmal lesions). Gliomas, craniopharyngiomas and other suprasellar tumors may be confused with lesions in the optic tract. CT scanning will show an isodense mass with contrast enhancement especially in chiasmal tumors. Hydrocephalus may be present with the intracerebral lesions. MR scans often show much greater spread due to local infiltration. Careful ophthalmological evaluation of fields and acuity is required in conjunction with CT scans for follow-up. Visual evoked responses may be required to assess vision in the young.

Prognostic features

Intracranial site carries a worse prognosis. Chiasmal tumors have a 10-year survival of around 50% compared with 90–100% for intraorbital tumors. Those with chiasmal tumors and preceding neurofibromatosis may have a better prognosis.

Management

The natural history of the optic gliomas is variable. Even without treatment some patients may remain stable for long periods of time while others may progress quite rapidly. Only surgical biopsy will confirm the diagnosis although CT or MR scanning is probably adequate for most. There may be a place for attempted surgical resection in those with isolated intraorbital lesions but deeper intracranial tumors need a biopsy to exclude other tumors which might be more radiosensitive. Complete resection is usually impossible. For optic nerve lesions there seems to be little difference in outcome between those who are observed compared with those given initial radiotherapy. The aim of radiotherapy even for optic nerve lesions is to reduce tumor mass to improve vision although it may improve survival for large chiasmal lesions. Radiotherapy, particularly with chiasmal lesions, may cause intellectual, neuropsychological or endocrine sequelae. Actinomycin and vincristine have been shown to arrest at least temporarily the progression of optic gliomata in up to 80% of cases, and to delay the need for radiotherapy to beyond 5 years for most patients.[176]

PINEAL TUMORS (0.5–2% of CNS tumors)

These fall into two categories:

1. 20–40% are pineal parenchymal tumors (pinealoblastomas or pinealocytomas) and occur in the first 10 years and more frequently in girls.
2. The remainder are germ cell tumors, seen much more commonly in boys and girls in the second decade of life.

Pinealoblastomas have all the appearances of medulloblastoma and are best categorized as PNETs, often showing some differentiation resembling retinoblastoma. Pinealocytomas are generally more differentiated. The germ cell tumors are a heterogeneous group. The commonest is the germinoma, then teratoma and the rarer embryonal carcinoma, choroid carcinoma and endodermal sinus tumor (see below). Pineal tumors spread locally and pinealoblastomas and germinomas may disseminate, but teratomas tend to remain localized. Systemic non-CNS metastases occur with pinealoblastoma, germinoma and the rarer embryonal carcinoma and choroid carcinoma.

Presentation

Raised intracranial pressure from third ventricular outflow obstruction is the most common presenting feature. Other signs will depend on the site and the degree of extension of the tumor. Encroachment on the midbrain will produce vertical gaze paralysis, on the thalamus will produce hemiparesis, incoordination, visual impairment and movement impairment, and suprasellar extension particularly in germ cell tumors will produce neuroendocrine disorders. CT scanning will identify the lesion but not differentiate the type since both germ cell and parenchymal tumors tend to have irregular mixed density mass lesions but with a fairly uniform contrast enhancement. Both of them may have calcification. The more mature teratomas often have a mosaic pattern with variable density and contrast enhancement with irregular calcification. CSF examination is needed following decompression particularly in pinealoblastoma and germinoma. Elevation of AFP in the CSF and possibly in the serum in germ cell tumors is a useful marker.

Prognosis

This is determined by histology with germinomas having the best prognosis at 60–85% 5-year disease-free survival, and teratomas 50%. Pineal parenchymal tumors fare badly with at least 50% dead within a year of diagnosis. The remaining rare germ cell tumors have an even worse prognosis. About 10% of pineal parenchymal tumors and germinomas show leptomeningeal spread. Extracranial metastases are rare but include bone, lung and nodes.

Management

Biopsy is recommended to clarify the diagnosis. It is associated with a high morbidity (though low mortality), with frequent impairment of vision. In well-circumscribed teratomas, excision may be possible but for the rest, where local infiltration is quite common, biopsy with some debulking and relief of hydrocephalus is all that can be achieved with surgery. The primary treatment for the majority is radiotherapy with whole brain irradiation in the region of 35–45 Gy and a boost of 10–15 Gy to the tumor area for germ cell tumors and pinealoblastomas. There is controversy as to who actually needs spinal irradiation. It should probably be judged by the presence or absence of cells in the CSF and MR appearances but some recommend routine whole neuraxis radiation in pinealoblastoma. There is no blood–brain barrier in the pineal region and drugs such as vinblastine, bleomycin, cisplatinum and VP16 have all been shown to have some efficacy in pineal tumors. The intensive chemotherapy used for non-CNS germ cell tumors including vinblastine, bleomycin and cisplatinum or carboplatin yield similar improved results for those with CNS tumors. A SIOP study evaluating reduced radiotherapy and combination chemotherapy for these tumors is ongoing.

CRANIOPHARYNGIOMA (about 6% of CNS tumors)

Two-thirds of these tumors occur before the age of 20 with a median age of 8 years. There is no sex difference. Most of the tumors are suprasellar but some occur in the sella itself. They may be solid, mixed or cystic with or without calcification. Although they are frequently well differentiated and benign histologically they cause erosion of surrounding tissues.

Presentation

Obstruction of the third ventricle and the foramen of Monro leads to hydrocephalus and raised intracranial pressure. The optic discs are often pale showing signs of atrophy from slow tumor growth. Papilledema is occasionally present. Other signs result from the tumor impinging on the optic chiasma producing visual disturbances (homonymous hemianopia or bitemporal hemianopia) or from pressure on the pituitary and the hypothalamus leading to hormone deficiency (growth hormone, adrenocorticotrophic hormone, thyrotrophin releasing hormone, TSH or ADH). Hormonal changes occur in 80–90% of patients. The patient may present with diabetes insipidus and short stature.

Diagnosis

Plain skull X-rays will identify the large distorted sella with or without calcification. CT scanning will show a cystic low density lesion with contrast enhancement and often considerable calcification. The MR scan may define the solid and cystic components of this tumor better and identify the surrounding anatomy.

Prognosis

Total resection and cystic tumors are favorable; large poorly resectable tumors and age under 5 years are adverse features.

Management[178]

For this low grade tumor with visual and neuropsychological disturbances the efficacy of treatment is often difficult to evaluate. With preoperative steroids to reduce pressure and vasopressin to control diabetes insipidus, morbidity and mortality have decreased. Seventy-five to eighty per cent of tumors can be completely removed with recurrence rates of 20–25% (most in the first 2 years). Morbidity is high with secondary bleeding and local tissue damage. Periodic CT or MR scanning plus endocrine follow-up are essential. If scans show no disease and no calcification postsurgery there is a 70% 10-year event-free survival. If there is residual tumor or calcification, radiotherapy (50–55 Gy local field) is required. Many now recommend subtotal resection and radiotherapy rather than radical surgery.[179] Intracystic radiocolloid injection has been used successfully in recurrent cystic lesions. No role has yet been established for chemotherapy.

CHOROID PLEXUS NEOPLASMS (3% of CNS tumors)

Most occur in the lateral ventricles and are intraventricular papillomas which secrete CSF, but they can seed. About 15% are slow-growing carcinomas which can reach huge dimensions and can truly metastasize.

Presentation

This is usually with raised intracranial pressure and hydrocephalus (they can produce CSF up to four times the normal rate) owing to ventricular obstruction with or without hemorrhage. Arachnoiditis may also occur. Other more specific neurological effects will depend on the site of the tumor. The differential diagnosis will include ependymomas and midline astrocytomas. A plain skull X-ray will show sutural diastases in 70% (20% of these patients are in their first year of life). CT scan will show hydrocephalus and an isodense to hyperdense intraventricular tumor with contrast enhancement, MRI will show where the fronds of the tumor extend into the ventricles.

Management

Surgery is the treatment of choice but there is a high mortality and morbidity. For papillomas, curative complete resection appears to be possible in between 75 and 100%. Shunting may be necessary to relieve persistent hydrocephalus. For the papillomas there is no need for further therapy. For carcinomas there is a worse prognosis with only an occasional long-term survivor. Radiotherapy has not been of benefit; chemotherapy may have a role but the optimal specific drug regimen has not yet been defined.

SUPRATENTORIAL PNETS (2–3% of CNS tumors)

This heterogeneous group of tumors may represent medulloblastomas or similar tumors in a supratentorial position. Ninety per cent occur within the cerebral hemispheres and less than 10% in the midline. Although they may appear well circumscribed there is frequently microscopic infiltration which may be quite extensive and there is a high risk of leptomeningeal spread.

Presentation

This is usually with raised intracranial pressure, seizures and motor signs. The time from symptom onset to diagnosis may be quite long (up to 10 months). CT scanning will show hydrocephalus plus the mass with or without calcification and cysts and with variable enhancement. Myelography and CSF examination will be required once the pressure has been relieved.

Management

This is by surgical reduction of bulk followed by craniospinal radiotherapy to the tumor bed in doses of 50–60 Gy. There is some evidence that dosages less than 45 Gy worsen prognosis but the whole craniospinal axis will require radiation. The prognosis is generally poor for the majority with 5-year survival in the region of 25%. Radiotherapy does appear to prolong survival. Chemotherapy is undergoing evaluation but as yet no clear-cut evidence in favor of specific agents or combinations has emerged. Cisplatinum or carboplatinum look most promising.

SPINAL CORD TUMORS

These comprise about 5% of primary CNS tumors and can occur throughout childhood. Two-thirds are astrocytomas and most of the rest are ependymomas. The majority are well differentiated and of low grade malignancy often with cystic change and slow growth with local infiltration. Leptomeningeal spread has a low incidence but multifocal disease may be seen in patients with neurofibromatosis.

Presentation

This is often insidious in onset with weakness, pain, sensory change, change in gait and eventually sphincter dysfunction. About 10% of patients have raised intracranial pressure secondary to either high cervical spinal canal obstruction or to spinal block and rise in protein. Plain X-rays are abnormal in about 50% of patients. MR scanning is the ideal modality to define spinal tumors.

Management

Biopsy is essential for diagnosis and wherever possible resection should be attempted using ultrasonography and laser scalpels. Careful follow-up of spinal growth and development is necessary in children. Where resection is complete, no radiotherapy is needed but if it is incomplete, dosages in the region of 45–50 Gy to the affected area are necessary.

Prognosis

For low grade astrocytomas survival appears to be about 55% at 10 years for those incompletely resected and treated with radiotherapy, but near 100% if resection is complete. For ependymomas of low grade malignancy 10-year figures vary between 50 and 70% but for high grade tumors progression and death is quite rapid. Consequently chemotherapy is now being explored.

NON-HODGKIN'S LYMPHOMA

Childhood non-Hodgkin's lymphomas (NHL) represent a heterogeneous group of disorders quite different from those seen in adults. They are almost invariably disseminated, diffuse not nodular, high grade malignancies of immature T or B cell lineage with frequent extranodal disease, marrow and central nervous system involvement. There is considerable worldwide variation in incidence (Table 22.1), and throughout the world NHL is more common in boys than girls. The highest incidence figures are reported from equatorial Africa with a gross excess there of B cell lymphomas usually of Burkitt type.

ETIOLOGY AND CELL BIOLOGY

The pattern of dissemination which determines the mode of presentation of NHL follows the layout of the lymphoid immune system. This consists of many different end stage functional cells as well as a wide array of precursor and stem cells. Children are constantly exposed to antigens but lack an immune memory bank with the consequence that a large proportion of their lymphoid cells are in a very active state undergoing molecular rearrangements to produce specific immunoglobulins and other factors required for the normal immune response. In B cells, genes which regulate the different components of immunoglobulin production have to be brought together and rearranged. In T cells the genes which control T cell antigen receptor molecules similarly need to be organized. The immunoglobulin heavy chain genes are on chromosome 14 (q32), the lambda light chain genes on chromosome 22 (q11), and the kappa light chain genes on chromosome 2 (p22). For B cells to function normally the rearrangements need to occur in an ordered sequence. The human T cell receptor alpha chain gene maps to the long arm of chromosome 14 (14q11–12) and harbours the T cell receptor delta genes between its V and J region gene sequences. The T cell receptor beta chain locus is on chromosome 7 (q35). The complete molecule requires an alpha chain from chromosome 14 and a beta from chromosome 7. In normal health the rearrangement process which produces the product of the T cell receptor gene is very similar to that for immunoglobulin gene rearrangements. However the enzyme Tdt is intimately involved in T cell rearrangements but is not found in B cell acute lymphoid leukemia or lymphoma. This can be used as distinguishing feature.

Malignancy arises within lymphoid cells secondary to deletion, mutation or translocation of these genes. There is increasing evidence that incriminates viruses at least in the genesis of some lymphomas. Products from the retroviruses HTLV1 and 2 rearrange genes within the host cell stimulating production of interleukin 2 and its receptor which can in turn activate T cell proliferation. Such proliferation provides the opportunity for a second hit which may be necessary in order to produce a fully malignant clone. HTLV1 appears to play a role in adult type peripheral T cell leukemia/lymphoma especially prominent in the Far East. However no viral inclusions have yet been clearly and repeatedly found in childhood T cell NHL. Much more common is the identification of Epstein–Barr virus particles in cell nuclei in endemic African Burkitt's lymphoma cells. The finding of such virus inclusion and high antibody titers especially to the viral capsid antigen of EBV in over 90% of B cell lymphomas in equatorial Africa contrasts with a much lower incidence of both raised titers and viral inclusions in patients with B cell NHL in temperate climates (15–20%).[180] However, there is increasing evidence of aberrant expression in sporadic cases. In sub-equatorial Africa malaria is endemic and this is thought to cause a continuous antigenic stimulus which alters responses to EBV infections which are also endemic (approaching 100% of children exposed by the age of 3 years). It is considered that EBV infection early in life probably enlarges the size of certain pre B and B cell populations and maintains them in a proliferative state rendering them much more likely to genetic change. Some have postulated that EBV may produce an immortal cell clone with genetic translocations already present. It is clear that with such a high prevalence of the virus particularly in tropical areas but also amongst adults in Europe that this virus alone cannot be the cause of Burkitt's lymphoma. Much speculation has occurred as to the role of malaria (a T cell suppressor and B cell mutagen), but also of malnutrition and other cofactors (e.g. the use of phorbol esters as herbal medicine) which result in T cell immunosuppression (reduced CD4:CD8 ratio and decreased number and function of EBV specific T cells) and B cell hyperplasia which can clearly potentiate the effects of the original EBV infection. During infection the number of EBV genome positive cells clearly is thought to rise increasing the risk of genetic changes including the characteristic translocation which involves the long arm of chromosome 8 (region q23–24) usually as a part of a t(8;14) translocation. There are many variants which include t(2;8)(p12;q24) and t(8;22)(q24;q11) seen in about 15% of all cases. The c-myc oncogene lies at the chromosome 8 breakpoint whilst the partner genes involved in these translocations are the heavy and light chain immunoglobulin genes. In all cases an immunoglobulin gene enhancer is placed close to the oncogene and induces its expression. In endemic cases the chromosome 8 breakpoint is upstream of c-myc whilst in sporadic cases it occurs within the oncogene or immediately upstream. However in all cases it would appear that deregulation of the oncogene not mutation seems to be the consequence of the translocation.[181] Deregulation of c-myc leads to progression through cell cycle and lymphoproliferation. Endemic Burkitt's lymphoma cases appear to have very low levels of surface immunoglobulin on their cells and sporadic cases high levels with evidence that the translocations in sporadic cases are at a later stage of B cell differentiation. Increasing understanding of the biology has also enabled technology to be applied to detect minimal residual disease using the polymerase chain reaction. What actually initiates the translocations is still not known but it does appear to be multifactorial.

The human immunodeficiency virus (HIV) produces profound T helper cell depression and predisposes to a variety of tumors including intermediate to high grade B cell lymphomas, Hodgkin's disease, T cell NHL and some pre T and pre B tumors especially Kaposi's sarcoma. Some of these lymphomas are polyclonal B cell proliferations similar to those seen after intense therapeutic immunosuppression. The very characteristic feature of HIV induced lymphomas is that they are very frequently extranodal especially of the skin. There has been considerable speculation about the high incidence of associated EBV positivity and the possibility that HIV infection may actually predispose to an EBV driven lymphoproliferative disease.[182]

Unlike the B cell lymphomas T cell lymphoma patients show much more heterogeneous chromosomal rearrangements. About 25% of T cell ALL involves a small deletion of the TAL1 gene on chromosome 1 sometimes as part of a t(1;14) translocation.

Anaplastic large cell lymphoma characteristically carries a t(2;5)(p23;q35) translocation and occasionally a t(1;5) translocation. There are patients with Hodgkin's disease who also have the 2;5 translocation. There may be intermediate states between anaplastic large cell lymphoma and Hodgkin's disease. To date no clear etiological link has been made between the gene rearrangements in T cell NHL or in anaplastic large cell lymphoma and any particular virus. As described earlier, a whole range of immune deficiency states are associated with the development of lymphomas as is post organ transplantation profound immunosuppression. Grierson & Purtillo[183] described an EBV associated lymphoproliferative condition inherited in an X-linked mode which also features hepatitis, encephalopathy, and marrow aplasia. Klinefelter's syndrome and neurofibromatosis type 1 have also been associated with development of NHL.

CLASSIFICATION

A confusing array of classifications exist for non-Hodgkin's lymphoma. In pediatric practice the Revised European/American Lymphoma (REAL) classification is now the scheme of choice (see Table 22.15). As can be seen from the table the predominant lymphomas are high grade B cell, precursor T lymphoblastic and anaplastic large cell.

Table 22.15 Revised European/American Lymphoma Classification (REAL)

1	Burkitt's (42%)* High grade B cell (4%) Burkitt-like
2	Precursor B cell (5%) Lymphoblastic
3	Precursor T lymphoblastic (20%)
4	Diffuse large B cell (3%) Primary sclerosing mediastinal (0.4%)
5	Peripheral T cell unspecified
6	Anaplastic large cell T or null types (15%)

* Percentages are from a review of over 200 cases registered with the UK Children's Cancer Study Group (Pinkerton R and Carter R – personal communication). There are some indeterminate and unclassifiable cases. Follicular lymphomas make up only 0.4% of series.

PRESENTATION

Though the scope for presentation is endless depending on the site of the primary lymphoid mass and features of dissemination such as fatigue, pain and anemia there are some very characteristic presentations.[184]

Abdominal primary

B cell lymphomas (either Burkitt or Burkitt-like) in Europe normally present with an abdominal mass. There are two recognizable types of presentation. Type 1 presents as a diffuse abdominal tumor often involving the omentum and mesentery plus infiltration into kidney, liver and spleen. Frequently the bone marrow and central nervous system are also involved. Unlike in Africa only a few cases present with jaw or neck masses even though occasionally orbital tumors do occur. In African Burkitt's 50% of African patients who have jaw primaries also have abdominal disease but a much lower involvement of the bone marrow is noted amongst them.[185] The second type (2) of presentation is with localized tumors of the bowel wall especially in the terminal ileum (thought to arise in Peyer's patches). These masses may lead to intussusception or bleeding sometimes with perforation of the bowel. They are often thought to have appendicitis or an appendix mass since they present with a right iliac fossa mass and pain. Type 2 presentation is much rarer than Type 1.

Mediastinal primary

Approximately 20% of all children with NHL in the UK present with a mediastinal mass with or without pleural effusions. Between two-thirds and three-quarters of all precursor T lymphoblastic lymphoma present in this way. There may be signs of superior vena caval obstruction with dysphagia, dyspnea and pericardial effusion. There may be associated neck and axillary lymph nodes and rarely abdominal lymph nodes. Much more common however is hepatospenomegaly along with bone marrow involvement (present in more than 50% of cases) and central nervous system disease. These patients are at especially high risk of developing respiratory obstruction and distress if general anesthesia is instigated for investigations.

Anaplastic large cell lymphoma

It is only in relatively recent times that this tumor has been recognized as a separate entity. Formerly many such tumors were classified as malignant histiocytosis. The most frequent presentation is with painful nodal swelling sometimes with apparent surrounding inflammation or much more generalized skin involvement (macules or generalized ichthyosis) and fever. The sort of B symptoms seen in Hodgkin's disease may be present and cause diagnostic dilemmas (see below).

Localized disease

Lymphoid swellings can occur anywhere but most commonly in the head and neck including Waldeyer's ring and the facial bones. Neck nodal tumors apparently have a lower risk of CNS spread. Other sites of origin include the pharynx (usually B cell origin) and also primary tumors of bone, skin, thyroid, testis (usually lymphoblastic), orbit, eyelid, kidney and epidural space have all been described. Bone lymphomas may be localized or quite disseminated and may be associated with hypercalcemia. Lymphoblastic lymphoma can present not with a mediastinal mass but with skin and/or bone disease. These tumors are usually of much more mature T cell phenotype. In contrast subcutaneous lymphoma sometimes seen in very young children is usually of precursor B cell type.

Central nervous system involvement

Primary intracranial lymphomas are rare although seen more frequently post organ transplantation. However CNS involvement as secondary spread from disease elsewhere is quite common particularly in lymphoblastic and advanced Burkitt's lymphoma. When present there are the characteristic features of headache, vomiting, papilledema, cranial nerve dysfunction and seizures. Rarely patients may have isolated CNS disease.

DIAGNOSIS

A full history and examination usually gives a good clue to the type of lymphoma and the extent of dissemination. All patients require a preliminary chest X-ray to exclude mediastinal mass and/or effusions. It must be performed prior to any anesthetic procedure. Imaging of lymphoid masses is best carried out by MRI particularly for tumors of the head and neck. However abdominal ultrasonography is the quickest and most efficient way to define liver, spleen and kidney involvement and extent of abdominal primaries without requiring sedation or anesthesia in young children. Either MRI or CT scanning can follow. Routine use of bone or gallium scanning is not recommended unless there is atypical disease or focal bone pain. All patients require to have bone marrow examination, from at least two but preferably four sites (ideally from two aspirates and two trephines). The specimens should be examined cytogenetically and immunologically as well as by routine cytomorphology. All patients also require examination of cerebrospinal fluid provided that there is no clinical evidence of raised intracranial pressure. If this is present then a CT or MRI scan should be carried out before lumbar puncture to exclude any focal deposit with consequent risk of brain shift. Particularly in lymphoblastic disease diagnosis can sometimes be made on cytological examination of tapped pleural fluid or bone marrow. However in the presence of any accessible localized disease particularly of peripheral lymphadenopathy excision biopsy should be carried out. If there is truly isolated mediastinal disease with no involvement of bone marrow or CSF material will need to be obtained preferably by percutaneous needle or mediastinoscopy. For abdominal primaries diagnosis should be attempted by cytological examination of ascitic fluid or by percutaneous needle biopsy. Unless there is an acute abdominal emergency (such as gastrointrastinal obstruction or intussusception) laparotomy should be avoided wherever possible to avoid what are really quite common sequelae of prolonged ileus and even ruptured abdominal wounds. Wherever possible the most accessible tumor deposit should be biopsied. Tumor material needs to be submitted obviously for routine histological diagnosis but also for full immuno-phenotyping profile and cytogenetics. Clinical patterns of presentation, histology, cytomorphology, immuno markers and cytogenetics usually facilitate very precise definition of the tumor. Initial blood tests should include obviously a full blood picture, but also liver and renal function tests and an electrolyte profile to monitor for tumor lysis. Lactate dehydrogenase serum levels which are thought to be significantly prognostic especially in B cell disease should be assessed pre treatment.

STAGING

Table 22.16 shows the most commonly used staging system for childhood NHL.[186] All primary mediastinal tumors and diffuse

Table 22.16 St Jude modified staging system for non-Hodgkin's lymphoma

Stage		Approximate by stage seen in UK
I	Single tumor (extranodal) or single anatomic area (nodal) (not mediastinum or abdomen)	5%
II	Single tumor (extranodal) with regional node involvement. Primary gastrointestinal tumor with or without involvement of associated mesenteric nodes only. On the same side of diaphragm: a) two or more nodal areas b) two single (extranodal) tumors with or without regional node involvement	20%
III	On both sides of the diaphragm: a) two single tumors extranodal b) two or more nodal areas. All primary intrathoracic tumors (mediastinal, pleural, thymic); all extensive primary intra-abdominal disease; all primary paraspinal or epidural tumors regardless of other sites	50%
IV	Any of the above with initial CNS* or bone marrow involvement** (< 25%)	25%

*CNS disease = unequivocal blasts > 5/mm^3 in a cytocentrifugal cerebrospinal fluid specimen ± neurologic deficits, e.g. cranial nerve palsies ± intracranial nodal deposits

**Arbitrary cutoff of 25% to distinguish leukemia from lymphoma. This may not be useful for all, e.g. in B cell NHL no difference in outcome between Stage III and IV disease up to 70% bone marrow infiltration

abdominal tumors are at least Stage III. The spread in NHL unlike Hodgkin's disease is not orderly and contiguous from node to node. There is no place for routine staging laparotomy in NHL nor for lymphangiography.

PROGNOSTIC FACTORS

Tumor load (and consequently stage) is the most significant prognostic indicator but also the treatment used. More precise diagnosis and selection of therapy accordingly has significantly improved survival. Each major category of NHL requires different forms of therapy. The speed of response to treatment especially in T cell NHL may predict for outcome. Elevated serum lactate dehydrogenase levels in Stage III B cell patients is an important indicator of poor prognosis. Stage I patients with orbital or Waldeyer's ring tumors fare worse than those with other localized nodal disease. Stage II localized abdominal tumors have a far better prognosis than similarly staged nasopharyngeal tumors. It is quite difficult to accurately stage patients with extensive skin and nodal disease which includes many patients with anaplastic large cell lymphoma.

TREATMENT

Many patients with lymphomas present with poor nutrition, concomitant infection and metabolic problems especially spontaneous tumor lysis. These require attention, and correction if possible before intensive therapy can be delivered. Prophylactic use of uricozyme has reduced the risks of therapeutic tumor lysis.[187] Chemotherapy is the preferred modality of treatment since all tumors already have, or potentially can disseminate.

CHEMOTHERAPY PROTOCOLS

Localized lymphomas (Stage I and II)

Localized NHL is best treated with short course therapy of not more than six months' duration. For Stage I and abdominal Stage II disease, Murphy[186] reported no need for CNS directed therapy. Eighty-five to ninety per cent event free survival can be achieved with short course pulsed therapy for low stage B cell lymphoma. Some groups have attempted to reduce the risk of late cardio-toxicity by limiting or omitting anthracyclines and of reducing the risks of alkylator infertility or of second tumor development by reducing anthracycline and alkylator dosages. Patte et al[188] reported 100% cure rates with only two pulses of cyclophosphamide based chemotherapy and Reiter et al[189] using three courses very successfully treated Stage I and IIa B cell lymphomas. The only exceptions are localized lymphoblastic tumors which appear to require more intensive and sustained therapy similar to that used for advanced lymphoblastic leukemia and lymphoma.[189,190]

Advanced stage B cell lymphomas

The best results are those reported by the SFOP and BFM groups.[188,189] Both groups used initial low dose cytoreductive therapy (cyclophosphamide, vincristine and prednisolone) in order to reduce tumor bulk before a more intensive induction regimen. The LMB protocol consists of high dose methotrexate, fractionated high dose cyclophosphamide, vincristine, prednisolone and adriamycin followed by a consolidation phase using continuous infusion cytosine arabinoside. CNS directed therapy is with high dose methotrexate and intrathecal therapy but not irradiation except for those with Stage IV disease involving the CNS at diagnosis. Event free survival has progressively improved over the last 20 years with therapy modified in duration and intensity but depending on stage. In recent times there has been a joint American, French and UK protocol stratifying disease by stage attempting to reduce intensity and subsequent toxicity for lower risk patients and giving very intensive therapy for those with the highest risk, in particular those with bone marrow involvement of greater than 70% and those with CNS disease at diagnosis. The initial response to the cytoreductive therapy has also proven to be a significant prognostic indicator. Application of such therapy even in the most advanced disease now carries with it over 80% chance of 5-year event free survival.

Advanced stage non-B cell lymphoma

Since the mid 1970s patients with lymphoblastic lymphoma usually of T cell origin (but a small percentage having precursor B cell disease) have been treated with leukemia type therapy.[189–191] The BFM Group have shown somewhat superior results because of their very sustained induction consolidation and maintenance therapy similar to that used for acute lymphoblastic leukemia. With such intensive treatment there seems to be very little difference in survival between Stage III and IV disease. The most significant adverse prognostic feature appears to be failure to respond early (as defined by the BFM Group for acute lymphoblastic leukemia). Such slow responders may benefit from early intensification. The BFM 90 protocol has transformed the previously observed pattern of ongoing relapses out beyond 4 years, to early relapses and virtually no late relapses. The French strategy is to test whether cranial irradiation can be avoided as CNS directed therapy in advanced T cell lymphoma by using moderately high dose systemic methotrexate. A European wide international protocol is now in development.

Anaplastic large cell lymphoma

This lymphoma is characterized by Ki antigen positivity and identification of the t(2;5) translocation. This has only been clearly defined and recognized over the last 20 years. It is still not clear whether this represents a single entity or a group of disorders since in some instances extensive skin involvement may resolve spontaneously whereas other patients progress rapidly and appear to require megatherapy and marrow transplantation.[192,193] The BFM Group[193] report 81% event free survival, with skin involvement and splenomegaly forming the most adverse features. As with T lymphoblastic leukemia there has been creation of a European Intergroup of investigators to create a trial using a prephase with vincristine, cyclophosphamide, and dexamethasone followed by a multiagent BFM type regimen (ifosfamide, etoposide, cytosine arabinoside, dexamethasone, and intrathecal therapy). There is a randomized question as to the dose of the systemic methotrexate between 1 g/m^2 and 3 g/m^2 and a second randomization as to the addition or not of weekly vinblastine therapy (which has been shown to be effective in recurrent or refractory disease). The duration of therapy is determined by stage.

Rarer forms of lymphoma

These include peripheral T cell lymphomas many of which have features in common with anaplastic large cell lymphoma.[194] These probably should be treated like anaplastic large cell lymphoma. Follicular lymphomas are extremely rare in childhood but appear to respond to CHOP (cyclophosphamide, adriamycin, vincristine and prednisolone) based regimens. However late relapse can occur, as it does in adults.

Immunosuppression/immunodeficiency related lymphoproliferative disease (LPD)

There are increasing reports of patients developing what is thought to be an EBV driven lymphoproliferation of B cell phenotype post severe immunosuppression, especially organ transplantation. In recent times the recognized strategy for dealing with them has first been to reduce immunosuppressive therapy and attempts to restore normal surveillance of infection. There is a clear correlation of the incidence of LPD with severity of immunosuppression. Antiviral therapy is only likely to have any effect at an early stage before gene rearrangements have occurred within the infected cells. It is not clearly always possible to reduce immunosuppressives in the post transplant situation, and the majority now appear to require some chemotherapy. Some respond to the use of cytoreductive therapy with cyclophosphamide, vincristine, and steroids. Those that don't appear to require intensive B cell lymphoma type therapy (Hann I – personal communication). Since the mortality is high for these patients use of targeted anti-B cell monoclonal antibodies[195] and the production of cytotoxic T lymphocytes against EBV infected cells are being tested.[196] It is too early to report on efficacy in children.

ALTERNATIVE STRATEGIES

Bone marrow transplantation has limited use in modern day therapy for NHL and should be reserved for those who have partial remission after intensive therapy, or those who relapse early but respond on reinduction with second line therapy.

Specific targeted monoclonal antibody therapy has been used in adult high grade lymphomas but not systematically in children. There may be a place for the use of antisense oligonucleotide therapy in patients with refractory or recurrent disease.

HODGKIN'S DISEASE

Hodgkin's disease has a peak incidence in teenagers and a second in old age (greater than 50 years). The early peak is peripubertal.

Epidemiological features include greater risk in: higher socioeconomic groups, siblings of patients, association with some immunological disorders (e.g. systemic lupus erythematosus, rheumatoid arthritis and ataxia telangiectasia); a pattern suggesting infective etiology. The Epstein–Barr virus has been linked to etiology, the virus being found in Reed–Sternberg cells in a significant percentage (at least 60%) of young cases especially boys and those with mixed cellularity subtype.[84–86, 197] The response to infection as determined by HLA alleles may play a role in susceptibility certainly in adults. What we don't know yet is whether Epstein–Barr virus is truly causative, contributory or a mere bystander.

CELL BIOLOGY AND CLASSIFICATION

The malignant cell in Hodgkin's disease is the Reed–Sternberg cell derived from an interdigitating reticulum cell involved in antigen presentation to T cells. Cell culture in the Reed–Sternberg cell produces a wide range of mediators and if this is similarly true in Hodgkin's disease it might explain the variable cellular patterns seen. Reed–Sternberg cells are not pathognomonic of Hodgkin's disease but are seen in some rarer non-Hodgkin's lymphomas, in EBV virus infection, and some carcinomas. Hodgkin's disease however cannot be diagnosed in the absence of such cells. They are large with abundant cytoplasm and multiple or multilobed nuclei, frequently with a prominent and characteristic halo around the nucleoli.

The Rye classification is universally used. Types 1 and 2 are commoner in young children. Prognosis appears to be related to the proportion of lymphocytes present in types 1–3.

1. *Lymphocyte predominance*: Reed–Sternberg cells may be quite scarce, fibrosis is rarely seen and the prognosis is very good.
2. *Mixed cellularity*: Reed–Sternberg cells are usually profuse (5–15 per high power field) often with fine fibrosis and focal necrosis.
3. *Lymphocyte depletion*: large mononuclear abnormal cells are often seen as well as Reed–Sternberg cells with few lymphocytes. Fibrosis and necrosis are common and often quite diffuse. This form is rarer in children.
4. *Nodular sclerosis*: lacunar cells are a characteristic finding with a thickened capsule and bands which divide the tissue into nodules. This histology is especially common in lower cervical, supraclavicular and mediastinal Hodgkin's disease of childhood.

Mixed cellularity is seen much more commonly in younger patients and in those from developing countries. Overall in the UK and North Europe nodular sclerosing and mixed cellularity types are seen in roughly equal proportions.

Non-random cytogenetic changes have been reported involving a range of chromosomes as well as the presence of an occasional t(2;5) translocation causing confusion as to whether the patient has Hodgkin's disease or anaplastic large cell lymphoma.

There is some correlation between patterns of presentation and histopathology with mixed cellularity and lymphocyte depleted forms usually presenting with more disseminated disease and nodular sclerosis classically presenting with mediastinal disease in adolescence. Lymphocyte predominant disease almost always presents with focal nodal disease characteristically in the neck or groin. Hodgkin's disease generally follows an orderly pattern of spread from node to contiguous node. When the spleen is involved, infiltration usually starts as a small nodule. Splenic enlargement itself does not necessarily mean that it is actually involved. Liver infiltration is usually focal. Progression of the disease from lymphocyte predominance to mixed cellularity does appear to occur followed by lymphocyte depletion if inadequate treatment is given.

CLINICAL PRESENTATION

In childhood most patients present with painless swelling of the cervical or supraclavicular nodes, which will feel firm or rubbery on palpation. They may be quite tender. Two-thirds of children have mediastinal involvement, which may be found coincidentally on X-ray but may compromise the airway and the patients present with dyspnea and/or wheeze. Involvement of the pleura or pericardium with effusions may worsen the chest symptoms. Axillary or inguinal node involvement is less common. The groin is involved in less than 5% of childhood cases. Hepatic and splenic disease is highly suggestive of advanced disease. Approximately 30% of young patients have non-specific features of tiredness and anorexia but very specific symptoms of fever, weight loss (more than 10%) and night sweating are designated as B symptoms and carry a worse prognosis. So for each stage it is important to define not only the extent of the disease but the presence or absence of such symptoms. Those with B symptoms need to be upstaged in terms of treatment delivered. It is not uncommon to have generalized pruritus and indeed unexplained pain on taking alcohol. These symptoms do not seem to affect prognosis. Anemia may be present either as a result of hemolysis or from iron utilization problems. A very few patients seem to have thrombocytopenia, again mediated through a platelet associated antibody. Lymphopenia when present prior to therapy is a sign of advanced disease. If the spleen is significantly enlarged hypersplenism can intervene. A number of patients may present with infection both before and during treatment due to underlying T cell dysfunction.

DIAGNOSIS

Differential diagnosis includes infective causes of lymphadenopathy (e.g. infectious mononucleosis, atypical TB, and other viruses) and non-Hodgkin's lymphoma particularly in lymphocyte predominant disease. Usually NHL has a more rapid onset and rapid tumor growth. Diagnostic investigations which are essential include:

1. Clinical assessment for any node or organ enlargement and documentation of any symptoms.
2. Standard posteroanterior (PA) and lateral chest X-ray. It is important to document the extent of the mediastinal mass since its dimensions determine whether the patient may require subsequent radiotherapy.
3. CT scan of chest, neck and abdomen to define precise dimensions and extent of disease. Although MR scanning may be better for neck masses, CT is more commonly used enabling scanning from neck through to the abdomen. In children there may be problems visualizing retroperitoneal nodes of 1 to 2 cm size due to lack of fat in children. Similarly the commonest site where disease may be missed is in the para-aortic area at the level of the pancreas. Sometimes ultrasonography will pick up abnormalities missed on CT scan in this area. Lymphangiography is now rarely performed but used to provide very clear visualization of pelvic and para-aortic nodes giving both size but also the filling pattern. MR scanning is probably superior to CT in the region of the pelvis.
4. Node biopsy to confirm diagnosis, subtype and to carry out molecular and EBV screening studies.
5. At least two bone marrow aspirates and two trephines are required to exclude infiltration certainly in patients with advanced disease and those with B symptoms.
6. Worthwhile initial blood tests include baseline full blood count, ESR or CRP (can be used to monitor response although non-specific), liver and renal function tests, EBV serology, baseline immune status for measles and chickenpox (infections which

can be quite a problem in Hodgkin's disease). Some centers use non-specific markers such as serum copper, or ferritin and interleukin 2 receptor levels. They are not in routine practice and are not specific for the tumor.

It is very rare now to carry out laparotomy and splenectomy (even in the presence of splenomegaly) is avoided wherever possible because of the risk of overwhelming sepsis. Invasive and potentially life threatening procedures like these can be avoided since the majority of patients receive chemotherapy not limited field irradiation. Table 22.17 shows the staging system most commonly used throughout the world. Now that chemotherapy is used in all but a very small number of localized Stage I patients, precise staging which involved laparotomy etc. is now avoided.

MANAGEMENT

Hodgkin's disease is very radiosensitive but its previous universal use was associated with unacceptable local tissue growth problems. Combined modality therapy was adopted to minimize the toxicity of both radiation and intensive chemotherapy but optimize cure. However evidence accrued that often the combination of alkylators such as procarbazine and radiation increased the risk of some late toxicity, very specifically second tumor formation and infertility. As a consequence modern therapy tends to contain radiotherapy in a dose range of 30–35 Gy only for those with very localized Stage IA disease where an involved field is included. Since such tumors are primarily in the neck there still is the consequence of developing compensated hypothyroidism (which if not treated with thyroxine can lead to thyroid adenomas and even carcinomas). Chemotherapy is substituted for irradiation for all but such very low stage disease. It is difficult to determine how many cycles of therapy are necessary for cure, if chemotherapy is used instead of radiotherapy for Stage I disease.

For patients with Stages II and IIIA the aim of therapy is to achieve cure with least long term sequelae. In Hodgkin's disease all the drugs utilized have some side-effects. It is a matter of balancing the potential toxicity of alkylating containing regimens such as the original MOPP (mustine, vincristine, procarbazine and prednisolone) or CLVPP (chlorambucil, vinblastine, procarbazine and prednisolone) where side-effects are potential infertility and second malignancies as against anthracycline containing regimens such as ABVD (actinomycin, bleomycin, vincristine and DTIC) where the major risks are of cardiorespiratory dysfunction. Most groups now use a hybrid chemotherapy approach, for example including three cycles of alkylating containing regimens and three of ABVD. Whether such strategy truly decreases long term toxicity is yet to be defined.[198] The tendency to use short course chemotherapy and involved field irradiation has now decreased worldwide. Although needed in adults it is far less clear whether radiation to residual mediastinal thickening post chemotherapy is required in pediatric patients.

The trend in advanced Stage IIIB and IV patients is to use more courses of therapy with/without radiation to an involved field for the primary mass.[199]

The current approach in the UK is to use for Stage II and III patients three courses of CHLVPP alternating with three courses of ABVD. If remission is achieved then the patient stops treatment. For Stage IV disease assessment occurs after four courses (two CHLVPP and two ABVD). If the patient is not in complete remission or very good partial remission (resolution or reduction of 50% or greater in any one axis of a measurable node mass) the patient comes off protocol and goes into a relapse therapy which includes high dose melphalan and peripheral stem cell rescue. If the patient does remit after four courses of therapy, four more are given. Consequently staging now determines duration of therapy rather than type. The speed of response appears to be related to prognosis. It is extremely difficult now to run randomized trials with low stage Hodgkin's disease where you would expect to obtain 5-year event free survival greater than 90%. It is only in Stage IV patients where the results have been disappointing (in the region of 50–60% 5-year survival) that greater effort is being applied to find new ways to deliver intensive chemotherapy.[200]

Table 22.17 Ann Arbor staging system for Hodgkin's disease

Stage I	Involvement of a single lymph node region (I) or of a single extralymphatic organ or site (I_E)
Stage II	Involvement of two or more lymph node regions on the same side of the diaphragm (II) or localized involvement of an extralymphatic organ or site and one or more lymphnode regions on the same side of the diaphragm (II_E)
Stage III	Involvement of lymph node regions on both sides of the diaphragm (III) which may be accompanied by involvement of the spleen (III_S) or localized involvement of extralymphatic organ or site (III_E) or both (III_{SE}).
Stage IV	Diffuse or disseminated involvement of one or more extra lymphatic organs or tissues with or without associated lymph node involvement

+B, presence of fever, night sweats or weight loss > 10% in previous 6 months; +A, none of above

NEUROBLASTOMA

Although most frequently presenting as a large abdominal mass, this tumor is metastatic in 70% of patients at diagnosis. The commonest primary sites are the adrenal gland 40%, other abdominal sites 25%, the chest 15%, pelvis 5% and neck 5%. The thorax is more frequently involved in those under 1 year. Neuroblastoma arises from primordial neural crest cells which form part of the sympathetic and rarely the parasympathetic nervous system. 1 in 250 neonates dying of other causes are found to have small foci of adrenal neuroblasts but disease occurs only in 1 in 10 000 live births. These foci may represent tumors in situ or may be a reflection of a normal stage of adrenal development which regresses in health but persists in malignancy. Spontaneous regression of malignant neuroblastoma to benign ganglioneuroma has been recorded particularly in infants with quite widespread disease (see below).

EPIDEMIOLOGY AND ETIOLOGY

Neuroblastoma occurs slightly more frequently in boys and occasional familial clusterings have been reported. Genetic rearrangement involving the short arm of chromosome 1 has been described and it is possible that up to 20–25% of cases may be heritable. Geographical variations may reflect genuine genetic or environmental factors or may be a reflection of low detection rates. Neuroblastoma occurs with increased frequency in Beckwith–Wiedemann syndrome, neurofibromatosis, nesidioblastosis and in fetal phenytoin syndrome.

PRESENTATION

The features of neuroblastoma are protean because of early dissemination and origin anywhere along the sympathetic chain.

Although there will always be a primary (often asymptomatic) this may not always be identified. Localized disease is most likely to be in the neck, or less commonly in the pelvis or chest. Neck lesions will present as a mass, while pelvic lesions often present as obstruction to the bowel or bladder outflow. Silent masses can occasionally be found on routine examination for other reasons. Most abdominal tumors have metastasized, most commonly to the bone marrow or liver or skin by the time of diagnosis. The commonest presentation is with a large firm abdominal mass often crossing the midline but with the features of marrow infiltration including anemia, bruising, fever, lethargy and irritability. Anemia is present in approximately 90% of cases even in the absence of marrow infiltration. Bony disease gives characteristic deep-seated intractable pain in one or more limbs and often causes a limp.

Proptosis and/or periorbital bruising is a characteristic but rare feature of Stage 4 disease due to infiltration either within the orbit or in the sphenoidal bone. Local extension through an intervertebral foramen can produce cord compression at any level in some 5% of patients. These patients nearly all need urgent treatment, either with radiotherapy, laminectomy or chemotherapy. Full neurological recovery can be expected in 50% of these patients, but recovery is unlikely if the presenting motor defect is severe.[201] Approximately 1–2% of tumors produce vasoactive intestinal peptide which produces intractable diarrhea associated with hypokalemia. Most (90%) tumors secrete catecholamines usually homovanillic acid (HVA) and vanillylmandelic acid (VMA), and although blood levels may be very high they do not normally cause hypertension. Hypertension does occur but is usually renovascular. Urinary levels of catecholamines are used to monitor disease. A syndrome of opsoclonus/myoclonus in which the patient has acute cerebellar and truncal ataxia with rapid eye movements may be seen. CNS disease is rare although increasingly described as length of survival improves.

Cervical disease often produces a unilateral Horner's syndrome. Large abdominal tumors involving the liver may present with elevation of the diaphragm and respiratory symptoms secondary to both pleural effusions and a splinted diaphragm but actual pulmonary disease is rare. Skin metastases present as non-tender bluish, mobile subcutaneous nodules and are characteristically seen in Stage 4S disease. In older patients even quite extensive abdominal masses may be missed and the patient presents with weight loss, change in behavior and vague generalized pain.

INVESTIGATIONS

The diagnosis must be confirmed and extent of disease evaluated.

Biopsy

All should have histological confirmation from the most easily accessible tumor deposit. In addition to routine histology, immunocytochemistry and molecular/genetic studies are required. Deletions of the short arm of chromosome 1 are found in 70–80% of near diploid cells (rarely 1p– is found in constitutional karyotype) and can assist in differentiation from other small round cell tumors. DNA content overall is of prognostic significance (pseudodiploidy is associated with advanced disease and poorer survival). MYCN amplification is associated with advanced disease and poor prognosis. Consequently, tumor cytogenetics, ploidy and MYCN amplification studies are all required. Histologically, neuroblastoma consists of small blue round cells with fibrillary bundles, hemorrhage, necrosis, calcification and attempts at rosette formation. Maturation to ganglion cells with fibrils may be diffuse (ganglioneuroma) or patchy (ganglioneuroblastoma). Table 22.18 shows ways in which small round cell tumors of childhood may be distinguished.

Bone marrow

Multiple site aspirates and trephines are necessary to exclude involvement since it is the commonest metastatic site. When present, infiltration may be very heavy and mimic ALL or show patchy clumps or rosettes. Monoclonal antibodies (e.g. UK13A) may identify equivocal infiltration.

Diagnostic imaging

CT, MR and ultrasound scans can all be used to define primary tumor extent. It is essential to have three-dimensional assessment of tumor size to document response accurately. MR is optimal to determine any spinal extension. Bony involvement should be assessed by technetium bone scan (the isotope may also be taken up by the primary). Iodine-131 (or -123) metaiodobenzylguanine (MIBG) scan taken up by secretory vesicles is frequently a good marker of disease. Plain bone X-rays may show mixed lytic and sclerotic areas especially in skull and long bones (especially around knees). There is often marked periosteal elevation leading to a misdiagnosis of osteomyelitis.

Urinary catecholamines

Eighty-five to ninety per cent of patients have detectable excess in their urine and the total levels of catecholamines and VMA and HVA can be used to monitor tumor response. Catecholamines should ideally be measured on 24-h specimens but can be done on spot specimens provided they are related to creatinine levels.

Blood tests

Full blood count, liver and renal function, serum ferritin (non-specific elevation associated with advanced disease) neuron-specific enolase (elevated in 95% of advanced but not localized disease) should all be performed. Serum levels of GD2 ganglioside can be a useful marker. Constitutional karyotyping should be arranged.

Biology

The molecular biology of neuroblastoma has been extensively studied. It is well established that amplification of the proto-oncogene MYCN is associated with higher stage tumors and a worse prognosis.[202] Deletion of the short arm of chromosome 1 (1p deletion), with its loss of a putative tumor suppressor gene is similarly associated with more advanced disease and disease progression.[203,204] Gain of the long arm of chromosome 17 (17q gain) is also a powerful negative prognostic factor.[205] Expression of the high affinity nerve growth factor (NGF) receptor, TrkA, and to a lesser extent the low affinity NGF receptor (LNGFR/p75), correlates with good outcome.[206,207] Expression of TrkB, the receptor for brain derived neurotrophic factor (BDNF), correlates with MYCN amplification and poor prognosis[208] whilst expression of TrkC, the receptor for neurotrophin 3 (NT-3), is associated with good outcome.[209] These correlations suggest a difference in differentiation state between those tumors with a favorable prognosis and those which do badly. On the basis of these markers patients can be divided into three prognostic groups. The first group consists of those whose tumors have a hyperdiploid or triploid karyotype, without MYCN amplification or 1p deletion and high expression of TrkA. These tend to be infants, less than 1 year of age, with stage 1, 2, or 4s tumors who have an excellent prognosis. The second group contains those whose tumors have a diploid or tetraploid karyotype, no MYCN amplification, but deletion of 1p and low expression of TrkA. This group tends to contain children over

Table 22.18 Useful markers in the differentiation of small round cell tumors of childhood

Tumor	Tdt	Cytoplasmic immunoglobulin	Markers now identified immunologically				Intermediate filament proteins			
			Actin	Myosin	Neuron-specific enolase	S100 protein	Desmin	Vimentin	Neurofilament	Cytokeratins
Rhabdomyosarcoma	–	–	+	+ (if differentiated type)	+/– (rare)	+/–	+	+	–	+/–
Neuroblastoma	–	–	–	–	+	+	–	–	+	–
Askin tumor	–	–	–	–	+	–/+	–	+/–	?	+/–
Peripheral PNET	–	–	–/+	–	+	+	-/+	+/–	+/–	+/–
Ewing's sarcoma 'typical'	–	–	–	–	–(+) (occasional)	–(+)*	–	+	–	+/–
Non-Hodgkin's lymphoma	+T -B	In B cell	–	–	–	–	–	+	–	–
ALL	+ (95%)	In pre-B (10–15%)	–	–	–	–	–	–	–	–

This battery of markers should be combined with specific antibodies to detect surface antigens, e.g. UJ13A for neuroectodermally derived cells or UJ181A from fetal brain cell origin.
(+)*, occasional in Ewing's sarcoma. ALL, acute lymphoblastic leukemia; PNET, primitive neuroectodermal tumor; Tdt, terminal deoxynucleotidy transferase.

the age of 1 year with Stage 3 and 4 disease who respond initially to chemotherapy but often relapse. They have an intermediate prognosis with 25–50% 5-year survival. The third group have tumors with diploid or tetraploid karyotypes, amplified MYCN, deletion of 1p, and absence of TrkA. These children have an appalling prognosis with a 5-year survival of 5%.[207]

STAGING

Brodeur et al[210] published an international neuroblastoma staging system (INSS) (Table 22.19) which has been widely adopted. Standardization has enabled comparison of treatment results which was difficult in the past. All previous criteria were based on clinical, radiological and bone marrow examination but now staging includes the division of Stage 2 into those with and without lymph node involvement which alters prognosis and may indicate the need for a change in therapy. The overall distribution by stage is approximately 10–15% Stage 1, 8–10% Stage 2, 15–20% Stage 3 and 60% Stage 4. In those under 1 year almost 30% have Stage 1 disease. Nearly 40% of infants (< 1 year) affected have localized disease compared with 20% of older children. Stage 4S (Stage 1 or 2 with dissemination limited to liver, skin and/or bone marrow) is almost exclusively seen in infants. Table 22.20 shows recognized prognostic features.

MANAGEMENT

Low risk group

(INSS Stage 1, 2 and 3, Stage 4 without bone, lung, pleural, or CNS metastases in infants, and INSS Stage 4S disease, without MYCN amplification)

Surgery only is recommended for Stage 1 and 2 disease (99% and 98% overall survival respectively) and for resectable Stage 3 disease in infants, in the absence of MYCN amplification. Chemotherapy is reserved for any recurrence and may be needed in 10% of Stage 1 patients and 20% of Stage 2.[211] Unresectable Stage 2 or 3 disease in infants in the absence of MYCN amplification can be managed with short non-intensive combination chemotherapy based on cyclophosphamide/vincristine (CO), etoposide/carboplatin (VP-CARBO) and cycophosphamide/doxorubicin/vincristine (CADO). A subset of Stage 2 patients with a poorer prognosis can be identified by MYCN amplification and age over 2 years.[212] These patients merit aggressive chemotherapy and should be regarded as high risk. Stage 4S disease is associated with spontaneous regression and good overall survival. However a group of infants who present at less than 2 months of age tend to have rapidly enlarging abdominal disease (either an abdominal primary or metastases in the liver) and a poorer prognosis. Whilst most patients with 4S neuroblastoma do not need treatment this group merit early combination chemotherapy[213,214] with VP-CARBO and CADO. A small group of infants with Stage 4 disease without bony metastases and without MYCN amplification, who would be categorized as 4S but for the presence of a large usually abdominal primary can also be treated with a similar expectant strategy and will regress spontaneously.

Table 22.19 New international staging system for neuroblastoma

Stage 1	Localized tumor confined to the area of origin, complete gross excision, with or without microscopic residual disease, identifiable ipsilateral and contralateral lymph nodes negative microscopically
Stage 2A	Unilateral tumor with incomplete gross excision, identifiable ipsilateral and contralateral lymph nodes negative microscopically
Stage 2B	Unilateral tumor with complete or incomplete gross excision, with positive ipsilateral regional lymph nodes, identifiable contralateral lymph nodes negative microscopically
Stage 3	Tumor infiltrating across the midline with or without regional lymph node involvement; or unilateral tumor with contralateral regional lymph node involvement; or midline tumor with bilateral regional lymph node involvement
Stage 4	Dissemination of tumor to distant lymph node, bone, bone marrow, liver and/or other organs (except as defined in 4S)
Stage 4S	Localized primary tumor as defined for stages 1 and 2 but with dissemination limited to liver, skin and/or bone marrow

Table 22.20 Prognostic features in neuroblastoma

Good	Intermediate	Adverse
Age < 1 year	Age > 1 year	Age > 1 year
INSS stage 1, 2, 4S	INSS stage 3, 4	INSS stage 3, 4
Single copy MYCN	Single copy MYCN	Amplified MYCN
Intact chromosome 1p	Deleted 1p	Deleted 1p
No gain of 17q	Gain of 17q	Gain of 17q
Hyperdiploid	Diploid/tetraploid	Diploid/tetraploid
High TrkA	Low TrkA	Low TrkA

Intermediate risk group

(Unresectable INSS Stage 2 and 3 without MYCN amplification and infants with Stage 4 with bone, lung, pleural, or CNS disease, but without MYCN amplification)

This group of patients is relatively small, only 15% of cases of neuroblastoma are Stage 3, and 15% of these will be high risk due to MYCN amplification. Combination chemotherapy alternating VP-CARBO and CADO is recommended with surgical resection of any remaining tumor.

High risk group

(Any child with INSS Stage 2 or 3 with MYCN amplification, infants with Stage 4 or 4S disease with MYCN amplification, Stage 4 disease over the age of 1)

Infants with disease above Stage 1 with amplification of MYCN do not do well in the absence of intensive therapy. Current European guidelines for this group of patients include chemotherapy with VP-CARBO and CADO followed by radiotherapy to the tumor site and myeloablative therapy with autologous bone marrow transplantation (ABMT). Children over the age of 1 year with Stage 4 disease constitute 40–50% of all patients with neuroblastoma. Without intensive chemotherapy the survival for this group of patients is < 5%. With intensive induction chemotherapy, high dose myeloablative therapy with stem cell transplantation and maintenance therapy with 13-cis retinoic acid the survival for this group has improved dramatically, but remains stubbornly stuck at around 30%.[215] Many different induction regimes have been utilized for high risk neuroblastoma; most involve cisplatin/carboplatin in combination with cyclophosphamide, etoposide and vincristine. In the US doxorubicin has usually been included. No schedule has been convincingly shown to be superior, although the best European results to date have been with the Rapid COJEC schedule (vincristine/cisplatin alternating with vincristine/carboplatin/ etoposide and vincristine/cyclophosphamide/ etoposide every 10 days for eight cycles) on ENSG 5 (5-year overall survival, 39.6%). The current European cooperative trial uses Rapid COJEC as induction therapy, followed by surgical resection of the primary tumor, ABMT with either busulfan/melphalan or carboplatin/etoposide/ melphalan as myeloablative therapy, 21 Gy of radiotherapy to the primary site, and 6 monthly cycles of 13-cis-retinoic acid. The use of immunological approaches including anti-G2 ganglioside antibodies and/or interferon are now under investigation as adjuvant therapy.

Since neuroblastoma is radiosensitive, a place for total body irradiation or targeted radiotherapy (radiolabelled metaiodobenzylguanidine – MIBG) in the above plan has been suggested. The optimal timing of such therapy remains unclear.

SCREENING

Since the prognosis for localized disease is good and that for advanced disease is so very poor and there is a readily obtainable marker for disease (urinary catecholamines) attempts have been made to carry out urinary screening of infants. Studies of screening in Japan and Canada have convincingly shown that it fails to detect Stage 4 disease in children over 1 year, and merely increases the number of previously asymptomatic and presumably spontaneously resolving cases detected.[216–219] Mass screening for neuroblastoma with urinary catecholamines thus cannot currently be recommended.

NEPHROBLASTOMA (WILMS' TUMOR)

The incidence of Wilms' tumor is approximately 1 in 10 000 live births with a very slight female preponderance (see Tables 22.1 and 22.2). The complex genetic picture is covered in the etiology section and Table 22.4. About 1% of patients have a family history of such tumors and it is likely that all bilateral (5% of all cases) and up to 20% of unilateral forms might be predominantly genetic in origin. The histological pattern seen in tumors does seem to correlate with the different genetic forms. Nephroblastomatosis is seen in various forms and may show different patterns with different forms of the tumor.

PRESENTATION

Presentation is usually with an enlarged abdomen and a mass although the child may be very well. The mass may be found coincidentally on routine examination. Fever is present in about 25% and may be due to unrelated causes, hematuria is seen in 25%, abdominal pain in 40% and hypertension in 5–10%. Usually the mass is smooth, non-tender and may be surprisingly large for the well-being of the child. Rarely, presentation is with peritonitis following rupture of the tumor.

INVESTIGATIONS

1. Plain abdominal films will show the soft tissue mass, peripheral calcification (less dense than in neuroblastoma) and displaced bowel. Non-invasive ultrasonography will define the mass and enable assessment of the contralateral kidney and vena caval patency. Ultrasound has replaced intravenous pyelography in most centers. The increasing availability of CT and MR scanning enables even more precise definition of tumor spread and anatomy. CT or MR are essential in bilateral disease and do assist operative decisions. PA and lateral chest X-rays must be carefully scrutinized for pulmonary metastases (the commonest secondary site). Equivocal shadows require CT scanning and this is mandatory in children who are to have immediate nephrectomy but who otherwise have Stage I disease (with subsequently confirmed favorable histology). Such patients if the chest is clear receive very short courses of vincristine only, but there is evidence that in the presence of CT nodules that upstaging and treatment with vincristine and actinomycin is required for their cure. Larger nodules visible on chest X-ray put the patient into true Stage IV.
   Bone scans are indicated if there is focal or diffuse bone pain or if histology confirms a clear cell sarcoma (bone metastasizing tumor). Rhabdoid tumors require CNS imaging for metastases or concomitant primary CNS tumors.
2. Peripheral blood and tumor cytogenetics plus molecular studies should be performed for the Wilms' tumor associated genes.
3. Very careful clinical review is required to exclude the congenital syndromes associated with Wilms' tumor formation.

HISTOLOGY

Tumors are separated into favorable and unfavorable categories.[220] There is little correlation between the very diverse histology and outcome except for the presence of large hyperchromatic nuclei with multipolar mitotic figures (anaplasia) which occur in about 5% of patients. This change is rare before 2 years of age and reaches a peak between 5 and 7 years. The presence of anaplasia in just one small focus within a tumor still conveys an adverse prognosis so multiple sectioning of all parts of any renal tumor is required. Formerly two other types of histology, namely clear cell sarcoma and rhabdoid tumor, were linked with anaplasia in the unfavorable group, but they are now recognized as quite separate entities. Clear cell sarcoma comprises 5–7% of childhood renal tumors and is associated with a very high risk of bony metastases (e.g. 76% of 38 cases described by Marsden et al[221]). These tumors are quite cystic and there are very characteristic cellular appearances with a fairly evenly spread fibrovascular network. With aggressive treatment these bone metastasizing tumors can be cured and therefore it is particularly important to recognize this even in a localized Stage I tumor, so that therapy can be altered accordingly.

Rhabdoid tumors comprise just 2% of childhood renal tumors, and are very malignant with a poor prognosis. They occur more in the first year of life and in younger males than either Wilms' or clear cell sarcoma. They metastasize to the brain and there is also an increased risk of developing a primary PNET (usually in the posterior fossa). These patients often have hypercalcemia. Anaplasia, clear cell sarcoma and rhabdoid histology account for more than 50% of deaths from renal tumors.[220]

PROGNOSIS

Stage and tumor histology (see Table 22.21 and above) influence outcome.[222] Sixty per cent of patients are of Stage I and II, 20% Stage III, and 10–20% Stage IV. In the UKCCSG first Wilms' tumor study (1980–1986) 10 year event free survival was 95% for Stage I, 87% for Stage II, 81% for Stage III, 62% for Stage IV and 73% for Stage V.[223]

The change in approach to treatment (see below) in comparison with historic reports means that comparisons of staging and outcome are becoming difficult.

Table 22.21 Staging system for nephroblastoma

Stage I	Tumor limited to one kidney and totally excised. The renal capsule intact with no rupture pre- or during surgery. No residual tumor is apparent beyond the margins of excision. Tumor may have been biopsied
Stage II	Tumor extension beyond the kidney but totally excised. The extension is regional referring to renal vessels outside kidney infiltrated or containing thrombus. There may be penetration through the capsule to the outer surface and into the perirenal soft tissue. Biopsy may have been performed with local flank spillage. No residual tumor beyond margins of excision
Stage III	Residual non-hematogenous tumor confined to abdomen. Any one or more of the following may be present: 1. Extension beyond surgical margins micro- or macroscopically 2. Diffuse peritoneal contamination by spread or spillage 3. Involved nodes (renal hilar nodes previously) 4. Tumor not fully resectable because of local infiltration into vital organs, e.g. liver
Stage IV	Blood-borne metastases, e.g. lung, liver, bone and/or brain
Stage V	Bilateral kidney tumors initially or subsequently

In particular the percentage of patients by stage and the outcome/stage are changing with increasing preoperative chemotherapy.

MANAGEMENT

Over the last 30 years there has been such a significant improvement in outcome for Wilms' patients especially those without metastases and with favorable histology. As a consequence the focus has been on reduction of potential sequelae and avoidance, e.g. of anthracyclines and alkylators. The aims of therapy are to cure without excessive toxicity in Stage I to III and improve long term disease control in Stage IV disease. Controversy still exists as to whether initial surgery or preoperative chemotherapy (formerly radiotherapy) is optimal. The International Society of Pediatric Oncology Studies have shown that presurgical therapy reduces the risk of tumor rupture, downstages tumors and consequently reduces the numbers requiring flank or whole abdominal irradiation. With such overall good survival for low stage disease, such considerations are of great importance. In the UK and USA except in Stage IV disease, the classic approach has been for initial surgical excision. With CT and MR scanning it is much easier to detect truly localized Stage I tumors which can be fully resected and where very limited postoperative chemotherapy (10 weeks of vincristine) can cure over 90% of patients. There may indeed be patients (under 1 year with Stage I disease) who do not require any postoperative chemotherapy but as yet these have not been clearly defined. For all other stages, following careful radiographic staging and exclusion of inferior vena cava or even cardiac thrombus, biopsy can and probably should now be followed by chemotherapy as follows (UKCCSG guidelines):

1. For initially localized tumors vincristine weekly × 4 doses plus actinomycin × 2 doses (in weeks 1 and 4) with reduced doses for those under 15 kg in weight. Surgery should be scheduled in week 5.
2. Postoperative chemotherapy for such localized tumors depends on staging. The first vincristine is given as soon postoperatively as bowel function is restored.
   Stage I (favorable histology) vincristine weekly × 4 more injections and actinomycin × 1 more. Total duration of therapy 10 weeks.
   Stage II (favorable histology) vincristine weekly × 10 more, actinomycin 6 weekly × 6 alternating with doxorubicin 6 weekly × 6. Total duration 42 weeks.
   Stage III (favorable histology) chemotherapy as Stage II but with interruption during weeks 9–10 when abdominal irradiation is given. (Total radiation doses now reduced to 20 Gy.)

These days primary nephrectomy is rarely performed except in Stage I disease. If it is and histology proves favorable, Stage I patients receive 10 weeks of vincristine and actinomycin, Stage II 26 weeks of vincristine and actinomycin, Stage III vincristine, actinomycin and doxorubicin for 31 weeks plus abdominal radiotherapy (given in weeks 2–4 postsurgery). For unfavorable histology, patients receive preoperative chemotherapy with three drugs and longer courses of therapy are used.

All Stage IV patients receive preoperative chemotherapy with three drugs.[224,225] Lung irradiation for pulmonary metastases may improve long term survival. For bilateral Stage V disease, the usual approach has been nephrectomy for the largest tumor and partial nephrectomy for the smaller but bilateral partial nephrectomies are now being considered.[223]

SPECIFIC LATE EFFECTS

Chronic nephritis and renal failure is clearly seen in the Denys–Drash syndrome but also following abdominal irradiation involving the contralateral kidney. Kidney shielding and reduced total dosage have lowered the risks. Scoliosis and asymmetrical soft tissue wasting were once very common. Fields including the full vertebral width have reduced bony anomalies and lower dosages reduced muscle atrophy. Hepatitis and especially late enteritis (vascular) have been reduced by lowering total abdominal dosage to 20 Gy from the previously used 30 Gy. An acute veno-occlusive syndrome is occasionally seen when right sided flank irradiation (liver involved) is combined with actinomycin or adriamycin (both should be avoided for 6 weeks post radiation). Lung irradiation for residual pulmonary metastases (or even whole abdominal) can cause an acute pneumonitis, fibrosis and impairment of lung function.[152] Meadows et al[125] described 24 second tumors amongst Wilms' tumor patients, with 22/24 having received radiotherapy and 10/24 chemotherapy and radiotherapy. As for Hodgkin's disease, increasingly attempts are made to avoid radiation combined with chemotherapy wherever possible, hence the increasing trend towards presurgical chemotherapy to reduce tumor rupture and the subsequent need for radiotherapy. Abdominal irradiation in young girls clearly does encroach upon breast bud tissue and a rising incidence of breast cancer has been described in long term survivors.

MESOBLASTIC NEPHROMA

This tumor forms only a small percentage of childhood renal tumors but it is the commonest in the neonatal period with a mean age at diagnosis of 3–4 months. It is a quite distinct entity from Wilms' tumor. The kidney may be large with no pseudocapsule. Hemorrhage, cysts and necrosis are rare but the tumor may appear to infiltrate into the normal kidney and into the perinephric connective tissue. The mass is most commonly felt coincidentally at the time of an examination for other reasons. Occasionally there is hematuria, hypertension secondary to a rise in renin and even congestive cardiac failure. Babies with this tumor can have increased risk of preterm delivery due to polyhydramnios. Prenatal diagnosis has been made using ultrasound. The differential diagnosis is between hydronephrosis and multicystic kidney. Ultrasound can distinguish between these but cannot distinguish a nephroma from nephroblastoma. The treatment of choice is nephrectomy; recurrence is rare and usually only in children presenting beyond 3 months of life. Adjuvant treatment is only required for recurrent or significant but rare renal rupture or if the patient is older than 3 months with marked cellular mitosis on histology. There are rare reports of mesoblastic nephroma metastasizing but doubt is cast as to whether the diagnosis was correct in those circumstances.

SOFT TISSUE SARCOMAS (STS)[226]

Sarcomas can arise from primitive mesenchymal cells anywhere in the body and can develop in bone, cartilage, muscle and fibrous tissue. They are the sixth most common form of childhood cancer.

RHABDOMYOSARCOMA (RMS)

These are the commonest soft tissue sarcomas and arise from tissue which imitates striated muscle. They make up over 75% of the soft tissue sarcomas. Males slightly predominate. There is no recorded worldwide variation in incidence. Bladder and vaginal rhabdomyosarcomas predominantly occur in infancy and in the young and are principally embryonal or botryoid in type. Older children most commonly have truncal and extremity lesions which more frequently have undifferentiated and alveolar histology. Intra-abdominal tumors can occur at any age.

Specific etiologic factors

Most cases of RMS are sporadic and of unknown etiology. However these tumors have been reported in association with congenital lung cysts, fetal alcohol syndrome, neurofibromatosis and Rubenstein–Taybi syndrome. Li & Fraumeni[23] first described the association of breast cancer and STS. Birch et al[227] reported that the risk of mothers having breast cancer when their child had STS was as high as 13.5-fold. This risk is due to germline mutations of the p53 tumor suppressor gene on chromosome 17. RMS has also been associated with the nevoid basal cell carcinoma syndrome (Gorlin) which results from a germline mutation of the human homologue of the Drosophila segment polarity gene, patched (ptc).[228] Mice heterozygous for ptc develop a Gorlin-like syndrome and have an increased incidence of RMS and this model offers some insight into the etiology of RMS.[229] The protein product of ptc is a membrane receptor that is involved in the regulation of sonic hedgehog (shh) and wnt-1 signalling. Shh and wnt-1 are very important in the induction of embryonal myogenesis, via expression of the developmental transcription factors Pax-3 and Pax-7.[230] Chromosomal translocations involving either Pax-3 (t(2;13)) or Pax-7 (t(1;13)) and the Forkhead (FKHR) transcription factor are seen commonly in alveolar RMS.[231] Thus a model is beginning to emerge in which abnormalities in the ptc/shh/Pax signalling pathway contribute to the development of RMS.[232]

Clinical presentation

Rhabdomyosarcomas can arise at any site in the body as mass lesions. They are usually non-tender and the presentation depends on the site of the tumor.

Head and neck (40% of all rhabdomyosarcomas)

About 10% of tumors arise in the orbit producing proptosis and ophthalmoplegia. These usually present early, before the tumor has metastasized. There is little lymphatic spread from the orbit and the prognosis is good. Parameningeal tumors (about 20%) arise from the nasopharynx, paranasal sinuses, middle ear, mastoid and pterygopalatine fossa, producing nasal airway and ear symptoms often with signs of secondary purulent or even bloody discharge. There is a high risk of cranial nerve or meningeal involvement by contiguous spread. If this has occurred, headache, vomiting and raised intracranial pressure may be the presenting features. These tumors frequently have hematological spread. Before the high risk of central nervous involvement was realized these patients had an extremely poor prognosis and treatment must include CNS detected therapy. Other head and neck sites including scalp, face, oral mucosa, oropharynx, larynx and neck do not carry the same risk of CNS spread and present as mass lesions; they tend to be of low stage and non-metastatic.

Genitourinary tract (20%)

These usually arise in the bladder and prostate (12%) presenting as a polypoid mass inside the bladder leading to hematuria, urinary obstruction or even extrusion of the tumor into the urethra in females. They tend to be localized. Prostatic tumors lead to bladder outlet obstruction. Constipation may arise from obstruction of the rectum. Bladder tumors tend to occur in younger patients. Prostatic tumors have a higher risk of dissemination (especially to the lungs). Vaginal and uterine rhabdomyosarcomas make up 2% of the total. Most are botryoid (grape-like) and present with a mucousy and sometimes bloody discharge, as would a foreign body from which they need to be distinguished. Paratesticular tumors make up about 6% of the total and usually present as painless swellings in the scrotum or inguinal canal – often with nodal involvement. The genitourinary tract tumors tend to have embryonal histology.

Extremity lesions

These comprise 20% of the total and present as mass lesions with or without pain. The majority have alveolar histology and some nodal involvement. Spread can be extensive locally and they metastasize both via lymphatics and blood.

Truncal (10%)

On the trunk the mass may reach massive proportions before diagnosis. Local recurrence and distant spread is more likely than lymphatic or nodal involvement.

Other sites (10%)

Intrathoracic and retroperitoneal tumors may reach large dimensions before diagnosis. Intrathoracic primaries may present with airway obstruction or other respiratory symptoms and abdominal tumors with gastrointestinal obstruction. Perineal lesions are rare but can present like an abscess or a polyp. They often have alveolar histology and nodal spread. Biliary tract and liver tumors are rare but can mimic hepatoblastoma and hepatocellular carcinoma though more frequently presenting with jaundice. Differential diagnosis for rhabdomyosarcoma includes almost any other tumor and may be infrequently mistaken for traumatic bruising and soft tissue damage. It is not uncommon for a history of trauma to bring a mass to the attention of the patient, family and doctors, but trauma is not thought to contribute to tumor causation.

Diagnosis

Careful assessment of primary tumor extent and regional node involvement (clinical and radiological with CT and MR scanning) is required as a baseline. A truly localized lesion should have a full excision biopsy attempted but most will have diagnostic biopsy, with material sent for routine histology, electron microscopy studies, extensive immunocytochemical staining (see Table 22.18), cytogenetics and DNA studies. In parameningeal sites, investigations should include full CNS visualization by CT or MR plus CSF examination if there is no evidence of an intracerebral mass lesion. All patients require PA and lateral chest radiographs (CT chest scans if the X-rays are equivocal), and bone scans. Bilateral marrow trephines and aspirates are required to exclude marrow involvement. Investigations should also include full blood count, assessment of liver and kidney function and blood levels of calcium, phosphate and uric acid.

Histological classification

Traditionally several forms of rhabdomyosarcoma were recognized.[233] Differences in classification of these tumors existed between North American and European pathologists and an attempt to produce a unifying classification based upon prognostic categories (International Classification of RMS) has been proposed.[234] This divides these tumors into three groups:

1. *Superior prognosis*: This consists of the botryoid and spindle cell subtypes of embryonal RMS. Both of these variants are uncommon, botryoid accounting for 6% of STS and spindle cell 3%. However both have an excellent prognosis; 95% 5-year overall survival (OS) for botryoid and 88% for spindle cell reported in the second Intergroup study (IRSII). Botryoid lesions are usually found at sites that allow growth into a cavity, normally in the genitourinary tract. They tend to have a distinctive macroscopic 'bunch of grapes' appearance, and microscopically a sub-epithelial layer of condensed tumor cells. Spindle cell RMS is of low cellularity and is almost exclusively formed of spindle-shaped cells. These tumors are normally paratesticular in site.
2. *Intermediate prognosis*: This group contains embryonal RMS. Histologically these consist of blastemal mesenchymal cells which tend to differentiate into cross-striated muscle cells. Considerable cytologic variation can exist. These tumors tend to be found in children less than the age of 10 years and in sites including head and neck, pelvis and retroperitoneum. In IRS II these patients accounted for 49% of STS and had a 66% 5-year OS.
3. *Poor prognosis*: This group contains alveolar RMS and the undifferentiated sarcomas. Alveolar RMS features a connective tissue stroma lined with tumor cells giving rise to the so-called alveolar pattern. This may not be present throughout the tumor, but any amount of alveolar tumor even within a predominantly embryonal RMS carries a worse prognosis and the tumor should be regarded as alveolar. Alveolar RMS tends to present in older patients in association with skeletal muscle, usually involving the extremities or the trunk. Undifferentiated sarcomas are usually diffuse and contain primitive mesenchymal cells which are negative for the antigenic markers of RMS. In IRS II, 31% of tumors were alveolar and 10% undifferentiated sarcoma; alveolar RMS had a 5-year OS of 54% and undifferentiated sarcoma 40%.

Although rhabdomyosarcoma is the commonest STS of childhood, other tumors including extraosseous Ewing's sarcoma, fibrosarcoma and peripheral primitive neuroectodermal tumors may need to be considered in the differential. Identification on light and electron microscopy of cross-striations will facilitate a specific diagnosis. Immunocytochemistry as outlined in Table 22.18 has enabled easier differentiation of rhabdomyosarcoma from other tumors.[235] Desmin is the most useful marker but caution is required for its interpretation. Multiple monoclonal antibodies may help to confirm the diagnosis. It is the pattern of positivity rather than any single marker which determines the diagnosis.

Staging

The system used by the Intergroup collaborators (IRS) is the most widely accepted (Table 22.22) but attempts are now being made to adapt the TNM system[236] and relate it to site and extent of disease. A new grouping system is being tested in most recent trials.

Prognostic variables

RMS is a heterogenous condition and several prognostic factors have been identified, in addition to the histological groupings described above. Both preoperative stage and post surgical extent of disease are important. For those with localized tumors, complete excision (Group I) yields better survival than those with microscopic residual tumor or regional extension (Group II). Even poorer survival is seen for those with macroscopic (Group III) residual tumor and the worst for those with metastatic disease (Group IV). In IRS III 5-year OS for Group I disease was 93%, whilst for Group IV disease it was only 30%.[237] The site of the primary influences the lag time between first symptoms and diagnosis, the likelihood of metastatic spread and the possibility of surgical excision, and is also related to histological type. Orbital tumors had a 5-year OS of 95% in IRS III, whilst 5-year OS for parameningeal tumors was only 70%, a difference that was still seen in IRS IV.[238] In all trials to date, alveolar histology confers a worse prognosis than embryonal (see above). Some data also exist to suggest that different molecular abnormalities may confer different prognoses. Event free survival amongst a group of patients with alveolar RMS having the Pax7-FKHR gene fusion was significantly better than for a group containing the Pax3-FKHR translocation.[239] Rate of response to treatment and achievement of complete response also closely predict for outcome.

Management

The outcome of treatment for RMS has improved steadily over the last 30 years. Overall survival was only 25% in 1970 but was 70%

Table 22.22 Intergroup rhabdomyosarcoma study clinical grouping system

Clinical group	Definition
I	A. Localized, completely resected, confined to site of origin B. Localized, completely resected, infiltrated beyond site of origin
II	A. Localized, grossly resected, microscopic residual B. Regional disease, involved lymph nodes, completely resected C. Regional disease, involved lymph nodes, grossly resected with microscopic residual
III	A. Local or regional grossly visible disease after biopsy only B. Grossly visible disease after > 50% resection of primary tumor
IV	Distant metastases present at diagnosis

by 1991. RMS is a rare tumor and expresses considerable heterogeneity in terms of histological subtype, location of primary tumor and extent of disease at presentation. The improvement in outcome for this condition has been achieved through cooperative studies; Intergroup Rhabdomyosarcoma Study Group (IRSG) in North America, and the SIOP Malignant Mesenchymal Tumor (MMT) studies in Europe. The major differences between these two groups' strategies lie in the intensity of initial therapy and the use of radiotherapy. IRS studies tend to give radiotherapy earlier and to a greater proportion of patients than MMT studies with the result that although overall survival is not significantly different, event free survival is better in IRS studies.[238] Both groups use a risk grouping strategy as the basis for treatment.

1. In IRS IV (1991–1997) patients with Group I (localized disease, completely resected) paratesticular and those with Group I or Group II (microscopic residual) orbit or eyelid tumors were treated with vincristine/actinomycin for 36 weeks, receiving radiotherapy if there was microscopic residual disease. This contrasts with the SIOP MMT 95 approach where all patients with localized disease without microscopic residue other than those with alveolar histology are treated with vincristine/actinomycin for 9 weeks without radiotherapy.
2. IRS IV standard risk patients were all those other than the group above without metastatic disease. These patients were randomized to receive either vincristine/actinomycin/cyclophosphamide (VAC), vincristine/actinomycin/ifosfamide (VAI), or vincristine/ifosfamide/etoposide (VIE) 3 weekly for 23 weeks and then VAC 3 weekly for a further 23 weeks. Radiotherapy was given at week 9 for all except stage I/II patients (i.e. all sites but without lymph node involvement) without microscopic residual disease. MMT 95 used a more complex strategy regarding this group, as they included patients with localized tumors that were incompletely resected, those with clinically localized tumor with extension beyond the tissue of origin detected at surgery but with complete resection, and those with vaginal, uterine or paratesticular tumor extending beyond the tissue of origin, whether completely or incompletely resected and excluding any patients with alveolar histology. These patients received IVA (ifosfamide/vincristine/actinomycin) 3 weekly for three courses and then were evaluated. If they had a PR = 50% they received a further three courses, if not they were switched to alternating carboplatin/epirubicin/vincristine (CEV) with ifosfamide/vincristine/etoposide (IVE). Those patients achieving a CR after six courses of IVA receive no further treatment. Those without a CR receive a further three courses of IVA and radiotherapy starting at week 18. Those patients switched to CEV/IVE that achieved a CR after six courses received a further three courses but no radiotherapy whilst those not in CR receive three more courses and radiotherapy.
3. MMT 95 defines a high risk group of non-metastatic patients containing all patients with incompletely resected localized tumors, all patients with tumor spread beyond the tissue of origin whether resected or not, other than the favorable sites described above, all patients with nodal disease, and all patients with alveolar histology. These patients were randomized between IVA and a six drug schedule combining vincristine, ifosfamide, epirubicin, etoposide, actinomycin and carboplatin (IVA/CEV/IVE). Patients were evaluated after three cycles. Those achieving PR = 50% continued with their allocated regime for three further courses. Those receiving IVA who did not achieve a PR were changed to CEV/IVE, those receiving the six drug regimen not achieving a PR received radiotherapy +/- surgery at week 8. Patients were re-evaluated at week 17. Those achieving CR received three further courses of chemotherapy but no radiotherapy. Those not achieving CR received chemotherapy and radiotherapy.
4. Both treatment groups recognize the need to treat patients with metastatic disease more intensively. In IRS III the survival for patients with metastatic disease was only 30%[234] and in MMT 89 was only 29%. Both groups have used the up-front window study as a means of evaluating the effectiveness of novel agents. In the IRS IV study single agents found to be effective when used alone were subsequently incorporated into the continuation chemotherapy regimen. Topotecan was shown to be highly effective in the treatment of newly diagnosed metastatic RMS[240] and IRS V is using a similar approach with irinotecan. MMT 98 uses the up-front window approach described above and follows this with the six drug regimen described above, the combination having been previously shown to be effective in this setting,[241] followed by nine cycles of maintenance chemotherapy with VAC. However MMT 98 also defined a high risk group of patients older than 10 years or those with bone or bone marrow disease who are treated with high dose sequential monotherapy (cyclophosphamide, etoposide, carboplatin) and nine courses of VAC as maintenance.

OSTEOSARCOMA

The childhood incidence of osteosarcoma is 2.4 per million for boys 0–15 years and 2.8 for girls in the UK representing about 2.5% of all tumors. However with a peak in the second decade of life there is a gradual reverse of the sex ratio giving a male preponderance during the second decade of 1.4:1.[242] The reported incidence is lower elsewhere (Tables 22.1 and 22.2). Osteosarcoma accounts for about 60% of malignant bone tumors in young people. It arises from primitive bone forming mesenchymal stroma. Ewing's sarcoma is slightly more common in the first decade of life.

ETIOLOGY

The peak age incidence is at the time of maximum growth spurt and osteosarcoma usually occurs at the metaphyses of the most rapidly growing bones (distal femur, proximal tibia, proximal humerus).

It has a slightly younger peak age for girls, corresponding to earlier onset of puberty. These features all point towards a relationship with rapid bone growth and a malignant transformation of rapidly proliferating bone forming cells. The question then is whether transformation is a spontaneous event or induced by other environmental factors. Trauma frequently draws attention to the tumor but is almost certainly not causative. Ionizing irradiation has been implicated in about 3% of all osteosarcomas secondary to therapeutic irradiation. Latency between initial treatment and onset of a secondary osteosarcoma is normally 10–15 years but recently more rapid onset has been reported with intensive first line chemotherapy. Osteochondromas and chronic osteomyelitis can predispose to tumor formation. There is a strong association with retinoblastoma. (Fifty per cent of the second tumors in heritable retinoblastoma are osteosarcomas both within and without the radiation fields.) The same chromosome 13 defect has been demonstrated in both tumors. It has been speculated that rapidly proliferating bone forming cells may be particularly susceptible to mitotic errors and lead to loss of heterozygosity at the Rb locus. A number of other familial clusterings have also been described, including in families with demonstrated p53 germline mutations. Many human osteosarcoma tumors do show rearrangements of p53 somatically.

PRESENTATION

Most osteosarcomas present with an associated soft tissue swelling. Symptom duration is usually about 2–3 months. A more delayed presentation is commoner in periosteal sarcomas when symptoms may be present for many months or even years. Distal femur (33–35%), proximal tibia (15%), proximal humerus (9–10%), mid-femur (5%) and proximal femur (4–5%) are the commonest sites. Axial flat bones can be affected especially in the pelvis and constitute 15–20% of all tumors. These sites tend to occur in older patients. Up to 20% of patients have metastases at diagnosis most commonly in the lungs. Spread is hematogenous and rarely lymphatic. Occasionally multifocal osteosarcoma is seen in childhood and this carries a very poor prognosis. Symptoms of weight loss, malaise and fever suggest the presence of metastases.

DIAGNOSIS

Plain X-rays of the primary tumor site usually show destruction of the normal trabecular pattern with irregular margins and no endosteal bone reaction. There is usually surrounding soft tissue swelling. Periosteal elevation and new bone formation is common, producing the classic X-ray appearances of Codman's triangle. The appearances are characteristic in about two-thirds of cases particularly in association with a metaphyseal site. The lesions are sclerotic in 45% of cases, lytic in 30% and mixed in 25%. In contrast, Ewing's sarcomas are usually diaphyseal, lytic and more often involve flat bones.

CT or MR scans are essential to define the extent accurately, especially within the medullary cavity, MR being superior to CT for this purpose. CT scanning of the chest is essential as plain X-rays may miss as many as 10–20% of small metastases. The presence of metastases requires a change in management. Ninety per cent of all metastases are within the lungs.

Bone scanning shows the extent and vascularity of the tumor, the latter frequently extending beyond the tumor. This frequently helps the surgeon attempting a safe excision and of course it also identifies any multifocal lesions or metastases within bone (10% of metastases).

Alkaline phosphatase, elevated in about 40% of cases, can be used as a non-specific marker, as can lactate dehydrogenase (LDH) (elevated in about 30% of patients), for tumor response.

Once the extent of the disease has been assessed a biopsy should be performed; most often an open biopsy is recommended with the site of incision carefully chosen to facilitate limb salvage and to enable the original wound to be excised as part of that procedure. A frozen section should be performed at the time of biopsy to ensure the adequacy of the tissue material obtained. The surgeon should always try to manipulate the limb as little as possible and to limit bleeding to decrease the risk of seeding of tumor. In addition to routine histopathology, ploidy studies are now proving helpful in prognostication.

PATHOLOGY

The characteristic features of osteosarcoma are a malignant sarcomatous stroma with variable tumor osteoid and bone formation. Differential diagnosis is with chondrosarcoma and fibrosarcoma which lack the production of osteoid. Chondrosarcomas tend to affect the trunk and proximal limbs and often have a longer history with metastases occurring late and less frequently. Both of these tumors do tend to occur in older patients.

A number of pathological types of osteosarcoma exist.[243] Amongst the commonest type in childhood is conventional osteosarcoma of which 50% are osteoblastic with active osteoid, 25% are chondroblastic with some differentiation to cartilage but osteoid is always present. Nevertheless it may be difficult to distinguish such a tumor from a true chondrosarcoma. Twenty-five per cent of tumors are fibroblastic and can be confused with fibrosarcoma but again osteoid is present. All of these tumors are of high grade malignancy. Quite uncommon in children but occurring at an older age are telangiectatic tumors where there is a lytic tumor with some calcification frequently looking like an aneurysmal bone cyst or giant cell tumor. A further tumor which causes confusion is malignant fibrohistiocytoma, which carries a poorer prognosis.

Parosteal tumors most frequently in the distal femur occur in older patients and often have a long history. They slowly encircle the whole bone with a risk of local recurrence but metastases are late. Periosteal tumors do not extend into the medulla and occur most commonly in the 10–15 age group especially in the upper tibia and are of high grade. Again local recurrence is common but metastases are late and rare. Finally there is a low grade intraosseous osteosarcoma which shows slow growth, local infiltration and a low metastatic rate.

STAGING

The usual scheme for bone tumor staging is to divide the tumors into 1) low grade, 2) high grade, and 3) metastatic with intramedullary or extramedullary primary.[244] However it is not of great use in children where almost all cases are high grade and extramedullary or metastatic. Ninety per cent of the metastases occur in the lung, with 10–30% also in bone. Osteosarcoma can rarely metastasize to the pleura, pericardium, kidneys, adrenal and brain. Lymph node involvement is rare. Pulmonary disease is the commonest cause of death.

PROGNOSIS

Overall between 50 and 60% of osteosarcoma patients achieve 5-year event free survival.[245] With surgery alone up until the early 1970s 5-year survival rates were under 20%. The best results reported are by the Memorial Sloan-Kettering Group who reported 70% disease free survival at 5-years.[246] However that study was not randomized. The extent of the disease is the most important inherent prognostic factor. Tumor size is also important. Involvement of more than one-third of affected bone, or for the tumor to be greater than 15 cm in diameter or extent of local infiltration all influence outcome.[247] Clearly multifocal tumors and those where there are skip lesions worsen survival. Those with metastases at diagnosis have a poorer prognosis and aggressive treatment including thoracotomies to remove the metastases has in recent years improved prognosis for such patients. Metastatic disease is suggested by significantly elevated LDH and alkaline phosphatase levels. Inherent favorable histological features include parosteal and intraosseous well-differentiated tumors; the telangiectatic type is unfavorable. Other favorable histological features include extensive lymphocyte infiltration of the tumor and near diploid tumors. Since total surgical removal appears to be essential for cure certain sites such as in the head and neck or vertebrae are extremely difficult to cure. In general the more distal the site the more favorable the outcome. Age under 10 is an adverse feature. Girls fare better than boys. The duration of symptoms suggests that slow growing tumors with long symptom intervals have a more favorable outcome.

MANAGEMENT

To achieve long-term survival adequate surgical removal is essential. Historically, this was achieved by amputation but most (80%) still developed metastases (50% within the first 6 months) with a 5-year event free survival of only 20% (15–20% at 10 years). Since so many died with metastases in the lungs it was assumed that the majority had micrometastases at diagnosis and therefore strategies were developed using primary chemotherapy post-biopsy to reduce tumor bulk, facilitate surgery and eliminate micrometastases.

The most effective agents in osteosarcoma are clearly cisplatinum, adriamycin and methotrexate, with the first two having been shown to be as effective as more complex regimens including high dose methotrexate in a randomized trial.[248] This trial compared cisplatinum and doxorubicin with cisplatinum, doxorubicin and high dose methotrexate. They showed no significant difference in survival between the two arms although disease free survival was higher in the two drug arm. A further trial was carried out comparing a multi-drug combination regimen with cisplatinum and doxorubicin only. Again no difference was identified. However equal efficacy with fewer drugs and potentially less toxicity has not translated into improved survival. We appear to be rather stuck at a 50–60% event free survival for non-metastatic osteosarcoma. Ifosfamide has been shown to be a promising agent with greater than 20% single drug efficacy in relapsed patients. However if used in combination with cisplatinum it compounds the nephrotoxicity of that agent. The degree of response to presurgical therapy (histologically) appears to relate to outcome. Some have recommended a change in chemotherapy postsurgery based on degree of tumor necrosis.[249,250] This practice has not yet been adopted worldwide. The aim of induction intensive chemotherapy is to reduce tumor bulk and optimize surgical resection at the same time as trying to sterilize micro-metastases. If at the time of surgery there is poor histological response a change in therapy might appear to be very logical. It may be more frequently incorporated into future regimens. A recent European osteosarcoma Intergroup study has been testing the concept of dose intensity using doxorubicin and cisplatinum with or without granulocyte colony stimulating factor. New approaches for osteosarcomas are required.

It is the norm now for limb salvage operation, wherever possible, to be carried out and provided preoperative planning, optimization of preoperative chemotherapy and postoperative intensive physiotherapy are incorporated into management there are very good outcomes for the majority of patients with such surgery. It is important when carrying out such surgery to inform patients what their limitations will be. Those who expect to have no disability whatsoever and no limitation on activity will be disappointed and frequently are psychologically disturbed. Conversely those who have to have an amputation if prepared for it well cope with it amazingly well.

Those patients presenting with metastatic disease in the chest or who acquire it after therapy can be salvaged with the use of second line intensive therapy, e.g. using ifosfamide and etoposide plus high dose methotrexate when they have initially received just cisplatinum and doxorubicin followed by thoracotomies to remove CT scan identified metastases as well as surgically identified lesions at the time of the operation. With these aggressive approaches to pulmonary metastases 30–40% of such patients may be alive 5 years from the time of relapse but their long term survival remains unclear but may be as high as 25%. Regular chest radiographs with follow-up CT scans in the presence of any suspicious lesions are required in the first few years after stopping initial therapy in all patients with osteosarcomas.

EWING'S SARCOMA[251]

This is the second most common malignant bone tumor of childhood with a peak age at 10–15 years. Worldwide variations are seen in Tables 22.1 and 22.2 with a low risk especially amongst American blacks and the Chinese. Although a few associated congenital features have been reported, there is no obvious pattern of inheritance. The primitive malignant cell may be of neural origin. A reciprocal translocation t(11;22)(q24, q12) resulting in an EWS-FL1 fusion oncogene has been identified in Ewing's, Askin tumors and peripheral primitive neuroectodermal tumors suggesting a common neural crest cell of origin. The hybrid gene transcripts can be employed as both a diagnostic marker and for monitoring residual disease. Further understanding of tumorigenesis will result from exploration of the DNA configuration. Although trauma (as for osteosarcoma) frequently brings the patient to medical attention, it is thought to be coincidental not causative.

PRESENTATION

The commonest presentation is with a painful swelling of an affected bone and adjacent soft tissue. In the presence of metastases tiredness, anorexia, weight loss and fever can be expected. Both X-ray appearances and the presence of fever may lead to the mistaken diagnosis of osteomyelitis and delay appropriate therapy. The most common sites are the pelvis, proximal humerus and femur but any bone can be involved. The axial skeleton is more frequently involved than with osteosarcoma where extremity lesions are commoner. In long bones, metaphyseal and diaphyseal sites are the rule. Rib primaries often present with pleural effusions and respiratory difficulties. Sacral tumors may present with sacral nerve compression and either limb or bladder signs and symptoms.

DIFFERENTIAL DIAGNOSIS

This includes osteomyelitis, arthritis, traumatic injury to bone, osteosarcoma, neuroblastoma, PNETs, lymphomas and even leukemia. Sometimes the precise definition of a small round cell tumor can be very difficult and often the diagnosis of Ewing's sarcoma is by exclusion of other tumor types. Few other tumors have a diffuse mass of undifferentiated round cells infiltrating into bone marrow and out into the soft tissues. Ewing's sarcoma does not have a collagenous stroma like most of the other tumors, and stains for reticulin will usually be negative. In rhabdomyosarcomas light and electron microscopy studies may identify cross-striations. PAS staining, immunocytochemistry and the use of monoclonal antibodies will prove useful in differentiating the different tumors.[235,252] Where the reciprocal translocation t(11;22) is present, PCR based diagnostic tests are now becoming available to definitively diagnose Ewing's sarcoma rather than in the past where it was a matter of excluding other tumors in order to reach the diagnosis.

DIAGNOSIS

Brain X-rays, MR scanning and CT are all required to determine the full extent of tumor particularly within the bone marrow as well as soft tissue component. Chest radiographs and CT scans are necessary to exclude metastases whilst bone scans help to determine the extent of vascularity. At biopsy adequate material must be obtained and all effort must be made to avoid a pathological fracture. Incision for biopsy must be in a place where if further definitive surgery is to take place the scar can be excised, as with osteosarcoma. A frozen section should be performed at the time of biopsy to ensure adequacy of material. It is usually possible to make a diagnosis on soft tissue rather than disrupting the bony component of the tumor. A battery of tests including light microscopy, electron microscopy and immunocytochemistry, cytogenetic studies and molecular studies may all be needed to make the diagnosis. In addition two bone marrow aspirations and two trephines from different sites should be performed to exclude marrow infiltration. There are no specific useful markers in the peripheral blood to assist in prognostication or markers of residual disease.

STAGING AND PROGNOSTIC FEATURES[251]

No staging system has proved universally acceptable. As for osteosarcoma the Enneking system is used by some.

The presence of overt metastases at diagnosis which occurs in about 15% of patients confers a poor prognosis, the most common site being lung, then bone and bone marrow. Lymphatic spread is much less common. There is a low incidence of cerebral disease both at diagnosis and subsequently but spinal and paraspinal spread is quite common and may cause cord compression. Bone and bone marrow metastases worsen the prognosis whilst patients with lung metastases at diagnosis, especially if treated aggressively, can be salvaged by intensive chemotherapy and lung irradiation with or without removal of pulmonary nodules.

Other prognostic features include site of the primary with distal extremity lesions being most favorable while pelvic and sacral tumor sites have a poorer prognosis and often greater volume. The humerus, femur and rib sites have an intermediate outlook.

The extent of soft tissue involvement significantly affects prognosis with a volume of 100 ml conferring a significantly worsened prognosis (only 17% 3-year disease free survival for those with large tumors compared to 75–80% for those with small ones).[253] Where tumors are isolated to bone, the prognosis is better than those with soft tissue involvement (where there is a 5-year survival of just 20%). Estimated LDH levels appear to predict poorer outcome. The initial response to chemotherapy may correlate with prognosis as it does for osteosarcoma. Girls seem to fare better than boys as do patients under the age 10 years.[251]

MANAGEMENT

Surgery

Poor long-term survival was obtained with surgery only. Improvement has resulted from the use of intensive chemotherapy coupled with local control obtained either with radical tumor removal or high dose radiotherapy. For all but the most localized tumors, biopsy is recommended followed by chemotherapy which may render the tumor totally resectable. There is some evidence that long-term sequelae, especially in the development of second tumors, are less common if chemotherapy and surgery are used rather than chemotherapy and radiotherapy. However, certain sites are not amenable to radical surgery and for them radiotherapy is essential. Amputation of certain bones, e.g. ribs or the small bones of the feet, are possible and associated with minimal loss of function. Proximal fibula lesions can be removed with the distal bone left to stabilize the ankle joint. By and large, attempts are made to treat all other long bone lesions with limb-sparing procedures involving removal of the bone segments, as for osteosarcoma, and replacement with increasingly ingenious prostheses. Sometimes regrettably amputation becomes necessary either when pathological fracture develops at a previous tumor site sterilized by radiotherapy or when soft tissue sequelae follow extensive radiotherapy.

Radiotherapy

Ewing's sarcoma is radiosensitive. Primary treatment must be with chemotherapy to control the almost inevitable dissemination. Local control can then be achieved with radiotherapy. If radiotherapy is given in the middle of a course of chemotherapy the subsequent therapy may be compromised, as a result for example, of myelosuppression secondary to extensive pelvic and spinal marrow irradiation. Consequently intensive early chemotherapy is essential to try to sterilize the tumor. The radiation fields should include the entire affected bone plus soft tissue extension with a 3–5 cm margin if possible although in the pelvis this may have to be reduced to 2 cm. Some benefit has been shown for the use of radiotherapy also to areas of gross metastatic disease, particularly the lung. Though its benefit cannot yet be fully validated total body irradiation and high dose chemotherapy with autologous marrow transplantation is now being tried in patients who have metastatic disease at diagnosis.

Chemotherapy

Initial drugs shown to be effective in Ewing's sarcoma were vincristine, doxorubicin and cyclophosphamide. Subsequent replacement of cyclophosphamide with ifosfamide and the addition of etoposide appears to be tolerable, though associated with significant short term sequelae including mucositis, profound neutropenia and regular febrile episodes. In most multicenter studies 3-year disease free survival is now in the region of 60–70% for distal extremity lesions, 30–35% for pelvic and proximity extremity disease and well under 20% for those with metastatic disease at diagnosis although those with lung disease may fare better than those with other, especially bony, metastases.

GERM CELL TUMORS

These tumors are derived from primordial germ cells and arise within the gonads and at a number of other midline sites in the sacrococcygeal, retroperitoneal, mediastinal, neck or pineal regions. Malignant germ cell tumors account for 3% of all childhood cancers. A number of structural chromosomal changes have been detected in germ cell tumors, most consistently an isochrome 12p, in about 80% of patients with testicular lesions.[254] A small number of families with multiple affected individuals have been reported. Klinefelter's syndrome is strongly associated with mediastinal tumors (20% of males so affected) and at other sites. 46XY gonadal dysgenesis is frequently complicated by germ cell tumors. Ataxia telangiectasia and Li–Fraumeni syndrome families have also been reported in association with such tumors.

TERATOMAS

These are tumors with tissue arising from all three germinal layers, with a lack of organization and variable maturation. They may be solid or cystic and are most often found in the sacrococcygeal region. There are three subtypes: mature, with well-differentiated tissues, e.g. brain and skin; immature, with embryonic components; and malignant with disorganized embryonic tissue and malignant germ cell elements (e.g. germinoma, choriocarcinoma, endodermal sinus tumor or embryonal carcinoma). In the newborn a sacrococcygeal teratoma may consist of either mature, immature or a mixture of both types of patterns. Neonatal tumors outside the sacrococcygeal region, e.g. in the nasopharynx, the jaw or the mediastinum, do not normally contain malignant components.

GERMINOMA (SEMINOMA IN TESTIS, DYSGERMINOMA IN OVARY)[255]

The commonest sites for these tumors in childhood are the ovary, anterior mediastinum and pineal region. Ten per cent of all ovarian and 15% of all germ cell tumors are germinomas and they are the commonest in undescended testicles. There is a characteristic histological appearance of large round cells, vesicular nuclei and clear eosinophilic cytoplasm. Serum levels of AFP and HCG levels are not elevated in pure germinoma.

EMBRYONAL CARCINOMA

This is a poorly differentiated tumor usually with an epithelial appearance (although it may look more like an anaplastic carcinoma with necrosis). Apparent pathological maturation to teratoma has been noted after chemotherapy. These tumors stain markedly for AFP and HCG. In pediatric practice it is rare to find the tumor in a pure form but more commonly in association with teratomatous and endodermal sinus tumor deposits. In young males, the commonest site is the testis.

ENDODERMAL SINUS TUMOR (YOLK SAC)

This tumor occurring alone or in combination with teratoma is the most common malignant germ cell tumor in childhood. The sacrococcygeal region is the usual site in infancy but later the ovary and testes are more frequently affected, although it can occur elsewhere. The tumors are often soft and friable with a papillary, reticular or a solid pattern.

CHORIOCARCINOMA

This highly malignant tumor is rare in childhood and arises from non-gestational extraplacental tissue. The commonest sites are the mediastinum, ovary and pineal region. Beta-HCG but not AFP is markedly elevated in serum. Histology shows large round cells with vesicular nuclei (cytotrophoblasts) and large, usually vacuolated, cells which form syncytia (syncytiotrophoblasts). Hemorrhage and necrosis are common.

GONADOBLASTOMA

This tumor is most frequently found in dysgenetic gonads. Thirty per cent of patients with gonadal dysgenesis develop a gonadoblastoma which is bilateral in 40% of cases. Local invasion is seen within the gonads but if elements of germinoma are present it is more likely to spread. AFP and HCG are not produced by this tumor.

POLYEMBRYOMA

This is a rare tumor of the ovary or anterior mediastinum. Both AFP and HCG are elevated. The tumor contains elements resembling small embryos.

Ovarian granulosa and theca cell and testicular Sertoli and Leydig cell tumors arise from the true sex cords and stroma of the developing gonad but are not classified as germ cell tumors.

Biochemical markers

Three markers may help with diagnosis and monitoring of therapy.

Alpha-fetoprotein

Alpha-fetoprotein (AFP) production from the yolk sac is maximal at about 12–15 weeks of gestation. Normal adult blood levels are not reached until 6–12 months postpartum. Tumor arising from the pluripotential germ cells of the yolk sac secrete high concentrations with the exception of pure dysgerminoma, pure choriocarcinoma, mature teratomas and gonadoblastoma. Monitoring of serum levels can be useful, especially for evidence of resistant or recurrent disease. Staining of tumor for AFP is a useful diagnostic tool.

Beta-human chorionic gonadotrophin

This glycoprotein is produced by specialized placental cells so that tumor with trophoblastic elements (choriocarcinoma and hydatidiform moles) have high levels. The half-life is extremely short (45 min) so rapid normalization occurs with tumor kill.

Lactate dehydrogenase isoenzyme 1

Elevation of this isoenzyme is seen in tumor derived from the yolk sac. It can be used to monitor response to therapy.

SACROCOCCYGEAL TERATOMAS

The incidence is 1 in 35 000 live births with 65% being benign, 30% malignant and 5–10% having an immature appearance. Approximately 40% of all germ cell tumors occur in this area. There is a marked female sex preponderance (70%). The mode of presentation will depend on the precise site of the tumor.

1. The buttocks with a minimal presacral component. This is the commonest site in the newborn (186 out of 398 in a series by Altman et al[256]). They are unlikely to be malignant but may become so if not fully excised.
2. External but with a significant intrapelvic component (138 out of 398 in Altman's series).
3. External with most of the mass intrapelvic extending into the abdomen (35 out of 398 in Altman's series). This is the group most likely to be malignant de novo.
4. Entirely presacral with no external component or significant pelvic extension (39 out of 398). These are likely to be missed clinically and more frequently give rise to constipation, less commonly to urinary frequency or lower limb weakness from sacral nerve compression. Any young child with a history of persistent constipation should have a rectal examination as well as careful pelvic ultrasonography or radiology.

In types 1, 2 and 3 the diagnosis is usually made on clinical grounds from the presentation of an external mass, although in type 2 the external component can be quite small and may be missed.

Diagnosis

The early detection and surgical removal of even a benign tumor is necessary because of the risk of subsequent malignant change. If the diagnosis is made before 2 months of age the chance of malignancy is low (10% in boys and 7% in girls). After 2 months, the risk of malignancy is over 60% in boys and 45–50% in girls. The estimation of AFP and HCG levels is mandatory and urinary catecholamines can be measured to exclude a pelvic neuroblastoma. CT or MRI scanning will delineate the tumor extent and relations, and determine the presence of any intraspinal component. Pulmonary metastases must be excluded.

Staging

Staging in this site is postsurgical. Stage I: a completely excised mass which was localized; Stage 2: an excised tumor which extended to adjacent structures or ruptured at surgery; Stage III: a mass which was resected but with residual microscopic (A) or macroscopic (B) tumor; Stage IV: a tumor with metastases.

MEDIASTINAL TERATOMAS

These almost always arise in the anterior superior mediastinum along the urogenital ridge which extends from C6 to L4. They are sometimes found coincidentally on chest X-ray or they may present with airway obstruction, cough, wheeze and dyspnea. Many histological types have been reported, ranging from pure teratoma to embryonal carcinoma and endodermal sinus tumor. Appearances on chest X-ray are of a well-rounded mass often with calcification. Sometimes teeth may be identified in a mature teratoma. CT or MR scanning is essential to determine the extent of the tumor. The differential diagnosis will include thymoma, cyst, lymphoma and neurogenic tumor. A full blood count including platelet count and bone marrow aspiration will exclude advanced stage lymphoma. AFP, HCG levels and urinary catecholamines should be measured. Ultrasonography of the abdomen is necessary to exclude an intra-abdominal mass. It is important to exclude other diagnoses because, for a mediastinal teratoma, complete surgical excision is necessary for cure whereas in other tumors (especially lymphomas) chemotherapy is the treatment of choice.

ABDOMINAL GERM CELL TUMOR

Most arise in the retroperitoneum but they can occur within the gastrointestinal tract, omentum or liver. In the stomach they may present as obstruction or hemorrhage and in the liver as a mass or jaundice. The retroperitoneum is the third commonest site after the sacrococcygeal and mediastinal regions in those under 2 years. Pressure from the mass causes pain, constipation or urinary difficulties. Ultrasonography and plain X-rays will often identify calcification or the presence of bone or teeth within the lesion. Investigations to distinguish other tumors should include abdominal ultrasound, CT scan and measurement of urinary catecholamines and serum AFP levels.

INTRACRANIAL TERATOMAS

These account for about 6% of germ cell tumors. Most arise in the pineal region but they can also arise in the suprasellar and infrasellar regions, more frequently leading to CSF pathway obstruction at third ventricular level. A wide variety of histological types including germinomas, embryonal carcinoma and pure teratoma are reported and it is important to distinguish between them since the treatment will be different. For teratoma, surgical excision is the treatment of choice; for embryonal carcinoma, which is more likely to be highly malignant, a biopsy is followed by intensive chemotherapy and radiotherapy.

Other sites for extragonadal germ cell tumors are the oral cavity, the pharynx, the orbit and the neck, collectively making up about 6% of germ cell tumors. These are mostly found at birth and are of benign histology though they can cause death from airway obstruction. Vaginal tumors, mostly of the endodermal sinus tumor type, usually present with bloody discharge. The differential diagnosis will be with rhabdomyosarcoma of botryoides type or a clear cell carcinoma.

GONADAL TUMORS

Ovarian tumor

These account for about 30% of all germ cell tumors; 65% are benign teratomas, 5% are immature teratomas and about 30% are malignant. In children epithelial carcinoma of the ovary is rare. Most malignant germ cell tumors within the ovary occur around the time of puberty. Presentation is usually with pain which may be acute, secondary to tumor torsion or necrosis or it may be chronic associated with some gastrointestinal upset such as nausea and vomiting. There may be fever. These tumors are not infrequently misdiagnosed as appendicitis and at laparotomy a mass is found within the ovary.

The mass may reach a surprising size with omental seeding before clinical symptoms related to the bowel or urinary tract bring the patient to attention. If beta-HCG secretion is marked, pregnancy may be misdiagnosed. The tumor can spread locally to the adnexae, throughout the abdomen (with ascites), to nodes or via the blood. Investigations of a suspected ovarian mass should include plain X-rays of the pelvis and abdomen plus ultrasonography. Malignant tumors less commonly show calcification. MR and CT scanning will give better identification of the exact extent and site of the tumor. Pulmonary metastases should be excluded. AFP levels will be elevated if the tumor is an endodermal sinus tumor or a teratoma and beta-HCG if it is an embryonal carcinoma or choriocarcinoma. Other potential sites for metastases include bones and brain.

Stage I tumors are localized to the ovary with no cells in the peritoneal fluid; Stage II extend beyond the ovarian capsule but only locally without invasion of retroperitoneal nodes (peritoneal fluid negative); Stage III has positive retroperitoneal nodes, cells in the ascitic fluid or abdominal extension; and Stage IV has extra-abdominal extension.

Testicular tumors[257]

These comprise about 7% of all germ cell tumors and about 70% of all testicular tumors in childhood. Eighty per cent are malignant and nearly 20% are pure teratomas. The most common malignant tumor is endodermal sinus tumor. The presentation is with a slowly growing painless testicular mass, with or without accompanying hydrocele (25%) and/or inguinal hernia (20%). These tumors may be misdiagnosed as either epididymitis or hydrocele. If the testis is undescended the risk of malignancy is 20–40 times greater. There may be an inherent problem within the testes since the risk of malignant change is also higher in the contralateral descended testis in a patient with unilateral cryptorchidism. Investigations include ultrasonography of the abdomen and pelvis with CT scanning of abdomen, pelvis and chest; and measurement of AFP and HCG levels. Einhorn's simple staging system for carcinoma of the testis is sufficient. Stage I is tumor localized to testis only; Stage II testis plus retroperitoneal nodes; and Stage III indicates supradiaphragmatic involvement.

MANAGEMENT

Benign germ cell tumors

The optimal treatment for mature teratomas is surgical excision and complete removal is necessary for cure. In the UKCCSG study 123 of 125 patients with mature or immature germ cell tumors had primary surgical resection and 114 of these needed no further treatment.[258] Six of these patients developed yolk sac recurrence which was successfully treated with combination chemotherapy. The AFP should be followed long term to identify any recurrence. External sacrococcygeal tumors require a transacral approach but if the pelvis is involved an abdominal combined approach is needed. Removal of the coccyx is essential if recurrence is to be avoided. Spillage from cysts must be avoided and the surgeon should ensure that there is no intraspinal extension of the tumor.

Immature germ cell tumors

Controversy exists about the ideal treatment of immature teratomas. For localized but immature forms, most authorities still recommend surgery and follow-up, as the diagnosis is often only made after tumor removal. The UK and US practice is to treat recurrence with chemotherapy if it arises; the POG experience in 68 children receiving surgery alone was of three recurrences, all salvaged with chemotherapy[259] and a 3-year disease free survival of 96.7%; the UK experience is of four recurrences out of 41 patients, three salvaged with chemotherapy.[258]

Malignant germ cell tumor

Einhorn et al[260] showed that cisplatinum, bleomycin and vinblastine (BVP) were superior to all previous chemotherapy for malignant ovarian and testicular germ cell tumors. More recently the UKCCSG has demonstrated that pulsed carboplatin, etoposide and bleomycin (JEB) is as effective and less toxic for all malignant extracranial non-gonadal tumors. Five-year event free survival was 87% and overall survival 95% in GC2 with JEB as compared with 46% and 63% respectively with the previous regime (GC1). Rates of renal toxicity and deafness in children treated on GC1 were 20% and 35% respectively, whilst on GC2 they were 0% and 10%.[261] The role of surgery has changed given the improvement in chemotherapy results. For all it is essential to have adequate material to make a reliable assessment of all cellular components of the tumor. For ovarian tumors wherever possible total excision without spillage should be attempted but extensive pelvic exenteration is contraindicated. If necessary, further surgery to remove residual disease after intensive chemotherapy is to be preferred. In localized testicular tumor, excisional biopsy is recommended through an inguinal approach, and for malignant tumor in that site, radical orchidectomy with high ligation of the cord. For all extracranial malignant germ cell tumors, other than stage I testicular tumors, intensive chemotherapy should be given. The current UK recommendation is to give 3 weekly JEB until the AFP is normal and then give a further two courses. For relapsing patients high dose chemotherapy with autologous bone marrow rescue have been used successfully in adult patients but there are few published pediatric data.[262]

RETINOBLASTOMA[263]

This malignant embryonal tumor occurs predominantly in the first 2 years of life (75% are diagnosed before 3 years). Its relative incidence varies considerably around the world, e.g. it accounts for 2.7% of tumors in the United Kingdom but 9.7% in the Ibadan registry and 9.4% in that from Madras (see Table 22.1). The increase in Africa and India is of non-genetic retinoblastoma and strongly suggests an environmental factor may be involved in etiology. The age standardized incidence rate in the UK is 7.5 per million children which amounts to between 40 and 50 new cases diagnosed per annum in the UK. There is no obvious sex difference in incidence. There is a family history in about 10% of cases, the remaining 90% appearing sporadic. However 20–30% of all tumors are bilateral and clearly 'genetic' (even if there is no family history) and about 10–12% of unilateral cases are also inherited. This means that overall about 40% are genetic or 'heritable' from an affected, surviving parent, from a non-affected carrier parent (sometimes they have regressed retinomas) or as the result of a new germinal mutation in the patient. Sixty per cent are 'non-hereditary' or 'non-genetic' and result from spontaneous somatic cell mutations (within retinal cells only). They are always unilateral and have no family history. Knudson[264] proposed that in the 'genetic' form the first mutation occurred prezygotically, while a second event triggered the tumor in the retina or in fact elsewhere in the body. In non-genetic tumors both events occur within the retinal cells. Carriers of the retinoblastoma gene (13q14) mutation can develop single or multiple retinal tumors and/or neoplasms at other sites. Indeed germline Rb mutations have been implicated in the development of osteosarcoma, small cell lung carcinoma, bladder and breast carcinoma and various soft tissue sarcomas. Abnormalities of the p53 gene do often occur concurrently with the inactivation of the retinoblastoma susceptibility gene.[265] The cloned gene encodes for a 928 amino acid protein, which is a nuclear phosphoprotein with DNA-binding activity, thought to play a critical role in cell growth regulation. Loss of both alleles at this locus is required for tumor formation. The wild type allele is probably a tumor suppressor gene. In view of all this knowledge, very accurate genetic counseling is possible from the mode of presentation, family history and search for evidence of the gene in parents. Any child of a surviving parent who had retinoblastoma has a 50% chance of developing a tumor. If normal parents have one affected child, the next one has a 1% risk if the first child had unilateral disease and 6% if it was bilateral. As with all tumor suppressor genes, sequencing has demonstrated heterozygous point mutations along the 27 exons of the Rb gene. Prenatal and postnatal prediction using such sequencing of this large gene, although cumbersome at present, clearly enables even more accuracy in terms of risk assessment.

Despite much research we do not know what causes the initial germline mutation in genetic retinoblastoma but such mutations may arise merely as a result of spontaneous mutations at a 'background' mutation rate.[266] New mutations appear to more frequently derive from the paternal allele, i.e. arise during spermatogenesis.[267,268] About 5% of retinoblastoma patients carry a constitutional deletion on the long arm of chromosome 13.[266] Sporadic non-hereditary retinoblastoma risk factors include older maternal and paternal age and paternal employment in the 'metal' industries.[269]

PRESENTATION

Nowadays most children are identified with the tumor still intraocular. The commonest presenting feature is leukocoria or the 'cat's eye reflex'. The tumor shows as a creamy to pinkish mass through the iris. Strabismus is common if the tumor arises in the macula. Occasionally, patients may show inflammatory changes or even a fixed pupil. A common reason for delay in diagnosis is a mistaken diagnosis of uveitis or endophthalmitis. The tumor is not painful unless there is secondary glaucoma or inflammation. If the involvement is unilateral the child will probably not complain of visual loss. Metastatic symptoms occur if the disease has spread outwith the orbit but this is rare at diagnosis these days in the UK. Most often parents note the eye abnormality and seek help. A full ophthalmological examination under general anesthetic is required (with pupillary dilatation). Ultrasonography, CT and MR scanning have enabled better visualization of the tumor. Skull X-rays may show calcification. Bone marrow aspiration and lumbar puncture should also be performed under general anesthetic (necessary for a good ophthalmological examination) to exclude dissemination. Hemorrhage and calcification are quite common and pieces of tumor may break off and seed either into the vitreous or elsewhere on to the retina. External layer disruption can lead to choroid involvement and a greater risk of blood-borne metastases. The iris may be pushed forward by a mass effect or the trabecular network infiltrated leading to glaucoma. Spread can occur along the optic nerve to invade the brain and CSF. Blood-borne spread commonly goes to bone, brain and other organs. Lymphatic spread to the preauricular and submandibular nodes is rare. A staging system based on size of tumor, site of tumor on the retina, extension to involve the choroid, optic nerve or vitreous and presence/absence of metastases is now employed.

MANAGEMENT

All patients require treatment in highly specialized multidisciplinary centers.

The general principles which guide therapy are:

1. For non-genetic tumors near 100% cure is possible by enucleation and insertion of an artificial eye.
2. Further treatment of non-genetic tumors is only indicated if there is evidence of extraorbital spread or if on histology, choroidal or nerve head infiltration is present. Most commonly chemotherapy is utilized and occasionally radiotherapy also needed.
3. For those with small unilateral lesions (less than 4 disc diameters) cryotherapy and photocoagulation offer an alternative, but very careful expert follow-up is required to ensure that the tumor is sterilized.
4. For 'genetic' disease, enucleation in unilateral disease, and the worse eye in bilateral disease, is usually performed.
5. With the high risk of tumors developing in the other eye with such genetic tumors, if not already present, radiotherapy and/or chemotherapy is used as well to try to conserve some vision in both eyes.
6. Vincristine, cyclophosphamide, adriamycin, ifosfamide, cisplatinum, carboplatin and etoposide have all been shown to produce shrinkage. Limited dosage JOE (carboplatin, vincristine and etoposide) has been used successfully with the least toxicity and lowest rate of secondary tumors to date, from any chemotherapy regimen. Careful attention must be paid to scheduling and total dosage.[270]
7. Even with bilateral disease, event free survival at 5 years can be 90% unless there is orbital or CNS invasion, but with germline Rb carriage it would appear that the development of secondary neoplasia is a very high risk over the ensuing 30–40 years.[22] All planned combined modality therapy should attempt to minimize the risk by avoiding for example combinations of irradiation and alkylators and careful attention to the dose and scheduling of drugs such as the topoisomerase 2 inhibitors.

LIVER TUMORS

Liver tumors make up about 1% of childhood malignancies; 60% are malignant, with hepatoblastoma being slightly more common than hepatocellular carcinoma (HCC). Forty per cent are benign hamartomas or hemangiomas. Both malignant types occur more often in males. Hepatoblastoma has a peak incidence at 18 months, and rarely occurs beyond 10 years while HCC has a median age of onset of 12 years. Predisposing conditions for hepatoblastoma are Beckwith–Wiedemann syndrome and hemihypertrophy (2% of cases) and indeed Wilms' and concurrent hepatoblastoma have been reported. Loss of heterozygosity at both 11p13 and 11p15.5 (see Wilms' tumor) has now been reported within some such hepatoblastomas. Other clonal anomalies, rare sibling pairs and an association with familial adenomatous polyposis (gene on 5q) strongly imply that a variety of gene disturbances can lead to tumor formation. Possible environmental associations have included maternal ingestion of oral contraceptives, and fetal alcohol syndrome. Hepatocellular carcinoma is associated with hepatitis B infection and patients have a greatly increased hepatitis B surface antigen carrier rate than controls. Recently hepatitis C has also been incriminated. Other causes of cirrhosis including hereditary tyrosinemia, alpha-1 antitrypsin deficiency, extrahepatic biliary atresia and progressive familial cholestatic cirrhosis all predispose to HCC. Prolonged use of anabolic steroids can induce adenomas and multifocal hepatocellular carcinomas. In young patients these are most often seen in Fanconi's anemia. HCC has also occurred in association with familial adenomatous polyposis, ataxia telangiectasia and neurofibromatosis.

Hepatoblastoma

This tumor usually presents as an abdominal mass in a child under 2 years with some having weight loss, anorexia, vomiting and pain but symptoms are less prominent than in hepatocellular carcinoma. Occasionally a tumor has ruptured and the patient presents with an 'acute' abdomen. Not infrequently the tumor is found during examination of a child with general malaise. Abdominal distension with a big liver is the most common finding. Jaundice is rare but the patient may be anemic. There may be splenomegaly and finger clubbing. Rarer associated features include sexual precocity if beta-HCG secretion is high, and up to one-third have severe osteopenia with bone pain and even vertebral fractures.

Hepatocellular carcinoma

Right upper quadrant distension is the most common presentation, often with features of underlying cirrhosis (or tyrosinemia). It is common to find splenomegaly with finger clubbing and spider nevi. Pain is more common than in hepatoblastoma as are nausea, vomiting, fever, weight loss and anorexia. These tumors may also rupture. Jaundice is reported in up to 25% of cases. There may also be associated thrombocytosis and polycythemia due to raised erythropoietin and probably thrombopoietin levels.

DIAGNOSIS

Ultrasound examination will define the liver mass, up to 10% of which may show calcification. Benign tumors tend to be poorly echogenic and much more commonly cystic. Ultrasonography is also useful to inspect the inferior vena cava, hepatic and portal veins. CT scanning shows lower attenuation in the tumor than in normal liver and can define the anatomic extent of the tumor. Both hepatoblastoma and hepatocellular carcinoma are deeply infiltrative and may be multicentric. MR scanning is superior to CT for definition of tumor margins. Hepatoblastoma occurs most commonly in the right lobe of the liver. Cooperation between radiologist and surgeon is likely to result in more reliable anatomical information. CT of chest is needed to exclude pulmonary metastases. Blood tests should include a full blood count and platelet count. Mild normochromic normocytic anemia is quite common but, particularly in hepatocellular carcinoma, increased erythropoietin production may lead to polycythemia. The platelets may be elevated in excess of 1000×10^9/L in childhood liver tumors. The most useful marker is AFP, produced exclusively in the liver in postnatal life. The normal adult range (3–15 ng/ml) is reached by approximately 1 year; the half-life is between 5 and 7 days and is raised in about two-thirds of patients with hepatoblastoma. It is less commonly elevated in those with embryonal type histology than in the fetal type and is useful for monitoring the course of the disease. Failure to fall along the usual gradient or a late rise suggests persistent or recurrent disease. This may occur prior to any clinical evidence of relapse. AFP levels are raised in about 50% of patients with hepatocellular carcinoma. In those with precocious puberty beta-HCG levels can be monitored for tumor response. Liver function should be evaluated and monitoring of calcium, phosphate and alkaline phosphatase levels are necessary particularly if there is any significant osteopenia. Hepatitis B serology is often positive in hepatocellular carcinoma but rarely in hepatoblastoma.

STAGING AND HISTOLOGY

Staging in Europe is based on the relationship between the tumor and the anatomy of the liver assessed preoperatively (the PRETEXT classification). Surgical resection is crucial for cure of hepatoblastoma, and this staging system aims to predict the anatomy of the healthy liver that will remain after resection and describes the number out of 4 sections of the liver involved. The presence of tumor beyond the liver, either of local spread to the vena cava and/or portal vein or distant pulmonary metastases is sufficient to categorize the disease as high risk. Biopsy of the tumor is usually necessary, although in children between 6 months and 3 years with a raised AFP it is not mandatory. Wedge biopsies, through a small abdominal incision, or 'true cut' biopsies from three separate sites are equally acceptable.

There are two morphological forms of hepatoblastoma: a pure epithelial (70%) of either fetal or embryonal cells, or a mixture of both, and a mixed tumor with mesenchymal tissue as well as epithelial elements.[271] Even osteoid production may be present in these. It is doubtful if the histological type truly predicts outcome, although which epithelial type (i.e. fetal or embryonal) predominates may determine resectability. Hepatoblastoma most often metastasizes to lungs and nodes at the porta hepatis and rarely to bone. Hepatocellular carcinoma similarly metastasizes to the lungs, nodes and later to bone.

MANAGEMENT

Hepatoblastoma

Hepatoblastoma requires total surgical excision for cure.[272] Preoperative chemotherapy, based upon doxorubicin and cisplatin, has been shown to produce tumor shrinkage and increases the number of patients whose tumors can be fully resected. Eighty to 100% of hepatoblastomas are chemoresponsive, and 67–80% will be resectable after this treatment.[273] The 3-year survival for this disease, as a result, is now 70%. In the first SIOP liver tumor trial (SIOPEL-1) all patients received preoperative chemotherapy regardless of initial resectability. The 3-year overall survival in this trial was 79%.[274] The presence of pulmonary metastases at diagnosis has been consistently found to be an adverse prognostic factor.[275] SIOPEL-1 also identified tumor affecting all four liver sections, extrahepatic tumor and multifocal tumor as poor prognostic factors. As a result in the current SIOP trial (SIOPEL-3) this group of patients are regarded as high risk and receive an intensive chemotherapy regimen alternating cisplatin with carboplatin/doxorubicin. The remaining patients are standard risk and receive either cisplatin as a single agent or cisplatin/doxorubicin. In SIOPEL-1 10 patients had liver transplantation because of unresectable disease; all but one of these patients were alive without evidence of disease at a median 3-year follow-up. The presence of pulmonary metastases at diagnosis is not a contraindication to transplantation, providing that these are no longer visible at the time of surgery; four of the successfully transplanted patients in SIOPEL-1 had pulmonary metastases at diagnosis.

Hepatocellular carcinoma

Historically less than 30% were amenable to primary surgical resection, and only one-third of these had long-term survival. Cisplatinum, doxorubicin and etoposide have all been shown to produce shrinkage. In the SIOPEL-1 study, preoperative therapy (cisplatinum, doxorubicin) was given to 40 patients of whom 12 had complete resection, and two incomplete. Seven of these patients were alive without disease at 10–46 months follow-up whilst 22 were still unresectable. Primary surgery should be performed for resectable disease and postoperative chemotherapy given on the high risk arm of SIOPEL-3. Those patients whose tumors are inoperable should be treated in the same way as high risk hepatoblastoma. Fibrolamellar hepatocellular carcinoma is more often circumscribed, and consequently more amenable to surgery. In multifocal non-resectable HCC in childhood, liver transplantation may also have a place; two patients were transplanted on SIOPEL-1, both were alive and disease free at 40 and 55 months follow-up.

HISTIOCYTOSES

This heterogeneous group of diseases causes confusion, exemplified by the wide range of conflicting classifications. Delineation is essential as the management required for each type is quite different. All of these conditions share an increase in mononuclear phagocytic cells (histiocytes derived from bone marrow). These cells accumulate in a variety of tissues. There are other conditions in which such cells also infiltrate the tissues including graft versus host reaction post transplantation, X-linked lymphoproliferative syndrome and some lipidoses.

In order to understand this group of conditions it is useful to look at the development of the histiocyte. The pluripotential marrow stem cell develops into a committed granulocyte and macrophage stem cell and these differentiate into colony-forming stem cells producing myelocytes and monocytes. When monocytes are produced they are released into the blood and undergo terminal differentiation into macrophages or histiocytes in many tissues, e.g. Kupffer cells in the liver and Langerhans' cells in the skin. Monocytes and these terminally differentiated cells can be divided into:

1. Antigen-processing or phagocytic cells. These include tissue histiocytes or macrophages, monocytes in the blood, lymph node follicle macrophages, sinusoidal histiocytes and epithelioid histiocytes.
2. Antigen-presenting or dendritic cells. These include dendritic reticulum cells in the node follicles, interdigitating reticulum cells in the node cortex and Langerhans' cells. These cells present antigen to the circulating T and B cells. All of the antigen-presenting cells and in particular Langerhans' cells have a strong affinity for class 2 antigens which the T4 or helper T cells recognize. In addition, Langerhans' cells contain structured organelles called Birbeck granules (these are rod-like structures with central striations and a terminal vesical expansion which looks like a tennis racket under electron microscopy).

CLASSIFICATION (Writing Group of the Histiocyte Society)[276]

In the group of conditions known as 'Langerhans' cell histiocytosis' the normal Langerhans' cell is immunologically stimulated to proliferate. This accumulation leads to a failure of normal immune mechanisms, including the development of autocytotoxicity (the body kills its own fibroblasts and red cells in culture) and an altered thymic appearance. In viral or other infections associated with hemophagocytic syndromes, the proliferation of histiocytes results from reaction to a foreign antigen or from excessive lymphokine production by lymphocytes. If the patient has an underlying or acquired T cell dysfunction (e.g. from the effects of infection), the lymphokine leads to continued proliferation and 'self'-phagocytosis. Primary erythrophagocytic lymphohistiocytosis, sometimes with a strong family also occurs (see below).

There is a further group of conditions in which there is a true neoplastic clonal proliferation of histiocytes. In some of these there may also be erythrophagocytosis. Table 22.23 shows the classification of histiocytoses.

Class 1 histiocytosis

The generic name Langerhans' cell histiocytosis (LCH) is used to encompass the entities formerly called eosinophilic granuloma (single or multiple), Hand–Schuller–Christian triad and Letterer–Siwe disease. These are proliferations probably secondary to defects of immunoregulation. Langerhans' cells seen in these conditions are identified by S100 protein sensitivity, T6 antigen surface expression and the presence of Birbeck granules (the key feature for diagnosis). The cells often have extra antigenic expression, especially to CD11 and at least 14 other monoclonal antibodies on their surface. In addition to the histiocytes in the granulomas within tissues, there will be variable numbers of eosinophils (especially in bone), lymphocytes and multinucleated giant cells. This group of conditions not surprisingly can present in a wide variety of ways from non-specific aches and pains to specific lytic bone lesions (either single or multiple), sometimes found quite coincidentally on X-rays, to widespread lymphadenopathy, hepatosplenomegaly and skin rash. Chronic otitis media, diabetes insipidus and weight loss are common in some forms particularly in young children.

Langerhans' cell histiocytosis does appear to be a monoclonal disorder. Very rarely indeed leukemias with dendritic cell phenotypes have been described. The old term 'histiocytosis X' has been modified into a form of staging system: Stage I, a single lytic bone lesion; Stage II, multiple lytic bone lesions (both of these were formerly called eosinophilic granulomata); Stage IIIA, bone plus soft tissue lesions, often associated with diabetes insipidus (pituitary involvement) or exophthalmos (previously termed Hand–Schuller–Christian triad); Stage IIIB, soft tissue only, which is the disseminated form previously termed Letterer–Siwe disease. These categories are not exclusive and overlap and progression is seen. Pathological staging includes breakdown of bony lesions into those with or without contiguous soft tissue involvement and/or involvement of immediately adjacent lymph nodes. Involvement of squamous mucous membranes is further classified on the basis of adjacent nodal involvement. It does appear that organ dysfunction is more important prognostically than mere organ involvement.[277]

Stage IIIB is most often seen in young infants and although overall Langerhans' cell histiocytosis has a low mortality, those aged under 6 months with such intensive soft tissue disease have a mortality of 50–60%. They often have wasting, adenopathy, hepatosplenomegaly, anemia and pancytopenia with red to purple skin lesions, a high incidence of seborrheic dermatitis and multiple organ involvement. Children under 2 years are at higher risk of dissemination and more advanced disease.

Seventy-eight per cent of all patients with LCH have bone lesions, whilst between 30 and 45% have skin and mucous membrane involvement, 25–30% pulmonary involvement, 25–30% hepatosplenomegaly, 30% lymphadenopathy, and 30% hemopoietic disorders. The pituitary is involved in about 15–20% of cases. It is quite common particularly in young children to have the generalized symptoms of fever, weight loss, lethargy and irritability. CNS involvement, and protein losing enteropathy, are rare associated conditions.

Bone lesions most commonly affect hematopoietically active bones including the skull, long bones, vertebrae (producing vertebral collapse or vertebra plana), mandible or maxilla (it is not uncommon to have gingival disease with even loss of teeth). Bone scans may identify such lesions but sometimes they can be missed but picked up preferentially by plain X-rays. Magnetic resonance imaging has identified lesions not seen either by X-rays or bone scans. Almost every bone in the body has at sometime been reported to show such lytic lesions. The skull is involved in nearly 50% of cases.

A wide range of skin lesions have been identified ranging from patterns similar to seborrhoeic dermatitis through nodular lesions, bronzing of the skin, and xanthomatous lesions.

The lungs may be identified as having infiltration but the patient may be asymptomatic. However the development of pulmonary dysfunction is an adverse sign. Similarly interruption of normal liver function particularly hypoalbuminemia is adverse and more likely to progress to fibrohistiocytic changes in the liver.

Anemia is not uncommon particularly in Stage III tumors and may be due to iron deficiency or secondary to infection. Other marrow suppression may also occur. However one always has to look for the possibility of developing erythrophagocytosis. The mere presence of an increase in macrophages within the bone marrow does not in itself worsen prognosis unless it is producing marrow dysfunction. Though rare apart from disorders of the hypothalamic pituitary system leading to diabetes insipidus, other CNS involvement can present with space occupying lesions and neurological dysfunction most often cerebellar pathway problems. Almost any other neurological feature can occur. Evidence of CNS deterioration is an unfavorable feature. These patients usually have multisystem disease and increased mortality.[278]

Definitive diagnosis of LCH depends on the characteristic pathological appearances with Birbeck granules and CD1A antigen positivity in the cells. Diagnosis is accepted although not definitive if there are the characteristic morphological appearances and any one

Table 22.23 Classification of histiocytosis syndromes in children

Class I	Class II	Class III
Langerhans' cell histiocytosis	1 Primary hemophagocytic lymphohistiocytosis (FHLH ± family history)	Malignant histiocytic disorders 1) Acute monocytic leukemia 2) Malignant histiocytosis 3) True histiocytic lymphoma
I Single bone	2 Secondary HLH (infection, malignancy, etc.)	
II Multiple bone	3 Other mononuclear phagocytosis (not Langerhans' cell)	
IIIA Bone + soft tissue		
IIIB Soft tissue only	4 Sinus histiocytosis + massive lymphadenopathy (Rosai–Dorfman)	
	5 Juvenile xanthogranuloma	
(Birbeck granules CD1A antigen positive S100 morphology)	6 Reticulocytoma	

Modified from the Writing Group of the Histiocyte Society 1987[276]

of two supplemental positive stains from 1) adenosine triphosphatase, 2) S100 protein, 3) alpha D mannosidase, 4) peanut lectin. All of this stresses the need for adequate and good sized biological samples for diagnosis.

In many cases of Langerhans' cell histiocytosis the disease appears to be self-limiting and what is clearly required is definition of the disease for which minimal intervention should be made and conversely that for which aggressive treatment is required.

For Stage I and II bone disease excisional biopsy or curettage for diagnosis with the intralesional injection of steroids is the treatment of choice. Local low dosage irradiation has been used for deposits which cannot easily be treated by curettage. Chemotherapy would appear to have little or no real place for such lesions unless multiple lesions are causing pain not cured by local curettage or irradiation or if there are lesions leading to significant dysfunction or fractures. Recently steroids have been used for multiple bony lesions, particularly those causing dysfunction sometimes with vinblastine followed by continuation therapy (with mecaptopurine, steroids and vinblastine).

For more advanced disease the International LCH Trial comparing vinblastine with etoposide has shown really no advantage for etoposide[279] and with the worry about development of second leukemias most now recommend the use of vinblastine with steroids for both multiple bony lesions if therapy is to be used and especially for those with additional soft tissue involvement but without signs of organ dysfunction. In this context those with diabetes insipidus or growth hormone deficiency are included. For patients with extensive dysfunction particularly of liver, lung, or hemopoietic system more aggressive chemotherapy has been used including the use of moderate dose systemic methotrexate in addition to prednisolone, mecaptopurine and vinblastine. In fact less than 15% of patients have such extensive organ dysfunction.[280] For those who respond to steroids and vinblastine with minimum late toxicity the outlook appears as good as with the use of more intensive therapy. The problem is how to manage progressive disease, especially in the very young. There is now a trial underway for such patients using high dose therapy including etoposide, cyclophosphamide and busulfan prior to allogeneic marrow transplantation (where there is a sibling match) and alternatively antithymocytic globulin, prednisolone and ciclosporin where there is no donor. Preliminary results are not encouraging. There has been some interest in the use of 2-chlorodeoxyadenosine but it is too early to say whether it will truly form part of the treatment for severe or refractory multisystem disease.[279,281]

Class II histiocytosis

Class II histiocytosis includes a whole range of non-malignant conditions in which normal macrophages and/or monocytes proliferate. These cells do not show atypical features or malignant change and lymphocytes may also be increased in numbers. In lymph nodes, total infiltration may be present and proliferation of the histiocytes may occur throughout the reticuloendothelial system. The familial type must be distinguished from infection-associated histiocytosis as the prognosis is very different. No Birbeck granules are seen in the cells of this form of histiocytosis. Other rare conditions are also placed into this class of histiocytoses (sinus histiocytosis with massive lymphadenopathy and Kikuchi's necrotizing lymphadenitis).

Hemophagocytic lymphohistiocytosis (HLH) consists of two quite different conditions. Primary hemophagocytic lymphohistiocytosis known as FHLH which may be familial or sporadic. The familial type is an autosomal recessive disease which is rapidly fatal. Clinically the patients present in the first 4 years of life with fever, weight loss, failure to thrive, hepatosplenomegaly, characteristic rash (yellow brown colour), central nervous system dysfunction (with coma and sometimes seizures), hyperlipidemia, low fibrinogen levels in the blood and cellular immune dysfunction. There may not be a family history and even where there is, this condition may be triggered off by infection. Secondary HLH is a similar proliferation with hemophagocytosis apparently arising from marked immunological activation by viral, bacterial or parasitic infections. A similar process has been reported in association with some malignancies and other conditions including rheumatoid arthritis, immunodeficiency and Chediak–Higashi syndrome.

Characteristic features of both forms are fever, splenomegaly, cytopenia affecting at least two of the three lineages in the peripheral blood, hypertriglyceridemia (fasting triglycerides greater than 2.0 ml/L or 3 standard deviations above the normal value for age) and/or hypofibrinogenemia (less than 1.5 g/L or 3 standard deviations below the normal level). Hemophagocytosis has to be identified in bone marrow, lymph nodes or spleen and there must be no malignancy.[282] In the primary form whether it be familial or sporadic, characteristic features are very low or absent natural killer activity, decreased T cell cytotoxicity capacity, very often the fibrinogen is very low and there is considerable disruption of the lipo-proteins. For the primary form though patients respond to high dose steroids (usually dexamethasone is preferred), vinblastine or etoposide and the use of intrathecal methotrexate (the risk of CNS disease seems to be high) the only curative therapy is with bone marrow transplantation. If there is no family related or unrelated donor, antithymocyte globulin, high dose methylprednisolone and ciclosporin have been tried. In the international trial designated HLH 94, the role of these agents is being tested.[282]

Infection associated hemophagocytosis (secondary) is most commonly associated with viruses including the human herpes virus 6, cytomegalovirus, adenovirus, parvovirus 19, herpes simplex, and measles. Again a range of therapies have been tried including the use of antibiotics, antiviral drugs such as aciclovir or ganciclovir along with corticosteroids and etoposide or vinblastine. Epstein–Barr virus infection has been incriminated as causative of some cases and although aciclovir has been used its efficacy in EBV is doubtful. Etoposide does appears to interfere with monocyte–macrophage function and may reduce toxicity of such infection related hemophagocytosis. It is not easy to assess those who will remit spontaneously and those who continue to progress.

Sinus histiocytosis and massive lymphadenopathy

This is more commonly seen in patients of African origin and presents with quite marked cervical lymphadenopathy, mediastinal enlargement and fever. There is a polyclonal increase in immunoglobulins and a neutrophil leukocytosis. In the vast majority the disease spontaneously regresses but just occasionally life threatening progression with superior caval syndrome requires either low dose radiotherapy or chemotherapy.

Class III histiocytoses

These are true malignant processes, and include:

1. Acute monocytic leukemia
2. Malignant histiocytosis with proliferation of macrophages intermediate between monoblasts and the fixed tissue histiocyte. There is a clear overlap between this condition and monocytic leukemia.
3. True histiocytic lymphoma is rare but can occur as a primary disease affecting any reticuloendothelial site as well as the skin and bone. Such lymphomas are very often classified as large cell immunoblastic lymphomas. In these malignant conditions the most useful cytochemical marker is non-specific esterase. Birbeck granules are not seen.

REFERENCES (* Level I Evidence)

*1 Stiller CA, Allen M, Bayne A, et al. UK national registry of childhood tumors England and Wales (1981–1990) in International Incidence of Childhood Cancer Vol II IARC. Scientific Publications 1998; 144:365–367.

*2 Sharp L, Gould A, Harris V, et al. UK Scottish Cancer Registry 1981–90 in International Incidence of Childhood Cancer Vol II IARC. Scientific Publications 1998; 144:369–371.

*3 Parkin DM, Kramarova E, Draper GJ, et al. (eds) International Incidence of Childhood Cancer Vol II IARC. Scientific Publications 1998; 144 Lyon.

*4 Kramarova E, Stiller CA, Ferlay J, et al. (eds) 1996. The international classification of childhood cancer. IARC Technical Report No 29, IARC, Lyon.

5 Birch JM, Marsden HB. A classification scheme for childhood cancers. Int J Cancer 1987; 40:620–624.

*6 McNally RJQ, Birch JM, Taylor GM, Eden OB. Temporal increases in the incidence of childhood peak precursor B cell ALL seen in North West England. Lancet 2000; 356:485–486.

*7 McNally RJQ, Cairns DP, Eden OB, et al. Examination of temporal trends in the incidence of childhood leukemia and lymphoma provides etiological clues. Leukemia 2001; 15:1612–1618.

*8 McNally RJQ, Kelsey AM, Cairns DP, et al. Temporal increases in the incidence of solid tumors seen in North West England 1954–98 are likely to be real. Cancer 2001; 927:1967–1976.

9 Stiller CA. Personal communication. From UKCCSG Annual Scientific Report; 2002.

10 Botting B, Crawley J. Trends and patterns in childhood mortality and morbidity In: The Health of our Children Decennial Supplement OPCS Series DS No 1995; 11:62–81.

*11 Coebergh JW, Capocaccia R, Gatta G, et al. Childhood cancer survival in Europe, 1978–1992: the EUROCARE study. Eur J Cancer 2001; 37:671–672.

12 Pizer B, Eden T. The treatment of childhood cancer. In: Southall D, Coulter B, Ronald C, et al. (eds). International child health care – a practical manual for hospitals worldwide. London: BMJ Books; 2002:302–313.

13 Eden OB. Therapeutic trials in childhood ALL: What's their future? J Clin Path 2000; 531:55–59.

14 Stiller CA, Eatock EM. Patterns of care and survival for children with acute lymphoblastic leukemia diagnosed between 1980 and 1994. Arch Dis Child 1999; 81:202–208.

*15 Stiller CA. Centralization of treatment and survival rates for cancer. Arch Dis Child 1988; 63:23–30.

16 Pritchard J, Stiller CA, Lennox EL. Overtreatment of children with Wilms' tumor outside pediatric oncology centres. BMJ 1989; 299:835–836.

17 UK Children's Cancer Study Investigators. The United Kingdom Childhood Cancer Study: objectives, materials and methods. Br J Cancer 2000; 825:1073–1102.

18 Stiller CA, Kinnier-Wilson LM. Down syndrome and leukemia. Lancet 1981; 2(8259):1343.

19 Zipursky A, Thorner P, de Harven E, et al. Myelodyplasia and acute megakaryoblastic leukemia in Down syndrome. Leukemia Res 1994; 18:163.

20 Miller RW, Fraumeni JF, Manning M. Association of Wilms' tumor with aniridia, hemihypertrophy, and other congenital malformations. N Engl J Med 1964; 270:922–927.

21 Call KM, Glaser J, Ho CY, et al. Isolation and characterisation of a zinc finger polypeptide gene at the human chromosome II. Wilms' tumor locus. Cell 1990; 60:509.

*22 Draper GJ, Sanders BM, Kingston JE. Second primary neoplasms in patients with retinoblastoma. Br J Cancer 1986; 53:661.

*23 Li FP, Fraumeni JF. Soft tissue sarcoma, breast cancer and other neoplasms. A familial syndrome. Ann Intern Med 1969; 71:747–752.

*24 Garber JE, Goldstein AM, Kantor AF, et al. Follow-up study of twenty four families with Li-Fraumeni syndrome. Cancer Res 1991; 51:6094–6097.

25 Birch JM, Hartley AL, Blair V, et al. Cancer in the families of children with soft tissue sarcoma. Cancer 1990; 66:2239–2248.

*26 Malkin D, Li FP, Strong LC, et al. Germline p53 mutations in a familial syndrome of breast cancer, sarcomas and other neoplasms. Science 1990; 250:1233–1238.

27 Birch JM, Aliston RD, McNally RJQ, et al. Relative frequency and morphology of cancers in carriers of germline TP53 mutations. Oncogene 2001; 20:4621–4628.

28 Dukes CE. The hereditary factor in polyposis intestini, or multiple adenomata. Cancer Rev 1930; 5:241.

*29 Gardner EJ. Follow-up study of a family group exhibiting dominant inheritance for a syndrome including intestinal polyps, osteomas, fibromas and epidermal cysts. Am J Hum Genet 1992; 14:376.

30 Fishel R, Lescoe MK, Rao MRS, et al. The human mutator gene homologue MSH2 and its association with hereditary non-polyposis colon cancer. Cell 1993; 75:1027.

*31 Mulligan L, Kwok J, Healey C, et al. Germline mutations of the RET proto-oncogene in multiple endocrine neoplasia type 2A. Nature 1993; 363:458.

32 Strong LC. Genetics, etiology and epidemiology of childhood cancer In: Sutow WW, Fernbach DJ, Vietti TJ (eds). Clinical pediatric oncology, 3rd edn. St Louis: Mosby; 1984:14–41.

33 Wood R. Seven genes for three diseases. Nature 1991; 350:190.

34 Woods C, Taylor AM. Ataxia telangiectasis in the British Isles: the clinical and laboratory features of 70 affected individuals. Q J Med 1992; 298:169.

35 Taylor AMR, Metcalfe JA, Thick J, Mak YF. Leukemia and lymphoma in ataxia-telangiectasia. Blood 1996; 87:423–438.

36 Savitsky K, Bar-Shira A, Gilad S, et al. A single ataxia telangiectasia gene with a product similar to PI-3 kinase. Science 1995; 268:1749.

*37 Joenje H, Oostra AB, Wijker M, et al. Evidence of at least eight Fanconi anemia genes. Am J Hum Genet 1997; 61:940–944.

38 Awan A, Taylor GM, Gokhale DA, et al. Increased frequency of Fanconi anemia group C genetic variants in children with sporadic AML. Blood 1998; 91(12):4813–4814.

39 Gatti RA, Good RA. Occurrence of malignancy in immunodeficient disease. Cancer 1971; 28:89–98.

*40 Gale KB, Ford AM, Repp R, et al. Backtracking leukemias to birth: identification of clonotypic gene fusion sequences in neonatal blood spots. Proc Natl Acad Sci USA 1997; 94:13950–13954.

*41 Wiemels JL, Cazaniga G, Daniotti M, et al. Prenatal origin of acute lymphoblastic leukemia in children. Lancet 1999; 354: 1499–1503.

42 Greaves MF. Childhood leukemia. BMJ 2002; 324:283–287.

43 Wiemels JL, Pagnamenta A, Taylor GM, et al. (and UK Childhood Cancer Study Investigators). Lack of function NAD(P)H: quinone oxidoreductase alleles are selectively associated with pediatric leukemias that have MLL fusions. Cancer Res 1999; 59:4095–4099.

44 Ross JA. Dietary flavonoids and the MLL gene: a pathway to infant leukemia? Proc Natl Acad Sci USA 2000; 97:4411–4412.

45 Alexander FE, Patheal SL, Biondi A, et al. Transplacental chemical exposure and risk of infant leukemia with MLL gene fusion. Cancer Res 2001; 61:2542–2546.

46 Strick R, Strissel PL, Borgers S, et al. Bioflavonoids do induce MLL cleavage and may contribute to infant leukemia. Proc Natl Acad Sci USA 2000; 97:4790–4795.

47 Wiemels JL, Smith RN, Taylor GM, et al. Methylene tetrahydrofolate reductase (MTHFR) polymorphisms and risk of molecularly defined subtypes of childhood acute leukaemia. Proc Natl Acad Sci USA 2001; 98(7):4004–4009.

*48 Thompson JR, Fitzgerald P, Willoughby MLN, Armstrong BK. Maternal folate supplementation in pregnancy and protection against common acute lymphoblastic leukemia in childhood: a case control study. Lancet 2001; 358:1935–1940.

49 Taylor GM, Dearden S, Payne N, et al. Evidence that an HLA-DQA1-DQB1 haplotype influences susceptibility to childhood common acute lymphoblastic leukemia in boys provides further support for an infection related etiology. Br J Cancer 1998; 785:561–565.

*50 Westerbeck RMC, Blair V, Eden OB, et al. Seasonal variations in the onset of childhood leukaemia and lymphoma. Br J Cancer 1998; 781:119–124.

51 Birch JM, Alexander FE, Blair V, et al. Space time clustering patterns in childhood leukemia support a role for infection. Br J Cancer 2000; 829:1495–1509.

52 Stewart A, Webb J, Giles D, Hewitt D. Malignant disease in childhood and diagnostic radiation in utero. Lancet 1956; ii:447.

53 Miller RW, Mulvihill JJ. Small head size after atomic irradiation. Teratology 1976; 14:355–357.

54 Yoshimoto Y, Kato H, Sihull WJ. Risk of cancer among in utero children exposed to A-bomb radiation 1950–84. Lancet 1988; 2:665.

*55 Gardner MJ, Snee MP, Hall AJ, et al. Results of a case control study of leukemias and lymphoma among young people near Sellafield nuclear plant in West Cumbria. BMJ 1990; 300:423–429.

*56 Dubrova YE, Nesterov VN, Krouchinsky NG, et al. Human minisatellite mutation rate after the Chernobyl accident. Nature 1996; 380:683–686.
57 Modan B, Ron E, Verner A. Thyroid cancer following scalp irradiation. Radiology 1977; 123:741–744.
*58 Upton AC, Albert RE, Burns FJ, Shore E. Radiation carcinogenesis. New York: Elsevier; 1986.
*59 Lyon JL, Klauber MR, Gardner JW, Udall KS. Childhood leukemias associated with fallout from nuclear testing. N Engl J Med 1979; 300:397–402.
60 Black D. New evidence on childhood leukemia and nuclear establishments. BMJ 1987; 294:591–592.
*61 Committee on Medical Aspects of Radiation in the Environment (COMARE) 1986/1988 Bobrow M (Chairman) HMSO Report 1 (West Cumbria 1986), HMSO Report 2 (Dounreay, 1988). London: HMSO.
*62 Committee on Medical Aspects of Radiation in the Environment (COMARE) 4th Report. The incidence of cancer and leukemia in young people in the vicinity of the Sellafield site, West Cumbria. London: HMSO; 1996.
*63 Heasman MA, Urquhart JD, Black RJ, Kemp IW. Leukemia in young persons in Scotland. A study of its geographical distribution and relationship to nuclear installations. Health Bull 1987; 45(3):147–151.
64 Kinlen LJ, Clarke K, Hudson C. Evidence from population mixing in British new towns 1946–85 of an infective basis for childhood leukemia. Lancet 1990; 336:577–582.
65 Greaves MF. Speculations on the cause of childhood acute lymphoblastic leukemia. Leukemia 1988; 1:120–125.
66 UK Childood Cancer Study Investigators. The United Kingdom childhood cancer study of exposure to domestic sources of ionising radiation: 1: radon gas. Br J Cancer 2002; 86; 1721–1726.
67 UK Childood Cancer Study Investigators. The United Kingdom childhood cancer study of exposure to domestic sources of ionising radiation: 2: gamma radiation. Br J Cancer 2002; 86; 1727–1731.
*68 Holman CDJ, Armstrong BK, Heenan PJ. Relationship of cutaneous melanoma to individual sunlight exposure habits. J Natl Cancer Inst 1986; 76:403.
69 Meier JR. Genotoxic activity of organic chemicals in drinking water. Mutat Res 1988; 196:211.
*70 Wertheimer N, Leeper E. Electrical wiring configurations and childhood cancer. Am J Epidemiol 1979; 109:273.
71 UK Children's Cancer Study Investigators. Exposure to power frequency magnetic fields and the risk of childhood cancer. Lancet 1999; 354:1925–1931.
*72 Feychting M, Ahlbom A. Magnetic fields and cancer in children residing near Swedish high-voltage power lines. Am J Epidemiol 1993; 138:467.
73 Melnick S, Cole P, Anderson D, Herbst A. Rates and risks of diethylstilbestrol related clear cell adenocarcinoma of the vagina and cervix. An update. N Engl J Med 1987; 316:514–516.
74 MacKinney AA, Booker HE. Diphenylhydantoin effects on human lymphocytes in vitro and in vivo. An hypothesis to explain some drug reactions. Arch Intern Med 1972; 129:988–992.
75 Tucker MA, Meadows AT, Boice JD, et al. Leukemia after therapy with alkylating agents for childhood cancer. J Natl Cancer Inst 1987; 78:459–464.
76 Ng A, Taylor GM, Eden OB. Treatment related leukaemia – a clinical and scientific challenge. Cancer Treat Rev 2000; 265:377–391.
77 Mulvihill JJ, Ridolfi RL, Schultz FR, et al. Hepatic adenoma in Fanconi anemia treated with oxymetholone. J Pediatr 1975; 87: 122–124.
*78 Golding J, Paterson M, Kinlen LJ. Factors associated with child cancer in a national cohort study. Br J Cancer 1990; 62:304–308.
*79 Roman E, Fear NT, Ansell P, et al. Vitamin K and childhood cancer: analysis of individual patient data from six case-control studies. Br J Cancer 2002; 86:63–69.
80 Kwa SL, Fine LJ. The association between parental occupation and childhood malignancy. J Occupational Med 1980; 22:792–794.
81 MacKenzie J, Perry J, Ford AM, et al. JC and BK versus sequences are not detectable in leukaemia samples from children with common acute lymphoblastic leukaemia. Br J Cancer 1999; 81:898–899.
82 MacKenzie J, Gallagher A, Clayton RA, et al. Screening for herpes virus genomes in common acute lymphoblastic leukemia. Leukemia 2001; 15:415–421.
83 Smith MA, Strickler HD, Granovsky M, et al. Investigation of leukemia cells from children with common acute lymphoblastic leukemia for genomic sequences of the primate polyoma viruses JC, BK and simian 40 viruses. Med Pediatr Oncol 1999; 33:441–443.
*84 Jarrett RF, Gallagher A, Jones DB, et al. Detection of Epstein–Barr virus genomes in Hodgkin's disease: relation to age. J Clin Pathol 1991; 44:844–848.
85 Mueller NE, Grufferman S. The Epidemiology of Hodgkin's disease. In: Mauch PM, Armitage JO, Diehl V, et al. (eds). Hodgkin's disease. Philadelphia: Lippincott Williams & Wilkins; 1999:Ch. 5.
86 Flavell KJ, Murray PG. Hodgkin's disease and the Epstein–Barr virus. J Clin Path/Molec Pathol 2000; 53:262–269.
*87 Taylor GM, Gokhale DA, Crowther D, et al. Further investigation of the role of HLA-DPB1 in adult Hodgkin's disease suggests an influence on susceptibility to different Hodgkin's disease subtypes. Br J Cancer 1999; 80:1405–1411.
88 Taylor JA, et al. Preliminary results of sequence based typing suggest that susceptibility to childhood Hodgkin's lymphoma in females is associated with HLA DRB1* 1501. Personal communication.
*89 Yoshida M, Miyoshi I, Hinuma Y. Isolation and characterisation of retrovirus from cell lines of human adult T-cell leukemia and its implication in the disease. Proc Natl Acad Sci USA 1982; 79:2031–2035.
90 Kushner BH, Yeung HWD, Larson SM, et al. Extending positron emission tomography scan utility to high risk neuroblastoma: fluorine-18 fluorodeoxyglucose positron emission tomography as sole imaging modality in follow-up of patients. J Clin Oncol 2001; 19:3397–3405.
91 Makin G, Dive C. Apoptosis and cancer chemotherapy. Trends Cell Biol 2001; 11: 522–526.
92 Rich T, Allen RL, Wyllie AH. Defying death after DNA damage. Nature 2000; 407:777–783.
93 Robert J. Resistance to cytotoxic agents. Current Opin Pharmacol 2001; 1:353.
*94 Davies HA, Lennard L, Lilleyman JS. Variable mercaptopurine metabolism in children with leukemia: a problem of non-compliance? BMJ 1993; 306:1239–1240.
95 Juliano RL, Ling V. A surface glycoprotein modulating drug permeability in Chinese hamster ovary cell mutants. Biochim Biophys Acta 1976; 455:152–162.
96 Roninson IB, Abelson HT, Housman DE, et al. Amplification of specific DNA sequences correlates with multi-drug resistance in Chinese hamster cells. Nature 1984; 309:626–628.
97 Kartner N, Evernden Porelle D, Bradley G, Ling V. Detection of P-glycoprotein in multi-drug resistant cell lines by monoclonal antibodies. Nature 1985; 316:820–823.
98 Goldie JH, Goldman AJ, Gudanskas GA. Rationale for the use of alternating non-cross-resistant chemotherapy. Cancer Treat Reports 1982; 66:439–449.
99 Hartmann O, Pinkerton CR, Philip T, et al. Very high dose cisplatin and etoposide in children with untreated advanced neuroblastoma. J Clin Oncol 1988; 6:44–50.
100 Bodey GP, Buckley M, Sathe YS, Friereich EJ. Quantitative relationships between circulating leukocytes and infection in patients with acute leukemia. Ann Intern Med 1966; 64:328–340.
101 Prentice HG (ed). Infections in haematology. Clinics in Haematology, Vol 133, 1984.
102 Pizzo PA. Fever in immunocompromised patients. N Engl J Med 1999; 341:893–900.
*103 Clarkson JE, Worthington HV, Eden OB. Interventions for preventing oral mucositis or oral candidiasis for patients with cancer receiving chemotherapy (excluding head and neck cancer) (Cochrane Review). In: The Cochrane Library Issue 3, 2001. Oxford: Update Software.
*104 Darbyshire P, Eden OB, Jameson B, et al. Pneumonitis in lymphoblastic leukemia in childhood. Eur J Pediatr Haematol Oncol 1985; 2:141–147.
*105 Gray M, Hann IM, Glass S, et al. Mortality and morbidity caused by measles in children with malignant disease BMJ 1987; 295:19–22.
106 Simpson RMcD, Eden OB. Possible interferon response in a child with measles encephalopathy during immunosuppression. Scand J Infect Dis 1984; 16:315–319.
107 Pinkerton CR, Williams D, Wooton C, et al. 5HT3 antagonist ondansetron – an effective outpatient antiemetic in cancer treatment. Arch Dis Child 1990; 65:822–825.
108 Zeltzer L, Le Baron S, Zeltzer PM. The effectiveness of behavioural intervention for

reduction of nausea and vomiting in children and adolescents receiving chemotherapy. J Clin Oncol 1984; 2:683–690.

109 Wang SC. Emetic and antiemetic drugs. In: Root W S, Hofmann F G (eds) Psychological pharmacology. New York: Academic Press; 1985; Vol 2:255–328.

*110 Hausdorf G, Morf G, Beron G, et al. Long term doxorubicin cardiotoxicity in childhood: non-invasive evaluation of the contractile state and diastolic filling. Br Heart J 1988; 60:309–315.

*111 Bielack SS, Erttman R, Winkler K, Landbeck G. Doxorubicin: effect of different schedules on toxicity and antitumor efficiency. Eur J Cancer Clin Oncol 1989; 25:873–882.

*112 Lipshultz SE, Colan SD, Gelber RD, et al. Late cardiac effects of doxorubicin therapy for ALL in childhood. N Engl J Med 1991; 324:808–815.

*113 Kremer LCM, Van Dalen EC, Offringa M, et al. Anthracycline-induced heart failure in a cohort of 607 children: long term follow-up study. J Clin Oncol 2001; 19:191–196.

114 Speyer JL, Green MD, Kramer E, et al. Protective effect of the bispiperazinedione ICRF-187 against doxorubicin induced cardiac toxicity in women with advanced breast cancer. N Engl J Med 1988; 319:745–752.

115 Hortabagyi GN, Frye D, Buzdar AU, et al. Decreased cardiac toxicity of doxorubicin administered by continuous intravenous infusion in combination chemotherapy for metastatic breast cancer. Cancer 1989; 63:37–45.

116 Weiss HD, Walker MD, Wiernik PH. Neurotoxicity of commonly used antineoplastic agents. N Engl J Med 1975; 291:75–127.

117 Pratt CB, Green AA, Horowitz ME, et al. Central nervous system toxicity following the treatment of pediatric patients with ifosfamide/mesna. J Clin Oncol 1986; 4:1253–1261.

118 Brock PR, Pritchard J, Bellman SC, Pinkerton CR. Ototoxicity of high-dose cisplatinum in children. Med Pediatr Oncol 1987; 16:368–369.

*119 D'Antiga L, Baker A, Pritchard J, et al. Veno-occlusive disease with multi-organ involvement following actinomycin-D. Eur J Cancer 2001; 37:1141–1148.

120 Ortega JA, Donaldson SS, Ivy SP et al. Veno-occlusive disease of the liver after chemotherapy with vincristine, actinomycin D, and cyclophosphamide for the treatment of rhabdomyosarcoma. Cancer 1997; 79: 2435–2439.

121 Bisogno G, de Kraker J, Weirich A, et al. Veno-occlusive disease of the liver in children treated for Wilm's tumor. Med Pediatr Oncol 1997; 29:245–251.

*122 Goldman SC, Holcenberg JS, Finklestein JZ, et al. A randomized comparison between rasburicase and allopurinol in children with lymphoma or leukemia at high risk of tumor lysis. Blood 2001; 97:2998–3003.

123 Eden OB, Black I, Mackinlay GA, Emery AEH. Communication with parents of children with cancer. Palliat Med 1994; 8: 105–114.

*124 Hawkins MM. Long term survival and cure after childhood cancer. Arch Dis Child 1989; 64:798–807.

*125 Meadows AT, Baum E, Fossati-Bellani F, et al. Second malignant neoplasms in children: an update from the Late Effects Study Group. J Clin Oncol 1985; 3:532–538.

*126 Meadows AT. Risk factors for second malignant neoplasms: report from the Late Effects Study Group. Bull Cancer 1988; 75: 125–130.

127 Tucker MA, D'Angio GJ, Boice JD, et al. Bone sarcomas linked to radiotherapy and chemotherapy in children. N Engl J Med 1987; 317:588–593.

*128 Pui C, Behm SG, Raimondi SC, et al. Second acute myeloid leukemia in children treated for acute lymphoid leukemia. N Engl J Med 1989; 321:136–142.

*129 Eden OB, Hann I, Harrison C, et al. Secondary acute myeloid leukemia in children treated for acute lymphoblastic leukemia on MRC trials 1980–1997. Blood 1998; 92(10) (suppl 183a).

*130 Nygaard R, Garwicz S, Haldorsen T, et al. Second malignant neoplasms in patients treated for childhood leukemia A population based cohort study from the Nordic countries. Acta Pediatr Scand 1991; 80:1220–1228.

*131 Neglia JP, Meadows AT, Robison LL, et al. Second neoplasms after acute lymphoblastic leukemia. N Engl J Med 1991; 325:1330–1336.

*132 Relling MV, Rubnitz JE, Rivera GK, et al. High incidence of second brain tumours after radiotherapy and antimetabolites. Lancet 1999; 354:34–40.

*133 Bessho F, Ohta K, Akunuma A. Dosimetry of radiation scattered to thyroid gland from prophylactic cranial irradiation for childhood leukemia. Pediatr Hematol Oncol 1994; 11:47–53.

134 Shaw MP, Wallace WHB, Eden OB. Spindle cell carcinoma of the tongue in a long term survivor of childhood acute lymphoblastic leukemia. Pediatr Hematol Oncol 1997; 14:79–83.

135 Shalet SM, Clayton PE, Price DA. Growth and pituitary function in children treated for brain tumors or acute lymphoblastic leukemia. Hormone Res 1988; 30:53–61.

136 Ogilvy-Stuart AL, Ryder WD, Gattamaneni HR, et al. Growth hormone and tumor recurrence. BMJ 1992; 304:1601–1605.

*137 Kirk JA, Raghupathy P, Stevens MM, et al. Growth failure and growth hormone deficiency after treatment for acute lymphoblastic leukemia. Lancet 1987; 1:1990–1993.

*138 Davies HA, Didcock E, Didi M, et al. Disproportionate short stature after cranial irradiation and combination chemotherapy for leukemia. Arch Dis Child 1994; 70:472–475.

139 Robson H, Anderson E, Eden OB, et al. Chemotherapeutic agents used in the treatment of childhood malignancies have direct effect on growth plate chondrocyte proliferation. J Endocrinol 1998; 157:225–235.

*140 Brennan BMD, Rahim A, Blum WF, et al. Hyperleptinanemia in young adults following cranial irradiation in childhood: growth hormone deficiency or leptin insensitivity. Clin Endocrinol 1999; 50:163–169.

*141 Brennan BMD, Rahim A, Adams JA, et al. Reduced bone mineral density in young adults following cure of acute lymphoblastic leukemia in childhood. Br J Cancer 1999; 79:1850–1863.

*142 Shafford EA, Kingston JE, Malpas JS. Testicular function following the treatment of Hodgkin's disease in childhood. Br J Cancer 1993; 68:1199–1204.

143 Shalet SM. Endocrine consequences of treatment of malignant disease. Arch Dis Child 1989; 64:1635–1641.

*144 Kun LE, Mulhearn RK, Crisco JJ. Quality of life of children treated for brain tumors: intellectual, emotional and academic function. J Neurosurg 1986; 58:1–6.

*145 Christie D, Leiper AD, Chessells JM, Vargha-Khadem F. Intellectual performance after pre symptomatic cranial radiotherapy for leukemia: effects of age and sex. Arch Dis Child 1995; 73:136–140.

146 Meadows AT, Evans AE. Effects of chemotherapy on the central nervous system: a study of parenteral methotrexate in long term survivors of leukemia and lymphoma in childhood. Cancer 1976; 37:1079–1085.

*147 Hill FGH, Vargha-Khadem F, Gibson B, et al. UKALL XI randomized trial of stratified CNS treatment and prospective neuropsychological assessment in childhood ALL. Blood 2000; 9: 466.

148 Meadows AT, McKee L, Kazak AE. Psychosocial status of young adult survivors of childhood cancer: a survey. Med Pediatr Oncol 1989; 17:466–470.

149 Malpas JS. Cancer: The consequences of cure. Clin Radiol 1988; 39:166–172.

150 Steinherz LJ, Steinherz PG, Tan CT, Murphy ML. Cardiac toxicity 4–20 years after completing anthracycline therapy. J Am Med Assoc 1991; 266:1672–1677.

*151 Shaw NJ, Tweeddale PM, Eden OB. Pulmonary function in childhood leukemia survivors. Med Pediatr Oncol 1989; 17:149–154.

*152 Shaw NJ, Eden OB, Jenney MEM, et al. Pulmonary function in survivors of Wilms' tumor. Pediatr Hematol Oncol 1991; 82:131–137.

*153 Attard-Montalto SP, Kingston JE, Eden OB, Plowman PN. Late follow-up of lung function after whole lung irradiation for Wilms' tumor. Br J Radiol 1992; 66:1114–1118.

154 Cohen ME, Duffner PK. Brain tumors in children. International Reviews of Child Neurology. New York: Raven Press; 1984: 1499–1503.

155 Rorke LB, Giles FH, Davis RL. Revision of the World Health Organization classification of brain tumors for childhood brain tumors. Cancer 1985; 56:1869–1886.

156 Coakham HB, Brownell B. Monoclonal antibodies in the diagnosis of cerebral tumors and cerebrospinal fluid neoplasia. In: Cavanaugh JB (ed). Recent advances in neuropathology. Edinburgh; Churchill Livingstone: 1986; Vol 3:25–53.

157 Packer RJ, Zimmerman RA, Bilanuik LT. Magnetic resonance imaging in the evaluation of treatment related central nervous system damage. Cancer 1986; 58:635–640.

158 Brunelle F. Noninvasive diagnosis of brain tumors in children. Childs Nerv Syst 2000; 16:731–734.

*159 Campbell JW, Pollack IF, Martinez AJ, et al. High grade astrocytomas in children: radiologically complete resection is associated with an excellent long term prognosis. Neurosurgery 1996; 38:258.

*160 Tait DM, Thornton-Jones H, Bloom HJG, et al. Adjuvant chemotherapy for medulloblastoma: the first multicentre controlled trial of the International Society of Pediatric Oncology (SIOP1). Eur J Cancer 1990; 26:464.
161 Habrand J-L, De Crevoisier R. Radiation in the management of childhood brain tumors. Childs Nerv Syst 2001; 17:121–133.
162 Kellie SJ. Chemotherapy of central nervous system tumors in infants. Childs Nerv Syst 1999; 15:592–612.
163 Harisiadis L, Chang CH. Medulloblastoma in children: a correlation between staging and results of treatment. Int J Radiat Oncol Biol Phys 1977; 2:833.
*164 Taylor RE, Bailey CC, Lucraft H, et al. Results of a randomized study of pre radiotherapy chemotherapy (carboplatin, vincristine, cyclophosphamide, etoposide) with radiotherapy alone in Chang Stage M0/M1 medulloblastoma (SIOP/UKCCSG PNET 3). Med Pediatr Oncol 2001; 37:191.
*165 Packer RJ, Goldwein J, Nicholson HS, et al. Treatment of children with medulloblastoma with reduced dose craniospinal radiation therapy and adjuvant chemotherapy: a Children's Cancer Study Groups Study. J Clin Oncol 1999; 17:2127–2136.
*166 Kortman RJ, Kuhl J, Timmerman B, et al. Postoperative neo-adjuvant chemotherapy before radiotherapy as compared to immediate radiotherapy followed by maintenance chemotherapy in the treatment of medulloblastoma of childhood: results of the German HIT '91 study. Int J Radiat Oncol Biol Phys 2000; 46:269–279.
*167 Evans AE, Anderson JR, Lefkowitz-Boudreaux IB, Finlay JL. Adjuvant chemotherapy of posterior fossa ependymoma: craniospinal irradiation with or without adjuvant CCNU, vincristine and prednisolone: a Children's Cancer Study Group Study. Med Pediatr Oncol 1996; 27:8–14.
168 Loftus CM, Copeland BR, Carmel PW. Cystic supratentorial gliomas: natural history, and evaluation of modes of surgical therapy. Neurosurgery 1985; 17:19.
169 Kaye AH, Walker DG. Low grade astrocytomas: controversies in management. J Clin Neurosci 2000; 7:475–483.
*170 Duffner PK, Kirschner JP, Burger PC, et al. Treatment of infants with malignant gliomas: the Pediatric Oncology Group experience. J Neurooncol 1996; 28:245–256.
*171 Finlay JL, Boyett JM, Yates AJ, et al. Randomized phase III trial in childhood high-grade astrocytomas comparing vincristine, lomustine and prednisolone with the eight-drugs-in 1-day regimen. J Clin Oncol 1995; 13:112–123.
*172 Kalifa C, Valtreau D, Pizer B, et al. High dose chemotherapy in childhood brain tumors. Childs Nerv Syst 1999; 15:498–505.
*173 Kaplan AM, Albright AL, Zimmerman RA, et al. Brainstem gliomas in children: a Children's Cancer Study Group review of 119 cases. Pediatr Neurosurg 1996; 24:185–192.
174 Hood TW, Gebarski SS, McKeever PE, et al. Stereotaxic biopsy of intrinsic lesions of the brain stem. J Neurosurg 1986; 65:172–176.
*175 Packer RJ, Boyett JM, Zimmerman RA, et al. Outcome of children with brainstem gliomas after treatment with 7800cGy of hyperfractionated radiotherapy: a Children's Cancer Study Group Phase I/II trial. Cancer 1994; 74:1827–1834.
*176 Jenkin RDJ, Boesel C, Ertel I, et al. Brainstem tumors in childhood: a prospective randomized trial of irradiation with or without CCNU, VCR and prednisone. A report of the Children's Cancer Study Group. J Neurosurg 1987; 66:227–233.
*177 Janss AJ, Grundy R, Cnaan A, et al. Optic pathway and hypothalamic/chiasmatic gliomas in children younger than age 5 years with a 6 year follow-up. Cancer 1995; 75:1051–1059.
*178 Amendola BE, Gebarski SS, Bermudez AG. Analysis of treatment results in craniopharyngioma. J Clin Oncol 1985; 3: 252–258.
*179 Habrand J-L, Ganry O, Couanet D, et al. The role of radiation therapy in the management of craniopharyngioma: a 25 year experience and review of the literature. Int J Radiat Oncol Biol Phys 1999; 44:255–263.
180 Gutierrez MI, Bhatia K, Barriga F, et al. Molecular epidemiology of Burkitt's lymphoma from South America: difference in breakpoint location and EBV association from tumors in other world regions. Blood 1992; 79:3261–3266.
*181 Rabbits T, Boehm T. Structural and functional chimaerism results from chromosomal translocation in lymphoid tumors. Adv Immunol 1991; 50:119–146.
182 Purtillo DT, Sakamoto K. Immunodeficiency as a factor in lymphomagenesis. Perspect Pediatr Pathol 1984; 8:181–191.
183 Grierson H, Purtillo DJ. Epstein–Barr virus infections in males with X linked lymphoproliferative syndrome. Ann Intern Med 1987; 106:538–545.
184 Magrath IT. Malignant non-Hodgkin's lymphomas in children. Hematol Oncol Clin North Am 1987; 1:577–602.
185 Burkitt D. A sarcoma involving the jaws in African children. Br J Surg 1958; 46:218–223.
186 Murphy SB. Classification. Staging and end results of treatment of childhood non Hodgkin's lymphoma: dissimilarities from lymphomas in adults. Semin Oncol 1980; 7:332–339.
*187 Patte C, Philip T, Rodany C, et al. High survival rate in advanced stage B-cell lymphomas and leukemias without CNS involvement with short intensive polychemotherapy. Results from the French Pediatric Oncology Society of a randomized trial of 216 children. J Clin Oncol 1991; 9:123–132.
*188 Patte C, Michon J, Behrendt H, et al. Updated results of the LMB 89 protocol of the SFOP (French Pediatric Oncology Society) for childhood B-cell lymphoma and leukemia (ALL) Ann Oncol 1996; 7:30 (abstract 96).
*189 Reiter A, Schrappe M, Parawaresch R, et al. Non Hodgkin's lymphoma of childhood and adolescence: results of a treatment stratified for biologic subtypes and stage. A report of the BFM group. J Clin Oncol 1995; 13:359–372.
*190 Patte C, Kalifa C, Flamant F, et al. Results of the LMT 81 protocol, a modified LSAs L2 protocol with high dose methotrexate on 84 children with non B cell lymphomas. Med Pediatr Oncol 1992; 20:105–113.
191 Eden OB, Hann I, Imeson J, et al. Treatment of advanced stage T-cell lymphoblastic lymphoma: results of the United Kingdom Children's Cancer Study Group protocol 8503. Br J Haematol 1992; 83: 310–316.
192 Paulli M, Berti E, Rosso R, et al. CD30/Ki-1 positive lymphoproliferative disorders of the skin – Clinicopathological correlation and statistical analysis of 86 cases. J Clin Oncol 1995; 13:1343–1354.
*193 Reiter A, Schrappe M, Tiemann M, et al. Successful treatment strategy for Ki-1 anaplastic large cell lymphomas of childhood: a prospective analysis of 62 patients enrolled in three consecutive Berlin–Frankfurt–Munster group studies. J Clin Oncol 1994; 12:899–908.
194 Saha V, Eden OB, Hann I, et al. Primary extrathoracic T cell non-Hodgkin's lymphoma of childhood. Leukemia 1995; 9:40–43.
195 Fischer A, Blanche S, Le Bidois J, et al. Anti B cell monoclonal antibodies in the treatment of severe B cell lymphoproliferative syndrome following bone marrow and organ transplantation. N Engl J Med 1991; 324: 1451–1456.
196 Papadopoulos BE, Ladanyi M, Emmanuel D, et al. Infusions of donor leucocytes to treat EBV associated lymphoproliferative disorders after allogeneic bone marrow transplantation. N Engl J Med 1994; 330:1185–1191.
197 Weiss L, Movahed LA, Warnke RA, et al. Detection of Epstein–Barr viral genomes in Reed–Sternberg cells of Hodgkin's disease. N Engl J Med 1989; 320:502–506.
*198 Bonadonna G, Zucali R, Monfardini S, et al. Combination chemotherapy of Hodgkin's disease with adriamycin, bleomycin, vinblastine and imidazole carboxamide versus MOPP. Cancer 1975; 36:252–259.
199 Schellong G, Hornig I, Bramswig J, et al. Favorable outcome of childhood Stage IV Hodgkin's disease with OPPA/COPP chemotherapy and additional radiotherapy. In: Proceedings of the International Society of Pediatric Oncology Abstract 132. 1987.
200 Eden OB. Lymphoma. In: Lilleyman JS, Hann IM, Blanchette VS (eds). Pediatric hematology, 2nd edn. Edinburgh: Churchill Livingstone; 1998:Ch. 28.
201 De Bernandi B, Pianca C, Pistamiglio P, et al. Neuroblastoma with symptomatic spinal cord compression at diagnosis: treatment and results with 76 cases. J Clin Oncol 2001; 19:183–190.
*202 Brodeur GM, Seeger RC, Schwab M, et al. Amplification of N-Myc in untreated human neuroblastoma correlates with advanced disease stage. Science 1984; 224:112–114.
*203 Caron H, Van Sluis P, De Kraker J, et al. Allelic loss of chromosome 1p as a predictor of unfavorable outcome in patients with neuroblastoma. N Engl J Med 1996; 334:225–230.
*204 Maris JM, Weiss MJ, Guo C, et al. Loss of heterozygosity at 1p36 independently predicts for disease progression but not decreased overall survival probability in neuroblastoma patients: a Children's Cancer Group Study. J Clin Oncol 2000; 18:1888–1899.
*205 Bown N, Cotterill S, Lastowska M. Gain of chromosome arm 17q and adverse outcome in

patients with neuroblastoma. N Engl J Med 1999; 340:1954–1961.

*206 Nakagawara A, Arima M, Azar CG, et al. Inverse relationship between Trk expression and N-Myc amplification in human neuroblastomas. Cancer Res 1992; 52:1364–1368.

*207 Nakagawara A, Arimanakagawara M, Scavarda NJ, et al. Association between high-levels of expression of the Trk gene and favorable outcome in human neuroblastoma. N Engl J Med 1993; 328:847–854.

208 Nakagawara A, Azar CG, Scavarda NJ, Brodeur GM. Expression and function of Trk-B and BDNF in human neuroblastomas. Mol Cell Biol 1994; 14:759–767.

209 Yamashiro DJ, Liu XG, Lee CP, et al. Expression and function of Trk-C in favorable human neuroblastomas. Eur J Cancer 1997; 33:2054–2057.

210 Brodeur GM, Seeger RC, Barrett A, et al. International criteria for diagnosis, staging and response to treatment in patients with neuroblastoma. J Clin Oncol 1988; 6:1874–1881.

*211 Perez CA, Matthay KK, Atkinson JB, et al. Biologic variables in the outcome of stages I and II neuroblastoma treated with surgery as primary therapy: a Children's Cancer Group Study. J Clin Oncol 2000; 18:18–26.

*212 Rubie H, Hartmann O, Michon J, et al. N-Myc gene amplification is a major prognostic factor in localized neuroblastoma: results of the French NBL 90 study. J Clin Oncol 1997; 15:1171–1182.

*213 Nickerson HJ, Matthay KK, Seeger RC, et al. Favorable biology and outcome of stage IV-S neuroblastoma with supportive care or minimal therapy: a Children's Cancer Group Study. J Clin Oncol 2000; 18:477–486.

*214 Katzenstein HM, Bowman LC, Brodeur GM, et al. Prognostic significance of age, MYCN oncogene amplification tumor cell ploidy, and histology in 110 infants with stage DS neuroblastoma: the Pediatric Oncology group experience – a Pediatric Oncology Group Study. J Clin Oncol 1998; 16:2007–2017.

*215 Matthay KK, Villablanca JG, Seeger RC, et al. Treatment of high-risk neuroblastoma with intensive chemotherapy, radiotherapy, autologous bone marrow transplantation, and 13-cis-retinoic acid. N Engl J Med 1999; 341:1165–1173.

216 Bessho F, Hashizume K, Nakajo T, Kamoshita S. Mass screening of infants with neuroblastoma without a decrease of cases in older children. J Pediatr 1991; 119:237–241.

217 Sawada T, Kidowaki T, Sakamoto I, et al. Neuroblastoma: mass screening for early detection and its prognosis. Cancer 1984; 53:2731–2735.

*218 Woods WG, Tuchman M, Robison LL, et al. A polulation-based study of the usefulness of screening for neuroblastoma. Lancet 1996; 348:1682–1687.

219 Yamamoto K, Hanada R, Kikuchi A, et al. Spontaneous regression of localized neuroblastoma detected by mass screening. J Clin Oncol 1998; 16:1265–1269.

220 Beckwith JB. Pathological aspects of renal tumors in childhood. In: Broecker BH, Klein FA (eds). Pediatric tumors of the genitourinary tract. New York: Alan Liss; 1988:25–48.

221 Marsden H B, Lawler W, Kumar B U. Bone metastazing renal tumor of childhood. Morphological and clinical features and differences from Wilms' tumor. Cancer 1978; 42:1922–1928.

222 Breslow NE, Beckwith JB. Epidemiological features of Wilms' tumor. Results of the National Wilms' Tumor Study. J Nat Cancer Inst 1982; 68:429.

223 Pritchard J, Imeson J, Barnes J, et al. Results of UKCCSG First Wilms' Tumor Study. J Clin Oncol 1995; 13:124–133.

*224 Mitchell C, Morris Jones P, Kelsey AM, et al. for the UKCCSG. The treatment of Wilms' tumor: results of the UKCCSG second Wilms' tumor study. Br J Cancer 2000; 83:602–608.

*225 Tournade MF, Com-Nogue C, de Kraker J, et al. Optimal duration of preoperative therapy in unilateral and non metastatic Wilms' tumor in children older than 6 months: results of the 9th International Society of Pediatric Oncology Wilms' Tumor Trial and Study. J Clin Oncol 2001; 19:488–500.

226 Arndt CAS, Crist WM. Common musculoskeletal tumors of childhood and adolescence. N Engl J Med 1999; 341:342–352.

227 Birch JM, Hartley AL, Marsden HB, et al. Excess risk of breast cancer in the mothers of children with soft tissue sarcomas. Br J Cancer 1984; 49:325–331.

228 Hahn H, Wicking C, Zaphiropoulos PG, et al. Mutations of the human homolog of Drosophila patched gene in the nevoid basal cell carcinoma syndrome. Cell 1996; 85:841–851.

229 Hahn H, Wojnowski L, Zimmer AM, et al. Rhabdomyosarcomas and radiation hypersensitivity in a mouse model of Gorlin syndrome. Nature Med 1998; 4:619–622.

230 Zahn S, Helman LJ. Glimpsing the cause of rhabdomyosarcoma. Nature Med 1998; 4:559–560.

231 Barr FG. Gene fusions involving PAX and FOX family members in alveolar rhabdomyosarcoma. Oncogene 2001; 20: 5736–5746.

232 Anderson J, Gordon A, Pritchard-Jones K, Shipley J. Genes, chromosomes, and rhabdomyosarcoma. Genes Chromosomes Cancer 1999; 26:275–285.

233 Marsden HB. The pathology of soft tissue sarcomas. In: D'Angio G J, Evans A E (eds). Bone tumors and soft tissue sarcomas. London: Edward Arnold; 1985:4–46.

234 Newton WA, Gehan EA, Webber BL, et al. Classification of rhabdomyosarcomas and related sarcomas. Pathologic aspects and proposals for a new classification – an Intergroup Rhabdomyosarcoma Study. Cancer 1995; 76:1073–1085.

235 Kemshead JT. Monoclonal antibodies. Their use in the diagnosis and therapy of pediatric and adult tumors derived from the neuroectoderm. In: Baldwin RW (ed). Monoclonal antibodies for cancer detection and therapy. London: Academic Press; 1985:281.

236 Lawrence W, Gehan EA, Hays DM, et al. Prognostic significance of staging factors of the UICC staging system in childhood rhabdomyosarcoma. A report from the Intergroup Rhabdomyosarcoma Study IRSII. J Clin Oncol 1987; 5:46–54.

*237 Crist W, Gehan EA, Ragab AH, et al. The third Intergroup Rhabdomyosarcoma Study. J Clin Oncol 1995; 13:610–630.

*238 Crist WM, Anderson JR, Meza JL, et al. Intergroup Rhabdomyosarcoma Study-IV: results for patients with nonmetastatic disease. J Clin Oncol 2001; 19:3091–3102.

239 Kelly KM, Womer RB, Sorensen PHB, et al. Common and variant gene fusions predict distinct clinical phenotypes in rhabdomyosarcoma. J Clin Oncol 1997; 15:1831–1836.

*240 Pappo AS, Lyden E, Breneman J, et al. Up-front window trial of topotecan in previously untreated children and adolescents with metastatic rhabdomyosarcoma: an Intergroup Rhabdomyosarcoma Study. J Clin Oncol 2001; 19:213–219.

*241 Frascella E, Pritchard-Jones K, Modak S, et al. Response of previously untreated metastatic rhabdomyosarcoma to combination chemotherapy with carboplatin, epirubicin and vincristine. Eur J Cancer 1996; 5:821–825.

242 Huvos AG. Bone tumors, diagnosis, treatment and prognosis. Philadelphia: WB Saunders; 1991.

243 Dahlen D, Unni K. Osteosarcoma of bone and its important recognisable varieties. Am J Surg Pathol 1977; 1:61–72.

244 Enneking WF, Spanier SS, Goodman MA. Current concept reviews: the surgical staging of musculo-skeletal sarcoma. J Bone Joint Surg 1980; 62 :1027–1030.

245 Lange B, Levine AS. Is it ethical not to conduct a prospectively controlled trial of adjuvant chemotherapy in osteosarcoma? Cancer Treat Rep 1982; 66:1699–1704.

246 Link M, Goorin A, Miser A, et al. The effect of adjuvant chemotherapy on relapse free survival in patients with osteosarcoma of the extremity. N Engl J Med 1986; 314:1600–1606.

247 Spannier SS, Shuster JJ, Vender Griend RA. The effect of local extent of the tumor on prognosis in osteosarcoma. J Bone Joint Surg 1990; 72 :643–653.

248 Bramwell VHC, Burgess M, Sneath R, et al. AS combination of two short intensive adjuvant chemotherapy regimens in operable osteosarcoma of limbs in children and young adults. J Clin Oncol 1992; 10:1579–1591.

249 Rosen G, Caparros B, Huvos AG, et al. Pre-operative chemotherapy for osteogenic sarcoma. Selection of post-operative adjuvant chemotherapy based on the response of the primary tumor to pre-operative chemotherapy. Cancer 1982; 49:1221–1230.

250 Jaffe N, Frei E, Watts H, Traggis D. High dose methotrexate in osteogenic sarcoma. A 5-year experience. Cancer Treat Rep 1978; 62: 259–264.

251 Jürgens H, Winkler K, Gobel U. Bone tumors. In: Pinkerton CR, Plowman PN (eds). Pediatric oncology, 2nd edn. London: Chapman & Hall; 1997 417–422.

252 Kemshead JT. Pediatric tumors: immunological and molecular markers. Boca Raton, Florida: CRC Press; 1989.

253 Gobel V, Jurgens H, Etspuler G, et al. Prognostic significance of tumor volume in localized Ewing's sarcoma of bone in children and adolescents. J Cancer Res Clin; Oncol 1987; 113:187–191.

254 Horwich A, Huddart R, Dearnely D. Markers and management of germ-cell tumors of the testes. Lancet 1998; 352:1535–1538.

255 Dehner LP. Gonadal and extragonadal germ cell neoplasia of childhood. Hum Pathol 1983; 14:493–511.

256 Altman RP, Randolph JG, Lilly JR. Sacrococcygeal teratomas. J Pediatr Surg 1974; 9:389–398.

257 Bosl GJ, Motzer RJ. Testicular germ cell cancer. N Engl J Med 1997; 337:242–253.

*258 Mann JR, Raafat F, Robinson K, et al. Mature and immature extracranial teratomas in children: the UK Children's Cancer Study Group's experience. In: Jones I, Appleyard P, Harnden P, Joffe JK (eds). Germ cell tumors. London: John Libbey; 1998; 237–246.

*259 Cushing B, Giller R, Cohen L, et al. Surgery alone is effective treatment of resected immature teratoma in children: a pediatric intergroup report. Med Pediatr Oncol 1996; 27:221.

260 Einhorn LH, Williams SD, Troner M, et al. The role of maintenance therapy in disseminated testicular cancer. N Engl J Med 1981; 305:727–731.

*261 Mann JR, Raafat F, Robinson K, et al. UKCCSG's germ cell tumor GCT studies: improving outcome for children with malignant extra-cranial non-gonadal tumors. Carboplatinum, etoposide and bleomycin are effective and less toxic than previous regimes. Med Pediat Oncol 1998; 30:217–227.

*262 Siefert W, Beyer J, Strohscheer I, et al. High-dose treatment with carboplatin, etoposide, and ifosfamide followed by autologous stem-cell transplantation in relapsed or refractory germ cell cancer: a phase I/II study. J Clin Oncol 1994; 12:1223–1231.

263 Kingston JE, Hungerford JL. Retinoblastoma. In: Pinkerton CR, Plowman PN (eds). Pediatric oncology, 2nd edn. London: Chapman & Hall; 1997:357–379.

264 Knudson AG. Mutation and cancer: statistical study of retinoblastoma. Proc Natl Acad Sci USA 1971; 68:820–823.

265 Stratton MR, Moss S, Warren W, et al. Mutation of the p53 gene in soft tissue sarcomas: association with abnormalities of the RB1 gene. Oncogene 1990; 5: 1297–1301.

266 Knudson AG, Meadows AT, Nichols WW, Hill R. Chromosomal deletion and retinoblastoma. N Engl J Med 1976; s295:1120–1123.

*267 Dryja TP, Mukai S, Petersen R, et al. Parental origin of mutations of the retinoblastoma gene. Nature 1989; 339:556–558.

268 Zhu XP, Dunn JM, Phillips RA, et al. Preferential germline mutation of the paternal allele in retinoblastoma. Nature 1989; 340:312–313.

*269 Bunin GR, Petrakova A, Meadows AJ, et al. Occupations of parents of children with retinoblastoma: a report from the Children's Cancer Study Group. Cancer Res 1990; 50:7129–7133.

270 Kingston JE, Hungerford JL, Madreperna SA, Plowman PN. Results of combined chemotherapy and radiotherapy for advanced intraocular retinoblastoma. Arch Ophthalmol 1996; 114:1339–1343.

271 Weinberg AG, Finegold MJ. Primary hepatic tumors in childhood In: Finegold MJ (ed) Pathology of neoplasia in children and adolescents. Philadelphia: Saunders; 1986:333–372.

272 Kalifa C, Lemerle J, Cailland MM, Valayer J. Resectability of childhood hepatoblastoma is improved by primary chemotherapy. Proc Am Soc Clin Oncol 1984; 3:308.

*273 Douglas EC, Green AA, Wrenn E, et al. Effective cisplatin based chemotherapy in the treatment of hepatoblastoma. Med Pediatr Oncol 1985; 13:187–190.

*274 Plaschkes J, Perilongo G, Shafford E, et al. Pre-operative chemotherapy – cisplatin (PLA) and doxorubicin (DO) PLADO for the treatment of hepatoblastoma and hepatocellular carcinoma: results after two years follow-up. Med Pediatr Oncol 1996; 27:256.

*275 Perilongo G, Brown J, Shafford E, et al. Hepatoblastoma presenting with lung metastases. Treatment results of the first cooperative, prospective study of the International Society of Pediatric Oncology on childhood liver tumors. Cancer 2000; 89: 1845–1853.

276 Chu T, D'Angio GJ, Favara B, et al. Classification of histiocytosis syndromes in children - from the Writing Group of the Histiocyte Society. Lancet 1987; 1:208–209.

277 Favara BE, Jaffe R. Pathology of Langerhans' cell histiocytosis. Hematol Oncol Clin North Am 1987; 1:75.

278 Grois NG, Favara BE, Mostleck GH, Prayer D. Central nervous system disease Langerhans' cell histiocytosis. Hematol Oncol Clin North Am 1998; 12:287–305.

*279 Ladisch S, Gadner H, Arico M, et al. LCH-1: a randomized trial of etoposide versus vinblastine in disseminated Langerhans' cell histiocytosis. Med Pediatr Oncol 1994; 23:107–110.

*280 Broadbent V. Favorable prognostic features in histiocytosis X: bone involvement and absence of skin disease. Arch Dis Child 1986; 61:1219–1221.

281 Arico M, Egeler RM. Clinical aspects of Langerhans' cell histiocytosis. Hematol Oncol Clin North Am 1998; 12:247–258.

282 Henter J, Arico M, Egeler RM, et al. HLH-94: a treatment protocol for hemophagocytic lymphohistiocytosis. Med Pediatr Oncol 1997; 28:342–347.

23

Gynecological diseases

Anne S Garden

INTRODUCTION

There has been a slight but definite increase in awareness of gynecological problems in children and adolescents in recent years. Some of the larger children's hospitals have dedicated gynecological clinics but the majority of girls and teenagers seen with such problems are still seen by general practitioners, pediatricians or gynecologists who have no particular knowledge or expertise.

There is a need for such a service – or at least for clinicians who have concerns to be able to access the expertise from such a service. Gynecologists do not always appreciate that girls are not just miniature women but have their own specific anatomy and physiology, as well as emotional and psychological makeup. Pediatricians often feel out of their depth dealing with sexual and hormonal problems. There is an additional issue in that while all our patients deserve to be treated with sensitivity, this is especially true for girls with gynecological problems. A painful, inappropriate examination may cause fears and phobias in young girls which will stay with them during their teenage years – and even into adulthood, with unfortunate effects on their future reproductive health.

A basic knowledge of female reproductive physiology is helpful in the management of girls with gynecological problems.

Prior to birth, high levels of estrogens produced by the placenta inhibit gonadotrophin release from the fetal pituitary. Following delivery and the loss of maternal estrogens a transient rise in neonatal gonadotrophin levels may result in neonatal ovarian activity. Such activity, however, is short-lived and both gonadotrophin and estrogen levels drop within a short time of delivery and remain so throughout childhood until just before puberty.

The high levels of circulating estrogens at delivery may cause secretion of milk from the neonatal breast and a white vaginal discharge to be present. The loss of the estrogens a few days after delivery may result in a vaginal bleed due to breakdown of the endometrium.

The high levels of circulating estrogens at delivery affect the appearance of the neonatal genitalia, causing the labia majora and minora to appear large and rounded and the hymen to appear edematous. These changes disappear with the loss of maternal hormones so that the labia majora become flattened, the labia minora thin and attenuated and the hymen less prominent. The hymenal changes are often the last to regress with the result that for the first year of life the hymen can appear quite prominent. The external genitalia of the girl then remain unchanged until the developments at puberty.

Hormonal changes begin to occur between the ages of 6 and 9 years with gonadotrophin-releasing hormone being released in a pulsatile fashion from the hypothalamus, initially during sleep. This results in release of gonadotrophins, initially luteinizing hormone (LH) but later also follicle stimulating hormone (FSH), from the pituitary. As the duration of gonadotrophin release becomes prolonged, the ovary responds with the release of estrogens.

Release of estrogens, along with the androgens produced by the female adrenal, causes the physical changes of pubertal development which were described by Tanner and his colleagues in the 1960s and 1970s. The first sign of female puberty is the appearance of the subareolar breast bud at the mean age of 10.8 years (range 8.8–12.8). Pubic hair growth occurs approximately 6 months later although in approximately one-third of girls it occurs before breast development.[1] Thereafter, pubertal development proceeds in a recognized sequence of events – increase in growth velocity; pubic and axillary hair development to Tanner Stage 4; breast development to Tanner stage 3–4; menstruation.[2] Although concern has been expressed about a recent apparent reversal of the decreasing age of menarche[3] which has been occurring since the nineteenth century, the evidence for this is slight. The median age of menarche in British teenagers is 13 years[4] with little geographic, social or ethnic variation. Ninety-five per cent of girls in the United Kingdom will have attained the menarche by the age of 15 and one in eight while still in primary school.

PROBLEMS AT BIRTH

AMBIGUOUS GENITALIA

The diagnosis, investigation and management of girls with ambiguous genitalia have been dealt with elsewhere.

Surgical correction of the genital abnormalities has traditionally been performed soon after birth, with the understanding that it is important to correct the appearance of the genitalia as soon as possible – and certainly before the girl reached her adolescent years.[5] More recently, however, clinicians have been questioning this management. Delaying corrective surgery until later years allows the girl herself to be involved in the decision making. Additionally, the growth of the structures and the estrogenization of the tissues makes the surgery easier, allowing, for instance, better dissection of the neural bundle during clitoridectomy, thus preserving function. Recent articles showing poor functional results at puberty in girls who had surgery performed in childhood have strengthened the argument that corrective surgery should be delayed until adolescence.[6]

HYDROCOLPOS

Hydrocolpos presents at birth with a bulging membrane visible on parting the labia at the introitus. Less commonly it may present as an abdominal mass rising out of the pelvis. It is caused by the failure of breakdown of the membrane which occurs at the junction of the Mullerian duct and the urogenital sinus. Fluid secreted under the influence of maternal hormones collects above the membrane. Treatment is by simple excision of the membrane. Failure to recognize that an abdominal/pelvic mass may be due to hydrocolpos may have serious consequences. Thirty-five per cent of neonates died after an unnecessary laparotomy for hydrocolpos in the only published series.[7]Although the paper is old it emphasizes the importance of making the correct diagnosis.

If the condition is not diagnosed in the neonatal period, resorption of the fluid causes the bulging membrane to disappear, the condition being subsequently diagnosed at puberty when the girl develops cryptomenorrhea (see below).

PROBLEMS IN EARLY CHILDHOOD

VULVOVAGINITIS

Vulvovaginitis is without doubt the commonest condition seen at a pediatric gynecology clinic – and has almost always been misdiagnosed and mismanaged before being referred.

Vulvovaginitis occurs because the anatomy and physiology of the genitalia of the prepubescent girl do not provide the resistance to bacterial infections found in the adult woman. In the prepubescent girl, the labia minora are, as has already been said, thin and attenuated. The changes in vaginal secretion which will occur at puberty, under the influence of estrogen (acidic vaginal secretions and the presence of Doderlein's bacilli), and which help prevent infection, are not present. This results in the girl being prone to bacterial infection. The common age of presentation, between the ages of 3 and 8 may be due to the girl being more responsible for her own personal hygiene at this age, although it is not uncommon to obtain a history of the condition being present well before the girl came out of nappies. The common organisms involved are *Haemophilus influenzae* and fecal flora.[8] Other organisms, particularly candida, are found much less commonly.

Girls with vulvovaginitis present with symptoms of vaginal irritation or pain, which can be quite severe, and vaginal discharge which can be quite profuse and is often described as green or brown in colour. Dysuria may also be present and the girl may well have been investigated for urinary tract infection before the correct diagnosis is made. Examination shows the labia to be inflamed and often excoriated. The state of the girl's hygiene should also be assessed. Careful inspection should also be undertaken to exclude dermatological conditions.

The differential diagnosis of vulvovaginitis includes other conditions which cause vulvar irritation or vaginal discharge which are mentioned below.

Management is usually limited to treatment for the relief of symptoms. The role of investigation is a vexed one. It is impossible to take an uncontaminated high vaginal swab in a young girl without a general anesthetic and no attempt should be made to do so. An introital swab may be helpful but interpretation may be difficult because of the presence of contaminants. The use of antibiotics in response to a specific swab result is limited as subsequent attacks are likely to be due to different organisms. Identification of specific bacteria therefore is usually of academic interest and is usually only required if there is a suspicion of sexual abuse or of a sexually transmitted disease.

Treatment, therefore, consists of advice regarding personal hygiene and clothing. Salt baths, with the girl being encouraged to sit for about 10 minutes in a basin of warm water to which two tablespoons of salt have been added, are often helpful particularly when the girl is sore. This may be followed by the use of an emollient cream such as E45 or Sudacrem which may also improve symptoms and provide a barrier especially to relieve pain on micturition. There is no place for antifungal therapy unless a *proven* candidal infection is present.

The use of estrogen cream has been advocated but its use is limited due to the risks of absorption.

One of the most important things which should be done is to explain to the mother why the condition has occurred along with reassurance as to how common it is and that it will improve as the girl approaches puberty. It is also important to stress that the girl will not have any long-term gynecological consequences.

BLOODSTAINED VAGINAL DISCHARGE

Bloodstained vaginal discharge is relatively uncommon. The commonest cause is a foreign body, but the diagnosis of genital rhabdomyosarcoma or other tumor must be excluded.

Foreign bodies in the vagina in this age group are not unusual and are not indicative of the child being psychologically disturbed, although a girl who repeatedly inserts foreign bodies into her vagina may well benefit from psychological referral.

Examination under anesthesia is mandatory. Imaging with ultrasound or X-rays will not pick up foreign bodies such as pieces of toilet paper or sponge. In any case, general anesthesia will be required to remove the object.

Genital rhabdomyosarcoma is an unusual tumor which may present with bloodstained discharge. It is dealt with more fully below.

VULVAR IRRITATION

Other common causes of vulvar irritation in this age group are:

- dermatological conditions;
- threadworms;
- non-specific vulvitis.

Dermatological conditions

Any dermatological condition such as eczema or psoriasis may occur on the vulva just as in any other part of the body. A family history of these conditions should raise the suspicion of the diagnosis.

A dermatological condition which is not uncommon in prepubertal girls is lichen sclerosus. This condition may occur anywhere on the body but is found on the vulva at the extremes of reproductive life – in the prepubertal girl and the postmenopausal woman. The etiology is unknown although genetic susceptibility and an autoimmune basis have both been suggested.[9] It presents with extreme irritation which is usually intermittent in nature. Examination shows characteristic appearances of shiny white (usually called pearly white) macules or papules which may coalesce into larger plaques. There are often associated hemorrhagic areas which may appear as bruising or as quite alarming hemorrhagic bullae. Ulcerated areas may also be present (Fig. 23.1). To the unaware, the condition may be suggestive of sexual abuse[10] and it has been suggested that lichen sclerosus is more common in girls who have been sexually abused.[11]

Treatment depends on the severity of the symptoms. If the irritation is severe, treatment with high potency steroids is required, the one used most commonly being clobetasol propionate 0.05%. In less severe cases or when the disease is asymptomatic an emollient cream is all that is required. As the condition may also involve the perianal skin, constipation is often a feature and laxative therapy may also be required. Most girls have complete remission of symptoms after 2 or 3 months[12] and the condition usually resolves completely before puberty. There is no risk of malignancy with lichen sclerosus in this age group unlike that debated in the postmenopausal group and it may be worth emphasizing that to parents, who in this age of the Internet, may be alarmed by the information they find there.

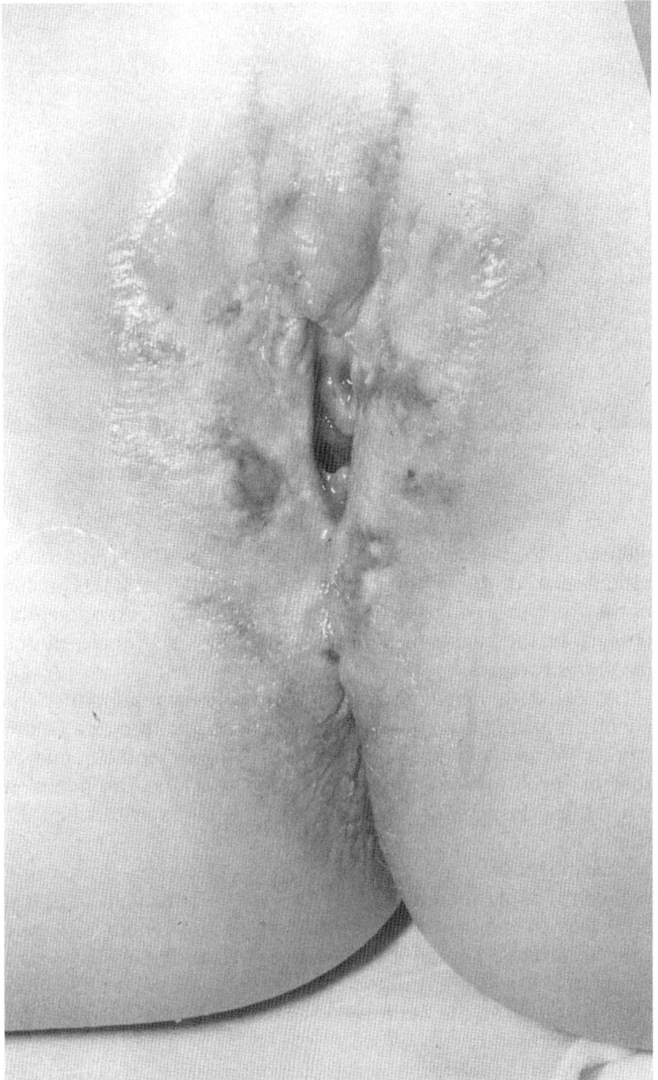

Fig. 23.1 Lichen sclerosus on the vulva of a prepubertal girl showing the classical appearances of pearly white areas with hemorrhage and ulceration.

Threadworms

Threadworms *(Enterobius vermicularis)* are common in this age group and although the most common presentation is with anal irritation, vulvar irritation may also be present or may be the only presenting symptom. Diagnosis is by a Sellotape test, the tape being applied to the perianal region overnight, removed in the morning and fixed to a glass slide. Examination of the slide will reveal ova and adult worms. Treatment is with mebendazole 100 mg as a single dose to all members of the family over the age of 2 years.

Non-specific vulvitis

Non-specific vulvitis is common but difficult to treat. Common precipitating factors are washing powder, fabric conditioners and bubble bath. Treatment is by identifying and removing the cause.

OTHER VULVAR DISORDERS

Vulvar warts

Vulvar or perianal warts (Fig. 23.2) present the dilemma of whether or not they are indicative of sexual abuse. They may well have been transferred quite innocently from the hands of a parent or childminder, or the child herself, and the situation requires sensitive handling. It has been suggested that DNA typing of the virus may be helpful but this is debatable except in cases of child abuse where a matching to genital warts from the alleged abuser will provide confirmation. Warts on the hymen are always significant.

Warts on the vulva, anal or perianal area are the most common sexually transmitted infection in adolescents.

Treatment is by cautery under general anesthesia or, in the older girl, by using podophyllin, taking care not to damage the surrounding skin. Adolescent girls with warts should be encouraged to attend for cervical screening.

LABIAL ADHESIONS

Labial adhesions are seen most commonly in girls under the age of 3 years and are thought to be secondary to chronic irritation. It is important to make the correct diagnosis. The child is commonly brought up by parents who are panic-stricken, having been told that their child has a congenital abnormality which will require major reconstructive surgery.

The difference between labial adhesions and congenital absence of the vagina is quite straightforward. In a girl with labial

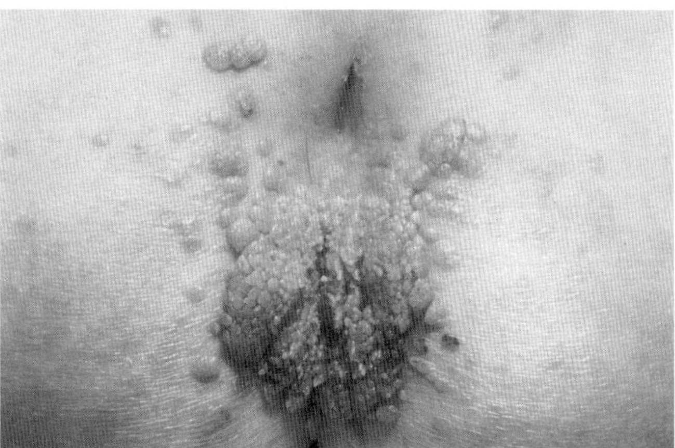

Fig. 23.2 Perianal warts in a young girl (reproduced by kind permission of Edward Arnold).

adhesions, the perineum is quite flat, with the fused labia preventing visualization of the urethra, clitoris or hymen (Fig. 23.3). The line of the fused labia can often be clearly seen. In a girl with congenital absence of the vagina, separation of the labia shows clearly the introital structures.

A girl with labial adhesions is usually asymptomatic, the condition having been noted by chance by the mother or a health worker. Occasionally, in a slightly older girl, the presentation may be that of incontinence, urine being trapped behind the adhesion when the girl is squatting on the toilet but being expelled when she stands up.

Treatment is simple with the use of estrogen cream used in a regimen of application twice daily for 2 weeks. This can be repeated cyclically as required until separation occurs. There is debate that treatment should be restricted to those girls who are symptomatic as the condition is a self-limiting one and resolves spontaneously as the child becomes older. There is no place for surgical separation.

The debate as to whether labial adhesions are diagnostic of, or more common in, girls who have been sexually abused is unresolved.[13]

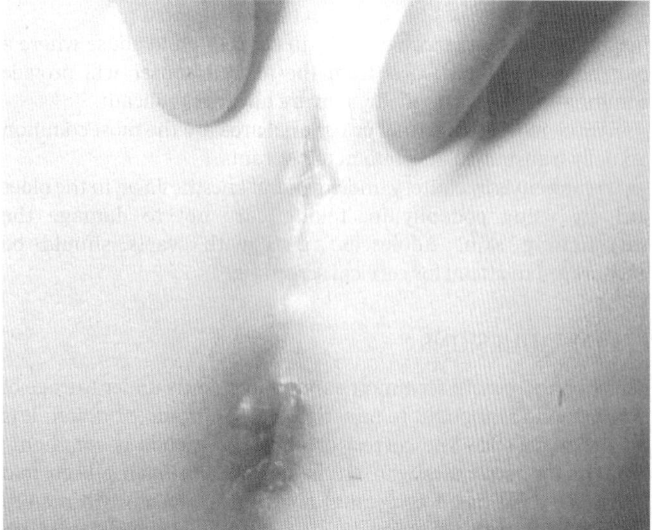

Fig. 23.3 Labial adhesions in a child of 18 months. Note the completely flat appearance of the perineum.

PROBLEMS OF PUBERTY

PRIMARY AMENORRHEA

Amenorrhea is usually considered as primary when the girl has never menstruated and secondary if she has not had a period for 6 months or more. Primary amenorrhea is usually subdivided into two groups – the girls who have no pubertal development in whom the problem is most likely due to a hormonal cause and those girls who have normal pubertal development in whom the cause is most likely an anatomical one. The causes of primary amenorrhea are shown in Table 23.1.

It is common practice to investigate girls with primary amenorrhea without pubertal development by the age of 14 and girls with primary amenorrhea and with normal pubertal development by the age of 16. More importantly, however, is the awareness that pubertal development is a continuum and that a break in the continuum is as, if not more, important than arbitrary cut-offs of age.

Primary amenorrhea without sexual development

Constitutional delay

Girls with constitutional delay may have a family history of the mother or sisters having late pubertal development. Investigations show low estrogen and low gonadotrophin levels. Bone age is delayed compared to chronological age. Reassurance is all that is required although girls in whom puberty is significantly delayed should be considered for induction of puberty.

Chronic systemic disease

Chronic diseases such as poorly controlled diabetes or hypothyroidism are not usually a diagnostic problem. Estrogen and gonadotrophin levels in these girls are low. Puberty follows control of the disease.

Absent ovarian function

Absent ovarian function may be due to primary or premature ovarian failure or to gonadal dysgenesis. The characteristic findings on investigation are high follicle stimulating hormone (FSH) and luteinizing hormone (LH) levels and low estrogen. Ovarian failure may also present as secondary amenorrhea depending on the stage of development at which the failure occurred. It is a devastating diagnosis to have to give any woman of reproductive years but worse for an adolescent girl and it requires sensitive handling.

The most common identified cause of premature ovarian failure in modern practice is subsequent to chemotherapy or irradiation for childhood or adolescent malignancy. The routine removal of ovarian tissue prior to therapy for use in future fertility therapy is still considered experimental.[14]

Other identified causes of ovarian failure in this age group are autoimmune, chromosomal (e.g. 46XXX, fragile X), metabolic

Table 23.1 Causes of primary amenorrhea

Without pubertal development
Constitutional delay
Chronic systemic disease
Absent ovarian function
Hypothalamic pituitary dysfunction
(Polycystic ovarian syndrome)
With pubertal development
Absent uterus
(Absent or imperforate vagina)

(e.g. galactosemia). Eight candidate genes for premature ovarian failure have been identified.[15]

Gonadal dysgenesis most commonly is associated with a 45X or variant karyotype (Turner's syndrome) but may also be found in girls with a 46XY karyotype (Swyer's syndrome or pure gonadal dysgenesis). Turner's syndrome is found in 1:2000 to 1:3000 of the female population. It is characterized by short stature and ovarian failure, the ovaries being only streaks of tissue (streak ovaries). However, only approximately 50% of girls with Turner's syndrome have the 45X karyotype on lymphocyte culture, the remainder being due to abnormal X chromosomes or mosiac karyotypes. Because of this, the phenotype varies greatly, but the main additional features include web neck, shield chest with wide-spaced nipples and wide carrying angle (Fig. 23.4). Delay in the diagnosis is often due to the failure to appreciate the variation in phenotype.

Hypothalamic pituitary dysfunction

Hypothalamic or pituitary causes of primary amenorrhea, such as craniopharyngiomas, hydrocephaly, Kallmann's syndrome or Laurence–Moon–Biedl syndrome are usually diagnosed prior to puberty and do not constitute a diagnostic problem as regards amenorrhea.

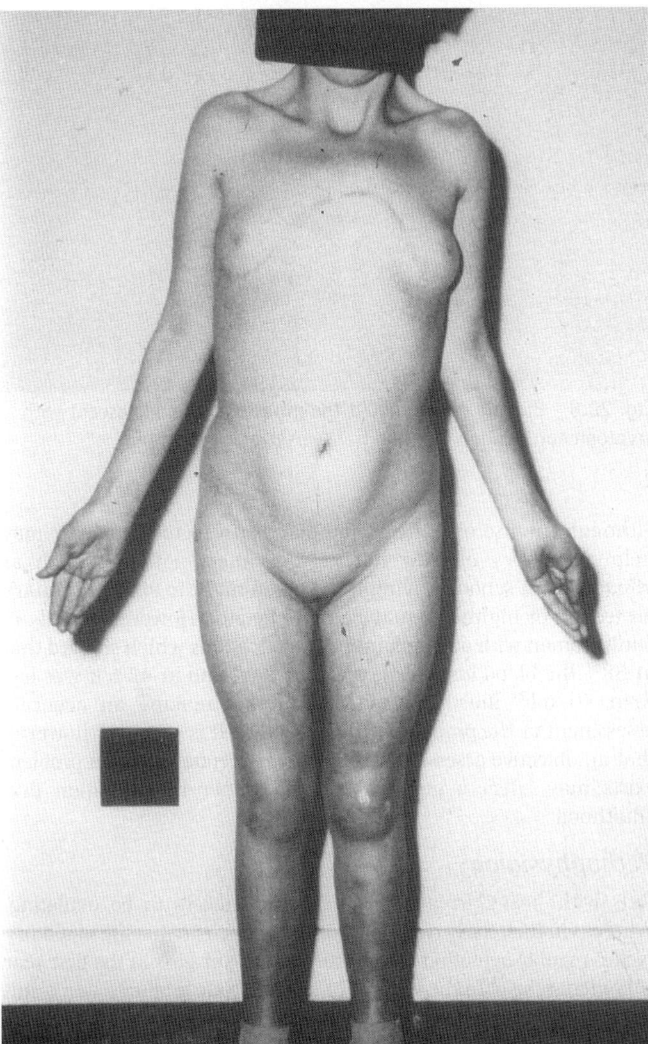

Fig. 23.4 Classical appearance of a girl with Turner's syndrome showing web neck, wide-spaced nipples and wide carrying angle. Mosaic conditions are common so that a wide variation in phenotype is seen.

Treatment

Treatment involves hormone replacement in such a way as to mimic the normal physiological response of the ovary. Obviously in girls with constitutional delay or those with chronic illness, development may proceed normally given time. However, while waiting for spontaneous development, adolescents may experience psychological stress or even bullying at school so induction of puberty should be considered and discussed even in this group.

Estrogen replacement should begin around the age of 10 or 11, unless it is wished to delay it for the administration of growth hormone in girls with Turner's syndrome. The initial dose should be 1 μg ethinyl estradiol increasing every 6 months to 2 μg, 5 μg and 10 μg. After this period of time a cyclical preparation of estrogen and progestogen should be introduced. Pediatricians have normally used one of the combined oral contraceptives for this purpose and certainly this is well tolerated and accepted by adolescents. However, use of one of the hormone replacement therapies has many advantages. The level of estrogen can be measured so that optimum dosage can be prescribed; estrogen is given throughout the 4 week cycle as opposed to the 3 weeks of therapy on the pill; the girl has the option of modes of delivery such as patches or tablets and she has the option of using one of the 'no-bleed' continuous combined preparations. However, it should be pointed out that while the combined oral contraceptive is free, a double prescription charge is payable on the cyclical hormone replacement therapy preparations which is a problem for older adolescents who have to pay for their prescriptions. In addition, it may not be acceptable because of peer pressure. Long-term treatment requires to be monitored for dosage and compliance to reduce the long-term risks of estrogen lack such as osteoporosis.

Primary amenorrhea with sexual development

Primary amenorrhea with normal development is usually due to an anatomical cause, either absence of the uterus (or more correctly the endometrium) or absence or blockage of the vagina which more correctly causes cryptomenorrhea.

Absence of the uterus

Absence of the uterus because of a congenital abnormality has two main causes – either as a result of failure of development of the Mullerian duct as in Rokitansky–Kuster–Hauser syndrome or as part of complete androgen insensitivity syndrome (CAIS).

Rokitansky–Kuster–Hauser syndrome. Girls with this condition are phenotypically normal, with a 46XX karyotype and normal ovaries. Associated renal tract abnormalities are found in 40% of patients and vertebral column abnormalities such as hemivertebrae or fused vertebrae in 12%. The degree of failure of development (Fig. 23.5) varies from total absence of Mullerian duct structures to varying degrees of uterine horn development, very occasionally including endometrium within a small blind uterine horn when the girl will present with severe cyclical abdominal pain (see cryptomenorrhea). It is not necessary to remove the rudimentary uterine horns unless endometrium is present. Vaginal reconstruction either by the use of dilators or surgically using a loop of bowel is required.

Complete androgen insensitivity syndrome (CAIS). Girls with CAIS have a 46XY karyotype. They are often slightly taller than average, have good breast development and sparse pubic and axillary hair. The condition arises as a result of the cells of the mesonephric duct and genital tubercle failing to respond to circulating androgens with

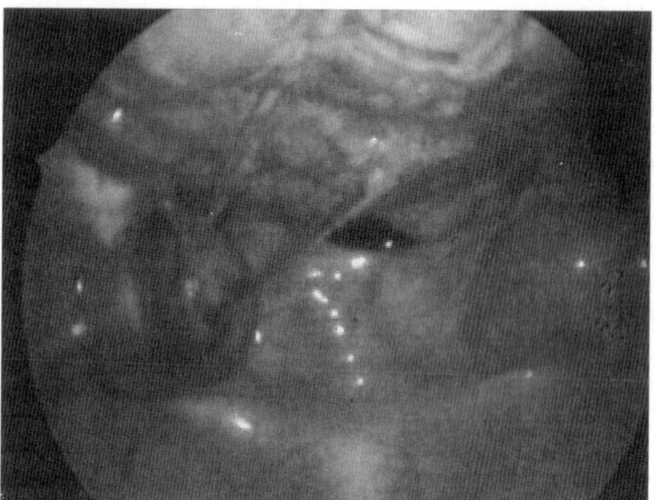

Fig. 23.5 Rudimentary uterine horns in a girl with Rokitansky–Kuster–Hauser syndrome (adhesions surrounding the left horn).

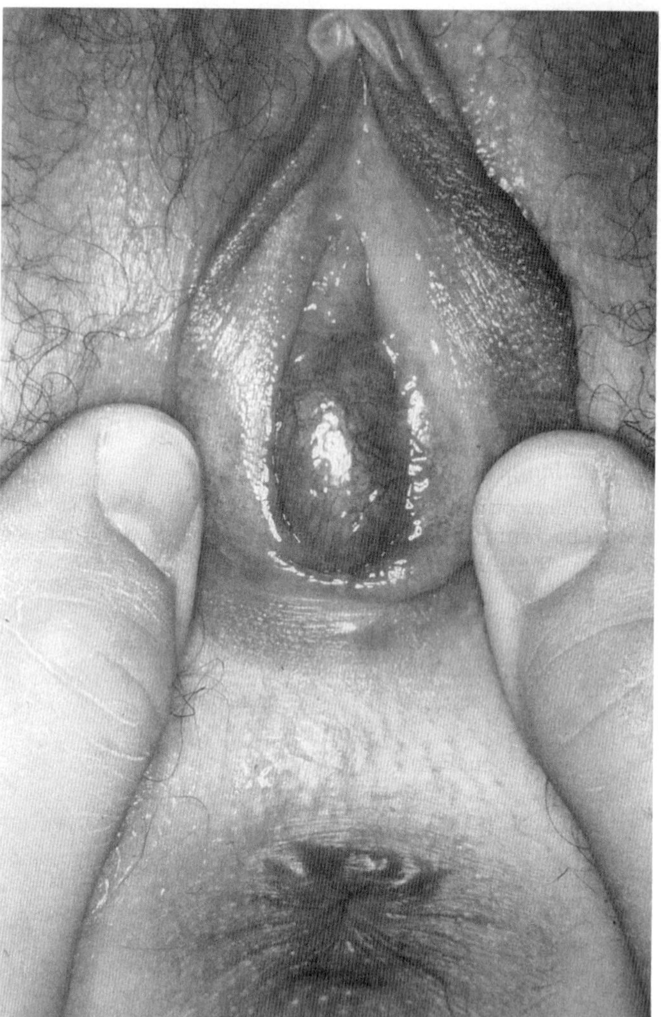

Fig. 23.6 Bulging membrane at the introitus of an adolescent with cryptomenorrhea due to a low transverse vaginal septum.

the resulting failure of development of male external genitalia. Production of Mullerian inhibitory factor (MIF) causes degeneration of the fallopian tubes, uterus and upper third of the vagina.

The condition is an X-linked disorder and a history of a sister or aunt with the condition may be obtained.

Treatment is by removal of the testes because of the 5% risk of malignancy[16] and vaginal reconstruction. Long term estrogen replacement is required to protect against osteoporosis.

Girls with CAIS and their families require sensitive management, particularly in regard to their sexual status.[17]

Cryptomenorrhea

Cryptomenorrhea or 'hidden menstruation' presents with amenorrhea in the presence of increasingly severe cyclical lower abdominal pain. The common blockage occurs at the lower end of the vagina, but higher lesions may occur.

In severe cases, the girl may present with acute urinary retention due to blockage of the urethra by the vaginal mass. Examination of the abdomen reveals a mass arising out of the pelvis, the size being dependent on the duration of menstruation. Examination shows the classical bulging blue membrane at the introitus on separation of the labia, if the blockage is a low one (Fig. 23.6). Treatment is by cruciate incision of the membrane.

More rarely, cryptomenorrhea may occur in the presence of menstruation when there is a blockage of a duplex genital tract in which case presentation is with severe dysmenorrhea.

PROBLEMS OF ADOLESCENCE

HEAVY PERIODS

A complaint of heavy periods is the commonest reason for seeing a teenager at a gynecological clinic. It is essential when seeing these patients that an accurate history is taken. A normal menstrual cycle is 28 days with a range of 23–39 days. The average blood loss per cycle is 40 ml with a normal range of 25–70 ml.[18] In practice, however, it is difficult to assess a girl's menstrual loss objectively in the absence of evidence such as anemia. Information about cycle length and duration is subjective and rarely helpful although the use of a menstrual diary or a pictorial chart[19] may help. A history of how her periods affect activities such as attendance at school, having to get up at night to change sanitary protection or nightwear may be more helpful. However, a study in adult women with a complaint of heavy periods which showed that in 68% the blood loss was less than 80 ml and in 42% it was less than 50 ml[20] illustrates the difficulty in making an accurate assessment of the problem through history. It is essential, however, that an objective assessment is made as acceptance that a problem exists may affect a girl's perception of her menstruation into adulthood.

Pathophysiology

Girls with heavy, irregular periods are unlikely to be ovulating. Whereas in their early twenties, 95% of women are having ovulatory cycles, regular ovulation only occurs in 15% of girls in the first year after menarche.[21] In the absence of progesterone produced as a result of ovulation, the endometrium continues to proliferate under the action of unopposed estrogen until the endometrium breaks down irregularly with resultant extremely heavy loss. Girls with regular heavy periods are more likely to be ovulating and the mechanism for the heavy loss is thought to be due to increased endometrial fibrinolysis[22] and an alteration in prostaglandin balance.[23]

Management

There is no place for bimanual vaginal or rectal examination of these girls. It is unlikely that there will be any pelvic pathology causing these symptoms and such an examination is only likely to upset these girls and result in their being put off from attending for future gynecological examination. If it is essential that an assessment is made of the pelvic organs, then pelvic ultrasound should be performed.

Full blood count should be performed. Thyroid function should only be assessed if there are features in the history or examination suggestive of thyroid dysfunction.[24,25] There is no indication in this age group for hysteroscopy or dilatation and curettage.

Girls who are not anemic and whose periods are not disrupting their school or personal life require reassurance only. Girls with heavy regular periods should be treated with tranexamic acid 1 g 6 hourly and mefenamic acid 500 mg 8 hourly.[26] Tranexamic acid has been shown to reduce menstrual flow by 54% and mefenamic acid to reduce menstrual flow by 20%.

In girls with irregular periods in whom it is thought that anovulation is the problem, treatment should be with cyclical progestogens, such as dydrogesterone, norethisterone or medroxyprogesterone, or the combined oral contraceptive pill. Treatment should continue for 6–12 months in the first instance before stopping, with the information that the medication is not curing anything, merely controlling symptoms until ovulatory cycles occur. Treatment should therefore be continued in the long term until the symptoms have settled.

Concerns about giving the combined oral contraceptive pill to adolescents are largely unfounded. The most common expressed are premature closure of epiphyses, which is unfounded as a girl producing enough estrogen to have heavy periods will already have closed epiphyses, and an increased risk of developing breast cancer. The risk of the latter has been defined by the Collaborative Group on Hormonal Factors in Breast Cancer[27] as being 0.5 excess cancers per 100 000 women when used in the ages 16–19.

PAINFUL PERIODS

Dysmenorrhea is another common symptom said to affect 60% of adolescents – 14% of them having symptoms severe enough to cause them to miss school.[28] Dysmenorrhea occurs in ovulatory cycles and is caused by increased levels of prostaglandins being released by the menstrual endometrium. The pain starts with the onset of menstruation, or just before, and lasts 24–48 h. It may be accompanied by nausea, vomiting, diarrhea, backache and pain in the thighs. Treatment is with one of the prostaglandin synthetase inhibitors, usually mefenamic acid 500 mg 8 hourly. The combined oral contraceptive pill is the treatment of choice for those girls who fail to respond to the prostaglandin synthetase inhibitors.

In girls who fail to respond to the combined oral contraceptive pill, underlying pathology should be excluded. The commonest underlying cause is endometriosis (Fig. 23.7) found in approximately 40% of adolescent girls investigated.[29,30] Treatment is with the combined oral contraceptive pill, progestogens, danazol and gonadotrophin releasing hormone (GnRH) agonists, the choice being made principally on the basis of the side-effects as they are equally effective in relieving pain.[31] Loss of bone mass is the main limiting side-effect of the use of GnRH agonists but has been shown to be reversible in adolescents.[32] GnRH agonists may be used with add-back estrogen/progestogen to prevent bone loss without apparent loss of effective therapy.[33]

The other condition that should be considered in girls who fail to respond to the combined oral contraceptive pill is cryptomenorrhea

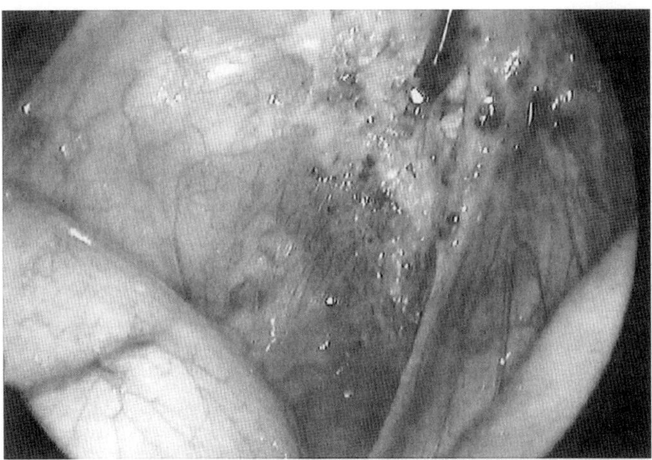

Fig. 23.7 Extensive endometriosis involving the right uterosacral ligament and pouch of Douglas in an adolescent girl.

in a patient with a duplex system. Ultrasound examination in such girls will be reported as showing an 'ovarian cyst' which is, of course, the blind uterine horn filled with menstrual blood. Depending on the level of the blockage, treatment is either by removing the vaginal septum blocking the uterus or removing the uterine horn. Endometriosis is often additionally present in these girls. Imaging of the renal tract should be performed as 47% of girls with Mullerian duct abnormalities have renal tract anomalies.[34]

SECONDARY AMENORRHEA

Secondary amenorrhea is defined as the cessation of periods for 6 months or more. The main causes are listed in Table 23.2.

Polycystic ovarian disease

Polycystic ovarian syndrome (PCO) presents with irregular periods or secondary amenorrhea and is associated with obesity, hirsutism, acne and anovulation. Endocrinologically it is characterized by LH hypersecretion and insulin resistance and a finding of an LH:FSH ratio of greater than three with slightly raised testosterone levels and low sex hormone binding globulin (SHBG). Ultrasound examination reveals a slightly enlarged ovary with hyperechoic stroma and 10 or more follicles of no greater than 10 mm around the circumference (Fig. 23.8). The ultrasound appearances alone are not enough to make the diagnosis being found in up to one-third of women.[35]

Treatment should emphasize the importance of weight loss through exercise and diet[36] as this reduces insulin resistance and is associated with improved regularity of menstruation, hirsutism and ovulation. It is also important as women with PCO have an increased risk of developing diabetes mellitus, or having a stroke or a transient ischemic attack.[37] Treatment otherwise is aimed at controlling the symptoms. In the case of secondary amenorrhea or irregular periods, this is achieved with the combined oral contraceptive pill.

Table 23.2 Causes of secondary amenorrhea

Pregnancy
Premature ovarian failure
Polycystic ovary syndrome
Pituitary disorders
Hypothalamic disorders

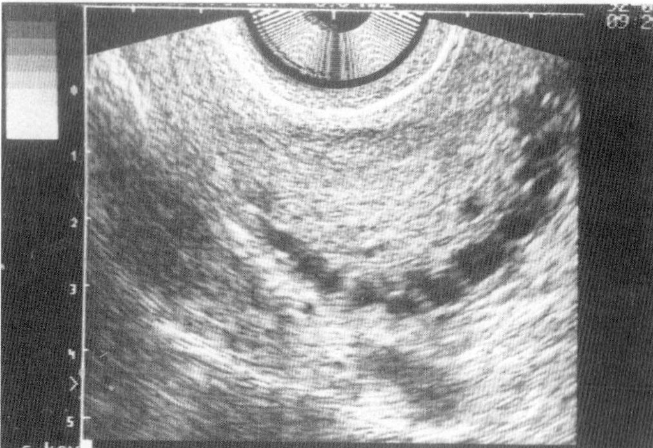

Fig. 23.8 Ultrasound appearances of polycystic ovarian syndrome.

Pituitary disorders

Pituitary disorders as a cause of secondary amenorrhea in adolescents is very rare.

Hypothalamic disorders

Girls who have a low body mass index (BMI) due to dieting, anorexia nervosa or excessive exercising will have amenorrhea secondary to hypothalamic dysfunction and low levels of gonadotrophin. Investigation reveals low levels of FSH, LH and estrogen. Menstrual cycles will normally resume when, or just after, the girl achieves normal weight. Management in the meantime, however, can be difficult as such girls often refuse replacement hormones as they fear putting on weight.

HIRSUTISM AND VIRILISM

Hirsutism is defined as the presence of excessive hair in a female in a distribution that is characteristic of an adult male. It is an extremely embarrassing and distressing condition for a teenager. Causes include ovarian disorders, adrenal disorders, drugs and hypothyroidism; polycystic ovarian syndrome is the most common.[38]

Examination should include careful recording of the extent of the abnormal hair growth as a baseline prior to treatment. Initial investigation is by hormone profile including FSH, LH, testosterone, SHBG, 17alphahydroxyprogesterone and the specific adrenal androgen dehydroepiandrosterone sulfate (DHEAS). Cortisol levels and thyroid function tests should also be assessed.

Treatment should be started as soon as possible as terminal hair growth can be difficult to stop once stimulated. Cosmetic treatments such as waxing, laser therapy or electrolysis should be used. Specific treatment depends on the cause. Ovarian or adrenal androgen secreting tumors should be removed. Late onset congenital adrenal hyperplasia is treated with dexamethasone.

Hirsutism due to polycystic ovarian syndrome is treated with the antiandrogen cyproterone acetate in conjunction with estrogen. Low dose cyproterone acetate may be given in the form of the combined oral contraceptive Dianette (Schering). Higher doses may be given in the reversed sequential regime initially described by Hammerstien. Cyproterone acetate 50–100 mg daily is given from days 5–14 in conjunction with Dianette from days 5–25. The dose of cyproterone acetate is then reduced to achieve the minimum dose required to control hair growth.

Spironolactone and finasteride have also been used for the treatment of hirsutism although neither is licensed for the treatment of hyperandrogenism.

FEMALE GENITAL MUTILATION

Female genital mutilation is a complex issue that raises concerns about competing cultural backgrounds, autonomy, health education and sexuality. It is practiced in many cultures but most widely in northern Africa and in the Arab peninsula. The age at which it is performed varies from culture to culture but most commonly around the ages of 7–9.

Immigration figures show that the number of women from communities that traditionally practice female genital mutilation is rising in the UK.[39] Girls from cultures where it is the practice for the procedure to be performed but who live in Britain probably have the operation performed in the country of their family.

Four main types are recognized.

Circumcision

This is the least extensive and involves cutting of the prepuce of the hood of the clitoris. In some countries this is known as 'Sunna'.

Excision

This involves removal of the clitoris and all or part of the labia minora with the remainder of the labia minora being stitched together leaving a small opening to allow urine and menstrual blood to be passed (Fig. 23.9).

Infibulation

This is the most extensive. It involves removal of the clitoris, labia minora and a substantial part of the medial aspect of the labia majora. The remainder of the labia majora are then pinned together to leave a small opening.

Intermediate

This involves removal of the clitoris and varying amounts of the labia minora and majora.

The most common problems likely to be seen by pediatricians in girls who have had circumcision performed are recurrent urinary tract infection and dysmenorrhea.

In Britain, female genital mutilation is illegal (Prohibition of Female Circumcision Act 1985) and is regarded as a form of abuse[40] and raises child protection issues. It differs from other forms of abuse in that it may be done with the best intentions for the future welfare of the child, there is no possibility of its repetition during childhood and it is approved by sections of the communities in which it is practiced. Measures may need to be taken under the Children Act 1989 if it is thought that a girl is at risk.

GYNECOLOGICAL TUMORS

Gynecological tumors are rare in childhood and adolescence – and malignant tumors particularly so. The commonest are ovarian lesions with tumors of the vagina and cervix being the next most common. Late presentation is a major problem, partly due in the case of ovarian lesions to the non-specific presenting symptoms, and partly due to the rarity of the tumors which may mean that clinicians have a low index of suspicion. The main presenting symptoms are non-specific lower abdominal pain, occasionally with vomiting. Vaginal bleeding may be the presenting symptom in estrogen secreting tumors.

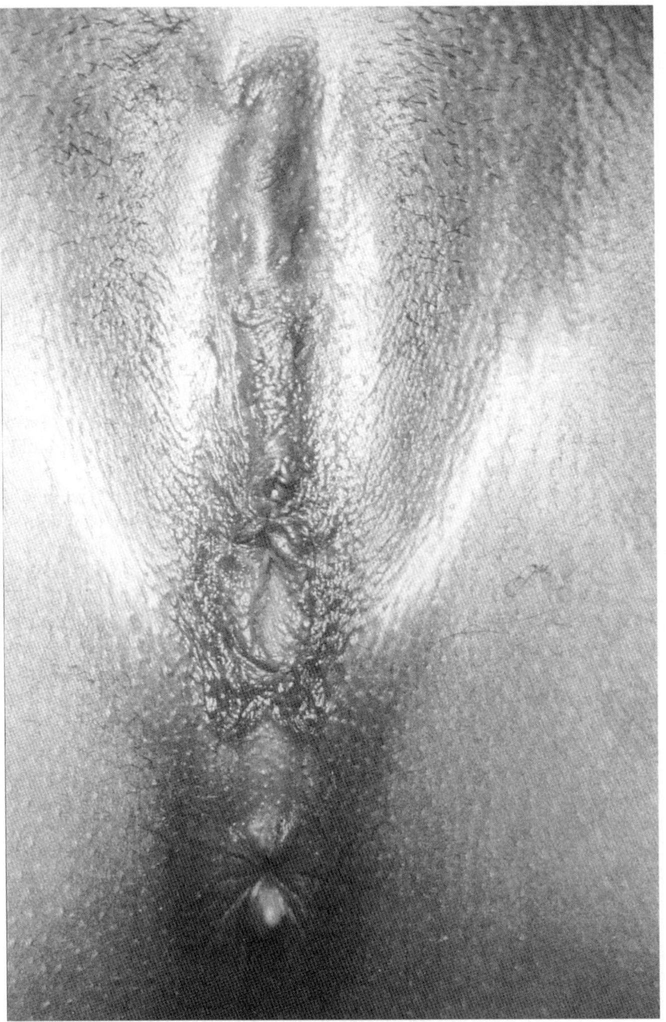

Fig. 23.9 Appearance of the external genitalia in an adolescent girl who has had excision of the genitalia (reproduced by kind permission of Edward Arnold).

BENIGN OVARIAN TUMORS

Follicular cysts are the most common, frequently being found incidentally as part of an ultrasound examination. Management for lesions less than 5 cm is simply by follow-up ultrasound examination to ensure that the cysts resolve. Larger cysts should be aspirated, either under ultrasound control or laparoscopically. If surgical removal is required, care should be taken to preserve as much of the normal ovarian tissue as possible.

Teratomas are the most common neoplasm. They arise from totipotential primordial cells and may contain tissue derived from all three tissue layers. The predominant tissue is usually ectodermal – i.e. sebum and hair – earning the common term 'dermoid cyst'. Treatment is by surgical removal, with conservation of as much ovarian tissue as possible, and close examination of the other ovary as 10–15% of these tumors are bilateral.

MALIGNANT OVARIAN TUMORS

Dysgerminomas are the most common malignant ovarian tumor in childhood and adolescence, 60% of these tumors being found in females under the age of 20. They are bilateral in 10–15% of cases. As they are usually of low malignant potential unilateral oophorectomy may be carried out, unless the girl has a Y chromosome – or part of one – in her karyotype when bilateral oophorectomy should be performed.

Other malignant tumors of the ovary such as immature teratomas, endodermal sinus tumors, embryonal carcinoma, mixed germ-cell tumors and granulosa cell tumors are less common.

OTHER MALIGNANT TUMORS

Genital rhabdomyosarcoma (previously known as sarcoma botryoides) is the most common genital tract neoplasm in children under the age of 16. The tumor occurs most commonly in the vagina, less commonly in the cervix and uterus. Vaginal lesions occur most commonly in girls under the age of 2 years, with lesions of the cervix and vagina being found most commonly in older girls and young adults.

The tumor presents with vaginal bleeding and bloodstained discharge and such symptoms should always be assessed by examination under anesthesia and should include cystoscopy and proctoscopy. Tumor tissue may also be passed vaginally. As the tumor is subepithelial the superficial appearance may be apparently benign and biopsy, taking care to ensure that deeper levels of epithelium are included, is required to make the diagnosis. There have been great advances in the treatment of genital rhabdomyosarcomas in recent years. Radical surgery used to be the norm but has been replaced with multimodal regimes using triple chemotherapy (vincristine, actinomycin D and cyclophosphamide), with or without radiotherapy. With this regime, the need for surgical resection has decreased over the years from 100% in the initial Intergroup Rhabdomyosarcoma Study Group (IRSG) to only 13% in the most recent study.[41]

TEENAGE PREGNANCY

The problems associated with teenage pregnancy are those associated with social deprivation rather than specifically related to young maternal age. The incidence of teenage pregnancies varies between countries and within countries. The Guttmacher Institute recently reported trend data on adolescent birth rates for 46 countries over the period 1970–1995. Lowest rates were reported from the Netherlands (12/1000 adolescents/year) with the highest among developed countries being the Russian Federation (< 100/1000 adolescents/year). Japan and most western European countries had rates of > 40/1000 adolescents/year.[42] Within the Netherlands, four times as many pregnant teenagers had non-Dutch ethnicity compared to all pregnant women.[43] Psychosocial problems, and the consumption of alcohol, cigarettes, marijuana, heroin and solvents are higher among pregnant teenagers than in the general teenage population.[44] Pregnant teenagers with higher levels of education are more likely to undergo termination of pregnancy than continue with the pregnancy.[45] There is some evidence that, in some areas, the difference in teenage pregnancy rates between more affluent and more deprived areas has widened over the last two decades.[46]

Antenatal problems reported in pregnant teenagers include pregnancy induced hypertension, anemia,[47] premature labour and low birth weight,[48] although some of these are also associated with social factors such as smoking and deprivation. There are no specific intrapartum problems faced by pregnant teenagers, high rates of spontaneous delivery with low rates of prolonged labour and cesarean section being consistently reported.[48] While no differences have been reported in outcome of first teenage pregnancy, a second teenage pregnancy is associated with three times the average risk of stillbirth.[49]

REFERENCES (* Level 1 evidence)

1 Tanner JM. Foetus into man, 2nd edn. Ware: Castlemead Publications; 1989:58–74.

2 Marshall WA, Tanner JM. Variation in the pattern of pubertal changes in girls. Arch Dis Child 1969; 44:944–954.

3 Dann TC, Roberts DF. Menarcheal age in University of Warwick young women. J Biosoc Sci 1993; 25:531–538.

4 Whincup PH, Gilg JA, Odoki K, et al. Age of menarche in contemporary British teenagers: survey of girls born between 1982 and 1986. BMJ 2001; 322:1095–1096.

5 Schnitzer JJ, Donahue PK. Surgical treatment of congenital adrenal hyperplasia. Endocrinol Metab Clin North Am 2001; 30: 137–154.

6 Alizai NK, Thomas DF, Lilford R, et al. Feminizing genitoplasty for congenital adrenal hyperplasia: what happens at puberty. J Urol 1999; 161:1592–1593.

7 Gravier L. Hydrocolpos. J Ped Surg 1969; 4:563–568.

8 Pearce AN, Hart CA. Vulvovaginitis: causes and management. Arch Dis Child 1992; 67:509–512.

9 Powell J, Wojarowska F, Winsey S, et al. Lichen sclerosus premenarche: autoimmunity and immunogenetics. Br J Dermatol 2000; 142: 481–484.

10 Muhlendahl KE. Suspected sexual abuse in a 10 year old girl. Lancet 1996; 348:30.

11 Warrington SA, de San Lazaro C. Lichen sclerosus et atrophicus and sexual abuse. Arch Dis Child 1996; 75:512–516.

12 Fischer G, Rogers M. Treatment of childhood vulvar lichen sclerosus with potent topical steroid. Pediatr Dermatol 1997; 14:235–238.

13 Berkowitz CD, Elvik SL, Logan MK. Labial fusion in prepubescent girls: a marker for sexual abuse? Am J Obstet Gynecol 1987; 156: 16–20.

14 Green DM. Preserving fertility in children treated for cancer. BMJ 2001; 323:1201.

15 Davison RM, Davis CJ, Conway GS. The X chromosome and ovarian failure. Clin Endocrinol 1999; 51:673–679.

16 Verp MS, Simpson JL. Abnormal sexual differentiation and neoplasia. Cancer Genet Cytogenet 1987; 25:191–218.

17 Goodall J. Helping a girl to understand her testicular feminisation. Lancet 1991; 337: 33–35.

18 Bayer SR, DeCherney AH. Clinical manifestations and treatment of dysfunctional uterine bleeding. JAMA 1993; 269:1823–1828.

19 Higham JM, O'Brien PMS, Shaw RW. Assessment of menstrual loss using a pictorial chart. Br J Obstet Gynaecol 1990; 97:734–749.

20 Cameron IT. Dysfunctional uterine bleeding. Bailliere's Clin Obstet Gynaecol 1989; 3: 315–337.

21 Apter D, Vihko R. Hormonal patterns of adolescent cycles. J Clin Endocrinol Metab 1978; 47: 944–954.

22 Dokery CJ, Sheppard B, Daly L, Bonnar J. The fibrinolytic enzyme system in normal menstruation and excessive uterine bleeding and the effect of tranexamic acid. Obstet Gynecol Reprod Biol 1987; 24:309–318.

23 Smith SK, Abel MH, Kelly RW, Baird DT. Prostaglandin synthesis in the endometrium of women with ovular dysfunctional bleeding. Br J Obstet Gynaecol 1981; 88:434–442.

24 Krassas GE, Pontikides N, Kaltsas T, et al. Menstrual disturbances in thyrotoxicosis. Clin Endocrinol 1994; 40:641–644.

25 Prentice A. Medical management of menorrhagia. BMJ 1999; 319:1343–1345.

*26 Bonnar J, Sheppard BL. Treatment of menorrhagia during menstruation: randomised controlled trial of ethamsylate, mefenamic acid and tranexamic acid. BMJ 1996; 313: 579–582.

*27 Collaborative Group on Hormonal Factors in Breast Cancer. Breast cancer and hormonal contraceptives: collaborative re-analysis of individual data on 53 297 women with breast cancer and 100 239 women without breast cancer from 54 epidemiological studies. Lancet 1996; 347:1713–1727.

28 Klein JR, Litt IF. Epidemiology of adolescent dysmenorrhoea. Pediatrics 1981; 68: 661–664.

29 Goldstein DP, deCholnoky C, Emans SJ, Leventhal JM. Laparoscopy in the diagnosis and management of pelvic pain in adolescents. J Reprod Med 1980; 24:251–256.

30 Vercellini P, Fedele L, Arcaini L. Laparoscopy in the diagnosis of pelvic pain in adolescent women. J Reprod Med 1989; 34: 156–160.

*31 Royal College of Obstetricians and Gynaecologists. The investigation and management of endometriosis. RCOG Guideline No 24. London: RCOG; 2000.

32 Fogelman I. Gonadotropin releasing hormone agonists and the skeleton. Fertil Steril 1992; 57:715–724.

33 Surrey ES. Steroidal and nonsteroidal 'add-back' therapy: extending safety and efficacy of gonadotrophin-releasing hormone agonists in the gynacologic patient. Fertil Steril 1995; 64: 673–685.

34 Fore SR, Hammond CB, Parker RT, Anderson EE. Urologic and skeletal anomalies in patients with congenital absence of the vagina. Obstet Gynecol 1975; 46:410–416.

35 Balen A. Pathogenesis of polycystic ovary syndrome – the enigma unravels? Lancet 1999; 354:966–967.

36 Pasquali R, Casimirri F. The impact of obesity on hyperandogenism and polycystic ovary syndrome in premenopausal women. Clin Endocrinol 1993; 39:1–16.

37 Wild S, Pierpoint T, McKeigue P, Jacobs H. Cardiovascular disease in women with polycystic ovary syndrome at long-term follow-up: a retrospective cohort study. Clin Endocrinol 2000; 52:595–600.

38 Baron JJ, Baron J. Differential diagnosis of hirsutism in girls between 15 and 19 years old. Ginekol Pol 1993; 64:267–269.

39 Forward (Foundation for women's health, Research and Development). Newsletter, November 1998.

40 Black JA, Debelle GD. Female genital mutilation in Britain. BMJ 1995; 310:1590–1594.

41 Andrassy RJ, Weiner ES, Raney RB, et al. Conservative surgical management of vaginal rhabdomyosarcomas: a 25 year review from the Intergroup Rhabdomyosarcoma Study III. J Pediatr Surg 1999; 34:731–734.

42 Singh S, Darroch JE. Adolescent pregnancy and childbearing levels and trends in developed countries. Fam Plann Perspect 2000;32: 14–23.

43 Van Enke WJ, Gorissen WH, van Enk A. Teenage pregnancy and ethnicity in the Netherlands: frequency and obstetric outcome. Eur J Contracept Reprod Health Care 2000; 5:77–84.

44 Quinlivan JA, Petersen RW, Gurrin LC. Adolescent pregnancy: psychopathology missed. Aust N Z J Psych 1999; 33:864–868.

45 Henderson LR. A survey of teenage pregnant women and their male partners in the Grampian region. Br J Fam Plann 1999; 25:90–92.

46 McLeod A. Changing patterns of teenage pregnancy: population based study of small areas. BMJ 2001; 323:199–203.

47 Konje JC, Palmer A, Watson A, et al. Early teenage pregnancies in Hull. Br J Obstet Gynaecol 1992; 99:969–973.

48 Van Eyk N, Allen LM, Sermer M, Davis VJ. Obstetric outcomes of adolescent pregnancies. J Pediatr Adolesc Gynecol 2000; 13:96.

49 Smith GC, Pell JP. Teenage pregnancy and risk of adverse perinatal outcomes associated with first and second birth: population based retrospective cohort study. BMJ 2001;323:476.

24

Inborn errors of metabolism

Edited by Robert D Steiner

INTRODUCTION

THE EVIDENCE BASE

There is great emphasis in medicine in general and indeed in this text on practicing evidence-based medicine (EBM). Randomized, controlled, clinical trials (RCTs) are the currency of EBM. Unfortunately, for rare disorders like the inborn errors of metabolism (IEM), there can be great difficulties in performing RCTs. There are too few potential subjects at any one or even several centers. There is often huge clinical heterogeneity so that generalizing results of RCTs might be inappropriate. Many IEMs show only very slow progression of disease, so that RCTs might need to be performed over years, rendering them costly and unwieldy. Furthermore, there may be a perception of treatment efficacy that makes recruitment of a control group difficult. This occurs in part because treatment of the IEMs has been based to a large degree on anecdotal evidence, empiric data and theory. Lorenzo's oil for adrenoleukodystrophy and supplemental cholesterol for Smith–Lemli–Opitz are examples of 'treatments' that have been accepted in the past without any real evidence of efficacy. Still, RCTs for IEMs are not impossible to perform. Recent examples include clinical trials for enzyme replacement therapy for Fabry disease and mucopolysaccharidosis (MPS) I. These trials, however, were funded by the pharmaceutical industry and it would have been very difficult if not impossible to carry these out without that funding. Unfortunately, the pharmaceutical industry until recently has shown little interest in these rare esoteric conditions, further hindering the development of RCTs for IEMs. Still, those of us in the metabolic disease community including our funding agencies have been remiss in not working together, as the oncologists have, in carrying out clinical trials at multiple centers. To be sure, for the reasons mentioned above, RCTs for cancers may not be as fraught with difficulties as RCTs for many IEMs, but there are certainly metabolic disorders for which RCTs could be designed and carried out reasonably easily at multiple sites. The community of metabolic disease professionals should take this as a challenge.[1]

An electronic search performed in January 2003 in EBM Reviews (Cochrane Central Register of Controlled Trials), using the search parameters 'title', 'original title', 'abstract', 'mesh headings', 'heading words' and 'keyword', revealed the following results:

- inborn errors of metabolism: 2 citations
- metabolic disease; 15 citations
- amino acid disorders: no citations
- lysosomal storage diseases: no citations
- lysosomal: 56 citations.

The results of the searches were reviewed, and very few of the 56 articles using the search term 'lysosomal' were reports of RCTs in English for lysosomal storage disorders.

The results of a manual search of the *Journal of Inherited Metabolic Disease* and the *Society for the Study of Inborn Errors of Metabolism Proceedings* for randomized clinical trials and controlled clinical trials in selected metabolic diseases are outlined in Table 24.1, demonstrating that there is a paucity of published trials relating to these conditions.

Useful references

The major reference on inborn errors of metabolism now is the four-volume textbook edited by Scriver et al;[2] it is the main resource for conditions discussed in this chapter. Other review texts and texts on laboratory diagnosis of metabolic disease are by Holton,[3] Fernandes et al,[4] Blau & Blaskovics,[5] Hommes[6] and Lyon et al.[7] The text by Clarke[8] is an excellent introduction to the subject and the new texts by Gilbert-Barness[9] and Nyhan & Ozand[10] are also excellent.

On-line Mendelian Inheritance In Man (OMIM) accessed through the Internet (http://www3.ncbi.nlm.nih.gov/Omim/), provides an invaluable list of virtually all known human genetic conditions.

Other useful contacts on the Internet include Genetests and Geneclinics (http://www.geneclinics.org). http://www.kumc.edu/gec/geneinfo.html is an excellent, fairly comprehensive Website on genetic diseases with very many useful links.

Other resources include 'Children Living with Inherited Metabolic Disease' (http://www.climb.org.uk/) and the National Organization for Rare Disorders (NORD), New Fairfield, CT, USA (http://www.rarediseases.org/).

GENETIC AND BIOCHEMICAL CONSIDERATIONS

The genome influences almost all disease. In the past 30 years, the boundaries between environmental, genetic and metabolic conditions,

Table 24.1 RCTs and CCTs in metabolic diseases identified through hand-searching JIMD* and SSIEM* by condition

Condition	Number of reports of trials identified by hand-searching JIMD		Number of reports of trials identified by hand-searching SSIEM conference proceedings		Total number of reports identified	
	RCTs	CCTs	RCTs	CCTs	RCTs	CCTs
Phenylketonuria	4	9	8	12	12	21
Menkes disease	0	0	0	2	0	2
Fabry disease	0	0	0	1	0	1
Galactosemia	0	1	0	1	0	2
Galactose-1-phosphate uridytransferase deficiency	0	1	0	0	0	1
Glycogen storage disease type 1A	0	1	0	0	0	1
Familial hypercholesterolemia	0	1	0	0	0	1
Hyperornithinemia	0	0	0	1	0	1
Homocystinuria	1	2	1	1	2	3
Total	5	15	9	18	14	33

*The search was performed using the Journal fo Inherited Metabolic Disease (JIMD) 1978–2000 and the Society for the Study of Inborn Errors of Metabolism (SSIEM) Proceedings published 1981–1982, 1987–1991 and 1995–2000.
CCT, controlled clinical trial; RCT, randomized clinical trial.
(From Poustie VJ. Dietary interventions for children with chronic disease. University of Liverpool: PhD thesis; 2003.)

never very clear, have become increasingly obscure; the inclusion of some conditions in this chapter may seem arbitrary but the principles and the diagnostic approaches that apply to standard metabolic disorders also apply to an increasing array of other genetic disorders. Over 400 conditions are discussed in this chapter; others, such as the metabolic endocrinopathies (Ch. 13) and the metabolic defects of leukocytes (Ch. 21), are presented elsewhere.

The Human Genome Project is resulting in very rapid identification of genes, their location and function. Some gene mutations are common in certain populations and rare in others but even the high incidences of Tay–Sachs, Gaucher disease and mild congenital adrenal hyperplasia in Ashkenazi Jews are caused by several different mutations, raising questions not only of founder effects but also of selective advantages. Expression of an enzyme activity usually represents the sum of the effect of two alleles. In Figure 24.1 the contribution of each allele is indicated (0–50) and the total enzyme activity is shown as a percentage. The mother (I-2) is heterozygous for an allele producing a non-functional protein and I-1 is heterozygous for a minor mutant. Individuals such as I-3, who is a compound heterozygote with 11% of residual function, might be totally asymptomatic, be mildly affected or may only exhibit problems when the enzyme is stressed. Such heterogeneity results in 0–100% of normal activity, giving rise to severe or mild cases of a disorder even within a single pedigree.

Methods to measure the biological activity of a protein in vitro usually involve highly unphysiological conditions so that the results do not always reflect the in vivo activity. For example, most assays for lysosomal diseases use artificial substrates. Occasionally healthy people have no activity against an artificial substrate in vitro. Conversely, it is possible to have normal activity against an artificial substrate in vitro but no activity against the natural substrate in vivo. Enzyme assays usually use very high levels of substrate or cofactor and it is probable that some mutant enzymes can give normal activity under such conditions in vitro although not in vivo (abnormal Km mutants). An example of this is seen in some vitamin-dependent diseases, when large doses of the vitamin cofactor improve the function of the enzyme. Similarly, the epitope of antibodies used in immunological assays may not involve the active site of the enzyme; immunological crossreactivity can therefore be present even though a mutant protein is functionally defective. Conversely a mutant protein can be functional but immunologically non-reactive.

Many enzymes have several distinct chemical forms in different tissues where different operating conditions may exist. Such *isoenzymes* may share some subunits but others are under separate genetic control. It is thus possible for a defect to occur in one tissue while normal activity is present in others. This must be remembered when leukocytes or cultured skin fibroblasts are used to diagnose an enzyme defect which is suspected to be present in other tissues. A further confounding fact is that some enzymes derive from a single gene but are matured to different forms in different tissues; an example is seen with an unusual form of acute intermittent porphyria in which the erythrocyte isoform is normal but the enzyme is deficient in the liver.

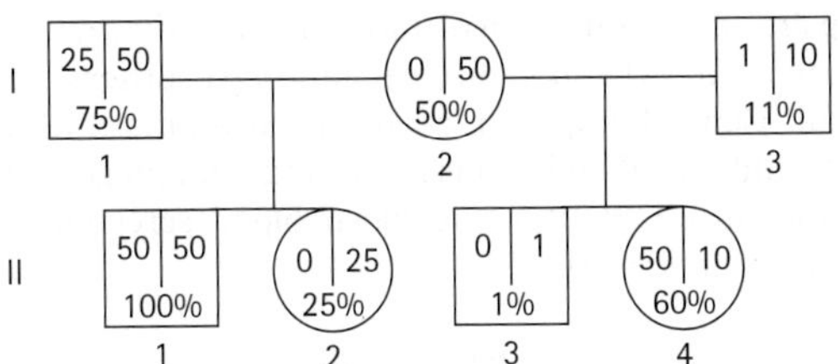

Fig. 24.1 Hypothetical pedigree showing the contribution of different mutant alleles to the total activity of an enzyme which is indicated as a percentage of the normal. Each normal allele contributes 50% of total normal function as seen in II-1. The index case II-3 has only 1% of normal activity. Case I-3 and even case II-2 might, under some circumstances, show evidence of the defect.

The potential metabolic consequences of an enzyme deficiency are illustrated in Figure 24.2. In phenylketonuria (PKU), for example, the metabolic derangements include inhibition of amino acid transport into brain cells, diminished synthesis of myelin and the aromatic amines and inhibition of normal pyruvate metabolism, but it is not known how the brain damage is actually caused. Phenotypic variations even within a single family are presumed to be due to different environmental exposures or to inherited differences in the other metabolic steps which are affected by the biochemical upset. Genotype/phenotype correlations are proving to be very difficult to predict.[11]

Heterozygotes

Since heterozygotes should produce reduced amounts of the normal protein, most usually show a mild biochemical abnormality if a specific test can be devised. For example, carriers of maple syrup urine disease have normal plasma amino acid levels and cannot be detected by amino acid tolerance tests, but reduced enzyme activity can be shown in their leukocytes with sensitive techniques. On the other hand, 80% of carriers for PKU can be identified by the phenylalanine:tyrosine ratio in fasting plasma or a phenylalanine tolerance test.

Inheritance patterns

Most metabolic defects are recessively inherited. In this chapter, the genetics of each condition will not necessarily be discussed unless they vary from this pattern.

CLINICAL CONSIDERATIONS

Incidences

At least 1–2% of individuals have a pathogenic metabolic disorder of which most, such as hyperuricemia and the hyperlipidemias, are of little clinical importance in childhood. Almost all of the conditions in this chapter are rare (~1:100 000–1:250 000); many are extremely rare (10^6–10^7). However, if there are 1000 diseases each occurring only one in a million, 1:1000 people will have one of them and for *each* of these conditions, 1:500 is a carrier! This rarity constitutes a major diagnostic stumbling block for clinicians.[12–14]

The commonest reasons for referral to our metabolic clinic in descending order are:

- suspected or confirmed lactic acidosis;
- suspected or confirmed metabolic neurological disorders, including non-specific development delay;

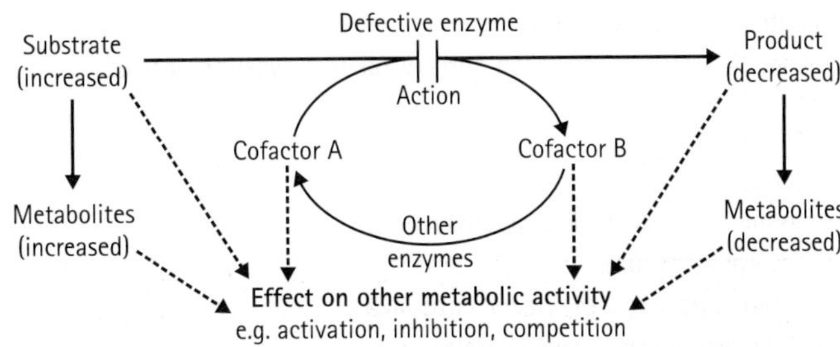

Fig. 24.2 Theoretical consequences of an enzyme deficiency.

- metabolic bone disease such as rickets (usually vitamin D resistant, X-linked hypophosphatemia);
- abnormal results from newborn screening;
- suspected or confirmed porphyria;
- failure to thrive or to grow;
- acute 'metabolic' crisis;
- visceromegaly.

CLINICAL FEATURES

Metabolic disorders should always be considered when patients present with puzzling or unexplained problems whether of growth, development or of specific organ pathology. They can disrupt the function of any organ and may present at any age to specialists in any clinical discipline. It is therefore impossible to prepare a comprehensive guide to assist in recognizing all these disorders, but some of the more usual characteristics of metabolic disorders are displayed in Table 24.2.

Metabolic screening

Because of this diversity and the fact that the symptoms of inborn errors of metabolism mimic non-genetic disorders, some kind of 'metabolic screen' is frequently done on blood or urine of potential cases in the hope that an abnormality may assist in the diagnosis. This screening is different from the newborn screen and varies in different centers but usually includes tests for sugars, MPS, amino acids and a variety of other compounds. Sometimes, organic acids and carnitine derivatives are included. It must always be remembered that these are only screening tests and that many disorders cannot be detected by them. In most centers, the cost of such testing is less than that of a computerized tomography (CT) scan.

Large-scale metabolic screening in subjects with neurodevelopmental delay and learning difficulties has led to the discovery of many new defects. Most are rare and the clinical variation even in diseases such as PKU can be considerable. When an unusual defect is associated with clinical symptoms it is tempting to assume that they are causally related. However, it is now clear that some are not consistently associated with clinical disease. Amino acid disorders once thought to cause neurodevelopmental delay but now considered probably benign include cystathioninuria, methionine adenosyl transferase deficiency, some hyperlysinemias, saccharopinuria, 2-ketoadipic aciduria, sarcosinemia, hyperprolinemia, hydroxyprolinemia, histidinemia, carnosinemia, urocanic aciduria, and beta-aminoisobutyricaciduria.

Table 24.2 Some common presentations of metabolic diseases

Neonatal symptoms – see Ch. 10
CNS symptoms
Developmental delay – static or progressive
Movement or psychiatric disorder
Seizures, neuropathy
Cerebral palsy – athetoid, ataxic, spastic, hypotonic
Growth failure/failure to thrive
Episodic symptoms such as anorexia, vomiting, lethargy, coma
Gastrointestinal – anorexia, vomiting, diarrhea, malabsorption
Hepatocellular damage/visceromegaly
Renal dysfunction – Fanconi syndrome, calculi
Ophthalmic – keratitis, cataracts, buphthalmos, retinopathy, optic atrophy
Auditory – nerve deafness
Muscular – cramps, myoglobinuria, weakness, wasting, loss of endurance
Cardiomyopathy
Osteodystrophies
Immune defects – leukocyte dysfunction
Dysmorphic features
Dermatologic – rashes, ulcers, cutis laxa
Metabolic acidosis, hypoglycemia

GENERAL THERAPEUTIC CONSIDERATIONS

Roughly 12% of metabolic diseases are markedly ameliorated by therapy; in about 54% treatment is partially effective, but in the remainder (34%), treatment has little effect.[15] These percentages continue to improve over the years, although the 12% of disorders markedly ameliorated has not changed significantly. The only treatment for most enzyme defects is either to induce activity, as in the vitamin-responsive conditions, or to counteract the biochemical disturbance by diet or, occasionally, with drug therapy. Enzyme replacement therapy is beginning to play a role. There is no assurance, however, that correction of the biochemical defect in some conditions will improve the symptoms since their basic cause is often not completely understood (Fig. 24.2). For example, in the Lesch–Nyhan syndrome, the blood urate is easily controlled with allopurinol, but the neurological symptoms are unchanged.

Parenteral administration of a protein requires that it must arrive at the site where it can function normally. Attempts to replace intracellular enzymes present formidable problems. In the first place, there must be adequate supplies of a stable, active product, which is non-allergenic. Secondly, the target cells must be able to take up the protein into the appropriate organelle, such as a lysosome, where it can function without being destroyed. Treatment of Hurler syndrome with infusions of fresh plasma is ineffective, which is not unexpected, but it is disappointing since cultured fibroblasts from Hurler and Hunter syndromes are mutually corrective in vitro. When some other lysosomal enzymes are infused, they are rapidly taken up by the liver, but not by the central nervous system (CNS). Infusion of genetically engineered human beta-glucosidase is dramatically effective in Gaucher disease but can cost more than *£50 000/year*. Similar therapy is in development (and approved for use in many European countries) for Fabry disease which lowers the abnormal plasma lipid and reduces symptoms. Experimental therapies for other lysosomal storage diseases are in clinical trials. Bone marrow transplantation offers the possibility of 'cure' of lysosomal disorders. While some reports are encouraging, the long term benefit is not known. Substrate inhibitors show promise as potential new therapies for lysosomal storage diseases (see pp. 1231). Liver transplantation for hepatocellular disorders, such as tyrosinemia type 1, alpha-1 antitrypsin deficiency, ornithine transcarbamylase (OTC) deficiency and Wilson's disease amongst others, has been successful. Gene therapy for adenosine deaminase deficiency is currently under trial and seems promising but real gene therapy is still in the future. Routine newborn blood screening tests are discussed in Chapter 10.

PEROXISOMAL DISORDERS

PEROXISOMES

Peroxisomes are single membrane-bound organelles found in most eukaryotic cells and are responsible for a variety of essential metabolic functions. Biosynthetic activities include synthesis of plasmalogens, which are important components of cell membranes and myelin, cholesterol, bile acids, glyoxylate and docosahexanoic acid (DHA). Additionally, two aminotransferases involved in gluconeogenesis are located in liver peroxisomes. Catabolic functions include H_2O_2-based cellular respiration, purine and pipecolic acid catabolism, alpha-oxidation of branched chain fatty acids (phytanic acid) and beta-oxidation of very long chain fatty acids (VLCFA; carbon chain > 22).[16,17]

Peroxisomal disorders can be classified into two categories: peroxisome biogenesis disorders (PBDs), which are associated with a general loss of peroxisomal function, and disorders associated with single enzyme deficiencies.

PEROXISOME BIOGENESIS DISORDERS

Clinical features

PBDs are a group of autosomal recessive genetic disorders with an incidence of approximately 1:50 000 which result from defects in peroxisome assembly.[16] Peroxisomes may be absent microscopically, or they may be in the form of 'peroxisome ghosts', remnant membrane structures which lack normal matrix enzymes. Clinically, this group of disorders is composed of three disorders which share clinical and biochemical features and represent a spectrum of disease severity: Zellweger syndrome (ZS), neonatal adrenoleukodystrophy (NALD) and infantile Refsum disease (IRD). Rhizomelic chondrodysplasia punctata (RCDP) is considered a partial PBD, with clinical and biochemical differences from the Zellweger spectrum of disorders.

ZS (cerebrohepatorenal syndrome) is the most severe phenotype and is characterized by neonatal hypotonia, seizures, psychomotor retardation, feeding difficulties, hepatomegaly, renal cysts, sensorineural deafness, and developmental brain abnormalities such as polymicrogyria, heterotopias and agenesis of the corpus callosum. Ocular abnormalities include corneal clouding, cataracts, glaucoma, nystagmus and pigmentary retinopathy. Characteristic craniofacial dysmorphism includes a high forehead, large fontanelles, midface hypoplasia, shallow orbital ridges, hypertelorism with upslanting palpebral fissures and epicanthal folds, posteriorly rotated ears with abnormal helices, anteverted nares and micrognathia. There is often radiographic stippling of epiphyses, most prominent in the patellar and acetabular areas. Pathological evaluation reveals absence of liver and kidney peroxisomes. Prolonged neonatal jaundice and liver disease[17–19] often complicate the neonatal period. Death usually occurs within the first year.

NALD and IRD are progressively milder clinical phenotypes. Infants with NALD show similar but less pronounced dysmorphic features as those seen in ZS. However, renal cysts, cataracts, and epiphyseal stippling are absent. In addition to neuronal migration abnormalities, a demyelinating process often occurs. Patients with NALD may initially show relatively normal development, followed by regression. NALD is also characterized by adrenal dysfunction, as well as liver disease. Of note, NALD is a completely separate disease entity from X-linked adrenoleukodystrophy (X-ALD), which is also associated with adrenal disease. While survival is increased relative to ZS, and may extend into the teen years, surviving children typically exhibit severe neurodevelopmental delay, with sensorineural hearing loss and blindness due to pigmentary retinopathy.[16]

IRD is characterized by often subtle dysmorphic facial features including midface hypoplasia, failure to thrive, hypotonia, psychomotor retardation, sensorineural deafness, pigmentary retinopathy, and neuronal migration abnormalities. There is no overt demyelination as seen in NALD. Occasionally, children with IRD present with bleeding due to a vitamin K-responsive coagulopathy.

RCDP has a different clinical presentation and is associated with more limited enzyme deficiencies. RCDP is associated with defects in only two peroxisomal metabolic functions: plasmalogen biosynthesis and branched chain fatty acid oxidation.[16] The most striking difference between RCDP and the Zellweger spectrum disorders is the presence of skeletal abnormalities which include rhizomelia (shortening of the proximal limbs), short stature, coronal clefts of vertebrae, metaphyseal splaying, kyphoscoliosis, joint contractures, and calcific stippling which disappears within the first year of life. As with the other PBDs, there is also characteristic facial dysmorphism, cataracts, sensorineural deafness, psychomotor retardation and feeding difficulty with severe failure to thrive. The majority of children with RCDP die before 2 years of age.

RCDP can be further classified based on enzymatic deficiency as type 1, 2 or 3. All types share a similar phenotype, however. Type 1 is associated with a peroxisomal receptor defect (PTS2) and deficiency of at least three peroxisomal enzymes; types 2 and 3 are each associated with single enzyme defects, dihydroxyacetone phosphate (DHAP) acyltransferase (DHAPAT), and alkyl-DHAP synthase, respectively.

Biochemical features

All disorders of peroxisome biogenesis share the same biochemical abnormalities, to varying degrees: elevations of plasma VLCFAs, phytanic and pipecolic acids, and decreased plasmalogen and DHA. Biochemical abnormalities seen in RCDP include elevated plasma phytanic acid and deficiency of erythrocyte plasmalogen. See Table 24.3 for a comparison of biochemical features.

Molecular genetics of peroxisome biogenesis disorders

PBDs are a genetically heterogeneous group, characterized by defects in peroxisome formation and global deficiencies of peroxisomal enzyme function. Cell fusion studies have established at least 12 complementation groups associated with the Zellweger spectrum, and a single complementation group associated with RCDP.[20] The genetic defect is now established in 11 of these complementation groups.[17] There are 11 PEX genes known to date which encode peroxisomal membrane proteins, targeting signals and receptors that are required for peroxisome assembly and protein importation.[16] Approximately 65% of patients with PBD have mutations in PEX1. A complete lack of PEX1 protein is associated with the Zellweger phenotype, while residual amounts are found in patients with NALD and IRD.[21]

Table 24.3 Biochemical abnormalities in selected peroxisomal disorders

	Plasma VLCFA	Plasma phytanic acid	RBC plasmalogen
Peroxisome biogenesis disorders (ZS, NALD, IRD)	Increased	Increased	Decreased
Rhizomelic chondrodysplasia punctata	Normal	Increased (type 1) Normal (types 2 and 3)	Decreased
X-ALD/AMN	Increased	Normal	Normal
Refsum disease (classical)	Normal	Increased	Normal

AMN, adrenomyeloneuropathy; IRD, infantile Refsum disease; NALD, neonatal adrenoleukodystrophy; VLCFA, very long chain fatty acid; X-ALD, X-linked adrenoleukodystrophy; ZS, Zellweger syndrome

Diagnosis

The possibility of a peroxisome biogenesis disorder should be considered in any infant with hypotonia and psychomotor retardation, particularly in association with retinopathy, sensorineural hearing loss and/or characteristic dysmorphic features. Specifically, these disorders should be considered in infants with both hearing loss and visual deficit.

The single most useful screening test is the measurement of plasma VLCFA, which is increased in all of the disorders of peroxisome biogenesis, but is normal in RCDP. Additional assays of plasma phytanic acid, pipecolic acid, plasmalogen, bile acid intermediates and essential fatty acids may also be useful in characterizing the metabolic status of the patient, but abnormalities of phytanic acid and plasmalogen may be age dependent.[16] Definitive diagnosis may require enzymatic studies in cultured fibroblasts, particularly in the differentiation of generalized PBD from a single enzyme defect, or in the characterization of RCDP.

Therapy

Treatment of individuals with PBDs has remained largely supportive and symptomatic, allowing for the prenatal onset of the multiple congenital anomalies present in PBDs. Bleeding tendencies may require treatment with vitamin K. Adrenal insufficiency may warrant correction with steroids. However, as individuals with milder phenotypes are surviving longer, there is active research into possible primary treatment. Because patients with PBDs have low levels of DHA, an important component of brain and retina, oral administration of DHA ethyl ester has been studied. In an open label study of 20 patients with PBD receiving daily doses of 100–500 mg of DHA ethyl ester, Martinez[22] reported normalization of DHA levels in plasma and erythrocytes, decrease in plasma VLCFA, improvement in liver function, vision improvement in half, and magnetic resonance imaging (MRI) findings suggestive of improvement in myelination. Unfortunately, randomized, controlled trials are lacking, and these initial promising results, level of evidence 4, must be interpreted with caution.[23] Another area of promising research involves the pharmacological induction of peroxisome number with sodium 4-phenylbutyrate (4PBA). In vitro studies of fibroblasts cells from PBD patients, as well as controls, showed a two- to threefold increase in peroxisome number cell lines treated with 4PBA. This correlated with an increase in peroxisome function, but only in NALD and IRD cells.[24]

DISORDERS ASSOCIATED WITH ISOLATED ENZYME DEFICIENCIES

While the enzymatic reactions localized to the peroxisome are numerous, there are currently recognized pathogenic disorders involving five primary metabolic pathways: fatty acid beta-oxidation, phytanic acid alpha-oxidation, etherphospholipid synthesis, isoprenoid synthesis and glyoxylate detoxification. Table 24.4 summarizes the clinical and screening biochemical abnormalities associated with the best characterized disorders in this group. The two most common disorders, X-ALD and Refsum disease, will be specifically discussed below.

X-LINKED ADRENOLEUKODYSTROPHY

Clinical features

X-ALD is an X-linked disease with an incidence in males of between 1:20 000 and 1:50 000. There are several distinct phenotypes, all of which can be seen within the same family. Childhood cerebral X-ALD accounts for approximately 35% of cases. It occurs in childhood with progressive neurological deterioration characterized by seizures, nystagmus, vision and hearing impairments, behavior and memory problems, and decreased school performance.

Table 24.4 Peroxisomal disorders due to single enzyme deficiencies

Metabolic pathway affected	Disorder	Clinical phenotype	Screening biochemical abnormality
Fatty acid beta-oxidation	X-ALD/AMN	Progressive neurodegeneration, adrenal insufficiency, myeloneuropathy (see text)	Increased VLCFA
	Acyl-CoA oxidase deficiency (OMIM 264470) Thiolase deficiency (OMIM 261510) Bifunctional protein deficiency (OMIM 261515)	NALD-like	Increased VLCFA
	2-methylacyl-CoA racemase deficiency (OMIM 604489)	Late onset neuropathy	
Phytanic acid oxidation	Refsum disease (OMIM 266500)	Retinitis pigmentosa, cerebellar ataxia, polyneuropathy	Increased phytanic acid
Etherphospholipid synthesis	DHAPAT synthase deficiency (OMIM 222765) Alkyl DHAP synthase deficiency (OMIM 600121)	RCDP	Decreased RBC plasmalogen
Isoprenoid synthesis	Mevalonate kinase deficiency (OMIM 251170)	Dysmorphic features, hepatosplenomegaly, hypotonia, cerebral atrophy, failure to thrive	Increased urinary mevalonic acid
Glyoxylate detoxification	Hyperoxaluria type 1 (OMIM 259900)	Recurrent nephrolithiasis and nephrocalcinosis	Increased urinary oxalic, glyoxylic and glycolic acids

AMN, adrenomyeloneuropathy; DHAP, dihydroxyacetone phosphate; DHAPAT, DHAP acyltransferase; NALD, neonatal adrenoleukodystrophy; OMIM, On-Line Mendelian Inheritance in Man; RCDP, rhizomelic chondrodysplasia punctata; VLCFA, very long chain fatty acid; X-ALD, X-linked adrenoleukodystrophy

Development is normal prior to the onset of neurological symptoms, typically between 4 and 8 years. School difficulty, behavioral disturbances and vision impairment are the most frequently reported initial symptoms.[25] As the disease progresses, dementia, blindness and quadriplegia develop, and death results. Adrenal insufficiency is present in at least 90%.[25] This rapidly progressive cerebral form is associated with an inflammatory, demyelinating process in the white matter, a leukodystrophy.

The second phenotype, adrenomyeloneuropathy (AMN) accounts for 35–40% of cases and presents either with Addison's disease or with signs of myelopathy with progressive polyneuropathy and bladder dysfunction in the second or third decade of life. Less common phenotypes include adults with adrenal insufficiency but without neurological abnormalities, adults who develop cerebral symptoms without evidence of myelopathy, and neurological abnormalities in approximately 15% of heterozygous females that can be confused with multiple sclerosis.

X-ALD is caused by a defect of X-ALD-protein (ALDP), a peroxisomal membrane adenosine triphosphate (ATP)-binding cassette transporter and is associated with increased levels of VLCFA in blood and tissues. The basis of the intrafamilial phenotypic variability is unknown, as there appears to be no genotype–phenotype correlation associated with mutations within the X-ALD gene.

Diagnosis

The diagnosis of X-ALD in affected males can be made by the measurement of elevated plasma VLCFA in the appropriate clinical scenario. Plasma VLCFA should therefore be measured in males of any age who develop Addison's disease. In heterozygous females, plasma VLCFA may be normal in 15%, so DNA analysis is required in some cases.[25] Approximately 85% of patients with the childhood cerebral form have characteristic abnormalities on brain MRI consisting of symmetric areas of increased signal in the parieto-occipital region on T2-weighted imaging.[25]

Therapy

Stem cell (bone marrow or cord blood) transplantation, if performed early in the course of the disease at the very earliest sign of CNS symptoms, has been shown to stabilize the progression of cerebral X-ALD. In a recent 5–10 year follow-up study of 12 patients with childhood onset cerebral X-ALD who had undergone bone marrow transplantation early in the course of the disease, Shapiro et al[26] showed MRI evidence for stabilization or even reversal of demyelination. Eight of the 12 children were functioning normally in school with no additional support. At this time, transplantation prior to the onset of any neurological signs or symptoms cannot be recommended since a fair proportion of affected males will not develop neurological symptoms, even without treatment. While oral therapy with 'Lorenzo's oil' (a 4:1 mixture of glyceryl trioleate and glyceryl trierucate) has been shown to normalize plasma concentrations of VLCFA in patients with X-ALD, the lack of well-controlled clinical studies has limited conclusions regarding clinical efficacy.[27] Studies have shown little effect of Lorenzo's oil in changing the course of cerebral forms of X-ALD, and a recent study showed no improvement in neurological or endocrine function when used in the treatment of milder forms.[28] Adverse effects include thrombocytopenia, and elevated liver enzymes.

New therapeutic approaches are currently under investigation, based on the observations of an improved ability of cultured fibroblasts derived from X-ALD patients to metabolize VLCFA in the presence of two agents, lovastatin and 4-phenylbutyrate. Two small open label observational studies have been published on the efficacy of lovastatin/simvastatin, but these failed to show clinical benefit, along with inconsistent reduction in plasma VLCFA.[29,30] There are currently no published randomized controlled trials.

REFSUM DISEASE

Clinical features

The cardinal manifestations of Refsum disease include retinitis pigmentosa, cerebellar ataxia and polyneuropathy.[31] The onset of symptoms is usually insidious and often begins with night blindness due to pigmentary retinopathy. The age of onset is very variable, ranging from childhood to the third or fourth decades. However, up to 40% of patients develop symptoms prior to 10 years of age and up to 75% by age 20.[31] The sensory-motor polyneuropathy associated with Refsum disease typically begins in the distal lower extremities and, if untreated, progresses to involve the upper extremities and trunk. Ataxia and cerebellar dysfunction usually become evident later than the retinal degeneration and polyneuropathy. Additional clinical features can include sensorineural hearing loss, anosmia, cardiac conduction abnormalities and cardiomyopathy and skeletal manifestations (epiphyseal dysplasia, shortening or elongation of the third or fourth metatarsals, hammer toes). Cardiomyopathy is a frequent cause of sudden death in untreated patients.

The underlying metabolic etiology for Refsum disease is a deficiency of phytanoyl-coenzyme A (CoA) hydroxylase, an enzyme that catalyzes an essential step in phytanic acid degradation. Deficiency of this enzyme results in the accumulation of phytanic acid. While the pathogenesis of Refsum disease has not been conclusively established, there is evidence that phytanic acid may play a role in modulation of gene expression.[31]

Therapy

Because phytanic acid is dietary in origin, therapy focuses on diets low in phytanic acid. Dietary intervention has resulted in stabilization or improvement in the peripheral neuropathy, auditory and visual deficits, changing the natural history of the disease.[31] In cases where plasma levels of phytanic acid are very high (> 100 mg/dl), plasmapheresis may be indicated to reduce levels more rapidly.

PURINE AND PYRIMIDINE DISORDERS

BACKGROUND

Purine and pyrimidine disorders were first reported in the 1950s as a cause of childhood nephrolithiasis. In 1967, the biochemical and enzymatic basis of a hereditary gout syndrome associated with severe neurological disease in children was reported, the Lesch–Nyhan syndrome.[32] Today, more than 25 defects of purine and pyrimidine metabolism have been identified, encompassing pediatric and adulthood disease entities. The extent of phenotypic (and genotypic) heterogeneity in these disorders is significant and they can present diagnostic conundrums for the clinician since they affect numerous systems, including hematological, neurological, musculoskeletal and renal. This phenotypic heterogeneity may relate to the integral position that the enzymes of purine and pyrimidine metabolism occupy in intermediary metabolism, providing the structural intermediates of DNA, RNA, cyclic nucleotides, purine sugars and pterins.

DISORDERS OF PURINE METABOLISM – CLINICAL FEATURES

Several of the disorders of purine biosynthesis (Fig. 24.3) present with marked hematological abnormalities. Adenosine deaminase (ADA) deficiency presents classically with severe combined

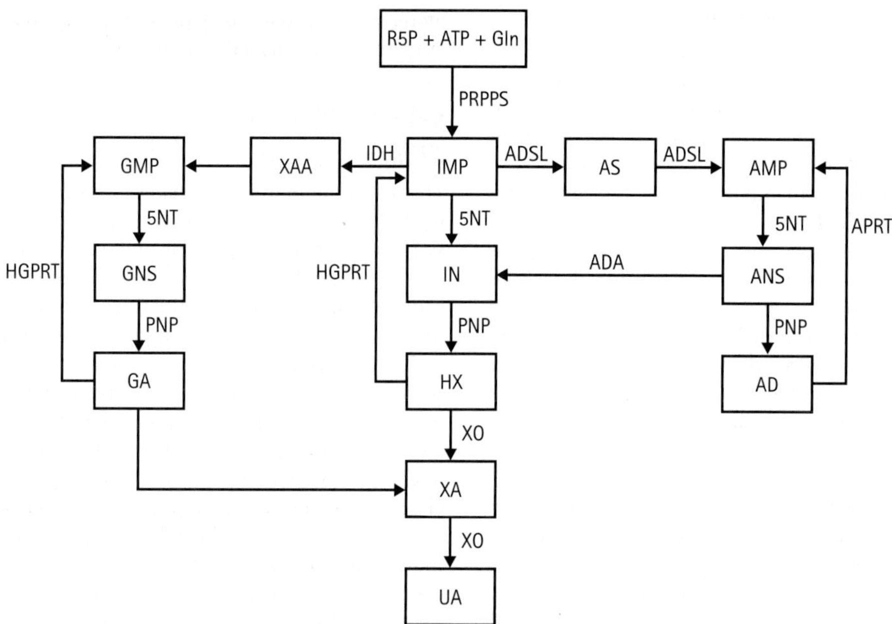

Fig. 24.3 Schematic overview of purine metabolism (not all steps are shown). R5P, ribose-5-phosphate; Gln, glutamine; PRPPS, phosphoribosylpyrophosphate synthetase; IMP, inosine monophosphate; 5NT, 5'-nucleotidase; IN, inosine; HX, hypoxanthine; XO, xanthine oxidase; XA, xanthine; UA, uric acid; ADSL, adenylosuccinate lyase; AS, adenylosuccinate; AMP, adenosine monophosphate; ANS, adenosine; PNP, purine nucleoside phosphorylase; AD, adenine; APRT, adenine phosphoribosyl transferase; ADA, adenosine deaminase; IDH, IMP dehydrogenase; XAA, xanthylic acid; GMP, guanosine monophosphate; GNS, guanosine; GA, guanine; HGPRT, hypoxanthine guanine phosphoribosyl transferase.

immunodeficiency (see Ch. 25) and lymphopenia.[33,34] Similarly, purine nucleoside phosphorylase deficiency manifests clinically with isolated T cell deficiency and predominantly normal immunoglobulins. Patients with both disorders are subject to unrelenting infection (candidiasis, varicella, etc.). For the remaining disorders of purine metabolism, the clinical picture features predominantly neurological and renal abnormalities, but may also involve the musculoskeletal system as well.

Patients with xanthine oxidase/dehydrogenase deficiency and the combined xanthine oxidase/sulfite oxidase or xanthine dehydrogenase/aldehyde oxidase deficiencies present with psychomotor retardation, convulsions and xanthine lithiasis owing to the extreme insolubility of xanthine.[35–37] In general, acute renal failure is the long term outcome. Purine precipitation in the lens can lead to ocular lens dissociation. Classical hypoxanthine-guanine phosphoribosyl transferase (HGPRT) deficiency (Lesch–Nyhan syndrome), an X-linked disorder, is a severe neurological disease that can manifest as cerebral palsy, including choreoathetosis, hypotonicity, self-injurious behavior and spastic quadriplegia. Uric acid accumulation may lead to crystalluria and acute renal failure. Similar findings may be seen in the Kelley-Seegmiller syndrome, where there remains partial activity of HGPRT.[38–41]

Adenine phosphoribosyl transferase (APRT) deficiency features a predominantly renal phenotype, with acute renal failure associated with lithiasis linked to the extreme insolubility of 2,8-dihydroxyadenine (2,8-DHA).[42] Calculi lead to a common complaint of abdominal and pelvic pain, recurrent urinary tract infection and hematuria. Similar features of gout and uric acid lithiasis can be seen in patients with phosphoribosyl pryophosphate (PRPP) synthetase hyperactivity. Patients invariably manifest developmental delay and ataxia, with dysmorphic appearance. Hereditary hearing loss may be associated with PRPP synthetase overactivity. Adenylosuccinate lyase (ADSL) deficiency features a clinical picture of psychomotor retardation, epilepsy and autism which may be associated with cerebellar hypoplasia.[43,44] Patients with ADSL deficiency accumulate a unique compound, succinylaminoimidazole carboximide riboside (so-called SAICAR) which can be identified by sensitive high pressure liquid chromatography (HPLC) methods, or more routinely identified using standard amino acid chromatography in the screening laboratory. In the latter, hydrolysis of urine samples with base leads to increases of aspartate and glycine related to SAICAR.

The remaining defects of purine metabolism exemplify the heterogeneity of these diseases. Myoadenylate deaminase (MDA) deficiency features musculoskeletal findings including muscle cramps, exercise intolerance and elevated creatine kinase activity, often associated with rheumatological disease.[45] Thiopurine methyltransferase (TPMT) catalyzes the conversion of thio-inosine monophosphate (IMP) to methylthio-IMP. Deficiency of TPMT does not become 'disease' until treatment of the patient with thiopurines, thus making TPMT deficiency a 'pharmacogenetic' disease.[46]

DISORDERS OF PYRIMIDINE METABOLISM – CLINICAL FEATURES

Disorders of pyrimidine metabolism (Fig. 24.4) are fewer than those of the purine pathway, but manifest a similar degree of phenotypic/genotypic heterogeneity. Three disease entities affect metabolism of uridine monophosphate (UMP), including UMP synthetase (UMPS) deficiency, UMP hydrolase 1 (UMPH 1) deficiency and UMP hydrolase (UMPH) superactivity.[32] UMPS deficiency is primarily a hematological disease, including megaloblastic anemia and T cell immunodeficiency (reminiscent of ADA deficiency), failure to thrive, crystalluria and intractable diarrhea. The offending compound in kidney is orotic acid. Similarly, UMPH 1 deficiency shows a characteristic non-spherocytic hemolytic anemia with basophilic stippling. Patients with UMPH superactivity manifest neurological sequelae, including developmental delays, seizures, hyperactivity and recurrent infection.

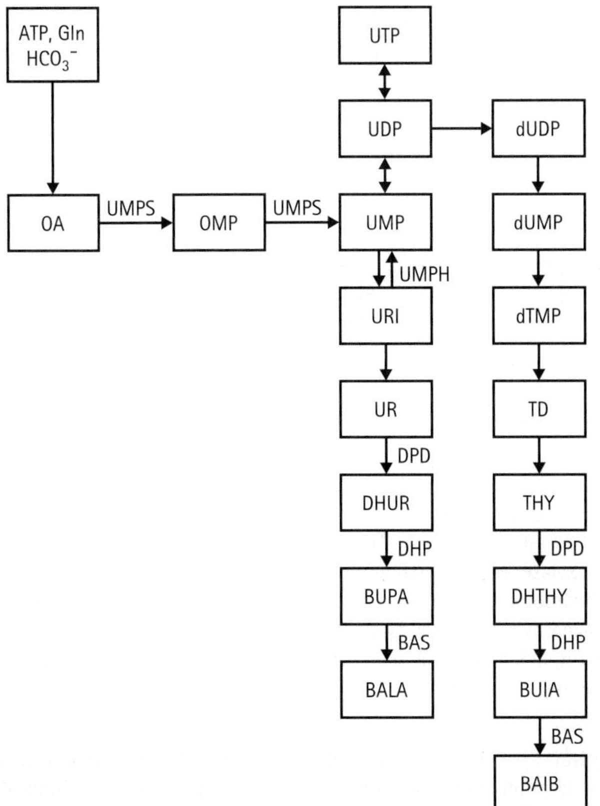

Fig. 24.4 Schematic diagram of pyrimidine catabolism (not all steps are shown). Gln, glutamine; OA, orotic acid; UMPS, uridine monophosphate synthetase; OMP, orotidine monophosphate; UMP, uridine monophosphate; UDP, uridine diphosphate; UTP, uridine triphosphate; dUDP, deoxyuridine diphosphate; dUMP, deoxyuridine monophosphate; UMPH, uridine monophosphate hydrolase; URI, uridine; dTMP, deoxythymidine monophosphate; UR, uracil; TD, thymidine; DPD, dihydropyrimidine dehydrogenase; THY, thymine; DHUR, dihydrouracil; DHP, dihydropyrimidinase (dihydropyrimidine amidohydrolase); DHTHY, dihydrothymine; BUPA, beta-ureidopropionic acid; BUIA, beta-ureidoisobutyric acid; BAS, beta-alanine synthase; BALA, beta-alanine; BAIB, beta-aminoisobutyric acid.

One of the more common defects of pyrimidine metabolism is dihydropyrimidine dehydrogenase (DPD) deficiency.[47] Phenotypically, neurological findings include psychomotor retardation, seizures, microcephaly, feeding difficulties, autistic features and hypertonia. DPD deficiency is another instance of 'pharmacogenetic' disease, in that treatment with the common anticancer 5-fluorouracil (5-FU) in patients with previously unrecognized DPD deficiency can lead to severe 5-FU toxicity.[48] Dihydropyrimidine amidohydrolase (DHP) deficiency also features a severe neurological disease with microcephaly, psychomotor retardation, spastic quadriplegia and seizures. Both DPD and DHP deficiencies manifest 'thymine/uraciluria', with accumulation of dihydrothymine and dihydrouracil in DHP deficiency. Thymine and uracil are detected using routine gas chromatography-mass spectrometry, or more accurately quantified employing HPLC.[47,48]

The final known disorders of pyrimidine metabolism are quite rare. In ureidopropionase deficiency (beta-alanine synthase; BAS) deficiency, the clinical picture of optic atrophy, dystonia and severe mental retardation is accompanied by excretion of the unusual metabolites beta-ureidopropionate and beta-ureidoisobutyrate.[49] These species can be detected by nuclear magnetic resonance (NMR) analysis, as well as using routine amino acid analysis with hydrolysis of the urine sample. Thymidine phosphorylase (TP) deficiency is a predominantly mitochondrial disorder featuring neurogastrointestinal myopathy (so called MNGIE, or mitochondrial neuropathy, gastrointestinal encephalomyopathy; see Mitochondrial disease section, p. 1219).[50]

DIAGNOSIS AND TREATMENT

Diagnostically, the defects of purine and pyrimidine metabolism can pose a significant challenge and sample referral must often be made to a handful of diagnostic specialist laboratories equipped for measurement of appropriate metabolites. Measurement of uric acid in urine may lead to suspicion, but complications of renal failure may cloud the diagnosis. Adequate, age related control ranges for uric acid must be established, since dietary intake of purines vary considerably around the world, and purine analogs are found in a number of foodstuffs (i.e. caffeine). Disorders associated with accumulation of insoluble purine bases (uric acid, xanthine and 2,8-DHA) should be included in the differential of the child presenting with acute coma or renal failure. Renal ultrasound may be invaluable in identification of crystal nephropathy (especially following acute infection).

Unfortunately, only a handful of the above disorders are amenable to treatment. Patients with hereditary orotic aciduria (UMPS deficiency) may be treated with uridine, and APRT deficient patients respond to allopurinol.[32] For the latter, tapering doses must be considered in end-stage renal failure. Treatment of ADA deficiency is via bone marrow transplantation or enzyme replacement therapy employing polyethylene glycol (PEG)-associated ADA; however, the latter may be cost prohibitive.[33] An alternate (and less expensive) approach is enzyme replacement therapy using erythrocyte encapsulated ADA. Limited reports have suggested clinical efficacy of ribose intervention for multiple acyl-Coenzyme A deficiency (MAD) and ADSL deficiencies.

NEUROTRANSMITTER DISORDERS

BACKGROUND – METABOLISM AND FUNCTION OF BIOGENIC AMINES

Biogenic amines include the catecholamines (dopamine, epinephrine and norepinephrine) and serotonin, which are derived from tyrosine and tryptophan via the activities of tyrosine and tryptophan hydroxylases (Figs 24.5 and 24.6).[51,52] Both enzymes utilize tetrahydrobiopterin, a product of guanosine 5′-triphosphate (GTP) metabolism, as a cofactor. The products of the hydroxylation reactions, 3,4-dihydroxy-L-phenylalanine (L-dopa) and 5-hydroxytryptophan, are further metabolized to active neurotransmitters via decarboxylation catalyzed by aromatic L-amino acid decarboxylase (ALAAD), a pyridoxine-dependent reaction. Dopamine is further metabolized to norepinephrine in noradrenergic neurones in a reaction catalyzed by dopamine beta-hydroxylase. Serotonin is converted to melatonin in the pineal gland.

Catechol *O*-methyltransferase and monoamine oxidase catalyze the breakdown of dopamine, serotonin and norepinephrine to homovanillic acid (HVA), 5-hydroxyindoleacetic acid (5-HIAA) and 3-methoxy-4-hydroxyphenylglycol (MHPG), respectively. The latter are the primary metabolites quantified in human cerebrospinal fluid (CSF) which are postulated to correctly reflect brain neurotransmitter metabolism. The biogenic amines control a host of critical processes, including (but not limited to) psychomotor function, memory, appetite, mood, and sleep, vascular tone and body temperature.[51,53]

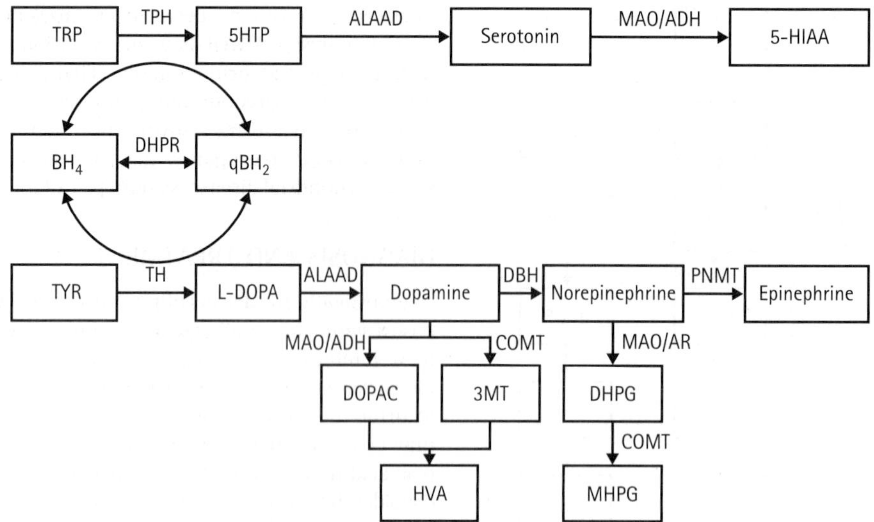

Fig. 24.5 Schematic diagram of catecholamine and serotonin metabolism. Not all steps are shown. TRP, tryptophan; TPH, tryptophan hydroxylase; 5HTP, 5-hydroxytryptophan; ALAAD, aromatic L-amino acid decarboxylase; MAO, monamine oxidase; ADH, aldehyde dehydrogenase; 5-HIAA, 5-hydroxyindoleacetic acid; BH_4, tetrahydrobiopterin; qBH_2, quinoid dihydrobiopterin; DHPR, dihydropteridine reductase; TYR, tyrosine; TH, tyrosine hydroxylase; L-DOPA, L-3,4-dihydroxyphenylalanine; COMT, catechol-*O*-methyltransferase; DOPAC, dihydroxyphenylacetic acid; 3MT, 3-methoxytyramine; HVA, homovanillic acid; DBH, dopamine beta-hydroxylase; AR, aldehyde reductase; DHPG, dihydroxyphenylglycol; MHPG, 3-methoxy-4-hydroxyphenylglycol; PNMT, phenylethanolamine-N-methyltransferase.

Thus, defects in the metabolism of neurotransmitters are expected to have severe, multisystem manifestations.

PRIMARY DEFECTS OF BIOGENIC AMINE METABOLISM – CLINICAL FEATURES

The primary defects of biogenic amine metabolism include tyrosine hydroxylase (TH), ALAAD, dopamine beta-hydroxylase (DBH) and monamine oxidase (MAO) deficiencies (Fig. 24.5). Isolated MAO-A has been described, as has a defect which includes deficiency of either MAO-A or MOA-B, or both, in conjunction with Norrie disease, the latter a syndrome of congenital blindness linked to malformed retinas.[51]

TH deficiency manifests oculogyric crises, Parkinsonian symptoms, tremor, hypokinesia, truncal hypotonia, irritability and tone alterations with marked hypotonia.[54] CNS catecholamine levels (dopamine, norepinephrine and adrenaline, as well as HVA and MHPG) are decreased while serotonin metabolism (5-HIAA) remains unaffected. Tetrahydrobiopterin and neopterin levels are normal, enabling distinction between TH deficiency and various forms of GTP cyclohydrolase (GTPCH) deficiency described below (a secondary defect of biogenic neurotransmitter metabolism).[55]

Patients with ALAAD manifest generalized hypotonia, paroxysmal movements, roving eye movements, cyanosis, heightened irritability, enhanced startle response, temperature instability and developmental delay. With age, the phenotype is that of an extrapyramidal movement disorder, frequently preceded by oculogyric crises and convergence spasm.[51] Metabolically, ALAAD results in central and peripheral deficiency of catecholamines, serotonin, HVA, MHPG and the serotonin metabolite 5-HIAA. Despite similarities in clinical findings, TH deficiency and ALAAD can be differentiated by an absence of hyperphenylalaninemia in ALAAD.[56]

Remaining primary defects of biogenic amine metabolism remain somewhat controversial. Orthostatic hypotension is the hallmark of DBH deficiency, which results in decreased norepinephrine production from dopamine.[57] The disease appears limited to adults, with retrospective case histories suggesting a neonatal period associated with ptosis, hypothermia, hypoglycemia and hypotension.[51] Catabolism of serotonin and catecholamines requires the actions of MAO-A and MAO-B.[58] Several males with a point mutation in the MAO-A gene on the X chromosome manifested borderline mental deficits and aggressive behavior.[51] Conversely, several males with X chromosome deletions including the Norrie, MAO-A and MAO-B genes manifested severe retardation, while brothers with an unusual deletion involving the

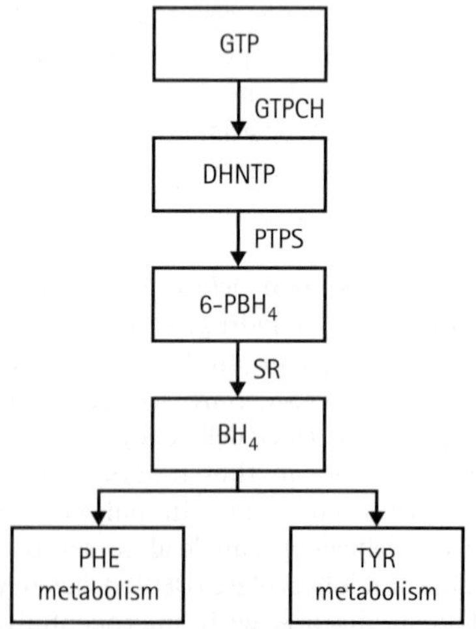

Fig. 24.6 Generation of tetrahydrobiopterin from guanosine triphosphate. Not all steps are shown. GTP, guanosine triphosphate; DHNTP, dihydroneopterin triphosphate; PTPS, 6-pyruvoyltetrahydrobiopterin synthase; $6\text{-}PBH_4$, 6-pyruvoyltetrahydrobiopterin; SR, sepiapterin reductase; PHE, phenylalanine; TYR, tyrosine. Tetrahydrobiopterin serves as bound cofactor in phenylalanine and tyrosine hydroxylase reactions, the first committed steps in the metabolism of both amino acids. Regeneration of tetrahydrobiopterin from quinoid dihydrobiopterin requires the action of pterin-4a-carbinolamine dehydratase (PCD), which is not shown.

Norrie gene and part of the MAO-B gene (but an intact MAO-A gene) had normal mental capacity. To date, no specific isolated abnormality of the MAO-B gene has been reported.

SECONDARY DEFECTS OF BIOGENIC AMINE METABOLISM – CLINICAL FEATURES

Secondary defects of biogenic amine metabolism encompass disorders in the production of tetrahydrobiopterin, including recessive and dominant forms of GTPCH deficiency, 6-pyruvoyltetrahydrobiopterin (PTPS) deficiency, sepiapterin reductase (SR) deficiency, pterin-4a-carbinolamine dehydratase (PCD) deficiency and dihydropteridine reductase (DHPR) (Fig. 24.6) deficiency. The clinical phenotype of recessive GTPCH, PTPS, DHPR and SR deficiencies includes progressive psychomotor retardation, altered tone, seizures, choreoathetosis, temperature instability, hypersalivation, microcephaly and irritability.[51] Patients with SR deficiency also manifest dystonic posturing, oculogyric crises and tremor.[59] PCD deficiency may not manifest significant clinical abnormalities, other than transient alterations in tone.

Autosomal dominant GTPCH deficiency (or so-called Segawa disease; dopa-responsive dystonia) manifests a syndrome of dystonia and Parkinsonism, with resting tremor, spasticity, postural instability, oculogyric crisis and a diurnal fluctuation of symptoms.[51] As the name implies, this form of the disease is amenable to intervention with L-dopa, leading to a complete resolution of symptomatology.

DIAGNOSIS

In general, CSF is required for measurement of biogenic amines and metabolites. This is available in only a handful of specialist laboratories in the USA and Europe. For primary abnormalities, TH deficiency results in low levels of catecholamines and related metabolites; ALAAD deficiency results in similar decreases accompanied by low CSF serotonin concentrations. Neurotransmitter precursors (5-hydroxytryptophan, levodopa and 3-*O*-methyldopa) also accumulate in ALAAD. CSF from patients with DBH deficiency shows low levels of norepinephrine with accumulation of dopamine, while patients with MAO-A deficiency manifest increased biogenic amines and *O*-methylated metabolites in CSF, with associated low concentrations of corresponding deaminated metabolites.

Blood phenylalanine can be a useful diagnostic marker for several of the secondary defects of biogenic amine metabolism, with elevated concentrations in PTPS, DHPR, PCD and recessive GTPCH deficiencies, but normal levels in SR deficiency and dopa-responsive dystonia. Further classification of these disorders requires accurate analysis of CSF pterins, HVA and 5-HIAA levels. In many cases, loading with phenylalanine and tetrahydrobiopterin followed by measurement of phenylalanine and its metabolites can provide important diagnostic information.[51] Measurements of blood and urine biopterins and serum prolactin may be useful, though hyperprolactinemia is non-specific.

TREATMENT

TH deficiency and dopa-responsive dystonia respond well to low dose L-dopa and carbidopa (Sinemet) combined with peripheral dopa-decarboxylase inhibitors.[60] Treatment of ALAAD is geared toward the correction of peripheral and central serotonin/catecholamine deficiencies, achieved by stimulation of the dopaminergic system with dopamine agonists combined with monoamine oxidase inhibitors to block breakdown of the small amounts of serotonin and catecholamines that are formed.[61,62] Application of dihydroxyphenylserine (which may be decarboxylated to norepinephrine) is aimed at correction of norepinephrine deficiency in DBH deficiency.[51]

Secondary defects of biogenic amine metabolism, which predominantly affect synthesis of tetrahydrobiopterin, are amenable to various interventions.[63,64] Dietary phenylalanine restriction is beneficial in DHPR and PCD deficiencies, but may also require tyrosine supplementation.[65,66] Autosomal recessively inherited GTPCH deficiency and PTPS deficiency are treated with tetrahydrobiopterin. Dopa-responsive dystonia and SR deficiency respond to application of L-dopa and carbidopa. Dietary supplementation of long chain polyunsaturated fatty acids may have therapeutic relevance in those disorders with hyperphenylalaninemia.[67]

AMINO ACID METABOLISM DISORDERS

GENERAL CONSIDERATIONS

The disorders of amino acid metabolism provide a significant challenge for diagnosis and management. Defects in amino acid catabolism represent the largest group, but abnormalities also exist in amino acid biosynthesis and transport. The clinical manifestations vary widely and involve many different organ systems (Table 24.5). Therefore, this group of single gene deficiencies must be considered in the differential diagnosis of many disease states. Systemic manifestations are common because of the presence of high levels of circulating small molecule metabolites and many of these abnormalities cause mental retardation.

The pyridoxine dependent transamination of the amino acid to the corresponding keto acid is an early step in the catabolism of most amino acids. Therefore, the accumulation of abnormal organic acids and systemic acidosis are the primary clinical manifestation of many disorders of amino acid metabolism (Table 24.5). Collectively, these conditions are a subgroup of the 'organic acidemias'.

This has important implications for the diagnosis of inborn errors of amino acid metabolism. While many disorders of amino acid metabolism can be diagnosed by quantitative analysis of plasma amino acids, the examination of urine organic acids is often the single most valuable diagnostic test. The more distal the enzyme deficiency lies in the degradation pathway, the more likely plasma amino acid levels are to be normal and urine organic acid analysis abnormal. Usually, both plasma amino acids and urine organic acids should be analyzed, if an inborn error of amino acid metabolism is suspected.

The nutritional characteristics of proteins and amino acids are discussed in Chapter 14. Hydrolysis of protein to oligopeptides and free amino acids in the gut is controlled by enzymes which may be defective as a result of a hereditary disorder (Ch. 17).

Figure 24.7 shows the possible metabolic fate of plasma amino acids which normally are maintained within narrow concentration limits, although they are also affected by nutrition, systemic diseases and hormones. Insulin and glucagon usually lower the plasma levels; conversely, many amino acids stimulate the release of insulin and other hormones. In obesity and early in fasting, the branched chain amino acids may be elevated. In starvation the essential amino acids are low and the non-essential amino acids may be elevated, although alanine, a major gluconeogenic substrate, is usually low. In sepsis, stress, renal failure and liver disease, there may be considerable changes, liver disease often causing marked elevation of methionine, phenylalanine and tyrosine. In early life, high protein intake and immature regulatory systems may cause major elevations of many amino acids. The level of free amino acids in intracellular fluid is about 10 times higher than in the plasma.

Table 24.5 Disorders associated with metabolic acidosis and/or organic aciduria. The major metabolite excreted is indicated either by the name of the disorder or by the compounds in parentheses

Branched chain amino acid disorders
Maple syrup urine disease (branched chain keto acids)
Methylmalonic acidemia
Propionic acid acidemia
Isovaleric acidemia
3-Methylcrotonylglycinuria
3-Methylglutaconic aciduria
3-Hydroxy-3-methylglutaryl-CoA lyase deficiency
Mevalonic acidemia
2-Methylacetoacetyl-CoA thiolase deficiency
3-Ketothiolase deficiency (3-hydroxybutyrate)
3-Hydroxyisobutyryl-CoA deacylase deficiency
Methylmalonic semialdehyde dehydrogenase deficiency (3-hydroxypropionate)
Other disorders
2-Ketoadipic aciduria
Glutaric aciduria types I and II
Crotonic acidemia
Oxalosis types I and II (glycollate, L-glycerate)
D-glyceric acidemia
5-Oxoprolinuria
Succinic semialdehyde dehydrogenase deficiency (4-hydroxybutyrate)
Succinyl-CoA:3-ketoacid CoA transferase deficiency
Threonine sensitive acidosis
2-Hydroxyglutaric aciduria
Barth syndrome (3-methylglutaconic acid)
Fanconi syndrome
The tyrosinemias (tyrosyluria) (succinyl acetone)
Renal tubular acidosis
Lactic/pyruvic acidosis
Multiple carboxylase and biotinidase deficiencies
Mitochondrial disorders
Krebs cycle disorders
Fructose 1,6-diphosphatase deficiency (lactate)
Glycogen storage disease type 1 (lactate)
Ketoacidosis as in diabetes mellitus
Carnitine depletion
Disorders of fatty acid catabolism
Disorders of ketone body utilization
Other disorders in which pathologic organic aciduria can occur
Urea cycle disorders (orotic acid)
Canavan's disease (N-acetylaspartate)
Phenylketonuria (phenylpyruvate)
Other acquired causes of acidosis include:
Poisoning: salicylate, methanol, benzyl alcohol, antifreeze, etc.
Ethanol
Starvation
Dehydration
Diarrhea
Reye's syndrome

In PKU, the blood phenylalanine concentration may be 20–60 times above normal. Conversely, a rise of alanine only 10–20% above normal may be the first indication of serious lactic acidosis or hyperammonemia. In some conditions, such as argininosuccinic aciduria and non-ketotic hyperglycinemia, the amino acid is excreted readily in the urine and blood levels may be only mildly abnormal, although in both these conditions the level is markedly increased in the CSF.

The quantity of amino acids in urine can vary over 10-fold in normal people and depends greatly upon age and nutrition. The levels are higher in infants but the range is so wide that normal values are hard to establish. Values expressed per unit volume are worthless and even when calculated per mg creatinine or per m^2, may be misleading. The predominant amino acids in urine (% of total amino acids in parentheses) are glycine (20–25%), taurine (5–15%), histidine (10–20%) and glutamine (7–10%). Normally, renal tubular reabsorption is nearly 100%, notable exceptions being histidine and glycine. In early infancy, many amino acids may be reabsorbed poorly, adult rates being reached by 3–6 months. Normal urine contains many metabolites arising from the diet, from drugs or from bacterial action in the gut; these compounds often pose diagnostic problems since many are detected on amino acid or organic acid analyses. The term *aminoaciduria* indicates that the urinary amino acid excretion is greater than normal. This can be due to raised levels in the blood caused by a defect of amino acid catabolism which increases the filtered load. Conversely, renal aminoaciduria occurs when there is defective reabsorption by the renal tubular cells. Excess of a single amino acid may saturate the renal absorption mechanism for others which share the same transport site and thus cause a competitive aminoaciduria.

In this chapter, the different disorders of amino acid metabolism are grouped by the biochemical pathways for different amino acids.

PHENYLALANINE-TYROSINE GROUP

Phenylketonuria

PKU is an autosomal recessive disorder of metabolism in which phenylalanine cannot be converted to tyrosine. Blood phenylalanine levels are elevated and phenylpyruvic acid is excreted in the urine. Since the advent of newborn screening programs, it has become evident that there are other varieties of hyperphenylalaninemias in addition to what has come to be known as classic PKU.

Clinical findings

In classic untreated PKU the most important clinical characteristic is neurodevelopmental delay. Most untreated patients are severely affected with intelligence quotients under 30 because persistently elevated phenylalanine levels are toxic to the CNS. The damage exerted by phenylalanine begins to become irreversible by 8 weeks after birth and therefore early screening and treatment are important. Phenylketonuric infants appear normal at birth, but early symptoms occur in over one half. Vomiting, irritability, an eczematoid rash, or a peculiar odor may also be present in the early months. The characteristic smell has been described as mousy, wolf-like, or musty, and has been correlated with excretion of phenylacetic acid in the urine. General physical development is usually normal. Over 90% of untreated patients are fair-haired, fair-skinned, and blue-eyed, but dark skin, hair, or irises do not exclude the diagnosis. Peripheral neurological findings are usually not prominent; but one-third have minimal signs, such as hyperactive deep tendon reflexes or hypertonicity. Seizures occur in about a quarter of the patients, predominantly in those most severely retarded. Electroencephalographic (EEG) abnormalities have been described in approximately 80% and CT or MRI scan may reveal cortical atrophy.

Clinical manifestations may also occur in patients treated early in life who then discontinued therapy later. Behavioral problems including restlessness, aggression and sleep disturbances are common.

Diagnosis and screening

Phenylalanine is normally converted to tyrosine by hepatic phenylalanine hydroxylase (PAH) which is undetectable in classic PKU.

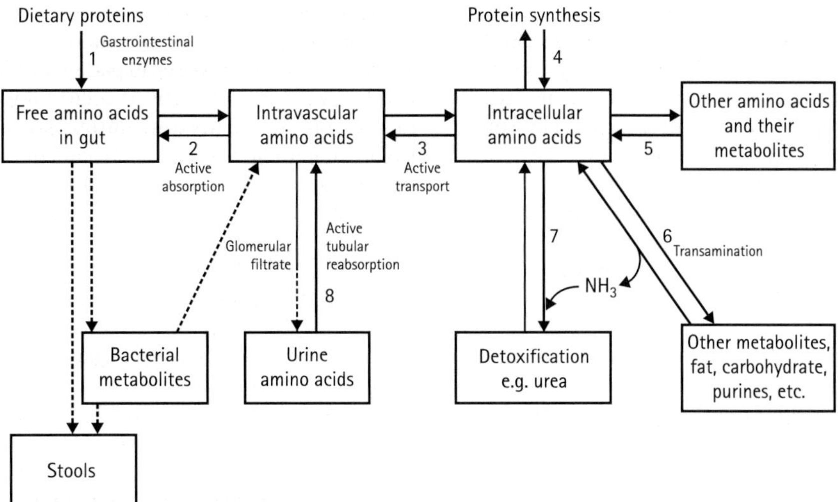

Fig. 24.7 Potential metabolic fate of amino acids. Numbers represent processes requiring active metabolism where congenital defects could occur. Dotted lines represent processes independent of metabolic activity.

In the absence of phenylalanine hydroxylase, tyrosine becomes an essential amino acid, and alternate pathways are used to metabolize phenylalanine. In PKU, phenylalanine and these metabolic products including phenylpyruvic acid and phenylacetic acid accumulate in body fluids. These compounds are not abnormal metabolites, but normal metabolites in abnormal amounts. Plasma phenylalanine concentrations range from 400 to 4800 μM (6 to 80 mg/dl) in untreated patients with PKU, in contrast to normal values of about 60 μM (1 mg/dl). Untreated patients with classic PKU virtually always have concentrations over 1200 μM (20 mg/dl) throughout infancy.

PKU should be diagnosed in the neonatal period. This is initiated through the routine screening of all infants after a few days of life, and after the initiation of feeding (see Ch. 10). Phenylalanine concentration is measured in blood collected from the heel onto filter paper in the newborn screening test.

After identifying patients from positive screening tests, the first step in diagnosis is quantitative analysis of the concentrations of phenylalanine and tyrosine in the blood. Many infants identified in the screening programs simply have delayed maturation of amino-acid metabolizing enzymes and may have as a clue, high tyrosine concentrations; they can be excluded and followed expectantly. The patient with classic PKU generally has a very rapid rise in serum concentration of phenylalanine on a normal diet to levels well over 30 mg/dl, and the concentration of tyrosine is low. About 1–2 % of patients with hyperphenylalaninemia do not have defects in PAH, but in biopterin synthesis or recycling (see below) and every PKU patient should be tested for this group of disorders.

PKU occurs in 1:10 000 to 1:20 000 persons. It is an autosomal recessive disease occurring around the world with a carrier frequency in most populations of ~1–2%. The gene for phenylalanine hydroxylase has been cloned and mapped to chromosome 12q24.1. Over 240 mutations have now been defined, but no single mutation accounts for a majority of patients. Carrier detection and prenatal diagnosis are possible with molecular genetic methods.

Treatment

All clinical manifestations of classic PKU can be completely prevented by restriction of dietary intake of phenylalanine. This has provided strong support for the concept that the clinical disease is an intoxication produced by the abnormal chemical milieu. Commercial preparations make long term treatment economically feasible and palatable. Dietary therapy readily lowers levels of phenylalanine in the blood; concomitantly, phenylpyruvic acid and its metabolic products disappear. Extensive experience indicates clearly that early diagnosis and consistent treatment will prevent the development of mental retardation.

The treatment of infants with a low phenylalanine diet is challenging and requires specialized expertise. The general approach is to reduce total natural protein intake and supplement essential amino acids as necessary for growth and development. This requires the use of special phenylalanine-free formulas. The phenylalanine tolerance must be individually established in each patient. Newly diagnosed babies are generally provided a diet containing ~40 mg/kg/day of phenylalanine. The blood levels are tightly monitored (i.e. twice weekly initially) and the diet is adjusted to maintain phenylalanine levels of 120–360 μM (2–6 mg/dl). If parental cooperation is good, this can be done in an outpatient setting and hospitalization is not necessary. Breast milk is relatively low in phenylalanine content and breast-feeding can be continued, but usually in conjunction with a phenylalanine-free supplement, replacing at least one daily breast-feeding with formula feeding. Frequent (at least weekly) monitoring of blood phenylalanine levels is recommended throughout infancy and early childhood.

All infants, including those with PKU, require a certain amount of phenylalanine; the minimal requirements are similar to those of normal infants. Patients with PKU may vomit or refuse feedings, and infections or other illnesses may complicate the metabolic state. If restriction of phenylalanine is too severe, chronically, tissue breakdown may occur and levels of phenylalanine increase; seizures may occur, and mental retardation and death are reported sequelae. There is general agreement that classic PKU must be treated; opinion on the other hyperphenylalaninemias, however, is divergent. We believe that it is advisable to treat any patient with blood phenylalanine levels over 500 μM (8 mg/dl) or who excretes phenylalanine metabolites in the urine.

It was formerly common to discontinue the dietary restriction of phenylalanine after a few years of age, but several studies have since shown that this leads to IQ loss and behavioral disturbances.[68] Therefore many metabolic centers now keep classic PKU patients on the diet life-long including adulthood. It also has been documented that many adult PKU patients who were not treated in childhood and who have severe learning difficulties nonetheless benefit from a low phenylalanine diet in terms of psychiatric manifestations of the disease.

Maternal PKU

High phenylalanine levels are exquisitely toxic to the developing fetal brain and thus the fetuses of mothers with PKU can be severely affected even though they usually do not have PKU themselves.[69] Affected children have microcephaly at birth and typically suffer severe, irreversible mental retardation, and sometimes have congenital heart defects. This outcome can be prevented if the maternal phenylalanine levels are maintained in a treatment range from the time of conception. Table 24.6 indicates the risk of damage to the fetus depending on maternal phenylalanine levels.

Hyperphenylalaninemia

Widespread screening of populations has led to the recognition that not all patients with hyperphenylalaninemia have classic PKU. It is now recognized that a variety of mutations in the hydroxylase gene lead to different clinically phenotypic variants with varying enzyme activity, level of phenylalanine, and tolerance to dietary phenylalanine.

Defects in the synthesis or recycling of biopterin (malignant PKU)

A group of patients with hyperphenylalaninemia have neurological symptoms which are progressive in spite of dietary treatment that maintained normal phenylalanine levels (malignant PKU).[70] These children have defects in the synthesis of tetrahydrobiopterin, the cofactor for phenylalanine hydroxylase, or the enzymes which regenerate tetrahydrobiopterin from dihydrobiopterin. Each of these defects results in deficient conversion of phenylalanine to tyrosine, even though the phenylalanine hydroxylase apoenzyme itself is normal. Tetrahydrobiopterin is also the cofactor for the hydroxylation of tryptophan and tyrosine, and its deficiency interferes with the synthesis of serotonin, dihydroxyphenylalanine (dopa), and norepinephrine. Severe neurological disease may occur with only mild hyperphenylalaninemia, suggesting that tetrahydrobiopterin levels may be relatively more adequate for phenylalanine hydroxylation than for that of tryptophan or tyrosine (see also pp. 1169 – section Neurotransmitter disorders). Affected patients have marked hypotonia, as well as spasticity and dystonic posturing. Some have seizures, myoclonus, and EEG abnormalities. Drooling is common. The delay in psychomotor development is usually profound. Defective biosynthesis of tetrahydrobiopterin can be diagnosed by blood and urine biopterin profiling. CSF neurotransmitter and biopterin levels and phenylalanine loading tests are often useful in diagnostic confirmation. Testing should be done routinely in all patients with hyperphenylalaninemia, because early treatment is vital. The diagnosis of specific enzyme deficiency can be confirmed in many cases by assay in cultured fibroblasts.

The treatment for this group of patients consists of phenylalanine restriction and the administration of biogenic amine precursors, such as 5-hydroxytryptophan and L-dopa, that do not require hydroxylation. Carbidopa is a necessary adjunct to prevent decarboxylation of these precursors before they reach the CNS. Tetrahydrobiopterin is used in patients with synthesis defects, but by itself may not be sufficient. It order to optimize the drug dosages, monitoring of neurotransmitter levels in CSF is indicated. Unfortunately, however, in some patients even early and aggressive therapy does not prevent progressive neurological deterioration and eventual death.

Table 24.6 Maternal phenylalaninemia: risk of damage to fetus according to maternal phenylalanine level

	Blood phenylalanine (mmol/L)		
	>1.25	0.65–1.2	<0.625
Spontaneous abortion (%)	24	22	8
Mental retardation (%)	92	53	21
Microcephaly (%)	73	57	24
Congenital heart disease (%)	12	11	0
Low birth weight (%)	40	52	13

Infantile Parkinsonism

An autosomal recessively inherited isolated deficiency of tyrosine hydroxylase causes severe Parkinsonism in infancy. A less severe form of the disease is termed Segawa syndrome or dopa-responsive dystonia. Dystonic posture or movement of one limb appears insidiously between ages 1 and 9 years. Intelligence is normal. This disorder can also be autosomal dominant. In these families the mutated gene is GTP cyclohydrolase I, involved in the biosynthesis of tetrahydrobiopterin. The diagnosis can be made by finding abnormally low levels of homovanillic acid in CSF. All forms of the disease respond to treatment with L-dopa (see also Ch. 20).

Tyrosinemia

The tyrosinemias are a group of disorders in which elevated quantities of tyrosine are found in body fluids. The most common form is transient tyrosinemia of the newborn resulting from delayed maturation of tyrosine-metabolizing enzymes. It is particularly common in premature infants. Tyrosinemia also occurs in scurvy and many forms of liver disease. In addition there are several genetic deficiencies of enzymes involved in tyrosine catabolism, all of which are autosomal recessive diseases.

Hepatorenal tyrosinemia (hereditary tyrosinemia type 1)

Clinical features

The liver and kidney are the primary organs affected in this disorder. Symptoms may begin early in infancy with an acute rapid course to demise, or they may progress more chronically. Most patients present with failure to thrive and liver dysfunction. Untreated, the liver disease is progressive causing cirrhosis, and icterus, ascites and hemorrhage often ensue. Patients display renal tubular acidosis of the Fanconi type and typical radiographic changes of rickets are often present. Neurodevelopmental delay is not a feature. Surviving patients have a high risk for developing hepatocarcinoma.

Diagnosis

This disease is caused by deficiency of fumarylacetoacetate hydrolase, the last enzyme in tyrosine catabolism. Biochemical alterations include elevated plasma concentrations of tyrosine and methionine and the excretion of tyrosyl compounds in the urine. The presence of succinylacetone in urine is diagnostic. Highly elevated blood concentrations of alpha-fetoprotein are seen, even before the elevation in tyrosine. Hypoglycemia may occur, and coagulation defects are common.

Treatment

The liver failure and renal Fanconi syndrome of hepatorenal tyrosinemia can be effectively treated with a new drug, 2(2-nitro-4-trifluoromethylbenzoyl)-1,3 cyclohexane dione (NTBC) which blocks tyrosine metabolism by inhibiting its second step (Fig. 24.8), and thus preventing the accumulation of toxic metabolites. NTBC raises blood tyrosine levels and thus needs to be combined with a diet low in phenylalanine and tyrosine. The prognosis of patients with this disease has vastly improved with this new therapy.[71,72]

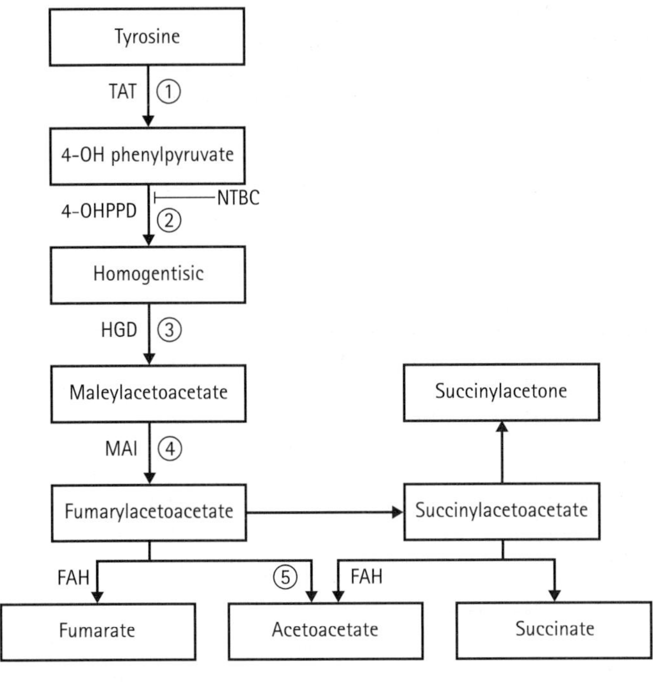

Fig. 24.8 The tyrosine catabolic pathway. The enzymes for each reaction are given on the left, the disease corresponding to its deficiency on the right. TAT, tyrosine aminotransferase; HPD, 4-PH phenylpyruvate dioxygenase; HGD, homogentisic acid dioxygenase; MAI, maleylacetoacetate isomerase; FAH, fumarylacetoacetate hydrolase.

The gene for fumarylacetoacetate hydrolase has been cloned and mutation analysis can be used for prenatal diagnosis and carrier detection. Hepatorenal tyrosinemia is common in the Canadian province of Quebec, where a single founder mutation is responsible for most cases.

Oculocutaneous tyrosinemia (tyrosinemia type 2)

Tyrosine aminotransferase, the first step of tyrosine degradation, is deficient in oculocutaneous tyrosinemia. The characteristic features of this disease are corneal ulcers or dendritic keratitis early in life and erythematous papular or keratotic lesions on the palms and soles. About 50% of patients display mental retardation, but this may be due in part to ascertainment bias. In addition, at least one patient has had mental retardation as a result of a contiguous gene deletion syndrome. Tyrosine itself is not hepatotoxic and the liver and kidney are not affected in this disorder. Plasma concentrations of tyrosine are higher than in other forms of tyrosinemia, and the urine contains large amounts of tyrosine metabolites. The lesions on the palms and soles and in the eyes relate directly to the accumulation of tyrosine. Both respond rapidly to treatment with diets low in tyrosine.

Tyrosinemia type 3

The second step in tyrosine catabolism is catalyzed by 4-hydroxyphenylpyruvate dioxygenase. Several patients lacking this enzyme have been identified and all suffer from mild psychomotor retardation, but no other organ systems are involved. Plasma tyrosine levels are elevated, but usually not to levels which cause corneal ulcers or hyperkeratosis. Treatment consists of a low tyrosine diet.

Alkaptonuria

Alkaptonuria results from defective activity of the enzyme homogentisic acid dioxygenase, the third enzyme in tyrosine degradation. However, blood tyrosine levels are not elevated and the disorder is characterized by the excretion of dark-colored urine. Fresh urine appears normal, but on standing and particularly after alkalinization, oxidation of homogentisic acid proceeds, and a dark brown or black pigment appears. This should permit the condition to be recognized early in life, but the diagnosis is usually first made in adult life during routine urinalysis or during investigation of arthritis. Persons with alkaptonuria are usually asymptomatic in childhood. After the third decade, deposition of brownish or bluish pigment is seen, particularly in the ears and sclerae. The deposition of pigment, which may be extensive in fibrous tissues, is referred to as ochronosis. Ochronotic arthritis, which occurs later, produces symptoms resembling rheumatoid arthritis or osteoarthritis, with limitation of motion; complete ankylosis is common.

Garrod's suggestion that the disorder results from absence in the liver of the enzyme that catalyzes the oxidation of homogentisic acid (Fig. 24.8) gave rise to the one-gene, one-enzyme hypothesis, the notion of inborn errors of metabolism and the field of biochemical genetics.[73]

SULFUR-CONTAINING AMINO ACIDS (Fig. 24.9)

Methionine plays an important role in methylation reactions. Some is resynthesized from homocysteine by two separate pathways, one of which interdigitates with folate metabolism and the 1-carbon pool. This pathway uses an enzyme which requires vitamin B_{12} as a cofactor, so that some defects of folate or vitamin B_{12} metabolism can cause accumulation of homocysteine. The disulfides, homocystine and cystine are formed from two molecules of homocysteine and cysteine, respectively. In proteins, two molecules of cysteine condense to form disulfide bonds which help to maintain the three-dimensional shape of the protein. Homocystine is not present in protein. Cystinuria and cystinosis are discussed on pp. 1189 and 1246, respectively.

Breast milk contains the sulfur-containing amino acid taurine which is also present in high levels in muscle, leukocytes and other tissues; it is frequently excreted in large quantities as a result of liver disease, a high protein intake, leukemia or endogenous protein catabolism. No primary defect of taurine metabolism is known and its role in metabolism is unclear.

Homocystinuria

Homocystinuria (elevated urinary levels of homocystine) is a hallmark of several disorders in the metabolism of sulfur-containing amino acids. The term is sometimes used to specifically indicate the classic form of the disease which is caused by defective activity of the enzyme cystathionine beta-synthetase (CBS). However, several other enzyme defects can also cause elevated homocysteine, including defects of B_{12} metabolism. Therefore homocystinuria is not a single disease, but a heterogeneous group of disorders. Plasma methionine, cystine and B_{12} levels as well as urine organic acids should be measured in all patients with homocystinuria.

Cystathionine beta-synthetase deficiency

This autosomal recessive enzyme defect is the most common cause of homocystinuria.

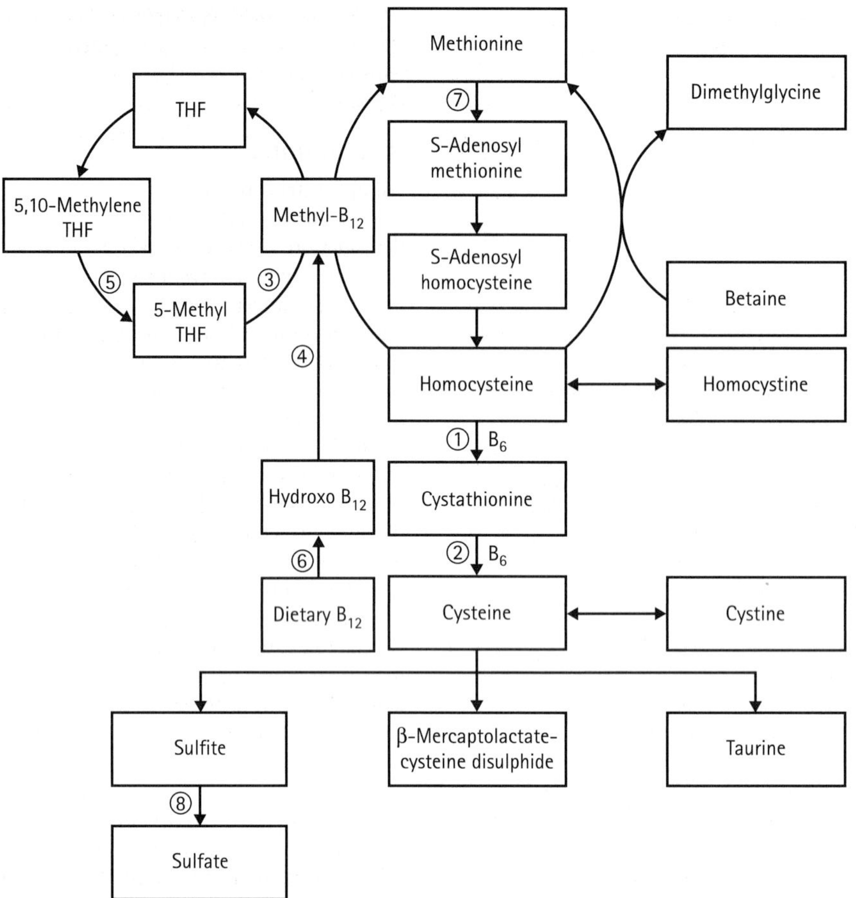

Fig. 24.9 Metabolism of the sulfur-containing amino acids. 1, Cystathionine synthase (homocystinuria); 2, cystathioninase (cystathioninuria); 3, 5-methyltetrahydrofolate-homocysteine methyl transferase; 4, cobalamin-activating system (homocystinuria and methylmalonic aciduria); 5, 5,10-methylenetetrahydrofolate reductase (homocystinuria); 6, gut absorption and reduction of vitamin B_{12} (homocystinuria and methylmalonic aciduria); 7, methionine adenosyltransferase (hypermethioninemia); 8, sulfite oxidase (sulfite oxidase deficiency). THF, tetrahydrofolic acid.

Clinical findings

The classic presentation of cystathionine beta-synthetase deficiency includes Marfanoid habitus, developmental delay, lens dislocation and predisposition for blood clotting. Presentation is usually in the first decade with the exception of embolism which may occur later. Homocystinuria is one of the few disorders of amino acid metabolism in which clinical manifestations tend to be progressive in adulthood, because many clinical manifestations result from thrombotic complications. Classic tests of clotting function are normal, but elevated homocystine levels cause increased platelet adhesiveness. The most characteristic feature of this disorder is subluxation of the ocular lens. Mental retardation is common, although not always present. Most patients have osteoporosis and skeletal abnormalities similar to those seen in Marfan syndrome. In homocystinuria, however, the joints tend to be limited in mobility rather than hypermobile. There is also lenticular subluxation in both conditions; however, in Marfan syndrome the lens is usually displaced upwards, whereas in homocystinuria it is displaced downwards and medially.

Diagnosis

The normal biosynthesis of the sulfur amino acid cysteine involves the demethylation of methionine to homocysteine, followed by its reaction with serine to form cystathionine. This latter step is catalyzed by the pyridoxine requiring enzyme cystathionine beta-synthetase. Homocystine is derived from the condensation of homocysteine to form the disulfide homocystine and is not normally detected in the usual assays of amino acids in body fluids. In CBS deficiency, elevated homocystine can be detected in both urine and blood. Levels of methionine are usually also elevated and levels of cystine are reduced. Because homocystine is unstable, testing should be done on fresh urine. Screening tests for homocystinuria using cyanide nitroprusside reagent are available, but are not completely sensitive. Measurement of blood total homocystine is useful. Because homocystinuria can be caused by several genetic defects, it is important to specifically confirm the diagnosis of CBS deficiency by measuring the enzyme in liver, cultured skin fibroblasts or lymphoblasts.

Importantly, CBS is a pyridoxine dependent enzyme and in many patients some activity can be restored by pharmacological doses of pyridoxine.

CBS deficiency is autosomal recessive and the gene has been cloned and mapped to chromosome 21q. Many disease causing mutations have been described and DNA based diagnosis can theoretically be used for prenatal detection of the condition.

Treatment

All patients should initially be treated with large doses (100–500 mg/day) of pyridoxine to determine their degree of vitamin responsiveness. If the homocystine levels normalize, no additional therapy may be needed. Those who do not respond may be treated with a diet low in methionine and supplemented with L-cystine. All patients should probably receive high doses of folic acid. In addition the compound betaine may be used to aid in the conversion of homocysteine to methionine.[74,75] Medications aimed at reducing platelet adhesiveness can be prescribed, but do not abolish all thromboembolic events. Oral contraceptives are considered by some metabolic disease specialists to be contraindicated in women with CBS deficiency due to the increased risk of thrombosis.

Other causes of homocystinuria

Homocystinuria may result from defects other than CBS. The most important of these is $N^{5,10}$-methylenetetrahydrofolate reductase (MTHFR) deficiency. It is associated with low rather than high plasma methionine levels. The deficient enzyme is involved in the recycling of homocysteine to methionine. The disorder lacks the eye and skeletal involvement of CBS deficiency, but shares a clotting propensity. Neurological features predominate this rare condition. The specific enzyme diagnosis can be made on cultured skin fibroblasts. Treatment is similar to CBS deficiency, but no pyridoxine is given and methionine may be supplemented rather than restricted in the diet. Folate administration may also be beneficial.

A mild form of MTHFR deficiency is associated with a thermolabile variant of the MTHFR gene. This can be easily diagnosed by DNA mutation analysis, and the test is offered by several clinical laboratories. The carrier frequency for the thermolabile variant is very high, and homozygous individuals may be clinically affected. The phenotype is hyperhomocystinemia, which can predispose to premature coronary or cerebrovascular disease. Hyperhomocystinemia of any cause is a risk factor for atherosclerosis, so that many commercial and university laboratories offer a test of total plasma homocystine. In addition to screening for individuals at risk for atherosclerosis who might benefit from administration of folate, B_6, and/or B_{12}, the test can detect true inborn errors of sulfur amino acid metabolism in those who have very high levels, and is a valuable test for monitoring response to therapy.

Homocystinuria and methylmalonic aciduria can occur jointly in disorders of vitamin B_{12} transport or metabolism because MetCbl is required for recycling of homocystine to methionine. These conditions are often associated with neurological deficits and have a guarded prognosis. For this reason it is important that every patient with homocystinuria has a urine organic acid analysis. If a vitamin B_{12} defect is found, B_{12} injections are used in addition to the usual treatments for homocystinuria.

The B_{12} defects will be discussed in more detail later in this chapter in the context of methylmalonic acidemia.

Cystathioninuria

Cystathioninuria, an inborn error of amino acid metabolism in which there is a deficiency of the activity of cystathionase, was first reported in two adults with mental deficiency. Subsequently, however, cystathioninuria has been found in a number of individuals with no clinical signs and is currently considered a benign variant.

Hypermethioninemia

Persistent hypermethioninemia occurs in methionine adenosyl transferase deficiency which appears to be benign.

Transient neonatal hypermethioninemia occurs in a small number of infants, most of whom are receiving a high protein intake. Although there are no known toxic sequelae, modest protein restriction seems warranted in view of the toxic effects of methionine in laboratory animals. It is also frequent in tyrosinemia type 1 and in hepatocellular damage from any cause.

Sulfite oxidase and molybdenum cofactor deficiency

The terminal step in the oxidative degradation of cysteine and methionine, the conversion of sulfite to sulfate, is catalyzed by the molybdenum-containing enzyme sulfite oxidase. Severe neurological diseases have been associated with deficiency in this system.

Clinical findings

Most patients present with neonatal neurological disease including severe hypotonia, seizures and myoclonic spasms. Symptoms are progressive and usually lead to early death. Patients with milder forms of the disease have progressive cerebral palsy and choreiform movements. Infantile hemiplegia has been reported and lens dislocation is a frequent finding even in neonates.

Diagnosis and treatment

Sulfite oxidase deficiency can be caused by a defect in the gene for this protein or by defects in the synthesis of the molybdenum cofactor required for its function. In all cases the disease is autosomal recessive in inheritance. Sulfite oxidase functions in the oxidative degradation of the sulfur containing amino acids cysteine and methionine. Deficiency results in increased amounts of sulfite, thiosulfate and S-sulfocysteine in the urine. These compounds are not readily detected during routine metabolic studies and the diagnosis needs to be suspected to initiate appropriate testing. The elevated urinary sulfite levels can be detected using commercial strip tests normally utilized for wine making, though this must be performed on a fresh sample. A test for urinary thiosulfate may be helpful, and specialized amino acid analysis may be useful for detection of S-sulfocysteine. However, the compound may be difficult to differentiate from other compounds so that care should be taken in this analysis. Mutations in two genes (MOCS1 and 2) can cause molybdenum cofactor deficiency resulting in absent aldehyde oxidase and xanthine dehydrogenase in addition to sulfite oxidase. Very low uric acid levels in blood and urine are a clue to this condition. In molybdenum cofactor deficiency the urinary excretion of hypoxanthine and xanthine is highly elevated, so a good test is the determination of urinary purines. Ophthalmologic examination is useful in diagnosis. The genes for all three proteins have been cloned and prenatal diagnosis can be performed.

Currently, no effective therapy is available.

DISORDERS OF THE GAMMA-GLUTAMYL CYCLE

The synthesis and recycling of the sulfur containing tripeptide glutathione involves a series of six enzymatic reactions termed the gamma-glutamyl cycle (Fig. 24.10). Deficiencies in several of these enzymes have been associated with disease. Pyroglutamic aciduria will be briefly discussed below.

Pyroglutamic aciduria (5-oxoprolinuria)

Pyroglutamic aciduria, or 5-oxoprolinuria, is caused by autosomal recessive deficiency of glutathione synthetase. Pyroglutamic acid is 2-pyrrolidone-5-carboxylic acid, a cyclized condensation product of glutamic acid or glutamine. It can be readily detected by urine organic acid analysis.

Clinically, the untreated disease is often characterized by neurological symptoms including spasticity, ataxia and mental retardation. Patients can experience episodes of acidosis and hemolysis. Glutathione deficiency has been considered the likely underlying cause of the disease and therapeutic attempts have been aimed at increasing cellular glutathione concentrations and antioxidant activity. Unfortunately this intervention does not

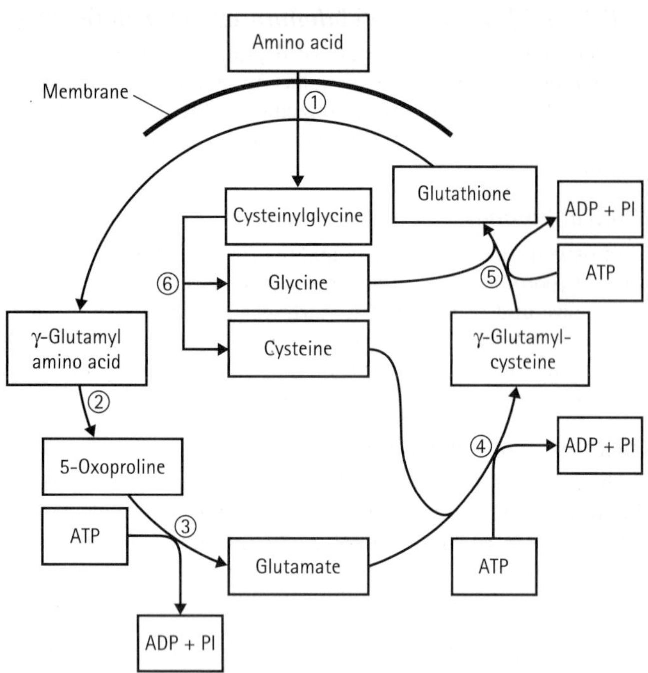

Fig. 24.10 The γ-glutamyl cycle. 1, Gamma-glutamyl transpeptidase; 2, γ-glutamyl cyclotransferase; 3, 5-oxoprolinase; 4, γ-glutamyl-cysteine synthase; 5, glutathione synthase; 6, peptidase.

completely eliminate neurological problems in severely affected patients. Drugs such as acetaminophen which require glutathione for detoxification should be avoided.

Treatment involves providing supplements to correct the metabolic acidosis in addition to supplying antioxidants, vitamin E and vitamin C. Bicitra may be used as an oral medication which can keep plasma bicarbonate levels in a normal range. Alternatively, bicarbonate itself may be used. Very large doses may be needed.

The prognosis is quite variable. On the basis of clinical symptoms, patients can be classified into three phenotypes: mild, moderate, and severe. Early supplementation with vitamins C and E may improve the long term clinical outcome. The early use of Bicitra or other buffers, vitamin C, and vitamin E may well allow normal development in some cases.

DISORDERS ASSOCIATED WITH HYPERAMMONEMIA

An average diet contains excess amino acids, the nitrogen of which is mostly excreted as urea. The enzymes of the urea cycle are active before birth. The first three steps of the pathway are mitochondrial so the full cycle requires the transport of ornithine into and the transport of citrulline out of the mitochondria. Arginine is an important regulator of the cycle since it induces N-acetylglutamate synthetase. N-acetylglutamate, in turn, activates carbamyl phosphate synthetase.

The urea cycle is only complete in the liver where urea is synthesized. Defects at all steps of the urea cycle have been described, the common feature of which is hyperammonemia. Some of the enzymes are present in other tissues where the enzymes must have other roles. In severe liver damage, hyperammonemia is sometimes found and may contribute to the cerebral symptoms of liver failure.

Clinical features

The clinical features of the different disorders associated with hyperammonemia are similar and therefore will be discussed as a group.

Patients with severe defects in the urea cycle often present in the newborn period with coma and acute metabolic crisis. Postnatal catabolic events and protein intake contribute to the metabolic derangement. In infancy, the symptoms are commonly episodes of poor feeding, vomiting, failure to thrive, lethargy, irritability or other neurological symptoms, all of which are aggravated by formula changes that increase protein intake and may be alleviated by reducing the protein content of the diet. Most babies with hyperammonemia are initially thought to be septic and therefore ammonia measurements are essential in any infant with sepsis symptoms but without an obvious source of infection. Respiratory alkalosis is a frequent, but often overlooked finding in hyperammonemia. Elevated blood ammonia levels cause an increased respiratory rate.

In older children, with, presumably, less severe mutations, symptoms often develop for the first time during weaning. Food intolerance or distaste for protein may be evident; some have failure to thrive, developmental or neurological problems with seizures, migraine, ataxia and abnormal EEG. Even adults may present with new onset of hyperammonemic symptoms particularly during times of high catabolic stress such as the postpartum period in women or during intercurrent illnesses such as infections, dehydration or surgery.

Transient neonatal hyperammonemia

Hyperammonemia is sometimes seen in infants receiving intravenous alimentation. In these cases it may be due to an inappropriately high nitrogen intake. Other infants with profound, but transient hyperammonemia have mostly been preterm; respiratory distress is usual. There are signs of progressive neurological damage with apnea, loss of reflexes and coma ensuing within 12–48 h of birth. Ammonia levels may be as high as 5000 μM/L. Liver function tests and amino acid studies may be normal, or glutamine may be normal in the face of hyperammonemia. If the condition is treated early and vigorously the babies rapidly improve and the prognosis is excellent. In infants who recover, the protein tolerance becomes normal and liver enzyme assays show no abnormality. The cause is unknown but rapid protein catabolism, mitochondrial dysfunction, maternal carnitine deficiency, and/or portocaval shunting may play a role.

Enzyme defects of the urea cycle (Fig. 24.11)

N-acetylglutamate synthetase deficiency (step 1)

This disorder, if it truly exists as an entity, is a rare autosomal recessive condition usually detectable in the first weeks of life. N-acetylglutamate does not participate directly in the urea cycle, but rather is an allosteric activator of carbamylphosphate synthetase (CPS). Thus, the absence of this compound results in secondary CPS deficiency. Several acyl-CoA derivatives of organic acids such as methylmalonyl-CoA, propionyl-CoA or valproic acid can inhibit N-acetylglutamate synthesis. This phenomenon explains the sometimes profound hyperammonemia that can occur in the 'ketotic hyperglycinemias' and valproic acid toxicity.

The treatment of this disease differs slightly from the other urea cycle disorders[76] in that carbamylglutamate can be used. This drug is structurally similar to N-acetylglutamate and hence can stimulate CPS activity. Arginine (1 mmol/kg/day) and carbamylglutamate (1.7 mmol/kg/day) were effective in controlling hyperammonemia at a protein intake of 2 g/kg/day. The number of recognized patients with this disorder is very low, and hence only single case reports of therapy are published.[77,78]

Carbamyl phosphate synthetase I (CPS) deficiency (step 2)

This enzyme is mitochondrial and provides carbamyl phosphate for the synthesis of urea. Deficiency (step 2) usually presents with

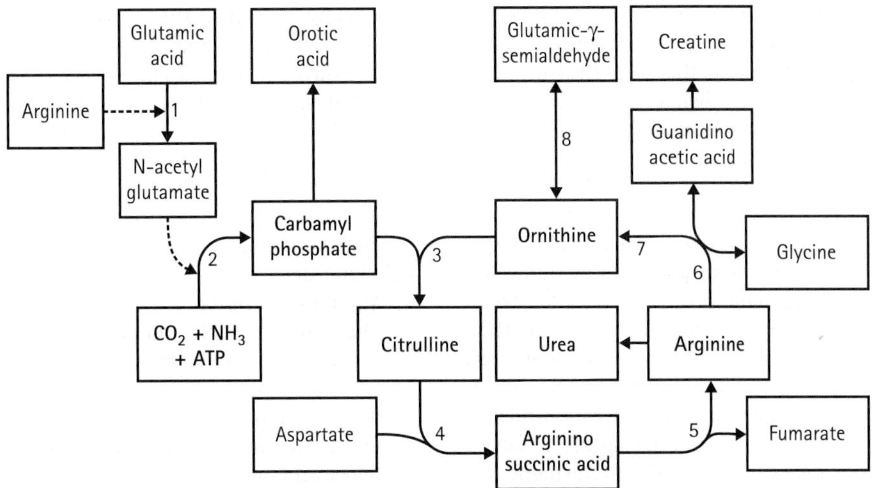

Fig. 24.11 The urea cycle. 1, N-acetylglutamate synthase; 2, carbamyl phosphate synthase; 3, ornithine transcarbamylase; 4, argininosuccinate synthase; 5, argininosuccinate lyase; 6, arginase; 7, ornithine uptake into mitochondria; 8, ornithine ketoacid aminotransferase.

severe neonatal hyperammonemia although other signs may present in infancy or childhood. Prenatal detection is possible. The disease is inherited in an autosomal recessive fashion. Carbamyl phosphate synthetase II is a separate enzyme in the cytoplasm and involved in the synthesis of pyrimidines.

Ornithine transcarbamylase (OTC) deficiency (step 3)

This is the most common urea cycle defect and it is an X-linked trait with many affected female carriers. Most affected males present as newborns in severe hyperammonemic crisis. About 20–30% are less severely affected and some have normal mental development and almost normal tolerance for protein except during stress. Some female carriers are totally asymptomatic while others have mild aversion or intolerance to protein and some have recurrent hyperammonemic crises which can be fatal. Even during crises, plasma amino acids are not grossly distorted; citrulline is very low, ornithine is normal but glutamine, alanine and sometimes lysine are increased in blood and sometimes in urine; during stress, orotic acid is usually increased in the urine. The combination of the typical clinical presentation, highly elevated urine orotic acid, normal urine organic acids, and blood amino acids showing only elevated glutamine and alanine, is diagnostic.

OTC can be assayed in liver or duodenal mucosa but not in fibroblasts. Enzyme activity from multiple liver biopsies from a single female carrier may vary widely, representing different degrees of inactivation of the mutant X chromosome in different areas. Most carriers can be detected by increased urine orotic acid from 0 to 8 and 8 to 16 h after a provocative challenge of allopurinol (100 mg/kg p.o.) either alone or together with 1.0 g protein/kg or L-alanine 0.5 g/kg p.o. DNA analysis can now detect most gene carriers and, when possible, is best for prenatal diagnosis and carrier detection.

Citrullinemia (step 4)

Citrullinemia is caused by autosomal recessive argininosuccinate synthetase (ASS) deficiency. The clinical severity of citrullinemia varies greatly, from death in the neonatal period to no symptoms at all, but many patients in the past were mentally retarded as a result of prolonged hyperammonemia with the first or subsequent episodes. Plasma and urine citrulline levels are markedly elevated, even between crises. The enzyme can be assayed in fibroblasts; prenatal diagnosis is possible. The ASS gene has been cloned and resides on chromosome 9q34.

Argininosuccinic aciduria (step 5)

Argininosuccinic aciduria is caused by deficiency of argininosuccinic acid lyase. Severe and mild cases of argininosuccinic aciduria are known and almost all patients have been developmentally delayed, even those who have not had prolonged coma with hyperammonemia. Trichorrhexis nodosa, an abnormal fragility of the hair, is found in some cases. The disease is easily diagnosed by chromatography of urinary amino acids since large amounts of argininosuccinic acid are excreted. Argininosuccinic acid is also found in the cerebrospinal fluid but is not as significantly increased in plasma. Citrulline will be elevated in plasma, but to a much smaller degree than in citrullinemia. The enzyme defect can be shown in several tissues including red blood cells. Prenatal diagnosis is available. Large supplements of arginine are added to the normal regimen since urinary argininosuccinic acid provides a major pathway for waste nitrogen disposal.

Argininemia (step 6)

Patients with argininemia (step 6) have autosomal recessive arginase I deficiency. Clinically, argininemia has a different presentation from the other urea cycle disorders. Profound hyperammonemia with coma is unusual in this condition. This disease usually presents with increasingly severe pyramidal tract signs starting within the first 2 years of life. It may mimic cerebral palsy. The plasma arginine is markedly raised. The urinary amino acid pattern may be similar to that seen in cystinuria, presumably caused by the high levels of arginine in the glomerular filtrate saturating the group reabsorptive site in the proximal renal tubules. Alternatively, urine amino acids may be normal or there may be a generalized aminoaciduria. Deficient arginase activity can be shown in the red blood cells of both patients and heterozygotes.

Hyperornithinemia

Two distinct disorders of elevated plasma ornithine levels exist, but only the HHH syndrome (hyperornithinemia with hyperammonemia and homocitrullinuria) has associated hyperammonemia. Most reported patients have had developmental delay and older patients tend to have spasticity. Symptoms may develop at any age. Excretion of ornithine, polyamines, orotic acid and glutamine may be increased. The primary defect is in the mitochondrial uptake of ornithine. Large, bizarre mitochondria may be present in the liver. Oral ornithine supplements have been reported to be beneficial. Homocitrulline can also be formed during pasteurization of milk and, if ingested, is excreted in the urine.

Gyrate atrophy

Hyperornithinemia in the absence of hyperammonemia also occurs in gyrate atrophy of the choroid and retina, caused by autosomal recessive deficiency of ornithine aminotransferase. The disease presents in adults without hyperammonemia but with a characteristic retinopathy, subcapsular cataract and progressive loss of peripheral vision leading to blindness by middle age. In children, small discrete circular patches of degeneration may be seen in the periphery of the retina; later these coalesce to form a characteristic lobular appearance which gives rise to the name. The electroretinogram (ERG) dark adaptation is abnormal. Plasma and CSF ornithine levels are markedly elevated. Ornithine ketoacid aminotransferase is deficient in several tissues, including cultured skin fibroblasts. Heterozygotes may be detected by oral ornithine loading tests (100 mg/kg) or by enzyme assay. Abnormal inclusions have been reported in muscle and bizarre, elongated mitochondria are present in liver. Direct toxicity of ornithine, low proline or lysine or low creatine have all been suggested as a cause of the retinal damage.

Pharmacological doses of vitamin B_6, the cofactor of the mutant enzyme may improve the biochemical and ERG findings in some but not all cases. Ornithine is not an amino acid contained in protein and hence cannot be directly restricted in the diet. Instead, long term arginine restriction can be used and improved visual function may result but such treatment is very hard to maintain.

Secondary hyperammonemias

Other causes of hyperammonemia include the following:

Liver disease (see Ch. 17)
Reye's syndrome (Ch. 17)
The ketotic hyperglycinemias (p. 1186)
Methylmalonic aciduria (p. 1186)
Propionic aciduria (p. 1186)
3-Ketothiolase deficiency (p. 1187)
3-Hydroxy-3-methylglutaric aciduria (p. 1187)
Familial lysinuric protein intolerance (p. 1188 – Amino acid transport disorders)
Neonatal glutaric aciduria type II (p. 1183 and Ch. 10)
Defects of fatty acid oxidation (p. 1196)
Valproic acid toxicity
Ureterostomy
Shock and after surgery

Diagnostic approaches

Assay of blood ammonia should be routine in any acutely sick child with neurological findings and in patients with mild, episodic symptoms. Hyperammonemia may be present in the fasting state but is sometimes induced only by a protein load. Elevations of the plasma ammonia of up to three times the normal limit are sometimes seen in severely ill infants, especially those with impaired hepatic function. In contrast, the ammonia levels in patients with primary hyperammonemia can be much higher and may exceed 1000 μM.

Great care must be taken in handling samples and in the assays– erroneously high values are common. When hyperammonemia is found, blood amino acids and urine organic acids should also be tested routinely. Raised levels of glutamine and alanine are usual and should always suggest this possibility. Patients with a defect at steps 3–6 of the urea cycle may exhibit orotic aciduria due to the diversion of carbamyl phosphate to the overproduction of pyrimidines.

An algorithm for the workup of hyperammonemia is provided in Figure 24.12.[79]

Treatment [80,81]

Every effort must be made to minimize catabolism for energy needs. Management of acute, severe hyperammonemic crises includes the following steps:

1. Maximal hydration p.o. or i.v. to enhance renal excretion.
2. Maximum tolerable non-protein caloric intake p.o. or i.v. Central venous access may be necessary to administer high concentrations of glucose (D20–D30).
3. Hemodialysis is the most effective method to rapidly remove ammonia and should be considered in any comatose hyperammonemic patient. Dialysis should not be delayed to await the effects of alternate pathway drugs (see below). Peritoneal dialysis can also be used, but is less effective.
4. Administer i.v. ammonia scavenging drugs. For sodium benzoate and sodium phenylacetate the loading dose is 250 mg/kg (or 5.5 g/m^2) given in 25–30 ml/kg of 10% dextrose solution over 90 min. The maintenance dose is 250 mg/kg/day (or 5.5 g/m^2/day) for each drug given as a 24 h infusion. In the USA, these medications have not been approved for general use by the Food and Drug Administration (FDA), so are considered investigational new drugs requiring informed consent for use. Great care in dosing and administration and monitoring must take place to avoid overdosing or serious complications such as acidosis from arginine-HCl.
5. Administer L-arginine-HCl i.v. The loading dose is 600 mg/kg (or 12 g/m^2) to be given along with the sodium benzoate and sodium phenylacetate as described above. The maintenance dose is 250 mg/kg/day (or 5.5 g/m^2/day).

The doses stated above are for acute hyperammonemia without a known enzyme defect. Arginine is very effective in reducing blood ammonia in citrullinemia and argininosuccinic aciduria and the high dose is aimed at these disorders. In patients with known defects in CPS or OTC, a lower dose is used for loading (200 mg/kg or 4 g/m^2) and maintenance (200 mg/kg/day or 4 g/m^2/day). In argininemia, no arginine should be used.

Maintenance therapy[81–83]

After the acute crisis, dietary protein is cautiously introduced starting at 0.5–0.75 g/kg/day. A mix of essential amino acids may be added. The protein intake is increased to the minimum daily requirement as tolerated. The ammonia scavenging drugs can be switched from i.v. to p.o. For chronic oral therapy sodium phenylbutyrate is preferred.[84] The dose is 450–600 mg/kg/day if < 20 kg and 10–13 g/m^2/day in larger patients. Arginine is used in patients with citrullinemia or argininosuccinic aciduria at 400–600 mg/kg/day (or 10–13 g/m^2/day). For CPS and OTC deficiency oral L-citrulline is preferred and is given at a dose of 170 mg/kg/day (or 3.3 g/m^2/day).

Liver transplantation has been successful in correcting the metabolic disease and preventing hyperammonemic brain damage in many patients.[85]

GLYCINE

Non-ketotic hyperglycinemia

Non-ketotic hyperglycinemia (NKH) is an inborn error of metabolism in which large amounts of glycine are found in body fluids, and there is no detectable accumulation of organic acids.

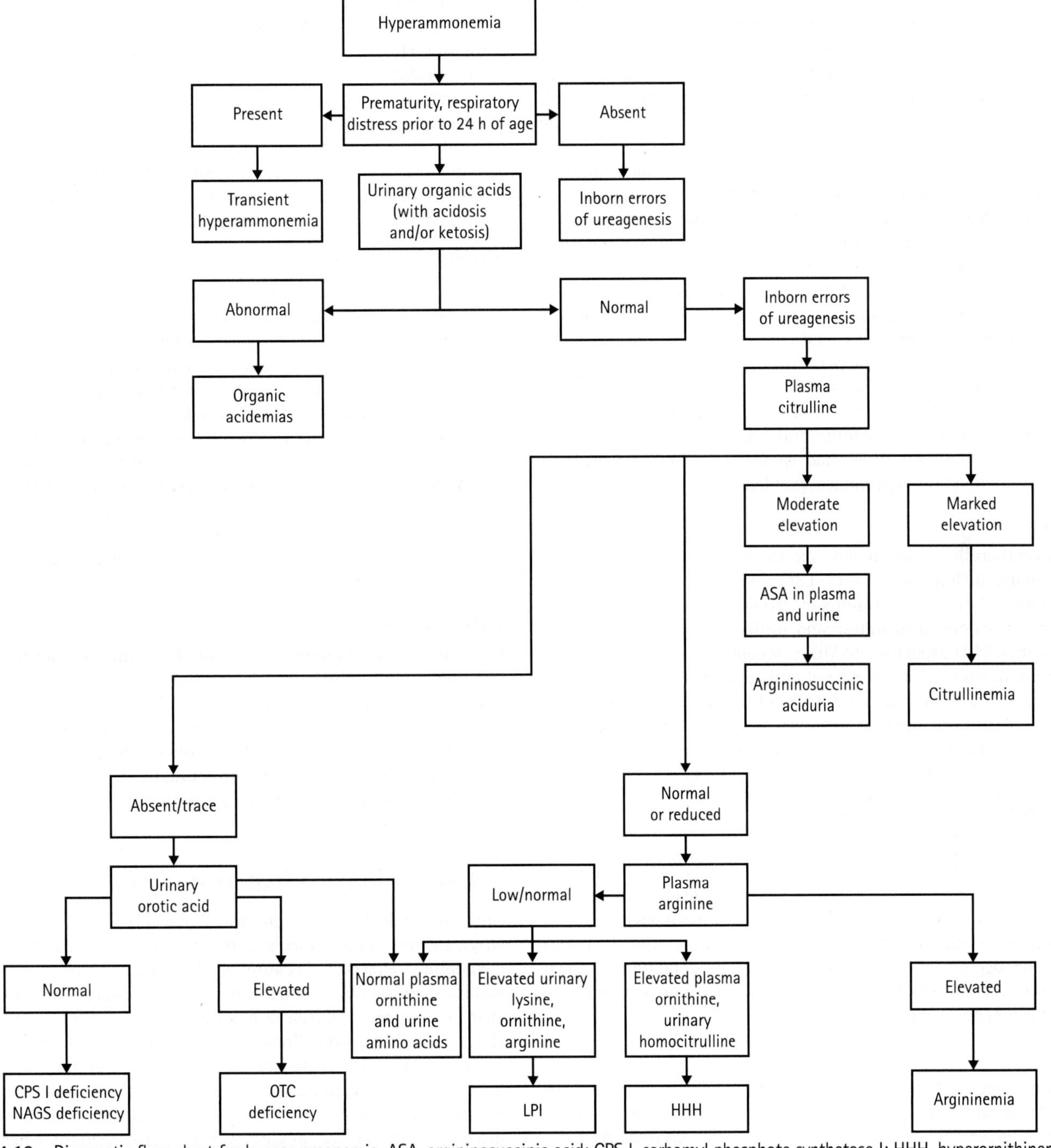

Fig. 24.12 Diagnostic flow chart for hyperammonemia. ASA, argininosuccinic acid; CPS I, carbamyl phosphate synthetase I; HHH, hyperornithinemia with hyperammonemia and homocitrullinuria; LPI, lysinuric protein intolerance; NAGS, N-acetylglutamate synthetase deficiency; OTC, ornithine transcarbamylase.

Clinical findings

NKH usually presents with intractable seizures in the neonatal period. Hypotonia, lethargy, hyperreflexia, hiccuping and myoclonic jerks are frequent. Many patients require assisted ventilation and death is a common outcome. The EEG is abnormal and displays a typical burst-suppression pattern. Most patients who survive have severe mental retardation. Patients with later onset forms have been described but are rare. In the infantile form of NKH, patients have an initial symptom-free interval and apparently normal development for up to 6 months. They then present with seizures and have various degrees of mental retardation. In the mild-episodic form, patients present in childhood with mild mental retardation and episodes of delirium, chorea and vertical gaze palsy during febrile illness. In the late-onset form, patients present in childhood with progressive spastic diplegia and optic atrophy, but intellectual function may be preserved and seizures have not been common.

Diagnosis

In NKH elevated glycine levels are found in all body fluids including blood, urine and CSF. In contrast to ketotic hyperglycinemia, plasma ketone levels are not elevated and no abnormal organic acids are found in the urine. Glycine levels are most elevated in the CNS and the ratio of CSF to blood glycine is used to make the diagnosis. Plasma glycine levels may, in fact, be normal, though urine glycine excretion is virtually always elevated. The ratio of the CSF concentration of glycine to that of the plasma is substantially higher in patients with non-ketotic hyperglycinemia than in hyperglycinemic patients with organic acidemia. Administration of valproate can interfere with the determination of this ratio.

The basic defect is in the glycine cleavage system which catalyzes the conversion of glycine to CO_2 and hydroxymethyltetrahydrofolic acid. The enzyme is multimeric with four distinct protein components designated P, H, T and L. All forms of NKH are autosomal recessive in inheritance. The genes for all four proteins have been cloned and mapped. Mutations in the P and T genes have been found with the P protein being most commonly affected. A single mutation is responsible for most cases in Finland.

Prenatal diagnosis can be performed by biochemical analysis of chorionic villus sample biopsies.

Non-ketotic hyperglycinemia can also be transient. Rare patients have presented with symptoms and laboratory tests consistent with classic NKH, but then had spontaneous reversal of both hyperglycinemia and neurological problems.

Treatment

Recently there has been modest success in the treatment of NKH, particularly in late onset cases. Large doses of sodium benzoate may reduce CSF concentrations of glycine and decrease seizures. Glycine is a neurotransmitter and anticonvulsants which block the N-methyl-D-aspartate (NMDA) receptor may be beneficial. Dextromethorphan has been used and resulted in some improved outcome.[86,87] Similarly, imipramine has had some beneficial effects. Classic NKH in our opinion, however, should not be considered a treatable condition, and consideration should be given towards allowing the lethal form to take its natural course.

Hyperoxaluria (oxalosis)

Clinical findings

Primary hyperoxaluria is a metabolic disorder in which large amounts of oxalate are excreted in the urine, leading to calcium oxalate lithiasis and nephrocalcinosis. Two distinct types are known with type 1 generally being more severe than type 2. When extrarenal deposits of calcium oxalate ensue, the condition is known as oxalosis. Renal failure is common and first signs or symptoms are often before age 5 years.

Diagnosis

Primary hyperoxaluria type 1 is caused by deficiency of the liver enzyme alanine:glyoxylate aminotransferase and type 2 by D-glycerate/glyoxylate reductase. Both types are characterized by hyperoxaluria, but in type 1 there is additional excretion of glycolic acid. In type 2 the urine contains high amounts of L-glycerate.

Oxalic acid is a dicarboxylic acid that forms a calcium salt of very low solubility. Oxalate in the urine is clearly of endogenous origin, and glycine is a precursor. Patients with hyperoxaluria may excrete 30 times as much oxalate as normal.

Both types of hyperoxaluria are autosomal recessive. The genes have been cloned and disease causing mutations have been identified. Prenatal diagnosis is available in highly specialized laboratories.

Treatment

This includes alkalinization of the urine, dietary restriction of calcium and a large fluid intake to improve the urinary flow. Rhubarb, spinach, beets and cocoa are foods high in oxalate and should probably be avoided, particularly in patients with gastrointestinal hyperabsorption of oxalate. Consultation with a dietitian is recommended. Only minimum daily requirements of vitamin C should be allowed. Some type 1 patients respond well to oral pyridoxine (200–500 mg/day), possibly by increasing conversion of glyoxylate to glycine. However, dietary and pharmacological treatment are often ineffective in the long term. Several patients have been successfully treated with combined hepatorenal transplantation.[88] Renal transplantation alone has been unsuccessful because systemically generated oxalate is deposited in the transplanted kidney.

Creatine deficiency

Two autosomal recessive diseases affect the biosynthesis of creatine from glycine and arginine via the intermediate metabolite guanidinoacetate. The deficient enzymes are arginine:glycine amidinotransferase (AGAT) and guanidinoacetate methyltransferase (GAMT). Clinically both disorders have neurological presentation with hypotonia, progressive movement disorder and seizures. Creatine levels are very low. Importantly, treatment with creatine monohydrate has been reported to reverse neurological symptoms.[89,90] Both the GAMT and AGAT genes have been cloned and disease causing mutations have been found. Very recently an X-linked disorder associated with creatine deficiency was described. It is caused by mutations in a creatine transporter (SLC6A8). The clinical symptoms consisted of developmental delay and hypotonia.

Sarcosinemia

Sarcosine is the N-methyl derivative of glycine. It is formed from dimethylglycine, which may be a product of betaine or choline. Sarcosine is not normally present in blood or urine in detectable amounts, although sarcosinuria may occur after the ingestion of lobster and some other foods. Sarcosine dehydrogenase deficiency causes sarcosinemia and has been found in individuals with short stature and mental retardation, but a causal relationship has not been established.

LYSINE, HYDROXYLYSINE, TRYPTOPHAN

Only one clinical disorder, glutaric aciduria type I, is caused by an enzyme defect in the catabolic pathway of lysine, hydroxylysine and tryptophan. However, because of some biochemical similarities, glutaric aciduria types I and II will be both considered here. A second form of glutaric aciduria, designated glutaric aciduria type II, is characterized by severe illness in the neonatal period. Organic acid analysis in type I reveals glutaric aciduria and glutaric acidemia. In type II there are, in addition, accumulations of a wide variety of organic acids, including adipic and ethylmalonic acids. In type I there is a specific defect in glutaryl CoA dehydrogenase, whereas in type II there is a general deficiency in the activity of many acyl-CoA dehydrogenases.

Glutaric aciduria type I

Clinical findings

Glutaric aciduria type I usually presents with neurological symptoms after a initial period of normal development and growth. There is typically acute neurological impairment associated with an illness. Afterward, the patient is often left with severe extrapyrimidal signs, with dystonia and choreoathetosis. Macrocephaly in early infancy is an alerting feature. Metabolic stress such as intercurrent infections can trigger ketosis, acidosis, liver dysfunction, vomiting and acute neurological symptoms such as seizures and coma. The neurological deficits can probably be prevented in children diagnosed and effectively treated before the first metabolic crisis.

Diagnosis

Glutaryl CoA is an intermediate in the catabolism of lysine, tryptophan, and hydroxylysine. Alpha-ketoadipic acid, the common product of all three amino acids, is oxidatively decarboxylated to form glutaryl CoA in a reaction catalyzed by alpha-ketoadipic acid dehydrogenase. Glutaryl CoA dehydrogenase, the enzyme deficient in glutaric aciduria type I is a mitochondrial flavin adenine dinucleotide (FAD)-dependent enzyme, which converts glutaryl CoA to crotonyl CoA. The cardinal characteristic is massive glutaric aciduria. 3-Hydroxyglutaric acid has been found in the urine of these patients.

Glutaric aciduria type I is autosomal recessive. The gene has been cloned, mapped to chromosome 12q and disease causing mutations have been found. Prenatal diagnosis can be performed on cultured amniocytes as well as by DNA based diagnosis.

Treatment

Therapy consists of protein restriction, especially lysine and tryptophan. In addition L-carnitine and riboflavin are used. Some success has been reported with the use of anticonvulsants which stimulate gamma-aminobutyric acid (GABA) receptors. Early treatment can significantly improve the neurological outcome. Aggressive management of intercurrent illness is critical.

Glutaric aciduria type II

Clinical presentation

The severe form presents in the neonatal period with hypotonia, hepatomegaly, acidosis and severe hypoglycemia in association with low ketone levels. A sweaty sock odor similar to isovaleric acidemia is often found. Congenital anomalies may be present and include cystic kidneys, hypoplastic genitals and facial dysmorphology. Death usually occurs despite treatment. Milder cases have also been described and may present with lipid storage myopathy or neurological symptoms.

Diagnosis

This disease is caused by autosomal recessive deficiency of electron transfer flavoprotein (ETF) or ETF-ubiquinone oxidoreductase (ETF-QO). These proteins are required for normal activity of several flavoprotein dependent dehydrogenases, including glutaryl CoA dehydrogenase (glutaric aciduria type I) and isovaleryl CoA dehydrogenase (isovaleric acidemia). The combined deficiency of several dehydrogenases results in the increased excretion of several organic acids in the urine, particularly glutaric and lactic acid, but also other dicarboxylic acids and hydroxy acids. Among the former are ethylmalonic, adipic, suberic and sebacic acids, as well as unsaturated suberic acids. Among the latter are gamma-hydroxybutyric, *p*-hydroxyphenyllactic, and gamma-hydroxyglutaric acids. Both gamma-hydroxyisovaleric (sweaty sock odor!) and gamma-hydroxyisocaproic acids are also found in the urine. The concentrations of the amino acids citrulline, lysine, ornithine and proline may be minimally elevated in plasma and urine. The lysinuria may be massive.

ETF has two subunits, alpha-ETF and beta-ETF. Mutations in the alpha-ETF gene located on chromosome 15q have been reported. Similarly, mutations in the ETF-QO gene, which is on chromosome 4q have been found. Prenatal diagnosis is possible by enzyme assay in cultured amniocytes and organic acid analysis of amniotic fluid.

Treatment

Treatment has only been truly beneficial in the milder, late onset cases. A diet high in carbohydrate (low fat, low protein) is used in conjunction with administration of L-carnitine and very high doses of riboflavin.

Other disorders of lysine metabolism

Deficiency of the bifunctional protein alpha-aminoadipic semialdehyde synthase causes familial hyperlysinemia. The clinical significance of this enzyme deficiency is controversial. Psychomotor retardation has been reported in many but not all affected individuals.

Individuals who lack 2-ketoadipic acid dehydrogenase excrete large amounts of 2-ketoadipic acid and 2-hydroxyadipic acid in their urine. The disorder is termed 2-ketoadipic acidemia. Although there are some case reports of neurological disease in this condition, other patients have been clinically normal.

Hydroxylysinemia has been found in several mentally retarded patients. The amino acid comes solely from collagen, where lysine is hydroxylated after incorporation into protocollagen. However, collagen metabolism was normal and the disorder was due to a defect in the metabolism of free hydroxylysine. A defect in lysine hydroxylation is found in Ehlers–Danlos syndrome type VI.

Hyperprolinemia and hydroxyprolinemia

Hyperprolinemia and hydroxyprolinemia are inborn errors of metabolism of the imino acids. Three distinct metabolic defects have been identified: proline oxidase is deficient in type I hyperprolinemia; 1-pyrroline-5-carboxylate dehydrogenase in type II hyperprolinemia; and hydroxyproline oxidase in hydroxyprolinemia. Although some patients with hyperprolinemia type II have been normal into adult life, it may be responsible for seizures in some patients.

BRANCHED CHAIN AMINO ACIDS (Fig. 24.13)

Defects in the degradation of the branched chain amino acids valine, leucine and isoleucine result in the accumulation of organic acid intermediates. High levels of these compounds are toxic, particularly to the CNS. These diseases are most readily detected by analysis of urine organic acids and in many cases there is a characteristic odor. There are many different enzymes involved in this pathway and autosomal recessive deficiencies have been described for many.

Several of the disorders of branched chain amino acid metabolism are associated with elevated plasma glycine levels and/or hyperammonemia. These disorders were historically termed 'ketotic hyperglycinemias'. They are discussed as a group in this chapter.

ORGANIC ACIDEMIAS

Many of the disorders of branched chain amino acids present with acidosis which is sometimes severe. These conditions represent an important subgroup of the organic acidemias. Diagnostic and therapeutic approaches to metabolic acidosis will be discussed first, followed by the description of individual disorders. Table 24.5 displays a list of disorders associated with metabolic acidosis.

Diagnostic approaches

Unexpectedly severe acidosis, with or without ketosis, in any infant should suggest the possibility of an organic acidemia. The blood pH may be normal or low, the PCO_2 is usually low and an anion gap or base deficit is to be expected. In some disorders, hypoglycemia is frequent and hyperammonemia or lactic acidosis reflects disturbed mitochondrial function. Hyperuricemia can be caused by inhibition of renal tubular secretion of uric acid by other organic acids. In the 'ketotic hyperglycinemia' syndromes (methylmalonic acidemia, propionic acidemia, isovaleric acidemia and 2-methyl-3-hydroxybutyric aciduria) the blood glycine is often raised; an elevated plasma glycine:alanine ratio is more consistent. The

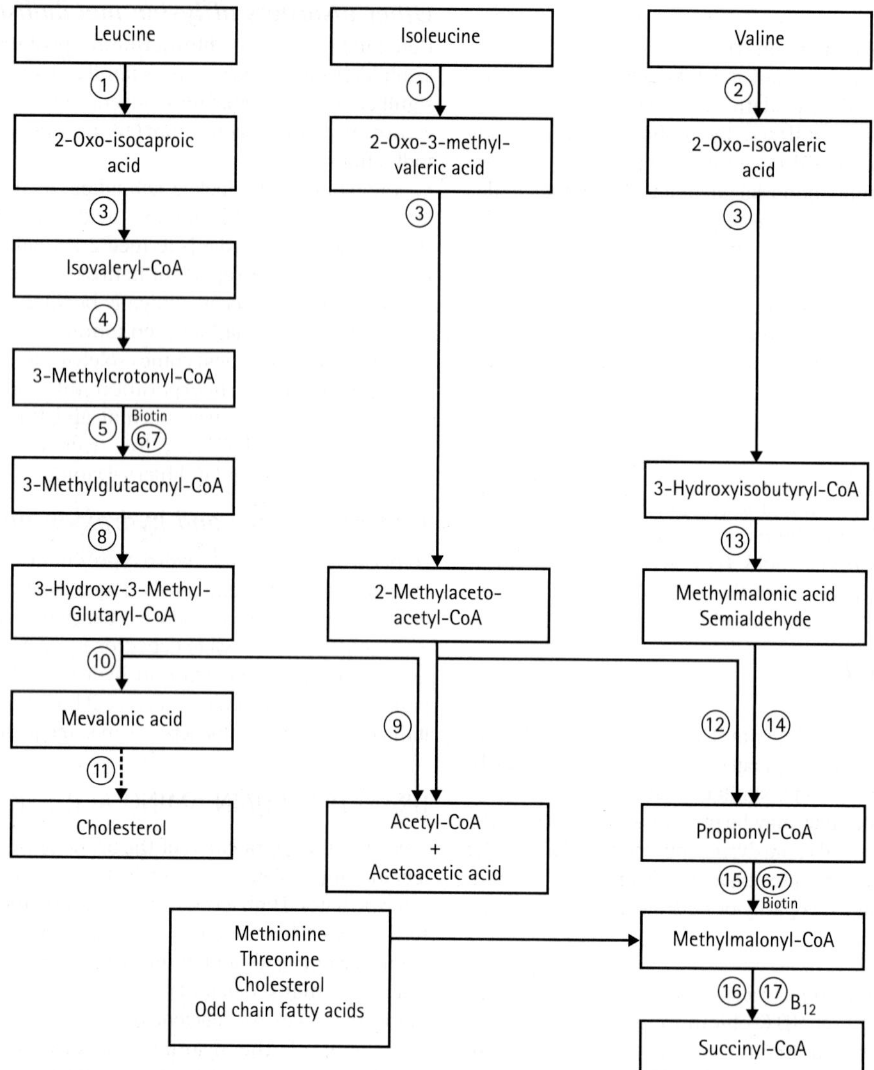

Fig. 24.13 Branched chain amino acid metabolism: numbers indicate known metabolic errors. 1, Leucine aminotransferase; 2, valine aminotransferase; 3, branched chain keto acid decarboxylase (maple syrup urine disease); 4, isovaleryl-CoA dehydrogenase; 5, 3-methylcrotonyl-CoA carboxylase; 6, biotinidase; 7, holocarboxylase synthetase; 8, 3-methylglutaconyl-CoA hydrolase; 9, 3-hydroxy-3-methylglutaryl-CoA lyase; 10, 3-hydroxy-3-methylglutaryl-CoA reductase; 11, mevalonate kinase; 12, 2-methylacetoacetyl-CoA thiolase (β-ketothiolase); 13, 3-hydroxyisobutyryl-CoA deacylase; 14, methylmalonic semialdehyde dehydrogenase; 15, propionyl-CoA carboxylase; 16, methylmalonyl-CoA mutase; 17, cobalamin defects.

neutropenia and thrombocytopenia seem to be related to the glycine levels. In contrast, in lactic acidosis, hyperalaninemia reflects increased transamination of pyruvate. The urine pH is low and the Acetest (Ames), Ketostix (Ames) or dinitrophenylhydrazine tests may be abnormal depending upon which metabolite is being excreted. Diagnosis can usually be made by identification of the organic acid pattern, or its glycine or carnitine conjugates, in blood or urine and can be confirmed by specific enzyme assay in tissues.

In milder cases, the diagnosis may be easily missed unless samples are obtained during an acidotic episode. Provocative tests with precursor amino acids have proved fatal and should rarely be used. *Blood and urine samples for metabolite identification should be taken from any child with unexplained acidosis.*

A number of organic acids may occur in the urine of sick, ketotic or acidotic children, presumably reflecting secondary metabolic disturbances. Lactate can reflect poor tissue perfusion and the *dicarboxylic acids* adipic, suberic and sebacic acids, 3-hydroxyisobutyric acid, 2-methyl-3-hydroxybutyric acid and 3-hydroxyisovaleric acid, as well as the ketone bodies, can all accumulate when lipolysis is increased, making it difficult to distinguish between primary or secondary effects on fatty acid breakdown.

Treatment

Since dehydration is associated with endogenous protein catabolism, it must be avoided; a urine output of 150–200 ml/kg/day or more, if tolerated, may help in the elimination of the metabolites. Before the abnormal metabolites are identified, the patient should receive a low protein and low fat diet with as many calories as can be tolerated i.v. or p.o. If this aggravates a lactic acidosis, the defect may be in the pyruvate dehydrogenase complex (Fig. 24.14). Once the abnormal metabolites are identified, their precursors are restricted in the diet to the limits of metabolic tolerance. Calories are then supplied from all other available sources. Thus in maple syrup urine disease, all three branched chain

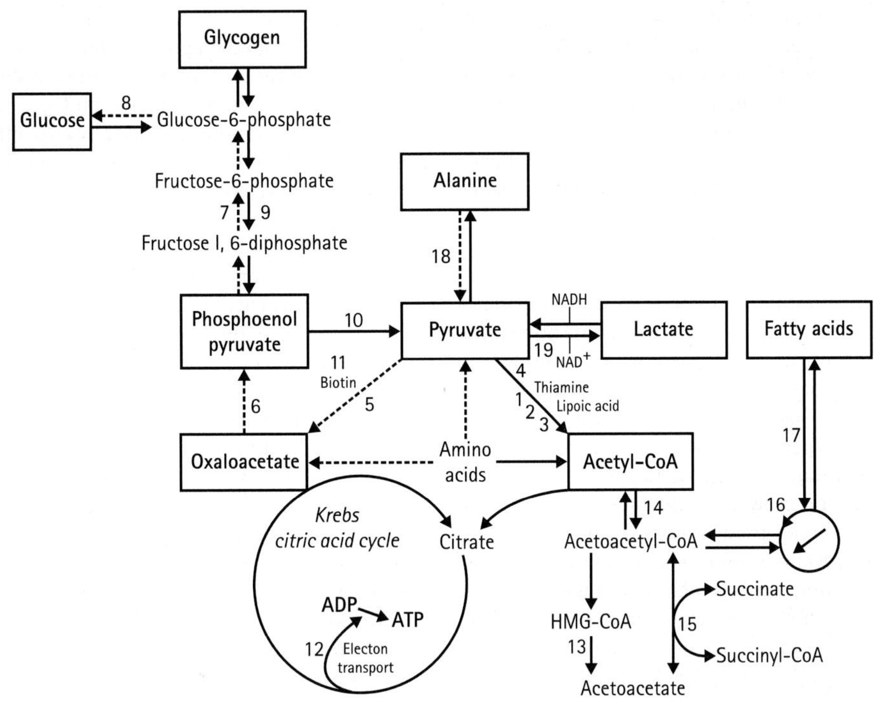

Fig. 24.14 Metabolic pathways involving lactate metabolism. Numbers indicate known metabolic defects. Dotted lines indicate gluconeogenic steps. 1, E_1 of pyruvate dehydrogenase (decarboxylase); 2, E_2 of pyruvate dehydrogenase; 3, E_3 of pyruvate dehydrogenase; 4, pyruvate dehydrogenase phosphatase; 5, pyruvate carboxylase; 6, phosphoenolpyruvate carboxykinase; 7, fructose 1,6-diphosphatase; 8, glucose-6-phosphatase; 9, phosphofructokinase; 10, pyruvate kinase; 11, biotinidase and holocarboxylase synthase; 12, electron transport chain; 13, 3-hydroxy-3-methylglutaryl-CoA-lyase; 14, acetoacetyl-CoA thiolase; 15, succinyl-CoA:3-ketoacid-CoA transferase; 16, beta-oxidation spiral; 17, liporotein lipase; 18, alanine:pyruvate aminotransferase; 19, lactic dehydrogenase.

amino acids are restricted, whereas in isovaleric acidemia only leucine needs to be controlled. Before the diagnosis is established, large doses of vitamin B_{12} (1–2 mg), pyridoxine (150–500 mg), thiamin (200–500 mg), folic acid (10–20 mg), biotin (10–20 mg), nicotinamide (100–500 mg) and riboflavin (100–500 mg) should be given in case the disorder is vitamin dependent. Once the definitive diagnosis is known, those not likely to be useful can be stopped. Abnormal quantities of any CoA derivatives combine with carnitine to make acylcarnitine derivatives which are excreted. This frequently causes profound secondary carnitine depletion which in turn aggravates the metabolic acidosis and may add muscle weakness, hypoglycemia, hepatocellular damage and cardiomyopathy. Initial treatment should include L-carnitine. In extreme cases, hemo- or peritoneal dialysis or continuous extracorporeal hemoperfusion should be used and a glucose/insulin drip may help to reverse endogenous protein catabolism. Of these, hemodialysis is most effective. Once the crisis is over, a diet appropriate to the particular disorder is cautiously reintroduced over several days.

Maple syrup urine disease (MSUD)

In maple syrup urine disease (branched chain ketoaciduria), major cerebral symptoms appear early in the newborn period, and the urine has an odor reminiscent of maple syrup. The branched chain amino acids–leucine, isoleucine and valine–are present in high concentration in the blood and urine, and the ketoacid analogs are found in the urine.

Clinical findings

Infants with MSUD appear well at birth. In the typical patient, symptoms begin after 3–5 days and progress rapidly in the absence of treatment to death within 2–4 weeks. Early manifestations include feeding difficulty, irregular respirations, or progressive loss of the Moro reflex. Severe hypoglycemia may occur. Characteristically these patients develop convulsions, opisthotonos, and generalized muscular rigidity with or without intermittent flaccidity. Death usually occurs after decerebrate rigidity develops. Cortical atrophy may be seen on CT or MRI scan, and the myelin is usually hypodense. This is consistent with the defective myelinization that has been observed at autopsy. The feature that distinguishes branched chain ketoaciduria from other cerebral degenerative diseases of infancy is the characteristic maple syrup, or caramel, odor of the urine, skin, ear cerumen or hair. The odor may become evident 1 or 2 days after birth and may persist, but varies in intensity and may not be detected at all in some specimens.

Milder forms of the disease occur; they represent variant mutations in the same enzyme complex as in classic MSUD. Ataxia and repeated episodes of lethargy progressing to coma occur without neurodevelopmental effects; these episodes may be precipitated by infection or anesthesia.

Diagnosis

Increased quantities of leucine, isoleucine, and valine are found in the plasma and urine. The presence of an abnormal amino acid, alloisoleucine, is diagnostic for MSUD. The catabolism of branched chain amino acids is initiated by a transamination reaction to generate the respective ketoacids which then undergo decarboxylation to CoA derivatives. The defect in MSUD is in this oxidative decarboxylation of the ketoacids which is catalyzed by a mitochondrial multienzyme complex similar to pyruvate dehydrogenase and alpha-ketoglutarate dehydrogenase. For this reason autosomal recessive mutations in four different genes can cause MSUD. Patients have been identified with defects in the E1alpha, E1beta, E2 and E3 subunits of the complex. The E3 subunit is shared by all three complexes and patients with defects in this gene have simultaneous deficiency of branched chain keto acid dehydrogenase, pyruvate dehydrogenase and alpha-ketoglutarate dehydrogenase. MSUD is rare in most populations with an incidence of ~1:150 000.

Treatment

Experience has now been accumulated in MSUD with prolonged use of special diets in which the intakes of leucine, isoleucine and valine are closely controlled. Concentrations of the branched chain amino acids in plasma can be maintained near normal limits. This therapy is difficult. Many patients have had permanent brain damage before treatment is started, but experience with siblings of previous patients, in whom very early diagnosis is possible, and with patients detected by neonatal screening programs, indicates that a normal IQ may be achieved. Commercial products are available that are useful in management. Intravenous solutions of amino acids that exclude the branched chain amino acids take advantage of protein synthesis to reduce concentrations of leucine and the other amino acids and reverse coma in acute episodes of metabolic imbalance. Rare patients have a thiamine responsive form of MSUD and therefore this vitamin should be tried in all cases.

KETOTIC HYPERGLYCINEMIAS

Secondary elevation of plasma glycine is found in some defects of branched chain amino acid metabolism particularly in propionic acidemia, methylmalonic acidemia and 3-ketothiolase deficiency. Because these conditions are also associated with ketoacidosis, they are grouped as the ketotic hyperglycinemias and contrasted to non-ketotic hyperglycinemia, a primary defect in the glycine cleavage system (see above). Urine organic acids should be analyzed in any patient with elevated plasma glycine.

Propionic acidemia

Clinical findings

This disease is characterized by recurrent episodes of metabolic acidosis with severe ketosis, similar to those observed in diabetic coma. There may be symptomatic hyperammonemia due to secondary inhibition of the urea cycle. Neutropenia, thrombocytopenia and osteoporosis severe enough to lead to pathological fracture may occur. Mental retardation is common in older patients. Symptoms begin as early as 18 h after birth, with vomiting, acidosis and ketonuria. Death has occurred with intractable acidosis, and it seems probable that other patients may have died unrecognized early in life. Convulsive seizures and EEG abnormalities may be found.

Diagnosis

The defect is in the enzyme propionyl CoA carboxylase, which catalyzes the formation of methylmalonyl CoA from propionyl CoA (Fig. 24.13). Propionyl CoA is formed in the catabolism of several essential amino acids (valine, isoleucine, methionine, and threonine), odd-chain fatty acids and cholesterol. These offending compounds can be remembered by the mnemonic 'VOMIT'. Propionic acidemia is most readily diagnosed by organic acid analysis of the urine for methylcitrate, 3-OH propionate, propionylglycine and others. Elevated quantities of glycine in the blood and urine may be suggestive. Patients frequently have an abnormal plasma carnitine profile with low free carnitine levels and an elevated fraction of short chain acyl-CoA carnitine. The defect can be demonstrated in leukocytes, in cultured fibroblasts and amniotic fluid cells. Prenatal diagnosis is possible using molecular techniques as well as analysis of amniotic fluid for abnormal metabolites.

The enzyme is multimeric and is composed of non-identical alpha and beta chains, encoded by two different genes. The mode of inheritance is autosomal recessive and families with mutations in both genes have been identified.

Treatment

Restricting dietary intake of protein reduces the frequency and severity of attacks of ketosis and acidosis which are produced by isoleucine, threonine, valine or methionine. Diets in which very small amounts of protein are supplemented with fat, carbohydrate or amino acids other than those listed above have been successfully used to treat propionic acidemia. The amounts of natural protein must be individually determined, but are usually under 1 g/kg/day; supplementation with amino acid containing medical food beverages are then necessary. Treatment with L-carnitine serves to reduce toxic quantities of propionyl CoA as well as reversing secondary deficiency of carnitine.[91] Episodes of intercurrent acidosis occurring with infection must be treated vigorously with large amounts of glucose, fluids and electrolyte, often including sodium bicarbonate and carnitine. Hyperammonemia can be life threatening. Dialysis may be needed during acute decompensation. Patients diagnosed early in infancy and raised according to these therapeutic principles have clearly improved survival and a favorable developmental outcome, though the severe form of this condition can be refractory to even the most aggressive treatment.

Methylmalonic acidemia

Clinical findings

Methylmalonic acidemia is a family of disorders in which methylmalonic acid accumulates in body fluids. The clinical manifestations are similar to those of propionic acidemia, and patients usually present with overwhelming illness in the first weeks after birth. Hyperammonemia, hypoglycemia and ketosis are prominent. Growth retardation may be striking. Convulsions and abnormalities of the EEG have been observed.

This disease is genetically heterogeneous and not all patients with methylmalonic acidemia have a primary defect in branched chain amino acid metabolism. An important second group of patients have a primary defect in vitamin B_{12} metabolism, which is an essential cofactor for methylmalonyl CoA mutase. These patients have lower plasma levels of methylmalonic acid than those with primary defects, they may not become ketotic and may have megaloblastic anemia. High plasma homocysteine levels may be present. Failure to thrive may be extreme and death can occur in early infancy. However, later presentations including in adults have been reported.

Diagnosis

Methylmalonic acid is found elevated in plasma or urine where it is not normally present in more than trace quantities. The urine also contains methylcitrate and plasma glycine may be elevated. Because plasma homocysteine levels may be elevated in patients with defects in B_{12} metabolism, this compound should be measured in every patient with methylmalonic acidemia. Blood concentrations of vitamin B_{12} are normal, except when B_{12} deficiency is the cause of elevated methylmalonic acid.

The defect in methylmalonic acidemia is in the same pathway as propionic acidemia (see above) and the same compounds are toxic. Methylmalonic acid is normally formed from methylmalonyl CoA, which is a product of the propionyl CoA carboxylase reaction (see Fig. 24.13). Methylmalonyl CoA is converted by methylmalonyl CoA mutase to succinyl CoA, which can then be metabolized through the citric acid cycle. The mutase enzyme has a vitamin B_{12} coenzyme, deoxyadenosylcobalamin (AdoCbl). The activity of methylmalonyl CoA mutase is defective in leukocytes, cultured fibroblasts, and amniotic fluid cells.

Impairment of methylmalonyl CoA mutase activity can be caused by mutations in many different genes. All defects are autosomal recessive. The enzyme itself is a dimer of identical subunits and isolated deficiency of the mutase can result from mutations in this gene or at two loci which are required for the biosynthesis of AdoCbl. Genetic defects which affect the transport or synthesis of both methylcobalamine (MeCbl) and AdoCbl cause additional alterations in homocysteine and methionine metabolism. The different defects in B_{12} metabolism and transport are designated as CblA, B, C, etc. The mutase locus and several of the Cbl genes have been cloned and mutations identified in some families. In order to provide accurate prognostic information and genetic counseling, it is essential that the exact cause of methylmalonic acidemia be determined if feasible.

Treatment

The treatment for patients defective in the mutase structural gene is similar to that of propionic acidemia described above. It includes L-carnitine supplementation as well as dietary protein restriction.[92] Liver transplantation has been shown to be beneficial.

Some methylmalonic acidemia patients with Cbl defects are responsive to injection of high doses of vitamin B_{12}. Those that do not respond may require specialized pharmacological and dietary management to control the elevated plasma homocysteine.

3-Ketothiolase deficiency

3-Ketothiolase (mitochondrial acetoacetyl-CoA thiolase) deficiency is a disorder of isoleucine metabolism in which 2-methyl-3-hydroxybutyric acid and tiglylglycine are excreted in the urine. 2-Methylacetoacetic acid, the compound immediately preceding the block, is found in the urine of some patients. The molecular defect is in the specific 3-ketothiolase that converts 2-methylacetoacetyl CoA to propionyl CoA and acetyl-CoA. Clinical manifestations and treatment are similar, but more mild than those of propionic acidemia. This condition is particularly difficult to diagnose because many of the abnormal metabolites are also found in patients which are ketotic for other reasons. The continued elevation of diagnostic metabolites between ketotic episodes indicates 3-ketothiolase deficiency.

Isovaleric acidemia

Isovaleric acidemia is a disorder of the catabolism of leucine that usually presents with severe illness in early life.

Clinical findings

Vomiting and acidosis are prominent, and patients have a characteristic pungent odor. The odor, first described as that of sweaty feet, is that of isovaleric acid. The clinical course is similar to propionic acidemia including acidosis, ketosis, and symptomatic hyperammonemia. Many patients die within a few weeks after birth.

In infants who survive the initial attack but remain untreated, there are recurrent episodes of vomiting, acidosis and ataxia, progressing to lethargy and coma. Acute episodes often occur with infections or after surgery. The odor is more likely to be appreciated during an episode of acute illness, but it may be absent. Mental retardation can be seen, especially among those diagnosed late, but normal IQ and good health are not uncommon. Patients with isovaleric acidemia also may have leukopenia, thrombocytopenia and anemia.

Diagnosis

Isovaleryl CoA is the product of the branched chain decarboxylase reaction in the catabolism of the ketoacid analog of leucine. It is catabolized by isovaleryl CoA dehydrogenase to 3-methylcrotonyl CoA. This enzyme is deficient in isovaleric acidemia. During acute episodes, concentrations of isovaleric acid in the serum and urine may be enormous. Assay for urinary isovalerylglycine is the most reliable approach to the biochemical detection of this disease, and this compound will be identified in routine urine organic acid analysis. The gene for this enzyme has been cloned and localized to chromosome 15q12-15.

Treatment

Acute episodes are treated by vigorous use of parenteral fluids that contain glucose and electrolytes. The acidosis may require sodium bicarbonate. Hemodialysis or peritoneal dialysis may be indicated to treat hyperammonemia and/or acidosis. Long term treatment requires restricting the dietary intake of leucine by lowering the intake of protein until the amounts of leucine ingested are just those necessary for growth. The observed conjugation of isovaleric acid with glycine permits the possibility of adjunctive treatment with exogenous glycine. Additionally L-carnitine and/or L-glycine is administered.[93] If treatment is begun early, the prognosis is good.

3-Hydroxy-3-methylglutaric aciduria

3-Hydroxy-3-methylglutaric aciduria is a disorder of leucine metabolism that leads to hypoketotic hypoglycemia as well as metabolic acidosis. The disease is particularly likely to be mistaken for Reye's syndrome (Ch. 17). Episodes of illness are likely to follow an acute infectious illness.

Clinical findings

Acute episodes of life threatening illness occur in early infancy with metabolic acidosis and hypoglycemia leading to coma.[95] Hyperammonemia can also occur. Persistent vomiting may be the first symptom. Coma and dehydration may lead to apnea and death unless vigorous measures of resuscitation, including mechanical ventilation, are used. Some patients have convulsions, and most patients have hepatomegaly. The acute episodes may be followed by mental retardation, neurological abnormalities, and cerebral atrophy.

Diagnosis

Concentrations of glucose may be strikingly low, but nevertheless there is no ketonuria; this distinguishes these patients from all others with organic acidemia. Liver function tests may be abnormal at times of acute illness. The organic aciduria is characteristic; in addition to large quantities of 3-hydroxy-3-methylglutaric acid, the urine contains 3-methylglutaconic acid and 3-methylglutaric acid, its reduction product. At times of acute illness the urine may also contain large amounts of lactic acid. The molecular defect is in 3-hydroxy-3-methylglutaryl CoA lyase, the last step in leucine catabolism. In addition, this enzyme is crucial for the formation of ketones in mammalian liver. The disorder is transmitted as an autosomal recessive trait. The gene has been cloned and mutations identified in patients.

Treatment

Management of the acute crisis requires large amounts of water, electrolytes, and glucose. Long term management depends on the avoidance of fasting and attendant hypoglycemia. Parents should bring the patient in early when the oral route is compromised by fasting or anorexia. A high carbohydrate diet is useful, and the intake of both fat (ketone precursors) and protein should be limited. L-carnitine has limited usefulness, because 3-hydroxy-3-methylglutaric acid does not form carnitine conjugates.

OTHER BRANCHED CHAIN ORGANIC ACIDURIAS

3-Methylcrotonylglycinuria due to isolated deficiency of 3-methylcrotonyl-CoA carboxylase, is similar to the presentation of isovaleric acidemia described above except there may be an odor similar to cats' urine. 3-Methylcrotonylglycine and 3-hydroxyisovaleric acid are excreted in large amounts in the urine but are not elevated in blood. A trial of biotin (10–20 mg/day) is indicated because most cases who excrete these metabolites have multiple carboxylase deficiency.

A defect of 3-methylglutaconyl-CoA hydratase (step 8) causes excretion of 3-methylglutaconic acid and 3-methylglutaric acid. The usual symptoms are progressive neurological deterioration in infancy, *without obvious metabolic acidosis*. However, hypoglycemia, metabolic acidosis and cardiomyopathy have also been reported although these could have been due to carnitine depletion. Other patients with 3-methylglutaconic aciduria but normal enzyme studies have presented with various symptoms of neurological deterioration including choreoathetosis, spasticity, optic atrophy, tapetoretinal degeneration and nerve deafness. Metabolic acidosis may be absent or marked and most such cases die. Some cases are associated with defects of the respiratory chain but in most, the primary enzyme defect is not known. Barth syndrome is a cardiomyopathy with neutropenia and 3-methylglutaconic aciduria. The gene for this X-linked disorder has been cloned, but its function remains unknown.

2-Methylbutyryl-CoA dehydrogenase deficiency is a newly reported defect of isoleucine metabolism. The clinical presentation included neurological symptoms in the newborn period along with mild acidosis and hypoglycemia. The abnormal metabolites included 2-methylbutyrylglycine and 2-methylbutyrylcarnitine.

MULTIPLE CARBOXYLASE DEFICIENCY

Biotin is an essential cofactor for many carboxylases including several involved in branched chain amino acid metabolism. For this reason pertubations of its association with these enzymes will cause deficiency of multiple different carboxylases.

Clinical findings

Neonatal and infantile forms of the disease are distinguished. The former generally presents with life threatening acidotic illness in the newborn period like that of propionic acidemia or methylmalonic acidemia. Symptoms include severe ketosis, acidosis, dehydration and coma. Death can occur unless vigorous treatment is instituted. Patients who survive the first days of life have alopecia totalis and an impressive red, scaly total body eruption. The infantile form presents later with periorificial dermatitis resembling acrodermatitis enteropathica, partial alopecia and neurological abnormalities such as ataxia, delayed mental development, and convulsions. Nevertheless, these patients too may develop life threatening acidotic episodes. Immunodeficiency may be found in either form of the disease and may involve T and B cell function.

Diagnosis

There are two distinct causes of multiple carboxylase deficiency. One is a deficiency of holocarboxylase synthetase and the other a deficiency of biotinidase. Holocarboxylase synthase catalyzes the association of biotin with the various carboxylases to form functional holoenzymes. Defects in this protein usually cause the severe, neonatal form of the disease. Biotinidase is involved in recycling of the vitamin and deficiency is usually clinically milder. Urine organic acid analysis is characteristic with excretion of 3-methylcrotonylglycine, 3-hydroxyisovaleric, methylcitric, 3-hydroxypropionic, and lactic acids. Tiglylglycine may also be found. The two forms of the disease can be distinguished by mutation analysis or by enzyme measurement in cultured fibroblasts. Biotinidase activity can be determined in blood samples.

Newborn screening for biotinidase deficiency is employed in several locations around the world because the disorder is readily treated and sequelae can be completely avoided. The incidence of complete deficiency is ~1:100 000.

The genes for both holocarboxylase synthetase and biotinidase have been cloned and mutations have been identified. The biotinidase gene maps to chromosome 3p25 and two alleles frequent account for ~50% of all mutations. Holocarboxylase synthetase deficiency is more rare than biotinidase deficiency and there are also two mutations which are more frequent. Prenatal diagnosis and successful prenatal treatment of affected fetuses has been reported.

Treatment

Patients with multiple carboxylase deficiency are exquisitely sensitive to exogenous biotin.[95] Doses of 10 mg/day are usually sufficient to reverse all of the findings, but some patients require more. Carnitine may be a useful adjunct to therapy.

AMINO ACID TRANSPORT DISORDERS

In the kidney and gut, amino acids are actively transported across cell membranes in five major groups (Table 24.7). In addition, there are other separate, but probably minor, transport systems.

Disorders of both group-specific and individual amino acid transport systems exist. In tissues other than kidney and gut there are similar, but not identical active transport processes, but only in lysinuric protein intolerance is any other tissue known to be involved. Renal transport defects result in specific patterns of aminoaciduria, when, if anything, the plasma levels of the same amino acids are

Table 24.7 Group systems of amino acid transport in kidney and gut and their disorders

Group	Disorder
1. (a) Cystine, lysine, ornithine, arginine	Cystinuria type I, II and III
(b) Lysine, ornithine, arginine	Dibasic aminoaciduria (i) Lysinuric protein intolerance (ii) Without protein intolerance
2. Glycine, proline, hydroxyproline	Iminoglycinuria
3. β-Amino acids, taurine	None known
4. Aspartic and glutamic acid	Dicarboxylic aminoaciduria
5. Neutral amino acids (e.g. glycine, alanine, valine, leucine, isoleucine, serine, threonine, cysteine, cystine, phenylalanine, tyrosine, methionine, histidine, tryptophan)	Hartnup disease

lower than normal. Plasma elevation of a single amino acid usually causes a single aminoaciduria, as in PKU, but a single amino acid may saturate the transport mechanism for all the other amino acids within the group causing a group aminoaciduria. For example, in hyperglycinemia, the imino acids (group 2) may be excreted.

Inherited defects of four group transport systems are known but they probably do not affect all cells. For example, the two types of iminoglycinuria imply that several genes must be required for amino acid transport in different tissues. *Dicarboxylic aminoaciduria* is also a benign trait.

Cystinuria

Although the disorder bears the name of only one amino acid, cystinuria is a disorder of transport of cystine and all of the dibasic amino acids, cysteine, ornithine, lysine and arginine ('COLA'). The gene defect is in the SLC7A9 gene, which encodes a subunit of a family of amino acid transporters expressed in kidney, liver, small intestine, and placenta. The condition is mainly important because cystine is very insoluble in normal urine and these patients tend to develop renal calculi at any age. About 1–5% of patients with renal stones have cystinuria. Cystine crystals, which are flat and hexagonal, may be found in the urine. The diagnosis is based upon the nitroprusside test and amino acid chromatography. The aim of treatment is to keep urine cystine levels in the range of maximum solubility (approx. 0.1 mmol/mmol creatinine). It consists of maintaining a urine flow of 2–3 L/m^2 per 24 h or more; 25% of the fluid intake should be taken during the night. Maximum alkalization of the urine to around pH 7.5 is important, since the solubility of cystine decreases markedly below that.

Isolated cystinuria, isolated dibasic aminoaciduria (lysine, ornithine, arginine) and isolated lysinuria have been reported, showing that partial transport defects within the group can also occur.

Lysinuric protein intolerance

Clinical features

In this disorder, most common in Finland, symptoms of hyperammonemia become evident following weaning, when food intolerance, diarrhea, vomiting, hypotonia, hepatosplenomegaly, sparse hair, osteoporosis and marked failure to thrive develop. Interstitial pulmonary fibrosis is a late feature and may prove lethal. Mental development may be normal.

Diagnosis

There is a defect in the renal and intestinal transport of lysine, arginine and ornithine, resulting in increased excretion in the urine and low levels in plasma. Cysteine transport is normal. The hyperammonemia may be explained by deficient transport of urea cycle substrates into liver cells. In addition to other treatment for hyperammonemia, supplementation with citrulline (2–10 g/day) is very beneficial.

Iminoglycinuria

Free imino acids are normally present in urine in the first 6 months but they fall to very low levels thereafter. A defect of proline, hydroxyproline and glycine transport has been found in both retarded and normal people; it appears to be benign. Gastrointestinal transport may be either normal or defective. Hyperglycinuria is marked but renal absorption of the imino acids may only be slightly reduced. Urine glycine normally varies within wide limits and accounts for up to 25% of the amino acids in urine. It is commonly seen in iminoglycinuria heterozygotes but also occurs in the ketotic and non-ketotic hyperglycinemias and in valproate therapy. Glycinuria with glucosuria can occur either alone or with vitamin D-resistant rickets, although the reason for this association is not known.

Hartnup disease

Hartnup disease is caused by defective transport in the kidney and usually the gut, of amino acids in group 5 (Table 24.7). The only constant feature is the characteristic aminoaciduria. The symptoms, if they occur, are those of pellagra which is due to tryptophan deficiency. They include photodermatitis, ataxia, psychiatric changes and mental deterioration, but these are usually intermittent and are only precipitated during protein deprivation or periods of stress. Symptoms usually lessen with age. Malabsorption of tryptophan results in diminished nicotinic acid synthesis, so that patients on a high protein or niacin-supplemented diet are without symptoms. Deficiency of the other amino acids causes no apparent problem. Treatment with oral nicotinic acid (25 mg/day) is effective.

Other amino acid transport defects

Methionine malabsorption in gut and kidney has been associated with mental retardation, convulsions, diarrhea and white hair. 2-Hydroxybutyric acid produced by gut bacteria gives a peculiar, beer-like body odor that gives rise to the name oast-house syndrome. Abnormal transport of several other amino acids may also occur. No treatment is known.

The blue diaper (napkin) syndrome is a rare isolated defect in gut absorption of tryptophan; gut bacteria degrade tryptophan to indoles which are then absorbed, metabolized in the liver and excreted in the urine. The defect may be associated with mental retardation, hypercalcemia and nephrocalcinosis. Urine from these patients intermittently contains the blue pigment indican.

MISCELLANEOUS DISORDERS

Carnosinemia

A number of patients with carnosinemia have been reported. Most have had abnormalities of the CNS, but further experience has revealed a number of completely normal people who have the same defect. Therefore, this metabolic curiosity probably does not cause human disease.

Histidinemia and urocanase deficiency

Histidinemia is a disorder of intermediary metabolism in which large amounts of histidine are found in blood and urine. The condition must be included in the differential diagnosis of PKU because it produces a positive ferric chloride test in the urine. Although there may be no clinical manifestations, more than half of these patients have speech retardation; mental and growth retardation also may occur. Relatively fair hair and blue eyes have been common.

Histidine is normally converted by histidase to urocanic acid, which is further metabolized to form iminoglutamic acid and ultimately glutamic acid. In histidinemia, histidine levels are increased in plasma, urine and CSF. Many patients also have hyperalaninemia. Deficiency of histidase (histidine-ammonia-lyase) has been demonstrated by direct assay of the enzyme in skin. Recent prospective studies have shown conclusively that histidinemia does not cause disease.

Rare case reports have associated autosomal recessive deficiency of the next enzyme in histidine metabolism, urocanase, with severe mental retardation and neurological deterioration.

Succinic semialdehyde dehydrogenase deficiency

Succinic semialdehyde dehydrogenase (SSADH) deficiency is a disorder in the catabolism of GABA, a neurotransmitter. GABA is transaminated to form succinic semialdehyde, which is then reduced by SSADH to succinate. In the presence of a block at this step, succinic semialdehyde is reduced to gamma-hydroxybutyric acid which accumulates in the urine, serum and CSF. Patients with this disease have variable degrees of ataxia and hypotonia, convulsions and mild psychomotor retardation. Gamma-hydroxybutyric aciduria is an interesting model disorder of metabolism because the basic defect leads to the accumulation of a compound of known neuropharmacological activity. Gamma-hydroxybutyric acid was originally developed by the pharmaceutical industry as an analog of GABA that could readily cross the blood–brain barrier and be used as an intravenous anesthetic. It had to be abandoned for clinical use because it produced convulsions and coma.

The gene for SSADH has been cloned and many disease causing mutations have been found. Prenatal diagnosis is available by enzymatic analysis of cultured amniocytes. Treatment is supportive and employs standard anticonvulsant drugs. Recent work with a murine model of SSADH deficiency suggests that treatment with taurine and/or antagonists of the GABA-B receptor may be of therapeutic benefit.[96]

GABA-transaminase deficiency

Deficiency of GABA transaminase has been reported in patients with progressive neurological deterioration, leukodystrophy and hypotonia resulting in eventual death. CSF levels of GABA and homocarnosine were highly elevated.

METAL METABOLISM DISORDERS

(Calcium and magnesium metabolism and the nutritional aspects of trace metals are discussed in Chapter 14.)

Similar to vitamins, metals function via association with proteins. Metals are required for a variety of functions, including electron transfer, oxygen binding and structural support. Although generally needed in trace quantities, inherited disorders which result in either a deficiency or overload state can have severe systemic consequences.

COPPER

Copper is a redox active metal which functions in electron transfer reactions. Copper dependent enzymes are found in a broad variety of metabolic pathways (Table 24.8).

In serum, over 90% of copper is bound to ceruloplasmin. Though historically ceruloplasmin was believed to function as a serum copper transport protein, its primary function is as a ferroxidase, which is required for normal iron homeostasis (see below). The circulating pool of copper which is available for utilization by the tissues is believed to be bound to histidine and other amino acids. An average adult has approximately 100 mg of copper in their body. Homeostasis is maintained via a balance between copper absorption from the gut and loss via biliary excretion. The two most common inherited disorders of copper metabolism affect either the absorptive (Menkes disease) or excretory (Wilson's disease) phases of copper homeostasis.[97]

Table 24.8 Copper dependent enzymes and their function

Cytochrome oxidase	Electron transport
Tyrosinase	Melanin biosynthesis
Peptidylglycine alpha-amidating monooxygenase	Activation of neuropeptides
Dopamine beta hydroxylase	Catecholamine biosynthesis
Lysyl oxidase	Collagen cross-linking
Cu-Zn superoxide dismutase	Protection from oxidative stress

Menkes disease

Menkes disease (~1:250 000) is an X-linked disorder resulting from a profound systemic copper deficiency. The Menkes disease gene (ATP7A or MNK) encodes an ATP dependent copper transporter (P type ATPase) which is expressed in nearly all tissues except the liver. The Menkes protein is required for the systemic absorption of copper from the gut and the placenta. It also functions in the transport of copper across the blood–brain barrier into the CNS. Lack of a functional Menkes protein results in the accumulation of high levels of copper in enterocytes and the placenta due to an inability to release copper to the systemic circulation.

Clinical features

Menkes disease results in severe developmental delay and failure to thrive. Drowsiness, lethargy, hypotonia, hypothermia and feeding difficulties are often evident within a few days of birth. The skin is soft and doughy. The most characteristic feature is the hair, which is sparse and depigmented, with a texture similar to steel wool, leading to the term 'Menkes kinky hair syndrome' (Fig. 24.15). The corkscrew-like microscopic appearance of the hair is termed pili torti. The clinical features are a direct result of the loss of function of copper dependent enzymes. Tyrosinase deficiency results in hypopigmentation of the skin and hair. Peptidylglycine alpha-amidating monooxygenase (PAM) is required for the activation of a large number of neuropeptides (e.g. gastrin, vasoactive intestinal peptide, melanocyte stimulating hormone, thyrotropin releasing hormone, cholecystokinin, vasopressin, corticotropin releasing hormone and calcitonin). PAM deficiency leads to a broad spectrum of neuroendocrine derangements.

Abnormalities of collagen due to lysyl oxidase deficiency cause osteoporosis, flared metaphyses and fractures, which may suggest battering; Wormian bones are also common. Arteries are often tortuous and may rupture. The ureters and the bladder wall are weakened and dilated. Deficiency of cytochrome oxidase and dopamine beta-hydroxylase result in CNS degeneration, characterized by abnormalities of myelin, and cerebral and cerebellar atrophy. Seizures are common. Rupture of weakened intracranial blood vessels frequently results in subdural hematomas. Death occurs commonly in the first decade.

Heterozygous females have normal levels of copper, ceruloplasmin, and catecholamines. Pili torti is present in approximately 50% of obligate carriers. Thus the absence of pili torti does not exclude carrier status.

A well characterized variant of Menkes disease associated with milder mutations in the ATP7A gene is the occipital horn syndrome also known as X-linked cutis laxa or formerly as Ehlers–Danlos syndrome type IX (see Ch. 27).

The occipital horn syndrome is a disorder of connective tissues characterized by lax skin and joints, bladder diverticula, inguinal hernias and arterial tortuosity. Ossification within the tendons which attach the trapezius and sternocleidomastoid muscles to the skull give rise to the pathognomonic occipital horns, which can be felt by palpation and demonstrated radiographically. Patients have a deficiency of lysyl oxidase activity as a result of the cellular defect in copper transport. Some patients also have symptoms of autonomic dysfunction, such as orthostatic hypotension, due to decreased dopamine beta-hydroxylase activity.

Diagnosis

The primary biochemical abnormalities are decreased serum levels of copper and ceruloplasmin. Abnormalities of catecholamine

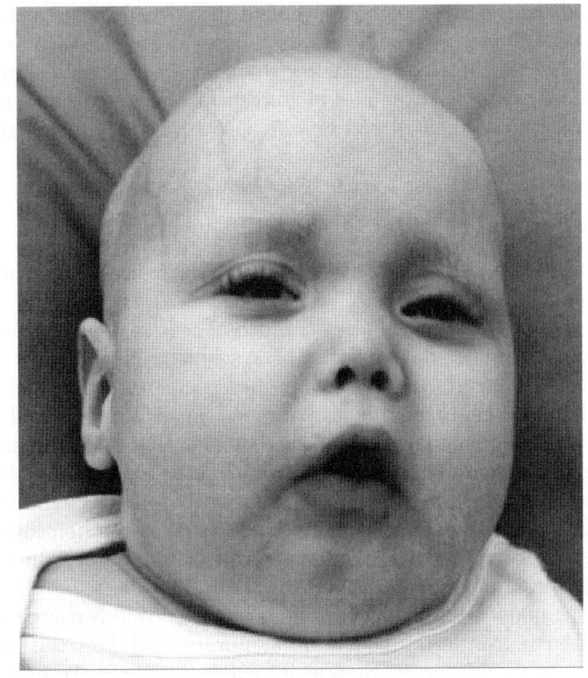
(a)

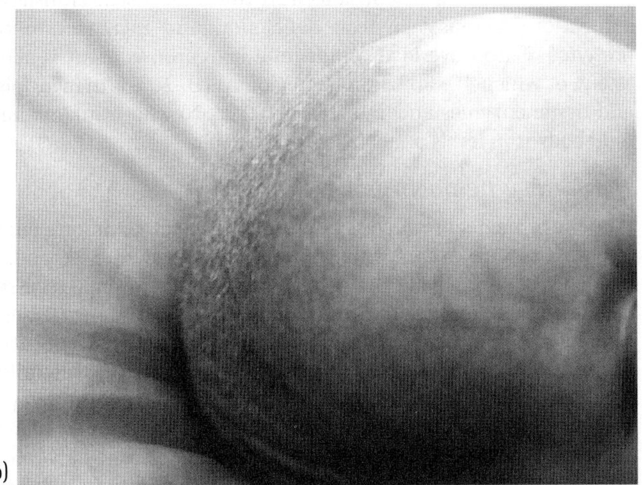
(b)

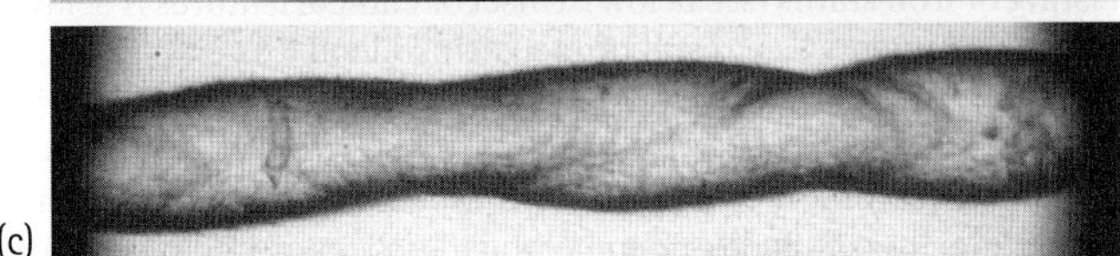
(c)

Fig. 24.15 Features and typical hair of Menkes syndrome.

levels secondary to dopamine beta-hydroxylase deficiency are also present, and can be used to confirm a suspected diagnosis. In neonates, analysis of plasma catecholamines is the preferred approach, as the levels of copper and ceruloplasmin are also low in healthy infants. Measurement of radioactive copper uptake by cultured fibroblasts is increased in Menkes cells, and can also be used for diagnosis. Because of the large number of mutations which have been identified in the Menkes gene, molecular diagnosis is not readily available.

Treatment

As a result of the defect in absorption of copper from the gut, oral copper supplementation is not effective. Parenteral administration of copper histidinate has been shown to improve neurological outcome when begun in the early neonatal period, however the patients still suffer from significant impairment. Improvement in seizure control has been observed following administration of copper histidinate. A single unsuccessful attempt at in utero copper treatment has also been reported. Long term follow-up of one series of treated patients demonstrated improvement in neurological status, but left significant residual connective tissue problems, leading the authors to conclude that the therapy should still be considered experimental.[98]

Wilson's disease

Wilson's disease is an autosomal recessive disorder caused by mutations in the ATP7B gene. The Wilson's disease protein is a copper transporting ATPase that is homologous to the Menkes disease protein. Like Menkes disease, Wilson's disease results from a defect in intracellular copper transport. The differences in clinical symptoms between Menkes and Wilson's diseases are a result of the different tissue distributions of the two proteins; the Wilson's protein is primarily found in the liver, whereas the Menkes gene is expressed in non-hepatic tissues. The Wilson's protein is required for the export of copper into the bile. It is also required for transport of copper into the Golgi apparatus for ceruloplasmin synthesis.

Clinical features

Wilson's disease, also known as hepatolenticular degeneration, primarily affects the liver and the nervous system, particularly the basal ganglia. Patients may present at any time from early childhood to the fifth decade. Pediatric patients most commonly present with liver disease, which usually becomes evident in the first or second decade. In childhood and early adolescence hepatosplenomegaly, jaundice and symptoms of hepatitis are the most common findings. Acute hepatic failure with a hemolytic anemia is a severe and often fatal presentation. Dystonia, characteristic of damage to the basal ganglia, may be seen in association with liver dysfunction, or may be the presenting sign. Indeed, children with Wilson's disease may present only with neurological manifestations without any evidence of liver disease. Deterioration of school performance and changes in mood and behavior may also be the first signs. After adolescence, the disease more commonly presents with neurological symptoms. Progressive extrapyramidal signs, including rigidity, dysarthria, dysphagia, drooling and intellectual deterioration may mimic Parkinson's disease. Psychiatric symptoms ranging from mania to depression, paranoia or anxiety can also be encountered. Occasionally, flapping tremor, schizophrenic behavior or the renal Fanconi syndrome may be the presenting feature. A brown or green ring around the corneal limbus in the eye – the Kayser–Fleischer ring – is caused by copper deposited in Descemet's membrane (Fig. 24.16), but is often not present in the first decade.

Diagnosis

Wilson's disease should be considered in any child with unexplained liver disease, neurological dysfunction or hemolytic anemia. The definitive test is the determination of liver copper content on a biopsy sample. In young presymptomatic patients liver copper content may be normal since the copper accumulates over time. Plasma copper and ceruloplasmin are usually low. However, ceruloplasmin levels can also be low in liver disease of other etiologies, as well as in patients with malnutrition. A normal ceruloplasmin does not rule out Wilson's disease. A Kayser–Fleischer ring is rarely present in pediatric patients presenting with hepatic disease but is more likely to be seen in the presence of neurological symptoms. MRI evaluation of

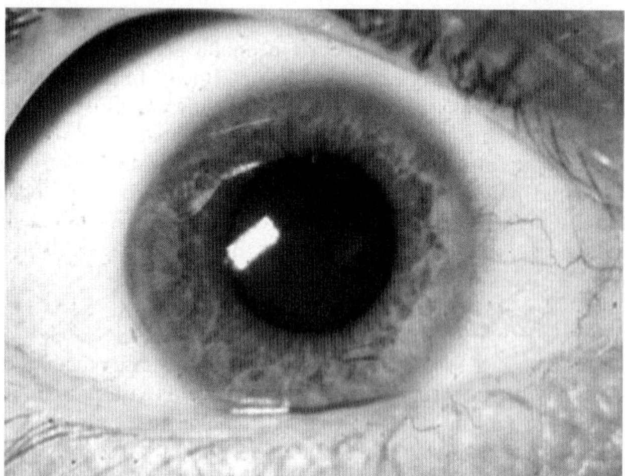

Fig. 24.16 Kayser–Fleischer ring caused by copper deposited in Descemet's membrane in a child with Wilson's disease.

the brain can be used to look for evidence of damage to the basal ganglia. A 24 h urine collection usually demonstrates an increased level of copper. 24 h copper excretion after a dose of D-penicillamine, which mobilizes copper stores, is also elevated in Wilson's disease. Some degree of Fanconi's renotubular syndrome is usual. The large number of disease causing mutations makes DNA diagnosis impractical at present.

Treatment

It is important to diagnose the disease early since treatment can prevent the onset of symptoms and results in striking clinical improvement. Chelation therapy with oral D-penicillamine to remove excess copper and limitation of dietary copper intake has historically been the most frequent approach to therapy. However, because of significant toxicity D-penicillamine use is decreasing. D-penicillamine should not be used initially in children with neurological dysfunction because of the risk of worsening of neurological dysfunction with onset of therapy. The efficacy of an alternative chelating agent, tetrathiomolybdate, is currently being evaluated. Oral zinc supplementation (zinc acetate: 25–150 mg/day in children) reduces copper absorption and is highly effective at reducing ongoing copper accumulation. Patients must be monitored by measurement of urinary copper excretion to avoid copper deficiency which can result from excessive treatment. The primary signs of copper deficiency in children are a hypochromic microcytic anemia and depressed white blood cell (WBC) count.[99]

Patients diagnosed with Wilson's disease should be referred to a center with experience in treatment.

Liver transplantation is indicated for progressive hepatic insufficiency associated with cirrhosis and in fulminant liver failure. Successful liver transplant results in complete correction of copper homeostasis and reversal of most neurological dysfunction.

Aceruloplasminemia is a rare autosomal recessive disorder due to mutations in the ceruloplasmin gene. Ceruloplasmin is a copper containing ferroxidase which is required for the mobilization of iron from reticuloendothelial cells into the systemic circulation. Expression of ceruloplasmin has also been demonstrated in astrocytes, where it functions in CNS iron metabolism. Accumulation of iron in the pancreas, basal ganglia and retina are responsible for the primary symptoms of aceruloplasminemia, which usually presents in the fourth decade of life. Clinical features include an extrapyramidal movement disorder, diabetes mellitus and retinal degeneration. Excess iron deposits are also seen in the liver. Plasma copper levels are low secondary to the ceruloplasmin deficiency. The abnormalities of iron metabolism result in a mild anemia and decreased serum iron level. No specific treatment is known.

IRON

The nutritional aspects of iron metabolism are discussed in Chapter 14.

Dietary iron which enters the mucosal cells of the gut has two possible fates. In the presence of systemic iron deficiency the majority of the iron is released into the systemic circulation where it is bound to transferrin. In iron overload states the majority of the iron which enters the mucosal cell is bound to ferritin and retained. This ferritin bound iron is subsequently lost through the sloughing of the mucosal cells into the gut lumen. There is no mechanism for iron excretion, therefore maintenance of normal iron homeostasis depends of the ability to regulate the rate of iron absorption from the gut in response to total body iron stores.

The major iron transport protein of the plasma is transferrin. After birth, transferrin is about 65% saturated with iron, this value falling to a norm of 20–30% as iron stores are used. Transferrin saturation decreases in iron deficiency, and increases in the presence of iron overload. Adult total body iron content is about 3–4 g, of which 40–60% is in hemoglobin, 10–20% is in myoglobin and tissue enzymes and 10–40% is stored. Newborn infants have total body iron levels of about 250–400 mg.

Hereditary hemochromatosis

Hereditary hemochromatosis is one of the most common genetic disorders of Caucasians, with a carrier frequency of 10% and an incidence of 2–3 per 1000. It is inherited as an autosomal recessive condition, and results from mutations in the HFE gene. Patients have total body iron levels which are 5 to 10 times normal (15–40 g) as a result of increased iron absorption from the gut. Only a few milligrams of iron are absorbed each day, resulting in a delay of symptom onset until adulthood in most cases. The disorder may be identified in children serendipitously during routine laboratory testing of iron status (see below). Onset of clinical features is delayed in female patients as a result of menstrual blood loss.

Clinical features

The most common symptoms are weakness, abdominal pain, arthralgia, loss of libido and impotency. Associated findings include hepatomegaly, increased pigmentation, diabetes mellitus and hair loss. The pathology in hemochromatosis is a direct result of tissue iron deposition, and is believed to be due to the iron catalyzed generation of toxic oxygen radicals.

Diagnosis

Patients with hereditary hemochromatosis have an elevated transferrin saturation (> 50%), which is present prior to the onset of clinical symptoms. Ferritin may also be elevated but is a less reliable indicator and may be elevated in other conditions. DNA based testing can also be done for hemochromatosis, with two common mutations (C282T and H63D) accounting for the vast majority of disease causing alleles. However, all patients homozygous for a mutation in the HFE gene will not demonstrate iron overload. Therefore treatment should be based upon measures of body iron status. Liver biopsy demonstrates increased iron which progressively increases with age; however this is rarely needed for diagnosis. Heterozygotes are sometimes mildly affected, and often can be identified by measurement of transferrin saturation and/or DNA analysis.

Treatment

Fortunately, the iron which accumulates in hemochromatosis can be readily mobilized, allowing for treatment via repeated phlebotomy. Each pint of blood removes around 200–250 mg of iron. The long term prognosis for patients who begin treatment before significant tissue damage occurs (hepatic cirrhosis, diabetes mellitus) is excellent, and in some reported series is no different from unaffected persons. However, much of the damage which occurs in hemochromatosis is irreversible, emphasizing the need for early diagnosis and treatment. Because of the high incidence and excellent response to early therapy, population screening for hereditary hemochromatosis has been considered.

Neonatal hemochromatosis

Neonatal hemochromatosis is a rare cause of neonatal liver failure. The etiology of this disorder is unknown, and may in fact be the end result of several different primary disorders. Elevated iron has been seen in the liver of neonates with viral infections [cytomegalovirus (CMV), echovirus], neonatal lupus, and inherited disorders of bile acid synthesis. The liver demonstrates cirrhosis, fatty infiltration and bile duct proliferation with hemosiderin deposits. The pancreas, adrenals, thyroid and myocardium may also be affected. There is no specific therapy, though liver transplant has been successfully employed.

Pantothenate kinase associated neurodegeneration

Pantothenate kinase associated neurodegeneration (PKAN) causes a progressive movement disorder with dystonia, chorea, athetosis and developmental deterioration. Death in the second decade is typical. The basal ganglia show extensive iron deposits. The disorder is caused by mutations in the PANK2 gene, which is believed to function in CoA biosynthesis.[100] There is at present no specific treatment.

Atransferrinemia

Atransferrinemia is a very rare autosomal recessive disorder due to mutations in the transferrin gene. Patients have a hypochromic anemia which is resistant to iron therapy but can be treated by infusion of plasma which contains transferrin. Excess iron accumulation occurs in the myocardium and liver.

NRAMP2 and HEPH

Recently two genes with a role in intestinal iron absorption have been identified via studies of mutant mouse strains. Mutations of either of these genes (NRAMP2 and HEPH) in the mouse result in an inherited iron deficiency anemia. No primary disorders of the genes have been described in human patients, but they have been implicated as modifier genes for hereditary hemochromatosis.

ZINC

Zinc is an essential element which functions as a cofactor for enzymes and plays a crucial structural role in a large number of DNA transcription factors. Hyperzincemia has been described in several members of a pedigree; the condition is benign and is probably due to an unusual zinc-binding protein in the plasma. Acrodermatitis enteropathica (see Ch. 28), is an inherited disorder associated with severe zinc deficiency. Typical symptoms include diarrhea, dermatitis, alopecia and failure to thrive. The primary defect is unknown, but it results in a decreased efficiency of zinc absorption from the gut. The symptoms respond completely to oral zinc sulfate supplementation.

MOLYBDENUM

Molybdenum is required for the function of three enzymes, xanthine oxidase, sulfite oxidase and aldehyde oxidase. The functional complex of molybdenum is called the molybdenum cofactor, and consists of a single metal atom in complex with a pterin. Molybdenum cofactor deficiency results in severe progressive neurological deterioration, seizures, dislocated lenses and early death. Serum uric acid is very low and the urine contains xanthine, sulfite and thiosulfate. Diagnosis can be made on the basis of low uric acid and an elevation of urine sulfite, which can be detected by dipstick in fresh urine. No successful treatment has been reported. (molybdenum cofactor deficiency is also discussed in the section on disorders of amino acid metabolism.)

THE PORPHYRIAS

The porphyrias are a heterogeneous group of disorders resulting from inherited or acquired abnormalities in heme biosynthesis.[101] The symptoms associated with these disorders result primarily from the accumulation of heme precursors, as opposed to heme deficiency. The tissues with the highest rates of heme biosynthesis are the liver and the erythroid bone marrow, leading to the frequent classification of porphyrias as either hepatic or erythropoietic. An alternative classification scheme for porphyrias is based upon the nature of their clinical symptoms. Acute porphyrias are characterized by symptom free periods alternating with episodic attacks. Non-acute or cutaneous porphyrias are characterized by chronic symptomatology.

Heme is biosynthesized in eight sequential steps, the first and last three taking place in the mitochondrion. The rate-limiting enzyme in heme biosynthesis is delta-aminolevulinic acid synthase (ALAS), which catalyzes the first committed step in the pathway, forming delta-aminolevulinic acid (ALA). The level of ALAS activity, and thus the rate of heme biosynthesis, is normally subject to feedback inhibition. An inherited deficiency in any of the enzymatic steps of the pathway results in a decreased rate of heme production and a loss of the normal feedback inhibition, resulting in the accumulation of symptom causing biosynthetic intermediates.

In the liver, large amounts of heme are required for the activity of the cytochrome P450 enzymes involved in metabolite and drug metabolism. Drugs that induce cytochrome P450 enzymes, such as phenobarbital, lead to an increased rate of heme production via elevation of the level of ALAS. In patients with acute forms of porphyria the increased rate of ALA synthesis results in a rapid rise in the levels of heme precursors and the onset of symptomatology. In contrast, the symptoms associated with the cutaneous porphyrias are primarily the result of the chronic accumulation of photosensitizing porphyrins in the skin. The specific symptoms in individual patients vary widely in all types of porphyria, depending on the nature of their specific disease causing mutation(s). Since an absolute block in heme biosynthesis would be lethal, all patients have some residual enzyme activity.

CLINICAL FEATURES

Acute porphyrias

The most common symptom of acute porphyria is severe abdominal pain, typically constant and poorly localized, and often associated with nausea, vomiting and constipation. Tachycardia is the second most common symptom. Dark urine, motor neuropathy and psychiatric symptoms including depression, anxiety, hallucinations and paranoia are also frequently observed. In severe cases, muscle weakness can lead to paralysis and respiratory compromise. Peripheral neuropathy may result in sensory changes and urinary retention. The symptoms of acute porphyrias are believed to result primarily from the effects of ALA and porphobilinogen (PBG) on the nervous system. Heme deficiency and free radical damage may also be contributory. Significantly, the symptoms of acute porphyrias are not associated with an inflammatory response, thus fever, an elevated WBC count and erythrocyte sedimentation rate (ESR) are not typical features.

Acute intermittent porphyria (AIP) is the most common of the acute porphyrias in the UK (1:10–20 000), it results from a 50% reduction in porphobilinogen deaminase (PBGD) activity. AIP is inherited as an autosomal dominant disorder, as are the two other common forms of acute porphyria, variegate porphyria and hereditary coproporphyria. Though rare in the general population, variegate porphyria has a prevalence of 1:3000 in Afrikaners. A very rare form of acute porphyria, aminolevulinic acid dehydratase deficiency porphyria is inherited as an autosomal recessive condition. In spite of its genetic basis, a family history of acute porphyria is frequently negative. Only 10–20% of patients who inherit the gene for AIP ever develop symptoms, which almost never occur before the onset of puberty.

Both endogenous and exogenous agents can trigger the onset of symptoms, the common feature being their induction of liver cytochrome P450s and a concomitant increase in the rate of liver heme biosynthesis. Precipitating factors include prescription and illicit drugs, fasting, smoking, alcohol and stress. The cyclical hormonal changes associated with menstruation as well as oral contraceptives can also precipitate attacks, resulting in a higher incidence of symptoms in females. A list of drugs that have been associated with symptoms is listed in Table 24.9. A more complete listing is available at the time of writing at the following web site (http://www.uq.edu.au/porphyria/) though the accuracy of the lists must be confirmed.

Patients with variegate porphyria and hereditary coproporphyria have neurovisceral symptoms similar to, but generally milder than those seen in AIP. In addition, variegate porphyria (and occasionally hereditary coproporphyria) can cause cutaneous photosensitivity and skin lesions similar to those seen in the non-acute porphyrias (see below). The symptoms of aminolevulinic acid dehydratase deficiency porphyria are highly variable in regards to both age of onset and severity. This variability likely results from heterogeneity in regards to the amount of residual enzyme activity in individual patients. In general the symptoms resemble those of AIP.

Diagnosis

Symptoms of acute porphyria in the prepubertal pediatric population are extremely rare, therefore more common causes of acute abdominal symptoms must first be excluded. In older patients with acute porphyria, symptoms suggestive of psychosomatic disease may predominate. A detailed inquiry for associated symptoms and possible history of affected relatives is essential. A history of photosensitive skin lesions in addition to the neurovisceral symptoms is highly suggestive of variegate porphyria and may be seen in hereditary coproporphyria. All types of acute porphyria result in marked elevations of urine PBG during an acute attack. Levels of urine ALA are also elevated to a lesser degree. An exception is in aminolevulinic acid dehydratase deficiency, where PBG levels are normal. Initial testing can be done on a single urine specimen, but requires special handling to avoid sample degradation, and referral to an experienced laboratory. A normal level of ALA and PBG on a spot urine sample taken during an acute episode effectively rules out acute porphyria as an etiology for the symptoms. In the presence of skin lesions total plasma porphyrins and fecal porphyrins should also be measured. Between episodes of AIP, levels of PBG typically remain elevated and can be quantitated via 24 h urine collection. Specific enzyme testing may be needed to confirm the diagnosis and to screen potentially affected family members. Minor elevations of porphyrins can be seen in a variety of disorders and care must be taken to avoid incorrectly making a diagnosis of porphyria in these patients.

Table 24.9 Some of the drugs and toxins which may aggravate acute porphyrias. The list is not exhaustive

Barbiturates	Oral contraceptives
Chloroquine	Pentazocine
Erythromycin	Phenytoin
Estrogens	Primidone
Ethanol	Sulfonamides
Griseofulvin	Theophylline
Ketamine	Trimethadione
Meprobamate	Valproic acid

Treatment

The onset of symptoms results from an increased demand for heme in the liver. Measures to reduce this demand include elimination of any drugs that may have contributed, infusion of heme, and i.v. fluids containing glucose. Infusion of a 10% glucose solution and correction of any electrolyte imbalances should begin immediately. Heme arginate (Normosang, Leiras) (3 mg/kg i.v. in a single daily dose) is given to inhibit the endogenous production of heme and thus decrease the rate of production of ALA and PBG. Nausea and vomiting can be treated with chlorpromazine or other phenothiazines. Pain should be managed aggressively, using narcotics if required during an acute episode. Symptoms usually resolve in several days so long term treatment with narcotics should not be necessary. Propranolol can be used for tachycardia and hypertension. Long term management includes the avoidance of precipitating drugs and a high carbohydrate diet (60–70% of total calories). Regular infusions of heme arginate may also be effective.

Non-acute porphyrias

In contrast to the acute porphyrias, the non-acute porphyrias usually have their onset in childhood, and symptoms are chronic rather than episodic. The primary symptom of these disorders is skin damage, which results from photosensitivity caused by the accumulation of porphyrins in the skin. In contrast to the acute porphyrias in which symptoms are usually triggered by drugs and endogenous metabolites, the cutaneous forms of porphyria are exacerbated by exposure to ultraviolet (UV) light.

Congenital erythropoietic porphyria (CEP) is a rare form of porphyria inherited as an autosomal recessive condition. The diagnosis may be first suspected following the observation of red tinted urine in the diaper. Accumulation of porphyrins in red cell membranes results in hemolytic anemia, which can cause severe in utero anemia and hydrops fetalis. Chronic anemia and splenomegally are characteristic features in older patients. Accumulation of porphyrins in the skin results in blistering and friability following exposure to UV light. Abnormalities of pigmentation, hypertrichosis and thickening of the skin occur with repeated damage. Recurrent skin infections can lead to loss of digits and scarring of the eyelids, nose and ears. Deposition of porphyrins in the teeth results in red discoloration called erythrodontia. The porphyrins that accumulate in CEP are fluorescent, and can be seen by long wave illumination of the teeth and red blood cells. The severe symptoms in this disorder often lead to a premature death.

Porphyria cutanea tarda (PCT) is the most common form of porphyria, and results from decreased activity of liver uroporphyrinogen decarboxylase (UROD). The primary manifestation of PCT is photosensitivity, which results in similar though somewhat milder symptoms than those in CEP. Mild elevations of liver enzymes are also characteristic. There are two forms of PCT; type I accounts for 80% of cases and is caused by an acquired deficiency of UROD. Type I PCT is the result of the sensitivity of UROD to a variety of hepatic insults, particularly iron overload. An association between hereditary hemochromatosis and type I PCT has been described. A reduction in UROD activity and symptoms of PCT can also be caused by alcohol use, hepatitis C, human immunodeficiency virus (HIV) infection, estrogens and smoking. Type II PCT is due to an inherited mutation in the UROD gene. Patients with type II disease have a 50% reduction in UROD activity; its inheritance is autosomal dominant. Patients with a homozygous deficiency of UROD have a more severe form of PCT called hepatoerythropoietic porphyria, which results in symptoms similar to those of CEP.

Erythropoietic porphyria (EP) is the most common inherited form of cutaneous porphyria. EP results from a reduction in ferrochelatase activity, and is inherited as an autosomal dominant disorder. Ferrochelatase catalyzes the final step of heme biosynthesis, the addition of Fe^{2+} to protoporphyrin. The cutaneous manifestations of EP include burning, itching, erythema and swelling. Chronic sun exposure and skin damage can lead to scarring, though this is usually less severe than in CEP and HEP. Occasional patients develop severe liver dysfunction secondary to porphyrin accumulation. A mild hypochromic anemia may be present, but hemolysis is uncommon.[102]

Diagnosis

In contrast to the acute porphyrias, which are characterized by the accumulation of ALA and PBG in the urine, most of the porphyrins that accumulate in the non-acute porphyrias are not highly water soluble and therefore are not primarily excreted in the urine. Initial screening of patients suspected of having a cutaneous form of porphyria can be done by analysis of total plasma porphyrins. Subsequent analysis of stool, urine and red blood cells may be required for specific disease identification.

Treatment

Because of the role of sun exposure in the pathophysiology of these disorders its avoidance is central to any treatment regimen. Special protective clothing and sunscreen lotions should be routinely utilized. Oral beta-carotene and cysteine may result in improved sun tolerance.[103] In CEP chronic transfusion therapy to suppress bone marrow heme production is an effective way to decrease circulating porphyrin levels. Chelation therapy is essential to avoid the complications of iron overload. Because of the sensitivity of UROD to iron, phlebotomy to lower liver iron levels is beneficial in all types of PCT. Low dose chloroquine treatment is also beneficial in PCT. The liver dysfunction in EP may be improved by a combination of oral bile acid supplementation to facilitate porphyrin excretion, and colestyramine to inhibit their reabsorption.

Liver transplantation has been performed in EP where it has been shown that porphyrins accumulate in the transplanted liver allograft, indicating that the erythroid bone marrow is the main source of porphyrins in this disorder.[104] Bone marrow transplantation in an animal model of EP resulted in a marked drop in tissue porphyrin levels, indicating that this approach may be helpful in EP patients. Successful gene therapy for the photosensitivity in EP has also been reported in the mouse. Several patients with CEP have been treated successfully by bone marrow transplant.[105,106] Gene therapy for this disorder is currently being developed.[107]

BILIRUBIN AND BILE ACID METABOLISM

The pathophysiology and differential diagnosis of jaundice are discussed elsewhere (Ch. 10) and only those conditions with a genetic defect in bilirubin metabolism are considered here.

UNCONJUGATED HYPERBILIRUBINEMIA

Crigler–Najjar syndrome

The type I variant of the Crigler–Najjar syndrome is an autosomal recessive condition characterized by complete absence of uridine diphosphate (UDP)-bilirubin glucuronyl transferase. It presents in the neonatal period with severe unconjugated hyperbilirubinemia (360–850 μmol/L or 21–50 mg/dl) and, unless repeated exchange transfusions are performed and continuous phototherapy instituted, kernicterus rapidly develops. Death frequently occurs during the first year but rarely the onset of kernicterus may be delayed until after the late teens. Heterozygotes have normal serum bilirubin levels but may have impaired glucuronidation of other substrates. Diagnosis is based on the exclusion of other causes of hyperbilirubinemia, normal liver histology, lack of bilirubin conjugates and absent enzyme activity. Treatment via the use of enzyme inducing agents such as phenobarbital is ineffective, however phototherapy and plasmapheresis can be used to lower unconjugated bilirubin levels. Liver transplantation is curative, and initial experience with hepatocyte infusion suggests that this may also be effective. Gene therapy is also being developed.

The type II variant of Crigler–Najjar syndrome is allelic with type I, and results from less severe mutations in the UDP-bilirubin glucoronyl transferase gene. It presents with jaundice usually in the first year of life but this may be delayed until childhood or later. The serum bilirubin may be intermittently raised to 80–360 μmol/L (5–21 mg/dl) and falls with phenobarbital treatment. Kernicterus is rare. Relatives may give a history of a similar pattern of jaundice.

Gilbert's syndrome

Gilbert's syndrome (~1:1000) is characterized by a mild, chronic and variable unconjugated hyperbilirubinemia (~50 μmol/L, 3 mg/dl). It is inherited as an autosomal recessive condition which is caused by mutations in the promoter region of the UDP-bilirubin glucuronyl transferase gene. Intercurrent infection, fasting, exertion and excessive alcohol intake may exacerbate the hyperbilirubinemia. Autosomal dominant inheritance has been described in some pedigrees, and males are more commonly affected than females.[108] The condition often remains undiagnosed until adulthood. Hepatic morphology is normal and kernicterus does not occur. The disorder is benign but if skin pigmentation is distressing, phenobarbital reduces the bilirubin level. Compound heterozygosity for a severe UDP-bilirubin glucuronyl transferase mutation and the promoter mutation seen in Gilbert's patients results in an intermediate phenotype. Molecular testing is currently available for the identification of mutations in the UDP-bilirubin glucuronyl transferase gene responsible for types I and II Crigler–Najjar syndrome, and Gilbert's syndrome.

PREDOMINANTLY CONJUGATED HYPERBILIRUBINEMIA

Dubin–Johnson syndrome

The Dubin–Johnson syndrome is an autosomal recessive disorder caused by a basic defect in the transport of conjugated bilirubin and other low molecular weight organic anions from liver cells into bile. Mild conjugated hyperbilirubinemia, 30–80 μmol/L (2–5 mg/dl) usually develops during adolescence but may be recognized in infancy; levels may reach as high as 340 μmol/L (20 mg/dl). At times, the stools may be acholic and the urine dark, the latter containing both bilirubin and urobilinogen. The patient may complain of generalized weakness, anorexia, nausea and of vague upper abdominal pain. The liver is enlarged in 50% of patients and may be tender. Infection, pregnancy or oral contraceptives may exacerbate jaundice. Serum transaminases, alkaline phosphatase and bile salts are normal. Cholangiographic dye is not well concentrated. Bromsulfthalein secretion is characteristically deranged; retention in plasma is normal at 45 min but is above normal at 90 min suggesting regurgitation of conjugated material from hepatocytes to plasma. Heterozygotes may show lesser abnormalities. Total urinary coproporphyrinogen is normal or slightly increased but the ratio of coproporphyrinogen I to coproporphyrinogen III is markedly elevated, and can be used to make the diagnosis. Characteristic coarse, blackish brown pigment, the nature of which is not understood, is present in the lysosomes of hepatocytes, particularly centrizonal areas. Hepatic structure is otherwise normal. Phenobarbital has variable effects but may improve the symptoms in some patients. Recently, mutations in the canalicular multispecific organic anion transporter (cMOAT), also known as MRP2, have been identified as the cause of Dubin–Johnson syndrome, which should allow for molecular testing in the future.

Rotor disease

Rotor disease is similar to the Dubin–Johnson syndrome in that the basic defect appears to be the transportation of conjugated bilirubin from hepatocytes into bile. The main difference is that, while the bromsulfthalein excretion is abnormal and shows a raised plasma value (greater than 25%) at 45 min, there is no secondary rise at 90 min. Total urinary coproporphyrinogens are markedly increased but the ratio of coproporphyrinogen I to coproporphyrinogen III is usually normal. Liver histology is normal with no pigmentation. Inheritance is autosomal recessive, the molecular basis for Rotor syndrome is unknown.

Benign recurrent intrahepatic cholestasis and Byler disease

Benign recurrent intrahepatic cholestasis is another, similar, self-explanatory disorder. Malabsorption, steatorrhea and biliary cirrhosis can occur. Liver function tests are as expected with elevated bile acids in blood. Inheritance is autosomal recessive. No specific treatment is known. Byler disease, which is usually fatal, is probably allelic.

DEFECTS IN BILE ACID METABOLISM

3-Beta-hydroxysteroid-Δ^5-oxidoreductase/isomerase and 3-oxo-Δ^4-steroid-5-beta-reductase

3-Beta-hydroxysteroid-Δ^5-oxidoreductase/isomerase and 3-oxo-Δ^4-steroid-5-beta-reductase are rare causes of cholestatic liver disease. Infants present with hepatitis resulting from the accumulation of abnormal bile acids, leading to cirrhosis and liver failure. They cannot be readily differentiated from other causes of aggressive liver disease with biliary obstruction in infants, except by sophisticated mass spectrometry techniques of urine and/or serum bile acids. Early treatment with chenodeoxycholic and cholic acids may be very effective and can be continued for years. Liver transplantation is required in advanced cases.

FATTY ACID OXIDATION DISORDERS (Fig. 24.17)

(in aggregate ~1:10–20 000)

After birth, fatty acids are the major fuel for cardiac and skeletal muscle, both at rest and during aerobic exercise. Following release from circulating or stored triglycerides by lipoprotein lipase (step 1), free fatty acids are bound to albumin in the plasma. After diffusing across the cell membrane, the long chain fatty acids, primarily palmitic and oleic acids, are converted to fatty acyl-CoA esters by an acyl-CoA synthase (step 3). Neither this step nor the transport systems into mitochondria seem to be required for medium or short chain fatty acids but these are usually minor metabolic pathways.

Transport into mitochondria requires L-carnitine, which is both endogenously produced and also comes from animal sources in the diet. Carnitine palmitoyl transferase (CPT)-I (step 4) forms fatty acylcarnitine conjugates that are transported into the mitochondria by a translocase (step 5). Once inside the matrix, the reaction is reversed by CPT-II and free carnitine and long chain fatty acyl-CoA are reformed (step 6).

Fatty acid beta-oxidation occurs in a repeating four-reaction cycle, each 'spiral' of the cycle releasing one molecule of acetyl-CoA (steps 7–12). The first reaction is performed by one of four acyl-CoA dehydrogenases, the choice of enzyme dependent upon the structure and chain length of the fatty acid substrate. Straight chain fatty acids of 12–18 carbons in length (C_{12-18}) are metabolized by very long chain acyl-CoA dehydrogenase (VLCAD), an enzyme that is bound to the inner mitochondrial membrane. Long chain branched or desaturated fatty acids are likely substrates for long chain acyl-CoA dehydrogenase (LCAD), an enzyme found within the mitochondrial matrix. Chain shortened fatty acids become substrates for either medium chain (C_{6-12}) or short chain (C_{4-6}) acyl-CoA dehydrogenases. All these reactions provide reducing equivalents and are coupled directly through electron transfer flavoprotein (ETF) and ETF: coenzyme Q (CoQ) oxidoreductase (ETF:QO) (steps 13–15) to CoQ of the electron transport chain. Three further enzymatic steps (steps 10–12) complete one cycle leaving a fatty acyl-CoA two carbons shorter for further beta-oxidation. For long chain fatty acids, steps 10–12 are all catalyzed by a single membrane bound enzyme complex called the trifunctional protein. For shorter fatty acids, three distinct mitochondrial matrix proteins individually catalyze the three remaining steps of the beta-oxidation cycle. Reducing equivalents generated in step 11 (3-hydroxyacyl-CoA dehydrogenase) are coupled to Complex I of the electron transport chain and used to generate ATP. Fatty acid oxidation in the liver produces the ketone bodies, acetoacetate and beta-hydroxybutyrate, which, under homeostatic conditions, are recycled to fatty acids for use in other tissues although they can be themselves directly metabolized by the brain for energy during prolonged fasting. In the liver, acetyl-CoA generated through fatty acid oxidation is a substrate for the citric acid cycle, sparing glycogen and preventing glucose depletion.

The transition from the continuous supply of glucose in fetal life to a mixed fuel system after birth requires efficient beta-oxidation, which is not usually stressed by the normal, frequent feeding schedules of newborn infants. It is often only when the time between feeding increases, or during a catabolic illness, that symptoms develop in patients with defects of fatty acid oxidation. When beta-oxidation is increased or disrupted, the dicarboxylic acids adipic (C_6), suberic (C_8)

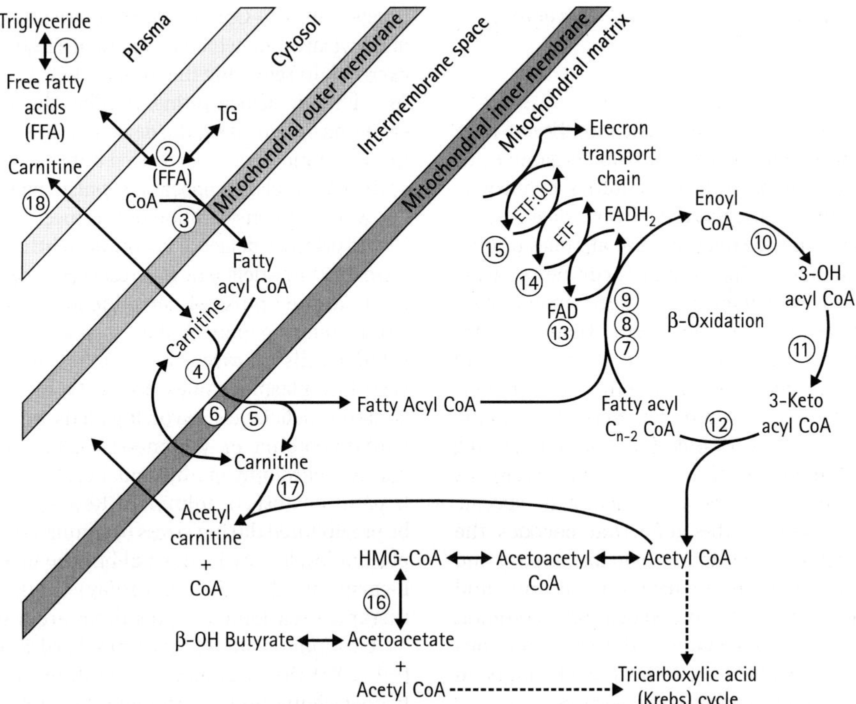

Fig. 24.17 Steps involved in fatty acid oxidation. 1, Lipoprotein lipase;* 2, fatty acid binding protein; 3, fatty acyl-CoA synthase; 4, carnitine palmitoyl transferase I (CPT-I);* 5, carnitine palmitoyl transferase II (CPT-II);* 6, fatty acyl carnitine translocase;* 7, long chain acyl CoA dehydrogenase (LCAD);* 8, medium chain acyl CoA dehydrogenase (MCAD);* 9, short chain acyl CoA dehydrogenase (SCAD);* 10, enoyl-CoA hydratase; 11, 3-hydroxyacyl-CoA dehydrogenase;* 12, thiolase; 13, flavin adenine dinucleotide (FAD);* 14, electron transfer flavoprotein (ETF);* 15, ETF: coenzyme Q oxidoreductase (ETF:QO);* 16, 3-hydroxy, 3-methylglutaryl CoA lyase (HMGCoA);* 17, carnitine acetyl transferase;* 18, carnitine transport.*
* Defects identified (see text).

and sebacic (C_{10}) are produced by omega-oxidation of the excess intermediates. Thus they are seen in fasting and in ketoacidosis from any cause, as well as in the disorders of fatty acid catabolism or ketone utilization. In addition to carnitine deficiency, at the time of writing this chapter at least 13 defects in fatty acid oxidation have been identified. Collectively, they appear to be relatively common. All are inherited in an autosomal recessive pattern, and specific gene defects have been identified for most of the disorders.

Clinical features

Disorders of fatty acid metabolism commonly present with one of three clinical phenotypes: sudden infant death, hypoketotic hypoglycemia in association with recurrent vomiting and hepatic encephalopathy, or recurrent rhabdomyolysis and myoglobinuria. The expected clinical phenotypes associated with the known disorders of fatty acid oxidation are presented in Table 24.10. Sudden infant death due to occult hypoglycemia often occurs in the setting of fasting or intercurrent illness, but sudden death may also occur in non-fasting neonates (particularly in infants with long chain fatty acid metabolism defects such as VLCAD deficiency) due to cardiac arrhythmias or cardiomyopathy. Long chain acylcarnitines or omega-oxidation products that accumulate within the cardiomyocyte may be responsible for triggering arrhythmia. More commonly, disorders of fatty acid metabolism cause episodes of lethargy with nausea and vomiting, hypoketotic hypoglycemia, progressive somnolence, and hepatic encephalopathy indistinguishable from Reye's syndrome (see Ch. 17). As many as one-third of the initial episodes may be fatal, the diagnosis of a fatty acid oxidation defect not being established unless appropriate perimortem metabolic studies are performed. Children who survive the initial metabolic crisis may have recurrent decompensation episodes prior to diagnosis. Young children who have suffered recurrent episodes may exhibit muscle weakness, hypotonia and developmental delay. Dysmorphic features and hypertrophic or dilated cardiomyopathy may occur in some of the disorders and CNS symptoms, when they occur, may be life threatening. Fatty acid metabolism defects may also present as exercise intolerance and recurrent episodes of rhabdomyolysis and myoglobinuria often with initial onset during adolescence or adulthood. Some cases may

Table 24.10 Clinical presentations of fatty acid oxidation disorders

Enzyme deficiency	Hepatic	Myopathic
Carnitine transporter		X
Carnitine palmitoyl transferase (CPT)-I	X	Rarely
Carnitine acyltranslocase	X	
CPT-II	X	X
VLCAD	X	X
MCAD	X	
SCAD	X	
LCHAD/MTP	X	X
SCHAD	X	X
Ketolytic defects	X	

Hepatic presentation – Recurrent Reye-like syndrome, hypoglycemia, acidosis
Myopathic presentation – hypotonia, recurrent rhabdomyolysis
LCHAD, long chain 3-hydroxyacyl-CoA dehydrogenase; MCAD, medium chain acyl-CoA dehydrogenase; MTP, microsomal triglyceride transfer protein; SCAD, short chain acyl-CoA dehydrogenase; SCHAD, short chain 3-hydroxyacyl-CoA dehydrogenase; VLCAD, very long chain acyl-CoA dehydrogenase.

remain permanently asymptomatic. Severe and mild cases of many of these disorders are recognized.

Diagnosis

Hypoketotic hypoglycemia is discussed below. The majority of fatty acid oxidation defects are detected by studies of urine organic acids and plasma carnitine status in patients with Reye's syndrome, myopathy, cardiomyopathy, unexplained liver disease or hypoglycemia. These patterns may be diagnostic at all times or only abnormal during metabolic stress. Plasma acylcarnitine or urine acylglycine profiles analyzed by tandem mass spectrometry often provide diagnostic patterns in these disorders. Histologically, microvesicular fat in the liver and myocytes are characteristic of carnitine depletion. Enzyme assays can usually be done on peripheral blood lymphocytes or cultured skin fibroblasts. Some fatty acid oxidation defects, such as medium chain acyl-CoA dehydrogenase (MCAD) or long chain 3-hydroxyacyl-CoA dehydrogenase (LCHAD) deficiency, are associated with specific disease-causing point mutations in the gene that encodes the enzyme in question. Mutation analysis, when available, is easy and quick to perform, less expensive than enzymatic testing, and absolutely diagnostic if the patient is homozygous for a common mutation. The common mutations associated with these conditions are responsible for most but not all cases, so negative findings on specific mutation analysis do not rule out these disorders.

Treatment

Optimal therapy for disorders of fatty acid oxidation has not been studied in any systematic manner and is generally based upon anecdotal experience. Avoidance of fasting and the ready provision of non-fat calories during stress, either orally or parenterally if needed, are critical. L-Carnitine (50–300 mg/kg/day orally or 50–100 mg/kg/day i.v.) is often prescribed to enhance urinary excretion of toxic fatty acid oxidation intermediates as carnitine conjugates,[109] but no controlled trials of carnitine supplementation have been performed to prove its clinical efficacy. The safety and efficacy of L-carnitine therapy in disorders of long chain fatty acid metabolism remain controversial. Carnitine supplementation in acute carnitine deficiency syndromes, such as cardiomyopathy secondary to a defect in the cellular carnitine transporter, is life saving.[110] For MCAD deficiency, a mildly fat restricted diet (30% of energy intake as fat) may be prudent. For defects in long chain fatty acid oxidation, further dietary long chain fat restriction may be useful with the guidance of an experienced nutritionist, and medium chain triglyceride (MCT) oil is an effective alternative fuel source.[111] Specific nutritional deficiencies including essential fatty acid deficiency (associated with hair loss, eczema and poor growth), fat soluble vitamin deficiency, vitamin B_{12} and iron deficiency may complicate extreme dietary fat restriction (total energy from fat < 20% of total energy intake); these parameters must be carefully and repetitively monitored during dietary therapy of fatty acid oxidation disorders.

SPECIFIC DISORDERS

Defects in the carnitine cycle

Carnitine derives partly from the diet and partly from endogenous synthesis. It can be depleted in liver or kidney disease, malnutrition and malabsorption. Low levels are usual in premature and neonatal infants and in pregnancy in which these lowered values are probably physiologically normal.

Marked depletion occurs either from renal loss (e.g. Fanconi's syndrome – see Ch. 16) or increased consumption (e.g. the organic acidemias or valproate therapy). The latter occurs because carnitine accepts any acyl-CoA ester and the resulting acylcarnitine, for example glutarylcarnitine which accumulates in the glutaric acidurias, is then excreted. In removing the toxic acyl-CoA esters, more carnitine is lost. In addition, acylcarnitines inhibit the renal reabsorption of free carnitine, aggravating the depletion. In such cases, plasma and urine free carnitine levels are reduced but the acylcarnitine values are high so that the total may appear normal. In plasma, an acyl:free ratio above 0.5 warrants consideration of this mechanism.

No primary defect of carnitine synthesis is currently known. The term 'primary deficiency' is reserved for patients in whom there is a defect in the uptake of carnitine into cells. Such *carnitine transport defects* may be pancellular or tissue specific in myocytes, renal tubular cells or, rarely, hepatocytes. Renal tubular losses produce very low plasma values and very high urine levels resulting in 'systemic deficiency', involving all tissues. Muscle depletion presents with hypotonia or weakness; cardiac depletion causes acute or chronic cardiomyopathy and hepatocellular depletion can cause hepatic steatosis or fulminant Reye's syndrome, any of which can be precipitated during stress or minor starvation. In other cases, the plasma levels may be normal but the involved tissues are deficient. L-carnitine (25–350 mg/kg/day) should be used as replacement therapy; occasionally higher doses are warranted.[110]

Carnitine palmitoyl transferase I deficiency (CPT-I) (steps 4 and 5) (~1:500 000) causes symptomatic fasting hypoketotic hypoglycemia and occasionally hepatocellular damage. The heart and muscle are rarely involved although plasma CPK can be high; severe rhabdomyolysis has only occasionally been observed. CPT-I isoforms specific to liver or to muscle have been detected in rat;[112] the fact that clinical symptoms associated with CPT-I deficiency are mostly restricted to a hepatic phenotype is probably explained by specific deficiency of the liver isoform of CPT-I. In CPT-I deficiency, total and free plasma carnitine are characteristically elevated; this observation is unique among all known fatty acid oxidation defects and is otherwise seen only in association with carnitine supplementation, renal insufficiency or cardiac muscle damage.

In *CPT-II deficiency*, an infantile form presents with severe hypoglycemia, myopathy and cardiomyopathy leading to death. Plasma carnitine is low with elevated acylcarnitines. A milder form presents with lipid myopathy, recurrent rhabdomyolysis and myoglobinuria in young adults. *Carnitine/acylcarnitine translocase deficiency* is clinically similar to infantile CPT-II deficiency.

Medium chain acyl-CoA dehydrogenase deficiency (MCADD) (step 8) (1:10–20 000)

Clinical features

This is the most common defect in fatty acid oxidation. The typical acute clinical presentation includes fasting- or illness-induced hypoketotic hypoglycemia, often associated with metabolic acidosis and hepatocellular dysfunction, that can progress to full-blown Reye's syndrome. Chronically, cardiomyopathy and/or signs of muscle carnitine depletion such as weakness or hypotonia can also occur and may be accompanied by fatigue or lethargy. As with all beta-oxidation defects, these problems are produced or aggravated by poor nutrition or the stress of even a minor illness and may be recurrent. The most severe presentation is of sudden death in the first months of life or even within the first few days after birth presumably due to occult hypoglycemia. In this scenario, an unexpected infant death may be mislabeled as sudden infant death syndrome (SIDS), especially if a detailed postmortem examination including metabolic testing is not performed.[113] This risk of sudden infant death, which can be prevented through avoidance of prolonged fasting, and the availability of a rapid neonatal screening test (see below), makes MCADD an ideal candidate for inclusion in newborn screening panels. On the other hand, some MCAD deficient individuals may never become symptomatic, presumably because they never develop carnitine depletion together with sufficient stress or because they carry mutations with relatively mild physiological effects. It is important to note however that the initial clinical manifestations of MCADD have occurred as late as adolescence or even adulthood.

Diagnosis

Characteristic medium chain fatty acid metabolites (adipic, sebacic and suberic acids), acylglycine and acylcarnitine conjugates (hexanoylglycine, suberylglycine, phenylpropionylglycine and octanoylcarnitine) are present in blood and urine. These metabolites are often detected by urine organic acid analysis especially during acute crises, but this test may be normal between decompensation episodes. Analysis of acylcarnitine conjugates by tandem mass spectrometry is more sensitive and is often diagnostic even between clinical episodes. This test can be performed on newborn filter paper samples as is now employed in a few routine neonatal screening programs. 80–90% of patients presenting clinically are homozygous for the A985G mutation in the MCAD gene, but the frequency of this mutation is lower in MCADD cases detected by newborn screening, suggesting that other MCAD mutations may be associated with only mild or subclinical disease.[114] Whether the likelihood of severe clinical manifestations can absolutely be predicted from genotype is still under evaluation.

Other defects of fatty acid oxidation

LCHAD is a component of a trifunctional enzyme that also comprises enoyl-CoA hydratase and CoA thiolase activities, the so-called trifunctional protein (TFP). LCHAD deficiency (step 11) appears to be the second most common of fatty acid oxidation defects and is frequently caused by homozygosity for a G1528C mutation in the TFP alpha subunit gene. Cases with other mutations in either the alpha or beta trifunctional protein subunit genes often exhibit deficiency of all three enzymatic activities associated with TFP; this may alter both the pattern of diagnostic metabolites and the clinical presentation. Long chain hydroxy acids are usually detectable by urine organic acid analysis during acute metabolic crises, but as in MCADD, acylcarnitine analysis to detect long chain 3-hydroxylated carnitine esters is often more sensitive. In LCHAD/TFP deficiency and in *very long chain acyl-CoA dehydrogenase deficiency* (VLCADD) (step 7), the clinical features are often similar to, but more severe than MCADD. Older patients may develop late onset cardiomyopathy or myopathy with recurrent myoglobinuria and patients are generally carnitine deficient. Pigmentary retinopathy and vision loss during childhood is a complication specific to LCHAD/TFP deficiency. In addition to fasting avoidance and ingestion of a fat restricted diet, treatment with dietary MCT oil and L-carnitine may be beneficial.[111] Acute fatty liver of pregnancy or the 'HELPP' syndrome occurs in many women who carry LCHAD deficient fetuses;[115] the pathophysiological mechanism of this complication is currently unknown.

Other defects include *short chain acyl-CoA dehydrogenase deficiency* (SCADD) (step 9), *short chain 3-hydroxyacyl-CoA dehydrogenase deficiency*[116] and *malonyl-CoA decarboxylase deficiency*. These disorders tend to cause failure to thrive, recurrent vomiting with or without hypoglycemia and/or ketosis, hypotonia, marked developmental delay, seizures and early demise. The urine organic acid profiles tend to suggest the site of the defects but confirmation requires detailed studies in fibroblasts or other tissues. Many individuals with clinical symptoms and biochemical evidence of SCADD have inherited variations in the SCAD gene that are also common in the normal population. In one study, 69% of 133 patients with biochemical findings of SCADD were either homozygous or compound heterozygous for two SCAD polymorphisms (G625C or C511T), yet 14% of the general population also carry these polymorphisms.[117] So, the exact pathophysiological relationship between the presence of these polymorphisms and clinical disease is as yet unclear.

Glycerol derives from hydrolysis of fats and, reversibly, from glycolysis, making it available for gluconeogenesis. Isolated *glycerol kinase deficiency* causes recurrent attacks of a Reye-like syndrome with vomiting, acidemia, CNS depression and hypotonia which are precipitated by a high fat intake or fasting. Milder cases are found by chance with pseudohypertriglyceridemia on routine multichannel blood testing. It also can be part of an X chromosome microdeletion syndrome which includes Duchenne muscular dystrophy, retinopathy and adrenal hypoplasia which usually dominates the clinical picture; note that glycerol in urine may derive from body lotions or suppositories. Frequent high carbohydrate feeding with mild fat restriction is indicated. *Glycerol intolerance* is a different condition associated with recurrent hypoglycemia and Reye-like attacks that may actually be a manifestation of fructose-1, 6-diphosphatase deficiency.[118]

Multiple acyl-CoA dehydrogenase deficiency (MADD)

MADD is actually a series of different disorders that are all associated with a defect in the entry of electrons into the electron transport chain (Fig. 24.18). This defect affects the handling of reducing equivalents generated from the metabolism of several amino acids and by numerous different acyl-CoA dehydrogenases, hence the name multiple acyl-CoA dehydrogenase deficiency. Defects of transport, processing or binding of FAD (step 13), ETF (step 14) or the ETF:QO (step 15) are all possible. Three forms are generally recognized with clinical overlap between groups and genetic heterogeneity within each group.

The severe form (MAD:S), also called *glutaric aciduria type II* is often lethal in the newborn period, secondary to profound acidosis, hypoglycemia, coma and multiple organ system involvement. A subgroup of these patients exhibit dysmorphic facial and other features, characteristic subependymal brain cysts, dysmyelination of brain and polycystic kidneys. Milder cases lack dysmorphism but usually exhibit severe failure to thrive, hypotonia, cardiomyopathy and liver damage. An unusual 'acrid' odor and the 'sweaty feet' odor of isovaleric acid are often described. The biochemical profile on urine organic acid analysis is generally diagnostic, with accumulations of

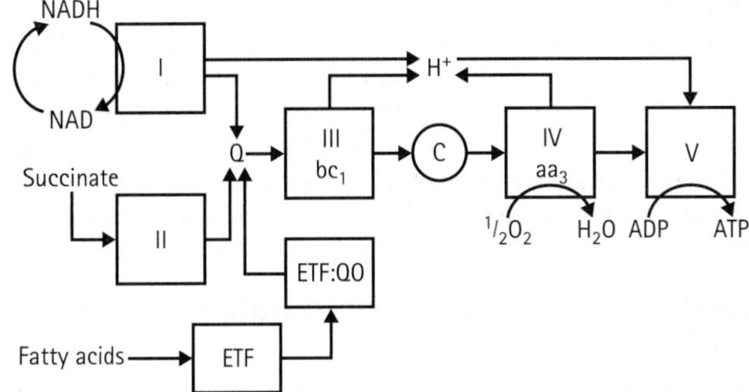

Fig. 24.18 The electron transport chain. I, Complex I, (NADH Co Q oxidoreductase); II, complex II, succinate Co Q oxidoreductase; III, complex III, ubiquinol cytochrome c reductase; IV, complex IV, cytochrome c oxidase; V, complex V, ATP synthase; Q, coezyme Q; C, cytochrome c; ETF, electron transfer flavoprotein; ETF:QO, electron transfer flavoprotein oxidoreductase. Electrons generated by complexes I, III and IV create the proton gradient which drives ATP synthesis.

ethylmalonic, glutaric, 2-hydroxyglutaric, adipic, suberic and sebacic acids, isovaleryl, isobutyryl- and 2-methylbutyryl-glycines with sarcosine often detected by urine amino acid screen.

A milder form of the disorder termed MAD:M (sometimes called ethylmalonic-adipic aciduria) may not even present until adulthood; the clinical presentation is generally similar to other acyl-CoA dehydrogenase deficiencies. The urine organic acid profile is simpler than in MAD:S, usually containing only ethylmalonic, adipic and methylsuccinic acids and hexanoyl and butyrylglycines. Dicarboxylic acids are abundant and sometimes disappear following riboflavin supplementation, giving rise to the original term *riboflavin-responsive dicarboxylic aciduria*. Unfortunately, a similar metabolite pattern may also be seen in isolated SCADD.

Defects of both ETF and ETF:QO dehydrogenase have been found in both forms of MAD. Generally, the severity of the enzyme deficiency correlates with the severity or type of disorder.

Some of these patients improve on riboflavin (100–300 mg/day) and carnitine (100–200 mg/kg/day).[119]

Disorders of ketone metabolism

Defects of ketone synthesis include *3-hydroxy-3-methylglutaryl-CoA synthase* (HMG-CoA synthase) and *3-hydroxy-3-methylglutaryl-CoA lyase* deficiency (HMG-CoA lyase). They are associated with a recurrent Reye-like syndrome with stress-related episodes of vomiting, lethargy, severe *hypoketotic* hypoglycemia, metabolic acidosis and characteristic patterns of urinary organic acids such as elevated 3-hydroxy-3-methylglutaric, 3-methylglutaric, 3-methylglutaconic and 3-hydroxyisovaleric acidosis. HMG-CoA lyase is the final step in leucine degradation but is also required for hepatic ketone body synthesis (step 9). Other patients with apparently similar biochemical findings have had normal enzyme activity. Growth failure, microcephaly, nerve deafness and basal ganglion lesions similar to Leigh syndrome (see p. 1223) distinguish these atypical cases from more typical patients with HMG-CoA lyase deficiency.

Defects of ketone utilization cause facile hyperketosis; they include deficiencies of *succinyl-CoA:3-ketoacid-CoA transferase* or of several different enzymes with *3-ketothiolase* activity. *2-Methylacetoacetyl-CoA thiolase* deficiency (step 12) can present with severe neonatal acidosis, intermittent episodes of ketoacidosis with lethargy and coma or may be asymptomatic. Developmental delay may occur. Hypoglycemia, ketotic hyperglycinemia and hyperammonemia are reported. The urine contains 2-methyl-3-hydroxybutyric acid, other organic acids and butanone. Acetoacetic and beta-hydroxybutyric acids can be greatly elevated, and the disease may mimic salicylism. The enzyme defect can be demonstrated in cultured skin fibroblasts. Deficiency of either of two other distinct 3-ketothiolases, *mitochondrial* or *cytosolic acetoacetyl-CoA thiolases*, seem to be associated with progressive neurological deterioration, neuropathy and extrapyramidal movement disorder. Lactic acidosis with abnormal lactate/pyruvate ratios and increased ketone body levels are usual. Treatment for these disorders is again based primarily upon avoidance of fasting.

Hypoglycemia as a presenting feature of metabolic disorders

The half-life of metabolic fuels in the plasma is about 100 s. Great variations in the rate of glucose consumption must be balanced by intricate hormonal controls and the coordinated release of fuels from glycogen, fat or protein. Often, hepatomegaly or acidosis suggests a metabolic diagnosis but, for the most part, inborn errors causing hypoglycemia require extensive metabolic testing. Hyper- or hypoketosis is often not recognized because blood and urine ketones must be measured at the time that the blood glucose is low (< 40 mg/dl (2.2 mmol/L)). In addition, free fatty acids, amino acids, carnitine and sometimes glycerol need to be measured *in samples obtained before any treatment has been given*. Urine for organic acids must also be obtained during the acute episode. Plasma acylcarnitine profiling is an additional valuable diagnostic tool in the case of hypoketotic hypoglycemia. If the initial blood amino acid, carnitine, and acylcarnitine analyses and urine organic acid analysis are not diagnostic, then starvation/fasting stress tests can be used to recreate an acute hypoglycemic episode. A diagnostic fasting study should only be performed in hospital with full emergency support available.[120]

Hypoglycemia with ketosis and/or acidosis

Ketotic hypoglycemia occurs frequently in small undergrown infants and children. Most cases are due to poor growth, poor nutrition with inadequate and/or infrequent feeding, but symptoms can sometimes occur even in apparently healthy, well fed infants. Lack of glycogen stores and of muscle protein for gluconeogenesis necessitate increased lipolysis. As a result, fatty acid intermediates and ketones readily accumulate in patterns that mimic hereditary defects of fuel homeostasis. In nutritional deprivation, plasma alanine and lactate are low and there is no response to an intramuscular glucagon challenge. The metabolic differential diagnosis includes glycogen storage disorders and defects of ketone utilization, pyruvate, the citric acid cycle and organic acid metabolism.

Hypoketotic hypoglycemia

Hypoglycemia with inappropriately low levels of blood ketones suggests a defect of fatty acid oxidation or of ketone production; it is also typical in hyperinsulinism. Measurement of serum free fatty acids during a hypoglycemic episode assists with the differential diagnosis; free fatty acid levels are suppressed in hyperinsulinism while they are elevated in fatty acid oxidation disorders.

CARBOHYDRATE METABOLISM DISORDERS

Disorders of digestion and absorption are primarily addressed in Chapter 17. In the gut, hereditary defects of *lactase, sucrose-isomaltase, trehalase* and *glucose-galactose absorption* are known.

In the kidneys, *renal glycosuria* is caused by a deficit in glucose reabsorption. *Pentosuria* is a benign condition, most common in Jewish people due to deficient L-xylulose reductase activity; xylulose is excreted in the urine where it reacts with Benedict's solution or Clinitest to give a false-positive test for glucose.

DEFECTS OF GLYCOLYSIS (Fig. 24.19)

In erythrocytes

Severe defects of glycolysis in erythrocytes are usually associated with hemolytic anemia (Ch. 21). Such conditions include defects of *glucose-6-phosphate dehydrogenase, hexokinase* (step 2), *glucosephosphate isomerase* (step 4), *phosphofructokinase* (step 5), *aldolase triose phosphate isomerase* (TPI) (step 7), *phosphoglycerate kinase* (PGK) (step 9), *diphosphoglycerate mutase* (step 10), *pyruvate kinase* (step 12) and *lactate dehydrogenase*. In contrast, deficiency of either *2,3-diphosphoglycerate (DPG) mutase* or *diphosphoglycerate phosphatase* causes mild erythrocytosis. Hemolysis can also be caused by defects of *glutathione metabolism* (see pp 1171 in amino acid section) and certain steps in purine and pyrimidine metabolism (see pp 1167 in purine/pyrimidine section) and *adenosine triphosphatase*. Another red cell enzymopathy is a deficiency of *6-phosphogluconate dehydrogenase* in the pentose monophosphate shunt. Finally, *cytochrome* b_5 reductase deficiency is often associated with methemoglobinemia and developmental delay.

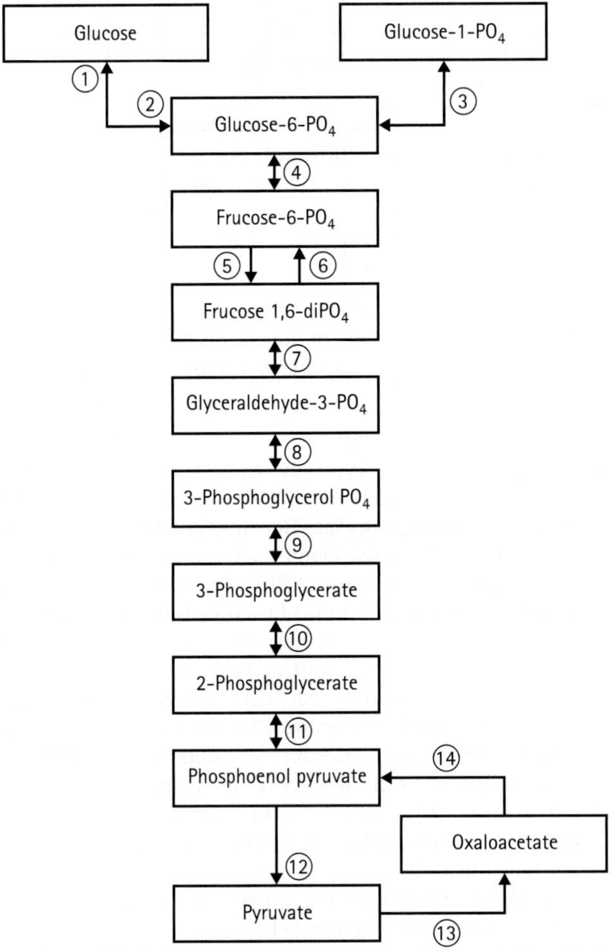

Fig. 24.19 The Embden–Meyerhof glycolytic pathway. 1, Hexokinase; 2, glucose-6-phosphatase; 3, phosphoglucomutase; 4, phosphohexose isomerase; 5, phosphofructokinase; 6, fructose-1,6-bisphosphatase; 7, triose phosphate isomerase; 8, glyceraldehyde-3 phosphate dehydrogenase; 9, phosphoglycerate kinase, 10, phosphoglyceromutase; 11, enolase; 12, pyruvate kinase; 13, pyruvate carboxylase; 14, phosphoenolpyruvate carboxykinase.

In the nervous system

Several of these disorders also cause neurological or muscular disease. Severe TPI deficiency is associated with severe, progressive neurological disease with both upper and lower motor neurone damage; the intellect is relatively well preserved. There is also a tendency to sudden death and increased susceptibility to infection. Severe PGK deficiency can cause developmental delay and attacks of behavioral and emotional abnormalities, movement disorders including hemiplegia and even coma that develop during hemolytic crises. *Glutathione reductase* deficiency has also been reported to cause a variety of neurological abnormalities, including myelopathy. About 15% of cases with *cytochrome* b_5 reductase deficiency have severe progressive neurological deterioration with microcephaly, athetosis and hypertonia in addition to methemoglobinemia. In all of these disorders, management of these neurological symptoms is unsatisfactory but should include avoidance of oxidant drugs.

In muscle – the metabolic myopathies

There is a large and growing number of metabolic myopathies, almost all of which involve energy metabolism. Since several are glycolytic disorders, the whole group is summarized here (Table 24.11).

Table 24.11 Metabolic myopathies

Glycogen storage diseases (GSDs)
Acid maltase deficiency (GSD type II), glycogen debrancher deficiency (III), glycogen brancher deficiency (IV), phosphorylase deficiency (V)
Glycolytic defects
Phosphofructokinase, phosphoglycerate kinase, phosphoglycerate mutase, glucosephosphate isomerase, lactate dehydrogenase, lactate transporter
Fatty acid oxidation disorders
Long chain fatty acid oxidation disorders (VLCAD, LCHAD/TFP deficiency), carnitine palmitoyl transferase deficiency, secondary carnitine depletion
Purine disorders
Myoadenylate deaminase deficiency
Mitochondrial defects
Defects in respiratory chain complexes I–IV, Luft syndrome (Complex V – ATPase deficiency), Krebs cycle defects, adenine nucleotide translocase defect, pyruvate dehydrogenase deficiency, defect in the malate–aspartate shuttle
Others
Periodic paralyses (hypo- or hyperkalemic), malignant hyperthermia secondary to ion channelopathies.

LCHAD, long chain 3-hydroxyacyl-CoA dehydrogenase; TFP, trifunctional protein; VLCAD, very long chain acyl-CoA dehydrogenase

Clinical features

The usual symptoms of these disorders are muscle weakness, lack of endurance and postexercise muscle pain or cramps; some are aggravated by fasting or a high fat diet. Muscle wasting, when present, is often due to disuse rather than to the intrinsic muscle disease. In glycolytic or fatty acid defects, excessive exercise leads to severe cramping and rhabdomyolysis with increased serum creatine phosphokinase (CPK) levels with recurrent myoglobinuria leading to severe renal damage. These disorders tend to present only in adolescence or later. Curiously, the disorders of the electron transport chain, which may occur at any age, are rarely associated with myoglobinuria, perhaps because the dyspnea from lactic acidosis is so marked that exercise capacity is too limited to result in much muscle cell damage.

Non-specific complaints of muscle weakness, lack of endurance or muscle cramps are very common and only 10–20% of such cases prove to have a real muscle disorder. Real cases are often not detected or evaluated for years or until a crisis such as rhabdomyolysis develops.

Diagnosis

The key to diagnosis of a metabolic myopathy is the initial clinical suspicion that a metabolic defect may be responsible for the exercise intolerance or other signs and symptoms exhibited by a patient. Physical signs including muscle wasting or hypertrophy and muscle weakness are supportive of the diagnosis, but their absence does not preclude a metabolic defect. Elevations of serum CPK levels suggest ongoing rhabdomyolysis; blood electrolyte abnormalities or lactic acidosis may suggest specific etiologies. Metabolic screening with plasma amino acid analysis, plasma total carnitine levels, plasma acylcarnitine profile by tandem mass spectrometry, and urine organic acid analysis may also yield the diagnosis. Physiological measurements of muscle function including electromyography

(EMG), ischemic forearm exercise testing, or treadmill exercise test, may assist with the diagnosis and will help assess exercise tolerance. Pathological elevation of lactate post exercise suggests a glycogen storage disease or mitochondrial defect. Blood ammonia levels normally rise with exercise; the lack of an increase in the blood ammonia with exercise suggests myoadenylate deaminase deficiency. Muscle tissue, obtained by needle or open biopsy, should *not* be preserved in formalin but submitted fresh or flash frozen for histochemical examination and enzymatic activity analysis which, when properly done, can indicate a number of enzymatic defects. Glycogen content is often increased in the glycogen storage diseases, the glycolytic defects and frequently in electron transport defects. The lipid content is usually increased in the lipid disorders and often in electron transport chain defects but not in carnitine palmitoyl transferase deficiency. Mitochondrial disorders may exhibit ragged-red fibers on histochemical analysis and abnormal mitochondria on electron photomicrographs. Necrotic changes are usually only seen after severe exercise, and for this reason muscle biopsy immediately following an acute rhabdomyolytic episode may not be informative. Sometimes, muscle histology including electron microscopy may be completely normal in metabolic myopathies.

In some research laboratories, intracellular levels of ATP, phosphocreatine and phosphate are measured in vivo by ^{31}P-NMR spectroscopy; this technique may be used to detect defects of energy generation and to monitor the effects of treatment.

Treatment

This is usually restricted to limiting exercise that should cease before symptoms are provoked. Mild aerobic exercise can be encouraged but rigorous training may be dangerous. In glycolytic and fatty acid disorders, 'carbo loading' may be useful and continuous intake of glucose during exercise is helpful; fasting and high fat diets should be avoided, especially before exercise. Anecdotal reports suggest that carnitine therapy (50–100 mg/kg/day) may help prevent rhabdomyolysis in certain fatty acid oxidation defects such as VLCAD deficiency.

DEFECTS IN GALACTOSE METABOLISM

The main source of dietary galactose is lactose (glucose-galactose disaccharide), the predominant carbohydrate in milk and most milk-based infant formulae, in which it provides a considerable amount of energy. Galactose is metabolized for energy mainly in the liver, but galactose cannot be utilized for energy directly and must be converted to glucose. Other tissues such as erythrocytes can metabolize galactose too; erythrocytes provide a convenient tissue for the evaluation of galactose metabolism in the sick neonate. The metabolic pathway of galactose is depicted in Figure 24.20.

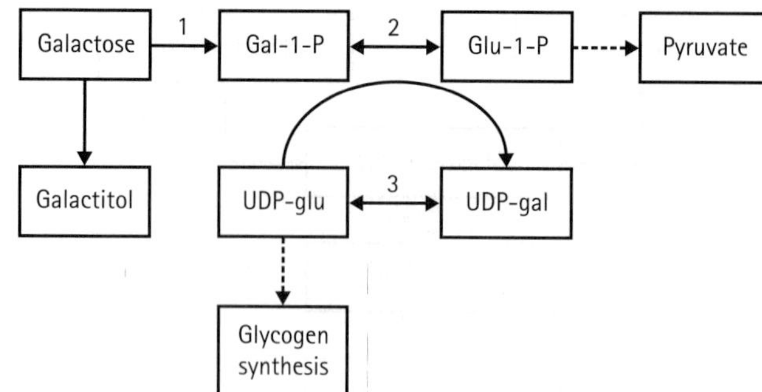

Fig. 24.20 Galactose metabolism. 1, galactokinase; 2, galactose-1-phosphate uridyltransferase; 3, uridine diphosphate galactose 4'-epimerase.

Galactose-1-phosphate uridyltransferase deficiency (galactosemia) (step 2)

Clinical features

Infants with severe transferase deficiency become sick soon after beginning to ingest milk. The severity of the presentation depends on the quantity of milk ingested (breast milk contains more lactose than milk-based formulae) and the presence of residual transferase activity in liver. Severe cases mimic sepsis and many do develop Gram negative (especially *Escherichia coli*) or beta-streptococcal sepsis. Prior to the availability of newborn screening and in areas where newborn screening for galactosemia is not yet routine, many transferase-deficient infants die from sepsis and/or liver failure without the diagnosis of galactosemia being entertained, the true cause of the infant's death not being revealed until the disease recurs in a subsequent sibling. Typically, transferase-deficient infants present within a few days after birth with vomiting, diarrhea, failure to thrive and persistent jaundice. Hepatosplenomegaly, progressive liver dysfunction with raised alanine aminotransferase (ALT) and aspartate aminotransferase (AST), hypoglycemia, anemia, coagulopathy with purpura and deficient clotting factors, and the biochemical findings of the renal Fanconi syndrome (see Ch. 16) are typical. Cataracts may be evident at birth or appear soon after. Edema, ascites, malnutrition, cachexia and septicemia usually presage a fatal outcome from hepatic failure within a few weeks if the condition is not treated. Mental retardation and behavioral abnormalities develop in the absence of treatment if the disease has a more protracted course. When residual enzyme activity is present, the course is less catastrophic, with failure to thrive and cataracts being the major features.

The acute abnormalities are rapidly corrected by complete elimination of galactose from the diet.[121]

However, long term complications are frequent, regardless of how early or how well the infant is treated. Overall, there is a slight reduction in intelligence and visual perceptual skills; 50% have dyspraxic speech, and hypergonadotropic hypogonadism with ovarian failure and often sterility occurs in approximately 80% of females. The causes of these late complications are unknown. Testicular function is unaffected.

Diagnosis

The simplest screening test is examination of the urine for reducing sugars (Clinitest) performed 24–36 h *after* the start of lactose-containing feeds. This test, however, is neither completely sensitive nor specific. The galactosemic infant who is ill and feeding poorly could have a falsely normal result. Alternatively, other reducing substances, such as antibiotics, in urine may cause a false-positive Clinitest reaction. It must be noted that the dipstick test for 'sugar' in urine commonly used in many clinical laboratories specifically detects glucose and will not react with galactose; this test cannot be used to screen for galactosuria. Newborn screening tests for blood galactose and galactose metabolites or by measurement of erythrocyte transferase enzyme activity (Beutler test) are in wide use in the USA and other countries, but often these results are only available after symptoms have already developed. The galactose metabolite galactose-1-phosphate (gal-1-P) is markedly elevated in cord blood enabling early detection in high risk infants. Vomiting or switches to non-lactose formulae may obscure the diagnosis and blood transfusion or exchange transfusion may negate the erythrocyte assays for gal-1-P and the enzyme. Any suspicious results are indications for initiating treatment, for quantitative assays of erythrocyte galactose and gal-1-P levels and confirmatory enzyme assays on erythrocytes or fibroblasts. Galactose tolerance tests should never be used when galactosemia is suspected.

The most obvious histological changes occur in the liver. There is fatty infiltration, fibrosis, bile duct proliferation and pseudoacinar arrangement of hepatic cells. The renal changes consist of widening of the proximal tubules and alterations of the tubular epithelium.

Transferase activity can be assayed in erythrocytes, cultured fibroblasts and chorionic villi. Many variants with lesser deficiencies of enzyme activity have been described; many of these cases are asymptomatic.

Variants

The commonest variant is the Duarte mutation for which about 1:25 people are carriers and have about 75% of normal enzyme activity. Duarte homozygotes have about 50% and Duarte/classical compound heterozygotes (who carry one Duarte and one galactosemia allele) have about 10–25% activity. Such cases often but not invariably have elevated blood gal-1-P and are often detected by routine newborn screening. If they drink lactose-containing formula or breast milk, gal-1-P remains high for months but usually falls to normal as lactose ingestion becomes a smaller portion of total energy intake. There is no evidence that the gal-1-P or other galactose metabolites are toxic in these cases or that there is any risk for any of the long or short term complications of classical galactosemia and opinion is divided as to whether galactose restriction should be recommended. Some authorities recommend non-lactose formula for the first year; others allow partial breast-feeding, while still others allow lactose intake to continue unrestricted. Often, clinical practice in this as in other controversial areas of medicine seems to be guided by medicolegal concerns.

Several other known mutations cause partial transferase deficiency and are associated with only mild galactosemia or are entirely asymptomatic. A specific mutation common to Blacks is associated with complete transferase deficiency in erythrocytes but 10% normal activity in liver and intestine and a mild galactosemia phenotype.

Treatment

In infants with the full-blown disease (i.e. complete transferase deficiency), elimination of dietary galactose corrects all of the acute problems within a few days if treatment is begun soon enough to prevent irreversible complications. Soy milk or synthetic formulae, which do not contain lactose, are supplied to the galactosemic infant. On the diet, weight gain ensues, residual liver damage is rare, and usually the cataracts resolve.[121]

Without question, the diet should be strictly followed if possible for the first several years. It is less clear how important strict galactose restriction is for older children. Some authorities believe that the diet requires life-long meticulous attention to detail, but the occurrence of long term complications from galactosemia including speech dyspraxia, tremor, ataxia and seizures does not appear to correlate well with dietary galactose exposure.[122] Once solid foods are introduced, it becomes more difficult to offer a truly galactose free diet. Many foods contain unlabeled lactose and even many fruits and vegetables contain galactose. Given the indigestibility of dietary fiber, the overall contribution of galactose from fruits and vegetables to the body galactose pool is unknown. In general, the list of foods to be avoided includes dairy products, some breads, sausage and candies which contain lactose, and other food products that list whey, casein or caseinates or milk solids as ingredients. Also, some medications may contain lactose. Such diets are very restrictive and can lead to eating disorders and serious parental anxiety. With the evidence that individuals with galactosemia synthesize significant quantities of galactose metabolites (see below), other authorities now believe that, after childhood, obsessive adherence is unnecessary and that small quantities of galactose are safe although deliberate and continuous high exposure is clearly contraindicated. Adults can tolerate small quantities of galactose without acute symptoms or obvious biochemical abnormalities; the long term safety of this is not known and some restrictions are clearly needed until further studies have been performed. Some children on a relaxed regime show deteriorating school performance and behavior problems. Life-long galactose restriction remains the standard of care.

Because cataracts may be present at birth, cord blood gal-1-P is often markedly elevated and because gal-1-P may also be increased in the mother's blood, prenatal restriction of galactose has been advocated. However, this seems to have no effect upon the long term outcome.[123] Heterozygote offspring of properly treated homozygous mothers appear to be completely normal.

Self-intoxication

About 12–24 mg/kg/day galactose is synthesized by these patients;[124] some galactose is essential for the synthesis of galactolipids and galactoproteins. Moreover, lactose is synthesized normally in the milk of a lactating mother. It is not surprising that, even with the use of strict galactose-free diets or parenteral nutrition, gal-1-P remains elevated in the blood of classical galactosemics. Galactose ingestion certainly raises the erythrocyte gal-1-P and this test is still used to monitor diet compliance; in view of the dual sources, elevated values may be misinterpreted.

Galactitol from free galactose is the likely cause of cataracts. The cause of the acute and the long term complications is not known; they have been attributed to gal-1-P toxicity but, by inference from the variants, this seems unlikely. Perhaps they arise from excess or depleted metabolites in the tissues.

Galactokinase deficiency

As soon as galactose is consumed by individuals with galactokinase deficiency, it accumulates in the blood and urine; some is reduced to the polyol galactitol which appears to cause cataracts because of osmotic swelling and disruption of lens fibers. Gal-1-P and UDP-galactose (UDP-gal) levels are normal and cataract is the only clinical abnormality directly related to the enzyme defect. Fetuses of affected females may also develop cataracts, as may heterozygotes in later life. A galactose-free diet is indicated and should be continued for life. Early treatment prevents cataracts or arrests their further increase. A similar diet has been proposed for heterozygotes but no long term studies have been reported. Prenatal diagnosis is possible.

Uridine diphosphate galactose-4-epimerase deficiency

This disorder occurs in two forms: confined only to erythrocytes or generalized deficiency affecting the liver as well. When it is confined to erythrocytes, epimerase deficiency is completely symptomless and needs no treatment. Generalized epimerase deficiency is clinically similar to transferase deficiency and galactose, gal-1-P and UDP-gal increase after galactose consumption. Dietary galactose restriction is followed by a drop of all three metabolites in the blood. UDP-gal is a critical substrate for the production of sphingolipids for the brain and dietary intake of approximately 1.5–2 g galactose/day is thought to be necessary to meet the requirement of UDP-gal while simultaneously preventing gal-1-P accumulation.

DEFECTS IN FRUCTOSE METABOLISM (Fig. 24.21)

The main dietary sources of fructose are fruits, fruit juices, vegetables, potatoes, honey and all products that contain fructose or

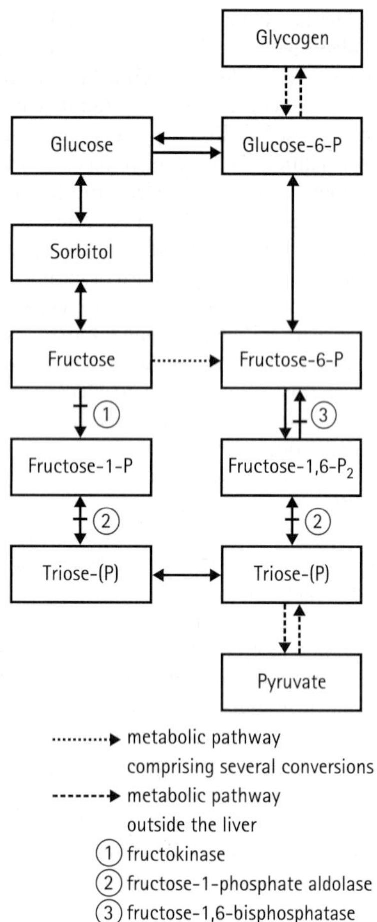

Fig. 24.21 The metabolism of fructose.

its disaccharide, sucrose (fructose-glucose). Another source is sorbitol, a fructose derivative, which is used as a sweetener in some foods, including some foods for diabetics. Sorbitol may be oxidized by the enzyme sorbitol dehydrogenase to fructose.

Fructose-1-phosphate aldolase deficiency (hereditary fructose intolerance) (step 2)

There are three aldolase isozymes, A, B and C, each with specific properties and tissue localization. In this condition, aldolase B is deficient; it is localized in liver, intestine and kidneys and normally cleaves fructose-1-phosphate (F-1-P) and fructose-1,6-diphosphate (F-1,6-P) into two trioses. These trioses are then substrates either for glycolysis or for gluconeogenesis. In hereditary fructose intolerance, F-1-P accumulates as soon as the patient ingests fructose; it is very toxic and it inhibits several enzymes of glycogenolysis and gluconeogenesis, causing rapid and profound hypoglycemia. Furthermore, the intracellular supply of phosphate is sequestered as F-1-P and this prevents the regeneration of ATP from ADP. Under these conditions, ADP is dephosphorylated to AMP and then further metabolized to uric acid.

Clinical features

Symptoms of intolerance develop as soon as fructose is ingested. This occurs usually after weaning, since breast milk and most infant formulas do not contain fructose, but symptoms can sometimes develop much earlier, at the first introduction of fruit or fructose containing infant formula (some soy formulas contain fructose), or when honey is misused as a pacifier. Acute symptoms include vomiting, diaphoresis, tremor, lethargy, convulsions and other manifestations associated with hypoglycemia. Chronic exposure to fructose leads to progressive liver damage with anorexia, failure to thrive, jaundice, hepatomegaly, splenomegaly, ascites, edema and hemorrhage. Aversion to sweets develops early in life and, by avoiding sweetened foods, most patients, if they survive infancy, unknowingly protect themselves from the toxic effects of fructose. Occasionally the condition is only diagnosed in adult life. Remarkably, the teeth often remain free of caries.

Diagnosis

Fructosemia is easy to diagnose if the association of acute symptoms with fructose ingestion is recognized. Metabolic abnormalities following acute fructose ingestion include hypoglycemia, hypophosphatemia, hyperuricemia and hypermagnesemia along with all the manifestations of renal Fanconi syndrome (see Ch. 16). The liver function tests are markedly abnormal and increased levels of some amino acids such as tyrosine and methionine are usual. These features occur only following fructose ingestion; their absence in a patient with fructose avoidance behavior does not eliminate the possibility of aldolase deficiency. Liver biopsy, during acute or chronic fructose ingestion, shows extensive abnormalities including focal areas of necrosis, fatty degeneration, proliferation of bile ducts, formation of pseudoacini and ultimately biliary cirrhosis.

The finding of a reducing sugar in urine following an episode of fructose ingestion is an important clue. When hereditary fructose intolerance is clinically suspected but not proven by the laboratory data, mutation analysis on DNA isolated from peripheral whole blood is a very useful confirmatory method. More than 80% of individuals of European descent with hereditary fructose intolerance can be identified by DNA analysis for a small set of common mutations in the aldolase B gene.[125] Importantly, this test currently screens only for specific mutations and is not an exhaustive search for changes in the entire aldolase B gene. In the future, sequencing of the entire aldolase B gene may be available. The fructose tolerance test can be dangerous and even fatal. This test carries a risk of significant metabolic decompensation should the patient have fructosemia, and probably should be avoided. If it is felt to be absolutely necessary, the test should be executed only in a hospital setting with full medical support available, with the advance knowledge and guidance of a metabolic disease specialist and only when the patient is clinically stable. A positive test is signaled by a rise of at least 50% in serum uric acid and a drop of 40–50% in the serum glucose and phosphate. In doubtful cases, enzymatic assay of a liver biopsy may be necessary.

Treatment

A strict fructose-free diet can prevent or arrest virtually all abnormalities and restore liver and kidney function to normal, except in cases of severe liver failure. The effects of the treatment are influenced by the age of the patient, the amount and duration of fructose ingestion and the residual aldolase B activity. Young infants are most susceptible to life threatening fructose toxicity. In older children, large amounts of fructose elicit acute symptoms, and continued exposure to small amounts, although insufficient to cause acute symptoms, may cause growth retardation. Successful treatment requires detailed knowledge of the fructose content of foodstuffs including processed foods.

Fructose-1,6-diphosphatase deficiency (step 3)

This enzyme is one of the unidirectional enzymes in the pathway of gluconeogenesis and is also important for the conversion of fructose into glucose. Fasting, fructose ingestion, or metabolic stress lead to hypoglycemia and increased protein and fat catabolism, resulting in the accumulation of lactate, pyruvate, alanine, ketone bodies and glycerol.

Clinical features

The symptoms of deficiency of this enzyme are similar to those of fructosemia or type 1 glycogen storage disease. They may develop in the neonatal period or later, provoked by insufficient food intake or by the inadvertent intake of fructose or sucrose. Dietary sugar ingestion usually is not the inciting event precipitating metabolic crisis, as these patients are not nearly as sensitive to fructose ingestions as are those with hereditary fructose intolerance. Fulminating lactic acidosis and hypoglycemia lead to hyperventilation, hypotonia, hepatomegaly, nausea, vomiting, lethargy and convulsions. Liver and kidney function may deteriorate and the course may be either severe and rapidly fatal or episodic, being exacerbated during acute metabolic stress.

Diagnosis

Hypoglycemia and lactic acidosis together with or without evidence of liver dysfunction demand metabolic investigation. Precipitation of problems by fructose may be a clue and characteristically, glycerol and glycerol-3-phosphate accumulate during hypoglycemia and are excreted in the urine. These metabolites derive from excessive proteolysis and fatty acid oxidation which increase to compensate for the lack of glucose. The lactic acidosis can be profound and recalcitrant to therapy. Liver histology may show fatty degeneration and fibrosis and the renal Fanconi syndrome may be apparent. All these are reminiscent of type 1 glycogen storage disease. A fasting test might elicit the above symptoms. Fasting, fructose or glycerol stress tests are not without risk, and should be avoided in most cases unless a metabolic disease specialist has been consulted and agrees a stress test is indicated. Definitive diagnosis requires enzyme assay of leukocytes or liver biopsy tissue. The leukocyte enzyme assay is fraught with difficulties.

Treatment

Treatment consists of frequent meals and the restriction of fructose, sucrose and sorbitol intake. Prolonged fasting must be avoided and early and aggressive treatment with glucose and bicarbonate intravenously may be necessary during infections. Sugar restriction does not need to be as severe as is indicated in hereditary fructose intolerance.

Other disorders of fructose metabolism

In *fructokinase deficiency* (essential fructosuria) (step 1), fructose metabolism is blocked in the liver, intestine and kidney and fructose levels in blood and urine are increased if the patient consumes fructose. The condition is benign and treatment is not required. Fructose malabsorption is reasonably common and is associated with fermentative diarrhea following quite modest fructose ingestion.

A defect of *aldolase A* detectable in fibroblasts is associated with non-spherocytic hemolytic anemia; some cases have had microcephaly and dysmorphic features.

DEFECTS IN GLYCOGEN METABOLISM: GLYCOGEN STORAGE DISORDERS AND ALLIED DISEASES (Fig. 24.22)

Several inherited enzyme defects interfere with the metabolism of glycogen. Defects in glycogen synthesis prevent or severely limit glycogen storage and are associated with postprandial hyperglycemia followed by fasting hypoglycemia. Defects in degradation often raise the glycogen content of the organ in which the enzyme is normally localized causing local tissue dysfunction. Glycogen is a giant polysaccharide in which glucose is stored in various organs but mainly in liver and muscle. Around 90% of the glucose molecules are linked in straight chains through alpha-1,4 bonds; about 8% are linked through alpha-1,6 bonds that form branching points. The usual glycogen concentration of the liver is < 5–7 g/100 g wet weight and in muscle < 2 g/100 g wet weight, these concentrations being influenced by factors such as the nutritional status, the pre- or postprandial condition of the patient and by hormonal stimuli. Therefore, quantitative glycogen analyses on tissue biopsies may be difficult to interpret, even in patients with glycogen storage diseases (GSD).

In liver, the major function of glycogen is to provide reserve glucose for export to other organs, mainly the brain. In contrast, muscle glycogen is only used as a fuel for ATP synthesis during muscle contraction. It follows that GSD involving the liver is usually characterized by fasting hypoglycemia, whereas the muscle defects are characterized by myopathy.

For the synthesis of glycogen (Fig. 24.22), glucose is phosphorylated to glucose-6-phosphate, then converted to glucose-1-phosphate. The enzyme glycogen synthase (enzyme 1) then catalyzes the polymerization of glucose-1-phosphate molecules into straight chain glycogen. Branching enzyme (enzyme 2) adds glucose-1-phosphate in alpha-1,6 linkages to form branch points.

In the initial step of glycogenolysis whether in liver or muscle, a phosphorylase enzyme cleaves glucose-1-phosphate molecules from the alpha-1,4 linkages of the outer chains. Liver phosphorylase (enzyme 3) is distinct from muscle phosphorylase (enzyme 4) and is activated by phosphorylase-beta-kinase (not shown) which in turn is activated by a cyclic AMP-dependent protein kinase. The activation

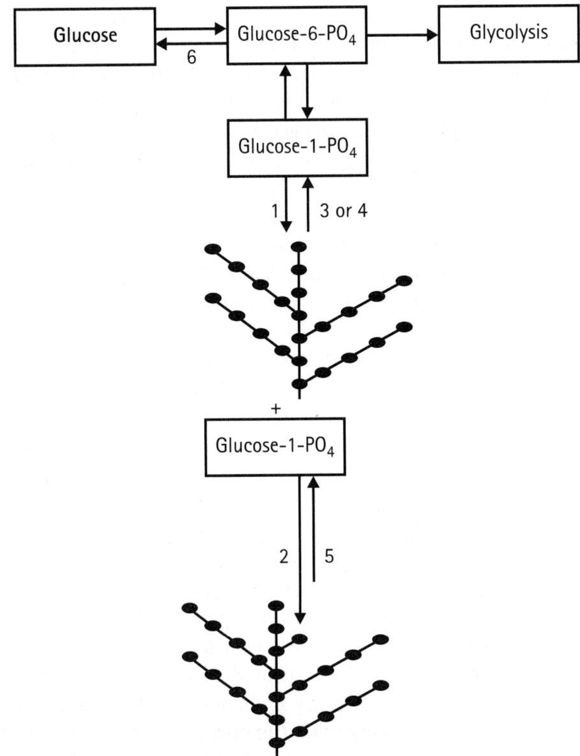

Fig. 24.22 Glycogen metabolism. 1, glycogen synthase; 2, branching enzyme; 3, liver phosphorylase; 4, muscle phosphorylase; 5, debranching enzyme; 6, glucose-6-phosphatase.

and inactivation of this cascade is mediated by hormones, mainly glucagon, insulin and adrenaline. Phosphorylase activity ceases as it nears a branch point; further degradation of the glucose polymer and removal of the branch point is mediated by debranching enzyme (enzyme 5). The product of glycogenolysis, glucose-1-phosphate, is converted to glucose-6-phosphate. In the liver, glucose-6-phosphate is predominantly dephosphorylated to glucose by glucose-6-phosphatase (enzyme 6). In muscle, glucose-6-phosphate is consumed as a substrate for glycolysis and ATP production.

This main pathway of glycogen degradation by phosphorylation and dephosphorylation in the cytoplasm is different from that in lysosomes. Pompe disease (GSD II), a disorder of excess lysosomal glycogen storage, results from inherited deficiency of lysosomal alpha-1,4-glucosidase. The severe phenotype of this disorder illustrates the importance of lysosome-mediated glycogen degradation.

Traditionally, the various glycogen storage disorders have been classified numerically or by eponym. Because, in the past, different numbers have been assigned to the same enzymatic defect, the specific enzyme nosology is preferable (Table 24.12). However, for historical reasons, both the numerical classification and the eponymic label are given for each disorder in this review. Two defects of glycogen synthesis are known, glycogen synthase (enzyme 1) deficiency and branching enzyme (enzyme 2) deficiency. For the disorders of glycogenolysis, the clinical phenotypes can generally be separated into two groups, hypoglycemia and hepatic dysfunction or skeletal myopathy, depending upon the normal tissue location of the missing enzyme. In the subsequent sections the glycogen synthetic defects will be described first followed by those disorders predominantly exhibiting a hepatic phenotype and then the glycogen storage diseases demonstrating primarily myopathic symptoms. Finally, the lysosomal storage disorder, Pompe disease, will be summarized. This condition is also discussed in the section on lysosomal storage diseases. The patterns of clinical presentation are related to the specific enzyme deficiencies (Table 24.13).

Table 24.12 Glycogen storage diseases, classification

Type	Deficient enzyme	Tissue involved	Main clinical findings
IA	Glucose-6-phosphatase	Liver, kidney	Hepatomegaly, hypoglycemia, lactic acidosis
IB IC ID	Glucose-6-phosphatase-related transport	Liver, leukocytes	IB additional immunologic abnormalities IC, ID?
II	Acid α-glucosidase (lysosomal)	Generalized	Infant form: cardiorespiratory failure. Later forms: myopathy
III	Debranching enzyme	Liver, muscle, heart	Hepatomegaly, hypoglycemia, myopathy
IV	Branching enzyme	Liver	Hepatosplenomegaly, cirrhosis
V	Phosphorylase	Muscle	Myopathy, exercise intolerance
VI	Phosphorylase system	Liver (muscle)	Hepatomegaly (myopathy)
VII	Phosphofructokinase and other defects of glycolysis	Muscle (erythrocytes)	Myopathy, exercise intolerance (hemolysis)
0	Glycogen synthase	Liver	Hypoglycemia

Glycogen synthase deficiency (GSD type 0)

Clinical features

This rare defect is usually grouped with the GSDs since it involves the same metabolic pathway. Failure to synthesize glycogen results in rapid and profound hyperglycemia after even quite modest meals. This is followed by a rapid and profound fall of the blood glucose when postprandial events normally turn to glycogenolysis to maintain blood glucose. Facile ketosis and postprandial hyperlactacidemia can be seen. The liver is not enlarged and its glycogen content is low. The enzyme defect can only be demonstrated in the liver. Diagnostic confirmation might also be possible by DNA studies.

Treatment

Treatment consists of small, frequent protein-rich meals and regular uncooked cornstarch feedings to prevent hypoglycemia and ketosis.

Branching enzyme deficiency (GSD type IV)

Clinical features

The main features of this disorder are marked hepatomegaly with progressive cirrhosis, splenomegaly, muscle hypotonia and weakness, hypo- or areflexia, retarded motor milestones, growth retardation and normal mental development. Death usually occurs in the first years of life, although liver transplant may prolong survival, and milder forms exist. Rarely, milder variants with myopathy are observed in adults and cardiomyopathy with heart failure may be the only presentation. The metabolic derangements

Table 24.13 Disorders of glycogen metabolism grouped according to symptom complex

Hypoglycemia or liver dysfunction	Liver and muscle symptoms	Skeletal myopathy
Glycogen synthase deficiency (type 0)	Glycogen branching enzyme deficiency (type IV)	Muscle phosphorylase deficiency (type V)
Glucose-6-phosphatase deficiency (type IA)	Glycogen debranching enzyme deficiency (type III)	Muscle phosphofructokinase deficiency (type VII)
Glucose-6-phosphate translocase deficiency (types IB and IC)		
Liver phosphorylase and phosphorylase b kinase deficiencies (type VI)		

Pompe disease (type II) is a lysosomal storage disease and as such exhibits a clinical phenotype distinct from those of other glycogen storage disorders.

are hypoglycemia, usually mild, increased transaminases and decreased clotting factors.

Diagnosis

The enzyme defect causes insufficient branching of the glycogen molecule and its prolonged inner and outer chains give it the appearance and properties of amylopectin. Apparently this abnormal glycogen is difficult to mobilize. It acts as a foreign body and glucose release from it is hampered. In contrast to the liver, muscle histology is usually normal in spite of absent enzyme activity in that tissue. The enzyme defect is expressed in many tissues including fibroblasts; antenatal diagnosis is feasible.

Treatment

Treatment is symptomatic and consists of frequent high carbohydrate feedings and, eventually, gastric drip feeding. This dietary treatment, however, does not prevent liver failure. Liver transplantation has been successful.

Glucose-6-phosphatase deficiency (GSD type IA: von Gierke's disease)

Clinical features

The most conspicuous clinical findings are a protruding abdomen because of marked hepatomegaly, hypotrophic muscles, truncal obesity, a rounded 'doll face' and short stature (Fig. 24.23). Because glucose-6-phosphatase activity is required for both glycogenolysis and gluconeogenesis, severe symptomatic hypoglycemia is frequent, often occurring during the night or after even short periods of reduced caloric intake. Even minor delays or reduction of carbohydrate intake may provoke hypoglycemic attacks that are accompanied by lactic acidosis. The liver may be enlarged at birth; its size increases gradually and may achieve a total span of 15–20 cm. Initially, the liver is smooth with a normal consistency, but by 10–20 years age, it becomes firmer and nodular due to the development of benign adenomas. Cirrhosis however does not typically develop. Severe hypertriglyceridemia is indicative of poor glycemic control and has occasionally been associated with acute pancreatitis. The spleen is normal in size, but kidneys are moderately enlarged. Easy bruising, epistaxis, and even frank hemorrhage after surgery or other event, may be troublesome due to impaired platelet function. Linear growth is retarded but truncal obesity is obvious; both are improved through judicious treatment. Cerebral function is usually normal so long as recurrent hypoglycemic damage is prevented. Left untreated, associated hyperuricemia frequently causes gout. Allopurinol is often prescribed to prevent this complication.

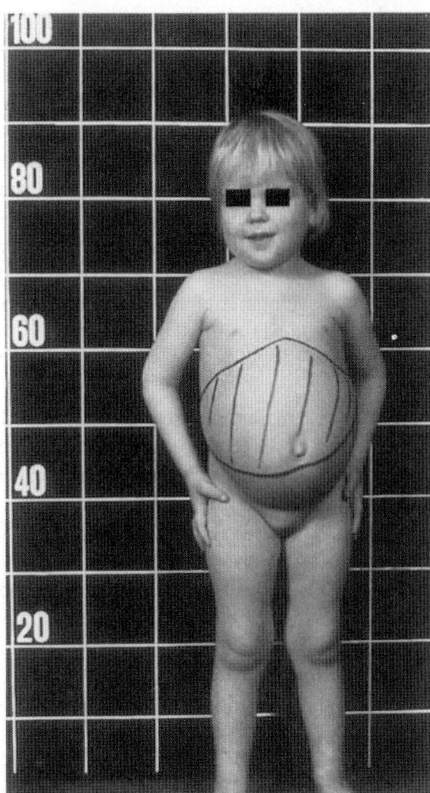

Fig. 24.23 The typical features of a patient with glucose-6-phosphatase deficiency.

Because of effective therapy preventing fatal hypoglycemia, the life expectancy of individuals with glucose-6-phosphatase deficiency has greatly improved, and consequently some late-onset complications have emerged. Rarely, hepatic adenomas become malignant, hyperuricemia and gout are now rare, but progressive focal glomerular sclerosis is a serious risk and can lead to renal failure. Anemia and osteopenia are also late-onset problems.

Metabolic derangements

Failure to dephosphorylate glucose-6-phosphate means that glucose production from both glycogenolysis and gluconeogenesis is blocked. However, the Embden–Meyerhof glycolytic pathway (Fig. 24.19) is intact and during fasting is intensified under hormonal stimulation. This increases lactate production which is useful since lactate can serve as a fuel to the brain. However, chronic lactic acidemia is usual and probably contributes to the retarded growth and osteoporosis. Excess acetyl-CoA is also produced and is converted into fatty acids and cholesterol; this probably underlies the hypertriglyceridemia, hypercholesterolemia and hyperprebetalipoproteinemia seen in most of these patients. Some of the excess glucose-6-phosphate is channeled via the pentose phosphate shunt to urate, thus explaining the hyperuricemia, which can be severe.

Diagnosis

In the past, oral glucose tolerance tests have been employed as a diagnostic aid. During this test, in GSD I patients, the blood lactate *decreases* from an initially high level to (near) normal. This is the opposite of the normal response. Oral glucose tolerance tests and fasting and other stress tests, however, can be hazardous. Assay of glucose-6-phosphatase activity in liver confirms the diagnosis and delineates the different forms of this syndrome. In the liver, fat accumulation often exceeds that of glycogen; this does not contradict the biochemical diagnosis. DNA mutational analysis is becoming more widely used as a diagnostic test for this condition. Antenatal diagnosis can only be done on fetal liver tissue or by DNA studies.

Treatment

Acute hypoglycemia should be treated with glucose 0.25 g/kg in 50–100 ml water orally or by intravenous bolus infusion; importantly, this should be followed immediately by an intravenous drip providing twice the normal glucose requirement (see below). Lactic acidosis usually resolves without the need for sodium bicarbonate since glucose administration suppresses lactate overproduction. Oral nutrition is reintroduced as soon as possible.

For maintenance, a high carbohydrate diet with 65–60% of the total energy as carbohydrates, 10% as protein and 20–25% as fat is used. Both lactose and sucrose intake should be restricted since neither galactose nor fructose can be converted to glucose because of the enzyme defect. Low-lactose, sucrose-free formulae are preferable if breast milk is not available. Maltose or dextrins can be added to give a total 65% energy as carbohydrate. Feedings should be administered at 2–3 h intervals around the clock before the age of 3 months, followed by a wider spacing from 3–6 months onwards. Gastric drip feeding at night is often introduced as early as possible using carbohydrate derived from glucose, maltose or glucose polymers to provide a constant supply of carbohydrate at 7–9 mg/kg/min for infants, 5–6 mg/kg/min for 1–6-year-olds and 4 mg/kg/min for older children. This treatment improves the clinical condition, decreases the liver size, suppresses the bleeding tendency and promotes growth.

Most older patients prefer to use uncooked cornstarch as a slow-release form of carbohydrate. Because of its thick consistency even mixed in water, it cannot be given via a gastric or nasogastric tube but can be given orally, between or together with meals and normalizes the blood sugar for several hours (Fig. 24.24); it is now considered a mainstay of therapy. Uncooked cornstarch can be started early in infancy though prior to about 1 year of age infants may not produce sufficient amylase to effectively metabolize the corn-starch. Early introduction of cornstarch may, however, induce earlier production of amylase. In any case, the mainstays of therapy are uncooked cornstarch and night-time enteral feeds and older children and adults usually can get by with uncooked cornstarch alone. Since disconnection of the tubing or pump malfunction in the GSD I patient receiving enteral feedings can be fatal, good equipment and alarms systems are crucial. Even optimum treatment may not correct the hypoglycemia, lactic acidosis and hyperlipidemia completely and some patients continue to grow poorly. Captopril is being evaluated for treating the renal disease; osteoporosis requires a generous calcium and vitamin D intake and periodic assessment of bone density. Hyperuricemia is treated with allopurinol. Liver transplantation has been successful. Granulocyte/macrophage cell stimulating factor (GM-CSF) is used in type IB.

Glucose-6-phosphate translocase deficiencies (GSD types IB and IC)

These are defects of translocases located on the luminal wall of the endoplasmic reticulum which normally allow entry of glucose-6-phosphate (GSD type IB) and exit of phosphate (GSD type IC). Both defects render glucose-6-phosphatase functionally inactive. A defect of the glucose translocase has not yet been described.

The clinical and metabolic symptoms and treatment of GSD IB are not discernibly different from GSD IA except for a grave propensity to immunological abnormalities. There is neutropenia and defective neutrophil and monocyte function; bacterial infections are frequent and may be fatal. Inflammatory bowel disease akin to Crohn's disease and myelogenous leukemia are added potential complications. The prognosis of translocase deficiency traditionally was worse than that of glucose-6-phosphatase deficiency because of the increased risk of metabolic derangements due to the frequent infections, but the introduction of GM-CSF as a treatment has improved the prognosis tremendously.

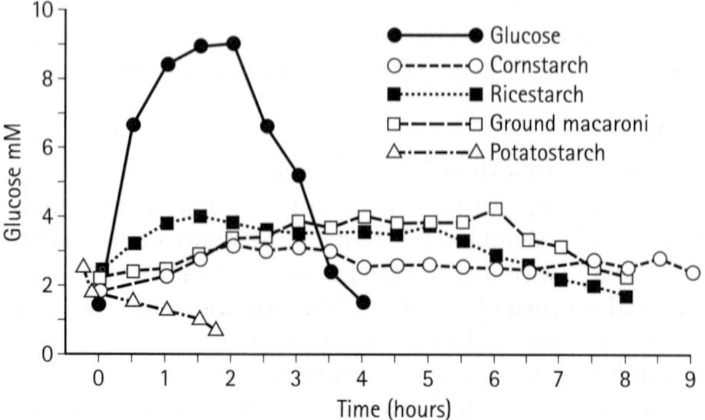

Fig. 24.24 Blood glucose curves of a patient with glucose-6-phosphatase deficiency after the ingestion of glucose or various uncooked starches, 2 g/kg body weight each.

Translocase 1 defect (GSD type IB) accounts for 12–15% of the total cases of glucose-6-phosphatase deficiency, whereas the translocase 2 defect is extremely rare.

Debranching enzyme deficiency (GSD type III; limit dextrinosis)

During glycogenolysis, this enzyme normally prunes the alpha-1,6, linkage branch points as the straight, alpha-1,4 links are being broken down by phosphorylase. When this does not happen, glycogen degradation stops at the branch points, leaving 'limit dextrin'. This abnormal glycogen may behave as a foreign body and elicit high transaminase levels, recurrent jaundice, fibrosis and even cirrhosis. Gluconeogenesis, however, is unimpeded and this drains glucogenic amino acids from muscle protein, presumably contributing to poor growth and muscle wasting. This also explains the observation that GSD III patients are not as prone to severe hypoglycemia as GSD I patients.

Clinical features

Two forms exist; one is confined to liver but the more common involves the muscles as well. In younger children the liver symptoms predominate and are very similar to glucose-6-phosphatase deficiency with hypoglycemia in the neonatal period or later or during decreased food intake or metabolic stress. The liver is markedly enlarged but the spleen and kidneys are not. Hypotonia, truncal obesity and a doll face develop and the patient may show retarded growth which gradually catches up later. Motor development is slow but mental development is usually normal. The liver has a normal consistency, but rarely cirrhosis may develop. Surprisingly, for unknown reasons, the liver size often returns to normal at or before puberty.

In the myopathic form, which has probably been underdiagnosed in the past, there is increasing muscle weakness and a slowly progressive distal muscle wasting, sometimes starting in childhood, sometimes in adult life. It may be accompanied by cardiomyopathy with left ventricular hypertrophy and electrocardiogram (ECG) abnormalities. These developments warrant close supervision of muscle function and regular ECG in all patients.

Diagnosis

Conspicuous findings during fasting are ketosis (not lactic acidosis), hyperlipidemia (mainly hypercholesterolemia) and hypoglycemia. An oral galactose tolerance test elicits a normal increase of blood glucose and an abnormal increase of blood lactate. A fasting glucagon test is characterized by an abnormally flat glucose response. These fasting tests can be dangerous.

The liver pathology shows an increase of reticulin fibers between hepatocytes and of fibrous tissue in portal tracts. In the myopathic form, the muscles show myofibrillary destruction and degeneration of the neuromuscular junctions.

Enzyme assay in liver or muscle is required to confirm the diagnosis of GSD III.

Treatment and prognosis

Treatment of the hepatic form is similar to that of GSD I except that restriction of galactose and fructose is not necessary as both can be converted normally into glucose. Although gastric drip feeding is not a prerequisite for glucose homeostasis at a later age, this treatment and extra protein may be useful in delaying or improving the myopathy. Thus, the diet for both forms of the disease should contain approximately 55–60% energy as carbohydrates, particularly starch, 15–20% energy as protein and 20–25% energy as fat, predominantly polyunsaturated. As for the prognosis, the late development of myopathy and cardiomyopathy remains a concern.

Liver phosphorylase and liver phosphorylase b kinase deficiencies (GSD type VI)

Phosphorylase b kinase is required to convert phosphorylase b (inactive) to the activated form and the kinase itself is regulated by another (cyclic AMP-dependent) kinase, the whole system being stimulated by hormones, particularly glucagon. The clinical heterogeneity of phosphorylase b kinase deficiency is due to the fact that it consists of four different subunits at least one of which is coded on the X chromosome. These two defects are discussed together because the clinical features and metabolic derangements are similar.

Clinical features

In early childhood, pronounced hepatomegaly, without splenomegaly and a protuberant abdomen due to muscle hypotonia are the most striking features; the liver enlargement resolves slowly and usually disappears at puberty. Equally, the muscle hypotonia and weakness, which initially cause slow motor development, also tend to improve. Growth and puberty are often delayed. Mental development is normal. There are exceptions to this usually mild course, particularly in phosphorylase b kinase deficiency, of which many variants exist. Rare cases have had combinations of hepatic symptoms and myopathy, fatal cardiomyopathy and even myopathy without hepatic symptoms. The X-linked form of phosphorylase b kinase deficiency is the most common and mildest form, and can present with isolated hepatomegaly in children.

Diagnosis

A tentative diagnosis is based on the pronounced hepatomegaly in contrast to the mild metabolic findings. Mild fasting hypoglycemia may develop; elevated serum transaminases, hypercholesterolemia and a marked tendency to fasting ketosis are evident at a young age, but normalize completely by puberty.

In the absence of galactosuria, an oral galactose test is abnormal as blood lactate increases excessively. Contrary to expectation, glucagon tests are not of much help as the increase of blood glucose is variable. Fasting or stress tests may be dangerous. Kinase defects can theoretically be detected in blood cells but assay of liver or muscle may be required in some cases.

Treatment

Treatment of this self-limiting disease is not necessary except for prevention of hypoglycemia which may require uncooked cornstarch. Use of polyunsaturated fat suppresses hypercholesterolemia. Severe forms of phosphorylase b kinase deficiency may be refractory to dietary treatment, and liver transplantation may be indicated for severe cases with liver failure.

Muscle phosphorylase deficiency (GSD type V; McArdle syndrome)

Clinical features

This disorder is characterized by increasing intolerance for strenuous exercise. During early childhood no symptoms occur except easy fatiguability. In adults, strenuous muscle activity is accompanied by severe cramps and may be followed by myoglobinuria, which can precipitate anuria and renal failure. In middle life, the fatigue increases and muscle wasting and weakness predominate. The serum CPK may be permanently or intermittently elevated.

Diagnosis

Muscle exercise is normally accompanied by release of lactate and of inosine, hypoxanthine and ammonia through the purine nucleotide cycle. In myophosphorylase deficiency lactic acid production is blocked and release of the purine nucleotide cycle compounds is exaggerated. The ensuing myogenic hyperuricemia is one of the characteristic features of defects of muscle glycogenosis. The semi-ischemic forearm exercise test gives abnormal results; it is carried out as follows: a blood pressure cuff is inflated above systolic pressure. A handgrip is formed and opened every second for 1 min. Prior to and for eight 1 min intervals after starting the exercise, venous blood is collected. Ammonia and hypoxanthine values rise abnormally but the normal increase in lactate is absent in this disorder and in other glycolytic defects in muscle, such as phosphofructokinase deficiency.

Phosphorylase activity must be assayed in muscle; liver phosphorylase is presumably normal, as is glucose homeostasis. DNA mutation analysis is useful in myophosphorylase deficiency as there are common mutations.

Treatment

Treatment is symptomatic and consists of the avoidance of strenuous exercise. 'Carbo loading' and a high protein diet are of some help and glucose should always be taken during exercise. Strenuous exercise is always a risk.

Muscle phosphofructokinase deficiency (GSD type VII)

Clinical features

The three clinical and metabolic characteristics of this rare disorder are myopathy, increased hemolysis and gout. The myopathy is similar to GSD type V and manifests itself in childhood by weakness, limitation of vigorous activity and exercise-induced cramps, accompanied by myoglobinuria; CPK is often raised. As in muscle phosphorylase deficiency, there is no rise of venous lactate after exercise and ammonia, inosine, hypoxanthine and urate are produced in excess. Continued myogenic hyperuricemia explains the gout.

Different isoenzymes of phosphofructokinase exist in various tissues. The absence of the M-subunit in erythrocytes results in hemolytic anemia. In muscles, however, the block in glycolysis may be partly compensated by increased fatty acid oxidation.

Treatment

Provision of extra glucose does not bypass the enzyme defect and is therefore of no help. This is different from muscle phosphorylase deficiency in which glucose enters the glycolytic pathway 'downstream' from the enzyme defect. A high protein diet and prevention of excessive activity are the only measures.

Lysosomal alpha-1,4-glucosidase deficiency (GSD type II: Pompe disease)

Deficiency of this enzyme, also called acid maltase deficiency (AMD), leads to a generalized glycogen storage disease. There are infantile, juvenile and adult forms. This defect is not in the regular cascade of glycogenolysis and is not associated with defects of circulating fuels in the blood.

Clinical features

Infantile AMD or Pompe disease is characterized by the rapid onset in the first months of life of profound muscle hypotonia, weakness, hyporeflexia, glossomegaly, massive cardiomyopathy without murmurs but no hepatomegaly except with cardiac failure. The infant is usually alert and the cerebral development is normal. The ECG shows a huge QRS complex, left or biventricular hypertrophy and shortened PR interval. The clinical course is downhill with cardiopulmonary failure or pneumonia leading to death in the first 2 years.

Childhood or adult forms with onset in the second to fourth decades are less severe and progress more slowly. The heart is not usually affected but motor milestones are delayed and weakness develops of limb girdle and truncal muscles, mimicking other chronic myopathies. Involvement of respiratory muscles ultimately causes ventilatory insufficiency with death usually between the second and fourth decade.

Diagnosis

The enzyme can theoretically be assayed in leukocytes but that assay is fraught with difficulties. More commonly, assay of the enzyme in muscle and/or fibroblasts is required. In the infantile form, glycogen-laden lysosomes are present in all organs except the kidneys and the cerebral cortex, being particularly abundant in anterior horn cells and motor nuclei of the brainstem. In the adult disorder, glycogen storage is absent in heart, brain and liver and varies greatly in different muscles. A second enzyme, neutral maltase, is produced by the kidneys and is also present in the leukocytes and must be differentiated during enzyme analysis. Antenatal diagnosis is possible.

Treatment

In the past, no effective therapy for Pompe disease has existed, and management has been primarily supportive. Recent results from experimental trials of intravenous recombinant alpha-glucosidase infusions are however very promising.[126,127]

Although this mode of therapy requires further investigation, the initial results suggest a promising future for the treatment of Pompe disease.

DISORDERS OF PLASMA LIPIDS AND LIPOPROTEINS

INTRODUCTION

Hyperlipidemia is relevant to the practice of pediatrics for several reasons. First, identification of secondary hyperlipidemia may alert the health care provider to the presence of an underlying condition, such as hypothyroidism. Second, familial disorders of lipid metabolism may be indicative of a genetic predisposition for cardiovascular disease, which might warrant additional testing of the entire family. Although coronary vascular disease is almost non-existent in pediatric patients, children with the rare disorder, homozygous familial hypercholesterolemia, have a high risk of myocardial infarction and death prior to the age of 20 years. Moreover, children with other forms of severe hyperlipidemia who have relatives with very early onset of cardiovascular disease may warrant initiation of treatment with lipid-lowering medication during childhood. Third, hyperlipidemia is an important complication of other metabolic disorders such as diabetes, obesity and the use of some medications. Fourth, children with defects in triglyceride metabolism resulting in severe hypertriglyceridemia have increased risk of pancreatitis, a potentially life threatening complication.

BASIC BIOCHEMISTRY

The primary lipids in plasma are triglycerides, cholesterol, and phospholipids. Other lipids that occur in small amounts in plasma include free fatty acids, mono- and diglycerides, steroid hormones (e.g. testosterone, estradiol, cortisol), sterol-derived vitamins (e.g. vitamin D), terpenes (e.g. vitamins A, E, and K) and sterols other than cholesterol (e.g. desmosterol). Because of their innate insolubility in aqueous media, lipids are transported in plasma as a constituent of lipoproteins or bound to plasma carrier proteins.

Triglycerides, which are composed of three fatty acid molecules covalently bound to a glycerol molecule, are synthesized in the liver from acetate or fatty acids and in the intestinal mucosa from absorbed dietary fat. Triglycerides are secreted into plasma in lipoproteins via the endogenous and exogenous pathways, as shown in Figure 24.25. Free fatty acids (non-esterified) are normally present in plasma in small amounts primarily bound to albumin and have a short half-life of 4–8 min, but the majority of fatty acids in plasma occur in the form of triglycerides and to a lesser extent in cholesteryl esters in lipoproteins. Release of free fatty acids and glycerol from adipose tissue triglyceride stores normally is increased during exercise, stress, and fasting as a consequence of increased activity of hormone sensitive lipase. Increased release of free fatty acids in patients with uncontrolled diabetes occurs as a result of the loss of insulin-mediated inhibition of phosphorylative activation of hormone sensitive lipase. A sustained increase in the delivery of free fatty acids and/or glucose to the liver, as occurs in uncontrolled diabetes, greatly stimulates hepatic synthesis of triglycerides, leading to hypertriglyceridemia. During hydrolysis of triglycerides, mono- and diglycerides are generated as intermediate products.

Fatty acids are classified on the basis of chain length and degree of saturation. Short chain fatty acids contain 2–6 carbon atoms, medium chain triglycerides 8–10 carbon atoms, and long chain fatty acids contain > 12 carbon atoms. Very long chain fatty acids normally are a minor component of the fatty acid pool, but these molecules accumulate in patients with peroxisomal disorders (see pp 1164). Saturated fatty acids (e.g. stearic acid, C18:0) contain no double bonds, whereas monounsaturated fatty acids (e.g. oleic acid, C18:1ω9) contain a single double bond and polyunsaturated fatty acids (e.g. linoleic acid, C18:3ω6) contain two or more double bonds. Unsaturated fatty acids are further subclassified into four classes, ω3 (e.g. linolenic acid), ω6 (e.g. linoleic acid), ω7 (e.g. palmitoleic acid), and ω9 (e.g. oleic acid), on the basis of the position of the first double bond from the methylene end of the molecule. The ω3 fatty acids found in marine oils and fish, such as eicosapentanoic acid (EPA, C20:5ω3)

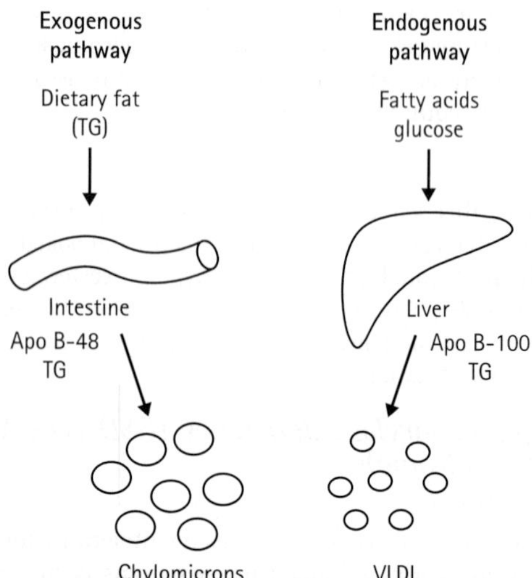

Fig. 24.25 Exogenous and endogenous sources of plasma triglycerides. TG, triglyceride; VLDL, very low density lipoprotein.

and docosahexanoic acid (DHA, C22:6ω3), have potent triglyceride-lowering effects when given in sufficient doses, may modulate immunity and platelet function, may have additional cardioprotective effects, and also may have a role in pre- and postnatal development of the brain and retina.

Cholesterol is synthesized from acetate by the liver and intestinal mucosa and released into plasma in lipoproteins. Other cell types also have the capacity to synthesize cholesterol in response to local cellular requirements, but the majority of such cholesterol does not appear in plasma. Current evidence suggests that a large proportion of cholesterol in high density lipoprotein (HDL) particles may be derived by receptor-mediated efflux from peripheral tissues. Although the majority of cholesterol in the body is synthesized endogenously, dietary cholesterol nonetheless influences the plasma cholesterol concentration by modulating hepatic secretion and uptake of cholesterol via transcriptional regulation of key enzymes and receptors. Delivery of dietary cholesterol to the liver inhibits proteolytic activation of sterol regulatory element binding protein-2 (SREBP-2), which is an agonist for the SRE in the regulatory sequence of the low density lipoprotein (LDL) receptor gene and other genes. Hence, increased intake of dietary cholesterol decreases hepatic expression of the LDL receptor, thereby contributing to hypercholesterolemia. Under normal conditions, about 40–50% of dietary cholesterol is absorbed. Cholesterol biosynthesis is regulated in the liver by the rate limiting enzyme, 3-hydroxy-3-methylglutaryl coenzyme A reductase (HMG-CoA reductase), which is the inhibitory target of 'statin' cholesterol lowering medications. A large amount of cholesterol and cholesterol derived bile acids circulate in the enterohepatic circulation, a pathway that consists of hepatic secretion of bile acids and cholesterol into the intestinal lumen via the bile duct followed by reabsorption of a portion of bile acids and cholesterol distally. The majority of cholesterol in plasma and tissues is esterified with a single fatty acid molecule to form cholesteryl esters.

The plasma phospholipids are primarily derived from hepatic and intestinal synthesis, but can be synthesized by many body tissues. Phospholipids are acylglycerols that contain phosphoric acid esterified to the C_3-hydroxyl group. The four major classes of phospholipids are phosphatidyl choline (lecithin), phosphatidyl serine, phosphatidyl ethanolamine, and phosphatidyl inositol. As a consequence of their polar structure, three of the four phospholipid classes form bilayers in aqueous media and are a critical component of cell membranes and the surface coat of lipoproteins. Phosphatidyl ethanolamine also is incorporated into cell membranes, but in isolation it has a tendency to form hexagonal complexes. As a consequence of the localization of phospholipids in the surface coat of lipoproteins, the phospholipid content of lipoprotein particles (expressed as a percentage of total weight) tends to be inversely proportional to the size of the particle.

The three main lipids, triglycerides, phospholipids and cholesterol, are transported in plasma as constituents of various lipoproteins that can be characterized on the basis of lipid composition, protein composition, particle size and density, and electrophoretic mobility. The various lipoprotein particles also differ in their origin and metabolic fate. The characteristics of the six major lipoprotein classes are shown in Table 24.14. The lipoprotein classes are sometimes subfractionated on the basis of density (e.g. HDL2a, HDL2b, HDL3; LDL1, LDL2, LDL3) or size [e.g. LDL pattern A (large) and B (small)], but subfractionation is unnecessary for most clinical situations. The protein moieties of lipoproteins, which are referred to as apoproteins (Table 24.15), contribute to the structure and metabolic fate of various lipoprotein particles. HDL particles also can be subfractionated on the basis of their apoprotein content into particles containing apo A-I without A-II [HDL(A-I)] and particles containing apo A-I and A-II [HDL(A-I/A-II)]. HDL(A-I) particles may be more cardioprotective than HDL(A-I/A-II) particles.

LIPOPROTEIN METABOLISM

Chylomicrons

Chylomicrons are synthesized by enterocytes in the small intestine and secreted into the thoracic duct in response to absorption of dietary fat. Dietary lipids undergo hydrolysis in the intestinal lumen, allowing absorption of the resulting fatty acids and glycerol by enterocytes. Fatty acids with chain length < 10–12 carbon atoms tend to be absorbed into the portal circulation, whereas other fatty acids are utilized by the intestinal mucosal cells for synthesis of chylomicrons. The enterocyte uses the hydrolyzed lipid products for the synthesis of triglycerides, cholesteryl esters and phospholipids, which are combined with a single apo B-48 molecule, apoproteins A-I, A-II, A-IV and some apo C-II and E to form chylomicrons. Chylomicrons are slowly released into the circulation via the thoracic duct, normally resulting in a peak increase in the concentration of plasma triglycerides 4–6 h after fat ingestion and a return to baseline after 8–10 h. After release into the plasma,

Table 24.14 Characteristics of plasma lipoproteins

Lipoprotein	Electrophoretic mobility	Density (g/ml)	Size (Å)	Lipid composition (% of total weight)	Major apoproteins	Origin
Chylomicrons	$alpha_2$	< 0.95	800–5000	2%P, 7%PL, 2%FC, 5%CE, *84%TG**	B-48, C-I, C-II, C-III, E, A-I, A-IV	Intestine
VLDL	pre-beta	0.95–1.006	300–800	8%P, 19%PL, 7%FC, 13%CE, *53%TG**	B-100, C-I, C-II, C-III, E	Liver
IDL	slow pre-beta (broad beta)	1.006–1.019	250–350	19%P, 19%PL, 9%FC, *29%CE, 23%TG**	B-100, E	VLDL, chylomicrons
LDL	beta	1.019–1.063	200–250	21%P, 22%PL, 8%FC, *37%CE,** 11%TG	B-100	VLDL, liver
Lipoprotein(a)	sinking pre-beta	1.06–1.08	200–300	33%P, 22%PL, 9%FC, *33%CE,** 3%TG	B-100, apo(a)	Liver
HDL	$alpha_1$	1.063–1.21	75–100	50%P, 23%PL, 4%FC, *18%CE,** 4%TG	A-I (70–75% of protein), A-II, (A-IV, D, CI-III, E)	Liver, peripheral tissues, intestine

CE, cholesteryl ester; FC, free cholesterol; HDL, high density lipoprotein; IDL, intermediate density lipoprotein; LDL, low density lipoprotein; P, protein; PL, phospholipid; TG, triglyceride; VLDL,very low density lipoprotein.
* Dominant lipid in each lipoprotein is in italic.

Table 24.15 The major plasma apoproteins

Apoprotein	Origin	Molecular weight	Metabolic function
A-I	Liver, intestine	28 000	Activates LCAT; ligand for ABC-A1 receptor, SR-B1, cubulin/megalin
A-II	Liver, intestine	17 500	May facilitate activation of hepatic lipase, may inhibit LCAT
A-IV	Intestine, liver	44 500	May facilitate LPL activation; satiety factor?
A-V	Uncertain		May be important determinant of plasma triglyceride concentrations
apo(a)	Liver	Variable	Covalently bound to apo B-100 in Lp(a) via sulfhydryl linkage; may adversely influence fibrinolysis and lipid deposition at sites of arterial injury
B-48	Intestine	264 000	Structural protein in chylomicrons
B-100	Liver	550 000	Structural protein in LDL and VLDL, binds to LDL receptor; critical for synthesis of VLDL and hepatic triglyceride secretion
C-I	Liver, adrenal	7000	Activates LCAT
C-II	Liver, (intestine)	9000	Activates LPL
C-III	Liver	9000	Inhibits C-II mediated LPL activation
D	Adrenal, kidney, pancreas, placenta, brain, intestine, spleen, testes	22 000 (29 000?)	May facilitate interlipoprotein and intercell lipid transfer; involved in brain lipid metabolism, activates LCAT
E (E2, E3, E4)	Liver, (intestine), CNS, peripheral tissues	34 000	Binds to LDL and apo E receptors, facilitates hepatic uptake of VLDL and chylomicron remnants
F	Liver		
J	Liver		Binds to megalin; found in amyloid
Transfer proteins	Liver	Variable	Transfer of lipids between lipoproteins

LCAT, lecithin-cholesterol acyltransferase; LDL, low density lipoprotein; LPL, lipoprotein lipase; SR-B1, scavenger receptor-B1; VLDL, very low density lipoprotein.

chylomicrons are rapidly remodeled and catabolized with a half-life < 15 min. Transfer of apo C and E from HDL to chylomicrons facilitates the hydrolysis of chylomicron triglycerides by lipoprotein lipase (LPL) and subsequent hepatic uptake of triglyceride-depleted chylomicron remnants via the LDL receptor-related protein (LRP), apo E receptor, and proteoglycan-mediated uptake pathways. During chylomicron degradation, fatty acids released by LPL in peripheral tissues can be utilized for energy or storage as triglycerides in adipose tissue. Apoproteins A-I and A-II and phospholipids are transferred to HDL during chylomicron catabolism.

Very low density lipoprotein (VLDL)

VLDL particles are primarily secreted by the liver, although there is evidence for intestinal secretion of VLDL. The rate of synthesis of VLDL is dependent on hormonal factors (such as insulin), time of day, background dietary composition, amount of adiposity (particularly visceral fat mass), and availability of substrate for triglyceride synthesis. Apo B-100 synthesis is essential for VLDL synthesis and secretion. During the initial steps of VLDL synthesis, apo B-100 is required on the endoplasmic reticulum to facilitate the aggregation of triglyceride and other lipids to form VLDL particles. Thus, lack of apo B-100, or the presence of truncation mutations in apo B-100, can suppress VLDL secretion. The metabolic pathways for VLDL particles in plasma are similar to those of chylomicrons, but VLDL particles also are remodeled by hepatic lipase and typically have a much longer half-life in plasma of 6–12 h. In addition, VLDL particles are sequentially metabolized to become intermediate density lipoprotein (IDL) particles and subsequently LDL particles. VLDL remnants can be taken up by hepatic LDL, apo E, and LRP receptors. The important role of apo E in hepatic clearance of VLDL from plasma is illustrated by the marked accumulation of VLDL and chylomicron remnants in patients with type III hyperlipidemia resulting from increased VLDL secretion and homozygosity for apo E2, a defective ligand for the apo E receptor and LRP.

Low density lipoprotein (LDL)

The majority of LDL particles in plasma are derived from intravascular catabolism and remodeling of VLDL particles. To a lesser extent, de novo synthesis of LDL does occur in the liver. Unlike chylomicrons and VLDL particles that can sequentially deliver fatty acids and other lipids to various tissues during catabolism, LDL particles primarily deliver cholesterol to tissues, which occurs via whole particle uptake by the LDL receptor or alternative pathways. Modified LDL particles may be taken up by scavenger receptors or oxidized LDL receptors. Transfer of cholesteryl esters from HDL to LDL is mediated in part by cholesteryl ester transfer protein (CETP) in the process of reverse cholesterol transport. Modification of LDL by LPL and hepatic lipase (HL) influences the size and density of LDL particles, as well as their atherogenicity. The normal half-life of LDL particles in plasma is 3–4 days. Although peripheral tissues can catabolize LDL particles, and steroidogenic endocrine tissues (e.g adrenal) take up proportionately large amounts of LDL per amount of tissue, the liver is the major site of LDL removal from plasma. Decreased numbers of functional LDL receptors in the liver resulting from genetic defects (i.e. familial hypercholesterolemia), hypothyroidism, or aging, lead to accumulation of LDL particles in plasma and hypercholesterolemia.

HDL and reverse cholesterol transport

HDL particles are believed to be the primary mediators of reverse cholesterol transport, the process whereby cholesterol is removed from peripheral tissues and delivered to the liver for disposal. Recent breakthroughs in our understanding of the rare genetic disorder, Tangier disease, have greatly advanced our understanding of the genesis and metabolism of HDL particles. In Tangier disease, the absence of functional ABC-A1 receptors results in dramatic reductions in the formation of HDL particles and a very low plasma HDL cholesterol concentration. This observation suggests that the acquisition of free cholesterol from peripheral tissues by apo A-I via the ABC-A1 HDL-receptor is a major source of HDL cholesterol in plasma. The earliest HDL particles in plasma are discoidal, but they become spherical after the accumulation of additional cholesterol and surface phospholipids. Most free cholesterol in nascent HDL particles normally is esterified in plasma by lecithin-cholesterol acyltransferase (LCAT) to form cholesteryl esters. Sequestration of additional cholesterol and further remodeling results in larger mature HDL particles typically in the HDL2 subfraction. CETP mediates the transfer of cholesteryl ester from HDL to VLDL and LDL for subsequent delivery to the liver via the LDL, apo E, and LRP receptors. HDL also can selectively deliver cholesterol directly to the liver via the scavenger receptor class B, type 1 (SR-B1) without uptake of the whole HDL particle. Cubulin is an additional HDL receptor that may mediate uptake of free apo A-I in the renal tubule. Megalin, a member of the LDL receptor family, also binds apo A-I and may mediate catabolism of HDL. After delivery of cholesterol to the liver at the terminus of the reverse cholesterol transport pathway, a portion of the cholesterol is utilized for bile acid synthesis by the rate-limiting enzyme CYP7A1 under the regulatory control of heterodimers of the nuclear retinoid X receptor (RXR) and farnesoid X (bile acid) receptor (FXR). Cholesterol and bile acids are secreted into the bile for subsequent excretion of a portion of the enterohepatic circulatory pool of cholesterol and bile acids in the feces. Additional cardioprotective effects of HDL may be related to antioxidant (related in part to paraoxonase) and anti-inflammatory properties.

Exercise, weight loss, alcohol intake, estrogen and phenytoin can increase plasma HDL cholesterol concentrations. Puberty in males (testosterone), weight gain, type 2 diabetes, hypertriglyceridemia, cigarette smoking, and a low fat diet can be associated with decreases in the plasma HDL cholesterol concentration. It is important to realize that the cardioprotective benefits from HDL are probably more dependent on the flux of cholesterol from peripheral tissues to the liver for disposal than on the absolute HDL cholesterol concentration. For example, increased removal of HDL cholesterol from plasma by overexpression of hepatic SR-B1 receptors in experimental animals lowers the plasma HDL cholesterol concentration, but reduces the risk of atherosclerosis. Conversely, deficiency of CETP in humans increases the plasma HDL cholesterol concentration to 150–200 mg/dl by blocking transfer of cholesteryl esters from HDL to VLDL and LDL, but this condition often is associated with increased risk for atherosclerosis. Thus, the relationship between risk for atherosclerosis and increases or decreases in plasma HDL cholesterol needs to be interpreted with an understanding of the potential effects of such changes on reverse cholesterol transport.

Lipoprotein(a)

Lipoprotein(a) [Lp(a)] probably is formed in plasma as a consequence of the covalent cysteine–cysteine disulfide linkage of circulating apo(a) to the C-terminal region of apo B-100 in LDL particles. More than 95% of apo(a) in plasma is found in Lp(a). The liver is the predominant site of apo(a) synthesis. Plasma concentrations of Lp(a) vary 100-fold in the general population, largely due to genetic factors resulting in > 70–80 % heritability of plasma Lp(a) concentrations. The genetically mediated apo(a) size polymorphism is an important determinant of the Lp(a) concentration, as reflected by the inverse association between the apo(a) size and the plasma Lp(a) concentration. Additional factors that can increase plasma Lp(a) concentrations are renal insufficiency, menopause, and dietary intake of trans fatty acids. Factors that may decrease plasma Lp(a) concentrations are postmenopausal estrogen replacement, treatment with niacin, anabolic steroids, and LDL apheresis (a process that removes apo B containing particles from plasma). High plasma concentrations of Lp(a) are associated with increased risk for cardiovascular disease, but the atherogenicity of Lp(a) may require the presence of elevated plasma concentrations of LDL cholesterol. The normal physiological function of Lp(a) is unclear, but it may be involved in the delivery of cholesterol and other lipids to sites of vascular injury. A deficiency syndrome is unknown, even among individuals with very low concentrations of Lp(a). The presence in apo(a) of multiple kringle four repeats with homology to plasminogen may contribute to alterations in fibrinolysis.

Enzymes and transfer proteins involved in lipoprotein metabolism

A variety of enzymes and transfer proteins serve important roles in lipoprotein metabolism, as shown in Table 24.16. Beginning in the small bowel, pancreatic lipase hydrolyzes dietary fats to release glycerol and triglycerides which can be absorbed by enterocytes. Within the enterocyte, microsomal triglyceride transfer protein (MTP) is involved in the formation of chylomicrons. MTP also is involved in formation of VLDL particles in the liver. Three additional enzymes are involved in intravascular metabolism of lipoproteins.

LPL and HL are bound by heparan sulfate to the vascular endothelium, where they are involved in hydrolysis of triglycerides (and phospholipids by hepatic lipase) in triglyceride-rich lipoproteins, remodeling of LDL, remnants, and HDL, and hepatic uptake of remnant lipoproteins. Heterozygous deficiency of LPL may be a subgroup of the familial disorder, familial combined hyperlipidemia, which is discussed below. Endothelial lipase is primarily a phospholipase that may be involved in HDL metabolism, placental lipid metabolism, and release of fatty acids from phospholipids for energy utilization.

CETP and phospholipid transfer protein (PLTP) are involved in the bidirectional transfer of lipids between lipoproteins. CETP plays an important role in reverse cholesterol transport by facilitating the transfer of cholesteryl esters from cholesterol replete HDL particles to VLDL and LDL for subsequent delivery to the liver for disposal. CETP deficiency results in very high plasma HDL cholesterol concentrations, but often an increased risk for atherosclerosis due to the block in reverse cholesterol transport. PLTP is involved in the transfer of surface phospholipids from shrinking triglyceride-rich lipoprotein particles during their catabolism.

Lipoprotein receptors

The number of recognized lipoprotein receptors has been expanding rapidly during recent years. These receptors are important for the

Table 24.16 Enzymes and transfer proteins involved in lipoprotein metabolism

Enzyme	Function
Pancreatic lipase	Hydrolysis of dietary fat in intestinal lumen
Hormone-sensitive lipase	Hydrolysis of triglycerides in adipose cells to release free fatty acids
Lipoprotein lipase	Hydrolysis of triglycerides in circulating VLDL and chylomicrons to release free fatty acids to peripheral tissues; uptake of triglyceride-rich lipoproteins
Hepatic lipase	Hydrolysis of triglycerides and phospholipids in VLDL and VLDL remnants, uptake of remnant lipoproteins, facilitation of SR-BI-mediated uptake of HDL cholesteryl esters by liver
Endothelial lipase	Hydrolysis of lipoprotein phospholipids, involved in HDL metabolism
Lecithin cholesterol acyltransferase (LCAT)	Catalyzes transfer of position 2 fatty acid from phosphatidyl choline to cholesterol in HDL to form cholesteryl esters
Acyl cholesterol acyltransferase (ACAT)	Catalyzes esterification of cholesterol to form cholesteryl esters in intracellular pools
Transfer protein	
Cholesteryl ester transfer protein (CETP)	Facilitates transfer of cholesteryl esters from HDL to VLDL and LDL
Phospholipid transfer protein (PLTP)	Facilitates transfer of phospholipids from triglyceride-rich lipoproteins to HDL, may facilitate recycling of HDL back to discoidal particles

HDL, high density lipoprotein; LDL, low density lipoprotein; SR-B1, scavenger receptor-B1; VLDL, very low density lipoprotein.

metabolism and uptake of lipoproteins by various tissues, as indicated in Table 24.17. The classic genetic disorder related to defective lipoprotein receptors is familial hypercholesterolemia, which is a consequence of a variety of types of mutation in the LDL receptor. It is anticipated that a myriad of genetic disorders related to mutations in lipoprotein receptors, lipolytic enzymes, and transfer proteins have yet to be identified.

HYPERLIPIDEMIA

The hyperlipidemias have traditionally been classified as Fredrickson types I–V on the basis of the type of lipoprotein particle that is increased in plasma (Table 24.18). Although the designation of hyperlipidemia as types I–V is still used, the descriptive quality of this classification diminishes its value as a clinical tool, since the classification rarely adds information that is not already apparent from the results of the fasting lipid profile. Additional problems with the utility of this classification arise because multiple disorders can result in the same lipoprotein phenotype. For example, both the genetic disorder familial hypercholesterolemia and hypothyroidism can be associated with type IIa hyperlipidemia. In addition, a single disorder may cause several different types of hyperlipidemia in different individuals, and the type of hyperlipidemia in a single individual can vary over time. This classification scheme, therefore, is particularly unhelpful in pediatrics. Moreover, the types I–V designation does not accommodate important disorders such as hypoalphalipoproteinemia, elevated Lp(a), or qualitative changes in lipoprotein particles such as small dense LDL. Thus, the Fredrickson types I–V classification of hyperlipidemia provides insufficient information regarding the etiology and metabolic characteristics of dyslipidemia in individual patients. The one exception to these comments is type III hyperlipidemia, which refers to a specific genetically mediated metabolic disorder that is described in more detail below.

The hyperlipidemias can be subdivided into primary hyperlipidemias (Table 24.19), resulting from inherited defects in lipid metabolism, and secondary hyperlipidemias resulting from acquired (often reversible) metabolic conditions (Table 24.20).

The best 'classification scheme' involves identifying the precise genetic and/or metabolic defect in an individual patient, although currently this is not often possible.

PRIMARY HYPERLIPIDEMIA (Table 24.19)

Familial hypercholesterolemia

Familial hypercholesterolemia is an autosomal dominant disorder that is caused by hundreds of different mutations in the LDL receptor, resulting in an absent or functionally defective receptor protein. Individuals heterozygous for such LDL receptor mutations typically have about half-normal levels of LDL-receptor expression in the liver and twice-normal plasma LDL-cholesterol concentrations. The elucidation of the molecular defects underlying familial hypercholesterolemia form the basis for the awarding of the Nobel Prize in medicine to Brown and Goldstein in 1985. The resulting hypercholesterolemia greatly increases the risk for atherosclerotic vascular disease, with about 50% of males developing myocardial infarction by the age of 50 years and 50% of females by the age of 60 years. The life-time risk for myocardial infarction is > 85% in untreated patients. In accordance with the concept that atherosclerosis is a generalized process that can affect multiple arterial trees, the risk for stroke and peripheral vascular disease also is increased in patients with this disorder, although myocardial infarction is the most common adverse outcome. In some families, other atherogenic factors, such as increased Lp(a), may accentuate the risk for vascular disease, resulting in earlier clinical expression of cardiovascular disease as early as the third decade. Homozygous familial hypercholesterolemia is associated with LDL cholesterol levels > 500–700 mg/dl and myocardial infarction and death in childhood without very aggressive treatment.

The primary physical manifestation of heterozygous familial hypercholesterolemia is tendon xanthomas, which are not always present and may not develop until the fifth or sixth decade. Children with heterozygous familial hypercholesterolemia commonly develop tendon and tuberous xanthomas. Treatment for homozygous familial hypercholesterolemia requires aggressive pharmacologic therapy (and possibly LDL apheresis), which should be provided in collaboration with a lipid disorders clinic. Liver transplantation has been used successfully in some patients to alleviate the severe hypercholesterolemia, but this aggressive intervention is itself associated with complications. It is possible that targeted gene therapy for delivery of normal LDL receptors to the liver may become feasible at some point in the future.

Familial defective apo B

This disorder is a subtype of familial hypercholesterolemia in which a defect in apo B-100 prevents binding of LDL to normal LDL receptors.

Table 24.17 Lipoprotein receptors

Receptor	Family	Ligand(s)	Function(s)
Low density lipoprotein (LDL)-R	LDL-receptor	apo B-100, E	Uptake of LDL, intermediate density lipoprotein (IDL) and very low density lipoprotein (VLDL) remnants
VLDL-R	LDL-receptor	apo B-100, E, reelin	VLDL uptake
apo E-R2	LDL-receptor	apo E, reelin	Uptake of apo E-containing lipoproteins
MEGF7	LDL-receptor		
LDL-R related protein (LRP)	LDL-receptor	apo E, LPL, PAI-1, tPA, lactoferrin, others	Uptake of VLDL and chylomicron remnants
LRP1B	LDL-receptor	Comparable to LRP	Comparable to LRP
Megalin	LDL-receptor	apo E, high density lipoprotein (HDL)	Endocytic uptake of retinoids and steroids
Scavenger receptor, class A, types I and II (SRA-I, SRA-II)	Scavenger receptor, class A	Acetylated LDL, oxidized LDL, polyanionic molecules, others	Uptake of modified lipoproteins and apoptotic and senescent cells by macrophages
CD36	Scavenger receptor, class B	Oxidized LDL, acetylated LDL, others	Uptake of oxidized LDL
SR-BI	Scavenger receptor, class B	LDL, HDL, acetylated LDL, oxidized LDL	Uptake of modified lipoproteins, selective uptake of HDL cholesteryl ester by liver
SR-BII	Scavenger receptor, class B	Modified lipoproteins	SR-BI splice variant
Lectin-like oxidized LDL receptor-1 (LOX-1)	??	Oxidized LDL	Uptake of oxidized LDL
ATP binding cassette subfamily A, member 1 (ABC-A1)	ABC transporter	apo A-I	Peripheral HDL receptor, mediates formation of nascent HDL from tissue derived cholesterol and apo A-I
Cubulin		apo A-I, intrinsic factor-vitamin B_{12} complexes	Uptake of apo A-I in renal tubule

R, receptor

Table 24.18 Descriptive classification of hyperlipidemia on the basis of lipoprotein accumulation

Type	Lipoprotein abnormality	Examples of possible etiologies	Lipid values
I	↑ Chylomicrons	Lipoprotein lipase (LPL) deficiency, apo C-II deficiency	↑↑ Triglyceride (TG), total cholesterol. 4–7% of TG level
IIa	↑ Low density lipoprotein (LDL)	Familial hypercholesterolemia, hypothyroidism	↑ Total cholesterol and LDL-cholesterol
IIb	↑ LDL and very low density lipoprotein (VLDL)	Familial combined hyperlipidemia, type 2 diabetes	↑ Total cholesterol, LDL- and VLDL-cholesterol and TG
III	↑ Remnants (IDL)	Homozygosity for mutant apo E2 + disorder of lipoprotein overproduction	↑↑ Intermediate density lipoprotein (IDL) and remnants, ↑ total cholesterol. TG
IV	↑ VLDL	Type 2 diabetes, familial combined hyperlipidemia, ethanol	↑ TG (< 1000 mg/dl), ↑ Total and VLDL cholesterol
V	↑ VLDL and chylomicrons	Type 2 diabetes, ethanol	↑↑ TG (> 1000 mg/dl), total cholesterol. 7–10% of TG level

Table 24.19 Primary hyperlipidemias and lipoprotein deficiencies

Disorder	Prevalence	Inheritance	Lipoprotein pattern	Genetic cause
Hyperlipidemias				
LPL deficiency	$1:10^6$	Recessive	Type I	LPL mutation resulting in absent or defective protein
apo C-II deficiency	Rare	Recessive	Type I	apo C-II deficiency
Familial hypercholesterolemia (heterozygous)	1:500	Dominant	IIa/IIb	Defective LDL receptor; hundreds of mutations. Homozygotes occur in $1:10^6$
Familial defective apo B	1:700–1000	Dominant	IIa/IIb	Glutamine < arginine 3500 in apo B-100 causes defective binding to LDL receptor. Phenotype similar to familial hypercholesterolemia
Polygenic hypercholesterolemia	1:100?	Polygenic	IIa/IIb	Unknown
Familial combined hyperlipidemia	1:100–200	Dominant	IIa/IIb,IV,V	Unknown, associated with increased apo B secretion. Single defects in a variety of genes may cause a common phenotype
Familial hypertriglyceridemia	1:200–500	Dominant	IV/V	Unknown
Type III hyperlipidemia (Broad-beta disease, dysbetalipoproteinemia)	1:5000–10 000	Usually recessive	III	Homozygosity for mutant apo E2 is permissive, but not sufficient Requires concurrent disorder of increased lipoprotein secretion Prevalence of E2/E2 homozygotes is about 1:100; most do not have hyperlipidemia
Sitosterolemia	≈ 40–50 cases	Recessive	IIa	Mutations in ABC-G5 and G8 sterol transporters
Cerebrotendinous xanthomatosis in 27-hydroxylase blocks	≈ 150 cases	Recessive	IIa/IIb	Defect bile acid synthesis
Lipoprotein deficiencies				
Tangier disease	< 100 cases	Recessive	Very low HDL-C	Defect in ABC-A1 (HDL receptor)
Abetalipoproteinemia	Rare	Recessive	Chol 20-30 mg/dl	Absence of apo B-100 with decreased or absent apo B-48; MTP mutations
Hypobetalipoproteinemia	1:1000–2000	Dominant	LDL-C 20-40 mg/dl	Apo B truncations
Chylomicron retention disease	Rare	Recessive	Low chol., TG	Inability to synthesize or secrete chylomicrons
Familial hypoalphalipoproteinemia	> 1:100–200	Dominant	HDL-C < 30 mg/dl	Apo A-I mutations, heterozygous ABC-A1 mutations
Fish eye disease	Rare	Recessive	–	Defect in LCAT activity
LCAT deficiency	Rare	Recessive	–	Absence of LCAT activity

HDL, high density lipoprotein; LCAT, lecithin-cholesterol acyltransferase; LDL, low density lipoprotein; LPL, lipoprotein lipase; MTP, microsomal triglyceride transfer protein; TG, triglyceride.

The most common mutation is a glutamine to arginine point mutation at amino acid 3500, but other mutations have been described.

Polygenic hypercholesterolemia

Polygenic hypercholesterolemia refers to a heterogenous group of prevalent disorders that clearly have a familial component presumably resulting from interactions between two or more genes. Polygenic hypercholesterolemia is probably the most common primary hyperlipidemia. The genetic basis for such disorders is unknown, but the elucidation of possible mutations is an area of intense interest since the genetic basis of most of the commonest monogenic disorders of lipid metabolism has been established.

Familial combined hyperlipidemia

Familial combined hyperlipidemia is a genetically heterogeneous disorder with a common phenotype characterized by hepatic overproduction of apo B-100 containing lipoproteins. The resulting hyperlipidemia is variable among affected family members and can vary over time in a given individual. The lipoprotein abnormalities often consist of increased plasma apo B in association with increased plasma concentrations of triglycerides (in VLDL) or LDL-cholesterol, or both. The plasma HDL cholesterol concentration often is reduced and the LDL particles often are characterized as small and dense LDL (e.g. pattern B) which is more atherogenic than more buoyant larger LDL particles. Patients with this disorder develop premature

Table 24.20 Examples of secondary dyslipidemias

Category	Condition	Lipoprotein abnormality
Dietary	Excess saturated fat/cholesterol	↑ cholesterol, ↑ low density lipoprotein (LDL)-C
	Very low fat	↓ LDL-C, ↓ high density lipoprotein (HDL)-C, possible ↑ triglyceride (TG)
	Excess calories	↑ TG, ↓ HDL-C
Endocrine	Diabetes	↑ TG if uncontrolled; abnormal lipoprotein composition in type 2
	Insulin resistance	↑ TG
	Hypothyroidism	↑ total cholesterol, ↑ LDL-C, ↑ TG
	Obesity	TG overproduction
	Cushing's syndrome	↑ TG, possible ↑ LDL-C
	Lipodystrophy	↑ TG
	Acromegaly	↑ TG
Drugs	Alcohol	↑ TG
	Thiazide diuretics	↑ LDL-C, ↑ TG
	Beta-adrenergic blockers	↑ TG, ↓ HDL-C
	Glucocorticoids	↑ TG, possible ↑ LDL-C
	Oral estrogen/tamoxifen	↑ TG
	Retinoic acid derivatives	↑ TG
	Ciclosporin	↑ total cholesterol, ↑ LDL-C
	Protease inhibitors	↑ TG (↑ total cholesterol, ↑ LDL-C)
Other	Renal failure/nephrotic syndrome	↑ total cholesterol, ↑ LDL-C, ↑ TG, ↑ lipoprotein(a)
	Cholestatic liver disease	↑↑ total cholesterol, ↑ lipoprotein X
	Lupus; myeloma; autoimmune disease	↑ TG
	Some glycogen storage diseases	↑ TG, ↑ LDL-C

myocardial infarction, stroke and peripheral vascular disease in mid-adulthood. It has been suggested that the hyperlipidemia phenotype of familial combined hyperlipidemia may not be expressed until young adulthood, which may prevent detection of this disorder in children. However, children in many families with familial combined hyperlipidemia may express the hyperlipidemia phenotype. The genetic basis for familial combined hyperlipidemia is unknown, but defects in multiple candidate genes are being sought. Heterozygous LPL deficiency appears to be one subtype of this disorder.

Familial hypertriglyceridemia

This disorder may be a subtype of familial combined hyperlipidemia, although the phenotype is one of hypertriglyceridemia with triglyceride concentrations usually < 1000 mg/dl. The results of older studies suggested this may be a benign condition other than the increased risk for pancreatitis during exacerbation of hypertriglyceridemia up to triglyceride concentrations > 1500–2000 mg/dl. The absence of coronary artery disease in a family with an autosomal dominant pattern of inheritance of hypertriglyceridemia is suggestive of this disorder, but the possibility of increased risk for coronary artery disease in affected individuals cannot be excluded. The genetic basis for this disorder is uncertain.

Type III hyperlipidemia

Type III hyperlipidemia, also known as broad beta disease or familial dysbetalipoproteinemia, is associated with homozygosity for the abnormal apoprotein E2 that is a poor ligand for triglyceride-rich lipoprotein receptors in the liver. Rare autosomal dominant forms of this disorder have been identified. Surprisingly, the prevalence of apo E2/E2 homozygosity is about 1% in the general population, but the prevalence of type III hyperlipidemia is only 1:5000–10 000. Thus, only 1–2% of individuals with the homozygous genetic abnormality in apo E develop type III hyperlipidemia. The expression of hyperlipidemia in this disorder typically requires a second metabolic disorder that causes overproduction of triglyceride-rich lipoproteins. Under normal conditions, the apo E2/E2 mutation alone is insufficient to cause hyperlipidemia, since alternative pathways exist for clearance of small amounts of triglyceride-rich lipoprotein remnants. However, in the setting of overproduction of triglyceride-rich lipoproteins, which occurs in hypothyroidism, obesity, high fat diet consumption, menopause, uncontrolled diabetes, familial combined hyperlipidemia, and other conditions, the clearance pathways become saturated, thereby resulting in the accumulation of atherogenic VLDL and chylomicron remnants. Patients with this disorder are susceptible to diffuse premature atherosclerosis. Treatment is directed to alleviation of factors causing lipoprotein overproduction.

LPL and apo C-II deficiency

LPL deficiency is an extremely rare condition present at birth that is thought to occur with a frequency of about $1{:}10^6$. Causes of LPL deficiency can include homozygous deficiency of functional enzyme, absence of the cofactor apo C-II, and dominant inheritance of a lipase inhibitor. The clinical manifestations of recurrent pancreatitis and eruptive xanthomas may not be recognized until late infancy or childhood, but the severity of hypertriglyceridemia and its complications are related to dietary fat intake. Plasma triglyceride concentrations may be > 3000 to 10 000 mg/dl in association with moderately increased plasma cholesterol concentrations. Lipemia retinalis often is visible when the triglyceride concentration is > 4000–5000 mg/dl, but it is much easier to examine the blood ex vivo after separation of plasma or serum from blood cells by centrifugation or standing. The plasma typically appears turbid when the triglyceride concentration exceeds 500–600 mg/dl. Plasma with a triglyceride concentration of 1000 mg/dl has the appearance of skim milk. Plasma with a triglyceride concentration > 2000–3000 mg/dl (2–3% fat) appears creamy, whereas levels > 5000–6000 mg/dl (5–6% fat) will have the appearance of whipping cream. The initial treatment during bouts of abdominal pain requires a very-low-fat diet containing no more than a few grams of dietary fat daily. Children with overt pancreatitis require hospitalization for intravenous hydration and cessation of oral intake. In stable children, the fat intake may be increased to 5–10 g/day, but higher levels of fat intake may be tolerated by some individuals. Medium chain triglycerides, which are absorbed into the portal circulation and do not contribute to chylomicron formation, may be used to improve the palatability of the low-fat diet. Older children may self-select a higher fat diet in parallel with the dietary habits of their peers, but the development of abdominal pain helps to attenuate such behavior. Pharmacologic therapy is generally unhelpful.

Tangier disease

Tangier disease is an extremely rare disorder that is characterized by the near absence of HDL cholesterol, very low plasma concentrations of apo A-I, and pathognomonic orange–yellow tonsillar enlargement, lymphadenopathy, and splenomegaly. The physical findings are a consequence of the accumulation of cholesteryl esters in the reticuloendothelial system. Premature atherosclerosis may occur in individuals with sufficient amounts of LDL cholesterol in plasma. The genetic basis for the disorder eluded investigators until the last few years when mutations in the ABC-A1 transporter protein were identified as the causative lesion. The unraveling of the genetic basis for the rare disorder revolutionized our understanding of HDL metabolism and helped to establish the important role of ABC-A1 as the peripheral HDL receptor. In Tangier disease, apo A-I is unable to sequester cholesterol from peripheral cells due to defective interactions of apo A-I with the ABC-A1 protein, resulting in a dramatic reduction in formation of HDL particles and increased degradation of apo A-I. LDL cholesterol concentrations typically are low, which diminishes the risk of cardiovascular disease, but premature atherosclerosis occurs in individuals with the highest LDL cholesterol concentrations.

Phytosterolemia/sitosterolemia

Phytosterolemia, also known as beta-sitosterolemia, is a rare autosomal recessive disorder first reported in 1974 that is associated with tendon xanthomas, premature atherosclerosis, and occasional hemolytic anemia. It can present as 'pseudohomozygous familial hypercholesterolemia' with LDL-C > 500 in childhood, and with xanthomas occasionally on the buttocks. Affected patients typically are very sensitive to diet-induced hypercholesterolemia due to enhanced intestinal absorption of cholesterol, as well as plant sterols. Sitosterol and other plant sterols, which are normally present in minimal amounts in plasma, accumulate in plasma of affected individuals. The disease is caused by defects in ABC-G5 and ABC-G8, which are sterol transporters that normally function to export non-specifically absorbed sitosterol and other plant sterols from the intestinal mucosa back into the intestinal lumen. The diagnosis can be established by identifying increased levels of plasma sitosterol, or possibly by screening for mutations in the genes for ABC-G5 and ABC-G8. A low cholesterol diet in combination with bile acid binding agents is helpful. Avoidance of dietary plant sterols is difficult, but affected individuals should avoid using over-the counter cholesterol-lowering margarines containing sitosterol (Take Control) or sitostanol esters (Benecol). A new selective inhibitor of cholesterol absorption, ezetimibe, is efficacious in patients with sitosterolemia and can also lower LDL-C in conditions other than sitosterolemia.

Cerebrotendinous xanthomatosis

Cerebrotendinous xanthomatosis is a rare autosomal recessive disorder that is characterized by development of xanthomas in tendons, the lungs, and brain in the setting of low or normal plasma cholesterol concentrations. Affected patients also develop progressive cerebellar ataxia, dementia, spinal cord paresis, diminished intelligence and cataracts. Dementia, ataxia and cataracts may be apparent between the ages of 10 and18 years, but milder cases may not be identified until later in adulthood. The primary abnormality is the accumulation in plasma of cholestanol resulting from homozygous deficiency of 27-hydroxylase, a key enzyme involved in hepatic bile acid synthesis and cholesterol oxidation. Treatment with chenodeoxycholic acid and HMG-CoA reductase inhibitors has beneficial effects on plasma cholestanol levels, but it may take years to diminish levels of cholestanol in the brain. Therefore, initiation of treatment as early as possible would be expected to provide the best outcome.

OTHER GENETIC AND METABOLIC DISORDERS

Generalized lipodystrophy

Patients with generalized lipodystrophy have minimal amounts of body fat which may be evident at birth or may be acquired in childhood or adulthood. The congenital form of this disorder often is familial whereas the acquired form commonly is sporadic. Children with generalized lipodystrophy tend to be tall, have advanced bone age, and have the appearance of increased muscle bulk. Insulin resistance associated with subsequent development of type 2 diabetes and hypertriglyceridemia are common. Treatment consists primarily of correction of the metabolic abnormalities.

Partial lipodystrophy

Partial lipodystrophy consists of several overlapping phenotypes that may be a consequence of several different metabolic disorders. The typical patient experiences progressive symmetrical loss of subcutaneous body fat most commonly from the face, with progressive involvement of the arms, trunk and hips. Other variations can involve preservation of subcutaneous fat in the face or patchy lipoatrophy. One unusual adult patient in the author's clinic has adiposity of her limbs in association with disproportionately diminished facial and truncal subcutaneous fat. The age of onset varies from 5 to 15 years of age, although the condition may not become clinically apparent until young adulthood. Girls are affected much more frequently than boys. Insulin resistance is common and can be severe, resulting in very high insulin requirements and possibly increased responsiveness to insulin-sensitizing thiazoladinediones in those who develop type 2 diabetes. Hypertriglyceridemia can be a consequence of insulin resistance and/or hyperglycemia.

AIDS and lipodystrophy

The advent of highly active antiretroviral therapy (HAART) for management of HIV infection and AIDS (see Ch. 25) has tremendously improved the longevity of patients with these afflictions, but has created a new metabolic disorder referred to as protease inhibitor-induced or HAART-associated lipodystrophy. The occurrence and severity of this condition is proportional to the duration of treatment and is related to the specific drugs being used. A loss of facial fat with a Cushingoid pattern of central adipose deposition and increased breast size in women are common. The lipodystrophy may be related in part to possible interactions between protease inhibitors and PPAR-gamma in adipose tissue. Insulin resistance, development of overt type 2 diabetes, and hypertriglyceridemia are common metabolic abnormalities in these patients. The hypertriglyceridemia is related in part to the insulin resistance ± hyperglycemia, but also may be mediated by other contributors to increased VLDL production and diminished triglyceride clearance. Regular physical activity may diminish the lipodystrophy as well as the abnormalities in glucose homeostasis and lipid metabolism. The optimal pharmacologic treatment for this condition is still uncertain, due in part to the potential for accentuation of risk for hepatotoxicity by many lipid-lowering medications.

Smith–Lemli–Opitz syndrome

Smith–Lemli–Opitz syndrome is an autosomal recessive disorder that is characterized by physical malformations (e.g. micrognathia, syn- and/or polydactyly, microcephaly, high forehead, low-set ears), mental retardation, other malformations and growth failure. Severely affected individuals may die at birth or in infancy, but survival into later adulthood is common in milder cases. The syndrome is caused by deficiency of the enzyme 7-dehydrocholesterol-Δ^7-reductase, the final enzyme involved in cholesterol synthesis. Plasma cholesterol concentrations are usually low and 7-dehydrocholesterol concentrations are increased. Brain development is presumably impaired due the lack of availability of cholesterol, but the possibility of toxicity secondary to increased levels of cholesterol precursors cannot be excluded. Increased dietary intake of cholesterol in egg yolk has increased plasma cholesterol and decreased 7-dehydrocholesterol concentrations in affected children, but irreversible defects are already present in some of these children at birth. Therefore, strategies to diminish complications from Smith–Lemli–Opitz syndrome will most likely require initiation of treatment early in gestation.

Mevalonic aciduria

Mevalonic aciduria is associated with dysmorphic features, failure to thrive, developmental delay, diarrhea, ataxia, recurrent fevers, and the presence of splenomegaly in 50% of cases. Mevalonate is the product of HMG-CoA reductase, the rate-limiting enzyme for cholesterol synthesis, and is a substrate for phosphorylation to form 5-pyrophospho-3-phosphomevalonate, as the next step in cholesterol biosynthesis. The diagnosis is established by determination of increased urinary mevalonic acid excretion, and confirmed by enzymatic assay in blood leukocytes or cultured skin fibroblasts. Treatment with cholesterol and possibly ubiquinone have been proposed, but have not been effective. A mild form of this condition, hyper IgD/periodic fever syndrome has been established to be also due to mevalonate kinase deficiency.

Barth syndrome

Barth syndrome is an X-linked disorder associated with cardiomyopathy, biventricular hypertrophy, systemic myopathy, neutropenia and growth failure associated with increased tissue lipid deposition. Plasma cholesterol and carnitine are reduced and levels of urinary 3-methylglutaconic and 3-methyglutaric acids are increased, presumably due to a defect in the mevalonic acid shunt component of the cholesterol synthetic pathway. Treatment with carnitine and possibly additional cholesterol have been proposed. Advanced cases may require cardiac transplantation.

Adrenoleukodystrophy

Adrenoleukodystrophy is an X-linked recessive disorder that is caused by a defect in peroxisomal membrane transport and beta-oxidation of very long chain fatty acids (see Ch. 13).

SECONDARY HYPERLIPIDEMIA

Secondary hyperlipidemia is the most common form of hyperlipidemia and can exacerbate primary hyperlipidemias. Excess intake of dietary saturated fat and cholesterol is the most common form of secondary hyperlipidemia which is prevalent in Western populations. Diabetes and hypothyroidism also are common forms of secondary hyperlipidemia. Additional types of secondary hyperlipidemia are described in Table 24.20.

Treatment

The cornerstone of treatment for all forms of hyperlipidemia is life-style modification consisting of decreased intake of dietary saturated fat and cholesterol, regular physical activity, and avoidance of excess body weight. A healthy diet typically is carbohydrate-based (complex carbohydrates) with increased amounts of fruits and vegetables, increased dietary fiber, and reduced amount of saturated and total fat and cholesterol. Although controversy still prevails regarding the optimal dietary composition, such a diet helps to minimize body weight, is replete with essential vitamins and phytochemicals, and helps to minimize most forms of hyperlipidemia. A low fat, low cholesterol diet such as the American Heart Association Step 1 diet is generally safe in children, but restrictive diets in children should not be prescribed without supervision of a dietitian and/or pediatric health care provider.

Drug therapy for treatment of hyperlipidemia is usually reserved for young adults unless there are compelling reasons for initiation of treatment in childhood. Concerns about possible unforeseen toxicity of lipid-lowering medications in growing children, the typically long delay in the onset of clinically significant vascular disease, and the imperfect association of hyperlipidemia in childhood with hyperlipidemia in adulthood, have supported the position of avoidance of drug therapy in general, in children. Important exceptions need to be considered, however. In the case of homozygous familial hypercholesterolemia, death from myocardial infarction often occurs in childhood in untreated individuals. Thus, aggressive drug and non-drug therapy is indicated in affected children. Among children with heterozygous familial hypercholesterolemia (or other severe conditions) with a very early onset of clinical cardiovascular events in relatives (e.g. before age 30), it often is advisable to initiate some form of treatment during childhood to prevent the accumulation of a heavy burden of atherosclerosis prior to adulthood. Bile-acid binding agents are believed to have the lowest risk for toxicity because they are not absorbed systemically, and they are approved for use in children, but such agents alone may lack efficacy. One study of children with familial hypercholesterolemia showed no evidence of toxicity in children receiving lovastatin 10–40 mg daily for 48 weeks. In children from very high risk families, it may be acceptable to treat with a low dose of a 'statin' in combination with a bile-acid binding agent and a healthy lifestyle, but the long term safety and benefit of such an intervention remain unproven. An experimental inhibitor of cholesterol absorption, ezetimibe, is currently under development that can reduce the LDL cholesterol concentration by 14–18% and may be useful in treatment of children. Drugs available for treatment of hyperlipidemia are outlined in Table 24.21. In the USA, the FDA has recently approved some statins for use in boys ≥ 10 years with heterozygous familial hypercholesterolemia and postpubertal girls with the same condition.

MITOCHONDRIAL DISEASE

INTRODUCTION

Mitochondria contain ~ 1000 enzymes and structural proteins, the great majority of which are encoded by nuclear genes, synthesized in the cytoplasm, and transported into the mitochondrial matrix. All the enzymes of the tricarboxylic acid and fatty acid oxidation cycles, the first three enzymes of the urea cycle and numerous others involved in intermediary metabolism are imported into mitochondria after initial cytoplasmic synthesis. Although defects in these enzymatic pathways occur and lead to various inborn errors of metabolism (e.g. organic acidemias, fatty acid oxidation defects), such disorders are not classified as mitochondrial disease. Mitochondrial disease is caused by dysfunction of the inner mitochondrial membrane respiratory (electron transport) chain with resultant decreased production of energy in the form of adenosine triphosphate.

Mitochondrial disorders have an overall incidence of approximately 1:8500 in children and are, therefore, as common as some forms of muscular dystrophy and more common than myotonic dystrophy.[128] These conditions may occur sporadically or be inherited in a Mendelian (autosomal recessive, dominant, X-linked) or maternal (mitochondrial) fashion. Children are commonly affected, but mitochondrial disease can present at any age, prenatal to adulthood and affect any organ system.[129]

THE RESPIRATORY CHAIN

The mitochondrial respiratory (electron transport) chain produces the majority of energy for eukaryotic cellular reactions through the process of oxidative phosphorylation (OXPHOS), in which the

Table 24.21 Drugs for treatment of hyperlipidemia*

Indication	Possible drugs
Elevated low density lipoprotein (LDL) cholesterol	'Statins' (lovastatin, simvastatin, pravastatin, fluvastatin, atorvastatin) Niacin Bile acid sequestrants (colestyramine, colestipol, colesevelam) Cholesterol absorption inhibitors
Hypertriglyceridemia (not type I)	Fibrates (gemfibrozil, clofibrate, fenofibrate) Niacin Fish oil (≥ 6 g daily in adults)
Type I hypertriglyceridemia (chylomicronemia)	Drugs not helpful. Treatment is very low-fat diet.
Combined hyperlipidemia (↑ LDL cholesterol and ↑ triglycerides)	'Statins' Niacin
Low high density lipoprotein (HDL) cholesterol	Niacin (most efficacious agent) Fibrates 'Statins' (less efficacious than niacin and fibrates)
Elevated lipoprotein(a)	Niacin

* Note: Most of these interventions have not been tested adequately for safety and efficacy in children.

reduction of oxygen to water is coupled to the production of the high energy phosphate compound adenosine triphosphate (ATP). Because the respiratory chain plays a critical role in generating cellular energy, mitochondrial disorders can cause dysfunction of any organ system, although the neuromuscular system is commonly involved. The respiratory chain consists of five inner mitochondrial membrane multi-subunit protein complexes (complexes I–V) that transport electrons down an electrochemical gradient using a variety of electron carriers, including iron–sulfur clusters, cytochromes and coenzyme Q_{10}. Electron transport between respiratory chain complexes is coupled to the extrusion of protons across the inner mitochondrial membrane by proton pump components of the respiratory chain. ATP is synthesized by complex V from adenosine diphosphate (ADP) and inorganic phosphate (P_i) using energy from the flow of protons back into the mitochondrial matrix from the intermembrane space (Fig. 24.26). Dysfunction of the respiratory chain causes decreased ATP production, as well as increased production of reactive oxygen species (free radicals) that further impair respiratory chain function and exacerbate the already diminished energy production. Decreased energy production and increased oxidative stress subsequently activate the mitochondrial membrane permeability transition pore, resulting in egress of apoptotic factors and cell death. Therefore, the pathogenesis of mitochondrial respiratory chain disorders is linked to decreased cellular energy production, increased generation of reactive oxygen species, and release of cellular apoptosis factors.[130]

The mitochondrial respiratory chain is formed and maintained by the coordinate interaction of two genomes, the mitochondrial and the nuclear. In other words, the genes encoding the proteins necessary for respiratory chain function are encoded by nuclear and mitochondrial genes. The mitochondrial genome consists of double-stranded circular DNA 16 569 base pairs long and encodes 13 OXPHOS subunits, 22 transfer RNAs (tRNAs), and 2 ribosomal RNAs (rRNAs) (Fig. 24.27). The nuclear genome encodes the remaining 71 respiratory chain subunits, as well as proteins responsible for the assembly and maintenance of the respiratory chain, ribosomal proteins, and enzymes responsible for mitochondrial DNA (mtDNA) replication. Only complex II (succinate dehydrogenase) is coded for entirely by the nuclear DNA (nDNA).

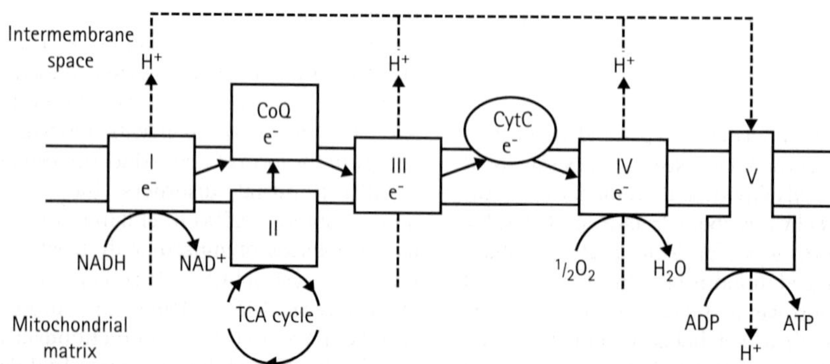

Fig. 24.26 The mitochondrial respiratory chain. The respiratory chain is embedded in the inner mitochondrial membrane and consists of five multi-subunit enzymes (complexes I–V). Electron transport down the chain (using transition metal compounds, flavins and coenzyme Q_{10}) is coupled to proton extrusion across an inner mitochondrial membrane by complexes I, III and IV, which creates an electrochemical gradient. Protons then re-enter the mitochondrial matrix through complex V and ATP is synthesized from ADP and inorganic phosphate. NADH (via complex I) and FADH2 (via complex II or coenzyme Q_{10}) donate electrons to the respiratory chain. Complex II (succinate dehydrogenase) is a critical enzyme in both the respiratory chain and tricarboxylic acid cycle and is encoded entirely by nDNA. The remaining complexes have both mtDNA- and nDNA-encoded subunits. CoQ, coenzyme Q_{10}; cyt b, cytochrome b; TCA, tricarboxylic acid.

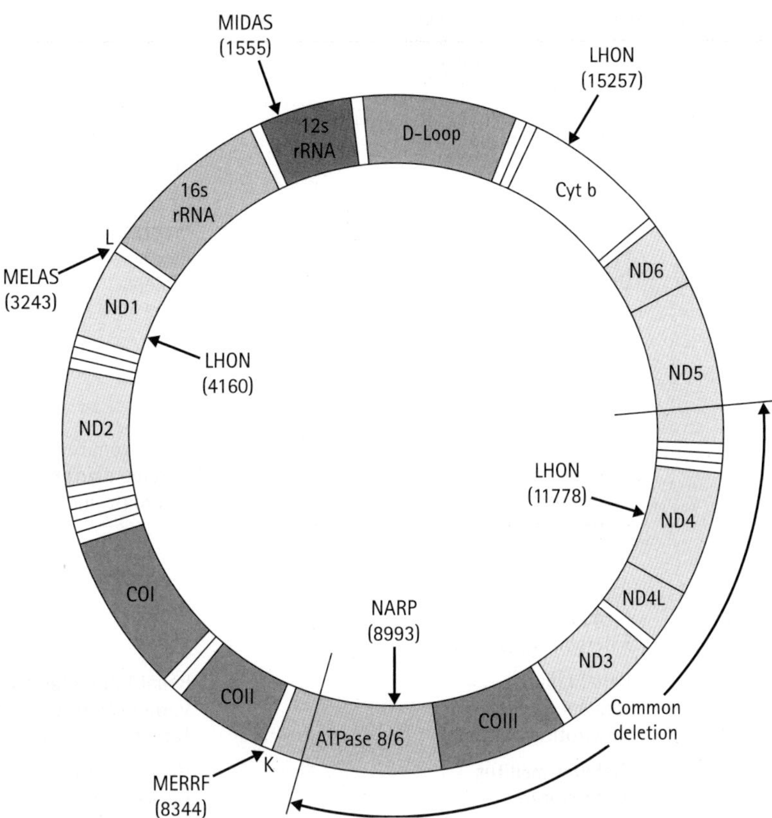

Fig. 24.27 Mitochondrial genome. Human mtDNA is a double-stranded, circular genome of 16 569 base pairs that encodes 13 OXPHOS subunits, 22 tRNAs, and two rRNAs. The locations of common mutations resulting in mitochondrial disease are shown, with the base pair positions given in parentheses. Different disease phenotypes may occur with the same mutation. For example, mutations at position 3243 have been reported in MELAS, PEO, cardiomyopathy and MIDD and 8344 mutations are associated with MERRF, deafness and cardiomyopathy, and PEO with myoclonus. On the other hand, different mutations may cause a similar clinical presentation (e.g. LHON). The common deletion is associated with KSS, PEO and PS. ATPase 8/6, complex V subunits; COIII, complex IV subunits; Cyt b, cytochrome b (complex III subunit); K, lysine tRNA; KSS, Kearnes-Sayre syndrome; L, leucine tRNA; LHON, Leber hereditary optic neuropathy; MELAS, mitochondrial encephalomyopathy, lactic acidosis and stroke-like episodes; MERRF, myoclonic epilepsy with ragged red fibers; MIDAS, maternally inherited deafness with aminoglycoside sensitivity; MIDD, maternally inherited diabetes and deafness; NARP, neurogenic weakness, ataxia, and retinitis pigmentosa; ND1-6, complex I subunits (7); PEO, progressive external ophthalmoplegia; PS, Pearson marrow-pancreas syndrome. White bars indicate position of mitochondrial tRNAs.

Each mitochondrion contains between 2 and 10 copies of mtDNA, and each cell contains a few to up to 1000 mitochondria, depending on the energy requirements of a given tissue. The mtDNA is inherited entirely from the ovum and mitochondria are distributed randomly to daughter cells during embryogenesis. Although sperm contain mitochondria, paternal mtDNA is not usually passed on to the embryo. If a mtDNA mutation arises in a cell, both mutant and normal mtDNA molecules will coexist in that cell, a condition known as *heteroplasmy*. The mutant and normal mtDNAs are then transmitted to daughter cells completely by chance, so that the proportion of normal to mutant DNA in each cell is determined stochastically. With repeated rounds of cellular division, there is a tendency for the proportion of intracellular mutant and normal mtDNAs to drift towards either completely normal or completely mutant in a given cell line (replicate segregation). The *threshold effect* refers to the expression of an abnormal phenotype (i.e. disease expression) only if the percentage of mitochondria harboring mutant mtDNA (mutant load) exceeds the proportion of normal mitochondria needed for the energy demands of a given tissue. In general, there is a greater likelihood of tissue dysfunction if a high percentage of abnormal mitochondria is present.[131] In most maternally inherited mitochondrial respiratory chain disorders, mutant mtDNA species typically coexist with normal mtDNA in a given cell (i.e. heteroplasmy is common in mitochondrial disorders). [*NB: Homoplasmic* mitochondrial disorders also exist (see LHON below).] The clinical phenotype and potential disease expression ultimately depends on the severity of the mutation, the percentage of affected mitochondria and the energy requirements of the involved tissues.

CLINICAL FEATURES OF MITOCHONDRIAL DISORDERS

Children with mitochondrial disease may present with a broad array of symptoms and signs, from hypotonia as a neonate to exercise intolerance in later childhood or adolescence (Table 24.22). The neuromuscular system is often prominently involved, because of the dependence of brain and muscle on oxidative metabolism. Nevertheless, mitochondrial disorders are typically multisystem diseases that affect virtually any tissue or organ system. Progressive dysfunction of seemingly unrelated organ systems may, in fact, provide the first clue to the presence of underlying mitochondrial disease.[129]

Although most children with mitochondrial disease are difficult to classify on the basis of their (usually diverse) features, a few

Table 24.22 Presenting clinical symptoms and signs in mitochondrial respiratory chain disorders

Brain and muscle	Hypotonia/hypertonia Weakness Seizures Stroke-like episodes Ataxia Exercise intolerance	Leigh syndrome, Alper syndrome Leukodystrophy Recurrent myoglobinuria Peripheral neuropathy Spinal muscular atrophy-like Elevated cerebrospinal fluid protein
Eye	Cataracts Pigmentary retinopathy Optic atrophy	Progressive external ophthalmoplegia Ptosis Diplopia
Ear	Sensorineural deafness Aminoglycoside induced ototoxicity	
Heart	Cardiomyopathy Cardiac conduction defect	
Gastrointestinal tract	Hepatic dysfunction/failure Exocrine pancreatic dysfunction Villous atrophy Gastroenteritis-like illness Failure to thrive	Cyclic vomiting Chronic diarrhea Valproate-induced liver failure
Bone marrow	Pancytopenia Megaloblastic anemia Sideroblastic anemia	
Kidney	Renal failure Fanconi syndrome Nephrotic syndrome	Renal tubular acidosis Vitamin D unresponsive rickets Tubulointerstitial nephritis
Endocrine system	Diabetes mellitus Short stature Hypoparathyroidism	Hypothyroidism Adrenocorticotrophin deficiency Infertility
Skin	Rashes Mottled pigmentation	Trichothiodystrophy Ichthyosis
Dysmorphology	Dysmorphic features	

classic clinical syndromes have been described in some patients with mtDNA point mutations or deletions, including Kearns-Sayre syndrome (KSS), mitochondrial encephalomyopathy lactic acidosis and stroke-like episodes (MELAS), myoclonic epilepsy and ragged red fibers (MERRF), maternally inherited diabetes and deafness (MIDD), and Leber hereditary optic neuropathy (LHON) (Table 24.23).[132,133] Even these somewhat distinct clinical syndromes have a degree of overlap in their symptoms and signs. Relatively common clinical presentations are discussed below, including lactic acidemia, Leigh syndrome, Alper syndrome, myopathy, cardiomyopathy, hepatopathy and renal tubular acidosis.

Lactic acidemia

Lactic acidemia is not an infrequent finding in any seriously ill child and may be caused by a number of conditions, acquired and genetic (Table 24.24). Poor tissue perfusion secondary to sepsis or inadequate cardiac contractility (congenital heart disease, cardiomyopathy), pulmonary hypertension, severe anemia, seizures, liver failure, toxins, and inborn errors of metabolism can all lead to an abnormal accumulation of blood lactate.

Children with persistent lactic acidemia, in whom acquired causes and metabolic disorders associated with clearly diagnostic metabolites have been excluded, are often described as having *primary (hereditary) lactic acidemia.* Primary lactic acidemia may present as an overwhelming, fatal disease in neonates or have a more mild course, with symptoms appearing at any age. A wide range of symptoms may be encountered, including hypotonia, seizures, cardiomyopathy, myopathy, renal tubular dysfunction and intermittent ketoacidosis. Although patients with a suspected mitochondrial disease or disorder of pyruvate metabolism may have elevation of blood lactate, it is important to evaluate such children with care (see Diagnosis of respiratory chain disorders below), because a number of metabolic disorders can cause similar increases of blood lactate (Table 24.24) (see also Organic acidemias, pp. 1183). It is sometimes difficult to determine whether the elevation in lactate is caused by a primary metabolic defect or is secondary to tissue ischemia in a very sick child who does not have an inborn error of metabolism. These two possibilities are also not mutually exclusive; an exogenous illness may constitute the initial environmental stress that unmasks an underlying inborn error of metabolism. Serial blood lactate levels may be useful in determining if the lactic acidemia is primary or secondary. In general, lactic acidemia corrects relatively quickly after the underlying cause is treated in acquired cases, but tends to persist if a metabolic disorder is present. This is a simplistic generalization, because even patients with proven metabolic disorders classically associated with an elevated lactate can have intermittent, or even absent, lactic acidemia. Spurious elevations of blood lactate may also occur as a result of a difficult blood draw and local tissue hypoxia. Every effort should be made to find the cause of the lactic acidemia including echocardiography and appropriate metabolic investigations (Table 24.25). Brain ischemia secondary to intracranial hemorrhage, for example, can also cause persistent lactic acidemia. In addition, some patients with unexplained lactic acidemia have

Table 24.23 Clinical features of mitochondrial encephalopathies*

Tissue	Signs and symptoms	KSS	MERRF	MELAS	MILS	NARP
CNS	Seizures	–	[+]	+	+	–
	Ataxia	+	[+]	+	±	[+]
	Myoclonus	–	[+]	±	–	–
	Psychomotor retardation	–	–	–	+	–
	Psychomotor regression	+	±	+	–	–
	Hemiparesis/hemianopia	–	–	+	–	–
	Cortical blindness	–	–	[+]	–	–
	Migraine-like headaches	–	–	[+]	–	–
	Dystonia	–	–	[+]	+	–
PNS	Peripheral neuropathy	±	±	±	–	[+]
Muscle	Weakness	+	+	+	+	+
Eye	Ophthalmoplegia	[+]	–	–	–	–
	Ptosis	+	–	–	–	–
	Pigmentary retinopathy	[+]	–	–	±	[+]
	Optic atrophy	–	–	–	±	±
Endocrine	Diabetes mellitus	±	–	±	–	–
	Short stature	+	+	+	–	–
	Hypoparathyroidism	±	–	–	–	–
Heart	Conduction block	[+]	–	±	–	–
	Cardiomyopathy	±	–	±	±	–
Gastrointestinal	Intestinal pseudo-obstruction	–	–	–	–	–
ENT	Sensorineural hearing loss	–	+	+	–	±
Kidney	Fanconi syndrome	±	–	±	–	–
Skin	Lipomas	–	+	–	–	–
Inheritance	Sporadic	+	–	–	–	–
	Maternal	–	+	+	+	+

* Boxes highlight the typical clinical features of each syndrome except for MILS, which is defined by neuroradiological findings. CNS, central nervous system; ENT, ear, nose and throat; KSS, Kearns–Sayre syndrome; MELAS, mitochondrial encephalomyopathy, lactic acidosis and stroke-like episodes; MERRF, myoclonus epilepsy with ragged red fibers; MILS, maternally inherited Leigh syndrome; NARP, neuropathy, ataxia and retinitis pigmentosa; PNS, peripheral nervous system. (Adapted from DiMauro et al 1999[132])

been found to have various brain defects including cerebral atrophy, agenesis of the corpus callosum, and brainstem and deep gray matter abnormalities. Head imaging by MRI (preferably with spectroscopy as MRS can quantify brain lactate) should be performed if the neurological examination is abnormal.

The above discussion refers to L-lactic acid accumulation. D-Lactic acidemia secondary to pathological intestinal bacterial overgrowth or associated with short bowel and blind loop syndromes may cause intermittent neurological symptoms, including dizziness and ataxia. D-Lactic acidemia is a cause of an unexplained elevation of the anion gap, because the D-stereoisomer of lactic acid is not typically detected by standard methods of lactic acid analysis. Specific testing for the D-stereoisomer of lactic acid is only available in a few specialized centers, but should be considered in patients with a persistent anion gap metabolic acidosis and normal metabolic screen (including L-lactate determination), especially if gastrointestinal pathology is present.

Leigh syndrome and Alper syndrome

Leigh syndrome (subacute necrotizing encephalomyelopathy) is a severe neurological disorder characterized by pyramidal and extrapyramidal symptoms, brainstem dysfunction, and a progressive course that typically presents in children aged 1–5 years. The Leigh syndrome designation does not imply a specific disorder, but rather is a clinical syndrome with several possible causes. Clinical features include hypotonia, weakness, ataxia, tremor, optic atrophy, ophthalmoplegia, retinitis pigmentosa and respiratory abnormalities. Bilateral basal ganglia lesions are a common neuroradiological finding. Symmetric necrotic lesions in the thalami, brainstem and posterior columns of the spinal cord are pathological features. Patients usually do not have ragged red fibers (RRF). Leigh syndrome is heterogeneous and may be caused by mtDNA, autosomal recessive, and X-linked disorders. The mtDNA mutations most commonly associated with Leigh syndrome are T8993G and T8993C, which affect a structural subunit of complex V and also cause neurogenic weakness, ataxia and retinitis pigmentosa (NARP). Mutations that alter mitochondrial tRNA structure (e.g. A3243G and A8344G) have more rarely been encountered in Leigh syndrome. A number of autosomal recessive nuclear gene mutations may also cause Leigh syndrome, including defects in specific components of respiratory chain complex I (NDUFS4, NDUFS7, NDUFS8) and complex II (Fp subunit).[134,135] Mutations in nuclear genes that code for proteins that are important in complex IV (cytochrome oxidase) assembly or stability [surfeit-1 (SURF-1) and SCO2] also cause Leigh syndrome.[136–138] Pyruvate dehydrogenase deficiency is an X-linked disorder that is another relatively common cause of Leigh syndrome. In general, the clinical course is similar in affected family members in whom Leigh syndrome is caused by a nuclear gene defect. A wide phenotypic spectrum, however, is typically encountered in Leigh

Table 24.24 The differential diagnosis of elevated blood lactate

Acquired causes	
Poor peripheral perfusion	Sepsis Cardiac dysfunction
Spurious elevation	Tight tourniquet/difficult blood draw Improper specimen handling (e.g. not on ice)
Seizures	
Liver failure	
Severe anemia	
Toxins*	Methanol, ethanol, ethylene glycol, salicylate poisoning
Inborn errors of metabolism	
Primary metabolic causes of lactic acidemia	
Pyruvate dehydrogenase complex deficiency	
Mitochondrial disorders	
Secondary metabolic causes of lactic acidemia	
Disorders of gluconeogenesis	Pyruvate carboxylase deficiency Phosphoenolpyruvate carboxykinase deficiency Fructose 1,6-bisphosphatase deficiency
Glycogen storage disease	Glucose-6-phosphatase deficiency Debrancher enzyme deficiency
Fatty acid oxidation defects	Medium chain acyl-CoA dehydrogenase deficiency Long chain 3-hydroxyacyl-CoA dehydrogenase deficiency
Biotin-responsive disorders	Multiple carboxylase deficiency (glutaric aciduria II) Biotinidase deficiency
Organic acidemias	Propionic acidemia Methylmalonic acidemia

* Lactic acidemia is not usually the predominant feature in toxin ingestion, but may be present.

Table 24.25 Evaluation of lactic acidemia

History	Traumatic delivery, infectious contacts, toxin/drug ingestion, family history of metabolic disease
Physical examination	Cardiac hemodynamic state, capillary refill*, ?hepatomegaly
Bedside tests	Blood pressure*, pulse oximetry*
Other studies	Chest X-ray, ECG, echocardiography, EEG, head imaging
Laboratory tests	Routine – complete blood count with differential, glucose, electrolytes, liver enzymes, BUN, creatinine, blood gases, serial lactate/pyruvate measurements, blood cultures (urine and CSF cultures if indicated), toxicology screen
	Metabolic studies – quantitative plasma amino acids, ammonia level, acylcarnitine profile, urine organic acids

* Decreased cardiac function (e.g. secondary to cardiomyopathy) may be present in patients with apparently normal perfusion, blood pressure, and cardiac examination.
BUN, blood urea nitrogen; CSF, cerebrospinal fluid; EEG, electroencephalogram; ECG, electrocardiogram;

syndrome families who harbor a heteroplasmic mtDNA mutation, with patients exhibiting a variety of clinical features from severe neurodegeneration with seizures to relatively mild behavior disorders.

Alper syndrome (progressive infantile poliodystrophy) is a neurodegenerative disorder with onset at 1–2 years and death in early childhood. Patients have lactic acidemia and a variety of symptoms, including myoclonic epilepsy, ataxia, hypo- or hypertonia, abnormal respirations and liver disease. Alper syndrome primarily affects the cerebral cortex and cerebellum, with lesser involvement of the basal ganglia and brainstem. A number of biochemical abnormalities that affect brain energy metabolism, e.g. respiratory chain complex deficiencies and tricarboxylic acid cycle defects, have been found in patients with Alper syndrome. Most cases appear to be autosomal recessive.

Mitochondrial myopathy

Hypotonia and muscle weakness are common presenting features in children with mitochondrial disease. The severity ranges from fatal infantile myopathy to more mild symptoms in later childhood or adulthood. Although severe lactic acidemia and multiorgan system failure may accompany severe infantile forms of mitochondrial myopathy, spontaneous remission has also been documented in early-onset disease.[139] Progressive weakness, exercise intolerance, myalgia and myoglobinuria may also occur. Numerous mtDNA (especially involving mitochondrial tRNAs) and nDNA mutations have been associated with myopathy.

Cardiomyopathy

Respiratory chain dysfunction is also a cause of cardiomyopathy in children and adults. A number of mtDNA point mutations and deletions, as well as nDNA defects, have been associated with cardiomyopathy. (Cardiac conduction defects are also relatively common in mitochondrial disease.) Patients usually have a concentric hypertrophic cardiomyopathy, but dilated forms are not uncommon. Heart pathology is often abnormal, showing fibroelastosis and interstitial fibrosis. Cardiomyopathy may be associated with a number of other clinical features, including neuromuscular disease, endocrine abnormalities and multiorgan system failure. The X-linked *Barth syndrome* is an important cause of congenital dilated cardiomyopathy in boys (see Nuclear genome defects below). Other nDNA mutations that affect the function of the respiratory chain may cause cardiomyopathy, in addition to causing neurological impairment (e.g. mutations in the SCO2 or frataxin genes, see Nuclear genome defects below).

Hepatic disease

Severe early onset liver failure and more indolent hepatic disease have been associated with various defects of the respiratory chain, often with multiple complexes being affected. Liver disease secondary to mitochondrial dysfunction may be associated with hypoglycemia, lactic acidemia, neuromuscular disorders, renal tubular dysfunction and other organ system involvement. Histopathology is non-specific, often showing steatosis, fibrosis and cholestasis. A general depletion of mtDNA and mtDNA rearrangements have been found in some patients with hepatic disease and respiratory chain dysfunction, but the molecular basis of the great majority of cases is unknown.

Renal disease

Renal tubular function is highly dependent on oxidative metabolism, so it is not surprising that kidney involvement is relatively common in mitochondrial disease. Proximal renal tubular dysfunction, manifesting as the *renal Fanconi syndrome*, is most frequently encountered, but the nephrotic syndrome, focal segmental glomerulonephrosis and chronic tubulointerstitial nephropathy have also been reported in patients with respiratory chain abnormalities (see Ch. 16). The Fanconi syndrome is characterized by proximal tubular dysfunction and subsequent urinary loss of glucose, protein, ions and amino acids. Children with mitochondrial disease may have only a partial Fanconi syndrome (e.g. mild aminoaciduria or renal tubular acidosis secondary to bicarbonate wasting). Initial symptoms may occur as early as the neonatal period, but milder disease may present in later childhood or adulthood. Kidney involvement is often associated with disease in other organ systems.

Endocrine disease

Diabetes mellitus, hypoparathyroidism, growth failure secondary to IgF1 deficiency, hypothyroidism, hypothalamic dysfunction and adrenocorticotropic hormone (ACTH) deficiency may occur in children with mitochondrial disease (see also Ch. 13). Diabetes secondary to respiratory chain abnormalities is typically associated with other clinical features including sensorineural hearing loss, cardiomyopathy, myopathy, renal tubular defects and neuropsychiatric disease (e.g. MIDD). Various mtDNA point mutations, including the A3243G tRNA mutation associated with MELAS syndrome, and mtDNA rearrangements have been associated with diabetes. Patients may present as neonates with ketosis, prominent hyperglycemia, and lactic acidemia or in later childhood or adulthood. *Pearson marrow-pancreas syndrome* (PS) is characterized by exocrine pancreatic dysfunction and refractory sideroblastic anemia with variable neutropenia and thrombocytopenia and is caused by a large mtDNA deletion. Diabetes may also occur in patients with PS. *Wolfram syndrome* is characterized by diabetes insipidus, diabetes mellitus, optic atrophy, and deafness (*DIDMOAD*). Wolfram syndrome in many cases is an autosomal recessive condition caused by mutations in the WFS1 gene which codes for a protein that localizes to the endoplasmic reticulum and is likely involved in membrane trafficking, protein processing, and/or calcium homeostasis, but has also been described in patients with mtDNA point mutations and deletions.[140]

Other clinical features

Although relatively common presentations of mitochondrial disease have been outlined above, patients often present in atypical ways at any age. Hydranencephaly, polyhydramnios and abnormalities of fetal tone have been detected prenatally.[141] Neonates may have severe hypotonia, seizures, congenital lactic acidosis, ketoacidotic coma and multiorgan system failure. Infants and children may have dysfunction of various organ systems in a seemingly unusual pattern. In addition to the presentations outlined above, patients have been described with various combinations of ophthalmological abnormalities (ptosis, optic atrophy, pigmentary retinopathy, cataracts), bone marrow depression, gastrointestinal illness (cyclic vomiting, chronic diarrhea, exocrine pancreatic dysfunction, intestinal pseudo-obstruction, failure to thrive), dermatological findings (mottled pigmentation, trichothiodystrophy), and even dysmorphic features (facial dysmorphism, microcephaly) (Table 24.22).

CLASSIFICATION OF MITOCHONDRIAL DISORDERS

Because the components of the respiratory chain are coded for by both the nuclear and mitochondrial genomes, inheritance of mitochondrial disorders may be either maternal or Mendelian in familial cases. Sporadic cases also occur as a result of new mutations in a given individual. Defects of mtDNA include point mutations, single deletions, insertions, and duplications or duplications/deletions. Defects of nDNA may affect specific respiratory chain subunits, intergenomic communication, OXPHOS coupling, mitochondrial substrate pores, protein importation or metal homeostasis (Table 24.26).[132]

Mitochondrial genome defects

Point mutations

MELAS, MERRF, LHON and NARP have each been associated with specific point mutations in mtDNA.[133] An A to G transition at base pair 1555 in the mitochondrial 12S ribosomal subunit gene causes *maternally inherited deafness with aminoglycoside sensitivity* (*MIDAS*). Mitochondrial disorders by nature show a considerable degree of overlap with respect to their clinical phenotypes; different mtDNA point mutations can result in similar clinical features, and, conversely, the same mtDNA mutation can lead to different findings in different patients. More that 100 pathological point mutations have been reported. Common mtDNA point mutation and deletion syndromes are compared in Table 24.26.

MELAS classically presents with stroke-like episodes and accompanying focal neurological deficits (which may be transient), headache, emesis, lactic acidosis and abnormal muscle morphology and respiratory chain function in later childhood and adulthood. Short stature, seizures, developmental regression, pigmentary retinopathy, deafness, diabetes mellitus and cardiomyopathy are variably present. Most patients (> 80%) with clinical features of MELAS have a heteroplasmic A3243G $tRNA^{Leu(UUR)}$ mtDNA mutation in muscle and, in most cases, blood. This same mutation has been associated with MERRF, progressive external ophthalmoplegia (PEO) and MIDD. Other point mutations in the same mitochondrial tRNA gene at positions 3252 and 3271 have also been described in MELAS. Many MELAS patients have a normal early childhood, but neurological symptoms occur by age 15 years in 80%. Multiple white matter lesions and basal ganglia calcification are common. Muscle histochemistry shows cytochrome c oxidase (COX) positive RRF and strong succinate dehydrogenase reactivity in blood vessels almost 90% of the time. Although biochemical studies may be normal, complex I deficiency,

Table 24.26 Classification of mitochondrial respiratory chain disorders

Defects of mitochondrial DNA (maternal inheritance)
Point mutations
MELAS, MERRF, LHON, NARP, MIDAS
Single deletions
KSS, CPEO, PS
Duplications or duplications/deletions
KSS
Defects of nuclear DNA (Mendelian inheritance)
Respiratory chain subunit disorders
Complex I deficiency
NDUFV1, NDUFS1, NDUFS2, NDUFS4, NDUFS7, NDUFS8 mutations
Complex II deficiency
Fp subunit of succinate dehydrogenase
Disorders of intergenomic communication
Respiratory chain subunit stability/assembly
SURF-1, SCO1, SCO2, COX10, BSC1L mutations
mtDNA replication
mtDNA depletion syndrome
multiple mtDNA deletions (autosomal dominant and recessive types)
thymidine phosphorylase deficiency (MNGIE)
Defective oxidative phosphorylation coupling
Luft disease
Mitochondrial substrate pores/translocase defects
ANT deficiency
VDAC deficiency
Malate/aspartate shuttle deficiency
Defects of mitochondrial protein importation
Chaperonins
hsp60
paraplegin (SPG7 mutations)
Mohr-Tranebjaerg syndrome (DDP1 mutations)
Defects of intramitochondrial metal homeostasis
Friedreich's ataxia (frataxin mutations)
X-linked sideroblastic anemia and ataxia (ABC7 mutations)
Wilson's disease (ATP7B mutations)
Other nuclear genome defects
Barth syndrome (G4.5/taffazin mutations)
Other neurodegenerative disorders
Alzheimer disease
Parkinson disease
Huntington disease
Amyotropic lateral sclerosis

ANT, adenine nucleotide translocator; CPEO, chronic progressive external ophthalmoplegia; KSS, Kearns-Sayre syndrome; LHON, Leber hereditary optic neuropathy; MELAS, mitochondrial encephalomyopathy, lactic acidosis and stroke-like episodes; MERRF, myoclonic epilepsy and ragged red fibers; MIDAS, maternally inherited deafness with aminoglycoside sensitivity; MNGIE, myoneurogastrointestinal disorder and encephalopathy; NARP, neurogenic weakness, ataxia and retinitis pigmentosa; PS, Pearson marrow-pancreas syndrome; VDAC, voltage dependent anion channel.

or partial combined deficiencies of complexes I, II and IV have been described.

MERRF is characterized by myoclonic epilepsy, myopathy and progressive cerebellar ataxia. Deafness is common, and optic atrophy, peripheral neuropathy and heart block may occur. Early development is usually normal, with onset of symptoms often occurring in the second or third decade. Mild to moderate elevations of lactate and creatine kinase may be present. Muscle biopsy shows prominent COX negative RRF and, most often, complex I and IV deficiencies. An A8344G mutation in the mtDNA $tRNA^{Lys}$ gene is the most common cause, although the common A3243G MELAS mutation, and other mtDNA point mutations may result in a similar phenotype.

LHON is one of the most common inherited causes of blindness in young men (incidence ~1:50 000). Although most pedigrees show only vision loss, non-ophthalmalogical features also occur and include encephalomyopathy, deafness, dystonia, ataxia, a multiple sclerosis-like illness and cardiac conduction defects. Males are affected in a 3:1 ratio over females, but the mechanism of this finding is not understood. A G11778A mutation in the ND1 subunit of complex I causes > 60% of cases, but ~20 different mutations in mtDNA have been associated with LHON. Usually, these mutations are present in a *homoplasmic* state, in contrast to the heteroplasmy present in most mitochondrial disorders.

NARP is characterized by proximal neurogenic weakness, pigmentary retinopathy, seizures, ataxia, sensory neuropathy and developmental delay. Mutations in mtDNA (T8993G and T8993C) causing dysfunction of the ATPase 6 subunit of complex V are associated with this condition. Leigh syndrome is often present when the mutant mtDNA load is particularly high (> 90%); patients may be described as having *maternally inherited Leigh syndrome* (*MILS*) in such cases. Head imaging may show cerebral or cerebellar atrophy, in addition to the typical features of Leigh syndrome. Biochemical findings on muscle biopsy may be normal and RRF or COX negative fibers are usually absent.

Single deletions

Large single deletions or duplications of mtDNA are most often sporadic, with patients having only a single type of abnormal mtDNA in their cells, theoretically arising from clonal expansion of a chance rearrangement event in oogenesis or early embryogenesis. The human oocyte contains approximately 100 000 mtDNA molecules, but only about 1000 will be passed on to the fetus. If a deleted and/or duplicated mtDNA molecule passes through this 'bottleneck', transmission to the fetus may result in mitochondrial disease.[142] KSS, PEO and PS are associated with sporadic mtDNA duplications/deletions in most instances.

Patients with KSS have onset of symptoms before 20 years, PEO, and pigmentary retinopathy, plus at least one additional feature including ataxia, heart block or CSF protein > 100 mg/dl. Proximal myopathy, areflexia, sensorineural deafness, stroke-like episodes, bulbar symptoms and lactic acidosis may occur. Up to 60% of muscle fibers are COX negative, with RRF in 5–20%. Nearly all patients have a mtDNA deletion. A particular mtDNA deletion that encompasses 4.9 kb from nucleotide 8482 to 13459 is present in ~40% of cases. This same 'common deletion' is also associated with isolated PEO or PS. PEO consists of ptosis, ophthalmoplegia and proximal weakness. Life span may be normal. The muscle pathological features are similar to KSS. PS presents in early infancy with a refractory sideroblastic anemia, variable neutropenia and thrombocytopenia, and exocrine pancreatic dysfunction. Diabetes mellitus, liver dysfunction and renal tubular dysfunction may occur. The 'common deletion' is present in up to 90% of total blood or bone marrow mtDNA, but may be quite low in muscle or fibroblasts. Muscle histology and biochemistry are often normal. The initial refractory anemia resolves in patients surviving infancy, but these children may develop KSS, with subsequent accumulation of deleted mtDNA species in muscle, and lessening of the proportion of mutant mtDNA in blood.[143]

Multiple deletions, duplications or duplications/deletions

Other major rearrangements of mtDNA include duplications, most commonly present in the context of duplications/deletions, and multiple deletions. While *single* mtDNA deletions and duplication/deletions often are sporadic, duplications/deletions may exhibit maternal inheritance and can be associated with a typical KSS phenotype or various other clinical presentations. *Multiple* deletions of mtDNA, on the other hand, exhibit Mendelian inheritance and are caused by defective signaling between the nuclear and mitochondrial genomes, with resultant defective mtDNA replication (see below).

Nuclear genome defects

Defects of nDNA that result in abnormal mitochondrial respiratory chain function are inherited in a Mendelian fashion and likely are responsible for the majority of cases of mitochondrial disease. Nuclear genome defects may cause dysfunction of:

1. specific respiratory chain subunits;
2. intergenomic communication between nuclear and mitochondrial genomes;
3. oxidation/phosphorylation coupling;
4. substrate pores or translocases;
5. mitochondrial protein importation; or
6. intramitochondrial metal homeostasis (Table 24.26).

Defects in specific nuclear respiratory chain subunit genes

The mitochondrial respiratory chain contains 13 subunits encoded by mtDNA and 71 encoded by nDNA. Defects in respiratory chain subunits encoded by nDNA are inherited in an autosomal recessive manner in most instances. Mutations in nuclear respiratory chain subunit genes have only been found in isolated complex I and complex II deficiencies. The first nuclear gene mutation shown to cause mitochondrial disease in humans was a mutation in the flavoprotein (Fp) subunit gene of succinate dehydrogenase (complex II) reported in two siblings with Leigh syndrome.[135]

Succinate dehydrogenase gene mutations have also been associated with familial cases of pheochromocytoma and paraganglionoma, highlighting an interesting link between mitochondrial dysfunction and hereditary cancer.[144,145] Mutations in the nuclear encoded complex I subunits NDUFS1, NDUFS7 and NDUFS8 have also been described in patients with complex I deficiency and Leigh syndrome. Mutations in complex I subunits NDUFV1 (leukodystrophy and myoclonic epilepsy), NDUFS2 (encephalomyopathy and hypertrophic cardiomyopathy), and NDUFS4 (mild combined complex I and III deficiencies) have also been reported.[134] A presumed nDNA complex I defect was present in an infant, born to consanguineous parents, who had clinical and biochemical features of long chain 3-hydroxyacyl-coenzyme A dehydrogenase deficiency, a defect of fatty acid metabolism.[146] This latter case highlights the interdependence of the mitochondrial respiratory chain and fatty acid oxidation cycle for normal function of either pathway.

Defects in intergenomic communication

Defects in respiratory chain complex activities may also be caused by nDNA mutations resulting in either aberrant subunit biogenesis/maintenance or mtDNA replicative errors. Most patients with isolated complex III deficiency have normal mtDNA and, therefore, must have nDNA defects. However, sequencing of nuclear encoded complex III subunit genes has not yet detected any mutations, leading to the hypothesis that non-structural nuclear genes responsible for the maintenance of complex III must exist. Indeed, mutations in BSCIL, an assembly gene for complex III, have recently been described in six patients with encephalopathy, renal tubulopathy and liver disease.[147] Similarly, sequencing of the 10 nuclear structural subunits of COX has failed to detect mutations in patients with isolated complex IV deficiency. In this case, nuclear mutations have been detected in the gene coding for the mitochondrial inner membrane protein SURF-1.[136,137] SURF-1 is postulated to be important in the assembly or stability of complex IV, although the mechanism of action is unknown. Patients with COX deficiency secondary to SURF-1 mutations present with Leigh syndrome. Mutations in the SCO1 and SCO2 genes result in impaired mitochondrial copper metabolism and subsequent defective COX activity, with patients having early onset encephalopathy, hypertrophic cardiomyopathy, hepatopathy, and ketoacidotic coma.[148,149] COX10 codes for hemeA:farensyltransferase, an inner mitochondrial membrane protein important in the biogenesis of COX. Siblings with mutations in the COX10 gene died by 3 years after a clinical course that featured progressive neurological deterioration and a proximal renal tubulopathy.[150] Although most known ATPase (complex V) defects have been inherited maternally, secondary to heteroplasmic T8993G or T8993C mutations, a patient with ATPase deficiency caused by a nuclear defect involved in the biosynthesis of complex V has also been reported. The patient was born to a consanguineous couple and presented with severe lactic acidosis, hypotonia, cardiomegaly and hepatomegaly and died from heart failure as a neonate.[151]

The nuclear genome codes for enzymes involved in mtDNA transcription, translation and replication. Therefore, defects in intergenomic communication may cause qualitative or quantitative alterations of mtDNA. Although all the genes responsible have not yet been identified, multiple mtDNA deletions (cf. single sporadic deletions) and depletion in the amount of mtDNA are also inherited in a Mendelian fashion.[152] Autosomal recessive and autosomal dominant forms of PEO are associated with multiple deletions of mtDNA. Linkage to chromosome 10 in a Finnish and a Pakistani family and chromosome 4 in Italian families underscore the heterogeneous nature of these defects. Furthermore, clinical variability exists between populations with autosomal dominant PEO; e.g. in the Finnish population PEO is associated with depression, whereas peripheral neuropathy, cataracts and ataxia are seen in Italian patients. Mutations in *adenine nucleotide translocator 1* (ANT1), the heart and muscle-specific isoform of the mitochondrial ADP/ATP transporter on chromosome 4, were found in six Italian families with autosomal dominant PEO.[153] Other genes responsible for autosomal dominant PEO include *polymerase gamma* (POLG) and the gene (located on chromosome 10) coding for a novel mitochondrial protein called Twinkle.[154,155] Mutations in OPA1, a gene that encodes a dynamin-related protein with GTPase activity that is targeted to mitochondria, cause a form of autosomal dominant optic atrophy (prevalence 1:12–50 000 in different populations) by interfering with mitochondrial function in an, as yet, undetermined manner. Most patients have a progressive loss of visual acuity in childhood.[156,157]

Multiple mtDNA deletions also occur in *myoneurogastrointestinal disorder and encephalopathy (MNGIE)*. MNGIE is characterized by a chronic intestinal pseudo-obstruction, ophthalmoplegia, peripheral neuropathy with 'stocking/glove' sensory loss, and myopathy. Deafness is common and developmental regression with white matter disease may be present. RRF, a partial COX deficiency, and neurogenic changes are seen on muscle histology.[158] Although the MNGIE clinical spectrum has been associated with a single base pair deletion in the mitochondrial $tRNA^{Thr}$ gene, MNGIE is most often caused by mutations in the nuclear thymidine phosphorylase gene and is inherited in an autosomal recessive fashion. Aberrant thymidine metabolism and subsequent impaired replication and/or maintenance of mtDNA occur secondary to thymidine phosphorylase deficiency. MNGIE patients typically have a depletion in the amount of mtDNA and ~50% have multiple mtDNA deletions.

The nuclear genome encodes the enzymes necessary for mtDNA replication and maintenance and a number of nDNA defects have been associated with a quantitative decrease in the amount of mtDNA. The mtDNA depletion syndrome is a heterogeneous autosomal recessive condition in which the concentration of mtDNA is decreased or nearly absent.[152] The clinical spectrum of mtDNA depletion syndrome is broad; a rapidly fatal congenital disorder with hypotonia or liver failure, an infantile myopathy, a spinal muscular atrophy-like condition, and later-onset disease with prolonged survival to early adulthood have been reported. Unlike most mitochondrial disorders, patients may have a relatively high elevation of creatine kinase, usually ~800–6000 IU/L. COX deficiency, with or without involvement of other respiratory chain enzymes, is common and RRF may be present, but are not invariably so. Deficiency of mitochondrial DNA polymerase gamma was found in a patient with Alper syndrome, epilepsy and fulminant hepatic failure with ~30% of the normal amount of mtDNA.[159] The mitochondria do not contain enzymes for de novo deoxyribonucleoside-5´-triphosphate (dNTP) synthesis and rely on dNTP salvage pathway enzymes, including thymidine kinase and deoxyguanosine kinase for mtDNA replication. Profound mtDNA depletion was present in patients with a severe myopathy, lactic acidemia and elevated creatine kinase levels (900–4000 IU/L) who had reduced activity of mitochondrial thymidine kinase and documented mutations in the thymidine kinase (TK2) gene.[160] A significant depletion of mtDNA (8–39% of controls) was found in three kindreds with early progressive liver failure and neurological abnormalities secondary to a single-nucleotide deletion in the mitochondrial deoxyguanosine kinase (dGK) gene.[161] Low levels of the nuclear encoded mitochondrial transcription factor A (mtTFA) were present in patients with mtDNA depletion, but is unclear whether this represents the primary defect or is simply a secondary phenomenon.[162] A decreased amount of mtDNA has also been reported in an autosomal recessive condition in which patients have a homozygous ~180 kb deletion of chromosome 2p16. Affected individuals had a unique constellation of features including facial dysmorphism, neonatal seizures, hypotonia, severe developmental delay, cystinuria and lactic acidemia.[163] Although the majority of cases of mtDNA depletion have autosomal recessive inheritance, the X-linked *mental retardation, epileptic seizures, hypogonadism and hypogenitalism, microcephaly, obesity (MEHMO) syndrome* has been associated with a decreased amount of mtDNA.[164] Some HIV patients treated with nucleoside reverse transcriptase inhibitors have mtDNA depletion and subsequent organ toxicity, possibly secondary to inhibition of DNA polymerase gamma by this class of drug.[165]

Defective oxidative phosphorylation coupling

Luft and colleagues reported the first patient with a mitochondrial disorder in 1962 and only one other case has since been described with this same disorder. Patients with Luft disease develop symptoms in childhood consisting of myopathy and euthyroid hypermetabolism, with increased body temperature, sweating, respiratory rate and heart rate. The characteristic pathological feature is uncoupling of skeletal muscle mitochondria with dissipation of the electrochemical gradient generated by the respiratory chain and subsequent decreased ATP production.[166]

Defects in mitochondrial substrate pores or translocases

In order for the mitochondrial respiratory chain to function properly, molecules involved in OXPHOS reactions, including ATP, ADP, phosphate and other ions, must cross the inner and outer mitochondrial membranes through protein channels. Dysfunction of the ANT, voltage-dependent anion channel (VDAC), and malate-aspartate shuttle may cause classic symptoms and signs of mitochondrial disease. ADP and ATP cross the inner mitochondrial membrane through the ANT. A child with shortness of breath, rapid fatigue, and lactic acidosis was found to have a muscle-specific deficiency of ANT by immunostaining.[167] (Mutations in ANT1 have also been associated with autosomal dominant PEO, see above.) VDAC (a.k.a. porin) is an outer mitochondrial membrane transporter that opens differentially for anions, cations and certain uncharged molecules at different transmembrane voltages. VDAC deficiency was documented in an infant with non-specific dysmorphic features, hypothalamic hypothyroidism and psychomotor retardation.[168] Investigation of a young adult with exercise induced myalgia documented a defect in the inner mitochondrial membrane malate-aspartate shuttle.[169]

Defects of mitochondrial protein importation

Proteins that are imported into mitochondria contain a leader sequence that acts as a targeting signal. They are then translocated into the mitochondrial matrix by import machinery consisting of chaperonins and translocases of the outer and inner mitochondrial membranes (*Tom and Tim complexes*). Point mutations in the leader peptide impair mitochondrial targeting and have been found in a number of intramitochondrial enzymes (e.g. ornithine transcarbamylase, methylmalonyl-CoA mutase, and the E1 alpha subunit of pyruvate dehydrogenase), but have not been detected in respiratory chain subunits.[170] The mitochondrial matrix chaperonin heat shock protein 60 (hsp60) ensures proper folding of imported proteins. Defective hsp60 synthesis was associated with decreased activities of multiple mitochondrial enzymes in a patient that died at age 2 days, after presenting with dysmorphic features, hypotonia and severe lactic acidosis.[171] Protein importation defects may involve the importation or processing of iron–sulfur clusters in some patients with complex II deficiency and have been reported in a patient with combined complex I–III deficiencies.[172] More recently, a defect in paraplegin, a ubiquitous inner mitochondrial membrane protein with proteolytic and chaperonin activities, was found in patients with *hereditary spastic paraplegia* (HSP). HSP is a heterogeneous disorder (autosomal dominant, autosomal recessive and X-linked forms exist) with a variable age of onset and prevalence of ~1:10 000. Patients classically have progressive weakness and spasticity of the lower limbs, but other features, including developmental delay, optic atrophy, retinitis pigmentosa, deafness, ataxia and ichthyosis, may be present. Mutations in SPG7 cause the production of aberrant paraplegin, an enzyme with homology to yeast ATP-dependent zinc metalloproteases. Muscle biopsies from two patients with HSP showed RRF, a finding consistent with impaired OXPHOS.[173] Finally, the X-linked neurodegenerative disorder *Mohr-Tranebjaerg syndrome* (DFN-1/MTS) is caused by mutations in the gene coding for the deafness/dystonia peptide (DDP), a protein which bears strong resemblance to the Tim subclass of mitochondrial transmembrane carrier proteins.[174] Mutations in the DDP1 gene are postulated to affect the biogenesis of the Tim23 complex, which is required for mitochondrial import of proteins responsible for the translocation, assembly, and integrity of the OXPHOS system. Patients with MTS have dystonia, spasticity, developmental delay, and progressive sensorineural hearing loss.

Defects in intramitochondrial metal homeostasis

The neurodegenerative disorders Friedreich's ataxia (FA), X-linked sideroblastic anemia and ataxia (XLAS/A), and Wilson's disease

(WD) are associated with aberrant intramitochondrial metal homeostasis, which may secondarily cause dysfunction of the respiratory chain.[175] FA is an autosomal recessive disorder caused by an expansion of a GAA triplet repeat in intron 1 of the gene frataxin. The frataxin gene product is targeted to mitochondria and is involved in iron homeostasis. FA patients have intramitochondrial accumulation of free iron, which impairs oxidative metabolism, possibly by interfering with the normal production of heme and iron–sulfur clusters.[176] Iron homeostasis is also altered in XLSA/A, a disorder characterized by non-progressive cerebellar ataxia and mild anemia starting in infancy or early childhood. The mitochondrial inner membrane iron transporter ABC7 is defective in XLSA/A.[177] WD is an autosomal recessive condition that features liver dysfunction and/or extrapyramidal symptoms. The WD protein localizes to the trans-Golgi network and a modified, cleaved, form of this protein is found in mitochondria.[178] WD gene (ATP7B) mutations result in intramitochondrial copper overload, mtDNA deletions and abnormal respiratory chain function. Recently, mutations in SCO1 and SCO2, nuclear genes that play a role in mitochondrial copper delivery, have been found in patients with COX deficiency (see Defects in intergenomic communication above). Although precise pathological mechanisms have not been elucidated, these examples highlight the importance of intramitochondrial metal homeostasis for proper functioning of the respiratory chain.

Other nuclear genome defects

Barth syndrome (3-methylglutaconic aciduria type II) is an X-linked disorder caused by mutations in the G4.5 (tafazzin) gene that is characterized by dilated cardiomyopathy, cyclic neutropenia, skeletal myopathy, short stature and abnormal mitochondria. Elevated urine 3-methylglutaconate, 3-methylglutarate and 2-ethylhydracrylate may be present, but are not invariably so. The G4.5 (tafazzin) gene is expressed at high levels in cardiac and skeletal muscle, but its exact function is unknown.[179]

OTHER NEURODEGENERATIVE DISORDERS

Mitochondrial respiratory chain dysfunction, with secondary generation of damaging free radical molecules, also appears to play a role in the pathogenesis of other neurodegenerative disorders including *Alzheimer disease* (AD), *Parkinson disease* (PD), *Huntington disease* (HD), and *amyotropic lateral sclerosis* (ALS).[180,181] Maternal (mitochondrial) inheritance may be present in some AD pedigrees. Platelets, cerebral postmortem samples and cybrid cell lines harboring mitochondria from AD patients may exhibit COX deficiency. An increase in free radical production in AD cybrids, which could, in theory, lead to an increase in mtDNA damage, has also been observed. However, to date mtDNA point mutations and/or deletions have not been unequivocally linked to the pathogenesis of AD. Although both mtDNA and nDNA encoded genes important in OXPHOS have shown reduced expression in AD, this may simply reflect physiological downregulation of the mitochondrial respiratory chain secondary to decreased neuronal activity.

A heteroplasmic mtDNA abnormality leading to a complex I defect may be responsible for some cases of PD. Some patients with PD have had low platelet and/or substantia nigra complex I activities. Complex I deficiency has also been postulated to lead to increases free radical production, with subsequent loss of the mitochondrial transmembrane potential and release of molecules important in cellular apoptosis.

HD is an autosomal dominant disorder caused by CAG repeat expansion in the IT15 gene encoding huntington. Excitotoxicity appears to play an important role in the pathogenesis of HD by generating nitric oxide and free radicals. Defects affecting several respiratory chain complexes, including combined complex II/III and isolated complex IV deficiencies, as well as deficiency of the tricarboxylic acid cycle enzyme aconitase, have been found in the caudate and putamen in HD patients.

Point mutations in the free-radical scavenging superoxide dismutase gene have been detected in ~25% of familial cases of ALS, suggesting that oxidative damage and increased free radical production may be responsible, in part, for disease pathogenesis. Furthermore, mild decreases in complex I and complex IV activities have been found in cell cybrids containing mitochondria from ALS patients. In addition, an out-of-frame five base pair microdeletion in the mtDNA COI subunit gene was reported in a patient with an unusual early-onset, rapidly progressive form of motor neurone disease. In this patient, COX deficiency was postulated to be linked to overproduction of free radicals.[182]

DIAGNOSIS OF RESPIRATORY CHAIN DISORDERS

Obtaining a meticulous pedigree is an essential part of the evaluation of any child with suspected mitochondrial disease. The family history may reveal classic maternal inheritance (matrilineal transmission to all offspring, with offspring having variable phenotypes) or Mendelian inheritance. However, the family history is often negative in cases of a spontaneous mtDNA mutation or an autosomal recessive condition. Targeted questioning for the presence of more subtle features of respiratory chain disorders, including hearing loss, vision problems, behavior abnormalities, migraines, diabetes mellitus and other endocrine disease, or short stature, should be routine.

In patients with neurological symptoms, brain MRI is routinely performed and EEG may be indicated depending on patient symptoms. Positron emission tomography (PET), single photon emission computed tomography (SPECT) and MRS have also been used in order to study the patterns of blood flow, lactate production, oxygen metabolism and glucose metabolism in brain and muscle in patients with mitochondrial disease. Because mitochondrial disorders can affect any organ system, screening tests to monitor ophthalmological, hearing, cardiac, liver and renal function are an essential part of the initial evaluation and subsequent management of patients.

Laboratory investigations include measurement of blood (and on occasion fibroblast) lactate and pyruvate levels. In the presence of lactic acidemia, an elevated blood lactate/pyruvate ratio > 20 is suggestive of a respiratory chain disorder, whereas a normal ratio is typical of an enzymatic block proximal to the respiratory chain (e.g. pyruvate dehydrogenase deficiency). (NB: A normal lactate/pyruvate ratio does not *exclude* the diagnosis of mitochondrial disease.) While the lactate/pyruvate ratio reflects the redox state in the cytoplasm, the beta-hydroxybutyrate/acetoacetate ratio is indicative of the intramitochondrial redox state, with a ratio > 1 suggestive of mitochondrial dysfunction. Although these ratios are commonly obtained by analyzing blood samples, confirmation of a suspected abnormality may be provided by measuring lactate and pyruvate levels in cultured fibroblasts. Elevated CSF lactate may be present in some patients with normal blood lactate. Highly elevated creatine kinase levels are unusual, but have been reported in the mtDNA depletion syndrome. Urine organic acid analysis may be normal, or show variable elevations of lactate, pyruvate, ketone bodies, tricarboxylic acid cycle intermediates or other organic acids, including ethylmalonic, malic, fumaric, 3-methylglutaconic, 2-ethylhydracrylic, 2-methylsuccinic and glutaric acids.[183] Orotic acid in urine may also be elevated. Urine amino acids may show a generalized aminoaciduria suggestive of the renal Fanconi syndrome (see Ch. 16). The fatty acid oxidation cycle and respiratory chain are interdependent on each other for the proper function of either pathway. Therefore, elevated dicarboxylic acids, more typically associated with fatty acid oxidation disorders, may also be present as a secondary phenomenon to a primary block in respiratory chain function. Because elevations of specific acylcarnitines are characteristic of fatty acid oxidation disorders, a plasma acylcarnitine profile may be useful in the differentiation of a fatty acid oxidation disorder from a defect in the respiratory chain. Carnitine levels may detect a secondary carnitine deficiency.

A muscle biopsy for histology, histochemical staining, mitochondrial morphology and biochemical analysis may be needed to establish a diagnosis of a respiratory chain disorder.[132] When mitochondrial disease enters the differential diagnosis for a child undergoing muscle biopsy, the specimen should be handled correctly to allow for the possibility of respiratory chain enzymatic testing. This should be discussed and arranged ahead of time. The modified Gomori trichrome stain detects abnormal red-staining subsarcolemmal collections of mitochondria. These RRF are considered to be a classic feature of mitochondrial disease. However, it must be emphasized that most respiratory chain disorders in children do not have associated RRF, and, therefore, the absence of RRF *does not* exclude the consideration of mitochondrial disease. Conversely, RRF and ultrastructurally abnormal mitochondria may be present in other conditions, including inflammatory myopathies, myotonic dystrophy and Duchenne muscular dystrophy.[132] Staining for succinate dehydrogenase (SDH) and COX activities is also routinely performed. SDH staining is a sensitive indicator of mitochondrial proliferation. COX staining is particularly useful in distinguishing mtDNA defects, which show a differential mosaic staining pattern with some fibers having activity (COX positive) and others without activity (COX negative), from nuclear defects that affect COX activity, in which fibers are uniformly COX negative.[132] In addition, COX positive RRF are seen in MELAS. Other non-specific histopathological findings of respiratory chain disorders include accumulation of glycogen and/or lipid, fiber-type variation, or neurogenic changes. On the other hand, muscle histology may appear entirely normal. Abnormal mitochondria, often with paracrystalline inclusions or alteration in shape and size, or an increased number of mitochondria may be apparent by electron microscopy, but such changes are non-specific.

Biochemical analysis of respiratory chain function using spectrophotometric or polarographic techniques is usually best performed on a muscle sample, because of the higher oxidative enzyme activities present in muscle. Complex I activity is also not reliably detected in fibroblasts. Some respiratory chain defects are only expressed in the affected tissue, so studies on lymphoblasts, liver tissue, or cardiac muscle may be needed in order to find a biochemical defect.[129] Biochemical analyses may reveal isolated deficiencies (e.g. specific complex I, cytochrome b, or COX deficiencies) suggestive of a new somatic mutation in a specific mtDNA respiratory chain subunit gene or a nuclear defect, or combined partial complex deficiencies suggestive of a mtDNA tRNA mutation. The absence of a biochemical defect does not exclude a diagnosis of mitochondrial disease, and may be seen, for example, in some cases of mtDNA mutations affecting mitochondrial tRNAs. The biopsy sample must be handled appropriately for respiratory chain studies, if reliable results are to be obtained.

When the family history, clinical presentation, and/or biochemical investigations suggest the presence of mitochondrial disease, it may be possible to detect a mutation by molecular diagnostic techniques. In cases where a nuclear gene is suspected, further investigations may only be available in specialized laboratories on a research basis. However, tests for common point mutations and deletions of mtDNA are available in some commercial labs. While many mtDNA point mutations and some deletions or duplications can be detected in blood, multiple mtDNA deletions or complex rearrangements may require analysis of a muscle specimen. If a specific mutation is not found, this does not exclude the presence of a mitochondrial disorder, because most laboratories only screen for a limited number of mtDNA mutations. Furthermore, the mutation may simply not be present in a high enough concentration to be detected in the assayed tissue. Overall, mtDNA deletions have been found in approximately 12% (11% single, 1% multiple) of patients with documented respiratory chain dysfunction, mitochondrial tRNA mutations in 16%, while the remainder are undiagnosed at the molecular level (possibly reflecting the presence of rare mtDNA or nDNA mutations that are not usually screened for).[184]

GENETIC COUNSELING (see Ch. 12)

Most children are diagnosed with mitochondrial disease on the basis of finding decreased enzymatic activity in one or more of the respiratory chain complexes and do not have a specific nDNA or mtDNA mutation identified. In these cases, it is difficult to provide accurate recurrence risk estimates, unless a particular mode of inheritance is suggested by the pedigree. However, even if maternal inheritance seems likely on the basis of family history, it may not be possible to provide a family with meaningful information regarding the likelihood of future children expressing features of disease. Because of the inherent characteristics of mitochondrial biology (heteroplasmy, replicative segregation, threshold effect), mitochondrial genetics is complex and genetic counseling is particularly challenging. In a given family with a mtDNA disease, future offspring may be more, similarly or less affected than the proband. Empiric recurrence risks have been estimated for some of the more common mtDNA disorders (NARP, MELAS, MERRF) based on maternal blood mutation loads.[131] The blood percentage of abnormal mtDNA in MELAS and MERRF does not correlate well with expression of clinical features, but there appears to be a good correlation with mutant load and outcome in NARP. Nevertheless, while counseling is relatively straightforward in NARP patients with either a very high or very low percentage of mutant mtDNA in maternal blood, great difficulty is encountered in less clear-cut patients with moderately high or low mutant loads. Single deletions in mtDNA are usually sporadic, but more complex deletion/duplications of mtDNA may be inherited (~5% transmission risk to offspring has been suggested in the latter case, but little data exist to support this figure). Multiple mtDNA mutations may be inherited in an autosomal dominant or autosomal recessive manner (see nDNA mutations above). Genetic counseling is more straightforward in cases of nDNA mutations causing mitochondrial disease; affected relatives tend to have similar features and classic Mendelian inheritance can be reviewed with the family.

Prenatal diagnosis of mtDNA disorders has been attempted by performing mutation analysis on amniocytes or chorionic villi. However, the mutant load in a prenatal sample does not necessarily predict the percentage of mutant mtDNA in most tissues at birth. It has been suggested that mutant loads $< 30\%$ or $> 90\%$ may predict a low or high probability, respectively, of having a child with clinical disease, although such a conclusion must be treated with caution at the present time because of the paucity of pregnancy outcome data in families with specific mtDNA mutations.[131] Molecular prenatal genetic diagnosis of oocytes, oocyte cytoplasmic transfer to dilute mutant mtDNA, and transfer of an unfertilized oocyte nucleus into an enucleated donor oocyte (followed by in vitro fertilization and reimplantation) are experimental techniques that may offer female carriers of a mtDNA mutation reproductive options in the near future.

Therapy for mitochondrial respiratory chain disorders

There is no proven specific therapy for children with respiratory chain disorders. Positive therapeutic outcomes have occurred in isolated cases treated with various combinations of L-carnitine, ascorbate, tocopherol, succinate, riboflavin, menadione, nicotinamide, thiamine, creatine, idebenone and coenzyme Q_{10}.[128] However, it is difficult to assess the efficacy of any therapy given the genetic heterogeneity and broad clinical spectrum present in mitochondrial disease. Succinate may be beneficial in patients with complex I deficiency, because of its ability to donate electrons directly to complex II. Coenzyme Q_{10} therapy has been shown to decrease blood lactate levels and may improve oxygen utilization in some patients.[185,186] Dichloroacetate (DCA), a stimulator of pyruvate dehydrogenase activity, is in clinical trials to test its utility in treating patients with lactic acidemia from a variety of causes, including mitochondrial disorders. DCA therapy has caused a decrease in blood lactate, improved brain oxidative metabolism on MRS, and amelioration of clinical symptoms in patients with mitochodrial disease.[187,188] Patients with mitochondrial disease may have uridine deficiency and supplementation with triacetyluridine has resulted in improved strength, growth, and renal tubular function in some patients. Vitamins and cofactors commonly used for the treatment of mitochondrial disorders are listed in Table 24.27.

Glucose oxidation is primarily aerobic in the liver, so patients with OXPHOS disorders may have relative difficulty in handling a large glucose load. A diet low in carbohydrate and without excessive calories may be beneficial in some patients with mitochondrial disease. In patients with secondary impairment of long chain fatty acid metabolism, avoidance of fasting and a diet low in long chain fats may be helpful.

Gene shifting has been proposed as a possible therapeutic approach in patients with heteroplasmic mtDNA mutations in muscle.[189] Resistance exercise training induces muscle damage and has the potential to stimulate dormant myoblast satellite cells to fuse with regenerating myofibers. In theory, myoblasts with normal mtDNA (and energy production) would be at a selective advantage and would more likely undergo such fusion. An increase in the ratio of wild-type to mutant mtDNA has been demonstrated in a patient undergoing such exercise training. Spontaneous improvement, with a decrease in the proportion of mutant mtDNA in muscle, has been observed in a patient with a mtDNA point mutation, giving further support to the theoretical possibility of this approach.[190] Aerobic exercise appears to increase oxidative capacity in patients with mtDNA mutations, possibly by inducing mitochondrial proliferation and the production of an increased amount of functional mtDNA, but the long-term outcome of such training is unknown.[191]

Experimentation has begun in the field of gene therapy for respiratory chain disorders. Potential approaches include:

1. complementation by cytosolic synthesis of mitochondrial proteins containing an appropriate targeting sequence, with subsequent translocation into mitochondria;
2. direct mitochondrial transfection of complementing DNA; and
3. sequence specific oligonucleotide or peptide-nucleotide conjugate targeting of mutant mtDNA.[192]

The first two approaches attempt to provide dysfunctional mitochondria with a normal copy of a missing or defective protein and could be used, for example, in disorders caused by a lack of a specific respiratory chain subunit. Peptide nucleic acids (PNAs) bind to DNA and interfere with DNA replication. In vitro studies using PNAs complementary to specific mtDNA point mutations or deletions showed specific inhibition of mutant mtDNA replication and increased proportion of wild-type mtDNA.[193] This technique would be especially beneficial in the treatment of mtDNA mutations that affect mitochondrial tRNA genes. Mitochondrial tRNA disorders tend to result in multiple respiratory chain deficiencies because of a general impairment of mitochondrial protein synthesis. Increasing the proportion of normal mtDNA copies in a heteroplasmic cell could potentially result in improved mitochondrial protein synthesis and overall mitochondrial function. These experimental approaches are exciting, but significant theoretical problems must be overcome before such therapy has practical implications for patients with mitochondrial disease. Prospects for studying the potential for gene therapy and other novel therapies to treat respiratory chain disorders have improved with recent reports of knock-out transgenic mouse models for mitochondrial disease and the creation of mice harboring heteroplasmic mtDNA mutations.[130]

Table 24.27 Vitamin, cofactor and drug therapy of mitochondrial disease

Medication	Mechanism	Dose
Ubiquinone (coenzyme Q_{10})	Bypass of complex I Free radical scavenger	5 mg/kg/day 30–250 mg/day in adults
Idebenone	Bypass of complex I Free radical scavenger	90–270 mg/day in adults
Carnitine	Corrects secondary deficiency	50–100 mg/kg/day Up to 3 g/day in adults
Dichloroacetate	Stimulates PDH activity	15–200 mg/kg/day
Succinate	Directly donates electrons to complex II	1–6 g/day
Thiamin (B_1)	PDH cofactor Stimulates NADH production	20–30 mg/kg/day 500–1000 mg/day in adults
Riboflavin (B_2)	Cofactor for complex I, complex II, ETF after conversion to FAD, FMP	10 mg/kg/day 50–1000 mg/day in adults
Nicotinamide	Increase NAD, NADH pool	20 mg/kg/day 100–1000 mg/day in adults
Ascorbate (C)	Antioxidant Bypass complex III when given with K_1 or K_3	25–100 mg/kg/day Up to 6 g/day in adults
Menadione (K_3)	Antioxidant Bypass complex III when given with ascorbate	40–80 mg/day
Creatine	Increases muscle phosphocreatine	Up to 10 g/day in adults

ETF, electron-transfer flavoprotein; FAD, flavin adenine dinucleotide; FMP, flavin monophosphate; NAD, nicotine adenine dinucleotide (oxidized); NADH, nicotine adenine dinucleotide (reduced); PDH, pyruvate dehydrogenase complex.

LYSOSOMAL STORAGE DISEASES

INTRODUCTION

Lysosomes are sac-like intracellular cytoplasmic organelles containing hydrolytic enzymes that digest a wide range of macromolecules thus acting as waste disposal units within cells. Lysosomal storage disorders (LSDs) result from deficiencies of one or more of these enzymes leading to the accumulation of substrates that are normally degraded within lysosomes. The majority of known LSDs arise from defects in sugar hydrolases that function in a very acidic lysosomal environment. These 'acid' hydrolases are synthesized and processed in the usual manner of protein synthesis and are then glycosylated in the Golgi, receiving specific mannose side chains that function as recognition sites which allow targeting, binding and uptake into lysosomes. Deficiency of any one of these enzymes causes lysosomal storage of its substrate(s) which then accumulate(s) mainly in the organs where they are synthesized (i.e. liver, spleen, bone and nervous system). This explains the varied organ involvement and symptomatology of these disorders. As the stored materials accumulate within the target cells, they lead to increasingly impaired function of the affected organs. Table 24.28 provides some examples of the accumulation of substrates in a particular tissue.

As of 2001, there were over 40 recognized LSDs corresponding to nearly every step in glycolipid catabolism.[194] A classification scheme is presented in Table 24.29. LSDs include glycolipidoses, mucopolysaccharidoses, glycogenoses, oligosaccharide and glycoprotein degradation disorders, disorders of transport of enzymes into lysosomes, neuronal ceroid lipofuscinoses, and defects of egress of products from the lysosomes. Accumulated substrates have a common structure – carbohydrate attached to a protein or a lipid. Figure 24.28 illustrates the biochemical pathways implicated in many of these disorders.

INCIDENCE AND GENETICS OF LSDs

On an individual basis, LSDs are rare with incidences ranging from about 1:50 000 to disorders with only a handful of case reports published. Some disorders affect up to 10 000 patients worldwide and, as a group, the overall incidence is estimated at 1:7000 to 1:10 000 births.[195,196] Some, particularly Tay–Sachs disease (TSD) and Gaucher disease are much more frequent in specific populations, (these two occurring with increased frequency in Ashkenazi Jews). All, with the notable exceptions of Hunter syndrome, Fabry disease and sialuria are inherited as autosomal recessive traits. Most of the disorders present in childhood. However, some of the disorders do not typically emerge until adult life and almost all have late-onset variants. For the most part, correlations of genotype to phenotype are still not completely understood although, for certain disorders such correlations are beginning to be understood. Thus, a single genotype may lead to a wide range of clinical severity, and in some cases, a single characteristic phenotype may be caused by different genotypes.

GENERAL CLINICAL FEATURES OF LSDs

Storage diseases characteristically have three clinical phases. In the first, which may last from weeks to decades, clinical findings are absent or occult. In the second, which can also be relatively acute or may evolve over decades as the disorder becomes progressively symptomatic, there is increasing evidence of specific tissue involvement. This leads to a third phase in which involved tissues begin to lose function; in those with nervous system involvement, there is progressive neuromuscular deterioration Occasionally, prenatal onset is manifested as non-immune fetal hydrops.

Table 24.28 Disease associated with tissue in which substrates accumulate

Tissue	Disease
Activated macrophages	Gaucher
Muscle	Pompe
Connective tissues	Hurler
Renal endothelium/epithelium	Fabry

GENERAL DIAGNOSIS OF LSDs

The first and perhaps most difficult step in diagnosis of LSDs is the recognition of signs and symptoms suggesting one of these disorders. LSDs should be considered in the following situations: family history of storage disease or a relative who died with signs or symptoms suggestive of LSD, developmental delay especially with regression (loss of developmental milestones), loss of fine motor control, coarse facial features, hepatosplenomegaly or isolated splenomegaly, leukodystrophy, ophthalmological abnormalities including but not limited to cherry red spot, corneal clouding, tortuosity of vessels, or ophthalmoplegia, dysostosis multiplex (characteristic skeletal changes apparent on radiographs), angiokeratomas and neonatal asctites/pleural effusions/hydrops fetalis. Classically, coarsening of the facies associated with neurological deterioration, dysostosis multiplex and/or visceromegaly should certainly lead the clinician to think of a 'storage disease' and request further evaluation.

Diagnostic evaluation at that point usually benefits from the assistance of an experienced clinical biochemist/biochemical geneticist or clinical geneticist because laboratory evaluation for these disorders involves a progressive cascade of biochemical and genetic testing. Mucopolysaccharides (MPS) and oligosaccharides can be screened, quantitated and identified in urine. There are specific enzyme assays for almost all the known disorders but some are only available in special research centers. Some enzymes can be measured in serum, while others require leukocytes or cultured skin fibroblasts. Occasionally, healthy individuals have low activity of one of the enzymes in vitro; it is assumed that their enzyme works normally against the natural substrates in vivo. Conversely, affected individuals occasionally have normal activity in vitro but presumably, inadequate function in vivo. Carrier testing is usually feasible but overlap between carrier range and normal range of enzyme activity and the possibility of partial defects and variants with 'normal' activity is always possible.

When the diagnosis may reasonably be thought to be in one of the classes of LSDs, it may be acceptable to perform a battery of appropriate screening tests, often in urine samples, but if a specific disorder is suspected, then it may only be necessary to perform the assay appropriate for the specific condition. When a LSD is suspected, but the clinical diagnosis is obscure, electron microscopic study of fibroblasts from skin, conjunctival or rectal biopsy, or even leukocytes may reveal the presence of lysosomal inclusions. This testing can then lead to further targeted analyses.

Virtually all of these disorders are amenable to prenatal diagnosis using chorionic villus samples or cultured amniocytes, though this is not a trivial undertaking and prior to requesting the testing, the laboratory offering the service should be contacted to confirm that it can be done.

GENERAL TREATMENT OF LYSOSOMAL DISEASES

There is currently no cure for any of these disorders. Specific therapeutic measures are discussed in the relevant disease sections. Extensive genetic counseling and family support are required.

For all the conditions with neurological deterioration, treatment is directed towards palliation and supportive measures such as

Table 24.29 Classification of the lysosomal storage diseases

Disease	Onset	Enzyme/defect
Sphingolipidoses		
GM_2-gangliosidosis		
type B Tay–Sachs	I,J,A	Hexosaminidase A (alpha chain)
type O Sandhoff	I,J,A	Hexosaminidase A and B (beta chain)
Gaucher disease	I,J,A	Glucocerebrosidase
Fabry disease	J→A	Alpha-galactosidase A
Niemann–Pick disease type A, B	I,J,A	Sphingomyelinase
Niemann–Pick type C	J→A	Defect in cholesterol esterification
Metachromatic leukodystrophy	I,J,A	Arylsulfatase A
MLD with 'normal' enzyme	J	Arylsulfatase A activator protein
Multiple sulfatase deficiency	I,J*	Multiple sulfatases
Krabbe disease	I,J,A	Galactocerebrosidase
Farber syndrome	I	Acid ceramidase
Mucopolysaccharidoses		
Hurler syndrome MPS I H	I,J*	Alpha-L-iduronidase
Hurler–Scheie MPS I H-S	J	Alpha-L-iduronidase
Scheie syndrome MPS I S	J*	Alpha-L-iduronidase
Hunter syndrome MPS II	I,J,A*	Iduronate sulfatase
Sanfilippo syndrome MPS III		
MPS IIIA	J*	Heparan-*N*-sulfatase
MPS IIIB	J*	Alpha-*N*-acetyl glucosaminidase
MPS IIIC	J*	Acetyl-CoA; alpha acetylglucosaminide acetyl-transferase
MPS IIID	J*	*N*-acetyl-glucosamine-6-sulfatase
Morquio syndrome (MPS IV)		
MPS IV-A	J*	Galactose-6 sulfatase
MPS IV-B	J*	Beta-galactosidase
Maroteaux–Lamy syndrome MPS VI	I,J,A*	Arylsulfatase B
Sly syndrome MPS VII	I,J*	Beta-glucuronidase
MPS IX	I,J	Hyaluronidase
Mucolipidoses		
Mucolipidosis II (I-cell disease)	I*	*N*-acetyl-glucosamine-I-phosphotransferase
Mucolipidosis III	J*	*N*-acetyl-glucosamine-I-phosphotransferase
Other lysosomal disorders		
Pompe syndrome (glycogenosis II)	I,J,A	alpha-D-glucosidase (acid maltase)
GM_1-gangliosidosis	I,J,A*	Beta-galactosidase
Aspartylglucosaminuria	J*	Aspartylglucosaminidase
Fucosidosis	I,J*	Alpha-fucosidase
Alpha-mannosidosis	I,J*	Alpha-mannosidase
Beta-mannosidosis	J*	Beta-mannosidase
Schindler disease	I,J*	Alpha-*N*-acetylgalactosaminidase
Disorders involving sialic acid		
Sialidosis type I	J,A*	Neuraminidase
Sialidosis type II (Mucolipidosis I)	I,J*	Neuraminidase
Galactosialidosis	I,J*	Neuraminidase and beta-galactosidase
Mucolipidosis IV	I*	Mucolipin 1
Infantile sialic acid storage disease, Salla disease	I,J,A*	Sialic acid egress from lysosomes
Sialuria	I,J,A	Impaired feedback on synthesis of sialic acid

* Conditions which usually have a 'Hurler-like' storage phenotype. I, infantile: symptoms or diagnosis usual within infancy; J, juvenile: symptoms or diagnosis usual within childhood; A, adolescents or adult: symptoms or diagnosis usually during or after adolescence.

physiotherapy and surgery to counteract feeding, pulmonary and orthopedic problems. Great care must be taken when considering surgery or other procedures in patients with LSDs since, with many, there is grave risk of cervical cord compression and atlanto-occipital dislocation. Anesthesia poses a special risk due to airway narrowing from tissue infiltation, possibile cardiopulmonary disease, and the need to position and stabilize the neck during induction. At present, stem cell (bone marrow or cord blood) transplantation is sometimes used in the hope that donor enzyme might be taken up by host cells and ameliorate or reverse the symptoms.[197–201] Enzyme replacement therapy (ERT) is now available for Gaucher disease and is in active clinical trials for MPS I, II, and VI, and Fabry disease, with still others under development.[202–207] These preparations must be given by regular infusion and are a prelude to true gene therapy. Substrate inhibition is another promising future therapy.[208,209]

THE SPHINGOLIPIDOSES

In sphingolipids, sphingosine is generally linked through its amino group to a variety of fatty acids containing 16–26 carbon atoms. Ceramide is a C-18 sphingosine linked to a fatty acid and therefore, is a long chain amino-alcohol base attached to carboxylic acid. (Fig. 24.29). Esterification through the hydroxyl group on the first carbon of ceramide is the basis for synthesis of many lipid compounds. Ceramide plus sialyloligosaccharides yields gangliosides. Ceramide plus phosphorylcholine yields sphingomyelins. Ceramide plus

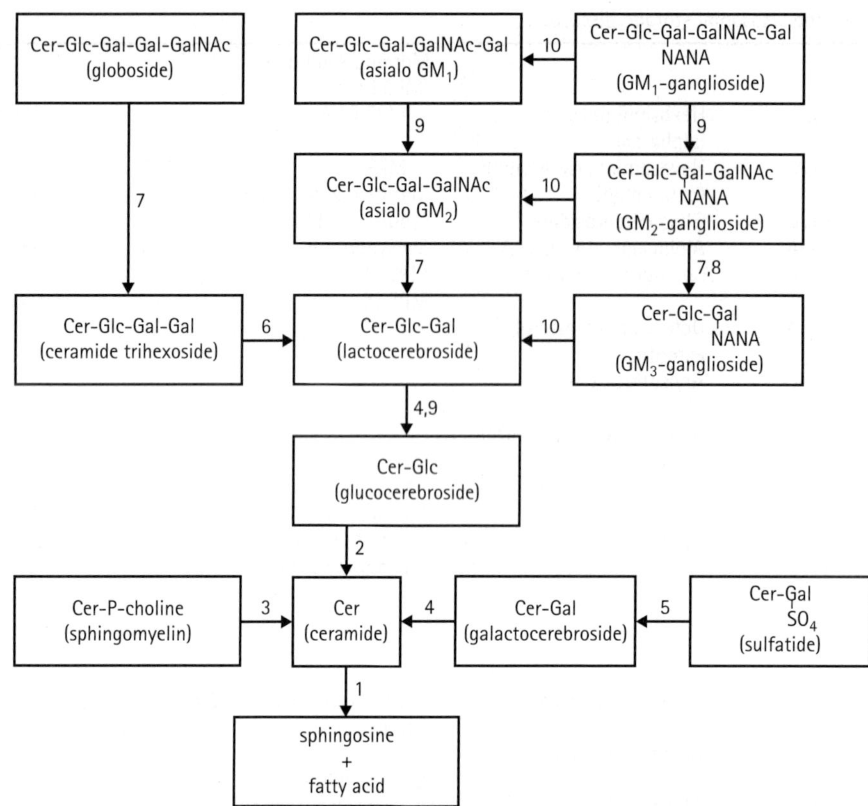

Fig. 24.28 Diagramatic representation of ganglioside and sphingolipid degradation, showing enzyme steps and metabolic blocks. 1, Ceramidase (Farber); 2, α-glucosidase (Gaucher); 3, sphingomylinase (Niemann–Pick); 4, galactocerebrosidase (Krabbe); 5, arylsulfatase A (metachromatic leukodystrophy); 6, α-galactosidase (Fabry); 7, total hexosamindase (Sandhoff); 8, hexosamindase A (Tay–Sachs); 9, β-galactosidase (GM_1-gangliosidosis); 10, α–neuraminidase (sialidosis).

monosaccharides or oligosaccharides yields neutral glycolipids. The glycolipidoses result from defective degradation of these compounds. The degradative pathway for higher gangliosides to sphingosine is depicted in Figure 24.28 in which the sites of known metabolic blocks are indicated. A basic understanding of these biochemical interrelationships is helpful in understanding the classification of the LSDs, in which these different compounds accumulate.

Although the sphingolipid storage diseases are closely related chemically, their phenotype varies considerably depending on the role of the individual metabolites or their precursors in different tissues. For example, glucocerebroside, which accumulates in the liver and spleen of patients with Gaucher disease, is derived from leukocytes which are particularly rich in membrane glycolipids. Gangliosides, on the other hand, are concentrated in neuronal membranes, particularly at nerve endings, thereby involving the gray matter of the brain.

TSD and Sandhoff disease: the GM_2 gangliosidoses

Gangliosides are glycosphingolipids consisting of a ceramide and an oligosaccharide side chain with sialic acid residues. TSD is a progressive neurodegenerative disorder characterized by the deficiency of beta hexosaminidase A (Hex A) and accumulation of ganglioside GM_2. There are two hexosaminidase (N-acetyl glucosaminidase) isoenzymes, acidic (Hex A) and basic (Hex B). Hex A cleaves terminal sugars from GM_2. Hex A is a heterodimer, and has subunits alpha and beta; Hex B has beta-beta subunits. Defects in the alpha subunit cause Hex A deficiency, TSD. Defects in the beta subunit cause Hex B deficiency, Sandhoff disease.

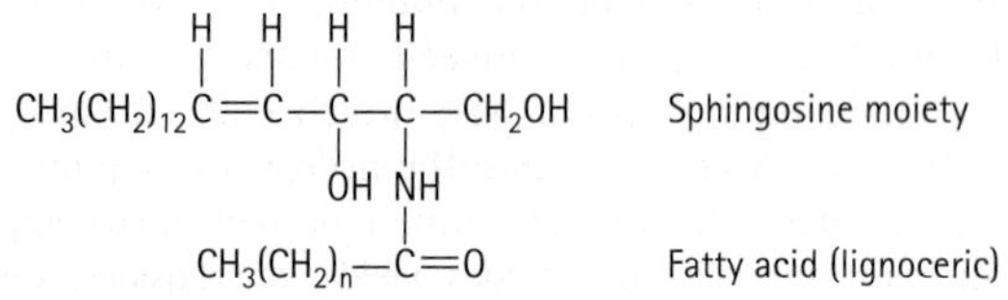

An activator protein (AP) mediates interactions between the substrate and Hex A/B. AP deficiency can also cause TSD.

$$
\begin{array}{ll}
CH_3(CH_2)_{12}\overset{H}{C}{=}\overset{H}{C}{-}\overset{H}{\underset{OH}{C}}{-}\overset{H}{\underset{NH}{C}}{-}CH_2OH & \text{Sphingosine moiety} \\
\qquad\qquad CH_3(CH_2)_n{-}C{=}O \ (\text{bonded to NH}) & \text{Fatty acid (lignoceric)}
\end{array}
$$

Fig. 24.29 Structure of a typical ceramide.

Clinical features

Classic infantile TSD is characterized by the gradual onset of progressive weakness, hypotonia, poor head control, decreasing attentiveness followed by paralysis, dementia, blindness and seizures. Although some motor skills may be achieved, most affected children never sit alone or crawl. An exaggerated startle response is very characteristic, but can also be seen in a few other LSDs. By 6 to 10 months, decreased attentiveness is obvious. A careful ophthalmological examination should reveal cherry red spots at the macula. The cherry red spot is a gray–white halo of lipid laden cells that creates the appearance of a central red spot. (Fig. 24.30). Upper and lower motor neurone signs are present. Seizures begin after 1 year, and macrocephaly is present by 2 years. The second year is characterized by continued deterioration leading to complete unresponsiveness, blindness, deafness and spasticity with decerebrate posture. Death occurs due to pneumonia by 3–5 years.

There are several variants of TSD, including juvenile, adult, and B1 (normal activity with artificial substrate) variants and activator protein defect. Late onset juvenile Hex A deficiency usually presents

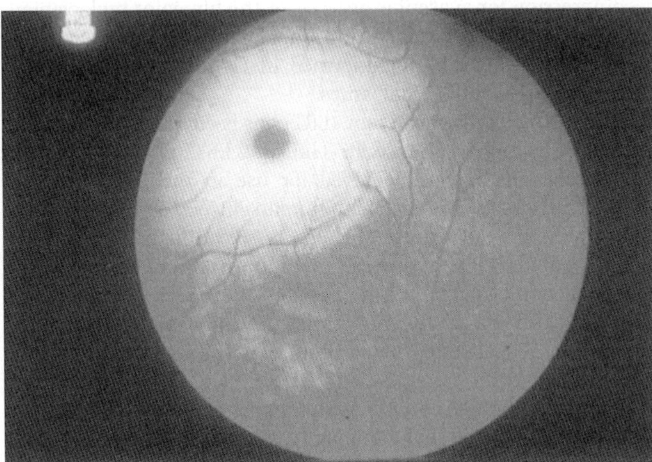

Fig. 24.30 Tay–Sachs disease. A cherry-red spot is seen at the posterior pole due to the presence of ganglioside in the ganglion cells of the macula. There are no ganglion cells at the fovea which presents as a red spot but the surrounding area appears white or milky in color.

between 2 and 10 years of age with ataxia, progressive spasticity, dementia, and increasing seizures. Most patients die as teenagers. Adult forms may also present first in childhood, and are often misdiagnosed as multiple sclerosis.

Infantile Sandhoff disease is clinically similar to infantile TSD but with the combined enzyme deficiency, there is more extensive extraneural involvement with mild visceromegaly and occasional foamy histiocytes in bone marrow or vacuolated lymphocytes in peripheral blood. Minor bony changes may also be present. There is no ethnic predilection. Juvenile and adult forms are also similar to their counterparts of TSD with delayed onset, slower progress and longer survival.

Activator protein deficiency is clinically identical to TSD except that hexosaminidase activities are normal when measured by conventional methods. At postmortem, the pathology is also identical. The defect is in a specific activator protein that facilitates the binding of GM_2-ganglioside to Hex A prior to degradation.

Diagnosis

For both TSD and Sandhoff disease, diagnosis is established by enzyme assay in serum, leukocytes or tissues. The diagnosis of Hex A deficiency requires demonstration of reduced Hex A and normal Hex B activity. Prenatal diagnosis for TSD is performed by enzyme activity in cultured amniocytes or chorionic villus samples. Molecular genetic testing, if feasible, provides even greater specificity.

Routine assays use artificial chromogenic or fluorogenic substrates that can give fallacious results in certain situations. Reference laboratories utilize sophisticated assays to identify unusual variants.

Vacuolated lymphocytes are not present in TSD but may be seen in Sandhoff. Urine oligosaccharides are normal in TSD variants but in the Sandhoff disorders, a number of unusual oligosaccharides have been identified. The pattern may be difficult to interpret.

Cherry red spots were once considered diagnostic of TSD, but can also be found in other forms of GM_2-gangliosidosis and variably in GM_1-gangliosidosis, Niemann–Pick disease, Farber disease and sialidosis. The TSD gene has been identified, and more than 70 mutations are described. There are three common mutations in Ashkenazi Jews, so that mutational analysis is sometimes used for diagnostic testing.

Population screening for TSD

TSD occurred in about 1:3500 Ashkenazi Jews prior to population screening, but only about 1:300 000 non-Ashkenazim; it is also common in French Canadians. Since about 1 in 27 Ashkenazim is a heterozygote (1 in 160 in non-Jews), widespread screening of serum Hex A for heterozygote identification is now common practice in selected populations. Carriers can then be given genetic counseling, including the option of prenatal testing for pregnancies. It is critical to note that pregnancy, certain medications and liver disease invalidate the normal serum test so that under these conditions a leukocyte assay is essential. In the International Tay–Sachs Prevention Program, 1 million people were tested, and the result was a dramatic decrease in TSD in the Jewish population. Since 1970, screening has reduced the incidence from approximately 60 cases per year to 3–5 cases per year in Jews in the USA.

Treatment

Supportive care is the only treatment option at present. There are currently no reports that bone marrow transplantation has been tried in humans, although animal studies show some encouraging preliminary results.[210] Platt and colleagues evaluated a potential strategy for treatment based on *N*-butyldeoxynojirimycin (OGT-918), an inhibitor of glycosphingolipid biosynthesis. TSD mice treated with this agent had no accumulation of GM_2 in the brain.[211]

Gaucher disease

Clinical features

Gaucher disease is the most prevalent of the lysosomal storage diseases. Three types of Gaucher disease have been described and are

Table 24.30 Clinical types of Gaucher disease

Clinical features	Type 1	Type 2	Type 3
Age at onset of signs/symptoms	Any	Infancy	Childhood
Splenomegaly	Mild to extreme	Moderate	Mild to extreme
Hepatomegaly	Mild to extreme	Moderate	Mild to extreme
Skeletal disease/bony crises	Absent to severe	Absent	Moderate to severe
Primary central nervous system disease	Absent	Significant	Mild to significant, increasing with age
Life span	Normal with enzyme replacement therapy	~2 years	2–60 years
Ethnicity	Panethnic	Panethnic	Panethnic
Demographic group	Ashkenazi Jewish		Norrbottnian
Frequency	~1/60 000 to 1/200 000 [~1/500 to 1/1000 Ashkenhazim]	<1/100 000	<1/50 000

summarized in Table 24.30. Type 1 is by far the most frequent. Common presenting signs include splenomegaly (typically 4–70 times the normal size) often with hypersplenism and bone marrow crowding leading to thrombocytopenia and/or anemia with easy bruising or bleeding especially menorrhagia and nosebleeds, less extreme hepatomegaly (1.5–10 times normal) is usual; bony lesions with or without symptoms; avascular necrosis of the hip in adults and growth retardation in children, or delayed puberty in adolescence. There are no neurological problems in type 1 Gaucher disease.

Gaucher disease is sometimes misdiagnosed as lymphoma, leukemia, bleeding disorders, osteomyelitis or Legg–Calvé–Perthes disease. Rarely, pulmonary hypertension, infiltrative lung disease, portal hypertension, and renal involvement are seen.

Type 2 presents with visceromegaly, strabismus, severe neurological dysfunction with spasticity, cortical thumbs, opisthotonos, failure to thrive, and cachexia. Type 3 is typically characterized by severe early onset massive visceral enlargement, and slowly progressive neurological dysfunction. Age at presentation for type 3 is later than type 2, and progression slower. The presentation, however, is variable, and some patients with type 3 do not have massive organomegaly.

Gaucher disease is panethnic but has an incidence of about 1 in 1000 in Ashkenazi Jews in whom it is much more common than in the general population.

Diagnosis

The most accurate diagnosis is by measurement of glucocerebrosidase activity in leukocytes. Abnormal results are often followed up by measurement of enzyme in another cell type such as fibroblasts, and/or by mutation analysis of the glucocerebrosidase gene. There are well established genotype/phenotype correlations, so that it is often possible to predict to some degree the potential severity of the condition by mutation analysis. Typical 'Gaucher cells' (Fig. 24.31) can be seen in bone marrow or liver but this finding is not necessary for establishing the diagnosis. High levels of total acid phosphatase and angiotensin converting enzyme in blood and/or increased levels of glucocerebroside in tissues are also found but are not considered diagnostic.

Treatment

In the past, supportive care included various combinations of iron and vitamin supplementation, transfusions, total or partial splenectomy and androgen therapy. Treatment for skeletal complications included pain management for bone crises, core decompression for avascular necrosis of the hip, joint replacement, fracture management and calcium supplementation. Bone marrow transplantation has been performed in Gaucher patients, but it carries high risk and ethical issues.[199]

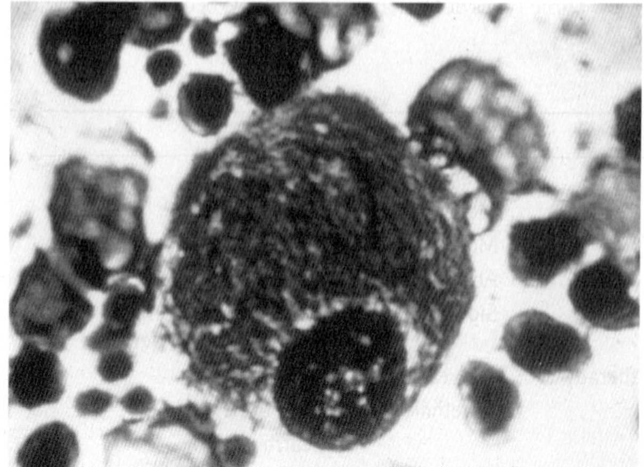

Fig. 24.31 Gaucher cell. Reticulendothelial-derived cell loaded with lipid storage material.

Enzyme replacement therapy (ERT) has become the treatment of choice for Gaucher disease.[202] The first ERT, placental derived glucocerebrosidase, was approved for use in the USA in 1991, followed in 1994 by a recombinant human glucocerebrosidase. At the time of writing, 2800 Gaucher patients in 55 countries worldwide are being treated. ERT improves anemia, thrombocytopenia and hepatosplenomegaly and can probably prevent bone crises and avascular necrosis of the hips if begun early enough. However, established skeletal changes may require 2–3 years for improvement to be noticeable.

Virtually all children with symptomatic Gaucher disease, even those with isolated splenomegaly, should be considered for treatment with ERT since presentation in childhood indicates moderate to severe disease. Asymptomatic adults are sometimes not treated because treatment requires intravenous infusions every 2 weeks, and is extremely expensive.[212] Figure 24.32a,b shows a typical response to ERT in a patient with Gaucher disease.

At the time of writing, an initial phase I gene therapy trial is currently in progress.[213,214] There is also continued research in different formulations and drug delivery methods. Substrate depletion, as discussed for TSD, may also prove helpful.[209] Although certainly not likely to replace ERT, it may be useful as adjunctive therapy.

Fabry disease

Fabry disease is caused by decreased alpha-galactosidase A activity, and intralysosomal accumulation of globotriasylceramide (GB-3) (also known as CTH, ceramide trihexosamide). The frequency of Fabry disease is estimated at 1:40 000–117 000 births. There is no apparent ethnic predisposition toward Fabry disease. There are an estimated 5000 known affected patients worldwide. Generally, each affected family has a unique gene mutation. The gene is on the X chromosome and Fabry disease is usually classified as an X-linked recessive condition, but that is inaccurate since most females, though rarely symptomatic in childhood, eventually develop symptoms showing slower and later progression than men.

Clinical features

Males are typically diagnosed in childhood, and, without dialysis or renal transplant, have a life expectancy of approximately 40 to 50 years. Skin, peripheral nervous system, heart, kidney and brain are the major sites of involvement. The most striking feature in children is attacks of acroparesthesia characterized by intense pain in the hands and feet; other evidence of peripheral neuropathy occurs somewhat later and includes impaired temperature perception and decreased vibratory sense. The diagnosis is often not made for many years until kidney involvement is evidenced first by proteinuria, followed years later by renal dysfunction, progressing to renal failure. CNS involvement may cause transient ischemic attacks and cerebrovascular accidents especially in elderly men. Autonomic nervous system involvement is characterized by dysautonomia, decreased vessel compliance, and hypo/anhydrosis. Hypertrophic cardiomyopathy is the most common cardiac manifestation. Angiokeratomas are clusters of dark, non-blanching, petechioid punctate lesions that are usually present in the 'bathing trunk' area, and especially the umbilicus or scrotum. Abdominal pain is not uncommon and gastrointestinal dysfunction can result in pain, diarrhea and mesenteric infarction. The eyes exhibit whorl-like corneal opacities, and tortuous retinal vessels and retinal vessel occlusion may occur. Constitutional difficulties may include fatigue,

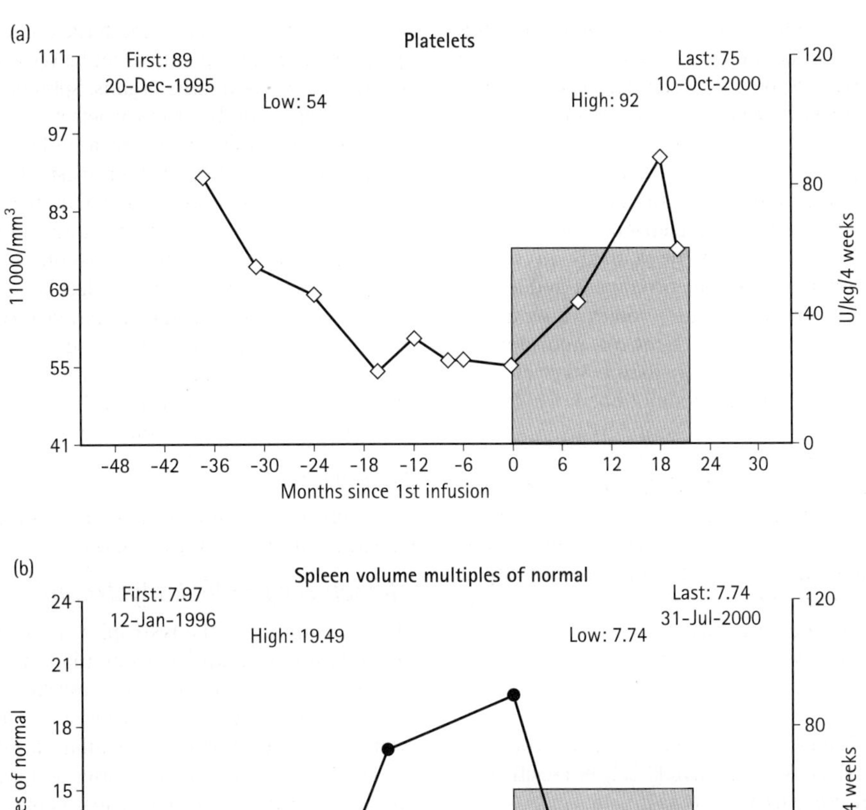

Fig. 24.32 Response of platelet count (a) and spleen volume (b) to enzyme replacement therapy (ERT) in a patient with Gaucher disease.

anhedonia, impaired social functioning, depression and an impaired quality of life. Females show later and slower onset of the same symptoms but rarely progress to renal failure. A small percentage of cases due to 'milder mutations' present with cardiomyopathy in adulthood but few, if any other problems.

Diagnosis

Decreased activity of alpha-galactosidase A in serum, leukocytes or other tissue is diagnostic. In urine, crystalline glycosphingolipids show birefringence under polarization microscopy and appear as characteristic 'Maltese crosses'. Histologically, lipid inclusions and capillary dilation can be seen in skin, and renal biopsies show lipid laden glomeruli. Lysosomal inclusions or vacuoles are present in almost all cell types.

Corneal changes that are virtually pathognomic for Fabry disease can be seen by slit lamp examination and since enzyme activity in females shows overlap between affected 'carriers' and non-carriers, ophthalmological examination may be the best diagnostic test for females in the absence of mutation data.

Treatment

Supportive treatment with analgesics is usually required and the pain may be so intense that narcotic pain medications are needed. In addition, phenytoin, neurontin, carbamazepine or other medications are often useful for pain. Renal dialysis and transplant are used for renal failure but the disorder progresses in other tissues. Two recombinant human alpha-galactosidase products are approved for use in several countries in Europe, but not yet in the USA where FDA approval is still pending.[203,204] Both products appear to offer a major breakthrough in the treatment for this disorder. One trial resulted in the successful clearing of lipid from the kidneys, heart, and skin and another reported a reduction of debilitating pain, and an increased number of days off pain medication.

Niemann–Pick disease types A and B

The common feature of these disorders is accumulation of sphingomyelin. Types A and B are due to primary defects of sphingomyelinase; type C is a completely different entity although the name is retained.

Clinical features

Type A is an acute neuronopathic variant; about 50% of affected patients have Jewish ancestry. Patients usually present in infancy with marked hepatosplenomegaly, failure to thrive and relentlessly progressive psychomotor regression. Typically, during the first 6 months, increasing hepatosplenomegaly is noticed. Lymphadenopathy is also often present. Neurological regression leads to hypotonia and muscular weakness with feeding difficulties. Recurrent vomiting and constipation may occur. A macular cherry red spot is seen in about 50% of affected patients, and there may be corneal and retinal opacification due to lipid deposits. Widespread infiltration of foam cells in the lungs may be detectable on radiographs. Xanthomas and a yellow–brown discoloration of the skin may be observed. Hypersplenism leads to microcytic anemia and thrombocytopenia. Most patients die in the first year or two of life.

Type B is a chronic non-neuronopathic disorder with variable onset in childhood or adult life. All patients have marked hepatosplenomegaly usually with hypersplenism. Patients may suffer general malaise and there may be a delay in sexual development. Lung infiltration may become prominent and lead to respiratory difficulties and cardiopulmonary failure but, unlike Gaucher disease, there is generally no bone or neurological involvement and cherry red spots are rarely found. Most affected children with type B Niemann–Pick live into adulthood.

Diagnosis

Deficient activity of sphingomyelinase in leukocytes or cultured fibroblasts is diagnostic. This enzyme is markedly deficient in the A variant, especially in fibroblasts. Type B patients may have significant residual activities (up to 15% of control), especially in fibroblasts. Foam cells (or 'sea-blue histiocytes') can be seen in bone marrow, liver and spleen, but their presence alone is not diagnostic, since they may be seen in other disorders.

Treatment

Liver transplantation has been used in the severe non-neuropathic cases. ERT is in early clinical trials. This will not likely be effective for type A, but is likely to prove very useful in type B.

Niemann–Pick type C

Niemann–Pick type C is a progressive neurodegenerative disease. It was historically grouped with Niemann–Pick type A and B, but it is a different condition altogether with a very different biochemical defect. Several other names have been given in the past to this condition including juvenile dystonic lipidosis, neurovisceral storage disease with vertical supranuclear ophthalmoplegia and juvenile Niemann–Pick disease with sea-blue histiocytes.

Clinical features

Onset may vary from infancy to late adult life; findings include vertical supranuclear ophthalmoplegia with impairment of upward gaze which is nearly a universal finding, progressive ataxia, dementia, dysarthria, dystonia and tremors, seizures, cataplexy and variable hepatosplenomegaly. School failure (intellectual impairment and impaired fine motor movements) and behavioral problems are common, neonatal hepatitis, sometimes with cholestasis, is often reported and rare cases develop liver failure. As the disease progresses, bulbar palsy, mental regression and encephalopathy set in but affected individuals seem to maintain a cheerful demeanor though they gradually lose contact with the environment. There is generally no cherry red spot. Death typically occurs after one to three decades of deterioration.

Diagnosis

Diagnosis is often significantly delayed, in part due to difficulties in diagnostic testing. On histological examination, foam cells or sea-blue histiocytes are found in many tissues. These are similar to those seen in Nieman–Pick types A and B, Wolman disease and cholesterol ester storage disease and are not specific and may be absent especially in cases without hepatosplenomegaly. Characteristic histiocytes stain with an unusual sea-blue color which gives rise to one of the names of this condition. Neuronal storage with a variety of inclusions may also be present. Skin and conjunctival biopsies usually show inclusions. Unesterified cholesterol, and secondarily, sphingomyelin, phospholipids and glycolipids are stored in excess in the liver, spleen and other organs. Sphingomyelinase activity may be low, but this is not the primary defect.

Cultured fibroblasts show a unique disorder of cholesterol processing – an accumulation of unesterified cholesterol in lysosomes. There is a characteristic pattern of filipin-cholesterol staining in cultured fibroblasts. (Filipin stains unesterified cholesterol.) Niemann–Pick type C cannot currently be diagnosed biochemically with a blood test, but as the molecular genetic basis has just been established, mutational analysis may prove useful diagnostically in the near future. Many cases are misdiagnosed for years as multiple sclerosis, Parkinson's disease, Leigh syndrome, or other mitochondrial disease although the vertical ophthalmoplegia is highly suggestive of Niemann–Pick type C. Prenatal diagnosis is offered in a few centers.

Treatment

No definitive therapy is currently available, but sphingolipid substrate inhibitors may prove useful.

Metachromatic leukodystrophy

Metachromatic leukodystrophy is caused by deficiency of arylsulfatase A leading to accumulation of lipid in neurones. Since sulfatide is a major constituent of myelin, progressive demyelination occurs, leading to a characteristic leukodystrophy. The most common presentations are late infantile and juvenile forms.

There are several arylsulfatases designated as A, B and C; the B enzyme is deficient in Maroteaux–Lamy syndrome (MPS VI) and arylsulfatase C is involved in steroid sulfatase deficiency. All three, as well as iduronate sulfatase, heparan N-sulfatase and N-acetyl-galactosamine-6-sulfatase, are involved in multiple sulfatase deficiency.

Clinical features

In the late infantile type, onset is usually between 1 and 2 years of age with learning difficulties and incoordination and gradually increasing signs of deteriorating psychomotor function with signs of cortical, cerebellar and peripheral nerve involvement. Increasing speech difficulties with dysarthria, ataxia and optic atrophy accompany marked mental and motor regression and within a few years the children are decerebrate, rarely surviving beyond 8 years.

Most patients with the juvenile form present before 6 years, but onset may be delayed past puberty. Subtle behavioral difficulties and declining school performance accompany or precede increasing signs of cortical and cerebellar dysfunction. Clumsiness progresses to ataxia, spasticity and increasingly obvious deterioration. The course is quite variable but most patients succumb by about 20 years of age.

An adult-onset form is rare and may emerge at any age, starting with behavioral or personality changes that may include paranoia, dementia or psychosis. Neurodegenerative signs and peripheral neuropathy become progressively more obvious. Most succumb after a prolonged course.

A defect of the enzyme activator, saposin B, results in a disease that is clinically indistinguishable from the usual cases except that the activity of arylsulfatase A is totally normal in vitro.

Diagnosis

Imaging of the brain shows symmetrical attenuation of white matter most prominent in the parietal and occipital regions. Peripheral neuropathy causes decreased nerve conduction velocity, especially in late infantile and juvenile types and raised protein levels in CSF. Peripheral nerve biopsy shows segmental demyelination with metachromatic material within Schwann cells and histiocytes.

Diagnosis requires enzyme assay in leukocytes or cultured fibroblasts. Assay of enzyme in urine is not reliable. Diagnosis of the activator protein deficiency form requires special sulfatide-loading experiments in cultured fibroblasts. Additionally, urine sulfatide excretion measurement may be helpful in diagnosing atypical cases of metachromatic leukodsytrophy.

The standard enzyme assay uses artificial substrates: values less than 10% of control occur in all types of metachromatic leukodystrophy; however, 2.5% of normal people have 'pseudodeficiency' due to a mutant enzyme with in vitro activity as little as ~20% of normal; these cases require mutational analysis. Because disease-causing and pseudodeficient genes can exist in the same family, prenatal diagnostic testing performed biochemically should always include a study of enzyme activity in the parents, as well as the proband. Chorionic villus tissue, if used for prenatal diagnostic testing, should be used with care due to the presence of high steroid sulfatase activity.

Treatment

Treatment is symptomatic; bone marrow transplantation has its advocates who claim that the process can be stopped within a year and that it will then start to reverse but these results remain to be validated in long term studies.[197]

Other sulfatase deficiencies

Multiple sulfatase deficiency affects several sulfatases and thus exhibits similarities with other LSDs particularily the mucopolysaccharidoses. Thus coarse features, stiff joints, hepatosplenomegaly and short stature are standard findings.

Arylsulfatase C (steroid sulfatase) deficiency causes X-linked ichthyosis and reduced activity in the placenta often results in delayed onset of labor. The gene is located on the Xp22.3-pter region and escapes X-inactivation. A contiguous microdeletion can also involve the Kallman syndrome locus.

Krabbe disease

Krabbe disease (infantile globoid cell leukodystrophy) is caused by deficiency of galactocerebrosidase (galactocerebroside beta-galactosidase or galactosylceramidase).

Clinical features

Krabbe disease is a rapidly progressive, invariably fatal disease. Most patients present between 3 and 6 months with pronounced irritability and increased sensitivity to stimulation. Progressive psychomotor retardation soon becomes obvious with increasing hyperactivity often accompanied by tonic spasms and spasticity. Peripheral neuropathy is evidenced by diminished deep tendon reflexes. There is usually no retinal degeneration nor cherry red spot, however, optic atrophy leads to blindness. Seizures become more frequent and patients rapidly deteriorate, most dying by 2 years of age. There is no visceromegaly and microcephaly is usual. Alternatively, macrocephaly may be found in some cases.

Late infantile, juvenile and adult forms occur but are less common. They are similar to the infantile form but with a more protracted course. The earlier the onset, the more aggressive is the neurological deterioration; later variants may present with loss of vision and hemiparesis.

Diagnosis

Specific enzyme assay in leukocytes or cultured fibroblasts is required for diagnosis. Leukodystrophy is apparent on brain CT scan or MRI and most patients have delayed nerve conduction velocity. CSF protein levels are usually raised in infants but may be normal in older patients.

Treatment

At this time treatment is experimental and limited to stem cell (bone marrow) transplantation in patients with only minimal neurological involvement.[215]

Farber disease

This very rare condition has a number of clinical phenotypes. However, most patients present in the first months of life with joint deformities, subcutaneous nodules and laryngeal involvement. Joints become swollen and painful and contractures then develop. Subcutaneous nodules develop and increase in size and number as the disease progresses; they tend to concentrate around joints or at pressure points. Laryngeal involvement leads to a characteristic hoarseness and both breathing and feeding difficulties develop. In most patients, this, with lung infiltration, usually causes death in the first year or two. Most of the difficulties result from a granulomatous infiltration that causes thickening of cartilaginous tissue. A few patients have had hepatosplenomegaly and macular cherry red spots. Some have a neonatal onset and marked hepatosplenomegaly whereas others have had some neurological involvement and occasionally significant psychomotor regression.

Diagnosis

Ceramidase deficiency can be found in cultured fibroblasts but this complex assay is not widely available. Ceramide levels are increased in the subcutaneous nodules.

MUCOPOLYSACCHARIDOSES

MPS or glycosaminoglycans (GAGs) are complex sugar/protein compounds that require at least 10 different enzymes for their degradation. Deficiency of any one leads to a specific disorder. The nature of the defects is shown in Figure 24.33. The GAGs include dermatan sulfate, heparan sulfate, keratan sulfate and chondroiton sulfate which, if incompletely metabolized accumulate in tissues and are excreted in urine. The pattern of excess GAG excretion may

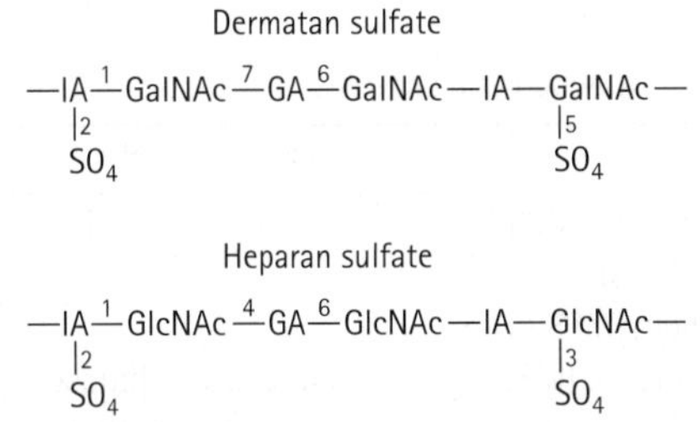

Dermatan sulfate

—IA —1— GalNAc —7— GA —6— GalNAc—IA—GalNAc—
(IA: 2-SO_4; last GalNAc: 5-SO_4)

Heparan sulfate

—IA —1— GlcNAc —4— GA —6— GlcNAc—IA—GlcNAc—
(IA: 2-SO_4; last GlcNAc: 3-SO_4)

	MPS
1. α-L-iduronidase	I
2. Iduronate sulfatase	II
3. Heparin-N-sulfatase	III-A
4. N-acetyl-α-glucosaminidase	III-B
5. Galactosamine-4-sulfatase (arylsulfatase B)	VI
6. β-glucuronidase	VII
7. N-acetyl-β galactosaminidase	

Fig. 24.33 Portions of polysaccharide chains of dermatan and heparan sulfate and nature of the defects in the various mucopolysaccharidoses.

be helpful in the diagnosis of MPS disorders. Lysosomal hydrolases are linkage specific, thus, alpha-L-iduronidase cleaves terminal alpha-L-iduronide from both dermatan sulfate and heparan sulfate which accounts for accumulation of both compounds in Hurler syndrome (Fig. 24.33).

The classification of these disorders is based on the symptoms, the enzyme deficiency, and type of GAG excreted (Table 24.31). MPS types are numbered from Roman numeral I to IX (i.e. MPS I, MPS IX). Some types have now been combined since they are caused by defects of the same enzyme, so that the designations MPS V and VIII no longer are used. Conversely, some types have letters after the numerals, to denote similar clinical conditions that are now known to be caused by different enzyme deficiencies.

Clinical features

Most of these disorders have a chronic and progressive course, generally characterized by coarse facial features, hepatosplenomegaly, corneal clouding, dysostosis multiplex (characteristic bone abnormalities on X-ray), cardiac valvular disease, stiff joints and later, cardiomyopathy. Sanfilippo syndrome is exhibited primarily as developmental regression, and developmental regression is a key feature of several of the MPS disorders. As in most LSDs, there is an initial period of normalcy, followed by insidious onset of signs and symptoms.

The radiographic features of these disorders are referred to as 'dysostosis multiplex'. The earliest findings are in the spine where often T12 and L1 exhibit a hooked vertebral body which progresses to a wedging with loss of anterior mass that results in a worsening gibbus deformity. Eventually, many of the lumbar vertebrae show similar findings that are due to defective ossification of the anterior superior portion of the vertebral body. Striking thoracolumbar platyspondyly occurs in MPS IV. There are obvious changes in the long bones, hands, ribs and clavicle; the basilar portions of the ilia are hypoplastic with flaring of the iliac wings. Dysplasia of the capital femoral epiphyses varies from severe in MPS VI to virtual absence of defect in MPS I – Scheie. Coxa valga and broad femoral necks are seen. There is macrocephaly. Thickening of the calvarium is most apparent over the occiput. The sella becomes J- or shoe-shaped. The optic foramina are enlarged. In addition to the skeletal changes, cardiomegaly is progressive and increased pulmonary markings are frequent.

Several forms of MPS have as a prominent feature CNS involvement and developmental regression. Hydrocephalus, blindness, hearing loss, carpal tunnel syndrome, obstructive airway disease, persistent rhinorrhea, recurrent upper respiratory infections, recurrent otitis media, inguinal and umbilical hernias, hirsutism and thick hair, and spinal cord compression are additional features of these disorders all being due to abnormal accumulation of the GAGs in the affected tissues.

Table 24.31 Mucopolysaccharidoses

Disease	Enzyme defect
Hurler syndrome (MPS I)	Alpha-L-iduronidase
Scheie (MPS I S)	
Hurler–Scheie (MPS I H-S)	
Hunter syndrome (MPS II)	Iduronate sulfatase
Sanfilippo A (MPS III)	Heparan *N*-sulfatase
Sanfilippo B	Alpha-*N*-acetylglucosaminidase
Sanfilippo C	Acetyl-CoA:alpha-glucosaminide acetyltransferase
Sanfilippo D	*N*-acetylglucosamine 6-sulfatase
Morquio (MPS IV A)	Galactose-6-sulfatase
Morquio (MPS IV B)	Beta-galactosidase
Maroteaux–Lamy (MPS VI)	*N*-acetylgalactosamine 4-sulfatase (arylsulfatase B)
Sly syndrome (MPS VII)	Beta-glucuronidase
MPS (IX)	Hyaluronidase

Diagnosis

Several simple urine screening tests are used for detecting increased excretion of GAGs; however, they are relatively insensitive, and non-specific. More useful is quantitation of total GAG excretion, and identification of specific GAGs excreted in urine. Definitive diagnosis of these disorders requires measurement of enzyme activity. Often this can be performed in leukocytes, but in some cases, cultured fibroblasts may be needed. When an MPS is clinically suspected and urine testing non-revealing, enzyme testing may still be warranted. Thus far, mutational analysis has not proven very useful in the diagnosis of MPS disorders nor in providing genotype/phenotype correlations. Hunter syndrome is an X-linked recessive trait but all of the others are autosomal recessive traits. Prenatal diagnosis by amniocentesis or chorionic villous sampling is routine for MPS I and II. The other disorders can also be detected prenatally, but such tests may only be performed in a few specialized laboratories. Carrier testing is possible, but is not always conclusive.

Treatment

There is currently no proven treatment for any of these disorders, although this situation is rapidly changing. Supportive and preventative measures are indicated. Behavioral difficulties may benefit from medications. Stem cell (bone marrow) transplantation may be effective in preventing progression of MPS I and VI and possibly other disorders; it should only be undertaken in specialized centers. ERT is in clinical trials for several of the MPS disorders.[205] Gene therapy is not yet available.

MPS I – Hurler, Hurler–Scheie, and Scheie syndromes

These conditions were earlier thought to be different disorders but they are now known to be caused by different mutations of the mutant gene encoding the enzyme alpha-L-iduronidase. In all, the accumulating GAGs are heparan and dermatan sulfate.

Clinical features

The frequency of MPS I – Hurler syndrome is 1:100 000 in the general population. Patients with MPS I – Hurler are usually diagnosed at 1–2 years of age, and typically have a life expectancy of 6–10 years. Major clinical manifestations include cardiomyopathy, hepatosplenomegaly, skeletal deformity, developmental regression, corneal clouding, hearing loss and dysostosis multiplex.

The frequency of MPS I – Hurler–Scheie syndrome is 1:115 000 in the general population. The condition is merely a more slowly progressive version of Hurler syndrome with one critical exception in that there is no CNS involvement. Patients are often diagnosed at age 2–5 years, with death occurring in the late 20s without treatment.

The frequency of MPS I – Scheie syndrome is 1:500 000 in the general population. MPS I – Scheie is characterized by joint stiffness with tendon compression syndromes (carpal tunnel syndrome), vision impairment (glaucoma), and aortic valve disease. There is normal growth and no CNS involvement, and life expectancy is normal. The differential diagnosis for MPS I – Scheie includes the acquired polyarthropathies and multiple epiphyseal dysplasias.

ERT for MPS I was first attempted in the 1970s but there were significant problems. A recent trial of ERT for MPS I included 10 patients (age 5 to 22 years) who were treated (eight Hurler–Scheie, one Hurler, one Scheie). There were positive results in reduction of organ size and other parameters.[205]

Hunter MPS II

MPS II – Hunter syndrome is caused by a deficiency of the enzyme iduronate sulfatase, and storage of the GAGs dermatan sulfate and heparan sulfate. Signs and symptoms are very similar to MPS I except that the corneae never become cloudy and a pebbly skin lesion, usually most apparent over the scapulae ('peau d'orange') is common. Severe cases usually die in the second decade. Symptoms in mild cases of MPS II include normal intelligence, short stature, and survival to the 20s to 60s. It is estimated that approximately 5000 patients worldwide have MPS II.

Diagnosis

Urine MPS excretion showing increased dermatan and heparan sulfate is suggestive. Measurement of iduronate sulfatase in leukocytes or cultured fibroblasts is the preferred diagnostic test.

Treatment

ERT is in very early clinical trials. Stem cell transplant has not been met with success in treatment of Hunter syndrome.

Sanfilippo syndrome MPS III A, B, C, D

All of the Sanfilippo syndromes are characterized by increased excretion of heparan sulfate. However, this may not be marked, so clinicians should never rely solely on a urine MPS screen to rule out this diagnosis; a high index of suspicion is necessary to establish a diagnosis.

MPS III A – Sanfilippo A is a result of heparan *N*-sulfatase deficiency. Symptoms include developmental regression, hyperactivity and behavioral difficulties including aggressive behavior, mild hepatosplenomegaly and, frequently, very mild bone changes. Coarsening of facial features in the MPS III disorders may be quite subtle or absent, making clinical diagnosis difficult. Life span is into the second to third decade.

MPS III B is caused by a deficiency of alpha-*N*-acetylglucosaminidase. MPS III C is a result of deficient acetyl-CoA: alpha-glucosaminide acetyltransferase and MPS III D is caused by *N*-acetylglucosamine 6-sulfatase deficiency. The symptoms in all three forms are similar to MPS III A.

Diagnosis

Urine GAG excretion is insensitive in testing for MPS III. Enzyme analysis in leukocytes or cultured fibroblasts is necessary.

Morquio syndrome A and B

Clinical features

MPS IV A – Morquio A is caused by deficiency of galactose-6-sulfatase.

Presentation is usually at 18–24 months with gait problems from genu valgum and coxa valga, kyphosis and growth failure. The trunk and neck are obviously short and the facies are broad, but without the coarseness of MPS I or II. In the upper limbs, especially the hands, there is joint laxity rather than contractures. By 6 years, the corneae are typically cloudy, there is progressive spinal deformity with lumbar lordosis, dorsal kyphosis and a barrel-shaped chest (Figs 24.34 and 24.35). Contractures of the knees and hips produce a jockey-like stance and the fingers are short and hypermobile with an ulnar deviation. Cardiac valvular lesions may occur. Intelligence is usually normal. An enamel dysplasia occurs that is not seen in other lysosomal storage diseases. Survival well into adulthood is usual, females seeming to fare better than males.

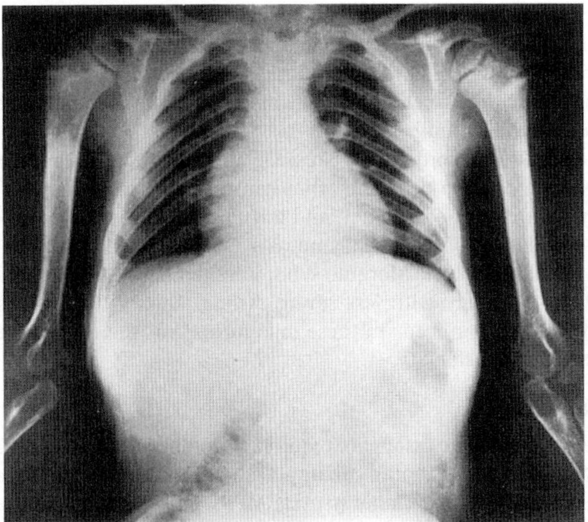

Fig. 24.34 Mucopolysaccharidosis IV. Crowding of ribs by dorsal kyphosis, imperfect modeling at shoulders and elbows.

A common and critical problem is odontoid hypoplasia with subluxation of C1 on C2. Myelopathy may occur acutely or insidiously, being precipitated by even minor trauma including flexion of the neck during anesthesia. Myelopathy may benefit from

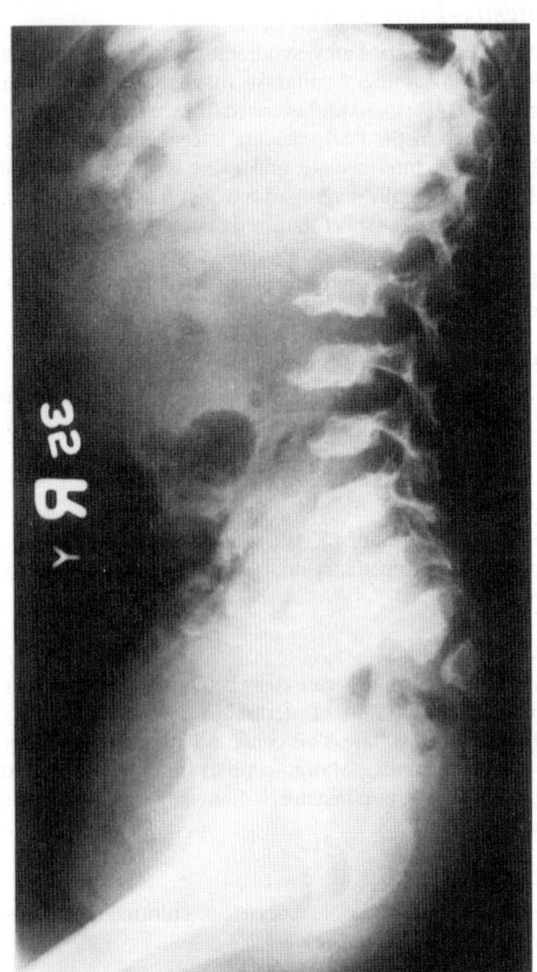

Fig. 24.35 Lateral view of the spine showing platyspondyly in mucopolysaccharidosis IV.

early treatment by surgical fusion of the spine or other orthopedic procedures, but the decision on whether to operate should be carefully considered by experts. Bracing alone is rarely satisfactory. Mechanically induced pulmonary insufficiency and valvular heart disease are eventually fatal.

MPS IV B – Morquio B is caused by deficient beta-galactosidase – the same enzyme deficiency that causes GM_1-gangliosidosis. The degree of enzyme deficiency, and the particular mutation involved determines the phenotype. Symptoms are similar to MPS IV A.

Mild forms of the Morquio syndromes, both MPS IV A and IV B are seen, usually with less severe skeletal changes. Atlantoaxial subluxation can occur in these mild forms, but there may not be atlantoaxial instability.

Diagnosis

Specific enzymatic assays are required to confirm the diagnosis. The GAGs affected are keratan sulfate and chondroitin 6-sulfate. In early childhood MPS IV is similar to other MPSs, but the evolving skeletal features soon become distinctive. A number of skeletal dysplasias with platyspondyly may resemble MPS IV; the spondyloepiphyseal dysplasias are easily confused, but corneal clouding and keratansulfaturia are absent.

Treatment

There is no accepted treatment for MPS IV, but these disorders may prove amenable to ERT.

Maroteaux–Lamy syndrome

MPS VI – Maroteaux–Lamy syndrome results from deficiency of N-acetylgalactosamine-4-sulfatase (arylsulfatase B). Dermatan sulfate is the GAG stored and excreted in excess. There are 50–300 patients known in the USA, yielding a frequency of 1:200 000 to 1:800 000. Mild, intermediate, and severe forms of the disorder are seen. MPS VI is usually diagnosed between 6 and 24 months. Signs and symptoms include short stature, dysostosis multiplex, stiff joints, corneal clouding and normal intelligence. Eventually, cardiac valvular disease occurs. In the severe forms life expectancy is into the second decade.

Diagnosis

Diagnosis is by determination of deficiency of arylsulfatase B in leukocytes or cultured fibroblasts. Urine GAG excretion showing excess dermatan sulfate is suggestive.

Treatment

A phase I clinical trial of ERT showed significant improvements in both primary and secondary endpoints.[216] Treatment at present is supportive.

Sly syndrome

MPS VII – Sly syndrome is caused by beta-glucuronidase deficiency, with resultant excretion of dermatan sulfate, heparan sulfate and chondroitin 6-sulfate. This condition is rare. Severe cases may have hydrops fetalis. Major clinical manifestations include dysostosis multiplex and hepatosplenomegaly with a wide variation in severity.

Diagnosis

Enzyme analysis in serum, leukocytes, or cultured fibroblasts is the diagnostic method of choice.

Treatment

Supportive measures represent currently the only available therapy.

Hyaluronidase deficiency (MPS IX)

Only one patient has been reported. Major findings were transient bilateral nodular soft tissue masses and painful generalized edema. The patient had mildly dysmorphic features, acquired short stature, normal joint movement and intelligence. Pelvic radiographs revealed multiple bilateral nodular, intra-articular soft-tissue masses, and acetabular erosions.

MUCOLIPIDOSES (ML-II AND ML-III)

These two conditions are allelic and due to a defect of N-acetylglucosamine-l-phosphotransferase which normally attaches phosphate to a polymannose side chain on the precursor proenzymes in the Golgi. As a result the lysosomal enzyme targeting and uptake system is dysfunctional and several lysosomal enzymes that were destined for uptake into lysosomes are elevated in serum, their electrophoretic patterns are altered and multiple enzyme deficiencies inside the lysosomes account for a heterogeneous accumulation of storage material. The gross cytoplasmic inclusions seen in cultured fibroblasts gave rise to the name 'inclusion (I)-cell disease' (clinical features shown in Fig. 24.36).

ML-II and ML-III are alternatively named I-cell disease and pseudo-Hurler polydystrophy. They are similar to severe and mild Hurler syndrome respectively. In type II, in contrast with most of the LSDs, features may be detectable at birth. ML-III is milder and is often diagnosed as polyarticular arthropathy for years before the true cause is recognized. In neither form is corneal clouding a feature. Clinical and radiological appearances are shown in Figures 24.36–24.38.

Diagnosis

Diagnosis is established based on the clinical findings associated with elevated levels of several lysosomal enzymes in serum.

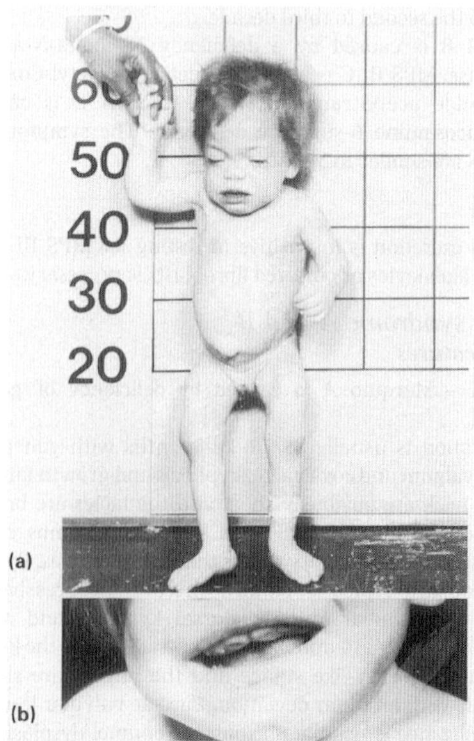

Fig. 24.36 Mucolipidosis II (I-cell disease) in an 18-month-old girl. (a) Facies and habitus, (b) gum hypertrophy.

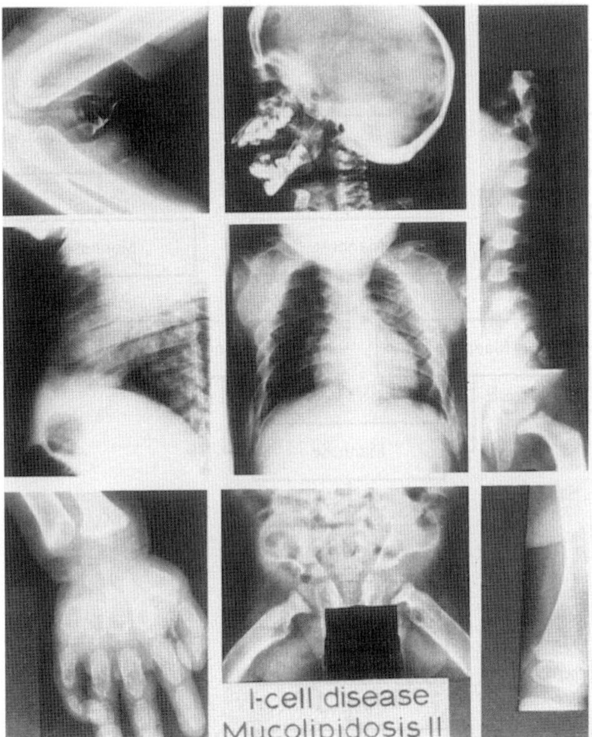

Fig. 24.37 Radiological changes in mucolipidosis type II in an 18-month-old girl.

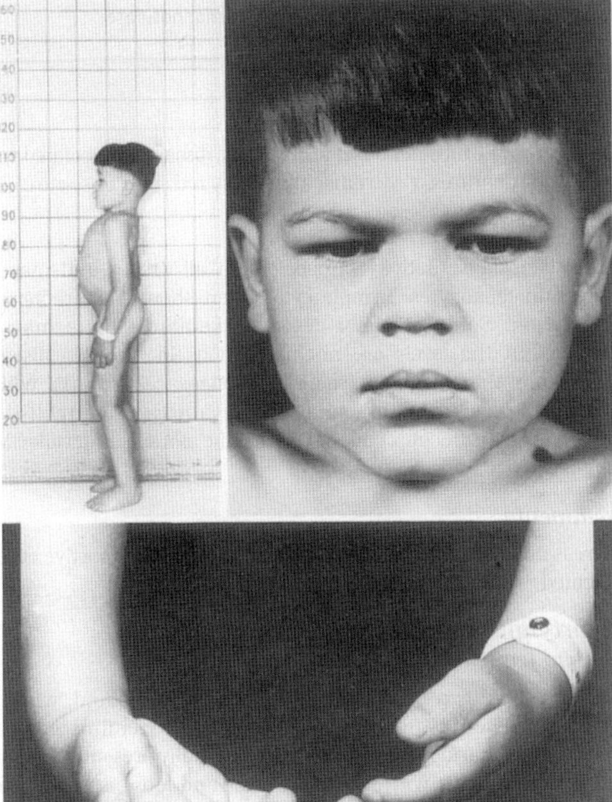

Fig. 24.38 Mucolipidosis III in an 11-year-old boy showing facies, dwarfed stature, barrel-shaped chest, lordosis and claw hands.

Measurement of the specific enzyme defect in these disorders is difficult, and may not be available as a clinical diagnostic test.

Treatment

There is no cure and no proven effective treatment for ML-II or ML-III.

POMPE DISEASE

The incidence of Pompe disease is 1:40 000–1:100 000. Pompe disease is caused by lysosomal acid maltase deficiency. Acid maltase catalyzes the cleavage of alpha-1,6 and alpha-1,4 linkages in glycogen and therefore completely hydrolyzes glycogen. It is present in all tissues, fibroblasts and lymphocytes. The worldwide prevalence is 5000 or more. The clinical presentation of infantile Pompe disease is a result of massive glycogen deposition in the liver, heart, and skeletal muscle and is sometimes alternatively classified as a glycogen storage disorder (see p. 1209).

Clinical features

Infantile Pompe disease manifests at age 2–5 months with variable hepatomegaly, cardiomegaly, hypotonia and weakness; death typically occurs at 1–2 years of age. Juvenile and adult variants of Pompe disease are recognized. Juvenile Pompe disease is diagnosed at age 2–5 years, with death around age 20. Adults are typically diagnosed in the third or fourth decade, and may have predominantly skeletal and not cardiac involvement. The myopathy in all types of Pompe disease is caused by the storage of glycogen in skeletal and cardiac muscle, leading to progressive muscle weakness and respiratory insufficiency.

Diagnosis

The diagnosis of Pompe disease can be suspected by characteristic ECG findings (shortened PR interval and large QRS complexes) and confirmed by demonstration of deficient acid maltase in cultured fibroblasts or muscle.

Muscle biopsy reveals glycogen freely dispersed in the cytoplasm and vacuoles that stain for glycogen [periodic acid-Schiff (PAS)+] and acid phosphatase. Increased glycogen content is usually found, though this is variable. Electron micrographs showing intralysosomal accumulation of glycogen are also highly suggestive, though not alone diagnostic of Pompe disease.

Prenatal diagnosis can be accomplished in cultured amniocytes or by chorionic villus biopsy by measurement of enzyme activity. Carrier testing shows significant overlap of enzyme activity in normals and carriers.

Treatment

ERT for Pompe disease is in early clinical trials. Enzyme derived from milk of transgenic rabbits was effective, as was recombinant human acid maltase from Chinese hamster ovary (CHO) cells.[206,207]

THE OLIGOSACCHARIDOSES, GLYCOPROTEINOSES

The glycoproteinoses are rare disorders in which different enzyme deficiencies result in accumulation of oligosaccharides that are excreted in excessive amounts in urine; some have ethnic predilections. The clinical presentations are often similar to a mild mucopolysaccharidosis but with no increased excretion of GAGs. The structures of two typical oligosaccharide chains are shown in Figure 24.39. As with all untreated lysosomal storage diseases, once the conditions manifest, they follow a steady downhill course. No specific treatment is available.

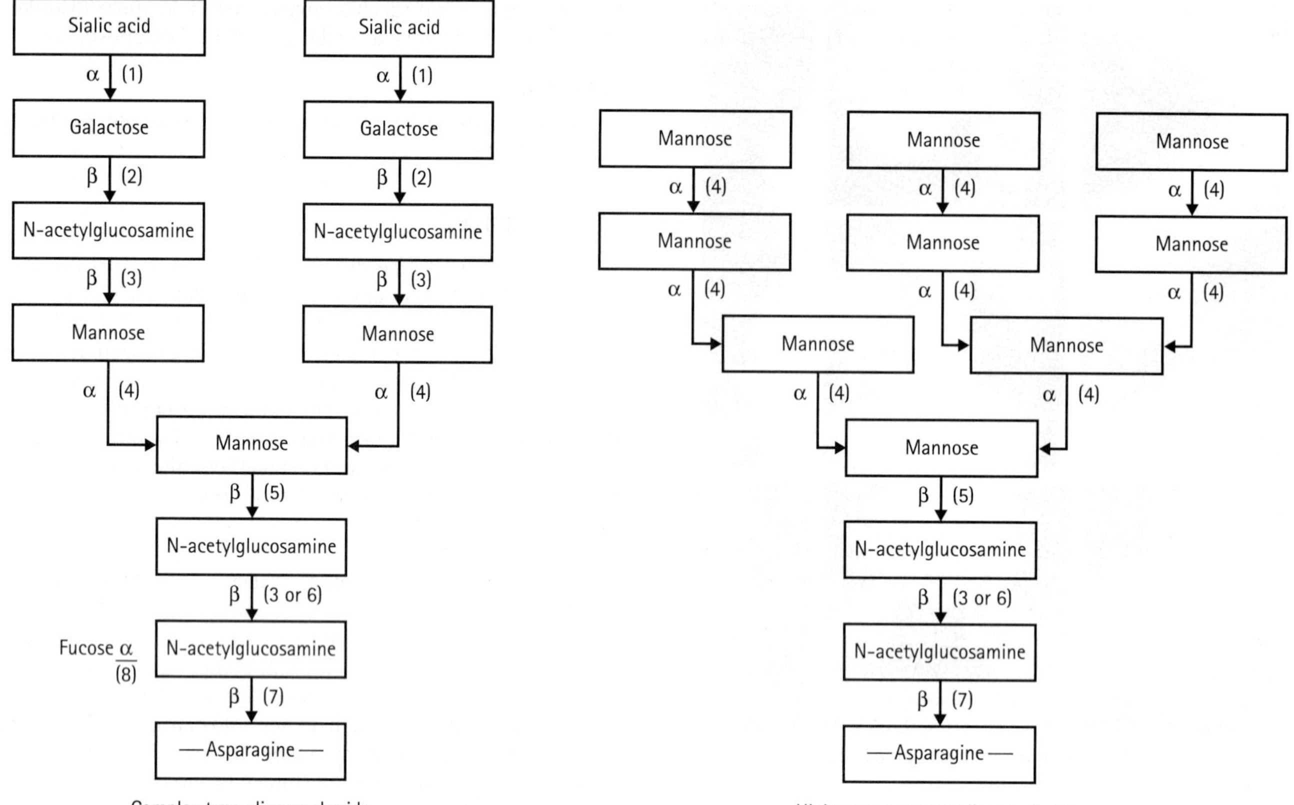

Fig. 24.39 Structures of two typical oligosaccharide chains as found on glycoproteins. Alpha and beta linkages are indicated and the specific degradative enzyme steps are numbered as follows: 1, α-neuraminidase; 2, β-galactosidase; 3, β-hexosaminidase; 4, α-mannosidase; 5, β-mannosidase; 6, endo-β-hexosaminidase; 7, aspartylglucosaminidase; 8, α-fucosidase.

GM_1-gangliosidosis (beta-galactosidase deficiency)

Three forms of GM_1-gangliosidosis have been described; the most common is the infantile form (type I). All patients have the same enzyme deficiency as do patients with Morquio type B (MPS IV B) and galactosialidosis (combined with neuraminidase deficiency).

Clinical features

Classic or infantile GM_1-gangliosidosis presents in the first months of life with increasing evidence of CNS damage, psychomotor retardation, failure to thrive and severe developmental delay. The facies are coarse with frontal bossing and hypertrophy of the gums, similar to that seen in the mucopolysaccharidoses. About 50% have a macular cherry red spot. Affected patients become blind and often exhibit an exaggerated startle response. Hepatosplenomegaly is usual and cardiomyopathy may develop. Dysostosis multiplex is prominent. By 1 year of age seizures are usual and continued deterioration results in respiratory failure with death by 2 years of age.

Juvenile GM_1-gangliosidosis (type II) has a later onset and the course is slower. Skeletal changes, hepatomegaly and cherry red spots are usually absent. Slowing of normal development starts around 1 year of age progressing to seizures, abnormal movements and progressive decline in function, leading to death between 3 and 10 years of age.

Adult GM_1-gangliosidosis (type III) with onset in the second or third decade, appears to be the least common variant but may be more frequent in Japan. Symptoms include slowly progressive dystonia, spinocerebellar degeneration and increasing cognitive deficits. None of the later onset forms of the disease is associated with dysmorphic features, visceromegaly, cherry red spots or seizures.

Diagnosis

Beta-galactosidase activity is deficient in all tissues and may be assayed in leukocytes. Lymphocytes often show a characteristic vacuolation. Some partially degraded keratan sulfate may be excreted but the levels are not as high as in Morquio disease. More often there is a characteristic oligosacchariduria which includes a specific octasaccharide. At autopsy, many tissues contain large histiocytes ballooned with the storage material, GM_1-ganglioside.

Treatment

There is no accepted treatment for this condition; supportive care is indicated.

Aspartylglucosaminuria

Clinical features

Most of the known cases have originated from Finland, where a very consistent phenotype somewhat reminiscent of mucopolysaccharidosis is found. Patients usually present between 1 and 5 years of age with coarse features and loose, sagging skin, often with prominent acne. Angiokeratomas are common. Growth is usually poor, often with radiographic evidence of mild dysostosis multiplex. Connective tissue involvement leads to joint laxity. Progressive mental deterioration and bizarre behavior become evident between 6 and 15 years with death 20–30 years later with pulmonary disease. About a third of patients have corneal opacities but there is generally no significant hepatosplenomegaly. Recurrent respiratory infections, urinary tract infections, hernia, clubfoot or planovalgus deformity, and strabismus are frequent.

Diagnosis

The deficient enzyme is aspartylglucosaminidase, which can be demonstrated in sonicates of white blood cells or fibroblasts. Most patients have vacuolated lymphocytes and lymphopenia and increased levels of glycoasparagines are found in urine on oligosaccharide analysis. Urine amino acid analysis with a method using Ninhydrin and chromatography may detect aspartylglucosamine, and be a useful, rapid adjunct to definitive diagnostic testing.

Treatment

Stem cell transplantation should be considered.[201]

Fucosidosis

Clinical features

Two major presentations are recognized: a severe form (type I) with onset between 3 and 18 months and type II with a less severe and more protracted course. The condition is rare.

Both types are similar to the MPS phenotype with skeletal abnormalities, coarse facial features, growth retardation, hepatosplenomegaly, cardiomegaly and mental retardation. Type I patients may never achieve their milestones and may never be able to sit unsupported. Type II patients have angiokeratomas identical to those seen in Fabry disease.

Diagnosis

Deficient alpha-fucosidase activity in leukocytes is diagnostic. Both types exhibit vacuolated lymphocytes and increased levels of Lewis A and B antigens in erythrocytes and saliva (these antigens characteristically contain fucose linked (1–>4) to N-acetyl-glucosamine). Oligosaccharide analysis of urine is helpful.

Treatment

Stem cell transplantation should be considered.[201]

Alpha-mannosidosis

Clinical features

Two phenotypes are described; both are rare. Type I presents between 3 and 12 months and type II between 1 and 4 years. The clinical features, however, are very similar and include mildly coarse MPS-like facial appearance, marked mental retardation, recurrent infections, impaired speech, hearing loss, corneal clouding, hepatosplenomegaly and dysostosis multiplex. There may also be marked hyperplasia of the gingiva similar to that seen in I-cell disease.

Diagnosis

Vacuolated lymphocytes are generally present in peripheral blood and bone marrow. Several mannose-rich oligosaccharides are found in urine but the urinary GAG pattern is normal. There is deficiency of a specific acid alpha-mannosidase, measurable in leukocytes.

Treatment

Stem cell transplantation should be considered.[201]

Beta-mannosidosis

Clinical features

The few reported severe cases have had seizures, quadriplegia and rapid decline to death. Symptoms have included mental retardation, angiokeratoma, feeding difficulties, recurrent infections, speech difficulties and hearing loss.

Diagnosis

Beta-mannosidase activity is markedly deficient in all tissues, and may be measured conveniently in leukocytes. Vacuolated lymphocytes are not present and the major storage substance is an oligosaccharide that may co-chromatograph with lactose.

Treatment

There is no proven treatment.

Schindler disease

Clinical features

This rare disorder is due to deficiency of alpha-N-acetylgalactosaminidase. Type I is an infantile onset neuroaxonal dystrophy with rapid deterioration starting about 1 year and leading to pancerebral damage, blindness and myoclonic seizures. There is no visceromegaly nor any peripheral storage cells.

Type II develops later, even in midlife. Angiokeratoma corporis diffusum, lymphedema and mild, progressive cerebral involvement are reported; inclusions may be seen in leukocytes and dystrophic axons are seen in rectal biopsies.

Diagnosis

Urinary oligosaccharides are abnormal. Enzyme assay, the definitive diagnostic test, can be performed in leukocytes.

The sialidoses

The sialic acids are a family of compounds derived from neuraminic acid. Neuraminidase deficiency occurs in several forms.

Clinical features

In type I (cherry red spot–myoclonus syndrome) debilitating myoclonic seizures and sometimes movement disorders develop, usually in the second decade and are accompanied by progressive visual loss associated with cherry red spots at the macula. Nystagmus, ataxia and seizures may occur. The intelligence is usually preserved until late and visceromegaly and bony abnormalities are mild or absent.

Type II (previously called mucolipidosis type I) is more severe and can present with fetal hydrops, neonatal ascites or in infancy. The phenotype is reminiscent of an MPS disorder with severe dysostosis, hepatosplenomegaly and developmental delay. Survival depends upon the severity of the symptoms.

Galactosialidosis is very similar to type II sialidosis. An early infantile form is characterized by coarse facies, macrocephaly, growth disturbance, hepatosplenomegaly, fetal hydrops, ascites, kidney and heart involvement, angiokeratomata, telangiectasia, seizures, myoclonus, ataxia, pyramidal tract signs, progressive neurological deterioration, cherry red spots, lens opacity, corneal clouding, hearing loss, dysostosis multiplex and foam cells. Late infantile cases present with somewhat less severe findings and slower progression. A late juvenile form is most common in Japan; symptoms develop more insidiously with survival into adult life.

Diagnosis

Alpha-neuraminidase activity is deficient in types I and II. The defect is best demonstrated in cultured fibroblasts. In galactosialidosis, there is a combined deficiency of neuraminidase and beta-galactosidase activity due to lack of a specific intralysosomal protein that protects these enzymes from degradation. In all three disorders, foam cells may be seen in bone marrow. Vacuolated lymphocytes are rare in type I but present in type II. Vacuoles and lysosomal inclusions in other cells may be marked. The urine contains several sialylated oligosaccharides that can be detected.

Treatment

Unfortunately, there is no treatment available for these conditions.

Mucolipidosis IV

Clinical features

ML IV is a rare neurodegenerative lysosomal storage disorder characterized by psychomotor retardation, corneal clouding, retinal degeneration and strabismus. There is wide variability in severity. This condition is one of the Jewish genetic diseases, and more than 80% of the patients described have been Ashkenazi Jewish. The carrier frequency in Ashkenazi Jews has been estimated at 1 in 100. The condition is described as a mucolipidosis, as there is storage of lipids and water soluble substances. Presentation is typically in infancy or early childhood, with severe psychomotor retardation that becomes evident by 2–3 years of age. There is no facial dysmorphism, visceromegaly or skeletal changes; retinal degeneration is usual. Patients can live well into the third decade, but the top developmental level reached is often 12–15 months. Iron deficiency anemia is common.

Diagnosis

There is no cellular metachromasia or mucopolysacchariduria although gangliosides and MPS accumulate in fibroblasts and inclusions can be seen in many tissues including conjunctiva. The defect lies in the MCOLN1 gene, and two mutations account for 95% of disease alleles in Ashkenazi Jews in a recent study. Therefore, if available, molecular genetic testing could be diagnostic. The defective protein, mucolipin 1, has unknown function.

Treatment

There is no treatment available for this condition.

Infantile sialic acid storage disease (ISSD), Salla diseases, sialuria

Clinical features

Four clinical entities present with intracellular accumulation and urinary excretion of sialic acid:

1. ISSD and Salla disease are probably allelic disorders, caused by mutations of a gene coding for a lysosome membrane transport protein.
2. Sialuria is a genetic error of impaired feedback inhibition in the synthesis of sialic acid.
3. Sialidosis is due to deficiency of lysosomal neuraminidase leading to storage of undegraded sialyloligosaccharides, or bound sialic acid.
4. Galactosialidosis is due to deficiency of a 32-kDa protective protein, and affected patients also excrete sialyloligosaccharides in urine.

ISSD is very rare, presenting with a severe 'Hurler' phenotype. Some patients have had punctate calcification of the epiphyses similar to Zellweger syndrome. There is also marked hypopigmentation with pale wispy hair. Growth retardation is common but there may only be mild radiological abnormalities. There is generally no corneal clouding but optic atrophy is common. Marked failure to thrive leads to death in the first years of life.

In Salla disease, symptoms emerge in the first year or two of life, but most patients live for decades. Symptoms include ataxia, athetosis and pyramidal signs. Many patients are exotropic and later, most develop mild 'storage' facies. There is usually no corneal clouding and the fundi are normal. Speech is primitive and most patients have a very low IQ. Growth retardation is usual, but apart from a somewhat thickened calvarium, the radiological picture is usually normal.

Sialuria is a separate condition presenting with developmental delay, visceromegaly and coarse facies. There is massive excretion of free sialic acid in urine but no lysosomal storage. It is caused by overproduction of sialic acid due to a failure in negative feedback control on uridine diphosphate N-acetyl-glucosamine-2-epimerase. Galactosialidosis and sialidosis are described earlier in this chapter.

Diagnosis

In the infantile disease there are prominent lysosomal vacuoles in lymphocytes and urinary free sialic acid levels are increased some 10-fold above normal in urine, leukocytes and fibroblasts. GAG excretion is normal but abnormal urinary oligosaccharides can be seen using a resorcinol reagent. Patients with Salla disease have similar but less severe findings. In sialuria, the cells contain non-lysosomal sialic acid in the cytosol. Prenatal diagnosis is possible and sialic acid is markedly raised in affected amniotic fluid in the infantile disease but not in Salla disease. Chorionic villus cells are vacuolated.

Treatment

There is no proven treatment.

CYSTINOSIS

Cystinosis occurs with an incidence of approximately 1 in 60 000 births. Cystinosis is a disorder of lysosomal transport in which there is intralysosomal storage of cystine in many tissues, secondary to deficient egress from the lysosomes. It is the most common cause of the renal Fanconi syndrome in childhood.

Clinical features

Children with infantile cystinosis present in the first year with tremendous water and salt craving, food refusal and failure to thrive, vomiting, lethargy, polyuria, irritability, anorexia and signs of progressive renal tubular and glomerular damage which can lead to death in the first decade. Growth failure is usually severe and rickets may be prominent. The skin is pale and the hair becomes blond due to inhibition of melanin formation; photophobia is common, probably due to a characteristic retinopathy combined with a crystal keratopathy. Progressive damage of the thyroid gland causes hypothyroidism and later, proximal myopathy and cerebral lesions may develop.

Milder variants present in childhood or adolescence with a slower progression of retinopathy and renal disease; there is also an adult form in which there is no renal damage, although cystine crystals are still present in the eye.

Diagnosis

The biochemical features of the severe form are those of the renal Fanconi syndrome with renal tubular acidosis, hypokalemia, hypouricemia, hypophosphatemia, glycosuria, proteinuria and aminoaciduria being prominent. Plasma amino acids, including cystine, are normal or low. The diagnosis may be confirmed by the demonstration of refractile corneal crystals seen on slit lamp examination (they can also be seen in bone marrow, lymph node, conjunctival or rectal biopsy) and by measurement of intracellular cystine levels in leukocytes or cultured skin fibroblasts (up to 100 times normal); levels in heterozygotes are typically 5–10 times normal. Histological examination shows severe damage of the proximal renal tubules. Cystinotic cells take up 35S-cysteine at about twice the normal rate but accumulate the disulfide, cystine, in greatly increased amounts.

Treatment

There is no cure. Therapy is directed towards correction of the fluid and electrolyte imbalances, acidosis, rickets and hypothyroidism. Dietary restriction of cystine and methionine, along with penicillamine, have no effect. Cysteamine or phosphocysteamine are the drugs of choice since they deplete intracellular cystine; they must be given every 6 h and the dose monitored by regular assay of leukocyte cystine; these drugs delay or prevent renal failure and other systemic consequences. Advanced renal failure is treated by renal transplantation; the transplanted kidneys do not express the cystinotic defect and have the same prognosis as kidneys transplanted for other reasons. The biochemical defect, however, continues in other tissues and long term complications, including a myopathy and central nervous system damage, are now recognized.

NEURONAL CEROID LIPOFUSCINOSIS (NCL)

Genetics

The neuronal ceroid lipofuscinoses are a group of disorders that, collectively, are one of the most common causes of progressive neurodegeneration in childhood. Recently, several of these disorders have been identified as lysosomal storage diseases. Infantile (Santavuori–Haltia) (CLN1), late infantile (Jansky–Bielschowsky) (CLN2), juvenile (Batten, Spielmeyer–Vogt) (CLN3), and adult (Kufs) (CLN4) onset forms are considered 'classic' clinical presentations but as many as 20% of cases are 'atypical' and CLN 4–8 are described in specific populations. Eight different gene loci are currently known; CLN1, 2, 3, 5 and 8 have been characterized but the molecular genetic and biochemical bases for CLN4, 6 and 7 remain unknown at the time of writing.[217] CLN1 codes for palmitoyl-protein thioesterase 1 and CLN2 for tripeptidyl peptidase 1. It is critical to recognize that even a single classical clinical variant can be caused by several different gene defects depending upon the severity of the mutations (Table 24.32).

Lipofuscin is an autofluorescent complex of lipid and protein that can be detected in lysosomes by electron microscopy.

Clinical

Common to all forms of NCL is the development of signs of neurological impairment that may be rapid or slow, followed by seizures, often myoclonic and overt deterioration, involving all brain functions, that leads inevitably to death. The younger the onset, the more rapid the progression. Infants may die within a year or two, but in the juvenile cases survival may be 10–20 years. In the juvenile form, the first symptom is often rapid loss of vision over a few months before any other signs of brain involvement are evident. Sudden onset of seizures can also precede overt deterioration. Cerebral atrophy is apparent by MRI even before the onset of symptoms. In adults, initial symptoms include psychiatric disorders, myoclonic seizures and signs of pyramidal involvement. In most of the forms, there is a characteristic pigmentary retinopathy; it is notably absent in at least one form of late infantile NCL reported from Finland. There is no dysmorphism nor visceromegaly.

Diagnosis

Early changes can be seen in visual evoked responses, ERG and MRI of the brain. Detailed ophthalmologic examination is useful. Diagnosis is based on detection of characteristic 'curvilinear' and fingerprint inclusions in lysosomes. The deposits are distinctive but with subtle differences in each subtype; rare cases show a granular appearance. In the late infantile and juvenile forms, the lipofuscin contains a large amount of subunit C of ATP synthase; in the infantile form the deposits do not contain this subunit, but rather, sphingolipid activator protein. The reason for the incorporation of these products is not known.

Table 24.32 Types and features of neuronal ceroid lipofuscinosis (NCL)

Major types	Frequency % of total NCL	Age of onset	Usual gene	Other reported genes
Infantile	~16	0–3 years	CLN1	
Late infantile	~50	2–8 years	CLN2	CLN 1,2,5,6,7
Juvenile	~30	4–10 years	CLN3	CLN1,2
Adult	~2	11–55 years	CLN4	

Deposits of lipofuscin can be found in most tissues but experts differ as to which tissue should be used for optimal chances of findings the lysosomal inclusions. In the juvenile form, many cases are diagnosed by electron microscopic examination of leukocytes, however, this is not always reliable; moreover, in some forms of NCL, the inclusions are sparse or absent in leukocytes. In addition to leukocytes, examination for inclusions may be performed in uncultured skin fibroblasts, rectal biopsy or in conjunctival biopsy. What may be most important in the selection of tissue to biopsy is the experience of the laboratory in working with the various tissues. Prenatal diagnosis can often be achieved through a combination of microscopic and/or biochemical and genetic studies.

Treatment

No definitive treatment is known to affect the outlook; treatment is purely supportive. Hematopoietic stem cell transplants have been reported in a few cases, but the results have, for the most part, been disappointing.

CONGENITAL DISORDERS OF GLYCOSYLATION

CONGENITAL DISORDERS OF GLYCOSYLATION TYPE I

Patients with congenital disorders of glycosylation (CDG) type I have defects in the N-glycosylation pathway caused by malfunction of cytoplasmic or endoplasmic reticulum enzymes responsible for oligosaccharide assembly or the attachment of oligosaccharides to proteins.[218,219] Screening for these disorders is performed by analyzing the glycosylation pattern of serum transferrin by isoelectric focusing (IEF), although a rapid mass spectrometry test has recently been described.[221] A typical electrophoresis banding pattern characterized by increased asialo- and disialotransferrin and decreased tetrasialo- and pentasialotransferrin is diagnostic of CDG type I. To date, seven different disorders have been associated with the CDG type I transferrin IEF pattern (CDG types Ia to Ig, Table 24.33).

Clinical features (Table 24.34)

CDG type Ia

Patients with CDG type I may present with a wide variety of clinical features, although neurological impairment is often the most striking finding.[221] CDG type Ia (phosphomannomutase deficiency) is by far the most commonly encountered entity, making up ~75–80% of CDG type I cases.[218] Although most reports have involved patients of northern European descent, CDG type Ia is panethnic in distribution. To date, > 300 patients with CDG type Ia have been detected worldwide.[222] Prominent neurological involvement (neonatal

Table 24.33 Congenital disorders of glycosylation types I and II

Disorder	Enzymatic or protein defect	Gene
CDG Ia	Phosphomannomutase	PMM2
CDG Ib	Phosphomannose isomerase	PMI
CDG Ic	Dolichol-P-Glc:$Man_9GlcNAc_2$-PP-dolicholglucosyltransferase	ALG6
CDG Id	Dolichol-P-Man:$Man_5GlcNAc_2$-PP-dolicholmannosyltransferase	ALG3
CDG Ie	Dolichol-P-mannose synthase	DPM1
CDG If	LEC35 protein	LEC25MPDU1
CDG Ig	Dolichol-P-Man:$Man_7GlcNAc_2$-PP-dolicholmannosyltransferase	ALG12
CDG IIa	N-acetylglucosaminyltransferase II	MGAT2
CDG IIb	Glucosidase I	GSI

CDG, congenital disorders of glycosylation; Glc, glucose; GlcNAc, N-acetylglucosamine; Man, mannose; P, phosphate; PP, pyrophosphate.

hypotonia, weakness, strabismus and cerebellar ataxia) and psychomotor retardation (IQs often in the 40–60 range) are common features, but intellectual regression does not occur.[223,224] Patients only rarely learn to walk without an aid and tend to have poor visuoperceptual abilities. A language disorder that affects articulation, expressive and receptive language is typical.[225] Other

Table 24.34 Clinical features of congenital disorders of glycosylation

Neurological	Hypotonia, developmental delay, hypo/areflexia, ataxia, seizures, stroke-like episodes, peripheral neuropathy, microcephaly, cerebellar hypoplasia, demyelination, epilepsy, demyelinating polyneuropathy
Ophthalmological	Strabismus, abnormal eye movements, optic atrophy, nystagmus, retinitis pigmentosa, iris or retinal colobomata, cortical blindness, corneal dystrophy
Gastrointestinal	Protein-losing enteropathy, failure to thrive, cyclic vomiting, hepatic dysfunction, liver fibrosis, intestinal villus atrophy, hypoalbuminemia, low protein C, protein S, antithrombin III, increased aspartate aminotransferase
Hematological	Coagulopathy, thrombosis, thrombocytopenia, thrombocytosis, decreased factor XI
Cardiological	Pericardial effusion, cardiomyopathy
Endocrinological	Hyperinsulinemic hypoglycemia, hypothyroidism, hypogonadism, hypoplastic genitalia
Renal	Nephrotic syndrome, renal tubular defects, hyperechogenic kidneys
Immunological	Recurrent infections, hypogammaglobulinemia
Orthopedic	Scoliosis, contractures, osteopenia, thoracic scoliosis
Other	Cholinesterase and pseudocholinesterase deficiency Craniofacial dysmorphy, inverted nipples, unusual fat distribution

relatively common neurological findings include hypo- or areflexia, seizures, stroke-like episodes and peripheral neuropathy. Some atypical CDG type Ia patients have relatively mild cognitive impairment.[226,227] Although cerebellar hypoplasia is a very common feature, a few patients with normal head MRIs have also been reported.

An unusual distribution of fat and inverted nipples are often present and may provide significant clues to the underlying diagnosis. Suprailiac and pubic fat pads are especially common, but abnormal trunk and extremity fat collections may also be noted. On the other hand, an unusual fat distribution may not be present in every case and fat distribution also tends to become more normal with time. Mild non-specific facial dysmorphic features may be noted. Some patients present with a severe neonatal illness with multiple organ-system involvement. Hypertrophic cardiomyopathy, pericardial effusion, liver disease, protein-losing enteropathy and the nephrotic syndrome may occur in variable degrees in such patients. Mortality in infancy is typically about 20%, although some centers have reported an even higher mortality rate in the first few years.[228] Failure to thrive, feeding difficulties, cyclic vomiting, recurrent infections and endocrinological problems (hypothyroidism, hyperinsulinism, hypogonadism) are relatively common findings. A pattern of thyroid function testing consistent with thyroid binding globulin deficiency is typical.

The primary defect in protein glycosylation causes a decreased concentration or activity of a number of serum glycoproteins including thyroid binding globulin, protein C, protein S, antithrombin III, factor XI, and cholinesterase. IEF or mass spectrometry analysis of serum transferrin shows characteristic abnormalities in most cases, but patients with CDG type Ia may rarely have normal transferrin studies. Confirmation of the diagnosis can be obtained by performing phosphomannomutase (PMM) enzyme studies on leukocytes or fibroblasts and/or direct DNA mutation analysis of the PMM2 gene. However, because fibroblast enzyme studies have given intermediate non-diagnostic PMM activity levels in some cases, leukocyte enzymology and DNA analysis are the preferred diagnostic methods.[227] Prenatal diagnosis in future pregnancies is straightforward if mutations have been found in a previously affected child. PMM enzyme analysis on amniocytes or a chorionic villus sample is also possible.[229] Therapy for CDG type Ia, in general, is supportive and aimed at specific complications (e.g. pericardiocentesis and steroids for pericardial effusion, intravenous hyperalimentation for severe feeding difficulty, diazoxide for hyperinsulinism). Attempts at treatment with oral or intravenous mannose have not been successful.[230,232]

OTHER FORMS OF CDG TYPE I

Only a limited number of CDG type I patients without PMM deficiency have been reported.[219,222,233] Although such patients (CDG types Ib to Ig) have different enzyme or protein deficiencies (Table 24.33), they share a similar transferrin IEF pattern to CDG type Ia. CDG type Ib (phosphomannose isomerase deficiency) is characterized by gastrointestinal illness (liver fibrosis, protein-losing enteropathy) *without* prominent neurological symptoms or cerebellar hypoplasia. Hyperinsulinemic hypoglycemia and a coagulopathy may also occur in CDG type Ib.[233,234] Although other forms of CDG do not appear to be responsive to mannose therapy, some patients with CDG type Ib have had a dramatic response to oral mannose supplementation (100–150 mg/kg dose daily in three to six doses) with correction of both clinical and biochemical abnormalities.[232] Children with CDG type Ic have similar, but typically more mild, neurological findings than in CDG type Ia and absent cerebellar hypoplasia. A single patient with CDG type Id has been reported with profound psychomotor retardation, acquired microcephaly, hypsarrhythmia, optic atrophy and corpus callosum atrophy. CDG type Ie has been found in four children with psychomotor retardation, epilepsy, hypotonia, failure to thrive, and mild dysmorphic features. Congenital ichthyosis, retinopathy, psychomotor retardation, hypertonia, and dwarfism were present in two siblings diagnosed with CDG type If. Severe hypotonia, feeding difficulties, psychomotor retardation, progressive microcephaly and facial dysmorphic features were reported in a single patient identified with CDG type Ig.[219] Aside from mannose supplementation in CDG type Ib, treatment is supportive.

CONGENITAL DISORDERS OF GLYCOSYLATION TYPE II

Patients with type II CDG syndromes have glycosylation defects similar to those observed in the type I disorders. Only four patients have been identified. Patients with CDG IIa show a type 2 pattern of serum transferrins (which includes a cathodal shift with increased amounts of mono- and trisialotransferrins). A single patient with CDG type IIb showed a normal pattern. All such patients have had a characteristic elevation of aspartate aminotransferase in serum.

Clinical features

CDG type IIa

Three patients have been reported who manifested severe mental retardation and a characteristic facial dysmorphy.[235,236] Blood levels of factor XI were significantly decreased.

CDG type IIb

A single patient with CDG type IIb has been reported. The phenotype included hypotonia, dysmorphic features, seizures and early death at 2.5 months of age.[237] Associated clinical findings included hypoplastic genitalia, respiratory insufficiency, thoracic scoliosis, demyelinating polyneuropathy and psychomotor retardation.

REFERENCES (* Level 1 evidence)

INTRODUCTION

1 Wilcken B. Rare diseases and the assessment of intervention: what sorts of clinical trials we use? J Inherit Metab Dis 2001; 24: 291–298.

2 Scriver CR, Beaudet AL, Sly WS, et al, eds. The metabolic and molecular bases of inherited disease, 8th edn. New York: McGraw Hill; 2001:2961–3062.

3 Holton JB, ed. The inherited metabolic diseases, 2nd edn. Edinburgh: Churchill Livingstone; 1994.

4 Fernandes J, Saudubray J-M, van den Berghe G, eds. Inborn metabolic diseases: diagnosis and treatment, 2nd edn. Berlin: Springer-Verlag; 1995.

5 Blau N, Blaskovics M, eds. The physician's guide to the laboratory diagnosis of inherited metabolic diseases. London: Chapman & Hall; 1996.

6 Hommes FA, ed. Techniques in diagnostic human biochemical genetics. A laboratory manual. New York: Wiley-Liss; 1993.

7 Lyon G, Adams RD, Kolodny EH. Neurology of hereditary metabolic diseases of children. New York: McGraw-Hill; 1996.

8 Clarke JTR. A clinical guide for inherited metabolic diseases. Cambridge: Cambridge University Press; 2000.

9 Gilbert-Barness E, Barness L. Metabolic diseases. Natick, MA: Eaton Publishing; 2000.

10 Nyhan WL, Ozand PT. Atlas of metabolic diseases. London: Chapman & Hall; 1998.

11 Alper JS. Genetic complexity in single gene diseases. BMJ 1996; 312:196–197.

12 Dionisi-Vici C, Rizzo C, Burlina AB, et al. Inborn errors of metabolism in the Italian pediatric population: a national retrospective survey. J Pediatr 2002; 140:321–327.

13 Applegarth DA, Toone JR, Lowry RB. Incidence of inborn errors of metabolism in British Columbia, 1969–1996. Pediatrics 2000; 105:e10.

14 Baird PA, Anderson TW, Newcombe HB, et al. Genetic disorders in children and young adults: a population study. Am J Hum Genet 1988; 42:677–693.

15 Treacy E, Childs B, Scriver CR. Response to treatment in hereditary metabolic disease. 1993 Survey and 10-year comparison. Am J Hum Genet 1995; 56:359–367.

PEROXISOMAL DISORDERS

16 Gould SJ, Raymond GV, Valle D. The peroxisome biogenesis disorders. In: Scriver CR, Beaudet AL, Sly WS, et al, eds. The metabolic and molecular basis of inherited disease, 8th edn. New York: McGraw-Hill 2001:2287–2324.

17 Suzuki Y, Shimozawa N, Imamura A, et al. Clinical, biochemical and genetic aspects and neuronal migration in peroxisome biogenesis disorders. J Inherit Metab Dis 2001; 24:151–165.

18 McKusick VA, ed. Online Mendelian Inheritance in Man. 2001. http://www3.ncbi.nlm.nih.gov/Omim/ed.

19 Raymond GV. Peroxisomal disorders. Curr Opin Pediatr 1999; 11(6):572–581.

20 Gould SJ, Valle D. Peroxisome biogenesis disorders: genetics and cell biology. Trends Genet 2000; 16(8):340–345.

21 Walter C, Gootjes J, Mooijer PA, et al. Disorders of peroxisome biogenesis due to mutations in PEX1: phenotypes and PEX1 protein levels. Am J Hum Genet 2002; 69:35–48.

22 Martinez M. Restoring the DHA levels in the brains of Zellweger patients. J Mol Neurosci 2001; 16:309–316.

23 Noetzel, MJ. Fish oil and myelin: cautious optimism for treatment of children with disorders of peroxisome biogenesis. Neurology 1998; 51:5–7.

24 Wei H, Kemp S, McGuinness MC, et al. Pharmacological induction of peroxisomes in peroxisome biogenesis disorders. Ann Neurol 2000; 47:286–296.

25 Moser HW, Smith KD, Watkins PA, et al. X-linked adrenoleukodystrophy. In: Scriver CR, Beaudet AL, Sly WS, et al, eds. The metabolic and molecular basis of inherited disease, 8th edn. New York: McGraw-Hill; 2001: 3257–3293.

26 Shapiro E, Krivit W, Lockman L, et al. Long-term beneficial effect of bone marrow transplantation of childhood-onset cerebral X-linked adrenoleukodystrophy. Lancet 2000; 356:713–718.

27 Moser HW. Treatment of X-linked adrenoleukodystroph with Lorenzo's oil. J Neurol Neurosurg Psychiatry 1999; 67:279–280.

28 Van Geel BM, Assies J, Haverkort EB, et al. Progression of abnormalities in adrenomyeloneuropathy and neurologically asymptomatic X-linked adrenoleukodystrophy despite treatment with 'Lorenzo's oil'. J Neurol Neurosurg Psychiatry 1999; 67:290–299.

29 Pai GS, Khan M, Barbosa E, et al. Lovastatin for X-linked adrenoleukodystrophy: clinical and biochemical observations in 12 patients. Mol Genet Metab 2000; 69:312–322.

30 Verrips A, Michel AAP, Wilemsen MD, et al. Simvastatin and plasma very long-chain fatty acids in X-linked adrenoleukodystrophy. Ann Neurol 2000; 47:552–553.

31 Wanders RJA, Jacobs C, Skjeldal OH. Refsum disease. In: Scriver CR, Beaudet AL, Sly WS, et al, eds. The metabolic and molecular basis of inherited disease, 8th edn. New York: McGraw-Hill; 2001:3303–3321.

PURINE AND PYRIMIDINE DISORDERS

32 Simmonds HA. Purine and pyrimidine disorders. In: Blau N, Duran M, Blaskovics ME, eds. Physician's guide to the laboratory diagnosis of metabolic diseases. London: Chapman & Hall; 1996:341–357.

33 Hershfield MS, Mitchell BS. Immunodeficiency diseases caused by adenosine deaminase deficiency and purine nucleoside phosphorylase deficiency. In: Scriver CR, Beaudet AL, Sly WS, et al, eds. The molecular and metabolic bases of inherited disease, 8th edn. New York: McGraw-Hill; 2001:2585–2626.

34 Apasov SG, Blackburn MR, Kellems RE, et al. Adenosine deaminase deficiency increases thymic apoptosis and causes defective T cell receptor signaling. J Clin Invest 2001; 108:131–141.

35 Raivio KO, Saksela M, Lapatto R. Xanthine oxidoreductases – role in human pathophysiology and in hereditary xanthinuria. In: Scriver CR, Beaudet AL, Sly WS, et al, eds. The molecular and metabolic bases of inherited disease, 8th edn. New York: McGraw-Hill; 2001:2639–2652.

36 Gille L, Staniek K, Nohl H. Effects of tocopheryl quinone on the heart: model

experiments with xanthine oxidase, heart mitochondria, and isolated perfused rat hearts. Free Radic Biol Med 2001; 30:865–876.

37 Ichida K, Matsumura T, Sakuma R, et al. Mutation of human molybdenum cofactor sulfurase gene is responsible for classical xanthinuria type II. Biochem Biophys Res Commun 2001; 282:1194–1200.

38 Becker MA. Hyperuricemia and gout. In: Scriver CR, Beaudet AL, Sly WS, et al, eds. The molecular and metabolic bases of inherited disease, 8th edn. New York: McGraw-Hill; 2001:2513–2536.

39 Jinnah HA, Friedmann T. Lesch-Nyhan disease and its variants. In: Scriver CR, Beaudet AL, Sly WS, et al, eds. The molecular and metabolic bases of inherited disease, 8th edn. New York: McGraw-Hill; 2001:2537–2570.

40 Hall S, Oliver C, Murphy G. Self-injurious behaviour in young children with Lesch-Nyhan syndrome. Dev Med Child Neurol 2001; 43: 745–749.

41 Allen SM, Rice SN. Risperidone antagonism of self-mutilation in a Lesch-Nyhan patient. Prog Neuropsychopharmacol Biol Psychiatry 1996; 20:793–800.

42 Sahota AS, Tischfield JA, Kamatani N, et al. Adenine phosphoribosyltransferase deficiency and 2,8-dihydroxyadenine lithiasis. In: Scriver CR, Beaudet AL, Sly WS, et al, eds. The molecular and metabolic bases of inherited disease, 8th edn. New York: McGraw-Hill; 2001:2571–2584.

43 Van den Berghe G, Jaeken J. Adenylosuccinate lyase deficiency. In: Scriver CR, Beaudet AL, Sly WS, et al, eds. The molecular and metabolic bases of inherited disease, 8th edn. New York: McGraw-Hill; 2001:2653–2662.

44 Ciardo F, Salerno C, Curatolo P. Neurologic aspects of adenylosuccinate lyase deficiency. J Child Neurol 2001; 16:301–308.

45 Sabine RL, Holmes EW. Myoadenylate deaminase deficiency. In: Scriver CR, Beaudet AL, Sly WS, et al, eds. The molecular and metabolic bases of inherited disease, 8th edn. New York: McGraw-Hill; 2001:2627–2638.

46 Evans WE, Hon YY, Bomgaars L, et al. Preponderance of thiopurine S-methyltransferase deficiency and heterozygosity among patients intolerant to mercaptopurine or azathioprine. J Clin Oncol 2001; 19:2293–2301.

47 Webster DR, Becroft DMO, van Gennip AH, et al. Hereditary orotic aciduria and other disorders of pyrimidine metabolism. In: Scriver CR, Beaudet AL, Sly WS, et al, eds. The molecular and metabolic bases of inherited disease, 8th edn. New York: McGraw-Hill; 2001:2663–2704.

48 Kuhara T, Ohdoi C, Ohse M. Simple gas chromatographic-mass spectrometric procedure for diagnosing pyrimidine degradation defects for prevention of severe anticancer side effects. J Chromatogr B Biomed Sci Appl 2001; 758:61–74.

49 Moolenaar SH, Gohlich-Ratmann G, Engelke UF, et al. Beta-ureidopropionase deficiency: a novel inborn error of metabolism discovered using NMR spectroscopy on urine. Magn Reson Med 2001; 46:1014–1017.

50 Nishino I, Spinazzola A, Hirano M. MNGIE: from nuclear DNA to mitochondrial DNA. Neuromuscul Disord 2001; 11:7–10.

Patient support group contacts and web-based resources for additional information
http://www.pacifier.com/~mstephe
http://www.peroxizome.org

NEUROTRANSMITTER DISORDERS

51 Blau N, Thony B, Cotton RGH, et al. Disorders of tetrahydrobiopterin and related biogenic amines. In: Scriver CR, Beaudet AL, Sly WS, et al, eds. The molecular and metabolic bases of inherited disease, 8th edn. New York: McGraw-Hill; 2001:1725–1776.

52 Bonafe L, Blau N, Burlina AP, et al. Treatable neurotransmitter deficiency in mild phenylketonuria. Neurology 2001; 57:908–911.

53 Rajput AH. The protective role of levodopa in the human substantia nigra. Adv Neurol 2001; 86:327–336.

54 Eells JB, Rives JE, Yeung SK, et al. In vitro regulated expression of tyrosine hydroxylase in ventral midbrain neurons from Nurr1-null mouse pups. J Neurosci Res 2001; 64:322–330.

55 Bonafe L, Thony B, Leimbacher W, et al. Diagnosis of dopa-responsive dystonia and other tetrahydrobiopterin disorders by the study of biopterin metabolism in fibroblasts. Clin Chem 2001; 47:477–485.

56 Blau N, Bonafe L, Thony B. Tetrahydrobiopterin deficiencies without hyperphenylalaninemia: diagnosis and genetics of dopa-responsive dystonia and sepiapterin reductase deficiency. Mol Genet Metab 2001; 74:172–185.

57 Cryan JF, Dalvi A, Jin SH, et al. Use of dopamine-beta-hydroxylase-deficient mice to determine the role of norepinephrine in the mechanism of action of antidepressant drugs. J Pharmacol Exp Ther 2001; 298:651–657.

58 Salichon N, Gaspar P, Upton AL, et al. Excessive activation of serotonin (5-HT) 1B receptors disrupts the formation of sensory maps in monoamine oxidase a and 5-ht transporter knock-out mice. J Neurosci 2001; 21:884–896.

59 Bonafe L, Thony B, Penzien JM, et al. Mutations in the sepiapterin reductase gene cause a novel tetrahydrobiopterin-dependent monoamine-neurotransmitter deficiency without hyperphenylalaninemia. Am J Hum Genet 2001; 69:269–277.

60 Haussler M, Hoffmann GF, Wevers RA. L-dopa and selegiline for tyrosine hydroxylase deficiency. J Pediatr 2001; 138:451.

61 Hwang WJ, Calne DB, Tsui JK, et al. The long-term response to levodopa in dopa-responsive dystonia. Parkinsonism Relat Disord 2001; 8:1–5.

62 Nutt JG, Nygaard TG. Response to levodopa treatment in dopa-responsive dystonia. Arch Neurol 2001; 58:905–910.

63 Trefz FK, Aulela-Scholz C, Blau N. Successful treatment of phenylketonuria with tetrahydrobiopterin. Eur J Pediatr 2001; 160:315.

64 Lindner M, Haas D, Zschocke J, et al. Tetrahydrobiopterin responsiveness in phenylketonuria differs between patients with the same genotype. Mol Genet Metab 2001; 73:104–106.

65 van Spronsen FJ, van Rijn M, Bekhof J, et al. Phenylketonuria: tyrosine supplementation in phenylalanine-restricted diets. Am J Clin Nutr 2001; 73:153–157.

66 Kalsner LR, Rohr FJ, Strauss KA, et al. Tyrosine supplementation in phenylketonuria: diurnal blood tyrosine levels and presumptive brain influx of tyrosine and other large neutral amino acids. J Pediatr 2001; 139:421–427.

67 Agostoni C, Scaglioni S, Bonvissuto M, et al. Biochemical effects of supplemented long-chain polyunsaturated fatty acids in hyperphenylalaninemia. Prostaglandins Leukot Essent Fatty Acids 2001; 64:111–115.

AMINO ACID METABOLISM DISORDERS

68 Smith I, Lobascher ME, Stevenson JE, et al. Effect of stopping low-phenylalanine diet on intellectual progress of children with phenylketonuria. BMJ 1978; 2:723–726.

69 Hanley WB, Clarke JT, Schoonheyt W. Maternal phenylketonuria (PKU) – a review. Clin Biochem 1987; 20:149–156.

70 Hyland K, Arnold LA, Trugman JM. Defects of biopterin metabolism and biogenic amine biosynthesis: clinical diagnostic, and therapeutic aspects. Adv Neurol 1998; 78: 301–308.

71 Lindstedt S, Holme E, Lock EA, et al. Treatment of hereditary tyrosinaemia type I by inhibition of 4-hydroxyphenylpyruvate dioxygenase. Lancet 1992; 340:813–817.

72 Holme E, Lindstedt S. Tyrosinaemia type I and NTBC (2-(2-nitro-4-trifluoromethylbenzoyl)-1,3-cyclohexanedione). J Inherit Metab Dis 1999; 22:665–666.

73 Garrod AE. The incidence of alkaptonuria: a study in chemical individuality. Lancet 1902; 2:1616.

74 Sakura N, Ono H, Nomura S, et al. Betaine dose and treatment intervals in therapy for homocystinuria due to 5,10-methylenetetrahydrofolate reductase deficiency. J Inherit Metab Dis 1998; 21:84–85.

75 Walter JH, Wraith JE, White FJ, et al. Strategies for the treatment of cystathionine beta-synthase deficiency: the experience of the Willink Biochemical Genetics Unit over the past 30 years. Eur J Pediatr 1998; 157 (suppl 2):S71–76.

76 Anon. Consensus statement from a conference for the management of patients with urea cycle disorders. J Pediatr 2001; 138:S6–10.

77 Guffon N, Vianey-Saban C, Bourgeois J, et al. A new neonatal case of N-acetylglutamate synthase deficiency treated by carbamylglutamate. J Inherit Metab Dis 1995; 18:61–65.

78 Hinnie J, Colombo JP, Wermuth, B, et al. N-acetylglutamate synthetase deficiency responding to carbamylglutamate. J Inherit Metab Dis 1997; 20:839–840.

79 Steiner RD, Cederbaum SD. Laboratory evaluation of urea cycle disorders. J Pediatr 2001; 138:S56–60; discussion S60–61.

80 Brusilow SW, Danney M, Waber LJ, et al. Treatment of episodic hyperammonemia in children with inborn errors of urea synthesis. N Engl J Med 1984; 310:1630–1634.

81 Batshaw ML, MacArthur RB, Tuchman M. Alternative pathway therapy for urea cycle disorders: twenty years later. J Pediatr 2001; 138:S46–54.

82 Brusilow SW. Phenylacetylglutamine may replace urea as a vehicle for waste nitrogen excretion. Pediatr Res 1991; 29:147–150.

83 Widhalm K, Koch S, Scheibenreiter S, et al. Long-term follow-up of 12 patients with the late-onset variant of argininosuccinic acid lyase deficiency: no impairment of intellectual and psychomotor development during therapy. Pediatrics 1992; 89:1182–1184.
84 Burlina AB, Ogier H, Korall H, et al. Long-term treatment with sodium phenylbutyrate in ornithine transcarbamylase-deficient patients. Mol Genet Metab 2001; 72:351–355.
85 Saudubray JM, Touati G, Delonlay P, et al. Liver transplantation in urea cycle disorders. Eur J Pediatr 1999; 158(suppl 2):S55–59.
86 Hamosh A, Maher JF, Bellus GA, et al. Long-term use of high-dose benzoate and dextromethorphan for the treatment of nonketotic hyperglycinemia. J Pediatr 1998; 132:709–713.
87 Wiltshire EJ, Poplawski NK, Harrison JR, et al. Treatment of late-onset nonketotic hyperglycinaemia: effectiveness of imipramine and benzoate. J Inherit Metab Dis 2000; 23:15–21.
88 Saborio P, Scheinman JI. Transplantation for primary hyperoxaluria in the United States. Kidney Int 1999; 56:1094–1100.
89 Stockler S, Holzbach U, Hanefeld F, et al. Creatine deficiency in the brain: a new, treatable inborn error of metabolism. Pediatr Res 1994; 36:409–413.
90 Stockler S, Hanefeld F, Frahm J. Creatine replacement therapy in guanidinoacetate methyltransferase deficiency, a novel inborn error of metabolism. Lancet 1996; 348:789–790.
91 Roe CR, Millington DS, Maltby DA, et al. L-carnitine enhances excretion of propionyl coenzyme A as propionylcarnitine in propionic acidemia. J Clin Invest 1984; 73:1785–1788.
92 van der Meer SB, Poggi F, Spada M, et al. Clinical outcome of long-term management of patients with vitamin B_{12}-unresponsive methylmalonic acidemia. J Pediatr 1994; 125:903–908.
93 Roe CR, Millington DS, Maltby DA, et al. L-carnitine therapy in isovaleric acidemia. J Clin Invest 1984; 74:2290–2295.
94 Gibson KM, Breuer J, Nyhan WL. 3-Hydroxy-3-methylglutaryl-coenzyme A lyase deficiency: review of 18 reported patients. Prenat Diagn 1995; 15:725–729.
95 Moslinger D, Stockler-Ipsiroglu S, Scheibenreiter S, et al. Clinical and neuropsychological outcome in 33 patients with biotinidase deficiency ascertained by nationwide newborn screening and family studies in Austria. Eur J Pediatr 2001; 160:277–282.
96 Hogema BM, Gupta M, Senephansiri H, et al. Pharmacologic rescue of lethal seizures in mice deficient in succinate semialdehyde dehydrogenase. Nat Genet 2001; 29:212–216.

METAL METABOLISM DISORDERS

97 Culotta VC, Gitlin JD. Disorders of copper metabolism. In: Scriver CR, Beaudet AL, Sly WS, et al, eds. The molecular and metabolic bases of inherited disease, 8th edn. New York: McGraw-Hill; 2001:3105–3126.
98 Christodoulou J, Danks DM, Sarkar B, et al. Early treatment of Menkes disease with parenteral copper-histidine: long-term follow-up of four treated patients. Am J Med Genet 1998; 76:154–164.
99 Brewer GJ, Dick RD, Johnson VD, et al. Treatment of Wilson's disease with zinc XVI: treatment during the pediatric years. Lab Clin Med 2001; 137:191–198.
100 Zhou B, Westaway SK, Levinson B, et al. A novel pantothenate kinase gene (PANK2) is defective in Hallervorden–Spatz syndrome. Nat Genet 2001; 28(4):345–349.

THE PORPHYRIAS

101 Anderson KE, Sassa S, Bishop DF, et al. Disorders of heme biosynthesis; X-linked sideroblastic anemia and the porphyrias. In: Scriver CR, Beaudet AL, Sly WS, et al, eds. The molecular and metabolic bases of inherited disease, 8th edn. New York: McGraw-Hill; 2001:2961–3062.
102 Gross U, Hoffmann GF, Doss MO. Erythropoietic and hepatic porphyrias. J Inherit Metab Dis 2000; 23:641–661.
103 Murphy GM (for the British Photodermatology Group). The cutaneous porphyrias: a review. Br J Dermatol 1999; 140:573–581.
104 de Torres I, Demetris AJ, Randhawa PS. Recurrent hepatic allograft injury in erythropoietic porphyria. Transplantation 1996; 61:1412–1433.
105 Zix-Kieffer I, Langer B, Eyer D, et al. Successful cord blood stem cell transplantation for congenital erythropoietic porphyria (Gunther's disease). Bone Marrow Transplant 1996; 18:217–220.
106 Tezcan I, Xu W, Gurgey A, et al. Congenital erythropoietic porphyria successfully treated by allogeneic bone marrow transplantation. Blood 1998; 92:4053–4058.
107 Pawliuk R, Bachelot T, Wise RJ, et al. Long-term cure of the photosensitivity of murine erythropoietic protoporphyria by preselective gene therapy. Nat Med 1999; 5:768–773.

BILIRUBIN AND BILE ACID METABOLISM

108 Schmid R. Gilbert's syndrome – a legitimate genetic anomaly. N Engl J Med 1995; 333:1217–1218.

FATTY ACID OXIDATION DISORDERS

109 Rinaldo P, Schmidt-Sommerfeld E, Posca AP, et al. Effect of treatment with glycine and L-carnitine in medium-chain acyl-coenzyme a dehydrogenase deficiency. J Pediatr 1993; 122:580–584.
110 Pierpont ME, Breningstall GN, Stanley CA, et al. Familial carnitine transporter defect: a treatable cause of cardiomyopathy in children. Am Heart J 2000; 139:S96–S106.
111 Gillingham M, Van Calcar S, Ney D, et al. Dietary management of long-chain 3-hydroxyacyl-CoA dehydrogenase deficiency (LCHADD). A case report and survey. J Inherit Metab Dis 1999; 22:123–131.
112 Kolodziej MP, Crilly PJ, Corstorphine CG, et al. Development and characterization of a polyclonal antibody against rat liver mitochondrial overt carnitine palmitoyltransferase (CPT I). Distinction of CPT I from CPT II and of isoforms of CPT I in different tissues. Biochem J 1992; 282:415–421.
113 Wang SS, Fernhoff PM, Khoury MJ. Is the G985A allelic variant of medium-chain acyl-CoA dehydrogenase a risk factor for sudden infant death syndrome? A pooled analysis. Pediatrics 2000; 105:1175–1176.
114 Andresen BS, Dobrowolski SF, O'Reilly L, et al. Medium-chain acyl-CoA dehydrogenase (MCAD) mutations identified by MS/MS-based prospective screening of newborns differ from those observed in patients with clinical symptoms: identification and characterization of a new, prevalent mutation that results in mild MCAD deficiency. Am J Hum Genet 2001; 68:1408–1418.
115 Ibdah JA, Bennett MJ, Rinaldo P, et al. A fetal fatty-acid oxidation disorder as a cause of liver disease in pregnant women. N Engl J Med 1999; 340:1723–1731.
116 Bennett MJ, Weinberger MJ, Kobori JA, et al. Mitochondrial short-chain L-3-hydroxyacyl-coenzyme A dehydrogenase deficiency: a new defect of fatty acid oxidation. Pediatr Res 1996; 39:185–188.
117 Corydon MJ, Vockley J, Rinaldo P, et al. Role of common gene variations in the molecular pathogenesis of short-chain acyl-CoA dehydrogenase deficiency. Pediatr Res 2001; 49:18–23.
118 Beatty ME, Zhang YH, McCabe ER, et al. Fructose-1,6-diphosphatase deficiency and glyceroluria: one possible etiology for GIS. Mol Genet Metab 2000; 69:338–340.
119 Mooy PD, Przyrembel H, Giesberts MA, et al. Glutaric aciduria type II: treatment with riboflavine, carnitine and insulin. Eur J Pediatr 1984; 143:92–95.
120 Saudubray JM, Charpentier C. Clinical phenotypes: diagnosis/algorithms. In: Scriver CR, Beaudet AL, Sly WS, et al, eds. The metabolic and molecular bases of inherited disease, 8th edn. New York: McGraw-Hill; 2001: 1327–1403.

CARBOHYDRATE METABOLISM DISORDERS

121 Waggoner DD, Buist NR, Donnell GN. Long-term prognosis in galactosaemia: results of a survey of 350 cases. J Inherit Metab Dis 1990; 13:802–818.
122 Kaufman FR, McBridechang C, Manis FR, et al. Cognitive functioning, neurologic status and brain imaging in classical galactosemia. Eur J Pediatr 1995; 154:S2–S5.
123 Irons M, Levy HL, Pueschel S, et al. Accumulation of galactose-1-phosphate in the galactosemic fetus despite maternal milk avoidance. J Pediatr 1985; 107:261–263.
124 Berry GT, Nissim I, Lin Z, et al. Endogenous synthesis of galactose in normal men and patients with hereditary galactosaemia. Lancet 1995; 346:1073–1074.
125 Tolan DR, Brooks CC. Molecular analysis of common aldolase B alleles for hereditary fructose intolerance in North Americans. Biochem Med Metab Biol 1992; 48:19–25.
126 Van den Hout H, Reuser AJ, Vulto AG, et al. Recombinant human alpha-glucosidase from rabbit milk in Pompe patients. Lancet 2000; 356:397–398.
127 Amalfitano A, Bengur AR, Morse RP, et al. Recombinant human acid alpha-glucosidase enzyme therapy for infantile glycogen storage disease type II: results of a phase I/II clinical trial. Genet Med 2001; 3:132–138.

MITOCHONDRIAL DISEASE

128 Chinnery PF, Turnbull DM. Epidemiology and treatment of mitochondrial disorders. Am J Med Genet. 2001; 106:94–101.

129 Munnich A, Rustin P. Clinical spectrum and diagnosis of mitochondrial disorders. Am J Med Genet 2001; 106:4–17.

130 Wallace DC. Mouse models for mitochondrial disease. Am J Med Genet 2001; 106:71–93.

131 Thorburn DR, Dahl H-HM. Mitochondrial disorders: genetics, counseling, prenatal diagnosis and reproductive options. Am J Med Genet 2001; 106:102–114.

132 DiMauro S, Bonilla E, De Vivo D. Does the patient have a mitochondrial encephalomyopathy? J Child Neurol 1999; 14(suppl 1):S23–S35.

133 DiMauro S, Schon E. Mitochondrial DNA mutations in human disease. Am J Med Genet 2001; 106:18–26.

134 Triepels RH, Van den Heuvel LP, Trijbels JM, et al. Respiratory chain complex I deficiency. Am J Med Genet 2001; 106:37–45.

135 Bourgeron T, Rustin P, Chretien D, et al. Mutation of a nuclear succinate dehydrogenase gene results in mitochondrial respiratory chain deficiency. Nat Genet 1995; 11:144–148.

136 Tiranti V, Hoertnagel K, Carrozzo R, et al. Mutations of SURF-1 in Leigh disease associated with cytochrome c oxidase deficiency. Am J Hum Genet 1998; 63:1609–1621.

137 Zhu Z, Yao J, Johns T, et al. SURF1, encoding a factor involved in the biogenesis of cytochrome c oxidase, is mutated in Leigh syndrome. Nat Genet 1998; 20:337–343.

138 Shoubridge EA. Cytochrome c oxidase deficiency. Am J Med Genet 2001; 106:46–52.

139 DiMauro S, Nicholson JF, Hays AP, et al. Benign infantile mitochondrial myopathy due to reversible cytochrome c oxidase deficiency. Ann Neurol 1983; 14:226–229.

140 Bespalova IN, van Camp G, Bom SJH, et al. Mutations in the Wolfram syndrome 1 gene (WFS1) are a common cause of low frequency sensorineurol hearing loss. Hum Mol Genet 2001; 10:2501–2508.

141 Castro-Gago M, Alonso A, Pintos-Martínez E, et al. Congenital hydranencephalic-hydrocephalic syndrome associated with mitochondrial dysfunction. J Child Neurol 1999; 14:131–135.

142 Poulton J, Macaulay V, Marchington DR. Mitochondrial genetics '98: is the bottleneck cracked? Am J Hum Genet 1998; 62:752–757.

143 Larsson NG, Holme E, Kristiansson B, et al. Progressive increase of the mutated mitochondrial DNA fraction in Kearns-Sayre syndrome. Pediatr Res 1990; 28:131–136.

144 Baysal BE, Ferrell RE, Willett-Brozick JE, et al. Mutations in SDHD, a mitochondrial complex II gene, in hereditary paraganglioma. Science 2000; 287:848–851.

145 Astuti D, Latif F, Dallol A, et al. Gene mutations in the succinate dehydrogenase subunit SDHB cause susceptibility to familial pheochromocytoma and to familial paraganglioma. Am J Hum Genet 2001; 69:49–54.

146 Enns GM, Bennett MJ, Hoppel C, et al. Mitochondrial respiratory chain complex I deficiency presenting with clinical and biochemical features of long-chain 3-hydroxyacyl-CoA dehydrogenase (LCHAD) deficiency. J Pediatr 2000; 136:251–254.

147 De Lonlay P, Valnot I, Barrientos A, et al. A mutant mitochondrial respiratory chain assembly protein causes complex III deficiency in patients with tubulopathy, encephalopathy and liver failure. Nat Genet 2001; 29:57–60.

148 Papadopoulou LC, Sue CM, Davidson MM, et al. Fatal infantile cardioencephalomyopathy with COX deficiency and mutations in SCO2, a COX assembly gene. Nat Genet 1999; 23: 333–337.

149 Valnot I, Osmond S, Gigarel N, et al. Mutations of the SCO1 gene in mitochondrial cytochrome c oxidase (COX) deficiency with neonatal-onset hepatic failure and encephalopathy. Am J Hum Genet 2000; 67:1104–1109.

150 Valnot I, von Kleist-Retzow JC, Barrientos A, et al. A mutation in the human heme A:faresyltransferase gene (COX10) causes cytochrome c oxidase deficiency. Hum Mol Genet 2000; 9:1245–1249.

151 Houstek J, Klement P, Floryk D, et al. A novel deficiency of mitochondrial ATPase of nuclear origin. Hum Mol Genet 1999; 8:1967–1974.

152 Suomalainen A, Kaukonen J. Diseases caused by nuclear genes affecting mtDNA stability. Am J Med Genet 2001; 106:53–61.

153 Kaukonen J, Juselius JK, Tiranti V, et al. Role of adenine nucleotide translocator 1 in mtDNA maintenance. Science 2000; 289:782–785.

154 Spelbrink JN, Li F-Y, Tiranti V, et al. Human mitochondrial DNA deletions associated with mutations in the gene encoding Twinkle, a phage T7 gene 4-like protein localized in mitochondria. Nat Genet 2001; 28:223–231.

155 Van Goethem G, Dermaut B, Löfgren A, et al. Mutation of POLG is associated with progressive external ophthalmoplegia characterized by mtDNA deletions. Nat Genet 2001; 28:211–212.

156 Alexander C, Votruba M, Pesch UEA, et al. OPA1, encoding a dynamin-related GTPase, is mutated in autosomal dominant optic atrophy linked to chromosome 3q28. Nat Genet 2000; 26:211–215.

157 Delettre C, Lenaers G, Griffoin J-M, et al. Nuclear gene OPA1, encoding a mitochondrial dynamin-related protein, is mutated in dominant optic atrophy. Nat Genet 2000; 26:207–210.

158 Hirano M, Vu TH. Defects of intergenomic communication: where do we stand? Brain Pathol 2000; 10:451–461.

159 Naviaux RK, Nyhan W, Barshop B, et al. Mitochondrial polymerase gamma deficiency and mtDNA depletion in a child with Alpers' syndrome. Ann Neurol 1999; 45:54–58.

160 Mandel H, Szargel R, Labay V, et al. The deoxyguanosine kinase gene is mutated in individuals with depleted hepatocerebral mitochondrial DNA. Nat Genet 2001; 29:337–341.

161 Saada A, Shaag A, Mandel H, et al. Mutant mitochondrial thymidine kinase in mitochondrial DNA depletion myopathy. Nat Genet 2001; 29:342–344.

162 Poulton J, Morten K, Freeman-Emmerson C, et al. Deficiency of the human mitochondrial transcription factor h-mtTFA in infantile mitochondrial myopathy associated with mtDNA depletion. Hum Mol Genet 1994; 3:1763–1769.

163 Parvari R, Brodyansky I, Elpeleg O, et al. A recessive contiguous gene deletion of chromosome 2p16 associated with cystinuria and a mitochondrial disease. Am J Hum Genet 2001; 69:869–875.

164 Leshinsky-Silver E, Naviaux RK, Zinger A, et al. MEHMO (mental retardation, epileptic seizures, hypogenitalism, microcephaly, obesity): a new X-linked mitochondrial DNA depletion syndrome. Mitochondrion 2001; 1:95–96.

165 White AJ. Mitochondrial toxicity and HIV therapy. Sex Transm Infect 2001; 77:158–173.

166 DiMauro S, Bonilla E, Lee CP, et al. Luft's disease. Further biochemical and ultrastructural studies of skeletal muscle in the second case. J Neurol Sci 1976; 27:217–232.

167 Bakker HD, Scholte HR, van den Bogert C, et al. Deficiency of the adenine nucleotide translocator in muscle of a patient with myopathy and lactic acidosis: a new mitochondrial defect. Pediatr Res 1993; 33:412–417.

168 Huizing M, Ruitenbeek W, Thinnes FP, et al. Deficiency of the voltage-dependent anion channel: a novel cause of mitochondriopathy. Pediatr Res 1996; 39:760–765.

169 Hayes DJ, Taylor DJ, Bore PJ, et al. An unusual metabolic myopathy: a malate-aspartate shuttle defect. J Neurol Sci 1987; 82:27–39.

170 DiMauro S. Mitochondrial encephalomyopathies: what next? J Inherit Metabol Dis 1996; 19:489–503.

171 Huckriede A, Agsteribbe E. Decreased synthesis and inefficient mitochondrial import of hsp60 in a patient with a mitochondrial encephalomyopathy. Biochim Biophys Acta 1994; 1227:200–206.

172 Hall RE, Henriksson KG, Lewis SF, et al. Mitochondrial myopathy with succinate dehydrogenase and aconitase deficiency. Abnormalities of several iron–sulfur proteins. J Clin Invest 1993; 92:2660–2666.

173 Casari G, De Fusco M, Ciarmatori S, et al. Spastic paraplegia and OXPHOS impairment caused by mutations in paraplegin, a nuclear-encoded mitochondrial metalloprotease. Cell 1998; 93:973–983.

174 Rothbauer U, Hofmann S, Muhlenbein N, et al. Role of the deafness dystonia peptide 1 (DDP1) in import of human Tim23 into the inner membrane of mitochondria. J Biol Chem 2001; 276:37327–37334.

175 Orth M, Schapira AHV. Mitochondria and degenerative disorders. Am J Med Genet 2001; 106:27–36.

176 Tan G, Chen L-S, Lonnerdal B, et al. Frataxin expression rescues mitochondrial dysfunctions in FRDA cells. Hum Mol Genet 2001; 19:2099–2107.

177 Allikmets R, Rashkind WH, Hutchinson A, et al. Mutation of a putative mitochondrial iron transporter gene (ABC7) in X-linked sideroblastic anemia and ataxia (XLSA/A). Hum Mol Genet 1999; 8:743–749.

178 Lutsenko S, Cooper MJ. Localization of the Wilson's disease protein product to mitochondria. Proc Natl Acad Sci USA 1998; 95:6004–6009.

179 Bione S, D'Adamo P, Maestrini E, et al. A novel X-linked gene, G4.5. is responsible for Barth syndrome. Nat Genet 1996; 12:385–389.

180 Beal MF. Mitochondrial dysfunction in neurodegenerative diseases. Biochim Biophys Acta 1998; 1366:211–223.

181 Schapira AHV. Mitochondrial dysfunction in neurodegenerative disorders. Biochim Biophys Acta 1998; 1366:225–233.

182 Comi GP, Bordoni A, Salani S, et al. Cytochrome c oxidase subunit I microdeletion in a patient with motor neuron disease. Ann Neurol 1998; 43:110–116.

183 Shoffner JM. Oxidative phosphorylation disease diagnosis. Sem Neurol 1999; 19:341–351.

184 Jaksch M, Kleinle S, Scharfe C, et al. Frequency of mitochondrial transfer RNA mutations and deletions in 225 patients presenting with respiratory chain deficiencies. J Med Genet 2001; 28:665–673.

185 Chan A, Reichmann H, Kögel A, et al. Metabolic changes in patients with mitochondrial myopathies and effects of coenzyme Q10 therapy. J Neurol 1998; 245:681–685.

186 Abe K, Matsuo Y, Kadekawa J, et al. Effect of coenzyme Q10 in patients with mitochondrial myopathy, encephalopathy, lactic acidosis, and stroke-like episodes (MELAS): evaluation by noninvasive tissue oximetry. J Neurol Sci 1999; 162:65–68.

187 De Stefano N, Matthews PM, Ford B, et al. Short-term dichloroacetate treatment improves indices of cerebral metabolism in patients with mitochondrial disorders. Neurology 1995; 45:1193–1198.

188 Saitoh S, Momoi MY, Yamagata T, et al. Effects of dichloroacetate in three patients with MELAS. Neurology 1998; 50:531–534.

189 Taivassalo T, Fu K, Johns T, et al. Gene shifting: a novel therapy for mitochondrial myopathy. Hum Mol Genet 1999; 8:1047–1052.

190 Kawakami Y, Sakuta R, Hashimoto K, et al. Mitochondrial myopathy with progressive decrease in mitochondrial tRNALeu(UUR) mutant genomes. Ann Neurol 1994; 35:370–373.

191 Taivassalo T, Shoubridge EA, Chen J, et al. Aerobic conditioning in patients with mitochondrial myopathies: physiological, biochemical, and genetic effects. Ann Neurol 2001; 50:133–141.

192 Collombet J-M, Coutelle C. Towards gene therapy of mitochondrial disorders. Mol Med Today 1998; 4:31–38.

193 Taylor RW, Chinnery PF, Turnbull DM, et al. Selective inhibition of mutant human mitochondrial DNA replication in vitro by peptide nucleic acids. Nat Genet 1997; 15:212–215.

LYSOSOMAL STORAGE DISEASES

194 Scriver C, Valle D, Sly W, et al, eds. The metabolic and molecular bases of inherited disease, 8th edn. New York: McGraw-Hill; 2001.

195 Applegarth DA, Toone JR, Lowry RB. Incidence of inborn errors of metabolism in British Columbia, 1969–1996. Pediatrics 2000; 105:e10.

196 Meikle PJ, Hopwood JJ, Clague AE, et al. Prevalence of lysosomal storage disorders. JAMA 1999; 28:249–254.

197 Krivit W, Shapiro E, Kennedy W, et al. Treatment of late infantile metachromatic leukodystrophy by bone marrow transplantation. N Engl J Med 1990; 322:28–32.

198 Hoogerbrugge PM, Brouwer OF, Bordigoni P, et al. Allogeneic bone marrow transplantation for lysosomal storage diseases. The European Group for Bone Marrow Transplantation. Lancet 1995; 345:1398–1402.

199 Ringden O, Groth CG, Erikson A, et al. Ten years' experience of bone marrow transplantation for Gaucher disease. Transplantation 1995; 59:864–870.

200 Krivit W, Aubourg P, Shapiro E, et al. Bone marrow transplantation for globoid cell leukodystrophy, adrenoleukodystrophy, metachromatic leukodystrophy, and Hurler syndrome. Curr Opin Hematol 1999; 6:377–382.

201 Krivit W, Peters C, Shapiro EG. Bone marrow transplantation as effective treatment of central nervous system disease in globoid cell leukodystrophy, metachromatic leukodystrophy, adrenoleukodystrophy, mannosidosis, fucosidosis, aspartylglucosaminuria, Hurler, Maroteaux-Lamy, and Sly syndromes, and Gaucher disease type III. Curr Opin Neurol 1999; 12:167–176.

202 Barton NW, Brady RO, Dambrosia JM, et al. Replacement therapy for inherited enzyme deficiency–macrophage-targeted glucocerebrosidase for Gaucher's disease. N Engl J Med 1991; 324:1464–1470.

203 Eng CM, Guffon N, Wilcox WR, et al. Safety and efficacy of recombinant human-galactosidase A replacement therapy in Fabry's disease. N Engl J Med 2001; 345:9–16.

204 Schiffmann R, Kopp JB, Austin HA 3rd, et al. Enzyme replacement therapy in Fabry disease: a randomized controlled trial. JAMA 2001; 285:2743–2749.

205 Kakkis ED, Muenzer J, Tiller GE, et al. Enzyme-replacement therapy in mucopolysaccharidosis I. N Engl J Med 2001; 344:182–188.

206 Van den Hout H, Reuser AJ, Vulto AG, et al. Recombinant human alpha-glucosidase from rabbit milk in Pompe patients. Lancet 2000; 356:397–398.

207 Amalfitano A, Bengur AR, Morse RP, et al. Recombinant human acid alpha-glucosidase enzyme therapy for infantile glycogen storage disease type II: results of a phase I/II clinical trial. Genet Med 2001; 3:132–138.

208 Platt FM, Neises GR, Reinkensmeier G, et al. Prevention of lysosomal storage in Tay-Sachs mice treated with N-butyldeoxynojirimycin. Science 1997; 276:428–431.

209 Cox T, Lachmann R, Hollak C, et al. Novel oral treatment of Gaucher's disease with N-butyldeoxynojirimycin (OGT 918) to decrease substrate biosynthesis. Lancet 2000; 355: 1481–1485.

210 Norflus F, Tifft CJ, McDonald MP, et al. Bone marrow transplantation prolongs life span and ameliorates neurologic manifestations in Sandhoff disease mice. J Clin Invest 1998; 101:1881–1888.

211 Platt FM, Reinkensmeier G, Dwek RA, et al. Extensive glycosphingolipid depletion in the liver and lymphoid organs of mice treated with N-butyldeoxynojirimycin. J Biol Chem 1997; 272:19365–19372.

212 Charrow J, Esplin JA, Gribble TJ, et al. Gaucher disease: recommendations on diagnosis, evaluation, and monitoring. Arch Intern Med 1998; 158:1754–1760.

213 Rosenberg SA, Blaese RM, Brenner MK, et al. Human gene marker/therapy clinical protocols. Hum Gene Ther 2000; 11:919–979.

214 Barranger JA, Rice R, Sansieri C, et al. Transduction and transplantation of mobilized CD34; significance for gene therapy of Gaucher disease. Am J Hum Genet 1997; 181(suppl)4:A35.

215 Krivit W, Shapiro EG, Peters C, et al. Hematopoietic stem-cell transplantation in globoid-cell leukodystrophy. N Engl J Med 1998; 338:1119–1126.

216 Harmatz P, Whitley C, Belan K, et al. A phase I/II double blind two dose group study of rhASB enzyme replacement therapy in patients with MPS VI (Maroteaux-Lamy syndrome). Am J Hum Genet 2001; 69(suppl):674, A2896.

217 Wisniewski KE, Kida E, Golabek AA, et al. Neuronal lipofuscinosis: classification and diagnosis. Adv Genet 2001; 45:1–34.

CONGENITAL DISORDERS OF GLYCOSYLATION

218 Freeze HH. Disorders in protein glycosylation and potential therapy: tip of the iceberg? J Pediatr 1998; 133:593–600.

219 Jaeken J, Carchon H. Congenital disorders of glycosylation: the rapidly growing tip of the iceberg. Curr Opin Neurol 2001; 14:811–815.

220 Lacey JM, Bergen HR, Magera MJ, et al. Rapid determination of transferrin isoforms by immunoaffinity liquid chromatography and electrospray mass spectrometry. Clin Chem 2001; 47:513–518.

221 de Lonlay P, Seta N, Barrot S, et al. A broad spectrum of clinical presentations in congenital disorders of glycosylation I: a series of 26 cases. J Med Genet 2001; 38:14–19.

222 Jaeken J, Matthijs G. Congenital disorders of glycosylation. Annu Rev Genomics Hum Genet 2001; 2:129–151.

223 Blennow G, Jaeken J, Wiklund LM. Neurological findings in the carbohydrate-deficient glycoprotein syndrome. Acta Paediatr Scand 1991; 375(suppl):14–20.

224 Jaeken J, Hagberg B, Stromme P. Clinical presentation and natural course of the carbohydrate-deficient glycoprotein syndrome. Acta Paediatr Scand 1991; 375(suppl):6–13.

225 Barone R, Pavone L, Fiumara A, et al. Developmental patterns and neuropsychological assessment in patients with carbohydrate-deficient glycoconjugate syndrome type IA (phosphomannomutase deficiency). Brain Develop 1999; 21:260–263.

226 van Ommem CH, Peters M, Barth PG, et al. Carbohydrate-deficient glycoprotein syndrome type 1a: a variant phenotype with borderline cognitive dysfunction, cerebellar hypoplasia, and coagulation disturbances. J Pediatr 2000; 136:400–403.

227 Grünewald S, Schollen E, van Schaftingen E, et al. High residual activity of PMM2 in patients = fibroblasts: possible pitfall in the diagnosis of CDG-Ia (phosphomannomutase deficiency). Am J Hum Genet 2001; 68:347–354.

228 Imtiaz F, Worthington V, Champion M, et al. Genotypes and phenotypes of patients in the UK with carbohydrate-deficient glycoprotein syndrome type I. J Inher Metab Dis 2000; 23:162–174.

229 Charlwood J, Clayton P, Keir G, et al. Prenatal diagnosis of the carbohydrate-deficiency glycoprotein syndrome type 1A (CDG1A) by a combination of enzymology and genetic linkage analysis after amniocentesis or chorionic villus sampling. Prenat Diagn 1998; 18:693–699.

230 Mayatepek E, Schröder M, Kohlmüller D, et al. Continuous mannose infusion in carbohydrate-deficient glycoprotein syndrome type I. Acta Paediatr 1997; 86:1138–1140.

231 Kjaergaard S, Kristiansson B, Stibler H, et al. Failure of short-term mannose therapy of patients with carbohydrate-deficient glycoprotein syndrome type IA. Acta Paediatr 1998; 87:884–888.

232 Niehues R, Hasilik M, Alton G, et al. Carbohydrate-deficient glycoprotein syndrome type Ib: phosphomannose isomerase deficiency and mannose therapy. J Clin Invest 1998; 101:1414–1420.

233 Babovic-Vuksanovic D, Patterson MC, Schwenk WF, et al. Severe hypoglycemia as a presenting symptom of carbohydrate-deficient glycoprotein syndrome. J Pediatr 1999; 135:775–781.

234 de Lonlay P, Cuer M, Vuillaumier-Barrot S, et al. Hyperinsulinemic hypoglycemia as a presenting sign in phosphomannose isomerase deficiency: a new manifestation of carbohydrate-deficient glycoprotein syndrome treatable with mannose. J Pediatr 1999; 135:179–183.

235 Jaeken J, Schachter H, Carchon H, et al. Carbohydrate deficient glycoprotein syndrome type II: a deficiency in Golgi localised N-acetyl-glucosaminyltransferase II. Arch Dis Child 1994; 71:123–127.

236 Cornier-Daire V, Amiel J, Vuillaumier-Barrot S, et al. Congenital disorders of glycosylation IIa cause growth retardation, mental retardation, and facial dysmorphism. J Med Genet 2000; 37:875–877.

237 De Praeter CM, Gerwig GJ, Bause E, et al. A novel disorder caused by defective biosynthesis of N-linked oligosaccharides due to glucosidase I deficiency. Am J Hum Genet 2000; 66:1744–1756.

25

Immunodeficiency

Andrew J Cant, Diana M Gibb, E Graham Davies, Catherine Cale, Andrew R Gennery

INTRODUCTION

The term 'immunity' is used to describe the state in which the immune system responds to a given antigenic challenge either in a useful (protective) sense or in a harmful way (allergy or hypersensitivity). The main role of the immune system is to repel invasion by microorganisms. Abnormalities in this system may result in an increased susceptibility to infection as well as other non-infective problems such as allergy and autoimmunity. Our increased understanding of the immune mechanisms used in handling microbes has led to a better understanding of both primary and secondary immunodeficiency.[1] Conversely, much has been learned of the intricacies of immune function from studying patients with immunodeficiency.

THE IMMUNE SYSTEM

The primary host defense against infection involves important innate factors. Whilst not part of the immunological system, physical and chemical barriers play an important role in pathogen exclusion by direct antimicrobial effects or the prevention of microbial attachment. Physical barriers such as epithelial surfaces and mucous membranes provide the first line of defense and are augmented by hair and cilia in conjunction with respiratory tract mucus secretions, stomach acids and other mucous membrane secretions. Commensal intestinal and skin flora produce antibiotics which act locally, excluding potential pathogens. The importance of such defenses is clearly demonstrated when they are significantly breached, for example bacterial sepsis following severe burns or repeated bacterial infection causing bronchiectasis in immotile bronchial cilia syndrome or in cystic fibrosis (see Ch.18). Although the role these barriers play in the initial defense is critical they will not be considered further in this chapter.

The immune system is comprised of cells and molecules adapted to protect the organism against infection. Cells develop from pluripotent stem cells in the fetal liver and bone marrow and circulate through blood and extracellular fluid. They signal to each other and interact via transmembrane receptors and peptide messengers, or cytokines, which interact with specific receptors on their target cells.

Cells, cytokines and receptors of the immune system

Surface molecules present on leukocytes and other cells of the immune system are known as leukocyte differentiation antigens and are identified by their reactivity with specific monoclonal antibodies. Monoclonal antibodies recognizing the same antigens are designated by CD (cluster designation or cluster of differentiation) numbers which designate the particular antigens that they recognize. Functional lymphocyte subsets are identified by their surface antigens. Other antigens classify cells according to their state of differentiation or activation. The more important surface antigens recognized by different CD antibodies are listed in Table 25.1. The functional roles of many of these surface antigens has been established.

Much of the immune response is mediated by soluble protein messengers (cytokines) secreted by leukocytes, organs such as the liver or vascular endothelium which regulate afferent and efferent immune responses, direct effector mechanisms and act as growth factors. The more important cytokines and their main effects are listed in Table 25.2. Many of these proteins have multiple and overlapping effects and are important in the innate and specific adaptive immune systems.

Cytokines interact with their ligands (or receptors) on the surface of the target cells. Most receptors belong to a family of cytokine receptors with common protein sequences. Receptors made up of more than one protein chain often share one or more chains common to other receptors. An example is the gamma chain of the interleukin-2 (IL-2) receptor which is shared with the receptors for IL-4, IL-6, IL-7, IL-9 and IL-15. Mutations in the gene for this chain result in X-linked severe combined immunodeficiency (SCID) (p. 1269).

Specific and non-specific mechanisms

Pathogens that breach the barrier defenses encounter two fundamentally different types of response (Fig. 25.1), firstly non-specific and then specific components of the immune system. Non-antigen-specific immune responses employ a limited number of receptors specific for conserved microbial structures, but are highly effective; phyllogenetically only vertebrates have needed to evolve more complex mechanisms. Elements of the response include neutrophil and mononuclear phagocytes, as well as humoral factors such as complement.

The specific (adaptive) immune system is distinguished by its ability to 'respond' to antigens by proliferation of antigen-specific T and B lymphocytes following presentation of antigen to their receptor by cells of the innate system. Such responses are then committed to 'immunological memory' resulting in more rapid and enhanced responses upon subsequent antigen exposure.

Non-specific and specific mechanisms are interdependent and many specific immune mechanisms exert their effects using the non-specific elements. Non-specific function is often greatly potentiated by factors produced by the specific immune response.

NON-SPECIFIC IMMUNE MECHANISMS

Humoral

Complement

One of the most important humoral defense systems is the complement system. The central component in this system (Fig. 25.2) is C3b, the active product of cleavage of the C3 molecule. C3b bound to an antigen acts as a powerful opsonin by interacting with C3b receptors on neutrophils and monocytes. C3 is cleaved either by the classical (antibody-dependent) pathway, which requires specific antibody–antigen interaction, or by the alternative pathway, in which microbial products, such as polysaccharides and endotoxin, directly activate another cascade of reactions involving serum protein factors B and D to form an alternative C3 convertase which is stabilized by factor P (properdin).

The fixing of C3b to the surface of a microorganism becomes self-amplifying, since C3b itself forms a component of the enzyme responsible for C3 cleavage. This is strictly controlled by a number of regulatory proteins. The later complement components C5–C9

Table 25.1 Leukocyte antigens

Designation	Main cellular expression	Properties/function
T cells		
CD1	Thymocytes. Langerhans' cells	Unknown
CD2	Mature T cells	Sheep erythrocyte (E Rosette) receptor; LFA-3 ligand
CD3	Pan T cell marker	Part of T cell receptor complex
CD4	Helper/inducer T cells	MHC class II receptor; HIV receptor
CD5	Mature T cells. B cell subset (B1)	Unknown
CD8	Cytotoxic/suppressor T cells	MHC class I receptor
CD25	Activated T cells	IL-2 α receptor
CD28	T cells	CD 80 receptor; T cell activation
CD38	Thymocytes Activated cells	Unknown
CD71	Activated T cells Thymocytes	Transferrin receptor
B cells		
CD19	Pre B and B cells	Unknown
CD20	Pre B and B cells	Unknown
CD21	B cells	Complement receptor (CR) 2 EBV receptor
CD22	Pre B and B cells	Unknown
CD23	B cells	Low affinity IgE receptor
CD40	B cells	Ig isotype switching
Surface immunoglobulin	B cells	Antigen receptor
Monocytes		
CD14	Monocytes	Receptor for lipopolysaccharide
NK cells		
CD16	NK, monocytes	Fc γ receptor III
CD56	PMN, NK and some T cells	Unknown
General		
CD11a	Leukocytes	Cell adhesion ICAM-I receptor
CD11b	NK cells, MΦ, PMN	CR3
CD11c	NK cells, MΦ, PMN	CR4
CD15	PMN	Lewis X antigen
CD18	Leukocytes	β_2 integrin associated with CD11 antigens
CD34	BM progenitor cells	L selectin ligand
CD35	Monocytes, PMN, B cells	CR1
CD43	All leukocytes	Sialophorin
CD45	All leukocytes	Tyrosine phosphatase. T cell activation. Variable isoforms – see text
CD58	All leukocytes	LFA-3; CD2 ligand
CD80	Activated B and T mono	CD28 receptor
HLA class I	All leukocytes	Antigen presentation
HLA class II	B, monocytes, activated T cells	Antigen presentation

Mϕ = macrophage; BM = bone marrow; PMN = polymorphonuclear cells

produce a membrane-attack complex which can lyse cell membranes, a mechanism particularly important in the handling of systemic neisserial infections.

As well as lysis and opsonization, the complement reactions generate pharmacologically and chemotactically active byproducts, such as the cleavage products C3a and C5a, for which there are cell surface receptors.

The major cell surface receptors for complement are the ligands for C3b and derivatives which are responsible for the most important functions of the system. Complement receptor 1 (CR1, CD35, Table 25.1) is found on neutrophils, monocytes, erythrocytes, B lymphocytes and glomerular epithelial cells. It recognizes C3b- and C4b-coated particles and facilitates phagocytosis. Erythrocyte CR1 helps clear circulating immune complexes. CR2 (CD21), found predominantly on B lymphocytes and recognizing C3d – the main C3b breakdown product, is believed to modulate activity of these cells. It is the receptor for Epstein–Barr virus (EBV). CR3 (CD11b/CD18) on phagocytic cells and on natural killer (NK) cells recognizes inactivated C3b (C3bi) and is important in phagocytosis. CR4 (CD11c/CD18) weakly binds C3bi. CR3 and CR4 are members of a family of adhesion molecules, the leukocyte integrins also involved in intracellular adhesion.

Mannan-binding lectin (MBL)[2]

This acute phase protein is a multimer of identical chains with structural similarities to first complement component, C1q. It binds to the sugar mannose, which is found on the surface of microorganisms, and facilitates opsonization of the organism perhaps by binding to MBL receptor on phagocytic cells, but mainly by activating the classical complement pathway, to fix C4 and C2, resulting in the generation of classical C3 convertase (Fig. 25.2). This can occur in the absence of C1 and antibody; consequently MBL is an important opsonin in the early stages of infection (before antibody production) and in young children (with immature ability to produce antibodies).

Other acute phase reactants

Serum levels of this diverse group of proteins, including clotting factors, amyloid proteins and C-reactive protein (CRP), rise rapidly at the onset of acute inflammatory responses. Their precise biological role is poorly characterized. CRP has some immune modulating effects and acts as a non-specific opsonin for bacterial phagocytosis.

Interferon

Alpha- and beta-interferons are proteins produced by virally infected cells. They render other cells immune to virus infection by producing an antiviral state. Interferons also increase NK cell activity, increase human leukocyte antigen (HLA) class I antigen expression on cells, and decrease cell growth including that of tumor cells. gamma-interferon, though having some antiviral effect, is primarily a cytokine, which upregulates immune responses particularly by enhancing intracellular killing of microorganisms such as mycobacteria.

Iron-binding proteins

Many bacteria require iron for growth, and decreasing its availability is one mechanism of defense used by the host. An avid iron-binding protein, lactoferrin, present in human milk reduces the growth of *Escherichia coli*. The reduction of serum iron, which occurs during infections, increases the bacteriostatic effect of serum.

Lysozyme

This enzyme with antibacterial properties is found in neutrophil lysosomes and in body secretions including tears and saliva.

Table 25.2 Principal cytokines

Cytokine	Other (previous) names	Produced by	Main actions
IL-1		Monocytes	Proinflammatory; fever; T cell activation
IL-2	T cell growth factor	T cells	T (mainly T_H1), NK cell activation/proliferation
IL-3	Multicolony stimulating factor	T cells	Proliferation of bone marrow progenitor cells
IL-4	B cell stimulating factor	T cells (T_H2)	T_H2 cell growth factor; B cell isotype switching especially to IgE
IL-5		T cells	T_H2 cytokine; activation and proliferation of eosinophils (and B cells)
IL-6		T, B cells monocytes	General cell growth and differentiation factor
IL-7	Lymphopoietin I	Bone marrow and thymic stroma	General cell growth factor
IL-8		T cells, monocytes, PMN	PMN activation, chemotaxis and adhesion
IL-9		T cells	T cell, mast cell growth and differentiation
IL-10	Cytokine synthesis inhibitory factor	T cells (T_H2) monocytes, mast cells	Inhibits T_H1 cytokine production
IL-11		Stromal cells	Growth factor similar in actions to IL-6
IL-12	NK stimulating factor	B cells, monocytes	Increases T and NK cell cytotoxicity; T_H1 growth and differentiation factor
IL-13		T cells (T_H2)	B cell isotype switching similar to IL-4
IL-14	High mol wt B cell growth factor	T, B cells	B cell growth and differentiation
IL-15		Stromal cells, monocytes	Similar actions to IL-2 (utilizes same receptor)
IFN α and β		Leukocytes-α Fibroblasts-β	Antiviral, antiproliferative Increased MHC expression, increased cytotoxic activity
IFNγ	Macrophage activating factor	T cells (T_H1) NK cells	Macrophage activation, increased MHC expression, T_H1 effects
TNF α	Cachectin	Monocytes	Proinflammatory
TNF β	Lymphotoxin	T cells	Proinflammatory
GM CSF		Leukocytes	Increased myelopoiesis, increased cytokine production by macrophages, proinflammatory
G CSF		Leukocytes	Increased granulopoiesis, activates PMN, reduces inflammatory cytokine production
M CSF		Monocytes, T, B cells	Increased monocyte growth and differentiation, increased cytokine production
TGF β		Platelets, monocytes	Suppresses inflammation and cell proliferation

IL = Interleukin; IFN = Interferon; TNF = Tumor necrosis factor; CSF = Colony stimulating factor; GM = Granulocyte macrophage; G = Granulocyte; M = Monocyte; TGF = Transforming growth factor; PMN = Polymorphonuclear cells; T_H1/T_H2 = T helper cells

Cellular non-specific immune mechanisms

Adhesion molecules

These molecules and ligands help cell-to-cell association, essential for normal immune and inflammatory responses. Found on all cells of the immune system and on vascular endothelium, their expression is tightly controlled during inflammatory responses by cytokines such as the interleukins, tumor necrosis factor alpha (TNF-alpha) and interferon gamma (IFN-gamma).

One group of adhesion molecules is the selectins. L selectin is constitutively expressed on neutrophils and monocytes and binds to its ligand, on the surface of vascular endothelium. E and P selectin expression on endothelial cells is induced during inflammation. These bind to ligands on leukocytes, an important one being a sialated carbohydrate called sialyl lewis x. Interaction between the selectins and their ligands results in the transient endothelial interactions of 'rolling' and margination which occur early in inflammatory reactions. Subsequently, L selectin is shed by the cells and expression of more tightly adherent molecules is upregulated.

The more firmly adhering molecules, called beta-2 intergrins, play a role in the firm adherence of neutrophils to endothelium and subsequent egress from the circulation. They have a fundamental role in cell–cell interaction, critical in the generation of immune responses, and cell effector functions such as cytotoxicity. Their expression is greatly upregulated by the proinflammatory cytokines such as TNF-alpha or IL-1 beta.

Effector cells

Phagocytic cells include neutrophils and monocyte/macrophages. Bacterial phagocytosis requires migration of neutrophils to the site of infection (chemotaxis). Products of the acute inflammatory response, including cleaved complement fragments (e.g. C5a), act as chemoattractants in this process. Chemotaxis is followed by adherence to the bacterium and ingestion (phagocytosis). This is aided by opsonization, particularly by immunoglobulin G (IgG) and complement (C3b), which bind to bacteria and also phagocyte cell surface receptors Fc gamma and CR1/3 respectively, but also C-reactive protein and soluble forms of fibronectin. Following

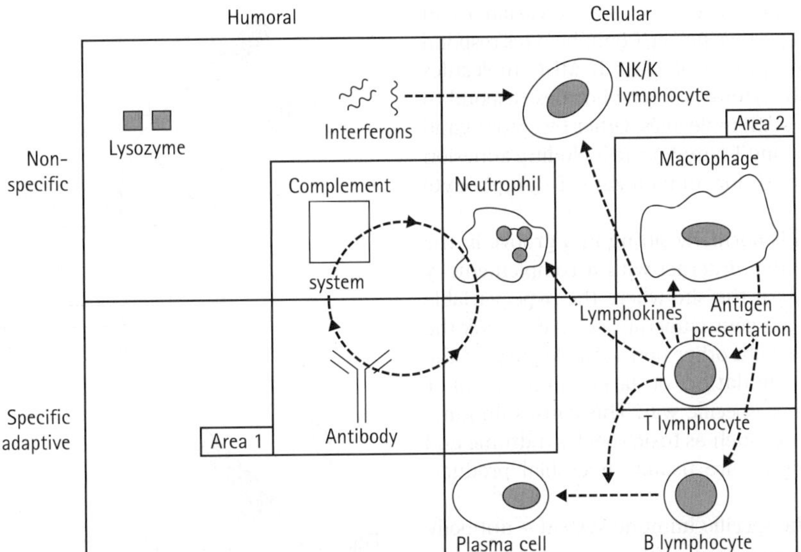

Fig. 25.1 Functional compartments of the immune system illustrating some of the more important interactions (dotted arrows). Area 1 mainly involved in handling pyogenic bacteria. Area 2 mainly involved with intracellular pathogens.

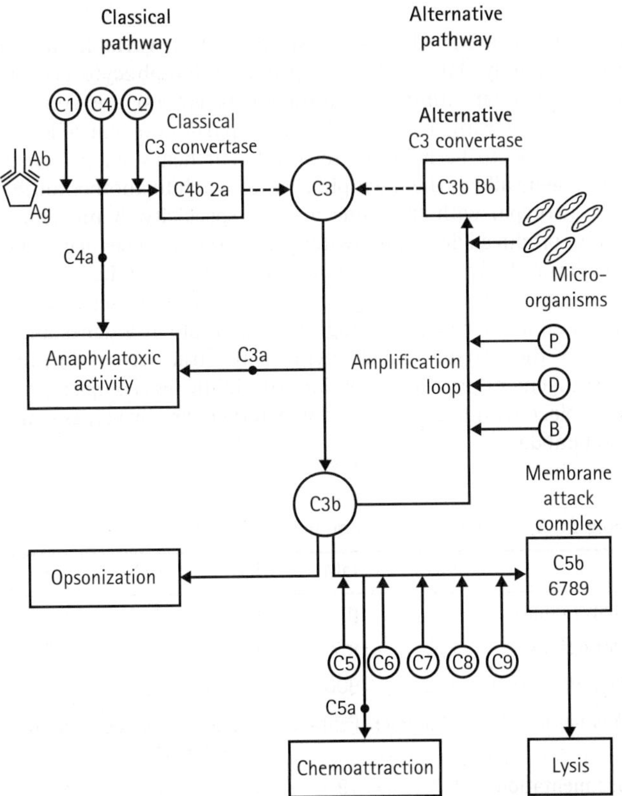

Fig. 25.2 The main features of the classical and alternative pathways of the complement system. Inactive cleavage and breakdown products are not shown.

phagocytosis, lysosomes rapidly fuse with the bacterium-containing phagosome exposing the bacterium to lysosomal enzymes (e.g. myeloperoxidase) which are involved in killing and digestion. The process is accompanied by the generation of hydrogen peroxide, superoxide and hydroxyl radicals which aid bacterial killing. Neutrophil numbers and function are enhanced by the inflammatory response.

Monocytes and macrophages ingest and kill extracellular bacteria in a similar fashion to neutrophils but more slowly and less efficiently. However, they are very important in defenses against intracellular microorganisms, including bacteria such as *Mycobacterium tuberculosis* and *Listeria monocytogenes*. Such pathogens are recognized directly by the cell surface mannose/fucose receptor interacting with microbial carbohydrate moieties such as mannose, or are opsonized and bound to Fc gamma or CR1/3 receptors. They are also cytotoxic against infected host cells or malignant cells. Macrophage activity is greatly enhanced by cytokines, particularly IFN-gamma, produced by T lymphocytes as part of the specific cell-mediated immune response.

NK cells are part of the non-T, non-B cell lymphoid population and recognize and kill tumor and virus-infected cells. They have surface receptors for the Fc fragment of IgG and, when 'armed' with specific IgG against a target cell antigen, kill by a process called antibody-dependent cellular cytotoxicity (ADCC). They also have killer-activating and killer-inhibitory receptors. Killer-activating receptors recognize a number of different cell surface molecules, and when engaged, issue a 'kill' message, normally over-ridden by the killer-inhibitory receptors engaging major histocompatibility complex (MHC) I molecules. Loss of MHC I expression due to viral cell infection or malignancy, removes the inhibitory control, resulting in cytotoxic cell killing.

SPECIFIC IMMUNE MECHANISMS

Specific responses are orchestrated by T and B lymphocytes, whose receptors are specific for the antigens presented to them. Binding of antigen to receptor leads to the generation of antigen specific effector immune mechanisms, such as antibody production or the generation of specific cytotoxic T lymphocytes.

Specialized cells of the macrophage series called antigen presenting cells (APC) and also B lymphocytes present antigens to T lymphocytes. APCs take up antigens, degrade them to small peptide fragments and then express them on the cell surface in association with the MHC molecules.[3] The T lymphocyte receptor (T cell receptor, TCR) will only recognize the peptide in association with a self MHC molecule. Some MHC polymorphisms provoke better responses than others, explaining part of the genetic variability in immune responsiveness. CD4 positive helper T lymphocytes respond to antigen bound within the groove of class II MHC molecules (HLA-DR) whilst CD8 positive cytotoxic T lymphocytes respond to antigen bound to class I (HLA-AB) molecules. Other receptor ligand interactions between the APC and T lymphocyte including adhesion molecules are also important for maximizing T lymphocyte stimulation.

When presented, antigen is normally sitting in a groove in the MHC molecule where it can then interact with a complementary groove in the TCR (Fig. 25.3) at the site where the hypervariable regions are expressed. Some antigens (superantigens) crosslink the presenting cell MHC molecule with other non-variable parts of the TCR chains, resulting in stimulation of large numbers of T lymphocytes in an antigen non-specific way. This causes immune mediated inflammatory diseases such as toxic shock syndrome and Kawasaki disease. Superantigens are usually microbial products such as exotoxins.

There are two arms of the specific immune system – antibody mediated and cell mediated.

Antibodies

These are immunoglobulins produced by B lymphocytes and their derivatives, plasma cells, in response to specific antigens. Antibodies produced against microbial antigens may follow exposure to the microbe or to a vaccine. Sometimes, specific antibodies may be present in the serum without prior exposure to the relevant antigen – so called 'natural' antibodies, resulting from cross-reactivity between antigens, particularly non-protein (polysaccharide) antigens.

The basic structure of the immunoglobulin molecule is shown in Figure 25.4. The variable region has a unique amino acid sequence, giving the antibody its unique specificity which ensures that there is an antibody complementary to every antigen that could be constructed. There are five main classes of immunoglobulin, each with its own structure and functions (Tables 25.3 and 25.4).

The immunoglobulin class or isotype is determined by the heavy chain. During B lymphocyte development, rearrangement of genes coding for the variable and constant parts of the immunoglobulin chain occurs (Fig. 25.5). One each out of the V, D and J heavy chain genes is rearranged to lie adjacent to the relevant heavy chain constant region gene, so that transcription produces a single protein with a constant and a variable portion. Approximately 10^{16} different specific T lymphocyte receptors (with a similar number of antibody receptors) are generated. Further rearrangement to bring a particular variable gene combination to lie adjacent to a different heavy chain constant region gene allows the B lymphocyte to switch to another antibody class (isotype) with the same antigen specificity. A mu chain is always produced first; class switching to other isotypes occurs later. Specific antibody diversity is created by the large number of possible combinations of variable region genes which can be selected and is increased further by a very high mutation rate in V genes and the effect of the enzyme TdT (deoxynucleotidyltransferase) during the rearrangement process. A similar but slightly less complex process takes place with light chains, of which there are two types – kappa and lambda.

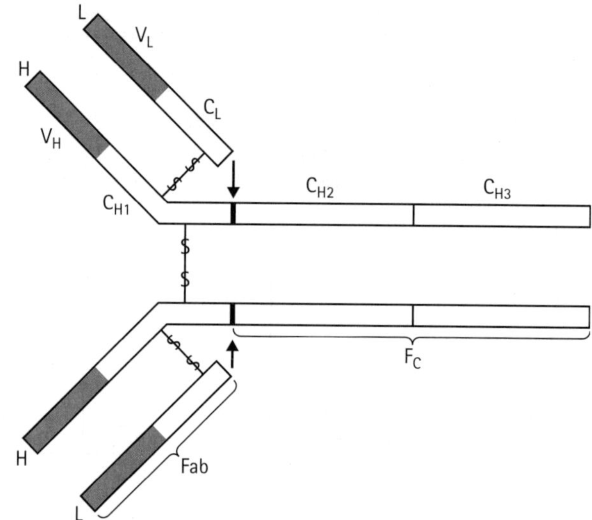

Fig. 25.4 Basic structure of an antibody molecule. Heavy (H) and light (L) chains comprise variable regions (V_H and V_L) – shown by solid bars – and constant regions (C_H and C_L) open bars. Constant region domains (C_{H1}, C_{H2} and C_{H3}) are shown. Arrows indicate site of pepsin-mediated cleavage to give Fc and Fab fragments.

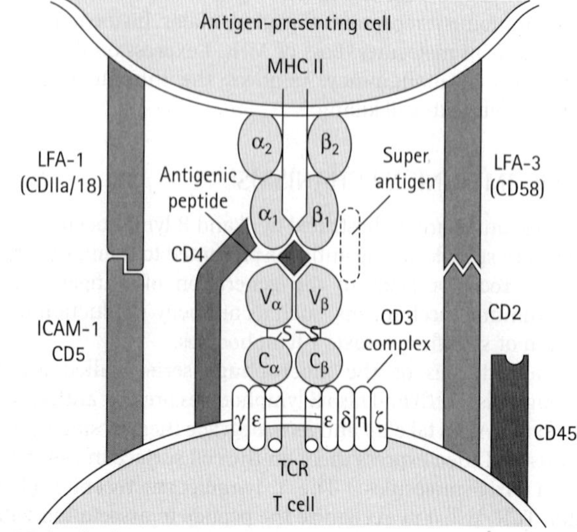

Fig. 25.3 Antigen presentation.

Table 25.3 Properties of serum immunoglobulins

	IgG	IgM	IgA	IgD	IgE
Heavy chain	γ	μ	α	δ	ε
Light chain	κ/λ	κ/λ	κ/λ	κ/λ	κ/λ
Mol wt (×10⁻³)	150	900	160–320	180	200
Polymeric status	Monomer	Pentamer	Monomer or dimer*	Monomer	Monomer
Sedimentation coefficient (Svedberg units)	6.7	19	7	7	8
Mean adult serum concentration (g/L)	12	1.5	3	0.03	0.001
Biological half-life (days)	23	5	7	2.8	2.3
Placental transfer	+	–	–	–	–

*Trimeric IgA may also occur. Secretory IgA is in dimeric form.

Table 25.4 Properties of IgG subclasses

	G1	G2	G3	G4
Mol wt ($\times 10^{-3}$)	150	150	165	150
% of total IgG (adults)	70	20	7	3
Biological half-life (days)	23	23	9	23
Complement-fixing ability	++	+	++	–
Fc receptor binding				
Monocytes	++	+/–	++	+/–
Neutrophils	++	+	+	+
Lymphocytes	+	+/–	+	+/–

IgM

This is the first antibody class produced in primary immune responses. For most antigens, there is a subsequent switching to other classes but for some, e.g. responses to the lipopolysaccharides of Gram negative bacilli, IgM remains the predominant class. Its large pentameric structure confines it to the intravascular space where it fixes complement.

IgG

This is the main class of antibody produced in secondary immune responses. Functions include opsonization, complement fixation leading to C3 opsonization and complement mediated lysis, neutralization of toxins or viruses, and participation in antibody-dependent cellular cytotoxicity. Though there is considerable overlap, the four subclasses of IgG tend to have different functions. In adults, antibodies to bacterial polysaccharides are predominantly of IgG1 subclass, but in children significant amounts are found in the IgG1 subclass. Responses to protein antigens are mainly in the IgG1 and IgG3 subclasses. The role of IgG4 is, as yet, unclear.

IgA

This is the main antibody in secretions, where it forms a dimeric molecule consisting of two IgA subunits joined by a J chain and associated with a protective secretory piece synthesized by epithelial cells. In addition to protecting mucous membranes and the gastrointestinal tract from infection, IgA may have a role in limiting food antigen uptake from the gut. Serum IgA is mainly in monomeric form, though dimeric and trimeric forms are also found.

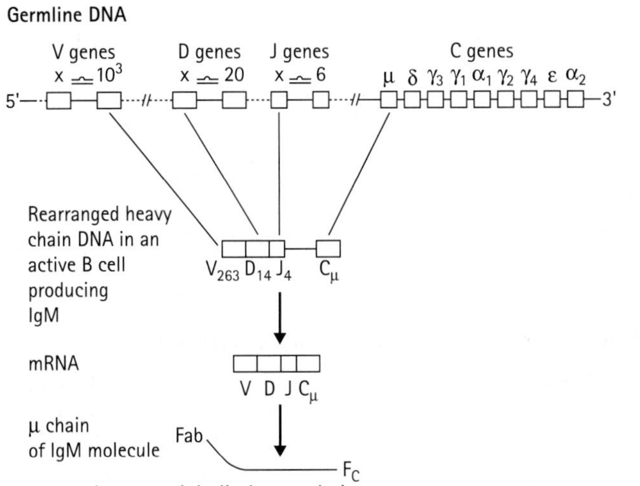

Fig. 25.5 Immunoglobulin heavy chain gene arrangements on chromosome 14 in germline configuration and showing an example of a rearrangement using V gene number 263, D_{14} and J_4 to produce a unique antigen binding site. In this example, the variable genes (V, D and J) have been combined with a μ constant region heavy chain gene ($C\mu$) to produce a complete μ chain of an IgM molecule.

IgD

This is mainly a surface molecule on the membrane of B lymphocytes which regulates B lymphocyte differentiation and maturation. Small amounts found free in plasma are not thought to have any biological role.

IgE

Mast cells and basophils have receptors for the Fc part of this molecule. Antigen binding may cause degranulation of the cells, triggering an immediate hypersensitivity response. Such reactions are often harmful rather than beneficial, but evolved as a mechanism for removing parasites.

Antibody production

Antibodies are produced by B (bone marrow derived) lymphocytes. Naive B lymphocytes have membrane antibody which acts as a receptor for antigen. B lymphocytes may be divided into two subsets on the basis of CD5 surface marker expression. B1 (CD5 +ve) lymphocytes predominate in fetal and neonatal circulations and produce a repertoire of antibodies against self antigens using a limited number of V region genes. They have a poorly understood role in immune regulation and self tolerance and may be increased in autoimmune disorders. B2 (CD5 –ve) lymphocytes are conventional B lymphocytes producing antibodies against foreign antigens.

The final stages of B lymphocyte differentiation require stimulation with the appropriate antigen leading (after final class switching) to maturation into plasma cells. The full process requires the cooperation of antigen-specific T helper (CD4 +ve) lymphocytes. Isotype switching from IgM production to the other antibody classes is critically dependent on T/B lymphocyte interaction via the CD40 antigen on B lymphocytes and its ligand expressed on activated T lymphocytes (CD40L, CD154). The responses to some antigens, e.g. bacterial polysaccharides, can result in limited antibody production without T lymphocyte help. There is no immunological memory generated in such responses.

Cell-mediated immunity

T (thymus-derived) lymphocytes predominate in immune responses to intracellular microbes and also regulate immune responses by secreting cytokines and growth factors.

T lymphocytes are generated from bone marrow derived stem cells, but acquire functional capabilities during a period of thymic maturation. Here the cells undergo a series of developmental stages including gene rearrangement to generate diversity in the variable domains of the TCR. They also become 'educated' with regard to self/non-self recognition so that self-reactive clones are deleted and only clones recognizing antigen in the context of self MHC are preserved.

The TCR, although not an immunoglobulin molecule, has a similar arrangement of constant and variable parts and the generation of diverse specificity is achieved along similar lines to the generation of antibody diversity in B lymphocytes. The TCR is a heterodimeric molecule with each chain having a constant and variable portion. The majority (> 90%) of mature circulating T lymphocytes express alpha and beta chains, the remainder are gamma and delta. Diversity is acquired in a method similar to that of the immunoglobulin molecule. Recombinase activating genes 1 and 2 (RAG1, 2) are critical for this gene rearrangement, and mutations in these genes lead to one form of T-, B- SCID (p. 1271).

During thymic maturation T lymphocytes also acquire important functional surface molecules. CD3 is constitutively expressed on T lymphocytes and is closely associated with the TCR (Fig. 25.3). Initially both CD4 and CD8 are expressed on the same cells, but during thymic maturation, one of the molecules is lost. Most gamma delta T lymphocytes do not express CD4 or CD8. Their precise function is unclear, but they seem to play a role in mucosal defense and gut antigen clearance and tolerance.

The primary effector cell in the adaptive response is the CD4+ T helper lymphocyte (Fig. 25.6). Once switched on by antigen presentation these cells develop in one of two ways: the T_{H1} route with production of IL-2 and interferon whose main role is in stimulating macrophage function and cell mediated immunity but also has effects on B lymphocytes including antibody class switching, particularly to IgG2. T_{H2} cells on the other hand produce predominantly IL-4 and IL-10 which promote antibody responses and class switching, particularly towards IgG1, IgG4 and IgE. Allergic responses and those against parasites are of T_{H2} type. Responses to an antigen may follow a T_{H1} or T_{H2} route depending on a complex set of circumstances. Once established these responses are self-amplifying in that production of IFN-gamma or IL-4 promotes T_{H1} and T_{H2} responses respectively and inhibits the other. There is much interest in learning more about these responses to allow therapeutic switching from T_{H2} to T_{H1} in allergic individuals.

The functions of T lymphocytes can be summarized as:

1. help and regulation of antibody production by B lymphocytes;
2. cytokine production which stimulates and regulates other non-specific immune effector cells;
3. secretion of growth and differentiation factors, e.g. colony-stimulating factors, B lymphocyte growth factors;
4. T lymphocyte-mediated specific cytotoxicity, e.g. against virus-infected cells or against foreign tissues.

Signal transduction

Once T and B lymphocytes have engaged antigen via their specific receptors they must activate to generate the next step in the immune response. This activation may take the form of increased transcription of the genes for surface receptors such as CD40 ligand and the IL-2 receptor on T lymphocytes, IL-2 production and preparation for cell division. The conveyance of the 'message' from the membrane receptors to the nucleus is called signal transduction (Fig. 25.7)[1] and its study in recent years has revealed several

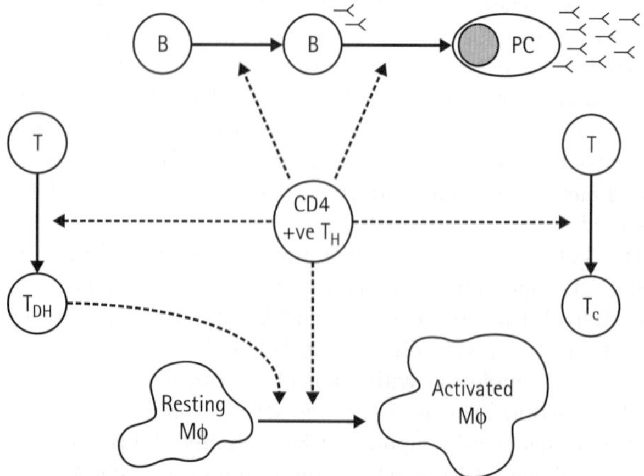

Fig. 25.6 Central role of CD4+ve T-helper (T_H) cell in immune responses. T_C = cytotoxic T-cell; T_{DH} = delayed hypersensitivity T-cell; Mϕ = macrophage; B = B-cell; PC = plasma cell.

inherited molecular defects resulting in failure of cell activation and thus immunodeficiency. Much is still to be learned about these processes. One of a number of pathways is described here.

Crosslinking of the TCR allows phosphorylation of the intracellular domains of the CD3xi chain which contains a specific antigen recognition activation motif (ARAM) to bind to the tyrosine kinase ZAP-70 and trigger a cascade of reactions involving protein tyrosine kinases and lipid kinases resulting in a release of intracellular calcium. This is critical for the activation and translocation of nuclear messengers (transcription factors) such as NFAT (nuclear factor of activated T lymphocytes) which induce transcription of activation genes including the IL-2 gene.

In B lymphocytes a similar cascade occurs with transmembrane proteins Ig alpha and Ig beta possessing a similar ARAM motif to the CD3xi chain of T lymphocytes. Full activation of T lymphocytes requires a number of signals apart from that via CD3 and the TCR. These come from CD28 engagement of its ligand CD80 on APC; LFA-1/ICAM interaction and the interaction of soluble IL-1 with its surface receptor.

THE DEVELOPMENT OF THE IMMUNE SYSTEM

PRENATAL DEVELOPMENT

The ontogeny of the cellular components of the specific immune system is summarized in Figure 25.8.[4] T and B lymphocyte development commences very early in the gestation of the human fetus. Cells capable of responding in mixed lymphocyte culture or to the mitogen, phytohemagglutinin, and recognizable NK cells are present in the fetal liver from as early as 6 weeks. Precursors of T and B lymphocytes are identifiable from 7–8 weeks and T lymphocyte precursors colonize the rudimentary thymus from the 9th week. By the second trimester, fetal blood sampling reveals circulating lymphocytes with mature T lymphocyte surface markers including the CD3, CD4 and CD8. Surface B lymphocyte markers, including surface immunoglobulin, are also expressed at this stage. Absence of these markers can be used for the antenatal diagnosis of SCID by fetal blood sampling (p. 1269).

Although the cellular elements of the specific immune system are present from early in gestation, their ability to respond to antigens, especially by making immunoglobulin, is limited until the time of birth.

The non-specific elements of the immune system also develop early in fetal life. Neutrophil precursors can be identified in the yolk sac. Mature neutrophils appear in the circulation in the second trimester but numbers are low until the onset of labor. C3 has been detected as early as 6 weeks of gestation. The serum levels of complement components, which are produced mainly by the fetal liver, rise slowly throughout fetal life.

THE IMMUNE SYSTEM IN THE NEWBORN

The newborn immune system exhibits a physiological immunodeficiency,[5,6] in full-term as well as preterm infants, but is more exaggerated in the premature and particularly marked in sick or stressed preterm infants. This accounts for the increased susceptibility to infection of the newborn, whether overwhelming group B streptococcal sepsis, or disseminated herpes simplex infection. Placentally transferred IgG partially offsets the deficiency. However, transfer of immunoglobulin (Fig. 25.9)[7] is a late event in gestation, and so preterm infants have significantly reduced levels; those at the limits of viability (23–24 weeks) have extremely low levels.

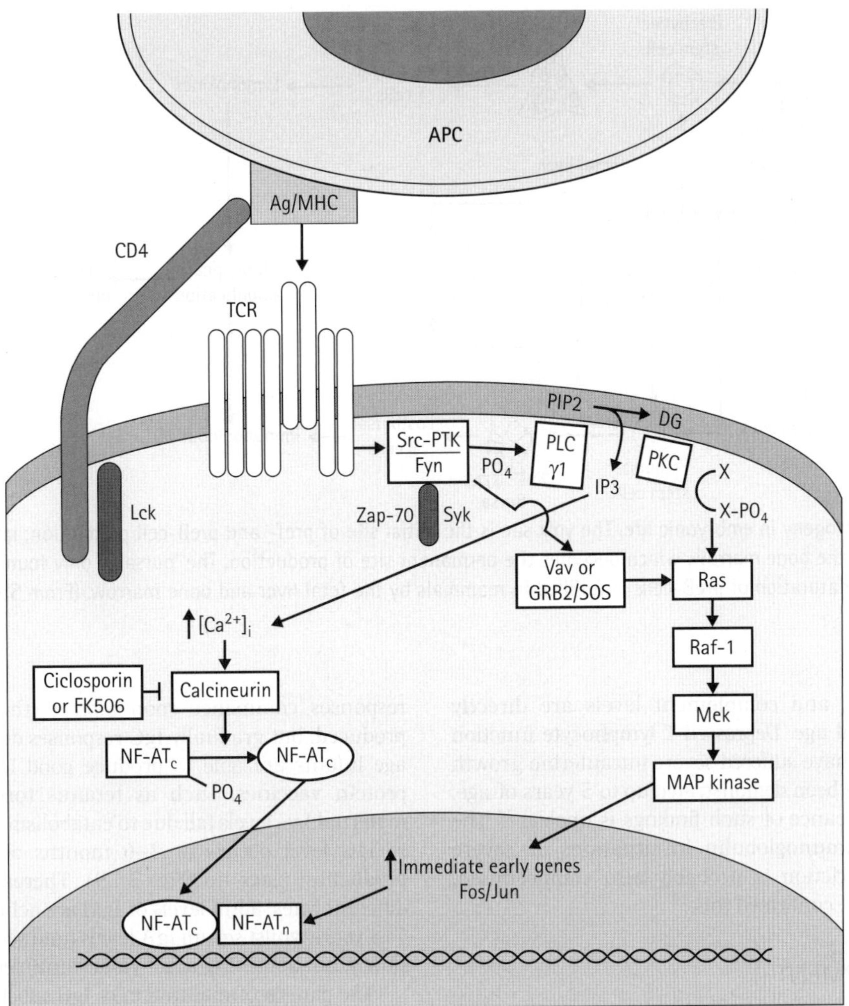

Fig. 25.7 Signaling pathways are induced following antigen-presenting cell/T-cell receptor interaction. APC = antigen-presenting cell; Ag-MHC = antigen/major histocompatibility class II interaction; Src-PTK = Src family protein tyrosine kinases; PIP2 = phosphatidyl-inositol bisphosphate; DG = diacylglycerol; PKC = protein kinase C; PLC-gamma1 = phospholipase C-gamma1; IP3 = inositol trisphosphate; NF-AT = nuclear factor of activated T cells; n = nuclear; c = cytosolic. (From Steihm 1996[1] with permission)

The protective effect of maternal immunoglobulin depends on the mother having IgG antibody to the appropriate antigens and, in the case of group B streptococcal sepsis, lack of maternal-type specific antibody to the relevant bacterial polysaccharides is a major risk factor. The newborn infant shows poor antibody responses especially to T independent antigens, poor ability to switch immunoglobulin isotypes and poor maturation of antibody affinity. Lymphoid cells, when cultured with B lymphocyte mitogens, produced a little IgM but no IgG or IgA (Table 25.5).[8] These poor responses are a function of intrinsic B lymphocyte immaturity and immaturity of antigen presenting cells. Diminished T lymphocyte expression of CD40 ligand reduces signaling to B lymphocytes via the CD40 receptor, and so depresses isotype switching.

T lymphocyte surface marker expression differs between neonates and adults. There is a high CD4:CD8 ratio, a high expression of the thymocyte antigen CD38 and low numbers of cells expressing the gamma delta T lymphocyte receptor. There is also a high proportion of B lymphocytes expressing the CD5 antigen (B1 cells). These differences resolve over the early months of life as a result of antigen exposure. Neonatal T lymphocytes have usually less than 10% of the CD45RO (memory) isoform and predominant expression of the CD45RA (virgin, naive) isoform. These proportions gradually reverse during childhood. Exposure to intrauterine infection may alter these neonatal patterns towards a more mature picture.

Neonatal T lymphocyte responses are poor in neonates largely because of the high proportion of naive T lymphocytes which are more difficult to stimulate. When adult naive cells are sorted and compared to neonatal cells the results are similar including IFN-gamma production. Nevertheless, the overall balance of neonatal T lymphocyte responsiveness is tilted towards T_{H2} rather T_{H1} response. This may contribute to the susceptibility to intracellular bacterial pathogens, such as *Listeria monocytogenes* or *Salmonella* species, since defenses to these pathogens rely on a T_{H1} pattern response.

Non-specific immune mechanisms are also immature at birth. Neutrophil bone marrow reserves are easily exhausted leading to neutropenia; chemotaxis and cell deformability may be reduced compared to values in adults or older children.[9] In contrast to the situation at other ages, neutrophil numbers and function have a tendency to deteriorate in the presence of infection or other stress.[10] Complement factor levels and function in a full-term infant are at approximately two-thirds of the adult level, and often below one-half in preterm babies. Alternative pathway factors are at relatively lower levels than classical pathway levels. The precise significance of these findings in predisposing to neonatal sepsis is not clear.

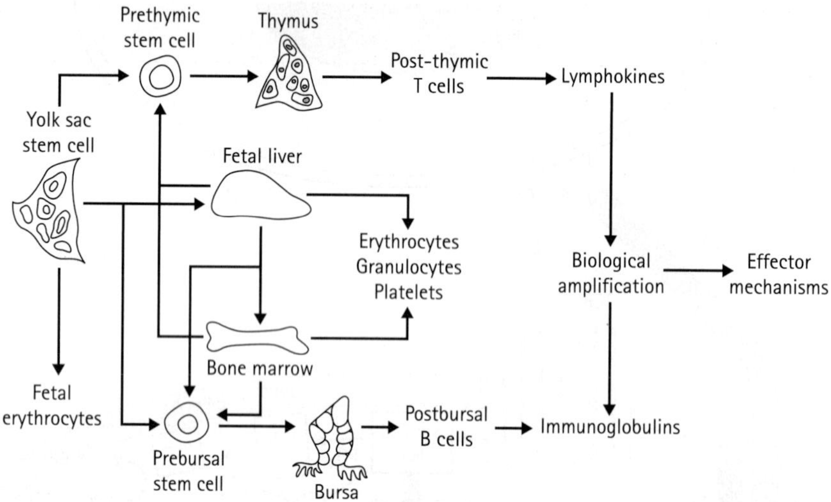

Fig. 25.8 T- and B-cell ontogeny in embryonic life. The yolk sac is the initial site of preT- and preB-cell production; later, the fetal liver produces these and, finally, the bone marrow, which becomes the permanent site of production. The 'bursa' is only found in avian species and its role in providing a site for maturation of preB-cells is fulfilled in mammals by the fetal liver and bone marrow. (From Steihm & Fulginiti 1980[4] with permission)

Low immunoglobulin and complement levels are directly proportional to gestational age. Depressed T lymphocyte function may occur in babies who have suffered severe intrauterine growth restriction. The latter have been demonstrated up to 5 years of age, though the clinical significance of such findings is unclear.[11] The placental transfer of immunoglobulin in situations of severe intrauterine growth restriction is probably also compromised, though not all studies have confirmed this.[12]

POSTNATAL DEVELOPMENT

Following birth the neonate is exposed to a wide variety of antigenic stimuli, which trigger immunological maturation regardless of gestational age. Immunoglobulin production and specific antibody responses commence soon after birth. Initially, mostly IgM is produced, but gradually IgG responses develop and by 2 months of age infants are able to produce good IgG antibody responses to protein vaccines, such as tetanus toxoid. During this period, maternal IgG levels fall due to catabolism, and a physiological nadir in IgG level occurs at 3–6 months of age before the infant's production picks up (Fig. 25.9). Thereafter isotype levels rise at different rates; adult levels of IgM are achieved by 4–5 years, IgG by 7–8 years whilst serum IgA levels (and secretory IgA) rise only very slowly, not achieving adult values until teenage years.

The pattern of maturation of IgG subclass levels also varies. IgG2 shows a prolonged physiological trough compared to IgG1 and IgG3 (Fig. 25.10).[13] Though antibody responses to most protein antigens mature early, responses to many polysaccharide antigens do not. Most

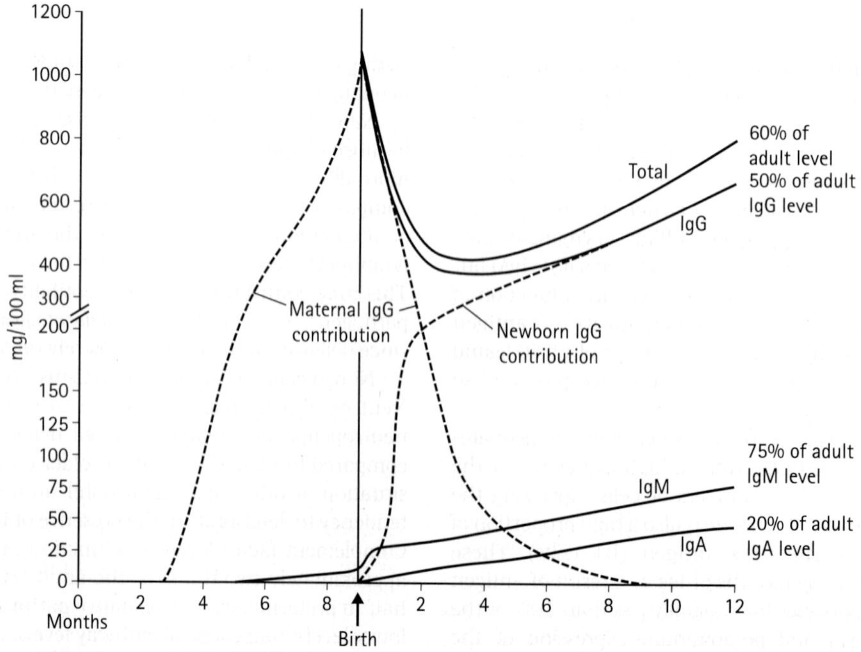

Fig. 25.9 Immunoglobulin levels in fetal life and in the first year postnatally. (From Miller & Steihm 1983[7] with permission)

Table 25.5 Protein A-induced plasma cell (PC) differentiation by newborn and adult lymphocytes (From Hayward & Lydyard 1979[8])

Source of lymphocytes	PC number/well × 10^{-3}		
	IgM	IgG	IgA
Adult	8.1	1.3	1.3
Newborn	0.3	0	0

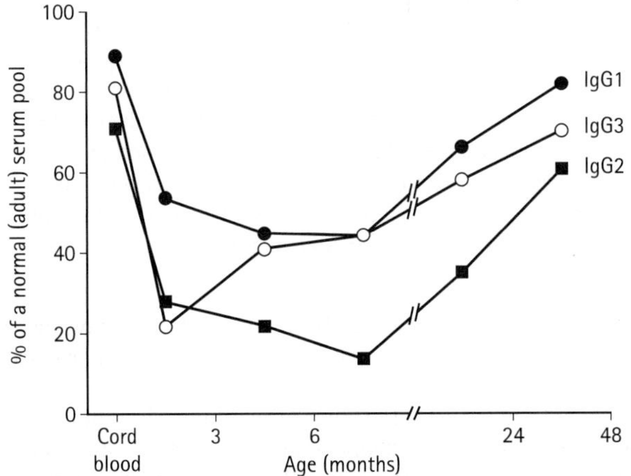

Fig. 25.10 Mean levels of IgG subclasses 1–3 in early life. Note the exaggerated fall and slow rise of IgG2 levels compared to IgG1 and IgG3. (Drawn from the data of Oxelius 1979[13])

antipolysaccharide IgG antibody in adults is found in the G2 subclass, while in young children the G1 subclass contains these. There is a high degree of susceptibility to polysaccharide-encapsulated organisms, such as pneumococcus in young children and a lack of responsiveness of children under the age of 18–24 months to pure polysaccharide vaccines, such as pneumococcal vaccine. Conjugation of the polysaccharide to a protein or peptide facilitates early responsiveness to both components as demonstrated by the high efficacy of Haemophilus influenzae type B (Hib) conjugate vaccine and the promising results with the new pneumococcal conjugate vaccines.[14]

T lymphocyte immunity appears to mature rapidly in the early weeks of life following antigen exposure. T lymphocyte expression of CD40 ligand improves as does cytokine production with the T_{H2}/T_{H1} balance shifting towards T_{H1}. However, the differences in T lymphocyte numbers and CD4:CD8 ratios between children and adults, and the unreliable responses of children to delayed hypersensitivity skin test antigens, such as *Candida* antigen, does suggest that maturation and development of the cell-mediated immune system continues through early childhood. Subtle immaturities in cell-mediated immunity probably account for the increased susceptibility of young children to tuberculosis (TB), and of young infants to invasive salmonellosis and listeriosis.

IMMUNODEFICIENCY DISORDERS: GENERAL PRINCIPLES

CLASSIFICATION AND GENETICS

Immunodeficiency may be due to a primary (inherited) or secondary (acquired) defect. The WHO working party on immunodeficiency[16] has classifed the primary disorders, and the main categories are listed in Tables 25.6A,B.[15,16] Figure 25.11[1] and Table 25.7[17] show the relative frequencies of the various disorders. The overall incidence of any significant immune deficiency disorder (excluding selective IgA deficiency) has been estimated at 1 in 10 000.

Many of the primary disorders have a genetic basis.[18–21] Identification of the responsible gene(s) has been achieved in an

Table 25.6A Primary immunodeficiencies – predominantly antibody deficiency (Adapted from Rosen et al 1999[16])

Immunodeficiency	Defect	Inheritance
X-linked agammaglobulinemia	Btk protein	XL
Autosomal recessive hyper-IgM syndrome	AID, CD40	AR
Common variable immunodeficiency	Unknown – some closely linked to C4 gene	Varied (occasionally AR or AD)
Ig heavy chain deletions	Deletion at Ig heavy chain locus (14q32)	AR
Ig kappa chain deletion	Mutation in Ig κ chain locus (2p11)	AR
Selective IgA deficiency	Unknown – some closely linked to C4 gene	Varied (occasionally AR or AD)
IgG subclass deficiency (± IgA deficiency)	Unknown	?
Antibody deficiency with normal immunoglobulin levels	Unknown	?
Transient hypogammaglobulinemia of infancy	Unknown	?

AD = autosomal dominat; AR = autosomal recessive; XL = X-linked

Table 25.6B Combined immunodeficiencies (Adapted from Rosen et al 1999[16])

Immunodeficiency	Defect	Inheritance
CD40 ligand deficiency (X-linked hyper-IgM Syndrome)	CD40 ligand	XL
Wiskott-Aldrich syndrome (WAS)	WAS protein	XL
X-linked lymphoproliferative disease	SLAM-associated protein	XL
DiGeorge anomaly	Developmental field defect chromosomal deletion (usually 22q11.2)	sporadic (some AD)
Cartilage-hair hypoplasia	RMRP gene	AR
Immunodeficiency with albinism		
1. Chediak-Higashi syndrome	Lyst gene	AR
2. Griscelli syndrome	Myosin 5a gene	AR
Ataxia telangiectasia	ATM protein	AR
Nijmegen breakage syndrome	NBS1 (nibrin) gene	AR

AD = autosomal dominant; AR = autosomal recessive; XL = X-linked

Table 25.6C Defects of phagocytic function (Adapted from Rosen et al 1999[16])

Immunodeficiency	Defect	Inheritance
XL chronic granulomatous disease	Killing defect gp91phox	XL
AR chronic granulomatous disease	Killing defect gp22phox, gp47phox, gp67phox	AR
Leukocyte adhesion deficiency type I	β integrin (CD18)	AR
Leukocyte adhesion deficiency type II	CD15	AR
Neutrophil G6PD deficiency	Neutrophil G6PD	XL
Myeloperoxidase deficiency	Myeloperoxidase	AR
AR severe congenital neutropenia	Elastase	AR
XL severe congenital neutropenia	WAS activating mutation	XL
Mycobactericidal defect	IFNγ receptor 1 deficiency	AR
	IFNγ receptor 2 deficiency	AR
	IL-12 receptor deficiency	AR
	IL-12 deficiency	AR

AR = autosomal recessive; G6PD = glucose-6-phosphate dehydrogenase; WAS = Wiskott–Aldrich syndrome; XL = X-Linked.

increasing number of conditions. Chromosomal aberrations may be found in some immunodeficiency disorders. Deletions of heavy chain constant region genes have been described in a minority of patients with immunoglobulin class or subclass deficiencies, while deletions on chromosome 18 (in some cases of IgA deficiency) and on

Table 25.6D Complement deficiencies (adapted from Rosen et al 1999[6])

Component	Inheritance	Main clinical associations
Clq	AR	SLE, MPGN, pyogenic infections
Clr*	AR	SLE
Cls*	AR	SLE
C4	AR	SLE
C2	AR	SLE, MPGN, HSP, pyogenic infections
C3	AR	Severe pyogenic infections
C5	AR	Neisserial infections, SLE
C6	AR	Neisserial infections, SLE
C7	AR	Neisserial infections, SLE
C8	AR	Neisserial infections, SLE
C9	AR	Neisserial infections (less marked than for C5–8 deficiency)
Factor D	?	Neisserial infections
Properdin	XL	Neisserial infections
C1 esterase inhibitor	AD	Hereditary angioedema
Factor H	AR	Pyogenic infections (less so than I deficiency), MPGN
Factor I	AR	Pyogenic infections

AD = autosomal dominant; AR = autosomal recessive; HSP = Henoch–Schönlein purpura; MPGN = membranoproliferative glomerulonephritis; SLE = Systemic lupus erythematosus, XL = X-linked. *NB* SLE is the most common immune complex disorder in complement deficiencies;
*Clr and Cls deficiency usually occur together.

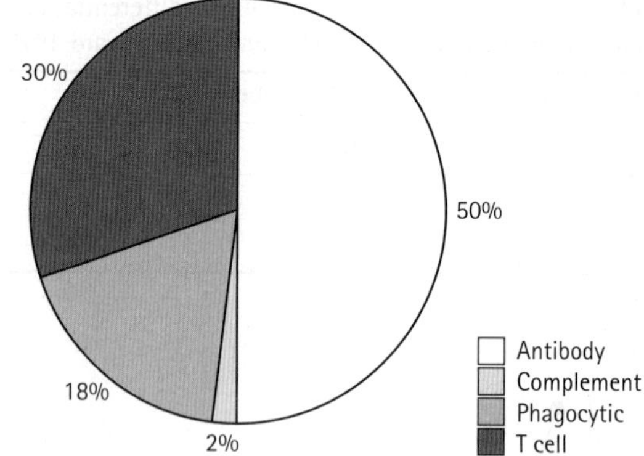

Fig. 25.11 Relative distribution of primary immunodeficiencies, based on combined experience from Japan, Switzerland and USA, excluding cases of asymptomatic selective IgA deficiency. T-cell deficiency group includes patients with combined cell-mediated and antibody deficiencies. (From Steihm 1996[1])

chromosome 22 (most cases of DiGeorge syndrome) have also been recorded. Immunodeficiency is often a feature of chromosomal breakage/repair disorders, such as ataxia telangiectasia.

The molecular basis of many of the primary immunodeficiency disorders has been elucidated. Usually several different mutations in the relevant gene have been described. Occasionally mutations at certain points have been found associated with partial forms of the disease, presumably because of some residual function of the protein concerned. Recognition of the molecular pathways involved enhances understanding of the immune response, and identification and clarification of precise molecular mechanisms enable more focused treatment of primary immune deficiencies, e.g. X-linked hyper-IgM used to be considered an antibody deficiency, although immunoglobulin replacement does not prevent liver disease secondary to *Cryptosporidium parvum* infection. Recognition that it is a primary T lymphocyte defect has lead to curative bone marrow transplantation in selected patients. Identification of the genes involved enables genetic diagnosis (including antenatal diagnosis) and involves a number of techniques including restriction fragment length polymorphism (RFLP) and single strand conformational polymorphism (SSCP) analysis.

DIAGNOSIS AND INVESTIGATION OF IMMUNODEFICIENCY

A careful history and examination should precede any laboratory tests as this will help determine which children should be investigated further and the nature and extent of investigations.

Table 25.7 Incidence of some primary immunodeficiencies (From Hosking & Roberton 1983[17])

Immunodeficiency	Incidence
Severe combined immunodeficiency	1 in 66 000
DiGeorge syndrome	1 in 66 000
Common variable immunodeficiency	1 in 83 000
Chronic mucocutaneous candidiasis	1 in 103 000
Chronic granulomatous disease	1 in 181 000
Selective IgA deficiency	1 in 500
X-linked agammaglobulinemia	1 in 103 000

HISTORY

Pregnancy and birth history may provide information regarding possible congenital infection, intrauterine growth retardation or prematurity, all of which are associated with immune defects. Delayed separation of the umbilical cord, in the absence of local infection, may suggest a neutrophil defect. Risk factors for human immunodeficiency virus (HIV) in the parents should be sought. Most children will present because of an infective problem. The age of onset of infections, their site, proven or suspected organisms and time to recovery with conventional treatments are all important considerations. An immunodeficient child is likely to have more infections which take longer to resolve or have an atypical course compared to other children. The type of organism involved, including the occurrence of atypical infections, should direct further investigations (Table 25.8). The occurrence of frequent upper respiratory tract infections (URTI) alone in a young child is not indicative of an underlying immune defect unless associated with frequent bacterial infections. There are a few studies on the frequency of URTI, but clinical experience suggests that up to eight upper respiratory tract infections per year is normal in the preschool years. When evaluating the number of infections, other factors such as parental smoking, attendance at daycare and anatomical problems should be considered. Infections with common organisms may run an atypical course in that they are unusually severe, e.g. hemorrhagic chickenpox, or they fail to respond to standard treatments, e.g. a bacterial pneumonia which fails to respond to appropriate antibiotic therapy. Alternatively, infections may be caused by uncommon (atypical) organisms which are in themselves highly suggestive of immunodeficiency, e.g. *Pneumocystis carinii* pneumonia.

The history should include inquiries about related problems which can be associated with immunodeficiency disorders. Failure to thrive is a common finding, and this may or may not be associated with diarrhea due to chronic or recurrent infection or autoimmune enteropathy. Evidence of end-organ damage, such as a cough productive of sputum consistent with bronchiectasis should also be sought. Allergic/atopic problems are common and may be unusually severe. Autoimmune and malignant diseases, though not common, have an increased incidence. Taking a careful family history may reveal other children with unusual or fatal infectious complications in keeping with an autosomal recessive or X-linked pattern of inheritance. A history of consanguinity should be sought. Some tactful inquiries to ascertain whether the parents have any risk factors for infection with the human immunodeficiency virus should be made as infection with this virus is often a differential diagnosis. In some disorders, e.g. IgA deficiency, there may be a family history of collagen vascular or other immunopathological disease. Older relatives who are carriers of or who are affected by milder variants of primary immune defects may have autoimmune manifestations (e.g. mouth ulcers and systemic lupus erythematosus variant in chronic granulomatous disease, CGD) or have a history of malignant disease (lymphoma in X-linked lymphoproliferative disease, XLP or Wiskott–Aldrich syndrome, WAS).

EXAMINATION

General physical examination should be directed towards potential sites of infection, including the throat, ears and sinuses and examination of the oral cavity and napkin area for candidiasis. The presence or absence of lymphoid tissue should be noted, as should cutaneous problems consistent with an immune defect. In more severe antibody states such as X-linked agammaglobulinemia, there is a lack of tonsils and lymphoid tissues. Signs of end-organ damage from infections, such as clubbing and respiratory abnormalities must be sought. Some diseases may have specific physical signs, such as oculocutaneous albinism in Chediak–Higashi syndrome, typical facies and/or cleft palate in DiGeorge syndrome, telangiectasia or neurological abnormalities in ataxia telangiectasia and disproportionate short stature in some forms of combined immune deficiency (see cartilage–hair hypoplasia below).

DIAGNOSTIC IMAGING

Radiological evaluation, directed by findings from history and examination, may be useful. The exception is in DNA repair defects (see below) where the effects of exposure to ionizing radiation may be harmful and X-ray and computerized tomography (CT) evaluation should be limited as much as possible. Magnetic resonance imaging (MRI) and ultrasound are safe alternatives.

Evidence of bony abnormalities may support a diagnosis of adenosine deaminase deficiency, Shwachman–Diamond syndrome or other dysplasias associated with immune defects. Dilatation of the common bile duct may be suggestive of sclerosing cholangitis, associated with a number of combined immune deficiencies especially X-linked hyper-IgM syndrome.[22] Careful review of chest X-rays may suggest bronchiectasis, and should prompt high resolution CT imaging. Although absence of a thymus on anterior posterior and lateral chest radiographs is consistent with a combined immune defect in infants and young children, thymic atrophy may also occur in response to stress (e.g. infection) and this finding is not diagnostic.

LABORATORY INVESTIGATION

Two main questions need to be addressed: which children to investigate, and how extensively to investigate selected children. The following should trigger investigation: family history consistent with immune deficiency, single infection with an unusual/opportunistic organism, single infection which is atypically severe, has an atypical course or occurs at an atypical age, recurrent minor bacterial infections [e.g. otitis media > two per year despite appropriate ear, nose and throat (ENT) management, resulting in significant school absence], or more than one episode of serious bacterial infection.

Table 25.8 Examples of association between infecting organisms and most likely type of immune defect

Organism	Candidate immune defect
Pneumococcus, Haemophilus influenzae	Antibody, complement
Staphylococcus	Neutrophil
Meningococcus	Complement
Gram negative bacteria	Neutrophil
Salmonella	Type-1 cytokine defects, cell-mediated
Cryptosporidium	Cell-mediated
Giardia lamblia	Antibody, cell-mediated*
Mycoplasma spp.	Antibody
Candida albicans	Cell-mediated, neutrophil, monocyte
Aspergillus spp.	Neutrophil
Herpes-viruses (e.g. CMV)	Cell-mediated
Enteroviruses	Antibody, cell-mediated
Other viruses (e.g. measles)	Cell-mediated
Mycobacteria (typical and atypical)	Type-1 cytokine defects
Bacille Calmette-Guérin (BCG)	Cell-mediated, type-1 cytokine defects

* particularly patients with HIV.

Laboratory investigations can be directed to a certain extent by the organism causing infection (Table 25.8) and the age of the child.

The laboratory investigations available range from those readily available in all centers, to highly specialized tests performed in a few research centers. Only a small proportion of children presenting with recurrent infections require complex investigation, and most can be adequately investigated using a few relatively straightforward tests.

Hematology

Much can be learnt from a full blood count and examination of a blood film. Modern analyzers can rapidly perform a white count and differential. Neutropenia is readily detected. If cyclical neutropenia is suspected, then twice weekly counts should be performed for 8 weeks as the nadir may be brief and easily missed. Bone marrow aspiration should be undertaken in neutropenic children to distinguish between failure of production and increased peripheral destruction, and also to exclude a myelodysplastic or malignant process. Neutrophilia in the absence of overt infection may be suggestive of a neutrophil adhesion defect or functional problem (e.g. CGD). Lymphopenia, using appropriate age related ranges (see Ch. 40), is highly suggestive of a combined immune deficiency of primary or secondary etiology,[23] although SCID can occur in the presence of a normal lymphocyte count. Nucleated red cells in infants and abnormal leukocyte morphology in sick children may render a manual differential necessary. Abnormal leukocyte granules are characteristic of Chediak–Higashi syndrome. Platelet volume is universally low in Wiskott–Aldrich syndrome, and is a rapid and very reliable diagnostic pointer.[24]

TESTS OF INNATE IMMUNITY

Complement

C3 and C4 can be routinely measured in pathology departments using nephelometry (see below); reference ranges for C3 are well defined. However, null alleles for C4 are present at a relatively high frequency in the population so that the significance of an isolated low C4 in an individual with recurrent infections is less certain. Furthermore, normal levels of C3 and C4 do not exclude deficiencies of other complement components. It is therefore better to assess the functional integrity of the complement pathway using assays which test the ability of patient serum to lyse sensitized red blood cells. All assays measure the intactness of one activation pathway plus the final common effector pathway (formation of the membrane attack complex). The species of red cell used in the assay and chelation of magnesium and/or calcium determines whether components of the classical pathway (CH50/CH100 or THC) or alternative pathway (AP50) are assayed. Deficiency in any one component will result in a failure of lysis. The commonest reason for failure of lysis is the presence of active infection, with consumption of complement components, or degradation of complement components if the sample is not separated and frozen within 2 h of venesection. However, if repeat testing shows a persistent abnormality, evaluation of individual complement components should be performed.

A third complement activation pathway has been defined recently which involves mannan-binding lectin.[25] Assay of serum concentrations by enzyme linked immunosorbent assay (ELISA) is available in some centers. Five polymorphic bases have been identified within the MBL gene which affect serum concentrations of the protein, which have differing frequencies in ethnic populations. Such analyses are currently a research tool.

Neutrophil function tests

Neutrophil function has three main components: chemotaxis, phagocytosis and activation of the respiratory burst. Neutrophil function tests are fraught with technical pitfalls, as neutrophils rapidly activate upon venesection and also die quickly. Historically a wide range of neutrophil function tests have been performed, although their validity is questionable. This particularly applies to assays of neutrophil chemotaxis, which should no longer be performed outside the research setting. Similarly, the Rebuck skin window, in which skin is abraded and covered with a cover slip to test neutrophil mobility, is no longer a routine part of clinical pediatric practice.

Chemiluminescence

This test evaluates the opsonizing capacity of patient serum, the ability of neutrophils and monocytes to phagocytose and activation of the respiratory burst. The use of autologous or third party serum can be used to distinguish defects in opsonization from defects in the respiratory burst. Phagocytosis of organisms by neutrophils and monocytes results in the activation of the respiratory burst and the production of oxygen free radicals. These react with oxidizable substances on microbes, such as unsaturated lipids, nucleic acids and peptides, to form unstable intermediates. When these intermediates return to their original state, light energy is emitted. This chemiluminescence is readily measured with a spectrophotometer or chemiluminometer. Such assays are now being superseded by flow cytometric assays (see below)

Nitroblue tetrazolium reduction test

Nitroblue tetrazolium (NBT) is a yellow dye that is readily taken up by phagocytes and, upon stimulation [for example with phorbol myristate acetate (PMA)] is reduced to the purple dye formazan by the oxidative burst. In normal individuals, at least 95% of neutrophils should contain a purple deposit in stimulated cells. In CGD, less than 1% of neutrophils reduce NBT. Carrier mothers of the X-linked disease can also be detected by this method as they show an intermediate level of NBT reduction (20–80%). (Fig. 25.12). In experienced hands, this is a rapid and sensitive test for CGD, but false normal results can be seen when the test is performed infrequently.

Flow cytometric assays of neutrophil function

Phagocytosis

Fluorescently labeled organisms can be used to assess the phagocytic ability of neutrophils. Although this assay is still primarily a research tool, it has the advantage of being able to study the phagocytic capability of the neutrophil to different organisms, and may help define the defect in undefined immune deficiencies. Comparison of phagocytosis with autologous and control serum can be used to assess opsonization.

Oxidative burst

Neutrophils take up dihydrorhodamine and activation of the respiratory burst by preincubation with PMA or other stimuli results in fluorescence within cells, which can be assessed using the flow cytometer. As with an NBT, carriers for CGD can also be detected (Fig. 25.13). The test has the advantage that more laboratories are experienced in the interpretation of flow cytometric readouts than reading slide NBTs and so false normal results are much less likely. It is, however, more sensistive than an NBT so neutrophil function defects other than CGD may also be detected.

Enzyme assays

Neutrophil killing defects may also occur in deficiency states of myeloperoxidase and glucose-6-phosphate dehydrogenase (G6PD), which can be assayed separately.

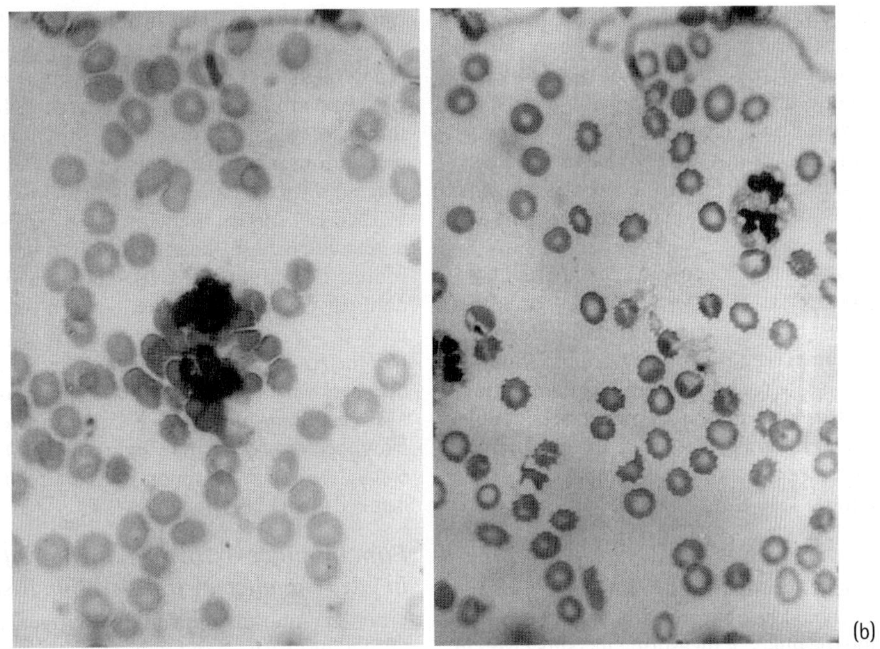

Fig. 25.12 Slide nitroblue tetrazolium (NBT) reduction test. (a) Normal subject. Neutrophils have taken up and reduced NBT to form a dense brown/black deposit. (b) Patient with chronic granulomatous disease. None of the cells has produced the deposit due to failure to reduce the NBT.

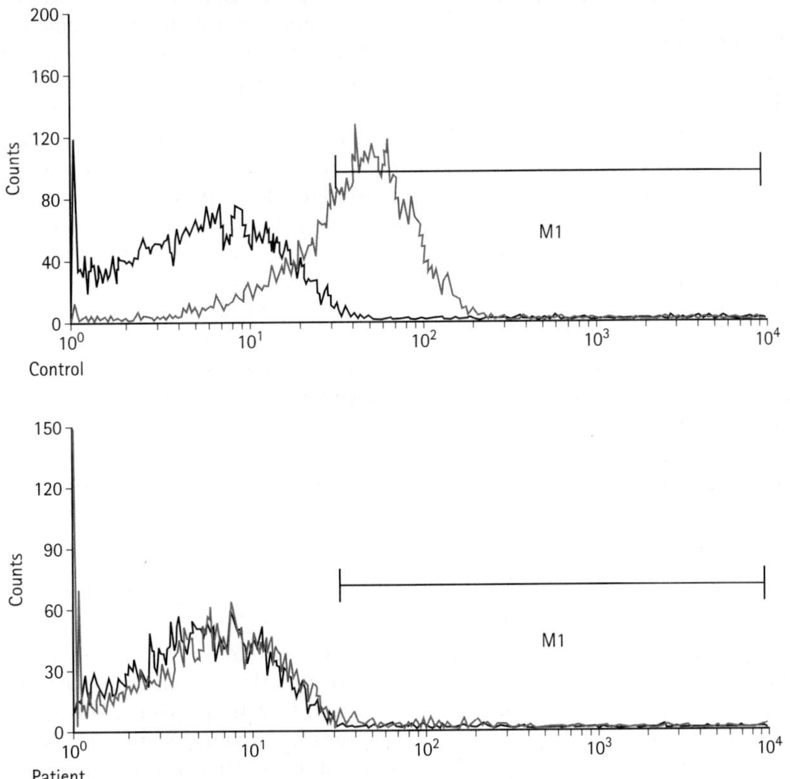

Fig. 25.13 Flow cytometric dihydrorhodamine oxidative burst assay. Both plots show isotype control and staining for common gamma chain using flow cytometry. The control has normal levels of expression, represented by a shift in the histogram peak. Surface expression is lacking in the patient enabling rapid molecular diagnosis of gamma chain deficient SCID.

ADAPTIVE IMMUNE SYSTEM

Test of humoral immunity

Immunoglobulins

IgG is the predominant circulating immunoglobulin. Smaller amounts of IgA, IgM, IgD and IgE are found in serum. IgG, A and M are routinely measured by nephelometry. This technique involves mixing of a known quantity of antibody to the test protein (in this case IgG, A or M) with serum containing an unknown quantity of the protein. Immune complexes form which will scatter light, the amount of light scattered being proportional to the quantity of protein within the sample. Results must be evaluated with reference to age specific normal ranges, as production of all five classes of immunoglobulin is low at birth and gradually matures over the first 5 years of life. Measurement of pediatric immunoglobulins may require different instrument settings. Immunoglobulin can be lost via the gut or urinary tract. Thus, low levels of Ig can only be attributed to a production defect if gut or renal losses have been excluded and the serum albumin is within the normal range. A number of catabolic states, such as myotonic dystrophy can also lower total immunoglobulin levels.

IgE is measured using a variety of techniques, including ELISA and automated solid-phase ELISAs. Measurement of IgE is indicated if hyper IgE (Jobs) syndrome is included in the differential diagnosis.

IgD is present in the serum in very low concentrations. It may be non-specifically increased as a part of multiple inflammatory reactions, but is not used as part of the routine assessment of immune deficiency. IgD is not routinely measured unless a periodic fever syndrome is suspected (see Ch. 26). It is commonly measured by radial immunodiffusion.

IgG subclasses

IgG subclasses are commonly measured by nephelometry or radial immunodiffusion. Results should be interpreted in the light of age specific normal ranges, and the utility of measuring IgG subclasses in children under 2 years of age, or if the total IgG is low is debatable. In addition, approximately 10% of the normal population have undetectable IgG4, and normal ranges should be adjusted to reflect this.

Measures of in vivo antibody responses

The ability of the immune system to produce functional antibody is more important than the amount of circulating antibody. Functional tests of IgG production rely on measuring antibody titers to antigens to which the child is known to have been exposed either naturally or by vaccination. Responses to protein antigens such as tetanus, diphtheria and the conjugated Hib vaccine are widely available. However, although normal ranges for antibody titers exist these are not well validated for antigens other than Hib, and may not be a true reflection of immunological memory. If antibody titers are low, booster vaccinations should be given to assess the memory response. In children over 2 years of age, administration of Pneumovax (23 serovalent polysaccharide vaccine) is useful to assess the ability to respond to carbohydrate antigens. Loss of this response may be the first sign of an evolving immune deficiency in patients with common variable immunodeficiency or WAS. Assessment of antibody responses to common respiratory viral pathogens and varicella zoster may also provide useful additional information, although negative tests in the absence of microbiologically proven disease are difficult to interpret.

The optimal test of in vivo antibody production is assessment of IgM and IgG responses and rate of clearance to a novel antigen whose clearance is dependent on opsonization by a specific antibody. The harmless bacteriophage psi X174 can be administered intravenously for this purpose, but this investigation is rarely used in current practice.[26,27]

Cell-mediated immunity

Humoral and cell-mediated immunity do not exist in isolation. Cell-mediated defects are likely to result in a degree of humoral immune deficiency as the latter is dependent on the former for help in making an antibody response with memory.

Quantification of cell numbers

Cell-mediated immunity can be assessed by measuring the number and function of cells. Lymphocytes can be enumerated using flow cytometry. This complex machinery uses fluid dynamics to separate cells into a single cell stream. Cells thus generated pass through beams of laser light and scatter the light with a pattern determined by their size and granularity. The scattered light is detected by photon multiplier tubes. The different light scatter properties of cells enable populations of neutrophils, monocytes and lymphocytes to be differentiated (Fig. 25.13). Lymphocytes can be characterized further by their cell surface markers. These can be tagged with monoclonal antibodies, whose fluorescent labels are excited by incident light beams. The number of cells staining with a particular monoclonal antibody can be expressed either as a percentage of the lymphocyte pool or as an absolute number. As with all immunological parameters, both proportions of different lymphocytes and absolute numbers vary with age and reference should be made to published age related normal ranges.[28] Approximately 60–80% of circulating lymphocytes are T lymphocytes, with 10–20% B lymphocytes and 5–15% NK cells. Common markers used to identify cell types are detailed (Table 25.9).

Functional tests of cell-mediated immunity

In vitro lymphocyte proliferation assays

When lymphocytes encounter antigen in vivo they respond by upregulation of activation markers and proliferation, without which an effective immune response cannot occur. This can be mimicked in vitro by culturing lymphocytes for a defined time period with an appropriate non-specific stimulus and using the incorporation of tritiated thymidine or a non-radioactive marker such as bromodeoxyuridine into the DNA of dividing cells as a surrogate measure of cell proliferation. A range of stimuli can be used. Plant lectins, e.g. phytohemagglutinin (PHA) and concavalin A, act as potent T lymphocyte mitogens and cause high levels of proliferation in normal cells. A more physiological assessment of proliferative capacity can be obtained using a monoclonal antibody to the T lymphocyte surface protein, CD3, which results in direct receptor stimulation or by using a recall antigen such as tetanus. Proliferation tests of in vitro B lymphocyte function, e.g. using Pokeweed mitogen and EBV, are rarely indicated in modern clinical practice. The results of responses to recall antigens need to be interpreted in the light of previous exposure, which reduces their clinical utility in children. Mixed lymphocyte cultures are a modification of lymphocyte proliferation assays where the stimulating cells are irradiated lymphocytes from an HLA disparate donor. Mixed lymphocyte culture (MLC) responses may be useful in assessing the suitability of donors prior to bone marrow transplantation.

Other measures of lymphocyte function

As well as dividing upon stimulation, T lymphocytes produce a range of cytokines (e.g. IFN-gamma and IL-2) and express activation markers on their surface (e.g. CD69, CD25, MHC II). The latter may be detected after only a few hours of incubation with an appropriate stimulus. Neither of these assays provides the same information as that given by formal proliferation assays. Rare immune defects have been described with aberrant cytokine production, and cytokine assays may be useful in this context.

In vivo tests: delayed hypersensitivity skin tests

Delayed hypersensitivity skin tests can be performed using a number of common antigens, including those derived from candida, streptococcus, mumps and tetanus toxoid. Induration at the site is indicative of an intact cell-mediated immune response to the test antigen, and make it unlikely that the patient has a significant cell-mediated immune defect. Responses are dependent

Table 25.9 Common markers used to identify cell types

Cell type	Detected with fluorescent monoclonal light antibody to
All T lymphocytes	CD3
T helper cells	CD4
Cytotoxic T lymphocytes	CD8
B lymphocytes	CD19 or CD20
Natural killer cells	CD16 and CD56 or CD57
Memory T lymphocytes	CD45RO
Naive T lymphocytes	CD45RA

on established memory and corticosteroids and some intercurrent viral infections may abrogate the response, all of which limit their clinical utility in children. They may, however, be useful in circumstances where in vitro lymphocyte proliferation assays are not readily available.

Definition of molecular defects

Protein assays

The genetic basis of an increasing number of immune deficiencies is now well defined; many occur because a surface or cytoplasmic signaling protein is absent or defective. In most cases a defect in the gene coding for the protein results in either no protein expression, expression of low amounts, or expression of abnormally sized protein. These abnormalities can be detected using a combination of Western blotting (Fig. 25.14) and flow cytometry.[29] These are highly specialized investigations and are only available in a limited number of centers. However, screening patients with a good clinical history by protein expression represents a considerable cost saving over genetic screening.

Genetics

In the presence of an appropriate history or abnormal protein expression, genetic analysis may be undertaken. Genes can be screened using single stranded conformational polymorphism analysis, but with increasing availability of automated sequencers, direct sequencing of genes is likely to replace this technology. It should be remembered however, that not all genetic differences between individuals result in clinical problems. Significant numbers of polymorphisms exist within the human genome which may have no clinical effects.

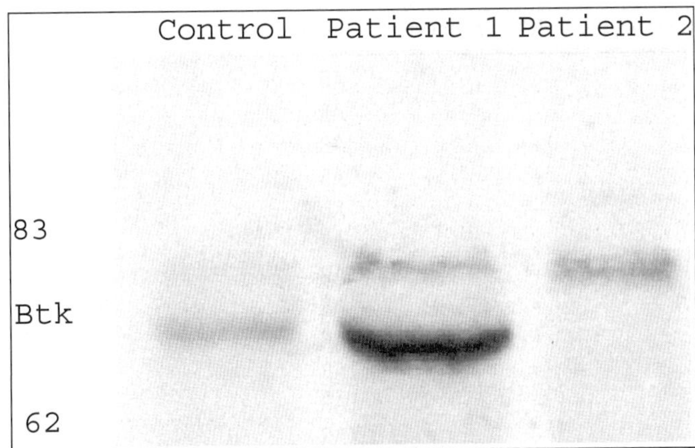

Fig. 25.14 Figure shows Western blotting for Btk protein, defective in X-linked agammaglobulinemia. Protein lysates are made from mononuclear cell extracts from peripheral blood. Btk is concentrated by immunoprecipitation with a Btk specific antibody. Immunoprecipitates are then subjected to electrophoresis, which separates the proteins on the basis of size. Gels are incubated with a second anti-Btk antibody to allow specific detection. Btk is seen in the control and patient 1, who lacked B cells but did not have X-linked agammaglobulinemia. Patient 2 lacked Btk expression, and a mutation in Btk was later defined.

Carrier testing

Appropriate genetic counseling should be offered to all families. Once mutations have been defined, parents can be tested for carrier status. In a number of conditions non-genetic tests may be useful in determining carrier status. These include the NBT in which intermediate numbers of neutrophils will reduce NBT in mothers who carry the mutation fox X-linked CGD, and intermediate levels of adenosine deaminase (ADA) in carriers of ADA deficiency. Females randomly inactivate one of their X-chromosomes in all cells. If a gene that is critical for the development of a particular cell lineage is carried on the X chromosome, this will result in apparent non-random X-inactivation as cells where the good gene is inactivated will fail to develop. Detection of non-random X-activation was historically a powerful tool for carrier detection, but as all the X-linked immune deficiencies have now had their genetic basis defined, the need to rely on non-random X-inactivation in the mother for carrier detection has been superseded. Carrier testing of siblings raises a number of ethical issues, and children should reach the age of informed consent before any tests are undertaken (see Ch. 4).

Antenatal diagnosis

Appropriate counseling by an individual conversant with the outcome of immune deficiencies in the modern era should be undertaken before antenatal diagnosis is undertaken. Due to the small risk of miscarriage, screening should only be offered to mothers in whom the result would determine whether the mother would terminate the pregnancy. The gestation at which antenatal diagnosis can be undertaken is influenced by the nature of the immune deficiency (see Table 25.10).

DISORDERS OF CELL-MEDIATED IMMUNITY: COMBINED IMMUNODEFICIENCIES

SEVERE COMBINED IMMUNODEFICIENCY (SCID)

Failure to develop normal T lymphocytes, usually due to specific gene defects affecting early T lymphocyte development or subsequent signaling pathways, leads to lymphocyte-mediated immunodeficiency. T lymphocytes are also critical for the maturation and function of B lymphocytes and so the more severe T lymphocyte deficiencies are nearly always accompanied by defective antibody responses resulting in a combined (lymphocyte-mediated and humoral) deficiency. In other combined immunodeficiencies single gene defects affect both B and T lymphocyte development. The severity of the humoral deficiency varies from a subtle defect of specific antibody response to complete hypogammaglobulinemia. Thus, it is unusual to find a significant primary T lymphocyte deficiency syndrome accompanied by normal humoral immune function. Combined immunodeficiency results from a large number of disorders with X-linked or autosomal recessive inheritance.[30] The molecular basis of many, but not all, combined immunodeficiencies has now been elucidated (Table 25.11). The most severe phenotype is termed severe combined immunodeficiency (SCID) and is associated with a profound T lymphopenia and panhypogammaglobulinemia with early death from infection. Whilst the usual clinical features of

Table 25.10 Antenatal diagnostic investigation and gestational age

	Type of sample	Gestational age	Analysis
Mutation defined	CVS	10–12 weeks	Restriction digest/sequence analysis
Linkage defined	CVS	10–12 weeks	Restriction digest/sequence analysis
X-linked	CVS	0–12 weeks	Karyotype*
Phenotype defined	Fetal blood sample	18–20 weeks	Microscopy for morphology
Cell morphology			
Lymphocyte distribution			Flow cytometry
			Functional assay as detected by disease (e.g. NBT for CGD)

*One in two male fetuses will carry the disease. CGD, chronic granulomatous disease; CVS, chorionic villus sample; NBT, nitroblue tetrazolium.

this group of diseases are well characterized, atypical presentations and 'leaky' forms with an attenuated phenotype are increasingly recognized. Circulating T lymphocyte numbers are usually low or absent but may be normal. In the classic SCID presentation, lymphocyte responses to mitogen are absent, but may be present in attenuated forms where immunoglobulin may also be produced. However tests of antigen specific T lymphocyte proliferation and antibody production are defective and there is cutaneous anergy. Patients usually have a limited diversity of T lymphocyte receptor and immunoglobulin gene rearrangements. Diagnosis may be more difficult in atypical patients. Identifying the molecular defect in specific patients with combined immunodeficiency or SCID is important for prognosis, treatment, genetic counseling and increasing our knowledge about these rare diseases. When identified, it is best to use the name of the underlying molecular defect.

General features of severe combined immunodeficiency

The presenting clinical features are characterized by early onset, persistent respiratory tract or gut infection and failure to thrive.[31] Affected babies appear well at birth but within the first few months of life fail to clear infection and fall progressively away from their birth centile. Chronic diarrhea and failure to thrive are due to persistent and sometimes multiple gastrointestinal viral infections, often with associated food intolerance. Persistent respiratory tract infections with respiratory syncitial virus or parainfluenza viruses are common with failure to clear virus accompanying persistent bronchiolitic-like signs. An insidiously progressive persistent respiratory infection with radiological evidence of interstitial pneumonitis should raise the suspicion of *Pneumocystis carinii* infection, often a copathogen with respiratory viruses. Other presentations include prolonged otitis media and invasive bacterial infections, particularly staphylococcal or pseudomonas septicemia and pneumonia, which may respond poorly to appropriate treatment. Severe invasive fungal infection is rare, but often fatal. Extensive, persistant superficial candidiasis is more common. Occasionally babies present with disseminated BCG or vaccine strain poliomyelitis virus. Children presenting within the first 6 months or so of life are more likely to have SCID or a severe T lymphocyte defect.

Non-infectious manifestations mainly result from graft-versus-host disease (GvHD) caused by the inability to reject foreign lymphocytes acquired either from the mother in utero or from

Table 25.11 Classification of severe combined immunodeficiency

Syndrome	T lymphocytes	B lymphocytes	NK lymphocytes	Inheritance
Reticular dysgenesis	–	–	–	AR
ADA deficiency	–	–	–	AR
RAG1, 2 deficiency	–	–	+	AR
Artemis deficiency (RS*)	–	–	+	AR
CgC deficiency	–	+	–	XL
JAK-3 deficiency	–	+	–	AR
IL-7Ra deficiency	–	+	+	AR
ZAP-70 kinase deficiency	CD4+	+	+	AR
MHC II deficiency	CD8+	+	+	AR
p56lck deficiency	CD8+	+	+	AR
IL-2/IL15Rb	CD8+	+	–	AR
Idiopathic CD4 lymphopenia	CD8+	+	+	AR
CD45 deficiency	+	+	+	AR
WHN gene deficiency	+	+	+	AR
Omenn's syndrome	+	–	+	AR
Non-host T lymphocytes (MFE or transfusion GvHD)	+	+/-	+/-	

ADA = adenosine deaminase; AR = autosomal recessive; CgC = common interleukin gamma chain; GvHD = graft-versus-host disease; IL-7Ra = interleukin 7 receptor alpha; JAK-3 = janus-associated kinase 3; MFE = maternofetal engraftment; RAG = recombination activating genes; WHN = winged-helix-nude; XL = X-linked; ZAP-70 = zeta-associated kinase-70.

unirradiated blood transfusion. Engraftment of transplacentally acquired maternal lymphocytes (maternofetal GvHD, MFGvHD) sometimes, but not always provokes GvHD, typically with a mild reticular skin rash with or without slightly deranged liver function tests. Its role in the gastrointestinal symptoms is not known. Surprisingly, up to 50% of children with SCID have clinically silent MFGvHD.[32] Fatal GvHD can follow transfusion with non-irradiated blood or with white lymphocyte or platelet concentrates. In these cases the skin rash is more severe and lymphadenopathy and hepatosplenomegaly may be present; here cases may be clinically indistinguishable from Omenn's syndrome (see below), but identification of maternal cells by karyotype or DNA fingerprinting will distinguish MFGvHD from Omenn's syndrome. EBV infection may lead to uncontrolled B lymphoproliferative disorders, similar to that seen in solid organ transplant recipients.

Examination usually reveals a wasted child (Fig. 25.15) who has dropped through the growth centiles, and with evidence of candidiasis and other infections. Skin rashes may be indicative of infection or GvHD. There is no clinically detectable lymphoid tissue. There may be hepatomegaly.

Investigations show severe lymphopenia from birth although in infancy a normal lymphocyte count is > 2.7×10^9/L, and if the normal adult lower limit of 1.0×10^9/L is quoted, the lymphopenia will be missed. Lymphocytic phenotyping shows severely depleted T lymphocyte numbers; B lymphocytes and NK cells may be present, or absent. Occasional variants show unusual patterns of immature T lymphocyte markers; in such cases maternal engraftment should be excluded. Mitogen responses, mixed lymphocyte reaction, in vitro antigen specific responses and delayed hypersensitivity skin testing to common antigens are usually absent. Immunoglobulin estimations show low levels of IgG, IgA and IgM but may be misleading as residual maternal IgG may give a falsely reassuring result and it can be difficult distinguishing IgA and IgM levels in SCID from the low levels seen in normal infants; furthermore some SCID infants make IgM, but this is not functionally active. Isohemagglutinins are a useful measure of in vitro IgM production and absence is significant. If SCID is suspected, lymphocyte phenotyping is more reliable than immunoglobulin estimation. Chest radiographs show an absent thymus, and hyperinflation and/or interstitial pneumonia, if infection is present. Typical cupping and flaring of the costochondral junction is also evident in patients with ADA deficiciency.

In children who die, postmortem examination reveals severely depleted lymphoid tissue, with nodes and thymus showing no lymphoid lymphocytes and absent Hassall's corpuscles in the latter. Plasma lymphocytes are absent.

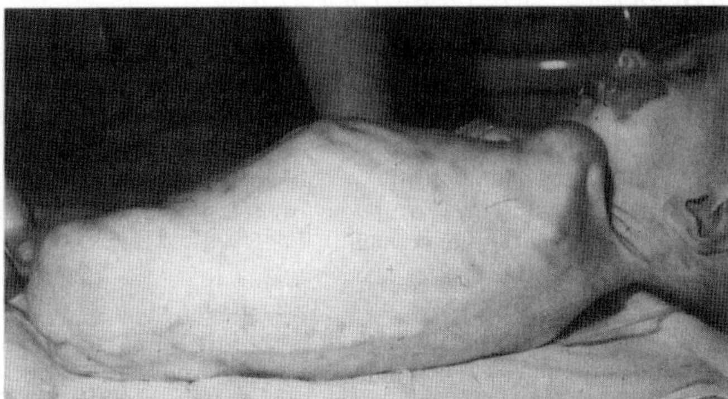

Fig. 25.15 Wasting in a child with severe combined immunodeficiency (SCID).

Without treatment, patients die from infection by about 12 months of age. Currently, the only curative treatment is bone marrow transplantation, although clinical gene therapy trials for common gamma chain deficiency are in progress. Supportive interim treatments include antibiotic prophylaxis with co-trimoxazole as antipneumocystis treatment, antifungal prophylaxis and antibody replacement (intravenous immunoglobulin). Live vaccines should be avoided. The diagnosis of SCID is a pediatric emergency, and suspected cases should be urgently referred to a designated treatment center for further assesment and treatment.

TYPES OF SEVERE COMBINED AND COMBINED IMMUNODEFICIENCIES

T negative B positive SCID

Common gamma chain deficiency (X-linked SCID)

The most common form of SCID is characterized by severe lymphopenia, absence of mature T and NK lymphocytes, but normal numbers of circulating B lymphocytes. It is caused by a deficiency of the gamma chain common to the IL-2, IL-4, IL-7, IL-9 and IL-15 receptors. The easiest form of SCID to treat, the first successful gene therapy was performed for this condition. Carriers show non-random skewed X inactivation of lymphocytes.

JAK-3 deficiency

This autosomal recessive form of SCID is phenotypically identical to the X-linked common gamma chain deficiency. It is due to mutations in the gene encoding Janus-associated-kinase 3, a protein which binds to the intracellular tail of the common gamma chain, and through which signals are transduced following cytokine binding.

IL-7Ralpha deficiency

This autosomal recessive form of SCID is characterized by a T− B+ NK+ phenotype, and has been described in a few patients.

T negative B negative SCID

Two forms of this autosomal recessive disorder have been described. Phenotypically they are identical, with absent T and B lymphocytes, but normal numbers of NK lymphocytes present. The first form is due to defects in the recombinase activating genes (RAG) which are necessary for the development of diverse T and B lymphocyte antigen receptors. In the second form cells cannot repair DNA normally following radiation damage and patients' fibroblasts show in vitro radiosensitivity. Recent studies have identified a defect in the artemis gene, which is necessary for rejoining DNA following TCR and B cell receptor (BCR) recombination. Whilst treatable by bone marrow transplantation, results are not as good as in the T-B+ form of SCID. 'Leaky' RAG defects have been shown in some patients with Omenn's syndrome.

Omenn's syndrome

Omenn's syndrome is characterized by a generalized erythematous rash, often with scaling and erythroderma, lymphadenopathy, hepatosplenomegaly, increased serum IgE levels with a marked eosinophilia and combined immunodeficiency.[33] Children usually present in early infancy but atypical forms may present towards the end of the first year of life, with the clinical features described, as well as diarrhea, failure to thrive and persistent infection. There are normally high numbers of oligoclonal activated poorly functional T lymphocytes of the T_{H2} phenotype but few if any B lymphocytes and low levels of immunoglobulin. The syndrome has been called a 'leaky' form of SCID in that small numbers of very abnormal

T lymphocytes 'leak' past the block in T lymphocyte development. The underlying defect, at least in some cases, is a mutation in the recombination activating genes.

In some families, one affected individual has presented with T– B– NK+ SCID whilst another has presented with Omenn's syndrome. The clinical picture may resemble SCID with maternofetal engraftment, when maternal T lymphocytes crossing the placenta cause a graft-versus-host disease-like reaction in an immunocompetent patient. Molecular genetic studies to identify the origin of the dermal infiltrative T lymphocytes can differentiate the two disorders. Activated oligoclonal lymphocytes in skin seemingly provoke Langerhans' cells to migrate to lymph nodes, liver and spleen where lymphoid tissue architecture is severely disrupted. It has been suggested that interferon gamma may ameliorate the clinical symptoms, but bone marrow transplantation is the only curative treatment.

Reticular dysgenesis

This rare form of SCID, inherited as an autosomal recessive trait, is characterized by defective lymphoid and myeloid differentiation. Bone marrow examination confirms the absence of myeloid precursors. Platelets and red lymphocytes are formed normally. There is some evidence that this is not a discrete entity, but due to other forms of SCID, complicated by severe maternal engraftment and bone marrow GvHD.[32] The absence of the non-specific cellular elements of the immune system makes the immune deficiency even more severe than in other forms of SCID. Clinical presentation often occurs earlier, as does the inevitable fatal outcome if immune reconstitution cannot be achieved.

Lymphocyte metabolism defects

ADA deficiency

This variety of SCID is due to a single gene defect which results in absence of the purine metabolic pathway enzyme, ADA.[34] Although the enzyme is expressed widely throughout the body, accumulation of adenosine and 2′-deoxyadenosine in immature lymphocytes is particularly damaging resulting in cell death. Patients typically present earlier than with other forms of SCID, with very low numbers of T, B and NK lymphocytes. Skeletal abnormalities (cupping deformities of the ends of the ribs, as well as abnormalities of the transverse vertebral processes and the scapulae) are reported in up to 50% of cases and can be correlated with histological changes.[35] Neurodevelopmental problems may also occur in some patients.[36]

Partial forms of ADA deficiency can occur and are associated with a milder immunodeficiency or even normal immune function. Occasional cases of ADA deficiency have been described, where inexplicably, immune function is normal. The diagnosis is confirmed by finding very low erythrocyte ADA activity and high levels of deoxyadenosine triphosphate (dATP) in the urine. First trimester antenatal diagnosis can be made by assaying ADA activity in chorionic villus sampling. Treatment is by bone marrow transplantation or by use of replacement polyethylene glycol-coupled ADA (PEG-ADA). Over several weeks immune function improves considerably and although not to full normality, often to a degree sufficient to keep the child free of infections and thriving. PEG-ADA has been used on a long term basis in those without a suitable donor. The disadvantages of this include the enormous cost, the continuing dependence on intensive medical input and concerns that the beneficial effects will not be maintained in the long term. Patients can develop antibodies against the bovine ADA but to date in most cases these have not been of great clinical significance.[37] Gene therapy has been tried in this condition.

Purine nucleoside phosphorylase (PNP) deficiency

Deficiency of the purine metabolic pathway enzyme, PNP, which results in combined immunodeficiency, is initially less severe than ADA deficiency though there is progression with age. It is an autosomal recessive condition, the gene for which is found on chromosome 9. The metabolites deoxyguanosine and deoxyguanosine triphosphate are particularly toxic for thymocytes resulting in a T lymphocyte deficiency with relatively preserved B lymphocyte function.[38]

The onset of symptoms is usually later than in ADA deficiency, and can be delayed for several years though most cases present in infancy with recurrent and severe infections, particularly with viruses and fungi, diarrhea and failure to thrive. There is a marked tendency to autoimmune disease, especially hemolytic anemia which can progress to red cell aplasia and a predisposition to GvHD following non-irradiated blood transfusion. Skeletal abnormalities do not occur, but neurodevelopmental problems are found in over half of all patients, particularly spastic paresis, disequilibrium and ataxia. There may also be more general neurodevelopmental and behavioral problems. In one series 20% of patients presented primarily with neurological disorder.[39]

Laboratory tests show a progressive fall in T lymphocyte numbers and function with time, poor in vitro mitogen responses and negative delayed hypersensitivity skin tests. Immunoglobulin levels and antibody responses are initially normal but in the late stages levels fall. Serum uric acid levels are very low. The diagnosis is confirmed by demonstrating absent PNP activity in red cells or fibroblasts and deoxyinosine and deoxyguanosine in the urine. Asymptomatic forms of the deficiency have not been reported. Prenatal diagnosis can be made by enzyme activity assays on chorionic villus samples.

The prognosis without corrective treatment is poor with most cases dying in early childhood. The risk of development of malignancy is high. Treatment with bone marrow transplantation is therefore indicated as early as possible. If successful this corrects the immunodeficiency but its effect on the neurological disease is uncertain. Enzyme replacement therapy with fresh irradiated red blood cells and other biochemical manipulations have not met with sustained success.

Other combined immunodeficiencies

Other rare immunodeficiencies have been described in only a few patients to date, with defects in other surface and signaling molecules. It is likely that these will become increasingly recognized as more laboratories are able to offer diagnostic testing. Other atypical or unusual presentations may be due to defects in molecules already described, or to as yet unidentified molecules or mutations.

ZAP-70 kinase defect (CD8 deficiency)

Defective signal transduction in T lymphocytes results from this autosomal recessive condition.[40] The defective kinase is important in T lymphocyte activation via the CD3/TCR complex.There is a marked effect on CD8+ lymphocyte development, resulting in a profound CD8+ lymphopenia which is the hallmark of this condition. Though CD4 lymphocytes are present in normal numbers, they are non-functional.

IL-2R defects

IL-2R alpha defects are characterized by CD25 deficiency, and lymphopenia. Elevated IgM and IgG with low IgA have been described. A patient with low T lymphocyte numbers and absent NK lymphocytes has recently been described with defects in the IL-2/IL-15R beta subunit.

CD45 deficiency

This immunodeficiency is characterized by low numbers of T lymphocytes that were unresponsive to mitogens, but normal B lymphocyte numbers. Immunoglobulin levels fell with time.

CD3 complex deficiencies

Defects in the gamma or epsilon chains of the CD3 complex have been described, leading to low numbers of poorly responsive T lymphocytes and low immunoglobulin levels.

IL-2 production defects

A rare disorder with normal or increased numbers of T lymphocytes which fail to secrete IL-2.

Other defects

Defects in nuclear factor of activated T cells (NF-AT) binding, and defective transmembrane calcium influx have also been described.

Defects in the winged-helix-nude gene have been described in a family with absent hair, dystrophic nails and low T lymphocyte numbers.

CD7 deficiency has been described. This molecule is thought to be important in early T lymphocyte development.

OKT4 deficiency is a defect in an epitope on the CD4 molecule recognized by a monoclonal antibody of that name. There is a mild immunodeficiency and a tendency to autoimmune disease.

Idiopathic CD4 lymphocytopenia

A marked depression in the CD4 positive lymphocyte count characterizes this condition. Most reports have been on adult patients, but it can be seen in children. It is best regarded as a primary immunodeficiency disorder[41] as strenuous efforts to look for a retroviral cause have proved negative and the epidemiology of the condition does not fit with a viral infection. Affected individuals may be highly susceptible to opportunistic infections. The nature of the defect is poorly understood. There is some evidence for defective lymphocyte homeostasis[42] and also evidence for restricted clonality in lymphoid populations.[43] There may well be a number of different causes.

Immunoglobulin levels and antibody responses may be normal. The natural history of this recently described condition is not yet well understood. The CD4 cell count seems to remain stable for a prolonged period in most patients rather than progressively declining as in HIV infection. Prophylaxis against *Pneumocystis carinii* infection should be given. A single case responding to treatment with pegylated IL-2 has been reported.[44] This merits further investigation in the most symptomatic cases.

MHC ANTIGEN DEFICIENCY

MHC CLASS II DEFICIENCY

Major histocompatibility complex (MHC) class II antigens (HLA DR, DP, DQ) are expressed on a limited repertoire of cells and present antigen to CD4+ T lymphocytes, which with the help of an appropriate second signal, leads to the activation of T-helper lymphocytes specific for that antigen and an effective immune response. Expression of MHC II in the thymus is also essential for positive selection of CD4+ T lymphocytes. Since HLAs are of vital importance for lymphocyte development and function, lack of MHC II expression, previously described as a variant of the 'bare lymphocyte syndrome', results in a profound susceptibility to viral, bacterial, fungal and protozoal infections.[3]

The disease is rare and is inherited in an autosomal recessive manner. Initial linkage studies demonstrated that the genetic lesions responsible for the disease lay outside the MHC II region on chromosome 6. It has subsequently been shown that MHC II deficiency can result from mutations in several different genes which code for a complex of regulatory factors controlling transcription of MHC II genes. The genes involved include MHC2TA, RFX5 and RFXAP.[45] The remarkable clinical and laboratory variability seen does not correlate with genotype.

The clinical picture resembles SCID, although sometimes infections develop slightly later. Intestinal and hepatic complications due to cryptosporodial infections are more common than in other immune defects. Neurological manifestations due to a range of viral infections are also well described. Coxsackie virus, adenovirus and poliovirus were the most frequently reported causes of meningoencephalitis.

The laboratory phenotype is very variable, but most patients will have a CD4 lymphopenia and hypogammaglobulinemia, but lymphocyte proliferation responses are usually normal. The diagnosis can be confirmed flow cytometrically by showing absent or significantly reduced levels of class II molecules, e.g. DR, on cells that constitutively express class II (B lymphocytes and monocytes).

Affected children require treatment with replacement immunoglobulin, co-trimoxazole and antifungal prophylaxis pending bone marrow transplantation, which is the definitive treatment although this has had limited success in comparison to other types of SCID.

MHC CLASS I DEFICIENCY

Although described before MHC II deficiency, SCID due to abnormal expression of the A, B and C components of the MHC I complex is much less common. MHC I is required for development of CD8 positive T lymphocytes, and affected children have low numbers of these cells. Mitogen responses are frequently normal. The genetic basis for the disease is mutations in TAP1 or 2.[46] These proteins are required for transport of antigen from the cytoplasm into the endoplasmic reticulum where they associate with MHC I. If the assembly of the antigen/MHC I complex cannot be completed due to antigenic lack, then the MHC is destroyed in the cytoplasm.

Clinically this disease has a milder phenotype than MHC II deficiency with symptoms often not beginning until late childhood. Recurrent respiratory tract infections leading to bronchiectasis and sinus problems are common. Gastrointestinal disease is rare. Unusual skin lesions thought to be due to vasculitis have been reported in a few patients.

Diagnosis is confirmed by showing absent HLA class I expression in peripheral blood. Treatment is directed towards prevention/limitation of lung disease with judicious use of antibiotics (directed by sputum cultures), physiotherapy and bronchodilators as required. Prophylactic continuous antibiotics are of unproven benefit, but may be helpful. The majority of cases do not require replacement immunoglobulin therapy or bone marrow transplantation.

COMBINED IMMUNODEFICIENCY FORMING PART OF OTHER SYNDROMES

DiGEORGE ANOMALY

This condition results from abnormal cephalic neural crest cell migration into the third and fourth pharyngeal arches in early embryological development. A microdeletion at chromosome 22q11.2 is present in 90% of cases while the remainder are associated with other chromosomal anomalies, particularly 10p–.

The 22q microdeletion is also found in velocardiofacial or Shprintzen syndrome, which should now be considered as a part of the same spectrum. DiGeorge syndrome belongs to a group of disorders which have been described as developmental field defects.[47] It is sporadic in occurrence, though familial cases, some associated with 22q chromosomal deletions, have been reported with a prevalence of 1 in 3000–4000 live births. The syndrome is extremely heterogeneous with partial forms more common than the complete phenotype. Whilst classically recognized by the triad of congenital heart defects, immunodeficiency secondary to thymic hypoplasia and hypocalcemia secondary to parathyroid gland hypoplasia, an expanded phenotype is increasingly recognized with dysmorphic facies (low-set, abnormally formed ears, hypertelorism and antimongoloid slant, micrognathia, short philtrum to the upper lip and high arched palate; Fig. 25.16), palatal abnormalities (cleft palate, velopharyngeal insufficiency), autoimmune phenomena, learning difficulties, (particularly speech delay), renal anomalies, neuropsychiatric disorders and short stature. Conotruncal heart defects are classically associated with the syndrome, but other defects are seen including tetralogy of Fallot, septal defects, pulmonary atresia, and aberrant subclavian vessels. Some patients have normal hearts.

Severe T lymphocyte immunodeficiency presenting with a SCID phenotype of profound lymphopenia and poor lymphocyte proliferation is rare and accounts for < 1.5% of cases. Humoral immunodeficiency is more common than previously thought, presenting with recurrent sinopulmonary infection, which may improve with time. Occasionally significant lung damage may occur due to repeated infection. Autoimmune features are increasingly recognized, including juvenile chronic arthritis and autoimmune cytopenias. The long term immunological outlook is not well defined, particularly in children with mild cardiac or palatal phenotypes.

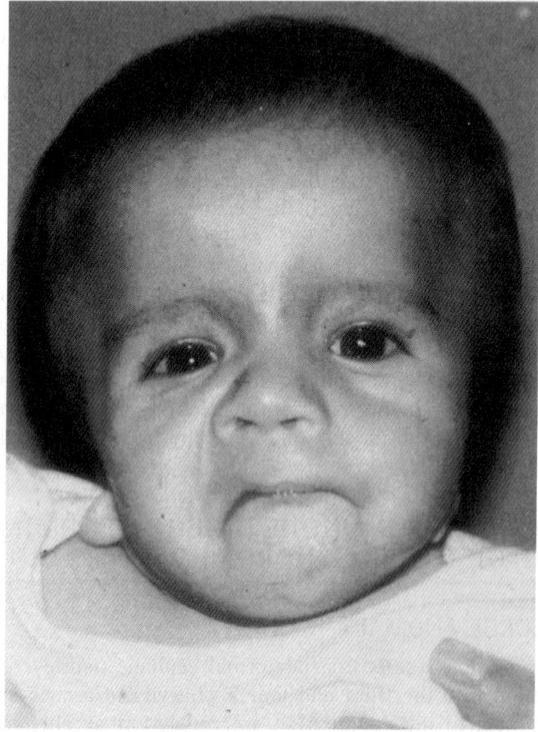

Fig. 25.16 Facies of a child with DiGeorge syndrome. (Courtesy of Professor CBS Wood. Reproduced with permission of the family.)

All children diagnosed with 22q11.2 deletion should have an immunological evaluation including lymphocyte subset analysis, T lymphocyte proliferative responses, immunoglobulin levels and specific antibody responses to vaccination antigens. Laboratory findings may show severe T lymphocyte depletion with poor mitogen responses or relatively normal findings. Previously considered a T lymphocyte defect, recent studies have shown that antibody responses, particularly to polysaccharide antigens, may be impaired. Immunoglobulin levels may be normal but hypogammaglobulinemia may develop, and minor humoral abnormalities are common. Chest X-ray shows lack of a thymic shadow.

In the severe phenotype, the cardiac problems are the main prognostic determinant. Blood products should be irradiated if T lymphocyte mitogen responses are poor. Patients with severe immune deficiency have been successfully treated with fetal thymus implants but bone marrow transplantation gives better results. In the partial phenotype with normal T lymphocyte function, the usual infant vaccination schedule can be followed and it is safe to give live vaccines such as oral polio vaccine, measles, mumps, rubella vaccine, or varicella zoster vaccine as long as the CD4 count exceeds 400/mm^3, and there are normal T lymphocyte mitogen responses. Demonstration of good antibody responses to tetanus and Hib vaccination give further reassurance that live vaccines can be safely administered.[48] Prophylactic antibiotics and occasionally intravenous immunoglobulin can be helpful, particularly for young children with recurrent infection due to humoral deficiency.

WISKOTT–ALDRICH SYNDROME (WAS)

Immunodeficiency, thrombocytopenia, eczema and an increased risk of autoimmune disorders and malignancy characterize this X-linked recessive condition. The gene responsible for WAS codes for a novel 501 amino acid protein, the Wiskott–Aldrich syndrome protein (WASP) which is only found in bone marrow derived cells. Mutations in the same gene are found in patients with X-linked thrombocytopenia (XLT), and more recently in X-linked severe congenital neutopenia.

Clinical features

The classical features of thrombocytopenia, recurrent infections and eczema vary in severity and in some patients the eczema is surprisingly mild. The condition usually presents in early life with bruising, petechiae and bleeding: thrombocytopenia and bleeding episodes may require platelet transfusions. In XLT, thrombocytopenia with small platelet volume is the only symptom, perhaps with mild eczema. In WAS, bacterial and/or viral infections of the upper and lower respiratory tract are common and opportunistic infection, such as *Pneumocystis carinii*, may occur. Herpes viruses, including herpes simplex and varicella zoster virus, are poorly handled and may cause severe and recurrent disease. Impetigo, cellulitis and skin abscesses are surprisingly common, molluscum contagiosum and viral warts may be very extensive. Infection exacerbates the bleeding tendency, and early death may result from bleeding. With increasing age, infective problems replace bleeding as the major cause of death. Immunization with polysaccharide and typhoid vaccines is ineffective and can cause severe, even fatal, reactions. The median survival is between 3 and 15 years. Autoimmunity, particularly autoimmune hemolytic anemia and vasculitis, and malignancy, particularly of the lymphoreticular system become more common with increasing age and in many cases are related to abnormal persistance of EBV infection.[49] Scoring systems have been used to distinguish the milder phenotype of XLT from classical WAS. Heterozygous female carriers are clinically normal and demonstrate non-random X-inactivation in all hemopoietic cells.

Laboratory tests

Thrombocytopenia with an abnormally small mean platelet volume (mean platelet volume < 5 fl) are pathognomic. The severity of immunodeficiency is variable, but affects cellular and humoral responses. T lymphopenia is progressive with depressed responses to mitogens and antigens and negative delayed hypersensitivity skin tests. Serum immunoglobulins show a characteristic pattern with a very low IgM, normal IgG and raised IgA and IgE. Antibody responses to tetanus, *Haemophilus influenzae* type B and *Pneumococcus* are often low, as are isohemagglutinin titers. The direct Coombs test is frequently positive, with or without a hemolytic anemia. *In vivo* neutrophil and monocyte chemotaxis is impaired. Electron microscopy shows greatly reduced numbers of microvilli on lymphocytes and platelets due to failure of the normal binding of actin bundles which is critical to the organization of the cytoskeleton. Lymphoid and myeloid cell lines are all affected so that phagocytes migrate poorly to sites of inflammation and do not put out normal filopodia, dendritic cells do not present antigen effectively, lymphocytes do not signal to each other normally and platelets form imperfectly from megakaryocytes.[50] WASP has a number of unique domains, suggesting multiple functions, which may explain the complex phenotype of a single gene mutation. Missense mutations in exons 1–3 which lead to normal or truncated sized protein result in the milder phenotype of XLT, whereas most other mutations result in the classic WAS phenotype.

Treatment

Acute bleeding episodes may be controlled by platelet transfusions (irradiated to prevent GvHD). Splenectomy and systemic steroids should be avoided if possible as they will increase the risk of infection. Topical steroids are required for the eczema. Intravenous immunoglobulin, with or without prophylactic antibiotics, reduces bacterial sinopulmonary infections and in high dose may help treat autoimmune phenomena.

With only these supportive measures the prognosis remains poor. Immunological and hematological reconstitution can be achieved by bone marrow transplantation and despite a higher risk of EBV-driven lymphoproliferative disorders, 5-year survival is 87% after HLA identical sibling donor bone marrow transplantation and 71% after unrelated donor bone marrow transplantation, although unlike HLA identical sibling BMT, results for unrelated donor bone marrow transplantation after 5 years of age are much poorer.[51]

X-LINKED HYPER-IgM SYNDROME (CD40 LIGAND DEFICIENCY)

X-linked hyper-IgM syndrome is a T lymphocyte immunodeficiency due to a defect in the gene encoding for the CD40 ligand glycopeptide (CD154) expressed on activated T lymphocytes. CD40L binds to CD40, expressed on B lymphocytes and monocyte/macrophage derived cells. Lack of binding prevents B lymphocytes immunoglobulin isotype switching from IgM to IgA, IgG and IgE as well as activation of Kupffer cells and pulmonary macrophages. Lack of IgA and IgG results in a similar clinical picture to XLA with sinopulmonary and invasive bacterial infection but in contrast to XLA, opportunistic infections also occur; failure of T lymphocytes to activate pulmonary macrophages results in *Pneumocystis carinii* pneumonia (Figs 25.17 and 25.18) whilst ineffective Kupffer cell function allows repeated infections of bowel, pancreas and biliary tree with *Cryptosporidium parvum* and similar organisms leading to

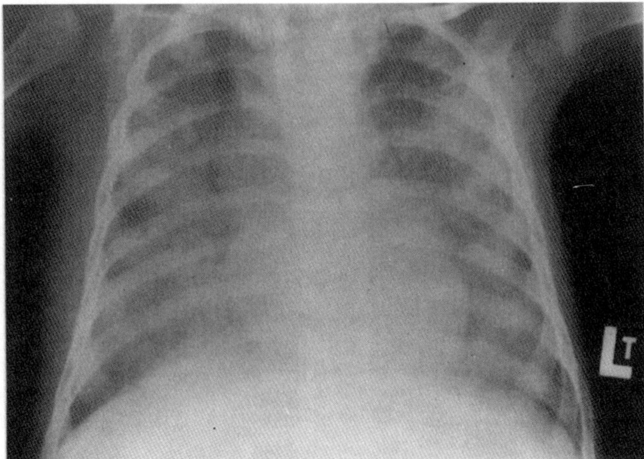

Fig. 25.17 Chest radiograph of a 6-month-old boy, presenting with *Pneumocystis carinii* pneumonia. The underlying immune deficiency was found to be immunoglobulin deficiency with hyper-IgM- syndrome.

sclerosing cholangitis, cirrhosis, pancreatitis and hepatic malignancy which becomes clinically apparent in the second or third decade. Neutropenia with oral ulceration is seen in as many as 66% of patients, and this together with low or absent IgA and IgG, and normal or raised IgM should suggest the diagnosis. Fatal CMV infection or enteroviral meningoencephalitis can occur and autoimmune phenomena are relatively common and include hemolytic anemias, thrombocytopenia, hypothyroidism, arthritis and liver disorders.[22]

Patients should receive co-trimoxazole as *Pneumocystis carinii* pneumonia prophylaxis and high doses of immunoglobulin replacement therapy are often required. With adequate replacement the rising IgM levels may normalize. The neutropenia sometimes responds to granulocyte-colony stimulating factor (G-CSF) and intravenous immunoglobulin (IVIG). All drinking water should be boiled. Azithromycin prophylaxis may also lessen the risks of *Cryptosporidium parvum* infection. Despite conventional treatment, many patients do not survive beyond the second decade of life, but a few patients with a common variable immunodeficiency-like clinical course and no biliary or liver disease are relatively well in middle life. Bone marrow transplantation is increasingly being recommended for this condition and combined bone marrow and liver transplantation has been successful.[52]

DEFECTS OF LYMPHOCYTE APOPTOSIS (AUTOIMMUNE LYMPHOPROLIFERATIVE SYNDROME, ALPS)

Apoptosis, or programmed cell death, is important for regulating immune responses once an infection has been countered. Defects in this process lead to marked autoimmune and lymphoproliferative features which characterize ALPS.[53] There are a number of pathways through which apoptosis can be induced; one of the most important is initiated through a cell surface molecule Fas (CD95). Ligation of this molecule initates a cascade of intracellular reactions culminating in apoptosis induced by proteolytic enzymes including caspases. Mutations in several molecules in this cascade result in molecularly distinct but clinically similar forms of ALPS (Table 25.12).

Most of the cases described have been heterozygotes though a few homozygous cases are also reported. The variablity of clinical severity and the occurrence of asymptomatic individuals makes estimation of the incidence of this condition very difficult.

(a)

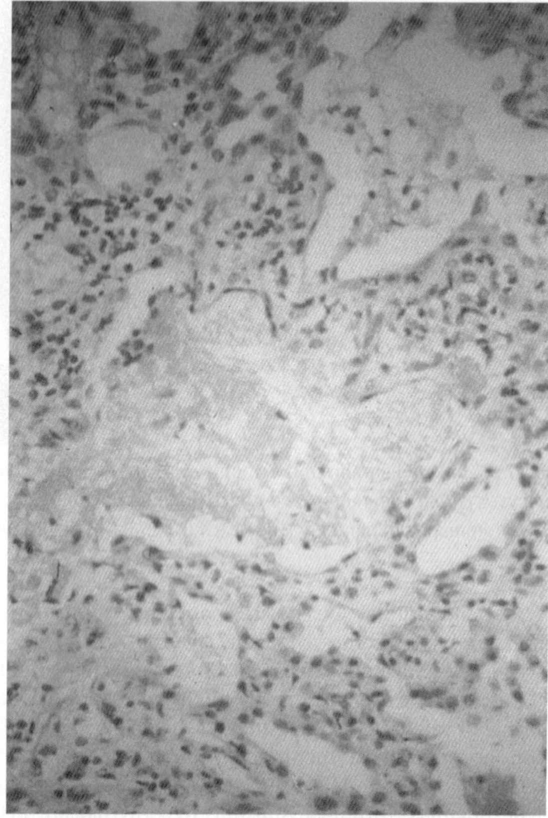

(b)

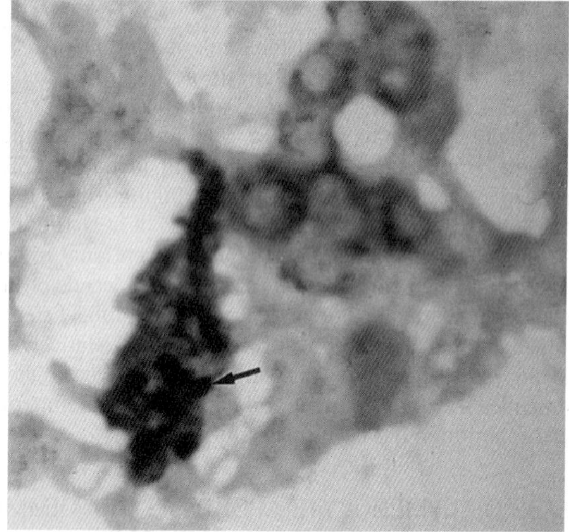

Fig. 25.18 Lung histology following open lung biopsy in the patient whose chest radiograph is shown in Figure 25.17. (a) Hematoxylin and eosin stain showing marked inflammatory infiltrate. (b) Grocott methanamine stain showing pneumocystis organisms (arrowed).

Clinical features

The age of presentation is variable. Many present in early childhood but adult presentation is also described. Asymptomatic cases may occur in the families of symptomatic individuals. Autoimmune disease most commonly affects the hemopoietic system but disease involving many other systems such as nervous, renal and dermatological also occurs. Lymphoproliferation often results in characteristically massive asymmetric lymph nodes in the anterior triangle of the neck, together with splenomegaly in nearly all cases and hepatomegaly in some. Malignant disease of the lymphoid system (both Hodgkin's and non-Hodgkin's) is reported with increased frequency but has probably been overdiagnosed because the histological picture of proliferation resembles malignancy: clonality studies distinguish the two.[54] Homozygous Fas deficiency has a more severe clinical phenotype, sometimes with prenatal onset resulting in hydrops.

Table 25.12 Different molecule types of ALPS

Type	Molecule affected
Ia	Fas (CD95)
Ib	Fas ligand
II	Caspase 10
III	Caspase 8
IV	Unknown

Laboratory features

Affected individuals will usually have high lymphocyte counts and normal or high immunoglobin levels. Autoantibodies are usually present. A universal feature is the occurrence of circulating CD3 positive T lymphocytes expressing the alpha/beta receptor but not expressing CD4 or CD8 (so-called double negative T lymphocytes) and usually constituting between 5 and 20% of the total CD3 cell count. Many of these cells also express HLA DR (which is normally only expressed on activated T lymphocytes). CD95 is not normally constitutively expressed on lymphocytes but is after activation with mitogens and failure of this expression can be demonstrated in type 1a ALPS after appropriate cellular activation. Apoptotic assays involving artificial ligation of CD95 with an antibody and then measurement of cell death can be used to confirm an ALPS defect. Mutation analysis of Fas, Fas L and the appropriate caspase genes will confirm the precise molecular diagnosis.

Treatment and prognosis

Autoimmune phenomena usually respond to standard treatments but there is a tendency for recurrence or the emergence of new autoimmune problems. Splenectomy for the control of hematological problems should be avoided if possible since there are reports of severe infective complications following this. However it may prove unavoidable in which case the usual infection prophylaxis measures should be adhered to. Corticosteriods may reduce the degree of lymphoproliferation but their use must be balanced against the risks of long term usage. Malignant disease is treated along standard lines but at the moment there are insufficient data to determine whether the response to treatment differs from non-ALPS patients. Bone marrow transplantation has been successful in patients with homozygous Fas deficiency but currently not enough is known of the long term prognosis to justify elective bone marrow transplantation in (milder) heterozygous cases, especially as some patients improve with age.

X-LINKED LYMPHOPROLIFERATIVE DISEASE

An X-linked immunodeficiency associated with fulminant fatal EBV driven infectious mononucleosis was first recognized in the Duncan kindred.[55] There are three common clinical presentations: fulminant infectious mononucleosis (58%), dysgammaglobulinemia, often evolving to common variable immunodeficiency (31%) and EBV driven B lymphocyte lymphoma, usually extranodal, and affecting the gastrointestinal tract or central nervous system (20%). Less commonly patients present with vasculitis, aplastic anemia, hemophagocytic lymphohistiocytosis or pulmonary lymphomatoid granulomatosis.[56] The prognosis is poor with 45–96% mortality, depending on the clinical presentation, and registry data indicate no survivors after 40 years of age. Most patients are well until infected with EBV, although other viruses may act as triggers. The gene responsible for the disease, SH2D1A in the Xq25 region of the X chromosome, was identified in 1998.[57] The gene encodes a small protein, SAP [signaling lymphocyte activation molecule (SLAM) associated protein] which appears critical for T lymphocyte and NK cell control of EBV-infected B lymphocytes but why this causes the clinical features is not yet understood.

Confirmation of the diagnosis involves demonstrating EBV genome in blood by polymerase chain reaction (PCR), together with the immune defects outlined above and an abnormal serological response to the virus with absent antibody response to EB nuclear antigen (EBNA). The mothers of affected boys also have abnormal EBV serology, with persisting very high titers against viral capsid antigen. Whilst the majority of cases appear to be triggered by EBV infection, EBV negative clinical cases have been described.[58] Protein analysis reveals absent or abnormal SAP protein in many cases, although a gene mutation is not apparent in up to 40% of patients, raising the possibility of mutations in intrinsic elements or other control proteins. Treatment with intravenous immunoglobulin on a regular basis as passive immunization against EBV is recommended in affected patients, particularly if hypogammaglobulinemia is present. Hemophagocytic lymphohistiocytic episodes may be treated with immunosuppression with ciclosporin. Correction of the disorder by bone marrow transplantation has been achieved and is the only curative treatment.

CHRONIC MUCOCUTANEOUS CANDIDIASIS

Chronic mucocutaneous candidiasis (CMC) describes a group of disorders characterized by chronic infection of skin, nails and mucous membranes by organisms of the genus *Candida*, most commonly *Candida albicans*. Recurrent and persistent candida of the mouth, napkin area, skin and nails is the hallmark of this condition, but the severity varies considerably and invasive disease almost never occurs. Failure of usually effective antifungal drugs to clear candida distinguishes CMC from other conditions that predispose to candida such as secondary immunodeficiency, steroid treatment or systemic antibiotics. Candidiasis is usually first noticed early in infancy and in severe cases gross esophageal involvement causes dysphagia, gastroesophageal reflux and failure to thrive whilst skin lesions may be extremely disfiguring and distressing (Fig. 25.19). As a patient becomes older candida may become less severe

In about half the patients there is an associated endocrinopathy (with, in order of frequency, hypoparathyroidism, Addison's disease, pernicious anemia, hypothyroidism and diabetes mellitus) which becomes apparent from the second to third decades onward. Cases may be familial or sporadic with recessive or dominant patterns of inheritance. Nail dystrophy and dental enamel hypoplasia associated with autoimmune endocrinopathy, suggest that CMC is part of autoimmune polyendocrinopathy, candidiasis, ectodermal dystrophy (APECED) which is inherited in an autosomal recessive manner. A minority of patients suffer from invasive bacterial sepsis, opportunistic infection, autoimmune hemolytic anemia, malabsorption and chronic active hepatitis. Bronchiectasis and restrictive lung disease can occur.[59]

The underlying defect is poorly defined and variable. There may be diminished T lymphocyte proliferation and cytokine production in response to candida antigens with impaired antibody production to polysaccharide antigens, and sometimes IgG2 subclass deficiency.[60]

Treatment with azole antifungals such as fluconazole can be very effective, even in severe cases, but often does not completely eradicate infection, or infection recurs on stopping treatment. Continuous treatment is necessary in severe cases. Bone marrow transplantation has been successful in very severe cases.

IMMUNODEFICIENCY AND SHORT-LIMBED DWARFISM

Abnormalities of T and B lymphocyte function are seen in a number of osteochondrodysplasias, including Shwachman syndrome where there is neutropenia and pancreatic insufficiency and Schimke immuno-osseous dysplasia which features radiographic changes of spondyloepiphyseal dysplasia, nephrotic syndrome and cellular immunodeficiency. Other short-limbed dwarfisms associated with immunodeficiency are less clearly delineated.

Cartilage–hair hypoplasia is the most well described variant, inherited in an autosomal recessive manner and mutations in the RMRP gene, which encodes endoribonuclease Rnase MRP (mitochondrial RNA-processing endoribonuclease RNA), have recently been described. Severe short-limbed short stature (–11.8 SD to –2.1 SD) with X-ray appearances of metaphyseal and spondyloepiphyseal dysplasia are always present and accompanied by sparse light hair in most patients. Severe anemia and

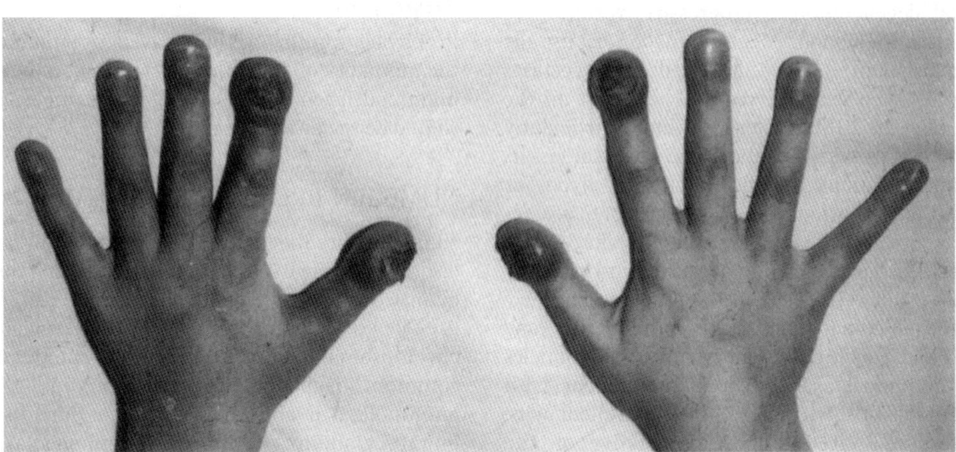

Fig. 25.19 Chronic mucocutaneous candidiasis.

Hirschsprung's disease are less common but well recognized associations, as are malignancies, notably lymphoma and skin carcinoma. The immunodeficiency is surprisingly variable; most have T lymphopenia, and impaired in vitro mitogen proliferative responses, but only half suffer recurrent infection.[61] However, some have IgA and/or IgG subclass deficiencies with frequent ear infections. Patients are excessively vulnerable to viral infections, particularly varicella zoster, EBV, and other human herpes virus infections and the risk of infective death is 300 times greater than normal.[62] Severely affected patients should be assessed for bone marrow transplantation which has been successful in correcting the immunodeficiency.

DNA REPAIR DEFECTS AND IMMUNODEFICIENCY

Recognition of a wide array of foreign antigens requires a huge number of genetically diverse lymphocytes, each bearing a unique receptor. These are created by rearranging the variable (V), diversity (D) and joining (J) gene segements that code for T or B lymphocyte receptor genes (VDJ recombination). This is initiated by introducing DNA double strand breaks between the gene segments, and then rejoining the rearranged segments using the cells' ubiquitous DNA repair machinary. In evolutionary terms, the immune system has utilized cellular DNA repair mechanisms to generate the diversity of specific immune responses. Without the ability to repair DNA damage, cells may apoptose or undergo malignant proliferation and so individuals with defective DNA repair mechanisms have a predisposition to neurodegeneration, developmental anomalies and cancer as well as defective immunity.[63] The mechanisms are complex with scope for many single gene defects to give rise to distinct clinical entities.

ATAXIA TELANGIECTASIA (AT)

This multisystem autosomal recessive disorder, the best known of the DNA repair disorders, is characterized by progressive cerebellar ataxia, oculocutaneous telangiectasiae, variable immunodeficiency and an increased risk of lymphoid malignancy and is associated with chromosomal instability, and cellular radiosensitivity. Diagnosis remains chiefly clinical and depends on the age of presentation. In the absence of a family history, it is usually detected by a pediatric neurologist on the basis of gait anomalies but before telangiectasiae appear it may be difficult to distinguish from other ataxia syndromes (see also Ch. 20). Ataxia and cerebellar signs are always present and usually appear in the second year, but may be delayed. Neurological degeneration is progressive, resulting in severe disability by late childhood. Mental function is usually preserved though retardation has been described. Telangiectases appear later, usually between 2 and 8 years of age, first on the bulbar conjunctivae (Fig. 25.20) but later elsewhere, particularly on the nose, the ears, and in the antecubital and popliteal fossae. Other cutaneous manifestations include patches of hypo- or hyperpigmentation, cutaneous atrophy and atopic dermatitis.

Gonadal atrophy occurs in both sexes, and growth failure is also prominent in the later stages. Cellular and humoral immunodeficiency affects 60–80% of cases but clinical manifestations are extremely variable. Recurrent sinopulmonary infection is common and may lead to bronchiectasis and clubbing. Lymphoreticular malignancies and, unusually for immunodeficiency, carcinomas, occur with increased frequency. Radiosensitivity means that treatment with radiotherapy is toxic and often lethal. Irrespective of the development of malignancy, survival beyond early adult life is unusual. Heterozygosity for the AT gene mutation confers an increased risk of developing breast cancer.

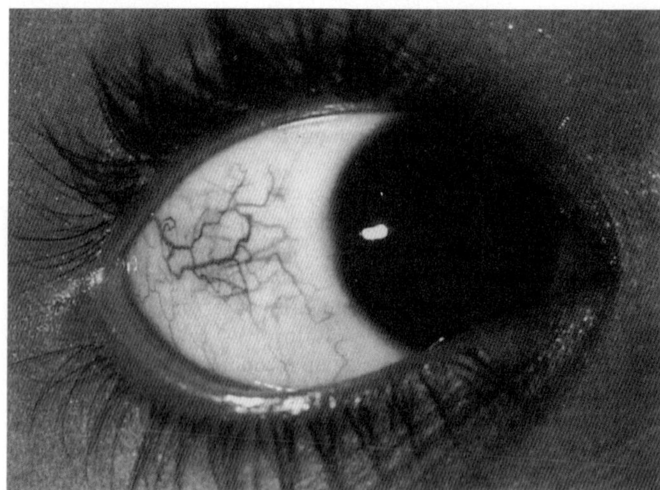

Fig. 25.20 Ataxia telangiectasia.

Laboratory features

Immunological findings are extremely variable. Low or absent levels of IgA, IgE, IgG, IgG2 and IgG4 subclasses are frequently found and antibody responses are particularly poor to polysaccharide and viral antigens. IgM may be raised and autoantibodies are sometimes found. Cellular immunodeficiency is characterized by defective thymic development and lymphopenia, predominantly of CD4+ T lymphocytes with an increase in the number of T lymphocytes bearing the gamma/delta receptor. Decreased mitogen and antigen responses can be demonstrated due to defective cytoplasmic to nuclear signaling. A raised alpha-fetoprotein (abnormal in 90%) supports the diagnosis, as does evidence of increased chromosome breakage on exposure to ionizing radiation. Patients are efficient at V(D)J rejoining, but have a high incidence of translocations at the sites of the T lymphocyte receptor and immunoglobulin heavy chain genes which may explain the immunodeficiency, and suggest a defect in detecting damaged DNA. This is in keeping with the discovery that the ATM gene found on chromosome 11q22.23 codes for a phosphatidyl kinase involved in meiotic recombination and cell cycle control.[64] This protein detects DNA damage and signals to proteins involved in DNA repair and cell cycle control;[65] it is absent or inactive in AT patients.

Treatment

Prophylactic antibiotics or intravenous immunoglobulin can reduce the morbidity of sinopulmonary infection in some patients. As the immunodeficiency is often progressive, the need for such treatment should be reviewed intermittently.

NIJMEGEN BREAKAGE SYNDROME

Nijmegen breakage syndrome (NBS), an autosomal recessive disorder described in the Dutch town of that name, is characterized by microcephaly with mild to moderate mental retardation, 'bird-like' facies, immunodeficiency, clinical radiation sensitivity and chromosomal instability. Bacterial sinopulmonary infection is common. Hypogammaglobulinemia is the most common immunological abnormality and a third of patients make no immunoglobulin. A CD4+ T lymphopenia with diminished T lymphocyte proliferative responses is also found.[66] A defect in the gene encoding nibrin has recently been identified as the cause of NBS.[67] Nibrin is part of a protein complex downstream of the ATM protein, and is part of the ATM signal transduction cascade. Absence of ataxia and telangiectasia, together with normal alpha-fetoprotein levels distinguishes NBS from AT. Treatment with antibiotic prophylaxis or IVIG can be helpful.

ATAXIA-TELANGIECTASIA-LIKE DISORDER

Patients with similar features to AT patients but with no mutation in the ATM gene have been described. In some, mutations have recently been found in the Mre11 protein, part of the complex with which nibrin associates and which is one of the complexes downstream from ATM.

BLOOM SYNDROME

This rare autosomal recessive disorder is associated with increased sister chromatid exchange, severe growth failure, increased malignancy and immunodeficiency. Affected individuals may develop facial telangiectases and facial photosensitivity. Recurrent bacterial sinopulmonary infections associated with hypogammaglobulinemia, most often low IgM, are the most common clinical manifestation of immunodeficiency, and may lead to bronchiectasis. The Bloom's protein, mutated in the disease, unwinds the DNA helix. The mechanism of the immunodeficiency is unclear.

DEFECTS IN DNA LIGASES

DNA ligases function in DNA repair. Defects in DNA ligases I and IV have been described in rare individuls with radiosensitive cell lines and combined immunodeficiencies.

FANCONI'S ANEMIA (see also Ch. 21)

Progressive bone marrow failure leading to pancytopenia is the main problem in this condition. There may also be skeletal malformations. Immune deficiency can occur, and selective IgA deficiency and T lymphocyte abnormalities have been recorded. At least seven genes are implicated in the disorder, encoding for proteins which form a complex, possibly involved in sensing DNA damage, and facilitating repair.[68]

XERODERMA PIGMENTOSA

Immune deficiency, predominantly involving NK cells may occur but is not a prominent feature. The mechanism of the immunodeficiency is unclear.

COMBINED IMMUNODEFICIENCIES AND RADIOSENSITIVITY

Some individuals with common variable immunodeficiency have radiosensitive lymphocytes. Rare individuals with uncharacterized combined immunodeficiencies also show radiosensitivity. The underlying defects are not understood.

OTHER IMMUNODEFICIENCIES

A number of syndromes have been described which include primary immunodeficiency as part of the phenotype. In some, the syndrome is well described, and in a few the underlying molecular defect has recently been elucidated. Most lack clear definition.

HOYERAAL-HREIDARSSON SYNDROME

This X-linked disorder is characterized by microcephaly, cerebellar hypoplasia, aplastic anemia and growth retardation. A progressive combined immunodeficiency, with hypogammaglobulinemia and lymphopenia is a well recognized association. Mutations in the dyskeratosis congenita gene (DKC1) have been found in some patients.

NETHERTON'S SYNDROME

This triad of generalized infantile erythroderma, diarrhea and failure to thrive may be associated with a variable immunodeficiency including mild lymphopenia. The clinical features are similar to those seen in Omenn's syndrome and SCID and maternofetal engraftment. Distinguishing these entities is important as the other conditions are treated by bone marrow transplantation, whereas Netherton's syndrome is not. Hair shaft abnormalities are diagnostic (bamboo hairs), and mutations in the serine protease inhibitor (PI) gene SPINK5 have been described.

ANHYDROTIC ECTODERMAL DYSPLASIA, INCONTINENTIA PIGMENTI AND DEFECTS IN THE NEMO GENE

X-linked anhydrotic ectodermal dysplasia has been associated with immunodeficiency. Patients present with sparse scalp hair, conical teeth and absent sweat glands. Some suffer from recurrent sinopulmonary infection, often with encapsulated organisms, and have poor antibody responses to polysaccharide antigens, or frank hypogammaglobulinemia. Incontinentia pigmenti is a rare X-linked dominant condition characterized by developmental abnormalities in skin, hair, teeth and the central nervous system. Previously thought lethal in male fetuses, rare male infants with a progressive combined immunodeficiency have been described.

Recently, hypofunctional mutations in the NEMO gene encoding a protein required to activate the transcription factor NF-kappaB have been described in male patients with both X-linked anhydrotic ectodermal dysplasia and incontinentia pigmenti suggesting that these conditions represent variants of the same disorder.[69]

THE IPEX SYNDROME

The immune dysregulation, polyendocrinopathy, enteropathy, X-linked syndrome is characterized by infantile ichthyosiform dermatitis, protracted diarrhea, insulin dependent diabetes mellitus and thyroiditis. Mutations in the FOXP3 gene have recently been described in affected patients. Bone marrow transplantation has been tried as a curative treatment.

ICF SYNDROME

ICF syndrome (immunodeficiency, centromeric instability and facial anomalies syndrome) is an autosomal recessive disorder in which there are characteristic structural chromosomal abnormalities in chromosomes 1, 9 and 16 in lymphocytes. Other cells do not show these changes. Affected children develop severe recurrent infections and have immunoglobulin deficiency, often with agammaglobulinemia but with normal T and B lymphocyte numbers.[70] T lymphocyte immunity is not normal and *Pneumocystis carinii* infection, severe viral warts and cutaneous fungal infection are described. The differential diagnosis is common variable immune deficiency (CVID). Mental retardation may occur but there is no increased risk of malignancy.

DEFECTS OF ANTIBODY PRODUCTION

X-LINKED AGAMMAGLOBULINEMIA (XLA, BRUTON'S DISEASE)

First described by Bruton in 1952,[71] this X-linked condition is due to an intrinsic defect which prevents the normal differentiation of B lymphocytes beyond the pre-B lymphocyte stage. The defective gene lying on the long arm of the X chromosome encodes a cytoplasmic enzyme, Bruton tyrosine kinase (btk). Affected boys classically show a complete failure to produce immunoglobulins and antibody responses, but cell-mediated immunity is normal. Milder phenotypes have been found though it has not proved possible to correlate severity with the many different mutations that have been found.

Clinical features

Typically, recurrent pyogenic infections commence in the latter half of the first year of life, after maternal IgG levels have declined. The diagnosis is often made surprisingly late; in one series, the average age at diagnosis was 3½ years without, and 2½ years with, a positive family history.[72] The situation may not have improved since then as a more recent audit of all forms of immunoglobulin deficiency in adults and children in the UK found an average delay of 6.26 years between onset of symptoms and diagnosis.[73]

Sinopulmonary infections are most common, but gastroenteritis, pyoderma, arthritis, meningitis and osteomyelitis may be presenting features (Table 25.13).[72] Common gastrointestinal pathogens include *Campylobacter jejuni* and *Giardia lamblia*.[74] Chronic conjunctivitis caused by *Pseudomonas* species may also occur. Recovery from viral infections is normal with the notable exception of those caused by enteroviruses (especially echoviruses) which can cause a chronic meningoencephalitis or dermatomyositis-like picture. Vaccine associated paralytic poliomyelitis has been reported with live vaccine. Pathogens in which cell-mediated immunity is thought to be important are not usually a problem, though occasional cases of *Pneumocystis carinii* infection have been reported. Other complications include a non-purulent arthritis affecting predominantly large joints. In some cases this has been shown to be due to mycoplasma infection. Neutropenia, alopecia totalis and amyloidosis are infrequent complications.

Laboratory findings

Once maternal IgG has declined, the usual pattern is one of absence or severe depletion of all serum immunoglobulin classes. It is not possible to demonstrate any antibody response to vaccines or to bacteriophage ΦX174. Circulating lymphocyte markers show a normal number of T lymphocytes, but absence of B lymphocytes. Bone marrow aspirate does, however, show pre-B lymphocytes (containing cytoplasmic mu chains). Lymph nodes show absent follicles and germinal centers. Plasma cells cannot be demonstrated at any site. Confirmation of the diagnosis can be made rapidly in over 90% of cases by demonstrating absence of the btk protein in cell lysates.[75] The finding of absent or abnormal btk in boys with partial antibody deficiency means that the condition should be considered in the presence of any form of antibody deficiency in boys, particularly if circulating B lymphocyte numbers are low. Foremost in the differential diagnosis of XLA is common variable immune deficiency. Table 25.14 lists some of the important differences between the two.

The mainstay of treatment is immunoglobulin replacement therapy (p. 1290). Infections may still occur especially giardiasis and chronic conjunctivitis. Chronic lung damage and sinus disease may also progress on treatment and for this reason vigorous and early antibiotic therapy should be used for respiratory tract infections. If the problems are recurrent despite increased doses of immunoglobulin, continuous prophylactic antibiotics may be required. A large series of patients treated before IVIG was available revealed a high incidence of chronic lung disease (75% of those over 20 years) even with treatment with intramuscular immunoglobulin (IMIG), and 17% of patients had died with a mean age of 16.9 years. With the widespread use of IVIG, lung disease seems less common and a recent sizeable retrospective study[76] found that the patients developing progressive lung and sinus disease while on treatment tended to be those with damage sustained before immunoglobulin therapy was commenced. These data emphasize the importance of early diagnosis and treatment for this condition. The same study also found that maintaining patients at higher IgG levels reduced the risk of lung disease but not of sinus problems.

Table 25.13 Presenting features in 96 patients with X-linked agammaglobulinemia (From Lederman & Winkelstein 1985[72])

Presenting feature	%
Ear, nose and throat infections (otitis media)	75 (59)
Lower respiratory tract infections (pneumonia)	65 (56)
Gastrointestinal infections (diarrhea)	35 (32)
Pyoderma	28
Arthritis (septic)	20 (8)
CNS infections (meningitis)	16 (10)
Septicemia	10
Neutropenia	10
Positive family history	26
Others: Failure to thrive; fever of uncertain origin; complications of immunization; osteomyelitis and dermatomyositis	<5% each

Diagnoses and figures in brackets indicate the predominant type of infection in each system and its overall incidence in the 96 patients.

Table 25.14 Comparison of X-linked agammaglobulinemia (XLA) and common variable hypogammaglobulinemia (CVH)

	XLA	CVH
Inheritance	X-linked	Mostly unknown (some may be AR or AD)
Age of onset	Infancy	Any age
Immunological defect	Antibody	Antibody +/– cell-mediated
Immunoglobulin classes	All decreased	One (usually IgM) or more often preserved
B cell numbers	Absent	Usually present
T cell numbers and function	Normal	Normal or decreased
Pyogenic infections	Yes	Yes
Opportunistic infections	Very rare	Yes
Autoimmune phenomena	Very rare	Yes
Chronic gastrointestinal problems	Rare	Common

AD = autosomal dominant; AR = autosomal recesive

X -LINKED AGAMMAGLOBULINEMIA AND SENSORINEURAL HEARING LOSS

Three unrelated boys with XLA were recently described with mutation confirmed XLA and progressive sensorineural hearing loss.[77] They all had large deletions in the terminal part of the btk gene which were believed to involve a contiguous gene coding the deafness, dystonia protein, DDP. Mutations in the latter gene have been associated with Tranebjaerg syndrome of deafness, dystonia and mental retardation. At the time of reporting the patients did not exhibit the other features.

HYPOGAMMAGLOBULINEMIA WITH GROWTH HORMONE DEFICIENCY

Very rarely hypogammaglobulinemia with low/absent B lymphocytes consistent with XLA has been described associated with isolated growth hormone deficiency. In the first case described no btk mutation was identified. In subsequent cases mutations in btk have been identified but the same mutations have also been found in boys without growth hormone deficiency. The relationship between the two conditions therefore remains enigmatic.

AUTOSOMAL RECESSIVE FORMS OF AGAMMAGLOBULINEMIA

When hypogammaglobulinemia is found in girls or when a patient's parents are consanguineous, one of the recently recognized autosomal recessive genetic defects affecting B lymphocyte differentiation should be considered. Mutations have been described so far in genes coding for: mu heavy chain, Ig-alpha (part of the signal transduction complex of the B lymphocyte antigen receptor), lambda 5 light chain, BLNK (B lymphocyte linker protein). These molecules are all required for early B lymphocyte development from pro-B lymphocyte to pre-B lymphocyte stage. Unlike XLA pre-B lymphocytes are therefore not detectable in marrow samples. Other families have also been described in whom the molecular defect is yet to be identified. In all cases the defect is B lymphocyte specific. The number of cases described is too small to draw firm conclusions but the clinical picture would seem to be similar to XLA, although patients with mu heavy chain deficiency may have more serious life threatening infections than those with XLA with an earlier onset of symptoms.[78]

IMMUNOGLOBULIN DEFICIENCY WITH TRANSCOBALAMIN II DEFICIENCY

Hypogammaglobulinemia due to a failure of terminal (antigen driven) B lymphocyte differentiation can result from congenital absence of one of the vitamin B_{12} carrier proteins, transcobalamin II. There is associated pernicious anemia. Parenteral high dose vitamin B_{12} corrects the immunological defect.

COMMON VARIABLE IMMUNE DEFICIENCY

Common variable immune deficiency (CVID) is a poorly defined entity characterized by the presence of quantitative or qualitative hypogammaglobulinemia. The incidence is described as between 1:10 000 and 1: 50 000 of the population and although the onset of symptoms is typically seen within the second or third decade of life it is increasingly being diagnosed in childhood.

Familial inheritance is seen in up to 25% of cases, but the variability of phenotype both within and between families suggests a polygenic inheritance. Selective IgA deficiency may be one end of the spectrum of this disease.[79] As the molecular basis of other immune deficiencies is being defined, it is clear that a number of patients with CVID have mild phenotypes of other immune deficiencies such as X-linked agammaglobulinemia, CD40 ligand deficiency or X-linked lymphoproliferative disease.[80,81] Autoimmune diseases, such as rheumatoid arthritis also have an increased incidence in these kindreds.

As with all patients with humoral immune defects, patients with CVID present with recurrent sinopulmonary and gastrointestinal infections. They are particularly susceptible to *Giardia lamblia*. They are also at risk from enteroviral infections, causing choriomeningitis in particular, and arthritis may result from chronic mycoplasma infection. Other clinical manifestations in this disease exemplify the inherent immune deregulation with an increased incidence of autoimmune disease, particularly autoimmune hemolytic anemia, thrombocytopenia and neutropenia. Non-malignant granulomatous lymphadenopathy, hepatosplenomegaly and involvement of the gastrointestinal tract is a frequent finding in a subgroup of patients,[82] and clinical differentiation from malignancy may be difficult although histologically lesions resemble those seen in sarcoidosis. These granulomata are normally sensitive to steroid treatment. Patients with CVID also have a significantly increased risk of lymphoreticular and gastrointestinal malignancies.

Laboratory findings

Hypogammaglobulinemia is the hallmark of these patients. This may vary from a failure of specific vaccine responses to panhypogammaglobulinemia. B lymphocyte numbers are frequently normal. A significant proportion of patients have T lymphocyte abnormalities, in particular a reversed CD4/8 ratio and a generalized lymphopenia.[83] Such abnormalities at presentation should prompt a search for other defined immune defects.

Treatment

The aim of treatment is prevention of further infections and consequent end-organ damage such as bronchiectasis. Mild phenotypes may require only prophylactic antibiotics. Significant degrees of hypogammaglobulinemia should be treated with immunoglobulin replacement therapy. If patients have significantly abnormal cell mediated immunity, they should be given prophylactic co-trimoxazole. Granulomatous lesions and autoimmune phenomena may respond to treatment with steroids.

OTHER HUMORAL IMMUNE DEFECTS

IgA DEFICIENCY

Studies on healthy blood donors have shown that 1 in 600–700 Caucasians have no demonstrable serum IgA. Deficiency of serum IgA is almost always associated with a lack of salivary IgA. The clinical significance of low IgA in isolation is unclear as the majority of affected individuals are asymptomatic. However in populations of patients with chronic lung disease and autoimmune diseases there is an increased incidence of IgA deficiency. As the majority of patients with IgA deficiency are well, the pathophysiology of disease in these individuals is probably multifactorial; other contributory elements may include IgG subclass deficiency and reduced levels of mannan-binding lectin. Selective IgA deficiency is part of the spectrum of CVID; both may be present in the same family and rarely patients with IgA deficiency progress to CVID. In an infant, low IgA may be the last manifestation of transient hypogammaglobulinemia to resolve. Acquired IgA deficiency (usually reversible) may occur as a result of drug therapies (e.g. penicillamine, phenytoin, sodium valproate, captopril). It has also been described in congenital infections and after hepatitis C infection.

Assessment of patients with IgA deficiency

If this is an incidental finding without a history of recurrent infections, an isolated low IgA is unlikely to be of clinical significance. If recurrent infections are present, further investigation should be undertaken, including assessment of IgG subclasses and specific vaccination responses. IgG subclass deficiencies occur in approximately 15% of cases.

Symptoms

Infective: Recurrent sinopulmonary infections are the commonest symptoms in young children. Middle ear infections can be troublesome, and recurrent lower respiratory tract infections may result in lung damage. In the majority of children the frequency and severity of infections improves with age, regardless of the IgA level. Gastrointestinal infections, in particular with *Giardia lamblia* have an increased incidence, but reports of increased numbers of urinary tract infections have not been substantiated.

Autoimmunity: There is a strong correlation between autoimmune disease of all types and IgA deficiency,[84] whether or not the latter is associated with infections. Mechanisms are poorly understood, but may include abnormalities in antigen handling.

Gastrointestinal disease: The increased incidence of gastrointestinal infection has been discussed above. There is also an increase in celiac disease in IgA deficiency, which may give a false negative test if the diagnosis of celiac disease is based on the presence of IgA antigliadin and endomysial antibodies.

Malignancy: There are multiple reports of lymphomas and gastric malignancies in patients with IgA deficiency, although the true incidence of this problem has not been well defined.

Treatment

Patients with significant symptoms may respond to prophylactic antibacterial treatment, particularly over the winter. Very occasional patients may require replacement immunoglobulin therapy. If they have a total IgA deficiency, they may have anti-IgA antibodies, which can result in severe anaphylactoid reactions if given IgA containing preparations (including IVIG or blood). The risks can be minimized by choosing an immunoglobulin preparation with the lowest IgA content.

IgG SUBCLASS DEFICIENCY

Many individuals with isolated subclass deficiencies are completely healthy. Immunoglobulin subclass deficiency is more likely to be associated with infection in patients who make poor specific antibody responses, particularly to polysaccharide antigens. The usefulness of IgG subclass measurement is therefore questioned by some authorities and assessment of results should occur in the context of clinical features and specific antibody responses.[85]

Criteria for diagnosis should include a normal total IgG with a subnormal level of one or more IgG subclasses.[16] As IgG1 is the predominant IgG subclass, low levels of IgG1 will result in low total IgG, and this should be defined as CVID. Although deletions of the corresponding gamma genes have been demonstrated in a few cases, a majority of patients suffer from a regulatory dysfunction, and the deficiencies are most often relative rather than absolute.[86]

IgG3 is the most common subclass deficiency in adults, with IgG2 predominating in children. IgG4 levels vary widely in normal individuals, with up to a fifth of the population having very low levels. The clinical significance of selective IgG1 deficiency is difficult to assess. IgG subclass deficiencies may be associated with IgA deficiency, be a part of the spectrum of the immune defect in combined or T lymphocyte immunodeficiency such as AT, or be an early manifestation of common variable immune deficiency.

Recurrent sinopulmary infections are the usual clinical presentation of a significant subclass defect. Most children can be effectively treated with prophylactic antibiotics, such as co-trimoxazole or a macrolide, over the winter months. Hearing loss and lung damage should be monitored. Very occasional children may require treatment with replacement immunoglobulin.

SELECTIVE ANTIBODY DEFICIENCY WITH NORMAL IMMUNOGLOBULINS

A small number of individuals have normal immunoglobulin levels, but fail to respond to specific antigens. The most frequent defect is a failure to respond to polysaccharide antigens (e.g. the polysaccharide pneumococcal vaccine, Pneumovax). The majority of individuals are normal, and clearly have other immune mechanisms that can compensate for this defect. A number, however, have recurrent sinopulmonary infections.

Lack of polysaccharide responses may also be seen in Wiskott–Aldrich syndrome, be normal in the first 2 years of life, or be an early manifestation of CVID. Children over the age of 3 years who are found to lack pneumococcal responses should be followed up until it is clear that they are not developing an immune defect.

DISORDERS OF PHAGOCYTIC CELLS

CHRONIC GRANULOMATOUS DISEASE

Chronic granulomatous disease (CGD) is an inherited defect of the phagocyte nicotinamide adenine dinucleotide phosphate (NADPH) oxidase enzyme complex which generates superoxide and other reactive oxygen species that are toxic to organisms ingested into phagosomes. The commonest gene defect, accounting for up to 60% of cases, is in the major membrane component gp91phox and inherited as an X-linked disease. Defects in the cytoplasmic components p67phox and p47phox are inherited in an autosomal recessive pattern, as are mutations in the second membrane component p22phox, the latter being very rare.

The disease has protean clinical manifestations, but the hallmark is acute, and potentially fatal, bacterial or fungal infection.[87] A subgroup of patients with some residual enzyme function may not present until adult life. A common manifestation is acute suppurative lymphadenitis in the neck, axilla or groin. Other frequent pyogenic infections include liver abscesses, osteomyelitis, arthritis, pneumonia, skin sepsis and perianal abscesses. Pathogens, such as *Staphylococcus aureus*, *Burkholderia cepacia*, *Aspergillus* species and *Serratia marcescens*, are common because they are catalase positive: this enzyme destroys any hydrogen peroxide produced by the organism within the phagosome. Infections with catalase negative organisms, such as *Streptococcus pneumoniae*, are rare. Fungal infection often manifests as pneumonia, but disseminated infection is frequently seen, with osteomyelitis and hepatic involvement. Once established, fungal infection is hard to treat and frequently fatal.

The occurrence of non-infectious granulomatous complications is increasingly recognized. These include inflammatory bowel disease, restrictive lung defects, genitourinary obstruction and cutaneous granulomata. Many children have colitis, which may be subclinical, manifested only as a persistent iron deficiency anemia and which histologically may be mistaken for Crohn's disease. These non-infective manifestations respond well to corticosteroid treatment.[88] Female carriers of the X-linked form have an increased incidence of autoimmune diseases and mouth ulcers.

Diagnosis is suggested by failure of reduction of nitroblue tetrazolium or dihydrorhodamine by neutrophils (see diagnosis section). In the X-linked form, mothers may have intermediate levels of dye reduction, consistent with non-random X-inactivation.

Treatment

The use of prophylactic antibiotics, in particular co-trimoxazole which is concentrated in neutrophils, has significantly reduced morbidity and mortality from bacterial infections in this disease.[89] Children should also be given oral antifungal agents as prophylaxis. Itraconazole is currently the best available agent, and early data suggest that it may be helpful in reducing the incidence of fatal fungal disease in these patients.[88]

Infections or unexplained fevers should be treated aggressively. IFN-gamma is a useful adjunctive treatment in severe bacterial or fungal infections. Although used as prophylactic therapy in the USA, in Europe it is mainly used for prophylaxis only after documented failure of oral antibacterial and antifungal agents.[87] White cell infusions may also be used as adjunctive therapy in severe infection. Registry data suggest that the outlook in early childhood has improved considerably in recent years, but considerable morbidity and mortality occurs and consideration should be given to bone marrow transplantation when a suitable donor is available.[90]

OTHER NEUTROPHIL DISORDERS

Neutropenia

This may result from reduced production in the bone marrow or increased peripheral destruction. These can be distinguished by the findings on bone marrow examination. Neutropenia most frequently follows decreased production induced by disease processes or drug treatments. Increased consumption may occur in autoimmune states, including those associated with immune deficiency. The degree of neutropenia will influence the clinical picture: neutrophil counts of less than 0.5×10^9/L carry a major risk of infection, whilst counts below 0.2×10^9/L are associated with a significant incidence of life threatening sepsis.

Cyclical neutropenia

Cyclical neutropenia is an autosomal dominant disorder in which cyclical decreases in hematopoiesis results in intervals of neutropenia and susceptibility to infection. This may occur approximately every 3 weeks (range 13–35 days). Patients are normally asymptomatic, but during the period of severe neutropenia, aphthous ulcers, gingivitis, stomatitis and cellulitis may develop. Death from overwhelming infection occurs in a small proportion of patients. Symptoms resolve over 3–4 days as the neutrophil count rises; counts taken after the onset of symptoms are likely to be normal. Mutations in the neutrophil elastase gene (ELA2) have been identified in patients with cyclical neutropenia.[91]

Severe congenital neutropenia

This was originally described by Kostman in 1956[92] as an autosomal recessive disease. Onset is within the first year of life with recurrent and life threatening infections. Symptoms include cellulitis, perirectal abscesses, peritonitis, stomatitis and meningitis. Examination of bone marrow shows an arrest at the promyelocyte to myelocyte maturation stage. More recently a small number of patients with congenital neutropenia have been defined who have mutations that result in overactivity of WASP (Wiskott–Aldrich syndrome protein)[93] or who have dysregulated expression of the GTPases RhoA and Rac2.[94]

Shwachman–Diamond syndrome

This rare autosomal recessive disorder is characterized by exocrine pancreatic insufficiency, skeletal abnormalities, bone marrow dysfunction and recurrent infections. Neutropenia occurs in all patients, whilst 10–25% of patients also have pancytopenia. There is an increased incidence of malignancy.

Treatment of neutropenia

Treatment with G-CSF results in increased counts and fewer infections in almost all patients with neutropenia not secondary to peripheral destruction. Concerns about the induction of leukemias with prolonged use have not been borne out, although pretreatment and annual bone marrow aspirates are recommended. Bone marrow transplantation may be indicated in selected cases.

Other enzymatic deficiencies resulting in neutrophil killing defects

Myeloperoxidase (MPO) deficiency is the commonest inherited disorder of neutrophils. Almost half of those affected have a complete deficiency, the rest have structural or functional defects in the enzyme. MPO is the primary component of azurophilic (primary) granules. The majority of patients with MPO deficiency are asymptomatic, a notable exception being diabetic patients with MPO deficiency, who appear to have a particular susceptibility to candidiasis.

Other enzyme defects are less common and include glutathione synthetase deficiency, pyruvate kinase deficiency and complete neutrophil G6PD deficiency (note: in the common red cell G6PD deficiency there is sufficient enzyme present in neutrophils for normal killing to occur). The phenotypes may be very mild, with variable numbers of bacterial infections. G6PD deficiency will result in an abnormal NBT test, otherwise the diagnosis is established by measurement of specific enzyme levels.

Neutrophil-specific granule deficiency

This rare disorder is characterized by recurrent skin and lung infections with staphylococci and enteric bacteria. The diagnosis can be confirmed by electron microscopy of patient neutrophils, which will show reduced or absent secondary granules. Specific stains will also demonstrate lack of the proteins that constitute the granules, including lactoferrin and vitamin B_{12} binding protein. Proteins that reside in azurophilic (primary) granules, such as lysozyme and myeloperoxidase are present. Neutrophils also show abnormalities in migration and nuclear morphology. Mice lacking the transcription factor CCAAT/enhancer binding protein have a similar phenotype, and case reports of patients with mutations in this gene have now been published.[95]

The clinical course of patients is variable. Treatment options include prompt institution of antibiotic therapy for infections and prophylactic antibiotic treatment. Bone marrow transplantation should be considered in patients with a severe phenotype.

Chediak–Higashi syndrome

Chediak–Higashi syndrome (CHS) is a rare autosomal recessive disease with partial oculocutaneous albinism, recurrent bacterial infections and the development of an accelerated lymphocyte and macrophage activation syndrome [similar to that seen in hemophagocytic lymphohistiocytosis (HLH) and X-linked lymphoproliferative disease (XLP)] in approximately 85% of patients, which is usually fatal. Variable neurological manifestations are also recognized. Characteristic giant lysosomal granules are seen in the cytoplasm of all cells containing these organelles, and are easily detected on a peripheral blood film. The gene for this disease codes for a regulator of lysosomal transport;[96] proteins normally transported through lysosomes enter these organelles but cannot exit, with subsequent lysosomal hypertrophy. In melanocytes this is thought to result in abnormalities of melanin transport and consequent albinism. In neutrophils degranulation of lysosomes cannot occur, with failure of release of bactericidal proteins into the phagosome and defective intracellular killing. The impaired NK cell function is not fully elucidated, whilst monocyte function is probably impaired because giant lysosomes interfere with intracellular motility systems leading to abnormal processing of MHC II in endosomes, and thus defective antigen presentation. The activation syndrome may result from failure to transport inhibitory molecules such as CTLA4 to the surface of leukocytes, with consequent failure of negative feedback mechanisms after T lymphocyte and macrophage activation. Common pathogens in CHS include *Staphylococcus aureus*, streptococci and pneumococci.

Treatment

Prophylactic co-trimoxazole should be given to prevent bacterial infection. The accelerated phase cannot be predicted, and patients should be closely monitored, particularly if febrile. Symptoms, signs, laboratory and clinical findings and diagnosis and treatment of the accelerated phase are as for HLH (see below). The only definitive treatment is bone marrow transplantation. This should be considered early if there is a matched sibling donor. The effects of bone marrow transplantation on later neurological problems are not known.

Griscelli syndrome

Individuals with Griscelli syndrome resemble those with CHS in that they have variable hypopigmentation of the skin and hair and recurrent pyogenic infections associated with absent delayed type cutaneous hypersensitivity and impaired natural killer cell function. Hypogammaglobulinemia can be seen as a secondary phenomenon. In contrast to CHS, large lysozomal granules are not seen and examination of their hair by electron microscopy shows large clumps of pigment, with the accumulation of mature melanosomes in melanocytes. Neurological abnormalities are absent in these patients. They do go on to develop an accelerated phase, which is fatal unless treated by bone marrow transplantation.[97] A candidate gene approach has identified the gene as MYO5A, which codes for myosin 5a.

Hemophagocytic lymphohistiocytosis (familial)

Hemophagocytic lymphohistiocytosis (HLH) is universally fatal without treatment. Patients present with high swinging fevers, hepatosplenomegaly and pancytopenia, and may appear septic. Laboratory findings include an acute phase response, elevated ferritin and elevated fasting triglycerides. Examination of bone marrow, cerebrospinal fluid, pleural effusions or ascitic fluid may demonstrate hemophagocytosis. This may be very difficult to find, and repeated sampling may be required. Hemophagocytosis may occur secondary to a number of infections, in particular viral infections and careful exclusion of infections by serology/PCR should be undertaken. A clinical syndrome resembling HLH may also occur in a number of immunodeficient states including Griscelli syndrome, CHS and XLP. Diagnosis of familial HLH should be suspected in an infant with an appropriate clinical picture. Older children are more likely to have secondary HLH.

Of patients with familial HLH, 20–30% will have a mutation in perforin, normally found in the granules of NK and cytotoxic T lymphocytes. The exact pathophysiology of the disease has not been elucidated, but it is thought that perforin may have a regulatory role, and absence leads to dysregulated immune activation.[98]

Treatment with a combination of chemotherapeutic agents, steroids, and monoclonal antibodies that deplete lymphocytes may induce remission, but bone marrow transplantation is required for cure.

Leukocyte adhesion disorders

To counter infection in tissues, leukocytes egress from the circulation toward sites of inflammation as described earlier in this chapter (p. 1256). Inherited defects in some of the cell surface molecules responsible for the process have been recognized.

Leukocyte adhesion deficiency type I

Deficiency of the 95 kd beta chain (CD18), common to the beta-2 integrin family of cell surface adhesive molecules leads to a profound immunodeficiency affecting the function of neutrophils, monocytes and certain lymphocytes, including T and NK cytotoxic cells.[99] Inheritance is autosomal recessive. Chemotaxis, adherence and phagocytosis are markedly depressed. Different mutations result in phenotypes of variable severity depending on the number of surface molecules that can be expressed. Occasional patients have also been described whose cells express normal levels of CD18 but have a mutation affecting the function of the molecule. This can be demonstrated by showing failure of expression of an activation epitope on the molecule. Although these molecules are involved in the lymphocyte interactions necessary for specific immune responses, these responses are preserved. Even the impaired lymphocyte cytotoxicity which can be demonstrated very clearly in the laboratory is of uncertain clinical significance. The clinical picture is almost entirely explained by the way in which leukocytes are attracted to areas of infection and can become fixed to the vessel walls at sites of inflammation in the usual way but cannot pass out into the tissues. This leads to blockage of small vessels and rapidly expanding necrotic lesions without pus. The beta-2 integrin family is also involved in the platelet function molecule Gp 2b3a and patients with a combined leukocyte and platelet defect have been found.[100]

Individuals affected by the most severe phenotype (< 1% expression) present in the first weeks of life with delayed umbilical cord separation (the cord fails to shrink down and may not separate until 3–4 weeks of age), together with rapidly progressive erosive perianal ulcers. Delayed umbilical cord separation does not seem to occur in patients with some expression of the molecule (usually in the range 2–10% of normal expression). In all forms there is excessive susceptibility to bacterial and fungal infections. Gingivitis and periodontitis are common and more deep seated infections of bone, respiratory and gastrointestinal tracts are often seen. Non-infective inflammatory lesions, particularly affecting the skin and resembling pyoderma gangrenosum, can occur in the partial forms of the deficiency and are often responsive to steroids.

Investigations almost invariably show a circulating neutrophilia (because of failure of the cells to migrate out of the circulation) and a profound neutrophil chemotactic defect. Diagnosis is confirmed by demonstrating the absence of the cell surface markers recognized by the anti-CD11/CD18 monoclonal antibodies.

In the severe form, early death from infection is the rule unless a successful bone marrow transplant can be performed. In the partial forms supportive and expectant management is pursued in the first instance but bone marrow transplantation may become necessary.

Leukocyte adhesion deficiency (LAD) type II

In this extremely rare disorder a defect of fucose metabolism results in a failure of fucosylation to generate sialyl lewis x (CD15s) and other ligand molecules to which the selectin molecules bind. This results in a failure of the 'rolling' type weak adhesion of leukocytes to endothelium which slows down the circulating leukocytes before beta-2 integrin binding can occur. There is a neutrophilia and neutrophil chemotaxis and migration from the circulation is severely impaired. There is no deficiency in specific immune responses. As in LAD I deficiency patients have a neutrophilia and suffer repeated bacterial infections and periodontal disease. Delayed umbilical cord separation is however not seen and other features peculiar to LAD II include mental retardation, short stature and the Bombay (hh) blood phenotype.[101]

Defects in the IL-12-dependent interferon-gamma pathway

Defects in the IL-12 dependent IFN-gamma pathway have recently been described in patients affected by persistent severe, invasive or intractable mycobacterial infections with bone and soft tissue abscesses complicated by persistant discharging sinuses. Implicated pathogens are usually BCG or poorly pathogenic enviromental non-tuberculous mycobacteria and are often fatal.[102] Invasive non-typhi salmonella infections have been described, and may be successfully treated with antibiotics. There may also be increased susceptibility to viral infection including human herpes viruses, respiratory viruses including respiratory syncitial virus and parainfluenza type 3. Infections result from a failure of upregulation of macrophage killing. The clinical picture depends on the precise molecular defect that is present. Defects have been described in a number of constituents of the IL-12/IFN-gamma pathway, including complete or partial IFN-gamma-R1 deficiency, IL-12p40 subunit deficiency, and complete IL-12b1 deficiency. The outcome of patients with complete IFN-gamma-R1 deficiency is poor, but bone marrow transplantation has been successfully attempted.

Hyper-IgE syndrome

This comlex disorder is characterized by extreme elevation of the serum IgE level (usually in the range 2000–40000 units/L); chronic dermatitis and repeated lung and skin infections occur.[102a] Jobis syndrome, so-called because of the presence of severe recurrent staphylococcal skin abscesses, was first described in fair-skinned red-headed girls with eczema and is almost certainly a variant of the hyper-IgE syndrome. Both sexes and all races are affected equally. Non-immunological features of the condition which are variably present include: abnormal coarse facies with a wide nasal bridge and large head; fragile bones leading to frequent fractures; joint laxity; a high incidence of scoliosis; and delayed resorption of primary dentition with consequent delayed eruption of secondary teeth.[102c]

While the immunological features can be explained as the consequence of a T cell regulatory defect, the other features are not easily explained. Abnormal bone and connective tissue turnover as a consequence of abnormal cytokine profiles has been postulated as a possible way of tying all the features together. The mode of inheritance is thought to be autosomal dominant with incomplete penetrance. The gene for the disorder has not been identified but studies on familial cases have found linkage to the proximal part of chromosome 4q.[102d]

Abscesses are said to be cold with little sorrounding inflammation but this is not always the case. *Staphylococcus aureus* is the predominant pathogen and can cause serious chest disease with pneumatoeles and chronic lung damage. Other bacteria, including streptococci and Gram negative bacilli as well as fungi such as *Candida albicans*, can also be problematic. In addition to the high IgE level, there is a profound neutrophil chemotatic defect. High titers of IgE antibody with specificity for *S. aureus, C. albicans* and tetanus toxoid may be found. The total IgE levels may fall in adulthood, sometimes to the normal range. In a significant proportion of patients there is a failure of antibody responses to polysaccharide antigens which contributes to the susceptibility to infection. Defective T cell responses and cutaneous energy have also been found in some patients. There is a evidence that histamine released from mast cells by the IgE may mediate the chemotactic defect via histamine receptors on neurophils.

The mainstay of treatment is long term antistaphylococcal antibiotic prophylaxis usually with flucloxacillin. Histamine 2 receptor blockers have been used, although their value is disputed. Gamma interferon treatment has been tried in a few patients but although there was some lowering of the IgE levels, there was no clinical benifit. Intravenous immunoglobulin therapy may be useful in those with a demonstrable antibody production deficit. Bone marrow transplantation failed to correct the disorder in the one patient in whom it was reported as being attempted despite sucessful engraftment of donor myeloid and lymphoid cells.[102e]

COMPLEMENT DISORDERS

PRIMARY INHERITED DEFICIENCIES

The main inherited deficiencies of complement components are listed in Table 25.6D (p. 1264). Severe disease is inherited in an autosomal recessive manner with absolute deficiency of a complement component due to gene defects in both alleles. However, heterozygosity results in approximately half normal levels of the protein which can sometimes be clinically important. A number of clinical patterns can occur depending upon which factor is deficient.

Autoimmune disease

A predisposition to autoimmune disease, particularly systemic lupus erythematosus and the other immune complex disorders, is a feature of most of the complement deficiency syndromes. Deficiency of C1q carries a very high risk with over 90% of patients in one series developing either systemic lupus erythematosus (SLE) or discoid LE.[103] Evidence, based on the finding that null alleles for a number of complement components (notably C2 and C4) occur with greater frequency in patients with autoimmune diseases such as SLE, suggests that heterozygosity for deficiency is also a risk factor. In general, the course of these diseases is similar to that in patients without complement deficiency.

Pyogenic infections

Recurrent pyogenic infections are a feature of complement deficiencies. Organisms such as streptococci and *Haemophilus influenzae* are the main problem as opsonization/binding of antibody and complement to bacteria is critical for their elimination. C3 deficiency is the most severe. Deficiency of the classical pathway components C1q and C2 and of factor D in the alternative pathway also predisposes to infection and the first two also carry a predisposition to autoimmune phenomena. Deficiencies of the alternative pathway control proteins, factors H or I lead to uncontrolled consumption of C3 resulting in increased susceptibility to pyogenic infections.

Neisserial infections

Deficiency of one of the later complement components, C5–C9 (leading to failure of membrane lysis), or of the control factor properdin (the only deficiency inherited in an X-linked manner) leads to a specific deficiency in handling neisserial species (*Neisseria meningitidis* and *N. gonorrhoeae*) but not to a generalized increase in susceptibility to pyogenic infections. There is a predominance of disease caused by rare serogroups of meningococci (W135, X, Y and Z) in these patients. In a Dutch study[104] complement deficiency (most commonly late components or properdin) was found in 33% of survivors of meningococcal disease due to rare serogroups compared to 2, 0 and 7% in patients who suffered Group A, B and C disease respectively. The disease is said to run a milder course in these patients. Recurrent attacks of meningococcal septicemia/ meningitis and severe invasive gonococcal disease are also associated with late complement deficiencies in factors 6–9. Late complement deficiencies are more common in individuals from the Middle East and Japan; C9 deficiency in Japan affects up to 0.1% of the population.[105] Screening for deficiencies should be undertaken in patients and their immediate families where there has been recurrent meningococcal disease due to common serogroups or single episodes caused by a rare serogroup. In the UK, screening children with single episodes of meningococcal disease due to common serotypes is unlikely to reveal a complement defect.[106]

Hereditary angioedema

Deficiency of the control protein, C1 esterase inhibitor (C1INH), leads to spontaneous episodes of localized edema (angioedema) without urticaria due to excessive release of proinflammatory breakdown products of complement. C1INH is also a negative regulator of the kallikrein pathway and edema may be due to the increased release of kinins. These occur spontaneously anywhere in the body but those affecting the upper airway are most serious and can be life threatening. Precipitating factors can include local trauma (including surgical procedures, endoscopy and dental work), exposure to extreme cold and emotional stress. Intra-abdominal swelling can occur causing pain and swelling which can be misdiagnosed as a surgical condition. There is a high incidence of SLE and related diseases. C4 levels are also persistently low due to excessive consumption (which occurs even between attacks) although C3 levels are normal. In most cases C1INH assay shows very low levels or absent protein but in approximately 15% of cases the protein is present but functionally defective. The condition is inherited in an autosomal dominant fashion. Episodes of visible swelling do not usually occur until the second decade of life, but younger children suffer from attacks of abdominal pain. Infusions of purified C1INH are effective in terminating attacks and should be used for all attacks affecting the head and neck and for intra-abdominal attacks which are running a protracted course. The concentrate should also be given prophylactically to cover surgical and dental procedures. For prevention of attacks, the treatment of choice after puberty is one of the 'retarded' androgenic steroids, such as danazol. In prepubertal children prophylactic use of tranexamic acid, a fibrinolytic agent which inhibits plasmin formation, is recommended. This raises functional C1INH levels sufficiently to prevent attacks and is relatively free of virilizing side-effects. Monitoring of liver function tests should be performed with long term usage.

SECONDARY COMPLEMENT DEFICIENCIES

Many immunopathological diseases can result in excessive complement activation and consumption. In SLE and other immune complex diseases, low levels of C3 and the early classical pathway components can occur. In acute nephritis, C3 levels are acutely depressed, while in membranoproliferative glomerulonephritis a more persistent depression of C3 levels occurs due to the presence of an autoantibody – C3 nephritic factor – directed against C3bBb, the alternative pathway C3 convertase. This autoantibody can also be associated with the condition partial lipodystrophy, with or without membranoproliferative glomerulonephritis. An increased susceptibility to pyogenic infections occurs when C3 levels are reduced below approximately 10%.

Gram negative sepsis, acute pancreatitis and acute vasculitis can all be associated with complement consumption.

INTERACTION OF ANTIBODY AND COMPLEMENT DEFICIENCIES

Deficiency of the early classical pathway complement components has been shown to be associated with poor antibody responses, presumably because of some immunoregulatory role of the complement factors. Later components are not implicated.

Alternative pathway opsonization is less efficient in the absence of specific antibody to bacterial surfaces. There is evidence that antibody may 'neutralize' surface molecules, such as sialic acid, which otherwise inhibit alternative pathway activation.

MANNAN-BINDING LECTIN (MBL) DEFICIENCY

MBL provides another antibody independent mechanism for opsonization of microorganisms by binding to mannose residues common on the surface of a number of different microorganisms.[107] Several allelic variants of the molecule are found and appear to be common findings in different populations. The variant affecting codon 54 is found in up to 20% of Caucasians while a variant at codon 57 has a frequency of 20–30% in West Africans.

The variant allelles affect the stability of MBL protein structure and so result in low serum levels of MBL in the heterozygous state and extremely low levels in those who are homozygous. Two promoter region polymorphisms also cause low levels of MBL.[108] It has been suggested that the persistence of such high frequencies of MBL deficiency in humans occurs because low levels may protect against certain parasitic infections.[2] This condition was formerly known as the yeast opsonization defect because of failure of serum from affected individuals to opsonize baker's yeast in a biological assay. Individuals with low levels have an increased incidence of bacterial infections particularly in early childhood before the ability to make high affinity antibodies is fully developed. They also have an increased incidence of autoimmune disease.[109] The true significance of MBL deficiency is much debated and may only be important when other 'minor' immunodeficiencies coexist.

DEFICIENCIES OF C3 RECEPTORS

The distribution and function of cell surface receptors for C3b and its derivatives have been described (p. 1254). Specific clinical syndromes have been attributed to deficiencies of some of these receptors. A dominantly inherited CR1 deficiency is associated with SLE and other immune complex disorders, presumably related to failure of the immune complex clearing function of this molecule.

Deficient expression of the CR3 receptor occurs as part of the leukocyte adhesion deficiency type I syndrome (p. 1284) since it is a member of the beta integrin family affected in this disorder though what contribution this makes to the overall clinical picture in that condition is unclear.

PAROXYSMAL NOCTURNAL HEMOGLOBINURIA

The membrane bound complement regulatory proteins DAF (CD55) and CD59 prevent the activation of complement on host cells. They are part of a family of proteins which are attached to the cell surface by a glycophosphatidylinositol anchor. A clonal defect in stem cells can result in abnormal expression which increases the susceptibility of cells especially red blood cells to complement mediated lysis. This can result in paroxysmal nocturnal hemoglobinuria.

MANAGEMENT OF COMPLEMENT DEFICIENCIES

Apart from C1 esterase inhibitor there are no specific replacement factor preparations. Fresh plasma infusions have been used prophylactically or can be reserved for the treatment of serious episodes of infection. Life-long prophylactic penicillin and meningococcal vaccination are advised in those complement deficiencies resulting in susceptibility to neisserial infections. A polyvalent vaccine (A, C, W135 and Y) should be given. Prophylactic co-trimoxazole can be used in deficiencies which result in an increased susceptibility to a wider range of organisms. Clinical monitoring may allow earlier diagnosis and treatment of autoimmune disorders should they emerge.

SECONDARY IMMUNODEFICIENCY

Secondary immunodeficiencies are more common than primary disorders and are easily overlooked. Increasing success in treating cancer and transplantation mean that more and more children receive immunosuppressive drugs (Table 25.15). Viral infections also depress immune function and specific aspects of immunity may be lost in other conditions, e.g. immunoglobulin deficiency secondary to protein-losing states, or complement consumption states. The causes of more generalized, and sometimes less well-defined, secondary immunodeficiency are discussed here.

Table 25.15 Some causes of secondary immunodeficiency

Drugs	
Corticosteroids	
Cytotoxic drugs	
Specific immunosuppressive – e.g. ciclosporin A, antilymphocyte globulin	
Miscellaneous – e.g. phenytoin	
Radiation	
Malnutrition	
Protein-losing states	
Nephrotic syndrome	
Gastrointestinal disease (especially intestinal lymphangiectasia)	
Burns	
Excessive immunoglobulin catabolism	
Myotonic dystrophy	
Metabolic disturbance	
Inherited	– galactosemia
	– glycogen storage disease
Acquired	– uremia
	– diabetes mellitus
Infections	
Viruses	– human immunodeficiency virus
	– cytomegalovirus, Epstein–Barr virus
Bacteria	– overwhelming infections
Protozoa	– e.g. malaria
Immune complex disorders – e.g. systemic lupus erythematosus	
Hyposplenism	
Congenital asplenia	
Sickle cell anemia	
Splenectomy	
Malignancy, esp. lymphoid	
Histiocytic disorders	
Langerhans' cell histiocytosis	
Hemophagocytic lymphohistiocytosis	
Miscellaneous	
Sarcoidosis	
Surgery and anesthesia	

INFECTION-INDUCED IMMUNODEFICIENCY

Many different infections have been shown to depress immunity. This is seen most commonly after viral infection[110] but chronic infection with other organisms can have similar effects. Examples include the depressed antibody responses in malaria infected children which correlates with the parasite load, or the T lymphocyte depression that complicates advanced mycobacterial disease and which may be due to the immunosuppressive effects of specific mycobacterial cell wall products.

Acute viral infection

Decreased numbers of circulating lymphocytes associated with markedly reduced T lymphocyte proliferative responses and cutaneous anergy are a 'normal' reaction to a wide variety of common acute viral infections. This was first recognized in measles infection by Von Pirquet in 1908. It has also occurred after live viral vaccines, including measles and oral polio. In some cases, it is due to direct infection of lymphocytes and/or macrophages. In others, there is an alteration in immunoregulation, most marked in acute infectious mononucleosis due to EBV infection in which there is B and T lymphocyte proliferation and a reversal of the normal helper: suppressor T lymphocyte ratios. Influenza and measles virus infections have also been shown to have non-specific depressive effects on neutrophil and monocyte function. The clinical importance of these observations is not always certain but in the developing world they probably account for the very high incidence of secondary bacterial infection after measles and the fatal downward spiral of infection and malnutrition that is commonly seen after measles.

Chronic viral infection

Congenital viral infection (and toxoplasmosis) results in an immune depression with specific failure of T lymphocyte reactivity, or tolerance, to the relevant agent and in some cases a more generalized depression of antibody responses and even hypogammaglobulinemia, sometimes of a pattern which mimics the hyper-IgM syndrome. Congenital cytomegalovirus and rubella infections can result in prolonged excretion of these viruses for several years. Other chronic viral infections, e.g. subacute sclerosing panencephalitis or persistent EBV infection, are associated with an ill-defined immune suppression, possibly partly due to an element of pre-existing immune incompetence. Hepatitis C virus infection is associated with acquired IgA deficiency.[111]

IMMUNODEFICIENCY DUE TO DRUGS AND RADIATION

Specific immunosuppressive agents

Antibodies to human lymphocytes (antilymphocyte globulin) or specific T lymphocyte subpopulations are used to treat idiopathic aplastic anemia, GvHD and graft rejection. They induce prolonged, profound lymphopenia and depress primary antibody and delayed hypersensitivity responses. B lymphocyte monoclonal antibodies have been used in the treatment of B lymphoproliferative disease in transplant patients, with some success.

Ciclosporin and tacrolimus are reversible calcineurin antagonists used in organ and bone marrow transplantation, affecting predominantly T lymphocytes, but also B lymphocytes and other cell types. They inhibit antigen processing as well as diminishing IL-1 and IL-2 production, and IL-2 receptor expression.

Corticosteroid drugs are less specific, but potent, immunosuppressive drugs.[112] The degree of immunosuppression induced is related to the dose, length of treatment course and probably varies between individuals. An equivalent dose of prednisolone 2 mg/kg/day for more than a week, or 1 mg/kg/day for greater than a month is generally considered immunosuppressive. Lymphopenia results from a diminution of recirculation of long-lived T lymphocytes. Cytotoxic function, mitogenic responses and delayed hypersensitivity responses are all depressed. With high-dose treatment for prolonged periods antibody responses, especially primary responses, also become impaired. Corticosteroids also affect recirculating monocytes and polymorphs, and microbicidal ability is depressed.

Cytotoxic drugs used in the treatment of leukemia and solid tumors have major immunosuppressive side-effects. Cyclophosphamide particularly affects B lymphocyte function and antibody production, but T lymphopenia (especially of CD4+ T lymphocytes) also occurs.

Azathioprine and 6-mercaptopurine suppress antibody production, particularly primary responses. T lymphocyte functions including delayed hypersensitivity responses are also depressed.

Methotrexate has potent anti-inflammatory activity and may also suppress antibody responses in higher doses.

Radiation therapy, particularly total body or total lymphoid irradiation, has profound and long-lasting effects on lymphocyte-mediated immune function and on antibody responses.

The most severe immunosuppressed states occur during bone marrow transplantation for malignant disease. In these cases, a combination of radiotherapy and chemotherapy is often used.

Clinical effects

The immunosuppressed child is susceptible to opportunistic infection, especially fungal infections and *Pneumocystis carinii* pneumonia (see Figs 25.17 and 25.18). After bone marrow transplant, there is a recognized pattern of susceptibility to different pathogens, depending on the elapsed time since the procedure (Fig. 25.21).[113] In the absence of neutropenia, susceptibility to pyogenic infections is less of a problem. 'Live' vaccines should be avoided, as should contact with cases of measles and chickenpox. Postexposure prophylaxis should be given when inadvertent exposure to these viruses occurs. Co-trimoxazole is effective as prophylaxis against *Pneumocystis carinii* pneumonia.

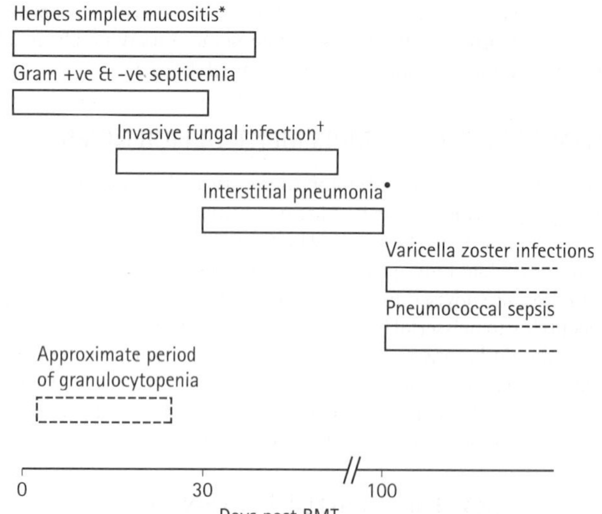

Fig. 25.21 Periods of maximal risk for various infectious complications after bone marrow transplantation with immunosuppression/marrow ablation. * Realighted infection; † predominantly *Candia* and *Aspergillus* species; • predominantly cytomegalovirus and *Pneumocystis carinii.* (Redrawn from Rogers 1985[113])

Other drugs

A variety of miscellaneous drugs may cause immunosuppression as part of their side-effect profile. The effects of phenytoin and other agents on IgA production is discussed in the section on IgA deficiency. Moderate or severe depression of neutrophil counts is a side-effect of a large number of drugs including antibiotics such as sulfonamides and flucloxacillin and results in a susceptibility to bacterial disease.

MALNUTRITION

Nutritional status, infection and immunity are closely linked, and nutritional deficiency can have profound effects on all aspects of the immune system. The most profound and wide-ranging effects are seen in protein calorie deficiency (Table 25.16), with changes in lymphocyte number and function, antibody production and quality, complement synthesis and phagocytosis.[114] There is increased susceptibility to TB, measles, *Pneumocystis carinii* as well as staphylococcal pneumonia, and Gram negative sepsis.

Specific nutritional deficiencies also affect immune function. Zinc deficiency, primary in acrodermatitis enteropathica, an autosomal recessive condition, in which specific zinc malabsorption occurs, or secondary to nutritional deficiency causes thymic atrophy, T lymphopenia, anergy, impaired cytotoxicity and decreased immunoglobulin production. Many immunological effects of zinc deficiency may be related to the critical role of zinc in intracellular zinc-finger-dependent transcription factors, and in DNA synthesis and lymphocyte proliferation. Treatment with zinc supplements reverses most effects. Iron deficiency, even without anemia, has subtle effects on T lymphocyte and phagocytic lymphocyte function. The clinical importance of this is not clear. Some studies have shown an increased frequency of infections which reverses with iron therapy, but others have not confirmed this. Vitamin A deficiency is associated with depressed T lymphocyte

Table 25.16 Main immunological effects of severe malnutrition

Cell-mediated immunity
T cell lymphopenia
Reduced CD4 cell numbers
Reduced CD4:CD8 ratio
Reduced delayed hypersensitivity responses
Reduced proliferative T cell responses to mitogens and antigens
Reduced lymphokine production
Antibody production
Polyclonal hypergammaglobulinemia
Decreased IgA in secretions
Increased serum IgE
Defective antibody responses
Reduced antibody affinity
Depressed function of antigen-presenting cells
Non-specific immune system
Depressed neutrophil bactericidal capability
Depressed levels of complement factors, especially C3

and humoral responses, and a dominant T_{H2} pattern of response. In populations at risk from malnutrition, vitamin A supplementation improves antibody responses to vaccines. In similar populations treatment with vitamin A during measles infection reduces mortality and has been shown to reverse some of the induced abnormalities in lymphocyte numbers and function.

VACCINATION OF THE CHILD WITH A POTENTIALLY IMPAIRED IMMUNE RESPONSE

Immunocompromised children are often more in need of the protection vaccination can offer because of their greater risk from infection, and yet are less likely to be vaccinated because of concerns about the underlying immunodeficiency. In general, live vaccine should be avoided in children with malignancy who are being treated with or have received chemotherapy within 6 months. Booster vaccines may be appropriate after completion of treatment. Children who have undergone bone marrow transplantation should be reimmunized 12–18 months post bone marrow transplantation providing immunosuppression has been stopped for 6 months or more and they do not have GvHD. Measles, mumps and rubella (MMR) vaccine should be given 6 months after commencement of the vaccination schedule. Vaccinations should be up to date before transplantation in those receiving solid organ transplants. As they remain on life-long immunosuppression following transplantation, live vaccines should be avoided. HIV infected children should receive killed polio vaccine, but MMR seems safe to give. Children with primary immunodeficiency should be immunized. Those with lymphocyte-mediated immunodeficiency should not receive live vaccines, all other forms of immunodeficiency can safely have live vaccine administered, except BCG in patients with CGD. Children on pharmacological doses of steroids (an equivalent dose of prednisolone 2 mg/kg/day for > 1 week, or 1 mg/kg/day for > 1 month) or other immunosuppressive therapy should not be given live vaccines. Conjugate pneumococcal vaccine should be given to children with asplenia, hyposplenia or nephrotic syndrome. Zoster-specific immunoglobulin should be given to those with significant immunosuppression who are chickenpox contacts and non-immune. Children receiving intravenous immunoglobulin treatment should not be vaccinated, as protective antibody is present in the immunoglobulin given.[115]

HYPOSPLENISM

Congenital asplenia, splenectomy and sickle cell disease are the major causes of hyposplenism in childhood. Finding Howell–Jolly bodies on a blood film or absence of a spleen on ultrasound are helpful when it is unclear whether the spleen is absent. Patients are at risk of pyogenic infection including pneumonia, septicemia or meningitis with polysaccharide encapsulated bacteria such as *Streptococcus pneumoniae* or *Neisseria meningitidis*. The absolute risk of infection of 0.42% per year is significant when viewed over a life time, and the risk is four times higher in young children with congenital asplenia where other aspects of immunity are less well developed. Young asplenic children also suffer infection with a greater range of pathogens including *Haemophilus influenzae* and Gram negative organisms. The immunodeficiency is multifactorial and probably largely functional. Factors thought to contribute include failure of clearance of opsonized bacteria in the spleen, lack of the B lymphocyte reservoir function, low levels of tuftsin (a bactericidal protein produced by the spleen) and low activity of the alternative pathway of complement. Defective alternative pathway complement activity was found in 10% of splenectomized and 16% of sickle cell patients. In older patients, IgG antibody responses to pneumococcal vaccine are similar to normal individuals although low serum IgM levels have been reported. Antipolysaccharide IgG levels decay more quickly.[116]

As pneumococcal infection is the most common severe infection, prophylaxis with penicillin is used in the UK, but alternative treatment may be necessary where penicillin-resistant pneumococci are common. In children below 4 years of age, the risks from other infections means a broader spectrum antibiotic such as amoxicillin (or co-trimoxazole) is recommended. Vaccination with conjugated *Haemophilus influenzae* type B and meningococcus C vaccines may diminish the risk but do not remove the need to give penicillin. The new conjugate pneumococcal vaccines may be particularly useful in this group of patients. Immunization should be performed prior to elective splenectomy. Antipneumococcal antibody levels should be measured annually, and patients revaccinated if levels are low.[117]

Much, but not all, of the increased susceptibility to infection in sickle cell disease stems from the hyposplenism which develops as the spleen is infarcted. In addition, sickle cell patients have impaired reticuloendothelial clearing capacity (due to chronic hemolysis) and focal tissue ischemia (as a result of sickling). As well as being susceptible to pneumococcus, these patients are also prone to Gram negative sepsis, including salmonella osteomyelitis. The risk of these problems is less in the variant form, hemoglobin SC (hemoglobin S, hemoglobin C) disease, but is still higher than background so prophylactic measures are still indicated.

TREATMENT OF IMMUNODEFICIENCY

SUPPORTIVE CARE

Children with immunodeficiency disorders often require the full spectrum of pediatric care. Particular attention needs to be paid to nutritional status and the management of dietary intolerances secondary to the gastrointestinal problems which frequently occur. Supporting the emotional needs of the family is also very important. Prevention and treatment of infections is the mainstay of supportive care.

GENERAL MEASURES FOR PREVENTION OF INFECTIONS

Newborns suspected of having a severe immunodeficiency disorder should be protected using isolation techniques, including limitation of the numbers of persons involved with care; individuals with respiratory or gastrointestinal symptoms of infection should avoid contact. Breast-feeding should be encouraged. Wherever the child is managed the importance of strict hand washing procedures cannot be overemphasized. If and when bone marrow transplantation with conditioning chemotherapy is embarked upon (see below), isolation in facilities with positive pressure filtered air supply is necessary mainly to reduce the risk of aspergillosis and droplet borne viral infections.

SPECIFIC MEASURES FOR PREVENTION OF INFECTIONS

Co-trimoxazole as prophylaxis against *Pneumocystis carinii* should be given for defects involving cell-mediated immunity mechanisms. For *Pneumocystis carinii* pneumonia (PCP) prophylaxis only, co-trimoxazole need only be given on 2 or 3 days a week. If this is not tolerated alternatives include dapsone or atovaquone. Inhaled pentamidine can be used in older children. Injectable pentamidine should not be used prophylactically because of the potential side-effects and possible reduced efficacy. Co-trimoxazole probably also reduces the incidence of pyogenic infections in these patients and those with phagocytic or humoral immune deficiencies and for this purpose it is usually given daily (dose 30 mg/kg/day in one or two doses). In circumstances of poor nutrition, increased bone marrow turnover and in all cases after bone marrow transplantation, weekly folinic acid supplements are given to lessen the risk of bone marrow depression without compromising the antimicrobial efficacy. Antifungal prophylaxis should be used in combined immunodeficiencies or phagocytic cell defects. In chronic granulomatous disease and other conditions where the risk of aspergillus infection is high, itraconazole is preferred. Otherwise fluconazole or non-absorbed agents such as nystatin are used.

Where the immune deficiency predisposes to infection with relatively few organisms, prophylaxis with a narrow spectrum antibiotic can be used, e.g. penicillin prophylaxis for the terminal complement deficiencies where only neisserial infection is a risk. Prophylactic antibiotics are most commonly used for patients with relatively minor humoral deficiencies such as symptomatic IgA deficiency. There is no scientific basis for the choice of antibiotic in these circumstances because of the great difficulty in performing a trial looking at efficacy. Co-trimoxazole has been widely used but concerns over potential side-effects have led to the use of other agents such as azithromycin which, because of its long half-life, can be given on 3 days out of every 14 and provides continuous prophylaxis against sinopulmonary bacterial infections. This is attractive, but less is known of its effects when given over many years. Cefixime is a further alternative given as a single daily dose. Antiviral prophylaxis with aciclovir is used in patients with cell-mediated immunodeficiency and previous herpes simplex infection. It is also used in the context of bone marrow transplantation to prevent herpes simplex and CMV reactivation.

Immunizations may be used judiciously if sufficient immune function is judged to be present to give an antibody response. 'Live' vaccines are contraindicated in combined immunodeficiencies and in the more severe antibody-deficiency states. Passive immunization is the basis of immunoglobulin replacement therapy (see below) and specific hyperimmune globulins are available for postexposure prophylaxis in patients with primary or secondary immunodeficiency exposed to chickenpox or hepatitis B. For measles exposure standard immunoglobulin is used. The role of immunoglobulins with high titers of anti-respiratory syncytial virus (RSV) or of monoclonal anti-RSV antibodies in protecting against RSV in children with primary immunodeficiencies during the winter season has not been evaluated and is unlikely to be formally investigated because of the rarity of these conditions. They may have a role in SCID patients before and during transplant bearing in mind that common cold symptoms in carers may be caused by this virus.

The prevention of complications of recurrent infections is most important. Evidence of middle ear disease which might lead to deafness should be sought and treated. Chronic lung disease leading to bronchiectasis is a serious complication, particularly of antibody deficiency states. Regular physiotherapy, with sputum cultures to direct appropriate antibiotic therapy and monitoring of pulmonary status are useful. Breakthrough infections threatening organ damage despite prophylactic antibiotics may be an indication for starting immunoglobulin therapy even if the tests show relatively minor abnormalities of humoral immunity. Serial measurements of lung function tests and judicious use of high resolution CT (HRCT) scanning may detect early damage or progression of existing damage. HRCT scans are contraindicated in disorders associated with increased radiosensitivity such as ataxia telangiectasia.

TREATMENT OF INFECTIONS

A policy of vigorous and early antimicrobial treatment of infections should be observed. Unusual agents may cause infection, and broader spectrum antimicrobial cover may therefore be needed. In neutrophil disorders it is particularly important to cover *Pseudomonas* and other Gram negative bacilli. Early treatment of an infection may be life saving, but its initiation should not detract from full attempts at identification of the causative agent. Invasive diagnostic procedures, such as bronchoalveolar lavage or, if this fails to produce a diagnosis, open lung biopsy, can be fully justified on the basis that they will facilitate precise and optimal therapy. The mainstay of treatment for systemic fungal infection remains amphotericin B, mostly used in its liposomal form to reduce toxicity and enable larger doses to be given. Promising new agents for treating invasive aspergillosis include voriconazole and caspofungin.

Antivirals such as the broad spectrum agent, ribavirin, and the anticytomegalovirus agents, ganciclovir and foscarnet, are particularly useful in the immunocompromised infant. Newer antivirals include cidofovir (for resistant CMV, adenovirus and severe molluscum contagiosum) and pleconaril for chronic enteroviral infections. The role of zanamivir in immunocompromised children with influenza has not been assessed.

BLOOD PRODUCT SUPPORT

Blood product infusions may be necessary in some disorders. In combined deficiencies and in patients undergoing heavy immunosuppression (as for bone marrow transplantation), all such products except intravenous immunoglobulin and fresh frozen plasma may contain viable leukocytes and should be irradiated with 2000–3000 rad to prevent possible GvHD. In those with no evidence of previous exposure to CMV, blood products should be obtained from CMV-antibody-negative donors. White cell infusions have a role in specific situations such as adjunctive therapy in poorly responding infections in patients with CGD and other neutrophil function disorders particularly if they are harvested from G-CSF primed donors.

SUPPORT FOR FAMILIES AND PATIENTS

Patient support organizations which are established in most high income countries are very helpful in providing information and advice and in helping families to meet others with the same (rare) diagnoses. In the UK the organization is the Primary Immunodeficiency Association (PIA) and has its own Web site (http://www.pia.org.uk/). Further information may be generally available on the Web but families should be warned that sometimes this is produced without reference to expert advice.

REPLACEMENT IMMUNOGLOBULIN THERAPY

This is the mainstay of treatment for the more severe antibody states and various combined immunodeficiencies. The need for IVIG must be evaluated on an individual patient basis. Absolute indications include quantitative defects (IgG less than the 95th percentile for age or less than 3 g/L in an older child) and qualitative defects (failure of response to booster vaccinations). Other indications include failure of antibiotic prophylaxis in a child with quantitatively minor Ig abnormalities (e.g. IgA and IgG subclass deficiency) and risk of end-organ damage (e.g. bronchiectasis) in a child with any degree of antibody deficiency. As immunoglobulin is a blood product, and there is a limited supply, new and existing uses should be carefully evaluated.

Risks of replacement therapy

Replacement immunoglobulin must contain the full range of protective antibodies in order to provide effective prophylaxis against infections. Unlike coagulation factors where the invariant protein needed can be made using molecular techniques, a polyclonal product cannot be generated by recombinant technology and human plasma has to be used as a source. To ensure that IVIG contains the full spectrum of protective antibody, preparations are made from pooled (5–100 000 donors) plasma donations, which increases the risk of transmission of an infectious agent.[118] Pools are screened for known agents (e.g. Hep B and C) and the process of cold ethanol precipitation, universally used for the fractionation of plasma, effectively kills some viruses, including HIV. New intravenous and subcutaneous products must include a further viral inactivation step such as pasteurization or nanofiltration before they are licensed. Older intramuscular (i.m.) preparations do not include these steps, and therefore carry an increased risk and their use should be phased out. The risk of transmission of variant Creutzfeldt–Jakob disease (vCJD) is theoretical and not quantifiable using modern techniques, but plasma is no longer sourced from the UK in an effort to minimize the risk. Taken together, these precautions have reduced the risk of infection to a very low level. Patients should be evaluated by PCR for hepatitis B and C prior to commencement of therapy, and require regular monitoring of immunoglobulin levels and liver function tests. Any elevation in liver function tests should prompt re-evaluation of their hepatitis status. Batch numbers of all products administered must be recorded to facilitate patient tracing if there is a problem with an individual batch. Switching between different preparations should be avoided unless there are good clinical reasons.

Mode of administration

The efficacy of replacement immunoglobulin therapy was established in the 1950s using i.m. preparations. However, this is painful and only limited volumes can be given so that adequate serum levels of IgG were rarely achieved. Improvements in manufacturing techniques in the 1980s meant IMIG was superseded by IVIG preparations. Large volumes of the latter could be given achieving better symptom control and trough IgG levels well within the normal range. Doses are in the range of 0.3 to 0.5 g/kg/3 weeks, infused over 2–3 h. Immediate reactions to IVIG are commoner than to the i.m. preparation and include nausea, vomiting, flushing, rigors and occasionally hypertension. These can normally be controlled by slowing the infusion rate. Rarely, anaphylactoid reactions occur, particularly in IgA deficient patients who may have anti-IgA antibodies.[119] Patients with known anti-IgA antibodies should be given a preparation with a low IgA content. In the 1990s subcutaneous (s.c.) administration of immunoglobulin was shown to be efficacious in adults[120] with far fewer side-effects, other than local reactions. The s.c. route is being more fully evaluated in children, but has advantages in terms of lack of need for venous access and ease of training parents for home therapy. However, given that only a limited volume can be given in one site, frequency of administration is normally increased.

REPLACEMENT THERAPY FOR COMBINED DEFICIENCIES

REPLACEMENT OF THYMUS FUNCTION

Fetal thymus and/or fetal liver (as a source of stem cells) transplants have been used for SCID with some limited success. Delayed immune reconstitution, severe infection, GvHD and lack of availability of fetal tissues together with significant improvement in bone marrow transplantation techniques has led to these procedures being abandoned.

BONE MARROW TRANSPLANTATION

Virtually all primary T lymphocyte and phagocyte immunodeficiency disorders are potentially correctable by bone marrow transplantation.[121] Patients with immediately life-threatening conditions, mainly SCID, are the largest group of patients treated by bone marrow transplantation. Improving results from bone marrow transplantation, together with an increasing understanding of the basis of the immunodeficiencies, and international registry data on their long term outcome has led to more conditions such as Wiskott–Aldrich syndrome, CD40L deficiency and CGD being treated by bone marrow transplantation (Table 25.17).

Early attempts at bone marrow transplantation using poorly matched donors were largely unsuccessful and so only transplants using HLA matched sibling donors were performed, an approach available only to about 20% of patients. Since the early 1980s, techniques have been developed to allow parent-to-child (haploidentical) grafts, by removing mature T lymphocytes that would otherwise cause fatal GvHD. These have become the most common bone marrow transplant procedure for patients with SCID.[122,123] Matched unrelated donor transplants are being increasingly used, particularly for non-SCID immunodeficiencies and peripheral blood and umbilical cord stem cells are sometimes used instead of bone marrow.

Complications of bone marrow transplantation

The five main complications of bone marrow transplantation are toxicity from conditioning agents, graft failure, graft rejection, GvHD, and infection which may be pre-existing due to immunodeficiency or be acquired after bone marrow transplantation. Rejection is less likely following transplantation with whole rather than T lymphocyte depleted marrow, but the risk of GvHD after whole marrow is greater. Graft rejection is unusual in SCID, but more likely in the NK+ phenotypes, or if clinically evident maternofetal engraftment is present.

Table 25.17 Primary immunodeficiency disorders which have been treated with bone marrow transplantation

Lymphocyte disorders
Severe combined immunodeficiency (including adenosine deaminase deficiency)
Wiskott–Aldrich syndrome
Omenn's syndrome
Nezelof syndrome
Major histocompatibility antigen class II deficiency
DiGeorge syndrome
Purine nucleoside phosphorylase deficiency
Cartilage–hair hypoplasia syndrome
X-linked lymphoproliferative disease
Hyper-IgM syndrome (CD40 ligand deficiency)
Mucocutaneous candidiasis
Immunodeficiency with partial albinism (Griscelli syndrome)
Phagocytic cell disorders
Chronic granulomatous disease
Leukocyte adhesion defect Type I
Congenital agranulocytosis
Chediak–Higashi syndrome
Familial hemophagocytic lymphohistiocytosis
IL-12-dependent interferon-gamma pathway defects
Hyper-IgE syndrome

Myeloablation with chemotherapy helps reduce the chance of rejection and may result in better engraftment quality. The risk of infectious complications is greatest in T lymphocyte depleted grafts where there is a prolonged period before functioning immunity develops.

GvHD primarily affects skin, gut and liver causing an erythematous maculopapular papular rash, watery diarrhea and jaundice. Diagnosis is clinical, but should usually be confirmed by biopsy of the affected organ. GvHD is rarely fatal but the associated severe acute inflammatory changes may be life threatening. The process itself causes further immunosuppression and bone marrow depression, which may cause delay or failure of graft maturation which, in turn, increases the risk from infection. Ciclosporin A is generally given as prophylaxis against GvHD with or without methotrexate. Corticosteroids and intravenous immunoglobulin are also sometimes used as GvHD prophylaxis, the latter also reducing the risk of infection. Acute GvHD is treated with immunosuppressive agents including high dose steroids, antitumor necrosis factor alpha, monoclonal antibodies and antithymocyte globulin, which further increase the infection risk. Chronic, ongoing GvHD is rarely a problem following bone marrow transplantation for immunodeficiency.

Infection after transplantation is discussed above (see secondary immunodeficiencies and Fig. 25.21).

Matched related donor bone marrow transplantation

Usually only sibling donors are matched, but when parents are consanguineous, other family members may be a full match. For severe combined immunodeficiency, HLA-matched grafts are relatively straightforward. Prior immunosuppression ('conditioning') is not usually required or can be minimal. GvHD can occur but is usually mild and self-limiting and prophylaxis is not usually given. Full and long-lasting immune reconstitution is usually achieved though in some cases B lymphocyte engraftment and therefore reconstitution of humoral immunity does not occur necessitating continuing immunoglobulin therapy. In recent years, the success rate in the European experience has been of the order of 90%.[124] Failure is usually related to the pre-existing condition of the child, rather than the technique.

Matched transplants for other conditions (where a residual immune system is capable of graft rejection) have a lower success rate, at least in part because of the need to give conditioning treatment, with the consequent risks of lung and liver toxicity and infection. Nevertheless, encouraging results have been reported[125] with overall survival of 81% since 1985.

Mismatched bone marrow transplantation

By removing all T lymphocyte lineage cells (back to the prethymic stage) from harvested bone marrow, GvHD can be prevented even in an HLA-mismatched situation. At first, T lymphocytes were removed by their propensity to bind to plant lectins, but now specific monoclonal antibodies are used that either remove T lymphocytes or positively select bone marrow stem cells in a semiautomated system. The resulting T lymphocyte-depleted, stem cell enriched marrow will constitute T lymphocyte immunity by producing precursor T lymphocytes which are 'educated' into a state of tolerance towards the foreign HLA haplotype in the new host. The fact that there is half matching of human luekocyte antigen allows most immune functions to proceed normally.

However, successful mismatched BMTs are not as easily achieved as matched ones. Even in SCID, the T lymphocyte-depleted bone marrow can be rejected (or fail to take), and to prevent this full conditioning therapy (marrow ablation) is often needed. Development of immune function is often slow (120 days before the appearance of T lymphocytes vs 42 days following matched antigen by bone marrow transplantation), and full immune reconstitution will take months. B lymphocyte function (antibody responses) is generally good following fully conditioned bone marrow transplantation,[126] although polysaccharide responses may remain poor. Failure to remove all the T lymphocytes can result in severe GvHD, which may require the use of immunosuppressive drugs. On the other hand absolute deficiency of T lymphocytes inhibits engraftment. The adding back of small numbers of T lymphocytes has been attempted to overcome this problem but it increases the risk of GvHD. The prolonged period of immunocompetence greatly increases the risk of opportunistic infections. In this group of transplants it has been shown that the use of high technology isolation facilities (such as laminar air flow) improves the outcome.

Despite these problems, refinements of the technique over recent years have resulted in continuing improvement in results, with success rates for SCID of around 78% for T lymphocyte depleted grafts, and > 90% for matched sibling donors.[123] Success is dependent on type of SCID, with better results for B+ SCID, than the B–phenotype.[122] Age at presentation also influences outcome, with very good results for those transplanted in the neonatal period, before they have contracted infections.[127]

The problems and risks of mismatched BMT have meant that it has been used less for non-SCID conditions. Nevertheless results are improving[125] with 47% survival in the post 1985 period in Europe. Interestingly, far better results were obtained in transplants for leukocyte adhesion deficiency type I than for other conditions.

Matched unrelated donor bone marrow transplantation

For many years there have been national and international registries of tissue typed volunteers willing to donate bone marrow, allowing the option of using phenotypically matched unrelated donors. There is considerable experience of this approach in the hematological field. Early results in SCID suggested that using mismatched haploidentical donors gave better results. However, with the increased sophistication of tissue typing techniques this may no longer be the case and unrelated donors are increasingly being used with similar results to those following mismatched bone marrow transplantation. Storage of screened umbilical cord donations is also performed. Advantages to using cord blood include high stem cell dose, no risk to the donor, less GvHD and 'instant' availability of a suitable unit. This is particularly important in treating infants with SCID where the delay involved in identifying, screening and harvesting an unrelated donor may mean new or worsening infection, decreasing the chance of successful transplantation. Relatively low stem cell dose/kg is less of a problem than for adult transplantation, particularly for infants with SCID.

Transplantation technique

This is relatively straightforward for donor and recipient. Under general anesthesia marrow is harvested by multiple punctures along the posterior iliac crest. If it is to be given unfractionated it is passed through a coarse filter to remove bone particles, the nucleated cells are counted and if necessary the volume adjusted. T lymphocyte depletion if required is done under strict aseptic conditions (details of this are beyond the scope of this chapter). A relatively new approach which avoids the need for bone marrow harvest is the technique of peripheral stem cell harvest which is increasingly being used and is under evaluation. Umbilical cord blood is harvested at time of delivery, and in families with known immunodeficiencies, directed cord donation is possible, targeted for potential future affected family members.

OTHER REPLACEMENT THERAPIES

Enzyme replacement

Some immunological reconstitution of immunological function can be achieved by administering replacement enzyme in ADA deficiency. Purified bovine ADA is conjugated with polyethylene glycol (PEG-ADA) and given by intramuscular injection. In the severe SCID phenotype this can significantly improve immune function, but regular treatment is needed and the long term outcome is not known. If a suitable donor is available, bone marrow transplantation seems the best treatment. However PEG-ADA may be useful in partial forms of the condition. Its role as an adjunct to transplantation is unclear.

Cytokines

Several cytokines and growth factors are available in recombinant synthetic form. Their widespread use in immunodeficiency disorders awaits evaluation. Gamma-interferon and IL-2 have been useful in improving cell-mediated immune function in deficiencies where their production was demonstrably absent.[128] Growth factors such as G-CSF or granulocyte-macrophage colony stimulating factor may be of benefit in phagocytic series defects. The use of IFN-gamma in chronic granulomatous disease has been discussed under the description of this disorder.

Somatic gene therapy

This has been attempted in adenosine deaminase deficiency using ADA transfected CD34 positive autologous cells. Some expression of the gene could be demonstrated but, to date, no consistent improvement in immunological or clinical parameters has been achieved. The first successful gene therapy was performed for common gamma chain deficiency,[129] ironically one of the easiest conditions to correct with bone marrow transplantation. Early results look encouraging, but detailed follow-up studies are required. A number of other conditions may be amenable to gene therapy, but progress has been slow, and at present bone marrow transplantation remains the treatment of choice.

HIV INFECTION

EPIDEMIOLOGY

The first cases of pediatric acquired immune deficiency syndrome (AIDS) were described in 1982 and the causative agent, HIV, was first isolated in 1983. Since then, an enormous amount has been learnt about the disease and for those rich countries that can afford them, antiretroviral therapies (ART) have had a major impact in reducing morbidity and mortality in HIV infected adults[130] and children,[131] as well as dramatically reducing transmission from mother-to-child.[132,133] However, the global HIV epidemic has continued unabated, with increasing gaps between rich and poor countries. African countries bear the brunt of the epidemic, with 70% of the estimated 40 million people living with HIV worldwide in 2001, living in sub-Saharan Africa (Fig. 25.22). Over half are women under 25 years of age and HIV seroprevalence among pregnant women in many sub-Saharan African countries is over 20%. As over 95% of pediatric infections are acquired from mother-to-child, this has major implications for HIV infection in children. In Africa, HIV has reversed gains in child survival and has lowered life expectancy. In addition, large numbers of children have become orphaned. By the end of 2000, UNAIDS estimated that there were over 12 million orphans in Africa who had lost their mother or both parents to AIDS,[134] and this was likely to double in the next decade, placing enormous strains on communities already devastated by the social and economic impact of so many young adults prematurely dying.

HIV is emerging as an increasing problem outside Africa. With over half of the world's population living in Asia/Pacific region and the HIV epidemic at a much earlier stage than in Africa, the explosive increase seen in the last decade is alarming. There was an increase from an estimated 0.5 million HIV infected adults and children in 1991, to 7.1 million in 2001[134] and India now has the largest number of HIV infected persons of any country except South Africa, with seroprevalence rates over 1% among pregnant women in six states[134] and around 10% in persons with TB. Worrying increases have also been observed in areas such as the Russian Federation, where the number of persons with HIV has risen over 10-fold between 1998 and 2001 making it the fastest growing HIV epidemic with intravenous drug use as a major risk factor.[134] HIV is being increasingly recognized in China, where until very recently, very little information was known about HIV prevalence.

Even in Western countries, prevention efforts appear to be stalling. Available information indicates that the number of newly infected people is no lower in 2001 compared with previous years, with 30 000 adults and children estimated to have acquired HIV in Western Europe and 45 000 in North America.[134] Overall HIV prevalence has risen slightly in both regions, also because ART is resulting in HIV infected individuals living longer, and also likely as a result of more people coming forward for testing (including in particular, pregnant women). Thousands of infections are still occurring through unsafe sex between men, where complacency may be attributed to the fact that in the age of ART, they no longer see their friends dying of AIDS. However, it is also true that transmission rates of HIV are likely to be lower from persons on highly active ART (HAART) who will have lower plasma concentrations of the virus.[135] In the USA, there remain an estimated 25% of persons with HIV who have not been diagnosed,[136] this proportion being higher in black African populations. The proportion of persons with undiagnosed HIV is higher in the UK. These persons are more likely to transmit HIV to their sexual partners.

By the end of 2001, there were an estimated 2.7 million children < 15 years old living with HIV infection worldwide, of whom 800 000 were newly infected and over half a million died during 2001 alone;[134] 87% live in sub-Saharan Africa.[134] Although contributing less than 1% of children infected with HIV worldwide, there are currently around 11 000 children living with HIV in North America and about 5000 in Western Europe.[134] With dramatic decreases in transmission rates from mother-to-child in developed countries, new pediatric infections usually occur only in countries where antenatal screening is not comprehensive and/or interventions to reduce mother-to-child transmission (MTCT) are not widely offered, or if the child is born elsewhere. It is not surprising that pediatric infections in many countries of the north are increasingly from countries with a high prevalence of HIV infection. In the UK, over 75% of seropositive newborns are delivered to mothers born in sub-Saharan Africa, and approximately one-third of HIV infected children were themselves born overseas. Similar patterns are being observed in many countries in Europe.

Romania has the largest number of HIV infected children in Europe, making up nearly half of the estimated 10 000 children living with HIV/AIDS in East and Western Europe.[134] The majority belong to a cohort of children who were uniquely infected with HIV through contaminated blood products and needles in the late 1980s. Although many have died, there remain a considerable number of these children now entering their teenage years in

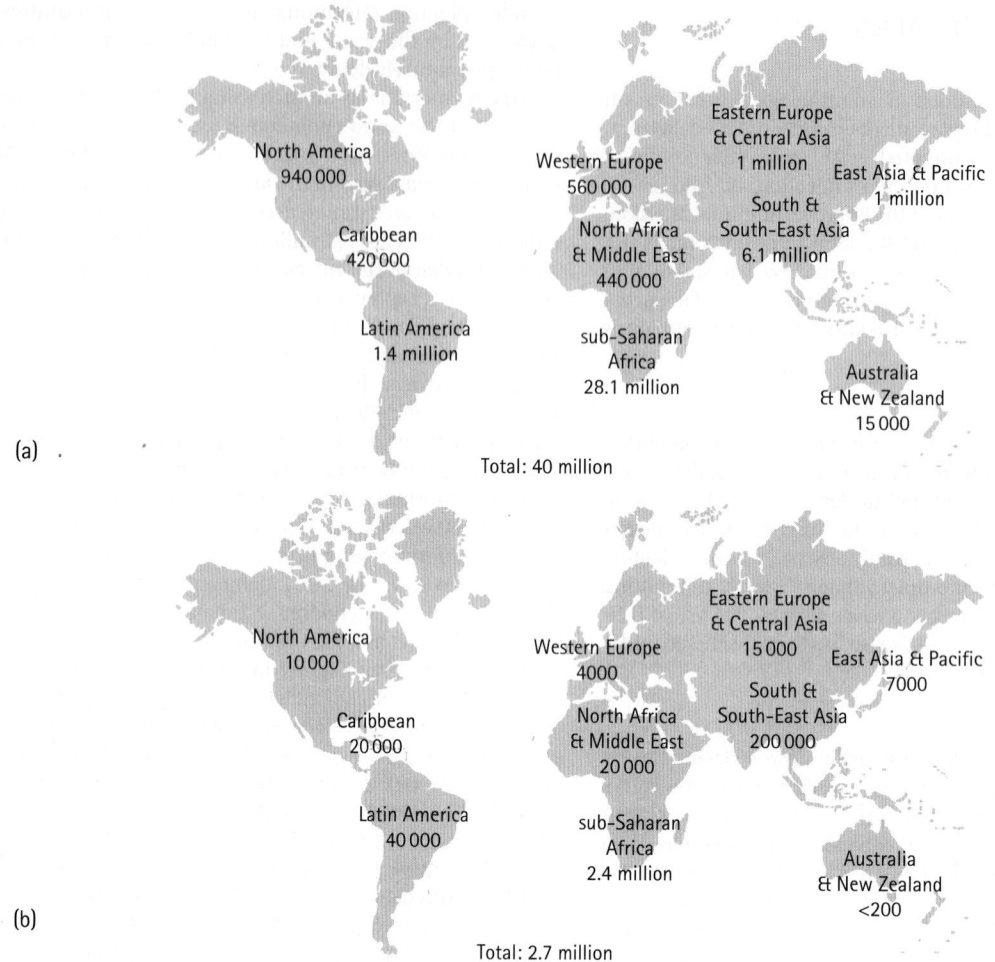

Fig. 25.22 (a) Adults and children estimated to be living with HIV/AIDS as of end 2001. (b) Children (< 15 years) estimated to be living with HIV/AIDS as of end 2001.

Romania. Maternal seroprevalence is about 0.3% in cities such as Costansa, on the Black Sea.

Surveillance for pediatric HIV infection

Unlinked anonymous monitoring of HIV through testing dried blood spots (Guthrie cards) collected on all newborns in many countries for metabolic screening, or antenatal bloods, can provide an unbiased estimate of the prevalence of HIV infection among women having live babies. This is a useful method of providing information about the extent of heterosexually acquired HIV infection in a population, particularly if monitoring is undertaken longitudinally. This might be done continuously, or if resources are scarce, it can be done intermittently (e.g. for 3 months each year). It is possible, while preserving full anonymity, to retain demographic information (e.g. mother's country of birth) which can then be very useful for documenting HIV seroprevalence among particular groups within a community as was done in North London, showing low HIV prevalence among women coming from Asian communities in 1998.[137] Data from anonymous serosurveys have also been combined with non-named confidential register data on HIV in pregnancy in order to provide an indication of the proportion of pregnancies being identified before or during pregnancy.[138] This can be a useful way to audit antenatal testing policy and provide local feedback to care providers (see below).

HIV antibody testing of Guthrie cards is being undertaken in the UK and covers 70% of births. In 2000, the prevalence of maternal infection was 1 in 240 births in inner London and 1 in 530 in outer London, the highest rates ever recorded; further rises were observed in 2001, particularly in outer London (Fig 25.23). The prevalence in England, outside London rose from 1 in 6500 in 1998 to 1 in 2100 in 2000, a nearly threefold increase. In Scotland, the rate was also 1 in 2100 in 2000, twice the rate in 1999 (Fig. 25.23).[139] This increase in the number of pregnant HIV infected women being reported in the last 3 years may in part reflect an increasing desire for HIV infected women who increasingly are already on HAART and clinically well, to have children in the new knowledge that the risk of MTCT can be very low. In London, three-quarters of seropositive newborns were delivered to mothers born in sub-Saharan Africa, and similar patterns are being observed in European countries such as France and Belgium. In Scotland, Ireland and southern Europe a higher proportion of seropositive children are still born to women with injecting drug use (IDU) as a risk factor, but here too the proportion of women acquiring HIV from heterosexual transmission is increasing.

There are over 600 children currently known to be living with HIV in UK and Ireland.[140] Over two-thirds reside in London and were born to women who acquired HIV in sub-Saharan Africa. With dispersal of refugees to other cities in the UK, this is changing. Similarly, whereas the majority of HIV infected children in Scotland and Ireland are still white children born to mothers with IDU as a risk factor for acquiring HIV, this is changing and

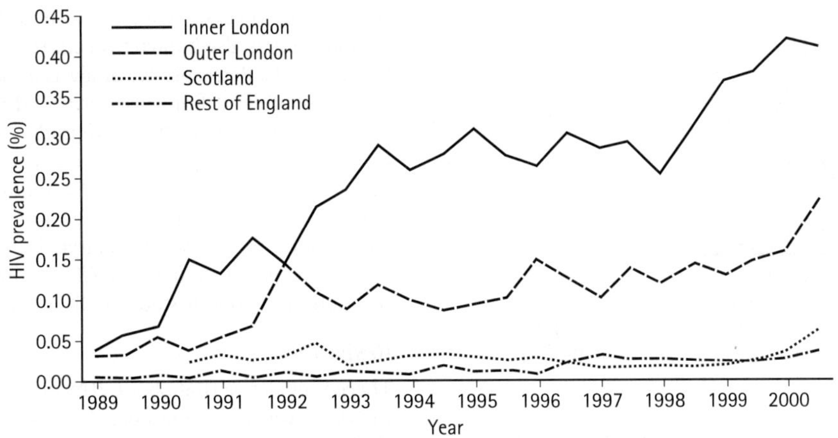

Fig. 25.23 Trends in prevalence of HIV infection in pregnant women by area of residence: 1989–2000. (From Unlinked Anonymous Surveys Steering Group 2001[139])

increasing numbers of mothers of more recently diagnosed HIV infected children acquired the disease through heterosexual contact, often abroad. Follow-up of infected children is being coordinated, along with follow-up of children in Europe participating in clinical trials [Paediatric European Network for Treatment of AIDS (PENTA)] through the Collaborative HIV in Paediatric Surveillance (CHIPS) Study which has over 600 children in follow-up and is coordinated through the MRC Clinical Trials Unit in London in collaboration with the Institute of Child Health (ICH) (penta@ctu.mrc.ac.uk; see Web site www.ctu.mrc.ac.uk/PENTA).

With the advent of HAART, children with HIV are living longer and the average age of the cohort of infected children in the UK and Ireland is now around 8 years, with a quarter of children being over 10 years of age. Children face issues which are similar to those facing other children with a chronic disease (such as the effect of the disease on growth and development and issues around long term adherence to therapy). There are additional issues about long term toxicity of HAART (particularly its effects on metabolic changes occurring in adolescence), social adjustment to a diagnosis which is stigmatizing and also affects other family members, and sexual health issues. These are new areas to be addressed by pediatricians involved in the care of HIV infected children, and require liaison with adult colleagues and coordination of services for adolescents.

MOTHER-TO-CHILD TRANSMISSION OF HIV

MTCT HIV transmission can occur during pregnancy, labor and during breast-feeding.[141] In the absence of breast-feeding, approximately two-thirds of transmission occurs around the time of delivery. The rate of MTCT in the absence of breast-feeding prior to the advent of interventions in Europe and the USA was around 15–20%, compared with around 30% in Africa. Most of this difference is due to breast-feeding which accounts for about one-third of transmission in Africa.[142] Factors independently affecting the rate of transmission include the maternal clinical status, HIV viral load and CD4 cell count, particularly at the time of delivery, prematurity, factors around delivery such as duration of rupture of membranes and mode of delivery[141,143] (Table 25.18).

In the last 5 years, rates of MTCT in resource-rich countries have fallen dramatically to 2% or less with strategies including use of antiretroviral therapy, elective cesarean section (CS) delivery and refraining from breast-feeding.[132,133,144]

Antiretroviral therapy to reduce MTCT

In 1995 the first placebo-controlled trials (the ACTG 076 trial) of zidovudine (ZDV) monotherapy given to the mother antenatally from a median of 26 weeks, by continuous intravenous infusion during labor, and then orally to the infant from birth for 6 weeks, resulted in a 67% reduction in MTCT in non-breast-feeding US and French HIV infected women compared with placebo.[145] This trial was followed by non-randomized studies to document the effect of ZDV monotherapy on MTCT in the clinical setting[132,133,144,146] and of non-randomized studies of double[147] and triple antiretroviral therapy. The results showed that ZDV was highly effective in reducing MTCT in the clinical setting and compared with historical controls, use of double therapy was superior to monotherapy.[147] With triple therapy, MTCT rates below 1% are achievable among women with undetectable HIV viral load at delivery.[148] Cohort studies have documented reductions in MTCT over calendar time with increasing use of triple HAART in pregnancy (Fig. 25.24).[133]

Since the initial ACTG 076 trial, a number of trials have been undertaken to simplify the 076 trial regimen and provide insight into the timing of MTCT. Although HIV RNA viral load reduction by ZDV did not appear to contribute substantially to the reduced MTCT in the ACTG 076 trial, the importance of low viral load around the time of delivery has been demonstrated in subsequent trials of MTCT.[149] However, it is not the only important factor and it is clear that ART reduces MTCT both by decreasing maternal viral load and by providing pre- and postexposure prophylaxis to the infant. In a recent individual patient meta-analysis of women with low HIV RNA of $< 10\,000$ copies/ml, the transmission rate was reduced from 10% to only 1% by the use of ZDV alone, which has only a

Table 25.18 Factors associated with mother-to-child transmission (MTCT) of HIV

- Without interventions, the rate of MTCT was 15–20% in Europe, and 25–40% in Africa
- Most MTCT occurs around the time of delivery
- Increased risk is associated with:
  - late stage maternal disease
  - invasive obstetric procedures
  - prematurity
  - breast-feeding

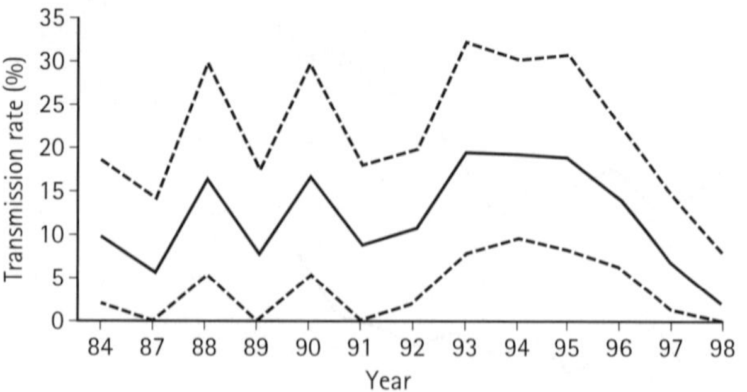

Fig. 25.24 Estimated vertical transmission rate (95% CI) in UK over time in non-breast-feeding women (From Duong et al 1999[133])

minimal effect on maternal viral load (reduction by only about 0.3 log copies/ml).[150] This suggests that postexposure prophylaxis to the fetus is also important, a factor borne out by the large impact on transmission of giving long acting nevirapine (NVP) to women during labor and to the baby.[151] Even if a woman has not received ART during pregnancy or delivery, ART given to the baby as soon as possible after birth is likely to have an effect on transmission. Guidelines for giving ART to pregnant women to reduce MTCT are available and are regularly updated.[152,153]

Reducing MTCT in resource-poor settings

Trials have taken place comparing different components of the ACTG 076 regimen and also evaluating other antiretroviral drugs. Most have taken place in resource-poor settings where an important goal was also to refine, simplify and reduce the costs of the initial ZDV regimen used in the ACTG 076 trial. A trial of ZDV monotherapy in non-breast-feeding women in Thailand showed that a 50% reduction of MTCT was possible with giving ZDV from 36 weeks' gestation, oral ZDV during labor and for 2 weeks to the baby.[154] However, another trial from Thailand also emphasized that starting ART at 28 weeks also added benefit compared with starting at 36 weeks,[155] suggesting that some in utero transmission may be prevented by ART. It is also true that if starting ART is left until 36 weeks, some women will go into premature labor having received minimal or no prelabor ART.

In more resource-poor settings, reductions in MTCT of around one-third were observed using a similar regimen among women in West Africa; benefit was maintained for 2 years despite the fact that these women were breast-feeding.[156,157] The short course ZDV regimens were considerably cheaper at around US$50 compared with the US$800–1000 for the ACTG 076 regimen, but this is still very expensive for resource-poor countries. Intrapartum ART alone does not appear to be useful[158] if given alone without postpartum prophylaxis to the baby. In the most exciting trial, HIVNET 012 undertaken in Uganda, a single 200 mg oral dose of the antiretroviral drug NVP, given to the mother in labor, followed by a single oral dose of 2 mg/kg to the infant at 48 h (total cost US$4), led to a 40% reduction in MTCT at 16 weeks compared with intrapartum and neonatal (for 1 week) oral ZDV.[151] Follow-up to 18 months has shown continued efficacy of around 40% despite breast-feeding for an average of 9 months.

Problems with ART to reduce MTCT

Mitochondrial dysfunction

Advances in the development of pharmaceutical interventions to reduce HIV MTCT are not without complications. In a French study of ZDV + 3TC, concerns were first raised about a possible link between mitochondrial dysfunction and perinatal exposure to antiretroviral nucleoside reverse transcriptase inhibitors (NRTIs).[159] This complication is also known to occur rarely in HIV infected individuals taking NRTIs. Retrospective analysis of other large cohort data failed to reveal other definitive cases.[160] Although concerns about the potential carcinogenicity and reproductive effects of ART as well as mitochondrial toxicity remain, current evidence suggests that the benefit of ART in dramatically reducing MTCT far outweighs potential harm. Many countries are now setting up long term surveillance to follow all children born to HIV infected mothers, whether exposed or not to ARTs in utero. In the UK this will be through the National Study of HIV in Pregnancy at the ICH.

Resistance

There is evidence that about 20% of women will develop resistance to NVP, even after one dose,[161] with unknown consequences for their own future therapy, therapy in future pregnancies or if used when they need treatment themselves. However this resistance fades with time and there is no difference in survival of babies with and without NVP resistance,[161] so it is likely that NVP will remain an important option for preventing vertical transmission in future pregnancies. This is an area for further research, but should not jeopardize the important role of NVP in reducing MTCT in resource-poor countries. However, in developed countries, adding NVP to other ART around the time of delivery in women with detectable viral load or giving NVP monotherapy is not recommended because of concerns about the development of resistance to all non-nucleoside reverse transcriptase inhibitor (NNRTI) drugs.[152,162]

Effect of mode of delivery on MTCT

Several cohort studies have shown that factors around delivery contribute importantly to MTCT. In a meta-analysis of 15 large studies including more than 5000 mother–child pairs from the USA and Europe, it was estimated that for every 1 h increase in time in labor with ruptured membranes, the risk of MTCT increased by 2%.[163]

From a meta-analysis of the studies and a randomized European trial, and also from a European controlled trial, it was also shown that among more than 8000 women, the risk of transmission was 50% lower in those whose babies were delivered by elective CS prior to membrane rupture, compared with those undergoing vaginal or emergency CS delivery.[164,165] This difference was maintained after adjusting for other risk factors and was independent of ZDV monotherapy administration. Subsequent cohorts have shown that reduction of MTCT to around 2% is possible with ZDV, elective CS delivery and not breast-feeding.[133,144] The question of how much additional reduction to transmission may occur if elective CS delivery is undertaken in women on combination ART with undetectable HIV RNA viral load around the time of delivery is unclear,[166] and is unlikely to be answered from controlled trials. However, as the risk is very low, most guidelines suggest that the women can undergo a normal vaginal delivery in this situation, but that membranes should not be ruptured prematurely, and interventions during labor delivery (e.g. use of scalp electrodes, instrumental delivery) should be avoided.[152,162]

Breast-feeding

HIV can be transmitted through breast milk.[167,168] Most transmission appears to occur early and factors including HIV viral content in colostrum, immaturity of the infant gastrointestinal tract in the neonatal period, and the contribution of breast and nipple complications (e.g. mastits and bleeding nipples which may increase the viral content of breast milk) all play a role. Breast milk transmission continues, however, throughout the duration of breast-feeding, posing extremely difficult dilemmas for policy in parts of the world where alternatives to breast-feeding are expensive, unsafe and culturally unacceptable, but where HIV prevalence is high.[169]

Currently the recommendation is that infants should continue to be breast-fed where infectious diseases and malnutrition are the main cause of infant mortality, as artificial feeding substantially increases the risk of illness and death.[169] Where infants of HIV infected mothers can be ensured uninterrupted access to nutritionally adequate safely prepared breast milk substitutes, they are at less risk of illness and death from non-HIV related illness and these mothers should therefore be encouraged not to breast-feed. Recent evidence from Durban, South Africa suggests that in their setting, exclusive breast-feeding may be the practice to be most encouraged and there is currently much discussion about the feasibility of advising HIV infected mothers to exclusively breast-feed for 4–6 months (which is anyway advocated for all women) and then wean as quickly as possible, as after this time the benefits of breast-feeding may be outweighed by the risk of HIV infection.[170] This strategy is likely to be more feasible than exclusive formula feeding which in many settings is likely to increase infant mortality from other infections, to be socially unacceptable and unaffordable and risk a 'spill over effect' on non-HIV infected mothers. Hopefully, larger prospective studies will help to clarify the effects of exclusive breast-feeding followed by early weaning after short course antiretroviral therapy on HIV transmission rates, and morbidity and mortality of HIV infected and uninfected babies. A randomized trial would be desirable but may not be feasible, as exclusive breast-feeding is advocated anyway in the early months of life, even if this advice is frequently not followed.

Other interventions to reduce MTCT

Other interventions that have been explored to reduce MTCT include trials of cleansing the birth canal and vitamin A supplementation during pregnancy. The rationale for the former is that the maximum risk of exposure appears to be around the time of delivery and therefore cleaning with chlorhexidine might reduce vertical transmission. However clinical trials have failed to show significant benefit with this approach.[171]

Observational studies suggested that low vitamin A levels were associated with increased MTCT.[172] However, results of randomized trials have failed to show a significant impact of supplementation with vitamin A on MTCT.[173]

ANTENATAL TESTING

In developed countries

The case for offering antenatal HIV testing is now overwhelming. A recommendation that HIV testing should be offered to all women in pregnancy has been successfully implemented in the USA and in most European countries, notably France, Italy and Spain where the prevalence of HIV in pregnant women was highest. In the UK, the universal offer of HIV testing during the antenatal period has been recommended in London because of high prevalence, since 1992. However, until 1999, it was recommended that antenatal HIV testing should only be offered to women considered at high risk (selective testing) outside London. An economic analysis was published in 1999 showing that a universal offer policy was cost effective throughout the UK provided that a high uptake of testing was achieved.[174] Department of Health guidelines (England and Wales) endorsing this approach were published in August 1999.[175] In low prevalence areas, up to 50 pooled samples can be tested for HIV antibody possibly also with hepatitis B in batches to reduce costs.[174]

During the 1990s, detection of previously undiagnosed HIV in pregnancy was low everywhere in the UK, but increased to about 50% in 1999 in inner London and further in 2000 and 2001 (Fig. 25.25). Whereas in most European countries and in the USA, a marked decrease in AIDS cases reported in infancy reflects the high proportion of pregnant women receiving appropriate care to reduce MTCT, this is only now beginning to occur in the UK (Fig. 25.26). Outside London, uptake of antenatal HIV testing is increasing more slowly and children first presenting with severe *Pneumocystis carinii* pneumonia (PCP) and cytomegalovirus (CMV) disease in early infancy continue to be seen as a result of perinatal transmission of HIV from mothers who are unaware of their own HIV infection.[176]

In resource-poor countries

In low income countries, ART to prevent MTCT is only one strand of a much more complex mesh of issues surrounding the prevention of vertical transmission.[177] With the available tools and knowledge that we have already, there is a strong argument for putting resources into providing antenatal diagnosis and the appropriate perinatal interventions. This undoubtedly requires a huge input of resources into the development of sustainable infrastructures in situations where antenatal care may currently be rudimentary.

Understandably, concerns have been raised that, rather than putting scarce resources into a 'magic bullet' of ART to pregnant women, efforts should be concentrated on the more difficult issue of preventing women getting infected in the first place. However, the setting up of a structure for antenatal testing and prevention of vertical transmission is proving to be a positive move, with increasing acceptance of HIV and paving the way for better care for women and families with HIV infection. In the last 12 months, most countries in southern Africa have started pilot schemes to offer antenatal HIV testing and ART to reduce transmission from mother to child.

ETIOLOGY AND PATHOGENESIS

HIV is a retrovirus. Transmission occurs through sexual intercourse, via infected blood and blood products and by transmission from mother-to-child. Many of the clinical features of HIV can be ascribed to the profound immune suppression because it infects cells of the immune system and ultimately destroys them. An understanding of the way it does this is helpful in interpreting tests used in monitoring the disease and helps explain the difficulties in developing a vaccine for HIV.

The virus predominantly infects a subset of the thymus-derived lymphocytes, carrying the surface molecule CD4, which binds the glycoprotein on the envelope of HIV called gp120. CD4 is also present on many monocytes and macrophages, and on Langerhans'

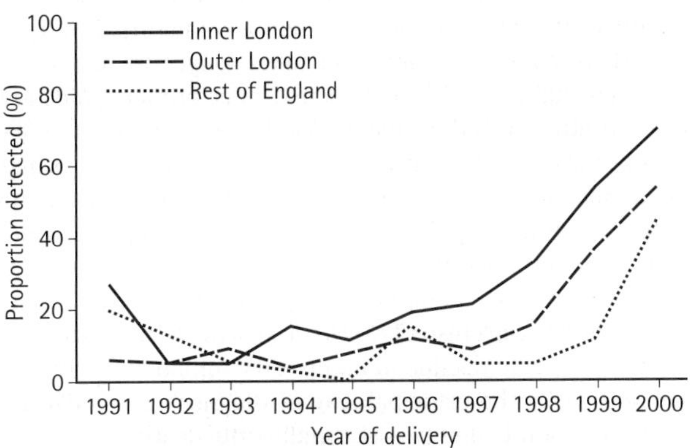

Fig. 25.25 Detection of previously undiagnosed HIV-infected pregnant women in England by calendar year.

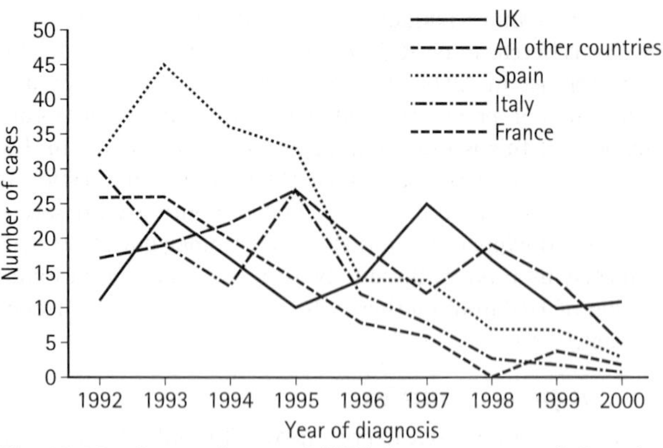

Fig. 25.26 Reported rates of AIDS diagnoses among infants in different European countries.

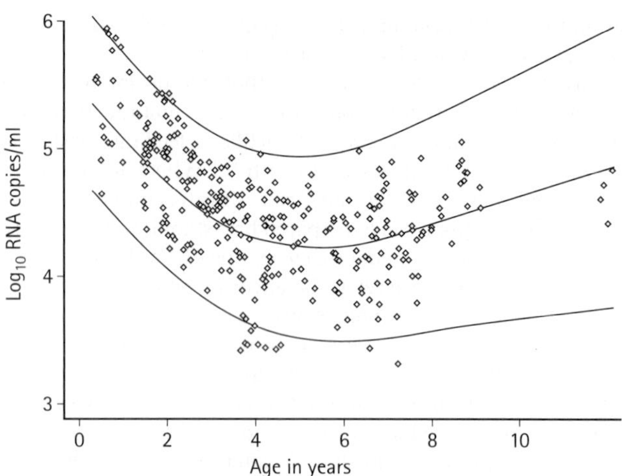

Fig. 25.27 Log_{10} HIV-1 RNA plotted against age in untreated HIV infected children (fitted line and 95% CI). (From Gibb et al 1998[184])

cells of the skin and dentritic cells of many other tissues. HIV also requires coreceptors to enter cells. Two of these which are of particular importance are CCR5 and CXCR4. These coreceptors are members of a family of receptors, expressed on the cells of lymphocytes, dentritic cells and cells of the rectal, vaginal and cervical mucosae which function as receptors for chemokines that orchestrate the migration and differentiation of leukocytes during immune responses. Virus strains able to infect primary macrophages (R5 tropic viruses) use CCR5 as a coreceptor and only these are detected early in infection, suggesting they are important for transmission. Further evidence for this comes from studies showing that individuals homozygous for a 32 pair deletion of CCR5 show increased resistance to being infected by HIV.[178,179] Both R5 and strains infecting T cells use CXCR4 as a coreceptor (T or X4 viruses) and they arise during the course of infection.

It is now recognized that CD8 cytotoxic lymphocytes (CTL) capable of killing HIV infected targets develop early in primary HIV infection and are very important in the initial control of viremia.[180,181] Among CD8 cells, rapid expansion of strong T cell responses to multiple viral epitopes has been shown to be associated with better control of viremia following primary infection in adults. The way in which CD8 T cells protect is by killing infected cells and producing CD8 T cell antiviral factor (CAF) which inhibits viral replication. The breadth and strength of the CTL responses are determined by the degree of CD4 specific helper response, which may be determined by the level of HIV viremia. In adults who fail to control viral load, CTL responses are narrower and less marked. Because HIV replication is very rapid and errors occur in reverse transcription, these mutants can evade CTL response (escape mutants) – i.e. the viral epitope mutates to 'escape' control by the CTL.

In infants in whom the immune system is immature, it may be that the CTL response is poorer and takes longer to develop,[182] allowing much higher viral load to persist after primary infection. This has been little studied in infants. Viral load rises over the first weeks after primary infection around the time of birth, and stays high throughout infancy. It then continues to fall in the absence of therapy over the next 3–5 years (Fig. 25.27)[183,184] to reach a 'set point' which is much later after primary infection than in adults (set point at about 6 months). On the other hand, infants have a highly active thymus which may 'work' to replenish CD4 cells destroyed by the virus.[185]

As viremia starts to decline in adults, HIV antibody production increases and forms the principal way of diagnosis in adults and older children, as antibodies persist usually until death.

Polyclonal activation of B cells also occurs resulting in high immunoglobulin levels in most children, commencing during infancy, although in those with rapid progression, hypogammaglobulinemia can also rarely occur. This polyclonal increase in immunoglobulin is in many cases non-functional and leads to increased susceptibility to bacterial infections.

There are reports of both adults and children being exposed to HIV and remaining uninfected; these individuals have had HIV specific CTL detected. In addition, individuals with strong CTL responses may have delayed disease progression (long term non-progressors).

The CD4 cell plays a central role in orchestrating the immune system and their destruction by HIV accounts for much of the immunosuppressive effect of the virus. Following fusion into CD4 and other cells, viral core material enters the host cell and the genetic material encoded in RNA is converted to DNA by reverse transcriptase. This DNA 'provirus' is then integrated into the host genome. HIV replicates at an enormous rate with $> 10^6$ particles being produced daily.[186] In addition, turnover of infected replicating CD4 cells is high, occurring approximately every 1.5 days. CD4 damage occurs both directly and through mechanisms resulting in apoptosis of infected cells. The exact role of both of these is still debated. HIV in resting memory and long-lived cells both in the immune system and in other tissues remains latent for long periods of time and is largely responsible for persistence of the virus despite the ability of HAART to decrease virus to undetectable levels in plasma. In 1996, with the advent of HAART there was great hope that the half-life of long-lived cells might be in the order of only a few years and that HIV eradication might be possible. Sadly this is not the case, and recent modeling exercises estimate the half-life of these long-lived infected cells to be around 70 years.[187] If HAART is stopped, even after plasma viral load has been undetectable for several years, HIV viral load rises again within 1–2 weeks. The virus also has a remarkable ability to mutate and develop resistance to antiretroviral drugs. Mutant virus may remain in latent cells for many years but re-emerge if that drug is again restarted in an individual.

Monitoring with CD4 and HIV RNA viral load

The most widely used markers for predicting disease progression in children, as in adults, are the CD4 cell count (or percentage) and viral load as measured by HIV-1 RNA in plasma.

Absolute CD4 counts are physiologically higher in young children compared with adults and there is great difference between and within individual variability.[188] CD4 percentages vary less with age, although are still higher at very young ages as can be seen from centile charts constructed from uninfected children born to HIV positive mothers (Fig. 25.28).[188] By around 7–8 years of age, the CD4 cell count number and range has fallen to nearer adult values. In children with HIV infection, as in adults, absolute lymphocyte counts and CD4 cell counts decrease with progression of the disease, but additional account has to made in children for changes with age. For this purpose, CD4 z-scores have also been proposed to monitor changes over time.[188] However, complexity in calculating these has impaired their use and in young children, most pediatricians follow the CD4% up until the age of around 6 years when increasing account should be taken of the total CD4 count. Using centile charts can be a useful way to follow both the CD4 count and percentage and is also useful for explaining immunological deterioration to parents, who may understand CD4 thresholds for their own disease, but find the concepts of change with age difficult in their children. Even accounting for age, by using CD4% or CD4 z-score, the predictive value of CD4 cell counts is not as good in children compared with adults. Whereas in adults, a CD4 cell count below 200 cells/mm^3 is a useful predictor of risk of developing Pneumocystis carinii pneumonia (PCP) and therefore used to determine the time to start prophylaxis against this disease, during infancy, neither CD4 count nor percentage is of any value in predicting PCP in infancy.[189] After infancy, however, a CD4% greater than 25% is considered evidence of minimal immunosuppression, 15–25% moderate, and < 15% severe immunosuppression and these form the basis of the Centers for Disease Control (CDC) immunological classification of HIV in children.[190] New information about the predictive value of both HIV RNA and CD4 cell counts, and how these vary with age, should soon be available from an ongoing meta-analysis (see below). Importantly, for the individual child, the rate of fall of CD4% and at older ages of CD4 cell counts, are of importance when deciding about when to start antiretroviral therapy.

Viral load as measured by HIV RNA is an independent predictor of HIV progression in adults after the 'set point' has been reached. Several different assays are available in kit form with quality control (Roche, Chiron and NASBA). The Roche PCR version 1.5 is widely used and now includes additional primers to ensure accuracy when measuring viral load in persons with different subtypes of HIV (e.g. subtype B is most the common virus subtype in white North Americans and Europeans but subtypes A and C are common in persons infected in Africa). With the Chiron assay there are fewer concerns about performance with different viral subtypes but it gives lower results than Roche or NASBA. Newer versions of all the assays tend to give higher results. It is important to be aware that assay variability may be as high as 0.7 log and that results need to be interpreted on a log scale. Repeating results is advisable if treatment decisions are being taken based on viral load results. All assays are less precise at values above 750 000 copies/ml but all assays are more robust at low levels down to a cut-off of 50 copies/ml.

In infants HIV RNA is very high after infection around the time of birth and remains much higher (often 1 million copies/ml or more) than observed in adults for the first 2 years of life.[183,185] In some children, the CD4% and count may remain high despite viral load between 100 000 and 1 million copies/ml which frequently gradually reduce by an average of about one log over the first 5 years of life in the absence of antiretroviral therapy (Fig. 25.29).[185,191] In analyses of cross-sectional studies with relatively small numbers, viral load and CD4 are both independent predictors of HIV progression in children, as in adults, but the positive predictive value is low.[192,193] A meta-analysis of longitudinal European and US data on nearly 5000 children is ongoing and may help to better define the predictive value of both these markers at different ages.

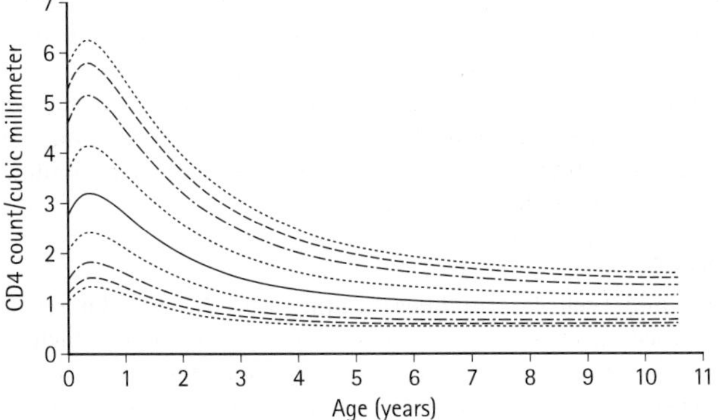

Fig. 25.28 CD4 lymphocyte counts in children by age: 3rd, 5th, 10th, 25th, 50th, 75th, 90th, 95th and 97th centiles. Created from data collected by the European Collaborative Study using the methods of Wade & Ades (1994)[188].

LABORATORY DIAGNOSIS

Enzyme linked immunosorbent assays (ELISA) for measuring HIV antibody are highly sensitive and specific for diagnosing HIV in adults and in children over 18 months of age. However, because of transplacental transfer of maternal antibody, all babies born to HIV infected women will have antibodies at birth which take a median of 10 months and a maximum of 18 months to clear. Therefore other direct techniques are required to diagnose HIV in young infants.

In Western countries, early diagnosis of HIV in infants has been improved significantly with the availability of polymerase chain reaction (PCR) techniques for detecting proviral DNA and RNA. Using these techniques, HIV infection can be definitively diagnosed in non-breast-feeding women in about 90% of infected infants by age 1 month and in virtually all by 6 months. HIV DNA PCR is the preferred virological method for initial diagnosis. In a meta-analysis, 38% (90% CI = 29–46%) of infected children had positive PCR DNA tests by age 48 h, rapidly increasing in the second week with 93% of infected children (90%CI = 76–97%) testing positive by 2 weeks of age.[194] Among women who have been taking HAART during pregnancy, there were fears that this might delay the diagnosis of an infected child; however, data to date suggest that this appears not to be the case, at least not if the woman has taken ZDV monotherapy.

HIV RNA tests may be more sensitive that DNA PCR for diagnosis, but limited data suggest lower specificity, just after birth. However, they may be used as confirmatory tests and give additional information about the degree of viremia. Culture of HIV is time consuming and expensive and is no longer routinely undertaken. The detection of p24 antigen, both standard and immune-complex dissociated, although highly specific, is not as sensitive as DNA PCR. Nevertheless, detection of acid or heat dissociated p24 antigen by ELISA is considerably cheaper than PCR tests and is also technically less demanding, making it more promising as a diagnostic tool for resource-poor settings; it is highly specific and reasonably sensitive.

Another laboratory clue that a child may have HIV infection is the presence of polyclonal hypergammaglobulinemia, which in the presence of CD4 lymphopenia should lead to a high suspicion of HIV infection, as it is more unusual in other immune deficiency diseases in childhood.

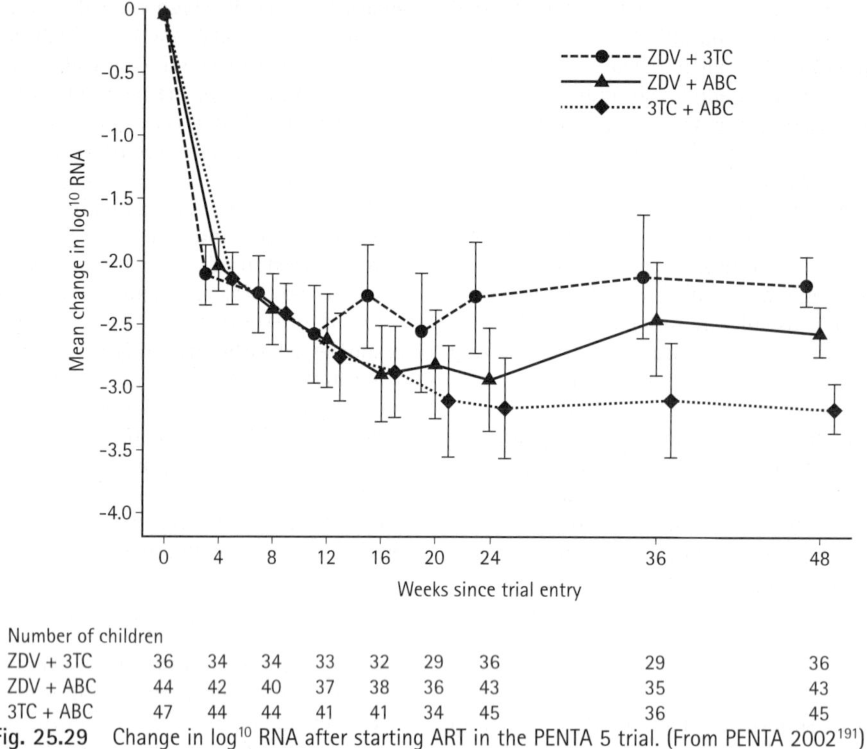

Fig. 25.29 Change in log^{10} RNA after starting ART in the PENTA 5 trial. (From PENTA 2002[191])

CLINICAL ASPECTS

HIV infected babies appear normal at birth with birth weight generally in the normal range. Therefore clinically one cannot usually detect any signs that a baby has HIV in the first days of life. Signs and symptoms develop over the first few weeks and most children have some evidence of infection by 12 months. Anecdotally, axillary lymphadenopathy may be an early sign that a baby is infected. However, there is a wide spectrum and some infected infants may have no clinical evidence of HIV and if the mother is unaware of her own HIV status, may not present to medical attention for several years.

As in adults, HIV may present with a spectrum of signs and symptoms in children. This is reflected in the revised CDC classification system for children (Table 25.19),[190] and important differences between adults and children are summarized in Table 25.20. In the absence of antiretroviral therapy or prophylaxis against PCP (see below), disease progression is faster than in adults, and cohort studies reported in the early 1990s that 15–20% of children progressed to an AIDS defining illness by 12 months of age.[195–197] Over half of this subset of perinatally infected children typically present with PCP at around 3–6 months of age. Data from prospective cohorts in Europe in the early 1990s reported overall survival rates in children on either no ART or only ZDV monotherapy of around 70% by 6 years and 50% by 9 years of age.[195–197]

Children with HIV infection frequently present with signs and symptoms that are common in general pediatrics and are non-specific. The most usual clinical features associated with HIV infection include persistent generalized lymphadenopathy (particularly axillary), hepatosplenomegaly, chronic or recurrent diarrhea, prelonged or recurrent oral or diaper candidiasis, fever, recurrent otitis or sinusitis and chest infections. Children may also present with a picture of idiopathic thrombocytopenic purpura with no other signs and may be more prone to developing eczema, extensive molluscum, and recurrent allergic iritis and rhinitis. A typical and quite specific presentation is non-tender bilateral parotid enlargement, which may be associated with generalized cervical lymphadenopathy and X-ray appearances of lymphocytic interstitial pneumonitis (LIP) with hilar lymphadenopathy (see below). Such children often also have allergic rhinitis, tonsilar and/or adenoid enlargement and may present with sleep apnea. Herpes zoster (shingles) in childhood is uncommon and suggests a defect in cellular immunity justifying an HIV test in the absence of other explanations.

Persistent or recurrent oral candidiasis after the neonatal period or neurological signs are more specific of HIV infection and have prognostic significance, as does failure to thrive and poor growth; all are indications of increasing immune deficiency. Conversely, thrombocytopenia does not indicate a poor prognosis and bilateral parotitis, lymphadenopathy and LIP (see below) are often associated with a relatively good prognosis. Details of the main AIDS (CDC stage C) presenting conditions are described below. Although the development of these conditions, along with immunological stage 3 disease has been shown to be predictive of a poor outcome, this varies. For example, conditions such as recurrent bacterial infections are associated with a better prognosis than HIV encephalopathy. Stage B disease includes a wide range of conditions with different predictive values.[190]

Infections

The T and B cell abnormalities resulting from HIV infection result in increased susceptibility to a wide range of organisms including fungi, mycobacteria, bacteria, protozoa and viruses. In a recent analysis of over 3000 HIV infected children participating in clinical trials in the USA *before* HAART became available, serious bacterial infections (rate 15.1/100 child-years; most commonly pneumonia 11/100 child-years) which occurred during all stages of HIV infection and *Mycobacterium avium-intracellulare* complex (MAIC)

Table 25.19 Centers for Disease Control classification system for children with HIV infection (From Galli et al 2000[190])

CATEGORY N: NOT SYMPTOMATIC

Children who have no signs or symptoms considered to be the result of HIV infection or who have only one of the conditions listed in Category A.

CATEGORY A: MILDLY SYMPTOMATIC

Children with two or more of the conditions listed below but none of the conditions listed in Categories B and C.

- Lymphadenopathy (≥ 0.5 cm at more than two sites; bilateral = one site)
- Hepatomegaly
- Splenomegaly
- Dermatitis
- Parotitis
- Recurrent or persistent upper respiratory infection, sinusitis, or otitis media

CATEGORY B: MODERATELY SYMPTOMATIC

Children who have symptomatic conditions other than those listed for Category A or C that are attributed to HIV infection. Examples of conditions in clinical Category B include but are not limited to:

- Anemia (< 8 g/dl), neutropenia (< 1000/mm^3), or thrombocytopenia (< 100 000/mm^3) persisting ≥ 30 days
- Bacterial meningitis, pneumonia, or sepsis (single episode)
- Candidiasis, oropharyngeal (thrush), persisting (> 2 months) in children > 6 months of age
- Cardiomyopathy
- Cytomegalovirus infection, with onset before 1 month of age
- Diarrhea, recurrent or chronic
- Hepatitis
- Herpes simplex virus (HSV) stomatitis, recurrent (more than two episodes within 1 year)
- HSV bronchitis, pneumonitis, or esophagitis with onset before 1 month of age
- Herpes zoster (shingles) involving at least two distinct episodes or more than one dermatome
- Leiomyosarcoma
- Lymphoid interstitial pneumonia (LIP) or pulmonary lymphoid hyperplasia complex
- Nephropathy
- Nocardiosis
- Persistent fever (lasting > 1 month)
- Toxoplasmosis, onset before 1 month of age
- Varicella, disseminated (complicated chickenpox)

CATEGORY C: SEVERELY SYMPTOMATIC

Serious bacterial infections, multiple or recurrent (i.e. any combination of at least two culture-confirmed infections within a 2-year period), of the following types:
septicemia, pneumonia, meningitis, bone or joint infection, or abscess of an internal organ or body cavity

- Candidiasis, esophageal or pulmonary (bronchi, trachea, lungs)
- Coccidioidomycosis, disseminated (at site other than or in addition to lungs or cervical or hilar lymph nodes)
- Cryptococcosis, extrapulmonary
- Cryptosporidiosis or isosporiasis with diarrhea persisting > 1 month
- Cytomegalovirus disease with onset of symptoms at age > 1 month (at a site other than liver, spleen, or lymph nodes)
- Encephalopathy (at least one of the following progressive findings present for at least 2 months in the absence of another concurrent illness :
    a) failure to attain or loss of developmental milestones or loss of intellectual ability, verified by standard developmental scale or neuropsychological tests;

Table 25.19 (Continued)

    b) impaired brain growth or acquired microcephaly demonstrated by head circumference measurements or brain atrophy demonstrated by computerized tomography or magnetic resonance imaging (serial imaging is required for children < 2 years of age);
    c) acquired symmetric motor deficit manifested by two or more of the following: paresis, pathologic reflexes, ataxia, or gait disturbance
- Herpes simplex virus infection causing a mucocutaneous ulcer that persists for 1 month; or bronchitis, pneumonitis, or esophagitis for any duration affecting a child > 1 month of age
- Histoplasmosis, disseminated (at a site other than or in addition to lungs or cervical or hilar lymph nodes)
- Kaposi's sarcoma
- Lymphoma, primary, in brain
- Lymphoma, small, non-cleaved cell (Burkitt's), or immunoblastic or large cell lymphoma of B-cell or unknown immunologic phenotype
- *Mycobacterium tuberculosis*, disseminated or extrapulmonary
- *Mycobacterium*, other species or unidentified species, disseminated (at a site other than or in addition to lungs, skin, or cervical or hilar lymph nodes)
- *Mycobacterium avium* complex or *Mycobacterium kansasii*, disseminated (at site other than or in addition to lungs, skin, or cervical or hilar lymph nodes)
- *Pneumocystis carinii* pneumonia
- Progressive multifocal leukoencephalopathy
- *Salmonella* (non-typhoid) septicemia, recurrent
- Toxoplasmosis of the brain with onset at > 1 month of age
- Wasting syndrome in the absence of a concurrent illness other than HIV infection that could explain the following findings:
    a) persistent weight loss > 10% of baseline
    OR
    b) downward crossing of at least two of the following percentile lines on the weight-for-age chart (e.g. 95th, 75th, 50th, 25th, 5th) in a child ≥ 1 year of age
    OR
    c) < 5th percentile on weight-for-height chart on two consecutive measurements, ≥ 30 days apart PLUS a) chronic diarrhea (i.e. at least two loose stools per day for ≥ 30 days) OR b) documented fever (for ≥ 30 days, intermittent or constant)

Table 25.20 Differences compared with adults

- Faster rate of disease progression, especially in infants (PCP and CMV)
- Lymphocytic interstitial pneumonitis and parotitis common
- More bacterial infections
- Encephalopathy presents differently
- Growth failure occurs as well as wasting
- Kaposi's sarcoma rare outside endemic areas
- Different immunology – Developing immune system in uninfected children
- Higher numbers and more variation of CD4 cells
- Decline to adult values in mid-childhood
- CD4% is less variable and so is used in children
- Different pattern of HIV RNA – decline of HIV viral load up to 5 years

CMV = cytomegalovirus; PCP = *Pneumocystis carinii* pneumonia

(1.8/100 child-years) which occurred in advanced disease, were among the most common infections.[198] PCP occurring at a rate of 1.3/100 child-years was also common and infants not on prophylaxis have particularly high susceptibility.

All infections occur at much higher rates than among HIV negative children. The rates of all infections are lower among adults on HAART, and there is anecdotal evidence that this is also the case among children (WM Dankner, personal communication, 2002). This is being evaluated in a Pediatric AIDS Clinical Trials Group (PACTG) study.

Opportunistic infections

Opportunistic infections, apart from PCP and primary disseminated CMV disease to which infants with rapidly progressive disease are particularly susceptible during the first 6 months of life, are usually a late complication of HIV infection and result from severe immunosuppression. The most common are esophageal candidiasis, multidermatomal varicella zoster, disseminated *Mycobacterium avium* complex (MAC), CMV infections, cryptosporidiosis, and more rarely, toxoplasmosis.[198] MAC should be considered in any child with advanced disease and unexplained fevers, weight loss and abdominal discomfort.

PCP infection and CMV

These infections are mentioned in greater detail as they present early, particularly in previously undiagnosed HIV infected babies, have a high mortality even in the era of HAART, and present differently in infants compared with older children and adults.

Among HIV infected babies who have not received PCP prophylaxis, PCP is a common first AIDS indicator disease, occurring most frequently in the first 6 months of life,[176,199,200] with reported survival rates of only 38–62%.[176,199,200] CMV is often isolated at the time of PCP diagnosis from HIV infected adults and in infants is more common if the mother breast-feeds.[176,200] In the UK, between 1989 and 1999, PCP was the commonest AIDS defining diagnosis, occurring in 68% of reported infected infants born in the UK and Ireland.[200] In almost all, the mother was unaware of her HIV diagnosis before the child developed PCP.

PCP in infants with HIV infection should be treated with high dose co-trimoxazole. An increased rate of reactions to co-trimoxazole has been reported with HIV infection in children, although interestingly this may be less common in black Africans[176] (Nunn, personal communication, 2002). Alternative therapies include pentamidine or atovaquone both of which may also be used for prophylaxis against PCP (see below). As well as supportive treatment including ventilation, high dose steroids are recommended for PCP and in a few reports have been shown to improve outcome in children as well as adults with PCP.[176] However, concerns have been expressed about the use of steroids in infants dually infected with PCP and CMV.[176,200] In infants, CMV is a primary infection and corticosteroids could adversely affect the course of CMV disease. Infants with PCP should certainly be investigated for CMV infection and retinitis, especially if they were breast-fed. In addition, anti-CMV therapy should be strongly considered in infants with PCP and evidence of CMV infection, especially in those who receive adjuvant corticosteroids. This strategy is already being followed in some London centers.[176,200]

As discussed above, CMV may present as pneumonitis as with PCP and the risk is higher in breast-fed infants.[176,200] In the UK based study, PCP was the commonest presentation among infants with HIV, and in many cases was presumptive, as lung biopsy was not undertaken. Among babies presenting with multisite CMV disease, retinitis occurred in nearly half, and should be actively sought. An association between CMV infection and HIV disease severity and progression has been hypothesized in children.[201]

Bacterial infections

Recurrent bacterial infections occur frequently in children with HIV infection including pneumonia, septicemia, meningitis, cellulitis, osteomyelitis, septic arthritis and skin and lymph node abscesses. The common causative organisms are similar to those seen in children with hypogammaglobulinemia and include pneumococci, non-typhi salmonellae, staphylococci, streptococci and *Haemophilus influenzae*, reflecting the B cell defect that accompanies destruction of the CD4 cells.

As noted above, despite the presence of hypergammaglobulinemia due to dysregulated polyclonal B cell activation, specific antibody responses are frequently absent either following infections or following immunizations. Studies of antibody levels following immunization with *H. influenzae* vaccine showed reduced levels in children with HIV infection compared with uninfected children, particularly in children with more progressive disease; in addition, at follow-up, antibody levels were not sustained.[202] Abnormal antibody function and avidity probably also play a role in the increased susceptibility to bacterial infections.

Lymphocytic interstitial pneumonitis

Lymphoid interstitial pneumonitis (LIP) is no longer included as a CDC stage C disease as it is associated with a better prognosis. It is characterized by multiple foci of proliferating lymphocytes in the lung interstitium and occurs in about 20–30% of vertically infected children, but is rare in adults or in children infected with HIV later in childhood. The cause of LIP is not clear. It may be an abnormal response to primary Epstein–Barr virus (EBV) infection. There are unsubstantiated data to suggest that it is more common in children of black African origin and may be due to early exposure to other pathogens such as EBV. Parotitis, prominent lymphadenopathy and very high immunoglobulin levels are frequently associated. It usually develops during the second year of life (and therefore should not be confused with PCP) and the child may have no clinical signs but persistent bilateral reticulonodular shadowing on chest X-ray. Alternatively in older children, clinical features may include chronic hypoxia and recurrent respiratory bacterial and viral infections with or without features of bronchospasm.[203]

The differential diagnosis includes other causes of interstitial pneumonitis including infection with *Mycobacterium tuberculosis*, which can be difficult to distinguish radiologically from LIP. Clinically a child with bilateral infiltrates due to TB would be highly symptomatic, as opposed to LIP which may be clinically silent. A definitive diagnosis of LIP requires lung biopsy but can be made presumptively on clinical grounds. The symptoms of LIP may respond to steroids, which was used in severe cases before the advent of HAART. Clinical and radiological features may regress over time with increasing immunodeficiency, in the absence of either steroids or antiretroviral therapy. The most important aspects of management include treating chest infections promptly, and treating bronchospasm if present with bronchodilators. Older children diagnosed late may already have chronic lung disease and present with a picture similar to cystic fibrosis (CF). Even with HAART, these children will continue to require treatment similar to those with CF, for recurrent chest infections, including antibiotic prophylaxis, regular physiotherapy and nutritional support.

HIV encephalopathy

Encephalopathy due to effects of HIV infection on the central nervous system is seen most frequently in the subgroup of children with rapid disease progression. The most common neurological manifestations are hypertonic diplegia, developmental delay (particularly affecting motor skills and expressive language) or acquired microcephaly.

Cranial imaging studies may show basal ganglia calcification and cerebral atrophy and MRI scans may show evidence of white matter damage. Seizures are not usually a feature of HIV encephalopathy, which does not tend to affect the gray matter. In older children, presentation is more similar to that observed in HIV dementia in adults and may include behavioral change and memory loss.

HIV encephalopathy is rarer with the advent of HAART, and particularly in children identified early with prospective follow-up. Even children in whom HIV is diagnosed late and who have signs of encephalopathy may respond well to HAART providing that neurological abnormalities have not been present for long.

Failure to thrive

Failure to thrive is a hallmark of HIV infection and is multifactorial in origin. In children, in addition to wasting, there is growth failure. Failure to gain weight in adults has been related most closely to decreased intake and the same is probably true for children.

Malignancy

The most common malignancy to occur in HIV infected children is non-Hodgkin's lymphoma (NHL). The incidence of lymphoma has been estimated to be about 1000-fold higher in HIV infected children compared with the normal population.[204] In HIV infected adults with access to HAART, some reduction in lymphoma risk has been reported for NHL and is also suggested for Hodgkin's disease,[205] but long term risks are as yet unknown, and may be related to duration of time spent in a state of immunosuppression. Success of treatment for lymphoma often depends on the state of immunosuppression. Response to standard chemotherapy may be good. Decisions such as whether to stop HAART therapy during chemotherapy need to be made on an individual basis taking account of the stage of HIV disease, ability of the patient to tolerate both ART and chemotherapy, as well as consideration of possible drug interactions.

Kaposi's sarcoma (KS), which is a common tumor in certain groups of adults with HIV, is associated with human herpes virus 8 (HHV8). It is uncommon in children except for those from endemic areas for the disease in Africa. As in adults cutaneous KS may regress with HAART alone,[205] but systemic disease may require additional treatment with liposomal daunorubicin. Cases have been reported of KS in both mother and child suggesting the MTCT of HHV8 may be responsible.[206]

MANAGEMENT

Recognition of testing

The recognition of HIV requires that the diagnosis is considered in any child presenting with a wide range of pediatric conditions. All pediatricians need to be able to hold a sensitive pretest discussion with caregivers explaining the benefit of early diagnosis, and the implications of a positive result for the family, including the fact that it will almost always indicate that the mother is HIV infected. To do this, there needs to be communication and collaboration with adult colleagues, and where HIV infection is rare in children, involvement of adult counselors and health advisors as and when appropriate (see below). This is in line with the new English Sexual Health and HIV Strategy published in July 2001.[207]

If a child is being adopted or entering long term foster care, consideration should be given to testing for HIV, hepatitis B and C; ideally maternal consent should be sought, to enable the mother to seek appropriate help for herself if any blood-borne viruses are detected, but if this is not possible, then the wishes of the adopting parents and welfare of the child should be of prime consideration.

Antiretroviral therapy

A detailed description of the many aspects of ART is beyond the scope of this chapter. This is a rapidly moving field with new drugs continually becoming available, and specialist input is required to manage children on ART. Guidelines for ART have been produced for adults[208,209] and children[210,211] and are regularly updated.

There are 16 drugs belonging to three different classes now available for treatment of HIV infection in adults (Table 25.21). In children, there is some lag in availability of drugs, particularly in the youngest children because of difficulties with development of appropriate formulations and undertaking of sufficient pharmacokinetic studies to assure correct dosing. However, increasingly, research is being undertaken in parallel in children, to ensure that pharmacokinetic and tolerability data are available in a timely manner. In addition to pharmaceutical company studies, there are two networks coordinating independent clinical trials in HIV infected children – the PACTG in the USA and the Paediatric European Network for Treatment of AIDS (PENTA, www.ctu.mrc.ac.uk/penta) in Europe. Both networks undertake trials addressing questions about management of ART in children (e.g. what to start with, when to switch, the value of resistance testing, etc.) as well as trials of specific drugs and drug combinations.

Combination ART has turned HIV into a treatable chronic disease of childhood. Until the mid-1990s, only one drug was available – zidovudine [ZDV, azidothymidine (AZT)]. Dual therapy was introduced in 1996/1997, following results of clinical trials in adults showing its superiority in terms of decreased disease progression to AIDS and mortality compared with monotherapy. Similar reductions in disease progression in children have been reported over calendar time but before the introduction of HAART, and can be attributed to increased use of prophylaxis against opportunistic infections, as well as use of double ART.[131,212] Triple (HAART) therapy became available for children in 1997/1998 and has led to further marked reductions in disease progression and mortality in HIV infected children in Europe and North America.[213] Eradication of HIV is not possible with current drugs and even after virus has been suppressed below the level of detectability in plasma (< 20 copies/mm^3 using HIV-1 RNA PCR) for several years in newly infected adults, after stopping therapy, HIV-1 RNA viral load rises promptly within 1–2 weeks. Most children on HAART remain clinically very well, thriving normally and asymptomatic. However, the complexity of life time administration of ART should not be underestimated. With increasing numbers of drugs available, yet

Table 25.21 Antiretroviral therapies

NRTIs	Protease inhibitors
– Zidovudine (ZDV)*	– Ritonavir †*
– Didanosine (ddI)*	– Nelfinavir †*
– (Dideoxycytidine*)	– Amprenavir ♦ †*
– Lamivudine (3TC)*	– Lopinavir ♦ †*
– Stavudine (d4T)*	– Indinavir ♦ †
– Abacavir (ABC)*♦	– Saquinavir ♦ †
Nucleotide TRIs	**Entry inhibitors**
– Tenofovir ♦ †	T-20 ♦ † (by injection)
NNRTIs	
– Nevirapine (NVP)*	
– Delavirdine ♦ †	
– Efavirenz (EFV) †*	

* Pediatric formulation
† Inadequate pharmacokinetic studies in infants
♦ Unlicensed in Europe

limited options for sequencing drugs within classes because of development of cross-resistance, it is important that expert consideration is given to when to start treatment, how best to sequence ART regimens, and how the whole family (other family members will often be on HAART as well) receive cohesive medical (generally outpatient) management, which is facilitated by attendance at a 'family-based' clinic (see below).

Monitoring HAART

As discussed above, CD4 cell count or percentage and HIV-1 RNA viral load in plasma are useful predictors of disease progression, although less so in children than in adults. In addition, they are used as surrogate markers for evaluating response to HAART, both as endpoint in clinical trials and for individual management of patients in clinical practice. Within 1 month of commencing HAART in children, the plasma HIV-1 RNA viral load substantially decreases (Fig. 25.29)[191] and the CD4 lymphocyte count starts to increase. There are differences between adults and children in both RNA and CD4 cell response to therapy. Infants with very high HIV-1 RNA viral load may take a longer time to reach an undetectable viral load,[214] possibly because children are starting from a higher viral load than adults. This higher baseline viral load seen in children may be one of the reasons that children have been reported to less commonly achieve an undetectable HIV RNA viral load.

Children's immune systems may also respond differently to HAART, due mainly to the fact that children have a much more active thymus than adults. Whereas in adults expansion of the CD45RO (memory cells) predominates, in children expansion is mainly of the CD45RA+ naive T cells which appear to be derived newly from the thymus.[185,215] Thus immune restoration in children may be more achievable than in adults, and studies are ongoing to further evaluate the quality of immune responses in children treated with HAART.

Most guidelines suggest that following HAART, children should have HIV-1 RNA viral load measured at 1 month and then both CD4 and viral load should be measured at 3 months to ensure that viral load is decreasing further and the CD4 cell count is starting to rise. Further measurements should be undertaken at least 3-monthly. Some centers perform tests more frequently although the benefits of more intense monitoring have not been evaluated in clinical trials. Weight gain and growth are also important.[216] Growth has been shown to be a sensitive marker of response to ART in HIV infected children, with significant differences reported in trials comparing different regimens, and reflecting HIV RNA response.[191] In the developing world with the advent of generic ART and cheaper drugs, and where the value of monitoring is being questioned because of cost, growth monitoring in children starting HAART may be a useful marker of response.

The goal of ART may vary according to the setting. Ideally, it is to achieve full virological suppression of HIV-1, associated with a restoration of both numbers and function of the immune system, alongside restoration of full growth and development potential for HIV infected children. This has to be balanced against the potential short and long term toxicity of ART and the effect of taking long term therapy on quality of life for the child, and family. Frequently and particularly in children, immunological and clinical responses to ART are good, but it is often more difficult to achieve full virological suppression of the virus. In such circumstances, the concern is the development of resistance which may jeopardize future treatment options (see below switching HAART).

When to start HAART

The PENTA 1 trial is the only trial addressing the issue of when to start ART in children, and, as in adults, showed no benefit from early therapy with ZDV monotherapy beyond about 6 months, due to the emergence of resistance.[212] There are no trials in adults or children addressing the question of when to start double or triple combination therapy. When HAART initially became available, guidelines based on a 'hit hard, hit early' approach recommended starting early in the disease course. Subsequently the development of cumulative adverse effects of long term HAART, as well as evidence of reasonable restoration of the immune system even when CD4 cell counts are low in adults and children, has resulted in adult guidelines being amended to start ART later in the disease course.[208,209] Guidelines for adults in the USA (currently start below CD4 350 cells/mm^3,[209]) have generally been more aggressive than UK (currently start all at CD4 cell count below 200 cells/mm^3 and consider for those between 200 and 350 cells/mm^3).[207]

In children, US guidelines have recommended starting HAART during infancy in all infants, if identified with HIV infection early in life.[210] Highly encouraging results have been reported with three or more drug combinations in selected, infected infants, which demonstrate that complete viral suppression and maintenance of entirely normal immune development can be achieved and sustained for at least 3 years.[217] However there are concerns about the lack of HIV specific immune responses seen,[217] and the problems of resistance and toxicity in those whose regimens fail.[218] Nonetheless, these successes in infants treated early with HAART, as well as studies of adults treated during primary infection, have provided a rationale for early aggressive therapy of infants. Another reason for promoting early treatment is that in infancy, viral load and CD4 cell counts are less predictive of outcome, and the anxiety this engenders tends to push towards starting HAART early as it can be difficult to distinguish the infant who will progress rapidly from the infant who remains asymptomatic for several years. However, the problem of inadequately defined pharmacokinetics for many drugs in infancy (and in particular, the PI class of drugs, such as nelfinavir in infants,[218]) and the likely adverse consequences of early prolonged therapy, particularly the long term adverse metabolic effects of lipid abnormalities (PI class of drugs) and mitochondrial effects (nucleoside analog class) are deterrents to such an approach. In addition, considerable support is required to enable families to sustain high levels of adherence long term. In Europe the approach is more cautious, and in the UK, children identified early in life are not necessarily started on HAART early, but if not, require very close observation. The differences between the US and European approach are summarized in Table 25.22.[210,211]

A number of factors need to be taken into account when starting ART in children, which rarely needs to be undertaken as an emergency (Table 25.22). Education of families, taking account of drugs other family members may be taking, as well as due care in choosing a regimen which the family can adhere to are important considerations. Frequency of dosing has been a major development and currently all drugs are given b.i.d. and the possibility of once daily regimens is becoming a reality. There is some evidence that adherence may be poorer among asymptomatic children who have never been ill. This disadvantage needs to be offset by the obvious desire to avoid children becoming seriously ill before starting ART. Educating parents and carers about following CD4 and viral load as predictors of progression at monitoring visits is important to ensure that a consensus between health professionals and the family is achieved about the right time to start therapy. Viral load and CD4% can fluctuate, and at least two or three values should be obtained. Time spent on preparing and educating the family before commencing ART is always important.

Older children presenting for the first time are a selected group who do not have rapid disease progression. For these children it is reasonable to monitor CD4 counts and only offer treatment if

Table 25.22 Antiretroviral therapy (ART) guidelines (US and European) for children

In children under 12 months	
US: Treat all	• Europe (draft):
	– Consider in all
	– Treat those with: symptoms (stage B or C)
	• RNA > 1 million copies
	• CD4% falling rapidly and/or < 25%
	• repeat surrogate markers to see trends
In children over 12 months	
US:	Europe (draft):
Start therapy in all (preferred approach) OR defer until	Clinical stage B or C
high or increasing RNA	CD4 < 25%
< 30 m – > 150 000	RNA > 100 000
> 30 m – > 20 000	
rapidly falling CD4	
clinical symptoms	
Indications for highly active ART (HAART)	
Clinical stage C (AIDS) or immunological stage 3 disease (CD4% < 15%)	
Consider if:	
Clinical stage B or CD4 < 20% or very high VL (> 6 log if age < 1 year, > 5 log if age over 1 year)	
Defer if:	
Stage N or A disease, and	
CD4 > 20%, and,	
VL (< 6 log if age < 1 year, and 5 log if age over 1 year)	
What HAART to start?	
Either:	2 NRTI + 1 PI (PI: NFV or Lopinavir/r) plus NRTI combinations: ZDV + ddI; ZDV + 3TC; ddI + d4T, d4T + 3TC; 3TC + ABC
Or:	EFV + 2 NRTI (if over 3 years)
	NVP + 2 NRTI (all ages)
Or:	3 NRTI: ZDV + 3TC + Abacavir

For definitions of stages see Table 25.19.

counts are declining steadily below 20% (Table 25.22).[211] In children over 9 or 10 years, CD4 guidelines for starting ART in adults and adolescents can increasingly be used. There is no consensus level of viral load above which treatment must be started in children.

Which ART to start

When starting HAART, most prescribers would initiate triple therapy with two NRTI drugs and one PI or one NNRTI. Quadruple combination therapy, sparing at least one class of drugs is another possible option as is the use of three NRTIs, particularly if the potent abacavir is included (see Table 25.22). The PI drugs are difficult to formulate into palatable suspensions for children compared with the NRTIs and NNRTIs. No data in children or adults provide evidence to conclude that PI containing or PI sparing regimens have greater long term clinical efficacy. This question is being addressed in ongoing clinical trials in both adults and children (see www.ctu.mrc.ac.uk/penta for details about the PEPACT1 trial which will be starting in 2002).

Data from the UK and Ireland CHIPS study[219] show that most children start HAART with a triple regimen and in approximately half, this is PI based and in the other half it is NNRTI based. The main PI used has been nelfinavir but increasingly this is being replaced by lopinavir. NVP is the main NNRTI in young children but efavirenz is increasingly being used in children over 3 years (the dosage for younger children is under study). The role of a triple NRTI based initial regimen has been less investigated in children but is increasingly used in adults as trizivir is available as a 'three-in-one' combination pill of ZDV, lamivudine and abacavir. However, no combination fluid formulation is available. Use of crushed whole or half tablets requires care as some pills (e.g. combivir, which contains ZDV and lamivudine have these drugs unevenly distributed through the tablet.

There is considerable variation in drug levels achieved even when using standard ART doses for size. The role of therapeutic drug monitoring (TDM) has not been clearly defined in pediatrics but is being increasingly undertaken and requires further research. TDM is definitely indicated where there is the possibility of drug interactions.

Adherence

It has become very clear from adult and pediatric studies that adherence is one of the principal determinants of both the degree and duration of virological suppression.[220] In one recent study, children whose caregivers reported no missed doses in the previous week, were more likely to have an undetectable viral load (50% vs 24%).[219] The reasons for non-adherence are complex and multifactorial. Adherence is difficult to assess in the clinic. No pediatric intervention studies aimed at improving adherence have been conducted, but one is planned through PENTA.

Changing therapy

Virological failure requires investigation into the potency of the regimen, including checking that the child is on the correct dose (which may be higher than the recommended dose in drug packet inserts[210,211]) and that the child has not outgrown their dose, checking for possibile pharmacokinetic interactions with other drugs or food, and checking on adherence. These should all be done before switching therapy.

There are concerns that virological failure may lead to resistance and therefore fewer options for second-line therapy, and eventually lead to immunological and subsequent clinical progression. Despite this, many pediatricians currently delay changing therapy if the child has no sign of clinical or immunological progression. Families and doctors often wish to continue the current regimen when the child is clinically and immunologically stable, and there is not an obvious easy palatable regimen to switch to. The choice of the new regimen will depend on the prior ART history, drug toxicity, availability of new drugs, and if available, maybe guided by resistance testing, although its role has not been fully defined.[221] A clinical trial to evaluate the role of resistance testing is currently ongoing in Europe (PENTA 8, PERA, ctu.mrc.ac.uk/penta).

Toxicity

Lipodystrophy (LD) is defined as abnormality in lipid metabolism resulting in dyslipidemia (high lipids) and body changes characterized by truncal obesity alongside disfiguring loss of fat on the face and in the periphery. It is associated particularly with the PI class of drugs and with stavudine (d4T). In the first major pediatric survey on LD, Babl et al[222] reported a 1% prevalence in PACTG centers in 1999. However, studies are hampered by the lack of a standard definition of LD in the growing child, and many reports are clearly subjective. Hyperlipidemia is being increasingly reported, but currently most clinicians are not changing ART therapy or treating with cholesterol lowering drugs. There are an increasing number of reports of bone demineralization, glucose intolerance, and lactic acidemia in children.[223]

As toxicity associated with long term continuous ART becomes more apparent, new strategies including structured treatment interruptions and immune therapies need evaluation in children as well as in adults and trials are planned in the USA and Europe. The former may also be important in providing more cost-effective ART to children in low- and middle-income countries.

Prophylaxis against opportunistic infections

Co-trimoxazole prophylaxis for prevention of PCP

There is good evidence from randomized trials in adults with HIV that co-trimoxazole is very effective at preventing PCP and this is the preferred drug to use. Dapsone or inhaled pentamidine can be used in the event of hypersensitivity to co-trimoxazole but they are less efficacious. The evidence for efficacy of co-trimoxazole in preventing PCP in infants with HIV is indirect, and comes from studies showing decreased PCP after the introduction of guidelines recommending starting all babies on co-trimoxazole.[133,224,225] Provided HIV infected mothers are identified during pregnancy, infants are recommended to be started on PCP prophylaxis from around 4–6 weeks of age onwards. Prophylaxis can be stopped once it has been established that the baby is uninfected. Infected children not on HAART should continue on prophylaxis throughout the first year of life, as CD4 counts are unreliable indicators of risk. Thereafter, it is not unreasonable to stop prophylaxis unless the CD4% is under 15%. As in adults, co-trimoxazole is the drug of choice. The dose is based on 900 mg/m^2 and can be given daily or three times weekly.

The MTCT rates are now so low in Europe and the USA that, coupled with the ability to exclude HIV infection by 3 months of age, the use of PCP prophylaxis has decreased. Many would suggest it can now be restricted to babies born to mothers who do not take interventions in pregnancy to reduce MTCT, or have a high risk of MTCT (e.g. because of detectable HIV RNA viral load at delivery) or babies where the mother is reluctant for the baby to be tested early in life.[152] Individual decisions about this need to be discussed with the family.

Recent guidelines for PCP prophylaxis in adults permit discontinuation of both primary and secondary PCP prophylaxis when the CD4 cell count is above 200 cells/μl for greater than 3 months in response to HAART. In pediatric practice, there is only limited evidence of safe discontinuation of primary prophylaxis when CD4 count has increased above 15% on HAART,[226] and clear guidelines have not been produced. In practice many pediatricians are discontinuing prophylaxis when CD4% is above 20–25%, and approximately half the children on HAART in the UK are not on PCP prophylaxis. In all children, whether or not they are on HAART, primary prophylaxis, guidelines recommend restarting co-trimoxazole when the CD4% falls below 15%. Life long secondary prophylaxis is still recommended for babies who have had PCP.[162] The need for this requires further study as in practice, with good immune reconstitution on HAART, many pediatricians are stopping it.

Prophylaxis against other infections

As a result of advances in antiretroviral therapy, there has been a shift in focus from diagnosing, managing and preventing opportunistic infections to restoring and maintaining cellular immunity with HAART and thereby preventing opportunistic infections.

HIV infected children who are contacts of individuals with open pulmonary TB should be carefully assessed, bearing in mind skin testing is frequently unhelpful because of anergy. If there is no evidence of infection, prophylactic isoniazid for 6 months, or isoniazid plus rifampicin for 3 months is recommended. Prophylaxis against *Mycobacterium avium-intracellulare* in children is not recommended because of adverse reactions and the potential for resistance and breakthrough on single agents such as rifabutin.

Primary prophylaxis against CMV is not recommended. With respect to secondary prophylaxis following CMV infection, infants who have had CMV usually reconstitute their immune systems very well obviating the need for secondary prophylaxis.

For most other established opportunistic infections, such as cryptosporidiosis for which there were few useful therapeutic options, the best treatment is HAART, which should be started as soon as possible if a child newly presents with HIV infection and an acute opportunistic infection. Immune reconstitution disease, which may occur particularly in severely immunocompromised children may make opportunistic infection symptoms worse initially. Supportive treatment for opportunistic infections such as cryptosporidiosis may be required alongside HAART.

LIP and chronic lung disease

Among HIV infected children now being diagnosed early in life, regular monitoring of HIV disease, prompt aggressive treatment of chest infections with antibiotic and physiotherapy, treatment of any bronchospasm with bronchodilators and inhaled steroids, and timely initiation of HAART, should all help to prevent chronic lung disease from developing, particularly in children with underlying LIP.

However, among older children who already have residual damaged lungs from early childhood infections before they started on HAART, and among those newly diagnosed who acquired HIV in other countries, chronic lung disease with bronchiectasis may continue to cause major problems even if the child responds well to HAART. Children in this situation need to be managed like children with other chronic lung disease (e.g. cystic fibrosis), with regular physiotherapy, increased nutritional support (which may require insertion of PEG for additional feeding), prophylactic oral or inhaled antibiotics, and prompt treatment of acute chest infections.

Immunizations

Children with HIV infection should be immunized according to normal schedules with both live and killed vaccines. The exceptions are that BCG is not advised for children with HIV infection in low prevalence areas because of the risk of dissemination. However, it should be given in areas of high TB prevalence and this, in the author's view, should include giving to babies born to African women in the UK who have a high rate of TB and may also return to Africa either to live or to visit. Inactivated polio vaccine (IPV) is to be preferred to live oral polio vaccine, because of theoretical concerns about paralytic poliomyelitis in contacts of children excreting live virus. However IPV may be difficult to obtain and in view of the low risk and low transmission rates, many units condone the use of oral polio vaccine. Pneumococcal polysaccharide vaccine has been recommended for HIV infected children over 2 years of age, but a trial of its use in adults with HIV in Africa showed no benefit. The new conjugate vaccine can be given to younger children and results of a trial in South Africa are awaited.

The efficacy of all vaccines is improved among children who have immune reconstitution following ART, and children immunized before starting ART in whom responses are inadequate should probably be revaccinated.

Passive immunization of symptomatic children with CD4% < 15% is recommended if they are in contact with varicella zoster virus (VZV) and are either VZV naive or have no detectable specific antibodies to VZV. Varicella zoster immunoglobulin (VZIG) ideally should be given within 72 h of contact. VZIG may prolong the incubation period to 28 days, so clinicians need to consider isolating these patients at clinic visits. Similarly normal human immunoglobulin should be given for susceptible symptomatic children in contact with measles.

Regular intravenous immunoglobulin infusions (400 mg/kg every 28 days) should only rarely be given to children with recurrent bacterial infections despite good compliance with co-trimoxazole prophylaxis, or those with proven hypogammaglobulinemia. Higher doses may be useful in the management of thrombocytopenia (0.5–1.0 g/dose every day, for 3–5 days). However, in the era of HAART, the number of children requiring such therapy de novo should be minimal.

Supportive care

Unlike most other severe chronic diseases of children, HIV simultaneously affects family members including the parents and other siblings. The parents' own health, their social isolation and feelings of guilt compound the difficulties of caring for a sick child. An effective well coordinated multidisciplinary team is required to address the changing needs of infected and affected children and their care givers. Continuity of care between inpatient and outpatient services, local referring hospitals and the community needs to be developed. Ideally adults and children should be treated in family based units.[227] All too often parents will ignore their own health needs because they put their children first.

Increasingly the work of the multidisciplinary team has shifted towards ways of helping families achieve long term adherence to HAART. As children survive longer, meeting the needs of adolescents and planning transition to adult clinics is placing new demands on services. The decision as to who should be informed should be tailored individually. Families may need help in explaining the diagnosis to older children. This needs to be undertaken at the child's pace, and is frequently most effectively achieved in gradual steps. It is not mandatory to tell staff at schools, as universal precautions should be employed for all children with injuries. The risks of transmission from casual contacts in school or daycare settings are virtually zero. Ensuring that adolescents are well informed and responsible before they become sexually active themselves is a priority and increasingly, pediatric family clinics in London are setting up specific adolescent clinics with their adult colleagues. Peer support for adolescents through organizations such as 'Teen Spirit' at 'Body and Soul' is important to help young people infected and affected by HIV to come to terms and live with their disease.

The multidisciplinary team should include a dietitian, as nutritional problems and growth faltering are not uncommon, even in the era of HAART, and particularly in children with chronic lung disease. Balanced supplements are sometimes required and enteral feeding through gastrostomy tubes may be necessary. Gastrostomy tubes have been used with success to allow unpalatable medicines to be given. However, with increasing choice of antiretorviral drugs, this should not often be required.

Pain management is of importance in late stage disease. Complementary therapies which are frequently used in adults in late disease, such as aromatherapy may be useful and require evaluation. With the continuing success of HAART, there are currently very few children in industrialized countries needing palliative or terminal care. However if new treatments and treatment strategies do not continue to become available, some children may run out of therapeutic options over the coming years, and this is already occurring in the USA.

Prevention remains the top priority in managing HIV infection in children. Reducing national perinatal transmission rates to below 2% is an achievable target that can only be realized if HIV infected mothers can be identified prenatally and offered appropriate interventions. This will require continued effort by health professionals, public health planners and community organizations.

REFERENCES (* Level 1 evidence)

1 Steihm RE, ed. Immunological disorders in infants and children, 4th edn. Philadelphia: WB Saunders; 1996.

2 Turner MW. Mannose-binding lectin: the pluripotent molecule of the innate immune system. Immunol Today 1996; 17:532–540.

3 Klein C, Lisowska-Grospierre B, LeDeist F, et al. Major histocompatibility complex class II deficiency: clinical manifestations, immunologic features, and outcome. J Pediatr 1993; 123:921–928.

4 Steihm ER, Fulginiti V. Immunological disorders in infants and children, 2nd edn. Philadelphia: Saunders; 1980.

5 Burgio GR, Hanson LA, Ugazio AG, eds. Immunology of the neonate. Berlin: Springer-Verlag; 1987.

6 Marshall-Clarke S, Reen D, Tasker L, et al. Neonatal immunity: how well has it grown up? Immunol Today 2000; 21:35–41.

7 Miller ME, Steihm ER. Immunology and resistance to infection. In: Remington JS, Klein JO, eds. Infectious diseases of the fetus and newborn infant. Philadelphia: Saunders; 1983.

8 Hayward AR, Lydyard PM. B cell function in the newborn. Pediatrics 1979;64(suppl): 758–764.

9 Hill HR. Biochemical, structural and functional abnormalities of polymorphonuclear leukocytes in the neonate. Pediatr Res 1987; 22:375–382.

10 Cairo MS. Neonatal neutrophil host defence: prospects for immunologic enhancement during neonatal sepsis. Am J Dis Child 1989; 143:40–46.

11 Ferguson AG. Prolonged impairment of cellular immunity in children with intrauterine growth retardation. J Pediatr 1978; 93:52-56.

12 Shapiro R, Beatty DW, Woods DL, et al. Serum complement and immunoglobulin values in small for gestational age infants. J Pediatr 1981; 99:139–142.

13 Oxelius VA. IgG subclass levels in infancy and childhood. Acta Pediatr Scand 1979; 68:23–27.

14 Choo S, Seymour L, Morris R, et al. Immunogenicity and reactogenicity of a pneumococcal conjugate vaccine administered combined with a *haemophilus influenzae* type B conjugate vaccine in United Kingdom infants. Pediatr Infect Dis J 2000; 19:854–862.

15 Rosen FS, Wedgewood RJ, Yang X, et al. Primary immunodeficiency diseases. Report of a WHO Scientific Group. Clin Exp Immunol 1995; 99(suppl 1):1–24.

16 Rosen FS, Eibl M, Roifman C, et al. Report of an IUIS Scientific Committee: primary immunodeficiency diseases. Clin Exp Immunol 1999; 118(suppl 1):1–28.

17 Hosking CS, Roberton DM. Epidemiology and treatment of hypogammaglobulinaemia. Birth Defects Orig Artic Ser 1983; 19:223–227.

18 [Anonymous]. Proceedings of the Jeffrey Modell immunodeficiency symposium. Advances in primary immunodeficiency disease. Clin Immunol Immunopathol 1995; 76: S145–232.

19 Buckley RH. Breakthroughs in the understanding and therapy of primary immunodeficiency. Clin Immunol 1994; 41:665–690.

20 Fischer A, Arnaiz-Villena A. Immunodeficiences of genetic origin. Immunol Today 1995; 16:510–514.

21 Puck JM. Molecular and genetic basis of X-linked immunodeficiency disorders. J Clin Immunol 1994; 14:81–89.

22 Levy J, Espanol-Boren T, Thomas C, et al. Clinical spectrum of X-linked hyper-IgM syndrome. J Pediatr 1997; 131:47–54.

23 Hague RA, Rassam S, Morgan G, et al. Early diagnosis of severe combined immune deficiency syndrome. Arch Dis Child 1994; 70: 260–263.

24 Ochs HD, Slichter SJ, Harker LA, et al. The Wiskott–Aldrich syndrome: studies of lymphocytes, granulocytes and platelets. Blood 1980; 55:243–252.

25 Gadjeva M, Thiel S, Jensenius JC. The mannan-binding-lectin pathway of the innate immune response. Curr Opin Immunol 2001; 13:74–78.

26 Pyun KH, Ochs HD, Wedgewood RJ, et al. Human antibody responses to bacteriophage ΦX174: sequential induction of IgM and IgG subclass antibody. Clin Immunol Immunopathol 1989; 51:252–263.

27 Ochs HD, Davis SD, Wedgewood JR. Immunologic responses to bacteriophage φX174

in immunodeficiency diseases. J Clin Invest 1971; 50:2559.

28 Comans-Bitter WM, de Groot R, van den Beemd R, et al. Immunophenotyping of blood lymphocytes in childhood. Reference values for lymphocyte subpopulations. J Pediatr 1997; 130:388–393.

29 Gilmour KC, Cranston T, Loughlin S, et al. Rapid protein-based assays for the diagnosis of T-B+ severe combined immunodeficiency. Br J Haematol 2001; 112:671–676.

30 Buckley RH. Primary immunodeficiency diseases due to defects in lymphocytes. N Engl J Med 2000; 343:1313–1324.

31 Fischer A. Severe combined immunodeficiencies (SCID). Clin Exp Immunol 2000; 122:143–149.

32 Muller SM, Ege M, Pottharst A, et al. Transplacentally acquired maternal T lymphocytes in severe combined immunodeficiency: a study of 121 patients. Blood 2001; 98;1847–1851.

33 Notarangelo LD, Villa A, Schwarz K. RAG and RAG defects. Curr Opin Immunol 1999; 11:435–442.

34 Hirschhorn R, Vauter GF, Kirkpatrick JA Jr, et al. Adenosine deaminase deficiency frequency and comparative pathology in autosomally recessive severe combined immunodeficiency. Clin Immunol Immunopathol 1979; 14:107–120.

35 Cederbaum SD, Kaitila I, Rimoin DL, et al. The chondro-osseous dysplasia of adenosine deaminase deficiency with severe combined immunodeficiency. J Pediatr 1976; 89:737–742.

36 Rogers M, Lwin R, Fairbanks L, et al. Cognitive and behavioural abnormalities in adenosine deaminase deficient severe combined deficiency. J Pediatr 2001; 139:44–50.

37 Hershfield MS. Immunodeficiency caused by adenosine deaminase deficiency. Immunol Allerg Clin North Am 2000; 20:161–175.

38 Cohen A, Grunebaum E, Arpaia E, et al. Immunodeficiency caused by purine nucleoside phosphorylase deficiency. Immunol Allerg Clin North Am 2000; 20:143–159.

39 Soutar RL, Day RE. Dysequilibrium/ataxic diplegia with immunodeficiency. Arch Dis Child 1991; 66:982–983.

40 Elder ME, Hope TJ, Parslow TG, et al. Severe combined immunodeficiency with absence of peripheral blood CD8+ T cells due to ZAP-70 deficiency. Cell Immunol 1995; 165:110–117.

41 Piketty C, Weiss L, Kazatchkine M. Idiopathic CD4 lymphocytopenia. Presse Med 1994; 23:1374–1375.

42 Fry TJ, Connick E, Falloon J, et al. A potential for interleukin 7 in T lymphocyte homeostasis. Blood 2001; 97:2983–2990.

43 Signorini S, Pirovano S, Fiorentini S, et al. Restriction of T lymphocyte receptor repertoires in idiopathic CD4 lymphocytopaenia. Br J Haematol 2000; 110:434–437.

44 Cunningham-Rundles C, Murray HW, Smith JP. Treatment of idiopathic CD4 lymphocytopaenia with IL 2. Clin Exp Immunol 1999; 116:322–325.

45 Masternak K, Muhlethaler-Mottet A, Villard J, et al. Molecular genetics of the Bare lymphocyte syndrome. Rev Immunogenet 2000; 2:267–282.

46 de la Salle H, Hanau D, Fricker D, et al. Homozygous human TAP peptide transporter mutation in HLA class I deficiency. Science 1994; 265:237–241.

47 Lammer EJ, Opitz JM. The DiGeorge anomaly as a developmental field defect. Am J Genet 1986; 2(suppl):113–127.

48 Driscoll DA, Sullivan KE. DiGeorge syndrome: a chromosome 22q11.2 deletion syndrome. In: Ochs HD, Smith CIE, Puck JM, eds. Primary immunodeficiency diseases; a molecular and genetic approach. Oxford: Oxford University Press; 1999:198–207.

49 Nonoyama S, Ochs HD. Characterization of the Wiskott–Aldrich syndrome protein and its role in the disease. Curr Opin Immunol 1998; 10:407–412.

50 Thrasher AJ, Kinnon C. The Wiskott–Aldrich syndrome. Clin Exp Immunol 2000; 120:2–9.

51 Filipovich AH, Stone JV, Tomany SC, et al. Impact of donor type on outcome of bone marrow transplantation for Wiskott–Aldrich syndrome: collaborative study of the International Bone Marrow Transplant Registry and the National Marrow Donor Program. Blood 2001; 97:1598–1603.

52 Notarangelo LD, Hayward AR. X-linked immunodeficiency with hyper-IgM (XHIM). Clin Exp Immunol 2000; 120:399–405.

53 Bleesing JHJ, Straus SE, Fleisher TA. Autoimmune lymphoproliferative syndrome: a human disorder of abnormal lymphocyte survival. Pediatr Clin North Am 2000; 47:1291–1310.

54 Straus SE, Jaffe ES, Puck JM, et al. The development of lymphomas in families with autoimmune lymphoproliferative syndrome with germline Fas mutation defective apoptosis. Blood 2001; 98:194–200.

55 Purtilo DT, Cassel CK, Yang JPS, et al. X-linked recessive progressive combined variable immunodeficiency (Duncan's disease). Lancet 1975; I:935–940.

56 Morra M, Howie D, Simarro Grande M, et al. X-linked lymphoproliferative disease: a progressive immunodeficiency. Annu Rev Immunol 2001; 19:657–682.

57 Coffey AJ, Brooksbank RA, Brandau O, et al. Host response to EBV infection in X-linked lymphoproliferative disease results from mutations in an SH2-domain encoding gene. Nat Genet 1998; 20:129–135.

58 Sumegi J, Huang D, Lanyi A, et al. Correlation of mutations of the SH2D1A gene and Epstein–Barr virus infection with clinical phenotype and outcome in X-linked lymphoproliferative disease. Blood 2000; 96:3118–3125.

59 Kirkpatrick CH. Chronic mucocutaneous candidiasis. Pediatr Infect Dis J 2001; 20: 197–206.

60 Lilic D, Calvert JE, Cant AJ, et al. Chronic mucocutaneous candidiasis. II. Class and subclass of specific antibody responses in vivo and in vitro. Clin Exp Immunol 1996; 105: 213–219.

61 Makitie O, Kaitla I, Savilahti E. Susceptibility to infections and in vitro immune functions in cartilage–hair hypoplasia. Eur J Pediatr 1998; 157:816–820.

62 Makitie O, Kaitla I. Cartilage-hair hypoplasia – clinical manifestations in 108 Finnish patients. Eur J Pediatr 1993; 152:211–217.

63 Gennery AR, Cant AJ, Jeggo PA. Immunodeficiency associated with DNA repair defects. Clin Exp Immunol 2000; 121:1–7.

64 Savitsky K, Bar-Shira A, Gilad S, et al. A single ataxia telangiectasia gene with a product similar to PI-3 kinase. Science 1995; 268:1749–1753.

65 Lavin MF, Shiloh Y. The genetic defect in ataxia-telangiectasia. Annu Rev Immunol 1997; 15:177–202.

66 Hiel JA, Weemaes CM, van den Heuvel LP, et al. Nijmegen breakage syndrome. Arch Dis Child 2000; 82:400–406.

67 Varon R, Vissinga C, Platzer M, et al. Nibrin, a novel DNA double-strand break repair protein is mutated in Nijmegen breakage syndrome. Cell 1998; 93:467–476.

68 Joenje H, Patel KJ. The emerging genetic and molecular basis of Fanconi anaemia. Nat Rev Genet 2001; 2:446–457.

69 Doffinger R, Smahi A, Bessia C, et al. X-linked anhidrotic ectodermal dysplasia with immunodeficiency is caused by impaired NF-kappaB signalling. Nat Genet 2001; 27:277–285.

70 Brown DC, Grace E, Sumner AT, et al. ICF syndrome (immunodeficiency, centromeric instability and facial anomalies): investigation of heterochromatin abnormalities and review of outcome. Hum Genet 1995; 96:411–416.

71 Bruton OC. Agammaglobulinaemia. Pediatrics 1952; 9:722–727.

72 Lederman HM, Winkelstein JA. X-linked agammaglobulinaemia: an analysis of 96 patients. Medicine 1985; 64:145–156.

73 Spickett GP, Chapel HM. Report on the audit of patients with primary antibody deficiency in the United Kingdom 1993–1996. Royal Victoria Infirmary. 1999

74 Hermaszweski RA, Webster ADB. Primary hypogammaglobulinaemia: a survey of clinical manifestations and complications. Q J Med 1993; 86:31–42.

75 Gaspar HB, Lester T, Levinsky RJ, et al. Bruton's tyrosine kinase expression and activity in X- linked agammaglobulinaemia (XLA). Clin Exp Immunol 1998; 111:334–338.

76 Quartier P, Debre M, De Blic J, et al. Early and prolonged intravenous immunoglobulin replacement therapy in childhood agammaglobulinaemia: a retrospective survey of 31 patients. J Pediatr 1999; 134:589–596.

77 Richter D, Conley ME, Rorher J, et al. A contiguous deletion syndrome of X-linked agammaglobulinaemia and sensori-neural deafness. Pediatr Allerg Immunol 2001; 12: 107–111.

78 Grunebaum E. Agammaglobulinaemia caused by defects other than btk. Immunol Allerg Clin North Am 2001; 21:45–63.

79 Vorechovsky I, Cullen M, Carrington M, et al. Fine mapping of IGAD1 in IgA deficiency and common variable immunodeficiency: identification and characterization of haplotypes shared by affected members of 101 multiple-case families. J Immunol 2000; 164:4408–4416.

80 Gilmour KC, Cranston T, Jones A, et al. Diagnosis of X-linked lymphoproliferative

disease by analysis of SLAM-associated protein expression. Eur J Immunol 2000; 30: 1691–1697.
81 Kanegane H, Tsukada S, Iwata T, et al. Detection of Bruton's tyrosine kinase mutations in hypogammaglobulinaemic males registered as common variable immunodeficiency (CVID) in the Japanese Immunodeficiency Registry. Clin Exp Immunol 2000; 120:512–517.
82 Spickett GP, Farrant J, North ME, et al. Common variable immunodeficiency: how many diseases? Immunol Today 1997; 18:325–328.
83 Cunningham-Rundles C, Bodian C. Common variable immunodeficiency: clinical and immunological features of 248 patients. Clin Immunol 1999; 92:34–48.
84 Liblau RS, Bach JF. Selective IgA deficiency and autoimmunity. Int Arch Allerg Immunol 1992; 99:16–27.
85 Shackleford PG. IgG subclasses: importance in pediatric practice. Pediatr Rev 1993; 14:291–296.
86 Pan Q, Hammarstrom L. Molecular basis of IgG subclass deficiency. Immunol Rev 2000; 178:99–110.
87 Fischer A, Segal AW, Seger R, et al. The management of chronic granulomatous disease. Eur J Pediatr 1993; 152:896–899.
88 Cale CM, Jones AM, Goldblatt D. Follow up of patients with chronic granulomatous disease diagnosed since 1990. Clin Exp Immunol 2000; 120:351–355.
89 Finn A, Hadzic N, Morgan G, et al. Prognosis of chronic granulomatous disease. Arch Dis Child 1990; 65:942–945.
90 Winkelstein JA, Marino MC, Johnston RB Jr, et al. Chronic granulomatous disease. Report on a national registry of 368 patients. Medicine (Baltimore) 2000; 79:155–169.
91 Horwitz M, Benson KF, Person RE, et al. Mutations in ELA2, encoding neutrophil elastase, define a 21-day biological block in cyclic haematopoiesis. Nat Genet 1999; 23:433–436.
92 Kostman R. Infantile genetic agranulocytosis. Acta Paediatr Scand 1956; 45(suppl):1–78.
93 Devriendt K, Kim AS, Mathijs G, et al. Constitutively activating mutation in WASP causes X-linked severe congenital neutropenia. Nat Genet 2001; 27:313–317.
94 Kasper B, Tidow N, Grothues D, et al. Differential expression and regulation of GTPases (RhoA and Rac2) and GDIs (LyGDI and RhoGDI) in neutrophils from patients with severe congenital neutropenia. Blood 2000; 95:2947–2953.
95 Lekstrom-Himes JA, Dorman SE, Kopar P, et al. Neutrophil-specific granule deficiency results from a novel mutation with loss of function of the transcription factor CCAAT/enhancer binding protein. J Exp Med 1999; 189:1847–1852.
96 Barbosa MDFS, Barrat FJ, Tchernev VT, et al. Identification of mutations in two major mRNA isoforms of the Chediak–Higashi syndrome gene in human and mouse. Hum Mol Genetics 1997; 6:1091–1098.
97 Klein C, Phillipe N, LeDeist F, et al. Partial albinism with immunodeficiency (Griscelli syndrome). J Pediatr 1994; 125:886–895.
98 Stepp SE, Dufourcq-Lagelouse R, Le Deist F, et al. Perforin gene defects in familial hemophagocytic lymphohistiocytosis. Science 1999; 286:1957–1959.
99 Crowley CA, Curnutte JT, Rosin RE, et al. An inherited abnormality of neutrophil adhesion: its genetic transmission and its association with a missing protein. N Engl J Med 1980; 302:1163–1168.
100 Inwald D, Davies EG, Klein NJ. Demystified...adhesion molecule deficiencies. Mol Pathol 2001; 54:1–7.
101 Etzioni A, Frydman M, Pollack S, et al. Recurrent severe infections caused by a novel leukocyte adhesion deficiency. N Engl J Med 1992; 327:1789–1792.
102 Remus N, Reichenbach J, Picard C, et al. Impaired interferon gamma-mediated immunity and susceptibility to mycobacterial infection in childhood. Pediatr Res 2001; 50:8–13.
102a Buckley RH. The hyper-IgE syndrome. Clin Rev Allergy Immunol 2001; 20:139–154.
102c Grimbacher B, Holland SM, Gallin JI, et al. Hyper-IgE syndrome with recurrent infections – an autosomal dominant multisystem disorder. N Engl Med 1999; 340:692–702.
102d Grimbacher B, Schaffer AA, Holland SM et al. Generic linkage of hyper-IgE syndrome to chromosome 4, Am J Hum Genet 1999; 65:735–744.
102e Gennery AR, Flood TJ, Abinun M, Cant AJ. Bone marrow transplantation does not correct the hyper IgE syndrome. Bone Marrow Transplant 2000; 25:1303–1305.
103 Bowness P, Davies KA, Norsworthy PJ, et al. Hereditary C1q deficiency and systemic lupus erythematosus. Q J Med 1994; 87:455–464.
104 Fijen CAP, Kuijper EJ, Bulte MT, et al. Assessment of complement deficiency in patients with meningococcal disease in the Netherlands. Clin Infect Dis 1999; 28:98–105.
105 Tedesco F, Nürnberger W, Perissutti S. Inherited deficiencies of the terminal complement components. Int Rev Immunol 1993; 10:51–64.
106 Hoare S, El-Shazali O, Clark JE, et al. Investigation for complement deficiency following meningococcal disease. Arch Dis Child 2002; 86:215–217.
107 Super M, Thiel S, Lu J, et al. Association of low levels of mannan binding protein with a common defect of opsonisation. Lancet 1989; ii:1236–1239.
108 Madsen HO, Garred P, Thiel S, et al. Interplay between promotor and structural gene variants control basal serum level of mannan-binding protein. J Immunol 1995; 155:3013–3020.
109 Davies EJ, Snowden H, Hillarby MC, et al. Mannose binding gene polymorphisms in systemic lupus erythematosus. Arthritis Rheum 1995; 38:110–114.
110 Lamelin J-P, Lenoir GM. Immunodeficiency secondary to viral infection. In: Chandra RK, ed. Primary and secondary immunodeficiency disorders. Edinburgh: Churchill Livingstone; 1983:204–218.
111 Ilan Y, Shouval D, Ashur Y, et al. IgA deficiency associated with chronic hepatitis C virus infection. Arch Intern Med 1993; 153:1588–1592.
112 Mukwaya G. Immunosuppressive effects and infections associated with corticosteroid therapy. Pediatr Infect Dis J 1988; 7:499–504.
113 Rogers TR. Prevention of infection in neutropenic bone marriw transplant patients. Antibiot Chemother 1985; 33:90–113.
114 Chandra RK. Nutrition and the immune system: an introduction. Am J Clin Nutr 1997; 66:460S–463S.
115 Skinner R, Cant A, Davies G, et al. Immunisation of the immunocompromised child. Best Practice Statement, London: Royal College of Paediatrics and Child Health; 2002.
116 Spickett GP, Bullimore J, Wallis J, et al. Northern Region asplenia register – analysis of first two years. J Clin Pathol 1999; 52:424–429.
117 Cavill I, for the Working party of the British committee for standards in haematology clinical haematology task force. Guidelines for the prevention and treatment of infection in patients with an absent or dysfunctional spleen. BMJ 1996; 312:430–434.
118 Chapel HM. Safety and availability of immunoglobulin replacement therapy in relation to potentially transmissible agents. Clin Exp Immunol 1999; 118(suppl):29–34.
119 Misbah SA, Chapel HM. Adverse effects of intravenous immunoglobulin. Drug Saf 1993; 9:254–262.
120 Chapel HM, Spickett GP, Ericson D, et al. The comparison of the efficacy and safety of intravenous versus subcutaneous immunoglobulin replacement therapy. J Clin Immunol 2000; 20:94–100.
121 Jabado N, Le Deist F, Cant A, et al. Bone marrow transplantation from genetically HLA-nonidentical donors in children with fatal inherited disorders excluding severe combined immunodeficiencies: use of two monoclonal antibodies to prevent graft rejection. Pediatrics 1996; 98:420–428.
122 Bertrand Y, Landais P, Friedrich W, et al. Influence of severe combined immunodeficiency phenotype on the outcome of HLA non-identical, T-cell-depleted bone marrow transplantation. J Pediatr 1999; 134:740–748.
123 Buckley RH, Schiff SE, Schiff RI, et al. Hematopoietic stem-cell transplantation for the treatment of severe combined immunodeficiency. N Engl J Med 1999; 340:508–516.
124 Fischer A, Landais P, Friedrich W, et al. European experience of bone-marrow transplantation for severe combined immunodeficiency. Lancet 1990; 336;850–854.
125 Fischer A, Landais P, Friedrich W, et al. Bone marrow transplantation (BMT) in Europe for primary immunodeficiencies other than severe combined immunodeficiency: a report from the European group for BMT and the European group for immunodeficiency. Blood 1994; 83:1149–1154.
126 Gennery AR, Dickinson AM, Brigham K, et al. CAMPATH-1M T-cell depleted BMT for SCID: long-term follow-up of 19 children treated 1987–98 in a single centre. Cytotherapy 2001; 3:221–232.
127 Kane LC, Gennery AR, Crooks BNA, et al. Neonatal bone marrow transplantation for severe combined immunodeficiency. Arch Dis Child (Fetal Neonatal Ed) 2001; 85:F110–113.
128 Cunningham-Rundles C, Kazbay K, Zhou Z, et al. Immunologic effects of low-dose polyethylene glycol-conjugated recombinant

human interleukin-2 in common variable immunodeficiency. J Interferon Cytokine Res 1995; 15:269–276.

129 Cavazzana-Calvo M, Hacein-Bey S, de Saint Basile G, et al. Gene therapy of human severe combined immunodeficiency (SCID)-xl disease. Science 2000; 288:669–672.

130 Palella FJ Jr, Delaney KM, Moorman AC, et al. Declining morbidity and mortality among patients with advanced human immunodeficiency virus infection. HIV outpatient study investigators. N Engl J Med 1998; 338:853-860.

131 de Martino M, Tovo PA, Balducci M, et al. Reduction in mortality with availability of antiretroviral therapy for children with perinatal HIV-1 infection. JAMA 2000; 284:190–197.

132 European Collaborative Study. HIV-infected pregnant women and vertical transmission in Europe since 1986. AIDS 2001; 15:761–770.

133 Duong T, Ades AE, Gibb DM, et al. HIV vertical transmission in the British Isles: estimates based on surveillance data. BMJ 1999; 319:1227–1229.

134 Joint United Nations Programme on HIV/AIDS. Report on the global HIV/AIDS epidemic. UNAIDS 2001. Available: http://www.unaids.org.

135 Pedraza MA, del Romero J, Roldan F, et al. Heterosexual transmission of HIV-1 is associated with high plasma viral load levels and a positive viral isolation in the infected partner. J Acquir Immune Defic Syndr 1999; 21:120–125.

136 Fleming P, Byers RH, Sweeney PA, et al. HIV prevalence in the United States, 2000. 9th Conference on Retroviruses and Opportunistic Infections, Seattle, US, February 2002; Abstract 11.

137 Ades AE, Walker J, Botting B, et al. Effect of the worldwide epidemic on HIV prevalence in the United Kingdom: record linkage in anonymous neonatal seroprevalence surveys. AIDS 1999; 13:2437–2443.

138 Cliffe S, Tookey PA, Nicoll A. Antenatal detection of HIV: national surveillance and unlinked anonymous survey. BMJ 2001; 323:376–377.

139 Unlinked Anonymous Surveys Steering Group. Prevalence of HIV and hepatitis infection in the UK 2000. London: Department of Health; 2001.

140 Royal College of Obstetrics and Gynaecology Newsletter 2002; 49.

141 Peckham C, Gibb DM. Mother-to-child transmission of the human immunodeficiency virus. N Engl J Med 1995; 333:298–302.

142 Dunn DT, Newell ML, Ades AE, et al. Risk of human immunodeficiency virus type 1 transmission through breastfeeding. Lancet 1992; 340:585–588.

143 Fowler MC, Simonds RJ, Roonsgpisuthipong A. Update on perinatal HIV transmission. Pediatr Clin North Am 2000; 47(1):21–38.

144 Mandelbrot L, Le Chenadec J, Berrebi A, et al. Perinatal HIV-1 transmission. Interaction between zidovudine prophylaxis and mode of delivery in the French perinatal cohort. JAMA 1998; 280:55–60.

145 Connor EM, Mofenson LM. Zidovudine for the reduction of perinatal human immunodeficiency virus transmission: Pediatric AIDS Clinical Trials Group Protocol 076 – results and treatment recommendations. Pediatr Infect Dis J 1995; 14:536–541.

146 Fiscus SA, Adimora AA, Schoenbach VJ, et al. Perinatal HIV infection and the effect of zidovudine therapy on transmission in rural and urban countries. JAMA 1996; 275:1483–1488.

147 Mandelbroot L, Landreau-Mascaro A, Rekacewicz C, et al. Lamivudine–zidovudine combination for prevention of maternal–infant transmission of HIV-1. JAMA 2001; 285: 2083–2093.

148 Cooper ER, Charurat M, Mofenson L, et al. Combination antiretroviral strategies for the treatment of pregnant HIV-1-infected women and prevention of perinatal HIV-1 transmission. J Acquir Immune Defic Syndr 2002; 29:484–494.

149 Mofenson LM, Lambert JS, Stiehm ER, et al. Risk factors for perinatal transmission of human immunodeficiency virus type 1 in women treated with zidovudine. Pediatric AIDS Clinical Trials Group Study 185 Team. N Engl J Med 1999; 341(6):385–393.

150 Ioannidis JP, Abrams EJ, Ammann A, et al. Perinatal transmission of human immunodeficiency virus type 1 by pregnant women with RNA virus loads <1000 copies/ml. J Infect Dis 2001; 183:539–545.

151 Guay LA, Musoke P, Fleming T, et al. Intrapartum and neonatal single-dose nevirapine compared with zidovudine for prevention of mother-to-child transmission of HIV-1 in Kampala, Uganda; HIVNET 012 randomized trial. Lancet 1999; 354:795–802.

152 Taylor G, Lyally E, Mercey D, et al. British HIV Association Guidelines for prescribing antiretroviral therapy in pregnancy. Sex Transm Infect 1999; 75:90–97. Available: http://www.BHIVA.org

153 Live document a. Public Health Service Task Force recommendations for the use of antiretroviral drugs in pregnant women infected with HIV-1 for maternal health and reducing perinatal HIV-1 transmission in the United States. Available: http://www.hivatis.org, 2001.

154 Schaffer N, Chuachoowong R, Mock PA, et al. Short-course zidovudine for perinatal HIV-1 transmission in Bangkok. Collaborative Oriental HIV Transmission Study group. Lancet 1999; 353:773–780.

155 Lallemant M, Jourdain G, Le Coeur S, et al. A trial of shortened zidovudine regimens to prevent mother-to-child transmission of human immunodeficiency virus type 1. N Engl J Med 2000; 343(14):982–991.

156 Dabis F, Elenga N, Meda N, et al. The DITRAME Study Group. 18-Month mortality and perinatal exposure to zidovudine in West Africa. AIDS 2001; 15:771–779.

157 Wiktor SZ, Ekpini F, Karon JM, et al. Short-course oral zidovudine for prevention of mother-to-child transmission of HIV-1 in Abidjan, Côte d'Ivoire: a randomised trial. Lancet 1999; 353:781–785.

158 The PETRA Study Team. Efficacy of three short-course regimens of zidovudine and lamivudine in preventing early and late transmission of HIV-1 from mother to child in Tansania, South Africa, and Uganda (Petra Study): a randomised, double-blind, placebo-controlled trial. Lancet 2002; 359:1178–1186.

159 Blanche S, Tardieu M, Rustin P, et al. Persistent mitochondrial dysfunction and perinatal exposure to antiretroviral nucleoside analogues. Lancet 1999; 354:1084–1089.

160 Dominguez K, Bertolli J, Fowler M, et al. Lack of definitive severe mitochondrial signs or symptoms among deceased HIV uninfected and HIV indeterminate children < 5 years of age, Pediatric Spectrum of Disease Project (PSD), USA. Ann N Y Acad Sci 2000; 918:236–246.

161 Eshelman SH, Mracna M, Guay LA, et al. Selection and fading of resistance mutations in women and infants receiving nevirapine to prevent HIV-1 vertical transmission (HIVNET 012). AIDS 2001; 15:1951–1957.

162 US Public Health Service/Infectious Disease Society of America. Guidelines for the prevention of opportunistic infections in persons infected with human immunodeficiency virus 2001. Available: http://www.hivatis.org/ trtgdlns.html#Opportunistic

163. International Perinatal HIV Group. Duration of ruptured membranes and vertical transmission of HIV-1: a meta-analysis from 15 prospective cohort studies. AIDS 2001; 15(3):357–368.

164 European Mode of Delivery Collaboration. Elective caesarean-section versus vaginal delivery in prevention of vertical HIV-1 transmission: a randomised clinical trial. Lancet 1999; 353:1035–1039.

165 International Perinatal HIV Group. Mode of delivery and the risk of vertical transmission of human immunodeficiency virus type 1. A meta-analysis of fifteen prospective cohort studies. N Engl J Med 1999; 340:977–987.

166 Read JS. Caesarean section delivery to prevent vertical transmission of human immunodeficiency virus type 1. Associated risks and other considerations. Ann N Y Acad Sci 2000; 918:115–121.

167 Leroy V, Newell ML, Dabis F, et al. International multicentre pooled analysis of late postnatal mother-to-child transmission of HIV-1 infection. Ghent International Working Group on Mother-to-Child Transmission of HIV. Lancet 1998; 352(9128):597–600.

168 Nduati R, John G, Mhori-Ngacha D, et al. Effect of breast-feeding and formula feeding on transmission of HIV-1: a randomized clinical trial. JAMA 2000; 283:1167–1174.

169 WHO Collaborative Study Team on the role of Breastfeeding on the Prevention of Infant Mortality. Effect of breastfeeding on infant and child mortality due to infectious diseases in less developed countries: a pooled analysis. Lancet 2000; 355:451–455.

170 Coutsoudis A, Pillay K, Kuhn L, et al. Method of feeding and transmission of HIV-1 from mothers to children by 15 months of age: prospective cohort study from Durban, South Africa. AIDS 2001; 15:379–387.

171 Gaillard P, Mwanyumba F, Verhofstede C, et al. Vaginal lavage with chlorhexidine during labour to reduce mother-to-child HIV transmission: clinical trial in Mombasa, Kenya. AIDS 2001; 15(3):389–396.

172 Read JS, Bethel J, Harris DR, et al. Serum vitamin A concentrations in a North

American cohort of human immunodeficiency virus type 1-infected children. National Institute of Child Health and Human Development Intravenous Immunoglobulin Clinical Trial Study Group. Pediatr Infect Dis J 1999; 18:134–142.

173 Fawzi WW, Msamanga G, Hunter D, et al. Randomized trial of vitamin supplements in relation to vertical transmission of HIV-1 in Tanzania. J Acquir Immune Defic Syndr 2000; 23(3):246–254.

174 Ades AE, Sculpher MJ, Gibb DM, et al. Cost-effectiveness of antenatal HIV screening in the UK. BMJ 1999; 319:1230-1234.

175 Department of Health (England & Wales) circular on antenatal testing Aug 1999. London: Department of Health; 2002.

176 Williams AJ, Gibb DM. *Pneumocystis carinii* pneumonia and CMV infection in HIV infected infants. HIV and AIDS, Current Trends March; 2002:1–5.5.

177 De Cock KM, Fowler MG, Mercier E, et al. Prevention of mother-to-child HIV transmission in resource-poor countries: translating research into policy and practice. JAMA 2002; 283:1175–1182.

178 O'Brien SJ, Moore JP. The effect of genetic variation in chemokines and their receptors on HIV transmission and progression to AIDS. Immunol Rev 2000; 177:99–111.

179 Wasik TJ, Bratosiewicz J, Wierzbicki A, et al. Protective role of beta-chemokines associated with HIV-specific Th responses against perinatal HIV transmission. J Immunol 1999; 162:4355–4364.

180 Hogan CM, Hammer SM. Host determinants in HIV infection and disease. Part 1: cellular and humoral immune responses. Ann Intern Med 2001; 134:761–776.

181 Soudeyns H, Pantaleo G. The moving target: mechanisms of HIV persistence during primary infection. Immunol Today 1999; 20:446–450.

182 Pikora CA, Sullivan JL, Panicali D, et al. Early HIV-1 envelope-specific cytotoxic T lymphocyte responses in vertically infected infants. J Exp Med 1997; 185:1153–1161.

183 Shearer WT, Quinn TC, LaRussa P, et al. Viral load and disease progression in infants infected with human immunodeficiency virus type 1. Women and Infants Transmission Study Group. N Engl J Med 1997; 336:1337–1342.

184 Gibb DM, Newberry A, de Rossi A, et al. HIV-1 viral load and CD4 count in untreated children with vertically acquired asymptomatic or mild disease – PENTA 1 Virology. AIDS 1998; 12: F1–F8.

185 Gibb DM, Newberry A, Klein N, et al (for the PENTA Steering Committee). Immune repopulation after HAART in previously untreated HIV 1-infected children. Lancet 2000; 355:1331–1332.

186 Ho DD. Perspectives series: host/pathogen interactions. Dynamics of HIV-1 replication in vivo. J Clin Invest 1997; 99:2565–2567.

187 Zhang L, Ramratnam B, Tenner-Racz K, et al. Quantifying residual HIV-1 replication in patients receiving combination antiretroviral therapy. N Engl J Med 1999; 340:1605–1613.

188 Wade AM, Ades AE. Age-related reference ranges: significance tests for models and confidence intervals for centiles. Stat Med 1994; 13:2359–2367.

189 Dunn D, Newell ML, Peckham C, et al (for the European Collaborative Study Group). CD4 T cell count as a predictor of *Pneumocystis carinii* pneumonia in children born to mothers infected with HIV. BMJ 1994; 308:437–440.

190 Galli L, de Martino M, Tovo PA, et al. Predictive value of the HIV paediatric classification system for the long term course of perinatally infected children. Int J Epidemiol 2000; 29:573–578.

191 Paediatric European Network for Treatment of AIDS (PENTA). Comparison of dual nucleoside–analogue reverse-transcriptase inhibitor regimens with and without nelfinavir in children with HIV-1 who have not previously been treated: the PENTA 5 randomised trial. Lancet 2002; 359:733–739.

192 Palumbo PE, Raskino C, Fiscus S, et al. Disease progression in HIV infected infants and children: predictive value of quantitative plasma HIV RNA and CD4 lymphocyte count. JAMA 1998; 279:756–761.

193 Mofenson LM, Korelitz J, Meyer WA, et al. The relationship between human immunodeficiency type 1 RNA level, CD4 lymphocyte percent, and mortality risk in HIV-1 infected children. J Infect Dis 1997; 175:1029–1038.

194 Dunn DT, Brandt CD, Krivine A, et al. The sensitivity of HIV-1 DNA polymerase chain reaction in the neonatal period and the relative contributions of intra-uterine and intra-partum transmission. AIDS 1995; 9:F7–11.

195 Tovo PA, De Marino M, Gabiano C, et al. Prognostic factors and survival in children with perinatal HIV-1 infection. Lancet 1992; 339:1249–1253.

196 Blanche S, Newell ML, Mayaux MJ, et al. Morbidity and mortality in European children vertically infected by HIV-1. The French Pediatric HIV Infection Study Group and European Collaborative Study. J Acquir Immune Defic Syndr 1998; 14:442–450.

197 Diaz C, Hanson C, Cooper ER, et al. Disease progression in a cohort of infants with vertically acquired HIV infection observed from birth: the Women and Infants Transmission Study (WITS). J Acquired Immune Deficiency Syndromes 1998; 18:221–228.

198 Dankner WM, Lindsey JC, Levin MJ and the Pediatric AIDS Clinical Trials Group 2001. Correlates of opportunistic infections in children infected with the human immunodeficiency virus managed before highly active antiretroviral therapy. Pediatr Infect Dis J 2001; 20:40–48.

199 Simonds RJ, Oxtoby MJ, Caldwell MB, et al. *Pneumocystis carinii* pneumonia among US children with perinatally acquired HIV infection. JAMA 1993; 270:470–473.

200 Williams AJ, Duong T, McNally LM, et al. *Pneumocystis carinii* pneumonia and cytomegalovirus infection in children with vertically acquired HIV infection. AIDS 2001; 15:335–339.

201 Chandwani S, Kaul A, Bebenroth D, et al. Cytomegalovirus infection in human immunodeficiency virus type 1-infected children. Pediatr Infect Dis J 1996; 15:310–314.

202 Gibb DM, Giacomelli A, Masters J, et al. Persistance of antibody responses to *Haemophilus influenzae* type b polysaccharide conjugate vaccine in children with vertically acquired human immunodeficiency virus infection. Pediatr Infect Dis J 1996; 15:1097–1101.

203 Sharland M, Gibb DM, Holland F. Respiratory morbidity from lymphocytic interstitial pneumonitis (LIP) in vertically acquired HIV-1 infection. Arch Dis Child 1997; 76:334–337.

204 Evans JA, Gibb DM, Holland FJ, et al. Malignancies in children with HIV infection acquired from mother-to-child transmission in the United Kingdom. Arch Dis Child 1997; 76(4):330–334.

205 Rabkin CS. AIDS and cancer in the era of highly active antiretroviral therapy (HAART). Eur J Cancer 2001; 37:1316–1319.

206 McCarthy GA, Kampmann G, Novelli V, et al. Vertical transmission of Kaposi's sarcoma. Arch Dis Child 1996; 76:455–457.

207 Kinghorn G. A sexual health and HIV strategy for England. BMJ 2001; 323:243–244.

208 British HIV Association Guidelines (BHIVA) for the treatment of HIV-infected adults with antiretroviral therapy. Available: http://www.bhiva.org, 2001.

209 Live document b. Guidelines for the use of antiretroviral agents in HIV infected adults and adolescents Available: http://www.hivatis.org, 2001.

210 Live document c. Guidelines for the use of antiretroviral agents in pediatric HIV infection. Available: http://www.hivatis.org, 2001.

211 Sharland M, di Zub GC, Ramos J, et al. PENTA guidelines for the use of antiretroviral therapy in paediatric HIV infection. Pediatric European Network for Treatment of AIDS. HIV Med 2002; 3(3):215–226. Available: http://www.ctu.mrc.ac.uk/penta

212 Paediatric European Network for Treatment of AIDS (PENTA). Five-year follow-up of vertically HIV infected children in a randomised double blind controlled trial of immediate versus deferred zidovudine: the PENTA 1 trial. Arch Dis Child 2001; 84(3):230–236.

213 Gortmaker SL, Hughes M, Cervia J, et al for the PACTG 219 team. Effect of combination therapy including protease inhibitors on mortality among children and adolescents infected with HIV-1. N Engl J Med 2001; 345:1522–1528.

214 Melvin AJ, Rodrigo AG, Mohan KM, et al. HIV-1 dynamics in children. 1999; 20:468–473.

215 De Rossi A, Walker AS, Klein N, et al. Increased thymic output after initiation of antiretroviral therapy in human immunodeficiency virus type 1-infected children in the Paediatric European Network for Treatment of AIDS (PENTA) 5 Trial. J Infect Dis 2002; 186(3):312–320

216 Lindsey JC, Hughes MD, McKinney RE, et al. Treatment mediated changes in human immunodeficiency virus (HIV) type 1 RNA and CD4 cell counts as predictors of weight growth failure, cognitive decline, and survival in HIV infected children. J Infect Dis 2000; 182:1385–1393.

217 Luzuriaga K, McManus M, Catalina M, et al. Early therapy of vertical human immunodeficiency virus type-1 (HIV-1) infection: control of viral replication and absence of persistent HIV-1 specific immune responses. J Virol 2000; 74:6984–6991.

218 Litalein C, Faye A, Compacnucci A, et al. on behalf of PENTA. Pharmacokinetics of nelfinavir and its active metabolite, M8, in infants less than 1 year old perinatally infected with HIV-1, in press, Pediatr Infect Dis J 2002.
219 Duong T, McGee L, Sharland M, et al on behalf of CHIPS. Effects of antiretroviral therapy (ART) on morbidity and mortality of UK and Irish HIV infected children. Arch Dis Child 2002; 86(suppl 1):A69.
220 Reddington C, Cohen J, Baldillo A, et al. Adherence to medication regimens among young children with human immunodeficiency virus infection. Pediatr Infect Dis J 2000; 19:1148–1153.
221 The Euro Guidelines Group for HIV Resistance. Clinical and laboratory guidelines for the use of HIV-1 drug resistance testing as part of treatment management: recommendations for the European setting. AIDS 2001; 15:309–320.
222 Babl FE, Regan AM, Pelton SI. Abnormal fat distribution in HIV-1 infected children on antiretrovirals. Lancet 1999; 353:1243–1244.
223 Vigano A, Sala N, Bricolli D, et al. HAART associated bone mineral loss through increased rate of bone turnover in vertically infected HIV infected children. 8th Conference on Retroviruses and Opportunistic Infections, Chicago, February 2001, Abstract LB 9.
224 Chokephaibulkit K, Wanachiwanawain F, Chearskul S, et al. *Pneumocystis carinii* severe pneumonia among human immunodeficiency virus-infected children in Thailand: the effect of primary prophylaxis strategy. Pediatr Infect Dis J 1999; 18:147–152.
225 Centers for Disease Control and Prevention. Revised guidelines for prophylaxis against *Pneumocystis carinii* pneumonia for children infected with or Perinatally exposed to human Immunodeficiency virus. MMWR 1995; 44(RR-4):1–11.
226 Urschel S, Schuster T, Dunsch D, et al. Discontinuation of primary *Pneumocystis carinii* prophylaxis after reconstitution of CD4 cell counts in HIV-infected children. AIDS 2001; 15:1589–1591.
227 Gibb DM, Masters J, Shingadia D, et al. A family clinic – optimising care for HIV infected children and their families. Arch Dis Child 1997; 77:478–482.

26

Infections

Edited by David Isaacs, J Brian S Coulter

CLASSIFICATION

Table 26.1 A classification of infections according to the system principally involved

	Bacterial	Viral	Protozoal	Fungal	Helminthic
General	Streptococcal Staphylococcal Diphtheria Brucellosis Tetanus Botulism Meningococcemia Tularemia Plague Bartonellosis Tuberculosis Atypical mycobacteria Leprosy Sarcoidosis Leptospirosis Rat bite fever Relapsing fever Syphilis Yaws Pinta *Pseudomonas pyocyanea* Legionnaires' disease Cat-scratch disease	Measles Chickenpox Influenza Q fever Mumps Poliomyelitis Rabies Cytomegalovirus Infectious mononucleosis Roseola infantum Erythema infectiosum Arbovirus gp A (e.g. Chikungunya) Arbovirus gp B (e.g. yellow fever, dengue, etc.) Arbovirus group C (e.g. sandfly fever) Rickettsiae (e.g. typhus fever) Lassa fever Marburg virus disease	Malaria Toxoplasmosis Leishmaniasis Trypanosomiasis	Aspergillosis Blastomycosis	*Mansonella perstans* *Mansonella ozzardi* *Schistosomiasis* *Inermicapsifer* *Madagascariensis*
Alimentary	Typhoid Paratyphoid Other salmonellae Bacillary dysentery Cholera (Gastroenteritis) Staphylococcal (enterocolitis: toxins) Tuberculosis *Escherichia coli*	Adenovirus (gastroenteritis) ECHO virus (gastroenteritis) Reovirus (gastroenteritis) Herpes simplex (ulcerative stomatitis) Coxsackie A (hand-foot-mouth disease) Cytomegalovirus (hepatic) Virus hepatitis A Virus hepatitis B Virus hepatitis C Arbovirus gp B (hepatic-yellow fever)	Amebiasis Acanthamebiasis Balantidiasis Giardiasis Leishmaniasis (visceral)	Moniliasis	Ascariasis *Enterobius vermicularis* Hookworm *Trichuris trichiura* *Strongyloides stercoralis* Trichinosis *Taenia saginata* *Taenia solium* *Hymenolepis nana, diminuta* *Dipylidium caninum* *Diphyllobothrium latum* Echinococcosis (hepatic) Schistosomiasis Liver flukes (hepatic) Intestinal fluke *Toxocara* *Oesophagostomum* sp. *Ternidens deminutus* Acanthocephala Capillariasis
Respiratory	Pertussis Pneumonia (pneumococcal: *Haemophilus influenzae*, group B streptococcal staphylococcal) Tuberculosis Atypical mycobacteria *Pseudomonas pyocyanea* (cystic fibrosis)	Measles Influenza Parainfluenza Respiratory syncytial virus Adenovirus Rhinovirus Psittacosis Ornithosis *Mycoplasma pneumoniae*	*Pneumocystis carinii*	Aspergillosis Blastomycosis Coccidioidomycosis Histoplasmosis Nocardiosis	Ascariasis Toxocara Echinococcosis Lung fluke (paragonimiasis) Strongyloides *Dirofilaria immitis*

(Cont'd)

Table 26.1 *Cont'd*

	Bacterial	Viral	Protozoal	Fungal	Helminthic
Neurological	Meningococcal *H. influenzae* Staphylococcal Pneumococcal Streptococcal Diphtheroids *E. coli* Proteus Pseudomonas *Listeria monocytogenes* Diphtheria Tuberculosis Botulism	Measles Herpes simplex, varicella-zoster Vaccinia Coxsackie A Coxsackie B ECHO virus Mumps Lymphocytic choriomeningitis Poliomyelitis Rabies (Guillain–Barré) (Infectious mononucleosis) Arbovirus gp A		Cryptococcosis (Torulosis)	Toxocara *Taenia solium* *Angiostrongylus cantonensis*
Skin and subcutaneous tissue	Erysipelas (staphylococci) Impetigo (streptococci) Rat bite fever Anthrax Bartonellosis Tuberculosis Leprosy Syphilis Yaws Pinta	Herpes simplex, zoster Varicella Smallpox Vaccinia Coxsackie A (hand-foot-mouth disease) Orf Molluscum contagiosum Rickettsiae (rickettsialpox)	Leishmaniasis (cutaneous)	Moniliasis Actinomycosis Aspergillosis Phycomycosis Sporotrichosis	Hookworm Dracunculosis Onchocerciasis Filaria, *Loa loa, Wuchereria bancrofti* Schistosomiasis Myiasis Strongyloides *A. braziliense* *A. caninum* Sparganosis
Genitourinary	Streptococci (*S. faecalis*) *E. coli* Proteus *Ps. pyocyanea* Staphylococci Gonorrhea Tuberculosis	Herpetic vulvovaginitis (Lymphogranuloma venereum)			Schistosomiasis
Upper respiratory tract	Streptococcal Diphtheria *H. influenzae*	Adenovirus Coxsackie A (herpangina) Parainfluenza Rhinovirus ECHO virus Reovirus		Rhinosporidioidosis	
Lymph glands and lymphatics	Diphtheria Plague Tuberculosis Atypical mycobacteria Sarcoidosis Cat-scratch disease	(Infectious mononucleosis) Rubella (Roseola infantum) (Lymphogranuloma venereum)	Toxoplasmosis Leishmaniasis (Splenomegaly) Trypanosomiasis		*Brugia malayi*
Blood (anemia)	Bartonellosis		Leishmaniasis Malaria		Toxocara Hookworm *Diphyllobothrium latum*
Ophthalmic and periorbital	Gonorrhea Tuberculosis	Adenovirus (conjunctivitis) TRIC virus (conjunctivitis) Trachoma Herpes simplex Acute hemorrhagic conjunctivitis	Trypanosomiasis (periorbital)		Toxocara
Muscle		Coxsackie B (e.g. myocarditis Bornholm)	Trypanosomiasis		Trichinosis

MORTALITY AND MORBIDITY IN INFECTIOUS DISEASE

THE GLOBAL PERSPECTIVE

Worldwide, infections as a disease category are responsible for the majority of deaths and loss of good health in children. It was estimated that in 1990, infectious diseases were responsible for 8.3 million of a total of 12.5 million deaths among a global child population (under 5 years of age) of 630 million.[1] Most of these deaths occurred in developing countries, where it is also estimated that five groups of infections: acute respiratory infections (ARIs), diarrheal diseases, congenital infections including human immunodeficiency virus (HIV), hepatitis B, and other congenital infections, malaria, and vaccine-preventable diseases including measles caused the death of more than 7 million children.[1,2] The relationship between infection, malnutrition and socially determined factors such as wars and orphanhood are subtle but important, as poor nutrition, poverty and social dislocation greatly multiply the impact of infections. To a considerable extent this explains why infections are so much more important as a cause of death and disability in resource-poor compared to industrialized countries. For the last 20 years, rising levels of HIV infection in resource-poor countries have added another multiplier, especially in sub-Saharan Africa. These relations are shown schematically in Figure 26.1, contrasting sub-Saharan Africa with South Asia in the mid-1990s.

Malnutrition underlies a substantial proportion of the deaths from diarrheal diseases, respiratory infections, measles and malaria, while HIV is of particular importance in sub-Saharan Africa. In contrast, in Western Europe and other industrialized countries, malnutrition plays little role as a cofactor for the effects of infection, except in children with serious constitutional diseases such as malignancies or congenital immunodeficiences. However, a growing population of immunocompromised children (very low birth weight babies, children with congenital immunodeficiencies, HIV infection and children on powerful immunocompromising therapies) represent an increasingly important source of deaths due to infections, often with organisms that are usually innocuous for immunocompetent children. It is estimated that infections are responsible for around 17% (37 000) of 214 000 deaths under 5 years old that take place among 78 million children annually in industrialized countries.[1] Proportionately, the burden of infections is far higher in primary care. In England and Wales, infectious diseases are responsible for 40% of all new episodes of illness presenting to general practitioners with annual rates of around 730 episodes per 1000 population. Rates are even higher for infants (children before their first birthday).[3]

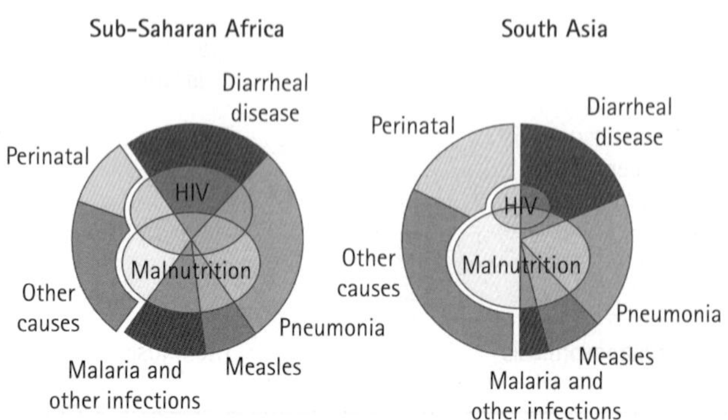

Fig. 26.1 Principal causes of death in children under age 5, sub-Saharan Africa and South Asia, circa 1995.

Mortality statistics and data on acute consultations need to be supplemented by estimates of the burden of disability (morbidity) and to allow for the varying implications of the disability or death of an individual at different ages. This can be done by use of a measure such as disability adjusted life years (DALYs).[4] Combining estimates of chronic disability and mortality statistics, this measure calculates the likely numbers of healthy years of life lost because of specific diseases and conditions and, by 'weighting', an allowance is made for the different significance of ill health and mortality among infants, elderly persons and adults providing for dependants. Estimates of the burden of disease experienced (Table 26.2)[1] further emphasize the importance of infectious disease in developing countries and the particular contribution to mortality in children under age 5 played by respiratory disease, diarrheal disease, the five vaccine-preventable diseases (diphtheria, measles, pertussis, polio and tetanus), and in older children by tuberculosis and intestinal helminths.[1]

HIV AND AIDS

Since the 1990s there has been an inexorable rise in the global importance of HIV such that by 2000 there were estimated to be 37.1 million persons worldwide infected with HIV, and half of all new cases were in young people, under 25 years old. The majority of childhood infections occur through mother-to-child transmission, with a smaller number from unscreened blood transfusions in resource-poor settings. The distribution of deaths varies dramatically by global region, with the highest numbers and rates in sub-Saharan Africa (Fig. 26.2). It is projected, for some of these countries, that HIV infection will reverse many of the improvements in child survival achieved in the latter half of the twentieth century (Fig. 26.3). HIV rarely kills children directly, but by lowering the child's immunocompetence it leaves the infected child increasingly vulnerable to other infections (Fig. 26.1) (see Ch. 25). Since the appreciation that the risk of mother-to-child transmission of HIV infection can be reduced to under 2%, screening for HIV infection has resulted in a fall in early AIDS cases

Table 26.2 Estimated distribution of burden of disease (combined mortality and chronic morbidity) in children in developing countries – 1990

	Total DALYs lost (million)			
	Age under 5 years		Age 5–14 years	
Perinatal conditions	13.5		Nil	
Communicable disease	63.3		33.9	
Congenital STDs (HIV and syphilis)		(2.0%)		(4.0%)
Diarrheal diseases		(32%)		(15%)
Tuberculosis		(1.0%)		(11%)
Other vaccine-preventable disease		(20%)		(18%)
Malaria		(8%)		(9%)
Intestinal helminths		Nil		(27%)
Respiratory infections		(35%)		(16%)
Non-communicable disorder	20.8		16.9	
Injuries	6.2		9.7	
Total	103.8		60.5	

Source: World Bank 1993[1].

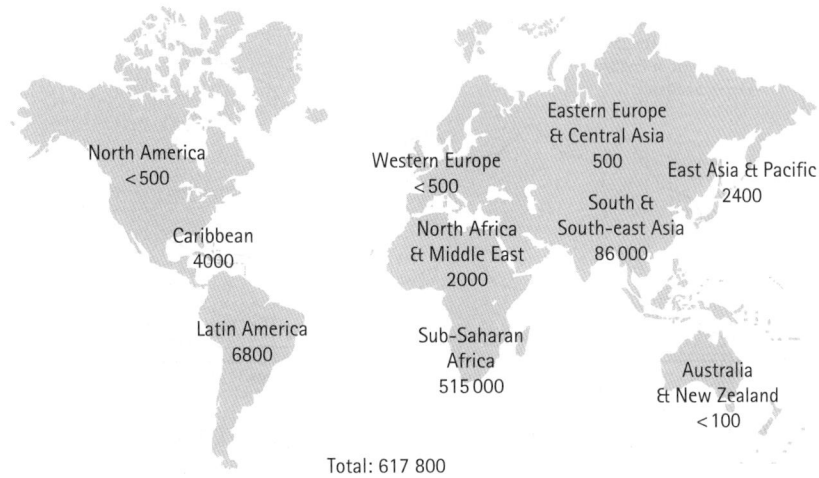

Fig. 26.2 New HIV infection in children globally and by region in 2001.

in France, Italy, Spain and the UK, the countries most affected in Western Europe. The fall was later in the UK, and only took place after it became policy that antenatal HIV testing be offered and recommended to all mothers as a routine part of antenatal care, circa 1998/1999 (Fig. 26.4).[5] The fall in early pediatric AIDS has taken place despite rising levels of HIV infection in mothers in the UK, notably in London, but also in the rest of the UK (Fig. 26.5).

THE UK

Infections remain an important cause of death in UK children. Conventional death registration data indicate that in 1996 infections were the main cause of death in 504 children, 252 infants and 252 older children (Table 26.3). The infant figure rises to 705 if sudden infant death syndrome is included.

Recent trends in a number of important infections are shown in Figures 26.4–26.14. Trends in vertically acquired HIV infection (Figs 26.4 and 26.5) have already been mentioned. The introduction of immunization against *Haemophilus influenzae* type b (Hib) in 1992 led to a dramatic decline in invasive infections attributed to this organism (Fig. 26.6). Conversely, there has been heightened awareness of meningococcal infections as the most important single cause of septicemic and meningitic infections in immunocompetent children.

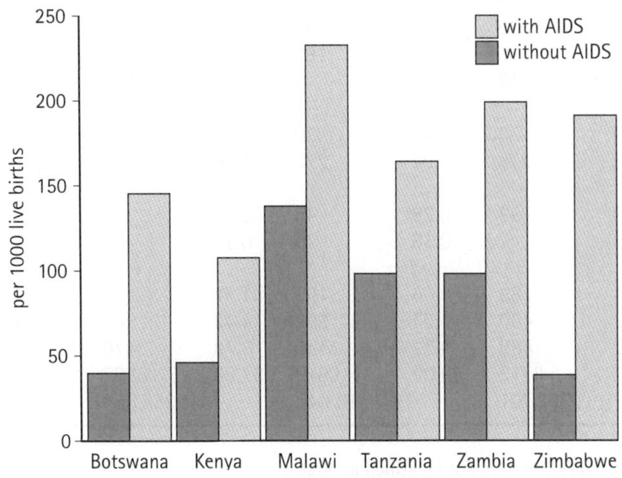

Fig. 26.3 Estimated impact of AIDS on under 5 child mortality rates – selected African countries, circa 2010.

The introduction of conjugate vaccine against type C meningococcal infections has resulted in a fall in cases attributed to this infection in the earliest targeted groups, the under 1-year-olds and teenagers (Fig. 26.7). Immunization was highly effective in reducing the incidence of measles in the 1970s (Fig. 26.8). However, measles vaccination only confers immunity in 90% of recipients and coverage is incomplete. Seroepidemiological investigations in England in the early 1990s indicated a growing number of susceptible (antibody negative) older children and hence an increasing risk of a substantial measles epidemic in school age children, with its inevitable morbidity and mortality.[6,7] A small epidemic took place in Scotland in 1993/1994[8] and to pre-empt further larger epidemics a UK-wide initiative immunized 8 million schoolchildren (90% of those eligible) in 1994. Transmission of indigenous measles was almost entirely interrupted and confirmed notifications fell dramatically. Hence the risk of an epidemic was averted, at least temporarily.[9] Small declines in measles, mumps and rubella (MMR) vaccination following parental concern have left some cohorts of children underprotected (Fig. 26.9) and a substantial epidemic of measles in Dublin in 1999 indicated what will inevitably happen if enough children are left unprotected.[10] Trends in whooping cough (pertussis) in the late 1980s and early 1990s, following the collapse of professional and public confidence in pertussis vaccine, are a reminder of what can happen if myths about immunization are allowed to prevail over science (Fig. 26.10).[11,12] Diphtheria and poliomyelitis declined dramatically in the UK following the introduction of immunization in the 1940s and 1950s

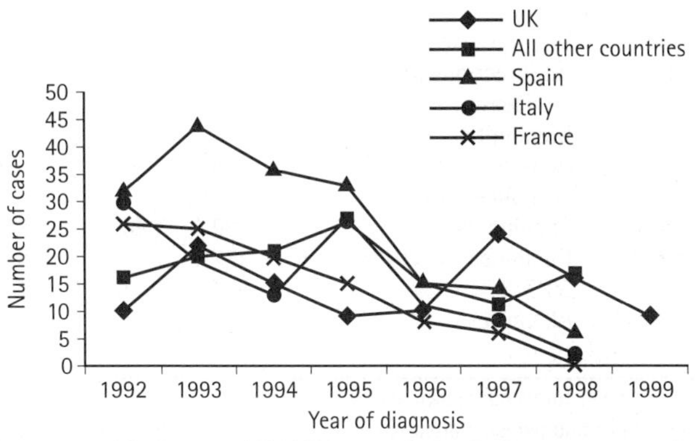

Fig. 26.4 Mother-to-child HIV transmission in European countries. AIDS cases in children aged less than 1 year at diagnosis.

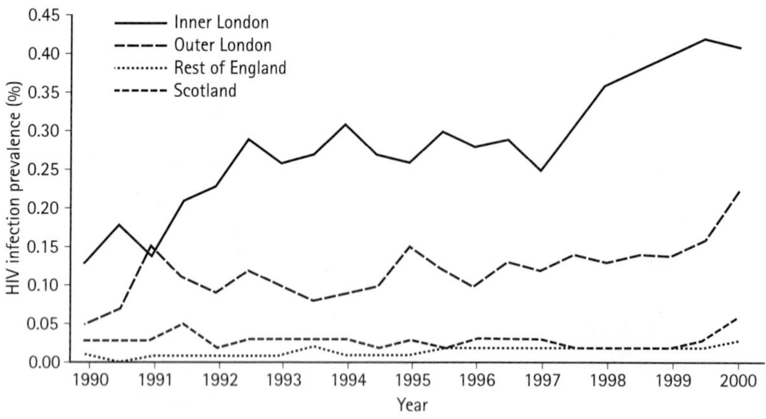

Fig. 26.5 Trends in prevalence of HIV infection in pregnant women in the UK by area of residence 1990–2000.

Table 26.3 Deaths due to infections in children aged 14 years and under; UK 1992–1996

ICD code	Disease	1992	1992	1993	1993	1994	1994	1995	1995	1996	1996
< 1											
			per 1000		per 1000		per 1000		per 1000		per 1000
001–009	Intestinal infectious disease	10	0.01	22	0.03	19	0.03	25	0.03	14	0.02
036	Meningococcal infection	36	0.05	41	0.05	30	0.04	39	0.05	34	0.05
038	Septicemia	19	0.02	20	0.03	20	0.03	35	0.05	25	0.03
030–041	Other bacterial disease*	59	0.07	70	0.09	56	0.07	79	0.11	67	0.09
045–079	Viral disease	6	0.01	12	0.02	12	0.02	11	0.02	10	0.01
001–139	All infectious and parasitic disease	81	0.10	117	0.15	98	0.13	129	0.18	105	0.14
320–322	Meningitis	27	0.03	38	0.05	21	0.03	30	0.04	35	0.05
466	Acute bronchitis and bronchiolitis	20	0.03	33	0.04	29	0.04	18	0.02	21	0.03
480–486	Pneumonia	60	0.08	102	0.13	96	0.13	83	0.11	91	0.12
Combined	Combined infections*	188	0.24	290	0.38	244	0.33	260	0.36	252	0.34
798	SIDS	504	0.64	491	0.65	463	0.62	412	0.56	453	0.62
All causes	All causes†	4961	6.30	4830	6.36	4649	6.20	4526	6.18	4466	6.09
Births	Population denominators (100 thousands)	787 400		759 470		750 201		731 912		733 367	
		1992	1992	1993	1993	1994	1994	1995	1995	1996	1996
<15											
			per 100 000		per 100 000		per 100 000		per 100 000		per 100 000
001–009	Intestinal infectious disease	15	0.13	24	0.21	23	0.20	29	0.26	17	0.15
036	Meningococcal infection	100	0.89	115	1.02	89	0.78	120	1.06	119	1.05
038	Septicemia	20	0.18	32	0.28	35	0.31	54	0.48	49	0.43
030–041	Other bacterial disease*			163	1.44	136	1.20	183	1.61	180	1.58
030–041 (excl 036, 038)	Other bacterial disease*	140	1.25	16	0.14	12	0.11	9	0.08	12	0.11
045–079	Viral disease	20	0.18	33	0.29	33	0.29	30	0.26	31	0.27
001–139	All infectious and parasitic disease	192	1.72	254	2.25	218	1.92	273	2.40	257	2.26
320–322	Meningitis	58	0.52	67	0.59	32	0.28	48	0.42	52	0.46
466	Acute bronchitis and bronchiolitis	35	0.31	50	0.44	41	0.36	28	0.25	35	0.31
480–486	Pneumonia	92	0.82	185	1.64	189	1.66	153	1.35	160	1.41
Combined	Combined infections*	377	3.37	556	4.92	480	4.23	502	4.42	504	4.44
798	SIDS	531	4.75	511	4.52	485	4.27	430	3.78	476	4.19
All causes	All causes†	7180	64.16	7096	62.77	6712	59.09	6519	57.38	6367	56.06
Pops		11 190 000		11 305 317		11 358 701		11 361 643		11 358 354	

* Contains other totals not shown above.

† All infectious and parasitic disease, plus meningitis, acute bronchitis and pneumonia. Excludes hepatitis not identified as viral.

Source: OPCS, General Register Office Scotland, and Department of Health and Social Services, Northern Ireland.

SIDS, sudden infant death syndrome.

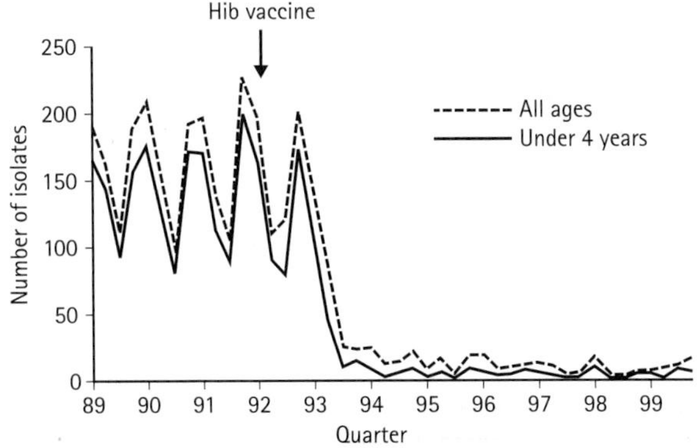

Fig. 26.6 Quarterly laboratory reports of Hib-CSF and blood isolates, 1989–1999.

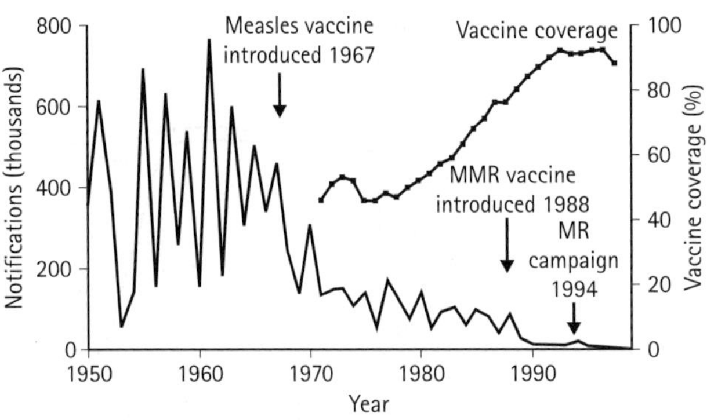

Fig. 26.8 Annual measles notification and vaccine coverage in England and Wales 1950–1999.

rather as it did for *Haemophilus* in the 1990s. In contrast, control of another vaccine-preventable illness, tuberculosis,[13] has been less successful with an overall rise in notifications in the 1990s, which particularly reflects trends in London (Fig. 26.11). Food poisoning has become the commonest notifiable infection in children. Sharply increasing trends in notified numbers of cases of food poisoning in the 1980s and 1990s were mirrored by trends in national laboratory reporting of salmonellosis. Since 1997, however, salmonella reports have declined while reports of *Campylobacter* spp. have risen (Fig. 26.12). Though numbers are far less than for campylobacter or salmonella, the emergence of *Escherichia coli* O157 since the 1980s is of concern because of the severe disease and specific renal pathology that often follows this infection (Fig. 26.13). Not all countries see this subtype of verocytotoxigenic *E. coli* (VTEC): in Australia for example the predominant subtype is *E. coli* O111.[14]

Sexually transmitted diseases are now appreciated to be a substantial problem among adolescents. Rates of gonorrhea have risen by 55% since 1995 (Fig. 26.14) with the highest percentage rise among adolescents.[15] The highest incidences of gonorrhea and chlamydia seen among genitourinary medicine clinic attenders are in females aged 16–19 years.[16] Chlamydia is the more important, because of its widespread distribution and serious sequelae of pelvic inflammatory disease, infertility and ectopic pregnancies. It is clear that the chlamydia infections seen in genitourinary medicine clinics are only a fraction of those prevalent in the teenage population.

General practitioner (GP) reporting provides the least-selected surveillance data in the UK on the nature and burden of infectious disease in children in the community, particularly on conditions such as chickenpox or influenza unlikely to be investigated microbiologically or to lead to hospital admission. These data show that respiratory tract infections (mainly upper tract infections)

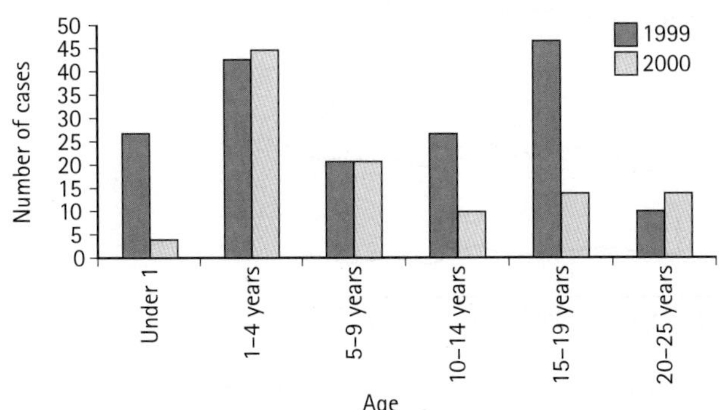

Fig. 26.7 Confirmed type C meningococcal infections – weeks 14–26, 1999 and 2000.

account for over 80% of new GP consultations for infectious diseases in children.[3]

EMERGING AND RE-EMERGING INFECTIONS

In the 1960s and 1970s it was a medical commonplace that improving social conditions and medical treatments were leading to a relentless decline in the importance of infectious diseases. Emerging and re-emerging infections such as HIV and tuberculosis (Figs 26.1 and 26.11), as well as high profile nosocomial outbreaks of legionnaires' disease and food poisoning in the UK, have changed medical opinion. In addition, the deliberate release of organisms such as anthrax has brought a new threat to health from infections.[17] It is now realized that infections remain important threats to the health of children and adults in every country. Following a lead from the United States Centers for Disease Control and Prevention (CDC), in 1995 the World Health Organization established a Division of Emerging Viral and Bacterial Disease Surveillance and Control (www.who.int/emc/index.html). Some countries and regional bodies (for example the European Union) have been establishing or strengthening infrastructures to detect and respond to emerging or re-emerging infections. Some emerging infections are new, or newly recognized pathogens (Table 26.4),[18] examples being human herpesvirus types 6 and 7 and variant Creutzfeldt–Jakob disease.[19] Others represent animal infections that have only recently come to affect humans, such as HIV and Lassa fever. Yet a third group are established infections whose incidence, pathogenicity or antimicrobial resistance has recently increased, for example dengue fever, methicillin resistant *Staphylococcus aureus* infection (MRSA) and tuberculosis (both drug-susceptible and multiply resistant *Mycobacterium tuberculosis*). Of particular importance to children are HIV, diphtheria, pertussis, *E. coli* O157 causing hemolytic uremic syndrome (HUS), and sexually transmitted infections in adolescents.

The reasons for emergence and re-emergence are almost as varied as the organisms themselves (Table 26.5).[20] Failure of public health programs can be an important cause. Diphtheria reappeared in the 1990s as an epidemic in Russia because of a collapse in vaccine production and the emergence of mistaken reasons among the public and professionals for refusing immunization. A similar phenomenon affecting pertussis occurred in the UK in the 1970s and 1980s from the mistaken impression that the vaccine was more dangerous than the disease (see Fig. 26.9).[11,21] Both *E. coli* O157 and various salmonellas have been spread efficiently through industrialized production and distribution of foods.[22] An outbreak of HUS due to contaminated commercial hamburgers occurred in the USA in 1993[23] and in 1995 an outbreak of gastrointestinal disease in children due to *S. agoma* in north London was traced to

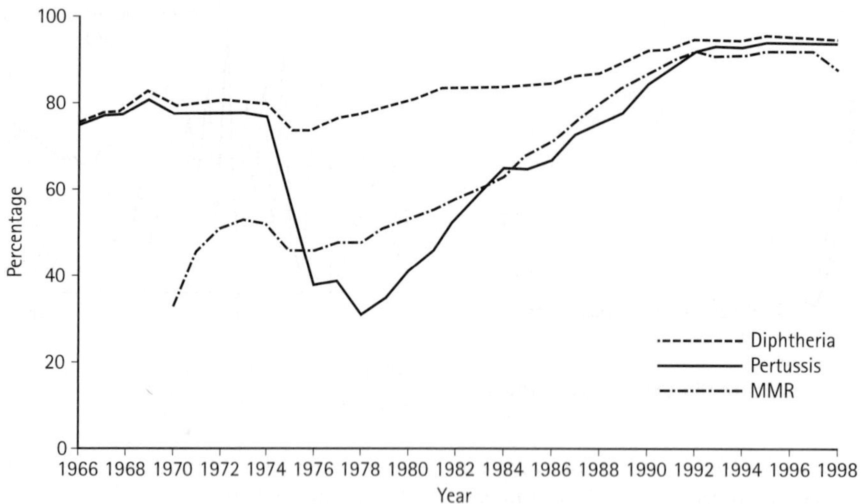

Fig. 26.9 2 Year vaccine coverage in England and Wales 1966–1998.

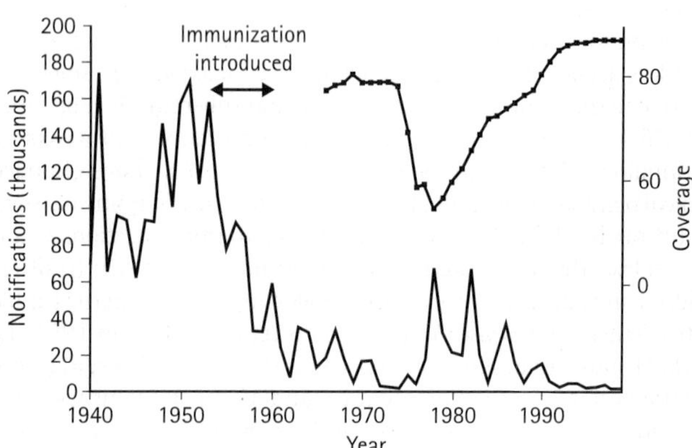

Fig. 26.10 Whooping cough cases and vaccine coverage in England and Wales 1940–1999.

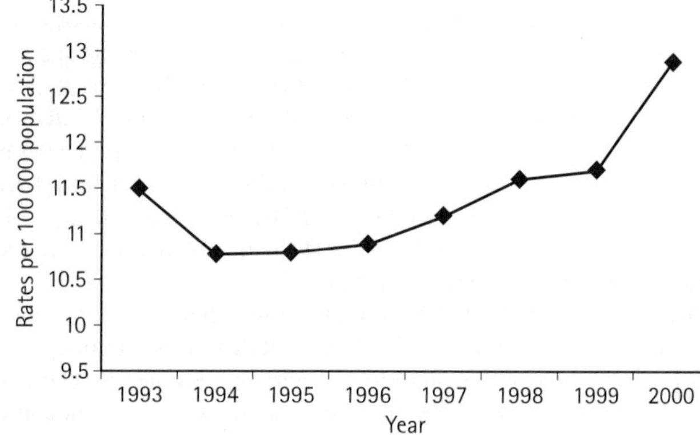

Fig. 26.11 Tuberculosis notification rates per 100 000 population in England and Wales 1993–2000.

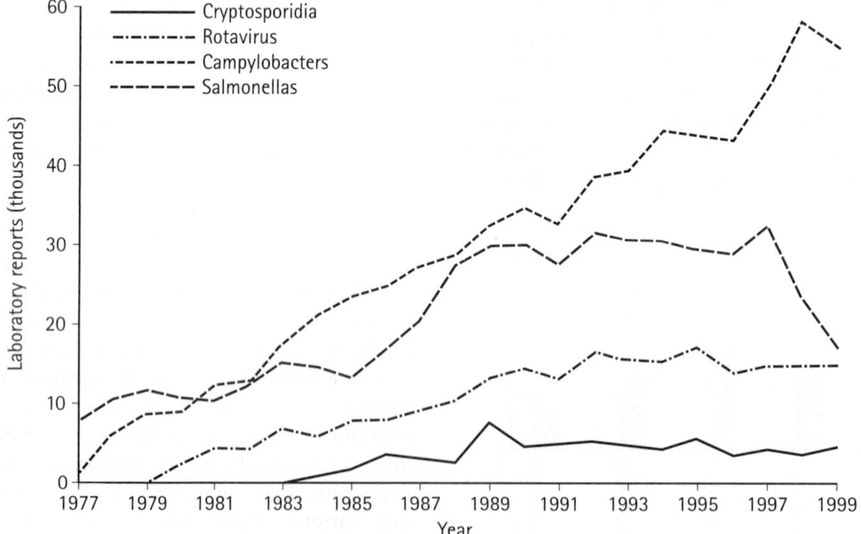

Fig. 26.12 Laboratory reporting of selected gastrointestinal pathogens in England and Wales 1977–1999.

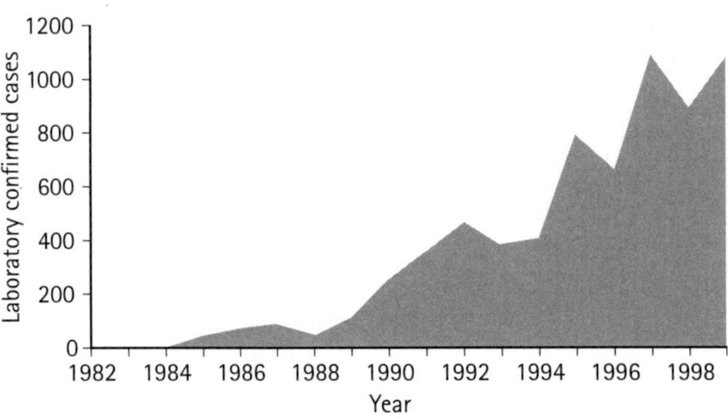

Fig. 26.13 Laboratory confirmed cases of VTEC O157 infection in England and Wales 1982–1998.

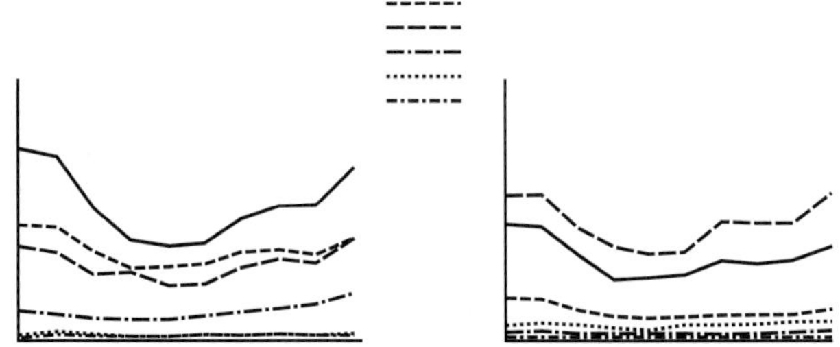

Fig. 26.14 Rates of uncomplicated gonorrhea seen in genitourinary medicine clinics by age group in the UK 1990–1999.

defective production in a factory in Israel. Changes in behavior can result in disease emergence. International trends towards earlier menarche and sexual debut are causing younger females to be exposed to STDs with a consequent rise in pelvic inflammatory disease, ectopic pregnancy and secondary infertility.[24]

EFFECTIVE INTERVENTIONS

In 1990, at a World Summit for Children government leaders including that of the UK, committed their administrations to 27 goals to improve the health and lives of children. There have been some major achievements towards these goals. More than 60 countries have reached their national goals of reducing mortality rates of children < 5 years by a third or more. Polio has been eradicated in more than 175 countries and deaths from diarrheal illnesses have been more than halved.[2]

Interventions designed to prevent or treat infections may be assessed by measuring their resulting health gain as healthy years of life and comparing their costs relative to other interventions. Thus it is possible to come up with 'best buys' for countries, and this has been undertaken for the developing world by the World Bank using the 'DALY' measure.[4] Interventions targeted against acute respiratory infections, diarrheal disease, malaria and the six vaccine-preventable diseases represent four of the six top interventions for health gain in children under age 5, and five out of six of those targeted at children aged 5–14 years[25] (Table 26.6). While new technologies and developments are necessary, greater health gains can come from the application of established interventions of proven effectiveness such as the early detection and treatment of acute respiratory infections, and the use of oral rehydration therapy (ORT) for gastrointestinal infections.[26] Immunization represents a success story. By 1990, the Expanded Program of Immunization (EPI) reached a goal of immunizing 80% of children in most countries with an estimated benefit of 3 million lives saved in 1995. A particular priority has been polio immunization. The EPI, supported by Rotary International had, by 1995, eliminated wild polio from 145 countries, including all of the Americas.[26] However, the 80% target remains unachieved in sub-Saharan Africa where overall immunization rates are static.

Table 26.4 New and emerging infections – New and newly recognized agents identified since 1973

Year of Report	Agent	Disease
1973	Rotavirus	Major cause of infantile diarrhea worldwide
1975	Parvovirus B19	Fifth disease; aplastic crisis in hemolytic anemia
1976	*Cryptosporidium parvum*	Acute enterocolitis
1977	Ebola virus	Ebola hemorrhagic fever
1977	*Legionella pneumophila*	Legionnaires' disease
1977	Hantaan virus	Hemorrhagic fever with renal syndrome (HFRS)
1977	*Campylobacter* sp.	Enteric pathogens distributed globally
1980	Human T cell lymphotropic virus-I (HTLV I)	T cell lymphoma leukemia
1981	*Staphylococcus* toxin	Toxic shock syndrome associated with tampon use
1982	*Escherichia coli* O157:H7	Hemorrhagic colitis; hemolytic uremic syndrome
1982	HTLV II	Hairy cell leukemia
1982	*Borrelia bugdorferi*	Lyme disease
1983	HIV	HIV disease including AIDS
1983	*Helicobacter pylori*	Peptic ulcers
1988	Human herpesvirus-6 (HHV-6)	Roseola infantum and encephalitis
1989	*Ehrlichia chaffeensis*	Human ehrlichiosis
1989	Hepatitis C	Parenterally transmitted non-A, non-B hepatitis
1990	Human herpesvirus-7 (HHV-7)	Roseola infantum and encephalitis
1991	Guanarito virus	Venezuelan hemorrhagic fever
1992	*Vibrio cholerae* O139	New strain associated with epidemic cholera
1992	*Bartonella (=Rochalimaea) henselae*	Cat-scratch disease; bacillary angiomatosis
1993	Sin nombre hantavirus	Hantavirus pulmonary syndrome
1994	Sabiá virus	Brazilian hemorrhagic fever
1995	Human herpesvirus-8 (HHV-8)	Kaposi's sarcoma
1997	Bovine spongiform encephalopathy (BSE) agent (a prion)	New variant Creutzfeldt–Jakob disease

(Modified from CDC Staff, 1997[18])

Table 26.5 Factors in infectious disease emergence and re-emergence relevant to child and adolescent health

Factor	Example of specific factors	Examples of disease
Ecological changes (including those due to economic development and land use)	Agriculture: dams, changes in water ecosystems; deforestation/reforestation; flood/drought; famine; climate changes	Schistosomiasis (dams); Rift Valley fever (dams, irrigation); Argentine hemorrhagic fever (agriculture); Hantaan–Korean hemorrhagic fever (agriculture); hantavirus pulmonary syndrome, southwestern US, 1993 (weather anomalies)
Human demographics, behavior	Societal changes and events: population growth and migration (movement from rural areas to cities); war or civil conflict; urban decay; sexual behavior; intravenous drug use; preference for 'fast foods'; use of high-density facilities	Introduction of HIV; spread of dengue; spread of HIV and other sexually transmitted diseases, meningococcal disease, cholera, increases in food poisoning (*Salmonella enteritidis)*
International travel and commerce	Worldwide movement of goods and people; air travel	'Airport' malaria; dissemination of mosquito vectors; rat-borne hantavirusues; antibiotic-resistant gonorrhea; introduction of cholera into South America; dissemination of O139 *V. cholerae*
Technology and industry	Globalization of food supplies; changes in food processing and packaging; organ or tissue transplantation; drugs causing immunosuppression; widespread use of antibiotics	Hemolytic uremic syndrome (*E. coli* contamination of hamburger meat), *S. agoma* in kosher snacks; transfusion-associated hepatitis (hepatitis B, C), opportunistic infections in immunosuppressed patients, Creutzfeldt–Jakob disease from contaminated batches of human growth hormone (medical technology)
Microbial adaptation and change	Microbial evolution, response to selection in environment	Antibiotic-resistant bacteria (multiply resistant *M. tuberculosis*), 'antigenic drift' in influenza virus; zidovudine-resistant HIV
Breakdown in public health measures	Curtailment or reduction in prevention programs; inadequate sanitation and vector control measures, immunization myths	Whooping cough in the UK, resurgence of tuberculosis in the US; cholera in refugee camps in Africa; resurgence of diphtheria in the former Soviet Union

Adapted from Morse 1995.[20]

Because of economic or social reasons there are at least some war-torn countries where polio elimination looks difficult or impossible. This makes the goal of global polio elimination, and its prize of release of resources currently committed to polio immunization, look difficult.[27]

SURVEILLANCE TO INFORM PUBLIC HEALTH ACTION

Given adequate resources and will, many infectious diseases can be prevented or contained, but eradication of all infection-related morbidity and mortality is unachievable as many microorganisms have extensive animal and environmental reservoirs. Interventions can prevent infections or ameliorate the effects of disease. Knowledge as to which interventions are effective must be combined with timely surveillance data on the epidemiology of infection and susceptibility so as to allow rational decisions to be made on resource allocation for public health action. Equally, surveillance provides the basis for health protection, for example in detecting and directing action on deliberate release of biological agents.[17]

Routine data for surveillance of the commoner infectious diseases in the UK are derived from mortality statistics, disease notifications and laboratory reporting (Table 26.7).[28] An infection may be made statutorily notifiable in the UK either because there is a need for rapid information for effective local control, or for the purpose of monitoring national immunization programs. Often taken for granted, these systems are among the best in the world. Routine reporting is supplemented by special surveillance systems for rare and/or more important infections such as HIV and congenital rubella syndrome. An example of this is active reporting by clinicians through the British Paediatric Surveillance Unit of the Royal College of Paediatrics and Child Health (RCPCH), whereby researchers combine reports from RCPCH members with data from other systems to give optimal coverage.[29] Surveillance of infectious disease mortality and morbidity in England and Wales is undertaken by the Office of Population, Censuses and Surveys (OPCS) and by the Communicable Disease Surveillance Centre (CDSC), the epidemiological arm of the Public Health Laboratory Service. CDSC and OPCS collaborate closely to obtain, analyze and interpret data from several sources which often overlap, but which

Table 26.6 Main cause of disease burden in children in demographically developing countries in 1990 and the cost-effectiveness of the interventions available for their control

Disease and injuries	Number of DALYs lost* millions (% total)	Main intervention	Cost-effectiveness ($ per DALY)
Respiratory infections	98 (14.8)†	Integrated management of the sick child	30–100
Perinatal morbidity and mortality	96 (14.6)	a. Prenatal and delivery care b. Family planning	30–100 20–150
Diarrheal disease	92 (14.0)	Integrated management of the sick child	30–100
Childhood cluster (diseases preventable through immunization)	65 (10.0)	Expanded Program on immunization (EPI) EPI-plus†	12–30
Congenital malformation	35 (5.4)	Surgical operations	High (unknown)
Malaria	31 (4.7)	Integrated management of the sick child	30–100
Intestinal helminths	17 (2.5)	School health program	20–34
Protein-energy malnutrition	12 (1.8)	Integrated management of the sick child	30–100
Vitamin A deficiency	12 (1.8)	EPI-plus†	12–30
Iodine deficiency	9 (1.4)	Iodine supplementation	19–37
Subtotal	467 (71.0)	–	–
Total DALYs lost	660 (100)	–	–

* DALYs lost (for specific diseases and the total) are taken from the 1993 World Development Report (World Bank 1993[1]).
† EPI-plus includes the six vaccines of the Expanded Program on Immunization (EPI), plus the vaccine against hepatitis B and vitamin A supplementation.

Table 26.7 The global balance sheet – child health 1990–2000

Goal	Gains	Unfinished business
Infant and under-5 mortality (U5MR): reduction by one-third in infant mortality and U5MR	More than 60 countries achieved the goal of U5MR At the global level, U5MR declined by 14%	U5MR rates increased in 14 countries (nine of them in sub-Saharan Africa) and were unchanged in 11 others Serious disparities remain in U5MR within countries: by income level, urban vs rural, and among minority groups
Polio: *global eradication* by 2000	More than 175 countries are polio free	Polio is still endemic in 20 countries
Routine immunization: *maintenance of a high level of immunization coverage*	Sustained routine immunization coverage at 75% [three doses of combined diphtheria/pertussis/tetanus vaccine (DPT3)]	Less than 50% of children under 1 year of age in sub-Saharan Africa are immunized against DPT3
Measles: *reduction by 95% in measles deaths and 90% in measles cases by 1995 as a major step in global eradication in the longer run*	Worldwide reported measles incidence has declined by nearly two-thirds between 1990 and 1999	In more than 15 countries, measles vaccination coverage is less than 50%
Neonatal tetanus: *elimination* by 1995	104 of 161 developing countries have achieved the goal Deaths caused by neonatal tetanus declined by 50% between 1990 and 2000	27 countries (18 in Africa) account for 90% of all remaining neonatal tetanus
Deaths due to diarrhea: *reduce them by 50%*	This goal was achieved globally, according to World Health Organization (WHO) estimates	Diarrhea remains one of the major causes of death among children
Acute respiratory infections (ARIs): *reduction of ARI deaths by one-third in children under 5*	ARI case management has improved at health center level The effectiveness of *Haemophilus influenzae* type b and pneumococcus vaccines is established	ARI remains one of the greatest causes of death among children Vertical, single-focus ARI programs seem to have had little global impact

Source: United Nations 2001[28]

are also complementary (Table 26.8). In Scotland, most surveillance is coordinated by the Scottish Centre for Infection and Environmental Health. Public health policy is coordinated by national departments of health and enacted by local specialists in public health medicine.

ACKNOWLEDGMENTS

In the preparation of this section the assistance of the following is gratefully acknowledged: the United Nations Special Program on AIDS, the European HIV Centre (EUROHIV) at INVS, Paris, the Office for National Statistics; Registrar General's Office, Scotland; Department of Health and Social Security, Northern Ireland; The Scottish Centre for Infection and Environmental Health, Glasgow; and the PHLS Communicable Disease Surveillance Centre, Colindale.

HOSPITAL INFECTION CONTROL: POLICIES AND PROCEDURES

It is essential that all hospitals have a strong infection control team. A model which works well is a team which consists of an infection control nurse practitioner and a clinical microbiologist or infectious disease physician. Feedback and support for the infection control team can be provided by an infection control committee consisting of representatives from medical administration, the surgical and medical staff, nursing and occupational health and safety, which should meet regularly. Each hospital should also have its own infection control policies and procedures manual that should be endorsed by the infection control committee. Infection control policies should be based on national infection control guidelines, such as those produced by the Hospital Infection Control Practices Advisory Committee (HICPAC) of the Centers for Disease Control in the USA, the National Health and Medical Research Council in Australia and the Public Health Laboratory Service in the UK. Full support (including financial) from the hospital executive is an essential component of a successful infection control program.

Table 26.8 Infectious disease morbidity and mortality: principal sources of data in the UK

Data source	Collected by	Type of information
Mortality data	OPCS, GRS, DHSS	Death entries from medical practitioners
Statutory notifications	OPCS, LGAs, SHHD, DH	Currently (1995) list of 39 IDs; selected because need for rapid local information for control, or to monitor national immunization program; clinical diagnoses
Laboratory reports	CDSC and SCIEH from PHLS and NHS laboratories	Wide range of microbiologically confirmed infections
General practitioners	RCGP from weekly returns from 40 practices	Wide range of infectious diseases presenting in general practice; clinical diagnoses
Computerized hospital discharge data	OPCS and SHHD individual HAs and HBs	All diagnoses categorized by ICD code; combination of clinical and microbiological
Consultant pediatricians	Royal College of Paediatrics and Child Health Surveillance Unit	Changing 'menu' of rare infections and infection-related disorders; specified case definitions

CDSC, Communicable Disease Surveillance Centre; DHSS, Department of Health and Social Security, Northern Ireland; GRS, General Registrar's Office for Scotland; HA, health authority; HB, health board; ID, infectious disease; LGA, local government authority; OPCS, Office of Population Censuses and Surveys; PHLS, Public Health Laboratory Service; RCGP, Royal College of General Practitioners; SCIEH, Scottish Centre for Infection and Environmental Health; SHHD, Scottish Home and Health Department.

The cornerstone of modern infection control is the concept of 'Standard Precautions'. As the name implies, these precautions should be standard practice for all patients whether or not they are known to be infectious. 'Standard Precautions' refers to hand washing *before* and after patient contact, and use of protective barriers such as gloves, gowns, plastic aprons, masks and eye protection when exposure to body fluids (*except sweat*) is a possibility. It also refers to careful handling of sharps and appropriate management of clinical waste. It does not include the routine use of single isolation rooms. Compliance with 'Standard Precautions' will help to prevent the spread of organisms that can be transmitted between patients on the hands of staff members and will also protect health care workers from exposure to blood borne pathogens such as HIV and hepatitis B and C.

Unfortunately, 'Standard Precautions' alone will not be adequate to prevent transmission of many infectious agents that affect children. In particular viral infections such as rotavirus, respiratory syncytial virus (RSV) and varicella pose a significant threat. The high risk of transmission of agents such as RSV result from children's lack of previous exposure (and hence immunity) to these infections and because they are usually suffering from primary infections which result in sustained, high levels of excretion of the virus.[30]

Chickenpox is highly infectious and may be spread by the airborne route. For this reason 'Additional Precautions' will need to be used and should include the use of a single room with negative pressure and external venting of air. It should be noted however, that hand washing remains the most important intervention to prevent the spread, even for airborne pathogens such as RSV infection.[31]

The specific 'Additional Precautions' required for an individual patient depends upon the type of organism they have and its mode of transmission. The decision to isolate a child in a single room may also be influenced by patient related factors. Young children who are mobile, but not yet able to control their impulsiveness, may require isolation in a single room if they are infected with organisms that are spread by direct contact. Isolation in a single room can be distressing for young children, but may be essential for containment of some infectious agents such as chickenpox. The seasonal nature of viral infections results in significant demands for pediatric isolation beds, particularly in the winter months. An inability to provide sufficient single rooms for these patients often results in the need to cohort patients with the same viral illness.

Although children's hospitals have traditionally had lower rates of multiresistant organisms compared to adult hospitals (possibly due to the relatively short duration of inpatient stay), this is now changing due to more intensive therapies, particularly those utilizing inserted foreign bodies and immunosuppressive chemotherapy.

Gram negative organisms such as extended spectrum beta lactamase producing enterobacteriaceae (ESBL) have been a particular problem in neonatal nurseries.[32] For organisms such as MRSA, it is considered desirable to manage children in single rooms, because of the risk of contamination of the local environment and because it is difficult to stop young children from interacting with other children on an open ward. Isolation in single rooms can pose significant problems for children with chronic illnesses who are admitted for prolonged periods. Sensible compromises, allowing children to go outside the hospital or into the hospital grounds, can relieve boredom and should not present a significant risk to other patients.

Immunization has dramatically reduced the requirement for isolation facilities in children's hospitals. Diseases such as measles and polio, which in the past placed huge demands on isolation beds, are now uncommonly seen in children's hospitals. The availability of varicella vaccine in many countries offers hope that chickenpox will also become an infrequent reason for isolation of children in hospitals in the future. Immunization with varicella vaccine of non-immune health care workers should be considered, both for the protection of staff and also to reduce the chance of cross infection to susceptible children by a staff member. The recent setback with rotavirus vaccine has unfortunately postponed the day when this too will become an uncommon nosocomial pathogen in children. Passive immunization with bovine serum colostrum has shown some efficacy in preventing transmission of rotavirus in pediatric hospitals.[33]

Routine surveillance of nosocomial infections remains an important mechanism to assess the efficacy of infection control measures and to help to monitor for outbreaks. The computerization of the clinical microbiology laboratory has greatly facilitated this process. Unfortunately many of the surveillance measures used in adult infection control practice, such as surgical site infection, may not be appropriate for pediatrics. It is important that meaningful surveillance measures for pediatrics are used, such as nosocomial rotavirus infection rates. Close communication with the microbiology laboratory is essential as changes in testing protocols for pathogens, such as rotavirus, can dramatically affect the frequency of positive surveillance results.

Some pediatric subspecialties, such as oncology and intensive care, are very dependent on antibiotic therapy for supportive care of their patients. The recent emergence of multiresistant pathogens such as vancomycin-insensitive *Staphylococcus aureus* (VISA) and multiresistant *Acinetobacter baumanii*, poses a significant threat to these medical specialties. Prudent use of antibiotics and effective infection control measures remain our most efficient tools to prevent the spread of these multiresistant organisms. It is essential that all pediatricians are familiar with the principles and practice of infection control in their institution.

PRINCIPLES OF ANTIMICROBIAL THERAPY

Although there are now literally hundreds of different antibiotics available worldwide, the mechanisms of action of antibiotics remain quite limited, and resistance via one mechanism may render inactive dozens of antibiotics in our antimicrobial arsenal. A clear understanding of the mechanism of action of antibiotics, and in particular mechanisms of antimicrobial resistance, will be helpful for the pediatricians of the future. The aim of this section is to provide pediatricians with a framework for appropriate decision making about the use of antibiotics. It should also provide a basic understanding of the mechanism of action of the antibiotics and mechanisms of antimicrobial resistance of the organisms that are relevant to day-to-day pediatric practice.

COMMON QUESTIONS WHEN PRESCRIBING ANTIBIOTICS

1. *Should I use an antibiotic at all?*
   Often antibiotic therapy is not necessary. One of the best examples of this in pediatrics is the treatment of otitis media. Only a small number of patients benefit from the use of antibiotics in this condition.[34,35] The choice of which patients to treat and which not to treat is however, more problematic. In mild episodes of otitis media, a watch and see approach would be prudent and could result in a dramatic reduction in the use of antibiotics in children in the community.
2. *Which antibiotic should I use?*
   There are two main situations in which antibiotics are chosen. The first is the empirical choice of antibiotics when the causative organism is not yet known and the second is in response to a positive culture result. When dealing with the empirical choice of antibiotics, it is important to know what common organisms are associated with the clinical scenario that you are faced with. It is also important to know what the local antibiotic resistance patterns are for these organisms. Clinical practice guidelines are often helpful in this situation. These guidelines may be written at a national, regional or hospital level. The degree of variability in the incidence of antibiotic resistance will determine which are the most appropriate guidelines to use. It is important to ensure that the guidelines that you use are appropriate for your local conditions and are up to date. It is beyond the scope of this chapter to discuss recommendations for empirical antibiotic choices but the reader is referred to an important reference for guidance.[36]
3. *Should I use more than one antibiotic?*
   There are several situations in which the use of a combination rather than a single antibiotic may be desirable.
   - The empirical therapy of conditions in which more than one pathogen may be responsible for a serious infection, e.g. neonatal meningitis, may require the combination of at least two different antibiotics in order to give adequate coverage until culture results become available. The use of ampicillin (to cover *Listeria monocytogenes* and group B streptococcus) and a third generation cephalosporin (to cover Gram negative organisms) is required in neonatal meningitis.
   - The second common reason is antibiotic synergy. Antibiotic synergy occurs when the combined effect of two antibiotics is greater than the sum of the individual action of each antibiotic on its own. One example of this is the treatment of enterococcal endocarditis. *Enterococcus* is relatively tolerant to the effects of penicillin antibiotics. This means that ampicillin will inhibit the growth of enterococcus but will not necessarily kill the organism. The addition of an aminoglycoside, such as gentamicin, results in potent killing of the organism (provided that the organism does not have an enzyme which will inactivate the aminoglycoside) and not just inhibition of growth. The mechanism of synergy occurs because beta lactam antibiotics increase the permeability of the cell wall to aminoglycosides (these are not normally able to easily enter streptococcal bacterial cells) which allows the aminoglycosides to reach their ribosomal targets.[37]
   - Improved outcome with combination therapy. This is seen with the treatment of *Pseudomonas aeruginosa* and other Gram negative infections in patients with bacteremia and neutropenia.[38]

- Prevention of development of antibiotic resistance. Although theoretically the combination of two antibiotics should reduce the chance of antibiotic resistance developing, this is not always the case. It is, however, true for certain infections such as the treatment of *Mycobacterium tuberculosis*. There is no justification for using this policy for all infections, and the trend now is towards single agent therapy unless good evidence exists for combined therapy.

4. *What route of administration should I use?*
This will depend upon the antibiotic, the patient, the organism and disease related factors. Some antibiotics, such as the glycopeptide vancomycin and aminoglycosides like gentamicin, are not well absorbed orally and must be given intravenously.[39] Neonates absorb oral antibiotics poorly, and parenteral therapy should be used in general. Some patients such as young infants, or patients who are vomiting, may tolerate antibiotics poorly and, therefore, require intravenous antibiotics for more serious infections. Some organisms such as *Ps. aeruginosa* have relatively high minimum inhibitory concentrations to many antibiotics, and require high doses of intravenous antibiotics to treat them. Infections of privileged sites, such as the cerebrospinal fluid (CSF), require high doses of antibiotics to achieve therapeutic levels at these sites, and such levels cannot be readily achieved by the oral route. Diseases such as meningitis require rapid therapy and therefore the intravenous route is preferred in order to obtain an immediate effect of the antibiotic.
5. *What dose should I use?*
The dose of antibiotic used is generally based on the pharmacokinetics of the drug, the site of the infection and the nature of the organism being treated. The dose may also depend on the route of administration. The bioavailability of some antibiotics can vary greatly depending on the route of administration. The oral dose may also need to be less than the intravenous dose because of the difficulty in tolerating high oral doses for some drugs (e.g. flucloxacillin). Generally, published doses should be used as outlined in therapeutic guidelines for the condition being treated.[37] Many of these guidelines will be based on published efficacy data.
6. *How often should I give the dose?*
This will depend on the pharmacokinetics and mechanism of action of the drug. Cell wall antibiotics such as penicillins and glycopeptides require a constant presence of the agent in order to maintain killing capacity. More frequent dosing, with relatively high antibiotic trough levels, will ensure that the concentration of antibiotic at the target site will remain above the minimum inhibitory concentration (MIC) of the organism for the majority of the dosing interval. The half-life of cell wall agents is therefore the principal determinant of the recommended dosing intervals. Aminoglycosides, on the other hand, have a significant postantibiotic effect. A postantibiotic effect means that these antibiotics have a persistent effect on the organism beyond the point at which the antibiotic concentration falls below the MIC of the organism.[40] This may allow less frequent dosing, e.g. once daily dosing, of these agents.
7. *Should I measure drug levels?*
If drug levels are to be measured it must be clearly understood why they are being measured and what clinical correlation exists between the drug levels and patient outcome. Often the reason for drug level monitoring is to prevent toxicity. This is particularly important for antibiotics with a relatively low therapeutic index (the ratio of the concentration required to give therapeutic benefit and the concentration that results in toxic side-effects). One of the best examples of this is aminoglycosides. There is general agreement that careful monitoring of antibiotic levels of these agents is important in order to avoid nephrotoxicity and ototoxicity. The use of therapeutic monitoring of aminoglycosides is particularly important in pediatric oncology patients who receive prolonged, repeated courses of aminoglycosides. They will also be exposed to other potent nephrotoxic and ototoxic agents. Routine monitoring of aminoglyoside levels in otherwise healthy children receiving aminoglycosides as empirical therapy for urinary tract infection, where the duration of therapy may be less than 48 h, does not seem warranted unless therapy is to be prolonged beyond this time.
8. *How long should I treat?*
This is one of the most commonly asked questions of the pediatric infectious disease physician and one with probably the least good clinical research to support the answers.[41] Convention dictates that we use fixed durations of therapy such as 5 days, 7 days, 10 days, 14 days, etc., which Radetsky[41] amusingly calls 'magic numbers' chosen because of their religious or anatomical significance. There are, however, few data to support many of these recommendations. Furthermore, in the past the popular advice was always to complete a long course of antibiotics in order to prevent resistance developing. This dogma is now being challenged and most experts now recommend using the minimum duration of therapy necessary to cure a patient of their disease. There is increasing recognition that our body's own immune system will often cure the disease and eradicate the organism provided antibiotics can tip the disease process in the host's favor. Penicillin resistance that now occurs in pathogens such as *Streptococcus pneumoniae* appears to have originated in our normal flora[42] and so the emphasis is now on minimizing the exposure of all organisms to antibiotics.

MECHANISMS OF ACTION OF ANTIBIOTICS

It is important to understand that there are only limited numbers of mechanisms that antibiotics use to kill organisms.

The six major targets for antibiotics include:

1. DNA synthesis – trimethoprim and sulfonamides, metronidazole;
2. DNA replication – fluoroquinolones (e.g. ciprofloxacin);
3. RNA synthesis – rifampicin;
4. protein synthesis – aminoglycosides, macrolides (e.g. erythromycin), lincosamides (e.g. clindamycin), chloramphenicol, tetracyclines and fusidic acid;
5. cell wall synthesis – beta lactam antibiotics (penicillins, cephalosporins and carbapenems), glycopeptides (e.g. vancomycin and teicoplanin);
6. cell membrane – polymyxins (e.g. colistin).

MECHANISMS OF RESISTANCE TO ANTIBIOTICS

Bacteria have a number of different strategies that are becoming increasingly effective in neutralizing the antibiotics that we use against them.

There are four major mechanisms of resistance to antibiotics:

1. reduced ability of antibiotics to reach the target: e.g. active efflux pumps or decreased permeability of the cell wall or membrane;
2. enzymatic inactivation of the antibiotic: e.g. beta lactamases, aminoglycoside inactivating enzymes such as adenyltransferases, acyltransferases and phosphotransferases;
3. alteration of the target: e.g. altered penicillin binding proteins, erythromycin resistance methylases;
4. alteration of local environment: e.g. formation of pus with altered pH.

Understanding these mechanisms of action and resistance is clinically relevant, because the acquisition of a single mechanism of resistance, e.g. an altered target such as a modified penicillin-binding protein, may render multiple antibiotics inactive within that class. Extrapolation of susceptibility results, using an understanding of the mechanisms of antimicrobial resistance is important, as it is impractical to test and report all known antibiotics for an individual clinical isolate.

COMMON EXAMPLES OF ANTIMICROBIAL ACTION AND RESISTANCE

Only the more common antibiotic resistance mechanisms and resistant organisms seen in pediatric practice will be described in this chapter.

PENICILLINS, CEPHALOSPORINS, CARBAPENEMS AND OTHER BETA LACTAM ANTIBIOTICS

Mechanism of action

Penicillin-binding proteins (PBPs) are enzymes that are involved in cell wall synthesis of bacteria. The principal mechanism of action of beta lactam antibiotics is to bind to these PBPs and to prevent them from catalyzing the formation of the bacterial cell wall.[43] Another major mechanism of action of penicillins is the activation of bacterial autolytic enzymes. The specificity of different beta lactam antibiotics for PBPs varies, which explains the differences seen in the activity of different beta lactam antibiotics for different bacterial species.

Mechanism of resistance

Beta lactamases (enzymatic inactivation of the antibiotic)

Beta lactamases are bacterial enzymes that are closely related to PBPs[44] and act as decoys for the PBPs of bacteria. Beta lactamase enzymes inactivate beta lactam antibiotics by disrupting the cyclic amide bond of the beta lactam ring of these antibiotics and forming acylenzyme intermediates. The acylenzyme intermediates that are formed are rapidly broken down, allowing the beta lactamases to inactivate additional beta lactam antibiotic molecules. Beta lactamases have varying specificity for different beta lactam antibiotics and beta lactam antibiotics also have varying stability against attack by different classes of beta lactamase. This explains the varying activity of different antibiotics against beta lactamase producing bacteria.

Altered PBPs (altered target)

By altering the principal target of beta lactam antibiotics, PBPs, bacteria can escape from the effects of these antibiotics. As beta lactam antibiotics often target more than one PBP, escape from the effect of these antibiotics may take decades to develop, as multiple proteins must be modified to have a significant effect on the MIC of the organism. The sharing of the DNA that encodes the altered PBPs between bacterial species can speed up this process. One of the most notable examples of this is methicillin resistance in staphylococci. The MecA resistance gene which encodes for a modified PBP2a (also known as PBP2´) has been transferred between different strains and species of staphylococci.[45] Many coagulase negative staphylococci, as well as some *Staphylococcus aureus* strains, now contain PBP2a. PBP2a has reduced affinity for all beta lactam antibiotics. The success of PBP2a is because it is still able to successfully participate in cell wall synthesis of the organism, allowing these strains to survive and grow in the presence of oxacillin. The PBP2a gene is highly conserved and it is clear that the PBP2a gene has been able to transfer itself between different strains and species of staphylococci. The resultant clones have then expanded due to their selective advantage and spread throughout the world.

Another important example of resistance due to altered PBPs is penicillin-resistant *Streptococcus pneumoniae.* The alteration in PBPs in *S. pneumoniae* is more complex than in staphylococci. The MIC of this organism increases with a stepwise alteration of as many as four of the six different PBPs,[46] in high level resistant strains. The relative affinity of different penicillin-binding varies for different beta lactam antibiotics.

Clinical relevance of beta lactam resistance

Example 1 – Extended spectrum beta lactamase (ESBL) producing Gram negative organisms. The ESBL beta lactamases have evolved from pre-existing beta lactamases in Gram negative organisms. Mutations of these beta lactamases have now resulted in their ability to hydrolyse third generation cephalosporins,[47] which until recently had been relatively stable to the effects of most Gram negative beta lactamases. One of the very concerning features of the ESBL genes that encode for the ESBL beta lactamases is that they can be transferred on mobile genetic elements such as plasmids. This allows these beta lactamases to readily spread between different strains of bacteria and indeed between different species. This may occur with tremendous rapidity, resulting in outbreaks of resistance genes (rather than just the clones of bacteria that contain them). This can confuse clinicians, who are used to recognizing antibiotic resistance outbreaks due to increased incidence of specific bacterial strains with a certain resistance profile. The outbreaks associated with ESBL gene transfer may involve more than one species of organism, which makes their recognition and detection very difficult.

Typically the ESBL beta lactamases are inhibited by clavulanic acid, but recent mutations have altered this typical pattern, making the laboratory detection of these beta lactamases (which had been dependent on this resistance pattern) more difficult. The specificity of different ESBL beta lactamases can vary greatly and may affect one type of third generation cephalosporin more than another. Most carbapenems (imipenem and meropenem) have remained stable to the effect of these ESBL beta lactamases and remain the cornerstone of therapy for these organisms. How long this will remain the case is yet to be seen. In order to predict susceptibility of Gram negatives in an individual institution, a local knowledge of the prevalence of these resistance mechanisms is essential.

Example 2 – Methicillin resistant staphylococci. Unlike the ESBL mechanism of resistance, methicillin resistance in staphylococci due to the presence of the MecA gene is highly predictable. The MecA gene, when present (and if expressed by the genome of the bacteria), renders the bacteria resistant to all beta lactam antibiotics of all classes including carbapenems. It is important to note the MecA gene is generally encoded in the chromosome of the bacteria. The MecA gene can be transferred to other strains, but the frequency of this occurrence is far lower than for the transfer of plasmids. As a result, the resistance seen in this case tends to be clonal expansion of bacterial strains rather than the rapid transfer of resistance elements (that can be seen with the ESBL genes). This can make early detection of outbreaks a little easier than with ESBL genes.

Example 3 – Penicillin resistant *Streptococcus pneumoniae*. Penicillin resistance in pneumococcus is a relative resistance rather than absolute resistance, and provided that the MIC of the organism can be exceeded sufficiently at the target site, penicillin therapy should be effective. Pneumococcus does not produce beta lactamases, and so agents such as amoxicillin/clavulanic acid have no additional benefit in treating these organisms compared to amoxicillin alone. The penicillin resistance in pneumococci is most clinically relevant in meningitis and otitis media. This is due to the difficulty in achieving high concentrations of antibiotics at the site of these infections. Even with high dose intravenous penicillin it may be difficult to achieve adequate levels of penicillin in the CSF in order to adequately kill penicillin-resistant strains of pneumococci. A similar situation occurs when treating otitis media with oral antibiotics, although high doses of oral amoxicillin, e.g. 80 mg/kg/day,[48] which is more efficiently absorbed may be successful.

Other foci of infection such as pneumonia may be adequately treated with high dose intravenous penicillin provided the MIC of the organism to penicillin is < 4 mg/L. Pneumococci that have reduced susceptibility to penicillin usually also have reduced susceptibility to third generation cephalosporins such as cefotaxime. Third generation cephalosporins may have different affinity for PBPs. This can lead to either higher or lower MICs to cefotaxime when compared to penicillin. Third generation cephalosporins, such as cefotaxime, have higher achievable levels in the CSF with inflamed meninges compared to non-inflamed meninges. Clinical failure with the use of third generation cephalosporins in pneumococcal meningitis caused by resistant strains has now been described.[49] The addition of vancomycin, with or without rifampicin, is now recommended for therapy of these strains when they cause meningitis.[36]

GLYCOPEPTIDE ANTIBIOTICS, E.G. VANCOMYCIN AND TEICOPLANIN

Mechanism of action

It is a common misconception that vancomycin is an aminoglycoside. It is a glycopeptide, and in no way related to aminoglycosides, and its mechanism of action is quite different. It acts by binding to the peptidyl-D-alanyl-D-alanine termini of peptidoglycan (cell wall) precursors.[50] This prevents cell wall synthesis of the organism. Gram negative organisms are inherently resistant to vancomycin, because of the impermeability of the outer cell membrane of bacteria to these large hydrophobic molecules.

Mechanism of resistance

The principal mechanism of resistance to glycopeptides is an altered target. Recently, resistance to glycopeptides in enterococci has been described. Two principal resistance phenotypes have been determined[51] – Van A and Van B. Van A encodes an enzyme which catalyzes the formation of D-Ala-D-lactate instead of the usual D-Ala-D-alanine precursor of the peptidoglycan cell wall. As vancomycin principally targets D-Ala-D-alanine residues, the organism has become resistant by altering the principal target of the antibiotic. The Van A phenotype demonstrates both vancomcyin and teicoplanin resistance. Van B has a similar mechanism of resistance but the enzyme is not induced by teicoplanin. Vancomycin will however, induce resistance and when this occurs, cross resistance to teicoplanin can occur.

Clinical relevance

Vancomycin resistant enterococci (VRE) have become common nosocomial pathogens in some parts of the world. These strains are often resistant to beta lactam antibiotics and may also contain aminoglycoside resistance genes. This has made infections such as endocarditis particularly difficult to treat. Enterococci themselves are not highly virulent pathogens and frequently the source of infection is a foreign body such as a central venous access device. Removal of the infected device may be curative and should always be considered early in order to prevent the development of endocarditis.

MACROLIDES (E.G. ERYTHROMYCIN) AND LINCOSAMIDES (E.G. CLINDAMYCIN)

Mechanism of action

Macrolides inhibit bacterial protein synthesis by binding to the 23S component of the 50S ribosomal subunit. They bind to a specific location on this ribosomal subunit. Lincosamides are structurally different from macrolides but target the same site in the ribosomal subunit.

Mechanism of resistance

The two most common mechanisms of resistance to macrolides are an altered target site and active efflux of the antibiotics. Resistance can develop to erythromycin by the acquisition of a methylase enzyme (Erm, i.e. Erythromycin resistance methylase) which methylates a specific adenine residue of the ribosomal subunit close to the target site of the antibiotic.[52] Macrolides potently induce this methylase, whereas lincosamides such as clindamycin only do so weakly or not at all. As a result of this, organisms such as pneumococcus that are resistant by this mechanism may appear susceptible in vitro to clindamycin. However if these isolates are exposed to erythromycin, the methylase is induced and cross resistance to clindamycin is induced. Resistance via this mechanism also confers resistance to streptogramin B. This mechanism is therefore often termed MLS_b (macrolide, lincosamide, streptogramin B) resistance. The second mechanism of resistance is confined to macrolides (without cross-resistance to lincosamides), and is due to an active efflux pump. The Mef (macrolide efflux) gene is responsible for this mechanism of resistance in *Streptococcus pneumoniae*.

Clinical relevance

It is important for clinicians to understand that cross resistance between macrolides and lincosamides can occur but does not occur in all isolates. It is important to clarify with your own microbiology laboratory whether cross resistance exists prior to using clindamycin in erythromycin resistant isolates of *Streptococcus pneumoniae*.

AMINOGLYCOSIDES, E.G. GENTAMICIN, TOBRAMYCIN AND AMIKACIN

Mechanism of action

Aminoglycosides bind irreversibly to the 30S ribosomal RNA subunit and in so doing prevent protein synthesis. In order for aminoglycosides to act they must be able to traverse the lipopolysaccharide coat of Gram negative organisms and they are thought do this principally via protein gateways called porins.

Mechanism of resistance

The two major mechanisms of resistance are enzymatic inactivation and altered permeability of the bacterial cell to aminoglycosides. The most common inactivating enzymes are phosphotransferases, acetyltransferases and adenyltransferases. These enzymes attach phosphate, acetyl and adenyl groups respectively onto aminoglycosides, and in so doing inactivate them. These inactivating enzymes are specific for different classes of aminoglycoside and so cross resistance between different classes of aminoglycosides does not always occur. Of concern is the fact that the genes that encode these enzymes are often located on mobile genetic elements such as plasmids and transposons. They form part of resistance gene cassettes and these cassettes may also contain other resistance elements such as ESBL genes. The second major mechanism of resistance is reduction in uptake of aminoglycosides by the bacteria. Although this was generally considered to be due to loss of porins (protein gateways for uptake of the molecules), this mechanism is now in question.[53] This results in an inability of the aminoglycosides to enter the bacterial cells and therefore reach their ribosomal target. Resistance due to decreased uptake of aminoglycosides can occur whilst on therapy and is particularly common in organisms such as *Pseudomonas aeruginosa*.

Clinical relevance

Rapid spread of aminoglycoside resistance genes, when combined with ESBL resistance mechanisms can lead to serious outbreaks of Gram negative organisms that are resistant to first line antibiotic therapy. Aminoglycosides and third generation cephalosporins have been the mainstay of empirical Gram negative therapy and the loss of effectiveness is an ominous sign that we are losing the war against resistant Gram negative organisms.

ANTIVIRAL AND ANTIFUNGAL THERAPY

A detailed description of this is beyond the scope of this chapter. Readers are referred to an excellent reference on these topics.[54]

CONCLUSION

Pediatricians of the twenty-first century will need a comprehensive understanding of antibiotics and mechanisms of resistance in order to rationally prescribe antibiotics in an era where resistance is the rule rather than the exception. The use of clinical practice guidelines is helpful in the prescribing of antibiotics but it is important to ensure that the guidelines used are up to date and relevant to the clinical setting in which the pediatricians find themselves practicing.

CLINICAL PROBLEMS: THE CHILD WITH FEVER

The most useful temperature measurement is the core or central temperature which has a normal range in young adults of 36.4–36.9°C, and fluctuation around these values of up to 0.4°C. Infants have a rectal temperature above 37°C which falls by about 0.8°C during sleep and rises before waking.[55] There is a circadian rhythm in childhood with the highest temperature at 6 p.m. The peripheral temperature is normally 0.5°C lower than that recorded centrally.[56] What is regarded as fever varies. Studies of infants define fever as a central temperature of greater than 38°C. Antipyretic agents have the same effect on fever of either bacterial or viral origin and the response should not be used as a distinguishing feature. The core temperature can be measured either rectally or orally using a mercury thermometer or electronic probe. Electronic tympanic membrane thermometers are only moderately accurate providing they are inserted correctly. Mercury thermometers for measurement of axillary (peripheral) temperature are now rarely used. A number of disposable strip thermometers are available for use on the forehead. They are simple to use but less accurate than mercury and electronic thermometers.

Although a central temperature reading is of value in the sick child, and measurement of the temperature difference between core and periphery is of particular value in the shocked patient, for most purposes a peripheral reading is adequate.

The commonest cause of fever in childhood is viral infection, usually resolving within a week of onset. Persistence of fever for longer demands thorough investigation; the term pyrexia or fever of unknown origin (PUO, FUO) is normally applied when fever has been present for 14 days.

FEVER IN THE NEWBORN

Fever during the neonatal period may be the presenting sign of bacterial infection. If investigation is delayed until other signs occur, such as lethargy, anorexia or apnea, infection may be far advanced before treatment is started. It is generally accepted that any febrile newborn should have cultures of blood, CSF and urine taken, and then should be started on empirical antibiotics.[57]

Viral infections, either congenital or acquired, may also be associated with fever. Babies who acquire herpes simplex virus (HSV) infection from their mothers at birth may present after 2–7 days with fever and non-specific signs of sepsis. It is unusual for Group B streptococcus to present this late, and HSV should be considered in the differential diagnosis. Clinical features may include skin, eye or mouth lesions, pneumonitis and hepatitis. Other viruses that commonly present with fever in the neonatal period include enteroviruses, influenza and respiratory syncytial virus.

FEVER DURING INFANCY AND CHILDHOOD

The commonest cause of fever in this group is viral infection and tends to be short lived. The challenge for the pediatrician is to determine whether the fever is the result of a viral or bacterial infection. In a series of 292 infants under 2 months old admitted to hospital with a history of fever, 19 (6.5%) were described as having serious bacterial infection, although five of the group were afebrile at the time of admission.[58] In a prospective study of children 3–36 months of age, pathogenic bacteria were isolated in blood culture from 60/519 (12%) with a fever greater than 39.5°C (method of temperature measurement not described). The risk of bacterial infection was found to be higher among infants with an elevated white blood count.[59]

The typical signs of viral upper respiratory infection include coryza, inflamed tympanic membranes, tonsillitis and fever. Bacterial tonsillitis and otitis media are difficult to differentiate from viral causes.

A good history and thorough examination are essential if a speedy diagnosis is to be achieved. Thus direct questions should be asked about the following:

1. previous immunizations;
2. family members with fever;
3. travel abroad;
4. consumption of unpasteurized milk (to exclude listeriosis, brucellosis), or raw eggs (*Salmonella* spp.);
5. history of congenital heart disease;
6. symptoms of this illness (abdominal pain, urinary frequency and dysuria);
7. signs noticed – rash, joint swelling.

Examination should take note of rash, lymphadenopathy, hepato- and splenomegaly, chest signs, heart murmurs, abdominal masses and tenderness. The bones and joints should be assessed for swelling and tenderness.

When fever has been persistent – over a week for instance – and no cause has been found, serious consideration should be given to hospital admission to confirm pyrexia and to initiate investigations. The physical signs and investigations required to exclude conditions producing FUO or PUO are given in Table 26.9.

However, certain basic investigations should be performed – of which urine and blood culture are the most useful.

FEVER AND NEUTROPENIA

The neutropenic child with fever is a similar clinical situation to the neonatal period, in that there is no time to wait for culture results. Antibiotics should be started after blood cultures have been taken. The antibiotics chosen must cover infections due to staphylococci and Gram negative enteric bacilli. Neutropenic children are also at risk of fungal infection, and empirical antifungal therapy is indicated if fever persists despite antibiotics and negative cultures.

CLINICAL PROBLEMS: THE CHILD WITH A RASH

In some cases a rash will be diagnostic, and in others the diagnosis will only be reached in conjunction with the history and appropriate investigations. Failure to recognize certain rashes could cost the life of a child, as in meningococcal infection or varicella in an immunocompromised child.

In establishing a diagnosis when an infectious cause is considered, certain information should be obtained by history as follows: prior infectious disease and/or rashes; recent contact with infectious disease; prior immunization; foreign travel; prodromal illness; fever.

In the general examination, note should be taken of the child's general state, the temperature, appearance of conjunctivae, ears and throat. Careful auscultation of the chest should be performed; all groups of lymph glands as well as liver and spleen should be examined.

Once this has been done interest should return to the rash which should be described carefully in its form (e.g. hemorrhagic, macular, papular):

1. macules – flat and impalpable;
2. papules – circumscribed, elevated lesions;
3. vesicles – circumscribed, elevated, fluid-filled, and normally less than 0.5 cm in diameter;
4. pustules – elevated lesions containing a purulent exudate;
5. petechiae and other hemorrhagic spots – cannot be blanched by compression and may be flat or raised; the term purpura usually refers to the larger lesions with a diameter greater than 0.5 cm.

The distribution may be an important clue to certain infections. Consideration may need to be given as to whether the rash is itchy, e.g. are there signs of scratching?

RASHES IN THE NEWBORN

In this age group rashes are common. Neonatal urticaria, or erythema toxicum, is characterized by a mixture of erythematous macules, and white or yellow papules. These usually develop over the first few days and may persist until the end of the second week. Staphylococcal infection of the newborn may be difficult to distinguish from neonatal urticaria. Although erythematous lesions are seen with staphylococcal infection, pustules and vesicles predominate. When there is uncertainty as to the diagnosis, a Gram stain of vesicle fluid should be performed. Plentiful polymorphs as well as Gram positive cocci should be seen in the presence of staphylococcal infection; eosinophils predominate in neonatal urticaria.

Vesicles are also seen in neonatal varicella and herpes simplex virus (HSV) infection. In the former, a history of maternal varicella will be elicited. In the latter, however, a history of past or current genital herpes is obtained in only a quarter of cases. The vesicles of HSV tend to be larger and less opaque than those of staphylococcal infection. Urgent treatment of neonatal HSV is essential, and diagnosis can be achieved by electron microscopy on vesicle fluid or by rapid viral identification tests such as immunofluorescence.

Other rashes associated with infection may be petechial or purpuric, as seen in congenital cytomegalovirus (CMV) or rubella, as a result of thrombocytopenia. In such cases the rash is usually just one of several clinical features of congenital infection.

RASHES IN INFANCY AND CHILDHOOD

These will be described under descriptive headings.

VESICULAR RASHES

Varicella

Lesions normally appear without a prodromal illness, and progress rapidly (within a few hours) from papules to vesicles surrounded by an erythematous base. Crops of vesicles appear over 3 days, predominantly on the trunk and proximal limbs. Vesicles may also develop on mucous membranes.

Herpes zoster

Lesions similar to those seen in varicella infection may develop over specific dermatomes or cranial nerves. Although the immunosuppressed are at increased risk from zoster, this condition is also seen in normal children.

Herpes simplex virus

Although infection is most commonly associated with gingivostomatitis during childhood, vesicles are seen on the skin in eczema herpeticum (Kaposi's varicelliform eruption). Pyrexia is followed by the appearance of crops of vesicles on the eczematous skin. Crops of lesions may occur over several days. Correct and rapid diagnosis is essential because untreated severe infection may be fatal.

Hand, foot and mouth

This is caused by enteroviruses, the commonest being Coxsackie virus type 16, and occurs in epidemics. It is associated with a papular–vesicular eruption of the mouth, hands, feet and sometimes buttocks.

Impetigo

This condition usually presents as a red macule and then becomes vesicular. The small vesicles burst to leave a honey-colored crust. Both streptococcal and staphylococcal impetigo occur commonly around the mouth but can occur elsewhere.

Molluscum contagiosum

This is caused by a pox virus. Flesh-colored papules with a central dimple are seen. Although firm initially they become softer and more waxy with time. Lesions are 2–5 mm in size and may occur anywhere. It is more severe in HIV infection.

Dermatitis herpetiformis

This occurs in children from 8 years upwards who develop recurrent crops of pruritic papulovesicles over extensor surfaces

Table 26.9 Causes of pyrexia of unknown origin

Disease	Signs	Investigations
Bacterial		
Brucellosis	Lymphadenopathy, splenomegaly	Antibody titers
Bacterial endocarditis	Murmur, splinter hemorrhages	Blood culture $\times$ 3, *Brucella, Coxiella* titers
Leptospirosis	Hematuria, jaundice, conjunctivitis	Blood culture, serology
Osteomyelitis	Bone swelling, tenderness, redness, immobility	Blood culture, bone aspirate culture, bone radioisotope scan
Pelvic abscess	Abdominal tenderness, tender mass rectally	Leukocytosis on full blood count
Pyelonephritis	Loin tenderness	Urine microscopy and culture
Tuberculosis	Pneumonia, meningitis	Tuberculin test, culture gastric washings $\pm$ cerebrospinal fluid, chest X-ray
Typhoid fever	Abdominal tenderness, rose spots, splenomegaly	Blood culture
Septic arthritis	Swelling, tenderness, immobility at single joint	Joint aspirate culture
Psittacosis	Chest crackles, tachypnea	Chest X-ray, serology
Listeriosis	Arthritis, meningism	Blood culture, cerebrospinal fluid culture
Virus		
Cytomegalic inclusion disease	Lymphadenopathy, hepatosplenomegaly	Urine culture etc., blood and urine PCR
Human immunodeficiency virus	Lymphadenopathy, failure to thrive, chronic infection, e.g. candida	T4/T8 lymphocyte ratio, HIV antibody, HIV PCR
Infectious mononucleosis	Tonsillitis, hepatosplenomegaly	Paul–Bunnell/Monospot, Epstein–Barr viral antibody
Hepatitis	Icterus, hepatomegaly	Hepatitis A, Hepatitis B serology, hepatitis B and C PCR
Parasite		
Malaria	Splenomegaly, hepatomegaly, encephalopathy	Thick or thin blood film
Toxoplasmosis	Cervical, supraclavicular lymphadenopathy	Smear from biopsy specimen, serology
Miscellaneous		
Crohn's disease	Abdominal tenderness and mass	GI endoscopy or barium study of GI tract. Exclude *Yersinia* and *Campylobacter* infection
Diabetes insipidus	Polyuria, polydipsia	Dilute urine following water deprivation
Juvenile rheumatoid arthritis		
1. Systemic	Fever, characteristic maculopapular rash, lethargy, arthritis, pericardial effusion	No diagnostic test
2. Monoarticular/polyarticular	Fever not a consistent sign	
Kawasaki disease	Cervical lymphadenopathy, bilateral conjunctival injection, red, fissured lips and tongue, maculopapular rash, swelling and desquamation of hands and feet	No diagnostic test
Malignancy Leukemia Lymphoma Neuroblastoma	Includes anemia, lymphadenopathy, splenomegaly Abdominal mass, bone pain	Full blood count, blood film, lymph node biopsy, bone marrow trephine, vanillylmandelic acid
Factitious fever (Munchausen by proxy)	Pyrexia only recorded by parent	None

including the elbows, buttocks and knees. Many of these children also have a gluten-sensitive enteropathy.

MACULOPAPULAR RASHES

Measles

Measles rash is blotchy, red or pink in color, raised in places, and starts behind the ears and on the face, spreading downwards. The lesions tend to become confluent on the upper part of the body and remain more discrete lower down. The rash fades, usually after 2–3 days. The skin becomes brown and although desquamation occurs this is not usually seen on the hands and feet as it is in scarlet fever.

Rubella

Rubella results in a pink rash which progresses caudally. The lesions are normally discrete and the rash develops more quickly and disappears earlier than in measles. Desquamation is not a characteristic.

Scarlet fever

The eruption is dark red and punctiform. The rash tends to be most prominent on the neck and in the major skinfolds. A distinctive feature is circumoral pallor as a result of the rash sparing the area around the mouth. As with measles, desquamation is seen but the hands and feet are involved. True scarlet fever is associated with inflammation of the tongue (white and red strawberry tongue). Scarlatina refers to the rash which may occur alone in milder streptococcal infection, and is often shortlived.

Kawasaki disease

Although several features are required for the diagnosis of this condition, which is of unknown etiology, the rash may be confused with that of scarlet fever. Discrete red maculopapules are seen on the feet, around the knees and in the axillary and inguinal skin creases. Desquamation of the hands and feet is a common feature (Fig. 26.15, Plate 26.15).

Erythema infectiosum or fifth disease

Infection caused by parvovirus B19 is associated with a rash which develops in two stages. The cheeks appear red and flushed, giving rise to a 'slapped cheek' appearance. A maculopapular rash develops 1–2 weeks later, predominantly over the arms and legs which, as it fades, appears lace-like.

Roseola infantum

The main cause is human herpesvirus 6 (HHV-6). Roseola infantum is characterized by a widespread morbilliform (measles-like) rash, seen in its most florid form on the trunk. The lesions tend to be discrete. As the rash appears the fever, which is normally present over the previous 4 days, resolves and the child looks well (in contrast to measles, in which the child is febrile and unwell when the rash appears).

Viral infections

Many viral infections, particularly those associated with the enteroviruses, may cause maculopapular rashes.

PETECHIAL AND PURPURIC RASHES

Meningococcal infection

The first sign of meningococcal septicemia may be a petechial or purpuric rash anywhere on the body and often localized (Fig. 26.16, Plate 26.16). On occasions these lesions may be preceded by or accompany a maculopapular rash which may blanch (Fig. 26.17, Plate 26.17). The petechiae will not blanch, and although it is conventional to make a microbiological diagnosis on blood culture and PCR bacteria can also be isolated from these lesions.

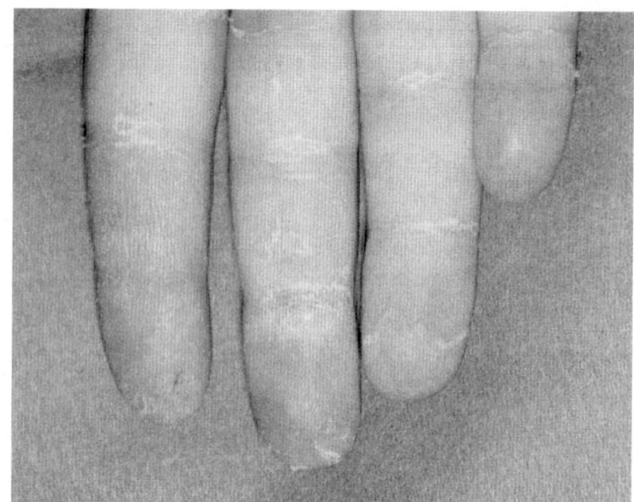
Fig. 23.15 Kawasaki disease: finger desquamation starting at the tips.

Meningococcal petechiae can be confused with those seen on the face around the eyes following events that result in a transient rise in venous pressure such as vomiting. Rarely petechial rashes are associated with septicemia caused by other bacteria particularly *Haemophilus influenzae*.

Henoch–Schönlein purpura

This condition often follows an upper respiratory tract infection but no single infective agent has been implicated. Hemorrhagic macules and papules develop on the buttocks and extensor surfaces of the limbs particularly the knees and ankles. The lesions come in crops and fade over a few days leaving a brown pigmentation.

Idiopathic thrombocytopenic purpura (ITP)

A purpuric rash sometimes associated with frank bleeding is seen in this condition. Even postinfective cases are referred to as ITP and rubella infection is considered to be the commonest cause.

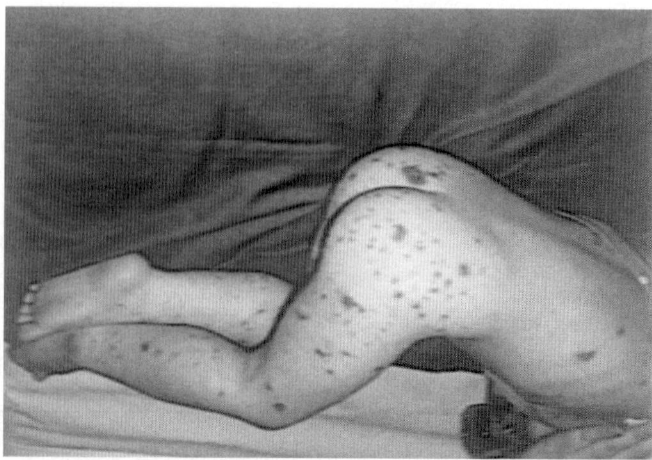
Fig. 23.16 Purpuric rash of meningococcemia. (Courtesy of Department of Medical Illustration, University of Aberdeen.)

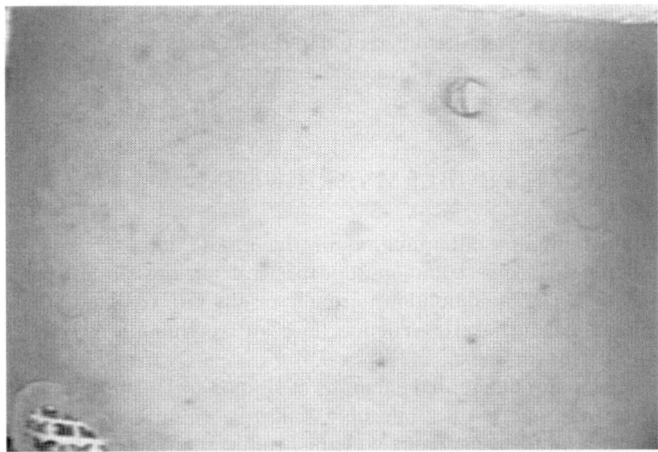

Fig. 23.17 Maculopapular/morbilliform rash of early meningoccemia. (Courtesy of Department of Medical Illustration, University of Aberdeen.)

Leukemia

Children with leukemia may present with a hemorrhagic rash as a result of thrombocytopenia but in addition, the pallor of severe anemia will usually be obvious.

CLINICAL PROBLEMS: FEVER AND INCREASED RESPIRATORY RATE

The combination of fever and rapid breathing is a common and important pediatric presentation. While the differential diagnosis is vast (Table 26.10), a serious underlying condition must always be considered, in particular sepsis (bacteremia or septicemia) and bacterial pneumonia. Fortunately, these serious conditions are uncommon and most infants and young children presenting with fever and increased respiratory rate simply have a relatively minor viral upper respiratory tract infection. In this situation, the respiratory rate is only mildly elevated and not associated with any other obvious signs of increased work of breathing (such as intercostal and/or subcostal retractions).

Table 26.10 Differential diagnosis of child with fever and increased respiratory rate

A. Serious infections:
- Bacteremia/septicemia
- Bacterial pneumonia (with or without parapneumonic effusion)
- Other focal bacterial infections (including meningitis, osteomyelitis, septic arthritis)

B. Less serious infections:
- Viral or Mycoplasma bronchopneumonia

C. Mild infections
- Viral upper respiratory tract infection (URTI)
- Viral bronchitis
- Viral exanthema

D. Fever and increased respiratory rate with upper airways obstruction (stridor)
- Viral laryngotracheobronchitis (viral 'croup')

E. Fever and increased respiratory rate with lower airways obstruction (wheeze)
- Acute viral bronchiolitis (usually due to respiratory syncitial virus)
- Asthma triggered by intercurrent viral URTI

Both the level of the fever and the degree of tachypnea are key indicators of a serious versus minor infection: the higher the level, the greater the likelihood of a serious bacterial infection. In addition, infants and young children with serious infections will have other features, both on history and physical examination, which will assist with the diagnosis. These include signs of marked increased work of breathing, and 'grunting' respirations with extensive bacterial pneumonia. Further, infants and young children with serious bacterial infections will look ill, with signs such as pallor, cyanosis, apathy, and altered level of consciousness. On the other hand infants and young children with a viral acute respiratory infection will have a history and physical evidence of a viral/coryzal illness with mild fever, clear rhinorrhea, conjunctival injection, redness of the tympanic membranes, sore throat and dry cough.

Clearly, the source or focus of infection must be thoroughly sought, both when taking the history and when performing the physical examination, in children presenting with this combination of symptoms. Recent contact with other children suffering from a viral infection (including one of the viral exanthemata) is vital information. Symptoms of a viral upper respiratory tract infection, or symptoms which localize the inflammation to a specific area of the respiratory tract, need to be elicited. This includes: a barking cough and inspiratory stridor indicating viral laryngotracheobronchitis (croup); coryzal symptoms plus acute history of significant cough (acute viral bronchitis); coryzal symptoms with acute wheeze, cough and shortness of breath (acute viral bronchiolitis in infants; acute asthma in older children).

A major symptom and sign to look for in children with fever and tachypnea is wheezing. In infants this is most likely to be due to acute viral bronchiolitis (usually due to respiratory syncytial virus), and in older children to an episode of acute bronchospasm (asthma) triggered by an intercurrent viral respiratory tract infection. In both these situations wheeze will be present, either audible with the ear or with a stethoscope. Generally, there will also be hyperinflation of the thoracic cage, tachypnea, and other signs of increased work of respiration. In infants with acute viral bronchiolitis, diffuse inspiratory crackles are generally audible throughout the chest plus the loud expiratory, musical wheezing.

Infants or children with viral or mycoplasma bronchopneumonia generally have other coryzal symptoms and signs in the ear, nose and throat plus a marked cough – which is often the major complaint. By contrast bacterial pneumonia presents with high fever, 'grunting' respirations and tachypnea, but no cough – particularly in the early phases of the illness.

The infant or young child with bacterial sepsis will generally have high fever (over 38.5°C), rapid respiratory rate, rapid pulse and will look ill. On close inspection, some of these children may have localized features of serious infection – such as meningitis, osteomyelitis, septic arthritis or endocarditis. Infants with a bacterial urinary tract infection will have very few localizing symptoms or signs apart from fever and mild elevation of respiratory rate.

In summary, there is a large differential diagnosis of the infant or young child presenting with a combination of fever and increased respiratory rate. This can range from a severe life-threatening illness to a trivial head cold. The latter is far more likely, and most will have only mildly elevated temperature and respiratory rate plus other symptoms and signs to indicate an intercurrent viral upper respiratory tract syndrome. On the other hand, a markedly elevated temperature and respiratory rate in a very sick child indicates a serious infection – particularly bacteremia/septicemia or bacterial pneumonia.

When in doubt, further investigations and/or a further period of observation is essential. These may include chest X-ray, blood cultures, lumbar puncture and blood or urine for bacterial antigen testing. In obviously sick infants and children, or those in whom a serious underlying bacterial infection is likely, appropriate antibiotics should be given while waiting for the results of the above testing.

CLINICAL PROBLEMS: COUGH AND FEVER

The presence of cough signifies irritation or stimulation of cough receptors in the upper or lower airways. This is most commonly secondary to inflammation from a viral infection of the upper or lower airways and will be accompanied by mild fever. Cough is also a feature of asthma, which is also often accompanied by fever, since the commonest trigger for an acute exacerbation of asthma in young children is an intercurrent viral upper respiratory tract infection (URTI).

Thus the combination of fever and cough suggests an infection somewhere in the respiratory tract and this is far more likely to be due to a virus, rather than bacteria. Diffuse, mild inflammation is typical of viral infection, while focal, severe inflammation is typical of bacterial infection in the respiratory tract. Indeed, one of the major distinguishing features between streptococcal pharyngitis and a viral URTI is the absence of cough and coryzal symptoms in streptococcal throat infections.

To determine the likely cause of cough and fever requires a comprehensive history and physical examination. Laboratory investigations may occasionally be required to further elucidate the cause.

If there is a past history of asthma the fever and cough are almost certainly due to episodic asthma or viral associated wheeze. If there is a past history of chronic bronchitis (frequent episodes of protracted cough with intercurrent viral acute respiratory infections) then it should be obvious from the history that the child is having a further episode of acute viral bronchitis.

Fever and cough due to an URTI should be readily distinguishable by the coryzal symptoms of rhinorrhea, conjunctival injection and a dry cough, but no increased work of breathing and no wheeze. While the child with viral laryngotracheobronchitis will have signs of a coryzal illness, the striking features will be the barking, 'croupy' quality of the cough and probable inspiratory stridor, particularly when the child is upset. When severe this inspiratory stridor will be associated with increased work of breathing (chest wall retractions, tracheal tug). Acute viral bronchitis is characterized by troublesome dry or wet cough in association with an acute respiratory infection. On auscultation there may be scattered coarse crackles (due to excessive airway secretions), which should clear following active coughing. Acute viral bronchiolitis is characterized by coryzal symptoms plus hyperinflation of the chest, loud wheezing, inspiratory crackles throughout both lung fields, and varying degrees of respiratory difficulty – in addition to fever and cough. Viral and mycoplasma bronchopneumonia will be characterized by coryzal symptoms, marked cough, increased work of breathing and widespread, scattered, inspiratory crackles.

A less common but important cause of cough and fever is foreign body inhalation – e.g. nuts and small parts of toys. Initially this is a dry cough often with wheeze and difficulty in breathing. If retained, the cough becomes loose and productive of purulent sputum. A child with a loose, productive cough and fever could also be suffering from chronic suppurative lung disease – bronchiectasis or chronic bronchitis. Most of these children will have some underlying problem (e.g. cystic fibrosis or immune deficiency).

In summary, fever and cough signifies some inflammatory process in the airways. This can range from a relatively uncomplicated viral upper respiratory tract infection due to rhinovirus through to viral or mycoplasma bronchopneumonia (Table 26.11). A major differential to consider is whether the fever and cough are due to an exacerbation of asthma in the child with underlying episodic asthma.

CLINICAL PROBLEMS: RHINITIS

Rhinitis implies inflammation of the nasal 'mucosa', and in children this is most commonly due to a viral upper respiratory tract infection. The inflammation normally results in a combination of rhinorrhea and nasal obstruction. Sneezing is commonly associated with these symptoms.

The major differential diagnosis of rhinitis secondary to a viral upper respiratory tract infection is allergic rhinitis. In children allergic rhinitis is generally perennial rather than seasonal and is characterized by its persistence for weeks or months – rather than the short term nasal symptoms of an acute viral infection. The symptoms of allergic rhinitis have a typical diurnal pattern (classically worse in the mornings) and there is absence of fever and other signs suggesting a viral upper respiratory tract infection (URTI). Nasal itch and sneezing are common as is clear rhinorrhea and nasal obstruction. There is often an associated allergic conjunctivitis, which can simulate a viral rhinoconjunctivitis. The child with allergic rhinitis generally has other signs of clinical atopy – particularly atopic eczema or bronchial asthma.

Vasomotor rhinitis is uncommon in young children and typically causes sudden onset (and sudden cessation) of clear rhinorrhea – often for only hours – but with recurrent episodes.

Other rarer causes of rhinitis include:

- foreign body – particularly small parts of toys and polystyrene beads (causes unilateral nasal symptoms);
- unusual infections (e.g. nasal diphtheria).

The distinction between acute viral rhinitis secondary to a viral infection and acute sinusitis is subtle and arbitrary. Most definitions base the distinction on duration of symptoms. Conventionally, acute sinusitis is the appropriate diagnosis if the nasal discharge is severe and persists for more than 10 days. These symptoms would generally be associated with cough and possibly bad breath.

Chronic sinusitis is arbitrarily defined as a persistent, mucopurulent nasal discharge for over 30 days. This is most commonly seen in children with underlying abnormalities of mucus, mucociliary clearance or immune function (e.g. cystic fibrosis, primary ciliary dyskinesia, agammaglobulinemia).

Drug therapy for rhinitis associated with a viral URTI is generally not required. However, in small infants the nasal obstruction and

Table 26.11 Causes of cough and fever

A. Acute respiratory tract infections:
- Viral upper respiratory tract infection (URTI)
- Acute viral bronchitis
- Acute viral laryngotracheobronchitis (viral croup)
- Acute viral bronchiolitis (infants)
- Acute viral bronchopneumonia
- Mycoplasma (bronchitis and bronchopneumonia)

B. Asthma syndromes:
- Classical bronchial asthma
- Wheezing associated respiratory infection (WARI)

C. Less common causes:
- Foreign body inhalation
- Suppurative lung disease (chronic bronchitis/bronchiectasis)

Table 26.12 Causes of rhinitis

Common
- Viral upper respiratory tract infection (acute viral nasopharyngitis – most commonly due to rhinovirus)
- Perennial allergic rhinitis

Uncommon
- Acute viral or bacterial sinusitis
- Vasomotor rhinitis

Rare
- Retained foreign body
- Uncommon infections (e.g. nasal diphtheria)

rhinorrhea may interfere with feeding and saline drops followed by suctioning of the drops ('nasal lavage') may be helpful, particularly immediately prior to feeds. Acute sinusitis is generally viral although secondary bacterial infection may occur. While there is some uncertainty as to whether or not antibiotics are indicated in this situation, there is little doubt that the color of the nasal discharge changes promptly with administration of antibiotics – but such treatment is best reserved for those who are more severely affected by the symptoms. Chronic sinusitis should be treated with antibiotics and prolonged courses (3 weeks) may be necessary.

Perennial allergic rhinitis in children warrants treatment particularly if the symptoms are severe. The most effective treatment is regular nasal topical corticosteroid (e.g. budesonide nasal spray).

In summary, while there are many possible causes for rhinitis (Table 26.12), most commonly it is the result of either a respiratory virus or allergic rhinitis.

CLINICAL PROBLEMS: NOISY BREATHING

Audible noises of respiration are common symptoms and signs in children. Clarification of the type of noise is critical with respect to identifying the most likely underlying cause. In general, noisy breathing signifies some obstruction to airflow and the specific type of noise – especially which phase of respiration – can greatly assist in determining the anatomic site of the airflow obstruction.

The types of noises identifiable are listed below in Table 26.13, together with the phase of respiration in which they are most audible, together with the usual anatomic site for the noise.

It is clear from the table that the noise is predominantly inspiratory when the obstruction is outside the thoracic cage (upper airways) and predominantly expiratory when the obstruction is inside the thorax (lower airways).

Table 26.13 Types of identifiable noises

Noise	Inspiration	Expiration	Site of obstruction
Snuffliness	++	±	Nasal
Snoring	++	±	Oronasopharynx
Stridor	+++		Extrathoracic trachea (subglottis/larynx)
Rattliness	++		Central tracheobronchial tree (trachea)
Wheeze		++	Small and medium sized intrathoracic airways
Grunting		+++	Alveoli

If a child has the noise when being examined then there is no difficulty determining its features. However, when the noise is from history alone this can create difficulties with respect to the terminology used by parents. In such instances, mimicking these noises will often assist with the accurate diagnosis. Alternatively, asking the parents to obtain tape recordings will enable clear identification of the type of noise.

There will generally be associated symptoms and signs with these noises, which will assist clinically in determining the exact site and cause for the obstruction. For example, the child with acute onset inspiratory stridor who also has an associated URTI and a barking cough is almost certainly suffering from acute viral croup (laryngotracheobronchitis). On the other hand, the child with grunting respirations who has high fever, looks toxic and unwell is almost certainly suffering from acute pneumonia.

The causes of the obstruction are numerous and are summarized in Table 26.14.

In summary, the child presenting with the problem of noisy breathing requires a comprehensive history and examination to determine the exact nature of the noise and to determine whether there are any associated symptoms or signs. By accurately determining the nature of the noisy breathing, the likely anatomic site of the obstruction can usually be determined, and this will greatly assist with the final diagnosis.

CLINICAL PROBLEMS: SUSPECTED MENINGITIS

Bacteria are still responsible for more than 2000 cases of meningitis in England and Wales every year. The mortality from these infections has declined in recent years, but there is disturbing evidence that the long term consequences of meningitis early in life may be worse than previously thought.

Table 26.14 Causes of obstruction

	Causes of noise	
	Acute	Persistent
Snuffle	Viral upper respiratory tract infection	Perennial allergic rhinitis
Snore	Acute tonsillitis/upper respiratory tract infection	Chronic enlargement of tonsils and adenoids
Stridor	Viral croup	Congenital subglottic stenosis or other fixed upper airway malformations
Rattle	Acute viral bronchitis	Cerebral palsy/CNS disorders ('sputum retention')
Wheeze	Asthma	Chronic small airways obstruction (e.g. cystic fibrosis)
Grunt	Acute bacterial (lobar) pneumonia Hyaline membrane disease (neonate)	Chronic interstitial lung disease (e.g. pulmonary fibrosis)

ETIOLOGY AND PATHOPHYSIOLOGY OF BACTERIAL MENINGITIS

The commonest route of meningeal infection is from the bloodstream, so the spectrum of pathogens causing meningitis is similar to that seen in bacteremia and sepsis. The introduction of the *Haemophilus influenzae* type b (Hib) polysaccharide-conjugate vaccine into the UK vaccination program has had a dramatic effect.[60] The incidence of Hib meningitis has dropped from around 2500 cases per year to less than 40 per year, and *Neisseria meningitidis* is now the commonest cause of community-acquired bacterial meningitis in the UK, followed by *Streptococcus pneumoniae*. The relative importance of these pathogens varies considerably with age (Table 26.15). In the neonatal period, Group B streptococcus is the prominent meningeal pathogen, followed by Gram negative bacilli, *S. pneumoniae* and *Listeria monocytogenes*. In children older than 3 months and in young adults, the most frequent cause of bacterial meningitis is *N. meningitidis* followed by *S. pneumoniae*. Infants between 1 and 3 months old are susceptible to *N. meningitidis* and *S. pneumoniae*, as well as the neonatal pathogens. The propensity of neonates to get meningitis is in part due to their immunological immaturity. Older children with congenital or acquired deficiencies in complement, immunoglobulin production, lymphocytes, neutrophils or splenic function are at increased risk from meningitis, sometimes due to atypical pathogens. A rare but serious form of bacterial meningitis is caused by *Mycobacterium tuberculosis*. This organism can affect patients of all ages and should be considered in any atypical presentation of meningitis, particularly patients presenting with an insidious illness.[61]

While meningitis often occurs in the context of systemic infections, it can also follow bacterial invasion from a contiguous focus of infection, such as the mastoids or paranasal sinuses, or from osteomyelitis of the skull. Skull fractures, craniospinal dermal sinuses, neurenteric or dermoid cysts, occult intranasal encephaloceles, or transethmoid meningoceles are also potential portals of entry for pathogens into the subarachnoid space.[62] The possibility of a cranial defect should be considered in children with recurrent meningitis. Neurosurgical procedures and the presence of ventriculoperitoneal shunts also provide routes for meningeal infection. In such cases, *Staphylococcus aureus* and coagulase negative staphylococci are more likely pathogens.

Bacterial invasion, of the cerebrospinal fluid (CSF), is followed by an outpouring of inflammatory cells, which cross the blood–brain barrier and enter the CSF. Inflammatory cytokines such as tumor necrosis factor, and interleukins-1, 6 and 8 are central to the inflammatory response. These mediators increase adhesion molecule expression on endothelial cells and leukocytes, which act in concert to facilitate the migration of cells into the CSF. Antibodies to adhesion molecules limit leukocyte migration and the consequences of meningeal infection.[63] The meninges become inflamed, swollen and covered by fibrino-purulent exudate. The thickest exudate is usually at the base of the brain. This leads to obstruction of the exit foramina of the fourth ventricle or the subarachnoid basal cisterns, restricting the CSF circulation to produce hydrocephalus. The ependymal lining of the cerebral ventricles may also be a site of intense inflammation (ventriculitis), causing ventricular enlargement and subsequent subependymal gliosis. A combination of cerebral vasculitis, thrombosis, cerebral edema and raised intracranial pressure leads to globally reduced cerebral blood flow and focal ischemia. This results in neuronal injury and cerebral damage, manifest clinically as coma, seizures and focal neurological signs.

CLINICAL FEATURES

The fully developed clinical picture of acute meningitis in children is sufficiently characteristic to be recognized without difficulty. More than 80% of children will have fever, vomiting, severe headache and signs of meningeal irritation. However, in the early stages of disease, and in young children, the symptoms and signs are often non-specific. Fever may be absent in up to 30% of individuals, and 20–30% do not have signs of meningism at presentation. Previous antibiotic therapy may also mask the significance of the presenting illness.[64]

Older children will often complain of headache or pain at the back of the neck, nausea and photophobia. The physical signs of meningeal irritation are neck stiffness and a positive Kernig test, which reflect inflammation of nerve roots of the spinal canal and adjacent sensory nerves. The most comfortable position for the patient is to lie with an extended neck and flexed hips and knees to reduce tension on the nerves emanating from the spinal cord. Neck stiffness can be detected by placing a palm of the hand on the supine child's occiput. Any attempt at flexing the child's neck will result in the lifting of the whole trunk. Kernig's sign is elicited with the child supine. The hip and knee joints are bent 90 degrees and then an attempt is made to extend the knee fully. In the presence of meningitis, there is resistance and severe pain as the sciatic nerve is stretched. A positive Brudzinski sign is involuntary muscular contraction causing leg flexion upon passive flexion of the neck, but is a less reliable sign of meningitis. Additional evidence of neurological involvement includes convulsions, which occur in 30% of children within 3 days of presentation, cranial nerve palsies (particularly III, IV, VI, and VII), delirium, drowsiness and coma.

In infants and toddlers, the symptoms are often those of a generalized illness. Irritability, lethargy, convulsions, refusal of feeds, vomiting, a high pitched cry and a bulging fontanelle should all alert the physician to the presence of meningitis. The 'typical' features of meningitis may be absent or difficult to interpret or elicit. When present they are often indicative of advanced disease.

Neisseria meningitidis is the commonest cause of bacterial meningitis in the UK (Table 26.15). More than 50% of patients

Table 26.15 Reports of isolates from the CSF to the Communicable Disease Surveillance Center (CDSC) in 1995 and 2000

		Age group				
	Year	1–11 months	1–4 years	5–9 years	10–14 years	15–24 years
Haemophilus influenzae	1995	14	12	4	2	4
	2000	5	10	1	1	2
Neisseria meningitidis	1995	220	278	112	90	253
	2000	231	220	105	86	219
Streptococcus pneumoniae	1995	60	29	13	7	9
	2000	53	27	4	9	14

infected with this organism will have a petechial rash, so a vigilant search for petechiae should be made in any child with features suggesting a diagnosis of meningitis. The whole skin surface should be carefully examined, since there may initially be only one or two petechiae. However it is also important to note that initially the rash of *N. meningitidis* may be maculopapular or urticarial in nature, and so an atypical rash should not be taken as evidence to exclude the diagnosis.

DIAGNOSIS

If meningitis is suspected, the diagnosis should be confirmed by lumbar puncture and examination of CSF. Over the last 10 years, there has been a move away from performing diagnostic lumbar punctures (LP) in patients presenting with suspected meningitis, since it is frequently argued that an LP will not affect patient management and may be hazardous. However, an LP offers immediate confirmation of the diagnosis, and allows appropriate treatment to be started, which may be particularly important in neonates and immunocompromised patients in whom the differential diagnosis is wide. Identifying the etiological agent and its antibiotic sensitivities may be crucial to administering the most appropriate antibiotics and providing important prognostic information.[64]

There are, however, specific and clear contraindications to LP in patients with meningitis.[65] These are:

1. signs of raised intracranial pressure with changing level of consciousness, focal neurological signs or severe mental impairment;
2. cardiovascular compromise with impaired peripheral perfusion or hypotension;
3. respiratory compromise with tachypnea, an abnormal breathing pattern or hypoxia;
4. thrombocytopenia or a coagulopathy.

An LP should also be avoided if it will result in a significant delay in treatment. The association between LP and cerebral tonsillar herniation has not been shown to be causal, and has not been reported in the absence of the specific contraindications listed above.

Lumbar puncture should be performed in the third to fourth lumbar space using a needle with a stylet, since use of a needle alone has been associated with the development of implantation dermoid cysts. CSF should be collected for microscopy and culture, bacterial and viral polymerase chain reaction (PCR), latex agglutination tests for bacterial antigens, protein and glucose. Blood cultures may also identify the etiological agent if an LP is not performed or fails to establish the cause of meningitis.

Analysis of the CSF leukocyte count, glucose and protein can usually establish a positive diagnosis of meningitis, but normal results do not necessarily exclude meningitis. The absence of cells may indicate very early meningitis before the migration of leukocytes into the CSF. Very high white cell counts of up to $20\,000/mm^3$ can be observed in bacterial meningitis, although the number of cells is usually less than $3000/mm^3$. There is a broad association between a predominance of polymorphonuclear leukocytes in the CSF and bacterial meningitis. However, lymphocytes may predominate in early or partially treated bacterial meningitis, in tuberculous meningitis and in neonates. In bacterial meningitis, CSF glucose is usually low with a CSF:blood ratio of less than 0.5, and protein is frequently raised to more than 0.4 g/L. Numerous studies have now shown that even after the administration of intravenous antibiotics, the diagnostic cellular and biochemical changes in the CSF may persist for at least 48 h. In the context of a negative Gram stain and CSF culture, the presence of bacterial antigens and PCR may prove invaluable for establishing a diagnosis of bacterial meningitis.

THE USE OF CT SCANS

Following the clinical diagnosis of bacterial meningitis, it has become common practice to arrange a computerized tomographic (CT) brain scan to exclude raised intracranial pressure prior to undertaking a lumbar puncture. This approach has three important drawbacks. Firstly, raised intracranial pressure (ICP) is very common amongst children with meningitis and clinically significant raised ICP cannot be ruled out by brain CT. Secondly, it is hazardous to transport patients to a CT scanner before they have been adequately stabilized. Thirdly, the inevitable delay in undertaking the CT scan requires that empirical antibiotics be given while awaiting the procedure, therefore impairing the diagnostic yield from a subsequent LP. Patients presenting with clinical signs of raised ICP are the minority, and these children should not undergo LP, regardless of the CT findings. CT scans can exclude lesions requiring neurosurgical intervention and identify conditions such as cerebral abscess or hydrocephalus requiring shunting. The diagnostic yield from a CT scan in children is, however, low and should not be allowed to compromise the procedures required for diagnosis and to initiate appropriate treatment.[64]

ANTIBIOTICS

Except in cases where the patient is well and the diagnosis very uncertain, antibiotics should be administered empirically while awaiting the result of the LP. The selection of the optimal antibiotic for the treatment of bacterial meningitis should be based on the following criteria: the spectrum of pathogens known to cause meningitis in different age groups (Table 26.15); the changing pattern of antimicrobial resistance;[66] the pharmacological properties of the antibiotics available and the results of therapeutic trials. In infants up to 3 months of age, a combination of ampicillin and cefotaxime is a logical choice, as cefotaxime provides cover for both neonatal and infant pathogens, and ampicillin is effective against *Listeria monocytogenes*. For the same reason, ampicillin should be included as part of empirical therapy for immunocompromised patients. Penicillin-resistant meningococci are emerging worldwide, as are chloramphenicol-resistant strains, but these have not yet resulted in treatment failures. Fortunately, almost all strains in the UK remain sensitive to the third generation cephalosporins.

In the USA, in excess of 25% of pneumococcal isolates are resistant to penicillin and this proportion exceeds 50% in countries such as Hungary, Spain and South Africa. Penicillin-insensitive strains of pneumococci are more likely to be resistant to third generation cephalosporins, and there have been documented cases of microbiological failure in the treatment of pneumococcal meningitis with third generation cephalosporins. In the UK, the level of penicillin resistance is increasing and is now more than 5% (Public Health Laboratory Service Data). In most UK cases, penicillin resistance is low level and cephalosporin resistance is rare and so a third generation cephalosporin (cefotaxime or ceftriaxone) is adequate for most community acquired meningitis in children over 3 months. The routine use of vancomycin for community acquired meningitis is not justified in the UK at the present time. However, vancomycin should be added to the treatment regimen for any patient coming from an area where high levels of penicillin resistance are endemic. The addition of rifampicin to vancomycin or the administration of vancomycin intraventricularly has been recommended by some authorities.[67]

THE ROLE OF CORTICOSTEROIDS

It is now widely accepted that much of the cerebral damage which occurs in bacterial meningitis is not caused by the invading organism itself but by the host mediated inflammatory response.[68] While a number of adjunctive anti-inflammatory agents have been suggested, only corticosteroids have been extensively tested in clinical trials. However, although several studies showed some improvement in morbidity (deafness or neurological deficit), these were largely conducted in children with *Haemophilus influenzae* type b meningitis, and this approach requires administration of corticosteroids either before antibiotic administration or at the time.[69] Data supporting the use of steroids in pneumococcal and meningococcal meningitis are lacking. With the emergence of pneumococcal antibiotic resistance, there is concern that limiting meningeal inflammation could actually delay sterilization of the CSF by agents such as vancomycin since these antibiotics cross the blood–brain barrier poorly, even when the meninges are inflamed. Selective administration of dexamethasone to patients who have a poor predicted mortality or morbidity may be a rational approach in the absence of more evidence of its efficacy.[64]

NEUROLOGICAL AND FLUID MANAGEMENT

Hyponatremia is frequently observed in patients with bacterial meningitis. While this is associated with elevated serum antidiuretic hormone (ADH), possibly suggesting inappropriate ADH secretion (SIADH), more recent studies indicate that SIADH is overdiagnosed.[70] Treatment of suspected SIADH with fluid restriction could potentially compromise circulating volume, and therefore cerebral blood flow. Circulatory shock should be treated aggressively, significant dehydration corrected carefully, fluid balance monitored frequently and maintenance fluids given with care.

Patients presenting with clinical signs of raised ICP require very careful fluid balance monitoring to help maintain adequate cerebral blood flow. Intubation and mechanical ventilation should be instituted early to facilitate oxygenation, allow adequate sedation and permit normalization of $PaCO_2$. Such patients should be nursed head up, and central venous catheters should not be placed in the neck. Intravenous mannitol may be useful for managing acute changes in intracranial pressure, and anticonvulsants for control of fits.[64]

COMPLICATIONS

Convulsions occur in 20–30% of children, usually within 72 h of presentation. The onset of late or persistent fits is associated with a poor prognosis. Subdural collections of fluid are common, particularly during infancy. They are usually sterile and rarely require aspiration unless there is evidence of increasing intracranial pressure, the presence of focal neurological signs, convulsions or persistent fever due to subdural empyema. Cerebral abscesses are rare outside the neonatal period. More frequent causes of persistent fever include intercurrent viral infection, ongoing inflammation and drug fever. In the absence of a definitive microbiological etiology, the combination of persistent fever and poor clinical condition may indicate that the meningitis is due to organisms resistant to the prescribed antibiotic therapy. A repeat LP should then be performed.

The commonest long term complication of meningitis is sensorineural deafness. All children should undergo audiological assessment after recovery from infection. The overall rate of deafness following meningitis is less than 5%. Hearing impairment is higher in cases of pneumococcal meningitis than in meningococcal infections. In a recent study of morbidity after an episode of meningitis in infancy, almost a fifth of patients had some degree of disability.[71] This figure is higher if subtle defects are included, such as behavioral problems, middle ear disease and squints. Morbidity was highest following neonatal meningitis and also after meningitis caused by *S. pneumoniae*, Group B streptococcus and atypical pathogens.

PREVENTION

Conjugate vaccines against *H. influenzae* type b (Hib) and *N. meningitidis* group C are now routinely given in the UK as part of the primary course of immunization at 2, 3 and 4 months. An effective vaccine against *N. meningitidis* group B is not yet available. Trials of conjugate pneumococcal vaccines are underway and may be introduced in the UK in the near future (see p. 1372).

When a child presents with meningococcal or Hib meningitis, other family members and close contacts are at increased risk of infection. Rifampicin (rifampin) is currently recommended for contacts of meningococcal disease (four doses of 10 mg/kg per dose 12 hourly) and *H. influenzae* type b (20 mg/kg per dose daily for 4 days). Decisions on who should receive prophylaxis can be difficult, and advice should be sought from the Consultant in Communicable Disease Control.

CLINICAL PROBLEMS: SEPTIC SHOCK

CLINICAL PROBLEMS

Despite the vast array of potential pathogens, the human host is remarkably resistant to life-threatening infection. Most pathogens are restricted by host defenses to their primary sites of invasion, with minimal clinical consequences. These first line defense mechanisms successfully intercept invading organisms in the majority of cases. On occasion, however, microbial invasion of the bloodstream can and does occur, even in apparently immunocompetent children, with potentially devastating consequences. The sequence of events following successful entry of microbes or microbial products to the circulation is complex, and depends both upon the virulent properties of the offending microorganism and the host response. Initial microbial invasion may be clinically silent and indeed may resolve without antimicrobial therapy. If, however, bacterial proliferation ensues, a systemic response is initiated in the host. This is referred to as SIRS (systemic inflammatory response syndrome) and is defined by the presence of abnormalities in two or more of the following: temperature, heart rate, respiratory rate and white blood count. SIRS can follow any severe insult including infection, trauma, major surgery, burns or pancreatitis, but when SIRS occurs in the context of infection, the patient is described as *septic*.

The term *severe sepsis* is used to describe a state characterized by hypoperfusion, hypotension and organ dysfunction, while the term *septic shock* is restricted to patients with persistent hypotension despite adequate fluid resuscitation and/or hypoperfusion even following adequate inotrope or pressor support.[72] In practice it can be difficult to divide patients neatly into these defined states, but the use of these terms serves to highlight the sequential nature of the events associated with microbial invasion, and will help in the evaluation of future clinical trials in septic patients.

MICROBIAL ETIOLOGY OF SEPSIS

In view of the multitude of potential pathogens with the capacity to cause disease, it is perhaps surprising that a very limited range of microorganisms is responsible for invasive infections in healthy children beyond the neonatal period. Three organisms predominate: *Streptococcus pneumoniae*, *Neisseria meningitidis* and *Haemophilus influenzae* type b.

The incidence of sepsis due to *H. influenzae* has been drastically reduced in countries with a vaccination program, but *S. pneumoniae* and *N. meningitidis* continue to cause severe and life-threatening infection in children with no predisposition to infection. Rarer causes of sepsis in healthy children include *Staphylococcus aureus*, Group A *Streptococcus* and *Salmonella* spp., and these may be associated with wound and skin infections or a history of diarrhea respectively. In vulnerable patient groups other pathogens are implicated. In neonates, Group B *Streptococcus*, *Escherichia coli*, other Gram negative bacteria, and *Listeria monocytogenes* are the usual causes of sepsis. In immunocompromised patients, Gram negative organisms, such as *Pseudomonas aeruginosa*, and fungi may be responsible. Any patient with an indwelling catheter is particularly at risk of sepsis from coagulase negative staphylococci and enterococci. With all of these organisms, the onset of bacteremia is a crucial event in the pathogenesis of sepsis, but invasion of the bloodstream is not necessary for bacteria to induce features of septic shock. Enterotoxins from staphylococci and streptococci are potent stimulators of T cell proliferation and activation, and can produce toxic shock syndromes, even in patients with an apparently localized focus of infection. Some viruses, including herpesviruses, enteroviruses and adenoviruses, can produce diseases which may be indistinguishable clinically from bacterial sepsis, particularly in neonates and infants.

PATHOPHYSIOLOGY OF SEPSIS

Over the last two decades it has emerged that it is the host response to microbial invasion which is predominantly responsible for the clinical features of sepsis and septic shock. Lipopolysaccharides (LPS) from Gram negative bacteria, and a variety of other microbial products have the capacity to stimulate the production of mediators from many cells within the human host. Tumor necrosis factor, interleukin 1 and interleukin 6 are just a few of the many inflammatory mediators reported to be present at high levels in septic patients. Recently, a family of receptors has been identified, which are able to transduce cellular signals in response to bacteria. These are known as human toll-like receptors (hTLR). This family of receptors consists of at least nine proteins, with hTLR4 acting as the principal mediator of LPS signaling, while other members of the family, such as hTLR2, can mediate signals induced by lipoproteins of mycobacteria and Gram positive bacterial peptidoglycans. It is the cytokines and inflammatory mediators produced in response to microbial stimuli which stimulate neutrophils, endothelial cells and monocytes and influence the function of vital organs, including the heart, liver, brain and kidneys. The net effect of excessive inflammatory activity is to cause the constellation of pathophysiological events seen in patients with sepsis and septic shock.

PRO- VERSUS ANTI-INFLAMMATORY MECHANISMS IN SEPSIS

The proinflammatory mediators produced in response to microbial invasion prime and activate cells to fight infection. However, the host also responds to proinflammatory stimuli by producing antagonists, known collectively as anti-inflammatory mediators. Interleukin 10 and soluble cytokine receptors or antagonists such as interleukin 1 receptor antagonist occur naturally, and act to limit the effects of proinflammatory cytokines. The balance between pro- and anti-inflammatory mediators is probably more critical than the levels of either alone. Patients who survive the initial inflammatory insult, but who still require assisted ventilation and intravenous support, have high levels of anti-inflammatory mediators. These patients are resistant to further proinflammatory stimulation, and may be more susceptible to nosocomial infections. Such patients may actually benefit from immune stimulation[73] to provoke the production of more inflammatory mediators, and the balance of pro- and anti-inflammation may prove crucial in therapeutic interventions. In the future, a clear characterization of the inflammatory status of septic patients may therefore be essential before adjuvant therapy is instituted (see below).

CLINICAL PRESENTATION AND DIAGNOSIS

The symptoms and signs of the initial phase of bacteremia are dependent upon the age and pre-existing health of the patient and the duration of the illness, as well as the causative organism. Bacteremia, with little inflammatory response, can be very difficult to diagnose clinically, because of the overlap in clinical presentation with common viral illnesses. A number of clinical parameters have been examined to try to estimate the probability of bacterial rather than viral infection: children with a bacteremic illness are more likely to have a fever of > 39°C and a white blood cell count (WBC) above 15×10^9/L or below 2.5×10^9/L. However, the specificity and sensitivity of these parameters for diagnosing bacteremia is low, and does not greatly add to the physician's general assessment of the child's condition.[74] Therefore frequent reassessment of the patient may be necessary if impending severe sepsis is to be recognized at an early stage. Non-specific signs, including lethargy, irritability, hypotonia, poor feeding, nausea and vomiting may be the earliest features of impending severe sepsis. Fever is not invariably present, and hypothermia may also occur, particularly in neonates and infants. Cardiovascular involvement with tachycardia or bradycardia, inadequate peripheral perfusion, prolonged capillary refill, cold extremities, peripheral edema, decreased urine output and evidence of shock may all be manifest as the systemic response to bacterial invasion progresses. Respiratory, gastrointestinal and neurological derangement may indicate systemic disease, or involvement of these specific organs in the infectious process. A petechial rash may be indicative of meningococcal disease, and in staphylococcal and streptococcal toxin-mediated shock, erythroderma, conjunctival and mucosal erythema and edema are usually present.

In all patients with suspected sepsis, blood cultures should be taken. The success of this procedure is dependent upon adequate blood inoculation of the culture media. If only a small volume of blood is available for culture, this should be added to the aerobic bottle, as few of the causative organisms will be anaerobes. Samples from potential sources of infection should be collected where appropriate. These include indwelling catheters, urine microscopy and culture, diagnostic radiology and aspiration for intra-abdominal sepsis, and lower respiratory tract secretions in ventilated patients, preferably by bronchoalveolar lavage. A lumbar puncture should be considered in patients with suspected meningeal involvement, but is contraindicated in the presence of shock, coagulopathy, reduced conscious level or focal neurological signs. Samples can also be analyzed by molecular microbiological techniques for bacteria, fungi and viruses, although these investigations are not always routinely available. In patients with suspected toxic shock syndrome, analysis of staphylococcal and streptococcal isolates for the presence of toxin production and of V beta T cell receptor repertoires can be helpful. WBCs, high or low, and markers of inflammation including C-reactive protein (CRP), procalcitonin and proinflammatory cytokine levels may be useful. However, none of these investigations is specific or diagnostic. Coagulation studies, hemoglobin, urea and electrolytes, glucose and liver function tests should be performed to help inform further management and guide fluid and electrolyte replacement and general support.

MANAGEMENT OF SEPSIS

RECOGNITION

Most cases of sepsis begin with the invasion of the bloodstream by a limited number of microbes. As the organisms multiply, often logarithmically, the host response intensifies and the condition of the patient deteriorates. The chances of a favorable outcome are greatly enhanced by initiating treatment at the earliest possible stage, so the most important aspect of sepsis management is the earliest possible recognition of the condition. In view of the diagnostic difficulties described above, it is imperative that otherwise healthy children presenting with non-specific features are observed carefully. Even if a health care professional considers the risk of impending sepsis to be low and the patient well enough to be at home, a detailed plan of management should be discussed with the family. The parents or guardians should have a clear understanding of the clinical features to observe and what actions to take if there is deterioration or failure to improve and a plan agreed for the clinician to review the child's condition. In patients at increased risk of bacteremia, such as neonates, immunocompromised children, children with neutropenia, or sickle cell disease, there should be a low threshold for initiating antimicrobial therapy.

ANTIMICROBIAL THERAPY

The choice of antibiotics is dependent upon the most likely pathogens and the particular antibiotic resistance patterns of the community or hospital. In otherwise healthy children without an obvious source, a third generation cephalosporin such as cefotaxime or ceftriaxone is appropriate. The emergence of antibiotic resistance precludes penicillin as adequate initial therapy. In more vulnerable populations other considerations apply. For example, in neonates, a third generation cephalosporin is frequently used together with ampicillin to treat *Listeria monocytogenes*, sometimes with the addition of an aminoglycoside for additional Gram negative bacterial cover.

Immunocompromised patients are vulnerable to infection with a wider spectrum of pathogens. Children with B cell and antibody deficiencies or with reduced or absent splenic function are at increased risk from encapsulated bacterial infections. Neutropenic patients are particularly susceptible to staphylococcal and Gram negative bacteria including pseudomonal infections. A combination of an antipseudomonal penicillin (e.g. piperacillin) with an aminoglycoside (e.g. gentamicin) is usually prescribed for this population. However, a glycopeptide (e.g. vancomycin) and antifungal therapy may be required if initial therapy fails to control the infection. Patients with sickle cell disease are at risk of salmonella septicemia, and may require treatment with ciprofloxacin. In patients with staphylococcal toxic shock syndrome, treatment with antistaphylococcal therapy is advisable, even though the total number of bacteria may be small. These are general guidelines and advice about local antimicrobial prescribing policies should always be sought.

SUBSEQUENT MANAGEMENT

The details of the emergency treatment of shock are covered in Chapter 35. Children will usually require transfer to a pediatric intensive care unit. Hypovolemia is invariably present due to fluid maldistribution, which occurs as a result of the release of vasoactive mediators by host inflammatory and endothelial cells. The loss of circulating volume is compounded by a loss of intravascular proteins and fluid due to endothelial dysfunction (capillary leak). Continuous monitoring of central venous pressure and urine output is required to guide fluid replacement. Large volumes of plasma or blood are normally required, and mechanical ventilation may be necessary to manage capillary leakage of fluid into the lungs.[75] The net effect of the host response to infection frequently leads to myocardial depression, necessitating the use of inotropic support. Severe peripheral vasodilatation compounds hypotension, and vasopressors may be required. Dysregulation of the coagulation and thrombotic pathways leads to widespread microvascular thrombosis and consumption of clotting factors. Treatment of disseminated intravascular coagulation (DIC) is largely symptomatic, with administration of fresh frozen plasma and platelets if bleeding occurs. While administration of antibiotics will prevent further bacterial proliferation, the concentration of microbial components, such as LPS and outer membrane proteins, may persist for some time. These will continue to cause inflammation and further deterioration in the patient's condition. Continuous reassessment and adjustment of supportive therapy is therefore required to optimize further management.

ADJUVANT THERAPY

The recognition that much of the pathology seen in sepsis is due to host-derived mediators has led to the development of numerous antagonists to offending bacterial and host components. Initial attempts to reduce the inflammatory response in sepsis used steroids. However, high doses of methylprednisolone were found to be detrimental in sepsis, and as a result, routine use of steroids in sepsis was abandoned. More selective agents were developed including antagonists of tumor necrosis factor, interleukin 1, platelet activating factor, and endotoxin. None of these has proved to be beneficial in large clinical trials. However, it is too early to discard these new forms of treatment, since a clearer understanding of the sequence of events in sepsis may identify subgroups of patients who might benefit from these interventions.

The use of high doses of intravenous immunoglobulin may be beneficial in toxic shock syndromes, and may be useful in other septic populations.[76] There is also evidence that administration of activated protein C can reduce mortality in adults with sepsis-induced organ failure.[77] This suggests that downstream inflammatory pathways, such as the protein C anticoagulation pathway, critical in thrombosis and hemostasis, may present potential targets for future interventions. Perhaps the most important recent development in critical illness concerns the modulation of endocrine pathways. The administration of growth hormone to critically ill adults was found to significantly increase mortality, whilst low doses of steroids and tight glycemic control appear to be advantageous.[78] The role of the endocrine axis in children with sepsis is still unclear but warrants further investigation in the future.

CONGENITAL AND NEONATAL INFECTIONS

SPECIFIC INFECTIONS

CONGENITAL RUBELLA

The association between rubella infection during pregnancy and congenital cataracts in the newborn was first made by an Australian ophthalmologist, Norman Gregg, in 1941.[79] The introduction of effective rubella vaccination programs has made congenital rubella syndrome an uncommon disorder in developed countries like the UK. However, there has been a small resurgence in the number of cases reported to the British Paediatric Surveillance Unit over the period 1996–2000, possibly due to falling vaccine coverage and immigration of non-vaccinated women.[80,81]

Both the risk of the fetal infection and the risk of sequelae vary with the gestation when maternal infection occurs. Transmission of the virus to the fetus occurs in 90% in the first 11 weeks, 50% from 11 to 20 weeks gestation, 37% 20–35 weeks, and 100% during the last month of pregnancy.[82] However, the risk of serious sequelae to the fetus after confirmed maternal rubella infection is greatest in early pregnancy, being 90% if infected < 11 weeks, 30% at 12–20 weeks and none thereafter, aside from some mild growth retardation.[82] The majority of infants with congenital rubella disease result from primary maternal rubella infection, although maternal reinfection may rarely result in an infant with anomalies.[83]

Clinical manifestation

The common manifestations of congenital rubella infection are shown in Table 10.124. Important clinical manifestations are disorders of the eye (microphthalmia, cataract, congenital glaucoma, retinitis), congenital heart disease [patent ductus arteriosus (PDA), peripheral pulmonary artery stenosis], and neurological sequelae (mental retardation, behavioral disorders, meningoencephalitis, convulsions). There may also be intrauterine growth retardation, microcephaly, thrombocytopenia, hepatosplenomegaly, purpuric skin lesions, pneumonitis and linear bone lesions. Only 68% of infected infants show signs at birth and up to 20% of these may die in infancy. A number of manifestations, however, present much later in life. These include hearing loss 87%, congenital heart disease 46–60%, mental or psychomotor retardation 30–50%, cataract or glaucoma 30–40%, diabetes mellitus, and thyroid dysfunction.

Diagnosis

Virus isolation, either from nasopharyngeal washing, urine or cerebrospinal fluid (CSF) is the most direct method of diagnosis, but may take many weeks. A positive rubella-specific immunoglobulin M (IgM) in a neonate and/or the detection of rubella RNA in urine or nasopharyngeal secretions by polymerase chain reaction (PCR) usually indicates recent postnatal or congenital infection, although false positive results do occur. A number of sensitive immunoassays are available for the detection of rubella-specific IgG. Rising or persistently stable levels of IgG from the newborn period to beyond 9 months of age confirm perinatal or congenital infection.

Management

There is no specific treatment for rubella infection. In countries where routine rubella vaccination has been used, the infection rate has been considerably reduced. Seronegative women of child-bearing age should be offered vaccination either after a pregnancy test or immediately postpartum. Rubella immunization of 13-year-old girls, which started in the UK in 1970, reduced the incidence considerably and the use of the measles, mumps and rubella (MMR) vaccine in the UK from 1988 has made congenital rubella rare.[80] Most new reports of congenital rubella in the UK are of infants born to mothers who were themselves born abroad and came to the UK after the age of schoolgirl immunization.

CYTOMEGALOVIRUS (CMV)

This is the most common congenital infection in Europe with a prevalence of 3–4 per 1000 births. CMV is a member of the herpesvirus family, and as such, establishes a latent infection after the initial infection and reactivates, especially under states of altered cellular immunity. It is ubiquitous in the community, although not highly infectious. It may be transmitted transplacentally or through genital secretions, saliva, breast milk or blood transfusion.

About 50% of women of child-bearing age in the UK remain susceptible to CMV infection and 1% of those susceptible at the beginning of pregnancy will have a primary infection during pregnancy. Like rubella, the greatest risk of fetal damage occurs after primary maternal infection. In about 50% of primary infections of the mother, the fetus will be infected, but only 10% of these infants will display symptoms at birth or through childhood. After a recurrent maternal CMV infection, there is a low risk of transmission to the infant (≤ 1%), with an equally low risk of sequelae.[84] However, some cases of infants with severe, symptomatic congenital CMV disease due to either maternal reinfection with a new CMV strain or reactivation of latent CMV infection during pregnancy have been reported.[85] Unlike rubella, fetal damage may follow primary infection or recurrent infection at any stage of pregnancy.

Clinical manifestations

The majority of infants with congenital CMV infection are asymptomatic. When symptomatic, the main clinical features are as shown in Table 10.123. The risk of neurological sequelae and intrauterine growth retardation in the fetus is greatest after infection in the first 20 weeks of pregnancy. Such effects include microcephaly, chorioretinitis, mental retardation, sensorineural hearing loss and intracerebral periventricular calcification. Infection in the second half of pregnancy usually results in visceral disease such as hepatitis, purpura, hyperbilirubinemia, and thrombocytopenia. Other effects include dental abnormalities and inguinal hernias. Pneumonitis is a common feature of postnatally acquired CMV infection, especially in the premature infant, but rarely follows true congenital infection. Those infants who have symptoms in the newborn period nearly always have subsequent handicap. Recently, it has been identified that the presence of microcephaly at birth is the strongest predictor of poor cognitive outcome in later life.[86] Of the infected infants who are asymptomatic at birth, up to 10% will have CMV-related problems by 3 years of age, the most common problem being sensorineural hearing loss.[87]

Perinatal CMV infection

Many infants acquire CMV infection through breast-feeding, or by contact with other infected secretions in the first weeks of life or, in hospitalized babies, through blood products. This usually results in an asymptomatic infection. The exception is premature infants, especially those with extremely low birth weight, or infants with cellular immunodeficiency in whom CMV infection may result in pneumonitis, hepatitis, thrombocytopenia, neutropenia and uncommonly gastroenteritis. In general, postnatal CMV infection does not result in long term sequelae, with the possible exception of babies less than 2000 g.[88]

Diagnosis

Diagnosis is based on isolation of the virus in the throat washings or urine. Cultures must be obtained within the first 3 weeks of life to distinguish congenital CMV infection from perinatally acquired infection. Demonstration of CMV-specific IgM antibody in neonatal serum is also suggestive of congenital infection, but it can only be detected in about 70% of infected newborns. Later in infancy, in the absence of clinical signs suggestive of congenital infection, laboratory methods alone will not make the distinction between CMV acquired during intrauterine life, and postnatal infection. Detection of CMV pp65 antigen in blood, or viral DNA by PCR are newer sensitive methods of diagnosis, but are usually not required for the diagnosis of congenital CMV infection.

Treatment and prevention

Intravenous ganciclovir has been used in a series of small clinical trials to try to reduce the risk and extent of central nervous system damage after symptomatic congenital CMV infection.[89,90] However, no firm conclusions about the efficacy of this treatment could be drawn due to the small sample sizes, and until more efficacy data are available, it is not routinely recommended. Ganciclovir therapy may be used to treat some congenitally infected infants with life-threatening CMV-related organ disease or retinitis involving the macula. Work is in progress towards production of a vaccine.

CMV is spread by intimate contact with infected secretions. Pregnant caregivers and hospital personnel should employ careful hand-washing after exposure to the secretions of a CMV-infected infant.

VARICELLA-ZOSTER (CHICKENPOX)

Congenital infection

Maternal varicella-zoster infection during the first 20 weeks of pregnancy may result in spontaneous abortion or fetal death in utero, or in an embryopathy characterized by dermatomal skin scarring and limb hypoplasia. There may also be disorders of the central nervous system (microcephaly, cortical atrophy) and eyes (cataracts, chorioretinitis), of the gastrointestinal tract and of the genitourinary tract. It is hypothesized that the damage results from in utero reactivation of varicella-zoster virus (VZV) or disseminated fetal infection.

Maternal infection in the second half of pregnancy may result in an asymptomatic primary fetal infection followed by herpes zoster in the first years of life in about 1% of exposed infants. A large prospective study from the UK and Germany of the effects of maternal VZV infection in pregnancy estimated the overall risk of embryopathy during the first 20 weeks of pregnancy to be 1%, with the highest risk of transmission of 2% being in the period 13–20 weeks.[91] Occasional cases resulting from maternal infection at 23 weeks have been reported.[92] Administration of varicella-zoster immunoglobulin (V-ZIG) to the mother may modify the course of chickenpox, but it has not been shown to alter the risk of transmission to the fetus.[93]

Perinatal infection

Maternal varicella that occurs in the period 5 days before delivery to 2 days after delivery may result in life-threatening, disseminated VZV infection in the infant due to transplacental passage of the virus in the absence of maternal antibody. If the onset of maternal infection is more than 7 days prior to delivery, there is usually sufficient passive transfer of antibody, unless the infant is less than 28 weeks gestation. Administration of V-ZIG to the infant has been shown to prevent or modify the course of the illness in most cases. However, as a significant number of infants will develop systemic VZV despite the administration of V-ZIG,[94] all infants with perinatal VZV exposure should be monitored closely for systemic disease, with prompt initiation of intravenous aciclovir should vesicles appear. Hospitalized infants with chickenpox should be placed in respiratory and contact isolation until the lesions have crusted, but breast-feeding can continue.

HERPES SIMPLEX VIRUS (HSV)

Neonatal HSV infection is invariably symptomatic and carries a high mortality if untreated. The incidence of disease ranges from 1:2500 live births in some parts of the USA[95] to 1:60 000 live births in the UK.[96] In the past, up to 75% of cases of neonatal infection were due to HSV type 2 and the rest due to type 1. More recently, the proportion of cases due to neonatal HSV-1 infection is increasing in the UK and elsewhere around the world possibly due to an increase in genital HSV-1 disease.[96] The infection is acquired from passage through an infected birth canal in 85% of cases, and is postnatally acquired from the oral lesions of an infected caregiver in 10–15% of cases. A true congenital syndrome is seen in < 5% of cases. The greatest risk for transmission (about 50%) is from a primary maternal infection when there has been insufficient time for seroconversion and transplacental transfer of antibody.[97] If a woman with a recurrent infection is shedding virus at delivery, the risk may be 5% or less. Cesarean delivery is not completely effective in preventing transmission to the infant.

Clinical manifestations

Neonatal HSV disease may manifest as lesions localized to the skin, eye or mouth (SEM), as encephalitis, as pneumonitis or as a disseminated multiorgan infection with or without central nervous system involvement. The age of presentation varies with the category of disease. In general, neonatal HSV disease usually presents in the first 3 weeks of life, but it may manifest at any time from day 1 to 4 weeks of life. About 50% of cases now present as SEM disease, possibly due to better awareness of the condition. The typical vesicular, ulcerative lesion usually occurs on the presenting part. Up to 70% of SEM disease will spread to the central nervous system or elsewhere without treatment, but is rarely fatal. Infants with SEM disease have 10% long term morbidity, with higher rates seen if there are frequent cutaneous recurrences in early life.

The disseminated form typically commences at about 1 week of age with a shock-like syndrome in the absence of positive bacterial cultures with thrombocytopenia, disseminated intravascular coagulation, hepatitis, jaundice, and sometimes encephalitis, and seizures. Skin lesions appear in 50% of these cases. Disseminated HSV infection may also present as an interstitial pneumonitis, usually presenting about day 3 of life. The mortality in this group is as high as 50% even with treatment, and over half of the survivors are left with long term sequelae (mental retardation, blindness, seizures, learning defects). The third group presents with central nervous system symptoms such as poor feeding, apnea, lethargy and seizures without visceral involvement, typically in the second to third week of life. It has been hypothesized that this group represents reactivation of an earlier asymptomatic infection. They have a 15% mortality, with severe long term central nervous system effects seen in 65%.[98]

Congenital infection

Intrauterine HSV infection may manifest as the presence of vesicles or scarring at birth, chorioretinitis, microphthalmia, microcephaly, hydranencephaly or cerebral atrophy on CT scan in the first week of life, organ calcification or organomegaly. The majority of reported cases are due to HSV-2. There is a high rate of early neonatal death and long term central nervous system sequelae.

Diagnosis

If neonatal HSV disease is suspected, viral swabs of skin vesicles, eyes, nasopharynx, and rectum should be sent for HSV culture and immunofluorescence or HSV PCR, CSF collected for routine examination, HSV PCR and culture, blood sent for liver function tests, platelet count and coagulation screen, and empirical therapy with systemic intravenous aciclovir promptly commenced. A chest radiograph may be indicated if respiratory distress is present. Imaging of the head by ultrasound or CT scan should be performed. Serological assays are usually not helpful in the acute diagnosis of neonatal HSV disease.

Treatment and prevention

Mothers with primary lesions should be delivered electively by Cesarean section while mothers with recurrent lesions, if they have a negative culture and do not have lesions or prodrome of infection, may be delivered vaginally. The use of invasive fetal monitoring and vacuum delivery should be avoided where possible in women with known genital HSV disease. Some suggest that the infant should be screened for infection by surface viral swabs at 48 h of life.

Aciclovir 60 mg/kg/day in three divided doses given intravenously should be commenced as soon as neonatal HSV disease is suspected. Many suggest it should be commenced empirically in the offspring of women with known primary genital HSV infection due to the high attack rate. The duration of therapy is for 14 days for SEM disease and for 21 days for all other categories or where a lumbar puncture could not be performed.[99] Topical therapy may be given in addition to systemic therapy for HSV eye disease under the direction of an ophthalmologist. The prognostic significance of persistence of HSV DNA at the end of therapy is currently under evaluation.

PARASITIC INFECTIONS

TOXOPLASMOSIS

Toxoplasmosis is a worldwide disease. In the UK between 20 and 40% of the population have been infected with this protozoan by adult life. The incidence of congenital toxoplasmosis in Europe is 1–10 in 10 000 newborns.[100]

Congenital toxoplasmosis infection usually occurs as a result of placental infection after a primary infection in a pregnant woman. Parasites form small focal lesions in the placenta, proliferate and are released as active forms into the fetal bloodstream. Rare cases of fetal transmission have been reported after preconception maternal infection in immunocompetent women,[101] presumably due to myometrial infection. It is generally accepted that women who bear a congenitally infected child do not have infected children in subsequent pregnancies, probably owing to persistence of immunity after the primary infection. Exceptions to this rule do occur, and it is suggested that the persistence of *Toxoplasma gondii* as cysts in the myometrium with liberation of active forms during pregnancy is one of the main infectious causes of repeated abortion in women. Congenital toxoplasmosis has been reported following reactivation in women with HIV infection, although it is a rare event, as shown by a European Collaborative Study.[102]

The risk of transmission and the clinical outcome after maternal toxoplasmosis infection vary with the trimester of pregnancy. Recently, up-to-date risk estimates of maternal transmission of toxoplasmosis during pregnancy have come from a large study of women with confirmed infection who were referred to a toxoplasmosis reference laboratory in France.[100] Infection in early pregnancy carried a low risk of transmission, that rose to 6% by 13 weeks, thereafter rising sharply to 40% at 26 weeks, and 72% at 36 weeks. If a fetus is infected, the risk of developing clinical signs (and the severity of disease) is greatest the earlier in pregnancy the infection occurs, falling from 61% at 13 weeks, to 25% at 26 weeks to 9% at 36 weeks.[100]

Clinical manifestations

Infection of the fetus with virulent strains early in pregnancy may produce fetal death and abortion; still later, severe fetal damage or stillbirth; and later still, a live-born infant with stigmata of congenital toxoplasmosis. However, up to 70% of infants with congenital toxoplasmosis are asymptomatic at birth. The most common single presenting feature is chorioretinitis and both eyes are involved in 40% of cases. Other important clinical features are given in Table 10.124. They include hydrocephalus, intracranial calcification, hepatosplenomegaly, jaundice, thrombocytopenia, and a maculopapular rash. Clinical sequelae of congenital infection, including visual disturbance, seizures and mental retardation may not manifest until later in life. The prognosis for patients with central nervous system involvement must be extremely guarded.

Diagnosis

This is usually based on *Toxoplasma* IgM and/or *Toxoplasma* IgA antibody test. The sensitivity of the IgM-ISAGA test is probably the highest. Persistently elevated *Toxoplasma* IgG beyond 12 months of life, and detection of *Toxoplasma* DNA by PCR in the placenta, neonatal blood or CSF may also be used to make the diagnosis. In the infant with suspected congenital toxoplasmosis, ophthalmological examination, hearing assessment, and central nervous system examination and imaging should also be performed.

Treatment

Infants diagnosed with symptomatic or asymptomatic congenital toxoplasmosis infection should be treated to reduce the incidence of long term sequelae such as chorioretinitis. Two synergistic antimicrobials, either sulfadimidine or sulfadiazine together with pyrimethamine, are used in various combinations. Prolonged treatment for up 12 months is required to reduce the risk of late reactivation in the eye.[103] Corticosteroids should be used in the presence of chorioretinitis or raised CSF protein. Many advise treatment of pregnant women with primary toxoplasmosis. A recent systematic review suggests that there are still insufficient data on whether this treatment is effective in preventing neonatal infection.[104]

Pregnant women should be educated to avoid ingestion of *Toxoplasma* cysts by adequate cooking of meat, washing of garden produce, and washing hands after contact with soil.

ENTEROVIRUSES (NON-POLIO)

Intrauterine, perinatal and postnatal transmission of enteroviruses [Coxsackie viruses group A and B, enteric cytopathogenic human orphan (ECHO) viruses, enteroviruses 68–71] have been documented, although there are no data available on the risks of transmission to the fetus or of sequelae, should this occur. While maternal enterovirus infection during pregnancy has not been conclusively proven to cause an embryopathy, there have been links between some specific maternal enteroviral infections and anomalies in the infant (Coxsackie B virus infection, with urogenital anomalies, Coxsackie B3 and B4 viruses, with cardiac anomalies, Coxsackie A9, with digestive anomalies).

Perinatal enteroviral infections generally cause asymptomatic infection or mild, non-specific illness, particularly if the baby acquires infection 'horizontally' from other babies. However, if a woman is infected just before or after delivery, severe disease may develop in the 'vertically' infected newborn, in the first week after birth. The mother may present with severe abdominal pain mimicking abruption, or with respiratory or gastrointestinal symptoms. The baby may present with one or more of the following: a sepsis-like syndrome [fever or hypothermia, anorexia, vomiting, lethargy, disseminated intravascular coagulation (DIC)] gastroenteritis (vomiting, diarrhea, fulminant hepatitis, pancreatitis), a neurological illness (aseptic meningitis, encephalitis or paralysis), a respiratory illness (pneumonitis, pharyngitis, laryngotracheobronchitis), with skin or mucosal manifestations (erythematous, maculopapular rash, herpangina, hemorrhagic conjunctivitis), cardiac disease (myocarditis, pericarditis). Some specific enteroviruses are associated with particular syndromes (see Enteroviruses. Severe ECHO virus infections are more likely to cause hepatitis with massive hepatic necrosis, DIC and death, while Coxsackie viruses are more likely to cause myocarditis and meningitis. Neonatal outbreaks of enterovirus 71 (EV 71) have recently been associated with neurological manifestations such as encephalitis, Guillain–Barré syndrome and neurogenic pulmonary edema.[105,106]

Diagnosis

Enteroviruses may be cultured from the nasopharynx, throat swab or feces. Serology is rarely helpful due to poor sensitivity. Detection of enterovirus nucleic acid in the CSF by PCR can be useful in the diagnosis of enteroviral meningitis.

Treatment

The new antiviral agent, pleconaril has been shown to have in vitro activity against a number of enteroviruses, but not EV 71.[107] In a small case series, treatment of severe neonatal enterovirus infection with oral pleconaril was associated with both virological and clinical improvement, but the sample size was too small to determine if this outcome was significant. Intravenous immunoglobulin has also been used to treat life-threatening disease, but its efficacy is unproven for this use.

BACTERIAL INFECTIONS: THE USE OF THE BACTERIOLOGY LABORATORY BY THE PEDIATRICIAN

The clinical microbiology laboratory specializes in the microscopic examination, isolation, identification and susceptibility testing of microorganisms. The quality of the specimen submitted influences the number and type of organisms isolated. Equally, the request form that accompanies the specimen should provide the laboratory with sufficient clinical information for the efficient processing of the specimen by the microbiology scientific staff and for interpretation of results by the clinician. In addition to basic demographic data, information regarding the child's condition, antibiotic treatment and immune status is of great importance to the processing laboratory. A great deal of clinical interpretation occurs at the microbiology bench level that determines how far organisms are worked up. Where unusual pathogens are suspected, details of recent travel or potential exposure should also be included in the clinical history provided.

The safety of laboratory personnel is a major consideration in microbiology laboratories. Although standard precautions are taken in the laboratory, which should prevent most infections from occurring in laboratory staff, there are still some organisms that may result in laboratory acquired infections in microbiology staff members despite these routine precautions. Notifying the laboratory in the clinical information provided about suspected Brucella infection, for example, is important.

THE NATURE, COLLECTION AND TRANSPORTATION OF SPECIMENS FOR BACTERIAL EXAMINATION

The laboratory often receives inadequate amounts of sample for microscopic examination and the multiple cultures that are required to isolate and identify the complete range of potential pathogens.

The 'ideal' specimen is aseptically obtained fresh pus, fluid or tissue that is rapidly and safely transported to the laboratory. Swabs represent a convenient and economic method of specimen collection, but they should not be sent on their own if fluid or pus can be obtained. Swabs without a buffer-type non-nutritive transport medium (Stuart's or Amies) should not be used, since they allow the specimen to dry out, with resultant loss of microbial viability. This is particularly important where clinically significant bacteria are present in low numbers, or fastidious organisms such as anaerobes are involved.

All specimens should be delivered to the laboratory as soon as possible. Where it is not possible for specimens to reach the laboratory in a timely fashion, they may be refrigerated, but it should be remembered that the results may be less than optimal. *Neisseria* species and anaerobic bacteria, in particular, may not survive refrigeration and these samples should be held at room temperature and processed as soon as possible.

BLOOD CULTURES

The detection of living microorganisms in the blood of a sick child has great diagnostic and prognostic importance. Obtaining blood cultures should be a consideration in any child who has a fever (greater or equal to 38°C) or hypothermia (less than or equal to 36°C), leukocytosis or fever and neutropenia (less than 1000 polymorphs/ml), or any combination of the above. In addition, blood cultures are complementary to cultures of urine and cerebrospinal fluid (CSF) in older children and neonates with suspected sepsis.

To detect bacteremia or fungemia, at least one viable microorganism must be present in the sample of blood cultured. The volume cultured is important in the detection of sepsis. In infants and young children 1–5 ml per culture and in older children 10 ml per culture give optimal recovery.[108]

A major problem in the interpretation of pediatric blood cultures is their contamination by skin microorganisms. To minimize this, the skin should always be cleaned, e.g. with 70% isopropyl alcohol, prior to venepuncture. Any blood culture isolate must be evaluated critically in relation to the clinical findings in the patient.

SPECIMENS FROM THE CENTRAL NERVOUS SYSTEM

Specimens of CSF must be collected aseptically and submitted to the laboratory in sterile containers. The wide range of microbiological, molecular and antigenic tests that are now available to detect infectious agents in CSF make it essential that an adequate volume of sample is collected. When the volume collected is small, the microbiology laboratory may be compelled to prioritize testing, and good communication with the laboratory by pediatricians is essential.

In the past, the only technique for rapid detection of microbes was direct microscopy. This has now been supplemented by identification of organism-specific nucleic acid sequences by polymerase chain reaction (PCR) techniques. PCR is particularly useful in the diagnosis of meningitis where antibiotic therapy may have been commenced prior to hospital admission.

Where there is a brain abscess, pus should be aspirated and sent immediately to the laboratory. Rapid transport and processing will help to maintain the viability of any anaerobes or other fastidious pathogens.

SPECIMENS FROM THE UPPER RESPIRATORY TRACT

In the case of the child with a sore throat, it is not clinically possible to distinguish a self-limiting viral infection from a specific bacterial infection, which requires antibiotic treatment. A precise diagnosis is best confirmed by laboratory testing. Diagnosis may be suspected by isolating a putative pathogen from the mass of indigenous commensal respiratory tract flora. Even so, the mere isolation of a potential pathogen should not necessarily be equated with the implication of the organism in the disease process; Lancefield group A, beta hemolytic streptococci, for example, can be isolated from throat swabs from carriers. Consequently, pediatricians must make initial diagnostic decisions on the basis of clinical probabilities rather than using the information received from the laboratories as absolute proof.

Tracheostomy and endotracheal tubes compromise the defense mechanisms which protect the lower airways, resulting in colonization within 24 h by Gram negative organisms and potential pathogens from the environment, regardless of the clinical status of the child. Interpretation of culture results requires careful correlation with clinical features.

Nasopharyngeal specimens are helpful in diagnosing infection with *Bordetella pertussis*. The specimen of choice for the diagnosis of whooping cough is mucus from the posterior nasopharynx, collected either by means of a flexible wire pernasal swab or suction catheter.[109] Since *Bordetella pertussis* is particularly susceptible to drying, it is advisable to employ the appropriate blood/charcoal transport medium if transport is delayed more than a few hours. A rapid immunofluorescent test may give a presumptive diagnosis but the sensitivity is relatively low and problems with specificity may occur. PCR for *Bordetella pertussis* is very sensitive and specific, and is being increasingly employed in routine clinical practice.

Middle ear infection is one of the most frequent infections of infants and young children. Cultures of throat and nasopharynx will yield commensals, but often do not reflect middle ear pathogens. Tympanocentesis is routinely used in some countries, but does not receive wide acceptance in others, in which antibiotic therapy is empirical.

SPECIMENS FROM THE LOWER RESPIRATORY TRACT

The significance of sputum culture results is largely dependent on the quality and source of the original sample and the organisms isolated. Some, such as *Mycobacterium tuberculosis*, are invariably pathogenic, whereas others such as pneumococci may be part of the normal commensal oropharyngeal flora. Some contamination is virtually inevitable with expectorated sputum and nasopharyngeal aspirates. Previous antimicrobial administration will further complicate matters. Ideally, specimens of expectorated sputum should be obtained with the help of the physiotherapist. Young children are usually unable to provide an adequate sputum sample and reliance on blood cultures (which have poor sensitivity) is necessary.

The diagnosis of the etiology of pneumonia in children is often difficult, since positive cultures from blood or pleural fluid are obtained in only about 10% of cases. Other than by deep tracheal suction, adequate respiratory tract specimens are difficult to obtain from children.

Specimens obtained by invasive procedures such as bronchoscopy, including aspirates, brushings and transbronchial biopsies, may be particularly useful where mycobacteria, legionellae and other opportunistic pathogens are implicated in immunocompromised patients with severe infection.

URINE SPECIMENS

Nowhere is the collection, storage and transport of specimens more important than in the laboratory diagnosis of urinary tract infections (UTIs). It must be remembered that interpretation of urine specimens relies on semiquantitative culture techniques. Urine is an excellent culture medium, and contaminating perineal bacteria can multiply in specimens standing at room temperature, invalidating the results of quantitative culture. Furthermore, the white cell count can be dramatically altered by prolonged delays in transport to the laboratory. Specimens that cannot be handled immediately should be refrigerated and examined within 24 h, or alternatively sample bottles containing boric acid should be used. The latter inhibits overgrowth of bacteria and preserves the pus cells for microscopic examination. Early morning specimens are ideal, as overnight incubation in the bladder yields high bacterial counts. Administration of large volumes of fluid in order to encourage the passage of urine may dilute the urine specimen and this must be taken into account when interpreting bacterial and white cell counts.

It is imperative that the accompanying request form contains details of the clinical diagnosis, and especially the method and time of collection and the use of antimicrobial therapy prior to collection. The method of collection, e.g. suprapubic aspirate, catheter or bag, may have a significant impact on level of workup of organisms and the interpretation of results by microbiology laboratory staff. Failure to provide information on collection method may result in significant pathogens being discarded by laboratory staff if more than one organism is obtained on culture, i.e. a mixed growth.

Depending on the age and clinical condition of the child, urine specimens can be collected by clean-catch midstream urine technique, from an in/out urinary catheter, or urine bag specimen or preferably suprapubic aspiration in babies.

The clean-catch midstream specimen largely reduces the risk of introducing infection but small numbers of urethral flora may be present which may still lead to erroneous results. Bag specimens of urine are particularly problematic and abnormal results should always be confirmed by an in/out urinary catheter or suprapubic aspirate in children who are either too young or not able to cooperate with the collection of an appropriate midstream specimen.

Suprapubic bladder aspiration is particularly helpful in confirming infection in neonates and small children. The investigation is almost always diagnostic, with any bacterial growth indicating bladder infection. Occasionally accidental contamination by penetration of the bowel can occur and usually results in mixed enteric flora.

In the untreated child, whether symptomatic or asymptomatic, pure cultures of $> 10^5$ bacteria/ml are usually indicative of infection. Mixed growths (which may include potential pathogens such as Gram negative enteric organisms) suggest the possibility of contamination, but it must be understood that this means that a UTI cannot be ruled out, and a carefully collected repeat sample is indicated.

Urine microscopy should always be performed to establish the presence or absence of white cells (pyuria). UTI may, however, occur without pyuria, particularly in neonates. The presence of pyuria does not confirm UTI either, because the rate of white cell excretion is increased in pyrexial children, and white cells may also appear in the urine as a result of local tissue inflammation, e.g. vulva, vagina or prepuce. A carefully collected repeat specimen will usually resolve this problem. Pyuria in the absence of a significant culture result should be investigated further. Repeated 'sterile pyuria' should raise the possibility of renal tuberculosis and a series of three consecutive early morning specimens of urine should be submitted for mycobacterial culture.

The rapid chemical screening dipstick tests for UTI such as the leukocyte esterase test for pyuria and the nitrite test for bacteriuria are helpful, and a child in whom both these tests are negative is unlikely to have a UTI. No screening tests, however, obviate the need for urine culture, to confirm UTI, to identify the causative organisms and to give sensitivities.

Bacteriological quantitative dip slides consist of a flat paddle, coated with selective and non-selective agar media, which is dipped into the urine, replaced in its container and incubated to give a rough quantitative estimate of the viable count.

SPECIMENS FROM THE INTESTINAL TRACT

The ideal specimen for the diagnosis of bacterial gastroenteritis is freshly passed feces. Specimens should be obtained as near to the acute onset of symptoms as possible and transported to the laboratory without undue delay. The yield of enteric bacterial pathogens from culture of feces is much greater than from rectal swabs, which are not ideal specimens.

While the immediate clinical concern in a child with acute diarrhea is appropriate rehydration, the identification of the infecting agent may provide invaluable information about possible clinical complications, infectivity, sources of infection, potential for spread to contacts, and the appropriateness of antibiotic therapy.

Given the frequency of mild gastrointestinal upset in children, attempts have been made to define clinical symptom complexes with a high predictive value for positive bacterial culture. The combination of watery stools, fever and blood, and the sudden onset of frequent diarrhea without vomiting have been positively associated.[110]

With the ever-increasing range of potential gastrointestinal pathogens, it is important that any relevant clinical and epidemiological information is noted on the request form. This information should include recent antibiotic therapy, consumption of seafood, recent overseas travel, attendance at day care or contact with unusual pets such as turtles, snakes or lizards (which may harbor salmonella species) and the immune status of the patient. This will ensure that the appropriate screening cultures are performed. It must be remembered that stool specimens are screened for specific pathogens using selective media. The range of pathogens sought varies from laboratory to laboratory. Close consultation with one's microbiology laboratory is essential to ensure that the laboratory tests for the pathogens of interest.

PROCEDURES FOR PROTOZOA AND HELMINTHS

The laboratory diagnosis of most protozoal and helminthic infections rests on the detection of the parasite or its cysts or ova in feces, urine (*Schistosoma haematobium*) or thick and thin blood films (malaria, babesiosis, trypanosomiasis and filariasis). Some filaria exhibit cyclical variation in parasitemia. Blood for detection of *Wuchereria bancrofti* should be collected around midnight. *Schisotoma haematobium* on the other hand is maximally excreted in the urine around midday. Consultation with the microbiology laboratory is essential to ensure appropriate specimens are submitted and appropriate testing conducted.

SEXUALLY TRANSMITTED DISEASE

The isolation of a sexually transmitted disease pathogen from a child is presumed to be evidence of sexual abuse.[111] The whole range of sexually transmitted diseases can be acquired, and specimens (swabs in charcoal transport medium) should be taken from pharynx, rectum and vaginal introitus. It is important to warn the laboratory if sexual abuse is suspected, as there will be a need to store any isolates for possible typing in the event of legal proceedings. If rapid antigen detection methods are used in such cases, the results should be interpreted with extreme caution, particularly where cultural confirmation is lacking. Recently PCR on urine for the detection of *Neisseria gonorrhoeae* and *Chlamydia trachomatis* has become widely available. Whilst PCR is a good screening method, it should not replace appropriately collected swabs and culture methods, as it does not provide reliable information about appropriate antibiotic therapy and its role in medicolegal proceedings still needs to be evaluated.

SEROLOGICAL DIAGNOSIS

Immunological techniques are used in the microbiology laboratory to measure the immune response to organisms, particularly those for which isolation by culture is not possible. They are also used to establish or confirm a presumptive diagnosis, to assess the level of protective immunity whether naturally acquired or vaccine-induced, or to indicate the etiological infective trigger of an ongoing immunological disease process, e.g. glomerulonephritis, reactive arthritis. The selection of the appropriate test and the timing of samples depend on the stage of the disease, the nature of the infectious agent and, in particular, the characteristics of the immunological response to that agent.

Serological diagnosis, based on antibody detection, is an indirect method of diagnosing an infection, is less reliable and cannot supplant isolation of the organism or direct antigen detection in tissues or fluid. The laboratory should be provided with adequate, pertinent detail to enable the appropriate test to be performed. Thus, in the child suspected of having a recent infection, or the newborn with possible intrauterine infection, it is necessary to measure specific IgM antibody. Otherwise, it is essential to obtain an early acute or baseline serum sample and an appropriately timed convalescent sample, in order to demonstrate a rising titer of IgG antibodies. As ever, the most efficient service will result from effective communication between the pediatricians and their laboratory counterparts.

MONITORING ANTIMICROBIAL THERAPY

Once the pediatrician has embarked on an antibiotic regimen, the microbiology laboratory can monitor the levels of the antimicrobial agent in blood and other body fluids to establish whether adequate therapeutic levels are being achieved or potentially toxic levels are present. This can be particularly important in neonates and young children, where there can be wide individual variation in the levels resulting from standard dosage, and when there is a narrow margin between therapeutic and toxic levels. In addition, in the management of bacterial endocarditis, it may be useful to assess the bactericidal effect of the patient's serum against the offending organism.

BACTERIAL INFECTIONS: BOTULISM

The name botulism derives from the Latin *botulus* for sausage, and was coined following an outbreak in Germany in 1793, in which 13 people who shared a large sausage became ill, and six died.

Botulism is an acute flaccid paralysis caused by botulinum toxin. The toxins responsible are exotoxins produced by *Clostridium botulinum*, an anaerobic spore-forming bacillus. They bind irreversibly to receptors on the presynaptic nerve terminal of the neuromuscular junction, blocking release of acetylcholine. They also bind to other cholinergic nerve synapses, resulting in atropinic manifestations such as pupillary dilatation and constipation, as well as hypotonia and cranial nerve palsies.[112] The blockage of acetylcholine release is permanent and irreversible. Later recovery is associated with sprouting of new nerve terminals.

Infant botulism, which has an insidious onset, is due to the baby ingesting spores of *C. botulinum* which germinate and result in gut colonization. The organism produces toxin, which is absorbed into the bloodstream via the gut. Classical botulism affects older children and adults and results from eating food already contaminated with preformed toxin.

Types A, B and E *C. botulinum* are associated with human disease. A and B are found in soil and E in fresh or salt water.

EPIDEMIOLOGY

Botulinum spores are ubiquitous in the soil, and contamination of food by soils is responsible for most human cases. Infant botulism is more common in babies living in rural areas or on a farm: in Australia cases occur when it is hot, dry and windy and spores may blow into the baby's mouth or into the water supply.[113] There is a particular association with babies, whose pacifiers were dipped in honey, but only 11 of 68 US babies reported with infant botulism had honey exposure.[114] Corn syrup ingestion (20 of the 68 babies) and breast-feeding were other risk factors. Breast milk is thought to generate favorable conditions for germination of spores.

Classical botulism results from ingestion of preformed toxin, which can only occur under anaerobic conditions. Canned or bottled foods, especially soil-contaminated vegetables, smoked fish and continental sausage are classic food vehicles. High temperatures are required to inactivate spores. If toxin production does occur, poisoning can be avoided by adequate cooking or reheating of the food, because the toxin is inactivated by moderate heat. Raw fish or fish products are also potential sources of botulinum toxin.

CLINICAL FEATURES AND DIAGNOSIS

Infantile botulism is characterized by an insidious onset of severe, progressive hypotonia, poor suck, constipation and bilateral ptosis. The pupils are often dilated and there may also be pooling of oral secretions, reduced facial movements and ophthalmoplegia. The gag reflex is often weak. Peripheral tendon reflexes are normal or diminished, but not usually absent.

The median age of onset is 2 months, with a range of less than 3 weeks to 12 months.[115] The differential diagnosis includes spinal muscular atrophy (absent reflexes, fasciculations), myotonic dystrophy [myotonia, electromyogram (EMG) pattern], wild-type or vaccine-associated paralytic poliomyelitis (asymmetric paralysis, CSF pleocytosis) and Guillain–Barré syndrome (ascending paralysis). The EMG in infant botulism shows denervation. The diagnosis is primarily based on clinical findings and EMG, and can be supported by detecting *C. botulinum* toxin in stools (by polymerase chain reaction or animal inoculation) and/or by growing *C. botulinum* from stool culture. An association between infant botulism and sudden infant death syndrome (SIDS) has been proposed, but is unproven.

Botulism in older children presents acutely with malaise, nausea, vomiting and dizziness, followed after hours (type E) or days (types A/B) by paralysis. This starts as ptosis, blurred vision, diplopia, dysphagia and dysarthria, then progresses to generalized paralysis with respiratory failure.

TREATMENT

Infant botulism is managed by protecting the airway and using artificial ventilation if required. Tracheostomy prolongs hospitalization.[115] Nasogastric tube feeds are usually well tolerated. Antibiotics such as penicillin do not speed recovery and gentamicin may exacerbate neuromuscular problems; antibiotics are only indicated for complications such as pneumonia. Botulinum immune globulin is available, but its use is not routine. Babies who require artificial ventilation recover after 3–4 weeks. With proper supportive care the outcome is excellent, with complete recovery the rule.

In older children, circulating toxin needs to be neutralized with antitoxin, in the form of botulinum immune globulin, as soon as possible. This has no effect on bound toxin, but it is always indicated as toxin may circulate for days. The remainder of the care is supportive of respiration, as for infant botulism.

BACTERIAL INFECTIONS: BRUCELLOSIS; UNDULANT FEVER

Brucellosis is usually caused by one of three organisms: *Brucella abortus, Brucella melitensis* or *Brucella suis*. All three are primarily diseases of domesticated animals (cattle, goats and pigs, respectively). The clinical picture ranges from clinically asymptomatic infection via acute brucellosis (with septicemic manifestations) to chronic brucellosis.

EPIDEMIOLOGY

Human brucellosis is mostly a disease of those who come into contact with infected animals in rural areas. Spread of infection from animal to animal occurs readily and the resulting illness is often chronic with long term excretion of the organism. Infection is transmitted to humans by infected milk or milk products and, less frequently, by direct contact or entry through skin. Person-to-person spread rarely occurs. Elimination of brucellosis in animal populations (by vaccination or slaughter policies) will eliminate new infections in humans. World Health Organization sources estimate 500 000 cases worldwide each year (childhood infections accounting for less than 10% of cases). In the UK there are about 20 patients each year, most with disease caused by imported *B. melitensis* infection of laboratory accident. The low incidence of brucellosis in children which results from milk-borne infection is unexpected and some have suggested that environmental exposure may be more relevant.

PATHOLOGY

Acute brucellosis is a septicemic illness, with seeding of organisms in the body, which may become apparent immediately or later after the systemic features have resolved. There is widespread reticuloendothelial system hyperplasia and focal manifestations may occur in many organs, particularly in the liver or spleen. Chronic brucellosis may follow acute brucellosis or begin insidiously. In chronic brucellosis the organisms usually remain intracellularly where they are relatively protected against host defenses and antibiotics.

B. melitensis often produces more invasive manifestations and debility than *B. abortus*, an important point to realize when generalizing about brucellosis. Those with low gastric acid levels are thought to be at particular risk of infection.

CLINICAL FEATURES

The incubation period of acute brucellosis is from a few days to a month.

With acute brucellosis symptoms develop rapidly with high fever, rigors, arthralgia and profuse sweating: patients often feel much iller than signs suggest but recovery follows in most. Fever has no particular pattern. Weight loss and secondary anemia may develop. If the patient does not recover then a state of chronic brucellosis ensues with vague irritability, malaise, fatigue, musculoskeletal aches and pains, headaches and depression. Fever may be intermittent, occurring every few weeks – hence the name 'undulant fever'.

Although chronic brucellosis is rarely life threatening the morbidity may be significant.

With both acute and chronic brucellosis suggestive signs may be prominent or absent – constituting a pyrexia of unknown origin. There may be hepatomegaly, splenomegaly or lymph node enlargement. Particularly with *B. melitensis* infection lymph nodes may suppurate and osteomyelitis or arthritis may develop.

Other rare, but potentially life-threatening manifestations include meningitis, endocarditis, peritonitis and encephalitis.

DIAGNOSIS AND DIFFERENTIAL DIAGNOSIS

Clinical diagnosis may be easy in areas where animal infection is endemic. In non-endemic areas clinical diagnosis may be difficult unless it is realized that patients have visited endemic areas or ingested milk products from endemic areas.

In acute brucellosis blood cultures may be positive, but the organisms are difficult to culture and cultures may take up to 2 weeks to become positive. Agglutination tests to detect IgM and IgG antibodies may be helpful but may be positive in asymptomatically infected patients in endemic areas. Nevertheless increasing titers are almost certainly diagnostic. Agglutination titers of greater than 1:160 in a patient with appropriate clinical features are very suggestive.

In chronic brucellosis blood cultures are rarely positive and bone marrow culture or, less often, liver or splenic biopsy culture may be necessary. If there is renal involvement urine cultures may be positive. Biopsy shows non-caseating granulomas.

If available, the presence of *Brucella*-specific IgM is diagnostic of acute brucellosis or of chronic brucellosis in an acute relapse, whilst *Brucella*-specific IgG indicates infection at some stage. Lymphocytosis with neutropenia may be found.

The differential diagnosis of acute brucellosis includes malaria, salmonellosis (including typhoid fever), tuberculosis, tularemia, rheumatic fever, infective endocarditis, Q fever, leptospirosis and non-infective conditions. If malaise and debility predominate, depression enters the differential diagnosis, as well as being a complication in its own right.

TREATMENT[116]

In acute brucellosis antibiotic treatment probably shortens the illness and reduces the risk of progression to chronic brucellosis. Opinions differ as to the optimal treatment: comparison of treatment results of *B. abortus* and *B. melitensis* infection are not necessarily valid. Most studies of children with brucellosis deal with children with *B. melitensis* infection. Regimens advocated include (either alone or in combination) co-trimoxazole, rifampicin or streptomycin. In chronic brucellosis suppression of intracellular infection may be attempted in the hope that the host's immunity will eventually eliminate or contain infection. Regimens advocated include protracted courses of the antibiotics used in acute brucellosis. Tetracyclines are useful but obviously cannot be used in children unless there is no alternative.

Single agent treatment carries a relapse rate of 5–40%, thought to be caused by inadequate killing rather than development of resistance.

Antipyretics, analgesics and antidepressant treatment may be indicated. Vaccination of humans with the live attenuated organisms used in animals is not practicable – and would certainly make subsequent interpretation of serological tests very difficult.

BACTERIAL INFECTIONS: CHOLERA

Cholera is an acute bacterial enteric disease characterized in its severe form with sudden onset, profuse painless watery stools, occasional vomiting, and, in untreated cases, rapid dehydration, acidosis, hypoglycemia and circulatory collapse. Cholera is caused by infection with *Vibrio cholerae* serogroup O1, which includes two biotypes - classical and El Tor – or *V. cholerae* serogroup O139 (non-O1). The clinical pictures are similar, because a similar enterotoxin is elaborated by these organisms that is critical in the pathogenesis. In any single epidemic, one particular type tends to dominate.

EPIDEMIOLOGY

During the nineteenth century, pandemic cholera spread repeatedly from the Gangetic delta of India to most of the world. During the first half of the twentieth century, the disease was confined largely to Asia. Since 1961, *V. cholerae* of the El Tor biotype has spread through most of Asia into eastern Europe, Africa and Latin America, assuming a worldwide distribution in developing countries. Sporadic imported cases occur among returning travelers or immigrants to high-income countries. Humans are the reservoir of infection, but other environmental reservoirs, such as small crustaceans, exist in association with brackish water or estuaries. Outbreaks occur as a result of ingestion of infected water, due to poor sanitation and hygiene, and, occasionally, as a result of ingestion of infected food especially shellfish.

The arrival of cholera in a region may be heralded by an epidemic of severe disease among all age groups – the presentation of large numbers of adults (as well as children) with severe dehydrating diarrhea should alert one to the possibility of a cholera epidemic. The initial outbreak may be explosive due to the short incubation period (1–5 days) and the ease of fecal–oral transmission in areas where standards of environmental sanitation and personal hygiene are low. Cholera may then become endemic, causing disease mainly in young children of less than 5 years. This is particularly likely with the El Tor biotype as, compared to classical, it has a longer carrier period (up to 2–4 weeks), a longer viability in water and a higher infection-to-case ratio. El Tor cholera has largely replaced classical cholera as the major pathogen of public health importance. However, *V. cholerae* O139 emerged as a cause of severe outbreaks in the Bay of Bengal region in 1992.

ORGANISM AND PATHOPHYSIOLOGY

V. cholerae are Gram negative curved rods measuring 1.5–3.0 × 0.5 µm. In culture, they may assume other forms such as spiral shapes. They possess somatic (O) antigens and flagellar (H) antigens that may be used to distinguish serological strains such as Ogawa, Inaba and Hikojima. In hanging-drop preparations, they are highly motile. The pathogenesis of diarrhea is mediated via an enterotoxin that consists of A and B subunits. The B subunit binds the toxin to surface receptors on the enterocyte and activates arachidonic acid metabolism. Once binding has occurred, the A subunit activates the enzyme adenylate cyclase to produce cyclic adenosine monophosphate (cAMP) which inhibits the absorption of sodium chloride and water. cAMP also stimulates secretion of sodium chloride and bicarbonate from the crypt epithelial cells. The excessive intestinal secretions accumulate in the intestinal lumen and are then expelled in the diarrheal stools. The severity of disease depends on the size of the infecting dose and the organism is easily destroyed by gastric acid. Thus, most patients with cholera are infected with large inocula of the organism or have relative achlorhydria. Breast-feeding is protective.

The electrolyte content of stools of patients with adult cholera, cholera in children and diarrhea due to other organisms is summarized in Table 26.16. Generally, stool osmolarity in pediatric cholera is isotonic with plasma. The stool sodium content of children with cholera is intermediate (~ 100 mmol/L) between that found in childhood diarrhea due to other organisms such as rotavirus (~ 30 mmol/L) or *Shigella* (~ 60 mmol/L) and that found in adult cholera (130–150 mmol/L). Stool potassium is higher in pediatric cholera (~ 30 mmol/L) compared to adult cholera (~ 15 mmol/L) and bicarbonate losses (~ 45 mmol/L) are also high. Cholera does not invade the gut mucosa but colicky abdominal pain and ileus may occur due to electrolyte disturbances such as hypokalemia and hypocalcemia with acidosis.

CLINICAL FEATURES

The majority of infections with *V. cholerae* are asymptomatic or mild and clinically indistinguishable from other causes of acute watery diarrhea. It has been estimated that in classical *V. cholerae* infection, the ratio of mild to severe cases is 1 to 1, while in an El Tor biotype outbreak, the ratio of mild to severe cases maybe as high as 7 to 1. The typical presentation of severe disease is of acute frequent diarrhea with copious, odorless, virtually colorless (described as 'rice-water') stools. Vomiting is common but fever is unusual.

Table 26.16 Relative electrolyte constituents of stools

	Sodium	Potassium	Chloride	Bicarbonate
Cholera in adults	+++	+	+++	+++
Cholera in children	++	++	++	++
Non-cholera infantile diarrhea	+	++	+	+

A similar presentation may occur in infants with rotavirus gastroenteritis. In older age groups, the presentation of acute diarrhea among a family group may be confused with food poisoning but severe vomiting which precedes diarrhea and marked abdominal pain are characteristics of food poisoning that are unusual with cholera.

The main clinical features of cholera are those due to severe water and electrolyte loss. Dehydration is commonly isotonic or hypotonic with typical sunken eyes, reduced skin turgor, thirst and dry mucous membranes. Hypovolemic shock may occur within hours of onset. Hypoglycemia is not uncommon and along with acidosis and hypovolemic shock, leads to deterioration in level of consciousness and occasional convulsions. Hypokalemia and hypocalcemia may also develop and cause colicky abdominal pain, paralytic ileus, muscle cramps and arrhythmias. In severe untreated cases, death may occur within a few hours, and the case fatality rate may exceed 50%; with proper treatment, the rate is < 1%.

DIAGNOSIS

Diagnosis is confirmed by isolating *V. cholerae* of the serogroup O1 or O139 from feces. If laboratory facilities are not close at hand, specimens should be transported to a central laboratory in special medium such as Cary-Blair transport medium.[117] For clinical purposes, a quick presumptive diagnosis can be made by darkfield or phase contrast microscopic examination of wet preparation and identification of the vibrios moving like 'shooting stars', inhibited by serotype-specific antiserum. For epidemiological purposes, a presumptive diagnosis can be based on the demonstration of a significant rise in titer of antitoxic and vibriocidal antibodies. In non-endemic areas, isolated organisms from initial suspected cases should be confirmed by appropriate biochemical and serological reactions and by testing the organisms for toxin production. In epidemics, once laboratory confirmation and antibiotic sensitivity have been established, not all cases need laboratory confirmation.

MANAGEMENT

The basis of therapy is replacement of water and electrolyte losses from the stool. In cases with no dehydration or mild dehydration, oral solutions will suffice but ongoing review is important. The World Health Organization oral rehydration solution (WHO-ORS) was developed for cholera management and the electrolyte content is appropriate replacement for these stool losses: 90 mmol/L of sodium, 20 mmol/L of potassium, 80 mmol/L of chloride, 30 mmol/L of bicarbonate and 111 mmol/L of glucose. Absorption is dependent on the glucose facilitated membrane transport of sodium. Other more complex substrates with a lower osmolality such as in cereal-based ORS (e.g. rice or sorghum-based) are safe and more effective at reducing fluid losses.[118,119] However, unless already available in a pre-packaged form, they may be logistically difficult to prepare in the acute epidemic situation.

Those with moderate dehydration have a fluid deficit of between 5 and 10% with decreased skin turgor, thirst, sunken eyes and tachycardia but an intact sensorium. Rehydration and maintenance may be oral or intravenous. Those with severe dehydration with fluid deficits of more than 10% will show all the above signs, together with peripheral cyanosis, drowsiness or coma and weak or absent peripheral pulses. Such patients require rapid rehydration with intravenous (or intraosseous) fluids. Ringer's lactate is the most appropriate widely available intravenous fluid for rehydration but normal saline may also be used. Provision must be made for ongoing stool losses and frequent review of fluid management is essential.

Electrolytes and blood glucose should be assessed at intervals to guide ongoing therapy. Potassium will need to be added (at least 20 mmol/L) if normal saline is used during the maintenance phase.

Antibiotics can shorten the duration of diarrhea, and in this way reduce fluid losses, and reduce vibrio excretion. Tetracycline is most commonly given in a dose of 50 mg/kg body weight per day in 6-hourly doses for 48 h. The first dose may be given 3 h after the onset of intravenous hydration. Children may also be given doxycycline (a single dose of 6 mg/kg) for 3 days; with such short courses, staining of teeth is not a problem. Tetracycline resistance is increasing in Asia and Africa. Alternative antibiotics include ampicillin, erythromycin or a single dose of ciprofloxacin.[119] Chemoprophylaxis for contacts has never succeeded in markedly limiting spread but is justified for close household contacts of an index case or if the outbreak is in a closed group, e.g. aboard ship. A single dose of doxycycline is preferable. Mass chemoprophylaxis of whole communities is never indicated and can lead to antibiotic resistance. Immunization of contacts is not indicated.

CONTROL AND PREVENTION

During an outbreak, a coordinated response is important.[117] An emergency treatment center should be established that is accessible to the community and appropriately supplied and staffed. Standardized treatment regimens and frequent review are essential for effective therapy. Early case-finding and management of household contacts should be organized. Educate the population at risk concerning the need to seek appropriate treatment without delay. Initiate a thorough investigation designed to detect the vehicle and circumstances (time, place, person) of transmission. Laboratory examination of implicated water or food sources and sewage will assist control measures. It may be necessary to educate the community by dissemination of important, factual information relating to water safety, food preparation and human waste disposal, and to obtain public support for control activities. Adopt emergency measures to ensure a safe water supply. Chlorinate public water supplies and chlorinate or boil water used for drinking, cooking and washing dishes and food containers. Provide appropriate safe facilities for sewage disposal.

Cholera will ultimately be brought under control only when water supplies, sanitation and hygienic practices attain such a level that fecal–oral transmission of *V. cholerae* becomes an improbable event. Active immunization with the current killed whole-cell vaccine is of little practical value in epidemic control or management of contacts of cases. This vaccine has been shown to provide only partial protection (50%) of short duration (3–6 months) in highly endemic areas. It takes 8–10 days to induce immunity and does not prevent asymptomatic infection and thus is not recommended. New vaccines are in various stages of evaluation including cheap oral vaccines that provide a higher level of protection and for longer.[119,120] These may prove to be useful and cost effective in cholera-endemic areas in the future.

BACTERIAL INFECTIONS: DIPHTHERIA

Diphtheria is an acute severe disease caused by exotoxin producing *Corynebacterium diphtheriae*. The organism usually infects the respiratory tract, but occasionally the skin or other mucous membranes. Whilst local disease at the primary site of infection may be severe, the most important clinical manifestations are often those at distant sites, following systemic absorption and dissemination of the extremely potent diphtheria exotoxin.

Having been one of the leading causes of pediatric mortality in Europe and the USA in the early twentieth century, the combined efforts of many scientific and clinical disciplines, culminating in the widespread introduction of mass immunization programs in the 1930s and1940s, have led to a dramatic decline in the incidence of diphtheria in the developed world (Table 26.17). However it remains endemic in many developing countries, and the recent major epidemic in the newly independent states of the former Soviet Union (over 50 000 cases reported in 1994) serves to remind us that the potential for serious outbreaks still exists across the globe.

HISTORY

Although epidemics of 'throat distemper' had occurred for several hundred years the French physician, Bretteneau, was the first to describe the unique clinical characteristics of the disease following the 1821 epidemic in France. He coined the term diphtheria, from the Greek root for leather or hide, to reflect the similarity in appearance of the typical pharyngeal membrane to a piece of leather. In the 1880s Loeffler grew the bacillus in pure culture, identified it as the causative agent of diphtheria (the first bacterium to be established as the etiological agent of any disease), and postulated that many of the severe manifestations were toxin mediated. This was confirmed by Roux and Yersin in 1888, and in 1890 von Behring demonstrated that an antiserum against the toxin prevented death in infected animals. Then 4 years later in Paris, human trials using antiserum raised in horses halved the mortality in foundlings with diphtheria. Work in the 1920s demonstrated that heat and formalin treatment rendered the toxin inactive whilst retaining its immunogenic capacity, paving the way for the implementation of mass immunization programs.

BACTERIOLOGY

Corynebacterium diphtheriae is a non-motile, unencapsulated non-sporulating Gram positive bacillus. The organism exhibits considerable pleomorphism in appearance, ranging from a classical club shape to long slender bacilli. However, although certain appearances are considered characteristic for *C. diphtheriae* on microscopy it is not possible to differentiate it reliably from other corynebacteria. It grows readily on ordinary nutrient agar, but is more easily identified by early growth on the nutritionally inadequate Loeffler's medium or on blood tellurite agar, on which growth of other throat organisms is inhibited. Conventionally three biotypes (gravis, intermedius and mitis) are recognized on the basis of differences in colonial morphology, fermentation reactions and hemolytic potential but latterly molecular techniques have proved to be more discriminating in differentiating between strains.

Toxin production, the major virulence factor of *C. diphtheriae*, depends on the presence of a lysogenic phage carrying the tox

Table 26.17 Diphtheria – England and Wales

	Cases	Deaths
1920	69 481	5648
1930	74 043	3497
1940	44 281	2480
1950	962	49
1960	49	5
1970	22	3
1980	5	0

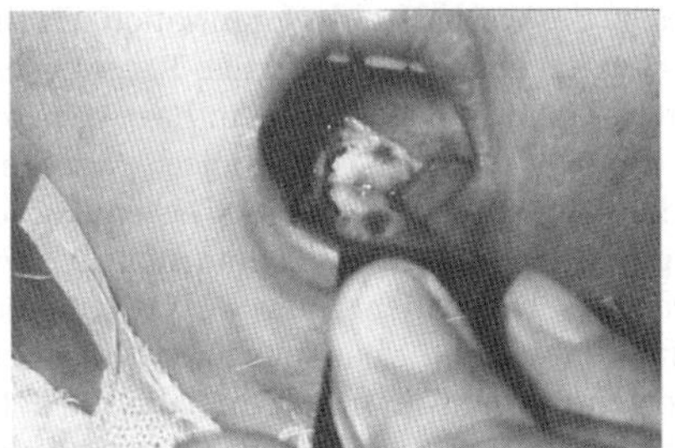

Fig. 26.18 Typical 'pseudomembrane' in a child with faucial diphtheria.

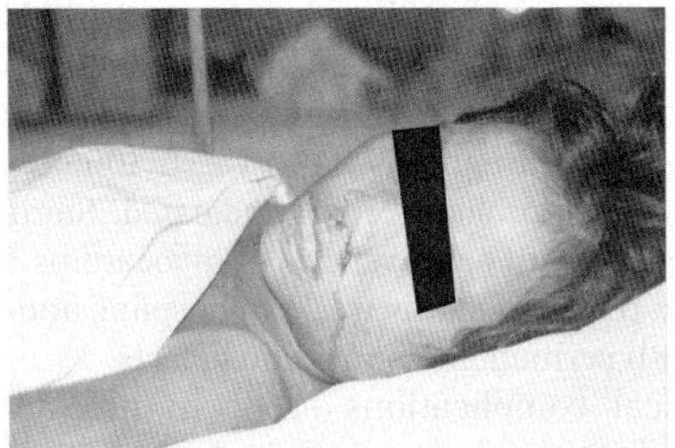

Fig. 26.19 Severe diphtheria showing brawny erythematous swelling of the neck (bull-neck) and serosanguinous nasal discharge.

structural gene, and is not related to biotype. Highly toxic strains may carry two or three tox^+ genes inserted into the genome. Gene expression is iron dependent; in an environment depleted of iron the gene regulator is inhibited, resulting in increased toxin production. Strains lacking the phage do not produce toxin, but conversion to toxigenicity by transfer of a tox^+ phage has been demonstrated in the laboratory, and is thought to occur in nature.[121] Elek's test, an immunoprecipitation assay, is traditionally used to demonstrate toxigenicity of individual strains, but more recently polymerase chain reaction (PCR) for the toxin gene has proved to be both sensitive and specific.[122] Rarely, non-toxigenic strains have been associated with significant invasive disease including endocarditis and osteomyelitis, suggesting that other virulence factors may exist.

PATHOGENESIS

In the absence of toxin production, *C. diphtheriae* is not generally a particularly invasive organism, usually remaining in the superficial layers of the respiratory mucosa and inducing only a mild inflammatory reaction. The toxin, a 58 kDa polypeptide, consists of two fragments; fragment B binds to specific receptors on susceptible cells allowing fragment A to enter the cell and catalyze the inactivation of elongation factor 2, thus inhibiting protein synthesis and leading to cell death.

At the site of infection, local toxin production induces tissue necrosis and the formation of a dense necrotic mass of fibrin, leukocytes, dead epithelial cells and organisms, closely adherent to the underlying mucosa (Fig. 26.18). Attempts to remove this 'pseudomembrane' often result in bleeding from the edematous submucosal layers. The membrane typically originates on the tonsils or posterior pharynx, but may occur anywhere in the respiratory tract and may spread widely to involve the whole of the tracheobronchial tree. Significant underlying soft tissue edema and cervical lymphadenitis occur, resulting in the typical 'bull-neck' appearance (Fig. 26.19), with severe respiratory compromise in some cases. Systemically absorbed toxin can affect all organs in the body, but the major clinical consequences generally involve the heart, kidneys and nervous tissue. After the toxin has become fixed to tissues there is a variable latent period before the cardiac and neurological effects become apparent, but the severity of these late complications usually reflects the severity of the initial infection and the extent of the membrane.

CLINICAL MANIFESTATIONS

The incubation period is typically between 2 and 5 days. The clinical manifestations depend on the site of the primary infection, the immunization status of the host, and the degree to which systemic absorption of toxin has occurred. The disease is conveniently classified into several clinical types, according to the site of primary infection.

Nasal diphtheria, in which the infection is limited to the anterior nares, is characterized by a serosanguinous or seropurulent nasal discharge associated with subtle membrane inside the nostrils, and sometimes excoriation of the external nares and upper lip. Absorption of toxin is limited and systemic complications rare.

Faucial diphtheria, involving the tonsils or posterior pharyngeal structures, is a more severe form of the disease. Anorexia, malaise, sore throat and low grade fever are followed after 1 or 2 days by the development of membrane, typically on one or both tonsils, extending variously to the uvula and soft palate or downwards to the larynx and trachea. The extent of the membrane correlates with the severity of the bull-neck, the degree of airway obstruction and the signs of acute systemic toxicity. In very severe cases, massive toxin absorption occurs resulting in cardiac and respiratory collapse, renal failure, and death within a few days. In many treated cases, the membrane sloughs off after 5–7 days and the patient recovers from the local infection, but remains at risk of the delayed cardiac and neurological problems.

Laryngeal diphtheria generally represents downward extension of the membrane from the pharynx and is correspondingly severe. Sometimes the membrane extends to involve the whole of the tracheobronchial tree, and in such cases, death is virtually inevitable. Occasionally, however, the membrane is limited to the larynx alone; symptoms include hoarseness, a brassy cough, progressive stridor and increasing respiratory distress. Alleviation of the airway obstruction by emergency tracheostomy often provides dramatic relief and, as absorption of toxin is limited in isolated laryngeal diphtheria, late complications are unusual.

Cutaneous, ocular, aural and genital diphtheria may all occur, but are rarely associated with significant toxin-mediated disease. The indolent non-healing ulcers of cutaneous diphtheria are common in the tropics and may serve as a reservoir for the organism, whilst at the same time inducing good immunity in the host.

COMPLICATIONS

Characteristically cardiac complications become evident during the second, or occasionally third, weeks of illness, and may be insidious in onset. Electrocardiogram (ECG) abnormalities such as subtle ST–T wave changes or first-degree heart block are detectable in many patients, but clinical dysfunction is apparent in between 10 and 25%. In these patients, the initial ECG abnormalities often progress to more complex conduction abnormalities including left bundle branch block, trifascicular block and complete heart block, prior to the development of clinical myocarditis.

Clinical signs include diminished heart sounds, a gallop rhythm, and varying degrees of congestive failure. A hypotensive low output state is a very poor prognostic sign, usually associated with major conduction disturbances, and suggests extensive myocardial damage. Cardiac pacing does not improve outcome in this group, although it may be helpful in those with predominant involvement of conducting tissue rather than heart muscle. Mild to moderate cardiac failure can usually be managed successfully with bed rest, oxygen, diuretics and angiotensin-converting enzyme (ACE) inhibitors. Ventricular and supraventricular tachyarrhythmias are common and thus digoxin is probably contraindicated. Steroids are of no benefit in the treatment or prevention of myocarditis.[123] Recovery is generally slow, requiring many weeks in hospital, and some patients may be left with permanent conduction defects.

Neurological complications occur in around 10–20% of patients, usually arising between weeks 3 and 8 of illness. They are typically bilateral, and motor, rather than sensory. Palatal paralysis is relatively common, manifesting as difficulty in swallowing with nasal regurgitation. Ocular and other cranial nerve palsies may follow, and if there is significant pharyngeal or laryngeal dysfunction there is a risk of aspiration. Later still, a peripheral polyneuropathy may develop, similar to, but usually more severe, than Guillain–Barré syndrome.[124] Recovery is slow, with persisting symptoms up to 1 year in some patients.

DIAGNOSIS

The diagnosis of diphtheria should be made on the basis of clinical findings, without waiting for laboratory confirmation, since any delay in treatment may have serious consequences for the patient. In developed countries where diphtheria is a rarity it may easily be missed. Differential diagnoses include infectious mononucleosis, herpetic tonsillitis, Vincent's angina, streptococcal pharyngitis and blood dyscrasias. A high index of suspicion is required, particularly in children without adequate immunization cover, and in those who have recently visited an area endemic for diphtheria.

TREATMENT

Neutralization of free toxin with diphtheria antitoxin is the cornerstone of therapy. Prompt administration of adequate doses is critical, since the antitoxin is only effective before the toxin enters cells. Prognosis is directly related to the duration of illness prior to administration of antitoxin. Empirical dosage recommendations, based on the site, extent and duration of disease are shown in Table 26.18.[125] Antitoxin is probably of no value in cutaneous disease, but a dose of 20 000–40 000 units is sometimes recommended. The antiserum is still raised in horses so, after preliminary sensitivity testing with 0.1 ml of a 1:1000 dilution of antitoxin, a single dose should be given to try to avoid sensitization to horse serum. Facilities for resuscitation must be available, even in the absence of a reaction to the test dose. If a reaction to the test dose does occur, the patient should be desensitized with progressively increasing doses of antiserum.

Antibiotic therapy should also be given to eliminate the organism and prevent spread. The organism is susceptible to a wide range of antibiotics, but penicillin and erythromycin are currently recommended by the World Health Organization. Erythromycin may be more effective at preventing carriage. Recently however, some clinical isolates resistant to erythromycin have been identified[126] so penicillin is probably the drug of choice; parenteral treatment (benzylpenicillin 25 000–50 000 units/kg/day or erythromycin 40–50 mg/kg/day) should be started immediately, later progressing to oral therapy as the patient improves. Antibiotics should be continued for 14 days, and the patient should be barrier nursed until eradication of the organism has been confirmed by culture of appropriate swabs. The disease is notifiable and all suspected cases should be reported immediately to the relevant authority, so that measures can be taken to minimize the likelihood of spread.

Supportive care is also important. Emergency tracheostomy may be life-saving in the initial stages of the illness. Regular ECG monitoring and careful clinical examination allow early detection of myocarditis and prompt management of conduction disturbances and heart failure. Secondary bacterial pneumonia may occur and should be treated with broad-spectrum antibiotics. Ventilatory and nutritional support may be required for long periods for those patients developing severe neurological complications.

PROGNOSIS

Before the introduction of antitoxin, antibiotics and routine immunization, the prognosis was grave, with mortality rates of 30–50%. Currently mortality rates of around 5–10% are usual,[127] with the majority of deaths in those with overwhelming disease at presentation or those who develop myocarditis. If antitoxin is administered within the first 72 h, severe disease and death are rare.

EPIDEMIOLOGY AND PREVENTION

Humans are the only known reservoir for *C. diphtheriae*. The principal modes of spread are by respiratory droplets from acute cases or asymptomatic carriers, or by direct contact with infected skin lesions. Vaccination with diphtheria toxoid (formalin inactivated toxin) is very effective at protecting against the effects of the toxin, but does not prevent infection with the organism. In the past, diphtheria was predominantly a disease of childhood, but during the recent resurgence in the former Soviet Union, many adults acquired the disease and the mortality was high in this group.[128] Waning immunity in the adult population, reduced immunization coverage in children, social unrest and population migration were some of the factors thought to have contributed to the epidemic.

The standard schedule for routine immunization should include a minimum of three doses of the triple vaccine [diphtheria, tetanus and pertussis (DTP)] during the first year of life, with a DTP booster at school entry, and a further booster at school leaving, using the low dose adult vaccine (Td).[129] Supplementary boosters should be given to high risk groups including health care workers, travelers to endemic areas, alcoholics and the homeless, and periodic boosters

Table 26.18 Dosage of antitoxin recommended for various types of diphtheria

Type of diphtheria	Dosage (units)	Route
Nasal	10 000–20 000	Intramuscular
Tonsillar	15 000–25 000	Intramuscular or intravenous
Pharyngeal or laryngeal	20 000–40 000	Intramuscular or intravenous
Combined types or delayed diagnosis	40 000–60 000	Intravenous
Severe diphtheria, e.g. with extensive membrane and/or severe edema (bull-neck diphtheria)	40 000–100 000	Intravenous or part intravenous and part intramuscular

for the general population may become routine in the future. Patients suffering from diphtheria should receive active immunization after recovery, since clinical disease does not always induce adequate antitoxin levels.

BACTERIAL INFECTIONS: *ESCHERICHIA COLI*

Escherichia coli was first described by Theodore Escherich in 1885. It is a Gram negative, non-spore forming, fimbriate bacillus which is motile by means of flagella (Fig. 26.20). Although *E. coli* is responsible for the vast majority of human infections there are four other species in the genus, *Escherichia blattae, Escherichia vulneris, Escherichia fergusonii* and *Escherichia hermannii*. *E. blattae* is an intestinal commensal of cockroaches and does not cause human infection, but the other three have been described as rare opportunists. In contrast *E. coli* is a major pathogen, both primary (Table 26.19) and opportunist. It is also the major aerobic Gram negative rod found in the human (and other animals) gastrointestinal tract at a concentration of approximately 10^8 colony forming units (cfu) per gram. It can be found in soil and water but this is invariably a result of fecal contamination.

The complete genome sequences of both *E. coli* K12 (a non-pathogenic laboratory strain) and *E. coli* 0157 are available.[130,131] *E. coli* K12 encodes some 4405 genes on a large circular chromosome of 4639 kilobase pairs. *E. coli* 0157 which causes hemorrhagic colitis and hemolytic uremic syndrome (HUS), has a larger genome with 1387 new genes encoded in clusters or islands not found in *E. coli* K12. *E. coli* K12 and *E. coli* 0157 share a common backbone but diverged some 4.5 million years ago.[132] Most of the differences result from acquisition of islands of genes. These islands encode pathogenicity determinants (pathogenicity islands), metabolic functions (metabolic islands) and several prophages (bacterial viruses whose genome has been incorporated into the bacterial chromosome). Other pathogenic *E. coli* such as

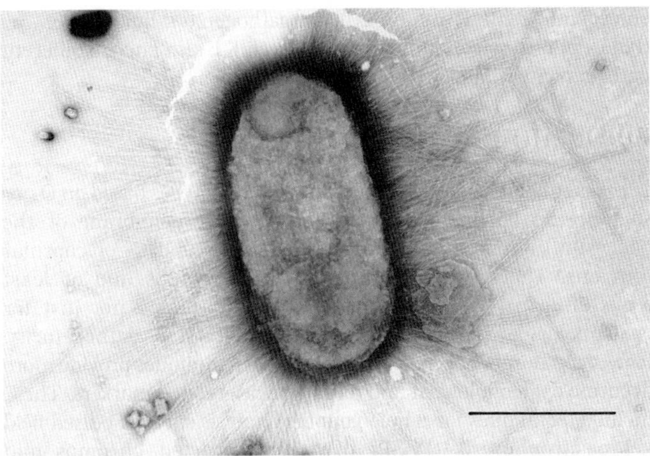

Fig. 26.20 Negative stain electron micrograph of *Escherichia coli* showing numerous fimbriae.

Table 26.19 *Escherichia coli* as a primary pathogen

	Serogroups	Pathogenicity determinants	Infection sites	Disease associations
GI tract				
Enterotoxigenic *E. coli* (ETEC)	06, 08, 015, 020, 025, 0128, 0139, 0148, 0153, 0159	CFA (pili), heat labile (LT) and heat stable (ST) toxins	Small bowel	Secretory diarrhea in travelers and children in developing countries
Enteroinvasive *E. coli* (EIEC)	028, 029, 0124, 0136, 0143	*Ipa* pathogenicity island on plasmid *ial*, adhesin	Large bowel	Mild dysentery in children in developing countries
Enteropathogenic *E. coli* (EPEC)	055, 086, 0111, 0119, 0125, 0126, 0127, 0128, 0142	Locus of enterocyte effacement pathogenicity island (LEE), *tir, eae*	Small and large bowel	Acute and chronic diarrhea in neonates and infants in developing countries
Enterohemorrhagic *E. coli* (EHEC)	026, 0111, 0128, 0157	*eae*A, *eae*B, verocytotoxins 1 & 2	Large bowel	Hemorrhagic colitis, hemolytic uremic syndrome, encephalopathy
Enteroaggregative *E. coli* (EaggEC)	044, 0111, 0121 but most are non-groupable	Adhesin, EAST-1	Small and large bowel	Acute and chronic diarrhea in children and travelers
Diffuse adhering *E. coli* (DAEC)	075 but most are non-groupable	Adhesins	Unknown	Perhaps a cause of diarrheal disease
Urinary tract				
P-fimbriate *E. coli* (PFEC)	01, 02, 03, K1	P-fimriae (adhesions) encoded on a pathogenicity island	Urinary tract, septicemia	Cystitis, pyelonephritis
S-fimbriate *E. coli* (SFEC)	01, 02, 03	S-fimbriae (adhesins)	Urinary tract, septicemia	Cystitis, pyelonephritis
Neonatal meningitis and bacteremia				
E. coli K1	01, 02, 03, K1	K1 capsule plus pathogenicity island function unclear	Urinary tract, meninges, septicemia	Urinary tract infection, meningitis, septicemia

enteropathogenic *E. coli* (EPEC), uropathogenic P-fimbriate *E. coli* (PFEC) and the neonatal pathogen *E. coli* K1 also encode different pathogenicity islands in their genomes.

EPIDEMIOLOGY

E. coli is subdivided into a large number of serotypes based on O- or somatic (on lipopolysaccharide on the outer membrane of the bacterium) antigens, H- or flagellar antigens and K- or capsular antigens. There are 167 different O-serogroups and at least 82 K-antigens.[133] Serogrouping is of importance not just for epidemiological purposes but also delineation of pathogenicity. However a number of molecular biological techniques provide more accurate epidemiological and pathogenicity related markers. These include techniques for whole genome analysis such as pulsed field gel electrophoresis (PFGE) of macrorestricted chromosomal DNA,[134] analysis of housekeeping genes (multilocus sequence testing; MLST) or of insertion sequence distribution (eubacterial repetitive intergenic consensus sequences; ERICS).

E. coli is part of the normal flora of most mammalian species. For example *E. coli* O157 is excreted asymptomatically by cattle but can be transferred to humans as a 'food-poisoning' to cause hemorrhagic colitis, HUS and encephalopathy. The uropathogenic PFEC and the neonatal pathogen *E. coli* K1 colonize the gastrointestinal tract[135] hence reaching their infective sites by ascending the urinary tract and by hematogenous spread respectively. In addition the commensal *E. coli* that do not possess defined pathogenicity determinants are important opportunist pathogens, for example post gastrointestinal surgery or in patients with indwelling urinary catheters. Finally the commensal *E. coli* are an important reservoir of antibiotic resistance genes that can be transferred to more pathogenic bacteria.[136]

ENTEROPATHOGENS

Enterotoxigenic *E. coli* (ETEC) are solely human pathogens although similar bacteria can cause diarrheal disease in domestic animals. They cause up to 25% of cases of diarrheal disease in children in developing countries and are a major cause of traveler's diarrhea (c. 80% of cases). Infection is usually acquired via food or water contaminated with human excreta. The infective dose is high (c. 10^7 cfu). Enteroinvasive *E. coli* (EIEC) are a minor cause of diarrheal disease, in most surveys being responsible for less than 5% of cases in children in the tropics. Enteropathogenic *E. coli* (EPEC) were responsible for epidemics of infantile diarrhea in UK and the USA in the 1940s and 1950s but are now found predominantly in neonates and infants in developing countries (in one study causing 11% of cases of infantile diarrhea). The infective dose is low ($< 10^4$ cfu) so direct person-to-person spread is also possible.

Enterohemorrhagic *E. coli* (EHEC) are most often acquired as food poisoning but since the infective dose is low ($< 10^2$ cfu) person-to-person spread in households and hospitals has been described. Enteroaggregative *E. coli* (EaggEC) are the most recently described group and are responsible for cases of acute and chronic diarrhea in children and traveler's diarrhea. It is particularly associated with chronic diarrhea in children in developing countries. The infective dose is unknown. It is still unclear what role diffuse adhering *E. coli* (DAEC) play in diarrheal disease and little is known of their epidemiology.

UROPATHOGENS

Most *E. coli* causing urinary tract infection fall into serogroups O1, O2, O4, O6 and O75, have thick capsules and express adhesins. Of particular importance are PFEC which bind to the P-blood group receptor. They colonize the intestine and in females the vagina, perineum and anterior urethra. From there they ascend to produce cystitis and pyelonephritis.

NEONATAL SEPSIS

E. coli K1 is responsible for 40% of the cases of neonatal bacteremia and 75% of the cases of neonatal meningitis that are due to *E. coli*. The incidence rate of *E. coli* neonatal meningitis in the USA is 1 case per 1000 live births. Infection is acquired from mother-to-baby at birth or baby-to-baby and staff-to-baby in neonatal intensive care units. Approximately 50% of women of child-bearing age have intestinal carriage of *E. coli* K1 and 70% of neonates born to carrier mothers will acquire carriage. The colonization to disease ratio is approximately 200–300 to 1.

PATHOGENESIS

ENTEROPATHOGENS

ETEC cause a non-inflammatory secretory small intestinal diarrhea. To do this they must colonize the upper small intestine by adhering to enterocytes using fimbriae (protein spikes) termed colonization factor antigens (CFA) in human ETECs. In addition they secrete one or both of heat labile (LT) and heat stable (ST) toxins. The LTs (I and II) are subunit toxins. They consist of five (toxophore) B subunits that carry and bind the toxin to ganglioside receptors on the enterocyte surface and one A (toxin) subunit. The A subunit is activated by cleavage to A1 which activates adenosine diphosphate (ADP) ribosylation of a regulatory subunit of adenyl cyclase. This results in activation of adenyl cyclase and raised intraenterocyte concentrations of cyclic adenosine monophosphate (AMP). This results in fluid and electrolyte secretion into the small intestinal lumen, and thus a voluminous watery diarrhea. LTI is very similar to cholera toxin. ST (a and b) are smaller (16–18 amino acids) and activate guanylate cyclase by mimicking guanylin, the endogenous modulator of cyclic guanosine monophosphate (GMP) signaling. How raised intracellular cyclic GMP levels induce diarrhea is unclear. EIEC cause colitis and an inflammatory diarrhea. They have similarity with *Shigella* spp. in that similar pathogenicity genes (on a pathogenicity island) are encoded as large plasmids in both genera. They attach to and invade colonic enterocytes (Fig. 26.21).

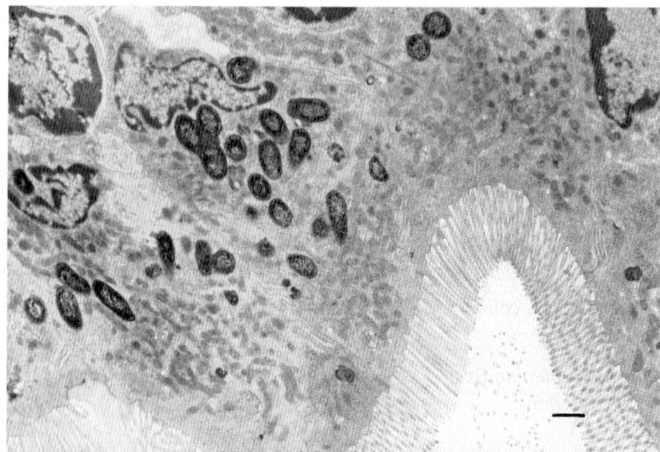

Fig. 26.21 Thin section electron micrograph of colonic enterocytes with numerous enteroinvasive *Escherichia coli* in the cytoplasm.

They can then migrate laterally from colonocyte to colonocyte. How this causes colonocyte death, loss of mucous membrane integrity and an inflammatory response is unclear but the initial stages might involve induction of colonocyte apoptosis.

EPEC produce specific ultrastructural lesions on the enterocyte surface termed attaching-effacement in which there is very close intimate attachment of the bacteria to the enterocyte surface with local loss of the microvilli (brush border) (Fig. 26.22). Although this lesion can be detected throughout the gastrointestinal tract it is the effect on the small intestine that is most important. EPEC initially adhere to the enterocyte surface by means of bundle forming pili. This then activates a chromosomal pathogenicity island called the locus of enterocyte effacement (LEE) which assembles a type III secretion system. Through this the bacterium injects effector molecules into the enterocyte. One is Tir (transferable intimin receptor) which inserts into the enterocyte membrane and acts as a receptor for a molecule (intimin) on the bacterial surface thus promoting intimate attachment of the bacterium to the enterocyte. Other effectors cause damage to the microfilaments of the terminal web causing loss of the microvilli (termed effacement). This causes a great loss of surface area for absorption and of the brush border disaccharidases sucrase, maltase and lactase, and leads to malabsorption and an osmotic diarrhea.

EHEC such as *E. coli* O157 have a pathogenicity island very similar to the EPEC LEE but their attaching effacement is confined to the terminal ileum and colon. In addition they elaborate verotoxins (VT) 1 and/or 2. These are subunit toxins with five B (toxophore) units and one A (toxin) unit. The B units carry, protect, and bind the A subunit to the enterocyte utilizing a globoside glycolipid receptor. The A subunit inhibits protein synthesis and is one of the most potent toxins known. VT-1 is identical to Shiga toxin and both it and VT-2 are encoded on promiscuous bacteriophages. This means that these toxin genes are widely distributed in enteric bacteria, but in order to produce disease, *E. coli* must have both LEE and VT. VT kills colonocytes causing hemorrhagic colitis. If VT enters the circulation it binds to receptors on endothelial cells, in particular, in the renal vasculature. This causes fibrin deposition, cell swelling and narrowing of the lumen of the vessel, and results in a microangiopathic hemolytic uremia or HUS.

EaggEC are so-called because they produce a 'stacked brick' appearance when adherent to cells in culture and each other. They adhere to both small and large intestinal mucosa by means of plasmid-encoded fimbriae (AAF/I, AAF/II). They elaborate toxins including EaggEC heat stable toxin-1 (EAST-1) which resembles ETEC ST and a plasmid encoded toxin (Pet) which induces mucin release, exfoliation of cells and crypt abscesses. Recently it has been shown that a novel flagellin from EaggEC induces the release of the inflammatory chemokine IL-8 from intestinal epithelial cells.

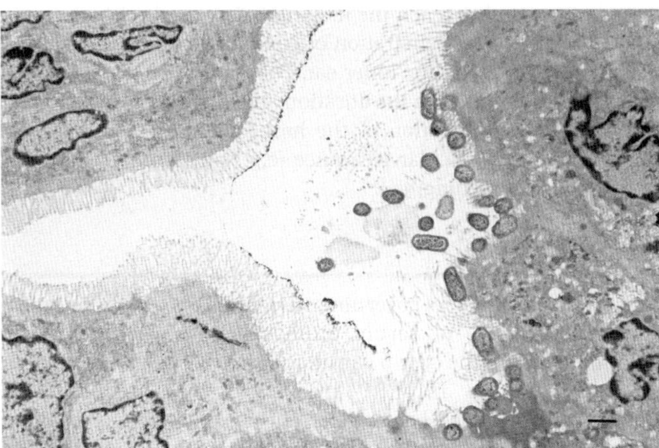

Fig. 26.22 Thin section electron micrograph showing enteropathogenic *Escherichia coli* closely adherent to duodenal enterocytes with loss of microvilli (attaching effacement).

PFEC have two pathogenicity islands in their genome which encode expression of fimbriae with a receptor binding molecule at their tip which recognizes the P-blood group antigen. This is a glycolipid with terminal digalactose residues and is expressed on most tissues including the epithelium of the urinary tract. Thus the bacteria are able to adhere and resist the flushing action of urine. How they induce inflammation is less clear but probably involves induction of cytokine and chemokine release.

E. coli K1 produces a thick capsule that allows it to evade the killing effects of neutrophils and complement. It, like the group B meningococcal capsule, is a homopolymer of N-acetyl neuraminic acid which is a self-antigen being expressed on neuronal tissue in particular. Further pathogenicity determinants are gradually being uncovered.

CLINICAL FEATURES

The clinical features associated with enteropathic *E. coli* are outlined in the Table 26.19. For a more detailed description of this and of urinary tract infections and neonatal sepsis see the appropriate sections.

DIAGNOSIS AND DIFFERENTIAL DIAGNOSIS

ENTEROPATHOGENS

For definitive diagnosis *E. coli* must be isolated from fecal samples. Although O-serogrouping was the method originally used to describe the different pathogenic types it is of little value except in outbreaks. For specific diagnosis the pathogenicity genes or their products must be detected. This is most conveniently done by polymerase chain reaction (PCR) and a number of multiplex PCR systems have been described; however none is commercially available.

UROPATHOGENS AND NEONATAL SEPSIS

Standard microbiological procedures are used to isolate *E. coli* from urine, blood or CSF. It is possible to demonstrate PFEC or *E. coli* K1 using specific antisera, although this is not entirely necessary.

TREATMENT, PROGNOSIS AND PREVENTION

ENTEROPATHOGENS

In general diarrheal disease should be managed by assessment of dehydration and appropriate rehydration. Antimicrobial therapy is not normally indicated and in some cases, for example with *E. coli* O157, might be harmful. However some infections with EPEC and EaggEC can produce persistent diarrhea and in such cases antimicrobial chemotherapy directed by in vitro sensitivity testing is appropriate.

The prognosis is good with full recovery without antibiotic therapy in most cases. There are no vaccines currently available, thus good hygiene and recognition of risk are the mainstay of infection prevention both in hospital and the community.

UROPATHOGENS

For uncomplicated infections short course (3–5 days) antimicrobial chemotherapy will suffice. If complicated by pyelonephritis or septicemia, longer duration of treatment will be needed. For prognosis prevention and follow-up see the appropriate section on urinary tract infection.

NEONATAL SEPSIS

For pre-emptive, empirical therapy see section on neonatal sepsis. This will need to be modified in the light of the local antimicrobial susceptibility patterns. No vaccine is available especially since the K1 capsule is a self-antigen.

BACTERIAL INFECTIONS: *HAEMOPHILUS INFLUENZAE*

GENERAL FEATURES AND EPIDEMIOLOGY

Haemophilus influenzae was first reported by Pfeiffer in 1892, but the sensational claim that it was the primary cause of epidemic influenza proved fallacious. None the less, the bacterium has a wide spectrum of pathogenic capabilities. A small Gram negative bacterium, it may be encapsulated or non-encapsulated (non-typable). In 1931 Pitmann[137] described six antigenically distinct capsular types, designated a to f. The possession of the capsule is an important virulence determinant and it is *Haemophilus influenzae* of capsular serotype b (Hib) that stands out as the most virulent strain, responsible for the great majority of invasive *Haemophilus* infections. Prior to the widespread use of effective vaccines against Hib, it was the major cause of bacterial meningitis and the predominant cause of epiglottitis in young children. In the Oxford region between 1985 and 1990 for example, the incidence of all invasive Hib disease was 36 cases/100 000 children < 5 years old.[138] Table 26.20 summarizes several characteristics relating to carriage and pathogenicity.

H. influenzae is among the bacteria normally found in the human pharynx and also colonizes the mucosae of the conjunctiva and genital tracts. Spread from one individual to another occurs by airborne droplets or by direct transfer of secretions. Exposure begins during or immediately after birth so that from infancy onwards, carriage of one or more strains for periods lasting from days to months is common. The presence of *H. influenzae* in cultures obtained from the upper (but not the lower) respiratory tract is therefore a common and normal finding. In about 3–5% of individuals, the organisms are encapsulated, most often with the serotype b antigen (in an unvaccinated population). Following widespread vaccination, however, carriage of type b strains has declined. In general, carriers of *H. influenzae*, whether colonized with encapsulated or non-typable organisms, remain healthy, but occasionally disease occurs. Two contrasting patterns of *H. influenzae* disease can be identified. The more serious in its consequences are invasive infections such as meningitis, septic arthritis, epiglottitis and cellulitis; these infections typically occur in young children, are associated with bacteremia and are caused by encapsulated type b strains. The second category includes less serious, but numerically more common, infections that occur as a result of contiguous spread of *H. influenzae* within the respiratory tract. *H. influenzae* is a common cause of otitis media (accounting for 23% of bacteria isolated by tympanocentesis),[139] sinusitis, conjunctivitis and lower respiratory tract infection. These infections are usually, but not invariably, caused by non-typable strains. These generalizations are not hard and fast; non-typable strains are a cause of neonatal sepsis, as well as sepsis and meningitis in infants and children.[140] They are a common cause of severe, acute lower respiratory tract infections (often accompanied by bacteremia) among young children living in the developing world[141] and are responsible for about 50% of all *H. influenzae* causing invasive disease in adults.[142] Epiglottitis, however, appears to be a syndrome associated overwhelmingly with serotype b. Brazilian purpuric fever is a rare disease caused by a non-typable *H. influenzae*, biotype *aegyptius*. This occurs in young children who present initially with a conjunctivitis and go on to develop a serious, potentially fatal form of septicemia which can mimic meningococcemia.

Table 26.20 Carriage and pathogenicity of *Haemophilus influenzae*

Strains	Common upper respiratory tract carriage rates	Principal manifestation of pathogenicity
Non-encapsulated (non-typable)	50–80%	Exacerbations of chronic bronchitis, otitis media, sinusitis, conjunctivitis Bacteremic infections rare
Encapsulated, type b (pre-vaccine)	2–4%	Meningitis, epiglottitis, pneumonia and empyema, septic arthritis, cellulitis, osteomyelitis, pericarditis, bacteremia Rarer manifestations include glossitis, tenosynovitis, peritonitis, endocarditis, ventriculitis associated with infected shunt tubing
Encapsulated, types a and c through f	1–2%	Rarely incriminated as pathogens

PATHOGENESIS

The host and microbial determinants of colonization by *H. influenzae* are poorly understood. In animal experiments infection is potentiated by viruses such as influenza. Adhesins facilitate attachment to mucus and to human epithelial cells and there are cell wall components that inhibit the normal ciliary function of respiratory tract epithelium. The primacy of type b capsule as a crucial factor in the pathogenesis of invasive disease has been well established. Lipopolysaccharide is also important in facilitating bloodstream survival and blood–brain barrier damage in experimental infections. In rat and primate models of *H. influenzae* type b meningitis, organisms were found to invade the submucosa of the nasopharynx and to reach the meninges as a result of bacteremia rather than by direct penetration of contiguous structures such as the cribriform plate or the inner ear. The occurrence of meningitis correlated strikingly with the duration and intensity of bacteremia; experimental manipulation of the host factors that decrease the efficiency of intravascular clearance (e.g. splenectomy) increased the incidence of meningitis.[143]

IMMUNITY

Among the host factors governing susceptibility to invasive type b infection, the role of serum antibodies to polyribosyl-ribitol phosphate (PRP), the type b capsular antigen, has been shown to be critical. Serum anti-PRP antibodies in conjunction with complement-mediated bactericidal and opsonic activity mediate protective immunity against systemic infections in humans. The sera of newborns and young infants (up until about 3 months old) generally have sufficient amounts of passively acquired antibody to afford protection. Thereafter, the natural decline of these maternally derived antibodies is followed by a period lasting until the age of 2–4 years when the levels of antibody are inadequate to provide protection. The delay in the acquisition of serum anti-PRP antibodies is characteristic of children less than 2 years old and is a major reason for the high attack rates of *H. influenzae* b invasive disease in early infancy. Although some infants may be exposed to type b *H. influenzae* through nasopharyngeal carriage, the antigenic stimulus for these antibodies may also be different commensal bacteria or ingested foods, which immunize through their crossreacting antigens. The role of local (mucosal) immunity and host defense against *H. influenzae* is poorly understood.

In an infant rat colonization model, anti-PRP antibodies given intranasally are able to prevent nasopharyngeal colonization by Hib. The same effect is seen when these antibodies are given intraperitoneally and a minimum effective serum level can be defined.[144] If it is assumed that anti-PRP antibodies function in a similar manner on the oropharyngeal mucosa of human children, both serum-derived IgG and locally produced IgA may reduce Hib carriage and thereby protect against invasive disease. Indeed, a recent clinical study has correlated protection against carriage of *H. influenzae* b in infants with vaccine-induced serum anti-PRP IgG antibodies of greater than or equal to 5 μg/ml.[145]

CLINICAL FEATURES

Meningitis is the most common, serious manifestation of invasive infection due to *H. influenzae* b. Antecedent symptoms of upper respiratory infection are common. The most common signs are fever and altered behavior – including poor feeding, vomiting, irritability and drowsiness. Thus, none of these clinical features distinguishes the child with *H. influenzae* meningitis from several other infectious diseases or other forms of meningitis. In particular, young infants have few specific signs; nuchal rigidity and a bulging fontanelle are typical, but often absent, early in the course of established meningeal infection. Seizures, cranial nerve involvement and coma may develop as the disease progresses and the effects of raised intracranial pressure, cerebral edema and vasculitis prevail. Subdural effusions are common but these very rarely require specific management and are usually sterile. Overall mortality for *H. influenzae* meningitis is currently less than 5% in developed countries but significantly higher, ranging from 22 to 40% in the developing world. Sequelae occur in 15–30% of those who survive; the commonest complication is sensorineural deafness.

Acute respiratory obstruction caused by involvement of the supraglottic tissue by *H. influenzae* b (epiglottitis or supraglottitis) is a potentially lethal disease of characteristically rapid onset. Typically, the child is aged 2–7 years and presents with sore throat, fever, dyspnea and dysphagia (causing pharyngeal pooling and then oral drooling of secretions). The child is restless and anxious and often adopts a characteristic posture in which the neck is extended and the chin is protruded in order to minimize airway obstruction. Abrupt deterioration leading to death within a few hours may occur if adequate treatment is not provided. The characteristic findings are supralaryngeal. The epiglottis is red and swollen and resembles a red cherry at the base of the tongue. Although an abrupt death is usually the result of acute airway obstruction, sudden collapse may result from less well defined mechanisms associated with acute toxemia. It should be emphasized that examination of the pharynx and larynx of a child in whom acute epiglottitis is suspected should only be attempted under conditions in which the airway can be secured immediately, otherwise the examination may precipitate respiratory arrest.

Invasive disease due to non-type-b encapsulated and non-typable *H. influenzae* is rarer but may present in a similar fashion. Presentation may also be similar in the rare group of children who develop invasive disease with *H. influenzae* b despite vaccination, 'vaccine failures'. In both groups, predisposing host factors such as immunodeficiency are frequent and should be sought.[140,146]

Confirmation of the clinical impression of invasive *H. influenzae* infection depends upon cultures of normally sterile fluids (e.g. CSF, blood, pleural or synovial fluid). Positive nasopharyngeal cultures are not helpful since carriage is common among healthy persons. Needle aspiration of the middle ear (tympanocentesis), maxillary sinus, the margins of an area of cellulitis or lung may occasionally prove helpful in selected cases, especially in a very sick child in whom no diagnosis has been established. Whenever practical, the results of Gram stain should be sought immediately; in up to 70% of cases of meningitis, CSF smears show the typical pleomorphic, Gram negative coccobacilli. Detection of capsular antigen in serum, CSF or concentrated urine by immunoassay (e.g. latex agglutination) may be useful, especially in children who have received prior antibiotic treatment. This test should be interpreted with caution, however, in those who have recently received Hib vaccine, as a false positive result is possible.

TREATMENT

Severe infections due to *H. influenzae* should be treated with parenteral third generation cephalosporins, for example cefotaxime or ceftriaxone. These agents also penetrate well into the CSF. Ampicillin resistance has emerged among both encapsulated and non-typable strains (in the range of 10–30% for European and USA strains). Resistance is almost always mediated by beta lactamases. This has particular relevance to the antibiotic management of less severe infections, such as otitis media and sinusitis. Although ampicillin/amoxicillin remains the antibiotic of choice, others such as amoxicillin-clavulanate or macrolides have become alternative first- and second-line choices.

The use of dexamethasone as adjunctive therapy in Hib meningitis can result in a reduction in sensorineural deafness.[147] Early administration, close to or even prior to the first dose of antibiotic is preferable. Elective intubation and antibiotics are usually mandatory in cases of epiglottitis.

PREVENTION

ACTIVE IMMUNIZATION

The first generation of vaccines against Hib consisted of the purified type b polysaccharide. A trial in 1974 in Finland demonstrated efficacy in children older than 18 months of age but not in younger infants, even when given two doses. No effect of the vaccine on nasopharyngeal carriage was observed.[148] This led to the development of a second generation of vaccines in which the immunogenicity of PRP is enhanced by covalent linkage of the capsular polysaccharide or oligosaccharides to protein to form conjugate vaccines. Currently, four conjugates are licensed for use in infants. Although differences in the immunogenicity of these vaccines have been observed, all elicit significantly enhanced antibody responses when compared to PRP and, in contrast to the latter, are found to prime for a secondary antibody response. Clinical trials and national surveillance have confirmed their efficacy in infancy.[149,150] An unexpected outcome has been a reduction in Hib colonization of the upper respiratory tract and this has contributed to the near elimination of Hib disease in countries where immunization has become routine. Unfortunately, on a global scale too few countries have had the resources to use this vaccine for routine immunization. Recent experience from The Gambia suggests that a dramatic effect on disease rates can be expected when vaccination is eventually implemented in developing countries.[151]

Children and adults who have an increased risk of invasive disease, e.g. those without spleens or with malignancy, should also receive *H. influenzae* b conjugate vaccines. These vaccines are safe and, in general, protective antibody responses are seen. It is good practice, however, to measure the antibody response to vaccination and to further boost those who do not respond.

Finally, the burden of disease due to non-typable *H. influenzae* strains is recognized and its prevention through vaccination increasingly desirable. Possible candidates for vaccines include various outer membrane proteins and lipopolysaccharide.

PASSIVE IMMUNIZATION

Individuals with congenital or acquired hypogammaglobulinemia are unduly susceptible to a variety of pathogens, among which infections due to *H. influenzae* are particularly frequent and troublesome. Replacement immunoglobulin therapy is the mainstay of treatment.

CHEMOPROPHYLAXIS

Young unimmunized or partially immunized children, living in the same household as a case of invasive *H. influenzae* b disease, are likely to be at significantly increased risk of secondary disease. In the prevaccine era secondary attack rates in household contacts were estimated to be 2–4% and in 'day-care centers' up to 1.3%. It is plausible that antibiotic treatment of such contacts could decrease this secondary attack rate. Rifampicin (20 mg/kg, maximum dose 600 mg/day), given orally once daily for 4 days, is effective in eradicating nasopharyngeal carriage. Treatment of household contacts (children and adults) where there are susceptible children (other than the index case) less than 4 years old should be considered, as should treatment of such children in nurseries who are contacts of a case. The course of Hib vaccines should also be completed. When a patient with *H. influenzae* b disease is to return from the hospital to a household with a susceptible child, treatment of the patient with rifampicin is also recommended prior to discharge.

BACTERIAL INFECTIONS: LEPROSY

EPIDEMIOLOGY

Worldwide, 4 million individuals have or are disabled by leprosy. Incidence however remains stable at around 800 000 new cases annually with high rates of childhood cases.[152] India dominates the global picture with 67% of the global caseload. Few childhood cases are seen in Europe and North America but in India childhood cases comprise at least 17% of the new case detection. In the UK all new leprosy cases have acquired their infection abroad. Average incubation times of 2–5 years and 8–12 years have been calculated for tuberculoid and lepromatous cases respectively. Age, sex, household contact and BCG vaccination are important determinants of leprosy risk. Leprosy incidence reaches a peak at the ages 10–11 and equal numbers of male and female cases are seen until puberty, after which there is an excess of male cases. Improved socioeconomic conditions, extended schooling and good housing reduce the risk of leprosy. HIV infection is not a risk factor for leprosy but may worsen leprosy nerve damage.

MICROBIOLOGY AND PATHOLOGY

Leprosy is caused by *Mycobacterium leprae*, an acid fast intracellular organism with the longest doubling time of all known bacteria (12 days) and cannot be cultivated on artificial media. *M. leprae* is a hardy organism, retaining viability for 5 months drying in the shade. The optimum temperature for growth is 27–30°C, which corresponds with the clinical observation of maximal *M. leprae* growth at cool superficial sites (skin, nasal mucosa and peripheral nerves). The *M. leprae* genome was recently sequenced and has a 3.27 Mb genome. Less than half the genome contains functional genes. 165 genes are unique to *M. leprae*, but functions can be attributed to only 29. *M. leprae* has lost many genes for carbon catabolism and many carbon sources (e.g acetate and galactose) are unavailable to it. The genome sequence is opening new possibilities for understanding the biological uniqueness of *M. leprae*.

Untreated lepromatous patients sneeze organisms into the environment. In Indonesia and Ethiopia *M. leprae* DNA has been detected in nasal swabs in up to 5% of the population. After entry via the nose, *M. leprae* is inhaled, multiplies on the inferior turbinates and then has a brief bacteremic phase before binding to Schwann cells and macrophages. The skin is unimportant in leprosy transmission. Bacilli are not excreted by the skin and are rarely found in the epidermis. Untreated lepromatous leprosy mothers excrete *M. leprae* in their breast milk, but treatment renders the bacteria non-viable.

PATHOLOGY

There are four important aspects to the pathogenesis of leprosy: bacterial load, the host immune response, the nerve damage and immune mediated reactions. Schwann cells and skin macrophages are infected early with granuloma formation. In established infection the host immune response determines not only the histological picture but also the clinical features of disease and the prognosis. The Ridley–Jopling spectrum describes the range of responses with tuberculoid and lepromatous poles. At the tuberculoid (TT) pole there is well-expressed cell mediated immunity and delayed hypersensitivity control of bacillary multiplication, with formation of epitheloid cell granulomas. In the lepromatous (LL) form there is cellular anergy towards *M. leprae* with abundant bacillary multiplication and unactivated macrophages. Between these two poles is a continuum, varying from the patient with moderate cell-mediated immunity (borderline tuberculoid, BT) through borderline (BB) to the patient with little cellular response, borderline lepromatous (BL).

Nerve damage occurs in small dermal nerves in skin lesions and peripheral nerve trunks. Acute immune mediated reactions are serious complications because they cause nerve damage. Reversal reactions (type 1) are episodes of delayed hypersensitivity occurring at sites of localization of *M. leprae* antigens. Erythema nodosum leprosum (ENL) (type 2) reactions are due to immune complex deposition.

CLINICAL FEATURES

Patients commonly present with skin lesions, weakness or numbness due to a peripheral nerve lesion, or a burn or ulcer in an anesthetic hand or foot. Borderline patients may present with nerve pain, sudden palsy, multiple new skin lesions or pain in the eye. Childhood cases are frequently detected in school surveys or as household contacts of adult leprosy patients. In an Indian study based on a survey area 30% of cases had a household contact with leprosy, usually a parent or grandparent.[153]

CARDINAL SIGNS

- Typical skin lesions, which are anesthetic at the tuberculoid end of the spectrum
- Thickened peripheral nerves
- Acid-fast bacilli on skin smears or biopsy

PRESENTING SYMPTOMS

Early lesions

Indeterminate lesions are slightly hypopigmented or erythematous macules, a few centimeters in diameter, with poorly defined margins. Hair growth and nerve function are unimpaired. The indeterminate phase may last for months or years before resolving or developing into one of the determinate types of leprosy.

Skin

The commonest skin lesions are macules or plaques; more rarely papules and nodules are seen.

Anesthesia

Anesthesia may occur in skin lesions when dermal nerves are involved or in the distribution of a large peripheral nerve. In skin lesions, the small dermal sensory and autonomic nerve fibers supplying dermal and subcutaneous structures are damaged causing local sensory loss and loss of sweating within that area.

Peripheral neuropathy

Peripheral nerve trunks are vulnerable at sites where they are superficial or are in fibro-osseous tunnels. Damage to peripheral nerve trunks produces characteristic signs with dermatomal sensory loss and dysfunction of muscles supplied by that peripheral nerve. The sites of predilection for peripheral nerve involvement are ulnar (at the elbow), median (at the wrist), radial, radial cutaneous (at the wrist), common peroneal (at the knee), posterior tibial and sural nerves (at the ankle), facial nerve (on the zygomatic arch), and great auricular in the posterior triangle of the neck.

THE LEPROSY SPECTRUM

Classifying patients according to the Ridley–Jopling scale is clinically useful. Table 26.21 gives the skin and nerve features of disease across the spectrum. There is also a simpler field classification of paucibacillary/multibacillary (Table 26.22) which guides the length of treatment. BB disease is unstable, BT leprosy may be associated with rapid, severe nerve damage. BL patients are at risk of both reversal and ENL reactions.

LL has an insidious onset. The earliest lesions are ill defined with shiny erythematous macules. Gradually the skin becomes infiltrated and thickened and nodules develop; facial skin thickening causes the characteristic leonine facies. Dermal nerves are destroyed and sensory loss develops in a glove and stocking distribution. Sweating is lost. Damage to peripheral nerves is symmetrical and occurs late in disease. Testicular atrophy results from diffuse infiltration and the acute orchitis that occurs with ENL reactions.

Most studies in childhood report all types of leprosy; incidence rates and proportion of lepromatous cases increases with age. Few children present under the age of 5.

EYE

Eye damage results from both nerve damage and bacillary invasion. Lagophthalmos results from paresis of the orbicularis oculi due to involvement of the facial (VIIth) nerve. Damage to the ophthalmic branch of the trigeminal (Vth) nerve causes anesthesia of the cornea putting it at risk of ulceration. Invasion of the iris and ciliary body makes them extremely susceptible to reactions.

DIAGNOSIS

Leprosy should be considered as a possible diagnosis in anyone with peripheral nerve or skin lesions who has lived in a leprosy endemic area. The diagnosis is clinical and based on finding a cardinal sign of leprosy, supported by the finding of acid fast bacilli on slit skin smears. Where resources permit, histological examination of a skin or nerve biopsy is ideal for accurate classification. Serological and polymerase chain reaction based diagnostic tests are not yet clinically useful.

SKIN EXAMINATION

The whole body should be inspected in a good light otherwise lesions may be missed, particularly on the buttocks in borderline disease. Skin lesions should be tested for anesthesia.

NEUROLOGICAL EXAMINATION

The peripheral nerves should be palpated systematically looking for enlargement and tenderness. Nerve function should be assessed by

Table 26.21 Major clinical features of the disease spectrum in leprosy

Classification	TT	BT	BB	BL	LL
Skin					
Infiltrated lesions	Defined plaques Healing centers	Irregular plaques Partially raised edges	Polymorphic Punched out centers	Papules, nodules	Diffuse thickening
Macular lesions	Single, small	Several, any size	Multiple, all sizes Geographic	Innumerable, small	Innumerable, confluent
Nerve					
Peripheral nerve	Solitary, enlarged nerves	Several nerves Asymmetrical	Many nerves Asymmetrical	Late neural thickening Asymmetrical anesthesia and paresis	Slow, symmetrical loss Glove and stocking anesthesia
Microbiology					
Bacterial index (0–6)	0–1	0–2	2–3	1–4	4–6

BB, borderline; BL, borderline lepromatous; BT, borderline tuberculoid; TT, tuberculoid

Table 26.22 Modified WHO recommended multidrug therapy regimens

Type of leprosy	Drug treatment: Monthly supervised	Drug treatment: Daily self-administered	Duration of treatment
Paucibacillary	Rifampicin 450 mg (or 10 mg/kg)	Dapsone 50 mg (or 1 mg/kg)	6 months
Multibacillary (MB)	Rifampicin 450 mg (or 10 mg/kg) Clofazimine 150 mg (or 3 mg/kg)	Clofazimine 50 mg (or 1.5 mg/kg) alternate days Dapsone 50 mg (or 1 mg/kg)	24 months
Paucibacillary single lesion	Rifampicin 450 mg, ofloxacin 200 mg, minocycline 50 mg (supplied in a single blister pack)		Single dose

WHO classification for field use when slit skin smears are not available:
- paucibacillary single lesion leprosy (one skin lesion);
- paucibacillary (2–5 skin lesions);
- multibacillary (more than five skin lesions).

In this field classification WHO recommends treatment of MB patients for 12 months only.

testing the small muscles of the hands and feet. Sensation on the hands and feet can be assessed and monitored using Semmes Weins monofilaments. These are now widely used in leprosy and diabetic clinics.

SLIT SKIN SMEARS

These should be undertaken from suspect lesions and standard sites (earlobes, arms and buttocks). Slit skin smears should be read by experienced technicians.

Outside leprosy endemic areas doctors frequently fail to consider the diagnosis of leprosy. Of new patients seen between 1995 and 1999 at The Hospital for Tropical Diseases, London diagnosis had been delayed in over 80% of cases.[154] Patients had been misdiagnosed by dermatologists, neurologists, orthopedic surgeons and rheumatologists. A common problem was failure to consider leprosy as a cause of peripheral neuropathy in patients from leprosy endemic countries. These delays had serious consequences for patients, with over half of them having nerve damage and disability.

DIFFERENTIAL DIAGNOSIS

SKIN

The variety of leprosy skin lesions means that many skin conditions need to be included in the differential diagnosis. In suspected tuberculoid lesions the presence of lesional anesthesia is crucial in differentiating leprosy from fungal infections, vitiligo, vitamin A deficiency and eczema. Single facial patches in children may be difficult to test for anesthesia and one may have to observe a lesion over some months. In lepromatous disease the presence of acid fast bacilli in smears differentiates leprosy nodules from onchocerciasis and post kala-azar dermal leishmaniasis.

NERVES

Peripheral nerve thickening is rarely seen except in leprosy. Hereditary sensory motor neuropathy type III is also associated with palpable peripheral nerve hypertrophy.

TREATMENT

The treatment of leprosy has six main components: chemotherapy, monitoring and treating nerve damage, management of reactions and neuritis, patient education, prevention of disability and social and pyschological support.

CHEMOTHERAPY

All children with leprosy should be given an appropriate multidrug combination. The first line antileprosy drugs are rifampicin, dapsone and clofazimine. Table 26.22 shows the drug combinations, doses and duration of treatment.

Rifampicin

Rifampicin is a potent bactericidal drug for *M. leprae*. Because *M. leprae* resistance to rifampicin can develop as a one-step process, rifampicin should always be given in combination with other antileprotics. Parents and children should be warned that their urine, sweat and tears will be red for 48 h after taking rifampicin.

Dapsone (DDS)

Dapsone (4,4-diaminodiphenylsulfone) is only weakly bactericidal. It commonly causes mild hemolysis but rarely anemia. Glucose-6-phosphate dehydrogenase deficiency is rarely a problem.

Clofazimine

Clofazimine has a weakly bactericidal action. It also has an anti-inflammatory effect, which has reduced the incidence of ENL reactions. Skin discoloration is the most troublesome side-effect, ranging from red to purple–black. The pigmentation usually fades slowly after stopping clofazimine. Clofazimine also produces a characteristic ichthyosis on the shins and forearms.

More than 10 million patients have been treated successfully with multiple drug treatment (MDT). Clinical improvement is rapid, toxicity rare and duration of treatment is shortened. Monthly supervision of the rifampicin component has been crucial to success. The three drugs used for MDT are donated by the drug manufacturers free of charge for distribution in blister packs (pediatric and adult) by WHO, Nippon Foundation and the International Federation of Anti-Leprosy Associations. At the end of 6 months treatment of borderline disease there may still be signs of inflammation, which should not be mistaken for active infection. The distinction between relapse and reaction may be difficult. WHO studies have reported a cumulative relapse rate of 1.07% for paucibacillary leprosy and 0.77% for multibacillary leprosy at 9 years after completion of MDT. *M. leprae* is such a slow growing organism that relapse only occurs after many years. However patients with a high initial bacterial load may be at greater risk of relapse and so require treatment until skin-smear negative.

Short course chemotherapy regimens have been tested for paucibacillary (PB) leprosy using either rifampicin in weekly doses or single dose chemotherapy using a combination of currently used drugs. So far all of these regimens have had higher relapse rates than the current WHO PB regimen. The fluoroquinolones (pefloxacin and ofloxacin) and the macrolide minocycline are all highly active against *M. leprae*, but because of cost are rarely used in field programs. A single dose of triple drug combination (rifampicin, ofloxacin and minocycline) has been tested in India for patients with single skin lesions and produced marked clinical improvement at 18 months in 52% of patients. Although the study had major flaws, and single dose treatment is less effective than the conventional 6 month treatment for PB leprosy, it is an operationally attractive field regimen and has been recommended for use by the World Health Organization.[155]

MONITORING AND TREATING NERVE DAMAGE

Nerve damage may occur before diagnosis, or during and after MDT. It may occur during a reaction or without overt signs of nerve inflammation (silent neuropathy). About 30% of newly diagnosed patients have nerve damage and at least 25% of multibacillary patients develop nerve damage during treatment. Children are at the same risk as adults of developing nerve damage and having reactions. Monitoring sensation and muscle power in a child's hands, feet and eyes should be part of the routine follow-up so that new nerve damage is detected early. Any new damage should be treated with a course of oral steroids starting with prednisolone 0.5 mg/kg/day and reducing by 0.1 mg/day each month. Response rates vary depending on the severity of initial damage but even when promptly treated nerve damage will only improve in 60% of cases.

MANAGEMENT OF REACTIONS AND NEURITIS

Reversal (type 1) reactions

Reversal reactions manifest clinically with erythema and edema of skin lesions and tender, painful peripheral nerves. Loss of nerve function may be dramatic and foot drop can occur overnight. Awareness of the early symptoms of reversal reactions by both patient and physician is important, because, if left untreated, severe nerve damage may develop. The peak time for reversal reactions is in the first 2 months of treatment. The treatment of reactions is aimed at controlling acute inflammation, easing pain, reversing nerve damage and reassuring the patient. MDT should be continued. If there is any evidence of neuritis (nerve tenderness, new anesthesia and/or motor loss) corticosteroid treatment should be started using the regimen given above.

Erythema nodosum leprosum type 2 (ENL) reactions

This complication affects only BL and LL patients and presents with crops of small pink, tender skin lesions on the face and the extensor surfaces of the limbs. In a cohort study from Hyderabad, India 31% of children with BL/LL disease developed ENL.[156] The patient is usually unwell with malaise and fever. Other accompanying signs are acute iritis and episcleritis, lymphadenitis, orchitis, bone pain, dactylitis, arthritis and proteinuria. This is a difficult condition to treat and frequently requires treatment with high dose steroids (1 mg/kg daily, tapered down rapidly) or thalidomide. Since ENL frequently recurs, steroid dependency can easily develop. Thalidomide (5 mg/kg daily) is superior to steroids in controlling ENL and is the drug of choice for young men with severe ENL. Unfortunately thalidomide is unavailable in several leprosy endemic countries despite its undoubted value. Clofazimine has a useful anti-inflammatory effect in ENL and can be used at 3 mg/kg daily for several months.[157] Acute iridocyclitis is treated with 4-hourly instillation of 1% hydrocortisone eye drops and 1% atropine drops twice daily.

Neuritis

Silent neuritis should be treated similarly to reversal reaction (see above). In the Hyderabad study 24% children developed neuritis.[156]

PATIENT EDUCATION

Patients and their parents deserve a clear explanation of the etiology, diagnosis and prognosis of leprosy. It should be emphasized that the infection is curable provided that they comply with the antibiotic regimen. It is important to stress that deformity is not an inevitable disease endpoint. It may be helpful to ask parents and older patients about their views of leprosy as there are many myths about leprosy, which can be dispelled. Lepromatous patients become non-infectious within 72 h of starting antibiotics. Patients and their families should be encouraged to lead a normal life and be reassured that family activities such as eating together, sharing baths and bed linen pose no risks to other family members. It should be emphasized that leprosy is not transmitted sexually nor is it hereditary.

PREVENTION OF DISABILITY

It is vital in preventing disability to create patient self-awareness so that damage is minimized. In a study from south India 33% of children presenting to a referral center had visible deformities.[158] The child with an anesthetic hand or foot needs to understand the importance of daily self-care especially protection when doing potentially dangerous tasks and regular inspection for trauma. For each patient it is helpful to identify potentially dangerous situations, such as cooking, radiators and hot food. Soaking dry hands and feet followed by rubbing with oil keeps the skin moist and supple.

An anesthetic foot needs the protection of an appropriate shoe. For anesthesia alone, a well-fitting 'trainer' with a firm sole and shock-absorbing inner will provide adequate protection. Once there is deformity, such as clawing, special shoes must be made to ensure protection of pressure points and even weight distribution.

Children should be taught to work out why an injury occurred so that the risk can be avoided in future. Plantar ulceration occurs secondary to increased pressure over bony prominences. Ulceration is treated by rest. In leprosy, ulcers heal if they are protected from weight-bearing. No weight-bearing is permitted until the ulcer has healed. Appropriate footwear should be provided to prevent recurrence.

Physiotherapy exercises should be taught to maximize function of weak muscles and prevent contractures. Contractures of hands and feet, foot drop, lagophthalmos, entropion and ectropion are amenable to surgery.

SOCIAL, PSYCHOLOGICAL AND ECONOMIC REHABILITATION

The social and cultural backgrounds of the patient determine the nature of many of the problems that may be encountered. The family may have difficulty in coming to terms with leprosy. The community may reject the patient. Education, confidence from family, friends and doctor, and plastic surgery to correct stigmatizing deformity all have a role to play.

PROPHYLAXIS

In non-endemic areas it is very unusual to see leprosy in contacts of leprosy patients. The last case of secondary transmission in the UK was reported in 1923. Household contacts of new patients should be examined for clinical signs of leprosy and advised to report any new skin lesions promptly and to tell their physicians that they have had contact with a known case of leprosy. In the UK, BCG vaccination is given to contacts under the age of 12; chemoprophylaxis is reserved for children under 10 years who are household contacts of lepromatous cases. They are given prophylaxis with rifampicin 15 mg/kg body weight given monthly for 6 months.[159] BCG gives variable protection, ranging from 80% in Uganda to 20% in Burma. In trials in Malawi and Venezuela adding killed *M. leprae* to BCG did not enhance protection.

BACTERIAL INFECTIONS: LEPTOSPIROSIS

Leptospirosis is a worldwide zoonosis transmitted to humans by infected urine of a wide range of domestic and wild animals: often the causative spirochetes are excreted asymptomatically for long periods of time.

Adults usually acquire infection because of occupational exposure: children may acquire infection by playing in areas contaminated with animal urine or by playing with the animals themselves.

PATHOLOGY

In the UK and USA the common serotypes of the genus *Leptospira* include *Leptospira icterohaemorrhagiae* (commonly acquired from rat's urine), *Leptospira canicola* (commonly acquired from dog's urine), *Leptospira pomona* (commonly acquired from pig's urine), *Leptospira hebdomadis* and *Leptospira ballum*. Correlation of named serotypes with specific syndromes is impossible because of the variability of illness produced by each serotype.

Leptospires gain entry to humans via ingestion, mucous membranes, skin abrasions or the conjunctivae. After entry, the organisms affect capillary epithelium and may cause capillary damage, hypoxia and hemorrhage into various organs. Liver damage may cause jaundice (although hemolysis may also play a part), renal damage may cause renal failure, central nervous system damage meningitis and encephalitis, and skeletal muscle involvement muscle pain. Blood clotting parameters are often not disordered enough to account for the hemorrhagic tendency. Illnesses may be biphasic with initial symptoms caused by leptospiremia and later symptoms by host immune responses.

CLINICAL FEATURES

The incubation period is probably from a few days to just under 3 weeks.

The clinical manifestations range through asymptomatic infection to multisystem disease. With clinical disease there is usually an abrupt onset of fever with several possible accompaniments:

1. muscular pains;
2. marked constitutional upset and hemorrhagic manifestations;
3. nephritic features usually without associated hypertension;
4. jaundice with or without hemorrhages;
5. jaundice with leukocytosis or a raised erythrocyte sedimentation rate (leukocytosis and a raised sedimentation rate are unusual in viral hepatitis);
6. meningitis with injected or hemorrhagic conjuctivae, or a lymphocytic meningitis with normal biochemical parameters: this syndrome is typically associated with *L. canicola* infection;
7. persistent fever lasting up to 3 or 4 weeks, perhaps without other signs;
8. jaundice with nephritis – Weil's syndrome, usually caused by *L. icterohaemorrhagiae* infection in which renal failure is a common cause of death (in contrast most patients with viral hepatitis have a low or normal blood urea and present with gradual-onset malaise and fever which usually remits once jaundice is apparent).

DIAGNOSIS AND DIFFERENTIAL DIAGNOSIS

Blood cultures may be positive in early illness, but some *Leptospira* resist standard culture and the diagnosis has to be confirmed by dark ground microscopy or by serology. Usually reactive antibody becomes detectable after the first week of illness. Agglutination and complement-fixation tests are often used. If there is a meningitic clinical picture the CSF is usually lymphocytic; the CSF biochemistry is often normal and CSF culture may be positive. Urine culture or dark ground microscopy may be positive once infection is established, and may remain positive for several weeks.

The differential diagnosis is very wide: if a zoonosis is suspected, Q fever or brucellosis are major contenders.

TREATMENT

Eradication of non-commercial animals (such as rats) or reducing potential exposure to animal urine is ideal. *Leptospira* are sensitive to penicillin, tetracyclines (which are contraindicated in renal failure and which, depending on the severity of illness, are contraindicated in children) and erythromycin. Usually high doses are given for 10 days. Early treatment is essential as antibiotics will do little to alleviate the immune-mediated elements of the illness. Isolation of patients is unnecessary as person-to-person spread is unlikely. Despite serious dysfunction of infected organs in acute illness, recovery is usually complete in survivors.

BACTERIAL INFECTIONS: LYME DISEASE

Lyme disease is a seasonal non-occupational bacterial zoonosis which is distributed throughout the temperate zones of the world.[160] It was first recognized in 1975 because of a geographic clustering of children with arthritis in Lyme, Connecticut.[161] It is now recognized that the causative agent is an arthropod-borne spirochete called *Borrelia burgdorferi* which is transmitted by the hard tick *Ixodes daminii* or related ixodid ticks depending on the geographical distribution, e.g. *Ixodes ricinus* is predominant in Europe.[162] The tick which has a wide range of hosts (deer, cattle, sheep, mice, squirrels, dogs) appears to prefer the white-footed mouse and white-tailed deer. Birds are now also recognized as reservoirs.

The anatomical location of tick bites appears important. Patients bitten on the head and neck had significantly more neurological manifestations, perhaps explaining the higher frequency of neuroborreliosis among children compared with adults.[163]

The illness is a multisystem disorder, which consists of a prodromal febrile illness with the characteristic rash of erythema chronicum migrans (ECM) and associated symptoms. Without antibiotic treatment a substantial number of patients will go on to cardiac, neurological and rheumatological sequelae. However, progression from early to late stage is not inevitable, even in the absence of antibiotic treatment. 'Incomplete' cases with minimal or absent rash can occur, and patients may have aseptic meningitis, facial palsy, carditis or arthritis as the first sign of disease.

ETIOLOGY AND VECTOR

In 1982 a previously unrecognized spirochete was isolated from *I. daminii* ticks that had been collected from Shelter Island, New York. This discovery was followed in 1983 by the successful culture of the spirochete named *B. burgdorferi* from patients with Lyme disease.

The main vector species are *I. ricinus* in Europe and the *I. scapularis* group in North America.[164] The lifecycle of the tick consists of larval, nymphal and adult stages. The larvae and nymphs primarily feed on rodents such as the white-footed mouse, the natural reservoir for *I. daminii*. The adults usually feed on large mammals like deer, sheep and horses. Furthermore, the growth of the vector population is promoted by deer and fails to occur in their absence. The nymphal stage, whose peak questing period is May through July, is primarily responsible for transmission of disease. As these immature ticks feed aggressively on more animal species they facilitate rapid transmission of the organisms and often escape detection by the human host because they remain very small, even after a feed.

EPIDEMIOLOGY

Lyme disease is the most common vector-borne disease among children with more cases in children than in adults. However, there is substantial regional variation in the incidence of Lyme disease although most cases appear to occur during the summer months. The estimated incidence in the USA in 1992 was 3.9 per 100 000 population with Connecticut having the highest incidence (53.6/100 000). These figures are undoubtedly underestimates as only a small proportion of cases are reported. In the UK, for example, the incidence of Lyme disease is not well documented although experience suggests that serious disease is not common. Children between the ages of 5 and 10 years appear to be at highest risk in endemic areas.

PATHOGENESIS

In early Lyme disease the spirochete is injected into the bloodstream or skin through tick saliva. It may also be deposited in fecal material on the skin, and from there the organism may invade the skin or blood. Following an incubation period of 3–32 days the organism migrates outwards in the skin to produce the classical immune-mediated lesion of ECM. It may also spread to the lymphatics or disseminate in the blood or organs such as the brain, heart or joints or to other sites to produce the secondary lesions of late-stage disease. The propensity to produce damage of a specific target organ appears to be determined by a number of factors including genospecies of *Borrelia* isolate as well as host factors such as human leukocyte antigen (HLA) phenotype. For example, *B. afzelli* is more common in patients with mainly dermatological manifestations, whereas *B. garinii* is more often associated with neurological complications. Furthermore, arthritis, which is a more common presentation of early or late Lyme disease in Europe as opposed to ECM in North America, is more commonly seen in patients with HLA-DR4 and -DR2.[165] There is also some evidence that patients with severe and prolonged illness, especially neurological or joint disease, have an increased frequency of the B cell alloantigen HLA-DR2.[166]

CLINICAL CHARACTERISTICS

Like other spirochetal infections the illness can occur in distinct stages which may overlap or occur alone without recalling earlier features.

EARLY MANIFESTATIONS[167]

Up to one-third of patients remember a tick bite which often leaves a non-specific small red macule or papule. About 1 week later this area expands to the pathognomonic warm, painless, erythematous, annular lesion called ECM which reaches a maximum diameter of 15 cm (larger areas up to 70 cm have been reported) and usually has a bright red outer border. In the largest community-based prospective study reported in children, 89% of those studied presented with a single or multiple lesions of ECM.[168]

This lesion, which resolves within 4 weeks without therapy, can occur at any site although the thigh, groin and axilla are particularly common. Concomitant signs and symptoms include high fever (particularly in children), malaise, regional lymphadenopathy, meningism, myalgia and migratory arthralgias. Most of the early clinical features are characteristically intermittent and fluctuating during a period of several weeks, before spontaneous resolution occurs. About 10% of patients have features suggestive of anicteric hepatitis. Cellulitis secondary to an infected insect bite is a common misdiagnosis.

Two uncommon skin lesions, acrodermatitis chronica atrophicans and lymphadenosis benigna cutis, which are rare both in children and in North America, are regarded as specific late skin manifestations in Lyme disease.[169]

LATE MANIFESTATIONS

These manifestations occur some weeks to months after the initial infection and the clinical features are dependent on the organ affected and the severity of damage.

In about 10–40% of patients, frank *neurological abnormalities* usually occur weeks to months after infection. The classical triad of early neurological disease includes a lymphocytic meningitis, cranial neuropathy, and radiculoneuritis. Neuroborreliosis in children most commonly presents as mild encephalopathy, lymphocytic meningitis and cranial neuropathy.[170] Radiculopathy, particularly in European children, and peripheral neuropathy both of which occur late in the disease are rare in children. Typically patients develop a fluctuating lymphocytic meningitis about 4 weeks after the onset of ECM often with superimposed cranial (especially facial) neuritis. Patients will have a CSF lymphocytic pleocytosis. Other less common neurological complications include ataxia, spastic paraparesis due to an acute myelitis, hemiparesis, optic neuritis, hydrocephalus, Guillain–Barré syndrome and a pseudotumor cerebri-like syndrome.

Cardiac disease, which is relatively uncommon in children, occurs roughly 5 weeks after the tick bite. The disease spectrum includes myopericarditis, cardiomegaly, left ventricular dysfunction and especially fluctuating degrees of atrioventricular block, which may progress to complete heart block. The latter may require temporary pacing. The duration of cardiac involvement is usually brief (3 days to 6 weeks) and self-limiting. The clinical features show similarities to rheumatic fever although valvular involvement has not been reported.

Arthritis is a common late sequela of Lyme disease occurring in up to 60% of patients within a few weeks to 2 years after the onset of illness. 20–40% of patients do not remember having ECM. The spectrum of Lyme arthritis ranges from subjective joint pains which are often migratory, to intermittent attacks of arthritis to chronic erosive disease (10%).[171] The commonest pattern of joint involvement is an acute asymmetric mono- or oligoarticular arthritis primarily affecting the large joints. Most commonly (> 90%) involved is the knee joint and the child typically presents with subacute effusion of the knee. The attacks of arthritis typically last for a few weeks to months and recur intermittently over several years. Fatigue is the commonest associated non-articular symptom, whereas fever or other systemic symptoms are unusual.

Numerous other rare manifestations have been associated with Lyme disease. These include ophthalmic complications (conjunctivitis, episcleritis, photophobia, uveitis), hepatitis, hepatosplenomegaly and testicular swelling. There is no clear evidence that *B. burgdorferi* causes congenital disease, although the existence of this rare syndrome cannot be ruled out.[172] Furthermore, transmission of Lyme disease in breast milk has not been documented.

DIAGNOSIS

The diagnosis is not always easy, given that symptoms may be non-specific, and serology may be misleading.[173] The hallmark for confirming the diagnosis is to obtain appropriate fluid or tissue for culture. Such tests are unlikely to be of value in everyday clinical practice and future diagnostic tests such as polymerase chain reaction (PCR) have not yet been adequately tested. Therefore, the diagnostic tests used most frequently are serological, and detect antibodies against *B. burgdorferi*. The most commonly used of these tests, which is now widely available as prepacked commercial kit, is the enzyme linked immunosorbent assay (ELISA). Unfortunately, this test yields many false positive reactions with other spirochetal infections, connective tissue diseases and certain viral infections.[172] There is also crossreactivity with antigens of spirochetes belonging to the normal flora. The immunoblotting technique currently offers the best means of validating a positive or equivocal ELISA in a patient with a low likelihood of Lyme, although this test is not widely available and its proper interpretation is as yet unclear.[174]

Currently the diagnosis of early Lyme disease, especially in the presence of skin lesions, is made on clinical and epidemiological grounds since serology (*B. burgdorferi* IgM) does not usually become positive until 3–6 weeks after the onset of the erythema migrans. Also, the antibody response may be aborted in patients with early Lyme who are treated promptly with an effective antimicrobial agent. The specific IgG antibody rises slowly and may not reach a level of diagnostic significance in early disease. It usually peaks months or years later, often when arthritis is present, and can persist for many years despite adequate treatment or cure. Furthermore, a substantial proportion of people who become infected by *B. burgdorferi* never have a clinical illness but have positive serology. Serological testing is not necessary for diagnosing typical ECM but is helpful in untreated atypical skin lesions, patients with acute meningitis, neuropathies and arthritis due to Lyme. The negative and positive predictive values of currently available serological tests are very much dependent on the pretest likelihood that a patient has Lyme disease. For example, a patient with ECM who lives in an endemic area has a very high probability of having Lyme even if the serological test is negative. Conversely, a patient with vague non-specific symptoms with a positive test is unlikely to have Lyme despite positive serology. Therefore, serological tests should not be used on patients with non-specific symptoms but clinicians should order serological tests for Lyme disease in selected groups such as those with clinical findings suggestive of Lyme or in highly prevalent areas so that the predictive value of the test is high.[172]

Notably the predictive value of positive serology in patients with erythema chronicum migrans as a single manifestation of Lyme disease is low.[175]

Patients reported to have Lyme disease who did not meet the United States Centers for Disease Control and Prevention (CDC) case definitions had increased symptoms and worsening quality of life indices, the implication being that such patients did not have Lyme disease.[176] A consensus paper noted that the risks of intravenous antibiotics in patients with non-specific complaints outweighed potential benefits.[177]

The differential diagnosis is wide but includes other tick borne diseases including ehrlichiosis and babesiosis.

TREATMENT

Since no clinical trials of treatment have been performed in children the recommendations for treatment have been extrapolated from adult studies (Table 26.23).[178,179] Lyme disease if treated early will respond well to antibiotic therapy, shortening the duration of illness and reducing the incidence of complications. The long term prognosis for this group as well as those treated for late Lyme disease is excellent.

PREVENTION

Acquisition of Lyme borreliosis can be reduced by simple practical methods such as wearing long trousers, tucking trousers into socks, wearing boots, promptly removing any attached ticks and impregnating clothes with DEET or permethrin. A vaccine is currently under development.

BACTERIAL INFECTIONS: MENINGOCOCCEMIA

Despite the recent introduction of an effective vaccine against group C organisms in the UK, *Neisseria meningitidis* is still the most frequent cause of septicemia in childhood, and affects otherwise healthy children of all ages after the neonatal period. In the UK, there are 2000–3000 microbiologically confirmed cases a year [180] with a further 2000 cases diagnosed on clinical grounds alone. In the last decade wider public awareness, better diagnosis and intensive care have improved the outcome, but mortality is still around 10%.

Table 26.23 The antibiotic therapy of Lyme disease

Skin	
Children > 8 years:	Tetracycline 40–50 mg/kg per day (max. 1 g) in divided doses p.o. for 10-30 days*
Children < 8 years:	Phenoxymethyl penicillin 50 mg/kg per day in divided doses p.o. for 10 days; or erythromycin 30 mg/kg per day p.o. for 10–30 days for penicillin-allergic children
Neurological	
Cefotaxime 100–200 mg/kg daily i.v. or i.m. for 14 days; or ceftriaxone 20–80 mg/kg daily†	
Benzylpenicillin 300 mg/kg i.v. by continuous infusion or 6 divided doses daily for 14 days is now considered to be second line therapy	
Cardiac	
First degree atrioventricular block – oral regimens, as for skin infection	
High degree atrioventricular block – benzylpenicillin G 300 mg/kg i.v., 6 divided doses daily for 14 days	
Joint	
Benzyl penicillin 300 mg/kg per day i.v. in divided doses for 14 days	
Benzathine penicillin intramuscularly or ceftriaxone may also be used.	
Aspirin or a non-steroidal anti-inflammatory drug may be added	

* Tetracyline is a drug of choice except in children < 8 years, because it is more effective than penicillin or erythromycin in preventing late sequelae (Steere et al 1983[178]).

† Cefotaxime or ceftriaxone have been found to be superior to penicillin in treating neurological complications, especially those that have failed to respond to penicillin (Pal et al 1988[179]).

N. meningitidis is a Gram negative diplococcus, which is surrounded by an outer polysaccharide capsule, an outer membrane and an underlying peptidoglycan layer. Pili or fimbriae extend through the capsule and are thought to play a role in the attachment to epithelial cells within the nasopharynx. Between 2 and 5% of the general population are colonized, but carriage rates may be much higher in outbreaks. The precise relationship between carriage and invasive disease remains unclear. Spread is predominantly by respiratory droplets from close contacts.

In Western Europe, the Group B organism is still the most commonly isolated strain but is closely followed by Group C organisms. In the UK, the introduction of a Group C conjugate vaccine has reduced the rate of Group C infections in the younger age group. Group A organisms have been responsible for large epidemics particularly in sub-Saharan Africa, and another serogroup, W135, has recently caused a number of infections in pilgrims returning from the Hajj.

In spite of high colonization rates, only a relatively small number of colonized individuals develop invasive disease. Progression from nasal carriage to bacteremia is thought to be influenced by both bacterial and host factors. Certain bacterial properties, such as the presence of a capsule, pili and lipopolysaccharide (LPS) structure are known to be associated with invasive disease. There are also some data to indicate that smoking, respiratory tract infections and mucosal injury may aid colonization. However, the most important host factor predisposing individuals to this infection is the presence of defects within the complement cascade. Deficiencies of terminal complement components C5–C9, properdin and mannose-binding lectin all lead to an increased incidence of disease, and sometimes recurrent disease.

Having gained access to the circulation, bacterial components including LPS cause a host inflammatory response with the release of proinflammatory mediators such as tumor necrosis factor, interleukin 1, interleukin 6 and 8. These cytokines influence a number of cellular and non-cellular functions including neutrophil, monocyte and endothelial cell activation, thrombotic and hemostatic pathway imbalance and complement activation. In addition, the organism can bind to vascular endothelial cells inducing adhesion molecule expression, with consequent leukocyte attachment and migration. Uninterrupted, this intense inflammatory process leads to tissue injury and ultimately to multiple organ failure and death.[181]

CLINICAL FINDINGS

There are two major clinical presentations of meningococcal disease: meningitis and septicemia. A proportion of patients will have evidence of sepsis and meningitis. Once in the bloodstream, however, *N. meningitidis* can localize to other sites including joints, bones, eyes, and heart. Most deaths occur in the predominantly septicemic form of the disease. The presence of meningitis is a good prognostic indicator, and may indicate that host defenses have contained the infection long enough for the bacteria to invade the blood–brain barrier. Sepsis commonly presents with non-specific symptoms of fever, vomiting, abdominal pain and muscle aches. These patients may also have a characteristic rash, which can occur anywhere and may be purpuric or morbilliform (Plate 26.17). The extent of the inflammatory response will influence other signs of sepsis or septic shock. In the early stages, fever, tachycardia and tachypnea may be present with the rash. Later signs of shock develop with poor peripheral perfusion, hypotension and oliguria. These are generally accompanied by an extensive purpuric rash and evidence of disseminated intravascular coagulopathy (DIC) (Plate 26.16). Recent evidence indicates that polymorphisms within the cytokine and hemostatic/thrombotic pathways can influence the severity of this disease. Hemorrhage into internal organs may occur. Classically this involves the adrenal glands in the Waterhouse–Friderichsen syndrome. In those who recover, skin necrosis or vascular occlusion may cause the loss of an extremity, though most small lesions heal with minimal scarring.

The predominantly meningitic form of the disease presents with symptoms and signs of meningitis with fever, vomiting, headache and neck stiffness. Patients with meningitis may develop convulsions, focal neurological signs, a depressed level of consciousness, coma and death due to raised intracranial pressure. As the organism gains access to the central nervous system (CNS) from the blood, the petechial rash may be present and helpful in the diagnosis.

Arthritis, pericarditis and pleural effusions may occur as autoimmune phenomena 5–10 days after the acute infection. This is due to immune complex formation and is self-limiting, but a large pericardial effusion may cause cardiac tamponade. A rare chronic form of meningococcal sepsis can occur and is characterized by anorexia, weight loss, fever, arthralgia or arthritis and skin rash. Erythema nodosum or bacterial endocarditis may occur.

In the differential diagnosis, other bacterial and viral infections, which cause purpura, must be considered. Anaphylactoid purpura and idiopathic thrombocytopenic purpura may cause similar purpuric rashes. A morbilliform rash may be confused with a drug eruption or a number of viral infections including measles. Subacute or chronic meningococcemia presents a greater challenge. The differential diagnosis must include the many causes of arthritis and fever in children. However, a petechial rash should be considered as diagnostic of meningococcal disease until proved otherwise.

LABORATORY INVESTIGATION

The diagnosis is established by recovery of *N. meningitidis* from the blood, petechial lesions or the CSF, but lumbar puncture is contraindicated in the presence of shock, coagulopathy, reduced conscious level or focal neurological signs. The practice of giving penicillin before hospital admission, to patients in whom meningococcal infection is suspected, which has saved lives, has also decreased successful culture of the organism. In these situations, meningococcal DNA may still be detected by polymerase chain reaction (PCR) in blood and CSF. Serology may confirm the clinical diagnosis retrospectively. The complete blood count may show a polymorphonuclear leukocytosis. Neutropenia is invariably present in severe disease, however, and indicates a poor prognosis (see below). There is usually also evidence of DIC with thrombocytopenia, a coagulopathy and intravascular fibrin and thrombosis within dermal vessels. The importance of platelets and neutrophils in this disease is highlighted in a number of studies, which show that reduced circulating numbers of both cell types is correlated with a worse outcome.

TREATMENT

The most important aspect of meningococcal disease management is recognition. As with other forms of bacterial sepsis, bacterial load is critical, with higher bacterial concentrations leading to a more severe inflammatory response and organ dysfunction. In patients with little capacity to limit bacterial growth within blood, a single bacterium may proliferate to more than a million organisms in under 8 h. Most deaths occur in patients with a bacterial load of more than a million organisms/ml. Early intervention with antibiotics will rapidly arrest bacterial growth and reduce levels of circulating LPS and other bacterial components. A third generation cephalosporin, such as cefotaxime or ceftriaxone, has become the standard therapy for the initial treatment of suspected meningococcal disease. Once the organism is isolated and sensitivity determined, penicillin can be used in the majority of cases. It is recommended that family doctors who see a patient with suspected meningococcal infection in the home give a dose of intramuscular penicillin immediately.

In shocked children, vigorous resuscitation is required. Volume expansion with plasma and/or 4.5% albumin (20 ml/kg and repeat as required) is the crucial first step. Emergency transfer to the regional intensive care unit is usually advisable as inotropic and vasopressor agents, artificial ventilation and hematological support are frequently required (see section on sepsis). In very severe disease, extracorporeal membrane oxygenation may be life saving.

New therapies, which alter the immune response or inflammatory cascade, are under investigation at present, but no such agents have been shown to be effective to date. However, as in other forms of sepsis (see section on sepsis), endotoxin and inflammatory modulation, activated protein C administration and endocrine manipulation may prove beneficial in the future.

PROPHYLAXIS

Prophylaxis against invasive disease should be given to the family and close contacts of the patient. Rifampicin, given in four doses over 2 days, has been shown to be effective in clearing the organism. A single injection of ceftriaxone, or an oral dose of ciprofloxacin, are appropriate alternatives.

In the UK, a conjugate meningococcal C vaccine has now been introduced with promising evidence of a decline in this organism in vaccinated individuals. Polysaccharide vaccines are available for *N. meningitidis* Groups A, C, Y and W135 for patients traveling to endemic areas. Trials continue on vaccines against *N. meningitidis* Group B.

PROGNOSIS

The mortality from acute meningococcemia remains high at around 10%, most deaths occurring in patients with very high bacterial loads. Survivors may suffer extensive tissue injury, sometimes requiring amputation and/or skin grafting. A number of prognostic scores have been developed, the most frequently quoted being the Glasgow meningococcal septicemia prognostic score. This is predominantly based upon clinical parameters such as blood pressure and coma, but as supportive care has improved, this score no longer accurately identifies patients at greatest risk of mortality. Other scores have now been developed which revolve around hematological parameters, and a simple score based on the product of the initial platelet and neutrophil count has been shown to be a better prognostic guide to mortality. This score may help to identify those patients at whom novel therapeutic agents should be targeted.[182]

BACTERIAL INFECTIONS: PERTUSSIS (WHOOPING COUGH)

Although theoretically vaccine-preventable, pertussis continues to be a significant health problem throughout the world. There are a number of reasons for this including:

- Immunization rates are low in some countries.
- The vaccine is not 100% effective and the immunity is transient.
- Because of potential adverse effects in older children and adults, the vaccine is not generally given to boost immunity.
- Because of the transient nature of the immunity many adults are non-immune and are now the major source of infection, particularly to prevaccinated or incompletely vaccinated infants.
- Because of perceived major adverse events from this vaccine, many parents and medical practitioners are wary about giving this vaccine. Further, they will often give an incomplete course of pertussis vaccination if there has been any (even minor) adverse events from earlier vaccinations.
- Infants are born with no passive immunity to pertussis. The non-immune status of neonates means they are highly vulnerable to this disease until vaccination is complete (generally at 6 months). Unfortunately, this is also the age group where the disease is most deadly.

PATHOGENESIS

Pertussis is a bacterial infection due to a Gram negative coccobacillus, *Bordetella pertussis*. Although this organism is sensitive to antibiotics (particularly macrolides), if the disease is already established, then antibiotics have little or no effect on the clinical course of the illness, except to render that patient non-infectious to others. This is an important public health issue and therefore it is crucial to diagnose index patients and to prescribe antibiotics to prevent further spread.

It is particularly crucial to diagnose pertussis *before* the development of the paroxysmal coughing phase, as antibiotics in this stage of the illness can substantially reduce the severity of the clinical illness. Although recognition in the preparoxysmal phase is difficult, diagnosis of index cases and treatment of any household contacts with any respiratory symptoms (particularly young children) with the appropriate antibiotics is warranted. Indeed, in a young unimmunized infant (less than 6 months), contact with a known pertussis case is absolute justification for immediate antibiotic treatment.

SPREAD

Droplet or aerosol spread is usual, and indirect spread (such as via fomites) is unlikely. The disease is highly infectious and over 80% of unvaccinated household contacts of a known case will develop the clinical illness.

CLINICAL FEATURES

There are several distinct phases of this illness (see Fig. 26.23). There is an initial early coryzal phase with upper respiratory tract symptoms and a dry, irritating cough. This phase lasts for up to 1 week and is abruptly followed by the paroxysmal phase. During the early paroxysmal phase, there are violent spasms of uncontrollable cough with facial flushing. These spasms persist for several minutes and are classically followed by an inspiratory whoop. Infants often vomit and may develop cyanosis with the cough, and a whoop may be absent in this age group. This phase of the illness can persist for up to 3 months.

Between the coughing spasms these children are strikingly well. Thus, pertussis is generally diagnosed on the basis of the history, unless a spasm has been observed. The number of spasms per 24 h is highly variable and generally peaks within the first 2–3 weeks of the illness before there is a very gradual reduction in the frequency and severity of the spasms.

In adolescents and adults the disease is highly modified, presumably reflecting their partial immune status. Thus, any adult with a troublesome cough, which has persisted for several weeks, should be suspected of having whooping cough. Epidemiological studies have repeatedly shown that adults are the major reservoir of

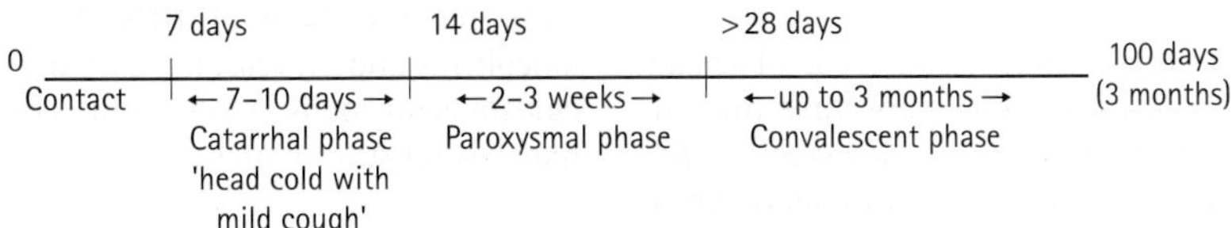

Fig. 26.23 Natural history of pertussis.

B. pertussis infection, particularly of young unvaccinated or incompletely vaccinated infants.

CASE DEFINITION

The current World Health Organization case definition is as follows: *B. pertussis infection* should be suspected if there is severe cough for greater than or equal to *2 weeks* (i.e. 'probable' pertussis). If *one* of the following are present *in addition* to the above, the child should be notified and treated:

- prolonged cough followed by apnea or cyanosis, and in the older child paroxysm followed by vomiting, inspiratory whoop or the presence of subconjunctival hemorrhages;
- exposure to suspected case in the previous 3 weeks;
- epidemic whooping cough in the area;
- a lymphocytosis of greater than or equal to 15 000/mm^3.

Cases can be confirmed by laboratory evidence of *B. pertussis* on culture, polymerase chain reaction or immunofluorescent antibody studies. Unfortunately, although culture has high specificity, its sensitivity is poor and false negatives are common.

EPIDEMIOLOGY

The disease is endemic in most developed countries despite widespread immunization programs. In addition to the endemic cases, there are frequent epidemic peaks, which classically occur every 2–5 years. The endemic nature of this disease presumably reflects the large reservoir of adults who develop a modified illness and infect infants and young children.

The true incidence of pertussis is difficult to determine because of the problems with accurate clinical diagnosis, the low sensitivity of positive microbiology, and uncertainty concerning serological testing methods. As well as underdiagnosis, there is almost certainly under-reporting of the condition in developed countries.

MORTALITY/MORBIDITY

The burden of disease reported by the World Health Organization is between 200 000 and 300 000 deaths per annum worldwide, with estimates of 20 million–40 million infections per annum worldwide.

The quoted mortality in developed countries for this disease is approximately 0.3%, and is slightly higher in infants under the age of 6 months (0.5%). Major complications resulting in prolonged morbidity include hypoxic encephalopathy and subsequent brain damage. Most of the morbidity and virtually all of the mortality is in infants under 6 months of age.

VACCINATION

Until recently, the standard vaccine used was a whole cell pertussis vaccine, which unfortunately had a reputation for being both relatively ineffective and potentially harmful. As a consequence, vaccination rates for pertussis have fluctuated widely and most countries observed major increases in the rates of pertussis when vaccine uptake was reduced.

Because of the widespread perception of a poor risk:benefit ratio with pertussis vaccine, complete coverage with pertussis in children less than 5 years of age was observed to be less than 50% in surveys in the USA and UK in the early 1990s.

The introduction of acellular vaccine, with high-quality studies showing excellent effectiveness and low adverse event rates, has dramatically altered the situation.[183] Most developed countries have seen almost total replacement of the whole cell vaccine with the acellular vaccine, with an anticipated increased coverage of complete vaccination in young children. However, to eradicate *B. pertussis* infection will require repeated booster vaccinations in adolescents and adults. The introduction of the acellular vaccine, which can be safely given to adolescents and adults, means eradication is now a real prospect.

VACCINE EFFICACY

The published data on vaccine effectiveness have been quite variable. For the whole cell vaccine this varied from approximately 35 to 98%. It was, nevertheless, clear that the whole cell vaccine did offer protection against the more severe disease, but did not confer long term immunity. Recent studies show that the efficacy of the acellular vaccine has ranged from 85 to 90%, with a much lower incidence of adverse events.

TREATMENT

In the paroxysmal phase, antibiotics are indicated to prevent the spread of infection. However antibiotics have little or no impact on the child's coughing illness. The usual antibiotic is erythromycin (or other macrolide) for 7–10 days.

In young infants, with severe and frequent spasms, admission to hospital and close observation is essential. Treatment revolves around experienced, high quality nursing care and includes avoidance of provoking spasms; close observation and treatment of spasms (with oxygen if necessary); minimal handling; and for uncontrollable spasms – endotracheal intubation and mechanical ventilation. Surprisingly, once the children are intubated the spasms of coughing completely subside and following extubation there is generally a rapid resolution of the coughing illness.

BACTERIAL INFECTIONS: YERSINIOSIS AND PLAGUE

YERSINIOSIS[184,185]

Yersiniosis is caused by two species of enteric bacteria, *Yersinia enterocolitica* and *Yersinia pseudotuberculosis*. A wide spectrum of clinical manifestations occurs, including acute watery diarrhea, mesenteric adenitis, extraintestinal infection and bacteremia. Postinfectious sequelae such as arthritis or erythema nodosum are also common.

MICROBIOLOGY AND PATHOGENESIS

Yersinia spp. are facultative anaerobic Gram negative coccobacillae which grow well on bile-containing media. There are three human pathogens within the genus, *Y. pseudotuberculosis*, *Y. enterocolitica* and *Yersinia pestis*. Over 50 serogroups of *Y. enterocolitica* have been described. *Yersinia* infections occur through invasion of the gastrointestinal tract via a membrane protein, invasin, which binds to a cell surface ligand. Multiplication may occur within intestinal epithelial cells and Peyer's patches, with the potential for systemic spread.

EPIDEMIOLOGY

Y. enterocolitica infection occurs globally but is most common in temperate regions. Yersiniosis is a zoonotic infection but usually causes food borne illnesses. The organism may be found in the gastrointestinal tract of a number of domestic and livestock animals. Infection of humans usually occurs after eating or drinking contaminated food or water; incompletely cooked pork is a major risk factor. Infection may also occur by person-to-person or direct animal-to-person contact. Most infections are sporadic but a number of specific outbreaks due to contaminated food or water have occurred. Infants and young children are more susceptible to infection with *Y. enterocolitica* than adults.

Infection with *Y. pseudotuberculosis* is less common, apart from in Japan. Infection results from contact with both sylvatic and domestic animals and a number of birds. It usually affects patients aged between 5 and 20 years.

CLINICAL FEATURES[186]

The incubation period for acute yersiniosis is 3–7 days. *Y. enterocolitica* infection most commonly presents as acute gastroenteritis in young children with diarrhea, fever, and abdominal pain, clinically indistinguishable from *Salmonella* or *Campylobacter* infection. Stools contain mucus, leukocytes and red blood cells. Patients may be symptomatic for up to 3 weeks and remain infectious over this period, due to shedding of organisms in the feces. Rare complications include diffuse ulceration of the small intestine and colon, perforation, intussusception and toxic megacolon.

Y. enterocolitica infection in older children most commonly causes mesenteric adenitis and terminal ileitis; this is also the most common manifestation of *Y. pseudotuberculosis* infection. The presentation mimics appendicitis. Diarrhea is unusual and the infection is usually self limiting. Ultrasound and/or CT may help by demonstrating a normal appendix and enlarged mesenteric nodes. The differential diagnosis includes acute appendicitis, or terminal ileal disease such as Crohn's or tuberculosis.

Y. enterocolitica bacteremia is rare and usually occurs in patients with other chronic medical conditions or immunosuppression. There is also a strong association with iron overload syndromes. Case fatality rates for *Y. enterocolitica* bacteremia range from 7.5 to 25%, but may reach 50% in patients with iron overload. Focal *Y. enterocolitica* infection can occur as a complication of bacteremia or occasionally in the absence of detectable bacteremia. *Y. pseudotuberculosis* bacteremia is much less common, but is also associated with chronic illness. Case fatality rates are extremely high in the immunocompromised population. In Japan, *Y. pseudotuberculosis* infection has been associated with renal failure in young children.

Secondary, immunologically mediated, postinfective complications may occur in up to 30% of patients following *Yersinia* infection. A reactive asymmetrical large joint polyarthropathy or erythema nodosum are the most common manifestations, occurring 1–2 weeks after the acute presentation. There is a strong association with the possession of HLA B27. Reiter's syndrome, glomerulonephritis and myocarditis have also been described. Synovial fluid culture is normally sterile. Joint symptoms of reactive polyarthritis may last for several months.

DIAGNOSIS

Definitive diagnosis of yersiniosis is by culture of the organism from stool, lymph nodes or blood. Isolation from stool may be optimized by using cold enrichment or cefsulodin-irgasan-novobiocin (CIN) agar. High titers of *Yersinia* antibodies in a previously healthy individual are suggestive of infection but fourfold rises in titer are rarely found. Interpretation of serology is also complicated by low titers following yersiniosis in infants or immunocompromised patients, a high background prevalence of positive serology in some populations and crossreactivity with *Brucella, Rickettsia* and *Salmonella* spp. Cultures are often negative by the time of appearance of postinfective symptoms.

Y. pseudotuberculosis may be found in sterile site samples, but is rarely isolated from stool. Serology is often the only mode of diagnosis available; antigens crossreact with those of *Y. enterocolitica*.

TREATMENT

Antimicrobial treatment does not shorten the course or severity of enterocolitis and is not indicated in uncomplicated cases. Localized infection, systemic disease, or enterocolitis in an immunocompromised patient should be treated. *Y. enterocolitica* is resistant to most penicillins and first generation cephalosporins; amoxicillin/clavulanate combinations are also unsuitable due to variable minimum inhibitory concentrations. Aminoglycosides, chloramphenicol, tetracycline, co-trimoxazole and fluoroquinolones have been most effective in clinical practice; third generation cephalosporins may also be effective. *Y. pseudotuberculosis* is sensitive to ampicillin and cephalosporins in addition to the drugs already discussed.

PLAGUE[187,188]

EPIDEMIOLOGY AND PATHOGENESIS

Plague is a zoonosis caused by *Y. pestis*. It occurs globally; over 4000 cases of plague were reported in 1997. Over 90% of cases currently occur in Africa, with epidemics in Madagascar and Tanzania; major active foci also exist in other parts of Africa, the Western USA, China and south-east Asia. Mammals, particularly rodents, act as host reservoirs. Fleas feed upon diseased hosts and organisms multiply within the midgut of the flea before being transmitted to humans or other mammals when the flea bites and regurgitates a blood meal. Human infection can also be acquired from direct contact with wild rodents or their predators (including cats) and person-to-person spread can occasionally occur in epidemics. Most human plague cases currently occur in rural settings with transmission from wild animals; epidemics in human settlements occur when domestic rat species become infected.

CLINICAL FEATURES

There are three main clinical forms of plague. *Bubonic* plague is most common. Bacteria multiply in regional lymph nodes following a flea bite, culminating 2–8 days later in systemic symptoms, fever, headache and malaise. Regional lymph nodes enlarge and become extremely tender with swelling and inflammation around the nodes: the bubo. Occasionally, pustules, eschars or papules occur at the site of flea bites. Most individuals develop a transient secondary bacteremia: in some this leads to septicemic or pneumonic plague.

Patients with *septicemic* plague present with Gram negative septicemic shock and may develop complications such as renal failure or disseminated intravascular coagulation (DIC). Septicemic plague occasionally occurs in the absence of buboes; this presentation is more common in children.

Pneumonic plague is usually a complication of bacteremia and presents with cough, fever and hemoptysis: the chest X-ray may show bronchopneumonia, consolidation or cavitation. Large numbers of bacteria may be exhaled with the potential for respiratory spread to cause primary pneumonic plague.

DIAGNOSIS

The patient's symptoms and an appropriate exposure history may lead to a clinical diagnosis of plague. Neutrophil counts are usually elevated and liver function tests may be abnormal. *Y. pestis* may be demonstrated on smears from blood, bubo fluid or CSF: fluorescent antibody techniques increase the sensitivity. Definitive diagnosis depends upon culture of the organism, which grows readily on standard media. Serological tests are useful in retrospective diagnosis of plague.

TREATMENT

Case fatality rates may reach 30–50% in untreated plague. Streptomycin (or gentamicin) is the traditional drug of choice; chloramphenicol and doxycycline have also been used successfully. Therapy is required for 10 days to prevent relapse; clinical improvement normally occurs within 3 days. Theoretically, fluoroquinolones may be useful to treat the rare strains with high level multidrug resistance, although clinical experience is limited.

PREVENTION

Plague vaccines are only usually administered to individuals at high risk in laboratories or field control teams: their efficacy against pneumonic plague is limited and frequent boosting is necessary. Public education, reducing flea bites and rodent exposure and avoidance of sick or dead animals are all measures that can help avoid infection.

BACTERIAL INFECTIONS: *PNEUMOCOCCUS*

Pneumococcus (*Streptococcus pneumoniae*) is a common cause of serious disease in children, particularly otitis media, pneumonia and meningitis. It is also a frequent cause of occult bacteremia.[189] *S. pneumoniae* are Gram positive oval cocci, and cause beta hemolysis (a green zone around the colony) on blood agar, and occur in pairs (diplococci) or short chains. Pneumococci can be characterized serologically by the capsular polysaccharides or by molecular biological techniques. A total of 84 pneumococcal serotypes have been characterized, but fewer than 10 are responsible for the great majority of infections in childhood.

EPIDEMIOLOGY

The pathogenicity of the pneumococcus is low and it may be recovered from the upper respiratory tract of up to 70% of healthy subjects. Pneumococcal disease is probably spread mainly by healthy carriers, but patient-to-patient and patient-to-doctor transfer has been documented. Children under 2 years have the highest rate of carriage, but why some infants develop disease whereas others remain unaffected is unknown. In developing countries, a high proportion of lower respiratory infection in young children is due to *S. pneumoniae*, and pneumococcal meningitis is associated with a high mortality (30–35%). Globally, *S. pneumoniae* is thought to cause over 1 million deaths in children under the age of 5 years.[190] The 'pneumonia season' in late winter and early spring has been attributed to indoor crowding with more opportunities for cross infection, but more probably it is due to damage to respiratory mucosal defenses from virus infections.

From the nasopharynx, pneumococci may reach the lungs or through impaired respiratory mucosa spread to the middle ear or meninges. Bacteremic spread to a variety of sites may occur, notably the joints.[191]

Antibiotics have reduced the severity and mortality of pneumococcal disease but have had little influence on disease incidence. The effect on morbidity has been disappointing. Infants with pneumococcal meningitis remain at considerable risk from neurological sequelae and the pneumococcus is more likely to cause permanent deafness than either the meningococcus or *Haemophilus influenzae*. Recurrent pneumococcal meningitis is occasionally seen when CSF leakage complicates skull fracture. Children with an absent or non-functioning spleen and children with impaired antibody production are at particular risk of serious pneumococcal infection.

DIAGNOSIS

In pneumococcal pneumonia there is usually tachypnea with grunting, inspiratory retractions, nasal flaring and cyanosis, but physical examination of the chest may be unhelpful and the radiological changes surprisingly few in the early stages of illness. Blood, CSF and urine cultures may be helpful in diagnosing pneumococcal disease particularly in preschool children. In bacteremic disease, the white blood cell count is often elevated to over 20×10^9/L. Recovery of the pneumococcus from the upper respiratory tract is unhelpful because of the frequency of the carrier state. Rapid methods of pneumococcal capsular antigen detection (e.g. countercurrent immunoelectrophoresis, latex agglutination) in CSF, pleural fluid and serum may be useful for rapid diagnosis, especially in children who have received antibiotics prior to culture.

TREATMENT

A worrying trend is the increasing antimicrobial resistance among *S. pneumoniae* worldwide.[192] Penicillin resistance is due to altered penicillin-binding proteins, not to beta lactamase production. Susceptibility to penicillin (usually the drug of choice), cephalosporin and macrolide antimicrobials can no longer be assumed. Penicillin remains the drug of choice for infections with penicillin-sensitive organisms. Where there is a high incidence of penicillin resistance, penicillin has still been shown to be effective for infections with penicillin-insensitive organisms, provided the child does not have meningitis. South African children hospitalized with pneumococcal pneumonia and treated with a penicillin fared equally well whether they had penicillin-sensitive or resistant organisms.[193] This is because it is possible to achieve local drug levels that exceed the minimum inhibitory concentration (MIC) of even resistant organisms. It is not possible, however, to achieve adequate CSF levels, and pneumococcal meningitis due to resistant organisms cannot be treated with penicillin. Many, but not all penicillin-resistant pneumococcal strains are also resistant to third generation cephalosporins. In areas of the world with high rates of penicillin resistance, initial treatment for proven or suspected pneumococcal meningitis includes vancomycin, to which all strains are currently sensitive.[194] This is often combined with a third generation cephalosporin such as cefotaxime or ceftriaxone until sensitivities are available. If the organism is penicillin sensitive, then penicillin should be used.

PREVENTION

PNEUMOCOCCAL VACCINE

A safe and effective 23-valent polysaccharide vaccine has been available for years, but remains relatively little used, even where strongly recommended.[195] Unfortunately the antibody response is not so reliable in young children, those with immunological impairment and those on treatment with immunosuppressive therapy. Antibody response is particularly poor in children under 2 years of age so that its potential for preventing pneumococcal meningitis is limited. Polysaccharide vaccines do not stimulate T cells, so do not induce a boostable memory response.[196]

Conjugate vaccines, in which the capsular polysaccharides from the commonest strains are conjugated to proteins, have been developed. These vaccines are T cell dependent, and so are immunogenic in infancy, and induce memory, so that the immunological response is boostable.[196] A randomized controlled trial of a 7-valent conjugate pneumococcal vaccine, given from 2 months of age, showed 97.4% protection against invasive pneumococcal disease.[197] A conjugate pneumococcal vaccine has been licensed in the USA and Australia since 2001, and is recommended for all American infants and for Australian Aboriginal children, who have a high incidence of pneumococcal invasive disease. At the present time, in the UK, polysaccharide pneumococcal vaccine is recommended[198] for the following children aged 2 years or older in whom pneumococcal infection is likely to be more common and/or dangerous:

- asplenia or severe dysfunction of the spleen, e.g. homozygous sickle cell disease and celiac syndrome;
- chronic renal disease or nephrotic syndrome;
- immunodeficiency or immunosuppression from disease or treatment (including HIV infection;)
- chronic heart, lung or liver disease;
- diabetes mellitus.

Note: Where possible, the vaccine should be given 4–6 weeks (but at least 2 weeks) *before* splenectomy and *before* courses of chemotherapy, together with advice about the risk of pneumococcal infection. If this is not possible, as for splenectomy following trauma, the vaccine should be given as soon as possible after recovery and before discharge from hospital. If not given before chemotherapy and/or radiotherapy its use should be delayed for at least 6 months after completion of treatment.

CHEMOPROPHYLAXIS

An alternative for children with functional or anatomical asplenia, for those receiving immunosuppressive therapy, or for infants under 2 years, is to give them continuous antibiotic prophylaxis, e.g. phenoxymethyl penicillin.[199]

EDUCATION

Patients at risk (or their parents) need to be educated about the risks and the importance of seeking medical help at the onset of illness. A MedicAlert bracelet should be used. A patient card and information sheet for asplenic or hyposplenic patients is available from: Department of Health, PO Box 410, Wetherby LS23 7LL. Advice is also available from The Splenectomy Trust, Swinbrook Post Office, Swinbrook, Oxfordshire OX18 4EE.

BACTERIAL INFECTIONS: *PSEUDOMONAS*

PSEUDOMONAS AERUGINOSA

Pseudomonas aeruginosa is a common contaminant of moist areas such as sink traps, water taps and ventilator and incubator humidification systems.[200] For epidemiological purposes, genomic typing of isolates can be performed by various techniques including the use of rare cutting restriction enzymes followed by pulsed-field gel electrophoresis. *Ps. aeruginosa* classically infects wounds and burns, producing pyocyanin, a blue pigment which discolors pus. Best known to pediatricians as a cause of lung infection in cystic fibrosis, *Ps. aeruginosa* can infect virtually any part of the body; infection is particularly likely to occur in the presence of congenital or acquired immunodeficiency, prematurity, neutropenia or white cell dysfunction, malignant disease and its treatment, transplantation, prolonged instrumentation of body cavities (e.g. tracheostomy, ventricular drainage, bladder catheterization, venous catheterization, peritoneal dialysis) and following puncture wounds. Some of the more common infections are as follows.

SEPTICEMIA

An important cause of septicemia in oncology and neonatal units, *Ps. aeruginosa* is seldom suspected as the infecting agent in children with no previous medical disorders, and antipseudomonas activity is not usually included in antibiotic protocols to cover presumed sepsis in such children. Even when appropriate antibiotic therapy is given, it has a high mortality.

MENINGITIS

Seen mainly in premature babies and in patients with ventricular drainage catheters, meningitis calls for immediate intravenous therapy with a suitable antibiotic, guided by the results of antibiotic sensitivities and, ideally, by the activity of the patient's own postantibiotic serum against the isolate.

EAR INFECTION

Ps. aeruginosa is commonly cultured from chronically infected ears (otitis externa) and mastoids, particularly in regular swimmers (swimmers' ear). Occasionally an aggressive and painful infection is produced which is difficult to eradicate and may require surgery.

EYE INFECTIONS

Keratitis commonly follows trauma, especially from the use of contact lenses, but may also occur in association with immunosuppression and prematurity. The response to apparently appropriate systemic and topical antibiotic therapy is often disappointing and keratoplasty may be necessary. *Ps. aeruginosa* also causes orbital cellulitis.

URINARY TRACT INFECTION

Urinary tract infection usually follows long term catheterization, but also occurs when chronic infection has impaired local tissue viability. The organism is a common commensal under the prepuce, and this should be suspected as the source of unexpected *Pseudomonas* bacteriuria.

PERITONITIS

Peritonitis following appendicitis, intestinal perforation or peritoneal dialysis may be caused by *Ps. aeruginosa*; failure to appreciate this possibility may result in inappropriate choice of antibiotics.

PNEUMONIA

Pneumonia caused by *Ps. aeruginosa* is common in cystic fibrosis, but also occurs in the presence of the predisposing factors already mentioned and following prolonged treatment of other bronchopulmonary infections.

OSTEOMYELITIS

Pseudomonas infection should be considered in osteomyelitis which fails to respond to the usual antibiotic therapy directed against *Staphylococcus aureus*. It is not always possible to isolate the organism from blood cultures, and antibiotic therapy may have to be broadened blindly.

SKIN INFECTIONS

Folliculitis occurs especially in users of whirlpool ('spa') baths. Skin infections are also seen where the skin of the foot has become macerated from prolonged immersion or the wearing of rubber footwear. Ecthyma gangrenosum, a more aggressive skin infection usually arising in children with one of the predisposing factors already mentioned, produces necrotic ulcerative lesions involving particularly the anogenital and axillary areas, and can be rapidly fatal.[201]

MANAGEMENT OF *PS. AERUGINOSA* INFECTIONS

The choice of antibiotic therapy will depend mainly on the laboratory sensitivity of the isolate;[202] many strains are sensitive to broad spectrum penicillins such as ticarcillin, aminoglycosides such as gentamicin, and third generation cephalosporins such as ceftazidime, all of which must be given parentally. Recently developed quinolones such as ciprofloxacin can be given orally, but resistant strains emerge with disappointing rapidity.

BURKHOLDERIA (PSEUDOMONAS) CEPACIA COMPLEX

Pseudomonas cepacia, now classified as the *Burkholderia cepacia* complex, has emerged as an important pulmonary pathogen in patients with cystic fibrosis and in children with chronic granulomatous disease.[203] It has also been reported as a nosocomial infection in a wide variety of tissues, commonly in relation to contamination of sterile solutions including disinfectants. When contaminated solutions are used for skin cleaning prior to blood culture, an erroneous diagnosis of sepsis ('pseudosepticemia') may be made. It is however unwise to assume that members of the *B. cepacia* complex are invariably contaminants; they can be aggressive pathogens producing pneumonia, bacteremia, endocarditis, meningitis and urinary tract infection.

B. cepacia complex species are even more resistant to antibiotics than *Ps. aeruginosa* but may be sensitive to trimethoprim. Of the newer antibiotics, meropenem is the most active agent.

BURKHOLDERIA (PSEUDOMONAS) PSEUDOMALLEI

Burkholderia pseudomallei causes melioidosis, is spread mainly by contaminated monsoon waters and is endemic in tropical areas of south-east Asia and Australia. The illness may include pneumonia among its features, but may also present with multiple metastic abscesses and 'imitate' other infections. Melioidosis has a high mortality, and responds better to intravenous ceftazidime than to conventional therapy with tetracyclines and chloramphenicol.[204]

OTHER *PSEUDOMONAS* SPECIES

Numerous species of *Pseudomonas* (e.g. *Pseudomonas fluorescens* and *Pseudomonas putida*), some renamed (e.g. *Stenotrophomonas maltophilia* and *Ralstonia pickettii*), are recovered from time to time from clinical microbiology specimens, particularly from immunocompromised or otherwise vulnerable patients.

PREVENTION OF NOSOCOMIAL *PSEUDOMONAS* INFECTIONS

Environmental measures, in particular thoroughly drying (and preferably sterilizing) equipment after cleaning, and scrupulous attention to the manufacturer's instructions for the storage and use of antiseptic solutions are important in curtailing hospital epidemics. Every effort should be made to isolate (or not to admit) patients who are known to be carriers of *Pseudomonas* spp.

BACTERIAL INFECTIONS: RELAPSING FEVER

Relapsing fever is caused by blood spirochetes of the *Borrelia* species. It is characterized by relapses occurring a week or so after remission. The epidemic form is caused by *Borrelia recurrentis* and is transmitted by the body louse, *Pediculus humanus corporis*, i.e. louse-borne relapsing fever (LBRF). The endemic form, which has a worldwide distribution (except for Australasia and the Pacific region) is caused by a variety of borreliae in complex with soft-bodied ticks of the genus *Ornithodoros*.[205] Notable examples are *Borrelia duttoni*, harbored by *Ornithodoros moubata* ticks, which inhabit cracks and crevices of earth and mud floors and walls of huts in East and central Africa and *Borrelia hermsii* harbored by *Ornithodoros hermsi* in rodent-infested nests in old log cabins in coniferous forests of western USA and British Columbia.[206] *O. moubata* is an exception in that it is confined to feeding on man, whereas for all other ticks involved in transmission of tick-borne relapsing fever (TBRF), the hosts are mainly rodents and possibly bats, and man is only infected incidentally. Where housing remains poor, TBRF continues to be an important health problem especially for pregnant women and young children as in parts of Tanzania, Rwanda, Zambia and the Democratic Republic of Congo.[207,208] Because of the similarity between the clinical features of TBRF and malaria, TBRF is frequently missed unless specifically looked for in patients presenting with fever.

Epidemics of LBRF have been recognized for centuries associated with mass movements of people due to wars, famine and earthquakes. A pandemic affecting millions of people occurred associated with the First and Second World Wars; mortality rates of up to 50–70% were estimated for the period 1920–1930.[209] Ethiopia is recognized as being a high endemic focus with occasional spread to neighboring countries such as The Sudan.[210] Poor migrant laborers sleeping in overcrowded unhygienic conditions maintain the transmission. Outbreaks in children were described associated with soldiers returning from a war in northern Ethiopia.[211]

TRANSMISSION

In LBRF, the louse is infected by *B. recurrentis* when it feeds on infected human blood. Infected hemolymph, released when the louse is crushed through scratching, penetrates abraded or intact skin giving rise to infection. Lice move from one host to another associated with a rise in temperature, death or discarded clothing, thus spreading infection.

In TBRF, infection is maintained in rodents by a variety of *Ornithodoros* ticks, with the exception of *O. moubata* which feeds only on man. Man is the only reservoir for *B. duttoni*. There is transovarial infection of borreliae from one generation of ticks to the next. Ticks feed at night and borreliae are transmitted to the host through saliva or coxial fluid. Ticks may remain infected with borreliae for years without feeding.

IMMUNITY

Borreliae can change their antigenic structure, termed antigenic variation, when they are sequestered in internal organs during afebrile periods. Waves of new antibodies to the antigenically modified spirochete are produced during relapse. Crisis occurs at the height of immunological activity or when spirochetes are destroyed by antibiotics, as in the Jarisch–Herxheimer reaction (JHR). In endemic areas, children generally have more severe disease than adults (with the exception of pregnant women) and natives tend to have milder disease than outsiders, suggesting a degree of acquired immunity.

CLINICAL FEATURES

Clinical features vary both geographically, depending on the type of borreliae causing disease, and between LBRF and TBRF. Clinical features may differ between children under 5 years and older children and adolescents. Generally, LBRF is a more severe disease and JHR are more common than in TBRF.

The incubation period is around 7 days (range 4–18 days). Initial symptoms include shaking chills, rapidly rising temperature, headache, neck pain, convulsions and abdominal pain. The skin is hot and dry. There is hepatosplenomegaly with local tenderness and guarding. Cough and tachypnea are common, and signs of bronchopneumonia may be detected (*Borrelia* may be detected in sputum). Jaundice and a bleeding tendency may complicate severe cases. A transient macular or purpuric rash may be present. Ocular complications include conjunctival suffusion and hemorrhage, and iridocyclitis. Neck stiffness, clouding of consciousness and delirium are common. There may be focal central nervous system complications such as hemiplegia or cranial nerve palsies. In untreated patients, crises occur at a mean of 3–6 days or immediately following administration of antibiotics, i.e. the JHR. A rigor is followed by hypotension, sweating and fall of temperature. This is a dangerous period, particularly in sick patients who may have a myocarditis. Relapse occurs within 7–10 days or longer and is more frequent in TBRF; the number of relapses is about 1–2 for LBRF and 3 for TBRF,[205] severity decreases with each relapse. Mean mortality rates in children are better recorded for TBRF. In a report of an outbreak of LBRF in Ethiopian children in the early 1990s, case fatality was 2%.[211] In a prospective study of 95 children admitted with TBRF in Tanzania, case fatality was 8.8%. Risk of death was highest for children under 1 year and those with anemia and pneumonia.[208] Neurological sequelae occur in a small proportion and include hemiplegia and deafness.

Pregnant women with relapsing fever have a higher density of blood spirochetes than non-pregnant women and there is a high incidence of abortion, preterm delivery and increased risk of maternal death.[207,212] With the short incubation period it is difficult to distinguish between congenital and intrauterine infection. Perinatal infection is associated with a high mortality. Symptoms are similar to other bacterial septicemias, and jaundice and splenomegaly are prominent features.[213]

DIFFERENTIAL DIAGNOSIS

In a child with fever and hepatosplenomegaly, the differential diagnosis is wide and includes malaria, typhoid fever, yellow fever, leptospirosis, leishmaniasis and rickettsial infections.

LABORATORY INVESTIGATIONS

A thick blood film stained with aniline dyes such as Giemsa, Wright or Field detects borreliae in about 70% of cases on initial smears.[205] Spirochetes may be detected with phase contrast or darkfield microscopy. Serology has limited value, due to false positive reactions. Paired titers may provide a retrospective diagnosis. Proteus OXK agglutinin titers are usually elevated. The leukocyte count may be normal or increased; there may be transient leukopenia during the crisis. Thrombocytopenia is common. Erythrocyte sedimentation rate (ESR) is usually high. CSF may show leukocytes (mainly mononuclear cells), a raised protein and spirochetes may be detected, especially in neonates. Liver transaminases may be increased whether or not serum bilirubin is raised. Leukocytes, red blood cells, casts and protein are frequently detected in urine and sometimes borreliae.

MANAGEMENT

Relapsing fever may be treated with a wide variety of antibiotics including tetracycline, penicillin, chloramphenicol, erythromycin and probably cephalosporins. In LBRF, a single dose of tetracycline will clear blood of spirochetes in 2–3 h. Failure to eradicate borreliae, particularly from the brain, in TBRF may result in relapse. Choice of antibiotics depends on age of the child, risk of JHR (higher in LBRF) and suitability for routine use in developing countries. Duration of treatment for LBRF is 1–2 days and TBRF 5–10 days. Penicillin is considered to result in a milder JHR, but risk of relapse is higher than with tetracycline. To reduce JHR in LBRF an initial dose of fortified procaine benzylpenicillin (procaine penicillin) (30 000 units/kg) is followed by a dose of oral or parenteral tetracycline (50 mg/kg) 12 h later.[211] For children less than 8 years, erythromycin (60 mg/kg) or chloramphenicol (70–100 mg/kg) and for pregnant women, erythromycin are alternatives. Delousing of the body and clothes is essential.

For TBRF in North America, a 10 day course of oral erythromycin 60 mg/kg/day or for children over 8 years tetracycline (50 mg/kg/day) is appropriate. Penicillin G 10 000 units/kg infused over 30 min may be given as initial treatment.

In developing countries, a practical treatment of TBRF for children and pregnant women is daily injections of fortified procaine benzylpenicillin (procaine penicillin) given for 5 days.[208]

The relapse rate may be around 5%, but relapsed cases are usually mild and respond to chloramphenicol or erythromycin.

Bed rest for 1–2 days and close monitoring of temperature and blood pressure are important, especially in the first 12 h after commencement of antibiotics. Fever should be controlled with antipyretics and cooling. Oxygen is required for respiratory distress. For sick children, intravenous hydration and volume replacement in shock are essential parts of management.

PREVENTION

Prevention of LBRF involves delousing, hygienic measures and use of dichlorodiphenyltrichloroethane (DDT). Prevention of TBRF involves community education, including replastering of walls and floors of huts, and advice about sleeping on beds, as opposed to on the floor, or on beds made of mud. Bed nets impregnated with insecticide, as used in prevention of malaria, may reduce the infection rate.[214]

BACTERIAL INFECTIONS: SALMONELLAE

Salmonellae are motile, Gram negative, non-spore-forming organisms. They can survive long periods in water, sewage, dried foodstuffs or in carcasses, and can withstand freezing. Their increasing prevalence in domestic animal produce, especially poultry and bovines, and their ability to develop resistance to antibiotics is a major health problem.

There are over 2000 serotypes of salmonellae. They can be divided into the following two categories.

1. Those that cause *enteric fever*: *Salmonella typhi* which is pathogenic only to man; *Salmonella paratyphi A*, *Salmonella schottmuelleri* (*Salmonella paratyphi B*), *Salmonella hirschfeldii* (*Salmonella paratyphi C*) which are primarily but not exclusively pathogenic to man. The term enteric fever includes typhoid and paratyphoid fever.
2. Those that cause *Salmonella* enteritis or salmonellosis; these salmonellae are primarily infectious to animals and may infect man, e.g. *Salmonella typhimurium* and *Salmonella enteritidis*. The infections are confined mainly to the bowel but they may result in septicemia, an enteric fever-type illness or metastatic abscesses, particularly in young infants or old people and those who are immunocompromised. Invasive disease is particularly associated with *Salmonella cholerae-suis* and *Salmonella dublin. S. typhimurium* accounts for the majority of infections throughout the world.

Two principal antigens, in the cell wall (O) and the flagellae (H), are used in the typing of *Salmonella*. A capsular polysaccharide antigen Vi is present in *S. typhi* and *S. paratyphi C*. It can block agglutination reactions with the underlying O antigen and so protect the bacillus from antibody.

SALMONELLOSIS

Salmonellosis is caused by non-typhoidal salmonellae. There has been a particularly dramatic increase in outbreaks of salmonellosis in the UK since 1980, and up to 80% of reported cases of food poisoning are due to *Salmonella*. These are associated with infections contracted abroad and with infected food, e.g. poultry, bovine and pig produce and, to a lesser extent, milk and dairy produce. Intensive farming methods, especially of poultry, and the addition of antibiotics to feeds is a major cause. In the UK, many chickens and turkeys reaching retail shops are colonized by salmonellae. Pet reptiles are important household sources of infection.

Infection may occur from handling meat, directly or with utensils, or through improper cooking, especially when frozen meat has not been allowed to thaw fully. Infection, especially *S. enteritidis*, which produces clinical disease in chickens, may pass to eggs from the ovary or oviduct of infected chickens, or through the shell if care is not taken when separating eggs from feces. *Salmonella* in eggs may resist boiling for 2–3 min, especially if the eggs have been stored in a refrigerator. Egg produce made from raw or improperly cooked eggs may be infected, e.g. homemade mayonnaise, egg powder, milkshakes and ice cream.

Spread between humans occurs from symptomatic or asymptomatic carriers who infect food, or less often by direct contact. A relatively large dose of *Salmonella* is required to cause infection, and this usually results from bacterial multiplication in food. Intrafamilial spread and spread through institutions is common, and outbreaks at restaurants, parties and picnics are frequently reported. Breast-feeding protects infants against infection, but occasionally a fully breast-fed infant may be infected by the mother.

In developing countries, where intensive rearing of food animals is not common, infection by chronic carriers and water-borne salmonellosis in sewage are more likely methods of spread.

PATHOGENESIS

The sites of invasion by salmonellae are usually the ileum and/or the colon. The bacilli can penetrate the mucosa to the lamina propria of the ileum without producing obvious damage to cells and invoke a mainly neutrophil response (as opposed to *S. typhi* which produces a monocytic response). Infection of the ileum results in a watery diarrhea, secretory in nature. Less commonly, invasion of the colon may produce a dysentery-type illness.

Under certain conditions there may be bloodstream invasion, resulting in an enteric fever-type illness, septicemia, or localized foci of infection, such as meningitis, osteomyelitis, septic arthritis, pyelonephritis or endocarditis. Systemic infection is particularly likely in infants less than 1 year old, malnourished infants, immunocompromised children, and conditions such as hypochlorhydria, hemoglobinopathies, especially sickle cell disease, schistosomiasis and malignancy. A focal lesion, e.g. in bone, may manifest itself long after the enteritis has ceased.

In sickle cell disease, infarction of the gut may allow salmonellae access to the bloodstream, from where they may invade infarcted areas of bone resulting in osteomyelitis. Also, the impaired opsonization and phagocytic activity in sickle cell disease may permit proliferation of bacteria, which exacerbates the infection.

People with schistosomiasis may harbor salmonellae, within the worm or perhaps the granuloma, which protects them from the body's immune system. There may be prolonged or intermittent fever with joint pains and malaise. Glomerulonephritis and an associated nephrotic syndrome may occur and are usually reversible with adequate chemotherapy, presuming there is no established glomerular disease (as occurs in *Schistosoma mansoni* infection). In *Schistosoma haematobium* infections there may be chronic *S. typhi* urinary excretion. Treatment should include appropriate chemotherapy for schistosomiasis and *Salmonella*.

Occasionally a cyst or infarcted area of the kidney or other organ may become a focus for chronic *Salmonella* infection.

CLINICAL FEATURES

The incubation period of *Salmonella* enteritis is 12–48 h. Symptoms in essentially healthy individuals include nausea, vomiting, abdominal pains and diarrhea. In mild cases there may only be diarrhea. The diarrhea may be secretory in nature with frequent high volume, watery stools resulting in hypotonic dehydration. Alternatively, the presence of blood and mucus may indicate a colitis. In severe cases, toxic megacolon and perforation may occur.[215] Fever is common and occasionally there may be an enteric fever-type illness. A reactive arthritis may occur and is associated with HLA-B27 histocompatibility antigens. Symptoms usually settle after 5–7 days but loose stools may continue for several weeks.

In infants less than 1 year old, especially neonates and infants under 3 months, septicemia with metastatic infections can occur. In a prospective study the incidence of *Salmonella* bacteremia was estimated to be 6% in children less than 1 year of age.[216] In systemic salmonellosis, gastrointestinal symptoms may not be prominent and the infection may be diagnosed only by blood culture.

Serious consequences of blood invasion in young infants are meningitis, osteomyelitis and failure to thrive. In older infants, bacteremia is usually associated with fever or toxemia, but infants less than 3 months of age may be afebrile.

Blood culture studies in sub-Saharan Africa have shown non-typhoidal *Salmonella* to be the commonest isolate from children < 5 years, especially those under 2 years; *S. typhi* was commoner in older children.[217,218] Associated clinical features in children with non-typhoidal *Salmonella* are cough, dyspnea, pneumonia, diarrhea, hepatosplenomegaly, malnutrition and malaria parasitemia. Extraintestinal disease is common, and meningitis has a mortality of over 50%. Conversely, *S. typhi* was found to be the commonest isolate in under-5s in the Indian subcontinent.[219]

DIAGNOSIS

Culture of *Salmonella* is more likely from feces than from a rectal swab. In suspected cases, repeat culture may be necessary as excretion of the organisms may be intermittent. Leukocytes are often seen, and red blood cells and mucus may be present. In *Salmonella* colitis, endoscopy may demonstrate a swollen edematous mucosa with mucus and areas of hemorrhage suggesting ulcerative colitis.

In invasive disease, blood, CSF, urine culture and culture of metastatic lesions such as bone will confirm the diagnosis. Blood culture is advised in infants < 3 months of age and immunocompromised children with *Salmonella*-positive stools, irrespective of the presence or absence of symptoms of bacteremia. There may be a variable increase in blood neutrophils.

MANAGEMENT

In cases of secretory-type diarrhea with hyponatremia, considerable volumes of normal and half-normal saline may be necessary to replace losses. In prolonged illness, with failure to thrive or in immunocompromised children, intravenous feeding should be considered before significant weight loss has occurred.

In healthy children, antibiotics do not alter the course of the disease and may result in prolongation of excretion of *Salmonella*.[220] Resistance of *Salmonella* to antibiotics is related to their ability to acquire drug resistance from other bacteria in the gut through plasmids and transposons.

Antibiotics are indicated in suspected *Salmonella* enteritis, pending blood culture results, for infants less than 3 months of age (particularly febrile infants and neonates), and immunocompromised children.[221]

For children with bacteremia, a third generation cephalosporin, cefotaxime or ceftriaxone, or one of the fluoroquinolones, e.g. ciprofloxacin, should be given for 7 days[217] (see section on Typhoid fever). Persistent bacteremia is common and 14 days' therapy or more may be required. Metastatic abscesses may require 4–6 weeks' treatment. The advantage of fluoroquinolones is excellent efficacy, particularly in eradicating intracellular infection with either parenteral or oral administration, and thus eradication of intestinal carriage.

Persistent excretion of *Salmonella* may occur for weeks or some months, especially in young infants. No action is necessary, except for advice regarding hygiene, e.g. when changing nappies and washing the hands of young children. No restriction of activities is necessary, if stools are normal.

TYPHOID FEVER

In England and Wales, from 1990 to 2000, there were on average 177 cases of typhoid fever, 129 cases of paratyphoid A, and 26 cases of paratyphoid B per annum, over two-thirds of which were contracted abroad, particularly in the Indian subcontinent.[222] Cases of paratyphoid C were rare. In many developing countries, where hygiene and sanitation are poor, typhoid fever is endemic and constitutes a major health problem.[223] It is considered that up to 80% of infections are mild or subclinical and thus hospital statistics grossly underestimate the prevalence. The classical features of typhoid fever are mainly found in school-age children and young adults. When *S. typhi* is isolated from young children the presentation is often atypical.[224]

S. typhi only infects humans. Subjects are infectious during the acute phase of the disease and when chronic infection of the biliary system, especially the gallbladder, occurs, persistent excretion of the bacteria in feces results. In patients with structural abnormalities of the urinary tract, such as those resulting from *Schistosoma haematobium* infection, there may be prolonged excretion of *S. typhi*.

EPIDEMIOLOGY

In technically advanced countries, typhoid fever is usually caused by contamination of food by a carrier. *S. typhi* can survive for long periods in food and can withstand freezing and drying. Outbreaks may occur from infected milk and ice cream, and in institutions a wide variety of foods have been infected when a carrier is involved with its preparation. Oysters and shellfish cultivated in contaminated sewage may be infected. In developing countries, flies and insects may transmit infection and a contaminated water supply may be the source of an outbreak. Contaminated ice may also be a cause. The infective dose is much smaller than in non-typhoidal salmonellosis.

PATHOGENESIS AND PATHOLOGY

After ingestion, the bacilli invade mainly the upper bowel, with minimal inflammation, and pass to the local lymphatics where they are taken up by macrophages. Their easy access through the bowel may be explained by *S. typhi's* ability to invade the gut without stimulating an acute inflammatory response or recruitment of neutrophils. If the macrophages have not been sensitized by a previous infection they are unable to kill the bacteria, which are then transported within the macrophages to the thoracic duct and thus to the reticuloendothelial system where the uncontained bacilli proliferate in the bone marrow, lymphoid tissue, liver and spleen. At this stage, marrow and blood culture will be positive. The degree of infection depends on the dose and virulence of the organism, the protective effects of gastric juice, and the host's immune response.

Proliferation of bacilli, which is enhanced by bile, continues in the bile ducts and especially the gallbladder, from where large loads of bacteria pass into the gut and may be cultured from a duodenal aspirate. The organisms are taken up by macrophages in Peyer's patches, particularly those in the ileum. By now, the macrophages have been activated by sensitized lymphocytes and an inflammatory reaction takes place. This results in swelling, necrosis and ulceration of Peyer's patches, which in most cases heal uneventfully. However, erosion of blood vessels may cause intestinal hemorrhage, and extension of the necrosis through the bowel wall may result in perforation. At this stage, which is usually 2–3 weeks after the initial infection, most of the bacteria are intracellular and so blood culture is less often positive, but continuous proliferation in the gallbladder results in shedding of large numbers of bacilli into the gut and stool culture becomes positive. Infection of urine reflects the bacteremia, and a quarter to one-third of patients may excrete *S. typhi* during the illness.

Within the body, reaction to the infection continues. Many tissues are affected including the liver, spleen, kidney, heart and lungs. Typhoid nodules, which are foci of macrophages and lymphocytes, can be detected in a number of organs. Cloudy swelling of the liver and kidney occurs and the enlarged spleen is packed with proliferating cells in the sinusoids and pulp. Toxemia is the most likely cause of organ dysfunction, as signs of inflammation are patchy, and is also probably responsible for the mental confusion. Glomerulonephritis and renal failure may occur and are, in some cases, due to immune complex disease.

Rarely, local suppurative infections may develop in bone, joints, lung, kidney and meninges. *S. typhi* osteomyelitis is commonly associated with sickle cell disease.

CLINICAL FEATURES

The incubation period is around 10–14 days and shorter in those receiving a high infecting dose of the organism. During the first week of illness there are vague influenza-like symptoms, namely fever, malaise, aches and pains and headache. Persistence of fever for over a week should alert one to the diagnosis. At this stage, common symptoms are headache, drowsiness, anorexia, vomiting, abdominal pain, diarrhea and cough; constipation may be a symptom in older children. On examination the temperature is often 39–40°C and may have a 'swinging' septicemic pattern. Occasionally, the temperature may be normal in moribund children and rise after resuscitation. Signs of toxemia and confusion are common. The respiration rate is often raised and non-localized wheeze and crackles may be heard in the chest. The pulse rate is raised and may be weak in late-diagnosed cases. A bradycardia relative to the level of temperature, common in adults, is usually not present in young children. Signs of heart failure may be present, especially if there is anemia and/or myocarditis. The abdomen is mild to moderately distended with vague non-localized tenderness. The spleen is enlarged in 20–30% of cases and the liver in a similar proportion. Rates of hepatosplenomegaly vary geographically and according to the duration of the disease. Meningism may be detected. Rose spots which are pink macules and fade on pressure may be seen, especially on the trunk. *S. typhi* may be cultured from them. They may appear in successive crops lasting 2–3 days. They have rarely been reported in children with dark skin.

In uncomplicated cases, treatment results in symptomatic improvement within 2 days and the temperature is usually normal within the week. The physical signs resolve in 2–4 weeks but the child may not regain full strength for 1–2 months.

S. typhi infection during pregnancy may cause abortion. Though transplancental infection occurs, perinatal infection is commonly due to infection during parturition.

In infants and young children, infection by *S. typhi* may present as a rapid septicemic-type illness with respiratory signs, seizures and meningism. Conversely, presentation may be milder in some infants compared to older children.[224]

In developing countries, the presence of nutritional anemia and malnutrition and diseases such as malaria, tuberculosis, sickle cell disease, schistosomiasis and leishmaniasis may complicate the diagnosis. In these diseases, splenomegaly is a common feature. The tendency to anemia in typhoid, which is commonly due to marrow depression, may be exacerbated by the above diseases, and also by glucose-6-phosphate dehydrogenase deficiency and the thalassemias. The association between *Salmonella* infections and sickle cell disease and schistosomiasis is described in the section on salmonellosis.

COMPLICATIONS

Perforation of the gut is one of the major complications. It appears to be less common in young children. It is commonest in the second to third week of the illness but may occur at any time. If it is observed in hospital, it is often associated with sudden deterioration, hypotension, tachycardia and abdominal rigidity. Sometimes perforation is less dramatic and presents more as an ileus. Occasionally, air is detected under the diaphragm in a child who is not particularly sick. Presumably, the perforation, being small, has sealed off spontaneously. Intestinal hemorrhage may accompany or occur independently of perforation. Other complications include pneumonia, myocarditis, heart failure, glomerulonephritis, renal failure, hepatitis, focal or generalized central nervous system disorders and meningitis. The association between septic osteitis and sickle cell disease has already been mentioned.

DIAGNOSIS

Blood culture is positive in 70–80% of cases in the first 7–10 days of the illness and in about half this number in the following 2–3 weeks and may still be positive after some weeks of illness. Culture of marrow is more often positive than blood, and both may remain positive despite previous or current antibiotic therapy. Early on, stool culture may be positive in 50% of cases and in over 70% later in the disease. Urine culture may be positive in 25–30% of cases. Thus, the combination of blood, stool and urine cultures should diagnose most untreated cases. Leukocytes, predominantly mononuclear, are usually detected in the stool and there is often some proteinuria.

The Widal test may be helpful but has its limitations. A high titer of O antibody (> 1:160) or fourfold rise in titer in a child in a non-endemic area who has not had a recent typhoid vaccination (within 1 year) is highly suggestive of typhoid fever. In endemic areas, H antibodies may be raised from previous infections and vaccination also results in a sustained raised H titer. Also, in endemic areas an anamnestic response of O antibody to non-typhoid illnesses may necessitate having a higher diagnostic level during the first week of illness. Conversely, O antibodies may fail to develop and, if present, fail to rise in confirmed typhoid fever. In tropical countries, immunosuppression by malaria may be a factor. Persistence of Vi antibodies may be used as evidence of carrier status, but they may be raised (> 1:5) in only 70% of cases. A number of rapid diagnostic tests including the enzyme linked immunosorbent assay (ELISA), antigen tests and polymerase chain reaction are being evaluated.[225]

Anemia is common and the white cell count is usually normal or low. There may be neutrophilia in young infants or when a pyogenic abscess is present. There is usually a decrease in eosinophil count. Thrombocytopenia may occur. The serum bilirubin is usually normal unless there is a hemolytic anemia, but serum transaminases are often raised. Hyponatremia is common.

MANAGEMENT

Correction and maintenance of fluid and electrolyte balance is important. Blood transfusion may be necessary. Care regarding overhydration is necessary in the presence of anemia, heart failure, nephritis and/or renal failure.

There is little to choose between chloramphenicol, co-trimoxazole (or trimethoprim), amoxicillin and furazolidone for treating typhoid fever when the organism is known to be sensitive. Chloramphenicol has a slightly higher chance of relapse, and does not treat the carrier state, but otherwise is a very effective and convenient drug, especially in developing countries, because of its low cost and good oral absorption. Chloramphenicol is given in a dose of 75 mg/kg/day. Therapy is continued for a minimum of 14 days; 21 days' duration significantly reduces the relapse rate.

Because of the emergence of multidrug resistance to *S. typhi*, alternative drugs need to be considered.[226] Ceftriaxone 60–80 mg/kg once daily for 7–14 days or until 3 days after defervescence is effective. Cefixime 20 mg/kg/day is an alternative for uncomplicated cases. Fluoroquinolones have the advantage of better tissue penetration, oral administration and eradication of the carrier stage. Relapse rates may be lower than with third generation cephalosporins. Ciprofloxacin 25 mg/kg/day intravenously, followed by 30 mg/kg/day orally is given for 7–14 days. Strains with reduced sensitivity to fluoroquinolones are increasing in developing countries. Fluoroquinolones, e.g. ciprofloxacin, are not licensed for children, owing to concerns regarding arthropathic effects on weightbearing joints in juvenile animals. However, these fears may be unfounded.[217,227]

Corticosteroids may be beneficial in some cases. A controlled trial of dexamethasone, 3 mg/kg followed by 1 mg/kg every 6 h for 48 h in severely ill patients, produced a significant reduction in mortality.[228] Perforation should be managed surgically, after full resuscitation with correction of electrolyte and fluid imbalance, and blood transfusion if necessary.[229] Procedures will vary according to circumstances and include simple oversewing of the perforation, or resection, especially in those with multiple perforations. Additional antibiotics to cover Gram negative organisms and anaerobes such as gentamicin and metronidazole should be given.

For clearance of infection, three consecutive stools should be cultured at weekly intervals after chemotherapy ceases. With adequate chemotherapy relapse is uncommon. Children may return to school when symptom-free; stools do not have to be culture-negative. Preschool children and children unable to practice normal hygiene may need to be excluded until clear of infection. Carriage of *S. typhi* for over 3 months indicates that the child may have become a chronic carrier, but this is uncommon in children. It may be associated with defective cell-mediated immunity to *Salmonella*. Ciprofloxacin or another fluoroquinolone should be given for relapse or chronic carriage.

PROGNOSIS

In the preantibiotic era, the mortality rate for typhoid fever for all ages was around 7–20% and in technically advanced countries is now < 0.5%. In developing countries, the overall mortality in children shows marked geographical variation. This may depend on age and stage of disease on admission, and management.

PREVENTION

Care should be taken in the handling of stools of infected children and attention paid to hygiene, particularly handwashing. Supervision of young and handicapped children is important.

There are two vaccines available for general use: parenteral Vi capsular polysaccharide and oral *S. typhi* Ty 21a vaccines. They provide approximately 50–70% protection.[230] A single dose of Vi polysaccharide vaccine is given by intramuscular or subcutaneous injection and side-effects are usually only local and mild. There may be a suboptimal response in children under 2 years. A reinforcement dose is required every 3 years. The Ty 21a vaccine is given for three to four doses on alternate days. It is not recommended at present for children under 6 years. In unexposed children, reinforcement courses need to be given every year.

The development of a Vi conjugate vaccine has potential for mass immunization of infants and children in low income countries.[231]

PARATYPHOID FEVER

Paratyphoid fever is similar to typhoid fever, but is usually milder with a shorter period of fever and a lower frequency of complications and mortality. The incubation period is often shorter and diarrhea is more common. However, in neonates and young infants complications and mortality may be high. It should be treated along the same lines as typhoid fever.

BACTERIAL INFECTIONS: SHIGELLA (BACILLARY DYSENTERY)

The term *bacillary* (as opposed to amebic) *dysentery* is used to describe infections of the gut by shigellae otherwise known as shigellosis. The bacillus was first described by Shiga in Japan in 1898. The organism he described was *Shigella dysenteriae* type 1, previously known as the *Shiga bacillus*, and is the most virulent of all the shigellae.

Shigellae are non-motile, Gram negative, non-spore-forming rods. The genus *Shigella* is subdivided into four species: *Shigella dysenteriae* (12 serotypes, the most important is type 1 (*Shiga*)), *Shigella flexneri* (eight serotypes), *Shigella boydii* (18 serotypes) and *Shigella sonnei* (one colicin type). Man and certain primates are the only hosts.

Although all four species may cause a wide spectrum of disease, generally *Sh. dysenteriae* is associated with severe, *Sh. sonnei* with mild and *Sh. flexneri* and *Sh. boydii* with intermediate severity. Host factors such as malnutrition and immunodeficiency may play a part and explain the vast difference in mortality between developing and technically advanced countries.

EPIDEMIOLOGY

Shigellae are important causes of diarrhea worldwide. They are transmitted by the fecal–oral route and are highly infectious. In the UK, *Sh. flexneri* and *Sh. sonnei* were of equal importance before the Second World War but, since the 1940s, *Sh. sonnei* is responsible for virtually all endemic infections. In the USA, 60–80% of reported cases are due to *Sh. sonnei* and the remainder to *Sh. flexneri*. Of course, imported infections may be of any type. Since the 1920s, *Sh. dysenteriae* 1 infection has been uncommon in Europe and North America, but it still causes devastating epidemics in developing countries. Since 1968 there have been major epidemics of drug resistant *Sh. dysenteriae* 1 in central America, south and south-east Asia and sub-Saharan Africa.[232] In developing countries, endemic disease is usually associated with *Sh. dysenteriae* and *Sh. flexneri* and is commonest during the hot humid and rainy seasons.

In industrialized countries, infection is commonest in preschool children, although less common in infants under 6 months of age. It is associated with poor hygiene and direct person-to-person spread. Outbreaks occur, particularly in playgroups and nursery schools, and also in institutions for the mentally handicapped of all ages. Outbreaks are commonest in late winter or early spring. In developing countries, in addition to the above, infection is associated with unprotected water and open latrines, and food- and waterborne transmission is common. Flies are also vehicles of transmission. Lack of soap and adequate water for washing after defecation are also factors. Breast-feeding has important protective factors against infection by shigellae.

Inoculi as small as 10–200 virulent organisms may be all that are required to cause disease. This explains the high infection rate through direct contact without the necessity for organisms to multiply in food, and contrasts with other bacteria such as salmonellae and *Escherichia coli*, which are usually food-borne infections. Liquid stools contain large numbers of organisms and are highly infectious and may contaminate lavatory seats, lavatory and door handles, etc., and fingers. Shigellae can survive on fomites for long periods, and *Sh. sonnei* may survive on wooden lavatory seats for over 2 weeks.

PATHOGENESIS AND PATHOLOGY

Infection by *Shigella* produces a spectrum of disease varying from a mild catarrhal inflammation of the rectum and pelvic colon associated with *Sh. sonnei*, to widespread devastating necrosis of the entire mucosa of the colon, as occurs with some *Sh. dysenteriae* infections.

Shigellae can survive gastric secretions for up to 4 h. Once they have overcome the surface immune defenses of the gut, they penetrate the epithelial cells and multiply in the submucosa and lamina propria of the colon and terminal ileum. The ability of cytotoxin to inhibit protein synthesis leads to cell destruction, resulting in mucosal inflammation and ulceration. The mucosa becomes swollen and covered in mucus and blood. In addition to blood, there is leakage of plasma proteins into the intestine. In severe cases, there may be widespread coagulation necrosis and destruction of the mucosa and, if the patient survives, there is often persistent colitis. Studies in experimental animals have shown that cytotoxin produced by *Shigella* binds to jejunal villus but not crypt cells, and inhibits villus cell sodium absorption which leads to fluid accumulation in the intestine.[233] This explains symptoms of watery diarrhea that occur in the initial stages of infection. In severe dysentery there is often a generalized systemic disturbance with neurological symptoms (described under Clinical features). No toxin responsible for extraintestinal disease has been identified, apart from the Shiga toxin, which is associated with the hemolytic uremic syndrome (HUS). Bacteremia occurs but is uncommon.

In endemic areas the HUS is a complication of *Sh. dysenteriae* 1, especially in young children, and is often associated with a leukemoid reaction. HUS usually occurs late in the course of the disease when active dysentery is resolving. Case fatality rates may be as high as 50%. There is structural and antigenic similarity between the Shiga toxin produced by *Sh. dysenteriae* and verotoxin produced by *E. coli* of O157:H2 (see section on HUS).

CLINICAL FEATURES

The incubation period is usually 1–3 days but may be up to 5–7 days for *Sh. dysenteriae* 1. The infection may be asymptomatic or associated with the passage of a few loose stools only, present as a secretory-type diarrhea, or dysentery of variable severity.

In the milder forms, as typified by *Sh. sonnei* or milder forms of *Sh. flexneri* infections, there are frequent loose stools for the first 24 h or so, which subside over the next 1–2 days and the stools are usually normal within a week. There may be macroscopic blood and mucus. Abdominal pain may be a prominent feature and may simulate appendicitis or, in young infants, intussusception until the diarrhea becomes apparent. Young children may become dehydrated during the acute watery diarrheal period. Infection of the newborn and young infants is uncommon but mortality may be high.[234] In the newborn it may be confused with necrotizing enterocolitis.[235]

Extraintestinal symptoms are an important feature of shigellosis, especially during the initial period, and sometimes occur before the diarrhea.[236] Convulsions occur in up to 45% of hospitalized children especially in those less than 5 years of age. They are usually associated with a rapidly rising temperature. Other central nervous system symptoms may occur, including headache, confusion, hallucinations, lethargy and meningism. Toxic encephalopathy though uncommon may be fatal.[237] Purulent meningitis is rare.

The etiology of central nervous system symptoms is not known. Release of a neurotoxin either from the bacillus or as a result of necrosis of bowel tissue would be a reasonable explanation, but this has not been demonstrated. Bacteremia is uncommon but is more likely in neonates and malnourished infants who are dehydrated and are often afebrile with protracted diarrhea.[238] It is associated with a high mortality. In developing countries measles is often complicated by *Shigella* dysentery. In HIV infected children, *Shigella* may cause prolonged relapsing disease.

Other complications include rectal prolapse, reactive arthritis, especially in HLA B27-positive children, rarely septic arthritis and myocarditis, infection of the vagina with bloody discharge, corneal infection, and urinary tract infection. Infection of the cornea is presumably due to contact with infected fingers.

Sh. dysenteriae and *Sh. flexneri* infections may be relatively mild, but in endemic areas, especially amongst populations with a high number of undernourished children, complications are common, are especially with *Sh. dysenteriae* 1. In addition to those described above they include severe hyponatremia, hypoglycemia, toxic megacolon, perforation, leukemoid reactions, disseminated intravascular coagulation and HUS.[239] Protracted diarrhea often associated with tenesmus is a major nutritional problem, especially if complicated by protein-losing enteropathy.

DIAGNOSIS

If the patient presents with fever and diarrhea without macroscopic blood in the stools, the diagnosis of *Shigella* infection may be suggested by the presence of large numbers of leukocytes accompanied by red blood cells in the stool. The association of central nervous system symptoms such as convulsions, encephalopathy or meningism may also suggest the diagnosis. If blood and mucus are present, *Campylobacter jejuni* or *Salmonella* infection should also be considered. In developing countries, parasitic causes such as amebic dysentery, a heavy *Trichuris trichiura* infection, or *Schistosoma mansoni* may be responsible for bloodstained stools.

Shigella do not survive long if allowed to dry, or when exposed to sunlight, and thus stools for culture should be inoculated promptly into culture media or put in an appropriate transport medium.

Blood culture should be undertaken in toxic patients, young infants and those who are immunocompromised.

MANAGEMENT

Dehydrated children, particularly young infants, will require correction of fluid and electrolyte balance, either orally or parenterally. Agents that suppress intestinal motility, such as diphenoxylate, loperamide and opium-containing preparations, are contraindicated as they may increase the severity of dysentery by delaying clearance of the organism.

Mild cases are self-limiting, last about a week and do not require chemotherapy. Severe cases with toxemia should be treated, especially in immunocompromised, malnourished or young infants. The choice of agents depends on the sensitivity of the organism in the community where the infection was contracted. In many developing countries there is multidrug resistance, including resistance to nalidixic acid. Suggested drugs are trimethoprim, ampicillin, pivmecillinam, cefixime, ceftriaxone or nalidixic acid given for 5 days. Amoxicillin is not effective. For multidrug resistant *Shigella*, one of the fluoroquinolones, e.g. ciprofloxacin, is presently the drug of choice. For discussion of use of fluoroquinolones in children see section on Typhoid fever.

In malnourished children nutritional support will be required and blood transfusion may be necessary.

PREVENTION

Children are most infectious during the acute phase of diarrhea. Occasionally they may excrete the organisms for some weeks. Chemotherapy decreases the duration of *Shigella* excretion and may be indicated in certain circumstances to reduce transmission. Hygiene, especially handwashing after defecation, is the main method of preventing transmission. Outbreaks in nursery schools and mental institutions are major problems. Rigorous attention to maintaining hygiene in lavatories, with adequate cleaning and disinfection, is required. Supervised washing of hands is essential. Management of outbreaks in the UK[240] and developing countries[239] has been outlined.

Natural immunity to *Shigella* is serotype specific and thus an effective vaccine needs to be polyvalent. Oral live and parenteral vaccines have been developed which produce protection against some type-specific *Shigellae*, but as yet no effective vaccine is in use.[241]

BACTERIAL INFECTIONS: *STAPHYLOCOCCUS*

Staphylococci are Gram positive cocci and include the coagulase positive *Staphylococcus aureus* which is responsible for most of the clinical problems. Coagulase negative staphylococci include *Staphylococcus saprophyticus*, a common cause of urinary tract infection and *Staphylococcus epidermidis*, a skin commensal, which has become an increasing problem with the use of intravascular and other implantable devices.

STAPHYLOCOCCUS AUREUS

Staphylococci are relatively resistant to heat and drying, enabling them to survive for some months on a variety of surfaces or in dust. Their pathogenicity depends on various cell wall components, enzymes and toxins. Catalase, coagulase, hyaluronidase, lipases and nucleases are cellular products with important enzymatic actions. The production of beta lactamases (penicillinases and cephalosporinases) is of particular clinical relevance as these enzymes effectively inactivate beta lactam antibiotics such as penicillin. Cephalosporins vary in their stability to beta lactamases but drugs such as flucloxacillin or amoxicillin-clavulanate remain useful. Staphylococci can express a variety of toxins. The enterotoxins and toxic shock syndrome toxin-1 can act as superantigens. The scalded skin syndrome of infants appears to be caused by 'exfoliative' toxins A and B (ET A and B).

Asymptomatic carriage of *S. aureus* is common, and the organisms can be found in the anterior nares and less often on the skin particularly the perineum and axillae. This can be a problem in hospitals, where staff and patients can become carriers of resistant staphylococci, and can have serious consequences in obstetric units, burns units and surgical wards. Immunocompromised patients on broad spectrum antibiotics are particularly at risk. Since the 1960s, the prevalence of methicillin resistant strains of *S. aureus* (MRSA) and epidemic MRSA (EMRSA) has increased both in hospital and in the community. Local hospital infection control strategies vary in terms of patient isolation, barrier nursing and 'decontamination programs' with detergent baths and topical use of mupirocin (pseudomonic acid) to the anterior nares. Serious infection can occur with MRSA, and although strains are generally sensitive to vancomycin and teicoplanin, there are now occasional reports of vancomycin-resistant *S. aureus* (VRSA) and vancomycin-intermediate *S. aureus* (VISA).

BACTEREMIA AND SEPTICEMIA

Septicemia and bacteremia with *S. aureus* is generally associated with a focus of infection such as osteitis, pneumonia or a severe skin infection and can be associated with intravascular devices such as Hickman catheter and prosthetic heart valves. Severe systemic upset with fever is common, and with prolonged illness, weight loss and anemia can occur. Staphylococcal bacteremia can progress to endocarditis with risks of damage to previously normal heart valves. Toxic shock syndrome can follow infection with a strain of *S. aureus*, which produces toxic shock syndrome toxin type 1 (TSST-1). This was particularly recognized with tampon usage but can occur with other foci of infection. Symptoms include fever, headache, diarrhea, myalgia and confusion. Clinical features include pyrexia, hypotension, a widespread erythematous rash, particularly on the hands and soles (which later desquamate) and mucosal involvement with conjunctivitis and red, inflamed lips. It is a multisystem disease with frequent renal impairment, hepatitis or thrombocytopenia.

Successful treatment depends on rapid institution of antistaphylococcal therapy and general supportive measures, including surgical drainage or removal of tampon, as indicated (Table 26.24). Eradication of staphylococci from indwelling devices such as central lines is unlikely with antibiotic therapy alone and removal of the infected device is usually required. Staphylococci are generally penicillin resistant and suitable antimicrobial agents include flucloxacillin, second generation cephalosporins, rifampicin and fusidic acid. Clindamycin or erythromycin may be useful in combination with fusidic acid, particularly if there is a history of penicillin allergy. Aminoglycosides, such as gentamicin, have antistaphylococcal action and can be used in combination with other antistaphylococcal agents. Vancomycin or teicoplanin is prescribed for more resistant organisms. Linezolid and quinupristin/dalfopristin are antibiotic options for the rare VRSA or VISA strains. Usually 2 weeks of therapy is sufficient for uncomplicated bacteremia.

SKIN INFECTION

Intact skin is a powerful barrier against staphylococcal infection and most skin infection is fairly minor resulting in boils, pustules,

Table 26.24 Antimicrobial therapy for *Staphylococcus aureus* infection

Parenteral				
Flucloxacillin or cloxacillin	i.v. or i.m.	1 month to > 12 years	12.5 mg/kg	6-hourly
Fusidic acid	i.v. only	1 month–12 years 12 years	6–7 mg/kg 500 mg	8-hourly diethanolamine fusidate
Vancomycin (infusion over 60 min, monitor levels)	i.v. only	> 1 month	15 mg/kg/day	
Oral				
Flucloxacillin		1 month–1 year 1–4 years 5–12 years > 12 years	62.5 mg 125 mg 250 mg 500 mg	6-hourly 6-hourly 6-hourly 6-hourly
Fusidic acid		1 month–1 year 1–4 years 5–12 years > 12 years	12.5 mg/kg 250 mg 250–500 mg* 500 mg*	8-hourly 8-hourly 8-hourly 8-hourly

* As sodium salt.

furunculosis, carbuncles, styes, paronychia and impetigo. Topical therapy with mupirocin or fusidic acid ointment should suffice for the treatment of impetigo. Large abscess formation may require surgical drainage. Children who are prone to recurrent minor staphylococcal skin infections should be investigated for possible nasal carriage as they may benefit from a course of mupirocin applied to the anterior nares, and if necessary other family members may also be treated. In children with recurrent staphylococcal skin infection, consideration should be given to screening for neutrophil abnormalities, although the vast majority of these children are immunologically normal.

Cellulitis, a more deep-seated, spreading infection of the skin is an indication for systemic antimicrobial therapy. Orbital cellulitis carries risks of cavernous sinus infection and should be treated promptly with high dose intravenous antibiotics.

The scalded skin syndrome is discussed in Chapter 28.

GASTROINTESTINAL INFECTION

Food poisoning

Foodstuffs such as cooked meat products, cream, custard and pastry can be a source of staphylococcal food poisoning. The organism can often be isolated from the food handlers involved, and often the food is found to have been undercooked and then refrigerated. Symptoms caused by the enterotoxin (which is heat stable) occur 2–5 h after consumption and result in an acute onset of sweating, abdominal pain, diarrhea and vomiting. The symptoms rarely last longer than a few hours but occasionally supportive therapy with intravenous fluids is required. Antibiotics are not helpful.

PNEUMONIA, OSTEITIS, MENINGITIS

These staphylococcal infections are discussed in Chapter 10.

STAPHYLOCOCCUS EPIDERMIDIS

With the increasing use of invasive procedures, this skin commensal has become an important pathogen particularly in the neonate and in the presence of indwelling catheters and shunts. Children with ventriculoatrial shunts may have bacteremia and ventriculoperitoneal shunts can lead to peritonitis. In this situation, eradication of infection with antimicrobial therapy may not be possible and relapse is common. Replacement of the infected device or catheter is, therefore, usually required.

Particularly in hospital-acquired infection, resistance to many antimicrobial agents is common. Resistance to vancomycin is rare, though, despite its widespread use in this setting.

BACTERIAL INFECTIONS: *STREPTOCOCCUS* AND *ENTEROCOCCUS*

The large family of streptococci can be responsible for a variety of disease and sequelae. Streptococci are Gram positive cocci, which tend to form chains. There are several classification systems based on serological or molecular biological techniques. A more traditional classification is based on the degree of hemolysis surrounding a colony on blood agar. Hemolysis can be complete (beta hemolysis), partial (alpha hemolysis) or absent (gamma hemolysis). Enterococci mostly cause alpha hemolysis but are now classified as a separate genus (*Enterococcus*).

The beta hemolytic streptococci are responsible for most of the streptococcal disease in humans and are among the most common bacterial infections of childhood. Streptococci belonging to the other two groups are mainly commensals of the pharynx or gastrointestinal tract and tend to be less virulent pathogens.

THE BETA HEMOLYTIC STREPTOCOCCI

Beta hemolytic streptococci can be further classified into Lancefield groups depending on the serological characterization of the polysaccharide layer of the cell wall. Most human disease is caused by group A streptococci (GAS), which include *Streptococcus pyogenes*. GAS can be further categorized into subtypes.

Beta hemolytic streptococci can produce disease by direct tissue invasion or by toxin production. Some strains have a hyaluronic acid capsule, which is non-antigenic and has an inhibitory effect on phagocytosis. The cell wall is a complex structure built upon a peptidoglycan matrix. There are a variety of antigenic determinants, including the protein M antigen, which confer further resistance to phagocytosis and may act as a superantigen. Streptococci lacking this antigen are generally avirulent. The T antigens are useful for epidemiological tracing. The polysaccharide layer determines the Lancefield group. Lipoteichoic acid is a further cell wall component, which influences membrane affinity and adherence to epithelial cells. Virulence also depends on the production of toxins. Several strains can produce the erythrogenic toxin, which causes the rash of scarlet fever. It is thought that toxins acting as superantigens may be important in the etiology of streptococcal toxic shock syndrome. The two streptolysins O and S are responsible for the hemolytic action of streptococci and the estimation of the antistreptolysin O (or ASO) titer can be useful in diagnosing streptococcal infection. Persisting high ASO titers are seen, for example, in rheumatic fever. Other extracellular products, which are possibly involved in spread of infection and the pyogenic process, include DNases, hyaluronidases and streptokinase. Streptokinase can be used therapeutically for thrombolysis.

EPIDEMIOLOGY

GAS are principally carried in the pharynx and asymptomatic carriage occurs in 15–20% of children. Infection is spread by direct contact or droplet spread and outbreaks may occur particularly in dormitory-type accommodation in winter months. Food- or waterborne outbreaks have been reported. There have been changing patterns in streptococcal disease worldwide. Scarlet fever, for example, is less of a clinical concern than previously, although over the last few decades there has been an increase in more severe invasive forms of disease such as necrotizing fasciitis.

IMMUNITY

In view of the antigenic variety of the streptococcal strains repeated streptococcal infection is possible. A child who has suffered from scarlet fever and developed antibodies to the erythrogenic toxin should be protected against further attacks of the syndrome.

CLINICAL FEATURES

The usual focus for GAS infection is the throat, and infection generally presents with symptoms and signs of acute tonsillitis. In children up to the age of 5 years the illness may be less specific. The incubation period is 2–4 days and the child usually complains of a sore throat and headache, is febrile and may have cervical lymphadenopathy. The pharynx may appear mildly inflamed or a more severe form of exudative pharyngitis may be present. Clinical discrimination from viral infection is not usually possible and uncomplicated carriage is always a possibility when streptococci are isolated from the throat swab. Classically, after 10 days of illness, a rise in the ASO titer will be apparent. Tonsillitis, otitis media, mastoiditis, sinusitis and the much rarer GAS pneumonia, empyema, meningitis and septicemia are described elsewhere. Scarlet fever and erysipelas are unique to streptococcal infection.

SCARLET FEVER

Scarlet fever is caused by infection with an erythrogenic toxin-producing strain of GAS. The usual portal of entry is via the pharynx and the syndrome classically follows acute streptococcal tonsillitis. However, a mild pharyngitis may be the portal, or the streptococci may gain access via broken skin following minor cuts, burns, surgical wounds or chickenpox infection.

Clinical features

The incubation period is usually 2–4 days and the illness may be of variable severity with sudden onset fever, headache, vomiting, sore throat and refusal to eat. In the past, severe illness was more common and delirium a frequent feature. The erythematous rash appears some 2 or 3 days after the onset of illness and classically is first seen in the axillae and groins with blanching on pressure (Figs 26.24 and 26.25).[242] Within 24 h the rash spreads to the trunk and limbs. The face may be flushed and circumoral pallor is a common feature. Pastia's sign – linear petechiae in the flexures – may be helpful diagnostically. After a week or so, desquamation usually occurs starting on the face, then the trunk and limbs. Initially the tongue appears swollen with a yellowish white coating and prominent papillae. This is known as the white strawberry tongue, which later becomes the red strawberry tongue as the coating disappears.

Untreated the illness runs its course within 10 days or less. A high fever and tachycardia are common.

Albuminuria is a common finding and a polymorphonuclear leukocytosis is usual.

Since the availability of antibiotic therapy, serious complications are rare. Immediate complications include cervical lymphadenitis with more rarely abscess formation necessitating surgical drainage. Acute otitis media may develop and without treatment further complications including mastoiditis, meningitis or cerebral abscess may ensue. Involvement of the paranasal sinuses can lead to suppurative sinusitis. Other recognized local complications include peritonsillar cellulitis or abscess formation, laryngitis and retropharyngeal abscess.

Rarely, bacteremic spread can lead to metastatic foci of infection, and bronchopneumonia is a further complication, which may lead to empyema or suppurative pericarditis.

The later complications, occurring about 2–3 weeks after the onset of illness, include rheumatic fever, acute glomerulonephritis

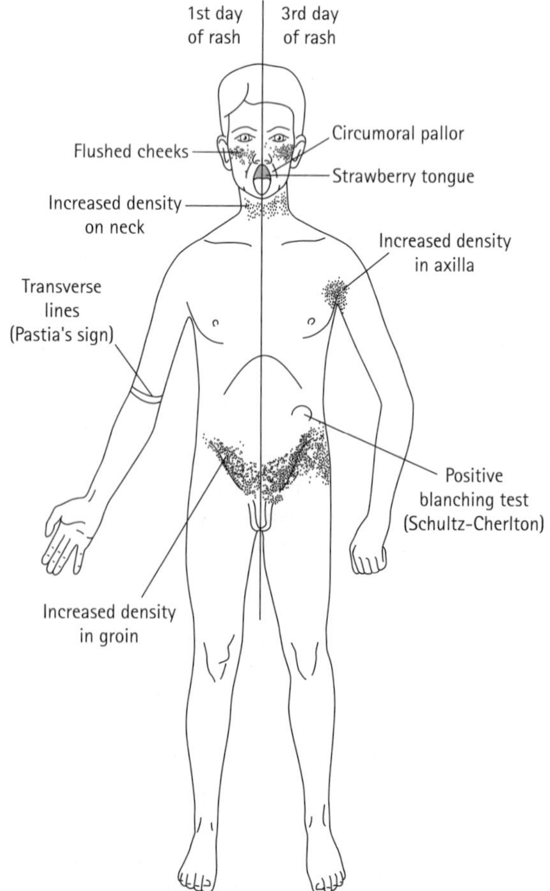

Fig. 26.24 The distribution and the development of rash in scarlet fever. (After Krugman & Ward 1968[242])

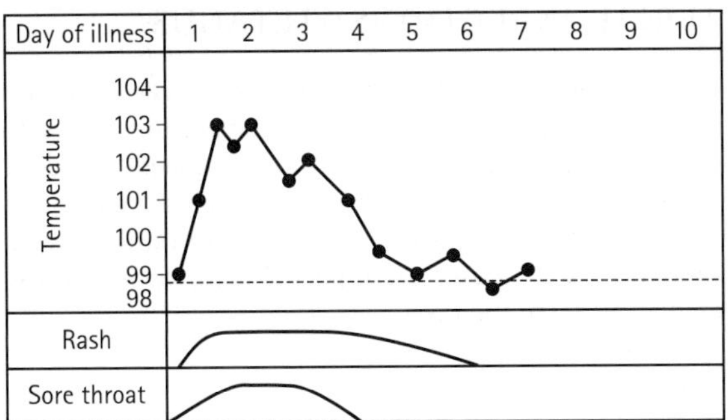

Fig. 26.25 The development of scarlet fever. (After Krugman & Ward 1968[242])

and erythema nodosum. Early antibiotic therapy should prevent such complications.

Differential diagnosis

Where acute tonsillitis is present the diagnosis is usually straightforward. With milder or subclinical pharyngitis the diagnosis may be less apparent and confused with other exanthemata. Measles is recognized by the prodromal catarrhal symptoms, diarrhea, conjunctivitis, the presence of Koplik spots and the different character and distribution of the rash. In rubella, the diffuse rash contrasting with the mild illness and the presence of predominantly occipital cervical lymphadenopathy are distinguishing features. Generalized lymphadenopathy with splenomegaly is often present in infectious mononucleosis; the blood film examination may reveal atypical mononuclear cells and Epstein–Barr virus (EBV) serology is positive. Other viral exanthemata run a shorter course and usually have leukopenia rather than polymorphonuclear leukocytosis.

Kawasaki syndrome (KS) may be difficult to differentiate. The rash, oral and peripheral changes are similar. The cervical lymphadenopathy of KS may be characteristically unilateral and matted, and the episcleritis with limbal sparing of KS is not usually seen in scarlet fever. In clinical practice, failure of a child with suspected scarlet fever to respond to antibiotics should arouse suspicion of KS.

A similar rash may be seen as a result of infection with toxin-producing *S. aureus*, but in the resulting syndrome of 'toxic shock' there is shock, and often an obvious focus of staphylococcal infection, and the rash tends to be more severe on the palms and soles.

Drug rashes particularly following antibiotic usage can be scarlatiniform (scarlet fever-like). The other features of disease are not usually present, however, and the rash fades with the cessation of therapy.

Prevention and treatment

The main aim of antimicrobial therapy is to eradicate the infection and thereby prevent the sequelae of local suppurative disease or later rheumatic fever and poststreptococcal glomerulonephritis (Table 26.25). Penicillin is the drug of choice for the treatment of GAS. In severe cases intravenous or intramuscular administration of benzyl penicillin may be required initially. In milder cases, oral phenoxymethyl penicillin for 10 days is usually sufficient. Erythromycin is a suitable alternative in cases of penicillin allergy. Ampicillin and amoxicillin should be avoided, as if mistakenly given in infectious mononucleosis they can cause a severe rash and constitutional upset.

It is unusual to get multiple cases of scarlet fever in a family, although uncomplicated streptococcal throat infection may develop in other children and this can be prevented by oral penicillin.

ERYSIPELAS

Erysipelas is a skin infection caused by any of the GAS, which can enter the skin through trivial wounds or abrasions. Children of all ages are susceptible and recurrent attacks often involving the same site can occur. Children with congenital lymphedema appear to be more at risk.

Clinical features

The illness may present with fever, malaise, vomiting and anorexia or the symptoms may be confined to the affected skin or occasionally the mucous membranes. A small erythematous patch may develop into a much larger area of affected skin, which becomes red, hot, painful, indurated and well demarcated by a raised edge. In infants, the periumbilical region is a common site, whereas in older children the extremities or the face are sites of predilection and both cheeks may be involved in a butterfly type of distribution. Facial erysipelas must be differentiated from the violaceous cellulitis caused by *Haemophilus influenzae* type b infection or the slapped cheek appearance of parvovirus B19 infection. Resolution of erysipelas starts centrally and may be followed by desquamation.

Blood cultures are frequently negative but after 10 days of illness there may be a rise in the ASO titer.

Erysipelas responds quickly to penicillin or erythromycin. It may be difficult to differentiate erysipelas from other soft tissue infection such as cellulitis, the more deep-seated infection caused mainly by staphylococcal infection, and in cases where doubt exists antistaphylococcal antimicrobial therapy should also be prescribed, e.g. flucloxacillin.

Table 26.25 Antimicrobial therapy for *Streptococcus pyogenes* infection

Parenteral				
Benzyl penicillin	i.m.	1–12 months	15 mg/kg	6-hourly
		1–4 years	150 mg	6-hourly
		5–12 years	300–600 mg	6-hourly
		> 12 years	600 mg–1.2 g	6-hourly
	i.v.	All ages	25–50 mg/kg	4 to 6-hourly
Erythromycin	i.v. only	1 month–12 years	8–12 mg/kg	6-hourly
Oral				
Phenoxymethyl penicillin		< 1 year	62.5 mg	6-hourly
		1–4 years	125 mg	6-hourly
		5–12 years	250 mg	6-hourly
		> 12 years	500 mg	6-hourly
Erythromycin		1 month–1 year	125 mg	6-hourly
		2–8 years	250 mg	6-hourly
		> 8 years	500 mg	6-hourly

STREPTOCOCCAL PYODERMA

Although most impetigenous lesions are caused by staphylococcal infection, localized purulent streptococcal infection of the skin (streptococcal impetigo or pyoderma) may result from secondary infection of wounds or burns. In children, particularly in the age range 2–5 years and living in tropical or subtropical climates, it mainly involves the lower limbs and may follow intradermal inoculation of streptococci by minor trauma or insect bites. Multiple lesions are common and begin as small papules, becoming vesicular with surrounding erythema. Pustule formation occurs and the lesions then enlarge and break down with formation of thick crusts. Systemic upset is not common but regional lymphadenitis is usually present. 10 days of penicillin therapy is advised although there appears much less risk of rheumatic fever with this type of infection.

Lymphangitis, characterized by red, linear streaks leading to the enlarged regional lymph nodes, may follow very minor skin infection or inoculation with streptococci. It may accompany cellulitis.

STREPTOCOCCUS AGALACTIAE

Streptococcus agalactiae, or Group B streptococcus (GBS), is a beta hemolytic streptococcus belonging to Lancefield group B (GBS) and is a major cause of neonatal infections, both early and late.

VIRIDANS GROUP STREPTOCOCCI

Viridans streptococci are usually alpha hemolytic but can be non-hemolytic. They are oropharyngeal commensals, and include the *Streptococcus mutans*, *Streptococcus salivarius*, *Streptococcus milleri*, *Streptococcus sanguis* and *Streptococcus mitis* groups. Even minor dental procedures can be complicated by a transient bacteremia, which is of no clinical consequence except for children with cardiac disease, either congenital heart disease, such as patent ductus arteriosus or bicuspid aortic valves, or acquired, such as rheumatic heart disease. Infective endocarditis is a risk in such cases. Regular dental care with additional antibiotic prophylaxis for dental procedures is advised for children who have a history of rheumatic fever or congenital heart disease.

ENTEROCOCCI

Enterococci are commensals of the intestinal tract. They can cause urinary tract infection particularly in cases of structural urinary tract abnormality or neurological dysfunction of the bladder such as in children with lumbar or sacral myelomeningocele. Enterococci, particularly *Enterococcus faecalis*, can also cause infective endocarditis and have emerged as a major cause of bacteremia in hospitalized patients. This group of organisms is often penicillin resistant, and determination of the antibiotic sensitivity is important. In endocarditis, combinations of antimicrobial chemotherapy are advised such as the synergistic combination of amoxicillin and an aminoglycoside such as gentamicin. Vancomycin is an alternative, but this treatment is threatened by the emergence of vancomycin resistant enterococci (VRE). Fortunately few of these isolates appear clinically relevant and the organisms are often no longer evident after cessation of vancomycin. There are concerns that VRE may cause more clinical problems in the future and drugs such as linezolid and quinupristin/dalfopristin are likely to be increasingly used in this setting.

BACTERIAL INFECTIONS: TETANUS

Despite the availability of an effective active vaccination since 1923 tetanus remains a major health problem in the developing world and is still encountered in the developed world. There are approximately 800 000 tetanus deaths each year, of which approximately 400 000 are due to neonatal tetanus.[243] Approximately 12–15 cases are reported per year in the UK and between 40 and 60 in the USA.

ETIOLOGY

Tetanus is caused by a toxin released following infection with *Clostridium tetani*, a Gram positive, spore forming, obligate anaerobic bacillus. Tetanus typically follows deep penetrating wounds where anaerobic bacterial growth is facilitated. The most common portals of infection are wounds on the lower limbs, postpartum or postabortion infections of the uterus, non-sterile intramuscular injections and compound fractures. Minor trauma can lead to disease and in up to 30% of cases no portal of entry is apparent.

Neonatal tetanus is caused by cutting of the cord with an unsterile instrument or application of fecal contaminated traditional concoctions to the cord.

EPIDEMIOLOGY AND PATHOGENESIS

Clostridium tetani is a ubiquitous inhabitant of the intestinal tract of many animals and commonly found in soil. The toxin binds to gangliosides on peripheral nerves, and the toxin is internalized. It is then moved by retrograde axonal transport to the central nervous system. The toxin prevents release of the inhibitory neurotransmitter [gamma aminobutyric acid (GABA)] into the synaptic cleft. The alpha motor neurones are therefore under no inhibitory control and undergo sustained excitatory discharge causing the characteristic motor spasms of tetanus.

PREVENTION

Tetanus toxoid is produced by formaldehyde treatment of the toxin. Immunogenicity is improved by absorption with aluminium hydroxide. In the UK and USA it is administered to children between 2 and 6 months (three doses at 4-week intervals) with boosters at 15 months in the USA and at 4 years in both countries. A further dose is recommended in both the USA and UK within 5–10 years. In order to maintain adequate levels of protection, additional booster doses should be administered every 10 years. Minor reactions to the tetanus toxoid are estimated to be 1 in 50 000 injections. Severe reactions such as the Guillain–Barré syndrome and acute relapsing polyneuropathy are rare. Neonatal tetanus can be prevented by immunization of women during pregnancy. Two or three doses of absorbed toxin should be given with the last dose at least 1 month prior to delivery. There is no evidence of congenital anomalies associated with tetanus toxin administered during pregnancy.[244] Maternal HIV and malaria infection may limit the transfer of protective maternal antibodies. For home deliveries, education of traditional birth attendants, midwives or female relatives in proper care of the umbilical cord, including provision of sterile cord-care packs, is also essential. Passive immunization with human or equine tetanus immunoglob-ulin shortens the course and may reduce the severity of tetanus. The equine form, widely available throughout the developing world has a higher incidence of anaphylactic reactions. In established cases patients should receive 500–1000 units/kg of equine antitoxin (newborn 5000 units) or 5000–8000 units (newborn 500 units) of human antitetanus immunoglobulin intravenously or intramuscularly. For prophylaxis 1500–3000 units equine or 250–500 units human antitetanus immunoglobulin should be given. Passive immunization should be administered as soon as possible after the injury because once the toxin is bound and internalized it will have no effect. In addition to passive immunization, active vaccination needs to be administered to all patients.

CLINICAL FEATURES

The incubation period (the time from inoculation to the first symptom) can be as short as 48 h or as long as many months after inoculation with *Clostridium tetani*. The period of onset is the time between the first symptom and the start of spasms. These periods are important in determining the prognosis; the shorter the incubation period or period of onset the more severe the disease. Trismus (lockjaw), the inability to open the mouth fully owing to rigidity of the masseters, is often the first symptom. Generalized tetanus is the most common form of the disease, and presents with pain, headache, stiffness, rigidity, opisthtonus, and spasms, which may lead to laryngeal obstruction. These may be induced by minor stimuli such as noise, touch, or by simple medical and nursing procedures such as intravenous and intramuscular injections, suction, or catheterization. The spasms are excruciatingly painful and may be uncontrollable, leading to respiratory arrest and death. Spasms are most prominent in the first 2 weeks; autonomic disturbance usually starts some days after spasms and reaches a peak during the second week of the disease. Rigidity may last beyond the duration of both spasms and autonomic disturbance. In neonatal tetanus the incubation period is around 3–10 days. Common presenting symptoms include difficulty in sucking and swallowing. Asphyxia, aspiration pneumonia and cardiorespiratory failure may result from prolonged severe spasms.

DIAGNOSIS AND DIFFERENTIAL DIAGNOSIS

The diagnosis is a clinical one, and is relatively easy to make in areas where tetanus is seen frequently, but it is often delayed in the developed world where cases are less common. The differential includes tetany, strychnine poisoning, drug induced dystonic reactions, rabies, and orofacial infection. In neonates the differential diagnosis includes hypocalcemia, hypoglycemia, meningitis and meningoencephalitis, kernicterus and seizures.

TREATMENT

In patients with a deep wound, thorough debridement and toilet are critical to reduce the anaerobic conditions in which the bacteria thrive. Common complications in tetanus are those of prolonged periods in intensive care. Secondary infections are a frequent complication, most commonly associated with the lower respiratory tract, urinary catheterization, and wound sepsis. Gram negative organisms, particularly *Klebsiella* and *Pseudomonas* are common. Meticulous mouth care, chest physiotherapy and regular tracheal suction are essential to prevent atelectasis, lobar collapse and pneumonia particularly as salivation and bronchial secretions are greatly increased in severe tetanus. Adequate sedation is mandatory before such interventions in patients at risk of uncontrolled spasms or autonomic disturbance and the balance between physiotherapy and sedation may be difficult to achieve. Energy demands in tetanus may be very high due to muscular contractions, excessive sweating and sepsis.[245] In severe tetanus, rigidity and muscle spasm may necessitate paralysis for prolonged periods.

SPECIFIC TREATMENT

Penicillin is the standard antibiotic therapy for tetanus. The dose is 100 000–200 000 units/kg/day (neonates 100 000 units/kg) intramuscularly or intravenously for 7–10 days. Metronidazole is a safe and effective alternative (see Prevention for administration of tetanus antitoxin). Autonomic disturbance with sustained labile hypertension, tachycardia, vasoconstriction and sweating is common in severe cases. Profound bradycardia and hypotension may occur and may be recurrent or a preterminal event. Diazepam has a wide margin of safety, has a rapid onset of action, and is a sedative, an anticonvulsant and a muscle relaxant. However it has a long cumulative half-life. Invariably, in the doses required to achieve adequate control of spasms, respiratory depression, coma, and medullary depression are common. Magnesium sulfate has been used both in ventilated patients to reduce autonomic disturbance and in non-ventilated patients to control spasms. There is very little information on follow-up of patients after tetanus. Enuresis, mental retardation and growth delay have all been reported after neonatal tetanus.[246]

In developing countries neonates are given paraldehyde 0.3 ml/kg or diazepam 1–2 mg/kg intramuscularly on admission and a nasogastric tube is passed to give expressed breast milk. If facilities for intravenous therapy are available diazepam may be given in a dose of 15–30 mg/day or more, in a continuous infusion. Alternatively a combination of chlorpromazine 2 mg/kg and diazepam 1–2 mg/kg may be given 4–6 hourly by nasogastric tube with additional parenteral doses of diazepam as required. Phenobarbital 5 mg/kg once or twice daily may be added to the above oral regimen to provide further control.

PROGNOSIS

The prognosis in tetanus remains serious despite the best available treatment. Globally the mortality rate in neonatal infection is approximately 60%. Prognosis is particularly related to standard of nursing care. Older children and adults have a mortality rate of 10–30% depending on the availability of basic intensive care facilities.

BACTERIAL INFECTIONS: TUBERCULOSIS

In technically advanced countries, morbidity and mortality from tuberculosis have declined progressively over the decades. This is associated with improved living conditions and medical care, particularly case finding and chemotherapy. However, it is still an important problem, especially in immigrant and minority groups. In some developing countries, the case rate has hardly changed and any decline is offset by an increase in population.

The majority of children infected by *Mycobacterium tuberculosis* are asymptomatic. However, in a small number, especially young children, the disease is serious or fatal, due to meningitis or disseminated disease, and survivors may be left with sequelae such as cerebral palsy, mental retardation, chronic lung or bone and joint disease.

MICROBIOLOGY

The 'tubercle bacillus' was first described by Robert Koch in 1882 and is now called *Mycobacterium tuberculosis*. However, the identification of the transmissible nature of tuberculosis is attributed to Jean Antoine Villemin in 1865. Mycobacteria derive their name from their mold-like appearance on culture. One of their unique characteristics is a highly complex, lipid-rich, cell wall which protects the bacillus from digestion by the lysosomal enzymes of macrophages and which, when stained, resists decolorization by acid alcohol. Like *Mycobacterium leprae*, but different from other mycobacteria, *M. tuberculosis* is an obligate parasite with total dependence on the living host.

The two major species of mycobacteria infecting man are *M. tuberculosis* and *Mycobacterium bovis*. *M. bovis* differs from the other types in its resistance to pyrazinamide. *M. tuberculosis* is aerophilic but *M. bovis* is microaerophilic (prefers reduced oxygen tension). Within the host, mycobacteria may lie dormant for many years.

M. tuberculosis is cultured on Lowenstein–Jensen medium and is slow growing, taking an average time of 21 days, and occasionally 1–2 months or longer. Growth of *M. tuberculosis* may be detected in 7–10 days using the Bactec radiometric or the Roche biphasic systems.

There are two major methods for direct identification in specimens: Ziehl–Neelsen stain and fluorescence microscopy. For fluorescence microscopy the specimen is stained with auramine–rhodamine. The latter is more rapid, more sensitive, and less likely to yield false positive results than the Ziehl–Neelsen method.

A number of serological tests have been developed using purified protein derivatives of *M. tuberculosis* by enzyme linked immunosorbent assay (ELISA) or solid-phase radioimmunoassays. However, many lack sensitivity and specificity especially for culture-negative cases and thus are not used for routine laboratory diagnosis.[247] Tests for antigen in CSF are useful but not routinely available. Gene probes can provide a rapid identification of mycobacteria once they have grown in culture. In adults, nucleic acid amplification (NAA) has approximate sensitivity of over 90% and specificity of 98% for smear positive respiratory specimens, but only 50–70% sensitivity for smear-negative specimens.[248] Sensitivity for non-respiratory is lower than for respiratory specimens, particularly for CSF. This is partly due to inhibitors especially in pleural, ascitic and CSF specimens. There are few studies in children and they are limited by numbers of confirmed or probable cases of tuberculosis.[249,250] Sensitivities for polymerase chain reaction (PCR) in gastric aspirates in children with confirmed or clinical pulmonary tuberculosis vary from 40 to 80% and generally are higher than culture. Sensitivity is increased by testing multiple samples. Specificity is reportedly 94–100%, although PCR may be positive in a third of children with tuberculous infection only. Sensitivities are no higher in bronchial alveolar lavage (BAL) than in gastric aspirates. PCR can differentiate between *M. tuberculosis* and environmental mycobacteria and PCR methods are available to detect rifampicin resistance. DNA fingerprinting is a valuable tool in studying transmission of tuberculosis.

EPIDEMIOLOGY

In studies of tuberculosis, differentiation has to be made between tuberculous infection (as evidenced by a positive tuberculin test) and disease. In tuberculous disease there is clinical, radiological or bacteriological evidence of infection. In the UK, people who are tuberculin positive, without demonstration of disease are not notified as having tuberculosis. The great majority of infected people remain asymptomatic. In England and Wales in 1949–1950, a national survey showed that nearly half of 14-year-old children were tuberculin positive. Today, less than 1% of 11- to 13-year-old children are tuberculin positive at routine school examination.

Three-quarters of tuberculosis cases occur in developing countries where 0.2–1% of the population are expectorating the tubercle bacillus. A rise in case rates in adults and children has been observed in countries with a high prevalence of HIV infection, especially sub-Saharan Africa.[251]

In technically advanced countries, where the prevalence of smear positive cases is small, the infection rate in children will be low and the majority of adults with tuberculosis will have endogenous reactivation. Conversely, in developing countries, the high prevalence of smear positive cases will result in a significant proportion of children and young adults developing primary tuberculosis, and exogenous reinfection in older adults will be common. However, despite the high prevalence of infection in these countries, up to 50% of 15-year-old adolescents may be tuberculin negative and thus prone to primary tuberculosis.

National surveys for England and Wales for the periods 1978–1979, 1983, 1988, 1993 and 1998 found 747 (estimate based on 6 month survey), 452, 308, 408 and 364 newly notified children under 15 years respectively (Communicable Disease Surveillance Center CDSC data – 1993 and 1998 national tuberculosis surveys). In 1998, rates (per 100 000) for children were highest for Black African (70.6) and Indian subcontinent (23.1) compared to Black Caribbean (9.0) and white (1.1) groups. Though rates for the Chinese group were high (82.1), cases were low (14).

The decline in the incidence of tuberculosis began in Europe before the introduction of BCG and chemotherapy. In the decade 1979–1988 there was an average reduction in notification rates in England of 7.2% per year. However, since 1988 there has been a 21% rise in notifications, with the highest increase in the London area.[252] Over 50% of cases were born outside the UK. There has also been a rise in notifications in parts of Europe and the USA. Factors associated with the rise in notifications in the US since 1987 include HIV infection, homelessness, immigration and decline in resources for tuberculosis control. The increase is focal, mainly confined to inner cities, and 80% of childhood cases are in minority ethnic groups. Multidrug resistance is a major problem. However, with increased support for tuberculosis control, the rise in cases has reversed in 1993–1994.[253]

The vast majority of cases of tuberculosis are caused by *M. tuberculosis*. *M. bovis*, which was an important cause of tuberculosis of the gastrointestinal tract, lymph nodes and bones, has virtually disappeared from technically advanced countries through eradication of tuberculosis in cattle and pasteurization of milk. In the UK before 1950, *M. bovis* was the cause of 33% of childhood and 10% of adult extrapulmonary disease. It is also considered to be an uncommon cause of tuberculosis in developing countries, except in communities where large amounts of raw milk are consumed, e.g. in cattle-herding tribes. In the UK it is still isolated from reactivated lesions in approximately 1% of adults.[254] *M. bovis* is resistant to pyrazinamide.

PATHOLOGY

The pathology of tuberculosis has been described by Miller.[255] The first response to the presence of the tubercle bacilli at the point of entry and in the regional nodes is a serous exudate. Soon neutrophils accumulate followed by macrophages. The macrophages ingest the bacilli. Some may be transformed into epithelioid cells, which contain more effective digestive enzymes in their lysosomes. Fusion of either the macrophages or epithelioid cells forms the characteristic multinucleate giant cells. Death of the cells in the center of the tubercle (granuloma) results in the appearance of caseation necrosis. Lymphocytes form a zone around the tubercle, and are particularly apparent during the second month of infection, which coincides with the development of tuberculin sensitivity. Healing takes place with the deposition of collagen fibrils by fibroblasts, which wall off the caseous area from healthy tissue. After 12 months or more, calcification may be seen, which remains for years but may be completely reabsorbed. It usually has a stippled appearance. Alternatively, healing may not occur, or the tubercle-containing dormant bacilli may reactivate after months or years. Extensive necrosis with caseation and liquefaction may develop. Liquefaction allows bacilli to survive, inhibits macrophage and lymphocyte function because of lack of oxygen, and prevents drug penetration. Activity and healing of the lesion may occur concurrently.

IMMUNOLOGY

The main defense against infection by the tubercle bacillus is cell mediated. The role of B cells is unclear.

Tubercle bacilli are readily ingested, but are not killed by macrophages, in which they multiply. Toxic substances and other properties in the lipid-thick cell wall protect the bacillus against lysosomal enzymes. CD4 T lymphocytes (T helper cells), when sensitized by tubercle bacilli, produce cytokines which activate macrophages and CD8 cytotoxic T lymphocytes (CTL). CTLs lyse cells containing mycobacteria and enable macrophages to kill their ingested bacilli. The positive effect of T helper cells may be countered by suppressor activity. In advanced disease or in the presence of a large bacterial load these suppressor effects may predominate, which may explain the anergy commonly seen in these children.

Defense against tuberculosis can be described as two components: one where cell-mediated immunity (CMI) controls the infection by activating macrophages which enables them to kill ingested mycobacteria; the other is delayed type hypersensitivity (DTH) which when the bacillary antigens reach high levels results in caseous necrosis of host tissues.[256] DTH is responsible for the tissue damage and caseation necrosis, characteristic of postprimary tuberculous disease. There is no correlation between the degree of hypersensitivity and resistance to tuberculosis. The balance between hypersensitivity and resistance will influence the manifestation of tuberculosis, i.e. the former will be associated with clinical and radiological signs of the disease, whereas with the latter there will be a paucity of signs. Improved knowledge of T helper cells has enhanced understanding of the above mechanisms.[257] Three types of T helper cells are recognized, Th_0 (naive cells), Th_1 and Th_2. Exposure of Th_0 cells to interleukin-12 (IL-12) or IL-4 drives them to differentiate into Th_1 cells or Th_2 cells respectively. Th_1 lymphocytes secrete IL-2, interferon-gamma (IFN-gamma) and lymphotoxin-alpha and stimulate type 1 immunity. It is characterized by phagocytic activity and DTH. IFN-gamma and lymphotoxin-alpha promote secretion of proinflammatory cytokines such as tumor necrosis factor-alpha (TNF-alpha). Th_2 cells secrete IL-4, IL-5, IL-9, IL-10 and IL-13 and stimulate type 2 immunity, which is characterized by high antibody titers. Type 1 and type 2 immunity cross regulate and suppress activity of the other. The immunological reactions to tuberculosis are not as clear cut in humans as in mice (in which much of experimental work has been undertaken), nor as in leprosy. It would seem, however, that in humans, a type 1 response is important in protective inflammation and mounting a DTH response, and a switch to a type 2 response is associated with the period of healing and granuloma organization. High or prolonged type 1 activity may result in excessive DTH reactions and tissue destruction associated with raised IFN-gamma and TNF-alpha levels. Conversely, failure to control infection, as in immunocompromised patients, is associated with increased type 2 activity. It is suggested that in humans, excessive tissue destruction may relate to mixed Th_1/Th_2 response whereby a factor produced by type 2 cells makes tissues very sensitive to TNF-alpha.[258] Other important factors include transforming growth factor beta (TGF-beta) produced by mononuclear phagocytes, which may have negative effects on Th_1 activity and 1,25 $(OH)_2$ vitamin D_3 which appears important for action of macrophages in controlling intracellular mycobacterial replication.

A number of primary factors influence the outcome of the immunological response, including the number of inhaled bacilli, their virulence and the immune response by the host. These are affected by secondary factors, e.g. age of the patient, infections such as measles, malnutrition, malignancy and immunodeficiency states. Children under 5 years and adolescents (especially females) are at higher risk of developing tuberculous disease.

PATHOGENESIS

The first infection by tubercle bacillus occurs most commonly by inhalation through the lungs, less often by ingestion through the alimentary tract (tonsils and ileum), and rarely by infection of an open wound on the skin. Infection of the mouth, skin and eyes may result from exposure to a dental surgeon with pulmonary tuberculosis. Enlargement of the regional lymph nodes occurs, which provides an indication of the site of primary focus.

PRIMARY INFECTION

The primary focus or site of entry in the lung is usually single and situated just under the pleura (*Ghon focus*) in a well-ventilated part of the lung. Because there is no acquired immunity, the bacilli multiply at the primary focus and in the regional lymph nodes. The primary focus and nodes form the primary complex. In most cases there is hematogenous and lymphatic dissemination throughout the body and to other parts of the lungs. Certain organs favor survival of the bacilli and these may later be affected by disease, e.g. apical and subapical regions of the lungs (*Simon focus*), where there is a higher oxygen tension, renal parenchyma, epiphyseal lines of bones, cerebral cortex and regional nodes. At about 4–8 weeks, acquired immunity develops, which coincides with sensitivity to tuberculoprotein, and this usually contains the infection. Multiplication of bacilli ceases and, in the great majority of cases, they either die or remain dormant indefinitely within the healing tubercle or macrophages. The tubercles, especially those which are large and are situated in the apical and subapical regions of the lungs, may become active again (reactivate) at any time during the person's life, if the balance between the organism and the host defense is upset.

In children, the primary focus in the lung is usually small or invisible on chest X-ray, but the regional nodes are enlarged and prominent. In contrast, regional nodes are usually not prominent in primary infection in adults.

The initial infection is usually asymptomatic. Occasionally a short period of fever and malaise may have been noted. Erythema nodosum may appear within a few weeks of the primary infection and coincide with tuberculin conversion. It is an allergic hypersensitivity reaction, which may be associated with high levels of circulating immune complexes. Phlyctenular conjunctivitis is another, though rare, manifestation of hypersensitivity.

If the infecting load of bacilli is large or the host defense inadequate there may be (Fig. 26.26):

1. extension of the lung focus;
2. softening of the regional nodes;

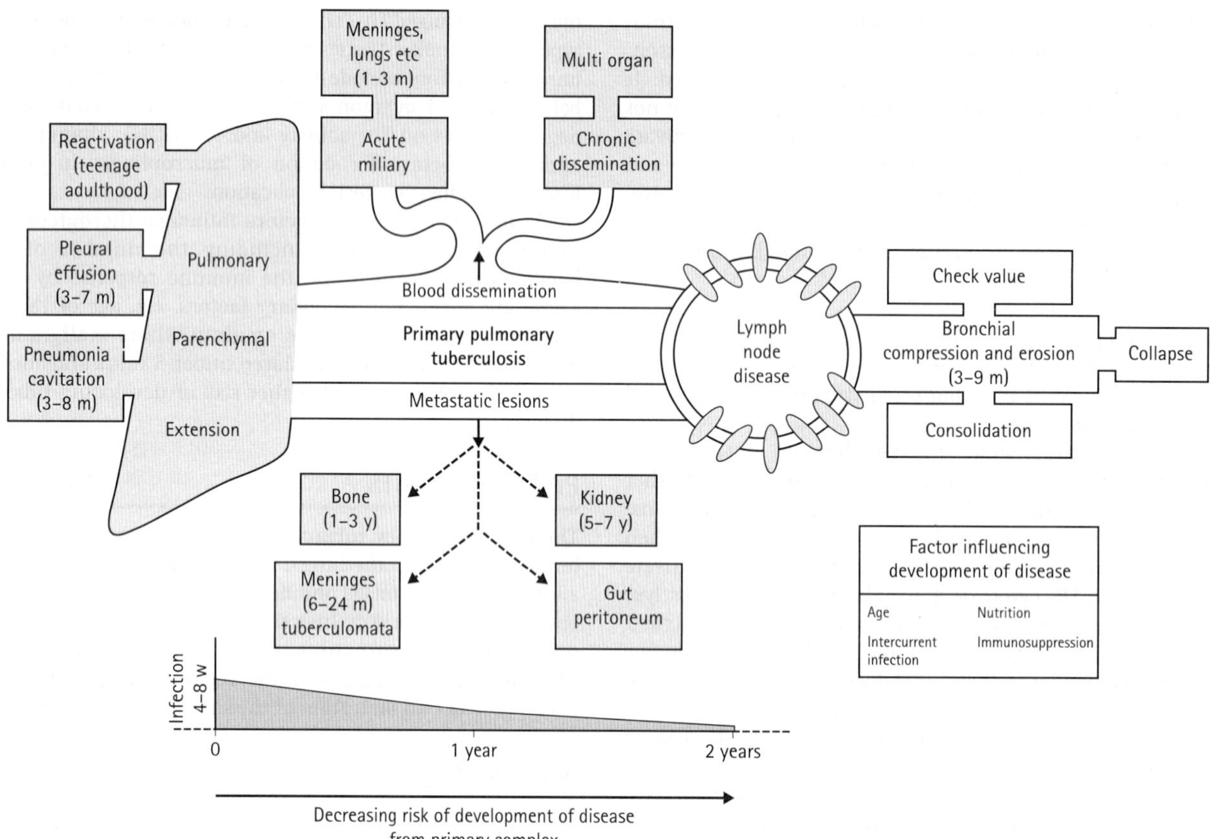

Fig. 26.26 Complications of primary pulmonary tuberculosis. Approximate interval between establishment of primary complex and development of complications in parentheses.

3. extension of foci in other parts of the body;
4. hematogenous spread with dissemination of bacilli throughout the body (miliary tuberculosis), or chronic low grade dissemination (cryptogenic tuberculosis).

In a newly infected person the risk of developing tuberculous disease is highest in the first 2 years following a primary infection (especially in the first year), and diminishing thereafter. The risk is greater in infants and young children and those with malnutrition or immunosuppression. Infants have a risk of 40% or more of developing disease compared with 5% for adults. Pulmonary disease, miliary tuberculosis and meningitis are usually manifest within 1 year of infection, especially in young children, whereas bone disease presents later (within 3 years), and renal disease usually much later (over 5–7 years).

POSTPRIMARY TUBERCULOSIS

Postprimary tuberculosis occurs when tuberculosis in a previously infected person becomes active and is characterized by strong resistance, which keeps the disease localized to the affected organ, and an active hypersensitivity state, which results in extensive tissue destruction and necrosis. The tubercle bacillus may have reached this area through blood spread following primary infection or via the airways in exogenous reinfection. For the latter, as the apices are not well ventilated, multiple exposure will usually be necessary.[259] It affects particularly the apical regions of the lungs, where the oxygen tension is higher. There is widespread caseation necrosis, liquefaction with cavity formation and healing by fibrosis.

Postprimary tuberculosis can develop from endogenous reactivation of a primary lesion, exogenous reinfection or both. Though sometimes termed 'adult'-type pulmonary tuberculosis, it may be seen in children.[260]

TUBERCULIN SENSITIVITY

The intradermal tuberculin test using old tuberculin was described by Charles Mantoux in 1908. A positive response results in induration within 72 h, associated with migration of activated lymphocytes and macrophages to the site of injection.

Different strengths of purified protein derivative (PPD-S) are available: 1 tuberculin unit (TU)/0.1 ml (1:10 000 solution), 5 TU/0.1 ml (1:5000 solution), 10 TU/0.1 ml (1:1000 solution) and 100 TU/0.1 ml (1:100 solution). The addition of Tween 80 to PPD reduces the adsorption to the walls of the syringe and multiplies the strength by a factor of 4–5. Thus, 1 TU with Tween 80 is approximately equivalent to 5 TU without it.[255] For surveys, 2 TU of PPD with Tween 80 is commonly used. In clinical practice, 5–10 TU PPD in 0.1 ml solution is used. In phlyctenular conjunctivitis or tuberculosis of the eye 1 TU is used initially as it is suggested that a stronger solution may result in a severe eye reaction. In the UK 10 units of the Evans vaccines PPD with Tween is used; in the USA and some other countries 5 TU PPD-S is the standard dose. 100 TU is rarely used as it may give a false positive response, more likely to be due to environmental mycobacteria.

TECHNIQUE OF TUBERCULIN TEST

If necessary, the skin may be cleaned with spirit and allowed to dry. The injection is given *intradermally* into the upper third of the flexor surface of the forearm with a 1 ml syringe and a small needle (short bevel gauge 25–27) producing a wheal of at least 5 mm. The result should be read at 48–72 h, but a valid result may be obtained at up to 96 hours. In strongly tuberculin positive subjects, a wheal may appear within 24 h. Rarely, lymphangitis or a systemic reaction may develop following the tuberculin test. If necrosis and ulceration develop, local hydrocortisone ointment may relieve the discomfort.

INTERPRETATION

The transverse diameter of induration is measured. In older children and adults, an indurated wheal of 5 mm or less is regarded as negative, 6–9 mm is likely to be associated with infection by environmental mycobacteria, and 10 mm or greater is indicative of infection by *M. tuberculosis*, unless the person has received BCG recently. *In infants and young children with clinical evidence suggestive of tuberculosis, those with malnutrition or immunosuppression or in close contact with a case, an intermediate reaction of 6–9 mm should be considered positive.* After BCG, the Mantoux response is usually less than 15 mm or Heaf grade 1–2. A Mantoux reaction of greater than or equal to 15 mm in any child is suggestive of sensitivity to *M. tuberculosis*.

A negative or weak response in the presence of tuberculosis may occur in the following conditions: 6–10 weeks after onset of infection, but before tuberculin sensitivity has developed, malnutrition, miliary or overwhelming tuberculosis, non-respiratory disease, especially tuberculous meningitis, tuberculosis in infants less than 6 weeks of age, recent viral infections such as measles and glandular fever, or whooping cough, recent immunization (within 6 weeks) against measles, mumps and rubella, immunosuppressive diseases including HIV, malignancy, and other debilitating diseases, and current treatment with immunosuppressive agents (including corticosteroids). In developing countries, the tuberculin test is often negative in children with tuberculosis, probably owing to immunosuppression due to malnutrition and/or overwhelming disease.

When the tuberculin test is negative in children with tuberculosis due to malnutrition, overwhelming infection or other causes, if it is repeated some months after treatment when the general condition of the patient has improved, it will usually be positive. However, a small proportion of children with culture-proven tuberculosis (perhaps 5%) are consistently negative, despite the absence of adverse factors such as malnutrition, overwhelming tuberculosis or other infections.[260] In children infected by *M. tuberculosis* (and those given BCG), tuberculin sensitivity may revert to negative over some years, particularly in those in whom there was not a strong initial reaction or who have had prompt treatment. This does not necessarily imply that they are not protected from reinfection. Repeated administration of tuberculin in subjects sensitized by BCG or tuberculosis may enhance tuberculin sensitivity (booster phenomenon).

MULTIPLE PUNCTURE TECHNIQUES

Multiple puncture tests such as the Heaf test are used to screen large numbers of children. Other tests include the Tine and Imotest. The Heaf test is the most reliable, but all doubtful reactions following multiple puncture techniques should be confirmed by a Mantoux test.

The Heaf gun has six needles arranged in a circle which puncture the skin through a strong solution of PPD (100 000 units/ml). The needles are set at 2 mm for children 2 years and over, and at 1 mm for those younger. Disposable heads or units are used which dispenses with the need for sterilization. The result may be read at any time from 3 to 10 days after the puncture, and is graded as follows: grade 1, at least four small indurated papules; grade 2, an indurated ring formed by confluent papules; grade 3, a disc of induration; grade 4, induration over 10 mm. Grade 1 is interpreted as unlikely to be associated with *M. tuberculosis* infection, grades 3–4 strongly support tuberculous infection and grade 2 is indeterminate. A grade 2 Heaf response is approximately equivalent to that of a positive Mantoux test of 5–14 mm using 10 TU and grade 3 or 4 to a Mantoux response of greater or equal to 15 mm.

BCG VACCINATION

BCG vaccine is an attenuated bovine strain of mycobacteria introduced by Calmette and Guérin in France in 1921 and originally given orally. It was first used in Sweden in 1927 and in England in 1948.

After intradermal injection of BCG, there is dissemination of small numbers of bacilli to internal organs, particularly the liver and lungs where granulomata develop. BCG sensitizes individuals so that when they are infected by *M. tuberculosis* multiplication of bacteria is curtailed and a granuloma develops quickly which walls off the infection. Systemic hematogenous dissemination is reduced, as also is secondary infection of the lung either from local extension of lesions or seeding from the blood. BCG vaccination does not prevent tuberculous infection; it particularly reduces the chances of disseminated disease and meningitis (and death), and, to a lesser extent, pulmonary disease.

INDICATIONS

In the UK, BCG vaccination is recommended for the following groups:[261]

1. schoolchildren between the ages of 10 and 14 years;
2. newly born babies, children or adults where the parents or the individuals themselves request BCG vaccination;
3. health service staff who may have contact with infectious patients or their specimens (it is particularly important to test and immunize staff working in maternity and pediatric departments in which the patients are likely to be immunocompromised, e.g. transplant, oncology and HIV units);
4. veterinary and other staff who handle animal species known to be susceptible to tuberculosis, e.g. simians;
5. staff of prisons, old people's homes, refugee hostels and hostels for the homeless;
6. contacts of cases known to be suffering from active pulmonary tuberculosis (see Prevention and contact tracing, and Management during pregnancy and of the newborn);
7. immigrants from countries with a high prevalence of tuberculosis, their children and infants, wherever born;
8. those intending to stay in Asia, Africa, central or South America for more than 1 month.

MASS CAMPAIGNS

In countries with a high prevalence of tuberculosis, BCG is given at birth or in early infancy. In countries such as the UK where there is a low prevalence of tuberculosis, it is given at 10–14 years.

CONTRAINDICATIONS

BCG vaccination is contraindicated in patients with immunosuppressive disorders, malignancy and those receiving corticosteroids or immunosuppressive treatment, and in generalized infective conditions. If eczema exists, vaccination should be given in an area free from skin lesions. An interval of

3 weeks should be allowed between administration of BCG vaccine and other live vaccines, with the exception of oral polio vaccine. BCG vaccination is not given to tuberculin positive subjects including those Heaf grade 2 or more.

The recommendations for BCG vaccination of infants born to mothers infected by human immunodeficiency virus (HIV) varies according to the prevalence of tuberculosis. In industrialized countries, BCG is contraindicated in HIV-infected infants, whether they are symptomatic or not. In countries where both HIV infection and tuberculosis are endemic, routine immunization of newborns is recommended.

TECHNIQUE

BCG is given to subjects whose Mantoux is less than 6 mm or who are Heaf grade 0 or 1. In people with a definite BCG scar, even if the tuberculin test is negative, revaccination is unnecessary. Newborns and infants up to the age of 3 months do not require a prevaccination tuberculin test. In developing countries, a prevaccination tuberculin test is not usually given at any age.

The vaccination is given by intradermal injection, usually into the left upper arm at the insertion of the deltoid muscle; 0.1 ml is given with a 1 ml syringe and a gauge 25–27 needle (as per Mantoux test). It is advised that newborn infants are given 0.05 ml because of the increased chance of local lymphadenopathy. Older infants may be given 0.1 ml. Proper technique is essential. The needle should be inserted for about 2 mm and a wheal of at least 5–7 mm produced. If resistance is not felt during injecting, the needle has been inserted too far (or the fluid has leaked externally) and it should be withdrawn. Injecting the vaccine subcutaneously may result in an abscess or large ulcer. BCG vaccination may also be given by the percutaneous multiple puncture technique using a modified Heaf gun (18–20 needles). It is more convenient and easier for newborn infants. A specific vaccine for percutaneous BCG should be used. A scar is detected less often than with the intradermal method but there are similar rates of conversion.[262] Study of efficacy of intradermal versus percutaneous BCG administration is required. Jet injectors are not advised because of the likelihood of mechanical fault. Normally a small papule develops at the site of vaccination within 2–6 weeks. Sometimes it may ulcerate and discharge but it usually heals after about 2–3 months, leaving a small scar (for management see Complications).

ACCELERATED BCG REACTION

If BCG vaccination is given to people infected by tuberculosis or who have received BCG previously, an accelerated reaction may result; a papule appears within 24–48 h, a pustule by 5–7 days, and a scab by 2 weeks. In malnourished children with tuberculosis, the Mantoux test is often negative but there may be an accelerated reaction to BCG. A papule of 5 mm or more appearing by the third day is regarded as positive. BCG is considered to be equivalent to 20–50 TU PPD. Because of the risk that a malnourished child has HIV infection, this practice is now not recommended.

COMPLICATIONS

Adverse reactions to BCG over 1% usually indicate incorrect dosage or bad technique. The commonest complication is abscess formation and the development of a large ulcer. Swelling of local lymph nodes with or without sinus formation is more likely in young infants. These complications usually result from an inadvertent subcutaneous injection. Excess volume of vaccine or the use of a vaccine with a higher potency may also be responsible. Both *Staphylococcus aureus* and/or the BCG mycobacterium may be cultured from the lesion.

Non-fluctuant enlarged nodes should be left untreated. Abscesses should be aspirated. If repeated aspiration of fluctuant nodes does not result in resolution they may be excised. Discharging ulcers should be cleaned with an antiseptic two or three times a day, left uncovered as much as possible, and, when necessary, a non-adherent dressing should be used. For ulcers that do not respond to these methods, isoniazid 6 mg/kg/day for 6 weeks usually results in healing. Hypertrophic or keloid scars may develop at the site of vaccination especially if given at sites other than insertion of the deltoid. Excision is not always successful. Local injection of triamcinolone at monthly intervals for three to four doses may result in atrophy.

Other rare complications of BCG vaccination include anaphylactic reactions, satellite lesions, bone lesions, meningitis or overwhelming infection. The latter usually occurs in immunodeficient infants.[263] Risk of complications in infants of HIV-infected mothers given BCG in the neonatal period is small; rarely disseminated BCG may occur.[264] Focal lesions such as osteitis may occur in apparently immunocompetent infants and in some cases has been associated with increased potency of the vaccine. This complication has been reported particularly from Sweden and Finland.[265,266] Osteitis may develop some years after vaccination. In HIV-infected infants, enlarged lymph nodes with sinus formation may develop months after the vaccination has apparently healed, coinciding with the onset of immunosuppression.

EFFICACY

The effectiveness of BCG in preventing tuberculosis, particularly disseminated disease and meningitis, has been demonstrated in a number of prospective trials and case control studies.[265] It also provides some protection against leprosy and Buruli ulcer. Protection is greatest within a few years after neonatal BCG vaccination and persists for up to 10 years. However, the results of studies vary between different communities and are influenced by factors such as the prevalence of and exposure to tuberculosis, distance from the equator, the prevalence of environmental mycobacteria, the administration and potency of the vaccine, and the age and nutritional status of the population.[267]

Schoolchildren in the UK vaccinated at around 13 years have demonstrated a consistent level of protection of about 75% persisting for 15 years.[268]

Two controlled trials of BCG in the newborn, one in North American Indians living in Saskatchewan, the other in Chicago, have shown 75–80% protection rate, and some case control studies have also demonstrated considerable protection.[269,270] BCG given a few months after birth may result in a better immunological response and have a lower complication rate.

In the northern hemisphere, BCG continues to provide substantial protection against tuberculosis overall and up to 80% for disseminated disease.[271] Some reasons for failure in warm climates are outlined above. Where there is a high prevalence of environmental mycobacteria, immunity to tuberculosis may not be enhanced by BCG.

TUBERCULIN SENSITIVITY AFTER BCG VACCINATION

When the technique and potency of vaccine is adequate, most vaccinated infants will have a scar and over 90% will be tuberculin positive. Tuberculin sensitivity (usually Heaf grade 1–2) will remain in most children for at least 5–12 years.[272,273] Preterm infants and those with severe intrauterine growth retardation may have a reduced response to BCG vaccination, possibly due to impaired cell-mediated immunity. Scars are less likely to persist in infants vaccinated in the neonatal period.

In developing countries, tuberculin sensitivity following neonatal BCG wanes considerably over the first few years. Most older children will be tuberculin negative or have low sensitivity.[274] Thus neonatal BCG should not affect the interpretation of the tuberculin test. In children recently vaccinated with BCG, who are in contact with a smear-positive case of tuberculosis, a Mantoux reaction of 15 mm or more or Heaf grade 3–4 should be interpreted as likely infection by *M. tuberculosis*. Repeat BCG vaccination is associated with larger tuberculin reactions.

NEW VACCINES

Vaccines are required which are more effective in preventing exogenous reinfection and in people already infected by environmental mycobacteria or in those who have received conventional BCG. Randomized controlled trials of administration of *M. vaccae* to adults on chemotherapy for tuberculosis have not demonstrated improved outcome.[275,276]

PREVENTION AND CONTACT TRACING

In the UK today, the majority of children in whom tuberculosis is diagnosed are detected through contact tracing of smear-positive cases of tuberculosis. Children with primary tuberculosis and patients with non-respiratory tuberculosis are rarely infectious. However, children with tuberculosis and their visitors should be segregated from the rest of the ward until family and visitors have been screened. Smear-positive adults who receive drug regimens which include rifampicin usually have a negative sputum culture within 2 weeks.

Procedures for control and prevention of tuberculosis in the UK have been outlined.[277] When a case of tuberculosis is diagnosed, household contacts should be screened. Children and young adults should have a tuberculin test and, when positive, a chest X-ray. Older adults and those who have received BCG vaccination should have a chest X-ray. If the tuberculin test is negative, it should be repeated after 6 weeks as the first test may have been done too early in the course of infection. Tuberculin negative subjects should be offered BCG. Tuberculin positive subjects with a normal chest X-ray should be given chemoprophylaxis (see below).

In the majority of cases of tuberculosis in young children, the source of infection is in the home. For older children it may be necessary to search outside the home, e.g. staff at school, a swimming pool attendant or a youth leader. In tuberculosis of the face or gums, the possibility of infection by a dentist should be considered.

CHEMOPROPHYLAXIS AND FOLLOW-UP OF CONTACTS

This section outlines the recommendations for chemoprophyaxis of contacts of a known case of tuberculosis.
Chemoprophylaxis is indicated for tuberculin-positive children (Heaf grades 2–4) with a normal chest X-ray, who have not had BCG. It should be considered in those with grade 3–4 who have received BCG. Guidelines for children < 2 years in close contact with smear-positive pulmonary disease are as follows :

1. *Without prior BCG*: give chemoprophylaxis irrespective of tuberculin test. Repeat tuberculin test after 6 weeks, if negative stop chemoprophylaxis and give BCG. If repeat tuberculin test is positive give full chemoprophylaxis if chest X-ray excludes disease.
2. *Prior BCG*: if tuberculin test is strongly positive (Heaf grade 3–4) give chemoprophylaxis. If tuberculin test is weak (Heaf grade 0–2), repeat in 6 weeks. If there is no change, no further action is required. If size of reaction increases, give full chemoprophylaxis if chest X-ray excludes disease. Routine follow-up chest X-rays are only required for those who are eligible for, but did not receive, chemoprophylaxis.

For chemoprophylaxis, isoniazid (INH) plus rifampicin (RIF) should be given for 3 months, or INH only 6 mg/kg/day should be given for 6 months. In young infants exposed to smear-positive patients, or in contacts at any age when the source is suspected to harbor INH-resistant *M. tuberculosis*, rifampicin may be added to INH and the combination given for 4–6 months. If INH resistance is confirmed RIF alone may be given for 6–9 months.[278]

SCHOOLS BCG PROGRAM

Children with a definite BCG scar or documented history of prior BCG vaccination do not require a Heaf test.

Children with Heaf grade 0 and 1 are given BCG; no action is required for those with grade 2; for Heaf grade 3–4 with normal chest X-rays, chemoprophylaxis is recommended for those with a history of contact with tuberculosis or residence in a high prevalence area within the preceding 2 years, and should be considered for others in high-risk groups.

CLINICAL FORMS OF TUBERCULOSIS

The commonest presentation of tuberculosis is respiratory disease followed by involvement of lymph nodes. However, unless culture of peripheral lymph node tissue is obtained, infection by environmental mycobacteria cannot be differentiated from that by *M. tuberculosis*. In the 1988 survey of childhood tuberculosis in England and Wales, non-respiratory lesions were present in approximately one-third of children, some of whom also had a respiratory lesion (Table 26.26). In developing countries, where the diagnosis is often late, non-respiratory disease is common, with or without respiratory disease. It is important to remember that tuberculosis can infect virtually any part of the body. Figure 26.26 shows an outline and a time scale of some of the complications of primary tuberculosis.

INTRATHORACIC TUBERCULOSIS

The distribution of respiratory and non-respiratory disease seen in children in England and Wales in 1988 is shown in Table 26.26.

Primary pulmonary tuberculosis

The primary complex consists of a focal lesion usually 1–2 cm in diameter which may be found in any part of the lung, and enlarged hilar nodes or, in heavier infections, the paratracheal nodes (Figs 26.27 and 26.28). Lymph node enlargement is particularly prominent in infants and young children. The primary complex is usually asymptomatic and discovered during contact tracing or a routine tuberculin test. Often the primary focus has resolved or is not visible and the diagnosis is based on enlarged regional nodes. Calcification of the focus and, more often, the nodes may occur after about 12 months, generally within 2–3 years of the infection, and remains an indication of previous infection. Calcification usually indicates healing of the tuberculous process, but healing and progression of the disease may continue concurrently. In many

Table 26.26 Clinical presentation of tuberculosis in children in England and Wales for 1988

Respiratory disease	n = 213	%	Non-respiratory disease*	n = 101	%
Pulmonary	166	78	Peripheral lymph nodes	61	60
Intrathoracic lymph nodes	55	26	Central nervous system	15	15
Pleural	12	6	Miliary	7	7
			Abdominal	7	7
			Bone and joint	6	6
			Other†	13	13

* 20 children had both respiratory and non-respiratory disease
† Other includes: genitourinary (3), pericarditis (1), abscess (2)
Source: Medical Research Council Cardiothoracic Epidemiology Group 1994[278a]

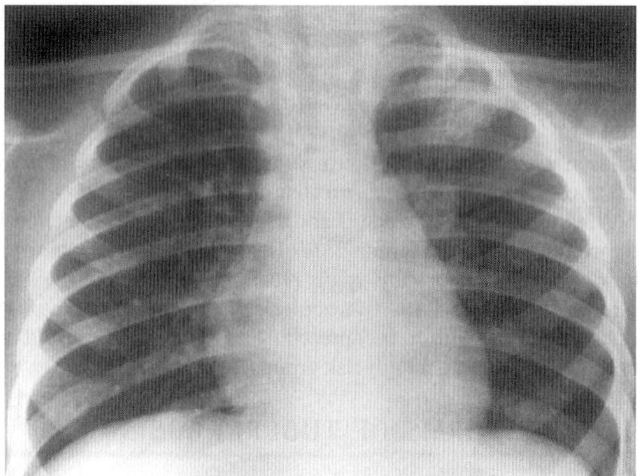

Fig. 26.27 Primary tuberculosis in a 2-year-old child. Primary focus in the left upper lobe with enlarged regional nodes.

cases the calcium slowly resolves leaving clear lung fields, which explains the common finding in adults where the tuberculin test is positive and the chest X-ray normal.

In older children and adolescents, the lung component is more prominent and commonly presents as an enlarging upper lobe infiltrate and cavitation, usually without lymph node enlargement, and is indistinguishable from postprimary tuberculosis. Pleural effusion is commoner at this age (Fig. 26.28).

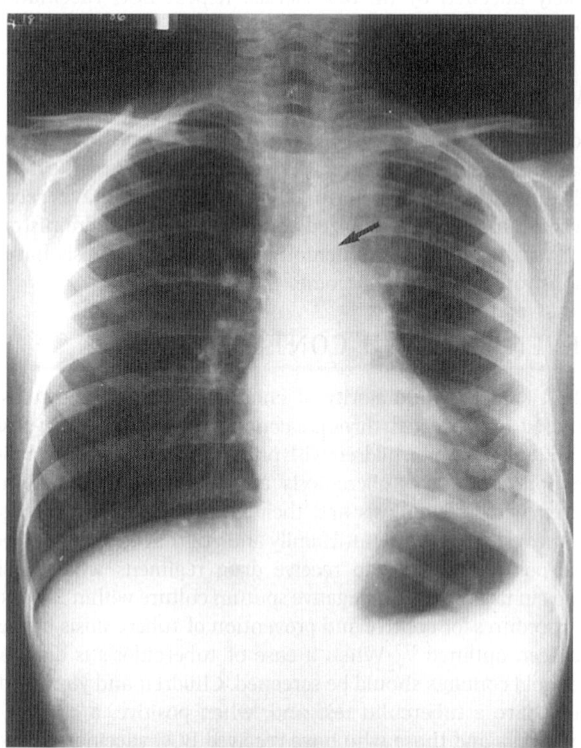

Fig. 26.28 A 10-year-old boy with primary tuberculosis. There is consolidation of the left upper lobe, displacement of the lower trachea and left main bronchus by enlarged nodes (→) and a pleural effusion.

Progression of primary tuberculosis

Progression of primary tuberculosis may result from extension of the pulmonary focus (progressive primary tuberculosis), or more commonly, softening of regional lymph nodes. Extension of the pulmonary focus may cause bronchopneumonia or rupture into the pleura resulting in pleural effusion. Tuberculous empyema may result from rupture of caseous material into the pleural space, which may be complicated by pneumothorax (pyopneumothorax). Evacuation of caseous material into a bronchus may result in the appearance of a cavity. Cavities in primary pulmonary tuberculosis are not uncommon in malnourished and debilitated infants with progressive primary tuberculosis.

Complications from enlargement or softening of regional nodes have a variety of manifestations. The bronchus may be compressed externally; more likely, the wall is eroded and caseous material either partly or completely blocks the lumen (endobronchial tuberculosis); or rupture of the wall results in bronchopneumonia. Partial obstruction may result in a ball–valve effect with lobar emphysema. This is often transient, because either the bronchus blocks completely or the material is coughed up with clearing of the obstruction.[279] More commonly, there is *segmental* collapse with or without consolidation. Rupture of caseous material into the bronchus may result in a predominantly allergic response with exudation, or, if there are a large number of bacteria present, a progressive tuberculous bronchopneumonia. The former may be associated with marked changes on chest X-ray but which clear spontaneously, whereas the latter, which is more often seen in debilitated children, may prove fatal if not treated. Spread of infected material into both main bronchi may result in bilateral bronchopneumonia.

Rarely, a caseous node may rupture into the trachea, resulting in bilateral obstructive emphysema or asphyxia, into the esophagus resulting in a fistula or the development of an esophageal pouch, or into the pericardium. Other complications from enlarged nodes include superior vena cava obstruction, and recurrent laryngeal or phrenic nerve compression.

There may be non-specific symptoms of irregular fever, anorexia, weight loss and, in severe or longstanding cases, the child may be marasmic. Compression of the bronchi may result in a spasmodic cough simulating whooping cough. When there is obstructive emphysema, the symptoms may be mistaken for asthma, though clinical examination will usually demonstrate signs of mediastinal shift. In longstanding cases, the child may present with clubbing of the fingers and bronchiectasis.

Adolescent tuberculosis

In adolescents, infection is usually in the upper lobes or the superior segments of the lower lobes, and is confined to the lungs with no hematogenous spread. In some cases it results from reactivation of a former primary lesion (postprimary tuberculosis) and, though usually associated with adults, it may occur in children and adolescents. Evidence of a previous primary pulmonary complex may be detected.[279] In other cases it is a primary exogenous infection. Common symptoms include a productive cough, especially in the morning, and there may be hemoptysis, fever, night sweats, malaise and weight loss.

Chest X-ray may show a variety of lesions including nodular or patchy shadows, cavities and various stages of healing with fibrosis and calcification. Both lungs may be affected and there may be a pleural effusion.

Diagnosis

The diagnosis of primary pulmonary tuberculosis is based on a positive tuberculin test (Mantoux > 10 mm) and enlarged nodes on chest X-ray with or without a pulmonary infiltrate. History of contact provides strong support. Enlarged lymph nodes may not be easily demonstrated; a lateral chest X-ray may be helpful. Persistent pulmonary infiltrate(s) in the presence of a positive tuberculin test is highly suggestive of tuberculosis.

Chest X-ray usually shows enlarged nodes with opacities more often in the right than left lung, due to collapse and/or consolidation. Bilateral disease may be seen in 25% of cases. In progressive disease, cavities may be seen. Lymph nodes may be detected on CT scan in children with normal chest X-rays.[280] In debilitated children, the tuberculin test may be negative. This is a common problem in developing countries where, in the absence of facilities for mycobacterial culture, the diagnosis is often based on the response to a trial of chemotherapy.

In older children with postprimary or adult type tuberculosis, diagnosis is made by smear and culture of sputum. For younger children, if sensitivities of the contact are not available or diagnosis is unclear, three early-morning gastric aspirations should be undertaken while the child is recumbent and has been fasted overnight. If the gastric aspirate (usually 5–10 ml) is very small or the tube is blocked, sterile water (< 20 ml) may be injected and after a few minutes aspirated. If there is delay in transporting the specimen to the laboratory, the acid should be neutralized (pH 7.0) by adding approximately 3 ml of sodium bicarbonate (100 mg/ml). Smear is seldom positive on gastric aspirates and in some cases it may be due to environmental mycobacteria. Culture is positive in no more than 30–50% of cases.[281,282] It is more likely to be positive in infants (75%) and those with extensive parenchymal disease.[283] However, it may be positive in children with only enlarged intrathoracic nodes and rarely in those with normal chest X-ray. Gastric aspiration undertaken in an ambulatory clinic has generally lower sensitivity for culture than when taken in the early morning. PCR is more sensitive than culture of gastric aspirates in identification of tuberculosis infection but does not differentiate from active disease (see Microbiology).

Laryngeal swabs or nasopharyngeal aspirates are useful for ambulatory clinics and when gastric aspiration is not possible.[284,285] Induced sputum is also valuable and may be undertaken in infants, or adolescents without productive sputum.[286,287] Bronchoscopy is no more sensitive for culture of *M. tuberculosis* than gastric aspiration.[288,289] Where diagnosis is important for management, biopsy of enlarged lymph nodes should be considered.

The blood count usually shows a normal white cell count. A raised ESR is associated with activity of the disease but otherwise has no diagnostic value.

A *pleural effusion* is due to an allergic response to the mycobacteria and thus the tuberculin test is usually strongly positive, except in very debilitated children. If large, or required for diagnostic purposes, it should be aspirated. The fluid is usually clear and straw-colored, but may be opalescent if there is a high cell count. Lymphocytes will be seen on microscopy, but early in the disease neutrophils may also be present. The protein content will be raised, > 40 g/L, and the glucose low, < 1.7 mmol/L. Mycobacteria are often not detected on direct smear, but in about half the cases they may be cultured, especially if a large volume of fluid is centrifuged. Mycobacteria are more likely to be cultured from an empyema. Pleural biopsy may also be taken for histology.

Management

Uncomplicated primary infection usually heals without treatment. The main purpose of chemotherapy is to prevent hematogenous spread and progression of disease, which is more likely in young, debilitated or malnourished children. Segmental collapse may occur despite chemotherapy, but tuberculous bronchopneumonia or pleural effusion is usually prevented. Radiological changes resolve slowly and 50% of children may still have evidence of the primary complex after 18 months. Lymph nodes may enlarge during chemotherapy, but there is usually no necessity to prolong therapy because of this.

Standard three-drug chemotherapy is isoniazid (INH), rifampicin (RIF) and pyrazinamide (PZA) for 2 months followed by INH and RIF for 4 months. Ethambutol (EMB) is added if drug resistance is suspected. If PZA is not given, INH + RIF should be given for 9 months. For alternative regimens see section on Chemotherapy. For hilar lymphadenopathy alone a three-drug regimen followed by INH + RIF for just 2 months or two drugs followed by INH + RIF for 6 months is adequate.[290]

Bronchial obstruction

Incomplete bronchial obstruction with air trapping and the development of *obstructive emphysema* may respond to corticosteroids (see Management). However, the transient nature of this lesion should be remembered, i.e. it may resolve or the bronchus may become completely obstructed. Complete obstruction will result in absorption collapse, and bronchoscopy should be performed to exclude other pathology, such as foreign body, and to suck out as much of the caseous material in the bronchial lumen as possible. Unfortunately, the obstruction may be difficult to visualize, especially in young infants.

Pleural effusion

The infective load in pleural effusion is low and responds quickly to treatment. The addition of corticosteroids may enhance the absorption of fluid but long term benefit regarding reduction of pleural thickening and adhesions has not been demonstrated.[291] In the presence of empyema, surgical drainage may be required.

Pericarditis

M. tuberculosis may reach the pericardium by lymphatic extension from mediastinal lymph nodes, direct extension from caseous lung tissue or lymph nodes, or from hematogenous spread. It is more common in developing countries.[292] In dry pericarditis, a loud pericardial rub may be heard. Occasionally, there is a large effusion, which may cause tamponade. An effusion will be detected by echocardiography. Pericardial aspirate is often bloodstained, and polymorphonuclear leukocytes may be seen in the early stages, after which lymphocytes predominate. *M. tuberculosis* may be cultured in over half the cases, and up to 75% using double strength Kirchner culture medium.[293] Diagnosis may also be made by culture and histology of a pericardial biopsy. Constrictive pericarditis may follow in spite of treatment.

Standard antituberculous treatment is given. Open drainage may prevent subsequent requirement for pericardial aspiration. Corticosteroids may enhance the rate of improvement, reduce the requirement for aspiration, but seem not to reduce the need for pericardiectomy.[293,324]

EXTRATHORACIC TUBERCULOSIS

About 25–35% of tuberculosis is non-respiratory, of which lymph node disease predominates (Fig 26.26). Non-respiratory disease usually results from hematogenous spread and arises from extension of a primary focus or extension of a regional node. Virtually any organ may be affected, and particularly in developing countries where non-respiratory disease is common, tuberculosis should be remembered in *any* unusual lesion where the diagnosis is not known. Some of the common types are described below. Tuberculosis may also affect the larynx, middle ear and mastoid bones. Middle ear disease may be associated with HIV infection. Virtually any part of the eye may be infected and tuberculosis should be remembered as a cause of an orbital mass. Tuberculosis of the skin may result from primary inoculation, from hematogenous dissemination, or from a cold abscess in an underlying structure.

Lymph node tuberculosis

Superficial lymph node tuberculosis commonly occurs in the cervical or supraclavicular, and, less often, the axillary or inguinal regions. As in primary tuberculosis of the lungs, the regional nodes enlarge in response to a focus. Less commonly, enlargement of a number of superficial lymph nodes results from hematogenous spread. The focus may be the tonsils, gums, lungs, or elsewhere. In cervical adenitis, the commonest focus is the upper lung fields. Enlarged axillary or inguinal nodes may be due to disseminated disease or infection of the skin. In the UK, in the majority of cases of white children with histological evidence of mycobacterial infection of the cervical glands, it is associated with environmental mycobacteria such as *M. avium-intracellulare. M. tuberculosis is* commoner in immigrant children.

Initially the nodes are discrete, mobile and non-tender, later becoming matted together. The primary node is the largest, with those draining it being progressively smaller. Without treatment, softening of nodes usually develops within 6 months of infection, and nodes may discharge forming a sinus or track along the fascial planes. Swelling and softening may occur in up to a third of patients during treatment or even years after the node is calcified and apparently healed. This phenomenon may be due to hypersensitivity to tuberculoprotein, released at intervals from the lesion, and does not necessarily indicate active infection.

The tuberculin test is usually positive and a chest X-ray should be taken to exclude pulmonary tuberculosis. Calcification within the node may be detected radiologically. Ultrasound or magnetic resonance imaging are helpful in confirming the lesion is a lymph node and in detection of caseous necrosis. Needle aspiration for smear and culture, or preferably excision biopsy, will usually confirm the diagnosis. All specimens, either from biopsy or aspiration, should be cultured as it is important to ascertain whether the infection is caused by *M. tuberculosis* or environmental mycobacteria. However, culture may be positive in only two-thirds of cases. The main differential diagnosis is from a cervical pyogenic abscess. Local viral or streptococcal infection of the tonsils may cause enlargement of existing tuberculous nodes. Other differential diagnoses include glandular fever, HIV infection, cat-scratch disease, malignancy or an infected branchial or thyroglossal cyst.

Treatment with standard chemotherapy is adequate. If softening of the node occurs, it may be aspirated. If excision is necessary, the primary node should be removed intact, or, if not feasible, as much of the caseous material as possible.[255] It is important to remember that cold abscesses are frequently of the 'collar stud' variety and that adequate drainage of the abscess in the deep fascia is necessary.

Disseminated tuberculosis

Hematogenous dissemination of small numbers of bacilli probably occurs in the majority of children with primary uncomplicated tuberculosis. In developing countries, a liver biopsy for an unconnected disease may show tuberculous granulomata in children not known to have had tuberculosis. These rarely become symptomatic. Massive hematogenous spread is referred to as acute miliary tuberculosis and if untreated is usually rapidly fatal. It may be associated with extension of caseous necrosis involving a blood vessel. It may be found at autopsy without being evident on chest X-ray. A more chronic form, cryptogenic disseminated, also occurs. In both forms, disease may develop in virtually any organ of the body.

Acute miliary tuberculosis

Acute miliary tuberculosis is commonest in young children and usually occurs within a year of the primary infection. The most important complication is meningitis. The onset is usually insidious. Presenting signs include pyrexia, dyspnea, anemia, hepatosplenomegaly and lymphadenopathy.[294] Anorexia and weight loss are common and variable degrees of malnutrition will be evident depending on the length of the illness. The lungs show a 'snowstorm' picture on chest X-ray. Rarely, respiratory failure with adult respiratory distress syndrome may develop. Choroid tubercles are pathognomonic of the disease. Cutaneous lesions include macules, papules, purpura and papulonecrotic tuberculides.

Except in the early stages, the diagnosis will usually be evident from a chest X-ray (snowstorm appearance). There may also be lobar infiltrates and hilar lymphadenopathy. The tuberculin test may be weak or negative in the early stages or if the child has severe debility. A lumbar puncture is essential in all cases to exclude meningitis. Bacteriological confirmation will be obtained in the majority of children, particularly from culture of gastric contents, and also CSF and urine. In difficult cases the diagnosis is sometimes made on liver, lung or marrow biopsy.

The differential diagnosis is wide depending on the geographical area. The lung disease may simulate tuberculous bronchopneumonia, HIV-related pulmonary disorders, Langerhans' cell histiocytoses, cystic fibrosis or idiopathic pulmonary hemosiderosis; and the systemic disease typhoid fever, systemic leishmaniasis, leukemia, collagen diseases and chronic malaria.

Acute miliary disease usually responds promptly to chemotherapy. Most deaths are related to meningitis and/or late diagnosis. A short course of corticosteroids will speed the resolution of symptoms, especially if there is alveolar capillary block. Standard chemotherapy is adequate. Prolonged (9 months) therapy may be required in complicated cases or meningitis.

Chronic disseminated (cryptic) tuberculosis

In chronic disseminated tuberculosis, small numbers of bacilli seed the bloodstream at intervals and produce metastatic foci in organs throughout the body. Apart from the lung lesions, there is usually generalized lymphadenopathy and often hepatosplenomegaly, and involvement of the pleural, pericardial and peritoneal cavities, bones and kidneys may occur. There may be multiple bone involvement with dactylitis or involvement of the skin with papulonecrotic tuberculides. In some cases the chest X-ray is normal and the primary site is unknown. A variety of hematological abnormalities may be seen, e.g. pancytopenia, or leukemoid reactions, which suggest leukemia or a lymphoma. The tuberculin test may be negative. Bone marrow biopsy may show necrotic foci with little cellular reaction but teeming with mycobacteria.

Treatment is similar to that of acute miliary disease. Corticosteroids may be of benefit in debilitated children.

Tuberculosis of the central nervous system

Tuberculosis of the central nervous system may have a variety of manifestations.[295] There may be generalized inflammation affecting brain and spinal cord; less commonly, single or multiple tuberculomata enlarge and present as an intracranial space-occupying lesion or rarely tuberculous disease may be confined to the spine.

Tuberculous meningitis

Tuberculous meningitis is commonest in children under 5 years of age, often occurring within 6 months and usually within 2 years of primary infection, but it may occur at any age. It results from rupture of one or more tubercles (Rich focus) into the subarachnoid space. The tubercle(s) is commonly situated in the subcortex of the brain, and less often in the meninges or spinal cord. Characteristically, the severe inflammatory response results in a thick gelatinous exudate and adhesions around the base of the brain with hydrocephalus and spinal block. Involvement of cranial nerves may result in single or multiple palsies. Arteritis may cause thrombosis and infarction of nervous tissue with permanent damage. Occasionally there is little exudate and the illness is termed *serous meningitis*. Spontaneous recovery without treatment has been described in some of the latter cases.

Symptoms develop over some weeks and may be grouped into stages, which give a guide to prognosis. Initially, the symptoms are non-specific and include irritability, malaise, anorexia, vomiting, constipation and low grade fever. Unless the child is a contact of tuberculosis or there is a high index of suspicion, the diagnosis is rarely made at this stage. Within a few weeks specific features in addition to the above become apparent: there is headache, disorientation, meningism, focal neurological signs, such as cranial nerve palsy, hemiplegia or visual defect, and seizures may develop. In young infants the fontanelle may be distended. Fundoscopy may demonstrate choroid tubercles, especially when there is miliary disease, papilledema or the development of optic atrophy. The third and often terminal stage is manifest by coma, a posture of decerebrate rigidity, dilated pupils, and the child is usually wasted.

Diagnosis. The diagnosis is based on CSF findings in association with a positive tuberculin test. There may be radiological evidence of pulmonary disease, or disease elsewhere in the body. The tuberculin test may be negative in over a third of cases, especially in the advanced stages when there is wasting. The differential diagnosis includes viral and partially treated pyogenic meningitis, cerebral abscess, subdural empyema, HIV disease, fungal infections, e.g. *Cryptococcus neoformans*, and unusual causes such as sarcoidosis, Lyme disease, leptospirosis, collagen diseases and malignancy.

The CSF is clear, unless there is a high cell count, when it may appear turbid. The cell count is usually less than 500/mm^3 and mainly lymphocytic, except in the very early stages when neutrophils may predominate. Neutrophils may also increase after commencement of chemotherapy. The protein rises to between 0.8 and 4 g/L and in spinal block may be well over 10 g/L and the CSF xanthochromic. The glucose is usually low. However, it should be remembered that the first lumbar puncture may be normal, that the cell count, protein and glucose levels may fluctuate from day to day, and that the cell count and protein may be lower in ventricular than in spinal fluid.[296] The chance of detecting tubercle bacilli microscopically is higher if a large amount of CSF is obtained and centrifuged; the success rate claimed varies from 30 to 90% depending on the care, volume of CSF and time taken in examining the fluid. Brain imaging will be abnormal in 75–100% of cases; usually there is hydrocephalus, also parenchymal disease, and basilar meningitis is typical. If raised intracranial pressure is suspected, CSF should be taken off slowly with a fine needle or from the ventricles. The CSF should always be cultured for mycobacteria, but is positive in less than half the cases. It may be possible to detect tubercle bacilli after chemotherapy has commenced. Occasionally, tuberculous meningitis (TBM) may be complicated by pyogenic meningitis. Studies of TBM, mainly in adults, have demonstrated sensitivities and specificities for PCR in CSF ranging from 33 to 100% and 88 to 100% respectively, and generally higher sensitivity than culture.[297]

Spinal tuberculosis

Spinal tuberculosis is usually secondary to downward extension of the tuberculous process, and usually occurs during treatment of tuberculous meningitis. There is pain and stiffness in the spine at the level of the lesion and symptoms are related to involvement of the spine or nerve roots. The CSF protein is high and there is evidence of a spinal block, which can be confirmed by magnetic resonance imaging (MRI) scan or a myelogram.

Rarely, diffuse tuberculous spinal subarachnoiditis may occur as a result of extension of a primary focus in the spine. It presents as a subacute, transverse or ascending myelitis with upper and lower motor neurone signs and may be mistaken for other causes of cord compression and polyneuritis.

Tuberculoma

A tuberculoma is a tuberculous focus, which enlarges within brain tissue without rupturing. It may be single or multiple. It may give rise to signs of raised intracranial pressure or a hemiplegia, or cranial nerve palsy if in the brainstem. A skull X-ray may show calcification. CT scan usually shows a hypodense mass and ring enhancement with contrast. MRI scan is more sensitive for detecting tuberculomata, infarcts and spinal lesions. Tuberculomata may expand weeks to months after commencing treatment for meningitis or pulmonary tuberculosis and result in raised intracranial pressure sometimes requiring surgical decompression.[298,299] This phenomenon which is termed 'paradoxical enlargement' may be a hypersensitivity response to release of tuberculoprotein and other antigens following destruction of the mycobacteria.

Management

The key to success in treating tuberculous meningitis is early diagnosis and immediate treatment. If there is doubt, antituberculous chemotherapy should be commenced, along with conventional antimicrobials for bacterial meningitis, if necessary.

Optimal chemotherapy is a combination of drugs with good penetration into the CSF and low toxicity. Standard chemotherapy is INH (15–20 mg/kg) and RIF (15–20 mg/kg) which are given for

9–12 months, with the addition of PZA (40 mg/kg) for the first 2 months of treatment. If drug resistance is suspected ethionamide 20 mg/kg, EMB [or streptomycin (SM)] should be added. A 6-month course may be adequate in most cases.[300]

A study of 99 children in Cape Town, of whom 96% had stage II or III, treated for 6 months with isoniazid 20 mg/kg, rifampicin 20 mg/kg, pyrazinamide 40 mg/kg and ethionamide 20 mg/kg had a satisfactory outcome with only one probable relapse.[301]

Drugs cross the blood–brain barrier more readily in the first 2–3 months of the disease when the meninges are inflamed. INH and PZA achieve high levels in the CSF, even when meninges are not inflamed. Ethionamide has adequate, RIF and EMB moderate to poor, and SM poor penetration across the meninges.[302–304] Ethionamide is useful for isoniazid-resistant *M. tuberculosis.* In children who are vomiting, INH, RIF and SM can be given parenterally and other drugs by nasogastric tube. Controlled trials on the value of corticosteroids in tuberculous meningitis have demonstrated benefit especially in stage II and III disease.[303,305–307] The rationale is based on their ability to reduce the inflammatory exudate and thus prevent the development of adhesions which result in internal hydrocephalus and basilar arachnoiditis. In South Africa, 141 children with stage II–III disease were randomized to receive prednisolone 4 mg/kg or placebo for one month.[306] The prednisolone treated group had a reduced mortality in stage III, a better cognitive function in survivors and a reduction in size of existing, and development of new, tuberculomata. Dexamethasone 0.6 mg/kg/day or prednisolone 4 mg/kg/day may be given for 2–3 weeks then tailed off over 2–3 months.

Serial brain imaging should be performed, depending on response to treatment, to detect cerebral edema and the presence or development of hydrocephalus or tuberculomata. In the presence of cerebral edema, controlled ventilation with monitoring of intracranial pressure may be indicated. Obstructive hydrocephalus is common and is not always clinically evident. If it is symptomatic, it should be treated by a ventriculoperitoneal shunt. In the initial stages, before the drugs have controlled the infection, the shunt may be exteriorized.

Spinal arachnoiditis with a CSF block may develop during treatment. If not improved by corticosteroids, release of pressure by surgery may be necessary.

Tuberculomata are treated on similar lines to meningitis. Most of the small and medium-sized lesions resolve completely with chemotherapy. Large lesions and those not responding to chemotherapy may require excision. Enlargement may occur during treatment of pulmonary or tuberculous meningitis, with the development of raised intracranial pressure or localizing signs such as cranial nerve palsy. It may settle without a change of treatment. Corticosteroids should be tried and, failing this, a ventriculoperitoneal shunt may be necessary. Most patients with unresolved tuberculomata have been given prolonged antituberculous therapy, e.g. 12–18 months or more.

Prognosis

The prognosis for meningitis is related to age of the child (young children have worse prognosis) and the stage of the disease at which therapy is commenced. The stages have been classified as follows:

Stage I: consciousness undisturbed; no, or only mild and focal, neurological signs.

Stage II: consciousness disturbed, but patient not comatosed or delirious. Mild or moderate neurological signs, such as paraparesis, hemiparesis, and cranial nerve palsies, may be present.

Stage III: patient comatose or delirious with mild, moderate or severe neurological signs.

In a study of 199 children in Hong Kong, complete recovery occurred as follows: stage I 96%, stage II 78% and stage III 21%. Of children in stage III, 17% died as opposed to 1% in stage II.[308] Resolution of neurological disability may continue for many months after commencement of therapy.

Abdominal tuberculosis

Abdominal tuberculosis usually results from swallowed sputum or *M. bovis*-infected milk, but may be associated with extension from thoracic nodes, hematogenous dissemination, and after the menarche may be an extension of pelvic tuberculosis. The primary focus is usually in the terminal ileum. Symptoms of disease in children are usually due to enlargement or softening of regional mesenteric nodes, and/or involvement of the peritoneum. In adults with cavitatory pulmonary disease, there may be a chronic enteritis and fistulo-in-ano resembling Crohn's disease or other inflammatory bowel disease.

Common symptoms are abdominal pain, fever, weight loss and abdominal swelling or there may be symptoms of intestinal obstruction. Enlarged mesenteric lymph nodes or a mass associated with adhesions of the omentum and intestines may be palpated, usually on the right side of the abdomen.

Peritonitis may be the dominant condition and is often unassociated with demonstrable pulmonary disease. It may result from extension of a mesenteric node or hematogenous spread. In the latter situation, rarely there may be a polyserositis with involvement of the pleura and pericardium. The ascitic fluid has a predominance of lymphocytes, and a protein concentration above 25 g/L (usually lower than in a tuberculous pleural exudate). Mycobacteria are not often identified and the culture may be positive in only a quarter of cases.

Diagnosis is made on the basis of a positive tuberculin test, peritoneal aspiration and bacteriological and histological examination of specimens obtained by laparoscopy, endoscopy, or at laparotomy. Ultrasonography and CT scan are useful for diagnosis and guidance for needle aspiration. Calcification may be detected on abdominal X-ray.

Treatment is by standard chemotherapy.

Tuberculosis of bones and joints

Tuberculosis of bones and joints results from hematogenous spread usually affecting a single or a few joints within 6–36 months of primary infection. The spine is affected in over half the cases (Pott's disease), followed by the knee, hip and ankle. In chronic disseminated tuberculosis, multiple large or small joints may be affected, with or without associated abscesses, or there may be dactylitis of one or both hands. Sometimes punched out cystic lesions are seen with few inflammatory changes affecting surrounding tissue. Lesions confined to the skull may resemble eosinophilic granuloma of bone, or, if associated with miliary disease, the systemic form of Langerhans' cell histiocytosis.

Infection usually starts in the well-vascularized metaphyses near the epiphyseal line of long bones, or, less commonly, in the synovium of the joint. Typically there is minimal periosteal reaction or new bone formation. Progression of the disease may result in destruction of the joint, and/or abscess or sinus formation. The cold abscess may track a considerable distance from the primary focus. For example, a cold abscess from the cervical vertebrae may present as a retropharyngeal mass or, from the lumbar vertebrae, as a psoas abscess pointing in the groin.

Treatment is by standard 6-month chemotherapy. However, if evacuation of necrotic sequestrum and abscesses is not adequate, which might prevent drug penetration, a longer course (9–12 months) may be necessary.[309] Ambulatory chemotherapy without surgery has been found the most satisfactory treatment for spinal disease in developing countries. Acute cord compression may respond to chemotherapy alone, but if the necessary technical expertise is available, early spinal decompression is the treatment of choice. A bone graft in cases of extensive destruction of vertebrae or weightbearing bones, such as the neck of the femur, may be necessary.

Genitourinary tuberculosis

Tuberculosis of the kidneys is uncommon in children as it usually presents 5–7 years or more after the primary infection, although it may occur sooner. The first symptom is dysuria and typically there is a sterile pyuria with or without red cells. There may not be any symptoms and even in advanced disease there may be very few leukocytes in the urine. Culture of urine for mycobacteria is usually positive.

Glomerulonephritis with immune complex disease complicating miliary tuberculosis has been described, and may be found to be more common if actively sought.[310]

Tuberculous epididymitis is seen in young boys and epididymo-orchitis in older boys.[255] The development of a cold abscess may be the first manifestation of disease. In girls, tuberculosis of the uterus or Fallopian tubes occurs after the onset of puberty and may be complicated by peritonitis.

Tuberculosis of the kidneys and genital tracts should be treated by standard chemotherapy.

MANAGEMENT DURING PREGNANCY AND OF THE NEWBORN

Active tuberculosis during pregnancy is associated with infection of the placenta in approximately half the cases; congenital tuberculosis is rare. The main considerations are of the mother during pregnancy and management of the infant at birth. Situations that may arise include a tuberculin positive woman with a normal chest X-ray, radiologically inactive disease with negative sputum cultures, or active disease.

The only commonly used drug absolutely contraindicated during pregnancy is SM because of its ototoxic effect on the fetus. INH and RIF are given for 6 months and PZA is added during the first 2 months of treatment. Pyridoxine supplements should be given with INH because of increased requirements during pregnancy.

At birth, if the mother has completed treatment or has inactive disease, the infant is given BCG. If she has active disease and/or is receiving treatment, the infant is given INH 6 mg/kg/day for 3 months and is then given a tuberculin test and chest X-ray. If these are negative INH may be stopped (presuming the mother is not infectious) and BCG given. Where it is doubtful that the mother will comply with treatment, as in developing countries, BCG may be given at birth and the infant also given INH for 3–6 months. The extent to which INH may interfere with BCG vaccination is not clear but is probably small.[311] It is not necessary to use isoniazid-resistant BCG.

If the tuberculin test is positive (> 5 mm), full investigation for tuberculosis should be undertaken. If no clinical or bacteriological evidence of disease is detected, INH should be continued for a total of 6 months. If disease is detected, full treatment as for congenital infection should be given.

Unless the mother has multidrug resistant tuberculosis she should not be separated from her child and should continue breast-feeding, once both are on appropriate chemotherapy. Small amounts of antituberculous drugs are excreted in breast milk, but they are not harmful to the infant. Consideration should be given to testing mother and infant for HIV infection

PERINATAL TUBERCULOSIS

Perinatal tuberculosis is uncommon, although increasing numbers are reported in areas where HIV/tuberculosis coinfection of women has risen.[312,313] Whether the infection is contracted before birth (congenital) or in the neonatal period is probably only of epidemiological significance. There are three possible routes for congenital infection:

1. transplacental, when the primary infection will be in the liver, or it may possibly bypass the liver through the ductus venosus and be detected in the lungs;
2. aspiration of infected amniotic fluid or infected material in the genital tract, when the lungs will be infected;
3. ingestion, when presumably the liver will be infected.

Symptoms of congenital infection may occur from birth up to 2 months of age with the majority presenting within 2–5 weeks. In neonatal infection, onset of symptoms is later (1–2 months). Common clinical features are respiratory distress, fever, hepatosplenomegaly, lymphadenopathy, poor feeding, and failure to thrive. There may also be skin lesions, ear discharge, jaundice and, in late diagnosed cases, meningitis. The tuberculin test is usually negative but may become positive 6 weeks or more after birth. Chest X-ray may show bronchopneumonia, sometimes resembling staphylococcal pneumonia, or miliary changes but may not be abnormal in the early stages. Mycobacteria are often isolated from gastric aspirates, also from tracheal aspirates or ear discharge. The diagnosis may also be made from CSF, or liver, lung or lymph node biopsy. PCR should be undertaken on all specimens. Placental histology or endometrial curettage may confirm a prenatal source of infection. The mortality is high in overwhelming or late-diagnosed cases and preterm infants.[314] Other bacterial or viral infections may be superimposed.

Treatment is with standard chemotherapy. If drug resistance is suspected, SM or kanamycin should be added for the first 2 months and then replaced by ethambutol. Duration of chemotherapy should be 9 months. There are no studies on the efficacy of chemotherapy for the newborn.

HIV INFECTION

There are no large studies of confirmed tuberculosis/HIV coinfection in children. In a cohort of 1426 HIV-infected children studied from 1989 to 1995 in New York City, 45 (3%) were diagnosed with tuberculosis compared to 5 (0.5%) of 1085 HIV-exposed uninfected children.[315] In sub-Saharan Africa there has been a marked increase in frequency of children treated for respiratory tuberculosis since the mid-1980s, associated with the rise in HIV infection, and 60–70% of cases may be HIV seropositive. However, because of confounding factors, including the high prevalence of HIV infection in mothers and of tuberculosis in the household, difficulty in confirming both HIV infection in infants and tuberculosis generally, and confusion with HIV-related pulmonary disease, the true incidence of tuberculosis/HIV coinfection is unknown.[316,317] What is clear is the high mortality in HIV-infected children treated for tuberculosis. For most cases there is no difference in the radiological features between HIV-infected and non-infected children with tuberculosis, except possibly a tendency for increased frequency of disseminated disease in the more immunosuppressed. Coinfection with systemic environmental mycobacteria is also a feature in the latter group. In children presenting with tuberculosis and HIV-related pulmonary disease with bilateral reticulonodular changes and hilar lymphadenopathy, the diagnosis of tuberculosis has to depend on methods other than radiology such as contact history, tuberculin test and culture of *M. tuberculosis*. Although the tuberculin test is often negative it should always be undertaken as it is positive (10 mm or more) in a substantial proportion of HIV-infected children, depending on their state of nutrition and immunosuppression.

Because of reports of slow eradication of *M. tuberculosis* and/or relapse, 9 months of chemotherapy is advised. For HIV-infected children with a positive tuberculin test and no evidence of tuberculosis, 12 months of INH chemoprophylaxis is advised. In HIV-endemic areas, SM should be avoided because of risks from unsterilized needles.[318] Thiacetazone may cause severe skin reactions in HIV-infected children and should be replaced by EMB.

GENERAL PRINCIPLES OF CHEMOTHERAPY

A 6 month short-course therapy is now standard for respiratory and most non-respiratory disease.[319] There are still differences of opinion regarding dosage of drugs especially INH, and the management of meningitis, bone or joint disease, HIV infection and drug resistance. In developing countries, the main constraint is the cost of drugs, especially RIF, which is essential for short-course regimens. Use of cheaper drugs may be a false economy, particularly in areas with a high incidence of drug resistance, as the longer the period of treatment, the more the chance of non-compliance. Duration of therapy need not exceed 1 year, except in unusual circumstances such as drug resistance or non-compliance. Intermittent therapy is useful where compliance may be in doubt and is cheaper, although probably only of practical value in areas where supervision is possible. Drugs are usually given twice or thrice-weekly. Directly observed therapy (DOT) is useful in overcoming poor compliance.[320]

Different drugs are effective (in order of efficacy) in:

1. killing actively dividing bacilli, e.g. in open cavities – INH, RIF and SM;
2. killing dormant, intermittently or non-dividing bacilli, e.g. in closed caseous lesions – RIF, INH; or within macrophages – PZA, RIF, INH;
3. suppressing drug resistant mutants – INH, RIF.

PZA is particularly active against bacteria inhibited by an acid environment (e.g. within macrophages and in areas of acute inflammation). Killing actively dividing bacilli and clearing the sputum of *live* infective bacilli can be accomplished rapidly but for *cure* or 'sterilization' a prolonged course of treatment is necessary to eradicate dormant and intracellular bacilli. Failure to do this may result in relapse. Mycobacteria may survive for years in a dormant state when metabolism is inhibited by low oxygen tension or low pH.

The most commonly used drugs are bactericidal, e.g. INH (the most potent), RIF, PZA, SM. INH can kill up to 90% of the bacillary population during the first few days of chemotherapy. Bacteriostatic drugs may be used along with bactericidal drugs to prevent emergence of resistance to the bactericidal drugs, e.g. EMB (bactericidal in large doses), ethionamide, thiacetazone and p-aminosalicyclic acid (PAS).

Standard regimen is INH + RIF for 6months, with addition of PZA for the first 2 months, and it is used for all types of tuberculosis. A longer duration of 9–12 months is advised for some types of disease as indicated in the respective sections. Other schedules are shown in Table 26.27. EMB is not advised for children under 5 years because of the possibility of optic neuritis, the symptoms of which they would be unable to report. However, it may have to be used for drug resistance. With a dose of 15 mg/kg it is unlikely that problems would arise.[278] Visual testing should be undertaken where possible. In Table 26.28 the drug dosage and common side-effects are shown. The recommended daily dose of INH is 6 mg/kg except for tuberculous meningitis when the dose should be 15–20 mg/kg. There is a large range of reported adverse reactions to tuberculosis chemotherapy.[321] They occur in 1–2% of patients and some of the commoner ones are shown in Table 26.28. They are uncommon in children and are usually apparent within 6–8 weeks of starting treatment. Peripheral neuropathy as a complication of INH is rare in children. Slow acetylators are at increased risk and pyridoxine will prevent it. Pyridoxine 10 mg is indicated only for children on meat- or milk-deficient diets, breast-feeding infants, malnourished children, and during pregnancy. Higher doses may interfere with the activity of INH.

The main complication is hepatic toxicity. Transient elevation of transaminases occurs in 7–17% of children taking INH, is dose-related and is more likely if RIF is also given. There are case reports of hepatocellular toxicity and death from INH therapy in children.[321] Unless there is pre-existing liver disease or high doses of these drugs are administered, e.g. in meningitis, there is no need to monitor serum transaminases. Parents should be asked to report persistent nausea, vomiting, malaise and especially jaundice. Children who are rapid acetylators do not have an increased risk of hepatitis when exposed to INH.

Cutaneous reactions, if mild, may not require cessation of treatment, but generalized hypersensitivity will. If toxicity occurs, all drugs should be stopped and reintroduced sequentially in the order INH, RIF and PZA in a small dose (approximately a quarter of the full dose) the first day, increasing to full dose over the next 2–3 days.[322]

The value of corticosteroids is their ability to reduce the host's inflammatory response if it is contributing to tissue damage or impairing function. Their use is discussed in the respective sections, and may be indicated in the following conditions: meningitis, spinal block, obstruction of bronchi by lymph nodes, miliary disease with alveolar capillary block, pleural effusion and pericarditis.[323] Prednisolone 1.5–2 mg/kg/day is given for 2 weeks and gradually tailed off over 6 weeks. Higher doses are given for meningitis.

In children, knowledge of drug resistance is usually obtained from culture and sensitivity of the contact. If drug resistance is suspected, four bactericidal drugs, e.g. INH, RIF, PZA and EMB or

Table 26.27 Drug regimens

Regimen	Duration
Standard daily	
HRZ(E)[†]: 2 months, then HR: 4 months	6 months
HR: 9 months	9 months
HRZ: 2 months, then HR: 2 months	4 months*
Intermittent thrice weekly	
HRZ: 2 months, then HR thrice weekly: 4 months	6 months
Alternative less potent daily	
HRZ: 2 months, then HE: 6 months	8 months
HRZ: 2 months, then HT: 6 months	8 months

H = isoniazid
R = rifampicin
Z = pyrazinamide
E = ethambutol
T = thiacetazone
[†]Add E if drug resistance suspected
*For hilar lymphadenopathy alone

Table 26.28 Recommended drugs for tuberculosis

Drug	Daily dose			Thrice weekly dose			Side-effects
	Children	Adolescents		Children	Adolescents		
		< 50 kg	> 50 kg		< 50 kg	> 50 kg	
Isoniazid (INH)	6 mg/kg p.o., i.m., i.v. 15–20 mg/kg (meningitis)	300 mg	300 mg	15 mg/kg (max 900 mg)	15 mg/kg	max 900 mg	Hepatic enzyme elevation, hepatitis, peripheral neuropathy, hypersensitivity
Rifampicin (RIF)	10 mg/kg p.o., i.v. 15–20 mg/kg (meningitis)	450 mg	600 mg	15 mg/kg (max 600 mg)	15 mg/kg	max 900 mg	Orange discoloration of secretions and urine (also contact lens), nausea, vomiting, hepatitis, febrile reactions, thrombocytopenia
Pyrazinamide (PZA)	30–35 mg/kg p.o. 40 mg/kg (meningitis)	1.5 g	2.0 g	50 mg/kg	2.0 g	2.5 g	Hepatotoxicity, hyperuricemia, arthralgia, gastrointestinal upset, skin rash
Ethambutol (EMB)	15–20 mg/kg p.o.*	15 mg/kg (max 2.5 g)	15 mg/kg (max 2.5 g)	30 mg/kg	30 mg/kg	max 2.5 g	Optic neuritis, skin rash
Streptomycin (SM)	15–20 mg/kg i.m.	750 mg	1.0 g	15–20 mg/kg	750 mg	1.0 g	Ototoxicity, nephrotoxicity
Thiacetazone	4 mg/kg p.o.	150 mg	150 mg	Not recommended	Not recommended	Not recommended	Gastrointestinal disturbance, vertigo, visual disturbance, hepatitis, agranulocytosis, exfoliative dermatitis in HIV infection
Ethionamide/ prothionamide	15–20 mg/kg p.o. (divided doses)	750 mg	1.0 g	Not recommended	Not recommended	Not recommended	Gastrointestinal disturbance, hepatotoxicity, allergic reactions

* In children under 5 years give 15 mg/kg

SM, should be given. If possible SM should be avoided because of the trauma of daily injections. In drug resistance, at *least two drugs* to which the mycobacteria are susceptible should be given. For INH resistance RIF, PZA and EMB are given for a 9–12 month course. For multiple drug resistance, e.g. to INH, RIF and SM, four or more drugs are required initially and treatment should continue for 12–24 months.[278,319] Depending on sensitivities, PZA and EMB are given with three or more second line drugs, e.g. ethionamide, ciprofloxacin, cycloserine or parenterally administered drugs, e.g. kanamycin, amikacin or capreomycin. DOT should be considered.

Patients should be seen monthly for the first 2–3 months to make sure of compliance and to monitor any problems with drugs. Chest X-ray should be repeated at 1–2 months, at the end of therapy and 3 or more months later. Resolution of pulmonary infiltrates may take over a year and lymphadenopathy (intra- or extrathoracic) 2–3 years. If adequate chemotherapy has been given, there is no need to prolong treatment; if relapse occurs or the patient stops treatment for a period, the same standard drug regimen should be given, preferably for 9 months' duration. If in doubt about activity of a pulmonary lesion, gastric aspirates or sputum should be obtained for microscopy and culture. Chest X-rays should be repeated every 6–12 months after cessation of therapy until stable.

Children with primary tuberculosis are rarely infectious and sputum is usually non-infectious after 2–3 weeks of chemotherapy and so they may return to school after this period.

BACTERIAL INFECTIONS: DISEASES CAUSED BY ENVIRONMENTAL MYCOBACTERIA

Mycobacteria may be divided into those associated with tuberculosis and leprosy and those causing disease associated with the environment, also referred to as non-tuberculous, or atypical mycobacteria (Table 26.29). The former (including *Mycobacterium leprae*) are highly infectious and are passed from person to person. Environmental mycobacteria, of which there are over 50 species, exist principally as harmless saprophytes in water, soil and vegetation, and also as pathogens in animals such as birds, reptiles and fish. Person-to-person transmission is extremely rare. Environmental mycobacteria generally prefer warm climates and the geographical distribution of the different species is quite variable. Water (fresh or salt) is probably a major vector, e.g. drinking, washing or aquatic sports, or by inhalation of aerosols.[325] The main portals of entry are probably through the skin or mucosa, and by inhalation or ingestion.

DIAGNOSIS

Environmental mycobacteria may be detected as commensals in sputum or gastric aspirates, swabs from wounds or abscesses, or in inadequately sterilized sputum pots. More definite proof of their pathogenicity is obtained when they are derived from a closed lesion, e.g. by aspiration or resection or the same strain of mycobacteria is repeatedly isolated. Differentiation between mycobacteria is by their cultural characteristics or by polymerase chain reaction (PCR). Histologically, it is usually not possible to differentiate lesions from the granulomata of tuberculosis, although non-tuberculous infection is more likely to show 'non-specific' inflammation with less prominent caseation. Variable numbers of acid-fast bacilli may be seen.

There may be a moderate reaction to the Mantoux test (purified protein derivative, PPD-S): 5–15 mm, less or no reaction.

Table 26.29 Mycobacteria and disease in humans

Pathogen	Disease
M. tuberculosis	
M. bovis (including BCG)	Tuberculosis
M. africanum	
M. leprae	Leprosy
Slow growing potential pathogens	
*M. avium**	
*M. intracellulare**	
*M. scrofulaceum**	
*M. kansasii**	
*M. malmoense**	
M. marinum	Swimming pool granuloma
M. ulcerans	Buruli ulcer
M. xenopi	
M. szulgai	
M. semiae	
M. gordonae	
M. haemophilum	
Rapidly growing potential pathogens	
*M. fortuitum**	Soft tissue abscess, wound infection and otolaryngeal infection
*M. cheloni**	
M. abscessus	

* Associated with cervical adenitis in children

M. avium, *M. intracellulare* and *M. scrofulaceum* are sometimes termed the MAIS complex; and *M. avium* and *M. intracellulare* as MAC

Differential intradermal tests with antigens prepared from specific environmental mycobacteria, e.g. *Mycobacterium avium*, *Mycobacterium intracellulare*, *Mycobacterium malmoense*, *Mycobacterium scrofulaceum* or *Mycobacterium kansasii* are more likely to produce a larger reaction than that with PPD-S. However, if the antigen is not specific for the infecting organism the reaction may be small or nil.

The commonest clinical problem due to infection by environmental mycobacteria in children is cervical adenitis. Other conditions include cutaneous infections, rarely pulmonary or otolaryngeal disease, osteitis, disseminated disease and meningitis.[326,327] In adolescents and adults, infection in the presence of pre-existing pulmonary disease (including cystic fibrosis) is the commonest association.

LYMPHADENITIS

There appears to be a relative if not an absolute increase in incidence of lymphadenitis due to environmental mycobacteria in areas of the world where tuberculosis is now uncommon, which may be partly due to decline in neonatal BCG vaccination.[328] A defect in the type 1 cytokine pathway could be a factor in some cases.[329] It usually presents in children aged between 1 and 5 years. The submandibular group of nodes is most often infected; other nodes in the neck include the tonsillar, preauricular and anterior cervical groups. It is usually unilateral. Outside the neck, infection of axillary, inguinal and epitrochlear nodes has been described. The area of entry is rarely identified, although occasionally a lesion on the tonsil or buccal mucosa is seen. Enlargement of preauricular nodes suggests that the eye might be a portal of entry in some cases. Enlargement of nodes is fairly rapid over some weeks to months, the overlying skin becoming erythematous prior to discharge of the abscess but is not usually warm unless secondarily infected. It is commonly mistaken for a pyogenic cervical abscess. A sinus may develop and later calcification may occur. Some nodes probably settle spontaneously. Infection by environmental mycobacteria should be considered when a submandibular or preauricular node enlarges in a young child from a background of low tuberculous endemicity in the presence of a normal chest X-ray and a negative or low grade sensitivity to PPD.

The treatment of choice is excision biopsy of the primary group of involved nodes.[326,330] A fluctuant abscess may be aspirated for diagnosis, but if possible aspiration should be avoided. Often the lesion is incised when mistaken for a cervical abscess, or it has discharged spontaneously. In these circumstances, as much necrotic material as possible should be removed and later, if necessary, the primary node excised.

Chemotherapy is not usually indicated as the disease is local and the usual mycobacteria causing disease, e.g. *M. avium* complex (MAC) and *M. malmoense* are commonly resistant to standard chemotherapy. However, if surgery is difficult, e.g. involvement of the parotid gland or closeness of the lesion to the facial nerve, incision and curettage together with antimycobacterial drug therapy should be considered. Suggested drugs are clarithromycin or azithromycin plus rifabutin or one of the following: ethambutol or ciprofloxacin for 6 months.[331] Occasionally longer treatment is required. A suitable regimen is azithromycin 10 mg/kg and rifabutin 6 mg/kg both given once daily. Azithromycin has the advantage of once daily treatment. Although there is little evidence of visual toxicity from ethambutol at a dose of 15 mg/kg in children, there seems little justification to give it if there are alternative drugs. There are no controlled trials on the value of single versus combined drugs or duration of therapy. Recurrence of disease in another site sometimes occurs and should be treated as usual.

OTOLARYNGEAL DISEASE

Chronic infection of the middle ear associated with tympanotomy tubes and chronic mastoiditis due to colonization by, particularly, rapidly growing mycobacteria, e.g. *Mycobacterium abscessus* and *Mycobacterium chelonei*, has been described. Debridement with removal of all diseased tissue and in the case of chronic mastoiditis securing maximum ventilation of the cavity is essential. Chemotherapy with appropriate drugs is given for 6 months. Treatment for *M. abscessus* and *M. chelonei* includes parenteral therapy with amikacin and cefoxitin or imipenem for a few weeks, followed by oral clarithromycin and/or ciprofloxacin, depending on sensitivities.[327,332]

SOFT TISSUE INFECTION

The most common soft tissue infections are 'swimming pool granuloma' and 'fish tank granuloma', both caused by *Mycobacterium marinum*. Local abscesses may follow infection by *Mycobacterium fortuitum* or *M. chelonei* at injection sites, trauma or surgery, and often present 3–4 weeks after infection although the incubation period may be much longer in deep infections. Regional nodes are not usually enlarged. Mycobacteria can usually be detected in the lesions. Management comprises debridement of diseased tissue, with chemotherapy reserved for extensive or deep-seated disease.

'Swimming pool granuloma' commonly affects children bathing in infected water on areas of abrasion such as the knees or elbows. Papules which may ulcerate appear on the affected areas; scab formation follows. Spontaneous healing occurs within a few months. If drug therapy is required, a single agent such as co-trimoxazole, clarithromycin or ciprofloxacin, or for more severe infections, rifampicin plus ethambutol are given for 3–6 months.

Buruli ulcer derives its name from a district in northern Uganda and is known as Bairnsdale ulcer in Australia where the causative agent (*Mycobacterium ulcerans*) was originally identified. It occurs in localized places in a number of tropical rain forest areas around swamps and river banks. It is transmitted through minor skin injury after contact with contaminated water, soil or vegetation. It starts as a subcutaneous nodule, often on a leg or arm, ulcerates and gradually progresses to a large ulcer with deep, undermined edges. Satellite nodules or ulcers may be present. Treatment requires wide excision, cleansing with antiseptic such as 0.5% silver nitrate, and immediate skin grafting. Application of heat to maintain the temperature of the ulcer above 40°C which inhibits growth of *M. ulcerans* may be successful. Chemotherapy is generally unrewarding, but may be tried along with surgery to assist healing.[333] Suggested drugs are clarithromycin, rifampicin or amikacin. BCG may give some protection.

PULMONARY DISEASE

Pulmonary disease due to environmental mycobacteria is rare in immunocompetent children. It presents similarly to pulmonary tuberculosis: primary complex, bronchial obstruction, bronchopneumonia or primary progressive disease.[334] The majority of cases are caused by MAC, less often by *M. kansasii* and, in some cases, by other mycobacteria such as *M. fortuitum*. Obstruction of a bronchus should be resected either at bronchoscopy or thoracotomy. Prolonged chemotherapy may be required.

In about 13% of patients with cystic fibrosis, environmental mycobacteria may be recovered from respiratory tract specimens.[335] Decision to treat with chemotherapy long term depends on a number of indications including: recovery of mycobacteria on serial specimens, reduction in lung function not responding to standard management, changes on chest X-ray compatible with superinfection and response to chemotherapy for mycobacteria. Choice of chemotherapy depends on cultures. Drugs may need to be continued for up to 2 years.[336]

DISSEMINATED AND EXTRAPULMONARY DISEASE

Disseminated disease is usually associated with severe immunological defects, especially AIDS. When bone disease occurs, it is usually disseminated osteomyelitis, but rarely, multifocal osteomyelitis without an apparent underlying immunodeficiency is seen. Infection of the meninges may also occur. A variety of inherited defects in the IL-12 dependent gamma interferon (IFN-gamma) output pathway with susceptibility to mycobacteria (especially environmental mycobacteria and BCG) and salmonella infections are recognized.[337] Some respond to IFN-gamma therapy.

In HIV infection, disseminated disease is usually seen in older children with a low CD4 count and advanced disease. MAC are the commonest mycobacteria. Trials are in progress regarding optimal chemotherapy. A suggested regimen is clarithromycin, ethambutol and rifabutin.[338] Other drugs include clofazimine, rifampicin, ciprofloxacin or amikacin.[332,336]

DRUG THERAPY

Drugs appropriate for environmental mycobacteria are outlined in Table 26.30. In vitro drug sensitivities may not predict clinical response, as minimal inhibitory concentrations are not known for many environmental mycobacteria. Duration of treatment and synergy between drug combinations are important factors. In

Table 26.30 Suggested drugs for environmental mycobacteria

Organism	Drugs
M. avium-intracellulare *M. scrofulaceum* *M. malmoense*	Clarithromycin (or azithromycin), rifampicin/rifabutin, ethambutol, ciprofloxacin, clofazimine, amikacin
M. kansasii	Rifampicin, ethambutol, ciprofloxacin, clarithromycin
M. marinum	Rifampicin, ethambutol, clarithromycin, TMP-SMZ, ciprofloxacin
M. fortuitum *M. chelonei* *M. abscessus*	Amikacin, cefoxitin, clofazimine, clarithromycin, ciprofloxacin, imipenem

TMP-SMZ, trimethoprim-sulfamethoxazole

general, neither isoniazid nor pyrazinamide are useful for environmental mycobacteria. Experience with many of the newer drugs is limited in children and it is important to be aware of side-effects particularly when used in combination, e.g. plasma levels of rifabutin may be increased by clarithromycin and fluconazole with a risk of uveitis.

BACTERIAL INFECTIONS: TULAREMIA

ETIOLOGY

This disease derives its name from Tulare, a county in California, where it was first discovered amongst ground squirrels by McCoy in 1911. It is caused by a small, intracellular, non-motile Gram negative coccobacillus *Francisella tularensis* which commonly causes disease in wild animals such as rabbits, hares, squirrels, foxes, rats and deer. There are four subspecies of the organism that are serologically identical but differ in biochemical properties and virulence.[339] *F. tularensis* subsp. *tularensis* represents over 90% of the isolates from North America and is highly virulent in man and rabbits. It is usually recovered from rodents and arthropods. *F. tularensis* subsp. *holartica*, the type most commonly found in Europe and Asia is less virulent in man and rabbits. It is usually isolated from aquatic animals. The other two subspecies have only rarely been associated with disease in humans.

EPIDEMIOLOGY

The organism can be isolated from a wide variety of wild mammals, from domestic animals such as sheep, cattle and cats, and from the arthropods that bite these animals such as ticks, fleas and deer flies. Human infection occurs after a bite from an infected arthropod, by contact with an infected animal, by ingestion of a diseased animal or contaminated water, or by inhalation of infected secretions. Humans are highly susceptible to the organism, with fewer than 50 organisms required for infection. Tularemia occurs throughout the northern hemisphere, with large outbreaks reported in North America, the southern part of the Soviet Republic, and northern Scandinavia. In the eastern part of the continental USA it occurs mostly in winter, related to the rabbit hunting season, whereas in the states west of the Mississippi River it occurs in summer when there is a preponderance of ticks. Human case-to-case contact has not been documented, though care must be taken in dressing discharging wounds. Tularemia is extremely infectious for laboratory workers, who must take exceptional care in the handling of infected material or cultures. Its high attack rate and virulence after inhalation has caused its frequent citation as a possible agent for bioterrorism.

PATHOLOGY

There is a local lesion at the portal of entry and, at times, disseminated lesions throughout the body. Entry is usually through the skin, but may be via the conjunctivae, the respiratory tract or rarely the gastrointestinal tract. Dissemination occurs via the lymphatics or blood and lesions may be found in the regional lymph nodes, and in many other parts of the body. The local lesion is a painful, erythematous papule often with central ulceration and regional lymph node enlargement. The lesions are granulomatous much like the lesions of miliary tuberculosis, but the center of the lesions is often necrotic and consists of polymorphonuclear leukocytes.

CLINICAL FEATURES

The incubation period ranges from 1 to 21 days but most cases occur 3–5 days after exposure. The severity of the disease depends on the route of entry, the subspecies involved, and the host's immune response. Children usually show more constitutional upset and less respiratory involvement than adults. Most frequently there is an abrupt onset of high fever, headache and malaise with or without regional adenopathy, chest X-ray changes, vomiting, and a cutaneous lesion at the site of entry. Sterile pyuria is also common. Rarely there may be pericarditis, osteomyelitis, meningitis, splenic abscesses or thrombophlebitis. Before antibiotics, reported mortality ranged from 7 to 30%. Six clinical syndromes have been described which occur according to the portal of entry. The commonest is the *ulceroglandular syndrome* characterized by a primary painful maculopapular lesion at the point of skin entry with subsequent ulceration and slow healing. This is associated with painful, acutely inflamed regional lymph nodes that may ulcerate and proceed to abscess formation. Other forms of the disease include *typhoidal* tularemia, with high fever and hepatosplenomegaly, *pulmonary* tularemia, with pneumonia, pleuritis and hilar adenopathy, *ocular* tularemia, in which the eyelids become edematous and painful, *oropharyngeal* tularemia, in which the tonsils are covered by a pseudomembrane, and a *glandular* form in which no portal of entry can be identified.[340]

DIAGNOSIS

The circumstances of the disease onset, especially a history of bite or scratch or exposure to wild animals, should readily suggest the diagnosis in endemic areas. There is a significant risk to laboratory personnel when handling specimens so the laboratory should be informed if tularemia is suspected. Serology is the usual means of establishing the diagnosis: a fourfold or greater rise in serum agglutination titer to *F. tularensis* is evident after the second week of illness. Non-specific, low titer crossreactions may occur to *Brucella*, *Proteus*, and *Yersinia* species. The organism can be cultured from infected sites on special media or by rodent inoculation, but this should be attempted only by personnel vaccinated against the organism. PCR-based methods may be used to distinguish subspecies,[339] but are not routinely available.

The differential diagnosis depends on the presentation, but includes causes of skin lesions with regional adenopathy such as cat-scratch disease, causes of prolonged fever including brucellosis and salmonellosis (especially typhoid), and causes of atypical pneumonia.

TREATMENT

Streptomycin is the historical drug of choice for treatment of severe tularemia. However, as it is not widely available, gentamicin is an effective alternative although treatment failures have been reported.[341] Chloramphenicol should be added for tularemic meningitis. Options for outpatient therapy of older children include tetracyclines or the quinolones, although relapses have been reported after completion of therapy with both drugs.[342] Treatment is usually for 6 to 10 days, the duration depending on the severity of the illness.

PREVENTION

In endemic areas, opportunities for arthropod bites should be minimized by wearing protective clothing and regular tick inspections. Prevention also involves avoidance of contact with infected or potentially infected animals and insect vectors, adequate cooking of potentially infected meat and the boiling of water from springs and streams.

In the USA, a live attenuated vaccine is available for those repeatedly exposed to the organism such as laboratory technicians.[343]

INFECTIONS DUE TO VIRUSES AND ALLIED ORGANISMS

THE USE OF THE VIROLOGY LABORATORY BY THE CLINICIAN

The virology laboratory has become an important resource to the clinician for many reasons. There is now an increased range of antiviral agents available that require a specific viral diagnosis to be made. In addition, the use of molecular techniques to determine 'viral load' has become common practice in the management of chronic viral illnesses such as those caused by hepatitis C virus or human immunodeficiency virus (HIV). There are also a number of new techniques available for the rapid diagnosis of viruses that allow specific diagnoses to be made in time to influence clinical decisions.[344]

However, the usefulness of the virologist to the clinician is often limited by lack of knowledge of the most appropriate specimens to submit to the laboratory. All too often the wrong specimens are sent, they are sent without viral transport media or at the wrong temperature, or they are collected too late in the illness to be of any use. It is essential that the virologist is given a full clinical account of difficult cases, which are best discussed in person or by phone. Determined efforts are also needed to ensure that convalescent samples of serum are sent at the appropriate time.

LABORATORY TECHNIQUES USED IN THE DIAGNOSIS OF CHILDHOOD VIRAL ILLNESSES

There is now a wide range of diagnostic techniques used in the virology laboratory. Some of these are listed in Table 26.31.

Table 26.31 Some laboratory techniques used in viral diagnosis

Direct microscopy	Electron microscopy Fluorescent antibody methods Presence of inclusion bodies
Virus isolation	Tissue culture Fertile hen's eggs Laboratory animals
Serological	Complement fixation Hemagglutination inhibition Neutralization Enzyme-linked immunosorbent assay Radioimmunoassay
Antigen detection	Immunfluorescence Enzyme-linked immunosorbent assay
Genome detection	Polymerase chain reaction

Virus isolation

Cell culture, the traditional method used to isolate viruses, is being superseded by molecular techniques. It is still necessary to provide an isolate for epidemiological studies, or antiviral susceptibility assays and to provide confirmation of the diagnosis made by a rapid technique. The type of morphological change (called cytopathic effect or CPE) and the speed at which these changes appear are usually characteristic for a particular virus. The diagnosis may be confirmed by virus-specific fluorescent antibody staining of the infected cell culture. The time to detect CPE ranges from 1 to 2 days for the diagnosis of herpes simplex virus (HSV) to over 3 weeks for the diagnosis of cytomegalovirus (CMV). Application of the shell vial culture method decreases the time required to detect slow-growing viruses such as CMV.

Antigen detection

Methods to detect viral antigens include immunofluorescence, enzyme-linked immunosorbent assay (ELISA), and immunoperoxidase staining. They are most useful for the detection of respiratory viruses in nasopharyngeal washings, or bronchoaveolar lavages, for HSV and varicella-zoster virus (VZV) from skin scrapings, for rotavirus in stool specimens, and for CMV in blood specimens. They do not depend on viability of the virus and are usually rapid, with a result available on the day the specimen was sent, but they may lack sensitivity.

Genome detection

Techniques to detect viral nucleic acid are rapidly becoming the cornerstone of diagnostic virology. Polymerase chain reaction (PCR) for detecting DNA from DNA viruses, or provirus from RNA viruses, and reverse transcriptase (RT-PCR) for detecting RNA from RNA viruses are sensitive and specific diagnostic techniques that amplify a specific region of the viral nucleic acid to a level at which it can be detected. It can be utilized to detect virtually any known virus for which part of the genome sequence is known. It can be scaled up to screen for a panel of viruses (multiplex PCR analysis), or utilized to quantify the number of viral particles in the specimen (quantitative PCR). It has allowed the number of viral copies (or 'viral load') to come into clinical decision making in the management of individuals with chronic hepatitis C infections and HIV. Its sensitivity is also its downfall, as very low levels of external contamination can easily result in false positive results. In addition, it is not always easy to determine the clinical significance of viral DNA in a specimen, as its presence does not always confirm that it is causing disease, or that it is in an infectious state.

Serology

A high proportion of virus diagnoses are made by serology. Even in those cases where a virus is isolated, the significance of the isolation is greatly enhanced where serological tests demonstrate a rising antibody titer to the agent in question. However, its usefulness is limited by the need to collect both an acute and convalescent specimen. Immunoglobulin M (IgM) assays are available to diagnose some virus infections on a single sample. Examples of these include CMV, hepatitis A virus, measles, rubella and mumps viruses, and *Mycoplasma pneumoniae*. In most cases, however, acute and convalescent sera are necessary to look for a rise in IgG antibodies. Infants under 6 months mount a relatively poor IgG response, and viral detection by isolation or an IgM response (if the assay is available) are the best ways to make a viral diagnosis.

THE NATURE, COLLECTION AND TRANSPORTATION OF SPECIMENS FOR VIROLOGICAL EXAMINATION

Blood specimens

Depending on the possible pathogen(s), blood specimens may be collected for PCR on serum or cells (usually on white blood cells), for antigen detection, or for serology. To perform PCR on white blood cells requires whole blood to be sent in a lithium heparin tube at room temperature. This must be coordinated with the laboratory, as ideally the cells should be extracted within 24 h of collection. Antigen assays, such as the pp65 antigen PCR for the diagnosis of CMV in immunocompromised hosts, are also usually done on the buffy coat. Clotted whole blood should be sent for PCR assays on plasma. For serology, an acute sample of clotted blood should be removed *as early as possible* in the illness and a convalescent sample sent 2–3 weeks later. Ideally at least 2 ml should be obtained, though lesser quantities have often to suffice in the case of infants. Provided the blood samples arrive in the laboratory within a day they will withstand cool atmospheric conditions; on no account should such specimens undergo freezing as this will provoke lysis of the erythrocytes. In the laboratory, serum will be separated from the clot and stored at −20°C pending examination. As a general rule blood is not a suitable medium from which to isolate viruses and blood viral culture is not a procedure that is routinely used.

Specimens from the upper respiratory tract

Nasal swabs may be taken for isolation of respiratory viruses but throat swabs have a more universal application. The latter should be taken in a vigorous manner in order to ensure that mucus and cellular material is wiped from the pharynx. In older children throat garglings can be obtained. Nasopharyngeal aspirates are particularly useful for the rapid diagnosis and isolation of respiratory syncytial virus and other respiratory viruses. Viruses which can be isolated from saliva include mumps, HSV and CMV.

After the collection of any specimen by swabbing, the swab should be immersed in the virus transport medium (VTM) supplied. Normally this will be contained in a small sterile bottle and, after immersion, the wooden shaft of the swab should be broken level with the neck of the container. The bottle cap should then be firmly replaced and the fluid gently agitated. Nasopharyngeal aspirates need not have VTM added unless there is a long transit time.

If the time interval between the collection of the specimen and delivery to the laboratory is under 2 h, ordinary room temperature is unlikely to produce significant loss in viability of the virus. For periods exceeding 2 h but less than 24 h, specimens should be retained at 4°C and transported in water-ice in a vacuum flask. Where greater delay is involved the specimen should be surrounded by solid CO_2 and packed in an insulated container. A notable exception to the above recommendations is any specimen suspected of containing respiratory syncytial virus; such specimens should not be frozen, but transported to the laboratory as soon as possible.

Specimens from the lower respiratory tract

Specimens may be obtained from the lower respiratory tract by bronchoalveolar lavage, usually in the setting of an immunocompromised child (early in the course of a pulmonary infection) or on the immunocompetent child with severe atypical pneumonia. Specimens should be sent both for routine culture (in VTM at 4°C) and for rapid diagnosis (a few drops in a container without VTM). The agents of psittacosis, Q fever and *Mycoplasma pneumoniae* may be recovered from specimens of sputum, and rhinoviruses have been grown from sputum.

Specimens from the intestinal tract

For the diagnosis of viral gastroenteritis, fecal specimens should be sent for antigen assays [e.g. enzyme immunoassay (EIA) or latex agglutination assays for rotavirus] without VTM. Examination of feces by electron microscopy and culture can produce a rich harvest of other viruses. Viral culture of the stools is particularly important in cases of suspected viral meningitis or encephalitis, but is not helpful in the diagnosis of viral gastroenteritis, as the common pathogens cannot be cultured in the laboratory. Often the infectivity is high and virus may persist within the specimen for over 24 h. As a result, fecal samples often withstand transport by mail. Rectal swabs are less suitable but may be employed where feces are not immediately available and urgent study of the case is desirable. Storage and transportation at room temperature is satisfactory providing the time interval does not exceed 24 h.

Specimens from the CNS

Techniques to detect viral nucleic acid are rapidly becoming the most important means of laboratory diagnosis of viral infections of the CNS. A sample of cerebrospinal fluid (CSF), approximately 1 ml in volume, should be submitted from cases of suspected viral infection of the CNS. It should be aseptically collected and placed in a sterile container *without* the addition of transport medium. Rapid transportation to the laboratory is desirable but, where the delay exceeds a few hours, the specimen should be placed in a thermos flask surrounded by water-ice. Further delay will necessitate the employment of solid CO_2 during transit (see above: respiratory specimens). Viral culture of CSF may be positive in primary HSV infections. During convalescence, virus-specific IgG in the plasma may be useful in the diagnosis of mumps, HSV encephalitis and in subacute sclerosing panencephalitis (SSPE).

Brain biopsy is occasionally indicated for diagnosis of severe encephalitis, where a diagnosis has not been made on molecular assays on the CSF or other specimens, or in the immunocompromised. It is essential that the virologist be consulted for each individual case to ensure that the specimens reach the laboratory rapidly and in the appropriate manner.

Specimens from the skin

Successful virus isolation is most likely to arise from samples of vesicle fluid but viruses may also be grown from, or seen in, pustular fluid, scabs and carefully taken scrapings from macules or papules. PCR is also available on tissue specimens in some laboratories. Fluid material should be collected from vesicles and pustules by puncturing their surface with a fine, sterile capillary tube. Scabs or crusts are removed by fine forceps and placed in a small sterile bottle. Scrapings from any lesion are carefully smeared on to scrupulously clean microscope slides. The material should be packed with care to prevent breakage, and contamination of the outside of the package avoided. Swabs should also be sent in VTM at 4°C for routine culture.

Urine specimens

Specimens of urine, preferably midstream, must be fresh and sent promptly without VTM to the laboratory. The specimen (approximately 10 ml in volume) should be collected in a screw-capped glass container and if delay in transportation exceeds a few hours, the container should be kept in contact with water-ice during transit. Urine may be used for PCR, antigen assays or culture depending on the suspected pathogen.

Other specimens

On occasion it may be desirable to submit specimens for examination from suspected viral lesions of the eye and genital tract. PCR may be performed on tissues after consultation with the laboratory, and virus isolation has also proved possible from mesenteric and other lymph glands as well as from serous exudates, such as ascites or pericardial fluid. The methods of collection and transportation are broadly as outlined above but a more detailed account is given in the appropriate section of the text.

Finally reference should be made to the obtaining of specimens at autopsy for virological examination. These require to be collected with scrupulous care so that contamination of the organs does not arise from instruments and other contacts. Each specimen should be collected with separate sterile instruments and careful labeling is essential. Contamination by fixatives such as formalin must be avoided.

THE PRACTICAL APPLICATION OF THE LABORATORY DIAGNOSIS OF VIRAL INFECTIONS

There are various situations in which laboratory diagnosis of viral infections is particularly valuable:

1. Rapid diagnosis of respiratory syncytial virus (RSV) infection is not only useful for clinical management, e.g. decisions on antibiotic use, but also for decisions about isolation of infected babies to prevent hospital-acquired infections.
2. Rapid diagnosis of HSV encephalitis can help rationalize the use of antivirals, e.g. aciclovir.
3. Rapid diagnosis of measles and VZV can help make decisions about the use of passive or active immunization to protect high-risk immunocompromised children who have been exposed.
4. Viral diagnosis can be important for epidemiological reasons, e.g. the example used previously of paralytic illness due to poliomyelitis or other enteroviruses.

THE EXANTHEMATA

MEASLES (MORBILLI AND RUBEOLA)

Measles is a viral disease of high infectivity, which presents with an acute catarrhal illness, fever, characteristic Koplik spots on the buccal mucous membranes followed by a distinctive maculopapular rash. There is a high incidence of serious complications of the respiratory and nervous systems. In large cities and towns, measles is most likely to occur in infants and preschool children, but in rural and less crowded urban areas the principal incidence is between the ages of 5 and 10 years. Measles is extremely rare under 3–4 months of age, because of protective maternal antibody, but authenticated cases have occurred.

In some countries measles outbreaks have shown a characteristic biennial periodicity but such a pattern is by no means universal and the introduction of active immunization has altered the natural epidemiology of the disease.

Mortality

In developing countries, where malnutrition is common, measles may have a mortality as high as 25% and produce serious complications.[345] Children are at increased risk of dying for a year after their measles due to impaired cellular immunity. Inhibition of macrophage production of interleukin-12, a cytokine important for driving cell-mediated immunity, by binding of measles virus to CD46, a cellular protein that regulates complement, is thought to be partly responsible for this immunosuppression.[346] Measles can cause devastating outbreaks when the virus is introduced into the naive populations such as on remote islands. Although the morbidity and mortality are lower in highly immunized, industrialized countries, outbreaks can still occur if a population of unimmunized children, usually preschool, is allowed to develop. In more exposed communities, measles is now comparatively mild and its morbidity and mortality lower, although several deaths still occur each year in the UK. Unimmunized children who contract measles are at particular risk, when in remission from acute leukemia or other conditions in which immunity is compromised.

Etiology

Measles virus is an RNA virus approximately 140 nm in diameter. It is a member of the paramyxovirus family, genus *Morbillivirus* and morphologically resembles the parainfluenza viruses. It is usually transmitted by droplet infection from the respiratory tract of a case before, or close to, the onset of the rash. Entry probably occurs through the respiratory tract but infection through the intact conjunctiva has been postulated. No antigenic variation has been described. An attack is usually followed by lifelong immunity and there is little or no authenticated evidence of second attacks of measles except in individuals with severe immunological defects. Subclinical infection can probably occur but is rare.

Clinical features

Measles has an incubation period of 8–14 days. A mild illness may occur at the time of infection but most cases develop a prodromal illness some 3–5 days before the eruptive stage. The main features of this illness are pronounced catarrh, characterized by a constantly running nose, conjunctivitis and a harsh dry cough. Fever and irritability are usually present and there may be a fleeting scarlatiniform or morbilliform rash. Koplik spots, the most pathognomonic sign of measles, appear during this stage and are seen as small, grayish white lesions on the buccal mucosa close to the posterior molar teeth; they are usually quite numerous but may be scanty or occasionally cover the entire lining of the cheek. They can be difficult to demonstrate and the angle of the inspecting light is critical; having faded, they are replaced by a dry, matte appearance on the mucosa, which has a ground-glass-like surface.

The true rash of measles (Fig. 26.29)[347] starts behind the ears and along the hairline. Fever, which will have lessened at the end of the prodromal period, may now rise again to 39–40°C (Fig. 26.30),[347] and the eruption spreads rapidly to involve the face. The lesions are maculopapular in character and of a dusky hue. Over the next 2 days the eruption spreads downwards and becomes generalized; marked confluence of the spots develops and this gives a blotchy appearance.

The extent and severity of the rash show wide variation. In some, especially the younger cases, the eruption may be unusually sparse and modification by maternal antibody has been suggested. There is frequently some degree of hemorrhage or diapedesis into the rash giving it a purpuric quality and subsequent skin staining. This should not be confused with the rare, and usually fatal, hemorrhagic measles in which extensive bleeding occurs into the skin and from the mucous membranes. In the immunocompromised child, the rash occasionally does not develop.

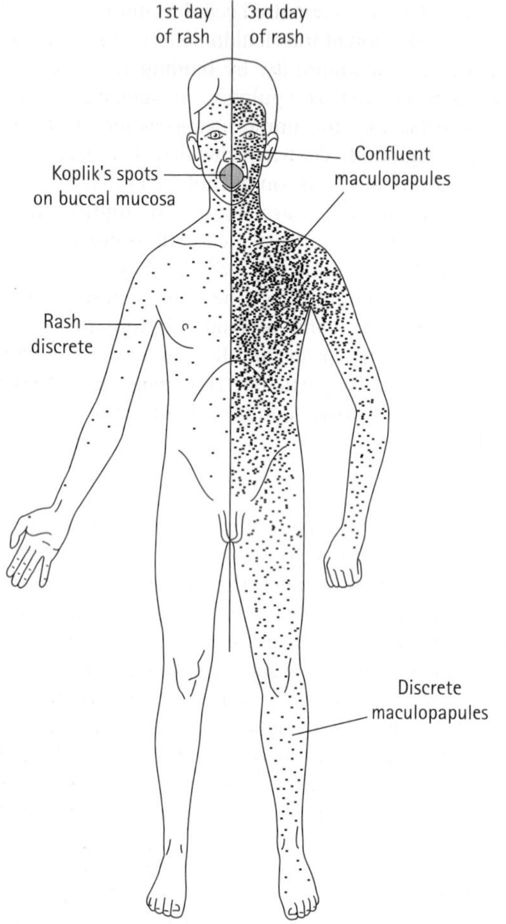

Fig. 26.29 The distribution and the development of rash in measles. (After Krugman & Ward 1968[242])

Fading of the rash can be surprisingly rapid but it usually disappears quite slowly, beginning to fade on the third day in the order of appearance; the rash may be largely gone from the face and upper trunk by the fourth day though persisting on the lower extremities. After a further 3–4 days a brownish staining appears, probably due to capillary hemorrhage and, on occasions, this staining can be very intense. In severe cases, a fine desquamation

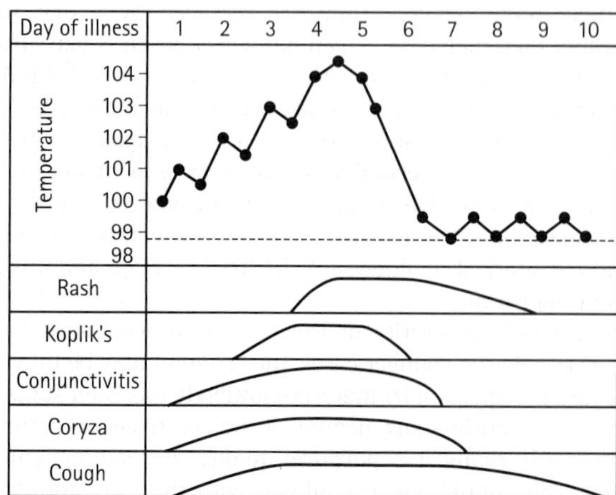

Fig. 26.30 The development of measles. (After Krugman & Ward 1968[242])

may occur at the site of the rash, but this does not usually involve the hands and feet like scarlet fever.

Complications

Respiratory

Measles virus always attacks the respiratory tract causing some degree of laryngotracheobronchitis. An element of bronchitis is universal and can be severe extending even to bronchiolitis; the latter can be complicated by acute mediastinal emphysema. Croup may be prominent. Viral damage may denude the respiratory tract of its protective lining and allow the aspiration of bacteria. Bronchopneumonia may result and the severity will depend on the nature of the aspirated material. Staphylococcal pneumonia can be life threatening.

In a few instances measles virus involvement of the respiratory tract may spread to the lung parenchyma, giving rise to the condition known as giant cell pneumonia. This complication may be prolonged, is often fatal and the illness may be accompanied by little or no rash. It is usually found in association with underlying disease such as immune deficiency HIV infection, leukemia, cystic fibrosis or Letterer–Siwe disease, particularly when there is impaired T cell function. In view of its atypical nature, this illness is often undiagnosed during life and the true diagnosis is made as a result of the autopsy findings.

Ophthalmic

Some degree of conjunctivitis and keratitis occurs in every case of measles. It is typically exudative, non-purulent and non-follicular and can be characterized by Koplik spots. When pseudomembranes or corneal ulcers occur they are the result of secondary bacterial infection. Optic neuritis and retinitis are associated with measles encephalitis.

Ear

Involvement of the middle ear used to be commonplace and could result in suppurative otitis media, chronic perforation or mastoiditis. The lessening severity of measles and prompt antibiotic treatment has reduced the incidence of these complications to a low level.

Gastrointestinal tract

Severe oral inflammation due to secondary infection by bacteria, *Treponema vincentii*, or thrush can occur but cancrum oris is only likely to be seen where malnutrition is rife. Cancrum oris (noma) is a gangrenous form of stomatitis, which commences with a dusky red spot on the inside and outside of the cheek. This rapidly spreads to form a sloughing gangrene of the gums and jaws and in extreme cases teeth may be shed. The breath develops a peculiarly foul odor and death can supervene.

Gastroenteritis is common in measles in non-industrialized countries and can be prolonged; it probably results from direct viral involvement of the gut with or without superinfection with organisms such as *Cryptosporidium*. Appendicitis can occur in measles though abdominal pain is more commonly due to associated mesenteric adenitis.

Enlargement of the spleen is more frequently encountered in measles than is generally realized.

CNS

Measles, with its pronounced constitutional upset and high fever, is often complicated by febrile convulsions. These are most commonly encountered at the start of the eruptive stage and either settle spontaneously or in response to simple sedation; they should not be assumed to be indicative of encephalitis.

True postinfectious encephalomyelitis occurs in from 1 in 1000 to 1 in 5000 cases of measles and has a mortality of about 10% and leaves about 15% with neurological residua. It normally presents after 7–14 days, when the rash is subsiding, but can commence earlier in the disease and rarely even before the rash. Drowsiness, fits, a recrudescence of fever, focal neurological signs and progressive coma suggest that severe cerebral involvement is occurring. In some cases the process may arrest at this juncture and be followed by rapid improvement; in others there is a steady deterioration and death. Between these extremes there are patients in whom recovery is slow and permanent cerebral damage likely.

Rarely subacute sclerosing panencephalitis may complicate measles infection, though not apparently measles immunization. In SSPE, measles virus becomes latent in the cerebrum following primary infection and is then reactivated, usually 5–10 years later, by some unknown stimulus. An alternative hypothesis suggests that a partially immune individual is reinfected by measles which then provokes this unique form of encephalitis. It is commoner in children in whom primary measles occurs before 1 year of age.

Others

Uncomplicated measles tends to produce a leukopenia, and significant thrombocytopenia is occasionally encountered. Epistaxis is a common and occasionally troublesome feature.

Lastly, there is a traditional belief that measles may activate, or predispose to, tuberculosis. This association now seems less common but authenticated examples still occur. Diagnostic difficulty is provided by the fact that measles may suppress the Mantoux reaction for several weeks.

Diagnosis

Provided the medical attendant is consulted at its inception, measles can be diagnosed on clinical grounds with a fair degree of accuracy. Difficulties can arise when an opinion is required later in the disease.

Neutralizing, complement-fixing and hemagglutination-inhibiting antibodies to measles develop during the illness and appropriate serological tests can confirm their presence. Detection of measles IgM on a single specimen is the simplest method for diagnosis. Measles IgM can be detected from 3 days after the onset of the rash for about a month. Sensitivity rates however, vary according to the type of assay used and the time after the onset of the rash, with the hemagglutination-inhibiting antibodies assay being the most sensitive and complement-fixation the least (87% and 37% of cases, respectively, 3 days after the onset of the eruptive phase).[348] The demonstration of a significant rise (fourfold or greater) in antibody titer to measles virus confirms the clinical diagnosis. The hemagglutination-inhibition and complement-fixation tests are usually employed, on account of the ease and rapidity with which they can be performed.

Measles virus can be isolated in primary tissue cultures of human kidney, human amnion or monkey kidney and several other tissue culture systems have been used. The growth rate of measles virus in tissue culture is relatively slow and serological tests will often yield a positive result before the virus has been isolated and identified. Immunofluorescence can be used to detect measles virus antigen in respiratory secretions if rapid diagnosis is needed.

During the late prodromal stage of the illness virus can be recovered from the nasopharynx, urine, conjunctival secretions and blood. By the second day of the rash, virus isolation becomes more difficult, though the urine may continue to contain virus for a further 2 days. In the immunocompromised child, there may be prolonged shedding of measles from the sites after the initial infection.[349]

In SSPE measles antibody in high titer is demonstrable in the serum many years after a typical attack of measles. Antibody may also be detected in the CSF and the ratio of this antibody to that in the serum may be of diagnostic significance. In SSPE the ratio of antibody in the serum to antibody in the CSF may be of the order of 50:1 and even lower ratios have been described. Brain biopsy can confirm the diagnosis of SSPE where facilities for electron microscopy and immunofluorescence are available.

Differential diagnosis

Kawasaki disease can cause a morbilliform rash with fever, conjunctivitis and lymphadenopathy and can be quite difficult to distinguish clinically from measles. The milder illness of rubella with its pinker rash and selective involvement of the suboccipital glands is usually distinguishable. The rash of infectious mononucleosis can cause confusion but its other clinical and laboratory features usually lead to the correct interpretation. Enteroviral infections associated with a rash are usually more transient and lack the catarrhal involvement. Influenza virus infections, both A and B, can occasionally cause a morbilliform rash with respiratory symptoms and fever. In roseola infantum, the rash is very like measles, but as it appears the fever falls and the child is well, in contrast to measles. Scarlet fever and drug eruptions have readily distinguishing features.

Treatment

There are currently no antiviral agents available with demonstrated efficacy in vivo against measles virus. Ribavirin has been shown to inhibit measles virus replication in vitro, and there are anecdotal reports of its use either intravenously or by aerosol to treat severe pneumonitis or encephalitis in the immunocompromised child.[350] However, this treatment remains experimental in the absence of data from a randomized controlled trial.

Amongst the earliest complications that may require treatment are croup and febrile convulsions. These are managed symptomatically (see Chs 18 and 20).

Secondary bacterial infection, superimposed on viral damage to the respiratory tract, will require treatment. Staphylococcal pneumonia is the most feared complication, and if bacterial pneumonia is suspected antistaphylococcal antibiotics should be used. Prophylactic antibiotics are unnecessary, as confirmed by a recent systematic review on the subject.[351]

Mastoiditis should not occur if adequate treatment of otitis media is given early, but if it does occur surgical drainage is required. Any sign of secondary infection of the conjunctivae should be treated with appropriate antibiotics and chloramphenicol eye ointment smeared on to the lids often proves efficacious.

It is rare for gastroenteritis to be so severe as to cause fluid and electrolyte depletion but where this occurs appropriate measures require to be taken. True appendicitis can present in the course of measles.

Postinfectious encephalitis requires intensive supportive treatment. Convulsions, which may be a particularly troublesome feature, should be treated with anticonvulsants. The use of corticosteroids remains controversial, but many clinicians feel such therapy warrants trial in severe cases whose progress is unsatisfactory.

Preventive measures

Quarantine

Because this disease is highly infectious and the maximum infectivity is before the rash appears, quarantine measures are frequently ineffective. However, any child who is suffering from a severe debilitating disease should be protected from exposure wherever possible. In the hospital setting, appropriate quarantine measures should be in place for up to 4 days after the onset of the rash while the child is infectious via the respiratory route. The immunocompromised child with measles should be placed on respiratory isolation for the duration of their illness.

Passive immunization

Passive immunization against measles has been an established procedure for many years and has proved highly effective. Normal human immunoglobulin (gamma globulin) is used (0.2 ml/kg intramuscularly for normal children, 0.5 ml/kg for immunocompromised children, maximum dose 15 ml). The use of passive immunization is particularly important when immunocompromised children, in whom active immunization is contraindicated, become exposed to measles.

Active immunization

In the early years of measles vaccines, an inactivated measles vaccine was used which not only failed to protect against infection but resulted in the children developing severe, atypical illness with giant cell pneumonitis when exposed to wild-type virus.

Live, attenuated measles vaccines are highly protective and have very few side-effects. Where they have been used to immunize whole populations acute measles, encephalitis and subacute sclerosing panencephalitis have virtually disappeared. In countries where immunization rates are relatively low, there are many cases of acute encephalitis with several children each year dying or handicapped as a result.[352] Measles vaccine is readily inhibited by maternal antibody and may be ineffective if given before 1 year of age. If it is wished to protect a child exposed to measles who has no contraindications to immunization and is over 1 year old, then measles vaccine is preferable to passive immunization. Many countries now give measles vaccine in conjunction with mumps and rubella vaccines (MMR) in the second year of life, and a second dose may be given at school entry or at 12–14 years old. The only contraindication to measles vaccine is immune deficiency (including high dose but not low dose steroids). Anaphylactic egg allergy is no longer considered to be a contraindication.[353] HIV infection is not a contraindication unless the patient is severely immunocompromised and on the contrary, as they are at high risk from wild-type measles virus, every attempt should be made to immunize HIV positive children against measles, whether or not they have symptomatic HIV infection.

RUBELLA (GERMAN MEASLES)

Rubella has been recognized as a distinct clinical entity for some time. Some of the original accounts of the disease emanated from Germany and because of this and a certain similarity to measles, the name of German measles became a popular, if ill-conceived, descriptive title. The disease has no relationship to measles. In its postnatally acquired form, rubella is characterized by its mild nature and relative freedom from complications.

Etiology

Rubella virus is an RNA virus of the Togaviridae family. It was first cultured and identified as recently as 1962. Since then it has proved possible to grow it quite readily on suitable tissue cultures, a factor that has considerably enhanced our knowledge of the disease. Transmission is primarily through droplet spread of infected nasopharyngeal secretions from a few days before to up to 14 days after the onset of the rash.

Incidence

The true incidence of rubella is difficult to assess as infection is subclinical in a sizeable proportion of cases; even the clinical illness itself has no pathognomonic features and this point is well substantiated in surveys of rubella antibody levels where the results show a poor correlation with the history of previously suspected infection. By early adult life as many as 90% of city dwellers may show serological evidence of previous rubella but the figure can be much lower in rural communities. Rubella is less common in preschool children than, for example, measles and in one survey less than 10% of children under 2 years showed evidence of previous infection, though this figure had risen to 25% between the ages of 2 and 5 years. By 12 years of age 80% showed evidence of antibody suggesting that the bulk of infection occurs between 6 and 12 years of age.

Clinical features

Rubella has an incubation period of 14–21 days, with an average of 17 days. In children it is rare to have a significant prodromal illness and the first indication of rubella infection is the appearance of a rash over the face (Fig. 26.31).[347] This soon spreads to cover the trunk and later the limbs. The basic lesions are fine, pink macules which, originally discrete, can soon coalesce over the face and trunk. The rash usually disappears within 2–3 days but may persist for as long as 5 days. Occasionally it has a duration measured in hours and in this instance can be readily missed. A biphasic type of rash, with complete regression in between, has been described and a small area of the eruption may persist on the medial aspect of the thighs after the main rash has subsided. Small purpuric spots sometimes appear on the soft palate but have no diagnostic significance as other infections are associated with a similar enanthem.

Lymph node enlargement is an important feature of the disease. It may appear as much as a week before the rash, though usually just before, and may persist for some time after the eruption has faded. The cervical, postauricular and suboccipital glands are most commonly involved, can be tender and are sometimes unassociated with any rash.

In adolescents and adults, especially female, prodromal symptoms are more likely and include malaise, headache, stickiness of the eyes, conjunctivitis and fever. In children the temperature rarely rises above 37.1–37.4°C but can attain 39.5–40.0°C in adults (Fig. 26.32).[347]

The clinical stigmata of congenital rubella are described in Chapter 10.

Complications

In general complications are unusual though a higher incidence is encountered in certain epidemics and some seem age dependent.

Polyarthritis may be a sequel of rubella. It usually commences when the rash has subsided, is more common after florid eruptions

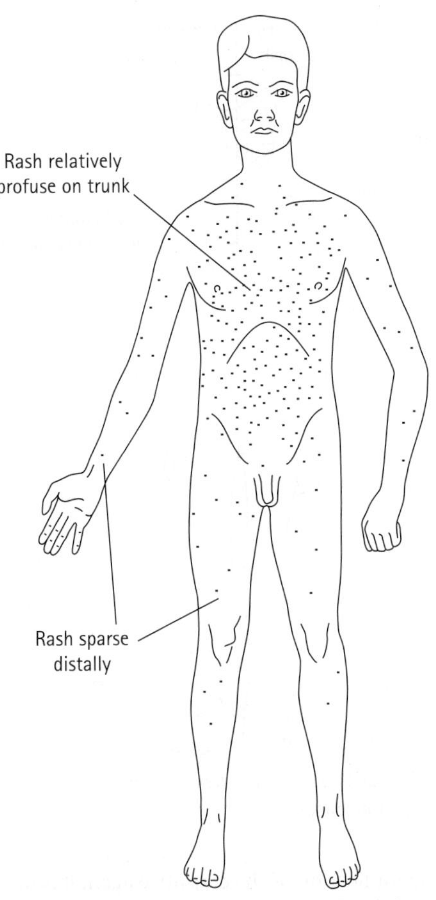

Fig. 26.31 The distribution and development of rash in rubella. (After Krugman & Ward 1968[242])

and occurs in adults, especially women, rather than in children. The small joints of the hands and the wrist joints are most often involved but the large joints can also be attacked. The condition usually resolves within 2 weeks.

Postinfectious encephalitis, myelitis and polyradiculitis may follow an attack of rubella and have a similar pathology to these syndromes when they occur after other infections. However, in rubella they appear to have a better prognosis.

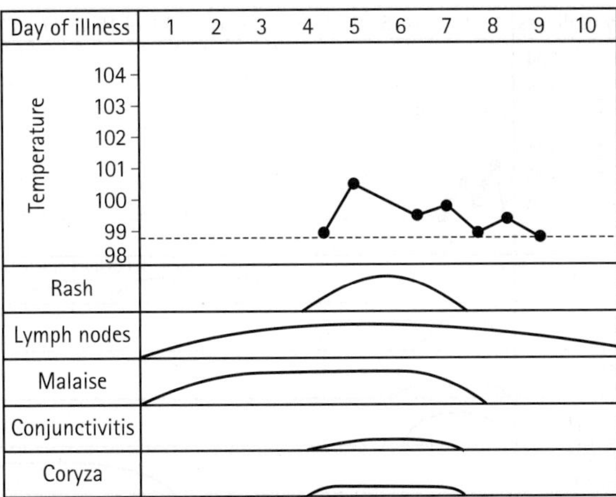

Fig. 26.32 The development of rubella. (After Krugman & Ward 1968[242])

Thrombocytopenia is quite common in the course of the illness and may become clinically manifest as purpura. Epistaxis, hematuria and melena can also develop. Some cases of so-called idiopathic thrombocytopenic purpura can be shown by laboratory tests to have resulted from subclinical rubella infection. Leukopenia is frequently found at the height of the illness and there may be an increase in plasma or Turk cells.

Diagnosis

Owing to the lack of pathognomonic features, one cannot rely on a clinical diagnosis of rubella and, whenever confirmation is important, laboratory tests (in the form of appropriate serological studies) should be used.

A serological diagnosis depends on the demonstration of a significant rise in antibody titer (fourfold or greater) when a sample of serum collected at the onset of the illness, and a further sample taken 2–3 weeks later, are compared.

Antibodies to rubella virus may be detected by hemagglutination-inhibition, neutralization, complement-fixation or radial hemolysis test. Nowadays, the hemagglutination test is generally preferred, owing to its reliability and the ease with which it can be performed.

Following infection both neutralizing and hemagglutination-inhibition antibodies persist, at a variable titer, for a long time whereas complement-fixation antibodies disappear more rapidly.

Virus may be recovered with relative ease from the nasopharynx during the last week of the incubation period and for up to 2 weeks thereafter. It is less readily isolated from the urine and blood. However, many laboratories do not offer viral culture for rubella.

Differential diagnosis

Rubella may be confused with many common exanthemata and other skin eruptions. Differentiation from measles, glandular fever and drug eruptions does not present great difficulty but scarlet fever can cause confusion. Enteroviral infections accompanied by a rash, especially those associated with ECHO virus infection, provide the greatest diagnostic challenge. The presence of the herald patch, the distribution over the trunk and the complete well-being of the patient help to distinguish pityriasis rosea.

Resort to laboratory tests is always desirable when doubt exists in regard to a suspicious rash in a pregnant woman or her contacts.

Treatment

There is no specific treatment for rubella. A rapid recovery is to be expected. Prodromal symptoms rarely cause trouble but analgesics may be needed when polyarthritis occurs. Neurological complications are managed along the usual lines for such conditions.

Prevention

As a general rule preventive measures are unnecessary in view of the mild nature of the disease. However, the situation is quite different in the case of women in early pregnancy and attempts to prevent rubella have traditionally been made by the intramuscular injection of normal human immunoglobulin. Evaluation of this procedure has proved difficult but cases of rubella, confirmed by laboratory tests, have occurred despite this use of immunoglobulin. Attenuated live rubella vaccines are now widely used and in general stimulate reasonable antibody levels. Opinions differ as to how they are best employed. Some recommend they are given to girls around puberty and non-immune pregnant women postpartum (selective immunization) while others believe children of both sexes should be given the vaccine in early childhood, usually in conjunction with measles and mumps vaccine as MMR, in an attempt to reduce the pool of infection in the community (universal immunization). Although terminations of pregnancy are frequently performed on pregnant women who have been inadvertently immunized there have been no cases of congenital rubella syndrome caused by the vaccine.

ERYTHEMA INFECTIOSUM (FIFTH DISEASE, SLAPPED CHEEK DISEASE)

This disease may occur at any time of year, but outbreaks in primary school children are classically in the winter and spring. Joint involvement may occur. Children with shortened red cell survival can develop profound anemia (aplastic crises). Infection during pregnancy can lead to hydrops fetalis.

Etiology

Erythema infectiosum is caused by parvovirus B19 (human parvovirus), a small, single-stranded DNA virus. Spread is by droplet infection, although, as the virus can be seen in plasma during infections, it could be transmitted by blood products. Erythrocyte precursors are particularly susceptible to the virus causing a mild fall in hemoglobin (of about 1 g/dl) in normal individuals but profound anemia in those whose red cell survival is already shortened.

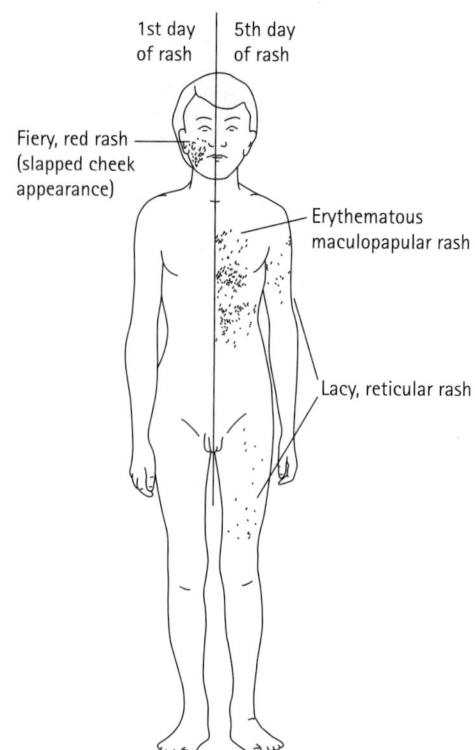

Fig. 26.33 The distribution and development of rash in erythema infectiosum (fifth disease).

Clinical features

B19 infection may be asymptomatic or may cause a mild febrile illness with rash. In children the first sign of infection is usually marked erythema of the cheeks or slapped cheek appearance often with relative circumoral pallor (Fig. 26.33). In volunteer studies, however, there is an initial febrile episode with headache, chills, myalgia and malaise associated with viremia and the rash appears about 7 days later (Fig. 26.34). Then 1–4 days after the slapped cheeks an itchy, erythematous, maculopapular rash develops on the trunk and limbs. As the rash on the limbs clears it leaves a lacy, reticular pattern. The rash may fluctuate over the next 1–3 weeks and a hot bath, for example, may lead to recrudescence of an evanescent rash.

Complications

Arthritis or arthralgia is more common in adults, but certainly can occur in children. It usually appears 1–6 days after the rash but there may be no history of rash at all. Arthritis is characteristically transient and asymmetrical, affecting wrists, knees, ankles, elbows and fingers, though it may persist for weeks or even months.

Children with a shortened red cell survival, such as those with sickle cell anemia, thalassemia major, hereditary spherocytosis or other hemolytic anemias, may have severe aplastic crises with hemoglobin levels falling as low as 1–2 g/dl and no reticulocytes.

Children with malignancy, particularly acute leukemia, or with HIV infection may develop prolonged anemia from chronic parvovirus B19 infection.

Infection during pregnancy can result in hydrops fetalis due to fetal anemia, which may be fatal, but no congenital syndrome has been described in babies of infected mothers who delivered at term.[354]

Encephalitis with or without neurological sequelae has rarely been reported after clinical erythema infectiosum, but as this was prior to the identification of the causative agent it is not certain that this is a true complication of B19 infection.

Diagnosis

Erythema infectiosum may closely mimic rubella, and the two diseases can circulate concurrently. The slapped cheek appearance with circumoral pallor can be mistaken for scarlet fever.

The diagnosis can be made serologically by demonstrating parvovirus B19-specific IgM on an acute serum sample, although it is always better to get a paired sample in case there is a late rise in antibody. The virus can be detected by electron microscopy in the plasma of patients with aplastic crises. This is particularly important in patients with sickle cell disease in whom severe

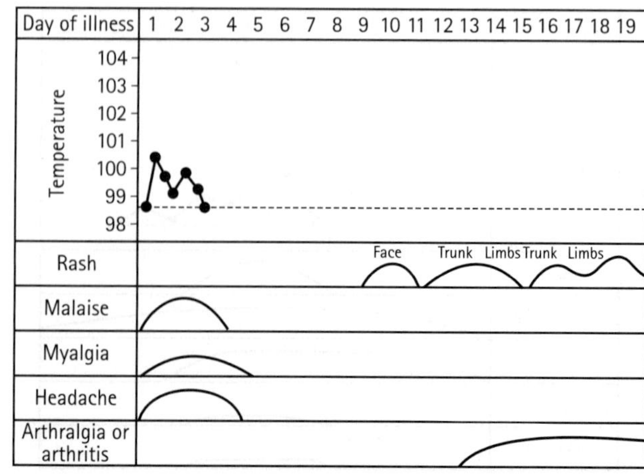

Fig. 26.34 The development of erythema infectiosum (fifth disease).

anemia might be due to sequestration or pneumococcal sepsis. DNA probes and PCR have been used to detect the viral genome in stillbirths with hydrops fetalis and to demonstrate persisting antigen in children with leukemia and chronic anemia.

Treatment

There is no specific treatment. Isolation of patients is unnecessary since they are no longer infectious when the rash appears.

Arthritis may require salicylates or non-steroidal anti-inflammatory agents. Children with aplastic crises may require blood transfusion until the red cell aplasia resolves spontaneously after 1–2 weeks.

ROSEOLA INFANTUM (SIXTH DISEASE, EXANTHEM SUBITUM, THREE DAY FEVER)

Roseola infantum is a common disease of infancy, characterized by fever and the appearance of an erythematous maculopapular rash as the fever defervesces. It may be confused with measles clinically. It is generally benign.

Etiology

A viral cause has long been postulated, since roseola was transmitted to a 6-month-old boy by injecting him with serum from a child with pre-eruptive roseola. There is good evidence that human herpesvirus 6 (HHV-6) is the main causative agent.[355,356] Seroconversion has been demonstrated in infants in association with clinical roseola, with modest rises in IgG but no IgM response, and the virus has been cultured from lymphocytes of affected children. HHV-7 is responsible for most clinical cases of roseola infantum which are HHV-6 negative.[357] These double stranded DNA viruses are members of the herpesvirus family, and as such, persist for the life of the host with frequent asymptomatic reactivation. There are two variant strains of HHV-6: type A and type B. Most of the primary infections in childhood are due to type B infection.

Clinical features

The illness starts abruptly with fever, and some anorexia and irritability although in general the child appears relatively well. Mild cough, coryza, diarrhea and vomiting rarely occur. The pyrexia of 38.9–40.6°C persists for 3–5 days, then falls precipitously as the rash appears (Fig. 26.35).[347] The rash is erythematous, with discrete macular or maculopapular lesions, and starts on the trunk and neck, sometimes spreading to the face and limbs. It lasts 1–2 days. Cervical lymphadenopathy is common and may sometimes be prominent: the suboccipital, posterior cervical and posterior auricular nodes are most commonly involved. There is no characteristic enanthem, although there may be pharyngitis, small exudative follicular tonsillar lesions, or small ulcers on the soft palate, tonsils and uvula.

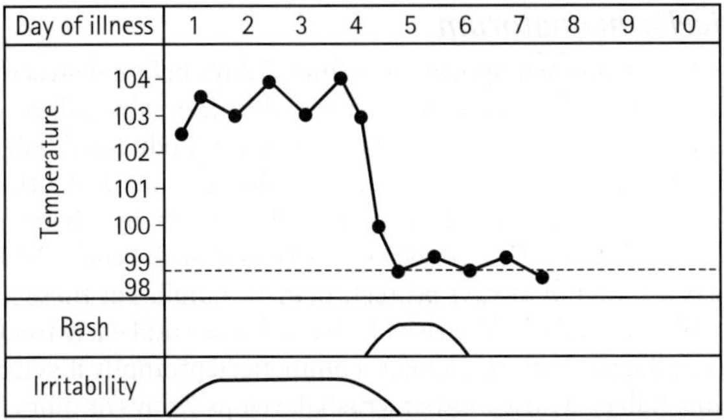

Fig. 26.35 The development of exanthem subitum. (After Krugman & Ward 1968[242])

For the first day or two of fever the white count is often elevated with a neutrophil leukocytosis, but then may fall as low as 3×10^9/L predominantly lymphocytes with an absolute neutropenia.

A number of clinical syndromes (bone marrow suppression, pneumonia, hepatitis, encephalitis) have been associated with reactivation of HHV-6 in the immunocompromised, although a causal link has been difficult to prove.[356]

Complications

Convulsions may occur in association with roseola. These are usually febrile convulsions but encephalitis has rarely been described, sometimes with severe residua such as hemiparesis or mental retardation. Rarely thrombocytopenic purpura may occur following roseola.[356]

Diagnosis

The diagnosis of roseola infantum is primarily clinical, although it can now be confirmed serologically. PCR assays to detect HHV-6 DNA are available, but cannot distinguish an acute infection from reactivation. The characteristic fever chart and discrete rash that does not become confluent distinguish roseola from other childhood exanthemata including measles. The rash may be confused with a drug rash if antibiotics have been given and a vaccine reaction may cause confusion if the illness comes on soon after immunization.

Treatment

There is no specific treatment. There are anecdotal reports of treatment of HHV-6 infection in immmunocompromised children with ganciclovir, but there is no evidence to support efficacy from clinical trials. Antipyretics may lessen the risk of convulsions, but if these occur, encephalitis should be considered and the child treated appropriately.

HERPESVIRUSES

CHICKENPOX (VARICELLA)

Chickenpox is a common and highly infectious disease caused by VZV, also known as HHV-3. In general it is a benign condition and has a virtually worldwide distribution. However, chickenpox is not endemic in some isolated areas and if introduced to such a community a more serious disease may occur. It can also prove fatal in neonates and sometimes in adults and can be fatal when contracted by a patient on immunosuppressive drugs.[358]

Immunity following chickenpox is usually life-long and second primary attacks are rare. Like all herpesviruses, however, the virus can remain latent and recur years later, in the case of VZV, in the form of zoster (shingles).

Etiology

Chickenpox is transmitted from person to person by direct contact, droplet or airborne spread; infection can also arise through articles recently contaminated by an infected person. Viral entry is through the upper respiratory tract mucosa or via the conjunctiva. Infectivity is maximal during the prodromal period 1 to 2 days before the eruption of the rash and has completely waned by the time the eruption becomes crusted. In the immunocompromised, infectivity may continue after crusting has occurred if new lesions continue to develop.

The causative agent, VZV, is a DNA virus. The virus particle is surrounded by a membrane and the approximate diameter of the capsid is 100 nm; it is readily seen under the electron microscope. The virus is highly specific for humans, and is very difficult to grow in culture in the laboratory.

Clinical features

Chickenpox is predominantly a disease of childhood and usually occurs between 2 and 8 years of age. Cases may occur in infancy. Peripartum intrauterine infection can lead to varicella neonatorum (see below) which, untreated, has a mortality up to 20%. Postnatal infection can cause classical chickenpox of a lesser severity occurring only in babies whose mothers have not had chickenpox.

Following an incubation period of 10–28 days, usually around 16 days, the disease starts with mild malaise and fever (Fig. 26.36).[347] In children prodromal symptoms may be absent and the illness begins with a rash. Older children and adults have more definite prodromata and symptoms include malaise, fever, headache, sore throat and backache.

The rash (Fig. 26.37)[347] commences as a crop of macules, which within hours pass through a papular stage to become vesicular; the vesicles persist for 3–4 days, becoming pustular and finally forming a crust. The spots are superficial and the vesicles may be round, oval, elliptical or irregular in shape; they are often surrounded by a red areola.

Evolution of the rash occurs by a series of crops, and lesions at different stages may be seen. The trunk is principally involved but spots also appear over the face, scalp and the proximal parts of the limbs. Lesions tend to be more abundant on covered rather than exposed parts of the body.

In mild cases the entire eruption may consist of a few spots; less often, the rash is almost generalized, extending to the distal parts of the limbs including the soles and palms. By the time of vesiculation there is often an intense pruritus. In some patients crusts can be very tenacious and 2–3 weeks may elapse before their separation is complete.

An enanthem is usually found and presents as vesiculation over the palate, tongue or buccal mucous membranes; the conjunctivae and vagina may be similarly affected.

Hemorrhagic chickenpox

In this there is usually a marked constitutional disturbance and high fever. Extensive bleeding into the vesicles develops and the lesions become black; areas of ecchymosis can appear on otherwise uninvolved skin. Bleeding may occur from mucous membranes and present as hematuria or melena. Both children and adults may contract this form of chickenpox and it has been particularly reported in patients receiving corticosteroids or cytotoxic drugs suggesting the importance of cell-mediated immunity as well as antibody in recovery from infection. It can be associated with profound thrombocytopenia (purpura fulminans) and is often fatal.

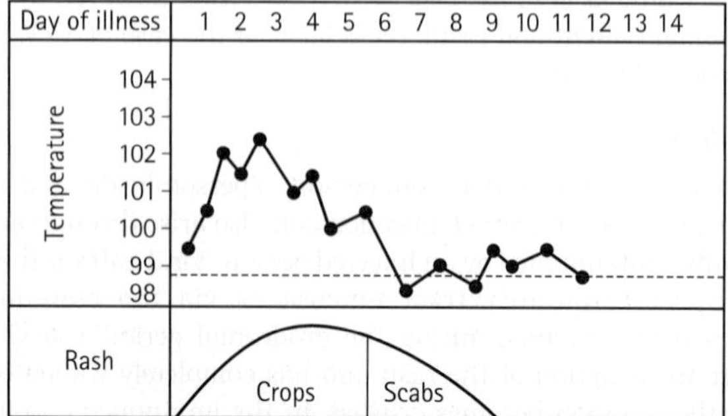

Fig. 26.36 The development of chickenpox. (After Krugman & Ward 1968[242].)

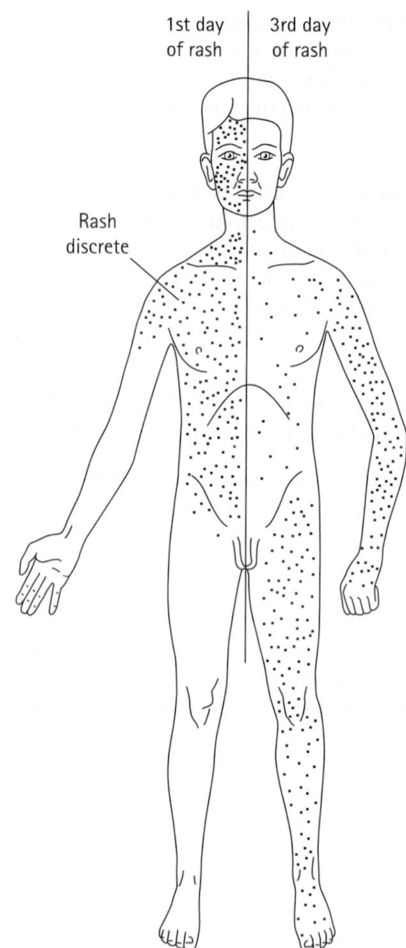

Fig. 26.37 The distribution of rash in chickenpox. (After Krugman & Ward 1968[242].)

Varicella gangrenosa

This form of the disease usually results from severe secondary bacterial infection (usually due to group A streptococci) of the vesicles which may extend down to muscle. These lesions are slow to heal and can leave considerable scarring. Occasionally this form of varicella appears to start ab initio before any apparent secondary infection.

Varicella neonatorum

If the maternal rash appears less than 7 days before delivery or up to 2 days after delivery there is a risk that the baby will receive a large inoculum of virus without maternal antibody. Such babies are at very high risk of disseminated disease with death from pneumonitis, and should be protected at birth by giving zoster immune globulin (ZIG) (reviewed in Heuchan & Isaacs 2001[359]). Since this does not always protect them,[360] families of these infants should be informed of the risk of severe disease and early treatment with acycloguanosine (aciclovir) commenced promptly if symptoms develop. Babies whose mother's rash develops 7 days or more before or 3 days or more after delivery are at low risk. Postnatally acquired chickenpox is nearly always mild although if the mother has not had chickenpox the use of ZIG should be considered for a neonate exposed to the virus.

Varicella bullosa

Bullous varicella may occur in children, the lesions developing into large bullae with a positive Nikolsky sign. It is due to superinfection with a toxin-producing *Staphylococcus aureus*, and the prognosis for full recovery without scarring is excellent. Treatment is with anti-staphylococcal antibiotics.

Complications

Sepsis

Secondary skin infection is the commonest complication. Abscesses may form locally or in regional lymph nodes. Cellulitis, erysipelas and scarlet fever can also develop. Bacteremic spread may give rise to pneumonia, osteomyelitis and septic arthritis. Common infecting organisms include group A streptococci and *S. aureus*.

Neurological

Postinfectious encephalitis can occur and usually starts as the rash reaches maturity. The most common manifestation is a pure cerebellar ataxia with an excellent prognosis. Complete recovery is virtually invariable, usually rapidly, though may rarely take some weeks. Acute disseminated encephalomyelitis (ADEM) is a more sinister but rarer form of postvaricella encephalitis with cerebral demyelination giving rise to long tract signs, cranial nerve lesions, convulsions, etc. Examination of the CSF may show a mild lymphocytic pleocytosis and slight elevation of the protein content. About 10% of cases of Reye syndrome occur secondary to chickenpox. Transverse myelitis, acute infantile hemiplegia and Guillain–Barré syndrome have been described complicating varicella.

Pneumonitis

Pneumonitis is usually seen in adults and immunocompromised children (and varicella neonatorum) and may present with acute respiratory distress or hemoptysis; diffuse nodular infiltration is seen on X-ray of the chest. The diagnosis is often obscure until the typical exanthem develops. Some cases die and, in those who recover, miliary calcification may be seen in the lung fields some years later.

In normal children, pneumonia complicating chickenpox is most likely to be bacterial, due to *S. pneumoniae*, group A streptococcus or occasionally *S. aureus*.

Others

Myocarditis, pericarditis, endocarditis, hepatitis and glomerulonephritis have rarely been reported. Appendicitis may also occur and can present before the eruptive phase; this sometimes leads to cross infection in pediatric surgical wards. Keratitis and conjunctivitis are rare and usually benign. Arthritis may mimic septic arthritis but the latter should always be excluded by examination of the joint fluid because septic arthritis can complicate chickenpox. If ampicillin is prescribed a drug eruption may occur as with EBV infection, probably as a result of drug–hapten interaction.

Congenital varicella

If the mother contracts chickenpox up to 20 weeks' gestation, there is about a 2% risk of the baby developing congenital varicella syndrome with cicatricial scarring of the limbs, cortical atrophy, hypoplasia of limbs, digital defects, retinitis or cataracts. Maternal chickenpox in the second 20 weeks of gestation may result in an inapparent primary infection in the fetus, and causes shingles in the first years of life in about 1% of exposed children.

Diagnosis

The clinical course of varicella and the nature of the rash are usually typical and a firm clinical diagnosis can be made. Rapid diagnosis can be by direct immunofluorescence (DFA) of cells scraped from the base of a vesicle and placed directly on a slide. DFA can also be performed on respiratory secretions obtained by nasopharyngeal aspirate or bronchoalveolar lavage for the diagnosis of infection in the immunocompromised.

VZV can be isolated from vesicle fluid collected during the first 3 or 4 days of the rash, but rarely from other sites. Tissue culture for varicella is not widely available. Detection of VZV DNA in body fluids or tissues by PCR is a sensitive technique that may be helpful in the diagnosis of VZV infection in the immunocompromised child.

A number of serological assays are available for diagnosis of past VZV infection that vary in their sensitivity. These have application in deciding if an exposed individual needs passive immunoprophylaxis. They can also be used to make a retrospective diagnosis of VZV infection if a significant rise in varicella IgG has occurred during the illness. In this setting, it is necessary to test two sera – an acute sample collected within a day or two of the onset of the illness and a convalescent sample collected 2 or 3 weeks later.

Differential diagnosis

Chickenpox can be confused with impetigo, scabies, dermatitis herpetiformis, eczema herpeticum or vaccinatum and erythema multiforme. In most of these the absence of the typical, centripetal distribution and cropping of varicella helps in the differentiation.

Treatment

General

No treatment is usually required and bed rest is probably unnecessary except in ill patients. Simple analgesics will control prodromal symptoms where these are troublesome. Aspirin should not be given because of the risk of Reye syndrome. Calamine lotion will normally soothe pruritus; if not, an antihistamine should be tried. If the enanthem is unusually severe careful oral toilet is needed and lesions on the conjunctiva should be protected from secondary infection. Treatment with aciclovir is indicated if infection develops in immunosuppressed cases, and in any patient with severe disease.

Sepsis

In convalescence simple antiseptics should control superficial skin infection. More severe sepsis will require appropriate antibacterial chemotherapy which should be guided by swabbing of the affected lesions and by cultures of the blood and of any pus. Flucloxacillin will adequately treat hemolytic streptococcal infection or staphylococcal infection until culture results are available.

Encephalitis

No specific treatment is available for the neurological complications and the usual supportive measures will be employed. Some clinicians favor the use of corticosteroids in severe cases despite the unhappy association of chickenpox with these drugs. It is argued that the encephalitis is of allergic origin and that by this stage of the illness there is sufficient antibody response to prevent further dissemination of the virus. In practice no serious untoward effects have been reported where steroids have been used in this condition although it is difficult to assess how much this therapy contributes to any recovery. Similarly the role of aciclovir in treating varicella encephalitis is unclear.

Others

Cases of severe varicella pneumonitis and profound thrombocytopenia have also been treated with aciclovir and corticosteroid drugs but an accurate evaluation of their benefit is impossible. Appendicitis should be treated surgically.

Prevention

The live attenuated Oka strain varicella vaccine is available in some countries for use in healthy children over 12 months of age or adults who have not had varicella. It has been shown to be highly effective (85–90% of children) in preventing clinical disease postexposure.[361]

The infectivity of chickenpox is such that the strictest isolation measures may fail to prevent its spread. In the community, it is usual practice to isolate a child from school or day care until the rash has become crusted. In the hospital setting, a child with active chickenpox should be quarantined in respiratory isolation while the rash remains vesicular.

Postexposure prophylaxis

In the case of patients who are receiving corticosteroid drugs or cytotoxic drugs, every effort should be made to prevent exposure to chickenpox and herpes zoster for reasons already described. If such exposure should occur then hyperimmune chickenpox gamma globulin (ZIG) has been shown to modify severity even if it does not always prevent the disease, and should be given. The use of ZIG in neonates has already been discussed. Chemoprophylaxis with aciclovir after exposure to the immunocompetent or immunocompromised individual has been observed to reduce the likelihood of clinical disease in a few small case control studies,[362–364] but this has not been assessed in a properly evaluated randomized controlled trial and is not routinely advocated.[365] Postexposure immunization with the Oka VZV vaccine has been shown to protect against or modify chickenpox in non-randomized cohort studies.[366] It is thought to be most effective if given within 5 days of exposure.

HERPES ZOSTER (ZOSTER: SHINGLES)

The clinical relationship between chickenpox and herpes zoster has long been recognized. The virus causing the two syndromes is identical, and is referred to as the varicella-zoster virus (VZV). Non-immune persons may develop chickenpox when exposed to herpes zoster but the converse rarely occurs. The inoculation of children with virus obtained from zoster patients has resulted in clinical chickenpox which has then spread to other children as chickenpox.

Following an attack of varicella, the virus survives in a latent form in the sensory root ganglia of the cord and brain, a situation with similarities to latent infection by HSV. After an interval of many years, but sometimes earlier, the virus becomes activated by local precipitating factors or by some depression of protective immunological mechanisms. Virus then spreads along the sensory root in question; adjacent motor areas of the cord, or other parts of the cerebrum, may become involved. A degree of systemic spread can also occur which provokes a modified form of chickenpox. Such modification may result from the antigenic stimulus provided by the reactivated virus, and the very high antibody levels found early in the course of herpes zoster support this impression.

Patients who develop zoster are usually elderly but the disease does occur in children and younger adults. In young children, pain is much less marked than in adults, and zoster is not suggestive of immune deficiency or malignancy. There is often a history of maternal varicella during pregnancy or early neonatal varicella: it is thought that varicella at a time of relatively poor immunity is more likely to result in childhood zoster. In a few instances, primary infection by the VZV appears to provoke zoster rather than chickenpox; the explanation is not known. On occasion zoster may also occur simultaneously with a primary attack of chickenpox.

For reasons alluded to above, zoster is seen quite frequently in persons suffering from leukemia or other malignant disease and can follow radiotherapy.

Clinical features

Zoster may start with constitutional disturbance or progressive pain over a particular dermatome, although in children zoster may be pain free. Clusters of macules and papules appear on the skin overlying the dermatome, rarely crossing the midline. These soon vesiculate and the vesicles formed may be larger than in chickenpox and tend to coalesce. Extensive crusting follows, which slowly separates to expose a raw, ulcerated area. This will bleed readily and is liable to secondary infection. Healing is slow and after months or years, vitiligo may develop and the involved skin is often anesthetic. Enlargement of the regional lymph nodes is very common.

Acute pain tends to subside as crusting sets in but extreme irritation and neuralgia may persist for months and even years (postherpetic neuralgia). In children the illness tends to be much milder, pain is mild or absent and recovery is considerably quicker.

In hospitals, one tends to find selected examples of zoster but more representative surveys show that thoracic segments are most commonly involved. However, zoster of the trigeminal nerve, and usually of the supraophthalmic division, is the commonest variety seen in hospital.

Geniculate herpes is of special interest and is frequently misdiagnosed; in this form of zoster, vesicles appear on the meatus and pinna of the ear. Pain may be experienced in the throat, in or behind the ear and taste may be lost over the anterior two-thirds of the tongue. Facial paralysis, sometimes permanent, may result. This condition is sometimes referred to as the *Ramsay Hunt* syndrome. A modified generalized rash over the trunk and face is seen in many cases provided examination is sufficiently diligent. Other features include involvement of the adjacent motor root with resultant paralysis which can be permanent, and meningitis, encephalitis or myelitis can be encountered.

Occasionally zoster occurs without any accompanying rash, the so-called zoster sine herpete.

Diagnosis

Prior to the appearance of the skin eruption diagnosis is difficult in children, in whom zoster is rather unexpected. Diagnoses such as pleurisy or fibrositis may be made but the difficulties are quickly resolved when the classical rash, along the line of a nerve, makes its appearance. Laboratory tests are referred to in the section on chickenpox.

Treatment

The illness is usually mild in children and simple analgesics such as paracetamol will usually control pain. Relief may follow the application of a dusting powder of zinc oxide or the use of cold sprays.

Supraophthalmic zoster requires special care. It is advisable to dilate the pupil with atropine and any break in the cornea may require treatment with topical antibiotics to prevent secondary bacterial infection. Topical idoxuridine is effective against ophthalmic VZV. The help of a qualified ophthalmologist is advisable.

In some instances, particularly severe zoster may show a dramatic response to treatment by corticosteroid drugs. However, their general use is not advised and they are best avoided in zoster affecting the eye and wherever any underlying immunological defect may be present. Aciclovir or vidarabine is only needed for immunocompromised children or those with severe zoster.

Prognosis

This is usually good in children. Postherpetic neuralgia is uncommon but may persist for a long time. Certain paralyses can prove permanent and impairment of vision has followed supraophthalmic zoster. Such complications are more commonly found in adult cases.

HERPES SIMPLEX

Primary infection by *Herpesvirus hominis* (HSV) usually occurs in early childhood and is generally subclinical. However, in a small percentage of children it may produce a variable clinical illness, the main features of which include localized vesiculation on some part of the body and a sharp constitutional reaction. Some children avoid infection altogether and may reach adolescence or adult life with no immunity to this virus. This is more likely to occur when they have been brought up in rural, as opposed to urban, areas and, as with many other viral infections, an attack in adult life can often be more severe.

An interesting feature of this virus is its ability to persist in a latent form once the primary infection, whether clinical or subclinical, has subsided. In some people, the virus becomes reactivated by certain non-specific stimuli at various times in their lives and the resultant clinical manifestations tend to differ from those seen with primary infection. Reactivation of HSV with asymptomatic shedding or less commonly clinical disease is a common event after the initial infection.[367]

Etiology

HSV is a DNA virus surrounded by a membrane and is approximately 150–180 nm in diameter. There are two strains, HSV types 1 and 2. HSV type 2 primarily infects the genital tracts of adults, and infection in the pregnant woman near term can result in serious infection in the newborn infant. HSV type 1 is primarily oral, although type 2 can cause oral disease and type 1 can infect the genitalia.

Clinical features: primary herpes

A variety of different syndromes may result from primary infection by HSV and are now described in detail.

Acute herpetic gingivostomatitis (ulcerative stomatitis)

This, the commonest manifestation, commences with a sharp constitutional reaction with high fever, malaise, anorexia and irritability. The patient, usually a young child, has difficulty feeding due to pain in the mouth. Inspection, often hampered by severe discomfort, reveals marked swelling and inflammation of the gums which may bleed at the merest touch. Deeper inspection will reveal the typical shallow ulcers, white in color, on such sites as the tongue, palate, gums, buccal mucosa and tonsils. In mild cases the ulcers are few; in more severe examples there may be a contiguous sheet of ulcers involving all the sites mentioned. Saliva tends to flow from the mouth and satellite lesions form down the chin or cheek where the child dribbles. Regional lymph nodes in the neck enlarge and fever will persist for several days. Mild cases subside rapidly but the worst may take up to 2 weeks before the local lesions disappear. Younger children may implant the virus onto other sites such as the sucked finger or perineal region, where vesiculation will develop. The isolation of HSV-2 from an oropharyngeal lesion in a child prior to puberty should raise the question of sexual abuse.

Perineal herpes (acute herpetic vulvovaginitis)

This is a less common primary manifestation, though it may be underdiagnosed in view of confusion with severe napkin and other eruptions in the same area. It is diagnosed far more often in girls, though primary perineal herpes sometimes occurs in boys. Some degree of constitutional upset will again herald the infection, to be followed by painful vesiculation over the perineum, which may extend into the vagina in girls. Lesions close to the external urethral orifice may cause difficulties with micturition and regional adenitis may develop. The lesions usually subside without scarring despite the likelihood of secondary infection. Reactivation occurs over the buttocks, thighs or perineum.

Traumatic herpetic infection

The intact skin appears relatively resistant to this virus but primary infection may arise over the site of abrasions and burns. An interesting variety is the herpetic whitlow of the finger which is sometimes seen in nurses who contract the infection by virus entering such lesions as needle puncture wounds or the abrasions that can result from opening glass phials – lesions that are common on the nurse's hand. Here again there may be a marked constitutional upset and regional lymphadenitis.

Acute herpetic keratoconjunctivitis

Primary herpetic infection of the eye is a serious presentation of this infection though relatively rare. The majority of cases are due to HSV-1, although HSV-2 eye disease may occur as a consequence of neonatal infection. Normally only one eye is involved and cases present with constitutional upset and pain. Marked reddening and edema appear on the affected conjunctiva, the cornea becomes hazy and the eye will usually close. Vesicles appear around the lids and a purulent discharge often occurs. So long as the infection remains superficial the condition will usually subside without complications in 10–14 days. Deeper involvement may give rise to keratitis disciformis, hypopyon keratitis or iridocyclitis, all of which may be followed by scarring; however, these are more commonly encountered in recurrent herpetic infection. Recurrent herpetic keratitis has been shown to be an immune-mediated phenomenon.[368]

Kaposi's varicelliform eruption (KVE) or eczema herpeticum

Children with eczema are prone to superinfection of the involved skin by a number of organisms including HSV. The disease starts with a particularly sharp constitutional upset and vesicles then appear on the skin and are most intense at the eczematous areas. An experienced observer may readily recognize the condition; more often the true diagnosis is unappreciated and extensive secondary infection accompanied by a marked serosanguinous discharge will develop. Further crops of vesicles may appear and the child's condition may deteriorate further. The most severe cases may be fatal without aciclovir therapy; in the remainder there is a slow recovery over a period of 3–4 weeks.

Primary herpetic meningoencephalitis

Previously considered an infrequent infection, modern virological techniques have shown that herpetic meningoencephalitis is more common than was believed. The signs of CNS involvement may appear shortly after a primary lesion at some other site but there is usually no clinical evidence to indicate the basic etiological agent. Cases may present as mild forms of aseptic meningitis or as a rapidly fatal form of encephalitis principally involving the temporal lobes. Confusion with a brain abscess or tumor may arise and in those who recover severe cerebral damage may persist. Neonatal herpes encephalitis classically presents with facial twitching and focal fits at 7–28 days, and there is rarely a history of skin lesions or maternal herpes.

Generalized herpetic infection

This form is normally confined to the newborn and occurs in infants with no protective maternal antibody. The source of the infection is usually the mother or rarely an attendant in the nursery or a relative. The condition presents with fever, hepatosplenomegaly and deepening jaundice, the infant becoming progressively weaker with vomiting and anorexia. The outcome is usually fatal and the diagnosis made at autopsy when typical inclusion bodies are found in the affected viscera. Visible involvement of the skin and mucous membranes is absent in most cases.

Neonatal infection

Skin, eye or mouth lesions may or may not precede the development of generalized or CNS herpes infection. Nevertheless there is a very high risk of progression from such isolated lesions, about 70% without treatment. The suspicion of neonatal HSV infection such as any vesicular lesion, pneumonitis starting on day 3 to 5 of life, or culture negative sepsis with or without thrombocytopenia, jaundice, or hepatitis should be treated as an emergency, and urgent direct immunofluorescence obtained on the vesicle fluid, CSF examination performed including detection of HSV DNA by PCR, and empirical intravenous treatment with aciclovir started. Duration of therapy is for 14 to 21 days, the longer course being required for proven encephalitis, or disseminated infection. The use of empirical oral aciclovir to suppress frequent recurrences after HSV-2 skin disease or either type of encephalits in the newborn is currently in clinical trial.

Clinical features: recurrent herpes

Exacerbations of latent HSV infection may be provoked by a variety of non-specific stimuli which include upper respiratory infections, any febrile illness, gastrointestinal upsets, overexposure to sunlight and emotional upsets. Drugs and certain foods have also been incriminated.

Whatever the excitant, recurrent herpes presents as a crop of tiny vesicles which are sometimes painful and after a few days will dry up to form a scab. They may erupt on almost any part of the skin or on the mucous membranes of the mouth, conjunctivae or genitalia. The most usual site is on the skin around the nose and mouth (cold sores). Exacerbations tend to recur at the same site in any particular individual. Recurrent herpes gives rise to little or no constitutional upset or fever but the excitant, such as lobar pneumonia, may do so.

Diagnosis

The clinical features are often diagnostic in themselves but resort to laboratory aid is of help in certain instances. The procedures most commonly employed are:

1. growth of the virus in tissue culture;
2. demonstration of viral antigens in the material by a fluorescent antibody technique;
3. detection of HSV DNA in CSF or other bodily secretion or tissue by PCR.

Other procedures that may be employed are:

4. demonstration under the electron microscope of herpesvirus particles in material taken from a lesion;
5. antibody estimations on acute and convalescent serum samples to show specific IgM or a significant rise in IgG during a suspected primary infection;
6. histological evidence of intranuclear inclusions and giant cells.

Primary herpes

The oral lesions of primary herpetic gingivostomatitis may be confused with a variety of conditions such as thrush, tonsillitis, Vincent's stomatitis, agranulocytosis and leukemia. Careful clinical and laboratory studies readily differentiate most of these but herpangina, due to infection by Coxsackie viruses group A, can cause genuine confusion; however, gingivitis does not normally accompany herpangina, but is common in herpetic infections. Virus studies may be needed in difficult cases. Herpetic vulvovaginitis is readily confused with ammoniacal dermatitis which has been secondarily infected. Impetigo of the vulva is usually accompanied by involvement elsewhere. Kaposi's varicelliform eruption (eczema herpeticum) may be confused with bacterial superinfection of eczema, with eczema vaccinatum and occasionally with varicella. Herpetic meningoencephalitis is difficult to diagnose on clinical grounds; usually virological studies are required to make a conclusive diagnosis.

Recurrent herpes

Recurrent herpes produces a fairly precise diagnostic picture, but on occasion can resemble herpes zoster. The absence of pain, lack of a definable, neurological distribution and differing nature of the vesicles should differentiate these conditions.

Treatment

As a rule, primary oral herpetic infections do not require other than supportive treatment. Severe examples of gingivostomatitis may have feeding difficulties due to pain, and careful coaxing will be needed to ensure adequate hydration; cleansing of the mouth is also difficult on account of this pain. Irritating acidic fluids should be avoided and diet restricted to cold, bland drinks during the most acute phase. Superinfection by *Candida* may occur but this usually responds to treatment by the local application of nystatin suspension; secondary bacterial infection rarely warrants any antibiotic therapy though this may be required in herpetic vulvovaginitis. Intravenous aciclovir should be reserved for children requiring hospital admission for intravenous rehydration.

Eye involvement is best managed by an experienced ophthalmologist. Herpetic infections are amongst the few viral diseases in which highly successful treatment by antiviral agents has been reported; topical 5-iodo-2-deoxyuridine (IDU) or aciclovir are effective in herpetic eye infections.[369] Intravenous aciclovir is the treatment of choice for herpes simplex encephalitis, for KVE and for any manifestations of HSV disease in a neonate.

CYTOMEGALOVIRUS INFECTIONS

Prior to 1950 cytomegalic inclusion disease (CID) was recognized as a fatal disease of infancy in which the diagnosis was invariably made at autopsy. A viral cause was always suspected and the discovery of large intranuclear inclusions in epithelial cells from stained urinary deposits lent support to this hypothesis. Subsequently the responsible virus was successfully grown in tissue cultures and the knowledge of cytomegalovirus (CMV) infections has greatly expanded in recent years. CMV is a DNA virus of the herpesvirus group and as such, after the primary infection, causes latent infection with frequent subclinical reactivations for the life of the host. It is ubiquitous in the community, and in the immunocompetent host usually results in asymptomatic infection.

Types

There are three main clinical syndromes produced by CMV. Firstly, infection in the newborn, usually acquired congenitally, results in the established picture of CID. Secondly, an illness may be produced in older children and adults which has similar clinical features to infectious mononucleosis. Lastly, there is increasing evidence of opportunistic infection by CMV in immunocompromised patients with human immunodeficiency virus infection, or post solid organ or bone marrow transplantation; it is postulated in these instances that the virus is transmitted through blood transfusion or that a latent infection becomes reactivated. Concurrent immunosuppressive therapy used in this field of surgery is an obvious factor of importance in disseminating the infection, regardless of the mode of entry.

It is also relevant to comment on the frequency with which healthy individuals may be found with antibodies to CMV in their blood or occasionally have the virus isolated from their urine, indicating that widespread subclinical infection by this agent occurs.

Clinical features

CID of infants is described in Chaper 10 (Infection and immunity in the newborn).

In older children and adults, CMV infection is usually asymptomatic. On occasion, it may present with fever, cough, headaches and pains which are usually situated in the back and limbs. The clinical picture is one of infectious mononucleosis, with lymphadenopathy, hepatosplenomegaly and sometimes jaundice. Examination of the peripheral blood reveals the presence of atypical lymphocytes, and there is a varying degree of derangement in liver function tests. Hemolytic anemia can occur, and cold agglutinins, cryoglobulins and antinuclear factor may be present. Ampicillin may cause a rash as in EBV infection. The suspected diagnosis is usually glandular fever, but this is not supported by the heterophil antibody test. CMV may produce a pneumonitis but this is usually seen in premature neonates with postnatally acquired infection or children suffering from underlying diseases such as chronic hepatic disorders, leukemia and other malignancies.

A febrile illness with features suggesting infectious mononucleosis may also be encountered in patients who have recently undergone open heart surgery or organ transplantation and investigation of obscure postoperative illness in such cases should include the possibility of CMV infection. In patients with immune deficiency, particularly AIDS patients, CMV may cause pneumonitis, hepatitis, encephalitis or myelitis, severe retinitis and colitis. Recently, HIV-infected children who acquire CMV during the first 4 years of life have been shown to have a more rapid progression to AIDS than those who remain CMV-negative.[370] CMV is a frequent cause of death due to hepatitis or pneumonitis in liver transplant patients and of graft rejection in renal transplant patients. The virus is usually acquired from the donor organ or blood products, although reactivation of latent host CMV may also occur.

Laboratory diagnosis

Histological lesions due to CMV infection are characterized by large cells containing intranuclear and cytoplasmic inclusion bodies; the inclusion-containing cells may be widely disseminated.

Rapid viral diagnosis using DNA probes or by early immunofluorescence testing of tissue cultures (so-called shell vial cultures) or detection of the CMV pp65 antigen in blood is particularly useful in the management of suspected CMV infection in immunocompromised patients.

A clinical diagnosis may be confirmed by:

1. isolation of the virus from urine, peripheral blood mononculear cells, or other secretions;
2. demonstration of a significant rise in antibody titer during the illness;
3. the presence of typical histological lesions in a biopsy specimen, e.g. liver;
4. typical inclusion bodies in cell deposits of fresh urine.

With improved virological techniques, efforts should always be made to grow CMV when CID is considered to be present. Suitable specimens are fresh urine samples and saliva swabs but these specimens must be delivered to the laboratory with minimum delay as the virus easily loses its infectivity. Isolation of the agent is usually carried out in tissue cultures of human fibroblasts.

Quantification of the amount of CMV DNA or antigen in blood or other secretions to monitor recurrence and allow early pre-emptive therapy in the immuncompromised child is currently being evaluated.[371]

Differential diagnosis

CID requires to be differentiated from other congenital infections such as rubella, syphilis, toxoplasmosis, disseminated herpes simplex and sepsis of the newborn. CMV infections acquired in later life may mimic a variety of febrile states but infectious mononucleosis is the most likely condition to cause confusion; where jaundice occurs infectious hepatitis, serum hepatitis and leptospirosis require exclusion.

Prevention

Blood products from CMV antibody negative donors should always be given to preterm neonates and immunocompromised patients, particularly post-transplant or HIV-infected patients. Alternatively, as the virus is cell associated, filtration or freezing of the donor blood to remove white cells also reduces the risk of acquired CMV infection.

Passive immunoprophylaxis of transplant patients with immunoglobulin is partially successful in reducing the risk of CMV infection. Seropositive CMV patients may reactivate when immunosuppressed, and interferon but not aciclovir reduces this risk.

Treatment

Ganciclovir, a derivative of aciclovir, has been successfully used to treat immunocompromised patients with CMV retinitis, enteritis and pneumonitis.[372] In adult patients, 70–80% cease excretion of CMV within a week, with the exception of marrow transplant patients with CMV pneumonitis of whom somewhat fewer respond. However, relapse occurs in about half when ganciclovir is stopped, it causes significant marrow suppression, the drug is incorporated into the host genome.

Foscarnet causes less marrow suppression, although transient renal impairment may occur. There are few controlled data on its use in CMV infections in childhood. Cidofovir is another antiviral agent with activity against CMV. Its use is in CMV retinitis or prophylaxis in the organ transplant population.

There are limited data available on the efficacy of intravenous ganciclovir to reduce or prevent clinical manifestations of congenital CMV disease.

Prognosis

Congenital CMV infection has a variable outcome. Normal individuals who contract CMV infection rarely suffer any sequelae, but in immunocompromised patients, blindness due to retinitis, graft rejection and death from pneumonitis, hepatitis and disseminated infection may occur.

EBV

EBV is the cause of infectious mononucleosis or glandular fever, a disease primarily of older children, adolescents and young adults. An almost identical syndrome can be caused by CMV and *Toxoplasma gondii* as well as EBV. An anginose form of glandular fever primarily affecting the tonsils is seen in younger children under 5 years of age. EBV is a DNA virus and like the other herpesviruses can persist in a latent state and reactivate. It has a worldwide distribution and is potentially oncogenic and has been linked with nasopharyngeal carcinoma, Burkitt lymphoma and other lymphomas, particularly in immunocompromised patients. It can also cause lymphoproliferative syndromes post-transplant or in the HIV-infected individual.

Etiology and epidemiology

Primary infection of the lymphoid tissue of the nasopharynx may be asymptomatic or may lead to symptomatic infection of lymph nodes. Humans are the only source of EBV and transmission is by the respiratory route and the virus is of low infectivity, usually requiring intimate oral contact. The 'kissing disease' refers to its spread among adolescents and young adults by this route. Epidemics are unusual. The virus persists in the nasopharynx and the uterine cervix. The virus primarily infects B lymphocytes but the atypical mononuclear cells seen in the blood film are activated T lymphocytes.

Clinical features

The anginose form of glandular fever is characterized by fever and sore throat with moderate or marked cervical lymphadenopathy. The tonsils are red and inflamed and there is often white exudative folliculitis. Other lymph nodes and spleen are rarely enlarged and the clinical picture is not readily distinguishable from acute streptococcal tonsillitis, except that EBV is more likely to cause palatal petechiae.

Glandular fever usually starts insidiously with malaise, anorexia and fever. Usually sore throat is a prominent symptom. Occasionally the patient merely has malaise and fever for 1–3 weeks with chills and sweats (febrile form of infectious mononucleosis) and presents with pyrexia of unknown origin. Generally, however, there is marked enlargement of posterior and anterior cervical lymph nodes, and the suboccipital, postauricular, axillary, epitrochlear and inguinal nodes may also be enlarged (glandular form). The tonsils may be inflamed with exudate and rarely this can be sufficient to impair swallowing and even breathing. Splenomegaly is usual and hepatomegaly may also be present, sometimes with jaundice.

Skin eruptions occur in about 10–15% of cases. The commonest is a widespread maculopapular rash but morbilliform, scarlatiniform, purpuric and urticarial rashes may occur. Ampicillin causes a particularly florid, confluent maculopapular rash in EBV infection, and this ampicillin rash may also be seen though less commonly in conjunction with other herpesvirus infections such as CMV and chickenpox.

In Duncan syndrome, or X-linked lymphoproliferative disease, affected males are unable to control EBV infection and develop generalized lymphadenopathy and hepatosplenomegaly which persists and is rapidly fatal. These patients usually have persistently high levels of IgG antibodies to the viral capsid antigen (VCA).

EBV may be responsible for the lymphoid interstitial pneumonitis that can occur in children with HIV infection, since the EBV genome has been demonstrated in lung biopsy specimens from these patients. It can also cause CNS and other lymphomas in patients with HIV infection.

Complications

Threatened obstruction of the airway may occur in the severe anginose variety especially when there is secondary edema in the neck. Neurological complications include aseptic meningitis, cranial nerve palsies (including Bell's palsy), encephalomyelitis, transverse myelitis and Guillain–Barré syndrome. Cardiac involvement may present as myocarditis or as transient arrhythmias. Other complications include pneumonitis, orchitis, rupture of the spleen, hemolytic anemia, thrombocytopenic purpura and various ocular manifestations; hepatic involvement has been referred to previously. A prolonged illness with fatigue and relapses over many months has occasionally been described in children, in association with raised EBV antibodies. Chronic EBV infection is not a common cause of the 'chronic fatigue syndrome' or myalgic encephalopathy (ME).

EBV is thought to be the cause of Burkitt lymphoma and of nasopharyngeal carcinoma, in both of which tumors the EBV genome can consistently be demonstrated.

Diagnosis

Five main points arise in the diagnosis of glandular fever – a suggestive clinical picture, typical changes in the peripheral blood, a positive heterophile antibody test, IgM antibody to EBV, and certain non-specific changes in other laboratory tests.

Blood changes

Most important is the presence of large, atypical mononuclear cells which have an irregular nucleus, whose cytoplasm contains vacuoles and with characteristic pale staining of the cellular cytoplasm. Often there is a leukocytosis of $10–20 \times 10^9$ cells/L and sometimes the predominant cells are initially polymorphonuclear. However, atypical monocytes and lymphocytes soon appear, or may be present from the outset, and these can represent from 5 to 50% of the total leukocyte count. Other changes in the blood include occasional cases where there is a leukopenia and rare instances of profound thrombocytopenia and transient autoimmune hemolytic anemia.

Heterophile antibody test (Paul–Bunnell reaction)

There is massive B cell activation in acute EBV infection resulting in an outpouring of non-specific antibodies. Frequently sheep red cell agglutinins (heterophile antibodies) develop by the second week of infectious mononucleosis but occasionally the appearance of these agglutinins may be delayed for 2 or 3 weeks, so an early negative test should be repeated.

Sheep red cell agglutinins are not specific for infectious mononucleosis and may occur in other conditions. However, by means of absorption tests using guinea pig kidney and ox erythrocytes the specificity of the test may be increased. The following are the salient features:

1. Antibodies present in infectious mononucleosis are not absorbed by guinea pig kidney but are absorbed by ox erythrocytes.
2. Antibodies found in normal serum are not absorbed by ox erythrocytes but they are absorbed by guinea pig kidney.
3. Antibodies found in serum sickness are absorbed by both guinea pig kidney and ox erythrocytes.

Agglutinins to horse erythrocytes may also be present in the serum of a patient suffering from infectious mononucleosis and in many laboratories a test based on the agglutination of horse erythrocytes is in use. This is the basis of the rapid slide test, the 'Monospot' test. This test may sometimes be negative early in the disease and if EBV is suspected should be repeated. The test is unreliable under 5 years of age owing to false negative results.

EBV antibody tests

The presence of specific EBV anti-VCA IgM antibody indicates a recent or current infection, whereas the presence of IgG antibodies to the VCA or nuclear antigen (EBNA) merely indicates an infection with EBV some time in the past. Only a small proportion of affected patients show a rise in IgG to VCA so the IgM test is preferred to show acute infection.

Non-specific laboratory tests

In well over half the cases, some derangement of liver function tests will be found. Most often there is mild or moderate rise in the serum alanine aminotransferase (AAT) or glutamic pyruvate transaminase (SGPT) level but the alkaline phosphatase and serum bilirubin levels may also rise. Usually these changes are transient but in cases with clinical evidence of hepatic involvement the derangement in liver function tests is more marked.

On occasion, a false positive Wassermann reaction occurs in infectious mononucleosis and high antistreptolysin 'O' titers may be found; the latter probably arise from an anamnestic reaction.

The detection of EBV DNA by PCR or in situ hybridization in saliva or tissue of an immunocompromised child may indicate a lymphoproliferative syndrome.

Differential diagnosis

Infectious mononucleosis may be diagnosed too readily. Young children with mild fever and lymph node enlargement in the neck are more likely to have a respiratory viral infection.

Cases that present with fever and little else may be confused with influenza, brucellosis or typhoid; those with a sore throat need to be differentiated from streptococcal tonsillitis, Vincent stomatitis, diphtheria, agranulocytosis and leukemia. Glandular enlargement may be mistaken for toxoplasmosis, CMV infection or reticulosis, and the icteric form of the disease has to be distinguished from infectious hepatitis, leptospirosis and, occasionally, from obstructive liver disease.

The skin eruption of glandular fever has produced confusion with measles, rubella, secondary syphilis and drug rashes.

In all the above situations careful attention to the five main diagnostic criteria will confirm or refute a suspected diagnosis of infectious mononucleosis.

Treatment

There is no specific treatment. Aciclovir has virtually no in vivo activity against EBV. The disease tends to be mild in children but simple analgesics may be required to ease pain and gargles to soothe the sore throat. There is increasing evidence that antibiotics can do more harm than good, as toxic skin eruptions appear to follow their use, and ampicillin is especially incriminated in this direction. However, in cases where significant secondary infection is fully substantiated, antibiotics may need to be employed. Corticosteroids can have a dramatic, symptomatic effect but should be strictly reserved for those cases where edema of the airway is severe or where life-threatening complications such as thrombocytopenic purpura or severe neurological involvement are encountered. Reduction of immunosuppression or bone marrow transplantation may be of value in the management of EBV-lymphoproliferative diseases.[373]

Prognosis

The prognosis is good and children recover more quickly than adults, though some cases run a protracted course and patients may take months to recover their full health. Death is rare and usually results from rupture of the spleen or severe neurological involvement. Recurrences in the immediate convalescent phase can occur but are usually short-lived.

VIRAL AND ALLIED INFECTIONS OF THE RESPIRATORY TRACT

Infections of the respiratory tract are frequent and ubiquitous. They are the most common cause of illness in almost any age group and have a predilection for the extremes of life. Agents that are capable of attacking one part or another of the respiratory tract include viruses, rickettsiae, mycoplasmas and fungi.

Respiratory infection frequently results from a combination of different organisms because, once the initial assault has damaged the defensive mechanisms within the air passages, secondary infection is readily superimposed. This often renders it difficult to deduce the primary cause. Nevertheless detailed studies on the etiology of acute respiratory tract infection indicate that up to 85% of such disease may be initiated by a virus.

In the ensuing account a description is given of the various viruses and allied organisms which play a significant role in the production of infective respiratory disease.

INFLUENZA

Influenza is an acute infectious disease of variable severity with an emphasis on general illness rather than on symptoms arising from the respiratory tract. It tends to occur in pandemic form every few years. In most instances the disease is a benign condition, but may have a devastating effect when it attacks immunosuppressed patients or those with chronic cardiorespiratory disease, when there is a high mortality.

Etiology

Influenza viruses are RNA viruses of the orthomyxovirus family. There are three antigenic types A, B and C. Infection by type C is relatively uncommon, results in mild or inapparent illness and does not produce epidemics. Type B virus produces more significant illness followed by reasonably effective immunity. Outbreaks or small epidemics may occur, especially in schoolchildren, but are often of a localized nature. Some variation in antigenicity of type B virus occurs and outbreaks appear sporadically at intervals of 3–6 years.

Most clinical, virological and epidemiological interest is focused upon type A viruses, as these produce the most noteworthy outbreaks or epidemics and, when major new variants emerge, pandemics. Pandemics have usually been identified by titles, which reflect the suspected geographical origin as indicated by titles such as 'Asian flu' or 'Hong Kong flu'. The World Health Organization has devised a more definitive classification of influenza viruses which reflects the nature of mutation more precisely.[374]

Structurally, influenza viruses comprise a central core of ribonucleoprotein with a covering envelope. From this envelope spikes containing hemagglutinins project and between these spikes the mushroom-shaped protrusions composed of neuraminidase.

Each basic type of influenza (A, B or C) has its own distinctive ribonucleoprotein consisting of the S or soluble antigen. Protein antigens on the viral surface are related to hemagglutinins (the H antigens) and to neuraminidases (the N antigens). In the case of type A viruses minor changes may occur year by year producing what is known as antigenic drift. However, at intervals usually exceeding a decade, major changes take place producing antigenic shift. The virtually new type A virus, which emerges, as a result of antigenic shift, has thus acquired the potential to produce a pandemic.

Strain designation of influenza viruses is, therefore, based on the following points:

1. identification of the S antigen – that is whether virus is type A, B or C;
2. the host origin – when isolated initially from man, no specific identification is recorded but, if from an animal source, a suitable suffix is appended;
3. the geographical origin;
4. the strain number and the subtype of the hemagglutinin and neuraminidase identified;
5. the year of isolation.

Without an appreciation of the relatively complex antigenic structure and its variation, an understanding of the epidemiology of influenza is difficult.[375] Furthermore, effective vaccination will require the use of vaccines whose antigenic components accurately reflect the strain of influenza virus prevalent at the time of use.

Epidemiology

Man is the principal reservoir of infection and the disease is transmitted by direct contact, through droplet infection and by articles that have been freshly soiled with discharges from the nose or throat of infected persons. Infectivity appears to persist for 4–5 days after the clinical onset of the disease. Occasional cases originate from animals, e.g. pigs or chickens. In view of the high infectivity of influenza and the rapidity of modern travel, an epidemic can soon develop pandemic proportions.

Pathogenesis

Influenza infection causes necrosis of ciliated respiratory epithelium and this commences in the nose and spreads downwards to the trachea and bronchi. Edema and leukocyte infiltration follow causing pharyngitis, tracheitis and bronchitis; in severe cases considerable exudation of blood and edema fluid may occur and enter the alveoli with resultant pneumonia.

Primary respiratory damage from influenza virus may in itself produce a severe illness, but secondary bacterial infection is more often the cause of fatal pneumonia; organisms such as *Staphylococcus aureus* and *Klebsiella pneumoniae* are particularly dangerous in this context.

Clinical features

The incubation period of influenza is short and ranges from 1 to 3 days. In children over 5 years of age there is a sudden onset of fever, headache and shivering, with pains in the limbs and back. Anorexia, listlessness and malaise may also be experienced and in some instances, particularly in children, nausea and vomiting may be unduly pronounced. Abdominal pain ('gastric flu') can be a prominent symptom. A dry, painful cough, discomfort in the throat, hoarseness and nasal discharge are usual.

The temperature may reach 39–40°C, but apart from signs of pharyngitis, objective physical findings are few and in uncomplicated cases clinical and radiographic examination of the chest is usually clear. Leukopenia will be found in uncomplicated cases and the ESR becomes moderately elevated.

The illness usually runs a short course and is followed by rapid improvement. Some patients experience a period of mental and physical lethargy in convalescence but seriously complicated cases are rarely seen outside epidemics.

In younger children and infants influenza A typically causes high fever (over 39°C) and upper respiratory tract infection with coryza, cough, irritability and pharyngitis. Otitis media, laryngotracheitis, bronchitis, bronchiolitis indistinguishable from that due to RSV, and pneumonia may all occur. Vomiting and diarrhea are frequent in infants. Febrile convulsions are frequent, as are fleeting erythematous rashes, which can be morbilliform. The risk of severe lower respiratory tract involvement is greater in immunocompromised children.

In neonates the picture is non-specific with apneic episodes, lethargy, poor feeding and impaired circulation. Outbreaks may occur in neonatal units.

Diagnosis

At epidemic times a clinical diagnosis of influenza has a high likelihood of being correct but such a diagnosis in a sporadic case can often be incorrect. Other respiratory viral infections and some quite unconnected diseases may present with a similar clinical picture and a specific diagnosis can only be based on definitive laboratory tests.

Virological confirmation of influenza can be established by serological studies or by demonstrating the presence of influenza virus. The latter can be isolated from pharyngeal swabs, nasal swabs or throat washing during the acute stage of the illness and can be grown in the amniotic cavity of chick embryos or in tissue cultures. Influenza may be isolated in monkey kidney tissue cultures. During epidemics immunofluorescence, using an antiserum to the epidemic strain to test nasopharyngeal secretions, can be used for rapid diagnosis. Complement-fixation neutralization and hemagglutination-inhibition tests are available for the serological study of antibody responses to infection with influenza. In all these tests it is desirable to show a significant (fourfold or greater) rise in antibody titer during the illness.

Complications

Viral complications such as myocarditis, polyneuritis, encephalitis and psychosis are rarely seen in childhood cases. Secondary bacterial infection of the respiratory tract is more likely, and pneumonia, otitis media and purulent sinusitis may occur. Death can result from severe overwhelming infection by influenza virus itself, though a fatal outcome is more likely to result from secondary bacterial infection. Acute myositis may be severe, particularly affecting the calves, with a raised serum creatine phosphokinase (CPK). Reye syndrome has sometimes followed influenza B infection.

Treatment

In mild cases this is essentially symptomatic. Bed rest is advisable and pain will be eased by simple analgesics such as paracetamol; troublesome cough should respond to codeine or similar preparations. Bacterial complications may require antibiotic treatment and wherever possible this should be guided by appropriate laboratory studies. Amantadine and rimantadine have been successfully used to treat severe infection in immunocompromised children or those with underlying chronic illnesses. The neuraminidase inhibitors are a new class of antiviral agents that have been shown to be effective in the treatment of severe influenza in high risk patients.[376,377] Zanamivir is an inhaled preparation, and oseltamivir is an oral preparation. Their use in childhood disease is still under evaluation.

Prophylaxis

The extreme infectivity of influenza renders such measures as isolation and quarantine virtually ineffective. There is evidence that killed virus vaccine can significantly reduce the incidence of influenza though the sudden emergence of a fresh A mutant may render it impossible to produce the specific vaccine in time to influence an outbreak. Annual influenza vaccination should be considered for the child over 6 months with chronic pulmonary or circulatory disorders, or with chronic renal disease or diabetes mellitus, or with immunosuppression (including HIV infection). Encouraging accounts of the use of amantadine in the prophylaxis of this disease have been reported and, more recently, the neuraminidase inhibitors have become available, but their exact value in preventing illness in children has still to be established.[378]

A cold-adapted live-attenuated vaccine is currently under investigation.

PARAINFLUENZA VIRUS INFECTIONS

The parainfluenza viruses are members of the *Paramyxovirus* group. They have some properties in which they differ from the influenza viruses and they appear more closely related to the agents of mumps and Newcastle disease. They are approximately 150–220 nm in diameter, and contain RNA.

Four antigenic varieties, called 1, 2, 3 and 4, are recognized though type 4 has an undetermined role in the production of disease in humans. Types 1, 2 and 3 have frequently been isolated from cases of acute laryngotracheobronchitis (croup), bronchitis, bronchiolitis and pneumonia occurring in infants and children; less often they have been isolated from cases of rhinitis and pharyngitis. They are undoubtedly the commonest cause of acute laryngotracheobronchitis in which other viruses, such as influenza A and ECHO viruses, play a lesser role.

Serological studies indicate that infection, especially with type 3, is a common event in preschool children. Type 3 infection is endemic and occurs at any time of the year. Type 1 infection tends to occur in summer or autumn outbreaks every second year while type 2 outbreaks are less predictable.

Laboratory diagnosis

Parainfluenza viruses can be isolated from nasal and pharyngeal swabs. The viruses are relatively labile so these swabs should be placed in virus transport medium and delivered to the laboratory with minimum delay. Antigen detection by immunofluorescence or ELISA is increasingly available. Serological diagnosis is rarely helpful, other than in epidemiological studies, because of heterotypic antibody rises among the three types and related viruses particularly mumps.

Treatment

There is no specific treatment available. Symptomatic treatment of laryngotracheobronchitis with steroids or adrenaline (epinephrine) for severe airways obstruction may be indicated. Ribavirin has been used to suppress infection in immunocompromised hosts.

RESPIRATORY SYNCYTIAL VIRUS INFECTIONS

Respiratory syncytial virus (RSV), first identified in 1956, is now recognized to be amongst the most important agents causing respiratory infection in infants and young children worldwide. RSV is an RNA paramyxovirus. The virus grows well in many tissue cultures. In contrast to members of the myxovirus group, to which it shows some resemblance, RSV has no hemagglutinins so does not cause hemagglutination, but produces a fusion protein which causes in vitro and in vivo fusion of cells to form syncytia. Only two antigenic strains of RSV have been described.

Clinical features

RSV has been found in association with several clinical syndromes including mild upper respiratory tract infection, croup, bronchitis, bronchiolitis and pneumonia. Its principal association is with acute bronchiolitis in infants below 1 year of age. Epidemics of RSV infection occur annually in late autumn and winter in temperate climates. Outbreaks are mainly found in urban communities. In tropical climates there is not such a clear-cut annual epidemic. Nosocomial infections can be a major problem in hospitals.

Bronchiolitis is described elsewhere and although infection by influenza viruses, parainfluenza viruses, mycoplasmas, adenoviruses and rhinoviruses may produce a similar picture, few clinical respiratory syndromes have so close an etiological association as bronchiolitis and RSV infection.

Neither maternal nor acquired antibody protect against RSV, so RSV can infect neonates. Reinfections throughout childhood are common, but successively milder. Toddler-age children may develop bronchitis or pneumonia, schoolage children more commonly develop otitis media while adults get a severe cold with sore throat.

Laboratory diagnosis

The ideal specimen is a nasopharyngeal aspirate of mucus. Rapid viral diagnosis by immunofluorescence (or ELISA) has greatly aided the management of infants with bronchiolitis. The virus can be isolated successfully in various tissue culture systems, but as it is relatively unstable it is recommended that the specimen should be inoculated directly into the cultures without previous freezing. If the specimen has to be stored for a few hours it should be kept in virus transport medium at 4°C.

Serology can be used in children over 6 months of age, usually by complement-fixation test on paired sera. Under this age there is often no IgG response.

Treatment

Treatment is primarily supportive with supplemental oxygen and/or fluids. Nebulized ribavirin may be indicated in proven severe RSV infection in infants at high risk, particularly those with pre-existing cardiopulmonary disease or immune deficiency.[379–381]

Prevention

Two agents have recently become available for the prevention of RSV in high risk infants (those born prematurely < 35 weeks' gestation, or those with underlying chronic lung disease, cardiac disease or immunosuppression). RSV intravenous immunoglobulin (RSV IVIG) from pooled donors is administered intravenously and palizumab is a mouse monoclonal antibody to the RSV protein that is given intramuscularly. Both are given monthly during the RSV season and have been shown to significantly reduce the number of cases of hospitalized RSV bronchiolitis in at-risk groups,[382–384] but are expensive. The cost effectiveness of these agents in the UK has been questioned based on local data.[385]

ADENOVIRUSES

The first isolation of an adenovirus took place in 1953 from fragmented human adenoids grown in tissue culture, hence the name. Subsequently a number of different strains, chiefly types 1, 2, 5 and 6, were isolated from cultures of tonsils and adenoids. Outbreaks due to these agents have been encountered in children at boarding schools, at summer camps and amongst those attending communal swimming pools; outbreaks in adults are mainly found in military recruits. The nature of the clinical illness produced shows considerable variation and overlap but some relatively specific syndromes are included.

Adenoviruses are DNA viruses. They are relatively stable to changes in temperature and pH. They are widespread in nature and have been isolated from monkeys, pigs, dogs, birds and cattle, as well as from man. They may persist for weeks or even months in the upper respiratory tract.

Clinical features

Adenovirus infections are principally diseases of childhood, occurring mostly in children under the age of 5. Furthermore, certain adenovirus types show a pronounced age association.

Amongst syndromes recognized to be associated with adenoviral infection are the following:

Acute febrile pharyngitis

This syndrome has a high endemic rate in infants and young children and mainly results from infection by types 1, 2 and 5. It can also occur in epidemic form when type 3 is usually involved.

Pharyngoconjunctival fever (PCF)

Most commonly associated with infection by type 3, and less frequently with types 7A and 14, this syndrome can also follow infection by types 1, 2, 5 and 6. Epidemics occur in children, some of which have been associated with swimming pool infection. Symptoms of the syndrome include sore throat, headache, myalgia, eye discomfort, abdominal pain and stiffness in the back. Examination of the throat often reveals a degree of pharyngitis, and follicular conjunctivitis, unilateral or bilateral, may be seen.

Acute respiratory disease (ARD)

Uncommon in children, ARD is usually found in military recruits. It is most commonly due to infection by types 4 and 7; less often by types 3 and 14. The main clinical features include pharyngitis, cough, hoarseness and chest pain.

Viral pneumonia in infants

Adenoviruses may cause severe pneumonia and outbreaks have been reported in hospital nurseries and fatalities have resulted. Types 3, 7 and 21 have caused the most severe cases. Infection may disseminate (see below) or may result in bronchiolitis obliterans, bronchiectasis and unilateral hyperlucent lung.

Ocular syndromes

Two specific ocular syndromes are associated with adenovirus infection. The first is called *epidemic keratoconjunctivitis* and is associated with type 8 infection; the second, *follicular conjunctivitis*, usually results from infection by type 3 and may expand into the fuller syndrome of pharyngoconjunctival fever.

Disseminated disease

Adenovirus types 7 and 21 are particularly prone to cause pneumonia and disseminate to involve the liver (hepatitis), heart (myocarditis or pericarditis) and CNS (meningitis or encephalitis). This is more likely in immunocompromised patients.

Gastroenteritis

Non-cultivable enteric adenoviruses (types 40 and 41), seen on electron microscopy of feces, have been associated with gastroenteritis.[386]

Laboratory diagnosis

Adenoviruses can be grown in a wide range of tissue cultures. These viruses are relatively stable and can readily be isolated from throat swabs and feces. In respiratory disease the specimen should consist of a pharyngeal swab, sent to the laboratory in virus transport media. Cytopathic effect may be slow to appear, so cultures should be incubated for at least 3 weeks before being regarded as negative.

Serological evidence of infection is by detecting complement-fixing antibodies to adenoviruses in acute and convalescent serum samples. Antigen detection by immunoassays and detection of viral DNA by PCR in body fluids may aid in diagnosis of adenovirus infection in the immunocompromised.

Treatment

Treatment is largely supportive. The new antiviral agent, cidofovir, has been used with some success in the treatment of severe adenoviral infections in children post bone marrow transplantation.[387]

MUMPS (EPIDEMIC PAROTITIS)

To mump is an old English word meaning to mope. Mumps is an acute infectious disease characterized by non-suppurative enlargement of the salivary glands, particularly the parotids. It results from infection by mumps virus, one of the myxoviruses, and is associated with an unusually diverse range of complications. Infection may be inapparent in as many as 30% of cases and the illness may present with a complication and no history of preceding salivary gland involvement.

Epidemiology and etiology

Mumps is an endemic disease of urban communities which occasionally occurs in epidemic proportions especially in certain closed communities. Spread is by droplet infection or from recently contaminated articles and close contact is required. The relatively high incidence in adults bears witness to the comparatively low infectivity of the disease, though when mumps is introduced into a naive community, a serious and widespread outbreak may follow.

The responsible agent is an RNA virus approximately 150 nm in diameter although considerable variation in size can occur. Man appears to be the only reservoir and the portal of entry is through the mouth or nose. Infectivity may extend from several days before the illness to several days after the first sign of salivary gland involvement. Virus has been isolated from the blood in the prodromal stage and from the urine up to 14 days after the commencement of clinical illness. It is not clear whether spread to the salivary glands occurs locally or through the bloodstream.

Clinical features

The main incidence occurs between 5 and 15 years of age and is relatively uncommon in younger children and in adults over 30 years.

The incubation period is between 14 and 21 days and the illness may commence with malaise, fever, headache and anorexia; these prodromal symptoms may be absent. Salivary gland involvement commences 1–2 days later and the parotid glands are the most frequently affected. Pain develops around the ear and a swelling appears which extends forwards from the lobe of the ear, downwards over the angle of the jaw and backwards behind the pinna, which is usually pushed outwards. The swelling may be so trivial as to escape casual inspection or be very marked and exquisitely tender. Often only one parotid is involved initially followed, in 75% of cases, by swelling of the other parotid 1–5 days later. Less often simultaneous and synchronous swelling of both parotids occurs.

Submandibular salivary gland involvement can easily be overlooked as the soft tissues under the jaw readily absorb such swelling, unless it is particularly marked, and it is often the concomitant swelling of the parotids that directs attention to it.

Sublingual involvement is much less common but is extremely painful and can be seen readily beneath the upturned tongue.

In addition to salivary gland involvement, the orifice of Stensen's duct may be swollen and the mouth rather dry. Fever is present in the majority of cases, may reach 40°C and persist for up to a week; in fact, cases without salivary gland involvement may present as examples of unexplained fever and recover without the true diagnosis being appreciated, though in others the later development of a typical pattern of complications may indicate mumps to be the cause.

There may be some degree of leukopenia in mumps though certain complications, such as meningitis and pancreatitis, may provoke a leukocytosis.

Complications

Complications are common and varied.

CNS

Aseptic meningitis is the commonest complication and may present before, coincidentally with, or after, the illness. The CSF will show a lymphocytic pleocytosis and the count may exceed 1000 cells/μl. The protein content may be moderately raised and the glucose level is usually normal. However, the latter is occasionally decreased in mumps meningitis and where no salivary gland enlargement occurs to indicate the diagnosis, confusion with tuberculous meningitis has occurred. Other less common complications include postinfectious encephalitis, myelitis and polyradiculitis. Although usually unilateral, bilateral nerve deafness, often complete, can also occur, as may transient facial paralysis. The virus is easily isolated from the CSF of patients with mumps meningitis, which is generally benign. The postinfectious encephalitis is, however, more severe; although complete recovery is usual, neurological sequelae and even death may occur. Virus can be grown from the CSF and an immune-mediated mechanism is likely.

Orchitis

This may occur in 20% of postpubertal males and in younger children can occasionally occur in an undescended testicle. The involvement is usually unilateral but even after severe orchitis sterility is rare, and cases with orchitis should be firmly reassured of the good prognosis.

Pancreatitis

A significant degree of pancreatitis is rare and this complication is overdiagnosed. Salivary gland enlargement by itself raises the serum amylase level but when the pancreas is significantly involved intense pain will occur with rigidity of the abdominal wall and there is often a marked leukocytosis.

Other complications

These include oophoritis, mastitis, bartholinitis, myocarditis, hepatitis, thyroiditis and thrombocytopenic purpura. An occasional case of diabetes mellitus has also been reported following mumps.

Laboratory diagnosis

Viral confirmation of mumps depends on isolation of the virus or the demonstration of a significant rise in antibody titer during the illness.

Mumps virus can be cultured from saliva swabs and urine during the acute illness and from the CSF in cases complicated by meningitis.

Serological tests are readily available to demonstrate a significant rise in antibody titer during the illness and the complement-fixation test is most commonly employed. In this test, two specific antigens, soluble (S) and viral (V), are often used. In general, antibody to S antigen rises earlier in the illness than antibody to V antigen, but whereas S antibody may only persist for a few months the V antibody is present for a very long period. Hemagglutination-inhibition and virus neutralization tests are also of help where available.

Differential diagnosis

In children the differential diagnosis is more limited than in adults as in the latter one may encounter more diseases that involve the salivary glands. Conditions that cause lymph node enlargement produce most confusion but careful clinical examination should resolve the difficulty. Pyogenic submandibular abscesses and glandular fever can prove more perplexing and in these instances the blood picture and serum amylase estimations can be helpful. Suppurative parotitis may be considered where there is overlying inflammation and where pus can be expressed from the appropriate salivary duct. Recurrent parotitis is quite common in children. It is not due to repeated attacks of mumps. Sometimes an underlying allergic disorder, sialectasis or duct calculi may be found. Other conditions which may require exclusion are tumors, Mikulicz syndrome, uveoparotid fever in sarcoidosis, HIV infection, tuberculosis and dental conditions.

Treatment

There is no specific treatment. Pain may be relieved by simple analgesics and the application of heat to the glands can prove soothing. The mouth should be kept clean and a fluid diet is needed until swelling subsides. Neurological complications are managed along customary lines though the diagnostic lumbar puncture in mumps meningitis often produces dramatic relief of headache. In orchitis the testes should be supported and ice bags may ease the discomfort; there is no evidence that corticosteroid drugs, stilbestrol or incision of the tunica albuginea significantly alter the course of this complication.

Prognosis

This is generally good and a fatal outcome exceedingly rare, although permanent brain damage and deafness have been described. Sterility is most unlikely and one attack of mumps appears to provide life-long immunity.

Prevention

Injections of human antimumps immunoglobulin have been used prophylactically and appear beneficial if given sufficiently early in the incubation period. Live vaccines are safe and produce a good antibody response with long immunity though the duration has not been fully substantiated. They can be used to immunize contacts, and are incorporated into the MMR vaccine for routine immunization in many countries.

COXSACKIE AND ECHO VIRUS INFECTIONS

Respiratory illness in association with these enteroviruses is usually of a mild character.

Certain *Coxsackie viruses* produce specific respiratory syndromes; some group A serotypes are identified as the cause of *herpangina* and certain group B viruses are the agents responsible for pleurodynia (Bornholm disease). Agents from both groups of Coxsackie viruses have been found in association with mild febrile respiratory disease and one strain, Coxsackie A21 (Coe virus), has been recovered with particular frequency from outbreaks in young servicemen.

ECHO viruses are not usually regarded as respiratory pathogens but they have been found in the throat or feces during upper respiratory disease. Amongst serotypes isolated in these circumstances are ECHO viruses types 6, 11, 19 and 20.

The laboratory diagnosis of infections due to Coxsackie and ECHO viruses is described in the section specifically devoted to these agents.

RHINOVIRUS INFECTIONS

Rhinoviruses are the main cause of the common cold. There are many serologically distinct types. They belong to the large group of picornaviruses, meaning small RNA viruses, but unlike Coxsackie and ECHO viruses they are acid labile at pH 3.

The common cold is probably the most ubiquitous infection in man and the illness tends to be more severe in children than in adults with an acute catarrhal inflammation involving the nose, nasopharynx and accessory sinuses. The onset is usually abrupt and is accompanied by a copious watery discharge, which may later turn mucopurulent even in the absence of bacterial superinfection. Little or no fever occurs and constitutional symptoms are mild.

Apart from their ability to produce the common cold, rhinoviruses have been found in association with acute wheezing episodes in children and with pneumonia.

Laboratory diagnosis

Nasopharyngeal aspirates in virus transport medium, nose swab or throat swab collected during the acute stage of the respiratory illness should be sent to the laboratory for the isolation of rhinoviruses. Serology is generally unhelpful. ELISA and PCR for rhinovirus have been developed but are not widely available.

CORONAVIRUSES

Human coronaviruses (HCV) are probably almost as frequent a cause of colds and acute upper respiratory tract infections as rhinovirus infections.[388] Coronaviruses have also been associated with wheeze and pneumonia.[389] The exact frequency of HCV infections has been difficult to ascertain because coronaviruses are difficult to grow and can often only be isolated in tracheal organ cultures. The diagnosis can be made by ELISA on respiratory secretions or serologically by detecting antibody to one of the two main serotypes, 229E and OC-43. PCR is not widely available.

REOVIRUS INFECTIONS

In 1954 a new group of respiratory-entero or reovirus agents was recognized. It had originally been thought to belong to the ECHO virus group. Since then three distinct types (1, 2 and 3) have been serologically differentiated though they share a common complement-fixing antigen.

Following these preliminary investigations reoviruses have been isolated from many different animal hosts in widely separated areas. These viruses have also been recovered from rectal and throat swabs taken from children suffering from mild respiratory disease, diarrhea, and occasionally fatal pneumonia.

The exact role of reoviruses in producing human disease is largely undetermined. However, the family Reoviridae also includes the agents named rotaviruses, which are associated with gastroenteritis, especially in children (see p.1434).

Laboratory diagnosis

Reoviruses can be isolated from pharyngeal swabs and nasal secretions but they are more commonly recovered from feces.

Acute and convalescent samples of serum are required for hemagglutination-inhibiting antibody titer estimations; a fourfold, or greater, rise in titer during the illness is evidence of infection with a reovirus.

Rotaviruses are difficult to culture and diagnosis depends on electron microscopic examination or ELISA tests on feces.

PSITTACOSIS

Psittacosis is a zoonosis contracted from birds or objects they have contaminated. It was originally considered that infection could only result from birds of the psittacine group (psittacosis) but it is now appreciated that infection may arise from many other birds, both wild and domesticated (ornithosis) and animals such as sheep and goats.

Chlamydia psittaci, the causative organism, belongs to the genus *Chlamydia*. This genus appears to occupy an intermediate position between viruses and rickettsiae. The organisms are obligate intracellular parasites, which show sensitivity to certain antibiotics.

Clinical features

The presentation is usually with high fever, chills, headache, myalgia, chest pain, anorexia and fatigue. A dry cough may become productive and fine rales are heard. The pulse may be relatively slow. There may be no history of bird or animal contact, but contact with a sick bird is suggestive. Chest radiography may show peri-hilar infiltrates, atelectasis or even consolidation. Children and adolescents seem less susceptible to psittacosis than adults. However, this may merely reflect the fact that less specific illness is produced in the young and the diagnosis may therefore be overlooked.

Laboratory diagnosis

A clinical diagnosis of psittacosis can be confirmed by serological tests or by isolation of the causative agent. The estimation of complement-fixing antibodies in acute and convalescent samples of serum is a reliable and popular test, which avoids the hazards involved in the isolation of a highly infectious agent, but it does not distinguish between other species of *Chlamydia*. The acute sample of serum should be collected as early in the illness as possible and a convalescent sample may be taken about 2 weeks after the onset of the illness; it is often worthwhile examining a third sample of serum obtained after a further 2 weeks. A fourfold, or greater, rise in antibody titer during the illness is indicative of infection with a member of the psittacosis–lymphogranuloma venereum group of agents.

The psittacosis agent can be isolated from blood in the early stages of the illness and later from pleural fluid and infected tissues. In the case of respiratory illness it is usual to send sputum or throat washings to the laboratory. Positive results may be available within a few days but it is frequently necessary to passage the material.

Sensitive immunoassays for *C. psitacci* are available in some reference laboratories.[390]

Prognosis

Spontaneous recovery is to be expected but where the diagnosis is confirmed during the clinical illness tetracycline (except in children less than 8 years old) or erythromycin should be given, as this may reduce symptoms and hasten convalescence.

CHLAMYDIA PNEUMONIAE

C. pneumoniae, previously called the TWAR agent (from Taiwan-associated respiratory agent) is closely related to *C. psittaci*, and crossreacts with it in complement-fixation serological tests. As the serological assays for *C. pneumoniae* are not widely available, this organism may be responsible for reported cases of person-to-person spread of psittacosis and cases with no history of bird or animal contact. During mass chest X-ray screening in Finland a number of young adults were identified with a single patch of pneumonic consolidation. They mostly had mild respiratory symptoms with dry cough, and were found to have antibodies to *C. pneumoniae*.[391] Serological surveys suggest it is a not uncommon cause of pneumonia in children, particularly in developing countries. Treatment is as for psittacosis.

CHLAMYDIA TRACHOMATIS

C. trachomatis, acquired by passage through an infected birth canal, can cause a pneumonitis usually at 3–11 weeks of age. There may be a history of maternal vaginal discharge and the infant may have had conjunctivitis. The infant is afebrile with a characteristic staccato cough. There are often rales and rhonchi on auscultation. About half the infants have otitis media with a pearly white tympanic membrane. The radiographic appearance is of diffuse pulmonary infiltrates with peribronchial thickening and focal consolidation. Definitive diagnosis is by culturing *C. trachomatis* or detecting antigen in a nasopharyngeal aspirate or conjunctival swab, or by detecting specific IgM by immunofluorescence. Presumptive evidence can be obtained by demonstrating characteristic inclusions on conjunctival scrapings if there is active conjunctivitis. Treatment is with erythromycin 40 mg/kg/day 6-hourly for 14 days but there may be chronic pulmonary sequelae. The parents should also be treated.

MYCOPLASMA PNEUMONIAE

For many years a distinct clinical entity known as *primary atypical pneumonia* was recognized but an exact basis could not be demonstrated. A specific viral causation was always suspected, and following Eaton's studies on this syndrome, a causative filterable agent (subsequently referred to as Eaton's agent) appeared to have been found. Later work has shown that *Mycoplasma pneumoniae*, a pleuropneumonia-like organism (PPLO) belonging to the distinctive genus of mycoplasmas, and not a virus, is responsible for some cases of primary atypical pneumonia.

Clinical features

M. pneumoniae may give rise to inapparent infection, mild upper respiratory tract infection, bronchitis, bronchiolitis, bronchopneumonia and bullous myringitis both in adults and children; furthermore, some childhood infections occur in epidemic form. *M. pneumoniae* may have an etiological role in some cases of Stevens–Johnson syndrome and can also cause myocarditis, pericarditis, arthritis and encephalitis. When it causes pneumonia, the radiological appearance may be of bilateral, diffuse reticular infiltrates or of consolidation including lobar consolidation.

Laboratory diagnosis

The isolation of *M. pneumoniae* can now be undertaken by many laboratories but the agent grows slowly and often the results of serological tests are available before the isolation and identity of the mycoplasma has been established. The agent can be isolated from sputum, throat washings or pharyngeal swabs.

For serological studies, acute and convalescent samples of serum should be collected. Various serological tests are available, but the complement-fixation test appears popular and reliable. A single high titer of IgG antibodies to *M. pneumoniae* on an acute serum sample may also be helpful since there is often a fairly long history before presentation. Detection of *M. pneumoniae* IgM by immunofluorescence does not distinguish an acute infection from one in the recent past, as the antibody may persist for many months.

Cold agglutinins are present in the serum in many cases and, although their detection is not specific for *Mycoplasma* infection, may be useful in acute management.

Treatment

M. pneumoniae displays sensitivity to certain antibiotics, particularly tetracycline (25–50 mg/kg/day) and erythromycin (30–50 mg/kg/day), and where a diagnosis is made during the active stage of illness, treatment by one of these drugs should be employed. Erythromycin is preferable in children under 9 years old in view of the potential toxicity of tetracycline. Other macrolides such as clarithromycin and arithromycin may also be effective.

Q FEVER (QUERY FEVER)

This disease results from infection by *Coxiella burnetii* and usually presents as an influenza-like illness with fever and headache, often followed by an atypical pneumonic illness. Unlike other rickettsial infections, Q fever is unaccompanied by a rash.

C. burnetii is an obligate intracellular parasite which is highly pleomorphic and contains both RNA and DNA. It is more resistant to chemical and physical agents than other pathogenic rickettsiae and is relatively sensitive to certain antibiotics and so has been reclassified into a subgroup of Proteobacteria.

The natural reservoir of *C. burnetii* is animals such as cattle, sheep and goats, as well as certain ticks, and the latter are probably involved in animal-to-animal spread. Infection in humans may arise from the handling of infected meat and placentae, the inhalation of infected dust in farmyards and from the consumption of infected raw milk. Cases are most likely to be found in farm workers, slaughtermen and shepherds; however, where milk is the vehicle of transmission, the disease may occur without any apparent occupational link and involve children.

Clinical features

Q fever is less commonly diagnosed in children than in adults because the illness produced in younger age groups is less severe and less intensively studied.

There is usually an incubation period of 2–3 weeks and the illness starts abruptly with fever, rigors, headache, malaise and weakness. In some instances the illness may terminate in approximately 1 week without any further progression but in most diagnosed cases the patient goes on to develop a cough and chest pain. Physical signs may be absent or minimal, though chest X-ray shows pneumonitis.

Severe cases may have symptoms for up to 3 weeks and radiological abnormalities can take a similar period to resolve. The surveying of contacts shows that inapparent infection can also occur. Occasionally Q fever presents with meningoencephalitis and in such instances diagnosis can be difficult.

Complications

The main complication is Q fever, or rickettsial, endocarditis. To date this has only been seen in people with pre-existing valvular disease of the heart and the clinical presentation is one of subacute bacterial endocarditis in which repeated blood cultures prove negative. Granulomatous hepatitis and bone granulomas have been described.

Laboratory diagnosis

C. burnetii can be isolated in laboratory animals or fertile hen's eggs. However, as it is a significant biohazard to laboratory workers, serological tests are preferred to confirm a clinical diagnosis, and a complement-fixation test or immunofluorescence is used on acute and convalescent sera. Detection of nucleic acid by PCR or hybridization techniques is also available.

Treatment

Prodromal symptoms require symptomatic treatment. Once the diagnosis is made tetracycline (25 mg/kg/day) should be given in standard dosage for 2 weeks. Chloramphenicol is the drug of choice in young children. Therapy should not be withheld where the diagnosis is retrospective and the patient has recovered; it is important to ensure eradication of the infection and avoid the possibility of chronicity. Endocarditis has a grave prognosis.

VIRAL INFECTIONS OF THE CNS

The viruses that may occasionally result in devastating neurological damage are more usually associated with a benign clinical illness or even subclinical infection. The reasons for this selective vulnerability remain unexplained but older theories of specific neurotropism have been largely disproved; in fact only a few viral agents such as rabies appear to have a particular predilection to attack the nervous system.

Viral infection of the nervous system may be established beyond question by the demonstration of specific viruses in neural tissue or in the CSF.[392] However, in certain instances of suspected viral infection no such proof has been forthcoming and in these instances it is postulated that an autoimmune or other immunological process takes place within the nervous system.

Against some of these diseases, such as poliomyelitis and rabies, immunization procedures are available and antiviral chemotherapy may have some part to play in the treatment of herpes simplex and certain types of encephalitis. In the main, however, treatment is symptomatic.

VIRAL MENINGITIS (ASEPTIC MENINGITIS, LYMPHOCYTIC MENINGITIS)

Meningitis may follow infection by a wide variety of viruses. Most frequently Coxsackie and ECHO viruses are involved, but cases may also arise following infection by the viruses of mumps, measles, lymphocytic choriomeningitis, herpes simplex, poliomyelitis, varicella-zoster and the *Arbovirus* (*Togavirus*) group.

The prognosis of uncomplicated viral meningitis is good and the pleocytosis stimulated in the CSF is usually, but not exclusively, lymphocytic in character. In fact, the terms viral and lymphocytic meningitis are sometimes used synonymously, but the latter term lacks accuracy as the pleocytosis may be entirely polymorphonuclear in the earliest days of attack. Perhaps benign, acute aseptic meningitis is a preferable descriptive title since certain non-viral infections, such as leptospirosis, can cause a similar picture in the spinal fluid. Enteroviral meningitis commonly occurs in the summer and autumn months in temperate climates but no such seasonal variation is seen in the tropics.

Clinical features

Viral meningitis is most commonly encountered in children up to the age of 10 years, although a sizeable proportion of cases is also encountered in adolescents and young adults. There is quite a marked male preponderance in early childhood cases. The clinical picture of viral meningitis may be variable. Where infection is due to such agents as mumps or measles, the well-defined stigmata of these diseases may suggest the actual virus responsible. Enterovirus type 71 has recently been associated with a number of outbreaks of hand, foot and mouth disease followed by severe neurological complications in young children, including brainstem encephalitis and pulmonary edema that appear to be immune mediated.[393,394] However, in many instances there is no pathognomonic clinical picture that permits the exact viral cause to be deduced. Certain enteroviral infections may produce a rash, but these are rarely so characteristic as to be diagnostic and detailed virological studies are required to elucidate the responsible agent.

In general, there is an introductory illness of short duration, and symptoms and signs of meningitis may follow immediately. In some, a short period of apparent recovery intervenes between the prodromal illness and nervous system involvement – a situation rather like the minor and major illness seen in poliomyelitis. The actual symptoms and signs simulate those of any other type of infective meningitis but are usually less pronounced. The progressive coma and marked toxicity of bacterial meningitis are usually absent and, in the average case, the full clinical picture together with analysis of the CSF permits broad division of the case into a bacterial or aseptic group, most of the latter being the result of viral infection.

The blood count is usually normal though an early leukocytosis or leukopenia may be noted. The CSF will usually be clear with a moderate increase in lymphocytes. The glucose level is usually within normal limits, with the exception of aseptic meningitis following mumps in which there may be some degree of hypoglycorrhachia. The protein content is modestly increased but rarely exceeds 100 mg/100 ml (1 g/L) of CSF.

Differential diagnosis

Although the epidemiological background and clinical features may suggest a likely etiological cause, a definitive diagnosis is dependent on detailed laboratory studies. Confusion can arise from leptospiral meningitis, cryptococcal infection, partially treated bacterial meningitis and tuberculous meningitis. Less often non-infectious conditions such as sarcoidosis, leukemia and other forms of malignant disease can produce CSF findings that are confusing.

Laboratory diagnosis

Detection of viral nucleic acid in the CSF by PCR analysis may aid in the diagnosis of aseptic meningoencephalitis due to enterovirus, VZV or HSV. For rabies, rubella, or mumps encephelomyelitis, virus may be isolated from throat swabs, feces, CSF or urine and the specimens should be inoculated into appropriate tissue cultures and, where indicated, into suckling mice. As the yield from CSF viral culture is low in viral meningitis it is particularly important to send a stool and throat swab for virus isolation. Serology is helpful in the diagnosis of meningoencephalitis due to mumps (IgM), measles, lymphocytic choriomeningitis, or arboviruses. Acute and convalescent samples of serum, preferably collected 3 weeks apart, should be tested for appropriate antibodies.

Treatment

With the exception of aseptic meningitis due to HSV and VZV, there is no specific treatment. Bed rest is desirable until symptoms and fever have settled as hasty mobilization may provoke paralytic disease in certain enteroviral infections. Where the clinical picture is unclear and bacterial infection is the possible cause of the presenting syndrome, empirical antibiotic treatment is justified until the situation becomes clarified by laboratory studies or further developments.

VIRAL ENCEPHALITIDES

See Chapter 20.

POSTINFECTIOUS MYELITIS

Some degree of myelitis may often be found in association with postinfectious encephalitis but on occasion may present as an isolated clinical syndrome.[395] It is rare and there is usually a latent interval between the initiating infection and the development of spinal cord involvement. Age distribution tends to follow the same pattern as postinfectious encephalitis, though in the case of rubella the age tends to be higher. The pathological changes are those associated with postinfectious neurological involvement, and direct viral invasion of the cord is rare except in infections due to polioviruses and enteroviruses. In one study of 911 cases of measles associated with neurological complications 877 showed encephalitis, 24 myelitis and 10 polyradiculitis; a similar distribution can be found for the neurological complications of rubella and chickenpox. Most recorded cases have followed specific exanthemata and the association seems well substantiated by the circumstantial evidence. Occasional reports of myelitis in association with other viral infections are difficult to evaluate as these reports often involve single cases and the association may have been fortuitous; nevertheless, there are good reasons to believe that other agents could play a role in this condition.

The prognosis is difficult to evaluate. Those developing ascending paralysis have a poorer outlook and most of the reported deaths are associated with this picture. Others may be left with permanent spastic paraplegia but those presenting with transverse myelitis often make an unexpectedly rapid and full recovery. The main differential diagnoses are Guillain–Barré syndrome and space-occupying or vascular lesions of the spinal cord.

POSTINFECTIOUS POLYNEURITIS (POSTINFECTIOUS POLYRADICULITIS, LANDRY–GUILLAIN–BARRÉ SYNDROME)

See Chapter 20.

LABORATORY TESTS APPLICABLE TO ENCEPHALITIS, MYELITIS AND POLYNEURITIS

Molecular techniques have significantly improved the ability to make a specific diagnosis in viral CNS infections. The differential diagnosis of viral encephalitis depends on the age and the immune status of the child. In the immunocompetent child, CSF should be collected and analyzed for routine examination, for viral nucleic acid by PCR, and for culture as outlined in the preceding section on viral meningitis, together with other specimens (saliva, blood, urine or stool) depending on the clinical history. In the immunocompromised child, the list extends to include the detection of CMV, EBV, and possibly human herpesvirus type DNA by PCR analysis.

A postmortem examination may confirm a clinical diagnosis of encephalitis, but during life the specific type can only be established by isolation and identification of the virus or by serological examination. Several viruses have been associated with encephalitis and consideration requires to be given to geographical and epidemiological factors in determining the possible causative agents.

Brain biopsy material may prove suitable for examination especially in the immunocompromised child. In the past, it was the gold standard for the diagnosis of herpes simplex encephalitis, but it has largely been superseded by PCR for HSV DNA. It may also be of value in some types of arbovirus infection and in the subacute sclerosing panencephalitis associated with measles. Acute and convalescent serum samples should always be collected and tested for a significant rise in antibody titer; guidance as to which antibodies to test in the serum will often be available from the associated clinical illness.

LYMPHOCYTIC CHORIOMENINGITIS

The agent, first recognized in 1934, was entitled lymphocytic choriomeningitis (LCM) virus. This virus is now classified as a member of the Arenavirus group. It occurs in mice.

Sporadic cases and small outbreaks of aseptic meningitis in man due to LCM have been reported in Europe and the USA in circumscribed areas where infected mouse colonies have been shown to exist.[396] Although originally suspected to be a common cause of aseptic meningitis, it is now known to have a very small role except in areas of endemic infection in mice.

Clinical features

The incubation period of LCM lies between 7 and 14 days. Any age group may contract the disease, if contact with the relevant infected mouse colonies occurs. The clinical picture and the abnormalities in the CSF are identical with those found in other types of viral meningitis and etiological diagnosis can only be made by laboratory studies. LCM can also cause mild respiratory illness and, rarely, pneumonia. Orchitis, myopericarditis, arthritis or alopecia may rarely occur. The prognosis is usually excellent though an occasional fatality has been reported in infants. No specific treatment is indicated, though control of infected mouse colonies should be undertaken by expert rodent exterminators.

Laboratory diagnosis

The LCM virus can be isolated from blood in the initial febrile phase of the illness, and from the CSF after the onset of meningitis. The virus can be propagated in young mice and in various tissue cultures.

Complement-fixing and neutralizing antibodies appear in the patient's serum following infection and a serological diagnosis can be made by demonstrating a significant rise in antibody titer during the illness. The antibodies tend to be produced rather late in the illness; as a result the convalescent serum sample for complement-fixing antibodies should be collected about the third week of the illness and that for neutralizing antibodies about 6 weeks after the onset of the disease.

RABIES (HYDROPHOBIA)

Rabies, the most feared of all zoonoses, has been a recognized disease of man since early times.[397] Spread to man may occur from a wide variety of warm-blooded animals which demonstrate variable susceptibility. Although this susceptibility is extremely high in such animals as foxes, jackals and wolves, it is only moderate in others including the dog. However, as man has a closer association with domestic animals, such as the dog, they provide a greater risk to him. In any particular geographical area, enzootic or epizootic infection may predominate in only one or two species of wild animal; in central and South America the dominant animal is the vampire bat, in Russia the wolf, in North America the bat and skunk, and in Europe the fox.

Certain areas of the world are currently free of rabies including Australia, New Zealand, certain Pacific islands, parts of Scandinavia and the UK. In an attempt to retain this position the movement of animals is governed by strict regulations including compulsory quarantine of animals, but such measures can be severely stretched. Enzootic rabies was eradicated from the UK in 1922 but fears exist that the current epizootic form amongst foxes in Europe, which has spread rapidly westwards over recent years, may result in the reintroduction of rabies.

Casual contact with a rabid animal should not produce infection in man as this will usually only follow a specific bite. However, infection can follow the licking of abraded skin or mucosa by an infected animal. It is also suggested that airborne infection from bats to man can occur within caves where such animals are roosting. In most instances suspicion will arise that the animal concerned is rabid especially where the furious form of the disease occurs. Should the less dramatic, dumb form occur, however, the true nature of the illness is not so readily suspected.

Clinical features

The incubation period may be as short as 10 days or as prolonged as 7 years but is usually between 1 and 3 months. Wounds on the hands, forearm and neck are especially dangerous and in them, or where there is extensive biting at any site, the incubation period may be shortened. Age may also be a factor and cases in young children tend to have a shorter incubation period.

The onset of clinical illness is heralded by a prodromal period, which may last from 2 to 7 days. Indefinite sensory changes may be experienced at the site of the bite together with such non-specific features as slight fever, headache, malaise, nausea and sore throat. Paresis and paralysis then develop and the muscles of deglutition go into spasm at any attempt to swallow (hence the term hydrophobia). Increasing depression and anxiety become apparent and the patient may become very withdrawn.

The disease may now enter a stage of excitement (furious rabies) with alternating manic activity and calm. The patient will remain lucid but fearful and the spasms in the throat become more violent. Cranial nerve palsies may develop and generalized convulsions become frequent. Death follows in virtually every case from either cardiac or respiratory arrest. Less often the picture is not so florid and a progressive ascending paralysis occurs giving rise to the so-called dumb form of the disease.

Clinical diagnosis

A classical case, following a significant bite, provides a clearly recognizable clinical picture. Otherwise, forms of viral encephalitis, bulbar poliomyelitis, hysteria and tetanus may produce similar features and cause diagnostic confusion. Encephalitis following antirabies vaccination with the old vaccines can occur and produce a similar picture to that of rabies itself, although this has not been recorded following the human diploid cell vaccine.

Laboratory diagnosis

Rabies virus is probably not a single antigenic species and four rabies-related viruses are recognized. These agents have a marked predilection for nervous tissue but multiply in other organs such as the salivary glands. Within the nervous system the main pathological process is an encephalomyelitis leading to the development of inclusion bodies particularly within the hippocampus. These inclusions are known as Negri bodies.

During life the laboratory diagnosis of rabies depends on testing such specimens as saliva, CSF, and conjunctival secretions by animal inoculation and immunofluorescent techniques. Viral antigens may be detected in skin biopsies. The rapidly fatal outcome, and the confusion which serum or vaccine can introduce, may render serological tests unhelpful.

If the suspected animal is available, it should be sacrificed, and the brain examined for rabies virus antigens by hybridization techniques.

After death, specimens of brain tissue should be inoculated intracerebrally into mice. The specimens should also be subjected to rabies immunofluorescent tests and examined for Negri bodies. These tests should yield results within 1–2 days. However, if they are inconclusive, the results of mouse inoculation must be awaited, and it may take up to 3 weeks to declare this test negative.

Treatment

The treatment of clinical rabies is largely symptomatic but intensive supportive therapy including artificial ventilation has been employed and at least two cases of proven rabies have survived following such measures. Appropriate steps must be taken to avoid possible spread to the attendants and to the immediate environment.

Postexposure prophylaxis

Local treatment of the wound. This can prove highly beneficial and should not be overlooked or delayed. Ideally wounds should be thoroughly cleansed using a 20% soap solution and, after washing any residual soap away with water, a 0.1% quaternary ammonium compound such as cetrimide should be applied. Alternatives include 40–70% alcohol or tincture and aqueous solutions of iodine. Should none of these agents be immediately available, extensive cleansing with clean water should be used as early as possible and the chemical agents employed when practicable. Primary suturing of the wounds should be avoided and human rabies immunoglobulin (HRIG) should be infiltrated into the tissue beneath the wound. If there is any suspicion of exposure to tetanus, appropriate prophylaxis against this disease should be instituted.

Special systemic treatment. The aim of prophylaxis by vaccination is to induce a rapid antibody response which may prevent clinical disease developing, and is safe and highly effective. Several vaccines are available for postexposure treatment and the site and frequency of injections will depend on the vaccine used. If the human diploid cell vaccine is used, vaccination should commence as soon as possible after the incident and injections should be given by deep subcutaneous or intramuscular injection on days 0, 3, 7, 14, and 28. As antibodies do not develop for some days, immunoprophylaxis with HRIG should be given intramuscularly as well as infiltrating the wound[398] of those not previously immunized, ideally within 24 h. Treatment may be discontinued if the suspected dog or cat remains healthy after observation for 5 days; other animals may require longer periods of observation.

Pre-exposure prophylaxis

Prophylaxis by the human diploid cell rabies vaccine may be used for those at high risk of contracting rabies, e.g. laboratory staff or veterinary staff in endemic areas. Immunization is not routinely recommended for those visiting endemic areas.

NEURODEGENERATIVE VIRUS DISEASES

Subacute sclerosing panencephalitis (SSPE)

This progressive CNS degenerative disorder is caused by measles virus. It is suspected that the disease reflects an abnormal immunological response to persisting measles virus or measles virus antigen. Children with SSPE make antibodies to most measles antigens but do not make antibodies to the matrix (M) protein. Whether this is important in permitting the virus to become latent is not known. Children with SSPE have high titers of antibody to measles virus by complement-fixation test in both serum and CSF.

The clinical features of SSPE are described elsewhere. Measles vaccination of a population leads to a decreased incidence of SSPE.

Rubella panencephalitis

Progressive panencephalitis may complicate both stable congenital and acquired rubella infections. The disease somewhat resembles SSPE, but in active rubella encephalitis there is detectable virus in the CSF, together with a pleocytosis and elevated protein. Rubella antibodies are present in both blood and CSF. The pathological picture is variable but usually one of a chronic meningoencephalitis with focal areas of degenerative vascular change.

Children present between 8 and 12 years of age with mental decline followed some months to years later by myoclonic jerks, chorea, ataxia, nystagmus and spasticity. The course is slower than SSPE and patients may survive 10 or more years.

Progressive multifocal leukoencephalopathy

This disease is a demyelinating disease caused by infection of astrocytes and oligodendrocytes with one of two papovaviruses, namely JC virus and simian virus 40 (SV40). The commoner of the two to cause disease, JC, is named after the initials of the first affected patient, a 38-year-old man with Hodgkin disease who developed progressive multifocal leukoencephalopathy.

All cases have been in patients who are immunosuppressed, e.g. postrenal transplant, have a malignant lymphoproliferative disorder or have a chronic disease such as tuberculosis or sarcoidosis. All areas of the brain and spinal cord may be affected. The usual presentation is early dementia with confusion, impaired cerebration and labile affect. There is often focal weakness progressing to hemiparesis and later bilateral long tract signs. Blindness, aphasia and ataxia are usual, with death occurring in less than 6 months. Detection of JC viral nucleic acid in the CSF by PCR analysis may be helpful in making the diagnosis of progressive multifocal leukoencephalopathy, but the sensitivity of the assay varies widely between laboratories.[344]

PRION DISEASES

Transmissible spongiform encephalopathies

The transmissible spongiform encephalopathies (TSE) of man are a rare, neurodegenerative, rapidly fatal group of disorders in which there is progressive degeneration of neurones with demyelination and gliosis of gray matter, causing a spongiform appearance of the brain, and the accumulation of a rare protein or prion (proteinaceous infectious agent). Their existence was first postulated by Pruisner in his analysis of the pathogenesis of scrapie in sheep.[399] Prions are thought to cause neuronal dysfunction and pathology when an alpha helical protease-sensitive form of the prion converts to a protease-resistant protein form associated with a structural predominance of beta sheet. Human TSE disorders include Creutzfeldt–Jakob disease (CJD), variant-Creutzfeldt–Jakob disease (v-CJD), Straussler–Scheinker disease, kuru, and fatal familial insomnia.[400] They closely resemble two animal diseases, scrapie and transmissible mink encephalopathy.

Kuru was the first TSE to be identified over 40 years ago. It was initially thought to be caused by a slow virus. In kuru, the cerebellum is most affected, and the disease is characterized by a progressive ataxia with a shivering tremor (the word 'kuru' means shivering). The incubation period is up to 20 years. It was acquired by the women and children of the Fore tribe in New Guinea who ate the brains of dead kinsfolk.

CJD is a progressive dementia with varying neurological features. Myoclonus, ataxic tremor, spasticity and parkinsonian features have all been described. CJD is sometimes familial. Cases have occurred in children who received human growth hormone from human pituitary extracts unwittingly infected with the agent and through brain and eye surgery.

The TSE of most relevance to pediatricians is v-CJD. It was first identified in the UK in 1996,[401] and there is evidence to suggest it is linked to exposure to tissues from cattle infected with bovine spongiform encephalopathy (BSE),[402,403] although the route of infection and indeed much about the natural history of this disease remains unclear despite analysis of the dietary history of people with v-CJD.[404] There appears to be a genetic component to the disease, as all patients identified to date are homozygous for methionine at codon 129 of the 'PRNP' gene.[400] v-CJD is distinguished from CJD by a younger age at onset, and some distinguishing clinical features such as a psychiatric presentation, altered pain sensation and the absence of the periodic electroencephalographic complexes seen in CJD. Neurological signs such as ataxia and myoclonus occur later in the illness than in CJD. Amyloid plaques and bilateral, increased thalamic densities may be seen on magnetic resonance imaging.

Treatment

No specific treatment for prion diseases is available. Supportive therapy is indicated for the sequelae of the neurodegeneration.

INFECTIONS DUE TO ENTEROVIRUSES

POLIOMYELITIS (INFANTILE PARALYSIS, ACUTE ANTERIOR POLIOMYELITIS)

Poliomyelitis is amongst the most feared of the communicable diseases. Documentation over the last century has recorded many epidemics of variable severity, with sporadic cases being reported at inter-epidemic periods. Furthermore, there are historical references which show that poliomyelitis has been a disease of man for many centuries, though these indicate that it has become more virulent since the late nineteenth century.

Modern epidemiological and virological surveys show that in the great majority of infected people poliomyelitis is a harmless subclinical event; nevertheless, severe epidemics can arise with remarkable rapidity and the mortality and morbidity that result demonstrate that the fear in which the disease is held is well founded.

Epidemiology

Man appears to be the main reservoir of polioviruses in nature and their proven presence in sewage, flies and food is probably of minor importance. In temperate climates, epidemics occur in summer months. Poliomyelitis has shown a change in its epidemiological pattern; the large epidemics of the early 1950s were associated with a higher attack rate in older children and in young adults. The clinical severity showed a parallel rise and these severe epidemics occurred in countries with a high standard of living. A possible explanation put forward for this change was that improved hygiene standards led to a diminished rate of subclinical infection in infancy. In view of this it became a matter of great urgency to provide effective immunization against poliomyelitis and it was fortuitous that developments in this field were so timely. The Expanded Program of Immunization of the World Health Organization with the goal of global eradication has led to a steady decline in the world incidence of poliomyelitis since 1973, and a 95% decline in cases worldwide.[405] Intense wild-type poliovirus activity is now limited to the Indian subcontinent and sub-Saharan Africa.[405] In the rest of the world, there are rare cases of vaccine-associated paralytic poliomyelitis attributable to the oral poliovirus vaccine.

Etiology

There are three strains, polioviruses types 1, 2 and 3, which show little antigenic overlap. They are particularly small, having a diameter of 25 nm, and contain RNA. Poliovirus type 1 has been associated with most of the major epidemics and shows the greatest propensity to cause paralytic forms of the disease, whereas type 2 causes sporadic cases or small outbreaks with a low incidence of paralysis; type 3 occupies an intermediate position. Certain factors appear to influence the virulence of polioviruses in the human host. Clinical severity is increased by age and pregnancy. Excessive muscular activity in a recently infected person makes a paralytic form of the disease more probable as do intramuscular injections into the limbs and other minor, traumatic procedures. Recent tonsillectomy predisposes to bulbar poliomyelitis and corticosteroid drugs can have an adverse effect. Antibody is clearly important as there is a higher incidence in patients with antibody deficiency.

The disease is spread by direct contact with infected persons through pharyngeal secretions and feces. Infectivity is probably maximal early, and oral–oral spread may be more common than fecal–oral spread. Rarely paralytic poliomyelitis may result from oral vaccine strains which revert to virulence.

Pathogenesis and pathology

Polioviruses enter the body via the oral route and multiply in the tonsillopharyngeal tissues and in the intestinal wall. From the former they pass to regional lymph nodes and infectivity of the pharyngeal secretions disappears rapidly. From the latter, viruses also pass to the appropriate regional lymph nodes but in this case there is continued excretion into the bowel. This is shown by the ease with which polioviruses can be isolated from the feces for weeks and sometimes months.

The viruses probably pass to the bloodstream from the infected lymph nodes and can be isolated from the blood on occasion. The mode of passage thereafter to the nervous system is not fully understood.

In man, the pathological lesions in the CNS are mainly found in the anterior horns of the spinal cord but the posterior horns and intermediate columns may be involved. The essential lesion is neuronal damage, and though some neurones will die, others may recover. Meningitis occurs, and in some cases there is an extensive encephalitis involving motor cells in the medulla and pons, the vestibular nuclei and the motor and premotor areas of the cerebral cortex. Sometimes the lesions are concentrated in the medulla with little damage at lower levels in the cord.

Clinical features

Poliomyelitis is highly infectious and has an incubation period of 1–3 weeks. Paralytic disease virtually only occurs in unimmunized children or adults, as the virus still circulates in the community. In countries where vaccination is not performed and where low economic standards obtain, poliomyelitis is still primarily a disease of infants and young children. Most people infected will have an inapparent illness, which can only be demonstrated by retrospective serological surveys or by examination of contacts in the course of an actual epidemic.

The minor illness

People infected by polioviruses may respond with a mild, insignificant illness whose features may include fever, anorexia, headache, lassitude and gastroenteritic symptoms. The title of 'abortive poliomyelitis' was sometimes used to describe this condition which is now more commonly referred to as the minor illness.

The major illness (non-paralytic or preparalytic poliomyelitis)

The major illness may immediately follow the minor or there may be a short gap of apparent recovery. Occasionally the minor illness does not occur.

In the preparalytic stage of the major illness, the symptoms simulate those of aseptic meningitis. The patient will experience headache, vomiting, malaise and fever. Later, pain and stiffness may be felt in the neck and back. Nuchal rigidity and a positive Kernig sign are usually elicited on examination. Patients may also complain of an aching pain and spasm in the limbs but this is rarely as marked a feature as older accounts of the disease suggest.

A lumbar puncture performed at this time will normally demonstrate a mild CSF pleocytosis (either polymorphonuclear or lymphocytic) and slight to moderate elevation of the protein content.

A variable percentage of cases presenting with this picture will gradually improve over the ensuing 7–10 days and thereafter make an uninterrupted recovery (non-paralytic poliomyelitis). Others, unfortunately, proceed to paralysis. Most paralytic cases pass through the preparalytic stage outlined above; the paralysis starting some 2–3 days later. Occasionally, paralysis comes on earlier or the preparalytic stage is absent.

Paralytic poliomyelitis

Spinal paralysis. The cervical and lumbar segments of the cord are most frequently involved and patchy, asymmetric paralysis in the limbs results. This may be trivial and can be confined to part of one muscle group when it is easily overlooked. Unilateral involvement of the dorsiflexors of the feet, of the quadriceps or of the deltoids is a common finding. The paralysis is of lower motor neurone type.

Spinal respiratory paralysis. This form is usually associated with rapid, severe limb paralysis, and neuronal damage may then extend through the central part of the cord. Paralysis of the abdominal muscles may show itself by weakness in the cough though lower intercostal involvement may be symptomless to the patient at rest and only evident to the examiner. Eventually such signs as tachypnea, tachycardia, cyanosis, a rising blood pressure and mental confusion will become apparent. In some instances the signs of increasing ventilatory failure are difficult to distinguish from those of bulbar involvement or encephalitis and these conditions can be simultaneously present.

Bulbar poliomyelitis. This form may be seen with unusual frequency in some epidemics and can be associated with recent tonsillectomy. Difficulty in swallowing is the cardinal sign and the subject is unable to clear mucus and saliva from the throat. There is a reluctance on the part of the patient to breathe deeply, in case secretions become aspirated into the lung. Such symptoms arise from pharyngeal involvement and further spread may occur manifesting itself in weakness of the flexors of the neck, facial paralysis, external ocular palsies and, occasionally, true laryngeal paralysis. Extension to the respiratory center, with totally irregular breathing and periods of apnea, has a grave prognosis and involvement of the circulatory center will result in circulatory collapse and an irregular, rapid pulse. Involvement of these vital centers is usually fatal.

Vaccine associated paralytic poliomyelitis (VAPP)

The World Health Organization defines VAPP as 'acute flaccid paralysis in a vaccine recipient 7 to 30 days after receiving oral polio vaccine, with no sensory or cognitive loss and with paralysis still present 60 days after the onset of symptoms'.[406] It occurs in about one case in every 750 000 first doses distributed,[407] and has lead to a reintroduction of the inactivated Salk vaccine into the routine immunization schedule in the USA.

Laboratory diagnosis

Isolation of the poliovirus from the patient is the method of choice. Polioviruses grow well in a variety of tissue cultures, and providing specimens are collected early in the illness, successful virus isolation is not difficult. Virus may be recovered from throat swabs during the early stages of the illness and from the feces for several weeks after the onset. CSF should be cultured for polioviruses but unlike Coxsackie and ECHO viruses, these are found infrequently.

Acute and convalescent samples of serum should be obtained and tested for a significant rise in antibody titer during the illness; tests for both complement-fixing and neutralizing antibodies are available.

Differential diagnosis

Non-paralytic poliomyelitis cannot be differentiated on clinical grounds from other conditions causing the syndrome of aseptic meningitis. Paralytic poliomyelitis may be confused with a variety of disorders including Guillain–Barré syndrome, botulism, localized paralysis following specific infections such as mumps or infectious mononucleosis, paralytic episodes in sickle cell disease, myasthenia gravis and familial periodic paralysis.

Particular forms of poliomyelitis can be specially confusing, such as isolated facial paralysis which may mimic Bell's palsy and bulbar paralysis which can be mistaken for tetanus. Pseudoparalysis may be found in acute rheumatism, osteomyelitis, fractures, scurvy, congenital syphilis and hysteria.

Emphasis must also be laid on the fact that a true poliomyelitis-like illness can follow infection by other enteroviruses such as Coxsackie, ECHO viruses and enterovirus type 71. Wherever possible the diagnosis of any case of clinical poliomyelitis should be supported by virus isolation and positive serological tests.

Complications, course and prognosis

Non-paralytic poliomyelitis

There are no complications of non-paralytic forms of poliomyelitis. However, unsuspected paralysis may be detected in cases of this type once they become mobilized and this is particularly seen in the back muscles, the strength of which is difficult to assess whilst the patient remains in bed.

Spinal paralytic poliomyelitis

Some recovery may occur in the first 4 weeks following paralysis. Improvement thereafter is much slower. In those muscles where the neuronal supply has been severely affected, permanent paralysis with extremely rapid wasting will result.

Spinal respiratory paralysis

At the height of the illness in this group various cardiac irregularities and even cardiac failure may be encountered and this may be a secondary effect from the respiratory complications or a direct effect of the virus on the myocardium.

Major complications include pneumonia, hypertension, urinary retention and constipation. Renal calculi are not uncommon.

Bulbar poliomyelitis

This form of poliomyelitis is of great seriousness if it spreads to the vital centers in the medulla. However, in those cases without involvement of these centers there is remarkably full and quite rapid recovery of the cranial nerves. Involvement of the diaphragm may be permanent.

Late effects (postpolio syndrome)

People with paralytic polio may develop new symptoms many years later, characterized by pain in muscles, weakness, fasciculation, breathlessness and problems with speech and swallowing. The mechanism is unknown.

Treatment

Spinal paralysis

The mainstay of therapy is physiotherapy, emphasizing passive movement and hydrotherapy if available. Paralytic limbs should be supported and splinting may prevent contractures.

Patients may remain fecal excretors of poliovirus for several weeks and isolation procedures must be used.

In children lack of growth in severely paralyzed limbs may lead to significant shortening, and skilled orthopedic advice is needed in such instances.

Spinal respiratory paralysis

Ventilatory support may be required and a constant watch for the incipient onset of respiratory insufficiency must be maintained; if these difficulties are diagnosed late, hypoxia may increase neuronal damage. Where respiratory paralysis is marked ventilation is best achieved by the use of intermittent positive pressure ventilation combined with tracheostomy.

Bulbar poliomyelitis

The milder examples of this condition, where the major defect is inability to swallow, can often be managed conservatively with nasogastric tube feeding and suction of secretions. These patients often do well and undergo spontaneous recovery in 2–3 weeks. More severe cases require tracheostomy. Even in these severe cases the prognosis is good and the tracheostomy can often be closed within a few weeks.

Prevention

Virtually all cases of paralytic poliomyelitis occur in children who have not been immunized. Poliomyelitis outbreaks are unlikely to occur in a community where there is a high level of protection by immunization and where that level is maintained. Active immunization can be produced by either killed virus vaccines (Salk type) or live attenuated virus vaccines (Sabin type). The former require to be given by injection and the latter by the oral route. A full primary course of either type involves three doses with a booster. In general, Sabin type vaccines result in higher humoral antibody levels, are easy and painless to administer and also produce local immunity in the gut. Children with immune deficiency are at increased risk of paralytic polio and must be immunized with the killed vaccine. Children with HIV infection can receive either live or killed vaccines, but if there is a relative at home with AIDS who might be infected by the vaccine virus, Salk (killed) vaccine should be given.

NON-POLIO ENTEROVIRUS INFECTIONS

The *Coxsackie* and ECHO viruses, non-classified enteroviruses and *polioviruses* are called enteroviruses and are classified with rhinoviruses into a larger group known as the *picornaviruses* (pico = small, RNA viruses). The agents in this group have a similarity in size, a similar nucleic acid core (RNA) and other common physical and chemical properties. Clinical and epidemiological studies show that the Coxsackie and ECHO viruses are widely distributed in man and can cause a considerable variety of clinical syndromes. However, they have not demonstrated the same propensity to produce such large and serious epidemics as polioviruses.

COXSACKIE VIRUS INFECTIONS

The existence of this group of viruses became apparent in 1948 when unidentifiable, filterable agents were isolated from the feces of two children in whom a clinical diagnosis of paralytic poliomyelitis had been suspected. These children resided in Coxsackie in New York State and the large group of similar viruses subsequently identified has been named after this town. At the present time there are approximately 30 different varieties of Coxsackie viruses and these have been classified into two groups, known as A and B; 24 of the strains have been allocated to group A and the remaining 6 to group B.

Some, but not all, viruses of the Coxsackie groups may be grown on suitable tissue cultures but all produce a characteristic histopathological effect when injected into suckling mice.

Coxsackie group A virus diseases

Relationship of group A viruses to disease

Viruses of this group may be isolated from a variable percentage of healthy individuals; as a result their isolation from a sick patient must not necessarily be construed as a diagnostic event.

Herpangina

This is one of the most clearly defined clinical syndromes caused by infection with Coxsackie A viruses. It is most commonly seen in infants and children, though can occur in adults. The onset is characterized by fever, anorexia and pain in the throat; other features include headache, abdominal pain and myalgia. Infection will normally derive from another human and the agent may be transmitted from nasal secretions as well as from the feces. The incubation period lies between 3 and 5 days and fecal infectivity may last for several weeks.

Local examination of the mouth will usually reveal hyperemia of the pharynx, and characteristic papulovesicular lesions, approximately 1–2 mm in diameter and surrounded by an erythematous ring, will be seen. Most commonly the lesions are present over the tonsillar pillars, soft palate and uvula though on occasion the tongue may be involved. It is rare to find more than five to six lesions and these soon enlarge and form shallow ulcers. The illness will usually subside within a week and few complications are found in children. Second attacks may result from infection by different antigenic strains. In a classical case the clinical picture is highly suggestive, but laboratory studies are required for full confirmation and at least nine different group A viruses are known to produce this syndrome.

CNS involvement

Aseptic meningitis is the most common clinical manifestation and may result from infection by several different Coxsackie A virus strains. As with other types of viral meningitis young children are most likely to be involved and a rather higher incidence is encountered in male children. There is usually no characteristic clinical picture that differentiates this from other causes of viral meningitis although in a few instances one of the more specific syndromes associated with group A infection may be simultaneously present. On occasion this group may also be associated with paralytic disease that is clinically indistinguishable from poliomyelitis; Coxsackie virus A7 is the most frequently implicated but other strains such as A9 have also been involved. Severe and fatal encephalitis has been described in only a small number of cases of Coxsackie A virus infection.

Hand, foot and mouth disease (HFM)

In 1957 there was a small epidemic in Toronto of an illness with certain characteristic features. These included the presence of vesicular lesions in the mouth as well as on the hands and feet. Virological studies on these cases indicated infection with Coxsackie virus A16 and in the ensuing years several similar outbreaks, including some from the UK, were reported. In the majority, Coxsackie virus A16 was once again the responsible virus though in some instances types A5 and A10 were responsible.

HFM disease usually presents with little or no constitutional upset. In babies, reluctance to feed may be an early sign and in older children a reluctance to eat. Examination of the mouth often shows some mild ulceration over the tongue and further examination indicates the pearly white vesicles, sometimes surrounded by a red halo, on the extremities. The lesions are mainly found over the ventral surface of the fingers and toes and have a characteristic distribution along the sides of the feet. Some cases also show a maculopapular rash over the buttocks, which may extend on to the thighs mimicking Henoch–Schönlein purpura. Fever may occur but it is rarely marked and there is little associated lymphadenopathy.

A fully developed case is extraordinarily characteristic and once seen is readily recognized thereafter. The mouth lesions can be confused with herpetic gingivostomatitis and herpangina as the peripheral lesions are painless, and may be overlooked. An occasional case has been confused with scabies.

Outbreaks of this syndrome are usually small and tend to occur in the summer months. Subclinical infection of family contacts can be demonstrated by the isolation of viruses from them and the prognosis is excellent.

The association between HFM disease caused by enterovirus type 71 and brainstem encephalitis is described below.

Miscellaneous Coxsackie A virus infections

Coxsackie A viruses have been isolated from children suffering from a febrile illness with a rash, from cases of pharyngitis and from cases of benign pericarditis. They have also been associated with mild undifferentiated respiratory tract infection, especially Coxsackie A21 virus (previously known as Coe virus), with acute febrile lymphadenitis, gastroenteritis, tracheobronchitis and pleurodynia.

Laboratory diagnosis

The isolation of most Coxsackie group A viruses is not difficult provided suitable specimens are sent to the laboratory. Suitable specimens include vesicle fluid, throat swabs, feces and CSF, depending on the clinical syndrome under investigation. Serological tests on acute and convalescent serum samples can be carried out but owing to the large number of serotypes this is not a practical procedure unless an agent has been isolated. The Coxsackie virus complement-fixation test frequently employed crossreacts with all enteroviruses and is not very sensitive. Detection of viral RNA by PCR is now generally available and more sensitive than culture.

Coxsackie group B virus diseases

Bornholm disease or epidemic pleurodynia

This disease, first recognized clinically over a century ago, is now known to result from infection with certain group B Coxsackie viruses. Children and young adults are usually involved and more severe cases occur in the latter.

After an incubation period of 2–4 days, the illness commences in a non-specific manner with fever, malaise and headache. However, the characteristic pain will soon follow and is principally experienced over the lower chest and may be associated with acute dyspnea. A clinical diagnosis of pleurisy may be made though no friction rub is audible and X-ray of the chest is clear. Pain may also be felt lower down the trunk and this may spread over the abdomen and simulate an acute surgical condition. Palpation over the affected muscles may reveal exquisite tenderness and this can have a band-like distribution suggestive of a neurological disorder or shingles.

In many instances the illness subsides within a few days but it may run a relapsing course and last for as long as 3–4 weeks. Several members of a family may be attacked in quick succession and show a wide variation in the severity.

Bornholm disease requires to be differentiated from pleurisy and pneumonia. Acute appendicitis and cholecystitis have been mimicked by an abdominal presentation but milder varieties, without significant pain, can be confused with influenza. In general, there is no significant leukocytosis and this may be helpful in the differentiation of pyogenic infection.

Outbreaks are small and often confined to family units. However, an epidemic can be more widespread and in these instances the correct clinical diagnosis may be made with reasonable accuracy. Nevertheless, full confirmation requires detailed virological assessment.

CNS involvement

The etiological role of the group B viruses in *aseptic meningitis* is fully established and all six types have been incriminated in this illness. The age incidence appears similar to that encountered in aseptic meningitis due to other viruses as indicated below. Clinical differentiation from other possible causes is impossible though pleurodynia is an occasional accompaniment. Severe and fatal encephalitis has been described in only a small number of cases as has mild paralytic disease.

Cardiac involvement

The clinical syndrome of *acute myocarditis* in infants and children has been variously described as idiopathic, isolated, Fiedler's or interstitial myocarditis. However, in the light of present knowledge, it has proved possible to make a definitive, causative diagnosis in an increasing proportion of such illness and the role of Coxsackie B viruses, and to a lesser degree some group A agents, has become firmly established.

Coxsackie B myocarditis of infancy

Coxsackie viruses B1–5 have been incriminated in this disorder though types B3 and B4 have been implicated most frequently. The illness usually commences within the first 2 weeks of life though older babies have been involved. Most neonatal cases are probably caused by vertical spread from an infected mother, and a maternal history of respiratory or gastrointestinal illness is common. Nursery outbreaks can also occur.

Clinical features (see Ch. 19) The onset is always sudden. Presenting symptoms include feeding difficulties, lethargy, fever, cyanosis, respiratory distress and shock. Cardiomegaly, tachycardia, hepatomegaly and electrocardiographic changes soon appear. Involvement may not be confined to the cardiovascular system. In up to one-third of cases central nervous signs such as convulsions, neck stiffness, coma and CSF disturbances are encountered.

The prognosis is poor, and up to 75% of cases die in spite of intensive therapy. At autopsy an intense inflammatory infiltration and necrosis is found in the myocardium and changes may also be found in the liver, pancreas, suprarenal glands, bone marrow and CNS.

Differential diagnosis. Myocarditis is a difficult entity to diagnose in a neonate. Most cases are initially considered to be some form of acute respiratory disorder (e.g. respiratory distress syndrome), other overwhelming infections or congenital heart disease.

Treatment. Infants with this condition require intensive nursing in hospital; oxygen, diuretics and digitalization may be required, although the heart is often very sensitive to digoxin and low doses may be needed.

Pericarditis and myocarditis due to Coxsackie B viruses in older children

Acute pericarditis in older children and adults is a syndrome where the causative role of Coxsackie B viruses (types B1–5) is well established. Less often, myocarditis may also occur in these age groups but, unlike infection in neonates, the prognosis is generally good. Clinical recovery is quite rapid and although the electrocardiographic changes can take some months to resolve, recovery seems complete and there is little evidence of any permanent cardiac damage. Rare cases of myocarditis are fulminant and fatal.

Miscellaneous Coxsackie B virus infections

Amongst other disorders found in association with group B viruses are mild respiratory tract illness, febrile illness with an exanthem and orchitis. They are also reputed to cause endocardial fibroelastosis, the infection of the fetus occurring in utero.

Laboratory diagnosis

The six types of Coxsackie group B viruses can be readily isolated in the laboratory either in tissue cultures or suckling mice. Virus can be grown from throat swabs, feces, CSF and in some cases from other organs, e.g. myocardium and testis. Acute and convalescent samples of serum should be sent to the laboratory so that, if present, a significant rise in antibody titer during the illness can be shown. Serological tests may be of special value if a Coxsackie group B virus has been isolated as in this instance the sera need only be tested for an antibody rise against this specific isolate. In all cases it is advisable to try to isolate a virus from the patient as early in the illness as possible. Detection of the presence of viral RNA by PCR is available in many laboratories.

ECHO VIRUS INFECTIONS

Agents of this group are so named after the initial letters of their original name, enteric cytopathogenic human orphan viruses. There are some 30 distinctive serotypes and their association with aseptic meningitis, encephalitis and paralytic diseases is well documented. They may also cause respiratory tract infections, gastroenteritis, myocarditis and exanthemata of a rather non-specific character. Subclinical infection with this group is common but clinical examples may present sporadically or in moderate sized epidemics.

A number of different types of ECHO viruses have been associated with each of the various clinical syndromes that this group may cause and most types have been found in association with more than one syndrome. A few of the identified types have not, as yet, been found in association with obvious disease. In general infection by this group of agents is relatively benign and, except in neonates, few fatalities have been described. They spread in a fashion similar to polioviruses and Coxsackie viruses.

Clinical syndromes

The most commonly associated disease is *aseptic meningitis*; this may be found sporadically or in epidemics. A considerable number of different ECHO virus types may be found in association with this syndrome but the age incidence once again follows the pattern found with infection by other viruses and this is referred to in greater detail later in this section. In general the prognosis is good and in many instances the cases are clinically indistinguishable from those produced by other viral infections. However, in some there is a rash and where this is seen in a reasonable proportion of cases in any outbreak of aseptic meningitis, it often indicates that an ECHO virus is responsible.

Sporadic cases of *poliomyelitis-like illness* with paralysis have been reported in which evidence of ECHO virus infection has been established; the involvement has usually been slight but instances of permanent residual paralysis are recorded. Cases of *encephalitis* due to ECHO viruses have also been reported and a fatal outcome has occasionally resulted. Children with antibody deficiency can get chronic ECHO virus infection of the brain and/or muscle.

Mild upper respiratory illness has been found in association with a few ECHO viruses, particularly types 11, 19 and 20. These agents may also cause gastroenteritis in infants and young children; fecal samples cultured from such cases have produced evidence of infection by ECHO viruses 5, 11, 14, 18, 19 and 20.

ECHO viruses have been isolated in association with sporadic cases of pleurodynia, pericarditis and myocarditis. However, as these agents may be cultured from many otherwise healthy people their etiological relationship should not necessarily be assumed.

Where rashes do occur as a result of ECHO virus infection they tend to be of a fine, maculopapular character, have a widespread distribution and fade rapidly. Generally there is no classical distribution or typical enanthem, although lesions may be papular, arranged in lines and located peripherally, the so-called papular acro-located syndrome (PALS).

Neonatal ECHO virus infection can cause disseminated infection with massive hepatic necrosis, disseminated intravascular coagulation, bleeding and usually death. Such severe cases are almost always acquired vertically and a maternal history of peripartum illness is usual. Although nursery outbreaks may occur most horizontal cases are relatively mild, although occasionally complicated by meningitis and myocarditis.

Laboratory diagnosis

The ECHO viruses can be readily isolated in various tissue culture systems, or enteroviral RNA detected by reverse-transcriptase PCR. Specimens usually required by the laboratory are CSF, throat swabs and feces depending on the clinical manifestations of the illness. Serological tests on acute and convalescent serum samples can be carried out to show a significant rise in antibody titer during the illness, but owing to the large number of different types of ECHO viruses it is usually not a practical procedure unless an agent has been isolated and identified. Some ECHO viruses cause hemagglutination, so in these cases hemagglutination-inhibiting antibodies can be estimated; otherwise it is usual to test for a rise in neutralizing antibody titer.

ENTEROVIRUSES TYPES 68–71

In addition to the spectrum of symptoms outlined above, this group of enteroviruses is also associated with specific syndromes. Enterovirus type 70 has been isolated from patients with acute hemorrhagic conjunctivitis. Enterovirus type 71 (EV71) is associated with hand, foot and mouth syndrome. In Australia, Malaysia, Taiwan and Japan, outbreaks of EV71-associated hand, foot and mouth disease in children have been followed by severe neurological symptoms such as brainstem encephalitis often with neurogenic pulmonary edema, and by Guillain–Barré syndrome, acute transverse myelitis, cerebellar ataxia, opsomyoclonus, benign intracranial hypertension and febrile convulsions.[393,394]

Treatment

No specific therapy is available. In a small, non-controlled case series, the antiviral agent pleconaril has been reported to be effective in improving survival after severe enteroviral infection in infants and immunocompromised children.[408] However, efficacy data from randomized controlled trials are as yet unavailable. Intravenous immunoglobulin has been used to treat both chronic enteroviral infection in immunodeficient children and severe neonatal enteroviral disease. Neither of these agents is reportedly effective against EV71-associated disease.[393]

VIRUSES AND THE GASTROINTESTINAL TRACT

Many viral agents may inhabit the intestinal tract without producing obvious clinical illness. As a result when such agents are cultured in the presence of gastrointestinal symptoms, their etiological role is difficult to establish. Nevertheless epidemiological studies in the recent past seemed to indicate that some agents, such as certain ECHO viruses, may be involved in outbreaks of diarrhea in infants. The picture has, however, changed in the last few years as a wide variety of new viral agents has been discovered by electron microscopy of feces. Notable amongst these are *rotaviruses* and *Norwalk-like viruses*.

GASTROENTERITIS

Amongst viral agents found in association with gastroenteritis are rotaviruses, Norwalk-like viruses, caliciviruses, coronaviruses, astroviruses, adenoviruses, stool parvoviruses and enteroviruses. The role of rotaviruses and Norwalk virus is more clearly established, but the other viruses can cause limited outbreaks of infantile diarrhea.

Rotaviruses were initially found on electron microscopy of duodenal biopsies taken from children with diarrhea in Australia in 1973. Since then these agents have been found to be common worldwide and their presence may be detected by a variety of methods. Several different human types have been identified as well as many animal varieties. Species specificity appears incomplete.

Between 1 and 7 days after infection, but usually within 2 days, the affected child starts to vomit and develops a low grade fever. Watery diarrhea soon follows and, although mucus may be seen in the stools, blood is rarely present. The vomiting stops after 1–2 days but diarrhea persists even if intravenous fluids are started with no oral intake. Non-specific respiratory symptoms may occur and, although the illness terminates in about 5–7 days, virus may be found in the stool for up to 10 days.

The peak age of attack is between 6 and 24 months of age, mainly from 9 to 12 months; there is a slight male preponderance. Asymptomatic cases will often be found in older members of the household. Neonatal infection occurs and has been associated with a clinical picture resembling necrotizing enterocolitis. However, neonatal infection is often subclinical, perhaps due to the presence of maternal antibody. It is suggested that breast-feeding can be protective.

Up to 50% of hospitalized cases of infantile gastroenteritis, and a somewhat lower proportion of community cases are caused by rotaviruses.[409] Transmission is by the fecal–oral route and, in temperate climates, it is mainly a winter disease although cases can occur throughout the year. Serological surveys show that up to 90% of children aged 3 years or over possess antibody to rotaviruses and surveys in the adult population show figures of up to 70%.

Treatment of gastroenteritis due to rotavirus infection is along standard lines (see p. xxxx). Fatalities are rare in industrialized countries and usually in otherwise debilitated children. A variety of complications have been found but the role of rotaviruses in their production is not firmly established.

A tetravalent rotavirus vaccine was licensed in the USA in 1998 and introduced into the routine schedule. It was then voluntarily withdrawn from the market in 1999, due to a possible rare association with intussusception, that was detected in postlicensing surveillance.[410]

The *Norwalk virus*, which was first discovered in 1972, and other caliciviruses are also known to produce gastroenteritis. Outbreaks have usually occurred in older children with secondary cases in adults, some involving schoolchildren and their teachers. These agents, first discovered in the USA and certain Far Eastern countries, are now found on a worldwide basis. After an incubation period of some 2 days the illness starts with nausea and vomiting. Diarrhea, abdominal cramps and fever follow in about half of those involved but symptoms usually abate within a day or so. Treatment is purely symptomatic.

Enteric adenoviruses are the second most important cause of viral diarrhea of infancy, in terms of hospitalization, and often cause prolonged diarrhea with or without vomiting. Astroviruses rarely result in hospital admission, but can cause winter vomiting and may cause rare outbreaks in hospitals.

INTUSSUSCEPTION

The etiology of this condition, which involves the invagination of a portion of the intestine into an adjacent portion, is not fully understood, but in some instances association with a recent infective illness appears to be present. Further investigation of this possible association in recent times has revealed evidence of infection of the intestinal tract by *adenoviruses* and this association appears to be encountered more often than one would expect to occur by chance. Furthermore, adenoviruses have been isolated from regional lymph glands in children found to be suffering from mesenteric adenitis and, as this condition is considered to be associated with the development of intussusception, the possible etiological role seems strengthened.

The association beween intussusception and live attenuated rotavirus vaccine is further evidence that intussusception may follow virus infections of the gastrointestinal tract.

OTHER CONDITIONS

Attempts to establish an association between viral infection and appendicitis have not proved very rewarding. Pancreatitis is a recognized complication of mumps and has occasionally been found in association with infection by Coxsackie viruses.

LABORATORY DIAGNOSIS

Various viruses have been associated with diseases of the gastrointestinal tract but the isolation of agents from clinically fit children is not infrequent, so caution must be used before incriminating a virus as the cause of a disease.

In general, the main pathogens responsible for viral gastroenteritis, rotavirus, enteric adenoviruses, caliciviruses and astroviruses cannot be readily isolated by culture.[344] Although these agents may be demonstrated in stools by negative staining electron microscopy this has largely been replaced by enzyme immunoassays for rotavirus and enteric adenoviruses.

OCULAR DISEASES CAUSED BY VIRUSES AND ALLIED ORGANISMS

It is now recognized that viral and chlamydial infections of the eye constitute a larger proportion of ocular disease than was formerly appreciated. In part this stems from the enormous advances in viral technology but many ocular diseases are now recognized to have a viral basis because chemotherapy has cleared secondary bacterial infection and revealed the true, underlying viral pathogenesis.

In most instances viral infection of the eye presents as part of a systemic infection which may manifest itself by direct tissue invasion or indirectly through neural involvement, as in the viral encephalitides. Examples of viruses that may act this way are CMV and HSV in the congenitally infected or immunocompromised. However, some viral infections seem to involve the eye selectively, and those include certain adenoviral infections, trachoma, inclusion conjunctivitis and acute hemorrhagic conjunctivitis.

ADENOVIRUS INFECTIONS OF THE EYE

Two main ocular syndromes are associated with adenovirus infection – *pharyngoconjunctival fever* and *epidemic keratoconjunctivitis*.

Pharyngoconjunctival fever

This condition may result from infection by several types of adenoviruses though type 3 is most commonly implicated. Clinically it may present as a follicular conjunctivitis, often with associated fever and pharyngitis, producing the recognized clinical entity of pharyngoconjunctival fever. The virus may infect one or both eyes causing an acute conjunctivitis with follicular hypertrophy and mild preauricular lymphadenopathy. A mild transient keratitis sometimes develops.

Children are most often affected and cases may occur sporadically or in epidemics, sometimes associated with swimming pools.

Epidemic keratoconjunctivitis

This disease presents as an acute keratoconjunctivitis with follicular hypertrophy of the conjunctiva and marked preauricular lymphadenopathy. A distinctive keratitis then develops and about a third of the cases have pseudomembranes.

Large epidemics may occur and adults are involved rather than children. Infection is usually due to adenovirus type 8 and spread may occur through ocular instruments, infected eye-droppers and contaminated solutions used in hospitals, first aid stations and surgeries. Complete recovery usually occurs but permanent impairment of vision can occasionally result.

Laboratory diagnosis

Ocular infection with an adenovirus can be confirmed by culturing the virus. Swabs or scrapings in virus transport medium should be sent to the laboratory for virus isolation. The adenoviruses are not difficult to propagate.

TRACHOMA AND INCLUSION CONJUNCTIVITIS

(See Chapter 10)

Agents of the genus *Chlamydia* are organisms with properties that are intermediate between viruses and bacteria, and they show sensitivity to certain antibiotics. *Chlamydia trachomatis* is the cause of trachoma, inclusion conjunctivitis, afebrile pneumonitis and lymphogranuloma venereum.

Trachoma

Trachoma is a specific form of keratoconjunctivitis which first involves the upper tarsal follicles. Later upper limbal changes appear followed by pannus formation and the development of Herbert's peripheral pits. The disease is mainly encountered in tropical areas where water is scarce. In such areas there is often a very high incidence. Permanent scarring and blindness may occur especially where adequate facilities for treatment are not available.

Infection occurs at an early age but the mode of transmission is still far from clear; all ages are affected but the disease is especially common in children and is often associated with secondary infection. Theories to explain the spread have included person-to-person contact, infection through fomites and dissemination by flies.

Treatment

Among drugs which may be used are sulfonamides, tetracycline and, less often, erythromycin. Opinions differ as to the efficacy and mode of treatment. However, where topical therapy is conscientiously applied over a period of several weeks, or even months, a good response can be anticipated. Some advocate supplementation by oral therapy.

Inclusion conjunctivitis

This condition is caused by certain strains of *Chlamydia trachomatis* that may reside in the genital tract and produce cervicitis or urethritis. There is a danger of spread to infants, resulting in inclusion blennorrhea, during their passage through the birth canal. Older children and adults may contract inclusion conjunctivitis from swimming pools that have been contaminated by urine or by discharge from the genital tract.

Treatment of inclusion conjunctivitis is also by sulfonamides or topical broad spectrum antibiotics. However, the response is quicker than in trachoma and treatment need not be so prolonged. The prognosis is also better and permanent scarring does not occur. Neonates with inclusion conjunctivitis should be treated with oral erythromycin 40 mg/kg/day 6-hourly for 14 days because of the risk of progression to afebrile pneumonitis.

Laboratory diagnosis

The agents are situated in the epithelial cells of the conjunctiva, and for successful culture epithelial scrapings or eye swabs in special transport medium should be sent to the laboratory. Cultural methods consist of inoculation of suitable tissue cultures and then after incubation, examination under the microscope for typical inclusion bodies. Direct microscopy on Giemsa-stained smears may reveal typical inclusions. ELISA antigen detection tests and PCR that avoid the need for culture and give a rapid diagnosis are increasingly being used.

ACUTE HEMORRHAGIC CONJUNCTIVITIS (APOLLO 11 DISEASE)

This condition was recognized as a clinical entity in 1969 at the same time as the Apollo 11 moon landing, and a virus, now classified as enterovirus type 70, has been isolated from the conjunctiva of affected patients. Extensive outbreaks have been reported from Africa, Pakistan, India and South America. The disease appears to have an incubation period of about 24 h and to be highly contagious in unhygienic and crowded conditions. The infection is of sudden onset with swelling, congestion, watering and pain in the eye. The most characteristic sign is subconjunctival hemorrhage of varying intensity, which may sometimes be accompanied by corneal keratitis. The disease is not influenced by antibiotics and symptoms usually subside within 1–2 weeks. The effect of oral pleconaril on this disease is still to be evaluated.

Laboratory diagnosis

Conjunctival scrapings or swabs should be sent to the laboratory where suitable tissue cultures can be used to isolate the causative agent.

VIRAL INFECTION OF THE LIVER

Acute inflammation of the liver may be caused by a number of viruses including hepatitis viruses A to F, CMV, adenoviruses, picornaviruses, HSV, EBV and the viruses of diseases such as yellow fever and rubella.

HEPATITIS A VIRUS INFECTION OR INFECTIOUS HEPATITIS (EPIDEMIC HEPATITIS, EPIDEMIC JAUNDICE OR CATARRHAL JAUNDICE)

This disease has an incubation period of 15–50 days (average 30 days) and is mainly found in young children. It is also quite common in older children and young adults but the attack rate declines with increasing age though a higher proportion of severe and complicated cases may be found in these older age groups. Pregnant women may contract a particularly severe form.

The distribution of infectious hepatitis is worldwide and epidemic periodicity varies greatly in different communities. Experimental studies indicate that the responsible agent, hepatitis A virus, is present in both blood and feces at the peak of the illness and persists in the feces for a relatively short time. Susceptible human volunteers have been fed filtered fecal extracts and virus could be found in the feces of those who developed jaundice from 14 to 26 days before the onset of icterus and for over a week thereafter. Furthermore, although at least two-thirds of the recipients displayed no clinical evidence of hepatitis, subclinical evidence of infection was found on serial examination by appropriate liver function tests. This indicates a ratio of 1:2 for clinical, as opposed to subclinical, infection and this impression is further substantiated by epidemiological studies in naturally occurring epidemics.

Although infectious hepatitis is mainly transmitted by the fecal–oral route through contamination of food and water, transmission may also occur from blood, urine, nasopharyngeal secretions and saliva. Large epidemics usually occur in institutions and closed communities and, in some of these, infection of a communal water supply has been responsible. Prevention of waterborne outbreaks of this type is difficult though carefully controlled super-chlorination may be effective. Outbreaks have also followed the ingestion of raw oysters and raw clams infected by sewage. Infection may also result from the use of imperfectly sterilized instruments, syringes and needles which have been contaminated by infected blood or blood products.

The diagnosis, differential diagnosis and detailed treatment of infectious hepatitis are referred to elsewhere (Chapter 17). Complement-fixation tests, immune-adherence hemagglutination,

ELISA and radioimmunoassay can be used to detect specific IgM and IgG antibody to hepatitis A virus; the presence of specific IgM antibody indicates a recent infection with hepatitis A virus. In the majority of childhood cases the illness is mild and treatment need not extend beyond simple bed rest and a moderate period of convalescence.

Mortality amongst otherwise healthy, well-nourished individuals is as low as 0.1–0.2% but can rise to 2 or 3% in those poorly nourished. Death may either be early from fulminating hepatitis leading to acute hepatocellular failure or occur considerably later from chronic liver damage.

Prevention

Killed vaccines are now available and are safe and effective,[411] and indicated for older children and adults at long term risk. Human normal immunoglobulin is effective prophylaxis and should be given to adult and child contacts of index cases and to people traveling to areas with poor sanitation for short periods.

HEPATITIS B (SERUM HEPATITIS, AUSTRALIAN ANTIGEN-POSITIVE HEPATITIS)

Hepatitis B is enormously important for a number of reasons: some 200 million worldwide carry hepatitis B virus (HBV), which is one of the most important causes of liver cirrhosis and hepatoma, the incidence of these being greatly increased in chronic carriers. Because of both vertical and horizontal transmission of the HBV infection is endemic in some parts of the world, notably the Far East where carriage rates may exceed 15%. About half of all carriers will die liver-related deaths.

The incubation period is 60–160 days, much longer than hepatitis A. Virus antigen can be detected in the blood up to 3 months before jaundice occurs and often for many years after clinical recovery. The virus is mainly transmitted via infected blood, and is highly infectious, far more so than HIV. Infected blood transfusions, needle sharing by intravenous drug abusers, tattooing and ritual scarification are all well-documented means of spread. The virus can be sexually transmitted and the incidence is high in many homosexual communities. Vertical spread is common and is thought to be mainly peripartum rather than transplacental, thus being largely preventable by intervention immediately after birth. Most vertically infected babies become chronic carriers. The virus is also found in breast milk, although breast-feeding has not been shown to be a clear risk factor for transmission. Clinical features of hepatitis B infection are discussed in elsewhere.

Etiology

In 1965 geneticists investigating inherited variations in human plasma proteins discovered an unusual protein antigen in the serum of an Australian aborigine. This antigen, originally called Australia antigen (Au), subsequently serum hepatitis antigen (SH) and now hepatitis B surface antigen (HBs), was found to be associated with hepatitis of long incubation. On electron microscopy of serum three particles are identifiable. Dane particles, 42 nm in diameter, are complete virus comprising an inner core containing double-stranded HBV DNA within a core antigen (HBc) and surrounded by an outer coat of surface antigen (HBs). A further antigen, the e antigen, a component of the inner core, may also be seen (see Fig. 26.38). The detection of e antigen in the absence of e antibody correlates with high infectivity. Subjects may be:

1. HBs antigen positive, with no e antigen or e antibody detected – these will be mainly chronic carriers;
2. HBe antigen positive, but e antibody negative – usually also HBs positive – suggests recent active infection and highly infectious;

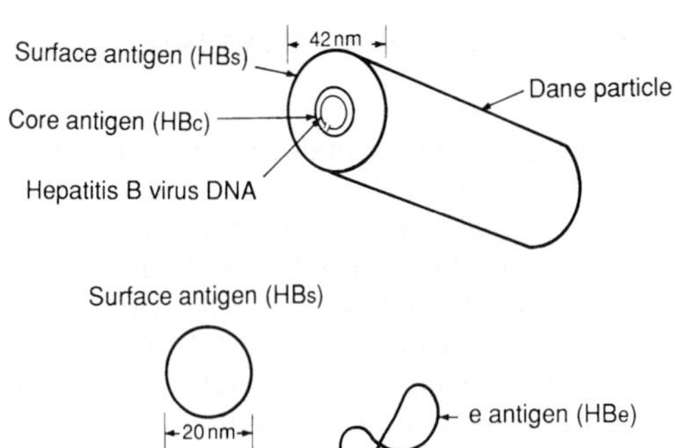

Fig. 26.38 Diagrammatic representation of electron microscopic appearance of hepatitis B virus.

3. HBe antibody positive – recovery phase, much less infectious.

Tests commonly used to detect the presence of HBV antigens and antibodies include hemagglutination tests and ELISA tests, which are often used to screen sera for surface antigen (HBs), and radioimmunoassays, which are more sensitive.

Detection of HBs antibody indicates either recovery from acute HBV infection or a response to immunization. Presence of HBc IgM antibody indicates acute HBV infection, while HBc IgG antibody is detected following infection but not immunization (which uses HBsAG).

Prevention

In many countries blood or blood product donations are routinely screened for surface antigen (HBs) and antenatal screening of all pregnant women or those from high-risk groups allows intervention to prevent vertical transmission. Great care should be taken handling blood and excreta from HBV-positive patients because of the high infectivity, although any person doing so should be immunized.

Passive immunization with specific immunoglobulin is given for accidental contamination with infected blood, e.g. in the laboratory or from a syringe and needle from a drug abuser. It is also given to babies of infected mothers as soon as possible after birth.

Recombinant DNA hepatitis B vaccines are now widely available. All health care personnel likely to come into contact with HBV-positive patients, i.e. doctors, dentists, nurses, midwives, students, laboratory staff, etc. should receive a course of three doses of the vaccine.

Babies of mothers who are in the above risk groups 1 (HBs positive) and 2 (HBe antigen positive) are at high risk of becoming chronic carriers without intervention. Indeed this will be the case in up to 90% of babies of HBe antigen-positive mothers. Such babies should receive both passive HBV-specific immunoglobulin and be actively immunized with hepatitis B vaccine. Babies of mothers in group 3 (HBe antibody positive) are at lower risk but may rarely develop acute hepatitis, and there is a risk of later horizontal transmission from the mother or an infected sibling. They should therefore be immunized and many would feel they should also receive specific immunoglobulin.

Many countries are now advocating universal neonatal hepatitis B immunization.

Treatment

Interferon alpha has been shown to have some antiviral effect in chronic carriers. Lamivudine has also been used in the treatment of chronic hepatitis B disease in adults,[412] but its use in children has not been fully evaluated.

HEPATITIS C (TRANSFUSION-ASSOCIATED NON-A, NON-B HEPATITIS)

It has been long known that hepatitis could be transmitted by blood transfusion in the absence of HBV, and the condition was previously called non-A, non-B hepatitis. The great majority of transfusion-associated hepatitis in which hepatitis B has been excluded are now known to be caused by hepatitis C virus, a flavivirus.

The structure of hepatitis C virus (HCV) was determined by molecular biology techniques in 1988, yet the virus is extremely difficult to grow. Serological tests have been developed to screen blood products, and PCR testing for the presence of viral nucleic acid is widely available.

HCV has an incubation period of around 30–60 days. Transmission is mainly via blood transfusion or by needle sharing between intravenous drug abusers. Screening of donated blood for the presence of hepatitis C antibodies has greatly reduced the risk from blood transfusion. HCV is more resistant to inactivation than HBV or HIV, and blood products such as intravenous immunoglobulin have occasionally transmitted HCV despite viral inactivation steps.

Vertical transmission from mother to fetus occurs in about 5% of pregnancies, and is thought to occur antenatally or perinatally almost exclusively in the setting of high maternal viral load in the serum. Maternal coinfection with HIV is associated with a higher risk of transmission.[413] HCV RNA and antibody have been detected in breast milk,[414] although breast-feeding has not been found to be conclusively associated with transmission to the infant by hepatitis C-positive women.[415] Nevertheless, a theoretical risk remains and the decision of a hepatitis C-positive woman whether to breast-feed should be made on an individual basis. The diagnosis of perinatally acquired HCV is usually based on the detection of HCV antibody and/or HCV RNA by PCR. The presence of maternal antibody makes interpretation of serological assays difficult in children less than 18 months. At 12 months, up to 10% of uninfected children remain HCV-seropositive, but this figure has dropped to < 0.1% by 18 months.[416] PCR for HCV RNA is sensitive over 1 month of age, and specific but is expensive. Any positive PCR test should be repeated to exclude false positive results, and because of the possibility of viral clearance.[416]

A high proportion of those infected with HCV become chronic carriers and may progress to cirrhosis. Interferon alpha therapy alone or with ribavirin is effective in reducing viral replication in around 40% of adult chronic carriers, though half of these responders will relapse when interferon is stopped. There is little experience in the use of these agents in HCV-infected children. Treatment may be considered for the child with severe hepatitis-C induced liver disease, which should be managed by a pediatric hepatologist.[417]

Children with hepatitis C infection should be immunized against hepatitis A and hepatitis B to protect against further insults to the liver.

DELTA AGENT (HEPATITIS D)

The delta agent is a defective RNA virus which requires HBV for its own synthesis. This is one of the most important examples of viral coinfection described. The delta agent was detected by immunofluorescence studies of liver cell nuclei of chronic HBV carriers. Delta antigen and antibody are detected by radioimmunoassay or ELISA and have never been demonstrated other than in association with HBV. The delta agent is most prevalent in intravenous drug abusers in Italy and the Mediterranean but has been detected worldwide. It appears to be a risk factor for acute hepatitis in drug abusers. About half of HBs-positive hemophiliacs in the USA and Italy have antidelta antibodies.

HEPATITIS E (ENTERIC NON-A, NON-B HEPATITIS)

Hepatitis E is the enterically transmitted form of non-A, non-B hepatitis and is transmitted by the fecal–oral route. It is of major importance in developing countries as a cause of hepatitis due to waterborne epidemics, which mainly affect young adults, but rarely children. It causes a high mortality, sometimes as high as 40%, in pregnant women. The viral genome has been cloned and sequenced, and serological tests and PCR assays are available.

HEPATITIS G

This single stranded RNA virus of the flavivirus family usually results in an asymptomatic infection. It can cause chronic infection, but rarely hepatitis. It has been documented in adults and children especially those whose mothers are coinfected with HCV or HIV.[418] It can be diagnosed by detection of viral RNA by PCR.

HEPATITIS – THE ROLE OF OTHER VIRUSES

Despite the ubiquity and prevalence of infectious and serum hepatitis, other viral infections may involve the liver.

CMV is known to attack the liver in 85% of newborn infants suffering from cytomegalic inclusion disease; the same virus may also cause hepatitis when older children or adults contract the acquired form of the infection. *Infectious mononucleosis*, due to EBV, is frequently accompanied by some degree of liver involvement; most often this will reveal itself as a mild derangement of liver function tests though some cases will manifest obvious jaundice. Infection by *arboviruses* may cause a similar picture, though amongst these yellow fever produces a more specific and severe form of hepatitis.

HSV infections of the newborn are serious and usually fatal, one pathological feature being an extensive hepatic necrosis. Neonatal echovirus hepatitis is often fulminant.

Lastly, there are instances where transient liver involvement has been found in a variety of viral infections including some due to ECHO viruses types 4 and 9, Coxsackie viruses, adenoviruses and lymphocytic choriomeningitis virus. In most the involvement has been extremely mild with full recovery, though in some severe hepatitis may occur.

MISCELLANEOUS INFECTIONS

ORF (CONTAGIOUS PUSTULAR DERMATITIS OF SHEEP, CONTAGIOUS ECTHYMA OF SHEEP)

This is a common and widespread viral infection of sheep and to a lesser extent of goats. In general infection is from animal to animal but virus can persist in the soil of affected pastures for several months. Lambs are most commonly involved and they develop a papulovesicular eruption on the mouth, lips and non-hair-bearing areas of the skin. Transmission to man is relatively rare and the main incidence occurs in springtime. The infection is most commonly encountered in shepherds, farm and abattoir workers. However, children can be infected owing to their liking for handling young lambs.

Orf virus is included amongst the poxviruses and has certain similarities to the virus of molluscum contagiosum. It can be grown with difficulty on tissue culture but is usually identified by electron microscopy. Scrapings from the base of the bullae are to be preferred to vesicle fluid in these studies.

Clinical features

Lesions, which are usually but not exclusively single, most commonly appear on the hand or forearm. Initially there is an area of infiltration presenting as brawny edema but this soon develops into a flaccid bulla. However, on puncture a rather clear serosanguinous fluid is obtained. There is little or no constitutional upset but the progression of the lesion is slow and may take 6–8 weeks before it finally heals. No specific treatment is available or required in view of the benign nature of the condition but it is wise to protect the lesion with dressings to counteract the possibility of secondary infection.

MOLLUSCUM CONTAGIOSUM

This viral disease (see also Ch. 28) is seen in children more often than in adults. The responsible agent is a DNA virus belonging to the pox group but serologically unrelated to vaccinia or variola; it is readily identified by electron microscopy of the curettings from a lesion or on the histological appearances of a biopsy. Transmission is by close contact but infectivity is low.

Clinical features

Molluscum contagiosum is unassociated with any constitutional upset and presents as a chronic viral infection of the epidermis. Lesions, which may be multiple, take the form of pinkish white or flesh-colored, dome-shaped nodules between 2 and 8 mm in diameter and some show a central depression or umbilication. They may appear on the face, arms, legs, buttocks, scalp or genitalia but sparing of the palms of the hands and the soles of the feet is a characteristic feature. Occasionally the margins of the eyelids are involved and chronic follicular conjunctivitis can supervene (Fig. 26.39, Plate 26.39). HIV infection may be associated with disseminated molluscum.

Treatment

The disease is benign and self-limiting. Treatment is advised only to prevent spread by auto-inoculation or to others. Treatment is simple and consists of the removal of the lesions with a sharp curette. Other methods include electro- or cryocautery. The lesions will usually heal without scarring and recurrence is rare.

TRANSFUSION TRANSMITTED (TT) VIRUS

TT virus is a DNA virus that was first identified in 1997 in the serum of a patient with post-transfusion hepatitis of unknown etiology.[419] To date, there has been no disease association with this virus. It can be detected in the serum of 2% of healthy blood donors in the UK, and can be transmitted by transfusion, by fecal–oral spread and vertically.[420]

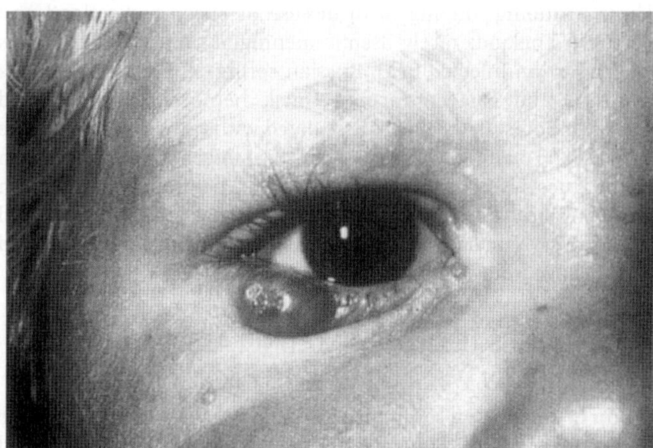

Fig. 26.39 Molluscum contagiosum.

LASSA FEVER

Lassa fever was first reported from Lassa in Nigeria in 1969. The Lassa virus shows some morphological and antigenic similarities to lymphocytic choriomeningitis virus. It is one of the arenaviruses and it is widely distributed throughout West Africa. It is one of five African viruses (yellow fever, Lassa, Ebola, Marburg and Congo-Crimean) that cause hemorrhagic fever (see p. 1440). The natural host is the rat *Mastomys natalensis*.

The virus is transmitted from person to person by close contact. It causes a diffuse serositis, hemorrhage and shock and is often fatal. Intravenous ribavirin reduces mortality from Lassa fever and is the treatment of choice. Additional treatment involves the use of plasma from a convalesced patient. For the adult 250–500 ml are used. Stocks of this are held in Nigeria, Sierra Leone, the London School of Hygiene and Tropical Medicine and the Communicable Disease Center, Atlanta, Georgia, USA. Strict isolation of patients is mandatory.

MARBURG VIRUS DISEASE (GREEN MONKEY DISEASE, VERVET MONKEY DISEASE, JO'BURG VIRUS DISEASE)

Marburg virus disease was first recognized in Germany in 1967 in personnel who had handled a consignment of African green monkeys (*Cercopithecus aethiops*) from Uganda. Outbreaks have occurred in Sudan and Zaire. The Marburg virus is long, rod shaped (rhabdovirus-like) and does not appear to possess antigenic affinity with other known viruses. Although the Marburg outbreak appeared to follow contact with African green monkeys no similar infections have been recognized as a result of other contacts with these monkeys and such monkeys suffer 100% mortality if experimentally infected. Thus the natural host or possible vectors are unknown.

The disease is highly infectious and carries a high mortality: 7 of the 31 Marburg cases died. Secondary cases appear to have a better prognosis than primary cases. There is as yet no protective vaccine. Strict isolation and barrier nursing of patients is necessary.

EBOLA VIRUS DISEASE

This disease is clinically indistinct from Marburg virus disease. The virus is morphologically identical to the Marburg virus, but antigenically distinct. The disease has been found in the Sudan and Zaire.

INFECTIONS DUE TO ARBOVIRUSES (TOGAVIRUSES)

The principal feature linking the viruses of this group is the fact that all are arthropod borne (hence the name) and well over 200 such agents have been recognized. Most viruses in this group are natural parasites of animals or birds and multiply in their arthropod vectors, the latter being unharmed in the process. Infection in the human may take several forms; most commonly encephalitis of varying severity results, but other diseases produced include yellow fever, dengue and sandfly fever. Arboviruses may also result in mild influenza-like illness. Children are particularly susceptible to this group of diseases. The arboviruses are further subdivided into a number of families: bunyaviridae (sandfly fever virus, Hantaviruses), togaviridae (western equine encephalitis virus, eastern equine encephalitis virus), flaviviridae (yellow fever virus, dengue viruses, West Nile virus), reoviridae and rhabdoviridae. They may also be classified according to the clinical syndromes they produce.

ARBOVIRUSES GROUP A

Some 20 arboviruses are included in this group of which the best known are the viruses of eastern and western equine encephalitis, and more recently West Nile virus;[421] these present in humans as aseptic meningitis or meningoencephalitis of varying severity. Children tend to be more seriously affected and death may result. Those who survive the illness may have permanent mental retardation, deafness, epilepsy and paralysis. Mortality may vary with age and the responsible virus; on average 5% of patients may die but this can be considerably higher following infection by certain agents of the group, reaching 74% in eastern equine encephalitis.

Other viruses of this group produce a mild dengue-like illness and most have their animal reservoir in wild or domestic birds. Their arthropod vectors are culicine and anophiline mosquitoes.

ARBOVIRUSES GROUP B

This, a larger group, can be divided into (1) *mosquito-borne* and (2) *tick-borne* sections. The best-known disease associated with the former is yellow fever; the latter are mainly associated with a variety of encephalitic illness.

Yellow fever (yellow jack)

Mosquito-borne, this disease has been a recognized clinical entity for over 300 years and in 1881 Carlos Finlay suggested that *Aedes aegypti* spread the infection. This theory was substantiated by the classical studies of Walter Reed and his colleagues working in Cuba.[422] Yellow fever occurs in parts of Africa, South America and central America but not Asia. The last cases of infection acquired in the UK occurred in the latter part of the nineteenth century, when ships arrived carrying infected *A. aegypti*.

Disease may vary from a mild fever to a fulminant hepatitis with jaundice, hepatic necrosis, hemorrhage and shock. In the jungle it is predominantly an adult disease. Where infection occurs in an urban community all ages and both sexes are equally affected.

There is no specific treatment.

Elimination of the responsible vector is of prime importance and infection has been eradicated from certain areas where this has been diligently performed. Vaccination with the 17 D attenuated strain of virus is compulsory for travel to endemic areas and immunity will usually last for up to 6 years. Complications of immunization are confined to an occasional case of benign encephalitis, usually encountered in young infants, and the vaccine is not recommended under 9 months of age if exposure to mosquitoes can be avoided.

Dengue fever (breakbone fever)

Mosquito-borne like yellow fever, this disease is caused by a virus from group B and the same vector, *A. aegypti*, is involved. The disease is widespread and is mainly found in warm areas, amongst which are Australia, Greece, Japan, India, Malaysia and Hawaii. So far, four antigenic varieties, known as types 1, 2, 3 and 4 have been described.

Clinical features

There is an incubation period of 5–9 days. The illness starts with high fever, malaise, headache, pain in the eyes, backache and excruciatingly painful limbs. Between the third and fifth days a maculopapular, scarlatiniform, or petechial rash appears and lasts up to 4 days; following this there is a rapid recovery. Occasionally, however, particularly in children the disease progresses to a severe hemorrhagic form, dengue hemorrhagic shock syndrome (DHSS), which may be fatal (see Hemorrhagic fevers below). It is thought that DHSS follows prior sensitization with a different strain of dengue virus, and is an example of antibody-mediated enhancement of disease.

Control

Eradication of the vector is desirable. Dengue viruses are poor antigens and this has frustrated efforts to produce effective vaccines.

HEMORRHAGIC FEVERS

A number of virus infections may occur in a hemorrhagic form, e.g. Lassa fever, yellow fever and measles. The arboviruses, particularly the Chikungunya (group A) and dengue (group B) viruses, are also prone to cause hemorrhagic disease. Hemorrhagic fever due to the mosquito-borne Chikungunya virus has been reported in Africa, India and Thailand. In south-east Asia hemorrhagic fever due to dengue virus is transmitted by the bite of the *A. aegypti* mosquito which is common in urban areas.

The hemorrhagic fevers affect mainly children in these countries, and patients develop fever, erythematous or petechial rashes, hepatosplenomegaly and bleeding which may be mild or severe. The majority of the patients recover but a certain number develop shock and die. Thrombocytopenia is common. In fatal cases there are gross effusions into the serous cavities, petechial hemorrhages on the surface of organs and bronchopneumonia. Treatment is symptomatic, and in shocked cases intravenous plasma together with the usual measures for collapsed patients should be administered.

Hemorrhagic fever with renal syndrome

This name is used for several similar conditions including Korean hemorrhagic fever and nephropathica epidemica occurring in Scandinavia, central Europe, Russia, China, Japan and Korea.[423] At least two viruses, Hantaan (Hantavirus) and Puumala, transmitted by arboviruses from rodents, are implicated. The clinical manifestations are of fever, shock, massive proteinuria followed by acute renal failure, and thrombocytopenia and bleeding with bruising, hematuria, hematemesis and melena. With supportive treatment the mortality is low.

TICK-BORNE ARBOVIRUS INFECTIONS

These including louping ill (a disease of sheep in Scotland and northern England; rarely aseptic meningitis can occur if man is infected by an infected tick), Russian spring–summer encephalitis (western and eastern forms), Omsk hemorrhagic fever and Kyasanur Forest fever. Illness associated with this group may range from aseptic meningitis to severe and even fatal encephalitis though the prognosis is better than with infection by group A strains. On occasion paralytic disease simulating poliomyelitis can occur and Omsk fever is usually characterized by bronchopneumonia and hemorrhage from various orifices.

ARBOVIRUSES GROUP C AND UNCLASSIFIED ARBOVIRUSES

Group C, comprising seven viruses, is responsible for influenza-like illness in parts of South America. Amongst the unclassified infections, sandfly fever is perhaps the best documented illness.

Sandfly fever (phlebotomus fever, papataci fever)

This illness results from infection by one of the unclassified arboviruses. It is relatively common in countries bordering the Mediterranean and occurs in parts of Africa, Russia, India and China. The responsible vector *Phlebotomus papatasii*, often called sandfly, is extremely small and may pass through mosquito nets. Infection in these sandflies may be a permanent feature owing to transovarian infection and no definite animal reservoir is known. Several different strains of virus have been isolated with established immunological variation.

Clinical features

The incubation period is 3–7 days. Onset is sudden and rigors may occur. Headache, pain behind the eyes, muscular aching and fever are typical features. Occasionally photophobia, neck and back stiffness occur and mimic meningitis. After 3 or 4 days there is an abrupt termination by crisis. Severe apprehension often accompanies this illness and acute depression may follow an attack for a short time; leukopenia is a common accompaniment. A clinical diagnosis is readily made in endemic areas or during an outbreak.

There is no specific treatment and the prognosis is good. Control is confined to attempts at eradication of the vector in its breeding grounds.

RICKETTSIAL INFECTIONS

Rickettsial infection in man produces a number of different diseases, spread over a wide geographical area. The resultant illnesses have certain basic similarities and all but one are characterized by some form of skin eruption. Definitive clinical diagnosis can be difficult and confirmatory laboratory tests are desirable. A simple classification of rickettsial infection is shown in Table 26.32.

Rickettsiae have biophysical properties that place them in an intermediate position between viruses and bacteria and are small coccobacilli, usually less than half a micrometer in diameter, with rigid cell walls. They contain both RNA and DNA but are obligate intracellular parasites and are sensitive to certain antibiotics.

LABORATORY TESTS

Procedures to isolate the causative organisms exist but should only be undertaken by a laboratory well equipped to deal with the risks involved. In view of the hazards involved in isolation, serological methods of diagnosis are usually employed.

The Weil–Felix agglutination reaction has been used for several years; this depends on the fact that patients with certain rickettsial infections develop agglutinins in their serum during the illness which agglutinate some strains of Proteus organisms, namely OX 19, OX 2 and OXK. There are now a number of other serological assays available in reference laboratories that specialize in the diagnosis of rickettsial infection. If possible, paired sera should be examined in the Weil–Felix test but agglutinins may appear as early as the fifth or sixth day after the onset of the fever and usually reach a peak during the second or third week. Detection of rickettsial DNA in the blood or tissue by PCR may allow the diagnosis to be made earlier in the illness.

TYPHUS FEVER (EPIDEMIC LOUSE-BORNE TYPHUS FEVER)

Historical writings suggest that typhus fever (classical or historic typhus) has been a scourge of humanity for many centuries. Typhus fever and war are inextricably linked. Although the responsible agent may be endemic in many parts of Europe, serious epidemics only arise during times of war or in their aftermath, due entirely to the increased infestation by lice that occurs in these periods. Epidemics occur chiefly in winter when people are crowded together for warmth and shelter, enhancing chances of spread of the louse. Following the 1914–1918 war it was estimated that 30 million cases of typhus occurred in Russia alone and some 10% of these probably died. In the 1970s large epidemics occurred in central Africa (Ruanda-Burundi).

The responsible organism is *Rickettsia prowazekii* and transmission is by the body louse *Pediculus corporis* or the head louse *Pediculus capitis*. The lice become infected by biting a human who is carrying the specific rickettsiae in the blood. Subsequent spread of the infection results from the infected feces of the lice rather than by an actual bite, and the irritation set up on the human body by the infestation results in the organisms being scratched into the skin. Infection may also result from the inhalation of louse feces in dust. At times fleas may act as a vector and also convey the infection through their feces.

Clinical features

The incubation period lies between 6 and 15 days. There are three main clinical phases – prodromal, invasive and eruptive.

Table 26.32 Rickettsial diseases: causal agents, vectors, reservoirs and differential Weil–Felix reactions

	Disease	Causal rickettsiae	Principal vectors	Animal reservoir	Geographic occurrence
Typhus	Epidemic (louse-borne typhus)	*R. prowazekii*	Lice	Man	Worldwide
	Brill–Zinsser disease	*R. prowazekii*	–	Man	Worldwide
	Endemic murine (flea-borne) typhus	*R. mooseri*	Fleas	Rats	Worldwide
	Scrub typhus (mite-borne) (Tsutsugamushi fever)	*R. tsutsugamushi*	Mites	Small rodents	Japan, South-east Asia, Pacific
Spotted fevers	Rocky Mountain spotted fever	*R. rickettsii*	Ticks	Small rodents	East and west USA
	Mediterranean fever (fièvre boutonneuse)	*R. conorii*	Ticks	Small rodents and dogs	Mediterranean, Caspian and Black Sea, Africa, South-east Asia
Rickettsialpox		*R. akari*	Mites	House mice	USA, Russia, Korea
Q fever	Query fever	*R. burnetii*	Occasionally ticks	Cattle Sheep Goats Bandicoots	Worldwide

Prodromal symptoms, which are not always present, include mild headache, lassitude, weakness and pyrexia. The invasive stage is characterized by a sharp rise in temperature, severe headache and generalized aching. Rigors may occur and the fever may reach 40.0–41.0°C. The pulse is rapid, the blood pressure reduced and a variable degree of prostration develops. A wide variety of additional symptoms and signs may be encountered including suffusion of the conjunctivae, facial flushing, photophobia, deafness, tinnitus, vertigo and cough.

The characteristic rash arises about the fifth day of illness and the initial lesions, comprising pinkish red macules, appear on the trunk and soon spread to the limbs. Most cases show sparing of the face, palms and soles. In mild cases the rash may develop no further but in the more severely ill the eruption becomes hemorrhagic or even purpuric. During this eruptive phase the mental state becomes dulled; stupor, delirium and coma may follow. Hypotension also becomes more intense and oliguria with azotemia is common. Severe cases will die between the 9th and 18th day of illness; those who recover slowly improve after 2 weeks, the mental recovery being more rapid than the physical. Typhus is usually accompanied by a leukopenia and normochromic anemia.

Complications

Bronchopneumonia, otitis media, skin sepsis, arterial thrombosis and gangrene are all encountered. Less often there may be areas of skin necrosis and secondary infection of the salivary glands. Prolonged hypotension has a grave prognosis.

Differential diagnosis

Typhus may be readily considered and diagnosed at epidemic times but sporadic cases can cause considerable confusion. Amongst diseases that may require differentiation are other rickettsial infections, typhoid fever, measles, malaria and meningococcal septicemia.

Treatment

In children 75–100 mg/kg/day of chloramphenicol or 50 mg/kg/day of tetracycline is used and treatment should continue until the temperature has settled for 48 h. Antibiotics should be reinstituted if there is clinical relapse.

Careful nursing and general supportive measures are required. A high protein diet is desirable and transfusion of blood or plasma may be needed. Electrolyte imbalance can readily occur and requires appropriate correction. Oxygen may be given for pulmonary complications and digoxin for cardiac failure.

Prognosis

The disease is rarely fatal in children, but about 10% of young adults and 60–70% of people over 50 may die.

Control

Killed vaccines prevent mortality though not necessarily infection. Scrupulous hygiene is desirable and insecticides should be used to eliminate lice: DDT, lindane and malathion have proved effective.

BRILL–ZINSSER DISEASE (RECRUDESCENT TYPHUS)

This condition represents a recrudescence of epidemic louse-borne typhus that occurs years after the primary attack. It is usually mild and the illness is drastically modified; skin rashes are usually absent and the prognosis is good. In view of its atypical clinical nature and the fact that a case may arise when no other typhus infection is occurring, diagnosis is difficult. Less marked reaction in the laboratory tests can also be misleading. However, if a diagnosis is made, treatment is along the lines employed for epidemic typhus. The real danger of Brill–Zinsser disease is to the community. If epidemiological factors are favorable, especially if the environment is heavily louse infested, an epidemic could arise from such a case.

MURINE TYPHUS (ENDEMIC FLEA-BORNE TYPHUS FEVER)

This disease is clinically similar to classical epidemic typhus but is milder and has a much lower fatality rate (2%); the management and treatment are also similar. The responsible agent is named *Rickettsia mooseri* and it is usually spread to man from its animal host by the rat flea (*Xenopsylla cheopis*).

Widely distributed throughout the world, the disease appears to be on the decline probably owing to stricter control of rats. It is commoner in summer when rats are more numerous and has a higher infection rate amongst persons in the food trade where rats may abound. Unlike lice which die from *R. prowazekii*, the rat flea is not killed by the multiplication of *Rickettsia mooseri* in its tissue. Control depends on flea eradication and extermination of rats.

SCRUB TYPHUS (TSUTSUGAMUSHI FEVER)

This disease, known by many different names according to the locality where it occurs, is transmitted to man by the bite of the larvae of different species of chigger-like mites; best known of these are *Trombicula akamushi* and *Trombicula deliniensis*. The responsible agent is known as *Rickettsia tsutsugamushi* and the cycle of infection involves chiggermite and various wild rodents. Clinical features are again like those of other rickettsial infections though fairly mild. A diagnostic finding in some is a small necrotic ulcer or eschar where the responsible mite has attached itself to the skin and introduced the infection. The disease occurs in the south-west Pacific and south-east Asia between Japan, the Solomon Islands and Pakistan.

Treatment is with chloramphenicol or tetracycline and the mortality is under 5%. Elimination of the disease is difficult and mite-infested areas are best avoided. Alternatively protective clothing, treated with a mite repellent, should be used. Vaccines have not proved effective in this condition.

ROCKY MOUNTAIN SPOTTED FEVER

This disease results from infection by *Rickettsia rickettsii* which is transmitted to man through a variety of ticks which are both the vector and the common reservoir for the responsible agent. Some rodents, dogs and sheep also act as additional but less prolific reservoirs. The clinical course has many similarities to classical typhus but the incubation period is often shorter (2–5 days in severe cases). Furthermore, the rash is usually more pronounced and frankly petechial. It can also be more widespread and may take some time to subside.

Complications, differential diagnosis and laboratory findings are also similar to epidemic typhus as is the treatment and management. Reported mortality rates have varied between 3 and 90% with an average, for all ages, of 20%. Despite its name this disease is now much more common in the eastern than the western USA. In the western USA adult males are most frequently attacked whereas in the east children are most commonly affected.

Control is difficult owing to the disseminated nature of the vector in the wild and where possible it is best to avoid tick-infested areas or to ensure that adequate protective clothing is worn.

TICK TYPHUS FEVERS (FIÈVRE BOUTONNEUSE)

There are three tick-borne spotted fevers caused by rickettsiae, which share the same group-specific antigen as *Rickettsia rickettsii*, the cause of Rocky Mountain spotted fever, but have distinct type-specific antigens.

Rickettsia conorii causes fièvre boutonneuse which is also called Mediterranean fever along the Mediterranean, Black and Caspian sea littorals; called Kenyan tick typhus and South African tickbite fever; and called Indian tick typhus in south-east Asia. *Rickettsia australis* causes Queensland tick typhus in eastern Australia. *Rickettsia sibirica* causes Siberian tick typhus which occurs throughout central Asia.

The main animal reservoir is dogs. These tick typhus fevers are clinically similar. A small, indurated lesion, the tache noire, develops at the site of the tick bite, and central necrosis gives way to eschar formation. There is regional lymphadenopathy. The tick typhus fevers are much milder than Rocky Mountain spotted fever, with a mortality under 1%. Antibiotic treatment is as for the latter disease.

RICKETTSIALPOX

Due to *Rickettsia akari*, this disease is usually transmitted to man by a mite and the house mouse is the main animal reservoir. Epidemics tend to occur where mice and mites are found together primarily in urban populations worldwide.

The illness is comparatively mild. The incubation period is 10–21 days. Fever is usual and a mild rash develops, most closely resembling adult chickenpox. Death is extremely rare. Tetracycline is the drug of choice.

Q FEVER (QUERY FEVER)

Q fever, caused by *Coxiella burnetii*, has clinical features quite unlike those of other rickettsial infections. The features are often those of respiratory or influenza-like illness with no rash (see p. 1425). Endocarditis can occur and children may present with fever of unknown origin.

PROTOZOAL INFECTIONS: MALARIA

Malaria is a disease of humans caused by infection with one or more of four species of protozoa of the genus *Plasmodium (Plasmodium falciparum, Plasmodium vivax, Plasmodium malariae* and *Plasmodium ovale)*. It is usually acquired through the bite of an infected female *Anopheles* mosquito, although it may also follow the transfer of infected blood as in blood transfusion, or transplacentally or by the use of contaminated syringes. Worldwide some 45 *Anopheles* species effectively transmit malaria, although the identity, behavior and importance of local vectors varies widely with geographic location. The most effective vector is probably *Anopheles gambiae* – a mosquito that is widely distributed in tropical Africa. *P. falciparum* is the most pathogenic of the malaria parasites and infections with it must always be regarded as serious and potentially life threatening. The other three species tend to cause less serious illness, although on occasion a lethal nephrosis may complicate *P. malariae* infections.

THE PARASITE LIFE CYCLE

Malaria parasites undergo a complex stage of asexual development in the human host and a stage of sexual development (sporogony) which occurs partly in man and partly in the mosquito vector.[424]

ASEXUAL DEVELOPMENT IN MAN

This begins with the introduction of infective forms (sporozoites) in mosquito saliva during the biting act. Sporozoites circulate for less than 60 min, eventually gaining access to parenchymal liver cells either directly or after passage through Kupffer cells. The invasion process may entail specific ligand/receptor interaction. Once within the hepatocyte, the sporozoite initiates the exoerythrocytic (EE) phase of asexual development during which it grows and undergoes repeated nuclear fission (schizogony) – eventually producing a cyst-like schizont filled with daughter parasites (merozoites). This phase usually proceeds without interruption and both the time taken to schizont maturity and the number of merozoites produced varies with the identity of the plasmodial species involved. *P. falciparum* completes its EE development fastest (about 5 days) and produces most merozoites per schizont (about 30 000). The other species are slower and less prolific, the respective values for *P. malariae*, for example, being about 15 days and about 15 000 merozoites. In two parasite species, *P. vivax* and *P. ovale*, some sporozoites initiate this uninterrupted EE stage of development but some do not. These latter, on entering hepatocytes produce small unicellular forms (hypnozoites) which persist without development for periods varying from several weeks to many months. Eventually the hypnozoites, activated by mechanisms as yet not known, resume growth and proceed to schizont maturation and merozoite liberation. Hypnozoites are currently widely believed to give rise to the relapsing parasitemias which characterize *P. ovale* and, particularly, *P. vivax* infections and which can occur even after drug treatment has effectively eliminated erythrocytic parasites. Hypnozoites do not develop in infections with *P. falciparum* and *P. malariae* and in these species recrudescence of parasitemia is generally considered to be due to persistent erythrocytic infection.

Merozoites liberated from EE schizonts are short lived and must find and enter a red blood cell within a few minutes. Within the erythrocyte each grows rapidly through ring form and uninucleate trophozoite stages eventually to form a schizont containing merozoites. On schizont rupture, the merozoites enter the bloodstream, attach to and penetrate fresh erythrocytes and again begin the cycle of erythrocytic asexual development. Attachment and penetration by merozoites are complex operations, which require specific ligand/receptor interactions. Erythrocyte invasion by *P. vivax* appears to require a ligand that is associated with Duffy blood group antigens, while attachment of *P. falciparum* merozoites to red cells requires one associated with sialic acid on the erythrocyte membrane. Age of the red cell also influences invasion by merozoites; *P. vivax* preferentially invades reticulocytes – a feature which tends to limit the density of parasitemia attained by this species – while *P. falciparum* can invade red cells of all ages.

The duration of the erythrocytic phase of asexual development and the merozoite yield per schizont vary with the plasmodial species. *P. malariae* has the longest cycle (72 h, i.e. quartan periodicity); the remaining species have cycles of about 48 h duration (i.e. tertian periodicity). *P. falciparum* has the greatest capacity to replicate and the merozoite yield of its schizonts is in the range 8–32. For the others the yields are 8–24 for *P. vivax*, 4–16 for *P. ovale* and 8 for *P. malariae*. The ability of *P. falciparum* to replicate rapidly in both the hepatic and erythrocytic phases of development partly accounts for the severity of the illness this species causes.

The time taken for parasites to become detectable in the peripheral blood following sporozoite inoculation is termed the prepatent period, while the time from infection to the onset of symptoms is termed the incubation period. While the two periods may be of equal duration, more usually the incubation period is about 2 days longer.

Late in its asexual erythrocytic cycle *P. falciparum* withdraws from the peripheral circulation and sequesters in deep vasculature. The phenomenon, which probably contributes importantly to the serious pathological effects that this *Plasmodium* causes, is effected by the binding of receptors on the surface of red cells infected with nearly mature parasites to ligands exposed on the surface of the endothelial cells lining deep blood vessels. Sequestration does not occur in the course of infections with the other plasmodial species that infect man.

SEXUAL DEVELOPMENT

In the course of blood stage schizogony in the human host some merozoites differentiate, by mechanisms which are not yet understood, to give rise to male and female sexual forms (gametocytes). In the case of *P. vivax*, gametocytes are formed early after the release of merozoites from the liver (before clinical symptoms), while *P. falciparum* gametocytes are generated after a number of erythrocytic cycles. Early treatment of fever with antimalarial drugs may therefore prevent gametocyte formation in *P. falciparum* but not in *P. vivax* infections. When mature, gametocytes circulate in the blood but do not undergo further development unless they are ingested by an anopheline mosquito during feeding. Once in the midgut of the mosquito, the female (macrogametocyte) escapes from the enclosing erythrocytic membrane and becomes a macrogamete. The male (microgametocyte) undergoes a process of exflagellation during which eight slender, uninucleate filaments (microgametes) are extruded and break free. Each microgamete seeks a macrogamete and, if successful, penetrates and fertilizes it. The two nuclei fuse and a zygote is formed. This is probably the only point in the life history of the parasite that genetic recombination occurs. The diploid zygote then undergoes meiosis and, as an ookinete, migrates to penetrate the epithelium of the mosquito midgut wall where it comes to rest on the external surface. There it rounds up, becomes an oocyst and begins a series of nuclear divisions. Oocyst maturity is reached after a period which is dependent on the identity of the plasmodial species and the ambient temperature to which the mosquito is exposed. It may be 1–4 weeks, or longer. At maturity the oocyst is filled with as many as 10 000 daughter parasites (sporozoites), each some 10–15 microns in length and feebly motile. The sporozoites escape at oocyst rupture and travel in the hemocelomic fluid to the salivary glands where they accumulate in the acinal cells to be discharged with saliva when the mosquito next feeds.

Infected humans constitute the only known source of mosquito infection for *P. falciparum*, *P. vivax* and *P. ovale*. For *P. malariae* some apes and monkeys may constitute reservoirs of infection in addition to humans.

EPIDEMIOLOGY

Despite widespread operations promoted by the World Health Organization between 1955 and 1975 with the aim of achieving global eradication, malaria remains probably the most prevalent, important, communicable disease throughout much of the tropical and subtropical world, the greatest burden of disease being in sub-Saharan Africa. It is estimated that 200–450 million episodes of febrile malaria occur annually in African children under the age of 5 years,[425] and the much-quoted estimate of around 1 million malaria deaths annually in Africa, > 75% of them in children, is supported by available evidence.[426] Over the past 25 years *P. falciparum* parasites have become increasingly resistant to chloroquine and other currently available antimalarial drugs. This development has greatly complicated the treatment and management of acute falciparum infections and has jeopardized effective chemoprophylaxis by drugs that are inexpensive and of low toxicity. As a result, travelers to endemic areas are at higher risk of contracting infections than perhaps at any time since the end of the Second World War. The consequence of this is that malaria must be considered as a possible diagnosis in all instances of illness – especially febrile illness – presenting in residents of temperate climate countries who have recently visited endemic areas.

Many factors influence the epidemiology of malaria. Atmospheric temperature is important. For successful development in the mosquito vector, *P. vivax* requires a sustained temperature of at least 16°C, while *P. falciparum* requires one of 20°C. The geographical limits of *P. vivax* transmission are thus more widely set than those of *P. falciparum*. Other factors relate to the identity and biology of the *Plasmodium*, the identity and behavior of the vector, the social and economic customs of human populations and the topography and climate of the region. It follows, therefore, that the epidemiological pattern of the infection is not uniform but varies considerably between and within countries.

Where transmission occurs the measurement of endemicity has, in the past, relied on establishment of spleen rates and parasite rates in children aged 2–9 years. Thus categories classified as hypo-, meso-, hyper- and holoendemic were characterized by both spleen and parasite rates of < 10%, 11–50%, constantly > 50% and constantly > 75% respectively. In hyperendemic areas spleens in adults were frequently enlarged; in holoendemic areas they were not (this observation was attributed to the greater acquisition of immunity in holoendemic areas).

However, the widespread use of antimalarial drugs in areas where malaria is endemic has adversely affected these classical indices of endemicity and they are less useful today than formerly. This change has prompted the use of seroepidemiological techniques in the identification of malaria transmission and the measurement of its intensity. These techniques detect and quantify specific malaria antibody in serum and establish age-specific profiles for prevalence and titer. Briefly, profiles which show little change with age denote low transmission while profiles showing values which rise rapidly with age denote high transmission.[427]

Epidemiologically malaria presents in two extremes, one of which is stable and shows little change from one year to another and the other which is unstable and may fluctuate violently in intensity at regular or irregular intervals. Stable malaria is most in evidence in areas where transmission rates are high; it is characterized by rates of mortality and morbidity which are high in infants and young children and which fall to low, even negligible, levels as age advances and effective immunity is acquired. Unstable malaria occurs where transmission rates remain low for periods of several years then suddenly increase greatly for climatic or other reasons; it is characterized by the occurrence of epidemics in which morbidity and mortality are conspicuous at all ages. Acquired immunity is not a feature of unstable malaria, save possibly at the end of a protracted epidemic period. Between the extremes of stability and instability, a range of intermediate epidemiological presentation occurs.

IMMUNITY

Malarial immunity may be innate, i.e. genetically determined, or acquired. Innate immunity may be due to a lack of ligands on the erythrocyte surface which bind to specific receptors on the merozoite surface at an essential stage in the invasion process, or to the presence of abnormal intramembranous erythrocytic components, which inhibit, but do not totally prevent, growth of the parasite within the red cell. An example of the former is the freedom from *P. vivax* infection that is apparent in people whose erythrocytes lack Duffy blood group antigens, while an example of the latter is the partial protection and survival advantage towards *P. falciparum* infections that heterozygosity for the sickle cell gene confers.[428]

Acquired immunity may be passive or active. Passive immunity due to the transplacental transfer of specific IgG malarial antibodies from mother to fetus probably accounts, at least in part, for the relative resistance to malaria that infants born in highly endemic areas show over the first few months of life. Acquired active immunity develops slowly in response to infection with malaria.[429] The first evidence is an ability to restrict the clinical effects of infection despite the persistence of high density parasitemia. This 'clinical' immunity is usually discernible in young children in highly endemic areas around the third to fourth year of life. Later, an ability to restrict parasite density develops and slowly strengthens throughout later childhood and adolescence to reach maximum expression in adult life. When fully developed, malarial immunity is species, strain and stage specific.

Acquired active immunity entails the collaboration of different cell populations, notably T cells, B cells and macrophages, during which specific and non-specific humoral factors are elaborated, which restrict parasite growth and replication.[430] Knowledge as to how this complex response is assembled and controlled remains incomplete. T cells play a central role and their recognition of, and response to, defined malarial antigens are probably controlled by immune response (Ir) genes. Sensitized T cells respond to antigen by replication and the secretion of lymphokines which promote further T cell replication and diversification, induce replication of B cells with antibody production and activate macrophages.

Specific malarial antibodies belong to the immunoglobulin classes G, M and A. They function by agglutinating parasites and parasitized cells, inhibiting interactions between host cell surface ligands and parasite receptors, mediating cellular cytotoxicity and phagocytosis and inhibiting sequestration of mature asexual erythrocytic forms of *P. falciparum* in deep vasculature. Antibodies do not kill parasites directly through the activation of complement. Natural malaria infection induces synthesis of a wide range of antibodies directed against specific parasite antigens. Thus antibodies with specificity for the antigens of sporozoites, EE forms, asexual blood stages and sexual stages can be detected and titrated in the sera of residents of endemic areas.

The killing of parasites, which is probably carried out mainly by activated macrophages and cytotoxic T cells, involves release from the host cells of toxic oxygen derivatives and occurs principally in spleen and liver. However, other killing mechanisms exist. Gamma-interferon released by sensitized T cells has been observed to kill EE stages in hepatic cells, while tumor necrosis factor (TNF) liberated from macrophages stimulated with endotoxin has been reported to inhibit replication of both EE and erythrocytic stages of the parasite.

PATHOLOGY

The pathogenic sequences which develop in malaria are attributable to events which arise during the asexual erythrocytic stage of development of the parasite in man.

Anemia is common and is due partly to the rhythmic invasion and destruction of erythrocytes by parasites and partly to additional mechanisms, such as dyserythropoiesis and immune hemolysis following sensitization of non-parasitized red cells.[431] Bone marrow changes in dyserythropoiesis include erythroblast multinuclearity, karyorrhexis, incomplete and unequal nuclear division and cytoplasmic bridging. The marrow may contain large amounts of stainable iron and show evidence of phagocytosis of defective red cell precursors by macrophages. Whether these changes are initiated by toxic substances liberated by the parasite, or represent the non-specific effects of macrophages rendered hyperactive by parasite antigens remains to be ascertained. The sensitization of uninfected red cells occurs commonly in malaria, often involves C3 and/or IgG and can be detected by the direct antiglobulin test (DAT) using specific antisera. DAT positivity of red cells, which is frequent in patients with falciparum malaria, has been found to be associated with enhanced blood destruction, but the association appears to be relatively uncommon.[431]

A characteristic feature of *P. falciparum* infections is the collection ('sequestration') of large numbers of late-stage parasites in the venules and capillaries of a variety of organs.[432] This results from the ability of this parasite, in the later stages of its development in the red cell, to display a number of proteins – known as *P. falciparum* erythrocyte membrane protein-1 (PfEMP-1) – on the red cell surface, by which the parasitized red cell attaches to host receptors on the microvascular endothelium.[433] PfEMP-1 is a family of proteins encoded by recently identified highly variable var genes.[434] It is possible that sequestration is augmented by adhesion between parasitized erythrocytes, a phenomenon that can be demonstrated in vitro.[435] Sequestration is believed to be the mechanism underlying some of the clinical complications of *P. falciparum* infection, including the coma and convulsions of cerebral malaria. It is not known how sequestration may lead to tissue dysfunction: one possibility is that the huge number of actively metabolizing parasites consume oxygen and glucose at the expense of neighboring tissue, or produce toxic metabolites, including lactate, that may affect cellular function. Another possibility is that sequestration stimulates the release of host transmitters, such as nitric oxide, that may have a local effect on blood flow or on the conduction of nerve impulses. Host cytokines, too, are released and these may make endothelial cells more adhesive for the surface of parasitized red cells, thus augmenting sequestration.[436]

Enlargement of the spleen and liver is common in acute and chronic infections and, on section, both organs are dark from the accumulation of malarial pigment (hemozoin). Evidence of phagocytosis of parasites, parasitized cells and hemozoin is usually present in the splenic pulp and in the sinusoidal macrophages and Kupffer cells of the liver.

In *P. falciparum* infections an acute diffuse glomerulonephritis may occur in which deposits of immunoglobulins, complement and malarial antigens are detectable in the mesangium and capillary loops. The condition is usually transient and resolves with appropriate antimalarial treatment. In *P. malariae* infections, however, a much more progressive and frequently lethal nephropathy may develop, again with evidence of antigen/antibody deposition. In children these lesions may progress despite antimalarial treatment to total glomerular sclerosis with secondary tubular atrophy. Clinically, the manifestations of a nephrotic syndrome develop with severe generalized edema and ascites accompanied by heavy proteinuria and hypoalbuminemia.

During pregnancy, *P. falciparum* may attain very high densities in the maternal placental blood and cause damage to the syncytiotrophoblast. Placental infection is associated with reduced infant birth weight and, in endemic areas, the association is most marked in first pregnancies. Occasionally, parasites cross the placenta, giving rise to congenital infection in the infant at or soon after birth. In endemic areas such infections seldom persist or cause disease in the neonate, but if the mother is a 'non-immune' individual, the baby may develop an illness with fever, anemia and jaundice.

Thrombocytopenia commonly occurs in *P. falciparum* infections for reasons that remain poorly understood. It usually occurs independently of changes in other measures of coagulation (prothrombin time, partial thromboplastin time) or to plasma fibrinogen concentrations and is usually unaccompanied by bleeding. Spontaneous bleeding may occur associated with disseminated intravascular coagulation (DIC), but this is an uncommon clinical feature of severe malaria in adults, and is rare in children.

PROPHYLAXIS

In recent years the development and spread of drug-resistant *P. falciparum* parasites together with increasing evidence that some antimalarial drugs are associated, albeit rarely, with serious side-effects have gravely compromised chemoprophylaxis. While *P. ovale* and *P. malariae* have shown no changes in drug susceptibility, *P. falciparum* parasites resistant to chloroquine and sometimes to a range of other drugs as well have developed and are now present in many endemic countries. In south-east Asia resistance of *P. vivax* to chloroquine has also been reported. The overall effectiveness of chemoprophylaxis, therefore, can no longer be guaranteed. When Fansidar (pyrimethamine–sulfadoxine) has been used as a weekly prophylactic drug, episodes of Stevens–Johnson syndrome and toxic epidermal necrolysis have occasionally occurred, some with fatal outcome. Maloprim (pyrimethamine–dapsone) has been associated with agranulocytosis and amodiaquine with neutropenia and hepatocellular dysfunction.[437]

These events have emphasized the need to limit contact between humans and mosquitoes as much as possible and advice to parents to this effect should be given. Protective measures include the wearing of clothing which effectively covers the arms and legs and the careful application of insect repellents [dimethylphthalate (DMP) or dimethyl-m-toluamide (DEET)] to exposed skin areas over periods of mosquito activity, the screening of houses, the use of knock-down insecticides in bedrooms before retiring, and sleeping under mosquito nets impregnated with permethrin.

When contemplating the need for chemoprophylaxis in particular instances, the physician should ascertain the risk to which the child is or will be exposed, the duration of exposure, the presence or absence of drug-resistant malaria in the area of residence and possible drug toxicity. Useful information on disease incidence and drug resistance in the malarious countries of the world is to be found in the periodic reviews published by the World Health Organization in its Weekly Epidemiological Record.

Children are highly susceptible to malaria, particularly *P. falciparum* infections, and the need for chemoprophylaxis must be seriously considered when they visit malarious areas. When the visit is short term, e.g. 1–2 months, and the risk of infection very low, chemoprophylaxis may be deemed unnecessary. In this event, however, the parents should be advised that the risk of infection does exist and that any illness, febrile or not, which occurs abroad, should be properly investigated to exclude malaria as a diagnosis. Any illness developing within 6 months of return from abroad should be reported to a physician as should details of the visit made.

Table 26.33 Age-related dosage of antimalarial drugs for chemoprophylaxis in children

Age	Fraction of adult dose
< 6 weeks	1/8
6 weeks–1 year	1/4
1–5 years	1/2
5–12 years	3/4
> 12 years	Adult dose

For children visiting or residing in areas where the risk of infection is other than very low, chemoprophylaxis should be prescribed.

Suggested chemoprophylactic regimens[438,439] are as follows:

1. Where only *P. vivax* malaria exists, prophylaxis should be by chloroquine proportional to an adult dose of 300 mg (two tablets) once weekly or by proguanil (Paludrine) proportional to an adult dose of 200 mg (two tablets) daily (see Table 26.33).
2. Where *P. falciparum* exists and is sensitive to chloroquine, chemoprophylaxis is as in 1 above.
3. Where chloroquine-resistant *P. falciparum* exists, chemoprophylaxis should be by mefloquine proportional to an adult dose of 250 mg taken once weekly; this is not advised for young children, for whom chloroquine plus proguanil should be used (doses as in 1 above).
4. Where chloroquine-resistant *P. falciparum* exists but where regimen 3 above is apparently ineffective, as is sometimes the case in south-east Asia, the choice of a prophylactic antimalarial can be a difficult problem. Local advice should be sought. For visits confined to cities, it may be best to take no drug prophylaxis. For visits to high-risk areas, options include Maloprim proportionate to an adult dose of one tablet (pyrimethamine 12.5 mg; dapsone 100 mg) once weekly plus chloroquine proportionate to an adult dose of 300 mg once weekly. (Maloprim should not be given to infants less than 6 weeks of age because of immaturity of several enzyme systems.) Doxycycline 100 mg daily, which is a useful prophylaxis for adults, is not suitable for children.

Chemoprophylaxis should be started 1 week before residence in an endemic area (to permit detection of early signs of idiosyncrasy or side-effects) and continued for 4 weeks after return. Parents should be advised to ensure that physicians attending illness in children after return from endemic areas are aware of the need to exclude a diagnosis of malaria. Similarly, parents who live in endemic areas and are visited from time to time by children being educated in non-endemic areas should ensure that guardians and school authorities are alerted to the need to exclude malaria as a diagnosis in any illness developing in the repatriated child.

CHEMOPROPHYLAXIS OF INDIGENOUS CHILDREN IN ENDEMIC AREAS

Large scale continuous prophylaxis is not recommended, the main reason being that it is economically and logistically almost impossible to achieve. Other theoretical but unproven disadvantages of mass chemoprophylaxis include interference with the development of acquired immunity, enhancement of the development and spread of drug resistance and risk of toxicity from long term drug usage. A modified form of partial chemoprophylaxis, more accurately termed intermittent therapy, has proved promising in one East African study, in which children given a therapeutic dose of sulfadoxine–pyrimethamine at 2, 3 and 9 months of age, irrespective of fever or parasitemia, had fewer episodes of malaria and of severe anemia than controls.[440] Continuous chemoprophylaxis is indicated in children who are homozygous for the sickle cell gene, because malaria may precipitate a crisis. There is no evidence yet (2001) that chemoprophylaxis against malaria improves life expectancy in children with HIV infection or AIDS.

VACCINATION

While much interest attaches to the development of malaria vaccines, a safe and effective one is not yet available. Several candidate vaccines, making use of antigens from various combinations of sporozoite, erythrocytic and sexual stages of *P. falciparum*, are undergoing development or clinical trials.

CLINICAL FEATURES

The manifestations of malaria in an individual are determined by the infecting species of *Plasmodium* and the resistance or immunity of the host.

Each of the four species of parasite causing human malaria may produce a febrile illness with non-specific symptoms including anorexia, malaise, headache, chills, rigors, sweating, irritability and failure to eat and drink. Symptoms begin about 10 days after the infective mosquito bite, but longer incubation periods are common, especially with the non-falciparum malarias, and sometimes the first symptoms are not experienced until months or years after exposure. Vomiting and cough are both common, but not severe, early symptoms; diarrhea is unusual. Febrile convulsions commonly complicate sudden rises of temperature in young children. The pattern of fever is irregular at first; the classical periodicity appears only if the illness is protracted and untreated, when *P. malariae* may cause quartan fever (72 h between spikes), *P. vivax* and *P. ovale* tertian fever (48 h intervals) and *P. falciparum* subtertian fever (less than 48 h intervals). The liver and spleen may become palpable during the first few days of fever; the spleen may become enlarged during the course of a single episode, and may become very large after repeated or untreated infections.

Anemia develops, its degree being greatest in those with the heaviest or most protracted infections. Minor abnormalities of hepatic enzymes may be found, but jaundice is unusual even in severe falciparum malaria.

The most important distinction between species in their clinical effects is in the capacity of *P. falciparum* to cause, in susceptible individuals, a rapidly progressive severe ('complicated') disease, which may be fatal. Most of the many deaths from malaria every year are due to *P. falciparum* infections in young children living in endemic areas.

In endemic areas the patient's first encounter with *P. falciparum* may be in utero. Parasitemia is common in pregnant women, and both placenta and cord blood may contain parasites at the time of delivery. Babies born to infected primigravid mothers may have a low birth weight but are otherwise unaffected. Parasitemia usually clears rapidly in the newborn, who remains relatively resistant to falciparum malaria for the first few months of life. Occasionally (rarely in endemic areas) the newborn goes on to develop congenital malaria, features of which may include fever, failure to feed, anemia, jaundice and hepatosplenomegaly. Severe disease begins to affect children in endemic areas after the first few months of life, and for the next few years. During this time the majority of children are increasingly able to tolerate parasitemia with few or no symptoms, and malaria-related mortality decreases later in childhood.

In areas where there is little or no malaria transmission, children are susceptible to infection and severe disease at any age, and congenital malaria is sometimes seen.[441]

ACUTE *P. FALCIPARUM* INFECTIONS

Falciparum malaria usually presents as a febrile illness similar to that caused by other species of malaria. In a proportion of patients, however, complications develop which may threaten life. The most important manifestations of severe malaria in children are altered consciousness, labored breathing (due to acidosis) and severe anemia. These features may occur singly or in any combination.[442] Hypoglycemia may accompany any of the above syndromes and is associated with increased mortality, especially when the hypoglycemia is profound.[443] Some of the organ complications of falciparum malaria which are common in non-immune adults are uncommon in children. Renal failure, pulmonary edema and disseminated intravascular coagulation are less likely to develop in children, and are not present in most of those who die of falciparum malaria.

Cerebral malaria (CM)

When impaired consciousness in a child with falciparum malaria cannot be explained by the presence of hypoglycemia, seizures or a transient postictal state, and no other causative disease is present, the term 'cerebral malaria' is used.

Clinical measurements of the depth of coma are helpful in defining severity.[444]

CM develops rapidly. In the majority of children febrile symptoms precede coma by 2 days or less; in some the interval is only a few hours. Most patients have been feverish, irritable, listless and unable to eat or drink prior to losing consciousness. Convulsions are common and sometimes herald the onset of coma. In CM there is no postictal recovery of consciousness as occurs after a febrile convulsion. Other symptoms that may precede coma include vomiting and cough; minor looseness of stool may occur, but severe diarrhea is unusual.

The rectal temperature may exceed 40°C, and is usually sustained during the first day or two of treatment. Occasionally a patient with CM may be afebrile when first examined, and rarely may remain so throughout the illness. Tachycardia is appropriate to the degree of fever, and the systolic blood pressure is normal in most patients. Dehydration is not clinically obvious, but vigorous fluid therapy in some patients leads to correction of acidosis and to improved tissue perfusion, suggesting that hypovolemia is commonly important. Respiration is rapid; in some patients breathing is stertorous, in others deep suggesting acidosis. About 5% of children with CM are jaundiced. The heart and lungs are normal on examination. The abdomen is soft; the liver may be moderately enlarged and the spleen may be palpable. In a minority of children with CM a shock-like state, with hypotension, cold peripheries and a wide core-to-skin temperature difference, may develop. Anemia is clinically apparent in some patients, and may develop during the course of illness in others.

The most striking clinical features are neurological. By definition the patient is unconscious and cannot be roused. Coma may be profound, the child being unable to withdraw from or localize a painful stimulus, and unable to moan or cry in response to pain. With less severe neurological impairment, motor and vocal responses to pain are retained but the patient is unable to watch or recognize familiar people. Corneal and pupillary reflexes are usually intact, but brainstem reflexes may be lost in the most severely ill. Retinal hemorrhages are common. Some of the most severely ill patients have papilledema.[445] Recently two further features have been identified that constitute a characteristic 'malarial retinopathy' not seen in other infections: these are areas of discrete retinal whitening, and a silver or white appearance of some of the smaller vessels, usually in a patchy distribution.[446]

In some patients the motor picture suggests decerebration or decortication, with symmetrical rigidity or posturing of limbs, which may be sustained or repetitive. These may represent underlying seizure activity. It is not uncommon for patients to be opisthotonic (see Fig. 26.40). Focal asymmetrical twitching movements of the face or of a limb may be witnessed, sometimes, but not invariably, proceeding to a generalized convulsion. These events are not associated with extremes of fever and cannot be regarded as febrile

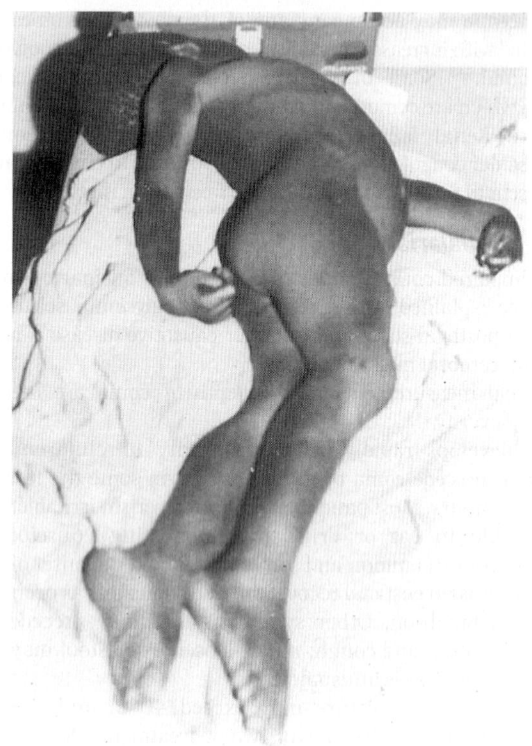

Fig. 26.40 Child with cerebral malaria showing opisthotonus.

convulsions. The plantar reflexes may be symmetrically abnormal. Abdominal reflexes are almost invariably absent.

The peripheral blood film reveals ring stages of *P. falciparum*. Occasionally parasites may be scanty, and rarely absent, in the blood film of a child with CM, perhaps as a result of the sequestration of mature parasites; parasitemia is usually revealed with repeated examination at intervals of a few hours. More commonly parasitemia is heavy: it is not uncommon for up to 20% of red cells to be parasitized, and in some patients the figure exceeds 50%. The packed cell volume may be normal or may be reduced; it usually falls further as the illness progresses. Life-threatening anemia may develop rapidly in patients with hyperparasitemia. Commonly the fall in hematocrit exceeds what would be predicted from the level of parasitemia. In the severely ill, red cells containing late trophozoite and schizont stages of the parasite, normally sequestered in deep capillary beds, may appear in the peripheral blood. The peripheral white cell count is normal in the majority of patients but may be elevated in the very ill. The most severely affected patients are acidotic. There are minor abnormalities of hepatic enzymes, and the plasma creatinine may be mildly elevated. Plasma sodium, potassium, chloride, phosphate and calcium concentrations may show mild abnormalities but are commonly normal. Plasma and cerebrospinal fluid (CSF) lactate levels are abnormally raised in some patients, commonly in association with hypoglycemia. CSF opening pressure is raised in most patients, and fluctuates over time.[447] The mean and distribution of opening pressures were similar in a series of patients with fatal and those with non-fatal CM, and the pathogenetic importance of raised intracranial pressure remains uncertain.[448] The CSF is clear with normal cell counts and protein concentration.

A significant proportion of patients with CM are hypoglycemic when first admitted to hospital.[443,449] These patients do not differ from others in their duration of preceding illness, fasting or coma, or by any distinctive physical signs, but they tend to be younger and are more likely to be profoundly unconscious, to exhibit motor abnormalities and to have elevated levels of lactate and alanine in the plasma.

Even with optimal treatment the mortality among children admitted to hospital with CM is 10–20%. The cause of death is not known, and in most cases cannot be attributed to renal, cardiac, pulmonary or hematological complications of malaria. Presenting features associated with an increased risk of death in children with CM include profound coma, age under 3 years, hypoglycemia, witnessed convulsions, motor abnormalities (hypertonicity, posturing), extreme hyperparasitemia (> 20% of red cells parasitized), acidosis, lactic acidemia and leukocytosis ($> 15 \times 10^9$ white blood cells/L).[444]

In patients who survive CM, the duration of coma after the start of treatment ranges from a few hours to several days, the average duration being about 30 h. The change from deep coma to full consciousness may be dramatically rapid, and usually occurs before the temperature has fallen to normal and before parasitemia has cleared. The great majority of children who survive CM make a full neurological recovery; 5–10% of patients, however, suffer neurological sequelae, including hemiparesis, spasticity and cerebellar defects, from which a gradual recovery is made in some patients over the subsequent months. Risk factors for the development of sequelae are the same as those associated with mortality. Areas of intracerebral infarction have been demonstrated by computerized tomography in some children with neurological sequelae after CM.[450] It is not yet known whether minor defects of motor or cognitive function may persist in some children recovering from CM.

Anemia

Anemia is a component of most episodes of malarial illness. In areas endemic for *P. falciparum* severe anemia (hemoglobin concentration < 5 g/dl) is an important clinical consequence of acute or recurrent malaria.

The history of fever and associated symptoms may be similar to that of any malarial illness, but it is common for a child to present without such symptoms, or for anemia to be identified when a child is examined for an unrelated complaint. Some children with severe malarial anemia develop respiratory distress, which is usually due to acidosis resulting from impaired tissue perfusion and oxygenation.[451] Less commonly, breathlessness is due to cardiac failure, with enlarging liver, and a gallop rhythm on auscultation of the heart.

Peripheral blood films reveal parasitemia and a normochromic normocytic or, in chronic infections, hypochromic anemia. The reticulocyte count is inappropriately low. Unconjugated bilirubin may be increased in the plasma, free hemoglobin may be present in plasma and urine, and the plasma haptoglobin concentration is usually decreased or absent in the acute stage of the illness. The bone marrow shows normoblastic erythropoiesis with minimal dyserythropoiesis and increased myeloid precursors.[431] Unless other diseases are present, serum and red cell folate values are normal. Serum iron may be normal or moderately reduced, but there is usually normal or increased stainable iron in the bone marrow.

After the start of treatment for acute malaria, the hemoglobin level falls further in proportion to, or in excess of, the degree of parasitemia. In endemic areas, many children have a positive direct antiglobulin test. Reticulocytosis begins within a few days, and the hemoglobin level rises rapidly in convalescence.

In endemic areas anemia is a common presenting sign in children who have *P. falciparum* parasitemia but no recent history of febrile illness. The role of malaria in the pathogenesis of the anemia is suggested by rapid improvement after antimalarial chemotherapy. In these patients the bone marrow may show severe dyserythropoiesis.

OTHER MANIFESTATIONS

P. malariae nephrotic syndrome

P. malariae infection if recurrent or prolonged may be complicated by a nephrotic syndrome characterized by non-selective proteinuria, unresponsiveness to steroid or cytotoxic treatment and relentless progression. Immunofluorescent studies suggest that the renal damage is due to the deposition of immune complexes on the glomerular basement membrane. Treatment with antimalarial drugs does not reverse the renal disease.

Hyper-reactive malarial splenomegaly

Some children with protracted or frequent *P. falciparum* infection develop hyper-reactive malarial splenomegaly, a condition in which massive enlargement of the spleen is accompanied by raised serum IgM, high titers of antimalarial antibody, and hepatic sinusoidal lymphocytosis. Splenomegaly resolves slowly with prolonged antimalarial treatment.

DIAGNOSIS AND DIFFERENTIAL DIAGNOSIS

Delayed diagnosis of *P. falciparum* malaria can have tragic consequences. In endemic areas it is a justifiable policy for all fevers without another obvious cause to be regarded as malarial and treated accordingly. In non-endemic areas a history of travel should alert the physician to the possibility of malaria, even if travel was many months or years ago. Malaria should be considered in the differential diagnosis of all fevers accompanied by cerebral complications, acidosis or anemia, and in patients with fever who develop hypoglycemia, acute renal failure, disseminated intravascular coagulation or pulmonary edema.

The diagnosis of malaria depends on finding the parasite in the peripheral blood. Thick smears stained with Field's or Giemsa stain, and thin films stained with Leishman's, Giemsa or a modified Field's stain, allow identification of the species and density of malaria parasitemia. There have been occasional, well-authenticated, reports of fatal falciparum malaria, in which blood films were repeatedly negative during life. Treatment should therefore not be withheld from a patient with an illness suggestive of malaria even if films are negative. In such patients blood films should be repeated at intervals during treatment, when parasitemia may be revealed. Serological methods of identifying malarial infection are valueless for individuals in endemic areas, and of limited use to the clinician seeing patients elsewhere. Serology identifies past or current infection, and may help towards diagnosis in a patient with recurrent fever in a non-endemic area in whom parasitemia cannot be found on repeated testing. Antigen-detecting test-strips and DNA probes can identify parasitemia; these methods are valuable in clinical and epidemiological research, but have not become standard methods for use in clinical practice.

TREATMENT

Malaria due to *P. falciparum* differs from disease due to other plasmodial species in two important respects: *P. falciparum* may cause severe and complicated disease, and the parasite may be resistant to chloroquine. In the patient with falciparum malaria treatment must therefore be undertaken urgently; complications must be foreseen, recognized and treated; and the antimalarial drugs must be chosen with care.

DRUG TREATMENT OF THE ACUTE ATTACK

The correct drug, dosage and route are important. In general, antimalarial drugs should be given by mouth unless the patient is too ill to swallow. Chloroquine is a safe and effective drug for sensitive parasites, and is the treatment of choice for non-falciparum malaria.

For severe or complicated falciparum malaria quinine is the drug of choice. If quinine is unavailable, quinidine as an equally effective alternative. Appropriate schedules for treatment are given in Table 26.34. In areas where *P. falciparum* is known to be partially quinine resistant, an additional drug may be given concurrently with quinine as soon as oral treatment is possible. The choice of additional drug should be guided by drug sensitivities of parasites in

Table 26.34 Drug treatment of acute malaria. In this table the first regimen listed in each section is the treatment of choice

Diagnosis	If patient can take oral drugs	If patient unable to take oral drugs
Malaria due to *P. vivax, ovale, malariae,* and uncomplicated CQ-sensitive falciparum malaria	Oral CQ: 10 mg/kg first dose then 5 mg/kg after 6, 24 and 48 h	CQ: 10 mg/kg over 8 h in saline or 5% dextrose; then 5 mg/kg by similar infusions × 3 (total 25 mg/kg in 32 h)
	Or: AQ, same doses	*Or*: CQ i.m. or s.c. 2.5 mg/kg 4-hourly to 10 doses. Substitute oral CQ when possible
Uncomplicated falciparum malaria of doubtful CQ sensitivity	S/P single dose (S: 25 mg/kg, P: 1.25 mg/kg) *Or*: oral AQ as above *Or*: oral MQ 15 mg/kg first dose, then 10 mg/kg after 8 h	As for complicated falciparum malaria
Severe or complicated falciparum malaria	QN: i.v., first dose* 16.7 mg/kg over 4 h in 5% dextrose, then 8.3 mg/kg over 2–4 h each, 8-hourly, until oral drug can be taken (viz. quinine 8.3 mg/kg 8-hourly) to complete 7-day course *Or*: QN i.m. 8.3 mg/kg 8-hourly as solution containing 60 mg/ml. Give supplementary glucose. Substitute oral quinine as soon as possible, 8.3 mg/kg 8-hourly to complete 7-day course *Or*: quinidine i.v. 7.5 mg/kg 8-hourly, each dose over 4 h in 5% dextrose, until oral treatment can be taken; this may be QN 8.3 mg/kg 8-hourly or quinidine 7.5 mg/kg 8-hourly. Total course 7 days	

* The first dose of i.v. quinine should be reduced to 8.3 mg/kg if the patient has received any quinine or mefloquine in the two preceding days.
CQ, chloroquine; AQ, amodiaquine; QN, quinine; MQ, mefloquine; S/P, sulfonamide-pyrimethamine combination, e.g. Fansidar. All doses of CQ, QN and quinidine refer to base, not salt (8.3 mg quinine base = 10 mg quinine dihydrochloride).

the area where the infection was contracted: options include pyrimethamine–sulfadoxine (Fansidar) in a single dose, equivalent to an adult dose of three tablets (see Table 26.33), or, in children over 10 years of age, tetracycline 250 mg 6-hourly for 5 days.

Both chloroquine and quinine may cause severe hypotension if given by rapid intravenous injection, but do not have this effect if infused slowly (over 3 or more hours). Parenteral quinine is known to stimulate the secretion of insulin from the pancreatic beta cells, but hypoglycemia in children being treated for malaria is usually due to the disease rather than to drug therapy.[443] If intramuscular quinine is used in the treatment of a comatose child, supplementary glucose must be given or the blood glucose level checked frequently.

Oral drugs should replace parenteral as soon as a patient can take them.

OTHER MEASURES

Hypoglycemia

This complication should be suspected in any child with impaired consciousness, convulsions, or acidosis, whether at the time of admission or during the course of treatment. Glucose should be administered as 25 or 50% solution by slow intravenous injection (0.5 g/kg). If 50% glucose is given, it is best diluted two- to threefold with normal saline before being infused over a few minutes. The blood glucose concentration must be measured again at hourly intervals until the patient's condition improves.

Convulsions

Hypoglycemia and hyperpyrexia should be corrected. Prolonged seizures should be treated with the optimal available drug regimen – drugs which may be used include lorazepam, diazepam, paraldehyde, phenytoin or phenobarbital, using drugs in sequence if convulsions prove refractory.

Acidosis

Deep or labored breathing due to acidosis is a common presentation of severe malaria in children. Possible contributory causes are dehydration, severe anemia, shock, repeated convulsions and hypoglycemia, all of which should be looked for and corrected in the acidotic child (see below under Anemia).

Hyperpyrexia

Hyperpyrexia (rectal temperature > 39°C) should be corrected by administration of oral or rectal paracetamol (15 mg/kg 4–6-hourly). However, the value of antipyretic measures in management of malaria has not been demonstrated.[452]

Severe anemia

Because of the increasing risk of transmission of human immunodeficiency virus by blood in parts of the world where malaria is endemic, blood transfusion should only be given if life-threatening anemia is present or can be predicted on the basis of the hematocrit and level of parasitemia on admission. Recent studies suggest that blood transfusion is particularly important for the child with severe anemia and respiratory distress.[453] Most children with severe malarial anemia who are breathless have acidosis rather than heart failure, and may be in urgent need of fluid volume replacement.[451]

Exchange transfusion has been advocated and successfully used for patients with hyperparasitemia, but no controlled trials have been done to prove the superiority of this measure. In countries with limited resources for blood transfusion and with high prevalence rates of HIV infection, exchange transfusion is not justifiable as a method for treating severe malaria.

Fluid therapy must be sufficient to correct hypovolemia, acidosis and oliguria. Pulmonary edema is rare in children with malaria, but the usual precautions are needed to avoid overhydration. Acute tubular necrosis is uncommon as a complication of falciparum malaria in children, but if it occurs peritoneal or hemodialysis may be required.

Antibiotics.

Some children with severe malaria are bacteremic, the proportion differing between studies and sites. In a series in Kenya the overall rate of bacteremia among 421 children with malarial coma or severe anemia was 8.6% and mortality was threefold higher in these patients than others, prompting the authors to recommend routine antibiotic treatment for patients with severe malaria.[454] Several studies indicate a specific association between severe malarial anemia (SMA) and non-typhoidal salmonella bacteremia, especially in infants and toddlers, suggesting that antibiotics should be considered in the management of SMA in very sick children and in those not responding to antimalarial and hematinic therapy. Policies for antibiotic use in various severe malaria syndromes may best be decided on the basis of local experience.

In a child with malarial coma, it may be impossible on physical examination to exclude a diagnosis of bacterial meningitis. Since asymptomatic parasitemia is common in endemic areas, parasitemia in the febrile unconscious child cannot be assumed to be the cause of the disease. Some clinicians prefer to perform a lumbar puncture in these circumstances, to clarify the diagnosis. If lumbar puncture is deferred because of the child's clinical condition, antibiotics should be given to cover the possibility of bacterial meningitis.

There is no place for heparin, dexamethasone or dextran in the treatment of CM.[455]

PRIMAQUINE

P. vivax and *P. ovale* malaria (unless acquired congenitally or by blood transfusion) may relapse if treatment does not include a drug to eliminate hepatic hypnozoites. Primaquine (0.25 mg/kg daily for 2 weeks) will achieve this, but is not worth giving in areas where reinfection is inevitable, and it should not be given to children under the age of 5 years. Primaquine causes severe hemolysis in patients with glucose-6-phosphate dehydrogenase deficiency; the red cell concentration of this enzyme should therefore be measured before the drug is given; if low, an alternative method of radical cure is weekly chloroquine for 6 months in prophylactic doses. Primaquine need not be given after malaria due to *P. falciparum* or *P. malariae*. Primaquine has the additional action of killing gametocytes of all species of malaria parasites; it therefore reduces transmission and is sometimes used for this purpose in areas of moderate endemicity.

MALARIA CONTROL

Since the epidemiology of malaria varies greatly between and even within countries, control measures which are effective in one area may prove ineffective in another. It is important, therefore, that national control programs be designed having regard to local epidemiological, social and economic circumstances. Vector control by residual insecticides remains valid in many countries despite the acquisition of resistance by mosquitoes in some areas. Its cost however restricts its use.

There are currently three principal methods of malaria control relevant to the well-being of children in areas of intense transmission:

1. *Prompt recognition and treatment of both mild and severe disease* at all levels of the health service, with referral to a larger health

facility when necessary. This requires appropriate diagnostic policies (often including presumptive diagnosis of fever as malarial) effective, safe and affordable treatment schedules, competent health staff, and health facilities that are accessible to the majority of people. Because health services are inevitably distant from the homes of many rural people, complementary strategies are needed, and several are being assessed. These include administration of antimalarial drugs for treatment or prevention by village health workers, the training of shopkeepers in appropriate prescribing and dosages (most first-line treatment for malaria in village communities is obtained from local grocery stores), and schemes to involve traditional healers in treatment or referral of patients with malaria.

2. *The use of insecticide-treated nets (ITNs) or curtains.* Several controlled trials and a meta-analysis have demonstrated that sleeping under ITNs can reduce all-cause child mortality in communities.[456] Inevitably there is concern that such results depend on the presence of a scientific team, providing materials and encouraging their use. A study in Tanzania showed a 27% increase in child survival among ITN users in the context of a bed-net program promoted by social marketing – i.e. without the involvement of an investigative team.[457] Impregnated nets and curtains therefore have a potentially important place in malaria control, which may depend on local culture and malaria transmission patterns. The need for annual re-impregnation of nets poses a challenge to sustainability; new methods (the 'permanet') may make reimpregnation unnecessary.
3. *Intermittent presumptive treatment (IPT) during pregnancy.* Pregnant women, especially primigravidae, are at increased risk of malaria, and placental malaria is associated with low birth weight and increased infant mortality. Provision of two or three therapeutic doses of an antimalarial drug such as pyrimethamine–sulfadoxine (Fansidar) between the fourth and eighth months of pregnancy, irrespective of symptoms or parasitemia, reduces placental malaria and improves birth weights.[458] IPT for pregnant women is now an instrument for control of malaria-induced morbidity in many endemic countries.

The success of any method or combination of methods of control is likely to be materially influenced by the degree to which the causes and consequences of malaria are appreciated by populations and by the willingness of communities to participate in, and even finance, specific operations.[455]

PROTOZOAL INFECTIONS: TRYPANOSOMIASIS

AFRICAN TRYPANOSOMIASIS: SLEEPING SICKNESS

Human African trypanosomiasis (HAT) is caused by two morphologically identical 'subspecies' of *Trypanosoma brucei* which are transmitted by the bite of the tsetse fly. Sleeping sickness is widely distributed in 36 countries in sub-Saharan Africa. Approximately 40 000 cases are reported annually to the World Health Organization, a significant underestimate of the true burden of disease.

T. b. gambiense occurs in west and central Africa and causes a disease which is slow in onset and progression (Gambian sleeping sickness). Infected humans can provide long term sources of infection for the tsetse and the *T. b. gambiense* disease may be largely an anthroponosis. Infection with *T. b. rhodesiense* occurs in east and southeast Africa and causes an acute illness that is often lethal within a few months (Rhodesian sleeping sickness). This form of the disease is a true zoonosis: infection is maintained within wild ungulate reservoirs. Both forms most commonly infect adults but any age may be affected; one study in a *T. b. gambiense* endemic area suggested infection was 2–3 times more common in adults than children.[459] In *T. b. rhodesiense* infections, children appear to develop meningoencephalitis more rapidly.

LIFE CYCLE

In the insect vector, stumpy trypomastigotes ingested with the blood meal transform into slender midgut forms of trypomastigotes. These eventually reach the salivary gland and transform via epimastigotes to the infective metacyclic trypomastigote. After inoculation the metacyclic trypomastigotes, on reaching the subcutaneous tissue of the host, are converted into long slender forms. Blood forms are polymorphic comprising slender and stumpy forms. The continual movement of the trypomastigote is activated by a flagellum and the fold of membrane which is lifted up by the motion of the flagellum – the 'undulating membrane'. Three 'subspecies' of *T. brucei* group exist: *T. b. brucei*, which is not infective to humans, cannot be distinguished morphologically from *T. b. rhodesiense* and *T. b. gambiense*. However, biochemical techniques, DNA analysis and isoenzyme characterization can distinguish different *T. brucei* populations. *T. b. rhodesiense* comprises two distinct zymodemes: the 'Zambezi' group in southern Africa and the 'Busoga' group in east Africa associated with more acute severe disease. *T. b. gambiense* is less variable.

EPIDEMIOLOGY

It is likely that all infections with human infective African trypanosomes proceed to sleeping sickness, which, if untreated, is invariably fatal. Recent evidence suggests that African trypanosomiasis is increasing as a human health problem. Substantial epidemics have recently occurred in Uganda, Mozambique, Angola and Zaire, partly because of breakdown of control measures and population movements due to civil unrest.

T. b. gambiense is restricted to West and central Africa and is transmitted by 'palpalis group' tsetse (*Glossina palpalis, G. tachinoides* and *G. fuscipes*), which inhabit dense vegetation along rivers and in forests. Vectors tend to feed on man near riverine vegetation at water collecting points and river crossings. The man–fly–man cycle of transmission may maintain the disease in the absence of an animal reservoir; infected individuals may be asymptomatically parasitemic for years. Although human infective parasites occur in both wild and domestic animals, especially in West African foci, their epidemiological significance remains uncertain.

T. b. rhodesiense is usually transmitted by 'morsitans group' tsetse (*Glossina morsitans, G. pallidipes* and *G. swynnertoni*) whose habitats are in East African woodland savanna and lake shores. Most infection is sporadic as in Tanzania when game hunters or honey gatherers are bitten by *G. morsitans* which transmit disease from the bushbuck host, or in southeast Uganda and western Kenya where fishermen are bitten by *G. pallidipes* on lake shores. More recently, large epidemics have occurred in western Kenya and in south-eastern Uganda with infections occurring in both sexes and all age groups. The vector is *G. f. fuscipes*, a 'palpalis group' tsetse which invaded *Lantana camora* thickets close to human habitation; domestic cows may play an important part in maintaining infection in such situations. Congenital infection with *T. b. rhodesiense* and *T. b. gambiense* does occur, but appears to be very rare. Imported trypanosomiasis is also relatively rare but an increased number of cases have been reported over the last 2 years in Europe and the USA as a result of exposure in game parks.

PATHOGENESIS AND PATHOLOGY

Pathological processes are similar but vary in intensity between *T. b. gambiense* and *T. b. rhodesiense*. Parasites inoculated into the subcutaneous tissue change into slender blood forms and multiply locally, forming a trypanosomal chancre, with edema and an infiltrate of polymorphonuclear leukocytes, lymphocytes and plasma cells. Parasites travel to regional lymph nodes where they also multiply and subsequently cause parasitemia 5–12 days after infection. Subsequently, waves of parasitemia occur, each differing in its surface antigens (particularly variant surface glycoprotein) as the parasite attempts to avoid the host immune response.

Hyperplasia of the reticuloendothelial system, with lymph node and spleen enlargement, occurs as a response to infection; lymph nodes may subsequently become atrophic and fibrotic. Morular cells (Mott cells) are found: plasmacytes that have an important role in the production of IgM. Blood parasites invade the CNS via the choroid plexus leading to the second stage of infection, a meningoencephalitis. Pathologically, a lymphocytic meningoencephalitis and focal vasculitis with perivascular infiltrates is found, particularly in the frontal lobes, pons and medulla. Parasites in the CNS are accompanied by changes in the CSF with a raised protein concentration and the presence of mononuclear cells, particularly lymphocytes. Parasites can also be identified in the CSF.

The succession of variable antigens induces a profuse production of IgM antibody, which reaches high levels in the serum and is also locally produced in the CNS by plasma cells and the morular cells of Mott. Immune complex damage (type III hypersensitivity) may explain less common lesions of the kidney, lungs, liver and heart. Expressions of cell-mediated immunity, induction of cell-mediated immunity and expression of humoral immunity have been shown to be impaired in *T. b. gambiense* infections in man.[460]

CLINICAL FEATURES

The trypanosomal chancre

The primary lesion (trypanosomal chancre) is a painful, erythematous and edematous swelling at the site of the bite that appears within 2 or 3 days. Skin vesicles and ulceration may develop and the chancre heals with residual scarring over 2–3 weeks. Chancres commonly occur in *T. b. rhodesiense* infection but are less common in *T. b. gambiense*. As the chancre develops, the regional lymph glands become enlarged and tender.

The hemolymphatic stage

Waves of irregular remittent fever, in association with the waves of parasitemia, occur 5–12 days after the bite. This is more severe in *T. b. rhodesiense* infections; in *T. b. gambiense* the hemolymphatic stage may be mild, subclinical or asymptomatic. Febrile episodes, sometimes with rigors, are accompanied by malaise, headache, muscular tenderness, joint aches and weight loss. An annular erythematous rash (circinate erythema) may be visible, particularly on the trunk in the fair skinned. Generalized lymphadenopathy may develop, especially in *T. b. gambiense*. Posterior cervical triangle lymphadenopathy, Winterbottom's sign, is seen in *T. b. gambiense* due to the predilection for *G. palpalis* to bite on the head. Edema may affect the ankles, feet or face, producing a dull expressionless facies. Irritability, insomnia and confusion may occur even in the early stage. The spleen and liver may enlarge. The serum albumin is low and bilirubin and transaminases may be raised. In the acute stage of *T. b. rhodesiense* infection, tachycardia is common; pleural or pericardial effusions may occur and myocarditis with arrhythmias or cardiac failure may lead to death. Hematological abnormalities may be seen in acute *T. b. rhodesiense*; a hemolytic, normocytic, normochromic anemia, severe thrombocytopenia and a hemorrhagic coagulopathy may all occur.

Meningoencephalitic stage

Meningoencephalitis is an inevitable consequence of human African trypanosomiasis. In *T. b. gambiense*, it tends to occur after months or years while in *T. b. rhodesiense* it occurs early, often during the febrile illness and progresses rapidly to a fatal outcome. A wide variety of neurological signs occur. Behavioral changes and sleep disturbances are often the first signs; inappropriate diurnal somnolence with insomnia and agitation at night are common. Patients become apathetic, lacking in attention and may exhibit trance-like states. Behavior becomes inappropriate, aggressive or overtly paranoid. Nutritional deficiencies, intercurrent infections and progressive emaciation result. Generalized weakness, unsteadiness of gait, expressionless facies, slurred speech, tremors of the limbs, hyperreflexia and delayed, deep hyperalgesia all occur. In advanced disease, focal epileptic attacks, profound ataxia and choreoathetosis and psychotic changes may be followed by coma and death.

DIAGNOSIS

Clinical diagnosis of African trypanosomiasis may be difficult; although the presence of a chancre is pathognomonic, the hemolymphatic stage must be differentiated from a wide range of febrile illnesses including malaria. Differential diagnosis of second stage disease includes other causes of meningoencephalitis, particularly cryptococcal and tuberculous meningitis in those with HIV, and psychiatric illness. Routine laboratory tests show a normal total white cell count, raised erythrocyte sedimentation rate (ESR), anemia, thrombocytopenia, low serum albumin and elevated serum IgM. A parasitic diagnosis must be attempted in all suspected of trypanosomiasis.

Parasitological diagnosis

In the early stages of *T. b. rhodesiense* infection, parasitological diagnosis is usually simple, as the concentration of trypanosomes in the blood or aspirates of trypanosomal chancres is high. Organisms can be seen by single or repeated microscopic examination of wet films or thick blood or aspirate fluid films stained with Field's stain or Giemsa. Blood film microscopy is less reliable in *T. b. gambiense*; repeated examination of blood films and concentration techniques are often required. However, organisms may readily be seen in fresh lymph node aspirates. Trypanosomes may also be identified in CSF, various effusions and marrow smears.

Concentration methods may increase the sensitivity of microscopy; microhematocrit centrifugation and microscopic examination of the area above the buffy coat are commonly used. The quantitative buffy coat technique (QBC®), a modification of the hematocrit method where motile trypanosomes are stained with fluorescent acridine orange and examined by fluorescent microscopy has proved to be a rapid and sensitive test.[461] The miniature anion exchange centrifugation technique MAEC[462] involves passing a sample of blood through an ion exchange column using a diethylaminoethyl (DEAE)-cellulose anion exchange column, in which red cells are held back and trypanosomes pass through into a collecting tube which is centrifuged and examined for motile trypanosomes. This is a sensitive technique but technically difficult in field conditions. Inoculation of blood, aspirates from lymph node or trypanosome chancre into laboratory rodents is valuable in *T. b. rhodesiense* infections but less so for *T. b. gambiense*.

Once trypanosomiasis is diagnosed or suspected, the CSF must be examined, preferably within 15 min of lumbar puncture. Increase in cell count (more than five cells/mm^3), protein elevation, CSF IgM or trypomastigotes in the centrifuged deposit indicate CNS involvement.

Immunodiagnosis

Immunodiagnostic tests utilized in human African trypanosomiasis include IFAT, ELISA, CFT and IgM estimation. IFAT is valuable in epidemiological investigation and screening of populations and suspects but provides only presumptive evidence of infection. A card agglutination test for trypanosomiasis (CATT), has been developed for the diagnosis of *T. b. gambiense*. This relies on the presence of common antigens not present in all foci of *T. b. gambiense*. The test provides a rapid field test for preliminary screening of populations in endemic areas. Positive serological tests require confirmatory parasitic diagnosis prior to treatment. Antigen detection techniques (card indirect agglutination test for trypanosomiasis, CIATT) have also been developed and appear to be sensitive and specific; they have potential for following the response to therapy.[463]

TREATMENT[464]

Treatment should be started as soon as possible after making a parasitological diagnosis although nutritional disturbances or intercurrent infection should also be treated as antitrypanosomal treatment may be toxic. Routine use of antihelminth and antimalarial drugs is common. Examination of the cerebrospinal fluid is mandatory to distinguish early stage from late stage disease, as CNS involvement requires different, more toxic therapy. Lumbar puncture should not be performed until at least one dose of suramin (or pentamidine) has been given to clear parasites from the blood and prevent inoculation into the CSF at the time of lumbar puncture.

Treatment of hemolymphatic trypanosomiasis

Suramin is effective in treatment of the hemolymphatic stage of both *T. b. rhodesiense* and *T. b. gambiense* disease and will rapidly clear the parasitemia in both early and late sleeping sickness. Pentamidine is the first line therapy for *T. b. gambiense* but is not effective against *T. b. rhodesiense*. Neither suramin nor pentamidine is effective in meningoencephalitis treatment.

Suramin

Suramin is given intravenously with a test dose of 5 mg/kg on day 1 followed by 20 mg/kg on days 3, 7, 14 and 21. Fever, nausea, vomiting and urticaria are common side-effects: renal toxicity may occur.

Pentamidine

Pentamidine is usually given intramuscularly at doses of 4 mg/kg base daily or on alternate days for 7 days. Intravenous administration avoids local side-effects but requires close supervision. Side-effects include syncope and hypotension, vomiting and abdominal pain, especially in the first half hour after administration. Peripheral neuritis is a rare complication and severe hypoglycemic reactions occur during the course of treatment. Adrenaline and glucose should be available when treatment with pentamidine is given.

Meningoencephalitic (late stage) trypanosomiasis

Melarsoprol

Melarsoprol (Mel B) is an arsenical compound which enters the CNS. Use is limited to late stage trypanosomiasis because of its toxicity. A variety of different treatment schedules have been used. In *T. b. rhodesiense* infection, melarsoprol is given in three or four courses, each course lasting 3 days and separated by 1 week, giving a total dose of 35–37.5 ml melarsoprol. Regimens which use lower doses initially and increase through four courses of treatment, may be less toxic.

A variety of other regimens have been advocated for treatment of *T. b. gambiense*, with rising doses over successive courses or a varied number of courses according to the degree of meningoencephalitis, determined by the CSF cell count. Shorter 10 day regimens have also been used for *T. b. gambiense* with no apparent loss of efficacy.[465]

Thrombophlebitis is a frequent complication of melarsoprol treatment; extravasation causes severe local reactions. The major side-effect is a *reactive arsenical encephalopathy* (RAE), which occurs in up to 5% of patients, usually after the third or fourth dose. The onset is usually sudden with neurological deterioration, confusion, convulsions and coma. It occurs more commonly in severe meningoencephalitis and is fatal in 10–50% of cases. In *T. b. gambiense* (but not *T. b. rhodesiense*) prophylactic prednisolone significantly reduces the incidence of RAE.[466,467] Other forms of toxicity which occur commonly with melarsoprol include agranulocytosis, aplastic anemia, thrombocytopenia and peripheral neuropathy. Melarsoprol should not be given as initial therapy to parasitemic patients; it may cause a Jarisch–Herxheimer-like febrile reaction after the first injection. Treatment normally leads to a striking improvement in the mental and physical condition of patients with sleeping sickness.

Difluoromethyl-ornithine (DFMO, eflornithine)

This drug has been used for the treatment of both early and late stage *T. b. gambiense* with good results. It is less effective in *T. b. rhodesiense*. The drug is given intravenously in a dose of 100 mg/kg 6-hourly for 14 days (4 g/m^2 for young children). Major side-effects are diarrhea and reversible marrow depression. Response rates vary from 73 to 97% with some geographical variability; attempts to shorten treatment to 7 days reduces the efficacy.[468]

Nifurtimox

Nifurtimox has occasionally been used in the treatment of arsenic-refractory *T. b. gambiense*; reported response rates vary from 50 to 80%.

Follow-up and relapse

Patients should be seen 3 months after treatment and followed up for 2 years to identify relapse, which normally presents as a chronic meningoencephalitis without a peripheral parasitemia and occurs in 5–20% of those treated. Follow-up should include routine lumbar puncture to identify rising levels of pleocytosis or protein estimations. Relapse in *T. b. gambiense* following treatment with suramin or pentamidine should be with melarsoprol; eflornithine can also be used in the treatment of relapse after melarsoprol therapy. Relapse in *T. b. rhodesiense* is usually treated with a second course of melarsoprol; nifurtimox may be effective, but more data are needed.

CONTROL OF SLEEPING SICKNESS

There are two major components of control activities, detecting and treating human cases and vector control. Sleeping sickness caused by *T. b. rhodesiense* is usually detected at fixed medical units in rural areas when patients present with the symptoms of early parasitemia (passive surveillance). In *T. b. gambiense*, limited clinical symptoms in the early stage means that active surveillance for infected individuals is necessary. Active surveillance may also be useful in *T. b. rhodesiense* epidemics. Blood film examination is used to screen for *T. b. rhodesiense* but in *T. b. gambiense*, gland aspiration and CATT tests are frequently used for initial population screening. Parasitological examination should then be performed; serologically positive but parasite negative individuals should be followed at regular intervals. Community education may play a large part in encouraging early diagnosis and reducing the number of parasitemic individuals. There is no role for mass community prophylaxis: it may mask second stage infections and lead to resistance.[464]

Vector control measures used have included destruction of tsetse habitats and insecticide spraying. Insecticide-impregnated (and/or odor-baited) traps have been very effective in reducing fly populations without the environmental problems associated with widespread application of insecticides.

AMERICAN TRYPANOSOMIASIS: CHAGAS' DISEASE

Chagas' disease is endemic throughout most countries of South and central America. It is caused by *Trypanosoma cruzi*, which is transmitted to humans by triatomine bugs. Acute *T. cruzi* infection is usually benign; its major public health and socioeconomic significance arises from the chronic stages of the disease. Around 16–18 million people may be infected and 2–3 million have chronic Chagas' disease.

LIFE CYCLE OF *T. CRUZI*

The organism occurs in three distinct forms: amastigotes which are found in tissues of mammalian hosts, epimastigotes found in the digestive tract of the triatomine bug and trypomastigotes found in mammalian blood. After ingestion by the vector, trypomastigotes change into and multiply as epimastigotes and in the succeeding 2–4 weeks develop into metacyclic trypomastigotes in the gut of the bug. Infective forms, excreted with the feces, enter through an abrasion in the skin or through an intact mucous membrane such as the conjunctiva. Within 1–2 weeks trypomastigotes enter and circulate in the bloodstream. After an undetermined period, the trypomastigote invades tissue cells, and is transformed into the amastigote.

EPIDEMIOLOGY

T. cruzi occurs in more than 100 mammalian species. The most frequent wild hosts are rodents and small marsupials. Many triatomine bugs are sylvatic and maintain infection among reservoir hosts. Three species have adapted to human dwellings: *Rhodnius prolixus*, *Triatoma infestans* and *Panstrongylus megistus*. Human infection usually occurs from transmission between man and domestic animals. Household populations of bugs may reach hundreds or thousands due to factors such as poor housing, thatched roofs and lack of wall resurfacing. Up to 40–50% of bugs may be infected in some locations. Most transmission occurs in rural populations but transmission in periurban areas is increasing as a result of the rapid urbanization occurring throughout much of South America.

Chagas' disease may also be acquired by blood transfusion, although widespread serological screening has decreased transmission considerably. Congenital disease is an important public health problem in rural areas of endemic transmission, occurring in up to 10% of seropositive women. It is associated with severe disease in early infancy including abortion, prematurity, and stillbirth.

PATHOGENESIS

In acute disease, parasites multiply at the site of the bite, which may lead to a chagoma, consisting of interstitial edema and focal inflammation. Parasites reach the blood but soon disseminate to enter cells, particularly histiocytes, neuroglia, smooth muscle, cardiac muscle and skeletal muscle cells. Amastigotes develop within cells to form pseudocysts. Pseudocyst rupture may lead to the development of acute inflammatory foci with tissue damage, such as the destruction of conducting tissue in the heart. A small proportion of individuals have acute complications, but in the vast majority, the inflammatory reaction subsides and parasitemia and multiplication of parasites in the tissues is reduced by the immune response. The mechanisms of the chronic complications of Chagas' disease remain uncertain; tissue damage, neuronal loss and an autoimmune response are all thought likely to be important.[469]

CLINICAL FEATURES

Acute Chagas' disease

Acute Chagas' disease is usually an illness of children, but can occur at any age. The acute phase of Chagas' disease is asymptomatic in over two-thirds of affected infants and children. If symptomatic, the acute phase lasts for 1–3 months and resolves spontaneously. Shortly after penetration of the connective tissue, parasites may elicit a local inflammatory reaction with marked edema at the site of the portal of entry (chagoma). The skin over the chagoma becomes hard and may desquamate. Romana's sign, unilateral eyelid edema and chemosis, is one of the classical syndromes associated with acute Chagas' disease, occurring when bug feces contaminate the conjunctiva.

After a period of 1–2 weeks, a febrile reaction develops, often associated with headache and myalgia. Vomiting, diarrhea, lymphadenopathy, moderate hepatosplenomegaly, and meningoencephalitis may all occur. Myocardial involvement may occur and varies from tachycardias and other dysrhythmias to myocarditis and cardiac failure; these complications may occasionally be fatal. Meningoencephalitis in the very young also has a bad prognosis. Lymphocytosis often accompanies the parasitemia.

Following the acute phase, if untreated, low level infection may persist asymptomatically for many years (sometimes termed indeterminate phase). Between 15 and 40% of these patients will develop chronic Chagas' disease.

Chronic Chagas' disease

Chronic symptomatic disease is rarely a pediatric problem, usually occurring between the ages of 15 and 50 years. It is characterized by the reappearance of clinical disease 10–20 years after infection. In adults, classical manifestations are the development of a biventricular congestive cardiomyopathy or cardiac rhythm disturbances. Complete right bundle branch block with left bundle hemiblock is the most common abnormality; atrioventricular block, extrasystoles and Stokes–Adams attacks also frequently occur. Inflammatory changes and destruction of parasympathetic ganglion cells in muscle may also eventually lead to megaesophagus and megacolon.

Congenital Chagas' disease

Congenital infection with *T. cruzi* probably occurs in between 2 and 10% of maternal infections. Infection is associated with abortion, stillbirth and death in early infancy in a high proportion. Clinical features include cardiac problems, megaesophagus, pneumonitis and meningoencephalitis. Transmission is also thought to occur through breast milk.

Chagas' disease in the immunocompromised

Chagas' diseases in immunocompromised individuals is an increasing problem in South America due to HIV infection and the use of immunosuppressive drugs in transplant patients. Reactivation of latent *T. cruzi* infection or transplantation of an infected organ can cause the recurrence of parasitemia and the development of disease. Intense myocarditis or severe neurological problems are the most common clinical manifestations if careful monitoring and pre-emptive therapy is not used.[470]

DIAGNOSIS

Parasitic diagnosis

A specific diagnosis, demonstrating *T. cruzi* in the peripheral blood, is usually easy in the early acute illness. The parasite appears as a C- or S-shaped trypomastigote with a prominent kinetoplast in Romanowsky-stained thick or thin films. Centrifugation steps on separated red cells or lysed blood increase the sensitivity of microscopic examination. Culture requires specialized media and is difficult to perform outside a laboratory. Xenodiagnosis is a method for detecting subpatent parasitemia in chronic infections (and occasionally in acute infection) by allowing triatomine bugs to feed on the individual patient: it is preferable to animal inoculation, which is unreliable. Bugs are then dissected to look for gut infection after 20–40 days. PCR methods have published sensitivities of 60–100% when compared with serology; the technique may be more sensitive in children than in adults. It may also be particularly useful in the early detection of congenital infection.[471]

Serological diagnosis

An initial IgM response and IgG response, which persists for life, may be detected by a number of serological tests, including complement-fixation test, indirect fluorescent antibody tests and enzyme-linked immunosorbent assays. Approximately 50% of individuals with positive serology will be also be positive using xenodiagnosis, but there is a poor specificity with false positive tests from other parasitic infections, particularly leishmaniasis, and autoimmune disorders.

There are particular difficulties in following the response to therapy; xenodiagnosis may be negative in those with low parasite burdens and serological tests often remain positive after parasitological cure. Recent studies suggest that PCR may be particularly useful in this situation.[472]

TREATMENT

Chemotherapy in Chagas' disease is problematic. Two drugs have been widely used: nifurtimox (8 mg/kg body weight daily for 60–90 days) and benznidazole (6–10 mg/kg body weight daily for 30 or 60 days). The latter is now more commonly used. Side-effects are more common in adults than in children and occur in 4–30% of cases; major manifestations are hypersensitivity reactions causing rashes and fever, vomiting and peripheral neuropathy. Treatment in acute disease suppresses parasitemia, shortens the course of the acute illness and helps to prevent complications and deaths from acute myocarditis or meningoencephalitis. However, elimination of parasites and prevention of chronic illness only occurs in 50–70% of patients.

The value of treatment in the indeterminate and chronic phase is less certain; results of clinical trials vary both geographically and according to the stage of the infection. Standard recommendations have been that chemotherapy is of no benefit. However, increasing evidence suggests that treatment of children with benznidazole in the indeterminate phase (chronic asymptomatic) leads to parasite clearance in around 60% (measured by negative serology or xenodiagnosis) and is associated with a reduction in the number of electrocardiogram (ECG) changes.[473,474] Both allopurinol and itraconazole have been used for treatment of chronic disease with parasitological cure in 40–50% and normalization of ECG abnormalities in 36–48% of individuals.[475] Further work is needed to evaluate the true value of chemotherapy in chronic disease. Heart failure is usually treated with vasodilators such as ACE inhibitors; digitalis may aggravate arrhythmias. Pacemakers are commonly implanted for heart block. A number of surgical procedures are used for megaesophagus and megacolon. Treatment of symptomatic congenital infection is often unsatisfactory. Recent evidence suggests that routine screening of babies of seropositive mothers with treatment of positive infants is a safe and effective approach.[471,476]

CONTROL

No vaccine exists for Chagas' disease; major preventative efforts center upon control of transmission. Chagas' disease is predominantly a disease of poverty, which is associated with poor quality housing and the inability to control domestic triatomine bugs. In recent years, control programs have been effective in countries in the southern cone of South America (Argentina, Brazil, Bolivia, Chile, Paraguay and Uruguay) with a reduction in incidence of between 60 and 99% from 1983 to 1997.[477] Seroprevalence surveys are used to indicate areas and dwellings at risk, and pyrethroid insecticides are used for the spraying of housing and peridomestic buildings; the use of fumigant canisters may also be useful. Community surveillance is then used to detect residual or new infections and further spraying performed. Housing improvements and health education help to promote sustainability. Programs to control blood transfusion transmission are based on routine serological testing and usually combine serological tests for HIV and hepatitis B as well as *T. cruzi*. In some circumstances the high prevalence of seropositivity for *T. cruzi* requires that seropositive blood has to be used and in these circumstances the addition of gentian violet 24 h before use appears effective and safe in preventing transmission.

PROTOZOAL INFECTIONS: LEISHMANIASIS

Leishmaniasis is caused by infection with a number of species of protozoan parasites of the genus *Leishmania*. It occurs in many parts of the world, including southern Europe and is particularly problematic in central and South America, the Middle East, South Asia, China and East Africa. An estimated 1–2 million new cases occur annually. Most forms of leishmaniasis are zoonoses, with rodent or canine reservoirs of infection; man and other vertebrate hosts become infected by the bite of sandflies (genera *Phlebotomus* and *Lutzomyia*). Clinical syndromes are determined by the infecting species. These range from self-limiting cutaneous lesions to potentially fatal visceral lesishmaniasis.

LIFE CYCLE AND PARASITE BIOLOGY

Leishmania are transmitted by sandflies of the genus *Phlebotomus* in the Old World and *Lutzomyia* in the New World. Sandflies take in blood from a minute hemorrhage made in the skin by their mouthparts. The aflagellate stage (amastigotes), taken in the blood meal, divide at least once before changing into the motile flagellate stage (promastigotes). These develop within the gut over 4–14 days and migrate forward to become inoculated when the sandfly attempts to take its next blood meal.[478] The intracellular stage in the vertebrate host (including man) is a small uninucleate ovoid body (2–5 μm long and 1–2 μm wide) containing a kinetoplast with a flagellar remnant and known as the amastigote (also referred to as the Leishman–Donovan body). The amastigote predominantly infects cells of the reticuloendothelial system and multiplies repeatedly by binary fission eventually destroying the host cell.

Parasite biology

Two major subgenera of importance in human leishmaniasis can be distinguished by the site of development within the sandfly vector: *Leishmania* subgenus *Leishmania* (*Leishmania donovani, L. mexicana, L. tropica* and *L. major*) and *Leishmania* subgenus *Viannia* (*L. braziliensis* complex).[479] Leishmania that infect man are morphologically similar apart from minor variations in size of amastigotes. However, isoenzyme profiles, DNA characterization, polymerase chain reaction (PCR), monoclonal antibody techniques and serotyping can all be used to distinguish species.[480] Culture of leishmania can be performed using specialized media. Some *Leishmania* species grow poorly in culture and culture characteristics have been used to differentiate *L. braziliensis,* which is slow growing, from *L. mexicana.*

The important leishmania affecting man and the clinical syndromes that they cause are summarized in Table 26.35.

VISCERAL LEISHMANIASIS (KALA AZAR)

Visceral leishmaniasis (VL) is caused by leishmania of the *L. donovani* complex (*L. donovani, L. infantum* and *L. chagasi*).

EPIDEMIOLOGY

L. donovani is endemic and epidemic in north-eastern India and Bangladesh, predominantly affecting young adults and children. Infection is confined to man and no animal reservoirs have been identified. The vector, *Phlebotomus argentipes,* is peridomestic and readily feeds on man. The parasite is similar in East Africa, where the disease is widespread with endemic foci and occasional epidemics, particularly in association with population movements and land development. Children are predominantly affected. Rodents are reservoirs of disease in Sudan, but no animal reservoir has been identified in Kenya. Transmission is often seasonal due to fluctuations in sandfly populations.

L. infantum is widely distributed through the Mediterranean littoral, southern Europe, the Middle East, southern regions of the former USSR and China. In endemic areas, children under 5 are predominantly affected although infection may occur at any age in visitors and in the immunosuppressed. The domestic dog is an important reservoir host; wild canine species and foxes also act as reservoirs.

L. chagasi in South and central America resembles *L. infantum* clinically and epidemiologically. Infection occurs in Amazonian Brazil, Bolivia, Paraguay, Argentina, Colombia and Venezuela.

Table 26.35 Summary of human leishmaniasis

Parasite	Geographical distribution	Animal reservoir	Disease
Visceral leishmaniasis (*Leishmania donovani* complex)			
L. donovani	India, Bangladesh, China	None	VL PKDL
	Kenya	(Dog)	VL PKDL
	Sudan and Ethiopia	Rodents	VL (CL) (MCL)
L. infantum	Mediterranean littoral, Central Asia, China	Canine sp.	VL (CL) VL CL
L. chagasi	Central and South America	Canine sp.	VL
Old World cutaneous leishmaniasis			
L. tropica	Middle East to India	(Dog)	CL (dry), LR
L. aethiopica	Ethiopia and Kenya	Rock hyrax	CL DCL
L. major	Africa, Middle East and Asia	Rodents	CL (wet)
American cutaneous leishmaniasis (*Leishmania mexicana* complex)			
L. mexicana	Mexico, Belize, Guatemala	Forest rodents	CL (DCL) Chiclero's ulcer
L. amazonensis	Brazil–Amazon basin	Forest rodents	CL DCL
American mucocutaneous leishmaniasis (*Leishmania braziliensis* complex)			
L. braziliensis	Brazil, Amazon forest, Peru, Ecuador, Bolivia, Venezuela, Colombia, Paraguay	Uncertain, forest animals	CL and MCL
L. guyanensis	North Amazon, Guyana	Sloth, lesser anteater	CL MCL
L. panamensis	Panama, Costa Rica	Sloth	CL (MCL)
L. peruviana	Western Andes	(Dog)	CL (Uta)

CL, cutaneous leishmaniasis; DCL, diffuse cutaneous leishmaniasis; LR, leishmania recidivans; MCL, mucocutaneous leishmaniasis; PKDL, post-kala-azar dermal leishmaniasis; VL, visceral leishmaniasis.

Children are predominantly affected and both domestic and wild canine species and foxes are reservoir hosts.

PATHOGENESIS

After inoculation into the skin, the promastigotes convert to amastigotes, in skin macrophages. These disseminate throughout the reticuloendothelial system and amastigote-laden macrophages are found in liver, spleen, bone marrow, lymphatic tissue and occasionally the skin. Progressive splenomegaly, hepatomegaly, anemia and thrombocytopenia result.

CLINICAL FEATURES

Subclinical or asymptomatic infection is common and protects against subsequent infection; clinical disease only occurs in 10–20% of infections. The clinical features of VL are similar throughout the world. A small cutaneous lesion may occur at the site of inoculation (a leishmanioma), but is often not observed. After a variable incubation period (usually 4–6 months), symptoms develop. Classical clinical features are a triad of fever, splenomegaly and anemia. However, the spectrum of VL ranges from an acute febrile infection with anemia, pancytopenia and splenomegaly to a protracted illness slowly progressing over 2 or more years with severe anemia and massive splenomegaly. *L. infantum* infections are usually more acute than infection with *L. donovani* but acute forms of *L. donovani* occur, especially in children. *L. infantum* may also cause simple cutaneous leishmaniasis in adults in southern Europe.

Fever is frequent, commonly remittent or intermittent, and may have a characteristic double diurnal periodicity. In very acute forms, fever is high, with prostration, toxemia and minimal splenomegaly. However, many patients remain active despite high fever and some patients with chronic infection may be afebrile for prolonged periods. Most patients develop progressive splenomegaly and hepatomegaly; in chronic infections, the spleen may be grossly enlarged, smooth and hard. Generalized or localized (often cervical) lymphadenopathy occurs in some geographical areas and may be present in the absence of hepatosplenomegaly or other features of VL.

Patients with chronic disease are pale and, especially in India, develop an earthy gray color with areas of hyperpigmentation (kala azar). In Africa, a diminution in skin pigmentation is more typical. Chronic VL leads to progressive wasting, nutritional skin changes and hair changes similar to those observed in kwashiorkor. Anemia and pancytopenia with associated immunosuppression leads to secondary infections such as pneumonia, bronchitis, meningitis and tuberculosis. Episodes of diarrhea are common and may be due either to secondary infection or submucosal infiltration with leishmania-laden macrophages. Patients are rarely jaundiced but dependent edema and ascites occur. Hemorrhagic features, especially recurrent epistaxis, are common; major or fatal hemorrhagic episodes may occur.

VL AND ACQUIRED IMMUNE DEFICIENCY SYNDROME

VL is an important opportunistic infection in HIV, particularly in southern Europe. Most cases occur in young adults but pediatric cases of coinfection have been reported. Both classical and atypical presentations with pulmonary, skin and gastrointestinal infection occur; fulminant infection without splenomegaly is also recognized. Leishmanial serology is frequently negative, but parasites are usually easy to find in appropriate samples.

LABORATORY FINDINGS

The hematological features of VL are characteristic. There is a moderate to severe normocytic, normochromic anemia with hemoglobin levels of 6–8 g/dl accompanied by a neutropenia and thrombocytopenia, commonly 80–100 × 10^9/L. Lymphocytes are usually in the normal range and circulating eosinophils reduced or absent from the peripheral blood. The serum albumin is reduced and there is a substantial elevation of immunoglobulins, predominantly IgG.

DIAGNOSIS[481,482]

A parasitic diagnosis may be made by microscopy or culture of bone marrow or splenic aspirates. Splenic aspiration is more sensitive and reasonably safe in the absence of disturbed hemostasis or thrombocytopenia. Marrow aspiration is preferable in children, acute illness or in the presence of thrombocytopenia or disturbed hemostasis. Leishmania may also be identified by examination of the buffy coat and in lymph node and liver biopsy specimens. Smears are fixed in methanol and stained with Giemsa or Leishman that stain the cytoplasm of the amastigote blue, the nucleus pink or violet and the kinetoplast bright red. Culture is generally less sensitive than direct smear examination, but will detect some smear negative cases.

Immunodiagnostic tests of value in the investigation of VL include IFAT, ELISA, CFT and direct agglutination tests (DAT). ELISA and DAT techniques are highly sensitive and specific. High titers are associated with active disease and fall slowly after treatment. The leishmanin skin test (a test of delayed hypersensitivity using leishmanial antigen) is invariably negative in active visceral disease. PCR techniques have been developed for the diagnosis of leishmaniasis, but their value in the diagnosis of VL is uncertain.

DIFFERENTIAL DIAGNOSIS

VL should be considered in the differential diagnosis of acute or chronic fever accompanied by hepatosplenomegaly and anemia, especially when there is a history of residence in an endemic area. Many other infections, including malaria, especially *Plasmodium malariae* infection, typhoid, brucellosis, relapsing fever and tuberculosis (which may coexist with visceral leishmaniasis) should be considered. Splenomegaly must be differentiated from schistosomiasis, tropical splenomegaly syndrome and lymphoma or leukemia.

TREATMENT[481,482]

Pentavalent antimonial compounds remain the treatment of choice for most cases of VL. Two preparations are in common use, sodium stibogluconate containing 100 mg antimony (Sb) per ml (Pentostam) and methylglutamine antimoniate containing 85 mg Sb per ml (Glucantime). Response rates are usually around 90%, but antimonial resistance, particularly in India, is an increasing problem; some regions report failure rates of up to 50%.

Sodium stibogluconate is administered by daily intravenous or intramuscular injection. The dose is 10–20 mg/kg Sb per day for 20–30 days. Children normally receive 20 mg/kg per day. Rapid extensive renal clearance occurs and dose adjustments should be made if renal function is poor. Common side-effects in adults include arthralgia, myalgia, biochemical and clinical pancreatitis, mild increase in liver enzymes and marrow suppression; the drug appears to be better tolerated by children.[483,484] Minor ECG changes are common; prolonged Q–T interval and dysrhythmias may occur in high dose regimens used for the treatment of antimony-resistant infections. Anaphylactic shock is a rare complication following administration. Sodium stibogluconate has been used in pregnancy without untoward effects on the fetus.

Amphotericin B in both conventional and lipid formulations has been proven to be effective in various regimens lasting for between 10 and 40 days depending upon geographical location and the immune status of the patient. Standard amphotericin B is now the first line of therapy in some areas of India. Lipid formulations are better tolerated and have the theoretical advantage of being preferentially taken up by macrophages, but expense precludes their use in many endemic countries.

Pentamidine is an effective drug in VL, but resistance appears to develop rapidly and relapse is not uncommon. The necessity for high dose prolonged regimens means that pentamidine may lead to more toxicity than antimonials. The drug is currently mainly used in areas of high resistance to antimonials or in patients who relapse.

Aminosidine (paromomycin) is an aminoglycoside that is active in the treatment of VL, but is less effective than antimonials as monotherapy. It is administered intravenously or by intramuscular injection at a dose of 14 mg/kg daily for 3–4 weeks. Combinations of aminosidine and antimonials may permit a reduction in the duration of therapy.

Miltefosine is a new oral drug, originally developed as an antineoplastic agent, that has good in vitro activity against all species of leishmania. Phase two trials in India suggested high efficacy in a 4 week regimen, even in those who had previously failed antimonial treatment; shorter courses may also be effective.[485,486] If phase three trials confirm these findings, the advantage of oral administration will make this a very important drug for endemic areas.

Supportive and symptomatic treatment is important in addition to chemotherapy. Intercurrent infections must be sought and appropriately treated and attention paid to correcting nutritional status and vitamin deficiencies. Patients with hemorrhage should receive vitamin K. Blood transfusions are often required for the treatment of anemia in children.

Response to treatment

Fever normally subsides and patients start to feel better in the first week of treatment. Hemoglobin and white cell counts improve over 2–4 weeks while the splenomegaly reduces more gradually over subsequent weeks or months. Patients should be followed-up for at least 1 year to detect relapse.

Relapse and non-responsiveness

Relapse normally occurs within 6 months and relapse rates vary considerably depending upon the geographical location and the initial treatment regimen. Initial treatment of relapse is usually with prolonged courses of sodium stibogluconate, but after repeated relapse, patients may become resistant to antimony treatment. Pentamidine, aminosidine, amphotericin B and liposomal amphotericin have all been used successfully to treat relapse. Systemic interferon gamma may be useful as an adjunctive therapy in resistant infections. HIV infected individuals are more likely to relapse and may need maintenance therapy.

Post-kala azar dermal leishmaniasis

Post-kala azar dermal leishmaniasis (PKDL) is most commonly seen in Indian VL (20%) and less often in African infections (1–5%). Following treatment of visceral disease, cutaneous lesions develop with symmetrical depigmented lesions especially on exposed surfaces. Lesions progress to become papular or nodular and mucosal surfaces may be involved with abundant leishmania (*L. donovani*) in lesions. Treatment with pentavalent antimonial compounds is effective although lesions also heal spontaneously.

CUTANEOUS LEISHMANIASIS

EPIDEMIOLOGY

L. tropica and *L. major* cause cutaneous leishmaniasis in the Middle East, Afghanistan, the southern Mediterranean, Sudan and sub-Saharan Africa. Clinical infection in endemic areas occurs mainly in children. *L. tropica* has a human reservoir and transmission is mainly urban whereas *L. major* occurs in rural areas with rodent reservoirs.

L. mexicana and *L. braziliensis* cause cutaneous leishmaniasis in central and South America. *L. mexicana* has a reservoir in forest rodents in central and South America and particularly affects the pinna of the ear in forest workers, notably chicleros (chewing gum collectors). *L. braziliensis* has a reservoir in domestic animals and forest rodents. Cutaneous lesions may progress to mucocutaneous leishmaniasis (espundia).

CLINICAL FEATURES

Clinical features of cutaneous leishmaniasis are similar throughout the world with some slight differences between species. Typically, after an incubation period of several weeks, a localized small raised cutaneous nodule occurs, surrounded by a zone of erythema often with fine papery desquamation. The lesion grows slowly and central shallow ulceration may occur. Lesions remain raised above the level of normal skin; ulcers are shallow and do not have undermined edges. Lesions continue to progress for 6–24 months followed by spontaneous healing eventually leaving a slightly depressed papery scar. Satellite lesions may develop and regional lymphadenopathy is found in some forms. Lesions may be single or multiple and are more common on the face, hands, feet or limbs. *L. tropica* tends to cause single lesions lasting for 1–2 years with very little tissue reaction and sometimes non-ulcerating lesions whereas lesions in *L. major* are often multiple with a greater degree of ulceration and tissue reaction. Spontaneous healing occurs in 50% of lesions by 3 months in *L. major* or *L. mexicana*, 10 months in *L. tropica* and much longer in *L. braziliensis*.

Diffuse cutaneous leishmaniasis (DCL)

In the Ethiopian highlands and western Kenya, *L. aethiopica* causes initial skin lesions similar to *L. tropica*. In very rare cases, leishmania disseminate throughout the skin to cause widespread, often symmetrical, lesions that resemble lepromatous leprosy. Similar syndromes occur in central and South America associated with *L. mexicana* and *L. amazonensis*. Cell-mediated immune responses to leishmania antigens are absent and the leishmanin skin test is negative.

Leishmania recidivans

This is an unusual form of cutaneous leishmaniasis found in the Middle East caused by *L. tropica*. The initial chronic skin lesion heals but then groups of lesions resembling lupus vulgaris occur around the healed scar. Leishmania amastigotes are difficult to find, but the leishmanin skin test is strongly positive.

Mucocutaneous leishmaniasis

L. braziliensis complex infections cause single, often self-healing, primary lesions of the skin. However, in a small proportion, probably less than 5%, subsequent metastatic spread to the oronasopharynx may occur (espundia). The time interval between initial infection and mucosal infection varies from a month to many years. The nasal septum is often involved initially causing symptoms of nasal stuffiness and epistaxis. Granulomatous lesions cause necrosis and destruction of cartilage and soft tissue and extend to involve the nose, mouth, tongue and soft palate. Lesions may ultimately involve the pharynx and larynx. Secondary infection is common and contributes to tissue destruction. Aspiration pneumonia occurs in the late stages and may be fatal.

DIAGNOSIS OF CUTANEOUS LEISHMANIASIS

The likelihood of finding parasites depends upon the infecting species and the stage of the lesion. Parasites are more numerous in early lesions and in *L. tropica* and DCL. Aspirates and slit smear preparation from the raised margins of a lesion, dermal scrapings and biopsies are all useful. Care should be taken to reduce the chance of bacterial contamination of samples. Multiple sampling and a combination of techniques increase the chances of a successful diagnosis. Samples should be examined microscopically and cultured on appropriate media. Impression smears should be made from biopsy samples. Although histology is less sensitive in detecting parasites, it is useful in excluding other causes of the lesion. Mucocutaneous disease is often difficult to diagnose due to the limited number of parasites. PCR may be helpful on lesion aspirates or biopsies and may distinguish between different species complexes. Species diagnosis may also be made on cultured parasites by isoenzyme analysis or other DNA diagnostic techniques.

The leishmanin skin test becomes positive during the course of infection and remains positive thereafter. It is particularly useful in travelers; in endemic areas, a high proportion of inhabitants is positive. It is negative in DCL and strongly positive in *L. recidivans*. Serodiagnostic tests are of limited value for the diagnosis of cutaneous disease but may be helpful for the diagnosis and follow-up of mucocutaneous disease.

There are a number of important differential diagnoses for cutaneous leishmaniasis including superficial mycoses such as sporotrichosis, cutaneous mycobacterial infections, yaws, syphilis, sarcoidosis and neoplasms. In mucosal disease, histoplasmosis, paracoccidioidomycosis and midline granuloma must also be considered.

TREATMENT

Many cutaneous leishmaniasis lesions heal spontaneously without specific treatment. Local treatment should include cleansing and antibiotics to control secondary infection and covering to prevent secondary contact lesions. Local infiltration with antimonials is used in some areas for treatment of early non-inflamed lesions to accelerate healing.[487] Topical paromomycin may be effective in *L. major* infection; success rates in other species are variable.[481,482] Oral agents such as allopurinol and imidazoles (ketoconazole, itraconazole) have been used for cutaneous leishmaniasis with generally disappointing results. Miltefosine may be effective orally for American cutaneous leishmaniasis.[488]

In *L. braziliensis* areas where mucocutaneous leishmaniasis occurs, all leishmanial lesions must be treated with prolonged systemic pentavalent antimonials (20 mg/kg stibogluconate for 20 days) to prevent metastatic spread. The clinical response may be poorer in children under 5.[489] Systemic therapy is also indicated for multiple or potentially disfiguring lesions of any species; shorter, lower dose courses may be adequate for *L. major* or *L. tropica*. Established mucocutaneous disease is difficult to treat and may require prolonged courses of systemic antimony or amphotericin. Diffuse cutaneous leishmaniasis is resistant to pentavalent antimonials but may respond either to combinations of aminosidine and antimonials or to prolonged courses of pentamidine.

CONTROL OF LEISHMANIASIS

Control centers upon vector control and reduction in the reservoir host. In central Asia, the simultaneous use of rodenticide and insecticide in gerbil burrows have reduced markedly the incidence of *L. major* infection: similarly, control of stray dog populations and residual insecticide spraying have reduced *L. infantum* infection in many areas. Effective control can be achieved by medical surveillance of the population at risk, when man is the major host reservoir. Insecticide spraying of houses is useful for peridomestic vectors such as in Indian visceral leishmaniasis. Control remains problematic in the vast forested areas of the Americas; the use of insecticides in tropical rain forests is impractical and control of the extensive reservoir of infected wild animals equally impossible. A number of candidate vaccines have been developed but clinical trials have been disappointing in both cutaneous and visceral leishmaniasis. A number of studies suggest that treated or untreated bednets reduce the risk of visceral leishmaniasis.[490]

PROTOZOAL INFECTIONS: TOXOPLASMOSIS

Toxoplasmosis is mainly of importance to pediatrics as a congenital infection where it may result in a number of defects including blindness or central nervous system abnormalities. Infection acquired after birth is usually only significant in those with underlying T cell immunodeficiencies. Occasionally, signs of congenital infection may not manifest until late in childhood or early adulthood.

The birth prevalence of congenital toxoplasmosis infection across Europe ranges from 1 to 10 per 10 000 newborns.[491] In the UK, only 10% of women show evidence of past infection with toxoplasmosis whereas in France, up to 55% of pregnant women show antibodies to toxoplasmosis on antenatal screening.

ETIOLOGY

The causative organism, *Toxoplasma gondii*, is, in its free active state, a small, crescentic protozoon, which is a strict intracellular parasite multiplying only within the cytoplasm of the nucleated host by binary fission or, probably more frequently, by internal budding (endodyogeny). The active form, responsible for acute infection, stimulates an immunological response by the host. At the same time, cyst forms of the parasite develop in any tissue, but chiefly in nervous tissue or striated muscle, and may persist for the life of the host.

PATHOGENESIS

T. gondii infects virtually all species of mammals, and several species of birds. The cat family is the definitive host. Cats usually acquire the infection after eating infected rodents, birds or uncooked meat. After primary infection, they shed millions of oocysts in their feces for up to 14 days. Oocysts may remain viable in soil for many months, and are not found on the cat fur, thus explaining the failure to link cat exposure with the risk of human toxoplasmosis infection.[492]

Humans are most commonly infected after ingestion of tissue cysts in raw or poorly cooked meat, or by ingestion of soil, food or water contaminated with oocysts. Infection from meat has been shown to be responsible for up to two-thirds of all new infections in pregnant women.[493] Traditionally pork, lamb, goat or game meats hold the highest risk for human infection, although undercooked beef has been shown to be a risk factor for toxoplasmosis seroconversion,[493] possibly due to combination with cheaper meats.[492] Congenital toxoplasmosis infection usually occurs as a result of placental infection after a primary infection in a pregnant woman. The risk of transmission and the clinical outcome after maternal toxoplasmosis infection vary with the trimester of pregnancy, with the first trimester having the lowest risk of transmission to the fetus but the highest risk of damage.

Transmission has also been rarely documented in children after blood or blood product transfusion, heart or bone marrow transplantation[494,495] and through infected breast milk.[496]

CLINICAL FEATURES

CONGENITAL TOXOPLASMOSIS

The clinical features of congenital toxoplasmosis in the newborn infant are described in Chapter 10.

ACQUIRED TOXOPLASMOSIS

Acquired infection with *T. gondii* is uncommon in the UK in children under 5 years. Serological surveys suggest a peak acquisition of infection in early and mid-teens. The disease is nearly always asymptomatic. The commonest manifestation if clinical signs do occur, is lymphadenopathy, particularly of cervical nodes, which may be accompanied by no ill health, or may be accompanied by fever and prostration, and resemble severe infectious mononucleosis. Muscle pain may also occur due, it is believed and occasionally confirmed, to infection of voluntary muscle. Acquired toxoplasmosis may also result in hepatosplenomegaly, lymphocytosis, and, rarely, pneumonitis, acute hepatitis, arthritis or cardiac arrhythmias (due to lesions in the region of the conducting system). The occurrence of cardiac failure due to toxoplasma infection of the mycocardium is conjectural. Isolated visual disturbance due to toxoplasmosis retinitis is usually due to reactivation of an undiagnosed congenital infection, although it can rarely occur after postnatal infection in the immunocompetent.[497]

Acquired toxoplasmosis infection has been documented in immunodeficient children with HIV infection, or post bone marrow or solid organ transplantation, but it occurs much less commonly than in adults. Toxoplasmosis in the immunocompromised child may manifest as encephalitis, pneumonitis or even a multiorgan systemic disease.

DIAGNOSIS AND DIFFERENTIAL DIAGNOSIS

Congenital toxoplasmosis should be considered a possible cause of generalized lymphadenopathy, hepatosplenomegaly, thrombocytopenia or severe and otherwise unexplained jaundice in the newborn. Cytomegalic inclusion disease, congenital rubella, neonatal hepatitis, rhesus incompatibility and congenital syphilis would also be considered. In later infancy and childhood, congenital toxoplasmosis enters into the differential diagnosis of hydrocephalus and of fits. Congenital toxoplasmosis should be considered as a possible cause of chorioretinitis whatever the stage of development of the lesions or age of the patient. It is believed that 25–35% of chorioretinitis is due to Toxoplasma infection. Chorioretinitis could also be due to congenital rubella or cytomegalovirus infection.

Acquired toxoplasmosis should be considered in any case of unexplained lymphadenopathy, particularly when maximal in, or confined to, the cervical region, whether or not it is accompanied by pyrexia. Lymph node enlargement in acquired toxoplasmosis may persist for several months, leading to the consideration of lymphoma and tuberculous lymphadenopathy in the differential diagnosis.

In the immunocompromised child, it enters the differential diagnosis for neurological disease (encephalitis, meningoencephalitis, brain abscess), for interstitial pneumonitis, and for myocarditis.

LABORATORY DIAGNOSIS

The most common laboratory aids to the diagnosis include serology, isolation of the organism, histology and the direct detection of *T. gondii* DNA in infected tissues or fluids by polymerase chain reaction (PCR). Other diagnostic methods used less commonly today include skin testing and the Sabin–Feldman dye test, which depends upon the inhibition by antibody-containing serum of methylene blue staining of laboratory cultures of *T. gondii*. The diagnosis of a congenital infection postnatally is discussed in Chapter 10.

Serological methods remain the most commonly used method for diagnosis. Acute infection in the older child or adult may be diagnosed by a fourfold rise in Toxoplasma-specific IgG by indirect immunofluorescence, or enzyme immunoassay. Toxoplasma-specific IgM can be detected by 2 weeks post infection, and usually declines by 6 months, but at times may persist for months (and occasionally over a year) after the initial infection. Thus the detection of Toxoplasma IgM may indicate either an acute or a recent past infection. Positive results should be confirmed by multiple tests in different laboratories, given a false positive rate of up to 2%. If timing of the infection is critical, as in the case of a pregnant woman, the presence of IgA and IgE antibodies to toxoplasmosis which decline more readily than IgM, and IgG avidity (high avidity suggests an infection > 12 months prior) may be helpful in differentiating an acute infection from a past infection. However, some suggest that even current serological assays cannot predict the time of infection within the first year after infection (reviewed in Petersen et al [498]).

The detection of *T. gondii* DNA by PCR in amniotic fluid is now commonly used for the prenatal diagnosis of congenital toxoplasmosis. Sensitivity rates of up to 90% have been reported, but there is a wide range in the quality of assays available, with false positive rates ranging from 0 to 10% reported in some laboratories (reviewed in Petersen et al[498]). Other applications of the assay are on cerebrospinal fluid, or peripheral white blood cells in the immunocompromised or congenitally infected infant.

Culture of *T. gondii* from lymph node biopsy material, amniotic fluid, placenta or, less often, from other tissue fluids is possible, although generally less widely used than serological methods. The organism can be cultured in suitable laboratory animals, particularly mice, embryonated eggs and tissue cultures. The most reliable of these procedures is that of intraperitoneal inoculation of mice. Histological examination of biopsy material is also of value, limited chiefly by the availability of suitable material. Cysts can be identified readily, but vegetative forms are recognized with difficulty.

In the immunocompromised child, such as those with HIV infection, the ability to document seroconversion to toxoplasmosis is impaired. A diagnosis must be made by demonstrating the organism by PCR, culture or histology in infected tissues, or presumptively by characteristic findings on imaging that respond to an empirical trial of antiparasitic therapy.

Dermal hypersensitivity to injection of a suspension of killed Toxoplasma is indicated by a delayed tuberculin type response. There is good correlation between a positive skin test and a positive dye test titer of 1: 8 or more. The test may be negative in very recent infections and is used chiefly in epidemiological surveys in man.

TREATMENT AND PROGNOSIS

Treatment of acquired toxoplasmosis infection in childhood is usually only indicated for active ocular infection or severe disease in other organs.

Treatment of congenitally infected infants is discussed later. Antibiotics, other than spiramycin, have proved to be of little value in the treatment of acute toxoplasmosis. Sulfonamides have proved disappointing and sulfones too toxic in the doses required. The most effective form of chemotherapy is a combination of pyrimethamine and sulfadiazine for a total duration of 3–4 weeks. The hematological toxic effects of pyrimethamine, due to its antifolic acid action, can be prevented or reversed by folinic acid. Spiramycin, though less toxic than the pyrimethamine and sulfadiazine combination, is clearly less effective. An alternative is the use of a combination of trimethoprim and a sulfonamide, e.g. co-trimoxazole. Life-long suppressive therapy with these agents is indicated for HIV-infected children after toxoplasmosis encephalitis.

In the pregnant woman, spiramycin may be given in early pregnancy for suspected primary toxoplasmosis to prevent transmission to the fetus, and after 17 weeks' gestation, pyrimethamine and sulfadiazine may be used for confirmed fetal infection to reduce the risk of transmission or complications in the child. However, a recent systematic review of randomized trials of antiparasitic treatment of toxoplamosis in pregnancy concluded that there was still insufficient evidence available to determine whether such treatment has a positive effect on clinical outcomes or risk of transmission.[499]

Chemoprophylaxis to prevent reactivation of toxoplasmosis should be considered in the significantly immunosuppressed child with HIV infection or prior to heart transplantation.

PROTOZOAL INFECTIONS: GIARDIASIS

The enteric protozoan *Giardia* is a major cause of diarrheal disease of humans and other animals including dogs and cats. Although frequently referred to as *Giardia lamblia* in the medical literature, this has no taxonomic validity. *Giardia duodenalis* is the species affecting most mammals including humans, companion animals and food animals.[500] Other recognized species are *G. agilis* in amphibians, *G. muris* in rodents, and *G. psittaci* and *G. ardae* in birds. The vegetative form of *G. duodenalis* or trophozoite is a pear-shaped flagellate protozoan 12–15 μm long and 5–9 μm wide (Fig. 26.41). It has two nuclei and four symmetrically arranged flagella originating from basal bodies at the anterior poles of the nuclei. The concave ventral surface has a ventral disc composed of microtubules, which are used by the protozoan for attachment to intestinal cells. The trophozoites are unusual among eukaryotes in having only a few rudimentary intracellular organelles.[501] The infective form is the cyst which is excreted in feces. It can survive water chlorination and for months in cold fresh water. The cysts are quadrinucleate, ovoid and 7–10 μm in length. The genome is small and consists of approximately 12 million base pairs on five chromosomes encoding an estimated 5000 genes.

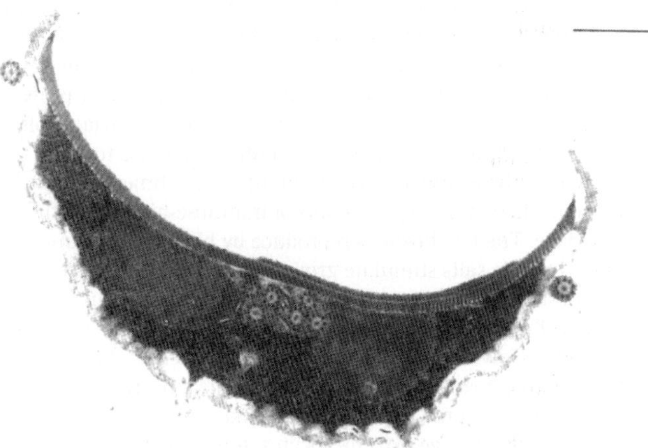

Fig. 26.41 Thin section electron micrograph of *Giardia duodenalis* showing the ventral disc and flagella in cross-sections.

EPIDEMIOLOGY

Giardiasis has a worldwide distribution and it is estimated that some 200 million people in Africa, Asia and Latin America have symptomatic infection and there are approximately 500 000 new cases each year.[502] It is an important cause of traveler's diarrhea and there is an increasing incidence of outbreaks in day care centers and crèches. Spread is fecal–oral especially when hygiene is poor. Waterborne spread is increasingly important and, since a number of animal species can harbor *G. duodenalis*, a proportion of cases could be zoonotic.[503] Cyst concentrations excreted in feces are 150–20 000/g but in contrast the infective dose is 10–100 cysts.

The impact of giardiasis is greatest in children, but prevalence rates are significantly higher in developing (20–30%) compared to industrialized (2–5%) countries. Recurrent and prolonged infections are not uncommon and some children may excrete cysts for long periods asymptomatically. Patients with hypo- or agammaglobulinemia are at particular risk of chronic giardiasis but HIV and AIDS do not apparently increase the risk greatly.

Recently it has been shown that strains infecting humans can be subdivided on the basis of 18S rRNA gene sequences into two major groups. These are called assemblages A and B and there are clusters of genotypes within the two assemblages.[500] Not only are these subdivisions useful for epidemiological purposes, but it also appears that assemblage A isolates tend to be associated with intermittent diarrhea and assemblage B with more severe persistent diarrhea.[504]

PATHOLOGY AND PATHOGENESIS

Histological changes in duodenal biopsies from cases of symptomatic giardiasis vary from entirely normal through partial, subtotal and total villous atrophy. Approximately 20–25% of patients will have normal villous architecture and less than 10% subtotal villous atrophy.[505] On electron microscopic examination there can be shortening and disruption of microvilli even in biopsies appearing normal on light microscopy.

Following ingestion, cysts are excysted by the sequential exposure to low pH in the stomach and higher pH in the duodenum, which activates giardial proteases.[506] Interestingly the newly excysted protozoa express different surface antigens (variant surface proteins, VSP) to those expressed by the trophozoite before it was encysted. The trophozoites then can be found free in the small intesinal lumen (here motility by flagella is important to prevent flushing out) and closely apposed to the enterocyte surface, often embedded in mucin. Most often their ventral surface is towards the enterocyte surface and it is thought that attachment is by the ventral disc; however they also have a mannose-binding lectin on their surface. The trophozoites reproduce by binary fission and it is thought that bile salts stimulate growth. Trophozoites encyst in the small intestine when they are at high cell densities and this is stimulated by high bile salt concentrations, lipid metabolites and neutral pH. How diarrhea is induced is not clear. Suggestions include the trophozoites acting as a mechanical barrier to prevent nutrient absorption (which is unlikely), structural and ultrastructural damage to enterocytes and malabsorption. The latter might result from small intestinal bacterial overgrowth, removal and use of bile salts by trophozoites and inhibition of intestinal proteases and lipases.

CLINICAL FEATURES

There are three clinical forms of giardiasis:

1. asymptomatic excretion of cysts;
2. acute diarrheal disease which is usually short and self-limited;
3. chronic diarrhea with malabsorption, weight loss and failure to thrive.

The asymptomatic carrier state can occur in children or adults but whether carriage follows symptomatic infection or carriage occurs with no prior disease is unclear. There is no information on whether the asymptomatic carrier has subclinical enteropathy. However it is clear that carriers can act as a reservoir of infection for others.

Acute giardiasis follows an incubation period of 3–20 days (mean 7 days) and the illness lasts 2–4 weeks, but can last as long as 7 weeks. Diarrhea (in over 90%) is the major feature and weight loss occurs in 60–70%. Other features are abdominal discomfort, flatulence, nausea and vomiting (in 30%). Approximately half the patients will have signs of steatorrhea. In patients with cystic fibrosis, giardiasis may worsen the malabsorption of fat and fat soluble vitamins.

A proportion of those with acute giardiasis (estimated to be about 30%) go on to develop chronic diarrhea most often with steatorrhea. Weight loss can be great with fat malabsorption in about 50%. In infants and young children this can cause failure to thrive. In some cases malabsorption of vitamins such as B_{12} or folate can lead to macrocytic anemia. Secondary lactase deficiency may occur and does not necessarily resolve with successful therapy.

DIAGNOSIS AND DIFFERENTIAL DIAGNOSIS

Giardiasis should be considered in cases of acute or chronic diarrhea. Specific diagnosis is by detection of the protozoan, its antigens or genome either in stool or duodenal fluid obtained by endoscopy, a nasoduodenal tube or a weighted nylon thread ('string-test'). Stool is the most appropriate specimen but more invasive specimen collection is indicated when there is a high index of clinical suspicion, but stool samples are repeatedly negative. Although trophozoites are shed in the initial phase of acute diarrhea, giardiasis is most often confirmed by detection of cysts on microscopy of wet-mount or formalin–ethylacetate concentrated stool samples. A single stool sample will detect giardiasis in 70% of cases and examination of three samples on separate days will detect it in 85%. The sensitivity of microscopy can be increased by using antigiardia fluorescent labeled antibody (direct immunofluorescence). In general antigen detection by ELISA is more efficient and cost effective.[507] There are a number of commercial kits available including one that can simultaneously detect *G. duodenalis*, *Entamoeba histolytica* and *Cryptosporidium parvum*.[508] Diagnosis by genome detection for example by PCR is at present experimental.

TREATMENT

There is no evidence of benefit in treating asymptomatic infection. At least five classes of drugs: nitroimidazoles (metronidazole, tinidazole), benzimidazoles (albendazole), acridine dyes (mepacrine), nitrofurans (furazolidine) and nitazoxanide are used for treating symptomatic giardiasis. A recent systematic review has concluded that drug treatment was associated with an improved cure rate (odds ratio 11.5; 98% confidence interval 2.3–58). Of the longer course regimens, metronidazole was the most effective (OR 2.4; 95% CI 1.2–4.4) with a smaller relapse rate. Of the single dose regimens, tinidazole which has a longer serum half-life than metronidazole was best.[509] Unfortunately there are few trials in children. The generally accepted regimen in children is metronidazole 15 mg/kg/day in three doses for 7–10 days. Mepacrine may be used as second line therapy (50 mg twice daily for children 1–5 years and 100 mg twice daily for children 5–10 years). Its use is limited by its bitter taste and induction of vomiting. In the USA furazolidine is preferred (metronidazole and tinidazole are not licensed for giardiasis). It comes as a suspension but is given four times daily (6 mg/kg/day) for 7–10 days and has a lesser efficacy than metronidazole.

CONTROL MEASURES

In nurseries, crèches and child care centers, personal hygiene should be emphasized. Hand washing by staff and children should be stressed especially after toileting and nappy changing. In outbreaks, attempts should be made to identify and treat all of those with symptomatic giardiasis. Those with symptomatic giardiasis should be excluded from work or nurseries until the diarrhea ceases. Although such infection control measures will decrease transmission, it must be remembered that routes other than direct person to person (e.g. waterborne, zoonotic) are possible. Recently, a vaccine has been licensed for the prevention of giardiasis in dogs and cats.[510] The vaccine which is made from killed whole trophozoite preparations proved highly effective. This could be of benefit to humans, firstly in decreasing an animal reservoir for zoonotic transfer and secondly by paving the way for a human vaccine.

PROGNOSIS

The prognosis is excellent except in immunocompromised children where relapse is common and treatment may need to be continued for prolonged periods. At the same time attention must be paid to adequate nutrition and the treatment of concurrent infections.

PROTOZOAL INFECTIONS: AMEBIC INFECTIONS

Amebae are characterized by two forms, the motile, feeding trophozoite and the cyst. The cyst has a rigid wall, resistant to environmental conditions, which allows it to survive for variable periods without feeding. The major ameba of importance to man is *Entamoeba histolytica*, which is anaerobic and an obligate parasite of the gut. It has to be differentiated from other non-pathogenic gut amebae, e.g. *E. dispar, E. coli* and *E. hartmanni*. There are a number of free-living aerobic amebae, which are found in the soil and feed on bacteria in muddy water. In dry conditions the cysts may be dispersed by wind. Species that are pathogenic to man and may cause meningoencephalitis are *Naegleria fowleri* and the opportunist *Acanthamoeba culbertsoni* and *Balamuthia mandrillaris*.

AMEBIASIS

Amebiasis is caused by *E. histolytica* and is transmitted by the fecal–oral route. Sewage contamination of water supplies, infection by food handlers and direct fecal contact from person to person, as may occur in mental institutions, have been identified as sources of infection. Transmission by sexual contact, especially among homosexuals, also occurs. It is worldwide in distribution, with a high prevalence in tropical countries where hygiene is poor.

E. histolytica cannot be differentiated from the morphologically identical but non-pathogenic *E. dispar*, except by using special methods including culture characteristics, isoenzyme analysis and molecular techniques, such as PCR. Recently introduced stool antigen tests may also differentiate the two amebae.[511] *E. histolytica* trophozoites characteristically demonstrate active erythrophagocytosis. *E. dispar* is more prevalent than *E. histolytica* and is most likely to be the species when 'amebic cysts' are detected in stools of asymptomatic subjects in any part of the world.

Why *E. histolytica* is activated to invade is not known. Malnutrition, pregnancy, ulcerative colitis, immunosuppression, corticosteroids, and intercurrent infection by bacteria or parasites may be precipitating factors. Inflammatory bowel disease should not be treated with corticosteroids until amebiasis has been excluded.

The majority of amebae detected in carriers in non-endemic areas are non-invasive and are probably *E. dispar*. The incidence of disease does not necessarily correlate with prevalence of infection. Invasive disease is reported, particularly from south-east Asia, Natal (South Africa), the west coast of Africa, Mexico and parts of South America. In the USA, infection is associated especially with children of Hispanic origin.

Rarely, amebic colitis or liver abscess may present within the neonatal period.

PATHOGENESIS AND PATHOLOGY

Infection occurs from ingestion of cysts, which, on digestion, release trophozoites in the intestine. The trophozoites feed on bacteria and fecal matter in the cecum and further down the colon. When they reach areas where the feces are more solid, they encyst and the cysts are passed in the stool. Trophozoites may be detected in the stool if there is no intestinal hurry, but the presence of either trophozoites or cysts is not necessarily indicative of invasive disease. However, the presence of hematophagous trophozoites (containing ingested red blood cells) is usually suggestive of invasion. Invasion is accomplished by lytic enzymes secreted by the trophozoites which result in tissue necrosis and erosion of blood vessels, but with a surprising lack of inflammatory response. Initial lesions are small superficial erosions. With progression, they penetrate the muscularis mucosae and may expand to produce flask-shaped ulcers. Further extension may result in intestinal perforation, but more commonly the parasite is carried to the liver in the portal vein, and rarely to other organs such as the lung, heart or brain. The colonic lesions may vary from small pinhead erosions confined to the cecum and rectosigmoid to extensive, deep, confluent ulcers extending throughout the colon. It is probable that the majority of amebae reaching the liver do not cause detectable disease. Possibly, an area of tissue necrosis is necessary for the disease to be established. As in the bowel, liver abscess is characterized by localized necrosis without much inflammatory response unless there is secondary infection.

CLINICAL FEATURES

The major organs affected in invasive amebic disease are the colon, the liver and adjacent organs, such as the right lung, pericardium and rarely the skin or eye.

Intestinal amebiasis

Intestinal amebiasis has a wide spectrum of severity. It may occur within a few weeks of infection or be delayed several months. There may be mild, intermittent diarrhea with blood and mucus accompanying the fecal material, usually with no systemic upset or fever. Severe, fulminating dysentery is associated with watery, bloodstained, mucoid stools resulting in dehydration, electrolyte disturbance and toxemia. Abdominal pain, tenesmus and tenderness may be present. Perforation, which is often multiple with slow leakage, and peritonitis may occur. Other complications include hemorrhage, ameboma, stricture, intussusception and rectal prolapse. Chronic or relapsing dysentery may occur unless the initial attack has been managed by adequate chemotherapy and nutritional support. Ameboma is a complication of previous amebic dysentery and presents as a tender mass in the cecum or colon.

Enlargement of the liver may occur without evidence of an abscess, presumably the result of toxic products transported in the portal vein from the diseased bowel.

Liver abscess and related disorders

Liver abscesses may be single or multiple and more often involve the right lobe. Multiple abscesses are common in young children (Fig. 26.42). The liver is tender and, if the abscess is situated anteriorly, a mass is commonly visible (Fig. 26.43). There is nearly always fever and usually anemia, leukocytosis and raised erythrocyte sedimentation rate (ESR). Jaundice is infrequent and serum transaminases are usually not raised. There is a history of previous, or evidence of concomitant, dysentery in only half the cases. In over two-thirds of cases elevation and immobility of the right diaphragm produces corresponding signs in the right lung.

Complications of amebic liver abscess include secondary bacterial infection, extension or rupture into the peritoneal cavity,

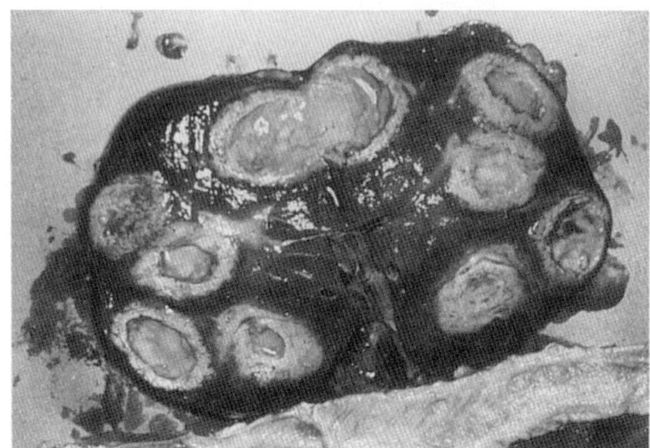

Fig. 26.42 Typical multiple amebic abscesses in the liver of an infant aged 8 months.

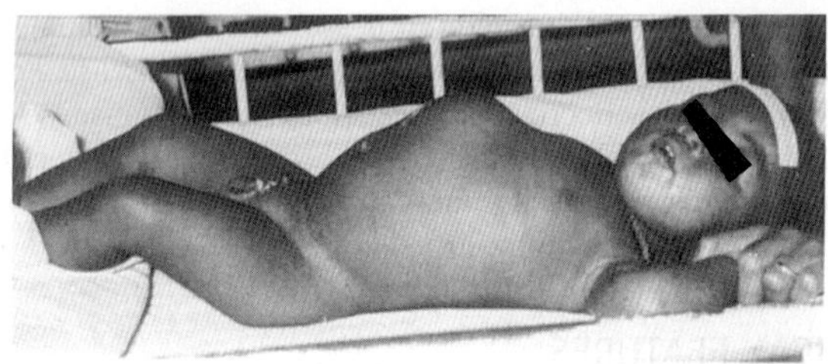

Fig. 26.43 An African infant of 10 months with a large amebic liver abscess presenting as a fluctuant mass in the epigastrium.

the pleural cavity and/or the lung. Involvement of the left lobe of the liver may result in a pericardial effusion or rupture into the pericardium. Rarely, there may be extension to abdominal organs including the stomach, gut or kidneys. Blood-borne spread may result in a brain or lung abscess.

Skin

Cutaneous amebiasis may be associated with rupture of a liver abscess, colostomy stomata or a laparotomy incision. In infants, amebic abscess of the perineum may result from direct contact with infected feces (Fig. 26.44).

DIAGNOSIS

The diagnosis of amebic dysentery is based on the finding of motile, hematophagous *E. histolytica* trophozoites in feces. Red cells, bacteria but few leukocytes are usually present. Examination of a freshly passed warm stool is important because, when the stool cools, the amebae stop moving and release the contained red cells in their vacuoles. Three or more stool examinations may be necessary and both direct and concentrated methods should be used. *E. histolytica* stool antigen test is more sensitive than microscopy. Endoscopy may demonstrate amebic ulcers, which are usually shallow, covered with a yellowish-gray exudate and contain numerous hematophagous trophozoites. Biopsy should be taken from the edge of the ulcer. The intervening mucosa is often relatively normal in appearance. Serum antibody titers may be raised in two-thirds of cases. In endemic areas, positive serology is suggestive in young children, but in older children does not distinguish between past and current infection.

The definitive diagnosis of amebic liver abscess is made by aspiration of bacteriologically sterile pus. The pus is usually gray–yellow at the first aspiration and only at subsequent aspirations takes on the pink or red–brown 'anchovy-paste' color. Amebae are seldom detected in necrotic material from the center of the abscess, but are more common in the walls of the cavity and thus are more likely to be detected in the last portions of the aspirate.

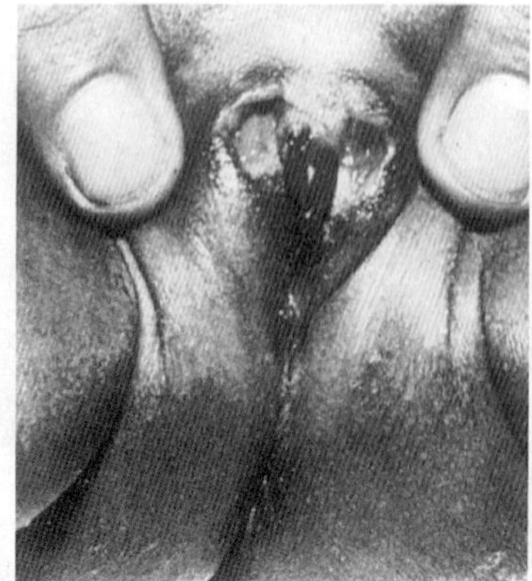

Fig. 26.44 Cutaneous amebiasis involving the vulva in an infant aged 5 months.

In most cases an ultrasound scan can localize and delineate the size of the abscess cavity. Ultrasound, CT and magnetic resonance have equal sensitivity in detecting amebic abscesses. Differential diagnosis includes pyogenic liver abscess, subphrenic abscess and hydatid disease. X-ray and screening may demonstrate a raised diaphragm with reduced movement and there may be an effusion or other signs of inflammation at the lung base. Usually there is a leukocytosis and a raised ESR. Antibody titers are usually high and may be detected in serum in over 95% of cases. A number of different methods are used including indirect hemagglutination, agar gel diffusion, fluorescent antibody test, counterimmunoelectrophoresis and ELISA. ELISA has high sensitivity and specificity and usually becomes negative 6–12 months after response to treatment, whereas indirect hemagglutination titers may remain raised for many years. For unknown reasons, infection is only detected in the stool in about one-third of cases, and usually only cysts are present.

MANAGEMENT

Chemotherapy of invasive amebiasis must include drugs, which can eliminate amebae both from the lumen of the bowel and the tissues. Metronidazole and tinidazole achieve both but are less effective as lumenal amebicides.

For asymptomatic patients, and following invasive disease, the lumenal amebicide diloxanide furoate 20 mg/kg/day in three divided doses for 10 days, is the treatment of choice. In endemic areas, older asymptomatic children are usually not treated, as reinfection is so common.

In symptomatic intestinal disease, metronidazole or tinidazole is recommended. Metronidazole 35–50 mg/kg/day in three divided doses orally is given for 5–10 days depending on the severity of the infection. Side-effects such as nausea and a metallic taste in the mouth may make compliance difficult. Alternatively, oral tinidazole 50–60 mg/kg is given as a single daily dose for 5 days. Both drugs may also be given intravenously. In severe colitis, correction of fluid and electrolyte imbalance is important, and gastric suction is necessary when there is ileus. Blood transfusion may be required. Broad spectrum antibiotics may be necessary if septicemia or other infection is suspected. Perforation of the bowel with leakage into the peritoneum may require surgery.

For liver abscess, metronidazole or tinidazole is usually effective and is given in doses similar to intestinal disease. In difficult cases, chloroquine 10 mg/kg/day in two divided doses may be added and given for 3 weeks. Diloxanide furoate should be given to eradicate the bowel infection.

Indications for aspiration of the abscess include: suspected pyogenic abscess (particularly when there are multiple lesions), a palpable mass, a markedly raised diaphragm, failure of symptoms to remit after 72 h of drug therapy, and abscess in the left lobe. Aspiration, by relieving the pressure within the liver tissues, allows better drug penetration of the abscess. Surgical evacuation may be necessary for multiple or inaccessible abscesses, or when secondary infection has occurred. For needle aspiration, a wide-bore needle with a three-way tap should be used and the abscess cavity evacuated fully. Aspiration is usually through the right chest wall at the point of maximum tenderness, or through the abdomen if the abscess is superficial. Aspiration should be guided by ultrasound scan. If repeat aspiration is required, or in the case of drug resistance, percutaneous catheter drainage for 24–48 h may be undertaken.[512]

Resolution of the abscess cavity may take many months. Follow-up should be arranged to ensure complete eradication of infection, otherwise relapse may occur.

Intrathoracic and intraperitoneal rupture of amebic liver abscesses usually respond to standard antiamebic chemotherapy.

NAEGLERIA AND *ACANTHAMOEBA*

Two distinct types of meningoencephalitis are caused by free-living amebae: primary amebic meningoencephalitis by *Naegleria fowleri* and granulomatous amebic encephalitis, usually by *Acanthamoeba culbertsoni* or the recently recognized *Balamuthia mandrillaris*.[513,514] *Acanthamoeba* infections of the cornea particularly associated with contact lenses are an increasing problem.

PRIMARY AMEBIC MENINGOENCEPHALITIS

This is an acute necrotizing meningoencephalitis, caused by *N. fowleri*, which gains access to the nasal cavities and results in direct invasion of the nervous system through the olfactory apparatus. There is usually a history of swimming under water or diving in warm fresh water or hot springs. In Nigeria, there are reports of infection from cysts, transmitted in dust, colonizing the nasal cavities of children.[515] The cerebrospinal fluid (CSF) has changes similar to bacterial meningitis, viz. a predominant neutrophil count, often accompanied by red cells, a raised protein (usually > 1 g/L) and low glucose concentration. Careful search for trophozoites should be undertaken on fresh CSF. Nasal secretions or washings should also be examined for amebae.

The course of the disease is usually rapidly fulminating within 3–6 days. Intravenous and intraventricular (through a reservoir) amphotericin is the main treatment. In addition miconazole is usually given by the intravenous and intrathecal route and rifampicin orally. Duration of therapy is 8–10 days.

GRANULOMATOUS AMEBIC ENCEPHALITIS

This is a slowly progressive disease, occurring usually in immunocompromised individuals. Sometimes no demonstrable defect may be apparent.[516] Infection by acanthamebae may result from swallowing or inhaling cysts, or by direct skin or corneal contact. The CSF shows a lymphocytosis, a raised protein and low or normal glucose. Acanthamoeba may be detected in histological specimens. Sometimes the trophozoites may be detected by wet mount of CSF and subsequently cultured. Serology may also be of value.

Severe brain damage may have occurred by the time the diagnosis is made. Suggested drugs for treatment include polymyxin B, pentamidine isetionate, co-trimoxazole, ketoconazole and flucytosine.

Successful outcome is more likely in immunocompetent children.

ACANTHAMOEBA KERATITIS

Most cases of acanthamoeba keratitis are associated with use of contact lenses, owing to a combination of abrasions of the cornea and contamination of the lens from washing in homemade solutions, especially fresh or tap water.

Treatment is difficult and often involves keratoplasty. Local application of 0.1% propamidine isetionate solution, 0.15% dibrompropamidine ointment and neomycin have been used. Local 1% clotrimazole may also be of value. Corticosteroids are required to control inflammation. Only fresh, sterile, commercial solutions should be used to clean contact lenses.

BALANTIDIASIS

Balantidium coli is a parasite of pigs, which may colonize the colon of man producing a disease similar to *E. histolytica*, but extracolonic disease does not occur. Treatment is with metronidazole or tetracycline for 8–10 days.

FUNGAL INFECTIONS

Fungi form a large and very diverse kingdom but only a small number are pathogenic for humans. Fungi are eukaryotes, that is, unlike bacteria, they have a nucleus and intracellular organelles. They also possess a cell wall composed of chitin. Infections are conveniently divided into superficial, subcutaneous and systemic or deep mycoses. In addition, there are an increasing number of opportunist fungi, which cause infection in immunocompromised children (Table 26.36).

Fungi can grow in a unicellular mode (yeasts) or in a multicellular mode when cells elongate and multiply to form long filaments called hyphae and collectively form a mycelium. Some fungi are dimorphic existing as a yeast at one temperature but forming multicellular hyphae at another. Rather confusingly some are given different names when in the different forms. Thus *Cryptococcus neoformans* is the name as a yeast and *Filobasidiella neoformans* is its hyphal form. *Actinomyces* and *Nocardia* spp. are not fungi but branching bacteria but are more conveniently included in discussions of fungal disease (Table 26.37). Treatment of subcutaneous and systemic mycoses is most often by antifungals such as polyenes (e.g. amphotericin B) or imidazoles (e.g. ketoconazole) (Table 26.37). To prevent repetition, information on dosage, mode of administration and side-effects and toxicity is included at the end of the chapter.

ACTINOMYCOSIS

ETIOLOGY

Actinomycosis is an infection with a worldwide distribution that affects humans and other animals such as cattle and canines. *Actinomyces* spp. are Gram positive, non-spore bearing, short or filamentous bacilli, which may exhibit true branching. Although *Aspergillus israelii* is the major pathogen, other species including *Actinomyces gerencserai*, *A. meyeri*, *A. naeslundii*, *A. odontolyticus*, *A. pyogenes*, *A. radicidentis* and *A. viscosus* do cause human infection. *Actinomyces* spp. can be found as commensals in the oral cavity, gastrointestinal tract and female genital tract.

PATHOGENESIS

Actinomyces spp. are incapable of invading normal tissues and thus require trauma to the mucous surface to initiate disease. This can result from mechanical (accidental or surgical) trauma, primary bacterial or viral infection or malignancy. In addition, this damage will produce injury that renders the tissue anaerobic which facilitates growth of the bacterium. Little is known of virulence determinants of *Actinomyces* spp. and for example, toxins have not

Table 26.36 Medically important fungi

Superficial mycoses		
	Dermatophytes (tinea capitis, tinea cruris, tinea pedis, tinea unguium, endothrix, ringworm)	*Epidermophyton floccosum* *Microsporum audouinii* (*M. gryseum*, *M. canis*) *Trichophyton rubrum* (*T. mentagrophytes*, *T. verrucosum*, *T. terrestre*, *T. violaceum*, *T. schoenleinii*, *T. tonsurans*)
	Pityriasis versocolor	*Malassezia* (*Pityrosporum*) *furfur*
	Black piedra	*Piedraia hortae*
	Tinea nigra	*Cladosporium werneckii*
	Candiosis (Mucous membrane)	*Candida albicans* (*C. tropicalis*, *C. parapsilosis*)
Subcutaneous mycoses		
	Sporotrichosis	*Sporothrix schenckii*
	Chromomycosis	*Phialophora verrucosa*, *Phialophora (Fonsecaea) pedrosoi*, *Cladosporium carrionii*
	Mycetoma	*Actinomadura madurae*, *Nocardia asteroides*, *N. brasiliensis*, *Streptomyces somaliensis*
	Rhinosporidiosis	*Rhinosporidium seeberi*
	Zygomycosis	*Basidiobolus haptosporus* *Conidiobolus coronatus*
Systemic mycoses		
	Histoplasmosis	*Histoplasma capsulatum*
	Cryptococcosis	*Cryptococcus neoformans*
	Blastomycosis	*Blastomyces dermatitidis*
	Coccidioidomycosis	*Coccidioides immitis*
	Paracoccidioidomycosis	*Paracoccidioides brasiliensis*
	Penicilliosis	*Penicillium marneffei*
Opportunist pathogens		
	Aspergillosis	*Aspergillus fumigatus*
	Candidosis	*Candida albicans* and other species
	Mucormycosis	*Mucor* spp.
	Pneumocystosis	*Pneumocystis carinii*

been detected. The commonest sites of actinomycosis are the cervicofacial region (60% of cases), abdomen (25%) and lungs (15%). In addition *A. naeslundii* and *A. viscosus* are associated with periodontal disease and *A. radicidentis* with dental radiculitis. In actinomycosis there is a dense cellular infiltrate with abscess and sinus formation. The small yellow particles (sulfur granules), characteristic of actinomycosis occur especially with infection due to *A. israelii*.

CLINICAL FEATURES

Actinomycosis is uncommon in children but a case series has been reported.[517] Cervicofacial actinomycosis presents as an indurated swelling in the mandibular region. Subsequently one or more sinuses develop. Less commonly, the tongue, pharynx, lacrimal glands or bone can be affected. Regional lymph nodes tend not to be affected. Local spread to cause brain or spinal cord abscesses has been reported. In these cases there is usually a mixed bacterial population.

Thoracic actinomycosis can occur by aspiration of oral bacteria, hematogenous spread, or local spread from cervical or abdominal lesions. Thus the initial focus can be in the bronchial tree or lung parenchyma. Subsequently multiple abscesses develop which form sinuses that traverse the chest wall. The main clinical features are chest pain, fever, productive cough and weight loss. Abdominal actinomycosis presents as fever with neutrophilia, and chronic abdominal pain and an inflammatory mass. Sinus formation is uncommon. Most often abdominal actinomycosis follows a perforated appendix.[518] Pelvic actinomycosis occurs most often in association with intrauterine contraceptive devices (the coil), and is thus very uncommon in children. Disseminated actinomycosis is uncommon in pediatric practice but has been reported.[519]

DIAGNOSIS AND DIFFERENTIAL DIAGNOSIS

Cervicofacial actinomysosis is part of the differential diagnosis of an indurated swelling of the mandibular region, especially if there is sinus formation. Specific diagnosis is by bacteriological culture of

Table 26.37 Subcutaneous and systemic mycoses

Disease	Causative organism	Geographical distribution	Predominant clinical features	Treatment
Actinomycosis	*Actinomyces israelii*	Worldwide	Abscesses and sinuses in face and neck, lungs, abdomen	Benzyl penicillin
Aspergillosis	*Aspergillus* species	Worldwide	Granulomata of lungs, skin or generalized, aspergilloma	Nystatin aerosol, i.v. amphotericin B or oral itraconazole or ketoconazole
North American blastomycosis	*Blastomyces dermatitidis*	North America	Granulomata of lungs or generalized	i.v. amphotericin B or oral itraconazole or ketoconazole
South American blastomycosis	*Paracoccidioides brasiliensis*	South America	Ulcerating granulomata of oropharynx, lungs or generalized	i.v. amphotericin B or oral itraconazole or ketoconazole
Chromoblastomycosis	*Cladosporium werneckii* *Fonsecaea compacta* *F. pedrosoi* *Phialophora verrucosa* *Rhinocladiella aquaspersa*	Tropics	Nodular, verrucose, tumors, plaque or cicatricial lesions of skin and deeper tissues	Surgery and i.v. amphotericin B, with 5-flucytosine, itraconazole or ketoconazole but mixed results
Coccidioidomycosis (San Joaquin Valley fever)	*Coccidioides immitis*	North and South America	Influenza-like illness. Progressive pulmonary or central nervous system infection in minority	i.v. amphotericin B or 5-flucytosine or i.v. miconazole or oral itraconazole
Cryptococcosis (torulosis)	*Cryptococcus neoformans*	Worldwide	Chiefly central nervous system infection, meningoencephalitis, or focal lesion but can cause pneumonia	i.v. amphotericin B or oral fluconazole
Histoplasmosis	*Histoplasma capsulatum*	Central USA	Granulomata in lungs, or in miliary distribution	i.v. amphotericin B or oral itraconazole or fluconazole
Moniliasis	*Candida* sp. usually *C. albicans*	Worldwide	Usually superficial infection. Systemic resembles septicemic illness	i.v. amphotericin B with or without 5-flucytosine or oral fluconazole
Mycetoma (Madura foot, maduromycosis)	Actinomycetoma *Actinomadura madurae* *A. pellotieri* *Nocardia brasiliensis* *N. madurae* *Streptomyces somaliensis* Eumycetoma *Madurella grisea* *M. mycetomatis* *Pseudallescheria boydii*	Tropics	Localized chronic infection involving skin, subcutaneous tissue and bone (nodule, sinuses and discharge) poor results)	Surgery (removal of lesions, amputation). Actinomycetoma: dapsone plus streptomycin, Eumycetoma: griseofulvin or imidazoles plus penicillin (but
Mucomycosis	*Mincor* spp. *Absidia corymbifera* *Rhizomusco* spp. *Rhizopus* spp.	Worldwide	Rhinocerebral, rhino-orbital, cardiac involvement, pulmonary, gastrointestinal, skin and soft tissue, bone involvement	i.v. amphotericin
Nocardiosis	*Nocardia asteroides* or *N. brasiliensis*	Worldwide	Pulmonary suppuration, occasionally central nervous system infection	Sulfonamides
Penicilliosis	*Penicillium marneffei*	South-east Asia	Generalized infection especially in immune compromised patients with skin, bone, liver, spleen and lung involvement	i.v. amphotericin and oral itraconazole
Pneumocystosis	*Pneumocystis carinii*	Worldwide	Acute or subacute pneumonia in children immunocompromised by HIV, malnutrition or cytotoxic drugs	Oral co-trimoxazole, nebulized pentamidine
Rhinosporidiosis	*Rhinosporidium seeberi*	India and Ceylon	Polypoid tumors of mucous membrane – nose, nasopharnx, conjunctival sac. Gelatinous lesions, bleeding easily. Diagnosis by microscopic examination of crushed fragments of polyp. Pulmonary and nasopalatal types with tissues destruction may occur in the patients subject to severe metabolic disturbance	Surgical removal

(Cont'd)

Table 26.37 *Cont'd*

Disease	Causative organism	Geographical distribution	Predominant clinical features	Treatment
Sporotrichosis	*Sporothrix schenckii*	Worldwide	Subcutaneous nodule (usually on hands or feet) which enlarges and adheres to skin and breaks down to form chronic ulcer. Satellite nodules develop by lymphatic spread. Usually localized but may be widely disseminated. Diagnosis by culture of exudates or scrapings or antibody tests. Extracutaneous forms involving muscles, lungs eyes, CNS, urinary tract and wide dissemination may occur	For lymphangitic form, potassium iodide 30 mg/kg/day up to maximum tolerance. For disseminated form i.v. amphotericin B or oral itraconzole

aspirated pus, sinus discharge, biopsy tissue or fine needle aspirations but care must be taken to avoid contamination by commensal bacteria. Cultures should be kept anaerobically at 35–37°C for up to 14 days. More rapid diagnosis can be obtained by examination of crushed sulfur granules stained by Gram stain where filamentous, branching or beaded Gram positive bacteria will be seen. It must be distinguished from other chronic suppurative lesions of the cervical region including chronic pyogenic osteomyelitis and tuberculosis. Thoracic actinomycosis may be confused with other chronic lung infection including bronchiectasis and pulmonary tuberculosis.[520] Culture of sputum, bronchial aspirates or biopsy material will confirm the diagnosis.

The mass of abdominal actinomycosis can mimic an appendix abscess, abdominal tuberculosis or intra-abdominal carcinoma.[519] Laparotomy with culture of pus or biopsy material will be necessary to establish the diagnosis. Serological diagnosis is unreliable.

TREATMENT AND PROGNOSIS

Benzyl penicillin is the treatment of choice. It is given in high doses, 1–6 mega units daily intravenously for 2 weeks at least, then orally for 6–8 months. This may be accompanied wherever possible with surgical drainage. For penicillin-allergic patients tetracycline and perhaps ciprofloxacin can be tried. The prognosis is generally good although thoracic actinomycosis in particular, may require even more prolonged and energetic treatment.

ASPERGILLOSIS

ETIOLOGY

Aspergillosis is a fungal infection with a worldwide distribution. There are over 90 *Aspergillus* species described and 19 have been associated with human disease. However, most infections are due to *Aspergillus fumigatus, A. flavus* and to a lesser extent *A. niger. Aspergillus* spp. are widely distributed in the environment and some cause infection in other animals. It is a member of the Eumycetes (true fungi) and produces a mycelium with a fruiting body, the conidium, from which spores are released into the atmosphere. The spores can be found in air sampled anywhere on earth.

EPIDEMIOLOGY AND PATHOGENESIS

Most disease manifestations involve the lung. In general, community-acquired disease tends to be non-invasive aspergillosis and hospital-acquired disease either non-invasive or invasive aspergillosis. In addition mycotoxins such as aflatoxin may contaminate cereals, groundnuts and other foods. Aflatoxin is a potent carcinogen but its role in human disease remains to be clarified. The non-invasive manifestations of aspergillosis are extrinsic allergic alveolitis (EAA), allergic bronchopulmonary aspergillosis (ABPA) and aspergilloma. In the former two, disease results from an allergic response to *Aspergillus* spp., a type III hypersensitivity response in EAA and type I in ABPA. An aspergilloma is a fungal mycelial ball that develops in a pre-existing lung cavity. In each case, the fungus is acquired by inhalation. Invasive pulmonary aspergillosis occurs in those immunocompromised by radiation, steroids or chemotherapy, especially if there is neutropenia. An increase in numbers of cases is often preceded by building work in, or in the vicinity, of the hospital, as this increases atmospheric contamination by aspergillus spores. Dissemination from invasive pulmonary aspergillosis can occur and can result in metastatic foci in most organs of the body.

CLINICAL FEATURES AND DIAGNOSIS

ABPA in pediatric practice is particularly associated with patients with cystic fibrosis, but may also occur in asthmatics. It presents insidiously with worsening bronchospasm and less commonly low grade fever. Up to two-thirds of patients expectorate brownish sputum, which contains aspergilli. Eight diagnostic criteria, (aspergillus precipitins, aspergillus specific IgE, chest radiographic infiltrates, blood eosinophilia > 500 mm^{-3}, *A. fumigatus* skin test, total serum IgE > 1000 ng/ml, bronchiectasis, cough and wheeze) are widely used,[521] but must be applied regularly to be of benefit.[522]

Invasive pulmonary aspergillosis occurs most often in the settling of relapse of the underlying condition or post bone marrow transplant[523] and presents with unremitting fever, new pulmonary infiltrates, dyspnea and unproductive cough. These together with hemoptysis and tachycardia can mimic pulmonary embolus. Massive hemoptysis is rare. Radiographic changes are variable, but most often, patchy bronchopneumonic infiltrates or nodular densities are seen. After 2–3 weeks cavitation may occur. Dissemination is clinically indistinguishable from bacterial septicemia in immunocompromised patients. The presentation of metastatic disease, which can occur almost anywhere, will depend on the site of infection. Specific diagnosis depends upon culture of aspergilli from the infective site but blood cultures are very rarely, if ever, positive. Since aspergilli are so frequently present in the environment it is also necessary to demonstrate tissue invasion by histological examination.

TREATMENT, PROGNOSIS AND PREVENTION

Allergic bronchopulmonary aspergillosis requires early therapy with oral corticosteroids and addition of high dose inhaled steroids may be of benefit. Recurrence is common. The natural history of aspergillosis is variable but only a minority resolve spontaneously. If there is evidence of some pulmonary invasion from the aspergilloma, antifungal therapy with amphotericin B or oral itraconazole may be beneficial. Surgical removal is necessary for example, if there is life-threatening hemoptysis; however, this does carry a risk of inoculating fungi into the field of surgery.

For invasive pulmonary or other aspergillosis surgical drainage, debridement or resection are most important with antifungal therapy acting as an adjunct. Amphotericin B is the gold standard for therapy, and addition of 5-flucytosine might be of benefit. Itraconazole given orally is licensed for therapy but long term administration will be needed. The prognosis is generally poor but it is difficult to distinguish the relative contributions of the aspergillosis and the underlying condition.

BLASTOMYCOSIS

ETIOLOGY

Blastomyces dermatitidis is a dimorphic fungus. It exists as a yeast in human infection and when cultured at 37°C but in a mycelial form at room temperature or in the environment. Two serotypes and several genotypes have been described. *Paracoccidioides brasiliensis* is also dimorphic. In human lesions, it is found as double-walled ovoid or round yeast 4–40 μm in diameter. In culture at 19–28°C or in the environment it has a mycelial form. Isolates of *P. brasiliensis* vary greatly in their ability to cause disease.

EPIDEMIOLOGY AND PATHOGENESIS

Although sometimes referred to as North American blastomycosis, *B. dermatitidis* infection has been reported in North and South America, Europe, Africa and Asia. Within North America it has been reported from midwest and south east USA and parts of Canada. It appears that the environment along waterways is an important reservoir and infection is probably acquired by inhalation. Humans and other animals can be infected but person-to-person transmission does not occur and children are rarely infected. *P. brasiliensis* infection was originally called hyphblastomycosis but is now known as South American blastomycosis, or, more correctly, paracoccidioidomycosis. It is limited to central and South America from Mexico to Argentina but most (80%) of cases are reported from Brazil. It is found in soil and is thought to be acquired by inhalation. It is rare in women, adolescents and children. Person-to-person transmission does not occur.

CLINICAL FEATURES

It is likely that most infections with *B. dermatitidis* are asymptomatic but, when clinically apparent, can range from acute self-limiting pneumonia to disseminated infection. Occasionally the acute pneumonia does not resolve and chronic pulmonary blastomycosis, which is clinically indistinguishable from pulmonary tuberculosis or histoplasmosis, occurs. Cutaneous lesions are the most frequent manifestations of disseminated infection. These begin as subcutaneous nodules or papules. They then become ulcerated with raised irregular borders and a crusted centre. Histologically these are granulomas.

P. brasiliensis cause a spectrum of disease ranging from acute pulmonary infection with or without mucocutaneous involvement to a progressive disseminated form with involvement of the mucocutaneous tissue, reticuloendothelial system and adrenals. It may also give a miliary appearance in the lung.

DIAGNOSIS AND DIFFERENTIAL DIAGNOSIS

Blastomycosis, although uncommon in children, should be suspected in patients from endemic areas with granulomatous and ulcerating lesions of the skin or mucous membranes especially if it is of long duration or there is involvement of other organs. Acute pulmonary blastomycosis is difficult to diagnose clinically, as it presents as an influenza-like illness or with pleuritic pain. The chronic form is indistinguishable from tuberculosis, histoplasmosis or coccidioidomycosis. Specific diagnosis is by demonstrating the presence of *B. dermatitidis*, by culture of lesions or sputum, and for superficial lesions, biopsy stained by methenamine silver (the yeasts may not stain by hematoxylin and eosin).

Paracoccidioidomycosis has similar differential diagnoses to blastomycosis. Since children may present with an acute or subacute form with large numbers of yeast in the reticuloendothelial system and fungemia, specific diagnosis can also be aided by blood culture.

TREATMENT AND PROGNOSIS

Without treatment the mortality rate of blastomycosis is over 60%. Amphotericin B is the mainstay of therapy but higher doses are needed. Treatment should continue until symptoms resolve and continue for 3–4 months thereafter. Even with this relapses occur in 10–20% of patients (up to 5 years later). Oral ketoconazole or better still itraconoazole appear as effective as amphotericin B but there are no trials directly comparing the regimens. Treatment should continue for at least 6 months. Ketoconazole is effective in 85% of cases of paracoccidioidomycosis and relapse rates are low (0–11%) if therapy is continued for at least 6 months. Itraconazole appears superior to ketoconazole.

CANDIDOSIS

ETIOLOGY AND EPIDEMIOLOGY

There are almost 200 *Candida* species and they have a worldwide distribution. They exist in budding yeast, hyphal or pseudohyphal forms (Fig. 26.45). *Candida albicans* is the commonest species found both as a commensal, particularly in the mouth, rectum, vagina or on skin, and as a pathogen. The others are found less commonly as commensals but *C. glabrata* can be found in the mouth, rectum or vagina and *C. parapsilosis* and *C. tropicalis* on skin. Infections occur particularly in neonates or immune compromised children, especially those with T cell defects.

PATHOGENESIS AND CLINICAL FEATURES

Different *Candida* spp. have differing virulence but *C. albicans* is the most competent pathogen. Virulence factors include adhesins, ability to switch from yeast to hyphal (invasive) forms, production

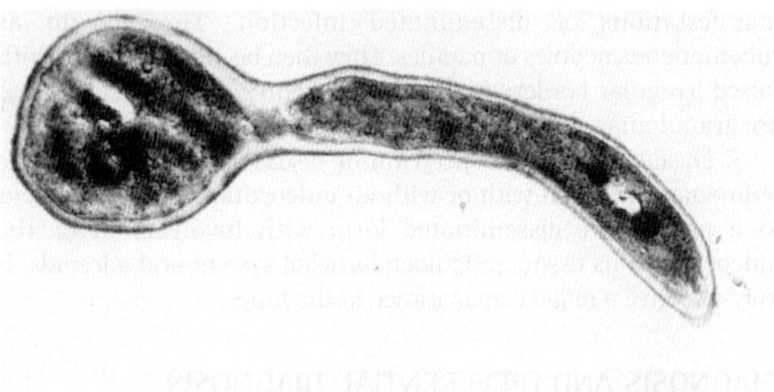

Fig. 26.45 A thin section electron micrograph of *Candida albicans* showing a pseudohypha (bar = 1 μm).

of proteolytic enzymes, antigenic variability and host mimicry. In addition to these however, there need to be breaches in the skin or mucosa, alterations in the normal flora (usually due to antibacterial therapy), or underlying conditions such as immune deficiency (congenital or iatrogenic), diabetes mellitus or implanted devices.

SUPERFICIAL CANDIDOSIS (THRUSH)

Oral thrush typically occurs in neonates with adherent gray–white plaques, which on removal reveal a raw red base. They are usually found on the tongue, gums or gingival mucosa but may extend into the esophagus or trachea, especially in HIV/AIDS. There may also be scaly macular or vesicular erythematous perianal lesions. In skin areas that are moist, occluded, or irradiated candidosis can occur as intensely erythematous intertriginous lesions. These can be papular, plaque-like or confluent with surrounding satellite lesions. Commonly involved sites include the axillae, inguinal regions, perineum and digital web spaces. *Candida* spp. can also cause onychomycosis which, unlike that due to dermatophytes, is painful.

CHRONIC MUCOCUTANEOUS CANDIDOSIS

This includes a heterogeneous group of patients with T cell deficits some of which are highly specific to *Candida* spp. Most cases present in infancy or early childhood with oral thrush or perineal candidosis which may become more widespread or just persist with localized lesions.

DEEPER CANDIDOSIS

Candidal infection of deeper tissues and organs occurs rarely in otherwise healthy patients. Oral or esophageal candidosis may be complicated by extension of infection to the intestine, typically with symptoms of diarrhea, abdominal pain and pruritus ani. The child may present with a celiac-like syndrome. In pulmonary candidosis the symptoms of fever and productive cough sometimes with hemoptysis are non-specific. On radiological examination, patchy consolidation is seen, and cavitation may occur with infections of sufficient duration. Pulmonary candidosis should be not diagnosed too readily on the evidence of culture of *Candida* from sputum, since the organism may be isolated in a proportion of healthy individuals, or particularly from hospital patients.

Disseminated *Candida* infection, although very uncommon in infancy and childhood, is thought to be increasing in frequency and has been reported in neonates, debilitated infants and children, particularly those treated with antibiotics or corticosteroids, or with diseases of the reticuloendothelial system, and in patients requiring prolonged intravenous therapy. Several *Candida* species have been isolated from such patients, whose clinical features are those of septicemia. Disseminated candidosis, which may be confirmed by blood culture, should be suspected when a septicemic illness supervenes in premature neonates, debilitated infants, or children in the course of antibiotic therapy, especially in the presence of a portal of entry for the organism such as an indwelling intravenous cannula.

The isolation of *Candida* from a specimen of urine obtained by suprapubic aspiration is highly suggestive of disseminated infection but must be interpreted in the light of other clinical data. Urinary tract infections with *C. albicans* do occur, especially in neonates or in association with indwelling urinary catheters. In neonates infection can ascend to produce fungal balls in the renal pelvis. The appearance of papular lesions on the skin containing *Candida* has been noted in preterm infants under such circumstances. Disseminated candidosis also raises the possibility of hypogammaglobulinemia.

Candida endocarditis, though rare, has been reported in childhood. Previously damaged heart valves are the site of localization of infection in a patient with disseminated *Candida* infection.

DIAGNOSIS AND DIFFERENTIAL DIAGNOSIS

Oral thrush can usually be diagnosed on observation of the typical lesion, which may be confused with deposits of milk. The latter can be scraped off without effort, revealing a normal mucosal surface. Candidal napkin rash may be confused with ammoniacal dermatitis, and, although it is common for the two lesions to coexist, the sharply demarcated edges of the former and its association with oral thrush should suggest the diagnosis. Confirmation of superficial candidosis is readily made by the finding of typical pseudohyphae on microscopic examination and by culture of the organism from swabs from superficial lesions. Yeast cells are not significant in feces as they occur in 15% of normal children but hyphal forms occur only with invasion of mucous membranes and their presence can therefore be taken as an indication of enteric candidosis.

The clinical and radiological features of pulmonary candidosis can be confused with a number of subacute and chronic bacterial infections of the lungs. The presence of characteristic predisposing circumstances should suggest the diagnosis, especially if pulmonary cavitation is present. Laboratory confirmation is best made by repeated sputum culture, or preferably, by culture of tracheal or bronchial aspirates.

In disseminated candidosis the organism can be isolated by blood or urine culture.

TREATMENT AND PROGNOSIS

Oral candidosis is best treated by local application of antifungal agents. Preparations in common use are suspensions of nystatin (100 000 units/ml) and miconazole (2% in a gel). Gentian violet (1% aqueous solution) is by far the cheapest but it is messy, may produce excoriation of buccal mucosa, and generally fails to eradicate the fungus from the lower alimentary tract and is now little used in Western countries. Nystatin and miconazole are probably equally effective. Nystatin is given in a dose of 1.0–2.0 ml dropped in the oral cavity 4 to 6 hourly for 7–10 days while miconazole gel is applied as 5.0 ml, two to four times each day.

Apparent failure of such treatments is seldom, if ever, due to the presence of antibiotic-resistant species of *C. albicans*. While resistance to nystatin and amphotericin B by *Candida* species other than *C. albicans* can readily be induced in vitro, only a minor degree of diminished antibiotic sensitivity can be induced in *C. albicans*. A dose of 1 ml of nystatin by oral instillation 6 hourly may be inadequate; higher and more frequent doses should be employed if the infection appears to be unresponsive. In perianal forms of candidosis of skin or nails, topical nystatin (100 000 units/g of ointment) or miconazole is effective. Oral therapy with either antibiotic is effective in candidal enteritis.

In the treatment of candidosis of deeper structures and organs, oral nystatin therapy is not recommended, since absorption from the gastrointestinal tract is poor. Oral ketoconazole may be effective. In pulmonary candidosis, nystatin may be administered by aerosol, e.g. 500 000 units in 15 ml distilled water. In systemic candidosis and candidal endocarditis and probably in pulmonary candidosis, the most effective treatment is the intravenous administration of amphotericin B. Recent reports have indicated that the liposomal amphotericin B (AmBisome) treatment is less toxic and at least equally effective.[524] Flucytosine has the advantages over amphotericin B of oral administration and lower toxicity. Many strains of *C. albicans* are resistant, however, and the drug cannot be administered parenterally to those patients too ill to take it by mouth. It should be reserved for those patients in whom amphotericin B has proved to be too toxic.

The prognosis of superficial candidosis is excellent; that of candidal enteritis has to be guarded. Disseminated candidosis carries a poor prognosis, largely related to the nature of the predisposing conditions. Meningeal candidosis, however, may run a surprisingly mild course.

CHROMOBLASTOMYCOSIS

ETIOLOGY, EPIDEMIOLOGY AND PATHOGENESIS

This is the commonest infection by the dematiaceous or black pigmented fungi. A number of fungi including *Fonsecaea pedrosoi*, *F. compacta*, *Phialophora verrucosa*, *Cladosporium carrioni*, *Rhinocladiella aquaspersa* and, less commonly, *Exophiala jeanselmei* cause chromoblastomycosis. Although most common in the tropics, cases have been reported from more temperate regions such as Europe and the USA. The habitat of each of the fungi is soil, decomposing vegetation and woodland. Humans most often become infected by traumatic implantation of such material for example when walking barefoot. Person-to-person transmission has not been described.

CLINICAL FEATURES, DIAGNOSIS AND TREATMENT

Chromoblastomycosis usually begins as a small pink papule which enlarges to a nodule. Over time it evolves to a scaly, fissured pink brownish plaque which eventually becomes verrucose. Eventually thick crusted hyperkeratotic masses occur which are prone to secondary infection, which can eventually, after many years, lead to lymphatic blockage and elephantiasis. The differential diagnosis includes blastomycosis, lupus vulgaris, leishmaniasis and tertiary syphilis. Specific diagnosis is by histological examination and isolation of the fungi which requires up to 6 weeks incubation at both 25 and 37°C. Treatment is difficult. For small lesions wide surgical excision is possible. Intraconazole for 6–24 months is effective in above 60% of cases. Amputation may be required.

COCCIDIOIDOMYCOSIS

ETIOLOGY AND EPIDEMIOLOGY

Coccidioides immitis is a dimorphic fungus, which exists as a mycelial saprophye in soil but as an endosporulating spherule in the human lung. Infection is acquired by inhalation of arthroconidia from soil and is particularly prevalent in the San Joquin Valley in California. Although most cases occur in and around this area, cases have been described in central (Guatemala, Honduras) and South (Venezuala, Colombia, Paraguay, Bolivia, Argentina) America. It may also occur when dust storms blow the arthroconidia into other areas.

PATHOGENESIS

Inhalation of arthroconidia results in a disease attack rate of about 40%. Once in the lungs the arthroconidia convert to the spherule-endospore phase within 3 days. This results in an initial influx of neutrophils and an inflammatory response which changes to a mononuclear cell infiltrate with granulomata once the spherule-endospore phase is well established. The spherules are too large (20–150 μm) to be ingested by neutrophils or even macrophages but they are important in defense presumably because they can engulf the released endospores (c. 2–5 μm). A brisk T_{H1} (T helper type 1) response is needed for recovery from infection.

CLINICAL FEATURES

Most often coccidioidomycosis is a somewhat prolonged influenza-like illness, often with pneumonia, which follows an incubation period of 1–3 weeks. In 90%, recovery is complete, the remainder are left with pulmonary cavities and nodules.[525] Non-pulmonary features include fever, malaise, headache, arthralgia, myalgia and skin rashes. Approximately 25% of patients develop erythema nodosum 6–16 days after onset of symptoms. In about 1% of patients, there is dissemination with skin (subcutaneous abscesses), bone, meningeal and even miliary manifestations. Dissemination is particularly found in immune compromised patients including cardiac allograft recipients (5% of those in Arizona) and those with HIV/AIDS.

DIAGNOSIS AND DIFFERENTIAL DIAGNOSIS

Coccidioidomycosis should be suspected in children in or from endemic areas, especially if non-white, who develop an acute febrile illness. Primary pulmonary coccidioidomycosis especially with erythema nodosum can be confused with primary tuberculosis and the postprimary nodular or cavitating disease with secondary tuberculosis. Diagnosis can be confirmed by culture of sputum, pus or blood (if disseminated), but the laboratory should be warned since this is a significant pathogen that will need special containment. The coccidioidin skin test (similar to tuberculosis) will become positive within 21 days of infection. Serological tests such as complement fixing titers are available and useful for confirmation of diagnosis.

TREATMENT AND PROGNOSIS

Primary coccidioidomycosis seldom requires more than symptomatic treatment. Amphotericin B, the most effective drug, should, in view of its toxicity, be reserved for severe primary or postprimary pulmonary disease. Intravenous amphotericin B therapy is, however, essential in disseminated coccidioidomycosis and, where there is infection of the central nervous system, may be given by intrathecal infection. Until recently, the only alternative form of therapy was intravenous miconazole but oral itraconazole has been shown to be of value and of relatively low toxicity.

The prognosis of primary coccidioidomycosis is excellent, while that of postprimary pulmonary disease is good. Disseminated coccidioidomycosis carries a poor prognosis, especially with meningeal infection, unless treated vigorously and at an early stage.

CRYPTOCOCCOSIS

ETIOLOGY AND EPIDEMIOLOGY

Cryptococcus neoformans exists as a yeast in mammalian infections and on artificial culture but in a mycelial form in the environment. *C. neoformans* has a worldwide distribution and there are two variants: *C. neoformans* var. *neoformans* and *C. neoformans* var. *gattii*. *C. neoformans* is subdivided into four serotypes (A–D). *C. neoformans* var. *neoformans* falls into serotypes A and D and var. *gattii*, serotypes B and C. The former is associated with soil, especially that contaminated by pigeon droppings and causes infection in patients immunocompromised by HIV/AIDS, chemotherapy or steroid administration. The latter is associated with the tropics and has been isolated from debris around *Eucalyptus camaldulensis*, the Australian red river gum tree. It causes infection in immunocompetent individuals. Although infection occurs in all age groups, children are less often infected.

PATHOGENESIS AND CLINICAL FEATURES

Infection is acquired, it is thought, by inhalation of the fungus but person-to-person transmission does not occur. Virulent strains of *C. neoformans* have a thick polysaccharide capsule (Fig. 26.46) that protects them from phagocytic killing by macrophages and neutrophils. In the lungs, it may cause pneumonia but this occurs in less than 15% of patients with cryptococcosis. Most often it passes through the lungs silently to infect at secondary sites. The major manifestation is chronic meningitis with headache, personality changes, dementia and focal neurological signs. It can be entirely asymptomatic early in the infection and especially in HIV/AIDS patients, neck stiffness and fever are not major presenting features (in less than 50% of cases). In approximately 15% of cases of cryptococcosis there is skin or bone involvement. The cutaneous manifestations can be acneiform, abscesses, ulcers, granulomas or plaques.

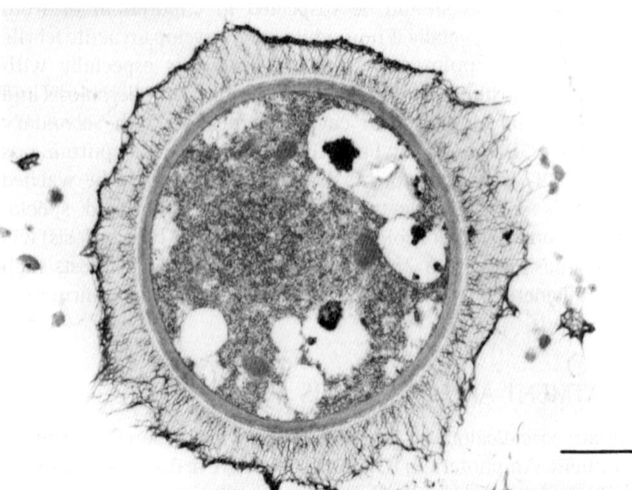

Fig. 26.46 A thin section electron micrograph of *Cryptococcus neoformans* showing its thick polysaccharide capsule (bar =1 μm).

DIAGNOSIS AND DIFFERENTIAL DIAGNOSIS

The specific diagnosis of cryptococcosis depends on demonstrating the presence of the fungus or its capsular antigen in CSF, blood or other infective sites. However, it must be remembered that *C. neoformans* can be present in sputum in the absence of disease. In CSF the cellular response varies. In AIDS patients, the cell count is low (< 5/mm^3) whereas in non-AIDS patients it ranges from 10 to 300/mm^3, but in each case there is a prevalence of lymphocytes (> 80%). On Gram stain *C. neoformans* will stain violet (Gram positive) however, the India ink stain is best for demonstration of the yeasts. This is a negative stain because the stain does not penetrate the yeast but shows it with its thick polysaccharide capsule against a black background. There are commercially available latex agglutination kits for detection of capsular antigen in CSF or serum. These can also be used to measure response to therapy. Finally *C. neoformans* can be cultured on suitable fungal culture medium. The differential diagnoses include other bacterial and viral causes of acute or chronic meningitis or meningoencephalitis in particular tuberculous meningitis, and for the skin lesions molluscum contagiosum, penicilliosis and histoplasmosis, especially in AIDS patients.

TREATMENT AND PROGNOSIS

For non-AIDS patients a combination of amphotericin B and 5-flucytosine for 6 weeks is curative in 75% of patients. In AIDS patients a number of regimens have been tried principally because relapse after cessation of therapy is high. Amphotericin B with or without 5-flucytosine for 2 weeks followed by 8 weeks of therapy with either fluconazole or itraconazole appears optimal in these cases. This is then followed by long term oral suppressive therapy with fluconazole. However with the advent of combination antiretroviral therapy for HIV/AIDS the outlook is much better.[526] In addition to frequent relapse, obstructive hydrocephalus is a major complication of cryptococcal meningitis.

HISTOPLASMOSIS

ETIOLOGY AND EPIDEMIOLOGY

Histoplasma capsulatum is another dimorphic fungus, which undergoes reversible morphological variation according to the environment in which it is placed. Its normal habitat is soil, especially below where birds and bats have roosted. Here it exists in a mycelial form with hyphae bearing macrocondia (8–14 μm diameter) and microconidia (2–5 μm), which are the infective forms. At temperatures above 35°C *H. capsulatum* grows as a yeast (2–3 × 3–4 μm) and this is the form found in human infections. Histoplasmosis is endemic in North America (especially the Ohio and Mississippi valleys) and Latin America, but cases have been reported from Europe and Asia. The taxonomy of *H. capsulatum* is currently under discussion. Three varieties are recognized: *H. capsulatum* var. *capsulatum*, *H. capsulatum* var. *duboisii* (which causes African histoplasmosis) and *H. capsulatum* var. *farciminosum* (which causes skin ulcers in horses and mules) but genetic analysis suggests *H. capsulatum* might harbor six species.[527] It is estimated that there are 200 000–500 000 cases each year worldwide. In endemic areas of the USA, it is estimated that 90% of the population have been exposed with frequent re-exposure.[528]

PATHOGENESIS AND CLINICAL FEATURES

Infection occurs when microcondia are inhaled. Most often this occurs when individuals disturb soil or dust containing microconidia, but they can travel for miles in the wind. In the lungs, the spores germinate to the yeast form, which elicits an influx of neutrophils, macrophages and lymphocytes and formation of granulomas. The yeasts are able to survive within macrophages,[529] and may persist for years within the reticuloendothelial system. Infection is more likely to progress, persist or disseminate if there is some abnormality of T cell function. Infection is also likely to disseminate in infants under 2 years,[530] but there is often an associated T cell defect. With exposure to a low infective dose, only 1% of patients develop clinical disease, but the rest have serological evidence of infection. With a higher inoculum only 10–50% are asymptomatic. Most clinically expressed infections are self-limited and include acute pulmonary histoplasmosis, mediastinal lymph node enlargement, pericarditis and rheumatological manifestations.

Approximately 80% of the symptomatic cases are of acute pulmonary histoplasmosis, which presents as a 'flu-like' illness with fever, chills, headache, myalgia and a non-productive cough. This usually resolves within a few weeks. More diffuse pulmonary disease leading to respiratory insufficiency can occur with a higher infecting dose. The rheumatological manifestations include erythema nodosum with arthralgia or frank arthritis, which can persist for months. Pericarditis occurs as an inflammatory complication of pulmonary disease. Chronic pulmonary histoplasmosis is very rare in children. It occurs mostly in middle-aged men with chronic obstructive airways disease. Disseminated histoplasmosis is a progressive illness with extrapulmonary spread of the fungus. It can occur following acute infection or years later. In infants it presents as fever, splenomegaly and/or hepatomegaly.[530] Subsequently shock, liver or renal failure and central nervous system involvement can occur. Cutaneous or mucosal granulomas in children in endemic areas should also be considered as possible histoplasmosis.

DIAGNOSIS AND DIFFERENTIAL DIAGNOSIS

Diagnosis requires a higher index of clinical suspicion in a child living in, or coming from an endemic region. Specific diagnosis requires a battery of tests including histology, antigen and antibody detection and fungal culture of bone marrow, spleen, lymph node, liver or bronchoalveolar lavage samples.[530] The histoplasmin skin test is not useful especially in those with T cell impairment and disseminated disease. The differential diagnosis includes pulmonary or miliary tuberculosis.

MYCETOMA[531]

Mycetoma is a chronic subcutaneous granulomatous disease caused by either fungi (eumycetoma) or branching bacteria (actinomycetoma). It has a worldwide distribution and is endemic in a belt between latitudes 15° S and 30° N, which encompasses Senegal, Sudan, Somalia, Mexico, India and parts of central and South America. In Sudan it is estimated that there are 300–400 new cases each year mostly in males aged 20–40 years, but children may rarely be affected. The clinical triad of subcutaneous nodules, sinuses and discharge is diagnostic. The differential diagnosis includes Kaposi's sarcoma, neurofibroma, malignant melanoma, syphilitic osteitis and bone tuberculosis, but specific diagnosis can be made by histological examination. Culture is difficult and takes a long time. Surgical treatment is to remove all affected tissue, which will involve amputation of affected feet or hands. Actinomycetoma can be treated with dapsone and streptomycin for 1 month. Medical treatment of eumycetoma is much more difficult. Griseofulvin, ketoconazole or itraconazole have had mixed success but treatment must be continued for 1–10 years.

NOCARDIOSIS

ETIOLOGY AND EPIDEMIOLOGY

Nocardia spp. are Gram positive, acid alcohol fast non-motile branching bacteria in the suborder *Corynebacterineae* that are closely related to the actinomycetes. There are 20 *Nocardia* spp. but most human infections are by *Nocardia asteroides* and less commonly by *N. farcinica* and *N. nova*. In tropical countries infection can also be by *N. brasiliensis* and *N. africana*.[532] They are environmental organisms living in soil and decaying vegetation. Person-to-person spread does not occur and although *Nocardia* spp. can cause infections in animals they are not zoonotic. Primary infections do occur but most infections occur in immune compromised individuals.

PATHOGENESIS AND CLINICAL FEATURES

Infection is acquired either by inhalation or direct inoculation into the skin. Characteristically *Nocardia* spp. produce abscesses and granulomas. Virulent strains of *N. asteroides* can evade phagocytic killing by inhibiting phagolyzosome fusion or acidification of phagosomes.[533,534] Dissemination is much more likely to occur if there is some form of immune compromise and has been reported in HIV/AIDS when it may involve the skin, kidneys and adrenals. In 5% of patients it involves the central nervous system either as diffuse meningitis or abscesses.

Pulmonary infection is found in 75% of patients with nocardiosis, alone or in association with disseminated infection, and may produce no symptoms. In other patients malaise, cough, fever and dyspnea may develop. Hemoptysis is an uncommon symptom. Involvement of the central nervous system may result in the clinical features of meningoencephalitis, or, if the lesion is a single abscess, of a localized intracranial or intraspinous tumor. Primary cutaneous nocardiosis can present as cellulitis or as an abscess with or without lymphadenitis and can be mistaken for *Streptococcus pyogenes* or *Staphylococcus aureus* infections.[535] *Nocardia* spp. are also pathogens in mycetoma.

DIAGNOSIS AND DIFFERENTIAL DIAGNOSIS

There are no typical symptoms and signs, and the pulmonary form may readily be confused with other suppurative lung conditions. Radiological examination of the chest similarly provides no characteristic features, the most common being patchy infiltration perhaps with cavitation. Specific diagnosis depends upon laboratory help but unfortunately *Nocardia* spp. are difficult to recognize and identify in the routine diagnostic laboratory, compounded by the fact that they are slow growing.

TREATMENT AND PROGNOSIS

Prior to the advent of the sulfonamides, nocardial infection was usually fatal, and at present the outlook is poor, partly because of the nature of the predisposing conditions and partly because of delay in diagnosis.

The treatment of choice is prolonged administration of sulfonamides or co-trimoxazole. Treatment may be necessary for several months, and may be combined with surgery. It is recommended that sulfonamides be given in a dose adequate to maintain a blood level of not less than 10 mg/100 ml.

Treatment with antibiotics, including benzyl penicillin and chloramphenicol, has been reported to be successful on occasions and, as indicated by sensitivity of the organism in vitro, may be given in addition to sulfonamides.

PENICILLIOSIS

This is an emerging infection which is the third commonest opportunist infection in HIV-infected patients in south-east Asia.[536] Most cases are due to *Penicillium marneffei* but occasional cases of *P. chrysogenum* occur.[537]

Approximately 80% of patients with penicilliosis are immunocompromised. It can present as cutaneous or disseminated infection or both. The skin lesions are usually umbilicated papules resembling molluscum contagiosum. Disseminated disease usually presents as fever, weight loss and anemia. Specific diagnosis is by isolation of the fungus from skin, bone marrow or blood. Mild to moderate disease can be treated with itraconazole or ketoconazole but severe disease will require amphotericin B. There are no controlled trials of therapy.

SPOROTRICHOSIS[538]

Sporotrichosis is caused by the dimorphic fungus *Sporothrix schenckii*. It grows as a saprophyte in decaying vegetation and infection occurs following traumatic inoculation into the skin. Some cases have been transmitted by domestic cat scratch.[539] It has a worldwide distribution but, for example, is the commonest subcutaneous mycosis in Latin America. Infection is often related to occupation (e.g. farmers, florists, gardeners) and most often in adults, although infections do occur in children.[540] The initial nodule at the inoculation site enlarges becoming red, pustular and ulcerating in turn. Extension occurs up the lymphatics to draining lymph nodes which themselves enlarge and drain to the skin. Spontaneous healing can occur but most often the lesions persist with gradual extension and scarring. Diagnosis depends upon demonstrating *S. schenckii* in lesions by immunohistochemistry or immunofluorescence. Fungal culture however, provides the definitive diagnosis. There are no controlled trials of therapy but oral itraconazole for 3 to 12 months has cure rates of 89–100%. Saturated potassium iodide (10 drops diluted in fruit juice three times daily) can be used in a resource poor setting but it is poorly tolerated. If disease is unresponsive to itraconazole it might be necessary to use amphotericin B.

ANTIFUNGAL CHEMOTHERAPY[541]

There are only a small number of antifungal drugs available for treatment of systemic mycoses and there are very few controlled trials to demonstrate efficacy with none in children. Most of the antifungals act on the fungal cell membrane by either chelating ergosterol (polyenes) or inhibiting its synthesis (imidazoles, triazoles). 5-Flucytosine is a nucleoside analog that inhibits fungal transcription.

POLYENES

Nystatin is a microcrystalline suspension so should not be given parenterally. It is very effective in treating superficial infections due to sensitive fungi and resistance has developed very slowly if at all. Amphotericin B is active against a wide range of fungi in vitro including *Candida* spp., *C. neoformans*, *H. capsulatum* and *Aspergillus* spp. However up to 40% of *P. marneffei* are resistant and the agents of chromoblastomycoses are usually resistant as are those causing eumycetoma.

For systemic mycoses amphotericin B must be given intravenously by slow infusion but can also be given intrathecally, intraventricularly or intraperitoneally. The lyophilized powder must be reconstituted in 5% dextrose solution (not saline which may cause it to precipitate) and is given as a slow infusion over 4–6 h at a concentration of 100 μg/ml. Usually treatment begins with a dose of 25 μg/kg/day with a gradual increase up to about 1 mg/kg/day as can be tolerated. A daily dose of 1.5 mg/kg/day should not be exceeded. For intrathecal use, doses of 100–500 μg or even 1 mg have been given to children according to weight and tolerance of the drug. Only 2–5% of the daily dose of amphotericin B is excreted in urine in the active form, and in experimental animals 20% is excreted in bile. The fate of the major part of the administered dose in unknown but there are reports of detection of the drug in liver, spleen and kidney 1 year after cessation of therapy. There are no trials delineating duration of therapy, but treatment is usually given for 1–3 months depending upon the rate of clinical and laboratory improvement. Amphotericin B has a high toxicity profile. During a 4–6 h infusion 50–90% of patients experience fever, chills, malaise, muscle and joint pains, nausea and vomiting. The major side-effect is nephrotoxicity, glomerular filtration rates fall by 40% in most patients and stabilize to 20–60% after multiple doses. Toxicity is manifest by increased blood urea and creatinine levels and the appearance of red cells, white cells and casts in the urine. If blood urea rises above 16.7 mmol/L or creatinine above 170 μmol/L treatment should be stopped until levels return to normal. Hematological side-effects occur in 75% of patients, most frequently a normochromic, normocytic anemia, and cardiac arrest, hepatotoxicity, neurotoxicity and allergic reactions do occur but are rare.

Encapsulating amphotericin B in liposomes (AmBisome, Abelcet) or in a colloidal dispersion (Amphocil) gives better tolerance and fewer side-effects in doses up to 3–5 mg/kg/day.

FLUCYTOSINE

5-Flucytosine is a fluorinated pyrimidine that was originally developed as an antineoplastic drug. Its mechanisms of action are, on conversion to 5-fluorouracil in the fungus, to act as an analog of uracil inhibiting protein synthesis and to inhibit thymidylate synthetase and thus DNA synthesis. It has a narrow spectrum of activity but is usually active against *C. albicans* and *C. neoformans*. However, resistance even in these fungi can develop. It is most often used in combination with amphotericin B. It is well absorbed orally and is usually given at 50–100 mg/kg/day in four divided doses in neonates and children. Although less toxic than amphotericin B, it can cause bone marrow suppression, cutaneous reactions (particularly in AIDS patients) and diarrhea. The risk of bone marrow suppression is greater with concomitant amphotericin B therapy and appears more likely in children. For these reasons, it is advisable to measure peak (2 h post oral or 30 min post intravenously) and trough (just prior to dose) serum levels twice weekly during therapy. Peak levels should not excede 100 mg/L and the trough is around 25 mg/L.

IMIDAZOLES

Of the licensed imidazoles, clotrimazole is solely a topical agent, ketoconazole can be given topically or orally and miconazole topically or intravenously. Miconazole has a broad range of antifungal activity in vitro but is less active against *Aspergillus* spp., *Hansenula anomala* and *Mucor* spp. It is particularly useful for topical application in dermatophyte infections and in oral and cutaneous candidosis. Intravenous miconazole should be considered in patients unable to tolerate amphotericin B and as an alternative to the latter drug in systemic infections with *Candida* resistant to flucytosine.

Recommended dosage for oral candidosis is 5 ml of miconazole gel (20%) two to four times per day. For systemic infections, an ampoule containing 200 mg of miconazole should be diluted with 5% dextrose or physiological saline solution and administered by slow intravenous infusion three times daily. In children, the total daily dose is of the order of 40 mg/kg body weight.

Toxic effects are in general less frequent and less severe than those encountered with amphotericin B therapy. They include gastrointestinal, mental and liver enzyme disturbances. The poor water solubility of miconazole necessitates the use of a lipophilic solvent causing major problems with venous irritation and occlusion.

Ketoconazole has an even better antifungal spectrum of activity. It is a less toxic alternative to amphotericin B but does cause gastrointestinal problems (in 3–40%) and hepatocellular damage (most often in females over 40 years). Its use has been reported in systemic candidosis, coccidioidomycosis and histoplasmosis. An appropriate dose is 3 mg/kg daily orally for a child and 200–400 mg once daily for an adult. Treatment should be maintained for 10 days, in the case of oral thrush, and for at least 1 month in the case of systemic infections. Less than 10% of either drug is excreted in urine, so they are of little use in urinary tract infections.

TRIAZOLES

The two major antifungals in this recently introduced class of drugs are fluconazole and itraconazole. Fluconazole has high bioavailability, and peak serum concentrations are similar by either the oral or intravenous routes. It is active against most *C. albicans* and *C. neoformans* but some other *Candida* spp. (e.g. *C. krusei*) are resistant. Its main clinical use is in treating cryptococcosis and candidosis. In children over 4 weeks, recommended doses are 3 mg/kg/day for mucosal candidosis, 6–12 mg/kg/day for systemic candidosis or cyptococcosis and 3–12 mg/kg/day for prophylaxis in neutropenic children. Neonates aged 2–4 weeks should be given similar doses but every 2 days and those aged 2 weeks and under every 3 days. Fluconazole is generally well tolerated with nausea, vomiting, abdominal pain and diarrhea in less than 5%. Asymptomatic elevation of hepatic aminotransferase enzyme occurred in 12% of children after 4 days of intravenous therapy.[542] About 80% of the drug is excreted by the renal route. Itraconazole has an even broader spectrum of activity being active against most *Candida* spp., *H. capsulatum, B. dermatitidis, C. immitis, P. braziliensis, P. marneffei, A. flavus* and *A. fumigatus*. It has an equally broad clinical use for infections by the above and in sporotrichosis, chromoblastomycosis and phatochromomycosis. For the latter two, response depends on the infecting fungus. The dose is 2.5–5 mg/kg daily by the oral route. The duration of therapy depends upon the infection being treated. It has a good safety profile but very little of the drug is excreted in urine.

HELMINTH INFECTION

Helminth or worm infections are worldwide although in warmer, moister areas, especially where standards of hygiene are low, the range of species and prevalence tends to be greater. In such parts, multiple infections are also often the rule. Because children tend to live more closely with nature and with their pets, many helminth infections are commoner in children than in adults. Reviews listing the estimated prevalences of the variety of worm infections in humans worldwide indicate that a vast health problem exists. New and emerging helminthzoonoses continue to be identified as discussed by McCarthy & Moore.[543]

Many tentative prevalence figures are undoubtedly underestimates and thus, referring to the trematodes alone, Rim et al[544] have concluded that there are more of these helminths infecting humans than any other group of animal parasites, with over 75 species of trematode infecting humans, mostly acquired from poorly prepared or cooked food.[545]

Helminth infections are by no means confined to tropical or developing countries and the increase in travel and of refugee movements in recent years has led to an increasing awareness in the developed world of the dangers of imported diseases.[546]

Helminth infections differ in most cases from those caused by viruses, bacteria or protozoa in that the clinical effects exhibited by the host are mostly related to the worm load carried, and the latter in turn is usually related to the infective dose. The controversy regarding the possible adverse effects of helminth infections and the value of antihelmintic treatment on cognitive function and learning or educational ability remains unresolved, but the concept may well be valid.[547,548]

The common parasitic helminths infecting humans include the Nematoda (roundworms) and Platyhelminthes (flatworms) which comprises the Trematoda (flukes) and Cestoda (tapeworms). Less commonly humans may be infected with such worms as the Acanthocephala (thorny headed worms).[549]

The control of human helminth infections usually depends on a detailed knowledge of the epidemiology and life cycles of the species concerned – the aim being to break the cycle. The following principles are utilized either alone or in combination, depending upon the species:

1. treatment of infected individuals, including mass treatment;
2. control of animal reservoirs where such exist;
3. hygiene, which includes education and provision of adequate and acceptable toilet facilities;
4. vector control where applicable;
5. the wearing of shoes where infection occurs from the soil through the skin;
6. instruction in food preparation and cooking;
7. immunization – a field which continues to be of great interest.

Of all the above, the most important method for the control of human helminthiases remains education combined with improved sanitation and personal hygiene. However, mass deworming may play an important role in the control of some helminthiases and, in relation to immunization, Maizels et al[550] have expressed the view that 'vaccines are the one major goal of the helminthological community'.

NEMATODES (ROUNDWORMS)

The nematodes or roundworms are non-segmented worms, round in transverse section with separate sexes. They possess both gut and body cavity (pseudocele). Roundworms especially important to humans include amongst others: *Ascaris lumbricoides, Toxocara canis, Enterobius vermicularis, Ancylostoma duodenale, Necator americanus, Trichuris trichiura, Strongyloides stercoralis, Angiostrongylus cantonensis, Oesophagostomum* spp., *Ternidens deminutus, Trichinella spiralis, Capillaria* spp., *Dracunculus medinensis, Onchocerca volvulus, Loa loa, Wuchereria bancrofti, Mansonella perstans, Mansonella ozzardi* and *Brugia malayi*.

ASCARIASIS

The intestinal roundworm *Ascaris lumbricoides* is cosmopolitan although variable in its distribution, thriving in a moist climate, be it temperate or tropical and especially under conditions of overcrowding. Ascariasis (like trichuriasis) does, however tend to have a lower prevalence and worm load at higher altitudes.[551] The adult ascarids, male and female, live in the lumen of the small intestine, maintaining only an intermittent attachment to the mucosa. The gravid female lays an average of 200 000 eggs each day. Newly excreted eggs may remain dormant for a long period; if conditions are suitable they develop into an infective stage in about 2 weeks, in which condition they can remain viable for months or years until ingested.[552] The hosts of these worms are humans, although cases of human infection with *A. suum*, the pig ascarid, have also been recorded. The life cycle of *A. lumbricoides* is depicted in Figure 26.47.

Clinical features

In fully 80% of cases the only manifestation of ascariasis in the human is the asymptomatic passage of eggs and adult worms in the stool. Symptoms, when they do occur, are related to three phases of the ascarid's life cycle:

1. invasion of larvae;
2. presence of a large adult worm load;
3. migration of adult worms from their normal habitat.

To this one may add symptoms associated with the development of true allergy to the ascarid.[553]

Ascariasis is potentially serious and can contribute to a significant proportion of abdominal emergencies in children.[554]

Larval pneumonitis

The initial migration of larvae through the intestinal wall and by way of the portal circulation to the lungs may, in the case of heavy infection, or if there have been repeated reinfections, cause a characteristic and often seasonal clinical picture.[555] The patient develops a dry spasmodic cough with intermittent wheezing and breathlessness, transient rhonchi and crackles in the lung fields; rarely, hemoptysis occurs. There may be malaise with fever as high as 40°C, discomfort over the liver, and urticarial rashes. Radiological examination of the chest reveals diffuse mottled opacities, peribronchial infiltration or areas of pneumonitis. Marked eosinophilia is present. Symptoms and signs subside after 2 or 3 weeks and the eosinophilia generally diminishes to 3–5% of the total white cell count. Chronic lung disease occasionally results from repeated larval onslaughts. Severe pulmonary infiltration with asthma, eosinophilia and raised IgE levels can result in children infected with *A. suum*, which may or may not become patent.

Worm load

Although some features of intestinal ascariasis are of an allergic or reflux nature, in the healthy child on a normal diet it is unlikely that the presence of a few ascarids will cause any significant disturbance.[555] A large worm load will, however, drain off a considerable proportion of a child's nutritional intake and *Ascaris* infection in children can be associated with impaired lactose digestion and absorption.[554] Cases of heavy infection are usually seen in underprivileged communities where nutrition is already inadequate. The combination of malnutrition, vitamin and iron deficiency, and the almost invariable presence of intestinal parasites of other types, make the part played by ascarids difficult to assess. However, studies in Columbia have shown steatorrhea and D-xylose malabsorption associated with heavy loads of *Ascaris* which improved after deworming. These children are ill, stunted and marasmic, with abdominal distension. Colicky abdominal pain is frequent. There may be low grade fever and a mass of worms can

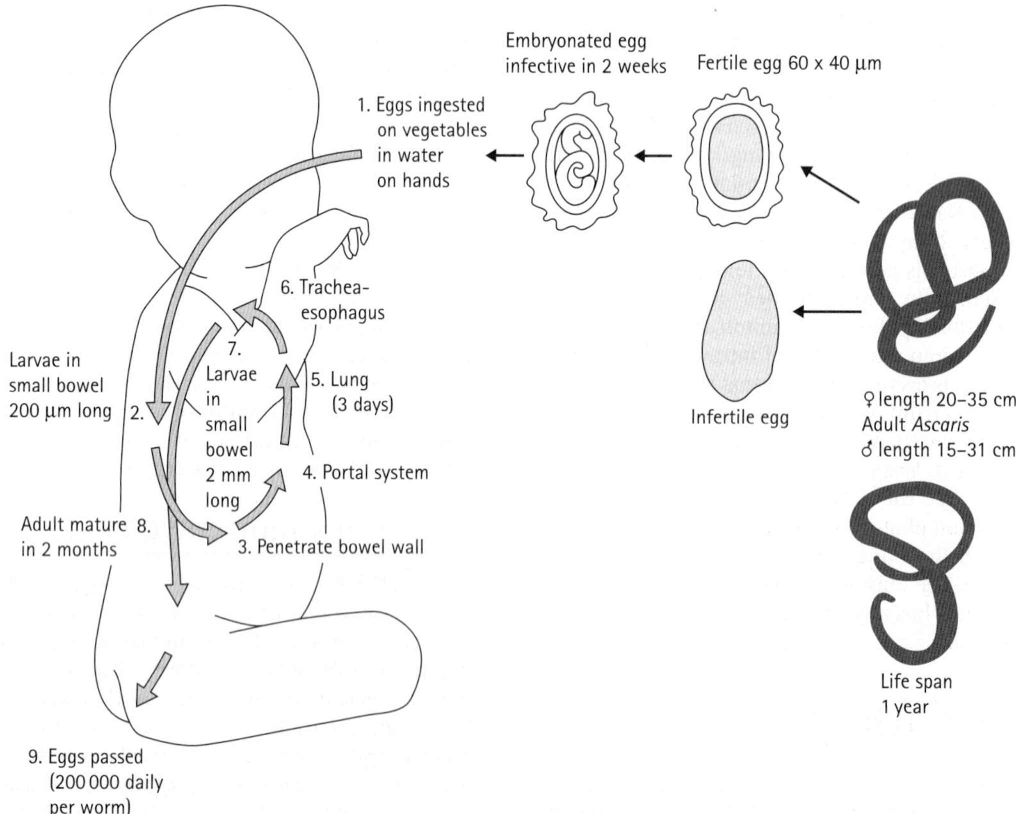

Fig. 26.47 Character and life cycle of *Ascaris lumbricoides*.

often be palpated abdominally. Toxins from ascarids may play a part in producing the chronic illness.

Intestinal complications associated with a heavy worm burden are frequently seen in hyperendemic areas.[556] A bolus of worms (usually both dead and living) may impact, particularly near the ileocecal junction (Fig. 26.48). A mass of ascarids may also precipitate temporary obstruction from spasm, cause inflammatory reactions and adhesions, or lead to volvulus or intussusception.

Migration of adult worms

Under certain circumstances, particularly with high fever, gastrointestinal upset or ineffectual antihelmintic therapy (e.g. the use of tetrachlorethylene for a concomitant hookworm infection), an ascarid may migrate from its normal habitat in the bowel and be vomited, or wriggle unaided, up the esophagus and emerge through the nose. Lodgment in the appendix or Meckel's diverticulum can result in obstruction and perforation. The common bile duct may be blocked by a roundworm, leading to severe upper abdominal pain, vomiting, tenderness and enlargement of the liver, a palpable gallbladder, and jaundice. Pancreatitis is a further complication. Other manifestations of the migrating ascarid include intestinal perforation with peritonitis, chronic peritonitis due to the presence of eggs, soft tissue or liver abscess, laryngeal impaction and even the passage of a worm per urethram. Ascarids also have a special propensity to congregate at the scene of incidental catastrophe – penetrating perforations, suture lines and into drainage or suction tubes.

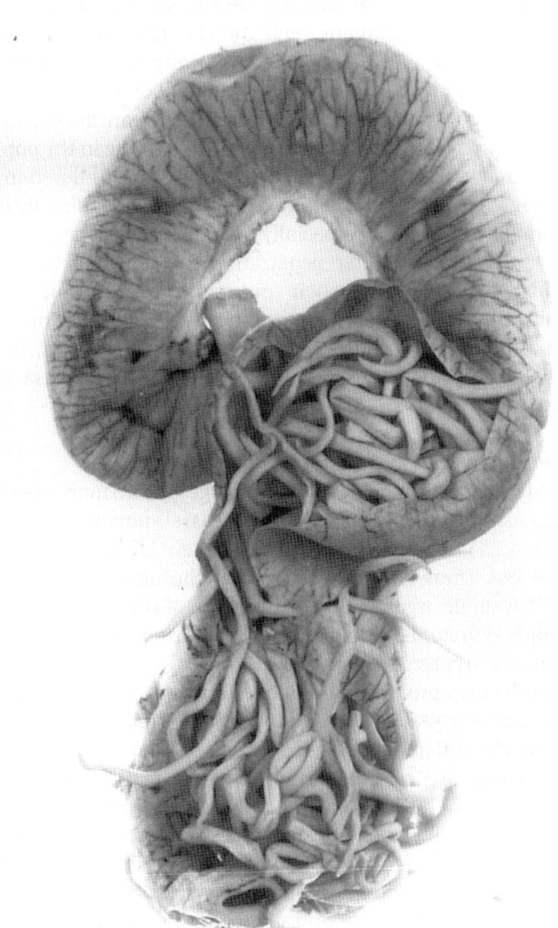

Fig. 26.48 Intestinal obstruction by *Ascaris lumbricoides* in a 14-year-old boy.

The development of roundworm sensitivity can produce a variety of allergic manifestations – nasal, pulmonary, dermal, or gastrointestinal.[555]

Diagnosis

Larval pneumonitis (Löffler's syndrome) is generally suspected by the presence of eosinophilia, but other parasites can produce this syndrome (Table 26.38), and proof of diagnosis can only be obtained if a larva is identified in the sputum. Adult worms may later be passed in the stool or seen on radiological examination (Fig. 26.49) of the abdomen using barium. Diagnosis, however, rests almost wholly on finding eggs in the stools (Fig. 26.50 a,b,c), except in the event of early infection or a population of purely male worms. Serological and intracutaneous tests are available but as yet are of little practical value although they have been used in epidemiological surveys.[557]

Treatment

No treatment is known to remove migrating larvae although some have claimed success using piperazine or pyrantel and the pneumonitis responds dramatically to prednisone.[555] Albendazole is a very valuable, broad spectrum anthelmintic with a wide activity against intestinal nematode species. It is generally well tolerated at doses recommended for these helminths and has, in fact, been designated as a 'WHO essential agent'. It is given at a dose of 400 mg as a single dose (200 mg for children < 10 kg).[552,555,558,559] An older but safe and effective treatment for established ascariasis is piperazine. Syrup is best and is given before the evening meal at a dosage of 75 mg/kg body weight to a maximum of 3.5–4 g.[560] If the bowels have not acted by the following morning a mild laxative is

Table 26.38 Worms and fly larvae giving rise to pulmonary infiltrations, visceral larva migrans and cutaneous larva migrans

	Pulmonary infiltration with eosinophilia	Visceral larva migrans	Cutaneous larva migrans
Ancylostoma braziliense			×
Ancylostoma caninum			×
Ancylostoma duodenale	Rare		
Angiostrongylus cantonensis		×	
Anisakis species		×	
Ascaris lumbricoides	×	Rare	
Ascaris suum	×	×	
Capillaria hepatica		×	
Dirofilaria species	×	×	
Fly larvae			
Dermatobia species		×	
Gasterophilus species			×
Hypoderma species			×
Gnathostoma species		×	×
Necator americanus	Rare		'Ground itch'
Schistosoma species			'Swimmer's itch'
Strongyloides stercoralis	×	Rare	'Ground itch'
Toxocara canis	×	×	
Toxocara cati	Uncertain	Uncertain	
Uncinaria stenocephala			×

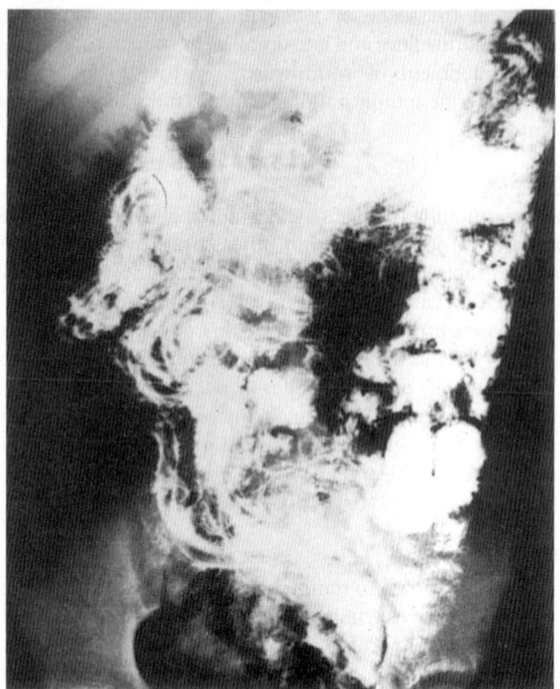

Fig. 26.49 *Ascaris lumbricoides.* Barium follow-through showing infestation in small bowel with worms coated with barium.

administered. The dose is repeated on the second evening. Worms are narcotized and eliminated by normal peristalsis. Nausea, vomiting, transient neurological disturbance and EEG changes have

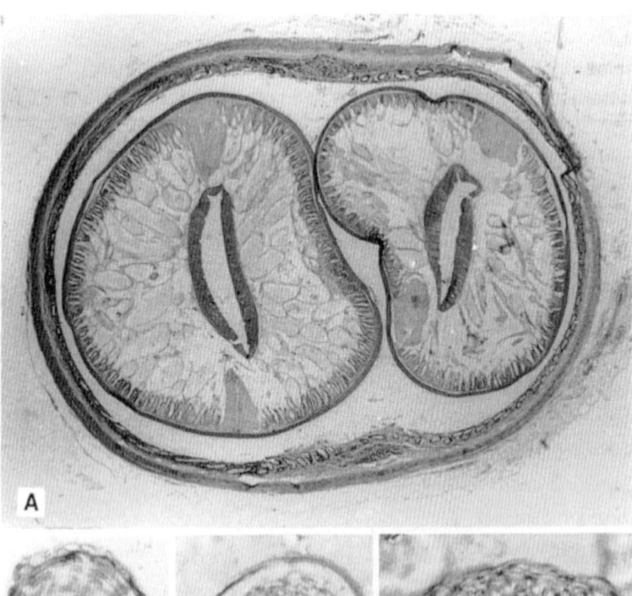

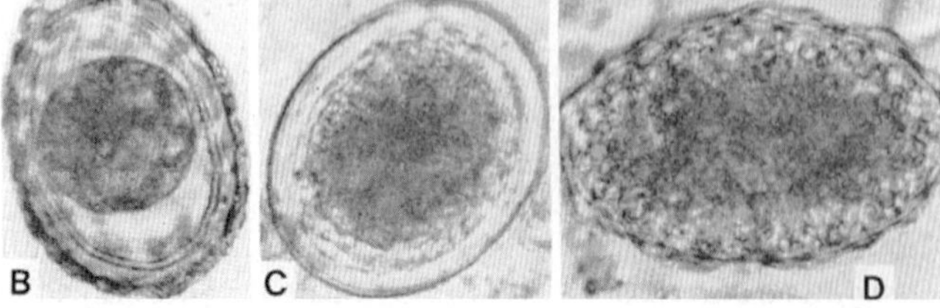

Fig. 26.50 (a) Pair of *Ascaris* in appendix (approx. × 10). (b) Fertilized egg of *Ascaris lumbricoides* (approx. × 600). (c) Decorticated fertilized egg of *A. lumbricoides* (approx. × 600). (d) Unfertilized egg of *A. lumbricoides* (approx. × 600).

been reported when the drug is given in excessive doses. Piperazine is contraindicated in the presence of liver and renal disease and where there is a history of neurological disease.[552,558]

Two anthelmintics highly effective in ascariasis and with minimal side-effects are pyrantel embonate/pamoate (Combantrin) (10 mg/kg, max. 750 mg) and mebendazole (Vermox) (100 mg twice a day for 3 days; children < 10 kg 50 mg b.d. for 3 days). Levamisole (Ketrax) 50–100 mg is also effective. Tiabendazole although effective, is better avoided owing to its side-effects.[561]

Where available, albendazole seems to be the drug of choice for ascariasis but, while results can be achieved quickly with chemotherapy, they are only temporary in the absence of other control measures. Prevention of ascariasis depends on improving living conditions and the sanitary disposal of feces, on preventing contamination of drinking water and raw vegetables, and on education in hygiene. There is evidence too, to indicate that the mass delivery of antihelmintic treatment to children may be an important option in the control of geohelminth infections, including ascariasis. The 1993 World Development Report of the World Bank,[562] includes mass deworming in its 'essential package of health interventions' and school-based mass delivery is singled out as one of the most cost-effective measures – a concept supported by studies such as that of Guyatt.[563]

TOXOCARA CANIS AND VISCERAL LARVA MIGRANS

Toxocara canis is a close relative of *Ascaris*. Its natural hosts are the young dog and the fox, in which it undergoes a cycle essentially similar to *Ascaris* in humans (Fig. 26.51). The cycle in dogs is complicated by the development of immunity with expulsion of adult worms by the animals at about 6 months of age. In pregnant bitches, however, this immunity is lost and dormant larvae in the tissues are reactivated or reinfection occurs, resulting in the puppies being infected in utero and being born with worms. Children ingest infective eggs from dirt contaminated with dog feces or directly from the animals themselves, especially young puppies or lactating bitches.[564] The larvae, after penetrating the intestinal wall, are incapable of completing their pulmonary migration in an unnatural host and wander aimlessly never to find their intestinal habitat. They pass through, or become encysted in liver, lungs, kidneys, heart, muscle, brain or eye, causing an intense local response from the tissue.

Clinical features

The child (most commonly 1–5 years of age) shows marked failure to thrive associated with pica (90% of cases), anemia (Hb below 9 g/dl in 45%), fever (80%) and enlargement of liver (65%) and spleen (45%). There is cough (80%), bronchospasm and wheezing (63%).[564] A single organ may bear the brunt of the infection so that pulmonary symptoms, or neurological abnormalities due to brain involvement (convulsions, disturbances of consciousness, hemiparesis) may predominate. Intense and persistent eosinophilia lasting months or years and reaching levels as high as 80×10^9/L is characteristic and may be the only abnormality found. Serum globulin levels are raised, particularly IgM, IgG and IgE, and elevated titers of anti-A and anti-B isoagglutinins have been described in 39% of cases. Transient chest shadows are recorded in about 50% of cases and the CSF may show an eosinophilia where the CNS is involved. The infection usually runs a chronic, benign course of 18 months or so and generally the prognosis is good, although deaths have been reported.

Ocular manifestations of toxocariasis may be the only evidence of the disease. The age of maximal ocular involvement is higher

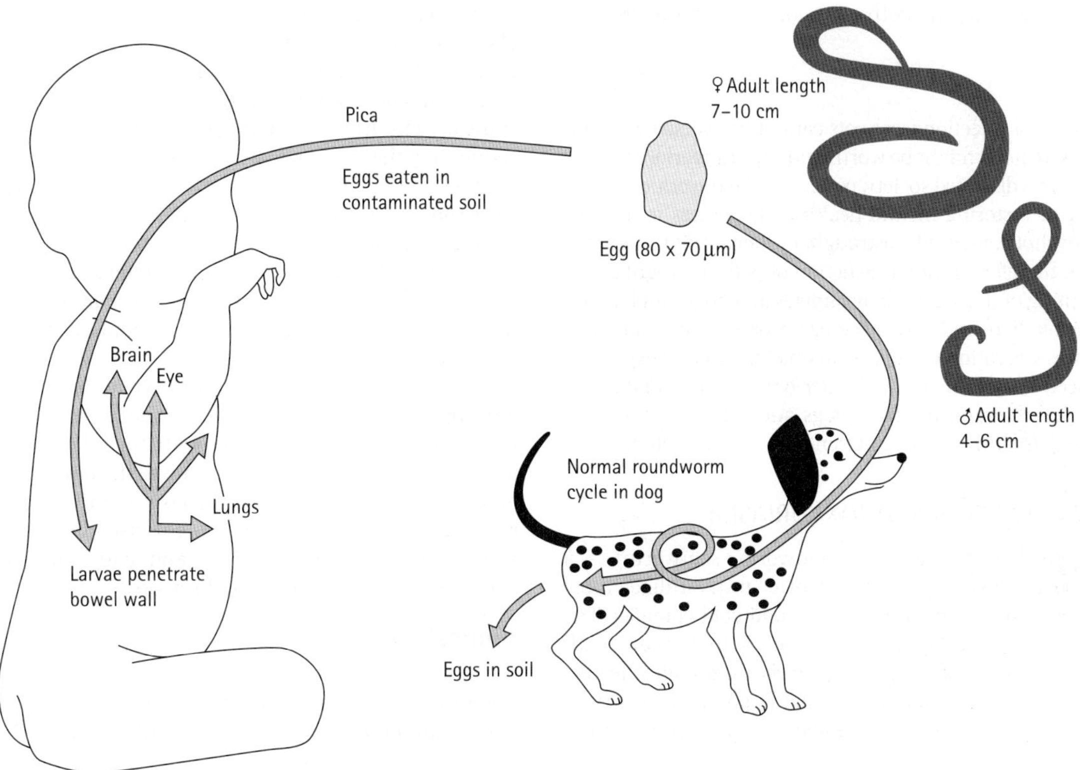

Fig. 26.51 Character and life cycle of *Toxocara canis.*

than that of systemic involvement, the average age being about 7–8 years. Loss of sight in the affected eye generally results, and usually only one eye is involved. A diagnosis of ocular toxocariasis should be considered when there is inflammatory detachment of the retina or retinitis of the posterior pole in a child, especially in one with geophagic habits, who has contact with young dogs. The diagnosis can be confused with retinoblastoma and this may lead to the unnecessary surgical removal of an eye in a child with ocular toxocariasis.

It appears, therefore, that there are two toxocaral syndromes in humans:

1. larvae in the eye presenting as granulomatous pseudotumors of the retina;
2. generalized toxocariasis with numerous larvae in the liver and other organs and associated with fever and eosinophilia.

Because ocular lesions are seldom found in the generalized forms, and because ocular disease is almost entirely confined to children, it has been postulated that ocular toxocariasis could be the manifestation of congenital infection of the child from an infected mother in a similar fashion to the transplacental infection of puppies. This hypothesis, if true, would have important implications for expectant mothers. Similarly, contact with cats or cat litter might entail risk of fetus-damaging infection due to toxocariasis from *Toxocara cati* as well as toxoplasmosis.

It has been suggested that the eosinophilia so often seen in children suffering from lead poisoning resulting from pica may well be due to concurrent *Toxocara* infection. Physicians managing children with lead intoxication should be aware of this possibility and treat the toxocariasis concurrently.

Undoubtedly, a similar clinical syndrome can be caused in children by filarial parasites of animal origin and by larvae of ther types[564] (Table 26.38). It still remains unclear whether *T. cati* (the cat roundworm) can be responsible for systemic larva migrans and warnings have been sounded that another dog ascarid, *Toxascaris leonina*, previously thought to be non-infective to humans, should be considered as a potential cause of visceral larva migrans.

Diagnosis

Acquisition of a puppy in the preceding year has proved to be a good suggestive indicator of *Toxocara* infection in symptomatic patients.[564] The diagnosis can only be established with certainty, however, by a biopsy (generally of the liver) or, undesirably and rather drastically, after enucleation of the eye. Skin tests and serological tests such as the indirect fluorescent antibody test and the *Toxocara enzyme immunoassay* (EIA) are available with the latter having a reported sensitivity of 78% and a specificity of 92%.[564,565] It is worth noting that 2–7% or more of symptomless adults and up to 23% of children with no symptoms may have detectable *Toxocara* antibodies.[564,566]

Fluoroscein angiography, ultrasound and CT scans are also described as useful adjuncts to diagnosis.[565]

Treatment

Diethylcarbamazine (Hetrazan, Banocide) (2 mg/kg three times per day for 7–10 days) is reportedly effective.[558,565] An alternative regimen is up to 6 mg/kg in divided doses for 3 weeks.[564] Repeated courses may be necessary and if respiratory distress or myocardial involvement develops, corticosteroids may be life-saving.

Tiabendazole (Mintezol) at a dose of 50 mg/kg per day for 3–5 days or 25 mg/kg for 1–4 weeks has also been recommended. It is especially useful for early ocular cases where diethylcarbamazine should not be used, as the cellular response it elicits could aggravate visual problems. Corticosteroids are also useful in controlling ocular lesions. Albendazole (400 mg twice daily for 3–5 days) has shown promise and flubendazole has also proved encouraging.[567]

Overall, however, the chemotherapy for toxocariasis remains unsatisfactory.

Prevention

While the dangers of infection from pets cannot be overstressed, this is a very emotive issue. It might be worth quoting Hungerford[568] who stated: 'In our stress distorted society, pets ... may be the critical factor in maintaining or restoring mental health or happiness to an only child, or to a psychotic, mentally distraught or lonely child or adult.'

The answer, therefore, is not destruction of pets, but regular and routine deworming of dogs, especially puppies and pregnant bitches, with mebendazole, fenbendazole, piperazine or pyrantel pamoate. Also important is education to impress upon children and expectant mothers the need to wash their hands after handling pets and not to allow dogs to lick them on the face. Dogs and cats should also be prevented from defecating where children play (sandpits etc.).

ENTEROBIUS VERMICULARIS (OXYURIASIS)

Enterobius vermicularis (threadworm, pinworm, seatworm) is a common parasite throughout the world but, unlike most nematodes, it is more prolific in temperate and cold climates. The incidence is highest in schoolchildren from 5 to 9 years with another peak at 30–49 years.[569] Boys and girls are equally affected. Enterobiasis is particularly common in highly populated districts, institutional groups, and among members of the same family. Incidences as high as 40–50% have been reported in London children and in institutions such as mental hospitals, prevalence may reach 90–100%. The absence of a prolonged developmental stage outside humans (Fig. 26.52) favors reinfection and transmission from child to child. Hands are contaminated by scratching the perianal area where eggs are deposited, and by contact with soiled underclothing, nightclothing or bedding. Infection is also acquired by inhalation of egg-containing dust, which may be disseminated from bedclothing by shaking, or movements of the sleeper. At room temperature eggs survive for 2–3 weeks. Furthermore, retroinfection may occur when the eggs hatch on the perianal area and larvae find their way back through the anus into the intestinal tract.

The usual habitat of the threadworm of both sexes is the cecum and adjacent appendix, lower ileum, and colon. The worms are free in the intestinal lumen or lie with their heads attached to the mucosa. The gravid females migrate to the lower colon and rectum and crawl through the anus to deposit thousands of sticky eggs on the anal verge and perineum at night, usually dying thereafter. It is worth emphasizing that dogs and cats play no part in the transmission of enterobiasis to humans.

Clinical features

Threadworm infection generally causes no symptoms whatsoever. The most common manifestation is pruritus of the perineal areas due to migration of the worms and the presence of eggs. Restless

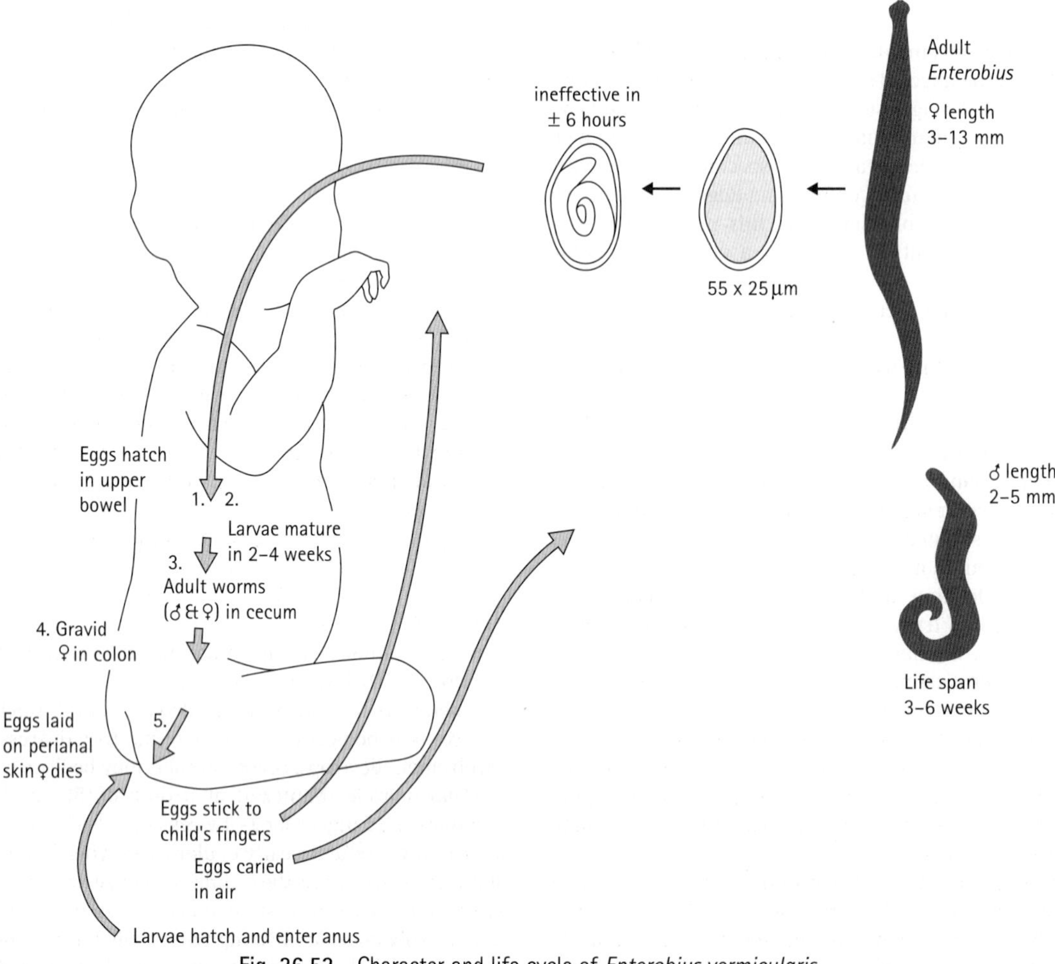

Fig. 26.52 Character and life cycle of *Enterobius vermicularis.*

sleep, nightmares, teeth grinding, and perhaps bed-wetting may result. In up to 20% of girls, vulval irritation and vaginal discharge are caused by threadworms and can persist for years [552] and night crying may be due to a threadworm in the vaginal introitus. Excoriation and pyogenic infection can follow from constant scratching.

It is most unlikely that threadworms play any significant part in causing the variety of symptoms commonly attributed to them. For example, threadworms are no commoner in children with recurrent abdominal pain than in those without pain. Similarly, threadworms are found as often in normal appendices as in appendices showing acute or chronic inflammation, so that they are not considered to play any material role in the production of appendicitis, although appendiceal blockage resulting in a simulated chronic appendicitis may occur at times.[569] Nail biting, nose picking, masturbation, convulsions, hyperkinesis and other behavior disturbances are also often erroneously ascribed to these parasites.

Very heavy infections can, however, result in catarrhal inflammation of the bowel from the attachment and irritation of worms, resulting in gastrointestinal disturbance. Intestinal obstruction has even been reported. Rarely, heavy infections have led to invasion of the bowel and appendiceal walls, peritoneum or viscera by larvae and immature worms. In their external migration gravid threadworms may occasionally crawl up the vagina into the uterus and Fallopian tubes or into the urethra and bladder depositing eggs in these sites with resulting, low grade salpingitis, cystitis or urethritis, and cases are on record of worms penetrating the intestinal wall, probably through a pre-existing mucosal breach, to reach the peritoneal cavity.

Enterobiasis may be associated with infection by the protozoan flagellate, *Dientamoeba fragilis* which is believed to be transmitted within the egg of the threadworm and may be a cause of diarrhea as discussed by Mills & Goldsmid.[570]

Eosinophilia is usually absent in enterobiasis but may occur in up to 12% of cases.

Diagnosis

Often the first evidence of infection is the discovery of the adult worms in the feces, particularly after enemas, or on the perineum. Worms may be clearly visible on proctoscopy. The most widely used and effective method of obtaining eggs from the perianal region is the adhesive cellulose tape method. The adhesive side of a piece of transparent tape is applied to the anus and surrounding skin – either directly or wrapped round a test tube – and the tape then transferred adhesive side down to a glass slide. The adhering eggs are clearly visible under a microscope (Fig. 26.53a). The test is best performed in the morning before bathing or defecation, and in view of the irregular migrations of gravid worms at least three examinations should be made on consecutive days. Eggs are found in the stools in only 5–10% of cases, but five perianal swabs reveal eggs in 97% of infections.

Treatment

A wide range of effective drugs are available for the elimination of threadworms. The drugs of choice at present are mebendazole (Vermox) and pyrantel embonate/pamoate (Combantrin, Antiminth). Combantrin is given at a dose of 10 mg/kg up to 750 mg by mouth as a single dose while mebendazole is given in a single dose of 100 mg (one tablet) stat. which is recorded as giving a cure rate of about 95% with no or very few side-effects.[552] Although some authorities advise that mebendazole should not be used in children under 2 years of age, Spicer et al[559] and others accept that a dose of 50 mg for a child of < 10 kg can be used. Albendazole is also reported as being effective,[571] being given at a dose of 400 mg orally (200 mg in children 10 kg or less). Neither mebendazole nor albendazole should be used during pregnancy.[559]

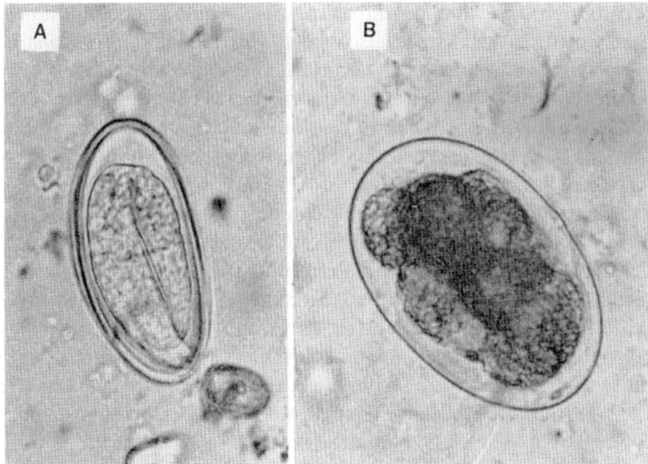

Fig. 26.53 (a) Fully developed egg of *Enterobius vermicularis* (approx. × 600). (b) Hookworm egg (approx. × 600).

Pyrantel is also very effective as a single dose treatment, giving cure rates of over 90% at doses of 10 mg/kg. Side-effects are usually mild (e.g. nausea and vomiting) and uncommon – about 3% of cases.[552,561]

Piperazine citrate (Antepar) and pyrvinium pamoate (Vanquin; Povan) are no longer in general use for enterobiasis, and tiabendazole (Mintezol), while efficacious, has unpleasant side-effects making the recommendation of the drug for enterobiasis inadvisable.

In general terms, treatment for most cases of threadworm is unnecessary, especially as reinfection of children is almost inevitable. However, if for clinical reasons, or to satisfy distressed parents treatment is deemed necessary, then whichever drug is used, the whole family must be treated and a second course should be given after 3 weeks. Intractable family infections can be controlled by the treatment of all family members with 100 mg (50 mg for children < 10 kg) mebendazole a week for 12 weeks.

Prevention of recurrence is extremely difficult, particularly in crowded communities and in humid temperate climates, which facilitate prolonged survival of eggs. Personal cleanliness is essential and this includes cutting of finger nails, regular washing of hands before meals and after using the toilet, washing the anal area on rising, and regular changing of underclothing and bed linen.

HOOKWORM (ANCYLOSTOMIASIS)

Ancylostoma duodenale (Old World hookworm) and *Necator americanus* (tropical hookworm) are morphological variants, tropical hookworm being rather smaller with many differences of fine morphology.

Hookworm occurs in most tropical and subtropical areas of the world, with *A. duodenale* distributed mainly around the Mediterranean littoral and *N. americanus* in south and central Africa and southern America. Both species are, however, widely distributed today in Asia as well as in most other tropical countries. In south-east Asia and Brazil, *A. ceylanicum* infections of humans occur as well and *A. malayanum* is yet another species from humans.[552] Hookworm is one of the world's chief causes of anemia.

A. braziliense, one cause of cutaneous larva migrans (Table 26.38) and a natural parasite of dogs and cats, is widely distributed throughout tropical and subtropical areas, while the common dog hookworm *A. caninum* is also widely distributed, and *Uncinaria stenocephala* infects dogs in temperate regions. These latter two species can also cause cutaneous larva migrans in humans and it is claimed that in northern Queensland in Australia, *A. caninum* may be a cause of eosinophilic gastroenteritis in humans as discussed by Smyth.[572]

The excreted egg, in favorable damp, shady conditions, hatches on the soil in about 2 days, releasing a rhabditiform larva which develops 8–10 days after hatching into the infective (filariform) larva. This larva penetrates the skin of the host, although *A. duodenale* is believed also to enter via the oral route, with fecally contaminated food and water and may infect by the transmammary and transplacental routes from infected mother to child.[573] The life cycle in humans from larval penetration to oviposition lasts about 5 weeks (Fig. 26.54). The adult worm may survive within its host for 7 years or longer.

The adult worms are attached to the wall of the jejunum, or, less commonly, the duodenum, by the buccal capsules, sucking blood from their hosts. Each worm may suck up to 0.5 ml of blood per day; thus heavy worm loads may result in a loss of 100–150 ml/day. Significant damage is therefore produced by hookworms, but clinical manifestations depend on the host's general resistance, on the worm load, and on the child's dietary intake and iron reserves.

Clinical features

Larval invasion

Penetration of the skin, usually of the feet or buttocks, by the filariform larvae may produce, within minutes, a series of wheals, which soon develop into an itchy, papular and vesicular eruption ('ground itch'). The rash may become ulcerative or pustular, but generally subsides within 10 days and the larvae do not wander within the skin as in the case of cutaneous larva migrans (see below).

Migration through the lungs

After penetration of the skin, larvae reach the small intestine via the heart and lungs as in ascariasis.

Respiratory symptoms are unusual in children except in the case of heavy or repeated infections, particularly of *N. americanus*, when there may be cough, sore throat, bloody sputum and pulmonary changes on X-ray (Table 26.38).

Adult worms in the intestine

A distinction should be made between hookworm infection (where patients carry a subclinical worm load) and hookworm disease, which results from heavy worm loads and inadequate diet. Where heavy infections occur, symptoms develop in 2–7 weeks after initial infection and consist of abdominal discomfort especially after meals, anorexia and sometimes nausea and vomiting. There may be intermittent diarrhea, general debility and undue tiredness. Once the adult worms are well established, there is little disturbance to the child, provided that the intake of iron, vitamins and protein keeps pace with the chronic blood loss produced by the parasites. When diet is inadequate and worm load heavy, severe hookworm disease results, characterized by profound iron deficiency anemia, hypoalbuminemic edema, cardiac failure and even death. It has been estimated that 100 worms will cause a daily loss of 4 mg of iron. A balanced diet easily compensates for this loss, but iron deficiency soon develops on a marginal dietary intake. Children with heavy hookworm infections are stunted, marasmic and anemic; the skin is dry and the face puffy. All aspects of development are retarded. An important concomitant which makes hookworm infection much more serious is sickle cell anemia.

A marked eosinophilia (40%) is characteristic of early hookworm infection. It reaches maximum intensity at about 3 months after initial infection and then diminishes gradually to levels of 5–20%. A partially effective protective immunity seems to develop in hookworm infection.[574,575]

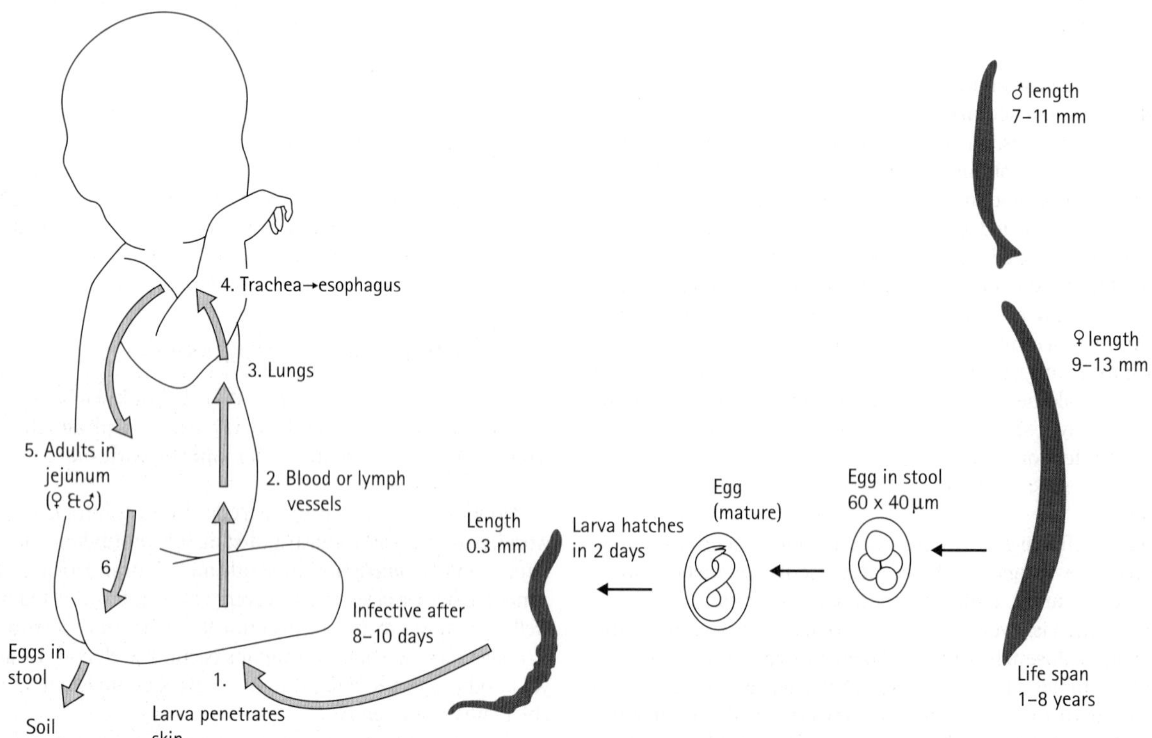

Fig. 26.54 Character and life cycle of hookworm.

Diagnosis

This depends on finding the eggs (Fig. 26.53b) in the feces and an egg count should be performed if a causal relationship with a concomitant iron deficiency anemia is to be established. An egg count greater than 2000 eggs/g of feces is generally considered to be of clinical significance.

In old stool specimens rhabditiform larvae are occasionally found and can be separated from those of *Strongyloides* by the short buccal chamber and larger genital primordium of the latter.

Eggs similar to those of hookworms can be recovered from humans infected with *Trichostrongylus* spp. and *Ternidens deminutus*. The eggs of the former species are more pointed than those of hookworm and the eggs of *T. deminutus* are significantly larger than those of the hookworm species. These infections can be treated as for hookworm.[576]

Treatment

Albendazole is reported to be effective against the migrating larval stages of the human hookworms, *A. duodenale* and *N. americanus*.[577] The avermectins (ivermectin) have shown promise against all stages of hookworm development, including migrating larvae.[552] Children with severe anemia, malnutrition, infection or heavy worm load should receive preliminary supportive treatment in the form of blood transfusion, high calorie and protein diet, vitamins and iron therapy before definitive treatment of the worms. A highly effective anthelmintic for hookworm infection is albendazole and at a single dose of 400 mg (200 mg for children 10 kg or less) which has also proved highly effective against a wide range of other intestinal helminths.[552,559] Albendazole is additionally reported to have ovicidal activity against hookworm, ascariasis and trichuriasis, making it especially valuable in integrated control programs for these infections.[577] Mebendazole (Vermox) also gives excellent cure rates for both species of hookworm at a dose of 100 mg twice a day for 3 days or 50 mg for children 10 kg or less – and with no side-effects.

Pyrantel embonate/pamoate (Combantrin) (11 mg/kg, max. 750 mg) is effective for *A. duodenale* given in a single dose regimen,[578] but for *N. americanus* needs to be given as a multiple dose treatment. Phenylene diisothiocyanate (Jonit) (adult dose: 100 mg every 12 h × 3) is reported to be equally effective against both *A. duodenale* and *N. americanus*.

Other well-tried treatments include bephenium hydroxynaphthoate and tetrachlorethylene. Bephenium hydroxynaphthoate (Alcopar) has proved highly successful against hookworm, but rather less so in *N. americanus* than in *A. duodenale*. The recommended dose is 2.5 g for children under 2 years, or 10 kg in weight, and 5.0 g in ages and weights above these figures. The drug should be taken when the stomach is empty and at least 1 h before food. The bitter taste can be masked by giving it in a sweet liquid. A second dose is only given if eggs continue to be passed. Side-effects are uncommon but include nausea and vomiting. In *N. americanus* the older treatment, tetrachlorethylene (TCE), is stated to be more effective. The dose is 0.1 ml/kg, with a maximum single dose of 5 ml. The dose can be repeated for up to three successive days. It should probably not, however, be given to very small, severely ill children, and is contraindicated in cases of liver disease. It is important to note here, however, that TCE must not be used for *Necator* when a concomitant *Ascaris* infection is present as it often results in the ascarids migrating up the bile duct and causing obstructive jaundice. In these cases, the ascarids must be treated before TCE is administered.

The preventive aspects of hookworm are complex and include education of the public into the mode of spread of the disease, provision and proper usage of latrines, improvement of diet, and, where the incidence is high, mass population treatment. The wearing of shoes will also help to prevent infection. Studies from Papua New Guinea by Quinell et al[578] suggest that host susceptibility differences may explain why different individuals are predisposed to heavy or light burdens. Interest is continuing regarding the possibility of vaccination against hookworm infection.[573,575,579]

CUTANEOUS LARVA MIGRANS (CREEPING ERUPTION, SAND WORM)

Clinical features

The larvae of the dog hookworms *A. braziliense*, *A. caninum* and *U. stenocephala*, together with certain other parasites (Table 26.38), produce in humans a skin eruption which differs from that caused by 'human' hookworms. The larva, after penetrating the epidermis, is unable to enter the blood or lymph streams and instead burrows just below the corium, traveling up to an inch a day. Papules mark the site of entry and advancing end of the larva and the tunneling causes linear, slightly elevated erythematous and serpigenous areas which itch intensely (Fig. 26.55). Vesicles may form along the course of the tunnels and scaling develops as the lesions age. The most common sites in children are the buttocks and the dorsa of the feet, but any area can be affected. The eruption generally disappears after 1–2 months, but may present for 6 months or longer.

Treatment

The time-honored treatment for cutaneous larva migrans in the past has been freezing of the area with ethyl chloride or similar refrigerant sprays. This is both extremely painful and ineffective. The larvae may be eliminated by a course of diethylcarbamazine (Hetrazan, Banocide) (5 mg/kg per day for 7 days), or tiabendazole (Mintezol) (50 mg/kg in two divided doses (max 1.5 g) twice daily for 3 days, the treatment being repeated at weekly intervals if necessary). Better cure rates, however, are achieved with topical tiabendazole, which can easily be made from the oral preparation if not commercially available. Ivermectin (children > 5 years) at a dose of 200 μg by mouth as a single dose or albendazole as a single oral dose (400 mg or 200 mg for a child < 10 kg) given daily for 3 days, is also listed by Spicer et al.[559]

TRICHURIS TRICHIURA (TRICHOCEPHALIASIS, WHIPWORM)

The whipworm, so called for its thin anterior lash-like end (Fig. 26.56), is widely distributed, being most common in hot, damp environs. The adult nematode frequents the cecum but can occur in

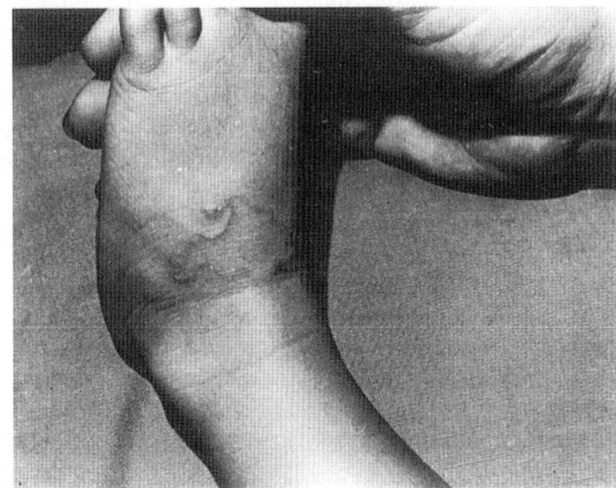

Fig. 26.55 Cutaneous larva migrans.

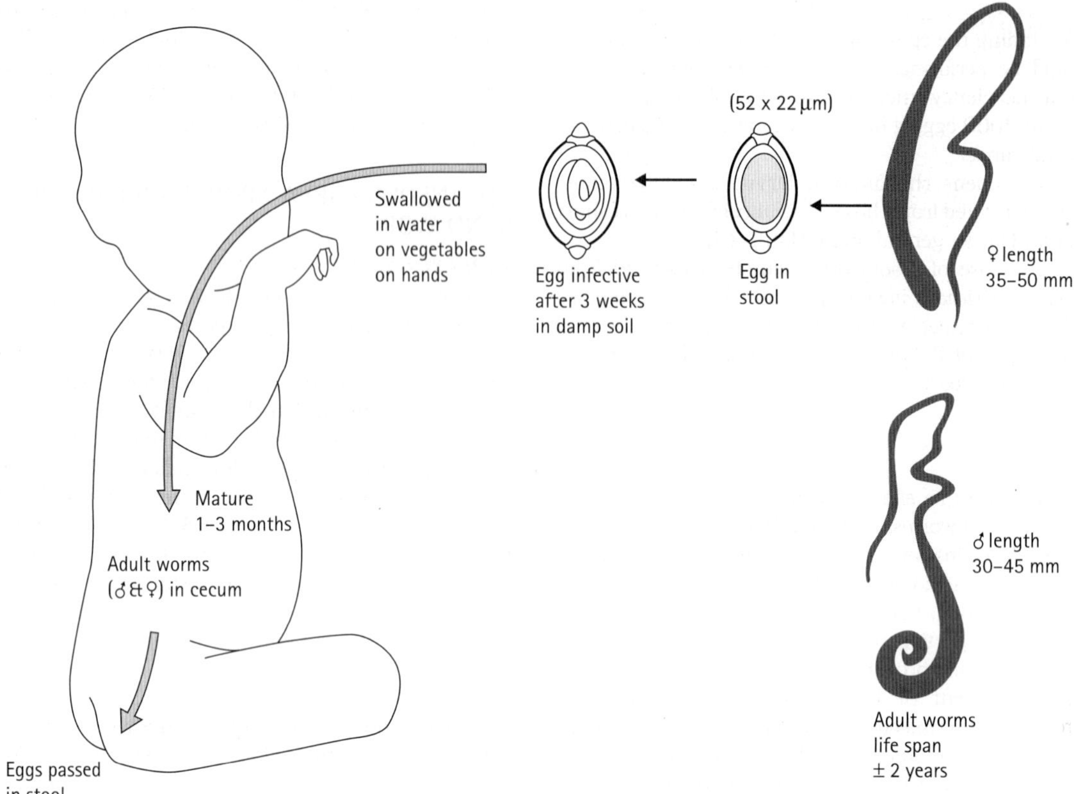

Fig. 26.56 Character and life cycle of *Trichuris trichiura*.

the appendix, colon or terminal ileum, its thin anterior extremity threaded or embedded in the mucosa. Children usually acquire whipworm by sucking fingers or objects contaminated with fecal-polluted soil containing infective eggs, but contaminated vegetables and fly-borne contamination are also important means of spread. Trichuriasis is by no means confined to the tropics[580] and may prove troublesome in mental institutions at times.

Trichuris vulpis, the dog whipworm, may occasionally infect humans as discussed by Milstein & Goldsmid.[566]

Clinical features

Whipworm infection is often asymptomatic but should not be underrated as a pathogen in humans.[580] Heavy worm loads may be responsible for intestinal symptoms, usually abdominal pain, which is most marked in the right iliac fossa, bloody diarrhea, tenesmus, and sometimes mild pyrexia. Appendicitis may also result. Excessive loads can lead to marked anemia, weight loss, and a picture closely resembling hookworm disease or amebic colitis. Clubbing of the fingers and toes is often seen in these children and is reversed with eradication of the infection. Rectal prolapse is a well-recognized complication. Trichuriasis often causes insidious disease and is frequently associated with growth retardation in children.[581]

Diagnosis

This is readily accomplished by finding the characteristic eggs (Fig. 26.57) in the stools. These eggs under suitable conditions in damp soil require about 3 weeks to mature to the infective stage. A barium enema may assist in diagnosis (Fig. 26.58).

Treatment

Albendazole at a dose of 400 mg, or 200 mg for children 10 kg or less, given by mouth for 3 days is the drug of choice,[559] but the very safe mebendazole (Vermox) which should be administered at a dose of 100 mg (50 mg for a child 10 kg or less) twice a day for 3 days is also highly effective.[552] If the child is suffering from diarrhea, the diarrhea should be controlled before the anthelmintic is administered, in order to achieve maximal efficiency. Difetarsone (Bemarsal) has been reported to be most useful in the treatment of whipworm – 2 g daily in divided doses for 10 days are given in adults. Oxantel pamoate is also reported to be effective at a dose of 15 mg/kg body weight.[552]

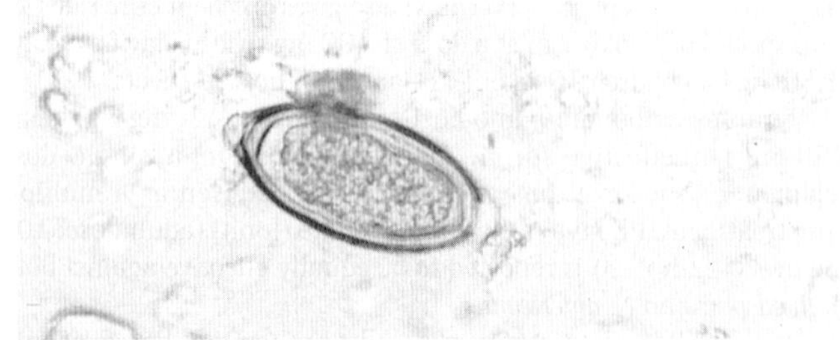

Fig. 26.57 Egg of *Trichuris trichiura* (approx. × 600).

STRONGYLOIDES STERCORALIS (STRONGYLOIDIASIS)

Strongyloides stercoralis (sometimes termed 'threadworm' in the American literature) has a human cycle closely resembling hookworm, except that internal autoinfection is common and a free-living cycle can occur if external conditions are favorable (Fig. 26.59). Strongyloidiasis is essentially an affliction of tropical or semitropical climates but its sporadic occurrence in temperate zones is recognized. The minute adult worms are to be found in the

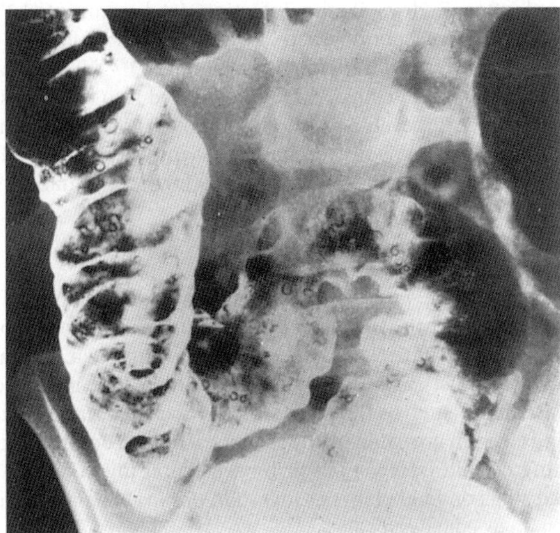

Fig. 26.58 *Trichuris trichiura.* Double contrast barium enema examination showing infestation and numerous small circular or sigmoid defects in barium coating of colon.

crypts of Lieberkuhn's glands in the upper part of the small intestine, where they burrow in the mucosa.

In central Africa, *Strongyloides fülleborni* is often found in humans and a similar species is reported to cause 'swollen belly syndrome' in infants about 6 weeks of age in Papua New Guinea.[582] The species in Papua New Guinea has been designated as *S. fülleborni kellyi* and infants can become infected in the first days of life, with children as young as 18 days of age being found to have patent infections – possibly owing to transmammary infection, as may also occur with *S. fülleborni* in Africa.[583]

Clinical features

Skin penetration by filariform larvae may be accompanied by a transient prickling sensation, but following heavy infection there is a pruritic petechial rash with local edema. Internal and external autoinfection frequently occurs, especially in immunodeficient patients or patients on immunosuppressant drugs or corticosteroids, larvae in the feces entering through the rectal mucosa or the skin in the perianal region. This gives rise to an often recurring eruption resembling cutaneous larva migrans (termed *larva currens*) but of shorter duration. Larvae may also re-enter through the anus. Generalized urticaria is sometimes seen as a result of hypersensitivity. Eosinophilia is common. Clinical manifestations of pulmonary migration of larvae are infrequent, but respiratory symptoms can occur and, rarely, chronic lung disease develops due to misguided larvae maturing within the lung.

In chronic strongyloidiasis the presence of the adult worms in the intestine is often asymptomatic.[584] A heavy worm load causes epigastric pain, episodes of acute appendicitis,[571] bowel upset often with bloody diarrhea, iron deficiency anemia, and debility. Infection can last for 20 years or more owing to constant internal and external autoinfection.[585] In immunocompromised patients, fatal

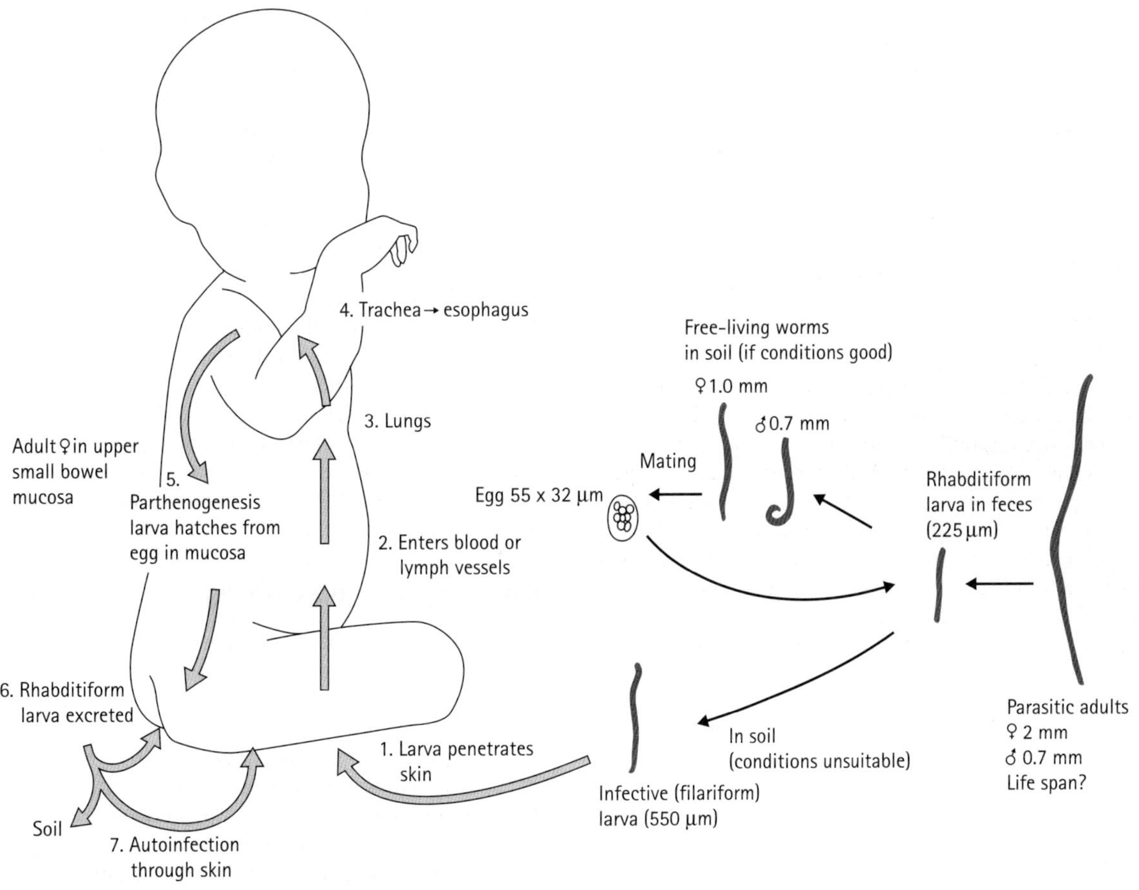

Fig. 26.59 Character and life cycle of *Strongyloides stercoralis.*

autoinfection can occur, but it is noteworthy that despite the HIV/AIDS pandemic in sub-Saharan Africa and elsewhere, *S. stercoralis* has not proved an important opportunistic pathogen.[576,584] *Strongyloides* hyperinfection syndrome carries a high mortality and may be complicated by Gram negative bacteremia in both immunocompromised and non-compromised individuals.[586,587]

Diagnosis

Considerable eosinophilia is usual and can be an important diagnostic indicator in some circumstances.[585] Diagnosis of *S. stercoralis* is established by demonstrating rhabditiform larvae (Fig. 26.60a) in fresh stools (repeat examinations may be necessary) or duodenal fluid. A most useful method for diagnosing *S. stercoralis*, giardiasis, and other upper intestinal parasites is duodenal drainage or the use of the duodenal capsule (Enterotest), or 'string test' of which a special pediatric size is available. The capsule, containing a length of thread and 3-ply nylon yarn, is swallowed while the protruding free end of thread is held at the mouth. The yarn within the capsule plays out, and within 3–4 h the line has almost invariably extended to the duodenum or jejunum. The gelatin capsule dissolves. The nylon yarn is then pulled back through the mouth and the adhering mucus examined for parasites.

In *S. fülleborni* infections, fully embryonated eggs (Fig. 26.60b) are passed in the feces. These are small, being about 50 × 36 μm in size and fully developed at time of passage.[576]

Treatment

Because of the dangers of autoinfection, especially in the immunocompromised, strongyloidiasis must always be treated when diagnosed.[588]

The treatment of choice for strongyloidiasis is now albendazole 400 mg b.d. orally for 3 days (children 10 kg or less 200 mg), repeated after 7 days if the infection is disseminated.[559,577] Ivermectin 200 μg/kg orally each day as a single dose for 1–2 days can also be used for children over 5 years of age.[559,588] Tiabendazole (Mintezol) which is effective (50 mg/kg divided into two doses and given morning and evening up to a total of 3 g daily max.) is an alternative.[559] It may, however, have most unpleasant side-effects. Ivermectin appears promising but requires further evaluation.[584]

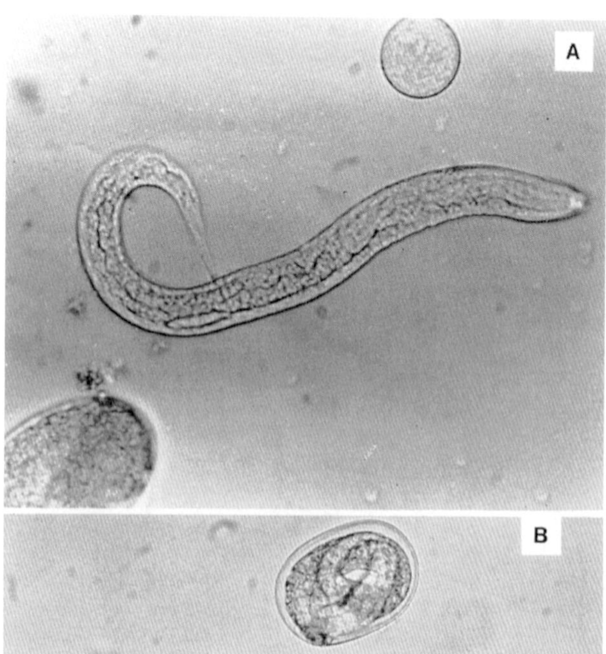

Fig. 26.60 (a) Rhabditiform larva of *Strongyloides stercoralis*. Note short buccal cavity and large genital primordium. Also in the field, an *Entamoeba* cyst and a hookworm egg (approx. × 600). (b) Egg of *Strongyloides fülleborni*. Note its small size. It contains a fully developed, motile larva when passed (approx. × 600).

ANGIOSTRONGYLIASIS

Angiostrongylus cantonensis is a natural parasite in the lungs of rats over a wide area of the world, with human infection being recorded from Indonesia, Papua New Guinea, northern Australia, Africa, the Pacific, south-east Asia, Cuba and Puerto Rico. The intermediate hosts are snails (such as the giant African land snail *Achatina fulica*) and slugs, which are eaten by the rodents. Humans become infected by eating certain edible snails or by accidental ingestion of small infected slugs on food plants or ingestion of paratenic (or 'carrier') hosts such as edible crustacea.[589]

In humans, larvae migrate to the brain causing a condition known as eosinophilic meningitis, with neck stiffness, photophobia, pyrexia, decreased consciousness and vomiting.

The diagnosis, in endemic areas, can be suspected when large numbers of eosinophils are found in the CSF in patients with a history of eating snails or perhaps crustacea. Occasionally adults or larvae of *A. cantonensis* may also be detected. A blood eosinophilia may also be present.

Surgical intervention may be necessary,[590] no effective treatment being presently available and may in any case be inadvisable as dead worms cause more clinical problems than live ones. However, mebendazole (100 mg b.d. for 5 days) together with corticosteroids (30–60 mg/day) is mentioned by Shorey et al.[565]

Other forms of angiostrongyliasis include an abdominal form caused by *A. costaricensis* in several Latin American countries. This species causes intestinal and liver lesions similar to those caused by *Toxocara*. It is usually diagnosed at surgery and has an epidemiology similar to *A. cantonensis*.[591]

HELMINTHOMA

The nodular worms belong to the genera *Oesophagostomum*, naturally occurring in simian and ruminant hosts, and the false hookworm, *Ternidens deminutus*, a natural parasite of non-human primates, are known in central Africa to cause human disease characterized by tumor-like granulomatous reactions in the wall of the colon.[592] Eggs of these species are hookworm-like but larger in size.[576]

The drug treatment of choice for the expulsion of the adult worm is mebendazole (Vermox) (100 mg twice a day for 3 days) and albendazole is promising.[576,592]

ANISAKIASIS (ANISAKIDOSIS)

This parasitic infection of humans is caused by the larval stages of some 30 genera of anisakid nematodes, of which the commonest are *Anisakis*, *Contracaecum* and *Terranova*.[571] These helminths are intestinal parasites of a range of fish-eating vertebrates, including dolphins, and the larval stages of the worm are found in intermediate hosts such as small fish (e.g. mackerel, herring, salmon), squid or octopus.[593,594] Humans become infected when they eat raw or undercooked fish.

The ingested worms live in the human gastrointestinal tract or penetrate the tissues, giving rise to abscesses or eosinophilic granulomata.

Clinically the infection may be asymptomatic or mild with nausea, vomiting, epigastric pain and often an eosinophilia, which may reach 41%. Death, although rare, may result from peritonitis following perforation of the gut.[593]

While the infection has for many years been recognized in Japan, an increase has been noted in the USA owing to better diagnostic techniques.[594] Diagnosis is established at laparotomy, by X-ray, or most reliably, by endoscopy. Serological tests for diagnosis include the radioallergosorbent test (RAST) and counterimmunoelectrophoresis.

The most effective treatment, where possible, is removal of worms from the stomach by endoscopy and prevention is best achieved by removal of worms from fish prior to eating and by thorough cooking of fish. No effective anthelmintic treatment is presently available[593] but Shorey et al[565] express the view that mebendazole might have some value.

TRICHINOSIS

The genus *Trichinella* contains at least four species of which the best known is *Trichinella spiralis*.[595] *T. spiralis* has a cosmopolitan distribution and the worm is usually transmitted to humans by inadequately cooked, infected pig meat, although outbreaks from other meat sources (e.g. horse meat) are recognized,[596,597] so that the disease may occur in outbreaks (Fig. 26.61). Trichinosis due to *T. spiralis* is rare in communities which shun pork and in those with vigilant agricultural control, but human disease, especially with other species (e.g. *T. pseudospiralis, T. nelsoni, T. bitovi* or *T. nativa*) may be associated with other species of animal. The adult *T. spiralis* naturally infects humans, pigs and rats, as well as other animals. Porcine infection usually results from the ingestion of either infected rats or garbage containing uncooked pork meat.

Clinical features

Human trichinosis is frequently mild or symptomless. Although symptoms may occur as early as 24 h following a pork meal, it is usually during the incubation period of 5–7 days or longer[598] in which the ingested larvae mature into adults, that a clinical picture resembling food poisoning develops – nausea, vomiting, diarrhea, and abdominal pain. This phase lasts about 5 days and is followed by signs and symptoms as the larvae enter the bloodstream and encyst in the muscle – a phase lasting a further 2–3 weeks. There is pyrexia, edema of the face and eyelids, splinter hemorrhages under the finger nails, tender lymphadenopathy, and myalgia, often extreme. Cough may occur and in severe cases the illness may suggest encephalitis or myocarditis. Marked eosinophilia is usual. Final encystment of the larvae occurs only in voluntary muscles particularly those of the diaphragm, throat, chest wall, extrinsic ocular apparatus and tongue, and patients may die of toxemia or myocarditis. The encysted larvae may live for many years.

Diagnosis

Diagnosis in the early stages can be made by finding worms in the feces, but in the later stages of the disease, diagnosis is established by muscle biopsy. Intracutaneous and fluorescent antibody tests, together with other serological procedures, are useful adjuncts.[565,598]

Treatment

Albendazole (400 mg for 3 days; 200 mg for children 10 kg or less) is the drug of choice. Mebendazole (200–400 mg t.d. for 3 days and then 400–500 mg for 10 days) is also cited by Shorey et al.[565]

There is evidence that tiabendazole (Mintezol) (50 mg/kg per day in two doses for 5 days; max. 3 g daily) rapidly kills off migrating larvae and relieves the symptoms.[558] If taken early, the drug also

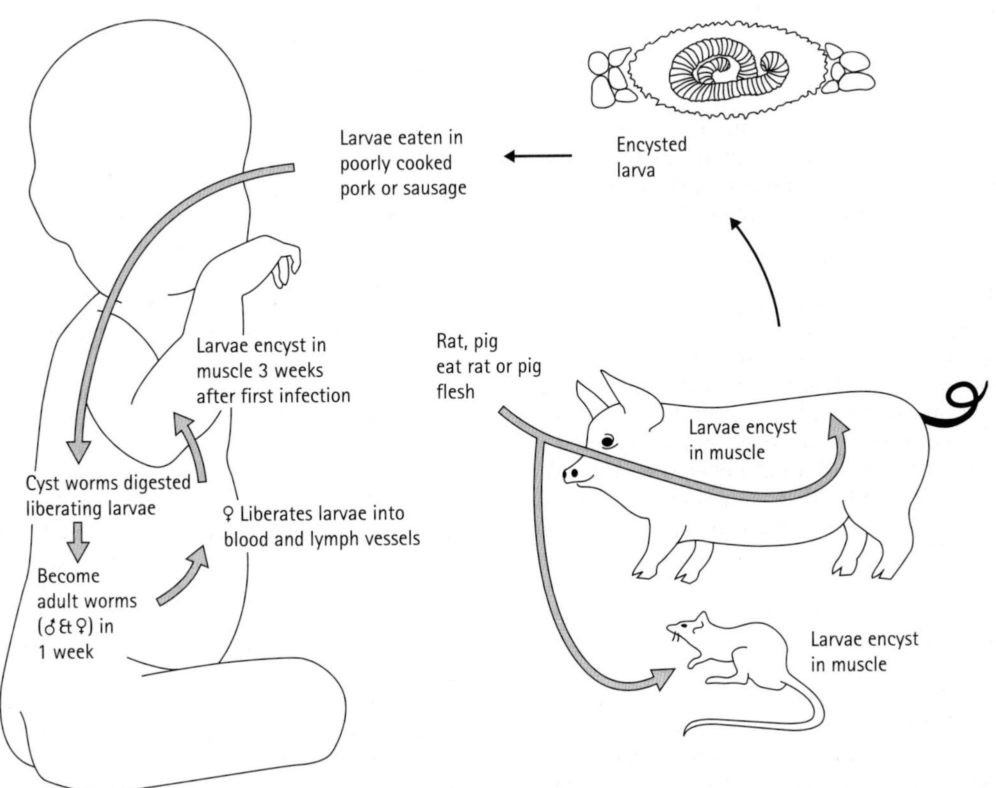

Fig. 26.61 Character and life cycle of *Trichinella spiralis*.

kills larvae in the bowel but is not lethal to the adult worms. Corticosteroids, previously recommended for the treatment of trichinosis, should be restricted to critically ill cases,[590] and then only used in conjunction with anthelmintics.

PARACAPILLARIA PHILIPPINENSIS (CAPILLARIASIS)

It has long been known that the nematode *Capillaria hepatica* can cause a visceral larva migrans-like syndrome in people who have eaten meat (e.g. infected liver) or sand containing the eggs of the worm. These children exhibit such symptoms as fever, eosinophilia, abdominal pain and hepatomegaly, with large numbers of typical eggs being found in the liver on histological examination.

Another species of the genus, *Paracapillaria philippinensis*, has also been shown to be an important cause of epidemic diarrhea in humans in south-east Asia, Asia and the Middle East. Clinical features in these cases include abdominal pain, malabsorption and diarrhea which is often severe and not uncommonly fatal (35%) without medical care.[599]

P. philippinensis is a parasite of the small intestine and it is believed to be a zoonotic infection involving birds and freshwater fish. Humans become infected by ingestion of eggs or infected raw fish, the usual intermediate host, and loads within the host may increase as a result of autoinfection.[571]

Capillaria aerophila is a zoonotic species found in the lungs of cats, and occasional human infections have been recorded.[565,571]

Diagnosis of capillariasis is based upon histology or finding eggs and larvae in feces. These eggs are like those of *Trichuris*, but the polar plugs are inset and the shells are striated or pitted. *C. hepatica* eggs can be found as spurious 'transit eggs' in feces of patients who have recently eaten infected liver.[600]

Treatment for capillariasis is tiabendazole (Mintezol) 25 mg/kg per day for 30 days or longer. Side-effects and relapses are, however, common.[599] Mebendazole and albendazole are also reported to be effective for the treatment of capillariasis.[571]

DRACUNCULOSIS (DRACONTIASIS)

Despite its bizarre mode of propagation, the guinea worm (*Dracunculus medinensis*) is widely distributed in equatorial Africa, the Middle East and India. However, with new international efforts to improve drinking water supplies, dracontiasis eradication may well be achievable.[601]

Clinical features

Children from the age of 2 years upwards may be infected by drinking water containing *Cyclops*, a tiny crustacean which is infected with the larvae of *Dracunculus*. During the asymptomatic incubation period, lasting approximately 1 year, the guinea worm matures in retroperitoneal tissues. The male, having fertilized the female, apparently dies. The gravid female, often over 100 cm in length by 1.5 mm in width, then migrates through the subcutaneous tissues to distal parts of the extremities, usually the lower limb, to form a large pruritic papule. This vesiculates and then bursts leaving a shallow ulcer. On immersion in water the worm's uterus prolapses through the ulcer releasing myriads of larvae. Occasionally adult worms may develop in ectopic sites.

Papule formation may be associated with a marked allergic reaction (vomiting, diarrhea, urticaria and bronchospasm).

Secondary infection of sinuses, subcutaneous cysts, sterile abscesses, and perarticular fibrosis with joint deformity are recognized complications. Calcified worms may be discovered on radiological examination.

Treatment

The ancient technique of repeatedly stimulating the parturient worm with cold water, grasping the uterus which then protrudes, and then cautiously winding the worm round a stick an inch or two per day is still used. However, drug treatments recommended for dracontiasis include the use of niridazole (Ambilhar) (25 mg/kg daily in two divided doses for 7–10 days) and tiabendazole (Mintezol) which has also been reported to be effective at a total dose of 25 mg/kg orally daily for 3 days.[558] Metronidazole (Flagyl) is also claimed to be highly effective at an oral dose for children of 25 mg/kg (max. 750 mg/day) daily in three doses for 5 days.[558,560]

FILARIASIS

Filariasis has been included among the diseases given priority by the United Nations Development Program/World Bank/WHO Special Program for Research and Training due to the huge number of people infected and the enormous burden of morbidity affecting whole communities in endemic regions.[602]

Humans are the primary hosts to several species of filariae, the adult worms living in the tissues. The adult female worms produce eggs, which hatch to release prelarval microfilariae. These are ingested by an appropriate blood-sucking arthropod vector, in which they undergo metamorphosis to form infective larvae. Important characteristics of the principal human filariae are shown in Table 26.39.

During the early stages of all filarial infections moderate to high eosinophilia is usual, but this gradually diminishes in those who have been infected for long periods. Apart from *Onchocerca volvulus* where microfilariae are found in skin snips, parasitological diagnosis is best achieved by using stained blood films or concentration techniques applied to peripheral blood. However, very promising and effective serological tests for the detection of circulating filarial antigen have been developed.

Onchocerca volvulus

Onchocerciasis is a filarial disease, which is transmitted to humans by bites from black flies of the genus *Simulium*. It is characterized by subcutaneous nodules, containing adult worms of *O. volvulus*, by skin eruptions due to microfilariae and by serious eye disease. The condition is only seen in central Africa and in central and parts of South America (Table 26.39) especially along the banks of fast flowing rivers, in which the flies breed.

Clinical features

Adolescents are most commonly affected but children down to 1 year of age may be afflicted.

Signs of disease begin to appear in 4–18 months and the commonest manifestation is the *Onchocerca* nodule. These subcutaneous fibrous nodules (onchocercomata), containing one or more adult worms in each, vary from a few millimeters to about 3 cm in diameter and become fully developed within a year of exposure. In Africa, they tend to occur most commonly in the pelvic region especially over the hips and on the buttocks, while in South America the head is more usually involved. Nodules do not generally give rise to much discomfort, but at times they may be painful, and secondary infection with abscess formation can occur. The number and size of nodules increase with intensity of the infection.

Typical skin lesions (onchodermatitis) consist of an intensely itchy papular dermatitis with edema in the early stages progressing to lichenification and atrophy ('lizard skin'). Large numbers of microfilariae are present in the skin and involvement may be generalized or limited to one area of the body. Transient urticaria is

Table 26.39 Types of filaria worms responsible for human disease

Type and distribution	Insect vector	Important features of microfilaria	Human adult worm location
Onchocerca volvulus, west, central and east Africa, Guatemala, Mexico, and Surinam	*Simulium* black flies	Do not occur in blood, but in skin as unsheathed intradermal microfilariae (microfilariae may penetrate eye)	Subcutaneous tissue
Mansonella perstans, tropical and subtropical areas mainly of Africa and South America	*Culicoides* midges	Occur in blood. Non-periodic. Unsheathed. Nuclear column extends into tip of thick blunt tail	Mesenteric, perirenal and retroperitoneal tissues
Mansonella ozzardi, South America	*Culicoides* midges	Occur in blood. Non-periodic. Nuclear column does NOT extend into tip of thin, pointed tail	Mesentery and serous body cavities
Wuchereria bancrofti, tropical and subtropical areas throughout the world	Many mosquitoes belonging to the genera *Culex*, *Aedes*, *Anopheles*, and *Mansonia*	Occur in blood. Nocturnal periodic. Sheathed. Nuclear column does NOT extend into tip of thin pointed tail	Lymphatic tissue
Brugia malayi, *B. timori*, East Indies and Southern Asia	Many mosquitoes belonging to the genera *Mansonia*, *Culex*, and *Anopheles*	Occur in blood. Nocturnal periodic. Sheathed. Nuclear column extends into tip of tail with single spaced nuclei in terminal bulb and subterminal swelling	Lymphatic tissue
Loa loa, west and central Africa	*Chrysops* flies	Occur in blood. Diurnal periodic. Sheathed. Nuclear column extends into tip of thick blunt tail	Subcutaneous tissue

often the only skin manifestation, and indeed the condition may be entirely asymptomatic despite the presence of microfilariae in the skin. General well-being is seldom disturbed.

Ocular lesions (river blindness) due to microfilariae penetrating the eyes represent the most serious feature of onchocerciasis and are a frequent cause of blindness in endemic areas. They occur especially when the disease is present in the upper half of the body and are commoner in South America. Children rarely show advanced ocular lesions, but hyperemia of the conjunctiva and nummular keratitis may be seen on occasions in older children. Any part of the eye can be involved.

Diagnosis

Diagnosis is best established by demonstrating microfilariae in skin snips and the adult worms on nodule biopsy. Serological tests, including tests for antigen, are also available in onchocerciasis but the work of Shelley et al[603] suggests that there may be some cross-reaction with other filarial species (e.g. *Mansonella ozzardi*) in areas where they coexist. Microfilariae are not uncommonly found in urine.

Treatment

Excision of nodules is recommended prior to chemotherapy, especially those near the eyes because of the danger of ocular involvement. Microfilariae are killed by diethylcarbamazine but the drug causes a temporary exacerbation of skin and eye lesions, tenderness of nodules, and enlargement of regional lymph glands. This reaction forms the basis for the Mazzoti test – a useful diagnostic procedure. Diethylcarbamazine should, therefore, be given in small doses initially (0.5 mg/kg three times daily) gradually increasing to 2 mg/kg (max. 150 mg/day) three times daily for 2–3 weeks. Severe reactions can be controlled with corticosteroids. Suramin (Antrypol) is lethal to the adult worms. A course consists of six doses of 20 mg/kg intravenously at intervals of 7 days. Regular urine tests should be made as the drug is nephrotoxic. Ivermectin is now accepted as the treatment of choice for onchocerciasis at a single dose of 150–200 μg/kg for both adults and children.[604–606] This treatment may need to be repeated every 3–6 months for 2–3 years.[565] Its use for mass treatment has given hope for the effective control of this disease. Amocarzine and albendazole are also being evaluated for efficacy in the treatment of onchocerciasis.[571]

Vector control would require the simultaneous application of control measures (spraying with appropriate insecticides) over whole river systems.

Loa loa

Loa loa is transmitted to humans by flies of the genus *Chrysops*, which, in turn, are infected by sucking human blood containing microfilariae. These are present in blood during the daytime, thus corresponding with the diurnal biting habits of most *Chrysops*. The disease is endemic in western and central Africa. Adult worms live in the subcutaneous tissues, the male being some 3 cm and the female 6 cm in length. They may remain viable for as long as 30 years.

Clinical features

Symptoms of loiasis are trivial. The most characteristic manifestation is a recurrent, painless, puffy, pink swelling, often referred to as a calabar, or fugitive, swelling. This lesion marks the journey of the adult worm in the subcutis. It develops over a period of 3–4 h and may acquire a diameter of 10 cm or more, before subsiding in a few days. The upper extremities and eyelids are most often involved and on occasions the thin worm may be seen rapidly traversing the bulbar conjunctiva and sometimes accompanied by periorbital edema. The appearance of the calabar swelling is frequently associated with fever and malaise. Eosinophilia is present.

Some patients remain afilaremic, no microfilariae being found in the peripheral blood despite intensive investigation.[607]

Treatment

Diethylcarbamazine is a highly effective remedy in loiasis. The recommended dose is 0.5 mg/kg three times daily for 2 days, and if no unfavorable reactions follow, the dose is increased to 3 mg/kg three times a day for a further 3 weeks. Mebendazole and ivermectin appear less effective.[607]

Wuchereria bancrofti and *Brugia malayi*

Infections by *Wuchereria bancrofti, Brugia malayi* and *B. timori* (termed 'lymphatic filariasis') occur in the tropics and in some semitropical areas, being transmitted by various species of mosquito. The adult female and male worms (some 85 mm and 40 mm in length respectively) attain maturity in the lymphatic system about 1 year following entry to the body, after which time the nocturnal periodic sheathed microfilariae are demonstrable in peripheral blood between 10 p.m. and 2 a.m. Some Pacific strains of *W. bancrofti* are non-periodic.

Clinical features

First infection may occur in children but the full clinical picture may take many years to develop. As with other filarial diseases, the early phases may be entirely asymptomatic or associated with florid allergic manifestations. The commonest manifestations of the mature filariae are acute and recurring lymphangitis. The affected lymph node, together with its afferent vessel, usually in the groin, are painful and tender. The lymphatic vessel becomes palpable and cord-like and is associated with a linear red streak in the overlying skin. This stage is often accompanied by pyrexia, malaise, nausea, and headache. Dreyer et al[608] believe that acute attacks of lymphatic filariasis can be divided into a number of clearly defined clinical syndromes. The acute attacks, which subside after several days, have a variable periodicity of weeks or months, gradually becoming less severe, often with persistence of residual subcutaneous swelling. Recurrent funiculitis may occur and involvement of intra-abdominal lymph nodes may give rise to the clinical picture of peritonitis. Chylous ascites, chyluria, varicose groin nodes, hydrocele and elephantiasis are classical end results but as they arise from chronicity over many years, emphasis on this aspect is out of place in a pediatric context. Nevertheless, early manifestations of chronic disease may sometimes appear in the late years of childhood.

Work by Hightower et al[609] has suggested that children born to mothers infected with *W. bancrofti* are more susceptible to this infection than those born to uninfected mothers.

Tropical eosinophilia syndrome. In some patients, an abnormal response to *W. bancrofti* infections results in a clinical picture which reflects a specific allergic sensitization to filarial antigens – a condition known as tropical pulmonary eosinophilia or tropical eosinophilia syndrome. These patients present with cough, asthma-like symptoms, respiratory distress and eosinophil counts of $3000/mm^3$ or greater. X-ray of the lungs usually shows extensive changes. An interesting feature of this syndrome is that patients do not develop a filaremia – hence the term 'occult filariasis'.

A similar condition can be caused by infection with *Brugia malayi* and perhaps by infection with non-human filariae.

Diagnosis

The clinical diagnosis based on symptoms can now be greatly aided by ultrasonography and lymphoscintigraphy.

The recovery of typical sheathed microfilariae in midnight blood slides and occasionally in urine will establish the diagnosis. Concentration techniques may need to be used to recover microfilariae from the blood.

In the case of tropical pulmonary eosinophilia, diagnosis is made clinically and confirmed by serology or rapid response to diethylcarbamazine.[610]

It is worth noting that visitors to endemic areas who contract lymphatic filariasis often do not develop a microfilaremia, which can make parasitological confirmation of the infection impossible. Thus the development of an EIA test (TropBio, Australia) to detect circulating filarial antigen has provided a major breakthrough in the diagnosis of lymphatic filariasis, the test for *W. bancrofti* being highly specific and very sensitive. So too, antigen detecting tests have been developed for *B. malayi*, including DNA detection from blood spots, which also show great promise and are very cost-effective.[611–613]

Treatment

Diethylcarbamazine rapidly removes circulating microfilariae but large doses are required to kill adult worms. The initial dosage should be 0.5–1.0 mg/kg (max. 25 mg/day) in divided doses daily for 3 days, followed by 1–2 mg/kg three times daily for a further 2–3 weeks.[558,560] There is often an acute exacerbation during therapy, for which antihistamines should be given. Ivermectin, which has significantly fewer side-effects than diethylcarbamazine, is also very effective in the treatment of lymphatic filariasis. It kills microfilariae but not adult worms and the single oral dose of 150–200 μg/kg should be repeated at yearly intervals. Ottesen et al[614] concluded that a single oral dose of ivermectin was a favorable method for controlling lymphatic filariasis and the review by Chodakewitz[606] has confirmed its value against *W. bancrofti*.

The use of yearly or 6-monthly doses of ivermectin or the regular use of salt, fortified with diethylcarbamazine, has proved invaluable in the control of lymphatic filariasis in endemic regions. Ultimately, however, the control of lymphatic filariasis will be an overall public health problem.[615] Control will be neither easy nor straightforward and Alexander et al[616] have shown that in the control of filariasis, even small areas omitted from a general filariasis vector control program due to, for example, difficult terrain, have the potential to disperse the infection. As Molyneaux[617] says: 'environment remains a key determinant in changing patterns of vector-borne infections. Changes are rapid and vectors have the capacity to change equally rapidly, a capacity not matched by health systems'. He further believes[617] that in future years, less time will be spent on developing new pesticides for insect vector control and that the emphasis will rather be placed on genetic approaches to make such insects less effective vectors.

Mansonella perstans and *Mansonella ozzardi*

Mansonella perstans has had many recent changes in its name[618] and is widely distributed in those tropical and subtropical areas which favor the habitat of the vector. The unsheathed microfilariae are transmitted by *Culicoides* midges from person to person, and the adult worms develop in the mesentery, perinephric and retroperitoneal tissues where they may survive for many years (Table 26.39).

Clinical features

This form of filariasis is often held to be harmless, but symptoms can be associated with infection, particularly in people visiting from non-endemic regions. Infection with these helminths may result in lethargy, arthralgia, urticaria and headache. Less frequently calabar-like swellings around the eye ('bung eye'), and pericardial or pleural effusions occur. Among indigenous inhabitants of endemic areas *M. perstans* is often asymptomatic.

The prepatent period from exposure to the appearance of non-periodic microfilariae in the blood is unknown.

Diethylcarbamazine is ineffective in treatment of the disease, but trichlorophone has been used with success in an adult dose of

10 mg/kg given every 2 weeks with a total of four doses. The judicious use of corticosteroids is valuable in severe cases. Mebendazole, or a combination of mebendazole (Vermox) and levamisole (Ketrax), has proved effective.

In rain forest areas of central Africa, a related species, *M. streptocerca*, infects humans. Microfilariae of this species are unsheathed and have a curled tail with nuclei extending to the tip. The adult and microfilariae of this species are found in skin, and diagnosis is by skin snips as for *Onchocerca*. Symptoms include a dermatitis, with macules and papules. Infection is more common in older people than in children.

M. ozzardi in South America is a species with many clinical similarities to *M. perstans*. In the past it too has been considered a commensal, but studies have suggested that this parasite may also not be as harmless as is often believed (Table 26.39).

Dirofilaria immitis

The dog heartworm is a common filarial nematode infecting dogs in most tropical regions of the world including parts of the USA and northern Australia. It is transmitted by mosquitoes.

Occasional human cases are diagnosed during serological surveys or on biopsy for investigations of pulmonary 'coin' lesions found on X-ray.[572] Cases of pleural effusion, intraocular infection and eosinophilic meningitis are also caused by *D. immitis* in humans. Most cases of dirofilariasis are recorded in adults, but clinical infections are seen at times in children and Hungerford[568] believes that dirofilariasis is much commoner in Australia than is believed at present.

As *D. immitis* infection in humans does not usually exhibit a filaremia, diagnosis is usually made on biopsy of a lung lesion or on removal of a worm from the eye. Skin tests or serological tests are unhelpful.

Other species of *Dirofilaria* are also recorded from humans, usually from subcutaneous tissue or from the conjunctival sac.

CESTODES (TAPEWORMS)

The cestodes are platyhelminths, which are dorsoventrally flattened, have no gut or body cavity and are hermaphroditic. Adult tapeworms have a characteristic morphology with a scolex armed with suckers and sometimes hooks, an unsegmented neck region and a long segmented strobila.

Life cycles are complex, with the adult tapeworms living in the gastrointestinal tract of the vertebrate definitive hosts and with larval stages occurring in a range of vertebrate or invertebrate intermediate host species. Larval forms vary from the free-living ciliated coracidium larva and worm-like procercoid and plerocercoid (sparganum) larvae of the pseudophyllidean tapeworms (e.g. *Diphyllobothrium latum*) to the cysticercoid, cysticercus (bladderworm) or hydatid larvae of the cyclophyllidean tapeworms.

Humans can become infected with a range of cestode species and mostly harbor the adult tapeworm although human infection with larval cestodes includes sparganosis (*Spirometra* sp.), cysticercosis (*Taenia solium*) and hydatidosis (*Echinococcus granulosus*).

The main cestodes relevant to humans are *Taenia saginata, Taenia solium, Hymenolepis nana, H. diminuta, Dipylidium caninum, Diphyllobothrium latum, Echinococcus* spp. and *Inermicapsifer madagascariensis*.

TAENIASIS

Taeniasis is caused by infection with adult *T. saginata* or *T. solium* (Table 26.40). In both these infections, the adult tapeworm is

Table 26.40 Characteristics of *Taenia saginata* and *Taenia solium*

	Taenia saginata	*Taenia solium*
Parasite		
Scolex	4 suckers only	Crown of hooklets and 4 suckers
Length	5–20 m	3–15 m
Lateral branches of uterus	15 or more	8–13
Intermediate host	Cattle	Pig, but occasionally man
Final host	Man	Man

found in the intestinal tract of humans – the only definitive host. The intermediate hosts harboring the larval stage (cysticercus) of the tapeworm are cattle in *T. saginata* (the beef tapeworm) and usually pigs in *T. solium* (the pork tapeworm). However, in the case of *T. solium*, in addition to pigs, a wide range of mammals, including humans, can harbor the cysticerci.

It has been suggested, that in the Asia–Pacific region, other but as yet incompletely defined, species of *Taenia* may infect humans.[619,620] One such species found in Indonesia, Taiwan and Korea morphologically resembles *T. saginata* but is acquired from pork and has been named *T. asiatica*.[545,571]

Infection with adult *Taenia* results from ingestion of infected meat and, as such, is not common in very young children.

Taenia saginata (the beef tapeworm)

The beef tapeworm is cosmopolitan, occurring in almost all countries where beef is eaten. It is especially common where local eating habits favor the consumption of raw or undercooked beef. The cysticerci in the beef can even survive salting and a moderate degree of drying.

The adult worm is harbored in the human intestine attached to the mucosa of the small intestine. It may reach 20–25 m in length and gravid proglottids (or segments), their uteri packed with eggs, break from the strobila singly or in chains of two to five segments, and either migrate actively out of the anus or pass out passively with the feces.

The proglottids crawl about on the ground releasing eggs, which are also liberated when the proglottid dies and disintegrates on pasture land. Eggs, lying on the grass, are ingested by grazing cattle (Fig. 26.62). The oncosphere (hexacanth) larva is released in the intestine, penetrates the intestinal wall using its six hooklets and is carried via the bloodstream to the heart and voluntary muscles, especially the tongue, shoulder and masseter muscles. Here it loses its hooklets, develops an inverted scolex with suckers but no hooks and changes into a bladderworm (or cysticercus) larva, termed *Cysticercus bovis*, over about 3 months. These cysticerci are about 8 × 5 mm in size and meat infected with them is commonly termed 'measly' owing to its spotted appearance.

When ingested, the cysticercus evaginates the scolex and elongates into the adult stage. Humans eating such 'measly' beef raw or undercooked thus become infected with adult tapeworm. Gravid segments are shed about 3 months after infection.

Epidemics of 'measles' in cattle have not uncommonly resulted from cattle grazed on pastures fertilized with untreated effluent from sewage outlets. Such cattle become infective in about 3 months after ingestion of eggs.

Clinical features

In most cases infection with *T. saginata* is quite symptomless, the only feature being the intermittent passing of segments. In 5–50%

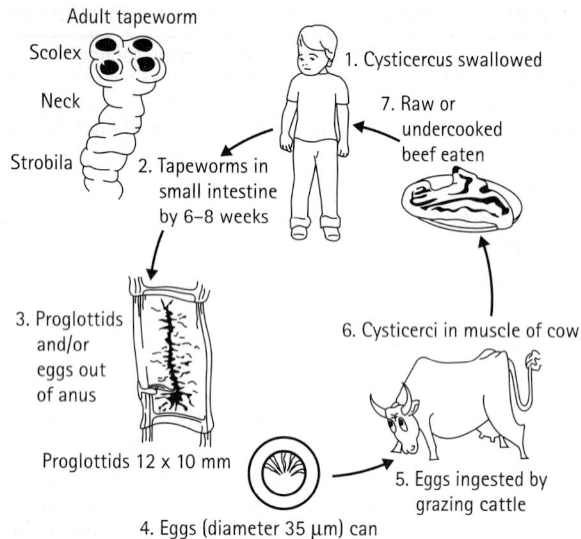

Fig. 26.62 Life cycle of *Taenia saginata.*

of cases, eosinophilia may occur while abdominal pain, weight loss, malaise, an increase or decrease in appetite and such allergic features as urticaria and pruritus ani may be seen.

Adult tapeworms absorb digested food through their cuticles and thus they compete for food with the host and in this process food deprivation and digestive upset may occur.

Rarely, intestinal obstruction results and at times proglottids wander into the appendix and, impacting there, may cause obstructive appendicitis.

Diagnosis

Diagnosis is generally made when proglottids are seen in the stool. These can readily be identified by pressing them between two glass microslides, and counting the number of uterine branches on each side of the central stem. In *T. saginata*, there are usually 15 or more primary uterine branches on each side.

In the cases where proglottids cannot be found, eggs (Fig. 26.63a,b) may be detected in the feces or on anal tapes as used for Enterobius, a process which is more effective for recovery of *T. saginata* eggs than stool examination. Eggs of *T. saginata* and *T. solium* are identical.

Treatment

The treatment of choice for *T. saginata* infection is now praziquantel as a single oral dose of 10–20 mg/kg.[558,559] Niclosamide (Yomesan) is also effective, being usually given without purgation at a dose of 1 g (11–34 kg) or 1.5 g (34 kg and over), which should be chewed

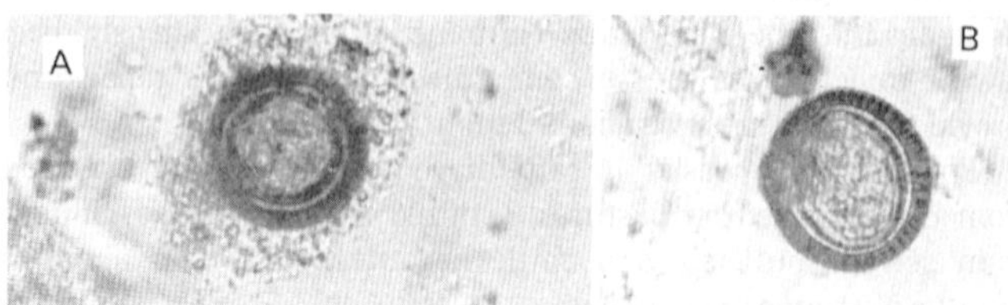

Fig. 26.63 (a) Complete egg of *Taenia* sp., the embryophore being surrounded by the remains of the vitelline cell. (b) Other egg has lost all traces of the vitelline cell and consists only of the oncosphere larva surrounded by its thick, striated embryophore (approx. × 600).

before swallowing.[558] The worm is passed in a partially digested state. Treatment can be followed, if desired, by a saline purge after 2 h.

Treated patients should be rechecked 3 months after treatment to assess cure. With modern anthelmintics it is not feasible to examine post-treatment stools for the scolex.

Prevention of *T. saginata* infection depends upon avoidance of consumption of raw or undercooked beef and hygienic disposal of human feces to prevent infection of cattle. Freezing of meat (–10°C for 10 days) is also reported to be effective in killing cysticerci.

Taenia solium (the pork tapeworm)

T. solium is widely distributed, but less so than the beef tapeworm. It is common, however, in Africa, Asia, Latin America and parts of eastern Europe.

The life cycle of *T. solium* (Fig. 26.64) is similar to that of *T. saginata* but with some very important differences. In both species humans comprise the only definitive host and may harbor one or more tapeworms. In *T. solium* infections humans become infected with the adult tapeworm after eating raw or undercooked 'measly' pork containing cysticerci. The range of intermediate hosts of *T. solium* is wider than that of *T. saginata* and besides pigs, can include the domestic dog. In fact, in areas where dogs form a significant part of human diet, they may serve as an important source of human *T. solium* infection. Humans too can become infected with cysticerci of *T. solium* (known as *Cysticercus cellulosae*) after ingestion of eggs – a condition termed cysticercosis.

The adult *T. solium* is, on average, a little shorter than *T. saginata*, reaching about 15 m in length. The scolex has both suckers and a double row of hooks. The cysticerci of both species are essentially similar, but again the invaginated scolex of *C. cellulosae* has hooks which are absent in *C. bovis*.

Clinical features

Taeniasis. Infection with the adult *T. solium* is much the same as with the adult *T. saginata* except that proglottids of the pork tapeworm are less mobile than those of the beef tapeworm and so such features as appendiceal blockage are rarer. Most cases are asymptomatic, but diarrhea and constipation have been recorded and a moderate eosinophilia may develop.

Cysticercosis. The greatest danger in infection with *T. solium* is the danger to others of infection with eggs via food or water (heteroinfection) and the danger to the patients themselves of

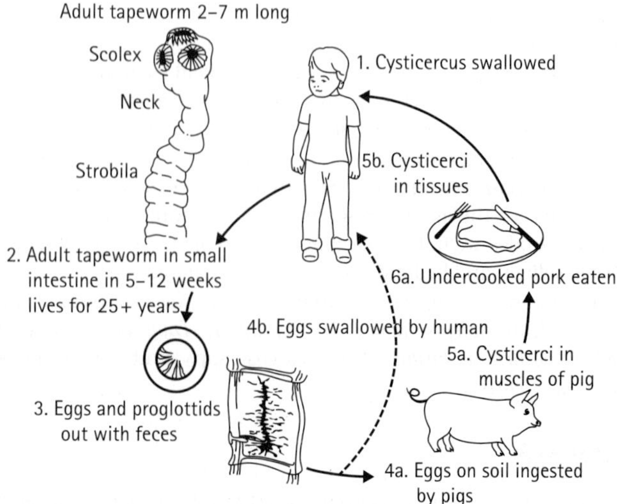

Fig. 26.64 Life cycle of *Taenia solium.*

autoinfection by external means (hand-to-mouth transfer of eggs) or internal means (vomiting up and reswallowing of proglottids).

The clinical effects of cysticercosis are essentially dependent upon the number and sites of the cysticerci. Cysticerci can develop almost anywhere in the body: beneath the skin (subcutaneous cysticercosis); in the myocardium; in the muscles; within the eye or in the brain (cerebral cysticercosis or neurocysticercosis). If within the ventricles of the brain the cysticerci can become greatly enlarged resulting in a racemose cyst.

Usually cysticerci do not cause clinical symptoms until they die, swell and calcify – a process which occurs about 3 years or longer after infection. Whether or not they cause symptoms is also dependent upon their site. In the muscles, heart or beneath the skin they are relatively benign but within the eye they can cause retinal detachment, loss of vision and even blindness, while if sited in the brain they may result in neurological disorders, personality changes or jacksonian-type epileptic convulsions. Neurocysticercosis is a common cause of epilepsy among Africans in southern Africa and although more common in adults, it has even been recorded in children as young as 3 years of age.[621] Death can follow hydrocephalus resulting from blockage of the ventricular spaces.

Diagnosis

Taeniasis. Diagnosis of infection with adult *T. solium* is established by the finding of eggs (indistinguishable from those of *T. saginata*) in feces (Fig. 26.63) or by the passing of typical gravid proglottids. The proglottids of *T. solium* have fewer than 13 lateral uterine branches on each side and so can be differentiated from those of *T. saginata* although some degree of overlap may occur. (*Note*: gloves must be worn when examining proglottids for counting of the uterine branches as eggs of *T. solium* are infective to humans.)

Cysticercosis. Cysticercosis can be diagnosed by palpation and biopsy of cysticerci if accessible and their microscopic examination after squashing between two glass microslides or after histological sectioning.

In patients in whom cysticercosis is clinically suspected confirmation can sometimes be obtained by radiology, where calcified cysticerci are visible as millet seed-shaped shadows in the muscles or small spotted areas on skull X-ray (Fig. 26.65a,b). X-rays are also useful in differentiating cerebral cysticercosis from CNS infection due to *Angiostrongylus, Gnathostoma* and *Paragonimus*.[622]

Eosinophils can at times be found in the CSF of patients with cerebral cysticercosis. About 25% of patients with cerebral cysticercosis will be found to harbor adult *T. solium* in their intestines or have a history of such infection.

Serological tests for blood or CSF are available for the diagnosis of cysticercosis.[622,623] In addition, tests have been developed to detect cysticercal antigen in CSF.

CT scans are of great value, not only for the diagnosis of cerebral cysticercosis, but also for an assessment of the length of infection and for post-treatment progress evaluation.[622,624,625]

Treatment

Treatment for *T. solium* is similar to that for *T. saginata* with praziquantel or niclosamide (Yomesan) being the drugs of choice.[626] Mepacrine or similar drugs which tend to cause nausea and vomiting should be avoided because of the danger of regurgitation of proglottids into the stomach and reswallowing them.

Cysticercosis. Albendazole (15 mg/kg) per day in 3 doses for 8–15 days is probably the treatment of choice for cysticercosis.[565] Although clinical studies have shown that praziquantel at a dose of 25–50 mg/kg in three divided doses for 14 days may be effective for

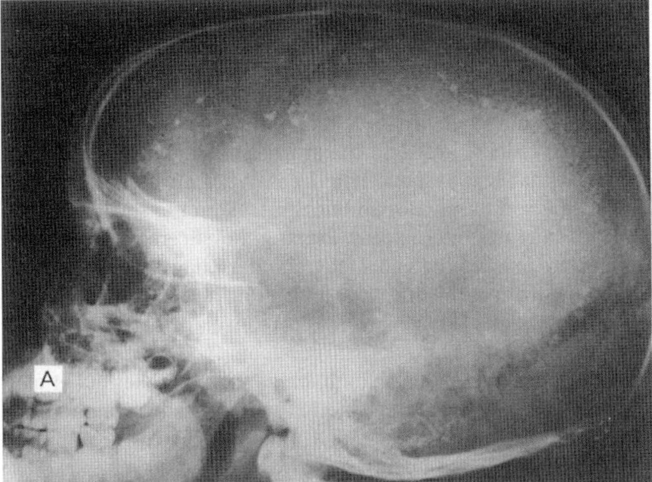

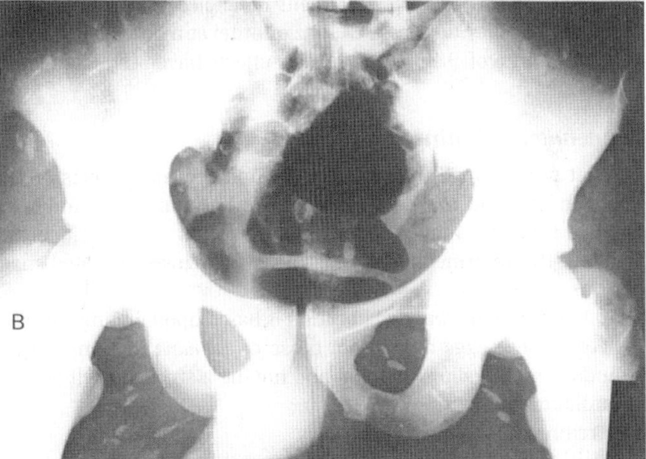

Fig. 26.65 (a) Cerebral cysticercosis. (b) Calcified cysticerci visible in the muscles in X-ray of pelvis.

the treatment of cysticercosis,[558,560,561,627] it is frequently associated with side-effects in neurocysticercosis and its use is thus not universally accepted in this situation.[558,628]

Reviews such as that of Salinas & Prasad[629] have concluded that 'There is insufficient evidence to assess whether cysticidal therapy in neurocysticercosis is associated with beneficial effects' and Shorey et al[565] also express caution in recommending that any decision regarding the need or advisabilty for chemotherapy in cases of cysticercosis requires careful consideration for each individual patient. The simultaneous administration of steroids may help reduce inflammatory complications which can follow the death of the cysticerci after anthelmintic treatment.[571]

Surgical removal of cysticerci is seldom feasible, especially if the cysticerci are numerous and deep seated.

Anticonvulsants to control fits, steroids to control raised intracranial pressure and occasionally surgery to control hydrocephalus may be required for controlling the fits in neurocysticercosis.

Prevention of *T. solium* infection and cysticercosis is essentially the same as for *T. saginata*. Cysticerci can be destroyed during cooking by heating the meat to 50°C.

Hymenolepis spp.

Two species of this genus of tapeworm infect man, *Hymenolepis nana* (the dwarf tapeworm) and *H. diminuta* (the rat tapeworm).

These are small tapeworms, reaching only 40 mm in length for *H. nana* and 40 cm in length for *H. diminuta*.

Hymenolepis nana

H. nana is harbored in the small intestine of the human (or sometimes rodent) host and the gravid proglottids disintegrate in the gut so that eggs pass out in the feces. When an egg is ingested by another person, it releases an oncosphere into the small intestine, and this burrows into a villus, forming a cysticercoid. It develops here before leaving the villus after about 14 days to grow into an adult tapeworm in the intestinal lumen (Fig. 26.66).

Because of its direct person-to-person mode of transmission, *H. nana* is a common tapeworm in developing countries and tends to be commoner in children than in adults. In fact, Goldsmid et al[630] recorded 18.7% of children infected with *H. nana* in a survey in Zimbabwe as opposed to only 3.8% of adults infected.

Diagnosis is based upon the recovery of characteristic *H. nana* eggs (Fig. 26.66) and the treatment of choice is praziquantel or niclosamide as for taeniasis.[561] Praziquantel at a dose of 25 mg/kg has a cure rate of 98.5% and no side-effects have been claimed by Schenone.[631]

Hymenolepis diminuta

The rat tapeworm, *H. diminuta*, is common in many parts of the world in rats and mice. Its intermediate hosts are fleas and flour beetles. Children may become infected when they accidentally swallow the intermediate host – often with insect-infested meal or flour.

Diagnosis of *H. diminuta* infection is based upon finding the eggs in feces. These eggs differ from those of *H. nana* in being larger, rounder, lemon yellow in color, and having a striated shell and no polar filaments.

Treatment is as for *H. nana*.

Neither *H. nana* nor *H. diminuta* causes serious clinical effects, but abdominal pain, diarrhea, loss of appetite and eosinophilia may occur when loads are heavy. One problem with *H. nana* is a build-up of worm load as a result of external autoinfection by ingestion of eggs.

Dipylidium caninum

This tapeworm is worldwide, commonly infecting both dogs and cats. The intermediate hosts are fleas, such as the common dog and cat fleas (Fig. 26.67a), which contain the cysticercoids, and infection of the final host occurs when the flea is swallowed. Children can become infected when they accidentally swallow a flea or when they are licked on the mouth by a dog, which has been 'fleaing' itself, and has cysticercoids on the tongue.

It is a relatively small tapeworm (20 cm long) and usually causes little discomfort, although at times diarrhea, fever, restlessness and even convulsions have been recorded.

Diagnosis is made when actively motile proglottids with two genital pores (Fig. 26.67c) are found by the mother on nappies or when typical egg capsules (Fig. 26.67b) are found in the feces on microscopic examination.

Niclosamide (Yomesan) is reported to be effective in treatment although in some cases repeated treatments with this drug have failed.

Diphyllobothrium latum

The fish tapeworm is one of the largest of the parasites of humans, the adult worm reaching 20 m or more. It is a common tapeworm of a variety of fish-eating mammals, including dogs and cats, in Scandinavia, the Baltic, South America, the Great Lakes of North America, parts of the Middle and Far East and Indonesia, while occasional cases are encountered in other parts such as Labrador and Australia.[571,626]

The scolex of this species has sucking grooves and eggs are shed from the gravid proglottids to pass out with the feces.

When the eggs fall into water, a ciliated coracidium larva develops and is released through the operculum into the water. This is ingested by the microscopic crustacean, *Cyclops*, in which a procercoid larva is formed. When the *Cyclops* is eaten by a fish,

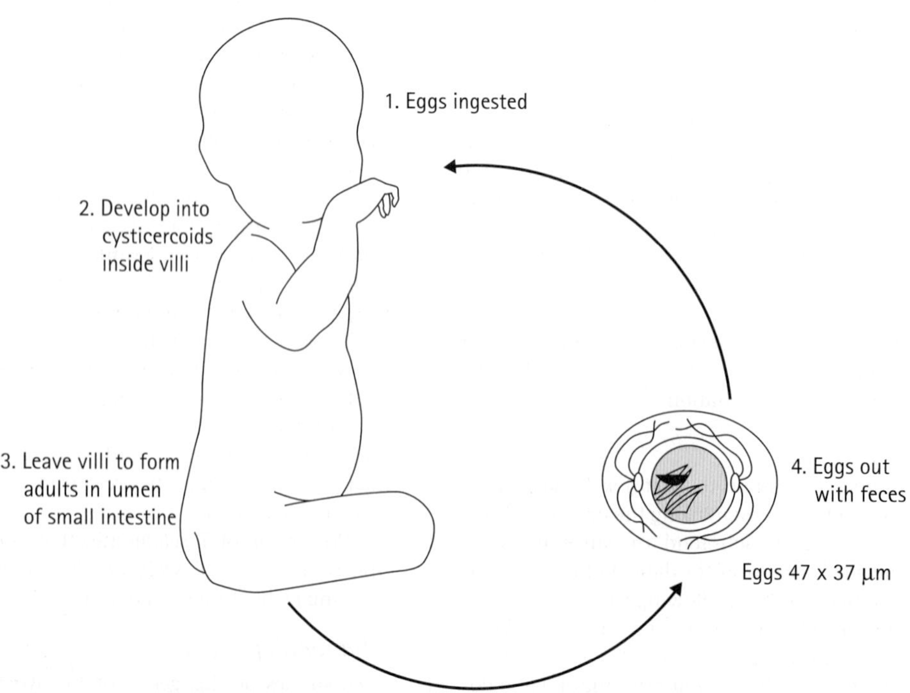

Fig. 26.66 Life cycle of *Hymenolepis nana*. Egg inset (approx ×600).

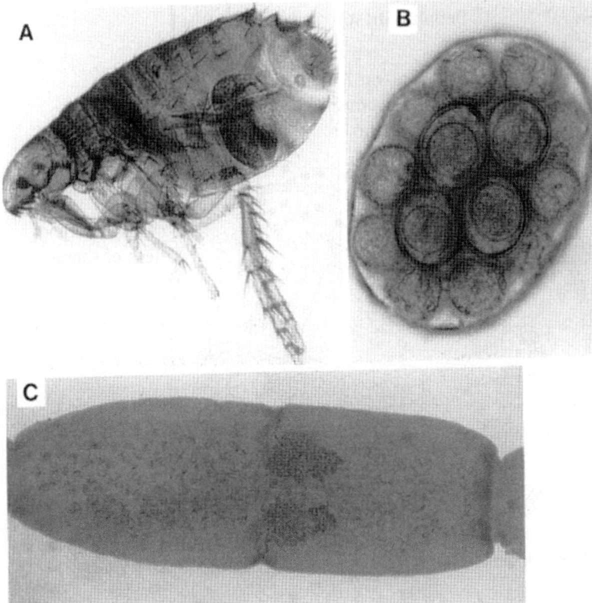

Fig. 26.67 (a) *Ctenocephalides* sp. – dog flea intermediate host of *Dipylidium caninum* (approx. × 50). (b) Egg capsule of *Dipyilidium caninum* (approx × 600). (c) Stained gravid proglottid of *Dipyilidium caninum.* Note characteristic double set of reproductive organs and twin genital pores (approx. × 20).

the procercoid changes into a plerocercoid (sparganum) larva in the muscles of the fish. Finally the life cycle is completed when the fish is eaten by the mammalian definitive host (Fig. 26.68), which may include humans.

Clinical effects of infection include, in heavy loads, diarrhea, abdominal pain, generalized weakness[626] and occasionally intestinal obstruction. *D. latum* is also recorded in Finland, as causing a megaloblastic (macrocytic) anemia in susceptible patients who have a genetic predisposition and who are on a diet deficient in vitamin B_{12}, by competition with the host for this vitamin – especially when

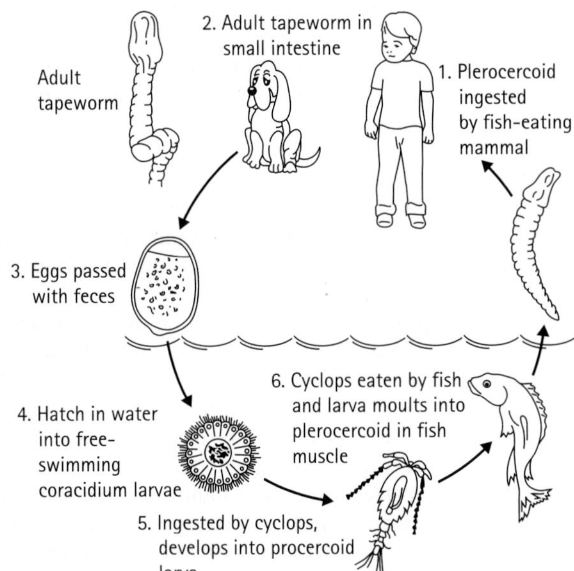

Fig. 26.68 Life cycle of *Diphyllobothrium latum.*

the worm is attached high up in the small intestine. Eosinophilia is not usually a feature of infection.

Diagnosis is based upon the finding of the typical operculate eggs in the feces (Fig. 26.69). Proglottids passed in the feces can be recognized by their centrally situated uterus and genital pore.

Treatments recommended are praziquantel 2.5–10 mg/kg orally as a single dose for people over 4 years. Niclosamide (Yomesan) 1 g orally as a single dose for children 11–34 kg is an alternative.[565] Whichever anthelmintic is used, concurrent vitamin B_{12} should also be given if the patient is anemic.

A common source of human infection is the eating of raw or smoked fish, so cooking of fish is an important factor in preventing infection of humans. Freezing fish (–10°C for 15 min) is also effective in killing plerocercoids.

The plerocercoids of certain species belonging to the related genus, *Spirometra*, the adults of which inhabit the intestines of dogs, can infect humans causing a condition called sparganosis. These elongated plerocercoid (sparganum) larvae can infect humans after ingestion of infected frogs or *Cyclops* with water (East Africa, North America) or by application of infected frog flesh to skin ulcers or eye wounds as poultices. Plerocercoids in the frog muscle migrate into the human flesh where they settle – a condition occurring in south-east Asia.

These spargana can encyst in any tissues. Perhaps the commonest manifestations are nodules about 2 cm in size under the skin with painful surrounding edema. They can be detected radiologically as elongated shadows and can usually be removed surgically if accessible. One species of sparganum can bud and proliferate so spreading through the tissues.

ECHINOCOCCOSIS (HYDATID DISEASE)

Echinococcosis (hydatid disease) in humans is caused by the larval stage of *Echinococcus granulosus* and to a much lesser extent by *E. multilocularis, E. oligarthrus* or *E. vogeli.*

The life cycle of *E. granulosus* is shown in Figure 26.70. The small adult tapeworms (Fig. 26.71a) live in the intestine of the dog and related canids. After ingestion of the eggs by the intermediate hosts, which are usually sheep, the larval tapeworms develop into hydatid cysts in the viscera. Humans also become infected when they ingest the tapeworm eggs, and children are particularly susceptible because of their, often intimate, contact with dogs. They may pick up eggs contaminating the animal's coat or from the dog's tongue after licking.

The infection is particularly common in rural sheep and cattle farming areas, especially where dogs are used for herding. It is widespread throughout Africa, Australasia, Asia, the Near East and South America and is also found in the Mediterranean, the USA and the UK.[546,632] *E. multilocularis* is widespread in the northern hemisphere, with human cases being common in parts of the former USSR, China, northern Japan, Alaska and central Europe including possible spread into eastern Germany.[632–634] Cycles involving wild animals are also found in certain parts of the world.

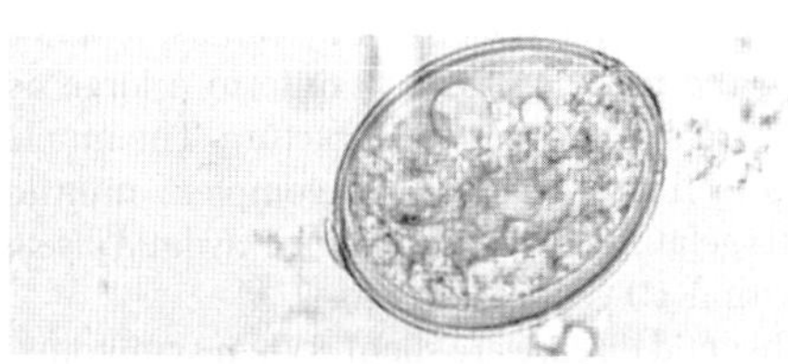

Fig. 26.69 Operculate egg of *Diphyllobothrium latum* (approx. × 600).

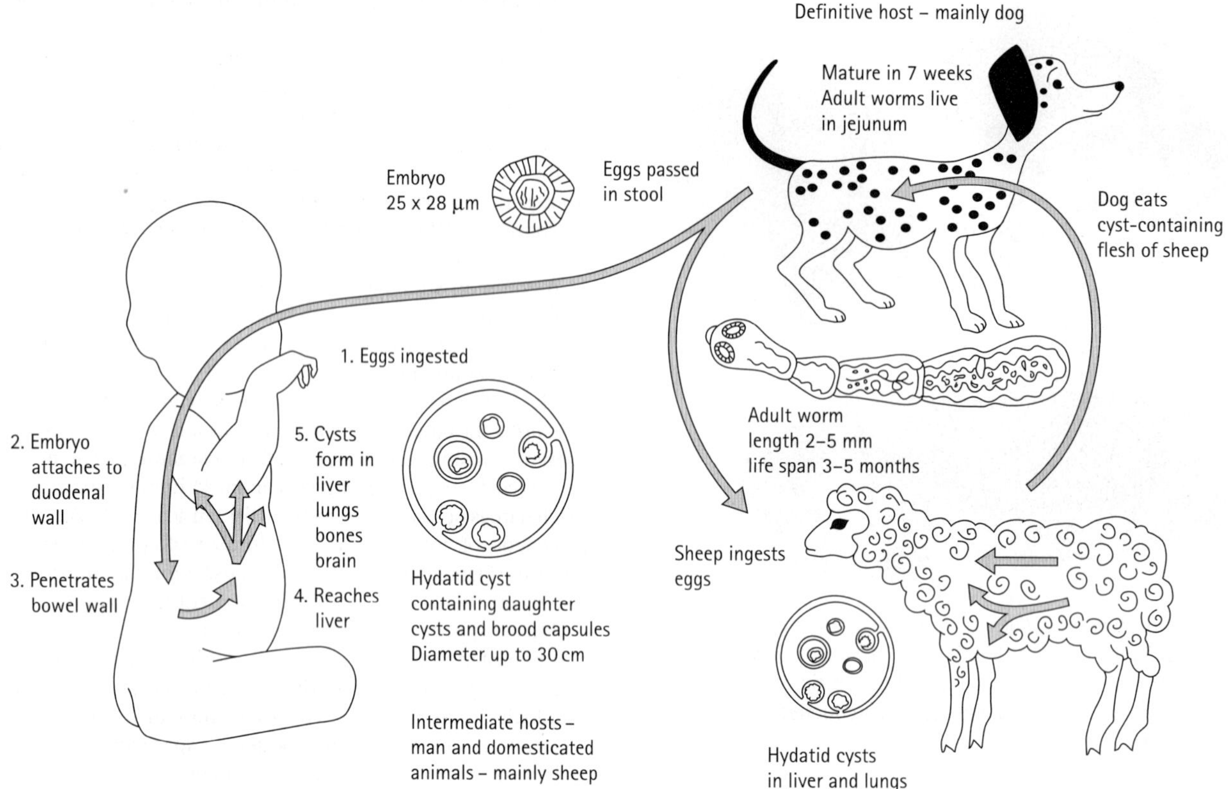

Fig. 26.70 Character and life cycle of *Echinococcus granulosus.*

In hydatidosis due to *E. multilocularis*, wolves, coyotes and foxes are the definitive hosts, and small field rodents serve as the natural intermediate hosts. Urban cycles involving the domestic cat and house mouse have been demonstrated.

The incidence of echinococcosis is decreasing in some areas owing to regular anthelmintic treatment of dogs and strict controls prohibiting the feeding of offal to dogs,[635] and global control has been mooted.[636]

Clinical features

Because development of cysts is slow, an infection acquired in childhood may only become clinically evident in adulthood, but manifestations of the disease in children are by no means uncommon. It has, in fact, been widely believed in the past that most hydatids detected in adults were acquired in childhood. Studies in Australia, however, have indicated clearly that adults are susceptible to infection and that the latent period between infection and diagnosis is, in many cases, only a few years.

The most frequent sites for cysts are the liver (Fig. 26.71b) and lungs (Fig. 26.71c). Spleen, peritoneum, kidneys, bone, orbital fossae, brain, heart and reproductive organs may also be invaded. In children, lung disease is reported to be the commonest form. Cysts sited in parenchymatous organs are large unilocular, well-circumscribed, fluid-filled structures in *E. granulosus* infections.

In bone, the parasite ramifies along bony canals, eroding bone and later involving the medullary cavity to form a large osseous cyst, which often results in spontaneous fracture. The much rarer *E. multilocularis* infection may produce complex, multilocular alveolar cysts with a gelatinous matrix. Alveolar hydatid disease has a 93% mortality within 10 years of diagnosis.[636]

Many cases of hydatid disease are silent. When symptoms occur they are usually those of a slow-growing tumor with pressure on, or blockage to the affected organ. Thus, recurrent pyrexia, paroxysmal cough, chest pain, hemoptysis and even expectoration of cyst fluid and membrane (should rupture occur into a bronchus) may occur as manifestations of pulmonary hydatidosis. Abdominal pain, vomiting, hepatomegaly and obstructive jaundice may indicate liver involvement. Intracranial localization produces symptoms and signs indistinguishable from those of a tumor – epilepsy, personality change, intellectual deterioration, signs of raised intracranial pressure or neurological abnormalities. Orbital cysts produce proptosis.

Sensitivity to cyst contents, resulting from slow leak of fluid, may develop with resulting allergic symptoms, notably urticaria. Severe anaphylaxis has been reported following rupture of a cyst, and secondary metastatic cysts may develop in other parts of the body following such rupture.

Diagnosis

Diagnosis depends initially upon clinical awareness of the condition – especially in patients from endemic areas. A moderate eosinophilia is almost invariably present in childhood cases, except during febrile illnesses.

Often an X-ray provides the first indication of hydatid disease especially in thoracic cases (Fig. 26.72). Ultrasound or CT scanning may be required to demonstrate the cystic nature of the lesion. Serological tests may be helpful in confirming diagnosis. The historic Casoni skin test gives variable results and should perhaps only be used where other serological tests are unavailable. Serological tests available include the indirect hemagglutination test, a hydatid ELISA test and the improved immunoelectrophoresis, Arc 5 test. The latter is considered by many to be the only reliable specific serological test available for hydatidosis, although false positives have been reported for this test in patients with certain

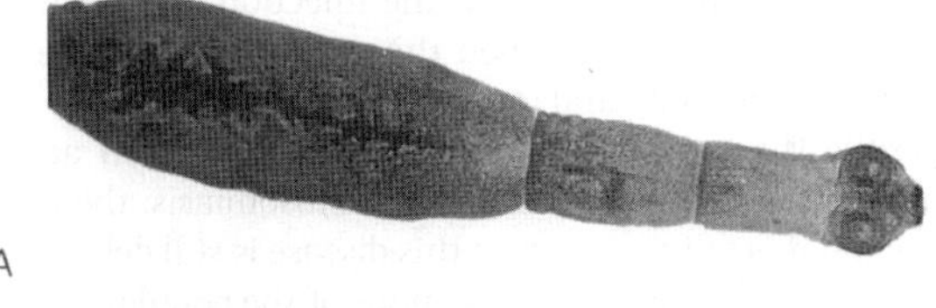

A

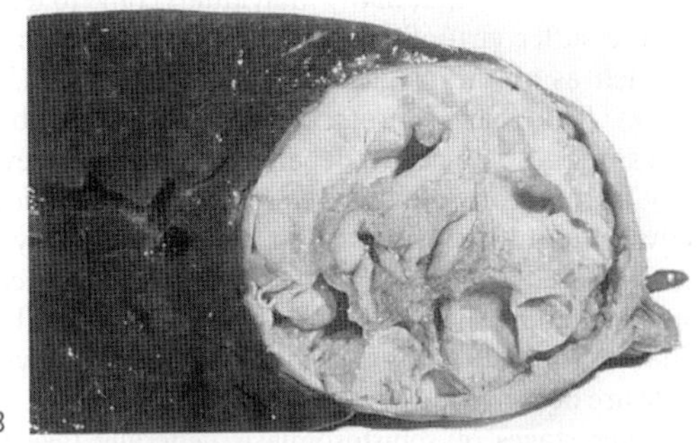

B

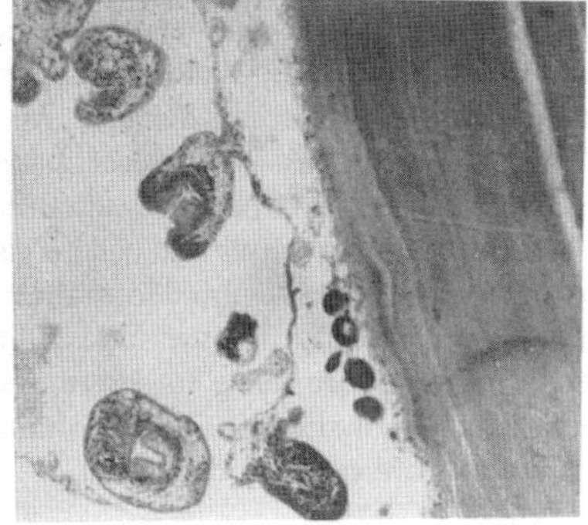

C

Fig. 26.71 (a) Adult *E. granulosus*. Note scolex and proglottids (approx. × 12). (b) Hydatid cyst in human liver. (c) Histological appearance of the wall of a pulmonary hydatid cyst.

types of tumors. The double diffusion Arc 5 test is reported to be even better.

It is worth remembering that pulmonary hydatids appear less serologically active than cysts in other parts of the body, and that after surgical removal of hydatid cysts, antibodies may be detectable in low titers for a while, but that sooner or later they disappear completely.

At times a cyst in the lung may rupture and diagnosis can then be made by finding hydatid sand or hooklets in the sputum.

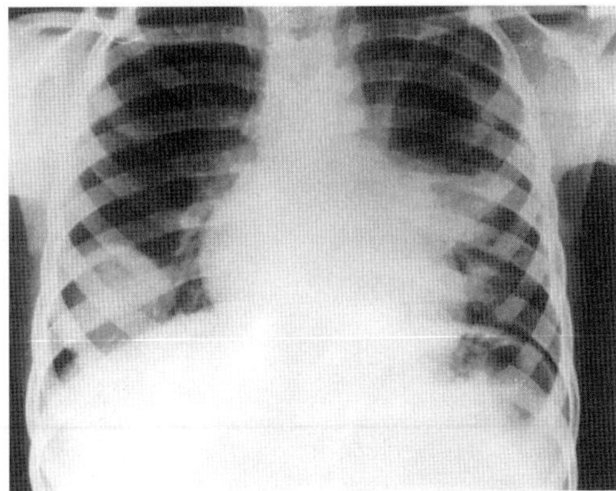

Fig. 26.72 Hydatid cysts in lung. Non-calcified cyst in right lung. Cyst in left lung has ruptured into a bronchus and contains fluid and air.

The latter are easily detected by using a standard Ziehl–Neelsen or auramine stain with UV microscopy, as they are intensely acid fast.

If hydatid cysts are suspected, aspiration must *not* be attempted because of the danger of anaphylaxis and metastatic spread.

If children vomit what appear to be hydatid cysts, care should be taken to confirm their nature microscopically by the presence or absence of a germinal membrane, as gel cysts, closely resembling small hydatids, can easily mislead the unwary. These gel cysts may be vomited, by children up to 2 years, after ingestion of commercial fruit gels containing carrageenan.

Treatment

Treatment is surgical, if cysts are accessible, but due precautions must be observed to prevent release of hydatid fluid and to sterilize cysts prior to removal, using formalin or 0.5–1% sodium hypochlorite (EUSOL).

Results of chemotherapy for hydatid cysts using mebendazole have been disappointing, but albendazole can be used as an adjunct to surgery or for the treatment of inoperable hydatids at a dose of 10 mg/kg daily for 8 weeks.[558,632] Albendazole can also be used in the treatment of infection with *E. multilocularis* but treatment of multilocular hydatidosis remains largely surgical drainage.[625]

Prevention

While highly successful control programs have resulted in decreases in the prevalence of hydatid disease in Tasmania and New Zealand, elsewhere the disease remains common and may even be spreading.[546,632,636]

Dogs should not be allowed access to offal, to limit canine infection, and their regular treatment with an effective teniafuge such as praziquantel (Droncit) is indicated. In endemic areas this deworming should be carried out every 2 months.

INERMICAPSIFER MADAGASCARIENSIS

I. madagascariensis is primarily a parasite of rodents with various arthropod vectors probably involved as intermediate hosts. Human infection, however, is common, especially in Africa, and it has been sporadically reported also from tropical and subtropical areas throughout the world, particularly Cuba where the parasite was introduced and has dispensed with its rodent reservoir.

This cestode has a rounded scolex containing four unarmed suckers and ranges up to 42 cm in length. The small, actively motile proglottids are shed in the stool and have the appearance of rice grains; they contain characteristic parenchmyatous egg capsules.

I. madagascariensis most frequently involves children between the ages of 1 and 5 years, and while the infection is usually asymptomatic, anorexia, asthenia, anemia and abdominal pain have occasionally been attributed to it. It has been found to be the most common tapeworm affecting white children in Zimbabwe and more cases in African children are coming to light as awareness increases.

Niclosamide (Yomesan) is the treatment of choice – one tablet (0.5 g) repeated in 1 h.

TREMATODES (FLUKES)

Trematodes are parasitic helminths belonging to the class Platyhelminthes (flat worms). Trematodes are dorsoventrally flattened worms, which have a gut, no body cavity and possess a dorsal and ventral sucker. Most are hermaphrodite, except the schistosomes. The flukes have a complex lifecycle involving various species of snail as intermediate hosts. Trematodes infecting humans include blood flukes (*Schistosoma*), liver flukes (*Fasciola, Clonorchis,*

Opisthorchis), intestinal flukes (*Fasciolopsis, Heterophyes, Metagonimus*) and lung flukes (*Paragonimus*).

BLOOD FLUKE INFECTION (SCHISTOSOMIASIS OR BILHARZIASIS)

Adult blood flukes live in the veins of the final host. There are three main species which infect humans: *Schistosoma japonicum, S. mansoni* and *S. haematobium. S. japonicum* is a zoonotic species found in the Far East. It frequents the superior mesenteric veins of humans and causes a more virulent and rapidly progressive illness than the other species, involving mainly the small and large intestine and liver. *S. mansoni* occurs in Africa, the Caribbean and South America, the worms living in the inferior mesenteric veins with resultant damage to the colon and liver. *S. haematobium* is found in the veins of the vesical plexus of humans throughout much of Africa, the Middle East and parts of India. In this infection, the disease predominantly affects the urinary tract.

The geographical distribution of the main schistosome species is shown in Table 26.41.[637] Other blood flukes less commonly recorded in humans include *S. intercalatum* (in Zaire), *S. bovis* (in North Africa and Iraq) and *S. mattheei* (in southern Africa). The latter two are zoonotic species of cattle and sheep. In south-east Asia, *S. mekongi* and *S. malayensis* are found.

The life cycle of the human blood flukes is shown in Figure 26.73.

Pathogenesis and clinical features

Humans are usually infected by direct penetration of the cercariae through intact skin. The pathological changes in schistosomiasis are produced by cercariae, schistosomulae, adult worms and eggs – by their physical presence, by virtue of metabolic products or from the body's immune response to the infection. The severity of the disease depends primarily upon the number of parasites that can gain entry to the body and mature.

Despite the wealth of knowledge that has been accumulated regarding the pathophysiology of schistosomiasis, the extent of ill health and mortality caused by this disease is still debatable.[638]

While in many areas, large sections of the population harbor the parasites, it is certain that many individuals come to terms with the disease and suffer virtually no morbidity owing to an interplay of factors such as immunological tolerance, worm load, and rate of reinfection. The role of protective immunity in schistosomiasis continues to be a subject of debate.[639] Increased prevalence and intensity of infection in childhood lend credence at least to some protective immunity playing a part.[640] The immunity involved in schistosomiasis is complex,[639] being described as concomitant immunity, whereby the adult worms are not affected by the hosts' immune responses to the infection although newly invading cercariae are destroyed.[641–644]

The later stages of schistosomiasis generally take many years to develop so that the spectrum of clinical disease in children is narrowed. Nevertheless, such late manifestations as portal hypertension, calcification of the bladder and even vesical carcinoma are by no means rare in adolescents living in hyperendemic areas. A further difference in the disease as it affects children compared with adults is related to the caliber of blood vessels. Because of the smaller and more tenuous venous plexuses and collaterals, schistosomes are less able to migrate in sites far removed from their normal habitat, as they do in older persons. The relative lack of immunity in young patients renders them more liable to severe systemic disturbance during the early stages of the disease. Determinants of infection in human communities are varied and involved.[645]

Table 26.41 Geographical distribution of schistosomiasis (After Warren & Mahmoud 1975[637])

	Distribution				
Species	Africa	Middle East	Asia	South America	Caribbean
S. mansoni	Egypt Libya Sudan South of the Sahara Malagasy Republic	Yemen* Aden* Saudi Arabia*		Brazil Surinam Venezuela	Puerto Rico Dominican Republic* Guadeloupe Martinique St Lucia
S. japonicum			Malaysia*¹ China Japan Philippines Sulawesi* Thailand* Laos*² Kampuchea*² Vietnam²		
S. haematobium	Widespread including Malagasy Republic and Mauritius‡	Lebanon Iran* Turkey Iraq Jordan Yemen Israel Saudi Arabia	India†		

*Very small focal areas.
†Focal distribution.
‡Limited foci have been reported in Portugal in the past.
¹ Species known as *S. malagensis*
² Species known as *S. mekongi*

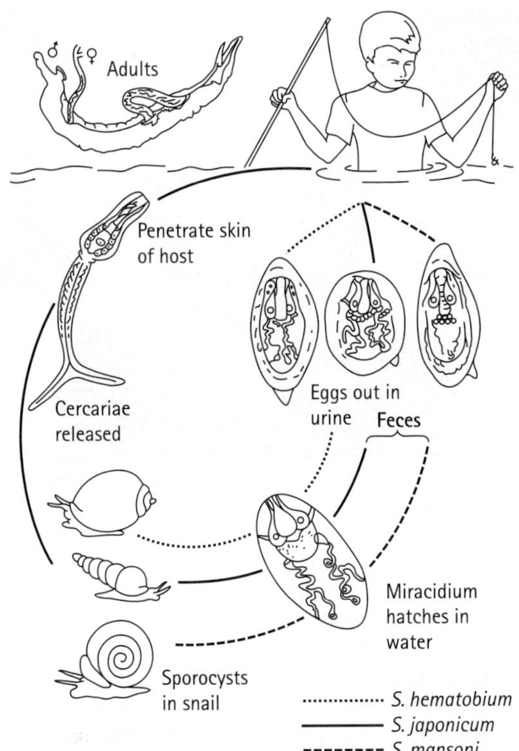

Fig. 26.73 Life cycle of schistosomes.

Clinical features can be related to the phase of parasitic invasion, and symptomatology is generally, but not always, proportionate to worm load. The pathogenesis of schistosomiasis is complex but it is essentially an immunological disease.[646–648]

Penetration of cercariae

At the time of penetration, within a few hours to a few days of exposure, a dermatitis termed swimmer's, or Kabure, itch may develop and last for 2–3 days. The condition is commoner in non-indigenous inhabitants. It can also be caused by avian or mammalian schistosomes, in countries where human schistosomiasis is unknown. For example it is quite common in Australia where it is sometimes termed 'pelican itch' and in the USA where it is known as 'seabather's eruption'. These latter cercariae, however, die while attempting to penetrate the skin. A prickly sensation is followed by intense itching and an urticarial, papular or occasionally vesicular rash appears, lasting from a few hours to several days.

Migratory/toxemic stage: the Katayama syndrome

Having passed through the skin, the cercariae lose their tails and the resulting schistosomulae enter the lymphatics, pass to the veins and travel to the heart and hence to the lungs to circulate freely in the systemic circulation. Many die, but those that gain access to the portal system reach the liver where they mature into adult male and female worms. Rarely, worms mature in other ectopic sites such as veins of the brain and spinal cord. Coupling takes place in the liver and the male transports the female against the flow of blood to their sites of predilection where egg laying begins. The prepatent period in schistosomiasis (i.e. from infection to egg laying) is normally about 5–9 weeks.

During the migratory stage of the life cycle with a crescendo just prior to egg laying, the patient may develop an illness known as the Katayama syndrome due to antigenic challenge by the parasitic metabolites in the non-immune host. Malaise, pyrexia, liver tenderness and splenomegaly occur. Eosinophilia is constant. Urticaria, joint and muscle pains, cough, abdominal discomfort and diarrhea may also occur. Encephalopathy, myocarditis and anaphylactoid purpura are reported complications.[571]

Katayama syndrome is commonest in *S. japonicum* infections but also occurs in *S. mansoni* when a previously uninfected individual is exposed to a heavy invasion by cercariae.

Early egg laying stage

Many eggs laid by female worms in the submucosal venules of the intestine or bladder pass through the tissues and are discharged in the feces (*S. japonicum* and *S. mansoni*) or urine (*S. haematobium*). This early egg laying stage may be associated with dysenteric symptoms or with dysuria, frequency and terminal hematuria.

Late egg laying stage – pathology of chronic schistosomiasis

Initially eggs pass through the tissues relatively easily but as infection progresses marked tissue reaction occurs. As a result of this, eggs can no longer pass through the tissues so readily, and many are swept back by the flow of blood to be deposited elsewhere.

The morbidity of chronic schistosomiasis is mainly related to the presence of eggs,[649] which initially stimulate a granulomatous reaction characterized by a pseudotubercle, rich in eosinophils (Fig. 26.74). This is followed by degeneration and calcification of the eggs with much reactive fibrosis. The principal pathological effects are as follows.

Genitourinary system. *S. haematobium* is the principal cause. The early bladder lesions usually occur on the trigone where deposition of phosphates round the egg deposits imparts a velvety appearance termed 'sandy patches'. Subsequent mucosal proliferation may produce multiple papillomata before ulceration, calcification (Fig. 26.75) and fibrosis lead to diminished bladder capacity. A similar process may involve the ureters, especially at their lower ends, leading to ureteric stricture and consequent hydronephrosis. This complication can also occur from vesical reflux in the absence of overt ureteric involvement. Vesical or ureteric calculi may occur. An important long term complication is the predisposition of the bladder affected by schistosomiasis to develop carcinoma, usually of squamous cell type. The pathogenesis of such bladder carcinoma in *S. haematobium* infection is complex and has still not been fully elucidated. While this is, of course, commonest in adults, it is recognized to occur in adolescents. Genital lesions are usually diagnosed after puberty. These include epididymo-orchitis (often with associated secondary hydrocele), salpingo-oophoritis and chronic cervicitis. Large schistosomal granulomata (bilharziomas) consisting of masses of eggs enveloped in granulation tissue (Fig. 26.74) may involve the skin of the perineum and vulva. The lesions have a warty papillomatous appearance and when situated at the urethral meatus such a lesion is indistinguishable from a caruncle. Cutaneous schistosomiasis may rarely involve other parts of the body, and bilharzial granuloma of the conjunctiva has even been described in children.

An extended bacteremia with *Salmonella typhi* or *S. paratyphi* can occur – including a prolonged urinary carrier state – in concurrent *S. haematobium* infections.

Bacteriuria is generally considered to be commoner in patients with *S. haematobium* than in uninfected controls.

Intestinal tract. Involvement of small bowel is usually only seen in *S. japonicum* infection but schistosomiasis of the colon may be due to both *S. japonicum* and *S. mansoni*. Eggs of *S. haematobium* may also be encountered in rectal snips taken from the lower part of the rectum. Mucosal involvement of the bowel gives rise to a similar

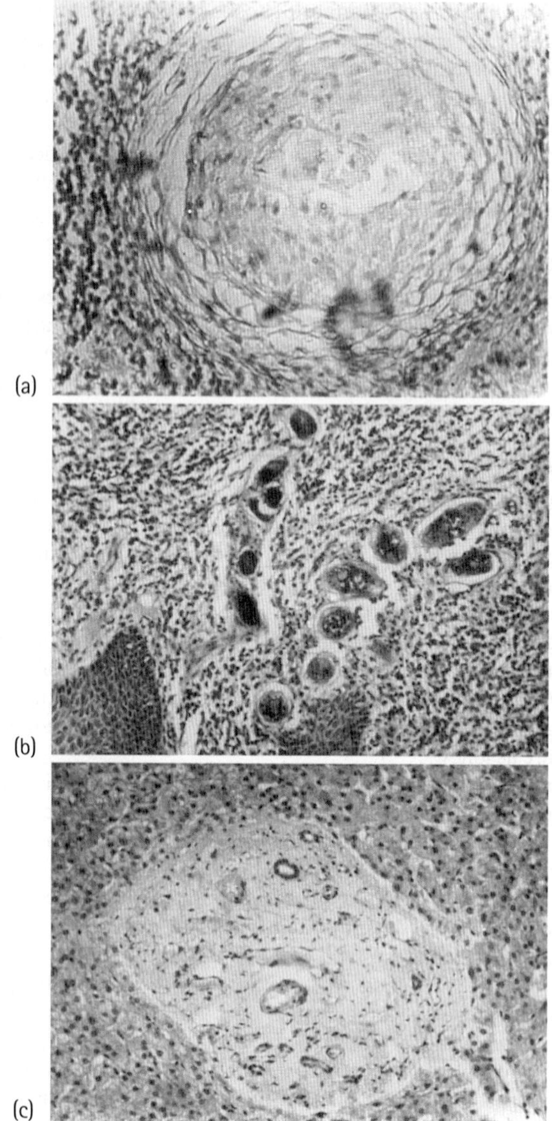

Fig. 26.74 (a) Schistosomal pseudotubercle. (b) Bilharzioma. (c) Liver biopsy showing collagenized periportal thickening due to schistosomiasis.

appearance to that seen in the bladder with a velvety roughening of the mucosa. This may be associated with dysentery in the early egg-laying phase of the disease, especially with *S. japonicum* infection. Gross lesions of the bowel are rare, but on occasions, papillomata, granulomata, ulcers, stricture and fistulae occur. The appendix is frequently involved and signs of chronic appendicitis are common, although acute obstructive appendicitis consequent upon fibrosis, is a rare complication.

Liver. Hepatic fibrosis may result from the presence of eggs of *S. mansoni* or *S. japonicum* with formation of granulomata and healing by fibrosis leading to thick tracts of periportal fibrous tissue traversing the liver in different directions. This 'pipe stem' fibrosis (Symmers' liver) gives the surface of the liver an irregular bosselated contour due to tethering of the capsule. In the later stage, eggs are scanty and may even be absent from biopsy material in which the essential features are of preserved liver architecture associated with gross thickening of the portal tracts by collagenized bands of fibrous tissue (Fig. 26.74). Kupffer cells usually contain schistosomal pigment. Liver involvement can lead to portal hypertension with ascites and splenomegaly, which is occasionally massive ('Egyptian splenomegaly'). Anemia is frequent and may be due to chronic hemorrhage from varices or to associated 'hypersplenism'. There is usually only mild impairment of liver function and thus the results of portal systemic shunting procedures usually give good results in selected cases. Splenectomy combined with lienorenal anastomosis is a helpful procedure if there is associated hypersplenism.

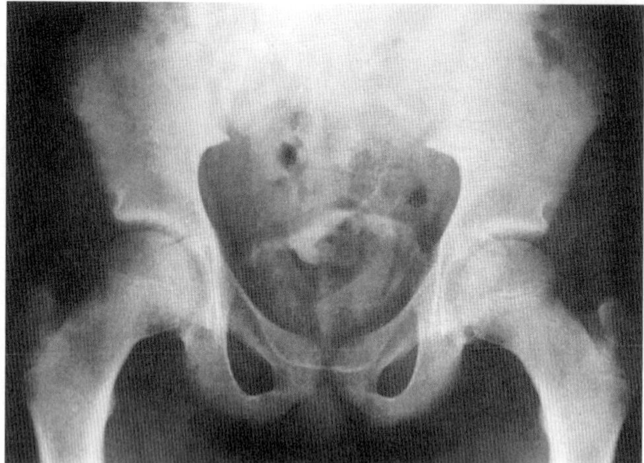

Fig. 26.75 X-ray showing bladder calcification due to schistosomiasis in a 10-year-old girl.

A relationship has been postulated between schistosome infection and carcinoma of the liver.

Cardiopulmonary systems. Lung involvement is usually the result of pulmonary embolization by eggs of *S. haematobium*. Though generally rare it is reported with some frequency from Egypt. Two forms of lung disease occur:

1. a bronchopulmonary form characterized by parenchymal egg granulomata – chronic bronchitis and bronchiectasis may result;
2. a cardiovascular form, which is due to occlusion of pulmonary arterioles by obliterative endarteritis resulting in Ayerza's syndrome with cor pulmonale.

Nervous system. Eggs may lodge in any part of the CNS, generally seeded there by gravid females ectopically situated in nearby veins. Migrating schistosomulae may also be arrested in the nervous system if treatment is administered during the early migratory phase of the disease. However, neurological complications are unusual in schistosomiasis, cerebral involvement being best known with *S. japonicum* and spinal cord lesions with *S. mansoni* and *S. haematobium*.

It has been claimed that school performance can be adversely affected by chronic schistosomiasis.

In patients infected with *S. mansoni*, glomerulonephritis has been reported due to the deposition of immune complexes (IgM and IgG) in the kidney.

Laboratory diagnosis

Confirmation of the diagnosis of active schistosomiasis can only be obtained by finding typical viable eggs (Fig. 26.76a,b,c). Eggs can be recovered by examination of urinary deposit (*S. haematobium*) or from stool (all other species) by direct smear (including a Kato smear), sedimentation or water centrifugation.[650] Flotation techniques are not satisfactory and formol ether concentration kills the eggs with the result that no report can be made on egg viability as judged by miracidial activity or flame cell activity. Confirmation of viability of the egg is important to differentiate active disease from past infection.

Egg recovery is not easy and as many as 20% of infected persons may not pass eggs. Repeated examination of stool and urine

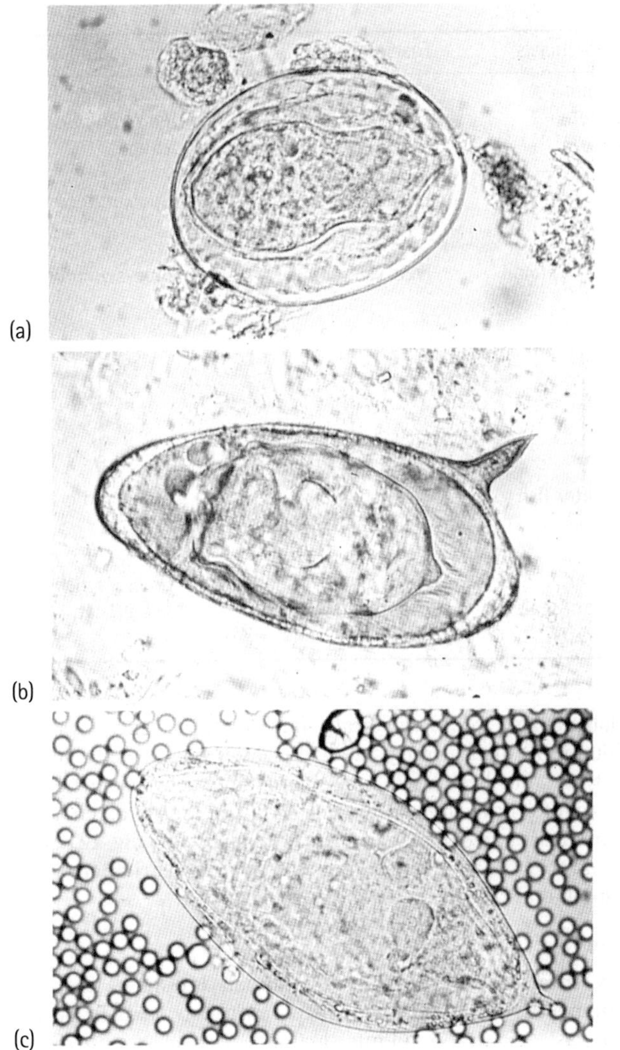

Fig. 26.76 (a) Egg of *Schistosoma japonicum* (approx. × 600). (b) Egg of *Schistosoma mansoni* (approx. × 600). (c) Egg of *Schistosoma haematobium* (approx. × 1000).

specimens, the latter collected at midday, is essential. If urine or stools fail to reveal eggs, a rectal snip may prove rewarding in *S. japonicum*, *S. mansoni* and *S. haematobium* infections. In fact a single rectal snip gives more positives than three urines and stools. Cystoscopy may be indicated where urinary symptoms are present, the cystoscopic picture depending on the worm load.

A type I response skin test and various serological tests are available. These may be negative in early disease and positive results indicate present or past infection, and therefore a positive result with these tests is not, in itself, an indication for treatment. However, these tests often provide good negative screens to exclude a diagnosis of schistosomiasis and are particularly useful in screening returned travelers from endemic regions.

The treatment of choice for all forms of schistosomiasis, and the only effective and safe treatment for *S. japonicum* infections, is praziquantel (Biltricide).[561,651–653] This drug is designated as a 'WHO essential agent', being extremely safe and highly effective when given as a single dose of 40 mg/kg (can be divided into two doses) for *S. haematobium* and *S. mansoni* and at a dose of 60 mg/kg divided into three doses and given in a single day for *S. japonicum*.[559,560,654]

Other treatments for schistosomiasis include hycanthone (Etrenol), mostly used against *S. haematobium* and given as a single intramuscular injection of 2.5–3.5 mg/kg. This drug can be hepatotoxic and deaths following its use are on record. Metrifonate (Bilarcil) is an organophosphorus compound, achieving a cure of about 60% in cases of infection with *S. haematobium*. It is not used for other species of schistosome. The dosage used for children is 7.5 mg/kg per fortnight for a total of three doses.[560] Although side-effects are minimal, some have been recorded. The drug does depress cholinesterase levels and caution is needed in cases where patients may require some form of surgery necessitating the use of the muscle relaxant, suxamethonium. Oxamniquine (Mansil) is only effective against *S. mansoni* infections. The dose regimen is 10–30 mg/kg given as a single or divided doses over 1–2 days after food.[558,560,654] High cure rates and few side-effects are recorded.[561] This drug is useful for treating children orally at a rate of 800 mg/m^3 body surface area per day in divided doses for 2 days. Antischistosome drugs such as the antimonials and niridazole (Ambilhar) have been superseded by the newer, more effective and safer compounds.

Prevention

Attempts to control schistosomiasis are complex and generally employ a two-pronged attack on the lifecycle of the fluke. The first is aimed at eliminating the snail population. Planned water systems for irrigation, which give a flow rate too high for survival of snails, is an ideal, but not always feasible method. Non-toxic molluscicides such as Frescon or Bayluscide have been found effective.

The experimental introduction of snail-eating predators and parasites has not proved to have any long term effect.

The second approach to control is aimed at preventing pollution of waterways by human excreta and involves public health education combined with provision of adequate and effective toilet facilities. In some control projects, mass treatment of infected humans has been used in conjunction with snail control. However, these aspects of prevention are ineffective in the case of *S. japonicum* which is extensively propagated by rodents. In *S. japonicum*, cercariae can be prevented from penetrating the skin by using topical applications of niclosamide or niclosamide-impregnated leggings.

Mass deworming, repeated chemotherapy and the provision of safe water supplies through pump systems have all been proposed for the control of schistosomiasis.[655]

By 1988, schistosome vaccines were entering phase 1 trials[656] and current research is continuing into the development of vaccines and chemoprophylaxis. The results to date appear to be encouraging, but there are concerns about the application of vaccine programs.[657–660]

OTHER TREMATODES

The lifecycles of these flukes involve a variety of snail hosts with infective metacercariae settling on plants or aquatic invertebrates or vertebrates[545] (Table 26.42).

Liver fluke infection

The main trematode infections of the liver are fascioliasis, caused by the cattle and sheep liver flukes *Fasciola hepatica* (temperate regions) and *F. gigantica* (tropical Africa, Asia and Hawaii); clonorchiasis caused by *Clonorchis* (*Opisthorchis*) *sinensis* in the Far East; and opisthorchiasis, caused by *Opisthorchis felineus* in parts of Europe and Asia or *O. viverrini* in Thailand.

Table 26.42 Lifecycles of intestinal and lung flukes

	Fascioliasis	Clonorchiasis	Opisthorchiasis	Fasciolopsiasis	Paragonimiasis
Adult fluke ↓	30 × 10 mm *F. hepatica* *F. gigantica* Liver	15 × 5 mm *Cl. sinensis* Liver	9 × 5 mm *O. felineus* *O. viverrini* Liver	50 × 15 mm *F. buski* Small intestine	12 × 6 mm *Paragonimus* spp. Lung
Egg ↓	Feces	Feces	Feces	Feces	Sputum/feces
Miracidium ↓	Free-swimming	Ingested by snail	Ingested by snail	Free-swimming	Free-swimming
Snail ↓	↓	↓	↓	↓	↓
Cercariae ↓					
Metacercaria ↓	Water plants	Freshwater fish	Freshwater fish	Water plants (water chestnut)	Crabs and crayfish
Definitive host	Plant eater: sheep, cow human	Fish eater: dog, cat, pig, human	Fish eater: dog, human, seals	Water chestnut eater: pig, human	Crab/crayfish eater: dog, cat, human

Clinical features

Infection with these flukes results when the metacercariae are ingested with aquatic plants (*Fasciola*) such as watercress to which the encysted metacercariae are attached, or in undercooked fish (*Clonorchis*; *Opisthorchis*).

Symptoms of liver fluke infection depend largely upon the worm load and mild infections are often asymptomatic. Heavier infections tend to produce a triphasic response with an initial phase of invasion being accompanied by irregular fever and eosinophilia. Diarrhea and urticaria are common and there may be tender hepatomegaly. This phase lasts for about 4 weeks and is followed by an asymptomatic latent period usually lasting several months before the stage of obstructive jaundice occurs. Rarely the parasites of *F. hepatica* may settle in ectopic sites such as the pharynx after eating raw liver and mature there with resulting local reaction. Pharyngeal fascioliasis is known in the Middle East as *halzoun*. Individual worms may migrate into the liver parenchyma resulting in liver abscess formation. Eosinophilia is often present and the ESR is usually raised.

In Thailand, cholangiocarcinoma has been found to be associated with infection by *O. viverrini*.[661]

Local prevalences are often dependent upon social customs and dietary habits and epidemic outbreaks of fascioliasis have been recorded.[546,661,662]

Diagnosis

The diagnosis is usually based upon the finding of typical operculate eggs in the feces (Fig 26.77) although in some infected patients stools are consistently negative for eggs. The finding of eggs of *Fasciola* in the feces must be regarded with caution as persons eating infected cattle or sheep liver can pass 'transit eggs' and this condition of spurious infection or false fascioliasis must be distinguished from true fascioliasis by the examination of repeat stool specimens.[600]

Treatment

On the whole, treatment of liver fluke infection remains unsatisfactory. For fascioliasis, treatment now consists of triclabenbazole 12 mg/kg orally once daily for 1–2 days.[565,590] Bithionol 50 mg/kg orally in divided doses on alternate days for 2–3 weeks has been used, and chloroquine, dehydroemetine and praziquantel have also been tried. Drug treatment of choice for clonorchiasis and opisthorchiasis is praziquantel 25 mg/kg t.d.s. for 1–2 days[558,560,561,590] although Hetol (1:4 bistrichloromethyl bensol) has also been shown to be promising.

Intestinal fluke infection

Many species of fluke infect the human intestinal tract[545,663] including the large intestinal fluke *Fasciolopsis buski* in parts of south-east Asia, the small intestinal fluke *Heterophyes heterophyes*, in the Nile Delta and Far East, and *Metagonimus yokogawai* in the Far East and eastern Europe.

Infection with these flukes results from ingesting metacercariae with aquatic vegetation (*F. buski*) or with raw or undercooked fish (*H. heterophyes* and *M. yokogawai*). As in the case of liver fluke infection, a local high prevalence may be caused by local eating habits.[545,662]

Symptoms of intestinal fluke infection may vary from a mild inflammatory reaction at the site of worm attachment in the small intestine to ulceration or abscess formation in the bowel wall, associated with severe bloody diarrhea.

Infections due to *F. buski* may result in vague abdominal symptoms, ascites and edema, probably as a result of protein-losing enteropathy and toxemia.[663] An eosinophilia may be present, and iron deficiency anemia is common in fasciolopsiasis.

Diagnosis

As with liver fluke infection, diagnosis is made by finding typical operculate eggs in the feces of infected patients (Fig 26.77).

Treatment

Intestinal fluke infections, especially that due to *F. buski*, can be treated with praziquantel in a dose of 25 mg/kg 8-hourly for 1 day.[558,560] Niclosamide (Yomesan) can also be used,[561] while tetrachlorethylene has been described as an effective and cheap anthelmintic.[571]

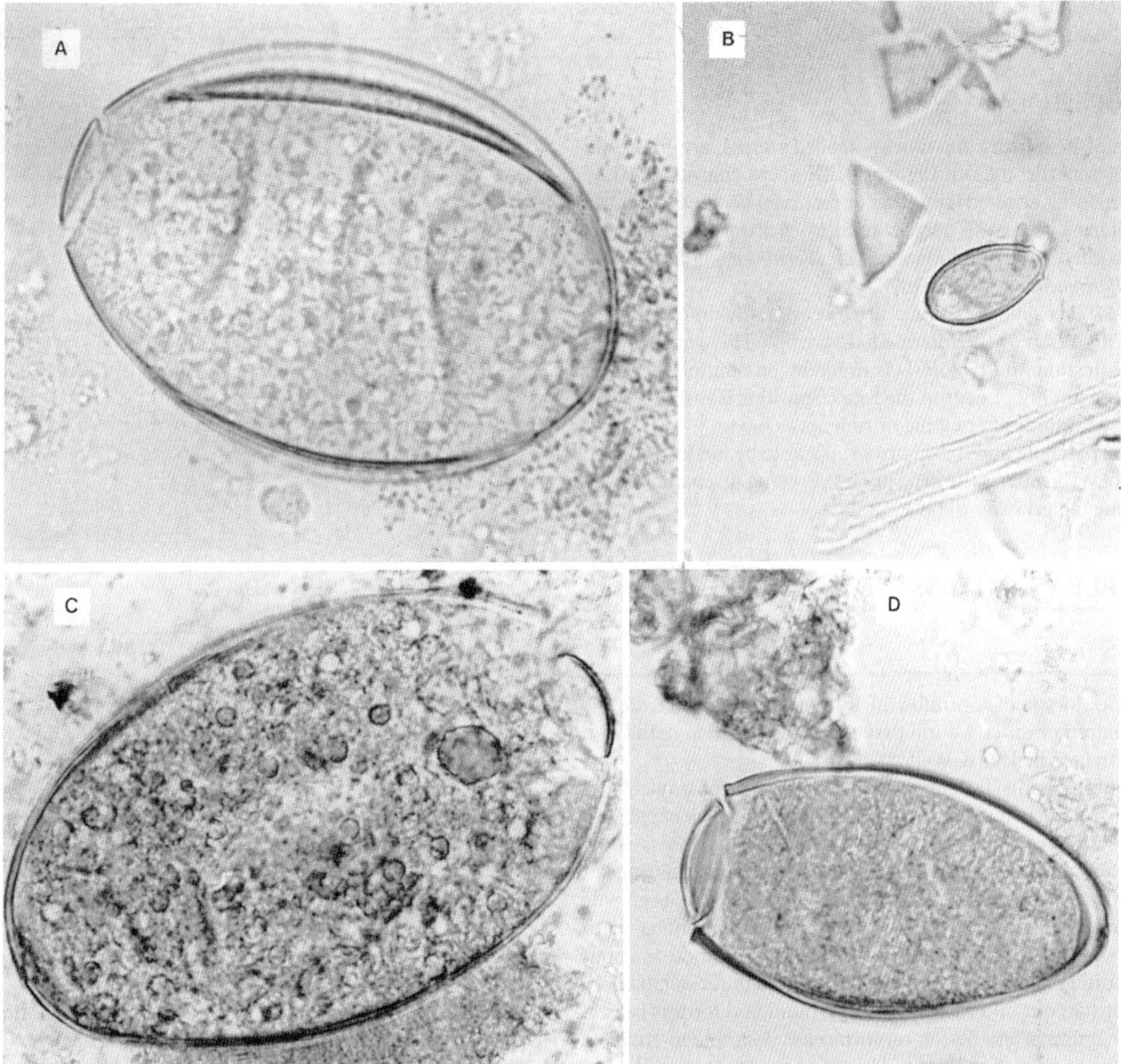

Fig. 26.77 Eggs of (a) *Fasciola hepatica* – ruptured to demonstrate operculum (approx. × 600); (b) *Opisthorchis sinensis* (approx. × 600); (c) *Fasciolopsis buski* – ruptured to demonstrate operculum (approx. × 600); (d) *Paragonimus westermani* (approx. × 600).

Lung fluke infection

Human lung fluke infection is caused by 11 species of the genus *Paragonimus*. In the Far East, south-east Asia and the Philippines, the species involved is *P. westermani* while in central and west Africa (and probably South Africa) the species is *P. africanus* or *P. uterobilateralis*. In the western hemisphere, *P. mexicanus* and *P. kellicotti* are the commoner species.[571]

Infection occurs with the ingestion of the metacercariae in crabs and crayfish. Again local high prevalences are largely dependent upon dietary habits and culinary practices of preparing and cooking the crustacean intermediate hosts.[545,662] However, an interesting epidemic is on record which resulted from the use of crab juice as an antipyretic for children suffering from measles.

Symptoms of lung fluke infection are often suggestive of pulmonary tuberculosis, which may also often be present concurrently. The onset is insidious with cough and chest pain. Hemoptysis is usual, with copious blood-tinged sputum containing many eggs. Bronchiectasis and pulmonary fibrosis are late results and finger clubbing is often present. An eosinophilia may occur and variable symptoms may result from flukes developing in ectopic sites, e.g. epilepsy, transverse myelitis and skin ulceration.

Diagnosis

The characteristic asymmetrical operculate eggs of *Paragonimus* may be recovered in sputum or feces (Fig. 26.77). X-rays and CT scans may prove useful and while serology is available, finding characteristic eggs in sputum or feces will establish a diagnosis of paragonimiasis.

Treatment

The drugs of choice are Bithionol (or Bitin) at a dose of 30–40 mg/kg in divided doses given orally every other day for 10–15 days, or the newer derivative of Bithionol, Bitin-S, given at a dosage regimen of 10–20 mg/kg every other day for 10–15 days. Praziquantel is also effective[558,560,561] and may be used in conjunction with corticosteroids if there is CNS involvement.[565]

Side-effects include diarrhea, nausea, vomiting and abdominal pain, but these are mild and soon subside.

ACANTHOCEPHALA

This group of helminths, the thorny-headed worms, are intestinal parasites of rats throughout the world. They are characterized by having a proboscis covered with rows of recurved hooklets and have as their intermediate hosts insects such as cockroaches. The only species recorded from humans are *Moniliformis moniliformis* and *Macracanthorhynchus hirudinaceus*.

Humans, especially children, are occasionally infected after accidental ingestion of the intermediate host.[549] The worms live in the small intestine and diagnosis is made by passing of the adult worms or the finding of eggs in the feces. Spurious transit eggs can be passed by humans after eating of rodents as food.

Pyrantel pamoate and tiabendazole appear to be ineffectual, and mebendazole (Vermox) is the drug of choice, being given at a dose of 100 mg (one tablet) twice a day for 3 days.

FLIES, FLEAS, MITES AND LICE

MYIASIS

Given access, larvae of a number of fly species may penetrate the skin of children or enter wound tissue as is discussed in detail in a review of myiasis by Hall & Wall.[664]

The tumbu, or putsi fly, *Cordylobia anthropophaga*, of tropical and subtropical Africa is but one of a large variety of flies capable of causing myiasis, which is the infestation of viable tissue by dipterous larvae or 'maggots'. Foci of infection with this species have recently been recorded in northern Europe.[665] The large pale brown tumbu deposits her eggs on shady soil contaminated with urine, or damp clothing, where they hatch to release larvae in about 3 days. Laundry placed out to dry is an ideal site for oviposition, especially if laid out on grass or on the ground and for this reason thorough ironing of clothes on all surfaces is desirable in endemic areas. The larvae penetrate intact skin where they grow rapidly, and unless removed, abandon the host in about 8 days to pupate.

The cutaneous lesions, which may be single or multiple, can occur on any part of the skin, particularly the waist area, back (Fig. 26.78a) and feet. The characteristic lesion is a tender, large, furuncular swelling with a central pore (Fig. 26.78b). Following application of petroleum jelly, the pore widens revealing movement of the posterior spiracles. The tough larva, about 0.5–1.0 cm in length, may then be squeezed out or grasped with forceps and extracted. Secondary infection of these lesions is rare.

In South America, the eggs and larvae of the tropical warble fly *Dermatobia hominis* may be transferred to the human skin by flies, mosquitoes or ticks and produce similar papular lesions.

Cutaneous myiasis is being increasingly recognized as an imported infection in many non-tropical areas.[665]

In areas of the world where sheep are farmed, the sheep nasal bot fly, *Oestrus ovis*, has been at times recorded as causing ophthalmomyiasis – a self-limiting but extremely painful condition.

Other larvae (e.g. those of *Gasterophilus*) may produce itching skin lesions related to the wanderings of the larvae or tender short-lived subcutaneous cystic swellings. *G. intestinalis* can cause intestinal myiasis.

Maggots in wounds tend to be related to the amount of necrotic tissue and their control to the maintenance of adequate wound toilet.

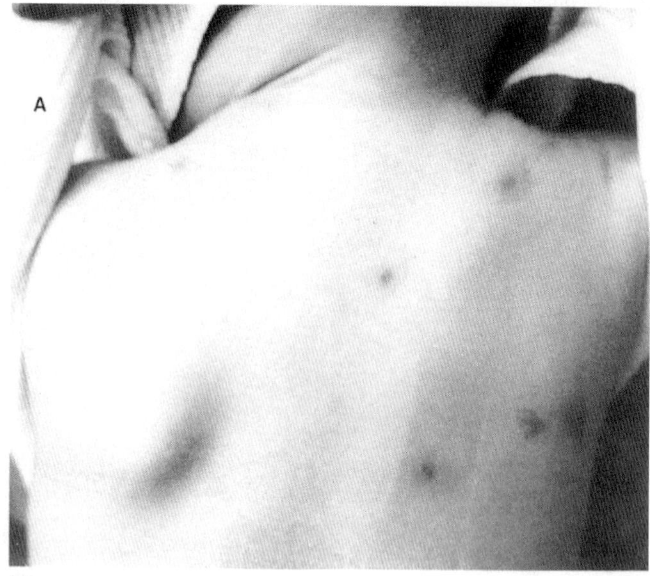

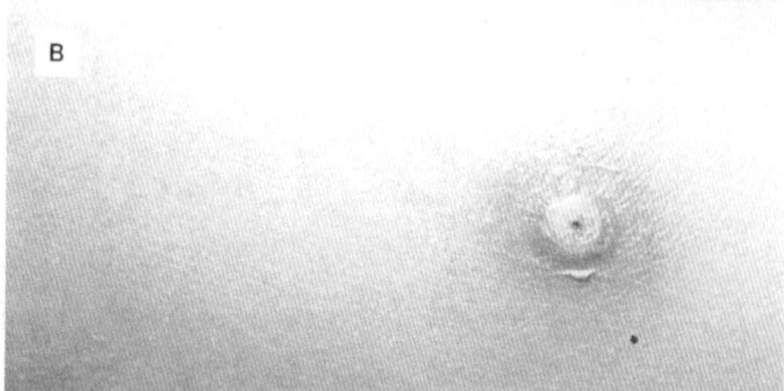

Fig. 26.78 (a) Child with multiple putsi lesions on back. (b) Lesion due to *Cordylobia anthropophaga* on leg to show characteristic appearance.

Myiasis may occur rarely in mucous membrane-lined orifices such as the mouth, anus and vagina and in the eye. One species *Auchmeromyia luteola* lives in cracks and crevices of floor in Africa, coming out at night to suck blood from the sleeping human host.

TUNGIASIS

Tungiasis is infection with the jigger (or chigoe) flea, *Tunga penetrans*. This flea, originally endemic to South America, has spread to central Africa and parts of India.

The young adult fleas live in soil or in the dust and cracks of earth floors of houses. After mating, the female flea penetrates the skin of the host (rodents, dogs, cats or humans). Here, she develops in the epidermis under the stratum corneum, her abdomen swelling tremendously with developing eggs. The lesion starts as a small black spot in the skin but then becomes inflamed and erythematous, developing into a pustule which may crust over or even form a suppurating ulcer if secondarily infected by bacteria. Lesions mostly occur on the feet, especially under the toe nails or between the toes (Fig. 26.79). Itching, pain and even regional lymphadenopathy are common.

Eggs are expelled by the female flea, fall to the ground and form free-living larvae and pupae in the soil.

Diagnosis is made by finding the flea in the lesion and carefully removing it. In unsuspected cases, diagnosis may be made after biopsy of the lesion and finding the fragmented flea in the lesion.

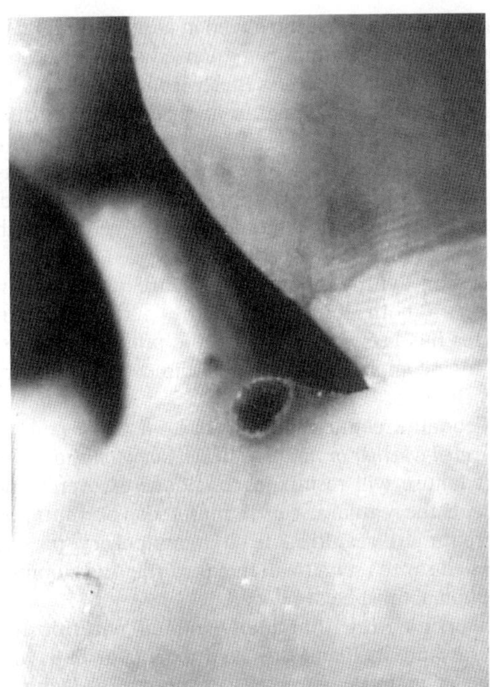

Fig. 26.79 Lesion due to jigger flea (*Tunga penetrans*). (Courtesy of Dr K. Ott)

Treatment consists of a careful removal of the flea, without rupturing it, using a sterile needle, followed by a cleaning of the wound with chloroform and a careful curetting of the affected area.

DEMODICIDOSIS

The hair follicle mite, *Demodex folliculorum* (Fig. 26.80) is one of the commonest parasites of the human skin, with infection rates of 25% or higher.

Human infection is probably acquired by direct person-to-person contact – often at a very young age (e.g. sucking babies infected from their mother). Human infection with other species of *Demodex* from animals has not been ruled out.

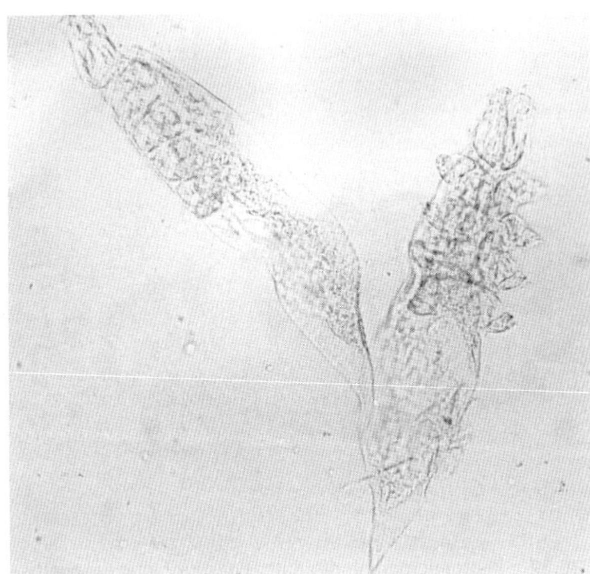

Fig. 26.80 *Demodex folliculorum* (approx. × 300).

The mites live in the pilosebaceous glands and hair follicles especially of the face, scalp, external ear and breast. They are common in the eyelids and mites can often be found clinging to removed eyelashes.

Clinically the condition may be asymptomatic or infected hair follicles may result in the formation of 'blackheads' with crops of red papules appearing often on the forehead. In heavy infestations, or in sensitized patients, dermatitis may follow, with scaling of the skin. Papulonodular demodicidosis may be associated with acquired immune deficiency syndrome in the form of a papulonodular rash of acute onset, usually localized to the head and neck.[666]

Diagnosis is established by finding the mites, often in seropurulent fluid expressed from the lesions, or in biopsied specimens of skin in which mites can be found.

Treatment consists of good hygiene, soap and water together with sulfur ointment or gamma-benzene hexachloride (lindane) if necessary.

SCABIES (see Ch. 28)

Scabies is a disease caused by the mite *Sarcoptes scabiei* (Fig. 26.81b). It is worldwide, being especially common in the underdeveloped areas of the world and in countries with a low standard of living. Scabies appears to sweep the world in cyclical pandemics.[665,667] It afflicts both rich and poor alike and is commoner in children. Most cases of human scabies are contracted from other infected humans, but occasionally animal strains of the scabies mite can infect humans.[668]

The gravid female mites burrow into the horny layers of the skin, forming tunnels (Fig. 26.81c) in which the eggs are laid. The female mite lives for about 1 month, laying two to three

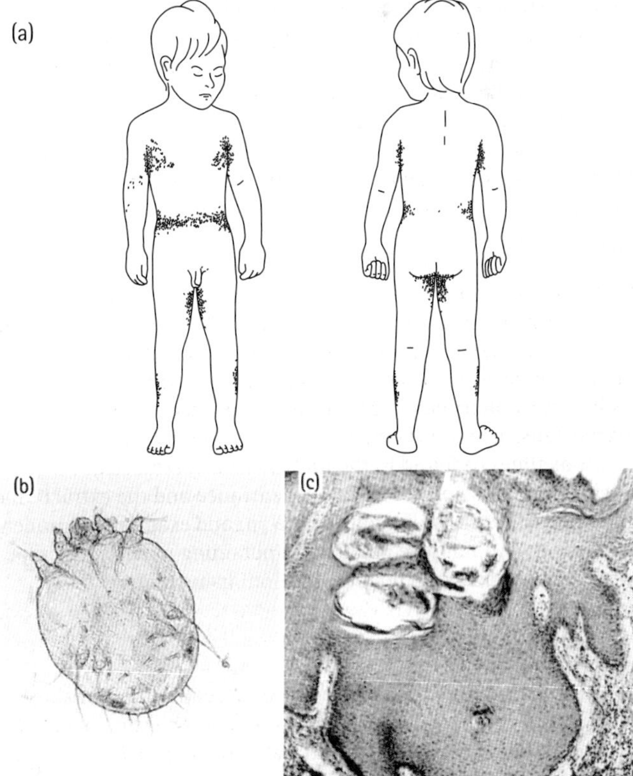

Fig. 26.81 (a) The distribution of the rash in scabies. (b) Adult *Sarcoptes scabiei* (approx. × 100). (c) Histological section of skin in scabies showing tunnels (approx. × 300).

eggs daily, which hatch in 3–4 days into six-legged larvae. These migrate to the surface and then burrow into the skin again and molt into eight-legged nymphs before becoming adults about 10 days after hatching. On average, each patient is infested with only 10–12 mites at any one time and much of the observed symptomatology is due to sensitization of the host to the mite and its products.[669,670]

CLINICAL FEATURES

Although the main sites infested can vary with the age of the patient, the commonest sites found to harbor mites include the hands (especially the sides of the fingers and the interdigital spaces), the wrists, the elbows, the feet, the penis and the scrotum, the buttocks and the axillae, with a lesser involvement of the body. The face is spared in most cases except in infants.[671]

The feeding activities of the mites and host sensitization result in itching and the development of an extensive rash, which does not correlate with the predilection sites of the mites (Fig. 26.81a).

The characteristic lesions of scabies are the burrows in the skin, but there may also be pruritic papules, vesicles and pustules. Often there is eczematization and crusting of the lesions, especially when they are secondarily infected by bacteria. Scabies lesions can provide an entry site for infection with Group A beta hemolytic streptococci and thus glomerulonephritis may follow scabies.[671]

Scabies may present in variable forms. Thus in the 'clean' and in patients on corticosteroids, scabies may present with minimal signs and symptoms. In young children, vesicles rather than tunnels are often the rule, while in some patients, the disease occurs in the nodular form. In mentally handicapped patients, debilitated patients and the immunosuppressed, crusted or 'Norwegian scabies' is sometimes seen and in HIV infected individuals, scabies can be particularly severe and persistent. In such cases the infestation is highly contagious and large numbers of mites can be found.

A common feature of scabies is the characteristic nocturnal itching, especially when the patient is warm in bed.

The infestation is transmitted by direct contact, including sexual contact. Fomites such as clothing and blankets generally play no part in the transmission of scabies.

DIAGNOSIS

Scabies is usually diagnosed clinically and should be considered as a diagnosis in any patient presenting with an itchy rash covering the whole body but sparing the face. In fact, scabies should be the first disease to be *excluded* in any patient presenting with such a rash.[670,672] Confirmation by the finding of mites is often difficult, even extensive lesions being associated with very few mites. Mites can sometimes be found in the tunnels after careful removal of the horny layers of skin over the tunnel entrance and the extraction of the shiny white glistening mite with a pin and examination under a microscope. An improved method of obtaining mites is to scrape a suspect lesion and then float the mite out using mineral oil.

TREATMENT

Treatment traditionally begins with a hot bath and a brisk scrub with a soft brush, but this is unnecessary or even inadvisable. Treatment of scabies involves the widespread application over the body of such topical preparations as benzyl benzoate (Ascabiol), gamma-benzene hexachloride (lorexane, lindane) or crotamiton (Eurax). Of these, benzyl benzoate is the classic treatment but its application causes an unpleasant stinging if used in full strength (25%). In children (and perhaps even in adults) it should be diluted to half strength, and in infants to quarter strength. Monosulfiram and crotamiton are possibly less effective but the latter is believed to be especially useful as it is said to have some antipruritic activity. Monosulfiram is sometimes used for treating scabies in children. Gamma-benzene hexachloride 1% (lindane) has in the past proved to be cheap and effective.[671] Gamma-benzene hexachloride should not be used in premature babies and should be used with care in pregnancy or in infants to 1 year of age.[673]

The newer synthetic pyrethroids are also effective.[670–672] Resistance to both lindane and the pyrethroids (including permethrin) has been recorded and the problem of resistance as opposed to incomplete treatment is discussed in the review of scabies by Burgess.[671]

For adequate treatment and control, *all members of the family must be treated whether or not they exhibit symptoms*, or relapses and treatment failure will result. In conditions of overcrowding and poor hygiene, the regular use of Tetmosol soap prevents reinfection.

Overtreatment resulting from a temporary persistence of symptoms due to sensitization and the development of a 'parasitophobia' must be avoided.

It is worth noting that many animal parasitic mites (e.g. *Dermanyssus* and *Ornithonyssus* from rodents or birds and mange mites from dogs and cats) as well as many free-living and non-parasitic mites can attack humans and cause an extensive rash with a severe dermatitis and an itchy allergic reaction resulting in the formation of papules, vesicles and skin blotches. This condition can be very distressing and infestation usually derives from pets, animals nesting in roofs, straw and other packing materials.[674]

The use of oral ivermectin may be required for the treatment of severe scabies but toxicity can be a problem.[670,671] The overall confusion in the literature relating to the effective treatment of scabies is really summarized in the conclusions drawn by Walker & Johnstone[675] in their analysis of the available literature. They found no difference in clinical cure rates between crotomiton and lindane or benzyl benzoate and sulfur and they concluded that 'The evidence that permethrin is more effective than lindane is inconsistent. Lindane, permethrin and ivermectin appear to be associated with rare but serious drug reactions'. More research is needed on the safety and effectiveness of ivermectin and malathion compared to permethrin, on community management, and on different regimens and vehicles for topical treatment.

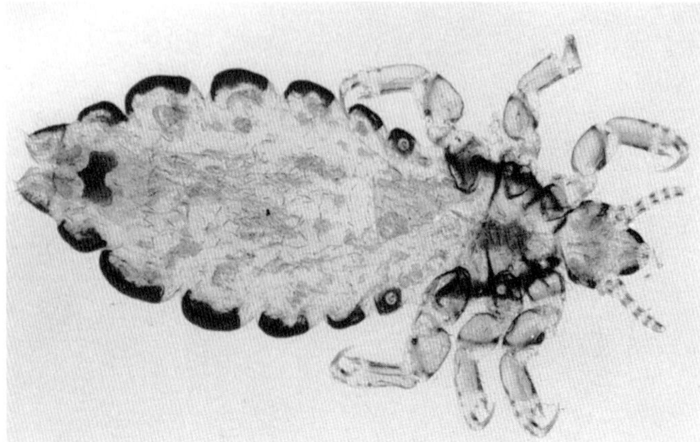

Fig. 26.82 Photomicrograph of adult *Pediculus humanus capitis* – the head louse (approx. × 50).

LOUSE INFESTATION

Humans can become infested with three types of lice: the head louse (*Pediculus humanus capitis*; Fig. 26.82), its morphologically identical, but behaviorally different variant, the body louse (*P. h. corporis*) and the crab or pubic louse, which forms a distinct species, *Pthirus pubis*. All three types are confined to humans worldwide and tend to be more prevalent in areas with poor living standards.[676]

PEDICULUS HUMANUS CAPITIS (THE HEAD LOUSE)

P. h. capitis is worldwide in distribution but tends to be commoner in colder countries. Its incidence is subject to unpredictable increases and decreases and with sporadic extensive pandemics. Prevalence figures vary from country to country and from year to year but vary from low percentage prevalences to prevalences of 60% or more amongst schoolchildren.[669,676]

Head lice tend to be confined to the scalp, but are occasionally found on other hairy parts of the body. The insects live close to the scalp and feed on blood which they obtain with their sucking mouthparts. After mating, the female louse lays six to eight eggs every 24 h. These eggs ('nits') (Fig. 26.83) are glued tightly to the hairs close to the scalp and hatch in about 7 days into a nymph, which feeds and passes through three nymphal instars before becoming adult in 10–11 days.[676]

Head louse infestation may be asymptomatic or, in heavily infested cases, may be manifested by scalp pruritus, loss of sleep, mild pyrexia and, with secondary bacterial infection, by cervical gland enlargement.

Pediculosis capitis is found in people of all age groups, but is commoner in children especially those aged 3–13 years, being maximal at 6–9 years. Although not directly correlated to hair length, head lice are commoner in girls than in boys. Both rich and poor alike are afflicted, but infestation is more frequently but not exclusively encountered in low socioeconomic areas.

While transmission is mostly by direct contact and is thus facilitated by overcrowding, many studies have suggested strongly that transmission can occur through shared headgear, hat and coat hooks, combs and brushes.

Head lice can only be controlled by regular inspection and treatment of infected cases *and all their family members*, whether or not lice or nits can be found in the latter.

In the past, DDT has been used for treatment, but its toxicity and resistance in the lice led to its replacement by gamma-benzene hexachloride (gamma BHC, gamma HCH; Quellada, lorexane; lindane). However, resistance is being recorded to HCH and this, plus its toxicity, has resulted in its being considered obsolete in many parts of the world.[669,677,678] It is being replaced by safer preparations such as carbaryl, malathion (Maldison, Prioderm) and the synthetic pyrethroids such as permethrin (Nix). Of these, malathion (a 0.5% preparation in a spirit base) is the most widely used. It is twice as safe as HCH and has the added but variable advantage of possibly being residual for at least a month, through bonding to the hair, and in being ovicidal, killing both lice and nits – a feature absent in HCH which is not ovicidal. Carbaryl is also said to be ovicidal but Burgess[679] has challenged this concept of an inherent ovicidal efficacy for malathion and carbaryl. Pyrethrins (Paralice) especially those in a mousse formulation (e.g. Banlice) may also be effectively used to treat head lice[676] with the third generation synthetic pyrethroids such as permethrin (Nix) proving the most promising.[677,678] Dodd[680] concluded that permethrin, synerized pyrethrum and malathion were all effective in headlouse treatment and that the choice between them will really depend on local resistance patterns. All these preparations are toxic to some extent and care should thus be exercised in their use, with particular care being taken to avoid accidental ingestion or contact with eyes. Both shampoos and lotions are available but lotions are far superior.[676,681,682] Developing resistance to headlouse preparations may prove a problem, albeit a sometimes controversial one.[676,680,683] Wargon[684] considers that ivermectin may be considered for the treatment of 'more difficult cases'.

The use of levamisole for pediculosis at a daily oral dose of 3.5 mg/kg for 10 days, although considered to be safe and economical by Namazi,[685] does not really seem to be a practical alternative to the more conventional methods of headlouse control.

Nits, although killed by malathion and carbaryl, remain tightly attached to the hairs and may have to be combed out with special fine toothed 'nit combs', although with ovicidal compounds this exercise is not necessary in louse treatment or control.

In the control of head lice, sterilization of clothing, bedding, combs, etc. is unnecessary, as insecticide treatment of the hair will provide sufficient protection from reinvasion by the short-lived lice that have strayed from the head.

In community control programs, antilouse preparations should be changed on a regular basis to prevent the emergence of resistance.

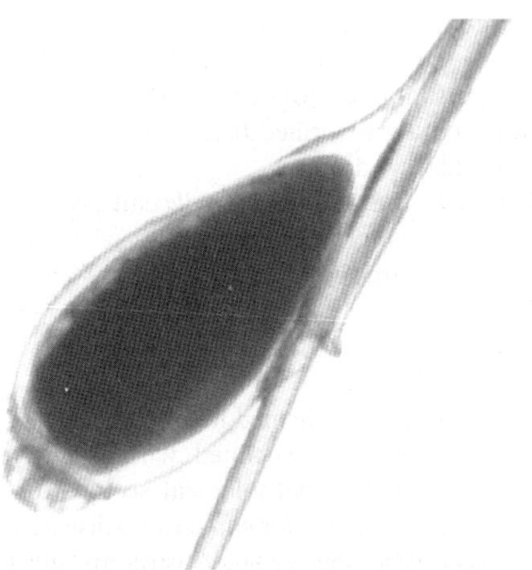

Fig. 26.83 Egg of crab louse (*Pthirus. pubis*) attached to hair (approx. × 60).

PEDICULUS HUMANUS CORPORIS (THE BODY LOUSE)

P. h. corporis is identical to the head louse in appearance, but differs in that it lives on the clothing and only visits the skin to suck blood. The eggs are glued to the clothing, especially the seams, and hatch in about 1 week to nymphs, which like those of the head louse, develop into adults in 7–10 days.

Body lice cause pediculosis corporis which may be characterized by the presence of feeding punctures appearing as small papules which, in sensitized patients, may become swollen, pigmented and hardened, a condition formerly known as vagabond's disease or *morbus errorum*.

Body lice are more limited to areas of overcrowding and poorer standards of living but may reach epidemic proportions during periods of social upheaval and unrest such as war, earthquakes, floods, etc. They are the vectors of epidemic typhus (*Rickettsia prowazekii*) and epidemic relapsing fever (*Borrelia recurrentis*).

Transmission of body lice is directly from person to person and from shared clothing and blankets. Control is with 0.5% malathion lotion or 5% carbaryl dust and treatment of clothing, blankets, etc.

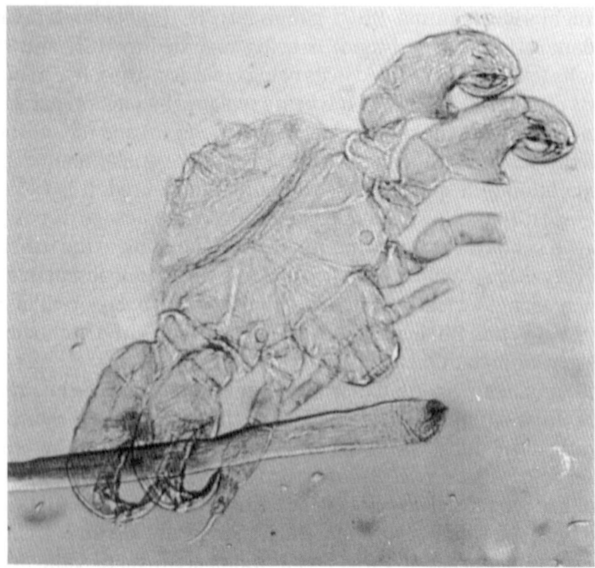

Fig. 26.84 Photomicrograph of nymph of *Pthirus pubis* tightly attached to hair (approx. × 100).

with methyl bromide fumigation, washing in hot water at 60°C or higher by heating in a domestic tumble drier for at least 5 min.

PTHIRUS PUBIS (THE CRAB OR PUBIC LOUSE)

Pth. pubis has a distinctive appearance and is usually found in the pubic region of humans only. It may also be found tightly attached to the hairs of the leg, the axilla or the beard (Fig. 26.84). Eggs are laid attached to hairs or even eyelashes (Fig. 26.85). It is usually transmitted during sexual intercourse and because of this, it is mostly found infesting adults. However, children can harbor the lice and even young children may become infected from heavily infested parents. Thus, toddlers are at times found to have phthiriasis, the lice being found attached to the eyelashes and even the hair of the forehead. The lice can survive for 9–44 h off the host and infestation from clothing and toilet seats is thus feasible, although unlikely.

Again, heavy infestations may result in itching and rarely, *maculae cerulae* or bluish spots due to repeated biting may be found.

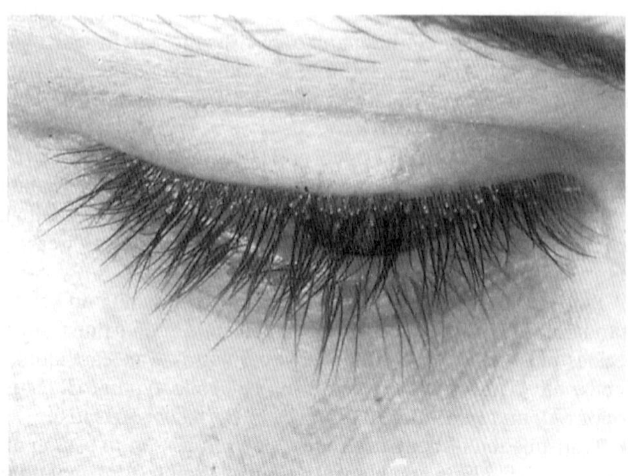

Fig. 26.85 Eggs of pubic louse on eyelashes.

Treatment is similar to that for head lice, namely the use of insecticides such as gamma-benzene hexachloride (lindane) as a lotion, shampoo or powder. This insecticide is toxic and treatment needs to be repeated, as it is not ovicidal. 0.5% malathion or carbaryl are safer and, being ovicidal, are more effective, but spirit base preparations should not be used. Pyrethroids are also effective and are widely used.

When on the eyelashes (Fig. 26.85) *Pth. pubis* should be dealt with by removal of individual lice or by treating each egg individually with a paint brush dipped in an ovicidal insecticide. Alternatively, the thick application of Vaseline twice daily for 8 days may be effective.[676] Laundering of clothing, sheets, etc. in hot water is advisable to prevent spread.

DISEASES TRANSMITTED BY ANIMALS

These are summarized in Table 26.43.[686]

CAT-SCRATCH DISEASE (CSD)

First described in 1950, cat-scratch is a relatively benign, widely encountered infection characterized by malaise, low grade fever and lymphadenopathy. About half of the patients with CSD develop a non-pruritic, erythematous primary lesion 3–30 days after getting a scratch. This lesion may form a small pustule but overall the infection usually resolves spontaneously in a few weeks. Rarely, complications can occur such as encephalitis, conjunctivitis (Parinaud's oculoglandular syndrome), neuroretinitis and thrombocytopenic purpura.[686–688] Contact with cats followed by skin lesions associated with a scratch or bite are found in the majority of cases. There may be a maculopapular rash. Chronic lymphadenitis may occur with the cervical lymph nodes frequently involved. Murano et al[689] reported a giant hepatic granuloma as associated with *Bartonella henselae* infection and suggested that this infection should be considered in the differential diagnosis of a large hepatic mass. Overall, systemic symptoms are unusual in CSD, but severe disease may occur in HIV positive patients. Isada et al[690] reported that in the USA, 22 000 cases of CSD occur annually with 10% requiring hospitalization.

ETIOLOGY

A proposed causative agent for CSD was identified in 1988 and named *Afipia felis* – a Gram negative, motile, oxidase-positive, non-fermenting bacillus.[686,691] The bacterium *B.* (formerly *Rochalimaea*) *henselae*, which is morphologically similar to *A. felis*, is in all probability more important in the etiology of CSD and the role of *A. felis* in the causation of CSD (if it has one) is small.[686,692] Kordick et al,[693] however, have described *B. clarridgeiae* as the cause of a cat scratch disease-like syndrome.

Other species of the genus *Bartonella* can infect humans but are not involved in causing CSD. The species of *Bartonella* and their disease associations are summarized in Table 26.44.

DIAGNOSIS

The diagnosis of CSD is confirmed if the history of cat contact and a primary skin lesion is associated with typical silver-staining bacteria identified on histopathological sections of lymph nodes, skin or eye lesions. A skin test for cat-scratch disease is available, but this is being superseded by serology using an indirect fluorescent antibody test for *B. henselae* which is said to be more sensitive.

Table 26.43 Diseases transmitted/harbored by dogs, cats and rodents*

Dogs	Cats	Rodents
Rabies	Rabies	Lassa fever
Ringworm	Cat-scratch fever (*Bartonella henselae*)	Hantavirus disease
Scabies	Ringworm	S. American arenavirus hemorrhagic fevers
Echinococcus granulosus infection	Scabies	Omsk hemorrhagic fever
Toxocara canis infection (larva migrans)	*Toxocara cati* (larva migrans)	Kyasanur forest disease
Leptospirosis	Pasteurellosis (*Pasteurella multocida*)	Group C virus disease
Canicola fever (*Leptospira canicola*)	Cutaneous larva migrans	E. Hemisphere sandfly fever
Leishmaniasis	Toxoplasmosis	Vesicular stomatitis fever
Dipylidium caninum	*Bartonella clarridgeiae*	Venezuelan equine encephalitis
Cutaneous larva migrans	*Capillaria aerophila*	Lymphocytic choriomeningitis
Dirofilaria immitis	Cutaneous dirofilariasis	Rat bite fever (*Spirillum minor*)
Capnocytophaga canimorsus (DF-2)	Paragonimiasis	Haverhill fever (*Streptobacillus moniliformis*)
Bartonella clarridgeiae	Q fever	Bubonic plague (*Yersinia pestis)*
Bartonella vinsonii	*Ctenocephalides felis*	Campylobacteriosis
Spotted fever (some forms)	Salmonellosis (gastroenteritis)	Salmonellosis (gastroenteritis)
Erlichiosis	Giardiasis	Leptospirosis (e.g. Weil's disease)
Cutaneous dirofilariasis	*Strongyloides* sp.	Endemic relapsing fever
Paragonimiasis	*Tunga penetrans*	Scrub typhus
Q fever		Murine typhus
Salmonellosis (gastroenteritis)		Rickettsialpox
Ctenocephalides canis		Spotted fever (some forms)
Giardiasis		Q fever
Diphyllobothrium latum		*Bartonella* spp.
Fasciola hepatica		*Babesia microti*
Lyme disease		Toxoplasmosis (where rodents are eaten)
Trichuris vulpis		Cutaneous leishmaniasis (some forms)
Strongyloides sp.		*Clonorchis sinensis*
Tunga penetrans		*Schistosoma japonicum*
		Multilocular hydatid
		Hymenolepis nana
		Hymenolepis diminuta
		Inermicapsifer madagascariensis
		Angiostrongyliasis
		Capillaria hepatica
		Monilliformis monilliformis
		Cordylobia anthropophaga
		Xenopsylla cheopis
		Tunga penetrans
		Dermanyssid mites
		Trombiculid mites

* Not all of these infections are directly transmissible to humans from the animal reservoir and in some cases the animal may only be an occasional reservoir for the infection. For details of these and other infectious diseases relating especially to control, the reference edited by Chin[684] is strongly recommended.

Table 26.44 Disease associations in the genus *Bartonella* in humans

Species	Disease association	Comments
B. henselae	Cat-scratch disease (CSD) Bacillary angiomatosis	From cat bite/lick
B. quintana	Trench fever Bacillary angiomatosis	From body lice
B. bacilliformis	Oroya fever, verruga peruana	*Lutzomyia* flies
B. elizabethae	Subacute endocarditis Neuroretinitis	
B. clarridgeiae	Subacute endocarditis CSD-like syndrome	From cats/dogs
B. vinsonii	Subacute endocarditis	Various subspecies From cats, dogs, rodents

TREATMENT

As most patients with this disease are not ill and spontaneous recovery is common, treatment is usually symptomatic. Antibiotics should be reserved for patients with severe disease. The most commonly used antibiotics are not effective and a recent review indicated that only four antimicrobial drugs are useful, with the oral drugs in decreasing order of efficacy being rifampicin (87%), ciprofloxacin (84%) and trimethoprim-sulfamethoxazole (58%). Intramuscular gentamicin was 73% effective.[694] Isada et al[690] while admitting that no controlled trials have been carried out in the treatment of CSD, report that erythromycin, doxycycline or co-trimoxazole, in that order, might be effective.

CAT-SCRATCH ENCEPHALOPATHY

CNS complications may develop from a few days to some weeks after the first evidence of illness, usually a mildly tender lymphadenopathy. Fever is not characteristic and may occur in only 50% of cases. Convulsions of varying severity will also affect about 50% of the children with encephalopathy, and they may remain lethargic or even comatose for several weeks. In the recovery phase, 'transient combative behavior' seems to be a characteristic feature of this particular type of encephalopathy. Changes in the CSF are neither consistent nor characteristic and peripheral blood counts are not helpful. In addition to the control of convulsions and supportive measures, the most important aspect of this encephalopathy is to establish the diagnosis and differentiate it from other causes of encephalopathy as quickly as possible to avoid extensive and invasive investigations. The prognosis is excellent with no evidence of lasting neurological impairment.[695]

RAT-BITE FEVERS

Rat-bite fevers comprise two separate and distinct infections, which are characterized by a relapsing fever usually following a rat bite. They are particularly prevalent in rat-infested communities of low socioeconomic status. Children living in such areas are at especial risk and may even be bitten by rats while asleep. Children may also become infected following the bite from a pet mouse or rat. *Streptobacillus moniliformis* (streptobacillary rat-bite fever; Haverhill fever; erythema arthriticum epidemicum) has been recorded worldwide, including from Europe and the USA while *Spirillum minus* (spirillary rat-bite fever; sodoku or sokosha) has also been reported worldwide, but mostly from Japan.[686] Streptobacillary rat-bite fever is a more common cause of fever following a rat bite than is the spirillary form.

STREPTOBACILLUS MONILIFORMIS

Streptobacillus moniliformis is a commensal in the rat nasopharynx and has also occasionally been recorded from other small mammal species such as squirrels, weasels and gerbils.[686,688,696] While transmission is usually through a rat bite, epidemic outbreaks in humans are believed to have resulted from ingestion of raw milk or water contaminated with rat urine or saliva.[686,688] The incubation period is usually 3 to 10 days, occasionally longer, during which a gastroenteritis may be present. The infected bite usually heals rapidly but a fever develops which is often relapsing and, although usually subsiding within 10 days or so, may continue for months if untreated. A generalized erythematous, morbilliform or even purpuric rash, particularly on the hands and feet, may develop and arthralgia (especially of the large joints) and sore throat, extreme prostration and headache may occur. Complications may include infective endocarditis, pericarditis and abscesses of soft tissue or brain.[686,697,698] The fatality rate may reach 10% if untreated.

Streptobacillary rat-bite fever needs to be differentiated from Coxsackie infections, meningococcal septicemia and erythema multiforme but infection can be confirmed by isolation of *S. moniliformis* from blood, infected joint fluid, abscesses or pustules. It should be cultured as a facultative anaerobe followed by subculture in a CO_2 atmosphere after 48 h. Isolation can also be achieved by inoculation of guinea pigs or laboratory mice. Serological diagnosis using an agglutination test is available and becomes positive in the second to third week of the infection. Penicillin, given as soon as possible after the bite, is effective as are cephalosporins, but strains resistant to penicillin, streptomycin and erythromycin have been recorded.

SPIRILLUM MINUS

Transmission of *Spirillum minus* is most commonly via the bite of an infected rat but can occur following the bite from other mammals including cats, which can serve as healthy reservoirs. Food contaminated by infected rat urine may also presumably cause infection.

The incubation period varies from 7 to 28 (mean 8) days after the bite, which may heal or become necrotic and chancre-like. Recurrent fevers occur at 5 to 10 day intervals, sometimes continuing for weeks in untreated patients, and may be accompanied by profuse sweating often with a marked flare up of inflammation at the site of the bite. Regional lymphadenopathy usually develops and a characteristic purplish, papular (or sometimes nodular) rash or urticaria may be present, especially on the chest and arms. Muscle pains, but rarely joint pains and arthritis, hyperesthesia and localized edema are additional signs. In severe cases, a meningoencephalitis with delirium may develop as may endocarditis and involvement of other organs. In untreated cases, the mortality may reach 10%, being associated with neuronal degeneration of the brain and degenerative changes in the liver and kidneys.

The differential diagnosis should consider other febrile infections, including those caused by spirochetes (such as relapsing fever), viruses, rickettsiae (such as the spotted fevers), bacterial infections (such as plague), tularemia and also malaria, in endemic regions. A puffiness of the face may suggest nephritis and children may present with persistent diarrhea and weight loss, which may further confuse the correct diagnosis. During febrile paroxysms there may be a leukocytosis and occasionally eosinophilia and anemia may be present. CSF pressure may be raised.

Diagnosis of spirillosis can be confirmed by detecting *S. minus* in lesion/tissue exudates, in an enlarged lymph node or, during a febrile episode, in peripheral blood by dark ground microscopy. Isolation by inoculation of guinea pigs, mice or laboratory rats is often successful. No specific serological tests are available.

Penicillin is the treatment of choice for spirillosis but streptomycin, erythromycin, chloramphenicol and tetracyclines (not during pregnancy or for children under 7–8 years of age) are also effective.

REFERENCES (* Level 1 evidence)

MORTALITY AND MORBIDITY IN INFECTIOUS DISEASE

1 World Bank. Investing in health, World Development Report. Oxford: Oxford University Press; 1993.

2 The United Nations Children's Fund. The state of the world's children. New York: United Nations Children's Fund (UNICEF); 2001.

3 Fleming D, Smith GE, Charlton J, et al. Impact of infections on primary care – greater than expected. Commun Dis Public Health 2002 5(1):7–12.

4 Murray CJL. Quantifying the burden of disease: the technical basis for disability-adjusted life years. In: Murray CJL, Lopez AD, eds. Global comparative assessments in the health sector. Geneva: WHO; 1994:3–19.

5 Cliffe S, Tookey P, Nicoll A. Antenatal detection of HIV: national surveillance and unlinked anonymous survey. BMJ 2001; 325:376–377.

6 Ramsay M, Gay N, Miller E, et al. The epidemiology of measles in England and Wales: rationale for the 1994 national vaccination campaign. CDR Rev 1994; 4:R141–R146.

7 Gay N, Miller E. Was a measles epidemic imminent? CDR Rev 1995; 5:R204–R207.

8 Christie P. Measles in Scotland. Commun Dis Environ Health Scotl 1994; 28(41):3–8.

9 Communicable Disease Surveillance Centre (CDSC). The national measles and rubella campaign – one year on. CDR Rev 1995; 5:237.

10 Cronin M, O'Connell T. Measles outbreak in the Republic of Ireland. Eurosurveillance Wkly 2000; 4:002101.

11 Gangarosa EJ, Galazka AM, Wolfe CR, et al. Impact of anti-vaccine movements on pertussis control. Lancet 1998; 351:356–361.

12 Nicoll A. Benefits, safety and risks of immunisation programmes. Interdisciplinary Sci Rev 2001; 26:20–30.

*13 Colditz GA, Brewer TF, Berkey JCS, et al. Efficacy of BCG vaccine in the prevention of tuberculosis. JAMA 1994; 271:698–702.

14 Elliott EJ, Robins-Browne RM, O'Loughlin EV, et al. Contributors to the Australian Paediatric Surveillance Unit. Nationwide study of haemolytic uraemic syndrome: clinical, microbiological, and epidemiological features. Arch Dis Child 2001; 5:125–131.

15 PHLS, DHSS & PS and the Scottish ISD(D)5. Collaborative group trends in sexually transmitted infections in the UK. 1990–1999. London: London Public Health Laboratory Service, 2000.

16 Nicoll A, Catchpole M, Cliffe S, et al. Sexual health of teenagers in England and Wales. BMJ 1999; 318:1321–1322.

17 Harling R, Twisselmann B, Asgari-Jihandeh N, et al for the Deliberate Release Team. Deliberate releases of biological agents: initial lessons for Europe from events in the United States. Euro Surveill 2001; 6(11):166–171.

18 Satcher D. Emerging infections: getting ahead of the curve. Emerg Infect Dis 1997; 1:1–6.

19 Verity CM, Nicoll A, Will RG, et al. Variant Creutzfeldt–Jakob disease in UK children: a national surveillance study. Lancet 2000; 356:1224–1227.

20 Morse SS. Factors in the emergence of infectious diseases. Emerg Infect Dis 1995; 1:7–15.

21 Begg N, Nicoll A. Myths in medicine. BMJ 1994; 309:1073–1075.

22 Gill ON, Sockett PN, Bartlett CLR, et al. Outbreak of *Salmonella napoli* caused by contaminated chocolate bars. Lancet 1983; 2:544–547.

23 Bell BP, Goldoft M, Griffin PM, et al. A multistate outbreak of *E. coli* 0157: H7-associated bloody diarrhea and hemolytic uremic syndrome from hamburgers. JAMA 1994; 272:1349–1353.

24 Wasserheit JN. Effect of changes in human ecology and behaviour on patterns of sexually transmitted diseases, including immunodeficiency virus infection. Proc Natl Acad Sci U S A 1994; 91:2430–2435.

25 Bobadilla J-L, Cowley P, Musgrove P, et al. Design, content and financing of an essential national package of health services. In: Murray CJL, Lopez AD, eds. Global comparative assessments in the health sector. Geneva: WHO; 1994:171–192.

26 United Nations Children's Emergency Fund. The state of the world's children 1996. Oxford: Oxford University Press; 1996.

27 Hull HF, Ward NA, Hull BF, et al. Paralytic poliomyelitis: seasoned strategies, disappearing disease. Lancet 1994; 343:1331–1337.

28 United Nations. We the children: end decade review of the follow-up to the World Summit for Children. Report of the Secretary-General, A/S-27/3. New York: United Nations; 2001.

29 Nicoll A, Lynn R, Rahi J, et al. Public health outputs from the British Paediatric Surveillance Unit and similar clinician-based systems. J Roy Soc Med 2000; 93:580–585.

HOSPITAL INFECTION CONTROL: POLICIES AND PROCEDURES

30 Hall C, Douglas RJ, Geiman J. Respiratory syncytial virus infections in infants: quantitation and duration of shedding. J Pediatr 1976; 89:115.

31 Hall C, Douglas RJ, Schnabel K, et al. Infectivity of respiratory syncytial virus by various routes of inoculation. Infect Immun 1981; 33:779–783.

32 Royle J, Halasz S, Eagles G, et al. Outbreak of extended spectrum beta lactamase producing *Klebsiella pneumoniae* in a neonatal unit. Arch Dis Child Fetal Neonatal Ed 1999; 80:F64–68.

33 Davidson GP, Whyte PB, Daniels E, et al. Passive immunisation of children with bovine colostrum containing antibodies to human rotavirus. Lancet 1989; 2:709–712.

PRINCIPLES OF ANTIMICROBIAL THERAPY

34 Paradise JL. Treatment guidelines for otitis media: the need for breadth and flexibility. Pediatr Infect Dis J 1995; 14:429–435.

*35 Glasziou PP, Del Mar CB, Sanders SL, Hayem M. Antibiotics for acute otitis media in children (Cochrane Review). In: The Cochrane Library, 1. Oxford: Update Software; 2001.

36 Therapeutic guidelines: Antibiotic, Version 11. Victoria: Guidelines Limited; 2000.

37 Davis BD. Bactericidal synergism between beta-lactams and aminoglycosides: mechanism and possible therapeutic implications. Rev Infect Dis 1982; 4:237–245.

38 Love LJ, Schimpff SC, Schiffer CA, et al. Improved prognosis for granulocytopenic patients with gram-negative bacteremia. Am J Med 1980; 68:643–648.

39 Schaad UB, McCracken GH, Nelson JD. Clinical pharmacology and efficacy of vancomycin in pediatric patients. J Pediatr 1980; 96:119–126.

40 Karlowsky JA, Zhanel GG, Davidson RJ, et al. Once-daily aminoglycoside dosing assessed by MIC reversion time with *Pseudomonas aeruginosa*. Antimicrob Agents Chemother 1994; 38:1165–1168.

41 Radetsky M. Duration of treatment in bacterial meningitis: a historical inquiry. Pediatr Infect Dis J 1990; 9:2–9.

42 Reichmann P, Konig A, Linares J, et al. A global gene pool for high-level cephalosporin resistance in commensal *Streptococcus* species and *Streptococcus pneumoniae*. J Infect Dis 1997; 176:1001–1012.

43 Waxman DJ, Strominger JL. Penicillin-binding proteins and the mechanism of action of beta-lactam antibiotics. Annu Rev Biochem 1983; 52:825–869.

44 Massova I, Mobashery S. Kinship and diversification of bacterial penicillin-binding proteins and beta-lactamases. Antimicrob Agents Chemother 1998; 42:1–17.

45 Ubukata K, Nonoguchi R, Song MD, et al. Homology of *MecA* gene in methicillin-resistant *Staphylococcus haemolyticus* and *Staphylococcus simulans* to that of *Staphylococcus aureus*. Antimicrob Agents Chemother 1990; 34: 170–172.

46 Laible G, Spratt BG, Hakenbeck R. Interspecies recombinational events during the evolution of altered PBP 2x genes in penicillin-resistant clinical isolates of *Streptococcus pneumoniae*. Mol Microbiol 1991; 5:1993–2002.

47 Sougakoff W, Goussard S, Gerbaud G, et al. Plasmid-mediated resistance to third-generation cephalosporins caused by point mutations in TEM-type penicillinase genes. Rev Infect Dis 1988; 10:879–884.

48 Block SL, Harrison CJ, Hedrick JA. Penicillin-resistant *Streptococcus pneumoniae* in acute otitis media: risk factors, susceptibility patterns and antimicrobial management. Pediatr Infect Dis J 1995; 14:751–759.

49 Bradley JS, Connor JD. Ceftriaxone failure in meningitis caused by *Streptococcus pneumoniae* with reduced susceptibility to beta-lactam antibiotics. Pediatr Infect Dis J 1991; 10:871–873.

50 Nagarajan R. Antibacterial activities and modes of action of vancomycin and related glycopeptides. Antimicrob Agents Chemother 1991; 35:605–609.

51 Arthur M, Courvalin P. Genetics and mechanisms of glycopeptide resistance in enterococci. Antimicrob Agents Chemother 1993; 37:1563–1571.

52 Weisblum B. Erythromycin resistance by ribosome modification. Antimicrob Agents Chemother 1995; 39:577–585.

53 Sawai T, Hiruma R, Kawana N. Outer membrane permeation of beta-lactam antibiotics

in *Escherichia coli*, *Proteus mirabilis*, and *Enterobacter cloacae*. Antimicrob Agents Chemother 1982; 22:585–592.

54 Kucers A, Crowe S, Grayson M, et al. The use of antibiotics. Part IV and part V, 5th edn. Oxford: Butterworth-Heinemann; 1997:1245–1881.

CLINICAL PROBLEMS: THE CHILD WITH FEVER

55 Wailoo MP, Petersen SA, Whitaker H, et al. Sleeping body temperatures in 3–4 month old infants. Arch Dis Child 1989; 64:596–599.

56 Morley CJ, Hewson PH, Thornton AJ, et al. Axillary and rectal temperature measurements in infants. Arch Dis Child 1992; 67:122–125.

57 Davies EG, Elliman DAC, Hart CA, et al. Manual of childhood infections. London: WB Saunders; 2001.

58 Bonadio WA, Hegenbarth M, Zachamason M. Correlating reported fever in young infants with subsequent temperature patterns and risk of serious bacterial infections. Paediatr Infect Dis J 1990; 9:158–160.

59 Bass JW, Steele R, Wittler R, et al. Antimicrobial treatment of occult bacteremia: a multicentre cooperative study. Paediatr Infect Dis J 1993; 12:466–473.

CLINICAL PROBLEMS: SUSPECTED MENINGITIS

60 Hargreaves RM, Slack MP, Howard AJ, et al. Changing patterns of invasive *Haemophilus influenzae* disease in England and Wales after introduction of the Hib vaccination programme. BMJ 1996; 312:160–161.

61 Garg RK. Tuberculosis of the central nervous system. Postgrad Med J 1999; 75:133–140.

62 Carrol ED, Latif AH, Misbah SA, et al. Lesson of the week: Recurrent bacterial meningitis: the need for sensitive imaging. BMJ 2001; 323:501–503.

63 van Furth AM, Roord JJ, van Furth R. Roles of proinflammatory and anti-inflammatory cytokines in pathophysiology of bacterial meningitis and effect of adjunctive therapy. Infect Immun 1996; 64:4883–4890.

64 Heyderman RS, Klein NJ. Emergency management of meningitis. J R Soc Med 2000; 93:225–229.

65 Tauber MG. To tap or not to tap? Clin Infect Dis 1997; 25:289–291.

66 Reacher MH, Shah A, Livermore DM, et al. Bacteraemia and antibiotic resistance of its pathogens reported in England and Wales between 1990 and 1998: trend analysis. BMJ 2000; 320:213–216.

67 Bradley JS, Scheld WM. The challenge of penicillin-resistant *Streptococcus pneumoniae* meningitis: current antibiotic therapy in the 1990s. Clin Inf Dis 1997; 24:S213–221.

68 Tauber MG, Moser B. Cytokines and chemokines in meningeal inflammation: biology and clinical implications. Clin Infect Dis 1999; 28:1–11.

69 McIntyre PB, Berkey CS, King SM, et al. Dexamethasone as adjunctive therapy in bacterial meningitis. A meta-analysis of randomized clinical trials since 1988. JAMA 1997; 278:925–931.

70 Powell KR, Sugarman LI, Eskenazi AE, et al. Normalization of plasma arginine vasopressin concentrations when children with meningitis are given maintenance plus replacement fluid therapy. J Pediatr 1990; 117:515–522.

71 Bedford H, de Louvois J, Halket S, et al. Meningitis in infancy in England and Wales: follow up at age 5 years. BMJ 2001; 323:533–536.

CLINICAL PROBLEMS: SEPTIC SHOCK

72 Sprung CL, Bernard GR, Dellinger RP. Guidelines for the management of severe sepsis and septic shock. Intensive Care Med 2001; 27(suppl 1).

73 Docke WD, Randow F, Syrbe U, et al. Monocyte deactivation in septic patients: restoration by IFN-gamma treatment. Nature Med 1997; 3:678–681.

74 Levin M, Klein N. Shock in the febrile child. In: Isaacs D, Moxon ER, eds. A practical approach to pediatric infections. New York: Churchill Livingstone; 1996:4425–4444.

75 Novelli V, Peters M, Dobson S. Infectious disease. In: Macnab A, Macrae D, Henning R, eds. Care of the critically ill child. London: Churchill Livingstone; 1999:281–298.

*76 Alejandria MM, Lansang MA, Dans LF, et al. Intravenous immunoglobulin for treating sepsis and septic shock (Cochrane Review). In: The Cochrane Library, 2. Oxford: Update Software; 2001.

77 Bernard GR, Vincent J-L, Laterre P-F, et al. Efficacy and safety of recombinant human activated protein C for severe sepsis. N Engl J Med 2001; 344:699–709.

78 Van den Berghe G, Wouters P, Weekers F, et al. Intensive insulin therapy in critically ill patients. N Engl J Med 2001; 345:1359–1367.

CONGENITAL AND NEONATAL INFECTIONS

79 Gregg NM. Congenital cataract following German measles in the mother. Trans Ophthalmol Soc Aust 1941; 3:35–46.

80 Tookey PA, Peckham CS. Surveillance of congenital rubella in Great Britain, 1971–1996. BMJ 1999; 318:769–770.

81 Rahi J, Adams G, Russell-Eggit I, et al. Epidemiological surveillance of rubella must continue. BMJ 2001; 323:112.

82 Miller E, Cradock-Watson JE, Pollock TM. Consequences of confirmed maternal rubella at successive stages of pregnancy. Lancet 1982; 2:781–784.

83 Best JM, Banatvala JE, Morgan-Capner P, et al. Fetal infection after maternal reinfection with rubella: criteria for defining reinfection. BMJ 1989; 299:773–775.

84 Boppana SB, Fowler KB, Britt WJ, et al. Symptomatic congenital cytomegalovirus infection in infants born to mothers with pre-existing immunity to cytomegalovirus. Pediatrics 1999; 104:55–60.

85 Boppana SB, Rivera LB, Fowler KB, et al. Intrauterine transmission of cytomegalovirus to infants of women with pre-conceptional immunity. N Engl J Med 2001; 344:1366–1371.

86 Noyola DE, Demmler GJ, Nelson CT, et al. Early predictors of neurodevelopmental outcome in symptomatic congenital cytomegalovirus infection. J Pediatr 2001; 138:325–331.

87 Fowler KB, McCollister FP, Dahle AJ, et al. Progressive and fluctuating sensorineural hearing loss in children with asymptomatic congenital cytomegalovirus infection. J Pediatr 1997; 130:624–630.

88 Paryani SG, Yeager AS, Hosford-Dunn H, et al. Sequelae of acquired cytomegalovirus infection in premature and sick term infants. J Pediatr 1985; 107:451–456.

89 Whitley RJ, Cloud G, Gruber W, et al. Ganciclovir treatment of symptomatic congenital cytomegalovirus infection: results of a phase II study. National Institute of Allergy and Infectious Diseases Collaborative Antiviral Study Group. J Infect 1997; 175:1080–1086.

90 Nigro G, Krzysztofiak A, Bartmann U, et al. Ganciclovir therapy for cytomegalovirus-associated liver disease in immunocompetent or immunocompromised children. Arch Virol 1997; 142:573–580.

91 Enders G, Miller E, Cradock-Watson J, et al. Consequences of varicella and herpes zoster in pregnancy: prospective study of 1739 cases. Lancet 1994; 343:1548–1551.

92 Chant KG, Sullivan EA, Burgess MA, et al. Varicella-zoster virus infection in Australia. Aust N Z J Public Health 1998; 22:413–418.

93 Heuchan AM, Isaacs D. The management of varicella-zoster virus exposure and infection in pregnancy and the newborn period. Australasian Subgroup in Paediatric Infectious Diseases of the Australasian Society for Infectious Diseases. Med J Aust 2001; 174:288–292.

94 Reynolds L, Struik S, Nadel S. Neonatal varicella: varicella zoster immunoglobulin (VZIG) does not prevent disease. Arch Dis Child Fetal Neonatal Ed 1999; 81:F69–70.

95 Gutierrez KM, Falkovitz HM, Maldonado Y, et al. The epidemiology of neonatal herpes simplex virus infections in California from 1985 to 1995. J Infect Dis 1999; 180:199–202.

96 Tookey P, Peckham CS. Neonatal herpes simplex virus infection in the British Isles. Paediatr Perinat Epidemiol 1996; 10:432–442.

97 Brown ZA, Selke S, Zeh J, et al. The acquisition of herpes simplex virus during pregnancy. N Engl J Med 1997; 337:509–515.

98 Whitley RJ. Herpes simplex virus infections of the central nervous system. A review. Am J Med 1988; 85(suppl 2A):61–67.

99 American Academy of Pediatrics. Herpes simplex. In: Pickering L, ed. 2000. Red book report of the Committee on Infectious Diseases. 25th edn. Elk Grove Village: American Academy of Pediatrics; 2000:309–318.

100 Dunn D, Wallon M, Peyron F, et al. Mother-to-child transmission of toxoplasmosis: risk estimates for clinical counselling. Lancet 1999; 353:1829–1833.

101 Vogel N, Kirisits M, Michael E, et al. Congenital toxoplasmosis transmitted from an immunologically competent mother infected before conception. Clin Infect Dis 1996; 23:1055–1060.

102 Dunn D, Gilbert R, Newell ML, et al. Low incidence of congenital toxoplasmosis in children born to women infected with human immunodeficiency virus. European Collaborative Study and Research Network on Congenital Toxoplasmosis. Eur J Obstet Gynecol Reprod Biol 1996; 68:93–96.

103 McAuley J, Boyer KM, Patel D, et al. Early and longitudinal evaluations of treated infants and children and untreated historical patients with congenital toxoplasmosis: the Chicago Collaborative Treatment Trial. Clin Infect Dis J 1994; 18:38–72.
*104 Peyron F, Wallon M, Liou C, Garner P. Treatments for toxoplasmosis in pregnancy (Cochrane Review). In: The Cochrane Library, 2. Oxford: Update Software; 2000.
105 McMinn P, Stratov I, Nagarajan L, et al. Neurological manifestations of enterovirus 71 infection in children during an outbreak of hand, foot, and mouth disease in Western Australia. Clin Infect Dis J 2001; 32:236–242.
106 Ho M, Chen ER, Hsu KH, et al. An epidemic of enterovirus 71 infection in Taiwan. Taiwan Enterovirus Epidemic Working Group. N Engl J Med 1999; 341:929–935.
107 Rotbart HA, Webster AD. Treatment of potentially life-threatening enterovirus infections with pleconaril. Clin Infect Dis J 2001; 32:228–235.

BACTERIAL INFECTIONS: USE OF THE BACTERIOLOGY LABORATORY BY THE PEDIATRICIAN
108 Szymczak EG, Barr JT, Durbin WA, et al. Evaluation of blood culture procedures in a pediatric hospital. J Clin Microbiol 1979; 9:88–92.
109 Onorato IM, Wassilak SGF. Laboratory diagnosis of pertussis – the state of the art. Pediatr Infect Dis J 1987; 6:145–151.
110 De Witt TG, Humphrey KF, McCarthy P. Clinical predictors of acute bacterial diarrhoea in young children. Pediatrics 1985; 76:551–556.
111 Beck-Sague C, Alexander ER. Sexually-transmitted diseases in children and adolescents. Infect Dis Clin North Am 1987; 1:277–304.

BACTERIAL INFECTIONS: BOTULISM
112 Midura TF. Update : Infant botulism. Clin Microbiol Rev 1996; 9:119–125.
113 Thomas DG. Infant botulism : a review in South Australia (1980–1989). J Paediatr Child Health 1993; 29:24–26.
114 Spika JS, Shaffer N, Hargrett-Bean N, et al. Risk factors for infant botulism in the United States. Am J Dis Child 1989; 143:828–832.
115 Schreiner MS, Field E, Ruddy R. Infant botulism : a review of 12 years' experience at The Children's Hospital of Philadelphia. Pediatrics 1991; 87:159–165.

BACTERIAL INFECTIONS: BRUCELLOSIS; UNDULANT FEVER
*116 Lubani MM, Dudkin KI, Sharda DC, et al. A multicenter therapeutic study of 1100 children with brucellosis. Paediatr Infect Dis J 1989; 8:75–78.

BACTERIAL INFECTIONS: CHOLERA
117 World Health Organization. Guidelines for cholera control. Geneva: World Health Organization; 1993.
*118 CHOICE Study Group. Multicenter, randomized, double-blind clinical trial to evaluate the efficacy and safety of a reduced osmolarity oral rehydration salts solution in children with acute watery diarrhea. Pediatrics 2001; 107:613–618.
119 Butler T. New developments in the understanding of cholera. Curr Gastroenterol Rep 2001; 3:315–321.
*120 Trach DD, Clemens JD, Ke NT, et al. Field trial of locally produced, killed, oral cholera vaccine in Vietnam. Lancet 1997; 349:231–235.

BACTERIAL INFECTIONS: DIPHTHERIA
121 Pappenheimer AM Jr, Murphy JR. Studies on the molecular epidemiology of diphtheria. Lancet 1983; 2:923–926.
122 Pallen MJ, Hay AJ, Puckey LH, et al. Polymerase chain reaction for screening clinical isolates of corynebacteria for the production of diphtheria toxin. J Clin Pathol 1994; 47:353–356.
123 Thisyakorn U, Wongvanich J, Kumpeng V. Failure of corticosteroid therapy to prevent diphtheritic myocarditis or neuritis. Pediatr Infect Dis 1984; 3:126–128.
124 Logina I, Donaghy M. Diphtheritic polyneuropathy: a clinical study and comparison with Guillain–Barré syndrome. J Neurol Neurosurg Psychiatry 1999; 67:433–438.
125 Bonnet JM, Begg NT. Control of diphtheria: guidance for consultants in communicable disease control. Commun Dis Public Health 1999; 2:242–249.
126 Kneen R, Giao PN, Solomon T, et al. Penicillin vs erythromycin in the treatment of diphtheria. Clin Infect Dis 1998; 27:845–850.
127 Quick ML, Sutter RW, Kobaidze N, et al. Epidemic diphtheria in the Republic of Georgia, 1993-1996: risk factors for fatal outcome among hospitalized patients. J Infect Dis 2000; 181(suppl 1):S130–137.
128 Galazka A. Implications of the diphtheria epidemic in the former Soviet Union for immunization programs. J Infect Dis 2000; 181(suppl 1):S244–248.
129 World Health Organization. Manual for the management and control of diphtheria in the European region. WHO regional office for Europe. Copenhagen: WHO; 1994.

BACTERIAL INFECTIONS: *ESCHERICHIA COLI*
130 Blattner FR, Plunkett G, Bloch CA, et al. The complete genome sequence of *Escherichia coli* K12. Science 1997; 277:1453–1474.
131 Perna NT, Plunkett G, Burland V, et al. Genome sequence of enterohaemorrhagic *Escherichia coli* O157: H7. Nature 2001; 409:529–533.
132 Reid SD, Herbelin CJ, Bumbaugh AC, et al. Parallel evolution of virulence in pathogenic *Escherichia coli*. Nature 2000; 406:64–67.
133 Whitfield C, Roberts IS. Structure, assembly and regulation of expression of capsules in *Escherichia coli*. Mol Microbiol 1999; 31:1307–1319.
134 Kariuki S, Gilks C, Kimari J, et al. Genotypic analysis of *Escherichia coli* strains isolated from children and chickens living in close priority. Appl Environ Microbiol 1999; 65:472–476.
135 Martindale J, Stroud D, Moxon ER, et al. Genetic analysis of *Escherichia coli* K1 gastrointestinal colonization. Mol Microbiol 2000; 37:1293–1305.
136 Kariuki S, Hart CA. Global aspects of antimicrobial resistant enteric bacteria. Curr Opin Infect Dis 2001; 14:579–586.

BACTERIAL INFECTIONS: *HAEMOPHILUS INFLUENZAE*
137 Pitmann M. Variation and type specificity in bacterial species of *Haemophilus influenzae*. J Exp Med 1931; 53:471–492.
*138 Booy R, Hodgson SA, Slack MPE, et al. Invasive *Haemophilus-influenzae*-type-b disease in the Oxford region (1985–91). Arch Dis Child 1993; 69:225–228.
*139 Kilpi T, Herva E, Kaijalainen T, et al. Bacteriology of acute otitis media in a cohort of Finnish children followed for the first two years of life. Pediatr Infect Dis J 2001; 20:654–662.
*140 Heath PT, Booy R, Azzopardi HJ, et al. Non-type b *Haemophilus influenzae* disease: clinical and epidemiologic characteristics in the *Haemophilus influenzae* type b vaccine era. Pediatr Infect Dis J 2001; 20:300–305.
*141 Shann F, Gratten M, Germer S, et al. Aetiology of pneumonia in children in Goroka hospital, Papua, New Guinea. Lancet 1984; 2:537–541.
*142 Farley MM, Stephens DS, Harvey RC, et al and the CDC Meningitis Surveillance Group. Incidence and clinical characteristics of invasive *Haemophilus influenzae* disease in adults. J Infect Dis 1992; 165(suppl 1):S42–S43.
143 Moxon ER, Zwahlen A, Rubin LB. Pathogenesis of *Haemophilus influenzae* meningitis: use of a rat model for studying microbial determinants of virulence. In: Sande M, Smith A, Root R, eds. Bacterial meningitis. Edinburgh: Churchill Livingstone; 1985:23–36.
144 Kauppi M, Saarinen L, Kayhty H. Anti-capsular polysaccharide antibodies reduce nasopharyngeal colonization by *Haemophilus influenzae* type b in infant rats. J Infect Dis 1993; 167:365–371.
*145 Fernandez J, Levine OS, Sanchez J, et al. Prevention of *Haemophilus influenzae* type b colonization by vaccination: correlation with serum anti-capsular IgG concentration. J Infect Dis 2000; 182:1553–1556.
*146 Heath PT, Booy R, Griffiths H, et al. Clinical and immunological risk factors associated with *Haemophilus influenzae* type b conjugate vaccine failure in childhood. Clin Infect Dis 2000; 31:973–980.
*147 Schaad U, Lips U, Gnehm H, et al. Dexamethasone therapy for bacterial meningitis. Lancet 1993; 342:457–461.
*148 Peltola H, Kayhty H, Virtanen M, et al. Prevention of *Haemophilus influenzae* type b bacteremic infections with the capsular polysaccharide vaccine. N Engl J Med 1984; 310:1561–1566.
*149 Booy R, Hodgson S, Carpenter L, et al. Efficacy of *Haemophilus-influenzae* type b conjugate vaccine PRP-T. Lancet 1994; 344:362–366.
*150 Heath PT, Booy R, Azzopardi HJ, et al. Antibody concentration and clinical protection after Hib conjugate vaccination in the United Kingdom. JAMA 2000; 284:2334–2340.
*151 Adegbola RA, Usen SO, Weber M, et al. *Haemophilus influenzae* type b meningitis in The Gambia after introduction of a conjugate vaccine [letter]. *Lancet* 1999; 354:1091–1092.

BACTERIAL INFECTIONS: LEPROSY
152 Leprosy – Global Situation. Wkly Epidemiol Rec 2000; 75:226–231.

153 Selvasekar A, Geetha J, Nisha K, et al. Childhood leprosy in an endemic area. Lepr Rev 1999; 70:21–27.
154 Lockwood DNJ, Reid AJC. The diagnosis of leprosy is delayed in the United Kingdom. Q J Med 2001; 94:207–212.
155 Lockwood DNJ. Rifampicin, ofloxacin and minocycline (ROM) for single lesions in leprosy. What is the evidence? Lep Rev 1997; 68:299–300.
156 WHO Technical Report Series. WHO expert committee on Leprosy. Geneva: World Health Organization; 1998.
157 Suman J, Reddy RG, Naser S, et al. Childhood leprosy – clinical presentation and the role of household contacts. Lepr Rev 2002 (in press).
158 Hammond PJ, Rao PS. The tragedy of deformity in childhood leprosy. Lepr Rev 1999; 70:217–220.
159 Department of Health and the Welsh Office. Memorandum on leprosy. London: The Stationery Office; 1997.

BACTERIAL INFECTIONS: LYME DISEASE
160 Schmid GP. The global distribution of Lyme disease. Rev Infect Dis 1985; 7:41–50.
161 Steere AC, Hardin JA, Malawista SE. Erythema chronicum migrans and Lyme arthritis. Cryoimmunoglobulins and clinical activity of skin and joints. Science 1977; 196:1121.
162 Muhlemann MF, Wright DJM. Emerging pattern of Lyme disease in the United Kingdom and Irish Republic. Lancet 1987; 1:260–263.
163 Berglund J, Eitrem R, Orristein K, et al. An epidemiological study of Lyme disease in Southern Sweden. N Engl J Med 1995; 333:1319–1324.
164 Anderson JF. Epizootiology of *Borellia* in *Ixodes* tick vectors and reservoir hosts. Rev Infect Dis 1989; 11(suppl 6):S1451–S1459.
165 Steere AC, Dwyer E, Winchester R. Association of chronic Lyme arthritis with HLA-DR4 and HLA-DR2 alleles. N Engl J Med 1990; 323:219–223.
166 Steere AC, Gibofsky A, Patarroyo M, et al. Chronic Lyme arthritis. Ann Intern Med 1979; 90:896–901.
167 Steere AC, Bartenhagen NH, Craft JE, et al. The early clinical manifestations of Lyme disease. Ann Intern Med 1983; 99:76–82.
168 Shapiro ED, Gerber MA. Lyme disease in children study group: Lyme disease in children. Sixth International Conference of Lyme Borreliosis, Bologna, Italy. 1994
169 O'Neill PM, Wright DJM. Lyme disease. Br J Hosp Med 1988; 40:284–289.
170 Garcia-Monoco JC, Benach JI. Lyme neuroborelliosis. Ann Neurol 1995; 37:691–702.
171 Steere AC, Schoen RT, Taylor E. The clinical evolution of Lyme disease arthritis. Ann Intern Med 1987; 107:725–731.
172 Shapiro ED. Lyme disease in children. Am J Med 1995; 98(suppl 4A):695–735.
173 Feder HM, Hunt MS. Pitfalls in the diagnosis and treatment of Lyme disease in children. JAMA 1995; 274:66–68.
174 Dressler F, Whalen JA, Reinhardt BN, et al. Western blotting in the serodiagnosis of Lyme disease. J Infect Dis 1993; 167:392–400.
175 Steere AC. Lyme disease. N Engl J Med 1989; 321:586–596.
176 Gardner P. Editorial. JAMA 2000; 283:658–659.
177 Lufti BJ, Gardener R, Lightfoot RW JR. Empiric antibiotic treatment of patients who are seropositive for Lyme disease but lack classic features. Clin Infect Dis 1994; 18:112.
178 Steere AC, Hutchinson DJ, Rahn DW, et al. Treatment of the early manifestations of Lyme disease. Ann Intern Med 1983; 99:22.
179 Pal GA, Baker JT, Wright DJM. Penicillin resistant borrelia encephalitis responding to cefotaxime. Lancet 1988; 1:50–51.

BACTERIAL INFECTIONS: MENINGOCOCCEMIA
180 Invasive meningococcal infections, England and Wales: Commun Dis Rep CDR Wkly [serial online] 2001 [cited 22 November 2001]; 11(2).
181 van Deuren M, Brandtzaeg P, van der Meer JW. Update on meningococcal disease with emphasis on pathogenesis and clinical management. Clin Microbiol Rev 2000; 13:144–166.
182 Peters MJ, et al. Early severe neutropenia and thrombocytopenia identifies the highest risk cases of severe meningococcal disease. Paediatr Crit Care Med 2001; 2:225–231.

BACTERIAL INFECTIONS: PERTUSSIS
183 Olin P, Rasmussen F, Gustafsson L, et al. Randomised controlled trial of two-component, three-component and five-component acellular pertussis vaccines compared with whole-cell vaccine. Lancet 1997; 350:1569–1577.

BACTERIAL INFECTIONS: YERSINIOSIS AND PLAGUE
184 Cover TL, Aber RC. *Yersinia enterocolitica*. N Engl J Med 1989; 321:16–24.
185 Naktin J, Beavis KG. *Yersinia enterocolitica* and *Yersinia pseudotuberculosis*. Clin Lab Med 1999; 19:523–536.
186 Larson JH. The spectrum of clinical manifestations of infections with *Yersinia enterocolitica* and their pathogenesis. *Contrib Microbiol Immunol* 1979; 5:257–269.
187 Perry RD, Fetherston JD. *Yersinia pestis* – etiologic agent of plague. Clin Microbiol Rev 1997; 35:66.
188 Smego RA, Frean J, Koornhof HJ. Yersiniosis I: microbiological and clinicoepidemiological aspects of plague and non-plague *Yersinia* infections. Eur J Clin Microbiol Infect Dis 1999; 18:1–15.

BACTERIAL INFECTIONS: *PNEUMOCOCCUS*
189 Gray BM, Dillon HC. Natural history of pneumococcal infections. Pediatr Infect Dis J 1989; 8(1) (suppl):S23–S25.
190 Obaro SK, Monteil MA, Henderson DC. The pneumococcal problem. BMJ 1996; 312:1521–1525.
191 Earley A, Richman S, Ansell BM. Pneumococcal arthritis mimicking juvenile chronic arthritis. Arch Dis Child 1988; 63:1089–1090.
192 Lister PD. Multiply-resistant pneumococcus: therapeutic problems in the management of serious infections. Eur J Clin Microbiol Infect Dis 1995; 14(suppl 1):18–25.
193 American Academy of Pediatrics. Committee on Infectious Disease. Therapy for children with invasive pneumococcal infections. Pediatrics 1997; 99:287–299.
194 Friedland IR. Comparison of the response to antimicrobial therapy of penicillin-resistant and penicillin-susceptible pneumococcal disease. Pediatr Infect Dis J 1995; 14:885–890.
195 Mayon-White RT. Pneumococcal vaccine. J Med Microbiol 1996; 44:397–398.
196 Ada G, Isaacs D. Vaccination: the facts, the fears, the future. Sydney: Allen & Unwin; 2000.
197 Black S, Shinefield H, Fireman B, et al. Efficacy, safety and immunogenicity of heptavalent pneumococcal conjugate vaccine in children. Pediatr Infect Dis J 2000; 19:187–195.
198 Department of Health (DoH). Immunization against infectious disease. London: HMSO; 1996.
199 Gaston MH, Verter JI, Woods G, et al. Prophylaxis with oral penicillin in children with sickle cell anemia: a randomized trial. N Engl J Med 1986; 314:1593–1599.

BACTERIAL INFECTIONS: *PSEUDOMONAS*
*200 Grundmann H, Kropec A, Hartung D, et al. *Pseudomonas aeruginosa* in a neonatal intensive care unit; reservoirs and ecology of the nosocomial pathogen. J Infect Dis 1993; 168:943–947.
*201 Boisseau AM, Sarlangue J, Perel Y, et al. Perineal ecthyma gangrenosum in infancy and early childhood: septicaemic and nonsepticaemic forms. J Am Acad Dermatol 1992; 27:415–418.
*202 Henwood CJ, Livermore DM, James D, et al. Antimicrobial susceptibility of *Pseudomonas aeruginosa*: results of a UK survey and evaluation of the British Society for Antimicrobial Chemotherapy disc susceptibility test. J Antimicrob Chemother 2001; 47:789–799.
*203 Govan JRW, Hughes JE, Vandamme P. *Burkholderia cepacia*: medical, taxonomic and ecological issues. J Med Microbiol 1996; 45:395–407.
*204 Chaowagul W. Recent advances in the treatment of severe melioidosis. Acta Trop 2000; 74:133–137.

BACTERIAL INFECTIONS: RELAPSING FEVER
205 Southern PM, Sanford JP. Relapsing fever: a clinical and microbiological review. Medicine 1969; 48:129–149.
206 Centers for Disease Control and Prevention. Outbreak of relapsing fever – Grand Canyon National Park, Arizona, 1990. Morb Mortal Wkly Rep 1991; 40(18):296–297, 303.
207 Goubau PF. Relapsing fevers. A review. Ann Soc Belge Méd Trop 1984; 64:335–364.
208 Barclay AJG, Coulter JBS. Tick-borne relapsing fever in central Tanzania. Trans R Soc Trop Med Hyg 1990; 84:852–856.
209 Bryceson ADM, Parry EHO, Perine PL, et al. Louse-borne relapsing fever: a clinical and laboratory study of 62 cases in Ethiopia and a reconsideration of the literature. Q J Med 1970; 39:129–170.
210 Salih SY, Mustafa D. Louse-borne relapsing fever: II Combined penicillin and tetracycline therapy in 160 Sudanese patients. Trans R Soc Trop Med Hyg 1977; 71:49–51.
211 Borgnolo G, Denku B, Chiabrera F, et al. Louse-borne relapsing fever in Ethiopian

children: a clinical study. Ann Trop Paediatr 1993; 13:165–171.
212 Jongen WVWM, Van Roosmalen J, Tiems J, et al. Tick-borne relapsing fever and pregnancy outcome in rural Tanzania. Acta Obstet Gynecol Scand 1997; 76:834–838.
213 Melkert PWJ, Stel HV. Neonatal *Borrelia* infections (relapsing fever): report of 5 cases and review of the literature. East Afr Med J 1991; 68:999–1005.
214 Talbert A, Nnange A, Molteni F. Spraying tick-infected houses with lambda-cyhalothrin reduces the incidence of tick-borne relapsing fever in children under five years old. Trans R Soc Trop Med Hyg 1998; 92:251–253.

BACTERIAL INFECTIONS: SALMONELLAE
215 Chao H-C, Chiu C-H, Kong M-S, et al. Factors associated with intestinal perforation in children's non-typhi *Salmonella* toxic megacolon. Pediatr Infect Dis J 2000; 19:1158–1162.
216 Torrey S, Fleisher G, Jaffe D. Incidence of *Salmonella* bacteraemia in infants with *Salmonella* gastroenteritis. J Pediatr 1986; 108:718–721.
217 Green S, Tillotson G. Use of ciprofloxacin in developing countries. Pediatr Infect Dis 1997; 16:150–159.
218 Graham SM, Molyneux EM, Walsh AL, et al. Nontyphoidal Salmonella infections of children in tropical Africa. Pediatr Infect Dis J 2000; 19:1189–1196.
219 Saha SK, Baqui AH, Hanif M, et al. Typhoid fever in Bangladesh: implications for vaccination policy. Pediatr Infect Dis J 2001; 20:521–524.
*220 Sirinavin S, Garner P. Antibiotics for treating salmonella gut infections (Cochrane Review). In: The Cochrane Library, 4. Oxford: Update Software; 2001.
221 St Geme JW, Hodes HL, Marcy SM, et al. Consensus management of *Salmonella* infection in the first year of life. Pediatr Infect Dis J 1988; 7:615–621.
222 Communicable Disease Surveillance Centre (CDSC) CDR Wkly. Available: http://phls.co.uk/publications 21 August 2001.
223 Edelman R, Levine MM. Summary of an international workshop on typhoid fever. Rev Infect Dis 1986; 8:329–349.
224 Mahle WT, Levine MM. *Salmonella typhi* infections in children younger than five years of age. Pediatr Infect Dis J 1993; 12:627–631.
225 Parry CM, Beeching NJ. Epidemiology, diagnosis and treatment of enteric fever. Curr Opin Infect Dis 1998; 11:583–590.
226 White NJ, Parry CM. The treatment of typhoid fever. Curr Opin Infect Dis 1996; 9:298–302.
227 Schaad UB. Pediatric use of quinolones. Pediatr Infect Dis J 1999; 18:469–470.
*228 Punjabi NH, Hoffman SL, Edman DC, et al. Treatment of severe typhoid fever in children with high dose dexamethasone. Pediatr Infect Dis J 1988; 7:598–600.
229 Richens J. Mangement of bowel perforation in typhoid fever. Trop Doct 1991; 21:149–152.
*230 Engels EA, Lau J. Vaccines for preventing typhoid fever (Cochrane Review). In: The Cochrane Library, 4. Oxford: Update Software; 2001.
231 Lin FYC, Ho VA, Khiem HB, et al. The efficacy of a *Salmonella typhi* Vi conjugate vaccine in two-to-five year-old children. N Engl J Med 2001; 344:1263–1269.

BACTERIAL INFECTIONS: SHIGELLA (BACILLARY DYSENTERY)
232 Kotloff KL, Winickoff JP, Ivanoff B, et al. Global burden of *Shigella* infections: implications for vaccine development and implementation of control strategies. Bull World Health Organ 1999; 77:651–666.
233 Keusch FT, Bennish ML. Shigellosis: recent progress, persisting problems and research issues. Pediatr Infect Dis J 1989; 8:713–719.
234 Huskins WC, Griffiths JK, Faruque ASG, et al. Shigellosis in neonates and young infants. J Pediatr 1994; 125:232–236.
235 Miron D, Sochotnick I, Yardeni I, et al. Surgical complications of shigellosis in children. Pediatr Infect Dis J 2000; 19:898–899.
236 Barrett-Connor E, Connor JD. Extraintestinal manifestations of shigellosis. Am J Gastroenterol 1970; 53:234–245.
237 Plötz FB, Arets HGM, Fleer A, et al. Lethal encephalopathy complicating childhood shigellosis. Eur J Pediatr 1999; 158:550–552.
238 Kligler RM, Hoeprich PD. Shigellemia. West J Med 1984; 141:375–379.
239 World Health Organization. Guidelines for the control of epidemics due to *Shigella dysenteriae*. CDR/95.4. Geneva: World Health Organization; 1995.
240 Newman CPS. Surveillance and control of *Shigella sonnei* infection. CDR Rev 1993; 3(5):R63–R70.
241 World Health Organization. New strategies for accelerating *Shigella* vaccine development 1997. Wkly Epidemiol Rec 1997; 72:73–80.

BACTERIAL INFECTIONS: *STREPTOCOCCUS* AND *ENTEROCOCCUS*
242 Krugman S, Ward R. Infectious diseases of children. St Louis: Mosby; 1968.

BACTERIAL INFECTIONS: TETANUS
243 Udwadia FE. Tetanus. New York: Oxford University Press; 1994.
244 Whitman C, Belgharbi L, Gasse F, et al. Progress towards the global elimination of neonatal tetanus. World Health State Q 1992; 45:248–256.
245 Silveira CM, Caceres VM, Dutra MG, et al. Safety of tetanus toxoid in pregnant women: a hospital-based case control study of congenital anomalies. Bull World Health Organ 1995; 73:605–608.
246 Anlar B, Yalaz K, Dizmen R. Long-term prognosis after neonatal tetanus. Dev Med Child Neurol 1989; 31:76–80.

BACTERIAL INFECTIONS: TUBERCULOSIS
247 Wilkins EGL. Antibody detection in tuberculosis. In: Davies PDO, ed. Clinical tuberculosis. London: Chapman & Hall; 1998:367–380.
248 Pfyffer GE. Nucleic acid amplification for mycobacterial diagnosis. J Infect 1999; 39:21–26.
249 Delacourt C, Poueda J-D, Chureau C, et al. Use of polymerase chain reaction for improved diagnosis of tuberculosis in children. J Pediatr 1995; 126:703–709.
250 Gomez-Pastrana D, Torronteras R, Caro P, et al. Diagnosis of tuberculosis in children using a polymerase chain reaction. Pediatr Pulmonol 1999; 28:344–351.
251 Dye C, Scheele S, Dolin PP, et al. Consensus statement: global burden of tuberculosis. JAMA 1999; 282:677–686.
252 Rose AMC, Watson JM, Graham C, et al. Tuberculosis at the end of the 20th century in England and Wales: results of national survey in 1998. Thorax 2001; 56:173–179.
253 Centers for Disease Control and Prevention (CDC). Tuberculosis morbidity – United States 1994. Morbid Mortal Wkly Rep 1995; 44:387–395.
254 O'Reilley LM, Daborn CJ. The epidemiology of *Mycobacterium bovis* infections in animals and man: a review. Tuber Lung Dis 1995; 76(suppl 1):1–46.
255 Miller FJW. Tuberculosis in children. Edinburgh: Churchill Livingstone; 1982.
256 Dannenberg AM. Immune mechanism in the pathogenesis of pulmonary tuberculosis. Rev Infect Dis 1989; II(suppl 2):369–378.
257 Spellberg B, Edwards JE. Type 1/type 2 immunity in infectious diseases. Clin Infect Dis 2001; 32:76–102.
258 Rook GAW, Herandez-Pando R. The pathogenesis of tuberculosis. Ann Rev Microbiol 1996; 50:259–284.
259 Smith DW, Wiegeshaus EH. What animal models can teach us about the pathogenesis of tuberculosis in humans. Rev Infect Dis 1989; II(suppl 2):385–393.
260 Steiner P, Rao M, Victoria MS, et al. Persistently negative tuberculin reactions. Am J Dis Child 1980; 134:747–750.
261 Department of Health (DoH). Immunization against infectious disease. London: HMSO; 1996.
262 Cundall DB, Ashelford DJ, Pearson SB. BCG immunisation by percutaneous multiple puncture. BMJ 1988; 297:1173–1174.
263 Casanova J-L, Jovanguy E, Lamhamedi S, et al. Immunological conditions of children with BCG disseminated infection. Lancet 1995; ii:581.
264 Talbot EA, Perkins MD, Silva SFM, et al. Disseminated Bacille Calmette-Guérin disease after vaccination: case report and review. Clin Infect Dis 1997; 24:1139–1146.
265 World Health Organization. Quality control for BCG vaccines by World Health Organization: a review of factors that may influence vaccine effectiveness and safety. WHO/EPI/GEN/89.3. Geneva: World Health Organization; 1989.
266 Kroger L, Korppi M, Brander E, et al. Osteitis caused by Bacille Calmette-Guérin vaccinations: a retrospective analysis of 222 cases. J Infect Dis 1995; 172:574–576.
267 Fine PEM. Variation in protection by BCG: implications of and for heterologous immunity. Lancet 1995; ii:1339–1345.
268 Sutherland I, Springett VH. Effectiveness of BCG vaccination in England and Wales in 1983. Tubercle 1987; 68:81–92.
269 Rodrigues LC, Diwan VK, Wheeler JG. Protective effect of BCG against tuberculous meningitis and miliary tuberculosis: a meta analysis. Int J Epidemiol 1993; 22:1154–1158.
270 Colditz GA, Berkey CS, Mosteller F, et al. The efficacy of Bacillus Calmette-Guérin

vaccination of newborns and infants in the prevention of tuberculosis: meta-analyses of the published literature. Pediatrics1995; 96:29–35.

271 Romanus V, Svensson A, Hallander HO. The impact of changing BCG coverage on tuberculosis incidence in Swedish born children between 1969 and 1989. Tuber Lung Dis 1992; 73:150–161.

272 Ormerod LP, Garnett JM. Tuberculin skin reactivity four years after neonatal BCG vaccination. Arch Dis Child 1992; 67:530–531.

273 Teale C, Cundall DB, Pearson SB. Heaf status 12 years after BCG vaccination. Tuber Lung Dis 1992; 73:210–212.

274 Menzies D. What does tuberculin reactivity after Bacille Calmette-Guérin vaccination tell us. Clin Infect Dis 2000; 31(suppl 3):S71–74.

***275** Durban Immunotherapy Trial Group. Immunotherapy with *Mycobacterium vaccae* in patients with newly diagnosed pulmonary tuberculosis: a randomised controlled trial. Lancet 1999; 354:116–119.

***276** de Bruyn G, Garner P. Mycobacterium vaccae immunotherapy for treating tuberculosis (Cochrane Review). In: The Cochrane Library, 4. Oxford: Update Software: 2001.

277 British Thoracic Society Joint Tuberculosis Committee. Control and prevention of tuberculosis in the United Kingdom: Code of Practice 2000. Thorax 2000; 55:887–901.

278 Swanson DS, Starke JR. Drug-resistant tuberculosis in pediatrics. Pediatr Clin North Am 1995; 42:553–581.

278a Medical Research Council Cardiothoracic Epidemiology Group. Tuberculosis in children: a national survey of notifications in England and Wales in 1988. Arch Dis Child 1994; 70:497–500.

279 Miller FJW. The natural history of primary tuberculosis. WHO/TB/84.144. Geneva: World Health Organization; 1984.

280 Delacourt C, Mani TM, Bonnerot V, et al. Computed tomography with normal chest radiograph in tuberculous infection. Arch Dis Child 1993; 69:430–432.

281 Khan EA, Starke JR. Diagnosis of tuberculosis in children: increased need for better methods. Emerging Infect Dis 1995; 1:115–122.

282 Starke JR. Diagnosis of tuberculosis in children. Pediatr Infect Dis J 2000; 19:1095–1096.

283 Vallejo JG, Ong LT, Starke JR. Clinical features, diagnosis and treatment of tuberculosis in infants. Pediatrics 1994; 84:1–7.

284 Thakur A, Coulter JBS, Zutshi K, et al. Laryngeal swabs for diagnosing tuberculosis. Ann Trop Paediatr 1999; 19:333–336.

285 Franchi LM, Cama RI, Gilman RH, et al. Detection of *Mycobacterium tuberculosis* in nasopharyngeal aspirate samples in children. Lancet 1998; 352:1681–1682.

286 Shata AMA, Coulter JBS, Parry CM, et al. Sputum induction for the diagnosis of tuberculosis. Arch Dis Child 1996; 74:535–536.

287 Zar HJ, Tannenbaum E, Apolles P, et al. Sputum induction for the diagnosis of pulmonary tuberculosis in infants and young children in an urban setting in South Africa. Arch Dis Child 2000; 82:305–308.

288 Abadco DL, Steiner P. Gastric lavage is better than bronchoalveolar lavage for isolation of *Mycobacterium tuberculosis* in childhood pulmonary tuberculosis. Pediatr Infect Dis J 1992; 11:735–738.

289 Somu N, Swaminathan S, Paramasivan CN, et al. Value of bronchoalveolar lavage and gastric lavage in the diagnosis of pulmonary tuberculosis in children.Tuber Lung Dis 1995; 76:295–299.

290 American Thoracic Society. Treatment of tuberculosis and tuberculosis infection in adults and children. Am J Respir Crit Care Med 1994; 149:1359–1374.

***291** Matchaba PT, Volmink J. Steroids for treating tuberculous pleuracy (Cochrane Review). In: The Cochrane Library, 4. Oxford: Update Software; 2001.

292 Hugo-Hamman CT, Scher H, De Moor MMA. Tuberculous pericarditis in children: a review of 44 cases. Pediatr Infect Dis J 1994; 13:13–18.

293 Strang JIG. Tuberculous pericarditis. J Infect 1997; 35:215–219.

294 Hussey G, Chisholm T, Kibel M. Miliary tuberculosis in children: a review of 94 cases. Pediatr Infect Dis J 1991; 10:832–836.

295 Starke JR. Tuberculosis of the central memory system in children. Semin Pediatr Neurol 1999; 6:318–331.

296 Donald PR, Schoeman JF, Cotton MF, et al. Cerebrospinal fluid investigations in tuberculous meningitis. Ann Trop Paediatr 1991; 11:241–246.

297 Pfyffer GE. Nucleic acid amplification for mycobacterial diagnosis. J Infect 1999; 39:21–26.

298 Hejazi N, Hassler W. Multiple intracranial tuberculomas with atypical response to tuberculostatic chemotherapy: literature review and a case report. Infection 1997; 25:233–230.

299 Ravenscroft A, Schoeman JF, Donald PR. Tuberculous granulomas in childhood tuberculous meningitis: radiological features and course. J Trop Pediatr 2001; 47:5–12.

300 Jacobs RF, Sunakorn P, Chotpitayasunonah T, et al. Intensive short course chemotherapy for tuberculous meningitis. Pediatr Infect Dis J 1992; 11:194–198.

301 Donald PR, Schoeman JF, Van Zyl LE, et al. Intensive short course chemotherapy in the management of tuberculous meningitis. International J Tuber Lung Dis 1998; 2:704–711.

302 Donald PR, Seifart HI. Cerebrospinal fluid concentration of ethionamide in children with tuberculous meningitis. J Pediatr 1989; 115:483–486.

303 Humphries M. The management of tuberculous meningitis. Thorax 1992; 47:577–581.

304 Ellard GA, Humphries MJ, Allen BW. Cerebrospinal drug concentrations and the treatment of tuberculous meningitis. Am Rev Respir Dis 1993; 148:650–655.

***305** Girgis NI, Farid Z, Kilpatrick ME, et al. Dexamethasone adjunctive treatment for tuberculous meningitis. Pediatr Infect Dis J 1991; 10:179–183.

306 Schoeman JF, Van Zyl LE, Laubscher JA, et al. Effect of corticosteroids on intracranial pressure, computed tomographic findings, and clinical outcome in young children with tuberculous meningitis. Pediatrics 1997; 99:226–231.

***307** Prasad K, Volmink J, Menon GR. Steroids for treating tuberculous meningitis (Cochrane Review). In: The Cochrane Library, 3. Oxford: Update Software; 2000.

308 Humphries MJ, Teoh R, Lau J, et al. Factors of prognostic significance in Chinese children with tuberculous meningitis. Tubercle 1990; 71:161–168.

309 Starke J, Correa AG. Management of mycobacterial infection and disease in children. Pediatr Infect Dis J 1995; 14:455–470.

310 Shribman JH, Eastwood JBJ, Uff J. Immune complex nephritis complicating miliary tuberculosis. BMJ 1983; 287:1593–1594.

311 Lancet Editorial. Perinatal prophylaxis of tuberculosis. Lancet 1990; ii:1479–1480.

312 Starke JR. Tuberculosis: an old disease but a new threat to the mother, fetus and neonate. Clin Perinatol 1997; 24:107–127.

313 Adhikari M, Pillay T, Pillay DG. Tuberculosis in the newborn: an emerging disease Pediatr Infect Dis J 1997; 16:1108–1112.

314 Mazade MA, Evans EM, Starke JR, et al. Congenital tuberculosis presenting as sepsis syndrome: case report and review of the literature. Pediatr Infect Dis J 2001; 20:439–442.

315 Thomas P, Bornschlegel K, Singh TP, et al. Tuberculosis in human immunodeficiency virus-infected and human immunodeficiency virus-exposed children in New York City. Pediatr Infect Dis J 2000; 19:700–706.

316 Couvadia HM, Jeena P, Wilkinson D. Childhood human immunodeficiency virus and tuberculosis co-infections: reconciling conflicting data. Int J Tuber Lung Dis 1998; 2:844–851.

317 Graham SM, Coulter JBS, Gilks CF. Pulmonary disease in HIV-infected African children. Int J Tuber Lung Dis 2000; 15:12–23.

318 World Health Organization. Treatment of tuberculosis: guidelines for national programmes. WHO/TB/97.220 Geneva: World Health Organization; 1997.

***319** British Thoracic Society: Joint Tuberculosis Committee. Chemotherapy and management of tuberculosis in the United Kingdom. Thorax 1998; 53:536–548.

***320** Volmink J, Matchaba PT, Garner P. Directly observed therapy and treatment adherence. Lancet 2000; 355:1345–1350.

321 Reed MD, Blumer JL. Clinical pharmacology of antitubercular drugs. Pediatr Clin North Am 1983; 30:177–193.

322 Ormerod LP, Skinner C, Wales J. Hepatotoxicity of antituberculosis drugs. Thorax 1996; 51:111–113.

***323** Dooley DP, Carpenter JL, Rademacher S. Adjunctive corticosteroid therapy for tuberculosis: a critical reappraisal of the literature. Clin Infect Dis 1997; 25:872–887.

324 Mayosi BM, Volmink JA, Commerford PJ. Interventions for treating tuberculous pericarditis (Cochrane Review). In: The Cochrane Library, 4. Oxford: Update Software; 2001.

BACTERIAL INFECTIONS: DISEASES CAUSED BY ENVIRONMENTAL MYCOBACTERIA

325 Grange JM. Mycobacteria and human disease. London: Edward Arnold; 1988.

326 Starke JR. Nontuberculous mycobacterial infections in children. Adv Pediatr Infect Dis 1992; 7:123–159.
327 Wolinsky E. Mycobacterial diseases other than tuberculosis. Clin Infect Dis 1992; 15:1–12.
328 Romanus V, Hallander HO, Wahten P, et al. Atypical mycobacteria in extrapulmonary disease among children. Incidence in Sweden from 1969 to 1990 related to changing BCG vaccination coverage. Tuber Lung Dis 1995; 76:300–310.
329 Nylen O, Berg-Kelly K, Andersson B. Cervical lymph node infections with non-tuberculous mycobacteria in preschool children: interferon gamma deficiency as a possible cause of clinical infection. Acta Paediatr 2000; 89:1322–1325.
330 Wolinsky E. Mycobacterial lymphadenitis in children: a prospective study of 105 non-tuberculous cases with long-term follow-up. Clin Infect Dis 1995; 20:954–963.
331 Powderly WG. Treatment of infection due to *Mycobacterium avium complex*. Pediatr Infect Dis J 1999; 18:468–469.
332 Starke JR, Correa AG. Management of mycobacterial infection and disease in children. Pediatr Infect Dis J 1995; 14:455–470.
333 Van der Werf TS, Van der Graaf WTA, Tappero JW, et al. *Mycobacterium ulcerans* infection. Lancet 1999; 354:1013–1018.
334 Dore ND, Le Souëf PN, Masters B. Atypical mycobacterial pulmonary disease and bronchial obstruction in HIV-negative children. Pediatr Pulmonol 1997; 26:380–388.
335 Oliver KN, Yankaskas JR, Knowles MR. Non-tuberculous mycobacterial pulmonary disease in cystic fibrosis. Semin Respir Infect 1996; 11:272–284.
*336 British Thoracic Society. Management of opportunist mycobacterial infections: Joint Tuberculosis Committee Guidelines 1999. Thorax 2000; 55:210–218.
337 Lammas DA, Casanova JL, Kumararatne DS. Clinical consequences of defects in the IL-12-dependent interferon-gamma (IFN-γ) pathway. Clin Exp Immunol 2000; 121:417–425.
*338 Gordin FM, Sullam PM, Shafran SD, et al. A randomised placebo-controlled study of rifabutin added to a regimen of clarithromycin and ethambutol for treatment of disseminated infection with *Mycobacterium avium* complex. Clin Infect Dis 1999; 28:1080–1085.

BACTERIAL INFECTIONS: TULAREMIA

339 Johansson A, Ibrahim A, Goransson I, et al. Evaluation of PCR-based methods for discrimination of *Francisella* species and subspecies and development of a specific PCR that distinguishes the two major subspecies of *Francisella tularensis*. J Clin Microbiol 2000; 38:4180–4185.
340 Jacobs RF, Condrey YM, Yamauchi T. Tularemia in adults and children: a changing presentation. Pediatrics 1985; 76:818–822.
341 Enderlin G, Morales L, Jacobs RF, et al. Streptomycin and alternative agents for the treatment of tularemia: review of the literature. Clin Infect Dis 1994; 19:42–47.
342 Johansson A, Berglund L, Gothefors L, et al. Ciprofloxacin for treatment of tularemia in children. Pediatr Infect Dis J 2000; 19:449–453.
343 American Academy of Pediatrics. Tularemia. In: Pickering LK, ed. Red book: Report of the Committee on Infectious Diseases. 25th edn. Elk Grove Village: American Academy of Pediatrics; 2000:618–620.

INFECTIONS DUE TO VIRUSES AND ALLIED ORGANISMS

344 Storch GA. Diagnostic virology. Clin Infect Dis J 2000; 31:739–751.
345 Rice AL, Sacco L, Hyder A, et al. Malnutrition as an underlying cause of childhood deaths associated with infectious diseases in developing countries. Bull World Health Organ 2000; 78:1207–1221.
346 Karp CL, Wysocka M, Wahl LM, et al. Mechanism of suppression of cell-mediated immunity by measles virus. Science 1996; 273:228–231.
347 Krugman S, Ward R. Infectious diseases of children. St Louis: Mosby; 1968.
348 Ozanne G, d'Halewyn MA. Performance and reliability of the Enzygnost measles enzyme-linked immuno-sorbent assay for detection of measles virus-specific immunoglobulin M antibody during a large measles epidemic. J Clin Microbiol 1992; 30:564–569.
349 Permar SR, Moss WJ, Ryon JJ, et al. Prolonged measles virus shedding in human immunodeficiency virus-infected children, detected by reverse transcriptase-polymerase chain reaction. J Infect Dis 2001; 183:532–538.
350 Mustafa MM, Weitman SD, Winick NJ, et al. Subacute measles encephalitis in the young immunocompromised host: report of two cases diagnosed by polymerase chain reaction and treated with ribavirin and review of the literature. Clin Infect Dis J 1993; 16:654–660.
*351 Shann F, D'Souza RM, D'Souza R. Antibiotics for preventing pneumonia in children with measles (Cochrane Review). In: The Cochrane Library, 4. Oxford: Update Software; 2001.
352 Noah ND. What can we do about measles? BMJ 1984; 289:1476.
353 Aickin R, Hill D, Kemp A. Measles immunisation in children with allergy to egg. BMJ 1994; 309:223–225.
354 Anand A, Gray ES, Brown T, et al. Human parvovirus infection in pregnancy and hydrops fetalis. N Engl J Med 1987; 316:183–186.
355 Yamanishi K, Okuno T, Shiraki K, et al. Identification of human herpesvirus-6 as a causal agent for exanthem subitum. Lancet 1988; i:1065–1067.
356 Jones CA, Isaacs D. Human herpesvirus-6 infections. Arch Dis Child 1996; 74:98–100.
357 Torigoe S, Kumamoto T, Koide W, et al. Clinical manifestations associated with human herpesvirus 7 infection. Arch Dis Child 1995; 72:518–519.
358 Meyer PA, Seward JF, Jumaan AO, et al. Varicella mortality: trends before vaccine licensure in the United States, 1970–1994. J Infect Dis 2000; 182:383–390.
359 Heuchan AM, Isaacs D. The management of varicella-zoster virus exposure and infection in pregnancy and the newborn period. Australasian Subgroup in Paediatric Infectious Diseases of the Australasian. Med J Aust 2001; 174:288–292.
360 Reynolds L, Struik S, Nadel S. Neonatal varicella: varicella zoster immunoglobulin (VZIG) does not prevent disease. Arch Dis Child Fetal Neonatal Ed 1999; 8:F69–70.
361 Vazquez M, LaRussa PS, Gershon AA, et al. The effectiveness of the varicella vaccine in clinical practice. N Engl J Med 2001; 344:955–960.
362 Asano Y, Yoshikawa T, Suga S, et al. Postexposure prophylaxis of varicella in family contact by oral acyclovir. Pediatrics 1993; 92:219–222.
363 Huang YC, Lin TY, Chiu CH. Acyclovir prophylaxis of varicella after household exposure. Pediatr Infect Dis J 1995; 14:152–154.
364 Goldstein SL, Somers MJ, Lande MB, et al. Acyclovir prophylaxis of varicella in children with renal disease receiving steroids. Pediatr Nephrol 2000; 14:305–308.
365 Ogilvie MM. Antiviral prophylaxis and treatment in chickenpox. A review prepared for the UK Advisory Group on chickenpox on behalf of the British Society for the Study of Infection. J Infect Dis 1998; 36(suppl 1):31–38.
366 Watson B, Seward J, Yang A, et al. Postexposure effectiveness of varicella vaccine. Pediatrics 2000; 105:84–88.
367 Lafferty WE, Coombs RW, Benedetti J, et al. Recurrences after oral and genital herpes simplex virus infection. Influence of site of infection and viral type. N Engl J Med 1987; 316:1444–1449.
368 Thomas J, Rouse BT. Immunopathogenesis of herpetic ocular disease. Immunol Res 1997; 16:375–386.
369 Schwartz GS, Holland EJ. Oral acyclovir for the management of herpes simplex virus keratitis in children. Ophthalmology 2000; 107:278–282.
370 Kovacs A, Schluchter M, Easley K, et al. Cytomegalovirus infection and HIV-1 disease progression in infants born to HIV-1-infected women. Pediatric Pulmonary and Cardiovascular Complications of Vertically Transmitted HIV Infection Study Group. N Engl J Med 1999; 341:77–84.
371 Sia IG, Wilson JA, Groettum CM, et al. Cytomegalovirus (CMV) DNA load predicts relapsing CMV infection after solid organ transplantation. J Infect Dis 2000; 181:717–720.
372 Meyers JD. Management of cytomegalovirus infection. Am J Med 1988; 85(suppl 2A):102–106.
373 Pondarre C, Kebaili K, Dijoud F, et al. Epstein-Barr virus-related lymphoproliferative disease complicating childhood acute lymphoblastic leukemia: no recurrence after unrelated donor bone marrow transplantation. Bone Marrow Transplant 2001; 27:93–95.
374 World Health Organization. Memorandum: a revision of the system of nomenclature for influeza viruses. Bull World Health Organ 1980; 58(4):585–591.
375 Lancet Editorial. Reinfection with influenza. Lancet 1986; i:1017–1018.
*376 Hayden FG, Treanor JJ, Fritz RS, et al. Use of the oral neuraminidase inhibitor oseltamivir in experimental human influenza: randomized controlled trials for prevention and treatment. JAMA 1999; 282:1240–1246.

*377 Lalezari J, Campion K, Keene O, et al. Zanamivir for the treatment of influenza A and B infection in high-risk patients: a pooled analysis of randomized controlled trials. Arch Int Med 2001; 161:212–217.

378 Poehling KA, Edwards KM. Prevention, diagnosis, and treatment of influenza: current and future options. Cur Opin Pediatr 2001; 13(1):60–64.

379 MacDonald NE, Hall CB, Suffin SC, et al. Respiratory syncytial virus infection in infants with congenital heart disease. N Engl J Med 1982; 307:397–400.

380 Hall CB, Powell KR, McDonald NE, et al. Respiratory syncytial virus infection in children with compromised immune function. N Engl J Med 1986; 315:77–80.

381 Isaacs D, Moxon ER, Harvey D, et al. Ribavirin in respiratory syncytial virus infection. Arch Dis Child 1988; 63:986–990.

*382 The PREVENT Study Group. Reduction of respiratory syncytial virus hospitalization among premature infants and infants with bronchopulmonary dysplasia using respiratory syncytial virus immune globulin prophylaxis. Pediatrics 1997; 99:93–99.

383 The IMpact-RSV Study Group. Palivizumab, a humanized respiratory syncytial virus monoclonal antibody, reduces hospitalization from respiratory syncytial virus infection in high-risk infants. Pediatrics 1998; 102:531–537.

*384 Wang EEL, Tang NK. Immunoglobulin for preventing respiratory syncytial virus infection (Cochrane Review). In: The Cochrane Library, 3. Oxford: Update Software; 2001.

385 Thomas M, Bedford-Russell A, Sharland M. Hospitalisation for RSV infection in ex-preterm infants – implications for use of RSV immune globulin. Arch Dis Child 2000; 83:122–127.

386 Brandt CD, Kim HW, Rodriguez WJ, et al. Adenoviruses and pediatric gastroenteritis. J Infect Dis 1985; 151:437–443.

387 Legrand F, Berrebi D, Houhou N, et al. Early diagnosis of adenovirus infection and treatment with cidofovir after bone marrow transplantation in children. Bone Marrow Transplant 2001; 27:621–626.

388 McIntosh K. Coronavirus. In: Mandell GL, Bennett JE, Dolin R, eds. Principles and practice of infectious diseases. New York: John Wiley; 1995.

389 Isaacs D, Flowers D, Clarke JR, et al. Epidemiology of coronavirus respiratory infections. Arch Dis Child 1983; 58:500–503.

390 Bas S, Muzzin P, Ninet B, et al. Chlamydial serology: comparative diagnostic value of immunoblotting, microimmunofluorescence test, and immunoassays using different recombinant proteins as antigens. J Clin Microbiol 2001; 39:1368–1377.

391 Heiskanen-Kosma T, Korppi M, Laurila A, et al. Chlamydia pneumoniae is an important cause of community-acquired pneumonia in school-aged children: serological results of a prospective, population-based study. Scandinavian J Infect Dis 1999; 31:255–259.

392 Grandien M, Olding-Stenkvist E. Rapid diagnosis of viral infections in the central nervous system. Scand J Infect Dis 1984; 16:1–8.

393 McMinn P, Stratov I, Nagarajan L, et al. Neurological manifestations of enterovirus 71 infection in children during an outbreak of hand, foot, and mouth disease in Western Australia. Clin Infect Dis J 2001; 32:236–242.

394 Ho M, Chen ER, Hsu KH, et al. An epidemic of enterovirus 71 infection in Taiwan. Taiwan Enterovirus Epidemic Working Group. N Engl J Med 1999; 341:929–935.

395 Boos J, Esiri ME. Viral encephalitis. Oxford; Blackwell; 1986.

396 Biggar RJ, Woodall JP, Walter PD, et al. Lymphocytic choriomeningitis outbreak associated with pet hamsters. Fifty-seven cases from New York State. JAMA 1975; 232:494–500.

397 Fishbein DB, Robinson LE. Rabies. N Engl J Med 1993; 329:1632–1638.

398 Bahmanyar M, Fayaz A, Nour-Salehi S, et al. Successful protection of humans exposed to rabies infection: postexposure treatment with the new diploid cell rabies vaccine and antirabies serum. JAMA 1976; 236:2751–2754.

399 Pruisner S. Novel proteinaceous infectious particles cause scrapie. Science 1982; 216:134–144.

400 Whitley RJ, MacDonald N, Asher DM. American Academy of Pediatrics. Technical report: transmissible spongiform encephalopathies: a review for pediatricians. Committee on Infectious Disease. Pediatrics 2000; 106:1160–1165.

401 Will RG, Ironside JW, Zeidler M, et al. A new variant of Creutzfeldt–Jakob disease in the UK. Lancet 1996; 347:921–925.

402 Hill AF, Desbruslais M, Joiner S, et al. The same prion strain causes vCJD and BSE. Nature 1997; 389:448–450, 526.

403 Scott MR, Will R, Ironside J, et al. Compelling transgenetic evidence for transmission of bovine spongiform encephalopathy prions to humans. Proc Natl Acad Sci USA 1999; 96:1537–1542.

404 Cousens S, Smith PG, Ward H, et al. Geographical distribution of variant Creutzfeldt–Jakob disease in Great Britain, 1994–2000. Lancet 2001; 357:1002–1007.

405 Hull HF, Aylward RB. Progress towards global polio eradication. Vaccine 2001; 19:4378–4384.

406 Halsey NA, Abramson JS, Chesney PJ, et al. Poliomyelitis prevention: revised recommendations for use of inactivated and live oral poliovirus vaccines. American Academy of Pediatrics Committee on Infectious Diseases. Pediatrics 1999; 103:171–172.

407 Burgess M, McIntyre PB. Vaccine-associated paralytic poliomyelitis. Commun Dis Intel 1999; 23:80–81.

408 Rotbart HA, Webster AD. Treatment of potentially life-threatening enterovirus infections with pleconaril. Clin Infect Dis J 2001; 32:228–235.

409 Isaacs D, Day D, Crook S. Child gastroenteritis: a population study. BMJ 1986; 293:545–546.

410 Morbidity and Mortality Weekly Report. Intussusception among recipients of rotavirus vaccine – United States, 1998–1999. Morbid Mortal Wkly Rep 1999; 48:577–581.

411 Goilav C, Zuckerman J, Lafrenz M, et al. Immunogenicity and safety of a new inactivated hepatitis A vaccine in a comparative study. J Med Virol 1995; 46:287–292.

412 Papatheodoridis GV, Hadziyannis SJ. Diagnosis and management of pre-core mutant chronic hepatitis B. J Viral Hepatol 2001; 8:311–321.

413 Resti M, Azzari C, Mannelli F, et al. Mother to child transmission of hepatitis C virus: prospective study of risk factors and timing of infection in children born to women seronegative for HIV-1. Tuscany Study Group on Hepatitis C Virus Infection. BMJ 1998; 317:437–441.

414 Ogasawara S, Kage M, Kosai K, et al. Hepatitis C virus RNA in saliva and breastmilk of hepatitis C carrier mothers. Lancet 1993; 341:561.

415 Jones CA. Maternal transmission of infectious pathogens in breast milk. J Paediatr Child Health 2001; 37:576–582.

416 Dunn D, Gibb DM, Healy M, et al. Timing and interpretation of tests for diagnosing perinatally acquired hepatits C virus infection. Pediatr Infect Dis J 2001; 20:716–717.

417 Jonas MM. Treatment of chronic hepatitis C in pediatric patients. Clin Liver Dis 1999; 3(4):855–867.

418 Hardikar W, Moaven LD, Bowden DS, et al. Hepatitis G: viroprevalence and seroconversion in a high-risk group of children. Viral Hepat 1999; 6(4):337–341.

419 Nishizawa T, Okamoto H, Konishi K, et al. A novel DNA virus (TTV) associated with elevated transaminase levels in posttransfusion hepatitis of unknown etiology. Biochem Biophys Res Commun 1997; 241:92–97.

420 Gerner P, Oettinger R, Gerner W, et al. Mother-to-infant transmission of TT virus: prevalence, extent and mechanism of vertical transmission. Pediatr Infect Dis J 2000; 19:1074–1077.

421 Mostashari F, Bunning ML, Kitsutani PT, et al. Epidemic West Nile encephalitis, New York, 1999: results of a household-based seroepidemiological survey. Lancet 2001; 358:261–264.

422 Monath TP. Yellow fever. In: Warren KA, Mahmoud AA, eds. Tropical and geographical medicine. New York: McGraw Hill; 1984.

423 World Health Organization. Haemorrhagic fever with renal syndrome. Bull World Health Organ 1983; 61:269–275.

PROTOZOAL INFECTIONS: MALARIA

424 Garnham PCC. Malaria parasites of man: life cycles and morphology (excluding ultrastructure). In: Wernsdorfer WH, McGregor IA, eds. Malaria. The principles and practice of malariology. Vol. 1 Edinburgh: Churchill Livingstone; 1988:61–96.

425 Breman JG. The ears of the hippopotamus: manifestations, determinants and estimates of the malaria burden. Am J Trop Med Hyg 2001; 64:1–11.

426 Snow RW, Craig M, Deichmann U, et al. Estimating mortality, morbidity and disability due to malaria among Africa's non-pregnant population. Bull World Health Organ 1999; 77:624–640.

427 Molineaux L. The epidemiology of human malaria as an explanation of its distribution, including some implications for its control. In: Wernsdorfer WH, McGregor IA, eds.

Malaria. The principles and practice of malariology. Vol. II. Edinburgh: Churchill Livingstone; 1988:913–998.
428 Miller LH. Genetically determined human resistance factors. In: Wernsdorfer WH, McGregor IA, eds. Malaria. The principles and practice of malariology. Vol. I. Edinburgh: Churchill Livingstone; 1988:487–500.
429 McGregor IA, Wilson RJM. Specific immunity acquired in man. In: Wernsdorfer WH, McGregor IA, eds. Malaria. The principles and practice of malariology. Vol. I. Edinburgh: Churchill Livingstone; 1988:559–619.
430 Allison AC. The role of cell-mediated immune responses in protection against plasmodia and in the pathogenesis of malaria. In: Wernsdorfer WH, McGregor IA, eds. Malaria. The principles and practice of malariology. Vol. I. Edinburgh: Churchill Livingstone; 1988: 501–513.
431 Weatherall DJ. The anaemia of malaria. In: Wernsdorfer WH, McGregor IA, eds. Malaria. The principles and practice of malariology. Vol. I. Edinburgh: Churchill Livingstone; 1988:735–751.
432 Boonpucknavig V, Boonpucknavig S. The histopathology of malaria. In: Wernsdorfer WH, McGregor IA, eds. Malaria. The principles and practice of malariology. Vol. I. Edinburgh: Churchill Livingstone; 1988:673–734.
433 Berendt AR, Ferguson DJP, Gardner J, et al. Molecular mechanisms of sequestration in malaria. Parasitology 1994; 108 (suppl): S19–S28.
*434 Baruch DI, Pasloske BL, Singh HB, et al. Cloning the *P. falciparum* gene encoding PfEMP-1, a malarial variant antigen and adherence receptor on the surface of parasitised human erythrocytes. Cell 1995; 82:77–87.
*435 Pain A, Ferguson DJP, Kai O, et al. Platelet-mediated clumping of *P. falciparum*-infected erythrocytes is a common adhesive phenotype and is associated with severe malaria. Proc Natl Acad Sci U S A 2001; 98:1805–1810.
436 Clark IA. Monokines and lymphokines in malarial pathology. Ann Trop Med Parasitol 1987; 81:577–585.
437 Cook GC. Prevention and treatment of malaria. Lancet 1988; 1:32–37.
438 Bradley DJ, Warhurst DC. Malaria prophylaxis: guidelines for travellers from Britain. BMJ 1995; 310:709–714.
*439 Croft A. Malaria: prevention in travellers. Clinical evidence issue 5. BMJ 2001; 505–519.
*440 Schellenberg D, Menendez C, Kahigwa E, et al. Intermittent treatment for malaria and anaemia control at time of routine vaccinations in Tanzanian infants: a randomised, placebo-controlled trial. Lancet 2001; 357:1471–1477.
441 Quinn TC, Jacobs RF, Mertz GJ, et al. Congenital malaria: a report of four cases and a review. J Pediatr 1982; 101:229–232.
*442 Marsh K, Foster D, Waruiru C, et al. Indicators of life-threatening malaria in African children. N Engl J Med 1995; 332:1399–1404.
*443 Taylor TE, Molyneux ME, Wirima JJ, et al. Blood glucose levels in Malawian children before and during the administration of intravenous quinine for severe falciparum malaria. N Engl J Med 1988; 319:1040–1047.
*444 Molyneux ME, Taylor TE, Wirima JJ, et al. Clinical features and prognostic indicators in pediatric cerebral malaria: a study of 131 comatose Malawian children. Q J Med 1989; 71:441–459.
*445 Lewallen S, Bakker H, Taylor TE, et al. Retinal findings predictive of outcome in cerebral malaria. Trans R Soc Trop Med Hyg 1996; 90:144–146.
446 Lewallen S, Harding SP, Ajewole J, et al. A review of the spectrum of clinical ocular fundus findings in *P. falciparum* malaria in African children with a proposed classification and grading system. Trans R Soc Trop Med Hyg 1999; 93:619–622.
*447 Newton CRJC, Crawley J, Sowumni A, et al. Intracranial hypertension in Africans with cerebral malaria. Arch Dis Child 1997; 76:219–226.
*448 Waller D, Krishna S, Crawley J, et al. Clinical features and outcome of severe malaria in Gambian children. Clin Infect Dis 1995; 21:577–587.
449 White NJ, Miller KD, Marsh K, et al. Hypoglycaemia in African children with severe malaria. Lancet 1987; 1:708–711.
*450 Newton CRJC, Peshu N, Kendall B, et al. Brain swelling and ischaemia in Kenyans with cerebral malaria. Arch Dis Child 1994; 70:281–287.
*451 English M, Sauerwein R, Waruiru C, et al. Acidosis in severe childhood malaria. Q J Med 1997; 90:263–270.
*452 Meremikwu M, Logan K, Garner P. Antipyretic measures for treating fever in malaria (Cochrane Review). In: The Cochrane Library, 4. Oxford: Update Software; 2001.
*453 Lackritz EM, Campbell CC, Ruebush TK II, et al. Effect of blood transfusion on survival among children in a Kenya hospital. Lancet 1992; 340:524–528.
*454 Berkley J, Mwarumba S, Bramham K, et al. Bacteraemia complicating severe malaria in children. Trans R Soc Trop Med Hyg 1999; 93:283–286.
455 World Health Organization. Severe and complicated malaria. Report of an informal technical meeting in Geneva, 1985. Trans R Soc Trop Med Hyg 1986; 80(suppl):1–50.
*456 Lengeler C. Insecticide-treated bednets and curtains for preventing malaria (Cochrane Review). In: The Cochrane Library, 1. Oxford: Update Software; 2001.
*457 Armstrong Schellenberg JRM, Abdulla S, Nathan R. Effect of large-scale social marketing of insecticide-treated nets on child survival in rural Tanzania. Lancet 2001; 357:1241–1247.
*458 Garner P, Gulmezoglu AM. Prevention versus treatment for malaria in pregnant women (Cochrane Review). In: The Cochrane Library, 3. Oxford: Update Software; 2000.

PROTOZOAL INFECTIONS: TRYPANOSOMIASIS
459 Triolo N, Trova P, Fusco C, et al. Report on 17 years of studies of human African trypanosomiasis caused by *T. gambiense* in children 0–6 years of age. Med Trop 1985; 45:251–257.
460 Greenwood BM, Whittle HC. The pathogenesis of sleeping sickness. Trans R Soc Trop Med Hyg 1980; 74:716–725.
461 Bailey JW, Smith DH. The use of the acridine orange QBC (R) technique in the diagnosis of African trypanosomiasis. Trans R Soc Trop Med Hyg 1992; 86:630.
462 Lumsden WHR, Kimber CD, Evans DA, et al. *Trypanosoma brucei*: miniature anion-exchange centrifugation technique for detection of low parasitaemias: adaptation for field use. Trans R Soc Trop Med Hyg 1979; 73:312–317.
463 Asonganyi T, Doua F, Kibona SN, et al. A multi-centre evaluation of the card indirect agglutination test for trypanosomiasis (TrypTect CIATT). Ann Trop Med Parasitol 1998; 92:837–844.
464 World Health Organization. Control and surveillance of African trypanosomiasis. Technical Report Series No 881. Geneva: World Health Organization; 1998.
465 Burri C, Nkunku S, Merolle A, et al. Efficacy of new, concise schedule for melarsoprol in treatment of sleeping sickness caused by *Trypanosoma brucei* gambiense: a randomised trial. Lancet 2000; 355:1419–1425.
466 Pepin J, Milord F, Guern C, et al. Trial of prednisolone for prevention of melarsoprol-induced encephalopathy in gambiense sleeping sickness. Lancet 1989; 1:1246–1250.
467 Pepin J, Milord F, Khonde AN, et al. Risk factors for encephalopathy and mortality during melarsoprol treatment of *Trypanosoma brucei* gambiense sleeping sickness. Trans R Soc Trop Med Hyg 1995; 89:92–97.
468 Pepin J, Khonde N, Maiso F, et al. Short-course eflornithine in Gambian trypanosomiasis: a multicentre randomized controlled trial. Bull World Health Organ 2000; 78:1284–1295.
469 Kierszenbaum F. Chagas' disease and the autoimmunity hypothesis. Clin Microbiol Rev 1999; 12:210–223.
470 Riarte A, Luna C, Sabatiello R, et al. Chagas' disease in patients with kidney transplants: 7 years of experience 1989–1996. Clin Infect Dis 1999; 29:561–567.
471 Russomando G, de Tomassone MM, de Guillen I, et al. Treatment of congenital Chagas' disease diagnosed and followed up by the polymerase chain reaction. Am J Trop Med Hyg 1998; 59(3):487–491.
472 Solari A, Ortiz S, Soto A, et al. Treatment of *Trypanosoma cruzi*-infected children with nifurtimox: a 3 year follow-up by PCR. J Antimicrob Chemother 2001; 48:515–519.
473 Sosa Estani S, Segura EL, Ruiz AM, et al. Efficacy of chemotherapy with benznidazole in children in the indeterminate phase of Chagas' disease. Am J Trop Med Hyg 1998; 59:526–529.
474 Viotti R, Vigliano C, Armenti H, et al. Treatment of chronic Chagas' disease with benznidazole: clinical and serologic evolution of patients with long-term follow-up. Am Heart J 1994; 127:151–162.
475 Apt W, Aguilera X, Arribada A, et al. Treatment of chronic Chagas' disease with itraconazole and allopurinol. Am J Trop Med Hyg 1998; 59:133–138.
476 Blanco SB, Segura EL, Cura EN, et al. Congenital transmission of *Trypanosoma cruzi*: an operational outline for detecting and treating infected infants in north-western Argentina. Trop Med Int Health 2000; 5:293–301.

477 Moncayo A. Progress towards interruption of transmission of Chagas' disease. Mem Inst Oswaldo Cruz 1999; 94 (suppl 1) :401–404.

PROTOZOAL INFECTIONS: LEISHMANIASIS

478 Lainson R, Shaw JJ. The role of animals in the epidemiology of South American leishmaniasis. In: Lumsden WHR, Evans DA, eds. The biology of the Kinetoplastida. Vol 2. London: Academic Press; 1979:1–116.

479 Lainson R, Shaw JJ. Evolution classification and geographical distribution. In: Peters W, Killick-Kendrick R, eds. The leishmaniases in biology and medicine, biology and epidemiology. Vol. 1. London: Academic Press; 1987:1–20.

480 Chance ML. The biochemical and immunological taxonomy of leishmania. In: Chang KP, Bray RS, eds. Human parasitic diseases. Vol. 1. Leishmaniasis. Amsterdam: Elsevier; 1985:93–110.

481 Berman JD. Human leishmaniasis: clinical, diagnostic, and chemotherapeutic developments in the last 10 years. Clin Infect Dis 1997; 24:684–703.

482 Herwaldt BL. Leishmaniasis. Lancet. 1999; 354:1191–1199.

483 Aronson NE, Wortmann GW, Johnson SC, et al. Safety and efficacy of intravenous sodium stibogluconate in the treatment of leishmaniasis: recent U.S. military experience. Clin Infect Dis 1998; 27:1457–1464.

484 Maltezou HC, Siafas C, Mavrikou M, et al. Visceral leishmaniasis during childhood in southern Greece. Clin Infect Dis 2000; 31:1139–1143.

485 Jha TK, Sundar S, Thakur CP, et al. Miltefosine, an oral agent, for the treatment of Indian visceral leishmaniasis. N Engl J Med 1999; 341:1795–1800.

486 Sundar S, Makharia A, More DK, et al. Short-course of oral miltefosine for treatment of visceral leishmaniasis. Clin Infect Dis 2000; 31:1110–1113.

487 Uzun S, Uslular C, Yucel A, et al. Cutaneous leishmaniasis: evaluation of 3,074 cases in the Cukurova region of Turkey. Br J Dermatol 1999; 140:347–350.

488 Soto J, Toledo J, Gutierrez P, et al. Treatment of American cutaneous leishmaniasis with miltefosine, an oral agent. Clin Infect Dis 2001; 33:57–61.

489 Palacios R, Osorio LE, Grajalew LF, et al. Treatment failure in children in a randomized clinical trial with 10 and 20 days of meglumine antimonate for cutaneous leishmaniasis due to *Leishmania viannia* species. Am J Trop Med Hyg 2001; 64:187–193.

490 Bern C, Joshi AB, Jha SN, et al. Factors associated with visceral leishmaniasis in Nepal: bed-net use is strongly protective. Am J Trop Med Hyg 2000; 63:184–188.

PROTOZOAL INFECTIONS: TOXOPLASMOSIS

***491** Dunn D, Wallon M, Peyron F, et al. Mother-to-child transmission of toxoplasmosis: risk estimates for clinical counselling. Lancet 1999; 353:1829–1833.

492 Dubey JP. Sources of *Toxoplasma gondii* infection in pregnancy. Until rates of congenital toxoplasmosis fall, control measures are essential. BMJ 2000; 321:127–128.

493 Cook AJ, Gilbert RE, Buffolano W, et al. Sources of toxoplasma infection in pregnant women: European multicentre case-control study. European Research Network on Congenital Toxoplasmosis. BMJ 2000; 321:142–147.

494 Michaels MG, Wald ER, Fricker FJ, et al. Toxoplasmosis in pediatric recipients of heart transplants. Clin Infect Dis 1992; 14:847–851.

495 Derouin F, Devergie A, Auber P, et al. Toxoplasmosis in bone marrow-transplant recipients: report of seven cases and review. Clin Infect Dis 1992; 15:267–270.

496 Bonametti AM, Passos JN, Koga da Silva EM, et al. Probable transmission of acute toxoplasmosis through breast feeding. J Trop Pediatr 1997; 43:116.

497 Montoya JG, Remington JS. Toxoplasmic chorioretinitis in the setting of acute acquired toxoplasmosis. Clin Infect Dis 1996; 23:277–282.

498 Petersen E, Pollak A, Reiter-Owona I. Recent trends in research on congenital toxoplasmosis. Int J Parasitol 2001; 31:115–144.

***499** Peyron F, Wallon M, Liou C, et al. Treatments for toxoplasmosis in pregnancy (Cochrane Review). In: The Cochrane Library, 2. Oxford: Update Software; 2000.

PROTOZOAL INFECTIONS: GIARDIASIS

500 Thompson RCA, Hopkins RM, Homan WL. Nomenclature and genetic groupings of *Giardia* infecting mammals. Parasitol Today 2000; 16:210–213.

501 Adam RD. Biology of *Giardia lamblia*. Clin Microbiol Rev 2001; 14:447–475.

502 World Health Organization (WHO). The World Health Report: Fighting disease, fostering development. Geneva: WHO; 1996.

503 Warburton ARE, Jones PH, Bruce J. Zoonotic transmission of giardiasis: a case control study. Commun Dis Rep 1994; 4:R33–R36.

504 Homan WL, Monk TG. Human giardiasis: genotype linked differences in clinical symptomatology. Int J Parasitol 2001; 31:822–826.

505 Farthing MJG. Giardiasis. In: Gilles HM, ed. Protozoal diseases. London: Arnold; 1999:562–584.

506 Eichinger D. Encystation in parasitic protozoa. Curr Opin Microbiol 2001; 4:421–426.

507 Aziz H, Beck CE, Lux MF, et al. A comparison study of different methods used in the detection of *Giardia lamblia*. Clin Lab Sci 2001; 14:150–154.

508 Sharp SE, Suarez CA, Duncan Y, et al. Evaluation of the Triage Micro Parasite Panel for detection of *Giardia lamblia*, *Entamoeba histolytica/Entamoeba dispar* and *Cryptosporidium parvum* in patient stool samples. J Clin Microbiol 2001; 39:332–334.

***509** Zaat JO, Monk T, Assendelft WJ. Drugs for treating giardiasis (Cochrane Review). In: The Cochrane Library, 2. Oxford: Update Software; 2000.

510 Olson ME, Ceri H, Morck DW. *Giardia* vaccination. Parasitol Today 2000; 16:213–217.

PROTOZOAL INFECTIONS: AMEBIC INFECTIONS

511 Petri WA, Singh U. Diagnosis and management of amebiasis. Clin Infect Dis 1999; 29:1117–1125.

512 Hanna RM, Dahniya MH, Badr SS, et al. Percutaneous catheter drainage in drug-resistant amoebic liver abscess. Trop Med Int Health 2000; 5:578–581.

513 Simon MW, Wilson HD. The amoebic meningoencephalitides. Pediatr Infect Dis J 1986; 5:562–569.

514 Ma P, Visvesvara GS, Martinez AJ, et al. *Naegleria* and *Acanthamoeba* infections: review. Rev Infect Dis 1990; 12:490–513.

515 Lawande RV. The seasonal incidence of primary amoebic meningoencephalitis in northern Nigeria. Trans R Soc Trop Med Hyg 1980; 74:141–142.

516 Singhal T, Bajpai A, Kabra V, et al. Successful treatment of *Acanthamoeba* meningitis with combination oral antimicrobials. Pediatr Infect Dis J 2001; 20:623–627.

FUNGAL INFECTIONS

517 Drake DP, Holt RJ. Childhood actinomycosis. Report of 3 recent cases. Arch Dis Child 1976; 51:979–981.

518 Schmidt P, Koltai JL, Weltzien A. Actinomycosis of the appendix in childhood. Pediatr Surg Int 1999; 15:63–65.

519 Hilfiker ML. Disseminated actinomycosis presenting as a renal tumor with metastases. J Pediatr Surg 2001; 36:1577–1578.

520 Goussard P, Gie R, Kling S, et al. Thoracic actinomycosis mimicking primary tuberculosis. Pediatr Infect Dis J 1999; 18:473–475.

521 Rosenberg M, Patterson R, Mintzer R, et al. Clinical and immunological criteria for the diagnosis of allergic bronchopulmonary aspergillosis. Ann Intern Med 1977; 86:405–414.

522 Cunningham S, Madge SL, Dinwiddie R. Survey of criteria used to diagnose allergic bronchopulmonary aspergillosis in cystic fibrosis. Arch Dis Child 2001; 84:89.

523 Baddley JW, Thomas P, Stroud D, et al. Invasive mold infections in allogeneic bone marrow transplant recipients. Clin Infect Dis 2001; 32:1319–1324.

524 Wong-Beringer A, Jacobs RA, Guglielmo BJ. Lipid formulations of amphotericin B: clinical efficacy and toxicities. Clin Infect Dis 1998; 27:603–618.

525 Smith CE, Beard RR, Whiting EG, et al. Variation of coccidioidal infection in relation to the epidemiology and control of the disease. Am J Public Health 1946; 36:1394–1402.

526 Rollot F, Bossi P, Tubiana R, et al. Discontinuation of secondary prophylaxis against cryptococcosis in patients with AIDS receiving highly active antiretroviral therapy. AIDS 2001; 15:1448–1449.

527 Kasuga T, Taylor JW, White TJ. Phylogenetic relationships of varieties and geographical groups of the human pathogenic fungus *Histoplasma capsulatum* Darling. J Clin Microbiol 1999; 37:653–663.

528 Deepe GS. Immune response to early and late *Histoplasma capsulatum* infections. Curr Opin Microbiol 2000; 3:359–362.

529 Kügler S, Sebghati TS, Eissenberg LG, et al. Phenotypic variation and intracellular parasitism by *Histoplasma capsulatum*. Proc Natl Acad Sci U S A 2000; 97:8794–8798.

530 Odio CM, Navarrete M, Carrillo JM, et al. Disseminated histoplasmosis in infants. Pediatr Infect Dis J 1999; 18:1065–1068.

531 Fahal AH, Hassan MA. Mycetoma. Br J Surg 1992; 79:1138–1141.

532 Hamid ME, Maldonado L, Eldin S, et al. *Nocardia africana* spp. nov., a new pathogen isolated from patients with pulmonary infections. J Clin Microbiol 2001; 39:625–630.

533 Spargo BJ, Crowe LM, Ioneda T, et al. Cord factor (α,α-trehalose 6,6'-dimycolate) inhibits fusion between phospholipid vesicles. Proc Natl Acad Sci U S A 1991; 88:737–740.

534 Black CM, Paliescheskey M, Beaman BL, et al. Acidification of phagosomes in murine macrophages: blockage by *Norcardia asteroides*. J Infect Dis 1986; 54:917–919.

535 Fergie JE, Purcell K. Nocardiosis in South Texas children. Pediatr Infect Dis J 2001; 20:711–714.

536 Duong TA. Infection due to *Penicillium marneffei*, an emerging pathogen: review of 155 reported cases. Clin Infect Dis 1996; 23:125–130.

537 Lopez-Martinez R, Neumann L, Gonzalez-Mendoza A. Case report: cutaneous penicilliosis due to *Penicillium chrysogenum*. Mycoses 1999; 42:347–349.

538 Bustamante B, Campos PE. Endemic sporotrichosis. Curr Opin Infect Dis 2001; 14:145–149.

539 Fleury RN, Taborda PR, Gupta AK, et al. Zoonotic sporotrichosis. Transmission to humans by infected domestic cat scratching: report of four cases in Sao Paulo, Brazil. Int J Dermatol 2001; 40:318–322.

540 de Lima Barros MB, Schubach TMP, Galhardo MCG, et al. Sporotrichosis: an emergent zoonosis in Rio de Janeiro. Mem Inst Oswaldo Cruz, Rio de Janeiro 2001; 96:777–779.

541 Lortholary O, Denning DW, Dupont B. Endemic mycoses: a treatment update. J Antimicrob Chemother 1999; 43:321–331.

542 Lee JW, Siebel NC, Amantea M, et al. Safety and pharmacokinetics of fluconazole in children with neoplastic diseases. J Pediatr 1992; 120:987–993.

HELMINTH INFECTION

543 McCarthy J, Moore TA. Emerging helminth zoonoses. Int J Parasitol 2000; 30:1351–1360.

544 Rim H-J, Forag HF, Sormani S, et al. Food-borne trematodes: ignored or emerging. Parasitol Today 1994; 10:207–209.

545 Goldsmid JM, Speare R. The parasitology of foods. In: Hocking AD, Editor-in-Chief. Foodborne microorganisms of public health significance, 5th edn. Sydney: AIFST; 1997.

546 Goldsmid JM. The deadly legacy. Sydney: University of NSW Press; 1988.

547 Nokes C, Bundy DP. Does helminth infection affect mental processing and educational achievement? Parasitol Today 1994; 10:14–18.

*548 Dickson R, Awasthi S, Demellweek C, et al. Antihelmintic drugs for treating worms in children; effects on growth and cognitive performance (Cochrane Review). In: The Cochrane Library, 4. Oxford: Update Software; 2001.

549 Bettiol S, Goldsmid JM. A case of probable imported *Moniliformis moniliformis* infection in Tasmania. J Travel Med 2000; 7:336–337.

550 Maizels R, Blaxter M, Kennedy M. Parasitic helminths: genomes to vaccines. Parasitol Today 1998; 14:131–132.

551 Flores A, Esteban J-G, Anler R, et al. Soil-transmitted helminth infections at very high altitudes Trans R Soc Trop Med Hyg 2001; 95:272–277.

552 Janssens PG. Chemotherapy of gastrointestinal nematodiasis in man. In: Vanden Bossche H, Thienpont D, Janssens PG, eds. Chemotherapy of gastrointestinal helminths. Berlin: Springer; 1985:183–406.

553 Lancet Editorial. Ascariasis. Lancet 1989; i:997–998.

554 Crompton D. Chronic ascariasis and malnutrition. Parasitol Today 1985; 1:47–52.

555 Pawlowski ZS. Ascariasis. In: Pawlowski ZS, ed. Baillière's clinical tropical medicine and communicable diseases. Vol 2.3. London: Baillière Tindall; 1987:595–615.

556 Crompton D. The prevalence of ascariasis. Parasitol Today 1988; 4:162–165.

557 Santra A, Bhattacharya T, Chowdhury A, et al. Serodiagnosis of ascariasis with a specific IgG 4 antibody and its use in an epidemiological study. Trans R Soc Trop Med Hyg 2001; 95:289–292.

558 Schneider J, Hughes J, Henderson A. Infectious diseases: prophylaxis and chemotherapy. Australia: Appleton & Lange; 1990.

559 Spicer J (Chairman). Therapeutic guidelines (Antibiotics). Version 11. Melbourne: Therapeutic Guidelines Inc; 2000.

560 Gustafsson LL, Beerman B, Abdi YA. Handbook of drugs for tropical parasitic infections. London: Taylor & Francis; 1987.

561 James SL, Gilles HM. Human antiparasitic drugs. Chichester: Wiley; 1985.

562 World Bank. Investing in health, World Development Report. Oxford University Press, Oxford; 1993.

563 Guyatt HL. Mass chemotherapy and school-based anthelmintic delivery. Trans R Soc Trop Med Hyg 1999; 93:12–13.

564 Gillespie SH. The epidemiology of *Toxocara canis*. Parasitol Today 1988; 4:180–182.

565 Shorey M, Walker J, Biggs B-A. Clinical parasitology. Melbourne: Melbourne University Press; 2000.

566 Milstein T, Goldsmid JM. The presence of *Giardia* and other zoonotic parasites of urban dogs in Hobart, Tasmania. Aust Vet J 1995; 72:154–155.

567 Rochette F. Chemotherapy of gastrointestinal nematodiasis in carnivores. In: Vanden Bossche H, Thienpont D, Janssens PG, eds. Chemotherapy of gastrointestinal helminths. Berlin: Springer; 1985:487–504.

568 Hungerford TG. Hazards from domestic pets. Aust Fam Phys 1977; 6:1503–1507.

569 Pawlowski ZS. Enterobiasis. In: Pawlowski ZS, ed. Baillière's clinical tropical medicine and communicable diseases. Vol 2.3. London: Baillière Tindall; 1987:667–676.

570 Mills A, Goldsmid JM. Intestinal protozoa. In: Doerr WS, Siefert G, eds. Tropical pathology. Vol. 8. Berlin: Springer; 1995:477–556.

571 Marty AM, Andersen EM. Helminthology. In: Doerr W S, Siefert G, eds. Tropical pathology. Vol. 8. Berlin: Springer; 1995:801–982.

572 Smyth JD. Rare, new and emerging helminth zoonoses. Adv Parasitol 1995; 36:1–47.

573 Crompton DH. Hookworm disease: current status and new directions. Parasitol Today 1989; 5:1–2.

574 Behnke JM. Do hookworms elicit protective immunity in man? Parasitol Today 1987; 3:200–206.

575 Pritchard DI. The survival strategies of hookworms. Parasitol Today 1995; 11:255–259.

576 Goldsmid JM. The African hookworm problem: an overview. In: Macpherson C, Craig P, eds. Parasitic helminths and zoonoses in Africa. London: Unwin & Hyman; 1991.

577 Reynolds JEF, ed. Martindale, the extra pharmacopoeia. London: The Pharmaceutical Press; 1996.

578 Quinell RJ, Griffin J, Nowell MA, et al. Predisposition to hookworm infection in Papua New Guinea. Trans R Soc Trop Med Hyg 2001; 95:139–142.

579 Hotez PJ, Le Trang N, Cerami A. Hookworm antigens: a potential for vaccination. Parasitol Today 1987; 3:247–249.

580 Cooper ES, Bundy D. Trichuriasis. In: Pawlowski ZS, ed. Baillière's clinical tropical medicine and communicable diseases. Vol 2.3. London: Baillière Tindall; 1987:629–643.

581 Cooper ES, Bundy D. Trichuris is not trivial. Parasitol Today 1988; 4:301–306.

582 Ashford RW, Barnish G. Strongyloidiasis in Papua New Guinea. In: Pawlowski ZS, ed. Baillière's clinical tropical medicine and communicable diseases. Vol 2.3. London: Baillière Tindall; 1987:765–773.

583 Ashford RW, Barnish G, Viney ME. *Strongyloides fuelleborni*: infection and disease in Papua New Guinea. Parasitol Today 1992; 8:314–318.

584 Genta RM. *Strongyloides stercoralis*: immunobiological considerations on an unusual worm. Parasitol Today 1986; 2:241–246.

585 Oliver NW, Rowbottom DJ, Sexton P, et al. Chronic strongyloidiasis in Tasmanian veterans – clinical diagnosis by use of a screening index. Aust N Z J Med 1990; 19:458–462.

586 Smallman LA, Young JA, Shortland-Webb WR, et al. *Strongyloides stercoralis* hyper-infestation syndrome with *Escherichia coli* meningitis: report of two cases. J Clin Pathol 1986; 39:366–370.

587 Pagliuca A, Layton D, Allen S, et al. Hyperinfection with strongyloides after treatment for adult T-cell leukaemia–lymphoma in an African immigrant. BMJ 1988; 297:1456–1457.

588 Grove D. Human strongyloidiasis. Adv Parasitol 1996; 38:252–309.

589 Cross JH. Public health importance of *Angiostrongylus cantonensis* and its relatives. Parasitol Today 1987; 3:367–369.

590 Chin J, ed. Control of communicable diseases manual, 17th edn. Washington: APHA; 2000.

591 Morera P. Abdominal angiostrongyliasis: intestinal helminthic infections. In: Pawlowski

ZS, ed. Baillière's clinical tropical medicine and communicable diseases. Vol 2.3. London: Baillière Tindall; 1987:747–753.

592 Polderman AM, Blotkamp J. *Oesophagostomum* infections in humans. Parasitol Today 1995; 11:451–456.

593 Bier JW, Deardorff TL, Jackson GJ, et al. Human anisakiasis. In: Pawlowski ZS, ed. Baillière's clinical tropical medicine and communicable diseases. Vol 2.3. London: Baillière Tindall; 1987:723–733.

594 Oshima T. Anisakis – is the sushi bar guilty? Parasitol Today 1987; 3:44–48.

595 Flockhart HA. *Trichinella* speciation. Parasitol Today 1986; 2:1–2.

596 Anonymous. Trichinosis outbreak associated with horsemeat. Parasitol Today 1986; 2:295.

597 Campbell WC. Trichinosis revisited – another look at modes of transmission. Parasitol Today 1988; 4:83–86.

598 Kociecka W. Intestinal trichinellosis. In: Pawlowski ZS, ed. Baillière's clinical tropical medicine and communicable diseases. Vol 2.3. London: Baillière Tindall; 1987:755–763.

599 Cross JH, Basaca-Sevilla V. Intestinal capillariasis. In: Pawlowski ZS, ed. Baillière's clinical tropical medicine and communicable diseases. Vol 2.3. London: Baillière Tindall; 1987:735–744.

600 Goldsmid JM. More than meets the eye: artefacts and pseudoparasites in faeces. Aust Microbiol 1995; 16:87–89.

601 Muller R. Guineaworm eradication – the end of another disease? Parasitol Today 1985; 1:39.

602 Nelson GS. Lymphatic filaria. In: Gilles HM, ed. Clinics in tropical medicine and communicable disease. Vol 1, no. 3. London: Saunders; 1986: 671–683.

603 Shelley M, Maia-Herzog M, Calvao-Brito R. The specificity of an ELISA for detection of *Onchocerca volvulus* in Brazil in an area endemic for *Mansonella*. Trans R Soc Trop Med Hyg 2001; 95:171–173.

604 Cupp EW. Treatment of onchocerciasis with ivermectin in Central America. Parasitol Today 1992; 8:212–214.

605 Whitworth J. Treatment of onchocerciasis with ivermectin in Sierra Leone. Parasitol Today 1992; 8:138–140.

606 Chodakewitz J. Ivermectin and lymphatic filariasis: a clinical update. Parasitol Today1995; 11:233–235.

607 Pinder M. *Loa loa* – a neglected filaria. Parasitol Today1988; 4:279–284.

608 Dreyer G, Medeiros Z, Netto M, et al. Acute attacks in the extremeties of persons living in an area endemic to bancroftian filariasis: differentiation of two syndromes Trans R Soc Trop Med Hyg 1999; 93:413–417.

609 Hightower AW, Lamine PJ, Eberhard MC. Maternal filarial infections – a persistent risk factor for microfilaraemia in offspring? Parasitol Today 1993; 9:418–429.

610 Partono F. Diagnosis and treatment of lymphatic filariasis. Parasitol Today 1985; 1:52–57.

611 Ganesh B, Kader A, Agarwal G, et al. A simple and inexpensive dot-blot assay using a 66-kDa *Brugia malayi* microfilarial protein antigen for diagnosis of bancroftian filariasis in an endemic area. Trans R Soc Trop Med Hyg 2001; 95:168–169.

612 Kluber S, Supali T, Williams S, et al. Rapid PCR-based detection of *Brugia malayi* DNA from blood spots by DNA detection test. Trans R Soc Trop Med Hyg 2001; 95:169–170.

613 Rahmah N, Lim B, Anuar AK, et al. A recombinant antigen-based IgG4 ELISA for the specific and sensitive detection of *Brugia malayi* infection. Trans R Soc Trop Med Hyg 2001; 95:280–284.

614 Ottesen EA, Vijayasekaran V, Kumaraswami V, et al. A controlled trial of ivermectin and diethylcarbamazine in lymphatic filariasis. N Engl J Med 1990; 322:1113–1117.

615 Molyneaux D, Neira M, Liese B, et al. Elimination of lymphatic filariasis as a public health problem. Trans R Soc Trop Med Hyg 2000; 94:589–591.

616 Alexander N, Bockarie M, Dimber Z, et al. Migration and dispersal of lymphatic filariasis in Papua New Guinea. Trans R Soc Trop Med Hyg 2001; 5:277–279.

617 Molyneaux D. Vector-borne infections in the tropics and health policy issues in the twenty-first century. Trans R Soc Trop Med Hyg 2001; 95:233–238.

618 Muller R. *Dipetalonema* by any other name. Parasitol Today 1987; 3:358.

619 Ito A. Cysticercosis in the Asian–Pacific regions. Parasitol Today 1992; 8:182–183.

620 McManus DP, Bowles J. Asian (Taiwan) *Taenia*: species or strain? Parasitol Today 1994; 10:273–275.

621 McKelvie P, Goldsmid JM. Childhood central nervous system cysticercosis in Australia. Med J Aust 1988; 149:42–44.

622 Jaroonvesama N. Differential diagnosis of eosinophilic meningitis. Parasitol Today 1988; 4:262–266.

623 Tillez-Giron E, Ramos MC, Dufour I. Detection of *Cysticercus cellulosae* antigens in cerebrospinal fluid by DOT enzyme-linked immunosorbent assay (DOT-ELISA) and standard ELISA. Am J Trop Med Hyg 1987; 37:169–173.

624 Camargo CA, Marshall WH. Radiological diagnosis of cysticercosis. Parasitol Today 1987; 3:30–31.

625 Craig PS, Rogers M, Alfan J. Detection, screening and community epidemiology of taeniid and cestode zoonoses. Adv Parasitol 1996; 38:169–250.

626 Kociecka W. Intestinal cestodiasis. In: Pawlowski ZS, ed. Baillière's clinical tropical medicine and communicable diseases. Vol 2.3. London: Baillière Tindall; 1987:677–694.

627 Kammerer WS. Chemotherapy of tapeworm infections in man. In: Vanden Bossche H, Thienpont D, Janssens PG, eds. Chemotherapy of gastrointestinal helminths. Berlin: Springer; 1985.

628 Moodley M, Moosa A. Treatment of neurocysticercosis: is praziquantel the new hope? Lancet 1989; 1:262.

*629 Salinas R, Prasad K. Drugs for treating neurocysticercosis (tapeworm infection of the brain) (Cochrane Review). In: The Cochrane Library, 4. Oxford: Update Software; 2001.

630 Goldsmid JM, Rogers S, Parsons GS, et al. The intestinal protozoa and helminths infecting Africans in the Gatooma region of Rhodesia. Central African J Med 1976; 22:91–95.

631 Schenone H. Praziquantel in the treatment of *Hymenolepis nana* infections in children. Am J Trop Med Hyg 1980; 19:320–321.

632 McManus DP, Smyth JD. Hydatidosis: changing concepts in epidemiology and speciation. Parasitol Today 1986; 2:163–167.

633 Craig PS, Desham L, Zhaoxun D. Hydatid disease in China. Parasitol Today 1991; 7:46–50.

634 Lucius R, Frosch M, Kern P. Alveolar echinococcosis: immunogenics and epidemiology. Parasitol Today 1995; 11:4–5.

635 Goldsmid JM, Pickmere J. Hydatid eradication in Tasmania – point of no return? Aust Fam Phys 1987; 16:1672–1674.

636 Gemmell MA, Lawson JR, Roberts MG. Towards global control of cystic and alveolar hydatid disease. Parasitol Today 1987; 3:144–151.

637 Warren KS, Mahmoud AAF. Algorithms in the diagnosis and management of exotic diseases. I. Schistosomiasis. J Infect Dis 1975; 131:614–620.

638 Mahmoud AAF, ed. Baillière's clinical tropical medicine and communicable diseases: schistosomiasis. Vol. 2.2. London: Bailliere Tindall; 1987.

639 Woolhouse MEJ. International Conference on Schistosomiasis. Parasitol Today 1993; 9:235–236.

640 Lancet Editorial. Immunity to schistosomiasis. Lancet 1987; i:1015–1016.

641 Hagan P, Williams HA. Concomitant immunity in schistosomiasis. Parasitol Today 1993; 9:1–6.

642 Terry RJ. Concomitant immunity in schistosomiasis. Parasitol Today 1994; 10:377–378.

643 Butterworth AE. Human immunity to schistosomiasis: some questions. Parasitol Today 1994; 10:378–380.

644 Greyseels B. Human resistance to schistosome infections. Parasitol Today 1994; 10:380–384.

645 Anderson RM. Determinants of infection in human schistosomiasis. In: Mahmoud AAF, ed. Baillière's clinical tropical medicine and communicable diseases. Vol 2.2. London: Baillière Tindall; 1987:279–300.

646 Colley DG. Dynamics of the human immune response to schistosomes. In: Mahmoud AAF, ed. Baillière's clinical tropical medicine and communicable diseases. Vol 2.2. London: Baillière Tindall; 1987:315–332.

647 Warren KS. Determinants of disease in human schistosomiasis. In: Mahmoud AAF, ed. Baillière's clinical tropical medicine and communicable diseases. Vol 2.2. London: Baillière Tindall; 1987:301–313.

648 Wyler DJ. Why does liver fibrosis occur in schistosomiasis? Parasitol Today 1992; 8:277–279.

649 Phillips SM, Lammie PJ. Immunopathology of granuloma formation and fibrosis in schistosomiasis. Parasitol Today 1986; 3:296–302.

650 Peters PAS, Kazura JW. Update on diagnostic methods for schistosomiasis. In: Mahmoud AAF, ed. Baillière's clinical tropical medicine and communicable diseases. Vol 2.2. London: Baillière Tindall; 1987:419–433.

651 Webster LT. Update on chemotherapy of schistosomiasis. In: Mahmoud AAF, ed. Baillière's clinical tropical medicine and communicable diseases. Vol 2.2. London: Baillière Tindall; 1987:435–447.
*652 Saconato H, Atalhah A. Interventions for treating *Schistosomiasis mansoni* (Cochrane Review). In: The Cochrane Library, 4. Oxford: Update Software; 2001.
*653 Squares N. Interventions for treating *Schistosomiasis haematobium* (Cochrane Review). In: The Cochrane Library, 2. Oxford: Update Software; 2000.
654 Jong EC, McMullin R. The tropical and travel medicine manual. Philadelphia: Saunders; 1995.
655 Tchuente LAT, Southgate VR, Webster BL, et al. Impact of installation of a water pump on schistosomiasis transmission in a focus in Cameroon. Trans R Soc Trop Med Hyg 2001; 95:255–256.
656 Capron A. Schistosomiasis: Forty years war on the worm. Parasitol Today 1998; 14:379–384.
657 James SL, Sher A. Prospects for a non-living vaccine against schistosomiasis. Parasitol Today 1986; 2:134–137.
658 Butterworth AE. Potential for vaccines against human schistosomes. In: Mahmoud AAF, ed. Baillière's clinical tropical medicine and communicable diseases. Vol 2.2. London: Baillière Tindall; 1987:465–483.
659 Butterworth AE, Wilkins HA, Capron A, et al. The control of schistosomiasis – is a vaccine necessary? Parasitol Today 1987; 3:1–3.
660 Coulson P. The radiation-attenuated vaccine against schistosomiasis in animal models. Adv Parasitol 1997; 39:272–336.
661 Haswell-Elkins MR, Sithithawarn P, Elkins D. *Opisthorchis viverrini* and cholangiocarcinoma in northwest Thailand. Parasitol Today 1992; 8:86–89.
662 Gillett JD. The behaviour of *Homo sapiens*, the forgotten factor in the transmission of tropical disease. Trans R Soc Trop Med Hyg 1985; 79:12–20.
663 Harinasuta T, Bunnag D, Radomyos P. Intestinal flukes. In: Pawlowski ZS, ed. Baillière's clinical tropical medicine and communicable diseases. Vol 2.3. London: Baillière Tindall; 1987:695–721.

FLIES, FLEAS, MITES AND LICE

664 Hall M, Wall R. Myiasis of humans and domestic animals. Adv Parasitol 1995; 35:257–334.
665 Goldsmid JM. The deadly legacy. Sydney: University of NSW Press; 1988.
666 Dominey A, Rosen T, Tschen J. Papulonodular demodicidosis associated with acquired immunodeficiency syndrome. J Am Acad Dermatol 1989; 20:197–201.
667 Christopherson J. Epidemiology of scabies. Parasitol Today 1986; 2:247–248.
668 Alexander JO'D. Arthropods and human skin. Berlin: Springer; 1984.
669 Robinson J. Fight the mite, ditch the itch. Parasitol Today 1985; 1:140–142.
670 Commens CA. The treatment of scabies. Aust Prescriber 2000; 23:33–35.
671 Burgess I. *Sarcoptes scabiei* and scabies. Adv Parasitol 1994; 33:235–292.
672 Commens CA. We can get rid of scabies: new treatment available soon. Med J Aust 1994; 160:317–318.
673 Chin J, ed. Control of communicable diseases manual, 17th edn. Washington: APHA; 2000.
674 Goldsmid JM. Unusual arthropod ectoparasitic infestations of man. Aust Fam Phys 1985; 14:386–388.
*675 Walker GJ, Johnstone PQ. Interventions for treating scabies (Cochrane Review). In: The Cochrane Library, 4. Oxford: Update Software; 2001.
676 Burgess I. Human lice. Adv Parasitol 1995; 36:271–342.
677 Meinking TL, Taplin D. Advances in pediculosis, scabies and other mite infestations. Adv Dermatol 1990; 5:131–152.
*678 Vander Steichele RH, Dezeure EM, Bogaert MG. Systematic review of clinical efficacy of topical treatments for head lice. BMJ 1995; 311:604–608.
679 Burgess I. Malathion lotions for head lice – a less reliable treatment than commonly believed. Pharmaceutical J 1991; (Nov 9) :630–632.
*680 Dodd CS. Interventions for treating headlice. (Cochrane review). In: The Cochrane Library, 2. Oxford: Update Software; 2001.
681 Goldsmid JM. The treatment and control of head lice: a review. Aust J Pharm 1989; 70:1021–1024.
682 Goldsmid JM, Langley J, Naylor P, et al. Further studies on head lice and their control in Tasmania. Austr Fam Phys 1989; 18:253–255.
683 Burgess I, Peock S, Brown CM, et al. Headlice resistant to pyrethroid insecticides in Britain. BMJ 1995; 311:752.
684 Wargon O. Treating head lice. Austr Prescriber 2000; 23:62–63.
685 Namazi MR. Levamisole: a safe and economical weapon against pediculosis. Int J Dermatol 2001; 40:292–294.

DISEASES TRANSMITTED BY ANIMALS

686 Chin J, ed. Control of communicable diseases manual, 17th edn. Washington: APHA; 2000.
687 Margileth AM. Cat scratch disease. Adv Pediatr Infect Dis 1993; 8:1–21.
688 Wilks CR, Humble MW. Zoonoses in New Zealand. Palmeston North: Veterinary Continuing Education; 1997.
689 Murano I, Yoshii H, Kurashige H, et al. Giant hepatic granuloma caused by *Bartonella henselae*. Pediatr Infect Dis J 2001; 20:319–320.
690 Isada CM, Kasten BL, Goldman MP, et al. Infectious diseases handbook, 3rd edn. Hudson: American Pharmaceutical Association, Lexi-Comp; 1999.
691 Brenner DJ, Hollis DG, Moss CW, et al. Proposal of *Afipia* gen. nov., with *Afipia felis* sp. nov. (formerly cat scratch disease bacillus), *Afipia clevelandensis* sp. nov. (formerly the Cleveland Clinic Foundation strain), *Afipia broomeae* sp. nov., and three unnamed genospecies. J Clin Microbiol 1991; 29:2450–2460.
692 Adal KA, Cockerell CJ, Petri WA Jr. Cat scratch disease, bacillary angiomatosis, and other infections due to *Rochalimaea*. N Engl J Med 1994; 330:1509–1515.
693 Kordick DL, Hilyard EJ, Hadfield TL, et al. *Bartonella clarridgeiae*, a newly recognized zoonotic pathogen causing inoculation papules, fever and lymphadenopathy (cat scratch disease). J Clin Microbiol 1997; 35:1813–1818.
694 Margileth AM. Antibiotic therapy for cat-scratch disease: clinical study of therapeutic outcome in 268 patients and a review of the literature. Pediatr Infect Dis J 1992; 11:474–478.
695 Carithers HA, Margileth AM. Cat scratch disease: acute encephalopathy and other neurologic manifestations. Am J Dis Child 1991; 145:98–101.
696 Stevenson WJ, Hughes KL. Synopsis of zoonoses in Australia, 2nd edn. Canberra: Commonwealth Dept of Community Services; 1988.
697 Hockman DE, Pence CD, Whittler RR, et al. Septic arthritis of the hip secondary to rat bite fever: a case report. Clin Orthop 2000; 380:173–176.
698 Rordorf T, Zuger C, Zbinden R, et al. *Streptobacillus moniliformis* endocarditis in an HIV-positive patient. Infection 2000; 28:393–394.

27

Disorders of bones, joints and connective tissues

Joyce Davidson, Andrew Gavin Cleary, Colin Bruce

Musculoskeletal symptoms are among the most common experienced by children and presented to pediatricians. Many pediatricians lack experience in the assessment of bones and joints in children and feel uneasy when presented with such symptoms. A comprehensive review of all conditions affecting the musculoskeletal system in childhood would not be possible within the scope of a single chapter. We have tried to cover in some detail those that are more commonly seen in pediatrics while also giving sufficient information to enable consideration of many of the more unusual conditions that may be encountered. We have also endeavoured to emphasize areas of recent progress.

ASSESSMENT OF THE MUSCULOSKELETAL SYSTEM

Clinical assessment of the musculoskeletal system is part of the routine pediatric examination but is unfamiliar to many pediatricians. A few simple screening questions and assessments can be used to determine whether an abnormality is likely to be present or not. If a child has no pain, swelling or stiffness of the joints, walks with a normal gait, and is able to keep up with his or her peers in normal activities then it is unlikely that a significant musculoskeletal problem is present. If there is any suggestion of a musculoskeletal problem then more detailed assessment is required. It must be remembered that some rheumatic conditions may present with constitutional symptoms such as a rash, fever or fatigue before the development of any musculoskeletal problems. This section describes a general approach to the examination of the musculoskeletal system. The more detailed assessment of individual problems is described in the relevant sections of the chapter.

A meticulous history and clinical examination is critical in the assessment and diagnosis of children with musculoskeletal disorders and will usually lead to the correct diagnosis. There are few tests that are diagnostically helpful: investigations are used to confirm clinically suspected diagnoses.

When assessing the musculoskeletal system in a child, knowledge of normal development is clearly important as normal findings vary considerably at different ages. For example a significant degree of joint laxity is normal in the young child and should not be confused with abnormal hypermobility.

HISTORY

As with many areas of pediatric practice the clinical history is often the most informative part of the assessment of the child. Information must be gleaned from both the parents/carers and the child. Even the very young child can contribute to the history when age-appropriate questions are used. Questions must be asked about musculoskeletal symptoms such as joint pain or swelling, muscle pain or functional difficulties and about relevant non-articular symptoms.

Non-articular symptoms

Children with musculoskeletal or rheumatic conditions frequently have prominent constitutional symptoms. Fever, fatigue, anorexia and weight loss are common to many inflammatory conditions but may also occur in infection and malignancy. Rashes may be characteristic of individual conditions and may be helpful diagnostically.

Pain

Pain is the most frequently reported musculoskeletal symptom, and musculoskeletal disorders are amongst the most common causes of pain seen in pediatric practice.[1] Detailed enquiry should be made into its location and characteristics including severity, precipitating and relieving factors, radiation and diurnal variation. It must be remembered that joint pain (arthralgia) is common in children and that most do not have serious pathology (Table 27.1). It should also be noted that not all children with a significant musculoskeletal problem will complain of pain.

Based on the history of the pain, its characteristics and associated features, musculoskeletal problems can be usefully divided into three broad categories: inflammatory, mechanical and idiopathic.

Inflammatory

Inflammatory symptoms are characteristic of arthritis but also occur in other conditions such as myositis. The hallmark of inflammatory symptoms is a relationship to immobility. The affected child is frequently worst first thing in the morning (morning stiffness) or after periods of inactivity ('gelling'). A young child with arthritis may be unable to walk first thing in the morning but be running around later in the day. Exercise will generally relieve the pain which is usually described as aching or uncomfortable rather than severe. Occasionally children with acute exacerbations of arthritis experience severe pain which may be sufficient to disturb sleep.

Inflammatory pain in arthritis is almost universally accompanied by objective evidence of persistent joint swelling without which the diagnosis of arthritis should not be made.

Mechanical

Symptoms in this category are, in contrast to inflammatory problems, generally exacerbated by exercise and relieved by rest. The characteristics of mechanical pain are variable but it tends to be described as more severe than that associated with arthritis. It is frequently of sudden onset rather than persistent and will resolve following a period of rest. Mechanical problems are more common in older children and adolescents and frequently affect the joints of the lower limb and the back.

Table 27.1 The differential diagnosis of joint pain in children

1. **Arthritis**
   Infective and reactive
   Juvenile idiopathic arthritis
   Other: autoimmune rheumatic disorders (e.g. systemic lupus erythematosus, dermatomyositis); vasculitis; miscellaneous
2. **Mechanical/degenerative**
   Trauma: accidental and non-accidental
   Hypermobility
   Avascular necrosis, osteochondritis and apophysitis, including Perthes, Osgood–Schlatter's and Scheuremann's
   Slipped capital femoral epiphysis
   Anterior knee pain
3. **Non-organic/idiopathic**
   Idiopathic pain syndromes – localized and diffuse
   Benign idiopathic limb pains (growing pains)
   Psychogenic
4. **Other**
   Osteomyelitis
   Tumors: malignant: leukemia, neuroblastoma
   benign: osteoid osteoma, pigmented villonodular synovitis
   Metabolic abnormalities: rickets, diabetes, hypophosphatemic rickets, hypo/hyperthyroidism
   Genetic disorders: skeletal dysplasias, mucopolysaccharidoses, collagen disorders

Associated symptoms are common. Joint 'locking' is frequently described. True joint locking, where there is a block to extension, is uncommon and may indicate a meniscal problem or patellar dislocation. Joint instability may occur with ligamentous laxity and a complaint of the knee 'giving way' is common with anterior knee pain. Joint swelling may occur with mechanical problems but is usually intermittent rather than persistent.

Idiopathic

Children and adolescents with the most severe symptoms frequently fall into this category where there is no identifiable organic pathology. They complain of severe, unremitting pain frequently associated with fatigue, poor sleep and significant functional impairment. Complaints of intermittent joint swelling are common but seldom corroborated on clinical examination, which is usually normal other than the described pain and tenderness.

Functional difficulties

It is important to enquire about the ability of the child to function normally both in activities of day-to-day living such as dressing and toileting and in more physically demanding activities such as sports. Such questions are informative in determining both the type of problem and its severity. It must be remembered that young children are particularly good at compensating for loss of function in one area by using another and absence of functional impairment does not imply absence of pathology. The most functionally disabled children at presentation tend to be those with idiopathic or non-organic problems.

Discriminating questions of function are useful in determining progress of disease and are now recognized as important in assessing response to treatment in conditions such as juvenile idiopathic arthritis. There are a variety of validated quantitative functional assessment tools now available for use in children with rheumatic disorders. These are reviewed in Duffy and Lovell.[2] The Childhood Health Assessment Questionnaire (CHAQ) first published in 1994[3] is perhaps the most widely used and has been validated for use in both arthritis and dermatomyositis[4] in children. It can be applied to all age groups, is simple to use and has been validated in a number of different countries and languages including a recent UK version.[5]

EXAMINATION

As with any system, examination of the musculoskeletal system of a child must be age appropriate and much information can be gained particularly in the younger child by observation of the child at play before attempting any more formal examination. Observing the child's general demeanour, gait and ability to get up and down off the floor is usually very informative. Ideally the musculoskeletal system should be examined in detail, with assessment of all joints and muscle groups. This is frequently impractical in the very young or the child who is in a lot of pain. The examination may need to be opportunistic, focusing initially on problem areas which will have been identified by initial observation of the child.

A screening examination (Table 27.2) may be appropriately used to identify children who merit more detailed assessment and can be easily incorporated into routine physical examination of any child.

General systemic examination

The child should be examined for evidence of any systemic features that may be relevant to musculoskeletal disorders. Rashes may be useful diagnostically and should be sought. Growth impairment is common in many chronic disorders and documentation of height and weight should be undertaken at all visits. Temperature, blood pressure and urinalysis should be measured where systemic involvement may occur.

Table 27.2 The screening musculoskeletal examination in a child

1. Extend the arms straight out in front then make a fist
2. Place palms and fingers together with wrists extended to 90°: 'prayer position'
3. Raise arms straight above the head
4. Turn neck to look over each shoulder
5. Walk normally, on tip-toe and on the heels
6. Sit cross-legged on the floor then jump up

A child who can perform all these actions without difficulty is unlikely to have a significant musculoskeletal problem

Gait

The gait should be carefully observed. This may help identify the nature and also site of the problem, particularly in the younger child who may find it difficult to localize pain.

A child who is unable to weight bear may have a serious disorder such as septic arthritis or a malignancy. A child with fixed flexion deformities at the hips will adopt an exaggerated lordosis to compensate. Weak hip and pelvic muscles will result in a waddling gait, while a painful hip or knee will result in an antalgic gait, where the child walks in such a way as to spend as little time as possible on the affected leg.

Examination of joints

Joints should be inspected, palpated and their range of movement determined. The results should be systematically documented. Preprinted tables or cartoon figures are frequently used for the documentation of joint abnormalities.

Inspection of joints yields useful information. The position of the joint and any limb deformity should be documented. The limb should be inspected for evidence of wasting of surrounding muscles or limb length discrepancy, resulting from overgrowth at an inflamed joint. Erythema or unusual laxity of the skin overlying the joint should be noted. Joint swelling is frequently obvious on inspection.

Following inspection the joint should be palpated looking for warmth, swelling or tenderness. Documenting the presence of joint effusions is important in assessing and diagnosing arthritis. It must be remembered that in some joints, e.g. the hips, effusions can not be detected clinically and must be searched for in other ways, e.g. using ultrasound (Fig. 27.1).

In many musculoskeletal conditions loss of joint range is one of the earliest objective signs of a problem. Examining for this requires experience, patience and a knowledge of the normal range of movement of the joints. Where the problem is clearly localized to a particular joint, the examination may focus on this area. If the child has evidence of a condition that may affect more than one area, e.g. a polyarthritis, a meticulous assessment of all joints should be made if possible. Arthritis in children is usually asymmetric enabling the contralateral joint to be used for comparison. Useful information can be obtained in many cases by simply comparing the two sides and documenting the loss of movement in the affected side.

Range of movement should be assessed both actively and passively. Assessment of active joint range involves observing the child moving the joints. Passive range is assessed by the examiner moving the joints through their full range. A useful sign of early arthritis in a joint is pain at the end of the range of passive movement. The child may deny pain but withdraw the limb consistently when pushed to the end of its range.

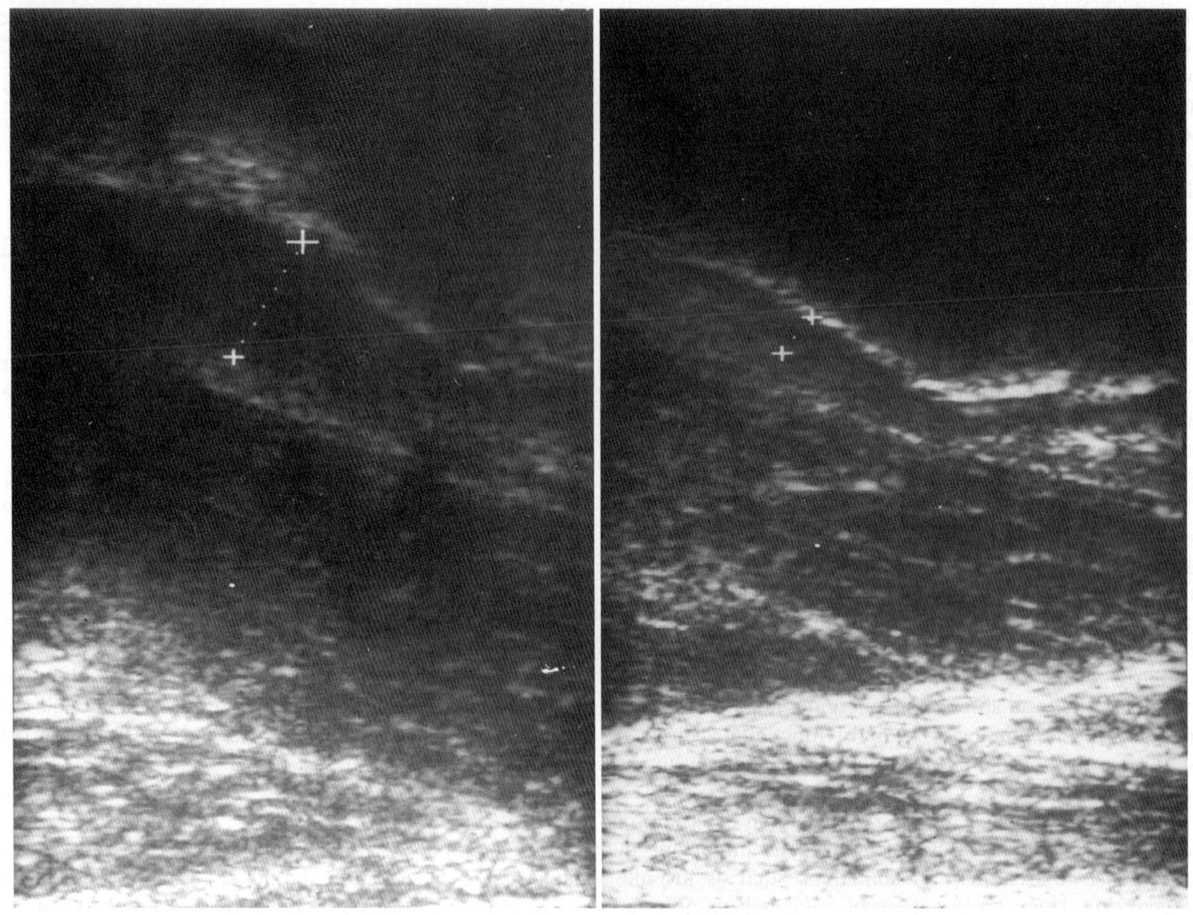

Fig. 27.1 (a) Hip ultrasound showing effusion; (b) normal hip for comparison.

Joints frequently forgotten, but important in the overall assessment of the child, are the sacroiliac joints, the temporomandibular joint and the cervical spine.

Examination of muscles

Assessment of muscles is also an essential part of the musculoskeletal examination. Muscle tenderness may indicate an underlying inflammatory process, while wasting and weakness may indicate a disorder of the muscle itself, of the surrounding joints or of the nervous system. Gait abnormalities or an inability to get up off the floor easily may be indicative of muscle weakness. The well-known Gowers sign where the child uses their hands to push off the body when attempting to stand is an indicator of proximal muscle weakness and not specific to any one group of disorders.

Muscle strength should be formally assessed using a standard scale for grading muscle strength. This requires experience in young children ensuring that clear, understandable instructions are given and taking care not to underestimate the strength of the younger child. A five point scale for grading muscle strength is familiar to most clinicians. In order to improve its sensitivity to change, + or – is frequently added in to the scale but this contributes to inaccuracies. A ten point scale may be more precise and is equally simple to use (see Table 27.3). Both have been shown to give valid results.[6]

In children with inflammatory myositis the childhood myositis assessment scale (CMAS)[7] is a validated method of quantitating muscle strength by scoring the child's ability to perform a variety of maneuvers. Its use in conjunction with manual testing of muscle strength gives reproducible scores which can be used to assess a child's progress and response to treatment.

CONGENITAL AND DEVELOPMENTAL PROBLEMS

In broad terms congenital abnormalities can be classified into:

1. failure of formation (transverse or longitudinal);
2. failure of differentiation;
3. duplication;

Table 27.3 Manual muscle testing: 5 and 10 point scales for grading of muscle strength

5 point scale	10 point scale	
0	0	No evidence muscle function
1	1	Slight flicker of contractility; no effective function
2	2	Movement with gravity eliminated
3	3	Movement against gravity
	4	Movement against gravity: unable to hold position
	5	Movement against gravity: able to hold position
4	6	Resists slight pressure
	7	Resists slight/moderate pressure
	8	Resists moderate pressure
	9	Resists moderate/strong pressure
5	10	Full power

4. overgrowth (or gigantism);
5. undergrowth (or hypoplasia);
6. congenital constriction band syndrome;
7. generalized skeletal abnormalities.

It is important to bear in mind that although congenital abnormalities may present as isolated deformities they may also occur in association with other abnormalities, sometimes as part of a recognized syndrome or generalized skeletal dysplasia.

SPINAL PROBLEMS

Congenital spinal problems

The child with a recognized vertebral anomaly must be fully assessed because associated abnormalities in other systems may be present as in the VATER (Vertebral, Anorectal, Tracheo-Esophageal, Renal, Radial) and VACTERL (Vertebral, Anorectal, Cardiac, Tracheo-Esophageal, Renal, Limb) syndromes. Deformities occurring as result of vertebral anomalies include scoliosis, kyphosis and lordosis.

Congenital spinal anomalies are classified into failure of formation or failure of separation of individual vertebrae or parts of vertebrae. Failure of separation is termed an unsegmented bar, the position of such a bar determining the deformity. With a lateral unsegmented bar the growth of the spinal column is tethered on that side, while continued growth on the opposite side leads to a progressive scoliosis. Failure of formation may involve the anterior, posterior or lateral side of a vertebra and once again the site will dictate the deformity. A hemivertebra on one side of the spinal column leads to extra growth on that side versus the side with the absent segment and a scoliosis may result (Fig. 27.2).

The treatment of the vertebral anomaly depends on its potential to lead to progressive deformity. Some abnormalities have only modest potential and two separate abnormalities may cancel each other out. Other anomalies or combinations have significant potential to progress and will need to be followed carefully and treated early if progressive deformity is to be prevented.

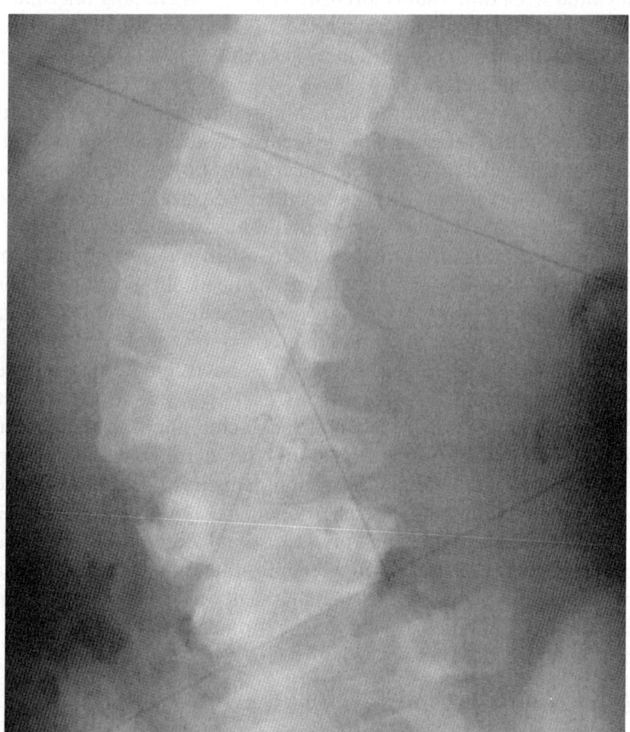

Fig. 27.2 Congenital hemivertebra resulting in scoliosis.

Idiopathic infantile scoliosis

This usually presents during the first 3 years of life and is distinguished from congenital scoliosis by the absence of a spinal malformation. In contradistinction to adolescent idiopathic scoliosis the condition is more common in boys and the convexity of the thoracic scoliosis is to the left in 90% of cases. The condition is often self-limiting but some cases do progress leading to poor cardiopulmonary development. These require prompt management. Prolonged molded plaster jacket treatment is often successful although some may require surgical treatment.

Congenital muscular torticollis

Congenital muscular torticollis is the most common cause of torticollis in the infant, resulting from a contracture of the sternocleidomastoid muscle. The etiology is unknown. Theories include in-utero crowding and muscle fibrosis following a compartment syndrome within the muscle as a result of compression of the neck during a difficult delivery. Clinically a non-tender 'tumor' or swelling can be palpated in the sternocleidomastoid muscle in the first 4–6 weeks, but subsequently regresses. Radiographs of the cervical region should be obtained if there is any suspicion of an underlying cervical abnormality.

Left untreated, plagiocephaly and facial asymmetry may develop. Treatment initially consists of passive stretching exercises together with encouragement of head rotation in the restricted direction by placing objects of interest towards that side. Passive stretching begun early can be expected to be successful in 90% of cases.[8] After the age of 1 year surgical treatment may be necessary. This involves division of the tight tendon and is best done before 4 years of age. Established facial deformity or a limitation of more than 30° of rotation usually precludes good results.

Klippel–Feil syndrome

Klippel–Feil syndrome is the result of failure of the normal segmentation of the cervical vertebrae so that two or more are joined forming block vertebrae. The etiology is unknown. The most consistent clinical finding is limitation of neck motion. Shortening of the neck is subtle.

Associated anomalies include facial asymmetry, torticollis or webbing of the neck in 20%. Sprengel's shoulder (a high riding scapula) occurs in up to one-third of patients and other associated abnormalities occasionally include ptosis of the eyelid, lateral rectus muscle palsy of the eye, facial nerve palsy, a cleft or high arched palate and abnormalities of the upper limbs including supernumery digits, hypoplasia of the thumb or even the entire upper limb. Abnormalities of the lower limbs are infrequent.[9] Affected patients should be screened for other abnormalities which include scoliosis or kyphosis in up to 60%, renal abnormalities in 30%, cardiovascular abnormalities in 14%, deafness or hearing impairment in 30%. Twenty per cent of patients demonstrate mirror motions (synkinesia) or involuntary paired movement of the hands.

UPPER LIMB PROBLEMS

Sprengel's shoulder

The scapula develops within the upper limb bud and descends to overlie the second to seventh thoracic vertebrae and ribs. Failure to descend fully gives rise to congenital elevation of the scapula; Sprengel's deformity. The condition is usually sporadic but is occasionally inherited in an autosomal dominant fashion. It is commoner on the left but can be bilateral. Radiographs of the chest and the cervical spine should be taken to rule out associated rib abnormalities and anomalies of the cervical vertebrae such as Klippel–Feil syndrome.

Shoulder elevation is usually only modestly limited and significant functional problems are rare. Treatment is directed towards maintaining the existing range of movement. Surgical procedures to remove the prominent superomedial tip of the scapula are purely cosmetic and do not improve shoulder function. Whilst procedures are described to bring about descent of the whole scapula they are associated with significant potential complications and long, sometimes ugly scarring.

Pseudarthrosis of the clavicle

This rare condition presents as a non-tender lump at about the midpoint of clavicle. When identified soon after birth it may be mistaken for a fracture, but should be distinguished by the absence of rapid callus formation and persistence of the pseudoarthrosis (Fig. 27.3). It should also be differentiated from cleidocranio-dysostosis where parts of both clavicles are deficient and associated anomalies are found in the skull, facial bones and pelvis. The clavicle develops from medial and lateral ossification centers and the condition may represent a failure of these centers to fuse.[10] Pseudoarthrosis of the clavicle is almost always seen on the right, thought to be a consequence of pressure attrition from the somewhat higher right-sided subclavian vessels.[11]

Shoulder and upper limb function is normally good on the affected side but the prominent lump is unsightly, and overhead activity may become uncomfortable in maturity. Unlike congenital pseudoarthrosis of the tibia and radius, the condition is not associated with neurofibromatosis and readily unites after excision and bone grafting. Surgery is best performed around the age of 4 years.

Radial club hand (preaxial absence)

Radial dysplasia is the commonest of the major longitudinal failures of formation (Fig. 27.4). It may present as partial or complete absence, bilateral or unilateral. When sporadic the etiology is unknown. The abnormality was seen previously in association with thalidomide when two-thirds of cases were bilateral.

Radial dysplasia is always associated with thumb hypoplasia, the thumb being small or completely absent. The spectrum of clinical abnormality can range from mild radial deviation of the wrist and minimal thumb hypoplasia, to complete absence of the preaxial structures including the thumb, the carpal and metacarpal bones and the radius with associated shortening of the ulna and a stiff elbow joint. The deformity is characterized by a weak, radially deviated wrist and a short forearm which grows to only one-half to two-thirds of normal length. The hand is usually correctable upon the wrist after birth and the elbow lies extended with reduced active and passive flexion.

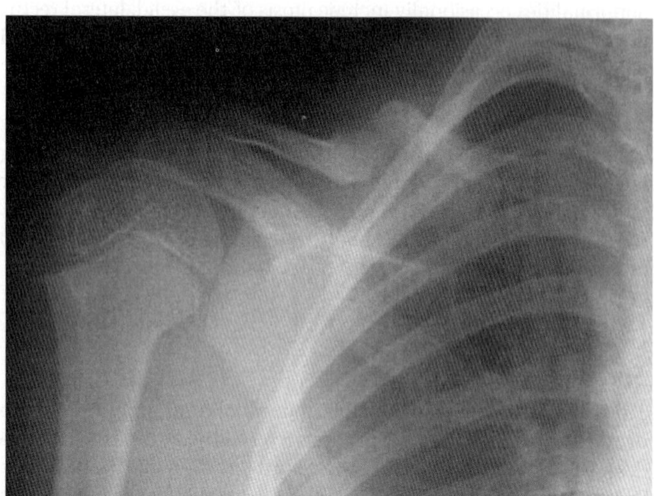

Fig. 27.3 Pseudoarthrosis of the clavicle.

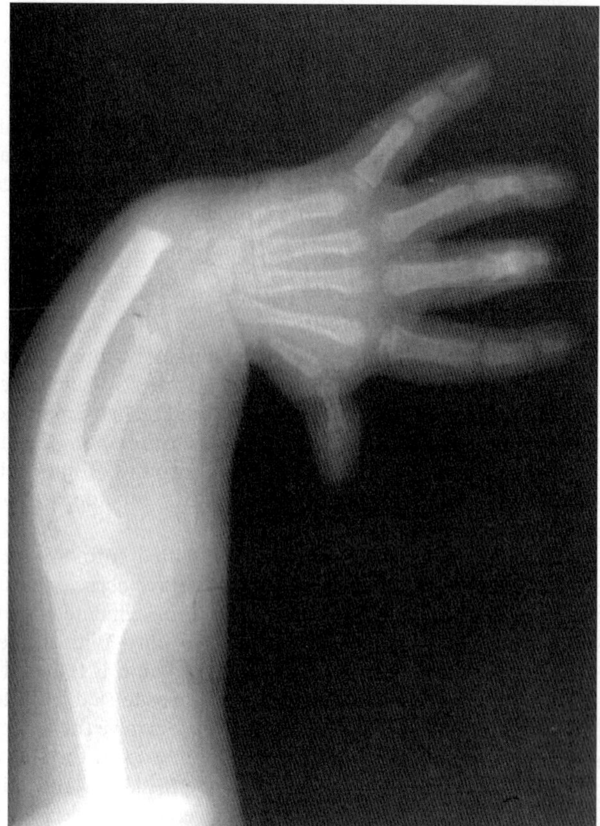

Fig. 27.4 Radial club hand.

Early passive stretching and splinting is indicated and should continue until a decision is made regarding surgical treatment. The standard surgical management is centralization of the carpus over the third metacarpal with subsequent pollicization of the index finger to replace the function of the absent thumb. Pollicization is the surgical shortening and rotation of an index finger to allow opposition with the other digits, so compensating for the absent thumb. Elbow mobility is a prerequisite for centralization procedures to ensure that hand to mouth movement is possible.

Radial deficiency can occur in isolation but is commonly associated with other congenital malformations. Forty per cent of patients with unilateral and 27% with bilateral radial club hand have associated malformations including those of the cardiac, genitourinary, respiratory, skeletal and neurological systems.[12] Syndromes associated with longitudinal radial deficiency include the VATER syndrome; the Holt–Oram syndrome (an autosomal dominantly inherited condition characterized by upper limb malformations and cardiac malformations); thrombocytopenia absent radius (TAR) syndrome (a recessively inherited disorder where thrombocytopenia is present at birth and usually improves with growth); and Fanconi's anemia.

Ulna club hand (postaxial absence)

This condition is rare, about ten times less common than absence of the radius. It is usually a partial absence of the lower two-thirds of the ulna and sometimes the postaxial rays. The absent bone may be represented by a fibrous remnant which becomes a deforming force during growth, leading to progressive ulnar deviation of the wrist and secondary curvature of the radius. As the forearm grows the radial bowing increases and the radial head may subluxate or dislocate proximally at the elbow joint.

Complete absence of the ulna is usually associated with a severe flexion contraction of the elbow and surgery has little to offer. In partial absence the deforming fibrous band can be excised to prevent progressive deformity. Other treatment strategies include ulna lengthening procedures as well as procedures to construct a so-called 'one bone forearm' where the proximal ulna is fused to the distal radius.

Congenital dislocation of the radial head

Congenital dislocation of the radial head is rare and usually occurs in isolation (Fig. 27.5). The condition frequency presents late, often not until school age, and may be difficult to distinguish from an overlooked post-traumatic dislocation. Radial head dislocation may also be acquired as a result of differential growth disturbance between the radius and ulna or secondary to conditions such as Madelung's deformity or familial osteochondromatosis. Features that suggest congenital rather than post-traumatic dislocation include a positive family history, bilateral involvement and the absence of a history of trauma. Radiographic features more typical of congenital dislocation include a small dome shaped radial head, a hypoplastic capitellum and ulnar bowing.

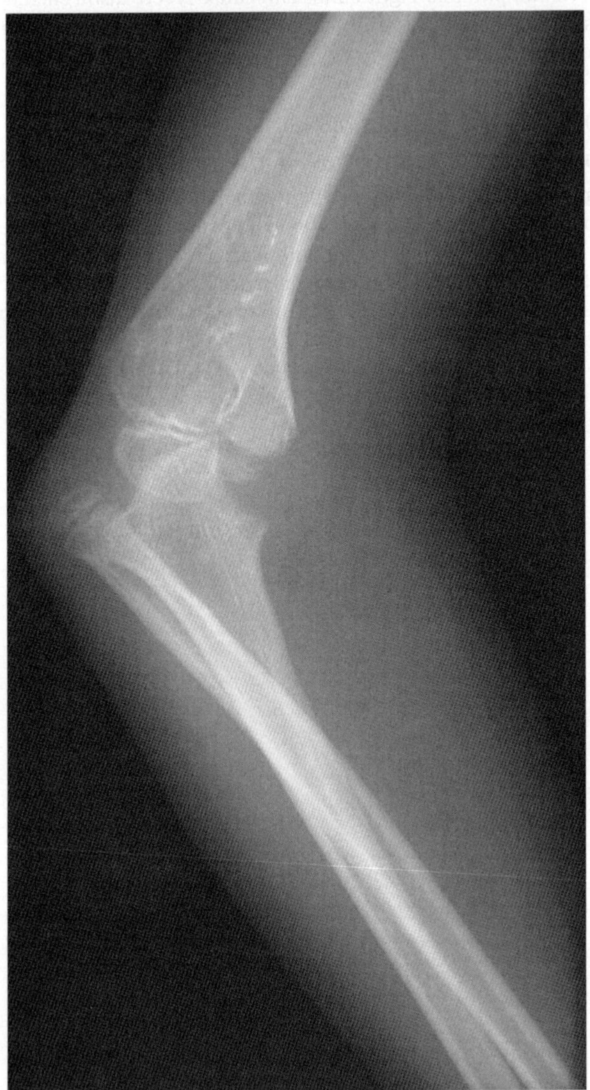

Fig. 27.5 Congenital dislocation of the radial head.

Children present during school years with limited elbow extension, a palpable mass (the radial head) or pain with athletic activities. The radial head is most commonly dislocated posterolaterally and can be palpated at the lateral side of the elbow joint.

If identified in children less than 2 years of age, consideration may be given to open surgical reduction of the radial head and annular ligament reconstruction. Though some promise is reported following this procedure the indications are yet to be properly defined, particularly the upper age limit at which surgery might be helpful.[13] Most children present beyond infancy and are best managed conservatively. If troubled by significant discomfort, management may include the removal of degenerate fragments of bone or excision of the entire radial head, a procedure to be approached with caution in the immature skeleton because of its association with progressive valgus deformity at the elbow and subsequent elbow, wrist and ulnar nerve problems.

Congenital radioulnar synostosis

Congenital synostosis of the proximal radius and ulna is a rare congenital abnormality caused by a failure of separation between the proximal radius and ulna (Fig. 27.6). Forearm rotation is therefore prevented and the hand fixed in a degree of pronation. Many children present late because of their ability to compensate for the absent rotation of the affected forearm with rotational hypermobility of the wrist and compensating shoulder movement. If the fixed pronation is more than 60° or if the condition is bilateral, children may present earlier with functional problems related to manual dexterity.

In the absence of functional limitation no treatment is required. Functional difficulties may lead to consideration of surgery to remove the abnormal fusion between radius and ulna but this has generally proved disappointing.

Congenital pseudarthrosis of the forearm

Congenital pseudoarthrosis of the forearm is very rare but affects the ulna more commonly than the radius. Like its more common counterpart in the tibia it is associated with neurofibromatosis and non-union after attempted reconstruction precludes successful treatment.

Madelung deformity

This wrist deformity results from an unexplained premature growth arrest of the ulnar aspect of the distal radial physis (or growth plate). Continued normal growth of the ulnar physis and the radial and dorsal aspects of the distal radial physis leads to progressive deformity. The distal ulna becomes more prominent and the distal radial articular surface becomes angulated towards the ulna. The carpus sinks into the developing gap between the radial and ulnar styloids.

Madelung's deformity usually occurs in girls and is most often bilateral. The condition is usually sporadic but may be inherited as part of dyschondrosteosis (Leri–Weill disease), and has been associated with a variety of conditions including Hurler's syndrome, Turner's syndrome, multiple hereditary exostoses and Ollier's disease. Damage to the growth plate from trauma or infection can also give rise to Madelung-like deformities.

Most patients do not present until adolescence when deformity and discomfort with activity are often marked. Treatment strategies

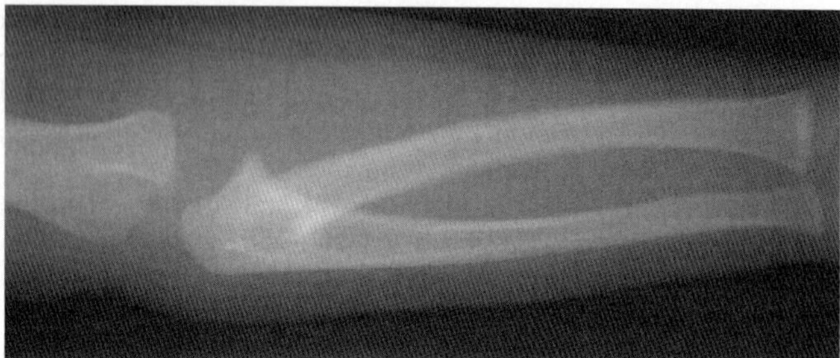

Fig. 27.6 Congenital radio-ulnar synostosis.

for these patients include corrective radial osteotomy and ulnar shortening or other procedures to remove or stabilize the distal ulna, which is frequently the site of pain and wrist degeneration.

Syndactyly

Syndactyly is classified as simple, if the failure of separation involves only skin, and complex, if other structures such as nail, bone, tendon, nerve or blood vessels have failed to separate. It is complete if the skin bridge is present to the distal tip of the finger. The interspace between the third and fourth fingers is most commonly affected with that between the first and second less frequently involved. Treatment depends upon the site and complexity, border digits being separated early to prevent progressive angulation. The separation of simple syndactyly can be expected to give excellent results.

Polydactyly

Polydactyly is classified as preaxial (thumb), central (index, middle) or postaxial (ring, little). Genetic transmission of polydactyly is common especially in native Africans, where postaxial duplication is predominant. The extra digit may be fully formed or vestigial. Before embarking on surgical correction it is important to determine which digit has the majority of intact parts and is therefore most suitable for reconstruction.

Camptodactyly

This is a flexion deformity affecting the proximal interphalangeal joint of the fingers and often inherited as an autosomal dominant trait. The precise etiology is unknown but it usually presents during periods of rapid growth, i.e. infancy and adolescence. In infants there is an equal sex distribution and any finger can be affected. Adolescent cases are more common and invariably affect the little finger, usually in girls. Treatment in infancy involves passive stretching and splintage and occasionally surgical release of soft tissues. In adolescence dynamic splintage may lead to modest improvement.

Clinodactyly

This is angulation of a digit in the radial or ulnar direction. Radial angulation of the tip of the little finger is the most common and often inherited as an autosomal dominant trait. Treatment is seldom necessary.

Trigger thumb

This is the commonest hand anomaly in infants and small children. It is something of a misnomer because the thumb does not really 'trigger' with sudden extension, as does the adult trigger finger, but is usually stuck in a flexed position. Clinically there is a palpable swelling in the thumb flexor tendon and flexor sheath on the volar aspect of the base of the thumb. About one-third of cases resolve spontaneously in the first year but later persistence makes spontaneous resolution unlikely. Surgical treatment to divide the entrance to the flexor sheath is simple and gives excellent results. It should be done before 4 years of age to avoid an increasing risk of a persistent flexion contracture.

Hypoplastic thumb

Thumb hypoplasia is a form of preaxial longitudinal failure of formation and like radial club hand is associated with congenital anomalies in other systems (e.g. VATER, VACTERL syndromes). It ranges from a mild anomaly where the thumb is fully formed but simply small, to complete absence of the thumb. In mild hypoplasia no treatment is necessary but if function is impaired by a tight thumb–index finger web space or thenar muscle hypoplasia, reconstructive surgery can be helpful. If the thumb is absent or unreconstructable pollicization of the index finger can be considered.

Constriction band syndrome

This condition occurs sporadically and is alternatively known as Streeter's dysplasia or amniotic band syndrome (Fig. 27.7). The etiology remains uncertain but constriction by intrauterine amniotic bands remains a hypothesis as well as localized failures of formation. Bands can be multiple and are asymmetric. Structures proximal to the band are normal but distally they may be deformed or even amputated. Tight bands can cause severe distal edema and vascular compromise with urgent 'Z'-plasty release required in the neonatal period.

LOWER LIMB PROBLEMS

Congenital abnormalities of the femur

Congenital abnormalities of the femur fall into two main groups: proportional hypoplasia of the whole femur and a deficiency of part or all of the bone. Both can be associated with more distal abnormalities, including absence of the anterior cruciate ligament at the knee and congenital abnormalities of the lower leg and foot.

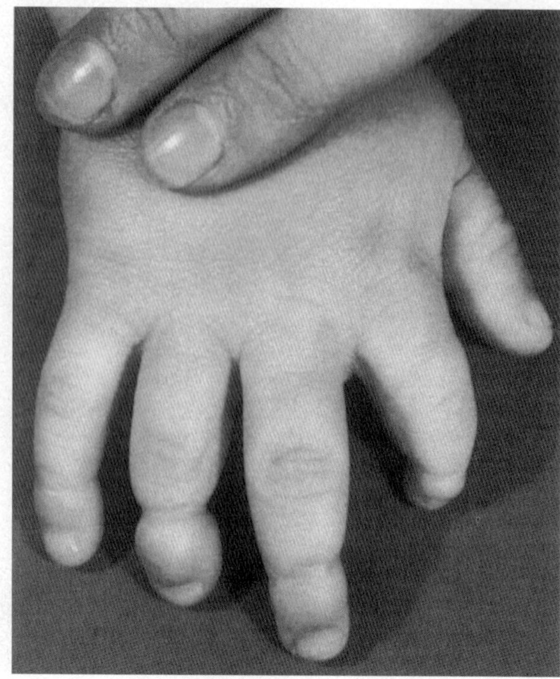

Fig. 27.7 Constriction band syndrome.

Children present with a limb length discrepancy either at birth or during early development. The femoral head and neck are radiolucent for the first 6 months of life even when no abnormality is present and ultrasonography provides a more reliable assessment.

Proximal femoral focal deficiency (PFFD)

PFFD or deficiency of the proximal part of the femur varies in severity (Fig. 27.8). Clinical examination typically reveals a position of flexion at the hip and the knee. Management of these children is complex and depends not only upon the potential limb length discrepancy, but also upon the stability of the hip joint and the presence of other associated limb problems.

Developmental coxa vara

The neck-shaft angle of the proximal femur measures a mean 144° in the first years of life, gradually falling to a mean 125° at maturity. Coxa vara is present when the neck-shaft angle falls below these parameters.

Coxa vara can be congenital, developmental or acquired as a consequence of a variety of conditions including developmental dislocation of the hip, slipped upper femoral epiphysis, Perthes disease, infection, trauma, tumors and metabolic disorders.

Congenital coxa vara is present at birth and commonly associated with other congenital musculoskeletal abnormalities.

Developmental coxa vara is a specific entity of unknown etiology and with an incidence of 1 in 25 000 births. There is an equal sex ratio and 30–50% of patients have bilateral disease. Most patients present between 1 and 6 years of age with a progressively deteriorating Trendelenburg gait, initially with no pain. Radiographs classically reveal coxa vara often with a neck-shaft angle of 90° or less and a vertically orientated physis (growth plate). A triangular piece of metaphysis outlined by an inverted 'Y' formed by the physis (or growth plate) on one side and radiolucent dystrophic bone on the other, is pathognomonic of the condition (Fig. 27.9). If left untreated the condition will lead to progressive degeneration, disability and pain. Valgus osteotomy to correct the deformity has been shown to be effective.[14]

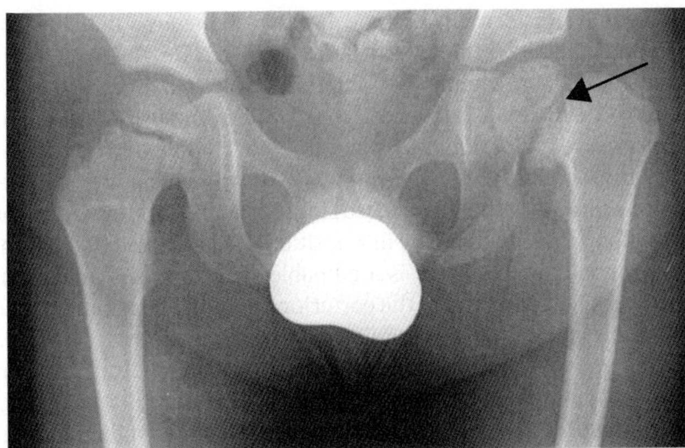

Fig. 27.9 Developmental coxa vara.

Developmental dysplasia of the hip (DDH) and congenital dislocation of the hip (CDH)

The term developmental dysplasia of the hip (DDH) encompasses the located hip with a shallow acetabulum (dysplasia), through subluxation, to frank dislocation. DDH is a more accurate term than congenital dislocation of the hip (CDH) and was introduced in recognition of the concept that a hip, located at birth, can become dislocated postnatally.[15] When dislocation of the hip presents at birth or in the neonatal period it is termed an early presentation. When dislocation presents beyond this period, commonly after 6 months, it is termed a late presentation. The term 'missed dislocation' should be avoided because it can be inaccurate. The term teratological dislocation is used to describe a dislocated hip in association with underlying problems such as arthrogryposis multiplex congenita or neuromuscular conditions such as myelomeningocele.

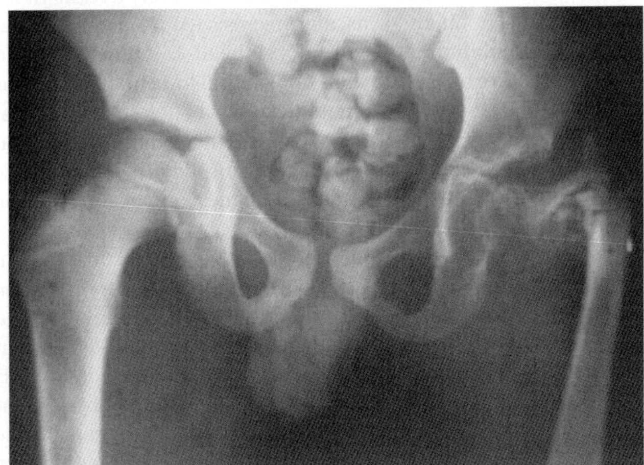

Fig. 27.8 Proximal femoral focal deficiency.

One in 60 neonates has hip instability demonstrable at birth,[16] although most of these hips stabilize spontaneously within the first weeks of life. Before the introduction of routine clinical screening in the UK the incidence of late dislocation was about 1–2:1000 live births. Screening has reduced but far from eradicated late presentation in the UK, a recent MRC trial showing the incidence to be at least 0.78:1000 live births.[17] There is considerable racial variation in the incidence of DDH. The incidence is very high in Navajo Native Americans, in the order of 50:1000 live births,[18] but very low in peoples of Chinese and African descent.[19, 20] DDH is six times more common in females than in males. It can present bilaterally but is usually unilateral and twice as common on the left.

Environmental factors both in utero, and after delivery can influence hip development. The most common fetal lie places the infant's left hip adducted against the maternal sacrum and it is thought that this might be the explanation for the predilection for the left side.[21] Breech position in utero is a significant risk factor for DDH,[22] as is oligohydramnios which limits fetal movement. Other conditions considered to be a result of intrauterine molding including metatarsus adductus and torticollis, are associated with DDH.[23] There is an increased incidence of hip dysplasia among first-born infants.[22] Postnatal influences include nursing habits such as swaddling. The infant hip and knee joints in utero are in a flexed position and normally have modest flexion contractures at birth. An attempt to straighten and adduct the limbs prematurely results in compression forces along the shaft of the femur, pushing the femoral head posterosuperiorly, where it is unstable. Cultural swaddling may in part explain the differing incidence of DDH between races. The hips are best allowed to rest in flexion and abduction, the position most infants naturally adopt.

Early diagnosis gives the best chance of a satisfactory outcome. Clinical examination to identify DDH should be part of routine infant examination. In the UK there is a nationwide clinical screening program that includes examination soon after birth, at 6 weeks and at 6 months. The first part of the examination is to determine whether the hip is in or out of joint. Clinical signs suggestive of dislocation include limited abduction, limb length asymmetry and asymmetric skin creases (Fig. 27.10). If the hip is considered to be in joint, its stability is evaluated with a Barlow maneuver. The hip is first placed in a vulnerable position of slight extension and adduction before longitudinal compression is applied along the shaft of the femur (Fig. 27.11a). The positioning is important because the hip is more stable and resists subluxation or dislocation if held incorrectly in a position of flexion and abduction. If the hip is unstable there is a palpable sensation of the femoral head riding posteriorly over the posterior rim of the acetabulum, the so-called 'clunk'. There is a similar sensation when compression is released and the femoral head returns to the acetabulum or if an Ortolani maneuver is used to reduce the joint. If the hip is considered to be dislocated, a gentle attempt can be made to return it to the acetabulum using an Ortolani maneuver. Once again positioning is important. The hip is held in 90° of flexion so that the femoral head is directly posterior to the acetabulum. Gentle traction is applied to the leg and the long fingers of the examiner's hand are placed on the greater trochanter where they gently lift the femoral head (Fig. 27.11b). If the dislocation is reducible the femoral head can be felt passing across the posterior lip of the acetabulum and into joint. Once in joint the hip can be gently abducted and flexed to a more stable position so that the reduction can be maintained.

These examinations are difficult and the introduction of clinical screening has not eradicated late presenting dislocations. The sensation of dislocation or reduction is difficult to elicit in the conscious child over about 3–4 months of age and thereafter limited abduction, or limb asymmetry are more reliable. After walking age the child with a unilateral dislocated hip stands either with the 'long' leg flexed at the knee or with the 'short leg' standing tiptoe to compensate for the length discrepancy. The child will walk with a limp, which can be a simple short leg gait, sometimes with a classical waddle or Trendelenburg gait pattern. Symmetry in bilateral dislocation can make these signs less easily identifiable. Radiographs reveal a subluxed or dislocated femoral head with a small ossific nucleus and a dysplastic acetabulum (Fig. 27.12).

Because of the shortcomings of clinical examination and the inability of radiographs to image the cartilaginous infant hip, ultrasound screening has developed. Population ultrasound screening has been introduced in Germany and parts of Europe but remains sporadic in the UK. Many units practice selective screening of infants at higher risk of DDH, which usually includes infants with a family history, a breech position in utero, a suspicious hip examination or who exhibit other structural examination abnormalities such as metatarsus adductus or torticollis. The investigation can result in false negatives and especially false positives, revealing 'abnormalities' of uncertain significance and resulting in very high treatment rates. Whilst it is widely acknowledged that ultrasound examination is an unequivocally useful tool to evaluate the progress of unstable and dislocated hips, its role as a screening tool for DDH in the UK remains controversial and its cost effectiveness is questioned.[24]

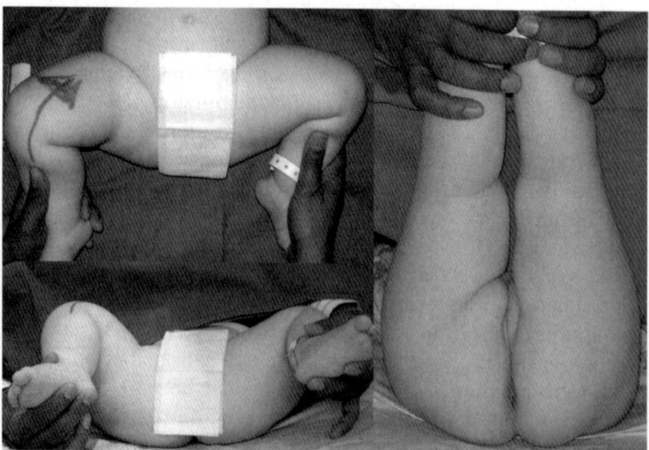

Fig. 27.10 Dislocated right hip showing limited abduction, asymmetric skin creases and short limb.

(a)

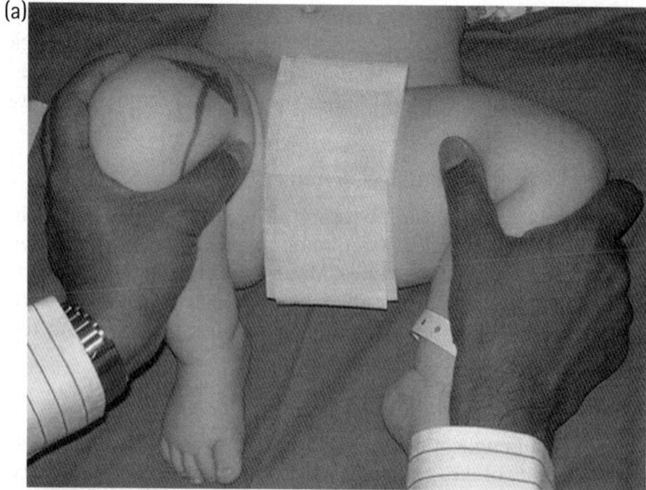

(b)

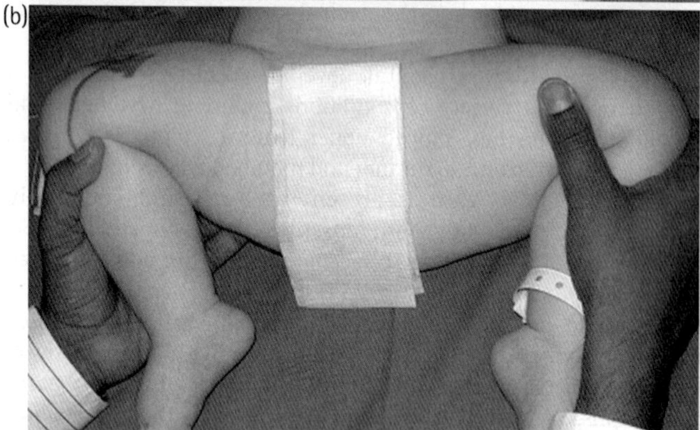

Fig. 27.11 (a) Barlow and (b) Ortolani maneuvers.

In general terms reduction of a dislocated hip becomes progressively more difficult the longer it has been dislocated. Treatment involves first reducing the hip and then keeping it in joint until it becomes stable. The chief complications of any treatment for DDH are redislocation and avascular necrosis (AVN) of the femoral head. The circulation of the femoral head is vulnerable and especially sensitive to pressure. It is known that forceful reduction or positioning of the hip in extreme flexion, abduction or internal rotation can apply excessive pressure to the femoral head and disturb the blood supply leading to AVN. In spite of avoiding these known causes AVN remains a troublesome complication in the management of hip dislocation (Fig. 27.13).

From birth to about 3–4 months the dislocated or subluxed hip will often reduce with a gentle Ortolani maneuver. In these circumstances the hip should be reduced and maintained in a position of gentle flexion and abduction until it becomes stable when released. There are a wide variety of splints available to maintain this position but the Pavlik harness (Fig. 27.14), a dynamic splint affording the infant some movement within a safe arc, is probably the most widely used. Use of the Pavlik harness is associated with a very low rate of AVN but injudicious use can still cause this complication.

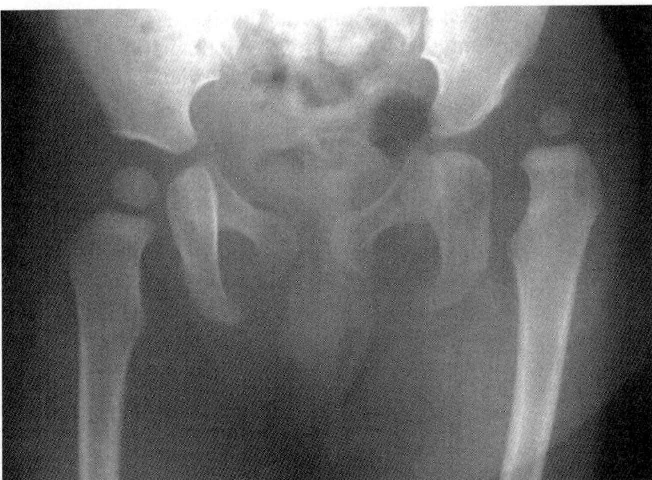

Fig. 27.12 Dislocated left hip with dysplastic acetabulum and small ossific nucleus.

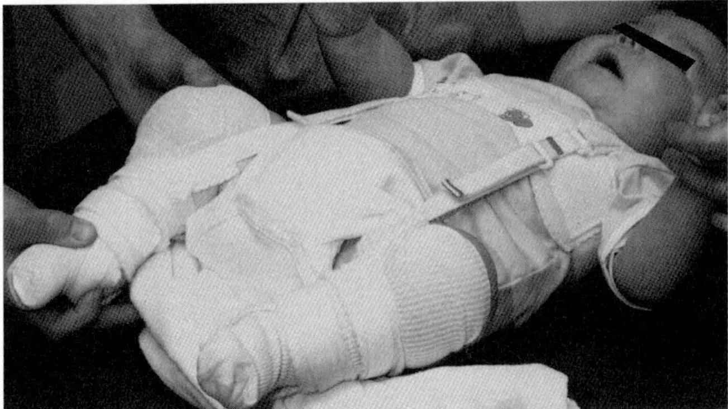

Fig. 27.14 Infant in Pavlik harness.

The harness is worn 24 hours a day and requires regular scrutiny to ensure proper fitting. Hip development can be followed by repeated ultrasound examination at 2–4 weekly intervals until normal with a clinically stable hip. Harness treatment typically lasts 12–16 weeks if the dislocation is identified early. The Pavlik harness is not practical in children older than about 6 months.

When children present between 4 and 6 months of age it can be difficult to be certain of an adequate reduction in the conscious patient and these infants are often examined under anesthesia. Radiopaque contrast is introduced into the hip joint during the examination and the resulting arthrogram outlines the cartilaginous femoral head and acetabulum so that a satisfactory reduction can be confirmed (Fig. 27.15). If there is any obstruction to proper location, or extreme force or positioning is required to maintain satisfactory location, closed (non-surgical) reduction is best abandoned in favor of a later open (surgical) reduction when the obstruction or resistance to location can be addressed operatively. If closed reduction is possible, immobilization in a stable position of gentle flexion and abduction can be achieved by a plaster of Paris hip spica cast, once again avoiding extreme or forced positions. It is common for the reduction to be confirmed by a later CT scan of the hips in the spica cast. Typically such children remain immobilized for between 6 and 9 months.

When children present after 12–18 months successful closed reduction becomes unlikely. The later a child presents the more likely they are to require a surgical open reduction and further secondary operations either to the femur or to the acetabulum to correct secondary problems, especially persistent acetabular shallowness (dysplasia). The long term prognosis for those presenting under 3–4 years nevertheless remains satisfactory. Presentation beyond 3–4 years inevitably leads to more difficult surgery and the outcome progressively deteriorates as the age at presentation increases. Surgical reduction after the age of 8–10 years is extremely difficult and if the problem is bilateral the child may be best left untreated. Such dislocations will cause gait abnormality but the affected individual may remain free of significant pain until early to mid adult life.

Congenital dislocation of the knee

This presents at birth with the knee severely hyperextended instead of in the normal flexed position (Fig. 27.16). The etiology is unknown

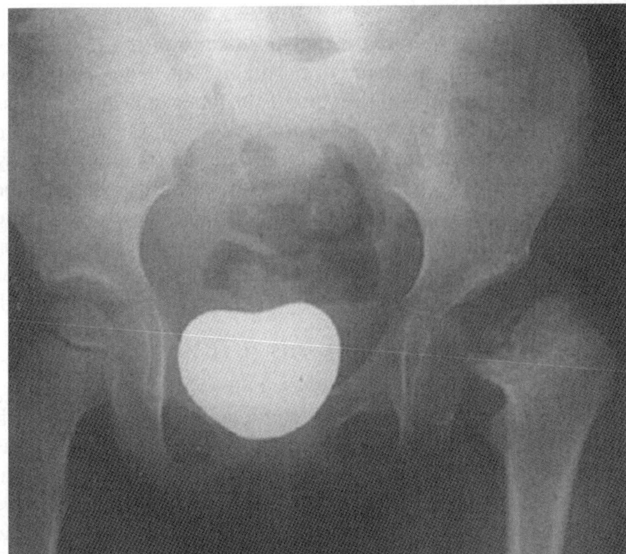

Fig. 27.13 Avascular necrosis after treatment for developmental dislocation of the hip.

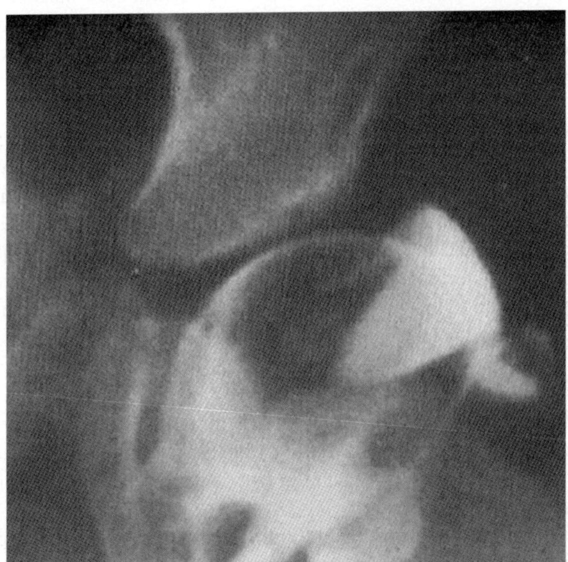

Fig. 27.15 Arthrogram showing a satisfactory closed reduction of a dislocated hip.

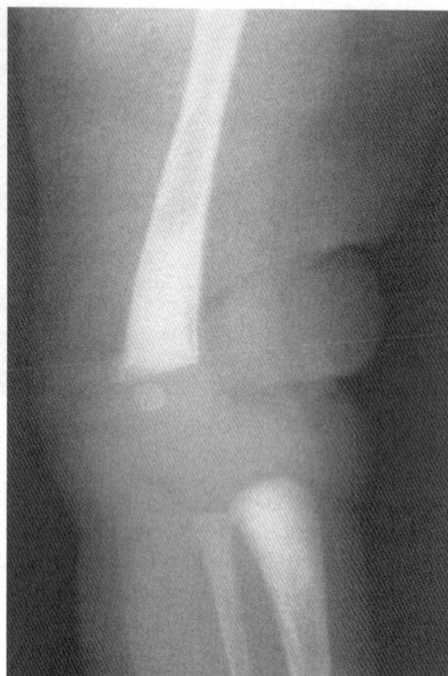

Fig. 27.16 Congenital dislocation of the knee.

but there is a high incidence of breech delivery[25] indicating a role for intrauterine positioning. Associated musculoskeletal abnormalities, especially subluxation or dislocation of the hip, are present in approximately 50%.[26] Plain lateral radiographs reveal anterior subluxation or dislocation of the tibia on the femur.

Treatment begins soon after birth with serial casting to gradually flex the knee and is often successful within a few weeks of birth. If conservative treatment fails there may be some underlying fibrosis of the quadriceps mechanism and open surgical release early in life can give good long-term results.

Tibial bowing

Tibial bowing at birth can take four characteristic forms. Broadly speaking the convexity of the bow points to the four points of the compass namely anteromedial, anterolateral, posterolateral and posteromedial. The first three directions are associated with relatively severe problems namely fibula hemimelia, pseudoarthrosis of the tibia and tibia hemimelia respectively. Posteromedial bowing of the tibia is relatively benign.

Posteromedial bowing of the tibia

Posteromedial bowing of the tibia is associated with a severe calcaneovalgus deformity of the foot.[27] The appearance can be alarming at birth. Initial treatment is directed towards passive stretching of the foot deformity sometimes with the addition of serial casting for severe deformities. The tibial bowing generally corrects rapidly in the first year of life although tibial length inequality may persist and require later orthopedic intervention.

Congenital fibula deficiency (fibula hemimelia)

The fibula is the most frequently congenitally deficient long bone. The deficiency can be modest and isolated. Severe fibula deficiency is more common and is associated with a generally dysplastic limb and other deformities.[28]

The choice of appropriate management can be extremely difficult. Modern prosthetics make amputation more acceptable and new methods of limb reconstruction, especially with the Ilizarov external fixator, make reconstruction more feasible. Amputation is recommended if the foot is non-functional, regardless of limb length, and if the length discrepancy is more than 30% even with a functional foot. Application of the appropriate management should be based on considerable clinical experience and tailored to the individual patient.

Congenital tibial deficiency (tibia hemimelia)

The child presents at birth with shortening of the tibia and a rigid equinovarus foot. The leg is bowed convex laterally. Other congenital limb abnormalities occur in as many as 75% of cases.[29] The tibia can be completely absent (Type I); absent in its distal portion but with a proximal portion remaining to form an articulation at the knee (Type II) (Fig. 27.17); or present but forming an abnormal distal tibiofibula diastasis or separation at the ankle (Type III).[30]

Management strategies range from prosthetics to reconstruction and once again, as in fibula hemimelia, considerable clinical experience is required to chart an appropriate course for each individual patient.

Congenital pseudoarthrosis of tibia

Congenital pseudoarthrosis of the tibia presents with anterior or anterolateral bowing at the junction of the proximal two-thirds and the distal one-third of the tibia. Up to 80% of cases are associated with neurofibromatosis.[31] The bone and its covering periosteum are abnormal at the site of the bowing and the fibula may also be involved in the pathology. Spontaneous fracture at the abnormality can occur and subsequently leads to persistent non-union or pseudoarthrosis.

Management should include the avoidance of fracture for as long as possible by the use of protective orthoses. Numerous methods have been used to encourage union at the fracture site with modest success. A Syme amputation of the foot followed by a below knee prosthesis remains a satisfactory long term solution although modern reconstructive techniques especially using the Ilizarov external fixator offer new solutions. The abnormal bone and periosteum at the site of the pathology can be excised and the remaining healthy bone lengthened.

Metatarsus varus

See section on Common orthopedic problems in childhood, page 1558.

Congenital talipes calcaneovalgus

This foot posture is frequent in newborns and in the majority of children is within the spectrum of normality. The foot is dorsiflexed so that the dorsum touches the shin. If the foot can be fully plantar flexed the condition is termed postural, requires no treatment and will resolve spontaneously. Occasionally the foot cannot be fully plantar flexed. Physiotherapy and/or splintage should be commenced promptly to stretch the tight anterior structures and should be successful within a few months in most cases. Sometimes, especially in resistant cases, there is an underlying neurological or skeletal explanation and this potential should always be considered.

Congenital talipes equinovarus (CTEV; congenital club foot)

Congenital talipes equinovarus is a common foot abnormality with an incidence of 1–2:1000 live births (Fig. 27.18). It is twice as common in boys, bilateral in up to 50%, and has a familial predisposition.[32] Unaffected parents with an affected son have a 1:40 chance of having another son with the disorder. The pathogenesis is unknown.

Clinically the hindfoot is in equinus and varus (inversion) and the heel is difficult to feel. The forefoot is adducted and plantarflexed

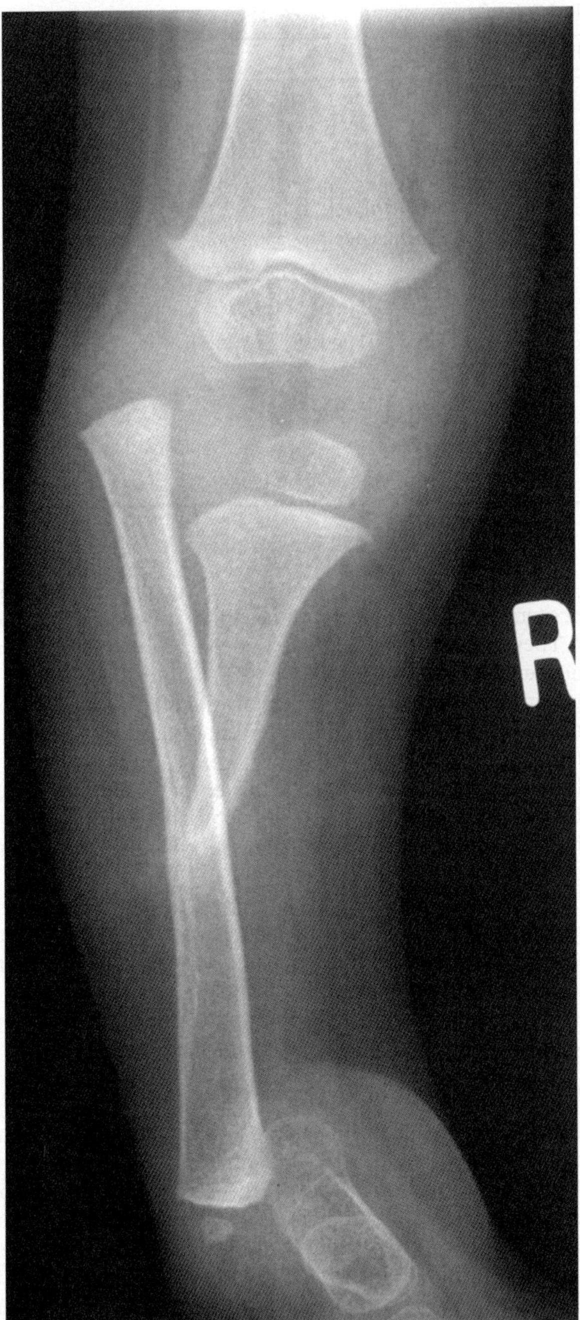

Fig. 27.17 Congenital tibial deficiency.

on the hindfoot giving a cavus or high arched appearance, and there is a deep transverse skin crease on the medial border of the foot. Internal tibial torsion is present and the foot and calf are often smaller than the opposite side. The navicular is medially displaced on the head of the talus. Passive correction to a neutral position is not possible.

A complete examination of the child is indicated to rule out potential neurological causes and associated conditions including DDH. Assessment of the severity and rigidity of the deformity at birth is difficult but is helpful to determine the likely success of conservative treatment or need for surgical correction. If the foot can be passively returned to neutral, conservative treatment can be expected to be successful in 90%. If fixed equinus is 0–20°, conservative treatment can be expected to succeed in 50% of cases; but if fixed equinus is more than 20°, conservative treatment can only be expected to be successful in 10%.[33] Even if clear from the outset that surgical treatment will be necessary, initial treatment with passive stretching and splintage should be used as passive stretching minimizes the extent of subsequent surgery. Conservative treatment techniques currently used include simple stretching, splinting with adhesive strapping, serial plaster casting or even continuous passive motion machines.

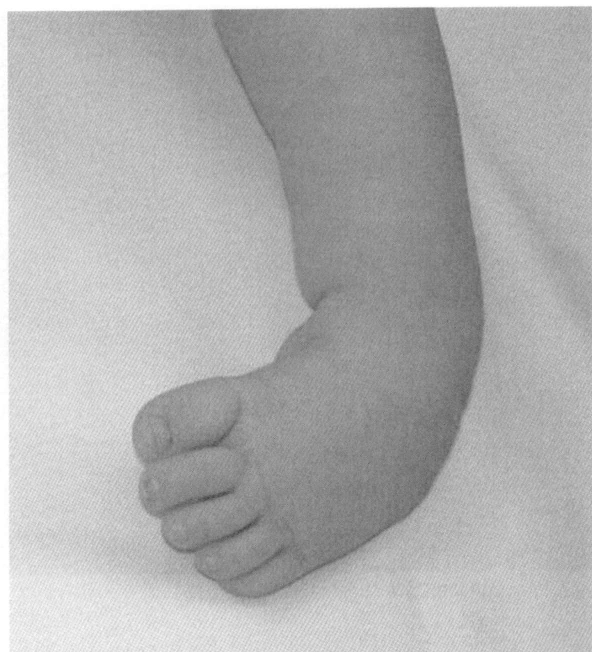
Fig. 27.18 Congenital talipes equinovarus.

Surgical correction involves the surgical release or lengthening of all tight joint capsules or tendons and the restoration of the normal alignment of the bones. The timing of surgery varies. It can be performed as early as 6–12 weeks of age but is often delayed until the foot is larger and easier to operate upon. Many offer surgery around the first birthday so that the child walks soon after the surgery thus applying corrective forces. Recurrence of deformity is a constant concern during the management of CTEV and secondary surgery to correct recurring deformity, especially forefoot varus, is not uncommon. Sometimes repeated recurrence occurs in spite of secondary operations: this can be successfully managed using Ilizarov external fixator techniques.

Congenital vertical talus

This is a rigid foot deformity that presents clinically as a 'rocker bottom' foot. In about 50%[34] the condition is associated with other congenital neuromuscular and genetic disorders like neural tube defects and arthrogryposis. The head of the talus is dislocated from its normal articulation with the navicular and takes on a more vertical position. Diagnosis is made with a lateral radiograph and the foot stressed into maximal plantar flexion. If the navicular remains dorsally dislocated on the talus, the diagnosis is confirmed (Fig. 27.19).

In addition to the vertical position of the talus and the tight anterior structures causing dorsal dislocation of the forefoot, the posterior structures are also tight resulting in fixed equinus of the hindfoot as in CTEV. The hindfoot and forefoot are therefore essentially broken over the vertically disposed talus giving the foot the characteristic 'rocker bottom' in severe cases.

Initial treatment is directed toward passive stretching and splinting of the foot into plantar flexion to stretch the tight anterior

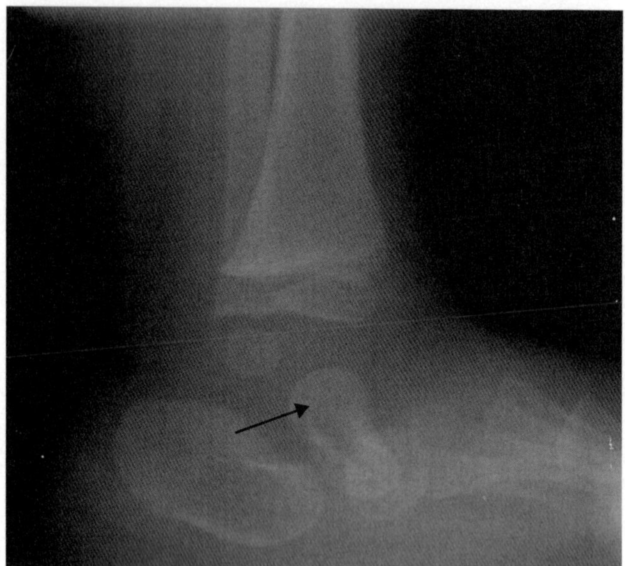

Fig. 27.19 Congenital vertical talus.

structures. Surgery is frequently necessary later to lengthen the tight anterior and posterior structures and to restore the normal alignment and relationship of the talus with the other bones of the foot.

INHERITED DISORDERS OF BONES AND JOINTS

Inherited disorders of bones and joints are rare but an important source of diagnostic confusion for the unwary as they may be easily confused with other disorders such as juvenile arthritis and Perthes disease. Most present with some combination of joint swelling or deformity; joint hypermobility or stiffness; and short stature. An awareness of these conditions will enable the correct diagnosis to be made. This ensures that appropriate advice and genetic counseling can be given and avoids the inappropriate use of drugs such as methotrexate in children who do not have an inflammatory arthritis.

This section is not intended to be an exhaustive review of a very complex area but describes some of the more common of the primary genetic disorders of bones and connective tissues, as well as identifying other genetic disorders in which bone and joint problems are a dominant feature. Many of these primary disorders of bones and connective tissues are now being associated with identifiable genetic defects, particularly of the collagen genes (Table 27.4). As these genetic defects are increasingly delineated it seems likely that the classification of these conditions will continually require to be updated. More detail of these disorders and their classification can be obtained from a number of excellent reviews.[35–38]

HYPERMOBILITY

Joint mobility follows a normal distribution in the population and is influenced by factors including age, sex and ethnicity. Infants and young children have joints that are more mobile than older children and adults but there are no good studies defining normal joint ranges in the very young. Females have a greater degree of joint laxity than males and hypermobile joints are much more common in certain ethnic groups, e.g. oriental. Hypermobility of the joints may be generalized or affect only one or two joints. Generalized joint hypermobility may occur as an isolated entity or as part of a number of well-recognized genetic syndromes.

Table 27.4 Genetic disorders of collagen synthesis

Collagen type	Condition
I	Osteogenesis imperfecta Ehlers–Danlos type VII Idiopathic juvenile osteoporosis
II	Stickler syndrome Kniest dysplasia Spondyloepiphyseal dysplasia congenita and tarda
III	Ehlers–Danlos types III, IV and VIII
IV	Ehlers–Danlos type VI
V	Ehlers–Danlos types I and II
VI	Cutis laxa
IX	Multiple epiphyseal dysplasia
X	Schmid's metaphyseal dysplasia
XI	Stickler syndrome type II

Adapted from Hall 2001[35]

The definition of hypermobility is based on clinical assessment. The criteria most frequently used are those defined by Beighton et al.[39] These assess joint laxity based on a number of clinical maneuvers:

1. passive dorsiflexion of the 5th metacarpophalangeal joint to 90°;
2. apposition of the thumb to the flexor aspect of the forearm (Fig. 27.20a);
3. hyperextension of the elbow to greater than 10° (Fig. 27.20b);
4. hyperextension of the knee to greater than 10°;
5. forward flexion of the trunk to place the palms of the hands flat on the floor with the knees extended.

Those experienced in examining young children will immediately realize that these measurements are not appropriate in the very young in whom these degrees of joint laxity are normal. There is a need for defining age related normal values but the Beighton scoring system has been shown to be valid in children over the age of 4 years when interpreted correctly.[40]

Benign hypermobility syndrome

Joint hypermobility is a normal variant and causes no symptoms in many individuals. In others it is associated with a variety of musculoskeletal symptoms as part of the 'benign joint hypermobility syndrome', BJHS.[38] Although labeled 'benign', affected individuals may have troublesome symptoms with significant morbidity. There is concern that it may predispose to the early onset of osteoarthritis in adult life.[41] It can be extremely difficult to differentiate BJHS from the milder variants of some of the genetic disorders such as Ehlers–Danlos syndrome.

The BJHS occurs more commonly in females than in males and appears to have an autosomal dominant mode of inheritance. Affected individuals may have a variety of symptoms including arthralgia, joint effusions, widespread muscle pain, low back pain, flat feet and recurrent dislocations. Recurrent sports injuries and back pain are commonly reported in older children and adolescents with BJHS[42] and there is an increased risk of developing chronic musculoskeletal pain syndromes.[43] Children with such symptoms should be carefully assessed for evidence of abnormal joint laxity.

Management consists initially of providing some explanation of the condition. Reassuring the family that the symptoms are real and have a physical basis, while assuring them that their child does not have arthritis is helpful for many. Physiotherapy and occupational therapy may be helpful but results are variable. Simple analgesics

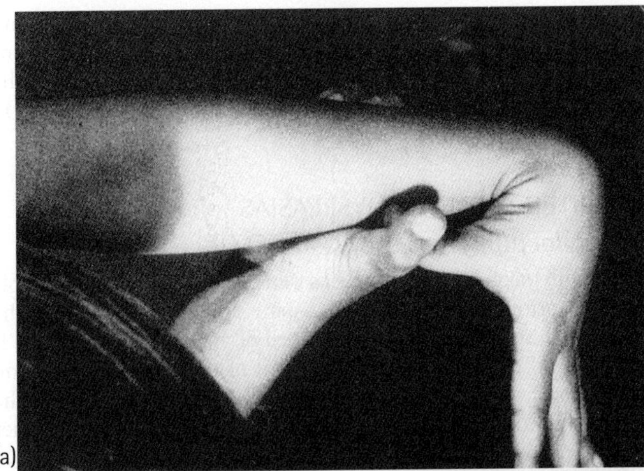

(a)

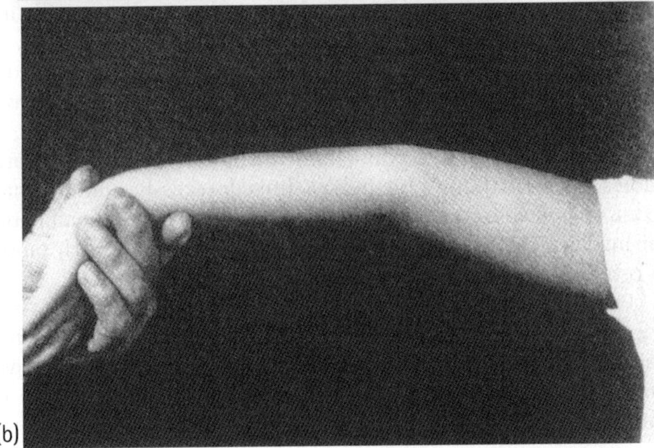

(b)

Fig. 27.20 Hypermobility: (a) apposition of the thumb to the flexor aspect of the forearm; (b) hyperextension of the elbow to greater than 10°.

are as effective as anti-inflammatory medication in most. Many affected children have significant flat feet and supportive footwear may improve symptoms.

INHERITED SYNDROMES WITH SIGNIFICANT HYPERMOBILITY

Ehlers–Danlos syndrome

Ehlers–Danlos syndrome (EDS) consists of a group of disorders of connective tissue characterized by joint hypermobility plus fragility and laxity of the skin. Ten types of EDS have been described, only some of which will be described here. These conditions are characterized by abnormalities in collagen genes resulting in the production of abnormal collagen and consequent tissue fragility. They vary both in severity and mode of inheritance and an accurate diagnosis is essential if patients are to be offered appropriate advice and counseling.

EDS type I, which is characterized by abnormalities of type V collagen with mutations in the COL5A1 gene, is inherited as an autosomal dominant condition. It results in what many think of as 'typical' EDS with soft, hyperextensible skin, 'cigarette paper' scars, easy bruising and marked hypermobility. EDS type II is similar to type I but less severe.

EDS type III, again inherited as an autosomal trait, causes familial joint hypermobility and minimal skin findings. It may be impossible to distinguish clinically from the benign hypermobility syndrome and there is an ongoing debate as to whether this division is purely arbitrary. The benign hypermobility syndrome can therefore be regarded as either one end of the normal spectrum of joint mobility or a mild form of EDS.

EDS IV, although much less common, is the form associated with serious involvement with a high incidence of rupture of the arteries, the colon or the pregnant uterus. This results from mutations in the COL3A1 gene which causes production of abnormal type III collagen. Although the inheritance is autosomal dominant approximately one-third are new mutations. The diagnosis can be confirmed by collagen studies of cultured dermal fibroblasts.

Management of EDS consists of patient education and support, with genetic counseling for the more severe forms. Physiotherapy together with advice regarding appropriate forms of exercise and footwear can be helpful. Children with severe hypermobility may have significant functional problems that cause difficulties, for example with handwriting at school.

Marfan's syndrome

Marfan's syndrome, also an inherited disorder of connective tissue, affects approximately 1 in 10 000 of the population. Inherited as an autosomal dominant trait it results from mutations in the gene on chromosome 15 which encodes for the glycoprotein fibrillin, a component of elastin fibrils in the extracellular matrix.[44]

Marfan's syndrome is characterized by tall stature, long extremities, fingers and feet, chest deformities, high arched palate and ocular abnormalities including lens dislocation. Joint hypermobility, although not diagnostic, is recognized frequently and there is a high incidence of spinal problems with the development of both scolioses and kyphoses. Mitral valve prolapse is common. Aortic valve disease and a tendency to sudden aortic rupture are of major concern.

Many individuals are only mildly affected and the diagnosis can be difficult. Diagnostic criteria are currently based on clinical features but recent reports suggest that this can now be supported by molecular analysis.[45,46]

Individuals with type 1 homocystinuria may have tall stature, a high arched palate and resemble Marfan's syndrome. Hypotonia occurs but the joints are stiff rather than hypermobile. Severe osteoporosis and mental retardation are characteristic.

Osteogenesis imperfecta

Osteogenesis imperfecta (OI) is a group of autosomal dominantly inherited collagen gene disorders typified by bone fragility and often associated with joint hypermobility. The underlying defects in these conditions are in the genes COL1A1 and COL1A2 which encode the peptide chains of type I collagen, the major structural protein of bone, ligament and tendon. Clinically the important features are those of an inherited osteoporosis. Radiological appearances range from mild osteoporosis with occasional fractures to a widespread skeletal abnormality with multiple fractures. In its most severe form, OI may be lethal in utero.

Types I and IV OI are the mildest form of the condition, presenting with recurrent fractures in infancy and childhood (Fig. 27.21). Spinal involvement results in short stature which may be marked. There is a tendency for the fracture rate to reduce after adolescence but become more severe again in later adult life. Type I is distinguished by the presence of the characteristic blue sclerae. Associated dentinogenesis imperfecta and joint laxity occur with variable frequency.

Type II OI is a severe, crippling and frequently lethal disease. Multiple intrauterine fractures occur and early death results from chest infections and pulmonary restriction caused by the widespread fractures.

Type III (Fig. 27.22) is the most severe non-lethal form causing severe bone fragility with marked joint hypermobility. Survivors of infancy are usually significantly disabled. Until recently there has been

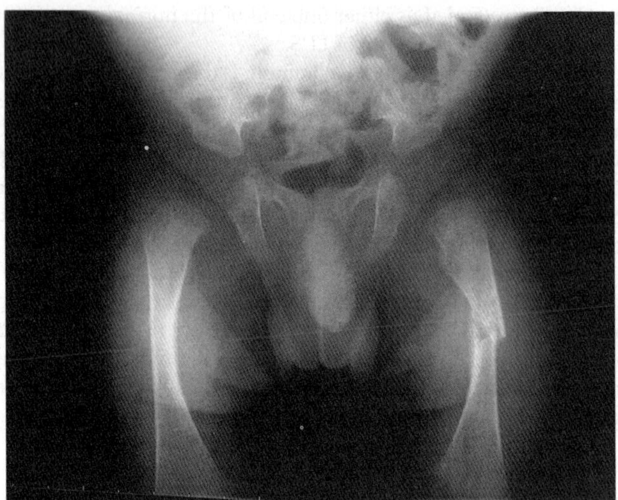

Fig. 27.21 Osteogenesis imperfecta type I.

no treatment for individuals with OI other than appropriate orthopedic management of fractures and supportive care. Expert physiotherapy and orthopedic input remain critical to optimal management of these children.[47] The development of the bisphosphonate group of drugs offers new possibilities for treatment. Treatment with intravenous pamidronate has been shown to result in reduced bone pain, a significant increase in bone density, a decreased number of fractures and an improved quality of life in affected children.[48] Given by intravenous infusion over 3 days every 3 months it is generally well tolerated although minor infusion reactions are common on the first of the 3 days. The role of the oral bisphosphates is as yet unclear.

Stickler syndrome

Stickler syndrome is an inherited disorder of connective tissues characterized by a typical facies with midface hypoplasia, high myopia with early onset, progressive hearing loss and arthropathy.

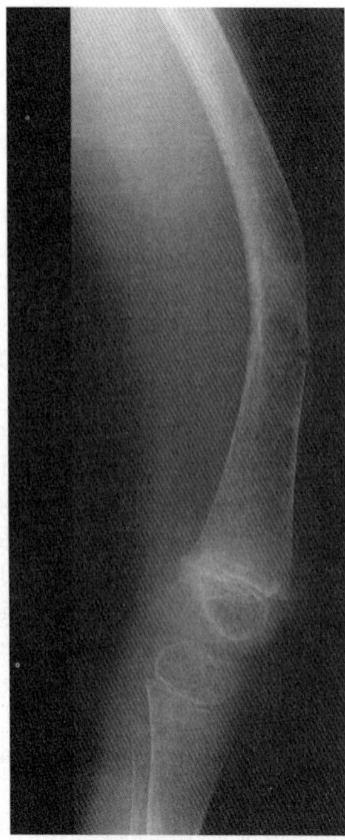

Fig. 27.22 Osteogenesis imperfecta type III showing recent fracture, severe osteoporosis and femoral deformity.

The joint problems include both generalized joint hypermobility and early degenerative joint disease. Retinal detachment is a serious complication of the syndrome. Mutations in the COL2A1 gene of type II collagen have been demonstrated in some families.

INHERITED SKELETAL DYSPLASIAS

Spondyloepiphyseal dysplasia (SED)

The spondyloepiphyseal dysplasias consist of a group of heritable disorders principally involving the spine and the epiphyses of the long bones. Several forms are described of varying severity. Type II collagen is the main protein component of articular cartilage and mutations of the COL2A1 gene are thought to result not only in the already mentioned Stickler syndrome but in a number of other disorders including the spondyloepiphyseal dysplasias.

SED congenita is an autosomal dominant condition with its onset at birth. Affected children may have delay in walking, a waddling gait and short stature. Limitation of range of motion affects elbows, knees and hips. Radiological investigation shows flattening of the vertebrae (Fig. 27.23) and coxa vara.

SED tarda results in symptoms which seldom present before adolescence. Although usually X-linked recessive, autosomal recessive and dominant forms have also been described. Spinal and hip involvement occur and the course is usually benign. Early onset of osteoarthritis occurs in adult life.

Progressive pseudorheumatoid arthropathy is a variant of SED (Fig. 27.24) which presents between 3 and 11 years of age with painful, swollen joints especially affecting the hands. Progressive joint contractures and short stature develop and the condition is unresponsive to standard antirheumatic medication.

Multiple epiphyseal dysplasia

This is one of the more common skeletal dysplasias and is inherited as an autosomal dominant trait. It presents in childhood with pain and stiffness and usually progresses to joint contractures and associated short stature. At first sight it may be confused with juvenile arthritis, but the absence of signs and symptoms of inflammation can distinguish the two. Radiology demonstrates irregularities of the end-plates of the mid-thoracic vertebral bodies, shortening of the metacarpals and flattening, sclerosis and fragmentation of the epiphyses at the hips and knees (Fig. 27.25).

Achondroplasia and hypochondroplasia

These disorders result from mutations of fibroblast growth factor receptor 3 (FGFR3) genes. Although inherited as an autosomal dominant trait, most cases of achondroplasia now occur as new mutations.

The classic form of achondroplasia causes severe disproportionate short stature. Affected individuals have normal or large heads with shortening of the limbs and an increased lumbar lordosis. The pedicles of the vertebrae are short which may lead to symptomatic spinal stenosis in adult life.

Hypochondroplasia is a milder form resulting from different mutations in the FGFR3 gene.

Trichorhinophalangeal dysplasia

This autosomal dominant disorder results from the deletion of multiple genes on chromosome 8. It is characterized by enlargement of the interphalangeal joints with a characteristic facial appearance. Affected individuals have a bulbous nose, hyperplastic nares, sparse, brittle hair and short stature. Radiographically the condition is characterized by cone-shaped epiphyses with short

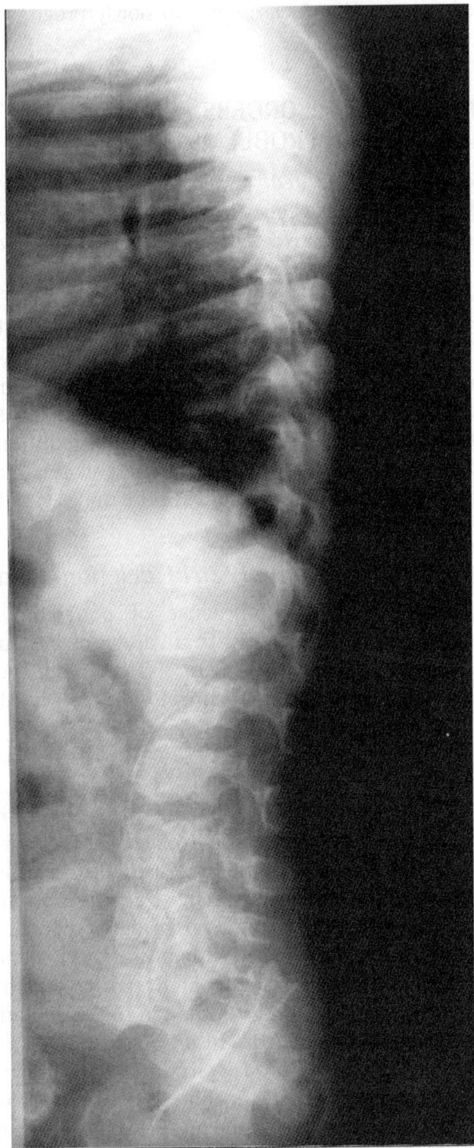

Fig. 27.23 Spondyloepiphyseal dysplasia congenita showing abnormal vertebrae.

metacarpals and metatarsals plus fragmentation of the epiphyses. Fragmentation of the femoral epiphyses may cause confusion with Perthes disease.

Storage disorders: the mucopolysaccharidoses (MPS)

The MPS are genetically determined deficiencies of enzymes involved in the metabolism of glycosaminoglycans. All are inherited as autosomal dominant conditions and a prominent feature of most is a skeletal dysplasia which affects particularly the hands, feet and vertebrae. In all of these conditions this may be the presenting feature. In the milder forms such as Scheie and Morquio syndromes the joint problems may dominate the clinical picture. In the more severe forms such as Hurler's syndrome the characteristic coarsening of the facial features is striking but this may take time to develop and flexion deformities of the fingers may be present earlier on.

For more detail on these conditions see Chapter 24. An awareness that they may present with skeletal symptoms will enable their early recognition, allowing appropriate genetic advice and counseling.

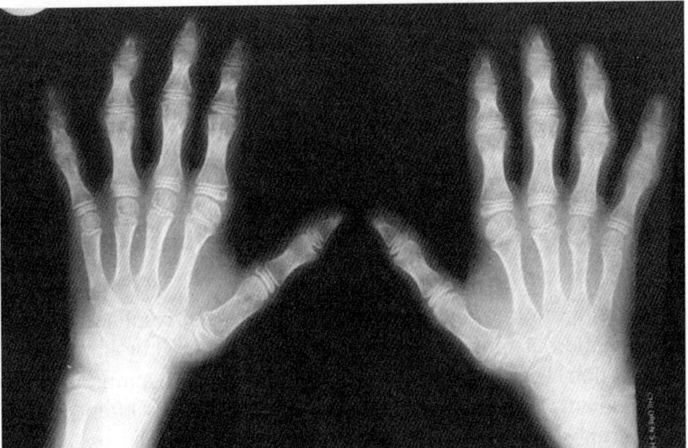

Fig. 27.24 Spondyloepiphyseal dysplasia tarda (progressive pseudorheumatoid arthropathy) affecting hands with obvious swelling of joints and bulbous ends to the phalanges.

OTHER INHERITED DISORDERS PRIMARILY AFFECTING THE MUSCULOSKELETAL SYSTEM

There are many other inherited disorders that primarily affect the musculoskeletal system and are currently difficult to categorize.

Osteopetrosis

This is a rare disorder resulting in frontal bossing, hypertelorism, exophthalmos and nasal obstruction which may be present from birth. It progresses during early childhood resulting in severe bleeding problems, recurrent fractures and early death. The disease is characterized by an increased density of the bones with metaphyseal flaring. Bone marrow transplantation may offer a cure.

Arthrogryposis

This refers to a number of disorders characterized by multiple congenital contractures.

Ollier's disease

Ollier's disease or multiple enchondromatosis becomes apparent during childhood when it presents with multiple juxta-articular outgrowths.

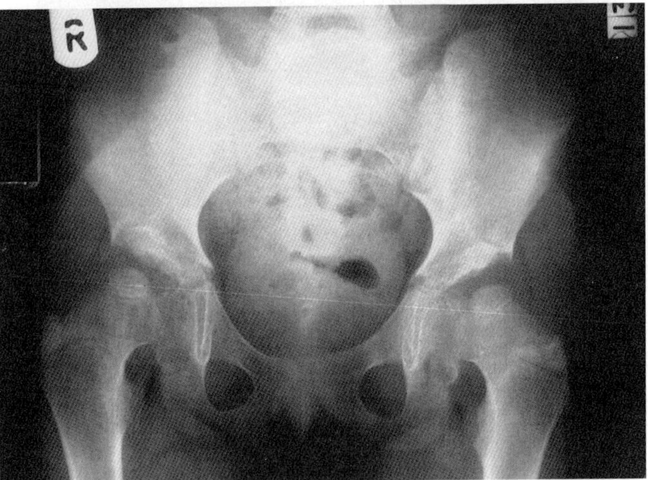

Fig. 27.25 Multiple epiphyseal dysplasia with bilateral hip involvement.

Idiopathic acro-osteolysis

This is inherited as an autosomal dominant trait and generally presents around 3 years with bony lysis which may affect the carpus or tarsus alone or occur in a more widespread pattern. The condition may mimic juvenile arthritis in that affected areas are warm and swollen. Radiographs show progressive bone lysis and destruction of affected joints.

Fibrodysplasia ossificans progressiva (FDP; myositis ossificans progressiva)

FDP is a rare autosomal dominant condition that results in painful inflammation of muscles and fascia, rapidly followed by fibrosis and calcification. The child may present with a swelling in a muscle or the development of a contracture, and the diagnosis is often elusive. Radiographs will show calcification in, and eventually ossification of, the muscles (Fig. 27.26a). The condition is characterized by congenitally short great toes (Fig. 27.26b), and sometimes thumbs, which may be useful diagnostically. Intermittent exacerbations are frequently precipitated by some trauma which may be very minor, to the affected muscle. The disease tends to slowly progress to severe disability.

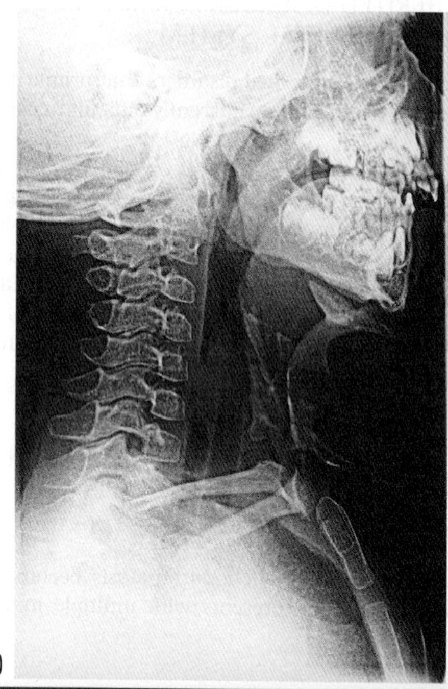

(a)

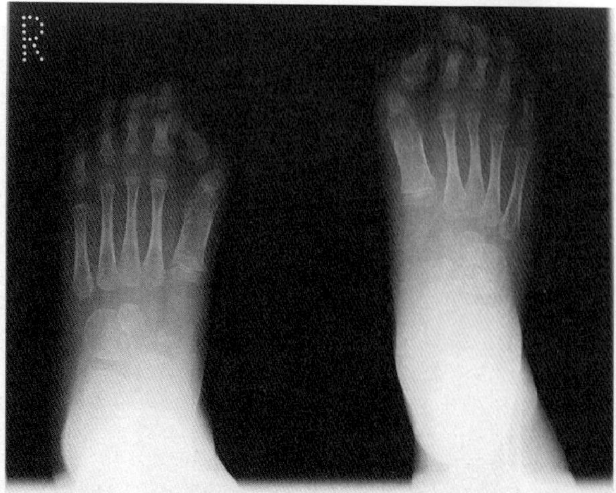

(b)

Fig. 27.26 Fibrodysplasia ossificans progressiva showing (a) ossification of anterior neck muscles and (b) dysplastic great toes.

OTHER INHERITED DISORDERS ASSOCIATED WITH MUSCULOSKELETAL PROBLEMS

There are many inherited conditions that may result in musculoskeletal problems. Some of the more important are outlined here. All are covered in more detail in other relevant chapters.

Down syndrome (trisomy 21)

Down syndrome is associated with a variety of musculoskeletal problems. In infancy generalized muscular hypotonicity may be striking and many affected individuals will remain significantly hypermobile with associated symptoms. Atlantoaxial instability is of major concern in Down syndrome. An inflammatory arthropathy is well recognized in affected children[49] and it is presumed that this in some way relates to the underlying identified immunological abnormalities.

Velocardiofacial syndrome (22q11 deletion syndrome)

This syndrome is a common cause of congenital cardiac malformations and is associated with a variety of immunological abnormalities, particularly impairment of T cell function. Perhaps as a consequence of this it is now known to be associated with an inflammatory arthritis.[50]

Cystic fibrosis (CF)

CF is associated with a variety of joint complaints.[51] With improved survival it is increasingly common to see teenagers with joint symptoms. Ciprofloxacin, an antibiotic used in cystic fibrosis, is known to cause arthralgia but this seems to be rare in young people. Many individuals with CF have arthralgias which may be troublesome but are not associated with any serious joint pathology. A few develop a recurrent acute arthropathy which can be extremely painful and distressing. Although the exact pathology is unclear it seems likely that this results from immune complex deposition[52] and the cutaneous vasculitis that may occur is presumed to have a similar mechanism. Non-steroidal anti-inflammatory drugs may be inadequate to control these acute symptoms and short courses of oral steroids may be required. In severe longstanding cystic fibrosis, hypertrophic pulmonary osteoarthropathy may develop as a cause for joint pain and swelling. This should be considered in an individual with marked clubbing of the fingers and severe pulmonary disease. Plain radiography will demonstrate the characteristic periosteal reaction.

Hemophilia

Hemophilia has previously been complicated by a destructive arthritis occurring as a consequence of recurrent bleeds into the joints. It is a tribute to advances in care in hemophilia and the use of prophylactic factor VIII that chronic hemophilic arthropathy is now seldom seen in developed countries. Hemophilia must still be remembered in the differential diagnosis when a young boy presents for the first time with a tense joint effusion. Joint aspiration will demonstrate blood and abnormal coagulation will be found.

Metabolic bone disease

Rickets usually presents with bone pain and bowing of the long bones. The most common cause is vitamin D deficiency (Fig. 27.27) but rickets may also result from a number of inherited disorders. Hypophosphatemic or vitamin D resistant rickets may be inherited as either an X-linked recessive or an autosomal disorder and is characterized by impaired parathormone dependent proximal renal tubular reabsorption of phosphate. Hypophosphatasia is a rare autosomal recessive disorder characterized by severe rickets and reduced serum levels of alkaline phosphatase.

Gout

Gout may result from either an increased production or a decreased excretion of urate and is extremely rare in childhood. There are a variety of inherited disorders of purine metabolism that may result in gout. Of these, familial juvenile hyperuricemic nephropathy is now known to be the most common.[53]

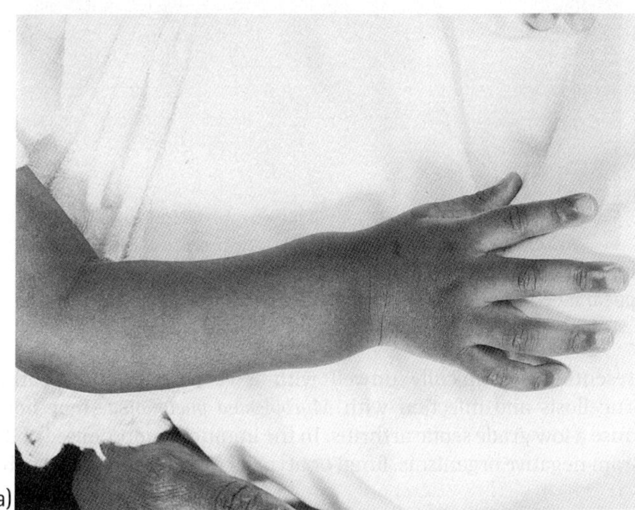

(a)

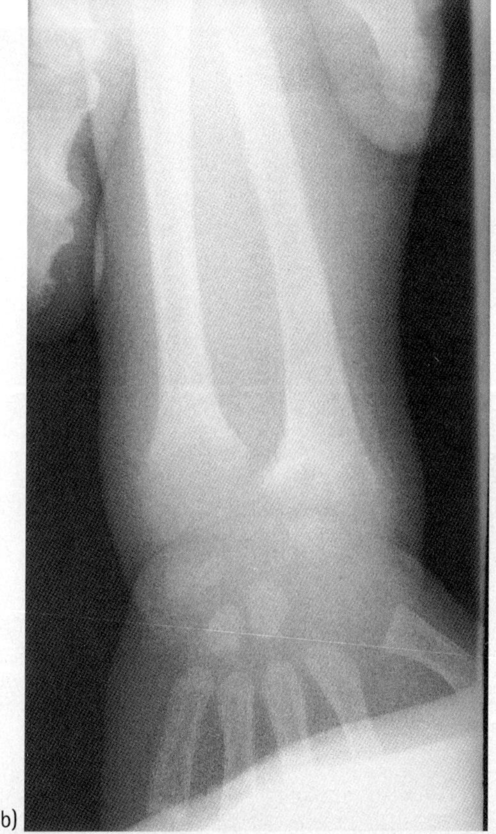

(b)

Fig. 27.27 Dietary rickets in a breast fed toddler: (a) clinical appearance; (b) radiological features with characteristic metaphyseal fraying.

Periodic fever syndromes

Familial Mediterranean fever (FMF) and other periodic fever syndromes may result in musculoskeletal symptoms especially arthralgia and myalgia. FMF may in addition cause a large joint arthropathy. These conditions are described in more detail in the section on the Differential diagnosis of systemic inflammatory disorders (p. 1579).

INFECTION IN BONES AND JOINTS

Bone and joint infections are relatively rare disorders in children, but may be associated with considerable morbidity and mortality unless rapidly recognized and adequately treated. The clinical features and etiology are age dependent within the pediatric population. Skeletal infections may result from direct bacterial invasion of a bone (osteomyelitis) or joint (septic arthritis). Direct infection with viruses and other infectious agents such as fungi and spirochetes may also occur. Other forms of arthritis, which are related to infection but distinct from septic arthritis are more common. Reactive arthritis occurs in response to infection elsewhere in the body especially the upper airway, the gastrointestinal or genitourinary tracts, and includes reactions to many viruses, streptococcal infections and other agents. In reactive arthritis the synovial fluid is, by definition, sterile and the arthritis is thought to result from immunological cross-reactivity between infecting agents and articular structures. Postinfectious arthritis is a term generally applied to a form of reactive arthritis resulting from the deposition of immune complexes in the joint as may occur following meningococcal infection.

The distinction between reactive arthritis and true joint infection is not always clear cut. With improvements in methods of detection of infectious organisms it may be that conditions previously considered reactive may be shown to be the result of true intra-articular infection.

SEPTIC ARTHRITIS AND OSTEOMYELITIS

Most frequently the result of hematogenous seeding of bacteria, septic arthritis and osteomyelitis may also result from extension of local sepsis, by iatrogenic inoculation (rare) or post trauma. Septic arthritis occasionally arises from contiguous spread from adjacent osteomyelitis, especially in the younger child, as a consequence of the anatomy where the metaphyseal–epiphyseal junction lies adjacent to the joint space.[54] In osteomyelitis the metaphyses of long bones or vertebral bodies are the commonest sites involved. Fever and pain are frequent symptoms, but a differential diagnosis including fracture, rheumatic fever, septic arthritis, bone infarction secondary to hemoglobinopathy, leukemia and bony neoplasm should be considered.[55] Osteomyelitis may be acute, subacute or chronic. Subacute osteomyelitis has a longer duration than acute and tends to result from infection with less virulent organisms. Chronic osteomyelitis may result from failure to identify or ineffective treatment of acute osteomyelitis.

In neonates the clinical features may be non-specific and include poor feeding, irritability and poor temperature control. The affected limb may become erythematous, tender and swollen, and there may be a paucity of spontaneous movement. Concomitant septicemia is commoner in this age group. In older children the features tend to be more localized when the peripheral skeleton is affected, but less so in the pelvis or spine. Gait abnormalities, in particular limp or refusal to walk are common if the leg is involved. A septic joint will exhibit the classical features of inflammation with swelling, pain, warmth and erythema. An affected hip is often held in flexion and external rotation; a knee in flexion.

Investigations

The full blood count may reveal thrombocytosis and neutrophil leukocytosis. Erythrocyte sedimentation rate (ESR) and C-reactive protein (CRP) are both likely to be elevated, although changes in the CRP tend to mirror the course of the infection more closely.[56]

The suspicion of septic arthritis should prompt microbiological analysis of both blood and synovial fluid. Multiple peripheral blood cultures should be taken prior to commencing antibiotics. Typical synovial fluid features on microscopy and a comparison with non-infective inflammatory arthritis are shown in Table 27.5.[57] Culture from bone may yield the organism in osteomyelitis.

Radiological investigations

Plain radiographs remain the primary imaging modality for suspected skeletal infections. In osteomyelitis soft tissue swelling and a periosteal reaction may be seen within a few days. Bony changes develop later (Fig. 27.28). In septic arthritis the early features are osteopenia of the epiphysis, increased joint space and soft tissue swelling (Fig. 27.29). Later in the disease destructive changes may be seen. Radionuclide bone scanning is sensitive at detecting areas of increased uptake, and may reveal multiple foci within the skeleton. However the specificity of this method, as with magnetic resonance imaging (MRI) and CT scanning, is low and the features may not distinguish septic from non-septic inflammatory lesions. Ultrasound (US) is a rapidly available and sensitive method for detecting effusions in the hip.

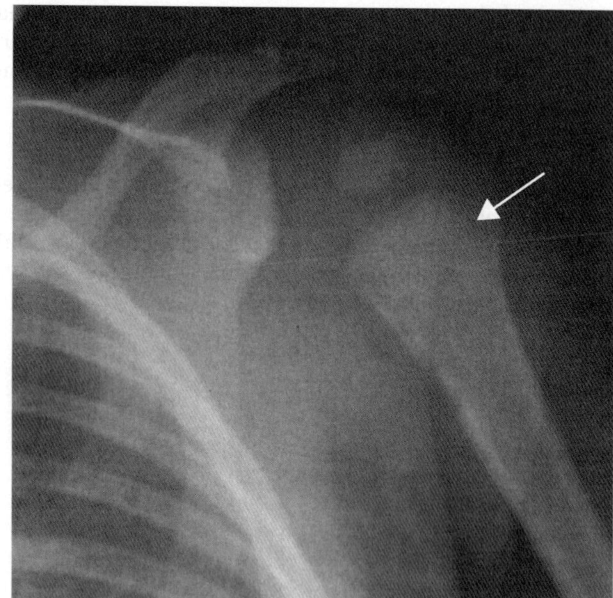

Fig. 27.28 Osteomyelitis of proximal humerus – 'moth eaten' appearance of bone and periosteal reaction.

Microbiology

The goal of microbiological analysis of synovial fluid or biopsy from an infected area of bone is isolation of the infective organism, and determination of appropriate sensitivities to refine the initial empirical antibiotic treatment. Approximately 75% of bone and joint infection in developed countries is currently caused by *Staphylococcus aureus*[58] and the primary source of the infection is rarely clear. The introduction of vaccination against *Haemophilus influenzae type b (Hib)* has dramatically reduced the incidence of septic arthritis caused by this organism. Previously the most common infecting organism in children under the age of 2 years, *Hib* is now a rare cause of skeletal infection in countries where the vaccine is readily available. In neonates *Group B Streptococcus* is a relatively common cause of skeletal infection. Group A beta-hemolytic streptococci (*Streptococcus pyogenes*) and *Streptococcus pneumoniae* are important causes at all ages.

Tuberculous arthritis is insidious in onset, and there is a tendency to sinus formation. If tuberculosis is suspected, synovial fluid and biopsy of synovial tissue should be sent for specific culture and also for analysis by the polymerase chain reaction (PCR). Gonococcal arthritis must be considered in the adolescent presenting systemically unwell with a very acute arthropathy. Brucellosis and infection with *Mycoplasma pneumoniae* may both cause a low grade septic arthritis. In the immunocompromised child Gram negative organisms, fungi or atypical mycobacteria need to be

Table 27.5 Comparison of synovial fluid analysis in children with infective and inflammatory arthritis

Characteristic	Normal	Juvenile idiopathic arthritis	Septic arthritis
Color	Yellow	Yellow	Serosanguinous
Clarity	Clear	Cloudy	Turbid
WBC count/mm^3	< 200	15–20 × 10^3	40–300 000 × 10^3
PMN count (%)	< 25	60–75	> 75

PMN, polymorphic nuerophil; WBC, white blood cell. Adapted from Shetty & Gedalia 1998[57]

(a)

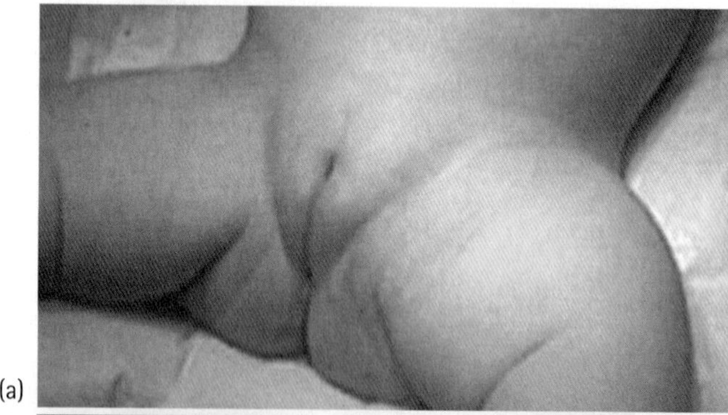

(b)

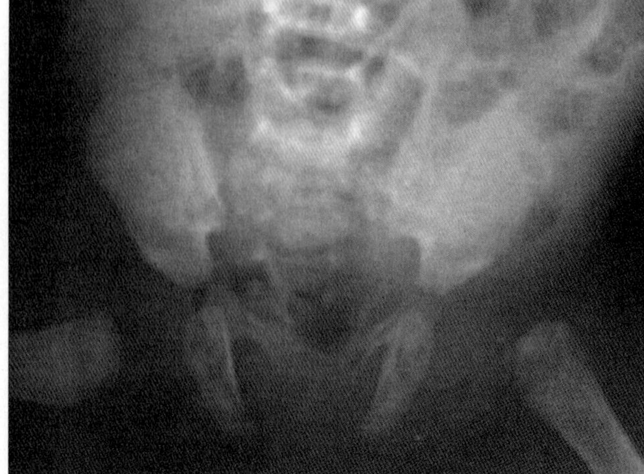

Fig. 27.29 Septic arthritis of the hip: (a) soft tissue swelling of thigh; (b) subluxation of the hip.

considered. Children with hemoglobinopathies are at increased risk of acute recurrent osteomyelitis with Gram negative bacteria such as *Salmonella, Shigella sonnei, Escherichia coli* and *Serratia species.*

Treatment

Treatment of skeletal infections is by a combination of medical and surgical therapy, although there are no controlled trials comparing medical management alone with combined medical and surgical treatment. Initial therapy is supportive with intravenous antibiotics for both osteomyelitis and septic arthritis. With concomitant septicemia management on the neonatal or pediatric intensive care unit may be necessary.

A septic joint should always be aspirated to confirm the diagnosis, allow microbiological studies and relieve pain. Irrigation of the joint at the time of aspiration has not demonstrated additional benefit[59] and there is no consensus on the benefits or otherwise of repeated aspirations or open surgical drainage. The exception to this is the hip where surgical drainage is mandatory to relieve pressure in the joint and minimize the risk of subsequent avascular necrosis. Surgical intervention is not always necessary in osteomyelitis[58] but may facilitate microbiological diagnosis.

The choice of antibiotic will depend on the clinical context and local guidelines, but in the child with previously normal immune function must include adequate staphylococcal cover. A summary of empirical antibiotic therapy in an immunocompetent child is shown in Table 27.6.

In the immunocompromised, flucloxacillin and cefotaxime are first line agents to provide adequate Gram negative cover. In the penicillin allergic child cefradine is an alternative, but if there is also cephalosporin allergy vancomycin should be considered. Cefotaxime or ciprofloxacin may be used in *Salmonella* osteomyelitis.[58]

The duration of antibiotic therapy is controversial. There has been a move towards greater use of oral antibiotics, beyond the initial stages of treatment, in recent years. Intravenous antibiotic therapy should be continued for a minimum of 3 days, then switched to oral for 3–4 weeks if fever has settled.[60] Intravenous administration of antibiotics for longer periods is necessary in the immunocompromised or neonate.

Outcome

With early recognition of the diagnosis and prompt treatment, the long-term outcome of skeletal sepsis in children is good. Growth disturbance may follow septic arthritis or osteomyelitis if the epiphysis has been involved, and these children will require prolonged follow-up. In the minority with articular damage permanent impairment of joint function and early osteoarthritis may ensue (Fig. 27.30). Inadequate or ineffective treatment of acute osteomyelitis may result in chronic osteomyelitis with necrosis and sequestration of the bone.

Table 27.6 Empirical antibiotic therapy in an immunocompetent child with skeletal sepsis

Age	Antibiotic	Dose
Neonate	Flucloxacillin Cefotaxime	50 mg/kg 8 hourly 50 mg/kg 8 hourly
Child < 2 years	Flucloxacillin Cefotaxime	50 mg/kg 6 hourly 50 mg/kg 6 hourly
Child > 2 years	Flucloxacillin Ampicillin	50 mg/kg 6 hourly 100 mg/kg 6 hourly

Adapted from Davies & Monsell 2000[58]

DISCITIS

Infection in the intervertebral disc is a condition related to osteomyelitis, with infection arising from the vertebral end-plates, but without resulting in osteomyelitis of the vertebral body. The condition is believed by many to be secondary to infection,[61] the organism most commonly responsible being *S. aureus*. It is considered by others to have a non-infective inflammatory pathogenesis.

The condition is more common in preschool age children and any disc may be involved. The most striking clinical feature is the refusal of the patient to flex the lumbar spine. The older child may have difficulty walking or limp, will have a stiff back and will complain of back pain associated with constitutional upset. The younger child will frequently refuse to walk and often will spontaneously adopt a prone position with extension of the lumbar spine for comfort.

The blood picture reveals a leukocytosis and raised ESR. Blood culture is usually negative although *S. aureus* may be identified in some. Culture of disc tissue is rarely indicated and frequently negative. The diagnosis is frequently made following radionuclide bone scanning. MRI will demonstrate clearly the inflammatory lesion within the disc (Fig. 27.31a). Plain radiographs eventually reveal disc space narrowing and varying vertebral end-plate damage (Fig. 27.31b).

Most children respond quickly to antibiotic therapy, initially intravenous and then oral, without the need for surgical intervention. Pain is managed symptomatically with analgesics and sometimes a short-term removable brace to unload the involved disc. Therapy is usually continued for 6 weeks. Failure to respond after approximately a week or deterioration in spite of treatment should raise concerns regarding the potential of an abscess that may need surgical drainage or an unusual organism such as

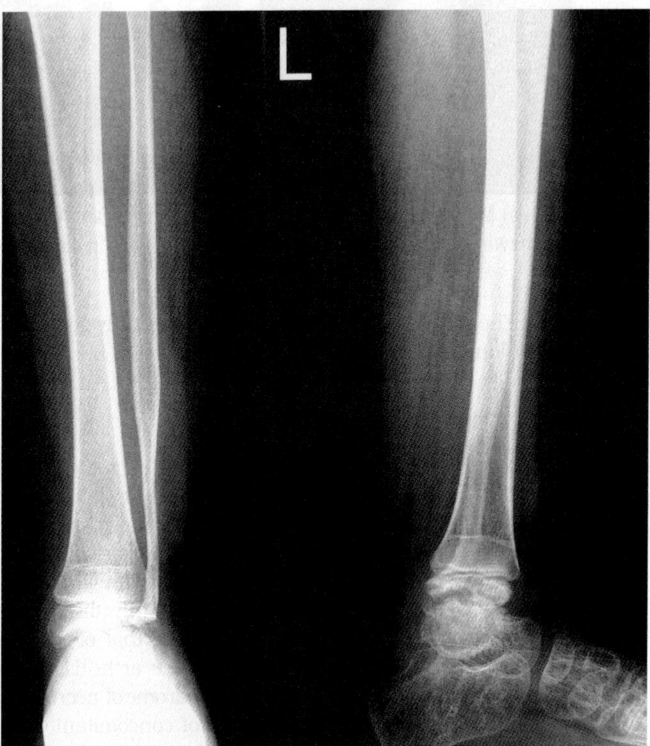

Fig. 27.30 Damage to ankle joint and distal fibula following disseminated staphylococcal sepsis with septic arthritis and osteomyelitis.

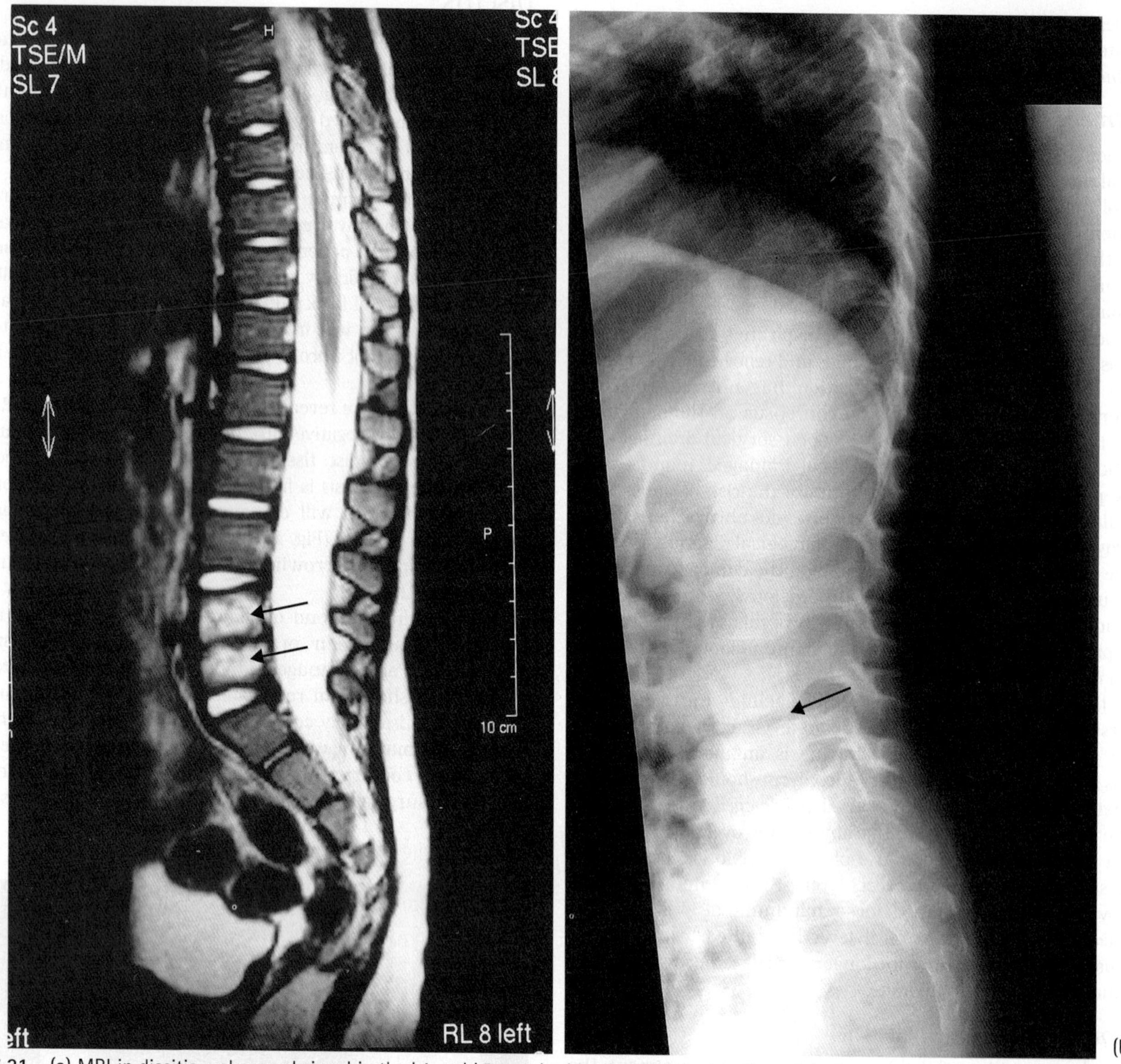

Fig. 27.31 (a) MRI in discitis – abnormal signal in the L4 and L5 vertebral bodies with destruction of the intervening disc space; (b) plain radiograph showing narrowing of L4/5 disc space following resolution of acute illness.

tuberculosis. The prognosis of juvenile discitis is generally good with no significant long term sequelae in the majority.

VIRAL INFECTION AND ARTHRITIS

Arthralgia is a common symptom of viral infection. In some cases a true septic arthritis results, with virus particles being isolated in the joint fluid. In others arthritis occurs as a reactive process with no evidence of infection in the joint. *Rubella*, particularly 'natural infection' but also post vaccination, is associated with arthritis.[62] *Parvovirus B19* (slapped cheek syndrome or Fifth disease) is occasionally associated with an arthritis similar to that of rubella. *Varicella* may be associated with a benign reactive arthritis, but is occasionally complicated by a potentially fatal syndrome of necrotizing fasciitis and toxic shock syndrome as a sequela of concomitant *Group A streptococcus* infection.[63] *Paromyxovirus* (mumps), *adenovirus*, *ECHO virus* and *Coxsackie B* virus may all be associated with arthritis.

Infection with the human immunodeficiency virus may be associated with a variety of rheumatological problems. These include arthralgias, septic arthritis, frequently fungal in origin, as a result of the immune deficiency, reactive arthritis, Reiter's syndrome and a seronegative spondyloarthropathy well described in affected adults.

REACTIVE ARTHRITIS

Transient synovitis of the hip

See section on Common orthopedic problems in childhood, page 1558.

Reactive arthritis associated with bowel and genitourinary infections

In children, as in adults, a reactive arthritis may develop after enteric infections with *Salmonella*, *Shigella*, *Yersinia* and *Campylobacter*, and post urethritis with *Chlamydia* in sexually active adolescents. The HLA B27 antigen is commonly found in children with this pattern of reactive arthritis which is frequently a peripheral, asymmetric lower limb arthritis. There may be associated dactylitis ('sausage digit' resulting from inflammation of both joints and tendon sheaths), tenosynovitis and involvement of the sacroiliac joints. There is usually a history of enteritis or urethritis within the preceding 4 weeks. Reiter's syndrome, a triad of arthritis, conjunctivitis and urethritis, is uncommon in children.

Treatment includes non-steroidal anti-inflammatory drugs in adequate doses. Occasionally systemic steroids are required to settle an acute arthritis. If the arthritis becomes chronic, intra-articular steroids and second-line agents including sulfasalazine and methotrexate may be considered as with other chronic arthropathies in childhood.

Rheumatic fever and post-streptococcal arthritis

Acute rheumatic fever remains prevalent in developing areas of the world. The disease arises as a complication of infection (pharyngo-tonsillitis) with *Group A beta-hemolytic Streptococcus pyogenes*. The modified Jones criteria are the basis for the diagnosis of acute rheumatic fever, and are shown in Table 27.7.

Inflammation in various tissues results in arthritis, carditis, a typical rash (erythema marginatum), subcutaneous nodules and a characteristic neurological syndrome, Sydenham's chorea. Pathologically, an immune mediated reaction occurs that culminates in a disseminated vasculitis. The pathognomic lesion, the Aschoff body, is seen on histological analysis of the heart.

Arthritis is a common clinical feature, tends to affect large joints and is flitting and self-limiting in nature. The rash associated with acute rheumatic fever is erythema marginatum, manifest by erythematous macular and non-pruritic serpiginous margins surrounding areas of normal skin. Sydenham's chorea (also known as St Vitus' dance) is caused by inflammation of the basal ganglia of the brain. It presents with involuntary movements of the extremities, muscular incoordination and emotional lability. Subcutaneous nodules may be seen on extensor surfaces of joints in the chronic phase of rheumatic heart disease.

Inflammation of the heart may affect all layers resulting in a pancarditis, and this manifestation accounts for the majority of the morbidity and mortality of acute rheumatic fever. Myocarditis leads to a resting tachycardia and electrocardiographic changes (prolonged P-R interval, heart block, arrhythmias). Endocarditis may result in valvular damage with murmurs arising from mitral and aortic regurgitation in the acute phase, and corresponding valve stenoses in the chronic stages of the disease. Pericarditis rarely occurs in isolation and is more usually seen with pancarditis. Rheumatic heart disease is discussed in more detail in Chapter 19.

Table 27.7 Modified Jones criteria for the diagnosis of rheumatic fever

Major criteria	Minor criteria
Polyarthritis common: flitting, large joints	Fever
Carditis common: pancarditis	Arthralgia
Chorea (Sydenham's) uncommon: persistent	Prolonged P-R interval
Erythema marginatum uncommon: macules evolving to serpiginous	Elevated ESR/CRP, leukocytosis
Subcutaneous nodules uncommon: extensor surfaces	Previous rheumatic fever

The diagnosis of rheumatic fever is made in the presence of either two major criteria or one major plus two minor criteria together with evidence of recent group A streptococcal infection (positive throat swab, elevated antistreptolysin O titer (ASOT) or other antistreptococcal antibodies).

Arthritis following Group A streptococcal infection is recognized in some children who do not fulfil the criteria for acute rheumatic fever. This post-streptococcal reactive arthritis differs from that of rheumatic fever in that it is non-migratory and more persistent. As with rheumatic fever recurrent episodes are recognized.

Treatment of both rheumatic fever and post-streptococcal reactive arthritis involves antibiotics to eradicate the streptococcus. Penicillin V is the antibiotic of choice, and should be given as a 10 day course. In penicillin allergic individuals, erythromycin is a suitable alternative. Non-steroidal anti-inflammatory drugs (NSAIDs) may provide symptomatic relief from the arthritis. Steroids are reserved for patients with pancarditis associated with congestive cardiac failure. In rheumatic fever prophylaxis against streptococcal infection is indicated for at least 5 years after the initial attack, and into adulthood in patients with carditis.[64] There is no consensus regarding the use of prophylactic penicillin in those with post-streptococcal arthritis but if attacks are recurrent antibiotic prophylaxis may prove beneficial. Additional prophylaxis for surgical or dental procedures is necessary in the chronic stage of rheumatic heart disease (see Ch. 19).

Lyme disease

The infectious spirochaete *Borrelia burgdorferi*, transmitted by the tick Ixodes, is responsible for Lyme disease. The regions where Lyme disease is seen most frequently are central Europe and north-eastern United States. The disease is manifest by cutaneous, articular, neurological and other systemic features. The most typical skin manifestation is erythema chronicum migrans. Early lymphocytic meningitis is commoner in children than in adults. The arthritis typically appears months to years after the original infection, and becomes chronic in up to 16%.[65] In the majority there is an episodic monoarthritis, but occasionally polyarthritis develops. Treatment with antibiotics is necessary, with ceftriaxone recommended at a dose of 50 mg/kg/day for 14–28 days.[65] Amoxicillin at a dose of 50 mg/kg/day for 28 days is an alternative, but compliance may be poorer due to the dosage regimen. Some authors recommend doxycycline, but not in children below the age of 8 years. Intra-articular steroids should be avoided until completion of antibiotic therapy.

Arthritis associated with meningococcal infection

Meningococcal disease may be associated with both a true septic arthritis occurring in association with the acute septicemic illness or a reactive arthritis seen in the post-acute phase. With improved survival rates from severe meningococcal septicemia a post-infectious, immune complex mediated arthritis is seen with increasing frequency, often in association with a recrudescence of fever and the development of a vasculitic rash.

JUVENILE IDIOPATHIC ARTHRITIS

Juvenile idiopathic arthritis (JIA) is not a single entity, rather a group of conditions with differing clinical and immunogenetic features. Synovitis, manifest as swelling within a joint, or limitation in range of joint movement with associated joint pain or tenderness and persisting for at least 6 weeks, is the essential clinical feature of all subtypes of JIA.

There have been many advances in the last decade of the twentieth century in aspects of JIA including new classification criteria, an improved understanding of immunogenetic pathways and new therapies. Standardized criteria for defining improvement in JIA have been developed,[66] and there has been the significant development of multicenter collaborative trials under the auspices of organizations such as the Pediatric Rheumatology International Trials Organisation (PRINTO).

Despite this progress JIA remains by definition a disease of unknown cause for which there is no curative treatment. However there is no doubt that the improved treatment options currently available are associated with an outcome that is now frequently favorable, allowing the young person with JIA to function normally in childhood and to undergo a normal transition into independent adulthood.

HISTORICAL OVERVIEW

Although possibly depicted in paintings from the Middle Ages, it was in the late nineteenth century that the first detailed descriptions of juvenile arthritis appeared, most famously by Still. He described chronic childhood arthritis, in particular the features of the systemic form later associated with his name, from personal clinical observation of 19 cases. Still also suggested that chronic arthritis in childhood may include more than one disease.

It was not until the latter half of the twentieth century that the view that childhood chronic arthritis represented a disease different from that seen in adults prevailed and distinct diagnostic criteria were developed. Classification criteria were developed in both Europe and North America in the 1970s and more recently a unified classification system has been proposed.[67]

CLASSIFICATION

There has been an important proposed change in the nomenclature of the chronic arthritides of childhood since the previous edition of this text. Previously two major but different classification criteria were in use, both based on the clinical onset pattern of the arthritis. The European League Against Rheumatism (EULAR) criteria used the term juvenile chronic arthritis (JCA) to describe the idiopathic arthritides of childhood.[68] The American College of Rheumatology (ACR) adopted the term juvenile rheumatoid arthritis (JRA).[69] Unfortunately although these two sets of criteria overlapped, they differed in several respects. Such differences continue to cause confusion for clinicians, scientists, patients and their families and undoubtedly impaired research into childhood arthritis. With this background, the Classification Taskforce of the Pediatric Standing Committee of the International League of Associations for Rheumatology (ILAR) proposed consensus criteria for the classification of childhood arthritis under the umbrella term juvenile idiopathic arthritis.[67] A comparison of these three sets of classification criteria is given in Table 27.8.

The ILAR criteria represent an important development. The fundamental goal of the classification committee was 'to develop criteria that would enable the identification of homogenous groups of children with chronic arthritis to facilitate research in immunogenetics and other basic sciences, epidemiology, outcome studies and therapeutic trials'.

Despite some concerns that children with similar clinical features may not in fact have disease with the same cause, and that a valid classification system can only be based on pathophysiology, many pediatric rheumatologists have embraced the ILAR criteria, although there remains the need for further evaluation and revision.

DIFFERENTIAL DIAGNOSIS

Juvenile idiopathic arthritis must be considered a diagnosis of exclusion. Any child presenting with musculoskeletal symptoms requires careful assessment by means of thorough history taking, meticulous clinical examination and judicious use of appropriate investigations. The age of the child and the clinical presentation will guide the diagnostic process. If the history and clinical examination confirm inflammatory joint disease then the differential diagnosis is different from the child with non-inflammatory features. Inherited disorders that present with true arthritis or other joint manifestations including stiffness and pain, are discussed in a previous section. The differential diagnosis of inflammatory arthropathies in childhood is shown in Table 27.9.

ETIOLOGY AND PATHOGENESIS

Epidemiology

Epidemiological studies have suggested that the basis of susceptibility to JIA is complex, comprising both genetic and environmental risk factors.

The incidence of childhood chronic arthritis is estimated to be 10–19.2:100 000 children in Europe and North America.[70] Despite methodological differences between studies there does appear to be a true variability in disease occurrence according to geographical factors. Ethnic differences in individual JIA onset patterns have also been reported, with African–American children more likely to have

Table 27.8 A comparison of classification criteria for the idiopathic inflammatory arthritides in childhood

ILAR	EULAR	ACR
Juvenile idiopathic arthritis Onset < 16 years Duration 6 weeks Subtypes: 1. systemic arthritis 2. oligoarticular arthritis —persistent —extended 3. polyarthritis; RF –ve 4. polyarthritis; RF +ve 5. enthesitis related arthritis 6. psoriatic arthritis 7. other arthritis	Juvenile chronic arthritis Onset < 16 years Duration 3 months Subtypes: 1. systemic arthritis 2. pauciarticular arthritis 3. polyarticular arthritis (excludes RF +ve disease: known as juvenile rheumatoid arthritis)	Juvenile rheumatoid arthritis Onset < 16 years Duration 6 weeks Subtypes: 1. systemic arthritis 2. pauciarticular arthritis 3. polyarticular arthritis (excludes spondyloarthropathies and psoriatic arthritis)

ACR, American College of Rheumatology; EULAR, European League Against Rheumatism; ILAR, International League of Associations for Rheumatology; RF, rheumatoid factor.

Table 27.9 Differential diagnosis of inflammatory arthritis in childhood

Infection:
Acute septic arthritis
Viral arthritis
Reactive/post-infectious arthritis
Juvenile idiopathic arthritis
Arthritis associated with inflammatory bowel disease
Other autoimmune rheumatic disorders:
Systemic lupus erythematosus
Juvenile dermatomyositis
Systemic sclerosis
Mixed connective tissue disease
Systemic vasculitis:
Henoch–Schönlein purpura
Kawasaki disease
Polyarteritis nodosa
Malignancy:
Leukemia
Neuroblastoma
Hematological:
Sickle cell anemia
Hemophilia
Immune deficiency
Genetic disorders:
Cystic fibrosis
Velocardiofacial syndrome
CINCA syndrome
Down syndrome
Stickler syndrome
Drug reactions
Trauma including non-accidental injury
Miscellaneous:
Sarcoidosis
SAPHO syndrome
Familial Mediterranean fever

CINCA, chronic infantile neurological, cutaneous and articular syndrome; SAPHO, synovitis, acne, pustulosis, hyperostosis and osteitis.

polyarticular onset disease compared to Caucasian children in whom oligoarticular onset is more common.[71]

Seasonal variations in disease occurrence in patients with subgroups of JIA have been reported. The disease subtype with the most frequently reported seasonal variation of onset is systemic JIA[72] and such studies lend support to the theory of environmental triggers, particularly infections. Many infective agents have been proposed, including influenza, parvovirus, rubella and Coxsackie virus, but to date there remains no conclusive evidence of a specific infective etiology.[73]

Overall, girls outnumber boys by approximately 2:1 in JIA. There are important variations within disease subtypes with girls outnumbering boys in oligoarthritis, polyarthritis and psoriatic arthritis, but a more even sex distribution in systemic JIA.[74] Boys significantly outnumber girls in the enthesitis related arthritis subtype (see below for definitions of subtypes). In children with uveitis the ratio of girls to boys is higher, up to 6.6:1.[75]

In Europe and North America a bimodal age of onset is frequently described. The early peak tends to be between 1 and 3 years and is largely accounted for by girls with oligoarthritis. The second peak occurs in later childhood, at approximately 9 years of age and is made up of roughly equal numbers of boys and girls. In certain parts of the world where the incidence of young girls with oligoarthritis is less, this bimodal distribution is not seen.

Genetics

JIA has been referred to as a 'complex genetic trait', albeit one in which there are now several consistent and strong associations.[76] Disease occurrence differences in epidemiological studies have generated the hypothesis that there are differences in genetic susceptibility. Studies of genetic polymorphisms in both adult and childhood chronic arthritis have frequently, but not exclusively, involved the major histocompatibility complex (MHC), following the original observation by Statsny in 1978 of an association with the HLA DRB1 locus in 80 patients with rheumatoid arthritis.[77] Human leukocyte antigen (HLA) genes are located within the major histocompatibility complex (MHC) on chromosome 6. The MHC class II loci DR, DQ and DP are particularly associated with JIA. Age related genetic susceptibility is suggested by the association of early childhood onset oligoarthritis with HLA A2, DR5, DR8, and DPB1*0201.[78] Oligoarthritis in older boys is associated with HLA B27, and to date this remains the only HLA association with any major relevance to routine clinical practice. Polyarticular JIA with a positive rheumatoid factor is associated with HLA DR4, as in adults with rheumatoid arthritis. A detailed review of HLA associations in JIA including theories on how HLA antigens are involved in disease pathogenesis is available elsewhere.[79]

Despite progress in this field the goal of an ideal disease classification based on a combination of clinical features and genetic markers remains in the future.

Cytokines

Cytokines, a family of soluble proteins involved in the regulation of the immune system, are produced by several classes of cells involved in the inflammatory process, and are responsible for regulating cell growth, differentiation and/or function and maintaining tissue homeostasis. In studies of synovial tissue from adults with rheumatoid arthritis, proinflammatory cytokines such as interleukin (IL)-1, and tumor necrosis factor (TNF)-alpha are elevated, and induce the release of tissue destroying metalloproteinases.[80] There has been great interest in the role of cytokines as mediators of the inflammatory response in JIA, both to further the understanding of the pathogenesis of the disease and also as potential targets for biological therapies.

Cytokines may have inflammatory or anti-inflammatory properties, and an imbalance between these two effects is fundamental in the pathogenesis of JIA. This imbalance may be a result of persistent antigen presence, or genetic imbalance in the cytokine network.[81] Examples of pro- and anti-inflammatory cytokines are shown in Table 27.10.

Table 27.10 Pro- and anti-inflammatory cytokines relevant in juvenile idiopathic arthritis

Pro-Inflammatory cytokines	Anti-Inflammatory cytokines
Interferon-gamma Interleukin-1 alpha and beta	Interleukin-1 receptor antagonist
Tumor necrosis factor-alpha	Interleukin-4
Lymphotoxin-alpha	Interleukin-10
Interleukin-6	Interleukin-13
Interleukin-12 (induces IFN-gamma)	Transforming growth factor-beta
	Soluble receptors (e.g. sTNFR and IL-1R) Interleukin-6

Adapted from Woo 1998[81]

The proinflammatory cytokine TNF-alpha occupies a central position in the cytokine network. TNF-alpha is produced by several cells throughout the body, including synovial cells, T-lymphocytes and mononuclear phagocytes, but in inflammatory arthritis its main site of origin is activated macrophages. TNF-alpha, with lymphotoxin-alpha (a related cytokine), is detected in synovial tissue in JIA and may amplify local inflammation and contribute to joint destruction.[82] TNF-alpha stimulates further proinflammatory cytokine production including IL-1 and IL-6.

JIA is a heterogeneous disease. It is not surprising then that studies have revealed differences in cytokine profiles between JIA subtypes. Rooney et al demonstrated an imbalance between TNF-alpha and its soluble receptor (sTNFR) in JIA, with different ratios in different subtypes, which may explain variations in resulting joint damage.[83] Children with extended compared to persistent oligoarthritis have evidence of a genetically determined lower IL-10 production.[84] As IL-10 is an important anti-inflammatory cytokine, this may explain why children with extended oligoarthritis tend to have more severe articular disease.

These observations and others have led to, and subsequently supported, the development of biological therapies particularly those targeted against TNF (see section on treatment).

CLINICAL FEATURES

Juvenile idiopathic arthritis remains a clinical diagnosis. The onset may be insidious over several months or much more rapid over a period of a few weeks. The presenting features vary according to the age and developmental stage of the child and the clinical subtype of the disease. In systemic arthritis and psoriatic arthritis, the relevant associated clinical features may precede the onset of the arthritis sometimes by many months.

The classical features of inflammation in a joint, namely swelling, heat, pain and loss of function, are paramount to the diagnosis of JIA. Marked erythema over the joint is suggestive of a more acute process such as reactive or septic arthritis. Rest may exacerbate symptoms, so children will complain of stiffness in the morning or after periods of inactivity. Pain is a feature of JIA, although it does not always correlate with disease activity and it should be noted that young children rarely complain specifically of pain. Tenderness may be elicited on passive movement of the inflamed joint.

Systemic upset is common in polyarthritis and a universal feature of systemic JIA. However even in children with oligoarthritis there may be subtle signs of systemic disturbance including vague malaise, anorexia, pallor, weight loss and sleep disturbance which may be underreported in the literature. Parents often report that their child is 'not quite their normal self'.

Oligoarthritis

Oligoarthritis is defined as arthritis affecting one to four joints during the first 6 months of disease, and is further subdivided into persistent oligoarthritis: no more than four joints throughout the disease course; and extended oligoarthritis: affects a cumulative total of five joints or more after the first 6 months of disease.

Oligoarthritis is the commonest onset pattern of JIA in Caucasian populations, accounting for approximately 50% of affected children.[74] This subtype is classically seen in preschool age girls (although does occur in boys) and in this age group is frequently associated with positive antinuclear antibodies (ANA) and an increased risk of silent uveitis. These children must be screened regularly by an ophthalmologist.

Oligoarthritis most frequently develops asymmetrically in large lower limb joints, especially the knee (Fig. 27.32) and the ankle, and occasionally in the upper limb. The initial presentation is frequently of a monoarthritis. In a child with a monoarthritis several differential diagnoses must be considered (Table 27.11). Any acutely painful, warm and swollen joint, with or without erythema, should raise the clinical suspicion of septic arthritis and examination of the joint fluid should be considered. JIA presenting with isolated hip disease is unusual and other causes of hip pain must be considered in the child with isolated hip symptoms.

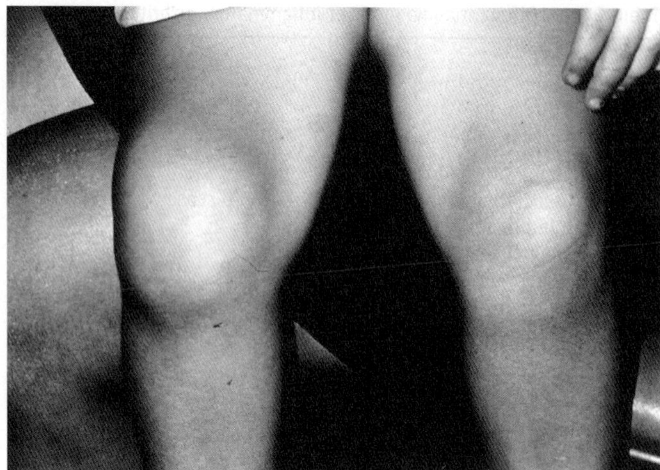

Fig. 27.32 Oligoarthritis showing marked swelling of R knee.

Oligoarthritis in preschool children is often insidious, but occasionally manifests over a short time period. The child may limp, especially after rest. The joint appears swollen and is warm, but rarely painful until passively moved through its full range. Examination of the knee may reveal a palpable effusion. With time, if unrecognized, flexion contractures may occur especially at the knee. Bony overgrowth of the joint may be seen and leg length discrepancy may develop due to overgrowth of affected limb (Fig. 27.33). Prompt recognition and treatment will prevent the development of such complications.

In a proportion of children with an oligoarticular onset there is an 'adding on' of involved joints beyond 6 months of disease-extended oligoarthritis. This polyarticular course is associated with a poorer outcome with an increased incidence of joint destruction.[85]

Table 27.11 Differential diagnosis of monoarthritis

Infection	Bacterial septic arthritis, osteomyelitis Direct infection with other agents including virus, fungi, spirochete Tuberculosis
Reactive arthritis	Response to infection elsewhere, e.g. post streptococcal, post viral, Reiter's syndrome, post dysenteric
Post-infectious arthritis	Articular deposition of immune complexes post meningococcal disease
Neoplastic disease	Acute leukemia, neuroblastoma Localized bone or cartilage malignancy
Hematological disease	Hemophilia, sickle cell disease
Trauma	Accidental and non-accidental injury
Miscellaneous	Vascular malformation Pigmented villonodular synovitis

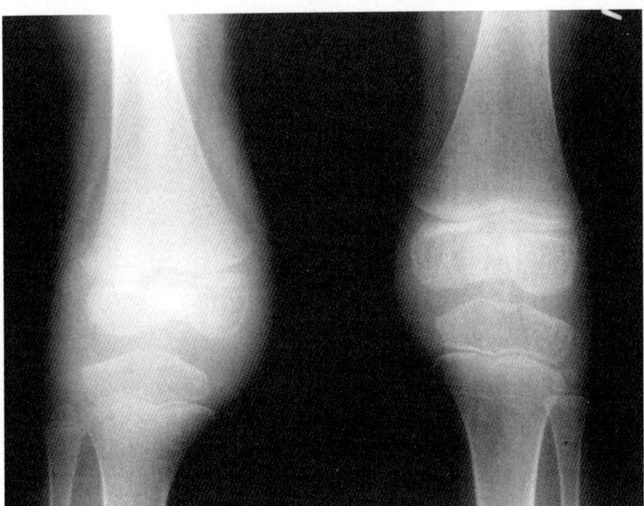

Fig. 27.33 Oligoarthritis – plain radiograph showing overgrowth of right knee.

Polyarthritis

This subtype of JIA is defined as arthritis affecting five or more joints during the first 6 months of disease. Polyarticular JIA is commoner in girls, and is further subdivided on the basis of testing for IgM rheumatoid factor into rheumatoid factor positive (seropositive) and rheumatoid factor negative disease. Seropositive JIA is rare, accounting for only 3% of all children with JIA, compared to 17% for seronegative polyarthritis.[74]

Children with seropositive polyarthritis are typically girls who develop disease in late childhood and adolescence. The arthritis is usually symmetrical affecting upper and lower limbs, in particular the small joints of the hands and feet. The test for IgM rheumatoid factor should be positive on at least two occasions 3 months apart. Rheumatoid factor positive polyarthritis represents an early manifestation of adult rheumatoid arthritis and may result in a poor outcome with destructive joint disease.

Seronegative polyarthritis (Fig. 27.34) has a variable clinical expression ranging from low grade grumbling disease to an aggressive polyarthritis. Compared to seropositive disease the peak age of onset is earlier in childhood, typically 6–7 years of age.

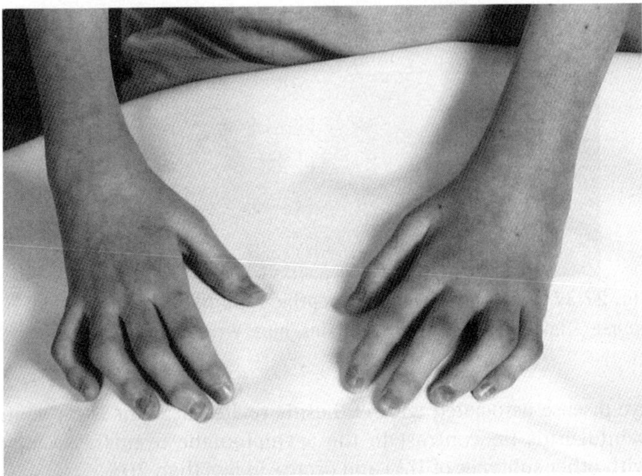

Fig. 27.34 Polyarthritis affecting wrists and the small joints of the hands.

Systemic arthritis

The systemic onset subtype accounts for 11% of all cases of JIA, often occurring in younger children with a median age of onset of 4.3 years and a male to female ratio of 1:1.2.[74] Systemic JIA is characterized by arthritis accompanied by a specific fever pattern. There are also a wide variety of extra-articular manifestations and children with systemic JIA have features that may be suggestive of sepsis and malignancy. These conditions require careful exclusion. Although mandatory to the diagnosis arthritis may not be present at the onset of the disease.

The fever of systemic JIA must be present for at least 2 weeks and documented to be quotidian, spiking once or twice a day, usually in the evening with return to baseline between pyrexial episodes (Fig. 27.35). The associated disease manifestations such as the rash are often much worse during the periods of fever, and the children are intensely miserable during these periods. In addition to fever and arthritis the diagnosis requires one or more of the following extra-articular features:

1. rash
2. generalized lymph node enlargement
3. hepatosplenomegaly
4. serositis.

The rash is pale pink and macular and is flitting in nature. It may occur in linear streaks and exhibits the Koebner phenomenon (Fig. 27.36). It most commonly occurs on the trunk, but can be generalized. Generalized lymphadenopathy occurs in the majority, and enlarged nodes are painless, rubbery and mobile. Hepatomegaly is common and splenomegaly present in approximately 50%. Serositis is often mild and asymptomatic but significant pericarditis is recognized and may require specific treatment including surgical drainage.

The pattern of arthritis associated with systemic JIA is variable, and it may not be apparent at the onset of the illness. Approximately one-third of children develop a polyarticular course with joint destruction within 2 years of disease onset (Fig. 27.37). Three patterns of disease progression have been described:

1. monocyclic – systemic disease with a single episode;
2. intermittent – recurrent fever and arthritis interspersed with periods of remission;
3. persistent disease activity with systemic and polyarticular phases.

Functional outcome is largely dependent on the nature of the arthritis course rather than that of the systemic features. Risk factors for an adverse outcome in systemic JIA are thrombocytosis, persistent fever and steroid dependency at 6 months.[86]

Psoriatic arthritis

In addition to children with psoriasis and arthritis (Fig. 27.38), this subgroup includes children with psoriasis or arthritis and at least two of the following:

1. dactylitis;
2. nail abnormalities – pitting or onycholysis;
3. family history of psoriasis confirmed by a dermatologist in at least one first degree relative.

In the UK, psoriatic arthritis accounts for 7% of all cases of JIA, is commoner in girls (male:female ratio 1:1.6) and has a median age of onset of 10 years.[74] Oligoarticular onset (with asymmetric involvement of large and small joints) is frequent and dactylitis (diffuse swelling of a finger or toe joint and periarticular tissues; Fig. 27.39) is a hallmark. Nail abnormalities may be seen, including nail pitting and nail dystrophy (onycholysis).

The arthritis precedes the psoriasis in as many as 75% of cases: 45% of children develop psoriasis within 5 years of onset of arthritis.[87] The outcome in psoriatic arthritis is variable, with both oligo- and polyarticular courses described.

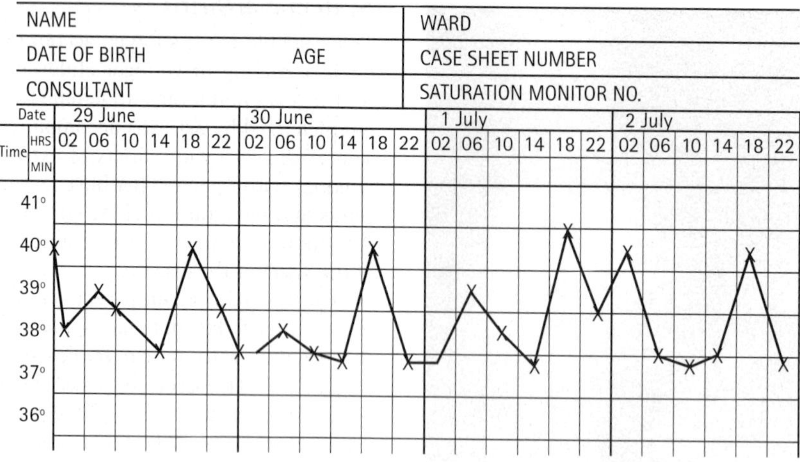

Fig. 27.35 Typical spiking fever in systemic JIA.

Fig. 27.36 Rash of systemic juvenile idiopathic arthritis.

Enthesitis related arthritis

Enthesitis is defined as inflammation of the insertion of tendons into bones. This new diagnostic group is intended to define those with disease related to the HLA antigen B27, and avoids the term juvenile spondyloarthropathy; inaccurate because of the rarity of spinal involvement in children.

Enthesitis related arthritis is defined as arthritis and enthesitis; or arthritis; or enthesitis with at least two of the following features:

1. sacroiliac joint tenderness and/or inflammatory spinal pain;
2. presence of HLA B27;
3. family history in at least one first or second degree relative of medically confirmed HLA B27 associated disease;
4. anterior uveitis that is usually associated with pain, redness, or photophobia;
5. onset of arthritis in a boy after 8 years of age.

The commonest joints involved are the peripheral large joints of the lower limb, in an asymmetrical distribution. It is rare for children to present with axial skeleton symptoms or signs, although a minority develop arthritis of the sacroiliac joints (Fig. 27.40) and subsequently ankylosing spondylitis in adulthood. There is a marked predominance of boys in this group, presenting after the age of 8 years. Enthesitis is a characteristic feature, often affecting the insertion of the Achilles tendon into the calcaneum, and is usually painful resulting in significant functional impairment. The eye disease associated with enthesitis related arthritis is an acute painful iritis (in contrast to the asymptomatic uveitis associated with other subtypes of JIA) and occurs in less than 20%.

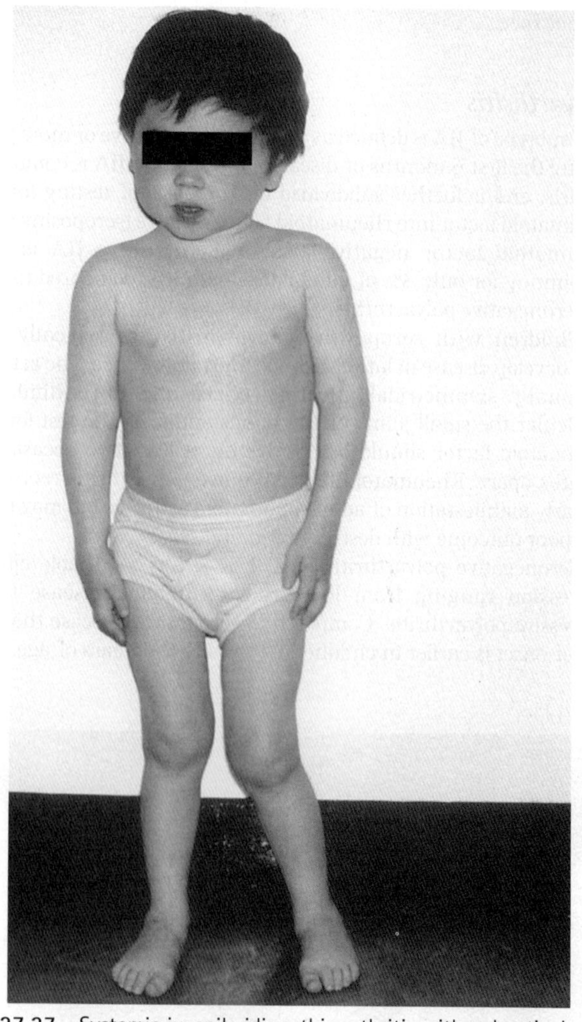

Fig. 27.37 Systemic juvenile idiopathic arthritis with polyarticular course – involvement of knees, ankles, hips, wrists and cervical spine.

Children with reactive arthritis and arthritis associated with inflammatory bowel disease (IBD) are by definition excluded

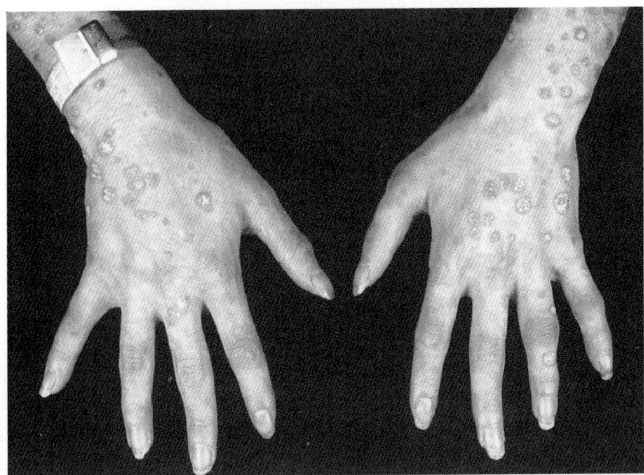

Fig. 27.38 Psoriatic arthritis.

from this diagnostic subgroup even if positive for HLA B27. Children with IBD can develop both axial and peripheral arthritis and enthesitis, in association with inflammatory eye disease, and as such share some of the features of the enthesitis related arthritis subtype of JIA. Indeed the arthritis may pre-date the onset of bowel symptoms. In the presence of HLA B27, children with IBD are also predisposed to sacroiliitis and ankylosing spondylitis.

Other arthritis

At present children are labeled 'other arthritis' if they have JIA but either do not fulfil criteria for any of the other categories or fulfil criteria for more than one of the other categories. This is a major new addition to the classification criteria and is included in recognition of the fact that not all children with arthritis are currently classifiable.

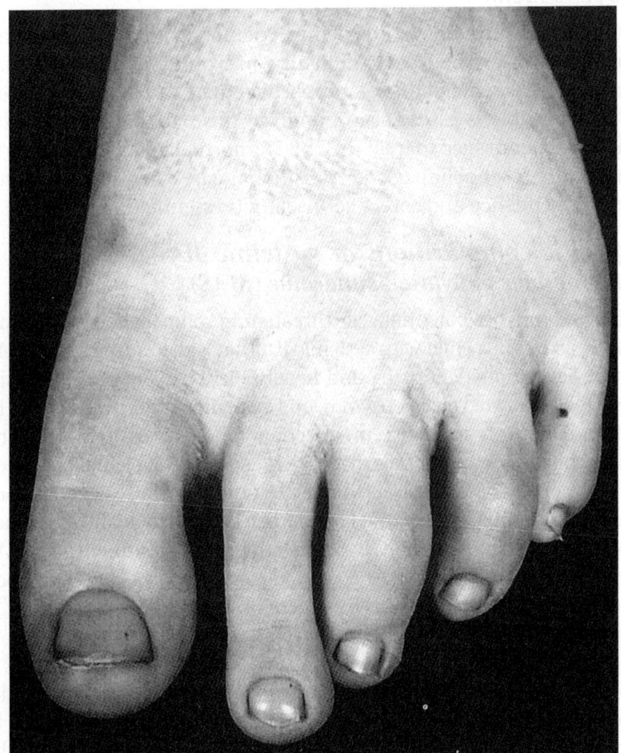

Fig. 27.39 Dactylitis – swelling of third and fourth toes.

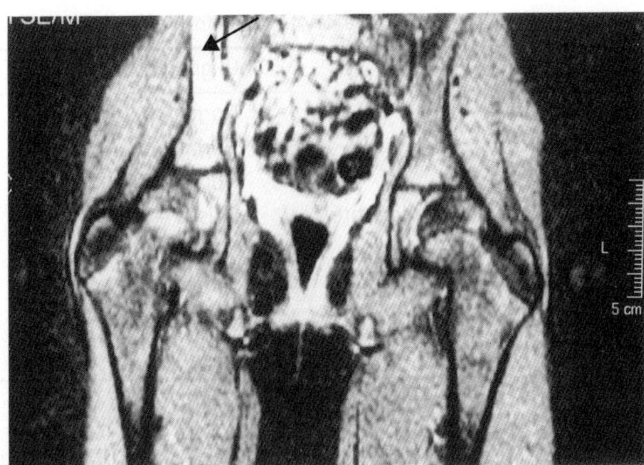

Fig. 27.40 Gadolinium enhanced MRI showing right sided sacroiliitis (note high signal on right compared to left).

INVESTIGATIONS

Judicious use of laboratory investigations may serve to support the diagnosis of JIA and aid with classification. Basic investigations will reflect the underlying inflammatory process but it must be remembered that a child may have JIA with normal inflammatory markers. The common findings are summarized in Table 27.12. Synovial fluid analysis is not required for diagnostic purposes in JIA.

Further investigations are dependent on the clinical picture. Anemia of chronic disease is especially marked in systemic JIA and leukocytosis and thrombocytosis are frequently seen. Non-specific hyperimmunoglobulinemia occurs in both polyarticular and systemic subtypes. Hypoalbuminemia and a mild transaminitis are common in systemic JIA and a disproportionately high serum ferritin may also be seen. Thrombocytopenia or leukopenia in systemic JIA may be an early manifestation of the macrophage activation syndrome (see section on Complications of JIA, below).

A positive antinuclear antibody in oligoarthritis is a risk factor for silent uveitis and will help to guide the ophthalmology screening program. Rheumatoid factor is only of clinical significance in the context of those children with a polyarthritis, especially when symmetrically affecting small joints. A positive test for HLA B27 may help classify the enthesitis related subtype.

Radiological investigations

Radiological imaging is not diagnostic in JIA but may aid in the exclusion of other diagnoses and is useful in following progress of the disease. Three stages of radiographic changes are seen on plain radiographs in JIA:[88] *early*: periarticular osteopenia; *intermediate*: cortical erosions, joint space narrowing and subchondral cysts and *late*: destructive joint changes with ankylosis, joint contractures, metaphyseal and diaphyseal changes and growth anomalies (Fig. 27.41).

Radionuclide bone scanning is sensitive in detecting areas of increased uptake within the skeleton, but will not differentiate between inflammation, infection or malignant disease. Ultrasound is a reliable method for detecting effusions, especially in the hip. It may have other indications, including guiding intra-articular injections and confirmation of popliteal cysts. Intravenous contrast (gadolinium-DPTA) enhanced magnetic resonance sequences are exquisitely sensitive at detecting inflamed synovium and particularly valuable in the assessment of inaccessible joints such as the hip, and complex joints such as the ankle, where it may be difficult to distinguish clinically between the tibiotalar and

Table 27.12 Common laboratory findings in the major juvenile idiopathic arthritis subtypes

Investigation	Oligoarthritis	Polyarthritis	Systemic disease
Hemoglobin	Normal	Low (anemia of chronic disease)	Low (anemia of chronic disease)
White cell count	Normal	Raised +	Raised +++
Platelets	Normal	Raised +	Raised +++
Erythrocyte sedimentation rate	Raised +	Raised ++	Raised +++
C-reactive protein	Normal	Raised +	Raised ++
Liver enzymes	Normal	Normal	Often raised
Antinuclear antibody	Often positive	Normal	Normal
Rheumatoid factor	Negative	Positive in subgroup	Normal

sub-talar joint (Fig. 27.42). Computed tomography (CT) is useful for visualizing certain joints, especially the sacroiliac joints.

COMPLICATIONS OF JIA: ARTICULAR

Articular complications are a direct result of synovial inflammation and can generally be minimized or prevented by optimizing control of the inflammatory process. Flexion contractures occur commonly and at a very early stage in JIA and if not treated intensively may become permanent. Overgrowth of affected limbs (Fig. 27.33) is a particular problem of oligoarthritis which may have serious long term complications. A discrepancy in lower limb length may result in a pelvic tilt and scoliosis in adult life. The temporomandibular joint (TMJ) may be involved in polyarthritis and specific features such as asymmetric mouth opening and micrognathia may be noted during clinical examination. TMJ involvement may result in both cosmetic and functional difficulties and appropriate advice from an interested maxillofacial surgeon should be sought.

COMPLICATIONS OF JIA: EXTRA-ARTICULAR

Uveitis

The incidence of uveitis in JIA overall is approximately 10%, although it is commoner in ANA positive oligoarthritis.[89] Two patterns of ocular inflammation are seen in JIA. An acute, painful iritis is seen in children with enthesitis related arthritis, and usually resolves rapidly with topical corticosteroid therapy. Chronic, asymptomatic anterior uveitis that may become sight threatening if not recognized and treated is especially common in preschool age girls with oligoarthritis. It is strongly associated with positive antinuclear antibodies. The presence of HLA DR5, and absence of HLA DR1 appear to be particular risk factors for its development.[90] The diagnosis requires slit-lamp examination by an ophthalmologist. Follow-up depends on the relative risk, but 3 monthly for 5 years followed by 6 monthly until adulthood is recommended for high risk children with oligoarthritis.

In many cases uveitis in children with JIA can be controlled with topical corticosteroids and short acting mydriatics. In refractory cases, or if there is significant steroid toxicity, methotrexate is the commonest second line agent in use, although there is some evidence for the use of ciclosporin and anti-TNF therapy.[91] Visual complications (synechiae, band keratopathy, cataract or glaucoma) may develop in up to 30% of cases, and significant visual loss has been reported in 11% although blindness is uncommon.[89]

Nutritional status and growth

Nutritional impairment is a recognized complication of JIA. The etiology of nutritional impairment in JIA is not fully understood, nor is it clear how frequently it occurs. Nutritional impairment affects the general well-being of the child and contributes to the growth disturbance that is a serious consequence of JIA in some children. Mid upper arm circumference (MUAC) and body mass index may be used as composite measures of nutritional status. For intervention to be appropriate further understanding of the cause of nutritional impairment is necessary.

Growth failure may occur in all subtypes of JIA but is particularly common in systemic onset disease. It relates not only to the use of systemic corticosteroids in treatment but to the disease process itself. There is some evidence supporting the benefit of human growth hormone (GH) in the treatment of children with JIA and growth failure, but this therapy must still be considered experimental.[92]

Osteoporosis

Osteoporosis is a significant long term complication of a variety of rheumatological disorders including JIA. This occurs as a consequence of the underlying inflammatory process; of inactivity; and as a consequence of steroid therapy. (See later section on osteoporosis, page 1584 for more detail.)

Psychosocial

Long term outcome studies have demonstrated a significant incidence of psychosocial difficulty in young adults with JIA. Attention to rehabilitation and early return to normal activities where possible is essential to minimize this. Families and schools must be encouraged to treat the child as normal and all should be in mainstream schooling. Good transitional care with an early focus on independence and career counseling is essential.

Specific complications of systemic JIA

Macrophage activation syndrome (MAS)

MAS is a rare but potentially life threatening complication of systemic JIA. Features in a child with systemic JIA that lead to suspicion of MAS are fever, lymphadenopathy and hepatosplenomegaly, pancytopenia, low ESR, elevated liver enzymes and coagulopathy.[93] MAS may be triggered by an intercurrent infection. The pathognomic feature, macrophages actively phagocytosing hematopoietic elements, is seen on the bone marrow aspirate. It must be noted that false negative bone marrow examinations may occur. Other laboratory features include hypertriglyceridemia and hyperferritinemia. Treatment of MAS consists of high dose corticosteroids and ciclosporin with good supportive care and vigorous treatment of concomitant sepsis.

Amyloidosis

With the improved treatment modalities available to suppress the inflammatory process amyloidosis is now fortunately rare in systemic JIA. The treatment of choice is chlorambucil but the prognosis with established amyloidosis remains poor.

(a)

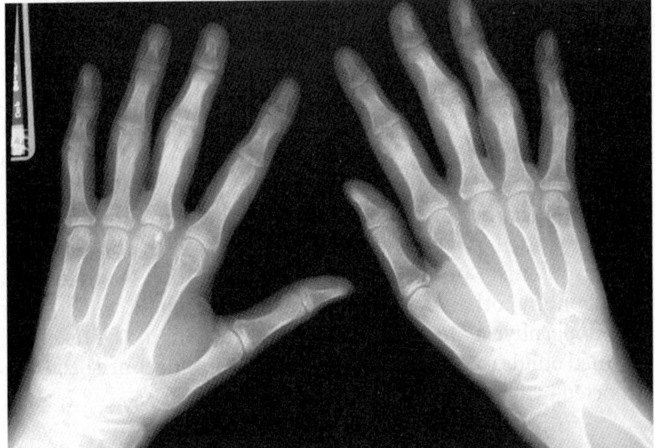

(b)

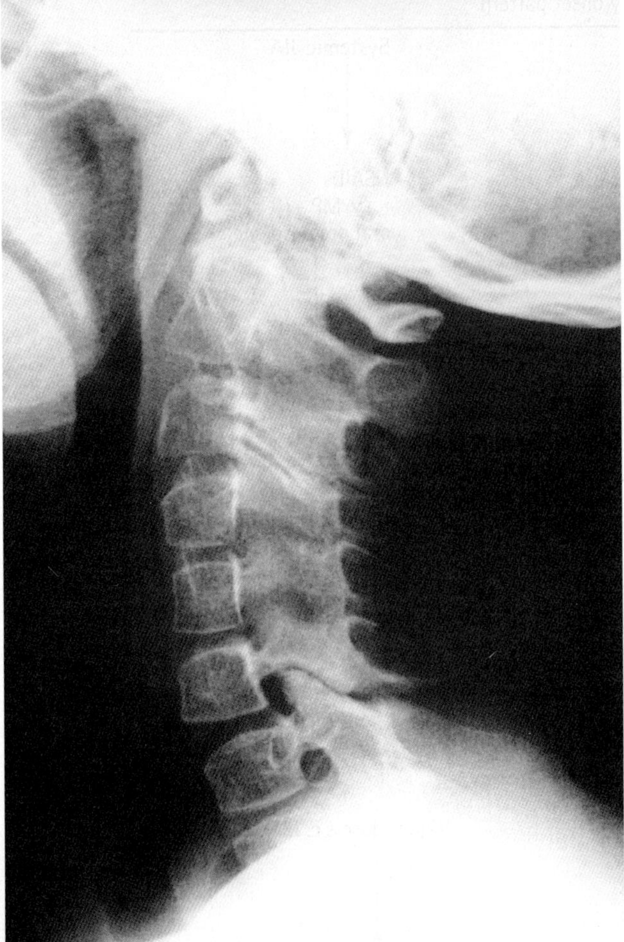

Fig. 27.41 Plain radiographs in juvenile idiopathic arthritis: (a) destructive changes of wrists with crowding of carpal bones; periarticular osteopenia and loss of joint space at proximal interphalangeal joints; (b) fusion in block of posterior elements of C2-C7.

MANAGEMENT OF JIA

The management of juvenile idiopathic arthritis, as with all chronic diseases of childhood, is based around a multidisciplinary team approach and is optimal where there is a dedicated team of professionals involved in the care of child and family (Table 27.13).

Adequate education of the child and family about the disease and possible therapeutic strategies is essential from the outset. The impact of JIA on the life of patient and family may be significant and good results depend on considerable commitment from all. Information and encouragement will empower patients and families to be involved in and committed to their treatment with improved compliance and better results. The provision of appropriate written information is helpful. Families are increasingly accessing the Internet for information and professionals must be prepared to deal with issues that may arise as a result.

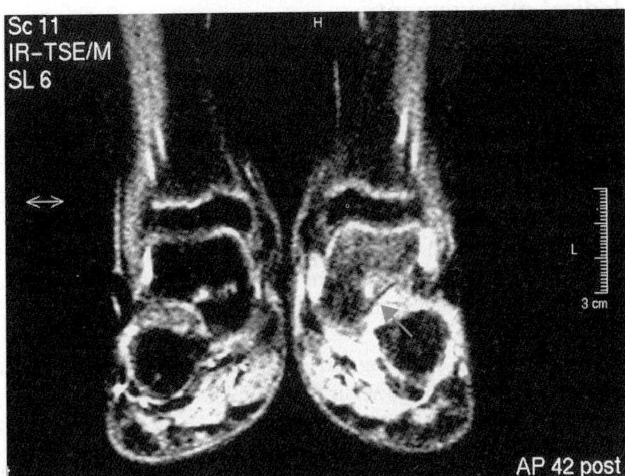

Fig. 27.42 Gadolinium enhanced MRI in juvenile idiopathic arthritis demonstrating synovitis of subtalar and talonavicular joints of the left foot.

Physiotherapy and occupational therapy

The aim of physiotherapy and occupational therapy is to maintain and restore joint function, to increase muscle strength and to facilitate normal development and independent living. Many different treatment strategies are available and vary with disease subtype and severity: specific therapy techniques are beyond the scope of this chapter. An occupational therapist may provide adaptations to the home or school environment to improve function in aspects of daily living if necessary. An occupational therapist or orthotist may provide splints where required to support inflamed joints. There is a trend to encourage more active therapy and confine splinting only to those children with severely affected joints, although policies vary between units.

Therapy input should be targeted selectively at those who need it. A child with a monoarthritis treated with intra-articular steroids early may not require any therapy input. With severe disease, physical and occupational therapy early in the disease may be associated with an improved outcome.[94]

Table 27.13 Members of the multidisciplinary team involved in the care of a child with juvenile idiopathic arthritis

Medical	Professions allied to medicine	Community
Pediatric rheumatologist	Physiotherapist	Family
Pediatrician	Occupational therapist	Friends
Ophthalmologist	Psychologist	School teacher
General practitioner	Social worker	Parental employer
Orthopedic surgeon	Dietitian	
Dental practitioner	Orthotist	
Radiologist	Podiatrist	

Medical management

The pharmacological management of JIA has evolved considerably in the last decade in terms of specific drugs and new strategies for their deployment. Current therapeutic approaches are aimed at attaining rapid remission of synovitis and maintaining it using drugs such as methotrexate early in the disease process. The traditional so-called pyramidal approach, starting with prolonged trials of non-steroidal anti-inflammatory drugs, and then slowly progressing through trials of various second-line agents and occasionally immunosuppressive therapies is now regarded as inappropriate as it leaves many children with uncontrolled disease for many months.

An algorithm showing an approach to pharmacological management of JIA is shown in Table 27.14.

Non-steroidal anti-inflammatory drugs (NSAIDs)

NSAIDs are widely used at diagnosis, provide good symptomatic relief and contribute to the control of the inflammatory process although this takes time to achieve. Table 27.15 lists the commonly used NSAIDs and the doses required to achieve anti-inflammatory effect. Drugs with once or twice daily regimens are likely to have better compliance particularly in older children.

Side-effects are uncommon in children. Gastrointestinal upset is relatively rare but when present may be relieved by the addition of a H_2 antagonist or proton pump inhibitor. Naproxen (and occasionally other NSAIDs) may be associated with scarring pseudoporphyria affecting the face and care should be taken in fair skinned children. Mood and behavior disturbances are occasionally reported by parents of young children on NSAIDs.

Table 27.14 Algorithm for the medical treatment of JIA by onset pattern

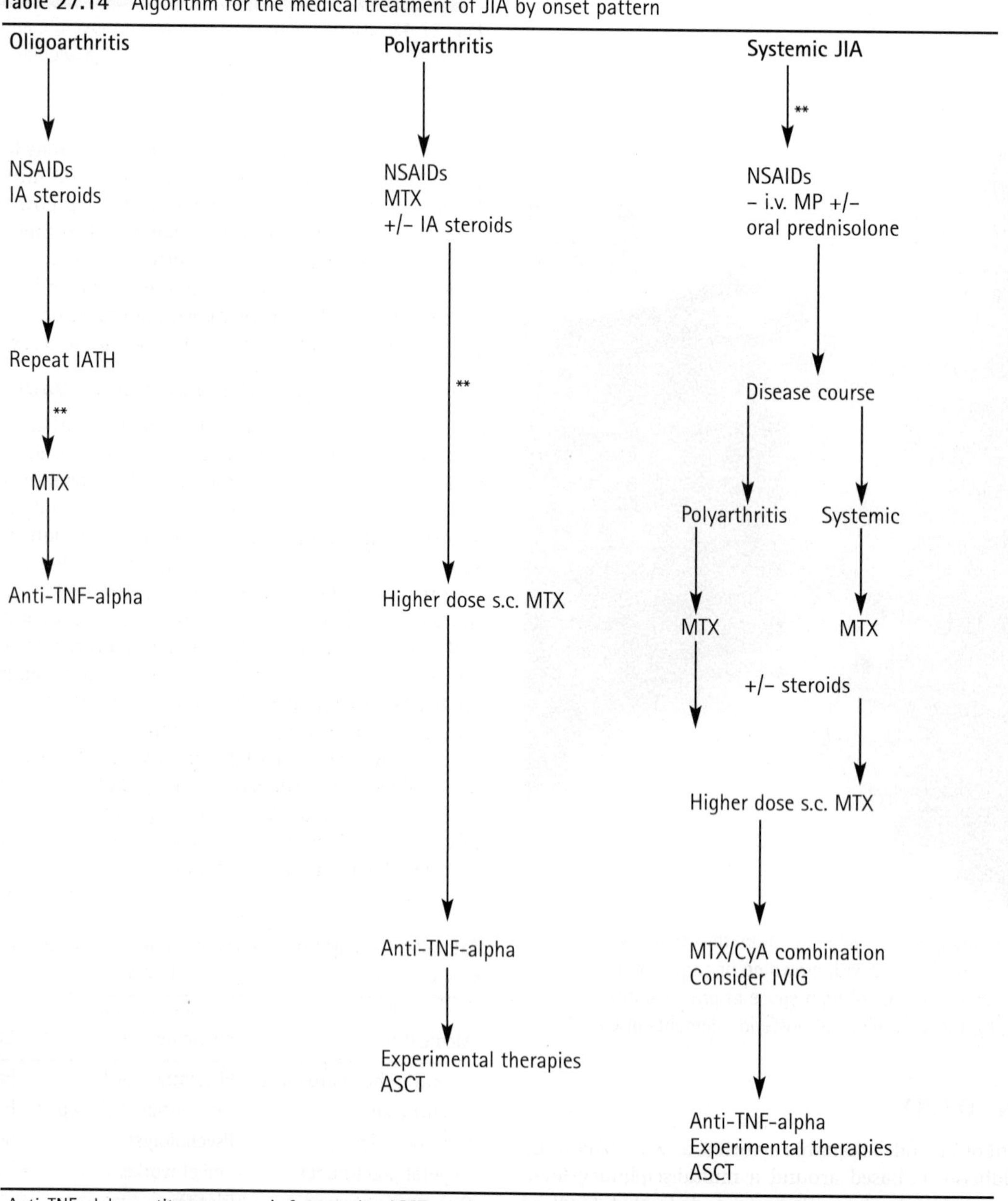

Anti-TNF-alpha, antitumor necrosis factor apha; ASCT, autologous stem cell transplant; CyA, ciclosporin A; IA steroid, intra-articular steroid; IATH, i.v. MP, i.v. methylprednisolone; IVIG, intravenous immunoglobulin; JIA, juvenile idiopathic arthritis; MTX, methotrexate; NSAIDs, non-steroidal anti-inflammatory drugs.

** Indicates stage requiring management in conjunction with regional pediatric rheumatology center.

Table 27.15 Non-steroidal anti-inflammatory drugs commonly used in children with juvenile idiopathic arthritis

Drug	Total daily dose		Times daily	Notes
Diclofenac	1–3 mg/kg		2–3	Max 150 mg/day *SR available*
Naproxe	10–20 mg/kg		2–3	Max 1 g/day
Ibuprofen	20–50 mg/kg		3–4	
Indometacin	1–3 mg/kg		2	Max 200 mg/day *SR available*
Piroxicam	< 15 kg	5 mg	once daily	*Sublingual preparation available*
	16–25 kg	10 mg		
	26–45 kg	15 mg		
	> 46 kg	20 mg		

SR, slow release.

The selective COX-2 inhibitors, rofecoxib and celecoxib, reduce the incidence of gastrointestinal complications in adults but have not been tested in children and are considerably more expensive than standard NSAIDs.

Corticosteroid therapy

The development and widespread use of effective second-line agents, particularly methotrexate, has dramatically reduced the number of children dependent on systemic corticosteroids and consequently the frequency of unacceptable toxicities associated with their chronic administration. Corticosteroids do still have a role in the management of JIA, in particular for remission induction and may be administered systemically by the intravenous and oral route, or locally by intra-articular injection.

Local corticosteroid therapy

Intra-articular steroid injections are effective, with a low risk of complications, in all subtypes of JIA, particularly oligoarthritis.[95] In oligoarthritis, intra-articular steroids may facilitate the withdrawal of NSAIDs. In polyarthritis, multiple intra-articular injections may be used simultaneously with the initiation of methotrexate therapy. The early use of intra-articular steroid injections and rapid resolution of synovitis provides pain relief, facilitates early physiotherapy and rehabilitation thus preventing joint contractures. When used early, and if necessary repeatedly, intra-articular steroids may prevent leg length discrepancy in oligoarthritis.[96]

Triamcinolone hexacetonide is the drug of choice for intra-articular injection in JIA. A typical regimen for dosage is 1 mg/kg for large joints (knees, hips and shoulders), 0.5 mg/kg in small joints (ankles, wrists and elbows) and 1–2 mg/joint for the small joints of the hands and feet.

In young children with JIA or if multiple joints are to be injected, intra-articular injection will need to be performed using general anesthesia. In older children, usually from the age of 7 years upward, the procedure can be safely and effectively carried out using a 50/50 mix of nitrous oxide and oxygen (Entonox®).

Subcutaneous atrophy at the injection site is the only common adverse effect, with the highest incidence in a single study of 8.3% of patients.[97] It can be minimized by good injection technique.

Systemic corticosteroids

A beneficial effect in all disease subtypes has been reported with the use of high dose 'pulses' of intravenous methylprednisolone as a remission induction agent.[98] The two commonest subtypes to be treated in this way are systemic arthritis and polyarthritis. Many regimes exist, but the usual dose of methylprednisolone is 30 mg/kg, administered either once a week for up to 6 weeks or on 3 consecutive days for 2 consecutive weeks.

Methotrexate

Methotrexate (MTX) is currently the drug of choice to treat persistent synovitis in children. MTX is a dihydrofolate reductase inhibitor, although its mechanism of action as an anti-inflammatory agent is not fully understood. In a double blind placebo controlled trial, MTX at a dose of 10 mg/m^2 was effective in polyarthritis.[99] MTX is effective in both extended oligoarthritis and systemic JIA.[100] The dose range for children is 10–30 mg/m^2. At doses higher than 10 mg/m^2 oral MTX is increasingly less well absorbed, so doses beyond 15 mg/m^2 MTX are often administered via the subcutaneous route. This is well tolerated by patients, and can be self-administered at home by patients or parents.

Common side-effects of weekly low dose methotrexate include nausea and vomiting, and transient elevation in liver enzymes. Mouth ulcers, bone marrow suppression and significant liver toxicity are rare.[98] Blood monitoring is mandatory whilst children take MTX, with most units recommending full blood count (FBC) and liver function tests (LFTs) fortnightly for 1 month, then monthly when on a stable dose. Abdominal discomfort may be exacerbated by concomitant administration of NSAIDs, and may be improved by either a H_2 antagonist or a proton pump inhibitor. Nausea may be relieved by the use of an antiemetic before the MTX but may be dose-limiting and is the most common reason for discontinuation of treatment. There is no consensus on the use of folic acid to minimize adverse effects in children on weekly low dose MTX.

Immunization with live vaccines is contraindicated during treatment with MTX. Children who are non-immune to varicella zoster should be treated with varicella zoster immune globulin if in contact with chicken pox. Methotrexate is teratogenic and liver toxicity may be increased with concomitant alcohol ingestion. Adolescents need specific counseling in these areas.

Other second line drugs in JIA

Sulfasalazine

Sulfasalazine is effective in oligo- and polyarticular JIA[101] but its use has been superseded by MTX in most centers. It is most frequently used as a second-line agent to treat enthesitis related arthritis. Sulfasalazine is given in doses of 50 mg/kg/day, in two or three divided doses. Adverse effects include rash, gastrointestinal upset (abdominal pain, anorexia, nausea, diarrhea) and headache. Elevated liver enzymes, leukopenia and hypoimmunoglobulinemia occur rarely.

Ciclosporin

The principal indication for the use of ciclosporin in JIA is in the macrophage activation syndrome. Some benefit has been reported in the treatment of systemic arthritis, predominantly in the control of fever and as a steroid-sparing agent, with less clear benefit in terms of control of synovitis.[102] Ciclosporin is started at a dose of

3–5 mg/kg/day. Serious adverse effects include hypertension, nephropathy and hepatotoxicity but are rare at these doses. Hypertrichosis and gingival hyperplasia occur more commonly and are particularly distressing for adolescent patients. Renal function, blood pressure, FBC and LFTs should be monitored.

Combination therapy

Combinations of drugs including MTX and sulfasalazine and MTX and ciclosporin, have been proposed in resistant cases but this practice has never been evaluated in controlled clinical trials.

Biological therapies

Following publication of the first study examining the use of anti-TNF therapy in JIA, there has been enormous interest in this form of therapy. Etanercept, a recombinant molecule comprising part of the human TNF receptor plus the constant region of immunoglobulin G1, binds to and inactivates both TNF-alpha and lymphotoxin-alpha. In a multicenter clinical trial of children with polyarticular JIA who had previously failed to respond to therapy with low dose methotrexate, 74% improved with etanercept.[103] Adverse effects were similar to those in the placebo group. Long term safety and efficacy data are not yet available. Active infection should be considered a contraindication. Etanercept is given at a dose of 0.4 mg/kg by subcutaneous injection twice a week.

Infliximab is a chimeric human–mouse monoclonal antibody that binds to and inhibits TNF-alpha. There are no controlled data on its use in JIA as yet. Anecdotal data suggest efficacy similar to that of etanercept. Infliximab is given by intermittent intravenous infusion and in combination with methotrexate. The role of anti-TNF therapies in systemic JIA is less clear than in polyarthritis.

Biologics are expensive and their use should be supervised by a pediatric rheumatologist within a tertiary care setting. The British Paediatric Rheumatology Group has developed national guidelines for the use of etanercept in the UK (unpublished data), now accepted by the National Institute for Clinical Excellence (NICE). The annual cost for etanercept is currently £8450, compared to £57 for MTX.[104] Following the successful development of anti-TNF therapy it seems likely that other biologic therapies will follow. An IL-1 receptor antagonist is under development and others will undoubtedly follow.

Other therapies

Intravenous immunoglobulin may occasionally be used in polyarthritis and systemic arthritis. Its use remains reserved for cases unresponsive to more conventional therapies. Cyclophosphamide has been used for severe resistent systemic onset disease. Hydroxychloroquine may prove of some benefit in seropositive patients. Gold is no longer used in JIA. Leflunomide, an oral dihydroorotate dehydrogenase inhibitor, has shown efficacy in adults with rheumatoid arthritis. There is anecdotal evidence of benefit in JIA but no controlled studies.

Autologous hemopoietic stem cell transplantation has been pioneered as a treatment for children with JIA refractory to conventional treatment.[105] Early results have shown promise, but optimum protocols for this treatment are still to be established.

Surgical management

Orthopedic surgery has a role in the management of severe JIA. Synovectomy is now uncommon but may be helpful. Soft tissue release may be useful for severe flexion contracture of hip or knee. Joint replacement should be avoided for as long as possible, but may be necessary in the older child with JIA with intractable pain associated with joint destruction.[75]

Transitional care

Young people with JIA entering transition into adulthood have specific medical and psychosocial needs, and many advocate that this process should be proactively managed. At present the provision of adolescent rheumatology care is patchy in the UK.[106] Models based upon specific adolescent clinics and active transfer into the adult health care are still to be developed in many geographical areas.

OTHER ARTHROPATHIES IN CHILDHOOD

Infections and JIA are the only common causes of arthritis in childhood. The differential diagnosis of inflammatory arthritis in children (see Table 27.9) is wide and other causes must be excluded as necessary. Many of these conditions are described elsewhere in the chapter.

COMMON ORTHOPEDIC PROBLEMS IN CHILDHOOD

Children present to the clinician with a wide spectrum of problems ranging from complaints relating to form, posture and gait to complaints of localized pain at various sites. This section covers the more common orthopedic explanations for such presentations.

COMMON PAINLESS COMPLAINTS

Normal variants

The shape and form of the lower limbs in children cause a great deal of parental anxiety. In spite of such concern, the majority of these children are normal[107] and sound knowledge of normal variation cannot be overemphasized. The most common causes for parental concern are flat feet, bow legs, knock knees, and in-toe gait. The chief objective when presented with such children is to exclude a pathological explanation. In broad terms unilateral 'deformities' are more suspicious of pathology than bilateral which frequently reflect normal physiological variation.

Toe walking

The commonest explanation for this presentation is habitual or idiopathic toe walking although other more serious explanations should be considered and excluded. A thorough neuromuscular evaluation is mandatory since toe walking may be a feature of muscular dystrophy, cerebral palsy, a tethered cord or indeed any neuromuscular disorder. Children with habitual or idiopathic toe walking persistently walk on the toes, but can be encouraged to adopt a more normal heel strike. They should be able to stand still with the heels to the ground. Treatment is directed towards constant encouragement to reinforce the normal heel–toe gait pattern, but occasionally serial casting is helpful to break a persistent habit or if true Tendo-Achilles shortening develops.

Flat feet

Most children who are brought for assessment of flat feet are normal. The clinician's responsibility is to exclude potential pathological causes such as congenital vertical talus, tarsal coalition or juvenile idiopathic arthritis.

The clinical assessment aims to determine if the flat appearance is flexible or rigid. Rigid flat feet are never normal, but flexible flat feet usually are. The feet should be observed weight bearing and walking if possible. Many infants have 'fat feet' rather than flat feet because a pad of fat in the sole of the foot hides the normal arch. Jack's test should be done. This requires the great toe to be dorsiflexed. As this is done a windlass mechanism tightens the planter fascia and draws the

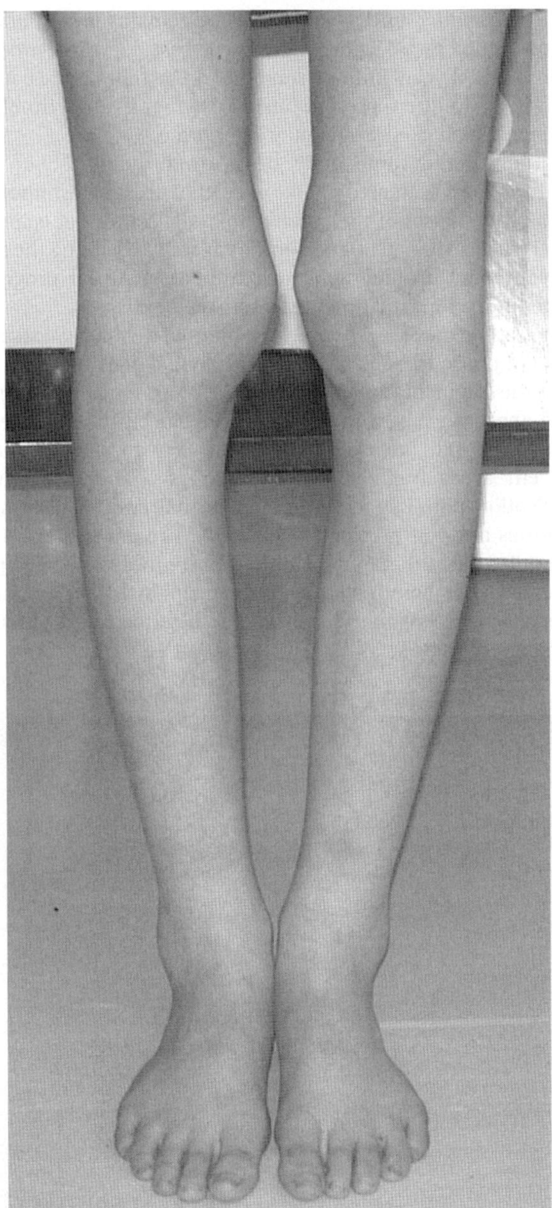

Fig. 27.47 'Squinting' patellae.

is sufficiently severe, derotation osteotomy is effective. Sometimes especially in adolescent girls external tibial torsion coexists: this compensates for the internal femoral torsion so that the feet point forwards but the patellae are left 'squinting' medially towards each other (Fig. 27.47). If treatment proves to be necessary in such patients, it will involve bilateral femoral and tibial osteotomies. This is a considerable undertaking and should not be approached lightly.

Tibial torsion

Internal tibial torsion is a common explanation for in-toe gait in the toddler age range. The degree of tibial torsion is assessed by measuring the thigh foot axis, as already described, or by measuring the angle between the coronal (or transcondylar) plane and a line joining the tips of medial and lateral malleoli at the ankle. In the term infant at birth, the medial malleolus usually lies behind the lateral malleolus. By walking age the malleoli are level on the coronal plane and by the time walking is well established the lateral malleolus is behind the medial. In other words the infant normally has relative internal tibial torsion, which gradually rotates externally with growth. Internal tibial torsion often coexists with bowing of the legs in infants and young children and may exaggerate the appearance of the bowing. No treatment is necessary or effective for physiological internal tibial torsion.

Excessive external tibial torsion is less common than internal tibial torsion and more likely to persist into adolescence.[110] Once again the only effective treatment for tibial rotational abnormalities is tibial osteotomy. Serious thought needs to be given before offering operative solutions as neither internal nor external tibial torsion have been shown to be risk factors for later degenerative change.

Metatarsus varus

Metatarsus varus or metatarsus adductus is medial deviation of the forefoot on the hindfoot. The subtalar and ankle joints are normal and the hindfoot is in neutral or slight valgus. This distinguishes the condition from clubfoot deformity where the hindfoot is stiff and in varus and equinus. The foot has a concave medial border which can be the cause of, or at least contribute to, an in-toe gait appearance.

The severity of the condition can be classified using the heel bisector as previously described. The condition is described as flexible if the forefoot can be passively overcorrected, partly flexible if it can be passively corrected to the midline and rigid if it cannot be returned to the midline. The natural history of metatarsus varus is of progressive spontaneous resolution. Consideration can be given to treatment if the deformity is rigid or partly flexible and serial casting has been shown to be effective.[111]

COMMON ORTHOPEDIC EXPLANATIONS FOR MUSCULOSKELETAL PAIN IN CHILDHOOD

Growing pains

Musculoskeletal pain in children is relatively common and usually benign. In evaluating children it is wise to remember that infection and neoplasia are amongst the myriad of potential explanations. Both commonly present in childhood as localized bone pain and must be given due consideration in the differential diagnosis.

The syndrome of benign 'growing pains' is common and is estimated to affect 4% of all children.[112] It usually presents in children between 4 and 8 years. It can occur in the upper but more frequently the lower limbs. The typical history is of a child who, after a busy day, complains of aching pains in the limbs, frequently in the thighs, shins or around the front or the back of the knees. The pain can be severe, even disturbing sleep, and usually settles after a variable period of parental rubbing of the affected limbs. The next day the child is fine and there are no sequelae. The natural history is of eventual resolution after 18–24 months but the course may be more protracted. The cause is not known. Treatment is primarily reassurance but can include stretching exercises if muscle fatigue is thought to be a factor.

Neck and back pain

See later section, page 1582.

The painful or irritable hip

The term irritable hip is not a diagnosis. It is the clinical presentation of hip pathology. The patient may present with symptoms ranging from severe pain with complete inability to weight bear to modest pain, localized to the hip or referred to the knee, with virtually no limp.

The most sensitive sign of hip joint pathology is subtle limitation of internal rotation, which should be carefully sought. Clinical examination of the hip is equally important when patients present with localized hip pain or with isolated thigh or knee pain. The potential for knee pain to be referred from the hip is frequently overlooked.

The commonest cause for an irritable hip in childhood is transient synovitis, but the differential is wide and includes infections, acute and chronic, including septic arthritis and osteomyelitis, Perthes disease and slipped capital femoral epiphysis (SCFE). Less common causes include the inflammatory arthritides such as juvenile idiopathic arthritis, idiopathic chondrolysis and neoplasms. Transient synovitis, Perthes disease, SCFE and chondrolysis will be discussed here. The other disorders are discussed elsewhere in the chapter.

Transient synovitis

This is the commonest cause for hip pain in children and it is estimated that about 3% of children will have at least one episode.[113] It is twice as common in boys and usually occurs between 3 and 8 years with a peak incidence around 6.[114] It is characterized by a transient period of hip joint irritability in a systemically well child. The etiology is unknown but hypotheses include trauma, allergic hypersensitivity or infection. In up to 70% of cases there is a history of either current or antecedent non-specific upper respiratory infection, and the most widely accepted explanation is that the condition represents a transient reactive synovitis.

Hip joint ultrasonography to identify a hip joint effusion is the most useful investigation, confirming that the hip joint is the source of complaint. The findings are non-specific and do not necessarily exclude other causes of an irritable hip. Radiographs and laboratory tests are normal or non-specific. Transient synovitis is essentially a diagnosis of exclusion and investigations are principally aimed at excluding other explanations for hip joint irritability. Pyogenic septic arthritis is the most important alternative diagnosis. The child with septic arthritis is usually systemically unwell with a high fever, a high white cell count and ESR and fails to improve with rest. The patient with an effusion due to transient synovitis is typically systemically well, may have a modest fever and mildy elevated ESR and improves with rest.

Treatment for transient synovitis is symptomatic. Skin traction has been popular but is now rarely recommended because positioning the hip in extension increases intracapsular pressure and pain. If traction is to be used the leg should be supported with the hip flexed. In practice it is more practical to let the child rest the limb in a position of flexion and external rotation for comfort, provided symptoms settle promptly.

Most cases resolve progressively over 5–10 days. Deterioration is more characteristic of septic arthritis and persistence of moderate or modest symptoms should raise suspicion of alternative explanations such as Perthes disease. Isotope bone scanning can be helpful in these circumstances to distinguish Perthes disease, characterized by reduced uptake, from transient synovitis and other inflammatory conditions where increased uptake is usual. A relationship between transient synovitis and the development of Perthes disease has been suggested but no direct causal correlation has ever been shown. It is safest to conclude that the only relationship is a similar mode of presentation, with an irritable hip.

Perthes disease (Legg–Calvé–Perthes disease)

Perthes disease is avascular necrosis of the femoral head epiphysis due to a disturbance of the epiphyseal blood supply. The disturbance can affect part or all of the femoral epiphysis and the extent of involvement is related to the ultimate prognosis. Despite enthusiasm for the notion that thrombophilia or hypofibrinolysis may be involved in the pathogenesis,[115] more recent work has proved less than encouraging and Perthes disease remains a condition of unknown etiology.[116] Eighty per cent of cases occur between the ages of 4 and 9 years and the condition is five times more common in boys.[117] Children present insidiously with an irritable hip syndrome which persists and may deteriorate.

Initially radiographs may be normal. Radionuclide bone scanning shows decreased uptake in Perthes disease, distinguishing it from other causes of an irritable hip. MRI can reveal epiphyseal necrosis earlier than plain radiographs as well as defining the extent of involvement. Radiographs will ultimately reveal progressive changes in the hip joint and the femoral epiphysis.

The pathogenesis is reflected in sequential radiological stages. In the initial phase there is increased epiphyseal density which gives way to the fragmentation phase (Fig. 27.48a), sometimes heralded by the appearance of a subchondral radiolucent line or 'crescent sign' (Fig. 27.48b) and eventually characterized by the appearance of lucent areas fragmenting the epiphysis. The reparative or reossification phase supervenes and normal bone density slowly substitutes areas of previous lucency. The process continues from the periphery of the epiphysis to the center until the healed phase is reached. The bony epiphysis once again has the consistency of normal bone but may have become deformed to a greater or lesser degree.

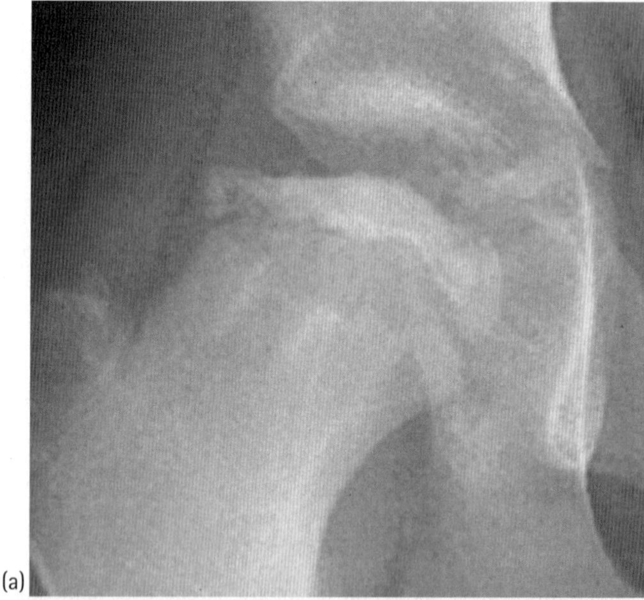
(a)

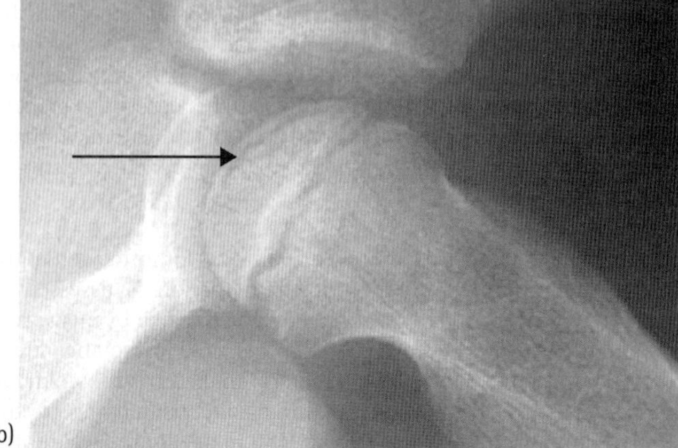
(b)

Fig. 27.48 Perthes disease: (a) stage of fragmentation and collapse; (b) crescent sign.

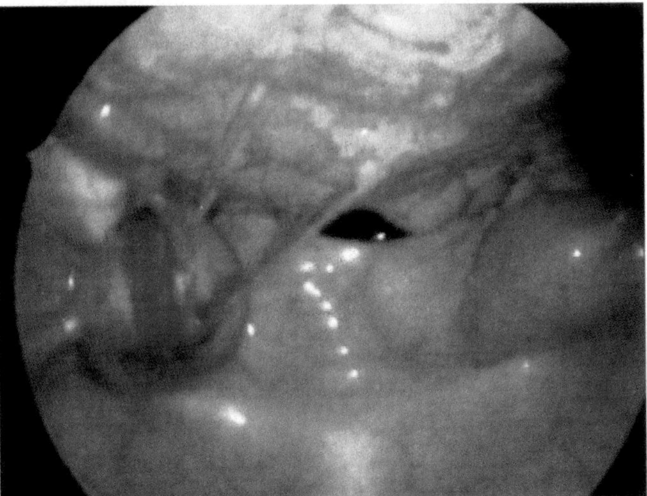

Plate 23.5 Rudimentary uterine horns in a girl with Rokitansky–Kuster–Hauser syndrome (adhesions surrounding the left horn) (see p. 1156).

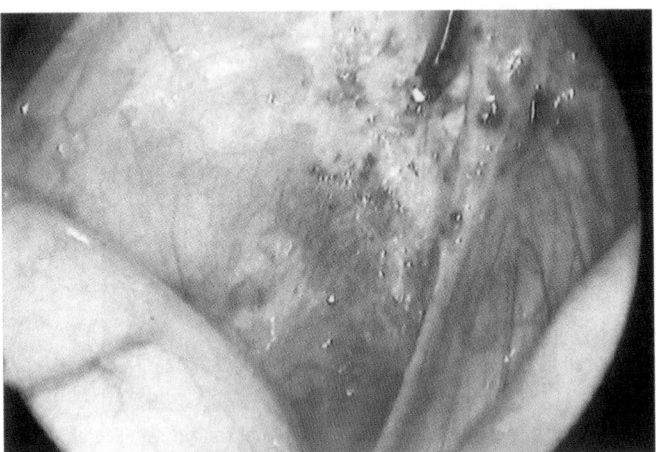

Plate 23.7 Extensive endometriosis involving the right uterosacral ligament and pouch of Douglas in an adolescent girl (see p. 1157).

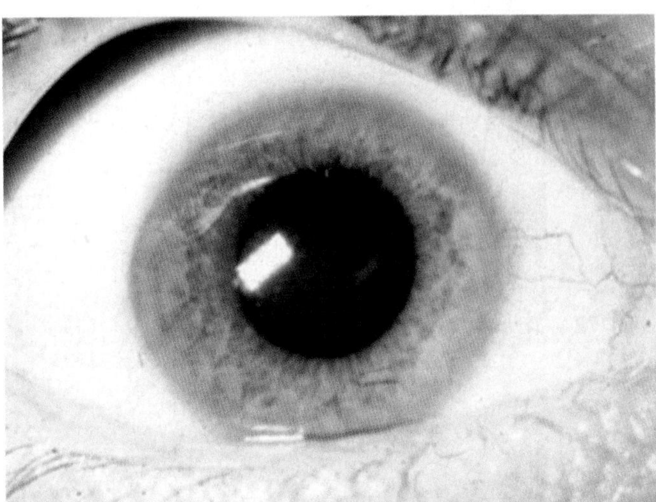

Plate 24.16 Kayser–Fleischer ring caused by copper deposited in Descemet's membrane in a child with Wilson's disease (see p. 1192).

(a)

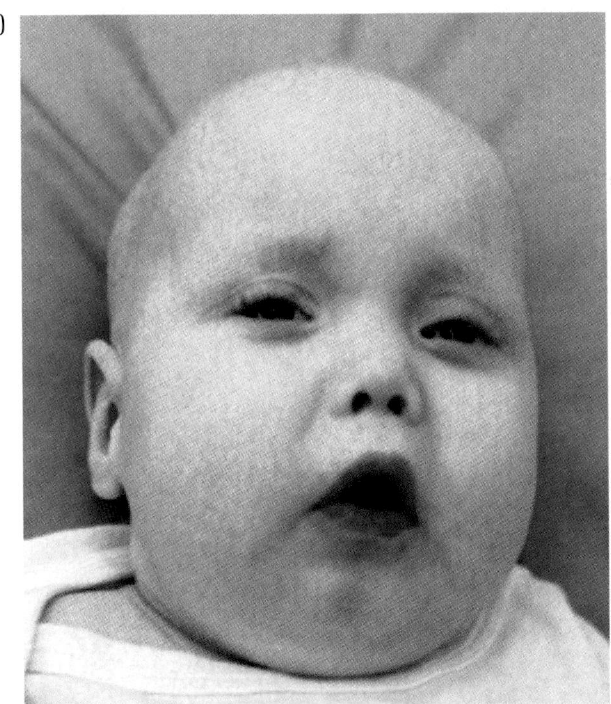

(b)

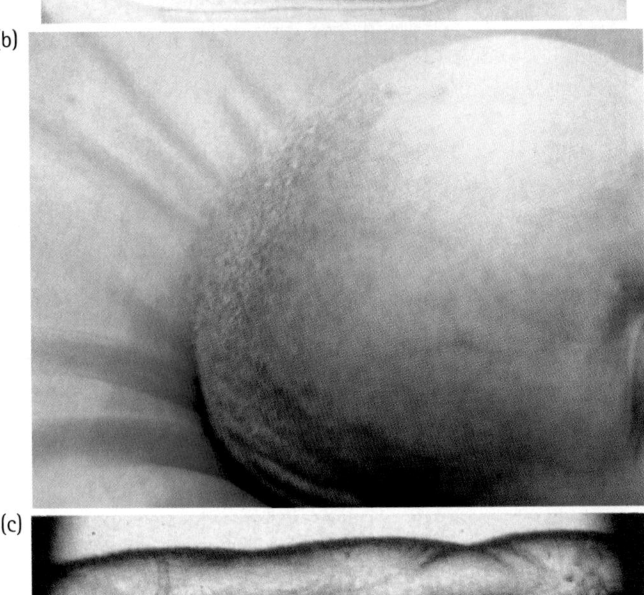

(c)

Plate 24.15 Features and typical hair of Menkes syndrome (see p. 1191).

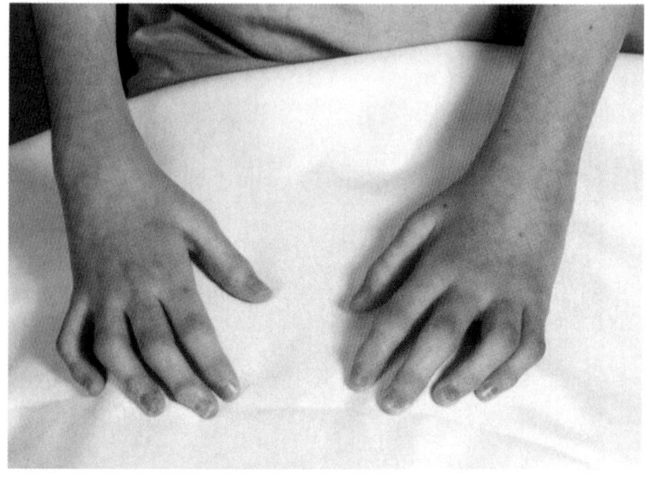

Plate 27.34 Polyarthritis affecting wrists and the small joints of the hands (see p. 1551).

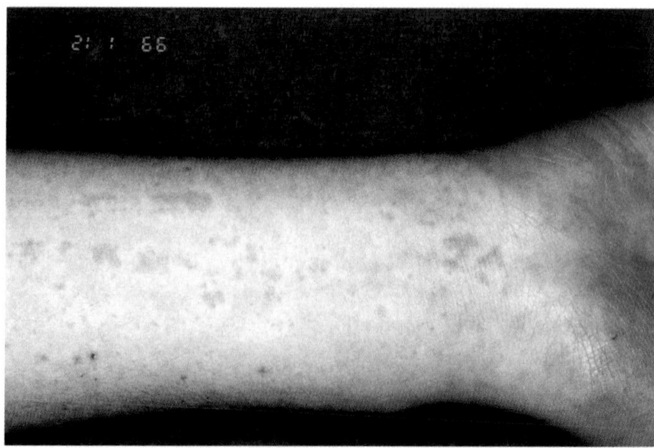

Plate 27.36 Rash of systemic juvenile idiopathic arthritis (see p. 1552).

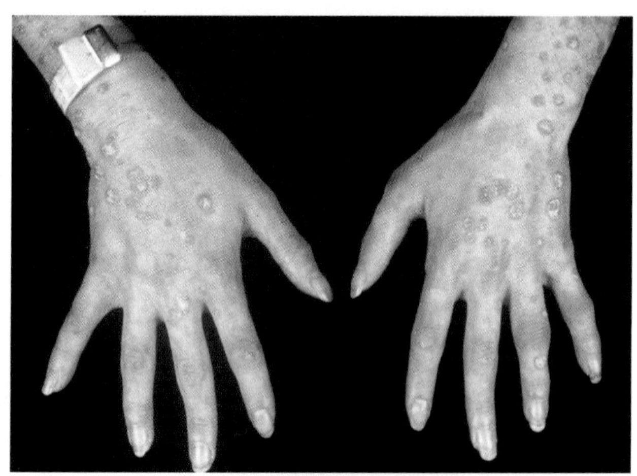

Plate 27.38 Psoriatic arthritis (see p. 1553).

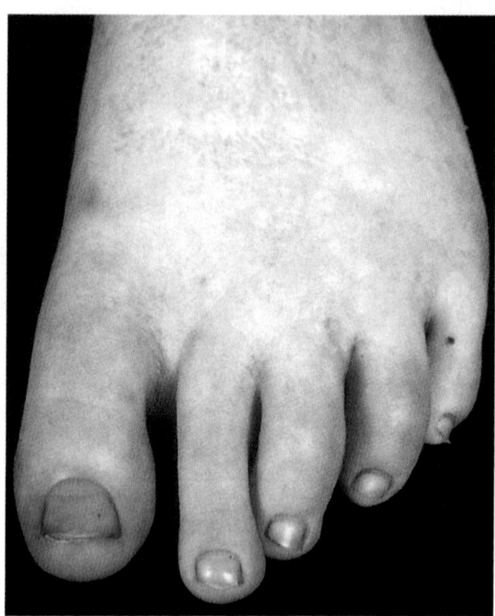

Plate 27.39 Dactylitis – swelling of third and fourth toes (see p. 1553).

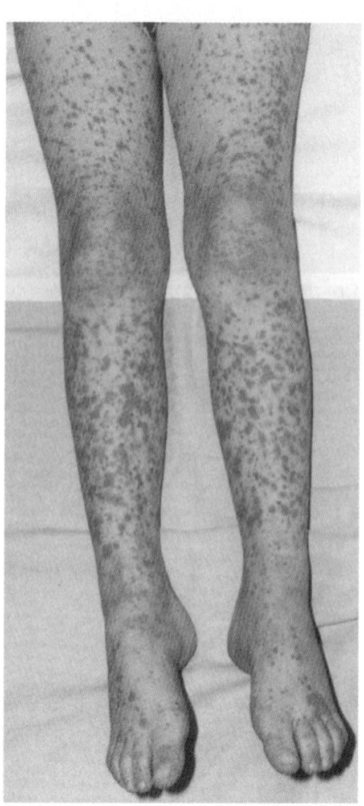

Plate 27.54 Rash of Henoch–Schönlein purpura (see p. 1568).

(a)

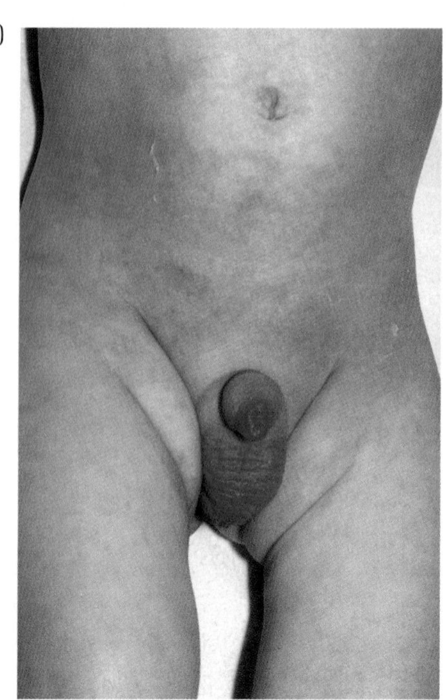

Plate 27.55 Kawasaki disease: (a) typical erythematous groin rash with peeling; (b) peeling of digits (see p. 1569).

(b)

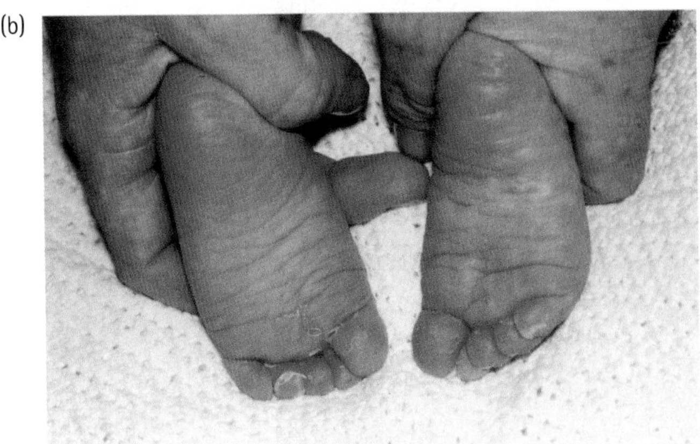

Plate 27.55 (b) Cont'd

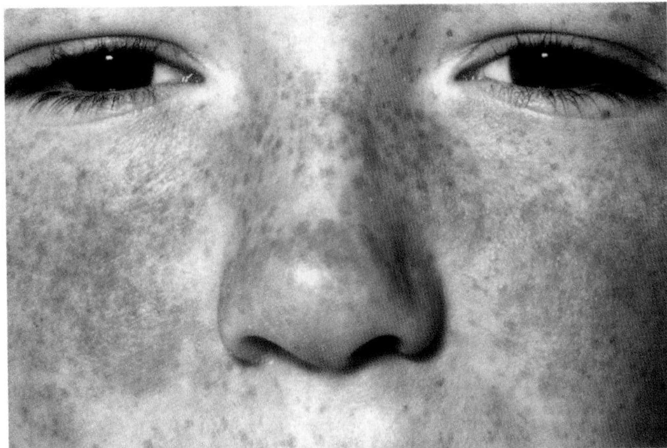

Plate 27.58 Typical facial rash in systemic lupus erythematosus – crossing the bridge of the nose and sparing the nasolabial folds (see p. 1572).

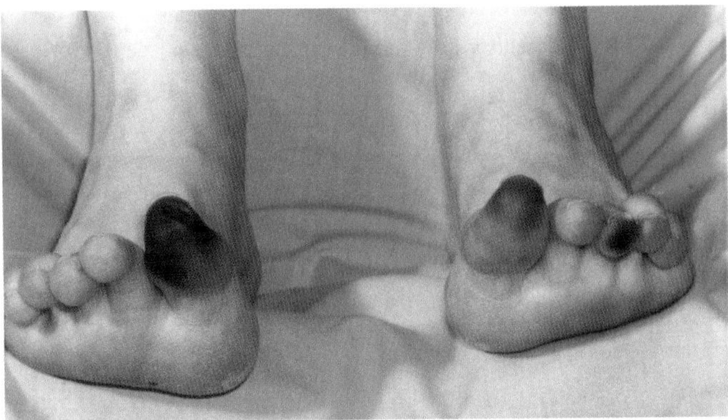

Plate 27.56 Gangrene of several toes in polyarteritis nodosa (see p. 1570).

(a)

(b)

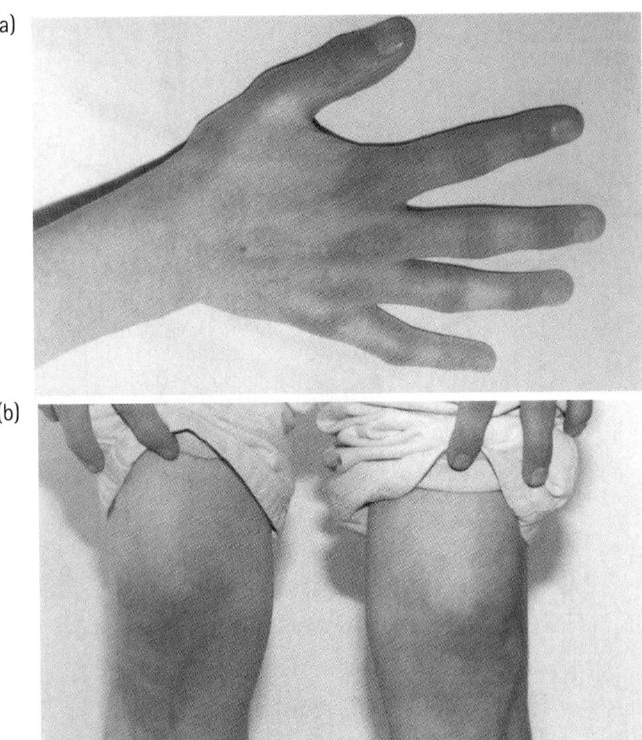

Plate 27.59 Typical rash of juvenile dermatomyositis with erythema over: (a) extensor aspects of metacarpophalangeal and proximal interphalangeal joints; (b) knees (see p. 1574).

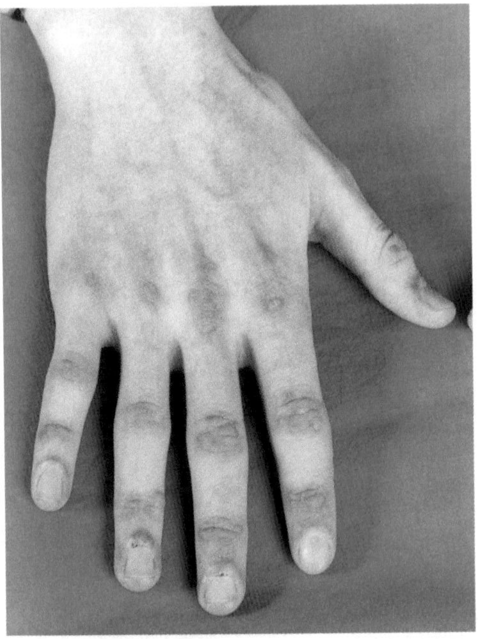

Plate 27.60 Juvenile dermatomyositis showing Gottron's papules and typical nailfold changes (see p. 1574).

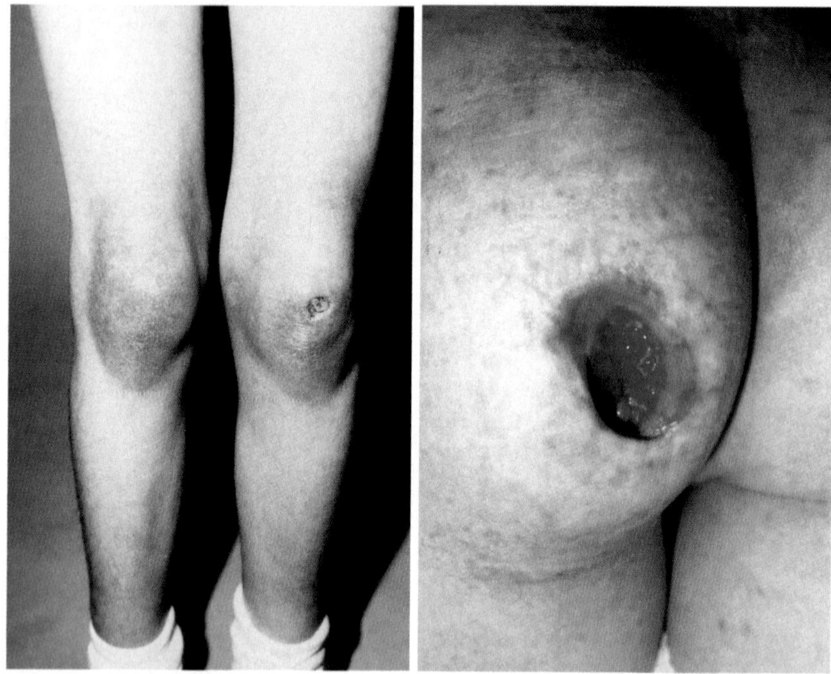

Plate 27.62 (a & b) Ulcerative vasculopathy in juvenile dermatomyositis (see p. 1575).

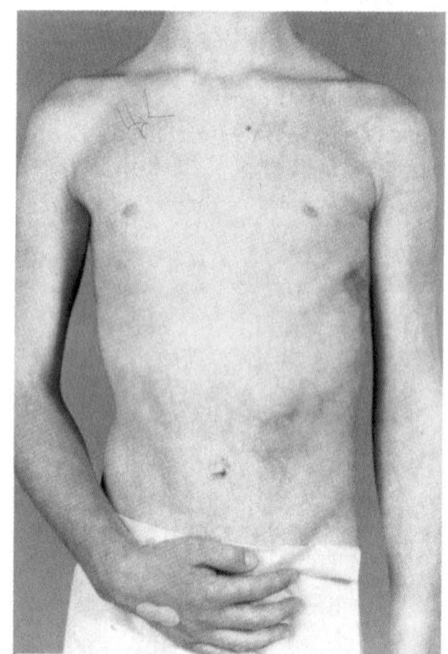

Plate 27.65 Morphea (see p. 1577).

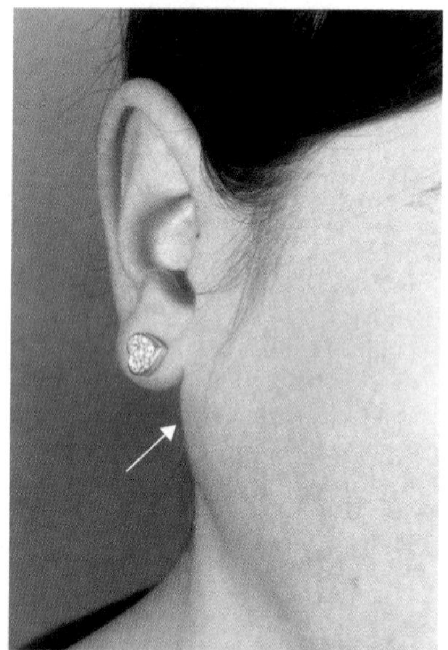

Plate 27.69 Sjögren's syndrome: (a) parotid swelling (see p. 1579).

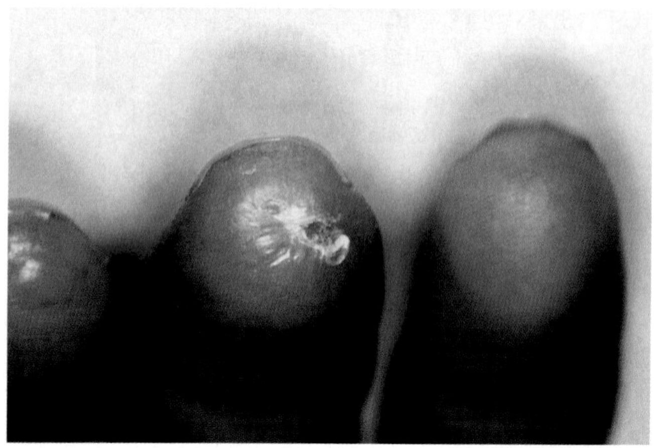

Plate 27.68 Digital pitting scars in systemic sclerosis (see p. 1578).

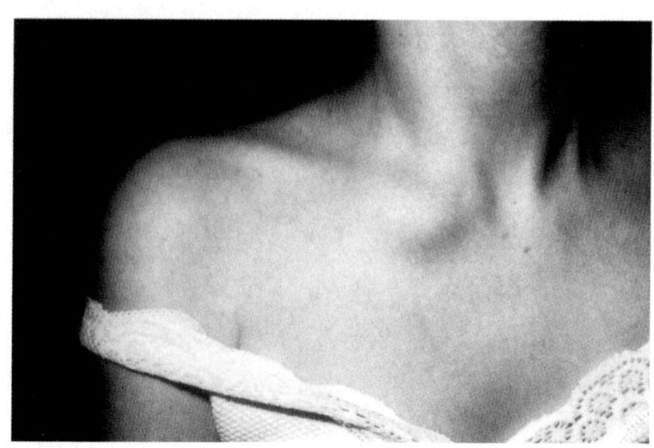

Plate 27.71 SAPHO syndrome: (b) hyperostotic lesion of right clavicle (see p. 1581).

Although Perthes disease can be bilateral in 10–12% of cases[118] radiographs characteristically reveal different stages of disease in the two sides. A similar appearance in both hips is very unusual and should raise suspicion of skeletal dysplasias such as multiple epiphyseal dysplasia (MED) (Fig. 27.25) and spondyloepiphyseal dysplasia (SED).

The progression from the initial phase to the end of the healed phase can take several years. During this time, especially during the fragmentation phase, the cartilaginous femoral head loses the support of its internal bony skeleton and becomes plastic, or able to change shape. The shape the femoral head becomes is determined by the extent of loss of support (or epiphyseal necrosis), and by the mechanical environment in which the plastic femoral head finds itself. The long term prognosis depends on how spherical the femoral head remains and how congruently it fits the acetabulum.

In early Perthes disease, when the femoral head remains plastic, the principle of treatment is the principle of 'containment'. The patient's own acetabulum is used as a template or mold to keep the femoral head spherical, or at least congruent. This can be achieved by the patient themselves if a good range of movement, especially abduction, is maintained. Alternatively, 'containment' treatment with an abduction brace or femoral or pelvic osteotomy is used to position the plastic part of the femoral epiphysis within the acetabulum. Clinical examination is a crucial part of patient assessment. If the patient maintains a good range of movement the soft femoral epiphysis will be constantly moving in and out of the acetabulum during day-to-day activity and will remain congruent. If on the other hand, range of movement is limited especially abduction, the femoral epiphysis will not be contained within the acetabulum and weight bearing forces will lead to flattening of the epiphysis and incongruity. Loss of range of movement is therefore a sinister clinical sign.

Radiological evaluation is easiest using the Herring grading system. Herring divided the epiphysis as seen on an anteroposterior (AP) radiograph into medial, middle and lateral columns. Only the lateral column is evaluated. The hip is classified as Herring A if there is no necrosis involving the lateral column, Herring B if the lateral column is involved but retains more than 50% of its original height and Herring C if it has lost more than 50% of its original height. The prognosis deteriorates from grades A–C. In concept if the lateral column is intact, the remainder of the femoral head is protected from weight bearing forces, but if the lateral column fails the whole femoral head is exposed to forces from above and will flatten.

Patients under 5 years at the onset of Perthes disease have a good prognosis. In this age group patients frequently maintain an excellent range of movement, even in the face of extensive epiphyseal necrosis on radiographs, and they essentially contain their own femoral head. They rarely require intervention, but should be constantly reviewed to ensure that a good range of movement is maintained. The good prognosis in this age range is also a reflection of the immature acetabulum with much growth remaining. If the femoral head does become aspherical as a result of the Perthes process, the acetabulum will grow to match.

In older children the acetabulum has less growth remaining, is less able to accommodate an aspherical femoral head and incongruity becomes progressively more likely. Clinical signs in older children (over 5–6 years) usually reflect the radiological extent of epiphyseal necrosis. If there is clinical loss of range of movement in this age group radiographs will usually reveal Herring grade C or B lateral column involvement. These findings usually dictate 'containment' treatment. In the past a wide range of abduction braces have been used but more recent reports question their efficacy.[119] There is a therefore a growing inclination to offer surgical containment because of emerging evidence that the results are better. Surgical containment is usually in the form of a varus femoral or a pelvic osteotomy. It is common practice for surgical candidates to undergo an examination of the joint under anesthetic and hip joint arthrography, to ensure that the epiphysis is containable before embarking on surgical treatment. Patients should be followed to maturity, mainly to ensure a significant leg length discrepancy does not develop. A modest leg length discrepancy is common; one requiring treatment unusual.

Once the Perthes disease is over and the femoral epiphysis is healed, it is no longer plastic. Hip pain can result if incongruity has developed. The objective of treatment now is restoration of functional congruity. Once again assessment commonly includes examination under anesthesia and arthrography. The principal problem encountered in a deformed incongruent joint is 'hinge abduction'. Because the femoral head is too big to enter the acetabulum during abduction, it levers itself out of the joint with the 'hinge' at the lateral lip of the acetabulum. This limits the patient's functional abduction. The problem can sometimes be helped with a valgus femoral osteotomy.[120]

Slipped capital femoral epiphysis (SCFE)

Slipped capital femoral epiphysis (SCFE) or slipped upper femoral epiphysis (SUFE) is the commonest hip disorder in the adolescent age range and is frequently the subject of medical negligence claims because of delay in diagnosis with potentially disabling consequences for the patient.

The capital femoral epiphysis is fixed to the femoral metaphysis by the proximal femoral growth plate or physis. If the cartilaginous physis is subjected to shear forces it can fail, usually through its hypertrophic zone and the femoral epiphysis will then 'slip' posteriorly on the metaphysis, either progressively or suddenly. A SCFE occurs when the load applied exceeds the resistance of the physis to slip. This can occur because the load is too great, because the physis is vulnerable or, most often, because of a combination of these factors.

Hormonal events during normal adolescence lead to relative widening of the physis and its hypertrophic zone during periods of rapid growth. The threshold at which the widened physis fails is lower than a normal physis making the adolescent vulnerable to SCFE. Any condition that widens the growth plate either because of increased growth or decreased ossification predisposes to SCFE and it has been associated with a variety of endocrine abnormalities including hypothyroidism, panhypopituitarism and hypogonadal conditions.[121] Treatment of short stature with growth hormone can also predispose and such children should be monitored carefully.[122] If a vulnerable physis is subjected to increased load, such as might occur in obesity, the risk of SCFE is further increased. 63% of affected individuals are over the 90th percentile for weight.

The incidence of SCFE is around 2:100 000 and its peak presentation is 9–15 years in girls and 10–16 years in boys, i.e. during the adolescent growth spurt. The condition is more common in boys than girls in a ratio of 1.5:1.0. If a case presents in a child outside the expected age range or in a child with an unusual body habitus more serious consideration should be given to an underlying endocrine or metabolic abnormality.

Careful radiographic interpretation is important if early detection of a slip is to be made. The AP radiograph is insufficiently sensitive and where a slip is considered possible a lateral radiograph should be obtained. The radiographic signs on the AP radiograph include subtle blurring and irregularity of the physis and slight loss of epiphyseal height. When the epiphysis slips a little further it is more obvious on the AP radiograph. A line, Klein's line,[123] drawn along the superior aspect of the femoral neck should cut off the lateral edge of the epiphysis but does not if the epiphysis has slipped. Minor degrees of slip are more easily seen on the lateral radiograph because the epiphysis primarily slips posteriorly (Fig. 27.49).

SCFE is classified into unstable (acute) slips or stable (chronic) slips.[124] A third category of a stable slip suddenly becoming unstable also exists (acute on chronic). The distinction between the different types of slip is important because the clinical presentation and the prognosis differ significantly.

In the stable slip the femoral epiphysis gradually and progressively slips posteriorly on the femoral metaphysis. The patient may have a limp but can weight bear and the presentation is essentially that of an irritable hip. Referred knee pain may be the patient's only complaint and a futile search for a local explanation at the knee is a common cause for delayed diagnosis. Pain, discomfort or reluctance when the hip is internally rotated is a subtle indicator of hip pathology and should always prompt further radiographic evaluation. Stable slips rarely if ever suffer the serious complication of avascular necrosis but can lead to significant proximal femoral deformity, limited range of movement, limb length discrepancy and premature degenerative change. If a stable slip remains undetected an unstable slip may supervene and seriously affect the prognosis. The keystone of management is early detection followed in most cases by fixation in situ with a cannulated screw. The principle of this treatment is to promote fusion of the growth plate to prevent further slippage and deformity. Osteotomies to correct deformity are controversial and are usually, though not always, deferred for 18–24 months to allow for remodeling. Persistent difficulties are unlikely to improve spontaneously thereafter.

There is usually no difficulty in diagnosing the unstable slip which occurs when the femoral epiphysis suddenly slips posteriorly off the femoral metaphysis. The patient presents in severe pain, unable to weight bear and the leg is held in external rotation. The rate of avascular necrosis in the unstable slip is around 47%.[124] The blood supply to the femoral epiphysis is vulnerable in the immature hip and the vessels passing along the femoral neck to the epiphysis are suddenly torn or stretched in the unstable slip. The avascular necrosis that follows may not be seen radiographically for some months, but if it occurs it is a devastating complication with no satisfactory treatment. The management of the unstable slip once again involves fixing the slipped epiphysis in situ to promote physeal fusion and to prevent further slippage and damage to the epiphyseal blood supply. No attempt is made to deliberately correct the unstable slip, for fear of further damage to the epiphyseal blood supply, but inadvertent reduction does take place during positioning for fixation in unstable slips and can be accepted. Once again the role of femoral osteotomies in the management of unstable slips is controversial.

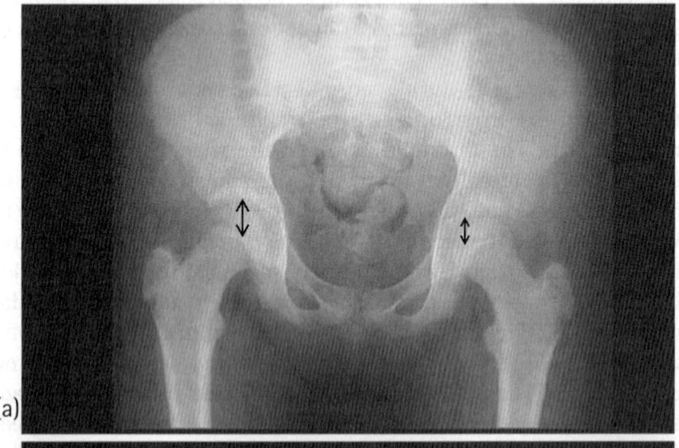

(a)

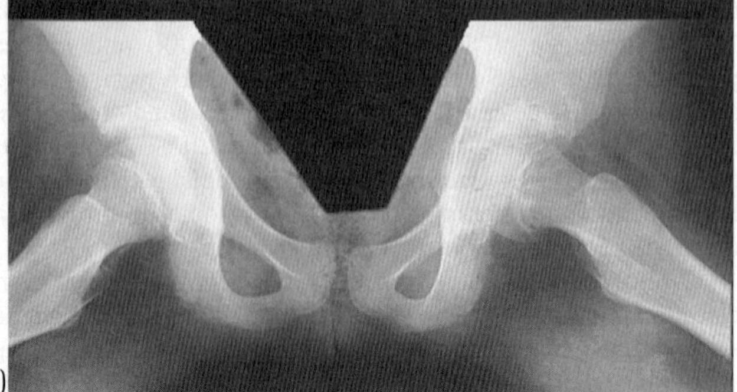

(b)

Fig. 27.49 Slipped capital femoral epiphysis: (a) AP radiograph; (b) frog lateral radiograph. Note the relative insensitivity of the AP radiograph – arrows demonstrate subtle difference in epiphyseal height.

The incidence of symptomatic bilateral SCFE averages around 25%, most contralateral slips occurring within 12 months of the original slip. Prophylactic fixation of the opposite side should be considered especially if the patient has an underlying endocrine or metabolic abnormality or in the young patient with some years of growth remaining. If the contralateral hip is not fixed the patient should be warned to return urgently at the first sign of hip or knee symptoms.

Idiopathic chondrolysis

This uncommon condition is characterized by the rapid and progressive destruction of articular cartilage from both sides of the affected joint with subsequent pain and stiffness. It is five times more common in girls than boys and is typically a condition of adolescents. Radiographs reveal narrowing of the affected joint space. Chondrolysis of the hip is of unknown etiology in most cases but has been reported in association with SCFE,[125] trauma, prolonged immobilization, and severe burns of the extremities.[126]

The natural history of chondrolysis includes an acute stage lasting 6–18 months with pain, inflammation, loss of range of motion and destruction of articular cartilage. Eventually the chronic stage emerges and can last from 3 to 5 years. During the chronic stage the hip may continue to deteriorate. Ultimately the hip may become pain free but stiff in a poor position, or pain free with partial or rarely complete return of motion and some restoration of the joint space.

The principles of treatment include control of any inflammation with therapeutic doses of NSAIDs and maintenance of motion with an aggressive physiotherapy program. Surgical release of persistent tendon contractures may be necessary in some patients and there are some encouraging results reported following aggressive subtotal capsulotomy and tendon release.[127] Some patients may ultimately come to hip arthrodesis in a functional position for the relief of pain.

Knee pain

Complaints of knee swelling, mechanical symptoms (giving way and locking) or pain are common in both children and adolescents. A knee joint effusion indicates intra-articular pathology and mechanical symptoms often indicate joint instability, loose bodies or meniscal pathology. Pain is either localized or diffuse. There are numerous explanations for localized knee pain in children including a variety of overuse and sport related problems (see later section, p. 1586). Referred knee pain is common and clinical examination of the hip is important in any patient presenting with unexplained knee pain.

Anterior knee pain (patellofemoral pain syndrome and chondromalacia)

Anterior knee pain is a descriptive term for diffuse pain at the front of the knee. It is a very common complaint in the adolescent age range and typically affects girls. The complaint is usually of a diffuse ache around the front of the knee at the patellofemoral joint (patellofemoral pain syndrome), which is worse after activity, after climbing up or down stairs and after sitting for prolonged periods with the knees in a flexed position. Chondromalacia is a term often used to describe this syndrome, but is really a pathological description of cartilage softening and degeneration, rarely present in young patients complaining of anterior knee pain.

The presentation of patellofemoral pain syndrome is fairly typical but evaluation should include reasonable steps to exclude other potential sources of pain. Lateral maltracking or subluxation of the patella is highly correlated with patellofemoral pain syndrome. Because the line of the quadriceps from the anterior superior spine to the tibial tuberosity passes to the lateral side of the knee joint, there is an inherent tendency for the patella to track to the lateral side of the trochlear sulcus in the anterior femur of the patellofemoral articulation. There are mechanisms to prevent such lateral maltracking, but these are sometimes inadequate. Pain at the lateral part of the articular surface of the patella can be a subtle consequence as can more overt subluxation or dislocation. Rotational malalignment also contributes to the problem and many patients will be found to have persistent femoral anteversion in association with compensatory external tibial torsion so that the feet point forwards but the patellae squint medially, the so called 'miserable malalignment'.[128]

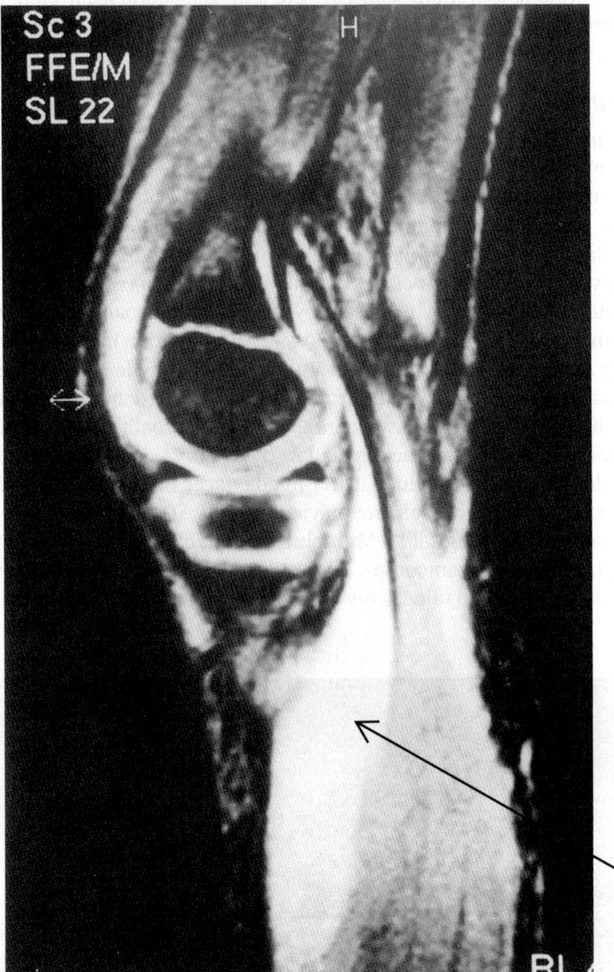

Fig. 27.50 MRI showing ruptured Baker's cyst – arrow indicates inflammatory fluid collection extending from the popliteal fossa into the calf.

The natural history of anterior knee pain is of slow resolution and most cases respond to non-operative treatment.[129] For many, reassurance is all that is necessary. Physiotherapy is helpful and activity modification may be necessary especially the avoidance of provoking sports. If there is evidence of maltracking some patients find a knee brace with a patella cut out, to hold the patella medially, is useful. An experienced physiotherapist can help with medial taping of the patella in combination with a program to stretch and strengthen quadriceps muscles. If symptoms are persistent and very troublesome in a patient with convincing maltracking surgical intervention in the form of a lateral retinacular release can be successful in 75% of cases.[130]

Discoid lateral meniscus

This is a congenital abnormality of the meniscus, which is the shape of a disc rather than the usual crescent. The discoid shape can be either complete, covering the whole lateral tibial platea, or partial forming a rather wider crescent than usual. Children present with mechanical symptoms of giving way, locking or snapping similar to patients with a meniscal tear. Radiographs of the knee sometimes reveal a lateral joint space that is wider than usual but MRI is the investigation of choice to demonstrate the extensive and thickened meniscus. Asymptomatic discoid menisci found incidentally should be left undisturbed. Symptomatic menisci can be successfully trimmed arthroscopically into a more normal crescent shape.[131]

Popliteal cyst

This common condition presents as a fluctuant transilluminable swelling in the popliteal fossa. The usual reason for referral is parental concern. The cysts are asymptomatic although they may ache with activity and fluctuate in size. They are typically found subcutaneously along the medial side of the popliteal fossa and are simple synovial lined cysts arising from the semimembranosus sheath.

Plain X-rays of the knee are normal and the cyst is best confirmed by ultrasound scan examination. No treatment is required other than reassurance since spontaneous resolution over months or years is usual.

Occasionally, usually in association with an inflammatory arthropathy, popliteal cysts may rupture presenting with calf pain and swelling, the ruptured 'Baker's cyst'. Ultrasound and MRI (Fig. 27.50) will distinguish this from other rare causes of calf pain and swelling in children.

Osteochondritis dissecans (OCD)

Osteochondritis dissecans most commonly involves the knee joint, but can affect the articular surface of any joint. For reasons that remain unclear an area of subchondral bone undergoes avascular necrosis. Etiological theories include trauma, ischemia, a genetic predisposition or a combination of these. Symptoms are usually vague and develop insidiously over several months. The overlying cartilage is initially intact but may subsequently develop degenerative change and break into a flap or a loose body causing the onset of mechanical joint symptoms, including locking, snapping or giving way. The most commonly affected part of the knee is the lateral part of the medial femoral condyle, although it can affect any part of the articular surface including the patella.

Radiographs usually reveal a lucent fragmented area in the subchondral bone (Fig. 27.51). In addition to the routine antero-posterior and lateral views of the knee, a tunnel view is useful because it visualizes the intercondylar notch region and the lateral part of the medial femoral condyle where the condition is most common. Magnetic resonance imaging is the investigation of choice

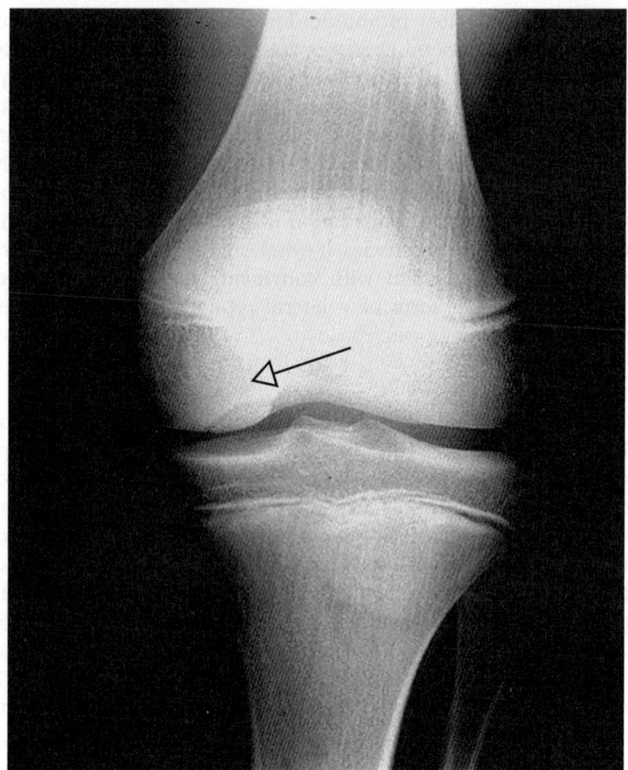

Fig. 27.51 Osteochondritis dissecans of the knee.

and not only delineates the bony abnormality but also provides some indication of whether the overlying cartilage is intact.

The prognosis of the condition is relatively good in young patients when the growth plate remains open but in adults and adolescents with a closed growth plate the prognosis is more guarded. Treatment should include activity modification to limit aggressive sporting activity, which may cause intact overlying cartilage to become loose. If there are no mechanical symptoms and MRI suggests that the overlying cartilage is intact, activity modification to limit symptoms is recommended until resolution which may take many months or even years. If there are mechanical symptoms or the MRI suggests the possibility of a breach or flap of the overlying cartilage, arthroscopic examination is recommended. Large flaps, especially on the weight bearing surface, should be fixed into position, although loose flaps are usually trimmed flush with the articular surface to prevent further mechanical symptoms and the base of the defect drilled to promote healing with fibrocartilage.

Kohler's disease

Kohler's disease or osteochondritis of the navicular presents in children around the age of 6 years. The radiographic appearance is that of fragmentation and flattening of the navicular (Fig. 27.52) but this radiological appearance may be a normal variant and is seen in asymptomatic children. The appearance is only considered pathological if there are associated symptoms of localized pain over the bone. Treatment of Kohler's disease is symptomatic. There is no evidence of any long-term sequelae.

Freiberg's disease

Freiberg's disease or osteochondritis of the metatarsal head is most common in the second metatarsal. It usually presents in adolescence with localized pain and radiographs reveal flattening and fragmentation of the metatarsal head. It is believed to be an avascular necrosis developing in a stress fracture[132] and is associated with local trauma as might occur in sport or in dancing. For reasons unknown the condition is much commoner in girls. Treatment is initially conservative but persistent local pain and limited dorsiflexion of the metatarsophalangeal joint may necessitate surgical debridement.

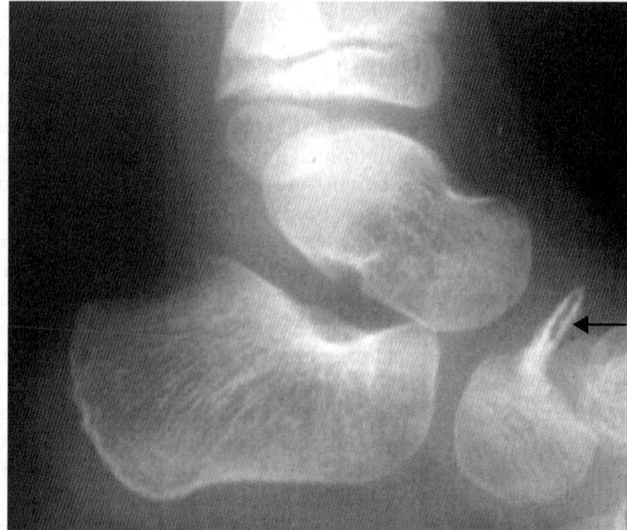

Fig. 27.52 Kohler's disease.

Tarsal coalition

Tarsal coalition is an abnormal cartilaginous, fibrous or bony connection between two or more tarsal bones. It is surprisingly common with a reported incidence of 2%. The condition is inherited as an autosomal dominant trait and the incidence in first-degree relatives is 39%.[133] Fortunately the majority of coalitions are asymptomatic. If symptoms develop they usually present during the late juvenile or early adolescent years when the coalition, which is initially cartilaginous, begins to ossify. The condition is characterized by a painful, rigid valgus foot and peroneal muscle spasm. Spasm may be continuous or intermittent, exacerbated by activity and relieved by rest.[134] The two commonest sites of coalition are between the calcaneus and the navicular (Fig. 27.53) and between the calcaneus and the talus, at the middle facet of the subtalar joint. Sixty per cent of calcaneonavicular and 50% of talocalcaneal coalitions are bilateral.[135] Multiple coalitions can rarely coexist in the same foot.[136] Calcaneonavicular coalitions begin to ossify between 8 and 12 years and talocalcaneal coalitions between 12 and 16 years.

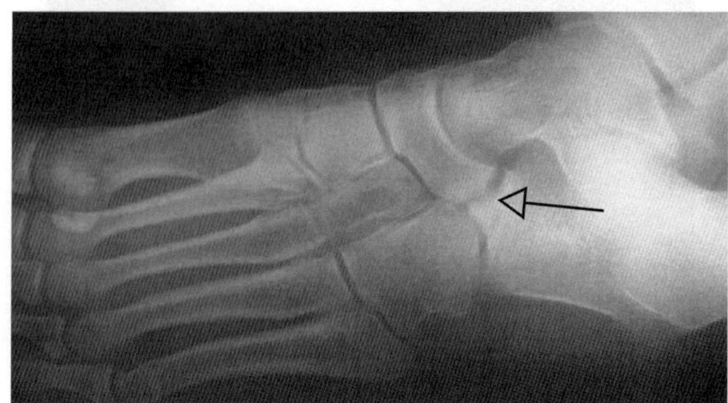

Fig. 27.53 Calcaneonavicular coalition.

Calcaneonavicular coalitions are most easily demonstrated radiographically with a 45° oblique radiograph of the foot. CT best demonstrates talocalcaneal coalitions. Secondary radiographic findings such as talar beaking should suggest the possibility of a tarsal coalition. Treatment is initially symptomatic with analgesia and immobilization. If conservative treatment fails, surgical resection of the abnormal coalition and interposition of fat or muscle to prevent recoalition has been shown to be successful in both calcaneonavicular[137] and talocalcaneal[138] coalitions. Generally, results are less satisfactory after talocalcaneal coalition resection and ultimately some patients come to a triple arthrodesis of the subtalar joint.

Adolescent hallus valgus

Hallux valgus or 'bunions' in adolescents is usually familial rather than the result of poor footwear. It is girls that usually present because of the appearance rather than because of functional problems or pain. There is often an associated bunionette of the fifth toe and patients often have a characteristically broad forefoot with varus of the first metatarsal (metatarsus primus varus). Surgery is best deferred until skeletal maturity is reached. Surgical treatment gives good results for symptomatic feet with a painful bunion but caution should be exercised in the pain free patient who may be disappointed if surgery leaves a better looking but painful foot.

VASCULITIS

Vasculitis is characterized by inflammation and necrosis of vessel walls. This may occur as a primary disorder, where the etiology remains unknown, or as a secondary phenomenon. Within the group of disorders known as the systemic vasculitides there are a variety of different conditions defined by the clinical pattern of the disease and the size of the vessels involved in the pathological process. Various systems have been proposed for the classification of these disorders, none ideal. The most widely used is that developed from the Chapel Hill Consensus Conference[139] which classifies the vasculitides on the basis of the size of the predominant vessels involved (Table 27.16). An alternative classification of pediatric vasculitis is shown in Table 27.17.[140]

Some of the childhood vasculitides are clearly defined, e.g. Henoch–Schönlein purpura and Kawasaki disease. However, there are many children with a systemic vasculitis in whom categorization is difficult due to overlapping clinical features. The importance of attempting to classify these conditions relates to their variable prognosis. Some are self-limiting while others require aggressive immunosuppressive therapy to try and minimize associated morbidity and even mortality. Prompt recognition of those requiring such treatment is perhaps more important than an exact diagnostic label but this would be facilitated by an improved classification system.

PRIMARY VASCULITIS

The only primary vasculitides seen with any frequency in childhood are Henoch–Schönlein purpura and Kawasaki disease. Rarer forms of primary vasculitis do occur and are important diagnoses to be aware of in order to avoid unnecessary delays in the instigation of appropriate treatment.

Henoch–Schönlein purpura

Henoch–Schönlein purpura (HSP) is the most common of the childhood vasculitides with an estimated incidence of 13.5:100 000.[141] It occurs most commonly in those under 10 years with a peak around the age of 5. In the majority of affected individuals it is a benign, self-limiting condition but it can be associated with significant morbidity and occasionally mortality if serious organ involvement occurs. It has been estimated that approximately 1% of children with HSP develop persistent renal disease with less than 0.1% having serious disease.[141]

Pathologically HSP causes a leukocytoclastic vasculitis. The etiology remains uncertain. The condition frequently appears to be triggered by an upper respiratory tract infection but no single causative agent appears to be responsible.[142] Although the pathology is poorly understood, there is much interest in the role of IgA. An elevated serum IgA may occur and the renal pathology overlaps with that seen in IgA nephropathy. Abnormalities in glycosylation of IgA1 have been identified in HSP and appear to be associated with renal involvement.[143]

HSP typically involves the skin, joints, GI tract and kidneys. The rash, characteristically a palpable purpura, affects the lower limbs (Fig. 27.54), buttocks, scrotum and elbows. More extensive involvement including rash affecting the face is not uncommon especially in younger children. An atypical rash which may even be urticarial may be seen in those under 2 years.

Arthralgia and even arthritis is common. The joint involvement is usually associated with marked periarticular swelling and is acute but self-limited. HSP does not cause a chronic arthropathy.

Table 27.16 Chapel Hill Consensus Conference classification of systemic vasculitis

Large vessel vasculitis *(aorta and major branches)*	Giant cell arteritis Takayasu's arteritis
Medium vessel vasculitis *(renal, hepatic, coronary and mesenteric arteries)*	Polyarteritis nodosa Kawasaki disease
Small vessel vasculitis *(venules, arterioles and capillaries)*	Wegener's granulomatosis* Churg–Strauss syndrome* Microscopic polyangiitis* Henoch–Schönlein purpura Essential cryoglobulinemic vasculitis Cutaneous leukocytoclastic vasculitis

*Associated with antineutrophil cytoplasmic antibodies
Adapted from Jennette et al 1994[139]

Table 27.17 A classification of systemic vasculitis in children

Polyarteritis	Polyarteritis nodosa Microscopic polyarteritis Cutaneous polyarteritis Kawasaki disease
Leukocytoclastic vasculitis	Henoch–Schönlein purpura Hypersensitivity vasculitis Mixed cryoglobulinemia
Granulomatous vasculitis	Wegener's granulomatosis Churg–Strauss syndrome Primary angiitis of the CNS
Giant cell arteritis	Takayasu's arteritis Giant cell arteritis
Miscellaneous	Behçet's disease Cogan's syndrome

Adapted from Lang 1999[140]

Gastrointestinal involvement with abdominal pain is one of the more troublesome symptoms of HSP and may be complicated by serious gastrointestinal bleeding, intussusception and rarely perforation of the bowel.[144] Renal involvement occurs in at least 50% of affected individuals and ranges from mild asymptomatic hematuria and proteinuria to a nephrotic/nephritic picture with hypertension and a rapidly progressive glomerulonephritis. The importance of HSP lies in the incidence of long term renal disease, and children with persisting urinary abnormalities require long term follow-up.

The diagnosis of HSP is clinical and usually straightforward. With an atypical course, the possibility of some other systemic vasculitis must be borne in mind but the distinction is seldom difficult. Urinalysis should be monitored throughout the course of the disease in all affected children to identify nephritis. Other laboratory investigation is unhelpful and unnecessary in most cases. Abdominal ultrasound may be useful in the assessment of gastrointestinal involvement: characteristic thickening of the bowel wall can be seen and intussusception ruled out where necessary. Evidence of serious or persistent renal involvement may be an indication for renal biopsy to assess the pathology and guide appropriate therapy.

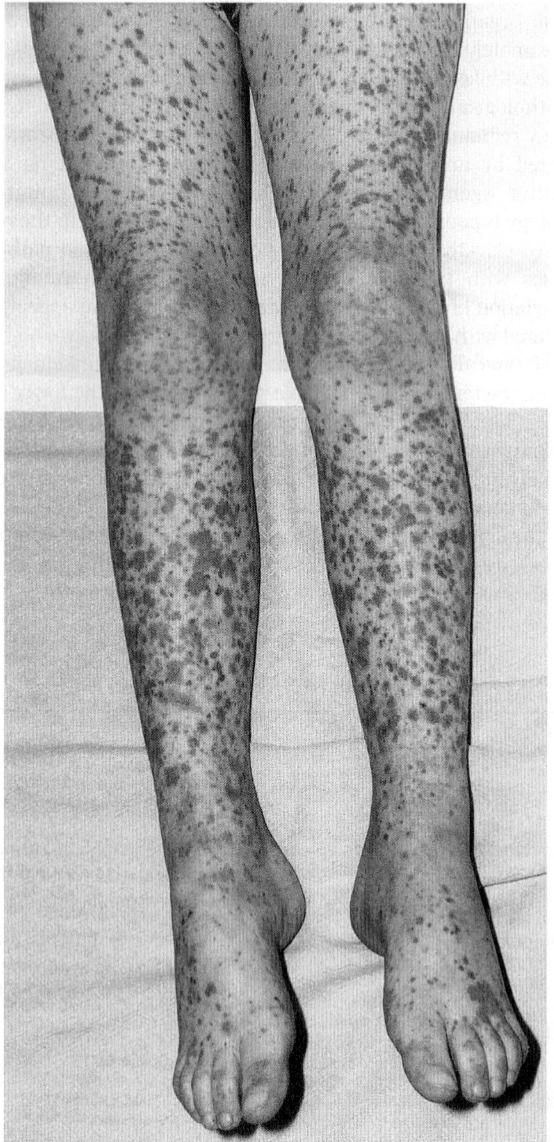

Fig. 27.54 Rash of Henoch–Schönlein purpura.

Management of HSP depends on its severity and the particular organ involvement in an individual. In most children it is mild and self-limiting although it may take a few weeks to settle. Recurrent attacks may be seen over a period of a few weeks or months. Most can be managed as outpatients with the parents being taught to test the urine for signs of renal involvement. Simple analgesia such as paracetamol may be adequate for joint and abdominal pain. More significant arthritis may respond to the use of NSAIDs although these must be used with caution if there is evidence of gastrointestinal involvement. Significant gastrointestinal involvement in HSP may be an indication for treament with steroids. There is much anecdotal evidence of improvement but no controlled trials. Management of renal involvement depends on its severity. Asymptomatic renal disease requires monitoring but no active therapy. There is uncontrolled evidence supporting the use of high dose steroids and immunosuppressive therapy where there is a rapidly progressive glomerulonephritis[145] but there are no controlled data. Debate continues around the issue of whether the incidence of serious renal sequelae can be reduced by the earlier administration of steroids.[146] There is a need for properly controlled studies in this area.[147]

Kawasaki disease

Kawasaki disease or Kawasaki syndrome, first described in Japan in 1967 by Tomisaku Kawasaki, is the other systemic vasculitis seen commonly in childhood. Originally thought to be a benign self-limiting illness it is now known to be a systemic vasculitis affecting medium sized vessels and with a particular predilection for involvement of the coronary arteries. This may lead to long term cardiac problems[148] and Kawasaki disease has replaced rheumatic fever as the most common cause of acquired heart disease in children in the developed world. Kawasaki disease predominantly affects children under 5 years with most cases, and most serious sequelae, affecting the under 2s.

As with all forms of primary vasculitis Kawasaki syndrome is poorly understood and its etiology unclear. Susceptibility to the disease appears to vary with race, children of Asian origin having a higher incidence than Caucasian populations. Recurrence is unusual but reported in around 3% of cases.[149] It occurs in mini-epidemics, its epidemiology therefore suggesting a role for infection in triggering the condition. Despite much research in this area, no single agent has been consistently associated with Kawasaki disease. There has been interest in the possible role of superantigens in triggering the syndrome in view of clinical similarities to toxic-shock syndrome and the identification of superantigen positive bacteria (both *Staphylococcus aureus* and *Streptococcus*) from a number of individuals with the syndrome.[150] This theory remains unproven to date. Although the trigger remains uncertain, immunological abnormalities are well documented in Kawasaki disease. Elevated levels of proinflammatory cytokines (TNF-alpha and beta; IL-1 and IL-6); upregulation of adhesion molecules (ELAM-1, ICAM-1 and VCAM-1) and more recently, elevated serum levels of macrophage colony-stimulating factor have all been demonstrated.[151]

The diagnosis is based on well-established clinical criteria (see Table 27.18). A definite diagnosis requires the presence of five of the six criteria or four plus documented coronary artery abnormalities. The problem in diagnosis lies with those children, commonly the youngest, who have 'atypical' or 'incomplete' Kawasaki syndrome.[152] These may only have two or three of the clinical criteria but go on to develop coronary artery involvement.

Table 27.18 Diagnostic criteria for Kawasaki disease

Criterion	Characteristics
1. Fever	5 days or more
2. Conjunctivitis	Bilateral, bulbar, non-suppurative
3. Lymphadenopathy	Cervical, tender, often unilateral > 1.5 cm diameter
4. Rash	Polymorphous
5. Changes in lips or oral mucosa	Dry, swollen, vertically cracked lips
6. Changes in extremities	Erythema of palms and soles; indurative edema hands and feet; membranous desquamation from finger and toe-tips in the post-acute phase

The current criteria may thus be insufficiently sensitive for diagnosis in the group at greatest risk of developing complications. A high index of suspicion is required to ensure that Kawasaki is not missed in the very young child.

The rash in Kawasaki syndrome is a polymorphous rash that usually occurs early in the disease course. Crusting, petechiae and vesicle formation are not typical of Kawasaki disease and should prompt a search for an alternative diagnosis. An erythematous rash affecting the groin and perineal area and which peels within 48 hours is characteristic (Fig. 27.55a). Involvement of the hands and feet consists of diffuse swelling and/or erythema of the palms and soles. Peeling of the digits (Fig. 27.55b) is well-known as a feature of Kawasaki but occurs relatively late in the subacute phase and is not diagnostically helpful. Kawasaki is a multisystem disease and can affect many organ systems (see Table 27.19 for other clinical features). Extreme irritability is very typical of the younger child.

As with most of the vasculitides, laboratory features are non-specific. Elevation of acute phase reactants is seen. Thrombocytosis may be marked in the subacute phase. A mild hepatitis is common, as is sterile pyuria. A lumbar puncture may be indicated in the febrile, irritable child and will show a mononuclear pleocytosis.

The importance of making the correct diagnosis lies in the fact that Kawasaki disease may result in dilatation and aneurysm formation of affected arteries, especially the coronary arteries. With treatment, the incidence of coronary artery involvement can be significantly reduced,[153] hence the importance of recognizing the condition at an early stage.

Untreated Kawasaki disease goes through three phases, acute, subacute and convalescent, the whole process lasting 6–8 weeks. Mortality from coronary artery involvement is 2%. With treatment the process can be switched off in the acute phase and the mortality reduced to 0.3%.

The recognition that the clinical features of Kawasaki disease were the result of an immunologically driven process led to the use of immunoglobulin in treatment with dramatic benefit. Treatment of acute phase Kawasaki disease with intravenous immunoglobulin has been clearly shown to reduce coronary artery involvement and hence mortality and morbidity.[153] A single infusion of 2 g/kg has been shown to be the optimal dose.[154] This is given with aspirin in high doses initially with reduction to an antiplatelet dose once defervescence occurs. Up to 20% of children with Kawasaki disease fail to settle following a first dose of intravenous immunoglobulin.[155] The dose can be repeated in the first instance. Those who fail to respond to treatment with a second dose or who have serious or life-threatening complications will usually benefit from high dose steroids.[156] The use of steroids in Kawasaki disease has been controversial over the years but there is sufficient anecdotal evidence to support their use in serious Kawasaki disease where they may be life saving.

All children with a definite diagnosis of Kawasaki disease require cardiac assessment to look for evidence of coronary artery involvement which will necessitate long term cardiology follow-up. Guidelines are available for long term follow-up[157] and the reader is referred to Chapter 19 for further information.

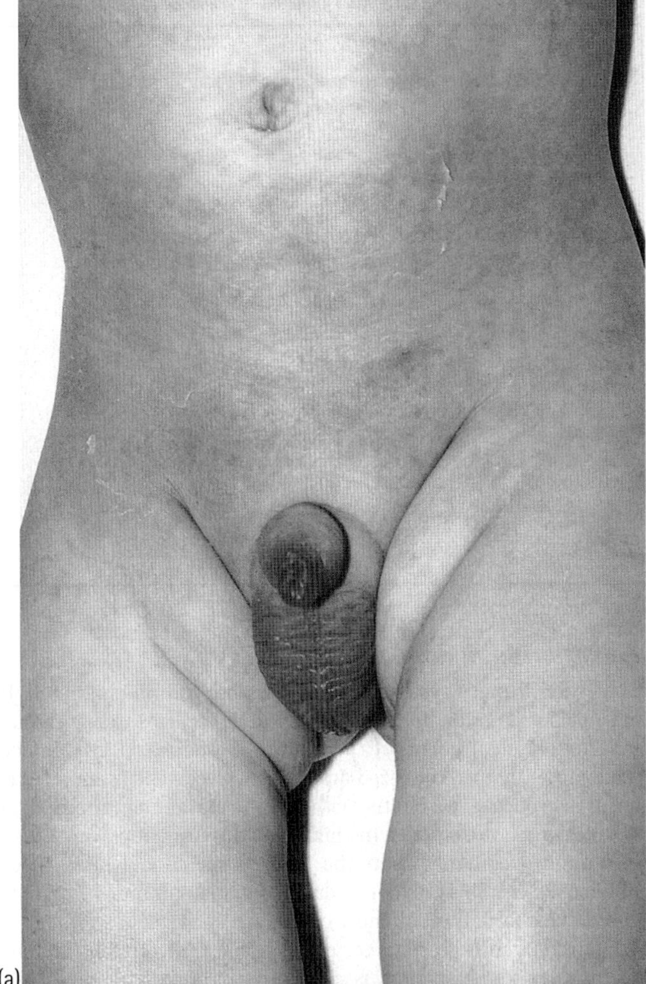
(a)

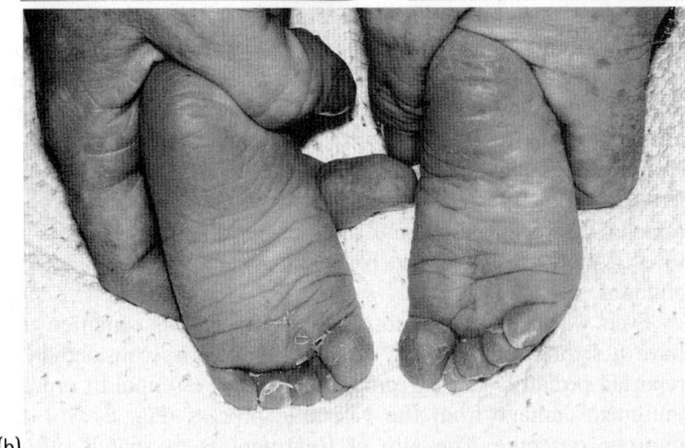
(b)

Fig. 27.55 Kawasaki disease: (a) typical erythematous groin rash with peeling; (b) peeling of digits

Table 27.19 Other features of Kawasaki disease

Cutaneous	Groin rash
Gastrointestinal	Diarrhea, vomiting, abdominal pain, Gall bladder hydrops Ascites
Joints	Arthritis Arthralgia
Renal	Sterile pyuria Proteinuria
Respiratory	Cough, rhinorrhea Pleural effusion
Cardiovascular	Pericardial effusion Myocarditis Murmurs, gallop rhythm Aneurysms of peripheral arteries
Neurological	Extreme irritability Convulsions Aseptic meningitis Facial palsy

Polyarteritis nodosa

The other primary systemic vasculitides are rare in childhood. In most pediatric series, polyarteritis nodosa is the least uncommon.

The classical form of polyarteritis nodosa (PAN) affects predominantly medium-sized arteries. Involved vessels are affected by a necrotizing vasculitis with the formation of aneurysmal nodules in the vessel walls. In childhood, this form of polyarteritis is seen more frequently than the microscopic kind which affects smaller vessels. This is in contradistinction to adult series where the microscopic form is much more common.

PAN frequently presents very non-specifically in childhood and a high index of suspicion is required to make the diagnosis. Presenting symptoms include unexplained malaise and fever, skin rash, abdominal pain, arthropathy and myalgia. Laboratory features are also very non-specific with the presence of anemia and raised inflammatory markers. Antineutrophil cytoplasmic antibodies (ANCA) are not associated with classical PAN.

The diagnosis is based on the presence of typical clinical features plus either characteristic abnormalities on biopsy of an affected tissue or abnormal angiography. Angiography is the investigation most likely to be diagnostically helpful in affected children.

Even with correct diagnosis and treatment this condition may have a significant mortality, although this varies considerably in reported pediatric series. Prompt treatment is essential in order to minimize damage from the vasculitic process (Fig. 27.56) and improve outcome. The aim of treatment is to switch off the inflammatory process. Unfortunately the rarity of these conditions in childhood means that there are no controlled studies. A combination of high dose steroids plus some other immunosuppressive drug is usually required. Cyclophosphamide is the drug of choice in most cases and can be used either orally or via intravenous pulses. Both are effective in inducing remission in PAN but intavenous pulse therapy has been associated with less toxicity than oral cyclophosphamide. Once remission has been attained, azathioprine has been shown to be as effective as cyclophosphamide for maintenance and is associated with less long term toxicity. Newer immunosuppressants such as mycophenolate mofetil may have a role to play. For those children who fail to respond to standard therapy with steroids and cyclophosphamide, there is anecdotal evidence that plasmapheresis may be useful. New experimental therapies such as stem cell transplantation may have a place in the management of disease resistant to other therapies.

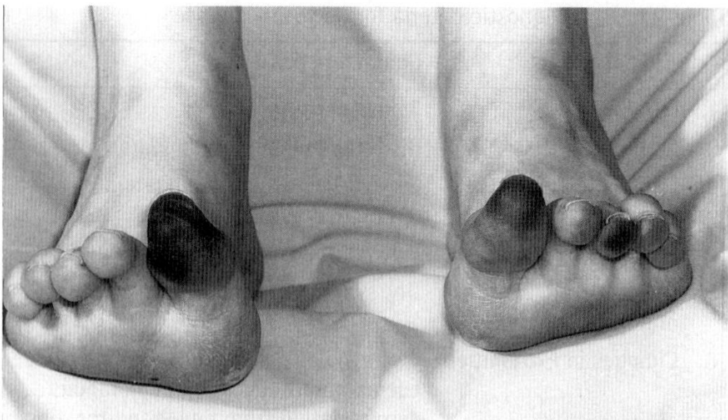

Fig. 27.56 Gangrene of several toes in polyarteritis nodosa.

Microscopic polyangiitis (MPA)

The microscopic variant of polyarteritis affects the smaller arteries and is less common than classical PAN in childhood, although there is some overlap between the two conditions. In adults this has been shown to have a worse prognosis and outcome than classical PAN. It is not clear whether this applies to pediatric cases. Renal involvement is common and frequently dominates the clinical presentation and course of this condition. As with other small vessel vasculitides, ANCA may be detectable. Management is similar to that of classical PAN.

Cutaneous polyarteritis

There are a group of children who present with a rash identical to that seen in PAN, sometimes associated with systemic upset, but with no evidence of major organ involvement. There is frequently evidence of previous streptococcal infection[158] and this is thought to play a role in the etiology. There is no evidence that this progresses to full blown PAN and it appears to be a separate entity. Prophylaxis with long term penicillin may prevent relapses.

Wegener's granulomatosis

Wegener's granulomatosis is rare in the pediatric population. Pathologically this is a necrotizing granulomatous vasculitis that predominantly affects the small vessels with a predilection for the upper and lower respiratory tract and kidneys. Although the exact pathophysiology is unclear, Wegener's granulomatosis is strongly associated with the presence of autoantibodies directed against proteinase 3 (c-ANCA). Whether or not these antibodies play a pathogenic role in the condition remains unclear. Wegener's may cause either localized or generalized disease. Steroids and cyclophosphamide are the mainstay of treatment in those with severe disease. With less serious involvement there may be a role for drugs such as methotrexate.

Churg–Strauss syndrome

This vasculitis is exceptionally rare in childhood. The clinical picture is of variable vasculitic features associated with asthma, eosinophilia and infiltrates on chest X-ray.

Takayasu's arteritis

Takayasu's arteritis, also known as 'pulseless disease', is rare in the UK but worldwide is one of the more common forms of systemic vasculitis affecting younger people. Pathologically it is a chronic giant cell arteritis which segmentally affects the large vessels particularly the aorta and its major branches. Following the initial inflammatory phase, stenosis of vessels leading to ischemia occurs.

During the active inflammatory phase of the disease, affected children may present with features of systemic upset such as fever, weight loss and myalgia. Often the disease presents with evidence of organ ischemia or hypertension.

The etiology of Takayasu's arteritis is unclear but genetic factors are important with evidence of racial variations in both incidence and disease expression. Infections and especially tuberculosis have been thought to play a role in triggering the disease but this remains unproven. Management is difficult. Steroids and methotrexate have a role in the active inflammatory phase. Once stricture formation has occurred, angioplasty and reconstructive surgery may be necessary.

Behçet's syndrome

Behçet's syndrome is an uncommon, poorly understood inflammatory condition in which at least some of the clinical features are the result of a vasculitis which can affect both arteries and veins. First described in 1937, Behçet's syndrome is characterized by aphthous oral ulceration, genital ulcers and uveiitis. Rare in the UK, Behçet's occurs much more commonly in eastern Mediterranean regions.

Behçet's disease is most commonly diagnosed in early adult life and is rare in childhood. The diagnosis is based on clinical features and may be difficult in children in whom recurrent oral ulceration may be the only manifestation for some years. Until other features become apparent, it may not be possible to confirm the diagnosis. The oral ulcers occur in crops lasting up to 2 weeks. They are painful and may cause the child to refuse to eat. Genital ulceration occurs frequently in children with Behçet's. Uveiitis, although common in affected adults, occurs less frequently in pediatric cases. Arthralgia and arthritis are common in children with Behçet's as is recurrent fever. Skin lesions seen most frequently in children are folliculitis and erythema nodosum. Gastrointestinal involvement may cause abdominal pain and diarrhea and is reported in approximately a fifth of affected children. CNS involvement, particularly meningoencephalitis, is seen in approximately 25%. Vascular involvement, which includes both venous and arterial thromboses and aneurysm formation, is potentially the most serious complication of Behçet's syndrome. Pulmonary vasculitis, although rare in affected children, is associated with a high mortality.

Significant vascular involvement is associated with a poor outcome and merits treatment with systemic immunosuppressive agents.[159] Colchicine[160] and thalidomide[161] have been shown to be effective for Behçet's syndrome where mucocutaneous lesions predominate.

Cogan's syndrome

This systemic vasculitis is extremely rare. It is characterized by the association of vasculitic features with interstitial keratitis and vestibuloauditory dysfunction.

SECONDARY VASCULITIS

Secondary vasculitis occurs quite commonly in children. It may be seen in the context of a child known to have some other autoimmune rheumatic disorder such as juvenile idiopathic arthritis or systemic lupus erythematosus (Fig. 27.57). Treatment is that of the underlying disorder.

Vasculitis may also occur in association with a variety of infections. These include bacterial infections, viruses such as

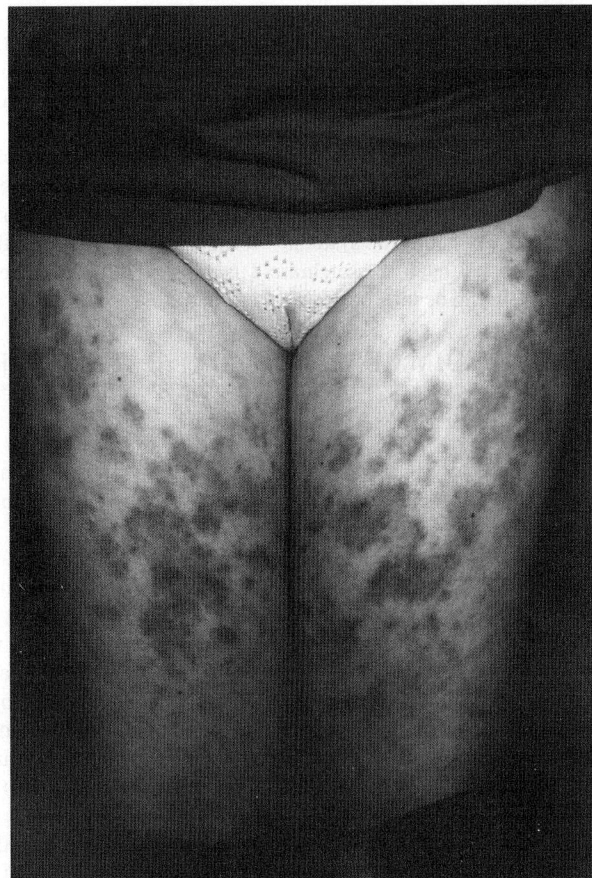

Fig. 27.57 Secondary vasculitis in a child with systemic lupus erythematosus.

Epstein–Barr virus and infections such as tuberculosis. Vasculitis is seen not uncommonly in association with meningococcal disease.

Drugs may also be associated with vasculitis which usually remits when the offending agent is withdrawn.

ANTINEUTROPHIL CYTOPLASMIC ANTIBODIES (ANCA)

Antineutrophil cytoplasmic antibodies (ANCA) were first described in association with Wegener's granulomatosis in 1985. Subsequent associations with MPA and Churg–Strauss syndrome have been documented and measurement of these antibodies has become part of the routine workup in a patient with suspected systemic vasculitis. Despite these recognized associations the clinical significance of these antibodies and their role, if any, in the pathogenesis of these conditions remains uncertain. A report of a positive ANCA must be interpreted with caution and in the context of the clinical problem. The initial screening test used to detect these antibodies is an indirect immunofluorescence method which documents the presence of the antibody and divides ANCA into three groups depending on the pattern of staining. Cytoplasmic or c-ANCA gives coarse granular staining of the cytoplasm; perinuclear or p-ANCA gives staining of the nucleus and perinuclear area; while atypical ANCA show no particular staining pattern. It must be remembered that the immunofluorescence test, although a good screening test, lacks specificity. The antigenic specificity of ANCA must be confirmed, usually by enzyme linked immunosorbent assays (ELISA). The number of antigens described as targets for ANCA is increasing.

The c-ANCA pattern, strongly associated with proteinase-3, is characteristically found in Wegener's granulomatosis. A positive p-ANCA, associated with antimyeloperoxidase, is more commonly seen in MPA. p-ANCA associated with other antigens and atypical ANCA are seen in many inflammatory conditions.

Although ANCA testing is commonly performed in a child with suspected vasculitis the result is not diagnostic. ANCA may be seen in many different clinical situations and a negative ANCA does not rule out the possibility of systemic vasculitis. A strongly positive c-ANCA directed against proteinase-3 is suggestive of Wegener's but results should be interpreted with caution.

OTHER AUTOIMMUNE RHEUMATIC DISORDERS

SYSTEMIC LUPUS ERYTHEMATOSUS

Systemic lupus erythematosus (SLE) is a multisystem systemic inflammatory disorder most commonly seen in young adult women but well recognized in the pediatric age group. It is rare in prepubertal children and seen more commonly in the teenage years. Most pediatric series show a peak at 11–14 years but this may reflect referral bias, with older teenagers being referred direct to adult clinics. Females predominates in adult series, making up 85–90% of all cases. In children males make up a larger percentage of cases with a male to female ratio of 1:4.5. There are no good epidemiological studies of lupus in children: estimates of incidence are in the region of 10–20 per 100 000 children (under 18 years) but this varies widely depending on the the ethnic mix of the population. Lupus is more common in non-Caucasian races.

SLE has been regarded as the prototype autoimmune disorder with the recognition that one of the hallmarks of the disease is the production of a variety of autoantibodies. The presence of antinuclear antibodies (ANA) is virtually universal in children with lupus, a fact which can aid in making the diagnosis. Despite this recognition, the pathophysiology of lupus and the role that these antibodies play in the disease remain poorly understood. The presence of antibodies against double-stranded DNA is associated with the development of glomerulonephritis in lupus and the deposition of DNA-anti-DNA immmune complexes is thought to play a role in the disease process. The role of other autoantibodies remains unclear.

Abnormalities in the functioning of most of the cells in the immune system have been documented in lupus. A genetic predisposition to the development of lupus exists as seen by a familial incidence of the condition.[162] Environmental triggers, including viruses, are thought to play a role in disease onset.

Lupus is a multisystem disorder which can present in many different ways and with many different features. This can make diagnosis difficult unless a high level of awareness of the condition exists. Delays in making the diagnosis are common with the mean time to diagnosis being estimated at over a year in most pediatric series. The diagnosis is based on a combination of clinical and laboratory features. Diagnostic criteria developed for use in adult patients (see Table 27.20) have been shown to be valid in a pediatric population.[164]

Lupus is extremely variable in both its clinical presentation and its severity. It ranges from a relatively mild condition characterized by a facial rash, joint pains and fatigue to a severe life-threating illness. The most common cause of mortality in lupus today is infection but CNS and renal involvement result in serious morbidity.

A wide variety of systems are involved in lupus. General systemic symptoms such as fevers, weight loss, fatigue, arthralgia and general malaise are common both at the onset of lupus in children and throughout the disease course. The fatigue may be profound, disabling and difficult to treat. The characteristic skin rash is the facial butterfly rash which crosses the bridge of the nose and spares the nasolabial folds (Fig. 27.58). Other rashes (e.g. vasculitic) may occur in SLE and many children with lupus exhibit marked photosensitivity.

Table 27.20 Revised American College of Rheumatology criteria for the classification of systemic lupus erythematosus

1. Malar rash
2. Discoid rash
3. Photosensitivity
4. Oral ulceration
5. Arthritis
6. Serositis:
   a. pleuritis
   b. pericarditis
7. Renal disorder:
   a. Proteinuria >0.5 g/24 h
   b. Cellular casts
8. Neurological disorder:
   a. Seizures
   b. Psychosis (other causes excluded)
9. Hematological disorders:
   a. Hemolytic anemia
   b. Leukopenia $< 4 \times 10^9$/L (two or more occasions)
   c. Lymphopenia $< 1.5 \times 10^9$/L (two or more occasions)
   d. Thrombocytopenia $< 100 \times 10^9$/L
10. Immunological disorders:
    a. Raised antinative DNA antibody binding
    b. Anti-Sm antibody
    c. Antiphospholipid antibodies
       i. Abnormal serum levels of IgG or IgM anticardiolipin antibodies
       ii. Positive test for lupus anticoagulant
       iii. False-positive serological test for syphilis present for at least 3 months
11. Antinuclear antibody present in raised titer

A person shall be said to have SLE if four or more of the 11 criteria are present (serially or simultaneously).
Adapted from Hochberg 1997[163]

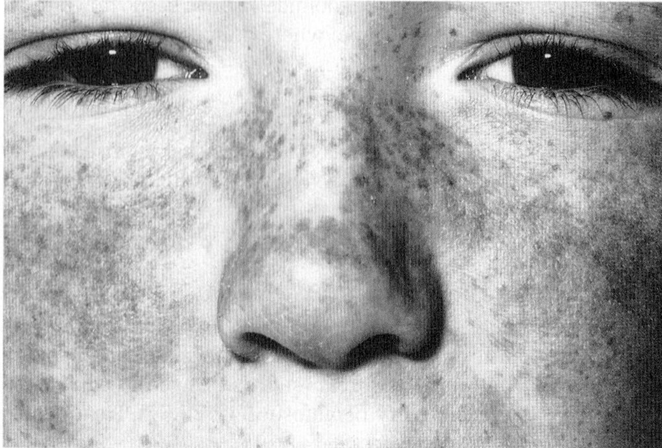

Fig. 27.58 Typical facial rash in systemic lupus erythematosus – crossing the bridge of the nose and sparing the nasolabial folds.

Alopecia is usually mild but can be severe with scarring. Raynaud's phenomenon is common. Hematological involvement is frequent in pediatric lupus which may present initially with what appears to be idiopathic thrombocytopenic purpura. CNS lupus is a cause of much long term morbidity and may manifest as seizure activity, psychosis, aseptic meningitis or headaches. Mood alteration is common and it may be difficult to separate organic CNS involvement from reactive symptoms due to coping with a chronic illness.

Renal involvement is frequent in childhood lupus and one of the major causes of morbidity. When present it tends to dominate the clinical picture. It may present as asymptomatic hematuria and proteinuria, hypertension, nephrotic syndrome or a rapidly progressing glomerulonephritis. Renal biopsy has an important role to play in determining the severity and therefore the likely outcome of the renal disease.

Children with lupus are at particular risk from infection which is now the most common cause of death. This is a result both from the disease process itself and from the use of immunosuppressive treatment regimens. Pneumococcal sepsis is a particular risk and pneumococcal vaccination is recommended.

Laboratory investigations are helpful both in the diagnosis and monitoring of SLE. Anemia occurs as a result of chronic disease or hemolysis. Thrombocytopenia and leukopenia are common. Characteristically the ESR is elevated while the CRP remains normal. Renal function needs to be monitored in those with renal involvement. A mild transaminitis is common but serious liver abnormalities are rare. Serum complement levels are reduced in most patients while serum immunoglobulin levels are non-specifically elevated. A positive antinuclear antibody (ANA) is found in virtually all patients and is a useful diagnostic tool. The ANA result must be interpreted in the light of the clinical picture as the specificity for lupus is low and children may have a positive ANA for many reasons. Antibodies against double stranded DNA and Sm (Smith antigen) are of greater specificity. Other autoantibodies such as anti-Ro, La and RNP may occur.

Management of lupus requires regular monitoring and attention to detail. Optimal management is in a multidisciplinary team setting with input from both a pediatric rheumatologist and a pediatric nephrologist. Drug therapy depends on disease severity and organs involved. Mild lupus can be managed with non-steroidal anti-inflammatories and hydroxychloroquine. Avoidance of sun exposure and the use of sunblock may also be helpful. Thalidomide has been used for severe mucocutaneous disease. More significant disease will require the use of moderate doses of steroids while severe disease which is life- or organ-threatening will require treatment with high dose steroids and immunosuppressive agents such as azathioprine and cyclophosphamide. Controlled studies in adults have shown the superiority of combinations of steroids and immunosuppressants over steroids alone[165,166] but there are no controlled studies in pediatric SLE. Treatment must be sufficient to suppress disease activity but aim to minimize toxicity where possible. The long term toxicity particularly of high dose steroid regimens is very significant and steroid side-effects are particularly unacceptable to teenage girls who are the group most affected by lupus. Recently there has been interest in the use of mycophenolate mofetil as a potentially less toxic alternative to cyclophosphamide.[167]

The ESR, urine protein level, levels of C3 and C4 and ds-DNA titer may all be used in monitoring disease activity and response to treatment but clinical assessment of disease activity remains the gold standard. A variety of assessment tools have been developed recently to allow quantitative assessment of disease activity in lupus. The SLEDAI (Systemic Lupus Erythematosus Disease Activity Index) and the BILAG (British Isles Lupus Assessment Group) indices have both been used in children and shown to be highly sensitive to changes in clinical disease activity.[168]

SLE is a serious disease and those who present in childhood have a high incidence of major organ involvement. Current treatment has markedly reduced the mortality but the long term morbidity remains high. Infection is the most common cause of death but renal death with the consequent need for dialysis and transplantation continues to occur in those with aggressive nephritis. Early diagnosis and optimal management should reduce this but the need for improved treatment protocols remains.

As survival rates from childhood lupus have improved it is clear that there is a high incidence of serious long term morbidity. CNS disease results in long term psychological sequelae in many. Osteoporosis results both from the disease and its treatment. Lupus is now known to cause a dyslipoproteinemia which is worsened by treatment with steroids and early onset coronary artery disease is a major complication of childhood lupus. Whether this can be altered by treatment of the lipid abnormalities is unknown.

Drug induced lupus

A number of drugs are well known to cause a lupus-like syndrome. The best known in children are the antiepileptic drugs phenytoin and carbamazepine and the antihypertensives hydralazine and captopril. A newly recognized addition to the list that is important in teenagers is minocycline, commonly prescribed for acne.[169]

Antiphospholipid syndrome

As with other autoantibodies such as ANA, antiphospholipid antibodies of low titer are seen not uncommonly in children. These are frequently thought to be epiphenomena of no clinical significance. Antiphospholipid antibodies are produced in around 30% of children with SLE but are frequently present in low titer and of dubious clinical significance: the level of antibody associated with a risk of developing a clinical problem is unknown. The antiphospholipid syndrome occurs where higher titers of antibodies are associated with coagulation abnormalities and thromboembolic events.

Antiphospholipid syndromes are usually secondary, frequently in association with SLE. Primary antiphospholipid syndromes have been described in childhood but are rare.

These antibodies should be looked for in any child presenting with unexplained thromboembolic phenomena. Anticoagulation is required where there is evidence of an associated thrombotic problem. The role of prophylaxis, with either low dose anticoagulation or aspirin, in children is unclear.

Neonatal lupus erythematosus

The neonatal lupus syndrome is defined by the presence of maternal autoantibodies to Ro and La which cross the placenta causing clinical abnormalities in the fetus and neonate. The characteristic skin rash, thrombocytopenia and hepatic abnormalities are usually self-limiting. The importance of the syndrome lies in its association with congenital heart block which may cause intrauterine bradycardia, cardiac failure and death. This syndrome usually affects pregnancies of women with only mild lupus or of healthy women subsequently found to have anti-Ro and La antibodies.

JUVENILE DERMATOMYOSITIS AND POLYMYOSITIS

The idiopathic inflammatory myopathies comprise a group of conditions characterized by unexplained inflammation of the muscles. In childhood, dermatomyositis is ten times more common than polymyositis.

Juvenile dermatomyositis (JDM) is a rare condition with an incidence of 1.9 per million children under 16 years in the UK.[170] Juvenile dermatomyositis can occur at all ages throughout childhood but with two peaks of presentation at 5–9 years and at 11–14 years. The condition is more common in females than males.

The etiology of JDM is unknown. In children, unlike adults, there is no association with malignancy. Both genetic and infectious factors may play a role. In the USA studies have shown an association with HLA-DQ1*501[171] implying a role for genetic factors in the etiology of this condition. More recently there has been interest in the role of TNF in the inflammatory myopathies and an over-representation of TNF-alpha-308A allele was found in a population of children with JDM.[172] A number of epidemiological studies have documented clustering of onset of cases, stimulating interest in the role of infectious agents in triggering the condition. No single agent has been identified. Once established, a variety of immunological abnormalities occur in children with JDM. Antinuclear antibodies are found in approximately 60%. Their specificity is for the most part unknown and in contrast to adults, myositis-specific antibodies (e.g. Jo-1; Mi) are seldom present. Active disease is associated with elevation of serum immunoglobulin levels, evidence of complement activation, lymphopenia and an increase in the percentage of B lymphocytes.

The diagnosis of JDM is based on criteria published by Bohan and Peters in the 1970s. A child is considered to have JDM if, having excluded other known causes, they have a characteristic rash plus three of the following four criteria: symmetrical proximal muscle weakness, elevated muscle enzymes, abnormal muscle histology and EMG changes. There is increasing use of modalities such as MRI to demonstrate inflammatory muscle changes. This may replace more invasive investigations in many patients and there is a need for a revision of these diagnostic criteria.

The rash in JDM is the first symptom in approximately 50% of children. A further 25% report a simultaneous onset of the rash and weakness while in the last 25% weakness precedes the rash. The typical rash affects the eyelids, knuckles and extensor aspects of the knees and elbows (Fig. 27.59). Erythema affecting the face and upper trunk may also be seen. The eyelid rash is violaceous in hue, while the lesions over the knuckles may have a hypertrophic appearance (Gottron's papules) (Fig. 27.60). Marked nailfold erythema is frequently seen and is indicative of the vasculopathy that characterizes JDM. Examination of the nail fold capillaries will show typical changes with capillary dilatation and areas of thrombosis (Fig. 27.60).

The other major feature of JDM is an inflammatory myopathy. This affects the proximal limb muscles, often first noticed by difficulty with climbing stairs or brushing hair. Muscle weakness may be severe and involvement of the neck flexors and abdominal muscles occurs in addition to those in the limbs. Weakness is frequently associated with complaints of muscle pain and tenderness. Myositis is confirmed by documenting abnormalities of muscle enzymes such as creatine kinase, aspartate aminotransferase (AST), alanine aminotransferase (ALT), aldolase and lactate dehydrogenase (LDH). It should be remembered that muscle enzymes may be normal despite active disease. EMG, muscle biopsy and MRI will show characteristic inflammatory change (Fig. 27.61).

JDM is a multisystem disease and although the main features are of skin and muscle involvement, many organ systems can be affected by the widespread vasculopathy. Dysphagia occurs as a result of disease affecting the esophagus while dysphonia results from involvement of the soft palate. Cardiac abnormalities are reported in up to 50%. Most are minor but cardiomyopathy can

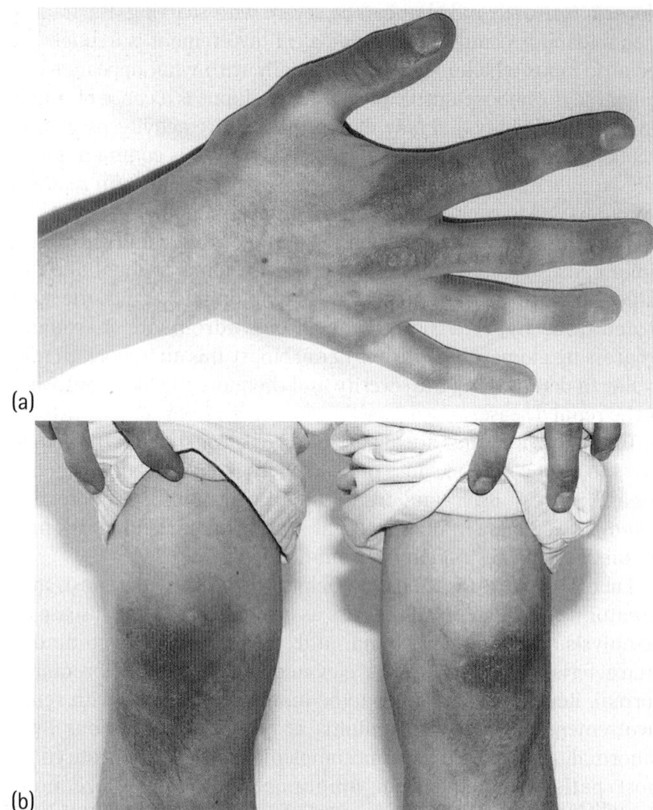

Fig. 27.59 Typical rash of juvenile dermatomyositis with erythema over: (a) extensor aspects of metacarpophalangeal and proximal interphalangeal joints; (b) knees.

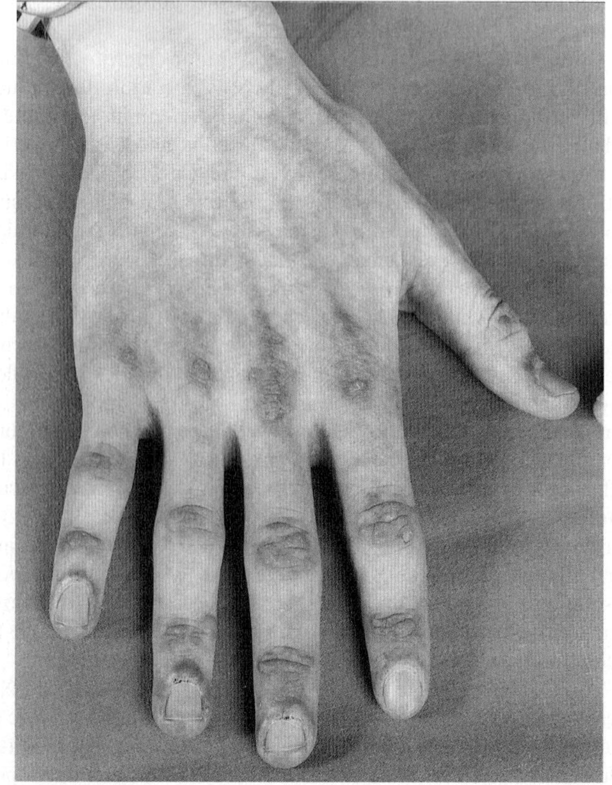

Fig. 27.60 Juvenile dermatomyositis showing Gottron's papules and typical nailfold changes.

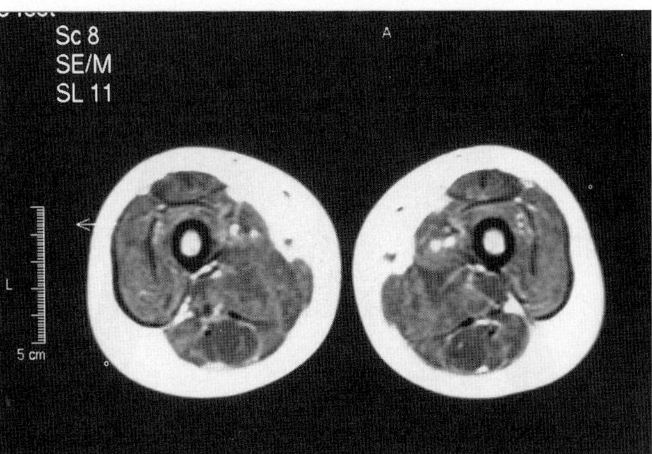

Fig. 27.61 Muscle MRI in juvenile dermatomyositis showing patchy, heterogeneous texture of the muscles typical of an inflammatory myopathy.

occur. Interstitial lung disease is uncommon but carries a poor prognosis.

Before the advent of steroids, JDM had a very poor prognosis. Thirty per cent of affected children died, 30% had severe chronic disease and only 30% recovered. Steroids and more recent developments in therapy have dramatically changed the outlook but this is still a disease with an associated mortality and significant morbidity. Traditionally three patterns of disease have been recognized. Some children have an acute monocyclic course which resolves with treatment; others a relapsing, remitting course while a third group have severe, unremitting chronic disease. In addition it is now recognized that there is a wide variety of clinical patterns seen within the overall label of JDM. Some children have predominantly muscle disease, others cutaneous. Some have both while a further group have evidence of a widespread vasculopathy with cutaneous ulceration (Fig. 27.62) and serious organ involvement.

Calcinosis of the muscle is a well-recognized complication of JDM (Fig. 27.63). It is at least in part related to disease severity and duration and its incidence can be reduced by prompt and appropriate treatment. In recent years it has been noted that lipodystrophy may complicate JDM (Fig. 27.64) and in some is associated with the development of insulin resistance. As with lupus, osteoporosis is a complication both of the disease and its therapy.

Treatment of JDM remains controversial. There is no consensus on the type, route of administration and duration of treatment and there are no randomized controlled trials. In uncomplicated JDM, oral prednisolone is the most commonly used treatment in a dose of 1–2 mg/kg/day, tapering over 12–18 months. In an attempt to get more rapid disease control and minimize toxicity from oral steroids, many now advocate initial treatment with pulse intravenous

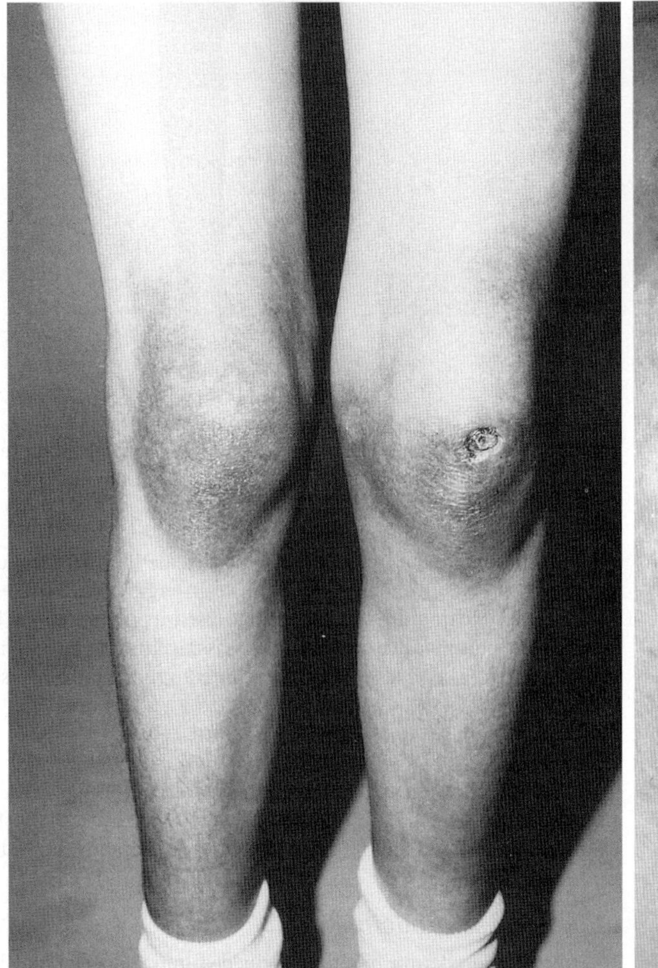

(a)

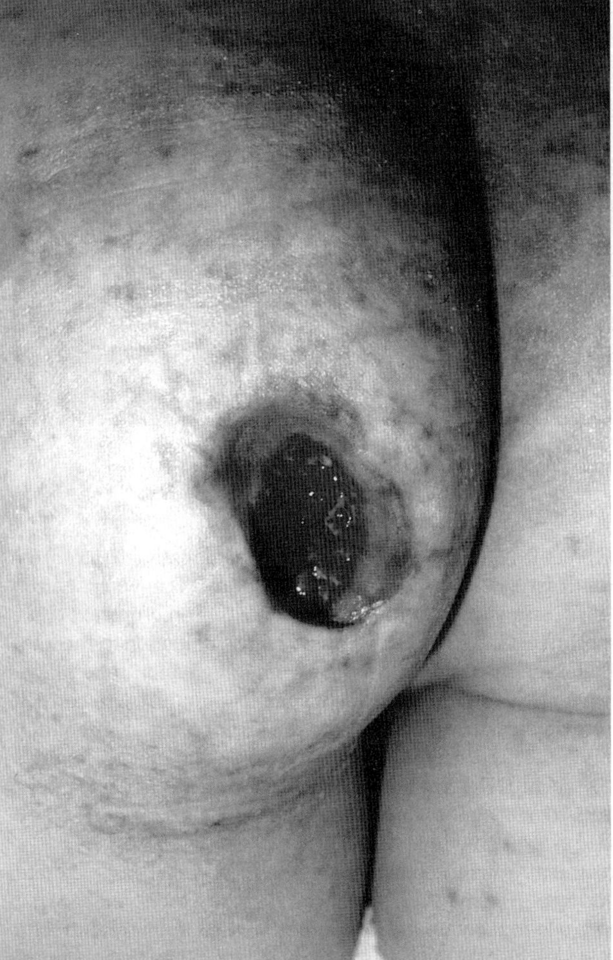

(b)

Fig. 27.62 (a & b) Ulcerative vasculopathy in juvenile dermatomyositis.

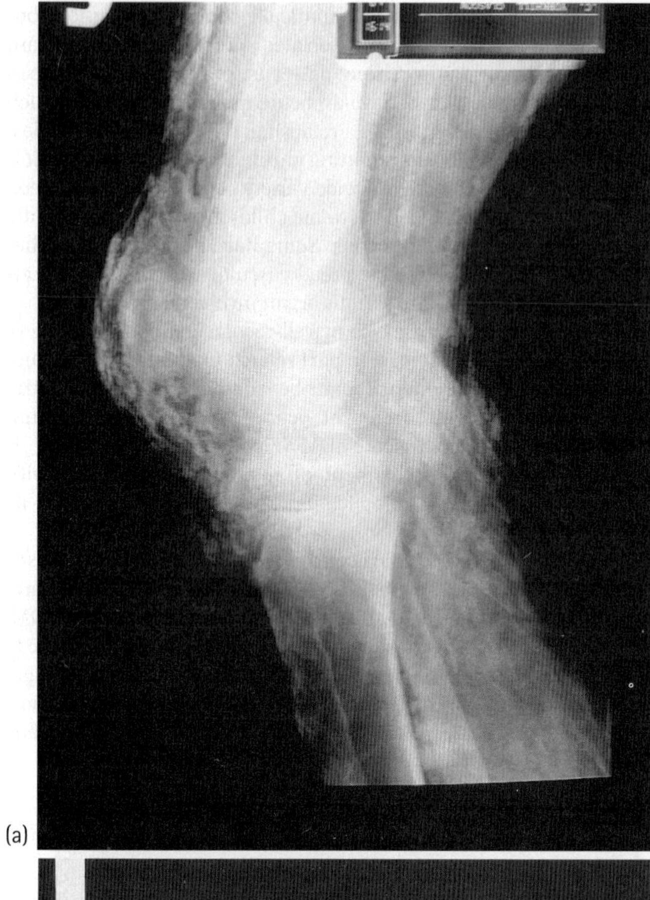

(a)

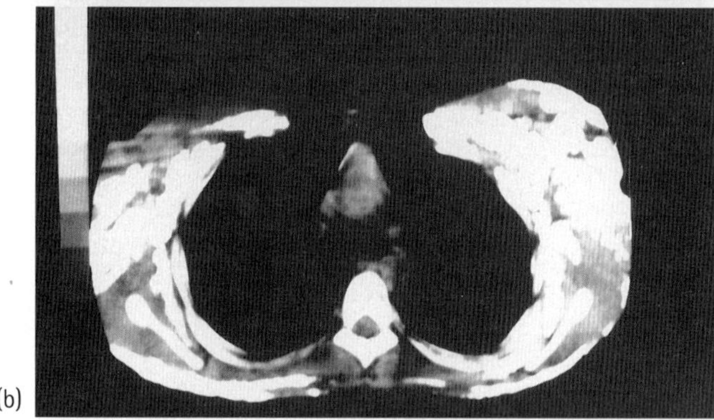

(b)

Fig. 27.63 Juvenile dermatomyositis with extensive calcinosis affecting: (a) lower limb (plain radiograph); (b) chest wall (CT scan).

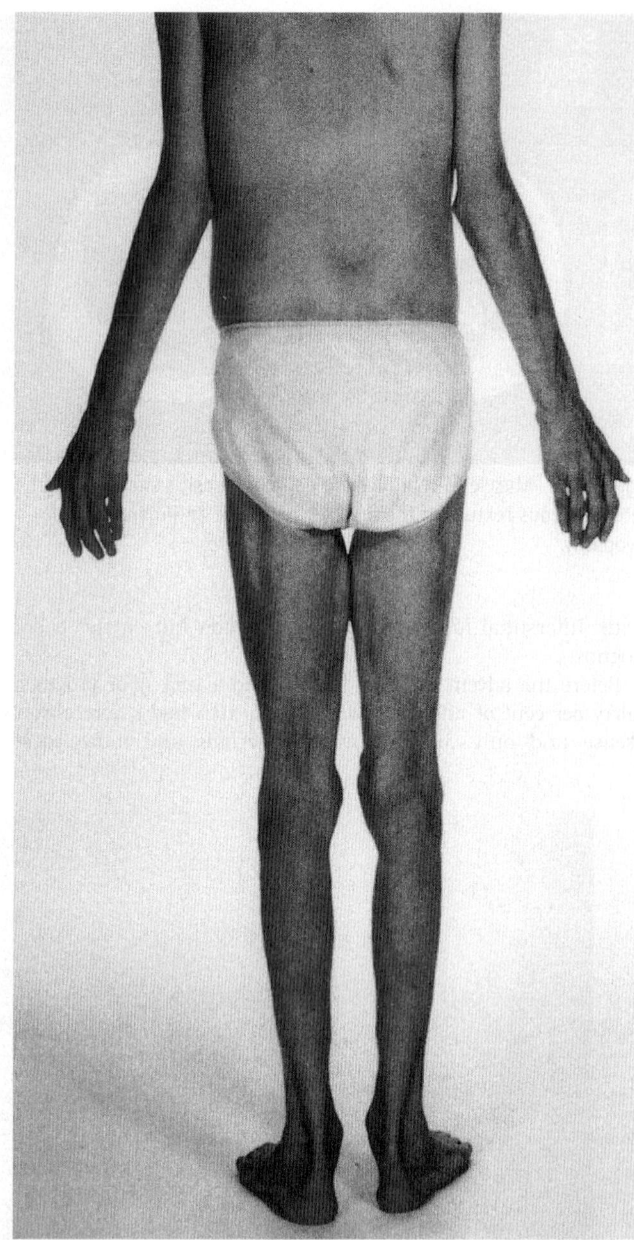

Fig. 27.64 Lipodystrophy in juvenile dermatomyositis – absence of subcutaneous fat in lower limbs.

methylprednisolone. Other drugs were traditionally reserved for those with severe or steroid resistent disease but it is now recognized that early use of an additional drug, either methotrexate or ciclosporin, results in reduced morbidity and a reduction in the total steroid dosage required. Intravenous immunoglobulin may play a role in some patients and cyclophosphamide may be indicated if there is evidence of significant vascular involvement or interstitial lung disease. There is interest in the use of new therapeutic options such as the anti-TNF drugs or stem cell transplantation in children who fail to respond to other therapies but these must still be regarded as experimental.

Treatment is adjusted depending on the clinical response but monitoring of JDM may be difficult. Levels of muscle enzymes are not a good guide to activity and should not be used to plan treatment. Clinical assessment is the gold standard and there have been various attempts to try and improve methods of doing this. The recently developed childhood myositis assessment scale (CMAS)[7] is a useful method for objectively assessing muscle strength. Serial scores can then be used to quantify changes in the disease process. MRI is being used as a non-invasive method of assessing muscle inflammation and again may be used serially to document progress of the disease.

SCLERODERMA IN CHILDHOOD

The scleroderma group of disorders is characterized clinically by thickening of the skin. This can occur in both localized and systemic forms, the former occurring much more commonly in pediatric practice.

Localized scleroderma

Localized scleroderma may be subdivided into morphea and linear scleroderma. Morphea lesions most commonly occur on the trunk and present as pale patches of thickened skin. When active there may be surrounding erythema and with time they become hyperpigmented (Fig. 27.65). They usually occur as isolated lesions and, although they may be cosmetically unpleasant, seldom cause other problems.

Linear scleroderma is of much greater concern. In this condition the child or parent may notice a band of skin discoloration in a linear distribution on a limb or on the face/scalp (when it is known as 'en coup de sabre'; Fig. 27.66). These lesions do not follow a dermatomal distribution and they are poorly understood. As with morphea, an erythematous color may indicate an active lesion. With time they may become hyperpigmented. These lesions may be associated with significant atrophy and undergrowth of surrounding structures or the affected limb (Fig. 27.67) causing significant cosmetic and functional difficulties.

Our lack of understanding of the underlying process in these conditions makes treatment difficult. There is anecdotal evidence that anti-inflammatory therapy can improve active lesions and a combination of steroid and methotrexate may be useful. Where a band of linear scleroderma crosses a joint, vigorous physiotherapy may be helpful in maintaining joint range.

Systemic sclerosis

The systemic sclerosis disorders are extremely uncommon in pediatric practice. Systemic sclerosis can be subdivided into diffuse cutaneous sytemic sclerosis (formerly known as progressive systemic sclerosis) and limited cutaneous systemic sclerosis

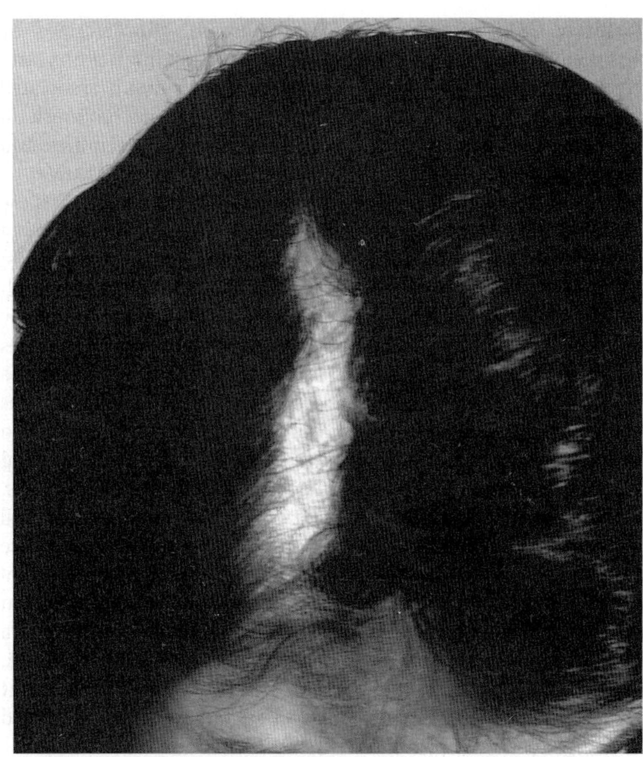

Fig. 27.66 En coup de sabre lesion.

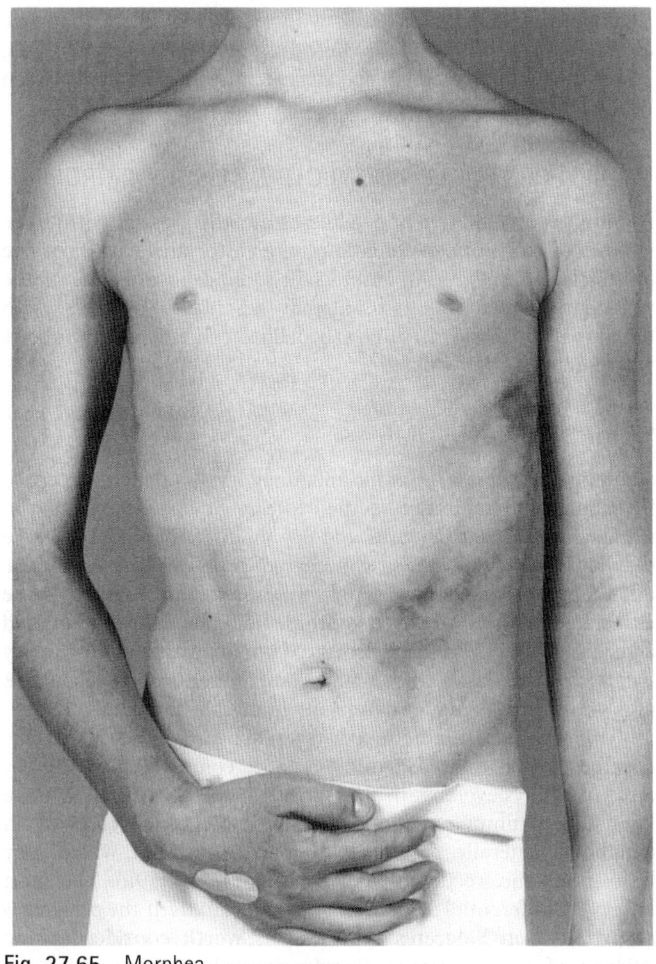

Fig. 27.65 Morphea.

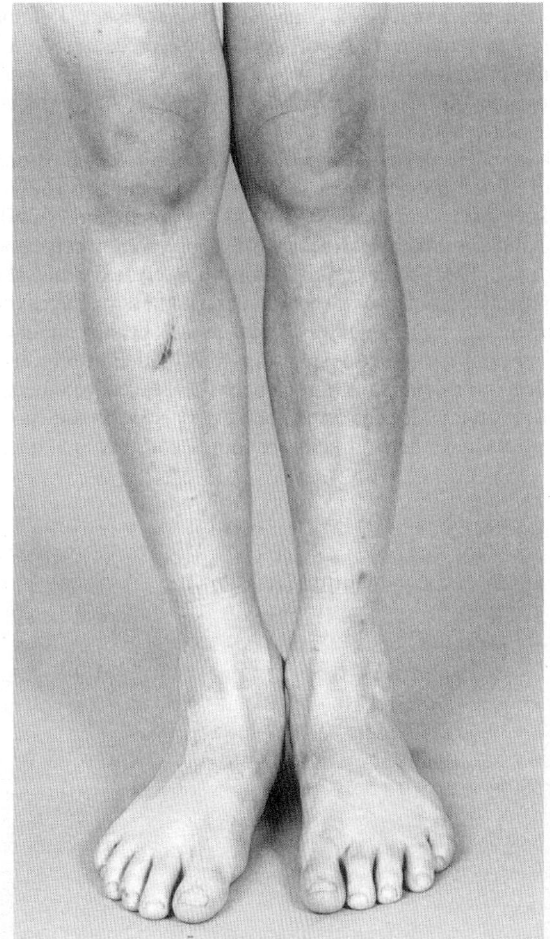

Fig. 27.67 Limb atrophy in linear scleroderma.

(formerly CREST syndrome). Diffuse disease, characterized by cutaneous involvement extending to the proximal limbs and trunk, progresses rapidly over the first few years and is associated with the presence of anti-Scl 70 antibodies. The hallmark of limited disease is skin involvement of the distal extremities and face only.

Raynaud's phenomenon is usually the first feature of these conditions and if not present the diagnosis is unlikely. A history of Raynaud's may be difficult to obtain in a young child. The earliest clinical finding is cutaneous edema usually affecting the hands which consequently feel firm on palpation. Biopsy at this stage will show inflammatory change in the subcutaneous tissue which becomes thicker and tighter. This results in stiffness of the extremities and the characteristic pinched appearance of the face. Joint contractures develop and the skin is very susceptible to minor trauma. Ischemia results in loss of the finger pulp and the typical digital pitting scarring (Fig. 27.68). Severe ischemia may result in the loss of digits. Subcutaneous calcification, pulmonary hypertension and esophageal disease are common in the limited form of the disease. Diffuse disease is characterized by early interstitial lung disease, gastrointestinal involvement, cardiac abnormalities due to small vessel obliteration and renal disease. The scleroderma renal 'crisis' which results from a critical reduction in renal blood flow causing cortical ischemia, activation of the renin–angiotensin system and malignant hypertension, was previously a fatal event but can now be treated with angiotensin converting enzyme (ACE) inhibitors.

The course of the disease depends on the subtype. Diffuse disease tends to be associated with a rapidly progressive course with major organ involvement. Limited disease may remain stable for many years before the development of pulmonary hypertension. Pulmonary, cardiac and renal involvement are the best predictors of a poor outcome. Although the mortality and morbidity of this condition remain high the prognosis for affected children has improved in recent years.

Management requires meticulous attention to detail. Protective measures are important in reducing ischemia of the digits. Avoidance of cold exposure, use of warm mittens and avoidance of smoking are important. Nifedipine, in a long acting preparation, is the drug of choice. Occasional patients with severe digital ischemia and impending gangrene will benefit, often impressively, from the use of intravenous prostaglandin. Emollients are helpful for dry skin while physiotherapy and splinting may benefit joint disease. Gastrointestinal symptoms may be helped by the use of omeprazole together with a prokinetic agent such as cisapride. Broad-spectrum antibiotics may help malabsorption secondary to bacterial overgrowth. ACE inhibitors given where there is any evidence of renal involvement will reduce the risk of a scleroderma crisis.

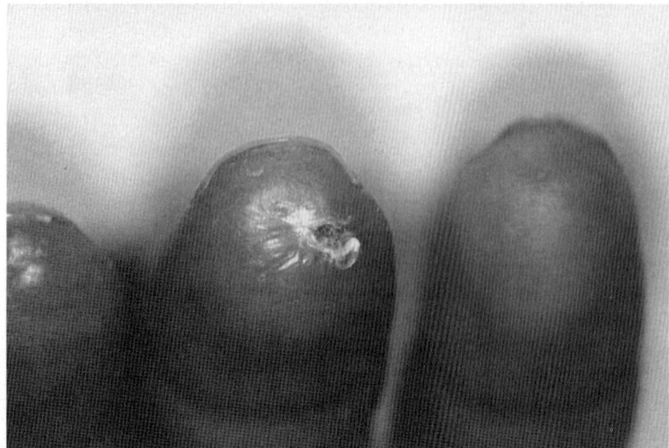

Fig. 27.68 Digital pitting scars in systemic sclerosis.

Immunosuppressive therapy is used where there is evidence of serious organ involvement and if used early enough may influence the course of the disease. Once fibrosis is well established it is likely to be irreversible. Monitoring to detect signs of organ involvement early is therefore vital if treatment is to have any possibility of success. Traditionally, treatment was with d-penicillamine but there is no evidence of benefit and the drug is associated with significant toxicity. Interest now lies in the use of powerful immunosuppressive regimens. Steroids, methotrexate, ciclosporin, cyclophosphamide, mycophenolate mofetil and antithymocyte globulin may all have a role. There is some anecdotal evidence suggesting that if used early steroids and cyclophosphamide will halt progression of the lung disease which is one of the major determinants of mortality. There are no controlled studies to date and little hard evidence on which to base treatment plans.

MIXED CONNECTIVE TISSUE DISEASE

Mixed connective tissue disease (MCTD) is an entity characterized by Raynaud's, swollen fingers and hands, myositis and a strongly positive antibody against RNP. Whether this is truly a separate disease or a subset of some other condition such as SLE is matter of continuing debate. Many individuals with MCTD would also fulfil diagnostic criteria for the diagnosis of SLE.

OVERLAP SYNDROMES

A number of patients are seen with features of more than one autoimmune disorder and are classed as having overlap syndromes. The most commonly seen in pediatric practice are overlaps between JDM or polymyositis and scleroderma.

UNDIFFERENTIATED CONNECTIVE TISSUE DISORDERS

A number of children and adolescents will present with some features of this group of conditions, often associated with a positive antinuclear antibody, but insufficient to be defined as one of the well-characterized conditions already described. Some will with time evolve into one of the clearly defined conditions while others will remain undifferentiated.

SJÖGREN'S SYNDROME

Sjögren's syndrome is a chronic inflammatory disorder characterized by lymphocytic infiltration of the exocrine glands and resulting in sicca symptoms, i.e. dry eyes and dry mouth. Sjögren's syndrome may be primary or secondary, occurring in association with some other autoimmune rheumatic disorder. Conditions known to be associated with Sjögren's syndrome include SLE, rheumatoid arthritis, MCTD, systemic sclerosis, dermatomyositis and primary biliary cirrhosis. Recognition is important as there is a significant risk of a lymphoid malignancy developing in the affected glands.

Although uncommon in pediatric practice, Sjögren's syndrome does occur. Secondary Sjogren's is more common than primary and usually develops in the context of a patient with a known autoimmune rheumatic disorder. Sjögren's syndrome in childhood generally presents with parotid swelling which may be troublesome, recurrent and painful (Fig. 27.69a). The most important differential diagnosis is viral sialedinitis. If the problem is recurrent then Sjögren's syndrome is worth considering and evidence of an autoimmune disorder should be sought.

(a)

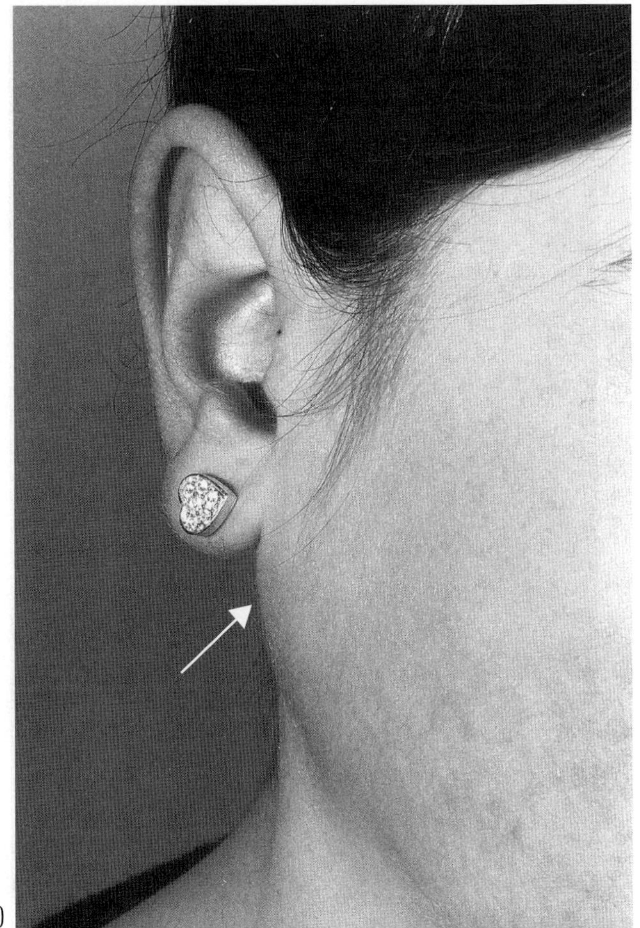

(b)

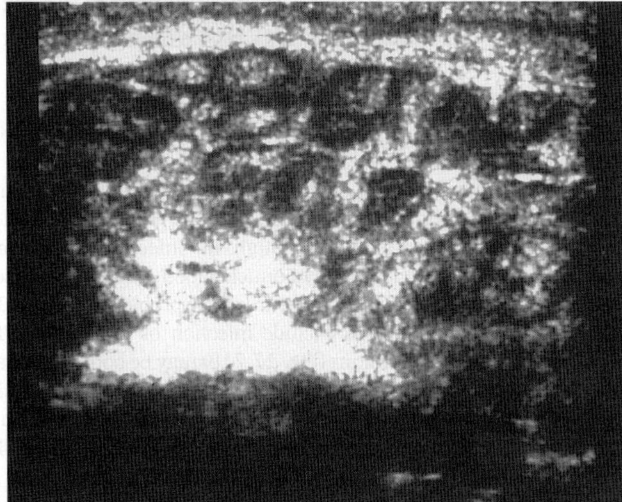

Fig. 27.69 Sjögren's syndrome: (a) parotid swelling; (b) abnormal echogenicity on ultrasound.

Although there are established criteria for the diagnosis of Sjögren's syndrome in adults these are difficult to apply in children. Parotid imaging may be difficult to interpret. Ultrasound may be the most useful imaging procedure as it is inexpensive, well tolerated and shows characteristic abnormalities (Fig. 27.69b). For the diagnosis to be made the parotid swelling should be accompanied by evidence of dry eyes, dry mouth, and the presence of autoantibodies.

Management of Sjögren's syndrome consists firstly of management of the underlying disorder. Artificial tears are used for dry eyes and a variety of preparations are available to relieve the dry mouth. Dental care must be meticulous as the lack of saliva predisposes to severe dental caries. Monitoring for the development of malignancy in the salivary glands is important.

RAYNAUD'S PHENOMENON

Raynaud's phenomenon was first described in 1862 as episodic digital ischemia provoked by factors such as cold or emotion. Classically in Raynaud's there is a triphasic color change. The digits initially blanche followed by cyanosis and then erythema on rewarming. For the diagnosis to be considered at least two of these phases must be present. In addition to the digits, changes may be seen in the ear lobes, tip of the nose and around the mouth.

Primary Raynaud's, where the phenomenon occurs in isolation in an otherwise healthy individual, is common in young women and frequently familial. Secondary Raynaud's occurs in conditions such SLE, systemic sclerosis and MCTD and is frequently the presenting feature of such illnesses.

All young people presenting with Raynaud's should have a careful evaluation including screening for the presence of antinuclear antibodies to exclude an underlying disorder such as SLE or systemic sclerosis. Any atypical features (year-round symptoms, digital ulceration) or the presence of antinuclear antibodies raise the possibility of secondary Raynaud's and the child or teenager should be followed up to ensure no further problems develop.

Primary Raynaud's will usually be controlled by symptomatic measures and protection from the cold. Unfortunately the use of warm gloves or mittens is unpopular in teenage years when primary Raynaud's may be troublesome. Nifedipine will often improve symptoms, the dose being titrated to clinical response and the development of side-effects.

ERYTHEMA NODOSUM

Erythema nodosum is seen not infrequently in children. The typical story is of the sudden onset of one or more tender, erythematous raised nodules or plaques on the anterior surface of the tibia. Pathologically this represents a septal panniculitis (inflammation within the subcutaneous fat). The nodules lie deep and may be easier to feel than to see. As they resolve they develop an ecchymotic appearance and lesions at varying stages of development are frequently seen. Resolution usually occurs over a 4–6 week period.

In the majority of cases, erythema nodosum is an acute process occurring in response to an infectious trigger. Recurrent or chronic erythema nodosum merits investigation for some underlying cause.

Most cases in children occur as a post-streptococcal phenomenon and are associated with markedly raised ASO titers. Other infections such as mycoplasma, viruses and tuberculosis must be remembered. Drugs including antibiotics and oral contraceptive pills may cause erythema nodosum. Rarely, but importantly, erythema nodosum may be the presenting feature of some systemic disorder such as inflammatory bowel disease, sarcoidosis or an autoimmune rheumatic disorder.

THE DIFFERENTIAL DIAGNOSIS OF SYSTEMIC INFLAMMATORY DISORDERS

A chronic systemic inflammatory process in a child may result from chronic infection, malignancy or a rheumatological disorder such as systemic onset juvenile idiopathic arthritis, SLE, JDM or a systemic vasculitis. There are a number of unusual conditions of unknown etiology that may present in this fashion and must be remembered in the differential diagnosis. Some are outlined in this section.

Familial Mediterranean fever and other periodic fever syndromes

Familial Mediterranean fever (FMF) principally affects individuals of eastern Mediterranean origin especially Sephardic and Iraqi Jews, Armenians and Levantine Arabs and is inherited as an autosomal recessive trait. It results from mutations of a gene on chromosome 16 that influences the production of a protein known as pyrin or marenostrum.[173] It is characterized by recurrent episodes of fever, serositis, arthralgia and synovitis of the large joints. Between attacks the joints return to normal. Untreated, it is associated with a high incidence of amyloidosis, the risk of which can be minimized by treating with colchicine.

Other periodic fever syndromes include the hyper-IgD syndrome which is characterized by recurrent fevers and an elevated immunoglobulin-D level. Mutations of the gene encoding mevalonate kinase have been identified in this condition.[174] Recently an autosomal dominant syndrome characterized by periodic fever has been found to result from a mutation of the TNF receptor 1.[175]

The chronic infantile neurological, cutaneous and articular (CINCA) syndrome

This rare disorder is of unknown etiology although familial cases have been described. The syndrome is characterized by the triad of rash, joint abnormalities and CNS involvement.[176] The rash which is urticarial and migratory usually appears in the first few months of life. Joint manifestations result from a disordered growth of cartilage (Fig. 27.70) and range from arthralgia and intermittent swelling to severe overgrowth of the epiphyses with loss of range of motion. Severe overgrowth of the patella is typical. Abnormalities of the central nervous system are universal and include chronic meningeal irritation and impairment of cognition. Laboratory examination shows non-specific elevation of inflammatory markers. Affected individuals have a characteristic facial appearance with frontal bossing, a hypoplastic midface and blond hair. There is no effective treatment and the course is generally one of persisting systemic inflammation, progressive joint deformity and CNS deterioration.

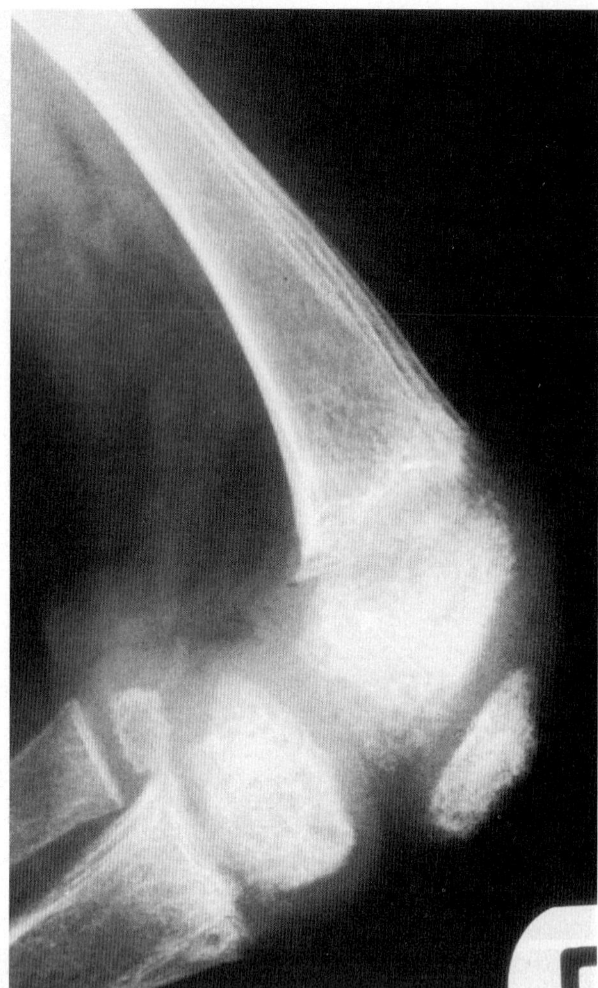

Fig. 27.70 Chronic infantile neurologic cutaneous and articular syndrome showing abnormal bone development.

Sarcoidosis

Sarcoidosis is an uncommon disorder in children and is characterized by a multisystem inflammatory process of unknown etiology. Two distinct disease patterns are seen although there are many cases where features overlap. In older children the pattern is very similar to that seen in adults with constitutional symptoms, lymphadenopathy and lung disease. In infants and young children a different pattern of disease is described with cutaneous involvement, arthropathy and uveiitis. Histologically the disease may result in the formation of granulomata. There is no single diagnostic test: serum levels of angiotensin converting enzyme are elevated in 80% but it should be remembered that levels are higher in normal children than in adults and pediatric standards are required. The Kveim test is no longer used.

Chronic recurrent multifocal osteomylelitis (CRMO) and SAPHO syndrome

The SAPHO syndrome is an inflammatory disorder of unknown etiology characterized by synovitis, acne, pustulosis, hyperostosis and osteitis. Many cases only have a few of these features and CRMO, which is characterized by multifocal osteitic lesions is thought to be part of the same spectrum of disease. The etiology is unknown. A family history of psoriasis is associated with SAPHO and an infectious trigger has been postulated, although no infecting organism is identified in most individuals. Radionuclide bone scanning is useful for demonstrating the multifocal nature of the problem (Fig. 27.71a). Biopsy may be necessary to exclude infection or malignancy. The hyperostostic clavicular lesions (Fig. 27.71b) may be both painful and cosmetically unsightly. Laboratory investigations may show mildly elevated inflammatory markers. Steroids and methotrexate are used to suppress the inflammatory process and most cases respond well.

CHRONIC PAIN SYNDROMES

Musculoskeletal pain is common in children and adolescents but generally shortlived and easily explained. A small group will develop unexplained disabling chronic musculoskeletal pain which poses a challenging diagnostic and management problem.

Pain is a universal phenomenon and in most cases a useful symptom, alerting the individual to tissue damage. Chronic pain differs in serving no useful function. Chronic pain occurring with no underlying physical disorder, or disproportionate chronic pain where the pain is out of all proportion to any known disease (the idiopathic pain syndromes) are perplexing conditions. Pain is by definition subjective and must therefore be accepted at face value.[177]

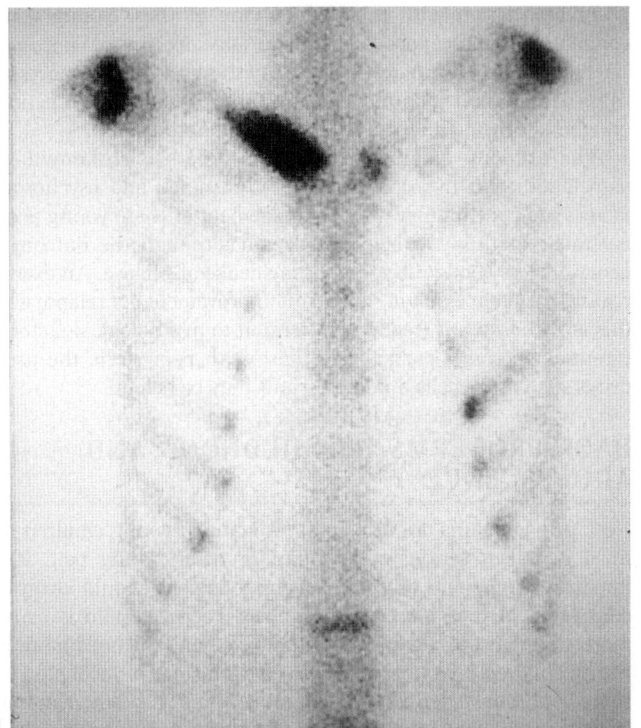

(a)

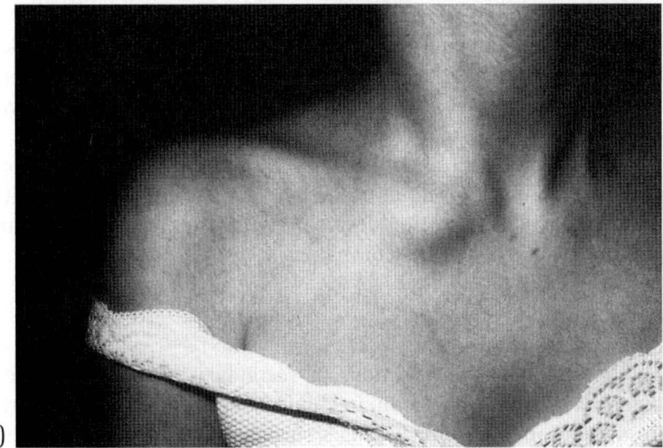

(b)

Fig. 27.71 SAPHO syndrome: (a) radionuclide bone scan demonstrating lesions in clavicle, rib and vertebra; (b) hyperostotic lesion of right clavicle.

The International Association for the Study of Pain[178] defines pain as 'an unpleasant sensory and emotional experience associated with actual or potential tissue damage, or described in terms of such damage... It is unquestionably a sensation in part of the body but is always unpleasant and therefore also an emotional experience.'

In all reported series, idiopathic pain syndromes predominantly affect girls. The age of onset peaks in the early adolescent years and these conditions are uncommon under 8 years.[179]

Children with idiopathic pain syndromes are among the most disabled children seen in pediatric rheumatology and orthopedic clinics. They complain of severe pain unresponsive to standard therapies and frequently have major functional limitations. It is often difficult for both the family and pediatrician to accept that there is no organic pathology and the diagnosis is often delayed while a prolonged series of investigations is undertaken. With the correct diagnosis and management many will do well and it is therefore important to recognize these conditions as early as possible. The diagnosis is by definition one of exclusion of underlying pathology. In most cases this can be done on the basis of a careful history and clinical examination and few investigations are necessary or helpful.

The terminology and classification system used to define the idiopathic pain syndromes in the literature is confusing and generally unhelpful in children. Pain syndromes in children differ in many respects from those described in adults and frequently fail to meet criteria required for clearly defined syndromes. Children with pain syndromes seem to divide into two distinct groups: those with localized pain and those with diffuse or generalized pain.[180]

LOCALIZED IDIOPATHIC PAIN SYNDROMES

The best example of a localized pain syndrome in children is reflex sympathetic dystrophy (RSD) also known as complex regional pain syndrome type 1, reflex neurovascular dystrophy, algodystrophy and Sudeck's atrophy. RSD is characterized by localized pain associated with evidence of autonomic dysfunction. In adults this syndrome usually follows immobilization of a limb following trauma. In children any preceding trauma is usually insignificant. It is presumed that the child stops using the limb in response to minor trauma and that subsequent changes are secondary to immobility, but the condition is poorly understood. Psychological factors are thought to be significant in the majority of children with the condition.[181] The child develops severe pain in the affected limb and rapidly becomes unable to use it. Hyperesthesia (an increased sensitivity to stimulation), allodynia (pain due to a stimulus that does not usually cause pain) and dysesthesia (an unpleasant abnormal sensation) are characteristic. The limb becomes cold, blue, diffusely swollen and at times may adopt bizarre postures (Fig. 27.72). Rarely, wasting and trophic changes will occur in longstanding RSD.

The diagnosis in most cases is straightforward as long as the physician is aware of the condition and considers it. The child presents with a single cold, extremely painful limb and complains of severe pain on even light touch. Frequently they are unable to tolerate even a sock on the affected foot. Despite their predicament many seem remarkably unconcerned (la belle indifference) unless asked to touch or use the painful limb. With an atypical history or a younger child, care must be taken to ensure that no underlying pathology (particularly malignancy) is missed. A blood count, ESR, plain radiograph and radionuclide bone scan are usually sufficient, the typical bone scan in established RSD showing reduced uptake in the affected limb (Fig. 27.73).

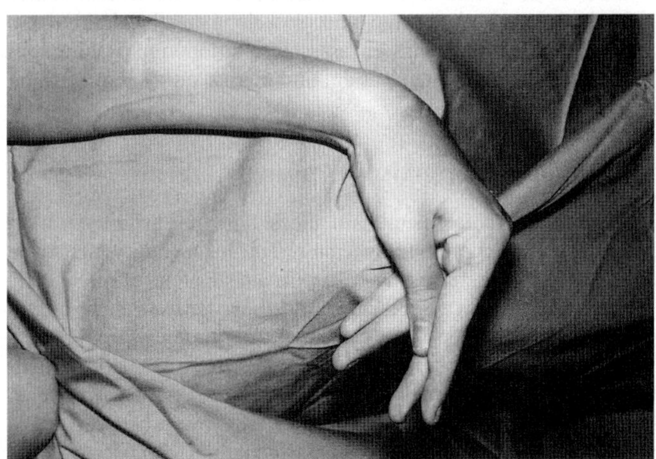

Fig. 27.72 Bizarre posturing of the hand in reflex sympathetic dystrophy.

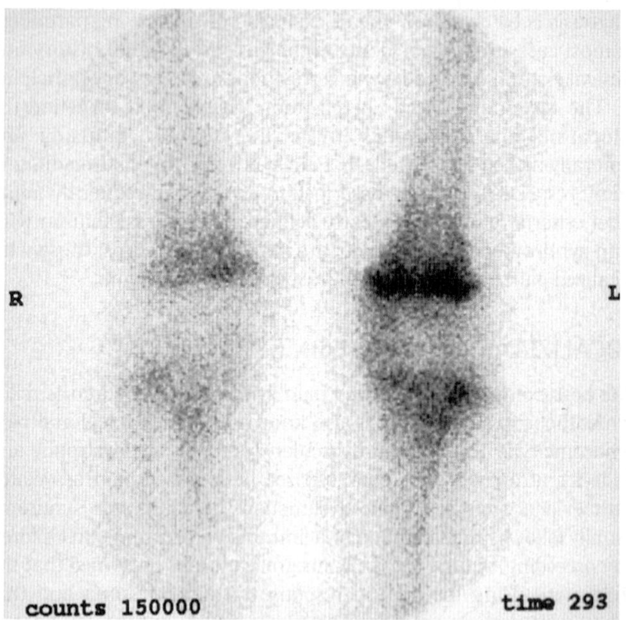

Fig. 27.73 Radionuclide bone scan in reflex sympathetic dystrophy showing reduced uptake in affected (R) compared to the normal (L) limb.

The management of these children depends on establishing trust. Many have seen multiple health professionals before a diagnosis has been reached;[182] this frequently leads to increasing psychosocial difficulty and a loss of faith in the medical profession. It is essential to successfully reassure both child and family that there is no underlying organic pathology while accepting their pain at face value. Once the diagnosis is made a simple explanation of the effect of immobilization on a limb is usually easily accepted and the role of 'stress' in contributing to this condition can be discussed. A combination of an individualized program of physiotherapy together with attention to psychological factors leads to full recovery in the majority.[179, 183] A few will require referral for formal psychiatric input. In the majority, once the family are aware of possible stressors the condition frequently resolves. RSD in many childen appears to be a 'cry for help' and a recognition of the problem will allow the child to recover. Sympathetic blockade and other treatment modalities used in affected adults are neither necessary nor helpful in the management of children and young people with RSD.

RSD is only one form of localized pain syndrome. Other individuals may have chronic musculoskeletal pain localized to one area of the body but without associated autonomic dysfunction. These syndromes are not clear cut and there is an overlap between such groups of patients.

DIFFUSE CHRONIC PAIN SYNDROMES

Widespread musculoskeletal pain affects a further group of young people, again predominantly female. The mean age tends to be slightly older than those with RSD with a peak at around 15 years. These patients can be subdivided into those with multiple tender points who meet criteria for the diagnosis of fibromyalgia and those without specific tender points. In our experience it is unhelpful to differentiate between the two groups or to use the term fibromyalgia. There are no significant differences between these groups and they differ in many ways from adults with fibromyalgia. It is more helpful to class all as simply having a diffuse chronic pain syndrome.

In association with their pain many of these young people complain of fatigue, poor sleep and, in some, feelings of depression. There appears to be an overlap between this group of teenagers and those with chronic fatigue syndrome, the exact diagnosis depending on whether the pain or the fatigue predominates.

The etiology of this group of disorders is unknown. An association with hypermobility has been noted and psychosocial factors are contributory.[184,185] Management of these young people is similar to those with localized pain although the outcome is generally less good with a higher incidence of relapse. An exercise regime will often result in significant improvement but relapse when this is withdrawn is frequent. Attention to psychological factors is essential. In some, particularly those with poor sleep, the use of drugs such as tricyclic antidepressants may be helpful.

BACK PROBLEMS IN CHILDHOOD AND ADOLESCENCE

Neck or back pains are unusual symptoms in young children and must be taken seriously. Persistent or deteriorating pain is an important complaint and tumors and infections should always be considered in the differential diagnosis. Localized pain is usually more suggestive of significant pathology than ill-defined pain, but young children are often unable to give a history of local pain and some conditions such as discitis may present with odd symptoms such as a gait abnormality or even abdominal pain.

In the adolescent population complaints of ill-defined pain without pathological explanation are common.[186] Nevertheless careful evaluation is important. Additional signs and symptoms such as torticollis, scoliosis, or neurological radicular symptoms will direct the approach to appropriate investigations.

As a rule of thumb, whilst pain, or pain provoking pathology, may cause abnormal spinal postures like torticollis or scoliosis, it is unusual for congenital or developmental explanations for spinal deformity to be responsible for pain.

TUMORS

Malignant neoplasms, primary or secondary, though rare, are a potential source of back pain in children. Primary tumors can arise from the bone, such as Ewing's sarcoma; from the hemopoietic tissue, such as the leukemias; or from the contained neurological tissue or its coverings. Only 3% of primary bone tumors occur in the axial skeleton and in children 60% of these are benign.[187] The most common benign lesions include osteoid osteoma or osteoblastoma, eosinophilic granuloma and aneurysmal bone cysts.

Osteoid osteomas typically involve the posterior elements and characteristically present with pain, especially night pain classically relieved by NSAIDs. Radiographs may show an area of sclerosis; radionuclide bone scanning will reveal intense focal uptake in the lesion. Subsequent CT scanning will identify a discrete lesion with a thick sclerotic rim and a lucent nidus of osteoid material at the center. Osteoblastoma is similar histologically to osteoid osteoma but larger. Aneurysmal bone cysts are typically expansile lytic lesions with a thin rim of cortical bone. Once again they usually occur in the posterior elements but may involve the adjacent pedicle or body. Eosinophilic granuloma usually affects the body of the vertebra which subsequently flattens giving the characteristic vertebra plana of Calvé's disease.

INFECTION

See section on Infection in bones and joints, page 1543.

TORTICOLLIS

Torticollis secondary to congenital and developmental problems is not usually accompanied by pain. In practice the commonest cause of painful torticollis in children is atlantoaxial rotatory displacement, but it is important to bear in mind that there are other explanations including infections, tumors, central nervous system abnormalities like syringomyelia, and ocular dysfunction.[188]

Atlantoaxial rotatory displacement

Typically the child awakes with a 'wryneck'. This commonly resolves without treatment over the course of a week but occasionally the posture persists when it is best described as atlantoaxial rotatory fixation. There is often associated muscle spasm of the long sternocleidomastoid muscle because of its attempts to correct the deformity, unlike congenital muscular torticollis where the contracted muscle is responsible for the deformity.

In most cases the etiology is not apparent although the condition can be caused by trauma or occur in association with recent upper respiratory tract infection. When subluxation occurs in association with inflammation of adjacent neck tissues or upper respiratory tract infection it is known as Grisel's syndrome. It is postulated that hyperemia of the atlantoaxial joints leads to variable ligament laxity and synovitis. Thickened synovial folds may subsequently impinge during rotation and lead to fixation.

Diagnosis in the acute stage is primarily based on the history. Radiological assessment is difficult because of the head posture, but in the anteroposterior film the anteriorly rotated lateral mass of C1 appears wider and closer to the midline than the posteriorly rotated lateral mass. Because of the difficulty in interpretation of plain radiographs, CT scanning or dynamic MRI is usually of more value for definitive diagnosis.

Atlantoaxial rotatory displacement with minimal subluxation and no encroachment of the vertebral canal is relatively benign. Greater degrees of subluxation are rare but do have potentially serious neurological complications because of increasing encroachment of the vertebral canal. Most cases resolve spontaneously with simple analgesia and a soft collar for support. If persistent the patient should be admitted for halter traction with analgesia and muscle relaxation. Halo traction is occasionally required, especially if presentation is delayed. If the displacement is fixed and significant there is potential compromise of the vertebral canal and surgical fusion is a consideration.

Paroxysmal torticollis of infancy

Paroxysmal torticollis of infancy is a rare episodic torticollis of unknown etiology. Episodes last for minutes to days with eventual spontaneous recovery. Two-thirds of affected children are girls, with an average age of onset of 3 months. Attacks usually occur in the morning, occurring 1–4 times each month and can be associated with trunk curvature, eye deviations and torticollis which may alternate sides on different episodes. The condition usually resolves over 12–24 months and requires no treatment.

Sandifer syndrome

This syndrome is the association of infant gastroesophageal reflux with posturing of the neck and trunk.[189] It is believed that the torticollis is the child's attempt to decrease the discomfort resulting from reflux.

JUVENILE DISCITIS

See previous section on Infection in bones and joints, page 1543.

Calcific discitis

This condition occurs in children with an average age of onset of 8 years. It is most common in the cervical spine and usually presents with the acute onset of neck pain and sometimes torticollis. Radiographs reveal calcified deposits in the affected nucleus pulposus. The etiology of the condition is unknown and treatment is symptomatic. The calcific deposits disappear in most patients by 6 months.

SCHEUERMANN'S KYPHOSIS

This condition can be responsible for a painful kyphosis. Patients present either with pain or an increasing round back deformity during adolescence (Fig. 27.74). The condition is more frequent in the thoracic but can also occur in the lumbar spine. There is usually a clear apex to the spinal deformity, which is relatively rigid distinguishing the condition from benign postural round back, which is flexible on extension. Lateral radiographs show vertebral wedging, end-plate irregularity and Schmorl node formation (herniation of intervertebral disc into the end-plate of an adjacent vertebra).

Treatment of the deformity with extension exercises and ocasionally extension bracing is usually successful. Surgical intervention for severe deformities is seldom required.

SPONDYLOLISTHESIS AND SPONDYLOLYSIS

Spondylolisthesis is the slipping forward of a vertebra on its neighbor below. It is classified into five types. Isthmic, and dysplastic types are most common in children: degenerative, traumatic and pathological types are unusual.

Isthmic spondylolisthesis occurs when a defect or lysis develops in the pars interarticularis (spondylolysis) and is most common in L5 and L4 (Fig. 27.75). This defect is usually the result of a stress fracture at the pars. Affected patients often give a history of sporting activity. The vertebra concerned, having lost its 'bony hook' on the vertebra below, is able to slip forward, although this probably only occurs in about 20% of cases of spondylolysis. Clinical examination of a significant slip reveals a step on palpation of the lumbar spine and so called 'heart shaped buttocks' because of the deformity.

Neurological radicular symptoms are rare but there is often associated hamstring spasm. The defect can be seen on oblique radiographs (the classical 'collar on the Scottie dog') but is best seen on reverse gantry CT scanning. If the slip is translated less than 30–50% symptoms can be treated by activity modification, analgesia and bracing. If symptoms settle the patient can be observed. Persistent symptoms, a slip of more than 50% or progressive slippage are all indications for surgical intervention. There are various surgical techniques but the principle is to fuse the unstable vertebra to its neighbor below.

Dysplastic (or congenital) spondylolisthesis is due to hypoplasia of the L5/S1 facet joint. This leads to instability of the L5 vertebra, which may subsequently slip.

ADOLESCENT DISC PROLAPSE

Disc prolapse is infrequent in children but occurs occasionally in adolescents when its presentation is somewhat different from adults. Stiffness is a more common symptom than back pain. There is commonly severe hamstring spasm with very limited straight leg raising and a spinal list (or tilt) is often present. The majority resolve without need for surgical intervention. If MRI shows a large sequestered fragment of disc material with significant symptoms, surgical excision may be considered.

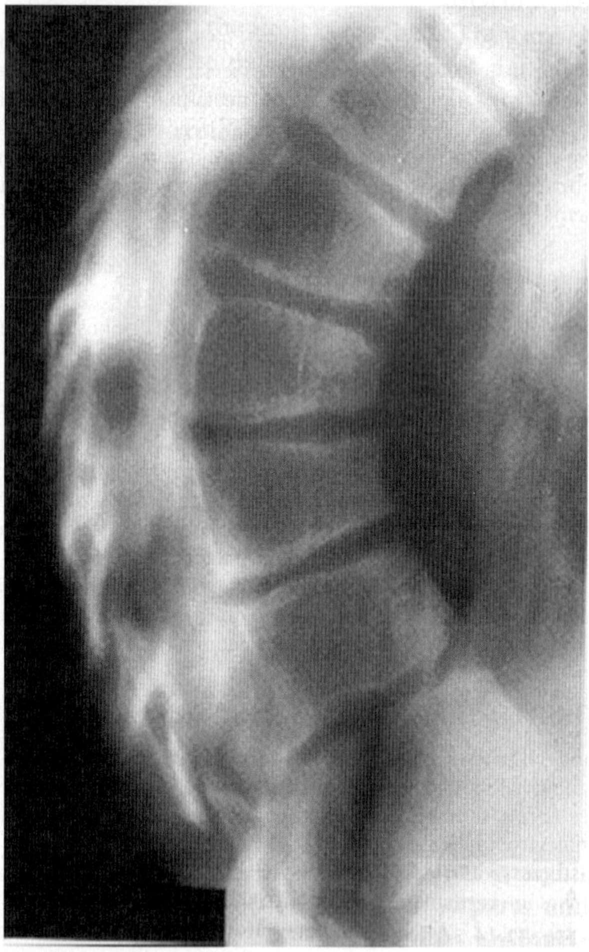

Fig. 27.74 Scheuermann's kyphosis.

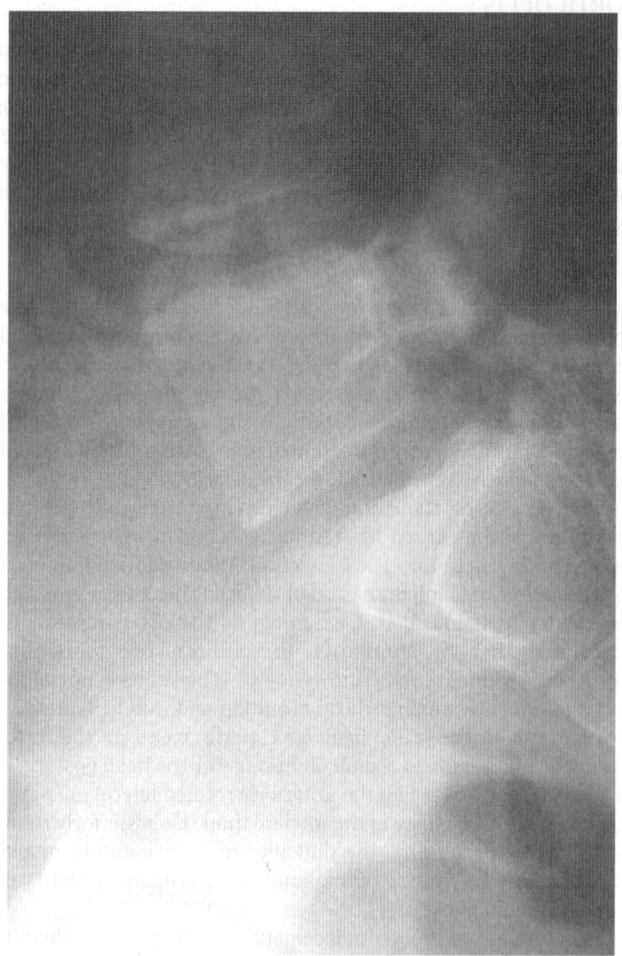

Fig. 27.75 Spondylolysis of L5.

OSTEOPOROSIS

Osteoporosis is a major health problem in the modern world and of major consequence in terms of its associated morbidity, mortality and health economics. The formation of bone structure occurs primarily during childhood and adolescence with 90% of the peak bone mass being accumulated during the years of longitudinal growth. At any given age, bone mass is the result of both the peak bone mass, i.e. that acquired during the growth years, and the rate of age-related loss which starts from around 30 years and accelerates in women after the menopause. Optimization of skeletal development during childhood and adolescence therefore has a role in the longer term reduction in osteoporosis. This becomes particularly important when caring for children with chronic diseases which may adversely influence bone formation.

Bone exists in a constant state of remodeling during which old bone is removed and replaced by new bone. Bone gain during childhood and adolescence, and bone loss in later life is therefore the result of a positive or negative balance between these two processes. This balance can be altered or disrupted by a variety of other factors. Bone structure is influenced by both genetic and lifestyle factors. It has been estimated that up to 80% of bone mineral density (BMD) can be accounted for by genetic factors with gender, race and body size being important determinants. A number of candidate gene polymorphisms have been identified that are significant in relation to bone mass. Of particular importance appear to be polymorphisms of the vitamin D receptor, estrogen receptor and collagen type 1 alpha-1 genes. Other polymorphic genes encoding for bone proteins, hormones and cytokines may prove significant and it seems likely that a great variety of genes are involved in determining bone mass and strength. Lifestyle factors have an important contribution to make, with diet and physical activity being particularly important. There is a relationship between the amounts of muscle and fat in the body and the amount of bone: any dieting that results in an excessive weight loss will be associated with bone loss. Nutritional factors such as dietary calcium and vitamin D are contributory and ensuring an adequate intake will optimize bone development. Physical activity has an importance influence on bone density and an adequate amount of weight bearing activity is essential for optimal bone growth.

The World Health Organization defines osteoporosis as 'a disease characterized by low bone mass and micro-architectural deterioration of bone tissue, leading to enhanced bone fragility and a consequent increased risk in fracture'. Categories of disease are based on the measurement of bone mineral density (BMD), with osteoporosis being defined as BMD more than 2.5 SD below the young adult mean value. Severe or established osteoporosis is defined as more than 2.5 SD below the young adult mean value in the presence of one or more low-trauma or fragility fractures.

These diagnostic criteria for osteoporosis have limitations. It must be remembered that they were developed in postmenopausal women and their applicability to other groups such as males and younger patients remains unclear. For such groups the relationship between BMD and fracture risk may be different and it is the fracture risk that is ultimately of importance. There are also difficulties inherent in the measurement of BMD in the growing child (see below) which may make the use of such definitions inappropriate. The definition of osteoporosis where fractures have not yet occurred is therefore somewhat arbitrary at present in children and young people. Further work is needed in this area.

ASSESSMENT OF BONE DENSITY IN PEDIATRIC PRACTICE

A high correlation exists between bone mineral density, bone strength and risk of fracture. The measurement of bone mineral density appears therefore to offer the most accurate method of quantifying fracture risk.

Conventional radiography is a relatively insensitive method of assessing bone mass and significant osteoporosis can only be diagnosed confidently when associated with a typical fracture. There has recently been interest in the use of ultrasound to assess bone density[190] and its acceptibility in pediatric practice may lead to further interest in this method in the future. Quantitative methods of CT scanning can be used to assess bone density but the tool most frequently used now, and generally regarded as the gold standard, is DEXA (dual energy X-ray absorptiometry) scanning.

DEXA scanning can be used to assess muscle mass, total and per cent body fat and bone mineral. DEXA measures both the bone mineral content and the bone mineral density. This has a number of pitfalls in pediatric practice and results must be interpreted with care.[191] The amount of bone mineral content is directly related to body size and it is necessary to correlate values with skeletal size. Reference standards for children in different population are not widely available, while genetic and racial difference in bone density make population based reference values essential.[192] In addition, machines vary considerably and calibration is important. With these provisos DEXA appears at present to be the method of choice for the assessment of bone density. Measurements are generally taken from the lumbar spine and proximal femur. Results should be expressed in terms of the number of standard deviations above or below the mean of an age-related control population (Z-score). DEXA provides a quantitative method that can be repeated serially to monitor change and assess the effects of treatment provided the results are interpreted with caution in the growing child or adolescent.

PRIMARY OR IDIOPATHIC JUVENILE OSTEOPOROSIS

Primary osteoporosis is rare in childhood. Juvenile osteoporosis occurs before or around puberty, affects both sexes and is of unknown pathophysiology. The child will present with pain in the back, hips and feet with evidence of fractures including vertebral crush fractures (Fig. 27.76). This is a self-limiting condition which resolves with puberty but treatment with pamidronate to reduce pain and increase bone density during the active phase may be helpful.

SECONDARY OSTEOPOROSIS IN CHILDHOOD

Osteoporosis in children usually occurs in relation to some underlying chronic disease or as a consequence of treatment with glucocorticoids.

Disease related

Osteoporosis is increasingly recognized as an important sequela of a number of chronic childhood disorders, contributing greatly to the long term morbidity. In the childhood rheumatic disorders such as juvenile idiopathic arthritis, dermatomyositis or systemic lupus erythematosus, osteoporosis occurs as a direct result of the underlying inflammatory process and prevention depends on optimal control of the disease process. Nutritional impairment, common in many children with chronic illness, may be contributory. Immobility or even relative inactivity in children with arthritis, chronic ill-health or conditions such as cerebral palsy may result in osteoporosis. Other unknown factors which are disease specific are clearly of importance, e.g. individuals with JDM or SLE are much more vulnerable than those with juvenile arthritis.

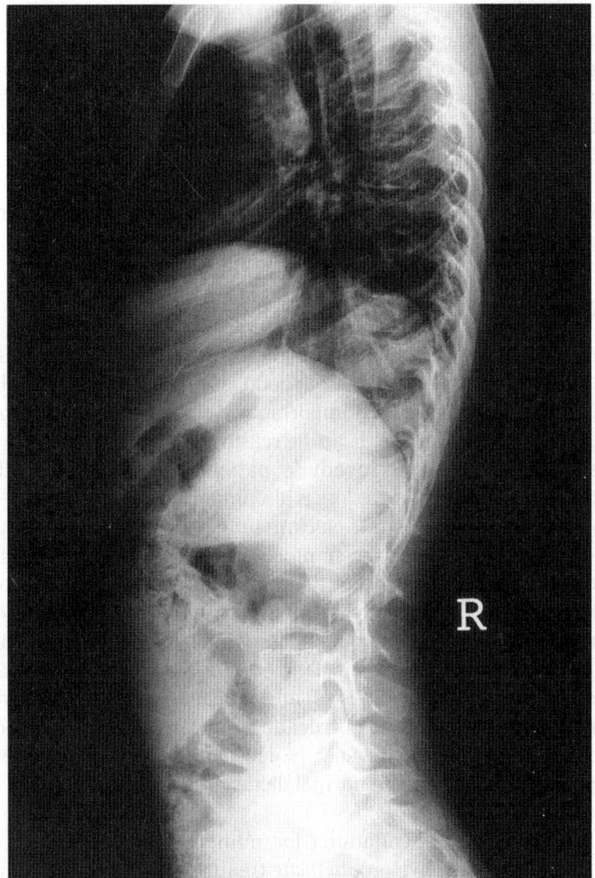

Fig. 27.76 Idiopathic juvenile osteoporosis – plain radiograph showing osteoporotic collapse of thoracic vertebrae.

Drug related

Glucocorticosteroids are widely used in the treatment of a number of common diseases in childhood including the rheumatic disorders, inflammatory bowel disease, asthma and nephrotic syndrome. Although clearly necessary for treatment their effect on bone mineral density can be significant. The adverse effects of steroids on bone metabolism are well known and result from a variety of actions of these drugs. They are known to induce renal calcium efflux and inhibit calcium uptake from the intestine, leading to a fall in serum calcium and secondary hyperparathyroidism. This increases bone resorption and reduces bone formation and is well documented immediately after commencement of treatment. The increase in bone resorption does not usually continue but the amount of new bone formation is reduced as a result of increased apoptosis of osteoblasts and contributes to ongoing bone loss. The bulk of the bone loss in steroid induced osteoporosis occurs in the first 6 months of treatment but overall the effect is related both to the total dose used and to the duration of therapy. There is considerable individual variation in the effect of steroids on bone density presumably as a result of genetic factors. Some individuals will tolerate a significant dose with little evidence of adverse effect whereas others will become significantly osteoporotic with minimal dosage regimens.

Other drugs such as methotrexate, heparin and thyroxine are known to reduce bone mineral density but none has been shown to have significant clinical effect in pediatric practice.

PROPHYLAXIS OF OSTEOPOROSIS IN CHILDHOOD

There is ongoing debate regarding the use of prophylactic measures to prevent osteoporosis in childhood. General advice regarding exercise and nutrition are important. Weight bearing exercise is clearly beneficial and with an increasingly sedentary lifestyle for many it is important to advise patients regarding this. The avoidance of severe weight loss is also important.

A diet with an adequate calcium intake is frequently lacking in adolescents. There has been much interest in the relationship between calcium intake and bone mineral acquisition and some evidence that calcium supplementation can increase bone mineral density. Any benefit shown in children and adolescents is transient and disappears when the supplementation is discontinued making it seem unlikely that this is of any longer term benefit. Current evidence supports the use of calcium supplements to improve bone mineralization where the diet is deficient[193] but the benefits of supplementing above the normal dietary recommended intake are unproven.

Current recommendations for adults are that patients on steroids should receive prophylactic treatment for bone loss. There are no recommendations for children. A recent survey of pediatric rheumatology units in the UK (unpublished data) showed no consensus on the use of prophylactic measures in the prevention of steroid induced osteoporosis. Some units advocate general advice only, some prescribe calcium supplements and others calcium and vitamin D for all children going on to long term steroids. At the moment there is no clear evidence on which to base a decision. There is clearly a need for studies in this area.

TREATMENT OF OSTEOPOROSIS IN CHILDHOOD

Until relatively recently, no specific treatments were available for osteoporosis. The advent of the bisphosphonates has altered our approach to the investigation and identification of at-risk children as there is now an effective treatment that can be used to reduce fracture risk.

The bisphosphonates are synthetic compounds whose main action consists of the inhibition of osteoclastic bone resorption. The newer bisphosphonates are thought to act directly on the osteoclast to induce apoptosis. There were initial concerns about the use of these drugs in children with rapidly growing bones and in women of child-bearing potential. They are of low molecular weight and therefore likely to be able to cross the placenta. Fetal bone turnover is high and these drugs could potentially cause substantial effects on skeletal development. Nonetheless the cost of untreated osteoporosis is such that these drugs are now well established for use in pediatric practice.

The first generation bisphosphonates such as etidronate have been associated with bone mineralization defects and have generally been superseded in pediatric practice by the newer drugs such as pamidronate and alendronate. Pamidronate is the established treatment for osteoporosis in children and adolescents and is generally well tolerated. It has the disadvantage of requiring to be given by intravenous infusion and there is therefore increasing interest in the use of an oral alternative such as alendronate.[194]

Where there is established osteoporosis with evidence of a fracture there seems little doubt that the use of these drugs is appropriate. With reduced BMD but no fracture, there is no clear agreement as to when children should be treated as the relationship between BMD and fracture risk is not clearly established. Most clinicians would agree that a BMD measurement more than 3 SD below the mean is likely to represent an increased fracture risk and would therefore merit treatment.

OVERUSE AND SPORT RELATED PROBLEMS IN CHILDREN

Active children frequently present with a variety of musculoskeletal symptoms that are a consequence of their activity. Such overuse syndromes can present in any child but become more common in the participants of organized competitive sport. While children are subject to the same injuries as adults their immature musculoskeletal system responds somewhat differently. Submaximal loading of musculoskeletal structures leads to tissue damage, followed by repair. Repeated submaximal loading results in tissue hypertrophy. Overuse syndromes are characterized by the development of inflammatory pain when tissue damage exceeds the rate of tissue repair. The structures involved can be the bones, the soft tissues or, most commonly the junctions where they converge. In children these junctions are weaker than either the tendons or ligaments: apophysitis and avulsion fractures are therefore more common than ligament or tendon rupture. In children tendon rupture is also rare because overuse typically results in inflammation of the tendon sheath (tenosynovitis) rather than the tendon itself (tendonitis), and tendon degeneration is rare in the young.

STRESS FRACTURES

Stress fractures are undisplaced fatigue fractures, which develop as a result of repeated loading. The lower limbs are most frequently affected, the metatarsals (march fractures) and the tibia being the most frequently involved bones.

Younger children and even toddlers can present with stress fractures but they are more common in adolescents where the proximal third of the tibia is the most frequent site, and running the most common explanation.[195] Symptoms of localized pain develop insidiously and are usually relieved by rest. Plain radiographs eventually show a localized periosteal reaction and increased density, but are frequently unhelpful at presentation.[196] Radionuclide bone scanning is a more sensitive investigation. Infection and tumors can present with similar features and should always be considered in the differential diagnosis.

Treatment involves protection from further trauma, which sometimes involves immobilization and always involves abstinence from the causative stress, usually running. Once symptoms have resolved a gradual return to activity can be begun.

EPIPHYSEOLYSIS

Repeated traction, compression, torsion and angular stress on the growth plate (physis) can lead to stress injury resulting in localized periarticular pain. Radiographs reveal widening of the growth plate and irregularity of the metaphyseal margin (Fig. 27.77). Involvement of the proximal humeral physis has been reported in baseball pitchers,[197] while female gymnasts have involvement of the distal radius.[198] Treatment involves modification of activity with

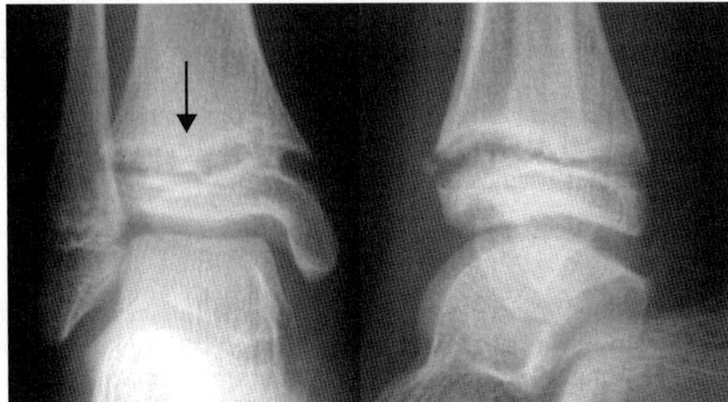

Fig. 27.77 Epiphyseolysis of distal tibia.

the epiphysis eventually returning to normal. Severe cases can be slow to resolve and premature physeal closure with subsequent wrist problems have been reported in gymnasts.[199]

OSTEOCHONDRITIS DISSECANS

See Common orthopedic problems in childhood, page 1558.

APOPHYSITIS

In the growing skeleton tendons join long bones at sites of ossification called apophyses. Apophysitis is inflammation at these junctions as a result of traction injury caused by the repeated pull of the attached tendon. Radiographs often reveal fragmentation and sclerosis of the apophysis with small, avulsed ossified fragments. Patients are usually in the adolescent age range from about 10–16 years. Symptoms usually begin insidiously, are made worse by activity and better by rest. Eponymous names are associated with the condition at some sites, but all are benign self-limiting conditions. The usual natural history is resolution by maturity. Treatment includes activity modification and symptomatic treatment. Occasionally in young athletes, explosive contraction of a muscle causes a tendon to pull off its whole attachment with a significant fragment of bone.

Pelvic apophysitis and avulsion fractures

The hip and pelvis can be the source of symptoms at the site of several apophyses. Sudden explosive contraction of the attached muscles can result in acute avulsion fractures of these apophyses and repeated submaximal trauma can result in the insidious development of symptoms. The iliac crest is the site of insertion of the abdominal muscles and can become painful as a result of trunk rotation such as when running. Other sites of apophysitis around the hip and pelvis include the insertion of sartorius at the anterior superior iliac spine (Fig. 27.78), the insertion of the rectus femoris at the anterior inferior iliac spine, the insertion of the gluteal muscles at the greater trochanter, the insertion of the psoas muscle at the lesser trochanter and the insertion of the hamstrings at the ischial tuberosity. Each of these conditions can explain pain in and around the hip region, but in the adolescent age range more serious explanations such as a slipped capital femoral epiphysis should always be considered.

Osgood–Schlatter's disease

Osgood–Schlatter's disease of the tibial tuberosity is the most common apophysitis, presenting in approximately 15% of teenage boys and 10% of teenage girls.[200] There is localized pain and swelling at the tibial tuberosity. Radiographs typically show fragmentation of the tibial tuberosity with avulsed fragments

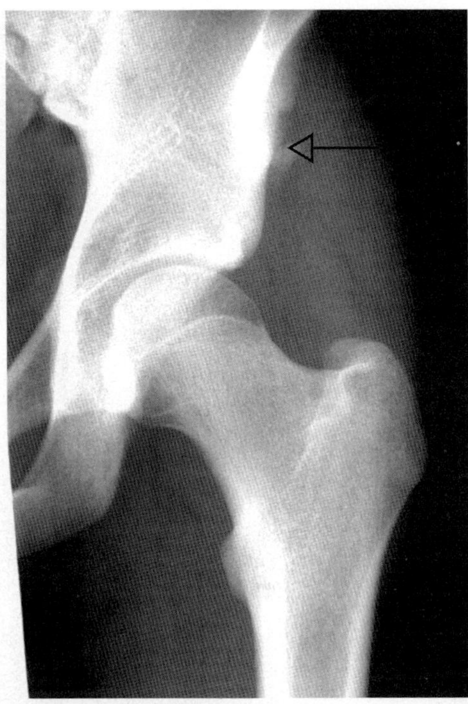

Fig. 27.78 Avulsion of anterior superior iliac spine.

(Fig. 27.80). Symptoms usually respond to activity modification. In the enthusiastic young athlete sport need not be prevented but simply modified. Occasionally symptoms do persist after maturity with up to 20% of mature patients complaining of discomfort when kneeling.[201] Treatment is seldom required or helpful, except if a loose ossicle persists, when excision can be curative.[202]

Sinding–Larsen–Johansson disease

Sinding–Larsen–Johansson disease is apophysitis at the lower pole of the patella. It is similar to Osgood–Schlatter's disease and the two conditions can coexist (Fig. 27.79). Treatment follows a conservative activity modification approach.

Sever's disease

Sever's disease is inflammation of the calcaneal apophysis, at the insertion of the Tendo-Achilles. Radiographs show increased density and fragmentation of the calcaneal apophysis, but this appearance is non-specific and can be seen in asymptomatic subjects. Treatment is conservative and a heel lift is sometimes helpful.

Iselin's disease

Iselin's disease is apophysitis at the insertion of peroneus brevis at the base of the fifth metatarsal. It should not be confused with fractures in the vicinity, which can follow acute trauma.

VALGUS OVERLOAD OF THE ELBOW

Valgus overload of the elbow occurs in a variety of throwing and batting sports and in activities where the upper limb is required to bear heavy loads such as in gymnastics. Perhaps the best example is the junior baseball pitcher – 'Little Leaguer's elbow'. Valgus stress of the elbow generates tension and distraction of the medial structures, including the medial collateral ligament and the medial epicondyle and compression of the lateral structures namely the capitellum and the radial head. The young athlete can develop problems in any of these areas.[203] The medial epicondyle may

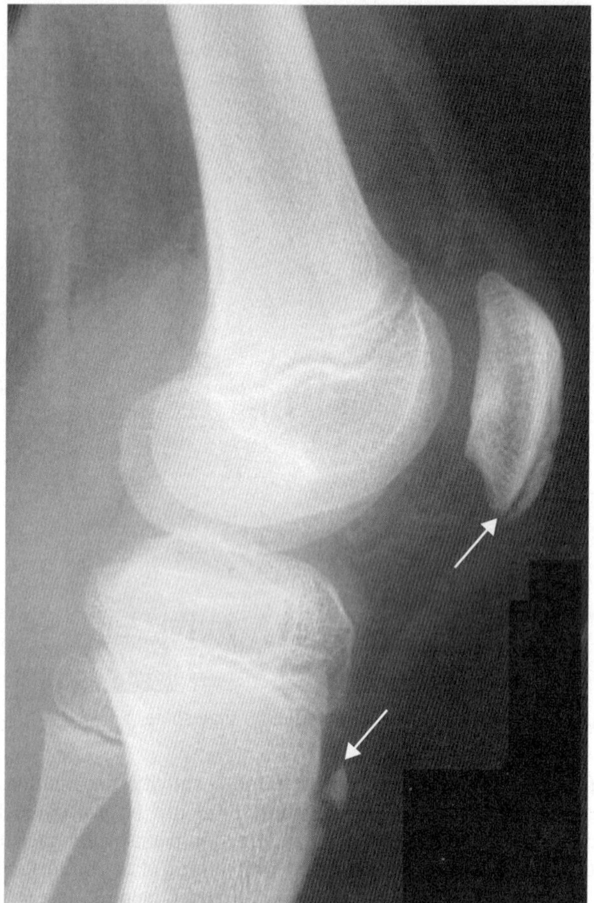

Fig. 27.79 Knee with coincidental Osgood-Schlatter's and Sinding-Larsen-Johansson disease.

become painful and prominent in a typical apophysitis-like presentation. Activity modification gives rise to resolution in most cases. Occasionally the medial epicondyle can be completely avulsed and if significantly displaced it should be reduced and fixed. The ossific nucleus of the capitellum may become fragmented with appearances similar to Perthes disease when the condition is referred to as Panner's disease. If the patient is young the prognosis for complete resolution is good. Older and adolescent patients can also develop subchondral defects, which are considered to be a form of osteochondritis dissecans (see Common orthopedic problems in childhood, p. 1558). Loose flaps or loose bodies can develop causing mechanical symptoms including elbow locking as well as pain. Treatment of the painful elbow usually involves activity modification but surgical debridement may be necessary if mechanical symptoms secondary to a loose body are present.

SNAPPING TENSOR FASCIA LATA SYNDROME

The iliotibial band is a broad condensation of the fascia on the lateral side of the leg running from the tensor fascia lata muscle at the iliac crest, across the greater trochanter of the hip and across the lateral side of the knee. When the leg is adducted at the hip and internally and externally rotated the iliotibial band can be pushed backward and forward by the passing greater trochanter beneath. The band is put under tension and then suddenly snaps back with a disconcerting clunk. If this occurs repeatedly a tender secondary trochanteric bursitis develops. The condition is more common in girls and the clunking is sometimes voluntary. Management includes stretching exercises, avoidance of the provoking movements and reassurance because some patients believe that their hip is dislocating. The condition sometimes presents in runners and if refractory to conservative management the iliotibial band can be lengthened by 'Z' plasty.

ILIOTIBIAL BAND FRICTION SYNDROME

This condition is caused by rubbing of the iliotibial band against the lateral epicondyle at the distal femur during repetitive knee flexion and extension. It usually affects runners and most cases are associated with a recent increase in activity.[204] Activity modification is the mainstay of treatment, sometimes including stretching exercises if the iliotibial band is thought to be tight.

ANTERIOR KNEE PAIN, PATELLOFEMORAL PAIN SYNDROME AND CHONDROMALACIA

See Common orthopedic problems in childhood, Page 1558.

MENISCAL INJURIES OF THE KNEE

Meniscal tears are unusual in young children unless there is an underlying meniscal anomaly such as a discoid meniscus (see Common orthopedic problems in childhood, p. 1558). In adolescence the incidence of meniscal tears begins to increase and the injury is most commonly sport related. Meniscal tears are usually the result of a twisting injury when a 'pop' is sometimes heard or felt, followed by knee swelling. There are few reliable clinical tests specific for meniscal tears but the patient may give a history of giving way and 'true' knee locking. 'True' locking specifically implies a block to full extension. If a tear is suspected, MRI is a sensitive investigation. In young patients the meniscus is more vascular than in the adult, especially at its periphery and is more likely to heal following injury. In recent years the vital role of the meniscus in load distribution and proper knee function has become recognized and preservation or repair of the injured meniscus, especially in young patients is important. Fortunately children and adolescents have a higher incidence of peripheral tears which, because of a good peripheral blood supply, are more amenable to successful repair.[205]

COLLATERAL AND CRUCIATE LIGAMENT INJURY OF THE KNEE

Ligament injury of the knee, and indeed of other joints, is rare in young children, becoming increasingly common as maturity is approached. Rupture of collateral and cruciate ligaments does sometimes occur, the mechanism of injury being similar to that in the adult. In the child ligaments are stronger than the bone to which they are attached, and mechanisms that would ordinarily lead to rupture of a ligament in an adult lead to avulsion of the underlying bone in the child. The best example is an avulsion fracture of the tibial eminence, the site of insertion of the anterior cruciate ligament. In general terms if avulsion fractures are significantly displaced from their origin management includes reduction and sometimes fixation.

BREASTSTROKER'S KNEE

Competitive breaststrokers can develop medial knee pain along the medial collateral ligament. The 'whip kick' technique, a modified frog kick, has been associated with the problem. Rest and avoidance of the technique is helpful.

'SHIN SPLINTS'

'Shin splints' is a term that has emerged to describe exercise induced shin pain in the athlete. It is a non-specific clinical presentation with a number of underlying pathological explanations. Radiographs are important to exclude serious explanations for bone pain such as infection or tumor and may identify other explanations such as stress fractures as described earlier.

Periostitis

Inflammation of the tibial periosteum or periostitis is a common cause for shin splints syndrome. It is characterized by pain along the posteromedial edge of the distal third of the tibia where the soleus muscle and its investing fascia originate. It is presumed to be a traction phenomenon and a variety of anatomical alignment variations such as forefoot pronation, genu valgum, femoral anteversion and external tibial torsion have been implicated as potential causes as well as poor footwear and training regimes.[206]

Radiographs sometimes show periosteal new bone along the posteromedial tibia and radionuclide bone scanning shows increased uptake in a longitudinal distribution in contradistinction to the transverse pattern of increased uptake seen in stress fractures.[207] Management should first involve an attempt to identify the underlying cause followed by conservative measures including footwear and activity modification to address the symptoms. Although surgical treatment has been described it should only be entertained as a last resort.[208]

Chronic compartment syndrome

Chronic compartment syndrome develops when muscle volume increases as a result of increased blood flow during exercise. The relatively unexpandable osseofascial compartment cannot accommodate the extra volume, and pressure within the compartment increases. When the intracompartmental pressure exceeds capillary filling pressure the muscles within the compartment develop ischemic pain. This usually resolves a short time after exercise stops. Some patients may experience a transient foot drop. Chronic compartment syndrome can present with 'shin splints' symptoms indistinguishable from periostitis.[208] Accurate diagnosis depends on measuring compartment pressures during exercise on a treadmill. All four compartments in the leg should be assessed although the most commonly affected compartment is the anterior compartment. Initial treatment involves a conservative approach with footwear and activity modification. Surgical treatment in the form of fasciotomy is reported to be successful in 90% of cases.[209]

Superficial peroneal nerve compression

Superficial peroneal nerve compression can also give rise to activity related shin pain. The superficial peroneal nerve emerges from the fascia of the lower third of the anterolateral part of the leg, to the subcutaneous plane where it travels distally, to supply sensory innervation to the dorsum of the foot. During exercise increased muscle pressure can compress the superficial peroneal nerve against the edge of the fascial hiatus where it emerges. This leads to exercise induced leg pain, sometimes with associated local pain at the hiatus in the fascia and altered sensation on the dorsum of the foot. In troublesome cases limited fasciotomy at the fascial hiatus is effective.

REFERENCES (*Level 1 evidence)

1 Goodman JE, McGrath PJ. The epidemiology of pain in children and adolescents: a review. Pain 1991; 46:247–264.

2 Duffy CM, Lovell DJ. Assessment of health status, function and outcome. In: Cassidy JT, Petty RE (eds). Textbook of pediatric rheumatology, 4th edn. Philadelphia: WB Saunders; 2001:178–188.

3 Singh G, Athreya BH, Fries JF, et al. Measurement of health status in children with juvenile rheumatoid arthritis. Arthritis Rheum 1994; 37:1761–1769.

4 Huber AM, Hicks JE, Lachenbruch PA, et al. Validation of the Childhood Health Assessment Questionnaire in the juvenile idiopathic myopathies. Juvenile Dermatomyositis Disease Activity Collaborative Study Group. J Rheumatol 2001; 28:1106–1111.

5 Nugent J, Ruperto N, Grainger J, et al. The British Version of the Childhood Health Assessment Questionnaire (CHAQ) and the Child Health Questionnaire (CHQ). Clin Exp Rheumatol 2001; 19:S163–S167.

6 Miller FW, Rider LG, Chung YL, et al. Proposed preliminary core set measures for disease outcome assessment in adult and juvenile idiopathic inflammatory myopathies. Rheumatol 2001; 40:1262–1273.

7 Lovell DJ, Lindsley CB, Rennebohm RM, et al. Development of validated disease activity and damage indices in the juvenile idiopathic inflammatory myopathies. II The Childhood Myositis Assessment Scale (CMAS): a quantitative tool for the evaluation of muscle function. The Juvenile Dermatomyositis Disease Activity Collaborative Study Group. Arthritis Rheum 1999; 42:2213–2219.

8 Binder H, Eng GD, Gaiser JF, et al. Congenital muscular torticollis: results of conservative management with long-term follow up in 85 cases. Arch Phys Med Rehabil 1987; 68:222–225.

9 Hensinger RN, Lang JR, MacEwan GD. The Klippel–Feil syndrome: a constellation of related anomalies. J Bone Joint Surg 1974; 56A:1246–1253.

10 Aldred AJ. Congenital pseudoarthrosis of the clavicle. J Bone Joint Surg 1963; 45B:312–319.

11 Lloyd Roberts GC, Apley AG, Owen R. Reflections upon the aetiology of congenital pseudoarthrosis of the clavicle. J Bone Joint Surg 1975; 57B:24–29.

12 Goldberg MJ, Bartoshesky LE. Congenital hand anomaly: aetiology and associated malformations. Hand Clin 1985; 1:405–415.

13 Sachar K, Mih A. Congenital radial head dislocations. Hand Clin 1998; 14:39–47.

14 Weighill FJ. The treatment of developmental coxa vara by abduction subtrochanteric and intertrochanteric femoral osteotomy with special reference to the role of adductor tenotomy. Clin Orthop 1976; 116:116–124.

15 Klisic PJ. Congenital dislocation of the hip. A misleading term: brief report. J Bone Joint Surg 1989; 71B:136.

16 Barlow TG. Early diagnosis and treatment of congenital dislocation of the hip. J Bone Joint Surg 1962; 44B:242–301.

17 Godward S, Dezateux C. Surgery for congenital dislocation of the hip in the UK as a measure of outcome of screening MRC working party on congenital dislocation of the hip. Lancet 1998; 351:1149–1152.

18 Coleman SS. Congenital dysplasia of the hip in the Navajo infant. Clin Orthop 1968; 56:179–193.

19 Hoagland FT, Kalamchi A, Poon R, et al. Congenital hip dislocation and dysplasia in Southern Chinese. Int Orthop 1981; 4:243–246.

20 Skirving AP, Scadden WJ. The African neonatal hip and its immunity from congenital dislocation. J Bone Joint Surg 1979; 61B:339–341.

21 Dunn PM. Prenatal observation on the etiology of congenital dislocation of the hip. Clin Orthop 1976; 119:11–22.

22 Carter CO, Wilkinson JA. Genetic and environmental factors in the etiology of congenital dislocation of the hip. Clin Orthop 1964; 33:119–128.

23 Kumar SJ, MacEwan GD. The incidence of hip dysplasia with metatarsus adductus. Clin Orthop 1982; 164:234–235.

24 Jones D. Topic for debate at the crossroads – neonatal detection of developmental dysplasia of the hip. J Bone Joint Surg 2000; 82B:160–164.

25 Niebauer JJ, King DE. Congenital dislocation of the knee. J Bone Joint Surg 1960; 42A:207–224.

26 Curtis BH, Fisher RL. Congenital hyperextension with anterior subluxation of the knee: surgical treatment and long-term observations. J Bone Joint Surg 1969; 51A:225–268.

27 Hoffman A, Wenger DR. Posteromedial bowing of the tibia. Progression in leg lengths. J Bone Joint Surg 1981; 63:384–388.

28 Farmer AW, Laurine CN. Congenital absence of the fibula. J Bone Joint Surg 1960; 42A:1–12.

29 Schoenecker PL, Capelli AM, Millar EA, et al. Congenital longitudinal deficiency of the tibia. J Bone Joint Surg 1989; 71A:278–287.

30 Kalamchi A, Dawe RV. Congenital deficiency of the tibia. J Bone Joint Surg 1985; 67B:581–584.

31 Jacobsen ST, Crawford AH, Millar EA, et al. The Symes amputation in patients with congenital pseudoarthrosis of the tibia. J Bone Joint Surg 1983; 65A:533–537.

32 Wynne Davies R. Familial studies and the cause of congenital clubfoot: talipes equinovarus, talipes calcaneovalgus and metatarsus varus. J Bone Joint Surg 1964; 46B:445–463.

33 Harrold AJ, Walker CJ. Treatment and prognosis in congenital clubfoot. J Bone Joint Surg 1983; 65B:8–11.

34 Hamanishi C. Congenital vertical talus: classification with 69 cases and new measurement system. J Pediatr Orthop 1984; 4:318–326.

35 Hall JG. Primary disorders of bone and connective tissues. In: Cassidy JT, Petty RE (eds). Textbook of pediatric rheumatology, 4th edn. Philadelphia: WB Saunders; 2001:739–761.

36 Raff ML, Byers PH. Joint hypermobility syndromes. Curr Opin Rheumatol 1996; 8:459–466.

37 Chalom EC, Ross J, Athreya BH. Syndromes and arthritis. Rheum Dis Clin North Am 1997; 23:709–727.

38 Grahame R. Heritable disorders of connective tissue. Baillieres Best Pract Res Clin Rheumatol 2000; 14:345–361.

39 Beighton P, Solomon L, Soskolne CL. Articular mobility in an African population. Ann Rheum Dis 1973; 32:413–418.

40 van der Giessen LJ, Lickens D, Rutgers KJ, et al. Validation of Beighton score and prevalence of connective tissue signs in 773 Dutch children. J Rheumatol 2001; 28:2726–2730.

41 Bird HA, Tribe CR, Bacon PA. Joint hypermobility leading to osteoarthrosis and chondrocalcinosis. Ann Rheum Dis 1978; 37:203–211.

42 Murray KJ, Woo P. Benign joint hypermobility in childhood. Rheumatology 2001; 40:485–487.

43 Gedalia A, Press J, Klein M, et al. Joint hypermobility and fibromyalgia in schoolchildren. Ann Rheum Dis 1993; 52:494–496.

44 Le Parc JM, Molcard S, Tubach F, et al. Marfan syndrome and fibrillin disorders. Joint Bone Spine 2000; 67:401–407.

45 De Paepe A, Devereux RB, Dietz HC, et al. Revised diagnostic criteria for the Marfan syndrome. Am J Med Genet 1996; 62:417–426.

46 Loeys B, Nuytinck L, Delvaux I, et al. Genotype and phenotype analysis of 171 patients referred for molecular study of the fibrillin-1 gene FBN1 because of suspected Marfan syndrome. Arch Intern Med 2001; 161:2447–2454.

47 Kocher MS, Shapiro F. Osteogenesis imperfecta. J Am Acad Orthop Surg 1998; 6:225–236.

48 Glorieux FH, Bishop NJ, Plotkin H, et al. Cyclic administration of pamidronate in children with severe osteogenesis imperfecta. N Engl J Med 1998; 339:986–987.

49 Yancey CL, Zmijewski C, Athreya BH, et al. Arthropathy of Down's syndrome. Arthritis Rheum 1984; 27:929–934.

50 Davies K, Stiehm ER, Woo P, et al. Juvenile idiopathic polyarticular arthritis and IgA deficiency in the 22q11 deletion syndrome. J Rheumatol 2001; 28:2326–2334.

51 Massie RJ, Towns SJ, Bernard E, et al. The musculoskeletal complications of cystic fibrosis. J Pediatr Child Health 1998; 34:467–470.

52 Wulffraat NM, de Graeff-Meeder ER, Rijkers GT, et al. Prevalence of circulating immune complexes in patients with cystic fibrosis and arthritis. J Pediatr 1994; 12:374–378.

53 McBride MB, Rigden S, Haycock GB, et al. Presymptomatic detection of familial juvenile hyperuricaemic nephropathy in children. Pediatr Nephrol 1998; 12:357–364.

54 Dagan R. Management of acute hematogenous osteomyelitis and septic arthritis in the pediatric patient. Pediatr Infect Dis J 1993; 12:88–93.

55 Sonnen GM, Henry NK. Pediatric bone and joint infections. Pediatr Clin North Am 1996; 43:933–947.

56 Kallio MJT, Unkila-Kallio L, Aalto K, et al. Serum C-reactive protein, erythrocyte sedimentation rate and white blood cell count in septic arthritis. Pediatr Infect Dis J 1997; 16:411–413.

57 Shetty AK, Gedalia A. Septic arthritis in children. Rheum Dis Clin North Am 1998; 24:287–304.

58 Davies EG, Monsell F. Managing osteoarticular infection in children. Curr Pediatrics 2000; 10:42–48.

59 Cassidy JT, Petty RE. Infectious arthritis and osteomyelitis. In: Cassidy JT, Petty RE (eds). Textbook of pediatric rheumatology, 4th edn. Philadelphia: WB Saunders; 2001:640–665.

60 Peltola H, Kallio-Unkila L, Kallio MJT, et al. Simplified treatment of acute staphylococcal osteomyelitis of childhood. Pediatrics 1997; 99:846–850.

61 Wenger DR, Bobechko WP, Gilday DL. Spectrum of intervertebal disc space infection in children. J Bone Joint Surg 1978; 60A:100–108.

62 Tingle AJ, Allen M, Petty RE, et al. Rubella-associated arthritis. I. Comparative study of joint manifestations associated with natural rubella infection and RA 27/3 rubella immunisation. Ann Rheum Dis 1986; 45:110–114.

63 Wall EJ. Childhood osteomyelitis and septic arthritis. Curr Opin Pediatr 1998; 10:73–76.

64 Dajani A, Taubert K, Ferrieri P, et al. Treatment of acute streptococcal pharyngitis and prevention of rheumatic fever: a statement for health professionals. Pediatrics 1995; 96:758–764.

65 Huppertz HI. Lyme disease in children. Curr Opin Rheumatol 2001; 13:434–439.

66 Giannini EH, Ruperto N, Ravelli A, et al. Preliminary definition of improvement in juvenile arthritis. Arthritis Rheum 1997; 40:1202–1209.

67 Petty RE, Southwood TR, Baum J, et al. Revision of the proposed classification criteria for juvenile idiopathic arthritis: Durban. J Rheumatol 1998; 25:1991–1994.

68 Wood PN. Nomenclature and classification of arthritis in children. In: Munthe E (ed). The care of rheumatic children. Basel: EULAR; 1978:47–50.

69 Brewer EJ, Bass JC, Cassidy JT, et al. Criteria for the classification of juvenile rheumatoid arthritis. Bull Rheum Dis 1972; 23:712–719.

70 Gare BA. Juvenile arthritis–who gets it, where and when? A review of current data on incidence and prevalence. Clin Exp Rheumatol 1999; 17:367–374.

71 Schwartz MM, Simpson P, Kerr KL, et al. Juvenile rheumatoid arthritis in African Americans. J Rheumatol 1997; 24:1826–1829.

72 Uziel Y, Pomeranz A, Brik R, et al. Seasonal variation in systemic onset juvenile rheumatoid arthritis in Israel. J Rheumatol 1999; 26:1187–1189.

73 Pugh MT, Southwood TR, Hill Gaston JS. The role of infection in juvenile chronic arthritis. Br J Rheumatol 1993; 32:838–844.

74 Symmons DM, Jones M, Osborne J, et al. Pediatric rheumatology in the United Kingdom: data from the British Paediatric Rheumatology Group National Diagnostic Register. J Rheumatol 1996; 23:1975–1980.

75 Cassidy JT, Petty RE. Juvenile rheumatoid arthritis. In: Cassidy JT, Petty RE (eds). Textbook of pediatric rheumatology, 4th edn. Philadelphia: WB Saunders; 2001:218–322.

76 Glass DN, Giannini EH. Juvenile rheumatoid arthritis as a complex genetic trait. Arthritis Rheum 1999; 42:2261–2268.

77 Statsny P. Association of the B-cell alloantigen DRw4 with rheumatoid arthritis. N Engl J Med 1978; 298:868–871.

78 Murray KJ, Moroldo MB, Donnelly P, et al. Age-specific effects of juvenile rheumatoid arthritis-associated alleles. Arthritis Rheum 1999; 42:1843–1853.

79 Albert ED, Scholz S. Juvenile arthritis: genetic update. Bailliere's Clin Rheum 1998; 12:209–218.

80 Choy ES, Panayi GS. Cytokine pathways and joint inflammation in rheumatoid arthritis. N Engl J Med 2001; 344:907–916.

81 Woo P. Cytokines in juvenile chronic arthritis. Bailliere's Clin Rheum 1998; 12:219–228.

82 Grom AA, Murray KJ, Luyrink L, et al. Patterns of expression of tumor necrosis factor alpha, tumor necrosis factor beta, and their receptors in the synovia of patients with juvenile rheumatoid arthritis and juvenile spondyloarthropathy. Arthritis Rheum 1996; 39:1703–1710.

83 Rooney M, Varsani H, Martin K, et al. Tumour necrosis factor alpha (TNFalpha) and its soluble receptors in juvenile chronic arthritis (JCA). Rheumatology 2000; 39:432–438.

84 Crawley E, Kon S, Woo P. Hereditary predisposition to low interleukin-10 production in children with extended oligoarticular juvenile

idiopathic arthritis. Rheumatology 2001; 40:574–578.
85 Flat B, Aasland A, Vinje O, et al. Outcome and predictive factors in juvenile rheumatoid arthritis and juvenile spondyloarthropathy. J Rheumatol 1998; 25:366–375.
86 Schneider R, Laxer RM. Systemic onset of juvenile rheumatoid arthritis. Bailliere's Clin Rheum 1998; 12:245–271.
87 Roberton DM, Cabral DA, Malleson PN, et al. Juvenile psoriatic arthritis: follow up and evaluation of diagnostic criteria. J Rheumatol 1996; 23:166–170.
88 Cohen PA, Job-Deslandre CH, Lalande G, et al. Overview of the radiology of juvenile idiopathic arthritis (JIA). Eur J Radiol 2000; 33:94–101.
89 Chalom EC, Goldsmith DP, Koehler MA, et al. Prevalence and outcome of uveitis in a regional cohort of patients with juvenile rheumatoid arthritis. J Rheumatol 1997; 24:2031–2034.
90 Giannini EH, Malagon CN, Van Kerckhove C, et al. Longitudinal analysis of HLA associated risks for iridocyclitis in juvenile rheumatoid arthritis. J Rheumatol 1998; 12:309–328.
91 Reiff A, Takei S, Sadehi S, et al. Etanercept therapy in children with treatment-resistant uveitis. Arthritis Rheum 2001; 44:1411–1415.
*92 Bechtold S, Ripperger P, Muhlbayer D, et al. GH therapy in juvenile chronic arthritis: results of a two-year controlled study on growth and bone. J Clin Endocrinol Metab 2001; 86:5737–5744.
93 Sawhney S, Woo P, Murray KJ. Macrophage activation syndrome: a potentially fatal complication of rheumatic disorders. Arch Dis Child 2001; 85:421–426.
94 Hackett J, Johnson B, Parkin A, et al. Physiotherapy and occupational therapy for juvenile chronic arthritis: custom and practice in five centres in the UK, USA and Canada. Br J Rheumatol 1996; 35:695–699.
95 Breit W, Frosch M, Meyer U, et al. A subgroup specific evaluation of the efficacy of intra-articular triamcinolone hexacetonide in juvenile chronic arthritis. J Rheumatol 2000; 27:2696–2702.
96 Sherry DD, Stein LD, Reed AM, et al. Prevention of leg length discrepancy in young children with pauciarticular juvenile rheumatoid arthritis by treatment with intra-articular steroids. Arthritis Rheum 1999; 42:2330–2334.
97 Job-Deslandre C, Menkes CJ. Complications of intra-articular injections of triamcinolone hexacetonide in chronic arthritis in children. Clin Exp Rheumatol 1990; 8:413–416.
98 Cassidy JT. Medical management of children with juvenile rheumatoid arthritis. Drugs 1999; 58:831–850.
*99 Giannini EH, Brewer EJ, Kuzmina N, et al. Methotrexate in resistant juvenile rheumatoid arthritis. N Engl J Med 1992; 326:1043–1049.
*100 Woo P, Southwood TR, Prieur A-M, et al. Randomized, placebo-controlled, crossover trial of low-dose oral methotrexate in children with extended oligoarticular or systemic arthritis. Arthritis Rheum 2000; 43:1849–1857.
*101 Van Rossum MA, Fiselier TJ, Franssen MJ, et al. Sulphasalazine in the treatment of juvenile chronic arthritis: a randomised, double blind, placebo-controlled, multicenter study. Dutch Juvenile Chronic Arthritis Study Group. Arthritis Rheum 1998; 41:808–816.
102 Gerloni V, Cimaz R, Gattinara M, et al. Efficacy and safety profile of cyclosporin A in the treatment of juvenile chronic (idiopathic) arthritis. Results of a 10-year prospective study. Rheumatol 2001; 40:907–913.
*103 Lovell DJ, Giannini EH, Reiff A, et al. Efficacy and safety of etanercept (tumor necrosis factor receptor p75Fc fusion protein; Enbrel) in children with polyarticular-course juvenile rheumatoid arthritis. N Engl J Med 2000; 342:763–769.
104 Drug and Therapeutic Bulletin (DTB) 2001; 39:49–52.
105 Wulffraat N, Royen A, Bierings M, et al. Autologous haemopoietic stem-cell transplantation in four patients with refractory juvenile chronic arthritis. Lancet 1999; 353:550–553.
106 McDonagh JE, Foster HE, Hall MA, et al. Audit of rheumatology services for adolescents and young adults in the UK. Rheumatology 2000; 39:596–602.
107 Roberts KP, Connor AN. Referrals to a children's orthopedic clinic. Health Bull 1987; 45:174–178.
108 Salenius P, Vankka E. the development of the tibiofemoral angle in children. J Bone Joint Surg 1975; 57A:259–261.
109 Greene WB. Infantile tibia vara. J Bone Joint Surg 1993; 75A:130–143.
110 Kling TF, Hensinger RN. Angular and torsional deformities of the lower limbs in children. Clin Orthop Rel Res 1983; 176:136–147.
111 Bleck ED. Metatarsus adductus: Classification and relationship to outcome of treatment. J Pediatr Orthop 1983; 3:2–9.
112 Naish JM, Apley J. Growing pains – a clinical study of non-arthritic limb pains in children. Arch Dis Child 1951; 26:134–140.
113 Landin LA, Danielsson LG, Wattsgard C, et al. Transient synovitis of the hip. Its incidence, epidemiology and relation to Perthes disease. J Bone Joint Surg 1987; 69B:238–242.
114 Haueisen DC, Weiner DS, Weiner SD. The characterisation of 'transient synovitis of the hip' in children. J Pediatr Orthop 1986; 6:11–17.
115 Glueck CJ, Crawford A, Roy D, et al. Association of antithrombotic factor deficiencies and hypofibrinolysis with Legg–Perthes disease. J Bone Joint Surg 1986; 78A:3–13.
116 Thomas J, Morgan G, Tayton K. Perthes disease and the relevance of thrombophilia. J Bone Joint Surg 1999; 81B:691–695.
117 Barker DJP, Hall AJ. The epidemiology of Perthes disease. Clin Orthop 1986; 209:89–94.
118 Van Den Bogaert G, De Rosa E, Moens P. Bilateral Legg–Calvé–Perthes disease: different from unilateral. Pediatr Orthop 1999; 8B:165–168.
119 Meehan PL, Angel D, Nelson JM. The Scottish Rite abduction orthosis for the treatment of Legg–Perthes disease: a radiographic analysis. J Bone Joint Surg 1992; 74A:2–12.
120 Quain S, Catterall A. Hinge abduction of the hip: diagnosis and treatment. J Bone Joint Surg 1986; 68B:61–64.
121 Loder RT, Wittenberg B, DeSilva G. Slipped capital femoral epiphysis associated with endocrine disorders. J Pediatr Orthop 1995; 15:349–356.
122 Weiner D. Pathogenesis of slipped capital femoral epiphysis: current concepts. J Pediatr Orthop 1996; 5B:67–73.
123 Klein A, Joplin RJ, Reidy JA, et al. Roentgenographic features of slipped capital femoral epiphysis. Am J Roentgenol 1951; 66:361–374.
124 Loder RT, Richards BS, Shapiro PS, et al. Acute slipped capital femoral epiphysis: the importance of physeal stability. J Bone Joint Surg 1993; 75A:1134–1140.
125 Heppenstall RB, Marvel JP, Chung SMK, et al. Chondrolysis of the hip joint. Clin Orthop Rel Res 1974; 103:136–142.
126 Pellicci PM, Wilson PD. Chondrolysis of the hips associated with severe burns. J Bone and Joint Surg 1979; 61A:592–596.
127 Roy PR, Crawford AH. Idiopathic chondrolysis of the hip. Management by subtotal capsulectomy and aggressive rehabilitation. J Pediatr Orthop 1988; 8:203–207.
128 Boucher JP, King MA, Lefebvre R, et al. Quadriceps femoris muscle activity in patellofemoral pain syndrome. Am J Sport Med 1992; 20:527–532.
129 Yates CK, Granna WA. Patellofemoral pain in children. Clin Orthop Rel Res 1990; 255:36–43.
130 Granna WA , Hinkley B, Hollingsworth S. Arthroscopic evaluation and treatment of patellar malalignment. Clin Orthop Rel Res 1984; 186:122–128.
131 Fugikawa K, Iseki F, Mikura Y. Partial resection of the discoid meniscus in the child's knee. J Bone Joint Surg 1981; 63A:391–395.
132 Gauthier G, Elbaz R. Freiberg's infraction: a subchondral bone fatigue fracture. Clin Orthop 1979; 142:93–95.
133 Leonard MA. The inheritance of tarsal coalition and its relationship to spastic flat foot. J Bone Joint Surg 1974; 56B:520–526.
134 Mosier KM, Asher M. Tarsal coalitions and peroneal spastic flatfoot. J Bone Joint Surg 1984; 66A:976–984.
135 Cowell HR. Diagnosis and management of peroneal spastic flatfoot. In: Instructional course lectures, The American Academy of Orthopedic Surgeons. St Louis: Mosby; 1975: 24:94–103.
136 Conway JJ, Cowell HR. Tarsal coalition: clinical significance and roentgenographic Demonstration. Radiology 1969; 92:799–811.
137 Gonzalez P, Kumar SJ. Calcaneonavicular coalition treated by resection and interposition of the extensor digitorum brevis muscle. J Bone Joint Surg 1990; 72A:71–77.
138 Kumar SJ, Guille JT, Lee MS, et al. Osseous and non osseous coalition of the middle facet of the talocalcaneal joint. J Bone Joint Surg 1992; 74A:529–535.
139 Jennette JC, Falk RJ, Andrassay K, et al. Nomenclature of systemic vasculitides. Proposal of an international consensus conference. Arthritis Rheum 1994; 37:187–192.
140 Lang BA. Systemic vasculitis. In: Isenberg DA, Miller JJ (eds). Adolescent rheumatology. London: Dunitz; 1999: 176–196.
141 Stewart M, Savage JM, Bell B, et al. Long term renal prognosis of Henoch–Schönlein purpura in an unselected childhood population. Eur J Pediatr 1988; 147:113–115.

142 Nielson HE. Epidemiology of Schönlein–Henoch purpura. Acta Pediatr Scand 1988; 77:125–131.

143 Allen AC, Willis FR, Beattie TJ, et al. Abnormal IgA glycosylation in Henoch–Schönlein purpura restricted to patients with clinical nephritis. Nephrol Dial Transplant 1998; 13:930–934.

144 Choong CK, Beasley SW. Intra-abdominal manifestations of Henoch–Schönlein purpura. J Pediatr Child Health 1998; 34:405–409.

145 Flynn JT, Smoyer WE, Bunchman TE, et al. Treatment of Henoch–Schönlein purpura with high dose corticosteroids plus oral cyclophosphamide. Am J Nephrol 2001; 21:128–133.

146 Szer IS. Henoch–Schönlein purpura: when and how to treat. J Rheumatol 1996; 23:1661–1665.

147 Wyatt RJ, Hogg RJ. Evidence-based assessment of treatment options for children with IgA nephropathies. Pediatr Nephrol 2001; 16:156–167.

148 Kato H, Inoue O, Kawasaki T. Adult coronary artery disease probably due to childhood Kawasaki disease. Lancet 1992; 340:1127–1129.

149 Yanagawa H, Nakamura Y, Yashiro M, et al. Update of the epidemiology of Kawasaki disease in Japan – from the results of the 1993–1994 nationwide survey. J Epidemiol 1996; 6:148–157.

150 Leung DYM, Meissner HC, Schlievert PM. The etiology and pathogenesis of Kawasaki disease – how close are we to an answer? Curr Opin Infect Dis 1997; 10:226–232.

151 Igarashi H, Hatake K, Shiraishi H, et al. Elevated serum levels of macrophage colony-stimulating factor in patients with Kawasaki disease complicated by cardiac lesions. Clin Exp Rheumatol 2001; 19:751–756.

152 Witt MT, Minich LL, Bohnsack JF, et al. Kawasaki disease: more patients are being diagnosed who do not meet American Heart Association criteria. Pediatrics 1999; E10:104.

*153 Newburger JW, Takahashi M, Burns JC, et al. The treatment of Kawasaki syndrome with intravenous gamma globulin. N Engl J Med 1986; 315:341–347.

*154 Newburger JW, Takahashi M, Beiser AS, et al. A single intravenous infusion of gamma globulin as compared with four infusions in the treatment of acute Kawasaki syndrome. N Engl J Med 1991; 324:1633–1638.

155 Wallace CA, French JW, Kahn SJ, et al. Intravenous gammaglobulin treatment failure in Kawasaki disease. Pediatrics 2000; E78:105.

156 Onouchi Z, Kawasaki T. Overview of pharmacological treatment of Kawasaki disease. Drugs 1999; 58:813–822.

157 Dajani A, Taubert K, Takahashi M, et al. Guidelines for long term management of patients with Kawasaki disease: report from the Committee on Rheumatic Fever, Endocarditis and Kawasaki disease, Council on Cardiovascular Disease in the Young, American Heart Association. Circulation 1994; 89:916–922.

158 David J, Ansell BM, Woo P. Polyarteritis nodosa associated with streptococcus. Arch Dis Child 1993; 69:685–688.

159 Kaklamani VG, Kaklamanis PG. Treatment of Behçet's disease – an update. Semin Arthritis Rheum 2001; 30:299–312.

*160 Yurdakul S, Mat C, Tuzun Y, et al. A double-blind trial of colchicine in Behçet's syndrome. Arthritis Rheum 2001; 44:2686–2692.

*161 Hamuryudan V, Mat C, Saip S, et al. Thalidomide in the treatment of the mucocutaneous lesions of Behçet's syndrome: a randomized, placebo – controlled, double-blind trial. Ann Intern Med 1998; 128:443–450.

162 Eroglu GE, Kohler PF. Familial systemic lupus erythematosus: the role of genetic and environmental factors. Ann Rheum Dis 2002; 61:29–31.

163 Hochberg MC. Updating the American College of Rheumatology revised criteria for the classification of systemic lupus erythematosus. Arthritis Rheum 1997; 9:1725.

164 Ferraz MB, Goldenberg J, Hilario MO, et al. Evaluation of the ARA lupus criteria data set in pediatric patients. Committees of Pediatric Rheumatology of the Brazilian Society of Pediatrics and the Brazilian Society of Rheumatology. Clin Exp Rheumatol 1994; 12:689–690.

*165 Gourley MF, Austin HA 3rd, Scott D, et al. Methylprednisolone and cyclophosphamide, alone or in combination, in patients with lupus nephritis. A randomized controlled trial. Ann Intern Med 1996; 125:549–557.

*166 Bansal VK, Beto JA. Treatment of lupus nephritis: a meta-analysis of clinical trials. Am J Kidney Dis 1997; 29:193–199.

167 Buratti S, Szer IS, Spencer CH, et al. Mycophenolate mofetil treatment of severe renal disease in pediatric onset systemic lupus erythematosus. J Rheumatol 2001; 28:2103–2108.

168 Brunner HI, Feldman BM, Bombardier C, et al. Sensitivity of the Systemic Lupus Erythematosus Disease Activity Index, British Isles Lupus Assessment Group Index and Systemic Lupus Activity Measure in the evaluation of clinical change in childhood-onset systemic lupus erythematosus. Arthritis Rheum 1999; 42:1354–1360.

169 Gough A, Chapman S, Wagstaff K, et al. Minocycline induced autoimmune hepatitis and systemic lupus erythematosus-like syndrome. BMJ 1996; 312:169–172.

170 Symmons DPM, Sills JA, Davis SM. The incidence of juvenile dermatomyositis: results of a nation-wide study. Br J Rheum 1995; 43:732–735.

171 Reed AM, Pachman LM, Hayford JR, et al. Immunogenetic studies in families of children with juvenile dermatomyositis. J Rheumatol 1998; 25:1000–1002.

172 Pachman LM, Liotta-Davis MR, Hong DK, et al. TNF alpha-308A allele in juvenile dermatomyositis. Association with increased production of tumour necrosis factor a, disease duration and pathologic calcifications. Arthritis Rheum 2000; 43:2368–2377.

173 The French FMF Consortium. A candidate gene for familial Mediterranean fever. Nat Genet 1997; 17:25–31. The International FMF Consortium. Ancient missense mutations in a new member of the RoRet family are likely to cause familial mediterranean fever. Cell 1997; 90:797–807.

174 Houten SM, Kuis W, Duran M, et al. Mutations in the gene encoding mevalonate kinase cause hyperimmunoglobulinemia D and periodic fever syndrome. Nat Genet 1999; 22:175–177.

175 McDermott MF, Aksentijevich I, Galen J, et al. Germline mutations in the extracellular domains of the 55 kDa TNF receptor, TNFR1, define a family of dominantly inherited autoinflammatory syndromes. Cell 1999; 9:133–144.

176 Prieur AM, Griscelli C, Lampert F, et al. A chronic, infantile, neurological, articular and cutaneous (CINCA) syndrome. A specific entity analysed in 30 patients. Scand J Rheumatol 1978; 66:57–68.

177 Turk DC, Okifuji A. Assessment of patients' reporting of pain: an integrated perspective. Lancet 1999; 353:1784–1788.

178 Merskey H. Pain terms: a list with definitions and notes on usage recommended by the ISAP subcommittee on taxonomy. Pain 1979; 6:249–252.

179 Sherry DD. Diagnosis and treatment of amplified musculoskeletal pain in children. Clin Exp Rheumatol 2001; 19:617–620.

180 Malleson PN, Al-Matar M, Petty RE. Idiopathic musculoskeletal pain syndromes in children. J Rheumatol 1992; 19:1786–1789.

181 Sherry DD, Weisman R. Psychologic aspects of childhood reflex neurovascular dystrophy. Pediatrics 1988; 81:572–578.

182 Murray CS, Cohen A, Perkins T, et al. Morbidity in childhood reflex sympathetic dystrophy. Arch Dis Child 2000; 82:231–233.

183 Cleary AG, Sills JA, Davidson JE, et al. Reflex sympathetic dystrophy. Rheumatology 2001; 40:590–591.

184 McBeth J, Macfarlane GJ, Benjamin S, et al. Features of somatisation predict the onset of chronic widespread pain: results of a large population-based study. Arthritis Rheum 2001; 44:940–946.

185 Aasland A, Flato B, Vandvik IH. Psychosocial factors in children with idiopathic musculoskeletal pain: a prospective, longitudinal study. Acta Pediatr 1997; 86:740–746.

186 Krist J, Ans D, Ottir G. Prevalence of self-reported back pain in school children: a study of sociodemographic differences. Eur J Pediatr 1996; 155:984–986.

187 Dreghorn CR, Newman RJ, Hardy G, et al. Primary tumours of the axial skeleton; experience of the Leeds Regional Bone Tumour Registry. Proceedings of British Scoliosis Society Meeting. J Bone Joint Surg 1989; 72B:338–339.

188 Williams CRP, O'Flynn E, Clarke NMP, et al. Torticollis secondary to ocular pathology. J Bone Joint Surg 1996; 78B:620–624.

189 Ramenofsky ML, Buyse M, Goldberg MJ, et al. Gastrooesophageal reflux and torticollis. J Bone Joint Surg 1978; 60A:1140–1141.

190 Njeh CK, Shaw N, Gardner-Medwin JM, et al. Use of quantitative ultrasound to assess bone status in children with juvenile idiopathic arthritis: a pilot study. J Clin Densitom 2000; 3:251–260.

191 Schonau E. Problems of bone analysis in childhood and adolescence. Pediatr Nephrol 1998; 12:420–429.

192 Leonard MB, Propert KJ, Zemel BS, et al. Discrepancies in pediatric bone mineral density refence data: potential for misdiagnosis of osteopenia. J Pediatr 1999; 135:182–188.

193 NIH Consensus Development Panel on Osteoporosis Prevention, Diagnosis and Therapy. Osteoporosis prevention, diagnosis, and therapy. JAMA 2001; 285:785–795.

194 Bianchi ML, Cimaz R, Bardare M, et al. Efficacy and safety of alendronate for the treatment of osteoporosis in diffuse connective tissue diseases in children: a prospective multicenter trial. Arthritis Rheum 2000; 43:1960–1966.

195 Orava S, Jormakka E, Hulkko A. Stress fractures in young athletes. Arch Orthop Trauma Surg 1981; 98:271.

196 Matheson GO, Clement DB, McKenzie DC, et al. Stress fractures in athletes. Am J Sports Med 1987; 15:46–58.

197 Barnett LS. Little league shoulder syndrome: proximal humeral epiphyseolysis in adolescent baseball pitchers. J Bone Joint Surg 1985; 67A:495–496.

198 Roy S, Caine D, Singer KM. Stress changes of the distal radial epiphysis in young gymnasts. Am J Sports Med 1985; 13:301–308.

199 Albanese S, Palmer A, Kerr D. Wrist pain and growth plate closure of the radius in gymnasts. J Pediatr Orthop 1989; 9:23–28.

200 Kujala UM, Kvist M, Heinonen O. Osgood–Schlatter's disease in adolescent athletes. Am J Sports Med 1985; 13:236–241.

201 Krause BL, Williams JPR, Catterral A. Natural history of Osgood–Schlatter's disease. J Pediatr Orthop 1990; 10:65–68.

202 Mital MA, Matza RA, Cohen J. The so-called unresolved Osgood Schlatter lesion. J Bone Joint Surg 1980; 62:732–739.

203 Brogden BG, Crow NE. Little leaguer's elbow. Am J Roentgenol 1960; 83:671–675.

204 Noble CA. Iliotibial band friction syndrome in runners. Am J Sports Med 1980; 8:232–234.

205 Cassidy RE, Schaffer AJ. Repair of peripheral meniscus tears: a preliminary report. Am J Sports Med 1981; 9:209–214.

206 Lutter LD. Runners knee injuries. AAOS Instr Course Lect 1984; 33:258–268.

207 Michael RH, Holder LE. The soleus syndrome. Am J Sports Med 1985; 13:87–94.

208 Mubarak SJ. The medial tibial stress syndrome. Am J Sports Med 1982; 10:201–205.

209 Detmer DE. Chronic compartment syndrome: diagnosis, management and outcomes. Am J Sports Med 1985; 13:162–170.

28

Disorders of the skin

Nigel P Burrows

INTRODUCTION

The skin comprises roughly 15% of the body weight. It is a complex organ which undergoes constant repair. Its main functions are:

1. a barrier to absorption and loss of fluid and electrolytes;
2. a barrier to external injurious agents and mechanical stress;
3. protection against ultraviolet light;
4. protection against pathogenic microorganisms;
5. regulation of body temperature;
6. as a sensory organ;
7. synthesis of vitamin D;
8. social (and sexual) communication.

To perform these functions, the skin requires a complicated structure. It consists of three layers:
1. epidermis, derived from ectoderm;
2. dermis, derived from mesoderm;
3. subcutis, derived from mesoderm.

The main function of the epidermis is to act as a barrier. The main barrier to fluid and electrolyte loss and to external injurious agents is the horny layer on the external surface of the epidermis: this is formed from flattened *keratinocytes* which originate from the basal layer of the epidermis and progress towards the exterior. *Melanocytes* are also found in the basal layer, and are differentiated from keratinocytes by darkly staining nuclei and clear cytoplasm: their main function is protection against ultraviolet radiation by distributing melanin throughout the basal layer. The amount of melanin determines the racial color. A third type of cell is the *Langerhans' cell*, found in the midepidermis which has been shown to be a dendritic antigen-presenting cell, and plays an important role in allergic contact eczema and forms part of the immune defense in the skin. A fourth cell has recently been described, the *Merkel cell*: the exact function of this cell has not been determined, but the present evidence suggests a sensory role.

The dermis is composed of collagen, elastin and reticulin within a matrix of ground substance. Blood vessels, sensory and autonomic nerves and nerve endings, hair follicles (pilosebaceous units) and sweat glands traverse the dermis. Temperature regulation is mainly effected by shunting of blood between the superficial and deep arteriolar and venular plexuses, modified by the glomus apparatus between the two plexuses which are under autonomic control. Secondary temperature regulation, which is particularly important where the ambient temperature exceeds 37°C, depends on evaporation from the eccrine sweat glands which are under adrenergic control.

The subcutis consists mainly of adipose tissue, whose main function is insulation of the body. In sites such as the sole of the foot, fibrous bands within the subcutis have a buffering and protective effect.

The skin appendages such as hair and nails are largely vestigial in the human; loss of either does not constitute any threat to the survival of the individual.

MANAGEMENT OF A SKIN PROBLEM IN A CHILD

It is important to take a detailed history either from the child or from the parents. History taking is similar to that in internal medicine, though the emphasis is different. Of particular importance are the following:
1. family history – many skin diseases are hereditary;
2. past history of the skin disease – conditions such as psoriasis and atopic eczema tend to be intermittent;
3. general health – some diseases (e.g. connective tissue diseases) are multiorgan problems;
4. previous treatment – both oral and topical: treatment may have modified the clinical picture (for better or for worse).

Examination of the child

The child should be undressed completely to allow full assessment of the condition. A general medical examination should also be performed. If a rash is present, note should be taken of the following points: (1) color, nature and distribution; (2) relationship of the rash to skin appendages, such as hair follicles and sweat ducts; (3) mucous membranes: some skin diseases have a banal appearance in the skin, but a characteristic appearance in mucous membranes, e.g. lichen planus, congenital syphilis; (4) examination of the hair and nails, as changes may give a clue as to the diagnosis.

TREATMENT OF SKIN DISEASES

As the skin is so accessible, it is sensible where possible to treat skin diseases with topical preparations. It is also important to introduce the active agent (e.g. steroid, antibiotic) in a suitable form or vehicle:
1. Lotions (solutions) are very useful for exudative rashes as 'wet dressings', where ointments and creams would 'float off', e.g. potassium permanganate.
2. Shake lotions (solution + 15–30% powder), e.g. calamine lotion.
3. Creams (oil–water emulsion). Bases such as cetomacrogol or aqueous cream are very acceptable to the patient, e.g. topical steroid creams.
4. Ointments such as petrolatum have a greasy base. They are useful for dry skin conditions, such as atopic eczema, e.g. steroid and antibiotic ointments.
5. Gels (semicolloids in alcohol base, which dry on the skin). Useful for scalp conditions.
6. Pastes (ointments + 15–30% powder). Used on linen dressings, e.g. tar paste.
7. Powders, e.g. antifungal foot powders, miticides.

NEVI AND OTHER DEVELOPMENTAL DEFECTS

MELANOCYTIC NEVI

Congenital melanocytic nevi (CMN)

These occur in 0.5–2% of the population (Figs 28.1 and 28.2). They are arbitrarily classified as small (less than 1.5 cm), medium (1.5–20 cm) or large/giant (greater than 20 cm or 5% or more of body surface), in estimated adult size. They occur at birth as raised, verrucose or lobulated nodules or plaques of varying shades of brown to black, sometimes with blue or pink components. They have an irregular margin and often long dark hairs and may become increasingly lobulated and hairy with time. Giant sized lesions may produce considerable redundancy of skin and often occur in a 'garment' or 'bathing trunk' distribution on the trunk and adjacent limbs. The very small CMN initially may be difficult to distinguish from café-au-lait macules. In patients with multiple large nevi an eruption of smaller ones (satellite nevi) may occur

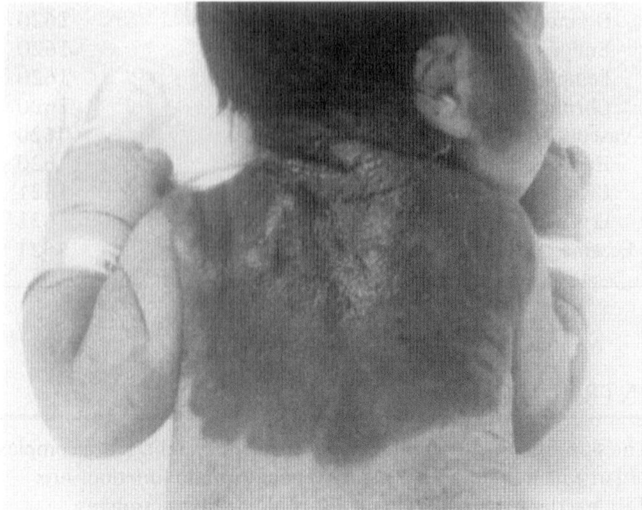

Fig. 28.1 Congenital melanocytic nevus.

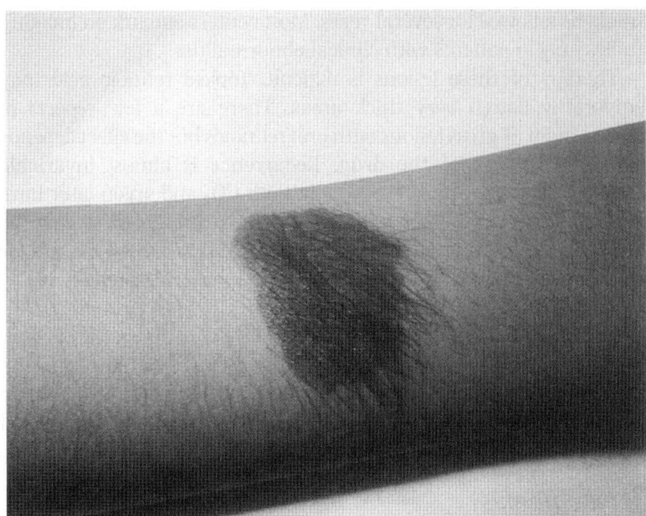

Fig. 28.2 Congenital melanocytic nevus.

over the first year of life. Once established, the nevi increase in size in proportion to the patient's growth. Although rare, large CMN on the scalp or dorsal spine, especially with satellite nevi, may be associated with symptomatic leptomeningeal melanocytosis (neurocutaneous melanosis) with a median age of onset of neurological symptoms at 2 years.[1] Furthermore, magnetic resonance imaging (MRI) scans detect leptomeningeal involvement in 30% of asymptomatic children with CMN in this distribution.[2]

Considerable controversy remains regarding the risk of development of malignant melanoma in CMN and hence the approach to management.[3] Malignancy can arise from the dermal as well as the junctional component of CMN. The incidence of malignancy in large nevi has varied from 2 to 31% in different series but most studies have been retrospective and biased. A long term prospective study based on the Danish birth register is probably the most reliable and a lifetime risk of 4.6% is calculated from it.[4] In a retrospective study which included a review of the world literature primary cutaneous malignant melanoma was diagnosed within a large CMN before the age of 5 years in 50% of cases. No melanoma developed in the satellite nevi. Melanoma also occurs in medium-sized and small CMN[5,6] but the exact incidence for small lesions is not known, though it is definitely lower than for large nevi. A recent study does not support the view of a significantly increased risk of melanoma in banal-appearing, medium-sized CMN, although median follow-up was short at 5.8 years.[7]

While small lesions, in which the malignancy risk is low and is usually postpubertal, can be easily excised, removal of large lesions in which the risk is much more significant is more difficult and with giant lesions may be impossible. In all cases the risk must be weighed against possible functional impairment and the morbidity of multiple operations. Many surgical procedures are available and are chosen depending on the site and extent of the lesions. Dermabrasion and laser therapy may improve the appearance of the nevus by removal of superficial pigment cells but the bulk of the lesion remains and the malignancy risk is not substantially reduced.

Acquired melanocytic nevi (AMN)

In a longitudinal study, 0.5% of babies had a CMN at birth and the number of melanocytic nevi in the same cohort at 1 year had risen to 35%.[8] These nevi continue to increase in number throughout childhood. They commence as brown or black macules, some of which become raised and enlarge laterally as they develop. They are usually of uniform color and well circumscribed. Histologically the flat lesions show clustering of nevus cells at the dermoepidermal junction (junctional nevus) and the raised ones also show intradermal nevus cells (compound nevus). Pure intradermal nevi are rare in children. The risk of melanoma arising from acquired melanocytic nevi is very low (less than 0.1%) and does not occur in childhood so their prophylactic removal in young patients is not justified.

Halo (Sutton's) nevi

A nevus may develop a depigmented halo (Fig. 28.3). The lesions are often multiple and are relatively common. The nevus may appear inflamed and often disappears leaving a white spot which may repigment years later. This is a completely benign change.

Atypical (dysplastic) nevi

Atypical nevi is the preferred term as dysplasia relates to histological features only. They are a subtype of acquired melanocytic nevi with characteristic clinicopathological features. They are a marker for the development of malignant melanoma, occurring in over 90% of patients with familial melanoma and over 10% of those with sporadic melanoma. These nevi differ from more typical AMNs by being larger (more than 5 mm diameter), having irregular and indistinct margins and irregular tan brown coloration, often with an erythematous component. They are predominantly macular, sometimes with a central elevated portion. They may appear in childhood as small typical appearing nevi which after puberty develop the atypical features. In adolescence and early adult life new atypical lesions may appear de novo. Atypical nevi may appear on the scalp in childhood. The final confirmation is based on the finding of some or all of a constellation of histopathological features of which the most important are nuclear atypia and a lymphocytic infiltrate.

Patients with multiple atypical nevi should be monitored with serial photography. Any mole showing significant alteration should be excised. Family members should be checked for the presence of atypical nevi or melanoma.

EPIDERMAL NEVI

Epidermal nevi are hamartomas arising from the basal layer of the embryonic epidermis that gives rise to skin appendages and keratinocytes. These nevi have been conventionally classified

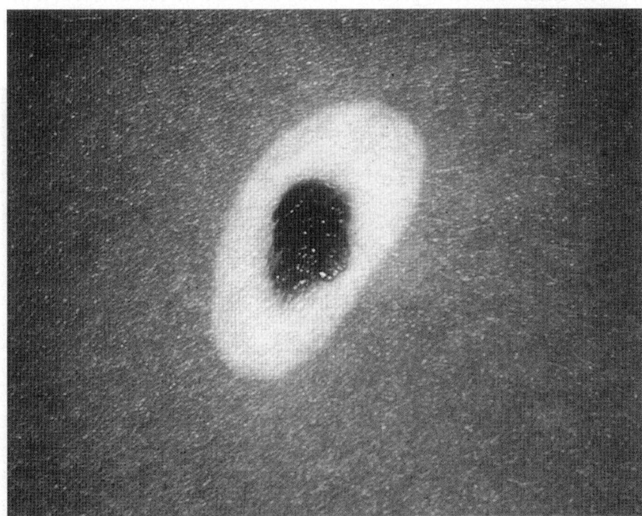

Fig. 28.3 Halo nevus.

according to the main tissue of origin (keratinocytic, sebaceous and follicular) although this is somewhat arbitrary as more than one cell type may be present.

Epidermal nevi can involve any area of skin and may be present at birth (particularly those on the head) or appear in the first few years of life (or exceptionally later). They may simply grow with the patient or can extend well beyond their original distribution over months or years. Extension occurs less often with nevi on the head and with nevi present at birth, whatever their location. It is now clear that the linear and swirled patterns taken by epidermal nevi follow the lines of Blaschko, which define the tracks of clones of genetically identical cells. All epidermal nevi can be explained on the basis of genetic mosaicism[9] with each type of nevus representing the cutaneous manifestation of a different mosaic phenotype. In most patients the nevus is the only detectable manifestation but in some patients there are associated abnormalities in other organ systems, particularly skeletal, neurological and ocular.[10,11] This association has been called the 'epidermal nevus syndrome'.[9,12]

Keratinocyte nevi often start as lightly pigmented streaks that thicken and darken with time to become verrucous. They usually spare the face and scalp. Up to 10% may show histological features of epidermolytic hyperkeratosis and biopsy is therefore recommended, if possible, due to the risk of parenting a child with bullous ichthyosis. Inflammatory linear verrucous epidermal nevi (ILVEN) usually present after 6 months of age with a linear pruritic and inflamed lesion often on the lower limb.

Sebaceous and verrucous nevi are closely related. The former most commonly occur on the scalp and face and have a yellowish color due to prominent sebaceous glands. They present as a hairless, often solitary linear plaque, usually flat in infancy and childhood and becoming verrucose at puberty. Sebaceous nevi (Fig. 28.4) are rarely (< 5%) complicated in adult life by basal cell or squamous cell carcinoma.

The follicular or comedonal nevus present as linear plaques with dilated follicular pores with comedones. The face is the commonest site but any involved site can be complicated in adolescence with acne-like cyst formation and scarring.

Skeletal abnormalities occur particularly with nevi of keratinocytic type on the limbs, and neurological and ocular abnormalities with nevi of sebaceous type on the head. The major clinical neurological features are seizures, developmental delay and hemiparesis. All patients with epidermal nevi should have a careful physical examination at presentation. Patients with linear nevi on the head who present in infancy and are normal on initial examination should be followed for several years. Most centers embark on imaging studies only in patients with clinical abnormalities.

Therapy of these lesions is difficult. Topical retinoic acid may temporarily flatten very thick areas. There are a few reports of improvement of gross lesions with oral retinoids but the effect depends on continued use of the drug. Recurrence is almost invariable following diathermy and cryotherapy. Both CO_2 and argon laser have been used, in some cases with good results though these may be temporary. Excision is appropriate for small and linear lesions and for irritating or cosmetically troubling areas of more widespread nevi.

VASCULAR NEVI

These can be divided into hemangiomas, which are proliferative vascular tumors, and vascular malformations which represent fixed collections of dilated abnormal vessels.[13]

Hemangiomas

Hemangiomas (Fig. 28.5) are usually not present at birth, undergo a fast growth phase and then, over a long period, tend to spontaneous resolution. Emerging evidence shows that hemangiomas share unique tissue-specific markers (e.g. GLUT-1) with placental microvessels suggesting a possible common origin.[14] The terms capillary (strawberry), cavernous and capillary–cavernous are misleading and should be abandoned in favor of the simple term hemangioma.

Clinical features

Superficial hemangiomas are usually not present at birth but appear in the first weeks of life as an area of pallor followed by a telangiectatic patch. They then grow rapidly into a lobulated, well-demarcated, bright red tumor. Rapid growth continues over the first 6 months; the growth rate then slows and further growth after 10 months is unusual. After a stationary phase signs of involution appear with the appearance of gray areas which enlarge and coalesce. The tumor becomes softer and less bulky and then disappears in 90% of cases by 9 years of age.

Deeper hemangiomas may occur alone or beneath a superficial lesion. They also usually appear after birth and undergo a growth phase which however may be less striking than that of the more superficial lesions. The overlying skin is normal or bluish in color. As they resolve they soften and shrink and complete disappearance occurs in many cases: occasionally some redundant tissue remains in the place of large lesions. Apparent deep hemangiomas which show no sign of resolution are now recognized as vascular malformations, usually of venous type, and are not hemangiomas at all.

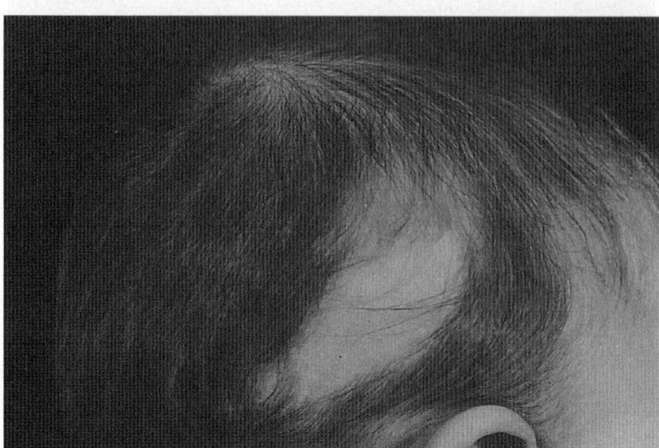

Fig. 28.4 Sebaceous nevus.

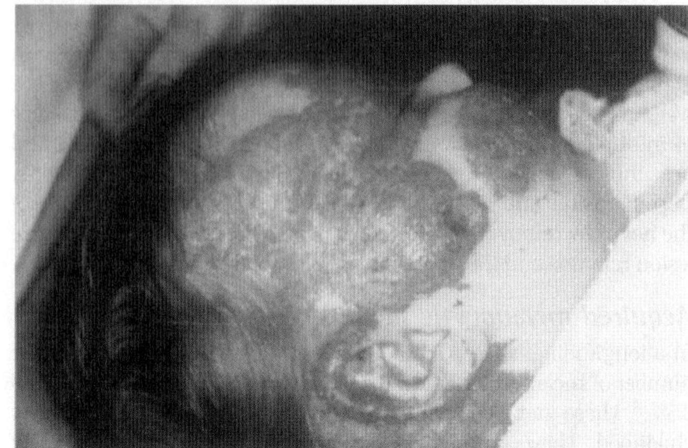

Fig. 28.5 Capillary (strawberry) hemangioma.

Complications

Ulceration may occur during the rapid growth phase of superficial hemangiomas. If secondary infection is controlled the ulcers usually heal in a few weeks but some scarring is inevitable. Ulceration of lesions on eyelids, lips or ala nasae can lead to full thickness tissue loss. Scarring following ulceration of lesions on or near the eyelids can result in a cicatricial ectropion and alopecia may be permanent after scalp ulceration.

Hemangiomas may encroach on vital structures. A hemangioma closing the eye for as little as 4 weeks in infancy can produce amblyopia. However, even without occluding the pupil an eyelid lesion, by pressing on the eye and producing a refractive error, can lead to failure of development of binocular vision and partial amblyopia. Large hemangiomas around the mouth may interfere with feeding and one blocking both nares can lead to respiratory difficulties while the child is being fed. A large deep hemangioma around the neck may displace the pharynx or trachea; the upper respiratory tract may also be directly involved with the hemangioma. The possibility of laryngeal involvement should be considered whenever there is a fast growing extensive lower face or neck hemangioma, particularly when there is accompanying intraoral involvement, and a lateral airways X-ray or MRI should be arranged. If there is stridor, an urgent laryngoscopy is mandatory. Even when traumatized, uncomplicated hemangiomas rarely bleed significantly.

Management

Simple observation and reassurance while awaiting natural resolution is the ideal approach for most hemangiomas. Serial photography and showing photographs of other resolving lesions are encouraging. Indications for active intervention are: an alarming growth rate; threatening ulceration in areas where serious complications could ensue; interference with vital structures; and severe bleeding. Oral corticosteroids are the treatment of choice. The optimal dose is not known but a meta-analysis suggests that 3 mg/kg or more for 6–8 weeks may give the best response.[15] Repeated courses should be avoided wherever possible. Intralesional steroids may shrink localized hemangiomas which fail to respond to steroids, and interferon-alpha has been effective in some life threatening cases although severe neurotoxicity, including spastic diplegia, has been reported.[16] Laser therapy has become an increasingly popular treatment modality for uncomplicated hemangiomas but without good evidence for effectiveness. Preliminary results from a randomized, controlled study of early pulsed dye laser treatment have shown no benefit of treatment at 1 year follow-up.[17] Life threatening hemangiomas have been treated with variable success with oral vincristine.[18] Cosmetic surgical procedures can improve the appearance when loose tissue remains.

PHACE syndrome

PHACE is an acronym to describe a constellation of features; posterior fossa brain malformations, facial hemangioma, arterial anomalies, cardiac anomalies (including aortic coarctation) and eye abnormalities. This syndrome should be considered in any infant presenting with an extensive facial hemangioma.[19]

Kasabach–Merritt syndrome (hemangioma–hemorrhage syndrome)

This is the rare association of thrombocytopenia with vascular tumors (Fig. 28.6). In children these are usually either large, deep hemangiomas, especially on limbs and around limb girdles, or diffuse hemangiomatosis. Thrombocytopenia is caused by entrapment of platelets within the lesions and is sometimes followed by disseminated intravascular coagulation (DIC). At first there may be bleeding into the hemangioma, which rapidly enlarges: widespread life threatening hemorrhage may follow. When bleeding is confined to the hemangiomas the approach should be conservative; in severe cases high dose systemic corticosteroids are indicated together with resuscitation, transfusion, and management of the DIC.

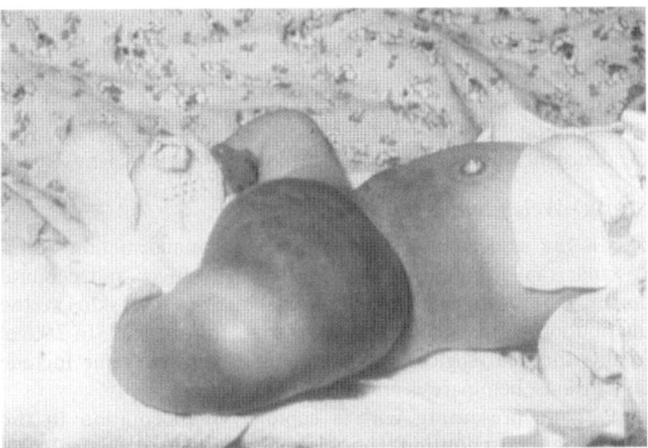

Fig. 28.6 Kasabach–Merritt syndrome.

Diffuse infantile hemangiomatosis

This is a condition with multiple small hemangiomas in a widespread distribution. A benign form has lesions limited to the skin but a potentially serious systemic form may occur with lesions in many organs, particularly liver, gastrointestinal tract, lungs and central nervous system with or, rarely, without cutaneous lesions. All patients with multiple cutaneous lesions should be carefully assessed with full blood count, chest X-ray, and examination for cardiac failure due to arteriovenous shunts and for bleeding from the gastrointestinal tract. An ultrasound or abdominal computerized tomography (CT) scan should be performed to exclude hepatic involvement and other organs may need to be further investigated. Angiography and technetium-labeled red blood cell scans can delineate further the extent of internal involvement.[20] With severe systemic involvement high dose corticosteroids are required along with management of cardiac failure and other complications, and active surgical intervention may be necessary in selected cases.

Vascular malformations

Vascular malformations are structural abnormalities and as such are present at birth, grow in proportion to the patient's growth and have no tendency at all to resolution. They can be further divided according to their vessel of origin into capillary, arterial, venous and lymphatic types and mixed entities with more than one vessel type may occur.

Capillary malformation (port-wine stain, nevus flammeus)

This is a vascular malformation composed of dilated mature capillaries. It is present at birth and shows no involution. Lesions may be unilateral or, less often, bilateral, and occur anywhere on the body, though they are most commonly found on the face. They are deep pink in infancy becoming more purple later. After puberty they may become raised and nodular. Good results can be achieved with the pulsed dye laser. Port-wine stains (PWS) must be distinguished from salmon patches at the nape of the neck (stork bite) and lesions on the eyelid or forehead (angel kiss). The facial lesions resolve in months whilst the occipital ones persist.

It is important to be aware that, even in the absence of Sturge–Weber syndrome, ocular complications can occur. If the PWS encroaches the upper eyelid glaucoma may occur. The incidence increases to over 30% if the lower eyelid is also involved.[21]

Sturge–Weber syndrome

This is the association of a facial capillary malformation and a vascular malformation of the ipsilateral meninges and cerebral cortex. The cutaneous lesion always involves the skin in the distribution of the first division of the trigeminal nerve.[22] In 20% of infants the neurological manifestations of the syndrome include convulsions, hemiparesis and mental retardation.

Patients presenting with a capillary malformation in the appropriate distribution should have early neurological and ophthalmological consultation and continued close follow-up. A CT scan may demonstrate the intracranial malformations in the first few months of life. Parallel streaks of calcification may be demonstrated radiologically after about 2 years of age.

Vascular malformations with limb hypertrophy

Klippel–Trenaunay syndrome refers to a Parkes–Weber syndrome (PWS), associated with ipsilateral overgrowth of a limb, with soft tissue and/or bony hypertrophy and venous varicosities. The condition arises predominantly due to venous malformations whereas PWS, with similar clinical features, is caused by arteriovenous fistulae. In both instances, deeper lymphatic abnormalities may also be present. In 15% of cases of Klippel–Trenaunay syndrome involvement may be bilateral. Treatment is generally unsatisfactory with few cases being amenable to surgical correction. Compression bandaging may help to some extent with the increased girth of a limb.

CONGENITAL APLASIA CUTIS

Aplasia cutis congenita (ACC) is a congenital absence of skin, usually localized but sometimes occurring as multiple lesions in a widespread distribution. The commonest form involves a localized oval, stellate or linear area at or near the midline of the scalp which presents as an ulcerated area which crusts (Fig. 28.7). Resolution occurs after some months to leave a scar that is usually atrophic but is occasionally hypertrophic. There is permanent alopecia at the site. Rarely the lesion is already scarred at birth.

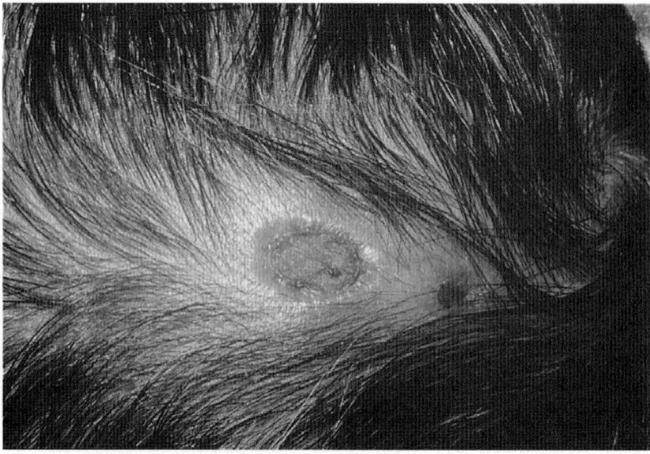

Fig. 28.7 Aplasia cutis.

The defect may involve not only skin but also subcutaneous fat and even bone. The bony defect will eventually heal but until it does there is a risk of meningitis. Deep aplasia may erode large vessels producing serious hemorrhage. A skull X-ray should be performed in all cases unless the lesion is obviously very superficial. Early management of scalp ACC is conservative with protection of the area and early treatment of secondary infection. Very deep lesions, however, may require skin and/or bone grafting. In later life scalp reduction techniques can be used to deal with the area of alopecia.

After the scalp the next commonest site is the lower limbs. When multiple lesions occur their distribution is often strikingly symmetrical and they may be covered with a shiny transparent membrane rather than being open erosions. Cases with extensive truncal and limb ACC are often associated with a fetus papyraceus at delivery, indicating the death of a twin early in the second trimester.

ACC-like lesions can occur on the lower limbs of patients with several types of epidermolysis bullosa probably resulting from intrauterine mechanical trauma. ACC may occur in a number of syndromes including trisomy 13, 4p– syndrome, 46XY gonadal dysgenesis and the Johanson–Blizzard syndrome. It may also be associated with a number of morphological abnormalities, particularly those involving the limbs.

DERMOID CYSTS

Congenital inclusion dermoid cysts typically present as asymptomatic subcutaneous swellings. Approximately 40% are present at birth with the rest appearing over the next 5 years. They arise due to entrapment of epithelium along embryonic fusion lines and occur particularly on the head and neck with predilection over the lateral eyebrow and dorsum of the nose. It is essential that adequate imaging investigations are performed prior to surgery as they may form deep tracts into underlying tissue.

HEREDITARY DISEASES

THE ICHTHYOSES

These are a group of inherited conditions with dry thickened skin of varying severity. The major ichthyoses comprise:

1. ichthyosis vulgaris (IV);
2. X-linked recessive ichthyosis (XLRI) (Fig. 28.8);
3. lamellar ichthyosis (LI);
4. congenital ichthyosiform erythroderma (CIE) (Fig. 28.9);
5. bullous ichthyosis (BI).

The histopathological and clinical features of the major ichthyoses are listed in Table 28.1. They are life-long disorders with little tendency to spontaneous improvement. The pathogenesis is unclear in most cases but several facts are known. IV and XLRI show a delayed shedding of stratum corneum cells. In XLRI there is a virtual absence of the enzyme steroid sulfatase from most tissues. In CIE there is an increased epidermal turnover and an abnormal stratum corneum lipid profile. In BI there is epidermal hyperproliferation and abnormal keratinization.

Management

Simple emollients such as aqueous cream may be adequate in IV. Keratolytics containing urea, propylene glycol or alpha-hydroxy acids may be more effective and useful in IV and XLRI but they may sting on fissured skin. The more severe ichthyoses often show little improvement with these topical agents. Oral retinoids may be very

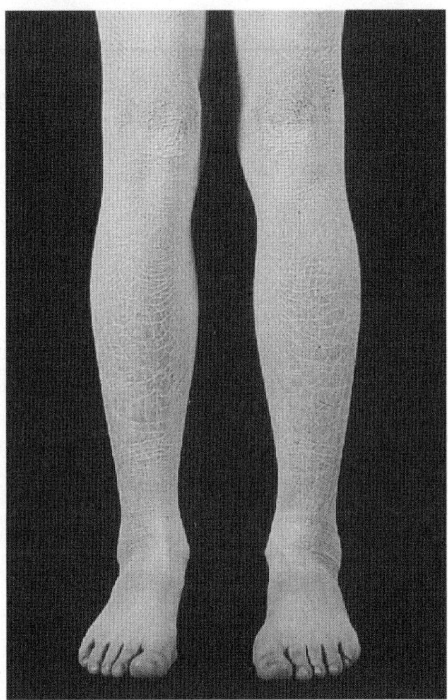

Fig. 28.8 X-linked ichthyosis.

helpful in CIE but their effectiveness must always be weighed against their potential side-effects, especially skeletal abnormalities and teratogenicity. In BI their usefulness is limited by their tendency to increase skin fragility. Detection and treatment of secondary bacterial infection is important in BI and topical disinfectants may reduce bacterial colonization and malodor.

Collodion baby

This is a descriptive term for the child who is encased at birth in a shiny tight membrane resembling collodion or plastic skin, producing ectropion and eclabium and fissuring (Fig. 28.10). The skin peels off in days or weeks. This may be a presentation of various conditions, particularly CIE (which overlaps with lamellar icthyosis), Netherton's syndrome and chondrodysplasia punctata. Rarely the membrane peels off to leave normal skin: this condition is called lamellar exfoliation of the newborn. Collodion babies show temperature instability and excessive fluid loss. Corneal exposure may result if the eyes are not covered and the eclabium may

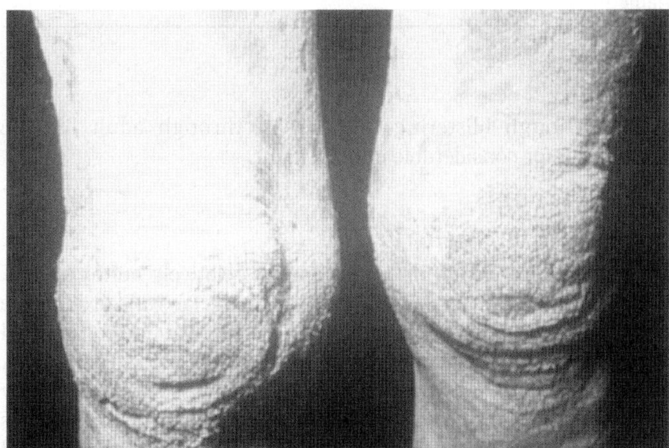

Fig. 28.9 Lamellar ichthyosis (congenital ichthyosiform erythroderma).

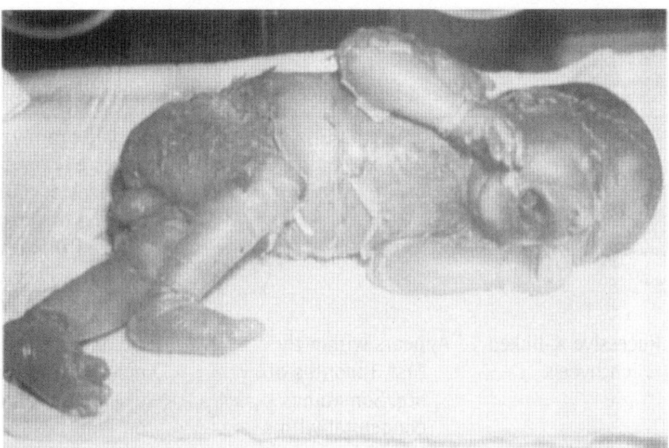

Fig. 28.10 Collodion baby.

necessitate squeeze bottle, tube or dropper feeding. As the fissures appear, secondary infection becomes a risk. The child should be nursed in a humidicrib with aseptic handling.

Harlequin ichthyosis

This may represent a phenotype of several disorders, all recessively inherited. Various abnormalities of keratinization and epidermal lipid metabolism have been demonstrated. At birth the child is covered in large dark plates of scale with severe ectropion and eclabium, deformed ears and claw hands and feet. Most die as neonates but the few who have survived have had a severe ichthyosiform erythroderma. (Note – this is different from the harlequin color change.)

Ichthyosis as part of other syndromes

Some of the syndromes of which ichthyosis is a part are listed in Table 28.2.

EPIDERMOLYSIS BULLOSA (EB)

This is a rare group of inherited diseases characterized by trauma-induced blistering of skin and mucosae. The prevalence is between 1/50 000 and 1/2 000 000 for the more common and rarer forms, respectively. Over 20 types are now identified, separated on the basis of inheritance, clinical features, immunohistochemistry, electron microscopic (EM) and molecular pathology. The split may be within the epidermis, at the dermoepidermal junction in the lamina lucida (junctional; Figs 28.11 and 28.12) or in the upper dermis (sublamina densa; Fig. 28.13). A classification is given in Table 28.3. The structure of the cutaneous basement membrane zone and the gene defects in epidermolysis bullosa are shown in Figure 28.14.

A firm diagnosis should always be established as soon as possible by EM and immunohistochemical analysis, if possible, of a new blister. This enables a prognosis to be given and a management plan to be established for present and future.

Epidermolysis bullosa simplex (EBS)

Localized EBS (Weber–Cockayne)

The blisters are often not noticed until the child starts to walk. It may be so mild that it does not present until adult life. However, morbidity can be such that daily activities are affected. Blisters develop on hands and feet and, as with all forms of EBS, they are often worse with increased temperatures in the summer months. Very occasionally other body sites are affected.

Table 28.1 Classification and features of the major ichthyoses

	Onset (and inheritance)	Clinical features	Complications and associations	Chrosomal/gene loci
Ichthyosis vulgaris	After birth but within the first year of life (AD)	Fine pale branny scales especially on extensor surfaces of limbs. Wide sparing of flexures of limbs. Trunk less severely involved. Face usually spared. Hyperlinear palms	Rarely corneal dystrophy, keratosis pilaris, atopy	1q21
Recessive X-linked ichthyosis	Appears within the first 3 months of life. Sometimes congenital with a thin shiny covering membrane (XLR)	Large dark adherent scales mainly on extensor surfaces of limbs. Scaling encroaches on limb flexures and axillae with narrow sparing. Trunk is diffusely involved. Sides of face often involved. Usually severe involvement of neck and thick scalp scaling. Palms and soles are uninvolved	Frequent corneal dystrophy (also in carriers). Cryptorchidism. Steroid sulfatase deficiency in most tissues including the amnion (which is derived from fetus). This placental steroid sulfatase deficiency may result in a failure of spontaneous onset of labor	Steroid sulfatase gene deletion (Xp22.3)
Lamellar ichthyosis	Usually at birth as 'collodion baby' (AR/AD)	Large dark plate-like scales. Mild to moderate erythroderma. The whole body surface is involved, including palms and soles	Ectropion. Blockage of external auditory meati with scale resulting in hearing loss. Block of nares with scale. Pyrexia from sweat duct obstruction. Failure to thrive. Alopecia	TGM1 gene mutations (14q11.2); also 2q33–35, 19p12–q12
Congenital ichthyosiform erythroderma	Usually at birth as 'collodion baby' (AR)	Fine white scale in most areas, sometimes larger and darker on lower legs. Mild to very severe generalized erythroderma. Whole body surface is involved including palms and soles	Similar to those of lamellar ichthyosis but of lesser extent	TGM1 gene mutations (14q11.2); also 3p21
Bullous ichthyosis (epidermolytic hyperkeratosis)	At birth with erythroderma and widespread blistering. After a few days the redness subsides and over early months the blistering tendency reduces (AD)	Thick dark warty scales from time to time to leave denuded areas with a red base. Blistering is rare after 1 year. The condition may be localized to extensor surfaces but is usually widespread although the face is usually spared. Palm and sole involvement is variable	Bacterial superinfection is a recurrent problem. Heavy bacterial colonization is inevitable. Maceration and offensive odor are major problems	K2e gene mutations (12q11–13)

AD, autosomal dominant; AR, autosomal recessive; XLR, X-linked resessive.

Generalized EBS (Koebner)

The onset of blisters is at birth or early infancy. They may be widespread but affect particularly areas of trauma such as hands, feet, knees and elbows. The oral mucosa is occasionally involved. Nails are not affected and there is no scarring. As with localized EB, secondary infection is the main complication. Life expectancy is normal.

Herpetiform EBS (Dowling–Meara)

Widespread blistering can be present at birth and severe cases may be mistaken for junctional EB. Transient milia develop at sites of grouped blisters. The hands and feet are especially affected, often leading to a palmoplantar keratoderma. Nail thickening is common. Oral, laryngeal and esophageal mucosal involvement is sometimes seen. Although blistering may persist through adult life the tendency is for considerable improvement.

Junctional EB

Generalized severe (Herlitz) EB

Blistering is present at birth and may be relatively minor at first. Slow wound healing is seen particularly on the face and around the nails. Typically affected babies have a hoarse cry due to mucosal involvement which is extensive and severe involving nasal, oral, esophageal as well as anogenital and urinary epithelium. Many infants die due to overwhelming sepsis. Survival to adolescence is rare but older children suffer from chronic sepsis, anemia and growth retardation.

Table 28.2 Syndromes associated with ichthyosis

Syndrome	Inheritance	Type of ichthyosis	Other major features	Molecular defects
Chondrodysplasia punctata	XLR	Onset may be as 'collodion baby'. Initially occurs as a diffuse redness and scaling. Later occurs in a whorled patchy distribution	Epiphyseal dysplasia, cataracts, follicular atrophoderma	XLR: Emopamil binding protein gene mutations
	XLD			XLD: Arylsulfatase E gene mutations
Sjögren–Larsson syndrome	AR	Generalized ichthyosis at birth. Later large dark scales most prominent in flexures	Mental retardation, spasticity	Aldehyde dehydrogenase family mutations
Chanarin–Dorfman syndrome (neutral lipid storage disease with ichthyosis)	AR	Ichthyosis simulating mild to moderate congenital ichthyosiform erythroderma	Lipid vacuoles in almost all cells. Normal serum lipids. Cataracts, deafness, developmental delay	Unknown
Refsum's syndrome	AR	Delayed onset of ichthyosis of mild form, simulating ichthyosis vulgaris	Failure to degrade phytanic acid. Retinitis pigmentosa, peripheral neuropathy, cerebellar ataxia	Phytanoyl-CoA hydroxylase gene mutations
Netherton's syndrome	AR	Erythroderma at birth. Late development of circinate migratory scaly lesions (ichthyosis linearis circumflexa) in widespread distribution. Some cases simulate congenital ichthyosiform erythroderma	Alopecia due to hair shaft abnormalities, especially trichorrhexis invaginata, atopic diathesis, developmental delay, generalized aminoaciduria	Serine proteinase inhibitor (SPINK 5) gene mutations

AR, autosomal recessive; XLD, X-linked dominant; XLR, X-linked recessive.

Generalized atrophic benign EB (GABEB)

Although in the initial stages the blistering has a similar pattern to Herlitz EB the child survives with a decreasing tendency to blister. Mucous membranes are involved but less so than the Herlitz form. The major feature of GABEB is alopecia which follows the blistering. Lesions may also heal with hyperpigmentation. The life span of the affected individual is normal.

Dystrophic EB

Dystrophic EB is characterized by skin fragility, blisters, scarring with milia formation and nail changes. The autosomal recessive form is more severe than the dominant disease with greater skin fragility and therefore more widespread blistering. Repeated blistering and scarring can lead to syndactyly of fingers, toes and club-like deformities of hands and feet with several digits encased together in a scar. Severe involvement of oral mucosa may lead to stricture formation in autosomal recessive patients. Laryngeal and tracheal involvement may threaten the airway. Hypoproteinemia is caused by constant loss of protein in blister fluid, malabsorption and malnutrition. In all cases the nails are thickened and often lost. Aggressive squamous cell carcinomas may arise in the scar tissues and metastatic disease is a major cause of death in adult patients with severe disease.

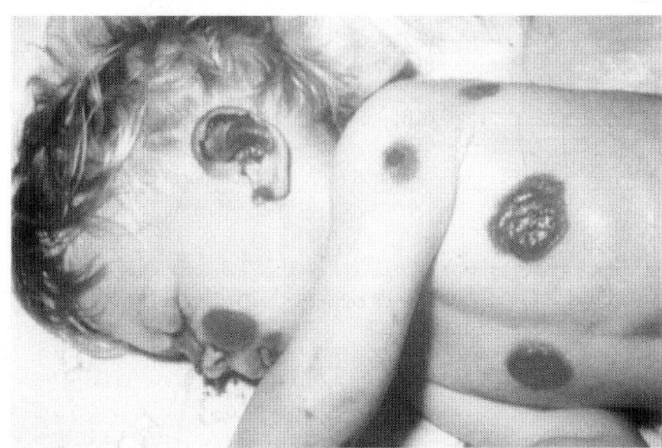

Fig. 28.11 Junctional epidermolysis bullosa.

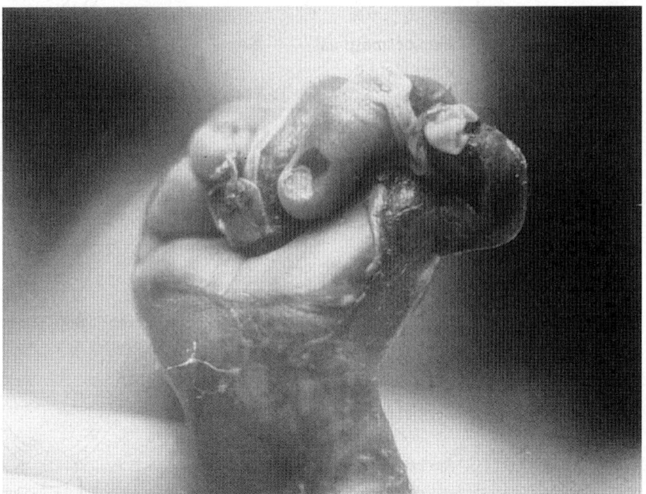

Fig. 28.12 Junctional epidermolysis bullosa.

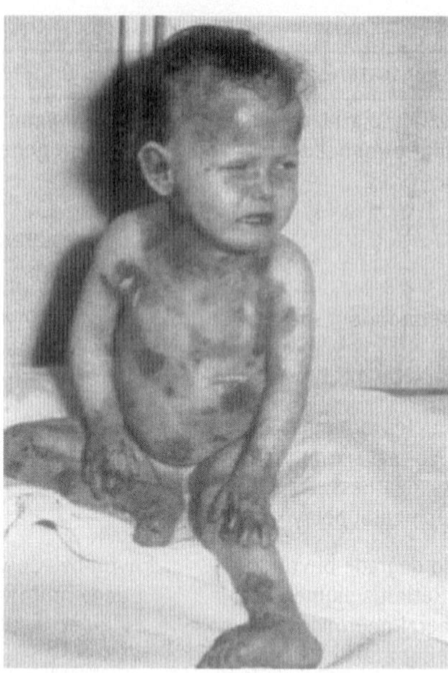

Fig. 28.13 Dystrophic epidermolysis bullosa.

Table 28.3 Classification of major types of hereditary epidermolysis bullosa

	Inheritance
INTRAEPIDERMAL BLISTER	
Epidermolysis bullosa simplex (EBS)	
Localized (hands and feet) EBS (Weber–Cockayne)	AD
Generalized EBS (Koebner)	AD
Herpetiform EBS (Dowling–Meara)	AD
EBS with muscular dystrophy	AR
LAMINA LUCIDA BLISTER	
Junctional epidermolysis bullosa (JEB)	
Generalized severe (Herlitz)	AR
Generalized atrophic benign (GABEB)	AR
JEB with pyloric atresia	AR
SUBLAMINA DENSA	
Dystrophic epidermolysis bullosa (DEB)	
Dominant DEB	AD
Recessive DEB (Hallopeau)	AR

AD, autosomal dominant; AR, autosomal recessive

Management

In mild epidermolysis bullosa simplex and dominant dystrophic cases advice is required regarding avoidance of trauma, a reduction of friction, appropriate clothing and footwear. New blisters should be pricked to drain them but not deroofed and various dressings of non-stick material are appropriate. Secondary bacterial infection is treated with topical or oral antibiotics.

In the severe forms with extensive neonatal blistering extreme care is necessary to avoid further skin damage. The infant should initially be nursed naked in a humidicrib lying on non-adherent material with barrier nursing to prevent infection. Blisters should be drained and antibacterial creams such as silver sulfadiazine applied to large erosions. Vaseline gauze or non-adherent plastic dressings should be used as required, secured with tubular gauze or by other means but never taped to the skin with adhesive. A nasogastric tube should never be passed.

Severe complications may require a multidisciplinary approach. In the UK advice, both medical and nursing, should be sought whenever appropriate, from regional centers with a particular expertise in EB. Where possible, one physician should coordinate the entire management program to provide stability and continuity. The family should be directed towards support organizations, which can offer practical advice, emotional support and companionship. Finally, genetic counseling of the parents and later the patient should be arranged at an appropriate time.

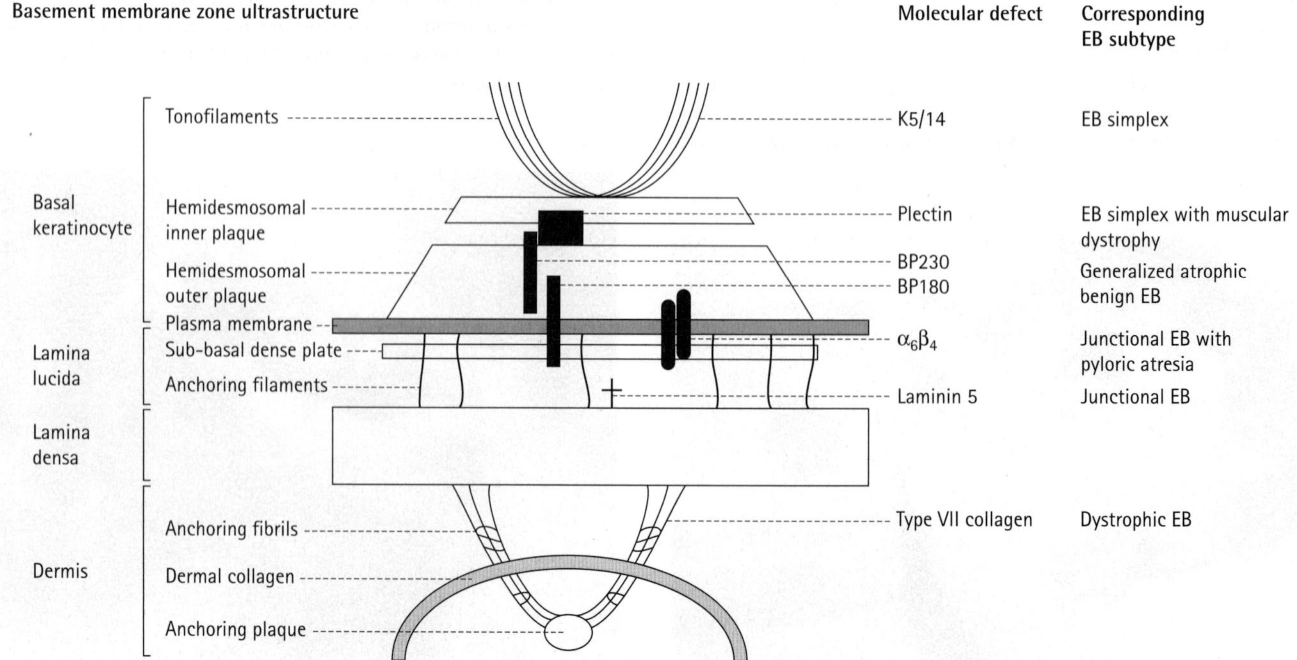

Fig. 28.14 Structure of cutaneous basement membrane zone and gene defects in epidermolysis bullosa.

ECTODERMAL DYSPLASIAS

The ectodermal dysplasias (Fig. 28.15) are a heterogeneous group of inherited conditions with a primary defect in two or more of the following: teeth, nails, hair, sweat glands or abnormalities in tissues of ectodermal origin, including eyes, ears, oral and nasal mucosa, melanocytes and central nervous system. A detailed classification of these syndromes has been produced.[23]

The major features of some of the more important ectodermal dysplasias are documented in Table 28.4.

Management

As these are disorders manifesting very diverse features, a multidisciplinary approach is essential.

If the scalp hair is very sparse the cosmetic benefit of a good wig may be invaluable. Primary and secondary dentitions can be assessed with dental X-rays in infancy in conjunction with a pediatric dentist experienced in these conditions. Early use of prostheses may prevent development of some of the structural facial abnormalities. Newer techniques include osseous implants into which prosthetic teeth can be fitted.

If hypohidrosis is extreme hyperthermia may result and may be severe and life threatening. Advice regarding activities, clothing and methods of cooling may be required.

Atopic eczema often accompanies hypohidrotic ectodermal dysplasia and will require the usual treatment. Many patients have dry skin and require emollients, and keratolytics may improve palmoplantar keratoderma.

All patients with eye abnormalities should be managed in conjunction with an ophthalmologist. Artificial tears are essential for dry eyes to prevent corneal damage. Reconstructive procedures will be required for atresia of nasolacrimal ducts and canaliculi. Severe respiratory infections complicate some of these syndromes and need antibiotics, physiotherapy and regular pediatric follow-up.

TUBEROUS SCLEROSIS

The tuberous sclerosis complex (TSC) is an autosomal dominant, neurocutaneous disorder characterized by the formation of hamartomata in many organs. Mutations in the hamartin gene (9q34) account for approximately half of the cases (TSC1) and the other half arise due to mutations in the tuberin gene (16p13) (TSC2).[24] Both genes act as tumor suppressor genes and around 60% arise due to spontaneous mutations. A small number of families are unlinked to either gene. Epilepsy occurs in 80% and mental retardation in 70%. Up to 20% of patients with infantile spasms will have TSC and should therefore have their skin examined. Other systemic abnormalities include retinal phacomata and a variety of hamartomata in renal tract, heart and other organs.

Dermatological features

The most pathognomonic features are angiofibromas (adenoma sebaceum), periungual fibromas, shagreen patches and ash leaf macules (Figs 28.16 and 28.17). The angiofibromas appear as 1–4 mm bright red papules in a centrofacial distribution. Sometimes they coalesce to form cauliflower-like masses. Their onset is usually between the ages of 3 and 10 years and they may become more

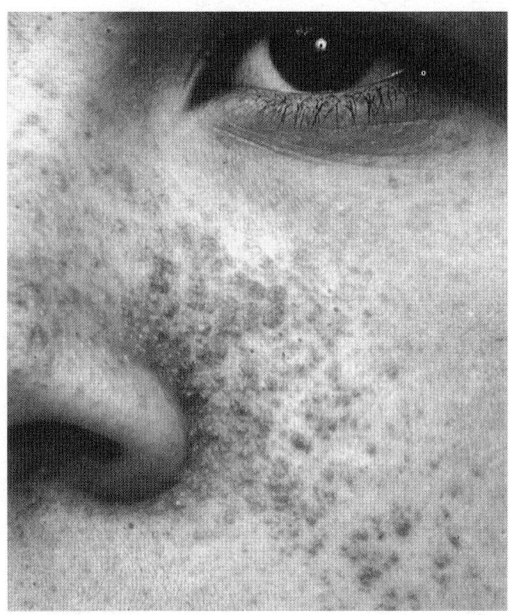

Fig. 28.16 Adenoma sebaceum: tuberous sclerosis.

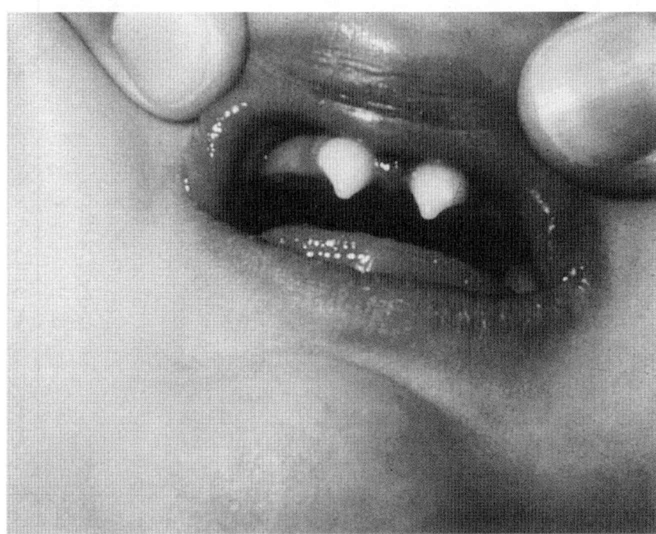

Fig. 28.15 Ectodermal dysplasia.

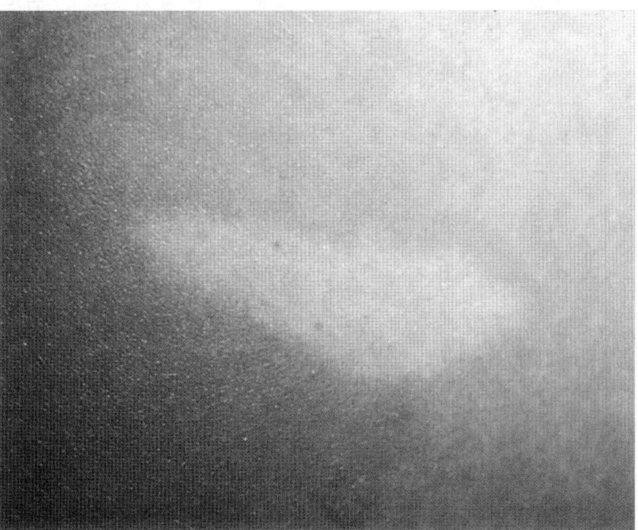

Fig. 28.17 Ash leaf patch: tuberous sclerosis.

Table 28.4 The ectodermal dysplasias

	1. Hypohidrotic ectodermal dysplasia (Christ–Siemens–Touraine syndrome)	2. Hidrotic ectodermal dysplasia (Clouson's syndrome)	3. Rapp–Hodgkin's syndrome	4. EEC syndrome (ectrodactyly ectodermal dysplasia and clefting)	5. AEC syndrome (ankyloblepharon ectodermal dysplasia and clefting) (Hay–Wells' syndrome)
Inheritance	X-linked recessive*	Autosomal dominant	Autosomal dominant	Autosomal dominant	Autosomal dominant
Hair	Hypotrichosis of scalp, body hair, eyebrows and lashes. Beard normal. Hair fine and fair	Hypotrichosis. Hair fine and dry	Sparse, coarse and stiff with hair shaft abnormalities	Sparse wiry hair	Severe hypotrichosis
Teeth	Hypodontia. Conical teeth	May be normal. Hypodontia, caries, widespaced teeth	Hypodontia, abnormally shaped teeth. Early caries	Hypodontia, abnormally shaped teeth	Variable hypodontia, abnormal shape, delayed eruption
Nails	Often normal. Sometimes fragile and occasionally dystrophic or absent	Thick, striated, discolored. Paronychia and nail loss. Rarely thin and brittle	Small and dysplastic	Thin, pitted and striated	Severe dystrophy. Short due to absence of distal nail plate
Sweating	Hypohidrosis often with hyperthermia	Normal	Hypohidrosis	Occasional hypohidrosis	Variable hypohidrosis
Skin	Smooth and dry, loss of dermatoglyphics, wrinkled and hyperpigmented around eyes, atopic dermatitis	Thick over finger joints, knees and elbows. Palmoplantar keratoderma	Dry and coarse. Thick over elbows and knees. Reduced dermatoglyphics	Dry and thin. Palmoplantar keratoderma	Large weeping areas at birth, later dry and scaly. May be recurrent scalp crusting. Palmoplantar keratoderma
Eyes	Hypoplasia of nasolacrimal duct, decreased lacrimal gland secretion, dry eyes, photophobia and corneal opacities	Usually normal. Occasionally premature cataracts	Atresia of lacrimal puncta producing epiphora, corneal opacities	Nasolacrimal duct stenosis, dacryocystitis, corneal scarring	Ankyloblepharon filiforme adnatum, nasolacrimal duct atresia
Facies	Variable. Thick lips, saddle nose, frontal bossing, maxillary hypoplasia. Occasionally abnormal ears	Normal	Cleft lip, hypoplastic maxilla. Microstomia. Prominent malformed ears	Cleft lip	Cleft lip often, microstomia, broad nasal bridge, sunken maxilla, abnormal pinnae
Mucosae	Poor development of mucous glands in gastrointestinal and respiratory tracts. Atrophic rhinitis, thick nasal secretion, recurrent chest infections, dysphagia. Dry mouth	Normal	Chronic rhinitis	Hoarseness due to abnormality of laryngeal mucosa	Filamentous bands in vagina, anal fissure
Miscellaneous	Absent or supernumerary nipples. Absent breast tissue in carriers. Asthma	Tufting of terminal phalanges with finger clubbing. Thickening of skull bones	Short stature. Cleft palate. Syndactyly	Cleft palate. Ectrodactyly (split hands and feet). Syndactyly	Cleft palate. Syndactyly

* Autosomal recessive variant is difficult to distinguish phenotypically

extensive at puberty. Numbers vary from a few to several hundred. Periungual fibromas appear around puberty as firm smooth flesh-colored papules in a periungual or subungual location. The shagreen patch is a connective tissue nevus comprising an accumulation of collagen as an irregularly thickened yellow–white plaque, usually in the lumbosacral area. It develops between the ages of 2 and 5 years. Ash leaf macules are depigmented macules, usually 1–3 cm in diameter but occasionally much larger. They are usually oval in shape, with a minority truly ash leaf shaped. They may be present at birth or appear during the first year. Large numbers may be present and they are best visualized under Wood's (ultraviolet) light.

Other dermatological features include fibromatous plaques on brow or scalp, intraoral fibromas, multiple fibroepithelial polyps around the neck and in the axillae and a variety of other depigmented lesions including numerous guttate macules and large dermatomal lesions. Poliosis and canities may also occur.

Patients who present with these characteristic skin signs should be referred for neurological assessment, skull X-ray and computerized axial tomography to demonstrate any intracranial lesions. Laser therapy may improve the cosmetic appearance of the angiofibromas.

INCONTINENTIA PIGMENTI

Incontinentia pigmenti (IP type 2) is a multisystem disorder inherited as an X-linked dominant trait and is usually prenatally lethal in males (Figs 28.18 and 28.19). It arises due to mutations (usually genomic rearrangement) in the NEMO gene (Xq28) and lesions probably occur through apoptosis of cells carrying the mutant gene.[25] There is increasing evidence that the 'sporadic type of IP' (IP type 1) represents a distinct disorder, hypomelanosis of Ito (q.v.), linked to Xp11. Neurological abnormalities occur in about 30% of cases and include epilepsy, mental retardation and spastic diplegia and tetraplegia. Ocular abnormalities are seen in 30% and include strabismus, cataracts, retinal vascular proliferation and retinal detachment. Over 80% of patients have dental abnormalities with partial anodontia and peg-shaped or conical teeth. A variety of skeletal abnormalities including limb reduction defects occur, and rarely cardiac abnormalities are seen.

Cutaneous lesions

The four cutaneous stages of this disease may follow each other in an orderly progression; however, there may be overlap, particularly in the earlier stages. Stage one comprises linear groups of vesicles which appear mainly on the limbs at birth or in the first days of life accompanied by a peripheral blood eosinophilia. They clear spontaneously over several weeks. Stage two is the verrucose stage with linear warty lesions appearing between 1 and 4 months of age: they occur particularly on the limbs, especially on dorsa of hands and feet, and resolve spontaneously after weeks or months. Stage three comprises streaks and whorls and splattered patterns of macular hyperpigmentation which appear on both limbs and trunk at 12–24 months of age. Lesions persist to early adult life. Stage four is typically seen in affected female adults as linear, hypopigmented, atrophic streaks on the lower legs. These lesions are permanent.

Other dermatological features of incontinentia pigmenti are cicatricial alopecia over the vertex of the scalp and nail dystrophy in 40%.

ACRODERMATITIS ENTEROPATHICA AND NUTRITIONAL ZINC DEFICIENCY

Acrodermatitis enteropathica is an autosomal recessive condition in which there is a defective absorption of zinc, possibly due to the absence of a specific carrier protein. An identical condition occurs in infants with nutritional zinc deficiency. This may occur as a result of prematurity with low zinc stores, particularly in bottle-fed babies (as there is a lower bioavailability of zinc in bovine milk as compared to breast milk), or as a result of low breast milk zinc. Zinc deficiency also occurs in acquired immunodeficiency disease, cystic fibrosis and other causes of malabsorption and in infants on parenteral nutrition solutions not containing adequate zinc.

Clinical features

The onset in the primary form occurs usually when the child is weaned or in the first few weeks of life in a bottle-fed infant. In the children with nutritional zinc deficiency the onset is usually at the time of the first growth spurt. Erythematous and crusted, sometimes vesicular and pustular lesions appear in an acral distribution particularly around nose, mouth and eyes (Fig. 28.20) and sometimes on tips of digits and the paronychial areas. An anogenital rash (Fig. 28.21) is also common and psoriasiform lesions may occur on knees and elbows and occasionally elsewhere. Secondary bacterial and candidal infection is common. In the primary form mucosal involvement with glossitis, cheilitis and conjunctivitis may occur, a nail dystrophy is usual, and alopecia and diarrhea may occur.

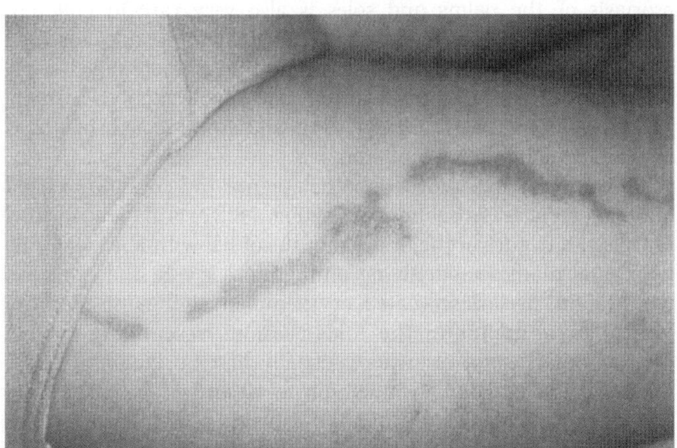

Fig. 28.18 Incontinentia pigmenti: pigmented stage.

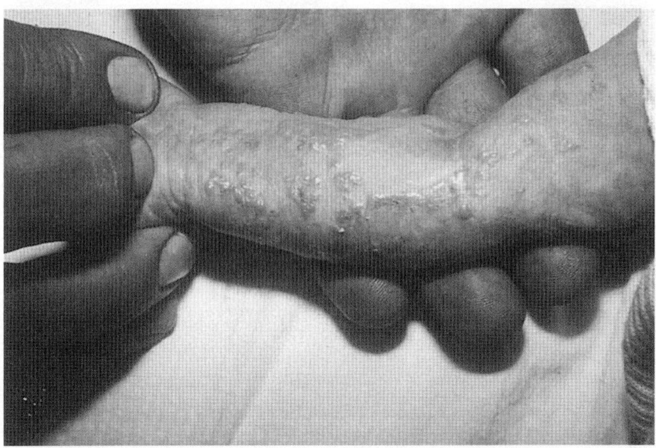

Fig. 28.19 Incontinentia pigmenti: vesicular stage.

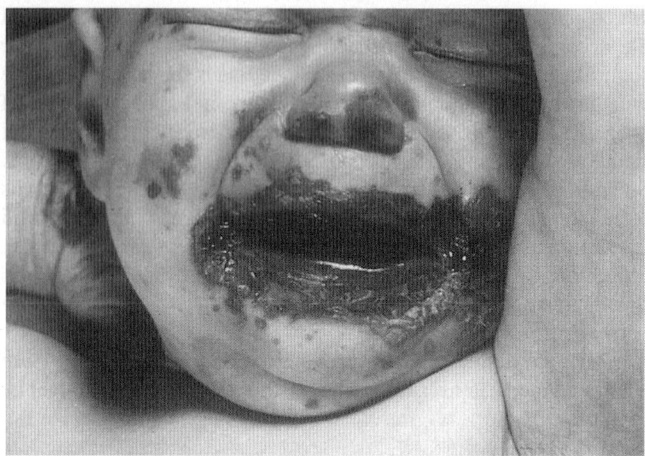

Fig. 28.20 Acrodermatitis enteropathica: mouth.

The diagnosis is confirmed by finding a low serum zinc (< 50 μg/dl). The condition responds rapidly to the administration of high doses of oral zinc as either zinc gluconate or zinc sulfate. This is required life-long in the primary form but only for a few weeks in the secondary variety.

NEUROFIBROMATOSIS

Neurofibromatosis is a very variable multisystem disorder which is described in detail in Chapter 20. Only the dermatological features will be considered here.

Pigmented lesions

The café-au-lait macule is the most common of these: most patients with neurofibromatosis have at least six macules of at least 1.5 cm in maximum diameter. They are usually oval or irregular in shape and most are 2–5 cm long. Some lesions may be present at birth and they increase in size and number during childhood. Eventually hundreds of macules may be present.

In 20% of cases small freckle-like pigmented macules occur in the axillae. These occur only in the presence of café-au-lait macules and the combination is of great diagnostic significance. Similar small pigmented macules may occur in a widespread distribution, especially in patients with large numbers of café-au-lait spots. Larger pigmented patches 10 cm or more in diameter may overlie plexiform neuromas.

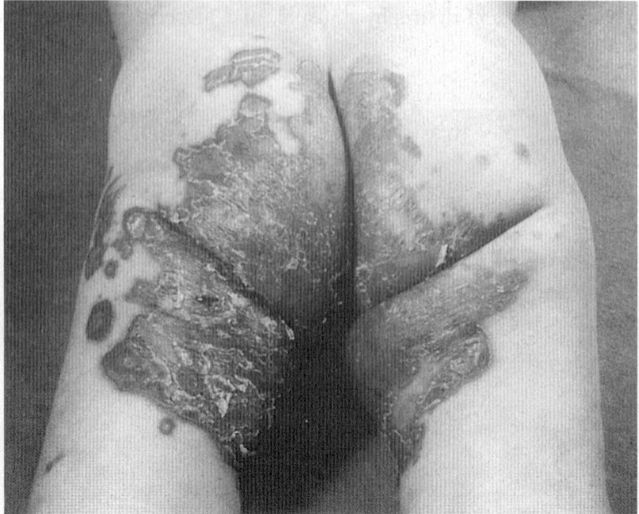

Fig. 28.21 Acrodermatitis enteropathica: buttocks.

Neurofibromas (mollusca fibrosa)

These are soft pink or skin-colored tumors, often sessile or pedunculated and characteristically indentable. They usually develop after puberty. Their distribution is widespread and up to thousands of tumors half to several centimeters in diameter may occur. Small firmer discrete nodules occur along the course of peripheral nerves. The plexiform neuroma is a larger diffuse elongated neurofibroma along the course of a peripheral nerve. These may be present at birth or develop later. There may be an overgrowth of skin and subcutaneous tissue associated with these lesions producing gross disfigurement as a giant pendulous tumor with a wrinkled surface.

PSORIASIS

A combination of epidemiological, family and human leukocyte antigen (HLA) studies indicate that psoriasis is a genetic condition. Its mode of inheritance is probably autosomal dominant with variable penetrance. Psoriasis appears by the age of 15 years in 30% of patients. Children may present with typical adult large erythematous plaques, with a thick silvery white scale, predominantly on the knees, elbows, buttocks and scalp but usually the plaques are smaller and with a finer scale. A common presentation is acute guttate psoriasis with the eruption of small papules in a widespread distribution, often following an intercurrent illness, particularly a streptococcal throat infection. A micropapular form of psoriasis occurs particularly in dark-skinned children with 1–2 mm papules most marked on the extensor aspects of the limbs. These lesions are usually skin colored until scratching demonstrates the white scale.

The face and intertriginous sites, such as retroauricular areas, axillae, groin, genital and perianal area, are commonly affected in children. Children presenting with vulvitis, balanitis and perianal itching may be found to have psoriasis. In these areas the typical scale is absent and the condition presents as a glazed erythema often with fissuring. Generalized pustular psoriasis is rare in children and has an explosive onset with sheets of pustules on a background of bright erythema accompanied by severe systemic toxicity. It may be the first presentation of psoriasis and settle spontaneously in a few weeks leaving normal skin. It often recurs and usually more typical psoriasis eventually supervenes. Pustular psoriasis of the palms and soles is also very rare in children. Acropustulosis, a glazed erythema studded with pustules followed by thick scaling and fissuring, involving one or more digits, is an occasional childhood presentation. Nail involvement is usually absent or minimal with minor pitting, and psoriatic arthropathy is extremely uncommon in children.

Controversy exists over whether or not the condition called 'napkin psoriasis' or 'sebopsoriasis' (Fig. 28.22) is in fact a form of psoriasis. It occurs in the first 3 months of life with a non-specific napkin dermatitis suddenly becoming more severe and extensive with bright, well-demarcated erythema involving most of the napkin area including the folds. Lesions resembling typical psoriasis then erupt elsewhere, usually first on face and scalp, then neck fold and axillae and finally trunk and limbs. In the scalp the lesions may appear similar to seborrhea. Evidence for this representing a form of psoriasis rather than dermatitis comes

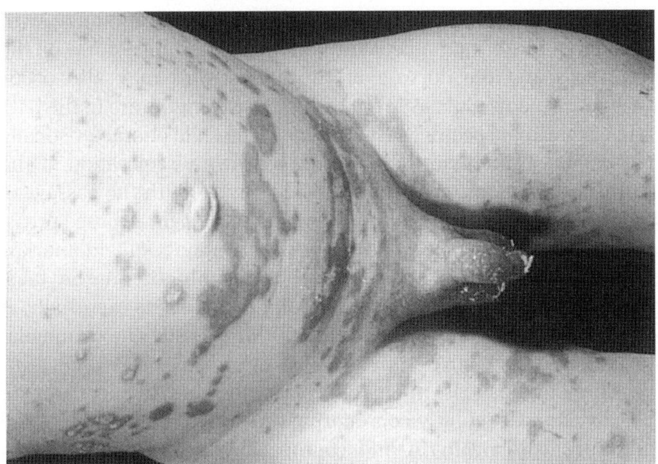

Fig. 28.22 Napkin psoriasis.

from the work of Andersen & Thomsen[26] who found a family history of psoriasis in 26% of patients compared with 4.9% of controls, and of Neville & Finn[27] who, on review of these patients at 5–13 years, found psoriasis in 17% with the expected rate being 0.4%.

In any child with a difficult napkin dermatitis responding poorly to conventional measures psoriasis should be considered, particularly if the lesions have well-defined margins and remain fairly fixed in position.

Management

Many systemic therapies (e.g. retinoids, methotrexate and ciclosporin) used in adults are inappropriate in children. As a general rule, psoriasis in children is better treated with tars than topical corticosteroids. They are often more effective, are safer for long term use, and rebound on their cessation is less of a problem. Tars may be irritant in infants, as they may be at any age when applied to the face or intertriginous areas. Useful preparations for guttate or small plaque psoriasis are coal tar and salicylic acid mixtures (equal parts 2–4%) in an aqueous cream base applied twice a day. A prospective, multicenter, double-blind study in children showed that the topical vitamin D analogue calcipotriol is effective and safe when using applied to less than 30% of the body surface area.[28] Whilst oral antibiotics and tonsillectomy have been advocated for patients with recurrent guttate psoriasis following recent streptococcal infection, there are no data to show they are beneficial.[29] For large plaque psoriasis in older children the adult regimes of topical dithranol with or without ultraviolet B (UVB) (preferably narrow band) are usually tolerated.

Patients with generalized pustular psoriasis require urgent hospitalization and close monitoring of fluid and electrolyte balance and evidence of infection. Wet compresses give symptomatic relief while awaiting spontaneous recovery. Tars are contraindicated and topical steroids must be used very cautiously due to the risk of considerable absorption. Palmoplantar pustulosis and acropustulosis usually respond slowly to tar preparations. Napkin psoriasis often clears quickly with hydrocortisone and anticandidal agents for the flexural areas and a weak corticosteroid elsewhere.

It is essential for the parents, and the child if old enough, to appreciate that psoriasis is a capricious recurrent disease which will require varying treatments depending on the site, nature and severity of the condition at different stages. Long term follow-up, preferably with the same practitioner, is important.

HEREDITARY PHOTOSENSITIVE DISORDERS

Photosensitivity is the cardinal feature of most of the porphyrias and occurs in other metabolic diseases including phenylketonuria and Hartnup disease. Severe photosensitivity also occurs in oculocutaneous albinism.

Xeroderma pigmentosum (XP)

This is a group of autosomal recessive conditions with a defect in the capacity to repair ultraviolet radiation (UVR)-damaged DNA (Fig. 28.23). In 80% of cases there is a defect in the initiation of DNA repair and nine genetically separate forms have been demonstrated. In the remaining 20% (XP variants) there is a defect in the S phase of DNA replication following UVR exposure.

Small and large pigmented macules are the earliest lesions and appear on exposed areas between the age of 6 and 24 months. Later telangiectases and small angiomas appear, and finally white atrophic lesions. Keratoses and keratoacanthomas are common, and malignant skin tumors can develop from as early as 3 or 4 years.

Photophobia and conjunctivitis are common. Ectropion and destruction of the eyelids by carcinoma can lead to exposure keratitis and pigmented macules and malignancies can occur on the conjunctivae. Other abnormalities in XP patients include short stature, hypogonadism, microcephaly, mental retardation, deafness, choreoathetosis and ataxia. The diagnosis can be confirmed by studying the DNA repair process following UVR in cultured fibroblasts obtained from a skin biopsy.

Patients must be protected from exposure to UVR up to 320 nm (which includes emissions from some fluorescent lights) by all possible means including opaque sunscreens, covering clothing, hats and sunglasses. Observation for and early treatment of malignancies is mandatory.

Bloom's syndrome

This is an autosomal recessive disorder most common in the Ashkenazi Jewish race, with a photosensitive rash, growth retardation and an increased risk of malignancy.

Reticulate telangiectatic erythema develops between 1 and 2 years at sun-exposed sites. Over 50% of patients demonstrate multiple widespread café-au-lait spots. There is a severe proportionate dwarfism. Deficiency of one or more classes of immunoglobulins (Ig) often occurs and these children suffer recurrent respiratory and

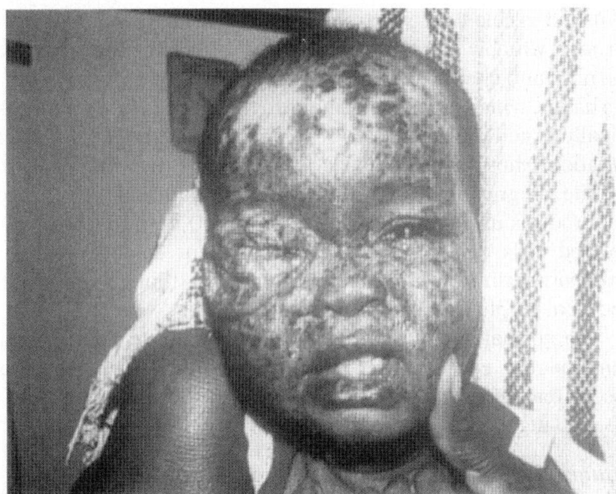

Fig. 28.23 Xeroderma pigmentosum.

gastrointestinal bacterial infections. Bloom's syndrome is one of the hereditary chromosomal breakage disorders and patients are at increased risk of malignancy, particularly leukemia but also lymphoma, squamous cell carcinoma and nephroblastoma.

Cockayne's syndrome

In this rare autosomal recessive condition a photosensitive eruption occurs with erythema and scaling in light-exposed areas, particularly on the face after the first year of life. Later the photosensitivity decreases but hyperpigmentation and atrophy remain in the affected areas. Subcutaneous fat atrophy occurs on the face and the eyes are sunken due to loss of orbital fat. There is dwarfism with disproportionally long limbs and large hands and feet. Mental retardation is common and cerebellar and upper motor neuron dysfunctions occur. Other features are optic atrophy, retinal degeneration and progressive deafness.

Rothmund–Thomson syndrome

The hallmark of this autosomal recessive syndrome is poikiloderma, particularly of the cheeks and hands. The first changes are seen between 3 and 24 months. Photosensitivity is usually transient and not severe. In some patients verrucose lesions develop in late childhood on the dorsum and sides of hands and feet, on palms and soles. Squamous cell carcinoma may occur on both verrucose and atrophic lesions.

The patients are often of short stature. Ocular abnormalities, particularly juvenile cataracts, occur in over 50% of cases. A wide variety of skeletal abnormalities occur and there have been several reports of osteogenic sarcoma. Mental development and life expectancy are usually normal.

Erythropoietic porphyrias

The porphyrias are an important group of diseases which result from enzyme deficiencies in the heme synthesis pathway. Two important examples cause photosensitivity in childhood, and both are inherited.

Erythropoietic protoporphyria

This autosomal dominant condition is associated with reduced ferrochelatase activity. It usually presents with photosensitivity which is relatively mild (cf. congenital erythropoietic porphyria). The child complains of burning of the skin either during or after exposure to sunlight, which may be followed by an erythematous rash in light-exposed areas. As the activating wavelengths are in the UVA and visible light spectra, the photosensitivity will also occur through window glass. Eventually small pock-like scars appear on the nose and cheeks, with thickening of the skin of the dorsum of the hands, which may give a clue as to the diagnosis. In due course, usually in adulthood, gallstones become a problem, and eventually hepatic cirrhosis may develop.

The diagnosis is confirmed by examination of the child's erythrocytes using a fluorescence lamp (400 nm radiation) when the red cells demonstrate a red fluorescent color. Erythrocyte protoporphyrin levels are markedly elevated, though the urinary and fecal porphyrins are normal.

The normal management of the child entails avoidance of the sun and the effective use of sunscreens (SPF 30+). In severe cases, treatment with beta-carotene may be helpful at a dosage of 50–200 mg daily to maintain serum levels of 0.5 mg/100 ml.

Congenital erythropoietic porphyria (Gunther's disease)

This autosomal recessive type of porphyria is rare. It results from uroporphyrinogen III synthase deficiency.

The child presents with severe light sensitivity in infancy, with erythema, blistering (subepidermal blisters) and ulceration of the face, ears and the dorsum of the hands. This may also occur through window glass as the activating wavelengths are in the UVA and visible light spectra (320–450 nm). The child characteristically passes pink urine, and there may be a brown discoloration of the teeth, which fluoresce red under Wood's light. With the passage of time, very marked scarring may develop in the light-exposed areas, particularly of the face and ears, which may result in marked disfiguration. Hypertrichosis may be prominent on the face. Fingernails may be lost, as may the tips of the digits eventually. A fatal outcome is usual in the second or third decade due to anemia, hepatic or renal failure.

The diagnosis is made by estimation of the erythrocyte porphyrins (particularly coproporphyrin) which are very high, the finding of uroporphyrin and coproporphyrin in the urine, and coproporphyrin and protoporphyrin in the feces.

Splenectomy, regular blood transfusions and oral superactivated charcoal have been used as treatments with variable success. Bone marrow/stem cell transplantation is currently the only known cure.[30] Management depends primarily on avoidance of the sun and the use of the most physical sunscreens (e.g. such as zinc oxide and titanium dioxide).

INFECTIONS AND INFESTATIONS OF THE SKIN

VIRUS INFECTIONS

Herpes simplex

Herpes simplex virus (HSV) infections are extremely common in children, and serological studies confirm that more than 90% of the population have been infected by adulthood (Fig. 28.24). The commonest type is HSV1, though HSV2 is more important in adulthood, being the cause of genital herpes. Four distinct presentations are recognized in childhood.

Neonatal herpes simplex virus infection

This is a potentially devastating infection usually contracted during delivery from infected vaginal secretions (HSV2) (Fig. 28.25). However, intrauterine and postnatal infection may occur. Approximately 50% of infected infants have skin lesions which are manifested as grouped blisters localized initially on the presenting part, usually the head, with the onset usually between the 4th and 8th days of life. The eruption may become widespread with

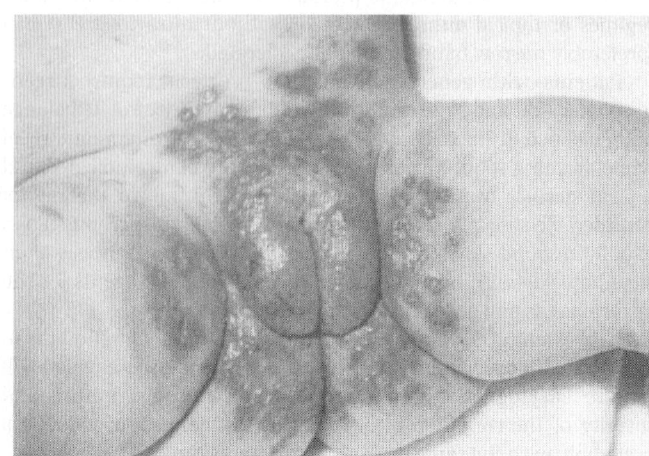

Fig. 28.24 Perineal herpes simplex.

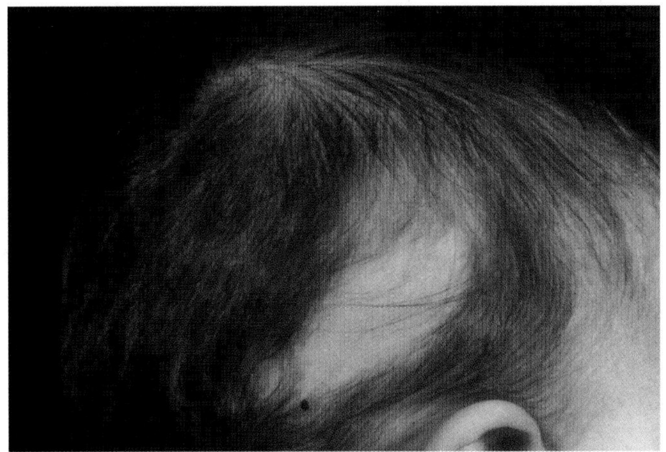

Plate 28.4 Sebaceous nevus (see p. 1598).

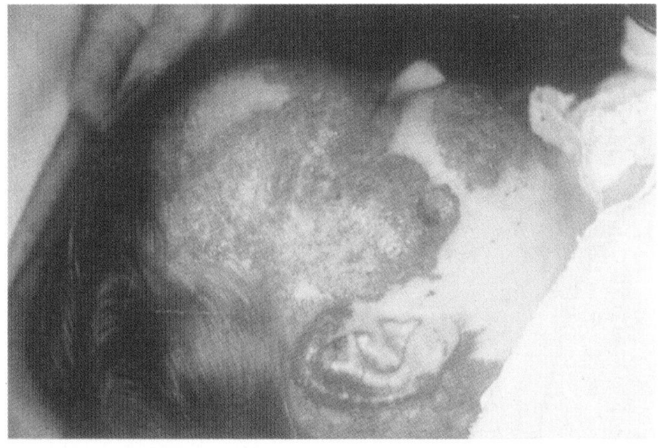

Plate 28.5 Capillary (strawberry) hemangioma (see p. 1598).

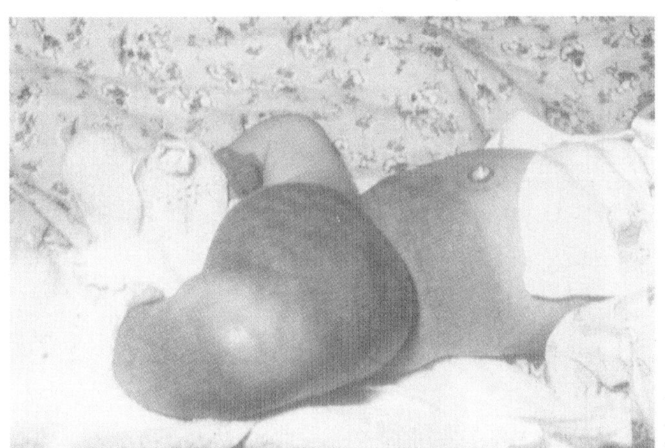

Plate 28.6 Kasabach–Merritt syndrome (see p. 1599).

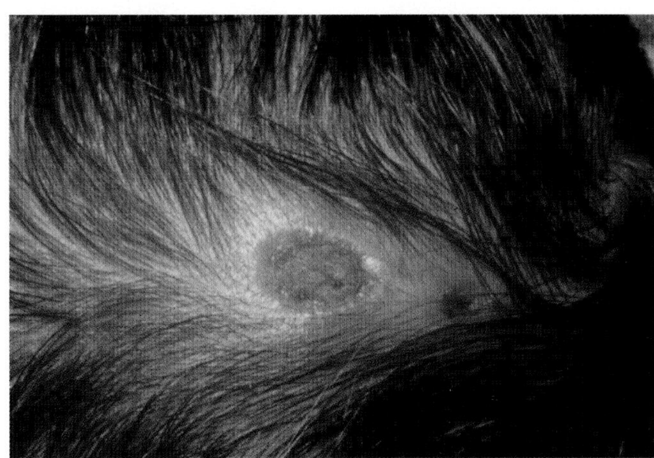

Plate 28.7 Aplasia cutis (see p. 1600).

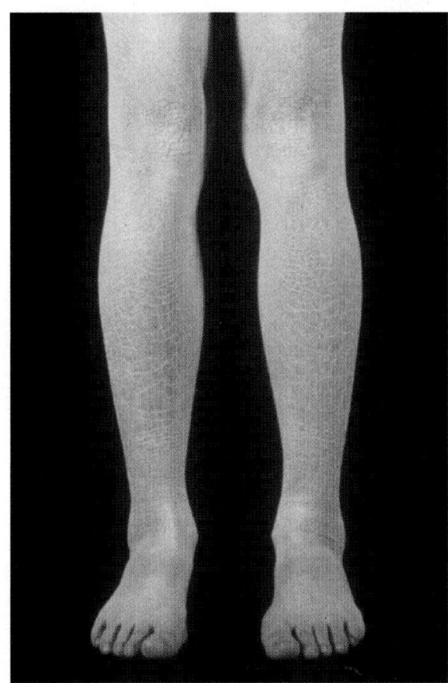

Plate 28.8 X-linked ichthyosis (see p. 1601).

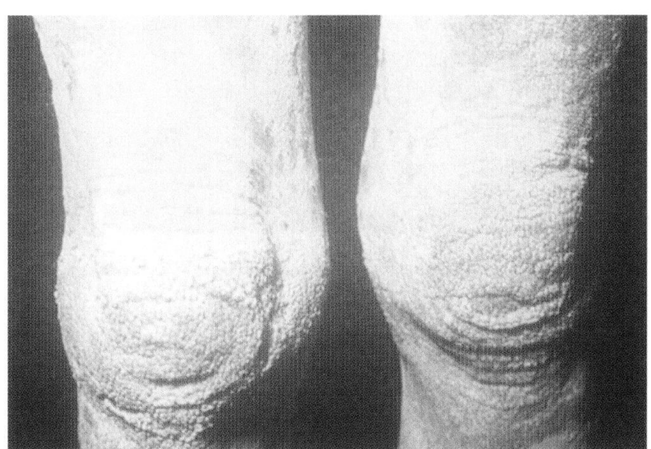

Plate 28.9 Lamellar ichthyosis (congenital ichthyosiform erythroderma) (see p. 1601).

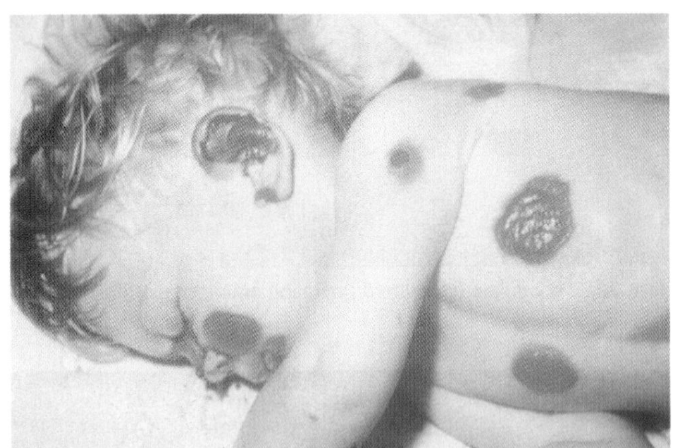

Plate 28.11 Junctional epidermolysis bullosa (see p. 1603).

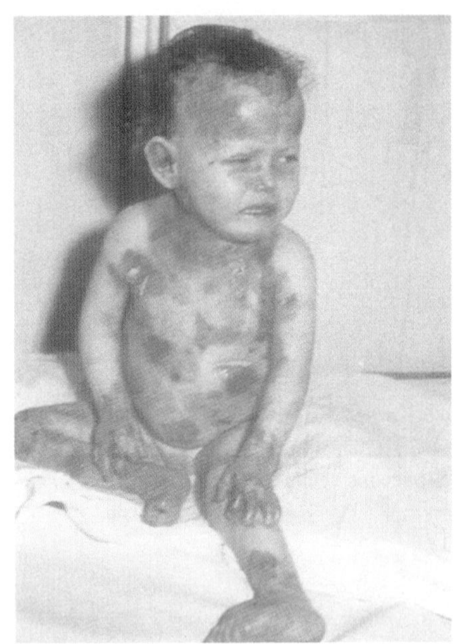

Plate 28.13 Dystrophic epidermolysis bullosa (see p. 1604).

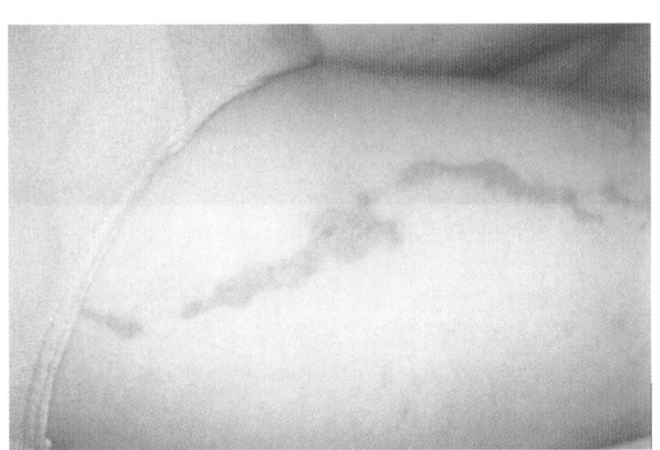

Plate 28.18 Incontinentia pigmenti: pigmented stage (see p. 1607).

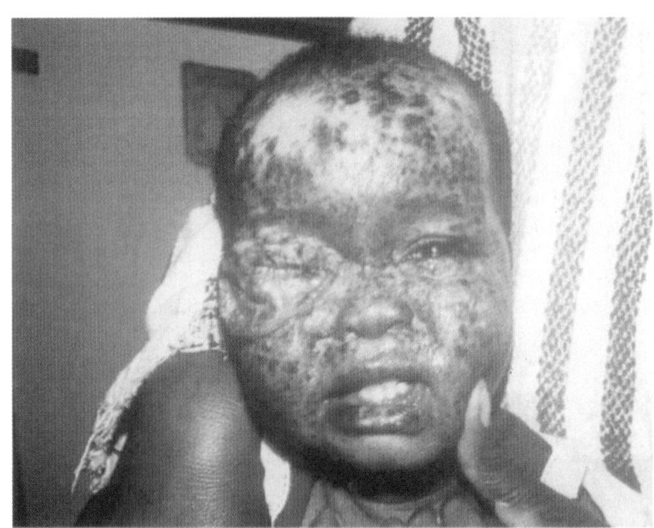

Plate 28.23 Xeroderma pigmentosum (see p. 1609).

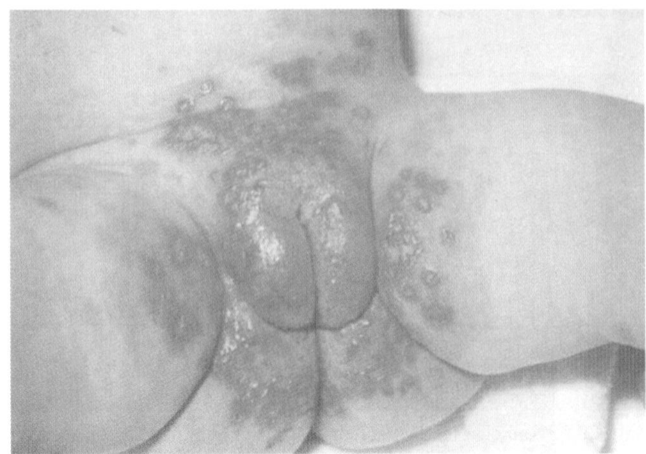

Plate 28.24 Perineal herpes simplex (see p. 1610).

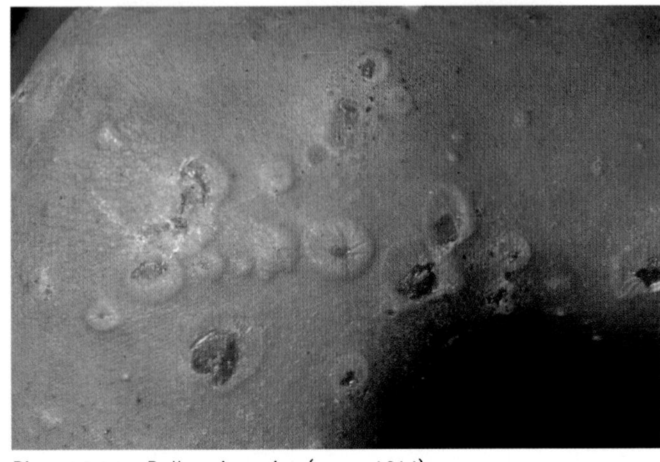

Plate 28.34 Bullous impetigo (see p. 1614).

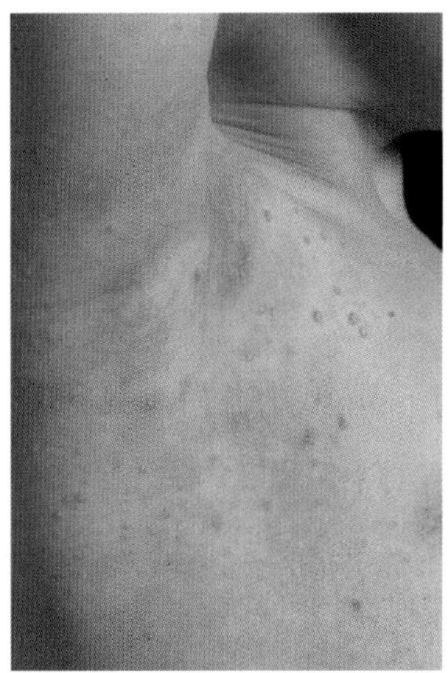

Plate 28.40 Scabies (see p. 1617).

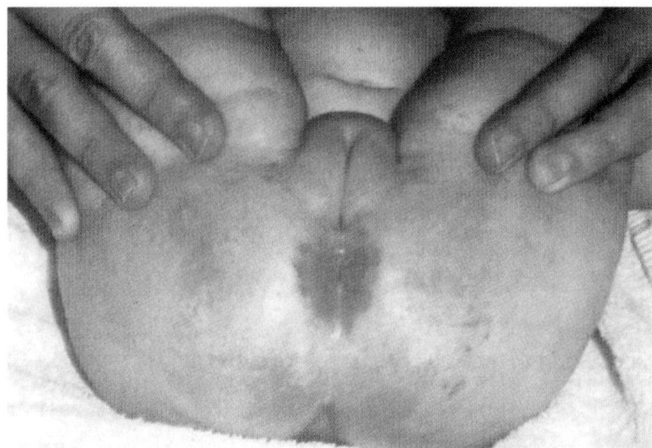

Plate 28.35 Perianal streptococcal disease (see p. 1615).

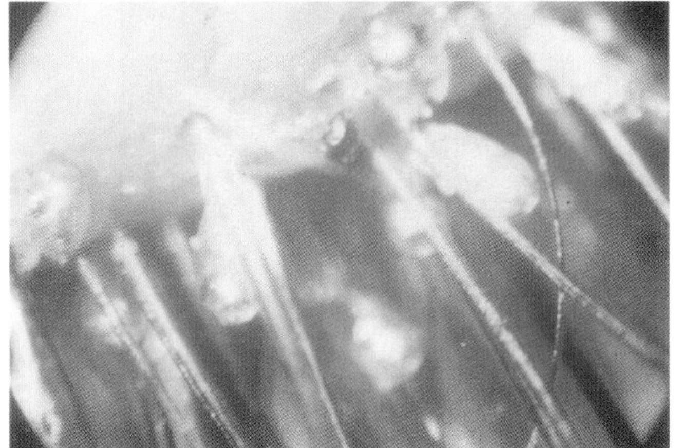

Plate 28.41 Pediculosis of eyelid (see p. 1618).

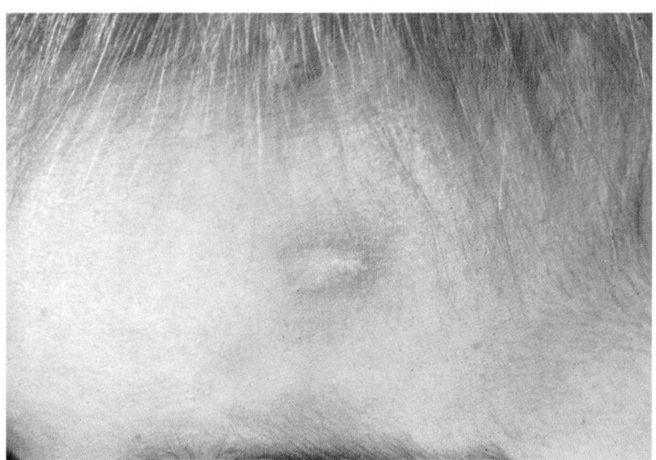

Plate 28.42 Mastocytoma (see p. 1619).

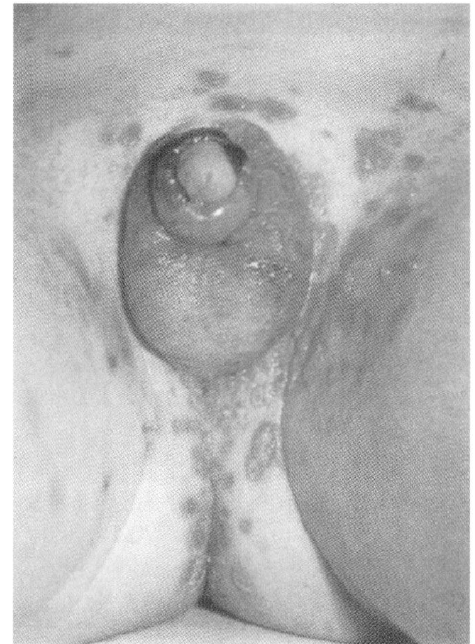

Plate 28.46 Chronic bullous disease of childhood (see p. 1621).

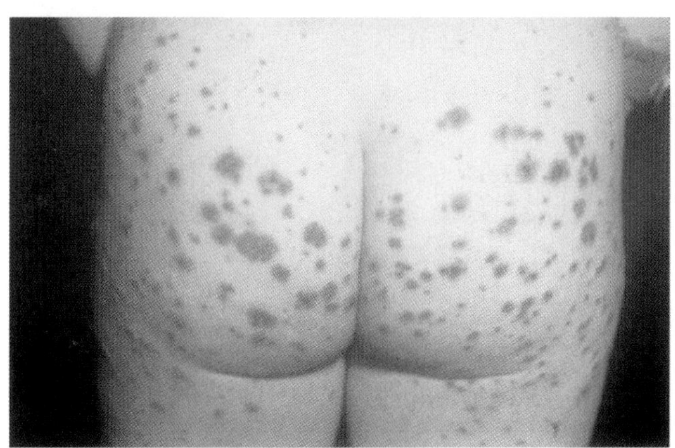

Plate 28.47 Henoch–Schönlein purpura (see p. 1621).

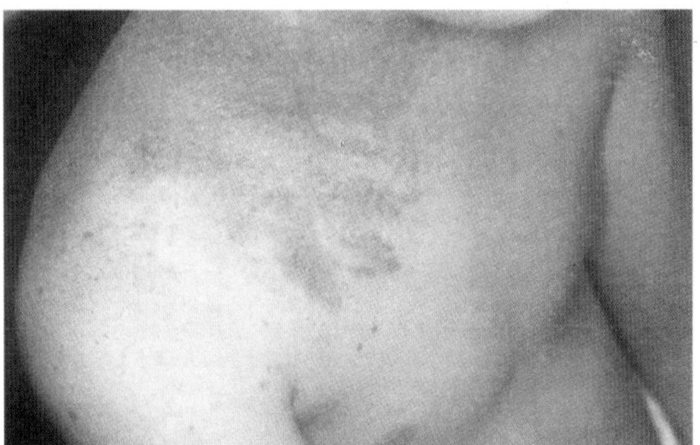

Plate 28.51 Plant (*Rhus*) dermatitis (see p. 1623).

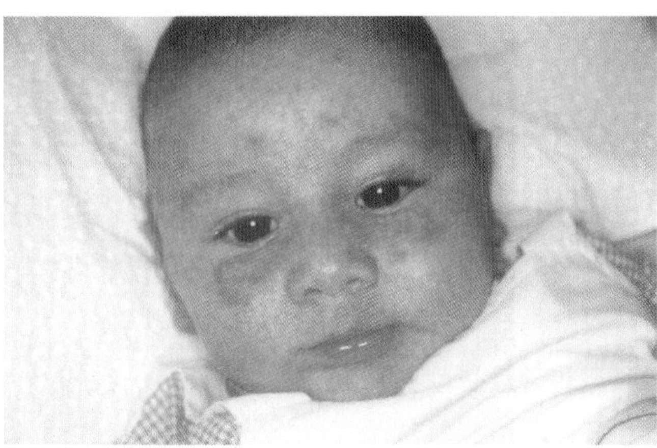

Plate 28.52 Neonatal lupus erythematosus (see p. 1623).

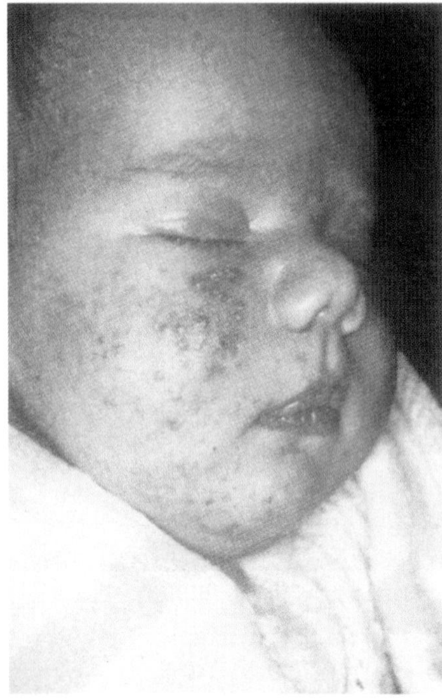

Plate 28.53 Pustular miliaria (prickly heat) (see p. 1626).

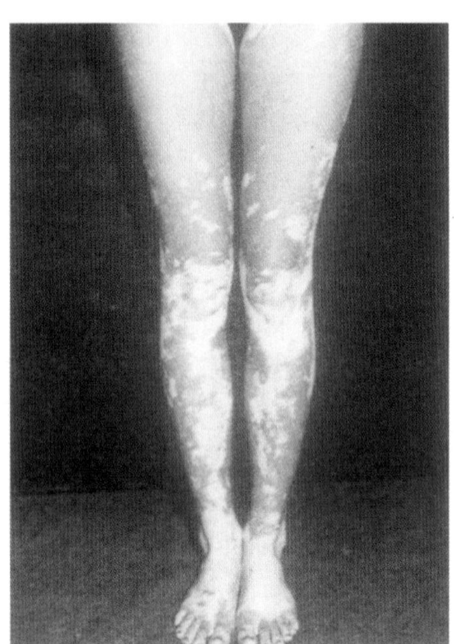

Plate 28.54 Vitiligo (see p. 1627).

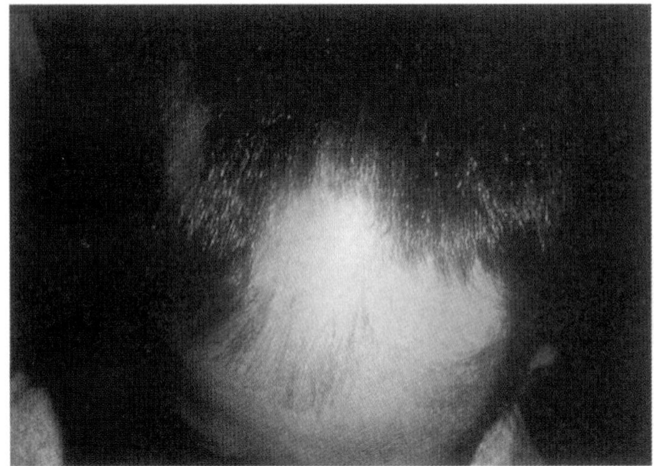

Plate 28.55 Alopecia areata (see p. 1628).

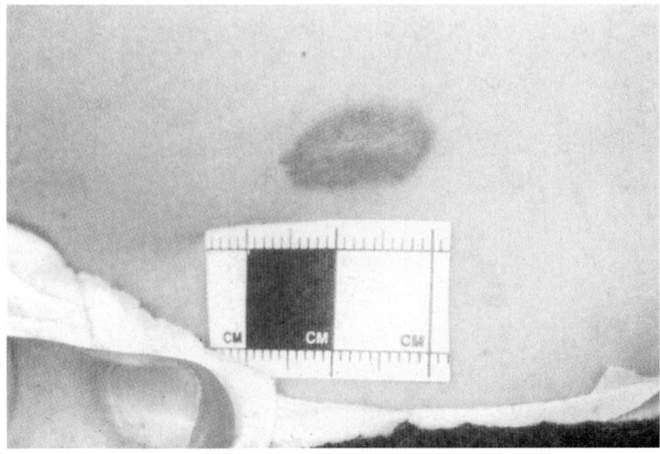

Plate 28.57 Juvenile xanthogranuloma (XTG) (see p. 1629).

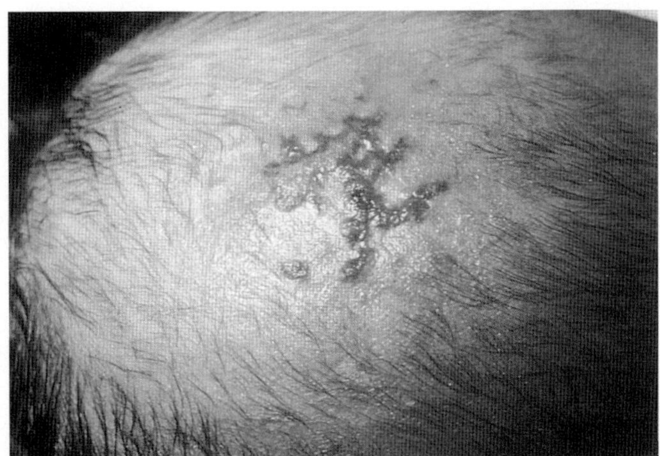

Fig. 28.25 Neonatal herpes on scalp.

individual lesions a few millimeters across coalescing to produce large erosions. A rapid immunofluorescence test on material from the blister base enables a diagnosis within a few hours. Culture of the virus takes several days. A rising titer of complement-fixing antibodies can be demonstrated comparing acute and convalescent sera.

The child with cutaneous neonatal herpes should be assessed urgently for the presence and extent of other organ involvement. Immediate treatment with intravenous aciclovir is indicated.

Primary herpetic gingivostomatitis

This is a common presentation of HSV infection in children (Fig. 28.26). The child is systemically unwell with a high fever and there is severe swelling, erosion and bleeding of the gums and the anterior part of the buccal mucosa. Posterior spread is rare but anterior spread to the lips and the facial skin often occurs. There may be considerable soft tissue swelling and prominent lymphadenopathy. The condition is extremely painful and the child often refuses to eat or drink, necessitating parenteral fluids as the condition may take up to 2 weeks to resolve. Having the child suck ice blocks helps clean the mouth, or large cotton wool swabs soaked with water can be used. Oral antibiotics may be required for secondary bacterial infection. Unless the condition is very severe systemic antiviral therapy is not usually required.

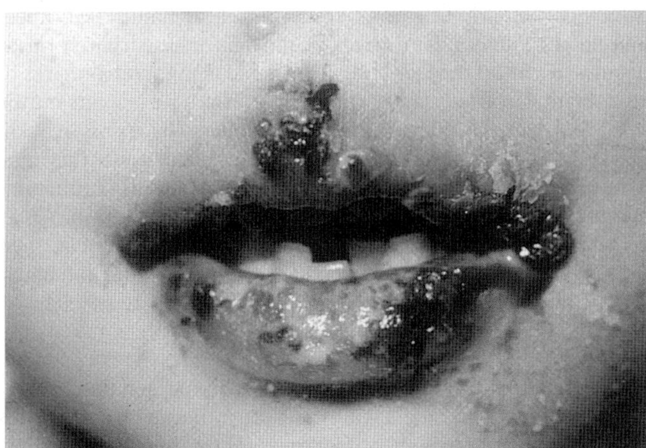

Fig. 28.26 Perioral herpes simplex.

Recurrent herpes simplex (herpes labialis)

Recurrent herpes simplex of the face, particularly around the lips (herpes labialis), is common in childhood. As in adults various factors, including fever and sun exposure, may reactivate the virus. Saline bathing of the lesions speeds resolution and prevents secondary infection. Topical antiviral agents are of limited value.

Disseminated herpes simplex (eczema herpeticum)

This occurs as a complication of atopic eczema and in immunosuppressed patients (Fig. 28.27). It may originate from a primary or recurrent infection, or from external reinfection. Spread is both on the surface of the skin and also by hematogenous dissemination. The lesions are vesicles or pustules 2–4 mm across which may spread with alarming rapidity and have a tendency to coalescence to produce extensive punched-out lesions. Topical steroids should be avoided as their application may spread the virus. Secondary bacterial infection should be treated with oral antibiotics. In most cases systemic aciclovir is indicated. Minor recurrences of HSV infection are seen in up to 20% of cases.

Varicella (chickenpox)

Chickenpox (Ch. 26) is caused by the same herpes virus which produces herpes zoster/shingles (the varicella zoster virus). The incubation period is from 9 to 23 days (mean 14–17 days). After a prodrome of 2–3 days a vesicular eruption develops at the sites of erythematous papules. They appear in crops over 2–4 days, initially on the trunk then face and limbs. Vesicles are often seen in the mouth and occasionally affect other mucous membranes. Pruritus and pyrexia are variable and resolution takes a little over 2 weeks. Complications (encephalitis, pneumonitis and hepatitis) are rare in otherwise healthy children and routine use of aciclovir is not recommended. A live attenuated vaccine is now licensed for prophylactic use in North America.

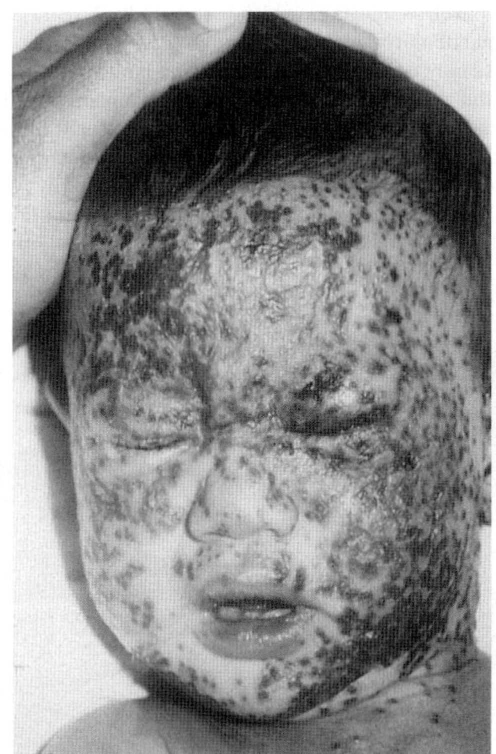

Fig. 28.27 Disseminated herpes simplex (eczema herpeticum).

Herpes zoster

It usually occurs when the virus, which has remained dormant in the cells of dorsal root or cranial nerve ganglia following an attack of chickenpox, reactivates, replicates and spreads along the nerves from these ganglia to infect areas of skin supplied by them (Fig. 28.28). Herpes zoster is much less common in children than in adults but it may occur as early as the first year of life. In children who develop zoster in the first 2 years of life, there is rarely a history of previous chickenpox in the child but often a history of maternal chickenpox during pregnancy.

Herpes zoster presents as a segmental blistering eruption on an erythematous base. Usually a single dermatome is affected but spread to one or two adjoining dermatomes may occur. The eruption is essentially unilateral though there may be minor spread to the opposite side on the trunk or brow. Up to 20 or 30 scattered lesions identical to chickenpox commonly occur. Infection involving the ophthalmic division of the 5th cranial (trigeminal) nerve may produce keratitis and uveitis, threatening vision. An important cutaneous sign of potentially dangerous herpes zoster ophthalmicus is blisters on the nose indicating involvement of the nasociliary branch. Blisters in the oral cavity occur with involvement of maxillary and mandibular divisions of the trigeminal nerve. Anogenital blistering and sometimes disorders of urination and defecation occur with involvement of sacral nerves. Scarring and postherpetic neuralgia are rare complications in children.

Management

This is directed at providing symptomatic treatment with wet compresses and appropriate analgesia, and dealing with any secondary bacterial infection. Early ophthalmological consultation is essential for ophthalmic zoster patients. Intravenous aciclovir is indicated in very severe cases, particularly of ophthalmic zoster and for all immunosuppressed patients.

Molluscum contagiosum

This is a poxvirus infection, which is rare under 1 year of age, and occurs particularly in the 2–5 year age group (Fig. 28.29). Outbreaks may occur among children who bathe or swim together and in the adolescent age group sexual transmission becomes important. The typical lesion is spherical and pearly white with a central umbilication, but they may vary from tiny 1 mm papules to large nodules over 1 cm in diameter. They occur on any part of the skin surface with common sites being the axillae and sides of the trunk, the lower abdomen and anogenital area. Rarely they occur on the eyelids where they may cause conjunctivitis and punctate keratitis. A secondary eczema often occurs around lesions, particularly in atopics, and scratching of this spreads the mollusca. Hundreds of lesions may be present in an individual patient. Secondary bacterial infection may occur producing crusting, erythema and suppuration. However, these same changes may be seen during spontaneous resolution which occurs in most within 6–9 months leaving normal skin or small varicelliform scars.

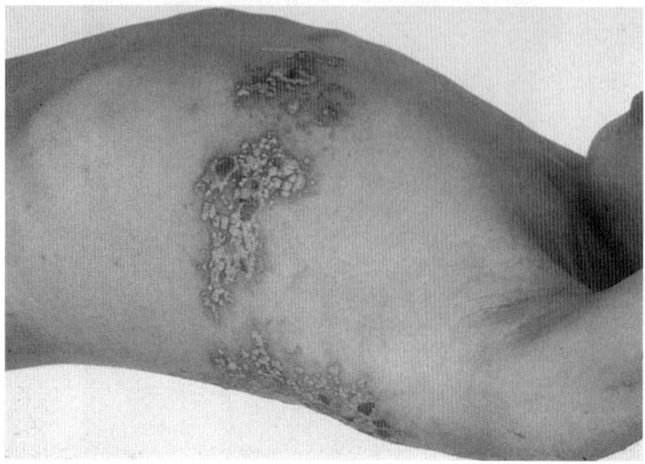

Fig. 28.28 Herpes zoster.

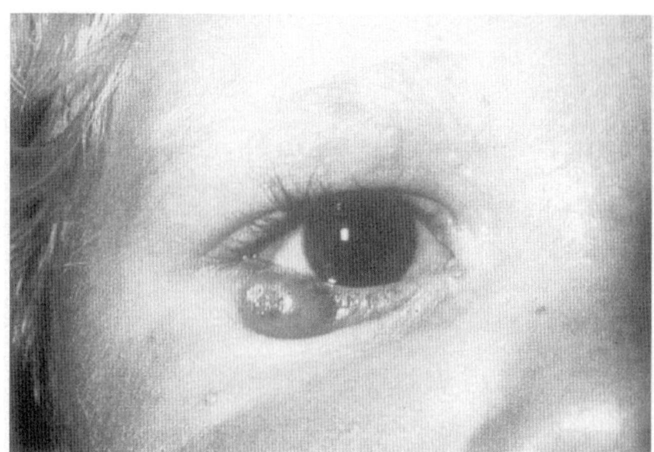

Fig. 28.29 Molluscum contagiosum.

Mollusca may clinically simulate warts or skin tags but they have a distinct histological appearance with lobulated downgrowths of epidermal cells containing intracytoplasmic inclusion bodies.

Management

With multiple small lesions in a young child spontaneous resolution should be awaited. No controlled trials exist for treatment of mollusca in childhood. However cryotherapy after application of anesthetic cream, topical therapy with salicylic acid, podophyllotoxin, cantharadin and more recently imiquimod or cidofovir have all been reported with variable success. Physical extrusion of the contents of larger lesions can also be undertaken and is usually best after anesthetic cream application. Up to 10% of cases develop eczema around the lesions which resolves when the mollusca clear. Spontaneous regression may be associated with secondary bacterial infection requiring a topical antibiotic.

Warts

Warts are benign tumors caused by infection with a variety of human papilloma viruses. The common wart (verruca vulgaris) occurs particularly at sites of trauma such as hands, feet, knees and elbows. Plane or flat warts, 1–3 mm pink or brown barely raised papules, occur on the face and often spread along scratch marks or cuts. Plantar warts occur particularly over pressure points on the soles and can be differentiated from calluses by a loss of skin markings over the skin surface. Unlike corns or callosities they tend to be painful on lateral pressure. Warts at mucocutaneous junctions often have a filiform or fronded appearance. Anogenital warts may be acquired from maternal infection during delivery, but their presence should always raise the suspicion of sexual abuse (Fig. 28.30).

Management

Various forms of treatment are available: they depend on the area, the type of wart and the age of the patient. Because spontaneous disappearance is common, aggressive treatment is usually inappropriate. A Cochrane review[31] of local treatments for

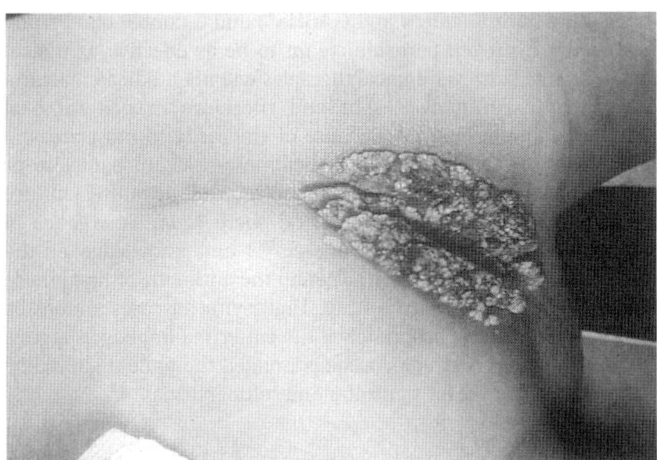

Fig. 28.30 Perianal warts.

cutaneous warts shows that there is very little good evidence on which to determine best practice. The best available evidence was for the use of topical salicylic acid preparations. Perhaps surprisingly cryotherapy was not found to be superior. Other currently used topical agents include glutaraldehyde and formaldehyde preparations. Podophyllotoxin is less irritant than podophyllin but both can be used for isolated anogenital warts. Facial plane warts may respond to retinoic acid preparations. Cautery or diathermy is useful for lesions on the lips or anogenital area but elsewhere recurrence is fairly frequent following their use and there is also a risk of producing a painful scar. The initial favorable response to oral cimetidine has not been replicated in double-blind placebo controlled trials.[32]

Papular acrodermatitis of childhood (Gianotti–Crosti syndrome)

Papular acrodermatitis of childhood was first described by Gianotti as an acrally distributed papular eruption occurring in young children due to the hepatitis B virus (Fig. 28.31). However, a similar eruption may occur with over a dozen different viruses and the condition is best regarded as a reaction pattern with multiple etiologies.[33]

This pattern of exanthem occurs particularly in children between 1 and 4 years of age. The rash comprises discrete firm red papules 1–5 mm in diameter, sometimes surmounted by vesicles. Pruritus is variable but not usually a significant feature. The lesions involve the limbs, particularly distally, and the face, with the trunk being essentially spared. The rash fades within 3–4 weeks. Lymphadenopathy is usually present but the child is often otherwise remarkably well, leading to such misdiagnoses as insect bites and papular eczema.

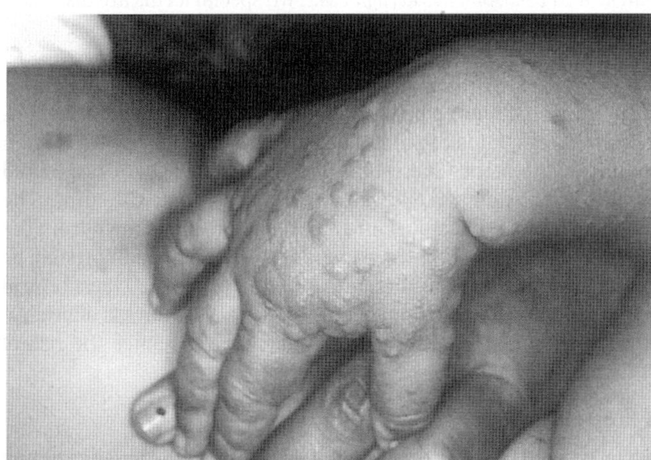

Fig. 28.31 Papular acrodermatitis of childhood.

Investigation should be aimed at excluding the more serious viral etiologies.

Pityriasis rosea

Epidemiological studies suggest a viral origin, now thought to be human herpes virus 7. It occurs in children and young adults and has no sexual or racial predilection (Fig. 28.32).

The eruption commences with the appearance of the so-called herald patch, typically a single round or oval scaly lesion 1–5 cm in diameter, flat or slightly raised with a tendency to clear in the center. It usually occurs on the trunk, neck or proximal limbs. Some 5–15 days later the secondary eruption appears comprising multiple, variably pruritic, dull pink, oval macules with a peripheral collarette of scale. The typical distribution is on trunk and proximal limbs but may be very extensive. The long axis of the lesions on the trunk runs parallel with the ribs giving a 'Christmas-tree' pattern. Rarer variants have lesions which are papular, urticarial, vesicular, purpuric or pustular but some of the typical lesions are usually intermingled. Lesions crop at 2–3 day intervals for 7–10 days and then spontaneous resolution occurs over several weeks. Sun exposure may speed this resolution and meanwhile symptomatic therapy can be used for the pruritus if this is troublesome.

BACTERIAL INFECTIONS

Staphylococcal and streptococcal infections of the skin are common in childhood. They take the following clinical forms:

Impetigo

This is a bacterial infection caused by *Staphylococcus aureus*), group A beta-hemolytic streptococcus (GABHS) or a combination of these

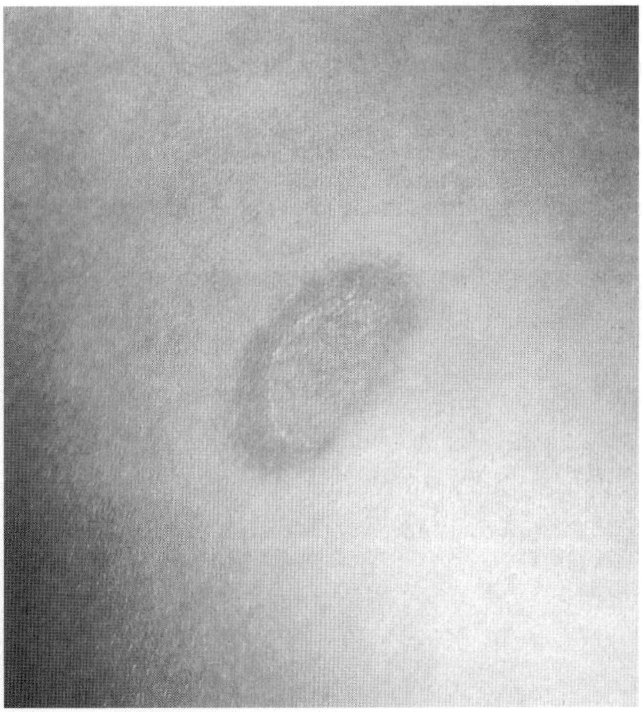

Fig. 28.32 Pityriasis rosea (herald patch).

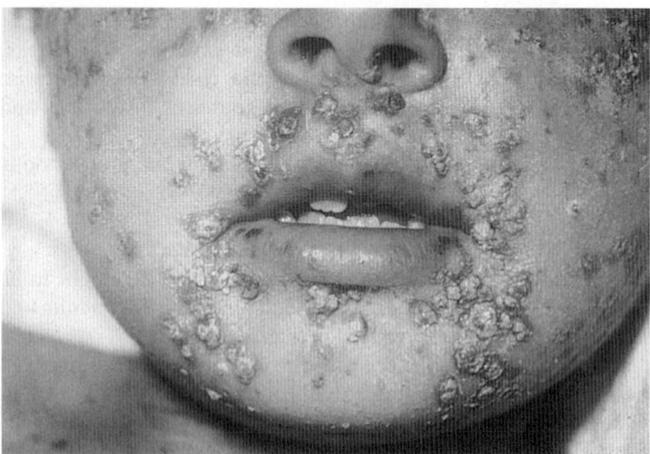

Fig. 28.33 Impetigo.

organisms (Fig. 28.33). Recently there has been a worldwide increase in the predominance of staphylococci in the causation of impetigo.[34,35] An increasing proportion of *S. aureus* isolates are resistant to methicillin (MRSA).

Impetigo occurs in two forms, bullous and more commonly non-bullous (or crusted). Bullous impetigo (Fig. 28.34) is always due to staphylococci. Blisters arise on previously normal skin and increase rapidly in size and number, soon rupturing to produce superficial erosions with a peripheral brown crust. The erosions continue to expand, sometimes clearing centrally to produce annular lesions. The condition is usually neither itchy nor painful. Non-bullous impetigo may be due to either organism or to a combination. The lesions begin with a small transient vesicle on an erythematous base. The serum exuding from the ruptured vesicle produces a thick soft yellow crust, below which there is a moist superficial erosion. The lesions extend slowly and remain much smaller than those of bullous impetigo. Impetigo is often superimposed on other skin diseases such as insect bites, scabies, pediculosis and atopic eczema. As impetigo is an intraepidermal infection, the condition does not scar although postinflammatory pigmentation can occur, particularly in dark-skinned patients.

Management

Impetigo is very contagious and the patient should, if possible, be isolated. A swab for culture and sensitivity testing should always be taken. Topical mupirocin is as successful as oral erythromycin in eradicating both *S. aureus* and GABHS[36] and a double-blind study has shown hydrogen peroxide cream to be as effective as topical fusidic acid.[37] However, topical therapies will not eradicate bacteria on clinically uninvolved skin and therefore in general oral antibiotics should be used. Because of the rarity in most areas of pure streptococcal impetigo, a penicillinase-resistant penicillin or erythromycin is the treatment of choice while awaiting culture results. In many areas of the world there is an emergence of erythromycin-resistant staphylococci[34,38] and knowledge of the local situation is important in selecting the antibiotic of first choice while awaiting sensitivity testing. Underlying diseases should be sought and treated appropriately if the pattern of impetigo suggests them. If a group A streptococcus is isolated the patient should be watched for 8 weeks for signs of glomerulonephritis.

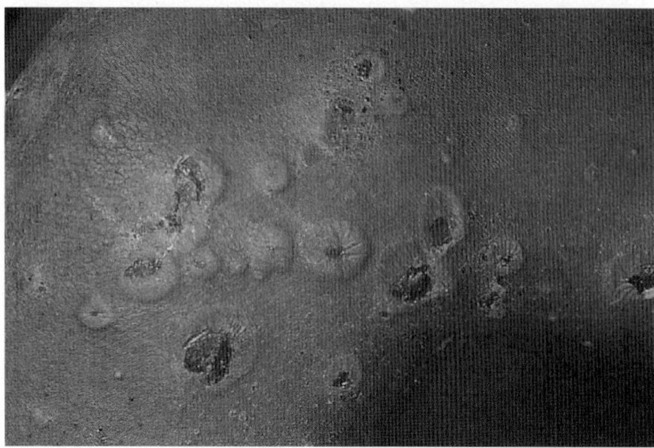

Fig. 28.34 Bullous impetigo.

Folliculitis

Superficial bacterial folliculitis is common in children. It is characterized by inflammation confined to the opening of the hair follicle whereas furuncles or boils are cutaneous abscesses, centered around usually ruptured, hair follicles. Both are caused by a wide variety of types and strains of *S. aureus* and predisposing factors are occlusion, friction, maceration and sweating. Patients with recurrent attacks are often found to carry the strains of *S. aureus* in their nose, axillae or perineum, or to be in close contact with another person who is a carrier. Folliculitis commences with perifollicular erythema with pustule formation that often ruptures to form a crust. Pruritus is common. Boils are larger, firm erythematous papules that evolve into fluctuant pus-filled nodules with central necrosis (pointing) and discharge.

Mild folliculitis is often self-limiting but can be treated with topical antiseptics. If the infection is persistent, or recurrent, topical or oral antistaphylococcal antibiotics should be given. Swabs should first be taken for culture from affected as well as *S. aureus* carriage sites. If necessary, other carriers who are in close contact should be identified and treated.

Cellulitis

This is an acute bacterial infection involving the subcutis as well as the dermis. The lesion is erythematous sometimes with a purple or blue hue. It is warm and tender and has a less well-defined edge than erysipelas. Fever and malaise, leukocytosis and lymphadenopathy are usually present. When cellulitis follows a wound or other break in the skin, group A beta-hemolytic streptococcus is the commonest cause. Other organisms involved in cellulitis include *Haemophilus influenzae*, *Streptococcus pneumoniae*, *S. aureus* and *Pseudomonas aeruginosa*. Two special forms are discussed below.

Perianal streptococcal disease

This occurs in children between 1 and 10 years of age (Fig. 28.35). The child complains of painful defecation and bright blood is often found on the stool. There is a well-demarcated, very bright red erythema extending out several centimeters from the anus. The anal rim is often macerated and fissured. GABHS is grown from the skin and often also from the patient's throat. The condition may be surprisingly resistant to therapy, recurring after 5–10 days of oral penicillin therapy: an initial course of at least 14 days is advisable. The addition of topical mupirocin may further reduce the risk of recurrence.[39]

Facial cellulitis

Facial cellulitis in young children often occurs in the absence of any break in the skin and is due to *H. influenzae* or *S. pneumoniae*

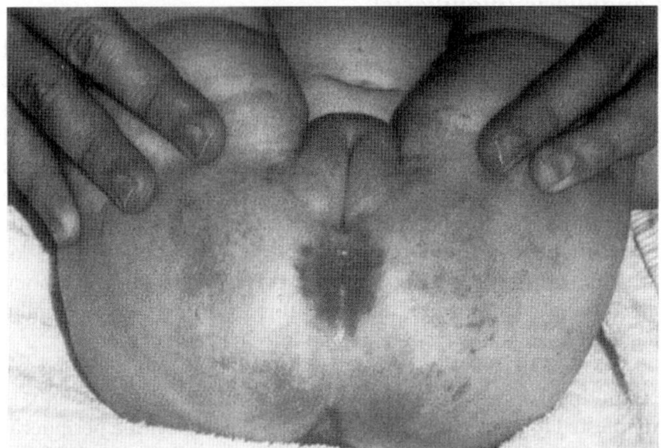

Fig. 28.35 Perianal streptococcal disease.

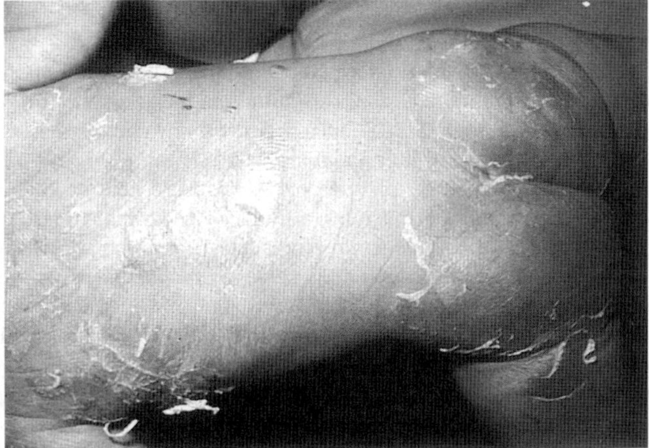

Fig. 28.36 Staphylococcal scalded skin syndrome.

accompanying an upper respiratory tract infection or otitis media. Cellulitis due to these bacteria often has a lilac-blue color. The condition may be complicated by bacteremia, septicemia and meningitis. In all cases of facial cellulitis cultures should be taken from nasopharynx, ears, blood and, if indicated, cerebrospinal fluid. Needle aspiration from the lesion after saline injection may provide material from which the organism can be cultured.

Intravenous cefotaxime, a third generation cephalosporin, is the initial treatment of choice until an organism is identified and sensitivity tests performed.

Erysipelas

This is an acute bacterial infection of the dermal connective tissue and superficial lymphatics caused most often by GABHS but occasionally due to other streptococci, *H. influenzae* and *S. aureus*. A brightly erythematous, hot, tender area with a rapidly spreading distinct edge develops. Superimposed bullae may occur. There is accompanying fever and malaise and a leukocytosis. Predisposing factors include lymphatic obstruction and a break in the skin due, for example, to a wound, bite or tinea infection. The episode produces a lymphangitis which further damages the lymphatics, and chronic lymphedema may result from and further predispose to recurrent erysipelas. Treatment involves rest and high doses of the appropriate antibiotic, usually penicillin V, orally or intravenously depending on the severity.

Staphylococcal scalded skin syndrome

Pathogenesis

The staphylococcal scalded skin syndrome (SSSS) is a widespread blistering disease caused by an epidermolytic toxin produced by certain strains of *S. aureus*, most often of phage group II, but occasionally phage group I or III (Figs 28.36 and 28.37). This toxin produces a superficial splitting of the skin with the level of split being high in the epidermis. Clinical disease occurs when there is sufficient toxin load produced from an infection with these organisms. The commonest sites of infection are the umbilicus (in neonates), the nose, nasopharynx or throat, the conjunctiva and deep wounds.

The condition commences with a macular erythema initially on the face and in the major flexures and then becoming generalized. The skin is exquisitely tender and the child draws back from contact. After 2 days flaccid bullae develop and the skin wrinkles and shears off. The exfoliation is most marked in the groin, neck fold and around the mouth and may involve the entire body surface but

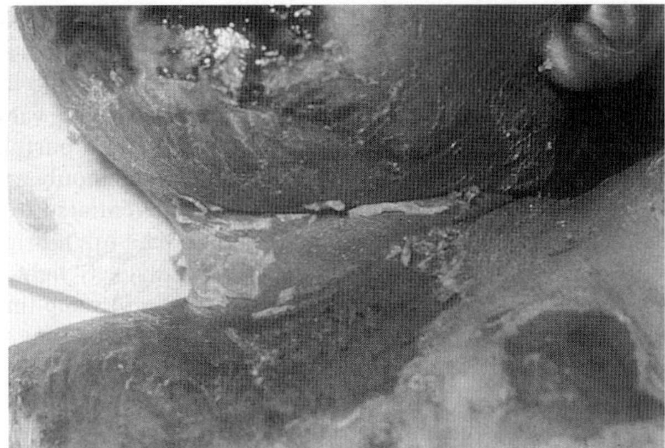

Fig. 28.37 Staphylococcal scalded skin syndrome.

mucosa remain uninvolved. The child is usually febrile but because of the superficial level of the split fluid loss is rarely significant. The erosions crust and dry and heal with desquamation over the next 4–8 days leaving no sequelae.

Diagnosis

Cultures from skin and blister fluid are usually negative. Cultures should be obtained from any area of obvious infection but, if none is apparent, from nasopharnyx and throat. The most important differential diagnosis is toxic epidermal necrolysis (TEN). In TEN the split is subepidermal and the blisters and erosions are usually hemorrhagic and mucosae are commonly involved. Microscopy of a Giemsa-stained section of the blister roof can detect the level of the split in the two conditions. Other conditions from which SSSS may be differentiated are scarlet fever, Kawasaki's syndrome and toxic shock syndrome, all of which show mucosal involvement and rarely demonstrate frank blistering.

Management

The child should be nursed with as little handling as possible. No topical agents should be applied. A penicillinase-resistant penicillin is the treatment of choice and should be given orally if possible. Insertion and securing of an intravenous line is very painful in these patients and should be performed only if oral antibiotics are refused or if rehydration is required in a child refusing oral fluids. Analgesia is often necessary in the early stages. Emollients are useful once the skin dries and desquamation commences.

FUNGAL INFECTIONS

Tinea

This is an infection due to dermatophyte fungi: the source of the fungus is an animal (e.g. dog, cat, guinea pig, cattle), the soil or another human (Fig. 28.38). Tinea occurs on any part of the skin surface and can involve hair and nails.

The classical features of tinea on the skin are itch, erythema studded with papules or pustules, annular or geographical lesions ('ringworm') with a tendency to central clearing and a superficial scale. Family members including pets are the usual source of infection. On the palms and soles erythema and increased skin markings may be the only signs. Between the toes maceration with a thick white scale is the main finding and an annular lesion may extend onto the dorsum of the foot. On the soles there are deep seated blisters or pustules which dry to produce brown crusts. Tinea is often unilateral and always asymmetrical, whereas eczema and psoriasis, which it may resemble, are often symmetrical in distribution. Nail tinea (onychomycosis) is uncommon in children but increases with age.

In the UK the principal dermatophytes causing tinea capitis are *Microsporum canis* and *Trichophyton tonsurans*. Both cause a combination of alopecia and inflammation with the hair loss being due to breakage of hair shafts. The inflammation varies from mild erythema and a fine dandruff-like scale to a pustular carbuncle-like lesion (kerion), which occurs most commonly with *T. violaceum*. Other causes of alopecia to be differentiated from tinea are trichotillomania (q.v.) and alopecia areata (q.v). Bright green fluorescence is seen under Wood's (ultraviolet) light in *Microsporum* infection of the scalp. Other varieties of scalp tinea produce no typical fluorescence and the Wood's light has no place in the diagnosis of tinea on the skin surface. The diagnosis of tinea is confirmed by scraping hairs or scales onto a slide, adding 20% potassium hydroxide and examining the specimen microscopically. Septate branching hyphae are seen in skin scales and spores are found in hair. The fungus can be cultured on appropriate media.

Topical antifungals (Whitfield's ointment, imidazole creams) may be satisfactory for small localized patches of tinea on the skin. Griseofulvin is the only antifungal licensed for oral treatment in children. It is effective against dermatophytes but in general a 3 month course is used with longer courses for nail tinea. Terbinafine is not yet licensed for children but a number of published studies have shown it to be safe and effective for tinea capitis.[40]

Candidiasis (moniliasis)

This is due to a yeast, *Candida albicans*. It occurs on both skin and mucosal surfaces and certain factors predispose to its establishment (Fig. 28.39). General predisposing factors in children include drug therapy with broad spectrum antibiotics, corticosteroids and immunosuppressives, diabetes and any disease which interferes with immunological competence. Local predisposing factors are particularly those which create a warm moist environment. Flexural areas are susceptible, especially in the presence of sweating, obesity and other skin disease. The oral mucosa in infancy also has a particular susceptibility to this infection which is usually acquired during passage through an infected birth canal.

On the general body skin, where candidiasis rarely occurs except in the presence of immunodeficiency, the infection is manifested by small round erythematous lesions with a peripheral overhanging scale. Occasionally small papules or superficial pustules occur, especially in the neonate. In flexural areas the typical picture is of a cheesy white material deep in the folds and satellite lesions with the typical peripheral scale. On mucosae a curd-like white material is superimposed on a red base. Acute or chronic paronychia may be seen, particularly in children that suck their fingers.

Chronic mucocutaneous candidiasis is a progressive candidal infection occurring in patients who have an inability to destroy candida due to a severe general immunodeficiency or due to a specific immunological defect. A variety of endocrinopathies may be associated with this syndrome. Initially, typical candida lesions become chronic and then become progressively hyperplastic, producing thick crusted plaques, even warty or horn-like lesions, occurring particularly around face and scalp, hands and feet. A nail dystrophy with thick crumbling nail plates and abundant subungual debris may occur and scalp hair may be lost. On the mucosae extensive thick white verrucose plaques occur.

The diagnosis of candidiasis is usually a clinical one which may be confirmed by microscopy and culture. Candida is frequently a secondary invader rather than a primary cause of skin disease and local and general predisposing factors should be eliminated. Once predisposing factors have been eliminated most localized infections respond well to topical agents including polyene antibiotics, nystatin and imidazole derivatives. Reduction of intestinal carriage with oral preparations is rarely necessary. Oral ketoconazole is useful in chronic mucocutaneous candidiasis and other candidal infections in the immunosuppressed.

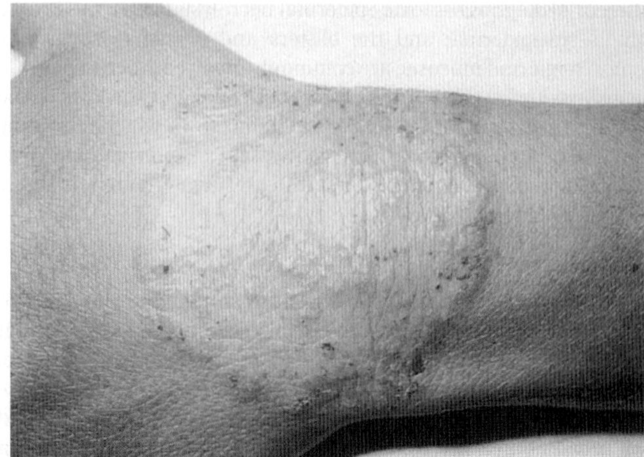

Fig. 28.38 Tinea.

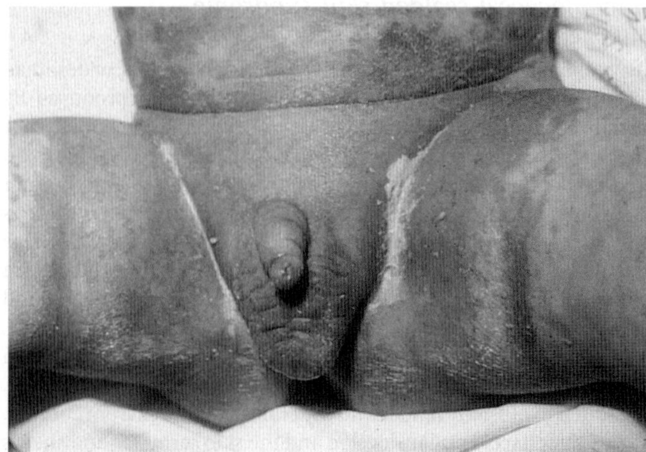

Fig. 28.39 Candidiasis.

Tinea versicolor (pityriasis versicolor)

This is an infection with *Pityrosporum* species which are part of the normal skin flora. It occurs mainly in tropical and temperate zones and usually affects adolescents and young adults. It presents as well-demarcated, asymptomatic or slightly itchy macules with a fine branny scale which is often only obvious on light scratching of the lesions. Primary macules 1–10 mm in diameter coalesce into larger patches. They occur in two colors, red–brown especially in the fair skinned and hypopigmented in darker skinned. In a partially tanned individual, lesions of both colors may be found. In young children, unlike adults, approximately 30% present with only facial lesions.[41]

Diagnosis is confirmed by microscopic examination of skin scrapings to which 20% potassium hydroxide has been added. Grape-like clusters of spores and short fragments of thick mycelia are seen. In its hypopigmented forms the condition must be distinguished from: (a) vitiligo, where the depigmentation is total and scale absent; (b) pityriasis alba where lesions are less well demarcated and some erythema may be seen; and (c) tuberculoid leprosy which is accompanied by anesthesia in the hypopigmented areas. The red–brown form has to be differentiated from seborrheic dermatitis, tinea and psoriasis, all of which lack the very fine branny type of scale.

Untreated the condition is persistent though some improvement may occur in winter. Various treatments are available. The treatment of choice is with topical imidazole creams. Alternatively two overnight applications of 2.5% selenium sulfide may be effective in the short term but relapse is frequent. With the depigmented form, whatever therapy is used sun exposure is required for full repigmentation.

ECTOPARASITIC INFESTATIONS

Scabies

This is due to *Sarcoptes scabei*, an eight-legged, oval-shaped mite less than 0.5 mm in length. The disease is transmitted by close physical contact.

A small number of mites burrow into the skin in certain sites, particularly between the fingers, the ulnar border of the hand, around the wrists and elbows, the anterior axillary fold, nipples and penis and, in infants, the palms and soles. The pathognomonic primary lesion, a typical burrow, is a 2–3 mm long curved gray line with a vesicle at the anterior end. Other lesions which mark the sites of burrows are small blisters or papules, larger blisters on the palms and soles of infants, scratch marks, secondary eczema and secondary bacterial infection. Eczema or impetigo in the target areas for scabies should always raise suspicion of this disease as should blisters on the palms and soles of infants.

Often more prominent than the evidence of burrows is the so-called secondary eruption of scabies. This presents as multiple, very pruritic, urticarial papules which are soon excoriated (Fig. 28.40). They occur particularly on the abdomen, thighs and buttocks. Young children may show a striking dermographism in the areas of scratch marks. When dermographism occurs in the first year of life scabies should always be suspected. Large inflammatory nodules may form part of the secondary eruption, occurring particularly on covered areas especially on axillae, scrotum, penis and buttocks. They may, however, be very widespread producing diagnostic difficulties. They may persist for months after effective scabies treatment.

The diagnosis of scabies is usually a clinical one but can be confirmed by demonstration of the mite. A burrow is scraped and the material smeared on a slide with potassium hydroxide for

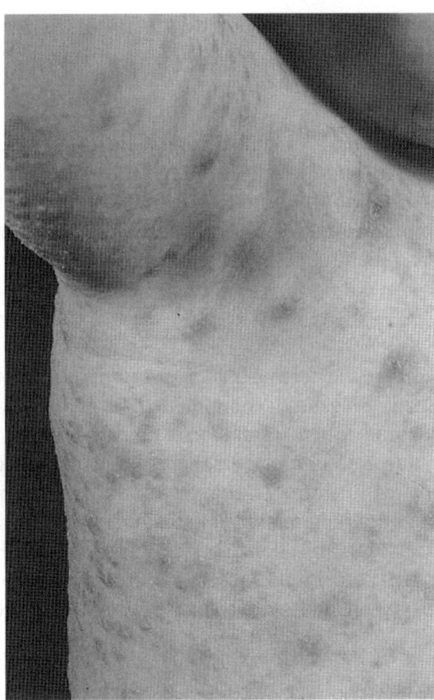

Fig. 28.40 Scabies.

microscopic examination. Burrows may be more easily identified by rubbing a thick black marking pen over suspicious areas and wiping with an alcohol swab leaving a burrow outlined with ink.

Management

The patient and all close contacts should be treated simultaneously. The treatment of choice is 5% permethrin cream[42,43]: it should be applied to all body surfaces from the neck down and left on overnight. A repeat application should be administered after 1 week. Bedclothes and clothing should be washed in the normal way with no disinfection required. An irritant dermatitis may follow scabies treatment, particularly in atopics, and may require emollients and topical steroids once the miticide therapy is fully completed. Persistent nodules may respond to topical corticosteroids and families should be warned that it can take up to 3 weeks before the pruritus subsides.

Pediculosis (lice)

Human lice are ectoparasites dependent on man for survival. They are wingless six-legged insects, gray–white in color or red–brown when engorged with blood. The head louse (*Pediculus humanus capitis*) and the body louse (*Pediculus humanus humanus*) have a 24 mm long slim body and three similar pairs of legs. The pubic louse (*Pthirus pubis*, crab louse) has a wider, shorter body 12 mm long and the second and third pairs of legs are larger than the first, producing a crab-like appearance. The nits or ova are seen as oval gray–white 0.5 mm specks firmly attached by a chitinous ring to hairs or clothing.

Pediculosis capitis

This is a very common infection, occurring in epidemics amongst schoolchildren. The infestation is most severe in and may be confined to the occipital area. It is very itchy and excoriations are seen but secondary eczematization and bacterial infection may mask the condition. Nits may be differentiated from epidermal scales and hair casts by their firm attachment and by fluorescence with a Wood's light. Occasionally the head louse infects the eyelashes in children (Fig. 28.41).

Pediculosis corporis

This is rare in children except in conditions of overcrowding and poor hygiene. The louse infects bedding and seams of clothing and nits are not found on the human. With body warmth the pediculi hatch and puncture the skin to produce small urticarial papules with hemorrhagic puncta. Pruritus is extreme and scratch marks are the main clinical sign.

Pediculosis pubis

The pubic hairs are the normal habitat of *Pthirus pubis* but it may also infect facial hair, eyelashes, general body hair and rarely the frontal margin of the scalp. Pubic infestation is usually sexually transmitted but bedding and towels may be responsible. Clinical signs may be minimal, even with severe itching, but excoriated papules and flat blue macules containing altered blood pigment may be seen as may evidence of secondary infection or eczematization. Eyelash infestation in children may occur from innocent close contact with an infected adult but the possibility of sexual abuse must always be considered.

Management of pediculosis

The management of pediculosis corporis involves removing the infestation from clothing with hot water laundering, hot electric drying, hot ironing or dry cleaning.

Permethrin shampoo is an effective pediculocide for scalp infestations but the efficacy as an ovicide is less certain and repeat application after a few days is recommended. Removal of nits with a fine comb can be facilitated by prior wrapping of the scalp for 1–2 h in a towel soaked in vinegar which softens the chitin.

Pediculosis pubis is treated with 5% permethrin cream applied for 12 h to all hairy areas in the anogenital region, repeated after 1 week. Sexual contacts should be treated simultaneously and all underclothing appropriately laundered.

Pediculosis of eyelashes is best treated with petroleum jelly applied thickly twice a day for a week.

URTICARIA AND ERYTHEMAS

URTICARIA

The most characteristic feature of urticaria (nettle rash or hives) is its transience. Erythematous swellings develop in the skin, which last for a few hours before disappearing. The urticarial wheals may be of variable size, and may have an obvious annular configuration. Angioedema (giant urticaria) is a variant of urticaria which affects the face and genital region and mainly involves the subcutaneous tissues with resultant gross swelling of the tissues.

Urticaria is common in all age groups, and is particularly so in children. In children, widespread urticaria is often the presenting feature of a number of viral infections, when it is accompanied by fever and malaise. It is due to increased permeability of capillaries or other small vessels, with resultant transudation of fluid. Several chemical mediators are involved, which are mainly released from mast cells: these include histamine, prostaglandins and leukotrienes. Mast cell degranulation results from both immune (IgE, complement) and non-immune mechanisms.

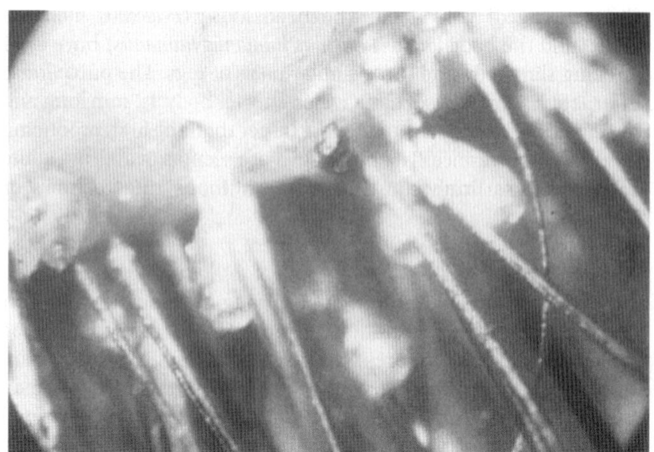

Fig. 28.41 Pediculosis of eyelid.

IgE-mediated urticaria and angioedema

Urticaria and angioedema following ingestion of food allergens is quite common in children with atopic eczema, and is often IgE mediated (confirmed by positive skin prick tests or radioallergosorbent tests). Swelling of the lips and tongue develops immediately after ingestion of the food, and contact urticaria may be seen if the food is in contact with the skin. If enough food allergen is ingested vomiting and diarrhea may occur, and the child may develop an asthmatic attack: generalized anaphylaxis may occur in a few children, especially with nuts. Widespread urticaria is common, usually occurring within 1 h of ingestion of the food, which may last for a few hours. Common foods involved in such reactions include hens' eggs, cows' milk, fish, nuts and soya. Food allergy is commonly outgrown by the age of 5 years although this is less likely for peanut and nut allergy.[44] IgE-mediated urticaria may also follow drug administration, particularly penicillin, and also insect stings, for example by bees or wasps.

Urticaria due to foods and drugs which is not apparently immunologically mediated

Certain foods such as strawberries, tomatoes and chocolate cause urticaria where no IgE-mediated mechanisms can be demonstrated. It seems likely that this is a direct effect on mast cells, and is similar to that caused by tartrazine (a common coloring in foods), benzoates and salicylates. Aspirin and morphine also commonly cause urticaria by a non-immunological mechanism.

Chronic idiopathic urticaria

This type of urticaria is not very common in children. The urticaria may recur repeatedly for a period of years, with often daily exacerbations.

Papular urticaria

This is a very common condition in children, and results from insect, flea or mite bites. In Britain dog, cat and bird fleas are the usual cause, but human fleas, bed bugs, mosquitoes and dog lice may be implicated. The child presents with papules and blisters on exposed skin such as the legs and arms. Each lasts for about 7–10 days before resolving.

It often takes the parents quite a lot of convincing of the cause of the condition. The family pet should be inspected and treated if necessary. In recurrent cases it is worth admitting the child to hospital upon which the child's rash will promptly disappear.

Treatment of urticaria

The management of a child with urticaria depends on the cause. If a food is implicated, this is usually fairly obvious, except perhaps in infants where skin prick testing may be helpful. Any food implicated should be withdrawn from the diet, though it may be possible to reintroduce it when the child is older. In chronic idiopathic urticaria, by definition no cause is found but certain ingested chemicals in foods (e.g. salicylates, benzoates, food colorings) may make it worse. A non-sedating H1 antihistamine can be given.

MASTOCYTOSIS

This refers to a group of conditions whose signs and symptoms are due to the infiltration of tissues by mast cells and to the release of the chemical mediators contained in these cells. Local effects include erythema and swelling of lesions on rubbing (Darier's sign), dermographism, pruritus, hemorrhage and blistering. General effects include generalized pruritus, fever and flushing; tachycardia and hypotension; headache and irritability; vomiting, diarrhea, increased salivation and peptic ulceration; rhinorrhea and bronchospasm; increased lacrimation; and a generalized hemorrhagic diathesis.

Mastocytosis may present in childhood or adult life. A retrospective review of 173 pediatric cases confirms that the different forms of the disease seen in childhood are mastocytomas, urticaria pigmentosa, diffuse cutaneous mastocytosis and rarely systemic mastocytosis.[45]

Mastocytoma

This is a round to oval flesh-colored to yellowish nodule or plaque usually present at birth or appearing in the first months of life (Fig. 28.42). Although usually solitary, some children develop a number of mastocytomas particularly on arms or trunk. They usually regress spontaneously over a few years but while present they urticate on rubbing, and blisters, which may be hemorrhagic, often occur in infancy. These children commonly have attacks of generalized flushing but other symptoms and signs of mediator release are rare.

Urticaria pigmentosa

Pigmented multiple macules, with occasional papules, nodules or plaques occur in a widespread distribution, particularly involving the trunk (Fig. 28.43). The onset is usually between 1 and 9 months of age. The lesions erupt over 1–2 months, then become static and finally in most cases resolve by adolescence. They are usually pruritic and may blister. Urtication occurs. There may be dermographism in nearby clinically normal skin. Generalized pruritus and flushing may occur, and less frequently other signs of mediator release.

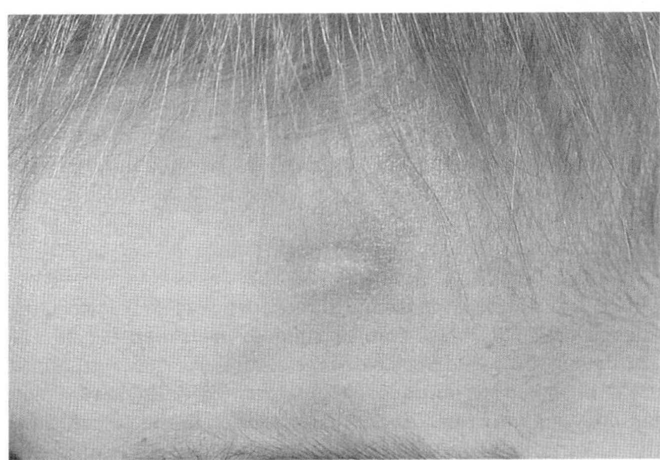

Fig. 28.42 Mastocytoma.

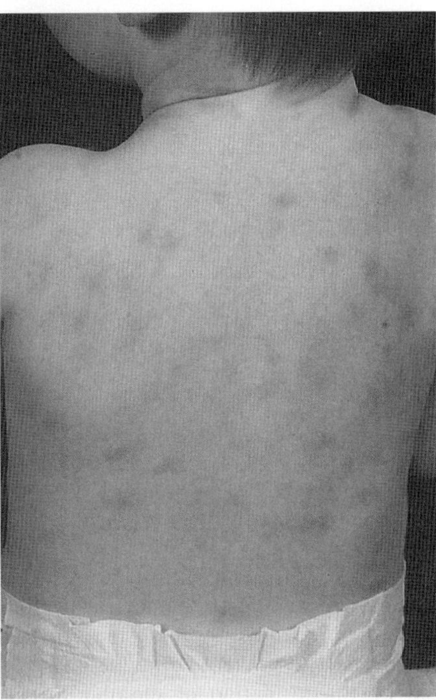

Fig. 28.43 Urticaria pigmentosa.

Diffuse cutaneous mastocytosis

This is a rare form of mastocytosis with the onset usually at birth. Massive mast cell infiltration into the skin produces a diffuse thickening with associated edema, erythema and blistering. The skin may have a leathergrain or peau d'orange appearance or be nodular or verrucose. The color is yellowish or red. Blistering is prominent and may be so severe that the presentation is that of a generalized bullous disease. The full spectrum of local and systemic symptoms and signs of mediator release may be seen. These are usually severe and disabling and may be life threatening. The cutaneous lesions tend to improve with time but some degree of infiltration usually remains.

Systemic mastocytosis

This implies the infiltration of mast cells into organs other than the skin, and not simply systemic features due to the release of mediators from cutaneous mast cell infiltrates. It is extremely rare in childhood and is almost always associated with diffuse cutaneous involvement in this age group. Hepatosplenomegaly and lymphadenopathy may occur; the cells may infiltrate renal parenchyma and gastrointestinal mucosa; skeletal involvement produces both osteoporotic and osteosclerotic lesions. Mast cell leukemia is a very rare complication.

Management

In general, mastocytosis is a self-limiting disease. If an isolated lesion is producing generalized flushing, excision can be considered. The patient should carry a list of agents (i.e. aspirin, morphine, codeine, d-tubocurarine, scopolamine, quinine, thiamin, procaine, polymixin B and radiographic contrast media) which stimulate mast cell degranulation and avoid these where possible. Physical trauma to the lesions should be avoided.

H1 antihistamines are rarely effective in controlling symptoms and signs of mediator release but combined with H2 blockers they may be more effective. In more severe cases oral disodium cromoglycate, ketotifen and nifedipine may be tried.

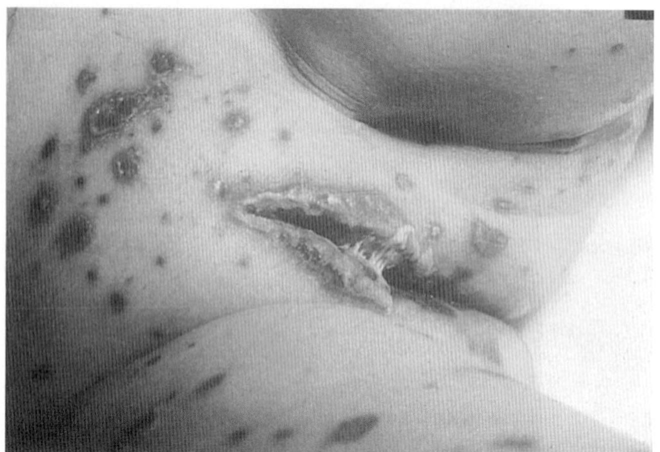

Fig. 28.44 Erythema multiforme, Stevens–Johnson: perineal.

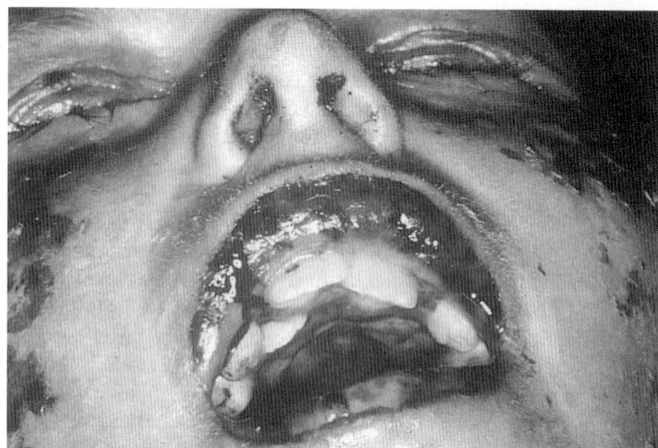

Fig. 28.45 Erythema multiforme, Stevens–Johnson: oral.

ERYTHEMA MULTIFORME

This is an uncommon condition in children which tends to follow herpes simplex infection, mycoplasma pneumonia and sulfonamide ingestion (Figs 28.44 and 28.45). Clinically, it is characterized by the formation of circular target lesions on the limbs, with a red periphery and blue (often bullous) center. Stomatitis and genital involvement are common. The rash of erythema multiforme, unlike urticaria, for which it is often mistaken is fixed with lesions lasting days as compared to hours in urticaria. The lesions may be widespread, and if extensive erosions are present at two or more mucosal sites the diagnosis of Stevens–Johnson syndrome (SJS) can be made. SJS in turn overlaps both clinically and histologically with toxic epidermal necrolysis. The rash of erythema multiforme usually fades within 10 days but may recur, particularly in the case of erythema multiforme following recurrent herpes simplex infections. No randomized controlled trials have been performed for treatment childhood erythema multiforme and there is therefore no evidence to recommend oral steroids. However, one double-blind, placebo-controlled study in adults found benefit with continuous aciclovir in recurrent erythema multiforme.[46]

VESICOBULLOUS DISORDERS

DERMATITIS HERPETIFORMIS

Dermatitis herpetiformis is associated with gluten-sensitive enteropathy (celiac disease), and in a study of 57 children only 3 (5%) had normal jejunal biospies.[47] Deposition of IgA in the dermal papillae of skin is the hallmark of the disorder.

It is rare before the age of 2 years, and presents with small intensely itchy blisters symmetrically on the elbows, knees, shoulders and buttocks. The correct treatment is a gluten-free diet, when the blisters, and small bowel mucosa, should resolve (permanently) within 2 years: concomitant treatment with dapsone or sulfapyridine is usually required.

BULLOUS PEMPHIGOID

This is a rare blistering disease, which results from the formation of IgG antibodies to the basement membrane zone of the epidermis. The child presents with large and widespread blisters, which may (as in chronic bullous disease of childhood) be most marked on the face and around the genitalia. The hands and feet are more frequently involved in children 1 year or younger compared to older age groups. The diagnosis is confirmed by immunofluorescence of skin biopsy or serum (with appropriate substrate) to demonstrate antibasement membrane zone antibodies. Treatment is with oral steroids, which should be tapered off as the condition allows. In most the disease is self-limiting.

PEMPHIGUS

Pemphigus is also rare in children, the most common types being pemphigus vulgaris and foliaceus. The blistering is less evident than in pemphigoid, though there may be widespread plaques and erosions. Over 50% of children with pemphigus vulgaris present with erosive stomatitis. The diagnosis is confirmed by immunofluorescence studies of skin and serum, which demonstrate IgG antibodies to the intercellular substance of the keratinocytes in the epidermis. Treatment is with oral steroids, as in pemphigoid.

CHRONIC BULLOUS DISEASE OF CHILDHOOD

It is most commonly seen in young children, with blistering which is around the mouth, neck and genital regions (Fig. 28.46) Genital blistering may be mistaken for herpes simplex infection. Immunofluorescence studies of skin show linear IgA deposition along the basement membrane zone of the epidermis with evidence of circulating IgA antibodies in up to 80%.

Treatment with dapsone or sulfapyridine usually clears the blisters very effectively. The disease is self-limiting, after months or years.

VASCULITIS

Vasculitis can be classified according to the size and nature of the vessel and the infiltrate.[48]

HENOCH–SCHÖNLEIN PURPURA

This is a distinct subset within the spectrum of leukocytoclastic (allergic) vasculitis that is relatively common in children (Fig. 28.47). The damage occurs to small blood vessels in the dermis, resulting in the development of purpura (often palpable) over the lower limbs, buttocks and forearms. Other organs involved in the vasculitis are the kidneys and intestinal vessels, resulting in proteinuria and hematuria, abdominal pain and gastrointestinal hemorrhage. In

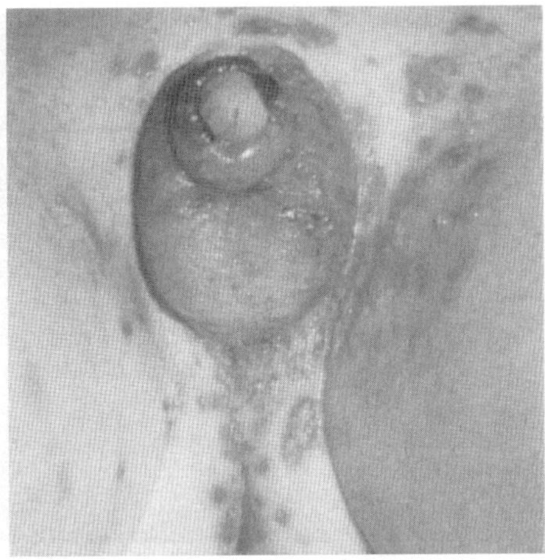

Fig. 28.46 Chronic bullous disease of childhood.

some arthralgia is also prominent. It usually follows a virus or respiratory infection, the vasculitis resulting from deposition of immune complexes in the vessels of the skin, kidneys and intestines, with complement activation and resultant polymorph infiltration. In Henoch–Schönlein purpura the immunoglobulin deposited is IgA, whereas in other types of vasculitis it is IgG.

The prognosis is very variable. In most children the condition is self-limiting; others may develop renal failure (usually treatable with dialysis or renal transplant) or may die of gastrointestinal hemorrhage.

URTICARIAL VASCULITIS

This is another variant of allergic vasculitis. The urticarial wheals last for several days, unlike those in 'classical' urticaria, where they last for a few hours. Urticarial vasculitis is often accompanied by arthralgia and skin lesions may resolve with purpura. A skin biopsy shows leukocytoclastic vasculitis, and complement studies may reveal low CH50 and C3 levels. It may result from drug ingestion or viral infection, or may be a feature of lupus erythematosus.

ERYTHEMA NODOSUM

This is rare in young children. It is a type of vasculitis affecting initially deep, dermal venules with subsequent development of a septal panniculitis. Clinically, erythematous nodules develop, usually on the shins though sometimes on the thighs and forearms.

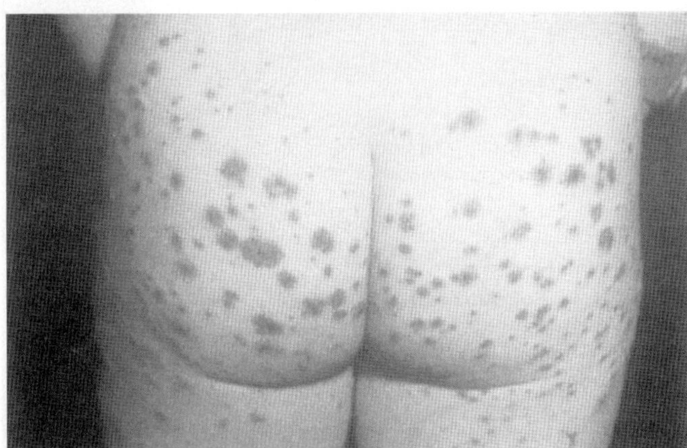

Fig. 28.47 Henoch–Schönlein purpura.

They last for about 2–3 weeks and are characteristically tender. They resolve leaving bruising, but then tend to recur in crops. Causes include streptococcal infections, sarcoidosis, tuberculosis and sulfonamide ingestion: often it occurs without obvious reason. Treatment is of the underlying cause. Usually it resolves spontaneously, but occasionally treatment with oral steroids is indicated.

ECZEMA AND DERMATITIS

Eczema and dermatitis are synonymous and are very often used interchangeably.

ATOPIC ECZEMA

Atopy is a genetically determined disorder with an increased tendency to form IgE antibody to inhalants and foods (see Ch. XX). There is increased susceptibility to asthma, allergic rhinitis and atopic eczema (Figs 28.48 and 28.49). Although eczema may begin at any age, in 75% of patients first signs are present by 6 months.

Clinical features

The characteristic clinical features are erythema, generalized dryness and itching which leads to excoriations and ultimately lichenification or thickening of the skin, particularly in children older than 2 years. Involvement of the whole cutaneous surface may occur but the predominant areas are the face in infants, extensor aspects of the limbs as the child begins to crawl, and the limb flexures in older children. In severe cases the whole skin may be erythematous and in these patients white dermographism is often a prominent feature: this indicates that the condition is likely to be unstable and difficult.

Complications

Patients with atopic eczema may develop secondary bacterial infection which presents either as impetigo or folliculitis, or simply as worsening eczema. Mollusca contagiosa appear more common, although there are no prevalence studies to confirm this. Atopic patients are at risk of developing severe widespread herpes simplex infections. The usual childhood immunizations are quite safe.

Management

A comprehensive systematic review of all treatments for atopic eczema has been recently published.[49] This review provides an up-to-date collection of all randomized controlled trials and summarizes the available data. It is clear that although emollients and topical steroids are the mainstays of treatment there are very few objective data to recommend their use. Despite this, clinical practice suggests that they are very helpful in the management of atopic eczema (see also Ch. 31).

Time should be taken in discussing factors that act as external irritants. Wool is a major irritant and should never be worn in direct contact with the skin. It is important to warn that wool contact may also occur with the parents' clothing, carpets, car seat and stroller covers, blankets and toys. Cotton material is always safe and cotton polyester combinations rarely irritate, but acrylic may be as troublesome as wool. Perfumed and medicated products, disinfectants and strong cleansers should be avoided. Soap in excess and bubble baths overdry the skin, so soap substitutes should be used.

It should be emphasized to parents that topical steroids are safe as long as these are used only where and when there is active eczema. In general, ointment bases, which are more emollient, are preferred. Only 1% hydrocortisone should be used on the face and in the groin but fluorinated steroids may be used elsewhere for short

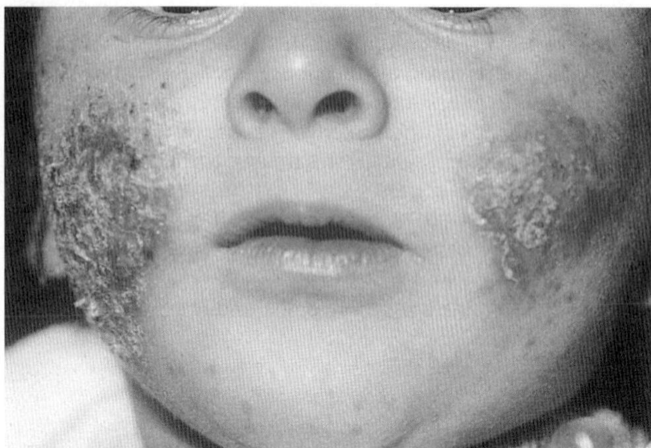

Fig. 28.48 Atopic eczema: facial in young infant.

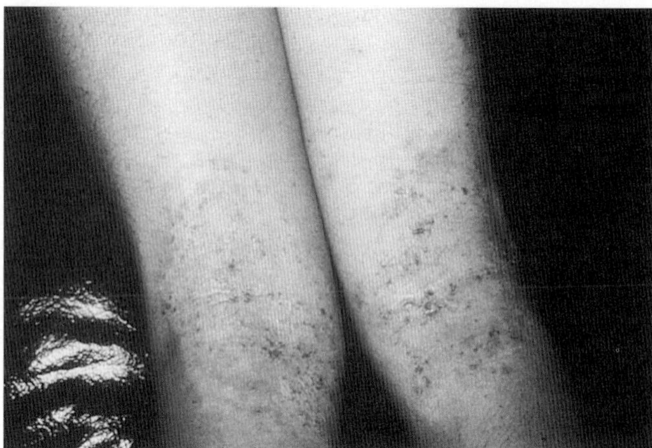

Fig. 28.49 Atopic eczema: flexural in older child.

periods. Patients and parents should be educated regarding the quantities of creams necessary to apply and guidance has been published.[50]

Second line therapy for severe cases or those not responding to routine treatment, includes paste bandages or wet wraps. The latter involves applying two layers of tubular cotton bandages over topical steroids and emollients on the skin. The inner bandage is soaked in warm water prior to application. These dressings increase the hydration of the skin, physically prevent scratching, immediately reduce itching and enhance the penetration of topical steroids. In infants only weak steroids should be used because of the risk of absorption. The use of dressings should be adequately supervised and used for no more than a few days at a time with topical steroids.

Obvious secondary bacterial infection should be treated with oral antibiotics. However, these are indicated in most patients with severe weeping eczema even in the absence of clinically obvious infection. Although current randomized controlled trial evidence does not support the routine use of antihistamines in atopic eczema many parents say that their child appears to be more comfortable at night with less scratching after a nocturnal dose of a sedative antihistamine. Oral steroids should be avoided because a severe rebound can occur on withdrawal and after several courses the eczema is rendered very unstable.

Third line treatments include phototherapy (narrow band UVB or psoralen plus UVA), ciclosporin (although not yet licensed in the UK for pediatric eczema)[51] and azathioprine. More recently topical FK506 (tacrolimus)[52] and topical pimecrolimus[53] look promising alternative therapies. A pilot study also suggests montelukast might be beneficial.[54]

Chinese herbal medicine (CHM) has been evaluated and 1 year follow-up of children treated with CHM showed good, sustained improvement in nearly 50% although 1 out of 37 developed abnormal liver function tests and 14 withdrew due to lack of efficacy or unpalatability.[55]

In children with a reported worsening of eczema after eating it is important first to take a careful history in order to exclude contact urticaria, a rapid development of redness and/or wheals at the site of contact with the food antigen. Foods which cause this reaction should be avoided. Otherwise no alteration to the child's diet should be considered unless the eczema has failed to respond to conventional topical therapy. Dietary manipulation in the management of refractory eczema is covered in Chapter 31. The role of the dust mite in these severe cases is covered in the same section.

There is increasing interest in the primary prevention of atopic disease. Probiotics are cultures of potentially beneficial bacteria and a randomized controlled trial of *Lactobacillus* GG was effective in the early prevention of atopic disease in children at high risk.[56]

As a child becomes older discussion about future careers is important as certain occupations are likely to aggravate the skin, such as hairdressing or car mechanics. It is important to develop a trusting and cooperative relationship with the patient and his parents as they will require much encouragement to help them cope with this distressing condition.

DISCOID ECZEMA (NUMMULAR ECZEMA)

In children this is often a manifestation of the atopic state. Well-defined patches of acute eczema occur in a strikingly symmetrical distribution (Fig. 28.50). In infants the commonest sites are the upper back and the tops of the shoulders; in older patients the extensor aspects of the limbs are particularly involved. The lesions may be very thick and exudative and they are very itchy. They have to be distinguished from tinea and impetigo which are less symmetrical and psoriasis which is rarely moist. The management involves emollients and topical steroids as for atopic dermatitis, with the continued use of emollient helping to prevent recurrences.

PITYRIASIS ALBA

This condition appears as poorly defined, slightly scaly, hypopigmented patches occurring particularly on the face and the

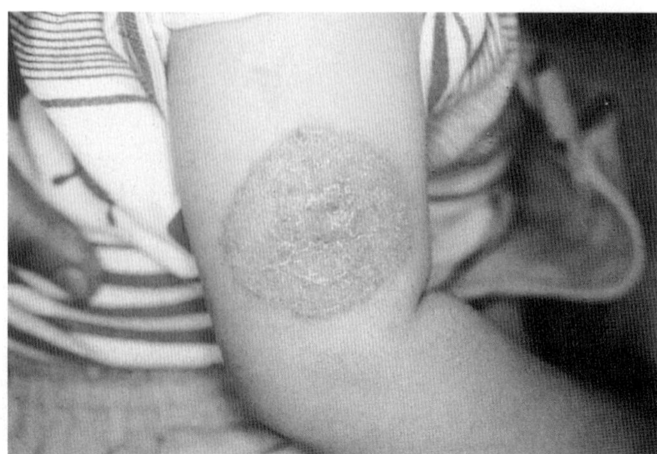

Fig. 28.50 Discoid eczema.

upper arms. It probably represents a very mild eczema which, however, produces a striking postinflammatory hypopigmentation. Occasionally some areas will show erythema and more definite eczematous changes. The condition is more common in atopics. The mild irritation and signs of mild eczema respond to emollients and weak topical corticosteroids but the hypopigmentation may be very persistent and require sun exposure over a prolonged period before repigmentation is complete. Most lesions clear by puberty. The condition should be differentiated from vitiligo where there is total depigmentation and no scale and from tinea versicolor which has very well demarcated lesions with very fine branny scaling.

SEBORRHEIC DERMATITIS

This is a condition of infancy and adult life; patients develop dermatitis at sites of greatest sebum production.

The rash has an erythematous background and a greasy yellow scale. In the flexures the scale may be absent and a glazed erythema the only sign. Scaling is particularly prominent on the scalp, producing the so-called 'cradle cap'. The main areas of involvement are scalp, glabella, behind and inside the ears, nasolabial folds, axillae and groin and in infants the neck and limb flexures. In the flexural areas candidiasis is commonly superimposed. The rash is usually asymptomatic.

Various conditions mimic seborrheic dermatitis including drug reactions (in children particularly due to phenytoin sodium), early psoriasis and Langerhans' cell histiocytosis. These should be considered when what appears to be a seborrheic dermatitis occurs at an unexpected age or fails to respond to therapy.

Seborrheic dermatitis usually responds quickly to weak topical corticosteroid preparations with the addition of an anticandidal agent for the flexural areas. On the scalp, sulfur and salicylic acid preparations left on overnight are usually more effective than corticosteroids. If the scale is very thick, warmed olive or paraffin oil can be used to soften it before the cream is applied. It should be emphasized that the disorder will tend to recur through infancy.

NAPKIN DERMATITIS

In all napkin dermatitis there is a combination of the elements of moisture, candidiasis and dermatitis, either seborrheic or primary irritant from the urine and feces. Miliaria or sweat duct occlusion is another common feature. The newer superabsorbent disposable napkins are often preferable to cloth napkins. A combination cream of 1% hydrocortisone and antimonilial agent is usually effective and a silicone or zinc barrier cream may be added to protect the skin against moisture. There will usually be a quick response to therapy but recurrences are to be expected.

ALLERGIC CONTACT ECZEMA

Allergic contact eczema is one of the main examples of delayed type hypersensitivity in the skin. It is much less common in children than in adults, probably due to lack of contact with sensitizing chemicals.

Clinically, allergic contact eczema is characterized by the development of erythema and small blisters (microvesiculation) at the site of contact with the allergen. The commonest allergen in children is nickel, which is contained in metal clips and studs (e.g. jeans studs) and in non-gold earrings. It seems likely that a number of children are sensitized following piercing of the ears, and by wearing costume jewelry earrings. Other contact allergens in children include plants such as *Rhus* (particularly in the USA and Australia) (Fig. 28.51), chemicals used in rubber production and topical medications such as neomycin and gentamicin.

Identification of the allergen is essential, and this is carried out by patch testing the child. The allergen is dissolved in a suitable vehicle (e.g. petrolatum) and applied in an aluminum chamber to the back of the child. This is removed at 48 h, and note of erythema and microvesication is taken; a further reading is performed at 96 h. Interpretation requires expertise, as not all reactions are necessarily specific delayed type hypersensitivity reactions.

CONNECTIVE TISSUE DISEASES (Ch. 27)

LUPUS ERYTHEMATOSUS (LE)

This is rare in children but neonatal lupus erythematosus is of considerable importance.

Neonatal lupus erythematosus

This occurs due to the passage of maternal antibodies through the placenta (Fig. 28.52), where the mother suffers from systemic LE, subacute cutaneous LE or the sicca syndrome. In 50% of cases the mother is asymptomatic but the vast majority have SS-A (anti-Ro) antibodies. The most important feature of neonatal LE is heart block of varying degrees. This is usually permanent, and without pacing there is a significant mortality (Ch. 19). Other features include autoimmune hemolytic anemia, thrombocytopenia, hepatitis, pneumonitis and splenomegaly.

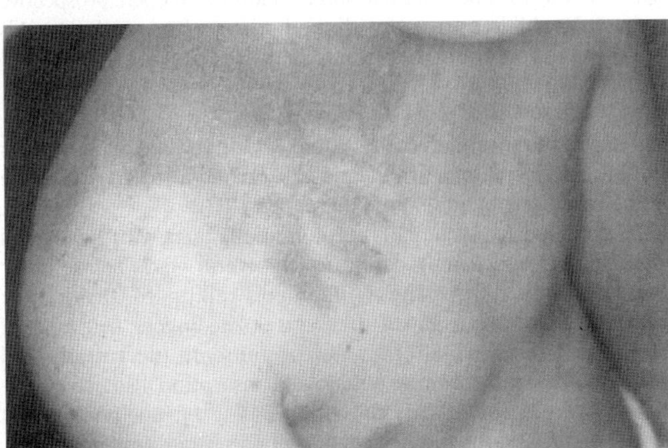

Fig. 28.51 Plant (*Rhus*) dermatitis.

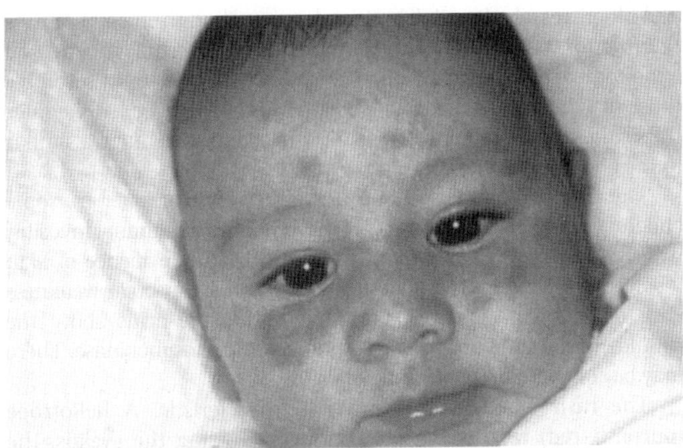

Fig. 28.52 Neonatal lupus erythematosus.

The skin lesions resemble those of subacute cutaneous LE in the adult, occurring on the face, neck and scalp, with erythematous macules or plaques with scaling. They are often present at birth, and disappear within the first year of life. There may also be photosensitivity. A skin biopsy will usually show the features of adult LE with liquefaction degeneration of the basal keratinocytes and a periappendageal lymphocytic infiltrate. Direct immunofluorescence is positive in 50% of infants, with a band-like deposition of IgG and complement at the dermoepidermal junction.

Treatment of the skin is with 1% hydrocortisone cream and protection from the sun.

Lupus erythematosus in the older child

This takes two main forms: systemic LE and discoid LE. It is thought that this is a spectrum of disease, as sometimes patients with discoid LE will progress to systemic LE and a proportion of those with discoid LE have circulating antinuclear antibodies, anemia, leukopenia and thrombocytopenia and other features such as Raynaud's phenomenon and arthralgia.

Discoid lupus erythematosus

This usually affects girls, who develop erythematous plaques on the face, the arms and dorsum of the hands. The most commonly affected parts of the face are the nose and the cheeks. Involvement of the scalp usually leads to scarring alopecia. Histological examination of the plaques shows characteristic liquefaction degeneration of the basal cell layer of the epidermis, and a periappendageal lymphocytic infiltrate in the dermis.

There may be mild anemia, leukopenia or thrombocytopenia and some children will have circulating antinuclear antibodies.

The prognosis is variable, as in some the plaques will resolve spontaneously whereas in others they tend to be persistent. Avoidance of sun exposure by the use of sunscreens and a hat is important.

Systemic lupus erythematosus

As in discoid LE, the systemic form is more common in girls. It is a multisystem connective tissue disease which often carries a poor prognosis, due to renal involvement. This is discussed fully in Chapter 27. The skin manifestations include a butterfly rash on the face, discoid plaques usually on the face, reticulate livedo most marked on the legs, panniculitis, vasculitic ulcers, cuticular hemorrhages at the fingernail folds, and alopecia.

DERMATOMYOSITIS

This is a rare connective tissue disease affecting the skin, muscle and blood vessels. Its etiology is unknown, though in some adults there is an association with carcinomas of internal viscera and lymphomas. The histological changes in the skin may resemble those of LE, though the dermal edema is more marked. In the later stages the dermis becomes sclerotic, and the picture may be similar to the changes in scleroderma.

The clinical manifestations are extremely variable. In some children the skin signs may be very prominent with minimal myositis, whereas in others there is polymyositis with little evidence of skin involvement. Myositis is manifested by a proximal muscular weakness with difficulty in climbing stairs and raising the arms above the shoulder girdle, and by a raised serum creatine phosphokinase. There may be concomitant fever and malaise.

The rash when present is very characteristic. A heliotrope (purplish–red) rash occurs on the face involving the eyelids, the forehead and upper cheeks. There may be marked edema of the hands and arms with an erythematous linear rash over the dorsum of the hands with nail fold telangiectasia. Erythema of the scalp may develop and there may be marked alopecia. Reticulate livedo is seen in some, and may lead to ulceration of the skin.

Calcification is common in children, affecting more than 50% of cases. It primarily involves the muscles, particularly around the pelvic and shoulder girdles, and may cause marked functional disability. It also occurs in the subcutaneous tissues, and there may be extrusion through the skin with ulceration.

The course of the disease is variable, but there is generally a good prognosis in children. Death may occur due to respiratory failure, difficulty in swallowing, or the side-effects of steroid therapy.

Treatment with oral corticosteroids is required with high doses of prednisone (1–2 mg/kg initially) tapering to a maintenance dose which should be carried on for months or years, till the serum creatine phosphokinase returns to normal and the signs of the disease have disappeared. Physiotherapy may be useful to prevent contractures.

SCLERODERMA

In children this may take two forms: morphea (localized scleroderma), which is relatively common, and systemic sclerosis which is very rare.

Morphea

This is a localized and benign form of scleroderma, though it can cause quite marked disfigurement. On histological examination, the dermis is at first edematous with swelling and degeneration of the collagen fibrils, with later thickening of the dermis and loss of appendages. The etiology of the condition is unknown.

The areas of morphea occur usually as either plaques or linear lesions of sclerosis in the skin. These are at first purplish in color, and later become white and waxy. Hairs are lost within the area, with loss of sweating. They occur on the trunk and limbs. When they involve a limb (usually linear lesions), they may involve muscles and bone leading to shortening of the limb.

A particular disfigurement which results from morphea is the so-called 'coup de sabre', which occurs in the frontoparietal area. This starts with contraction of the skin over the affected area with development of an ivory plaque with hyperpigmentation at the edge and telangiectatic vessels coursing over it. The resulting groove may extend downwards, affecting the mouth and mandible. The tongue may be atrophic on the affected side, and there may be marked alopecia. There is marked facial asymmetry with consequent disfigurement.

There is no effective treatment for morphea but intralesional triamcinolone may be helpful in some children. An open, prospective study of 10 children treated with methotrexate and corticosteroids showed a median time to response in nine patients of 3 months.[57]

Systemic sclerosis

This is very rare in children. The etiology is unknown, but as similar changes may be seen in graft versus host reactions, it may be some sort of rejection phenomenon.

In the majority of patients the condition starts with Raynaud's phenomenon which may continue for several years before other manifestations occur. These include: swelling of the hands; sclerodactyly with atrophy of the pulps of the fingers; calcinosis of the finger pulps which may be prominent; ulceration; and gangrene. In some, terminal phalangeal absorption also occurs.

Later, other features occur with beaking of the nose, radial furrowing around the mouth which becomes smaller, macroglossia, esophageal dilatation and stricture, and abnormal colonic peristalsis.

The prognosis is variable, and depends on internal organ involvement, though most patients continue with the condition for many years with increasing deformity. No formal trials have evaluated the wide range of potential immunosuppressive therapies.

LICHEN SCLEROSUS

The etiology of lichen sclerosus is unknown but may show some overlap with morphea. It has a predilection for genital and perianal skin. It is more common in females and usually presents with itch although in children may be asymptomatic. In its early stages the appearances are of erythema and excoriations with subsequent development of well-defined pale atrophic areas. The lesions often occur in a figure of eight pattern around the vulva and anal region. This condition may be misdiagnosed as sexual abuse. In approximately 10% extragenital lesions will also be present. In boys, the usual history is of balanitis and tightening of the foreskin which can progress to phimosis (balanitis xerotica obliterans). Potent topical steroids are the treatment of choice.[58] The overall prognosis is good but for cases that persist long term follow-up is recommended because of the risk of malignant change in adults.

IDIOPATHIC PHOTOSENSITIVITY ERUPTIONS

Before considering a child to have an idiopathic photosensitivity eruption, it is important to exclude one of the hereditary diseases (q.v.), and photosensitive drug eruptions which are common and may be caused by a number of drugs (notably sulfonamides, tetracyclines and phenothiazines).

POLYMORPHIC LIGHT ERUPTION (PLE)

About 20% of patients with PLE present before the age of 10 years. A delayed reaction occurring several hours or the next day after exposure to the sun results in erythema, burning and itching, followed by papule and plaque formation. With avoidance of sun exposure this reaction will settle but will usually relapse when the child is exposed to the sun again. It usually presents during the summer, but in some children it is most marked in the spring and early summer, with remission of the symptoms in midsummer with 'hardening' of the skin. Juvenile spring eruption is probably a localized variant of PLE with papules and vesicles confined to the helices of the ears.

Most children with PLE continue into adulthood with it. Action spectrum studies are usually normal, and are therefore unhelpful. Prevention of PLE depends on adequate topical photoprotection with sunscreens. In those children with severe PLE, photochemotherapy with oral psoralen and UVA light may be helpful.

ACTINIC PRURIGO

This condition is clinically similar to PLE but is now recognized to be a separate entity. It is significantly associated with the haplotype HLA-DR4/DRB1*0407.[59] Actinic prurigo nearly always develops in early childhood and 80% of patients are female. There is usually progressive improvement in adolescence.

Clinically all exposed sites are affected, including face, lips, neck, ears, arms, dorsum of hands and lower legs. In the majority there is also involvement of covered skin, though to a lesser extent. It is worse during summer months but very often persists even in winter. In most cases there is a family history and there is also a strong association with atopy.

Action spectrum studies are abnormal in the majority with sensitivity to both UVA and UVB; however, in some children these studies are normal. Treatment is similar to that of PLE, but thalidomide has also been found to be particularly effective in this condition.

HYDROA VACCINIFORME

This is a very rare condition which invariably starts in childhood. On exposure to sunlight the child develops tingling and erythema followed by blistering and umbilicated papules on the face, ears, arms and dorsum of hands. These lead to crusting and varioliform scars.

Action spectrum studies are abnormal with sensitivity mainly involving UVA. Treatment is generally unsatisfactory, though broad spectrum topical sunscreens may be helpful.

SKIN DISEASES OF THE NEONATE

ERYTHEMA TOXICUM NEONATORUM

This is a transient condition of unknown etiology occurring in up to 70% of neonates. The onset is from birth to 14 days but most cases start between day 1 and day 4. The commonest lesions are erythematous macules and papules but in some cases pustules appear. Lesions occur anywhere on the body surface except palms and soles but with a predilection for face and trunk. In cases present at birth, lesions are more acrally distributed and are often pustular. A peripheral blood eosinophilia is present and smears from pustules demonstrate sheets of eosinophils. The condition usually resolves in 2–3 days but, rarely, may persist for several weeks.

Recognition of this entity is important to avoid unnecessary investigations of serious neonatal infections.

TRANSIENT NEONATAL PUSTULAR DERMATOSIS

This is a benign condition in which superficial pustules are present at birth; it is rare for further lesions to develop postnatally. The pustules rupture within 24 h, developing a brown crust that separates after a few days to leave normal skin or a hyperpigmented macule in dark-skinned individuals. Lesions occur mainly on chin, upper anterior trunk, lower back and buttocks. They are asymptomatic and the infant is otherwise well. Lesions are sterile on culture enabling differentiation from important neonatal infections. If hyperpigmented macules occur, they resolve over 3–4 months.

ACROPUSTULOSIS OF INFANCY

This is a benign condition of unknown etiology occurring in otherwise healthy infants. The onset is usually in the neonatal period but may be delayed for some months. Recurrent crops of papules which quickly evolve into 2–4 mm vesicopustules occur, most commonly on the palms and soles and dorsa of hands and feet. Initially each crop takes 1–2 weeks to settle and new crops occur every 2–3 weeks. As time goes on the crops occur less frequently and the episodes are less severe and of shorter duration. Lesions are pruritic but are accompanied by no systemic symptoms. The condition finally resolves by 2–3 years.

The disease must be differentiated from other neonatal pustular conditions including herpes simplex, impetigo, scabies and candidiasis. Cultures of the lesions of infantile acropustulosis are sterile. A clinically identical condition can occur also as a postscabetic reaction in infants who have been successfully treated for scabies.

Topical therapy is usually ineffective. Oral antihistamines can be used if pruritus is severe.

MILIA

These represent retention cysts of the pilosebaceous follicles. They occur in approximately 50% of neonates as firm pearly white 1–2 mm papules particularly on the face. They usually disappear by 4 weeks of age. Epstein's pearls are epidermal cysts on the palate present in the majority of newborns. Persistent milia may be a marker for certain syndromes including Bazex's syndrome, orofaciodigital syndrome type I and Marie–Unna hypotrichosis.

SUBCUTANEOUS FAT NECROSIS OF THE NEWBORN

This is a necrosis of subcutaneous fat in the newborn probably induced by ischemia. It occurs usually in healthy full-term infants. Often, however, there is a history of a difficult labor and delivery with such complications as prolonged labor, fetal distress, perinatal asphyxia due to meconium aspiration or other cause and forceps delivery. The condition has also been reported in an infant following hypothermic cardiac surgery.

The lesions appear between the second and third weeks of life as non-tender, firm, skin-colored or red–purple nodules or plaques occurring particularly on buttocks, shoulders, upper back, proximal limbs and cheeks. New nodules may develop over several weeks. They usually disappear spontaneously without complication in several months leaving no trace. However, sometimes they become fluctuant, ulcerate or calcify. In patients with calcified lesions hypercalcemia may develop.

Fluctuant lesions should be aspirated, secondary infection should be dealt with if it complicates ulcerated lesions, and serum calcium levels should be monitored in the presence of calcified lesions. Otherwise management involves observation and reassurance.

CUTIS MARMORATA (CONGENITAL LIVEDO RETICULARIS)

This term usually refers to a transient benign physiological vascular reaction occurring in both premature and full-term infants as a response to minor cooling. A blue or purple discoloration in a marbled or reticulate pattern occurs on trunk and limbs. It lasts minutes to hours but reverses quickly on warming the infant. The tendency to the condition lasts for weeks or months.

There are a number of important conditions which may be associated with more severe and persistent cutis marmorata. These include Down syndrome, trisomy 18, homocystinuria, de Lange syndrome, neonatal lupus and congenital hypothyroidism. A nevoid vascular disorder, cutis marmorata telangiectatica congenita, presents with reticulate purple lesions but the distribution is often segmental rather than generalized and atrophy and ulceration may occur in the affected areas.

MILIARIA (PRICKLY HEAT)

This is a sweat retention phenomenon common in young infants. Unlike the equivalent condition in older persons it can occur in the absence of fever or significant occlusive factors. An obstruction of unknown etiology occurs within the intraepidermal portion of the eccrine sweat duct with retention of sweat behind the block. Lesions commence as red macules on which are superimposed 2–3 mm papules, vesicles or pustules (Fig. 28.53). Secondary infection can occur but most commonly these pustules are sterile. Characteristically the pattern and severity of the condition alter significantly from day to day enabling differentiation from infantile acne and infective conditions. Lesions occur most commonly on the face but scalp, neck and upper trunk are other common sites. The condition is also prone to occur under plastic napkins and napkin covers.

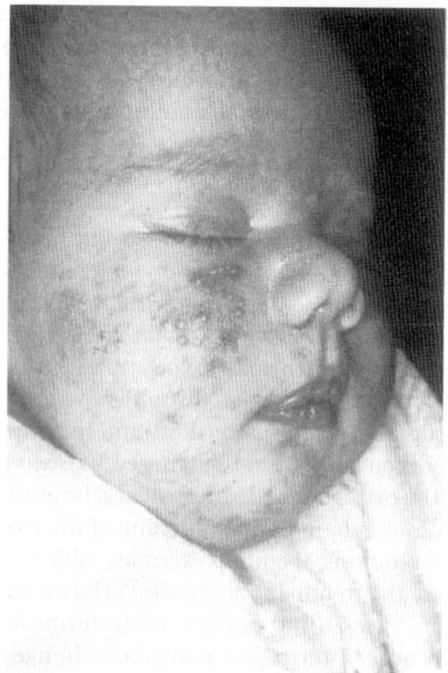

Fig. 28.53 Pustular miliaria (prickly heat).

Management involves keeping the child as cool as practicable, avoidance of contact with non-porous materials such as nylon and plastic, and of occlusive topical agents. The parents should be reassured that this is a transient condition and is uncommon after 6 months of age.

HARLEQUIN COLOR CHANGE

This is a vascular phenomenon probably caused by an immature autonomic regulatory mechanism. When the neonate is lying on one side the lower half of the body is red and the upper half is pale with a clear midline separation. This color change is transient and can be reversed by altering the infant's position. It is a very transient phenomenon and is rare after the first few days of life. It does not indicate any significant neural or vascular abnormality.

INFANTILE ACNE

This condition commences at about 3 months of age with lesions particularly on the cheeks. Open comedones predominate but closed comedones, papules, pustules and even cysts can occur. Deeper lesions may produce significant scarring. Untreated the condition usually lasts 2–3 years. In patients with a strong family history of acne the condition may be more severe and there may be difficult acne at puberty. Hormonal abnormalities are rarely found in these patients and investigation is indicated only in cases which are unusually severe, prolonged or unresponsive to therapy. Most patients respond well to topical retinoic acid used at night-time. If pustules are present topical clindamycin can be added and intralesional steroid injection is indicated for the rare large cyst. Isotretinoin has been successfully used in a handful of severe cases.

DISORDERS OF HYPOPIGMENTATION

OCULOCUTANEOUS ALBINISM

The term oculocutaneous albinism (OCA) refers to a group of autosomal recessive conditions with an absence or severe reduction in the pigmentation of skin, hair and eyes. In ocular albinism only ocular pigmentation is defective. Individuals with type I OCA have mutations in the tyrosinase gene and mutations in the P gene accounts for type II OCA. Type I OCA is further divided into IA if the mutation leads to absence of tyrosinase, and therefore, total lack of pigment, or Type IB if tyrosinase activity results in yellow hair and slight tanning ability. In general type II OCA is less severe than type I OCA.

Patients with severe OCA are unable to live a normal life due to their extreme photosensitivity and visual deficits (nystagmus, photophobia and visual loss). The child should be directed towards hobbies, sports and other activities which are performed indoors, and there should be early counseling regarding appropriate future careers. When outside, covering clothing, hats and broad spectrum sunscreens will be necessary. Patients should be examined regularly for the development of solar-induced premalignant and malignant lesions to which they are significantly more susceptible due to the lack of protective cutaneous pigmentation.

Several non-allelic syndromes exist with variable degrees of albinism and other associated features. Chediak–Higashi syndrome is characterized by incomplete OCA, photophobia and immunological defects leading to recurrent infections. Hermansky–Pudlak syndrome patients have partial pigmentation and a defect in platelet function causing a bleeding diathesis. The Cross syndrome refers to patients with reduced skin pigment in association with mental retardation.

VITILIGO

This is possibly an autoimmune disease. Though specific antimelanocyte antibodies cannot be demonstrated by immunofluorescence, complement-fixing antibody to melanocytes has been shown in some patients. It is well recognized that patients with vitiligo frequently have thyroid, gastric and adrenal autoantibodies (Fig. 28.54). Vitiligo causes complete depigmentation of the skin (unlike tinea versicolor and pityriasis alba), due to absence of melanocytes and melanin in the epidermis. Vitiligo is common in adults, and is not rare in children. The depigmentation is usually symmetrical but localized, although in some patients the condition progresses to involve almost the whole body. Spontaneous repigmentation occurs more in children than in adults. In those that do not repigment topical corticosteroids can be tried although fluorinated steroids should not be used for prolonged periods. Photochemotherapy with topical or oral psoralen may be helpful in the older child although complete repigmentation rates are disappointing. The efficacy of PUVA (oral administration of psoralen and subsequent exposure to UVA) has been shown in adults to be enhanced by concurrent topical calcipotriol.[60] Otherwise stains may be applied to the depigmented skin to minimize disfiguration.

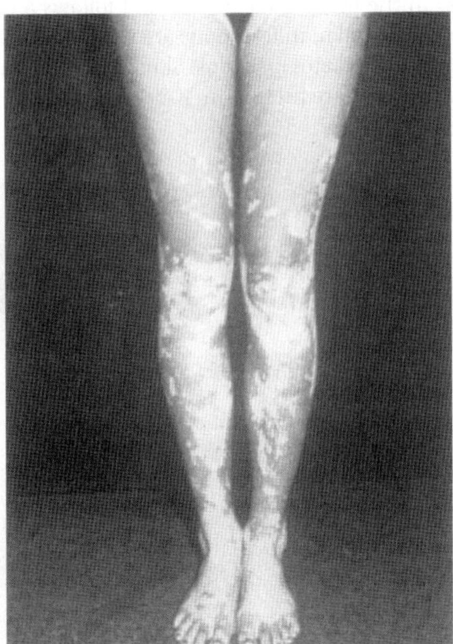

Fig. 28.54 Vitiligo.

PIEBALDISM

Congenital leukoderma occurs due to mutations in the KIT proto-oncogene. Piebaldism is an autosomal dominant condition most commonly presenting with a white forelock and leukoderma of the underlying scalp skin. Other common sites of involvement include the anterior trunk and mid-area of the limbs. Neurological abnormalities have been associated in a small number of patients. Leukoderma may also be a feature of Waardenburg's syndrome.

NEVUS DEPIGMENTOSUS

Usually solitary, nevoid patches of hypopigmentation are present at birth and can involve any body site. A decrease but not absence of pigment helps differentiate nevus depigmentosus (achromic nevus) from vitiligo. The differential diagnosis also includes ash leaf macules seen in tuberous sclerosus but these are often multiple and smaller. Systemic abnormalities have only been rarely reported.[61]

HYPOMELANOSIS OF ITO

There is convincing evidence that hypomelanosis of Ito does not represent a distinct entity but is rather a symptom of many different states of mosaicism.[62] Incontinentia pigmenti type 1, which was subsequently shown to be hypomelanosis of Ito, is a sporadic condition associated with an X/autosome translocation involving Xp11.

Unilateral or bilateral macular hypopigmented whorls, streaks, and patches of hypopigmentation present at birth along the lines of Blaschko. Although some features are similar to those of classic incontinentia pigmenti the preceding inflammatory stage is absent. Abnormalities of the eyes and the musculoskeletal and central nervous systems occur in some.

DISORDERS OF HAIR LOSS

The normal transition from vellus to terminal hair in the newborn may be delayed up to 1 year giving the false impression of diffuse congenital alopecia. Genuine inability to grow normal hair can be seen in a number of genetic conditions including the ectodermal dysplasias and hair shaft abnormalities. The latter group may be detected by light microscopy of the affected hair and includes trichorrhexis nodosa which occurs as an isolated problem or in Menkes' syndrome; trichothiodystrophy, characterized by sulfur-deficient, brittle hair; trichorrhexis invaginata (bamboo hair) usually associated with Netherton's syndrome; monilethrix (beaded hairs due to keratin mutations) and pili torti which describes flattened and twisted hairs.

LOOSE ANAGEN SYNDROME

Diffuse or occasionally patchy hair loss is seen typically in fair-haired girls aged 2–9 years. The hair is a little unruly. Loose anagen syndrome is often familial and is diagnosed by an increased number of anagen hairs present when plucked from the scalp. The features become less prominent into adult life.

TELOGEN EFFLUVIUM

This refers to hair loss following the abrupt transformation of anagen hairs to the telogen phase during which they are shed. Normally 80–90% of hairs are in anagen but up to half may change in synchronization to telogen. This results in hair loss 3–4 months after the initiating event which may be 'stress', severe illness or certain drugs, e.g. anticoagulants, retinoids, etc.

ALOPECIA AREATA

It seems likely that at least in some patients with this condition the process is due to autoimmunity, though conclusive proof is lacking (Fig. 28.55). There is an increased incidence of autoantibodies and autoimmune diseases. There is also an increased incidence of atopy, and atopic children are more likely to develop total alopecia. A family history of alopecia areata is present in 5–25% of cases.

Most children develop discoid areas of alopecia in the scalp with peripheral exclamation hairs, and these areas regrow hair normally in due course. In some children, however, particularly those with an ophiasifom distribution of hair loss (involving the temples and occipital region), the condition is progressive to become total and regrowth is much less likely. There are also nail changes, with fine pitting and horizontal depressions known as Beau's lines. Although alopecia areata is not a life threatening condition, it is obviously distressing for children and parents.

There is no effective treatment for alopecia areata at present. Intralesional steroids may cause some local hair growth but this has no permanent effect on the course of the alopecia. In older children, short contact dithranol treatment may induce hair growth but the result is rarely cosmetically acceptable. There is no evidence as yet that topical minoxidil is helpful.

TRICHOTILLOMANIA (HAIR PULLING)

Trichotillomania is more common in girls. The alopecia is patchy with variable hair lengths in the affected region usually located on the contralateral side to the child's handedness. Hair ingestion may lead to bowel symptoms. Trichotillomania is most often an isolated symptom with a good prognosis following appropriate psychological support. However, follow-up until resolution is important to avoid missing more severe psychological disease.

THE HISTIOCYTOSES

Histiocytes include circulating monocytes and tissue macrophages as well as the dendritic cell system (antigen presenting cells). The histiocytoses have been classified into class I (Langerhans' cell histiocytosis), class II (proliferative histiocytoses of mononuclear phagocytes other than Langerhans' cell) and class III (malignant histiocyte disorders).[63]

CLASS I LANGERHANS' CELL HISTIOCYTOSIS (HISTIOCYTOSIS X)

This condition is rare (Ch. 22), and the cells involved are Langerhans' cells which contain Birbeck granules, and express CDI markers. Although historically four types are recognized on the basis of clinical organ involvement, clinicians should be aware that the presentations may overlap and the disease may progress from one subtype to another.[64]

Letterer–Siwe disease

This usually presents in the first year of life (Fig. 28.56). Discrete yellow–brown papules develop on the scalp, face, upper trunk and flexures, with a distribution mimicking seborrheic eczema. Purpura and crusting of the lesion may become evident. In some children mucous membranes are also involved, with gingivitis and oral and genital ulceration.

Signs of systemic involvement become manifest, with hepatosplenomegaly, lymphadenopathy and anemia. Chest X-ray shows miliary shadowing and bone scans may show osteolytic areas. Treatment with steroids and cytotoxic drugs has reduced the mortality and slowed the progression.

Hand–Schüller–Christian disease

This is a more benign form of histiocytosis X, which usually presents within the first 5 years of life and follows a chronic non-fatal course. The usual manifestations are radiological bone defects, exophthalmos and diabetes insipidus. Skin lesions similar to those in Letterer–Siwe disease are present in 30%.

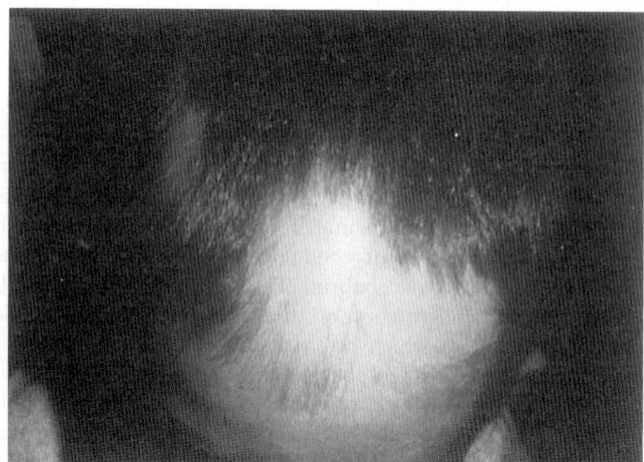

Fig. 28.55 Alopecia areata.

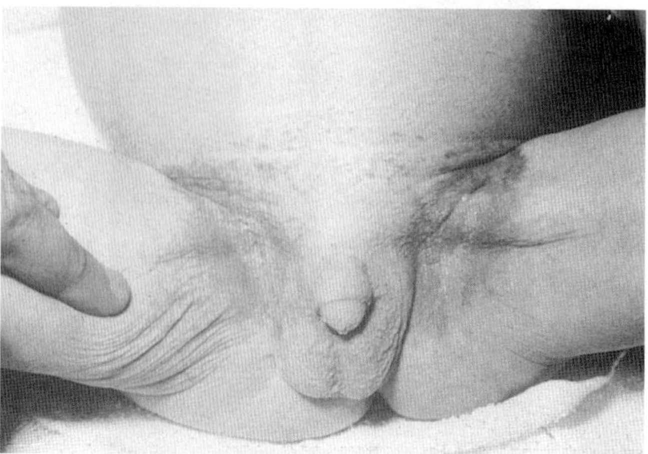

Fig. 28.56 Letterer–Siwe disease.

Eosinophilic granuloma

This is the most benign form of histiocytosis X. It commonly presents within the first 5 years of life, and skin involvement is rare. When it does occur, yellowish or brownish papules are found on the scalp and trunk in a distribution similar to the other forms of histiocytosis X. Spontaneous resolution usually occurs.

Congenital self-healing histiocytosis

This usually affects skin only with lesions that are nodular or may mimic chickenpox. If this is the case spontaneous resolution occurs within months.

JUVENILE XANTHOGRANULOMA (JXG)

JXG is an example of a benign self-limiting non-Langerhans' cell histiocytosis (class II) (Fig. 28.57). Histologically lesions are characterized by histiocytes with foamy macrophages and multinucleated giant cells. Despite its name and appearance JXG is not associated with lipid disorders. Lesions are occasionally present at birth but typically before 1 year. They are domed-shaped nodules with a red and then orange color often located on the head and neck. Single lesions are more common but if multiple lesions are present up to 10% have ocular involvement which may lead to glaucoma.

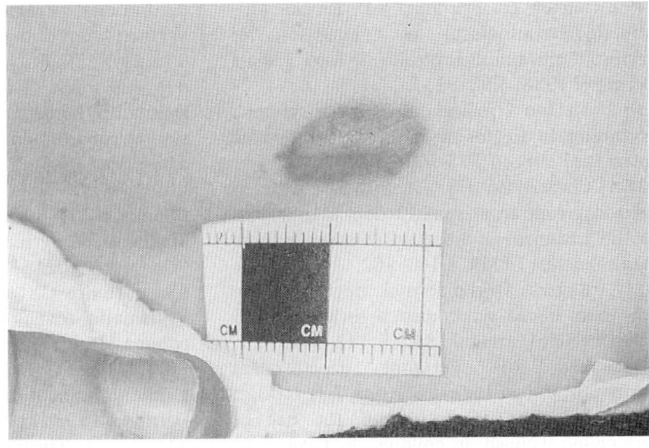

Fig. 28.57 Juvenile xanthogranuloma (XTG)

REFERENCES (* Level 1 evidence)

1 DeDavid M, Orlow SJ, Provost N, et al. Neurocutaneous melanosis: clinical features of large congenital melanocytic nevi in patients with manifest central nervous system melanosis. J Am Acad Dermatol 1996; 35:529–538.

2 Foster RD, Williams ML, Barkovich AJ, et al. Giant congenital melanocytic nevi: the significance of neurocutaneous melanosis in neurologically asymptomatic children. Plast Reconstr Surg 2001; 107:933–941.

3 Anon. Management of congenital melanocytic nevi: a decade later. Pediatr Dermatol 1996; 13:321–340.

4 Lorentzen M, Pers M, Bretteville Jensen G. The incidence of malignant transformation in giant pigmented nevi. Scand J Plast Reconstr Surg 1977; II:163–167.

5 Illig W, Weidner F, Hundeeker M, et al. Congenital nevi < 10 cms as precursors to melanoma. Arch Dermatol 1985; 121:1274–1281.

6 Rhodes AR, Sober AJ, Calvin L, et al. The malignant potential of small congenital nevocellular nevi. J Am Acad Dermatol 1982; 6:230–241.

7 Sahin S, Levin L, Kopf AW, et al. Risk of melanoma in medium-sized congenital melanocytic nevi: a follow-up study. J Am Acad Dermatol 1998; 39:428–433.

8 Goss BD, Ansell PE, Bennett V, et al. The prevalence and characteristics of congenital pigmented lesions in the newborn babies in Oxford. Paediatr Perinatal Epidemiol 1990; 4:448–457.

9 Happle R. How many epidermal nevus syndromes exist? J Am Acad Dermatol 1991; 25:550–556.

10 Solomon LM, Esterly NM. Epidermal and other organoid nevi. Curr Probl Pediatr 1975; 6:1–56.

11 Rogers M, McCrossin I, Commens C. Epidermal nevi and the epidermal nevus syndrome. J Am Acad Dermatol 1989; 20:476–488.

12 Rogers M, Dorman DC, Gapes M, et al. A three year study of impetigo in Sydney. Med J Aust 1987; 147:59–62.

13 Enjolras O, Mulliken JB. The current management of vascular birthmarks. Pediatr Dermatol 1993; 10:311–333.

14 North PE, Waner M, Mizeracki A, et al. A unique microvascular phenotype shared by juvenile hemangiomas and human placenta. Arch Dermatol 2001; 137:559–570.

*15 Bennett ML, Fleischer AB, Chamlin SL, et al. Oral corticosteroid use is effective for cutaneous hemangiomas. Arch Dermatol 2001; 137:1208–1213.

16 Dubois J, Hershon L, Carmant L, et al. Toxicity profile of interferon alfa-2b in children: a prospective evaluation. J Pediatr 1999; 135:782–785.

*17 Batta K, Goodyear H, Moss C, et al. Randomised controlled trial of early pulsed dye lasser (PDL) treatment of uncomplicated childhood haemangiomas. (Abstract) Br J Dermatol 2001; 145(suppl 59):29.

18 Payarols J, Pardo Masferrer J, Gomez Bellvert C. Treatment of life-threatening infantile hemangiomas with vincristine. N Engl J Med 1995; 333:69.

19 Metry DW, Dowd CF, Barkovich AJ, et al. The many faces of PHACE syndrome. J Pediatr 2001; 139:117–123.

20 Esterly NB, Margileth AM, Kahn G. The management of disseminated eruptive haemangiomata in infants: special symposium. Pediatr Dermatol 2001; 1:312–317.

21 Stevenson RF, Thompson HG, Marin JD. Unrecognized ocular problems associated with port wine stain of the face in children. Can Med Assoc J 1974; 11:953–955.

22 Enjolras O, Riche MC, Merland JJ. Facial port wine stains and Sturge Weber syndrome. Pediatrics 1985; 76:48–51.

23 Freire-Maia N, Pinheiro M. Ectodermal dysplasias: a clinical and genetic study. New York: Alan R Liss; 1984.

24 Cheadle JP, Reeve MP, Sampson JR, et al. Molecular genetic advances in tuberose sclerosis. Hum Genet 2000; 107:97–114.

25 Smahi A, Courtois G, Vabres P, et al. Genomic rearrangement in NEMO impairs NF-kappaB activation and is a cause of incontinentia pigmenti. The International Incontinentia Pigmenti (IP) Consortium. Nature 2000; 405:466–472.

26 Andersen SL, Thomsen K. Psoriasiform napkin dermatitis. Br J Dermatol 1971; 84:316–319.

27 Neville EA, Finn OA. Psoriasiform napkin dermatitis – a follow up study. Br J Dermatol 1975; 92:279–285.

*28 Oranje AP, Marcoux D, Svensson A, et al. Topical calcipotriol in childhood psoriasis. J Am Acad Dermatol 1997; 36:203–208.

*29 Owen CM, Chalmers RJG, O'Sullivan T, et al. Antistreptococcal interventions for guttate and chronic plaque psoriasis (Cochrane review) In: The Cochrane Library, 3. Oxford: Update Software; 2001.

30 Shaw PH, Mancini AJ, McConnell JP, et al. Treatment of congenital erythropoietic porphyria in children by allogeneic stem cell transplantation: a case report and review of the literature. Bone Marrow Transplant 2001; 27:101–105.

*31 Gibbs S, Harvey I, Sterling JC, et al. Local treatments for cutaneous warts: systematic review. Br Med J 2002; 325:461–464.

32 Karabulut AA, Sahin S. Is cimetidine effective for nongenital warts: a double-blind, placebo-controlled study. Arch Dermatol 1997; 133:533–534.

33 Caputo R, Gelmetti C, Ermacora E, et al. Gianotti–Crosti syndrome: a retrospective analysis of 308 cases. J Am Acad Dermatol 1992; 26:207–210.

34 Coskey RJ, Coskey LA. Diagnosis and treatment of impetigo. J Am Acad Dermatol 1987; 17:62–63.

*35 Barton LL, Friedman AD, Portilla MG. Impetigo contagiosa: a comparison of erythromycin and dicloxacillin therapy. Pediatr Dermatol 1988; 5:88–91.

*36 McLinn S. Topical mupirocin vs. systemic erythromycin treatment for pyoderma. Pediatr Infect Dis J 1988; 7:785–790.

*37 Christensen OB, Anehus S. Hydrogen peroxide cream: an alternative to topical antibiotics in the treatment of impetigo contagiosa. Acta Derm Venereol 1994; 74:460–462.

38 Rogers M. Epidermal nevi and the epidermal nevus syndromes: a review of 233 cases. Pediatr Dermatol 1992; 9:342–344.

39 Krol AL. Perianal streptococcal dermatitis. Pediatr Dermatol 1990; 7:97–100.

40 Jones TC. Overview of the use of terbinafine (Lamisil) in children. Br J Dermatol 1995; 132:683–689.

41 Terragni L, Lasagni A, Oriani A, et al. Pityriasis versicolor in the pediatric age. Pediatr Dermatol 1991; 8:9–12.

*42 Schultz MW, Gomez M, Hansen RC, et al. Comparative study of 5% permethrin cream and 1% lindane lotion for the treatment of scabies. Arch Dermatol 1990; 126:167–170.

*43 Taplin D, Meinking TL, Chen JA, et al. Comparison on crotamiton 10% cream (Eurax) and permethrin 5% cream (Elimite) for the treatment of scabies in children. Pediatr Dermatol 1990; 7:67–73.

44 Hourihane JO, Roberts SA, Warner JO. Resolution of peanut allergy: a case control study. BMJ 1998; 316:1271–1275.

45 Hannaford R, Rogers M. Presentation of cutaneous mastocytosis in 173 children. Australas J Dermatol 2001; 42:15–21.

*46 Tatnall FM, Schofield JK, Leigh IM. A double-blind, placebo-controlled trial of continuous acyclovir therapy in recurrent erythema multiforme. Br J Dermatol 1995; 132:267–270.

47 Reunala T, Kosnai I, Karparti S, et al. Dermatitis herpetiformis: jejunal findings and skin response to gluten free diet. Arch Dis Child 1984; 59:517–522.

48 Ryan TJ. Cutaneous vasculitis. In: Champion RH, Burton JL, Burns DA, et al, eds. Textbook of dermatology. Oxford: Blackwell Science; 1998:2155.

49 Hoare C, Li Wan Po A, Williams H. Systematic review of treatments of atopic eczema. Health Technol Assess 2000; 4:37.

50 Long CC, Mills CM, Finlay AY. A practical guide to topical therapy in children. Br J Dermatol 1998; 138:293–296.

51 Zaki I, Emerson R, Allen BR. Treatment of severe atopic dermatitis in childhood with cyclosporin. Br J Dermatol 1996; 135(suppl 48):21–24.

52 Boguniewicz M, Fiedler VC, Raimer S, et al. A randomized, vehicle-controlled trial of tacrolimus ointment for treatment of atopic dermatitis in children. Pediatric Tacrolimus Study Group. J Allergy Clin Immunol 1998; 102:555–557.

*53 Wahn U, Bos JD, Goodfield M, et al. Efficacy and safety of pimecrolimus cream in the long-term management of atopic dermatitis in children. Pediatrics 2002; 110(1):e2.

*54 Pei AY, Chan HH, Leung TF. Montelukast in the treatment of children with moderate-to-severe atopic dermatitis: a pilot study. Pediatr Allergy Immunol 2001; 12:154–158.

*55 Sheehan MP, Atherton DJ. One-year follow up of children treated with Chinese medicinal herbs for atopic eczema. Br J Dermatol 1994; 130:488–493.

56 Kalliomaki M, Salminen S, Arvilommi H, et al. Probiotics in primary prevention of atopic disease: a randomised placebo-controlled trial. Lancet 2001; 357:1076–1079.

57 Uziel Y, Feldman BM, Krafchik BR, et al. Methotrexate and corticosteroid therapy for pediatric localized scleroderma. J Pediatr 2000; 136:91–95.

58 Dalziel K, Millard PR, Wojnarowska F. The treatment of vulvar lichen sclerosus with a very potent corticosteroid (clobetasol proprionate 0.05%) cream. Br J Dermatol 1991; 124:461–464.

59 Grabczynska SA, McGregor JM, Kondeatis E, et al. Actinic prurigo and polymorphic light eruption: common pathogenesis and the importance of HLA-DR4/DRB1*0407. Br J Dermatol 1999; 140:232–236.

*60 Ermis O, Alpsoy E, Cetin L, et al. Is the efficacy of psoralen plus ultraviolet A therapy for vitiligo enhanced by concurrent topical calcipotriol? A placebo-controlled double-blind study. Br J Dermatol 2001; 145:472–475.

61 Dahr S, Kanwar AJ, Kaur S. Nevus depigmentation in India: experience with 50 patients. Pediatr Dermatol 1993; 10:299–300.

62 Donnai D, Read AP, McKeown C, et al. Hypomelanosis of Ito: a manifestation of mosaicism or chimerism. J Med Genet 1988; 25:809–818.

63 Chu T, D'Angio GJ, Favara B, et al. Histiocytosis syndromes in children. Lancet 1987; i:208–209.

64 Komp DM. Concepts in staging and clinical studies for treatment of Langerhans' cell histiocytosis. Semin Oncol 1991; 18:18–23.

29

Disorders of the eye

Brian W Fleck

INTRODUCTION

Pediatric ophthalmology deals with large numbers of children with relatively minor health problems (5% of children have strabismus or amblyopia), and a smaller group of patients with sight threatening diseases that require extensive investigations and medical and surgical therapies. Close liaison with pediatricians, especially pediatric neurologists, is vital when dealing with this second category of patients.

NORMAL VISUAL DEVELOPMENT

The visual system in neonates is immature, especially during the first 3–6 months of life. Preferential looking grating measurements of vision reach 6/6 level at 3 years.[1] However this test is dependent on complex sensory and motor responses. Cortical VEP estimates of visual acuity give a 6/6 response by age 6–8 months.[2] Stereopsis develops between the ages of 2 and 6 months.[3] Binocular fusion also develops at this age.[4]

THE CRITICAL PERIOD OF VISUAL DEVELOPMENT

Early visual experience is critical to the development of synaptic connections in the primary visual cortex.[5] Input from each eye 'competes' for cortical connections.[6] The visual outcome of congenital cataract surgery is poor if visual rehabilitation is delayed beyond 3 months of age. The visual outcome of surgery for uniocular cataract is less satisfactory than that for binocular cataract,[7] as the normal eye dominates synaptic development.

THE PLASTIC PERIOD OF VISUAL DEVELOPMENT

While the critical period of visual development is at age 0–3 months, the visual system remains plastic until the age of 8–12 years. Interrupted visual development below the age of 6 years[8] may lead to permanent reduction of visual acuity even after the causative abnormality has been removed. This is termed amblyopia. The younger the age at which developmental interruption happens, the greater the degree of amblyopia that may occur. Once again uniocular defects produce a greater effect than binocular defects, because of competition effects at the occipital cortex. Amblyopia may be treated during the plastic period of visual development – up to age 8–12 years.

CLINICAL ASSESSMENT

CLINICAL HISTORY

A parent's, or grandparent's, concern for an infant's vision is usually reliable. At around 6 weeks an infant will smile in response to visual stimuli, and delay of this developmental stage is significant. Visually directed reaching commences at age 2–3 months.

In older children perceptual visual difficulties related to central nervous system (CNS) disease may go undetected unless a careful history is taken. Useful questions to ask include:

- Does the child have difficulty identifying objects within a 'busy' or 'fast moving' environment?
- Does the child have difficulty recognizing faces?
- Does the child have difficulty recognizing abstract shapes?
- Does the child have difficulty visualizing moving objects?
- Does the child have difficulty with orientation either in unfamiliar environments or familiar environments?
- Does the child have difficulty with color identification?

VISION ASSESSMENT

In infants and very young children observed visual behavior will give useful qualitative information about visual function. A visually alert infant will fixate on and follow the movement of small objects of interest held by an examiner. Each eye is tested separately by covering one eye with a hand or eye patch. If a child will not tolerate uniocular testing then some useful information may be obtained from binocular testing. However poor vision in one eye will not be detected by binocular testing.

QUANTITATIVE MEASUREMENTS OF VISUAL ACUITY

'Visibility' refers to the ability to identify a single object such as a sweet, thread on a carpet, or airplane in the sky.

'Resolution' refers to the ability to distinguish between two points or lines. Visual acuity tests measure resolution. Clinical tests of visibility such as Stycar balls, Catford drum, etc. may significantly overestimate results obtained with resolution tests and should be interpreted with caution.

PREFERENTIAL LOOKING ACUITY CARDS

An infant will 'prefer' to look at an object of interest rather than at a blank background. Black and white stripes (gratings) of varying widths ('spatial frequency') are used as the stimulus (Fig. 29.1). The tester uses a series of test cards, each of which has two test areas – one

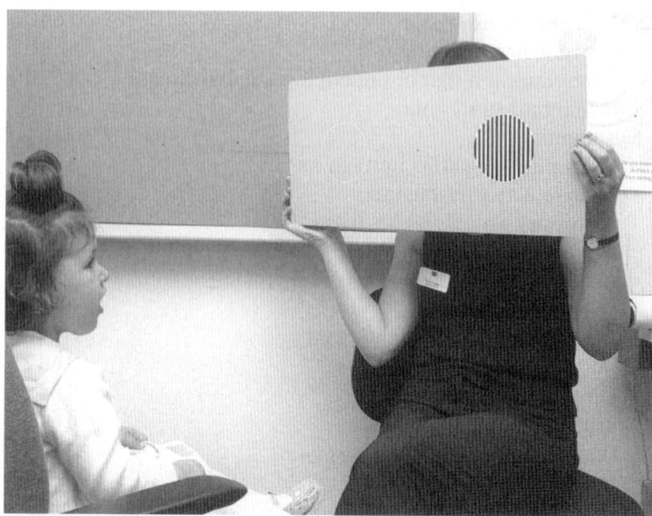

Fig. 29.1 Forced choice preferential looking test (Keeler cards). The tester peeps through a hole in the card and is forced to choose which target area the child looks at.

blank and one a test grating. The tester observes which area the infant looks at. The test is repeated a number of times, using varying stripe widths. The narrowest stripe width (lowest spatial frequency) consistently looked at by the infant is a measure of the infant's visual resolution. Preferential looking tests may be successfully used in most infants, but are of less interest to 18–24-month-old children.

Cardiff cards use black and white stripes shaped into interesting pictures (Fig. 29.2). These are useful in children aged 1–3 years. The child will look at the picture if the black and white stripes are sufficiently wide to be observed (resolved).

OPTOTYPE TESTS

From the age of 3 years upward more traditional 'optotype' visual acuity symbols may be used. Kay pictures use simple line drawings (Fig. 29.3). The Sheridan Gardiner test uses letters. A limited range of letters is used so that the child may match the shape of the letter rather than name it (Fig. 29.4). A letter placed among a line of other letters is less easily observed than a single letter. This phenomenon is termed 'crowding'. The Snellen visual acuity chart, as used in adults, is therefore preferred in children aged 4–5 years and upwards. Charts that use lines of letters arranged in log unit size are preferred for research studies – LogMAR charts (Fig. 29.5).

VISUAL FIELDS

Visual field testing may be undertaken in infants and toddlers by introducing an object of interest from either side and observing the response. In children aged 2–5 years two observers may undertake a slightly more detailed visual field assessment (Fig. 29.6). The child sits on the lap of a parent. An observer sits approximately 1–2 m in front of the child. A second observer stands behind the parent and child. The second observer slowly brings an object of interest into the field of vision of the child. The child will turn to look at the object when it comes into the observable visual field. Binocular testing is more easily performed than uniocular testing. In most cases the suspected abnormality is in the posterior visual pathway, with homonymous defects.

In children aged 6 years upwards, Goldman visual field testing may be possible. This type of detailed visual field testing requires considerable concentration by the child. The child must fix on a central point in the testing bowl and a spot of light is brought in from the peripheral field of vision (Fig. 29.7). The child presses a buzzer when the spot of light comes into view. The test is very operator dependent. Testing is normally performed uniocularly, and accurate and reproducible charting of visual field defects related to optic nerve and CNS disease may be obtained.

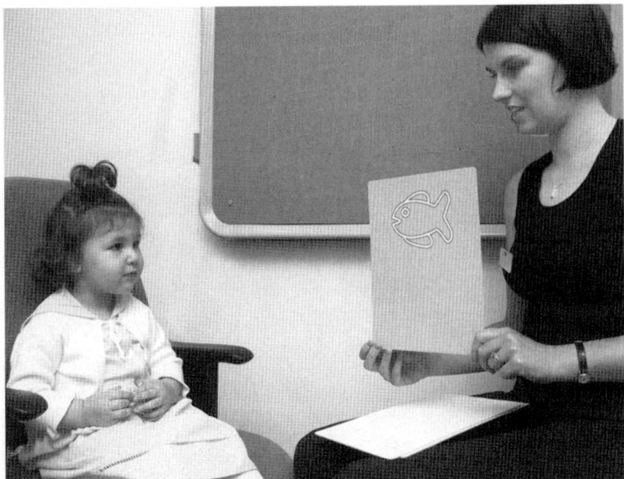

Fig. 29.2 The tester observes whether the child looks at the top or bottom half of the test card. The images are randomly distributed to the top halves and bottom halves of the test cards. The test is normally performed at 50 cm or 100 cm.

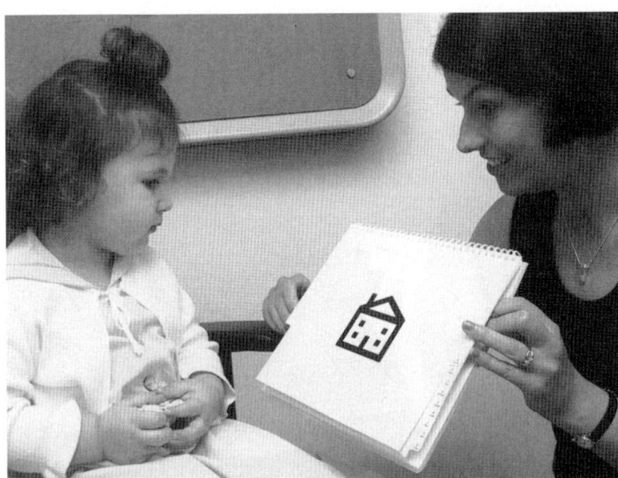

Fig. 29.3 Kay picture optotypes. The test is normally performed at 3 m or 6 m.

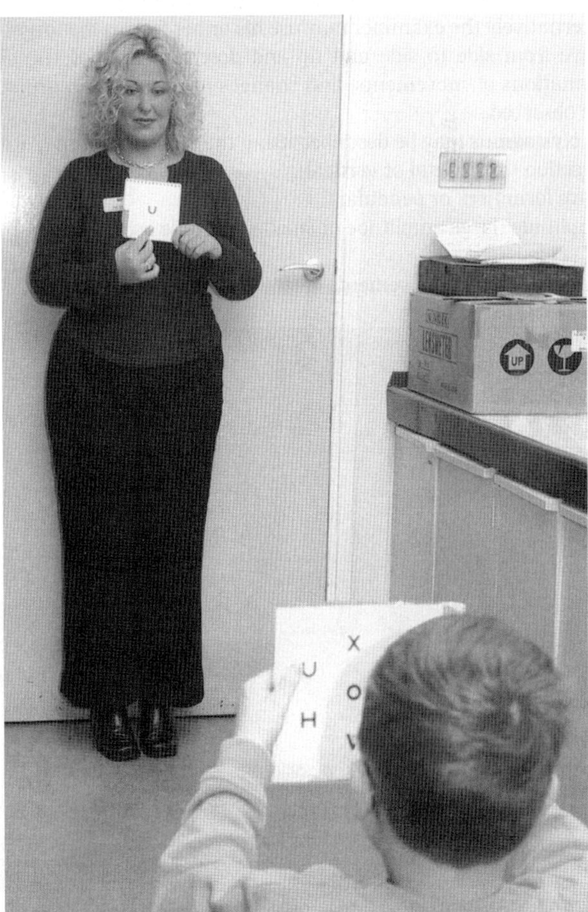

Fig. 29.4 Sheridan Gardiner optotypes. The test is usually performed at 6 m and the child matches the test letter to the key card.

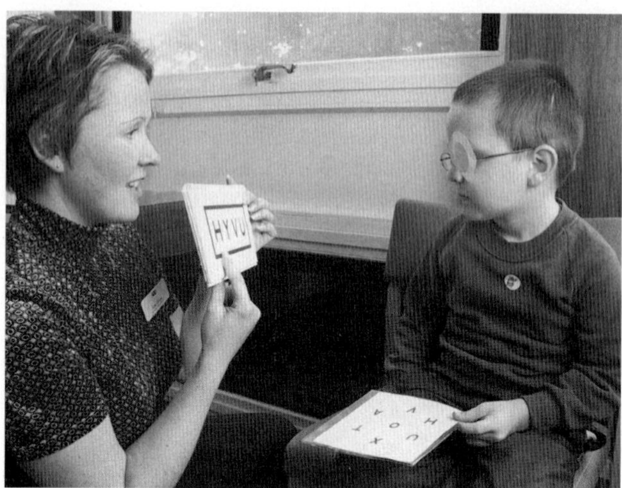

Fig. 29.5 LogMAR optotypes (Glasgow cards). The test is usually performed at 6 m and the child matches the test letter to the key card. Reduced vision due to 'crowding' is detected as the test letter is placed within a row of letters.

CLINICAL EYE MOVEMENT TESTING

The cover test may be performed in order to detect a strabismus. When the straight eye is covered the strabismic eye quickly moves in order to take up fixation (Figs 29.8 and 29.9).

The range of eye movements may then be observed. The child is asked to observe an interesting target moved by the examiner. Alternatively the examiner may use his or her face as the target and move from side to side and up and down in front of the child. Limitations of movements, and changes in palpebral fissure width are observed.

Nystagmus may be described using the pneumonic 'DWARF':
*D*irection (horizontal or vertical),
*W*ave form (jerk or pendular)
*A*mplitude (large amplitude or small amplitude oscillations)
R
*F*requency (rapid movements or slow movements).

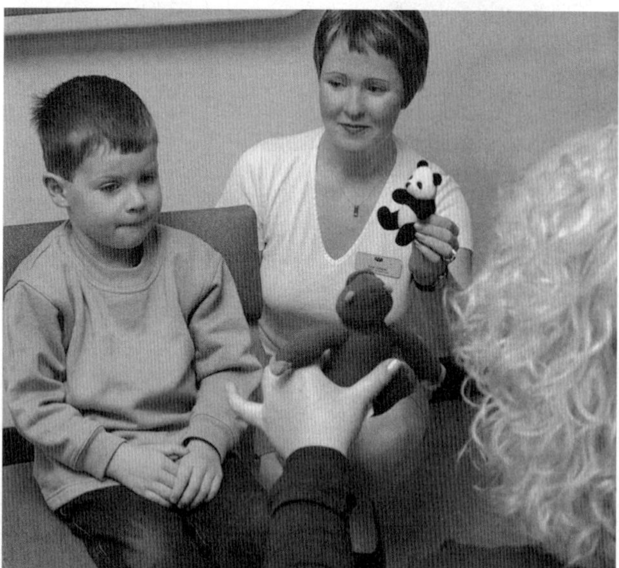

Fig. 29.6 Binocular visual field testing. Observer 1 maintains interest while observer 2 brings the test object (panda) into the child's visual field from behind. The child turns to look at the test object when it becomes visible.

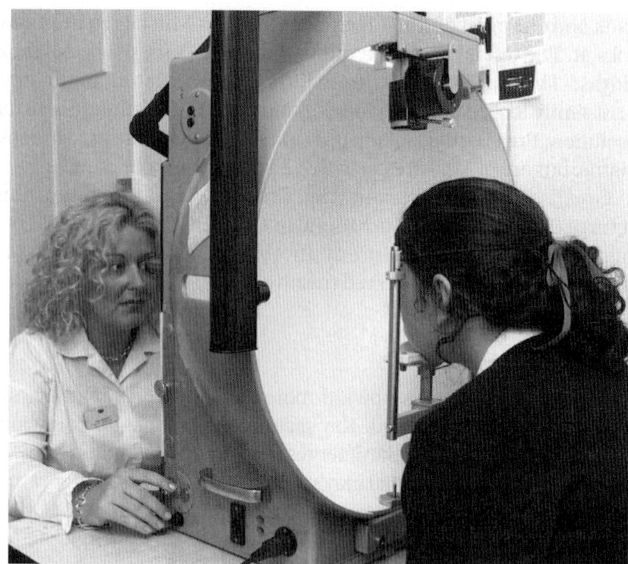

Fig. 29.7 Goldman visual field testing. The tester observes the eye fixing behavior of the child. The child fixes on the center target within the bowl and presses a buzzer when the test spot of light becomes visible in the peripheral visual field.

The direction of nystagmus movements is recorded as the direction of the fast phase (jerk) of the oscillation.

While some information on nystagmus movements may be obtained by clinical observation, much more detailed information may be obtained by analysis in an eye movement laboratory. Eye movements are analyzed using electro-oculography, infrared tracking and video observation.[9] Such laboratories are in general limited to research centers.

EXTERNAL EYE EXAMINATION

The eyelids, conjunctiva, cornea and iris may be observed using a torch. Ophthalmologists use magnification in the form of a slit lamp microscope to allow detailed examination of these structures (Fig. 29.10). Where there is a suspicion of a corneal epithelial abrasion or other corneal epithelial disease a drop of fluorescein dye

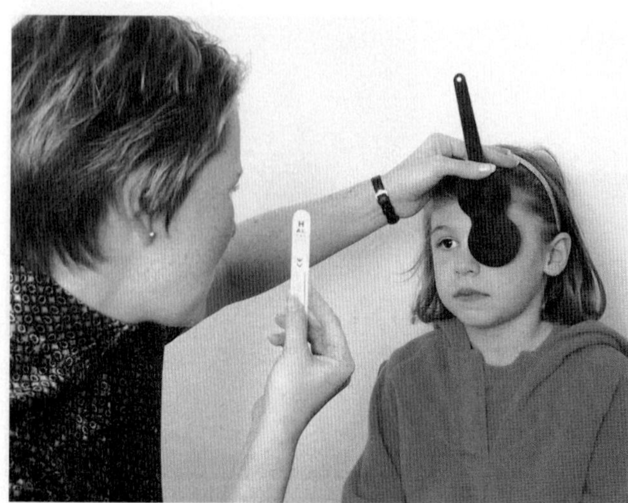

Fig. 29.8 Cover test. The child fixes on a test target at 6 m or 50 cm. The normal eye is covered. The strabismic eye then moves in order to take up fixation. Small flicks of movement may be easily detected, allowing diagnosis of small angled deviations.

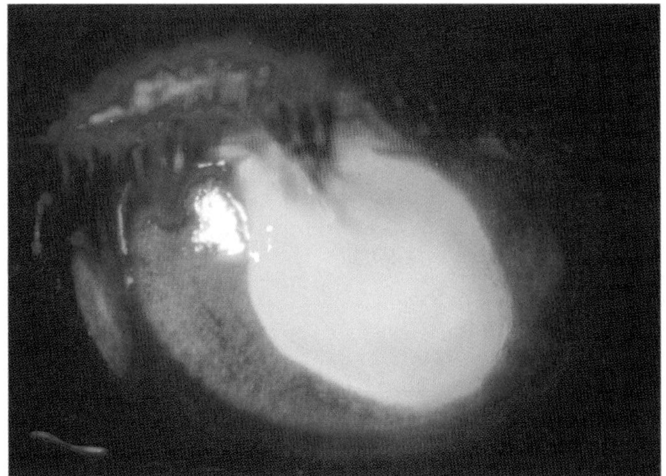

Plate 29.11 Yellow/green fluorescein staining of an area of cornea abrasion visualized using blue light (see p. 1636).

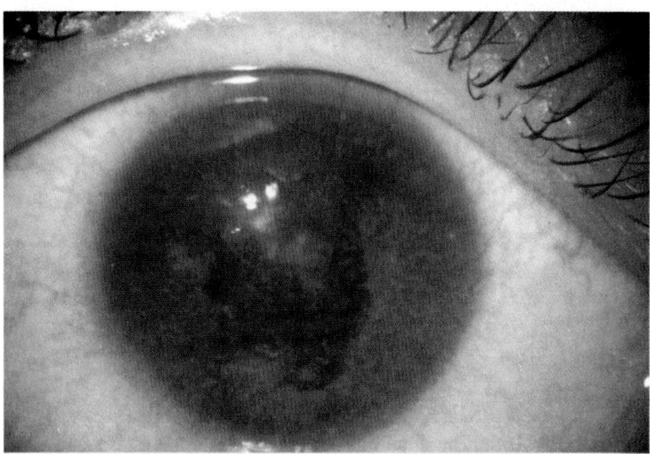

Plate 29.24 Aniridia. No iris tissue is seen. There is fibrovascular pannus covering the peripheral cornea in this case (see p. 1641).

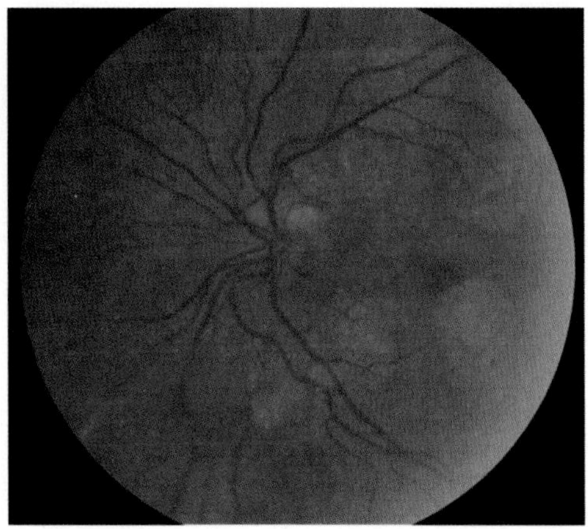

Plate 29.25 Hypoplastic disc. Optic nerve hypoplasia. The optic disc is anatomically very small in this case, with severely reduced vision (see p. 1643).

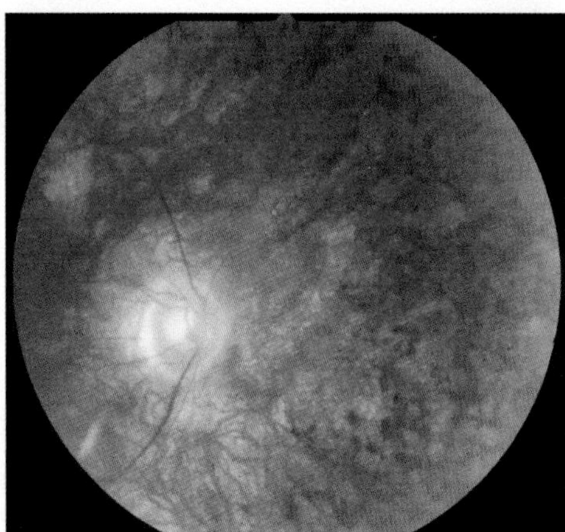

Plate 29.26 Retinitis pigmentosa. Typical 'bone spicule' pigmentation is seen in the mid periphery of the fundus (see p. 1644).

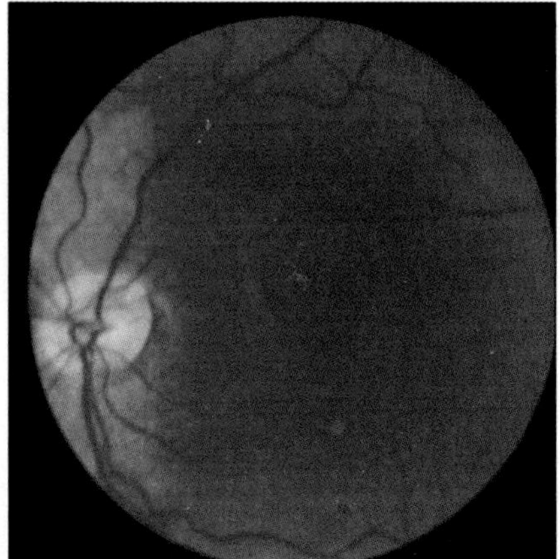

Plate 29.27 Retinal cone dystrophy with typical 'bull's eye' pigmentation at the center of the macula (see p. 1644).

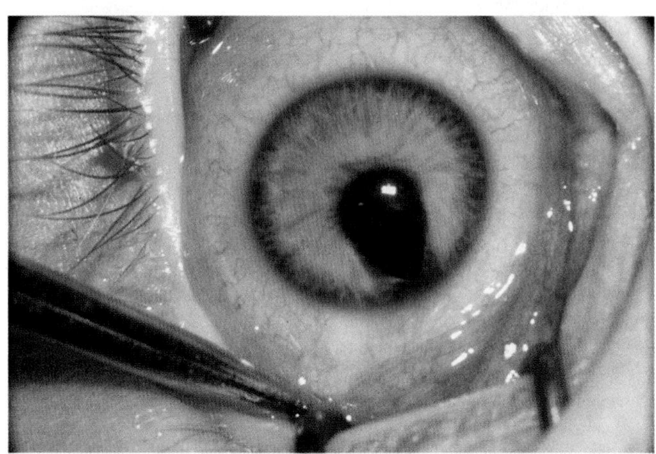

Plate 29.33 Coloboma of the inferior iris (see p. 1647).

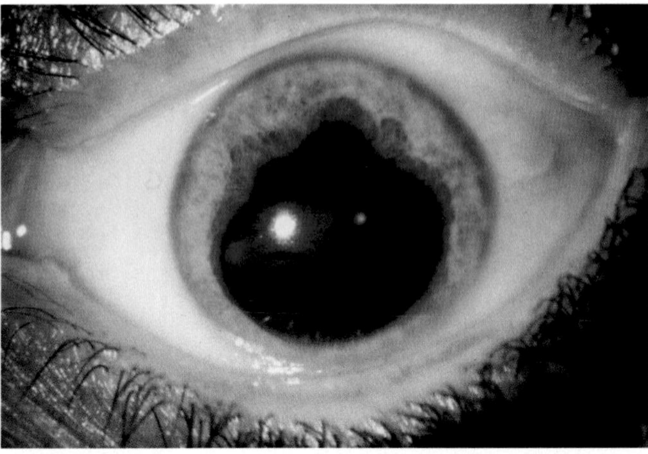

Plate 29.35 Iritis. The pupil has been dilated and adhesions between the iris and lens (posterior synechiae) are seen (see p. 1648).

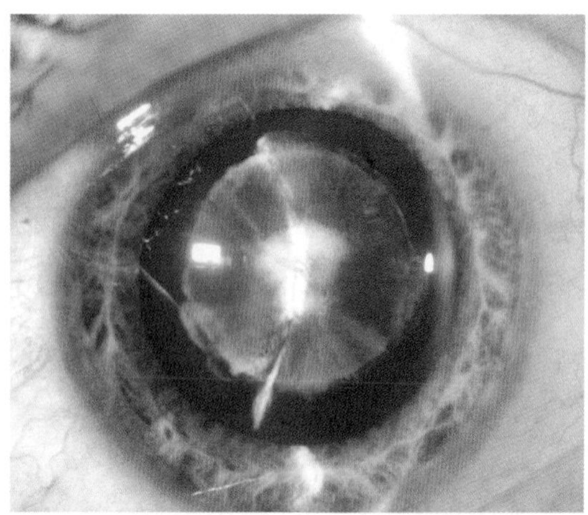

Plate 29.36 Congenital cataract. This is a partial, lamellar cataract with relatively good vision. Surgery in infancy was not needed in this case (see p. 1649).

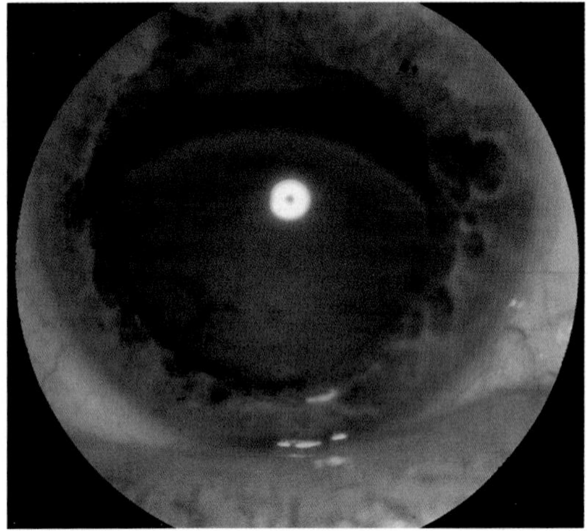

Plate 29.37 Subluxed lens (see p. 1649).

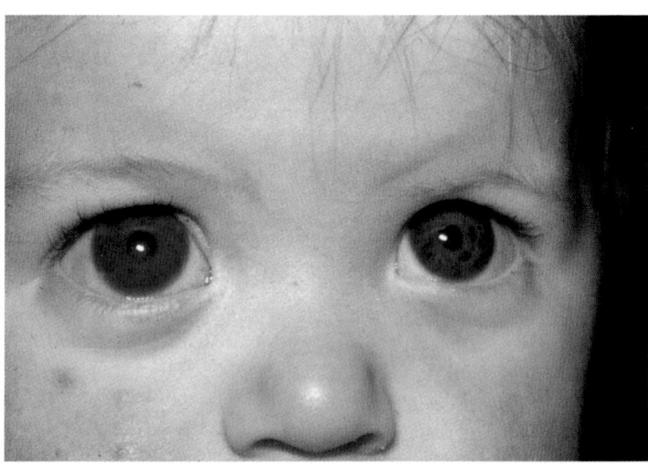

Plate 29.38 Congenital glaucoma. Note enlarged corneas. This child had goniotomy surgery performed in infancy, which satisfactorily controlled the intraocular pressures (see p. 1650).

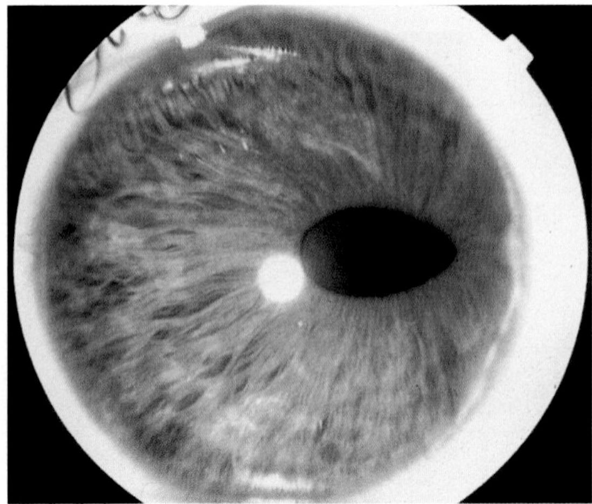

Plate 29.39 Reiger's syndrome. Note posterior embryotoxon and abnormal pupil shape and position (corectopia) (see p. 1650).

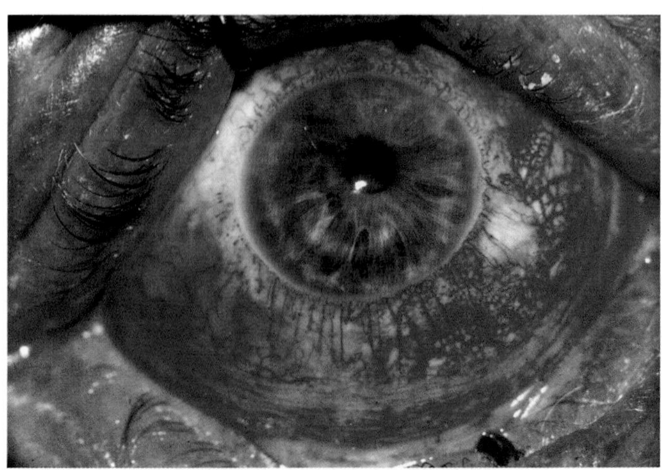

Plate 29.40 Sturge–Weber syndrome. Note eyelid port wine stain, and abnormal scleral blood vessels (see p. 1650).

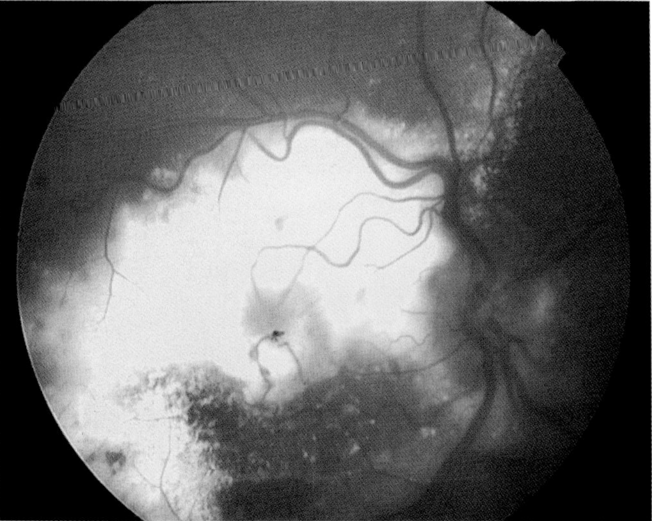

Plate 29.41 Coats' disease. Massive subretinal lipid exudation is seen at the macula, with severely reduced visual acuity (see p. 1650).

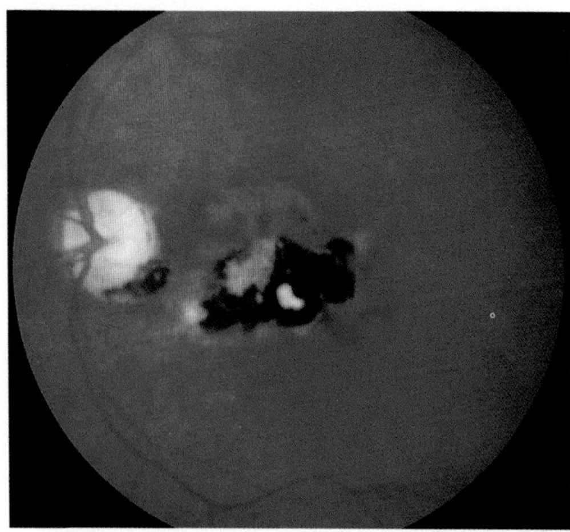

Plate 29.44 Toxoplasmosis. Pigmented scar at macula. No active inflammation present (see p. 1652).

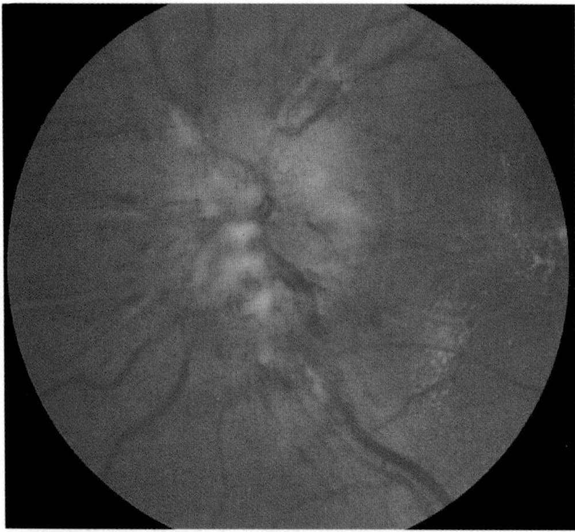

Plate 29.45 Severe papilledema with hemorrhages and exudates (see p. 1652).

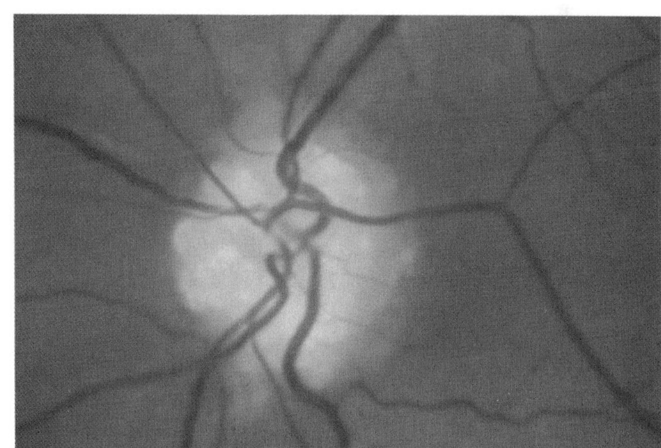

Plate 29.47 Optic disc drusen (see p. 1653).

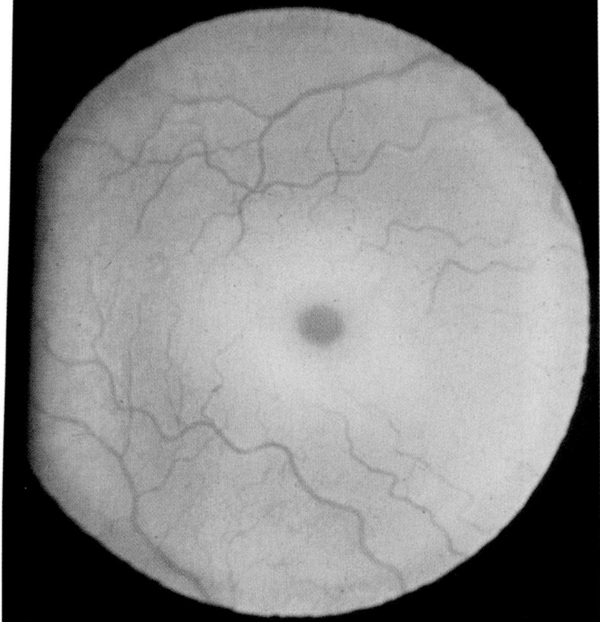

Plate 29.49 Cherry red spot due to Tay–Sachs disease (see p. 1654).

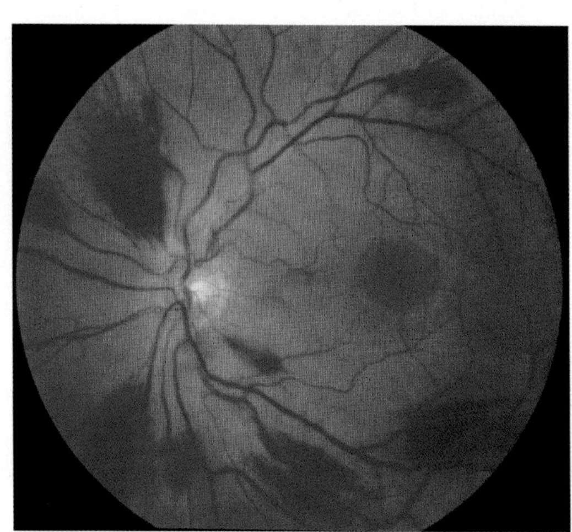

Plate 29.50 Retinal hemorrhages related to leukemia (see p. 1655).

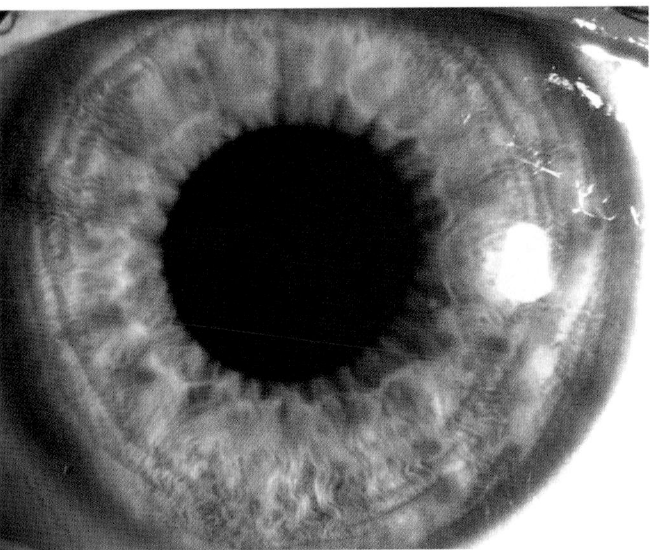

Plate 29.51 Lisch nodules of the iris. Multiple pigmented nodules are easily visualized against the background of a lightly pigmented iris in this case (see p. 1655).

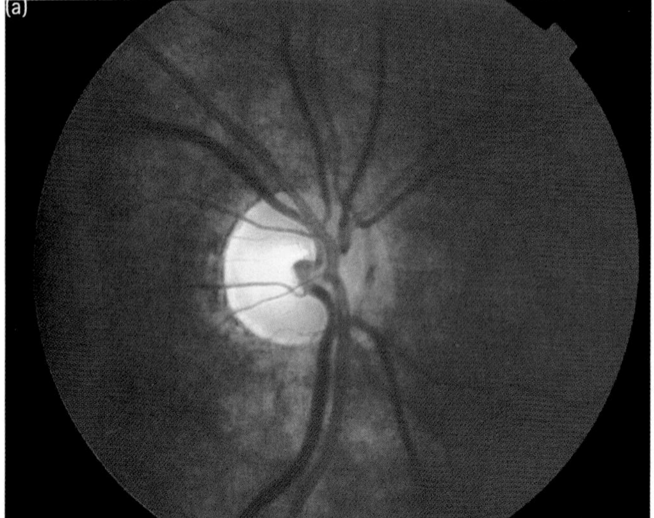

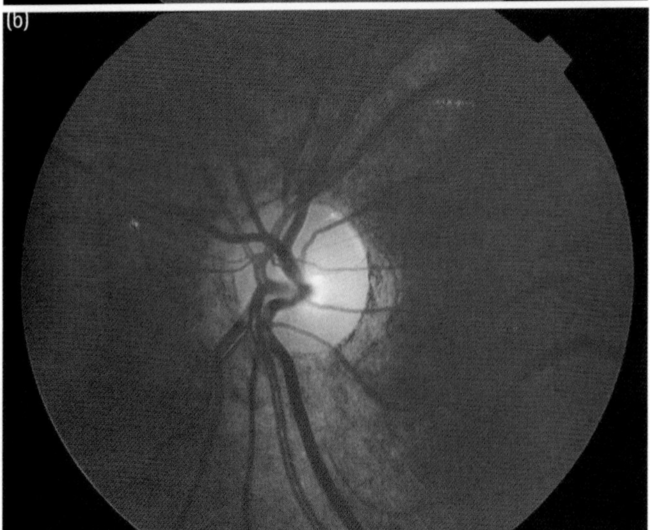

Plate 29.52 (a) Right optic disc showing pallor on the temporal side. MRI scan showed optic nerve glioma. (b) Normal left optic disc (see p. 1655).

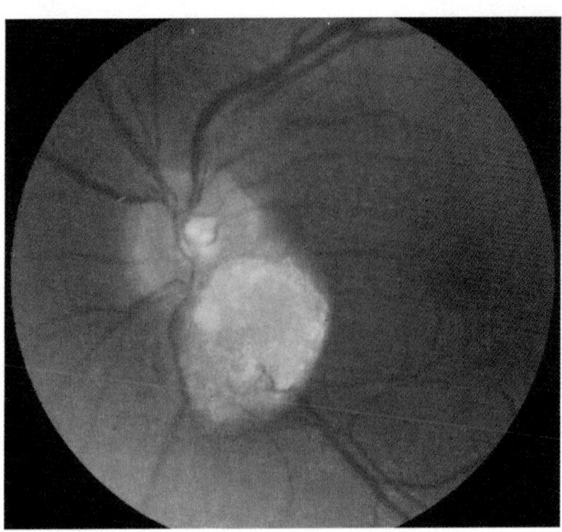

Plate 29.53 Large multinodular retinal hamartoma adjacent to optic disc in a case of tuberous sclerosis (see p. 1656).

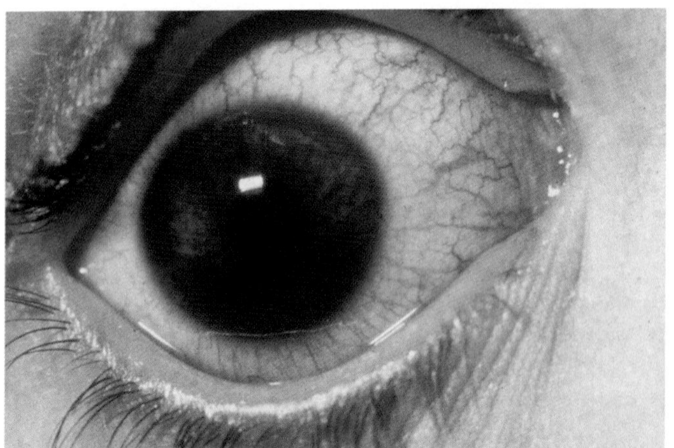

Plate 29.54 Hyphema. Blood in the anterior chamber obscures the iris. (see p. 1656).

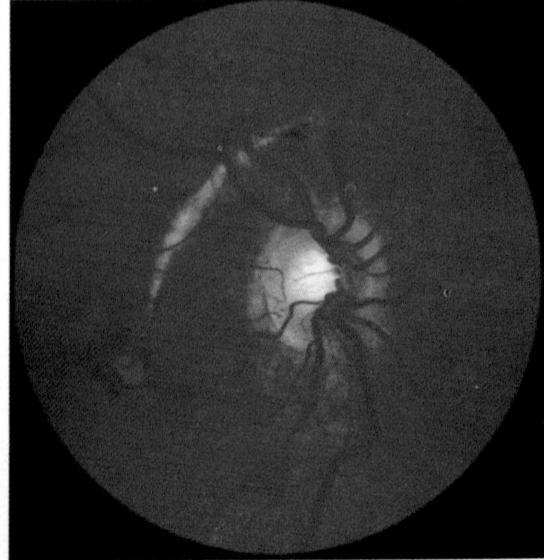

Plate 29.55 Choroidal rupture. Blunt force has caused a curved tear in Bruch's membrane deep to the retinal pigment epithelium. There is additional pigment scarring at the macula (see p. 1656).

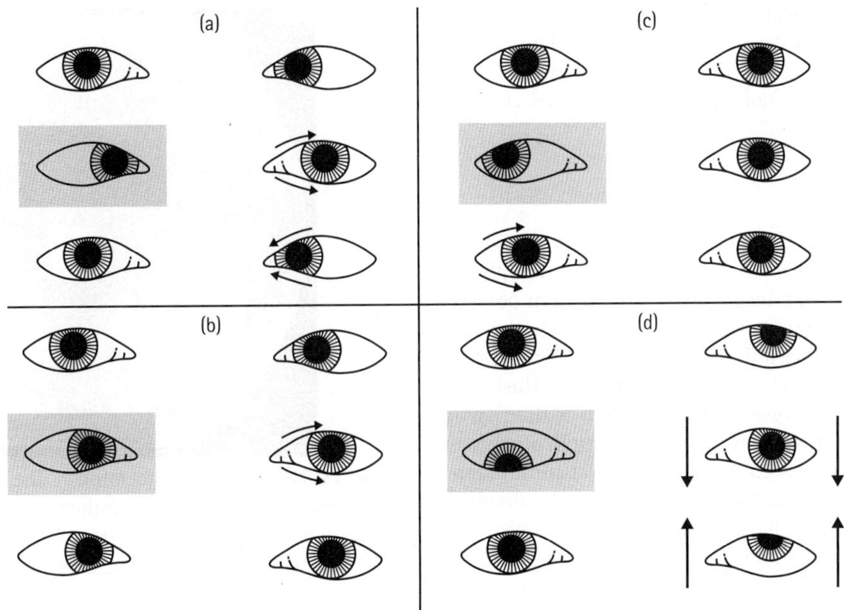

Fig. 29.9 The cover test for squint. Where there is no squint and there is normal binocular vision, both eyes maintain steady fixation on a distant object. There will be no deviation when one or other eye is covered and this is the basis of a cover test. When there is a latent or manifest squint some deviation will be observed on occluding one or other eye. (a) In manifest convergent squint the squinting eye is turned in and the non-squinting eye maintains fixation. If the squinting eye is occluded in the cover test there will be no variation in the angle of squint, but when the non-squinting eye ('fixing eye') is occluded it converges and the squinting eye takes up fixation. When the occluder is removed the original position of the eyes is resumed. (b) In alternating convergent squint either eye can maintain fixation while the other eye is turned in. If the squinting eye is occluded there is no alteration in the angle of deviation, but when the 'fixing eye' is occluded the opposite eye fixes the distant object and the previously straight eye converges. The former position is not resumed when the occluder is removed and the previously squinting eye maintains fixation (and the previously straight eye converges) until the occluder covers the originally squinting eye, when the originally fixing eye takes up position. (c) In latent squint both eyes will fix distant object but when one eye is covered it deviates. When the cover is removed the eye with the latent squint resumes fixation. The other eye does not shift or lose fixation while the opposite eye is being covered or uncovered. (d) The cover test is used to diagnose vertical squint as in horizontal squint, e.g. in left hypertropia the left eye is elevated (or the right eye depressed) and when the fixing eye is covered the opposite eye moves vertically to take up fixation.

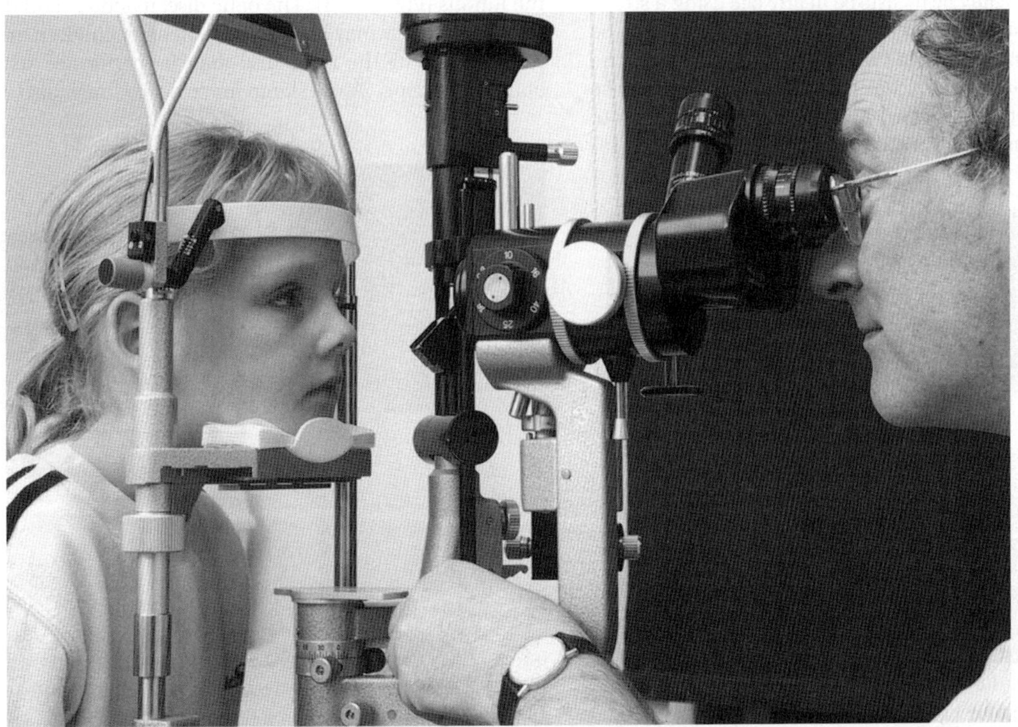

29.10 The slit lamp is a binocular microscope with an illuminating light in the form of a slit. This enhances stereoscopic viewing of tissues.

may be instilled and the corneal epithelium may be observed using a blue light (Fig. 29.11). Any defects in the corneal epithelium will absorb fluorescein and these areas will fluoresce yellow.

Corneal signs such as posterior embryotoxon may be visualized with a slit lamp (Fig. 29.12).

PUPIL REACTIONS

The relative size of the pupils should be observed. Slight asymmetry of pupil size may be observed as a normal variant. A torchlight may then be shone in each eye and the direct response to light observed. The light is then alternately shone in each eye, with the torch swinging backwards and forwards from eye to eye. This tests for relative afferent pupil defect. When the torch is shone in the healthy eye, the pupil constricts. However when the torch is then swung across to the eye with a sensory defect the pupil of this eye paradoxically dilates. This is because limited neural stimulation is produced by light shining in the defective eye and the dominant effect is the withdrawal of light from the healthy eye. Pupil dilatation in both eyes results and is observed in the defective eye. Motor pupil defects such as those seen following anticholinergic eye drop instillation or a III nerve palsy result in an absent pupil reaction to any stimulus.

PUPIL RED REFLEX

The transparency of the 'media' of the eye may be observed by observing the red reflex. When the media are transparent a beam of light directed from a direct ophthalmoscope will be observed to produce an orange-red reflection of the fundus, observable in the pupil area (Fig. 29.13). When cataract or vitreous opacity is present the red reflex will be dark or absent. A white reflex in the pupil area is an important pathological sign of possible underlying retinoblastoma or other significant ocular pathology.

RETINOSCOPY

The focusing of the eyes may be measured at any age using a streak retinoscope. Anticholinergic eye drops are instilled to dilate the pupil and relax the ciliary muscle so that there is no accommodation. In Caucasians cyclopentolate 1% eyedrops may be used, with measurements performed 30 minutes after instillation. In Asians and Africans it may be necessary to use atropine 1% eyedrops or ointment, instilled on two or more occasions a number of hours before the examination. A streak of light is directed into the pupil area and movement of the pupil light reflex is observed when the streak of light is moved from side to side. A test spectacle lens is then held in front of the eye and the process is repeated (Fig. 29.14). The power of the lens that neutralizes movements of the pupil light reflex gives a measure of the focusing of the eye.

OPHTHALMOSCOPY

Finally the fundi may be examined with the pupils dilated. Fundus examination of infants and young children is difficult with a direct ophthalmoscope. Ophthalmologists prefer to use an indirect ophthalmoscope. The light source is worn on the head and a convex lens is held in front of the eye in order to produce a focused image of the fundus (Fig. 29.15). The optic disc, macula, retinal vessels and retinal periphery may be examined. In older children, more detailed examination of the optic disc may be performed using a direct ophthalmoscope. A slit lamp microscope may also be used, in

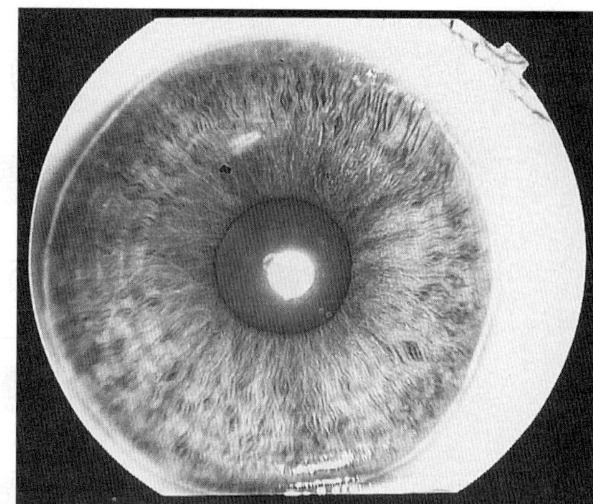

Fig. 29.12 Posterior embryotoxon. The edge of the basement membrane of the corneal endothelium is visible as a fine white line just inside the edge of the cornea. This is termed posterior embryotoxon. This line is normally more peripheral, and therefore not visible.

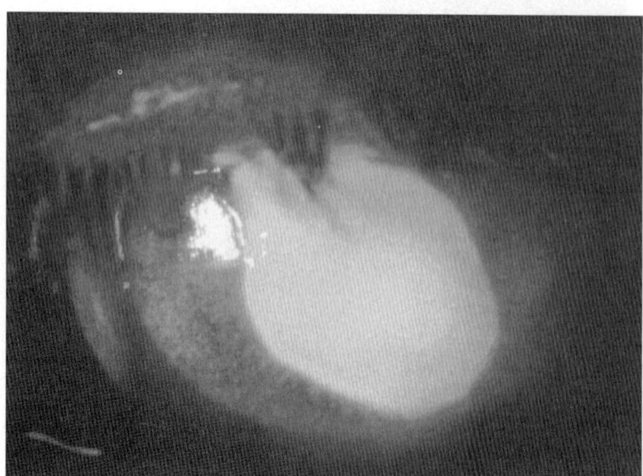

Fig. 29.11 Yellow/green fluorescein staining of an area of cornea abrasion visualized using blue light.

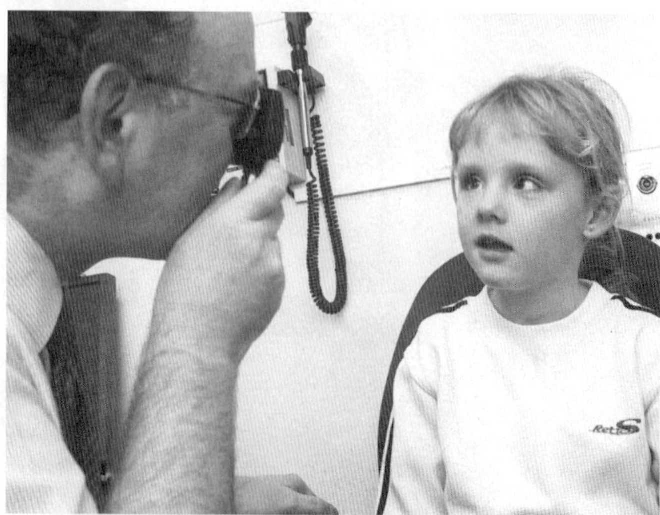

Fig. 29.13 Pupil red reflex testing using a direct ophthalmoscope. This is normally performed in a dimly lit room.

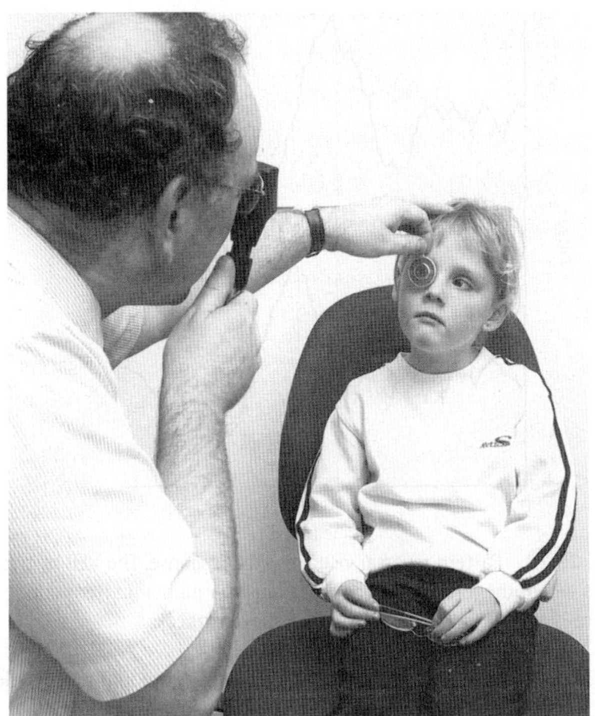

Fig. 29.14 Retinoscopy measurement of eye focusing.

conjunction with a high powered convex lens. This allows a detailed stereoscopic examination of the optic disc.

SPECIALIZED METHODS OF EXAMINATION

ULTRASOUND

Ultrasound imaging may be used to examine the retina when the media are opaque due to cataract or other pathology (Fig. 29.16). The diameter of tumors such as retinoblastoma may be measured. High definition ultrasound scans may be used to image the optic nerve head and optic nerve. Optic nerve head drusen may be detected. Widening of the cerebrospinal fluid (CSF) space around the optic nerve may be helpful in the diagnosis of raised intracranial pressure with papilledema.[10]

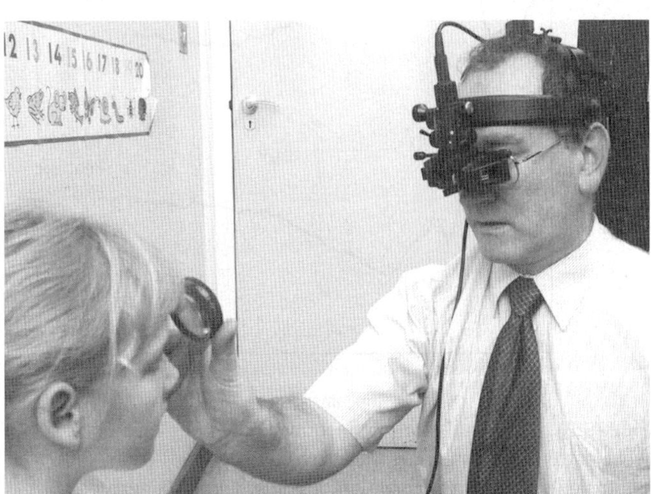

Fig. 29.15 Binocular indirect ophthalmoscope examination of the fundus.

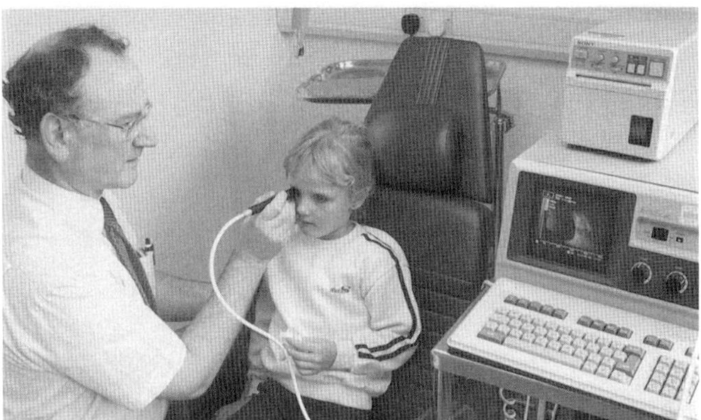

Fig. 29.16 Ocular ultrasound examination.

FUNDUS FLUORESCEIN ANGIOGRAPHY

Angiogram photographs of the retinal blood vessels may be obtained using intravenous or oral fluorescein dye (Fig. 29.17). This technique may be of value in assessing retinal vascular disease, retinal inflammatory disease and optic disc abnormalities. In the presence of optic disc edema, capillaries on the surface of the optic disc are dilated and leaky (Fig. 29.18). Optic nerve head drusen 'autofluoresce'– angiogram fluorescence is seen in the absence of fluorescein dye.

ELECTROPHYSIOLOGY STUDIES

Studies of the visual system using visually evoked potentials (VEP), and of the retina using the electroretinogram may be of great diagnostic value in infants and young children with reduced vision. The stimulus for a VEP is a flash of light or a reversing pattern of black and white squares (Fig. 29.19). Pattern onset stimulation may be used as an alternative to pattern reversal. Uniocular testing and hemifield testing may be performed. The occipital cortex response is detected using electroencephalogram (EEG) electrodes. Delayed VEP response following stimulation of one eye may indicate optic nerve demyelination on that side, while reduced amplitude may indicate reduced axonal function as in optic nerve hypoplasia (Fig. 29.20). In albinism there is increased chiasmal nerve crossing and this produces asymmetrical occipital lobe responses to uniocular stimuli.

VEPs may be used in vision laboratories as a method of visual acuity testing in infants. Statistical analysis of a rapid sequence

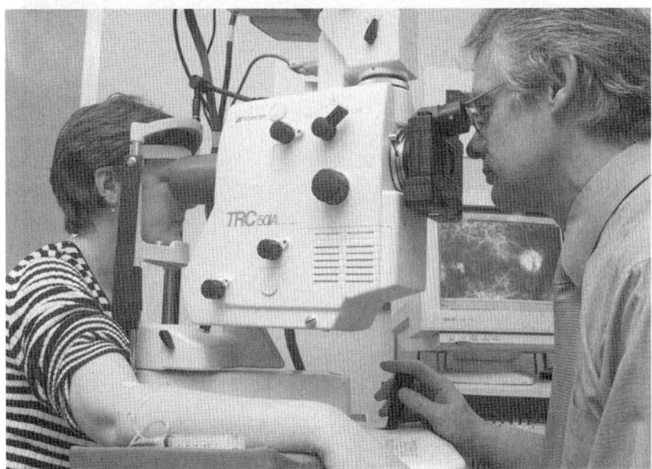

Fig. 29.17 A digital fundus camera images the retina following intravenous injection of fluorescein dye.

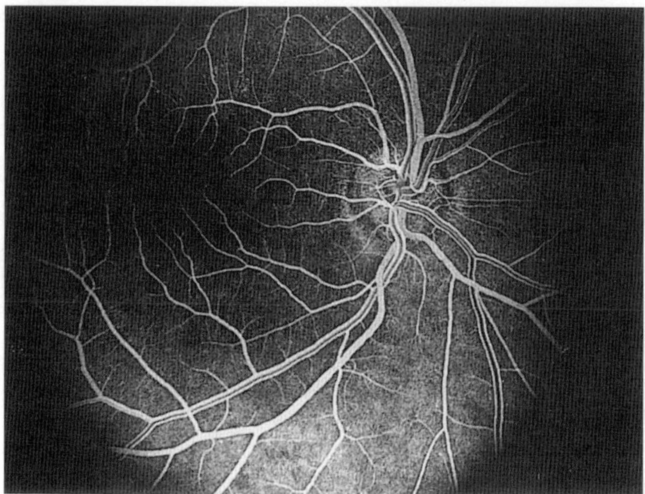

Fig. 29.18 Fluorescein dye is seen in the retinal arteries and capillaries 12 s after intravenous injection. Dye is starting to return to the veins.

('sweep') of checker pattern sizes is used to produce an estimate of visual acuity.

The electroretinogram (ERG) gives information about retinal function. The stimulus is a flash of light. The response is detected by skin electrodes on the eyelids or by ocular contact electrodes.[11] Ocular contact electrodes require anesthesia or sedation in young children but may be performed using local anesthetic eye drops in older, cooperative children. The electrical response is generated in the retina – the 'a' wave by the photoreceptors and the 'b' wave by the inner retina. Cone function and rod function may be analyzed separately by using a range of test strategies in which the background illumination is varied and the light flash stimulation is varied. Rod responses are measured using dim flash stimuli after dark adaptation (scotopic responses). Cone responses are measured in normal lighting conditions (photopic responses) (Fig. 29.21). 30 Hertz flicker stimuli are used to isolate cone responses. The individual components of the ERG are best seen in the bright flash response following dark adaptation. Diseases which predominantly affect rod function produce abnormal scotopic ERG responses, diseases which predominantly affect cone function produce abnormal photopic and 30 Hz flicker ERG responses, and diseases which predominantly affect the inner retina predominantly affect ERG b waves.

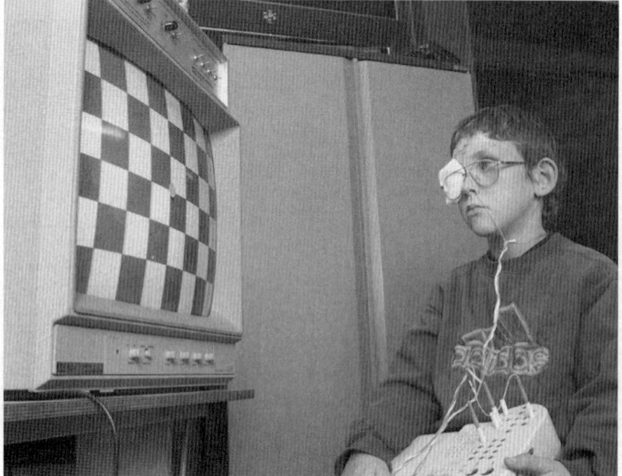

Fig. 29.19 Visually evoked potential examination using a reversing checker pattern stimulus.

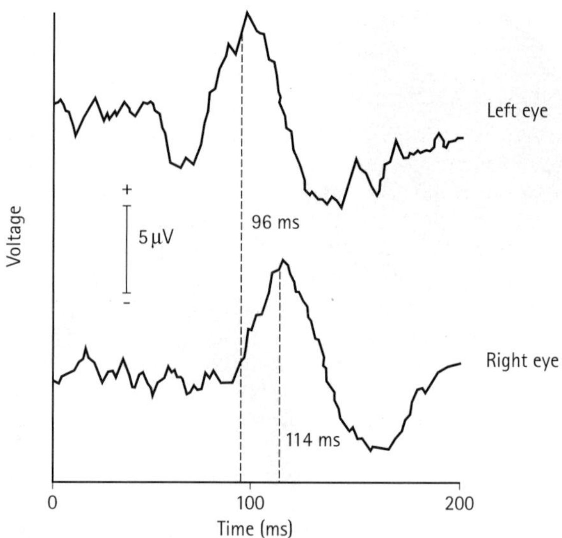

Fig. 29.20 Pattern reversal visual evoked response. The VER of two eyes where the left eye (upper trace) shows a normal pattern and there is a slight delay in the right eye (lower trace).

REFRACTIVE ERRORS AND AMBLYOPIA

REFRACTIVE ERRORS

Refractive errors may be treated with spectacles. However the presence of a refractive error may also be of diagnostic value. For instance Leber's congenital amaurosis is often associated with hypermetropia,[12] and Marfan's syndrome[13] with myopia.

In hypermetropia, additional accommodation is used to maintain clear focus. This may lead to excessive convergence of the eyes and is a common cause of convergent squint. In myopia,

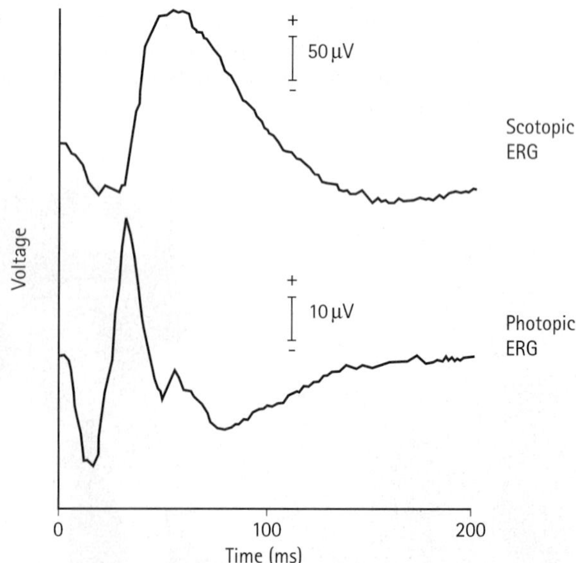

Fig. 29.21 A normal electroretinogram (ERG) showing the typical wave pattern and amplitude. The electroretinogram is taken under photopic (light adapted) conditions and scotopic (dark adapted) conditions. The wave pattern is reduced or abolished in various pathological conditions of the retina.

distance vision is blurred but near vision is in focus. Astigmatism refers to irregular focusing due to the corneal surface being very slightly oval shaped rather than perfectly spherical.

Most infants are slightly hypermetropic, and there is a trend towards reducing hypermetropia with age.[14] Myopia is rare in young children. When high degrees of myopia do occur an underlying disease such as homocystinuria[15] or Marfan's syndrome[13] should be considered. While refractive errors are relatively uncommon among schoolchildren in developing countries,[16] the incidence of myopia among schoolchildren is rapidly increasing in developed countries.[17,18] This may be related to increased near work,[19] and is not influenced by spectacle wear.[20]

Children with cerebral palsy are more likely to be hypermetropic and have reduced accommodation range. The threshold for spectacle prescription is therefore lower in children with cerebral palsy.

AMBLYOPIA

When one eye is more hypermetropic than the other, accommodation produces a clear image in the more normal eye. However the retinal image in the more hypermetropic eye remains blurred, as accommodation amplitude is under bilateral neural drive. Untreated, occipital cortex synaptic connections related to this eye will remain under-developed.[21] This is termed anisometropic amblyopia.[22]

When a squint develops, the brain suppresses vision from the squinting eye in order to avoid diplopia. However continued suppression leads to failure of development of synaptic connections in the occipital cortex and once again the affected eye becomes amblyopic – strabismic amblyopia.[21] Anisometropic and strabismic amblyopia may coexist.[23]

The treatment of amblyopia is to first treat the underlying cause with spectacles. Occlusion of the normal eye is then used to drive development of synaptic connections relating to the amblyopic eye (Fig. 29.22).[24,25] Atropine eyedrops may be used to blur vision in the normal eye, as an alternative to occlusion (atropine penalization.)

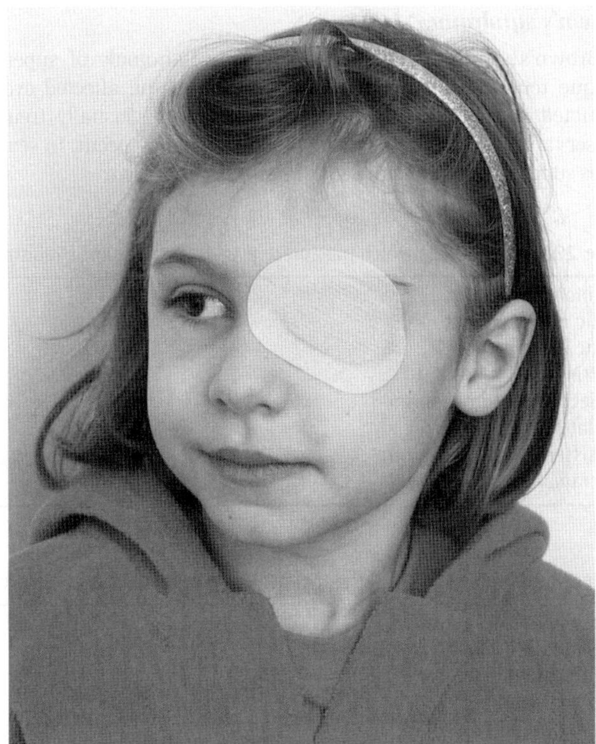

Fig. 29.22 Occlusion treatment

Community visual screening programs are used to detect amblyopia.[26] These are particularly necessary for the detection of anisometropic amblyopia, which is generally asymptomatic.[26] Visual acuity measurements in each eye detect reduced vision in the amblyopic eye and lead to referral for assessment and treatment. Screening may also detect small angled strabismus with amblyopia.[26] Photographic techniques, which use pupil light reflex patterns to measure refractive errors, are currently under development as an alternative approach to community screening.[27]

STRABISMUS

TERMINOLOGY

The term 'strabismus' and 'squint' are used interchangeably. 'Strabismus' is preferred. The prefix 'eso' is used for convergent deviations, and 'exo' for divergent deviations. 'Hyper' refers to upward deviation of an eye and 'hypo' to downward deviation. A 'tropia' is a manifest strabismus, which is present in binocular viewing conditions and is detected using the cover test. A 'phoria' is a latent strabismus, which is only apparent when binocular viewing is disrupted. The word 'deviation' is used to include both tropias and phorias. In 'concomitant' strabismus the deviation angle is the same in all directions of gaze. In 'incomitant' strabismus the deviation angle may be greater in one direction of gaze – for example in the direction of action of a paretic muscle. Adduction refers to medial movement of one eye, towards the nose, and abduction to lateral movement of one eye. 'Primary position' refers to the straight-ahead viewing position.

'Pseudosquint' refers to the appearance of apparent esotropia due to wide epicanthic skin folds. No true ocular deviation is present when a cover test is performed.

There are three common types of concomitant strabismus in childhood.

INFANTILE ESOTROPIA

This type of convergent strabismus becomes apparent at age 3–4 months (Fig. 29.23). In most cases there is no associated neurological abnormality. However infants who have developmental

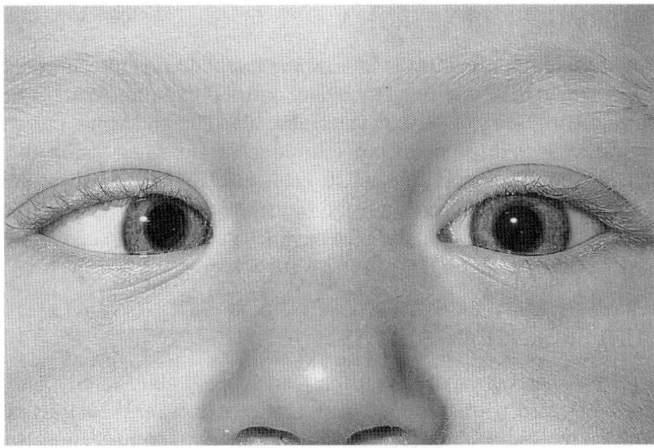

Fig. 29.23 Infantile esotropia. The right eye was converging when the photograph was taken.

neurological problems are at increased risk of developing infantile esotropia. The typical characteristics of infantile esotropia are a large angled convergent strabismus, which alternates between the two eyes. There is no amblyopia as each eye is in use part of the time. There is no significant refractive error in most cases although hypermetropia is present in some cases. There is no binocular function. The lateral recti may appear to be weak, as the infant habitually tends to use the right eye to look to the left side and vice versa ('cross fixation'). This may lead to the suspicion of bilateral VI cranial nerve weakness.

An unusual type of nystagmus may be present, termed manifest latent nystagmus. In this form of nystagmus, the nystagmus is exaggerated by covering one eye. The uncovered eye develops a jerking nystagmus with the jerk towards the side of the fixing eye. Manifest latent nystagmus is specific to infantile esotropia and its clinical recognition may lead to the avoidance of unnecessary neurological investigation.

When present, hypermetropia should be treated with spectacles. Very early surgery, performed before the age of 12 months, improves binocular function outcome.[26–30] However high levels of stereopsis are rarely achieved.

ACQUIRED ESOTROPIA

Children who are hypermetropic habitually use extra accommodation in order to maintain clear focus. As accommodation and convergence reflexes are linked, this may lead to excessive convergence. Loss of control of convergence will lead to a convergent strabismus. The treatment is to promptly recognize the problem and promptly provide full spectacle correction.[23,31,32] This may reverse the condition. However if the strabismus does not fully reverse with spectacle wear occlusion treatment for amblyopia followed by surgical treatment may be necessary. The use of preoperative prism spectacles improves the accuracy of surgical outcome.[33]

A late onset acquired esotropia may be mistakenly diagnosed as an acute VI nerve palsy. Patients with acute onset of esotropia should be assessed by an ophthalmologist as this may lead to prompt curative spectacle treatment rather than to a series of neurological investigations. Conversely concomitant convergent strabismus may be a presenting feature of VI nerve weakness due to a brainstem glioma, raised intracranial pressure or other pathology. A high index of suspicion for underlying neurological disease must therefore be maintained.

INTERMITTENT EXOTROPIA

The third common cause of strabismus in children is intermittent exotropia. In this condition binocular control is maintained at times but at other times one eye deviates laterally. The child may partly close the deviating eye in order to concentrate when using the straight eye. Vision is normal in each eye. Usually there is no significant refractive error and no treatment is needed unless the child is significantly symptomatic, in which case surgical correction may be undertaken.

CONVERGENCE WEAKNESS

Weakness of convergence is usually an isolated abnormality, and can be treated with orthoptic convergence exercises. Weakness of both convergence and accommodation may develop in teenagers, and is generally self-limiting. Prolonged periods of study, and stress related to prolonged periods of study, may partly be responsible for symptoms. In some cases correcting spectacles may be needed in addition to orthoptic exercises.

STRABISMUS AS A SIGN OF UNDERLYING ORGANIC DISEASE

All cases of strabismus should be promptly assessed, as both convergent and divergent strabismus may be a presenting feature of more serious underlying disease (Table 29.1). Mild VI cranial nerve weakness can cause apparently concomitant strabismus.

INCOMITANT STRABISMUS

Weak lateral rectus function is the most common cause of incomitant strabismus. VI cranial nerve weakness should be suspected in all cases (Table 29.2).

Incomitant strabismus syndromes

Duane's syndrome

In Duane's syndrome VI cranial nerve innervation of the lateral rectus muscle is variably defective, and an anomalous branch of the III cranial nerve supplies the lateral rectus muscle. On attempted adduction of the eye the medial rectus and lateral rectus muscle both contract and the eye retracts into the orbit, with narrowing of the palpebral aperture. On attempted abduction there is variable lateral rectus weakness, which may be mistaken for VI cranial nerve palsy caused by aquired neurological disease.

Surgical treatment is reserved for those children who develop a significant compensatory head turn (towards the side of the affected eye), or strabismus in primary position.

Moebius syndrome

Moebius syndrome consists of congenital absence of cranial nerve nuclei, including the VI and VII nerve nuclei. Abduction is absent in each eye, and there is bilateral facial palsy.

Brown's syndrome

In Brown's syndrome there is a congenital anomaly of superior oblique tendon and trochlea function. When the affected eye is adducted it shoots downwards. The condition is usually treated conservatively as some spontaneous recovery may occur. In severe cases superior oblique tenotomy surgery is performed.

Table 29.1 Conditions which may present with concomitant strabismus

Retinoblastoma
Optic nerve hypoplasia
Optic atrophy:
Primary
Secondary to neoplasm
Unilateral cataract
Persistent fetal vasculature
VI cranial nerve weakness

Table 29.2 Causes of true or apparent VI nerve weakness in children

VI cranial nerve paresis:
Raised intracranial pressure
Brainstem glioma
Moebius syndrome
Duane's syndrome
Esotropia (abduction is usually normal)

Congenital superior oblique tendon laxity

Weakness of superior oblique function in children (and adults) is more commonly caused by congenital laxity of the superior oblique tendon than by IV cranial nerve paresis. Typically there is a compensatory head tilt to the side opposite to that of the abnormal tendon. This may be mistaken for neck muscle induced torticollis. Eye movement examination reveals weakness of the affected superior oblique, with secondary overaction of inferior oblique function. Surgery may be performed if there is a significant compensatory head posture, or strabismus in primary position. The lax tendon may be tucked, or the overactive inferior oblique muscle may be weakened by recession surgery.

NYSTAGMUS

CONGENITAL IDIOPATHIC NYSTAGMUS

In congenital idiopathic nystagmus the onset of nystagmus occurs between the ages of 2 and 3 months. Some cases are familial – dominant, recessive and X-linked inheritance has been described. An underlying vision defect should be excluded. Typically the nystagmus is horizontal and the amplitude is greater on looking to one side and less on looking to the other side (null zone). Head nodding may be present. Ocular examination is otherwise normal and there are no neurological abnormalities. The ERG and VEPs are normal. On follow-up, near vision develops to a relatively normal level. There is moderate reduction of distance vision and some modification of the classroom environment is often helpful. Treatment consists of spectacle correction of refractive errors. Surgical treatment is occasionally useful if there is a well-defined null zone that can be moved into a more central position by adjusting the position of the horizontal recti muscles.[34]

SENSORY DEFECT NYSTAGMUS

Infants with congenital nystagmus may have an underlying vision defect. In most cases an ocular abnormality is present and a systematic approach to ocular and electrophysiological examination is required. A differential diagnosis is given in Table 29.3. As a general rule posterior visual pathway defects do not result in nystagmus,[35] although periventricular leucomalacia may cause nystagmus.[36]

ALBINISM

Albinism refers to a group of conditions, which may be divided into oculocutaneous albinism (OCA) and ocular albinism (OA). The ocular abnormalities found are common to all forms of albinism. In addition to defective iris and fundus pigmentation, abnormalities include: reduced vision and photophobia; nystagmus; strabismus; delayed visual maturation; foveal hypoplasia; and abnormal chiasmal crossing. More than 90% of fibers cross at the chiasm, resulting in cortical asymmetry of VEP responses. Iris translucency varies from very pink irises in tyrosinase negative OCA, to relatively minor defects of iris pigmentation which may only be detected by slit lamp transillumination performed in a dark room. Most forms of OCA are autosomal recessive. Two rare forms of OCA are associated with systemic disease – increased susceptibility to infection in Chediak–Higashi disease, and frequent bruising due to platelet dysfunction in Hermansky–Pudlak syndrome.

In ocular albinism typical ocular abnormalities are present, but skin and hair color are normal. OA1 is X-linked, and is frequently misdiagnosed as congenital idiopathic nystagmus.

Refractive errors should be corrected with spectacles, and photophobia reduced with tinted spectacles and peaked hats. Mainstream education, with some attention to the classroom environment, and normal educational attainment may be anticipated in almost all cases.

Table 29.3 Causes of sensory congenital nystagmus

Albinism
Leber's amaurosis
Aniridia
Optic nerve hypoplasia
Retinal cone dystrophy

ANIRIDIA

Aniridia is an autosomal dominant condition caused by mutations in the PAX 6 homeobox gene. Gene expression is variable in familial cases – relatively small iris defects may be the only abnormality found in some family members.

About 30% of cases are sporadic, with deletions at 11p13. Sporadic cases have a high incidence of associated abnormalities, including Wilm's tumor, genitourinary abnormalities and mental retardation. Up to 30% of sporadic cases develop Wilm's tumor by age 3 years, and 3 monthly abdominal examinations or abdominal ultrasound examinations are required until age 5 years.

Aniridia represents a defect of neural crest cell development. In addition to the striking absence of iris tissue, with only very rudimentary stubs of iris tissue present, the following ocular abnormalities are frequently seen: nystagmus, fibrovascular corneal pannus, refractive errors, glaucoma, cataract, foveal hypoplasia and optic nerve hypoplasia (Fig. 29.24). Foveal hypoplasia refers to poorly differentiated foveal structures – in extreme cases major retinal blood vessels may cross the normally avascular fovea. Corneal disease may be due to defective limbal stem cells, and can respond well to stem cell grafts. Glaucoma surgery outcomes are limited by conjunctival scarring – tube surgery with antimetabolite augmentation is usually required. Cataract surgery is also complicated, because of absent iris tissue and weak lens zonules. Progressive loss of vision over decades is usual in aniridia patients.

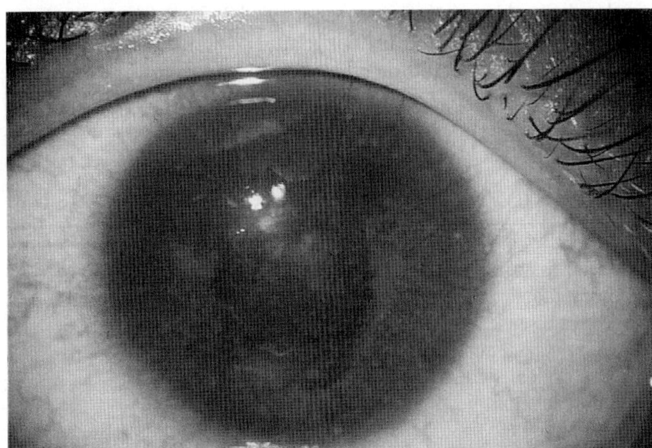

Fig. 29.24 Aniridia. No iris tissue is seen. There is fibrovascular pannus covering the peripheral cornea in this case.

ACQUIRED NYSTAGMUS

Acquired nystagmus in childhood always requires prompt ophthalmic and neurological assessment. A differential diagnosis is given in Table 29.4. Vertical nystagmus may consist of downbeat nystagmus, associated with craniocervical junction abnormalities, or more rarely upbeat nystagmus, associated with brainstem and cerebellum lesions. Urgent brain imaging is usually indicated.

SPASMUS NUTANS

Spasmus nutans is a syndrome of infancy with nystagmus, head nodding and torticollis. Investigation to exclude an intracranial tumor is required. The syndrome resolves after 12–18 months and the diagnosis is one of exclusion, made retrospectively.

THE APPARENTLY BLIND INFANT

Infants with poor visual behavior require urgent assessment by an ophthalmologist. Treatable disease such as cataract must be dealt with promptly in order to avoid the development of irreversible amblyopia. In most cases the cause is apparent following ophthalmic examination. Ocular defects which may cause bilateral congenital blindness are given in Table 29.5.

In some cases there may be no ocular abnormality evident, or only very subtle defects are found (Table 29.6). In these cases electrophysiological and neurological investigations may be required.

DELAYED VISUAL MATURATION (DVM)

Delayed visual maturation refers to visual unresponsiveness from birth that subsequently improves.[37] The diagnosis is one of exclusion and is always retrospective. The onset of visually stimulated smiling is delayed, clinical pupil responses are normal and there is no nystagmus. The underlying defect may be subcortical, with secondary cortical mediated effects.[38] Four types are recognized.

- Type 1 – DVM as an isolated anomaly. Vision improves to normal levels at age 10–20 weeks and there are no significant sequelae (mild neurodevelopmental sequelae have been detected in some cases).
- Type 2 – DVM with severe, permanent neurodevelopmental problems. Vision improves after 6–18 months, but remains subnormal.
- Type 3 – DVM associated with infantile nystagmus or albinism. Nystagmus is absent during the period of blindness, but develops when vision improves at age 10–25 weeks.
- Type 4 – DVM with severe congenital structural ocular abnormalities (excluding albinism). Vision improves during the first 1–2 years of life but remains severely subnormal.

Table 29.4 Causes of acquired nystagmus in children

Suprasellar tumor
Posterior fossa tumor or malformation
Neurometabolic:
Leigh's disease
Organic acidemias
Urea cycle disorders
Aminoacidopathies
Neurolipidoses
Batten's disease
Peroxisomal disorders

Table 29.5 Ocular defects which may cause bilateral congenital blindness

Whole globe	Anophthalmos Microphthalmos
Cornea	Sclerocornea Peter's anomaly (associated glaucoma and cataract)
Lens	Cataract
Retina	Retinal detachment (e.g. following retinopathy of prematurity) Retinal dysplasia (e.g. Norrie's disease) Retinal folds Chorioretinal coloboma Chorioretinitis scarring Cherry red spot in storage diseases (e.g. Tay–Sachs disease)
Optic atrophy	Prenatal: Infection Asphyxia Cerebral malformations Perinatal: Asphyxia Postnatal: Meningitis/encephalitis Compression (e.g. hydrocephalus, craniopharyngioma) Retinal diseases Genetic (e.g. autosomal dominant optic atrophy
Optic nerve hypoplasia	
Optic disc colobomas	

CEREBRAL VISUAL IMPAIRMENT (CVI)

Infants and children with CVI often have a clear history of severe CNS insult. Causes are given in Table 29.7.

Infants and children with CVI have normal ophthalmic examination, with preserved pupil responses. Nystagmus is not present.[35] The VEP may be normal or abnormal. The visual defect may be total initially, but there is variable improvement with time, dependent on etiology and severity. Most children achieve some navigational vision. Recovery may take from a few hours to 2 years. Full recovery has been reported after head injury and cardiac arrest, but is less likely after bacterial meningitis and does not occur in children with neurodegenerative disorders.

LEBER'S AMAUROSIS

Leber's amaurosis (isolated infantile rod–cone dystrophy) is an autosomal recessive congenital retinal dystrophy. Vision is absent or severely reduced from birth and the ERG is markedly reduced or absent.

Table 29.6 The blind infant with apparently normal eyes

Delayed visual maturation
Cerebral visual impairment
Leber's amaurosis
Retinal cone dystrophy
Optic nerve hypoplasia
Oculomotor apraxia

Table 29.7 Causes of cerebral visual impairment

Prenatal	CNS malformations Intrauterine infections Maternal toxemia
Perinatal	Neonatal asphyxia Intracerebral hemorrhage Hypoglycemia Meningitis Encephalitis
Postnatal	Trauma (accidental and non-accidental) Cardiac arrest Meningitis Encephalitis Neurodegenerative disorders Cortical vein thrombosis Hydrocephalus shunt failure

The pupils may show a sluggish afferent response. Refraction shows significant hypermetropia. The fundus appearances are normal or near normal. The disease is static in some cases, and progressive in others.[39] The term Leber's amaurosis should be reserved for cases of isolated infantile rod–cone dystrophy. Several genes have been identified.[40] While no active treatment is possible at present, laboratory models of gene therapy are under development.[41]

Infantile rod–cone dystrophy is one component of a number of congenital syndromes (Table 29.8), and the diagnosis of Leber's amaurosis should only be made after exclusion of other recognized syndromes. Hearing, neurological, renal and metabolic abnormalities should be sought.

CONGENITAL RETINAL CONE DYSTROPHIES

Achromatopsia and blue cone monochromatism present with reduced vision, nystagmus and photophobia in infancy. The electroretinogram is abnormal, especially for cone functions, but the fundus appearances may be normal. The conditions are not progressive.

Congenital stationary night blindness is a non-progressive congenital abnormality of rod function of the retina. Vision is particularly reduced in dim lighting conditions.

OPTIC NERVE HYPOPLASIA (ONH)

ONH is not inherited, and most cases are idiopathic. Insults in early embryonic development have been associated with ONH – maternal diabetes, maternal alcohol and substance abuse. OHN may occur in isolation or in association with failure of development of the anterior midline structures of the brain (septo-optic dysplasia), hydranencephaly, porencephaly, cerebral atrophy or leucomalacia. ONH also occurs in aniridia. Mutations in the homeobox domain HESX1 have been identified in a small number of patients with septo-optic dysplasia.[42]

Table 29.8 Syndromes associated with infantile rod–cone dystrophy

Cerebellar vermis hypoplasia, e.g. Joubert's syndrome
Deafness, e.g. Usher's syndrome type 1, peroxisomal disorders
Renal disease, e.g. nephronophthisis
Skeletal abnormalities
Peroxisomal disorders, e.g. Zellweger syndrome
Mitochondrial cytopathies, e.g. hydroxyacyl-CoA dehydrogenase deficiency
Amino acid disorders, e.g. methylmalonic aciduria

Cases may be unilateral, bilateral or asymmetric. There is a spectrum of severity ranging from complete blindness with very tiny optic nerve structures to virtually normal vision with very minor degrees of ONH.

The optic disc appearances vary (Fig.29.25) and include:

- variably small optic disc;
- peripapillary pigmented ring (double ring sign);
- slightly tortuous retinal vessels;
- associated optic atrophy;
- segmental disc hypoplasia.

Mild cases present with reduced vision in one or both eyes, or with strabismus. Mild degrees of optic nerve hypoplasia may be misdiagnosed as amblyopia, and cases of amblyopia which do not respond well to occlusion treatment should always be carefully examined for the presence of subtle optic nerve hypoplasia.

Severe bilateral cases are more likely to have associated neuroendocrine dysfunction. Hypoglycemia may occur in the neonatal period. Magnetic resonance imaging (MRI) scanning is useful as a predictor of later neuroendocrine dysfunction and also allows assessment of optic nerve size. Growth, thyroid and gonadotrophic hormones may be defective.

OCULOMOTOR APRAXIA

Absent saccadic eye movements may be mistakenly interpreted as defective visual function. The ERG is reduced in some cases,[43] further increasing the possibility of misdiagnosing Leber's amaurosis.

ACQUIRED VISUAL LOSS IN CHILDREN

Acquired visual loss at any age requires urgent investigation. Uniocular visual loss may result in the development of strabismus. Binocular visual loss will lead to impaired visual behavior and, in older children, a complaint of reduced vision. In most cases, acquired visual loss is due to retinal, optic nerve or neurological disease (Table 29.9). When the cause is not evident on ophthalmic examination, neurological, electrophysiological, and neuro-imaging assessment will be needed.

CATARACT

Bilateral cataract developing in later childhood is rare. Metabolic disorders such as diabetes mellitus and disorders of galactose metabolism should be excluded.

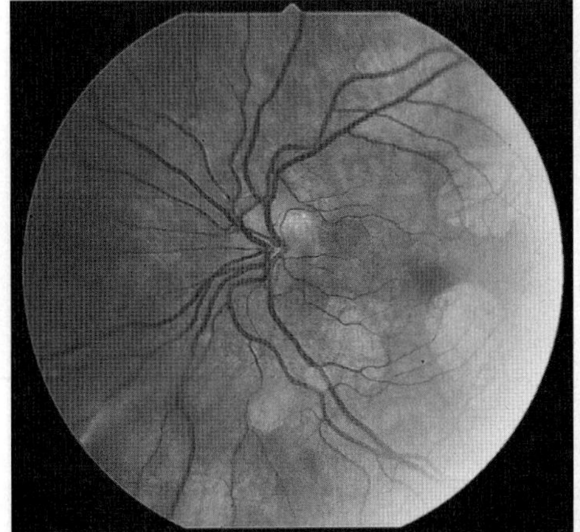

Fig. 29.25 Hypoplastic disc. Optic nerve hypoplasia. The optic disc is anatomically very small in this case, with severely reduced vision.

Table 29.9 Causes of visual loss in children evident on ophthalmic examination

Cataract	Metabolic disease		
Retina	Retinal dystrophies	Rod–cone dystrophies X-linked juvenile retinoschisis Stargardt's disease/fundus flavimaculatus	
Optic atrophy	External compression	Hydrocephalus Tumor	 Craniopharyngioma Other suprasellar tumors
	Intrinsic tumor	Glioma	Neurofibromatosis type 1
	Retinal diseases		
	Genetic	Autosomal dominant optic atrophy	
	Demyelinating diseases		

RETINAL DYSTROPHIES

This term refers to genetic abnormalities of the retina or retinal pigment epithelium, which lead to reduced retinal function. They may be non-progressive, as in the congenital cone dystrophies discussed above, or progressive. Rod dysfunction presents with reduced vision, especially in dim lighting conditions. Cone dysfunction presents with reduced vision, photophobia, and reduced color vision. Fundus examination may show pigmentary disturbance. When the rods are predominantly affected, black spiky blotches of pigment are seen in the retinal periphery (bone spicule pigmentation) (Fig. 29.26). This appearance lead to the historical term 'retinitis pigmentosa'. When the cones are affected pigmentation at the macula, often in a ring shape (bull's eye) (Fig. 29.27), may be present. The diagnosis is made on clinical grounds, supported by electroretinogram abnormalities of rod and cone functions.

Most types of retinal dystrophy are currently not treatable. Two rare forms of rod–cone dystrophy of childhood are amenable to treatment. In Refsum's disease serum phytanic acid levels are raised. Dietary intervention will improve the prognosis for vision and also reduce morbidity due to other systemic features of the disease. In abetalipoproteinemia, there is acanthocytosis of the red cells on a blood film, with absent plasma beta-lipoproteins. Vitamin and dietary treatment will improve the prognosis.

X-LINKED JUVENILE RETINOSCHISIS

In X-linked juvenile retinoschisis there is progressive loss of visual acuity due to schisis (splitting) of the nerve fiber layer at the fovea. In some cases there is more extensive splitting of the retina in the retinal periphery. The ERG a wave is normal, but the b wave is reduced. The disease presents at age 5–10 years, and the prognosis is relatively good as disease progression is very slow.

STARGARDT'S DISEASE

Stargardt's disease is an autosomal recessive disease with onset in late childhood. Symptoms are limited to reduced visual acuity, with no symptoms of night blindness or of photophobia. Typically there are creamy fishtail shaped flecks in the retina (fundus flavimaculatus) with additional retinal pigment epithelium atrophy at the macula (Fig. 29.28). Fundus fluorescein angiography may be helpful in the diagnosis of early cases. There is a characteristic 'dark choroid' appearance due to reduced transparency of the retinal pigment epithelium. Phenotype variation is related to different mutations in the ABCR gene.[44]

The disease progresses until visual acuity is reduced to about 6/60.[45]

AUTOSOMAL DOMINANT OPTIC ATROPHY

The finding of reduced vision and optic atrophy should lead to prompt neurological and neuroimaging investigations. In autosomal dominant optic atrophy neurological investigations are normal. There is reduced visual acuity, some reduction of color vision, reduced visual field sensitivity between fixation and the blind spot ('centrocaecal scotoma'), reduced amplitude pattern VEP, and

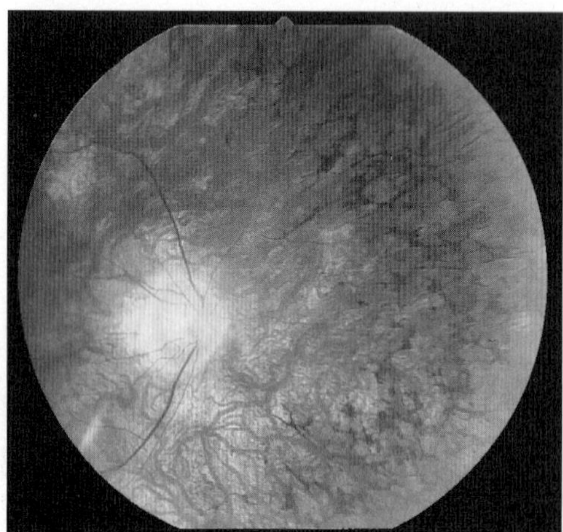

Fig. 29.26 Retinitis pigmentosa. Typical 'bone spicule' pigmentation is seen in the mid periphery of the fundus.

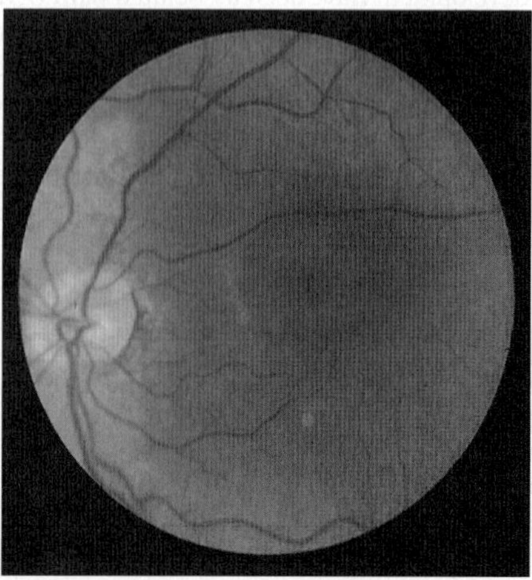

Fig. 29.27 Retinal cone dystrophy with typical 'bull's eye' pigmentation at the center of the macula.

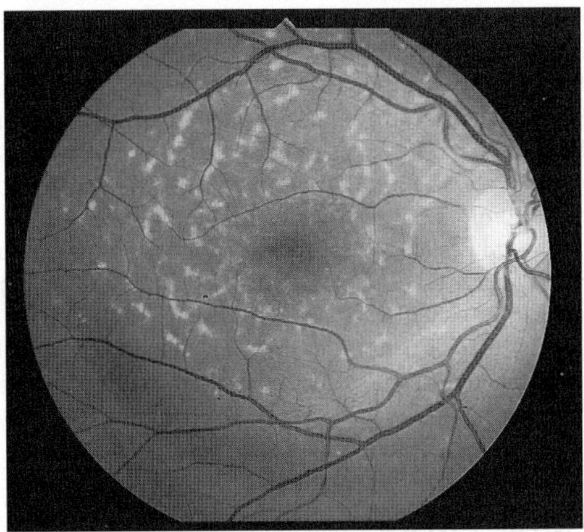

Fig. 29.28 Stargardt's disease. Typical creamy fishtail shaped flecks are seen in the fundus. There are no macular pigment changes in this case.

variable pallor of the temporal part of the optic disc. Visual loss is not severe, and progression is very slow.

CHILDHOOD VISUAL LOSS WITH NO ABNORMALITY ON OPHTHALMIC EXAMINATION

BATTEN'S DISEASE (NEURONAL CEROID LIPOFUSCINOSIS)

The neuronal ceroid lipofuscinoses (NCL) are a group of autosomal recessive neurodegenerative lysosomal storage diseases. While classification by age of disease onset has been helpful in the past, more precise molecular genetic diagnosis is now possible. To date eight genes have been identified – CLN1–8. Diagnosis is made using electron microscopic examination of lymphocytes, skin biopsy or conjunctival biopsy. Characteristic osmiophilic inclusions are seen, which may be 'fingerprint', curvilinear or granular in appearance. Biochemical enzyme function studies and molecular genetic analysis of CLN2 and CLN3 genes further refine diagnosis.[46] Prenatal and presymptomatic diagnosis may be offered to families.

The juvenile onset form of Batten's disease may present with visual loss. Neurological degenerative symptoms may not develop for up to 3 years later. The diagnosis must therefore be considered in any child aged 4–10 years with visual loss, that cannot be explained on ophthalmic examination. The fundi may initially appear normal. The ERG is reduced, especially the b wave. Later a 'bull's eye' pigmentary disturbance develops at the macula. The disease is progressive, with epileptic seizures and dementia. While no treatment is available at present rapid progress in molecular understanding of the disease may lead to gene therapies.

FUNCTIONAL VISUAL LOSS

A relatively common cause of apparent reduction of vision in young teenagers is 'functional' visual loss. Symptoms are precipitated by stress. Typically the child complains of blurred vision. On examination there are no objective abnormalities. The diagnosis can be made if the child is 'tricked' into giving normal visual acuity test results by using neutralizing combinations of spectacle lenses or other means. Having made the diagnosis, psychological counseling may be helpful. Underlying problems at school or in the home may be detected. The prognosis is usually good, as the underlying psychological disturbance tends to be relatively minor. When a positive diagnosis cannot be made, follow-up and investigations to exclude other causes of visual loss are necessary.

ORBITAL DISEASE

CONGENITAL ABNORMALITIES OF SKULL DEVELOPMENT

A number of craniosynostoses have ocular features. Crouzon's, Apert's and Pfeiffer's syndromes result in shallow orbits, which can lead to corneal exposure. Hydrocephalus is common in these conditions and regular optic disc examination is required. Visual loss may also occur because of amblyopia secondary to refractive errors and strabismus.[47] Complex horizontal and vertical strabismus patterns are frequently present. Strabismus surgery may be considered after corrective skull surgery has been performed.

SYMPTOMS AND SIGNS OF ORBITAL DISEASE

Symptoms of orbital disease include reduced vision, diplopia and altered appearance. Signs include proptosis which may be axial (forward protrusion of the eye in the axis of the orbit) or non-axial. The pattern of non-axial proptosis gives useful clues to the site of orbital disease. For instance, if the eye is deviated laterally, it is likely that the site of orbital disease will be medial. Eye movements may be reduced. Visual acuity may be reduced and there may be sensory abnormalities of pupil reactions.

PRESEPTAL CELLULITIS

Preseptal cellulitis refers to eyelid cellulitis that does not extend beyond the orbital septum into the orbit. The eye appears normal and vision remains normal. While the infection may be related to local skin infection or local skin trauma, this form of cellulitis is commonly secondary to upper respiratory tract infection with *Haemophilus influenzae* or *Streptococcus aureus*. Blood cultures should be obtained. An orbital computerized tomography (CT) scan may be indicated when severe eyelid swelling prevents adequate eye examination.[48] Treatment is with intravenous antibiotics.

ORBITAL CELLULITIS

True orbital cellulitis is much less common than preseptal cellulitis. The orbit becomes inflamed with proptosis of the eye, reduced eye movement and reduced vision. Most cases are secondary to ethmoidal sinusitis. *H. influenzae* is the most common organism responsible. Blood cultures should be performed and an orbital CT scan should be performed. Treatment is with intravenous antibiotics. Visual acuity should be monitored. An otolaryngologist should be involved in all cases as urgent sinus drainage may be needed in order to protect vision.

ORBITAL TUMORS

Capillary hemangioma, venous–lymphatic malformations and dermoid cysts are the most common orbital masses in infants and children under the age of 2 years.

Capillary hemangiomas grow rapidly during the first 6 months of life, stabilize, and then regress at age 3–8 years. Superficial lesions are a typical 'strawberry' color (Fig. 29.29), deeper lesions have a bluish appearance. They may enlarge during crying. The diagnosis may be made clinically, and CT or MRI scans may be used to delineate the extent of the lesion. Visual loss is usually related to amblyopia,[49] but can be due to optic nerve compression or corneal exposure. Amblyopia may be due to covering of the pupil, or astigmatism in the axis of the lesion. Treatment is conservative in most cases, with spectacle and occlusion treatment for amblyopia. However larger lesions may require early intervention as part of the treatment of amblyopia. Intralesional depot steroids may be used,[50] as may dye laser. Surgery is normally deferred until maximal spontaneous regression has occurred at about age 8 years.

Venous–lymphatic malformations present with proptosis in childhood, which may be abrupt if bleeding occurs into a cystic space. While the lesions consist of venous-like vascular channels they are not directly connected to the venous system and therefore do not enlarge with the Valsalva maneuver. They may be delineated by CT or MRI scan. Unlike capillary hemangiomas they do not regress with age. However surgical intervention is unsatisfactory and most lesions are best treated conservatively.

Dermoid cysts may be superficial or deep. Superficial lesions are most often found at the upper outer angle of the orbit. Having excluded a deeper component to the lesion by clinical examination, ultrasound examination or CT scan, excision may be performed. Deeper lesions tend to present with proptosis, at a later age. Conservative treatment is often appropriate, as they must be fully excised during surgery. Spillage of their contents may cause severe inflammation.

Rhabdomyosarcoma is the commonest malignant orbital tumor of childhood and usually develops between the ages of 4 and 12 years. The tumor enlarges rapidly with increasing proptosis, mild redness and edema of the eyelids and reduced eye movements. The diagnosis is made by biopsy, and as much tissue as possible should be removed for examination. A direct approach to the lesion should be performed, as tumor seeding may occur in the biopsy track. Treatment has been defined by the Intergroup Rhabdomyosarcoma Studies (IRS).[51] Depending on clinical stage, chemotherapy with or without radiotherapy is the initial treatment. Orbital exenteration may be needed if primary treatment fails.

EYELID ABNORMALITIES

Coloboma refers to a condition where part of the upper eyelid does not develop in first branchial arch syndromes. Oculoplastic reconstructive surgery may be required to avoid corneal exposure.

Epiblepharon refers to the presence of a fold of skin near the lower eyelid margin, which may cause inturning eyelashes (Fig. 29.30), most commonly affecting Chinese infants. The natural history is spontaneous resolution during the first 1–2 years of life and surgery is reserved for exceptionally severe cases.

Blepharitis refers to inflammation of the eyelid margins. This is a relatively common condition in older children and in adults. Hot bathing and eyelid margin toilet using cotton tipped buds may be effective. When secondary staphylococcal infection is present, treatment with topical fucidic acid cream is indicated.

A *tarsal cyst* is a retention cyst of an oil producing meibomian gland of an eyelid. These cysts resolve spontaneously over a period of months and surgical drainage is indicated in the minority of cases in which significant eye discomfort is present.

CONGENITAL PTOSIS

Dystrophic changes of the levator muscle of one or both upper eyelids will result in drooping of the upper eyelid, termed ptosis (Fig. 29.31). Congenital III nerve palsy or Horner's syndrome should be excluded. Congenital Horner's syndrome is associated with neuroblastoma and urine vanillylmandelic acid (VMA) should be measured. The jaw winking (Marcus Gunn) phenomenon should be sought – lateral movements of the jaw produce synkinetic movements of the ipsilateral upper eyelid.

If the pupil is occluded by ptosis, prompt surgery is indicated in order to prevent amblyopia. However in milder cases corrective surgery is best deferred until later childhood, when better cooperation with surgical measurements may be obtained, leading to a better cosmetic result. Surgery generally involves advancement or resection of the levator aponeurosis.

LACRIMAL SYSTEM

Congenital dacryocystocele is a cystic swelling of the tear sac present at birth. Typically a bluish cystic lesion is present deep to the skin in the tear sac area. Frequently there is associated cystic dilatation of nasal mucosa at the exit of the tear duct in the inferior meatus, which can lead to breathing difficulties in bilateral cases. Spontaneous resolution may occur at an early stage. However secondary infection and breathing difficulties are relatively common, and probing of the nasolacrimal ducts, with or without excision of intranasal cystic tissue is indicated when early spontaneous resolution does not occur.[52]

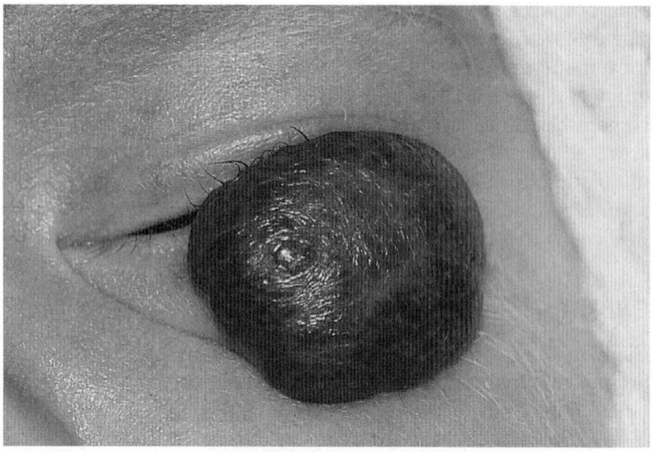

Fig. 29.29 Capillary hemangioma of the lower eyelid.

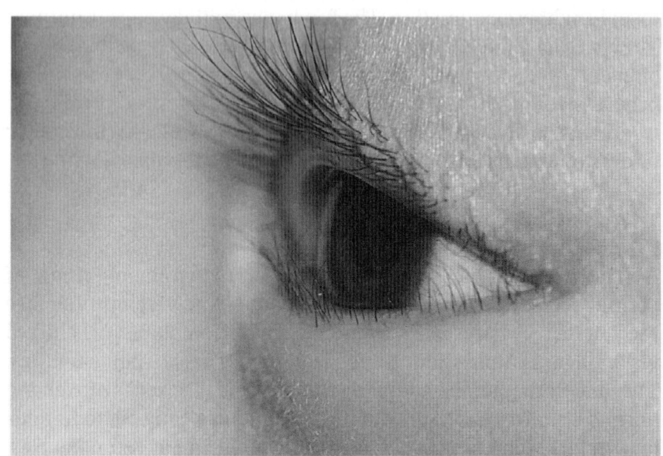

Fig. 29.30 Epiblepharon.

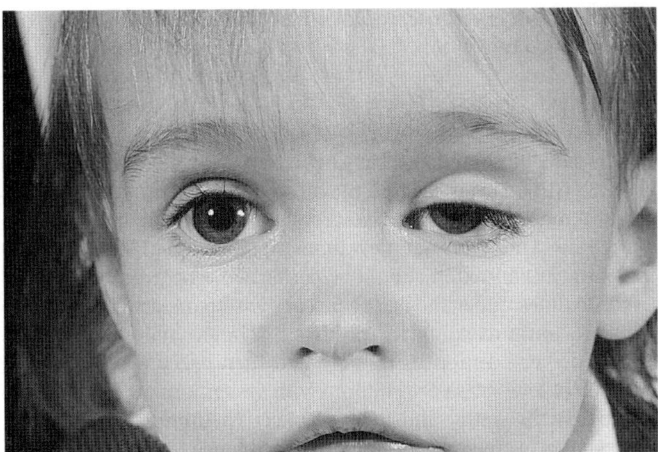

Fig. 29.31 Congenital ptosis of the left upper eyelid due to levator muscle dystrophy.

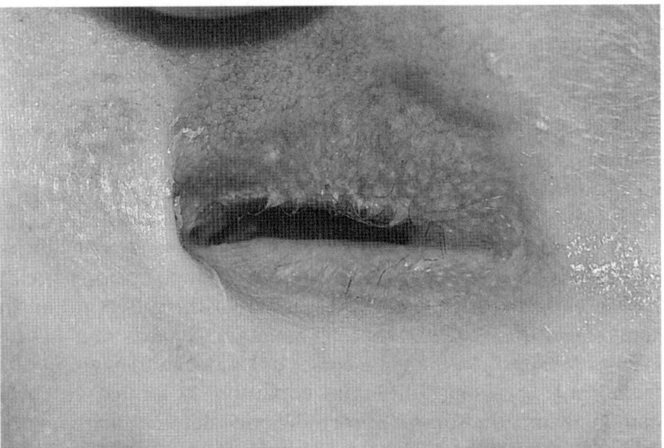

Fig. 29.32 Anophthalmos. No identifiable ocular structures are apparent.

CONGENITAL NASOLACRIMAL DUCT OBSTRUCTION

The nasolacrimal duct commonly has a persistent membranous occlusion at the distal end of the duct. This leads to watering (epiphora) of the affected eye or eyes. Epiphora is almost always first noticed during the first month of life.[53] The fluorescein dye disappearance test is useful in diagnosis. A drop of fluorescein dye is placed in the conjunctival sac and the time taken for dye to clear is observed.[54] The natural history is spontaneous resolution of watering during the first 1–2 years of life.[53] If watering persists beyond the age of 2 years, probing of the nasolacrimal duct may be undertaken.[55] While waiting for spontaneous resolution, the eyes should be bathed if they become sticky. Topical antibiotics need only be used if signs of active tissue inflammation are present.

LACRIMAL OBSTRUCTION IN OLDER CHILDREN

In some children, epiphora persists despite probing. In these cases intranasal anatomical abnormalities may be found.[56] Endoscopic exploration with silicone intubation of the lacrimal system is effective in 60–70% of cases. Where severe anatomical occlusion of the nasolacrimal duct is present, dacrocystorhinostomy surgery may be required. However epiphora in older children is more often due to allergy or upper respiratory tract infection than to nasolacrimal duct occlusion.[57]

CONGENITAL ABNORMALITIES OF EYE DEVELOPMENT

The whole eye may be absent at birth (anophthalmos) (Fig. 29.32) or may be small (microphthalmos).

Orbital growth is partly stimulated by the volume effect of the eye. Orbital growth is reduced if an eye is removed during early childhood. Orbital prostheses are therefore used to enhance orbital growth in cases of anophthalmos or severe microphthalmos.

Microphthalmos is commonly associated with coloboma due to embryonic optic fissure closure defects. Typically the inferior part of the iris is absent along with the inferior choroid and retina (Fig. 29.33). The optic disc may or may not be involved. Microphthalmos and coloboma may be isolated abnormalities, associated with chromosomal syndromes such as trisomy 13 or cat eye syndrome, or associated with a single gene defect such as CHARGE syndrome. Epidemiological studies have failed to link microphthalmos to other environmental teratogens.

CONJUNCTIVITIS

Neonatal conjunctivitis has been discussed in Chapter 10. Bacterial infection, viral infection, chlamydial infection and allergy may cause conjunctivitis in older infants and in children.

Bacterial conjunctivitis produces a purulent discharge and is generally treated with a topical broad spectrum antibiotic such as chloramphenicol. Viral conjunctivitis produces a watery discharge with a mucous component and is generally self-limiting. Chlamydial neonatal infection has been discussed in Chapter 10. In hot dry countries with limited water supplies flies cause endemic chlamydial conjunctivitis – trachoma. Conjunctival scarring leads to dry eyes and eyelid scarring. Secondary corneal scarring follows, and remains a common avoidable cause of blindness worldwide. Treatment is by improved water supply and hygiene, and community use of tetracycline eye ointment.

Chronic allergy in the form of vernal keratoconjunctivitis results in morbidity due to ocular discomfort and visual loss. Corneal scarring may be present along with papillary inflammation of the tarsal conjunctiva. Treatment is with mast cell stabilizers such as sodium cromoglycate, and with steroid eye drops. Topical steroid eye drops may cause glaucoma and cataract. Close supervision by an ophthalmologist is required. Topical steroid eyedrops are also used in the acute phase of Stevens–Johnson syndrome.

Conjunctival dryness (xerosis) and corneal melting are features of vitamin A deficiency. Acute deficiency signs may be precipitated

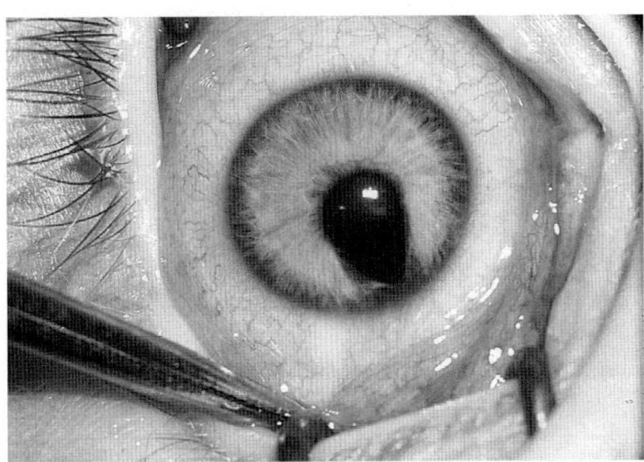

Fig. 29. 33 Coloboma of the inferior iris.

by intercurrent respiratory or gastrointestinal infection and urgent treatment with high doses of vitamin A is then needed.

CORNEAL DISEASE

Corneal scarring due to trachoma and vitamin A deficiency remains the leading cause of childhood blindness in developing countries.

In developed countries herpes simplex corneal infection is a relatively frequent cause of morbidity. Prompt treatment with topical aciclovir is usually sufficient to clear the infection, but in some cases areas of chronic inflammation and scarring of the cornea develop. Epidemics of adenovirus keratoconjunctivitis occur from time to time. While the condition is limited to viral conjunctivitis in most cases, some individuals develop inflammatory infiltrates deep to the corneal epithelium. Cautious use of topical steroids provides symptomatic relief, and reduces scarring.

Congenital corneal opacities due to dystrophies or as part of Peter's anomaly or sclerocornea are relatively rare. In bilateral cases corneal transplant surgery may be indicated. As with congenital cataracts, surgical treatment must be undertaken early if visual loss due to amblyopia is to be avoided. Corneal transplant surgery in infants, and the necessary intensive aftercare, are very demanding of the surgeon and the family and treatment is best undertaken in specialized referral departments.

Congenital limbal dermoids (Fig. 29.34) may occur in isolation or as part of a number of syndromes. They may be excised in early childhood.

Keratoconus is a corneal dystrophy with onset in teenage years. There is often a history of atopy, and eye rubbing may play a part in the etiology. Keratoconus is also seen in children with retinal dystrophies who have developed habits of eye poking and eye rubbing.

Initially the cornea appears structurally normal, but a progressive increase of astigmatism develops. With progression the central part of the cornea becomes slightly cone shaped on slit lamp examination. The disease may stabilize at this stage, or progress to more marked cone development, with thinning and scarring of the central corneal stroma. Episodes of acute edema ('acute hydrops') may occur, due to the development of splits in Descemet's membrane (the basement membrane of the corneal endothelium). The edema settles spontaneously as the splits heal.

Mild cases of keratoconus are treated with spectacle correction. As the corneal surface becomes more irregular specialized contact lens fitting may be needed to correct abnormal focusing. Corneal transplant surgery is reserved for cases where contact lenses do not produce adequate vision.

UVEITIS

Uveitis screening is necessary in children with juvenile idiopathic arthritis (JIA). This is because the intraocular inflammation may be asymptomatic in its early stages, but untreated, may lead to glaucoma and cataract development (Fig. 29.35). Slit lamp screening examination should be performed. The group at highest risk is females under the age of 5 years with pauciarticular disease who are antinuclear factor positive.[58] These children should be screened every 3 months initially and then every 6 months. The children at lowest risk are children with systemic onset JIA, juvenile spondyloarthropathy and juvenile onset rheumatoid arthritis. In these cases, screening is only required once, at disease onset. Children at intermediate risk with other categories of JIA should be examined every 6 months. Screening should continue for 5 years.[59] When iritis is detected, topical steroids may be used. Supervision of treatment by an ophthalmologist is needed because of the risks of glaucoma and cataract development due to the inflammation or due to the steroid treatment.

CATARACT

Congenital cataract remains a major cause of childhood blindness worldwide (Fig. 29.36). In developed countries severe visual handicap due to congenital cataract is now rare because of improvements in surgical management.[60] The key is early detection and early surgery in order to avoid amblyopia.[61–64]

Two-thirds of cases of congenital cataract are bilateral and one-third unilateral.[65] Cataract is an isolated finding in 60% of bilateral cataract cases.[65] The causes of congenital cataract are given in Table 29.10. Every infant with congenital cataract should be examined for dysmorphic features or evidence of metabolic disease. The parents should be examined for evidence of cataract as autosomal dominant cataracts may vary in disease expression.

Surgery should be performed within the first 6–8 weeks of life in order to ensure that optical rehabilitation has been completed by the age of 3 months.[64] Delayed detection and treatment will lead to irreversible visual loss due to amblyopia.[64] In bilateral cases the surgery is performed on one eye initially, with surgery to the second eye a few days later. There is controversy as to whether plastic intraocular lens implants should be used in neonates.[66,67] The use of

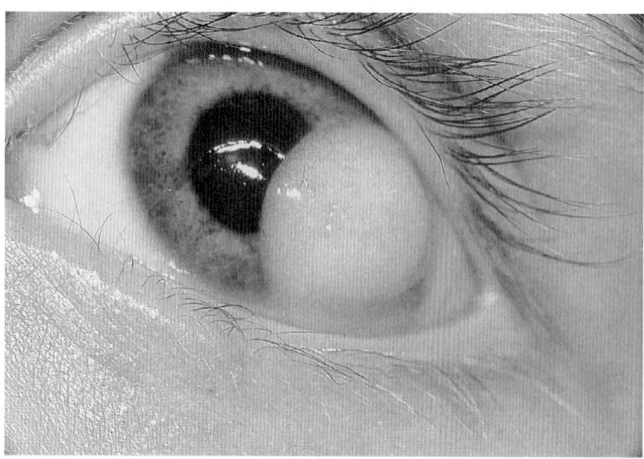

Fig. 29.34 Limbal dermoid.

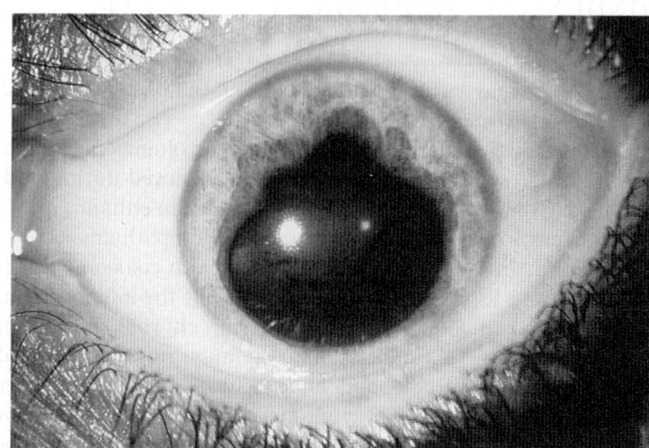

Fig. 29.35 Iritis. The pupil has been dilated and adhesions between the iris and lens (posterior synechiae) are seen.

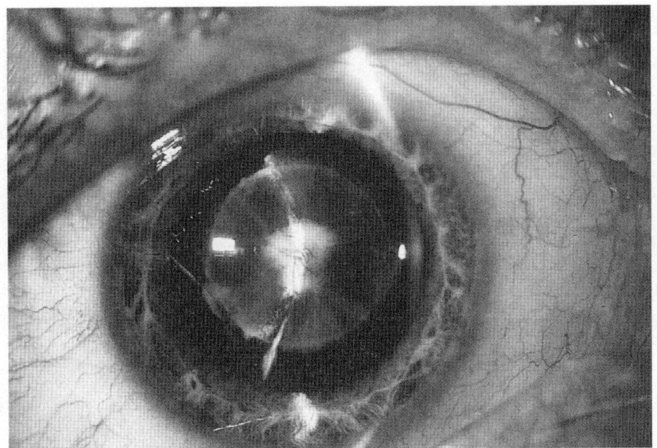

Fig. 29.36 Congenital cataract. This is a partial, lamellar cataract with relatively good vision. Surgery in infancy was not needed in this case.

implants produces lesser degrees of refractive error. However surgical complication rates are higher and revision surgery is more often required when implants are used. An alternative to primary intraocular lens implantation is the use of contact lenses for primary optical correction.[68] This results in fewer operative complications and fewer revision procedures. Long wear soft contact lenses are normally used although there is a risk of infection and corneal ulceration when contact lenses are used in this way.

LENS SUBLUXATION

The most common cause of lens subluxation (Fig. 29.37) in children is Marfan's syndrome.[69] The lenses tend to be subluxed from an early age and there is rarely any significant progression with time.[13] For this reason a single screening examination in early childhood is sufficient to detect lens subluxation and regular follow-up is generally not required. The differential diagnosis includes homocystinuria[69] and plasma homocystine levels should be measured.[15]

When lens subluxation occurs, treatment may be either optical or surgical. Surgical treatment generally involves removing the subluxed lens and using contact lenses for optical correction.[70]

Table 29.10 Causes of congenital cataracts

Idiopathic		
Isolated inherited	Dominant, recessive, X-linked	
Inherited syndrome	Chromosomal	Trisomy 21,13,18 Turner's Translocation 3;4 and 2;14 Cri du chat 5q15.2
	Mitochondrial diseases Lowe's oculocerebrorenal syndrome Ectodermal dysplasia	
Metabolic	Galactosemia Galactokinase deficiency Hypocalcemia Hypoglycemia Mannosidosis	
Prenatal infection	Rubella Toxoplasma Herpes simplex Varicella	
Trauma	Accidental Non-accidental	
Ocular associations	Microphthalmos Aniridia Persistent fetal vasculature Peter's anomaly Endophthalmitis	

GLAUCOMA

PRIMARY CONGENITAL GLAUCOMA

Primary congenital glaucoma typically occurs in boys between the age of birth and 2 years. Some cases are autosomal recessive and there is a 1 in 20 empirical recurrence risk in siblings. The presenting signs may be present in one or both eyes. Watering, photophobia and enlargement of the corneas occur (Fig. 29.38). The diagnosis is made by performing an examination under anesthetic and measuring the intraocular pressure. Intravenous or intramuscular ketamine sedation is preferred for these examinations as ketamine produces a small, predictable rise in intraocular pressure. In contrast inhalational anesthetics produce a variable lowering of intraocular pressure. Treatment is surgical and demanding. Multiple operations may be required and surgical treatment is better undertaken in a pediatric glaucoma referral center.

SECONDARY GLAUCOMAS

Glaucoma may be secondary to other congenital ocular abnormalities. These include Reiger's syndrome (Fig. 29.39) and aniridia. Glaucoma may develop secondary to iritis in patients with JIA. A particularly difficult form of childhood glaucoma is aphakic glaucoma in children who have had congenital cataract surgery. Complex surgical treatment may be required.

Glaucoma may develop in Sturge–Weber syndrome, especially if the upper eyelid has a port wine stain lesion (Fig. 29.40).

RETINAL DISEASES

Retinal disorders, which cause bilateral visual loss in children, have been described above.

COATS' DISEASE

Coats' disease is a primary retinal telangiectatic disease in which leaky vessels cause progressive accumulation of fatty deposits in

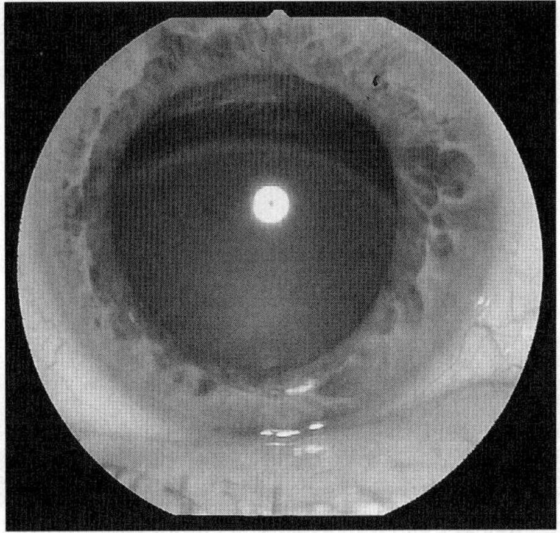

Fig. 29.37 Subluxed lens.

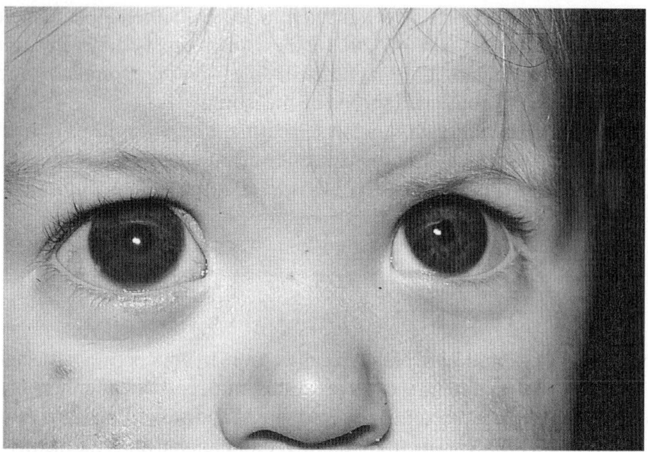

Fig. 29.38 Congenital glaucoma. Note enlarged corneas. This child had goniotomy surgery performed in infancy, which satisfactorily controlled the intraocular pressures.

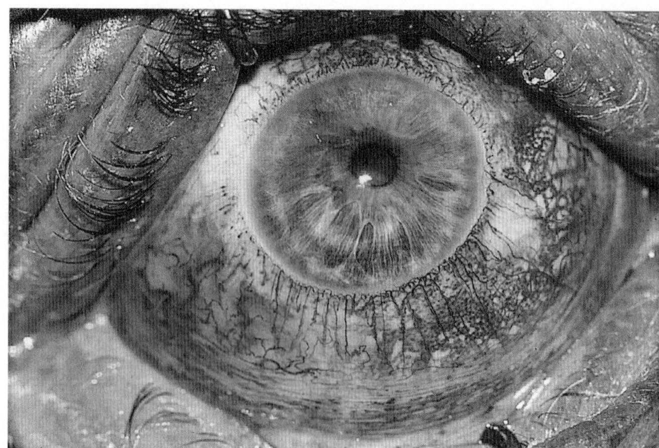

Fig. 29.40 Sturge–Weber syndrome. Note eyelid port wine stain, and abnormal scleral blood vessels.

the subretinal space (Fig. 29.41). Treatment with laser therapy or cryotherapy can reduce serous leakage and improve visual prognosis.[71–73] The condition is diagnosed at a median age of 5 years, is more common in males and is almost always unilateral.[74] There are no systemic associations.

RETINOBLASTOMA

Retinoblastoma is a malignant neuroblastic tumor of the retina, which normally develops during the first 2 years of life. Approximately 50% of cases are heritable, with a mutation of the RB1 tumor suppressor gene. In these cases, additional somatic mutations of allelic RB1 genes in retinal cells lead to loss of tumor suppressor function and neoplasia occurs. Tumors are usually multiple. Approximately 50% of heritable cases have a family history of retinoblastoma; the remainder represent new germline mutations.

In cases in which there is no germ-cell mutation, two mutations are needed to produce neoplasia in a retinal cell.[75] In these cases, the tumor is almost always solitary, with slightly later onset than heritable cases (median age 24 months compared to 12 months). However 15% of cases with solitary tumors have an underlying germ-cell mutation.

Presenting signs include leucocoria (white pupil) and strabismus.

The diagnosis is made clinically. Typically the tumors have a creamy white appearance, are moderately vascular, and have areas of calcification (Fig. 29.42). The tumors tend to grow out from the retina into the vitreous ('endophytic') or grow underneath the retina ('exophytic'). Rarely the tumor diffusely infiltrates the retina.

The differential diagnosis includes Coats' disease, tuberous sclerosis, retinal hamartomas, Norrie's disease (retinal dysplasia), toxocara infection, and, in diffuse cases, endophthalmitis. Rarely a benign form of retinoblastoma – 'retinoma' – may occur. The age of onset is older, retinal pigment epithelium changes are seen surrounding the elevated gray retinal mass, and the tumor remains non-progressive.

When the optic nerve is clinically in contact with retinoblastoma tissue, assessment will include examination of the CSF and a CT scan of the brain and orbits. The CT scan will delineate the extent of the tumor, and exclude a coexisting pineal tumor ('trilateral retinoblastoma'). The most common route of spread is along the optic nerve. In advanced cases blood spread to bone marrow may occur.

An ocular oncology team in specialized referral centers should undertake management.

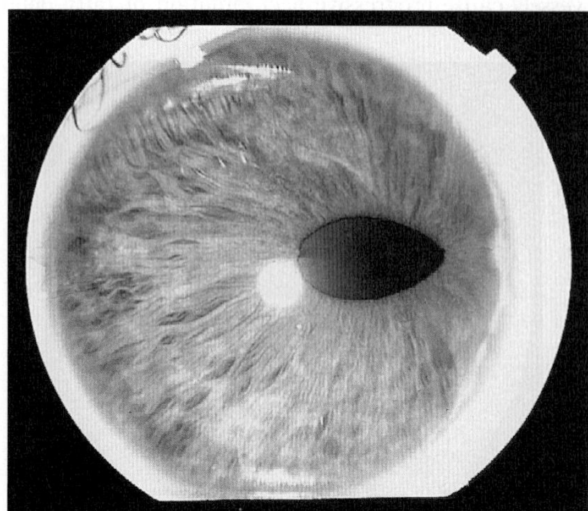

Fig. 29.39 Reiger's syndrome. Note posterior embryotoxon and abnormal pupil shape and position (corectopia).

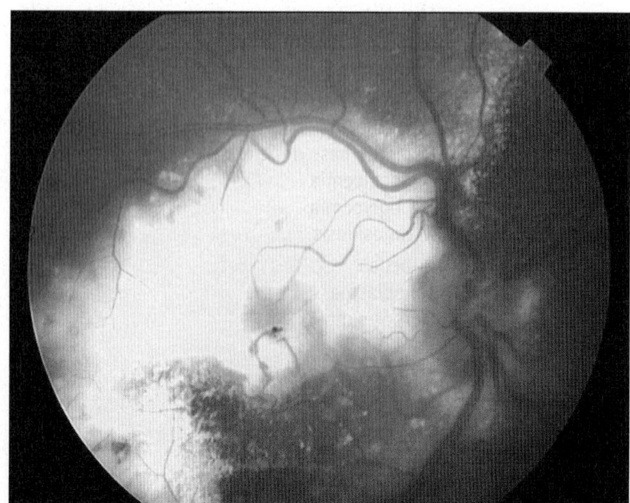

Fig. 29.41 Coats' disease. Massive subretinal lipid exudation is seen at the macula, with severely reduced visual acuity.

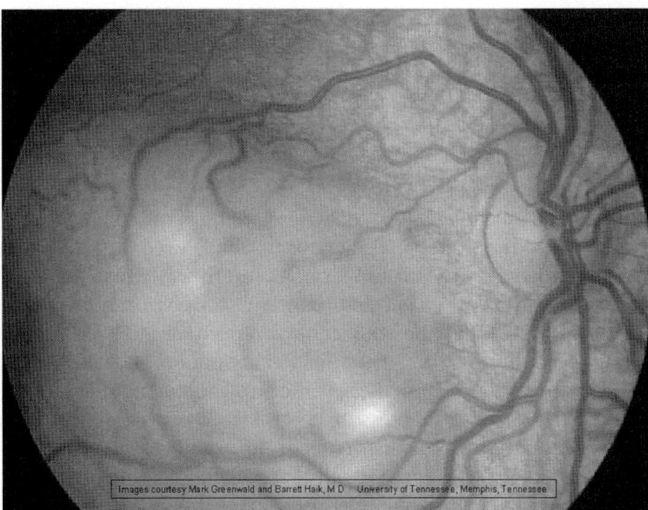

Fig. 29.42 Retinoblastoma. Creamy white tumor. Image taken with 'Retcam' digital fundus camera.

A range of treatment modalities may be used. Primary enucleation surgery is indicated for advanced disease (Fig. 29.43). A long length of optic nerve should be removed with the eye, and a primary orbital implant placed within the muscle cone. Less extensive disease may be treated by external beam radiotherapy, or a scleral radioactive plaque.

Chemotherapy is now the first line treatment for unilateral cases which have been detected at an early stage, and for the more normal eye of bilateral cases following enucleation of the severely affected eye. Six cycles of cisplatin, etoposide and vincristine are given. Ciclosporin may also be given in order to reduce multidrug resistance. Additional treatment modalities are required in some cases. These include retinal laser therapy and retinal cryotherapy.

Frequent follow-up examinations are performed in order to detect tumor regression, and to look for new tumors, which develop in 10% of cases. If there has been no evidence of local or metastatic disease for 3 years after local disease control, cure is very likely. Long term survival is over 95%.

Heritable cases will transmit the defective RB1 gene to 50% of offspring, with 90% penetrance. The risk of disease is therefore 45%. The siblings of cases and the offspring of cases should have regular retinal examinations. This includes cases of solitary tumor, as 15% of these cases have an underlying germline mutation. The initial examination may be performed without general anesthetic soon after birth. Examinations under anesthetic are then performed every 2–4 months until age 2 years, and 4–6 months until age 5 years. Further examinations without anesthetic are then performed 6 monthly until age 5 years. At each examination the peripheral retina must be fully visualized using scleral indentation. Identification of RB1 mutations within families now allows molecular identification of at-risk individuals. Intensive screening may then be limited to individuals with RB1 mutations.

The product of the RB1 gene is the retinoblastoma protein pRB. RB1 mutations normally result in no detectable pRB production. pRB is a phosphoprotein which is involved in cell cycle control and inhibits cell proliferation. Its function is tissue specific – RB1 mutations increase the risk of retinoblastoma, pineal tumors (which presents with hydrocephalus), osteogenic sarcoma (especially in the orbit following ocular radiotherapy for retinoblastoma), other sarcomas, and some carcinomas. However the RB1 gene does not predispose to other childhood neoplasias such as leukemia. All heritable cases require long term oncology follow-up.

TOXOCARA INFECTION

Toxocara infection of the retina may occur in early childhood either in subclinical infection or as part of a systemic illness. The nematode dies within the eye and antigen release incites a

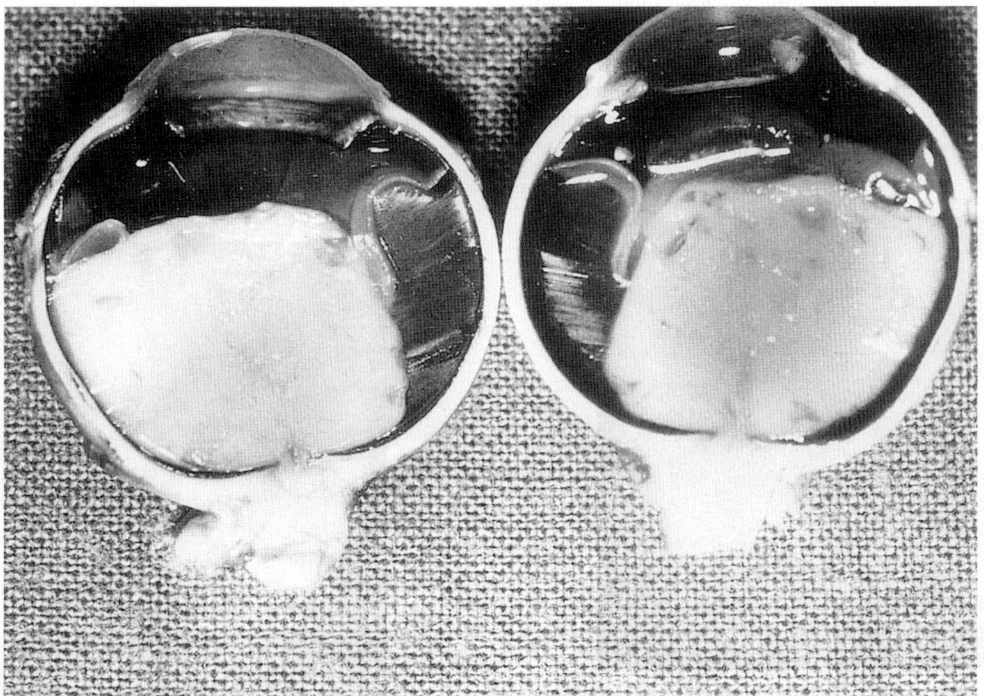

Fig. 29.43 An enucleated eye showing a large retinoblastoma causing detachment of the retina and almost filling the vitreous cavity.

profound inflammatory reaction. This leads to an isolated area of fibrosis with associated retinal traction. No active treatment is possible.

TOXOPLASMA INFECTION

The congenital toxoplasmosis syndrome includes chorioretinitis, intracranial calcification, seizures, hydrocephalus, microcephaly, hepatosplenomegaly, jaundice, anemia and fever.

However toxoplasma infection acquired in the late prenatal period, or postnatally may remain quiescent for many years and then reactivate. The individual may have no neurological or systemic features of toxoplasma infection. At the time of infection recurrence an area of scarring of the choroid and retina is seen, with an adjacent area of retinal and vitreous inflammation (Fig. 29.44). The symptoms are reduced vision and floaters. A number of antimicrobial treatments may be used. Azithromycin may be used as monotherapy. Alternatively triple therapy with sulfadiazine, pyrimethamine and folinic acid may be given. Clindamycin may be used but there is a risk of pseudomembranous colitis. When antimicrobial therapy is given, very close follow-up is needed as death of the organisms may lead to increased inflammation due to antigen release. For this reason oral steroid treatment is often given 24–48 h after commencement of antimicrobial treatment.

DISEASES OF THE OPTIC NERVE

OPTIC ATROPHY

The causes of optic atrophy have been discussed above. Significant optic atrophy leads to reduced visual acuity, reduced color vision, and constricted visual fields.

OPTIC DISC EDEMA

Optic disc edema with severe visual loss

Optic disc edema due to demyelinating diseases (optic neuritis) results in profound visual loss. In children the most common pattern is of bilateral optic neuritis in girls. The discs are swollen, but hemorrhages and exudates are rare. An afferent pupil defect is present. Spontaneous, complete recovery over a period of days is usual, but high doses of systemic steroids may be given in order to expedite recovery. There are usually no long term neurological sequelae and the condition should be regarded as an entity separate from multiple sclerosis.

Inflammatory causes of optic disc edema include uveitis secondary to connective tissue diseases.

Optic disc edema without severe visual loss

The most significant cause of optic disc edema is raised intracranial pressure and the term papilledema is normally used in these cases. Papilledema may cause no visual symptoms. However in more severe cases brief periods of visual disturbance (visual obscurations) occur, and urgent investigation and control of intracranial pressure is required in these cases. Visual field examination shows enlarged blind spots in almost all cases. Paracentral scotomas may also be found. Poor intracranial pressure control leads to progressive loss of axons, with progressive constriction of the visual fields.

In its mildest form, papilledema causes slight blurring of the optic disc margins superiorly and inferiorly. As severity increases a larger portion of the optic disc circumference becomes blurred and the optic disc develops a pink appearance. In severe cases hemorrhages and exudates (nerve fiber layer infarcts) are present (Fig. 29.45).

In mild cases the diagnosis may be aided by fluorescein angiography. In mild optic disc edema the capillaries on the surface of the optic disc are dilated and leak fluorescein dye (Fig. 29.46). High definition ultrasound examination of the optic disc and orbital optic nerve may allow detection of enlargement of the CSF space within the optic nerve sheath.[76]

The differential diagnosis of papilledema includes hypermetropia and optic disc drusen. Moderately severe hypermetropia leads to small 'crowded' optic discs, which may have blurred edges and may be elevated. Optic disc drusen are deposits of amyloid tissue deep within the optic discs, leading to apparent swelling of the optic discs (Fig. 29.47). Drusen may be diagnosed using fluorescence photography or ultrasound examination.

CNS VISUAL IMPAIRMENT

VISION PROBLEMS ASSOCIATED WITH CEREBRAL PALSY

CNS disease is the most common cause of visual impairment in children.[60] Severe cerebral visual impairment has been discussed above. Less severe visual impairment is frequently found in children

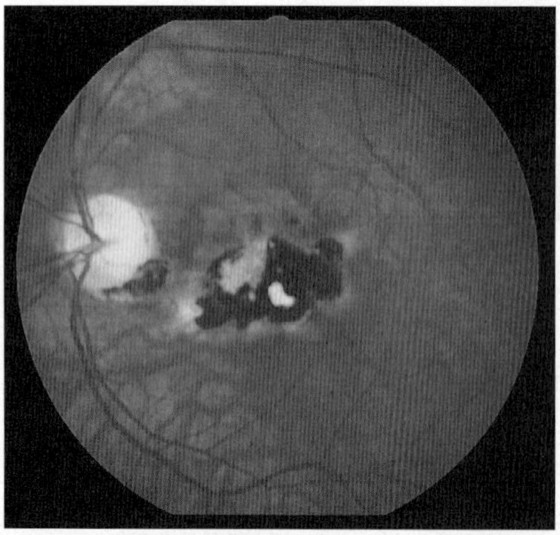

Fig. 29.44 Toxoplasmosis. Pigmented scar at macula. No active inflammation present.

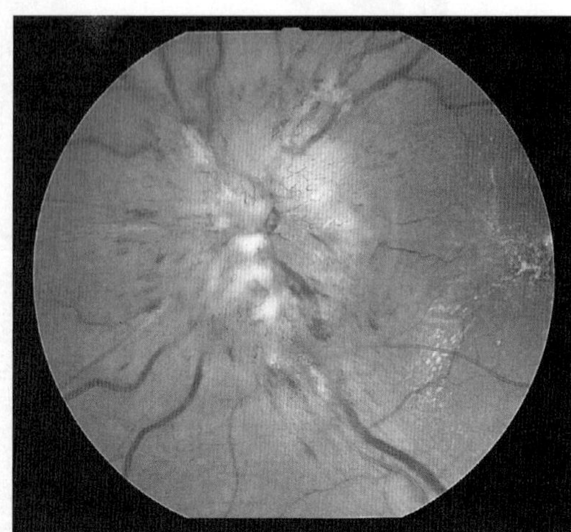

Fig. 29.45 Severe papilledema with hemorrhages and exudates.

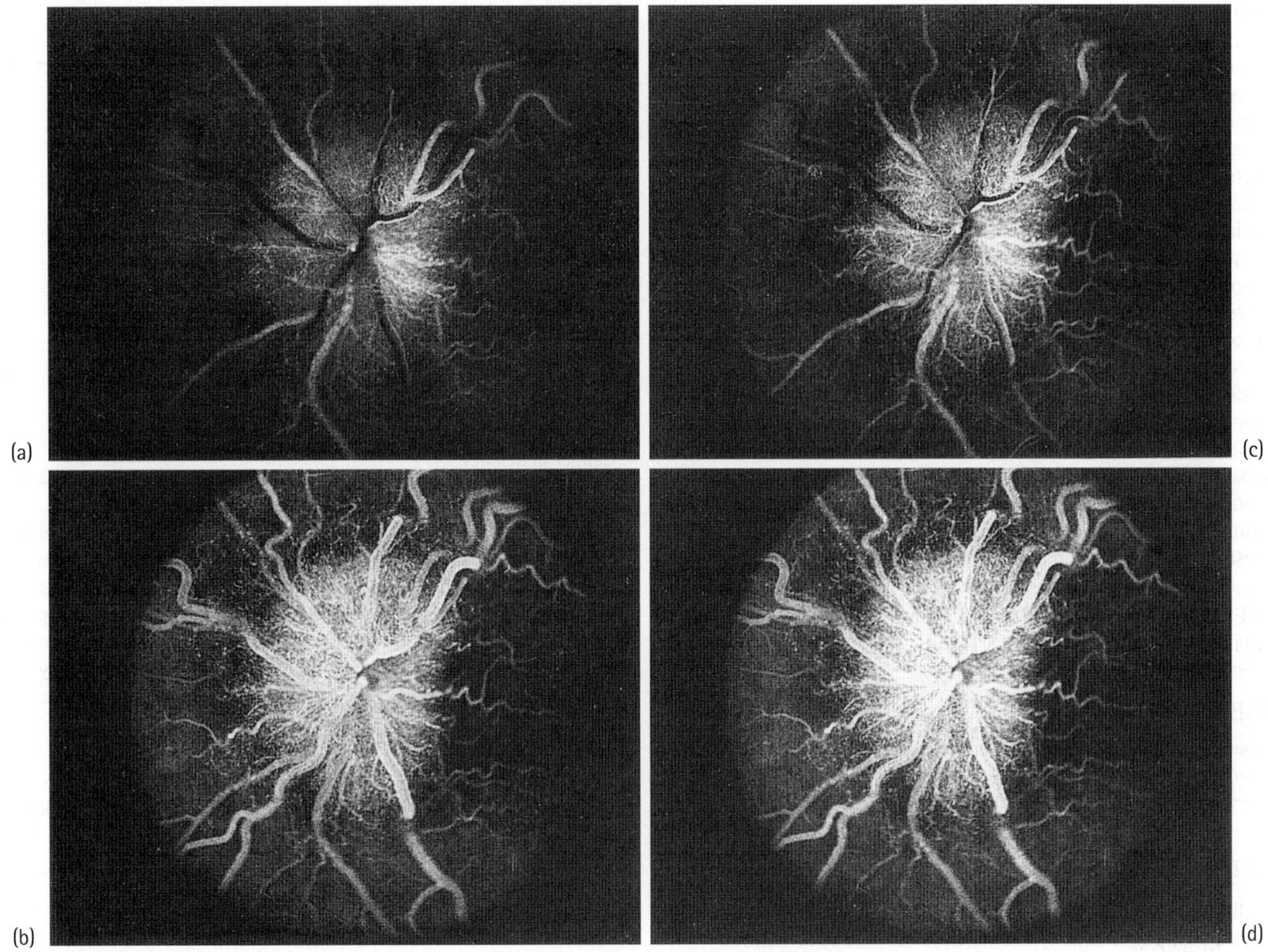

(a) (c)

(b) (d)

Fig. 29.46 Fundus fluorescein angiogram showing dilated capillaries on the optic disc surface.

with cerebral palsy and may be under-recognized. Visual acuity may be reduced, visual field defects may be present, and refractive errors and reduced accommodation may produce blurred vision. Perceptual defects of higher visual functions may be present. A structured history as suggested above may reveal specific perceptual defects. Neuroimaging may help map functional deficits to anatomical abnormalities in some cases.

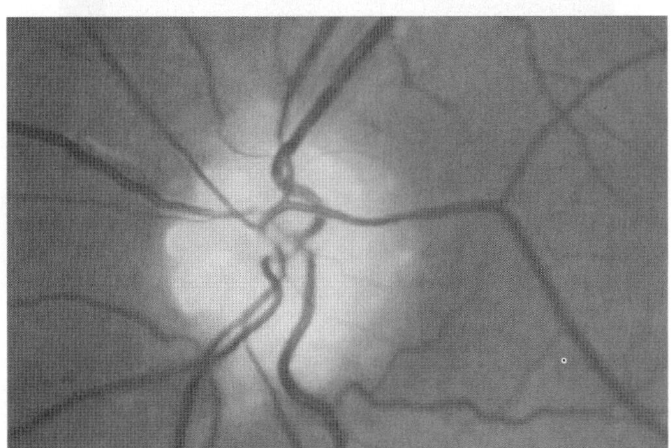

Fig. 29.47 Optic disc drusen.

Behavioral strategies may be developed in order to reduce the impact of specific perceptual defects. Spectacles to correct hypermetropia and accommodation deficits are often helpful. Symptoms due to inferior visual field loss may be aided by using a tilted work board so that the child may look directly at written material rather than looking down.

PERIVENTRICULAR LEUCOMALACIA

Prematurity may lead to visual loss due to retinopathy of prematurity or cerebral visual impairment.[36,77] Typically, severe grades of periventricular hemorrhage may be accompanied by periventricular leucomalacia. Symptoms emerge in these children at about the age of 2–5 years. Reduced visual acuity, inferior visual field defects, nystagmus, and diplegia may be present.[36] The optic discs show an enlarged physiological cup, which may be due to transynaptic degeneration of fibers synapsing in the lateral geniculate bodies.

Cortical visual processing capacity may be limited, leading to difficulties in visualizing a 'busy' or rapidly changing environment.

SHAKING INJURIES

Shaking injuries commonly produce extensive retinal hemorrhages and an ophthalmologist should be involved in the diagnostic process. Possible mechanisms include raised venous pressure and direct shearing forces within the retina and at the vitreoretinal interface. Typically hemorrhages are extensive, covering the whole retina from the optic disc to the ora seratta (Fig. 29.48). The hemorrhages are present deep within the retina (dot hemorrhages), on the surface of the retina (flame-shaped hemorrhages within the nerve fiber layer) and on the surface of the retina (preretinal hemorrhages). Vitreous hemorrhage and traction retinal detachment may be present in more severe cases.

Flame-shaped surface retinal hemorrhages tend to clear within 1–2 weeks, although deep retinal hemorrhages and preretinal and vitreous hemorrhages may persist for a number of weeks. The differential diagnosis is given in Table 29.11[78] and includes birth hemorrhages and retinal hemorrhages secondary to blood clotting disorders.[79] Retinal hemorrhages do not occur as a part of accidental head injury unless trauma is severe.[80] A few small retinal hemorrhages have been found in case series following seizures,[81] and following cardiopulmonary resuscitation.

No specific treatment is indicated for retinal hemorrhages secondary to shaking injury. On follow-up, long term visual loss is more often due to associated brain and optic nerve injury than to retinal injury.

Table 29.11 Differential diagnosis of retinal hemorrhages in an infant with suspected shaking injury (After Taylor 2000[78])

Non-accidental shaking injury
Accidental injury (severe trauma)
Leukemia
Coagulation disorders
Retinopathy of prematurity
Birth hemorrhages
Maternal cocaine ingestion
Extracorporeal membrane oxygenation (ECMO)
Sickle cell retinopathy
Subarachnoid hemorrhage (Terson's syndrome)
Intracranial vascular malformations
Neonatal arterial hypertension
Glutaric aciduria type 1
Meningococcal meningitis
Severe papilledema with raised intracranial pressure
Copper deficiency

THE EYE IN RELATION TO MEDICAL PEDIATRICS AND CLINICAL GENETICS

DIABETES MELLITUS

Diabetic retinopathy is exceptionally rare before puberty. Retinal screening examinations should be carried out annually from puberty. Cataract may develop as an acute feature of diabetes mellitus.

CYSTINOSIS

Small crystals may develop in the corneal epithelium, which may be painful. Treatment with cysteamine eye drops may be helpful.[82]

NEUROMETABOLIC STORAGE DISEASES – EYE SIGNS

Cherry red spot

In Tay–Sachs disease (GM2 type1) ganglioside accumulation in retinal ganglion cells leads to a 'cherry red spot' appearance (Fig. 29.49). The central fovea has no overlying ganglion cells and remains a red color due to the underlying choroidal circulation. The surrounding retina is a milky white color due to ganglioside storage in the ganglion cells. The ERG is normal, but the VEP is reduced. A cherry red spot is also seen in Niemann–Pick disease type A (sphingomyelinase deficiency) and neuraminidase deficiency (sialidosis types 1 and 2). With disease progression the cherry red spot fades as ganglion cells die and optic atrophy develops.

Corneal clouding

Corneal clouding develops in:

- mucopolysaccharidoses, all of which show corneal clouding, except MPSII and MPSIII;
- mucolipidoses;
- fucosidosis;
- mannosidosis.

WILSON'S DISEASE

Copper deposition in the peripheral cornea may be detected on slit lamp examination.

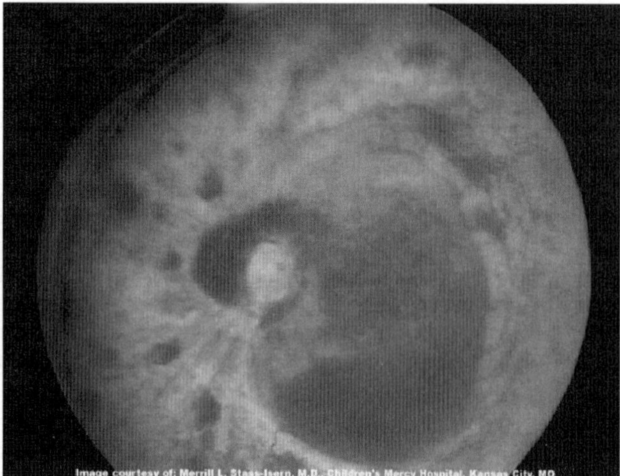

Fig. 29.48 Retinal hemorrhages following non-accidental shaking injury in an infant. Image taken with 'Retcam' digital fundus camera.

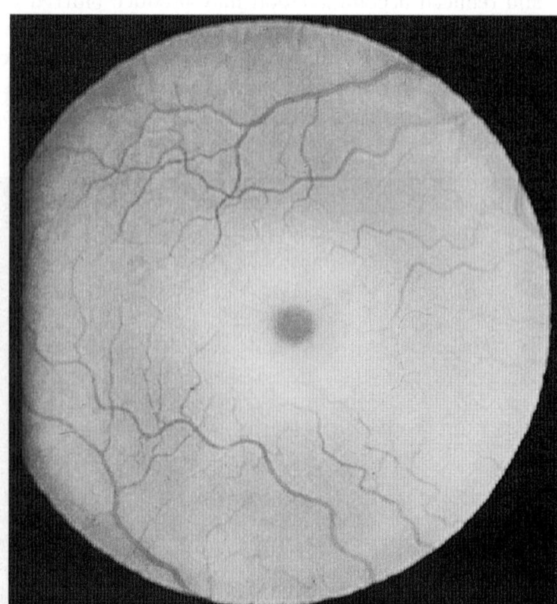

Fig. 29.49 Cherry red spot due to Tay–Sachs disease.

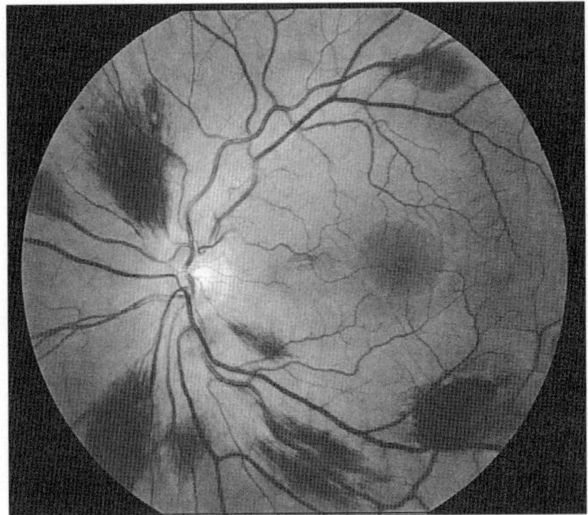

Fig. 29.50 Retinal hemorrhages related to leukemia.

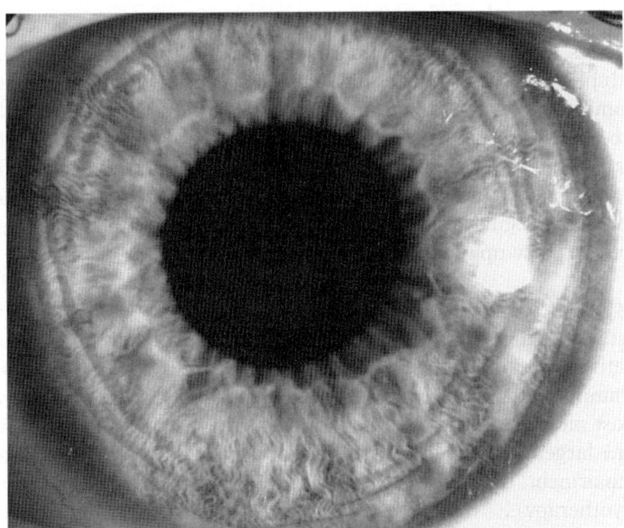

Fig. 29.51 Lisch nodules of the iris. Multiple pigmented nodules are easily visualized against the background of a lightly pigmented iris in this case.

OPHTHALMOLOGY CHANGES IN LEUKEMIA

Retinal hemorrhages may be found in severe anemia and leukemia (Fig. 29.50). The iris may act as a sanctuary site following chemotherapy for lymphoblastic leukemia. During remission periods, disease recurrence may occur in the iris, with clinical effects similar to those seen in iritis. Clinical suspicion and, if necessary, iris biopsy, will allow the correct diagnosis to be made. Treatment with further chemotherapy, and with radiotherapy to the irises, is indicated.

OPHTHALMOLOGY AND THE CLINICAL GENETICIST

The ophthalmologist may be asked to look for diagnostic signs in a range of inherited syndromes.

Marfan's syndrome

Screening for lens subluxation may be requested. A single examination in early childhood is usually sufficient as lens subluxation develops early in life and there is rarely any significant progression with time.[13]

Neurofibromatosis

The ophthalmologist may provide diagnostic information in cases of suspected neurofibromatosis types 1 and 2 (NF1, NF2). Lisch nodules of the iris will be present in over 90% of children aged 5 years or more who have NF1 (Fig. 29.51). However these nodules are less common in younger children. Children with confirmed NF1 also require regular screening examinations for optic nerve gliomas and optic chiasma gliomas. Screening examinations include measurement of visual acuity, color vision, pupil reactions, visual field measurements and optic disc examination (Fig. 29.52). Gliomas, when present, may present with visual failure and/or proptosis. Vision may fluctuate, deteriorate or remain stable for many years. When there is consistent deterioration of visual function, active treatment may be considered. In younger children this will consist of chemotherapy with etoposide and cisplatin. In older children, radiotherapy may be considered.

Neurofibromas typically involve the upper eyelid, and there is an association with glaucoma in these eyes.

In NF2, posterior subcapsular cataract is present in more than 50% of cases and is a useful diagnostic sign. Combined hamartoma of the retina and pigment epithelium is a less common ocular association of NF2.

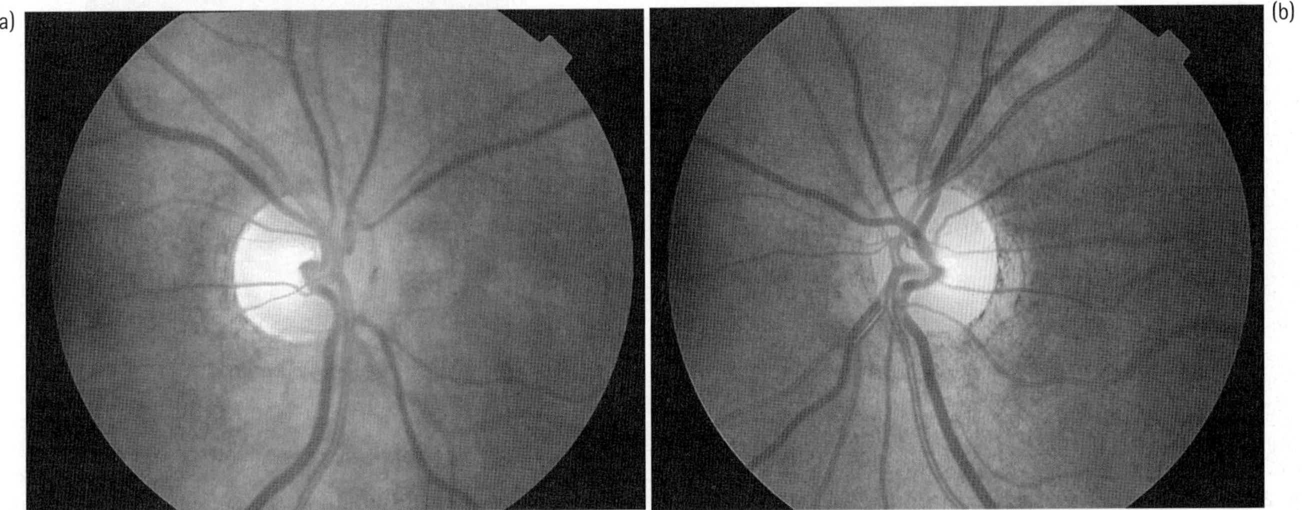

Fig. 29.52 (a) Right optic disc showing pallor on the temporal side. MRI scan showed optic nerve glioma. (b) Normal left optic disc.

Tuberous sclerosis

Fundus examination for retinal hamartomas should be performed in children with seizures and delayed cognitive development. Hamartomas will be found in approximately 50% of patients with tuberous sclerosis.[83] These may appear as minimally elevated smooth translucent retinal lesions anywhere in the fundus, or as yellowish multinodular masses near the optic disc (Fig. 29.53). The lesions do not change significantly with time and do not cause significant visual defect. Follow-up examination is generally not required.

Von Hippel–Lindau disease

Retinal angiomas are the earliest and the most common clinical features of von Hippel–Lindau disease. Careful annual fundus examination is required in order to detect early lesions, which are most often found in the mid periphery. The lesions tend to grow, and larger lesions leak serous fluid, which may lead to visual impairment. Early lesions should therefore be treated with laser or cryotherapy.

Screening retinal examinations are needed for patients with known von Hippel–Lindau disease, and for presymptomatic family members who are known to have a mutation of the von Hippel–Lindau gene (3p25–26).

OCULAR TRAUMA

Significant ocular trauma remains a relatively common occurrence in children. Examination of an injured child requires patience, and examination under anesthetic is often preferred, especially when there is a suspicion of ocular perforation. Foreign bodies tend to lodge in the corneal epithelium, or become trapped underneath the upper eyelid. Corneal abrasions may be more easily detected by instilling a drop of fluorescein dye. A prophylactic topical broad spectrum antibiotic should be prescribed when the corneal epithelium has been damaged. Eyelid lacerations should be carefully repaired, with particular attention to correct apposition of lacerations that involve the eyelid margins. Small ocular lacerations may result in a distorted pupil, with prolapse of iris tissue at the perforation site.

Non-perforating blunt injuries most frequently present with hyphema – blood within the anterior chamber (Fig. 29.54). The intraocular pressure should be measured, and treated if elevated. Topical steroid and mydriatic eyedrops are given to treat associated iritis. Follow-up examinations are required in order to detect fundus abnormalities and traumatic glaucoma. Permanent visual loss is most often due to choroidal rupture (Fig. 29.55) or retinal detachment.

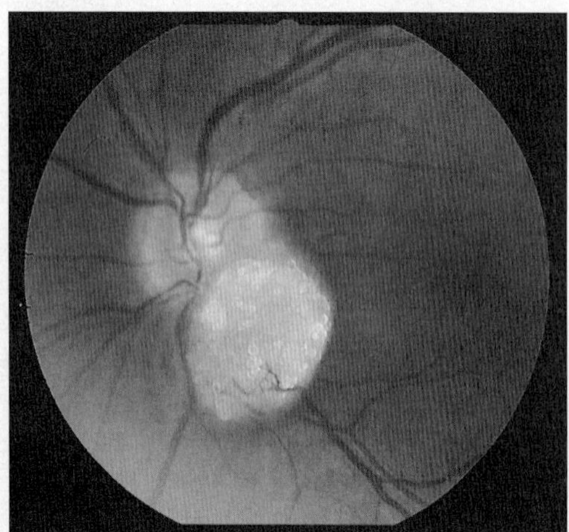

Fig. 29.53 Large multinodular retinal hamartoma adjacent to optic disc in a case of tuberous sclerosis.

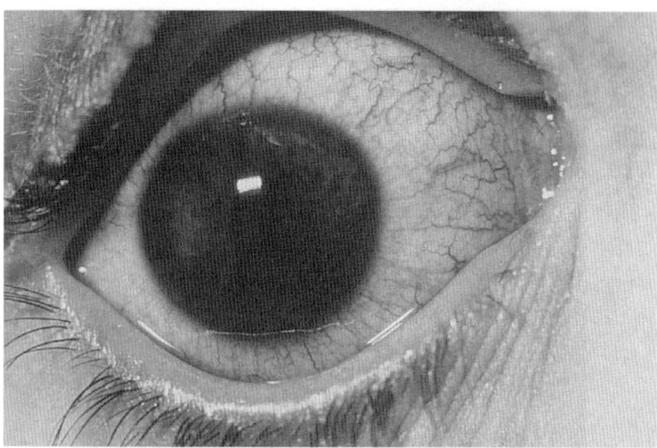

Fig. 29.54 Hyphema. Blood in the anterior chamber obscures the iris.

MANAGEMENT OF THE VISUALLY IMPAIRED CHILD AND THEIR FAMILY

The diagnosis of visual impairment in an infant or child may be devastating for a family. Parents are often in a state of shock when bad news is given and an early review consultation is helpful in order to further discuss the implications of the diagnosis. Visual impairment in infants has secondary effects on general development, and appropriate use of sound and tactile stimuli by the parents will improve developmental progress. Considerable social and educational support will be needed in addition to medical interventions. Local and national parent support groups are available and should be used.

EDUCATION OF VISUALLY IMPAIRED CHILDREN

Many children with visual impairment may be satisfactorily educated in a mainstream school, provided that adequate additional teaching resources are made available. Simple measures such as positioning of the child within the room and satisfactory lighting

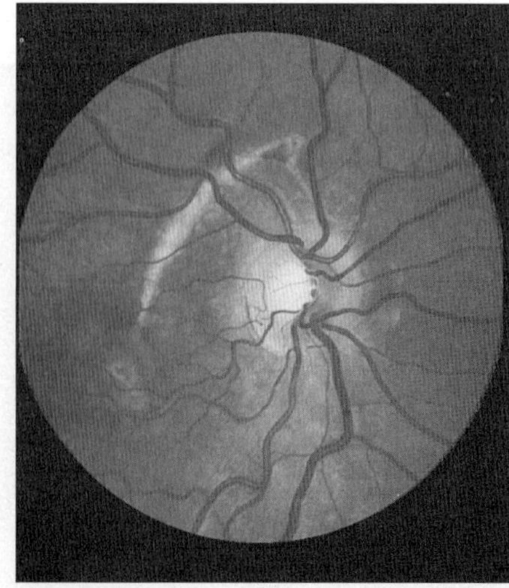

Fig. 29.55 Choroidal rupture. Blunt force has caused a curved tear in Bruch's membrane deep to the retinal pigment epithelium. There is additional pigment scarring at the macula.

should be considered. Enlarged text is required for some children. Developments in computer technology are of great benefit to many visually impaired children.

Low vision aids

Children with moderately reduced vision may benefit from the use of magnifying optical aids. These include simple handheld magnifiers, illuminated magnifiers, spectacle mounted magnifiers and distance monocular telescopes.

Braille

Braille supplemented by audiotape and speech recognition computer software enables many severely visually impaired children to progress to tertiary education.

REFERENCES (* Level 1 evidence)

1 Teller DM. Assessment of visual acuity in infants and children: the acuity card procedure. Dev Med Child Neurol 1986; 28:770–790.

2 Norcia AM. Vision testing by visual evoked potential techniques. In: Isenberg SJ, ed. The eye in infancy, 2nd edn. St Louis: Mosby; 1994:157–173.

3 Birch EE. Stereopsis in infants and its developmental relation to visual acuity. In: Simons K, ed. Early visual development, normal and abnormal. Oxford: Oxford University Press; 1993:224–236.

4 Birch EE. Preferential looking assessment of fusion and stereopsis in infants aged 1–6 months. Invest Ophthalmol Vis Sci 1991; 32:820.

5 Wiesel T. Single cell response in striate cortex of kittens deprived of vision in one eye. J Neurophysiol 1963; 26:1003–1017.

6 Wiesel T. Comparison of the effects of unilateral and bilateral eye closure on cortical unit responses in kittens. J Neurophysiol 1965; 28:1029–1040.

7 Vaegan TD. Critical period for deprivation amblyopia in children. Trans Ophthalmol Soc UK 1980; 99:432–439.

8 Keech RV. Upper age limit for the development of amblyopia. J Pediatr Ophthalmol Strabismus 1995; 32:89–93.

9 Jacobs M, Harris C, Shawkat F, Taylor D. The objective assessment of abnormal eye movements in infants and young children. Aust N Z J Ophthalmol 1992; 20:185–195.

10 Salgarello T, Tamburrelli C, Falsini B, et al. Optic nerve diameters and perimetric thresholds in idiopathic intracranial hypertension. Br J Ophthalmol 1996; 80:509–514.

11 Kriss A. Skin ERGs: their effectiveness in paediatric visual assessment, confounding factors, and comparison with ERGs recorded using various types of corneal electrode. Int J Psychophysiol 1994; 16:137–146.

12 Lambert SR, Kriss A, Taylor D, et al. Follow-up and diagnostic reappraisal of 75 patients with Leber's congenital amaurosis. Am J Ophthalmol 1989; 107:624–631.

13 Maumenee IH. The eye in Marfan syndrome. Trans Am Ophthalmol Soc 1981; 79:684–733.

14 Watanabe S, Yamashita T, Ohba N. A longitudinal study of cycloplegic refraction in a cohort of 350 Japanese schoolchildren. Cycloplegic refraction. Ophthalmic Physiol Opt 1999; 19:22–29.

15 Cruysberg JR, Boers GH, Trijbels JM, et al. Delay in diagnosis of homocystinuria: retrospective study of consecutive patients. BMJ 1996; 313:1037–1040.

16 Pokharel GP, Negrel AD, Munoz SR, et al. Refractive error study in children: results from Mechi Zone, Nepal. Am J Ophthalmol 2000; 129:436–444.

17 Rose K, Smith W, Morgan I, et al. The increasing prevalence of myopia: implications for Australia. Clin Exp Ophthalmol 2001; 29:116–120.

18 Villarreal MG, Ohlsson J, Abrahamsson M, et al. Myopisation: the refractive tendency in teenagers. Prevalence of myopia among young teenagers in Sweden. Acta Ophthalmol Scand 2000; 78:177–181.

19 Kinge B, Midelfart A, Jacobsen G, et al. The influence of near-work on development of myopia among university students. A three-year longitudinal study among engineering students in Norway. Acta Ophthalmol Scand 2000; 78:26–29.

*20 Ong E, Grice K, Held R, et al. Effects of spectacle intervention on the progression of myopia in children. Optom Vis Sci 1999; 76:363–369.

21 Choi MY, Lee KM, Hwang JM, et al. Comparison between anisometropic and strabismic amblyopia using functional magnetic resonance imaging. Br J Ophthalmol 2001; 85:1052–1056.

22 Weakley DR Jr. The association between nonstrabismic anisometropia, amblyopia, and subnormal binocularity. Ophthalmology 2001; 108:163–171.

23 Weakley DR Jr, Birch E, Kip K. The role of anisometropia in the development of accommodative esotropia. J AAPOS 2001; 5:153–157.

24 Cleary M. Efficacy of occlusion for strabismic amblyopia: can an optimal duration be identified? Br J Ophthalmol 2000; 84:572–578.

25 Flynn JT, Woodruff G, Thompson JR, et al. The therapy of amblyopia: an analysis comparing the results of amblyopia therapy utilizing two pooled data sets. Trans Am Ophthalmol Soc 1999; 97:373–390.

26 Kvarnstrom G, Jakobsson P, Lennerstrand G. Visual screening of Swedish children: an ophthalmological evaluation. Acta Ophthalmol Scand 2001; 79:240–244.

27 Tong PY, Enke-Miyazaki E, Bassin RE, et al. Screening for amblyopia in preverbal children with photoscreening photographs. Ophthalmology 1998; 105:856–863.

28 Shirabe H, Mori Y, Dogru M, et al. Early surgery for infantile esotropia. Br J Ophthalmol 2000; 84:536–538.

29 Birch EE, Fawcett S, Stager DR. Why does early surgical alignment improve stereoacuity outcomes in infantile esotropia? J AAPOS 2000; 4:10–14.

30 Birch E, Stager D, Wright K, et al. The natural history of infantile esotropia during the first six months of life. Pediatric Eye Disease Investigator Group. J AAPOS 1998; 2:325–358.

31 Mulvihill A, MacCann A, Flitcroft I, et al. Outcome in refractive accommodative esotropia. Br J Ophthalmol 2000; 84:746–749.

32 Coats DK, Avilla CW, Paysse EA, et al. Early-onset refractive accommodative esotropia. J AAPOS 1998; 2:275–278.

*33 Prism Adaptation Research Group. Efficacy of prism adaptation in the surgical management of acquired esotropia. Arch Ophthalmol 1990; 108:1248–1256.

34 Spielmann A. Clinical rationale for manifest congenital nystagmus surgery. J AAPOS 2000; 4:67–74.

35 Fielder AR, Evans NM. Is the geniculostriate system a prerequisite for nystagmus? Eye 1988; 2(Pt 6):628–635.

36 Jacobson LK, Dutton GN. Periventricular leukomalacia: an important cause of visual and ocular motility dysfunction in children. Surv Ophthalmol 2000; 45:1–13.

37 Lambert SR, Kriss A, Taylor D. Delayed visual maturation. A longitudinal clinical and electrophysiological assessment. Ophthalmology 1989; 96:524–528.

38 Cocker KD, Moseley MJ, Stirling HF, et al. Delayed visual maturation: pupillary responses implicate subcortical and cortical visual systems. Dev Med Child Neurol 1998; 40:160–162.

39 Dharmaraj SR, Silva ER, Pina AL, et al. Mutational analysis and clinical correlation in Leber congenital amaurosis. Ophthalmic Genet 2000; 21:135–150.

40 Gerber S, Perrault I, Hanein S, et al. Complete exon–intron structure of the RPGR-interacting protein (RPGRIP1) gene allows the identification of mutations underlying Leber congenital amaurosis. Eur J Hum Genet 2001; 9:561–571.

41 Acland GM, Aguirre GD, Ray J, et al. Gene therapy restores vision in a canine model of childhood blindness. Nat Genet 2001; 28:92–95.

42 Dattani ML, Martinez-Barbera J, Thomas PQ, et al. Molecular genetics of septo-optic dysplasia. Horm Res 2000; 53(suppl 1):26–33.

43 Moore AT, Taylor DS. A syndrome of congenital retinal dystrophy and saccade palsy—a subset of Leber's amaurosis. Br J Ophthalmol 1984; 68:421–431.

44 Fishman GA, Stone EM, Grover S, et al. Variation of clinical expression in patients with Stargardt dystrophy and sequence variations in the ABCR gene. Arch Ophthalmol 1999; 117:504–510.

45 Armstrong JD, Meyer D, Xu S, et al. Long-term follow-up of Stargardt's disease and

fundus flavimaculatus. Ophthalmology 1998; 105:448–457.
46 Wisniewski KE. Pheno/genotypic correlations of neuronal ceroid lipofuscinoses. Neurology 2001; 57:576–581.
47 Newman SA. Ophthalmic features of craniosynostosis. Neurosurg Clin N Am 1991; 2:587–610.
48 Goldberg F, Berne AS, Oski FA. Differentiation of orbital cellulitis from preseptal cellulitis by computed tomography. Pediatrics 1978; 62:1000–1009.
49 Stigmar G, Crawford JS, Ward CM, et al. Ophthalmic sequelae of infantile hemangiomas of the eyelids and orbit. Am J Ophthalmol 1978; 85:806–813.
50 Kushner BJ. Intralesional corticosteroid injection for infantile adnexal hemangioma. Am J Ophthalmol 1982; 93:506.
*51 Maurer HM, Gehan EA, Beltangady M, et al. The intergroup rhabdomyosarcoma study – II. Cancer 1993; 71:1904–22.
52 Paysse EA, Coats DK, Bernstein JM, et al. Management and complications of congenital dacryocele with concurrent intranasal mucocele. J AAPOS 2000; 4:46–53.
53 MacEwen CJ, Young JD. Epiphora during the first year of life. Eye 1991; 5:600.
54 MacEwen CJ. The fluorescein disappearance test (FDT): an evaluation of its use in infants. J Pediatr Ophthalmol Strabismus 1991; 28:302–305.
*55 Young JD, MacEwen CJ, Ogston SA. Congenital nasolacrimal duct obstruction in the second year of life: a multicentre trial of management. Eye 1996; 10(Pt 4):485–491.
56 MacEwen CJ, Young JD, Barras CW, et al. Value of nasal endoscopy and probing in the diagnosis and management of children with congenital epiphora. Br J Ophthalmol 2001; 85:314–318.
57 Maini R, MacEwen CJ, Young JD. The natural history of epiphora in childhood. Eye 1998; 12(Pt 4):669–671.
58 Kanski JJ. Screening for uveitis in juvenile chronic arthritis. Br J Ophthalmol 1989; 73:225–228.
59 Southwood TR, Ryder CA. Ophthalmological screening in juvenile arthritis: should the frequency of screening be based on the risk of developing chronic iridocyclitis? Br J Rheumatol 1992; 31:633–634.
60 Fleck BW, Dangata Y. Causes of visual handicap in the Royal Blind School, Edinburgh, 1991–2. Br J Ophthalmol 1994; 78:421.
61 Bermejo E, Martinez-Frias ML. Congenital eye malformations: clinical–epidemiological analysis of 1,124,654 consecutive births in Spain. Am J Med Genet 1998; 75:497–504.
62 Horton JC, Hocking DR. Timing of the critical period for plasticity of ocular dominance columns in macaque striate cortex. J Neurosci 1997; 17:3684–3709.
63 Rahi JS, Dezateux C. National cross sectional study of detection of congenital and infantile cataract in the United Kingdom: role of childhood screening and surveillance. The British Congenital Cataract Interest Group. BMJ 1999; 318:362–365.
64 Taylor D, Vaegan, Morris JA, et al. Amblyopia in bilateral infantile and juvenile cataract. Relationship to timing of treatment. Trans Ophthalmol Soc UK 1979; 99:170–175.
65 Rahi JS, Dezateux C. Congenital and infantile cataract in the United Kingdom: underlying or associated factors. British Congenital Cataract Interest Group. Invest Ophthalmol Vis Sci 2000; 41:2108–2114.
66 Markham RH, Bloom PA, Chandna A, et al. Results of intraocular lens implantation in paediatric aphakia. Eye 1992; 6(Pt 5): 493–498.
67 Lambert SR, Fernandes A, Drews-Botsch C, et al. Multifocal versus monofocal correction of neonatal monocular aphakia. J Pediatr Ophthalmol Strabismus 1994; 31:195–201.
68 Aasuri MK, Venkata N, Preetam P, et al. Management of pediatric aphakia with silsoft contact lenses. CLAO J 1999; 25:209–212.
69 Fuchs J, Rosenberg T. Congenital ectopia lentis. A Danish national survey. Acta Ophthalmol Scand 1998; 76:20–26.
70 Halpert M, BenEzra D. Surgery of the hereditary subluxated lens in children. Ophthalmology 1996; 103:681–686.
71 Budning AS, Heon E, Gallie BL. Visual prognosis of Coats' disease. J AAPOS 1998; 2:356–359.
72 Ridley ME, Shields JA, Brown GC, et al. Coats' disease. Evaluation of management. Ophthalmology 1982; 89:1381–1387.
73 Shields JA, Shields CL, Honavar SG, et al. Classification and management of Coats' disease: the 2000 Proctor Lecture. Am J Ophthalmol 2001; 131:572–583.
74 Shields JA, Shields CL, Honavar SG, et al. Clinical variations and complications of Coats' disease in 150 cases: the 2000 Sanford Gifford Memorial Lecture. Am J Ophthalmol 2001; 131:561–571.
75 Knudson AG. Mutation and cancer: statistical study of retinoblastoma. Proc Natl Acad Science U S A 1971; 68:823.
76 Aldave AJ, Shields CL, Shields JA. Surgical excision of selected amblyogenic periorbital capillary hemangiomas. Ophthalmic Surg Lasers 1999; 30:754–757.
*77 Fleck BW. Therapy for retinopathy of prematurity. Lancet 1999; 353:166–167.
*78 Taylor D. Unnatural injuries. Eye 2000; 14:123–150.
79 O'Hare AE, Eden OB. Bleeding disorders and non-accidental injury. Arch Dis Child 1984; 59:860–864.
80 Buys Y, Levin A, Enzenauer R, et al. Retinal findings after head trauma in infants and young children. Ophthalmology 1992; 99:1718–1723.
81 Tyagi AK, Scotcher S, Kozeis N, et al. Can convulsions alone cause retinal haemorrhages in infants? Br J Ophthalmol 1998; 82:659–660.
82 Bradbury JA, Danjoux JP, Voller J, et al. A randomised placebo-controlled trial of topical cysteamine therapy in patients with nephropathic cystinosis. Eye 1991; 5(pt 6):755–760.
83 Rowley SA, O'Callaghan FJ, Osborne JP. Ophthalmic manifestations of tuberous sclerosis: a population based study. Br J Ophthalmol 2001; 85:420–423.

30

Disorders of the ear, nose and throat

David L Cowan, Alastair IG Kerr

THE EAR

CONGENITAL ABNORMALITIES

MICROTIA/ANOTIA/MEATAL ATRESIA

The auricle forms from six tubercles of His. Malformations include microtia, a misshapen auricle, or anotia, the absence of the auricle. Both may be associated with accessory auricles, which are small residual tubercles that may lie sometimes over the cheek without function. Either of these congenital abnormalities of the auricle may be associated with meatal atresia, the absence of the bony meatus. They are commonly associated together in a variety of congenital conditions and syndromes. They may present as a unilateral problem, e.g. first arch syndrome, or as a bilateral problem, e.g. craniofacial dysostosis or Treacher Collins syndrome. If the deformity is a unilateral one it is extremely important to investigate the normal ear to ensure that the hearing is normal on the unaffected side. Assuming the normal ear has normal hearing, then surgical or other intervention on the affected side becomes purely cosmetic. If the condition is bilateral, then the degree of conductive hearing loss should be established and, in the first instance, a bone conduction hearing aid fixed by a head band should be fitted at an early age. With the advent of osseus integrated bony implants, this bone conduction hearing aid should be replaced by an implant aid when the skull is thick enough to sustain this (usually aged 3 to 4). Surgical attempts to construct a patent meatus have not been successful and have been abandoned but rib graft reconstruction of the pinna is becoming increasingly popular from the cosmetic point of view. An alternative to this is an osseus integrated prosthesis.

MEATAL STENOSIS

Meatal stenosis may occur either as a congenital abnormality or as a result of chronic otitis externa. Down syndrome children have very narrow external auditory meati and they often have middle ear problems. This sometimes makes the fitting of grommet tubes impossible and hence careful monitoring of their hearing is important.

OSSICULAR ABNORMALITIES

Congenital abnormalities of the ear ossicles are rarely seen in isolation and are usually associated with some other manifest congenital abnormality. Attempts at surgical repair of ossicles in children are not normally advisable and any bilateral hearing deficit should be treated by a hearing aid.

INJURIES/FOREIGN BODIES

Direct trauma to the auricle may produce a hematoma and is commonly seen in sporting injuries. The hematoma should be aspirated and a pressure bandage applied to avoid the cosmetic abnormality known as 'cauliflower ear'.

PERFORATIONS OF THE TYMPANIC MEMBRANE

This can be caused either by an object inserted into the ear or alternatively by pressure, e.g. in non-accidental injury where a slap across the ear can cause a perforation of the drum due to the pressure of the air column in the narrow meatus. This form of injury is also seen in explosions or in diving accidents. Head injuries may be associated with perforation of the eardrum and also leakage of cerebrospinal fluid.

Treatment of perforation of the eardrum is conservative; the ear is kept dry and in the great majority of traumatic perforations the eardrum will heal spontaneously. This healing may take several months but no attempt at surgical intervention should be considered for at least 6 months.

95% of traumatic tympanic membrane perforations will close spontaneously

WAX

It is normal for wax to be present in ears and as a general rule this causes no problems unless the wax is impacted into the external auditory meatus by the use of cotton buds. The superficial squamous epithelial cells in the external meatus have a natural flow pattern outwards, so that wax will be naturally extruded from the ear and hence, if the wax is kept soft by the use of simple olive or almond oil drops, syringing of the ears should not be required. As a general rule it is preferable not to syringe children's ears as they will find it uncomfortable and it will interfere with the natural extrusion process.

INFECTIONS OF THE EARS

OTITIS EXTERNA

This condition does not occur as commonly in children. The basis of treatment is aural toilet and the application of a topical antibiotic, with or without steroids, either on a small gauze dressing, which is preferable, or, alternatively, administered as eardrops. The skin of the meatus is often swollen and extremely tender and aural toilet may have to be carried out under a general anesthetic.

FURUNCULOSIS

A furuncle in the external meatus will produce an acutely painful ear which is tender to the touch. It is often associated with a tender lymph node over the mastoid tip and hence the combination is often mistaken as an acute mastoiditis. In acute mastoiditis, the maximum area of tenderness is rarely, if ever, over the mastoid tip. Treatment of furunculosis is oral antibiotics and local dressings.

ACUTE OTITIS MEDIA

This occurs commonly in infants and children as the eustachian tube is shorter, relatively wider and more horizontal than in the adult and also because children have adenoids which are close to the opening of the eustachian tube: hence, acute otitis media is a common accompaniment to upper respiratory tract infections and other infections. Clinically, the condition will present as an acutely painful ear, usually bilaterally, and the child will be fevered and may develop febrile convulsions.

The eardrum if inspected will appear either acutely inflamed or bulging, with obvious pus behind it, and the pain is due to the build-up of mucopurulent secretions in the middle ear. The first-aid treatment is analgesics/antipyretics, and antibiotics. Antibiotics provide only a small benefit for acute otitis media in children.[1] A Cochrane review[2] compared the outcome of short acting antibiotics for 5 days with short acting antibiotics for 8–10 days and concluded that 5 days of short acting antibiotics (ceftriaxone or azithromycin) is effective. If the eardrum perforates, the pain will subside. In the vast majority of patients the drum will heal once the infection has settled. The treatment of infants and children with recurrent attacks of acute otitis media is either by repeated use of antibiotics or by surgical intervention. In young children, whose adenoids have not developed, the insertion of ventilation tubes (grommets) in the tympanic membranes will prevent recurrent attacks of acute otitis media. In older children who have significant adenoids, their removal will reduce further attacks of otitis media.

Acute otitis media is the commonest cause of otalgia with fever in children

ACUTE MASTOIDITIS

Acute mastoiditis still occurs but not nearly as frequently as it used to, due to the use of antibiotics for acute otitis media. Clinically, the child with acute mastoiditis will present with an acutely tender swelling in the postauricular region with the area of maximum tenderness being over the surface marking of the mastoid antrum which is at the level of the top of the tragus. If looked at from behind, the auricle will be seen to be projecting outwards from the skull due to the loss of the postauricular sulcus and this is most commonly due to the collection of subperiosteal pus. The ear may or may not be discharging. The child will usually be in considerable pain and will be febrile. Treatment is admission, administration of intravenous antibiotics and analgesics and careful monitoring of the pulse and temperature for 24–48 h. If the postauricular swelling is increasing or if the temperature is not settling in that time, then surgical drainage of the subperiosteal pus and drilling away of the diseased cortical bone should be undertaken under general anesthesia. Acute mastoiditis rarely becomes a recurrent problem nor does it lead to chronic otitis media or cholesteatoma formation.

Postaural subperiosteal swelling with a protruding pinna is pathognomonic of acute mastoiditis

CHRONIC OTITIS MEDIA

Chronic otitis media is associated with a permanent perforation of the tympanic membrane. There are two quite distinct groups: tubotympanic disease and attico/antral disease.

Tubotympanic disease

Usually such children have had recurrent attacks of otitis media which have either been inappropriately treated or which have resulted in a permanent residual anterior central perforation of the tympanic membrane. The clinical presentation is of intermittent quite profuse painless mucopurulent discharge from the ear. The profuse discharge occurs in association with an upper respiratory tract infection or following the child swimming or getting the ear wet. If treated with oral antibiotics, the discharge should cease. The hearing loss will be minimal. Effective antibiotic treatment of tubotympanic disease is required and the child should keep the ear dry. Closure of the perforation by myringoplasty using a temporalis fascia graft is not advisable until the child has gone at least 6 months without any discharge from the ear and this will rarely be before the age of 8 or 9.

Attico/antral disease

These children have a continuous painless moderate purulent or bloodstained discharge from the ear. There may be middle ear granulations. This discharge will often be foul-smelling as the commonest organism is *Pseudomonas pyocyaneas*. This form of chronic otitis media does not usually respond to antibiotics and is more serious as it is usually associated with cholesteatoma in the mastoid antrum or mastoid cell system which may erode the ossicles and cause a significant hearing loss. If cholesteatoma is identified in the ear by suction clearance, under general anesthesia, then mastoid surgery is indicated as facial nerve palsy or cerebral complications will occur if the cholesteatoma is not cleared completely from the mastoid system.

REFERRED OTALGIA

Referred pain in the ear may be from the tonsils, sinuses or teeth, all of which must be considered in a child who has unexplained otalgia.

SECRETORY OTITIS MEDIA

This is a very common condition in childhood which can occur at any age but is found most commonly between the ages of 4 and 6 years. It is commoner in boys. It is alternatively called non-suppurative otitis media, seromucinous otitis media, exudative otitis media, or simply 'glue ear'. Children with secretory otitis media commonly present with a hearing loss due to the collection of fluid in their middle ears. Cytologically, the fluid contains polymorphonuclear leukocytes, macrophages and cell debris but no ciliated columnar cells or eosinophils. The fluid is invariably sterile and various searches for viruses have proved negative. Biochemically, the fluid contains glycoproteins and nucleoproteins and this gives the fluid its thick tenacious quality.

Natural history

Classically, a child with secretory otitis media will present with painless insidious bilateral conductive deafness, which if measured audiometrically, will not be greater than 40 decibels. Fluid will classically collect without prior middle ear infections and often the child does not remark on the loss of hearing. The problem may not be identified until routine audiometric testing is done at school. The fluid collects due to blockage of the eustachian tube. If children are left for up to 12 weeks, 30–40% of them will drain their fluid and their hearing will return to normal. Alternatively, a distinct group of children who have recurrent otitis media which has been treated appropriately by antibiotics develop a collection of sterile fluid in the middle ear which does not drain down the eustachian tube, presumably due to edema of the mucosa.

Prevalence

At any one time, 1 child in 100 will have secretory otitis media, and approximately 10% of children under 10 years will have had secretory otitis media.

Secretory otitis media is the commonest cause of conductive deafness in childhood

Diagnosis

Diagnosis is usually made by taking a careful history from the parents and/or the teachers, who are seeing the child on an everyday basis. Otoscopic examination will reveal an abnormal eardrum which may be retracted, bulging, dull, blue/yellow in color, or have air–fluid level or bubbles visible behind it. Puretone audiometry will reveal a conductive hearing loss which is usually bilateral and worse in the lower frequencies than the higher frequencies but never greater than 40 decibels. Impedance audiometry will give a flat tympanogram with a negative middle ear pressure and a greatly reduced tympanic membrane compliance.

Etiology

The underlying cause is believed to be some abnormality of eustachian tube function and, certainly, children with cleft palate, and hence impaired eustachian tube function, have a greatly increased risk of having secretory otitis media. Children with chronic secretory otitis media do have persistent negative middle ear pressure due to eustachian tube malfunction and this results in the loss of the elastic layer of the tympanic membrane with atelectasis or atrophy of the membrane. Adenoids blocking the eustachian tube orifice in the nasopharynx have long been associated with this condition and so their removal is often undertaken as a form of treatment. However, children without adenoids still get secretory otitis media and therefore there must be more complex factors involved. Attempts to associate nasal allergy with secretory otitis media have never been substantiated and apart from the already mentioned age and sex factors, the only other recently proven etiologic factor is passive smoking within the home environment.[3] Because the eustachian tube is situated so centrally, it is extremely difficult to investigate its function in these children, and hence the etiology remains obscure.

Treatment

The treatment of secretory otitis media remains controversial. The policy of watchful waiting for 12 weeks has been mentioned and should be pursued. Parents of children with secretory otitis media are the first to notice when the hearing loss recurs and are always the quickest to demand treatment. Children tend to accept what is given to them and rarely complain when the condition recurs, although their behavior may alter. Another symptom not uncommonly seen in children with secretory otitis media, that of loss of balance, may also improve following treatment with a 30–40% chance of spontaneous recovery. Many suggest that surgical treatment should not be undertaken as the condition may resolve spontaneously with time. However, there is no doubt that some young toddlers who are slow to talk may turn out to have secretory otitis media, or that the schoolchild with secretory otitis media may present with poor oral work in comparison to his written work.

Attempts to treat the condition medically with long term, low dose antibiotics and/or local or oral decongestants have never convincingly been proven to be effective and any positive results may well be due to the natural history of the condition and the spontaneous recovery in some children. A Cochrane review[4] of treating children with this condition with systemic or topical nasal steroids concluded there was no evidence of any long term benefit and this should not therefore be recommended. If clearance of the fluid does not occur within 2 months then the only available treatment is surgical.

Surgery consists of myringotomy (drainage of the fluid) and insertion of ventilation tubes (grommets). This should be combined with adenoidectomy if a child presents with symptoms of enlarged adenoids (chronic mouth breathing, snoring, etc.). Adenoids are very small at birth but grow to a maximum size between the ages of 4 and 8 and it is in this group that adenoidectomy maybe required. By ventilating the middle ear, grommet tubes reduce negative middle ear pressure and hence prevent atelectasis of the tympanic membrane.

Children with grommet tubes are advised not to immerse their head under water, either in the bath or in the swimming pool. If children insist on diving deep in the swimming pool, then either a commercial earplug or cotton wool impregnated with petroleum jelly may be inserted into the ears to prevent water reaching the tympanic membrane. Classically, grommet tubes remain in place in the eardrums from 6 months to 1 year, but the range may be from 2 months to 2 years. Apart from infection, there are no long term complications from the use of grommet tubes.

Surgery for secretory otitis media should only follow 3 months of watchful waiting

---

Outcomes

The number of children with chronic otitis media has fallen since treatment of secretory otitis media has been more active. As far as the final hearing goes, the long term results appear to be reasonably good, although these have not been totally scientifically delineated.

DEAFNESS

Secretory otitis media will produce a conductive deafness of up to 40 decibels which can affect speech and language development.

A child with a hearing handicap should be identified as having conductive deafness or sensorineural deafness (nerve deafness). In conductive deafness the disability is not so severe and often there may be a surgical or medical method of treating it. Sensorineural deafness in children is not uncommon. In developed countries, the incidence of bilateral significant sensorineural deafness is 1 in 1000 live births. 'Significant loss' is a loss of between 25 and 35 decibels in the better ear. It is the high frequency component of the loss that is usually important. If the loss in the better ear is at a level of 30 decibels when averaged over the four frequencies 500 Hz, 1 kHz, 2 kHz and 4 kHz, then the child will require some kind of amplification to attain normal speech and language.

Significant bilateral sensorineural deafness has an incidence of 1 in 1000 live births

---

CAUSES OF SENSORINEURAL DEAFNESS

Hereditary prenatal causes

There are large numbers of syndromes in which deafness is a recognized factor:

Waardenburg syndrome. This autosomal dominant condition with variable expression consists of some or all of the following characteristics: unilateral or bilateral sensorineural deafness (20% of cases); hypertrichosis of the eyebrows which meet in the midline; heterochromia of the irises; or a white forelock.

Klippel–Feil syndrome. A short neck limits head movements, the hairline is low at the back, there may be paralysis of the external rectus muscle in one or both eyes and there is sensorineural hearing loss which may be severe.

Alport's syndrome is X-linked dominant and affects boys more severely than girls. There is severe progressive glomerulonephritis and a progressive sensorineural loss which does not show itself until the boy is about 10 years old.

Pendred's syndrome is autosomal recessive and causes simple goiter at about the age of 4–5 years. There is an associated deafness which is often severe.

Refsum's syndrome consists of ichthyosis, ataxia, retinitis pigmentosa, night blindness, mental retardation and a sensorineural deafness.

Usher's syndrome is autosomal recessive. There is retinitis pigmentosa with contraction of the visual fields and a severe sensorineural loss which may be progressive.

Jervell and Lange-Neilsen syndrome is autosomal recessive with a cardiac arrhythmia and a profound sensorineural deafness. These children may present with syncopal attacks and if untreated, these attacks can be fatal.

The inheritance of deafness is well recognized and in some children with recessive inheritance, the sensorineural hearing loss may be progressive. Non-hereditary prenatal deafness is due to maternal illness, especially in the first trimester of pregnancy. Cytomegalovirus infections, toxoplasmosis, glandular fever and rubella are the most common, while parental syphilis and the taking of certain ototoxic drugs by the mother may cause deafness in the baby.

Ototoxic drugs that should be specifically avoided during pregnancy are the aminoglycosides, quinine and to a lesser extent salicylates and alcohol.

Perinatal causes of deafness are basically related to prematurity and hypoxia. With the advances in neonatology, when extremely immature babies with complex neonatal problems are now surviving, the number of children with significant bilateral deafness sometimes associated with other abnormalities, and often related to hypoxia, is increasing. The cochlea is particularly sensitive to lack of oxygen. As neonatology improves further, the numbers of children with perinatal deafness will hopefully reduce.

Early diagnosis of sensorineural deafness is vital for acquisition of speech and language

---

Postnatal causes

Middle ear problems cause conductive deafness and the causes of these have already been discussed. Sensorineural loss may result from head injury, from the use of ototoxic drugs and as a result of specific infections. Parents whose children get repeated attacks of acute otitis media are often concerned that significant sensorineural loss may result, but this is extremely rare.

Measles and mumps. Measles and mumps remain the specific infections that can cause significant sensorineural hearing loss. Luckily, mumps, although it will cause a profound sensorineural loss, generally only produces a unilateral loss, while the increasing use of the measles/mumps/rubella (MMR) vaccine will reduce the incidence of deafness from these infections.

Meningitis. Meningococcal or pneumococcal meningitis may give severe bilateral sensorineural hearing loss which will be permanent and may progress in severity following recovery from the meningitis. All children who have recovered from bacterial meningitis should have their hearing tested and monitored.

In summary, only about 50% of children with significant bilateral sensorineural loss have an identifiable cause.

DIAGNOSIS OF DEAFNESS

The first 2 years of life are absolutely vital for the acquisition of speech and language and hence the early detection of significant hearing loss in a baby is vital.

No child has no islands of hearing at all and with early detection and appropriate amplification the chances of the child learning to speak are greatly increased. The ideal would be to have a quick, simple, objective test that could be done on every child during the first 24 h of life and the long term aim is to develop a system for universal neonatal screening. This should be done measuring otoacoustic emissions followed up by automated brainstem testing. At present this is being piloted in several centers in the UK.

Only 50% of children with sensorineural deafness have an identifiable cause

---

SUBJECTIVE AUDIOMETRY

Distraction audiometry

This is still a reliable, efficient method of testing which requires the minimum of equipment. The disadvantage is that it cannot be performed until the child is holding his head up unsupported. In the UK this is carried out by the health visitor as one of the routine screening tests at 7 or 8 months.

Conditioned audiometry

As the child gets older, he can be conditioned to perform a specific task in response to the input of sound.

Puretone audiometry

This is the main method of testing but cannot be done until the child will tolerate wearing headphones and can be relied upon to respond accurately to puretone sounds.

OBJECTIVE AUDIOMETRY

Brainstem evoked response audiometry

This is the most reliable form of objective audiometry and can be performed at any age. Disadvantages are that it takes a considerable time, it is not frequency specific, and the child will have to be lying quietly or else sedated for it to be performed satisfactorily. In some multiply-handicapped children it may have to be done under general anesthetic.

Otoacoustic emissions

This is a quick, efficient and very simple form of objective audiometry that is increasingly being suggested as the most useful test for screening children. Its disadvantage is that it does not distinguish between conductive deafness and sensorineural deafness and that any children who fail the otoacoustic emission test usually have to then progress to brainstem evoked response audiometry.

Impedance audiometry or tympanometry

This is a simple test that measures the compliance of the eardrum and the pressure of the air in the middle ear. It is ideally suited for identifying secretory otitis media patients and is useful in screening outpatients who have failed their routine school audiometric testing.

TREATMENT OF DEAFNESS

Treatment of conductive deafness has been discussed elsewhere in this chapter. There is no medical treatment for sensorineural deafness and treatment is based on prophylaxis. Genetic counseling and preventive measures such as immunization are important to avoid some causes of sensorineural hearing loss. As neonatology advances and hypoxia becomes less common, the incidence of deafness amongst ex-premature infants will be reduced. Sensorineural hearing loss is not normally progressive but in some congenital conditions it is, and so careful monitoring of the child's hearing is vital once the diagnosis has been made.

The mainstay of treatment remains amplification by some form of hearing aid. A large range of hearing aids is now available for children with sensorineural hearing loss and it is extremely important that the degree of handicap and the shape of the audiogram is known before the hearing aid is prescribed. Nowadays the hearing aid can be customized to the child's actual specific hearing loss.

THE PHONIC EAR

Teaching the deaf has been revolutionized by the advent of the phonic ear. This is a radio-aid type of hearing device where the mother or the teacher wears a microphone and a transmitter and the child wears the radio receiver. This means the child can sit anywhere in the class and be in direct radio contact with the teacher and hence the degree of amplification can be greatly enhanced. Many children with quite severe hearing handicap can therefore now be educated in their own local school rather than having to go to specific schools for the hearing impaired.

COCHLEAR IMPLANTS

This is the latest and most powerful form of hearing aid in which a small fenestration is made surgically in the basal turn of the cochlea and 22 electrodes on a very delicate wire are inserted into the cochlea itself. At present, these devices are extremely expensive and require considerable expertise and a huge amount of time for each individual electrode to be specifically tuned to the child's needs. This can only be done in highly specialized centers and children requiring these devices at present are only those who are deriving nothing whatsoever from the standardized hearing aid systems described above. Thresholds for recommending cochlear implantation are gradually dropping and although initially they were thought to be of most value in children with acquired deafness, it is now accepted that children with profoundly congenital deafness will derive great benefit. Surgery should be performed at as early an age as possible (usually aged 2–3). Cochlear implant has been one of the most exciting developments in pediatric audiology.

Cochlear implants are only required for a very small number of profoundly deaf children

THE NOSE AND SINUSES

THE NOSE

The nose functions as an air conditioner for the lower respiratory tract. It achieves this by cleaning, warming and humidifying the inspired air. The turbinates (Fig. 30.1) project from the lateral wall, increasing the surface area and causing turbulence. This allows heat and fluid exchange and causes any particles to be deposited on the lining of the nose in the sticky mucus which then passes posteriorly and is swallowed. The function of the paranasal sinuses is unknown.

FOREIGN BODIES

These present as foul-smelling and sometimes bloodstained unilateral nasal discharge. They occur most often in children between the ages of 2 and 4 years, and are usually bits of foam rubber or toys which they have inserted themselves. It is rare for them to cause lower respiratory tract infections and the treatment is removal of the foreign body.

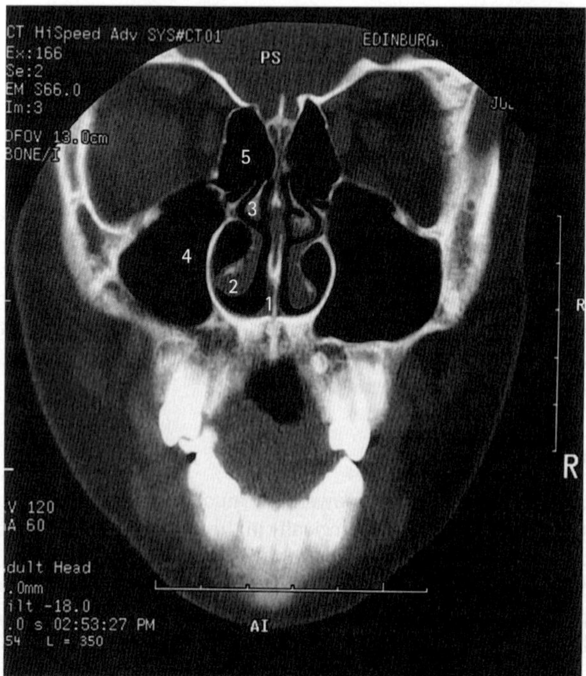

Fig. 30.1 Normal coronal CT scan of an 11-year-old boy showing: (1) nasal septum; (2) inferior turbinates; (3) middle turbinates; (4) maxillary sinuses; (5) ethmoid sinuses.

This can be done in a treatment or outpatient area if a headlight and appropriate instruments are available and the child is cooperative. Often, however, it has to be done under a general anesthetic.

Unilateral foul-smelling nasal discharge in a young child is pathognomic of a nasal foreign body

FRACTURE OF THE NOSE

The nose is the commonest bone in the body to be broken. In children nasal fractures are less common than in adults as the nasal bones are smaller and the tissues more pliant.

Nasal fractures result from direct trauma. Initially, there is swelling over the bridge of the nose and around the eyes which takes 5–7 days to subside. It is then possible to see whether the nasal bones are deviated, when manipulation under general anesthetic to straighten them is usually advised. Manipulation must be carried out within 21 days of the injury otherwise the bones become fixed.

Hematoma of the septum presents as severe blockage of the nose after an injury. This inevitably becomes infected resulting in development of a septal abscess and destruction of cartilage and requires surgical drainage and a broad spectrum antibiotic for 10 days.

EPISTAXIS

This is very common at any age. The bleeding can be spontaneous or secondary to mild trauma and usually arises in Little's area, in the anterior part of the nasal septum. Epistaxis can occur in leukemia or patients with bleeding disorders (e.g. hemophilia or thrombocytopenia) but is rarely the presenting feature of these conditions. First aid treatment consisting of pinching the anterior cartilaginous portion of the nose with the child upright is usually successful. If there are repeated episodes, nasal cautery is indicated.

Epistaxis in a child usually comes from Little's area at the front of the nose and can be controlled by local pressure

After identifying the source of bleeding, local anesthetic, 5% topical lidocaine (lignocaine) with 0.5% phenylephrine hydrochloride, (co-phenylcaine) is applied using cotton wool or a spray. The area is then cauterized using a silver nitrate stick. In severe cases not responding to cautery, admission with nasal packing and intravenous fluid replacement may be required.

RHINITIS

This is extremely common and is characterized by swelling and inflammation of the lining of the nose, often accompanied by clear or purulent rhinorrhea.

Viral rhinitis (the common cold or coryza)

This occurs very commonly with a pyrexial illness, runny nose, throat discomfort, sneezing and occasional earache. Treatment is symptomatic – analgesics and antipyretics as required. There is no proven place for decongestants in this condition. Viruses which have been identified as causing the common cold include rhinovirus, reovirus and adenovirus.

Viral rhinitis may be the precursor of laryngotracheobronchitis or pneumonia. A simple cold will normally last for 7–10 days and the child will not be unwell.

Bacterial rhinitis

This usually presents as purulent discharge following acute rhinitis. Antibiotics are rarely required unless the nasal blockage becomes worse or systemic symptoms such as fever and headaches occur when adenoiditis or sinusitis should be suspected. In some children there is a constant low grade bacterial rhinitis variable in severity, where no definitive underlying cause can be found. This can be associated with poor diet, damp housing and parental smoking. The underlying problem is thought to be lowered local nasal immunity. Most children with this condition will improve spontaneously from about the age of 8 years onwards. Immotile cilia syndrome is a rare cause and will often be associated with lower respiratory tract disease.

Allergic rhinitis

This usually occurs in children over 5 years old. It presents as sneezing, associated with clear rhinorrhea, nasal blockage and can be accompanied by conjunctivitis and sore throat. Seasonal rhinitis usually occurs in the summer and is caused by allergy to pollens. Perennial rhinitis can occur at any time of the year and can be associated with exposure to extrinsic allergens such as animals (e.g. cats or dogs) or housedust mite.

The diagnosis is made from the history. On examination, the nasal lining will usually be slightly pale and swollen. Confirmation of the allergic basis can be made by carrying out skin testing or sending serum immunoglobulin E assay.

Treatment is, if possible, by removal of the allergen but if this is not possible (e.g. seasonal rhinitis), a non-sedating antihistamine such as loratidine, supplemented by occasional use of a nasal steroid spray such as beclometasone may be helpful. Allergy to housedust mite and housedust is increasingly recognized as a cause of rhinitis and allergic asthma. Treatment consists of cutting down the allergen in the bedroom by use of sprays or antiallergic sheeting. Non-sedating antihistamines and sometimes a short course of steroid sprays are also useful in combating this condition.

Non-allergic rhinitis (vasomotor rhinitis)

This presents as nasal blockage and catarrh and is differentiated from allergic rhinitis by negative allergy testing. Treatment is by antihistamine and decongestant combinations and occasionally by steroid sprays for 2 months. Where there is no response to medical treatment, surgical diathermy or laser reduction of the inferior turbinate can be carried out.

NASAL SEPTAL DEVIATION

This can be traumatic but is more commonly developmental. Slight deviation is common and causes no symptoms, but more severe deviation will cause nasal obstruction, sometimes on both sides, occasionally with external nasal deformity. There may be associated allergic or vasomotor rhinitis. Surgery is only indicated for significant nasal blockage and is usually performed only in older children as surgery in young children can cause deformity which increases with age.

DISEASES OF THE PARANASAL SINUSES

The paranasal sinuses (maxillary, ethmoid, frontal and sphenoid; Fig. 30.1) are all derived from the nasal cavity and are lined by respiratory epithelium. The maxillary sinuses are small at birth and do not attain significant size until 4 or 5 years of age. The ethmoid sinuses are well developed at birth, but the frontal sinuses do not develop until 9 or 10 years old. The sphenoid sinuses rarely cause symptoms in childhood.

There is slight inflammation of the sinus mucosa in all forms of rhinitis and when the ostium to the sinus gets blocked, secretions are retained and purulent sinusitis develops. Treatment with antibiotics and local decongestants opens up the ostium and allows the sinuses to drain.

MAXILLARY SINUSITIS

This is rare under the age of 6 and it usually follows influenza or parainfluenza. The nose becomes very congested, there is copious purulent catarrh and there may be associated headache and fever. The commonest organisms found are *Pneumococcus* and *Haemophilus influenzae*. Diagnosis is on suspicion and the finding of purulent catarrh in the nose and throat. Treatment is by ephedrine nosedrops, combined with a broad spectrum antibiotic such as amoxicillin or erythromycin for 1 week. X-rays are indicated when there is no response to the appropriate antibiotics, at which time surgical drainage may occasionally be required.

ETHMOIDITIS

This is a potentially serious condition which occurs in children from 3 years upwards. It usually follows an upper respiratory tract infection. The symptoms are of frontal headache and pain around the eye with fever and nasal blockage. Examination shows periorbital swelling and tenderness with marked inflammation. If there is abscess formation it is usually subperiosteal and this causes lateral displacement of the globe. The clinical diagnosis is now confirmed by a computerized tomography (CT) scan. Urgent treatment with parenteral broad spectrum antibiotic and ephedrine nose drops is required with surgical drainage if there is abscess formation.[5] If the condition is not treated or inadequately treated, extension of the infection can result in the serious complication of cavernous sinus thrombosis or intracranial abscess.[6]

Periorbital infection often arises from infection of the ethmoid or frontal sinuses and should be treated vigorously

---

FRONTAL SINUSITIS

This is less common than ethmoiditis and presents in children over 10. Like ethmoiditis, it is potentially serious with a risk of spread to involve the orbit or intracranial structures. It usually occurs after a cold or flu and causes severe frontal headache associated with inflammation and tenderness over the frontal sinus. Nasal symptoms are often minimal. Diagnosis and treatment are similar to that for ethmoiditis. Spread can occur inferiorly to involve the eye.

NASAL POLYPS

These present as unilateral or bilateral nasal blockage. Examination of the nose will show a pale, fleshy usually mobile structure. Most common is a unilateral antrochoanal polyp arising from the maxillary antra. These grow into the nose and down into the nasopharynx often causing total obstruction of one side with purulent catarrh. They are benign and treatment is removal.

Ethmoidal polyps are less common and cause nasal blockage and catarrh. Ethmoidal polyps occur in children with cystic fibrosis, when the histology is different from the usual 'allergic type'. Treatment is removal under general anesthetic.

CHOANAL ATRESIA

This rare anomaly is due to failure of breakdown of the nasobuccal membrane which normally occurs at 6 weeks' fetal development. The incidence is 1 in 8000 and unilateral atresia is commoner than bilateral. Of the cases, 50% are associated with the CHARGE syndrome – choanal atresia with ear, eye, heart and genital defects.

Gasping respiration in a neonate is suggestive of choanal atresia

Bilateral choanal atresia is a neonatal emergency. The nose breathing neonate may gasp and make significant respiratory efforts but becomes hypoxic and requires airway support. Some cases may mouth breathe, but then have difficulty when feeding. The diagnosis is by suspicion, by inability to pass a catheter along the nose and confirmation by endoscopic examination. The treatment consists of establishment of an airway either oral or orotracheal. A CT scan is carried out to determine the characteristics and extent of the atresia. Reviews using CT studies suggest that most atresias contain both bony and membranous components. Corrective endoscopic surgery is carried out as soon as is practicable.[7]

DISEASES OF THE NASOPHARYNX

ADENOIDS (NASOPHARYNGEAL TONSIL)

These are part of the Waldeyer's ring of lymphoid tissue which protects the upper airway. Adenoids are normally small at birth but enlarge from 18 months and regress normally at 8–9 years.

Adenoid hypertrophy

Since all children have adenoids, obstruction is a result of either a relatively small nasopharynx or large adenoids. Persistent enlargement causes snoring and often results in children having upper respiratory tract infections which last for 3–4 weeks instead of for 7–10 days. Such children usually mouth breathe and have hyponasal speech. There is an association between enlarged or infected adenoids and middle ear disease.

Adenoid hypertrophy is suspected with the above history and on the finding of a patent anterior nasal airway. Confirmation of adenoid size can be carried out by a lateral soft tissue X-ray of the neck (Fig. 30.2). In mild or intermittent cases, treatment is reassurance that the adenoids will go away. Surgery should be reserved for more persistent problems.

Adenoiditis

Adenoiditis occurs with viral infections and exacerbates nasal blockage. It can be quite severe in a small child with fever and purulent nasal discharge. A broad spectrum antibiotic for 5 days is indicated in severe cases.

Adenoidectomy

Removal of the adenoids is indicated for:

1. airway obstruction in a small child (see airway obstruction, tonsillitis);
2. severe persistent nasal obstruction;
3. recurrent acute otitis media;
4. otitis media with effusion.

A multicenter randomized controlled trial run by the MRC Institute of Hearing Research (TARGET – Trial of alternative regimes for glue ear treatment), which incorporates the effect of adenoidectomy on otitis media with effusion, is nearing completion and should provide evidence for or against adenoidectomy in this condition.

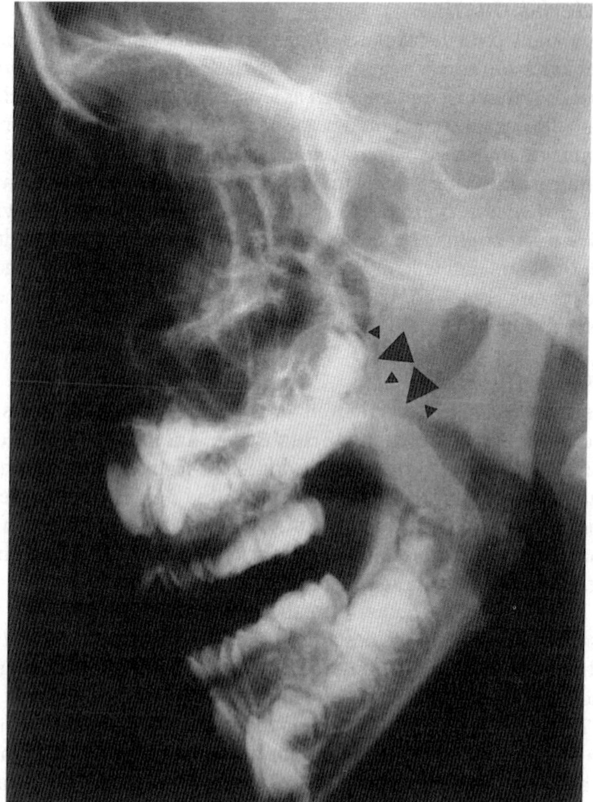

Fig. 30.2 Lateral soft tissue X-ray of a 4-year-old boy showing enlarged adenoids occluding the postnasal airway (arrowed).

Primary or secondary hemorrhage occurs in about 1 case in 200.

ANGIOFIBROMA

This is a benign tumor of the back of the nose and nasopharynx which presents in males in their early teens. Its symptoms are of nasal blockage with epistaxis. If expansion is rapid, cranial nerve compression can occur. The diagnosis is confirmed by endoscopy and a CT scan. Treatment is by surgery initially, radiotherapy being reserved for intracranial extension.

PHARYNGITIS

This is very common and usually of viral origin. It is a common presenting symptom of many upper respiratory tract infections, including the common cold, and may also precede the exanthemata of rubella or measles. There is generalized inflammation of the pharynx and often rhinitis. Treatment is supportive with antipyretics and analgesics as necessary.

TONSILS

The palatine tonsils, like the adenoids, are part of the body's defensive mechanism and serve to protect the upper airway from infection. Their removal, however, causes no subsequent immunological problems, nor is it associated with any deleterious long term effect.

Acute tonsillitis

This is commonest between the ages of 3 and 8, but can occur at any age. Of the cases, 50% are viral and 50% are bacterial with the beta-hemolytic streptococcus commonest, although *Staphylococcus aureus*, *Pneumococcus* and *H. influenzae* are also implicated.

The onset is abrupt, with pain in the throat, associated shivering and a pyrexia up to 39°C. The pain may be severe and radiate to the ears. Swallowing is acutely sore and solid food is refused, although fluids may be accepted. The disease progresses over 48 h, even with antibiotic therapy, and the swelling of the throat and the tonsils may give dysphagia for fluids and even for saliva which may dribble from the mouth. Speech may become thick and muffled and there is often painful enlargement of cervical glands.

On examination, the mucosa of the pillars of the fauces and soft palate are congested and as the disease progresses the tongue becomes coated and the breath become offensive. The tonsils are swollen and inflamed, with a purulent exudate. In severe cases, edema of the palate and the uvula may make the voice muffled and thick. Sometimes in streptococcal infections a scarlatiniform rash appears over the body.

Investigation

Throat cultures showing Group A beta-hemolytic streptococcus may confirm the diagnosis but a negative culture does not rule it out. There is also a high asymptomatic carrier rate of this streptococcus.[8] Throat swabs should not be carried out routinely in sore throats [Scottish Intercollegiate Guidelines Network (SIGN) guidelines].[9]

Rapid antigen testing, e.g. antistreptolysin O titer, although widely used and although showing a high specificity, shows a low sensitivity compared both with throat culture and clinical assessment.[10,11] Rapid antigen testing should therefore not be carried out routinely in sore throat (SIGN guidelines).

Differential diagnosis

1. *Infectious mononucleosis.* This occurs in older children and is often accompanied by marked lymphadenopathy in the neck and other areas. The child is miserable with throat discomfort due to generalized congestion of the throat and swelling of the tonsils. Serological confirmation can resolve doubt and treatment is supportive with analgesia and fluids.
2. *Viral pharyngitis.* In this condition, the child is less ill and has other symptoms, e.g. blocked-up nose.
3. *Herpangina.* This self-limiting condition due to Coxsackie virus has papular, vesicular and ulcerative lesions on the anterior pillars of the fauces, the palate and the tonsils.
4. *Moniliasis.* White patches are present on the tongue and on the tonsils and pharynx. This is usually associated with immunodeficiency but can occur after antibiotic therapy.

Treatment

In mild tonsillitis, analgesia, usually paracetamol, and adequate fluid intake is all that is required. It has been traditional in more severe cases to give penicillin V for 7–10 days. Erythromycin has been used where there is penicillin sensitivity. Amoxicillin or co-amoxiclav if given to a child with mononucleosis will result in an extensive skin rash. Parenteral penicillin may be required in persistent cases. The child should be encouraged to drink and eat a soft diet if possible. There is no clear evidence that the use of antibiotics in tonsillitis expedites symptomatic improvement, prevents rheumatic fever or glomerulonephritis or reduces the occurrence of suppurative complications, e.g. quinsy (SIGN guidelines).

There is no good evidence that antibiotics for tonsillitis alters the course or severity of the acute episode

Complications of tonsillitis

1. *Peritonsillitis.* Inflammation spreads outwith the tonsillar area and the child develops increasing pain and fever, often with significant swelling of the soft palate. Parenteral penicillin for 3–4 days can be changed to oral medication as the fever and pain subside.
2. *Peritonsillar abscess (quinsy).* When peritonsillitis localizes, an abscess can form. Although this condition is less common in children, it still presents as a serious and potentially lethal complication. It occurs during or just after an acute attack of tonsillitis presenting with increasing pain and swelling, usually on one side of the throat, with marked dysphagia and often otalgia. The child will have difficulty in opening his mouth. Examination can be difficult because of trismus but will show the affected tonsil to be very red, covered in pus and pushed medially. In addition, there will be gross swelling and redness of the palate and marked cervical lymphadenopathy on the ipsilateral side. If untreated, the abscess can spread to give rise to a parapharyngeal abscess with the risk of spread to the base of the skull or even into the superior mediastinum. The treatment is drainage under general anesthetic and can be a hazardous procedure. If it is not certain that pus is present, intravenous penicillin or erythromycin is given with fluids and analgesics.
3. *Airway obstruction.* This usually occurs in children aged 2–3 as a result of chronic hypertrophy of the adenoids and tonsils. The child breathes noisily at night and often during the day. Occasionally the parents will volunteer that the child stops breathing for short periods during the night and this can cause them some understandable alarm. At other times more direct questioning is required to elicit this symptom. If untreated, this relatively common complication of tonsillitis can lead to chronic hypoxia, pulmonary hypertension and, in severe cases, cor pulmonale. Where there is any suggestion of airway obstruction, the child should undergo a sleep study with monitoring of the oxygen saturation. If there are episodes of desaturation, indicative of sleep apnea, and there is no other cause for the airway obstruction, adenotonsillectomy usually cures the condition.[12] Such children should be admitted to the high dependency unit on the night of surgery and their breathing pattern should be monitored. In some more severe cases the respiratory drive is depressed and they may need oxygen until the respiratory drive returns to normal.
4. *Rheumatic fever and glomerulonephritis.* These are very rarely seen now as a complication of tonsillitis.

Indications for tonsillectomy

The following are indications for tonsillectomy (enlargement of the tonsils on their own is not an indication for their removal):

1. Airway obstruction is an absolute indication in small children with persistent noisy breathing and suspected or proven sleep apnea. The adenoids will also be removed.
2. Suspicion of other pathology, e.g. lymphoma, is also an absolute indication. There is usually a change in the architecture of the tonsil which would suggest lymphoma.
3. Two or more attacks of peritonsillar abscess.[13]
4. Recurrent acute tonsillitis. By this is meant five or six attacks of definite tonsillitis in 1 year. (SIGN guidelines). This number has been arrived at arbitrarily.[14] There has been no completely randomized trials of surgery versus conservative treatment.

Complications of tonsillectomy

A primary hemorrhage occurs within the first 24 h in 0.5–1.0% of children. Usually this is in the first 6 h after surgery and the child will start coughing up blood or, if unrecognized, may vomit a variable quantity of blood. After fluid replacement the child is returned to the operating room where the bleeding vessels are identified and controlled by diathermy or ligature. A secondary hemorrhage occurs after 7–10 days. Often the child's throat will have started to become sore again and he then becomes aware of blood coming into his mouth. These children should be admitted, crossmatched and intravenous access obtained. A broad spectrum antibiotic such as amoxicillin is administered and local treatment consisting of hydrogen peroxide gargles and, occasionally, local adrenaline swabs can be carried out. If the bleeding persists, return to theatre for ligature of the vessels or in rare cases packing of the tonsillar fossa.

DISORDERS OF PHONATION

DYSPHONIA

Dysphonia, or difficulty in producing sound, is usually associated with laryngeal disease (hoarseness). Some children have weakness or roughness of their voice in the course of an upper respiratory tract infection, this being a manifestation of laryngitis. Following recovery the voice usually returns to normal and no further investigation is required. Persistent hoarseness should be investigated and this can only be done by visualization of the larynx with a fiberoptic endoscope passed along the nose, into the nasopharynx. This can be done in the clinic where the child is cooperative but where this is not possible, examination under a general anesthetic is indicated to define the pathology.

The causes of hoarseness in children are as follows:

1. *Vocal nodules.* These occur at the junction between the anterior third and posterior two-thirds of the vocal cords. They are usually secondary to voice abuse and in loud and noisy children are known as 'screamers' node. Small nodules can improve with speech therapy or if the nodules grow, surgery involving microscopic dissection is indicated. Histology shows hypertrophic squamous epithelium with underlying edema of Reinke's space.
2. *Polyps of the larynx.* These occur spontaneously or following intubation and cause variable hoarseness. They are removed under general anesthetic.
3. *Laryngeal papillomas.* These are a rare cause of hoarseness associated with maternal genital warts (papilloma virus). They present as persistent hoarseness, sometimes with aphonia and occasionally airway obstruction. Treatment is by removal and multiple operations may be required. They do not become malignant but can spread into trachea and in rare cases, into bronchus.
4. *Unilateral vocal cord paralysis.* This can follow surgical or non-surgical trauma to the neck, or occur following viral infections including mononucleosis. The voice may be breathy if the cord is abducted or well maintained if the cord is medialized. The diagnosis is usually made on fiberoptic endoscopy, and treatment consists of speech therapy.

APHONIA

Complete loss of voice can occasionally occur with laryngeal pathology, e.g. papillomas, and in most cases the larynx should be visualized. Complete aphonia in an otherwise healthy child should be viewed with suspicion. Functional or 'hysterical' aphonia occurs after emotional or physical trauma, e.g. tonsillectomy. It usually affects older children and in most cases is self-correcting. Occasionally a laryngoscopy may have to be carried out to establish the diagnosis, but usually explanation of the problem together with counseling will suffice.

REFERENCES (* Level 1 evidence)

THE EAR

*1 Glasziou PP, DelMar CB, Sanders SL, Huyem M. Antibiotics for acute otitis media in children (Cochrane Review). In: The Cochrane Library, Issue 4. Oxford: Update Software; 2002.

*2 Kozyrskyj AL, Hildes-Ripstein GE, Longstaffe SEA, et al. Short course antibiotics for otitis media (Cochrane Review). In: The Cochrane Library, 1. Oxford: Update Software; 2001.

3 Maw AR, Parker AJ, Lance GN, et al. The effects of parental smoking on outcome after treatment for glue ear in children. Clin Otolaryngol 1992; 17:411–414.

*4 Butler CC, van der Voort JH. Oral or topical nasal steroids for hearing loss associated with otitis media with effusion in children (Cochrane Review). In: Cochrane Library, 1. Oxford: Update Software; 2001.

THE NOSE AND SINUSES

5 Arjmand EM, Lusk RP, Muntz HR. Acute sinusitis, children and the eye. Otolaryngol Head Neck Surg 1993; 109:886–894

6 Bluestone CD, Stool SE. Paediatric otolaryngology. WB Saunders; 1982:793–796.

7 Brown OE, Pownell P, Manning SC. Choanal atresia: a new anatomic classification and clinical management applications. Laryngoscope 1996; 106:97–101.

8 Feery BJ, Forsell P, Guylasekharam M. Streptococcal sore throat in general practice – a controlled study. Med J Aust 1976; 1:989–991.

*9 SIGN - Scottish Intercollegiate Guidelines Network. Management of sore throat and indications for tonsillectomy. SIGN publication 34; 1999.

10 Lewey S, White GB, Lieberman MM, et al. Evaluation of the throat culture as a follow up for an initially negative enzyme immunosorbent assay rapid streptococcal antigen detection test. Paediatr Infect Dis J 1988; 7:765–769.

11 Burke P, Bain J, Lowes A, et al. Rational decisions in managing sore throat: evaluation of a rapid test. BMJ 1988; 296:1646–1649.

12 Strading JR, Thomas G, Warley ARH, et al. Effect of adeno-tonsillectomy, on nocturnal hyponaemia, sleep disturbance and symptoms in snoring children. Lancet 1990; 335:249–253.

13 Wolf M, Euen-Chen I, Talmi YP, et al. Tonsillectomy following peritonsillar abscess. Int J Paediatr Otolaryngol 1995; 31:43–46.

*14 Paradise JL, Bluestone CD, Bachman RZ, et al. Efficacy of tonsillectomy for recurrent throat infection in severely affected children. Results of parallel randomised and non-randomised clinical trials. N Engl J Med 1984; 310:674–683.

31

Allergic disorders

Timothy J David, Peter D Arkwright

DEFINITIONS AND EXPLANATION OF TERMS

The widespread misuse of the word allergy causes confusion. It is essential to have a definition or explanation of terms.

ALLERGY

Allergy is a reproducible adverse reaction to an extrinsic substance mediated by an immunological response, irrespective of the precise mechanism. The substance provoking the reaction may have been ingested, injected, inhaled or may merely have come into contact with the skin or mucous membranes. The terms allergy and hypersensitivity have the same meaning and are interchangeable.

ATOPY

There is no good definition of atopy. The term was introduced to describe the 'asthma and hay fever group' of diseases. Subsequently atopy has been redefined as an hereditary predisposition to the production of IgE antibody, an unsatisfactory oversimplification. The atopic diseases comprise asthma, atopic eczema, allergic rhinitis, allergic conjunctivitis and some cases of urticaria. The association between food allergy and these atopic diseases is so strong that there is a case for considering food allergy as an atopic disease, although this usage has not yet been widely adopted.

ANAPHYLAXIS

The term anaphylaxis is usually reserved for an allergic reaction associated with severe, life-threatening circulatory and/or respiratory compromise.

FOOD INTOLERANCE

Food intolerance is a reproducible adverse reaction to a specific food or food ingredient, and it is not psychologically based. Food intolerance occurs even when the subject cannot identify the type of food which has been given. This definition does not take into account dosage. Clearly any food in vast excess will cause a reproducible adverse reaction. Such events are not generally covered by the term food intolerance.

IMMUNE MECHANISMS

Immune mechanisms determine the timing of allergic responses. Both humoral and cellular responses mediate allergic reactions to allergens.

HUMORAL IMMUNE MECHANISMS MEDIATING ALLERGIC REACTIONS

Acute type I hypersensitivity reactions (Gell and Coombs classification) result from allergen specific production of IgE antibodies by B lymphocytes. These IgE antibodies then stimulate the degranulation of mast cells in the dermis of the skin and the submucosa of the respiratory and gastrointestinal endothelium. A number of inflammatory mediators released from cytoplasmic granules (including histamine) cause the clinical features of the disease (acute allergic reactions). Fluid secretion results in the visible cutaneous urticaria and increased watery discharge characteristic of allergic rhinitis and conjunctivitis. Histamine also causes pruritus which results in rubbing and scratching. Other inflammatory mediators result in smooth muscle hyperactivity (bronchospasm, vomiting and diarrhea). These reactions characteristically occur within minutes of exposure to the allergen. Reactions with an onset hours after allergen exposure are in general not IgE mediated. The radioallergosorbent (RAST) and skin prick tests for diagnosis and antihistamines for treatment are only of value in acute reactions.

IgG autoantibodies directed at the FεR on mast cells have recently been found to cause chronic urticaria in some patients (idiopathic or intrinsic urticaria). The inflammatory mediators are the same as with type I hypersensitivity reactions and symptomatic treatment with antihistamines is often effective. In these cases specific triggers will not be found and the disease is more appropriately classified as autoimmune disease.

Unlike urticaria, angioedema is not thought to be mediated by histamine, but rather by other inflammatory effectors released from mast cells, especially kinins which have vasoactive properties. In urticaria the inflammatory edema is in the superficial dermal tissue, while in angioedema the swelling is mainly in the deeper subcutaneous layers. Kinin-mediated angioedema will not respond to antihistamines and may require treatment with other medicines including adrenaline (epinephrine) and glucocorticoids. Subcutaneous, respiratory and gastrointestinal tract angioedema is characteristic of hereditary angioedema, which is due to an inherited deficiency of C1 esterase inhibitor. It is solely mediated by kinins and is never associated with urticaria. Thus angioedema in combination with urticaria rules out hereditary angioedema.

CELLULAR IMMUNE MECHANISMS MEDIATING ALLERGIC REACTIONS

T lymphocyte hyperactivity associated with cytokine-mediated inflammatory changes in surrounding tissue and chemokine-initiated infiltration of tissue by auxiliary inflammatory cells, especially eosinophils, may also mediate allergic disease. These are typified by atopic dermatitis in the skin, asthma in the respiratory tract and cow's milk intolerance in the gastrointestinal system. The reactions come on more slowly over a number of hours or days rather than minutes. RAST and skin prick tests are unhelpful and often associated with false positive and negative reactions. These reactions are not mediated by histamine and therefore anti-histamines have no effect on the inflammatory process. In the case of atopic dermatitis and asthma, glucocorticoids which act by inhibiting cytokine release and other cellular immune responses are the treatment of choice. In cow's milk intolerance, avoidance of the allergen cures the disease.

T lymphocytes mediating either autoimmune or allergic diseases in transplant donors may be transferred to recipients during bone marrow or solid organ transplantation. Normal tolerance to allergens controlled by regulatory T cells in recipients may in some cases be inhibited by immunosuppressive agents such as tacrolimus. Thus it is that food intolerance can develop after transplantation, either through the transfer of donor lymphocytes within the transplanted organ from a food intolerant donor[1] or as a result of immunosuppression.[2]

A summary of the types of immune mechanism mediating allergic reactions and the clinical spectrum of diseases is given in Table 31.1. It should be noted that reversible airway obstruction (asthma) may be mediated by both humoral and cellular immune mechanisms. The pathogenesis and mechanisms of allergic disorders are reviewed in more detail elsewhere.[3–6]

TIMING OF THE ALLERGIC RESPONSE

When the airways, skin or conjunctivae are challenged by a single dose of allergen, a reaction can be classified as immediate, late, dual (that is both immediate and late), or delayed. The timing of these responses has been used to formulate hypotheses as to their immunopathogenesis (e.g. the Gell and Coombs types I to IV classification). However, these classifications mainly serve a didactic purpose, and may not relate to inflammation in disease. A single provocation with a large dose in the laboratory may differ greatly from the real life continuous or repeated exposure to smaller doses of allergens. In a study of patients with asthma who experienced only a late reaction after inhalation of low doses of allergen, the

Table 31.1 Clinical spectrum of allergic disease based and immune responses aimed at allergen avoidance and removal

Body interface		
Skin	Respiratory tract	Gastrointestinal tract
A. Diseases		
Urticaria (humoral) Atopic eczema (cellular)	Rhinoconjunctivitis (humoral) Asthma (humoral/cellular)	Food intolerance (humoral/cellular)
B. Protective responses against allergens		
Pruritus (rubbing/scratching) Hyperkeratosis (barrier)	Copious secretions Sneezing and coughing Bronchospasm (prevent/reduce further exposure)	Vomiting and diarrhea

inhalation of a higher allergen dose resulted in a dual reaction.[7] Most allergic reactions are not confined to a single Gell and Coombs type and usually involve a combination of mechanisms far more complex than such categorizations imply. A common error is to assume the presence of one type of reaction based on the timing of events. Thus immediate reactions (e.g. anaphylaxis) are often wrongly equated with a type I reaction. Another example is that most late bronchial reactions after allergen provocation are not type IV reactions, but inflammatory consequences of a type I reaction. The pathogenesis and mechanisms of allergic disorders are reviewed elsewhere.[3,4,6,8]

HYGIENE HYPOTHESIS

The prevalence of atopic diseases (atopic dermatitis, asthma and allergic rhinitis) has doubled over the last few generations.[9] These diseases are largely a problem of developed countries such as the United Kingdom, United States of America, Australasia and Canada. Within these countries, the affluent within these communities (social class I and II) are most commonly affected. Because this increase in prevalence has occurred over only a few generations, it must be due to environmental rather than genetic causes. The hygiene hypothesis is one possible explanation for these observed changes.[10] It suggests that the increase in allergic diseases has paralleled a reduction in morbidity and mortality from infectious diseases. Infectious triggers of the immune system may have previously promoted a generally non-atopic phenotype.

Evidence for this comes from two main sources. Firstly, a Japanese study of 867 children over the age of 12 years showed a clear negative relationship between delayed hypersensitivity responses to tuberculin and the presence of asthma.[11] Secondly, a number of studies performed in Switzerland, Austria and Germany have provided convincing evidence that growing up on a farm with regular contact with farm animals protects against allergic sensitization and the development of childhood allergic diseases.[12]

With reduced exposure to infectious agents, the immune system of predisposed individuals veers towards allergic responses. What is often less appreciated is that as well as a rise in allergic diseases, there has also been a noticeable increase, over the last few generations, in some autoimmune conditions, such as multiple sclerosis, Crohn's disease and insulin-dependent diabetes mellitus. Other autoimmune diseases have either shown little change in prevalence (ulcerative colitis) or a reduced prevalence (rheumatoid arthritis). Taken overall, modern society seems to be associated with a generalized increase in immune hypersensitivity, rather than just an increase in allergic disease. The exact mechanisms leading to this increase in immune hypersensitivity are still unclear.

Whatever the underlying mechanism leading to an increased immune hypersensitivity to both allergic diseases, some usually innocuous substances seem to be more potent in promoting allergic reactions than others. The next section reviews common allergens, most of which are protein antigens.

TYPES OF ALLERGEN[12a]

PLANTS

Plants are a cause of adverse reactions in the skin, but most reactions are not allergic. The major mechanisms of adverse reactions are allergic contact dermatitis (e.g. poison ivy, chrysanthemum, primula), irritant contact dermatitis (e.g. buttercup), pharmacological effects (e.g. stinging nettles), and phytophotodermatitis (e.g. giant hogweed).

Grass pollen

There are hundreds of species of grass, but a relatively small number account for most cases of pollen allergy. These are timothy grass, red top grass, blue grass, orchard grass, sweet vernal grass, meadow grass, Bermuda grass, rye grass and cocksfoot. With the exception of Bermuda grass, skin prick testing demonstrates extensive cross-reactivity between these grass species.[6] Pollen grains are only released during the day. Pollen counts are highest in the morning and early afternoon, and on hot, dry days. Wind can transport pollen many miles, and in cities the pollen count can remain high well into the evening. The timing of the peak pollen counts depends on the geographical location, the type of grass, and the weather conditions. In temperate regions in the northern hemisphere, a peak from mid-May to mid-July is usual.

Weed pollen

While grass pollens are the major trigger of allergic rhinitis and conjunctivitis in the UK, in North America the major cause are pollens of the various species of ragweed. Other weeds of importance in other places are mugwort, sagebrush, cocklebur, English plantain, Lamb's quarter, goosefoot, Russian thistle and burning bush. Peak levels of weed pollen occur in late summer and the autumn.

Tree pollen

Many deciduous trees produce pollen, usually in the spring. Birch pollen in Scandinavia, Japanese cedar pollen in Japan, and mountain cedar pollen in North America are all important causes of allergic rhinitis and conjunctivitis.

Fungal (mold) spores

Molds require a high relative humidity for growth, and reproduce by the production of spores. Yeasts are unicellular molds. Molds are ubiquitous. Exposure to molds is continuous rather than seasonal, and, as with house dust mites and in contrast to grass pollen, the extent to which a patient's symptoms can be attributed to mold allergy is often unclear. Occasionally the history may suggest mold allergy, e.g. symptoms occurring after being in a barn or raking leaves.

Outdoor molds

Cladosporium, *Alternaria*, *Fusarium*, smuts and rusts (and to a lesser degree *Aspergillus*, *Penicillium*, *Mucor*, *Didymella* and *Sporobolomyces*) are the most important outdoor causes of mold allergy.[13] The major sources of exposure are rotting leaves, straw, hay, grass, grain and flour. Wet weather favours mold growth. Some spores (e.g. some species of *Cladosporium* and *Alternaria*) are released in sunny and windy conditions, but others (e.g. *Fusarium*, *Phoma*, *Basidiomycetes*) are released by processes that require free water, and high levels of these particles occur with rainfall, dew, fog and the relatively damp conditions which prevail during darkness. Light intensity and duration can also affect spore production in certain molds, and in *Cladosporium* species, for example, a dark interval appears necessary to ensure the formation of a single spore crop in each 24-h period. Thus circadian trends in humidity, temperature, air speed and light interact to produce a diurnal and nocturnal pattern of spore distribution. In addition, the type of vegetation affects the local air spora. Temperate grasslands and grain-growing areas are particular sources of the spores of *Alternaria* and *Cladosporium*. Forests abound with wood-rotting molds, and large orchards can raise levels of airborne yeasts.

Indoor molds

Aspergillus and *Penicillium* are the two molds most commonly cultured from houses, especially from basements, inaccessible crannies and bedding.[13] These molds are often called storage fungi because they are common causes of rot in stored grain, fruits and vegetables. In contrast to most molds which require a relatively high moisture content (22–25%) in their substrate, *Aspergillus* can thrive on substrates with a lower moisture content (12–16%). *Penicillium* is the green mildew seen on articles stored in basements. Roquefort, Stilton and other blue cheeses owe their sharp aroma to veins of the bluish-green mold *Penicillium roquefortii* and Camembert and Brie are ripened from the outside by a coat of white *Penicillium camemberti* mold. The major sources of exposure to indoor molds are damp cellars, poorly ventilated bathrooms, wallpaper on cold walls, window frames (condensation), artificial humidifiers, damp textile materials, and stored food.

Latex

Natural latex is produced by nearly 2000 species of plants. Although attempts have been made to extract latex from different plant species, so far only the rubber tree *Hevea brasiliensis* is commercially valuable as a source of natural rubber. Whether natural rubber latex collected from the rubber trees of Malaysia is different from that collected in Thailand or elsewhere is not known. The total protein content in natural rubber latex varies between 1 and 2%, and it is these proteins or peptides that are responsible for allergic reactions to latex. Allergy to latex rubber is unusual in that it commonly involves sensitization to multiple constituent proteins. Different groups of patients appear to be sensitized to different groups of latex proteins.[14] The major rubber proteins are hevamines (proteins with chitinase and lysozyme properties), and hevein, a fungotoxic protein with considerable structural homology with wheat germ agglutinin and other plant lectins.

ANIMALS

Mammalian pets

The sources of allergens are dander (epidermal scales), hair, feathers, saliva and urine.

HOUSE DUST

House dust mites

The predominant house dust mite in Europe is *Dermatophagoides pteronyssinus*, but in the USA the dominant species is *Dermatophagoides farinae*. These mites feed from desquamated human skin scales, which are mainly shed in the bed and bedroom. The amount of skin shed by one person in a day provides enough food to supply thousands of mites for months, and the decisive factors which influence the number of mites are air humidity and temperature. The optimum conditions for mites are 70–80% relative humidity and an ambient temperature of 26°C. Mites cannot reproduce when the relative humidity falls below 60%, and cannot survive for more than a few days in a relative humidity of below 40% if the temperatures is above 25°C. The lack of mites at higher altitudes (e.g. alpine resorts) is due to the lower relative humidity. The mite antigen is predominantly found in mite fecal pellets which are of a similar size to pollen grains. It appears that the majority of house dust mite allergens are enzymes involved in digestion which become entrapped within the fecal pellet. Mites are found in bedding, mattresses, carpets, cuddly toys and upholstered furniture. They are also found in carpets and upholstered furniture in other parts of the house. Moisture from human skin causes particularly humid conditions in beds and bedding which creates favourable conditions for mite survival. The relationship between the season and mite density in houses is attributable to seasonal changes in the ambient indoor humidity. In temperate areas, the number of mites is lowest in the winter, when central heating dries the indoor air.

Storage mites

The most important species are *Glycophagus*, *Tyrophagus*, *Lepidoglyphus* and *Acarus*. They do not cross-react with the *Dermatophagoides* species. Storage mites are common in farm stores (e.g. stored hay), granaries, warehouses and places where food is stored. They are infrequent in houses unless the same room is used for cooking, eating and sleeping, as can happen with dwellings in the tropics.

INSECTS

Stinging insects

The medically important Hymenoptera are bees, wasps, hornets, yellow jackets, fire ants and harvester ants.[6] Hymenoptera venoms are complex mixtures of enzymes, peptides and other vasoactive substances. Thus reactions to insect stings can be immunological, pharmacological, or both.

Biting insects

Allergy to the salivary secretions of biting insects is common. Local immediate and delayed allergic reactions to bites from fleas (papular urticaria), mosquitoes, sandflies, deerflies and horseflies are common.

Inhalant allergens from insects

Inhalant allergies to moths, butterflies, bees and beetles have all been described in those exposed to them as a result of a hobby.

FOODS

Foods as allergens are discussed in the section on food intolerance.

INHERITED PREDISPOSITION

Atopy is by definition the genetic predisposition to develop allergic reactions to otherwise innocuous substances. Twin studies suggest that the genetic component accounts for approximately 80% of the predisposition to atopic dermatitis, asthma and allergic rhinoconjunctivitis. It also accounts for about 82% of the predisposition to peanut allergy. Many other allergies (other food allergies, latex allergy, etc.) are associated with the asthma–hay fever group of atopic disease and thus are likely to have a similar genetic predisposition. The risk of atopic disease in the general community is approximately 10%, but this increases to 50% if one parent is affected and up to 75% if both parents are affected.

Although numerous candidate genes have been implicated in the development of atopy, including major histocompatibility genes (HLA-D), genes coding for cytokines which are overexpressed in allergic diseases (IL-4 cytokine gene cluster), genes involved in IgE mediated responses (FcεRI-α) and response to hormones (α-adrenergic receptor), evidence linking any one of these genes as a major cause of clinical atopy is lacking and the search for alternatives continues.

CLINICAL SPECTRUM OF DISEASE

Clinical features of allergic disease occur mainly at the three major interfaces between the body and its environment: the skin, upper and lower respiratory tract and gastrointestinal system. This subdivision, although paralleling the types of pediatric specialists to whom such patients will be referred (namely dermatologists, respiratory physicians and gastroenterologists), is artificial. Moreover in some ways it may be unhelpful to characterize allergic diseases in this way. For instance, acute allergic reactions to ingested food may manifest not only as vomiting and diarrhea, but in some cases solely as cutaneous urticaria and in others as acute pharyngeal angioedema or bronchospasm or in yet other cases with clinical features related to all three systems. Allergic disease is primarily a systemic illness with many overlapping features. Only by understanding the underlying immune mechanisms of the presenting clinical problem can a logical approach to investigations and treatment strategies be devised.

SKIN

Urticaria

Acute urticaria

Acute urticaria is the result of a variety of causes (often not identified) and mechanisms. The proportion of cases in which a cause is found varies; in childhood the most common is a viral infection. Urticaria may develop during an illness or within 1–2 weeks after the illness, and remain a problem for a few days or weeks. Immediate allergic reactions to foods are the other major cause of acute urticaria. A parent notices, for example, that whenever a child eats fish his lips swell and he develops an urticarial rash. Fish is avoided, and the problem disappears. Occasional lapses of avoidance either demonstrate continued intolerance or, with time, loss of symptoms. Cases which come to medical attention are mostly severe (e.g. associated with laryngeal edema), atypical, or associated with other disorders notably atopic eczema. The common foods incriminated (egg, cow's milk, fish, nuts, tomatoes and fruit) are similar to those which cause allergic contact urticaria (see below), the difference being that children are in general more likely to touch raw foods than to eat them, and raw foods are on the whole more likely to trigger urticaria than cooked foods.

Allergic contact urticaria

This is an immediate allergic reaction, and should not be confused with contact dermatitis which represents a delayed reaction. Although certain foods, such as raw egg, cow's milk, raw potatoes, raw fish, apples and nuts are particularly common causes, any food containing protein could in theory cause allergic contact urticaria. In addition to erythema and urticarial wheals, where the food is taken by mouth the symptoms often include itching or tingling of the lips. The tissues and secretions of pet mammals are also common causes of allergic contact urticaria in childhood. Other causes are chemicals, a number of drugs applied topically, and a few vehicles contained in topical medicaments.[15]

Irritant contact urticaria

Common causes are plants such as stinging nettles or creatures such as jellyfish, moths and caterpillars. Chemicals are a major cause of irritant contact urticaria, and the relevant chemicals are widely used in food, medicines and cosmetics.

Chronic urticaria

Chronic urticaria is rarely allergen-IgE mediated. In over 70% of cases no cause can be found. Screening laboratory tests are of no value unless indicated by the history and examination. Recently, there has been some evidence to suggest that a significant percentage of adults have an autoimmune basis, with IgG autoantibodies being found to FcεR on mast cells. In 25% of these cases (especially adult females) thyroid autoantibodies have been found and 10% of cases have abnormal thyroid function tests. The prevalence of autoimmune urticaria in children is presently unclear.

In the majority of cases of chronic (i.e. lasting more than 2 months) urticaria, no cause is found and the disorder spontaneously improves over a period of 6–12 months. Most studies implicating food additives are seriously flawed,[16] but genuine cases of additive-provoked urticaria do exist, and this has been documented under double-blind placebo-controlled conditions for sodium benzoate, tartrazine, sunset yellow, amaranth, indigo carmine, monosodium glutamate and sodium metabisulfite.[17] Aspirin has also been shown to provoke urticaria.[17] In persistent and troublesome urticaria it is worth performing a trial of complete food additive avoidance for an arbitrary period of 4 weeks. If the urticaria disappears then it is simple to perform challenges with individual additives.[17]

If urticaria persists in one place for over 48 h, leaves residue (e.g. hyperpigmentation), is associated with purpura or systemic manifestations (arthritis, fever, etc.) one should consider an underlying vasculitis (urticarial vasculitis). Skin manifestations are typically recurrent episodes of urticaria-like wheals, often associated with arthralgia (50%) and angioedema (40%). In addition to the skin, the respiratory (20%), renal (5–10%) and gastrointestinal (20%) systems are most frequently involved in the disease, which is probably an immune complex mediated process. Urticarial vasculitis is most commonly an acquired idiopathic phenomenon but may occur in association with other disorders, most often systemic lupus erythromatosus (SLE), Sjögren's syndrome and serum sickness. As with other autoimmune diseases, 60–80% of patients are female. Investigations should include a skin biopsy with immunofluorescent staining for immunoglobulin deposits. The most common laboratory abnormalities reported are an elevated ESR, hypocomplementemia and circulating immune complexes. Measurement of serum complement is useful prognostically, as hypocomplementemia is associated with more serious systemic involvement. There is no universally effective therapy for urticarial vasculitis, but commencing treatment with antihistamines and proceeding through non-steroidal anti-inflammatory drugs (NSAIDs), to colchicine, dapsone or hydroxychloroquine. If these medications do not achieve control, systemic steroids and azathioprine can be tried.

The causes of urticaria and angioedema (see below) are listed in Table 31.2.

ANGIOEDEMA

Unlike urticaria, where the inflammatory edema is in the superficial dermis, in angioedema the swelling is mainly in the deeper subcutaneous and submucosal layers. Angioedema is usually painful rather than pruritic and commonly affects the face and extremities. In the upper respiratory tract it is associated with swelling of the lips, tongue, and pharyngeal tissues which may lead to life-threatening upper airway obstruction. Angioedema of the gastrointestinal tract usually manifests as abdominal pain. The major mediators of angioedema are plasma kinins (e.g. bradykinin), the activation of which is inhibited by C1 inhibitor and other protease inhibitors. Angioedema is associated with urticaria in 80% of cases; in the remaining 20% of cases angioedema occurs without any urticaria.

HEREDITARY ANGIOEDEMA

The most important differential diagnosis of allergy-induced angioedema is hereditary angioedema, because the prognosis and management of this condition is different. In the past, the mortality rate for attacks involving the upper airways exceeded 25%.

Table 31.2 Classification of urticaria and angioedema

Urticaria
1. Local irritants: plants, jellyfish, chemicals
2. Direct mast cell activation: opiates, antibiotics, curare, contrast media
3. Agents altering arachidonic acid metabolism: aspirin/NSAIDS, benzoates
3. IgE mediated: allergen mediated (pollens, dander, foods, worms, molds, Hymenoptera venom, drugs) physical (cold: consider cryoglobulinemia, solar: consider SLE and porphyria, exercise, cholinergic, vibration)
4. IgG mediated: viral infections, autoimmune (associated with other autoimmune diseases, especially thyroid disease), urticarial vasculitis
5. Idiopathic
Angioedema
1. Complement inhibitor deficiency: hereditary angioedema
2. Complement activation vasculitis, infections, serum sickness
3. Angiotensin converting enzyme inhibitors

Subcutaneous, respiratory and gastrointestinal tract angioedema characteristic of hereditary angioedema is due to an autosomal dominantly inherited deficiency of C1 esterase inhibitor. Swelling of the gastrointestinal mucosa results in nausea, vomiting, diarrhea and severe pain that can mimic a surgical emergency. The subcutaneous swellings are disfiguring but not erythematous, pruritic or painful. The angioedema is solely mediated by kinins and never associated with urticaria. That is why angioedema in combination with urticaria rules out a diagnosis of hereditary angioedema. Interestingly the pulmonary vascular tree is spared, probably because the cells lining the pulmonary vessels have surface enzymes that inactivate bradykinin and other kinins. Symptoms can last from 1 to 4 days and most patients have one or more attacks per month.

The diagnosis of hereditary angioedema should be considered if (1) angioedema occurs without urticaria; (2) atypical pattern of angioedema (hands, feet, abdomen rather than face); (3) family history (but 20% are sporadic); (4) abdominal symptoms. There are two types of disease: type 1 (85% of cases) due to absent C1 inhibitor and type 2 (15% of cases) where there are normal or elevated levels of C1 inhibitor antigen, but the protein is dysfunctional.

Investigations in suspected cases should include measurement of CH50, C1 inhibitor levels and function and C4.

Unlike allergen-mediated urticaria and angioedema, antihistamines, adrenaline (epinephrine) and steroids are of little or no use in the treatment of hereditary angioedema. C1 esterase inhibitor concentrate which should be available in all casualty departments is the treatment of choice for laryngeal edema and severe abdominal attacks. If the concentrate is not available fresh frozen plasma may be used. Danazol can be used as prophylaxis in postpubertal children and non-pregnant adults. In younger children the plasmin inhibitor tranexamic acid is an alternative. Angiotensin converting enzyme (kininase II) inhibitors may precipitate attacks by blocking bradykinin degradation.

ALLERGIC ASPECTS OF ATOPIC ECZEMA

We do not know what proportion of children with atopic eczema will benefit from antigen avoidance regimens. All advice in this area is empirical.

The management (see also Ch. 28) can be divided into first line approaches (e.g. use of emollients and topical steroids,[18] recognition and treatment of bacterial and viral skin infection,[19,20] use of sedating H_1 antihistamines at night), and if these are unsuccessful, possibly some form of antigen avoidance regimen.

The situations in which antigen avoidance should be considered are:

1. **Severe disease.** Exclusion diets are highly disruptive to family life, and are potentially nutritionally hazardous,[16] so it makes little sense to employ a diet when the condition is mild (under 10% of the skin surface area affected) and easily controlled with simple topical therapy. Such diets may be appropriate if 25% or more of the skin is affected.
2. **History.** A history of immediate urticarial or gastrointestinal reactions to foods is common. It is unproven whether the regular administration of a food which after a single exposure causes urticaria leads to the worsening of atopic eczema, but it seems reasonable to avoid foods for which there is a clear history of an immediate allergic reaction.
3. **Multiple atopic disorders in infancy.** The occurrence of more than one atopic disorder appears to increase the possibility of an important allergic element. This is especially true if atopic features such as eczema, asthma or rhinitis are accompanied by gastrointestinal symptoms such as persistent loose stools or vomiting.
4. **Age.** Elimination diets are simpler to administer and control in infancy and results are better at this age.
5. **Severe eczema in exclusively breast-fed infants.** In one study, in 6 of 37 breast-fed infants eczema improved when the mother avoided cow's milk protein and egg and relapsed when these were reintroduced.[21] It was impossible to predict which baby would respond to maternal dietary exclusion, and it is reasonable to try maternal avoidance of cow's milk and egg in an infant with eczema who is being exclusively breast-fed. Other foods can provoke eczema in this way, but their detection depends on parental suspicion followed by avoidance and challenge.

ANTIGEN AVOIDANCE IN ATOPIC ECZEMA

Diets

The important principles underlying any elimination diet are:

1. The diet should in the first instance be tried for a defined period of time (e.g. 6 weeks in patients with eczema) and not just imposed indefinitely.
2. At the end of this period the patient should be reassessed to see if the diet has been helpful. If it has not, then the diet should be discontinued. If the diet has helped, and the parents and doctor feel that the therapeutic benefit outweighs the inconvenience of the diet, then the items omitted should be reintroduced one by one (in eczema at the rate of about one new food every 5–7 days).
3. The help of a dietitian is important, to ensure that specific food items have been properly excluded from the diet, and to ensure the nutritional adequacy of the diet.[22–24]

There are four varieties of dietary exclusion. All are empirical, and the details of which items are excluded may vary. Infants and toddlers are far more likely to benefit than teenagers.

Half-hearted attempts to 'have a go'

The very small quantity of food which can provoke an adverse reaction means that the 'try cutting down his milk' type of tinkering with the diet is most unlikely to succeed. The advantage of a carefully conducted diet is that even if it fails, at least the parents will be satisfied in the knowledge that it was tried properly.

Complete avoidance of known triggers

A trial of rigorous avoidance of known or suspected triggers is a logical first step. It is common to see a child with a clear history of intolerance to a food, but where the food is being incompletely avoided. An example would be a child with a history suggesting cow's milk protein intolerance who is avoiding cow's milk but consuming products which contain whey or casein, or who is receiving goat's milk.

Cow's milk and egg avoidance

The main place for this diet is in infancy. The chances of a useful clinical benefit are small.

Avoidance of 10 common food triggers

The patient avoids approximately 10 common food triggers, plus foods for which there is a history of intolerance. The foods usually chosen for exclusion are cow's milk, egg, wheat, fish, legumes (pea, bean, soya, lentil), tomato, nuts, berries and currants, citrus fruit and food additives (for a discussion of these see separate section below). The chances of a useful clinical benefit are small.

The few-foods diet (oligoantigenic diet)

This consists of exclusion of all foods except for five or six items. These items should not include a food for which there is a history of intolerance. Such diets comprise a meat (usually lamb or turkey), three vegetables (e.g. potato, rice, and carrot or a brassica – cauliflower, cabbage, broccoli or sprouts), a fruit (usually pear) and possibly a breakfast cereal (e.g. Rice Krispies). There are scanty data on the outcome of few-foods diets. In one study, a few-foods diet was associated with marked improvement in 50% of patients (median age 2.9 years, range 0.4–14.8) with atopic eczema, but after 12 months' follow-up, the results were the same (marked improvement) in the group that improved, the group that failed to improve, and the group that tried a diet but were unable to cope.[25] In another study, 85 children (median age 2.3 years, range 0.3–13.3 years) with atopic eczema were randomly allocated to receive a few-foods diet supplemented with either a whey hydrolysate or a casein hydrolysate formula, or to remain on their usual diet and act as controls, for a 6-week period.[26] After 6 weeks, there was a significant reduction in all three groups in the percentage of surface area involved and skin severity score. Sixteen (73%) of the 22 controls and 15 (58%) of the 24 who received the diet showed a greater than 20% improvement in the skin severity score. This is the only controlled study of a few-foods diet, and it failed to show benefit. However, the drawback to these two studies is the relatively high median age and the wide age range, which is important because it is general experience that the best results for elimination diets are in infants. Given the tendency for most children with food hypersensitivity to grow out of the problem by the age of 3 years, the inclusion of substantial numbers of older children in these studies biased the results against finding benefit from a diet.

Elemental diet

The application of an inpatient regimen of 4–6 weeks of a so-called elemental diet (e.g. Elemental 028, Vivonex or Tolerex) is the ultimate test of whether food intolerance is relevant or not, but until more data are available this approach must be regarded as experimental.[27] The drawbacks comprise the lack of a guarantee of success, family disruption associated with 2–3 months' hospitalization, loose stools (due to hyperosmolarity of the formula), weight loss and hypoalbuminemia.

House dust mite and pet avoidance

House dust mites and pets are of major importance as triggers in atopic eczema, and it is increasingly recognized that an important reason for a lack of therapeutic response to an elimination diet is failure to avoid them. However, the number of patients who experience benefit solely from the avoidance of pets or mites appears to be small. As with elimination diets, there is no test which predicts benefit from avoidance measures. Some patients with atopic eczema are worse during the pollen season or after grass has been cut, but avoidance is impossible.

ALLERGIC ASPECTS OF ASTHMA

There is no doubt that exposure to various triggers can provoke or worsen asthma in certain patients. However, there is a lack of objective investigations to establish the qualitative importance of allergy. For example, it is impossible to state, for asthmatic children of any specific age, in what proportion exposure to an animal provokes an attack of asthma, or what proportion will benefit from removal of a household pet. The management of the allergic aspects of asthma is largely empirical. Some triggers are allergens, but others are not, so it is misleading to think of asthma solely as an allergic disease. Some triggers, in addition to causing airway smooth muscle contraction, also cause an increase in the non-specific responsiveness of the airway smooth muscle. Non-allergic triggers are discussed in Chapter 18.

Importance of allergic triggers in asthma

It is unknown whether the complete avoidance of all potential triggers, were this possible (which it plainly is not), would abolish asthma or merely cause improvement. The disappearance of asthma following the removal of household pets and their antigenic traces (exceedingly difficult to achieve) is a poorly documented but occasionally striking phenomenon. Observations of children with unusually severe asthma who are sent to alpine resorts, where the exposure to house dust mites and pets is greatly reduced or abolished, are that somewhere between one- and two-thirds become completely asymptomatic and can discontinue all therapy. Return home is followed by relapse in most patients. In the past it was believed that this improvement was due to separation from parents and 'family tension', but the current doctrine is that the benefit is due to the avoidance of inhaled allergens. A history may help identify intermittent triggers which provoke attacks, but may not identify allergens to which the patient is regularly exposed and which are responsible for maintaining the asthmatic state (e.g. house dust mites).

Investigations

Skin tests, RAST tests and provocation tests (see above) are unhelpful. A trial of specific allergen avoidance is the only logical approach.

Trigger avoidance

It is impossible to avoid cold weather, exercise, laughing and crying. Viral infections, pollens and fungal spores are ubiquitous, and total avoidance is impossible without unacceptable restrictions.

Home interventions for dust mite avoidance have three goals: to reduce live mite populations, to reduce mite allergen levels, and to reduce human exposure to both. The general principles of reducing house dust mites[28] are as follows:

Reducing indoor relative humidity

Dust mites maintain their water balance primarily by absorbing water from the air. Maintaining relative humidity below 50%, using high-efficiency dehumidifiers and air conditioning in high humidity climates, is recommended because ambient relative humidity is a key factor that influences dust mite prevalence. Depending upon the temperature, mites die of dehydration in 5–11 days when continuously exposed to a relative humidity of 40–50%.

Using encasements

Encasing mattresses and pillows in specially manufactured protective coverings is effective in reducing exposure to dust mites and their allergens. Encasements may be made from plastic, vapour permeable materials, finely woven fabrics, or non-woven synthetics.

Washing, drying, and dry cleaning of bedding materials

Washing sheets, pillow cases, blankets and bed quilts at least weekly in hot water (55°C or higher) kills mites and removes most allergens. Adding benzyl benzoate (0.03%) to the wash cycle also kills mites, as does tumble drying items if a temperature above 55°C is maintained for 10 min. Dry cleaning kills mites but does not destroy all allergens.

Replacing carpets, draperies and upholstery

By collecting detritus and holding moisture, these furnishings provide an ideal habitat for mite breeding. In humid climates it makes sense to replace carpets by hard surfaces, fabric upholstery can be replaced by vinyl or leather covering, and curtains can be replaced by blinds or shades.

Vacuuming carpets

Where carpet cannot be removed, vacuuming carpets at least weekly using vacuum bags with two layers or a high-efficiency particulate air filter is recommended. Regular vacuum cleaning removes surface mites and allergens but not deeply embedded allergens, and it does not reduce the number of live mites. Steam cleaning usually does not penetrate deep enough and by leaving residual water may actually promote mite population.

Freezing soft toys and small items

Freezing (–17°C to –20°C) soft toys and small items such as pillows for at least 24 h kills mite populations. These items then need washing to remove dead mites and allergens.

Air cleaning and air filtration

In undisturbed spaces these methods, which are not recommended, capture little mite allergen, because mite allergens are usually associated with particles that may become airborne but settle quickly.

Chemicals

Experiments have been conducted with a variety of acaricides such as benzyl benzoate, sumethrin, permethrin, disodium octaborate tertahydrate and tannic acid. Controlled studies have given mixed results; some show a reduction in mite allergen concentration and others show insufficient reduction.

Since a large proportion of a child's life is spent in the bedroom, measures to reduce exposure to house dust mites must be focused on the bedroom, but it is unclear whether the implicit assumption that mites in other parts of the house are less important is true. Near complete avoidance of dust mites is theoretically possible in the bedroom but entails expense and an obsessional attention to detail:

1. Place the mattress and pillow in a plastic bag or vapour-permeable cover and seal.
2. Replace a divan bed base (which cannot be completely sealed in a cover) by a non-upholstered wooden or metal base.
3. Remove woolen blankets, eiderdowns, quilts and duvets, even if made of synthetic materials, and replace with cotton or acrylic blankets which are hot washed (at least 130°F, 55°C) weekly.
4. If there is more than one bed in the bedroom, then the above precautions must be applied to all beds.
5. Remove floor carpet, and replace with flooring which can be wet mopped.
6. Remove upholstered furniture, teddy bears and similar furry creatures to another room.
7. Remove toys and clothing, other than items kept enclosed in a cupboard, to another room.
8. Remove all items on horizontal surfaces such as bedside tables, book shelves, window sills, tops of cupboards, so that these areas can be damp dusted daily.
9. Retain curtains, to be washed every 3 months. Do not replace with venetian blinds, which are more likely to accumulate dust.
10. Remove mobiles and lamp shades which cannot be wiped free of dust.

Measures for the rest of the house are lower priority. Ideally, the whole house is changed to minimize the sites in which mites can grow. This requires removal of all carpeting and replacement by polished flooring, removal of all upholstered furniture, and ensuring that all window blinds are washable.

Many parents and doctors would regard such measures as unacceptably restrictive, and such an extreme approach can only be justified in unusual cases where either there is a clear history that house dust mites play an important part or where conventional drug therapy has failed to control severe disease.

Avoidance of pets and pet antigens is theoretically possible but often unpopular or unacceptable to the family. Removal of the animal itself is insufficient, and if the level of pet antigen in the household is to be adequately reduced then also required are intensive carpet and furniture cleaning. Complete removal of cat antigen is especially difficult (if not impossible), and because of its adhesion to wall surfaces[29] requires washing of the walls.

Role of antigen avoidance in management of asthma

There are no objective data upon which to base clear recommendations, with the result that there are differences of opinion about the relevance of antigen avoidance. The cornerstone of the treatment of asthma is drug therapy, supplemented where possible or relevant by the avoidance of triggers. Even with the most enthusiastic approach to the identification and avoidance of triggers, it is rare for this alone to abolish symptoms. The major triggers which are at least potentially avoidable are house dust mites and pets. Since there is no clinical or laboratory test which can accurately identify those patients who will benefit from antigen avoidance, the only logical approach is to attempt a defined trial period of avoidance, including an assessment after an agreed period of time (e.g. 3 months) as to whether there has been any benefit.

HAY FEVER (SEASONAL ALLERGIC RHINITIS)

The incidence and peak months of hay fever depend upon the proportion of the population who are atopic and the type of pollen (e.g. grass, birch tree, ragweed, mugwort) which is prevalent.[30]

The severity of the symptoms varies with the daily pollen count. The symptoms are multiple consecutive sneezes, rhinorrhea, nasal blockage, itching of the eyes, itching of the soft palate and referred itching in the ears [attributed to the common innervation (the glossopharyngeal nerve) of the ear and the pharyngeal mucosa]. Asthmatic symptoms sometimes coexist with attacks of hay fever.

The diagnosis is based on the occurrence of the above symptoms each year during the pollen season. No investigations are required. Avoidance of pollen is impossible outdoors, and staying indoors during good weather is unjustifiable in view of the safe and effective therapy which is available. Non-sedating H_1 antihistamines are by far the simplest treatment for mild cases, given either at the onset of attacks or regularly during the pollen season. An advantage of H_1 antihistamines is that they also help eye symptoms, but they are less effective for nasal symptoms than prophylactic topical steroids. Prophylactic treatment, which is required for the more troublesome cases, comprises:

1. Sodium cromoglycate: for greatest benefit this needs to be applied to the nasal mucosa at least four times a day. It is much less effective than steroids. The main use is as eye drops, given 6-hourly.
2. Inhaled steroids: fluticasone (once daily), beclometasone or budesonide (twice daily) are highly effective in most cases. A combination of steroids and non-sedating H_1 antihistamines is of greater benefit than steroids alone, and is logical in troublesome cases.
3. Oral decongestants (e.g. pseudoephedrine) cause central nervous system stimulation, or drowsiness if combined with a sedating H_1 antihistamine, and are not very effective. Topical vasoconstrictors are unsatisfactory except for short-term use (e.g. air travel).
4. The short-term advantage of systemic steroids (short course of oral prednisolone or depot injection of a microcrystalline ester such as methylprednisolone acetate) may be offset by the small risk of fatal chickenpox resulting from temporary immunosuppression.[31–33]

PERENNIAL RHINITIS

Perennial rhinitis can be classified[30] as:

1. **Perennial rhinitis (known allergic trigger).** This accounts for most children with perennial rhinitis. If the patient has been exposed to the causative allergen in the last few days, then eosinophilia will be seen in a nasal smear in 80% of patients. Prophylactic topical sodium cromoglycate or steroids are effective. The important triggers are house dust mites or pets.
2. **Perennial rhinitis (no identifiable allergic trigger, but nasal eosinophilia present).** The cause is unknown, but the condition can sometimes be provoked by non-allergic mechanisms, e.g. alcoholic beverages. Prophylactic topical steroids are effective.
3. **Perennial rhinitis (no identifiable allergic trigger, and no nasal eosinophilia).** This mainly affects adults, and the etiology is unknown. The anticholinergic effect of sedating H_1 antihistamines (e.g. triprolidine) may be helpful.

ALLERGIC CONJUNCTIVITIS

Allergic conjunctivitis can be seasonal or perennial. The major symptom is itching. Rubbing gives immediate but only short-lasting relief, and this is followed by more itching and worsening inflammation of the conjunctivae. Sometimes this leads to a sensation that there is a foreign body present. In seasonal allergic conjunctivitis, allergen (pollen) avoidance is impossible. In perennial conjunctivitis, the identification and avoidance of allergens (e.g. house dust mites, pet animals) is as empirical as it is in asthma. The management of allergic conjunctivitis is mainly pharmacological.

Symptomatic treatment

For immediate relief it is helpful to apply a crushed ice compress. This can be accompanied by either topical application of H_1 antihistamine with vasoconstrictor eye drops (xylometazoline and antazoline eye drops give effective symptomatic relief but cause quite marked transient stinging), or oral quick-acting, non-sedating H_1 antihistamines (e.g. loratadine).

Prophylactic treatment

This consists of either regular administration of oral H_1 antihistamines or 6-hourly sodium cromoglycate eye drops. Topical steroids should only be used under the supervision of an ophthalmologist, for there is a danger of enhancement of herpes simplex corneal infection and a risk of producing glaucoma.

VERNAL KERATOCONJUNCTIVITIS

This is a rare, severe chronic inflammation of the conjunctiva which may last 5 years or more. The characteristic feature is the presence of cobblestone-like papillae on the upper tarsal conjunctiva. The papillae do not themselves cause symptoms, and may be present when the disease is inactive. Exacerbations of conjunctivitis are often seasonal, during which keratitis may develop. The majority of patients have atopic eczema or asthma, but it is rare to find a trigger (allergic or otherwise). Approximately 85% of patients are boys, and the onset of the disorder is below the age of 10 years in about three-quarters of patients. The condition tends to start in the spring (this is the meaning of the word vernal), and the symptoms are itching, rubbing, a burning sensation, redness, a discharge and ptosis. During an exacerbation keratitis is common, causing photophobia and reduced visual acuity, and sometimes leading to an ulcer which may in turn cause permanent loss of vision. The management, which should always be supervised by an ophthalmologist, consists of topical steroids for exacerbations, topical antibiotics for secondary infection, and acetylcysteine eye drops if there is a thick discharge. Topical sodium cromoglycate alone is only of benefit in the mildest cases.

BEHAVIOR PROBLEMS

Both hospital and community-based double-blind placebo-controlled studies have repeatedly failed to confirm any validity in the idea that food or food additives cause behavioral problems in otherwise healthy individuals.[16,34] The avoidance of food additives seems to have only a very short-lived beneficial effect on hyperkinesis and other behavior problems, and any benefit from additive avoidance diets is likely to be a placebo response. One source of confusion has been the presence of atopic disease. If a food additive makes eczema or asthma worse, then the concentration span and behavior may also be expected to suffer, but there is no evidence that this is anything other than an indirect effect.

FOOD INTOLERANCE

The prevalence of food intolerance is unclear, although it is greater in infants than in adults, particularly atopic children. The difficulties in establishing the prevalence of food intolerance are the individual variation in tolerance of feelings and symptoms, the unreliability of unconfirmed parental observations, and the lack of definition of what constitutes a reaction to food. All eating causes reactions, for example satiety, the urge to defecate, a feeling of warmth, and weight gain. In the present context we are dealing with unwanted reactions, but families vary in their tolerance of events.

The prevalence of reported food intolerance in children ranges widely from 6 to 18%,[35] a problem with these figures being that only about a third of parental reports of food intolerance can be confirmed when tested by blind food challenge.

The prognosis for food intolerance is good. A prospective study showed that the offending food or fruit was back in the diet after only 9 months in half the cases, and virtually all the offending foods were back in the diet by the third birthday.[36] The mechanisms for food intolerance may be immunological (food allergy), metabolic (e.g. lactase deficiency), pharmacological (e.g. vasoactive amines), toxic (e.g. lectins in red kidney beans), irritant (e.g. curry) or unknown.

Intolerance to cow's milk protein, egg, soya, fish, nuts and food additives are discussed below. Intolerance to most other foods can occur; these are mainly responsible for immediate allergic reactions. Skin prick and RAST tests are generally unhelpful. Where there is doubt about a specific food intolerance, the only reliable way to confirm or refute the diagnosis is to perform a food challenge. The management consists of avoidance.

Cow's milk protein intolerance

Cow's milk protein intolerance is a heterogeneous disorder. The most common antigens in cow's milk are α-lactoglobulin, casein, α-lactalbumin, bovine serum albumin and bovine α-globulin. Digestion may result in the production of additional antigens. The marked antigenic similarity between cow's and goat's milk proteins explains why most children with cow's milk protein intolerance are intolerant to goat's milk.[37] Intolerance to carbohydrates present in cow's milk and milk formulae is dealt with in Chapter 14.

The quantity of cow's milk required to produce an adverse reaction varies. Some patients develop anaphylaxis after ingestion of less than 1 mg of casein, α-lactoglobulin or α-lactalbumin. In contrast, Goldman et al[38] showed that 29 out of 89 children (33%) with cow's milk intolerance did not react to 100 ml of milk but only to 200 ml or more. The median reaction onset time in those who reacted to 100 ml milk challenges was 2 h, but the median reaction onset time in those who required larger amounts of milk to elicit reactions was 24 h.

Most cow's milk formula-fed infants with cow's milk protein intolerance develop symptoms in the first 3 months of life. The age of onset of the first symptoms in breast-fed babies depends on the age at which cow's milk is first introduced. A few breast-fed infants develop symptoms during breast-feeding, because of the presence of cow's milk protein in the mother's breast milk. In fact a high proportion of infants with cow's milk protein intolerance react adversely to traces of cow's milk protein in their mother's milk.[39,39a]

Prevalence studies of intolerance to cow's milk protein vary from 1.9 to 7.5%. The most detailed recent study estimated a point prevalence of cow's milk protein intolerance in children with parentally perceived reactions at the age of $2\frac{1}{2}$ years was 1.1% (CI 0.8–1.6).[40]

Symptoms of cow's milk protein intolerance

There is no single symptom or pattern of symptoms which is pathognomonic of cow's milk protein intolerance. Vomiting is a common immediate symptom. Frequent loose stools occur in 25–75% of patients. In an uncommon but florid picture, infants can present with heavily bloodstained loose stools, sometimes accompanied by mucus, giving rise to the clinical description of food-allergic colitis. Malabsorption may mimic celiac disease with bulky fatty stools, abdominal distention and poor weight gain, and protein-losing enteropathy may be an associated feature. In such cases a jejunal biopsy usually shows some degree of villous atrophy. Acute abdominal pain (often but not always accompanied by vomiting or loose stools) can be a striking symptom. The acute presentation of blood in the stools and abdominal pain may mimic intussusception.

Discomfort, crying or irritability are common and major features of cow's milk protein intolerance in infancy, but it is not clear whether this represents painful hyperperistalsis of the gut or discomfort associated with vomiting or other symptoms. They may occur in conjunction with other symptoms, particularly gastrointestinal symptoms, or they may occur alone. These symptoms usually commence within an hour of cow's milk protein ingestion, although this is not always noted by the parents, partly because irritability from one feed can merge into that caused by the next feed. Crying or screaming are non-specific symptoms in infants, are often accompanied by drawing-up of the legs, and have a number of causes including hunger, tiredness, infection or pain. Many studies of colic as a possible symptom of cow's milk protein intolerance fail to define the term colic, to record associated symptoms that might suggest cow's milk protein intolerance, and to record any temporal relationship between symptoms and milk ingestion.

Wheezing, coughing or rhinitis are common symptoms of cow's milk protein intolerance, and are usually seen in combination with other symptoms such as atopic eczema or vomiting. The acute onset of stridor is occasionally seen within a few minutes of cow's milk ingestion, and indicates angioedema of the larynx or trachea. A persistent perioral erythematous rash, urticaria or eczema can be features of cow's milk protein intolerance. Anaphylactic shock is a rare but potentially fatal feature of cow's milk protein intolerance. The symptoms usually develop within minutes of ingestion of cow's milk protein, but anaphylaxis may be delayed for as much as 9 h after ingestion of cow's milk.[22]

Patients with cow's milk protein intolerance may be intolerant to other foods. In one hospital-based series of 100 children with cow's milk protein intolerance, over 50% exhibited intolerance to one or more other foods.[41] Approximately 8–14% of children with intolerance to cow's milk protein are also intolerant to soya protein.[42]

Clues to the diagnosis of cow's milk protein intolerance in the history

1. Symptoms occur, or are made worse, soon after ingestion of cow's milk protein. Multiple affected systems (e.g. gut, chest and skin) make the diagnosis more likely; single symptoms make it most unlikely.
2. Symptoms date from the time, or soon after the time, that breast-feeding was stopped or cow's milk protein was first introduced into the diet. (NB Feeding changes often coincide with the onset of atopic disease, and do not prove a cause and effect relationship.)
3. A family history of cow's milk protein intolerance.
4. The presence of severe atopic disease in an infant under the age of 12 months.
5. The observation that spilling cow's milk onto non-eczematous skin causes an urticarial rash.

Making the diagnosis of cow's milk protein intolerance

Most patients whose symptoms commence within an hour of cow's milk ingestion have a positive skin prick test, but most of those whose symptoms occur more slowly have negative skin prick tests. As is the case with most other examples of food intolerance, skin prick tests and RAST tests are unhelpful because of the high incidence of false positive and false negative results. A jejunal biopsy is unnecessary because it cannot replace the need for milk elimination and challenge, and the histological changes seen in the small intestine are not diagnostic for cow's milk protein intolerance.

The procedure required to diagnose cow's milk protein intolerance is:

1. A period of avoidance (2 days for those with symptoms occurring within an hour of milk ingestion; 14–28 days for those with delayed-onset symptoms) causing loss of symptoms.

2. Recurrence of symptoms on reintroduction of cow's milk protein.
3. Loss of symptoms after second withdrawal of cow's milk protein.
4. Continued abatement of symptoms with continued avoidance of cow's milk protein.

This strategy must be accompanied by regular attempts to reintroduce cow's milk protein, for example yearly, to see if the patient has grown out of the intolerance.

Failure of cow's milk exclusion

The reasons why a trial period of cow's milk elimination may fail are:

1. The patient has an alternative cause for the reported symptoms.
2. The period of elimination was too short.
3. Foods containing cow's milk protein have not been fully excluded from the diet.
4. The patient is intolerant to the cow's milk substitute which has been given. This is common with goat's milk or sheep's milk. About 8–14% of patients with cow's milk protein intolerance are also intolerant to soya. A smaller proportion are intolerant to whey hydrolysate formulae (these vary in their antigenicity), and there are rare cases of intolerance to casein hydrolysate formulae (Pregestimil or Nutramigen).
5. Coexisting or intercurrent disease, e.g. gastroenteritis.
6. The patient is intolerant to other items which have not been withdrawn from the diet or the environment.
7. The patient's symptoms are trivial and have been exaggerated, or alternatively do not exist at all and have either been imagined or fabricated by the parents. Complete fabrication of symptoms by parents is rare, but the mistaken belief that a child's symptoms are attributable to food intolerance is common.

Milk challenge procedure

A challenge with cow's milk protein is done either to confirm the diagnosis or to see if the patient has grown out of the intolerance. If it is known that the child can tolerate small amounts of cow's milk at home then a formal challenge in hospital is not required, and the parents can continue to increase the quantity of cow's milk given at home.

WARNING! ANAPHYLAXIS! It is vital to remember that during cow's milk protein challenge, symptoms may appear that had not been present previously. The real worry here is anaphylactic shock. In Goldman et al's original study, 3 of 89 patients developed anaphylactic shock as a new symptom during milk challenge.[38] In a further 5, anaphylaxis had been noted prior to milk challenge. Any strategy for cow's milk protein challenges has to take into account the risk of anaphylaxis.

Procedure for patients with no history of anaphylaxis after cow's milk ingestion

Prior to the challenge procedure described below, firmly rub some cow's milk onto the patient's skin with a piece of gauze or cotton wool and observe for 15 min for urticaria. If this occurs, do not proceed with the challenge, continue cow's milk protein avoidance, and repeat direct skin tests in 12 months.

For the first 60 min of the procedure, a nurse, doctor or parent should be present; the patient must not be left alone. The observer is looking for signs of an adverse reaction, which are:

rash around the mouth
urticarial rash
sneezing
vomiting
irritability and pallor
wheezing or coughing
loose stools
STRIDOR
COLLAPSE.

After the first 60 min, the patient should be checked half hourly, provided a parent is present, or quarter hourly if no parent is present. The observer needs to know that the signs above are being sought, and that it is just as important to remove the clothes and look for an urticarial rash as it is to perform the usual nursing observations of the temperature, pulse and respiration rate.

If any of the above signs appear, no further cow's milk should be given, and in the event of a rash, wheezing, stridor or collapse a doctor should be summoned.

During the challenge, apart from the cow's milk being given, the patient should remain on a cow's milk protein-free diet.

The challenge procedure itself is:

1. Place one drop of ordinary cow's milk on the patient's tongue, and observe for 15 min.
2. If no reaction, give 5 ml of cow's milk and observe for 15 min.
3. If no reaction, give 10 ml of cow's milk and observe for 15 min.
4. If no reaction, give 30 ml of cow's milk and observe for 15 min.
5. If no reaction, give cow's milk freely, and give cow's milk protein-free solids as normal at meal times. Provided this does not exceed the usual intake volume, ensure the patient has taken at least 200 ml of cow's milk.

It is unclear how long observation in hospital should be continued. Rare cases are described in which severe reactions have developed late (e.g. 9 h after starting challenge) so parents must be warned that a reaction may develop later in the day, when the child is at home.

If any adverse reaction occurs, as well as stopping further cow's milk it is essential to monitor the patient very closely, as such patients are at special risk of suffering severe and possibly fatal collapse without warning. One may need to keep an infant in hospital overnight where a challenge has had to be stopped because of an adverse reaction. Such infants require close monitoring, including the use of an apnea alarm.

Procedure for patients with previous history of anaphylaxis after cow's milk ingestion

Serious consideration should be given to whether a cow's milk challenge is really necessary. If it is being done to confirm the diagnosis it is best omitted, because the risks of misdiagnosis are likely to be outweighed by the hazards of the challenge procedure. If the challenge is being done to see if the patient has grown out of cow's milk protein intolerance, then the author's recommendations are:

1. Ensure that 12 months have elapsed since the previous positive challenge or anaphylactic reaction.
2. Prior to the challenge procedure outlined above, firmly rub some cow's milk onto the patient's skin with a piece of gauze or cotton wool and observe for 15 min for urticaria. If this occurs, do not proceed with the challenge, continue cow's milk protein avoidance, and repeat direct skin tests in 12 months.
3. If there is no urticarial reaction (a red flare without a wheal does not count as a reaction), proceed with milk challenge as described above.

Natural history of cow's milk protein intolerance

Cow's milk protein intolerance often lasts only a few months, and in many cases it has disappeared completely by the age of 12 months, hence the need for milk challenge at the age of 12 months in patients who were diagnosed in infancy. Most children become tolerant to cow's milk protein by the age of 3 years, although some degree of intolerance persists, occasionally into adult life, in a small number of patients.

Cow's milk-free diets

Cow's milk exclusion means the avoidance of all foods which contain cow's milk protein. A dietitian will be able to provide an appropriate diet sheet containing an up-to-date list of milk-free manufactured foods. Beef avoidance is unnecessary as the coexistence of intolerance to cow's milk and beef is unusual. Infants on a cow's milk-free diet require a cow's milk substitute. The choice is between formulae based on soya, whey hydrolysate, casein hydrolysate (Pregestimil or Nutramigen) or amino acids (Neocate). Goat's, sheep's and ass's milk are inadvisable because of the high incidence of cross-sensitivity, their high solute content, and the risk of serious gastrointestinal infections due to unhygienic methods of collection and distribution. Non-infant formulae soya-based milks are unsuitable because of their low calcium, vitamin and energy content.[16] If an infant is intolerant to both soya and casein hydrolysate, the options are donated human milk, a comminuted chicken-based formula, an elemental diet, or in exceptional circumstances intravenous feeding. After infancy, the rare cases of intolerance to all milk substitutes are dealt with by introducing milk-free solids with added calcium supplements (e.g. calcium and ergocalciferol tablets which contain 97 mg calcium or 2.4 mmol of Ca), effervescent calcium gluconate tablets (2.25 mmol elemental calcium per tablet) or calcium gluconate BPC tablets (1.35 mmol elemental calcium per tablet). Even where a soya or casein hydrolysate infant milk formula is provided, the calcium intake may fall below the recommended requirements.[23,42a] The importance of such low intakes of calcium is unknown, but there may be special risks for patients with atopic eczema. In these children intestinal absorption may be impaired because of an associated enteropathy, the absence of lactose from the diet may impair calcium absorption, and there is a risk of vitamin D deficiency and consequently diminished gastrointestinal calcium absorption in children with atopic eczema who are kept out of sunlight.[23]

EGG INTOLERANCE

The major allergens in egg white are ovalbumin, ovomucoid and ovotransferrin, and all three are also present in much smaller quantities in egg yolk. Cooking reduces the allergenicity of eggs by 70%. Almost all children with egg intolerance can tolerate cooked chicken. The eggs of turkeys, duck and goose contain similar allergens to hen's eggs.

Egg intolerance is very common, and one population-based study found the estimated point prevalence of intolerance to egg in children aged $2\frac{1}{2}$ years was 1.6% (CI 1.3–2.0%), with an upper estimate of the cumulative incidence by this age of 2.6% (CI 1.6–3.6).[43] It is most common in the first 6 months of life, and the most frequent presentation is the rapid onset of symptoms minutes after an infant is given egg for the first time. Reactions occur within an hour of eating egg, and consist of an erythematous rash around the mouth, swelling and urticaria of the oral mucosa and angioedema of the face, sometimes with wheezing, stridor, conjunctivitis, rhinitis, vomiting, loose stools and in severe cases anaphylaxis. Those with immediate reactions also exhibit urticaria after skin contact with egg.

The diagnosis of egg intolerance is made from the history. Skin prick tests and RAST tests are unhelpful because of false positive and false negative results, and on the rare occasions when the diagnosis is in doubt it can only be confirmed by challenge, which would normally comprise ingestion of increasing quantities of hard boiled egg. The management is to exclude egg from the diet.

Egg intolerance is not a contraindication to measles or measles–mumps–rubella (MMR) vaccination because modern measles vaccines are grown on fibroblasts and do not contain detectable quantities of egg protein. Studies have shown that MMR vaccine can be safely given to children with egg allergy.[44–46] The majority of life threatening allergic reactions to MMR vaccine have been reported in children who are not allergic to eggs, and these are mainly explained by IgE-mediated gelatin allergy.[47]

The same may not apply to other vaccines such as influenza vaccine, which is grown in the allantoic cavity of chick eggs and which does contain traces of egg protein. However a recent study has shown that individuals with egg allergy can safely receive influenza vaccine in a two-dose protocol when the vaccine preparation contains no more than 1.2 mcg/ml egg protein.[48]

In the majority of cases, egg intolerance has disappeared by the age of 3 years. Where the presentation is after the age of 12 months, which is unusual, the duration of intolerance may be longer, and is occasionally life-long.

SOYA INTOLERANCE

Soya protein is a common constituent of flour, and is widely distributed in manufactured foods including bread, pastry and sausages. Soya protein is also commonly employed as a meat extender and found in sausages, hamburgers and pie fillings. Soya and other beans can cause flatulence, abdominal pain and loose stools, which are due to the action of intestinal bacteria on poorly digestible oligosaccharides, mainly raffinose and stachyose.

Soya protein intolerance is less common than cow's milk protein intolerance. The clinical features and management of the two disorders are the same, but the widespread use of soya in manufactured foods means that soya protein avoidance is more difficult than cow's milk protein avoidance.

FISH AND SHELLFISH INTOLERANCE

Fish and shellfish constitute a large proportion of dietary protein for many of the world's coastal populations. The prevalence of seafood allergy is not firmly established, but seafoods are reported among the foods most commonly inducing allergy after milk and eggs. Fish allergies are common in children, whereas shellfish allergy appears to be more prevalent in adults. Fish allergens are highly cross-reactive on in vitro testing with the exception of tuna fish, in keeping with the clinical association between codfish allergy and allergy to hake, carp, pike and whiting but not tuna. Parvalbumins (e.g. Gad C 1), a family of vertebrate muscle calcium chelating proteins are major fish allergens. Crustacae protein allergens, which are less well characterized, are also highly cross-reactive on in vitro tests and patients who are allergic to prawns are also likely to be allergic to crab, shrimp and lobster. Molluscs such as mussels and oysters are much more likely to be eaten and therefore to cause problems in adults.

Although most reactions to fish are caused by ingestion, reactions can also occur as a result of inhalation of fish aeroallergens at fish markets or when fish is being cooked.[49] Reactions to food aeroallergens are either respiratory (asthma) or in the skin (urticaria). The latter has been labeled as 'osmylogenic urticaria'; 'osmyls' are minute particles given off by odoriferous substances.[50] Aas[51] has reported from Norway that fish antigens could be found in house dust in most homes where fish is often eaten, and he suggested that this was a likely source for sensitization to fish.

Anaphylaxis caused by the unexpected presence of casein after consuming salmon has been reported.[52] Casein has been recently introduced in the processing of salmon, posing a threat to individuals who are intolerant to cow's milk protein.

FRUIT INTOLERANCE

Technically, fruit is the fleshy or dry ripened ovary of a plant, enclosing the seed or seeds: thus apricot, bananas and grapes, tomatoes and cucumbers, almonds, chestnuts and coconuts should be considered as fruit. All fruit have been known to cause allergic reactions. However a few groups of fruit (nuts and legumes) are most commonly implicated in causing reactions.

INTOLERANCE TO PEANUT AND OTHER NUTS

What is a nut?

There is much confusion amongst non-botanists (this includes the public at large and doctors) as to what does or does not constitute a nut. Whereas most nuts come from trees, peanut, the most common nut to cause allergic reactions, is in fact a legume, and the seed pod grows underground. As far as allergic reactions are concerned, the key information is not the precise botanical origin or plant family but the degree to which the nut does or does not provoke allergic reactions. Allergic reactions to peanuts, walnuts, pecans, brazil nuts, hazelnuts, cashew nuts, pistachio nuts, almonds and macadamia nuts are all well recognized. In contrast, allergic reactions to coconuts, pine nuts, oyster nuts, sweet chestnuts and horse chestnuts are only very rarely reported.

Epidemiology and importance

Peanuts or ground nuts are a major cause of allergic reactions. The prevalence of peanut intolerance in Western countries is approximately 0.5%. In a recent US survey,[53] it was estimated that the prevalence of peanut and/or tree nut intolerance was 1.1% (95% CI, 1.0–1.4%).

In a recent US survey, it was noted that peanut and tree nuts accounted for 20 out of 32 (72%) total fatalities due to food-induced anaphylaxis.[54] Similar trends have been found in the UK.[55]

The main source of exposure to peanut and its products is consumption, but peanut oil (also known as arachis oil) has been used in some injectable, oral and topically applied pharmaceutical preparations. Because of concern that percutaneous absorption of peanut protein could cause sensitization to peanut, efforts have been made in recent years to remove arachis oil from topically applied pharmaceutical products.

The incidence of peanut intolerance is higher in siblings of affected individuals; in one study, 3 out of 39 siblings (7%) had peanut intolerance.[56] The concordance rate for peanut allergy in monozygotic twins is 64% compared with 7% in dizygotic twins, providing evidence for a strong genetic predisposition.[57] Nearly all patients who have had fatal or near fatal reactions to nuts have other atopic diseases, especially asthma, but often also atopic dermatitis and allergic rhinitis. The severity of the asthma in these fatalities is variable and may be relatively mild. Asthma has in the past been thought of as a risk factor for the development of potentially severe reactions, but this is probably misleading and it is likely that asthma and peanut allergy are simply different manifestations of the same atopic disease process.

Peanut processing and its effects

The prevalence of peanut intolerance in China is much lower despite a high rate of peanut consumption. The method of frying or boiling peanuts, as practiced in China, reduces the allergenicity of peanuts compared with the method of dry roasting practiced widely in Western countries.[58] Roasting uses higher temperatures that apparently increase the allergenic property of peanut proteins, and this may help to explain the difference in prevalence of peanut allergy observed in the two countries.[58]

Untreated peanut oil contains peanut protein and consumption risks provoking adverse reactions in individuals with peanut intolerance. However processed and refined peanut oil, which has been subjected to degumming (separation of oil and water by centrifugation at 30–50°C), refining with alkali and further centrifugation at 60–70°C, bleaching with filters at 110°C, and deodorization with steam under vacuum at 230–260°C, does not contain peanut protein, and in one study refined peanut oil failed to provoke a reaction in any of 60 individuals with peanut intolerance.[59,59a] However the marked variation in the degree of processing of peanut and other nut oils means that there will be marked variation in the nut protein content of various different types of refined nut oils.[60] It is worth noting that peanut oil may be used in the pharmaceutical industry, and has been used, for example, in vitamin A and D solutions.

Different cultivars of peanut are grown in many different parts of the world, but peanuts of different varieties from different parts of the world all appear to contain similar antigenic proteins.[61]

Cross-reactivity

In a study of 122 children with allergic reactions to peanuts and tree nuts, 68 had reactions to peanut alone, 20 to tree nuts alone, and 34 had reactions to both peanut and at least one tree nut.[62] Of those reacting to tree nuts, 34 had reactions to one, 12 to two, and 8 to three or more different tree nuts, the most common being walnut, almond and pecan. One should note, however, that there is an inherent selection bias in non population-based studies of this sort which emanate from allergy clinics, for it is probable that those with intolerance to multiple foods are more likely to be referred in the first place.

Although there is extensive cross-reactivity between peanuts and other legumes on skin prick testing and RAST testing, clinically important cross-reactivity is rare on food challenge and thus intolerance to peanut should not lead to automatic avoidance of other legumes.[63]

Clinical features

In the above mentioned study of 122 children, 89% of reactions involved the skin (urticaria, angioedema), 52% the respiratory tract (wheezing, throat tightness, coughing, dyspnea), and 32% the gastrointestinal tract. Two organ systems were affected in 31% of, and all three in 21% of reactions. Accidental ingestions were common (30–50% over a 5 year period), and on average the symptoms after accidental exposure were generally similar to those at initial exposure.[62]

Modes of accidental ingestion include sharing food, hidden food ingredients,[64] cross-contamination (in kitchen utensils or in food manufacturing), and school craft projects using peanut butter.

The threshold dose required to produce a reaction varies. In one study of 14 individuals with peanut intolerance, the lowest dose of peanut to produce a convincing reaction was 2 mg, although individuals with peanut intolerance sometimes report short-lived symptoms after doses as low at 100 mcg.[59,59a] It is not uncommon for peanut intolerant individuals to experience local allergic reactions after being kissed by someone who has eaten peanut.

This is not specific for peanut intolerance; the same phenomenon is seen in individuals who are intolerant to other foods.

Acute allergic reactions to peanuts have been seen in 1 week old neonates, and thus in some children, sensitization must occur in utero. At present there is no definitive evidence to suggest that avoidance of peanuts during pregnancy and lactation will prevent the development of peanut allergy in the child. However, given the evidence that traces of foodstuffs commonly enter breast milk, there is some logical basis for a mother from an atopic family avoiding consuming nuts during lactation.

The severity of any reaction is in part related to the quantity of nut eaten. When patients with peanut intolerance are followed-up, and experience a further reaction resulting from accidental ingestion, most follow-up reactions are less severe than the index reaction.[65] Those who present with a mild index reaction are less likely to develop a severe follow-up reaction, and on the basis of this observation it has been questioned whether those with a mild reaction require preloaded adrenaline (epinephrine) syringes.[65]

Diagnosis

Skin prick tests and RAST tests have a notoriously poor specificity and positive predictive value and therefore cannot be used to show that an individual will have clinical symptoms on ingestion of peanuts. In addition, these tests cannot indicate the severity of symptoms.

Negative skin prick tests and RAST tests correlate rather better with absence of peanut intolerance, but false negatives, even in those with severe reactions, can occur,[66–68] making both skin prick tests and RAST tests unreliable diagnostic tools. If the history is unclear, then the only reliable way to make the diagnosis of nut intolerance is to perform a food challenge.[68,69,69a]

Natural history

Whilst most children fairly rapidly grow out of most food intolerances, nut intolerance has always been regarded as an exception, being life-long in most cases. Recent claims that up to 20% of patients outgrow intolerance to peanut have been based on studies of patients whose original diagnosis of nut intolerance was questionable, and there has not yet been a single published case of disappearance of intolerance in an individual proven to have intolerance by blind challenge. There probably are a few genuine cases in which nut intolerance is not permanent,[70] but they are rare.

Management

The management of nut allergy consists of education on avoiding the allergen plus three treatment options – antihistamine for mild reactions, antihistamine plus inhaled adrenaline (epinephrine) for moderate reactions, and antihistamine, adrenaline (epinephrine) inhaler and adrenaline (epinephrine) autoinjector for severe reactions. In the UK adrenaline (epinephrine) inhalers (Medihaler Epi) are unavailable, and this means that adrenaline (epinephrine) autoinjectors may need to be considered for some UK patients who have had moderately severe reactions.

Peanuts are cheap, readily available and are often used as a substitute for other nuts. For these reasons, even if there are no features of clinical cross-reactivity, patients who have peanut intolerance should in general avoid all tree nuts.

Treatment of peanut intolerance by hyposensitization using injections of peanut extract is poorly tolerated and unsatisfactory.

FOOD-PROVOKED EXERCISE-INDUCED ANAPHYLAXIS

In simple exercise-induced anaphylaxis, exercise is followed by hypotension, accompanied by a varying combination of cholinergic urticaria (widespread tiny 1–3 mm wheals with variable erythema which last 30–60 min and occur in association with sweating) and angioedema of the face and pharynx. In a curious but well-described variant of this disorder, attacks only occur when the exercise follows within a couple of hours of the ingestion of specific foods such as celery, shellfish, peaches or wheat.[71] The mechanism of this rare food-dependent exercise-induced anaphylaxis is obscure but in these patients a simple double-blind food challenge performed without exercise will fail to validate a history of food intolerance.

INTOLERANCE TO FOOD ADDITIVES

Food additives include coloring agents, preservatives, antioxidants, emulsifiers, stabilizers, sweeteners, other flavour modifiers and a large miscellaneous group of other agents. The scale of use of additives in food comes as a surprise to most people, and it is understandable that many should find these substances vaguely menacing. An obsession with food that is natural overlooks both the large number of toxic substances naturally occurring in food[72] and the fact that most substances which provoke food intolerance are naturally occurring, such as eggs, cow's milk and nuts. There is an enormous discrepancy between the public's perception of food additive intolerance and objectively verified intolerance. In one study, 1372 of 18 582 people living in High Wycombe claimed to suffer from food additive intolerance, but double-blind challenges confirmed this in only two subjects, who were both shown to react adversely to the coloring agent annatto, which caused headache in one and abdominal pain in the other.[73]

Tartrazine and benzoic acid

Tartrazine is a yellow coloring agent, and one of the group of azo dyes. It is used as a coloring agent in a wide range of foods and medicines. Benzoic acid and the related benzoates retard the growth of bacteria and yeasts, and are used as food preservatives. Small quantities occur naturally in certain foods such as cranberries and bilberries. Double-blind placebo-controlled studies have demonstrated that tartrazine can provoke urticaria, asthma or rhinitis in a small number of atopic subjects.[16] Similar studies have shown that benzoates can provoke urticaria. There is a lack of objective information about whether benzoates can provoke asthma. Tartrazine or benzoate intolerance can be identified by history (particularly unreliable in suspected food additive intolerance), elimination and challenge. It is possible that repeated administration of tartrazine or the benzoates leads to tolerance, and the severity of adverse reaction may not always be severe enough to warrant avoidance.

Sulfites

Sulfur dioxide and the sodium or potassium salts of sulfite or metabisulfite are widely used as food preservatives. Dried fruit is commonly treated with sulfur dioxide, and high levels of sulfite are sometimes found in wine, beer and salads in restaurants. Sulfites are sometimes used as preservatives in parenteral preparations of drugs, including several drugs used for the intravenous or inhalational treatment of asthma. Double-blind placebo-controlled studies have demonstrated that the oral administration of sulfite solutions can provoke bronchoconstriction in 35–70% of children with asthma.

A history of worsening of pre-existing asthma after consuming artificial drinks, eating in a restaurant or inhalation or injection of a drug containing sulfite raises the possibility of sulfite intolerance. Skin tests are unhelpful, and the diagnosis can only be confirmed by challenge, employing increasing doses of sulfite so as to establish the patient's threshold dose which can provoke asthma. Knowledge of the threshold enables the patient to avoid only those foods with a relatively high sulfite level, making a very restrictive diet unnecessary.

Other food additives

Evidence for harmful effects to children from other food additives does not exist, apart from those additives which can provoke urticaria (see above) and a single case of orofacial granulomatosis (Melkersson–Rosenthal syndrome) provoked by carmoisine, sunset yellow and monosodium glutamate.[74]

LATEX ALLERGY

Sources of latex

Latex is used in the manufacture of a number of products in general and medical use, including gloves, catheters, condoms, balloons, rubber bands, toys and tyres. About 90% of harvested rubber is processed by acid coagulation at pH 4.5–4.8 into dry sheets or crumbled particles for manufacture of extruded rubber products (rubber thread); compression, transfer, or injection moulded goods (rubber seals or diaphragms); or pneumatic tyres. The remaining 10% of harvested rubber is non-coagulated and ammoniated; it is used in the manufacture of rubber gloves and other 'dipped' products, such as condoms and balloons. Dipped rubber products are responsible for most allergic reactions to natural rubber latex.[6]

Latex antigens can be leached from rubber gloves by normal skin moisture, with subsequent adsorption onto cornstarch powder inside the gloves. Latex allergen can also be adsorbed to powder inside gloves that have not been worn. When the gloves are donned or discarded, the cornstarch particles with adsorbed latex allergens become airborne and can sensitize nearby persons by inhalation or can evoke symptoms in previously sensitized persons.

The cow's milk protein casein is compounded into some brands of surgical and household gloves, and this may be responsible for glove-related reactions in patients who are intolerant to casein.

Predisposing factors

Atopy is a significant risk factor in the development of latex allergy with two-thirds of affected patients being atopic. Latex allergy is one disease that may affect providers of health care services more frequently than patients themselves. Health care workers who are atopic and wear latex gloves are at high risk. Other high risk workers include housekeepers, doll manufacturers and tyre plant workers. High risk patient groups are those requiring multiple surgical procedures. Individuals with spina bifida are at increased risk of latex allergy as a consequence of undergoing repeated neurological, urological and orthopedic procedures, or by early, repeated contact with rubber urinary catheters, and rubber gloves during removal of fecal impactions. The reported prevalence of latex allergy in spina bifida has varied from 18 to 64%.[6]

Reasons for increasing prevalence of latex allergy

There are a number of possible reasons for the large increase in the prevalence of this disorder.[14] One is the increased use of gloves owing to the risk of hepatitis and AIDS. Another is the replacement of mineral talc powder by cornstarch powder. Mineral talc is heavy and only transiently airborne, and has a high capacity to act as an allergen eliminator by binding firmly to latex allergens.

Cross-reactions

Cross-reactions may occur between proteins in latex and various foods such as avocado,[75] bananas and chestnut; the so-called 'latex-fruit syndrome'.[76,77] Cross-reactions may also occur with the weeping fig *Ficus benjamani* which is increasingly used for indoor decoration. The existence of cross-reacting allergenic structures in plant-derived products such as latex, fruit and enzymes may explain extensive allergenic reactivity. Because of the frequency of cross-reactions, some authorities have recommended that children who are at risk of developing latex allergy should avoid bananas and weeping figs, but this advice has not been objectively evaluated.

Clinical manifestations

The most common reaction to latex products is non-immunological, *irritant contact dermatitis*, the development of dry, irritated areas on the skin caused by the effects of repeated hand washing, detergents or sanitizers, or powders added to gloves. *Allergic contact dermatitis* appears 1–2 days after contact with the offending product such as rubber gloves, shoes, sports equipment and medical devices. The dermatitis is a cell-mediated delayed-type hypersensitivity reaction to low molecular weight accelerators and antioxidants in the rubber product. Examples of rubber product components that cause contact dermatitis are thiurams, carbamates, benzothiazoles, thioureas and amine derivatives. *Contact urticaria* is the most common early manifestation of rubber allergy, particularly in latex-sensitive health care workers. Symptoms, such as redness, itching, and wheal-and-flare reactions at the site of glove contact, often mistakenly attributed to glove powder or hand washing, are IgE-mediated and appear 10–15 min after putting on gloves. Inhalation of latex allergen-coated cornstarch particles from powdered gloves can cause *rhinitis* and *asthma* in latex allergic individuals, mainly adults who manufacture gloves and health care workers. Latex allergic individuals can experience *anaphylaxis*, occasionally fatal[78] in a variety of medical care situations and as a result of blowing into balloons or using rubber-handled squash racquets. Finally, latex allergic individuals can react to food that has been contaminated by latex, for example by food handlers wearing latex gloves.[79]

Diagnosis of latex allergy

Diagnosis depends on the clinical history, coupled with examination and laboratory tests. Because there are many latex allergens, it is not known whether when performing a skin prick test or RAST test all or some of the appropriate epitopes are present in the latex solution. Latex specific IgE tests result in up to 25% false negatives and 27% false positive results and must be interpreted with caution. Latex allergens for skin prick testing are available, but adverse reactions are more common than for other allergens and the rate of systemic reactions after latex testing can be as high as 1/200 skin tests.

Management

The mainstay of management is avoidance, especially of powdered latex gloves which are the major contributors of transferable allergen.[80]

ANAPHYLAXIS

In this chapter, and in the clinical situation, the term anaphylaxis or anaphylactic shock is taken to mean a severe life-threatening reaction of rapid onset, with circulatory collapse or respiratory compromise. In the past the term anaphylaxis was used to describe any immediate allergic reaction caused by IgE antibodies, however mild, but such usage fails to distinguish between, for example, trivial urticaria and a life-threatening event. The mechanisms are believed to be IgE mediated (e.g. penicillin or insulin allergy), the generation of immune complexes (e.g. reactions to blood products), a direct (not involving antigens or antibodies) effect on mast cells or basophils causing inflammatory mediator release (e.g. reactions to radiocontrast media) and presumed abnormalities of arachidonic acid metabolism (e.g. anaphylactoid reactions to aspirin). It is possible to theoretically differentiate between anaphylaxis (immunologically mediated reactions) and anaphylactoid (non-immunologically mediated) reactions. Previous sensitization is required for the former but not the latter.

The major causes of anaphylactic shock are drugs (e.g. penicillin, muscle relaxants), heterologous antisera (used for the prophylaxis and treatment of tetanus, diphtheria, rabies, snake bites and botulism), radiographic contrast media, the administration of blood products, hyposensitization injections, venoms from stinging insects (honeybee, wasp, hornet, yellow jacket) and foods (especially egg, cow's milk, nuts, fish and shellfish). Although delayed (12 h or more) anaphylactic reactions can occur, most cases of anaphylaxis produce symptoms within minutes after exposure to the causative agent. In general, the sooner the symptoms occur the more severe is the reaction. The first symptoms are feeling unwell, feeling warm, generalized pruritus, fear, faintness and sneezing. In severe cases these early symptoms are quickly (in seconds or minutes) followed by loss of consciousness, and death from severe bronchospasm, suffocation (edema of the larynx, epiglottis and pharynx) or shock and cardiac arrhythmia.

DRUG TREATMENT OF ANAPHYLAXIS

Anaphylaxis not associated with circulatory failure/arrest

Epinephrine (adrenaline) 10 mcg/kg (0.1 ml/kg of a 1:10 000 solution), given intramuscularly is the drug and route of choice for most patients with anaphylaxis associated with life-threatening respiratory compromise (Project Team of the Resuscitation Council (UK) (1999). An alternative is 0.01 ml/kg of a 1:1000 solution, which would be applicable to larger children or older patients. Subcutaneous administration results in slower rates of systemic absorption than via the intramuscular route and is therefore not recommended.

Preloaded epinephrine syringes are available for use in the community. Min-I-jet 1 ml 1:1000 epinephrine with a 6 mm needle is for subcutaneous injection, requires assembly before use and the dose will need to be adjusted before administration. Thus it is less suitable than the EpiPen or the Anapen, which are spring-loaded devices with a concealed needle giving a single dose of 0.3 ml of 1:1000 or 1:2000 epinephrine (0.15 or 0.30 mg) as a deep intramuscular injection. The simplicity of use and concealed needle makes this the most popular option with many patients.

The junior EpiPen or Anapen (0.15 mg) are suitable for children of 15–30 kg; above this weight the adult EpiPen or Anapen (0.3 mg) should be used. It will rarely be appropriate to issue epinephrine for children below 15 kg.

Epinephrine has a short half-life, and if necessary the intramuscular injection is repeated at 5 min intervals. Repeated (i.e. more than one) epinephrine injections are required in approximately 10–40% of patients with anaphylaxis, and therefore it is advisable to prescribe two preloaded epinephrine syringes per patient. Intravenous administration of epinephrine has been associated with acute strokes and is therefore to be avoided in most situations.

Only 20% of fatal/near-fatal anaphylactic reactions to foods occur at home. The remainder occur at school, at the home of friends, and at restaurants[81] and thus it is essential that if a preloaded epinephrine syringe is prescribed, it is available where the patient is and that there is someone around who is trained in its use. Thus for schoolchildren it is important that two preloaded epinephrine syringes are available at the school and that teachers have appropriate training in the recognition of anaphylaxis and the use of the epinephrine syringe.

Indications for use of preloaded epinephrine syringes

A major factor predisposing to fatalities in cases of food anaphylaxis was the delay in recognition and instigation of medical treatment. In general it is recommended that a preloaded epinephrine syringe should be given at the first signs of upper airway obstruction, wheeziness not relieved by a bronchodilator inhaler or if there is any faintness. Allergic reactions are frightening and are often associated with panic attacks, which may mimic or exacerbate the symptoms and signs of anaphylaxis. This often makes it difficult to differentiate between clinical features of allergy and acute anxiety.

Indications for preloaded epinephrine syringe prescribing

The indications for prescribing preloaded epinephrine syringes vary from center to center, and the topic is highly controversial.[82] Some authorities recommend, for example, that all children with peanut intolerance should be issued with epinephrine syringes, however mild the previous reactions, on the basis that the next reaction could be life-threatening. Others are concerned that epinephrine syringes are vastly overprescribed, and should only be used in very selected cases.[83] Unfortunately it is not possible to predict which individuals are likely to get severe reactions, except to say that those who have had previous severe reactions are those at greatest risk. The possible role of asthma as a risk factor has already been discussed above in relation to peanut allergy. Fatal or near-fatal anaphylactic reactions are rare (approximately 1 per 1 000 000 per year), often occur in places where the prescribed preloaded epinephrine syringe is not available, where there is no one trained in its use, or in some cases the reaction occurs so rapidly as to lead to circulatory arrest which is unlikely to respond to intramuscular epinephrine (see section on anaphylaxis associated with circulatory failure/arrest below). Most non-venom and non-medication induced allergic reactions respond to antihistamines. Alas there is no guarantee that treatment with epinephrine will be life saving, and there are well-documented cases in which death has occurred despite the correct use of epinephrine syringes.

Preloaded epinephrine syringes

Advantages

Efficacy

Most effective acute treatment for anaphylaxis not associated with (i) circulatory failure or (ii) large airway obstruction due to angioedema

Provides reassurance for the patient and relatives

Disadvantages

Rarity: risk of death from anaphylaxis is approximately 1/1 000 000, i.e. very rare indeed

May not work: Anaphylaxis associated with circulatory failure is not likely to respond, and some cases of anaphylaxis will prove fatal even if epinephrine is given early

Can cause anxiety: having to carry an epinephrine syringe everywhere causes considerable anxiety to some patients, relatives, carers and teachers. Exclusion from school trips and social outings have in some cases been associated directly with prescription of a preloaded epinephrine syringe to children

Lack of warning signs: fatal reactions are sometimes not associated with warning signs

Side-effects: preloaded epinephrine syringe use for anaphylaxis has caused death from arrhythmias and strokes
Availability: preloaded epinephrine syringes are often not available at the emergency (i.e. reactions away from home, patient not carrying epinephrine)
Need for training: inadequate training may prevent adequate recognition of anaphylaxis or use of preloaded epinephrine syringe

Based on the current difficulties associated with the use of a preloaded epinephrine syringe, if it is prescribed, it is recommended that the following conditions are met.

1. Appropriate training should be given to the patient, their relatives, teachers and work colleagues (see below)
2. Preloaded epinephrine syringes should be available at all times, not just at home but also at school, when visiting friends and during all leisure activities
3. All trainees should undergo periodic retraining and reassessment.

Information which should be given to users of preloaded epinephrine syringes

As mentioned above, training of patients and their relatives in the correct use and safe handling of the preloaded epinephrine syringe as well as regular annual review of technique is essential. Table 31.3 lists the information that should be covered at training sessions.

The date on which training was given, the people trained, the epinephrine dose and a list of the information given to the patient and the relatives should be documented in the clinical notes. Allergy clinics might use a standardized preloaded epinephrine syringe checklist form, signed and dated by the prescribing doctor, with copies added to the clinical notes, sent to the GP and given to the patient.

Nebulized epinephrine and other treatment modalities

Nebulized epinephrine is no longer recommended as treatment of anaphylaxis in the UK because the metered-dose aerosol (Medihaler-epi) has been withdrawn from the market. Bronchoconstriction is best treated with a nebulized alpha 2-agonist (e.g. salbutamol or terbutaline). Intravenous fluid boluses are often required in addition to epinephrine for treatment of hypotension. A number of 20 ml/kg boluses may be required. After injection of epinephrine, an H_1 antihistamine, for example chlorphenamine (chlorpheniramine) should be administered, and may be continued for 48 h to prevent recurrences of the reaction. Steroids take some hours to be effective and are unhelpful in the immediate treatment of anaphylaxis, but are of possible benefit in preventing a secondary relapse. Further management consists of avoidance of the cause, and in the case of insect venom stings consideration of hyposensitization.

Table 31.3 Information which should be covered at preloaded epinephrine syringe training sessions

A. *Instructions should be given to the parents and if old enough the patient on the following:*
How to recognize an anaphylactic reaction
When to use the preloaded epinephrine syringe(s)
Where and how to inject the epinephrine
How to dispose of the used preloaded epinephrine syringe
What to do if the epinephrine is injected incorrectly
When to use other medicines
Always to seek medical help if having a reaction
When to replace the preloaded epinephrine syringe

B. *The preloaded epinephrine syringe should be checked and the parents/patient told:*
To keep the preloaded epinephrine syringe in the original pack
Label with the patient's name
Store safely
Store at room temperature
Always keep accessible for an emergency

Anaphylaxis associated with circulatory failure/arrest

If the patient has life-threatening circulatory compromise with no palpable peripheral pulse, then intramuscular epinephrine is unlikely to effective, as it will not be adequately absorbed. In patients with circulatory failure, basic life support must be commenced, followed by the injection of *intravenous* epinephrine (at an initial dose of 0.1 ml/kg of a 1:10 000 solution) as per the asystole protocol for advanced pediatric life support (APLS). Great vigilance is needed to ensure that the correct strength of epinephrine is used; anaphylactic shock kits need to make a very clear distinction between the 1 in 10 000 strength normally used for intravenous use and 1 in 1000 strength used for intramuscular use. Intravenous administration of epinephrine for treatment of patients with anaphylaxis has been associated with death from acute strokes and ventricular fibrillation, and is therefore to be avoided in anaphylaxis not associated with circulatory failure.

Medication for non-life threatening allergic reactions

H_1 antihistamines are very useful in controlling symptoms of non-life-threatening allergic reactions such as acute and chronic urticaria and allergic rhinitis and conjunctivitis. Antihistamines can be divided into two groups (Table 31.4). The older sedating antihistamines are very effective, but because they cross the blood–brain barrier they are sedative and therefore may adversely affect children's learning ability. In an effort to reduce the sedative side-effects of these drugs, a new generation of non-sedating antihistamines has been developed. Some of these non-sedating antihistamines (in particular astemizole, terfenadine) are associated with life-threatening arrhythmias (*torsades de pointes*) by inhibiting potassium ion channels in cardiac tissue. Astemizole and terfenadine are therefore no longer available. Mizolastine which is still available has been associated with an increased risk of ventricular fibrillation when given together with other drugs (analgesics, antiarrhythmics, sotalol).

Doxepin is classed as a tricyclic antidepressant, but also has anti-H_1 and H_2 antihistamine activity (75× more potent than diphenhydramine and 6× more potent than cimetidine). It may be a useful therapeutic adjunct in older children with urticaria not controlled with traditional antihistamines.

DRUG ALLERGY

Epidemiology

Prospective studies have estimated that the incidence of serious adverse drug reactions in hospitalized patients is 6.7% and the incidence of fatal drug reactions is 0.32%.[84] Whereas most adverse drug reactions are non-allergic in nature, 6–10% may be attributed to an immune mechanism involving either antibodies or T cells.[85] Drug reactions that are immunologically mediated (1) require a period of sensitization, (2) occur in a small proportion of the population, (3) are elicited at drug doses far below the therapeutic range, and (4) in most instances subside after drug discontinuation.

Table 31.4 H_1 antihistamines used in the treatment of allergic reactions

Antihistamine	Route of administration
Classical/sedating	
Chlorpheniramine (Piriton)	oral/parenteral
Promethazine (Phenergan)	oral/parenteral
Trimeprazine (Vallergan)	oral
Newer non-sedating	
Astemizole*	
Terfenadine*	
Acrivastine (Semprex)	oral
Cetirizine (Zirtek)	oral
Desloratadine (Neoclarityn)	oral
Fexofenadine (Telfast)	oral
Loratadine (Clarityn)	oral
Mizolastine (Mistamine)	oral
Antazoline (Otrivine-Antistin)	eye drops
Azelastine (Optilast)	eye drops
Levocabastine (Livostin)	eye drops
Azelastine (Rhinolast)	nasal spray
Levocabastine (Livostin)	nasal spray
Antazoline (Wasp-Eze)	topical skin ointment
Mepyramine (Anthisan)	topical skin ointment

*May cause cardiac arrythmias especially torsades de pointes

The mean age of allergic drug reactions is approximately 40 years, allergic drug reactions in childhood being much less common than in adults.[86] Many patients who are said to have drug allergies are not allergic to the drug. For instance, 80–90% of patients who report a penicillin allergy are not truly allergic when assessed by skin testing, and virtually all patients with a negative skin test result can take penicillin without serious sequelae.[87] In children, most of the reactions that coincide with drug administration are exanthema which are usually due to the underlying disease.

Clinical spectrum of disease

True allergic reactions are restricted to a limited number of syndromes that are generally accepted as allergic in nature, such as anaphylaxis, Stevens–Johnson syndrome, angioedema and urticaria, contact sensitivity and various exanthema, among others. Skin reactions are the most frequent symptoms of adverse drug reactions, occurring in nearly 80% of patients and are most commonly observed with ampicillin, amoxycillin and co-trimoxazole. Beta-lactam antibiotics are the most frequent pharmacological group involved in allergic drug reactions. NSAIDs, minor analgesics and other antibiotics (e.g. co-trimoxazole) are other drugs implicated. Anesthetic agents may cause immediate type allergic reactions: muscle relaxants are implicated in 60% of cases, suxamethonium being responsible for 39% of these.[88]

Drug antigenicity

Only a few drugs such as large peptides (e.g. insulin), papain, streptokinase and foreign antisera can directly induce an immune response. The majority of drugs are simple chemicals of low molecular weight which are not immunogenic unless combined with serum or tissue proteins to form an immunogenic complex. Thus most drugs that cause hypersensitivity reactions must first be made immunogenic by being haptenated onto proteins, a process that occurs as the drug is metabolized. The cytochrome P450-dependent oxidation pathway in the liver is an important enzyme involved in the production of these reactive drug intermediates that covalently bind to serum and membrane proteins. Penicillin is an exception, as it may haptenate proteins directly without previous metabolism.[89] Acylation of serum proteins results from an amine bond formed from the hydrolysed beta-lactam ring of the antibiotic.[90]

Diagnosis and management

Diagnosis of drug allergy is largely based on history (Table 31.5) and examination. Although diagnostic testing methods exist, overall they are still of limited practical value for the clinician who is evaluating a patient with suspected drug allergy. One major problem that affects the use of diagnostic tests for drug allergies is that, except for penicillin, the immunochemistry of most drugs is still not known. In most instances the definitive test for drug allergy is rechallenge. This must be approached with caution, as it may precipitate anaphylactic reactions.

In children where the use of a particular drug is essential and there are no alternatives, hyposensitization can be used to induce tolerance in a highly sensitized patient. The procedure is performed by the cautious administration of incremental doses of the drug to the patient over a period of hours to days. The drug can be administered either by oral or intravenous route. The starting dose for the procedure can be determined by performing intradermal skin tests with the native drug at a dose that does not cause a non-specific. Typically, doses are doubled every 15–30 min and vital signs, physical examination, and peak flow values are regularly monitored. It is critical that the individuals involved with the hyposensitization procedure understand that it can have serious consequences. While anaphylactic reactions rarely occur if conservative protocols are used, health care personnel must be prepared to treat anaphylaxis if it does happen.[91]

Penicillin and cephalosporin allergy

Anaphylactic reactions occur in 0.004–0.015% of penicillin courses and are mostly seen in adults between the ages of 20 and 49 years.[92] Anaphylactic reactions to cephalosporins are also uncommon occurring in 0.0001 to 0.1% of cases.[93] The frequency of allergic reactions within 24 h of cephalosporin administration to patients with a history of penicillin allergy is only 2–6%. Thus available data suggest that the vast majority of patients who are allergic to penicillin tolerate cephalosporins without significant reaction.[87] A history of atopy does not generally place an individual at increased risk for a type I penicillin reaction.

Degradation products of penicillin may bind with tissue or serum proteins to form an immunogenic complex which can elicit an immune response. Penicillin allergy is attributed either to the benzylpenicilloyl hapten (the so-called 'major' determinant because 95% of tissue-bound penicillin is in this form), or to a group of

Table 31.5 Important questions to ask in the history of a patient with suspected drug allergy

1. What drugs were administered, by what route and at what dose?
2. For what reason was the drug administered?
3. How long after starting the drug did the reaction commence?
4. What was the nature of the reaction?
5. What treatment if any was required for the reaction?
6. What happened when the drug was discontinued?
7. Has the patient taken the drug (or similar drugs) before and after the reaction? If so what was the result?
8. How old was the patient at the time of the reaction?

compounds collectively called the 'minor' determinants which are paradoxically responsible for many of the most severe allergic reactions. Adverse reactions to penicillin can be most simply classified by the timing of their occurrence. Immediate reactions occur within 1 h of administration and are usually directed against the minor determinant antigens. Life-threatening reactions occurring beyond 1 h of penicillin administration are rare.

The clinical features include urticaria, laryngeal edema, bronchospasm and anaphylactic shock. Accelerated reactions occur 1–72 h after penicillin administration, have the same clinical features as immediate reactions, and are usually directed against the major determinant. Late reactions, the mechanisms of which are generally less well understood, occur more than 72 h after drug administration. They comprise such disorders as a maculopapular (measles-like) rash, urticaria, serum sickness, erythema multiforme, hemolytic anemia, thrombocytopenia and neutropenia. Rarely, late reactions are due to the new development of an immediate or accelerated reaction. Only 3.5% of patients with a maculopapular rash associated with penicillin administration had adverse reactions to oral challenge with penicillin.[94] Maculopapular eruptions caused by penicillin may subside spontaneously despite continuing use of the drug and may not recur on re-exposure, presumably as many of these exanthema are due to the infectious disease rather than the antibiotic.

Ampicillin can provoke the same allergic reactions as other penicillins, but in addition is associated with a particularly high incidence of a non-allergic maculopapular rash, beginning a week or more after starting therapy.

An inquiry about possible penicillin allergy is mandatory prior to an injection of penicillin. However, not all patients with penicillin allergy give a history of previous penicillin administration. In these patients either the history is incorrect and the patient has received penicillin therapy, or sensitization has occurred through inadvertent exposure to penicillin in other sources such as food, milk or even soft drinks. Where there is a history of penicillin allergy, the choice is either to withhold antibiotics or to avoid the use of penicillins, cephalosporins or imipenem, which like the penicillins contains a beta-lactam ring and which shows extensive cross-reactivity with penicillin. Almost all deaths from anaphylaxis have resulted from injection of the drug, and the oral route has only been associated with a handful of fatal cases.

The penicillin skin test has no place in the management of patients without a clinical history of a type I penicillin allergy, and is unnecessary in the face of a bona fide history of a life-threatening type I reaction in which cases the drug should be avoided. In cases where the history is suggestive of a milder type I hypersensitivity reaction, a negative result to skin testing is associated with tolerance to penicillin in 98% of cases. In contrast, a positive skin test result should lead to avoidance of this antibiotic, or use only after hyposensitization.[87] There are no clinically useful skin tests or IgE tests for use in patients with suspected cephalosporin allergy. On the very rare occasions in childhood (e.g. endocarditis) when treatment with penicillin is essential, then it is possible to hyposensitize the patient by oral and then continuous intravenous administration,[95] but this procedure carries a risk of fatal anaphylaxis. The protection from hyposensitization is short lived, although it is possible to maintain a state of hyposensitization by long-term administration of a low dose.

Aspirin - non-steroidal anti-inflammatory drug allergy

The prevalence of aspirin intolerance is around 5–6%. Up to 20% of the asthmatic population is sensitive to aspirin and other non-steroidal anti-inflammatory drugs (NSAIDs) and present with a triad of rhinitis, sinusitis and asthma when exposed to the offending drug. Chronic persistent inflammation is the hallmark of patients with aspirin-induced allergy. Fifty per cent of the patients with aspirin-induced allergy have chronic, severe, corticosteroid-dependent asthma, 30% have moderate asthma that can be controlled with inhaled steroids, and the remaining 20% of patients have mild and intermittent asthma. Up to 25% of hospital admissions for acute asthma requiring mechanical ventilation may be due to NSAID ingestion.[96]

Aspirin allergy is now thought to be at least partly due to a deviation of the arachidonic acid metabolic pathway towards the production of excessive inflammatory leukotrienes (especially LTC_4) and away from the production of anti-inflammatory prostaglandins (PGE2). Leukotriene-modifying drugs (montelukast, zileuton) have been found to attenuate but not abolish aspirin-induced bronchial reactions in aspirin-induced allergy patients. Salmeterol, a long acting alpha2-agonist has also been found useful in the management of aspirin-induced allergy.

DIAGNOSIS OF ALLERGY - TAKING A HISTORY

The lack of really useful laboratory tests for allergy (see below) means that there is no substitute for a careful history.

Important questions when taking a history for allergy

The history should include questions about:

1. when symptoms occur;
2. where symptoms occur;
3. when or where the patient is free of symptoms;
4. the presence of other allergic symptoms;
5. family history of allergy or atopic disease.

Other clues from the history

1. ***The symptoms are worse at night.*** Both asthma and eczema are often worse at night, but it is wrong to equate all nocturnal symptoms with house dust mite allergy, as there are other possible explanations. Circadian rhythms affecting airway caliber, bronchial reactivity[97] and cortisol secretion account for some of the increase in symptoms at night in asthma. In eczema, heat, tiredness and low cortisol secretion may contribute to nocturnal symptoms. In theory a high concentration of house dust mite antigen found in some bedrooms could contribute to nocturnal symptoms in asthma, rhinitis or atopic eczema, but in one large study there was no association between worsening at night or on waking and the presence of house dust mite allergy.[98] Only improvement in the symptoms following the complete avoidance of house dust mites in the bedroom (very difficult to achieve – see below), and recurrence of symptoms on re-exposure, will prove the point. A study of the symptoms associated with house dust mite allergy showed that a history of symptoms being provoked during domestic activity that stirs up house dust (bedmaking, dusting, vacuuming, emptying a vacuum cleaner bag, sweeping, shaking out bedding) when house dust mite antigen becomes airborne, is probably the only reliable pointer to house dust mite allergy.[98]
2. ***The symptoms are worse at certain times of the year.*** The usual inference is that the symptoms are attributable to a seasonal allergen. Sometimes the history is convincing. For example, where sneezing and conjunctivitis occur each year in June and July on sunny days when the grass pollen count is high, it is highly probable that the symptoms are attributable to allergy to

grass pollen. Often, the history is not so easy to interpret. For example, a worsening of asthma in August, September or October is often difficult to explain. Possibilities include allergy to inhaled molds, an increase in the number of house dust mites in the autumn, changes in the weather, or catching viral respiratory infections when returning to school after the summer holidays.[99,100]

3. ***The symptoms are worse in certain weather conditions.*** The reasons for attacks of asthma after a thunderstorm or heavy rainfall are not fully understood. Allergy to inhaled fungal spores, a fall in the barometric pressure, a sudden fall in air temperature, and release of allergenic starch granules from ruptured pollen grains are all possible explanations.
4. ***The symptoms improve when the patient is away from home (e.g. on holiday).*** Improvement in atopic eczema when the patient goes on holiday is frequently noted, but the reason is usually obscure. In one study[101] there was a significant correlation between improvement in eczema and a more southerly holiday location; improvement was common in holidays taken in the Mediterranean or further south (63/92 – 69%), while holidays in northern Britain were more likely to be associated with deterioration (27/100 – 27%) than improvement (13/100 – 13%). The absence of pets or house dust mites may be the explanation in some cases, although the improvement which occurs on holidays (the disease often virtually disappears) is far greater than the modest improvement which can be seen after admission to hospital in the same patients. Exposure to sea water, sunlight or lack of stress are believed by some parents to be the explanation for such improvement, but there is no evidence to support these ideas. The improvement or complete disappearance of asthma at high altitude resorts, seen in some patients, is generally attributed to the absence of house dust mite and pet animal antigens.
5. ***The presence or absence of a family history of atopic disease.*** Patients with atopic disease often have a positive family history of atopic disease, though atopy is so common in the normal population (wheezing in 21%, eczema in 12% and hay fever in 4% of all children in the UK by the age of 5 years)[102] that a positive family history is a rather non-specific finding. In an apparently atopic child, the absence of a positive family history is more important, and should make the physician reconsider a diagnosis of atopic disease.
6. ***Multiplicity of symptoms.*** Allergic symptoms are usually multiple. It is important to inquire if the patient has other symptoms or signs that may be allergic in origin, in addition to the presenting complaint, and these features are: wheezing, sneezing, pruritus, urticaria, perioral erythema, eczema and conjunctivitis. Several symptoms may coexist. Unilateral symptoms, whether nasal, ocular or respiratory, suggest the presence of a non-allergic condition.
7. ***Symptoms occurring after exposure to pets.*** Several situations cause confusion:
   a. The patient who is noted to have an immediate allergic reaction when stroking or being licked by, for example, a dog, but who is otherwise apparently able to live in the same house as the animal without obvious immediate allergic reactions; delayed reactions or enhanced bronchial reactivity may be overlooked.
   b. The patient who apparently experiences an immediate allergic reaction to, for example, certain cats but not others; again, delayed reactions or enhanced bronchial reactivity may be overlooked.
   c. The patient whose atopic disease predates the acquisition of a pet animal; the animal could still be an important trigger continuing to provoke the disease.
   d. The patient who had a pet animal some years before the onset of symptoms; the animal could still be an important trigger.
   e. The patient's symptoms did not improve when the pet was sent to live elsewhere for a few weeks; sufficient pet antigen to provoke disease may still be present in the household.

   A major source of confusion is that parents equate allergy with immediate reactions, and are unaware that constant exposure to pet antigen in the home tends to cause chronic rather than acute symptoms. Many patients who are allergic to pets react to minute traces of the animal, for example a few hairs on someone's clothing, and this explains why the disease in question fails to improve after the pet is removed from the household. For therapeutic trials to be meaningful, extensive cleaning of carpets, upholstered furniture, clothing and bedding is necessary to remove the allergen.
8. ***Food intolerance.*** Food intolerance is generally associated with multiple symptoms, and it is rare for a single symptom (e.g. asthma, rhinitis, abdominal pain) to be caused by food intolerance. Parents commonly overvalue food intolerance as a cause of symptoms. In one study, double-blind food challenges provoked symptoms in only 27 of 81 (33%) of children whose parents had reported food intolerance.[103]

Unqualified reports of allergy

It is unhelpful to write 'allergy' in a patient's notes without any description of the evidence for the diagnosis. Many untoward events are wrongly labeled as allergies. For example, there are several reasons why penicillin administration may be followed by an adverse event, but few justify a diagnosis of penicillin allergy. A rash during antibiotic therapy may be caused by an underlying infection, or by a coloring agent or preservative included in a liquid preparation of the antibiotic. Loose stools are likely to be due to an underlying viral infection or a disturbance of the gut flora, but it is common to find this described by parents as an allergy to the antibiotic. The incorrect and careless labeling of a child as having penicillin allergy may rob the patient of penicillin treatment for life. Common and similar examples are the patient said to be allergic to cow's milk, in whom inquiry reveals that this is based not on observation of the patient but on the fact that someone has placed the child on a cow's milk-free diet, or the patient said to be allergic to something solely on the basis of skin or blood tests.

Simple cause and effect

The interpretation of the observation that exposure to a single item (e.g. a cat) is followed within minutes by an obvious adverse event (e.g. sneezing and orbital edema) should be quite simple, but there are pitfalls. The history is more reliable if it is based on the parents' unprompted original observations. The parents' observations may be especially unreliable because:

1. There is a strong emotional underlay, e.g. strong attachment to a family pet, leading to underdiagnosis of allergy because the family do not want to part with the animal.
2. In the case of food intolerance, double-blind studies have repeatedly shown parental histories to be particularly unreliable (see below).
3. In the case of behavioral symptoms, there is a widespread but mistaken belief in the importance of adverse reactions to foods or food additives.[34]
4. A parent's report of alleged allergic reactions may have been fabricated (factitious illness).

In general, the quicker the onset of the allergic reaction, the more reliable is the history. A history of the same allergic symptoms after repeated exposure to an allergen is more reliable than a report of a single episode.

DIAGNOSTIC TESTING FOR ALLERGY

There is no ideal test which will predict with certainty whether avoidance of a specific allergen will improve or abolish symptoms in an individual patient. Some of the problems are due to difficulties intrinsic to the test, but some are inherent in the complex nature of atopic disease. Take, for example, a child with asthma who develops sneezing, conjunctivitis and angioedema of the orbit immediately after playing with a cat, and who has a positive skin prick test and positive RAST test to cat dander. Clearly it is logical that the child should avoid cats, but there is no guarantee that cat avoidance will help the patient's asthma. The reasons for the failure of allergen avoidance are discussed later, but can be summarized as:

1. the allergen was incompletely avoided
2. the allergen was only one of several factors provoking the patient's disease
3. the allergen was irrelevant to the patient's symptoms.

It is unrealistic to expect any clinical or laboratory test to cope with the first two of these problems. The best that can be hoped for is that a test will help establish the potential clinical relevance of a particular allergy. Regrettably, the currently available tests, described below, all suffer from serious limitations.

SCRATCH, PRICK AND INTRADERMAL SKIN TESTS

The principle of these skin tests is that the skin wheal and flare reaction to an allergen demonstrates the presence of mast-cell-fixed antibody. This is mainly IgE antibody, although in theory it could also be IgG4 antibody. IgE is produced by plasma cells primarily in lymphoid tissue in the respiratory and gastrointestinal tract, and is distributed via the circulation to all parts of the body, so that the sensitization is generalized and therefore can be demonstrated by skin testing. Age influences the reaction, and a child under 2 years of age produces much less reaction than an older child.

Short-acting antihistamines (H_1 receptor antagonists) must be discontinued at least 5 days prior to skin testing. However, astemizole and certain other non-sedating antihistamines are long acting, and suppression of the wheal and flare response has been noted as much as 5 months after their discontinuation. Because of the variability of cutaneous reactivity, it is necessary to include positive and negative controls whenever skin prick tests are performed. The negative control solution should consist of the diluent used to preserve the allergen extracts. The positive control solution usually consists of histamine, and is mainly used to detect suppression of reactivity, for example caused by H_1 antihistamine medication.

Scratch testing

A drop of allergen solution is placed on the skin which is then scratched so as to superficially penetrate the skin. The scratch test introduces an inconstant amount of allergen through the skin and is therefore poorly standardized and produces results which are too variable for routine clinical use.[104,105]

Prick testing

A drop of allergen solution is placed on the skin which is then pricked with a plastic lance, and the result read after 15 min. The negative control should be negative, unless the patient has dermographism. The histamine control should be positive, unless the patient has recently received H_1 antihistamines, which would invalidate negative skin test results. The flare is ignored, and the diameter of the wheal is measured. Later reactions may occur, but their significance is unclear. Prick tests can also produce variable results, but the introduction of standardized precision lances for prick testing has made the method potentially more reproducible.

The interpretation of skin prick tests is difficult. There is a lack of agreed definition about what constitutes a positive reaction.[106] Most definitions of a positive reaction are based on the absolute diameter of the wheal, with arbitrary cutoff points for positivity at 1 mm, 2 mm or 3 mm. The problems with the interpretation of prick test results in an individual patient are:

1. Skin prick test reactivity may be present in subjects with no clinical evidence of allergy.[104,105]
2. Skin prick test reactivity may persist after clinical evidence of allergy has subsided (e.g. Ford & Taylor[107]).
3. Skin prick tests may be negative in some patients with allergies. For example, skin prick tests are negative in 13–17% of those with rhinitis provoked by pollen.[108]
4. False negative results may occur in infants and toddlers. The wealing capacity of the skin is diminished in early infancy, and when wheals are produced they are smaller than in later life, so that the criteria for a positive wheal must be adjusted.[105] There are no age-related guidelines for what constitutes a positive reaction.
5. There is a poor correlation between the results of provocation tests and prick tests.
6. Skin prick tests for foods are especially unreliable.[16] A positive result using a raw food antigen does not necessarily mean that the cooked food will cause a reaction.
7. False negative skin prick tests can occur after anaphylaxis.[66]

The results of skin tests cannot be taken alone, but need to account for the history and physical findings.[105,109] From a carefully taken history one might suspect a particular allergen, and the finding of a positive prick test would increase the likelihood that the allergen was causing symptoms. Few people, however, would be prepared to ignore a strong history of allergy in the face of a negative prick test, yet it is illogical to regard the prick test as significant when it confirms the history and to disregard it when it fails to do so. The contentious issues in clinical practice are whether a child with atopic disease will benefit from attempts to avoid household pets, house dust mites or certain foods, but skin prick tests are unreliable predictors of response to such measures.

Intradermal testing

Intradermal testing is painful, can cause fatal anaphylaxis, and is only performed for limited reasons and then only if a preliminary skin prick test is negative.[110] Intradermal tests are more sensitive than skin prick testing, and also produce more false positive reactions. As with skin prick testing, there is a lack of agreement as to what constitutes a positive reaction. The number of false positive reactions makes the interpretation of the results of intradermal testing even more difficult than skin prick testing.

Skin patch testing

Patch testing is used to identify causative allergens in suspected allergic contact dermatitis, and is discussed elsewhere.[111]

Measurement of circulating IgE antibody

In vitro tests for circulating allergen-specific IgE antibody (e.g. RAST tests) avoid possible confounding variables in skin testing, namely IgE affinity for mast cells, their tendency for degranulation, and skin reactivity to released mediators. Thus, in theory, the in vitro test should be more reliable than skin testing. However, the clinical interpretation of in vitro IgE antibody tests is subject to most of the same pitfalls as the interpretation of skin prick testing. Additional problems with IgE antibody tests are:

1. Cost.
2. The IgE antibody concentration in the plasma varies with allergen exposure. A few patients with allergic rhinitis are RAST negative before the pollen season, but become positive after the pollen season.
3. A very high level of total circulating IgE (e.g. in children with severe atopic eczema) may cause a false positive result.
4. A very low level of circulating IgE may be associated with false negative results.
5. A very high level of IgG antibody with the same allergen specificity as IgE antibody can cause a false negative result.
6. For each allergen, the test differs in the degree to which it is influenced by elevated total serum IgE.
7. In vitro IgE assays are slightly less sensitive than skin testing.

In vitro tests for IgE antibody are only preferable to skin testing where the patient has had a very severe reaction to the allergen in question (because of the small risk of anaphylaxis with skin testing), where the patient has widespread skin disease (e.g. atopic eczema), where the skin shows dermographism, or when H_1 antihistamines cannot be discontinued.

Provocation challenge tests

With the exception of food challenges in patients with suspected food intolerance, provocation tests (bronchial, nasal, conjunctival) have little place in routine clinical practice but have been helpful in the study of the pathophysiology and pharmacology of atopic disease. The results suffer from the same major limitation as the results of skin or IgE antibody testing, which is that a positive result from an allergen challenge by no means proves that the allergen is contributing to the patient's disease.

Blinded oral food challenge

The test comprises the oral administration of a challenge substance, which is either the item under investigation or an indistinguishable inactive (placebo) substance. Neither the child, the parents nor the observers know the identity of the administered material at the time of the challenge. Food challenges are subject to a number of pitfalls:

1. There is a danger of producing anaphylactic shock, even if anaphylactic shock had not occurred on previous exposure to the food.[22,38]
2. Difficulties arise if a cooked food is used for testing and the patient is only sensitive to a raw food, or vice versa. Cooking reduces the sensitizing capacity of cow's milk, and intolerance to raw but not cooked egg, potato and fish are well described.
3. It is unclear what dosage of different foods is required to exclude food intolerance. The dosage used in studies employing encapsulated foods is inevitably limited. Larger quantities of food may cause an adverse reaction when smaller quantities do not. For example, Hill et al[69] found that whereas 8–10 g of milk powder (corresponding to 60–70 ml of milk) was adequate to provoke a response in some patients with cow's milk protein intolerance, other patients (with late-onset symptoms) required up to 10 times this volume of milk daily for more than 48 h before symptoms developed.
4. Failure to randomize the order of placebo with active substance or to employ a double-blind placebo-controlled methodology are errors common to many studies, especially those of food additives in chronic urticaria.
5. A food challenge performed during a quiescent phase of the disease may fail to provoke an adverse reaction. For example, in chronic urticaria intolerance to salicylates is confined to patients with active disease.
6. The regular administration of salicylates to patients with salicylate intolerance quickly leads to a state of tolerance to salicylate. It is possible, although unproven, that a similar phenomenon occurs with certain food additives. Thus a double-blind challenge performed while a patient is regularly consuming a foodstuff may fail to provoke an adverse reaction.
7. Where food intolerance exists in children with atopic dermatitis, it is common for the patient to be intolerant to several foods. The removal of only one offending item may fail to help the patient and reintroduction may not provoke deterioration.
8. In some situations, factors other than a food are necessary for positive challenges to occur. For example, in a subgroup of patients with exercise-induced anaphylaxis, symptoms only occur if exercise follows the ingestion of a particular food.[71] Exercise or the food alone fail to provoke symptoms.

HYPOSENSITIZATION

Hyposensitization by injection

Hyposensitization comprises the regular injection of allergen extracts with the objective of reducing or abolishing the patient's reaction to the allergen. The mode of action of hyposensitization is poorly understood. The drawbacks to hyposensitization injections are:

1. lack of significant clinical benefit;
2. the need for multiple injections;
3. the need for prolonged (many years) treatment for benefit to be maintained;
4. the risk of fatal anaphylaxis, particularly but not exclusively in subjects with asthma.

Because of the risk of death from anaphylaxis (26 deaths in the UK between 1967 and 1986) the Committee for Safety of Medicines (CSM) in the UK has concluded that hyposensitization should only be used for (1) life-threatening allergy to bee or wasp venom (rare in childhood); and (2) seasonal allergic hay fever (which has not responded to anti-allergy drugs), caused by grass or tree pollen, using licenced products only. In patients with hay fever, those who also have asthma should not be treated with desensitizing vaccines as they are more likely to develop severe adverse reactions. Hyposensitization must only be performed in hospitals with full facilities for cardiopulmonary resuscitation, and patients need to be monitored for 1 h after injections. There is inadequate evidence of benefit from hyposensitization to other allergens such as house dust mite, animal danders and foods and hyposensitization to these allergens is not recommended.

Intolerance to carbamazepine (skin rash) has been successfully treated by the oral administration of 0.1 mg daily and doubling the dose every 2 days, with a delay in increments if any skin rash appears. It is probable that intolerance to a number of other drugs could be approached in the same way,[112] though there is a risk with some drugs (e.g. penicillin, see above) of provoking anaphylaxis. Oral desensitization has been achieved in a small number of children with food intolerance, but carries the risk of anaphylaxis and must be regarded as experimental.

On the very rare occasions in childhood (e.g. endocarditis) when treatment with penicillin is essential, then it is possible to hyposensitize the patient by oral and then continuous intravenous administration,[95] but this procedure carries a risk of fatal anaphylaxis. The protection from hyposensitization is short lived, although it is possible to maintain a state of hyposensitization by long-term administration of a low dose.

Oral hyposensitization

There are a number of anecdotal reports describing successful oral hyposensitization to foods, particularly cow's milk.[113,114] However there are no objective data on the safety or efficacy of this approach, which plainly risks causing anaphylaxis. There are a number of recent claims that sublingual hyposensitization may be a viable alternative to injection hyposensitization. The limited available data suggest that this approach may work, may offer some logistic advantages, and may be safe, but on current evidence sublingual hyposensitization requires further evaluation before it can be recommended for use in routine practice[115] and as yet no licenced preparations are available.

PREVENTION OF ATOPIC DISEASE

Since it was reported that breast-feeding protects against atopic eczema, the notion that atopic disease can be prevented by breast-feeding has been surrounded by confusion. Not one study of this subject is without serious defect, and those from the greatest enthusiasts for breast-feeding are often the most flawed. Objections to previous studies include:

1. ***Observer bias.*** Doctors known to be protagonists of breast-feeding decided whether infants had eczema or not in the full knowledge of whether the baby was breast- or bottle-fed.
2. ***Non-blind ascertainment of history.*** Interviewers asking for feeding history are likely to be biased if they know of the child's outcome (i.e. atopic status). Knowledge of the outcome tends to create an association between exposure and outcome where none exists. Feeding histories must be taken by someone who knows nothing about the child, and should be taken before the outcome is known.
3. ***Reliance on prolonged maternal recall.*** A history taken years after the feeding period is prone to error regarding both the duration and exclusivity of breast-feeding. Prospective studies avoid this problem.
4. ***Adequate exclusivity of breast-feeding.*** If breast-feeding is protective it may be through exclusion of foreign proteins like egg or cow's milk, or protection may be due to protective substances in human milk. The consumption of other foods during breast-feeding may interfere with the protective effect of breast-feeding. Unless breast-feeding has been exclusive for a period of time, it is difficult to test the preventative effect of breast-feeding.
5. ***Definition of atopic diseases.*** The conditions being investigated must be carefully defined. There should be close agreement between the observations of two observers and between the observations of the same observer at different times. Skin rashes, wheezing and sneezing all have numerous causes. Not all are atopic.
6. ***Sufficient duration of breast-feeding.*** Brief exposure to human milk may not be expected to provide long-term protection against subsequent atopic disease. If breast-feeding is protective, then the longer the duration of breast-feeding the greater would be the expected protection against atopic disease.
7. ***Assessment of disease severity.*** Misleading information based on the failure to differentiate between minor and major forms of disease. Studies compared the total incidence of diseases such as eczema or asthma in babies fed different ways, but parents fear *severe* cases. The protective effect of breast-feeding is unlikely to be all or none, so that if there is a genuine protective effect there should be some dose–response relationship. The demonstration of a graded degree of outcome in response to varying duration of breast-feeding would strengthen the inference that breast-feeding prevented the outcome.
8. ***Controls*** are essential to exclude confounding variables such as family history of atopic disease, racial origin, social class, exposure to pets and so on. Atopic mothers may, for example, preferentially breast-feed in the hope of preventing atopic disease. This tends to bias the results against a protective effect of breast-feeding, because the breast-fed infant would then be at greater genetic risk of developing atopy.
9. ***Adequate follow-up is essential.*** Breast-feeding may simply delay the age of onset of disease. Thus a follow-up study lasting 12 months might show a protective effect, but a 24-month follow-up might show no protective effect. Delaying the age of onset might be beneficial or harmful.

Contrary to the current received wisdom that breast-feeding is protective, it is increasingly being recognized that ingested food antigens can pass into human milk.[16,21,39,39a] Maternal avoidance of the food in question is followed by remission of atopic disease in the infant, and re-exposure followed by relapse. Some studies from Scandinavia have served to further undermine belief in the protective effect of breast-feeding, exclusive or otherwise. A prospective study from Finland showed a steadily *increasing* incidence of atopic disease the longer a mother exclusively breast-fed her infant.[116] A prospective study of breast-fed babies from Sweden showed that those who had been exclusively breast-fed in the first few days of life were *more likely* to develop atopic disease than those who were given supplementary cow's milk feeds for the first few days of life and then breast-fed.[117] Finally, a follow-up study of 69 preterm infants showed that the 38 infants fed exclusively with human milk to the age of 4 months had significantly more allergic symptoms than the 31 infants fed with adapted cow's milk formula from birth.[118]

Several studies have examined the effect of the inhalant environment in early infancy on the subsequent manifestations of allergic disease, by comparing the month of birth of patients with immediate skin reactions to specific allergens to the month of birth of a reference population.[119] A relationship between the month of birth and the subsequent development of an allergy has been claimed for birch tree pollen, grass pollen, ragweed pollen and house dust mites, but the evidence is far from clear. The inference has been made (but never substantiated) that allergy to these items could be avoided by ensuring that the birth of a child takes place shortly after the seasonal disappearance of the allergen, thereby avoiding sensitization in infancy.

REFERENCES (* Level 1 evidence)

1 Legendre C, Caillat-Zucman S, Samuel D, et al. Transfer of symptomatic peanut allergy to the recipient of a combined liver-and -kidney transplant. N Engl J Med 1997; 337:822–824.
2 Nowak-Wegrzyn AH, Sicherer SH, Conover-Walker MK, Wood RA. Food allergy after pediatric organ transplantation with tacrolimus immunosuppression. J Allergy Clin Immunol 2001; 108:146–147.
3 Mygind N. Essential allergy. Oxford: Blackwell Scientific; 1986.
4 Chapel H, Haeney M. Essentials of clinical immunology, 2nd edn. Oxford: Blackwell Science; 1988.
5 Kay AB (ed). Allergy and allergic diseases. Oxford: Blackwell; 1997.
6 Middleton E, Reed CE, Ellis EF, et al. Allergy. Principles and practice, 5th edn. St Louis: Mosby; 1998.
7 Ihre E, Axelsson IGK, Zetterstrom O. Late asthmatic reactions and bronchial variability after challenge with low doses of allergen. Clin Allergy 1988; 18:557–567.
8 Holgate ST, Church MK. Allergy. London: Gower Medical; 1993.

9 Fleming DM, Crombie DL. Prevalence of asthma and hayfever in England and Wales. BMJ 1987; 294:279–283.
10 Cookson WO, Moffatt MF. Asthma: an epidemic in the absence of infection? Science 1997; 275:41–42.
*11 Shirakawa T, Enomoto T, Shimazu S, Hopkin JM. The inverse association between tuberculin responses and atopic disorder. Science 1997; 275:77–79.
12 von Ehrenstein OS, von Mutius E, Illi SL, et al. Reduced risk of hay fever and asthma among children of farmers. Clin Exp Allergy 2000; 30:187–193.
12a Aalberse RC. Structural biology of allergens. J Allergy Clin Immunol 2000; 106:228–238.
13 Bush RK, Portnoy JM. The role and abatement of fungal allergens in allergic disease. J Allergy Clin Immunol 2001; 107:S430–S440.
14 Frankland AW. Latex-allergic children. Pediatr Allergy Immunol 1999; 10:152–159.
15 Fisher AA. Contact dermatitis, 3rd edn. Philadelphia: Lea & Febiger; 1986.
16 David TJ. Food and food additive intolerance in childhood. Oxford: Blackwell Scientific; 1993.
*17 Supramaniam G, Warner JO. Artificial food additive intolerance in patients with angio-oedema and urticaria. Lancet 1986; 2:907–909.
18 David TJ. Atopic eczema. Prescribers J 1995; 35:199–205.
19 David TJ, Longson M. Herpes simplex infections in atopic eczema. Arch Dis Child 1985; 60:338–343.
20 David TJ, Cambridge GC. Bacterial infection and atopic eczema. Arch Dis Child, 1986; 61:20–23.
*21 Cant AJ, Bailes JA, Marsden RA, Hewitt D. Effect of maternal dietary exclusion on breast fed infants with eczema: two controlled studies. BMJ 1986; 293:231–233.
22 David TJ. Anaphylactic shock during elimination diets for severe atopic eczema. Arch Dis Child 1984; 59:983–986.
*23 Devlin J, Stanton RHJ, David TJ. Calcium intake and cows' milk free diets. Arch Dis Child 1989; 64:1183–1184.
*24 Mabin DC, Sykes AE, David TJ. Nutritional content of few foods diet in atopic dermatitis. Arch Dis Child 1995; 73:208–210.
*25 Devlin J, David TJ, Stanton RHJ. Six food diet for childhood atopic dermatitis. Acta Dermatovenereologica 1991; 71:20–24.
*26 Mabin DC, Sykes AE, David TJ. Controlled trial of a few foods diet in severe atopic dermatitis. Arch Dis Child 1995; 73:202–207.
27 Devlin J, David TJ, Stanton RHJ. Elemental diet for refractory atopic eczema. Arch Dis Child 1991; 66:93–99.
28 Arlian LG, Platts-Mills TAE. The biology of dust mites and the remediation of mite allergens in allergic disease. J Allergy Clin Immunol 2001; 107:S406–S413.
29 Wood RA, Mudd KE, Eggleston PA. The distribution of cat and dust mite allergens on wall surfaces. J Allergy Clin Immunol 1992; 89:126–130.
30 Mygind N. Nasal allergy, 2nd edn. Oxford: Blackwell Scientific; 1979.
31 Kasper WJ, Howe PM. Fatal varicella after a single course of corticosteroids. Pediatr Infect Dis J 1990; 9:729–732.
32 Clogg DK. Varicella in children receiving steroids for asthma: risks and management. Pediatr Infect Dis J 1992; 11:419–420.
33 Rice P, Simmons K, Carr R, Banatvala J. Near fatal chickenpox during prednisolone treatment. BMJ 1994; 309:1069–1070.
*34 David TJ. Reactions to dietary tartrazine. Arch Dis Child 1987; 62:119–122.
35 Buttriss J (ed). Adverse reactions to food. The Report of a British Nutrition Foundation Task Force. Ch 4, Epidemiology of food intolerance and food allergy, Oxford: Blackwell Science; 2002:57–65.
36 Bock SA. Prospective appraisal of complaints of adverse reactions to foods in children during the first three years of life. Pediatrics 1987; 79:683–688.
37 Bellioni-Businco B, Paganelli R, Lucenti P. Allergenicity of goat's milk in children with cow's milk allergy. J Allergy Clin Immunol 1999; 103:1191–1194.
38 Goldman AS, Anderson DW, Sellers WA, et al. Oral challenge with milk and isolated milk proteins in allergic children. Pediatrics 1963; 32:425–443.
39 Järvinen K-M, Mäkinen-Kiljunen S, Suomalainen H. Cow's milk challenge through human milk evokes immune responses in infants with cow's milk allergy. J Pediatr 1999; 135:506–512.
39a Järvinen K-M, Suomalainen H. Development of cow's milk allergy in breast–fed infants. Clin Exp Allergy 2001; 31: 978–987.
40 Eggesbø M, Botten G, Halvorsen R, Magnus P. The prevalence of CMA/CMPI in young children: the validity of parentally perceived reactions in a population-based study. Allergy 2001; 56:393–402.
41 Hill DJ, Ford RP, Shelton MJ, Hosking CS. A study of 100 infants and young children with cow's milk allergy. Clin Rev Allergy 1984; 2:125–142.
42 Zeiger RS, Sampson HA, Bock SA, et al. Soy allergy in infants and children with IgE-associated cow's milk allergy. J Pediatr 1999; 134:614–622.
*42a David TJ, Waddington E, Stanton RHJ. Nutritional hazards of elimination diets in children with atopic eczema. Arch Dis Child 1984; 59:323–325.
43 Eggesbø M, Botten G, Halvorsen R, Magnus P. The prevalence of allergy to egg: a population-based study in young children. Allergy 2001; 56:403–411.
44 Aickin R, Hill D, Kemp A. Measles immunisation in children with allergy to egg. BMJ 1994; 309:223–225.
45 Lakshman R, Finn A. MMR vaccine and allergy. Arch Dis Child 2000; 82:93–97.
46 Khakoo GA, Lack G. Recommendations for using MMR vaccine in children allergic to eggs. BMJ 2000; 320:929–932.
47 Nakayama T, Aizawa C, Kuno-Sakai H. A clinical analysis of gelatin allergy and determination of its causal relationship to the previous administration of gelatin-containing acellular pertussis combined with diphtheria and tetanus toxoids. J Allergy Clin Immunol 1999; 103:321–325.
48 James JM, Zeiger RS, Lester MR, et al. Safe administration of influenza vaccine to patients with egg allergy. J Pediatr 1998; 133:624–628.
50 Derbes VJ, Krafchuk JD. Osmylogenic urticaria. Arch Dermatol, 1957; 76:103–104.
51 Aas K. Fish allergy and the codfish model. In: Brostoff J, Challacombe SJ (eds). Food allergy and intolerance. London: Baillière Tindall; 1987:356–366.
52 Koppelman SJ, Wensing M, de Jong GAH, Knulst AC. Anaphylaxis caused by the unexpected presence of casein in salmon. Lancet 1999; 354:2136.
53 Sicherer SH, Muñoz-Furlong A, Burks AW, Sampson HA. Prevalence of peanut and tree nut allergy in the US determined by a random digit telephone survey. J Allergy Clin Immunol 1999; 103:559–562.
*54 Bock SA, Muñoz-Furlong A, Sampson HA. Fatalities due to anaphylactic reactions to foods. J Allergy Clin Immunol 2001; 107:191–193.
55 Pumphrey RSH, Stanworth SJ. The clinical spectrum of anaphylaxis in north-west England. Clin Exp Allergy 1996; 26: 1364–1370.
56 Hourihane JOB, Dean TP, Warner JO. Peanut allergy in relation to heredity, maternal diet, and other atopic diseases: results of a questionnaire survey, skin prick testing, and food challenges. BMJ 1996; 313:518–521.
57 Sicherer SH, Furlong TJ, Maes HH, et al. Genetics of peanut allergy: a twin study. J Allergy Clin Immunol 2000; 106:53–56.
*58 Beyer K, Morrow E, Li XM, et al. Effects of cooking methods on peanut allergenicity. J Allergy Clin Immunol 2001; 107:1077–1081.
*59 Hourihane JOB, Bedwani SJ, Dean TP, Warner JO. Randomised, double blind, crossover challenge study of allergenicity of peanut oils in subjects allergic to peanuts. BMJ 1997; 314:1084–1088.
*59a Hourihane JOB, Kilburn SA, Nordlee JA et al. An evaluation of the sensitivity of subjects with peanut allergy to very low does of peanut protein: a randomized, double-blind, placebo-controlled food challenge study: J Allergy Clin Immunol 1997; 100:596–600.
60 Teuber SS, Brown RL, Haapanen LA. Allergenicity of gourmet nut oils processed by different methods. J Allergy Clin Immunol 1997; 99:502–506.
61 Koppelman SJ, Vlooswijk RAA, Knippels LMJ, et al. Quantification of major peanut allergens Ara h 1 and Ara h 2 in the peanut varieties Runner, Spanish, Virginia, and Valencia, bred in different parts of the world. Allergy 2001; 56:132–137.
62 Sicherer SH, Burks AW, Sampson HA. Clinical features of acute allergic reactions to peanut and tree nuts in children. Pediatrics 1998; 102(1):e6.
63 Bernhisel-Broadbent J, Sampson HA. Cross-allergenicity in the legume botanical family in children with food hypersensitivity. J Allergy Clin Immunol 1989; 83:435–440.
64 Steinman HA. 'Hidden' allergens in foods. J Allergy Clin Immunol 1996; 98:241–250.
65 Ewan PW, Clark AT. Long-term prospective observational study of patients with

peanut and nut allergy after participation in a management plan. Lancet 2001; 357:111–115.
66 Aalto-Korte K, Mäkinen-Kiljunen S. False negative SPT after anaphylaxis. Allergy 2001; 56:461–462.
67 Pucar F, Kagan R, Lim H, Clarke AE. Peanut challenge: a retrospective study of 140 patients. Clin Exp Allergy 2001; 31:40–46.
68 Armstrong D, Rylance G. Definitive diagnosis of nut allergy. Arch Dis Child 1999; 80:175–177.
69 Hill DJ, Ball G, Hosking CS. Clinical manifestations of cows' milk allergy in childhood. I. Associations with in-vitro cellular immune responses. Clin Allergy 1988; 18:469–479.
69a Hill DJ, Heine RG, Hosking CS Management of peanut and nut allergies. Lancet 2001; 357:87–88.
70 Kelso JM. Resolution of peanut allergy. J Allergy Clin Immunol 2000; 106:777.
71 Kidd JM, Cohen SH, Sosman AJ, Fink JN. Food-dependent exercise-induced anaphylaxis. J Allergy Clin Immunol 1983; 71:407–411.
72 Harris JB. Natural toxins. Animal, plant, and microbial. Oxford: Clarendon Press: 1986.
73 Young E, Patel S, Stoneham M, et al. The prevalence of reaction to food additives in a survey population. J R Coll Physicians Lond 1987; 21:241–247.
74 Brehler R, Theissen U, Mohr C, Luger T. 'Latex-fruit syndrome'. Frequency of cross-reacting IgE antibodies. Allergy 1997; 52: 404–410.
*75 Chen Z, Posch A, Cremer R, et al. Identification of hevein (Hev b 6.02) in Hevea latex as a major cross-reacting allergen with avocado fruit in patients with latex allergy. J Allergy Clin Immunol 1998; 102:476–481.
76 Sweatman MC, Tasker R, Warner JO, et al. Oro-facial granulomatosis. Response to elemental diet and provocation by food additives. Clin Allergy 1986; 16:331–338.
77 Tücke J, Posch A, Baur X. Latex type I sensitization and allergy in children with atopic dermatitis. Evaluation of cross-reactivity to some foods. Pediatr Allergy Immunol 1999; 10: 160–167.
78 Pumphrey RSH, Duddridge M, Norton J. Fatal latex allergy. J Allergy Clin Immunol 2001; 107:558.
79 Franklin W, Pandolfo J. Latex as a food allergen. N Engl J Med 1999; 341:1858.
*80 Heilman DK, Jones RT, Swanson MC, Yunginger JW. A prospective controlled study showing that rubber gloves are the major contributor to latex aeroallergen levels in the operating room. J Allergy Clin Immunol 1996; 98:325–330.
*81 Pumphrey RSH. Lessons for management of anaphylaxis from a study of fatal reactions. Clin Exp Allergy 2000; 30:1144–1150.
82 Patel L, Radivan FS, David TJ. Management of anaphylactic reactions to food. Arch Dis Child 1994; 71:370–375.
83 Unsworth DJ. Adrenaline syringes are vastly over prescribed. Arch Dis Child 2001; 84:410–411.
*84 Lazarou J, Pomeranz BH, Corey PN. Incidence of adverse drug reactions in hospitalized patients: a meta-analysis of prospective studies. JAMA 1998; 279:1200–1205.
85 DeShazo R, Kemp S. Allergic reactions to drugs and biologic agents. JAMA 1997; 278:1895–1906.
86 Boguniewicz M, Leung DY. Hypersensitivity reactions to antibiotics commonly used in children. Pediatr Infect Dis J 1995; 14:221–231.
*87 Salkind AR, Cuddy PG, Foxworth JW. Is this patient allergic to penicillin? An evidence-based analysis of the likelihood of penicillin allergy. JAMA 2001; 285:2498–2505.
88 Gueant JL, Aimone-Gastin I, Namour F. Diagnosis and pathogenesis of the anaphylactic and anaphylactoid reactions to anesthetics. Clin Exp Allergy 1998; 28(Suppl 4):65–70.
89 Gruchalla R. Understanding drug allergies. J Allergy Clin Immunol 2000; 105:S637–S644.
90 Parker CW, Shapiro J, Kern M, Eisen HN. Hypersensitivity to penicillenic acid derivatives in human beings with penicillin allergy. J Exp Med 1962; 115:821–838.
91 Gruchalla RS. Acute drug desensitization. Clin Exp Allergy 1998; 28(Suppl 4):63–64.
92 Idsoe O, Guthe T, Willcox RR, De Weck AL. Nature and extent of penicillin side-reactions, with particular reference to fatalities from anaphylactic shock. Bull World Health Organ 1968; 38:159–188.
93 Kelkar PS, Li JT. Cephalosporin allergy. N Engl J Med 2001; 345:804–809.
94 Green GR, Rosenblum AH, Sweet LC. Evaluation of penicillin hypersensitivity: value of clinical history and skin testing with penicilloyl-polyserine and penicillin G. J Allergy Clin Immunol 1977; 60:339–345.
95 Stark BJ, Earl HS, Gross GN, et al. Acute and chronic desensitization of penicillin-allergic patients using oral penicillin. J Allergy Clin Immunol 1987; 79:523–532.
96 Babu KS, Salvi SS. Aspirin and asthma. Chest 2000; 118:1470–1476.
97 Sly PD, Landau LI. Diurnal variation in bronchial responsiveness in asthmatic children. Pediatr Pulmonol 1986; 2:344–352.
98 Murray AB, Ferguson AC, Morrison BJ. Diagnosis of house dust mite allergy in asthmatic children: what constitutes a positive history? J Allergy Clin Immunol 1983; 71:21–28.
99 Khot A, Burn R, Evans N, et al. Biometeorological triggers in childhood asthma. Clin Allergy 1988; 18:351–358.
100 Storr J, Lenney W. School holidays and admissions with asthma. Arch Dis Child 1989; 64:103–107.
101 Turner MA, Devlin J, David TJ. Holidays and atopic eczema. Arch Dis Child 1991; 66:212–215.
102 Butler NR, Golding J. From birth to five. A study of the health and behaviour of Britain's 5-year-olds. Oxford: Pergamon; 1986.
103 May CD, Bock SA. A modern clinical approach to food hypersensitivity. Allergy 1978; 33:166–188.
104 Lessof MH. Skin tests. In: Lessof MH, Lee TH, Kemeny DM (eds). Allergy: an international textbook. Chichester: John Wiley; 1987:281–287.
105 Bousquet J, Michel FB. In vivo methods for study of allergy. Skin tests, techniques, and interpretation. In: Middleton E, Reed CE, Ellis EF, et al. (eds). Allergy. Principles and practice. St Louis: Mosby; 1993:573–627.
106 Lessof MH, Buisseret PD, Merrett J, et al. Assessing the value of skin tests. Clin Allergy 1980; 10:115–120.
107 Ford RPK, Taylor B. Natural history of egg hypersensitivity. Arch Dis Child 1982; 57:649–652.
108 Pepys J. Skin testing. Br J Hosp Med 1975; 14:412–417.
109 Patterson R. Allergic diseases. Diagnosis and management, 3rd edn. Philadelphia: Lippincott; 1985.
110 Bernstein IL. Proceedings of the task force guidelines for standardizing old and new techniques used for the diagnosis and treatment of allergic diseases. J Allergy Clin Immunol 1988; 82(suppl):487–526.
111 Wilkinson JD, Rycroft RJG. Contact dermatitis. In: Champion RH, Burton JL, Ebling FJG (eds), Rook/Wilkinson/Ebling textbook of dermatology. Oxford: Blackwell Scientific; 1992:611–715.
112 Battersby NC, Patel L, David TJ. Increasing dose regimen in children with reactions to ceftazidime. Clin Exp Allergy 1995; 25:1211–1217.
113 Wüthrich B. Oral desensitization with cow's milk in cow's milk allergy. Pro! Highlights in Food Allergy, Wüthrich B, Ortolani C (eds). Monogr Allergy 1996; 32:236–240.
114 Bauer A, Ekanayake Mudiyanselage S, Wigger-Alberti W, Elsner P. Oral rush desensitization to milk. Allergy 1999; 54:894–895.
115 Frew AJ, Smith HE. Sublingual immunotherapy. J Allergy Clin Immunol 2001; 107:441–444.
116 Savilahti E, Tainio VM, Salmenpera L, et al. Prolonged exclusive breast feeding and heredity as determinants in infantile atopy. Arch Dis Child 1987; 62:269–273.
117 Lindfors A, Enocksson E. Development of atopic disease after early administration of cow milk formula. Allergy 1988; 43:11–16.
118 Savilahti E, Tuomikoski-Jaakkola P, Jarvenpaa AL, Virtanen M. Early feeding of preterm infants and allergic symptoms during childhood. Acta Pediatr 1993; 82:340–344.
119 Zeiger RS. Development and prevention of allergic diseases in childhood. In: Middleton E, Reed CE, Ellis EF, et al. (eds). Allergy. Principles and practice. St Louis: Mosby; 1993: 1137–1171.

32

Accidents, poisoning and SIDS

Jo Sibert, John M Goldsmid, Peter J Fleming

POISONING IN CHILDHOOD

Poisoning in children may be accidental, non-accidental, and iatrogenic or, in older children, deliberate.

ACCIDENTAL CHILD POISONING

Epidemiology

Accidental poisoning is predominantly seen in children under the age of 5 years but older children may be involved if they are developmentally delayed. The peak age is between 1 and 4 years. More boys than girls take poisons accidentally. Some children die from poisoning each year, but the number of deaths has fallen over recent years, probably because of better treatment and because of the child-resistant container (CRC) regulations. There are also less tricyclic antidepressants prescribed. Though the number of deaths are few, many more children are admitted to hospital for treatment and observation and even more present to hospital accident and emergency departments. Many of these are sent home directly because they have taken relatively non-toxic substances.

Substances taken

Children may take a variety of substances accidentally. These are conveniently divided into medicines (prescribed and non-prescribed), household products and plants. The majority of children who take poisons do not have serious symptoms. Medicines may be of low toxicity, e.g. the oral contraceptive pill or antibiotics; intermediate toxicity, which may cause symptoms in young children; or potential high toxicity. Many of the household products children take may be relatively non-toxic, but a few such as caustic soda, soldering flux and paint stripper may cause serious harm. The commonest household product that children take is white spirit and turpentine substitute. About 10% of these children have patchy chest X-ray changes. In developing countries paraffin (kerosene) poisoning is a particular problem as it is used as a cooking fuel and is often kept in open containers. These incidents are common in poor social circumstances and in summer and are probably largely related to thirst. Kerosene may cause serious aspiration pneumonitis and death.

A child may eat a poisonous plant accidentally or a group may sample a plant, such as laburnum, together. Most plants are relatively non-toxic, e.g. cotoneaster, rowan or sweet pea. However, some such as arum lily, deadly nightshade or yew can cause serious symptoms.

Etiology of accidental child poisoning

Perhaps surprisingly, the availability of poisons does not appear to be a major factor in accidental child poisoning. There is evidence that family psychosocial stress and behavioral problems, such as hyperactivity, predispose towards child poisoning[1] and these family and personality findings have importance for the prevention of child poisoning.

Preventing child poisoning

Education

A campaign in Birmingham, UK, to publicize accidental child poisoning and to encourage the return of medicines concluded 'that publicity, storage and destruction of unwanted medicines have little preventive value'. A New Zealand study evaluated placing 'Mr. Yuk' stickers on poisons together with a campaign to prevent child poisoning. No reduction in poisoning admissions was found. The link between accidental child poisoning and family psychosocial stress and hyperactivity make it unlikely on theoretical grounds that education will be effective. Families under stress will be unlikely to remember safety propaganda.

Child-resistant containers

Child-resistant containers (CRCs) were first suggested in 1959 by Dr Jay Arena in Durham, North Carolina. These containers were evaluated in a community in the United States by Scherz[2] and found to be successful. They were then introduced into the United States for aspirin preparations, with successful results. Following this work in the US, child-resistant closures were introduced by regulation in 1976 in the United Kingdom for junior aspirin and paracetamol preparations. This resulted in a fall in admissions of children under 5 years with salicylate poisoning.[3] In 1978 CRCs were introduced by regulation for adult aspirin and paracetamol tablets. Child-resistant containers or packaging are now a professional requirement by the Royal Pharmaceutical Society and are regulated for a number of household products (e.g. white spirit and turpentine substitute).

Other methods of preventing child poisoning

Lockable medicine cupboards have been suggested for the prevention of child poisoning. On theoretical grounds they are unlikely to be effective as parents under stress are less likely to remember to put their medicines away or lock the cabinets. Making household products unpalatable with bitter chemical agents (e.g. Bitrex – denatonium bromide)[4] is a possible preventive measure to child poisoning. Serious accidental poisoning might also be prevented by a reduction in the prescribing of toxic drugs. This has been done for barbiturates and tricyclics and might also be done for quinine and vaporizing solutions.

DELIBERATE SELF-POISONING IN OLDER CHILDREN

A number of older children take poisons deliberately. They may take medications as a response to an emotional crisis (mainly adolescent girls) or ingest excess alcohol (predominantly adolescent boys). They form one end of an age spectrum of overdose in adults.

NON-ACCIDENTAL POISONING (see also Ch. 34)

The recognition of non-accidental poisoning as an extended syndrome of child abuse was made in 1976. These children are deliberately poisoned by their parents and may present with bizarre or unusual symptoms rather than poisoning directly. A number of medicines or household products may be given to children including salt in feeds to babies. These cases probably form part of the syndrome of factitious illness in childhood or the Munchausen syndrome by proxy.

TREATMENT OF CHILD POISONING

Management of accidental poisoning in childhood

General

The majority of children who present to hospital after accidental poisoning do not have serious symptoms. There are nevertheless a few children who have taken a significant poison and who are potentially ill or are ill. We should clearly like to prevent unnecessary admissions to hospital whilst maintaining safety. A way round this dilemma is to classify the substance the child has taken into one of four categories: low toxicity, uncertain toxicity, intermediate toxicity or potential high toxicity. After classification children can be either sent home, observed in the accident and emergency department or admitted for observation or treatment. THE POISONS INFORMATION CENTER SHOULD BE CONTACTED IF THERE IS ANY DOUBT ABOUT THE TOXICITY OF A SUBSTANCE A CHILD HAS TAKEN OR THE TREATMENT THAT IS NEEDED. A list of some of the poisons commonly taken accidentally by children is shown in Table 32.1.

Older children who have taken poisons deliberately and cases of iatrogenic poisoning and non-accidental poisoning should all be admitted to hospital.

The parents of all children who present with accidental poisoning should be given advice regarding the storage of medicines and household products. The health visitor should be contacted in all cases, remembering that family psychosocial stress is often linked with accidental poisoning in childhood. There may be specific problems, which need medical or social help.

Emptying the stomach

It used to be standard practice to empty the stomach in cases of accidental poisoning in childhood. This has come under review and emesis using ipecacuanha pediatric mixture (ipecac) is now not used.[5] Gastric lavage was largely abandoned some years ago. It may be needed in certain cases, such as iron poisoning, for substances to be instilled into the stomach. The stomach should never be emptied in cases of hydrocarbon ingestion, such as paraffin or white spirit, or with corrosive substances such as caustic soda.

Activated charcoal

Activated charcoal is being increasingly used in the management of childhood poisoning. Activated charcoal absorbs toxic materials in the gut by offering alternative binding sites. Its routine use is limited by its poor acceptance by children. Activated charcoal may not be effective more than 1 h after ingestion.[6] Two preparations are available, Medicoal 5 g sachets and Carbomix 50 g. Activated charcoal has been used for a variety of drugs including aspirin, carbamazepine, digoxin, mefenamic acid, phenobarbital, phenytoin, quinine and theophylline. It is particularly useful in tricyclic antidepressant poisoning.

Accidental poisoning with substances of low toxicity

Children who have taken substances of low toxicity can be allowed home after assessment. Their parents should be given advice regarding storage of medicines and the general practitioner should be contacted. If there is doubt over what substance has been taken, a child should be admitted for observation.

Accidental poisoning where there is uncertainty of toxicity

If there is any doubt about the toxicity of a substance a child may have taken, the Poison Information Center should be contacted day or night:

London – Guy's Hospital	Tel. 0207 407 7600 or 0207 635 9191
Edinburgh – Royal Infirmary	Tel. 0131 536 1000
Cardiff – Llandough Hospital	Tel. 02920 709901
Belfast – Royal Victoria Infirmary	Tel. 01232 240503

Some children arrive in hospital having taken unknown tablets or household products. Often research with the pharmacist

Table 32.1 Guide to toxicity of substances taken in accidental child poisoning

Low toxicity
Medicines
Antibiotics (except ciprofloxacin, sulfasalazine and chloramphenicol)
Antacids
Calamine
Oral contraceptives
Vitamin preparations which do not contain iron
Zinc oxide creams
Household products
Chalks and crayons
Emulsion paints and water paints
Fabric softeners
Plant food and fertilizers
Silica gel
Toothpaste
Wallpaper paste
Washing powder (except dishwasher powder)
Plants
Begonia
Cacti
Cotoneaster
Cyclamen
Honeysuckle
Mahonia
Rowan
Spider plant
Sweet pea
Intermediate toxicity
Medicines
Cough medicines (most)
Fluoride
Ibuprofen
Laxatives
Lidocaine (lignocaine) gel
Paracetamol elixir
Salbutamol
Household products
Alcohol-containing colognes, aftershaves and perfumes
Bleach
Detergents
Disinfectants (most)
Nail varnish remover
Paints (oil based)
Pyrethrins
Rat or mouse poison
Talc
Window cleaners
Plants
Berberis
Fuchsia
Holly
Pyracantha
Potentially toxic
Medicines
Benzodiazepines
Carbamazepine
Codeine-containing cough medicines
Clonidine
Digoxin
Diphenoxylate (Lomotil)
Hyoscine
Iron
Mefenamic acid (Ponstan)
Metoclopramide
Mianserin (Bolvidon)
Paracetamol tablets
Phenytoin
Quinine
Salicylates
Theophyllines
Tricyclic antidepressants (including dothiepin and amitriptyline)
Household products
Acids
Alcoholic beverages
Alkalis
Bottle-sterilizing tablets
Camphor and camphorated oil
Carbon monoxide
Cetrimide
Disc batteries
Essential oils (e.g. real turpentine, pine oil, citronella and eucalyptus)
Methylene chloride (paint stripper)
Organochloride insecticides
Organophosphorus insecticides
Paradichlorobenzene mothballs
Paraquat
Petroleum distillates (white spirit, paraffin, turpentine substitute)
Phenolic compounds
Slug pellets (metaldehyde)
Plants
Arum lily
Deadly nightshade
Laburnum
Philodendron
Yew

will help. If there is doubt the child should be admitted for observation.

Intermediate toxicity

Children who have taken substances of intermediate toxicity accidentally should be observed for a period in hospital (usually up to 6 h) until one can be confident that significant symptoms are not going to occur. This observation can be undertaken in many cases in an accident and emergency department which has a section for children or for short periods in the pediatric ward or day unit. If there are adverse factors, particularly social factors, children should be admitted to hospital for longer periods.

Accidental poisoning with potentially toxic substances

Children who have taken substances of potential toxicity should be admitted to hospital for observation and treatment.

Treatment of individual poisons

Table 32.1 shows the toxicity of the substances which are most frequently taken accidentally by children under 5.

Deliberate poisoning in older children

Deliberate poisoning in older children should be treated differently from accidental poisoning in younger children. These children form one end of the age spectrum of overdose in adults and such children are more likely to take significant amounts of poison. Substances that can be regarded as having intermediate toxicity when taken accidentally should be regarded as potentially toxic when taken deliberately.

Poisoning in older children should be recognized as a serious symptom and an indication of child and family disturbance. Children who deliberately take poisons show more disturbed family relationships than children referred for psychiatric help for other reasons. They have a high level of psychiatric symptoms, especially depression. All children who take poisons deliberately should be admitted to hospital and should be assessed by a child and adolescent psychiatrist. Many will need educational, psychological and social work help as well as psychiatric assessment.

CHRONIC POISONING

Lead poisoning

Lead is a serious poison for children. Its toxic effects are due to its combination with sulfhydryl groups of essential enzymes resulting in disturbances in carbohydrate metabolism, cell membrane transport, renal tubular absorption and other body processes. The blood level at which toxic effects become evident varies from child to child but in general major symptoms are unlikely if the whole blood lead level is less than 2.5 μmol/L (52 μg/100 ml). It is probable that behavioral and learning difficulties may result from exposure to only moderately elevated lead levels between 1.4 and 2.9 μmol/L. Low level fetal lead exposure at less than 1.4 μmol/L may also affect mental development. Children in the United Kingdom may be poisoned by sucking or chewing lead paint. Lead from burning batteries, lead shot for fishing and lead from old water pipes are other potential sources. Children from the Indian subcontinent may be poisoned by *surma*, the lead-containing eye make-up used even in young babies.

Clinical features

Children who are poisoned by lead are likely to present with pica (compulsive eating of substances other than food), anorexia, abdominal pain, irritability and failure to thrive. Severe lead poisoning may present with neurological symptoms including drowsiness, convulsions and coma from lead encephalopathy. Lead poisoning may also present as progressive intellectual deterioration.

The diagnosis is made by elevated blood lead levels and anemia with hypochromia and basophilic stippling. There may also be increased bone density with transverse bands at the ends of the long bones on radiological examination.

Treatment

The source of lead should be identified and removed. Chelating agents should be used to form non-toxic lead compounds. In mild cases D-penicillamine should be used orally in two daily doses of 10 mg/kg. In severe cases sodium calcium edetate (EDTA) should be used, 40 mg/kg by i.v. infusion over 1 h twice daily for up to 5 days. Each gram of EDTA should be diluted in 100 ml normal saline. The effectiveness of EDTA can be enhanced by the deep i.m. injection of dimercaprol 2.5 mg/kg 4-hourly for 2 days, 2–4 times on the third day, then 1–2 times daily until recovery.

Mercury poisoning

This once common disorder was called 'pink disease' because of the color of the extremities or 'acrodynia' because of the accompanying pain. It was largely due to the use of mercury-containing teething powders which have now been withdrawn. There was anorexia, loss of weight and hypotonia as well as the characteristic painful red or pink extremities. A differential diagnosis of this condition is the red extremities of neglected children. Treatment of mercury poisoning is by the deep i.m. injection of dimercaprol 5 mg/kg 4-hourly for 2 days, 2.5 mg/kg twice daily for the third day and once daily for the next 10 days.

Chronic boric acid poisoning

Chronic boric acid poisoning was a major problem in the 1940s and 1950s. It was caused by ingestion of boric acid used either as a treatment for nappy rash or as a pacifier. It presented with convulsions, vomiting and diarrhea.

NOTES ON POISONING WITH INDIVIDUAL SUBSTANCES

Intermediate toxicity

Medicines

Cough medicines. Most cough medicines do not cause serious symptoms in the doses available to children. Medicines based on antihistamines may cause drowsiness and anticholinergic effects. Drowsiness will usually not need treatment but if coma occurs resuscitative measures should be used. Medicines based on codeine should be regarded as potentially toxic.

Fluoride. Fluoride has a rapid action but is seldom toxic in the quantities taken by children. Symptoms include vomiting, nausea and abdominal pain.

Ibuprofen. Ibuprofen and other non-steroidal anti-inflammatory agents only seldom cause symptoms in children. Symptoms may include gastrointestinal irritation, kidney and liver damage. Oral fluids should be encouraged.

Laxatives. Serious symptoms after laxative ingestion are rare. If diarrhea occurs it occurs quickly. Occasionally patients may need intravenous fluids. The child should be observed for serious symptoms for a short time.

Lidocaine (lignocaine) gel. Local anesthetics such as lidocaine (lignocaine) are toxic in overdose, causing convulsions and circulatory collapse. Significant amounts of lidocaine (lignocaine) gel are seldom ingested accidentally by children.

Paracetamol elixir. Paracetamol elixirs such as Calpol are sweet and sickly in large doses and serious accidental poisoning is very rare. There is insufficient paracetamol in most small bottles of elixir to cause problems. Blood levels should be checked 4 h after the ingestion if more than 150 mg/kg has been taken. Treatment (see potential toxicity section below) is only needed if the serum paracetamol level is above 200 mg/L at 4 h (or in rare delayed cases in children above 50 mg/L at 12 h). In most cases children can be discharged after a period of observation.

Salbutamol. There may be peripheral vasodilatation, muscle tremors and agitation. Serious symptoms are rare although severe hypokalemia and arrhythmias have been seen.

Household products

Alcohol-containing perfumes, cologne and aftershave. Symptomatic cases are rare. Asymptomatic children can be allowed home after a short period of observation to make certain they do not become drowsy.

Bleach. Ingestion of household bleach causes fewer problems than would be expected.[7] Ipecac or lavage should not be used. Milk or antacids can be given orally. Local lesions in the mouth can be treated symptomatically and in the few cases where significant esophageal involvement is possible, endoscopy can be undertaken.

Detergents (anionic). Dishwashing liquid and shampoo are only toxic in large doses. Vomiting occurs in large doses. A period of observation may be needed.

Disinfectants. Serious cases are unusual.

Nail varnish remover (acetone). Observation for a period should be all that is needed but nausea and vomiting may occur, going on to coma if large amounts are taken.

Paints (oil based). Unless the paint has lead in it, the only problems that occur are caused by the petroleum distillate base. The stomach should not be emptied. In practice children do not seem to take significant amounts.

Pyrethrins. These insecticides are not usually a hazard if ingested or inhaled accidentally. The child should be observed for a short period.

Rat or mouse poison. The common ingredients of rat or mouse poison (warfarin or dichlorolose) are usually non-toxic in the doses taken by children. The exact type of poison should be identified using the poisons center and in most cases the child can be sent home after a short period of observation.

If large amounts of warfarin are ingested vitamin K can be used but this is not needed in most cases.

Talc. Talc is only toxic if inhaled. It may cause retching and choking due to pulmonary edema. Cases of ingestion only need a short period of observation to make certain inhalation did not occur.

Window cleaner. Most are non-toxic unless aspirated. The cleaner should be identified using the poisons center. In most cases the child can be sent home after a short period of observation.

Plants

Berberis. Very occasionally causes confusion, epistaxis or vomiting. The child should be observed for a short period.

Fuchsia. Unlikely to cause problems although potentially toxic. Observe for a short period.

Holly. Unlikely to cause problems although potentially toxic due to ilicin and theobromine.

Pyracantha. This causes nausea and vomiting but is unlikely to cause problems. The child should be observed for a short period.

Potential toxicity

Medicines

Barbiturates. May cause coma and hypotension. Cases are becoming less common, as they are less frequently prescribed. Activated charcoal can be used.

Benzodiazepines – tranquilizers and hypnotics such as diazepam (Valium) and nitrazepam (Mogadon). These can cause drowsiness and coma, but problems are unusual in accidental ingestion. In very young children respiratory depression may need treatment with artificial ventilation.

Carbamazepine. This drug has some anticholinergic activity. Paradoxically convulsions and violent reactions may occur as well as cardiac problems such as heart block. Activated charcoal is useful to adsorb carbamazepine.

Codeine-containing cough medicines. If significant amounts are taken there can be respiratory depression, for which the antagonist naloxone can be used (10 μg/kg i.v.)

Clonidine. Clonidine can cause bradycardia, hypotension, coma and gastrointestinal upset. The use of atropine and dopamine infusion for the hypotension is controversial and supportive treatment (including assisted ventilation) may be adequate for even the most severe cases.[8]

Digoxin. Digoxin can be a serious poison in children, with only a few tablets being fatal. Activated charcoal is useful. These children should be monitored very closely, probably in an intensive care unit, with careful ECG monitoring. Beta-blockers such as propranolol should be used in severe cases, with atropine if there is heart block. The serum potassium should not be allowed to go too low or too high. Digoxin-specific antibody fragments are now available for the reversal of life-threatening overdosage (Digibind, Wellcome).

Diphenoxylate (the active constituent in Lomotil, the antidiarrheal agent). This compound has an opiate-like action, which causes prolonged respiratory depression. Treatment is with the opiate antagonist naloxone (10 μg/kg as i.v. bolus). There may be a transient improvement followed by relapse and cases should be observed for at least 36 h and repeated doses of naloxone given as necessary.

Hyoscine. Hyoscine may cause dilated pupils, dry mouth, tachycardia and delirium due to anticholinergic effects. Observation will be all that is needed with most patients.

Iron. Iron is a potentially very serious poison, initially causing vomiting and hematemesis, but going on to acute gastric ulceration and shock. Later convulsions and cardiac arrhythmias may occur. Iron tablets may be detected by X-ray of the abdomen. Further treatment should be aimed at preventing additional absorption of the iron, by the use of the chelating agent desferrioxamine methylate, instilled into the stomach (5–10 g in 50–100 ml of liquid). Desferrioxamine should also be used parenterally (15 mg/kg/h to a maximum of 80 mg/kg) in all cases where a potentially toxic amount of iron may have been taken. The severity of a poisoning episode can be judged by the serum iron level. Levels above 16.1 mmol/L at 4 h indicate significant poisoning.

Mefenamic acid (Ponstan). This drug rarely causes problems in young children. Activated charcoal is effective. Convulsions can be treated with diazepam.

Metoclopramide (Maxolon). In overdose this drug causes extrapyramidal signs, drowsiness and vomiting. If extrapyramidal signs develop antiparkinsonian drugs such as procyclidine can be used.

Mianserin (Bolvidon). Mianserin has milder anticholinergic effects than the tricyclic antidepressants. Serious problems are uncommon. Drowsiness is the most common symptom.

Paracetamol (acetaminophen). Serious accidental ingestion of paracetamol is rare in children because the tablets are bitter and difficult to swallow and the elixir is too sweet to take in toxic quantities. Serious paracetamol poisoning may cause hepatocellular necrosis. Patients at risk of liver damage can be identified by measurement of blood levels 4 h after the ingestion. Treatment is needed if the serum paracetamol level is above 1.32 mmol/L (200 mg/L) at 4 h (or in rare delayed cases in children, 0.33 mmol/L at 12 h). Treatment is with oral methionine (at a dose of 1 g 4-hourly) for four doses. *N*-acetylcysteine intravenously is an alternative particularly in children who are vomiting or who present after 12–24 h when methionine is ineffective.

Phenytoin. Phenytoin ingestion may cause ataxia and nystagmus. Activated charcoal can be used.

Quinine. Quinine is a significant poison in children and has caused several deaths. It is used for night cramps. Quinidine and chloroquine are also toxic. Activated charcoal can be used.

Salicylates. Severe poisoning is now rare as aspirin preparations are no longer used for children because of the dangers of Reye's syndrome. Hyperventilation is an early sign of significant salicylate poisoning due to stimulation of the respiratory center with resultant respiratory alkalosis. There may also be a metabolic acidosis. In severe cases there is disorientation and coma.

The severity of a poisoning episode can be judged by salicylate levels. Toxicity can occur at levels above 2.2 mmol/L (300 mg/L) in children. In asymptomatic and mild cases nothing more needs to be done apart from encouraging fluid and electrolyte replacement and giving vitamin K. Activated charcoal is useful. Forced alkaline diuresis can be used in moderate to severe cases but its use is controversial and alkalinization of the urine is the important thing rather than the induction of excessive urine flow. Peritoneal dialysis can also be effective.

Theophylline. Theophylline can cause restlessness, agitation, vomiting, convulsions, coma, hypotension, hypokalemia and ventricular tachycardia. Activated charcoal can be used. Convulsions can be treated with diazepam.

Tricyclic antidepressants. Tricyclic antidepressants such as amitriptyline are serious poisons for young children. They may cause cardiac effects such as sinus tachycardia, hypotension and conduction disorders and death by their direct effect on the myocardium. There may be blurred vision and dry mouth from the anticholinergic effects. There may also be central effects of agitation, confusion, convulsions, drowsiness, coma and respiratory depression. Activated charcoal should also be used.

There is no specific antidote for tricyclic ingestion. The ECG should be monitored for cardiac arrhythmias. No treatment is indicated if there is adequate tissue perfusion and blood pressure. Metabolic acidosis should be corrected. Convulsions should be treated with diazepam. Life-threatening arrhythmias should be treated with propranolol. As tricyclics are protein bound active methods of elimination such as hemodialysis do not remove significant amounts of the drug.

Household products

Acids. Acids tend to cause inflammation and ulceration at the pylorus rather than the esophagus. This may lead to stenosis. Emesis or lavage should not be undertaken and chemical antidotes should not be given as the heat of the chemical reaction may increase injury. The extent of the injury should be assessed by endoscopy at an early stage. Steroids should be used to suppress the inflammation (prednisolone 2 mg/kg/day).

Alcoholic beverages. These may cause severe hypoglycemia. Blood alcohol levels are useful in management. Hypoglycemia should be detected by frequent blood glucose measurements, and prevented and treated by intravenous glucose infusions.

Alkalis. Alkalis such as caustic soda and dishwasher powder can cause burns to the mouth and esophageal ulceration, leading to stricture: review by esphagoscopy and treatment with steroids have improved the outlook for this condition. Emesis or lavage should not be undertaken, nor any chemical antidotes as the heat of the reaction may increase injury. The extent of the injury should be assessed by endoscopy at an early stage. Steroids should be used to suppress the inflammation (prednisolone 2 mg/kg/day).

Bottle-sterilizing tablets. Bottle-sterilizing tablets contain a bleach-like substance (sodium dichloroisocyanurate). They effervesce with water to make a sterilizing solution. If this reaction takes place in the mouth considerable damage can take place with edema and ulceration. Cases need to be monitored for their airway patency and intravenous fluids may be needed. Monitoring for esophageal involvement by endoscopy may be needed in some cases. The use of steroids is logical in severe cases.

Camphor and camphorated oil. These are dangerous poisons for children. They are absorbed quickly and because they are lipid soluble, enter the brain causing delirium, rigidity, coma and convulsions. Convulsions should be treated with diazepam.

Carbon monoxide. Hemoglobin has an affinity for carbon monoxide over 200 times greater than for oxygen. Carboxyhemoglobin will reduce the amount of hemoglobin available to carry oxygen and also hinders oxygen release. The incidence of carbon monoxide poisoning has fallen since house gas no longer contains this substance. Carbon monoxide poisoning should be treated with 100% oxygen over a period of several hours. Hyperbaric oxygen should be considered in severe cases if it is available.

Cetrimide. Cetrimide is a cationic detergent and can be caustic when concentrated. The stomach should not be emptied. If problems with ulceration occur steroids should be used. Cetrimide may also have depolarizing muscle-relaxing effects leading to breathlessness.

Disk or button batteries. Mercury cell, alkaline manganese and silver cell batteries contain a strong alkali (usually potassium hydroxide) as a main ingredient. Mercury cell batteries contain toxic amounts of mercury. Silver cell batteries generally contain less toxic ingredients than the other types. Worn batteries are less toxic than new ones.

Disk batteries can cause problems if they lodge in the gut and become corroded and release their contents. They may cause ulceration or perforation from caustic injury if lodged in the esophagus or stomach and should be removed endoscopically if they lodge there. If they go beyond the stomach they are usually passed without problem. Their progress should be monitored by abdominal X-ray. Mercury levels should be measured when appropriate. If the battery shows signs of leaking or breaking it should be removed surgically.

Essential oils. Essential or volatile oils contain mixtures of cyclic hydrocarbons, ethers, alcohols and ketones. They include turpentine, pine oil, citronella and eucalyptus as well as such things as Karvol capsules. Their toxicity varies, with real turpentine (not to be confused with turpentine substitute) being very toxic. Symptoms of essential oils include vomiting, drowsiness and convulsions. Ipecac should not be used.

Methylene chloride (paint stripper). This is a very serious poison for children. It is caustic and may cause damage to skin, stomach, mucous membranes and pharynx. Vomiting, dizziness, confusion, toxic myocarditis and hemoglobinuria may occur. Methylene chloride is metabolized to carbon monoxide and carboxymethemoglobin concentrations may be elevated for several days. The stomach should not be emptied. Fluids should be given to dilute the methylene chloride. High-flow oxygen should be given if carboxyhemoglobin is present.

Organochloride insecticides. These include DDT, dieldrin and lindane. Symptoms include excitability, muscle twitching and convulsions. Activated charcoal is valuable.

Organophosphorus insecticides. A wide range of compounds which include malathion. They act by inhibiting cholinesterase in the blood. Symptoms include confusion, nausea, vomiting, wheezing and convulsions. If symptoms appear atropine (i.v.) 0.05 mg/kg and pralidoxime 20–60 mg/kg as required, depending on the severity of the poisoning, should be given by slow i.v. injection and repeated if needed.

Paradichlorobenzene mothballs. Most cases of accidental ingestion do not have serious symptoms. Ingestion may cause nausea and vomiting and cyanosis may develop due to methemoglobinemia. This should be treated with methylene blue.

Paraquat. Paraquat weedkiller is available in two forms: a concentrated form (Gramoxone) available only to farmers and horticulturists and a granular form (Weedol) which contains only 2.5% paraquat. Accidental ingestion of the concentrated form is rare and ingestion of the granular form rarely causes serious problems. Paraquat causes local ulceration and in severe cases a proliferative alveolitis. Treatment should be to prevent absorption by Fuller's earth or bentonite.

Petroleum distillates, e.g. kerosene, turpentine, white spirit and turpentine substitute. These substances may cause a pneumonitis from lung aspiration. Ipecac or lavage should not be used. Kerosene poisoning is a particular problem in the Third World. Rhonchi are the most common physical sign and X-ray changes are common.

Treatment in mild cases is symptomatic, together with the use of prophylactic antibiotics. Corticosteroids are often used, but clear evidence of their effectiveness is lacking. Severe cases may need oxygen and intensive respiratory care.

Phenolic compounds. These include cresols, menthols, phenols and hexachlorophene. Coal tar vaporizing solution contains cresol. They may cause local corrosive damage and there may be cerebral symptoms. Activated charcoal can be used.

Slug pellets (metaldehyde). Slug pellets contain about 3% metaldehyde which is toxic in children and 4 g is said to be fatal for a child. Experience suggests that problems do not arise after accidental ingestion. The child should be observed for 4–6 h to check for serious symptoms such as flushing, salivation and convulsions. Convulsions should be treated with diazepam.

Plants

Arum lily. Causes gastrointestinal side-effects and later CNS manifestations.

Deadly nightshade (atropa). This plant has an atropine effect causing photophobia, visual disturbance, dryness of mouth, flushed skin, etc. If there are symptoms a slow intravenous injection of physostigmine can be used.

Laburnum. Causes vomiting, diarrhea and nausea. Although quite commonly taken, serious problems are very rare.[9]

Philodendron (Swiss cheese plant) and Dieffenbachier. This plant has a local caustic action due to oxalic acid and may cause a sore mouth and laryngeal edema. Steroids may be useful in severe cases.

Yew. Causes gastrointestinal side-effects and later CNS manifestations. There may be severe hypotension.

INJURIES TO CHILDREN (UNINTENTIONAL)

MORTALITY FROM INJURIES

Injuries to children are important to the pediatrician. They are the most frequent cause of deaths in children over 1 year of age in Western countries and thus are a challenge to any efforts to reduce mortality in childhood. Mortality rates in OECD (Organization for Economic Cooperation and Development) countries are shown in Table 32.2.[10] In Britain, nearly twice as many children aged 5–14 years die from injuries as from malignant disease.

Road traffic injuries remain the most frequent cause of death by injury in children in Britain and Europe (Fig. 32.1).[10] Particularly important are deaths to child pedestrians but children also die on bicycles and in cars.

Many children drown. Deaths from conflagrations and complications of burns and scalds have been highlighted with house fires due to foam furniture. There has been a reduction of the number of children dying from injuries over the years. This is probably due to improvements in the environment and the general care of children as well as better treatment (Fig. 32.2).[10]

MORBIDITY FROM INJURIES

Injuries are a significant cause of handicap in children. Head injuries, which may follow pedestrian, cycle or passenger road traffic accidents, falls or child abuse are the major cause of handicap following injury. Children may also be brain damaged following near-drowning or suffocation episodes. Cosmetic damage following burns, scalds and road traffic accidents may be psychologically damaging to the child. The child may be emotionally scarred by remembering the actual accident or from the effects of the subsequent hospital admission and treatment.

Childhood injuries are a frequent cause of attendance at accident and emergency departments. Nearly 30% of children attend our Department in a year in Cardiff and although the majority of these injuries are relatively trivial, amongst them there are serious injuries. Childhood injuries are also a frequent cause of admission to hospital.

WHERE TO TREAT CHILDHOOD INJURIES?

Children should be treated in the best possible environment after an injury and if this is the accident and emergency department, it should not be hostile to the child. Children should not be managed in the same areas as seriously ill, violent or disturbed adults and this means separate waiting areas and accommodation. Such areas should have a bright, welcoming decor with toys. This can be provided at low cost in most accident and emergency departments.

GENERAL PRINCIPLES IN TREATING CHILDHOOD INJURIES

Injured children may need the care of many separate specialties. After a road traffic injury, for instance, a child may need orthopedic surgeons, pediatric surgeons, plastic surgeons, neurosurgeons and anesthetists as well as the pediatrician. There should be a multidisciplinary coordinated approach between everyone caring for these children. In some cases, such as after head injuries in

Table 32.2 Number of child injury deaths, 1991–95

	Child injury deaths 1991–95	Share of injury deaths in all deaths (%)	Lives saved with Sweden's child injury death rate
Australia	1715	42	786
Austria	608	42	269
Belgium	781	40	337
Canada	2665	44	1233
Czech Republic	1138	42	638
Denmark	334	36	120
Finland	368	43	133
France	4701	41	2004
Germany	5171	38	1949
Greece	666	40	211
Hungary	982	36	507
Ireland	357	39	133
Italy	2563	28	405
Japan	7909	36	2617
Korea	12 624	53	9996
Mexico	29 745	30	21 965
Netherlands	864	30	186
New Zealand	519	47	324
Norway	294	37	93
Poland	5756	44	3507
Portugal	1524	40	1071
Spain	2643	33	931
Sweden	391	33	–
Switzerland	537	40	246
UK	3183	29	454
USA	37 265	49	23 555
OECD total	125 303	39	73 872

The table shows the total number of injury deaths among 1–14 year olds during the 5 years 1991–95. The OECD totals exclude Iceland (37 deaths), Luxembourg (34 deaths) and Turkey. Were Turkey to have had the average child injury death rate of other OECD members over the period, another 12 500 deaths would have been added to the total.

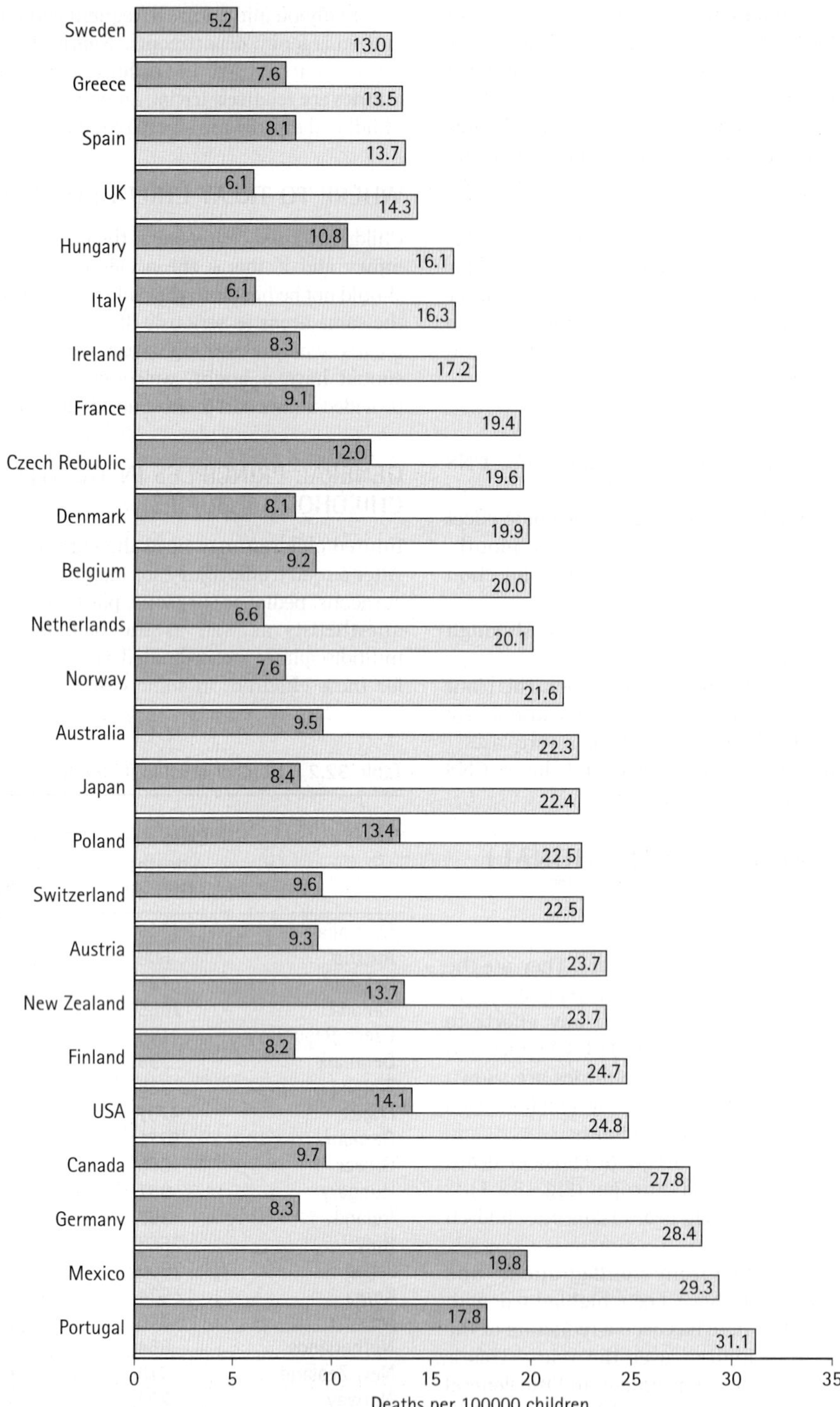

Fig. 32.1 Rate of child injury deaths in the 1970s and 1990s. The longer bars show annual deaths per 100 000 children aged 1–14 in 1971–75 (the basis for the ranking) and the shorter bars show the rates in 1991–95. Reproduced with permission from UNICEF, 'A league table of child deaths by injury in rich nations', Innocenti Report Card No. 2, February 2001. UNICEF Innocenti Research Centre, Florence.

children, clear plans for patterns of care need to be discussed and agreed in advance.

After an injury the interests of the whole child and family should not be forgotten. Children can be emotionally scarred not only by the episode itself but also by painful and insensitive treatment. Parents often feel guilty and may anyway have been under stress before it happened. Follow-up of children should pay attention not only to the injury itself but also to the psychological sequelae. Particular attention to reintegration into school may be required.

ETIOLOGICAL FACTORS IN CHILDHOOD INJURIES

Social factors are important in childhood injuries. Road traffic injuries to children are five times more common and deaths in

UK	6.06	2.91	0.39	0.66	0.26	0.80
Italy	6.14	3.30	0.46	0.18	0.51	0.50
Netherlands	6.59	3.42	1.24	1.26	0.24	0.56
Greece	7.64	4.71	0.56	0.35	0.41	0.26
Spain	8.12	4.02	1.12	1.30	0.39	0.33
Germany	8.32	3.64	1.33	1.62	0.39	1.07
Japan	8.36	3.04	1.93	1.48	0.33	1.12
France	9.05	3.81	0.81	0.47	0.39	1.58
Australia	9.53	4.37	1.97	0.68	0.22	0.85
Canada	9.68	4.33	1.26	1.01	0.20	1.45
Czech Republic	11.95	4.64	2.23	0.34	0.61	1.61
Poland	13.41	5.89	2.84	0.36	0.60	1.14
USA	14.06	5.76	1.74	1.65	0.23	2.74
Mexico	19.75	6.05	3.30	0.62	1.09	2.90
Korea	25.57	12.59	5.14	0.91	1.18	1.08

Fig. 32.2 Injury deaths in large countries. The figure shows annual death rates for all injuries and for the five major identified causes among 1–14 year olds in 1991–95, expressed per 100 000 children. The table is restricted to the 15 most populous OECD member states (excluding Turkey). These countries account for 95% of the deaths shown in Table 32.2. Dark grey denotes the worst performing countries, light grey the average performers and white the best. Reproduced with permission from UNICEF, 'A league table of child deaths by injury in rich nations', Innocenti Report Card No. 2, February 2001. UNICEF Innocenti Research Centre, Florence.

house fires 16 times more common in the poorest families compared to the well off. Similar social class gradients are seen in other injuries to children with the disadvantaged children having more injuries. The reasons are complex. Poorer families usually live in more dangerous environments; for example, it is much easier for a child to have a road accident if his house opens straight onto a main road in the inner city than if he lives in a detached house with a garden. Pyschosocial stress factors are also involved in the etiology of many childhood injuries particularly road traffic injuries and accidental childhood poisoning.

The question of personality in childhood accidents and whether children can be injury prone is difficult. It is much more likely that injury proneness is related to the environment, both physical and social, rather than to personality factors. It is probably more correct to speak of an injury-prone community than an injury-prone child.

PREVENTION OF CHILDHOOD INJURIES

The prevention of injuries is an important public health issue. They are unlikely to be prevented by campaigns covering all types but well-researched multidisciplinary action on individual types of accident can be successful. In preventing a particular injury a methodological approach is needed: looking first at the size and nature of the problem, then deciding what preventive solutions are possible, implementing them on a small scale and then introducing them more widely when they have proved to be effective.

There are three main strategies for injury control: education of children and parents, changing the environment and enforcing changes in the environment by law. Research suggests that whilst in some fields, such as teaching children to swim, education is important, most successes in prevention have followed environmental changes and that educational campaigns by themselves are only of limited value.

Research evidence in childhood injury prevention

Evidence in child injury prevention is more difficult to obtain than in many fields of pediatrics and child health. Injury prevention is often a part of public policy and randomized control trials (RCTs) are difficult to construct and undertake. Nevertheless increasingly researchers are overcoming these difficulties and there are increasing numbers of RCTs in the literature. There have also been valuable systematic reviews.[11]

Environmental change in child injury prevention

Environmental change can prevent injuries. This has been shown in the use of child-resistant containers to prevent childhood poisoning, child safety seats to prevent injury in passenger car accidents, fencing private swimming pools to prevent drowning and by flame-proofing of nightdresses to prevent burns. Sometimes an environmental measure, such as seat belts for cars, is effective but is not fully used by the population and has to be enforced by law.

Health education and childhood injuries

A number of studies have shown that education campaigns to prevent accidents to children by themselves are ineffective. A program directed at the parents of children to reduce home accidents (the Rockwood County study) made no difference in accident rates between control and target families. There was little evidence that the 'Play it Safe' television programs made any impact on accident rates in children.[12] An education campaign with posters and literature in Cardiff only sensitized the population to trivial accidents.[13] There is evidence, however, that health visitors visiting the home giving specific attention to accident prevention can make a difference in the way that families behave, in particular with regard to the installation of safety equipment.

Health education therefore must be directed either on a one-to-one basis by people such as the health visitor or general practitioner or to educate public opinion to institute environmental change. For instance, parents can be educated that safe playground equipment is needed for their children. They can then press the local authority to act.

Action on childhood injuries

In England in 1977 Donald Court and Hugh Jackson were instrumental in the formation of the Child Accident Prevention Trust (CAPT). Other similar organizations exist in other countries such as Safe Kids in the USA and Kidsafe in Australia. These organizations bring many disciplines together to foster action and research on injuries to children.

As well as national action on injury prevention and control local action is needed. In Sweden, public health physicians led by Stangström from the Karolinska Institute in Stockholm developed local action through the concept of Safe Communities. The First World Injury Control Conference in 1989 approved a manifesto for Safe Communities: 'Safety – a universal concern for all'.[14] Further World Conferences have confirmed this.

The basis of any program of injury control is surveillance. This needs close liaison between the community pediatrician and the accident and emergency department. Once an injury has happened it may happen again. For instance, a dangerous balcony that allowed a fall should be repaired straight away, together with others like it.

INJURIES TO CHILDREN AT PLAY AND RECREATION

Playground injuries

Play is vital for children in their physical development and their ability to make social relationships. Although children of course play at home and in organized groups, many play in playgrounds provided by local authorities and private organizations. Playgrounds provide an alternative to playing in dangerous places such as the road and need to be as safe as possible. Pediatricians will wish to influence playground safety in their districts by lobbying the local authority. There has been much work developing safer equipment and surfaces and producing acceptable safety standards. This has been done in Europe, America and Australia. These standards and safety features in modern playgrounds have been developed in the laboratory using road crash adult cadaver data on head injury. They include safety surfaces, modifying equipment and maintenance.

Impact-absorbing surfaces have been introduced to lessen the severity of a head injury from falling from equipment onto a hard surface. These may be bark, sand or special impact absorbing rubberized surface. Looking at overall injury presentations Mott and her colleagues[15] found that Cardiff children suffered significantly more injuries on playgrounds with concrete surfaces than those with bark or rubber. Rubber was the safest surface with injury risks half that of bark and a fifth of concrete.

Equipment is also important. The majority of injuries in playgrounds are now equipment related. Swings, slides, climbing frames and roundabouts are all commonly involved in playground accidents. They all can be designed for better safety.[16] Certain items of equipment may involve particular risk. The risk from falls from monkey bars was twice that from climbing frames and seven times that on a swing or slide. There were significantly fewer fractures from climbing frames with maximum fall heights under 1.5 meters ($p < 0.05$).[15]

There is a question of whether these safety features, surface and equipment, actually prevent injuries, as there has been little systematic surveillance. There have been two case control studies[17,18] that provide reasonable evidence that interventions can work. It does appear that head injuries are prevented in modern playgrounds but it may be that modern surfaces are not protective against arm fractures.

Sports and recreational injuries

The whole ethos of preventing injuries to children during sport and recreation is a difficult one. Clearly, one cannot protect children from all risks in recreational activity, which is important in physical development and the development of personality. On the other hand, one does not want to expose children to unnecessary risk.

There has been little research on the risks of various sports, in particular whether rugby or soccer are dangerous for boys. A study in Wales[19] suggested that rugby may cause more injuries than soccer, in particular to the upper part of the body. There is also the danger of neck injuries and paraplegia with rugby. The risk can be reduced by sensible supervision and other safety measures. Hill and mountain climbing expeditions need careful supervision by experienced guides and teachers if disasters are to be prevented. Rugby teams should be of similar age and ability and referees should pay particular attention to collapsing the scrum.

DOG BITES

Dog bites to children are extremely common and as many as 1 in 100 children a year presents to an accident and emergency department with this problem. In America and Britain, many of the accidents occur in the home or with dogs well known to the children. However, a significant number of children are bitten in public areas, particularly play areas. The majority of dog bites are minor, but severe lacerations, particularly facial lacerations, may occur. There are a few deaths, mainly children exposed to guard dogs. There has also been concern about potentially dangerous breeds of dog kept in the home. A randomized control trial has shown an educational intervention was effective in modifying children's behavior with dogs.[20]

Significant dog bites should be debrided and sutured. It is usual to give tetanus prophylaxis, but routine antibiotics are not needed. In many countries, particularly in India, the danger of rabies is present.

HORSE ACCIDENTS

Horse riding is a common leisure pursuit, particularly in girls around puberty. Horse-riding accidents are one of the few types of accident that are more common in girls than boys, with the peak incidence in 10–14-year-olds. The few deaths each year usually result from severe head injuries. Just under half of horse accidents arise from a fall leading to head injuries, limb fractures and occasionally spinal injuries. Some children get kicked and some are crushed by horses falling on them. Horses also sometimes bite and butt children and tread on their feet.

Many injuries to children on horses are caused by inexperience on the part of the rider, particularly when the horse is startled in traffic. Injury during competitions is rare. Good supervision and teaching are important in prevention and horse and rider should be matched. Good head protection is vital in preventing serious head injury. Many traditional riding hats offer little protection for the rider and British Standard protective hats should be used.

THERMAL INJURIES IN CHILDREN

Thermal injuries occur particularly in children under 5 years old from deprived backgrounds. They are a significant cause of accidental death in childhood. The majority of children die in conflagrations in private dwellings often in conditions of poverty. Many children die from gas and smoke inhalation rather than by direct heat. There have been striking reductions in the number of children who have died from fire in recent years. Despite this, the death rate from fires is unacceptably high. A major component of the reduction has been the fall in the number of deaths from the ignition of clothing following flame-proofing regulations and the reduction of open fires. House fires are a particular problem in poor families.

As well as being an important cause of death in childhood, burns and scalds cause significant morbidity from long-term scarring and psychological damage. Scalds, most of which are in children under 5, cause over half the admissions to hospital from thermal injuries. Children are scalded most commonly from a cup or a mug but significant numbers are scalded from teapots and kettles and from hot bath water. Bath scalds are usually caused by unsupervised children falling in the bath[21] but the differentiation between accident and abuse can be difficult.

As well as in house fires, children are burnt from small igniting sources such as matches, outdoor fires, space heating and cooking equipment. Firework accidents have been reduced with the discontinuation of certain types of firework, the restriction in the minimum age of people to whom fireworks are sold and the limitation of time fireworks are available in the shops to a few weeks before 5 November.

The prevention of injuries from house fires

Many conflagrations are caused initially by smoking. Accidents involving open fires have fallen with the introduction of central heating but they still remain a problem with poor families. Fireguards should be used with young families and should conform to BS 6539. Injuries and deaths due to flammability of nightdresses have lessened with the Night-dress (Safety) Regulations in 1967. Many children have died in house fires because of the flammability of upholstered furniture and from the toxic fumes produced when it burns. There is now legislation in the UK to ban the foam which causes dangerous fumes and replace it with a safety foam. The full effects of this legislation will take many years to come through because of the long life of furniture in homes.

Smoke detectors are widely used in many countries and found to be effective, particularly for children.[22,23] They have an important role in the prevention of injury from house fires and their use should be enforced both in public and private housing. The effectiveness of education programs to use smoke alarms has been less clearly established. In a recent systematic review of controlled trial interventions to promote smoke alarms DiGuiseppi and Higgins[24] suggest only modest potential benefits from education to promote smoke alarms. Smoke alarm promotion through the child surveillance program may be more effective. Most effective of all would be regulations to have wired alarms in all housing, particularly in social housing. Giving away smoke alarms will not necessarily increase the prevalence of functioning alarms.[25]

The prevention of scalds in children is more difficult. A wider use of mugs and the elimination of unstable cups should be encouraged. A number of children injure themselves from spillage from kettles and these injuries can be avoided by the use of coil or short electric kettle flexes without large expense. Some children scald themselves by pulling saucepans down from cookers, incidents that could be prevented by reducing access to the cooker and by using cooker guards. Reducing the temperature of the hot water in domestic systems could prevent bath scalds. This can be done in two ways: reducing the thermostat temperature in domestic hot water tanks and, more expensively, by thermostatically controlled mixer taps. However, there is little evidence that the distribution of devices to control hot water temperatures is effective.[26]

ARCHITECTURAL ACCIDENTS AND FALLS

There has been an increasing recognition that safety is an important consideration in the design of homes where children live. Many falls, glass accidents and burns can be prevented by good design. A dialog between architects and those treating injuries on safer design for children in new houses is needed. Practical design guidelines are now available.

Falls

Falls cause some deaths in childhood but are also the commonest cause of presentation to the accident and emergency department. They have a varied etiology. They may be on one level, such as falling on the pavement, at home or in the school playground. Younger children may be dropped, fall from furniture or fall down the stairs. The danger of falls from baby walkers has been highlighted and they can no longer be advised for children's use.[27] Older children fall from trees, cliffs and mountains, play equipment and buildings. Poor window catches and design allow a number of accidents, particularly in high-rise flats. The introduction of safety catches or window guards will reduce these. In New York City a program providing free window guards (The Children Can't Fly Program) has been successful in preventing window falls in a poor area of New York.[28]

Falls downstairs are a particular problem for toddlers. Much can be done to prevent them, by better stair design and stair gates. The use of stair gates can be encouraged by the health visitor, and a Safe Community program. Open stairs with wide gaps between balustrades may be esthetically beautiful, but are dangerous for young children. In 1985 UK building regulations were changed to make certain that a 100 mm sphere could not be passed through any opening or guard to a flight of stairs.

Glass injuries

Falls through glass may cause severe lacerations to hands, wrists and arms, and occasionally the face. Severe damage may result from injury to arteries, nerves and tendons, and internal injuries may also be found, with the bowel sometimes protruding from the abdominal wall. There may be uncontrolled arterial bleeding. There are also cases of scarring and permanent disability from nerve damage.

The child is usually injured by glass in doors or by low-level glazing. A typical story would be a child falling downstairs into a glass door. The sharp, jagged parts of the glass may cause severe lacerations to any parts of the body, particularly the upper limbs. First aid to severe bleeding from glass injuries is best done by pressure on the wound, using a pad after the glass has been removed. In some cases, quite extensive surgery is needed.

The whole problem of glass injuries in childhood could be prevented by the use of safety glass. There are a number of types of glass or plastic that can be used in building. Annealed flat glass breaks easily into shards and annealed wire glass cracks easily with exposed wires. Safety glass is either laminated, which absorbs impact and is resistant to penetration, or toughened tempered glass that shatters into small cuboid pieces. Other safe alternatives to annealed flat glass are polycarbonate sheet or plastic safety film. Laminated glass is only about 1.8 times more expensive than annealed flat glass. Safety glass is covered by the building regulations in the UK.

ROAD TRAFFIC INJURIES

Road traffic injuries cause more deaths and severe disability in children than any other type of injury. This presents a major challenge in prevention and treatment to all those who work in the field.

Pedestrian road traffic injuries

Pedestrian road traffic injuries are particularly common in the inner city and in children from socially deprived families. Fatality rates are correlated with the prosperity of the area. Psychosocial stress is an important factor in road traffic injuries and the interaction of a poor environment with stress is probably involved in many injuries.

Children under 10 years are particularly at risk from pedestrian road traffic injuries. Boys between 5 and 8 years are at maximum risk as they are unable to estimate the speed or dangers of traffic. Parents may overestimate the ability of their children to handle traffic and let them go out on the road unsupervised. Sharples et al[29] looking at deaths from head injuries in the northern region, found that 72% of these deaths occurred between 3 p.m. and 9 p.m. and mostly to boys playing after school.

Environmental change and child pedestrian road traffic injuries

The most effective means of preventing pedestrian road traffic injuries is by modification of the environment. Residential areas can be redesigned to give priority to pedestrians and to separate them from traffic. The speed of traffic can be reduced by speed bumps and safe crossings can be provided. There is now good evidence that area-wide engineering schemes and traffic-calming schemes reduce injuries.[11] The provision of play areas will reduce the number of children on dangerous streets. The Safe Community approach is a way of introducing traffic calming.

Education and child pedestrian road traffic injuries

It is possible to teach some children pedestrian skills. One approach is designating safer routes to school. Two randomized trials[30,31] have shown improvements in children's ability to find safe places to cross the road. There is little evidence that these programs have actually gone on to prevent injuries. Roberts et al[32] concluded that safety and traffic education are unlikely by themselves to prevent road traffic injuries. School-based traffic clubs have not been shown to be effective.

Passenger injuries

The protection of children in cars from serious injury and death must be an important part of any child safety program. A major part of such protection is the development of child-restraint systems and seat belts. Much of the research on seat belts has been on adult passengers. There is good evidence that seat belts are effective in preventing death and serious injury. The Transport and Road Research Laboratory found that no child died in a 2-year period when in a restraint whereas 264 non-restrained children were killed in that period. Child-restraint systems have the unexpected bonus of improving children's behavior and this probably improves driving standards. The problem is getting children to use them.

In young children and babies the barrier to the use of child restraints has in many cases been cost and child-restraint loan schemes have been developed to help poorer families. They appear to be an effective strategy to increase the number of children safely transported in cars.[11] However a RCT of demonstrating restraint use did not appear to increase correct use.[33]

Educational campaigns used to persuade children to wear seat belts have had mixed results. Miller and Pless[34] found no significant differences in seat belt usage however Macknin et al[35] found a campaign effective in the short-term. Most countries have believed that legislation is needed to ensure seat belt usage. Serious injuries fell by 20% following the 1983 legislation in the UK compelling the wearing of seat belts in front seats. A systematic review[11] of nine studies in the US evaluating seat belt legislation concluded that it was associated with reductions of injuries and death and increases the numbers of children using restraints. Many children remain unrestrained however. Enforcement of car passenger restraint increases observed restraint.

Bicycle injuries

Bicycles play an important part in the life of most children, particularly boys between 3 and 12 years. Bicycle injuries are a significant cause of death and disability in children. There are factors in bicycle design which are vital to safety; for example, the high-rise bicycle that was introduced into Britain in the late 1960s and early 1970s had features that made it more dangerous than standard models.

The prevention and reduction in severity of bicycle injuries may involve education and environmental change. There is now some evidence that bicycle skills training can improve riding behavior. van Schagen and Brookhuis[36] in a RCT in the Netherlands showed improved behavior in the intervention children.

The use of helmets is now accepted as a key part of preventing bicycle injuries. There are at least five case control studies that show the effectiveness of cycle helmets in preventing head injury. A key case control study was by Thompson et al[37] in Seattle where cyclists were shown to have an 85% reduction in their risk of head injury by wearing helmets. What is more difficult is getting children to wear them. One RCT[38] showed no difference in helmet wearing after an intervention. In some places, such as parts of Australia and the US, helmets have been introduced by legislation with a reduction in injuries.

DROWNING AND NEAR-DROWNING IN CHILDHOOD

Drowning is the third most common cause of death in children from injury in the UK. In 1988/89 Kemp and Sibert[39] reviewed drowning deaths and near-drowning and in 1998/9 they reviewed what progress had been made in 10 years.[40] Overall drowning deaths had fallen significantly from 149 to 104. Many more boys drown than do girls (75% in both series) which reflects their different behavior patterns. Most were less than 5 years of age. Approximately the same numbers of children are admitted after near-drowning than drown. Many near-drowning cases admitted to hospital are seriously ill and have to be admitted to the intensive care unit. Drowning incidence rates are much higher in warmer parts of the world such as California or Australia than in the UK.

Modes of drowning by development and by site

Children can drown indoors and outdoors, and in deep or shallow water. Drowning and near-drowning in childhood can be divided by the site where the injury takes place, each site having a definite age range and corresponding to a stage in child development:

- Babies and developmentally delayed older children may drown when they are unable to sit up in the water. A typical example is bath drowning. A similar mechanism applies to older children who have epileptic fits.
- Toddlers and children with autistic spectrum disorder may wander off to unprotected water. Examples are garden ponds, domestic swimming pools and open water.
- Older children may be playing near any open water, they fall in and are unable to rescue themselves in that situation.
- Older children may be swimming with no lifeguard or inadequate lifeguard. Examples are open water, public and private pools.
- All ages of children may drown from boats.
- All ages, particularly babies, may be drowned deliberately.

Bath drownings

Bath drownings mainly occur in the babies or older disabled children. They can drown in quite shallow water and should not be left unattended. The possibility of non-accidental drowning should be remembered in young children.[41] Accidental bath drownings occur in children under 2 or those with disability. Children with epilepsy continue to die in the bath and they should always shower.

Garden pond drownings

Garden pond drownings occur in toddlers. The numbers of children dying has increased in the UK probably because of the increased number of water features in gardens. Children can drown in quite small shallow ponds. The commonest story is of an unsupervised toddler in a neighbor's garden or when visiting friends or relatives. Toddlers can also drown in pails, farm slurry pits, cattle troughs and puddles.

Domestic and private swimming pools

Toddlers and young children are also in danger when wandering off unsupervised into domestic swimming pools. Unsupervised children may either fall into the pool or crawl under the covers. These drownings are a particular problem in warm affluent countries. Children may also drown in private pools without supervision in hotels and holiday camps.

Public pools

Deaths from public pool drownings are a minor problem in the United Kingdom following health and safety regulations introduced in 1985 which insist that there is a high level of supervision of children in such pools.[42] Drownings in public pools are at a level of one per year in the UK, a tribute to the level of supervision.[39,40] Many of the children who are admitted to hospital after nearly drowning in public baths have had effective poolside resuscitation.

Rivers, canal, lakes and sea

Drowning in rivers, canals and lakes is predominantly a problem of older boys who play unsupervised and get into trouble in deep water.[39] Many are non-swimmers. The numbers have fallen over the 10 years 1988/1989–1998/1999. These numbers of boys correspond to the number of boys in Australia who drown in creeks. A few children drown at sea in England and Wales, some from falling into docks, some lost at sea in boating accidents and some drowned from the beach.

Pathophysiology of drowning and near-drowning

The excellent prognosis for some children rescued from apparent death has encouraged a better understanding of the pathophysiology of drowning. The majority of deaths from drowning, even amongst competent swimmers, occur within 10 meters of a safe refuge. This suggests that some physiological disturbance associated with the initial immersion is in many cases responsible for incapacitation. There may also be some pathological reason why a child drowns, such as epilepsy.

The survival of some children after a long period of immersion may be due to the vestigial diving reflex (active in diving mammals) where the peripheral circulation is shut down with a profound bradycardia and the brain receives the majority of the cardiac output. There is work to show, however, that the diving reflex is not active in humans.[43] Harries[44] has suggested that survival for prolonged periods under water is because the circulation fails as a secondary event some time after the immersion and because of the protective effect of hypothermia. Orlowski[45] has used the term 'ice water drowning' rather than 'cold water drowning' as a review of the world's medical literature revealed that all the cases with a good outcome after very prolonged immersion occurred in water with a temperature of 10°C or less. This suggests also that it may be the hypothermia that is protective. A child is not dead until he or she is warm and dead.

Complications and sequelae of near-drowning

There is some controversy over how many children suffer severe brain damage after resuscitation following a near-drowning episode. Studies in the USA have shown that fixed dilated pupils and coma predicted those patients who would die or have neurological deficit after severe submersion incidents. These studies may have referred to children drowning in the relatively warm pools found there. In contrast, in Britain some children do survive normally after severe submersion incidents despite being admitted to hospital unconscious with fixed dilated pupils.[46] Of 64 nearly drowned children unconscious on admission, 31 had normally reactive pupils and all but three (all of whom had severe pre-existing neurological disease and had secondary drowning complications) made a full recovery. Of the 33 patients with fixed dilated pupils on admission 10 children made a full recovery, 13 died and 10 sustained severe neurological deficit in the form of a spastic quadriplegia with profound learning difficulties. Spontaneous respiratory effort on admission was associated with normal survival. Pupils that remained dilated 6 h after admission and fits continuing 24 h after admission predicted a poor outcome. The prognosis for near-drowning episodes in warm water seems worse than for those occurring in cold or ice water.[45] Many children who have had a severe hypoxic episode following near-drowning will develop cerebral edema, which may contribute to the ultimate brain damage suffered by these casualties.

Salt and fresh water drowning

There has been discussion about different mechanisms occurring in salt and fresh water drowning in children because of experimental animal data showing hemolytic crises following aspiration of fresh water in large volumes into the lungs. In practice, humans aspirate much smaller volumes and fears of hemolytic crises have proved to be unfounded. It may be that secondary drowning is more serious in salt water than in fresh water. The differences between salt and fresh water drowning in children are less important than those between warm and cold water drowning.

Aspiration pneumonia

A proportion of children who nearly drown aspirate water and develop a pneumonia with secondary infection. This is rarely a serious complication unless the child has developed brain damage.

Secondary drowning

Secondary drowning is a phenomenon in which respiratory deterioration occurs with pulmonary edema, between 1 and 72 h after the original incident. Harries[44] suggests that this complication occurs only in the first 24 h and approximately 5% of near-drownings are affected. There may be a worse prognosis in salt water than in fresh water near-drownings. The alveolar membrane dysfunction is probably due to surfactant deficiency and should be treated by adequate intermittent positive pressure ventilation. The value of corticosteroid treatment is unproven, but they are often prescribed.

Treatment

The aims of treatment of a nearly drowned child are to restore adequate ventilation and circulation, prevent further heat loss and to correct acid–base status. Apart from correcting the acidosis directly these can usually all be achieved at the waterside. Simple first aid with mouth-to-mouth resuscitation, covering and warming are vital. Many children may vomit during resuscitation so it is important to ensure a clear airway throughout the resuscitation procedure. As some apparently dead children may recover fully from near-drowning episodes, it is wise to attempt to resuscitate all apparently dead, drowned children. This is particularly the case in cold or ice water.

All children who may have inhaled water should be admitted to hospital. The presence of crepitations is helpful in deciding whether there has been aspiration. Children who have adequate ventilation and no apparent sequelae should be reviewed for 24 h for signs of secondary drowning and supraventricular cardiac arrhythmias. They should have chest physiotherapy. Secondary drowning should be treated by positive end expiratory pressure and intermittent positive pressure ventilation.

Severely ill children who cannot maintain adequate oxygenation initially should be admitted to an intensive care unit where they can be mechanically ventilated. Those children who have neither respiration nor cardiac output should be ventilated, have external cardiac massage and have their acidosis corrected.

If the core temperature is below 28°C consideration should be given to slow rewarming although 'the optimal treatment of these children is unproven'.[45] The effect of hypothermia, barbiturate therapy and monitoring and regulating intracranial pressure in hypoxic/ischemic brain injury has been studied by Bohn et al.[47] They found that these measures provided little benefit and recommended that therapy should be directed at maintaining cerebral perfusion and adequate oxygenation. Children who appear dead after exposure to drowning at very low temperatures should not be pronounced brain dead until they have been brought up to a near normal core temperature.

Prevention

Most drowning accidents occur with children too young to be able to swim. Preventing bath accidents in babies should be part of the health visitor's program of education with mothers. It should be emphasized that it is unsafe to leave young children unsupervised in the bath even for short periods. Parents should also be told about the dangers of drowning in garden ponds and families with young children are well advised to fence or cover these. Much could be done to insist on protecting children from access to these ponds particularly in garden centers. There is evidence that fencing with self-shutting gates, which prevents children from having access to domestic pools, can prevent drowning. In Canberra, private swimming pools have to be fenced by law but there was no such legal sanction in Brisbane at the time of one study: only one child died in the Australian capital from a swimming pool accident over a 5-year period, compared with 55 in Brisbane. Fencing has now been introduced by regulation into Australia, South Africa, New Zealand and parts of the US.

To be unable to swim probably increases the risk of drowning. Teaching children to swim may reduce the number of deaths among 5–14-year-olds. Certainly, there has been an overall fall in the number of deaths of children from drowning which has coincided with better swimming training. A number of older children drown whilst swimming unsupervised in rivers, lakes and creeks: this unsupervised swimming should be discouraged but is impossible to prevent. The reduction in serious drowning in public swimming pools incidents with health and safety regulations has been most welcome.[39] This supervision at the waterside should remain a high priority for local authorities and should be extended to private pools and open water where swimming is common. Life jackets and buoyancy aids are important in helping to prevent children who use boats and canoes from drowning if they fall overboard. Getting children to wear them is difficult but boat and canoe clubs can insist that their members wear them.

Accidental suffocation, choking and strangulation in childhood

Accidental mechanical asphyxia is a significant cause of death in children. Nixon and his colleagues[48] reviewed deaths registered as choking, suffocation or strangulation in a total population study for the 2 years 1990–1991 in England and Wales. Some of these incidents are not true accidents and there may be problems of classification, with inhalation of vomit, non-accidental injury and the coexisting diagnosis of SIDS. Nixon et al found an overall annual incidence of 0.7 per 100 000 children at risk with two modal peaks at less than 1 year of age and in the early teenage years because of boys being found hanged. Children die from choking, on food and on non-food items. Few children now suffocate on a toy and that emphasizes the importance of Standards for Toy Safety. They also die from inhalation of vomit often associated with medical conditions. Children also die from strangulation. They may be younger children who are strangled by cords, clothing and accessories and by poorly maintained cots. Parents of young children should be discouraged from using poorly maintained cots, telephone wires or window cords near cots or necklaces or dummy cords when in cots. There may also be boys found hanging; this may be deliberate but are probably mainly not true suicide.

POISONOUS ANIMAL BITES AND STINGS

In an overview of poisonous animal bites and stings published by the World Health Organization, it was stated that in excess of 100 000 deaths result worldwide each year from bites by snakes, stings from scorpions and from anaphylactic reactions to insect stings.[49]

SNAKE BITES

Snakes are the most widely distributed of the reptiles, and different species, often with highly individual features, predominate in different countries. Overall, there are 2.5 million snakebites each year, with a fatality rate of between 1.5 and 3%.[49,50] Environmental change in some parts of the world has resulted in changes in the pattern of snakebite – as for example in parts of Africa, where prolonged drought has reduced vegetation cover, favoring the spread of *Echis ocellatus*, and resulting in more bites.[49] Clinicians have to concern themselves primarily with the characteristics and venomous effects of the poisonous snakes in their own area. Of the nearly 3000 known varieties only some 300 are of medical significance.

Adder bites (Europe)

There is only one poisonous species of snake in Britain, the common viper or adder (*Viper berus*), and its bite seldom causes death in an adult, although young children very occasionally die as a result. The fully grown adder may be 50–60 cm in length and is recognized by the dark zigzag band which runs along the center of the back, although rarely the snake may appear uniformly black. It is a shy creature, living in clearings, the edges of woods, moors and low lying damp ground, and normally disappears quickly on the approach of people. It is only likely to bite if disturbed unexpectedly.

Clinical features

When the amount of venom injected is small, as is usual in a defensive bite, there may be few signs or symptoms, but fear often causes transient pallor, sweating or vomiting. With moderate poisoning there may be local swelling increasing over 1 or 2 days to involve the whole limb. This swelling resolves within a few weeks. In more serious cases, a burning pain is experienced at the place bitten, usually an extremity. Vomiting may begin within a few minutes of the bite (often accompanied by diarrhea) and may continue for up to 48 h. Shock is likely with weakness, sweating, thirst, coldness, absent pulse, hypotension, drowsiness and occasionally loss of consciousness. Swelling of the face, lips and tongue may occur, Soon hemorrhagic discoloration and swelling appear and may gradually extend up the limb. Bleeding may occur from gums, wound and infection sites. With recovery, discoloration slowly changes from blue to green and finally to yellow before disappearing. The child generally recovers quickly from the initial collapse but in severe poisoning there may be persistent or recurrent hypotension. Full recovery may take 1–6 weeks.

Treatment

When a child is bitten by a snake, the reptile should be killed for identification, *if this can be done without risk of further bites*. The bite should not be incised but merely covered with a clean handkerchief or cloth. The patient should be kept quiet and the limb maintained at rest by splinting, helping to retard absorption of venom. The child and his parents should be reassured about the expected outcome and taken to hospital as quickly as possible. On admission to hospital paracetamol may be given for the pain, chlorpromazine if required for vomiting and an antihistamine drug for the swelling. In hospital, blood pressure should be monitored hourly, and bleeding time should be recorded; the white cell count (raised), serum creatine phosphokinase (may be raised), serum bicarbonate (may be low) and ECG should be determined twice daily. Antibiotics and tetanus antitoxin are not required routinely. Antivenom (two ampoules) should be given if there is evidence of systemic poisoning especially hypotension, bleeding or ECG changes. It should be given diluted with isotonic saline, by slow intravenous infusion, over a period of 30–60 min with adrenaline (epinephrine) ready in case of need. The antivenom is produced in Zagreb and can be obtained in Britain from Regent Laboratories Ltd., London NW10 6PN. Before antivenom arrives or if a history of allergy contraindicates its use, blood transfusion may help to combat collapse.

Tropical and subtropical snakes

Morbidity and mortality from snake bites are highest in those areas where snakes have adapted to farm, plantation and village life and live in close proximity to large human populations. Examples are the Indian cobra, krait and Russell's viper in South-East Asia, and some pit vipers in Latin America.

Land snakes may be classified according to the presence or absence of poisonous injecting fangs, and their position when present in the snake's mouth (Table 32.3). Sea snakes, of which there are some 50 species, have characteristic flattened tails and short front fangs.

Although the Elapidae include many highly venomous varieties, these usually retreat when approached by humans and are generally non-aggressive unless cornered or molested. The large family of Colubridae contains only a few snakes of medical significance and these are rarely the cause of bites in humans. The Viperidae, on the other hand, are broad sluggish snakes which hold their ground and may easily be trodden on (puff adder) or touched, on or in the ground or among rocks (rattlesnake, burrowing adder, berg adder). These snakes, despite their sluggishness, strike with great rapidity and power, virtually stabbing their victim with frontally situated large fangs which are swung forward during the strike.

Many non-venomous snakes are capable of inflicting bites which are liable to become infected, sometimes with exotic bacteria, such as *Arizona* species.

Snake venoms broadly correspond with the families shown in the table. They are complex mixtures of toxins and enzymes and effects depend upon which of these predominate. Viper (and some cobra) venoms are mainly cytotoxic. Elapid venoms produce neurotoxic effects, as do varieties of tropical rattlesnake (*Crotolinae*). Venoms are complex with varying mixtures of neurotoxins, myotoxins, procoagulants, anticoagulants and nephrotoxins.[50] The venoms can also cause hemolysis, hemorrhage and coagulation disturbances.

Colubrid (boomslang) venoms are hematoxic and anticoagulant, while hydrophiid (sea snake) venoms are mainly myotoxic. Nephrotoxic properties have also been demonstrated in puff adder, sea snake and rattlesnake venoms.

Children are particularly at risk in areas where snakes are common because of their love of outdoor pursuits, together with their curiosity and carelessness. However, it is important to realize that the majority of bites from snakes are not caused by venomous species. In these circumstances two distinct puncture marks are not seen and the bites are irregular and lacerated to a greater or lesser degree, with little local swelling or pain. Even venomous species do not always inflict clinically significant envenomation as the bite may be deflected by clothing or the venom stores of the snake depleted. When envenomation has occurred, symptoms tend to be more severe in children because of their smaller size relative to the volume of injected venom.

Despite popular belief, while sudden collapse and death may occur (e.g. Australian brown snake, death adder), signs of systemic envenomation in even the most poisonous snake bites seldom occur before 30 min. The earliest features are often those due to fright – shock, pallor, sweating, vomiting, weak pulse and faintness. Severe pain and swelling at the site of the bite, with rapidly spreading

Table 32.3 Classification of snakes

Group of snake	Features of groups	Common examples and habitat	Principal action of venom
Viperidae	Mobile front fangs	Viperinae Puff adder, widespread in Africa Gaboon viper, central and southern Africa Berg adder, southern Africa Russell's viper, Asia and Indonesia Saw-scaled viper, India, Iraq, North Africa European viper (adder), Europe, Asia, Japan Crotalinae (pit vipers) Cottonmouth mocassin, south-eastern United States Fer-de-lance, Mexico and South America Jaracara, South America Rattlesnakes, Mexico, southern and western United States Taiwan Habu, south-eastern China	Cytotoxic (tropical rattlesnakes and berg adder are mainly neurotoxic)
Elapidae	Fixed front fangs	Cobras, widespread in Africa and Asia Mambas, east, central and southern Africa Rinkhals, southern Africa Indian krait, India, Burma, Malaya, Indonesia Tiger snake, Brown snake, Australia Death adder, Australia and New Guinea Coral snake, southern United States	Neurotoxic (king cobra also has cytotoxic effect)
Colubridae	Back fangs	Boomslang, Herald snake, Vine snake } widespread in Africa	Hematoxic
Hydrophidae (sea snakes)	Short fixed front fangs	Beaked sea snake and many other species, mainly in Pacific. A few varieties in Indian Ocean	Myotoxic
Non-venomous	Fangless	House snake, Grass snake } cosmopolitan Python, Africa, Asia	Nil

edema, are the first signs in most viperine and some cobra bites. Later large blisters may form around the bite and painful lymphadenopathy develops. Sometimes there is extensive bruising in superficial and deeper tissues. Within 5 or 6 h the whole limb may be tensely swollen. There is thus a profound local cytotoxic effect and subsequent systemic disturbance is largely due to this tissue damage rather than to circulating venom. Necrosis of superficial or deep tissues may be seen. 'The intravascular clotting–fibrinolysis syndrome', with resultant hemolytic anemia, hemorrhagic manifestations and hemoglobinuric nephrosis, can complicate the bite.

In heavy envenomation, especially by puff adders and Gaboon vipers, bloody saliva may be expectorated, and sudden death may follow due to circulatory collapse. Notable exceptions in this family of snakes are the hemorrhagic reactions seen in bites from saw-scaled and Russell's vipers and the neurotoxic effects occurring in tropical rattlesnake and berg adder bites.

Elapid bites generally cause much less local reaction, but have profound systemic effects which are predominantly neurotoxic. African elapids such as cobras may, however, cause significant local tissue necrosis[51] and in a review of bites from the Australian copperhead, one-third showed significant local effects.[52] The first symptoms of snakebite are usually ptosis, rapidly followed by strabismus, slurred speech and dysphagia, with drooling saliva. There is confusion and hypersensitivity to tactile stimuli. If untreated, respiratory paralysis may result in death within 15 h. In survivors there are no neurological sequelae. In the case of mamba bites, the first systemic symptoms are combined with a sensation of tightness and pain across the chest. Violent abdominal pain sometimes occurs after krait and coral snakebites. Local blistering may be seen after envenomation by some cobras and a burning sensation at the site is often described. Local pain after snake bites is, however, extremely variable. Hematuria and hemoglobinuria may occur as may hemorrhage or menorrhagia.

Some elapids, such as the spitting cobra, or rinkhals, of southern Africa, are able to eject venom with considerable force and accuracy at the victim's head. Should this enter the eyes, a very severe keratoconjunctivitis is produced which may lead to blindness.

The boomslang is the only venomous snake in the large family of Colubridae which is a significant hazard to humans. Fortunately bites from this species are rare, usually occurring in those handling or working with snakes. There is little or no local reaction apart from mild burning pain but severe headache about 1 h after the bite is a regular and unexplained phenomenon. Colubrid venoms contain mainly fibrinolysins and hemorrhagins which result in severe, systemic defibrination and generalized hemorrhage, widespread cutaneous bruising especially at sites of trauma, and free bleeding from fang punctures. There may be massive intestinal, urinary tract or intracranial hemorrhage leading to death. As mentioned earlier, the venom of certain vipers and also some elapids (such as the Papuan black snake) produces similar hemorrhagic effects.

Sea snakes do not attack in water if unmolested. Most bites result from handling the snake when caught in fishing nets. The bite shows no local reaction and minimal pain[53] and in most sea snake bites no envenomation occurs.[54] Initial symptoms, due to a myotoxin, are seen after a latent period of 30–120 min. There is muscular pain, stiffness and trismus followed by ptosis and progressive weakness which may threaten respiratory function. Myoglobinuria, renal tubular necrosis and acute renal failure may ensue.

Hadley et al[55] found thromboelastography to be a good predictor of severity in snakebite in children. They felt that, although it did not supersede clinical observation in the management of snakebite in children, it did allow stratification into high and low risk categories.

Treatment

The only effective treatment for a case of envenomation by a poisonous snake is the administration of antivenom, preferably intravenously. The use of antivenom, especially polyvalent antivenom, carries a substantial risk of anaphylaxis and serum sickness because of its foreign protein content, but there is no doubt that the benefits of antivenom treatment far outweigh the risks.[49,51] Its administration in every case of snake bite is, however, dangerous, wasteful and unnecessary. As only a minority of bites are due to poisonous snakes, it is obviously of paramount importance, as an initial step, to identify the snake accurately, or at least to decide into which group it falls. Much can be deduced from the color and shape of the snake, manner and circumstances of striking, the situation of the bite and presence or absence of fang marks. For instance, the puff adder, responsible for 95% of poisonous snake bites in Africa, is encountered on paths or in grassy terrain, and almost always strikes at the feet or ankles. On the other hand, cobras often attack when they are surprised near outbuildings or chicken runs. They rear up prior to striking and bites are frequently inflicted above the knees or even on the trunk or upper limbs.

As many victims of snake bites are not within easy access of clinic or hospital, it is most important to lay down firm and easily understood guidelines which can be applied to a layman on the spot:

1. *Symptoms* developing within the first half hour of a bite are almost always due to fear and its effects – and not to envenomation. The patient should be calmed and reassured, and encouraged to lie down quietly so as not to disseminate the poison by restless body movements. The affected limb should be kept horizontal at this stage and gently splinted to avoid movement. A mild analgesic (paracetamol) should be given and a placebo injection of saline has been found of value in older patients to allay anxiety.
2. *Bites* from non-venomous snakes should be thoroughly cleansed with a dilute antiseptic solution, any loose teeth removed, and a light dressing applied. Tetanus toxoid (or antitetanus serum if applicable) should be administered within 24 h to all cases of snake bite and broad spectrum antibiotics should be given at the first indication of possible infection.
3. *Signs* of significant envenomation generally develop from half to 2 h after the bite. These may be local in the case of viperine bites, with swelling and pain, or systemic in the case of elapid and some other snakes, with varying manifestations including vomiting, abdominal pain and neurotoxic symptoms, as noted earlier.[51] They call for urgent administration of antivenom: get the patient to a hospital or a trained person to the patient, so that it can be given intravenously. If this is not possible, the antivenom should be administered intramuscularly (see below). Sprivulis and Jelinek[51] advise that multiple doses of antivenom may be required. Premedication with parenteral antihistamine and low dose subcutaneous adrenaline (epinephrine) (0.003–0.007 mg/kg) prior to administration of antivenom will prevent anaphylaxis. This should be followed by a 5-day course of prophylactic oral corticosteroids to avoid delayed serum sickness.[56,57] Sprivulis and Jelinek[51] recommend that a short course of oral steroids may reduce the incidence of serum sickness, particularly in children and in patients receiving polyvalent or multiple doses of monovalent antivenom.
4. *Tourniquets:* under no circumstances should a tourniquet be applied in the case of viper or colubrid bites. The local effects and subsequent complications are aggravated by compression. However, where highly venomous snakes with pronounced systemic effects are incriminated (e.g. cobras, mambas, crotalids and sea snakes), and especially if there are already signs of systemic toxicity, a tourniquet is sometimes applied to the affected limb above the bite to prevent further absorption. It should be broad and tightly applied to constrict arteries and veins. The tourniquet should be completely released for 90 s every 15 min, and finally removed after 1 h. The time of initial application should be clearly marked on the patient. There is no place for the application of a tourniquet more than 1 h after a bite or if antivenom has been given. Australian experience with elapid bites has much to recommend it. Thus it has been found that for this group of snakes, rather than using a tourniquet, venom movement can be effectively delayed for long periods by the application of a firm crepe bandage to the length of the bitten limb combined with immobilization by a splint. It is worth noting here that this 'pressure immobilization' method may be used for all elapid snake bites and some other types of bites or stings such as those from bees, wasps, or ants in sensitive subjects, and funnel-web spider bites.[51,56,58] It can also be used for sea snake bites.[53] However, exceptions when the method should *not* be applied include ant, bee and wasp stings in normal, non-sensitive subjects, red-back spider bites and jellyfish stings.[56] Where pressure immobilization is impractical (e.g. a bite on the body), then infiltration around the bite site with diluted adrenaline (epinephrine) is suggested by Sprivulis and Jelinek.[51]
5. *Suction:* suction apparatus is available in many commercial snake bite kits, and if used immediately may be of help in withdrawing venom from fang punctures. Suction by mouth, however, entails a definite risk of absorption of venom through the oral or intestinal mucous membranes. In general, suction is not recommended for snakebite.[49]
6. *Incision:* most authorities now condemn the use of deep incisions over fang marks as a first aid measure. Superficial incisions, if made within minutes of the bite, may be of possible benefit in enhancing removal of venom, when coupled with efficient suction but again, in general, its use is not recommended.[49]
7. *Other local measures*, such as freezing, injection of antivenom, EDTA or other agents into the bite and application of permanganate crystals to incised wounds, have no place in the management of snake bites, and can only serve to aggravate tissue damage.

Antivenom

Some 30 centers in different countries manufacture antivenom appropriate to local varieties. Polyvalent antisera generally cover most bites encountered, but in the case of certain snakes (e.g. boomslang) monospecific antisera are required. Antivenom is preferably given intravenously but the intramuscular route may be necessary when a doctor is not available. If more than 2 h have elapsed since the bite, the allergic status of the patient should be tested with a small intradermal test dose. A positive skin test constitutes a relative contraindication to its use, but this must be assessed according to the clinical condition of the patient. Adrenaline (epinephrine) should always be at hand to combat possible anaphylaxis. It is advisable to give a corticosteroid, such as hydrocortisone, prior to antivenom as this tends to modify serum reactions as well as having anti-inflammatory and antihypotensive effects.

Once a decision to administer antivenom has been reached, it must be given in adequate dosage[59] especially in the case of children and thus it must be emphasized that the dosage for children is the same as that for adults.[49] Antivenom is undoubtedly best given in an intravenous drip, diluted in about four times its volume of normal saline over a period of half an hour. A recommended initial intravenous dose is 40 ml. This should be repeated every 4 h if clinical response is not satisfactory and if necessary up to 200 ml should be given within the first 24 h. When large doses are used, steroids should be continued to modify possible serum sickness reactions. With the use of i.v. antivenom administration, the incidence of anaphylactoid reactions does increase, but these reactions respond quickly to prompt adrenaline (epinephrine) injection. If a doctor is not available, the usual dose that can be tolerated intramuscularly is about 20 ml.

In the case of ophthalmia due to a spitting cobra, the affected eye should be well washed with water or other bland fluid before diluted antivenom is instilled.

Venom detection ELISA kits (CSL Diagnostics, Australia), suitable for field use, are available in some countries such as Australia for venom detection and species identification in snakebite washings, blood or urine.[51,59] Thus in Australia, it is recommended that snakebite wounds are **NOT** washed as part of initial first aid technique.[51]

Further supportive care

Unless it has been shown with the passage of some hours that the bite is trivial all cases of poisonous snake bite require admission to hospital.

If severe bulbar or respiratory paralysis has developed, airway suction, oxygen and assisted respiration with or without tracheostomy are indicated.

Management of acute renal failure should be anticipated by adequate intravenous replacement, careful monitoring of input and output, urinalysis and measurement of plasma urea and electrolytes.

Hemorrhagic manifestations require careful appraisal with a coagulation profile as hemorrhagins (Russell's viper), fibrinolysins (boomslang) or intravascular clotting (puff adder) can be responsible. Intravenous vitamin K, blood transfusion, fresh plasma, or fibrinogen, low molecular weight dextran, heparin or alpha-aminocaproic acid may be required according to circumstances.

In the event of severe local swelling, the limb should be kept elevated. Bullae should not be burst as this increases the likelihood of infection. Skin or fascial release to ease jeopardized circulation, debridement of necrotic tissue, and subsequent grafting or amputation are not uncommonly required, especially in untreated puff adder bites.

In an interesting analysis of deaths from snake bites Sutherland[60] has emphasized that snake bite deaths result from:

1. victims not being observed for an adequate period – suspected snake bite victims should be observed for at least 12–24 h after the bite;
2. antivenom being withheld despite clear indication of systemic envenomation;
3. giving the wrong antivenom – often more than once;
4. giving too little of the correct antivenom or not giving more antivenom if signs and symptoms reoccur.

Prevention

1. Treat all snakes with respect.
2. Endeavor to know the snakes in your area.
3. Watch out in summer months particularly after first rains. Be careful when walking at night; use a torch.
4. Wear boots and leggings or at least shoes and socks when walking in the bush (80% of human snake bites are on the legs and 55% on the ankle and foot).
5. Avoid thickly bushed country, long grass, etc.
6. Do not panic and run away when confronted by a snake; movement will attract attention whereas the snake is likely to move off if you keep still.
7. Keep an appropriate anti-snakebite kit with you.

It has also been found important in Australia to emphasize the need to believe a child who claims to have been bitten by a snake.[61]

INSECTS, SPIDERS, TICKS, BEETLES, SCORPIONS, CENTIPEDES AND CATERPILLARS

Hymenoptera stings

All stinging insects, such as bees, wasps, hornets and ants, are included in the order Hymenoptera. Bee venom contains many toxic fractions, the most important being mellitin which alters capillary permeability, causes local pain, hemolyzes red cells, and lowers blood pressure. The venom also contains antigenic components which are capable of invoking an allergic response in the form of hypersensitivity in a significant proportion of the population if subjected to a subsequent challenge. Cross-antigenicity may occur between wasp and bee stings and even on occasions, the rare stings by bumblebees.

In Australia serious clinical problems are becoming more common owing to severe allergy to jumper ant (*Myrmecia pilosula*) and bull ant (*Myrmecia pyriformis*) bites and stings.

The management of insect stings has been well reviewed by Reisman.[62] In general terms, uncomplicated stings require no treatment, apart from mild analgesics. Bee sting barbs should be carefully removed with a flat blade, taking care not to express further venom, which will happen if the sting is grasped with forceps. It has been claimed that meat tenderizer, available in most kitchens, applied in a dilute solution (a quarter teaspoon mixed with 1 teaspoon of water), rubbed into the sting relieves all pain within seconds. In sensitive individuals, however, even a single sting may result in acute anaphylactic shock with urticaria, hypotension, tachycardia and sweating, glottic edema, or bronchospasm. Prompt treatment is vital. Adrenaline (epinephrine) is indicated. In the case of laryngeal edema, hydrocortisone should be injected intravenously. Tracheostomy may be life saving in the event of severe edema of the glottis.

Skin tests to detect hypersensitivity to Hymenoptera stings are unreliable. However, children who are known to react in a hypersensitive manner should undergo desensitization with a carefully planned immunization schedule, using polyvalent Hymenoptera antigen. Immunotherapy may become more reliable with the development and use of pure venom immunization and phospholipase A, when and if it becomes available. However, children appear to exhibit considerably less frequent severe side-effects to stings than adults. Accordingly Valentine et al[63] conclude that immunotherapy is unnecessary for most children allergic to insect stings.

Bee venoms also possess hemolytic properties and multiple stings, usually in excess of 100, may result in significant hemolysis with acute anemia and subsequent renal failure. Cases of massive bee stings should be admitted to hospital and carefully observed for early signs of these complications, where prompt treatment can be instituted and renal failure minimized to ensuring a high urine output. Biphasic renal failure has been known to occur with early renal failure due to hemolysis and a second episode of azotemia about 10 days later, corresponding with a depressed serum complement C3 level and nephritic changes on renal biopsy – a phenomenon probably representing a serum sickness reaction caused by a large volume of foreign protein.

Studies in Australia have shown that 'Stingose' (an aqueous solution of 20% aluminum sulfate and 1.1% surfactant) is an effective, wide-acting first aid treatment to counteract the venoms of insects, marine invertebrates and plants when applied topically soon after the bite or sting.

The application of ice packs to insect stings (and platypus stings in Australia) will help to relieve local pain.[64]

Spider bites

Only a small fraction of the several hundred genera of spiders contain poisonous species and Alexander[65] has discussed these in detail. The most important medically are *Latrodectus* and *Loxosceles* with *Latrodectus mactans* (the black widow spider of the USA and button spider of South Africa) and *L. geometricus* (the brown widow spider) being the commonest species, being widely distributed throughout the warmer areas of the world. In Australia, *L. hasseltii* (red-back spider) and in New Zealand, *L. katipo* (katipo spider) are found.[58]

Only the aggressive females are hazardous to humans. They have black or dark velvety globular bodies about 15 mm in length with orange-red markings often in the shape of an hourglass on the ventral surface of the abdomen. They tend to spin their webs in dark places, such as under lavatory seats, hence the number of bites which occur on the buttocks or genitalia. *Latrodectus* venoms (alpha-latrotoxin) possess neurotoxic properties and cause stimulation of neuromuscular junctions. Following a bite from *Latrodectus*, there is a very variable local reaction. Signs of systemic envenomation occur between 20 and 200 min later. There is often a regional lymphadenopathy within 30 min of the bite, followed by severe muscular pains involving the limbs and trunk with tightness around the chest and abdominal rigidity which may mimic an acute abdomen. Hyperreflexia is often present. Death is rare, even in untreated cases, but when it occurs, is usually due to respiratory or cardiac failure. Treatment is aimed at relieving muscular spasm. It is worth noting, however, that only about 25% of people bitten, progress to systemic envenomation.[58] Calcium gluconate 10% (5–10 ml by slow i.v. injection) is effective in depressing the excited neuromuscular junctions. However, specific *Latrodectus* antivenom is available in most endemic areas,[59] and in cases of severe envenomation it should be given intravenously (5 ml) and if necessary repeated. If the victim shows only a mild local reaction and no systemic effects are detectable after 24 h then antivenom should not be given.[60] The possibility of adverse serum reactions although uncommon should be borne in mind and adrenaline (epinephrine) and corticosteroids should always be at hand. The use of premedication remains controversial.[58]

The genus *Loxosceles* includes many long-legged spiders occurring throughout Latin America as well as in focal areas elsewhere. The venom is cytotoxic and a bite is accompanied by severe local pain rapidly followed by marked edema, which may progress to necrosis. Treatment is aimed at controlling the local reaction. Parenteral antihistamines have been shown to decrease both the pain and the swelling.

In Australia, the Sydney funnel web spider (*Atrax robustus*), and various species of the genus *Hadronyche* are the cause of serious spider bites each year. These are large aggressive spiders which rear up before attacking when disturbed. They have a complex venom (robustoxin) and with multiple bites being the rule, considerable pain and panic ensue. In cases where systemic envenomation develops, airway obstruction may occur due to muscle spasm, excessive salivation, and vomiting. Loss of consciousness may occur and death can result from respiratory failure.

In management of bites from this spider, atropine and diazepam have proved useful, but repeated doses may have to be given. Encouraging results have been obtained in the development of a funnel web spider venom antagonist.

There is some evidence that the bite of the white-tailed spider, *Lampona cylindrata*, in Australia can cause chronic non-healing skin ulcers.[58,66] Other dangerous spiders in Australia are the wolf spider (*Lycosa* spp.) and the mouse spider (*Missulena occatoria*).[58]

Tick bites: tick paralysis

Ticks are the vectors of a number of human diseases in both tropical and temperate regions. These include the tick bite fevers, certain arbovirus diseases and Lyme disease due to *Borrelia burgdorferi*.[67] However, as well as this role in the transmission of infectious diseases, dealt with elsewhere, tick bites may have other unpleasant effects.

Engorging ticks should be encouraged to detach themselves, by applying a lubricant such as liquid paraffin, before gently extracting them. They should never be hastily pulled off, as the tick's mouthparts may be retained in the skin. This may subsequently give rise to a granuloma composed of a dense dermal granulomatous reaction associated with overlying pseudoepitheliomatous hyperplasia, which on occasions may be so marked in biopsy material that it can lead the unwary pathologist to an erroneous diagnosis of squamous carcinoma. On other occasions, the bite may lead to ulceration which is slow to heal. It remains covered by a necrotic, black eschar which takes many days to separate.

Certain ticks of the genera *Ixodes, Dermacentor, Haemaphysalis, Rhipicephalus* and *Hyalomma* produce a neurotoxin in their saliva which may cause 'tick paralysis'. The condition is commoner in children than in adults and particularly tends to afflict girls, probably because their longer hair hides the tick engorging on the scalp or neck, often with little or no local discomfort. A period of irritability occurs several days after the tick has been present. This is followed by ascending symmetrical flaccid paralysis. Initially there is difficulty in walking and standing.[65] Within a day or two, paralysis spreads up from the legs to involve the trunk, arms and neck. Bulbar involvement causes dysphagia, slurring of speech and may result in death from respiratory failure. A local paralysis of the face, for example, may result when the tick is attached to the eardrum. Sensory changes are minimal although there may be paresthesia in the paralysed limbs. The cerebrospinal fluid remains normal. Mortality may reach 11%, although death is uncommon if the engorging tick is removed.[60] Tick paralysis should be considered in the differential diagnosis of Guillain–Barré syndrome and it can mimic poliomyelitis.[65] Rapid and complete recovery usually attends the removal of the offending tick, although sometimes neuroparalysis may become transiently worse after removal of the tick. In Australia a canine antitick antivenom is available[59] and has been used in children with promising results.

Tick bites can also cause a severe life-threatening anaphylactic reaction in sensitized patients.

Beetles

Two large families of beetles, found in many parts of the world, produce urticating toxins. These are the Staphylinidae (rove beetles) and the Meloidae (blister beetles).

In Africa, and parts of Asia, America and Europe, rove beetle dermatitis due to the genus *Paederus* poses a difficult problem. When the tiny beetles are brushed off the skin, or crushed, an irritant toxic principle, pederin, is released. This causes blistering 1–2 days later. The blisters vesicate in 2–8 days and have a tendency to spread as a result of the release of fluid. Thereafter, the lesions flatten and dry out with subsequent peeling. On occasions the blistering is accompanied by systemic symptoms, with headache, fever, myalgia and arthralgia. A severe conjunctivitis, commonly known as 'Nairobi eye' results if pederin comes into contact with the eyes.

Several genera of Meloidae, including *Lytta* ('Spanish fly'), produce a vesicant, cantharidin, which is falsely credited with aphrodisiac properties, but which is toxic if ingested.

Treatment of dermatitis due to rove or blister beetles relies on the topical application of compresses, such as magnesium sulfate, and eye lesions should be bathed with isotonic saline.[65]

The condition termed 'Christmas eye' in Australia is as yet of undetermined origin. It may prove to be due to an orthopteran of some type, but a blister beetle seems more likely.

Scorpion stings

Scorpions have a single caudally placed sting with which they can inject venom. Some varieties, such as the genus *Parabuthus*, are dangerous especially to young children. Serious stings are characterized by hypersensitivity and severe pain at the site of the sting, paresthesia and myalgia in the affected limb, quickly followed by generalized weakness, muscle spasm, epigastric pain, excessive salivation and rhinorrhea, excitement, coma, convulsions and respiratory failure, often fatal. Less venomous varieties, or stings in older subjects, result in only local pain and swelling, sometimes with lymphangitis. Nausea, vomiting and headache may also occur, and pancreatitis is a reported complication.

Treatment

In India, it has been noted that scorpion stings in children can have a high mortality rate unless adequate symptomatic and specific therapy are given. Prompt application of a tourniquet will slow the spread of venom. Ice packs applied to the sting site may help to reduce pain and limit local circulation. Scorpion antivenom is available and can be life saving in severe envenomation; 10 ml should be given intramuscularly, as soon as possible, keeping adrenaline (epinephrine) and corticosteroids on hand in case of anaphylaxis. When antivenom is not available, general supportive treatment is needed and subcutaneous atropine and intravenous calcium gluconate have been reported to be effective. The need for assisted respiration must be anticipated. In milder stings, immersion of the affected part in very hot water alleviates the pain, but injection of a local anesthetic into the site may be required.

Centipedes

Bites from centipedes can cause considerable pain and swelling, and sometimes local ulceration and spreading lymphangitis result.

Caterpillars (lepidopterism)

The fine, spiny, venom-containing hairs of some species of caterpillar induce a very painful urticarial or vesicular dermatitis. This may be acquired by actual contact with the larva or from hairs blown in the wind. Where caterpillars are very prolific, severe symptoms may occasionally be induced in children, with extensive rashes, fever, vomiting and even paralysis. Hairs are best removed by applying adhesive tape to the site. Immersion in a very hot bath is soothing, and analgesics may be required. There is little evidence for the development of an allergic response from repeated exposure. Shock syndrome can follow stings from caterpillars of *Megalopyge* and can be treated with subcutaneous 1:1000 adrenaline (epinephrine) solution twice a day if necessary.[65]

STINGS FROM VENOMOUS MARINE ANIMALS

Stings from venomous marine animals can be a major health problem in many parts of the world, including Australia, Papua New Guinea, South-East Asia, Asia and the Far East, the Mediterranean, North and Latin America, the Caribbean and even Russia.[68] As might be expected, the problem is greatest in tropical waters and its magnitude can be gauged by figures from Australia where, over the summer months of 1990–1991, more than 18 000 people were treated for marine stings[69] while in the USA, in Chesapeake Bay alone, about 500 000 jellyfish envenomations occur each year.[70]

Although mostly seasonal, the problem of marine stings in the waters of northern Australia is so significant that it often precludes swimming during the summer months, except in areas protected by special nets – termed 'stinger enclosures'.

Overall, the most common cause of jellyfish stings is coelenterates of the genus *Physalia*, the common blue bottle or Portuguese man-of-war. Stings from these animals occur in the water or on the beach and, especially with the short-tentacled species, can be painful for up to an hour or so, but are not usually life threatening.[64] Stings from the multiple-tentacled species, however, can be severe and rare fatalities are on record.[64,69]

The so-called 'nematocyst dermatitis' from the blue bottle jellyfish is often exacerbated by the tentacles sticking to the skin, with subsequent discharge of the nematocysts causing ongoing pain and discomfort.

Treatment of blue bottle stings consists of gentle washing off of the attached tentacles with water (not vinegar) and then covering the affected area with a plastic bag containing ice and water to alleviate the pain.[64]

By contrast, stings due to the seawasp or box jellyfish (*Chironex* spp.) are excruciatingly painful and are associated with a significant mortality. Thus stings by this species in northern Australia have resulted in over 300 cases between 1984 and 1994, with in excess of 80 deaths being recorded from these stings in the twentieth century in Australia – often only minutes after the sting has occurred in the water.[66,71]

The bodies of people stung by this jellyfish are often covered with long red wheals which, if the victim survives, can result in permanent scarring.[64] Reactions to the sting may, however, in some cases, be delayed for some time.[69] The toxin of this species has three modes of action – it damages the skin, attacks the red blood cells and, most importantly, can affect the heart and respiration.[66,71]

The treatment for *Chironex* stings is the immediate application of vinegar by pouring it liberally over the affected area to prevent further nematocyst discharge. In severe cases, CPR can be life saving[71] and the use of a specific *Chironex fleckeri* antivenom produced by the Commonwealth Serum Laboratories in Melbourne, Australia is beneficial.[53,59] The recommended dosage should not be reduced for children.[69]

It is worth reiterating that vinegar is essential to inhibit the discharge of further nematocysts but will not reduce pain and, paradoxically, may initially increase pain. Compression-immobilization bandaging may be helpful.[53,72]

In Australia, a third type of jellyfish sting is the so-called 'Irukandji sting' which is caused by a minute carybdeid jellyfish (*Carukia barnesi*) and which can result in severe joint pains, low back pain, trunk pain, headache, shivering, sweating, hypotension and cardiac involvement.[53,66,71] Stings usually occur in the water in the afternoon and the jellyfish, being so small, is often not seen.

Treatment for the pain in Irukandji syndrome involves the use of ice packs, and 20 mg i.v. furosemide (frusemide) proved beneficial in one case.[69] Again the application of vinegar may help prevent further envenomation from undischarged nematocysts.[71]

Other jellyfish known to cause stinging of humans include the large carybdeids ('firejellies') in Tomoya or Morbakka stings; the 'hairjelly' or 'sea blubber', *Cyanea*, and *Pelagia noctiluca*, the 'mauve blubber'.[64,71]

There are, of course, a large number of other potentially dangerous marine animals, including stingrays, the blue ringed octopus, sea urchins, starfish, stonefish and lion fish amongst others. The management of such a diverse range of envenomations is obviously beyond the scope of this chapter, but the topic has been well reviewed by Williamson et al,[68] Pearn[71] and Auerbach.[73]

THE SUDDEN INFANT DEATH SYNDROME (SIDS)

DEFINITION AND HISTORICAL PERSPECTIVE

Sudden unexpected deaths in infancy have been recognized since antiquity. Historically, many were attributed to overlaying, and in some countries legislation was enacted in an attempt to prevent babies being taken into bed with parents, particularly if they had been drinking alcohol.[74] In some societies parents were accused of infanticide. During the twentieth century, as more babies in Western countries slept in cots, and overall infant mortality rates fell, it became clear that certain infant deaths, unexpected by history, remained unexplained after detailed postmortem examination.[75,76] Whilst a small proportion of such deaths were (and remain) a result of deliberate parental actions, in most there is no suspicion of such actions, and the consistent epidemiological features of the condition (e.g. age incidence, seasonality) make such a cause inherently very unlikely for the great majority.[77]

In 1969, at a conference in Seattle, a definition was drawn up for the sudden infant death syndrome (SIDS):

> *The sudden death of an infant or young child, which is unexpected by history and in which a thorough postmortem examination fails to demonstrate an adequate cause for death.*

Many subsequent attempts have been made to improve upon this definition, particularly emphasizing the need for a review of the clinical history and the circumstances of death. At the 3rd SIDS International Meeting in Stavanger in 1994 a modified definition was proposed, which whilst retaining the inherent simplicity of the original definition, includes caveats to cover these concerns:

> *The sudden death of an infant, which is unexplained after review of the clinical history, examination of the circumstances of death, and postmortem examination.*

Whilst the cause or causes of such deaths remain unknown a more precise definition is unlikely to be achieved.[78]

The human definition, that of a family who put a loved and apparently healthy baby down to sleep only to find him or her a few minutes to a few hours later dead with no adequate explanation for the death even after detailed investigation, is the one with which the clinical pediatrician must struggle to cope and try to provide comfort, support and information to the family.

INCIDENCE

The reported incidence of SIDS varies widely between countries and over time. During the 1970s the incidence apparently rose in the United Kingdom and many other Western countries. This rise was attributed to diagnostic shift, in that the diagnosis of SIDS was not a registerable cause of death in the United Kingdom until 1971. Throughout the 1980s the incidence of SIDS in the United Kingdom remained between 1.6 and 2.2 per 1000 live births. In some countries (e.g. New Zealand) the rates were consistently higher, at 3–4 per 1000 live births, and in others (e.g. Hong Kong) much lower, at 0.2 per 1000 live births or less. The recognition in the late 1980s of the contributory role of prone sleeping position, and the implementation in many countries of campaigns to reduce the risk of SIDS (see below) has led to a remarkable fall in incidence, to 0.4 in the United Kingdom in the year 2000, and 1.4 in New Zealand. In Sweden the SIDS rate rose during the 1970s and 1980s to a peak of around 1.1/1000 births, falling again after a risk reduction campaign in 1992 to a level of 0.3/1000 live births in 1999, a level virtually the same as in 1973.[79] In the USA the SIDS rate, previously between 1.2 and 1.4 per 1000 live births, fell after a risk reduction campaign in 1994 to 0.87 in 1995, and 0.77 in 1997.[80]

EPIDEMIOLOGY, RISK FACTORS AND RISK REDUCTION CAMPAIGNS

Epidemiological features of SIDS

A number of characteristic and consistent features of SIDS have emerged from studies in various countries over the past 30 years, notably a characteristic age distribution, with very few deaths in the first 2 weeks after birth, a peak at 2–3 months and less than 10% of deaths occurring after 7 months; an excess of deaths in male babies and (until recently) a marked seasonality, with more deaths in the winter months, particularly in temperate or colder regions. This excess of deaths in the colder months, when the incidence of viral upper respiratory tract infections is highest, has led to an interest in the role of infection in the etiology of SIDS. Whilst many babies who die suddenly and unexpectedly have been apparently well in the preceding few days, an increased proportion compared to matched control infants have had signs or symptoms suggestive of minor viral infection.[81,82] In a population-based case control study of the role of viral infection in SIDS, Gilbert et al[83] did not find a significant excess of viral infections in the infants who died, but found that the combination of heavy wrapping and the presence of a viral infection was a major risk factor. Infants who had started or completed their courses of immunization were shown, in studies from New Zealand[84] and the UK[85] to be at a lower risk of SIDS, with no evidence that immunization reactions of any type led to an increased risk. The introduction of the accelerated immunization schedule (in 1990) and the Haemophilus influenzae b (hib) immunization (in 1992) in the UK were associated with marked falls in the incidence of SIDS.

The association between infant mortality and socioeconomic deprivation has been recognized since the nineteenth century, and the marked excess of SIDS in the most deprived groups in society has been noted in several epidemiological studies, though similar patterns occur in other causes of infant mortality.[86,87] SIDS occurs within all socioeconomic groups, but certain factors have consistently been found to be associated with increased risk, notably young maternal age, high parity, maternal smoking or drug abuse, short gestation, low birth weight for gestation, multiple births and male sex. The fall in SIDS rate that has followed the 'Back to Sleep' campaign in the UK was more marked in the less socially deprived groups, with the consequence that SIDS is now even more strongly associated with socioeconomic deprivation than previously.[77,88] In a large population based study of unexpected infant deaths Leach et al[88] showed that almost all of the risk factors associated with SIDS were similarly associated with infant deaths that, although unexpected, were fully explained (e.g. from infection). Three factors differed: i) the characteristic age distribution of the SIDS deaths, ii) a much higher prevalence of maternal smoking amongst the SIDS families, and iii) a higher incidence of minor anomalies amongst the explained deaths. Socioeconomic factors, whilst of value in identifying populations at increased risk of SIDS, and thus potentially suitable for inclusion in studies of possible pathophysiological processes, are not (with the exception of smoking and drug abuse) within the power of the parents to change, and are thus of limited value in any attempt to reduce the incidence of the condition. Certain other factors (e.g. breast or bottle-feeding, maternal alcohol intake) may act as markers of lifestyle or socioeconomic status, and have less consistently been found to have independent effects on the risk of SIDS.[77,89] Whilst considerable attention has been focused on the subsequent siblings of SIDS victims as a group at increased risk of SIDS, large scale population-based studies have not confirmed a greatly increased risk for such infants independent of environmental or childcare factors (which are likely to remain constant within families, and may thus lead to an apparently increased risk for successive infants in the same family).[90] Fleming et al[77] showed that, for an infant in a family in which anyone smoked the risk of SIDS was 1 in 700, compared with 1 in 5000 if nobody smoked. Similarly for an infant in a household with no waged income, the risk was 1 in 500, compared with 1 in 2000 if there was a waged income. For an infant of a mother aged less than 27 years, and parity 2 or more, the risk was 1 in 567, compared with 1 in 882 for a mother over 27 or parity of 1. For families with all three factors, the risk of SIDS was 1 in 214, compared with 1 in 8543 where none was present – i.e. a 40-fold difference in risk.

A family history of a previous unexplained infant death must raise the possibility of an underlying metabolic disorder or an abnormality of physiology, which should be carefully sought, both at the postmortem examination and after the birth of any subsequent children. A history of a previous unexpected infant death, particularly if preceded by one or more apparent life threatening episodes (ALTE) may also raise the question of imposed upper airway obstruction or other form of abuse. The care and investigation of families in which such abuse is suspected remains controversial, but should follow the same broad guidelines as all cases of suspected child abuse, with early, careful multiagency involvement, and great care to protect not only the well-being of the child but, if possible, the family structure (see Apparent life-threatening events). [77,91–94]

Potentially modifiable factors

Over the past decade attention has increasingly been given to a number of factors in the infant's pre- and postnatal environment which affect the risk of SIDS and *are* potentially amenable to change. Studies in Hong Kong, Holland, England, New Zealand and Australia have shown the strong association between the prone sleeping position and the risk of SIDS.[89,95–99] Heavy wrapping, a warm environment, soft bedding and covers which can slip over the baby's head have all been implicated as risk factors.[77,89,97,100–103] These studies have drawn attention to the importance of pre- and postnatal exposure to tobacco smoke as a risk factor for SIDS.[77,104,105] In New Zealand, but not in the UK, breast-feeding had a protective effect independent of associated sociocultural factors.[77,106–108] Bedsharing by parents with their baby was initially identified by the New Zealand cot death study group as a risk factor for SIDS, but more detailed analysis of their data showed that this was only the case for parents who smoked,[109,110] findings subsequently confirmed in the United Kingdom and in the USA.[77,108,111,112] Blair et al[112] showed that the increase in risk of SIDS for infants sleeping with a parent was particularly associated with parental alcohol intake, excessive tiredness, and the infant being under a duvet, in addition to parental smoking. Sharing a sofa was associated with a particularly high risk. He suggested that it was more appropriate to consider bedsharing as an environment in which certain conditions could lead to increased risk (as for cot sleeping infants) rather than an inherently dangerous sleeping environment for infants. Indeed for infants over 14 weeks of age, and infants of non-smoking parents he found no evidence of any increased risk from bedsharing. These suggestions are supported by the work of McKenna,[80,113] an anthropologist who has studied the interactions between mothers and babies during bedsharing, and suggests that, under certain circumstances, these interactions may be protective, and reduce the risk of SIDS.

Risk reduction campaigns

The recognition of the apparent importance of the potentially modifiable risk factors led in the late 1980s and early 1990s to the introduction in several countries (e.g. New Zealand, the UK, Australia, Holland, Norway) of campaigns to change infant care practices in order to reduce the risk of SIDS.[114] Such campaigns have all included attempts to stop babies being placed in the prone position to sleep, and information on the adverse effects of exposure to tobacco smoke. Some have included advice on avoiding overheating, illness care, promotion of breast-feeding and avoidance of bedsharing. These campaigns have all been followed by a dramatic fall in the incidence of SIDS, which has been largely attributed to the avoidance of the prone sleeping position.[99,115–118] In the USA, the implementation of a concerted risk reduction campaign in 1994 was followed by a significant fall in the SIDS rate by the end of 1995 (see above).

SIDS after a risk reduction campaign

Few studies have so far been published on the epidemiology of SIDS after risk reduction campaigns, but data from the Confidential Enquiry into Stillbirths and Deaths in Infancy[77,88,93,105,108] show that in the UK, whilst some factors remain unchanged (e.g. male preponderance), others have changed significantly (e.g. there has been a marked reduction in the seasonal occurrence). The time that the death was discovered in this study was between 5 and 10 a.m. for almost 70% of the deaths. With the marked reduction in prevalence of prone sleeping, the overall incidence of SIDS has fallen (as noted above), but for those infants put down to sleep prone the risk of SIDS remains approximately eight times higher than for those who are supine. The side sleeping position, whilst safer than the prone position, carries approximately twice the risk of the supine position. The use of bedding (particularly duvets), which can slip over the baby's head was found to be a major risk factor. Exposure to tobacco smoke, either before or after birth, is now identified as the single largest potentially avoidable factor, with a population attributable risk estimated at 60% (i.e. it may be responsible for this proportion of the deaths). The use of a pacifier (dummy) was associated with a significantly reduced risk of SIDS, though for infants who usually used a pacifier, failure to use one on a particular occasion was associated with an increased risk.[119] Some studies have shown pacifier use to be associated with decreased prevalence and durations of breast-feeding, whilst others have shown no effect.[119] Studies in the laboratory[120] have shown that pacifier use is associated with decreased digit sucking, and that the physiological effects of both types of non-nutritive sucking are similar, with increased oxygen saturation, decreased respiratory rate, and modulation of sleep states, though no identifiable effects upon breast-feeding frequency were seen in this study. North et al[121] showed a strong association between pacifier use and increased prevalence of minor infections in infancy.

The evidence linking some of the risk factors and SIDS is now very strong, amounting in the case of sleeping position and parental smoking to evidence of a *causal* relationship. This is not to say that all (or even a high proportion of) babies put to sleep prone or exposed to tobacco smoke will die as SIDS, but that these factors exert their effects somewhere in the pathway of causality, so that removing the factor will have a major influence on the incidence of SIDS. The ways in which risk factors are related to the process or processes which lead to death are largely unknown, though a number of hypotheses have been proposed.

PATHOLOGY AND THE MEDICOLEGAL SYSTEM

In England and Wales all sudden unexpected deaths must be reported to the coroner, who will order that certain basic information be collected (usually by the police or the coroner's officer) and that a postmortem examination be carried out. The coroner's main responsibility is to ensure that deaths due to non-natural causes are identified. In Scotland the Procurator Fiscal has a similar role to that of the coroner. The quality of the postmortem examination has varied widely in the past, but the adoption in 1993 by the Royal College of Pathologists of a recommended minimum standard for such examinations has led to increased consistency and quality of postmortems in the United Kingdom.[93] The Confidential Enquiry into Stillbirths and Deaths in Infancy (CESDI) Report and the Allitt enquiry[122] both strongly recommend that most if not all such examinations be carried out by pathologists with particular expertise in pediatric pathology. From the data collected in the CESDI study Berry has described an 'evidence-based' autopsy protocol, less complex than the original Royal College of Pathologist's protocol, and not involving the retention of any whole organs.[77] The CESDI Report also emphasized the importance of obtaining a detailed clinical history (usually by a pediatrician) from the parents of all infants dying suddenly and unexpectedly. This history should be obtained if possible *prior* to the postmortem, as it may be of importance in helping to direct the pathologist's attention to particular features. The importance of multiagency working after sudden deaths of infants or children (as in suspected child abuse) has also been emphasized, and recent experience has shown that joint home visits by a pediatrician and a member of the police Child Protection Team may be very helpful in facilitating appropriate care of bereaved families, whilst ensuring the legal requirements of the coroner's system are met.[77]

Understanding and interpretation of the available information for the family is helped by holding a multidisciplinary case discussion meeting a few weeks after the death, which should usually be attended by the pathologist, the general practitioner, the health visitor and the pediatrician. The value of such meetings has been emphasized by the Report of the Confidential Enquiry into Stillbirths and Deaths in Infancy.[77,93]

At postmortem examination or the multidisciplinary case discussion meeting, a proportion of infant deaths which were sudden and apparently unexpected are found to have a complete explanation (e.g. overwhelming infection, inborn error of metabolism, non-accidental injury). Such deaths, which together comprise between 10 and 30% of all sudden deaths in infancy, should not therefore be classified as SIDS, but as deaths due to the identified cause. For comparative purposes information should be collected on all unexpected deaths, including both SIDS and those deaths that were fully explained.[77,93]

Certain other findings are relatively common, and, whilst not giving an explanation for the death, do suggest that the infant may not have been completely well before death (e.g. viral upper respiratory tract infection, otitis media). Such deaths do come within the definition of SIDS, but should be separately identified for purposes of classification.[83,93] In the remaining cases, no evidence of pathological processes that may have contributed to the death is identified, but certain features are commonly seen which are characteristic of babies dying as SIDS. Such findings include liquid heart blood, and petechial hemorrhages on the serosal surfaces of intrathoracic organs. The presence of bloodstained fluid at the nose or mouth is common, as is intra-alveolar pulmonary hemorrhage and recent population-based studies have shown that these features are *not* particularly associated with conditions in which asphyxia (either natural or imposed) is a possibility. Both are more common in younger infants.[123,124] Postmortem hypostatic staining may give information on the position in which the baby died if the baby lay in this position for a number of hours after death. It is important that skeletal X-rays are carried out to look for possible bony injuries, and that samples are taken for detailed microbiological and histological examination. Electrolyte determination of the vitreous humor may identify biochemical abnormalities present at the time of death.

NORMAL DEVELOPMENTAL PHYSIOLOGY AND POSSIBLE PATHOPHYSIOLOGICAL PROCESSES

The precise series of events that occurs during sudden infant death is not known; nor is it known whether there is a single final common pathway or a number of possible pathophysiological pathways. The characteristic pathological findings outlined above have been interpreted as suggesting that respiratory failure is the final event in the majority of cases, perhaps preceded by one or more episodes of tissue hypoxia of variable severity.[125]

Recent evidence from infants who died suddenly and unexpectedly whilst undergoing cardiorespiratory monitoring and recording[126] showed that, in these cases at least, the first abnormal event was a sudden severe, prolonged bradycardia, followed by cessation of breathing.

The observation by Steinschneider[127] that prolonged episodes of apnea were recorded from some infants who had presented with apparent life-threatening events, and that such episodes were also identified in infants whose siblings had died as SIDS, led to the 'apnea hypothesis' of SIDS. This postulated that the final event in most, if not all, SIDS victims was apnea, and that infants at risk of dying in this way were likely to have repeated apneic episodes prior to death. Several large studies have failed to find any evidence to support this hypothesis, and Southall et al,[128] in a large, population-based prospective study, found that none of those infants identified as having episodes of prolonged apnea in the first week or at 6 weeks subsequently died as SIDS. None of the infants in this study who died as SIDS had previously shown prolonged apnea. Despite this lack of supporting evidence, the use of 'pneumograms' to identify infants with prolonged or frequent apnea, who were then deemed to be at increased risk of SIDS, was widespread, particularly in the USA until recently. The use of apnea monitors or more complex monitoring and/or recording devices (including measures of oxygenation) for infants identified by any technique as being at high risk of SIDS has not to date been shown to be of value in reducing the death rates for such infants[129] (see Investigation of ALTE). Similarly there is no evidence that the use of apnea or other monitors is of any direct value in the care of subsequent siblings of infants who have died as SIDS (p. 1719).

The absence of supporting evidence for the 'apnea hypothesis' does not rule out a defect of cardiac or respiratory control as an underlying part of the pathophysiology of SIDS. A number of studies have shown apparent differences in cardiac or respiratory pattern between normal control infants and those who subsequently died as SIDS, though such differences are relatively subtle, and of no value in identifying individual infants at particular risk.[130,131] The very strong association between SIDS and sleep or presumed sleep has led to the suggestion, supported by some experimental evidence, that a part of the final common pathway to death may be a defect in the process of arousal.[132]

During the first few months after birth complex developmental changes occur in a number of physiological systems, including the control of respiration, and thermoregulation. The effect of spontaneous and imposed disturbances on the pattern of respiration changes with age; prolonged and highly oscillatory responses to spontaneous deep breaths or brief exposure to increased CO_2 are most common at around 2–3 months of age. The presence of spontaneous oscillatory patterns of breathing (periodic breathing) is a normal feature of respiration in infants, particularly at this age.[133]

There are characteristic changes in the organization of the sleep–wake cycle over the same time period, with a marked increase in the amount of time spent in quiet sleep at around 8–12 weeks of age, and evidence that some infants who die as SIDS may have immaturity of these processes. Many physiological control systems behave differently according to the infant's sleep state, e.g. control of respiration, heart rate, arousal and thermoregulation.[134,135]

There is an increase in daytime and a decrease in night-time rectal temperature during early infancy. Rectal temperature changes little during night-time sleep in the newborn period but around the age of 8–16 weeks a characteristic pattern appears, with a relatively abrupt fall to below 36.5°C soon after sleep followed by a plateau and then a gradual rise in the early morning prior to waking. This pattern develops earlier in infants who are breast-fed, female, first-born and from more affluent families; infants gaining weight most rapidly mature later.[136]

The insulation provided by bedding and clothing, and room temperature have only a small effect upon infant rectal temperature during nocturnal sleep. Bottle-feeding or parental smoking individually did not affect rectal temperature but in combination, bottle-fed babies exposed to smoke had rectal temperatures 0.1°C higher for the entire night. In infants sleeping at home, the prone position is associated with an increased rectal temperature for some or all of the night.[137]

Daytime metabolic rate increases rapidly during early infancy[135] but little is known about nocturnal maturation during this period. By 3 months of age the infant excretes approximately 50% more heat per unit surface area than in the first week after birth. The 3-month-old infant is thus better adapted to dealing with cold stress than the newborn, but may be more vulnerable to the effects of heat stress.[138,139]

In a prospective study of normal infants, the metabolic rate during infection varied with age. In infants less than 3 months of age the metabolic rate commonly fell at the time of an infection, and fever was unusual, whilst in older infants the metabolic rate usually increased, and fever was more common.[140] In infants of all ages developing viral infections, the fall in temperature during the night was reduced 3–7 days before clinical signs of illness appeared. During this prodrome parents often reported that their infants were 'not right'. When clinical signs of infection appeared the fall in rectal temperature during the night returned to that expected for the infant's age, and few infants became pyrexial.[141] These observations suggest that changes of body temperature (and possibly metabolic rate) occur in the absence of significant clinical signs of illness and may fit with the concept of SIDS occurring in the prodromal phase of infection. This would fit the observations of recent signs or symptoms suggestive of infection but the lack of objective postmortem evidence of established infection in many infants.[81,82,92,142]

The concept of unrecognized illness preceding death and possibly leading to reduced weight gain prior to death has been the basis for the use of weighing scales as a means of monitoring infant well-being and perhaps allowing early identification of such illness. However, Brookes et al[143] did not find any evidence of poor weight gain preceding SIDS in a large population-based study. In a more recent study, Blair et al showed that the use of conditional growth charts allowed the identification of infants whose growth was less good than expected from their birth weight, and that such relative growth failure was associated with significantly increased risk of SIDS.[144]

Blackwell et al[145] have suggested a possible mechanism by which the prone sleeping position, heavy wrapping and the presence of a viral infection might predispose to the development of a secondary bacterial infection, with release of inflammatory mediators, particularly tumor necrosis factor, into the pharynx, leading to rapid and potentially lethal development of shock.

Exposure to tobacco smoke before or after birth may impair the development of autonomic function (as assessed by the infant's blood pressure response to changes in position from horizontal to a 60% head-up tilt),[146] and may also contribute to deficient arousal in infants during hypoxia.[147]

Inborn errors of metabolism, particularly defects of fat oxidation (e.g. medium chain acyl-CoA dehydrogenase deficiency), have been reported in a small proportion of infants dying suddenly and unexpectedly, but probably account for only 1–3% of the total of apparent SIDS deaths.[148]

One current view of SIDS envisages a 'triple-risk' model of the pathophysiology. This suggests that infants compromised by the effects of antenatal or perinatal factors (e.g. poor fetal growth, maternal smoking, perinatal asphyxia) may go through a period during their development in which one or more physiological systems (e.g. respiratory or cardiac control, arousal, thermoregulation) is vulnerable. The effect of a stressor (e.g. infection, thermal stress, hypoxemia) during this vulnerable period may be to cause failure of the vulnerable system. SIDS would thus be seen as the result of exposure to an exogenous stressor(s), during a critical developmental period, in vulnerable infants. Such a model may allow understanding of the ways in which many apparently unrelated factors may combine to contribute to the risk of death, particularly in infants predisposed by prenatal factors such as poor fetal growth, exposure to tobacco smoke, etc. Such a model does not imply that all such deaths occur as the result of the same insult or follow the same pathophysiological pathway, nor does it imply that all infants who die will necessarily have been identifiably compromised in utero or in the perinatal period.[149,150]

SUPPORT FOR BEREAVED FAMILIES

The death of a child is perhaps the worst tragedy that can befall any family. To lose a child suddenly, unexpectedly and with no subsequent explanation for what happened may impose unbearable stress on parents, surviving siblings and the extended family. Because of the circumstances of the death, and the inevitable involvement of the coroner and/or the police, many families bereaved in this way suffer the additional torture of the spoken or unspoken suspicion that they may have, deliberately or accidentally, contributed to the cause of their baby's death.

Families bereaved by the sudden unexpected death of their babies have special needs, which health care professionals must recognize and provide for. Almost inevitably, parents feel guilty because of some perceived imperfection that they recall in the way in which they cared for their infant. In their anxiety to reassure parents, health care professionals may sometimes fail to listen effectively to what the parents are trying to say. There is no point in reassuring parents that they did all the right things in the care of their baby unless you have first listened in detail to exactly what they did and what happened.

Bereaved parents need and deserve a sensitive, compassionate, caring approach from professionals. They need to be given time to be together as a family, perhaps for the last time, but should not be made to feel isolated by being left alone for long periods in a strange place such as an accident and emergency department. If resuscitation attempts have been made in the A & E department, it is important that doctors and nurses realize that it is not necessary to leave the endotracheal tube in place after death. If there has been a concern that it was not correctly placed and that this contributed to the death, then the tube position should be checked carefully and documented by an experienced clinician (preferably not the person who inserted the tube) prior to its removal.

Parents must be given clear, simple information (preferably written) on what will happen, and what will be required of them (e.g. registration of the death). They need to know that a postmortem examination will be performed, and they need to know, in sensitive terms, what that will involve. At the postmortem tissue samples will be taken for histological examination, and, on occasions whole organs (notably the brain) may need to be removed for fixation prior to sampling for histological examination. It is important that the doctor caring for the family is aware of what samples are taken, and that the family are given the opportunity to have this information should they wish to know. If the pathologist deems it necessary to retain a whole organ the family must be given the options of either arranging for respectful disposal of the organ at a later date, allowing the organ to be retained for diagnostic, research or teaching purposes, or of delaying the funeral (for 4–6 weeks) until the organ is returned to the body. Some families may have similar concerns about the tissue samples taken for diagnostic purposes. The law on this subject is complex, and at present unclear. A review of the rules governing such tissue or organ samples is currently being conducted in the UK. Whatever the outcome of this review, it is important that the family are given appropriate information.

The family need to know exactly where their baby will be, and when and how they will be able to see him or her.

As soon as possible after the death, often whilst parents are still holding their baby, in their home or in the accident and emergency department, they should be given the opportunity to talk at length about what has happened. Experience in the Avon Infant Mortality Study and the CESDI study[77,93,153] has shown the importance of this initial sensitive but detailed 'debriefing'. This interview should usually be carried out by an experienced senior doctor (pediatrician or general practitioner) or senior nurse, and careful notes recorded immediately afterwards. A visit to the home, to allow the parents to show the pediatrician exactly where the death occurred, and show the precise circumstances of the death may also be of great value, both in terms of aiding understanding of the events, and of helping the 'debriefing' process for the parents. This 'death scene' assessment must be very carefully documented, and must be followed by the opportunity for the family to talk to a sympathetic and experienced clinician about the issues raised for them. The pediatrician may carry out this assessment together with a Child Protection police officer,[77] but the emotional needs of the family must be given the highest priority. Information obtained at these interviews may be of particular importance to the pathologist, in helping to direct specific investigations at the postmortem examination. It may also be of particular value in helping the parents to start to come to terms with the death of their baby. The parents may have particular questions or concerns about what they believe may have happened, and eliciting this information early may allow the pathologist to give an answer. Unless the circumstances of the death or the postmortem findings are unusual or suspicious, the great majority of SIDS deaths are not followed by an inquest. Usually the coroner will issue a death certificate very shortly after the pathologist gives an initial report, which should usually be within 48 hours of the death.

If the baby who died was a twin, consideration should be given to whether the family would be helped by admitting the surviving twin to hospital for a few days. Whilst the real risk of death of the second twin is probably small, the family are likely to be very worried about this, and may find it easier to express their grief if they feel that the surviving twin is safe. For other families keeping the surviving twin at home may be important.

Arrangements should be made for an experienced doctor (usually a consultant pediatrician) to see the family again, preferably at home, with their general practitioner or health visitor, within a few days, to talk through the preliminary results of the postmortem examination, to give information on what is known about SIDS, and to try to answer their questions. This meeting will also give an opportunity to talk about the effects of grief on the members of the family (including siblings and grandparents), and their close friends. It may be the first opportunity which the members of the primary care team have had to talk in detail about what has happened with the parents and to establish their very important role in providing continuing support. For most families at least one further visit from the pediatrician will be appropriate, again usually with a member of the primary care team. A recent study[151] showed the importance of this follow-up from both the primary care team and the pediatrician, but showed that for the majority of families this support was not made available. As noted above, a multidisciplinary case discussion and future care planning meeting a few weeks after the death, attended by the pediatrician and the primary care team, at which the clinical history, postmortem findings and special needs of the family are discussed is of great value, and should be implemented as a routine.[77,93] Dent has described a valuable assessment tool, for use by professional caring for such families, in identifying the particular needs of individual family members, and providing appropriate, focused support.[152]

Parents should be given information on national and local parents' support groups* and on parent befriending schemes run by volunteers from those groups.

CARE OF THE NEXT INFANT

A further value of a multidisciplinary case discussion meeting is in planning appropriate care for the family should they decide to have a further baby. Approximately 80% of bereaved families have another baby within 3 years, and parents will be very worried about the risk to the next baby. The real risk of SIDS for the next

* The Foundation for the Study of Infant Deaths (FSID)
11–19 Artillery Row, London SW1 1RT
24 hour Helpline for bereaved families: 020 7233 2090

baby is approximately the same as if the baby who died were still alive. That is not to say that the risk is the same as for the rest of the population, since many risk factors (particularly those relating to socioeconomic factors) will still be present.

Bereaved families should be given the opportunity to discuss their concerns and have their questions answered during a subsequent pregnancy, and to be seen on one or more occasions after the baby's birth by a pediatrician with a particular interest in the care of such infants. In many areas of the United Kingdom the CONI (Care of Next Infant) program of the FSID may provide some additional help for such families. As noted above, there is no evidence that the use of any type of monitoring device is of direct value to the baby, but as part of a support package for the parents the use of a monitor may be of value for some families.[153,154]

REFERENCES (* Level 1 evidence)

1 Sibert JR. Stress in families of children who have ingested poisons. BMJ 1975; ii:87–89.

2 Scherz RG. Prevention of childhood poisoning. Pediatr Clin North Am 1970; 17:713.

3 Sibert JR, Lyons RA, Smith BA, et al. Preventing deaths by drowning in children in the UK: have we made progress in 10 years? Population based incidence study. BMJ 2002; 324:1070–1071.

4 Sibert JR, Frude N. Bittering agents in the prevention of accidental poisoning: children's reactions to denatonium benzoate. Arch Emerg Med 1991; 8:1–7.

5 Krenzelok EP, McGuigan M, Lheur P. Position statement: ipecac syrup. American Academy of Clinical Toxicology; European Association of Poisons Centres and Clinical Toxicologists. J Toxicol Clin Toxicol 1997; 35(7):699–709.

6 Chyka PA, Seger D. Position statement: single-dose activated charcoal. American Academy of Clinical Toxicology; European Association of Poisons Centres and Clinical Toxicologists. J Toxicol Clin Toxicol 1997; 35(7):721–741.

7 Craft AW, Lawson GR, Williams H, Sibert JR. Accidental childhood poisoning with household products. BMJ 1984; 288:682.

8 Yagupsky P, Gorodischer R Massive clonidine ingestion in a 9 month old infant. Pediatrics 1983; 72:500–501.

9 Bramley A, Goulding R. Laburnum 'poisoning'. BMJ 1981; 283:1220–1221.

10 UNICEF. A league table of child deaths by injury in rich nations. Innocenti Report Card No. 2. Florence: UNICEF Innocenti Research Centre; 2001.

*11 Towner E, Dowswell T, Mackereth C, Jarvis S. What works in preventing unintentional injuries in children and young adolescents? An updated systematic review. London: NHS Health Development Agency; 2001.

12 Williams H, Sibert JR. Medicine and the media. BMJ 1983; 286:1893.

13 Minchom P, Sibert JR. Does health education prevent childhood accidents? Postgrad Med J 1984; 60:260–262.

14 World Health Organization. Manifesto for Safe Communities. First world conference on accident and injury prevention, Stockholm, 1989.

15 Mott A, Rolfe K, James R. Safety of surfaces and equipment for children in playgrounds. Lancet 1997; 348:1874–1876.

16 Chalmers DJ, Marshall SW, Langley JD. Height and surfacing as risk factors in falls from playground equipment: a case-control study. Inj Prev 1996; 2:98–104.

17 Sibert JR, Mott A, Rolfe K. Preventing injuries in public playgrounds through partnership between health services and local authority: community intervention study. BMJ 1999; 318:1595.

18 Roseveare C, Brown J, Barclay-McIntosh J, Chalmers D. An intervention to reduce playground hazards. Inj Prev 1999; 5:124–128.

19 Hughes DR, Evans RC, Sibert JR. Sports injuries to children. Br J Accid Emerg Med 1986; 1:4–13.

*20 Chapman S, Cornwall J, Righetti J, Sung L. Preventing dog bites in children: randomized controlled trial of an educational intervention. BMJ 2000; 320:1512–1513.

21 Yeoh C, Nixon JW, Dickson W, et al. Patterns of scald injuries to children in the bath. Arch Dis Child 1994; 71:156–158.

22 Runyan CW, Bangdiwala SI, Linzer MA, et al. Risk factors for fatal residential fires. N Engl J Med 1992; 327:859–863.

23 DiGuiseppi C, Roberts I. Smoke alarm ownership and house fire death rates in children. J Epidemiol Community Health 1998; 52:760–761.

*24 DiGuiseppi C, Higgins JP. Systematic review of controlled trials of interventions to promote smoke alarms. Arch Dis Child 2000; 82:341–348.

*25 DiGuiseppi C, Roberts I, Speirs N. Smoke alarm installation in inner London council housing: cross sectional study. Arch Dis Child 1999; 81(5):400–403.

26 Katcher M, Landry G, Shapiro M. Liquid crystal thermometer use in pediatric office counseling about tap water burn prevention. Pediatrics 1989; 83:766–771.

27 Glendill DNS, Robson WV, Cudmore RE, Tavistock RR. Baby walkers – time to take a stand. Arch Dis Child 1987; 62:491–494.

28 Spiegal CN, Lindaman FC. Children can't fly: a program to prevent childhood morbidity and mortality from window falls. Am J Public Health 1977; 67:1143–1147.

29 Sharples PM, Storey A, Aynsley-Green A, Eyre JA. Causes of fatal childhood accidents involving head injury in northern region, 1979–86. BMJ 1990; 301:1193–1197.

*30 Thomson J, Ampofo-Boeteng K, Pitcairn T, Grieve R. Behavioural group training of children to find safe routes to school. Br J Educ Pyschol 1992; 62:173–183.

*31 Thomson J, Whelan K. A community approach to road safety education using practical training methods. The Drumchapel Project. Road Safety Report No. 3. London: Department of Transport 1997.

32 Roberts I, Ashton T, Dunn R, Lee-Joe T. Preventing child pedestrian injury: pedestrian education or traffic calming? Aust J Public Health 1994; 18:209–212.

*33 Christopherson E, Sosland-Edelman D, LeClaire S. Evaluation of two comprehensive infant car seat loaner programs with one-year follow-up. Pediatrics 1985; 76:36–42.

*34 Miller J, Pless I. Child automobile restraints: evaluation of health education. Pediatrics 1977; 59:907–911.

*35 Macknin M, Gustafson C, Gassman J, Barich D. Office education by pediatricians to increase seat belt use. Am J Dis Child 1987; 141:1305–1307.

*36 van Schagen IN, Brookhuis K. Training young cyclists to cope with dynamic traffic situations. Accid Anal Prev 1994; 26:223–230.

37 Thompson R, Rivara FP, Thompson DC. A case control study on the effectiveness of bicycle safety helmets. N Engl J Med 1989; 320:1361–1367.

*38 Cushman R, Down J, MacMillan N, Waclawik H. Helmet promotion in the emergency room following bicycle injury A randomized trial. Pediatrics 1991; 88:43–47.

39 Kemp AM, Sibert JR. Drowning and near drowning in children in the United Kingdom. Lessons for prevention. BMJ 1992; 304: 1143–1146.

41 Kemp AM, Mott AM, Sibert JR. Accidents and child abuse in bathtub submersions. Arch Dis Child 1994; 70:435–438.

42 Health and Safety Commission. Safety in swimming pools. London: Sports Council; 1988.

43 Ramey CA, Ramey DN, Hayward JS. Dive response of children in relation to cold water drowning. J Appl Physiol 1987; 63:665–668.

44 Harries M. Drowning and near drowning. BMJ 1986; 293:123–124.

45 Orlowski JP. Drowning, near drowning and ice water drowning. JAMA 1988; 260:390–391.

46 Kemp AM, Sibert JR. Outcome for children who nearly drown: a British Isles study. BMJ 1991; 302:931–933.

47 Bohn DJ, Biggar WD, Smith CR, et al. Influence of hypothermia, barbiturate therapy and intracranial monitoring on morbidity and mortality after near-drowning. Crit Care Med 1986; 14:529–534.

48 Nixon JW, Kemp AM, Levene S, Sibert JR. Suffocation, choking and strangulation in childhood in England and Wales: epidemiology and prevention. Arch Dis Child 1995; 71:7–14.

49 World Health Organization. Poisonous animal bites and stings. WHO Weekly Epidemiol Rec 1995; 44:315–316.

50 White J. How to treat snakebite. Pt1 Australian Doctor March, 2001 (Supplement).

51 Sprivulis P, Jelinek G. Snakebite. In: Cameron P (ed). Textbook of adult emergency medicine. Edinburgh: Churchill Livingstone; 2000:649–651.

52 Scharman E, Noffunger V. Copperhead snakebites: clinical severity of local effects. Ann Emerg Med 2001; 38:55–61.
53 Banham NDG. Marine envenomation. In: Cameron P (ed). Textbook of adult emergency medicine. Edinburgh: Churchill Livingstone; 2000:655–657.
54 Heatwole H. Seasnakes. Sydney: University of NSW Press; 1987.
55 Hadley GP, McGarr P, Mars M. Role of thromboelastography in the management of children with snakebite in southern Africa. Trans R Soc Trop Med Hyg 1999; 93:177–179.
56 Sutherland S. Antivenom use in Australia. Med J Aust 1992; 157:734–739.
57 Tibballs J. Premedication for snake antivenom. Med J Aust 1994; 160:4–7.
58 Jelinek G, Spider bite. In: Cameron P (ed). Textbook of adult emergency medicine. Edinburgh; Churchill Livingstone; 2000:652–655.
59 White J. CSL antivenom handbook: CSL Diagnostics; Melbourne 1995.
60 Sutherland S. Venomous bites and stings. Med Aust 1978; 6:402–412.
61 Sutherland S. First aid for snakebite in Australia. Parville: CSL Diagnostics; 1979.
62 Reisman RE. Insect stings. N Engl J Med 1994; 331:523–527.
63 Valentine MD, Schuberth KC, Kagey-Sobotka A, et al. The value of immunotherapy with venom in children with allergy to insect stings. N Engl J Med 1990; 323:1601–1603.
64 Sutherland S. Poisonous Australian animals. Victoria; Hyland House: 1992:64.
65 Alexander JOD. Arthropods and human skin. Berlin; Springer:1984.
66 Sutherland S. Venomous creatures of Australia. Melbourne: Oxford University Press; 1982:127.
67 Piesman J. Emerging tick-borne diseases in temperate climates. Parasitol Today 1987; 3:197–199.
68 Williamson J, Fenner P, Burkett J, Rifkin J, (eds). Venomous and poisonous marine animals. Sydney; University of NSW Press:1996.
69 Fenner P, Williamson J, Burnett J. Some Australian and international marine envenomation reports, 1995.
70 Fischer PR. The danger of marine envenomations. Travel Medicine Adviser Update 1995; 5:32–33.
71 Pearn J. The sea, stingers, and surgeons: the surgeon's role in prevention, first aid and management of marine envenomations. J Pediatr Surg 1995; 30:105–110.
72 Beadnell CE, Rider TA, Williamson JA, Fenner PJ. Management of a major box jellyfish sting. Med J Aust 1992; 156:655–658.
73 Auerbach PS. Marine envenomation. N Engl J Med 1991; 325:486–493.
74 Norvenius G. Is SIDS a new phenomenon? In: Rognum TO (ed). Sudden infant death syndrome. New trends in the nineties. Oslo; Scandinavian University Press; 1995: 11–14.
75 Templeman C. Two hundred and fifty eight cases of suffocation of infants. Edinb Med J 1892; 38:322–329.
76 Limerick SA. Sudden infant death in historical perspective. J Clin Pathol 1992; 45(suppl):3–6.
77 Fleming PJ, Blair PS, Bacon C, eds. Sudden unexpected death in infancy. The CESDI SUDI Studies. London: The Stationery Office; 2000.
78 Rognum TO, Willinger M. The story of the 'Stavanger definition' In: Rognum TO (ed). Sudden infant death syndrome. New trends in the nineties. Oslo: Scandinavian University Press; 1995: 21–22.
79 Alm B, Norvenius SG, Wennergren GJ, et al. Changes in the epidemiology of sudden infant death syndrome in Sweden 1973–1996. Arch Dis Child 2001; 84:24–30.
80 Byard RW, Krous HF. Sudden infant death syndrome. London Arnold, 2001.
81 Ward-Platt M, Blair PS, Fleming PJ, et al. Sudden unexpected death in infancy. A clinical comparison of explained and unexplained deaths – how healthy and how normal? Arch Dis Child 2000; 82:98–106.
82 Cole TJ, Gilbert RE, Fleming PJ, et al. Baby check and the Avon Infant Mortality Study. Arch Dis Child 1991; 66:1077–1078.
83 Gilbert RE, Rudd PT, Berry PJ. Combined effect of infection and heavy wrapping on the risk of sudden infant death. Arch Dis Child 1992; 67:272–277.
84 Mitchell EA. Smoking: the next major and modifiable risk factor. In: Rognum TO (ed). Sudden infant death syndrome. New trends in the nineties. Oslo: Scandinavian University Press; 1995:114–118.
85 Fleming PJ, Blair PS, Ward Platt M, et al. The accelerated immunisation programme in the UK and sudden unexpected death in infancy. BMJ 2001; 322:822–825.
86 Taylor JA, Sanderson M. A re-examination of the risk factors for the sudden infant death syndrome. J Pediatr 1995; 126:887–891.
87 Spencer N. Poverty and child health. Oxford: Radcliffe Medical Press; 1996.
88 Leach CEA, Blair PS, Fleming PJ, et al. Epidemiology of SIDS and explained sudden infant deaths. Pediatrics104: (electronic pages) e43 (http://www.pediatrics.org/cgi/content/full/4/e43)
89 Fleming PJ, Blair P, Bacon C, et al. The environment of infants during sleep and the risk of the sudden infant death syndrome: results of the 1993–5 case-control study for the confidential enquiry into stillbirths and deaths in infancy. BMJ 1996; 313:191–195.
90 Irgens LM, Oyen N, Skjaerven R. Recurrence of sudden infant death syndrome among siblings. Acta Paediatr 1993; 389 (suppl 82):23–25.
91 RCPCH. The fabricated or induced illness report. London: Royal College of Paediatr and Child Health; 2001.
92 Department of Health. Safeguarding children in whom illness is fabricated by carers with parental responsibilities. www.dohgov.uk/qualityprotects/info/publications/childprot.htm, 2001.
93 National Advisory Body for CESDI. Annual Report for 1994. London: Department of Health; 1996.
94 Meadow R. Unnatural sudden infant death. Arch Dis Child 1999; 80:7–14.
95 Lee NNY, Chan YF, Davies DP, et al. Sudden infant death syndrome in Hong Kong: confirmation of low incidence. BMJ 1989; 298:721.
96 Jonge GA, Engleberts AC, Koomen-Liefting AJM, Kastense PJ. Cot death and prone sleeping position in The Netherlands. BMJ 1989; 298:722.
97 Fleming PJ, Gilbert R, Azaz Y, et al. Interaction between bedding and sleeping position in the sudden infant death syndrome: a population based case control study. BMJ 1990; 301:85–89.
98 Beal SM, Finch CF. An overview of retrospective case control studies investigating the relationship between prone sleeping position and SIDS. J Paediatr Child Health 1991; 27:334–339.
99 Mitchell EA, Brunt JM, Everard C. Reduction in mortality from sudden infant death syndrome in New Zealand: 1986–92. Arch Dis Child 1994; 70:291–294.
100 Ponsonby AL, Dwyer T, Gibbons LE, et al. Factors potentiating the risks of sudden infant death syndrome associated with the prone position. N Engl J Med 1993; 329:377–382.
101 Kemp JS, Nelson VE, Thach BT. Physical properties of bedding that may increase the risk of sudden infant death syndrome in prone-sleeping infants. Pediatr Res 1994; 36:7–11.
102 Wilson CA, Taylor BJ, Laing RM, et al. Clothing and bedding and its relevance to sudden infant death syndrome: further results from the New Zealand Cot Death Study. J Paediatr Child Health 1994; 30: 506–512.
103 Williams SM, Taylor BJ, Mitchell EA, et al. Sudden infant death syndrome: insulation from bedding and clothing and its effect modifiers. Int J Epidemiol 1996; 25:366–375.
104 Mitchell EA, Stewart AW, Clements M. Immunisation and the sudden infant death syndrome. BMJ 1995; 310:88–90.
105 Blair P, Fleming PJ, Bensley D, et al. Smoking and sudden infant death syndrome: results of the 1993–5 case-control study for the confidential enquiry into stillbirths and deaths in infancy. BMJ 1996; 313:195–198.
106 Ford RP, Taylor BJ, Mitchell EA, et al. Breast feeding and the risk of sudden infant death syndrome. Int J Epidemiol 1993; 22:885–890.
107 Gilbert RE, Wigfield RE, Fleming PJ, et al. Bottle feeding and the sudden infant death syndrome. BMJ 1995; 310:88–90.
108 Fleming PJ, Blair P, Bacon C, et al. The environment of infants during sleep and the risk of the sudden infant death syndrome: results of the 1993–5 case-control study for the confidential enquiry into stillbirths and deaths in infancy. BMJ 1996; 313:191–195.
109 Scragg R, Mitchell EA, Taylor BJ, et al. Bed sharing, smoking and alcohol in the sudden infant death syndrome. BMJ 1993; 307:1312–1318.
110 Scragg R, Stewart AW, Mitchell EA. Public health policy on bed sharing and smoking in the sudden infant death syndrome. NZ Med J 1995; 108:218–222.
111 Klonoff-Cohen HS, Edelstein SL, Lefkowitz ES, et al. The effect of passive smoking and tobacco exposure through breast milk on sudden infant death syndrome. JAMA 1995; 273:795–798.

112 Blair PS, Fleming PJ, Smith IJ. Babies sleeping with parents: case-control study of factors influencing the risk of the sudden infant death syndrome. BMJ 1999; 319:1457–1462.

113 McKenna JJ, Thoman E, Anders T, et al. Infant–parent cosleeping in evolutionary perspective: implications for understanding infant sleep development and SIDS. Sleep 1993; 16:263–282.

114 Stewart AJ, Mitchell EA, Tipene Leach D, Fleming PJ. Lessons from the New Zealand and United Kingdom Cot Death Campaigns. Acta Paediatr Scand 1993; 389(suppl):119–123.

115 Wigfield R, Fleming PJ, Berry PJ, et al. Can the fall in Avon's sudden infant death rate be explained by the observed sleeping position changes? BMJ 1992; 304:282–283.

116 Irgens LM, Markestadt T, Baste V, et al. Sleeping position and sudden infant death syndrome in Norway 1967–91. Arch Dis Child 1995; 72:478–482.

117 Dwyer T, Ponsonby AL, Blizzard L, et al. The contribution of changes in the prevalence of prone sleeping position to the decline in sudden infant death syndrome in Tasmania. JAMA 1995; 273: 783–789.

118 Wigfield RE, Fleming PJ. The prevalence of risk factors for SIDS: impact of an intervention campaign. In: Rognum TO (ed). Sudden infant death syndrome: New trends in the nineties. Oslo: Scandinavian University Press; 1995: 124–128.

119 Fleming PJ, Blair PS, Pollard K, et al. Pacifier use and SIDS – results from the CESDI SUDI case-control study. Arch Dis Child 1999; 81(2):112–116.

120 Pollard K, Fleming PJ, Young J. Night time non-nutritive sucking in infants aged 1 to 5 months: relationship with infant state, breast feeding, and bed- versus room-sharing. Early Hum Dev 1999; 56:185–204.

121 North K, Fleming PJ, Golding J. Socio-demographic associations with digit and pacifier sucking at 15 months of age and possible associations with infant infections. Early Hum Dev 2000; 60:137–148.

122 Clothier C. The Allitt Enquiry: independent enquiry relating to deaths and injuries on the children's ward at Grantham and Kesteven General Hospital during the period February to April 1991. London: HMSO; 1994.

123 Becroft DMO, Thompson JMD, Mitchell EA. Nasal and intrapulmonary haemorrhage in sudden infant death syndrome. Arch Dis Child 2001; 85:116–120.

124 Blair P, Fleming PJ, Ward Platt M. Babies sleeping with parents and sudden infant death syndrome. BMJ 2000; 321:1019–1020.

125 Naeye RL. Sudden infant death. Sci Am 1980; 242:52–58.

126 Meny RG, Carroll JL, Carbone MT, Kelly DH. Cardiorespiratory recordings from infants dying suddenly and unexpectedly at home. Pediatrics 1994; 93:44–49.

127 Steinschneider AS. Prolonged apnea and the sudden infant death syndrome: clinical and laboratory observations. Pediatrics 1972; 50: 646–654.

128 Southall DP, Richards JM, de Swiet M, et al. Identification of infants destined to die unexpectedly during infancy: evaluation of predictive importance of prolonged apnoea and disorders of cardiac rhythm or conduction. BMJ 1983; 286:1092–1096.

129 Keens TG, Ward SL. Apnea spells, sudden deaths and the role of the apnea monitor. Pediatr Clin North Am 1993; 40: 897–911.

130 Schectman VL, Harper RM, Kluge KA, et al. Cardiac and respiratory patterns in normal infants and victims of the sudden infant death syndrome. Sleep 1988; 11:413–424.

131 Schectman VL, Harper RM, Kluge KA, et al. Heart rate variation in normal infants and victims of SIDS. Early Hum Dev 1989; 19:167–181.

132 Hunt CE. Impaired arousal from sleep: relationship to sudden infant death syndrome. J Perinatol 1989; 9:184–187.

133 Fleming PJ, Levine MR, Long AM, Cleave JP. Postneonatal development of respiratory oscillations. Ann NY Acad Sci 1988; 533:305–313.

134 Schectman VL, Harper RM, Wilson AJ, Southall DP. Sleep state organization in normal infants and victims of the sudden infant death syndrome. Pediatrics 1992; 89:865–870.

135 Azaz Y, Fleming PJ, Levine M, et al. The relationship between environmental temperature, metabolic rate, sleep state and evaporative water loss in infants from birth to three months. Pediatr Res 1992; 32:417–423.

136 Lodemore MR, Petersen SA, Wailoo MP. Factors affecting the development of night time temperature rhythms. Arch Dis Child 1992; 67:1259–1261.

137 Tuffnell C, Petersen S, Wailoo M. Prone sleeping infants have a reduced ability to lose heat. Early Hum Dev 1995; 43:109–116.

138 Fleming PJ, Levine MR, Azaz Y, Wigfield R. The development of thermoregulation and interactions with the control of respiration in infants: possible relationship to sudden infant death. Acta Paediatr Scand 1993; 389(suppl): 57–59.

139 Sawczenko A, Fleming PJ. Thermal stress, sleeping position and the sudden infant death syndrome. Sleep 1996; 19:S267–270.

140 Fleming PJ, Howell T, Clements M, Lucas J. Thermal balance and metabolic rate during upper respiratory tract infection in infants. Arch Dis Child 1994; 70:187–191.

141 Jackson JA, Petersen SA, Wailoo MP. Body temperature changes before minor illness in infants. Arch Dis Child 1994; 71:80–83.

142 Gilbert RE, Fleming PJ, Azaz Y, et al. Signs of illness in babies preceding sudden unexpected infant death. BMJ 1990; 300:1237–1239.

143 Brookes JG, Gilbert RE, Fleming PJ, et al. Postnatal growth preceding sudden infant death syndrome. Pediatrics 1994; 94:456–461.

144 Blair PS, Nadin P, Cole TJ, et al. Weight gain and sudden infant death syndrome. Arch Dis Child 2000; 82:462–469.

145 Blackwell CC, Weir DM, Busuttil A, et al. Infection, inflammation and the developmental stage of infants: a new hypothesis for the aetiology of SIDS. In: Rognum TO (ed). Sudden infant death syndrome. New trends in the nineties. Oslo: Scandinavian University Press; 1995:189–198.

146 White M, Beckett M, O'Regan M, Matthew T. The effect of maternal smoking in pregnancy on autonomic function in infants. In: Rognum TO (ed). Sudden infant death syndrome. New trends in the nineties. Oslo: Scandinavian University Press; 1995:174–176.

147 Lewis KW, Bosque EM. Deficient hypoxia awakening response in infants of smoking mothers: possible relationship to sudden infant death syndrome. J Pediatr 1995; 127:691–699.

148 Holton JB, Allen JT, Green CA, et al. Inherited metabolic disease in the sudden infant death syndrome. Arch Dis Child 1991; 66:1315–1317.

149 Filiano JJ, Kinney HC. A perspective on neuropathological findings in victims of sudden infant death syndrome: the triple-risk model. Biol Neonate 1994; 65:194–197.

150 Harper RM, Kinney HC, Fleming PJ, et al. Sleep influences on homeostatic functions: implications for sudden infant death syndrome. Respir Physiol 2000; 119:123–132.

151 Dent A, Condon L, Blair P, Fleming PJ. A study of bereavement care after a sudden and unexpected death. Arch Dis Child 1996; 74:522–526.

152 Dent A. Family support after sudden child death. Community Pract 2002; 75: 469–473.

153 Stewart AJ, Fleming PJ, Howell T. Follow-up support for families with subsequent children. Health Visitor 1993; 66:244–247.

154 Stewart AJ, Fleming PJ. Bereavement care for families. Health Visitor 1993; 66: 207–209.

33

Psychiatric disorders in childhood

Peter Hoare

INTRODUCTION

Child psychiatry is concerned with the assessment and treatment of children's emotional and behavioral problems. These problems are very common with prevalence rates of 10–20% in several community studies. The majority of disturbed children are not seen by specialist psychiatric services, but by general practitioners, community doctors and pediatricians along with other professionals such as teachers and residential care staff. Consequently, knowledge about the range and variety of emotional and behavioral problems shown by children is important for all doctors involved in the care of children. The everyday work of the pediatrician provides clear evidence of the stressful effects of illness on the children and family's psychological well-being and adjustment.

Psychiatric disturbance in childhood is most usefully defined as an abnormality in at least one of three areas: emotions, behavior or relationships. It is *not* helpful to regard these abnormalities as strictly defined disease entities with a precise etiology, treatment and prognosis. Rather, it is preferable to regard them as deviations or departures from the norm, which are distressing to the child or to those involved with his welfare. (The male gender is used throughout this chapter wherever this could refer to either gender as the alternative wording is cumbersome and unwieldy.) Although child psychiatric disorders do not conform to a strict medical model of illness, it does not mean that these disorders are trivial or unimportant. Some disorders such as autism or conduct disorder have major implications for the child's development and adaptation in adult life.

In childhood, the distinction between disturbance and normality is imprecise. Isolated symptoms are common and not pathological. For example, many children will occasionally feel sad, unhappy or have temper tantrums. This does not mean that they are disturbed. Disturbance is characterized by the number, frequency, severity and duration of symptoms rather than by the type of symptomatology. In addition, disturbed children rarely present with unequivocal pathological symptoms such as hallucinations or delusions, whereas symptoms such as unhappiness and lying are common and not diagnostic. In clinical practice, it is often more important to establish why the child is the focus for concern rather than to adopt the more narrow perspective of whether the child is disturbed or not.

Another important feature of psychiatric disturbance in childhood is that several, as opposed to single, factors contribute to the development of disturbance. This makes assessment and treatment more difficult, so that an essential prerequisite for successful treatment is the correct evaluation of the relative contribution of the different etiological factors. Etiological factors are usually categorized into two groups, constitutional and environmental. The former includes heredity factors, intelligence and temperament. The three major environmental influences are the family, schooling and the community. Another factor, physical illness or handicap, if present, can have a profound effect on a child's development and vulnerability to disturbance.

Three other considerations are of general importance in understanding children's behavior: the situation-specific nature of behavior; the impact of current stressful events; and the role of family. Children's behavior varies markedly in different situations, that is it is situation specific. For instance, a child may be a major problem at school but not at home, or vice versa. Consequently, there may well be an apparent discrepancy between accounts of the child's behavior from the parents and from the teachers. The most likely explanation for this discrepancy is that the demands and expectations upon the child in the two situations are different. It is therefore essential to obtain several independent accounts about the child's behavior wherever possible in order to derive a more accurate and realistic assessment of the problem. This situation-specific nature of the behavior has implications for treatment, as it is important to explain to parents and to teachers the reasons for the discrepancy, thereby lessening the likelihood of misunderstanding.

Children are immature and developing individuals whose capacities and coping skills change markedly during childhood. Childhood is also a period of life characterized by change, challenge and the necessity for adaptation. Consequently it is not surprising that symptoms of disturbance may arise at times of stress when the demands on the child are excessive. Recent research[1] has shown that life events are associated with an increased psychiatric morbidity among children, a finding similar to that reported for adults. Some stresses such as the birth of a sibling or starting school are of course normal and inevitable, whereas others, such as marital break-up or life-threatening illness, are serious with long term implications for the child's well-being.

The child may, however, cope successfully with the stress, thereby enhancing self-esteem and confidence. Alternatively, the child may be overwhelmed, responding with the development of symptomatic behavior. The latter may involve regressive behavior (i.e. behaving in a more immature, dependent fashion), or more specifically maladaptive (e.g. aggression, excessive anxiety or withdrawal). A crucial feature of assessment is the identification of stressful factors that may be contributing to the problem, as this will influence treatment strategies and also the prognosis.

The family is the most potent force for the promotion of health as well as for the development of disturbance in the child's life. Assessment of parenting qualities, the marital relationship and the quality of family interaction are essential components of child psychiatric practice. It is a frequent observation that it is the parents who are disturbed and not the child. One consequence of this observation is that in many cases the focus of treatment is likely to be the parents, or the whole family, rather than the child. Indeed, in many instances the main emphasis of treatment is the promotion of normal healthy family interaction as much as in the amelioration of disturbed behavior.

Finally, many disturbed children do not complain about their distress nor admit to problems, but rather it is their parents or other adults involved with their care who bring the child to the attention of professionals. Disturbed children more commonly manifest their distress or unhappiness indirectly through symptoms such as abdominal pain, aggression or withdrawal. Direct questioning of the child during the initial interview is unlikely to reveal the true extent of the child's feelings or the degree of his distress. Sensitive observations during the interview and the use of indirect techniques such as play are necessary to elicit a more accurate view of the child's feelings. This is only likely to be successful once a relationship of trust has been established between the child and the doctor.

NORMAL AND ABNORMAL PSYCHOLOGICAL DEVELOPMENT

Children are developing individuals. They are not small adults. A 2-year-old is very different from a 12-year-old, whereas an adult aged 25 may not differ that much from a 35-year-old. During childhood, the child undergoes a remarkable transformation from a helpless, dependent infant to an independent self-sufficient individual with his own views and outlooks, capable of embarking on a career and living separately from his family. Knowledge about the *mechanisms, processes* and *the sequences* underlying these events is necessary in order to understand the nature of psychological disturbance in childhood. This knowledge also helps to define more clearly what is age-appropriate behavior and to distinguish the pathological from the normal. This section has three parts: developmental theories, developmental psychopathology and personality development.

DEVELOPMENTAL THEORIES (Table 33.1)

It is useful to define some terms at the outset, as they are often used interchangeably. *Growth* refers to the incremental increase of a characteristic; *maturation* is those phases and products of

Table 33.1 Summary of cognitive, emotional and social development

	Age in years				
	0	2	6	9	12+ upwards
Cognitive	*Sensorimotor*	*Preoperational*	*Concrete operational*		*Formal operational*
(Piaget)	Differentiates self from objects Begins to act intentionally Achieves object permanence	Learns to use language and to represent objects by image and words Thinking is egocentric (unable to see other viewpoint) and animistic (everything has feelings including inanimate objects)	Thinking is more logical and less egocentric Achieves conservation of number (age 6), volume (age 7), mass (age 8) Able to arrange objects in rank order		Able to think in abstract manner about propositions and hypotheses
Emotional	*Oral*	*Anal*	*Phallic*	*Latency*	*Genital*
(Freud)	Main concern is initially with satisfaction of basic needs such as hunger Later on, attachment to care giver	Cooperative activity with caregiver Satisfaction with increased self-control and achievement	Learns to interact with peers, often leads to rivalry Aware of own sexuality causing Oedipal conflict, resolved by identification with the same sex parent Conscience begins to form	Reduced sexual interest with main concerns about peer relationships and position within peer group	Revival of earlier conflict, especially sexual conflict Four main tasks: separation from parents, sexual role, career choice, identity
Social and personality development	Social smiling (8 weeks) Attachment (6 months) Stranger anxiety (10 months)	Cooperative play (3 years)	Strong preference for same sex friends with stereotyped expectations (6–7 years)	Enduring relationships (8 years onwards)	
	Erikson's stage of trust vs mistrust	*Erikson's stage of autonomy vs shame and doubt*	*Erikson's stage of initiative vs guilt*	*Erikson's stage of industry vs inferiority*	*Erikson's stage of identity vs role diffusion*

development that are mainly due to innate or endogenous factors; *development* is those changes in the nature and organization of an organism's structure and behavior that are systematically related to age. Many behaviors (for example walking and talking) have a substantial maturational component, whereas others (for instance emotional and social development) are strongly influenced by environmental factors. The continuous interaction between maturational and environmental factors throughout childhood helps to mould the personality development of the child.

Developmental theories tend to focus on at least one of the following areas: cognitive, emotional and social. They differ widely in theoretical orientation, in supporting empirical evidence and in the relative importance attributed to experience in influencing development. No single theory is satisfactory, so that most clinicians utilize some parts of the various theories to explain different aspects of development. The theories are usually described as stage theories, implying that they regard development as a series of recognizable phases of increasing complexity through which the child progresses.

Cognitive development

In 1929, the Swiss psychologist Piaget proposed a comprehensive theory about cognitive development. Many of his conclusions were based on experiments conducted on his own children over a number of years. Piaget has had a tremendous impact on educational concepts and teaching, particularly in primary schools over the last 30 years. More recently, the theoretical basis and validity of Piaget's conclusions have been questioned by further empirical studies.[2] Despite these criticisms, his views remain the most useful account of cognitive development.

Piaget's theory is set within a biological framework. In order to survive, the individual must have the capacity to adapt to the demands of the environment. Cognitive development is the result of interaction between the individual and the environment. Four factors influence cognitive development: increased neurological maturation, enabling the child to appreciate new aspects of experience and to apply more complex reasoning as he gets older; the opportunity to practice newly acquired skills; the opportunity for social interaction and to benefit from schooling; and the emergence of internal psychological mechanisms or *structures* that allow the child to construct a successively more complex cognitive model based on maturation and experience.

Piaget describes two types of intellectual structure, *schemas* and *operations*. The former are present at birth, the latter arise during childhood. *Schemas* are internal representations of some specific action, for instance sucking or grasping, whereas *operations* are internal rules of a higher order which have the distinctive feature that they are *reversible*, as, for example, multiplication is reversible by division. There are two ways whereby the child adapts his cognitive structure to the demands of the environment, *assimilation* and *accommodation*. The former refers to the incorporation of new objects, thoughts and behavior into existing structures, whereas the latter describes the change of existing structures in response to novel experiences. The child attends and learns most when his environment has a degree of novelty that challenges his curiosity but is not so strange that it becomes too confusing.

Piaget describes four main phases: *sensorimotor, preoperational, concrete operational* and *formal operational*. The age range given for each stage is the average, though this can vary considerably depending upon intelligence, cultural background and socioeconomic factors. However, the order is assumed to be the same for all children. Schemas predominate in the sensorimotor and preoperational stages, whereas operations predominate in the concrete operational and formal operational stages.

Sensorimotor (birth–2 years). Initially, behavior is dominated by innate reflexes such as feeding, sucking and following, hence the name for this period. Gradually, the infant realizes the distinction between *self* and *non-self*, namely where his body ends and the world outside begins. The infant also realizes that his behavior can influence the environment, so that intentional and purposeful behavior begins. Finally, the infant achieves *object permanence* whereby he recognizes that an object still exists even although it is no longer visible.

Preoperational (2–7 years). Language development greatly facilitates cognition, so that the individual begins to represent objects by symbols and words. Thinking is, however, *egocentric* and *animistic*. The former refers to the child's tendency to regard the world solely from his own position along with the inability to see a situation from another point of view. Animistic thinking describes the child's tendency to regard everything in the world as endowed with feelings, thoughts and wishes. For instance, the moon is watching over you when you sleep, the child says 'naughty door' when he bangs into the door.

The child has problems with the principles of conservation for number, volume and mass. The essential principle underlying conservation is that the number, volume or mass of an object are not changed by any visual alteration in their display or appearance. For instance, the child readily believes that the more widely spaced of two rows of counters has more counters than a denser packed row, or that there is more water in a tall beaker when it has been poured there from a shorter, more squat beaker.

The child also believes that every event has a preceding cause, rejecting the concept of chance or coincidence. Again, the child's moral sense is rigid and inflexible, so that punishment is invariable, irrespective of the circumstances. The child's concept of illness is radically different from that of the adult, with illness seen as a consequence for misdeeds, a punishment for a misdemeanour.

Concrete operational (7–12 years). Thinking becomes more logical and less dominated by immediate perceptual experience or by changes in appearance. Conservation of number, volume and mass is successively achieved during this period. The child becomes less egocentric, capable of seeing events from another person's standpoint. The child is able to appreciate and utilize reversibility, for example if 2 and 2 equals 4, then 4 minus 2 must equal 2.

Formal operational (12 years and upwards). This stage represents the most complex mode of thinking. Its main characteristics are the ability to think in an abstract fashion, to formulate general rules and principles and to devise and test hypotheses, an approach similar to that used in mathematics or in a scientific investigation. An example of such reasoning is the following: Joan is fairer than Susan; Joan is darker than Anne. Who is the darkest? (Answer: Susan). Prior to the formal operational stage, the child would require the aid of dolls to solve this problem. It should be pointed out that not everyone achieves this stage of thinking, even as an adult! The content of thinking also alters markedly with an emphasis on the hypothetical, the future and ideological issues.

Critical comment on Piaget

Recently, the Piagetian model has been criticised extensively for the lack of evidence to support the existence of the internal structures necessary for the concrete and formal operational stages. Alternative non-Piagetian explanations for a child's inability to carry out conservation tasks successfully before a certain age have also been put forward.[3] These criticisms are substantial, but they do not detract from the major conceptual contribution that Piaget has made to knowledge about cognitive development in children.

Recent developments in cognitive theory

Psychologists and psychiatrists have become increasingly interested in the development and application of cognitive theory to the understanding and treatment of psychiatric disorders.[4,5] The main principles underlying this theory are that an individual's beliefs about (i) himself, (ii) the future and (iii) the world influence his mood and behavior, an idea similar in some ways to the Piagetian concept of schemas. When a person is depressed, his thoughts are self-defeating and he commits certain cognitive errors. Two common types of cognitive errors are *personalization* and *dichotomous thinking.* The following two statements are examples of these two errors respectively: 'The reason my parents separated is all because of me' and 'I'm no good at tennis, so I'm bound to be useless at any other sport'.

A major extension of these ideas in childhood is the notion of the *self-concept.* By the age of 6 or 7 years, most children have very definite and clear ideas about themselves and their qualities. For example, they are able to compare themselves to other children with respect to popularity, attractiveness, scholastic ability, and so on. Self-concept is a construct similar to that of a schema in Piaget's theory. Another important facet of self-concept is the favorable or unfavorable evaluation that the child makes of himself, an aspect called *self-esteem.* Children with high self-esteem appear to do better in school, regard themselves as in control of their own destiny, have more friends and get along better with their families.[2]

Emotional and social development

Sigmund Freud developed the most comprehensive theory about emotional development, while Erikson[6] (also a psychoanalyst) applied psychoanalytic concepts within a social and cultural framework. Freudian theory emphasizes the biological and maturational components of development with an invariable sequence to development for everyone. Like Piaget, it is a stage or phase theory with the individual progressing successively through each phase. A major criticism of Freudian theory is that its concepts do not lend themselves readily to scientific investigation, so that it is difficult to prove or disprove the validity of the theory.

Freud proposed that an individual goes through five stages prior to adulthood, namely *oral, anal, phallic, latency* and *genital.* These terms refer to the major developmental task or potential conflict that the individual has to achieve or resolve during this period. Table 33.1 describes the important features of the different stages, e.g. during the phallic stage, the Oedipal crisis arises. At this time (around 3–4 years), the child becomes aware of his own sexual feelings and also that he is attracted in a sexual manner to the parent of the opposite sex. Moreover, the child is simultaneously aware that the parent of the same sex is a rival for the attention of the other parent. The conflict arises because the child is caught between the desire for one parent and the wrath of the other. The conflict is successfully resolved by the child identifying with the parent of the same sex, thereby eliminating the rivalrous feelings.

Erikson's major contribution has been to place psychoanalytic concepts in a social and cultural dimension (see Table 33.1). For Erikson, the most important task for the individual is to achieve a coherent sense of identity, a balanced and mature appraisal of one's abilities and limitations, with a recognition of the importance of previous experience and with realistic expectations for the future. Such a task occupies the individual throughout his life time. The individual passes through a series of developmental stages, all of which are polarized into two extremes, one successful and adaptive and the other unsuccessful and maladaptive. The two poles of the first stage are *trust* and *mistrust.* The former refers to the child's belief that the world is safe, predictable, and that he can influence events towards a favorable outcome, whereas a sense of mistrust implies a world that is cruel, erratic and unable to meet his needs. The role of the caregiver, usually the mother, is crucial to the achievement of a successful outcome. Erikson also believed that the individual carries forward the residues of earlier stages into the present, thereby giving the past an influence on contemporary behavior. Erikson's writings are a compelling and coherent account of development. A major weakness is, however, the lack of empirical evidence to support the conclusions.

Development of social relationships[2]

A characteristic of human beings is their predisposition to establish and maintain social relationships. Although Freud and Erikson refer to social relationships, it is only with the recent elaboration of attachment theory by Bowlby[7] and by Ainsworth[8] that a plausible theory for this phenomenon has been described. Attachment theory proposes that social relationships develop in response to the mutual biological and psychological needs of the mother and the infant. Mother–infant interaction promotes social relationships. Each member of the dyad has a repertoire of behavior that facilitates interaction: the infant by crying, smiling and vocalization; the mother by facial expression, vocalization and gaze. A mother can regulate the infant's state of alertness, for instance rocking or stroking to soothe the child, whilst talking or facial expression stimulates the child.

The term *attachment* describes the infant's predisposition to seek proximity to certain people and to be more secure in their presence. Bowlby maintained that there is a biological basis for this behavior, as it has been found extensively in other primates as well as in most human societies. It has considerable survival and adaptive value for the species, as it enables the dependent infant to explore from a secure base and also to use the base as a place of safety at times of distress. From 6 months onwards, infants develop selective attachment to people, usually the mother initially, but not exclusively to her. This first relationship is regarded as the prototype for subsequent relationships, so that its success or failure may have long term consequences. Clinicians distinguish between *secure attachment* and *anxious attachment,* with the former referring to healthy and the latter to potentially unsatisfactory relationships.

Bonding refers to the persistence of relationships over time, namely the child's capacity to retain the relationship despite the absence of the other individual. Much of the infant's behavior promotes the development of attachments by ensuring close proximity and interaction with the mother. These ideas have many implications for obstetric and pediatric practice, for the reduction of stress associated with hospitalization and for possibly explaining the origins of non-accidental injury to children.

Other aspects of development

Gender and sex role concepts

Gender identity is a part of self-concept, but the development of the child's understanding about 'boyness' or 'girlness', the sex role concept, is a more elaborate process. Children usually acquire *gender identity* (correctly labeling themselves and others) by about age 2 or 3 followed by *gender stability* (permanence of gender identity) by about 4. *Gender constancy* (gender identity unalterable by change in appearance) appears around 6 years, similar to other conservation-like concepts. Children show clear evidence of sex role stereotyping from an early age, with an excessively rigid concept for a brief period around 6 or 7 years. Freudian theory explains these findings on the basis of identification whereby the child imitates the same sex parent, thus acquiring appropriate sex-typed behavior. Alternative explanations emphasize the importance of social reinforcement and of cognition whereby the child acquires a schema about the respective roles and behavior of boys and girls.

Moral development

The acquisition of moral or ethical values is an important aspect of the socialization of children. Freud and Piaget have both described how this process happens. Freudian theory maintains that the superego or conscience develops during the phallic stage around 4–5 years. At this time, the child is identifying strongly with the same sex parent in order to resolve the Oedipal conflict and in consequence acquires parental values and prohibitions. In contrast, Piaget hypothesizes a much more gradual or stage-like sequence to the acquisition of moral values. The child around 3 years old bases his judgment on the outcome rather than the intention of an act, with an emphasis on punishment following on from a misdemeanour. Subsequently, the child adopts a more conventional morality based upon conformity with family values. Finally, the adolescent derives a personal value system that combines his own idiosyncratic values with those of his family and of society with the intention of achieving the 'greatest good for the greatest number'.

DEVELOPMENTAL PSYCHOPATHOLOGY

This long-winded phrase refers to two important dimensions necessary to evaluate children's behavior: first, whether the behavior is age appropriate (the developmental aspect), and second, whether the behavior is abnormal (the psychopathological). For example, separation anxiety is a normal phenomenon among children between 9 months and 4 years approximately, whereas it would be abnormal in a child aged 6 years.

The threefold division of disturbance into abnormalities of behavior, emotions or relationships provides a useful way to analyze disturbance. Many behavioral problems can be conceptualized in terms of deficits or excesses. For instance, children with encopresis or enuresis can be regarded as having failed to acquire the skills necessary for toileting. Similarly, the aggressive child is showing excessive belligerent or assertive behavior at an inappropriate time. This approach also has implications for treatment, as the latter is often based on behavioral techniques designed to increase certain behaviors or alternatively to eliminate others.

Anxiety is central to the understanding of emotional disturbance. It has physical manifestations such as palpitations or dry mouth as well as psychological such as fear or apprehension. Anxiety is a normal, indeed essential, part of growing up. It may occur in many situations: in response to external threat; new or strange situations; in response to the operation of conscience. Anna Freud[9] developed the concept of *defense mechanisms* to explain how the individual dealt with excessive anxiety. This response is entirely healthy and appropriate in many situations, only becoming maladaptive when it is used exclusively or excessively, thereby preventing the individual from learning how to cope with a normal amount of anxiety. Common defence mechanisms include *denial, rationalization, regression,* and *displacement.* Denial is the process where the child refuses to accept the psychological implications of a particular event or situation. For instance, a child refuses to admit to stealing, even when the theft is obvious, as the resultant loss of self-esteem and the sense of guilt make this impossible. Rationalization is when the child attempts to justify or minimize the psychological consequences of an event. 'I don't really like football, so that I am not bothered about playing for the team' is an example of the way in which the child may deal with a failure to gain selection for the school team. Regression occurs when a child behaves in a more developmentally immature manner, often at times of stress, for example becoming enuretic at the start of primary school. Displacement is the transfer of hostile or aggressive feelings from their original source on to another person, for instance getting angry with a sibling rather than with an adult.

Social relationships are often impaired among disturbed children. This may be a primary failure in some instances, such as autism, or more commonly a secondary phenomenon. Children with neurotic or conduct disorders are usually isolated and unpopular with their peer group as they have either excluded themselves or have alternatively been excluded as a result of their deviant behavior. In addition, the behavior usually brings them into conflict with parents or other adults such as teachers.

PERSONALITY DEVELOPMENT

Childhood is the time during which personality is formed. Wordsworth's aphorism 'the child is father to the man' is substantially true. Personality is a broad concept referring to the enduring and uniquely individual constellation of attributes that distinguish one person from another. It comprises cognitive, emotional, motivational and temperamental attributes that determine the individual's view about himself, his world and the future. Throughout childhood, the various elements interact with each other to mold the child's personality. Moreover, this process occurs in the context of the child's life experiences, particularly within the family, and also subsequently in the world outside the family. Healthy personality formation is an important prerequisite for satisfactory adjustment during childhood and also during adult life.

Personality is influenced by two main factors, constitutional and environmental, whilst a third, illness or handicap, if present, can have a profound effect on the child. Constitutional factors include intelligence and temperament. The former describes the individual's ability to think rationally about himself and his environment, while the latter refers to the individual's characteristic style or approach to new people or situations, his level of activity and prevailing mood. These temperamental traits influence the child's response to his environment and also shape the range and variety of his experiences.

The main environmental influences are the family, schooling and the community. The family is the most powerful force for promoting healthy development as well as for causing severe disturbance in a child's life. Families fulfil many functions for children including: the satisfaction of basic physical needs such as food and shelter; the provision of love and security; the development of social relationships with adults and peers; the promotion of cognitive and language skills; the experience of appropriate role models and socialization; and the acquisition of ethical and moral values.

Schooling has three main roles for children: the attainment of scholastic skills; the promotion of peer relationships; and the acceptance of adult authority outside the family. The community through the quality of housing and the availability of resources also has a considerable influence on the child's development. Finally, physical handicap or illness, when present, exert a major effect on personality development. This arises not only from the direct restrictions or limitations that they may impose on the child's abilities or activities, but more commonly and importantly, through indirect effects on the child's self-esteem, from overprotectiveness by the parents and from poor social relationships with siblings and peers.

Figure 33.1 is a diagrammatic representation of an interactive model of personality development that incorporates the ideas discussed in this section. As shown in Figure 33.1, constitutionally determined temperamental traits have a direct effect on personality and behavior, with the environment also exerting a similar impact. Environmental and temperamental factors have direct effects on the self-concept which in turn shapes and modifies the personality as

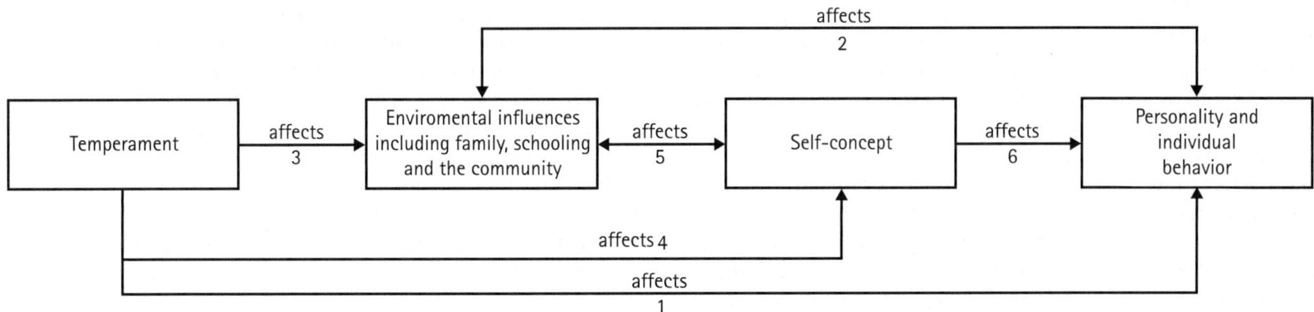

Fig. 33.1 Interactive model of personality development.

well as the environment. These interactive processes continue throughout childhood in a dynamic manner to produce a final product, an individual.

GENERAL FEATURES OF PSYCHIATRIC DISTURBANCE

DIAGNOSTIC CLASSIFICATION

A single cause is rarely responsible for the development of disturbance. The usual pattern is for several factors to be involved with a broad distinction into constitutional and environmental factors. The important constitutional factors are intelligence and temperament, whilst current life circumstances, the family, schooling and the community are the major environmental influences. One consequence of this multiple causation is that it is not possible to devise a diagnostic classification on the basis of etiology, as the relative contribution of each factor is often unclear.

Diagnostic practice is therefore descriptive or phenomenological, with three main categories of abnormality: *emotions*, *behavior* and *relationships*. In addition, these abnormalities should be of sufficient severity that they impair the individual in his daily activities and/or cause distress to the individual or to those responsible for his well-being. A commonly used definition of disturbance is as follows: an abnormality of emotions, behavior or relationships which is sufficiently severe and persistent to handicap the child in his social or personal functioning and/or to cause distress to the child, his parents or to people in the community.

The two commonest systems are the ICD-10[10] and DSM-IV.[11] DSM-IV is used extensively in North America, whereas ICD-10 is popular in the UK. The two systems have similar underlying principles with an emphasis on a clinical–descriptive approach to diagnosis. An important difference between ICD-10 and DSM-IV is that the latter allows for more than one diagnosis, whereas ICD-10 prefers a single diagnosis. The following list shows a convenient way to classify the important psychiatric syndromes in childhood:

1. conduct disorders;
2. emotional disorders;
3. mixed disorders of conduct and emotions;
4. hyperkinetic disorders (ICD-10) or attention deficit hyperactivity disorder (DSM-IV);
5. disorders of social functioning;
6. tic disorders;
7. pervasive developmental disorders;
8. miscellaneous disorders – encopresis, enuresis, sleep disorders and eating disorders.

Conduct disorder is characterized by severe, persistent, socially disapproved of behavior such as aggression or stealing that often involves damage to or destruction of property and is unresponsive to normal sanctions. The main feature of emotional disorder is a subjective sense of distress, often arising in response to stress. This group is further divided into phobic, anxiety, obsessional, conversion states and severe reactions to stress. Many disturbed children show a mixture of emotional and behavioral symptoms, so that a mixed category is clinically useful. An important source of confusion between the two classificatory systems is the terminology relating to hyperkinetic disorders in ICD-10 and attention deficit hyperactivity disorder in DSM-IV. Although both systems have the same core features (overactivity, impulsivity and inattention), the different names imply the two systems regard the main abnormality differently, namely hyperactivity for ICD-10 and inattention for DSM-IV. The situation is further complicated by the popular usage of another term to describe this group of disorders, namely attention deficit disorder (ADD). Disorders of social functioning comprise conditions such as selective mutism and attachment disorders. Pervasive developmental disorders include autistic spectrum disorder, Rett's syndrome and childhood disintegrative disorder. The miscellaneous group contains a diverse group of problems such as encopresis, enuresis and developmental disorders. Other important but uncommon conditions such as schizophrenia and mood disorders are categorized in a similar fashion to that for adults, providing that the diagnostic criteria are fulfilled.

EPIDEMIOLOGY OF DISTURBANCE

Epidemiology has been an important research interest in the UK for the past 30 years. It has provided accurate information about the frequency and distribution of disturbance throughout childhood and adolescence,[12] the differences between urban and rural areas,[13] the effects of illness and handicap on vulnerability to disturbance,[14] as well as providing clues about the relative importance of various etiologic factors.[13]

Most studies have shown prevalence rates of between 10 and 20% depending on the criteria for deviance. The first and most influential study was the Isle of Wight study (IOW) carried out by Rutter and his colleagues.[12] Using a strict definition of disorder, they found rates of approximately 7% among 10–11-year-old children. Follow-up of these children into adolescence indicated a prevalence rate of around 7% with more than 40% of the children with conduct disorder still having major problems. Disorders arising for the first time during adolescence were more adult like in presentation, with a preponderance of females. Over 80% of the disorders were in the emotional, conduct or mixed categories. Emotional disorders were more common among girls with anxiety as the commonest type. By contrast, conduct disorders, and to an important extent mixed disorder, were more common among boys with an association with specific reading retardation. A comparative study of 10-year-olds living in London[13] showed a rate of disturbance over twice that on the IOW. This study also showed that the difference in prevalence rate was entirely accounted for by the increased frequency of predisposing factors among children and their families in London compared with those on the IOW. These factors were family discord, parental psychiatric disorder, social disadvantage and inferior quality of schooling.

The IOW study[14] also showed that children with chronic illness or handicap had much higher rates of disturbance than healthy children. For instance, children with a central nervous disease such as epilepsy or cerebral palsy had a rate over five times that of the general population, while children with other illnesses such as asthma or diabetes were twice as likely to be disturbed as healthy children. A more recent epidemiological survey (carried out by the Department of Health in the UK[15]) on 10 000 children aged 5–15 years found a very similar prevalence and range of disturbance to the IOW study, namely an overall prevalence rate of 10% with conduct disorder (5%), emotional disorder (4%) and attention deficit disorder (1%) the main diagnostic categories. The survey also confirmed that adverse social circumstance, chronic illness and learning difficulties were still important risk factors for disturbance.

Studies of preschool children, most notably by Richman et al,[16] have found that about 20% of children have significant behavior problems with 7% classified as severe. Follow-up studies of these children indicated that about 60% persisted, most commonly among overactive boys of low ability. An important association was found between language delay and disturbed behavior. Finally, problems were more likely to persist when there was marital discord, maternal psychiatric ill health and psychosocial disadvantage such as poor housing or large family size.

ASSESSMENT PROCEDURES

Assessment is more time consuming in child psychiatry than in other branches of pediatrics. It has three components: history taking and examination; psychological assessment; information about the child and family from other professionals.

HISTORY TAKING AND EXAMINATION

This has many similarities to traditional methods, though with important modifications. Interview skills are essential to elucidate, understand and treat emotional and behavioral problems in children. Points of general importance include: clarification about the nature of the problem and the reason for referral; obtaining adequate factual information; observing and eliciting emotional responses and attitudes about past events and about behavior during the interview; establishing trust and confidence from the child and family; providing the parents with a summary of problems and a provisional treatment plan at the end of the initial interview.

There are no absolute rules about interviewing, indeed flexibility is essential. However, the following guidelines are useful:

1. The interview room should be large enough to seat the family comfortably and also to allow the children to use the play material in a relaxed manner.
2. Avoid having a desk between the interviewer and the family, i.e. put the desk against the wall of the interview room.
3. Do not spend the interview writing down notes but rather encourage eye-to-eye contact, taking the minimum notes necessary.
4. The play material must be suitable for a wide age range and include crayons and paper, jigsaws, simple games, books (provides a rough estimate of reading ability), doll's house, play telephones and miniature domestic and zoo animals.
5. The play material should be gradually introduced as appropriate and not left around in a haphazard manner.
6. Interview parents and young children together.
7. Older children and adolescents like to be seen separately from parents at some point during interview.
8. Older children and adolescents are able to talk about problems openly once trust in the interviewer has been established.
9. Too direct questions usually elicit denial from the child, so that open-ended questions are preferable.

The interview should provide information about the following (italic type indicates essential facts):

1. *Presenting problem(s). Frequency. Severity. Onset. Course. Exacerbating/ameliorating factors. Effect on family. Help given so far.*
2. Other problems or complaints
   - General health: eating, sleeping, elimination, physical complaints, fits or faints
   - Interests, activities and hobbies
   - *Relationship with parents and sibs*
   - Relationship with other children, special friends
   - Mood – happy, sad, anxious
   - Level of activity, attention span, concentration
   - Antisocial behavior
   - *Schooling. Attainments, attendance, friendships, relationship with teachers*
   - Sexual knowledge, interests and behavior (when relevant).
3. *Any other problems not previously mentioned*
4. Family structure
   - *Parents. Ages.* Occupations. *Current physical and psychiatric state.* Previous physical and psychiatric history
   - Sibs. Ages. Problems
   - Home circumstances.
5. Family function
   - Quality of parenting. Mutual support and help. Level of communication and ability to resolve problems
   - Parent–child relationship. Warmth, affection and acceptance. Level of criticism, hostility and rejection
   - Sibs' relationship
   - Pattern of family relationships.
6. Personal history
   - Pregnancy and delivery
   - Early mother–child relationship. Postpartum depression. Early feeding patterns
   - Temperamental characteristics. Easy or difficult, irregular, restless baby and toddler
   - Developmental milestones
   - *Past illnesses and injuries. Hospitalization*
   - Separations greater than 1 week
   - Previous schooling.
7. *Observation of child's behavior and emotional state*
   - *Appearance. Nutritional state, signs of neglect or injury*
   - Activity level. Involuntary movements. Concentration
   - Mood. Expressions or signs of sadness, misery, anxiety
   - Reaction to and relationship with the doctor. Eye contact. Spontaneous talk. Inhibition and disinhibition
   - Relationship with parents. Affection/resentment. Ease of separation
   - Habits and mannerisms
   - Presence of delusions, hallucinations, thought disorder.
8. Observation of family relationships
   - Patterns of interaction
   - Clarity of boundaries between parents and child

- Communication
- Emotional atmosphere of family. Mutual warmth/tension, criticisms.

9. Physical examination
   - Screening neurological examination
     - Note any facial asymmetry
     - Eye movements. Ask child to follow a moving finger and observe eye movement for jerkiness, incoordination
     - Finger–thumb apposition. Ask child to press the tip of each finger against the thumb in rapid succession. Observe clumsiness, weakness
     - Copying pattern. Drawing a man
     - Observe grip and dexterity in drawing
     - Observe visual competence when drawing
     - Jumping up and down on the spot
     - Hopping
     - Hearing. Capacity of child to repeat numbers whispered 2 m behind him
   - Further medical examination (if relevant).

Formulation

At completion of the assessment, the clinician should be able to make a formulation. This is a succinct summary of the important features of the individual case. The formulation consists of the following: statement of main problems; diagnosis and differential diagnosis; relative contribution of constitutional and environmental factors to the etiology; probable short term and long term outcome; further information required (including special investigations); initial treatment plan. The formulation should be included in the case notes, thereby providing the clinician with a record of his views at referral.

PSYCHOLOGICAL ASSESSMENT

Psychological assessment carried out by a child psychologist is a valuable part of the overall assessment of a child's problems in some situations. It can provide information about three aspects of development: general intelligence, educational attainments and special skills. Assessment is usually based upon the administration of standardized assessment tests. These are either norm referenced or criterion referenced. The former compares the child's ability with other children of the same age, whereas the latter is on a pass/fail basis, for instance whether he can tie his shoelaces. Ideally, the test items should have good discriminatory value (distinguish between children of different ability), be reliable (give similar results when repeated) and valid (in agreement with other independent evidence). An important aspect of the assessment is that the tasks are carried out in a standardized fashion, thereby increasing reliability and validity.

INTELLECTUAL ABILITY

DEVELOPMENTAL ASSESSMENT IN INFANCY AND EARLY CHILDHOOD

The commonly used tests are the Bailey's Scales,[17] Griffiths Mental Development Scales[18] and the Kaufman Assessment Battery for Children (K-ABC).[19]

ASSESSMENT OF GENERAL INTELLIGENCE AMONGST SCHOOL-AGE CHILDREN

The most popular test is the Wechsler Intelligence Scale for Children — Revised Form (WISC-R).[20] This covers an age range from 6 to 16 years. Usually 10 subtests are undertaken, measuring different aspects of the child's ability. Commonly, the tests are divided into 'verbal' and 'performance' categories yielding a 'verbal intelligence quotient (IQ)' and a 'performance IQ'. The 'verbal' subtests commonly used are *information, comprehension, arithmetic, similarities* and *vocabulary*, whilst the 'performance' tests are *picture completion, picture arrangement, block design, object assembly* and *coding*. Each subtest has a mean score of 10, so that combining the 10 tests gives a 'full scale' IQ of 100 with a standard deviation of 15. The 'normal' distribution of the test scores means that it is possible to state that 66% of children will be within the IQ range 85–115, 95% within IQ range 70–130, 99% within IQ range 55–145. Other tests used include the Stanford–Binet[21] and the British Ability Scales (BAS).[22]

EDUCATIONAL ATTAINMENT

There are two commonly used reading tests, the WORD (Wechsler Objective Reading Test)[23] and the Neale Analysis of Reading Ability.[24] The former measures basic reading, comprehension and spelling skills, whilst the latter provides information about speed, accuracy and comprehension of reading. The scores on the Neale test can be transformed into reading ages of so many years and months, for instance 6 years 11 months. The subtest scores of the WISC-R or the BAS can be used as a guide to mathematical ability.

Specific skills

Reynell development language scale,[25] Bender Motor Gestalt Test and the Vineland Social Maturity Scale are examples of tests to assess the child's acquisition of certain abilities and skills. These are often helpful with some specific problems.

Limitations of assessment

Caution should always be exercised in the interpretation of test results. It is wrong to attribute undue significance to a single result, most often done with the IQ score. Many factors influence test results including fatigue, poor testing conditions and the use of inappropriate tests. The results should be evaluated in the context of the overall assessment and the report from the child psychologist. A great deal of harm, upset and distress can arise for a child when he is incorrectly classified or labeled as too able or too dull on the basis of an unreliable psychological assessment.

Additional information

A distinctive feature of child psychiatry practice is the importance attached to obtaining independent evidence about the child's behavior. This is for two reasons: first, a child's behavior varies from one situation to another, so that it is helpful to have information about the child's behavior in several contexts; second, parental accounts of the child's behavior are likely to be distorted in many cases, as it is the parents who are disturbed rather than the child. Consequently, an important part of assessment is to obtain reports from other professionals involved with the family such as schools, health visitors or general practitioners. Another common practice is the use of questionnaires to supplement information provided by referrers and other more formal reports. Several questionnaires[16,26] have been devised to assess different age ranges and have satisfactory psychometric properties. Until recently, the most extensively used questionnaires for school-age children in the UK have been the Rutter parents' and teachers' scales, also known as Rutter A and Rutter B respectively. These scales have established reliability and validity as well as classifying children into neurotic or emotional, conduct or antisocial and mixed categories. Over the past five years, the Strengths and Difficulties Questionnaire (SDQ)[27] has become more popular, as it assesses pro-social behavior as well as disturbed behavior.

DISORDERS IN PRESCHOOL CHILDREN

Except for rare but severe disorders such as childhood autism, psychiatric disorders in this age group are mostly deviations or delays from normality rather than a psychiatric illness as such. Moreover, the child's behavior and development are so influenced by the immediate surroundings that it is often the environment rather than the child that is responsible for the problems.

ETIOLOGY

Four types of factors contribute to problems in varying degrees in the individual case: temperamental factors; physical illness or handicap; family psychopathology; and social disadvantage. The New York Longitudinal Study[28] showed clearly that children with certain types of temperamental characteristics, the so-called 'difficult child' and the 'slow to warm up child' profiles, were more likely to develop problems. Again, physical illness or handicap can reduce activity, directly or indirectly affect developmental progress and increase parental anxiety, all of which potentiate the likelihood of behavioral disturbance. Parental psychiatric illness, marital disharmony and poor parenting skills are examples when disturbance in the parents adversely affects the child's behavior. Several authors[16,29] have shown high rates of depression among mothers with preschool children. Social disadvantage such as poor housing or inadequate recreational facilities increases the risk of disturbance among preschool children.[16]

FREQUENCY OF PROBLEMS

Table 33.2[30] shows the prevalence of common problems among 3- and 4-year-olds in the general population.

Problems are mainly about eating, sleeping and elimination, with a marked decrease in wetting and soiling over the 1-year period. Affective symptoms such as unhappiness and relationship problems are much less common, but probably more significant. Community studies[16] indicate that 20% of children are regarded by their mothers as having problems with 7% rated as severe.

Table 33.2 Problem behaviors in 3- and 4-year olds

Behavior	3-year-olds (%)	4-year-olds (%)
Poor appetite	19	20
Faddy eater	15	24
Difficulty settling at night	16	15
Waking at night	14	12
Overactive and restless	17	13
Poor concentration	9	6
Difficult to control	11	10
Temper	5	6
Unhappy mood	4	7
Worries	4	1
Fears	10	12
Poor relationships with siblings	10	15
Poor relationships with peers	4	6
Regular day wetting	26	8
Regular night wetting	33	19
Regular soiling	16	3

From Richman & Lansdown 1988.[30] ©John Wiley & Sons Limited. Reproduced with permission.

COMMON PROBLEMS

This section discusses those problems that are particularly frequent among the preschool child, whilst others such as soiling which occur in older children as well are discussed later in the chapter.

Temper tantrums

They usually arise when the child is thwarted, angry or has hurt himself. They can occur in isolation or as part of a wider problem. They comprise a variety of behaviors, including screaming, crying, often with collapse onto the floor and banging of feet. A child can be aggressive towards other people around him, but the child rarely injures himself. Most tantrums 'burn themselves out', so that specific intervention is not necessary. If it is, then the following points are useful: if necessary, restrain from behind by folding arms around child's body; minimize any additional attention to the child; and only respond and praise when behavior is back to normal.

Feeding problems

Feeding problems range in severity from a minor problem such as the finicky child to the severe disabling problem of non-organic failure to thrive. Minor problems will usually respond to patient and attentive listening to the parents' concerns, counseling and specific advice. Severe non-organic failure to thrive (prevalence 2%) is a complex problem requiring comprehensive assessment and a large amount of time and resources to remedy.[31] Several factors are responsible in most cases including poor mother–child relationship, often in the context of more widespread emotional and social deprivation, and factors in the child, including temperamental factors and an aversion to feeding. *Pica*, the ingestion of inedible material such as dirt or rubbish, is a normal transitory phenomenon during the toddler period. Persistent ingestion is found amongst mentally retarded, psychotic or socially deprived children. Lead poisoning, though always mentioned, is a possible but uncommon danger from pica.

Sleep problems

These are common with up to 20% of 2-year-olds waking at least five times per week.[16,32] The two most frequent problems are reluctance to settle at night and persistent waking up during the night. Several factors contribute to the problem including adverse temperamental characteristics in the child, perinatal problems and maternal anxiety. It is also important to distinguish between those factors responsible for the onset of the problem and those for maintaining the problem. Medication such as alimemazine (trimeprazine) and promethazine are frequently prescribed, but side-effects often outweigh any advantages. Their only real indication is to provide a brief respite for the parents as well as ensuring that the child has an uninterrupted night's sleep. The most successful management is a behavioral strategy (see Treatment section). Richman & Landsdown[30] provide a useful summary of these techniques. More recently, there have been case reports of the successful use of melatonin to treat sleep disorders among visually and neurologically impaired children.[33] This has now been extended to other groups of children with sleep problems with some success. (Sleep problems in older children are discussed in the Miscellaneous section.)

PSYCHIATRIC ASPECTS OF CHILD ABUSE[34]

Originally this was restricted to the 'battered baby syndrome', but it has now been extended to include physical abuse, sexual abuse, emotional abuse and neglect. This section will concentrate on the psychiatric aspects in childhood as other sections discuss diagnostic (see Ch.5) and adolescent issues (see later in the chapter). It is also important to remember that the different aspects of child abuse are frequently present in the same child and family and that many comments about the detection, management and treatment apply equally to all aspects of child abuse.

PHYSICAL ABUSE

Diagnostic awareness and suspicion are the key elements in the detection and recognition of physical abuse. The following list summarizes the common characteristics of abused children and their families, although the most important factor to recognize is that child abuse can occur in any family irrespective of social class, ethnic group or religious affiliation.

Common characteristics of abused children and their families

Risk characteristics of the abused child:

1. product of unwanted pregnancy;
2. unwanted child in the family;
3. low birth weight;
4. separation from mother in neonatal period;
5. mental or physical handicap;
6. habitually restless, sleeplessness or incessantly crying;
7. physically unattractive.

Risk characteristics of the parent(s):

1. single parent;
2. young;
3. abused themselves as a child;
4. low self-esteem;
5. unrealistic expectations of the child and his development;
6. inconsistent or punishment-orientated discipline.

Risk characteristics of social circumstances:

1. low income or unemployment;
2. current stress such as housing crisis, social isolation;
3. domestic friction, exhaustion or ill health;
4. large family.

Management

Most cases of child abuse do not require the involvement of a child psychiatrist, as the principal concerns are the protection of the child, practical support for the family and help with parenting skills. The child psychiatrist can make a useful contribution in two ways: firstly, to act as an outside consultant on various aspects of management and treatment to the other professionals and agencies working with the family; and secondly to provide individual and/or family therapy for the child, the parents or the family depending upon the assessment.

In addition to the immediate effects, child abuse may have medium term and long term sequelae. Many abused children continue to be exposed to emotional abuse and neglect throughout their childhood, so that they often show symptoms of disturbance such as unhappiness, wariness, untrusting, low self-esteem and poor peer relationships. This childhood experience in turn predisposes abused children to become abusing parents when adults.

SEXUAL ABUSE

This has become a major public and pediatric concern over the past decade. Several factors have contributed to the increased concern: it is a common event affecting 12–17% of females and 5–8% males according to several epidemiological surveys,[35] it is traumatic for the child giving rise to major distress at the time of its occurrence; but equally importantly acts as a predisposing factor for psychiatric disorder later on in life. Indeed, a history of sexual abuse in childhood is a very common finding among women referred to adult psychiatric services.

Complex psychological processes contribute to the development of psychopathology, as attitudes to sexuality are shaped in a dysfunctional manner by the abuse. Also, the individual has a sense of betrayal, powerlessness and stigmatization leading to shame, guilt and low self-esteem. One consequence of this process is that sexual abuse can present in a wide variety of ways from the physical (e.g. vaginal discharge) to the psychological such as anxiety, aggression or encopresis. It is therefore crucial to be aware that unexplained or atypical symptoms may be the presenting complaint for a child with a current or past history of sexual abuse.

The child psychiatry team has a more clearly defined role in the management of sexual abuse, as interviewing skills, psychotherapeutic expertise and the use of specialist equipment (anatomically accurate dolls) are often necessary at the detection and also during the treatment stage of management. Detailed accounts of this work, including the use of the anatomical dolls, are well described in several books (the Great Ormond Street child sex abuse team[36]) and the APSAC Handbook.[34]

EMOTIONAL ABUSE

This term has been introduced to describe the severe impairment of social and emotional development resulting from repeated and persistent criticism, lack of affection, rejection, verbal abuse and other similar behavior by the parent(s) to the child. Affected children display a variety of symptoms: low self-esteem; limited capacity for enjoyment; severe aggression; impulsive behavior.

NEGLECT

This varies markedly, ranging from relative inadequacy and incompetence in providing basic shelter, love and security for the child to a severe failure in the provision of basic essentials, often combined with emotional and social deprivation.

MUNCHAUSEN'S SYNDROME BY PROXY[37]

This remarkable variant of physical abuse often occurs against the same background of parental psychopathology and social disadvantage as other forms of abuse. The role of the child psychiatrist is usually confined in most cases to offering counseling for the parents and/or family therapy when indicated.

PERVASIVE DEVELOPMENTAL DISORDERS[38,39]

Historically, these disorders were classified under childhood psychoses, as they are severe and disabling with clear-cut abnormalities. However, autistic children do not experience hallucinations or delusions, key features of a psychotic disorder, and moreover have had the abnormalities from early infancy.

For these reasons, ICD-10 and DSM-IV have separated out childhood autism and related conditions from other psychotic conditions in childhood into a new diagnostic category called pervasive developmental disorders. In clinical practice, most people recognize that autistic disorders comprise a spectrum of disabilities (autistic spectrum disorders) with childhood autism at the severe end and Asperger's syndrome at the mild end. Rett's syndrome and disintegrative disorder are also included in the pervasive developmental disorders category.

CHILDHOOD AUTISM

Kanner's[40] original description of 11 children with 'an extreme autistic aloneness' has not been improved upon with its astute observation of 'inability to relate in an ordinary way to people and to situations' and 'an anxiously obsessive desire for the maintenance of sameness'. Subsequently, opinions have fluctuated about the diagnosis, etiology and treatment. Most authorities now agree that three features are essential to the diagnosis: general and profound failure to develop social relationships; language abnormalities; and ritualistic and compulsive behavior. Additionally, these abnormalities should be manifested before 30 months.

Prevalence

Previous epidemiological studies in childhood have found prevalence rates of 4 per 10 000 increasing to 20/10 000 when individuals with severe mental retardation and some autistic features are included. Boys are three times more affected than girls. However, a much more recent study[41] found a rate of 16 per 10 000 for autistic disorder and 64 per 10 000 for other pervasive developmental disorders. It remains to be seen whether these new findings are replicated elsewhere. There is no serious evidence for the suggestion of a link with vaccination.[42]

Clinical features

Impaired social relationships

Parental recollections of infancy often reveal that as an infant the child was slow to smile, unresponsive and passive with a dislike of physical contact and affection. Contemporary social deficits include the failure to use eye-to-eye gaze and facial expression for social interaction, rarely seeking others for comfort or affection, rarely initiating interaction with others, a lack of empathy (the ability to understand how others feel and think) and of cooperative play. The children are aloof and indifferent to people.

Language abnormalities

Language acquisition is delayed and deviant with many autistic children never developing language (approximately 50%). When present, language abnormalities are many and varied, including immediate and delayed echolalia [repetition of spoken word(s) or phrase(s)], poor comprehension and use of gesture, pronominal reversal (the use of the third person when 'I' is meant) and abnormalities in intonation, rhythm and pitch.

Ritualistic and compulsive behavior

Common abnormalities are rigid and restricted patterns of play, intense attachments to unusual objects such as stones, unusual preoccupations and interests (timetables, bus routes) to the exclusion of other pursuits and a marked resistance to any change in the environment or daily routine. Tantrums and explosive outbursts often occur when any change is attempted.

Other features

Autistic children often exhibit a variety of stereotypies including rocking, finger twirling, spinning and tiptoe walking. They are often overactive with a short attention span. Of autistic children 70% are in the retarded range of intelligence with only 5% having an IQ above 100. Occasionally, some have remarkable abilities in isolated areas, for instance computation, music or rote memory. About 20% will develop epilepsy during adolescence, though not usually severe.

Association with other conditions

Autistic behavior occurs in some patients with a diverse group of conditions including the fragile X syndrome, rubella, phenylketonuria, tuberous sclerosis, neurolipoidoses and infantile spasms.[43] More recently, Rett's syndrome, with its marked autistic features, has been described.[44]

Etiology

Most people favor an organic basis as neurological abnormalities are common, and because of the association with epilepsy and various neurological syndromes, the increased rate of perinatal complications and a greater concordance rate among monozygotic compared with dizygotic twins.[43,45] Application of new investigative techniques such as computerized axial tomography (CAT) scan, magnetic resonance imaging (MRI) and positron emission tomography are beginning to reveal abnormalities in the frontal lobe region, with distinctive deficits on tests of executive function.[46] The relationship between autism and the fragile X syndrome is also unclear, as the different rates in the various studies may be a reflection of the degree of mental handicap rather than of any etiological significance. A most interesting psychological perspective on the autistic deficit is provided by the work of Baron-Cohen[47] and Hobson.[48] On the basis of sophisticated cognitive experiments with autistic children, they propose that the primary deficit in autism is a lack of empathy, namely an inability to perceive and interpret emotional cues in social situations.

Recent suggestions of a link with immunization, particularly related to the mumps component of MMR vaccine have not been substantiated by more careful scientific and epidemiologic review.[42]

Treatment

The explanation of the diagnosis is a vital first step in helping parents to accept the presence of handicap with the consequent lessening of the parental guilt about etiology. Counseling and advice are likely to be necessary throughout childhood. Lord & Rutter[43] suggested that treatment aims should have four components: the promotion of normal development; the reduction of rigidity and stereotypies; the removal of maladaptive behavior; and the alleviation of family stress. Behavioral methods, including operant conditioning and shaping (see Behavioral treatment section), are the most likely ways to achieve some success with the first three aims, whilst counseling is important for the fourth. Special schooling, where the child's special social and educational needs are recognized, is very beneficial, sometimes on a residential basis. Drugs do not have an important part in management.

Outcome

Many autistic individuals are unable to live independently with only 15% looking after and supporting themselves as adults. Many were placed previously in institutions for the mentally handicapped, though government policy now favors community care. Autistic children with an IQ of at least 70, receiving proper education and coming from middle-class families do better than other groups.

In most individuals there is some improvement in social relationships, though many are still handicapped. Parents often find it helpful to join a voluntary society such as the National Society for Autistic Children.

OTHER PERVASIVE DEVELOPMENTAL DISORDERS

Asperger's syndrome/schizoid personality

This condition, originally described by Asperger,[49] shows some similarities to childhood autism in that there is an impairment of social relationships with a lack of reciprocal social interaction and a restricted repertoire of interests and activities. However, the children differ diagnostically from those with childhood autism in two important respects: there is no general intellectual retardation; and the language development is normal. Other characteristics include male preponderance and poor motor coordination with marked clumsiness. The condition is now regarded as one of the autistic spectrum disorders[39] with the impairment in social relationships persisting into adult life.

The term 'schizoid' personality of childhood was coined by Wolff & Chick[50] to describe a small number of children with unusual but distinctive personality characteristics, similar in some ways to children with Asperger's syndrome. These 'schizoid' children were described as aloof, distant and lacking in empathy. Other features include: obstinate and aggressive outbursts when under pressure to conform, often at school; undue rigidity; excessive sensitivity to criticism; and unusual interests to the exclusion of everything else. More recently, Wolff[51] has argued from follow-up studies of these children that they form a separate diagnostic category, the schizoid personality of childhood, similar to but distinct from childhood autism and Asperger's syndrome. As adults, Wolff[51] found that they showed features of the schizotypal disorder.

Rett's syndrome

In 1966 Rett described 22 mentally handicapped children, all girls who had a history of regression in development and displayed strikingly repetitive movements of the hands. He thought that the children were autistic with progressive spasticity, and proposed that diffuse cerebral atrophy was the underlying cause. A more recent review[44] has indicated this syndrome is more common than previously thought with a prevalence rate of 1 per 15 000 among girls.

Clinical features

The condition which has only been described in girls shows a characteristic clinical picture: a period of normal development up to around 18 months followed by a rapid decline in developmental progress and the rapid deterioration of higher brain functions.

Over the following 18 months, there is evidence of severe dementia, a loss of purposeful hand movements, jerky ataxia and acquired microcephaly. After this rapid decline, the condition may stabilize with no further progression for some time. Subsequently, more neurological abnormalities appear including spastic paraplegia and epilepsy.

Etiology

Rett originally believed that high levels of ammonia were responsible for the condition, though subsequent studies have not confirmed this observation. The most commonly proposed explanation is that it is due to a dominant mutation on one X chromosome, and that the condition is non-viable in the male.

Prognosis

The majority of children are left profoundly retarded with severe neurological impairments. Many succumb to intercurrent infections or to the underlying neuropathological disorder.

Disintegrative disorder

Clinical features[43,52]

This term refers to a group of conditions characterized by normal development until around 4 years of age followed by profound regression and behavioral disintegration, loss of language and other skills, impairment of social relationships and the development of stereotypies. It can follow on from a minor illness or from more definite neurological disease such as measles encephalitis. The prognosis is poor due to the underlying degenerative pathology in many cases. Most individuals are left with severe mental retardation.

Other related conditions

Many children with mental retardation show some autistic features. In clinical practice, it is often difficult to know whether they fulfil the criteria for pervasive developmental disorder in addition to that for intellectual retardation. It is clear that there is a wide diversity in the severity of these 'autistic features', so that it is often arbitrary whether the label childhood autism is applied to these children. Many of them also show features of hyperactivity and aggression. For these reasons, ICD-10 has made two additional categories, overactive disorder associated with mental retardation and stereotyped movements and secondly, pervasive developmental disorder unspecified.

EMOTIONAL DISORDERS

The primary abnormality is a subjective sense of distress due to anxiety that can be expressed overtly as in anxiety disorders or covertly as in somatization or conversion disorders. This group of disorders is similar in many respects to neurotic disorders in adults. They are further divided into the following categories: anxiety and phobic states; obsessional disorders; conversion disorders, dissociative states and somatization disorders; and reaction to severe stress and adjustment disorders. Many children often show a mixed pattern of symptoms, so that a clear-cut distinction into a single category is not possible. The DOH 2000 study[15] found a prevalence rate of 4.0% with an equal gender prevalence. Prognosis is generally favorable as many problems arise from an acute stress, so that the problems should resolve once the stressful effects lessen.

ANXIETY STATES

Clinical features

This is the commonest type of emotional disorder. Anxiety has physical and psychological components with the former referring to palpitations and dry mouth, while the latter to the subjective sense of fear and apprehension. Somatic symptoms, particularly abdominal pain, are common. Again, many symptoms represent the persistence or exaggeration of normal developmental fears, ranging in severity from an acute panic attack to a chronic anxiety state over several months. Predisposing factors include temperamental characteristics, overinvolved and overconcerned parents and the 'special child syndrome'. The latter refers to children who are treated differently by their parents. This may arise in several circumstances, for instance the child is much wanted, previous ill health during pregnancy or infancy, resulting in 'anxious' attachment between the child and parents. In turn, 'anxious' attachment may lead the parents to inadvertently reinforce normal fears and anxieties.

Treatment

Several approaches, including individual, behavioral and family therapy, are used, often in combination depending upon the assessment and formulation. The newer SRIs (serotonin reuptake inhibitors) such as buspirone have been shown to be effective in clinical trials, and are preferable to benzodiazepines.

PHOBIC STATES

Clinical features

Phobias are common and normal among children. For instance, toddlers are fearful of strangers, whereas adolescents are anxious about their appearance or weight. Pathological fears often arise from ordinary fears that are exacerbated by parental and/or social reinforcement. A phobia is defined as a fear of a specific object or situation, for instance dogs or heights. Its characteristics are that it is out of proportion to the situation, is irrational, is beyond voluntary control and leads to avoidance of the feared situation. This avoidance behavior is the main reason the fear is maladaptive as it leads to increasing restriction and limitation of the child's activities.

Treatment

A behavioral approach using graded exposure to the feared situation is the most commonly used treatment. The rationale of this approach is that continued exposure to the feared stimulus reduces the anxiety associated with the stimulus, thereby decreasing avoidance behavior. The success of this method often depends on the ability of the therapist to devise a treatment program that combines gradual exposure without inducing too much anxiety. Occasionally, anxiolytic drugs are used in conjunction with this behavioral approach.

SCHOOL REFUSAL[53]

This term, also known as school phobia, refers to the child's irrational fear about school attendance. It is also known as the masquerade syndrome as it can be present in a variety of disguises, including abdominal pain, headaches or a viral infection. The child is reluctant to leave home in the morning to attend school, in contrast to the truant who leaves home but does not arrive at school. It occurs most commonly at the commencement of schooling, change of school, or the beginning of secondary school.

Most cases can be understood in terms of the following three mechanisms, often in combination: first, separation anxiety, whereby the child and/or the parent are fearful of separation, of which school is an example; second, a specific phobia about some aspect of school such as travelling to school, mixing with other children, or some part of the school routine, for instance some subjects, gym, or assembly; third, an indication of a more general psychiatric disturbance such as depression or low self-esteem. The latter is more frequent among adolescents. Typically, most school refusers have good academic attainments, are conformist at school, but oppositional at home. School refusal can present acutely or insidiously, often becoming a chronic problem in adolescence.

Treatment

The initial essential step is to recognize the condition itself, namely to avoid unnecessary and extensive investigations for minor somatic symptoms or to advise prolonged convalescence following minor illness. For the acute case, early return to school with firm support for the parents and liaison with the school is the most successful approach. For the more intractable cases, extensive work with the child and parents, along with a graded return to school is advisable. A specific behavioral program for the phobic aspects may be necessary as well as the use of anxiolytic drugs in some instances. The chronic problem often requires a concerted approach, sometimes involving a period of assessment and treatment at a child psychiatric day or inpatient unit. Many clinicians use family therapy to tackle the major relationship problems that exist in some cases.

Outcome

Two-thirds usually return to school regularly, whilst the remainder, usually adolescents from disturbed families, only achieve erratic attendance at school at best. Follow-up studies have found that approximately one-third continue with neurotic symptoms and social impairment into adult life.

OBSESSIVE–COMPULSIVE DISORDERS[54] (Fig. 33.2)

Definition

An obsession is a recurrent, intrusive thought that the individual recognizes is irrational but cannot ignore. A compulsion or ritual is the behavior(s) accompanying these ideas, the aim of which is to reduce the associated anxiety.

Clinical features

Most children display obsessional symptoms to a minor degree at some time, for instance avoiding cracks on paving stones or walking under ladders. They have no significance. It is when the behavior interferes with ordinary activities that it amounts to a disorder. Common obsessional rituals are hand washing and dressing. Obsessional thoughts often have a foreboding quality, for instance that 'something could happen' to a parent or sibling, that he might die, or get run over. The rituals are maintained, though maladaptive, because they produce temporary reduction in anxiety. Commonly, the child involves other members of the family in the performance of rituals, so that the child assumes a controlling role within the family. The disorder is rare (community prevalence 0.3%) but commoner among older children and adolescents with an acute or gradual onset. In addition to anxiety symptoms, many children have depressive features.

Treatment

Behavioral methods, particularly response prevention, are successful in eliminating the obsessive–compulsive behavior. Response prevention consists of training the child to become aware of the cues that trigger the symptom and then using distraction techniques to make the performance of the ritual impossible. Recent clinical trials[54] have shown that SRIs such as paroxetine or sertraline are effective in their own right, but more importantly are very valuable as part of a combined medication–behavioral treatment package. Involvement of other members of the family, whether specifically in family therapy or to assist the child in the elimination of rituals, is necessary. Some cases require inpatient admission.

Outcome

Two-thirds do well with the remainder continuing to have problems, usually in a fluctuating fashion.

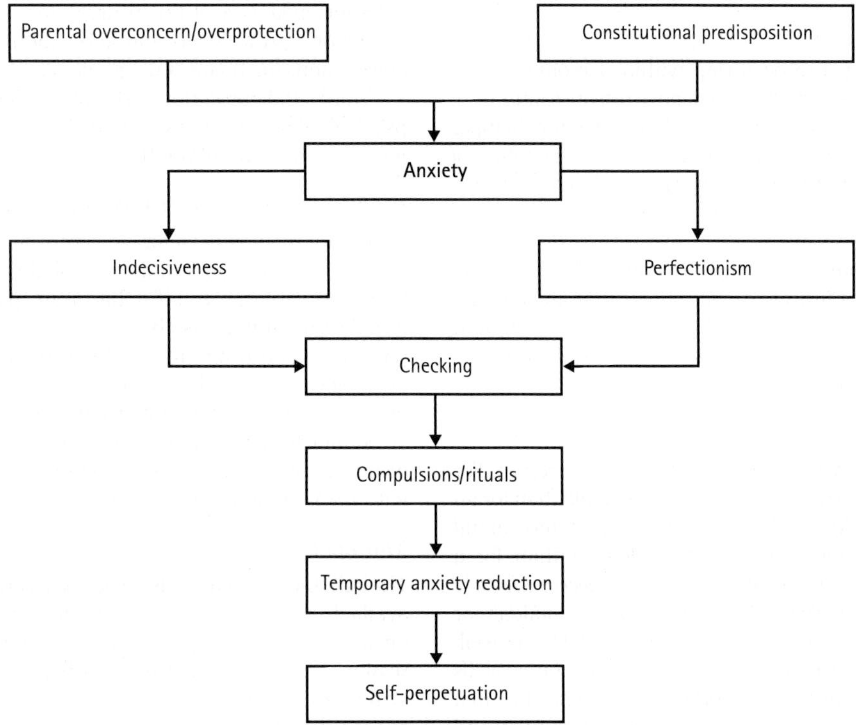

Fig 33.2 Development of obsessional systems.

CONVERSION DISORDERS AND DISSOCIATIVE STATES

Clinical features

These are rare in childhood. Conversion disorder is the development of physical symptoms, usually of the special senses or limbs, without any pathological basis in the presence of identifiable stress and/or affective disturbance. The emotional conflict is said to be 'converted' into physical symptoms which is less threatening to the individual than the underlying psychological conflict. A dissociative state is the restriction or narrowing of consciousness due to psychological causes, for example amnesiac or fugue states. It is, however, extremely dangerous to diagnose the condition solely by the exclusion of organic disease, as follow-up studies have found that a minority subsequently develop definite organic illness. There should always be positive psychological reasons to explain the development of the symptoms. Common reasons include major life events or stresses for the child, a similar illness among other family members/peers or an underlying depressive disorder.

Minor degrees of these disorders are extremely common and frequently occur as a transitory phenomenon during the course of many illnesses. The more general term 'abnormal illness behavior', similar to the physician's phrase 'functional overlay', has been coined to describe the situation when the individual persists with or exaggerates symptoms following on from an illness.

Treatment

Successful treatment depends upon the recognition that the symptoms are 'real' for the child. Psychic pain is just as distressing as physical pain. Anger and confrontation are unhelpful. A firm sympathetic approach with little attention to the symptom per se as well as avoiding rewarding the symptom is the best strategy. Allow the child to give up the symptoms with good grace, often providing the child with some face-saving reason for improvement. Identify and treat any affective disturbance. The outcome is good for the individual episode, though other psychological problems may persist.

SOMATOFORM DISORDERS[55]

(See adolescent section for chronic fatigue syndrome.)

Clinical features and management

Many children complain of somatic symptoms that do not have a pathological basis. Common symptoms are abdominal pain, headaches and limb pains with community prevalence rates of approximately 10%. This condition is usually managed by general practitioners, though it sometimes results in a referral for a specialist opinion. Management involves the minimum necessary investigation to exclude any pathology, the identification of any stressful circumstances and a sensitive explanation of the basis for the symptoms. The prevention of restrictions and the active encouragement of normal activities are essential.

When the somatic symptoms are persistent, chronic and involve several systems of the body, the International Clasification of Diseases (ICD) and Diagnostic and Statistical Manual of Mental Disorders (DSM) use the term somatization disorder. Whilst it is doubtful whether this disorder occurs in childhood, there is no doubt that persistent unexplained physical complaints are a common reason for children being taken to see the doctor. In many cases, there is clear evidence of underlying anxiety or recent stressful events.

REACTION TO SEVERE STRESS AND ADJUSTMENT DISORDERS

This group of disorders arises in response to an exceptionally stressful event or to a significantly adverse life change. The clinical features of the different syndromes vary considerably with a preponderance of affective symptoms in most cases.

Adjustment disorder

Definition

This is a maladaptive response occurring within 3 months of an identifiable psychosocial stressor. The maladaptive response must be of sufficient severity to impair daily activities such as schooling, hamper social relationships and be greater than expected given the nature of the stressor. Finally, the reaction must not last longer than 6 months.

Clinical features

By definition, the symptoms vary with ICD and DSM recognizing more than six categories. Clinical practice shows that anxiety and depressive symptoms, often combined, are the most frequent categories. Common stressors include parental divorce, unemployment, family illness or family move.

Predisposing factors

Age has different effects depending on the type of stressor. For instance, separation is more upsetting for a younger child than for an adolescent, whereas a loss of or change in a heterosexual relationship is far more important for an adolescent than for a younger child. Boys are also more vulnerable to the adverse effects of stress than girls. Temperamental characteristics such as 'difficult' or 'slow to warm up' style probably influence susceptibility as well. Again, the child's previous experience and repertoire of coping skills affect the response to the current stressor. For instance, if the child has successfully coped with adversity in the past, resilience and ability to withstand the present situation are enhanced. Finally, the family, particularly the parents, can magnify or minimize the impact of a stressor, dependent on their resourcefulness and coping style.

Outcome

By definition, the disorder can only last for 6 months, after which time the diagnostic category must change. The more important clinical consideration is not the change in diagnostic category, but the adverse effect that chronic or repeated stresses can have on the child's long term adjustment.

Post-traumatic stress disorder (PTSD)[56]

The 'epidemic' of disasters that some UK children have been involved with over the past 20 years (the capsize of the Herald of Free Enterprise, the sinking of the cruise ship Jupiter, the PanAm Lockerbie air crash and the crushing disaster at the Hillsborough football stadium) has made clinicians acutely aware of this syndrome. Clinicians are now familiar with the wide symptomatology often found, and have also become involved in treatment programs to reduce the distress both in the immediate aftermath and also in the long term.

Definition

This disorder arises following exposure to a stressful event of an exceptionally threatening or catastrophic nature that would cause pervasive distress in almost anyone. The events include accidents or disasters as well as more personal traumas such as witnessing a murder, a rape or torture. In clinical practice, children who have been sexually abused commonly present with symptoms falling within the diagnostic category of PTSD.

Clinical features

These include 'flashbacks'(the repeated re-enactment of the event with intrusive memories, dreams or nightmares); a sense of detachment, 'numbness' and emotional blunting; irritability, poor concentration and memory problems. Following disasters, many survivors often experience an increased awareness of danger, a foreshortened view of the future ('only plan for today'), a feeling of 'survivor' guilt (self-reproach about own survival, whilst companions died) and acute panic reactions.

Yule[56] indicates that 30–50% of children show significant psychological morbidity following disasters with symptoms persisting for several months.

Individual vulnerability factors

Important modifying factors are probably age, previous experiences, current life situation and the availability of help. Though cognitive immaturity may protect the child from appreciating the implications of a disaster, it may also be a disadvantage, as the child may not be given the opportunity to talk about the event. The child's previous experience of stressful events and their outcome, successful or otherwise, are likely to influence the response to the disaster.

Similarly, coexisting adverse circumstances such as family disharmony or school problems reduce the child's capacity to cope with the new situation.

Management

Though most research is anecdotal rather than systematic, the available evidence[56] suggests that postdisaster 'debriefing' sessions on an individual or group basis are helpful. Specific counseling sessions to help a child deal with phobic, anxiety or depressive symptoms are frequently necessary as well. Cognitive/behavioral approaches are particularly suitable for this pattern of symptoms.

MOOD DISORDERS

See adolescent section.

CONDUCT DISORDER

Clinical features

This is usually defined as persistent antisocial or socially disapproved of behavior that often involves damage to property and is unresponsive to normal sanctions. The IOW study[14] found a prevalence rate of 4% when the mixed disorder category was included as well, with a marked male predominance (at least 3:1). There is no independent criterion for deviancy as social and cultural values determine the seriousness or otherwise attached to antisocial behavior. Consequently, most clinicians would add the criterion of impairment, namely an adverse effect on the child's daily life or development, before applying the diagnostic label of conduct disorder.

Common symptoms include temper tantrums, oppositional behavior, overactivity, irritability, aggression, stealing, lying, truancy, bullying and wandering away from home/school. Delinquency (a legal term for a person committing an offence against the law) is a frequent feature among older children and adolescents. Stealing, vandalism, arson and firesetting are common forms of delinquency (male : female 10:1).

Traditionally, a distinction has been made between socialized and unsocialized behavior. The former describes behavior that is in accord with peer group values, but contrary to those of society, for instance antisocial gang behavior such as stealing and vandalism. Unsocialized antisocial behavior implies more disturbed behavior as it is often done alone against a background of parental rejection or neglect and poor peer relationships. Learning difficulties, especially specific reading retardation, occur more commonly among children with conduct disorders. This is a further reason why schooling is unpopular and a source of discouragement for these children. Additionally, many children with conduct disorder have affective symptoms such as anxiety or unhappiness, as well as low self-esteem and poor peer relationships. When these symptoms are prominent, it is often appropriate to classify the disorder as mixed, implying both emotional and behavioral symptomatology.

Etiology

Four factors, the family, the peer group, the neighbourhood and constitutional, make some contribution in most cases, but the family is usually the most important. Families of children with conduct disorder are characterized by a lack of affection and rejection, marital disharmony, inconsistent and ineffective discipline, parental violence and aggression. The families are often of large size, which aggravates the problems of supervision and care. Constitutional factors present in some cases include low intelligence and learning difficulties, along with adverse temperamental features such as overactivity and impulsiveness. Oppositional peer group values are an important feature in older children and adolescents. Many children with conduct disorder live in areas of urban deprivation with poor schooling. The intractable and chronic nature of these problems is a major reason for the continuation of conduct disorder into adolescence and adult life.

Treatment

Help for the family, either by counseling for the parents or by family therapy, is often used. More recently, specific intervention programs aimed at promoting positive parenting have been developed with good outcomes in the short term at least.[57] Educational support through remedial teaching or the provision of special education can be important in some cases. For many families however, the role of psychiatric services is limited with practical support with rehousing in order to alleviate social disadvantage the most important contribution.

Prognosis

Continuity into adult life is common with over 50% having problems as adults. Bad prognostic features are many and varied symptoms, problems at home and in the community and antiauthority and aggressive attitudes.

HYPERACTIVITY AND ATTENTION DEFICIT SYNDROMES[39,58]

Clinical features

Considerable controversy surrounds the diagnostic terms hyperkinetic disorder (HKD), attention deficit hyperactivity disorder (ADHD) and attention deficit disorder (ADD). HKD is the category used by ICD-10, which is the diagnostic system mainly used in the UK. This emphasises the importance of pervasive overactivity (i.e. present in all situations) as a diagnostic feature. By contrast, North American psychiatrists use DSM-IV that has the diagnostic category of ADHD. The latter stresses inattentiveness as a key symptom rather than overactivity. The different diagnostic practices probably explain the wide variation in prevalence rates (from 1 to 10%) found in epidemiological studies. Despite the difference in terminology, the two systems agree upon the same three core features, *overactivity*, *impulsivity* and *inattentiveness*.

Current UK practice has changed radically over the past 10 years, so that most UK psychiatrists use the term ADD rather than HKD. One consequence of this change has been the dramatic increase in the prescription of methylphenidate with the annual rate rising from 180 000 in 1991 to 1.5 million by 1995.

Another controversy concerns the existence of comorbidity among children with ADD symptoms, which in turn is linked to the conceptual argument about whether disorders are categorical or dimensional. Traditional UK clinical practice prefers a single as opposed to several concurrent diagnoses. For instance, if a child was overactive, they would be classified as HKD or conduct disorder, but not both. By contrast, North American practice allows, or even encourages, more than one diagnosis, namely the overactive child could have ADD and conduct disorder. Unfortunately, current evidence is unable to provide a definite answer about the best approach. This difference in diagnostic approach is another reason for the divergent prevalence rates in epidemiological studies.

In conclusion, it is probably best to regard overactivity as a symptom rather than a diagnostic term that can occur in many clinical situations: a symptom of ADHD, HKD or ADD; a feature of many children with conduct disorder; a reflection of developmental delay on its own or in association with general intellectual retardation; one extreme of normal temperamental variation; an uncommon response to high anxiety or tension; a symptom of childhood autism; and rarely, as a reaction to some drugs, for example barbiturates or benzodiazepines.

Treatment of attention deficit disorder

The recent MTA study[59] and the NICE report[60] have provided the clearest evidence and guidance respectively about the most effective treatment package. Most people would advocate a multimodal approach involving drug treatment, psychoeducational, parenting skills program and individual or group work with the child. The MTA study showed that 80% of children improved significantly on methylphenidate with improvement persisting over the 14-month trial period. There appeared little convincing evidence that a combined approach involving drug and behavioral treatments significantly improved the outcome, but it must be remembered that the MTA study was carried out in the USA where diagnostic practices are different.

Methylphenidate (up to 60 mg daily in divided doses) is the commonest prescribed drug in the UK, whereas dexamfetamine (up to 30 mg daily) is more popular in the USA and Australasia. Both drugs are equally effective with a similar side-effect profile, but dexamfetamine has a longer time course of effect. Stimulant drugs seem to work through an increase in dopamine levels in the frontal lobes. The common side-effects of both drugs are loss of appetite and night-time insomnia with abdominal pain, headache, tearfulness and tics less common. It is debatable whether stimulants have any long term effect on growth or the exacerbation of tics, but careful monitoring is advisable.

Tricyclic antidepressants such as imipramine or nortriptyline are also an effective alternative treatment, and are used when the child is unresponsive to stimulants, side-effects are disabling or there is a depressive component to the child's symptoms. There are also open label studies with clonidine, particularly for aggressive symptoms, but there have been case reports of sudden death due to cardiac arrhythmias, so that an electrocardiogram (ECG) prior to commencement of treatment is essential. Pemoline, which has the considerable advantage as a once daily dosage, has now been withdrawn in the UK on account of fears about hepatic toxicity.

Behavioral techniques, parental counseling and the alteration and manipulation of the child's environment, particularly at school, to reduce and minimize distraction are important components of most treatment programs. An alternative approach adopted by some clinicians has been the use of exclusion diets on the basis that the child is allergic to certain substances, commonly tartrazine. Evidence for the efficacy of these exclusion diets other than as a placebo response is unconvincing, though Egger et al,[61] using a sophisticated methodological design, showed that children with severe hyperactivity and mental retardation did respond. It is, however, unclear whether these results would apply to children of normal intelligence with less severe problems who make up the majority of children with ADD.

Outcome

Hyperactivity and attention deficits lessen considerably by adolescence, though other major problems such as learning difficulties and behavior problems persist. A substantial minority continue to have problems in adult life, mainly of an antisocial nature. There is also increasing evidence for the efficacy of methylphenidate in adults in whom the diagnosis of attention deficit disorder had been missed in childhood or who have continued on treatment from childhood.[62,63]

DISORDERS OF ELIMINATION

ENURESIS

This term refers to the involuntary passage of urine in the absence of physical abnormality after the age of 5 years. It may be nocturnal and/or diurnal. Bed wetting continuously, though not usually every night, since birth is termed primary enuresis, whereas when there has been a 6 month period of dry beds at some stage, recurrence of bed wetting is termed secondary or onset enuresis. Diurnal enuresis is much less common than nocturnal, but more common among girls and among children who are psychiatrically disturbed. Depending upon definition, approximately 10% of 5-year-olds, 5% of 10-year-olds and 1% of 18-year-olds will have nocturnal enuresis. The majority of children with nocturnal enuresis are not psychiatrically ill, though a substantial minority, approximately 25%, have signs of psychiatric disturbance.

Etiology

A combination of individual factors such as positive family history (approximately 70%), low intelligence, psychiatric disturbance and small bladder capacity along with environmental factors such as recent stressful life events, large family size and social disadvantage are present in most cases.

Treatment

It is important to exclude any physical basis for the enuresis by history, examination and, if necessary, investigation of the renal tract. Assuming no physical pathology, the most important initial step is to minimize the handicap, namely to point out to the parents the very favorable natural outcome of the condition, and to relabel the child's enuresis as immaturity rather than laziness or wilfulness. A star chart, the accurate recording of enuresis plus positive reinforcement for dry nights, provides an accurate baseline as well as a successful treatment in its own right. An enuresis alarm is successful with older cooperative children. The success of this approach is probably because the child becomes more aware of the sensation of a full bladder along with the encouragement from parents for dry nights. The modern alarms are extremely compact, and do not require a pad placed between the sheets, thereby increasing patient compliance considerably. It is useful to combine a buzzer with a star chart. Drugs such as desmopressin and imipramine are very effective at stopping enuresis, though their major limitation is that the enuresis returns when they are stopped. Most pediatricians believe it is wrong to prescribe potentially lethal drugs such as imipramine for a benign condition such as enuresis, so that desmopressin is the preferred drug treatment.

SOILING AND ENCOPRESIS

Most children are continent of feces and clean by their fourth birthday. Encopresis is usually defined as the inappropriate passage of formed feces, usually onto the underwear, in the absence of any physical pathology after 4 years of age. Soiling, the passage of semi-solid feces, is often used synonymously with encopresis. Symptoms vary widely in severity, ranging from slight staining of underwear to encopresis with the smearing of feces onto the walls. It is uncommon with a community prevalence among 8-year-olds of 1.8% for boys and of 0.7% for girls. Psychiatric disturbance is common among children with encopresis. Enuresis may also be present.

Clinical features (Fig. 33.3)

Figure 33.3 shows a convenient way to classify encopresis with a broad distinction between children who retain feces with eventual overflow incontinence and those who deposit feces inappropriately on a regular basis. Some children have never achieved continence, a situation called continuous or primary encopresis, whilst others have had periods of cleanliness followed by relapse, the so-called discontinuous or secondary encopresis. Figure 33.3 also lists the common different patterns of interaction found among children with encopresis and their parents. For instance, children with retentive encopresis have often been subjected to coercive and obsessional toilet training practices, so that the encopresis is seen as a reaction, often of anger or aggression, towards this practice. Similarly, many children with continuous non-retentive encopresis come from disorganized chaotic families where regular training and toileting are not the norm. Again, encopresis can arise in some children as a response to a stressful situation. Finally, encopresis can reflect poor parent–child relationship, often longstanding and usually associated with other aspects of psychiatric disturbance. The clinical picture is often, however, not as clear-cut with the different elements each making some contribution. There may be a previous history of constipation and occasionally of anal fissure.

Treatment

A physical etiology such as Hirschsprung's disease must be excluded before commencement of psychiatric treatment. The assessment must include an account of previous treatments and most importantly, the current attitude of the parents and the child to the problem. Treatment has two aims, the promotion of a normal bowel habit and the improvement of the parent–child relationship. Initially, a bowel washout and/or microenemata may be necessary to clear out the bowel. Judicious use of bowel smooth muscle stimulants (Senokot), stool softeners (Dioctyl) and bulk agents (lactulose) is helpful for the child with retention. Again, suppositories are often useful from time to time. This should also be combined with parental and child education about the dietary importance of fiber. The psychological component includes behavioral (star chart) and individual psychotherapy to gain the cooperation and trust of the child along with parental counseling or family therapy to modify attitudes and hostile interactions between the child and his parents.

Prognosis

Encopresis usually resolves by adolescence, though other problems may persist. Occasional case reports of persistence into adult life have been published.

MISCELLANEOUS DISORDERS

DEVELOPMENTAL DISORDERS

Language disorders (See also Ch. 20)

Children with language disorders are more vulnerable to disturbance, mainly because of the associated anxiety and

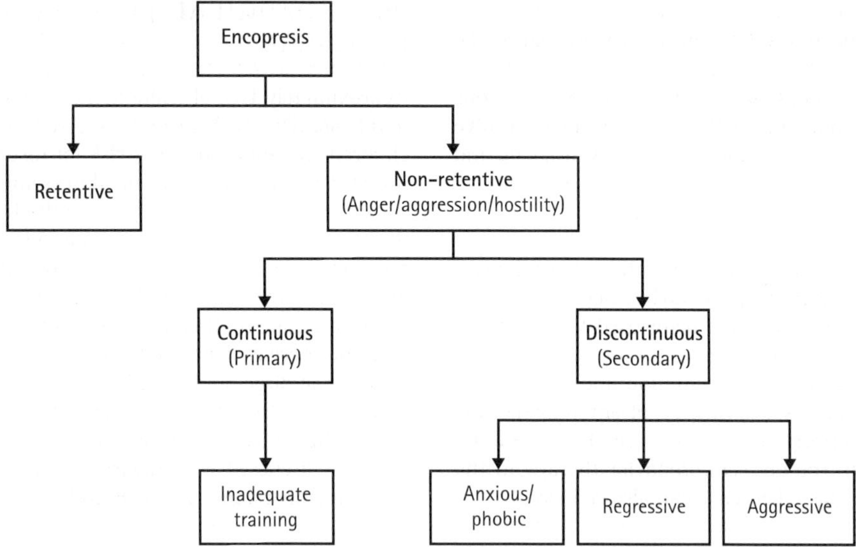

Three patterns are common:
- Child with primary encopresis
- Child with retentive encopresis
- Child with secondary encopresis

Fig. 33.3 Types of encopresis and their psychopathology.

embarrassment caused by the disorder. Specific language delay (5–6/1000) is twice as common in boys as it is in girls, with a strong association with large family size and lower social class. Richman et al[16] found that approximately 25% of 3-year-olds with specific language delay had behavioral problems.

Stuttering, an abnormality of speech rhythm consisting of hesitations and repetitions at the beginning of syllables and words, is a normal, though transitory phenomenon, occurring at around 3–4 years of age. When it persists (approximately 3% of the general population), often due to inadvertent parental attention, it leads to anxiety and low self-esteem.

Selective mutism

This is not strictly a language disorder, as the main problem is the child's refusal to talk in certain situations, most commonly at school, rather than an inability to speak. Mild forms of the disorder are common but transitory, usually at the commencement of schooling, while the severe form has a prevalence rate of about 1 in 1000. Other features include a previous history of speech delay, excessively shy but stubborn temperament and parental overprotectiveness.

A combination of behavioral and family therapy techniques to promote communication and the use of speech is most commonly used, though some cases require inpatient assessment. Fluoxetine had been shown to be effective in an open trial of children with selective mutism and comorbid anxiety disorder.[64] Prognosis is good for approximately 50%, with failure to improve by the age of 10 years a poor prognostic sign.

Reading difficulties

Though mainly of educational concern, the pediatrician or child psychiatrist may get involved because of the associated behavioral or emotional problems. The two main types are first, general reading backwardness, when the retardation is a reflection of generalized intellectual delay, and second, specific reading retardation when the attainment in reading is significantly behind the expected level after controlling for age and intelligence. The problem is 'significant' when the delay is at least 2 years. Dyslexia is a concept similar to specific reading retardation, implying a neuropsychological substrate for the specific reading difficulties. The use of this term is contentious, so that the more bland expression, specific reading retardation, is preferred by many clinical psychologists.

The etiology is multifactorial, involving genetic, social, perceptual and language deficits. A noteworthy feature is the strong association between specific reading retardation and conduct disorder with the behavior problem most likely arising secondary to the frustration and disillusionment associated with the reading difficulty. Treatment involves a detailed psychometric assessment of the problem by a psychologist followed by an individualized remedial program carried out by a specialized teacher in collaboration with the psychologist. Help with the behavioral problem is also necessary in order to prevent more serious problems arising during adolescence.

HABIT DISORDERS

Tics and Tourette's syndrome

Tics are rapid, involuntary, repetitive muscular movements, usually involving the face and neck, for instance blinks, grimaces and throat clearing. Simple tics occur as a transitory phenomenon in about 10% of the population with boys outnumbering girls three to one and with a mean age of onset around 7 years. They range in severity from simple tics involving head and neck through to complex tics extending to the limbs and trunk and finally to Tourette's syndrome. The latter comprises complex tics accompanied by coprolalia (uttering obscene words and phrases) and echolalia (the repetition of sounds or words). Like stammering, tics are made worse at times of stress and may be exacerbated by undue parental concern. The differential diagnosis of tics in childhood is principally from chorea where the movements are less coordinated and predictable, not stereotypic in form and cannot be suppressed.

Other features of tics are a positive family history and a previous history of neurodevelopmental delay. Many tics resolve spontaneously, but those that persist can be extremely disabling and difficult to treat.

Treatment

Several approaches are used singly or in combination, depending on assessment. Medication is effective, but should be reserved for severe cases. Haloperidol is the most common drug used for Tourette's syndrome, but pimozide and clonidine are alternative drugs. Many children with simple tics respond to explanation and reassurance along with advice for the parents. Individual and/or family therapy may be indicated when anxiety and tension are clearly making important contributions to the problem. Behavior therapy in the form of relaxation and/or massed practice can also be helpful.

Prognosis

Simple tics have a good outcome with complete remission, whereas in Tourette's syndrome the condition fluctuates in a chronic manner with 50% continuing with symptoms into adult life.

SLEEP DISORDERS (See Preschool children section)

Night terrors

The usual pattern is for the child to wake up in a frightened, even terrified state, not to respond when spoken to, nor appear to see objects or people. Instead, he appears to be hallucinating, talking to and looking at people/things not actually present. The child may be difficult to comfort with the period of disturbed behavior and altered consciousness lasting up to 15 min, occasionally longer. Eventually the behavior settles, with or without comfort, and the child goes back to sleep, awakening in the morning with no recollection of the episode. The latter point is invaluable in helping to allay parental anxiety about the episodes. Night terrors arise from stage 4 or deep sleep. The peak incidence is between 4 and 7 years with a continuation of 1–3% into older children. It is also helpful to identify and ameliorate any identifiable stresses that may occasionally contribute to the problem. Lask[65] described an apparently successful novel behavioral approach relying on waking the child 15 min prior to the expected time of the night terror. Drugs such as benzodiazepines or tricyclics have also been used successfully.

Nightmares

These are frightening or unpleasant dreams, occurring during REM (rapid eye movement) sleep. The child may or may not wake up but there will be a clear recollection of the dream if he does wake up and also in the morning. There is no period of altered consciousness or inaccessibility as in night terrors. Again, daytime anxieties and/or frightening television programs in the evening may be contributory factors.

Sleep walking (somnambulism)

The child, usually aged between 8 and 14 years, calmly arises from his bed with a blank facial expression, does not respond to attempts at communication and can only be awakened with difficulty. The child is in a state of altered consciousness at the deep level of sleep (stages 3 or 4). Any contributory anxiety should be treated as well as giving the parents some advice about the safety and protection of the child during these episodes.

PSYCHOLOGICAL EFFECTS OF ILLNESS AND HANDICAP

Approximately 15% of children have some form of chronic illness or handicap. The IOW study[14] showed clearly that this group of children was much more at risk for disturbance, namely a rate of 33% for children with chronic illness affecting the central nervous system and of 12% for children with chronic illness not affecting the central nervous system compared with 7% among the general population. The IOW study also showed that children with chronic illness or handicap had the same range of disorders as other disturbed children, thereby implying that the mechanisms involved with this increased morbidity are probably indirect and non-specific rather than direct and specific to each illness or handicap. Illness or handicap imposes psychological stress on the child and family not only at the time of diagnosis but also in the long term. These effects are now discussed with regard to the child himself and to other family members, though the two effects interact with each other.

EFFECTS ON THE CHILD

Three aspects are important: the acquisition of skills and outside interests; the development of self-concept; and the development of adaptive coping behavior. Many illnesses or handicaps inevitably restrict the child's ability or opportunity to acquire everyday skills and to develop interests and hobbies. For example, the child with cerebral palsy is by definition motor handicapped, the dietary restrictions of diabetes, the exercise limitations of asthma and the avoidance by children with epilepsy of some activities such as cycling or swimming. Additionally, educational problems are common among this group of children for a variety of reasons including increased absence from school, specific learning difficulties, especially among children with epilepsy, and low expectations of parents and teachers.

Illness and handicap can adversely affect the child's self-concept in several ways through the effects on the child's body image and self-esteem. Many children have a distorted view of their body believing the handicap to be very prominent or disfiguring. These ideas can often be reinforced by comments from parents or peers. Self-esteem can also be impaired due to a faulty cognitive appraisal of the situation and to a pessimistic attitude to the situation. This leads the child to have a low self-esteem with a gloomy view about his illness and his prospects for the future. This is particularly likely and also potentially very disabling among older children and adolescents.

Successful adaptation to a disability depends on the acquisition of a range of coping behaviors and defence mechanisms to lessen anxiety to an acceptable level. Effective coping strategies include rationing the amount of stress into containable amounts, obtaining information, rehearsing the possible outcomes of treatment and assessing the situation from several viewpoints. Parents, nursing staff and pediatricians have an important role in promoting this repertoire of skills for children with a disability. Additionally, defence mechanisms such as denial, rationalization and displacement can be helpful for the child during the initial stages of adjustment to the illness or disability.

EFFECTS ON THE PARENTS

The parents can respond in various ways in the short term and also in the long term. Most parents eventually achieve some degree of adaptation, though for a minority maladaptive behavior patterns emerge and are prominent. The common reaction is overprotection whereby the parent(s) is unable to allow the child to experience the normal disappointments and upsets inevitable during childhood, so that the child leads a 'cotton wool' existence. Less frequently, the parent(s) may be rejecting and indifferent to the child because the child's disability is so damaging to the parents' self-esteem or because the disability has exacerbated an already precarious parent–child relationship. Overprotection and rejection are sometimes combined together in the parental reaction to the child's disability.

The parents may also find it difficult to provide appropriate discipline and control, as they irrationally fear that such control may aggravate the child's illness. For example, parents of children with epilepsy may think that thwarting the child's wishes may induce an epileptic fit.

Finally, the stress of coping with the child's illness may exacerbate parental marital disharmony, though in a minority it may paradoxically unite them as they face the adversity together.

EFFECT ON SIBLINGS

This can manifest itself in several ways: the oldest sibling may be given excessive responsibility such as looking after the handicapped sib; the sibs may lose friendships because they are reluctant to bring their friends home in case their handicapped sibling is an embarrassment; and finally, the sibling's own developmental needs may be neglected with consequent resentment and frustration.

BREAKING BAD NEWS TO PARENTS

This distressing but inevitable aspect of pediatrics comes in various guises such as the birth of a child with Down syndrome or with the diagnosis of cystic fibrosis. Unfortunately, most undergraduate and postgraduate training includes very little teaching about this important subject. Though the details vary for each case, the following general principles are important:

1. Information should be given by the most senior and experienced doctor involved with the child's care.
2. Both parents must be seen together if at all possible, as this reduces misinformation and allows the parents to be mutually supportive from the outset.
3. Allow adequate time for the interview (not 10 min at the end of a ward round).
4. Privacy is essential not only as a matter of courtesy and dignity but also because it allows parents to express their emotions more freely.
5. Begin the interview by asking the parents to tell you what they know about the problems.
6. Tell parents frankly and honestly in simple and non-technical language the nature of the problem, explaining the reasons for the investigations and the basis for the diagnosis.
7. Encourage the parents to ask questions (by asking them some open-ended questions).
8. Emphasize the positive as well as the negative aspects of the diagnosis, for instance the child will be able to have physiotherapy and special equipment, will be able to go to school and to receive effective control for pain.
9. Facilitate the expression of emotions by the parents, namely respond sympathetically and sensitively to the parent(s)' distress and crying.
10. Make a definite offer of a further appointment to talk things over again.
11. Many parents find it helpful to continue the discussion with a nurse or social worker after the interview.

REACTIONS TO HOSPITALIZATION

Admission to hospital is a common experience during childhood with approximately 25% admitted by the age of 4 years. For most children, this is a short admission for a brief treatable illness, whilst a minority (approximately 4%) remain in hospital for at least a month. While most parents and their children cope successfully with the admission, some, particularly those with repeated admissions for minor illnesses, show evidence of disturbance which may in turn have been the reason why the child was admitted in the first place.

Admission to hospital can have adverse effects in the short term as well as in the long term. The contributory factors can be grouped under three headings: the child and family; the nature of the illness; the attitudes and practices of the hospital and its staff. Important factors within the child and family include age, temperament of the child, previous experience of hospital, previous parent–child relationship and current family circumstances. Children aged between 1 and 4 years are particularly stressed by separation from familiar figures. Similarly, children with adverse temperamental characteristics, such as poor adaptability or irregularity of habits, are more vulnerable. If the child had a favorable experience when in hospital previously, this will ease the burden for any subsequent admission. If the parent–child relationship was poor prior to admission, hospitalization is likely to exacerbate this problem because of the additional stress. Adverse family circumstances, for instance financial, may also be aggravated by admission.

The nature of the illness, particularly the associated pain or the necessity for painful procedures, influences the child's response. Again, an acute admission is likely to be more stressful than an elective procedure.

The attitudes of the staff and hospital practices can minimize considerably the distress for the child. Helpful and favorable aspects include good rooming-in facilities, adequate preparation for painful or unpleasant procedures, nursing and medical staff trained to minimize distress and to offer comfort when required. The ward should be organized so that parents and sibs are encouraged to visit as well as ensuring the ready availability of playleaders and teachers. Medical and nursing staff should also have access to social work resources as well as to psychological and psychiatric services. Finally, joint liaison between the medical and psychiatric team and the establishment of a staff support group to enable staff to discuss their own anxieties about working in a stressful environment are likely to be beneficial.

TREATMENT METHODS

Several factors are usually responsible for the development of disturbance, so that it is unlikely that one treatment method will resolve the problem. All treatment approaches also rely upon common elements that are not only necessary but also essential for a successful outcome. These elements include active cooperation between the therapist and the child and family, agreement between them about the aims of treatment, and a mutual trust to enable these aims to be achieved. Again, the relative efficacy of different treatments is not clearly established, so that the choice of treatment is often a reflection of the therapist(s)' training and experience rather than an absolute indication in any particular instance. Careful analysis of the following elements is therefore necessary in order to devise an effective treatment program:

1. Individual
   - Physical illness or handicap

- Intellectual ability
- Type of symptomatology

2. Family
   - Developmental stage (for instance a family with preschool children or one with adolescents)
   - Psychiatric health of parents
   - Marital relationship
   - Parenting qualities
   - Communication patterns within the family
   - Ability to resolve conflict
   - Support network, for instance availability of the extended family
3. School
   - Scholastic attainments
   - Child and parents' attitude to the authority of the school
   - Peer relationships
4. Community
   - Quality of peer relationships and of role models
   - Neighborhood and community resources.

The formulation of the problem along these four dimensions provides the basis to decide the suitable treatment program.

The three main types of treatment approach available are *drug treatment, the psychotherapies* and *liaison* or *consultation work.* The latter refers to the common practice whereby the child psychiatrist or a member of the psychiatric team does not have direct contact with the referred child, but rather helps those involved with the child to understand and modify the child's behavior. Psychotherapies are those treatments that use a variety of psychological techniques to ameliorate disturbance. They include individual therapy, behavior therapy, family therapy and group therapy as well as counseling and advice for parents.

Drug treatment[66]

This has increasing importance in child psychiatry. Table 33.3 summarizes the important indications and side-effects of various drugs used in child psychiatry.

Psychotherapies

These are a very common treatment approach in child psychiatric practice.

Individual psychotherapy[67]

Though there are several theoretical orientations, including psychoanalytic[68] and Rogerian,[69] the therapist has nevertheless the same therapeutic tasks. These are: to develop a trusting, non-judgmental relationship with the child; to enable the child to express his feelings and thoughts; to understand the meaning of the child's symptoms, including his behavior during the therapeutic session; and finally to provide the child with some understanding and explanation for his behavior. The indications for individual psychotherapy are not clearly established, though most usually it is for children with a neurotic or reactive disorder rather than for those with a constitutionally based disorder. For younger children the medium for communication is play such as sand play or through drawing, whilst for older children verbal exchange and discussion are possible.

Behavioral psychotherapy[70]

This approach is based upon the application of the findings from experimental psychology, particularly learning theory, to a wide range of problems such as enuresis, encopresis, tantrums and aggression. Its characteristics are as follows:

1. Define problem(s) objectively with reference to the Antecedents, the Behavior itself and the Consequences (the ABC approach).
2. Emphasis on current behavior rather than on past events.
3. Set up hypotheses to account for the behavior.
4. Pretreatment baseline to determine the frequency and severity of the problem.
5. Devise behavioral programs on an individual basis to test the hypothesis.
6. Evaluate outcome of treatment programs.
7. Tackle one problem at a time.

As with other psychotherapies, success depends upon the establishment of a trusting relationship with the patient and the close

Table 33.3 Drug treatment in child psychiatry

Drug	Usage	Comment
Anxiolytics	Anxiety/phobic conditions	Short term adjunct to behavior treatment
Neuroleptics		
Phenothiazines (e.g. chlorpromazine)	Schizophrenia /ADD	Extrapyramidal side-effects common
Butyrophenones (e.g. haloperidol)	Complex tics/Tourette's syndrome	Extrapyramidal side-effects common
Newer antipsychotics (e.g. risperidone/olanzepine)	Schizophrenia	Fewer side-effects
Tricyclics		
imipramine/nortriptyline	Second line of treatment for ADD	Useful when an affective component present
clomipramine	Obsessional compulsive disorder	Long term usage often necessary
SRIs (fluoxetine, paroxetine, sertraline)	Probably first choice for depressive disorder	Better compliance with fewer side-effects
Stimulants		
methylphenidate/dexamfetamine	ADD	80% effective. Side-effects closely monitored
Hypnotics (melatonin)	Persistent sleep disorder	Sometimes used for sleep problems associated with ADD
Lithium	Recurrent bipolar affective disorder	Close supervision of blood level and for signs of toxicity
Laxatives (e.g. bulk-forming (methylcellulose), stimulants (senna), softener (dioctyl))	Encopresis with constipation	Facilitates formation and passage of feces
Central alpha-agonist (e.g. clonidine)	Unresponsive Tourette's syndrome	Sedation and rebound hypertension

ADD, attention deficit disorder; SRIs, serotonin reuptake inhibitors supervision of the treatment program together with the involvement of teachers and parents in many cases.

Cognitive behavioral therapy (CBT)[71]

This is used increasingly with older children and adolescents for a variety of conditions including anxiety, depression and anorexia nervosa. The central premise is that the individual's cognitive distortions are responsible for the symptoms and the disorder, so that therapy is designed to change cognitions through a collaborative approach between the therapist and the patient. Usually the treatment lasts about 12 sessions. The early part of the treatment is devoted to teaching the patient to recognize their cognitive distortions, and then training them to devise alternative and more healthy interpretations of the situation. This is combined with 'homework tasks' between sessions in order to put into practice the new ideas or responses to situations that they find difficult.

Family therapy[72]

This is a popular treatment approach now. The rationale underlying family therapy is that the child's disturbed behavior is symptomatic of the disturbance within the family as a group. There are many different theoretical approaches and techniques,[72] but all usually involve interviewing the whole family on each occasion for about 1 h. Most family work is short term, lasting about 6 months, with approximately monthly sessions. The emphasis is on current behavior, verbal and non-verbal, observed during the session rather than on past events. The main aim is to improve communication within the family, so that dysfunctional patterns of behavior are replaced by more healthy and adaptive behavior.

Group therapy

Older children and adolescents often benefit from group therapy when the aim is to improve interpersonal relationships, particularly with the peer group, using a variety of theoretical models (for instance psychodynamic and social skills).

Supportive psychotherapy and counseling

The former is frequently used for the child with chronic illness or handicap when the focus may be the child or the parents. It is especially beneficial at the time of diagnosis and also in the long term when the implications of the disability become more evident. Parental counseling is also used to help the parents understand their child's behavior problems, the factors that may have led to them and that are responsible for their continuation, along with an emphasis on the parent–child relationship and the improvement of parenting skills. Counseling may therefore help the parents to devise and implement a behavioral program to modify the child's behavior as well as to promote normal development.

Liaison and consultation psychiatry[73]

This is a collaborative approach between the child psychiatry team and the professionals directly involved with the child, for instance hospital staff, teachers or residential care staff, in order to help these professionals to understand the child's disturbed behavior, their own possible contribution to the problem and to suggest ways to improve the situation. Although the child psychiatrist may see the referred child in the first instance, subsequent contact is usually with the staff rather than with the child. This approach can also include the establishment and supervision of a staff support group whose aim is to look at the attitudes and emotional responses of the staff towards the behavior shown by the children under their care.

PYSCHIATRIC DISORDERS IN ADOLESCENCE

This section has two parts, adolescent psychological development and adolescent psychiatric syndromes.

ADOLESCENT DEVELOPMENT

Adolescence is the transition between childhood and adult life. Four maturational tasks must be accomplished successfully to ensure a favorable outcome:

- the attainment of independence;
- the establishment of a sexual role and orientation;
- the self-control of aggressive and oppositional impulses;
- the achievement of self-identity.

Though these tasks are not necessarily complete nor entirely resolved by the end of adolescence, the adolescent should have made substantial progress with these tasks. Three tasks, independence, sex role and orientation, self-control of aggressive and oppositional impulses, refer to specific aspects of psychological development, whereas the fourth, self-identity, is a global term referring to that sense of uniqueness or individuality that distinguishes one person from another. Erikson[6] believed that the attainment of a stable self-identity during adolescence is the prerequisite for successful adult adjustment. Important components of self-identity for Erikson are 'sexual identity' and 'career identity'. The Eriksonian unsuccessful outcome of adolescent conflict is 'identity diffusion' with the person lacking clear goals and direction in the fulfilment of individual ambition.

Adolescent development is commonly divided into four phases:

1. the preadolescent phase (11–13 years);
2. early adolescence (13–15 years);
3. mid adolescence (15–17 years);
4. and late adolescence (18 years onwards).

The main features of the preadolescent phase are the onset of biological puberty and an increased interest in peer relationships and teenage pursuits. Early adolescence is characterized by the critical questioning of parental values combined with an uncritical acceptance of peer group views. The establishment of a separate sexual and social identity occurs during mid adolescence. The individual explores and develops their own gender and sexual role. The development of social relationships outside the family enables the individual to have their own social network as well as altering the basis of their relationship with their parents. Later adolescence is focused on the career or work choice along with the expression of the sexual role through more satisfying and enduring relationships.

DETERMINANTS OF ADOLESCENT ADJUSTMENT

Though the same general factors influence development and adjustment in adolescence as in earlier periods, brief mention will be made of those that are of particular relevance.

Previous childhood experience(s)

Unsatisfactory earlier experience(s) and relationships, particularly the child–parent(s) relationship, are major factors affecting predisposition to adjustment during adolescence. The individual's capacity to withstand the inevitable stresses of adolescence and also their resilience are greatly impaired when the outcome of earlier experiences was unsatisfactory. Adverse childhood experience is an important vulnerability factor in adolescent breakdown.

Family psychopathology

Parental psychopathology such as marital disharmony or parental psychiatric illness has a powerful influence on children's behavior throughout childhood, but even more so during adolescence, when conflicts over discipline, control and autonomy are normal and unavoidable. Parental disagreements and disunity on these matters greatly exacerbate the difficulties.

Schooling

Common problems are: academic failure with scholastic subjects; poor motivation and disillusionment with schooling; conflicts over authority with teaching staff.

Peer group

Peer group values and pressure exert enormous influence on the adolescent, so that contact with and membership of a deviant peer group can lead to major problems in school, for instance truancy, or in the community, for instance delinquency or vandalism.

Chronic illness or handicap

The normal adolescent drive for self-appraisal and self-identity leaves the disabled or handicapped adolescent feeling isolated and different from their peers, a most distressing experience. Early childhood feelings of acceptance and tolerance by peers are replaced by those of exclusion and separateness with a reluctance or inability to gain peer group acceptance. The adolescent often deals with these feelings of anger and frustration by denial or minimalization of the seriousness of his condition. This can result in poor compliance with medication or reckless exposure to dangerous situations.

INTERVIEWING AND ASSESSMENT OF ADOLESCENTS

Though the earlier part of the chapter discussed the general principles of interviewing and assessment, it is helpful to mention some specific points relating to adolescence. Flexibility in approach is essential for successful interviewing. In general, the older the adolescent and the more serious or intimate the problem, the greater the necessity for a separate interview with the adolescent. Usually, this is combined with a family interview in order to complete the assessment.

Many adolescents are reluctant, confused or anxious attenders, so that the clinician must clarify and explain the purpose, sequence and duration of the assessment procedures at the outset. Respect for the adolescent's maturity, the right to privacy and confidentiality must be acknowledged clearly. The distinction between 'family business' and 'individual business' must be emphasized to the adolescent and to the parents. Adolescent anxieties about 'seeing the shrink' or being 'treated like a child' must be addressed and talked through. The individual interview may allow the clinician to conduct a thorough assessment of the mental state, though careful phrasing of questions about sexual or psychotic phenomena is essential in order to avoid a dismissive denial and a further increase in anxiety and confusion.

Silence and refusal to talk during the interview are common and often difficult to overcome. The clinician can use three tactics to deal with this problem: it can be pointed out that the silence is just as difficult for the interviewer as it is for the adolescent; there will be the opportunity and time to talk through difficult topics now or alternatively on another occasion; and finally, to terminate the interview when necessary to prevent prolonged or undue tension.

Family interviews are often not only part of the assessment procedure but also of the treatment plan. Sometimes however, it is more appropriate to interview the parents and the child together rather than the whole family.

ADOLESCENT PSYCHIATRIC SYNDROMES

These are divided into three categories: those disorders persisting from earlier childhood; new disorders arising during adolescence; and those disorders with features special to adolescence. Prior to the discussion of these topics, brief comment will be made about the prevalence of psychiatric disorders in adolescence.

Prevalence

This varies widely from 10–20% depending upon the population studied, the diagnostic criteria and the age group. Most studies do however show a consistent pattern with respect to gender ratio, urban versus rural differences and the range of clinical syndromes. In contrast to earlier childhood when psychiatric disorder is more common among boys, the adolescent period shows a shift towards an equal gender ratio in early adolescence followed by a subsequent female preponderance in late adolescence and adult life. Prevalence rates in urban populations are at least twice that for rural populations. Schizophrenia, major affective disorder, suicide and attempted suicide, anorexia and substance abuse all begin to appear with some frequency during adolescence, whereas encopresis or enuresis decrease markedly.

PERSISTENT CHILDHOOD DISORDERS

Childhood disorders are more likely to continue into adolescence when one or more of the following are present: a major constitutional factor to the syndrome; the adverse circumstances responsible for the onset of the disorder are still present; and perpetuating or maintaining factors are prominent. The follow-up study of 10-year-old children in the IOW study[13] showed that 40% of the disorders had persisted into adolescence with a strong continuity for boys with conduct disorder and associated educational problems. This section now discusses the factors responsible for the persistence of some disorders into adolescence from earlier childhood.

Conduct disorder

The oppositional and defiant character of conduct disorder means that it is very likely to be exacerbated by the rebellious and antiauthoritarian nature of ordinary adolescent behavior. Childhood predictors of persistent conduct disorder are: early onset of symptoms; extensive and varied symptomatology; and the severity of aggressive behavior. Adverse temperamental characteristics combined with continued exposure to deviant family psychopathology such as deficient and ineffective parenting, marital disharmony or parental psychiatric illness are thought to be important factors maintaining the conduct disorder. The persistence of the frequently associated learning disorders is another source of frustration and disillusionment for the adolescent, producing conflict with the teachers and reluctance to attend school.

Emotional disorders

Generally, emotional disorders have a good prognosis, often because they arise in response to some identifiable but remedial stress. Consequently, emotional disorder persisting into adolescence implies a more serious underlying cause. The school refusal syndrome is the most likely condition to show continuity from early childhood. It may reappear at the transfer from primary to secondary school, or early on during secondary schooling. Previous history of separation difficulties, for instance at the start of nursery or primary school and/or an overdependent relationship between the child and parent(s), are commonly found. The increased necessity for independence, autonomy and assertiveness at secondary school may prove too much for the vulnerable adolescent.

Childhood autism

The overt autistic-like behavior and overactivity prominent in younger children with the disorder often decrease during adolescence, but the majority are still profoundly impaired in social and communication skills with a marked apathy and lack of empathy. Educational and learning disabilities are very evident. Epilepsy also develops in about 15% of individuals with a greater risk when severe mental retardation is also present.

Attention deficit disorder

The overactivity usually decreases during adolescence, but persistent problems with antisocial behavior, impulsivity, recklessness, distractibility and learning disorders mean that the adolescent with ADD is likely to remain disturbed.

NEW DISORDERS ARISING DURING ADOLESCENCE

These can be divided into two categories, those related to the stress of adolescence and major adult-like disorders arising in adolescence.

Stress-related adolescent disorders

During adolescence, the distinction between normal and abnormal behavior is often imprecise, so that it is more important to understand why the adolescent's behavior is such a cause of concern rather than whether the behavior fulfils the criteria for a disorder in a diagnostic classification system. In many cases, conflict often arises between the adolescent and the parents over independence and control issues. Allied with the pressure from peers, this often leads the adolescent to engage in antisocial or conduct disordered behavior. Delinquency, vandalism and out of control behavior are common, sometimes mixed with a pattern of alcohol or drug abuse. Persistent antisocial disorder often culminates in criminal behavior and arrest by the police. Coexistent family problems with a limited capacity to resolve issues also contribute to the severity of the disorder. Eventually, it may be necessary for the adolescent to leave the family home and to provide him with alternative care arrangements, for instance with foster parents or community carers. Another solution sometimes adopted by the adolescent is to run away from home. Although the majority of runaways eventually return home, a minority stay away and become involved with the homeless subculture found in large cities.

The common neurotic or emotional responses to adolescent stress are affective symptoms such as irritability, lability of mood and anxiety symptoms, particularly related to social situations or mixing with peers. The latter may sometimes lead to marked social withdrawal. School refusal may sometimes present for the first time during early adolescence when it represents a combination of adolescent stress and the revival of an earlier overdependent parent–child relationship. The increased need for independence and autonomy posed by the demands of secondary school precipitates an avoidance response to school attendance from the adolescent. The anxiety symptoms often masquerade themselves as physical complaints such as headaches or abdominal pain. The prompt exclusion of organic pathology with a minimum amount of investigation is essential in order to prevent the secondary elaboration of physical symptomatology. Delay in the recognition of the underlying psychological basis for the problem greatly exacerbates the difficulties. The prognosis is not good for a significant minority of adolescents with up to a third failing to maintain regular school attendance. Poor prognosis is usually a sign of more serious underlying family psychopathology. Follow-up studies into adult life have shown that anxiety or agoraphobic symptoms are present in about 20%.[53]

Obsessive–compulsive disorder sometimes begins during adolescence when its occurrence can be seen as a maladaptive response to the stress of adolescence. There is often a history of earlier childhood obsessional and anxiety traits. The key element in the maintenance and exacerbation of the disorder is usually the willingness of the family to participate in the ritualistic behavior. SRIs such as sertraline and fluvoxamine have been shown to be effective in reducing obsessive–compulsive symptoms, but more importantly are particularly effective when combined with cognitive-behavior therapy.[74]

Major adult-like disorders arising in adolescence

Three categories of disorder, schizophrenia, mood disorders and anorexia nervosa, begin to occur with increasing frequency during adolescence.

Schizophrenia[75]

This is a rare disease during childhood. Even during adolescence, it has a frequency of less than 3 per 10 000. Symptoms are usually classified into two groups, positive and negative. Positive symptoms comprise delusions (fixed, false beliefs), hallucinations (a perceptual experience in the absence of the relevant sensory stimulus) and distortions of thinking (thought insertion and withdrawal). Negative symptoms include social withdrawal, emotional blunting, apathy, lack of motivation, poverty of speech and slowness of thought. The usual presentation is insidious rather than florid with a gradual social withdrawal and increased internal preoccupation. Dysphoric symptoms are common, so that a diagnosis of affective disorder is sometimes made. The adolescent is often able to conceal his bizarre ideas from parents and peers. However, it is the presence of increasingly unpredictable and erratic behavior that indicates something more serious is occurring. The possibility of drug misuse is an important alternative diagnostic possibility.

Etiology

There is good evidence of a genetic component with approximately 20% of relatives having the disease.[75] The Maudsley long term follow-up study of early onset psychosis[75] showed that one-third had significant premorbid social difficulties affecting the ability to make and retain friends. There was also a downward shift in intelligence with a mean IQ of 85. The disorder tends to run a chronic course with only a minority making a full symptomatic recovery – only 12% of patients in the Maudsley study were in remission at 6 months. The best prognostic indicator was the clinical state at that time.

Treatment

It must be comprehensive including drug treatment with antipsychotics, individual and family therapy as well as help with education. Traditional antipsychotics such as chlorpromazine and haloperidol are effective, particularly for positive symptoms, but extrapyramidal side-effects and drowsiness adversely affect compliance. Consequently, the newer antipsychotics such as risperidone and olanzapine with their low side-effect profile are now the drugs of first choice. When treatment with first line drugs is ineffective, serious consideration should be given to clozapine. This drug has been shown to be effective for treatment resistant schizophrenia in adults, and promising case reports have been published for adolescents. There must be careful screening and monitoring for side-effects, particularly for blood dyscrasias, when clozapine is used.

Finally, bad prognostic features include poor premorbid functioning, negative symptoms and a long period of untreated illness.

MOOD DISORDERS[76,77]

This section has the following parts: depression as a symptom; depressive disorders; bipolar affective disorder; and suicide and attempted suicide.

Depression as a symptom/syndrome

Depression has been recognized as a syndrome in adults for a long time because of its characteristic constellation of symptoms, response to treatment and outcome. The depressed mood or dysphoria has qualities other than just simple sadness or unhappiness. Rather, it is the inability to derive pleasure or satisfaction from daily life (anhedonia) or to be able to respond emotionally to ordinary events. Other features of the syndrome are cognitive disturbances, behavioral changes and alterations in physiological functions. The cognitive disturbances are primarily cognitive distortions around oneself (self-blame, self-reproach, guilt and worthlessness), the world (helplessness and despair about one's life situation) and the future (hopelessness and despondency about the future). The behavioral changes range from marked agitation to withdrawal and stupor, while the physiological changes are poor appetite, weight loss and disturbed sleep pattern.

In adolescence, depression can present in the following ways: as a transient mood state; as a symptom in other psychiatric disorders, for instance anxiety states; as a symptom in physical illnesses, for instance infectious mononucleosis; and as part of a symptom complex in major depressive disorder. Epidemiological studies have shown an increasing prevalence of depressive symptomatology from childhood to adolescence. Rutter et al[78] found that adolescents had experienced feelings of misery and depression (40%), self-deprecation (20%) and suicidal thoughts (7%) at one time or another.

Depressive disorders

Both the ICD and DSM classifications now state that depression in children and adolescents should have the same features as that in adults. They recognize the following core features: abnormal depressed mood for at least 2 weeks; marked loss of interest or pleasure in almost all activities; decreased energy or increased fatigue. Additional features include: loss of confidence and self-esteem; unreasonable feelings of guilt or self-reproach; suicidal thoughts; poor concentration and indecisiveness; psychomotor agitation or retardation; sleep disturbance; and loss of appetite.

Etiology

There is no adequate theory for child or adolescent depression, but there is some support for the two main theories, genetic and environmental. Evidence for a genetic component comes from twin studies, adoption and family studies, though the size of the effect is not known. Environmental theories range from the traditional psychoanalytic perspective to the adverse impact of life events to the cognitive theory of Beck et al.[79] The latter regards the individual's negative view of himself, the world and the future as the cause of the depression, though clearly these cognitions could be seen as a consequence of the depressed mood rather than the cause.

Assessment

This involves detailed and sensitive interviewing of the adolescent, usually alone, as well as assessment of the adolescent and the family. Family assessment is useful for two reasons: the adolescent's behavior can be seen in the context of current family functioning; and other sources of stress for the adolescent or family may be identified. Physical symptoms are frequently found among depressed adolescents, though the findings are not specific as anxious adolescents often have physical symptoms as well. The differential diagnosis must involve the distinction between normal sadness or unhappiness, other psychiatric conditions with depressive symptomatology, for instance anorexia nervosa, or physical illnesses such as infectious mononucleosis or influenza.

Treatment

A comprehensive treatment package is most likely to be most effective. Components include drug treatment, individual and family therapy and the reduction or lessening of stressful circumstances. The relative emphasis and sequence of treatments are dependent upon assessment.

Drug treatment is most likely to be effective for adolescents who are most severely affected and have a disturbance of physiological functions such as appetite, sleep or weight. SRIs are the drugs of choice because of the low side-effect profile. Emslie et al[80] have shown the superiority of fluoxetine to placebo in a well conducted randomised control trial.

The purpose of individual therapy varies widely depending on the assessment and therapeutic style of the clinician. The common aims of an individual approach are: to establish a trusting relationship with the adolescent; to enable the adolescent to feel understood and accepted; and to allow the adolescent to disclose his concerns and anxieties including suicidal thoughts. Beyond these core aims, the therapeutic approach is varied, ranging from the psychodynamically insight-orientated psychotherapy to the cognitive–behavioral.

Work with the family is often undertaken more to improve communication between members of the family rather than to specifically treat family dysfunction. Family sessions are extremely useful at the start of treatment as a way to discuss events of emotional significance that may have happened recently but have not been talked through, for instance a family illness or a bereavement. These sessions also provide the opportunity to discuss ways to reduce any overt source of stress or anxiety for the adolescent. Common sources of stress include lack of friends, bullying or teasing at school and the adolescent's sense, usually distorted, of academic failure at school.

Bipolar disorder or manic-depressive psychosis

ICD and DSM use similar criteria for the diagnosis of bipolar disorder whether in adolescents or adults. The following points summarize the main diagnostic criteria of ICD and DSM:

- A disorder characterized by repeated episodes, that is two or more, in which the subject's mood and activity are significantly disturbed. This disturbance consists on some occasions of an elevation of mood with increased energy and activity (mania or hypomania), and on others of a lowering of mood with decreased energy and activity (depression).
- Recovery is characteristically complete between episodes.
- Manic episodes usually begin abruptly, lasting from 2 weeks to 4 or 5 months, whilst depressive episodes often last longer.

Clinical features

A hypomanic or depressive episode is equally common as the first manifestation of a bipolar illness with subsequent episodes more likely to be hypomanic than depressive. A depressive episode shows similar features to other depressive illnesses except that it tends to be more severe with a pronounced disturbance in physiological functioning and frequent suicidal thoughts.

The main feature of the hypomanic episode is an elevated, expansive or irritable mood with the other aspects understandable in terms of the elevated mood. The common features are: increased physical activity or physical restlessness; increased talkativeness; difficulty in concentration and distractibility; less need for sleep; increased sexual energy; mild spending sprees or other types of reckless behavior; and increased sociability or overfamiliarity. A manic episode causes severe disruption to the individual's life. The increased talkativeness becomes a 'pressure of speech' with flight of ideas (rapid switching of ideas based on a literal rather than a logical association, for instance rhyming or punning). The social disinhibition and recklessness can have a devastating effect on the individual's life. Cases with early onset have a worse prognosis with more frequent episodes, rapid cycling and a greater risk of suicide.

Though uncommon, several organic conditions can mimic a hypomanic episode. These include infections (encephalitis), endocrine (hyperthyroidism), neurological (repeated seizures, head trauma), brain tumor (meningioma, glioma), medication (steroids) and substance misuse [alcohol and amfetamine/lysergic acid diethylamide (LSD) misuse].

Management

A depressive episode should be managed in a similar manner to other depressive episodes, that is SRIs, individual and family support. Electroconvulsive therapy (ECT) may need to be considered for a severely depressed and/or suicidal patient.

The hypomanic episode is often harder to manage, as it usually requires inpatient admission, measures to ensure the safety and protection of the patient and also drug treatment. The most useful drug for an acute episode is haloperidol (dosage 0.05 mg/kg/day in three divided doses). It is usually necessary to supplement this medication with anti-Parkinsonian drugs such as trihexyphenidyl (benzhexol) or orphenadrine. An acute dystonic reaction such as an oculogyric crisis or acute torticollis can occur when treatment is commenced. Consequently, it is essential to observe closely the initiation of the medication.

Lithium carbonate is also effective in the acute episode, though its effect has a slower onset. Lithium is more useful as a prophylactic medication for individuals who have had several episodes. Its introduction should be carefully supervised and monitored. There have however been no controlled trials of the effectiveness of lithium in the prevention of further episodes in children or adolescents. Lithium has however been shown to be less effective among individuals with a rapid cycling disorder, features common among adolescents with bipolar disorder. Other drugs such as carbamazepine and sodium valproate have been used in the treatment of previously drug resistant manic episodes in adults, but there is insufficient evidence to evaluate their efficacy for adolescents with bipolar disorder.

Prognosis

Most individuals usually recover from an acute episode. For individuals with repeated episodes, poor prognostic features include the absence of a precipitating factor, a family history of recurrent illness and the continuation of some symptoms between acute episodes.

SUICIDE

This is extremely rare below the age of 12 years with an increase during adolescence to approximately 30 cases per million per year.[81] It is more common in males with no trend in social class. Males tend to use violent methods such as hanging or jumping from high buildings or bridges, whilst females have a preference for self-poisoning. Shaffer & Piancentini[81] identified four types of personality characteristics among adolescents who commit suicide: irritable and oversensitive to criticism; impulsive and volatile; withdrawn and uncommunicative; and perfectionist and self-critical. They also found that some evidence for an increased psychiatric disturbance in the family and that a 'disciplinary crisis' was the most common reason precipitating the suicide.

Attempted suicide

This is common with a rate of 4 per thousand per year among 15–19-year-olds. Females are three times more likely than males to make an attempt with an excess among lower socioeconomic groups. Not surprisingly, the families show evidence of marital disharmony, maternal psychiatric ill health, particularly depression, and paternal personality disorder. About 50% of adolescents show some evidence of psychiatric disorder, usually depression. In older adolescents, there is often a history of alcohol or drug misuse and running away from home. Social isolation and poor peer relationships are also common.

The most common method is an overdose of non-opiate analgesics such as aspirin or paracetamol, probably related to their easy availability. The severity of the overdose varies markedly from a few tablets taken impulsively to swallowing the contents of a bottle of analgesics. The attempt often follows a row with a boyfriend or a serious dispute with the parents over discipline. The adolescent may have threatened to take an overdose on previous occasions, and about 50% have consulted their general practitioner in the month prior to the overdose.

A crucial part of management is the assessment of future suicide risk. This depends on three factors, the circumstances of the attempt, the patient's current mental state and their attitude to the future. Detailed questioning about events prior to the attempt are necessary as well as a 'blow by blow' account of the attempt. The latter includes information about the degree of planning, whether anybody else was present and any action taken after the attempt. The identification of any difficulties at home or at school is also important.

The presence of significant depressive symptoms and pessimism about the future are predictors of continued suicide risk. It is important to enquire whether the overdose has altered the adolescent's or family's attitude to their current difficulties and their resolve to improve the situation. An assessment of the coping strategies and the capacity for change within the family is important in order to make a more realistic judgment about the future. Finally, there should be some agreement about future plans and any further contact between the adolescent, the family and the relevant professional agencies.

Treatment depends on the assessment and clinical judgment. The majority of adolescents do not require specialist psychiatric follow-up, though clearly they must know how to access psychiatric services in order to arrange further help when necessary. The indications for more specialized help include: the seriousness of the attempt; the presence of definite depressive disorder or persistent suicidal ideas; poor family circumstances and social support; and the limited capacity of the family for change. A small number may require inpatient psychiatric care, particularly the older adolescent. Follow-up psychiatric contact often involves individual counseling for the adolescent as well as family sessions to improve communication and the capacity to resolve disagreements.

There have been few systematic follow-up studies, though clinical impression suggests that those with definite psychiatric disorder or adverse social or family circumstances are more likely to be 'repeaters'.

Anorexia nervosa and related disorders[82]

Anorexia nervosa is a disorder of older female adolescents with a prevalence rate of 1% among 15–19-year-olds. It does however occur among prepubertal children. The core features are:

- self-induced starvation and weight loss;
- a strong desire to be thinner with a marked fear of weight gain;
- a distorted body image (for instance feeling fat when emaciated);
- a BMI (body mass index) < 17.5.

Clinical features

The presentation is varied, sometimes mimicking physical illness or the consequences of weight loss and starvation. The history is of prolonged self-imposed starvation. Dieting often begins following a chance remark about size or shape, or alternatively as a group behavior with other adolescent girls. Food portions at mealtimes are reduced, and some meals such as breakfast or lunch are skipped entirely with the total elimination of high calorific foods such as sweets, puddings or cakes. The individual derives satisfaction from the weight loss, which in turn is a further incentive for weight loss. Parents and other adults are often complimentary and pleased at this initial weight loss. More extreme and rigid dieting is then self-imposed to meet the target for further weight reduction. Appetite and hunger pains are prominent, but the prospect of further weight loss is a powerful motivator. Only when the illness is well established does the anorexia and nausea over food become apparent. Interest and participation in exercise and athletic activities often parallel the dieting in the belief that these activities will enhance weight loss. Later on, excessive laxative use begins in order to reduce weight further.

Despite an increasingly thin physique, the adolescent refuses to accept her emaciated status, still believing and perceiving herself as fat or overweight. The distorted body image is often the first indication to the parents that the adolescent has a serious illness. Increasing arguments over food and its consumption combined with an implacable refusal to eat convince the parents that urgent medical help is required. Often, the adolescent is initially referred to a pediatrician or an endocrinologist in order to exclude a physical basis to the problem rather than accepting a psychological basis for the weight loss.

Physical examination usually shows an individual who is bright and alert despite the evident emaciation. Prominent cheekbones, sunken eyes, bones protruding through the skin, dry skin and hair with blue cold hands and feet are common features. Severe emaciation is accompanied by the appearance of fine downy hair or lanugo hair on the face, limbs and trunk with a slow pulse rate, low blood pressure and hypothermia. Most biochemical investigations are normal, but low gonadotrophin levels with high growth hormone and cortisol levels are sometimes found. Although anorexia is the most likely diagnosis, other psychiatric conditions such as depression, obsessive–compulsive disorder or schizophrenia may need to be excluded.

Etiology

Almost as many theories have been proposed as the number of people who have researched the condition with individual, family or societal factors prominent in most explanations. Review of the premorbid personality characteristics of anorexics shows them to be conformist, conscientious, compliant and high achieving. Issues over autonomy and independence are core issues for anorexics with control over food intake the only available means to preserve self-identity and independence. Similar conflicts over autonomy and independence have been observed among families with an anorectic member, but whether this is cause or effect is unclear. Again, over the past 40 years, society's view about female attractiveness has veered towards the thin end of the spectrum, so that the 'pursuit of thinness' is a major issue for many women.

Management

The severity of the condition varies widely, so that treatment includes outpatient and inpatient management with an emphasis on a 'multimodal' approach. The latter implies that a variety of treatment strategies such as individual, family or cognitive therapies are used, often concurrently or sequentially, dependent on assessment. Recognition and acknowledgement of the problem are the first crucial steps in management. The nature and seriousness of the condition highlighted by the avoidance of food and the irrational ideas about eating must be explored thoroughly in order to establish a therapeutic alliance with the adolescent and the family. Only when the latter has occurred is it possible to commence a specific treatment program.

The next stage is the alteration of eating habits in order to restore weight and to correct nutritional deficiencies. Advice and collaboration with the dietician are important from the outset, particularly for any nutritional deficiencies. A target weight, usually around the average for the age and height, should be agreed upon along with the appropriate daily calorific intake to ensure its attainment. Only minimal concessions to food fads or preferences should be allowed with a standard protocol for regular weight checks.

If the patient is in hospital, the nursing care and support are the most important aspects of management. The nursing staff have to win the cooperation of the adolescent for the treatment plan. They must also be vigilant about food hoarding and surreptitious vomiting. Treatment programs usually involve a graded series of privileges dependent upon satisfactory weight gain. Once the target weight is attained, the diet should be modified, so that age appropriate weight gain continues. Inpatient programs often involve nursing staff supervising family meals at home during weekend leave.

Working with the family has two aims: to provide educational advice about the disorder; and to improve communication patterns within the family. Individual and group work is also useful, but drug treatment is not indicated unless there is a specific treatable disorder such as comorbid depression. Russell et al[83] in a randomized intervention study into the effectiveness of family versus individual therapy found that family therapy was better than individual therapy in the prevention of relapse among anorexics under 18 years of age who had had the illness for less than 3 years. An important limitation of this study was that only 65% of the 80 patients completed the intervention program.

In many ways, the easiest part of the treatment program, particularly with inpatients, is the restoration of weight loss. A more challenging aspect is the restructuring of the adolescent's and family's attitude to food and their pattern of interaction. Regular supervision, support and contact are essential to maintain progress and keep up morale. Very often a compromise has to be made between an ideal resolution of the problem and a realistic appraisal of the adolescent's and family's capacity to change.

Outcome

Results from follow-up studies vary widely according to inclusion criteria, outcome measures and length of follow-up. Despite these problems, outcome appears to fall into three categories, one-third good, one-third intermediate and one-third poor. There is a 10% mortality in the long term with malnutrition and suicide accounting for most deaths. Poor prognostic factors are an early age of onset, coexistent psychiatric disorder and poor family functioning.

BULIMIA NERVOSA

This has three key features – recurrent binges and purges, a lack of control and a morbid preoccupation with weight and shape. It is rare in the prepubertal period, but becomes increasingly common in older adolescents and young adults when it is often associated with depression. Most patients are of normal weight. The most serious medical concern is potassium depletion from frequent vomiting. The patient's lifestyle is often chaotic, so that the first aim of treatment is to establish some structure and boundaries for the patient. Dependent on assessment, a combination of individual, cognitive–behavioral and family work is appropriate in most cases.

Two new types of eating disorder have recently been described, *food avoidance emotional disorder* and *pervasive refusal syndrome*. The former is a disorder of emotions in which food avoidance is a prominent symptom along with other affective symptoms such as depression, anxiety or phobias. There is often a previous history of food fads or food restrictions, but the symptoms do not meet the criteria for anorexia nervosa. The validity and independence of this syndrome has however not yet been established.

Pervasive refusal syndrome is a severe life-threatening syndrome characterized by pervasive refusal to eat, drink, talk, walk or engage in any self-care skills. The patients are markedly underweight with an adamant refusal to eat or drink, which ultimately becomes life threatening. Although they fulfil some criteria for anorexia nervosa, the pervasiveness of the symptomatology makes this diagnosis inappropriate. They require prolonged and extensive inpatient nursing care in order to maintain vital body functions. Most patients have been girls with some suggestion that previous traumatic sexual abuse, often involving violence, may have been responsible for the precipitation of the disorder. Most make a satisfactory physical recovery, but the long term psychiatric adjustment is not yet known.

SPECIAL TOPICS

CHRONIC FATIGUE SYNDROME[84]

This has attracted widespread media coverage because of the controversy surrounding etiology and treatment. It is usually defined as a severe disabling fatigue affecting physical and mental functioning accompanied by myalgia, mood and/or sleep disturbance. Accurate prevalence figures are difficult to obtain, but are probably about 1 in 2000. Clinic samples tend to be adolescents aged between 11 and 15 years with more girls and from a higher socioeconomic grouping.

Two-thirds of patients have had a previous viral infection, but not usually of the Epstein–Barr type. This leads to fatigue which results in a reduction in physical activity leading to more fatigue on undertaking any physical activity. The situation is reinforced by parental and personal beliefs about causation, so that a state of inactivity and fatigue become established.

Management involves a thorough assessment to exclude comorbid psychiatric disorder such as depression, but keeping investigations to an agreed minimum. The establishment of mutual trust and a collaborative approach with the adolescent and the parents are essential to a good outcome. Individual cognitive and family work combined with a structured incremental rehabilitation strategy (a graded exercise program) are the best way to make progress and limit further incapacity. A coordinated plan for school and social reintegration is also necessary.

Outcome is varied depending on the initial severity, but three-quarters have made a reasonable recovery after 2 years.

SUBSTANCE MISUSE

This ranges from the readily available and legal substances such as tobacco or alcohol to the more uncommon and illegal substances such as heroin or cocaine. Though the latter give rise to more public concern, there is little doubt that cigarette smoking and excessive alcohol consumption have a far more deleterious effect on the health of the population as a whole. A recent survey of over 7000 15- and 16-year-olds in the UK[85] found that almost everyone had drunk alcohol, 30% had smoked cigarettes in the previous 30 days and 43% had at some time used illicit drugs. High levels of smoking were associated with a poorer school performance, and smoking was more common among girls. Adolescents are however only rarely referred to psychiatric services because of their smoking or alcohol habits.

Solvent abuse (glue sniffing)

Ashton[86] reviewing the available literature, estimated that 5–10% of adolescents have at some time inhaled solvents with 0.5–1% regular users. Since 1971, the death rate from solvent overdose has risen from two per annum to over a 100 per annum recently. Solvent abusers have the following characteristics: male gender; peak adolescent usage between 13 and 15 years; and more common among lower socioeconomic groupings, minority ethnic groups and disrupted families.

Inhaled substances include many everyday items such as adhesives, aerosols, dry cleaning fluids and cigarette lighter fuel. The substances are inhaled through paper bags, saturated rags or direct inhalation. It is often done as a group activity in the socio-economically disadvantaged areas of large cities, with regular solitary sniffing a cause for more serious concern. The immediate effect is euphoria followed by confusion, perceptual distortion, hallucinations and delusions. The regular user is often able to titrate the 'sniffs', so that a pleasantly euphoric state is maintained for several hours. The characteristic appearance of red spots around the mouth is highly suggestive of solvent abuse.

Sudden death during inhalation can occur from anoxia, respiratory depression, trauma or cardiac arrhythmia. The latter accounts for over half the deaths, whilst anoxia, usually from inhalation of vomit, is responsible for over 10% of deaths. Accidents or suicide attempts during the intoxication are another cause of death, particularly with toluene adhesives. Long term effects include neurological damage (peripheral neuropathy, encephalopathy, dementia and fits) as well as renal and liver damage.

Most solvent abusers do not come into contact with psychiatric services, unless they are referred following hospital admission with acute intoxication. School-based educational programs and community-resource initiatives are more likely to be beneficial in the long term. The encouragement of retailers and shop owners to enforce the restrictions on the sale of solvents is also useful. A number of solvent abusers are referred for psychiatric assessment, usually when the abuse is seen as part of more widespread individual or family psychopathology. In the long term, most adolescents do not persist with the habit, but a minority progresses onto more addictive drugs such as heroin or cocaine.

Other substances

These include 'soft' drugs such as cannabis (marijuana) or 'hard' drugs such as amfetamines, cocaine, heroin, LSD and designer drugs such as 'Ecstasy'. The effects are euphoric and relaxing in the short term, but apathy and inertia occur with chronic use. Most individuals do not progress from cannabis to other more seriously addictive drugs, and its consumption is not indicative of underlying psychological disturbance.

Hard drug consumption is a far more serious problem with deleterious effects on physical and psychological well-being and also from the risk of physical or psychological dependence. In addition to euphoric and pleasurable effects, most of these drugs can produce acutely distressing symptoms such as panic, fright or hallucinations. This can result in suicidal behavior or an increased risk of accidents. Long term use, for example with amfetamine or cocaine, can precipitate a florid psychotic episode with hallucinations, usually visual, and paranoid delusions. Psychological withdrawal symptoms such as an unbearable craving for a 'fix' and physical withdrawal symptoms such as nausea, vomiting and diarrhea make stopping the drug extremely difficult. Physical neglect and malnutrition are also common and exacerbate the problems. The necessity for a regular supply of the drug means that the individual resorts frequently to stealing or crime to support the addiction. The practice of needle-sharing is a major health hazard with HIV infection a strong possibility. Referral of the adolescent to a specialist treatment center and support for the parents are essential to prevent the serious social and psychological problems inevitable with long term drug misuse.

SEXUAL PROBLEMS

Two topics are discussed: sexual abuse and sexual offenders in adolescence; and gender identity disorders.

Sexual abuse and sexual offenders in adolescence[34]

Sexual abuse can present in two ways, direct disclosure of abuse or indirect manifestations of abuse. The same principles of practice and management apply to adolescents as to children (see child section of the chapter), but some special features are important. Open disclosure by the adolescent is often accompanied by the plea for complete confidentiality and no further action. Clearly this guarantee cannot be given, and the adolescent must be counseled about the necessity for an open investigation and the need for a child protection conference.

Indirect manifestations of abuse are twofold, sexually related behavior and psychiatric symptomatology. Sexually related manifestations include pregnancy, venereal disease and promiscuity. The latter often arises because the adolescent relates too readily to adults in a sexual manner as a result of the earlier experience of sexual abuse by an adult. Paradoxically, the promiscuous behavior may also lead some adults to disbelieve the adolescent's claims of abuse or that the adolescent was responsible for the initiation of the sexual contact. Psychiatric presentations of abuse are numerous with distress a prominent feature. Common presentations include depression, deteriorating school performance or attendance, suicidal behavior and running away from home.

Help for the sexually abused adolescent has two aims, the protection of the adolescent from further abuse and the provision of therapy to lessen the psychological trauma of the abuse. The first aim is usually achieved by ensuring that the perpetrator is no longer living at home and/or does not have contact with the adolescent. A wide range of therapies is used including individual counseling and support, family therapy or group therapy. Group therapy has become extremely popular recently. This approach has several advantages; the adolescent realizes that other adolescents have had a similar experience; the adolescent has the opportunity to discuss and share their feelings with other adolescents who are in a similar predicament; and the adolescent may feel less stigmatized. The group approach is probably less successful when the predominant feeling of the adolescent is betrayal. In this instance, it is more useful to offer individual psychotherapy to enable the adolescent establish trust with the therapist, so that disclosure and discussion can occur in a confidential setting.

A more recent development has been the provision of treatment strategies for adolescents who have committed sexual offences. The latter include exhibitionism or indecent exposure as well as sexual abuse of other, usually younger, children. The treatment program(s) involves an assessment of the offender's sexual knowledge and attitudes as well as their social skills and relationships. Treatment programs use a variety of approaches, often in combination, including social skills training, sex education and cognitive–behavioral approaches.

GENDER IDENTITY DISORDERS[87]

Society's attitudes towards sexuality have been changing in recent years, so that a more open discussion about sexual values and behavior is possible with greater tolerance and less stigma associated with homosexuality whether in males or females. Homosexual behavior in some form or another is quite common during the preadolescent and adolescent years occurring in approximately 20% of boys and 10% of girls. It appears to be a transitory pattern of behavior as adult estimates of male and female homosexuality are 3 and 1.5% respectively. Whilst homosexuality per se is most unlikely to be a reason for psychiatric referral, occasionally anxiety and depression associated with doubts about the homosexual role are sufficiently severe to warrant referral.

Clinicians are more likely to be involved with children or adolescents who have a gender identity disorder. A core distinction is made between individuals who display anomalous gender role behavior and those with gender identity disorder. Anomalous gender role behavior is the individual's preference for interests, activities and clothes normally associated with the opposite gender. For example, effeminate boys prefer girls' style of clothing and to play with dolls, whilst 'tomboy' girls like aggressive contact games and boys' style of clothing.

By contrast, the essential feature of the gender identity disorder is the persistent wish to be of the opposite gender. This is confirmed by the frequent expression of this wish and by extensive anomalous gender role behavior including cross-dressing. During adolescence, referral is often sought for problems associated with cross-dressing, homosexual behavior and social ostracism from peers. Transsexualism or the wish for permanent change of gender assignment can also become an issue.

The search for etiological factors in gender identity disorder has not been fruitful with no convincing evidence for chromosomal, physiological or endocrine abnormalities. Most clinicians believe that several psychosocial factors acting in combination are responsible. The initial parental tolerance of the anomalous sexual behavior followed by subsequent acceptance and reinforcement is a common finding among referred patients together with an overdependent mother–child relationship.

Treatment strategies for gender identity disorder include individual and family therapy, parental counseling and behavior therapy. The most important aspect of treatment is to define and agree goals with the parents and the child. Clinic studies[88] indicate that the earlier treatment is commenced the better the prognosis. Behavioral programs with attainable short-term goals are much more likely to be successful than more ambitious plans. Minimizing anomalous gender behavior such as cross-dressing and the promotion of gender appropriate behavior are the basis of the intervention strategies. Treatment of coexisting individual and family psychopathology is also beneficial. Finally, the long term follow-up of 66 effeminate boys[88] found that three-quarters were bisexual or homosexual as adults.

PSYCHIATRIC ASPECTS OF MENTAL RETARDATION IN CHILDHOOD

INTRODUCTION

Child psychiatrists are likely to become involved with children who have mental retardation in several different ways. Sometimes they are responsible for the provision of the specialist medical care for these children, but more commonly they are asked for advice from other professionals about the emotional and behavioral problems that are quite frequent in this group of children.

TERMINOLOGY

Many terms such as mental subnormality and/or mental handicap have been used in the past. ICD and DSM use IQ or mental age as the basis for classification. IQ is defined as mental age/chronological age × 100. The mean or average IQ is therefore 100 with a standard deviation of 15. The normal or Gaussian distribution of intelligence means that approximately 2.5% of individuals are 2 standard deviations below the mean, corresponding to an IQ of 70. This is usually taken as the dividing point between the normal range of intelligence and mental retardation. ICD and DSM have four categories of mental retardation: mild (IQ 50–69 approximately); moderate (IQ 35–49 approximately); severe (IQ 20–34 approximately); profound (IQ less than 20). The other important defining criterion is that there should be evidence of social impairment and limitation in the individual's daily activities and self-care skills.

PSYCHIATRIC DISORDERS IN CHILDREN WITH MENTAL RETARDATION

Prevalence

The IOW study[14] found that approximately one-third of children with mental retardation showed signs of disturbance with the rate rising to 50% among moderate to severely retarded children. The children exhibited the same range of disturbance as children of normal ability but in addition three disorders were much more frequent: childhood autism, pervasive hyperkinetic disorder and severe stereotyped movement disorder. Self-injurious behavior and pica were also more frequent.

Etiology

It is important to distinguish between the factors responsible for disorders occurring in mildly mentally retarded children and those with moderate to severe retardation. Children with mild mental retardation probably have the same risk factors as children of average ability, but to a greater extent, that is adverse temperamental characteristics, specific learning disorders and family psychopathology. The latter is particularly important, as parents of children with mild mental retardation are also likely to be within the lower range of intellectual ability. Consequently, their parenting capacity may be limited with inconsistent discipline and control prominent features. In addition, this may be combined with marital disharmony and socioeconomic disadvantage, so that the vulnerability to psychiatric disturbance is considerably increased among this group of children.

By contrast, brain damage is an important causative factor among children with severe mental retardation. Several studies[12,14] have found that half the children with moderate to severe mental retardation have demonstrable brain damage. This increases the risk of psychiatric disturbance in several ways: loss of specific functions or skills; active disruption or dysfunction of normal brain activity; and the increased risk of epilepsy. Children with moderate to severe mental retardation are also more likely to have specific learning difficulties that further increase vulnerability. In addition, adverse temperamental characteristics such as impulsivity, distractibility or overactivity are more common among this group of children. The psychosocial consequences of handicap for the child and the family also make a factor in some cases, though its importance is difficult to quantify.

PSYCHIATRIC SYNDROMES SPECIFICALLY ASSOCIATED WITH MODERATE TO SEVERE RETARDATION

Childhood autism

Of children with childhood autism, 80% have an IQ less than 70. Many clinicians distinguish between individuals who have classical childhood autism from those with severe mental retardation and some autistic features. The latter include stereotypies, mannerisms and deficits in comprehension and expressive language. These symptoms, which are quite common among many retarded children, tend to occur in isolation, so that the individual does not fulfil the diagnostic criteria for childhood autism. Clinical practice and research findings do not however provide clear cut criteria to decide the dividing line between childhood autism and severe mental retardation with autistic features. Consequently, clinicians tend to have their own personal preferences in terminology and classification.

Autistic behaviors are also features of some syndromes associated with mental retardation such as tuberous sclerosis, rubella, fragile X syndrome and infantile spasms. In some cases, for instance rubella, the autistic behavior seems to be a response to the coexisting sensory deficit rather than the separate occurrence of childhood autism. Finally, individuals with the extremely uncommon neurodegenerative diseases such as subacute sclerosing panencephalitis or with disintegrative disorder often show autistic-like stereotypic behavior.

Hyperkinetic syndrome/attention deficit disorder

Like autistic behavior, overactive or hyperkinetic behavior is common among children with severe mental retardation. In most cases, the overactivity occurs in some situations but not in others, with the overactivity reflecting an immaturity in behavior and language skills. A much smaller but nevertheless significant number of children with severe mental retardation do show pervasive hyperactivity with other features of that syndrome including distractibility, impulsivity and aggressive behavior.

Stereotypic and self-injurious behavior

Stereotypic movements such as body rocking or hand-flapping have been reported as frequently as 40% in mild to severely mentally retarded children. Self-injurious behavior such as headbanging, biting of limbs or eye gouging is much less common but more potentially harmful and also difficult to eradicate. It often arises in an individual of very limited ability whose surroundings and immediate environment provide little or minimal stimulation. The Lesch–Nyhan syndrome is particularly associated with the development of self-mutilating behavior.

Murphy[89] reviewed the treatment methods for these intractable and destructive behaviors. Protective devices such as helmets, treatment with major tranquilizers such as haloperidol and behavioral approaches have all been used with some success. A real disadvantage with drug treatment is that once started it is difficult to stop, so that the individual can remain on a drug for several years, often with an increasing dose over time. A behavioral approach is more likely to produce long lasting benefits, but it is more time consuming to carry out and more demanding of staff cooperation.

Pica

The ingestion of inedible substances is a transitory phenomenon among normal toddlers and is even more common among children with severe mental retardation. The main adverse consequence of this behavior is lead intoxication from the licking of objects. Fecal smearing and ingestion can occur among some severely retarded children, particularly those with an additional sensory handicap such as blindness.

MENTAL RETARDATION SYNDROMES ASSOCIATED WITH SPECIFIC BEHAVIORAL CHARACTERISTICS

Traditionally, children with certain mental retardation syndromes have been said to show a characteristic behavioral or personality profile, though contemporary opinion is more sceptical about such association.

Down syndrome

Children with this syndrome are often described as sociable, musical, contented and easy going, features they share with their siblings. Overall, these children have a slightly increased rate of disturbance with a minority showing aggressive and oppositional behavior, usually associated with Down syndrome due to a translocation trisomy.

Phenylketonuria

Untreated, these children develop severe mental retardation with autistic and hyperkinetic behavior prominent. Successful dietary treatment usually results in normal growth and development, but treated children have a greater risk of psychiatric disturbance with overactivity, distractibility and restlessness common.

Lesch–Nyhan syndrome

This sex-linked disorder of purine metabolism, occurring only in boys, is associated with an extrapyramidal movement disorder including chorea and athetosis, severe mental retardation and self-injurious behavior. The latter is extremely difficult to treat and eliminate.

Prader–Willi syndrome

The main behavioral feature is the explosive outbursts associated with dietary restriction frequently imposed to control the voracious appetite and accompanying obesity.

Hydrocephalus

Children with hydrocephalus were previously described as showing the 'cocktail party' syndrome. This is characterized by a verbosity to their speech and a superficiality or shallowness to the content of their conversation. The early detection and treatment of hydrocephalus has now produced a reduction in morbidity, so that these features are less commonly seen.

Management

Many professionals including pediatricians, teachers and psychologists are likely to be involved in the provision of care for children with mental handicap and their families. A multidisciplinary approach to assessment and treatment is vital. Different aspects of management are important at various stages during the child's life.

Breaking the news

This topic is discussed more fully in the child section of the chapter, so that only brief comments are made here. The ability to communicate bad news in a sensitive manner is a skill rarely taught to medical students or junior doctors. Many parents complain justifiably that the initial interview with the doctor was unsatisfactory and distressing. Tact, sympathy and time are essential to enable the parent(s) to begin to grasp and understand the implications of the situation. Honest discussion combined with an emphasis on the hopeful aspects are the important prerequisites for a satisfactory interview.

Promotion of normal development

Parents should be encouraged from the outset to develop the social, self-care and educational skills of their child to the maximum. A 'normalization' and 'optimalization' strategy is the basis to the approach. Specific treatment packages, for example the Portage scheme, are helpful in enabling the parents to set realistic targets for their child.

Treatment of medical and behavioral problems

Advice from neurologists, physiotherapists and occupational therapists is important in the management of the neurological deficits frequently present among this group of children. Behavioral problems are managed in a variety of ways including medication (for hyperactivity and aggressive outbursts), protective devices (for excessive headbanging) and operant or time-out procedures (for maladaptive behavior).

Educational needs

Parents need advice from an early stage about the most appropriate educational provision. A specialized preschool nursery is vital, and should be combined with a plan for later special educational placement. Some children may benefit from attendance at schools for children with communication or autistic-like disorders.

Genetic counseling

This is clearly essential for all parents, especially when a specific syndrome is identified.

Long term casework and support

Clinical experience and practice suggest that many families find this type of help invaluable in the long term. The identification of a key professional worker who coordinates the care plan for the child is very useful. A social worker or a professional from a voluntary organization with counseling skills is often the person best placed to fulfil this role.

Outcome

Treatment programs with their emphasis on maximizing potential, minimizing adverse effects and integrating the child into the community are the best approach. Despite cognitive impairment, behavior problems can be reduced by treatment programs, and families learn to adapt satisfactorily. The policy of the UK Government is to close institutions for individuals with mental retardation and to integrate them into the community in order to promote better long term adjustment.

REFERENCES (*Level 1 evidence)

1 Goodyer I. Life experiences. Development and childhood psychopathology. Chichester: Wiley; 1990.
2 Bee H. The developing child, 9th edn. New York: Harper; 1999.
3 Matthews S. Cognitive development. In: Bryant P, Colman A, eds. Developmental psychology. London: Longman; 1994.
4 Hawton K, Salkovskis P, Kirk J, et al. Cognitive behaviour therapy for psychiatric problems: a practical guide, 2nd edn. Oxford: Oxford University Press; 1995.
5 Zealley A, Johnstone E, Freeman C. Companion to psychiatric studies, 6th edn. Edinburgh: Churchill Livingstone; 1998.
6 Erikson E. Childhood and society. London: Penguin; 1965.
7 Bowlby J. Attachment and loss, vol 1: Attachment. London: Hogarth Press; 1969.
8 Ainsworth M. Attachment: retrospect and prospect. In: Parkes C M, Stevenson-Hinde J, eds. The place of attachment in human behaviour. New York: Basic Books; 1982.
9 Freud A. The ego and the mechanisms of defence. London: Hogarth Press; 1936.
10 World Health Organization. The ICD-10 classification of mental and behaviour disorders: clinical descriptions and diagnostic guidelines. Geneva: World Health Organization; 1992.
11 American Psychiatric Association. Diagnostic and statistical manual of mental disorders, 4th edn. Washington: American Psychiatric Association; 1994.
12 Rutter M, Tizard J, Whitmore K. Education, health and behaviour. London: Longmans; 1970.
13 Rutter M, Yule B, Quinton D, et al. Attainment and adjustment in two geographical areas. III. Some factors accounting for area differences. Br J Psychiatry 1975; 126:520–533.
14 Rutter M, Graham P, Yule W. A neuropsychiatric study of childhood. Clinics in Developmental Medicine, nos 35/36. London: SIMP/Heinemann; 1970.
15 Meltzer H, Gatward R. Mental health of children and adolescents in Great Britain. London: The Stationery Office; 2000.
16 Richman N, Stevenson J, Graham P. Pre-school to school: a behavioural study. London: Academic Press; 1982.
17 Bailey N. Bailey's scales II. San Antonio: Psychological Corporation; 1993.
18 Huntley M. Griffiths mental development scales from birth to two years. London: Association for Research on Infant and Child Development; 1996
19 Kaufman A, Kaufman N. Kaufman assessment battery for children (K-ABC). Circle Pines: AmGuidance Service; 1983.
20 Wechsler D. Manual for the Wechsler intelligence scale for children, 3rd UK edn (WISC-III UK). Kent: Psychological Corporation; 1992.
21 Thorndike R, Hagen E, Sattler J. Stanford–Binet intelligence scale, 4th edn. San Antonio: Psychological Corporation; 1986.
22 Elliott C. British ability scales, 2nd edn (BASI II). Windsor: National Foundation for Educational Research/Nelson; 1996.
23 Rust J. Wechsler individual achievement tests. San Antonio: Psychological Corporation; 1995.
24 Neale MD. Neale analysis of reading ability test, 2nd edn. Windsor: National Foundation for Educational Research/Nelson; 1989.
25 Reynell J. Reynell developmental language scales. 2nd revision. Windsor: National Foundation for Educational Research; 1985.
26 Achenbach T. Integrative guide for the 1991 CBCL/4–18, YSR and TRF profiles. Burlington: University of Vermont; 1991.
27 Goodman R. The strengths and difficulties questionnaire: a research note. J Child Psychol Psychiatry 1997; 38:581–586.
28 Thomas A, Chess S, Birch H. Temperament and behaviour disorders in childhood. New York: New York University Press; 1968.
29 Brown G, Harris T. Social origins of depression. London: Tavistock; 1978.
30 Richman N, Lansdown R. Problems of pre-school children. Chichester: Wiley; 1988.
31 Skuse D, Wolke D, Reilly S. Failure to thrive. Clinical and developmental aspects. In: Remschmidt H, Schmidt M, eds. Child and youth psychiatry, European perspectives. Vol. II Developmental psychopathology. Stuttgart: Hans Huber; 1992.
32 Morrell J. The infant sleep questionnaire: a new tool to assess infant sleep problems for clinical and research purposes. Child Psychol Psychiatry Rev 1999; 4:20–26.
33 Jan J, Espezel H, Appleton P. The treatment of sleep disorders. Dev Med Child Neurol 1994; 36:97–107.
34 Briere J, Berliner L, Buckley J, et al. The APSAC handbook on child maltreatment. Thousand Oaks: Sage Publications; 1996.
35 Stevenson J. Treatment of sequelae of child abuse. J Child Psychol Psychiatry 1999; 40:89–112.
36. Bentovim A, Elton A, Hildebrand J, et al. Sexual abuse within the family. London: Wright; 1988.
37 Eminson M, Postlethwaite R. Munchausen by proxy: a practical approach. Oxford: Butterworth-Heinemann; 1999.
38 Cohen D, Volkmar F. A handbook of autism and pervasive developmental disorders. Chichester: Wiley; 1997.
39 Gillberg C. Clinical child neuropsychiatry. Cambridge: Cambridge University Press; 1995.
40 Kanner L. Autistic disturbances of affective contact. The Nervous Child 1943; 2:217–250.
41 Chakrabarti S, Fombonne E. Pervasive developmental disorders in pre-school children. J Am Med Assoc 2001; 285:3094–3098.
42 Farrington CP, Miller E, Taylor B. MMR and autism: further evidence against a causal association. Vaccine 2001; 19:3632–3635.
43 Lord C, Rutter M. Autism and other pervasive developmental disorders. In: Rutter M, Taylor E, Hersov L, eds. Child and adolescent psychiatry: modern approaches, 3rd edn. Oxford: Blackwell; 1994.
44 Hagberg B. Rett's syndrome – clinical and biological aspects. London: MacKeith Press; 1993.
45 Rutter M, Schopler E, eds. Autism: a reappraisal of concepts and treatment. New York: Plenum Press; 1988.
46 Pennington B, Ozonoff S. Executive functions and developmental psychopathology. J Child Psychol Psychiatry1996; 37:51–88.
47 Baron-Cohen S. Mindblindness. London: MIT Press; 1995.
48. Hobson P. Autism and the development of mind. Hove: Lawrence Erlbaum; 1993.
49 Asperger H. 'Die Autistischen psychopathen' im kindesalter. Arch Psychiatr Nervenkrank 1944; 117:76–136.
50 Wolff S, Chick J. Schizoid personality in childhood: a controlled follow-up study. Psychol Med 1980; 10:85–100.
51 Wolff S. Schizoid personality in childhood and adult life III: The childhood picture. Br J Psychiatry 1991; 159:629–635.
52 Corbett J, Harris R, Taylor E, et al. Progressive disintegrative psychosis of childhood. J Child Psychol Psychiatry 1977; 18:211–219.
53 Berg I. Absence from school and mental health. Br J Psychiatry 1992; 161:154–166.
54 Shafran R. Obsessive–compulsive disorders in children and adolescents. Child Psychol Psychiatry Rev 2001; 6:50–58.
55 Garralda E. Somatisation in children. J Child Psychol Psychiatry 1996; 37:13–33.
56 Yule W. Posttraumatic stress disorder. In: Rutter M, Taylor E, Hersov L, eds. Child and adolescent psychiatry: modern approaches, 3rd edn. Oxford: Blackwell; 1994.
57 Webster-Stratton C, Herbert M. Troubled families – problem children. Chichester: Wiley; 1993.
58 Taylor E, Sergeant J, Doepfner M, et al. Clinical guidelines for hyperkinetic disorder. Eur Child Adolesc Psychiatry 1998; 7:184–200.
*59 MTA Co-operative Group. Fourteen-month randomised clinical trial of treatment strategies for attention deficit hyperactivity disorder. Arch Gen Psychiatry 1999; 56:1073–1086.
*60 NICE report. The clinical effectiveness and cost effectiveness of methylphenidate for hyperactivity. London: NICE; 2000.
*61 Egger J, Stolla A, McEwan L. Controlled trial of hyposensitisation in children with food-induced hyperkinetic syndrome. Lancet 1992; 339:1150–1153.
62 Bierderman J, Faraone S, Spencer T, et al. Patterns of comorbidity, cognition, and psychosocial functioning in adults with attention deficit hyperactivity disorder. Am J Psychiatry 1993; 150:1792–1798.
*63 Spencer T, Wilens T, Biederman J, et al. A double-blind crossover comparison of methylphenidate in adults with childhood-onset attention deficit hyperactivity disorder. Arch Gen Psychiatry 1995; 52:434–443.
64 Dummit E, Klein R, Tancer N, et al. Fluoxetine treatment of children with selective mutism. J Am Acad Child Adolesc Psychiatry 1996; 35:615–621.
65 Lask B. Novel and non-toxic treatment for night terrors. BMJ 1988; 297:592.
66 Kutcher S. Child and adolescent psychopharmacology. Philadelphia: Saunders; 1997.

67 Lanyardo M, Horne A. A handbook of child and adolescent psychotherapy. London: Routledge; 1999.

68 Freud A. The psychological treatment of children. London: Imago; 1946.

69 Reisman JM. Principles of psychotherapy with children, 2nd edn. New York: Wiley; 1973.

70 Herbert M. ABC of behavioural methods. Leicester: British Psychological Society; 1996.

71 Kendall P. Child and adolescent therapy: cognitive–behavioral procedures. New York: Guilford Press; 1999.

72 Gorrell Barnes G. Family therapy. In: Rutter M, Taylor E, Hersov L, eds. Child and adolescent psychiatry: modern approaches, 3rd edn. Oxford: Blackwell; 1994.

73 Lask B. Paediatric liaison work. In: Rutter M, Taylor E, Hersov L, eds. Child and adolescent psychiatry: modern approaches, 3rd edn. Oxford: Blackwell; 1994.

74 King R, Leonard H, March J, et al. Practice parameters for the assessment and treatment of children and adolescents with obsessive–compulsive disorder. J Am Acad Child Adolesc Psychiatry 1998; 39(suppl):27S–47S.

75 Hollis C. Adolescent schizophrenia. Adv Psychiatric Treat 2000; 6:83–92.

76 Goodyer I. The depressed child and adolescent: developmental and clinical perspectives. Cambridge: Cambridge University Press; 1995.

77 Park R, Goodyer I. Clinical guidelines for depressive disorders in childhood and adolescence. Eur Child Adolesc Psychiatry 2000; 9:147–161.

78 Rutter M, Graham P, Chadwick O, et al. Adolescent turmoil: fact or fiction? J Child Psychol Psychiatry 1976; 17:35–56.

79 Beck A, Rush A, Shaw B, et al. Cognitive therapy of depression. New York: Wiley; 1979.

***80** Emslie G, Rush J, Weinberg W, et al. A double blind, randomised, placebo-controlled trial of fluoxetine in child and adolescents with depression. Arch Gen Psychiatry 1997; 54:1031–1037.

81 Shaffer D, Piancentini J. Suicide and attempted suicide. In: Rutter M, Taylor E, Hersov L, eds. Child and adolescent psychiatry: modern approaches, 3rd edn. Oxford: Blackwell; 1994.

82 Lask B, Bryant-Waugh R. Anorexia nervosa and related eating disorders in childhood and adolescence, 2nd edn. Hove: Psychology Press; 1999.

***83** Russell G, Szmulker G, Dare C, et al. An evaluation of family therapy in anorexia nervosa and bulimia nervosa. Arch Gen Psychiatry 1987; 44:1047–1056.

84 Wright B, Partridge I, Williams C. Management of chronic fatigue syndrome in children. Adv Psychiatric Treat 2000; 6:145–152.

85 Miller P, Platt M. Drinking, smoking and illicit drug use among 15 and 16 year olds in the United Kingdom. BMJ 1996; 313:394–397.

86 Ashton C. Solvent abuse: little progress after twenty years. BMJ 1990; 300:135–136.

87 Di Ceglie D. Gender identity disorder in young people. Adv Psychiatric Treat 2000; 6:458–467.

88 Zucker K, Bradley S. Gender identity disorder and psychosexual problems in children and adolescents. New York: Plenum Press; 1995.

89 Murphy G. Update-self-injuring behaviour in the mentally handicapped. Assoc Child Psychol Psychiatry Newsletter 1985; 7:2–11.

34

Adolescent medicine

Russell Viner

WHAT IS ADOLESCENCE?

Strictly speaking, adolescence is the period between childhood and adulthood. But finding a useful definition of adolescence is difficult. Biologically it is the time of sexual maturation and the completion of growth. More than mere biology, adolescence is psychosocially the period between childhood dependency and being a functionally independent autonomous adult. Theorists have viewed adolescence in different ways; Freud saw adolescence as the period of recapitulation of the childhood Oedipal complex, while Erickson claimed that the struggle between Identity and Role Confusion typified the adolescent stage of development.[1]

Chronological definitions abound and are more pragmatic in allowing us to identify who is or is not an 'adolescent'. The World Health Organization for example defines adolescence as the second decade of life, from 10 to 20 years of age, but also defines a category of 'youth' as being 10–25 years.[2] However, chronological definitions take little account of the developmental changes of adolescence and their temporal variation, failing to apply to certain cultures or to those who are early or late developers. Because of this, some have suggested that adolescence is merely a social construct, a rite of passage that is culturally and socially invented.[3] These claims ignore the biological changes of puberty and the psychological developments driven by increasing central nervous system (CNS) maturation and myelination. The most useful definition of adolescence is that it is a period between the ages of 10 and 25 years of biopsychosocial maturation, leading to functional independence in adult life.

WHY IS A SPECIAL MEDICAL APPROACH NEEDED FOR ADOLESCENTS?

Adolescence, the period between childhood and adulthood, is increasingly recognized as a life period that poses specific challenges for treating disease and promoting health. In working with adolescents, the treatment of disease, the prevention of ill health and the promotion of healthy behaviors are played out against a background of rapid physical, psychological and social developmental changes – changes that produce specific disease patterns, unusual symptom presentations, and above all, unique communication and management challenges. At no other time of life are the physical and the psychosocial elements of illness and behavior so inextricably intertwined as in adolescence. This can make working with adolescents difficult. However given the right skills (which can be learned!) practicing medicine with young people can be extremely rewarding and fruitful. These skills are not only for those who work solely with young people, but are needed by all those in pediatric practice.

The reasons for a distinct approach to medicine with adolescents are outlined below.

1. ADOLESCENTS ARE A LARGE CLIENT GROUP

One argument for considering adolescents differently from children is sheer numbers; young people between 10 and 20 years of age make up between 12 and 15% of the population in most developed countries (13% in the UK), a client group as large as children under 10 in the UK (Fig. 34.1). Projections suggest that the adolescent population will grow by 8.5% between 1998 and 2011.[4] While adolescence is generally considered to be a healthy period, health resource use by young people is higher than in late childhood.[5] Most adolescents visit their general practitioner (GP) each year:[6] around 30% have a chronic condition that requires some health resource utilization;[7] mental health resource use is higher than in childhood;[8] and hospital bed use is higher during adolescence than in late childhood.[9]

2. ADOLESCENTS HAVE A UNIQUE EPIDEMIOLOGY OF DISEASE AND HEALTH RISK

The second argument for a special approach to adolescent health is that young people have a distinct epidemiology of disease and health risk. The diseases that are unique to adolescence are small in number (Table 34.1). But both disease and health behaviors in adolescents present a unique constellation of symptoms and problems not found in children or adults. Those practicing with adolescents must be familiar with both persisting or late-onset 'pediatric' diseases and with early-onset 'adult' diseases. In each, ongoing adolescent development produces characteristic symptom patterns and management problems that meld the biological with the psychosocial in unique ways. For example, type I diabetes has its peak age of incidence around 12–14 years, and the growth hormone excess of puberty and the psychosocial challenges of chronic illness self-management produces poorer metabolic control during adolescence than at any other age.[10] Furthermore, puberty itself accelerates the progression of diabetic complications such as nephropathy.[11] Cancer during adolescence is remarkable for its threat of mortality to a personality with a newly developing sense of identity and place in the world, but also in its combination of 'late' presentation of pediatric type cancers such as rhabdomyosarcoma, medulloblastoma and 'age-specific' cancers of adolescence, e.g. bone tumors and early onset 'adult-type' carcinomas.[12]

3. INCREASING SURVIVAL FROM AND INCIDENCE OF CHRONIC ILLNESS IN YOUNG PEOPLE

Increases in the prevalence of chronic illness amongst adolescents is changing the pattern of pediatric practice, and it is likely that young people will in the future make up a larger part of the pediatric workload. This has been driven by an increasing incidence of common chronic illnesses such as asthma and diabetes, but also by increasing survival from congenital diseases previously fatal in childhood. Cohort studies in the UK show a 70% increase in the prevalence of wheezing illness at age 16 years between 1974 and 1986 with further rises apparent in the 1990s.[13] Recently almost 20% of UK 12–14-year-olds used asthma medications in the past 12 months.[13] Diabetes in 10–14-year-olds has increased by almost 24% Europe-wide during the past 10 years,[14] and the incidence of type II diabetes has risen dramatically in adolescents, particularly in minority ethnic populations.[15]

Advances in the last 20 years in the treatment of metabolic conditions, cystic fibrosis and congenital heart disease have produced new cohorts of young people surviving into adolescence and early adulthood.[16–18] The prevalence of cystic fibrosis over 15 years of age in the UK more than doubled between 1977 and 1985,[19] and currently over 85% of children with chronic illness survive to adult life.[18]

4. HEALTH BEHAVIORS ARE LAID DOWN IN ADOLESCENCE AND CONTINUE INTO ADULT LIFE

One of the most compelling arguments for a focus on adolescent health is that adolescence is a time when new health behaviors are laid down, behaviors that track into adulthood and will influence health and morbidity life-long. Health behaviors in childhood are dominated by parental instruction and shared family values. During adolescence young people begin to explore alternative or 'adult' health behaviors, including smoking, drinking, drug use, violence and sexual intimacy. The continuities between adolescent initiation of health behaviors and adult behavior are well documented. Regular smoking rates rise from 1% at 11 years to 24% at 15 years,[20] and over 90% of adult smokers began in the teenage years.[21] Depression and its related mental health problems are rare in childhood, but rise through puberty to adult levels in late adolescence.[22,23]

Equally importantly, health behaviors concerning exercise and food are laid down in adolescence and track into adult life. Adolescent obesity predicts adult obesity,[24] which is strongly and independently predictive of cardiovascular risk,[25,26] and cardiovascular risk in young adulthood is highly related to the degree of adiposity as early as age 13 years.[24]

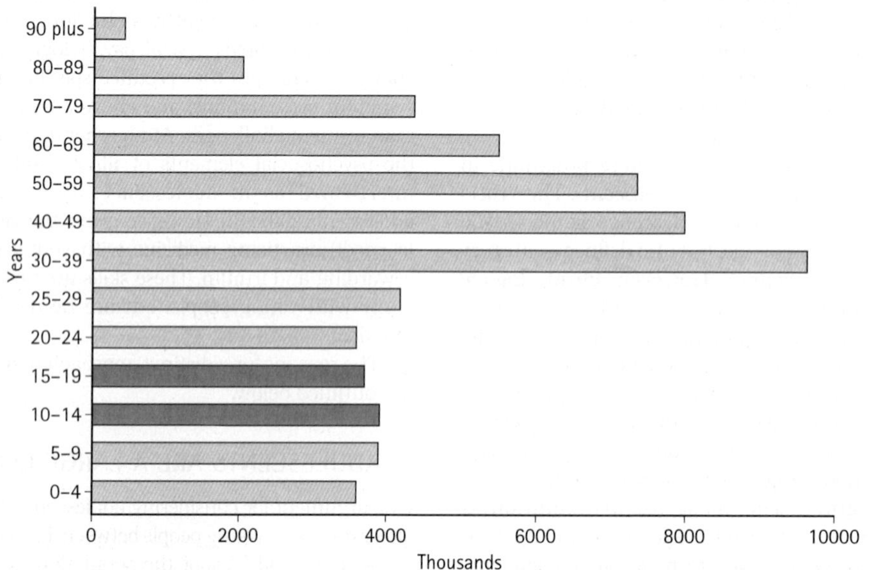

Fig. 34.1 UK population by age, mid 2000 (ONS)

Table 34.1 Disorders unique to adolescence or with onset predominantly in adolescence

Disorders
Disorders of puberty and pubertal growth
Adolescent idiopathic scoliosis
Juvenile idiopathic arthritis – subtypes
Adolescent acne
Eating disorders (anorexia nervosa, bulimia nervosa)
Mental disorders, e.g. conduct disorder, adolescent psychosis

5. ADOLESCENTS HAVE UNIQUE NEEDS IN THE MANAGEMENT OF HEALTH AND ILLNESS

Dynamic and continued development in every aspect of a young person's life during adolescence means that young people have distinct needs in the management of illness and health. In clinical interactions with younger children, management decisions are made 'adult to adult' by health professionals in consultation with parents, and day-to-day disease management is generally undertaken directly by parents. When working with adolescents, the wishes, desires, knowledge base, capabilities and rights of the young person involved must also be taken into account – as must the fact that these wishes, desires, knowledge, capabilities and rights are constantly evolving and changing! Different approaches are required to all aspects of the doctor–patient relationship. Specialized clinical communication skills are needed to take an accurate history, bearing in mind new life domains not applicable to children (sex and drugs) and adding communication and engagement of the young person to the standard pediatric communication with the family. Physical examination of adolescents requires consideration of privacy and personal integrity as well as requiring additional skills such as pubertal assessment, breast examination and possibly genital examination. The effective treatment of illness in adolescence requires adept management of the issues regarding adherence (compliance), consent and confidentiality, and relationships between the young people and their family.

6. INCREASING SOCIAL MORBIDITIES AND MORTALITY LEVELS

Perhaps the most cogent argument for specific attention to adolescent health lies in the public health arena. The causes of mortality and morbidity in adolescents are distinct from both children and adults as environmental or social causes of mortality (e.g. accidents and suicide) make up a larger proportion of total adolescent mortality than at any other age (Fig. 34.2). In most public health priority areas, including cardiovascular risk (obesity, diabetes, smoking), mental health (suicide) and sexual health [teenage pregnancy and sexually transmitted diseases (STDs)], the extent of problems in young people is stable or increasing rather than diminishing. Suicide rates amongst older male teenagers doubled over the last three decades of the twentieth century and remain high.[27] Obesity has doubled amongst teenagers in the past 10 years, leading to the emergence of type II diabetes as a significant clinical and public health problem.[28,29] While smoking rates have fallen amongst teenage boys, rates amongst teenage girls have risen over the past 20 years. Earlier sexual debut and increased rates of high-risk sexual activity have lead to high rates of teenage pregnancy and STDs in countries with poor sexual and relationship education such as the UK and USA. Given explicit evidence of the continuities between adolescent and adult health risk behaviors, adolescent morbidity trends argue strongly for urgent attention

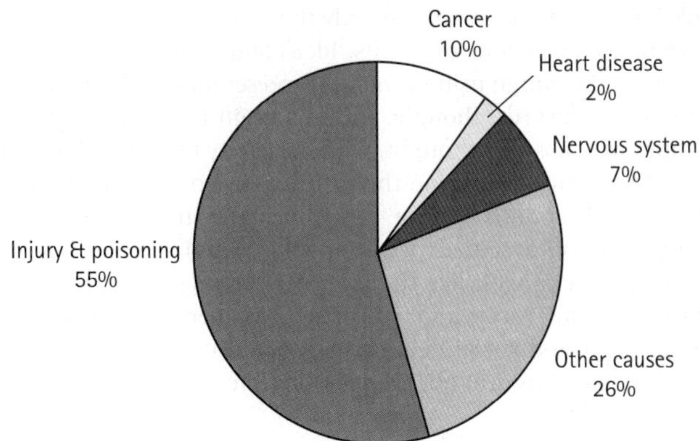

Fig. 34.2 Causes of mortality in young people (15–19 years) in the UK, 1997.

to adolescent health and the development of targeted adolescent-specific interventions.

ADOLESCENT DEVELOPMENT

All clinical interactions with adolescents must be seen against the dynamic background of continued development. For example, chronic illness management issues can be quite different between a 13-year-old boy in very early puberty who has poorly developed abstract thinking and a 16-year-old girl who is sexually mature, at final height and has well-developed adult cognitive skills. The developmental tasks or events of adolescence are outlined in Table 34.2. While we group development for convenience into early, mid and late adolescence, it is important to remember that the timing and tempo of biological, psychological and social development each proceeds independently in each individual, although each strand can influence the others. Those who are pubertally early developers may be late in developing cognitive skills or vice versa, and it is imperative to assess biological and psychosocial maturity separately. Gender issues are important here, as the timing of biological and psychosocial maturation is subtly different in boys and girls.

BIOLOGICAL CHANGES

The biological changes of adolescence are puberty, the pubertal growth spurt, and accompanying maturational changes in other organ systems. The processes and timing of puberty and pubertal assessment skills are outlined in Chapter 13. The defining event of puberty in girls is menarche. The mean age at menarche showed a dramatic decline in most developed countries through the first half of the twentieth century, stabilizing in the 1960s at 12.8 years in the USA and 13.2 years in the UK.[30] Despite recent controversy, the evidence is clear that there has been no change in the age of menarche in the USA or the UK over the past 40 years.[31]

As well as completion of linear growth and sexual maturation, other biological systems develop their final adult form during adolescence. These include maturation of enzyme systems such as cytochrome P450 systems, accretion of peak bone mass, and the development of sexually dimorphic adult patterns in blood lipids, hemoglobin and red cell indices.

PSYCHOLOGICAL DEVELOPMENT

Psychological changes in thought patterns and cognitive ability are driven by increasing maturation and myelination of the adolescent brain.[32] Between the ages of 6 and 11 years, children generally think concretely, understanding only the immediate and short-term consequence of actions or events. Ideas and concepts can only be manipulated through using concrete representations. From the age of 12 years onwards, thought patterns begin to change to formal operational or abstract thought, with the ability to manipulate ideas rather than things, imagine the future, and conceive of multiple outcomes of actions. These capacities are important for the development of a settled personal and sexual identity.[33] These psychological changes, like the biological changes of puberty, are universal to all races and cultures. However, the majority of psychological and social development is culture specific, varying with social and cultural norms regarding the roles of children and adults in society.

SOCIAL DEVELOPMENT

The social changes of adolescence are outlined in Table 34.2. Biological and psychological changes occur within the context of an individual's social environment. The essential social tasks of adolescence are developing a sense of personal identity, moving from dependence to independence, and developing mature relationships with peers. These challenges exist across all cultures; however the timing of changes and the point at which successful completion is expected varies greatly between cultures.[34] In Western societies, adolescence commonly extends over many years, with its endpoints marked by relative financial independence after the completion of education. In contrast, in some societies, the social rights and responsibilities of adulthood are conferred at initiation ceremonies or rites.

IMPLICATIONS OF ADOLESCENT DEVELOPMENT FOR HEALTH

It is the reciprocal impacts of adolescent development on disease management and health related quality of life that pose the greatest challenges of adolescent medicine. This is especially true in chronic conditions (Table 34.3). A chronic illness or disability of any type may retard normal adolescent development, producing pubertal and growth delay, delayed social independence, poor body and sexual self-image and educational and vocational failure. Doctors, including both pediatricians and adult physicians are poor at monitoring growth and pubertal development in adolescents with chronic illness, and attention is required to growth in chronic illness well into the early 20s.[35]

Being chronically ill, having a visible disability, or being required to adhere to difficult treatment regimens is difficult at all ages – but particularly so during adolescence. Alienation from the peer group and absence from school cause social isolation, failure of socialization and ultimately, educational and vocational failure. The importance of thinking proactively about helping young people with chronic illness or disability develop independent adult living and vocational skills has been shown in longitudinal follow-up studies.[36]

Table 34.2 Developmental tasks of adolescence

	Biological	Psychological	Social
Early adolescence	Early puberty Girls Breast bud and pubic hair development (Tanner stage II) Initiation of growth spurt Boys Testicular enlargement, beginning of genital growth (stage II)	Thinking remains concrete but with development of early moral concepts Progression of sexual identity development: development of sexual orientation – possibly by experimentation Possible homosexual peer interest Reassessment and restructuring of body image in face of rapid growth	Realization of differences from parents Beginning of strong peer identification Early exploratory behaviors (smoking, violence)
Mid adolescence	Girls Mid to late puberty (stage IV–V) and completion of growth Menarche (stage IV event) Development of female body shape with fat deposition Boys Mid puberty (stages III and IV) Spermarche and nocturnal emissions Voice breaking Initiation of growth spurt (stage III–IV)	Emergence of abstract thinking although ability to imagine future applies to others rather than self (self seen as 'bullet-proof') Growing verbal abilities; adaptation to increasing educational demands Conventional morality (identification of law with morality) Development of fervently early vocational plans held ideology (religious/political)	Establishment of emotional separation from parents Strong peer group identification Increased health risk (smoking, alcohol, drugs, sexual exploration) Heterosexual peer interests Early vocational plans Development of an educational trajectory; early notions of vocational future
Late adolescence	Boys Completion of pubertal development (stage V) Continued androgenic effects on muscle bulk and body hair	Complex abstract thinking Post-conventional morality (ability to recognize difference between law and morality) Increased impulse control Further completion of personal identity Further development or rejection of ideology and religion – often fervently	Further separation from parents and development of social autonomy Development of intimate relationships – initially within peer group, then separation of couples from peer group Development of vocational capability, potential or real financial independence

Table 34.3 Reciprocal effects of chronic illness or disability and adolescent development

Effects of chronic illness or disability on development	Effects of developmental issues on chronic illness or disability
Biological Delayed puberty Short stature Reduced bone mass accretion	Biological Increased caloric requirement for growth may negatively impact on disease parameters Pubertal hormones may impact upon disease parameters (e.g. growth hormone impairs metabolic control in diabetes)
Psychological Infantilization Adoption of sick role as personal identifier Egocentricity persists into late adolescence Impaired development of sense of sexual or attractive self	Poor adherence and poor disease control due to: Poorly developed abstract thinking and planning (reduced ability to plan and prepare using abstract concepts) Difficulty in imagining the future; self-concept as being 'bullet-proof' Rejection of medical professionals as part of separation from parents Exploratory (risk-taking) behaviors
Social Reduced independence at a time when independence is normally developing Failure of peer relationships then intimate (couple) relationships Social isolation Educational failure and then vocational failure; failure of development of independent living ability	Associated health risk behaviors Chaotic eating habits may result in poor nutrition Smoking, alcohol and drug use often in excess of normal population rates Sexual risk-taking, possibly in view of realization of limited life span

Conversely, adolescent development issues impact upon the management of illness and disability. Poor adherence to medical regimens and poor disease management are virtually developmentally 'appropriate' in adolescence. Immature abilities to imagine future consequences allied with a concept of themselves as 'bullet-proof' means that the prevention of long-term complications of illness is a poor motivator for compliance. Additionally, medical advice may be rejected as part of a young person's growing independence from parents, particularly in chronic pediatric illnesses where medical staff have become medical 'parents'. Adherence and disease control are also put at risk by the developmental need to explore possible modes of future behavior, no matter how dangerous (usually derogatively referred to as 'adolescent risk-taking'). Health risk behaviors such as smoking, alcohol and drug use are as common in adolescents with chronic illness or disability as in the general population.[37]

Developmental issues in adolescent medicine are becoming more important, as the burden of chronic illness in adolescence increases as larger numbers of chronically ill children survive into the second and third decades.

RESILIENCE AND RISK IN ADOLESCENT HEALTH

Morbidity in adolescence is generally understood to result from 'risk-taking', impulsivity, the rejection of parental values and the testing of boundaries. But the standard conceptions of adolescents as risk-takers with poor future thinking abilities have been shown to be largely false.[38] Most adults take as many risks and have equally poor future thinking abilities as the majority of young people. Indeed, mental health problems, drug use and sexual risk-taking is comorbid in the same way in adults as occurs in adolescents.[39,40] That adults seem to take fewer risks is largely because they have learned the consequences of their risk-taking more effectively. It is more helpful to understand so-called 'risk-taking' behaviors in young people as developmentally appropriate 'exploratory behaviors', i.e. young people exploring the diversity of possible adult behaviors open to them – behaviors that they may or may not continue as adults.

Once these behaviors are understood to be largely developmentally motivated, it becomes unsurprising that interventions based upon education about 'risk' behaviors show very poor results.[41] Large studies of adolescent behavior and health show convincingly that health risk behaviors of all types (substance misuse, sexual risk, suicide, injuries and violence) occur together, and are strongly associated with deprivation and ethnicity.[42] Conversely, high family, community and school support ('connectedness' or 'social capital') are protective against most health risk behaviors in adolescents.[42] Identifying such 'resilience' or protective factors is now the focus of public health interventions with young people, and known protective factors for different behaviors are outlined in Table 34.4.[40,42–54]

The search for protective factors applies equally to clinical management of acute or chronic illness in young people. In young people with poor control of a chronic illness, it is traditional to search for causes of poor control and why things go wrong. In a young person with recurrent hospital admissions with asthma, for example, causes of exacerbations may be a lack of education or lack of a crisis plan, or psychological problems including non-adherence and manipulation of the treatment regimen. In some cases, it may be more fruitful to examine 'what has helped' and what has kept the young person out of hospital between admissions. This 'solution-focused' approach, asking young people what resources they have used to stay well between exacerbations, can be very effective in treating poor chronic illness control.[55]

THE MANAGEMENT OF ILL HEALTH IN ADOLESCENCE

Most doctors (with the notable exceptions of neonatologists and geriatricians) have adolescents in their practice. But many are not comfortable or skilled in dealing with adolescents. US studies suggest that only around a third of physicians and pediatricians actually like working with adolescents and that around another third have very little interest in adolescent care.[56]

The effective management of young people with acute or chronic illnesses requires a non-judgmental communication style, knowledge of adolescent development and an awareness of consent and confidentiality issues, and an ethnographic approach which

Table 34.4 Identified risk and protective factors for adolescent morbidities and health behaviors

Behavior	Risk factors	Protective factors
Smoking	Depression[43] Alcohol use[44] Disconnectedness from school or family[42,44] Difficulty talking with parents[44] Minority ethnicity[45,46] Low school achievement[42] Peer smoking and high peer popularity[47]	Family connectedness[42] Perceived healthiness[44] Higher parental expectations[42] Low school smoking prevalence[47]
Alcohol and substance use	Depression[45] Low self-esteem[42] Easy family access to alcohol[42] Ethnicity[45] Working outside school[42] Difficulty talking with parents[44] Risk factors for transition from occasional to regular use are cigarette smoking, availability, peer use and other risk behaviors[48]	Connectedness with school and family[42] Religious affiliation[42]
Teenage pregnancy	Disadvantage Urbanicity Low educational expectations[49,50] Lack of access to sexual health services[51,52] Drug and alcohol use[53]	Religious affiliation[54] Parental connectedness and expectations[42,50]
Sexually transmitted diseases (STDs)	Psychological disturbance[40] Substance use[40]	

aims at understanding the health beliefs and contexts in which the young people manage their disease.

COMMUNICATION WITH YOUNG PEOPLE

Consultations with adolescents differ from pediatric consultations in that the young person forms a more important and more problematic third party in the decision-making process. In working with young people, we must communicate not with another adult, but with a personality undergoing rapid psychological and social changes who may or may not share an adult's understanding of society nor adult cognitive abilities to decide between treatment alternatives in the light of future risk.

Effective clinical communication is a basic health right for young people, as well as being necessary for effective disease management. Yet adolescents report that they frequently find communication with doctors unsatisfactory, with doctors often seen as remote and judgmental figures whose confidentiality cannot be trusted.[57] Communication with adolescents requires an understanding of the cognitive and social developmental level of the young person and a non-judgmental understanding of the social contexts of that individual's health behaviors. Important elements of effective communication with young people are outlined in Table 34.5.

The standard pediatric consultation (doctor communicates with parents) and the standard adult consultation (doctor communicates solely with patient) are both inappropriate in dealing with adolescents. Best practice is to see young people both together with their parents and by themselves. While this is time consuming, it is essential for taking an accurate history, understanding the young person's motivations and goals, and for getting accurate information on health risk behaviors such as smoking, drinking, drugs and unsafe sex.[58]

Frameworks have been developed for best practice in clinical settings with young people, the most well known being the HEADSS approach which reminds clinicians to cover the important domains of Home life, Education, Activities, Drugs, Sexuality and Suicide (depression and self-harming) when interviewing any young person (Table 34.6).[59] But having a framework is not enough; the key skills required for effective communication with young people

Table 34.5 Practical points for communicating and working with adolescents

- Assure confidentiality – both in the clinical interaction and in the clinical/hospital set up.
- See young people by themselves as well as with their parents. The best strategy for getting the parents out of the room is warning families when you first see them that you routinely see adolescents by themselves as a way of respecting their rights as a young person.
- Be empathic, respectful and non-judgmental and try to avoid taking the 'expert' position. Treat the young person as the expert in their own condition, with the doctor as the medical advisor. Find out what the young person's goals are for their treatment and health, and negotiate matching treatments to their health goals.
- Try to communicate and explain concepts in a developmentally appropriate fashion. This is particularly important in health promotion. For young adolescents, concentrate on concrete 'here-and-now' issues and avoid abstract discussions, particularly about possible future health risks. You may need to repeat the information in a different form as they mature cognitively.
- Be yourself and don't be 'cool' or use youth language. Young people don't want you as a friend, they want a knowledgeable doctor whom they can respect and trust.
- Provide an emotionally and physically safe environment. A gender balance amongst staff is important, particularly where physical examinations are undertaken.
- Take a full psychosocial history when seeing young people for the first time, for example using the HEADSS protocol (Table 34.6).

REFERENCES (*Level 1 evidence)

1 Cooklin A. Psychological changes of adolescence. In: Brook CDG, ed. The practice of medicine in adolescence. London: Edward Arnold; 1993:8–24.

2 World Health Organization. The health of young people. Geneva: WHO; 1993.

3 Rutter M. Changing youth in a changing society. Cambridge MA: Harvard University Press; 1980.

4 Social focus on young people. London: The Stationery Office; 2000.

5 MacFaul R, Werneke U. Recent trends in hospital use by children in England. Arch Dis Child 2001; 85:203–207.

6 Kari J, Donovan C, Li J, et al. Adolescents' attitudes to general practice in North London. Br J Gen Pract 1997; 47:109–110.

7 Health Survey for England: The Health of Young People '95–97. London: The Stationery Office; 1998.

8 College Research Unit. National in-patient child and adolescent psychiatry study (NICAPS). London: Royal College of Psychiatrists; 2001.

9 Viner RM. National survey of use of hospital beds by adolescents aged 12 to 19 in the United Kingdom. BMJ 2001; 322:957–958.

10 Greene S. Diabetes in the young: current challenges in their management. Baillieres Clin Paediatr 1996; 4:563–575.

11 Lawson ML, Sochett EB, Chait PG, et al. Effect of puberty on markers of glomerular hypertrophy and hypertension in IDDM. Diabetes 1996; 45:51–55.

12 Michelagnoli M, Viner RM. Commentary: care of the adolescent with cancer. Eur J Cancer 2001; 37:1523–1530.

13 Kaur B, Anderson HR, Austin J, et al. Prevalence of asthma symptoms, diagnosis, and treatment in 12–14 year old children across Great Britain (international study of asthma and allergies in childhood, ISAAC UK). BMJ 1998; 316:118–124.

14 Variation and trends in incidence of childhood diabetes in Europe. EURODIAB ACE Study Group. Lancet 2000; 355: 873–876.

15 Fagot-Campagna A, Pettitt DJ, Engelgau MM, et al. Type 2 diabetes among North American children and adolescents: an epidemiologic review and a public health perspective. J Pediatr 2000; 136:664–672.

16 Siegel D. Adolescents and chronic illness. JAMA 1987; 257:3396–3399.

17 Newacheck P, Taylor W. Childhood chronic illness: prevalence, severity and impact. Am J Public Health 1992; 82:364–371.

18 Gortmaker S, Sappenfield W. Chronic childhood disorders: prevalence and impact. Pediatr Clin North Am 1984; 31:3–18.

19 British Paediatric Association Working Party on Cystic Fibrosis. Report on cystic fibrosis 1988.

20 Goddard E, Higgins V. Smoking, drinking and drug use among young teenagers in 1998. London: The Stationery Office; 1999.

21 US Department of Health and Human Services. Preventing tobacco use among young people: a report of the Surgeon General. Washington DC: US Department of Health & Human Services, Centers for Disease Control & Prevention; 1994.

22 Harrington R, Fudge H, Rutter M. Adult outcomes of childhood and adolescent depression. Arch Gen Psychiatr 1990; 47:465–473.

23 Angold A, Costello E, Worthman C. Puberty and depression: the roles of age, pubertal status and pubertal timing. Psychol Med 1998; 28:51–61.

24 Steinberger J, Moran A, Hong CP, et al. Adiposity in childhood predicts obesity and insulin resistance in young adulthood. J Pediatr 2001; 138:469–473.

25 Hubert HB, Feinleib M, McNamara PM, et al. Obesity as an independent risk factor for cardiovascular disease: a 26-year follow-up of participants in the Framingham Heart Study. Circulation 1983; 67:968–977.

26 Osmond C, Barker DJ. Fetal, infant, and childhood growth are predictors of coronary heart disease, diabetes, and hypertension in adult men and women. Environ Health Perspect 2000; 108(suppl 3):545–553.

27 McClure GM. Suicide in children and adolescents in England and Wales 1970–1998. Br J Psychiatry 2001; 178:469–474.

28 Reilly JJ, Dorosty AR. Epidemic of obesity in UK children. Lancet 1999; 354:1874–1875.

29 Fagot-Campagna A, Narayan KM, Imperatore G. Type 2 diabetes in children. BMJ 2001; 322:377–378.

30 Eveleth P, Tanner J. Worldwide variation in human growth. Cambridge: Cambridge University Press; 1990.

31 Viner R. Splitting hairs. Arch Dis Child 2002; 86:8–10.

32 Paus T, Collins DL, Evans AC, et al. Maturation of white matter in the human brain: a review of magnetic resonance studies. Brain Res Bull 2001; 54:255–266.

33 Leffert N, Petersen AC. Patterns of development during adolescence. In: Rutter M, Smith DJ, eds. Psychosocial disorders in young people. London: John Wiley; 1995:67–103.

34 Muuss RE. Theories of adolescence. New York: McGraw Hill; 1996.

35 Ghosh S, Drummond H, Ferguson A. Neglect of growth and development in the clinical monitoring of children and teenagers with inflammatory bowel disease: review of case records. BMJ 1998; 317:120–121.

36 White PD. Transition to adulthood. Curr Opin Rheumatol 1999; 11:408–411.

37 Hargrave DR, McMaster C, O'Hare MM, et al. Tobacco smoke exposure in children and adolescents with diabetes mellitus. Diabet Med 1999; 16:31–34.

38 Males M. Adolescents: daughters or alien sociopaths? Lancet 1997; 349(suppl 1): I13–I16.

39 Cohen ED. An exploratory attempt to distinguish subgroups among crack-abusing African–American women. J Addict Dis 1999; 18:41–54.

40 Ramrakha S, Avshalom C, Dickson N, et al. Psychiatric disorders and risky sexual behaviour in young adulthood: cross-sectional study in birth cohort. BMJ 2000; 321:66.

41 Lister-Sharp D, Chapman S, Stewart-Brown S, et al. Health promoting schools and health promotion in schools: two systematic reviews. Health Technol Assessment 2001; 3:1–6.

42 Resnick MD, Bearman PS, Blum R, et al. Protecting adolescents from harm. Findings from the National Longitudinal Study on Adolescent Health. JAMA 1998; 278:823–832.

43 Windle M, Windle RC. Depressive symptoms and cigarette smoking among middle adolescents: prospective associations and intrapersonal and interpersonal influences. J Consult Clin Psychol 2001; 69:215–226.

44 Health and health behaviour among young people. Health behaviour in school-aged children: A WHO cross-national study (HSBC) international report. Copenhagen: WHO; 2000.

45 Kelder SH, Murray NG, Orpinas P, et al. Depression and substance use in minority middle-school students. Am J Public Health 2001; 91:761–766.

46 Alexander CS, Allen P, Crawford MA, et al. Taking a first puff: cigarette smoking experiences among ethnically diverse adolescents. Ethn Health 1999; 4:245–257.

47 Alexander C, Piazza M, Mekos D, et al. Peers, schools, and adolescent cigarette smoking. J Adolesc Health 2001; 29:22–30.

48 Coffey C, Lynskey M, Wolfe R, et al. Initiation and progression of cannabis use in a population-based Australian adolescent longitudinal study. Addiction 2000; 95:1679–1690.

49 Hogan DP, Sun R, Cornwell GT. Sexual and fertility behaviors of American females aged 15–19 years: 1985, 1990, and 1995. Am J Public Health 2000; 90:1421–1425.

50 Lammers C, Ireland M, Resnick M, et al. Influences on adolescents' decision to postpone onset of sexual intercourse: a survival analysis of virginity among youths aged 13 to 18 years. J Adolesc Health 2000; 26:42–48.

51 DuRant RH, Jay S, Seymore C. Contraceptive and sexual behavior of black female adolescents. A test of a social–psychological theoretical model. J Adolesc Health Care 1990; 11:326–334.

52 Porter LE, Ku L. Use of reproductive health services among young men, 1995. J Adolesc Health 2000; 27:186–194.

53 Raine TR, Jenkins R, Aarons SJ, et al. Sociodemographic correlates of virginity in seventh-grade black and Latino students. J Adolesc Health 1999; 24:304–312.

54 Coyne-Beasley TS, Choenbach VJ. The African–American church: a potential forum for adolescent comprehensive sexuality education. J Adolesc Health 2000; 26:289–294.

55 Christie D, Fredman G. Working systemically in an adolescent medical unit: collaborating with the network. Clin Psychol 2001; 3:8–11.

56 Klitsner I, Borok G, Neintstein L, et al. Adolescent health care in a large multispecialty prepaid group practice: who provides it and how well are they doing? West J Med 1992; 156:628–632.

57 Royal College of General Practitioners and Brook. Confidentiality and young people. London: Royal College of General Practitioners; 2000.

58 MacKenzie RG. Approach to the adolescent in the clinical setting. Med Clin North Am 1990; 74:1085–1095.
59 Goldenring JM, Cohen E. Getting into adolescent heads. Contemp Pediatr 1988; July:75–90.
60 Sanci LA, Coffey CM, Veit FC, et al. Evaluation of the effectiveness of an educational intervention for general practitioners in adolescent health care: randomised controlled trial. BMJ 2000; 320:224–230.
61 Taylor SJ, Whincup PH, Hindmarsh PC, et al. Performance of a new pubertal self-assessment questionnaire: a preliminary study. Paediatr Perinat Epidemiol 2001; 15:88–94.
62 Oppong-Odiseng AC, KHeycock EG. Adolescent health services – through their eyes. Arch Dis Child 1997; 77:115–119.
63 Burack R. Young teenagers' attitudes towards general practitioners and their provision of sexual health care. Br J Gen Pract 2000; 50:550–554.
64 Ford CA, Millstein SG, Halpern-Felsher BL, et al. Influence of physician confidentiality assurances on adolescents' willingness to disclose information and seek future health care. A randomized controlled trial. JAMA 1997; 278:1029–1034.
65 Churchill R, Allen J, Denman S, et al. Do the attitudes and beliefs of young teenagers towards general practice influence actual consultation behaviour? Br J Gen Pract 2000; 50:953–957.
66 British Medical Association. Consent, rights and choices in health care for children and young people. London: BMJ; 2001.
67 Kyngas HA, Kroll T, Duffy ME. Compliance in adolescents with chronic diseases: A review. J Adolesc Health 2000; 26:379–388.
68 Eiser C. Psychological effects of chronic disease. J Child Psychol Psychiatry 1990; 31: 85–98.
69 Sawyer S, Blair S, Bowes G. Chronic illness in adolescents: transfer or transition to adult services? J Paediatr Child Health 1997; 33:88–90.
70 Rosen D. Between two worlds: bridging the cultures of child health and adult medicine. J Adolesc Health 1995; 17:10–16.
71 Viner RM. Transition from paediatric to adult care. Bridging the gaps or passing the buck? Arch Dis Child 1999; 81:271–275.
72 Dowsett EG, Colby J. Long-term sickness absence due to ME/CFS in UK schools. J Chron Fatigue Syndr 1997; 3:29–42.
73 Report of the CFS/ME Working Group. Report to the Chief Medical Officer of an Independent Working Group. London: Department of Health; 2002.
74 Pawlikowska T, Chalder T, Hirsch SR, et al. Population based study of fatigue and psychological distress. BMJ 1994; 308: 763–766.
75 Fukuda K, Straus SE, Hickie I, et al. The chronic fatigue syndrome: a comprehensive approach to its definition and study. Ann Intern Med 1994; 121:953–959.
76 Garralda E, Rangel L, Levin M, et al. Psychiatric adjustment in adolescents with a history of chronic fatigue syndrome. J Am Acad Child Adolesc Psychiatry 1999; 38:1515–1521.
77 White PD, Thomas JM, Crawford DH, et al. Incidence, risk and prognosis of acute and chronic fatigue syndromes and psychiatric disorders after glandular fever. Br J Psychiatry 1998; 173:475–481.
78 Chronic fatigue syndrome: Report of a joint working group of the Royal Colleges of Physicians, Psychiatrists and General Practitioners. London: RCP; 1997.
79 NHS Centre for Reviews and Dissemination. Interventions for the management of CFS/ME. Effective Health Care 2002; 7:1–12.
80 Chalder T, Tong J, Deary V. Family cognitive behaviour therapy for chronic fatigue syndrome: an uncontrolled study. Arch Dis Child 2002; 86:95–97.
81 Lim A, Lubitz L. Chronic fatigue syndrome: successful outcome of an intensive inpatient programme. J Paediatr Child Health 2002; 38:295–299.
82 Carter BD, Edwards JF, Kronenberger WG, et al. Case control study of chronic fatigue in pediatric patients. Pediatrics 1995; 95:179–186.
83 Coleman J. Key data on adolescence. Brighton: Trust for the Study of Adolescence; 1999.

35

Emergency care

Tom Beattie, Gale Pearson

PEDIATRIC ACCIDENT AND EMERGENCY CARE

A pediatric emergency medical service (PEMS)

In an ideal world there would never be a critically ill or injured child. We do not live however, in an ideal world and consequently for the foreseeable future there will be a substantial requirement to provide for the treatment of these children. In order to provide optimum care for these children a seamless structure of continuous care is essential. There are few centers in the world where this seamless care exists. Where it has been achieved however, outcomes for critically ill and injured children have been positively influenced.[1,2]

The continuum of pediatric emergency care is best summarized in Figure 35.1. Within this there should be the desire to keep as many children as possible out of institutions and maintain their care within the home and community environment for as much of the time as possible.

THE HOME SETTING

For the first 5 years of life most children spend the bulk of their time within the home and community environment. The majority of children coming into contact with emergency medical services do so as a result of infection or injury.

Most children will experience upper and lower respiratory tract infection with considerable frequency between the ages of 0 and 5 years. After this age it is much less frequent. Much of this illness can be treated within the home providing parents have sufficient confidence and education. Most illness in this age group will be viral and will require little more than supportive measures such as antipyretic therapy and encouraging fluid intake. However, there is an increasing demand for this type of treatment to be obtained from family doctors or emergency departments. The disintegration of the nuclear family is one factor increasing this demand on medical time particularly in primary care. Recent evidence has indicated that attenders at emergency departments for minor illness and injury come from deprived areas of the community.[3] The reasons for this are complex but probably relate to coping mechanisms, education and general inability to cope.

In a small number of cases bacterial infection will be present which require antibiotic therapy. In an even smaller number significant infectious disease such as meningitis, septicemia and osteomyelitis will be present. A small number of children with viral illness will get further complications such as a febrile seizure or superimposed bacterial infection may supervene. If parents are unaware of these problems they will lose confidence in managing illness within the community.

An education program which teaches parents how to deal with febrile illness must also alert them to the dangers of bacterial illness which requires antibiotic treatment with or without a stay in hospital. Within this education program it is important to differentiate the needs of the infant under 3 months of age from that over 3 months of age. The response of the younger child to infection is totally different from that of older children and adults and parents should be aware of how to get advice for these children should the need arise.[4] This is a difficult task as even health professionals using clinical decision tools cannot reliably detect children with significant infection.[5–7]

Despite the frequency of infections, injuries are still the leading cause of morbidity and mortality between the ages of 1 and 5 years. Most of these accidents occur within the home setting, which includes the garden and its surroundings. Burns and scalds, poisonings, falls from a height, finger tip injuries and near drowning account for the majority.

One of the means to tackle the toll wrought by injury in this age group is an integrated accident prevention program within an emergency medical system. The components of such an accident prevention system include:

1. accident surveillance;
2. data analysis;
3. identification of problems;
4. development of strategies;
5. implementation of strategies;
6. accident surveillance.

In many ways this is a typical audit cycle. It relies on collaboration among emergency physicians, general practice, public health medicine, educationalists and health promotion agencies. These should bring their respective skills together in a coordinated fashion.

At present injury surveillance is patchy with much information being derived from inpatient databases. These are inaccurate and only reflect 10% of total accidents which occur.[8] Without meaningful measures of injury severity these data are at best a reflection of current medical practice. A good example of this is the documentation of poisoning. Many children who are poisoned can be safely dealt with in the home without ever coming to hospital

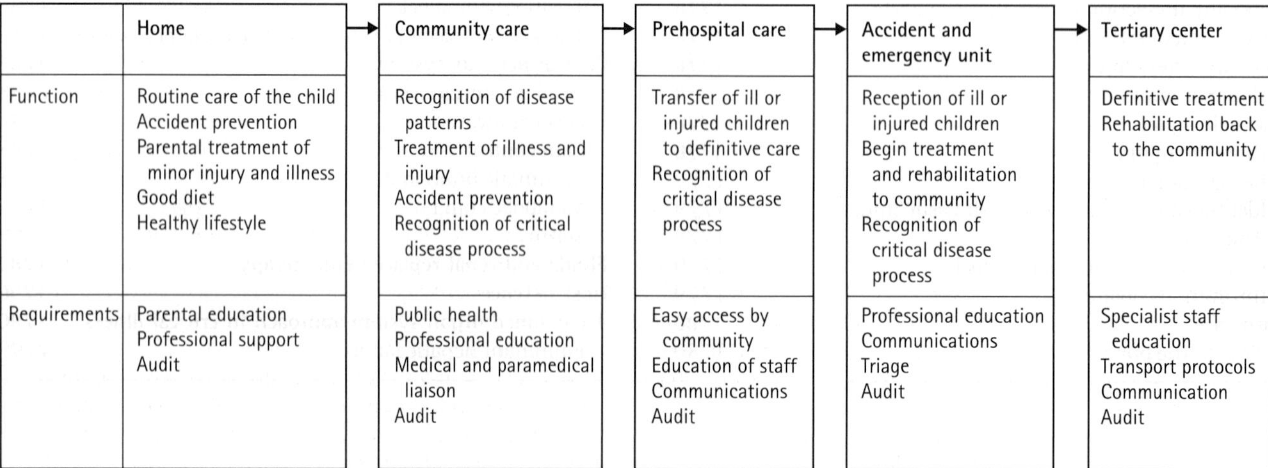

	Home	Community care	Prehospital care	Accident and emergency unit	Tertiary center
Function	Routine care of the child Accident prevention Parental treatment of minor injury and illness Good diet Healthy lifestyle	Recognition of disease patterns Treatment of illness and injury Accident prevention Recognition of critical disease process	Transfer of ill or injured children to definitive care Recognition of critical disease process	Reception of ill or injured children Begin treatment and rehabilitation to community Recognition of critical disease process	Definitive treatment Rehabilitation back to the community
Requirements	Parental education Professional support Audit	Public health Professional education Medical and paramedical liaison Audit	Easy access by community Education of staff Communications Audit	Professional education Communications Triage Audit	Specialist staff education Transport protocols Communication Audit

Fig. 35.1 Components of a pediatric emergency medical system: continuum of care.

provided adequate medical advice can be given and monitored by telephone. If this advice is not available then many children will present to hospital. They will present to the emergency room where their treatment will depend on the experience and confidence of the staff working in that department. Insecure, ill taught and junior staff will tend to admit because they are unsure of what to do. Senior staff, experienced and confident will be able to manage many of these children on an outpatient basis. In an institution staffed in the former manner poisonings determined from inpatient stay will be at a high level whereas those in an institution managed in the latter manner will be lower. This has nothing to do with the incidence of the poisoning but all to do with medical practice. Simply by changing medical practice one can demonstrate an apparent fall in the incidence of poisoning when in fact the incidence remains high. Failure to take cognisance of these matters when developing accident surveillance will lead to inappropriate preventive measures.[9]

Effective data surveillance should start with a minimum data set. This minimum data set should aim to capture a small, important amount of information on every child who presents.[10] If too much information is to be documented staff will tend not to collect it and parents will get irritated because they feel that their child should be treated rather than them answering questions. Typically it should include age, sex, postcode and proxies for social class and/or deprivation. Some idea as to the causation should also be included. One way of doing this is to use international classification of disease E codes.[11] This is universally accepted and is adequate for most things. This could be further refined to having the most common injuries already precoded. Similarly some ideas to the most common diagnoses using a system such as the International Classification of Disease codes (ICD) could also be included on discharge. If this information were to be collected on all children one would very rapidly develop a very suitable accident surveillance system that could be expanded as the need arose.

DATA ANALYSIS AND PROBLEM IDENTIFICATION

Once an accurate database is in place that gathers details on a substantial proportion of injury occurring within the community then problem areas can be identified. This can be on the basis of deprivation or need; clustering; type of accident e.g. fall, poisoning; type of injury e.g. fracture or head injury. Once analyzed this information can then be made available to the relevant health education agencies who can then implement parts three and four of the audit cycle.

DEVISING A STRATEGY

Before any strategy can be devised to protect against childhood accidents three components have to be addressed:

1. the child;
2. the family;
3. the environment.

Tackling any of these on their own will fail if it does not concomitantly address the problems inherent in the other two areas. It is well recognized that some children are more accident prone than others. Is this because the family is poor or the environment is poor? Or is it that that child is inherently more prone to injury for reasons of clumsiness, poor eyesight/coordination? Attention deficit and hyperactivity disorder is an example of a behavioral problem which might be expected to be associated with injury and this is the case.[12] To date many accident prevention programs have been simplistic with individuals working in isolation without the complete umbrella of a PEMS.

IMPLEMENTING A STRATEGY

Before a strategy can be successful the lessons learnt from commercial advertisers has to be learned. Simply repeating the same message ad infinitum leads to message fatigue. The message must be appropriate to the target audience and must take note of all the above factors. In addition the target audience must be identified and targeted effectively.

RE-AUDIT

It is important to measure any effect of the prevention campaigns against the initial database. Failure to do so may lead to inappropriate and ineffective campaigning being continued indefinitely. If there has been no diminution in the levels of injury that one has targeted then the strategies need to be re-evaluated in the light of the data analysis and message.

COMMUNITY EDUCATION

In order for the child to be cared for within the home as effectively as possible, ideally not accessing emergency medical services, a substantial amount of effort must be paid to community education. However, the target audience has not been well defined. Does one, for instance, tackle children in junior school or senior school in an effort to help future generations? Should one address the problem at antenatal classes where there is a substantial chance that one will reach an interested mother and perhaps the father? Is it appropriate to address the issue of safety in the postnatal period when one is almost certainly not going to get the father present? These issues need to be addressed as a matter of urgency if child accident prevention is to be taken forward in a meaningful manner.

COMMUNITY CARE

Within the context of a PEMS, community care should be directed at disease prevention. There will however, be a significant proportion of children who have transient episodes of acute illness requiring medical intervention. Interspersed with these will be children with chronic disability who will have more sophisticated needs for emergency care than their able bodied peers.

To work effectively there needs to be a network of experienced general practitioners and community pediatricians working alongside health visitors, district nurses, midwives and other paramedical staff. The public health system working alongside ensures good sanitation and maintenance of water supplies. Attention to housing and overcrowding are also all-important issues in the prevention of disease and illness. Surveillance by public health physicians and public health laboratories can identify trends in disease. Many infectious diseases, e.g. mycoplasma infection, occur in a cyclical fashion. Disease reporting can help identify when these infections are imminent and serological testing can help confirm that they have actually arrived. This will alert practitioners to the common disease that may be in the community setting at any given time and may help avoid unnecessary hospital admissions by the correct use of antibiotics.

The health professionals within the community have several roles. The first is disease prevention, primarily in terms of immunization and accident prevention. Where immunization has been effective many diseases have all but been eradicated. This is in danger of disappearing with recent changes in attitude to immunization. The recent scare regarding possible links with autism and bowel disease has led to concern about the safety of the combined measles/mumps/rubella (MMR) vaccination.[13] That this link has yet to be proven has not yet convinced a section of the public. This has led to a small but significant decrease in herd immunity, possibly opening the way for a measles epidemic in particular.[14,15]

Health professionals in the community should be able to give advice to parents on disease and accident prevention. They should also be able to recognize situations where family dynamics are breaking down making accidents and child abuse more common.

Within the community one of the more vital functions is recognition of the child who has a disease process that is not suitable for treatment in the community but needs further care within a hospital setting. A good example of this is bronchiolitis. Many cases of bronchiolitis will be cared for in the community with children getting supportive care and advice. However, family practitioners should be in the position to identify the child at risk from significant airway distress, e.g. not feeding, a respiratory rate over 55 or apneic attacks.[16] In this situation the child needs to get to hospital for further treatment that may include high-dependency and/or intensive care. Equally the community services should be able to identify the child who may not be so ill but where the family circumstances mean that the child is not going to be capably looked after at home. Situations where this may occur include poverty, mother who is not coping because of two or three other small children, single parents or families of drug abusers. In these situations even though the child may not warrant admission for medical reasons, the social factors may indicate the child needs to be transferred for inpatient care. Community practitioners are much better placed to identify these problems than hospital based staff.

PREHOSPITAL CARE

Prehospital care is a link between home and the community on one hand and the hospital based services of accident and emergency and tertiary level care on the other. The function of prehospital care is to transfer ill or injured children to places of either advanced or definitive care. Two issues predominate within the prehospital care setting:

1. access;
2. education.

To be effective prehospital care has to be easily accessed by all members of the community, e.g. in the UK dialling '999' gains access to the ambulance service. This universal national access code available to all and free of charge is probably the most effective component in the prehospital setting.

Education is also vital. The role of practitioners in prehospital care has got to be fully defined. It must be relevant to the PEMS within which the prehospital care is practiced. It will differ between urban and rural areas in terms of decisions to 'stay and play' and 'scoop and run'. It must be remembered that the absolute numbers of true pediatric emergencies (illness or trauma) is relatively rare, particularly compared to the adult population. The skills needed to carry out emergency care effectively require time to attain and practice to maintain.[17] An integrated pediatric emergency medical system can best evaluate the needs of its catchment area and train the prehospital care staff accordingly. Where short distances are envisaged and transfer times are rapid then training needs may be less demanding with concentration on simple airway, breathing and circulation skills. In rural areas where transport times may be prolonged advanced life support skills may be necessary.[18] Where land-based transport is adequate, training in driving skills may be required. However, should air medical transport by helicopter or fixed wing aircraft be necessary as a routine then training in aviation medicine and the associated problems will need to be included in the training package.

There is increasing evidence that prehospital life support should include effective, simple measures. Gausche et al showed that prehospital intubation had no benefit on outcome, and worryingly might increase mortality and morbidity.[19–21] This poses a dilemma for rural practitioners in particular. Urban and semiurban situations have clear guidance that in an emergency intubation should not be attempted in the field. Rather they should concentrate on bag–valve–mask ventilation with good, simple airway-opening maneuvers and transport of the child to the nearest pediatric unit. In rural and remote areas, or in situations where weather or geography make transport impossible, advanced airway care may be needed. The rarities of this, combined with the complexity of skills needed, make maintenance of skills difficult. Innovative and practical solutions have to be found, but there is no doubt that this will lead to increasing costs. Similarly the value of intravenous access has been questioned.[22] In particular the value of delaying at scene must be set against potential benefits. In this study Teach et al found no such benefit and some possible harm, either from delay at scene or inappropriate fluid administration.

Inner city areas with significant drugs problems may well have a high incidence of penetrating trauma which will require an emphasis to be placed on treatment of such injuries within that setting.[23]

THE ACCIDENT AND EMERGENCY UNIT SERVICES

Pediatric accident and emergency departments fall into three broad categories:

1. those attached to specialist pediatric hospitals which treat only children;
2. those attached to large district or teaching hospitals which have combined pediatric and adult populations;
3. those attached to small community or cottage hospitals treating relatively small numbers of patients overall.

Within each of these three settings various problems exist.

The dedicated pediatric unit is usually situated in a large conurbation, often attached to a university or medical school. It will provide child and family centered care of an exceptionally high order. Major injury and illness will often be much less than that in a comparable adult population so there will have to be significant emphasis on education directed at the recognition of illness and the development of resuscitation skills to facilitate optimum care of ill and injured children. Retention of these skills is also a major issue which needs to be addressed.[24,25]

In a unit that combines pediatric and adult patients, general resuscitation skills and teamwork will be much more practiced but in contrast recognition of pediatric illness and skill in treatment may be deficient. The ability to provide a child and family centered approach is often more difficult than in the purely pediatric setting.

The cottage hospital may benefit from being able to provide care closer to the patient's home but illness recognition and resuscitation skills may be poor unless teaching programs are available. This may require that staff rotate to busy units at regular intervals to update and recertify in pediatric skills.

A computer-based model of a typical region with various types of hospital postulates that all types of hospital are necessary to enable children to receive optimal care. This presupposes that skills are present and are updated regularly in each setting and that facilities for children are maintained.[26]

In all settings with the regular turnover of staff inherent with movement of junior doctors and nursing staff, regular resuscitation updates (e.g. pediatric advanced life support courses) are essential. Staffing and training in departments that have children attending should build in adequate time for training and staff development to ensure that skills are maintained at an optimum level.

Within these settings certain basic concepts need to be addressed.

There should always be dedicated facilities for the reception and treatment of children, removed from the sights and sounds of the adult world. Children are often already frightened and distressed by being in hospital and every effort should be made to keep them as calm and content as possible. An attractive child friendly environment should facilitate this. Examination rooms should have sufficient toys and pictures to enable efficient distraction therapy to be practiced. Play leaders are an invaluable resource to aid this process.

Resuscitation rooms should be fully equipped with all the various equipment that is required for pediatric resuscitation. Children change shape and size with age. A full knowledge of how this occurs and the clinical implications are important. It is almost impossible to accurately recall all the weights of children at various age groups. Drug and fluid therapy is usually done on a dose per weight basis. It is important to avoid calculations in 'the heat of the moment'. It is all too easy to place a decimal point in the wrong place and either over or underdose children. For this reason charts should be available or tapes laid out on beds so that rapid determination of dosage depending on the weight/length of the child can be established. These charts will also have details of the correct size of endotracheal tube, the length to which the tube should be cut and various other parameters necessary for effective pediatric resuscitation.[27,28]

Typical equipment required in the resuscitation room is shown in Table 35.1.

The staff working within such an environment must be familiar with recognition of the sick child and similarly be comfortable with all aspects of pediatric care.

Parents often arrive at the accident and emergency department with other siblings. The presence of play leaders will help entertain these children and enable the distressed relatives to be with the sick

Table 35.1 Equipment to provide emergency care for children: equipment for the resuscitation room

Airway
Guedel airways – 000→3
Endotracheal tubes – 2.5→8 uncuffed, 7→10.5 cuffed
Introducers
Laryngoscope handles
Laryngoscope blades – straight and curved
Yankauer suction catheters
Argyle suction catheters
Suction device (with backup)
Cricothyroid puncture set (this may be commercial or 'homemade')
Jet insufflation system

Breathing
Round masks
Triangular masks
Bag–valve–mask device with pressure limiting device set at 30–40 cm H_2O
Reservoir bag
O_2 supply (with backup)
Ayres T-piece circuit (or equivalent)
Chest drains 10→32G
Drainage tubing and jars for underwater seal

Circulation
Intravenous cannulae 24→14F
Central venous cannulae and Seldinger introducer wire
Intraosseous cannulae 17F
Giving sets
Blood warmer
Infusion pumps
Defibrillator with facility for synchronized DC version capable of variable energy delivery

Disability
Cervical collars
Spinal boards
Arm and leg splints

Monitoring equipment
Pulse oximeter
Cardiac monitor
Blood glucose test machines
Blood gas analyzer

Other
Tapes for i.v. lines, ETT tubes, chest drains
Syringes 1 ml, 2 ml, 5 ml, 10 ml
3-way taps
Connection tubing
Suture material

Other (contd)
Suture packs
Chest drain packs
Urinary catheters
Nasogastric tubes
Clock
Warmth

Drugs
Epinephrine (adrenaline) – 1:10 000 and 1:1000
Atropine
Lidocaine (lignocaine) – 1%, 2%
Sodium bicarbonate – 1.84%, 4.2%, 8.4%
Morphine
Naloxone
Glucose – 50%, 25%
Glucagon
Diazepam (as emulsion)
Phenytoin
Adenosine
Disopyramide
Beta-blocker
Thiopental
Suxamethonium
Atracurium
Mannitol – 10%, 20%
Beta 2-agonists – nebulizer solution
Ipratropium – nebulizer solution
Beta agonists – i.v. solution
Aminophylline
Hydrocortisone
Procyclidine

Fluids
Normal saline
Plasma

If neonates are expected the following equipment should also be available in addition:
Resuscitaire
Heat source
Warm towels/wraps
Umbilical catheters

or injured child. Quiet rooms should be laid aside so that bereaved or distressed relatives can be alone in their time of distress though a staff member should always be available for this if required. Facilities should be available to enable nappy changing and breast-feeding to occur in private.

The function of staff in the accident and emergency unit is to receive all ill and injured children and to institute treatment in a timely and appropriate fashion depending on the urgency of the condition (triage).

The nursing staff usually perform triage but medical staff could also perform this task. Objective triage is difficult in the pediatric population. There are few objective pediatric scales that can be related to all types of presenting problems, medical, surgical, trauma or other. Much triage therefore is subjective and will in part depend upon the volume of work. A well child presenting at a quiet time will very often get through the system more rapidly than an ill child presenting at a busy time. It is imperative that staff working within the accident and emergency unit are able to recognize the child who has a disease process which, if left untreated, will lead to serious incapacity or death. Key recognition skills relate to respiratory and circulatory compromise.

In parallel, skills are needed to:

1. open and secure an airway;
2. ensure that oxygenation is maintained;
3. ensure that circulation is maintained.

The frequency with which these skills are practiced will depend on the population served and the effectiveness of the home, community and prehospital services. Communities which have poor home safety, poor community immunization rates and primitive public sanitation can expect to deal with large numbers of ill or injured children.

Where numbers are small maintenance of recognition skills can only be maintained by appropriate teaching programs, for example pediatric advanced life support (PALS). PALS courses were introduced into UK in the early 1990s. Roberts et al[29] have demonstrated increased survival since these were introduced. Cause and effect have still to be reconciled.

Once a child has been received through the accident and emergency unit and the airway, breathing and circulation have been stabilized, the child needs to be transferred from the accident and emergency unit to a place of definitive treatment. Often this will be via an imaging facility to surgery, and from there to an intensive care setting. To complete the emergency medical system, a system of safe transfer to and from each of these areas needs to be established. Even if the accident and emergency department is within the tertiary care center transfer to the scanning suite or the intensive care unit can be fraught with danger if not performed expertly and efficiently.

A transport team therefore should be a priority development in any pediatric emergency care system so that there can be safe transfer to the tertiary care center for definitive treatment.

Both within the accident and emergency setting and the tertiary care unit rehabilitation is important. This will enable the ill or injured child to regain its place as effectively as possible within the home/community setting.

APPROACH TO THE MANAGEMENT OF THE SEVERELY ILL OR INJURED CHILD IN THE ACCIDENT AND EMERGENCY DEPARTMENT

Most ill children will be brought to hospital by the prehospital services. In these situations airway care and circulatory support will have been instituted according to local training and policy guidelines. In addition there will be an element of warning so that the resuscitation team can be gathered and tasks allocated.

As it is very easy for parents or by-standers to pick up smaller children, children who are severely ill or injured will often be brought to hospital unannounced and unexpected in private transport.

Consequently the components of the resuscitation team should be established in advance. It is important that one doctor is in charge to coordinate the resuscitation and decide on the priorities for care, with other staff in complementary roles.

INITIAL ASSESSMENT

Rapid assessment of the airway, breathing and circulation is mandatory (primary survey).

AIRWAY

The airway can be described as open, maintainable or unmaintainable. An open airway is defined as one with no obstruction present. This includes the absence of secretions, stridor, gurgling or other noises. An open airway needs no further management at this stage but this should be kept under review.[30,31]

A maintainable airway is defined as one which can be kept open with simple measures such as positioning; chin lift/head tilt (or jaw-thrust only if trauma to the cervical spine is a possibility); the use of an oropharyngeal airway; or the use of gentle suction.

An unmaintainable airway is one which is still at risk despite these simple measures necessitating either intubation or the creation of a surgical airway (cricothyrotomy).

The airway should be maintained at this stage by the simplest effective measures available. Intubation must only be carried out by experienced operators who can intubate with skill in a timely fashion. Any attempt taking longer than 30 s should be abandoned and the child oxygenated with a bag–valve–mask device pending a second attempt.

All sick or injured children require high flow oxygen. This should be administered using a facemask if the airway is open and maintainable. Otherwise artificial ventilation should be established using a bag–valve–mask device (see below).

BREATHING

The efficacy of breathing can be assessed only after the airway has been opened. The rate, volume and symmetry of respiration should be assessed by observation and auscultation.

Respiratory compromise can be characterized by either an increasing or decreasing work of breathing.

Increased work of breathing

Increasing respiratory rate
Increasing heart rate
Use of accessory muscles in respiration
Flared nostrils
Intercostal/sternal recession
Decreasing level of consciousness

Decreased work of breathing

Decreasing respiratory rate
Poor respiratory effort
Poor lung expansion

If breathing is absent, or diminished, ventilation using a bag–valve–mask device should be instituted as soon as possible. Absent breath sounds and hyper-resonance to percussion on one side should lead one to consider a pneumothorax. This should be immediately drained using a needle thoracostomy. The needle should be inserted into the midclavicular line in the second intercostal space pending the insertion of a formal chest drain. Once inserted the needle should be left in place until the chest drain is working properly. If signs of respiratory compromise are present supplemental oxygen should be administered in the highest rate available.

CIRCULATION

A central pulse should be palpated at this stage. The carotid pulse should be palpated lateral to the thyroid cartilage and medial to the sternocleidomastoid muscle in a child. In an infant the brachial pulse should be palpated in the upper arm.

If there is no pulse palpable (or pulse is less than 60 beats/min) cardiac massage should be started at a rate of 80–100 beats/min. If a pulse is palpable look for other signs of circulatory embarrassment.

Circulatory embarrassment

Circulatory embarrassment can be identified by the following physical signs:

Rising pulse
Weakening peripheral pulses
Increasing capillary return (greater than 2 s)
Increasing peripheral core temperature difference
Decreased urine output
Altered level of consciousness

All children with circulatory embarrassment (and all children who are severely ill or injured) should have intravenous (i.v.) access established as soon as possible. Failure to establish peripheral i.v. access within a few minutes in children who are in circulatory distress should lead one to insert an intraosseous needle into the tibia or femur. If signs of circulatory embarrassment or shock are present, fluid should be administered as a 20 ml/kg bolus.

Recent meta-analysis has suggested that crystalloid fluids are to be preferred.[32] Certainly UK practice has been to use colloid, e.g. plasma, but crystalloid has been widely used elsewhere. The quality of the literature makes it difficult to make a definitive decision as to best initial fluid resuscitation, but the Cochrane database review recommends avoiding albumin outwith controlled studies.

Blood pressure (BP) is an unreliable sign of circulatory compromise in children. Up to 40% of the circulating blood volume needs to be lost before the blood pressure will fall. A falling blood pressure is a late sign and indicates a failure of compensatory mechanisms to maintain perfusion to vital areas. Once BP falls, early and urgent treatment is indicated if permanent harm is to be avoided.

While the medical staff are assessing the airway, breathing and circulation, the nursing staff should help get the child undressed and should attach a cardiac monitor and a pulse oximeter.

As a result of this initial assessment one should find oneself in one of the following situations:

1. a child in cardiac arrest;
2. a traumatized child who requires further trauma orientated resuscitation;
3. an unstable child with continuing airway, breathing or circulatory compromise associated with underlying pathology.

CARDIAC ARREST

Cardiac arrest is rare in the pediatric population. Common causes include sudden infant death syndrome, trauma, drowning and asphyxia.[33]

Cardiac arrest in children is primarily asystolic in nature. Occasionally electromechanical dissociation [(EMD) also known as pulseless electrical activity (PEA)] or ventricular fibrillation (VF) is present.[33] It is important to begin resuscitation as above but consider definitive drug and fluid therapies as indicated by the underlying rhythm.

The outcome of cardiac arrest in children is dismal, particularly when it occurs in the community.[34] Children who sustain cardiac arrest in the emergency department have a better outcome than those who arrest in the community, but worse than those who arrest in hospital.[35] Prolonged hypoxia, hypoglycemia and acidosis in addition to the underlying disease process, all contribute to cell death particularly in the myocardium and brain making restoration of vital functions difficult. Even if cardiac function is restored the prolonged insult to the brain usually leaves the child with permanent and usually profound neurological deficit.

ASYSTOLE

Asystole is characterized by a pulseless, apneic child associated with no complexes on the cardiac monitor. It is important to confirm that this is so by going through the following procedure;

1. turning up the gain on the cardiac monitor;
2. ensuring that all the connections are made;
3. checking that the monitor is not connected to 'paddles'.

The recommended sequence for dealing with asystole is found in Figure 35.2.[36]

PULSELESS ELECTRICAL ACTIVITY (PEA) [PREVIOUSLY KNOWN AS ELECTROMECHANICAL DISSOCIATION (EMD)]

PEA is associated with a pulseless, apneic child and often bizarre complexes on a cardiac monitor. This may be associated with underlying pathology such as pneumothorax, cardiac tamponade, electrolyte imbalance, hypovolemia and hypothermia. Treatment should be aimed at correcting these underlying disorders. An algorithm for treating EMD can be seen in Figure 35.2.

VENTRICULAR FIBRILLATION (VF)

VF is much rarer in children than in adults. Recent reports have indicated that it might be more frequent than once suspected.[37,38] An algorithm for treating ventricular fibrillation can be found in Figure 35.2.

STOPPING RESUSCITATION

The decision to terminate resuscitation can be difficult. Children who have been poisoned, drowned or who are hypothermic should have active resuscitation continued for considerable time. This will usually occur within the intensive care setting with continuing resuscitation during transit. Post-traumatic cardiac arrest has a very poor prognosis and prolonged attempts at resuscitation should be avoided. Similarly sudden infant death syndrome should not lead to unduly prolonged resuscitation attempts.

APPROACH TO THE SEVERELY INJURED CHILD

Major trauma is a relatively rare occurrence in the pediatric population compared to the adult population. Of children who die, 80% will be dead on arrival of the paramedical team at the scene, a fact which

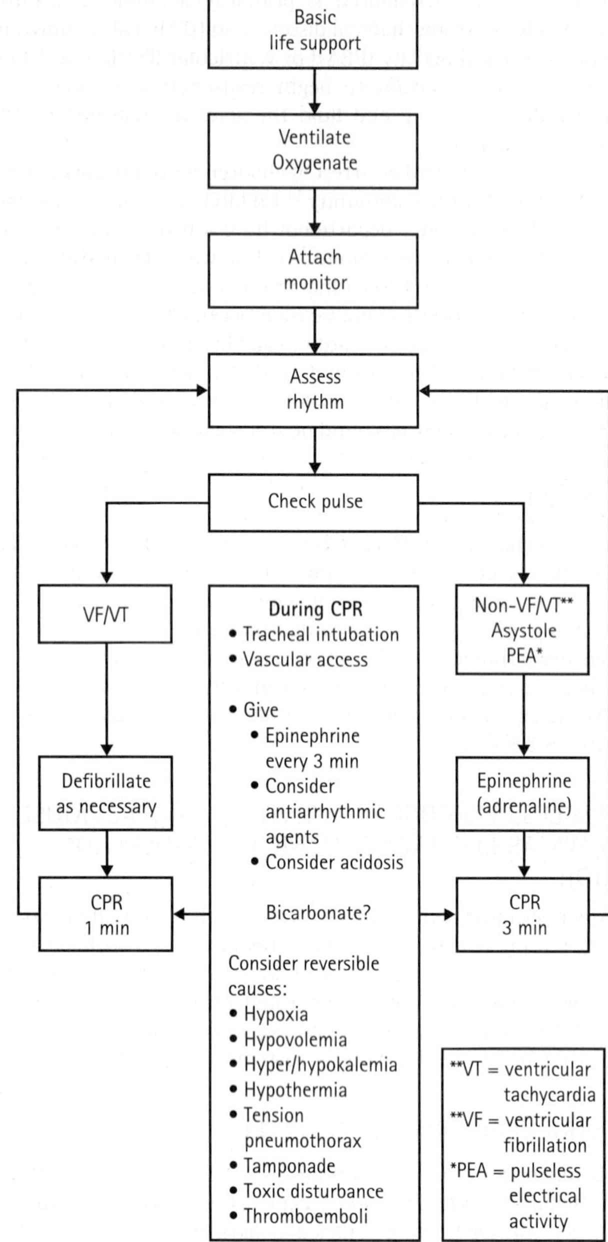

Fig. 35.2 Algorithm for management of pediatric cardiac arrest. (Adapted from Resuscitation Council (UK)[36] with permission)

makes accident prevention all the more important. The role of paramedical intervention at the scene has been discussed earlier.

As with other forms of illness care of the airway, breathing and circulation are of paramount importance. *One of the major differences however, is that traumatized children are at risk of having damage to the spinal column, particularly the cervical spine.* In particular this means that one has to be able to perform airway-opening maneuvers without excessive movement being involved in the cervical spine area. Measures such as chin lift without head tilt are important. Oropharyngeal airways are important adjuncts to the process.

SCIWORA

SCIWORA is an acronym for Spinal Cord Injury WithOut Radiological Abnormality. This is a rare finding but has a potentially horrendous outcome.[39]

PATHOPHYSIOLOGY

Relative laxity of spinal ligaments associated with underdevelopment of the articular facets of the vertebrae in the spinal column allow excessive movement to take place during severe hyperflexion/extension injuries. This results in compression of the spinal cord with subsequent damage. The column will return to its normal anatomy without any evidence of fracture or subluxation being present. Normal X-rays therefore in an unconscious child should not lead one to assume that there is no possibility of spinal cord injury.

IMPLICATIONS FOR CLINICAL PRACTICE

If the child is awake and is able to move all four limbs then SCIWORA is unlikely to be present.[39] However, in those children who have an altered level of consciousness, SCIWORA must be suspected. In these children full spinal column immobilization measures must be implemented until such time as the spine can be cleared either radiologically or clinically. Simple measures to immobilize the spine will include: use of sand bags or other similar sized objects to immobilize the head; taping the head to a spinal board; and immobilizing the head on the shoulders using hands and arms. The airway should be assessed and opened in the simplest way possible and this should be carried out without moving the cervical spine (see above).

BREATHING

Breathing abnormalities are common following trauma. Causes include pneumothorax, hemothorax, rib fractures and gastric dilatation. Children with traumatic injuries should be given supplemental oxygen and any specific underlying disease treated as appropriate. A pneumothorax should be decompressed by needle thoracostomy (above). Gastric dilatation should be decompressed by a gastric tube. If a basal skull fracture is suspected the gastric tube should be passed orally rather than nasally to avoid inadvertent placement in the brain!

CIRCULATION

Problems with circulation may be due to hypovolemia, tension pneumothorax or cardiac tamponade. Hypovolemia is the most common, particularly after intra-abdominal injuries. Small babies may become hypovolemic from an intracerebral bleed but this is unusual and other causes must be sought. Some of the signs of hypovolemia are mimicked by trauma: in particular altered level of consciousness and poor peripheral pulses. A low blood pressure is a sign of great importance, indicating the need for urgent fluid replacement.

Intravenous cannulae should be inserted into large veins, ideally avoiding fractured limbs. At the same time blood should be taken for laboratory analysis. If the child is stable and blood is not required urgently a simple 'group and save serum' is all that is required. Where the child is unstable blood will be required urgently. Ideally this blood should be fully grouped and cross-matched but occasionally O-negative blood will be needed. If sufficient blood is obtained the rest can be sent for full blood count, serum amylase and possibly urea and electrolytes. The value of each in managing the child will depend on the nature of the injury, underlying illness and laboratory policies.

DISABILITY

Most head injuries are minor with the incidence of intracranial bleed being much less in the pediatric population than in the adult population.[40] As part of the first assessment one does not need to assess a complete coma score, e.g. the Glasgow Coma Scale. It is sufficient to document whether the child is *A*wake, responding to *V*erbal stimuli, responding to *P*ainful stimuli or *U*nresponsive (the AVPU scale). Pupillary reflexes may be documented but at this stage they will not alter management significantly. While the medical team are assessing airway, breathing, circulation and disability the nursing team should undress the child, apply a cardiac monitor and a pulse oximeter and prepare to assist with airway and i.v. access procedures. Surgical trays should be made available if required.

SECONDARY SURVEY

Once the airway, breathing and circulation have been addressed a full secondary survey of the child should be carried out. Every part of the body will be examined both visually and by palpation. Judicious use of plain X-ray, ultrasound and computed tomography (CT) will aid the diagnostic process. Minor injuries that may have been missed on the first brief survey will be detected and will lead to further treatment and investigation. Injuries that are commonly detected during the secondary survey include bleeding from the ear and nose, small pneumothoraces, gastric dilatation and minor fractures to the peripheries.

HEAD INJURY

Head injury is a significant cause of morbidity and mortality in the pediatric population.[41] The relatively large head changes the center of gravity and the head is one of the most commonly injured parts of the body in the pediatric population.

The causes of significant head injury include falls from a height, motor vehicle accidents and non-accidental injury.

While most children who sustain significant head injury will lose consciousness it should be borne in mind that hypoxia, hypovolemia or both are significant causes of altered level of consciousness. Sharples et al[42] have shown that children transferred to a central neurosurgical unit with head injury were more likely to die as a result of associated hypoxia and/or hypovolemia due to respiratory or circulatory distress than death from the head injury. It must be questioned whether these children actually needed to be transferred at all as the head injury was often a relatively minor part of the problem. It is extremely important to exclude respiratory or circulatory problems before diagnosing intracranial problems as the cause of the altered level of consciousness.

The role of the accident and emergency department in managing head injury is straightforward but it is important to grasp the concept of primary and secondary brain injury.

Primary brain injury occurs at the time of impact. Any damage done at this stage is usually irreversible. Secondary brain injury occurs early due to an extra insult, commonly hypoxia, hypovolemia and brain edema. Later infection, hydrocephalus and seizures may contribute substantially. The management of these later problems will fall to inpatient teams, but emergency staff need to be aware of their role in identifying circumstances where and when they are likely to occur. There is a complex relationship between the primary injury and these other secondary factors. As a result of the initial injury there will be a degree of swelling secondary to a normal inflammatory response. Localized brain injury which might occur if the child has been hit with a hard object such as a golf club or hammer, will result in a reasonably localized injury. Here the inflammation will be localized and will not cause generalized brain edema. At the other extreme is the small baby who is exposed to vigorous shaking (non-accidental injury). Here there will be diffuse brain injury with generalized inflammation throughout the brain. Postmortem examinations in this situation reveal multiple hemorrhages and diffuse brain edema which is often progressive and unstoppable. This malignant cerebral edema is almost impossible to treat and is usually the cause of significant morbidity and mortality associated with 'shaken baby syndrome'.[43,44] Most cases of head injury fall between these two extremes.

If the initial insult is associated with loss of consciousness then hypoxia will almost certainly follow as a result of an obstructed airway, usually from the tongue obstructing the oropharynx, or from vomitus entering the lungs. This will in turn cause cerebral anoxia with resultant cell damage and death and lead to a generalized inflammatory response with a variable degree of cerebral edema being present. The same situation will occur with other causes of hypoxia, e.g. pneumothorax, pulmonary contusion.

A decrease in perfusion pressure to the brain secondary to hemorrhage or other cause of hypovolemia will result in failure to deliver glucose and oxygen to the brain leading to an equivalent situation. Again as the inflammation increases the intracranial pressure also increases and unless there is adequate circulatory drive to perfuse the brain, a vicious circle ensues.

The primary role of the accident and emergency department therefore is to ensure that the airway is open; that ventilation is maximized and that oxygen saturations are maintained between 95 and 100%; and to maintain circulation to enable cerebral perfusion to be normalized if possible.

By the time the child gets to accident and emergency a degree of intracranial swelling may already have taken place. In the early stages this will usually be due to an intracranial hematoma. Extradural, acute subdural or intracranial bleeds can all produce considerable pressure effects. It is important to recognize that children can sustain an extradural hematoma in the absence of fractures to the middle meningeal region in contrast to the adult population and normal skull X-rays therefore can be misleading.[45] The role of the accident and emergency department is to ensure the airway, breathing and circulation are maximized and that any other life threatening injury is identified and controlled. Only then should the child be transferred to the scanning suite when the formal diagnosis can be made. There will often be a dilemma between surgical hemostasis (e.g. from a ruptured liver or spleen) and management of significant intracranial hematoma. It is imperative in these situations to control the circulation and to ensure brain perfusion is maximized to reduce the effect of secondary brain injury from hypoxia and/or hypovolemia. This tension is not easy to resolve and takes considerable experience and seniority to ensure the correct sequence of events occurs.

With CT there is often evidence of raised intracranial pressure and no evidence of intracranial bleed. In this situation one is dealing with cerebral edema and several mechanisms exist to try to reduce the pressure including hyperventilation to maintain a $PaCO_2$ of about 4 kPa; use of mannitol or furosemide (frusemide) (or other loop diuretic) and sedative techniques such as barbiturate anesthesia. It should be noted that most of these measures only work on a normal brain and are of little benefit at best.[29] Use of these agents should be discussed with the neurosurgeon.

The accident and emergency department is responsible for identifying basal skull fractures by clinical examination. Physical signs that indicate a basal skull fracture include 'panda eyes' (racoon eyes), blood or cerebrospinal fluid from the nose or ears or 'Battle's sign' (bruising over the mastoid process). Basal skull fractures are open fractures and there is a high risk that infection will supervene. This will usually supervene between 12 and 24 h but may be later. The use of antibiotics for the management of basal skull fractures is controversial. There is no clear evidence that antibiotics will reduce the chance of meningitis but this should be discussed with the local neurosurgical unit.[46] Many children will have seizures subsequent to the head injury. This can result in hypoxia with the inherent risks discussed above. After supplying oxygen and assisting ventilation the fit should be stopped using diazepam 0.2 mg/kg. Assessment of the level of consciousness is now difficult and these child should undergo CT scanning. Phenytoin 15 mg/kg may be used to reduce subsequent seizures after discussion with the neurosurgical unit.

Once a child has had a secure airway established, oxygenation is maximized and circulation and perfusion restored to normal, the child should be transferred for definitive diagnosis to the CT suite under stringent transfer conditions. Transfer from the safety of the resuscitation room should not be commenced until full transfer protocols have been instituted. Transfer from the accident and emergency setting to the scanning suite is just as dangerous as travelling from one center to another.

THORACOABDOMINAL INJURIES

Thoracoabdominal injury is relatively rare in the pediatric population compared with the adolescent and adult population. Most injuries are blunt although increase of firearms has meant that penetrating thoracoabdominal trauma is rising.[23] Many children with major thoracic injuries will die before reaching hospital although improvements in prehospital care may mean that an increasing number may survive. Injuries that fall into this category include traumatic dissection of the aorta and massive tension pneumothorax.

TRAUMATIC DISSECTION OF THE THORACIC AORTA

This is typically caused by rapid deceleration injury and most children will die in the prehospital phase. If they survive to reach hospital the diagnosis can be suspected by the presence of a widened mediastinum on a chest film associated with fractures of the upper ribs. It is best confirmed by either arteriography or CT. If suspected the child should be transferred to a thoracic surgical center.

TENSION PNEUMOTHORAX

Tension pneumothorax is treated by the insertion of a large bore needle into the second intercostal space on the affected side. Signs of tension pneumothorax include signs of respiratory distress; distended neck veins and absent breath sounds on the affected side. Once the pneumothorax is drained using the needle a formal chest drain should be inserted and connected to an underwater seal as soon as possible. Drainage of a pneumothorax on one side may reveal the presence of a lesion on the other side and this should be treated appropriately.

MODERATE CHEST INJURY

The use of seat belts and seat restraints has led to an increase in chest wall bruising due to the seat belt physically restraining the child. Children who have seat belt abrasions to the chest and abdomen have been subjected to quite considerable deceleration forces. While the mostly likely thoracic injuries will be fractured clavicle with or without a fractured sternum, it should be borne in mind that underlying myocardial contusion is possible. This is extremely difficult to detect clinically. The presence of slightly abnormal electrocardiograms (ECGs) and raised cardiac enzymes are unreliable. If there is any doubt the child should be admitted for a period of observation with continuous cardiac monitoring.

Fractured ribs are rare in the pediatric population. If seen in the infant or toddler group non-accidental injury should be suspected. Management is required for relief of pain. If there are more than three ribs fractured on one side the child should to be admitted to an intensive care unit for intercostal blocks to be administered. Bilateral rib fractures may lead to a flail chest but this is rare in children.

ABDOMINAL INJURY

Blunt trauma is the usual cause. Penetrating trauma increases in frequency as children get older. Blunt trauma can result in hemorrhage and loss of perfusion from rupture to solid organs such as spleen, kidney and liver; or peritonitis from injury to the bowel and pancreas. With each of these a strong index of suspicion is needed as early on the child can have minimal abdominal signs, but will subsequently develop significant problems. This is particularly so of pancreatitis and bowel perforation where peritonitis can take between 6 and 12 h to develop.

Intra-abdominal hemorrhage should be considered in any child who shows evidence of circulatory collapse following trauma. Clinical diagnosis is unreliable and imaging is almost certainly indicated particularly if the child is stable. Ultrasound is a useful screening tool. In skilled hands small amounts of free fluid can be detected. If free fluid is present then CT with contrast is indicated. Children who are unstable should have intra-abdominal bleeding suspected and treated according to the accompanying diagram (Fig. 35.3). Hepatic and splenic trauma will usually be treated conservatively provided the child remains stable.[47] A full evaluation of the solid organs should be made using computed tomography if any injury is suspected on ultrasound examination.

SEAT BELT INJURY

A seat belt usually involves three point fixation with a lap belt and harness. If children are restrained using a lap belt alone and are involved in a high speed collision there is a reasonable chance they will sustain a hyperflexion injury of the torso. This will usually result in intra-abdominal injury with a significant hepatic or splenic component. This will often be associated with a degree of spinal instability with fractures occurring in the L_1, L_2 region of the lumbar spine.[48] Any child who has a significant lap belt injury to the midabdominal region should have spinal injury suspected and should have full spinal immobilization carried out until the spine has been fully cleared both radiologically and clinically (see SCIWORA as above).

ORTHOPEDIC INJURY

It should be stressed that orthopedic injuries are a long way down the order of treatment. Priority should be given to airway, breathing and circulation prior to doing anything with orthopedic injuries.

Orthopedic injury following trauma is common. Within the accident and emergency department there are three aspects that should be considered:

1. recognition of the fracture;
2. identification of associated soft tissue injury which may cause compromise to the limb;
3. splintage and analgesia.

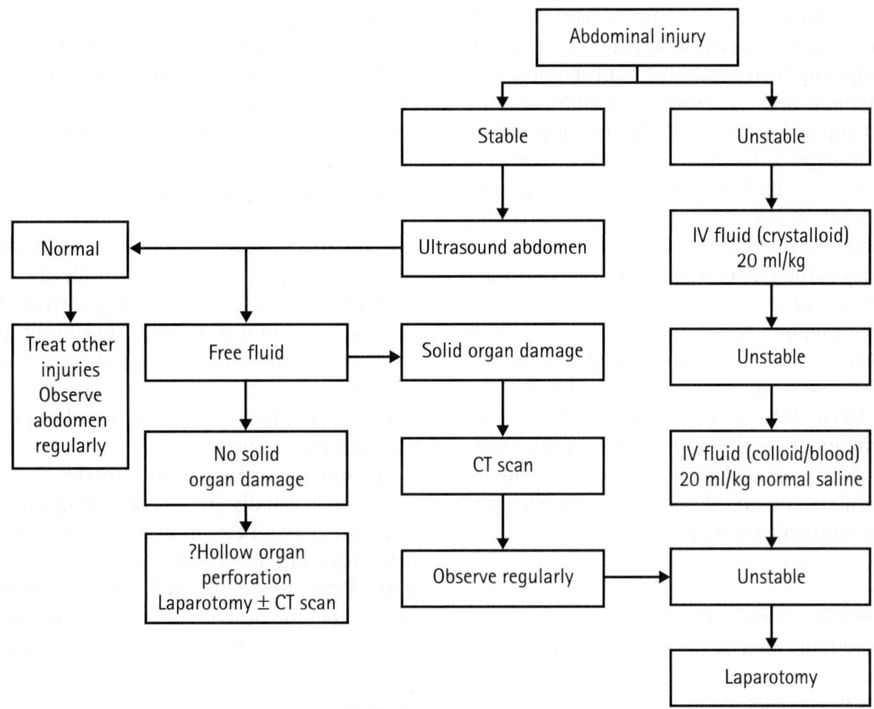

Fig. 35.3 Management of blunt abdominal trauma.

RECOGNITION OF THE FRACTURE

If a bone is bent, it is broken! Of more concern is the occult undisplaced fracture. Such fractures can bleed into tight fascial compartments with subsequent compartment syndrome. Vascular compromise is particularly common with fractures of the elbow, where the brachial artery may be involved, and the tibia. If there is any concern about the presence of an occult fracture the area should be X-rayed to either confirm it or rule it out.

With all fractures the distal pulses should be palpated and distal neurological function should be checked. If the perfusion is adequate distal to the fracture site then all that is needed is for the limb to be splinted until life threatening conditions such hypoxia or hypovolemia are corrected. Nerve injuries need to be noted and examined further when the child is stable.

IDENTIFICATION OF ASSOCIATED SOFT TISSUE INJURY

Soft tissue injuries associated with fractures include:

1. tissue loss;
2. open wounds;
3. vascular damage;
4. nerve damage;
5. tendon damage.

Tissue loss and open wounds associated with fracture will lead to infection in the bone if not adequately treated and debrided. The accident and emergency department is not the place to start this process but the wound should not be ignored. It is sufficient to assess the distal pulses and neurological function and as long as these are intact, dress the wound with a disinfectant dressing and leave further management to the orthopedic department. Broad spectrum antibiotics effective against Gram positive, Gram negative and anaerobic organisms are important. Local policies determine which antibiotics are given. Tetanus prophylaxis is also important if the patient is not fully immunized.

ANALGESIA

Analgesia in children with long bone fracture is greatly under used. There is often a fear of masking intra-abdominal injury or of aggravating conscious level with head injury. Both of these are inadequate reasons to withhold analgesia in a child who is in considerable pain. Two methods of analgesia exist in this situation:

1. local and peripheral nerve block;
2. intravenous opiate.

LOCAL AND PERIPHERAL NERVE BLOCK

The femur is most amenable to this management strategy. Successful block can be obtained by infiltrating a long acting anesthetic such as bupivacaine around the femoral nerve where it passes under the inguinal ligament lateral to the femoral artery. This will take 5–10 min to work [and can be preceded by a more fast acting local anesthetic such as lidocaine (lignocaine) or prilocaine]. If epinephrine (adrenaline) is used great care must be taken not to inject epinephrine (adrenaline) into the femoral artery which is adjacent to the nerve. Some authors advocate the use of sciatic nerve block for tibial fractures. To be effective however, this requires sophisticated equipment which is not always available within the accident and emergency setting.

INTRAVENOUS OPIATE

In trauma situations opiate analgesia should always be given intravenously. Recent reports on the efficacy of intranasal diamorphine should be treated cautiously. These reports compared intranasal diamorphine against intramuscular.[49,50] There is no place for the intramuscular route as absorption is unreliable. Whether i.v. opiate will be replaced by intranasal has yet to be established.

The weight of the child should be estimated by whatever means possible and the appropriate dose of opiate obtained. This should be further diluted to 10 ml. This can then be titrated 1 ml at a time over a period of 10 min to maximal effect. As soon as the child becomes settled the administration can be stopped and a further bolus given at intervals to maintain analgesia. Usually at this stage the pain drive will be sufficient to keep the child awake and to counteract any possible diminution of level of consciousness. If there is any concern subsequently about the ability to assess either level of consciousness or the abdomen then naloxone can be used to reverse the opiate. This is rarely necessary.

Once analgesia has been administered then the fractured limb should be splinted until the child can be brought to theater by the orthopedic surgeons. Splintage is an important consideration for analgesia in injured children. One of the major challenges for pediatric emergency departments is the absence of commercially available splints suitable for all the different shapes of children. Often these have to be fashioned on an ad hoc basis from plaster of Paris or some other newer synthetic casting material.

BURN CARE

Burns are a common problem in children. Two broad issues need to be addressed:

1. the burn injury (by whatever cause);
2. complications such as smoke inhalation, hypothermia, toxic shock syndrome.

Although both issues can occur together, usually one or the other is the main problem on initial presentation to the accident and emergency department. There are many etiologies for burn injury (Table 35.2). No matter what the cause, the approach to a burn injury is the same. The airway, breathing and circulation should be assessed and looked after as in all previous circumstances. Once these have been addressed it is important to identify the size of the burn. Management of the burn will depend on the following factors:

1. area involved;
2. depth of the burn;
3. site of the burn.

AREA OF THE BURN

Small burns, i.e. less than 5% of total body surface area (TBSA), can be managed on an outpatient basis provided that the burn is superficial, does not involve a significant area and there are no complications present.

Treatment will consist of analgesia, usually oral, and dressings according to local policy. One method of dressing the burn is to use tulle gras impregnated with mupirocin, which is an effective anti-staphylococcal agent. Once the burn is greater than 5% TBSA analgesia requirements will usually necessitate admission and i.v. opiate will be required. Whether the wounds are dressed or left open is dependent on local practice. Once the burn is greater than 10% TBSA then the child will need i.v. rehydration according to local formulae, e.g. Muir and Barclay formula.

Table 35.2 Causes of burn injury

1. Wet heat	Scald
2. Dry heat	Flame Hot surface
3. Radiation	Ultraviolet (sunburn) Iatrogenic (as radiation treatment in oncology)
4. Chemical	Acid Alkali Corrosive
5. Electrical	

DEPTH OF THE BURN

Burns can be classified into superficial, partial thickness and full thickness. Superficial burns include those with erythema only or with small amounts of blistering. Partial thickness burns are those that have a significant area of blistering, with either blisters intact or spontaneously burst. Full thickness burns present as white avascular areas that are insensitive to touch (it is not usually very kind to touch burns in children and inspection is usually all that is required for diagnosis).

In reality a mixture of superficial, partial thickness and full thickness is usually present depending on the burning agent and the duration it has been in contact with the skin. In general all full thickness burns should be referred to a plastic surgeon for immediate assessment and treatment. Partial thickness burns may be suitable for outpatient care if they do not extend over a large surface area. Treatment is as discussed above.

SITE OF THE BURN

Burns to the face, airway, mouth, pharynx, buttock and perineum, hands and feet and any circumferential burn to either the trunk or a limb need to be treated with a great deal of caution. Burns in any of these areas need to be referred to a burns specialist for inpatient treatment. Burns to the face and airway in particular, may require admission to an intensive care unit as the risk to the airway is quite considerable.

COMPLICATIONS OF BURNS

In the accident and emergency department it is important to identify those children with complications such as smoke inhalation, hypothermia or those with burns possibly from non-accidental injury.

SMOKE INHALATION

Smoke inhalation is a complex entity with several mechanisms:

1. inhalation of toxic fumes such as carbon monoxide and/or cyanide;
2. local action of soot and other organic particles;
3. chemical burns from acids and other compounds.

Carbon monoxide poisoning and cyanide lead to asphyxia due to red cells being unable to release oxygen. It is the leading cause of death following house fires. Children who are suspected of having carbon monoxide poisoning should be resuscitated with 100% oxygen. If cyanide poisoning is suspected then treatment with standard cyanide kits is suggested either with dicobalt edetate if the child is comatose and asystolic or sodium nitrate and thiosulfate solutions if the child is comatose but still perfusing.

Bronchial lavage may be considered if particulate matter or acids are considered to be present in the airway.

The net result of the contamination is a fulminant inflammatory process leading to significant pulmonary edema. This can be of insidious onset and consequently all children who are suspected of having had smoke inhalation should be admitted for a period of observation until such time as they are proved normal.

MANAGEMENT OF THE UNSTABLE CHILD WITH UNDERLYING PATHOLOGY

After securing the airway, breathing and circulation, the real challenge is to identify the actual disease process and the etiological factors that have led to the presentation so that the most appropriate therapy can be given.

The standard approach of taking a history and then doing a physical examination is often inappropriate. The history available at this stage can be scrappy and imprecise. Most information will be gained from a detailed physical examination. This is best done in a systematic fashion, excluding groups of illnesses in turn.

Patterns of illness include:

1. infection and life threatening infection;
2. seizure disorder and coma;
3. metabolic abnormalities;
4. cardiac lesions;
5. respiratory disorders;
6. surgical pathology;
7. poisoning.

INFECTION

Life threatening infection is relatively rare in the Western world where vaccination and immunization are widespread. Diseases such as diphtheria and epiglottitis have been almost eradicated with effective vaccination but in areas where vaccination is less good or has waned these diseases continue to form important causes of mortality. Meningococcemia continues to be one of the most important life threatening infections to appear acutely to the accident and emergency department.

When dealing with infection three broad age groups have to be considered:

1. those aged 0–3 months;
2. those aged 3 months–3 years;
3. those aged 3 years and over.

Children aged 0–3 months

Neonates and young infants have many of the problems related to infection. The symptoms with which these children present are many and varied.[51,52] They include going off feeds, failure to thrive, jitteriness and irritability. While many of these children will have an infection, other causes have to be considered. These include congenital anomalies such as congenital heart disease or inborn errors of metabolism or surgical causes such as intussusception and obstructed hernia.

Physical signs such as neck stiffness and bulging fontanelles are unusual in this age group as are blood parameters such as white cell count and preponderance of neutrophils to lymphocytes. Clinical suspicion therefore is the mainstay of diagnosis and if there is any doubt children should have blood cultures taken and antibiotic treatment started. These children are usually admitted until such time as the diagnosis is reached.

Children aged 3 months–3 years

The children at the lower end of this spectrum will still be prone to neonatal illness. Viral illness is more common than bacterial illness in this age group but underlying bacterial illness or bacteremia should still be considered. However, it is still important to recognize the child who is toxic, and who is 'not right'.[52,53] Physical signs are more precise, with these children often being pyrexial, tachycardiac and tachypneic. Signs such as neck stiffness are more reliable in the diagnosis of meningitis. Signs of chest infection, osteomyelitis and septic arthritis may be easier to detect.

Children aged 3 years and over

Significant bacterial disease is relatively rare in this age group but includes chest infection, septicemia, urinary tract infection and orthopedic infection. Meningitis and meningococcal septicemia are still relatively rare. Abdominal conditions are easier to diagnose in these children because these children are better able to communicate symptoms.

Meningococcal disease

Infection with *Neisseria meningitidis* is one of the most significant causes for a child to be critically ill. Often starting as a vague non-specific illness at any age this infection can kill within hours. The florid purpuric rash is often not present initially, more often developing from a subtle finding in the early stages. In the community, treatment should consist of intramuscular benzyl penicillin and urgent transfer to hospital with supplemental oxygen by mask. In the accident and emergency department i.v. access and fluid replacement will be added. Fluid volumes of 60 ml/kg may be needed (in 10–20 ml/kg bolus) to restore perfusion. A cephalosporin (e.g. cefuroxime or cefotaxime) will be added to penicillin to control infection. Prompt transfer to the intensive care unit should be arranged when inotropic agents may be added to the management.

Management of life threatening infection

These children should be resuscitated and blood taken for full blood count, urea and electrolytes, blood glucose and culture. Chest X-ray, urine culture and lumbar puncture may also be indicated. Care should be taken not to perform lumbar puncture on children who are unconscious as this may produce herniation of the brain through the tentorium with resultant brain death.

Intravenous antibiotics should be administered according to local sensitivity patterns and protocols. Children should be admitted to a high dependency or intensive care unit where inotropic support may be needed.

SEIZURE DISORDER

The list of underlying pathologies for patients presenting with seizure disorders is vast. Most will either be due to idiopathic epilepsy, a febrile seizure disorder or secondary to metabolic defects such as hypoglycemia or electrolyte disorder. Trauma should also be considered. Treatment should be aimed at stopping the seizure and at the same time trying to identify underlying treatable causes such as hypoglycemia and electrolyte imbalance. If fever is present this should be reduced as rapidly as possible.

Management of seizure disorder in the emergency situation

First line treatment is i.v. diazepam, 0.2 mg/kg to a maximum 0.6 mg/kg intravenously. This should be followed (if the seizure is not stopped) by a slow i.v. administration of phenytoin 10–15 mg/kg under ECG control. At this stage if the child is still fitting then consideration must be given to reducing intracranial pressure, paralysis and ventilation in order to control the seizure with additional anticonvulsants. Such management will need an intensive care/high dependency unit.

Blood sugar should always be tested by strip testing. If the blood sugar is low this may reveal an underlying metabolic disorder. Further blood should be taken along with urine to help diagnose metabolic anomalies if present and the child given 25% glucose 1–2 ml/kg.

COMA

Comatose children are particularly at risk of obstructing their airway so great care must be given to maintaining this. Once the airway is secured the underlying causes such as poisoning, epilepsy, head injury or other trauma, hypoglycemia or intracranial infection should be investigated. Treatable causes should be identified and treated appropriately and the child transferred to a high dependency area as soon as possible. This may involve transfer via CT scanning if intracranial lesion is suspected. If trauma is suspected, particularly non-accidental injury, the child should be treated as with any other trauma victim and resuscitated aggressively prior to transfer.

METABOLIC ABNORMALITIES

Diabetic abnormalities, either hypo- or hyperglycemia, are the commonest to present. Small babies may present critically ill as a result of an inborn error of metabolism. While these are relatively rare they should be suspected in any child who presents close to the neonatal period, particularly if there is an intercurrent infection suspected. A strong clue to this might be the presence of hypoglycemia. Diabetic emergencies should be treated as detailed under the diabetic section (Ch. 13).

CARDIAC LESIONS

Children with cardiac lesions present in one of two ways:

1. in heart failure;
2. in cardiac arrest.

Heart failure is often due to progression of cardiac abnormalities. Underlying disease processes such as renal failure may have to be considered. Supraventricular tachycardia is the commonest underlying cardiac dysrhythmia to cause heart failure, particularly in the younger age groups. The treatment of heart failure should be aimed towards maximizing oxygenation and reducing the fluid load. Any underlying dysrhythmia should be treated appropriately according to local guidelines. The child should be transferred to a high dependency area as soon as possible where future treatment can be monitored and inotropic support given if necessary.

The management of cardiac arrest is described earlier (p. 1775). The underlying causes may include hypertrophic cardiomyopathy or dysrhythmia.

RESPIRATORY DISORDERS

Common respiratory disorders to present include asthma, bronchiolitis, croup and foreign body in the airway. Recognition of respiratory distress/failure has been considered earlier. All children with respiratory disease should have oxygen delivery maximized and treatment directed to the underlying cause.

If it is suspected that a foreign body is wedged in the airway, the Heimlich maneuver or chest thrust maneuver may be necessary depending on the level of consciousness of the child.

SURGICAL CAUSES

Surgical causes of collapse are often forgotten in the accident and emergency department particularly in the younger age group. Intussusception and obstructed herniae commonly cause symptoms such as vomiting. This vomiting is not typical of that of gastroenteritis; it may only consist of one or two vomits. After that the child becomes unduly collapsed. Intussusception in particular can present with a child who is deathly pale but without much else in the way of physical signs. The classic signs of redcurrent jelly stool and a palpable mass are often absent.[54]

Pyloric stenosis may present with a dehydrated alkalotic child if the vomiting has been profuse.

If a pubertal girl presents in a collapsed state, two diagnoses should be considered – drug overdose (either intentional or accidental) and ectopic pregnancy. These may be related, i.e. the pregnancy is the reason for the overdose. In both situations resuscitation is vital. Pregnancy may be the result of child sexual abuse and this should be treated, if suspected, along local guidelines.

POISONING (see Ch. 32)

Poisoning in children is commonest between the second and third year of life. Children who are poisoned usually present with minimal signs or symptoms. The role of the accident and emergency department is to identify the child who is at risk of either airway or circulatory collapse and to deal with these problems accordingly. All doctors working in accident and emergency should have a good working knowledge of pharmacology of medications that are both prescribed and bought over the counter. The knowledge of the potential side-effects will help in determining which children can be discharged and those which need to be admitted for further care.

The role of gastric decontamination in this age group is difficult. The current trend is to move away from gastric lavage which is a particularly unpleasant process. The role of syrup of ipecacuanha has also been challenged. There is evidence to suggest that it will only be effective (if at all) if administered within 1 h of the ingestion. The current vogue is for decontamination using charcoal. Most children will actually drink charcoal despite it looking unpleasant and this probably is the method of choice for all children who actually require gastric decontamination.

Specific antidotes are available for only a few poisons. Staff working within the accident and emergency department should be familiar with these and their usage.

SAFE TRANSFER

All categories of ill and injured children will initially require transfer to the accident and emergency department. Subsequent to this they will need to be transferred from the resuscitation room to facilitate further investigation and/or treatment. This may be in-house or sometimes between facilities. There should be considerable liaison between the intensive care unit and the accident and emergency department to ensure that this transfer is safe and as fast as possible. Treatment and resuscitation may need to be continued throughout the transfer. In particular care to the airway, breathing and circulation will be mandatory. People experienced in all aspects of care who are able to intervene en route if required must manage the transfer.

CONCLUSION

The pediatric emergency medical system has many facets, all of which need to be coordinated to provide for the streamlined care of sick or injured children. The aim should be prevention if at all possible. If prevention is not possible then facilities must exist for the efficient care of all children within a seamless emergency medical structure capable of providing all aspects of emergency care and rehabilitation back to the community.

PEDIATRIC INTENSIVE CARE

INTRODUCTION

Pediatric intensive care is a specialist field which has roots in pediatric medicine and anesthesia and to a lesser extent, surgery. Intensive care is distinguished from high dependency or ward care by the level of observation and the level of intervention required by the patients. Close observation is assured by:

- The numbers of staff: at least one nurse per patient and at least one doctor awake and working on the unit at all times;
- The skill level of staff: only experienced pediatric intensive care nurses are allowed to work at the bedside and the resident medical staff have to have advanced resuscitation and airway skills. There are high levels of supervision from senior staff.

Higher levels of intervention take the form of:

- Continuous physiological monitoring: this will often involve additional circulatory access such as arterial and central venous lines but may also include a variety of other techniques, for example more invasive hemodynamic monitoring, indwelling oximetric catheters, intracranial pressure monitoring;
- Intensive care dependent techniques of organ-system support: the term 'intensive care dependent' meaning that it would be inappropriate to contemplate undertaking such support for a critically ill child without the level of monitoring and supervision available on the pediatric intensive care unit. Examples include mechanical ventilation, inotropic or mechanical circulatory support and renal replacement therapies such as hemofiltration.

Pediatric intensive care units cater for critically ill children from birth to 16 years of age but the age distribution is heavily skewed towards the lower age range. The median age of admissions is frequently less than 1 year and the mean is usually around 3 years. The units are predominantly geared towards emergency admissions since typically only about 30% of admissions are booked in advance in association with elective surgery or other procedures. The case mix bears comparison with the predominant causes of death in pediatrics, which themselves change with age. Infections and congenital abnormalities along with their attendant surgery figure prominently in young patients, whereas malignancy and trauma are commoner in older patients. Of admissions, 40% occur in the context of congenital heart disease whether they are new presentations, elective admissions after surgery or emergency admissions for other causes such as respiratory infection complicating pulmonary edema. Otherwise primary respiratory problems account for about 20% of admissions with strong seasonal and geographical variations. Major trauma also displays seasonal variation (lower in winter and highest during summer holidays) but accounts for up to 15% of admissions overall. Neurological problems (other than trauma) make up less than 10%. The contribution of other diagnostic categories is more varied, depending upon the allocation of neonatal surgical patients and other services. Survival rates amongst critically ill children are generally high (about 92% of admissions) compared to the intensive care of other age groups. The length of intensive care stay is another skewed distribution (most are of very short duration, median circa 24 h) but the mean varies from 2 to 4 days depending principally on the quality of local 'step down' (high dependency) facilities. This average length of stay is comparatively short compared to neonatal and adult intensive care.

Many intensive care admissions are critical emergencies and decisions to admit the patient under these circumstances are not difficult or often disputed. However, the apparently abrupt decline in a patient's condition is frequently the manifest decompensation of a process or processes that have been proceeding for some time and hence could, at least in theory, have been identified in advance. The final common pathway of cellular hypoxia/ischemia and organ dysfunction that leads to death in children is initiated by circulatory or respiratory failure and ends in asystole. Successful resuscitation from arrest is unlikely and the outcome when a cardiac output is restored is still very poor. The potential benefits of intensive care are therefore best realized by pre-emptive intervention to avert probable further deterioration.

Hence it is important to learn to recognize the sick child. Firstly, recognize ominous diagnoses for which the likely course of the disease is known (e.g. purpura fulminans in meningococcal septicemia). Alternatively, try to realize the severity of illness from basic clinical signs. Work on a system by system basis taking respiration and circulation first. The two key questions are:

1. How much work is being done? which then indicates a second question – how sustainable is this level of physiological effort? and
2. How effective is it? since ineffective effort will need to be supplemented sooner rather than later.

For example the work of breathing can be assessed by the respiratory rate, tidal volume and the apparent ease or otherwise of chest expansion. Look for the use of accessory muscles and the strain involved. Breathing may be difficult due to poor compliance or airway obstruction (listen for inspiratory stridor or expiratory wheeze) and there may be subcostal, intercostal, costal or sternal recession, tracheal tug or head bobbing, etc. Assess the effectiveness of breathing by the adequacy of chest expansion, the amount of oxygen required to avoid desaturation, conscious level, heart rate, presence of sweating and adequacy of peripheral perfusion as well as measurements of oxygen saturation and formal blood gases. Remember that cyanosis is a preterminal sign in respiratory failure and that premature infants respond to stress (including hypoxia) with bradycardia rather than the tachycardia otherwise expected first.

Once compensatory mechanisms have been exceeded, a precipitate and rapid deterioration occurs. Hence it is also very important to use recent *trends* in physiological observations as an indication of the patient's current condition and likely progress. Early intervention is far more likely to be successful and the use of thresholds for action usually causes delay even if they are based upon age appropriate norms and reference ranges.

In the acute presentation of critical illness, the ultimate cause (i.e. the diagnosis) may not be apparent. Hence a treatment plan may have to be devised that addresses all the possibilities until further information becomes available. The sequence of priorities is to Resuscitate, then Diagnose and Treat, i.e. *Resuscitation comes first*. If immediate resuscitation is not necessary, still concentrate on physiology/pathophysiology (in terms of work and effectiveness) to decide how and when to instigate specific organ system support and monitoring. Then proceed with investigations that may lead to more specific treatment. The ultimate diagnosis may be made over a broad timeframe and the patient may sometimes have left intensive care before the whole clinical picture is apparent.

POSTRESUSCITATION STABILIZATION AND TRANSFER

The initial resuscitation of acutely ill children is often described as being followed by a period of 'postresuscitation stabilization'. This may be prolonged and you may find it necessary to defer some aspects depending upon the resuscitation priorities. For example in severe trauma the resuscitation can involve emergency surgery after which the patient is moved to the intensive care unit. At this point reassess the patient and complete a secondary survey. The resuscitation may have also created problems that need to be identified and dealt with. Studies suggest that medically significant complications due to cardiopulmonary resuscitation are rare in children (< 3%). Those complications that have been reported include retroperitoneal hemorrhage, pneumothorax, pulmonary hemorrhage, epicardial hematoma, and gastric perforation.

Once resuscitation is complete or nearing completion, prepare the patient for longer term intensive care by revision/augmentation of airway and vascular access. For example oral intubation may need changing to nasal and if necessary replace intraosseous access with a central venous line and peripheral intravenous cannulae. An arterial line may be required. Good intensive care is about doing simple things well. Hence procedures such as the style of intubation, the manner of endotracheal tube fixation and the method of securing drips should all be controlled by unit protocol unless otherwise contraindicated. For example routine, non-essential revision of the intubation is unwise if the airway was precarious initially or if intubation was difficult to achieve. But in all other circumstances, especially if the patient is to be transferred, the most stable and familiar techniques should be employed.

Oxygenation is the highest priority but adequate minute volume must be provided to clear carbon dioxide. Assess both by serial measurements of arterial blood gases. Acidosis may have metabolic consequences such as hyperkalemia (a compartment shift) or pharmacological effects such as failure to respond to catecholamines. It may aggravate symptoms of poisoning with drugs that are weak acids. Correct any respiratory acidosis by increasing minute volume particularly if the $[H^+]$> 63 nmol/L (pH < 7.2). Treat the cause of any metabolic acidosis in preference to giving bicarbonate, since without treatment of the cause the acidosis will recur. Intravenous bicarbonate may be indicated to compensate for recognized bicarbonate losses (e.g. ileostomy fluid) or to recruit a pharmacodynamic response (e.g. if there is a poor response to inotrope therapy due to acidosis) but otherwise runs the risk of increasing the work of breathing (through CO_2 production) and aggravating intracellular acidosis ($CO_{2(aq)}$ and H^+ ions diffuse into cells more rapidly than bicarbonate).

A normal blood pressure is not a sufficient assessment of the cardiovascular system. Determine the adequacy of the circulation by assessing end organ (cellular) function using markers like urine output, mental state, degree of metabolic acidosis or serum lactate levels. Remember that resuscitation may have compensated for the presenting problem rather than resolved it. Furthermore a variety of other problems are common after acute resuscitation. Look for dilutional anemia, which can arise as a consequence of large intravascular volume boluses having been given during resuscitation. Give red cell transfusion priority if oxygen delivery is critical or compromised (one possible cause of metabolic acidosis). Also establish an appropriate ongoing intravenous fluid and electrolyte regime at this point which includes maintenance requirements, metered replacement of any deficit and comprehensive replacement of ongoing losses. If inotropic or chronotropic support is required then use titratable infusions of short acting agents in preference over longer acting agents whose effects may persist when the current hemodynamic state changes. Measure the blood glucose level since hypoglycemia is common and not detectable by clinical observation in the obtunded, sedated or otherwise critically ill child. The risk of hypoglycemia is increased in smaller and younger patients as a consequence of low glycogen reserves and a high basal metabolic rate. The dose of glucose in acute hypoglycemia is 0.5 g/kg. This dose must be followed by repeated assessment of the blood glucose level to check that a therapeutic effect has been achieved and that the resulting level is maintained. The normal maintenance requirement for babies is 6 mg/kg/min.

For all but the most straightforward of resuscitation scenarios the patient then requires further management on an intensive care unit. For all but the simplest cases this should be a specialist pediatric intensive care unit particularly if it is difficult to anticipate what the length of intensive care unit stay will be or if it is likely to be more than 24 h. Transfers within hospital or between hospitals usually occur after stabilization and are conducted without undue haste by a retrieval team from the pediatric intensive care unit. The use of a skilled and trained transfer team substantially reduces critical incidents and morbidity. The need for such transfer is entirely predictable and so detailed protocols should be prepared in advance including specified indications and provision for more urgent movement. Training in intensive care transport must be practical and is best provided by supervised episodes accompanying a skilled team. Trainees must become familiar with the modes of transport used and must attain higher levels of proficiency in equipment maintenance and repair than are necessary for clinical staff within a hospital environment. This is because technical backup is not available during transfers.

RESPIRATORY SYSTEM

INDICATIONS FOR MECHANICAL VENTILATION

One of the commonest reasons for arranging intensive care admission is a decision to start mechanical ventilation. Infants and children have less respiratory reserve than adults, which leads to a relatively high incidence of respiratory failure during severe illness. Respiratory support may be indicated:

- to secure the upper airway;
- to reduce the work of spontaneous breathing;
- to supplement gas exchange in respiratory disease;
- to achieve desirable hemodynamic effects;
- as an incidental requirement during sedation or anesthesia;
- due to neurological disease with or without respiratory complications.

If the patient has adequate airway protection reflexes it may be possible to provide mechanical support with minimal sedation and without intubation.[55] Select such patients carefully on their own merits. Successful nose mask or face mask ventilation requires a degree of patient cooperation and a pressure controlled device with the capacity to deliver high flows to compensate for any leak. Negative pressure devices, whether tank or cuirass, have the disadvantage of obstructing access to the patient. So called 'non-invasive' ventilation should only be provided in an environment where anesthetic and airway skills are readily available.

TECHNIQUE OF INTUBATION

The purpose of recognizing sick children is to enable appropriate early intervention. Hence intubation is usually performed as part of the induction of anesthesia. There are two basic approaches to the administration of an anesthetic: intravenous (usually a rapid sequence induction) and inhalation. Anesthetic skills, equipment and assistants are required for both. Rapid sequence induction is the preferred approach for most situations especially when regurgitation and aspiration of stomach contents are potential problems. It is contraindicated when the airway is compromised or when intubation may be difficult. In which case inhaled anesthetics are used.

Use a straight bladed laryngoscope to view the larynx in infants because its position is high (at the level of the C4 vertebra) and anterior compared to the adult. The large, soft, sigma shaped epiglottis can be kept under the blade if it obscures the laryngeal inlet. In older children, use a curved blade and lift away from you (as opposed to rotating) for a better view of the vocal cords. Once beyond puberty the larynx has assumed its adult position.

Use non-cuffed tubes in prepubertal children because the larynx has a gradually tapering shape narrowest in the subglottic region (behind the cricoid cartilage). The tube should be small enough to permit a small leak of air under pressure giving reassurance that excessive pressure is not being exerted on the subglottic tracheal mucosa where damage would otherwise lead to scarring and subsequent stenosis. After puberty the vocal cords are the narrowest part of the airway so use cuffed tubes in more mature children. The ideal position of an endotracheal tube tip is at the level of the sternoclavicular junction on the chest X-ray. In infants the trachea bifurcates at the level of T2. The tip of the tube will move significantly when the neck is flexed (moves down) or extended (moves up).

Always attempt to preoxygenate the patient and make sure that you are proficient in airway intervention techniques because any interruption in ventilation in babies and infants very quickly leads to hypoxemia. Their high metabolic rate means faster consumption of oxygen and greater carbon dioxide production. Furthermore normal ventilator settings must include the routine use of positive end expiratory pressure because atelectasis occurs early and at a higher volume relative to the functional residual capacity of older children and adults.

CHOICE OF VENTILATOR

Ventilators differ in relation to their power source, cycling characteristics, method of generating gas flow and the provision of gas supply for spontaneous breaths. The 'cycling' label is attached to the parameter (pressure, time, volume or flow) that determines when inspiration stops and expiration starts.

The choice of cycling method will affect the behavior of the ventilator as the patient's condition changes (Table 35.3).

The method by which gas flow is generated affects the choice of 'control' mode (e.g. pressure control and volume control) and hence the pattern of pressure and flow over time during inspiration. The terms 'support' or 'assist' are applied to modes where the breath is initiated by the patient then detected and supported by the ventilator. 'Mandatory' or 'control' breaths are initiated by the ventilator and may be blended with 'support' (e.g. synchronized intermittent mandatory ventilation with pressure support).

Table 35.3 Ventilator cycling

	Low compliance/high airways resistance	High compliance/low airways resistance
Volume cycled	V_T becomes a smaller % of cycled volume PIP increases	i.t. becomes short PIP falls
Pressure cycled	i.t. and V_T both fall V_T increases	i.t. becomes very long
Flow cycled	i.t. and V_T both fall	i.t. and V_T both rise
Time cycled	No effect	No effect

i.t., inspiratory time; PIP, peak inspiratory pressure; V_T, tidal volume.

For neonates there is a historical preference for using continuous flow, pressure regulated, time cycled ventilators. They are less susceptible to the fluctuations in tidal volume that are generated by the disparity between tidal volume and total gas volume in the ventilator circuit. They also do not generate large pressure fluctuations when the patient is uncoordinated with the ventilator and can function in the presence of a modest leak around the endotracheal tube. However, when compliance changes (e.g. as muscle relaxants wear off, or disease severity worsens) large changes in delivered tidal volume occur. Despite being intrinsically sensitive in the detection of circuit disruption, older models may not be capable of detecting absent tidal volume (endotracheal tube blockage). They must therefore be used in combination with an apnea monitor.

For older patients there is a historical preference for volume controlled ventilation. Nevertheless improved technology is making it easier and sometimes more appropriate to ventilate smaller patients with such devices. However, even with newer models, when compliance changes or airway obstruction develops, airway pressure escalates and the effective tidal volume is reduced as gas is compressed in the ventilator tubing.

VENTILATOR SETTINGS

Oxygenation is critical. Since oxygen is poorly soluble in water, the important factors in oxygen uptake across the lung are:

- the amount of blood flow (e.g. the cardiac output);
- the hemoglobin concentration;
- the effective surface area of the lung (after the effects of shunt, deadspace and ventilation–perfusion matching);
- the diffusion gradient for oxygen.

All of the above can be manipulated independently but the ventilator is only used for the last two. To increase the diffusion gradient for oxygen, increase the inspired oxygen concentration. The effective surface area of the lung can be increased (within limits) by increases in tidal volume and mean airway pressure. Some components of shunt may be relatively fixed and not respond to changes in ventilation. It is important not to overventilate under these circumstances. Deadspace is proportionately more significant at low tidal volumes. Ventilation–perfusion matching changes with posture and positioning of the patient as well as other changes in ventilation technique.

Carbon dioxide diffuses easily across respiratory membranes and comes in and out of solution easily. Hence the rate limiting step in removal across the lung is the speed with which equilibrated (alveolar) gas is replaced with fresh gas, i.e. the alveolar minute ventilation. Use tidal volume and respiratory rate to influence the minute volume and create responses in arterial carbon dioxide level. At low tidal volumes deadspace is more significant and reduces the effectiveness of each tidal volume in clearing carbon dioxide. There are therefore limits to how much a reduction in tidal volume can be compensated by increasing respiratory rate.

Wherever possible, choose ventilator settings that can be considered therapeutic, such as the use of higher levels of positive end expiratory pressure in pulmonary edema to reduce alveolar water content or in bronchomalacia to maintain patency of the conductance airways. Lung volume and $[H^+]$ (via carbon dioxide partial pressure; PCO_2) can also be used to manipulate pulmonary vascular resistance. The amount of work required to breathe is increased when compliance is poor or when airway resistance is high. Try to adapt ventilator settings to match the disease state and avoid complications such as gas trapping (dynamic hyperinflation), for example allow a long expiratory time if the patient has bronchospasm.

CONSEQUENCES OF VENTILATION

Endotracheal intubation and mechanical ventilation are not natural processes and are associated with hazards, which can be minimized by appropriate attention to detail. Choose the correct size and length endotracheal tube. Take care to ensure that the inhaled gases are humidified to 100% relative humidity at body temperature. Avoid high pressures and tidal volumes. Any ventilator settings that induce overinflation are likely to induce or aggravate lung injury although the specific settings involved will differ between restrictive and obstructive diseases. Peak pressure is far more dangerous than end expiratory pressure and many of the problems previously associated with peak pressure are as much to do with the associated high end inflation lung volume and tidal volume as anything else. Previously injured lungs are more susceptible to ventilator induced lung injury and if the disease is not homogenous it may be the less severely diseased segments that receive the greater insult.

NEWER VENTILATION STRATEGIES

In recent times the concept of minimizing the stress of mechanical ventilation has become pivotal in the ventilation of patients with respiratory disease. The appeal of novel approaches to ventilation is often based upon their potential (even if unproven) abilities in this respect. The simplest approaches include improved coordination between the ventilator and the patient. More complex approaches are aimed at providing increasing degrees of 'lung rest'. The conventional and best validated method of providing lung rest is extracorporeal membrane oxygenation (ECMO) which is a modified form of cardiopulmonary bypass. ECMO can be used to achieve total lung rest (gas exchange during prolonged apnea) and the circuit can be configured to provide pulmonary (venovenous cannulation) or cardiopulmonary support (venoarterial cannulation).

Examples of ventilation strategies with proposed benefits in terms of reducing ventilator associated lung injury include:

- Permissive hypercarbia: where (pressure limited) minute ventilation is minimized in the hope of reducing lung stress. To perform this technique, once hypoxia is overcome, allow arterial carbon dioxide levels to rise to limits dictated by the associated rise in hydrogen ion concentration (e.g. ≤ 63 nmol/L correlating with pH ≥ 7.2). Over time, metabolic compensation allows higher and higher carbon dioxide levels to be tolerated.[55–58]
- High frequency oscillation: these devices use the continuous distending pressure (mean airway pressure) to recruit and maintain lung volume. Gas exchange is achieved by a high frequency vibration (6–12 Hz). Minimal tidal volumes (less than deadspace) result from the amplitude of the vibration, which itself is highly attenuated within the respiratory tract, hence minimizing shearing forces.[56] Use the amplitude (ΔP) preferentially to control the partial pressure of carbon dioxide in arterial blood ($PaCO_2$). The fall in tidal volume as frequency increases attenuates carbon dioxide removal which is otherwise highly efficient.
- Inhaled nitric oxide[59–61]: in responsive patients, ventilation perfusion mismatch can be reduced by NO which causes vasodilatation in ventilated areas. Some cases of pulmonary hypertension may also respond.
- Liquid ventilation (usually in the form of perfluorocarbon assisted gas exchange)[62]: this technique involves first gradually replacing the functional residual capacity of the lung by slow instillation of perfluorocarbon during conventional ventilation. This causes bulk distension of the alveoli and considerable recruitment of lung volume. Subsequent tidal ventilation with 100% oxygen is more effective as the low surface tension at the perfluorocarbon : gas interface improves compliance.
- Intratracheal pressure release ventilation[61,63]: where expiratory flows are augmented increasing respiratory efficiency at lower tidal volumes and lower mean pressures.

WEANING VENTILATION

Improving respiratory function is reflected in the behavior of the patient and the ventilator. In the latter case the effects depend upon the mode of ventilation employed at the time. Improved compliance or airways resistance during volume controlled ventilation causes airway pressures to fall. With pressure controlled ventilation under the same circumstances, tidal volumes increase and the partial pressure of oxygen in arterial blood (PaO_2) may rise as the $PaCO_2$ falls. Effective tidal volume can be usefully expressed in relation to deadspace using end tidal carbon dioxide measurements. In flow cycled ventilator modes such as pressure support, the inspiratory time decreases as compliance improves. Close observation of the patient and regular blood gas measurement allows you to respond to these changes.

Start to deliberately wean patients from mechanical ventilation when the pathology or indication for ventilation is resolving or finished. The speed of successful weaning is dictated by the adequacy of the response and the skill lies in getting the best performance out of the partially dependent patient. The patient must be able to take over ventilation without excess energy expenditure, and there must be adequate respiratory muscle strength, hemodynamic stability and a good nutritional state. Only extubate electively when the patient:

- is hemodynamically and metabolically stable;
- is making effective efforts to breathe;
- is sufficiently awake and alert;
- has protective airway reflexes.

Prior to extubation, always ensure that there is adequate provision of equipment, medication and staff to deal with complications such as laryngospasm which might require urgent reintubation.

CARDIOVASCULAR SYSTEM

Another common reason to arrange intensive care admission is the need to perform invasive monitoring of the circulation using arterial or central venous lines. This need arises:

- as a wise precaution in case of potential instability, e.g. after major surgery or other trauma;
- in the treatment of shock such as during large volume fluid losses/replacement;
- when blood pressure is excessively high or low;
- when vasoactive drugs are being administered by infusion.

RECOGNITION OF SHOCK

Do not rely on blood pressure in the first instance or alone to assess the circulation. Shock is defined as inadequate perfusion of tissues (in particular oxygenation) and its severity is assessed in terms of end organ function. When flow measurements are available, the global delivery of oxygen to the tissues can be calculated as the product of the oxygen content of arterial blood and the cardiac output. But not all of this oxygen is available to the tissues. Factors that influence the distribution of blood also apply and may be particularly affected by disease. The two most sensitive and clinically useful organs in the assessment of the circulation are the brain and the kidney. Altered conscious level is an important sign of shock and up to the point of acute renal failure, urine output is a good marker of renal perfusion. The patient with severe cardiovascular dysfunction (shock) generally has peripheral pulses that are difficult to feel, poor capillary refill, cool extremities, decreased urine output and altered sensorium. A *low blood pressure is a preterminal sign* since blood pressure can be maintained by intense vasoconstriction even in the presence of a markedly reduced circulating volume. The fall in blood pressure thus represents decompensation and is out of control.

It is important to monitor fluid losses and replacement accurately. In the short term this can be approximated by the fluid balance but remember to extend the comparison over days. Weigh the patient regularly and match your impressions with clinical and laboratory observations.

RECOGNITION OF HEART FAILURE

Heart failure is distinguishable from shock. It is a more chronic condition in which the heart fails to respond adequately to its preload and hence fails to obey its normal Starling relation. There may be diastolic or systolic dysfunction or both and the problem may apply to specific ventricles or regions of myocardium. Fluid retention results from 'back pressure' as well as humoral responses to a reduced cardiac output. Although true heart failure can occur in children, most patients with signs that would represent heart 'failure' in an adult are in fact displaying the manifestations of a left to right shunt. These patients may have positively athletic cardiac function.

RECOGNITION OF CONGENITAL HEART DISEASE

Suspect congenital heart disease especially and most importantly in neonates with shock or cyanosis but also in patients with:

- murmurs;
- pulmonary edema;
- rhythm disturbances;
- abnormally severe symptoms from respiratory disease;
- failure to thrive.

Right to left shunts cause cyanosis and rarely cause murmurs because they are relatively low volume shunts occurring at low pressure. Left to right shunts cause pulmonary and ventricular volume overload. The loudness of the murmur is to some extent inversely proportional to the size of the shunt. Sustained high pulmonary blood flow causes pulmonary hypertension. Ventricular outflow tract obstruction (pressure overload) tends to cause ventricular hypertrophy. Ventricular hypertrophy is associated with decreased ventricular compliance (diastolic dysfunction). Congenital heart disease can produce many combinations of defects, which also evolve according to the loading forces they create.

It is essential to recognize duct dependent lesions. These present early in the neonatal period. Duct dependent pulmonary flow presents with cyanosis and duct dependent systemic flow with heart failure and/or shock in the first week of life. Both require an infusion of prostaglandin (typically 20 ng/kg/min) and urgent evaluation by a pediatric cardiologist.

TREATMENT OF SHOCK

The first line in cardiovascular resuscitation and support is an intravascular volume bolus of 20 ml/kg. Such preload augmentation should increase stroke volume and therefore blood pressure even if heart failure is suspected as well as shock. The most common cause of an inadequate response to this treatment is that the magnitude of the problem has been underestimated and inadequate fluid volumes have been used. Hence the protocol for repeating the boluses of intravenous fluid at least twice if there is an inadequate response. However, do not give excessive amounts of intravascular volume if heart failure is present. In rapid large volume resuscitations the central venous pressure is a useful guide to how the volume is being handled by the circulation. Palpating the liver edge can also help, hepatic engorgement suggests right ventricular volume overload.

Both myocardial contractility (and hence stroke volume) and heart rate are increased by catecholamines. The first line inotropic support started after the second or third fluid bolus is usually adrenaline (0.05–0.5 μg/kg/min) or dopamine (2–10 μg/kg/min). Cardiac output can also be influenced by manipulation of afterload (end systolic ventricular wall tension) for example by agents which affect the systemic vascular resistance. The term 'systemic vascular resistance' refers to a global approximation of the resistance of the circulation to blood flow. It is calculated after measuring cardiac output by dividing the pressure drop across the circulation by the measured blood flow. Reduction of afterload may improve cardiac output in conditions where there is a left to right shunt. Increases in afterload (e.g. using alpha adrenergic agents) are an important component of support in shock states such as septic shock when characterized by a low systemic vascular resistance.

The intrinsic response of the cardiovascular system both to disease and resuscitation depends upon the age of the patient and the nature and stage of palliation of any congenital heart disease as well as any intercurrent disease. The fetal circulation is characterized by the fetal connections, a high pulmonary vascular resistance and a low systemic vascular resistance. The neonatal (transitional) circulation is characterized by the potential persistence of all the fetal connections other than the umbilical vessels, reactive pulmonary vasculature and limited inotropic and chronotropic reserve; that is to say reduced capacity to increase contractility in response to catecholamines and a poor return in terms of cardiac output for increases in heart rate (despite a rate dependent cardiac output in bradycardia). The neonatal heart also displays muted (e.g. to potassium) or accentuated (e.g. to calcium) responses to various electrolytes and drugs compared to later life. In infancy and childhood the myocardium adapts progressively to its new loading conditions and develops an increased reserve to beta adrenergic stimulation.

In refractory shock, i.e. failure to respond to intravascular volume loading, it is crucially important to get accurate monitoring of the circulation. Then consider the following possible explanations:

- Overestimation of the filling pressures: both central venous and pulmonary capillary wedge pressures are heavily influenced by thoracic pressure and hence positive pressure ventilation. Use the end expiratory values in your evaluation.
- Systolic cardiac dysfunction: depression of the contractile state of the myocardium can occur with a range of common disorders, for example sepsis, acidosis, hypoglycemia, hypoxia or hypocalcemia. In addition, drugs (especially antiarrhythmics) can also decrease the contractile state. A hydrogen ion concentration greater than 63 (pH < 7.2) can decrease the effectiveness of catecholamines and may need to be corrected.
- Diastolic dysfunction: when the compliance of the myocardium is poor as can occur alongside depression of systolic function or more independently as a result of congenital heart disease, the end diastolic volume does not increase normally in response to fluid challenge, whilst the end diastolic pressure increases markedly. Poor myocardial compliance is aggravated by catecholamines.

- Extrinsic cardiac compression: tamponade can restrict atrial and therefore ventricular filling resulting in a low end diastolic volume and low cardiac output despite high measured filling pressures. Echocardiography rapidly detects pericardial fluid and in extremis, given a compatible history, a pericardial tap may be indicated as part of resuscitative efforts.

The problem may be specific to one ventricle, particularly in congenital heart disease. It is often wise to request the opinion of a pediatric cardiologist in patients with refractory shock. Left ventricular preload is commonly inferred from left atrial pressure after cardiac surgery or pulmonary capillary wedge pressure under other circumstances. Swan–Ganz catheters are available which are small enough to use in patients as young as 18 months.

THERAPEUTIC EFFECTS OF VENTILATION IN CIRCULATORY FAILURE

Patients in significant shock should be intubated and ventilated. Since this will probably involve the induction of anesthesia, take care to pick the right moment. There is no substitute for experience in these sorts of judgments. Anesthetic agents have cardiovascular side-effects and the best approach is usually to optimize resuscitation before anesthetic induction. In contrast when patients are deteriorating rapidly and are likely to continue to do so, early ventilatory support is a priority. Patients in shock require less anesthetic to suppress the central nervous system but they take longer to respond to intravenous injections of anesthetic agents because of the reduction in effective blood flow.

Positive pressure ventilation can have a variety of hemodynamic effects most of which are therapeutic for patients with normal anatomy but who have cardiovascular instability. The right ventricular preload is reduced by the rise in intrathoracic pressure. Left ventricular preload may be decreased as a consequence or increased as pulmonary venous blood is encouraged to leave the lung. The dominant effect can often be inferred from the systemic arterial pressure trace looking for effects reminiscent of a Valsalva maneuver or the opposite during inspiration. Left ventricular afterload is reduced by the effects of raised intrathoracic pressure on the ventricle and by encouraging diastolic arterial flow out of the thorax. The effects on right ventricular afterload depend upon the pervading pulmonary vascular resistance. Further cardiovascular benefits in terms of the treatment of shock are achieved by the decreased work of breathing and decreased oxygen consumption associated with sedation and paralysis. Reduction in alveolar water content can also improve lung compliance and oxygenation.

There are a wide variety of situations in pediatric intensive care where cardiopulmonary interactions dictate management, for example patients with high pulmonary vascular resistance and right to left ductal shunts, patients with univentricular physiology or patients with cavopulmonary connections and hence passive pulmonary blood flow as a result of cardiac surgery. Patients with low or critical pulmonary blood flow may have extraordinarily compliant lungs and experience symptomatic reductions in cardiac output during positive pressure ventilation. Patients with high pulmonary blood flow have predictably non-compliant lungs.

CENTRAL NERVOUS SYSTEM

LEVEL OF CONSCIOUSNESS

Determine the patient's level of consciousness in a reproducible fashion. Describe the stimulus required to elicit a response and then describe the organization or sophistication of that response. At lower and lower levels of consciousness, greater stimuli (voice then pain) achieve less organized reactions. The commonest nomenclature used to describe this relationship is the Glasgow coma score which breaks the responses into three groups: 'eyes' (4 point scale), 'vocalization' (5 point scale) and 'motor' responses (6 point scale). There are a variety of adaptations for preverbal or intubated patients. The AVPU classification distinguishes patients who are *A*lert, respond to *V*oice, respond only to *P*ain or who are *U*nresponsive. Painful stimuli administered peripherally can elicit spinal reflexes and mislead the unwary as to the sophistication/localization of the response. Avoid this by causing pain in a cranial nerve distribution, e.g. by pressure under the supraorbital ridge and documenting the response particularly of any limb movement. Patients who respond only to deep pain (Glasgow coma score ≤ 8) or who are unresponsive (Glasgow coma score 3) are unlikely to have adequate airway protection reflexes and are likely to require intubation.

LEVEL OF AWARENESS

Sedation (hypnotic) agents obtund the patient, i.e. induce mental blunting often with amnesia. They are used to induce stupor so that symptoms and treatments are better tolerated. Sedation is usually provided by continuous or intermittent doses of benzodiazepines. Although these agents dull the responses they do not induce normal sleep and are not analgesics.

PAIN CONTROL

Analgesia is a high priority in intensive care and the need to provide adequate analgesia is arguably increased by the use of sedative or anesthetic agents. Conscious children naturally use distraction and play as coping mechanisms for dealing with pain and distress. They can be encouraged in their efforts by diversion therapy. Stress and anxiety amplify children's apparent distress. Anything that can minimize such stress such as the presence of a parent, a full stomach, or a degree of sedation is to be encouraged. Assessment of pain control may be difficult; first because of the patient's age and communication skills and secondly because of appropriate sedation which impedes the response even to age-appropriate pain assessment tools. It is best to anticipate and assume that pain is present and to treat it accordingly with a morphine infusion.

TRAUMATIC BRAIN INJURY

In severe diffuse brain injury, particularly that caused by trauma, cerebral edema worsens over the first 24–48 h and is accompanied by a loss of the capacity to autoregulate cerebral blood flow. It therefore becomes highly important to keep parameters that influence cerebral blood flow as stable as possible. These include the cerebral perfusion pressure, the $PaCO_2$, the PaO_2, regional metabolic demand and autonomic activity.

'Neuroprotective' intensive care should be instigated after significant brain injury (e.g. Glasgow coma score < 12). The intention is to minimize secondary brain injury but as yet there are no therapeutic approaches outside those aimed at adequate perfusion and oxygenation of the brain. The strategy includes:

- elective sedation;
- mechanical ventilation with strict attention to adequate oxygenation and avoiding hypercarbia (keep $PaCO_2$ within the normal range);
- cranial CT scan in the early *postresuscitation* phase of management to determine the need for neurosurgery and the subsequent management of raised intracranial pressure;

- nursing with the head midline and with a 30 degree upwards head tilt and avoid stresses that increase intracranial pressure;
- circulatory support to maintain the cerebral perfusion pressure.

Maintenance of the cerebral perfusion pressure requires intracranial pressure monitoring. This enables the detection of raised intracranial pressure as well as allowing one to determine the adequacy of cerebrovascular autoregulation. Intraventricular drains are preferred for this purpose firstly because they are more reliable than the alternatives. The second advantage of an intraventricular drain is that it enables venting of cerebrospinal fluid to control recalcitrant peaks of intracranial pressure from other causes such as cerebral edema. The treatment of raised intracranial pressure depends upon the cause. Neurosurgery may be required for space occupying lesions such as hematomata. Hydrocephalus can be treated via the intraventricular drain. However, the first line treatments for cerebral edema are medical maneuvers designed to reduce the cerebral water content (fluid restriction or infusion of hypertonic saline or mannitol). If raised intracranial pressure is problematic or unresponsive then barbiturates (thiopental) should be used for sedation since these agents uncouple the relationship between cerebral blood flow and the metabolic consumption of oxygen. The use of barbiturates may necessitate increased use of pressors to maintain the cerebral perfusion pressure. The ultimate management for raised intracranial pressure that cannot be lowered by medical means is craniectomy (removal of bone flaps to allow cerebral expansion at lower pressure).

Anticonvulsants should be given in traumatic brain injury particularly if any component of contusion or hemorrhage is seen in the brain substance on CT scan. Breakthrough seizures may only be detected by hemodynamic or pupillary signs and should be confirmed/monitored by electroencephalogram (EEG) or alternative electrophysiological monitoring and treated aggressively. The natural tendency to become pyrexial should be counteracted by therapeutic cooling to normothermia in order to prevent increases in cerebral metabolic oxygen demand. The possible merits of cooling to varying degrees of hypothermia are currently under investigation.

The duration of neuroprotective intensive care is usually judged by the behavior of the intracranial pressure over time. A minimum period of 24 h after injury is wise since cerebral swelling increases over this period. Imaging techniques such as CT and magnetic resonance imaging (MRI) are insensitive when detecting raised intracranial pressure. After 10 days any opportunity to prevent secondary brain injury has probably passed and patients should be woken and weaned from support.

METABOLIC COMA

Many components of neuroprotective intensive care are routinely transferred from traumatic brain injury where their justification is far from complete, to other forms of encephalopathy where there is even less evidence of their utility. Whilst loss of cerebrovascular autoregulation may occur in both conditions, in metabolic coma the insult is cytotoxic rather than vasogenic and cerebral edema is frequently more persistent. Metabolic and infective causes of coma may also be preceded by delirium which is not a feature of traumatic brain injury.

SEIZURES

The diagnosis of 'status epilepticus' is made on the basis of the duration of continuous or consecutive seizures (30 min or more). The protocol for resuscitation of patients in status epilepticus culminates in barbiturate coma after a further 30 min of progressive treatment with lesser measures. This is usually achieved by intravenous induction and maintenance of anesthesia with thiopental and followed by transfer to the pediatric intensive care unit. Subsequent treatment on the intensive care unit depends upon the cause and prior duration of the seizures. Make rigorous attempts to detect potentially treatable causes such as hypoxia, fever, hypoglycemia, hypocalcemia, infection (do not perform a lumbar puncture in the acute phase after protracted seizures), poisoning, trauma, raised intracranial pressure and kernicterus.

Seizures that lasted for less than 2 h before admission are unlikely to be complicated by secondary cerebral edema and it is worth allowing sedation to wear off so that the patient can wake up and be extubated. The longer the history the greater the risk of complications such as cerebral edema, hyperthermia and rhabdomyolysis. Don't forget to perform fundoscopy to detect papilledema and to watch patients carefully for signs of hypertension or bradycardia (since the third component of Cushing's triad – hypoventilation – is masked by anesthesia and mechanical ventilation). A cranial CT may be warranted and if cerebral edema is present give mannitol and consider intracranial pressure monitoring.

Seizures that recur or persist on the intensive care unit can be highly problematic and the mortality and morbidity are appreciable. Persistent seizures imply an unresolved cause so comprehensive investigation is necessary. In recalcitrant cases it can be worthwhile monitoring the EEG during the acute phase of a new treatment to ensure that a sustained period of burst suppression has elapsed before trying to wean the dose of anticonvulsant. Trials of pyridoxine in infants with resistant seizures should also be monitored by EEG. If no diagnosis or specific treatment is forthcoming a variety of drug regimens can be tried to reach a state of seizure control without excessive obtundation. It is not appropriate to sedate patients to the point of anesthesia and nurse them on an intensive care unit when their seizures are due to an incurable or degenerative condition.

FLUIDS AND RENAL REPLACEMENT THERAPY

Fluid and electrolyte balance are covered elsewhere in the text. In general terms the tendency to fluid retention and edema in critical illness make fluid regimes on intensive care highly restrictive once intravascular volume is assured. There is also a low threshold for the use of diuretic and renal replacement therapies on the pediatric intensive care unit.

There are two approaches to conventional renal replacement therapy: peritoneal dialysis and extracorporeal circulation. In childhood the peritoneum has a greater surface area proportional to body mass making peritoneal dialysis more effective than it would be in older patients. Short term renal replacement therapy can also be provided by hemofiltration. The favored venovenous approach to hemofiltration minimizes the hemodynamic consequences of this approach. A variety of techniques are available. Water removal can be achieved by ultrafiltration without replacement fluid. Solute clearance is enhanced by higher ultrafiltration rates in which the solutes are removed by bulk flow. The high ultrafiltration rates are achievable when providing replacement fluid. It is this approach that is termed 'hemofiltration'. Hemodiafiltration is an attempt to increase solute removal by additional diffusion but this can be achieved with high volume hemofiltration (e.g. with prefilter administration of replacement fluid) or dialysis. The removal of larger molecules (e.g. protein bound moieties) from the circulation can be achieved by plasmafiltration.

These modalities are used in many more situations than just renal failure.[64–66] Renal replacement techniques are occasionally used electively, e.g. to allow large volume transfusions of clotting factors prior to liver transplantation in fulminant hepatic failure. They are also used therapeutically in inflammatory conditions such as the systemic inflammatory response syndrome (e.g. after cardiopulmonary bypass or in severe sepsis) and Guillain–Barré syndrome. Plasmafiltration and plasmapheresis have also been tried in a variety of 'desperate diseases' such as lupus nephritis and polymyositis, though with no evidence of benefit. The liver replacement device Molecular Adsorbents Recirculating System (MARS™) represents an alternative to plasmafiltration in the attempt to clear protein bound toxins. It uses adsorbent membranes and recycles the albumin it uses but its clearance profile has not been shown to be greater than plasmafiltration. Pediatric patients require smaller quantities of albumin replacement during plasmafiltration than adults because smaller exchange volumes are used.

HOST DEFENCE

Infections are a major cause of mortality in young children and immune suppressed individuals such as transplant recipients and those receiving cytotoxic chemotherapy. The invasive treatments and monitoring techniques used in intensive care increase the chances of nosocomial infection as do debilitating illnesses themselves. However, liberal antibiotic policies are a major stimulus for the generation and selection of multiresistant organisms. Normal intensive care procedures do not require antibiotic prophylaxis. Reserve antibiotic treatment for patients who have had procedures that do require prophylaxis, e.g. abdominal surgery, those with proven infection or those for whom the consequences of delay in treatment pending culture results are unconscionable. Use acute phase reactants and other tests (which predict positive cultures with varying degrees of success) to aid in decisions to withhold antibiotic treatment as well as decisions to commence.

A COMBINED ORGAN SYSTEM APPROACH TO CRITICAL ILLNESS

To conclude this section there follows a logical approach, consistent with the points covered above, to a disease with multiple organ system problems, in this case fulminant hepatic failure.

FULMINANT HEPATIC FAILURE

The typical history of patients with fulminant hepatic failure is one of nausea and malaise, followed by jaundice and coagulopathy (unresponsive to vitamin K). The most rapidly progressive cases develop hypoglycemia, metabolic acidosis and hyperammonemia in association with coma before jaundice is detected. There is no definitive treatment available and management depends upon supportive care, with liver transplantation in selected cases. Currently most patients receive *N*-acetyl cysteine in the acute phase. The mortality without transplantation is 50–80% but rises to more than 90% when there is severe encephalopathy or coagulopathy. Early transfer to a specialist center with a transplant program is therefore advisable. In many patients the cause is never identified despite extensive investigation and if hepatic failure is severe enough, the diagnosis is largely academic unless it is likely to recur in a transplanted liver or contraindicate treatment by transplantation. The intensive care priorities follow the ABCD (airway, breathing, circulation, disability) approach.

Comatose patients (grade IV encephalopathy) will require intubation for airway protection and ventilation. Avoid nasotracheal intubation because of the coagulopathy. Cardiac output, blood pressure and hemoglobin concentration must all be sustained in order to preserve cerebral oxygen delivery. Ventilate with a modestly increased fractional inspired concentration of oxygen (FiO_2) even if the patient does not have pulmonary complications. Hemodynamic instability is common, often a low systemic vascular resistance and variable cardiac output. Use invasive cardiovascular monitoring (at least central venous pressure and arterial lines) and anticipate a need to use inotropic agents with alpha agonist activity (e.g. noradrenaline). Remain vigilant to detect hypovolemia due to occult/acute hemorrhage.

Identify treatable causes of coma such as hypoglycemia or subclinical status epilepticus. Hypoglycemia specifically should be anticipated, appropriately supplemented with intravenous dextrose (without compromising the fluid restriction) and closely monitored. A CT scan can be useful to exclude cerebral hemorrhage as the cause of acute neurological deterioration. Cerebral edema is present in 75% of patients with grade IV encephalopathy. Assume that cerebrovascular autoregulation is impaired. It may be possible to measure intracranial pressure but intraventricular catheters and intraparenchymal bolts both require aggressive correction of coagulopathy first and even then the risk of bleeding may not be returned to normal. Furthermore such a strategy would mask an important marker of liver function (the prothrombin time). Nevertheless ventilate to a low normal $PaCO_2$ and assume that cerebral bloodflow will bear a linear relationship with cerebral perfusion pressure. Use pressor support to a level that implies that the cerebral perfusion pressure is likely to be adequate and avoid potential rises in intracranial pressure by a policy of minimal handling, nursing with head midline and a 30 degree head up position. Elective paralysis prevents coughing and straining but makes it difficult to identify status epilepticus without EEG monitoring. Minimize cerebral oxygen demand principally by recognizing and controlling seizures, and avoiding hyperthermia. Barbiturate coma may be preferred and is induced by thiopental infusion in doses sufficient to cause a burst suppression EEG.

Plasmafiltration may temporarily improve encephalopathy. Efficacy has not been proved and it has not been shown to alter outcome. In larger patients MARS™ will probably use less albumin but has not been formally compared to plasmafiltration. Attempts to alter gut pH and flora to reduce the number of urea splitting organisms present are also theoretically justifiable.

Impose a therapeutic fluid restriction (e.g. 50% of normal) even to the point of hypernatremia as high as 150 mmol/L. This may require the use of high concentration dextrose solutions to provide adequate carbohydrate. Mannitol is not likely to have a dramatic effect on cerebral edema since the insult is cytotoxic and therefore ongoing. Concurrent renal failure aggravates fluid overload and complicates both the management of cerebral edema and the correction of coagulopathy. Avoid mannitol if there is oliguric renal failure. Treatable causes of prerenal failure such as hypovolemia or hypotension due to hemodynamic instability should be corrected but you should have a low threshold for hemofiltration particularly if there is a metabolic acidosis.

Since the prothrombin time is the best prognostic liver function test, only correct coagulopathy with fresh frozen plasma (± cryoprecipitate) if there is a therapeutic indication such as bleeding, the need to establish intracranial pressure monitoring, or imminent surgery. Supplement the platelet count if it falls below 50 when the patient is also coagulopathic.

Treat metabolic complications as they arise. Seek the cause of metabolic acidosis rather than treating blindly with bicarbonate. Increased lactate production due to impaired oxygen delivery/extraction and impaired metabolism can impair the response to inotropes and recurs inexorably if the cause cannot be treated. Recurrent acidosis can be treated without causing hypernatremia by moderate volume hemofiltration using a bicarbonate buffered replacement fluid.

Secondary sepsis is likely as a consequence of invasive treatment, gut translocation of organisms and impaired cellular and humoral immunity. Maintain a high index of suspicion for infection if the patient's clinical condition fluctuates. This approach should be extended to starting blind therapy with broad spectrum antimicrobial and antifungal agents when dramatic changes in clinical condition occur.

REFERENCES (* Level 1 evidence)

1 Haller JA Jr, Shorter N. Regional pediatric trauma center: does a system of management improve outcome? Z Kinderchir 1982; 35(2):44–45.

2 Haller JA Jr, Shorter N, Miller D, et al. Organization and function of a regional pediatric trauma center: does a system of management improve outcome? J Trauma 1983; 23(8):691–696.

3 Beattie TF, Gorman DR, Walker JJ. the association between deprivation levels, attendance rate and triage category of children attending a children's accident and emergency department. Emerg Med J 2001; 18(2):110–111.

4 Morley CJ, Thornton AJ, Cole TJ, et al. Baby Check: a scoring system to grade the severity of acute systemic illness in babies under 6 months old. Arch Dis Child 1991; 66(1):100–105.

5 McCarthy PL, Lembo RM, Baron MA, et al. Predictive value of abnormal physical examination findings in ill-appearing and well-appearing febrile children. Pediatrics 1985; 76(2):167–171.

6 Baker MD, Avner JR, Bell LM. Failure of infant observation scales in detecting serious illness in febrile, 4- to 8-week-old infants. Pediatrics 1990; 85(6):1040–1043.

7 Wilson D. Assessing and managing the febrile child. Nurse Pract 1995; 20 (11 pt 1):59–60, 68–74.

8 Currie CE, Williams JM, Wright P, et al. Incidence and distribution of injury among schoolchildren aged 11–15. Inj Prev 1996; 2(1):21–25.

9 Beattie TF. An accident and emergency based child accident surveillance system: is it possible? J Accid Emerg Med 1996; 13(2):116–118.

10 Rodewald LE, Wrenn KD, Slovis CM. A method for developing and maintaining a powerful but inexpensive computer data base of clinical information about emergency department patients. Ann Emerg Med 1992; 21(1):41–46.

11 Ribbeck BM, Runge JW, Thomason MH, et al. Injury surveillance: a method for recording E codes for injured emergency department patients. Ann Emerg Med 1992; 21(1):37–40.

12 DiScala C, Lescohier I, Barthel M, Li G. Injuries to children with attention deficit hyperactivity disorder. Pediatrics 1998; 102(6):1415–1421.

13 Wakefield AJ, Murch SH, Anthony A, et al. Ileal-lymphoid-nodular hyperplasia, non-specific colitis, and pervasive developmental disorder in children. Lancet 1998; 351(9103): 637–641.

14 Anonymous. Fall in MMR vaccine coverage reported as further evidence of vaccine safety is published. Commun Dis Rep CDR Wkly 1999; 9(26):227, 230.

15 Fombonne E, Chakrabarti S. No evidence for a new variant of measles-mumps-rubella-induced autism. Pediatrics 2001; 108(4):E58.

16 Isaacs D. Bronchiolitis. BMJ 1995; 310(6971):4–5.

*17 Su E, Schmidt TA, Mann NC, Zechnich AD. A randomized controlled trial to assess decay in acquired knowledge among paramedics completing a pediatric resuscitation course. Acad Emerg Med 2000; 7(7):779–786.

18 Grossman DC, Hart LG, Rivara FP, et al. From roadside to bedside: the regionalization of trauma care in a remote rural county. J Trauma 1995; 38(1):14–21.

*19 Gausche M, Lewis RJ, Stratton SJ, et al. Effect of out-of-hospital pediatric endotracheal intubation on survival and neurological outcome: a controlled clinical trial. JAMA 2000; 283(6):783–790.

20 Gausche-Hill M, Lewis RJ, Gunter CS. Design and implementation of a controlled trial of pediatric endotracheal intubation in the out-of-hospital setting. Ann Emerg Med 2000; 36(4):356–365.

21 Cooper A, DiScala C, Foltin G, et al. Prehospital endotracheal intubation for severe head injury in children: a reappraisal. Semin Pediatr Surg 2001; 10(1):3–6.

22 Teach SJ, Antosia RE, Lund DP, Fleisher GR, et al. Prehospital fluid therapy in pediatric trauma patients. Pediatr Emerg Care 1995; 11(1):5–8.

23 Cummings P, Grossman DC, Rivara FP, Koepsell TD. State gun safe storage laws and child mortality due to firearms. JAMA 1997; 278(13):1084–1086.

24 Wheeler DS. Emergency medical services for children: a general pediatrician's perspective. Curr Probl Pediatr 1999; 29(8):221–241.

25 American Academy of Pediatrics, C o P E M, P. American College of Emergency, et al. Care of children in the emergency department: guidelines for preparedness. Pediatrics 2001; 107(4):777–781.

26 Sacchetti A, Brennan J, Kelly-Goodstein N, Graff D. Should pediatric emergency care be decentralized?: an out-of-hospital destination model for critically ill children. Acad Emerg Med 2000; 7(7):787–791.

27 Oakley PA. Inaccuracy and delay in decision making in paediatric resuscitation, and a proposed reference chart to reduce error. BMJ 1988; 297(6652):817–819.

28 Luten RC, Wears RL, Broselow J, et al. Length-based endotracheal tube and emergency equipment in pediatrics. Ann Emerg Med 1992; 21(8):900–904.

*29 Roberts I, Schierhout G, Alderson P. Absence of evidence for the effectiveness of five interventions routinely used in the intensive care management of severe head injury: a systematic review. J Neurol Neurosurg Psychiatry 1998; 65(5):729–733.

30 Tepas JJ 3rd, Mollitt DL, Talbert JL, Bryant M. The pediatric trauma score as a predictor of injury severity in the injured child. J Pediatr Surg 1987; 22(1):14–18.

31 Tepas JJ 3rd, Ramenofsky ML, Mollitt DL, et al. The Pediatric Trauma Score as a predictor of injury severity: an objective assessment. J Trauma 1988; 28(4):425–429.

*32 Schierhout G, Roberts I. Fluid resuscitation with colloid or crystalloid solutions in critically ill patients: a systematic review of randomised trials. BMJ 1998; 316(7136): 961–964.

33 Eisenberg M, Bergner L, Hallstrom A. Epidemiology of cardiac arrest and resuscitation in children. Ann Emerg Med 1983; 12(11):672–674.

34 Hassan TB. Use and effect of paediatric advanced life support skills for paediatric arrest in the A&E department. J Accid Emerg Med 1997; 14(6):357–362.

35 Teach SJ, Moore PE, Fleisher GR. Death and resuscitation in the pediatric emergency department. Ann Emerg Med 1995; 25(6): 799–803.

36 Resuscitation Council UK. www.resusc.org.uk

37 Mogayzel CL, Quan L, Graves JR, et al. Out-of-hospital ventricular fibrillation in children and adolescents: causes and outcomes. Ann Emerg Med 1995; 25(4):484–491.

38 Quan L, Mogayzel C. Ventricular fibrillation in pediatric cardiac arrest. Ann Emerg Med 1995; 26(5):658–659.

39 Ferguson J, Beattie TF. Occult spinal cord injury in traumatized children. Injury 1993; 24(2):83–84.

40 Teasdale GM, Murray G, Anderson E, et al. Risks of acute traumatic intracranial haematoma in children and adults: implications for managing head injuries. BMJ 1990; 300(6721):363–367.

41 Brookes M, MacMillan R, Cully S, et al. Head injuries in accident and emergency departments. How different are children from adults?' J Epidemiol Community Health 1990; 4(2):147–151.

42 Sharples PM, Storey A, Aynsley-Green A, Eyre JA. Avoidable factors contributing to death of children with head injury. BMJ 1990; 300(6717):87–91.

43 Barlow KM, Milne S, Aitken K, Minns RA. A retrospective epidemiological analysis of non-accidental head injury in children in Scotland over a 15 year period. Scott Med J 1998; 43(4):112–114.

44 Barlow KM, Minns RA. The relation between intracranial pressure and outcome in non-accidental head injury. Dev Med Child Neurol 1999; 41(4):220–225.

***45** Thillainayagam K, MacMillan R, Mendelow AD, et al. How accurately are fractures of the skull diagnosed in an accident and emergency department. Injury 1987; 18(5):319–321.

46 Villalobos T, Arango C, Kubilis P, Rathore M. Antibiotic prophylaxis after basilar skull fractures: a meta-analysis. Clin Infect Dis 1998; 27(2):364–369.

47 Aseervatham R, Muller M. Blunt trauma to the spleen. Aust N Z J Surg 2000; 70(5):333–337.

48 Moir JS, Ashcroft GP. Lap seat-belts: still trouble after all these years. J R Coll Surg Edinb 1995; 40(2):139–141.

***49** Wilson JA, Kendall JM, Cornelius P. Intranasal diamorphine for paediatric analgesia: assessment of safety and efficacy. J Accid Emerg Med 1997; 14(2):70–72.

***50** Kendall JM, Reeves BC, Latter VS. Multicentre randomised controlled trial of nasal diamorphine for analgesia in children and teenagers with clinical fractures. BMJ 2001; 322(7281):261–265.

51 Baraff LJ, Oslund SA, Schriger DL, Stephen ML. Probability of bacterial infections in febrile infants less than three months of age: a meta-analysis. Pediatr Infect Dis J 1992; 11(4):257–264.

52 Baraff LJ. Outpatient management of fever in selected infants. N Engl J Med 1994; 330(13): 938–939, discussion 939–940.

53 Baraff LJ, Lee SI. Fever without source: management of children 3 to 36 months of age. Pediatr Infect Dis J 1992; 11(2):146–151.

54 Macdonald IA, Beattie TF. Intussusception presenting to a paediatric accident and emergency department. J Accid Emerg Med 1995; 12(3):182–186.

55 Plant PK, Owen JL, Elliott MW. Non-invasive ventilation in acute exacerbations of chronic obstructive pulmonary disease: long term survival and predictors of in- hospital outcome. Thorax 2001; 56(9):708–712.

56 Bohn D. Lung salvage and protection ventilatory techniques. Pediatr Clin N Am 2001; 48(3):553–572.

57 Hickling KG. Low volume ventilation with permissive hypercapnia in the Adult Respiratory Distress Syndrome. Clin Intensive Care 1992; 3(2):67–78.

58 Laffey JG, Kavanagh BP. Carbon dioxide and the critically ill – too little of a good thing? Lancet 1999; 354(9186): 1283–1286.

***59** Finer NN, Barrington KJ. Nitric oxide for respiratory failure in infants born at or near term. Cochrane Database Syst Rev 2000; 2:CD000399.

60 Kinsella JP, Abman SH. Inhaled nitric oxide: current and future uses in neonates. Semin Perinatol 2000; 24(6):387–395.

61 Hirschl RB. Respiratory failure: current status of experienced therapies. Semin Pediatr Surg 1999; 8(3):155–170.

62 Wiedermann HP. Partial liquid ventilation for acute respiratory distress syndrome. Clin Chest Med 2000; 21(3):543–554.

63 Kolobow T, Giacomini M, Reali-Forster C, et al. The current status of intratracheal-pulmonary ventilation (ITPV). Int J Artif Organs 1995; 18(10):670–673.

64 Reeves JH, Butt WB, Sathe AS. A review of venovenous haemofiltration in seriously ill infants. J Pediatr Child Health 1994; 30(1):50–54.

65 Reeves JH, Butt WW, Shann F, et al Continuous plasmafiltration in sepsis syndrome. Plasmafiltration in Sepsis Study Group. Crit Care Med 1999; 27(10):2098–2104.

66 Schetz M. Non-renal indications for continuous renal replacement therapy. Kidney Int Suppl 1999; 72:S88–94.

36

Surgical pediatrics

Gordon A MacKinlay

Pediatric surgery encompasses a wider range of surgery than any other surgical specialty. It is confined to an age group rather than an organ system. In the older child, adult surgeons may deal with some commoner problems.

Congenital problems presenting in the neonatal period or later, together with other conditions peculiar to childhood, should be treated in a specialist center by trained pediatric surgeons backed by pediatric anesthetists, pediatric radiologists, pediatric pathologists and experienced nursing staff specifically trained in the care of children. In a general hospital the child should be nursed on a children's ward and if there is no pediatric surgeon, care should be provided by the surgeon who is treating the child *together* with a pediatrician.

In the case of the neonate, a particular surgical challenge is encountered not only in the requirement for a meticulous surgical technique but also in careful pre- and postoperative management. The reward is the prospect of a full three score years and ten survival compared with the commonly sought 5-year survival in many aspects of adult surgery.

The presence of an anomaly requiring surgery is often detected antenatally by ultrasound, enabling discussion with the parents, obstetrician, pediatric surgeon and neonatologist. The parents can thus be prepared and reassured, where possible, that although an abnormality has been detected it can be treated. They can visit the surgical neonatal unit, meet the staff and, where appropriate, the timing of delivery may be planned to facilitate optimal transfer of the baby to the awaiting surgical unit or direct to the operating theater. Pregnancy is a time of potential parental stress and unless great care is taken in explaining the possible consequences of an antenatally diagnosed anomaly their anxiety will be increased.

NEONATAL SURGERY

RESPIRATORY PROBLEMS

Whilst respiratory distress in the newborn is primarily the domain of the neonatologist some causes may be surgical and early referral to a pediatric surgeon may be of lifesaving importance.

CAUSES OF RESPIRATORY DISTRESS IN THE NEWBORN

1. Upper airway
   a. choanal atresia
   b. nasal encephalocele
   c. tumors of the nasopharynx
   d. Pierre Robin syndrome
   e. macroglossia
   f. hemangio/lymphangiomata of oral cavity
   g. laryngotracheoesophageal cleft
   h. laryngeal web
   i. laryngeal stenosis
   j. hemangioma of larynx

k. laryngomalacia
l. tracheomalacia
m. tracheal stenosis
n. cystic hygroma
o. cervical teratoma

2. Intrathoracic
a. congenital lobar emphysema
b. cystic adenomatoid lung malformation
c. bronchogenic and lung cysts
d. enterogenous cysts
e. pneumothorax
f. sequestration of lung
g. vascular ring
h. congenital heart disease
i. diaphragmatic hernia
j. eventration of the diaphragm
k. esophageal atresia and tracheoesophageal fistula.

Choanal atresia is obstruction of the posterior nares by a bony or occasionally membranous septum. If bilateral it is a neonatal emergency, as babies are obligate nasal breathers. An oral airway will overcome this problem until the obstruction is relieved.

An oral airway is also of benefit in *Pierre Robin syndrome* where there is a hypoplastic mandible and central cleft palate, the tongue falling posteriorly to occlude the glottis. An airway can be maintained in position for several weeks, the baby being fed nasogastrically or via a gastrostomy. A tracheostomy may be easier to manage and is maintained until the mandible grows. It also facilitates repair of the cleft palate which is associated in the majority of cases.

A *laryngeal web*, if complete, leads to death in utero. If partial, the symptoms may merit emergency tracheostomy. *Laryngomalacia* leads to inspiratory stridor which usually resolves in the first 2.5 years of life. *Tracheomalacia* is commonly associated with esophageal atresia. It has been postulated that the hypertrophied upper pouch, containing swallowed liquor, compresses the developing trachea, preventing the normal growth of tracheal rings. The problem increases postoperatively sometimes making it impossible to extubate these babies. The diagnosis may be confirmed radiologically by lateral screening of the neck, observing the anteroposterior narrowing of the trachea with inspiration. Aortopexy, suturing the aorta to the back of the sternum, thus pulling the pretracheal fascia and hence the anterior tracheal wall forward, is sometimes of benefit. Prolonged intubation may allow time for the tracheal rings to become more supportive but may itself lead to subglottic stenosis. Tracheostomy is required in some cases.

Congenital lobar emphysema leads to overexpansion of a lung lobe with compromise of ventilation. Half the cases present within days of birth, the remainder in the first few months of life. The most common cause is bronchomalacia of the associated bronchus although some cases may be caused by external compression. The baby may present with feeding difficulties due to dyspnea. The diagnosis is made radiologically and the most commonly affected lobes are the left upper lobe or the right middle lobe. Treatment is lobectomy in severe cases but in many conservative management is appropriate.

Cystic adenomatoid lung and *congenital lung cysts* can present in much the same way as lobar emphysema. Their expansion produces respiratory distress. Congenital cysts tend to be unilocular and solitary. *Cystic adenomatoid malformation* is due to excessive overgrowth of bronchioles with multiple cysts lined by cuboidal and ciliated pseudostratified columnar epithelium. The left lower lobe is commonly affected and the appearance may antenatally or even postnatally be mistaken for a diaphragmatic hernia. Treatment is resection of the affected lobe.

Pulmonary sequestration is a mass of lung tissue not communicating with the bronchial tree and which receives its blood supply from an anomalous systemic vessel. It may be within the substance of the lung (intralobar sequestration) or completely separate (extralobar). Areas of sequestration are thought to arise from an extra bronchopulmonary bud of the foregut. They most commonly occur in the left lower lobe and the blood supply comes direct from the aorta, above or below the diaphragm. The anomalous blood supply may be identified by ultrasound techniques avoiding the need for angiography. The condition usually presents with respiratory infections, more commonly after the neonatal period. The treatment is resection.[1]

Diaphragmatic hernia

Diaphragmatic hernia may be congenital or acquired, the latter usually being traumatic in origin. Congenital diaphragmatic hernia arises due to an abnormality in the formation of the diaphragm between the fourth and tenth weeks of fetal life.

The commonest herniation is the Bochdalek type, a posterolateral defect, possibly a failure of closure of the pleuroperitoneal canal. It has been postulated that the primary anomaly is in the developing lungs which fail to induce diaphragmatic closure and this may explain hypoplasia in the contralateral lung. A hernia through the foramen of Morgagni is less common in neonates. This defect is retrosternal, to the right or left of the midline. The third site for herniation is the esophageal hiatus – the so-called hiatus hernia.

The true incidence of congenital diaphragmatic hernia is difficult to ascertain as so many die at birth, others present as live births and others after the neonatal period. This lesion represents 8% of major fatal congenital anomalies noted in a British perinatal mortality survey (present in 1 in 2200 of all births). In Edinburgh the incidence is 1 in 7000 live births, other series report 1:4000–1:10 000.

Some cases are now detected antenatally by ultrasound but the majority present with respiratory distress – cyanosis, dyspnea and tachypnea – either immediately after birth or within a few hours. Occasionally, particularly on the right side, the presentation may be later, the defect being present at birth but actual herniation of abdominal content occurring as a postnatal event. The later the onset of symptoms, the better the prognosis. Examination reveals a scaphoid abdomen, bowel sounds on auscultation of the affected side of the chest and a shift of the apex beat to the right in the case of a left-sided hernia. The right side is less common, perhaps due to plugging by the liver, but if a defect is present here it tends to be large with herniation of the liver as well as bowel.

Once air has been swallowed after birth a chest X-ray confirms the diagnosis, showing gas filled loops of bowel on the affected side of the chest with displacement of the mediastinum to the opposite side (Fig. 36.1).

Treatment

A nasogastric tube is passed to reduce the gaseous distention of the bowel with air. In the past the surgical repair of the hernia was a true emergency, it being felt that the sooner the hernia was reduced the more easily the lungs could expand. Babies were operated on virtually regardless of condition and the survival rates were poor. It has been shown that respiratory mechanics, far from improving, frequently deteriorate as a result of repair of the hernia. The role of urgent surgery has thus been re-evaluated. It has always been known that the babies with the least hypoplastic lungs fared better. These also tend to be the cases that present after hours rather than immediately at birth. Now an initial, non-surgical approach to diaphragmatic hernia has been adopted in most centers with the aim of improving pulmonary function and reducing pulmonary

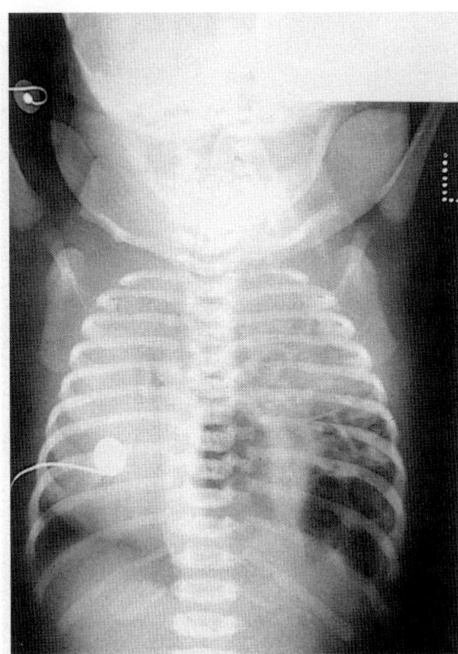

Fig. 36.1 Diaphragmatic hernia (left-sided Bochdalek defect).

vascular resistance.[2,3] After diagnosis the baby is intubated and hyperventilated to reduce the $PaCO_2$ to < 4.7 kPa (< 35 mmHg) and paralyzed. Metabolic acidosis is corrected with bicarbonate therapy. A chest X-ray is taken to verify the endotracheal tube position and exclude a pneumothorax. A preductal arterial line (radial) is sited for blood gas and pressure monitoring. The ventilatory index (mean airway pressure × respiratory rate) is calculated and this should be < 1000 with a $PaCO_2$ < 5.3 (< 40 mmHg) prior to surgery. If the index is higher, high frequency oscillatory ventilation is instituted. Tolazoline may be administered to reduce pulmonary vascular resistance and prevent shunting through the ductus arteriosus. In some centers extracorporeal membrane oxygenation (ECMO) is used for prolonged support with variable results. Whatever the method of stabilization preoperatively, it must be carried out in a surgical unit as it is the pediatric surgeon who must be in a position to determine the timing of surgery.

Operative treatment

An abdominal approach is usually preferred with a transverse upper abdominal incision on the side of the hernia. The bowel and other organs are reduced and the defect in the diaphragm examined. If the defect is large a patch of prosthetic material may be used. Repairing a defect under tension merely reduces lung compliance. An underwater seal drain is positioned prior to completion of the repair.

Postoperatively, support is maintained until the baby can be weaned from the ventilator. A few patients who require little or no ventilatory support preoperatively may be extubated immediately. Of the remainder the mortality rate still remains around 50%, although it is hoped that the change in preoperative management will improve the outlook.

Eventration of the diaphragm

This is due to a deficiency in the muscle of the diaphragm. The thin layer becomes attenuated and bulges up into the thorax. Extensive eventrations are similar to diaphragmatic hernia presenting in the neonatal period. Smaller eventrations present later and require localized plication.

Esophageal atresia

Atresia is absence or closure of a normal body orifice or passage (Greek *a* = negative, *tresis* = hole). A fistula is an abnormal communication between two epithelial surfaces.

Esophageal atresia is a congenital defect of unknown etiology, the great majority of cases being associated with a tracheoesophageal fistula. The incidence is approximately 1 per 3000 live births. Many babies with esophageal atresia are premature and of low birth weight. The lower the birth weight, the greater the mortality. More than half the babies presenting with esophageal atresia have associated congenital abnormalities. Commonly associated are vertebral, anorectal, cardiac, tracheoesophageal, renal and limb anomalies (VACTERL). This was formerly known as the VATER complex. The anatomical varieties of esophageal atresia and related disorders are illustrated in Figure 36.2.

Clinical features

Maternal hydramnios is so common that all babies born to a mother with hydramnios should have a tube passed to assess the patency of the esophagus. In cases with esophageal atresia the tube will be

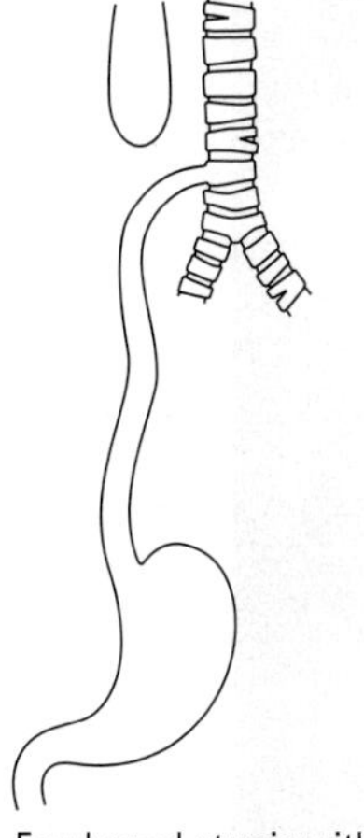

i. Esophageal atresia with distal tracheoesophageal fistula (85%)

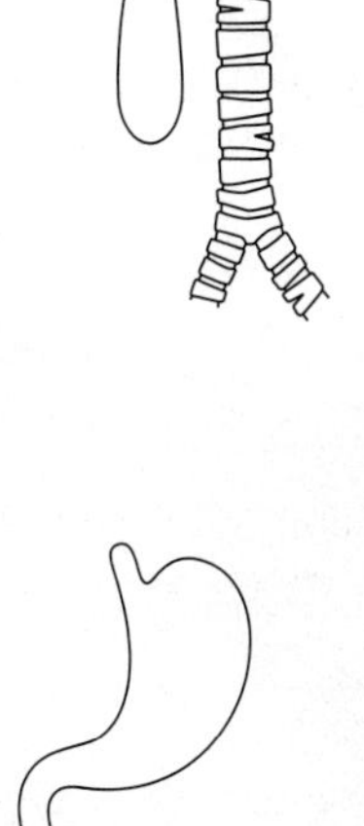

ii. Esophageal atresia without fistula; stomach small and distal esophagus usually short (10%)

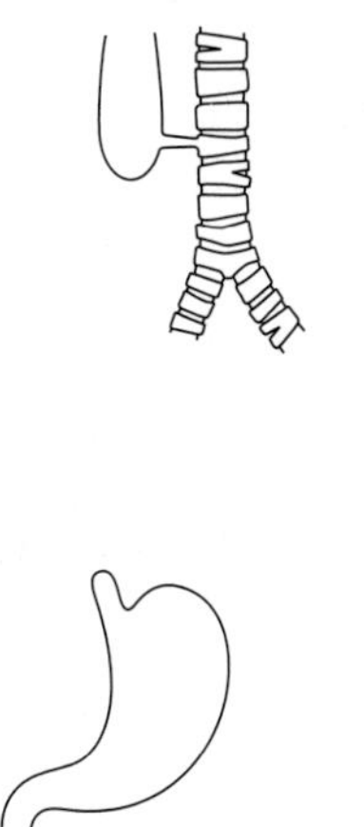

iii. Esophageal atresia with proximal tracheoesophageal fistula (2%)

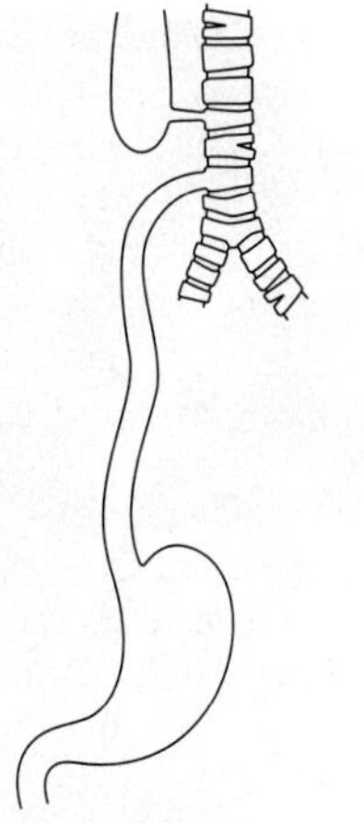

iv. Esophageal atresia with both proximal and distal tracheoesophageal fistula (1%)

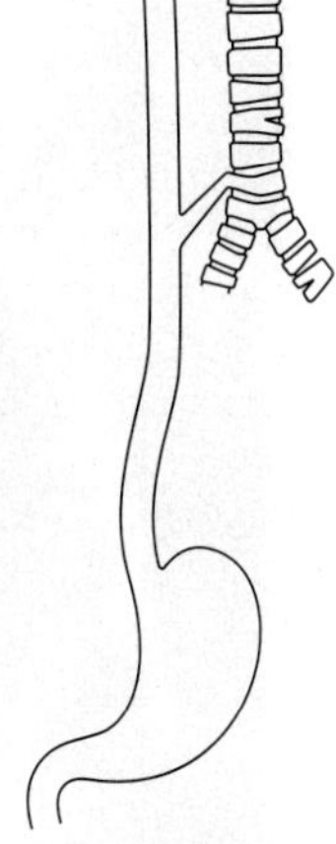

v. Tracheoesophageal fistula without esophageal atresia (2%)

Fig. 36.2 Esophageal atresia and tracheoesophageal fistula.

arrested about 10 cm from the lips. If the diagnosis is not made in this manner then the baby will be noted to froth at the mouth, choke, cough or become dyspneic and cyanosed. These symptoms will be exacerbated by attempts to feed the baby. The patency of the esophagus should then be tested by a firm tube of at least 10 or 12 FG, which should be passed orally. Acid secretions aspirated from the tube may have refluxed through the fistula so radiological confirmation of the position of the tube is necessary if suspicion is high.

A Replogle tube is a double lumen plastic catheter which can be passed via the nose into the upper esophageal pouch, enabling continuous suction to be applied without causing damage to the mucosa. Suction is applied to the end of the catheter, air passing along the finer of the two lumina as secretions are aspirated. If the latter are particularly thick, careful irrigation may be carried out via the finer lumen tube.

A plain chest X-ray with gentle pressure on the Replogle tube enables the distal extent of the pouch to be ascertained. The presence of air in the stomach and bowel confirms the presence of a distal tracheoesophageal fistula (TEF) (Fig. 36.3). In the case of atresia without a fistula there is absence of air in the stomach (Fig. 36.4). Occasionally there may be associated duodenal atresia, but providing there is a TEF, then the gas pattern should clarify this (Fig. 36.5).

Some surgeons like to use 1–2 ml of contrast to define the upper pouch but there is great danger of spillage into the tracheobronchial tree and the procedure is unnecessary. Preoperatively, apart from adequate aspiration of the upper pouch, opinions differ as to the best position in which to nurse the baby. Some advocate the Trendelenburg (head down) position to prevent aspiration of secretions but this may lead to reflux of gastric content via the fistula into the lungs (especially the right upper lobe). Others, to prevent this, advise a head up position. A horizontal and semiprone position reduces the incidence of right upper lobe collapse and seems satisfactory.

Treatment

In the commonest type of anomaly (with a distal TEF), surgery does not have to be performed immediately in the middle of the night but can be safely left until the following day. If pneumonitis is present, it is justifiable to delay treatment for 24 h or more to allow chest physiotherapy and appropriate antibiotics to be administered. A right posterolateral thoracotomy is made and, via an extrapleural approach, the fistula is divided and repaired and an end-to-end anastomosis between the proximal and distal esophagus is made in a single layer. A fine transanastomotic silastic tube is passed nasogastrically prior to completion of the anastomosis so that early nasogastric feeding can be instituted. In some centers the operation can be safely performed thoracoscopically.

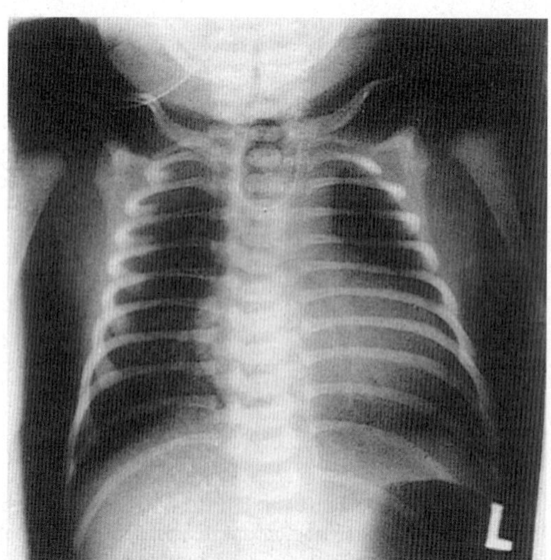

Fig. 36.3 Esophageal atresia with distal tracheoesophageal fistula.

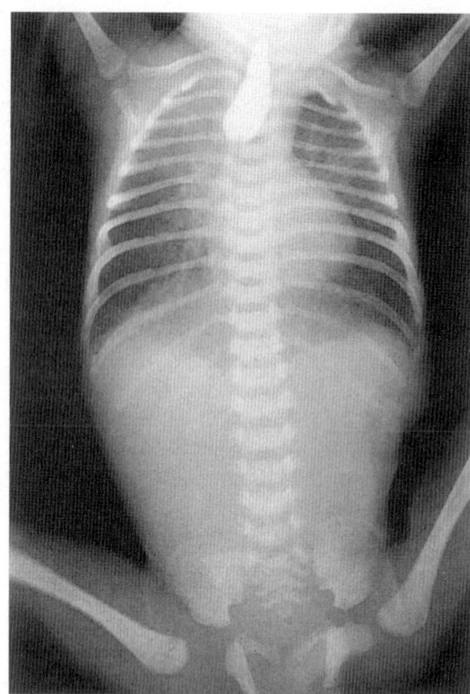

Fig. 36.4 Esophageal atresia without TEF.

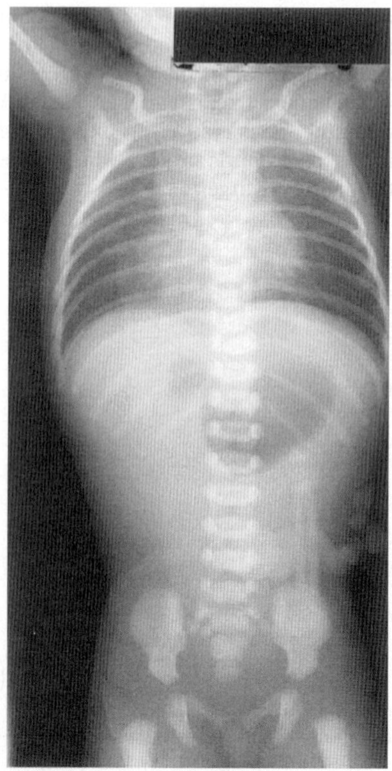

Fig. 36.5 Esophageal atresia with duodenal atresia.

On the fifth postoperative day a contrast swallow is performed to confirm patency of the anastomosis and exclude leakage at this site. If leakage is present it can safely be managed conservatively if an extrapleural approach has been followed. Anastomotic stricture, if it occurs, is treated by esophagoscopy and bougienage or balloon dilation under X-ray control. Most children, following a successful repair, have a persistent brassy cough or 'seal bark' which may last for 1 or 2 years. This is probably due to a degree of tracheomalacia.

Dysphagia due to abnormal motility in the esophagus both above and below the anastomosis may be due to vagal nerve damage or, more probably, an intrinsic abnormality associated with the lesion. This, like the seal bark, usually resolves by the age of 2 years.

Cases of esophageal atresia without a fistula are best managed initially by gastrostomy and aspiration of the upper pouch via a Replogle tube. In my experience, delayed primary anastomosis can be achieved after 3 months of regular stretching of the upper pouch by the nursing staff using a Nelaton catheter at feed times. Once there is radiological evidence of a gap of less than 3 cm, as visualized with a metal bougie in the lower pouch (passed per gastrostomy) and a radiopaque tube in the upper pouch, surgery can be carried out. Postoperatively, the infants are electively paralyzed and ventilated for up to 7 days to relieve the tension on the anastomosis, a technique also of value in tight anastomosis in the common type of atresia with a distal fistula.[4] Others favor construction of a cervical esophagostomy followed by gastric transposition or colonic interposition to bridge the gap between the upper pouch and the stomach.

H-type tracheoesophageal fistula

These occasionally present in the first few weeks of life with coughing or cyanosis on feeding. More commonly they present much later with recurrent chest infections, a history of coughing on feeds, and sometimes abdominal distention. Because the fistula runs obliquely upwards from esophagus to trachea, the flow of esophageal content into the trachea is limited and intermittent. The diagnosis is made at a contrast swallow under screening. Treatment is surgical division of the fistula, usually via a cervical approach.

DUODENAL OBSTRUCTION

Duodenal obstruction may be intrinsic (atresia, membrane, stenosis or annular pancreas) or extrinsic (Ladd's bands with or without volvulus of the midgut).

Intrinsic duodenal obstructions (Fig. 36.6)

The etiology of duodenal atresias and other intrinsic duodenal obstructions differs from that of intrinsic obstructions in the remainder of the small intestine. It appears to be a failure of luminal development due to an early insult and there are often associated abnormalities. Down syndrome is present in 30% of cases. In 10% there is esophageal atresia, and a further 10% have anorectal anomalies. Cardiac and renal anomalies may also be associated. Cardiac abnormalities are particularly common in those with Down syndrome.

Atresia or stenosis usually affects the second or occasionally the third part of the duodenum.

Complete obstructions present with vomiting within 24 h after birth. The vomitus may or may not be bile stained, depending on whether the obstruction is proximal or distal to the ampulla of Vater. In those with bile stained vomitus the meconium, if passed, may also be normally bile stained as there may be openings of the bile duct proximal and distal to the obstruction via Wirsung's and Santorini's ducts.

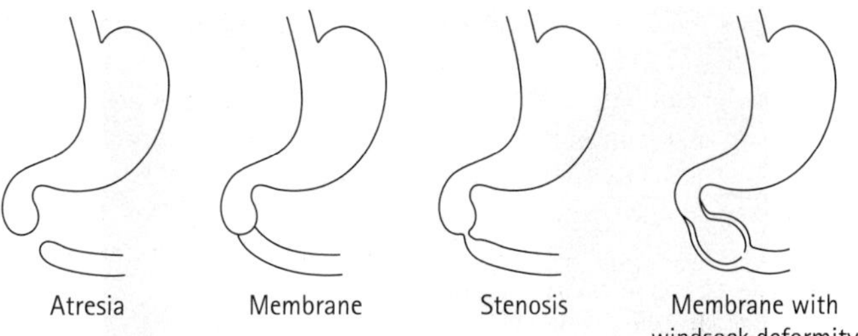

Fig. 36.6 Duodenal anomalies.

In maternity units where passage of a nasogastric tube is a routine soon after birth, aspiration of more than 20 ml of fluid may be indicative of a duodenal or small bowel obstruction.

Abdominal distention, if any, is confined to the upper abdomen due to obstruction of the stomach and duodenum.

The diagnosis is confirmed by a plain erect X-ray which demonstrates the characteristic 'double bubble' appearance of air–fluid levels in the stomach and duodenum (Fig. 36.7). The double bubble may also be detected antenatally, ultrasound detecting fluid distention of the stomach and duodenum.[5] An incomplete obstruction, stenosis, or membrane with a small hole in it may allow air to pass through to the rest of the bowel, thus masking the double bubble (Fig. 36.8), but a contrast study confirms the presence of obstruction (Fig. 36.9). Sometimes the diagnosis may be delayed several months or even a year or two if sufficient food can pass through.

Treatment

If there is any delay in diagnosis of a duodenal obstruction then any resulting metabolic disturbance must be corrected preoperatively. At laparotomy a duodenoduodenostomy is the procedure of choice (Fig. 36.10), or for a stenosis or membrane a duodenoplasty may be

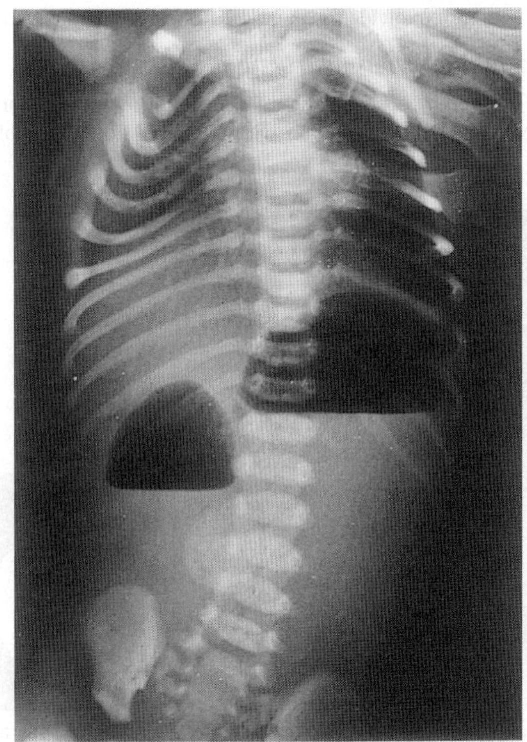

Fig. 36.7 'Double bubble' in duodenal atresia.

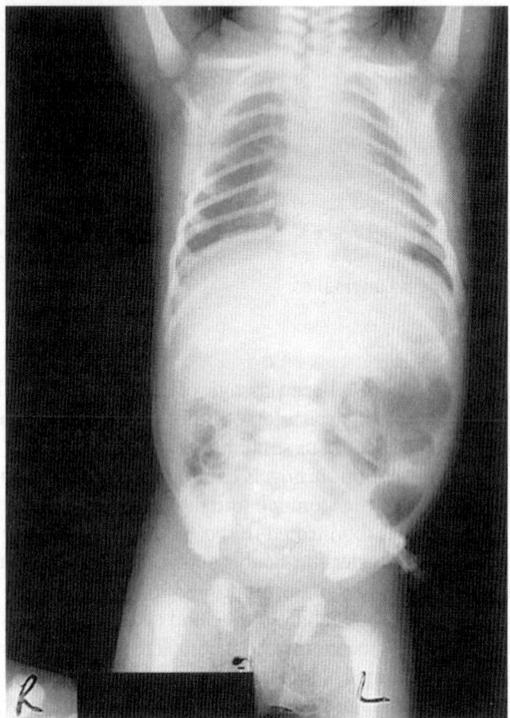

Fig. 36.8 Plain film of baby soon after birth.

performed, opening the duodenum lengthways across the obstruction and closing it transversely. Resection of a diaphragm must be undertaken cautiously to avoid damage to the ampulla of Vater.

An annular pancreas (Fig. 36.10a) is caused by the failure of the normal migration of the ventral bud to join the dorsal one. It is rarely a true ring around the duodenum but more commonly associated with an intrinsic obstruction within the duodenum (membrane or stenosis). A duodenoduodenostomy is performed with no attempt to divide the pancreas for fear of fistula formation.

Extrinsic duodenal obstruction

Ladd's bands may obstruct the duodenum, occasionally alone but more commonly in association with a midgut volvulus (volvulus

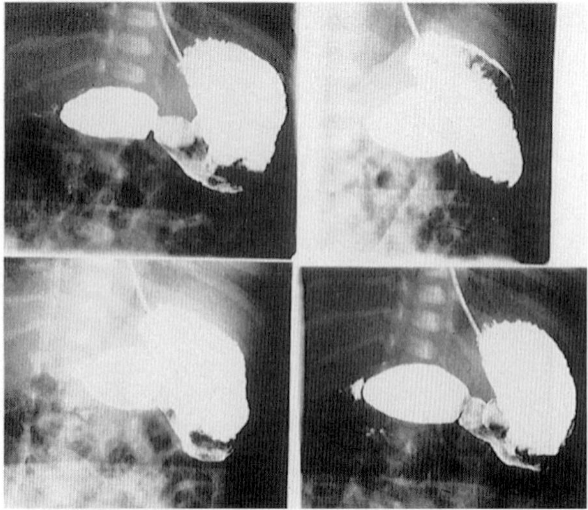

Fig. 36.9 Upper gastrointestinal contrast study on same baby as Figure 36.8.

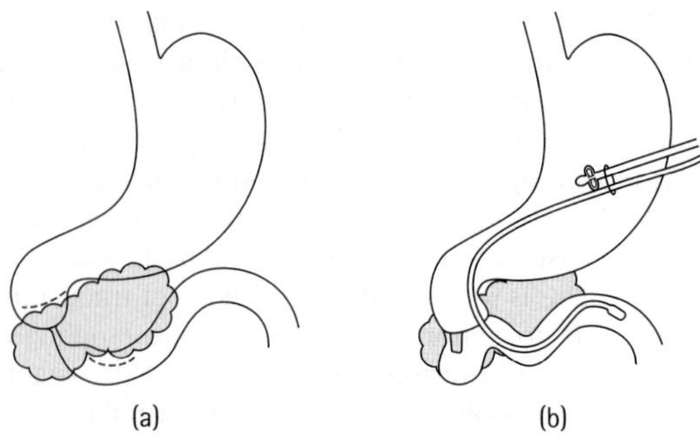

Fig. 36.10 (a) Annular pancreas with intrinsic duodenal membrane. (b) Duodenoduodenostomy with gastrostomy and transanastomotic silastic feeding tube.

neonatorum). Such a volvulus may present in the neonatal period or at any age and arises due to an incomplete, or malrotation of the bowel. By the sixth week of intrauterine life the gut tube elongates to a greater extent than can be accommodated in the developing abdominal cavity and thus herniation through the umbilical ring occurs. During the next month the bowel undergoes an anticlockwise rotation returning to the abdominal cavity by the tenth week. By the time the stomach has rotated to the left, the duodenal C-loop has formed and the small bowel, followed by the large bowel, returns to the abdomen. The cecum and ascending colon pass to the right of the abdomen, the latter becoming retroperitoneal. The small bowel mesentery is then fixed between the duodenojejunal flexure and the ileocecal region. Failure of the cecum and ascending colon to reach their normal position results in a short base to the midgut mesentery and peritoneal bands passing from the cecum (in the midline or to the left side) to the right posterior abdominal wall. These bands (Ladd's bands) obstruct the duodenum. In addition, the short base to the mesentery allows a midgut volvulus to arise, the bowel rotating in a clockwise direction, and resulting in duodenal obstruction. A plain X-ray will show a double bubble and usually a small amount of gas in the bowel more distally. Contrast studies may confirm the diagnosis. An upper gastrointestinal study may show a duodenal obstruction and a typical coiled spring sign. An enema may show an anomalous position of the cecum.

Once any electrolyte or acid–base disturbance is corrected, laparotomy must be performed without delay to avoid ischemia of the midgut.

SMALL BOWEL OBSTRUCTION

This may arise due to an abnormality directly associated with the bowel itself (intrinsic), pressure from without (extrinsic), or obstruction within the lumen (intraluminal).

Intrinsic anomalies

These are mainly atresias, membranes, stenoses and duplications of the bowel. Atresias may arise anywhere along the length of the bowel, being most common in the distal ileum and rarely seen in the colon. Their likely cause is an interruption of the mesenteric vessels in utero. These vary from membranous obstruction in continuity, those with or without an associated gap in the mesentery and multiple atresias, to the so-called apple peel type deformity with extensive loss of mesentery and bowel, the distal small bowel receiving its blood supply from the middle colic vessels through a precarious continuity between marginal arcades (Fig. 36.11).

The bowel proximal to the obstruction is distended and hypertrophied and distally the bowel is collapsed, often with a

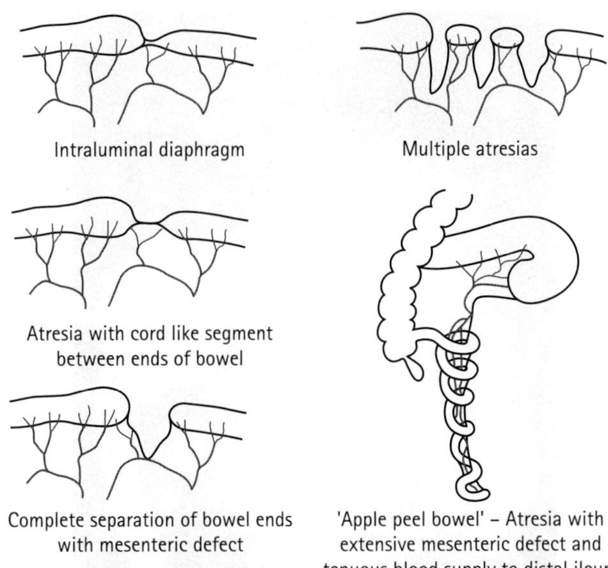

Fig. 36.11 Small bowel atresias.

microcolon (unused) although babies with obstructions of this kind may pass meconium of normal appearance. The latter is dependent on the timing of the vascular accident in utero.

The diagnosis is confirmed by plain X-ray which will show a number of distended loops of small bowel with air–fluid levels in an erect view (Fig. 36.12). The level of obstruction can be estimated by the number of distended loops. There will be absence of air distal to a complete obstruction.

Contrast studies have a limited role in the diagnosis of such obstructions unless to exclude intraluminal or functional conditions.

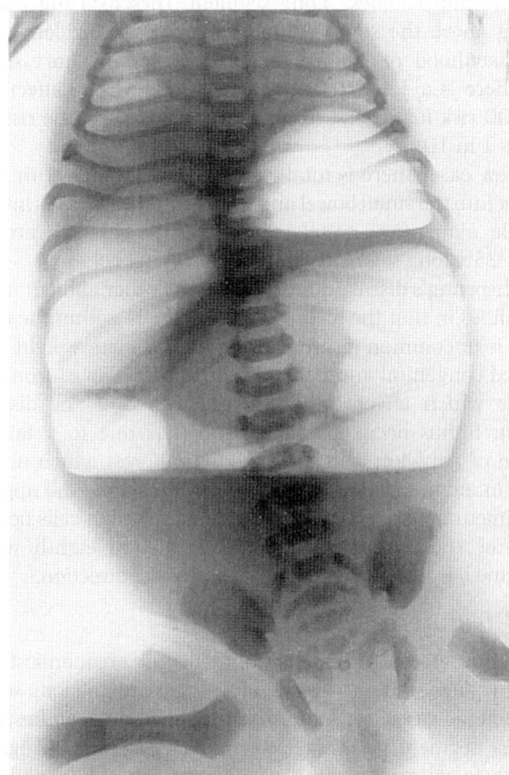

Fig. 36.12 Jejunal atresia.

Treatment

Preoperative treatment involves passage of a nasogastric tube and correction of electrolyte imbalance by appropriate administration of intravenous fluids. If the diagnosis is established early there is little or no requirement for intravenous resuscitation.

Operative treatment involves laparotomy, resection or tapering of grossly dilated bowel proximal to the atresia (to prevent problems of postoperative peristaltic inertia) and then anastomosis between the dilated proximal bowel and the collapsed distal bowel.

Duplications

Duplications of the alimentary tract can occur at any level from mouth to anus. A length of bowel may be duplicated, the two segments sharing a common blood supply and muscular wall yet having separate mucosal linings. They may or may not communicate, and it is the non-communicating type that tends to form a short cystic segment which, by accumulation of secretions within it, leads to intestinal obstruction. Such duplications may be palpable as a cystic intra-abdominal mass which together with the signs of intestinal obstruction lead to the diagnosis. Ultrasound and contrast studies may be of value.

Treatment. The treatment usually involves a localized bowel resection but if the duplication is extensive in length or at a site such as the ileocecal junction, the mucosa of the duplicated segment should be dissected out, thus avoiding extensive resection or loss of the ileocecal valve.

Extrinsic anomalies

Extrinsic anomalies leading to intestinal obstruction include hernias (inguinal or internal), localized volvulus, bands, vitellointestinal remnants and mesenteric cysts.

An incarcerated inguinal hernia is the commonest cause of intestinal obstruction at any age. The inguinal region must thus be carefully examined when any patient, neonate or older, presents with intestinal obstruction. Internal hernias are rare and can only be identified at laparotomy.

Localized volvulus may arise in relation to bands, duplication cysts and vitellointestinal remnants. Treatment at laparotomy varies according to the causative factor and the condition of the affected bowel. Mesenteric cysts may lead to local volvulus or may present as a palpable cystic mass. They are treated by resection.

Intraluminal anomalies

Intraluminal causes of intestinal obstruction include meconium ileus, milk curd obstruction and meconium plug syndrome.

Around 10% of patients with cystic fibrosis present in the neonatal period with obstruction of the distal ileum (meconium ileus). The distal few centimeters of ileum contain pale gray 'rabbit pellets' of inspissated meconium proximal to which is a segment containing hard green-black meconium and, more proximally still, distended loops containing tarry fluid meconium and air. Distal to the obstruction is a microcolon and usually no meconium is passed, presenting signs being abdominal distention and bile stained vomiting within a few days of birth.

Plain abdominal films show gross abdominal distention with few fluid levels and often a ground glass appearance (of air bubbles in the viscid meconium) in the right iliac fossa. Sometimes there are signs of calcification from perforation and leakage of meconium antenatally.

Volvulus of the hypertrophied distended bowel may also lead to atresia, or perforation may occur after birth.

The presence of meconium ileus has no relationship to the subsequent 'severity' of the cystic fibrosis.

Conservative management

Treatment can be either conservative or operative. Conservative management involves the administration of a gastrografin enema under fluoroscopic control. Gastrografin with 0.1% Tween 80, a detergent, added as a wetting agent has a high osmolarity of 1900 mOsm/L and acts by drawing fluid into the bowel, thus freeing the inspissated meconium in the distal ileum. It is essential, therefore, that the baby is adequately hydrated and an intravenous infusion must be in progress. If necessary the procedure may be repeated after 24 h. If there is calcification the procedure is best avoided for fear of reperforation.

Surgical management

For cases in which there are complications such as perforation or signs of meconium peritonitis (calcification) or after failed gastrografin enema, operative treatment is required. Laparotomy is performed via an upper transverse abdominal incision. Intestinal resection is necessary for bowel that is grossly dilated or of doubtful viability. A Bishop Koop ileostomy is usually performed. This is a Roux-en-Y anastomosis between the end of the proximal limb of ileum and the side of the distal limb, bringing the end of the latter out of the abdomen as an end ileostomy in the right iliac fossa. This acts as a safety valve through which the distal ileum can be irrigated. In the case of continued obstruction the stoma will function. Once it is relieved, bowel contents pass the natural way.

Milk plug or mild curd obstruction also occurs in the distal ileum and may be due to the administration of inappropriately concentrated artificial milk feeds, or possibly a transient low bile acid excretion. The management is similar to that described above.

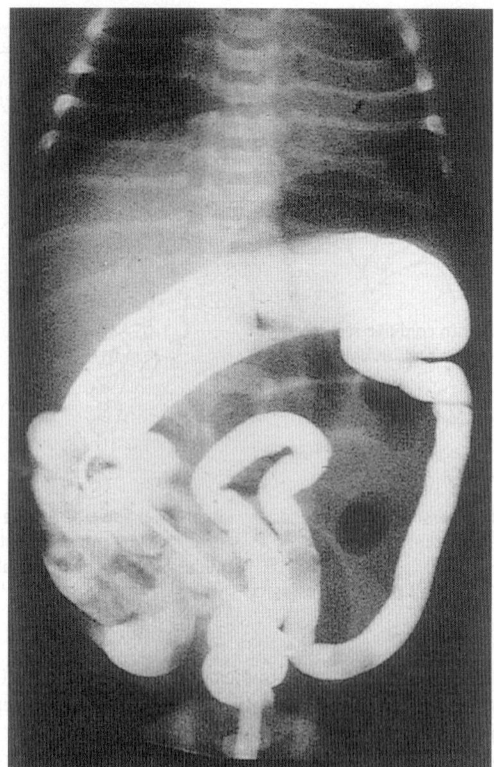

Fig. 36.13 Small left colon syndrome.

MECONIUM PLUG SYNDROME/SMALL LEFT COLON SYNDROME

Meconium plug syndrome must not be confused with meconium ileus. It is sometimes described as small left colon syndrome. The distal colon or rectum is plugged by sticky gray-white mucus distally with sticky meconium above it. The presentation is usually at about 2 days with a history of failure to pass meconium. There is evidence of low intestinal obstruction with generalized abdominal distention, frequently with a history of bile stained vomiting and X-ray showing gaseous distention. There are multiple fluid levels present in the majority of cases.

The diagnosis is made by contrast enema. Initially barium is used to exclude Hirschsprung's disease, but then changed to water-soluble contrast when the appearance of a meconium plug is seen in a narrowed left colon. The colon is usually narrow up to the splenic flexure where it becomes dilated (Fig. 36.13). It has been postulated that there is a discrepancy in the activity of the parasympathetic supply from the vagus nerve (supplying the bowel to two-thirds of the way across the transverse colon to the splenic flexure) and the sacral parasympathetics which supply the remainder. Whatever the etiology, the enema invariably proves to be therapeutic with satisfactory evacuation of meconium. The abdomen in most cases decompresses over 24 h and feeds can then be introduced. If bowel evacuation is not normal then Hirschsprung's disease must be excluded.

HIRSCHSPRUNG'S DISEASE[6]

Hirschsprung, a Danish pediatrician, described two patients who died at 7 and 11 months from constipation associated with gross abdominal distention and a highly dilated hypertrophied colon full of feces. There is absence of ganglion cells in the myenteric plexuses (both Auerbach's and Meissner's) of the most distal bowel and extending proximally for a variable distance. Aganglionosis involving only the rectum or rectosigmoid is often termed 'short segment' Hirschsprung's disease and affects males five times more commonly than females. 'Long segment' Hirschsprung's disease, extending above the sigmoid, has an equal sex incidence and a greater likelihood of siblings being affected. In short segment disease there is a 1 in 20 risk that brothers will be affected and a 1 in 100 risk for sisters. In long segment disease the risk to all siblings is 1 in 10.

In a few cases there is total colonic aganglionosis with disease extending into the small bowel and in extremely rare cases involving the whole alimentary canal. At least 70% of cases are short segment, 25% long segment and about 5% total colonic.

Hirschsprung's disease differs from many other alimentary tract abnormalities in that the birth weight is usually within the normal range. It is uncommon in premature and low birth weight babies. Associated congenital anomalies are uncommon apart from Down syndrome which affects 1 in 20. The cause of the disease is unknown. It has been postulated that it is due to a failure of migration of ganglion cells from the neural crest which normally proceeds in a craniocaudal direction having entered the upper end of the alimentary tract.[7] Differentiation of ganglion cells occurs in the wall of the gut between the seventh and eighth week of intrauterine life and proceeds in a craniocaudal direction.

Clinical features

Usually the symptoms of Hirschsprung's disease are manifest within the first few days of life. This is certainly the case in all long segment or total colonic cases but some short segment cases and especially 'ultrashort' segment cases may present later, even into old age.

Failure to pass meconium within the first 24 h, abdominal distention, bile stained vomiting and reluctance to feed are the main symptoms. Diarrhea may be the presenting feature of Hirschsprung's enterocolitis, a devastating complication of the condition which has a high mortality. The etiology of Hirschsprung's enterocolitis is unknown but apart from diarrhea it is associated with gross abdominal distention and circulatory collapse. A rectal examination results in the explosive passage of flatus and loose stool, deflating the abdomen.

Diagnosis

A plain abdominal X-ray shows distended small and large bowel, sometimes with multiple fluid levels on an erect film. A barium enema is best carried out without a previous rectal examination as then the narrow aganglionic bowel with dilation proximally is demonstrated. A delayed film at 24 h, again avoiding an invasive rectal examination, shows retained barium and often a clear indication of the level of disease with a cone-shaped transition zone between normal bowel above and the narrowed aganglionic distal segment.

Definitive diagnosis is by rectal biopsy. A suction biopsy is adequate to confirm the absence of ganglion cells in the submucosal plexus, specimens being taken at 1 and 3 cm above the dentate line. Histochemical staining will demonstrate excessive acetyl cholinesterase activity in abnormal nerve trunks and absence of ganglion cells.

Treatment

Once the diagnosis is made, bowel washouts may be sufficient to maintain bowel decompression prior to a laparoscopically assisted pull through procedure. Others prefer a defunctioning stoma, proximal to the diseased bowel. A definitive procedure is then carried out when the infant is 3–12 months of age, depending on the surgeon's preference. It usually consists of excision of the aganglionic bowel and a 'pull through' procedure.

If enterocolitis supervenes (and it can even happen after a definitive procedure, especially if an aganglionic segment remains), then rapid replacement of lost fluid by a suitable electrolyte solution, often preceded by plasma, is required. This should be combined with saline bowel washouts using a two tube technique, one to run saline in, preferably above the aganglionic segment, the other at a slightly lower level to allow evacuation. Broad spectrum antibiotics are usually administered prophylactically although infection has not been shown to be the precipitating factor. Enterocolitis is certainly the most lethal complication of Hirschsprung's disease.

UROLOGICAL PROBLEMS IN THE NEONATE

Posterior urethral valves

The commonest obstructive uropathy in male children is valvular obstruction of the posterior urethra. Occasionally the diagnosis is made on antenatal ultrasound. A large proportion of cases present in the first 2 weeks of life, the majority in the first 6 months and the remainder, whilst usually becoming apparent in the first few years, may present as late as early adult life.

The neonate may present with retention of urine or dribbling and a palpably distended bladder with or without infection or uremia. Later presentation is usually with incontinence or infection.

The valves are classically folds of mucosa attached just below the verumontanum and attempts to void lead to apposition of the valves. The obstruction leads to dilation of the posterior urethra, the bladder, the ureter and renal pelvis.

As micturition commences in the fetus in the first trimester, the back pressure on the kidneys may lead antenatally to severe damage – renal dysplasia. Occasionally the bladder hypertrophy is such that reflux no longer occurs but the ureters remain dilated and tortuous.

Diagnosis

A micturating cystourethrogram (MCU) is diagnostic in this anomaly, demonstrating the gross dilation of the posterior urethra and usually the refluxing dilated ureters and bilateral hydronephrosis.

Treatment

Disruption of the valves is required. This may be effected by pulling the inflated balloon of a Fogarty catheter across the valves or by delicately disrupting them with a Whitaker hook. A resectoscope can be used transurethrally and the valves either fulgurated or, to avoid a deep destruction of tissue, cut with a cold knife. If renal function is particularly poor, temporary drainage via bilateral cutaneous ureterostomies (preferably ring ureterostomies) may be required.

Prune belly syndrome (triad syndrome)

This consists of deficiency of the anterior abdominal wall muscles, cryptorchidism and urinary tract deformities. The abdominal muscular deficiency is mainly in the lower abdomen, the whole abdominal wall taking on the wrinkled appearance of a prune (Fig. 36.14). The ribs may be flared outwards at the lower costal margin and respiratory infections are common.

Surgery is best avoided unless there is significant renal impairment. In severe cases ring ureterostomies may be required, followed at a later date by tapering and reimplantation of the

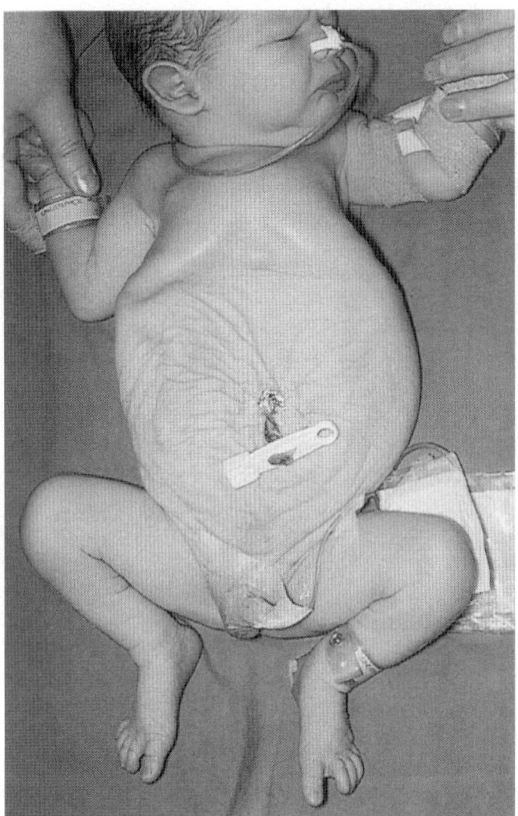

Fig. 36.14 Prune belly syndrome.

ureters, trimming of the bladder, orchidopexies and excision and repair of the lower anterior abdominal wall. Some cases have a functional urethral obstruction which may require urethrotomy. Other cases show urethral stricture or even a diverticulum at the site of the prostatic utricle.

Urachal anomalies

The urachus in the embryo connects the bladder to the allantois. It is normally obliterated to form the median umbilical ligament. It may, however, persist as a patent urachus in the neonate, requiring repair. Occasionally the two extremities of the urachus close, leaving a cyst in the middle which becomes filled with secretions and may present as a mass or more commonly, when it becomes infected, as an abscess.

Bladder exstrophy (ectopia vesicae)

This is part of a range of lower abdominal wall defects, ranging from epispadias, through exstrophy of the bladder, to the even more catastrophic vesicointestinal fissure or cloacal exstrophy.

In bladder exstrophy there is a lower abdominal wall anomaly in which there is wide separation of the pubic bones, the bladder surface being flat and exposed with the two ureteric orifices clearly visible (Fig. 36.15). In the male there is complete epispadias with a strip of urethral mucosa on the dorsum of a short broadened flattened penis. In the female there is also an epispadiac urethra with a bifid clitoris and separation of the labia anteriorly at the level of the vaginal orifice.

The bladder is best repaired soon after birth. If necessary, bilateral iliac osteotomies enable the pubic bones to be better approximated thus facilitating the repair. Careful construction of the bladder neck is vital to achieve subsequent continence, and in the male later repair of the severe epispadiac deformity is required. If the bladder repair is unsuccessful it may be necessary to carry out a urinary diversion procedure.

EXOMPHALOS AND GASTROSCHISIS

These are two distinct conditions of different etiology. Although formerly exomphalos was believed to be more common, gastroschisis is now seen more frequently. Antenatal diagnosis of both conditions by ultrasound examination is now almost routine. Gastroschisis also gives rise to an elevated maternal serum alpha-fetoprotein and distinction from other anomalies such as neural tube defects is by ultrasonography. Gastroschisis is not an indication for termination of pregnancy whilst exomphalos major, with its high incidence (30–40%) of associated anomalies, may be.

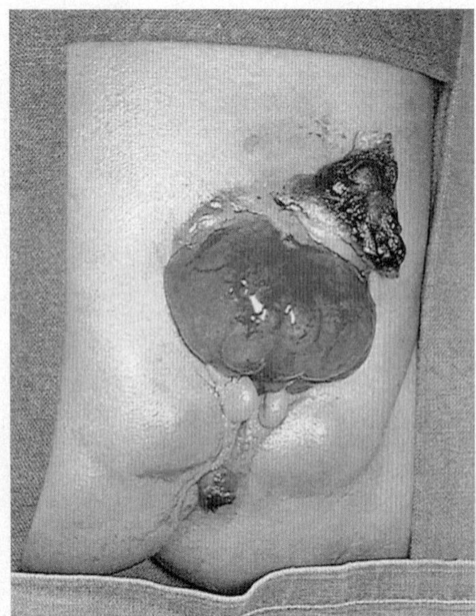

Fig. 36.15 Ectopic vesicae.

Exomphalos

Exomphalos (omphalocele) is a herniation of intra-abdominal contents through the umbilical ring into the umbilical cord. Defects less than 4 cm in diameter are classified as *exomphalos minor* (Fig. 36.16). There are rarely associated abnormalities in this group.

Exomphalos major (Fig. 36.17), on the other hand, commonly has coexisting abnormalities and a defect greater than 4 cm in diameter, presumably arising through failure of development of the anterior abdominal wall prior to herniation of the midgut loop. In a large defect, not only the intestines (small and large) herniate but also the liver, spleen, stomach, bladder and even ovaries and fallopian tubes in the female. Incomplete or malrotation of the bowel is common and the associated abnormalities often include cardiac defects; 20% of cases are anencephalic. In the *Beckwith–Wiedemann* syndrome there is exomphalos, macroglossia and gigantism. The baby is large for his gestational age with an exomphalos, a big tongue and large solid viscera. There is also a facial nevus flammeus in the center of the forehead and odd indentations in the ear lobe (Fig. 36.18). There may also be pancreatic hyperplasia leading to severe neonatal hypoglycemia.

An *omphalocele* is usually covered by a sac composed of the fused layers of amniotic membrane and peritoneum. The sac may rupture ante-, intra- or postpartum.

Treatment

In a large omphalocele, conservative management may be appropriate in the neonatal period. The danger of mercury poisoning has led to the recommendation that 0.5% mercurochrome in 65% alcohol solution be used for only 48 h, applying the solution 2 hourly. A simple alcohol solution should then be applied daily until an eschar forms. Epithelialization of the sac from the periphery results over the ensuing weeks. It may take 3–4 months before the infant can be discharged home, returning for later surgical repair of the ventral hernia. Other methods of treatment include mobilization of skin around the defect and skin coverage or coverage with prosthetic material and later repair of the

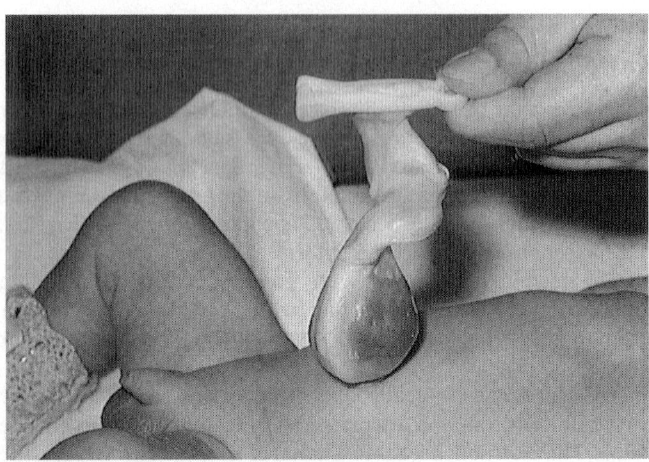

Fig. 36.16 Exomphalos minor.

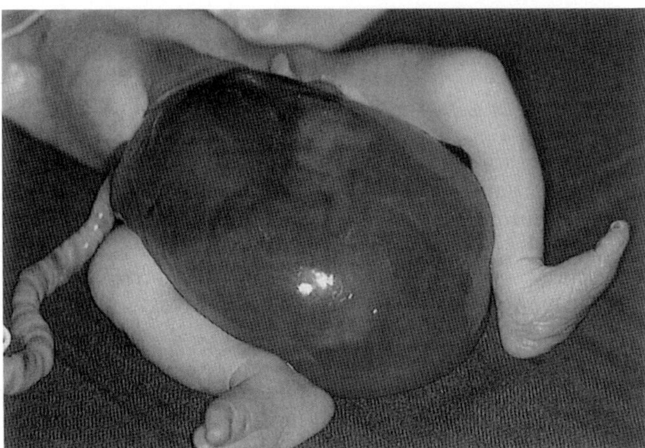

Fig. 36.17 Exomphalos major.

ventral hernia. If the defect is small enough then, with stretching of the anterior abdominal wall, primary repair may be possible as in gastroschisis (see below). In cases with an apparently simple herniation through a small defect into the umbilical cord it is tempting to twist the cord to reduce the contained bowel into the abdominal cavity, then simply ligate the cord. Such a temptation must be strongly resisted as all too frequently there is a Meckel's diverticulum or another cause of adherence of the bowel to the sac and serious damage may result. Formal surgical repair is always indicated.

Gastroschisis

Gastroschisis is a complete defect through all layers of the anterior abdominal wall extending up to about 3 cm in length and usually lying to the right of a normally attached umbilical cord (Fig. 36.19). It is almost as though a short transverse incision had been made with a scalpel antenatally. The etiology is unknown.

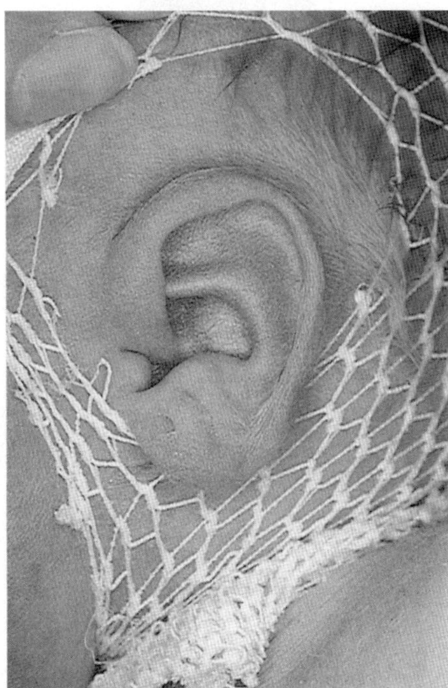

Fig. 36.18 Earlobe indentations in Beckwith–Wiedemann syndrome.

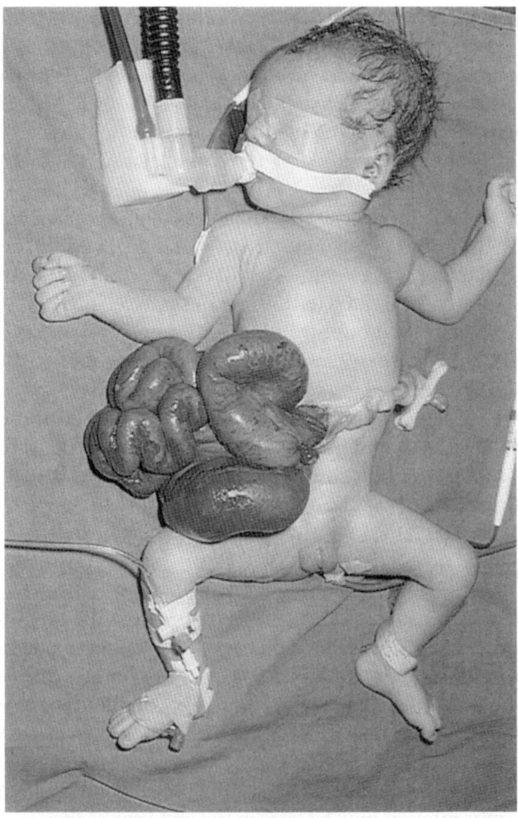

Fig. 36.19 Gastroschisis.

Almost all the small and large bowel are eviscerated through the small defect – in most instances from stomach to rectum inclusive. Other organs are rarely apparent. The eviscerated bowel is markedly thickened, apparently foreshortened, matted together and often covered with a confluent gelatinous layer like 'gut in aspic'.

If possible, delivery should be in a perinatal center close to the regional pediatric surgical center. The decision whether to deliver the baby with exomphalos or gastroschisis by cesarean section or vaginally is an obstetric one. The results of treatment of the baby are not significantly improved by cesarean delivery.

At delivery it is essential that the baby is placed in a plastic bag extending to above the level of the defect and leaving the head and, if necessary, the upper limbs exposed. The bowel must not be allowed to become contaminated, the baby being transferred in a transport incubator directly to the pediatric surgical operating table and the baby extracted from the bag aseptically, by the surgeon, once anesthesia is induced. The passage of a nasogastric tube prior to transfer reduces bowel distention and resulting ischemia if the anterior abdominal wall defect is very small. Transport in a polyethylene bag helps reduce hypothermia which would otherwise result from heat loss by evaporation. These babies rapidly drop their temperature from 37°C to 35°C when exposed for even a few minutes to site an intravenous infusion. The application of warm saline soaked swabs is not a good idea as they rapidly cool, increasing the heat loss.

Treatment

Providing the temperature has been adequately maintained and no fluid loss has occurred, direct transfer to the operating table for primary repair will achieve the best results. The anterior abdominal wall is slowly and gently, yet vigorously, stretched manually.

Once the abdominal cavity has been sufficiently enlarged the bowel can be returned under minimal tension and the defect closed with an absorbable purse-string suture. It is essential that the baby is left with a reasonable umbilicus and this is achieved by leaving the cord intact with or without a further purse-string suture to the skin. The defect is usually so small that the umbilicus is not eccentric in position.

Postoperatively, ventilatory support is often required for a few days. In addition a prolonged ileus necessitates intravenous nutrition for days or in some cases even weeks. The prognosis in gastroschisis cases treated in this manner is excellent.

On occasion the bowel wall is too thickened to allow complete reduction and in these cases a silastic 'silo' is constructed, the content being reduced gradually over succeeding days.

Some surgeons now choose to reduce the bowel in the incubator without anesthesia and this avoids the need for assisted ventilation. A new 'silo' device that can be applied without anesthesia has also recently become available.

SACROCOCCYGEAL TERATOMA

The sacrococcygeal teratoma is the commonest teratoma presenting in the neonatal period. They tend to be large and protrude from the space between the anus and the coccyx (Fig. 36.20). The lesion is usually covered in skin but the most protuberant part may be necrotic due to vascular compromise. The tumor may also extend up into the pelvis and a large retrorectal component is palpable in all cases. In a presacral teratoma there is no protrusion behind the anus and the presentation may be later in the first year of life.

The tumor may be both solid and cystic in nature. A very large tumor may give rise to dystocia and if diagnosed antenatally is best delivered by cesarean section.

Treatment is excision within the first few days of life. A double 'chevron' incision is made with the baby in a prone position and with careful excision and reconstruction of the pelvic floor which, despite its gross stretching, recovers normal function (Fig. 36.21). Excision of the coccyx is an essential component of the operation as failing to do so may predispose to the development of a yolk sac tumour.

There is usually an elevated alpha-fetoprotein level in the baby at birth and this should decline appropriately following excision. Even benign tumors should be followed up into adulthood as recurrence of benign or malignant elements may occur.

ANORECTAL ANOMALIES

Congenital anomalies of the anus and rectum are reported to occur in 1 in 1800 to 1 in 10 000 live births. In Edinburgh the incidence is 1 in 3100. There is a wide spectrum of anomalies and many attempts have been made to classify them.

An anatomical approach simplifies matters (Table 36.1).[8] The lesions are grouped according to whether the end of the rectum is above levator ani, *high* (supralevator), or below, *low* (translevator). There is also an *intermediate*, partially translevator group. The essential component of the levator ani in these malformations is the puborectalis sling which is the key to fecal continence.

In the male a high lesion commonly communicates with the urethra whereas in the female, with the genital tract intervening, the fistula is to the vagina. A low lesion may open onto the skin of the perineum, or in the male, track forwards along the median raphe of the scrotum (Fig. 36.22), or in the female, towards the vestibule. In addition, a severe cloacal anomaly may arise in girls with urethra, vagina and rectum opening into a common channel. Anal stenosis may arise in either sex and presents with the passage of toothpaste-like motions.

Fig. 36.20 Sacrococcygeal teratoma.

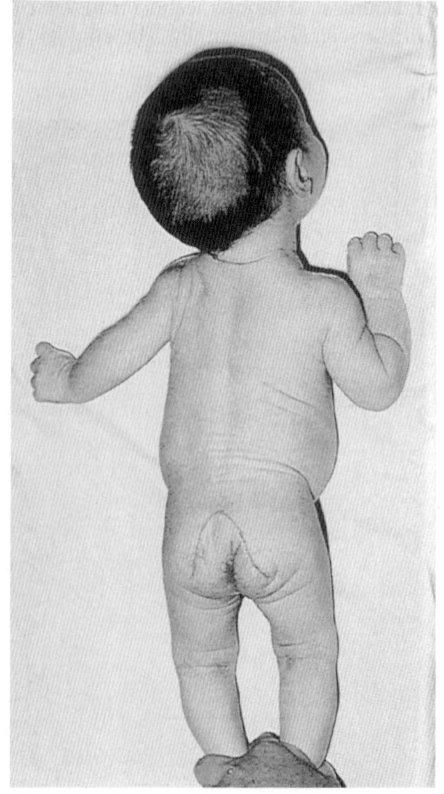

Fig. 36.21 Postoperative appearance of Figure 36.20.

Table 36.1 Classification of anorectal malformations (Stephens 1984[8])

Female	Male
High	*High*
Anorectal agenesis:	Anorectal agenesis:
With rectovaginal fistula	With recto-prostatic-urethral fistula
Without fistula	Without fistula
Intermediate	*Intermediate*
Rectovestibular fistula	Rectobulbar urethral fistula
Rectovaginal fistula	
Anal agenesis without fistula	Anal agenesis without fistula
Low	*Low*
Anovestibular fistula	
Anocutaneous fistula	Anocutaneous fistula
Anal stenosis	Anal stenosis
Cloacal malformations	
Rare malformations	Rare malformations

Treatment

Anal stenosis is treated by graduated anal dilation with Hegar's dilators. A low lesion with a long subcutaneous tract should have the latter opened and an anoplasty performed. An anovestibular fistula can also be managed by a cutback procedure. This may result in rather close proximity of anal and vaginal openings (shotgun perineum) but the perineum develops as the child grows, separating the orifices. To avoid this appearance some prefer to transpose the anal opening to a more normal site.

High and intermediate lesions, and low lesions where the diagnosis is not at first obvious, require a defunctioning colostomy in the neonatal period. A sigmoid colostomy will enable subsequent adequate washouts of the distal loop, a procedure that is especially important in lesions communicating with the urinary tract. Prophylactic antibiotics are also required in such cases.

Once the colostomy is established, formal contrast studies via the distal loop (distal loopogram) define the level of the lesion accurately. Definitive repair is then deferred for a few weeks or months depending on the preference of the surgeon. The procedure of choice is the posterior sagittal anorectoplasty described by de Vries & Pena,[9] requiring meticulous technique and a thorough understanding of the anatomy. Some now perform a laparoscopically assisted pull through.

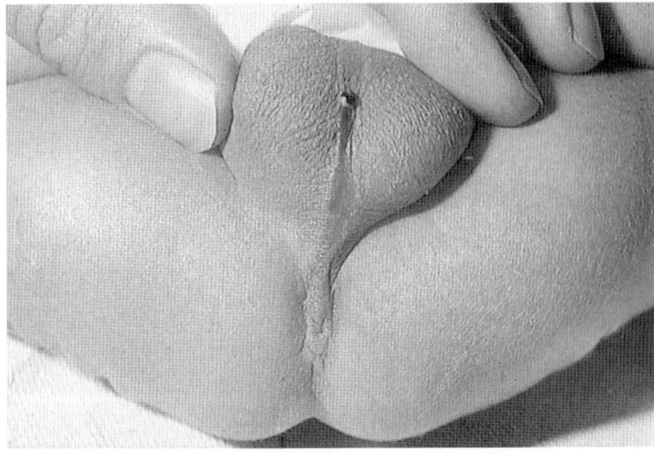

Fig. 36.22 Low anorectal anomaly.

NEONATAL NECROTIZING ENTEROCOLITIS (NEC)

This condition is described in detail on page 285. Presenting as it does with abdominal distention and bile stained vomiting, it is occasionally considered that the baby has intestinal obstruction but the presence of blood in the stool and pneumatosis intestinalis, often with portal venous gas, are pathognomonic of NEC. The management is conservative, wherever possible with nasogastric decompression, intravenous feeding and broad spectrum antibiotics. The criteria for surgical management include pneumoperitoneum, persistent and increasing abdominal tenderness and continued clinical deterioration despite appropriate medical management. Operative management includes resection of necrotic bowel and stoma formation. Occasionally localized drainage under local anesthesia is of value in extremely ill babies, with appropriate intervention at a later date. Conservatively managed survivors often develop intestinal strictures requiring later resection. Asymptomatic strictures identified on contrast studies are best kept under review, reserving surgery for symptomatic cases.

BILIARY ATRESIA

Biliary atresia is a condition in which the extrahepatic bile ducts are grossly non-patent. The condition is characterized by obstructive jaundice. There has traditionally been a division into 'correctable' biliary atresia, where only the distal ducts are occluded, and 'non-correctable', in which the proximal ducts are occluded.

Presentation is with jaundice persisting beyond the first 2 weeks of life. Appropriate tests are carried out to exclude causes of hepatocellular disease (hepatitis A, hepatitis B, toxoplasmosis, rubella, cytomegalovirus, herpes, syphilis, listeriosis, galactosemia, fructosemia, alpha1-antitrypsin deficiency, etc.). It is vital not to waste too much time awaiting the results of all tests as delay in treatment of biliary atresia will adversely affect the progress. Suspected cases must therefore be referred early to a center capable of undertaking the necessary investigation and surgery. Ultrasound will rarely show a gallbladder and may show increased hepatic parenchymal echoes in biliary atresia. An isotope liver scan using a ^{99m}Tc iminodiacetic acid (IDA) radiopharmaceutical will demonstrate good hepatic uptake but no excretion into the bowel at 24 h. In hepatocellular jaundice there is a decrease in hepatocyte clearance.

Some surgeons prefer to do a percutaneous liver biopsy which may be strongly indicative of biliary atresia, but others proceed directly to operative cholangiography if there is a positive IDA scan. This is carried out through a small transverse right upper abdominal incision. The gallbladder is often small and fibrotic making a cholangiogram impossible. Occasionally patency of the cystic duct and common bile duct may be identified and, rarely, biliary hypoplasia.

Treatment

The procedure of choice for extrahepatic biliary atresia is Kasai's hepatic portoenterostomy. This was first described in Japanese in 1959 and only in 1968 in English.[10]

Kasai reports satisfactory bile drainage in 80% of cases. In other series this ranges from 35 to 75% (personal small series 75%). Many will develop portal hypertension and cholangitis (various modifications of Kasai's procedure are carried out to reduce this complication). Liver transplantation is of great value in cases that fail to achieve or maintain bile drainage following the Kasai procedure.

SURGERY OF THE INFANT AND CHILD

HEAD AND NECK, FACE AND MOUTH

Embryological

Branchial

Sinuses, fistulae, cysts and cartilaginous elements may be apparent at birth or may be noted in infancy or later in childhood. These anomalies arise from the first and second pharyngeal arches and clefts. First cleft remnants are rare and include a tract from the external auditory canal to the upper lateral neck. They may present with recurrent abscesses in the neck, and treatment involves excision of the whole tract, usually a sinus, being blind ending at the external auditory canal. Abnormal development of the first arch results in cleft lip and palate, abnormal shape of the pinna, and deafness due to malformation of the malleus and incus.

Second branchial remnants are more common. In theory sinuses should be more common than fistulae but the reverse is true and cysts are the least common, often presenting in adult life. Fistulae have a skin opening over the anterior border of the lower third of the sternomastoid. This may be noted to discharge clear mucus. The tract passes upwards between the internal and external carotid arteries to open in the tonsillar fossa.

The length of this tract often necessitates two incisions to facilitate its removal, one being at the skin opening and the other parallel to it, at a higher level, to follow the tract through the carotid bifurcation.

Branchial cysts manifest themselves as they slowly enlarge with secretions, appearing in late childhood or young adulthood. They tend to lie deep to the anterior border of the upper third of the sternocleidomastoid muscle. They may become infected. The treatment is excision.

Cartilaginous branchial remnants may appear along the anterior border of sternocleidomastoid. They do not usually have an associated tract and are excised purely for cosmetic reasons.

Thyroglossal cysts

These are more common than branchial remnants. The thyroid develops as a diverticulum from the floor of the pharynx leaving it attached to the foramen cecum (at the junction of the anterior two-thirds, and posterior one-third of the tongue) by a stalk, the thyroglossal duct, which is normally completely reabsorbed. The tract of a persistent thyroglossal duct should developmentally be ventral to the hyoid bone but differential growth results in part of the duct reaching its deep surface. A thyroglossal cyst arises typically in the midline of the neck anteriorly, or occasionally just to one or other side of the midline. By virtue of its attachment to the thyroglossal duct the cyst moves on swallowing or protrusion of the tongue (Fig. 36.23a, b and c). The cyst is usually at the level of or just below the hyoid bone but can be anywhere along the line of the duct. Surgery is best performed when the lesion is diagnosed, as infection may arise and lead to difficulty in complete excision. The operation involves not only removal of the cyst but the body of the hyoid and the tract must be followed up to the level of the foramen cecum. Failure to do this is likely to lead to recurrence.

Dermoid cysts

These usually occur at sites of embryological fusion. These may be in the midline. A dermoid cyst in the neck may be mistaken for a thyroglossal cyst although it will not move on swallowing or protrusion of the tongue. A common site is the external angular dermoid cyst in the eyebrow area at the outer angle of the eye. Occasionally there may be a dumbbell extension intracranially. They occur if ectodermal cells become buried beneath the skin surface during development. An inclusion dermoid cyst may similarly arise secondary to trauma.

Cystic hygroma

Commonly arising in the neck, these fluid filled lesions of lymphatic origin may be found elsewhere, including the axilla and groin or, rarely, on the trunk. They are either present at birth, sometimes being diagnosed on antenatal ultrasonography, or may appear within the first 2 years or sometimes later. Usually arising in the posterior triangle of the neck, they may sometimes be very large indeed extending into the floor of the mouth and tongue where complete excision may prove difficult, leading to disfigurement and

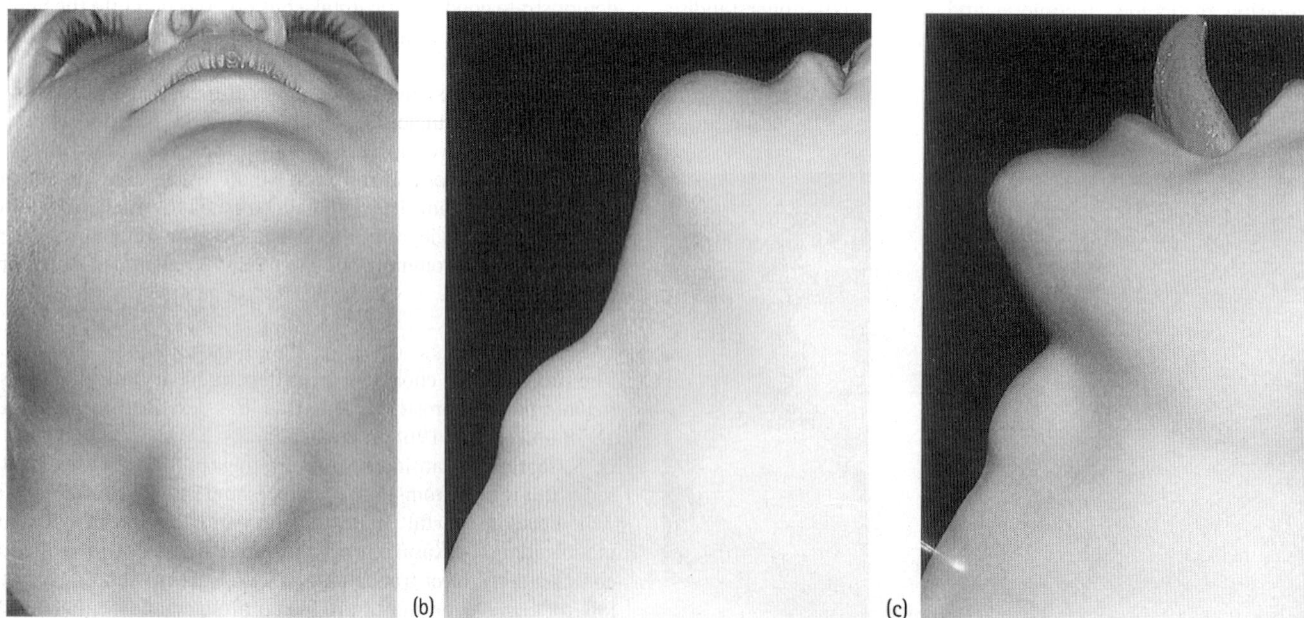

Fig. 36.23 (a) Thyroglossal cyst; (b) and (c) show elevation on tongue protrusion.

occasionally to the need for a tracheostomy. Infection leads to difficulty with subsequent surgery, which is thus best performed soon after diagnosis. Aspiration of the cysts and injection of a streptococcal derivative 'OK432' is a new treatment that is proving to be an effective alternative to surgery.[11]

Salivary gland enlargement

This may arise secondary to a calculus in a duct (the submandibular duct in particular). Parotid duct calculi are rare but recurrent swelling of the gland may be due to sialectasis, seen on a sialogram as dilated duct radicles. The treatment is to advise the sucking of acid drop sweets to promote salivary flow and at the same time massaging the gland from back to front. If infection supervenes then antibiotics must be administered.

Ranula (Latin rana *= frog)*

This is a sublingual cyst which may be small or may fill the floor of the mouth. It may be related to a salivary or mucus gland. It is thin walled and contains clear viscid fluid. Care is required not to damage the submandibular duct during its excision and marsupialization is often safer.

Tongue tie

A short lingual frenum leads to maternal anxiety regarding future problems with speech. Speech therapists confirm that there will be no speech problem and others that the anterior third of the tongue will grow and a normal appearance will result. Tongue-tie may lead to difficulty with breast-feeding. Division of the tongue-tie in a baby prior to appearance of dentition is a simple procedure for a surgeon in the outpatient clinic. In the older child, general anesthesia is required. Tongue tie may occasionally present beyond the first 2 years and I personally believe in division, as all children deserve to be able to stick their tongue out – if only to lick an ice cream!

Cervical lymphadenopathy

Cervical lymph nodes are readily palpable in most children. Lymphoma is rare, but persistent painless enlargement of a cervical node is best diagnosed by excision biopsy although it is reasonable to administer an antibiotic in doubtful cases and re-examine the child in 2 weeks. Cat scratch disease, toxoplasma and both tuberculosis and atypical mycobacterial infections may occur and usually affect jugulodigastric and submandibular nodes.

In mycobacterial infections, nodes may feel fixed to deeper tissues and to skin and may caseate and discharge. Sinus formation may result from abscess rupture or incomplete excision. Antituberculous chemotherapy is necessary once the diagnosis has become established.

Acute suppurative cervical lymphadenitis usually results from an upper respiratory tract infection. Early administration of antibiotics may lead to resolution without abscess formation but if an abscess does form it should be allowed to point before drainage. Kaolin poultices seem old fashioned but are still of value in this process.

Sternomastoid tumor

This is the commonest cause of torticollis in childhood (other causes include hemivertebrae, acute fasciitis, cervical adenitis and ocular muscle imbalance). The cause of this lesion is unknown. It is more common in babies born by breech presentation and was considered to be a result of trauma to the muscle during delivery. It seems likely, however, that it arises in utero, resulting in breech presentation. Within the muscle there is an area of endomysial fibrosis with atrophied muscle fibers surrounded by collagen and fibroblasts. The infant presents usually at 2–3 weeks of age with a hard swelling within the substance of sternocleidomastoid. The shortening of the muscle makes the infant look upwards and to the opposite side. It is important to commence physiotherapy as soon as the diagnosis is made. The parents are taught how to stretch the muscle by rotating the head towards the side of the tumor. These stretching exercises should be carried out twice daily and must continue for at least the first year, diminishing in frequency thereafter. Failure to treat adequately leads to shortening of deeper cervical structures and craniofacial asymmetry. Surgical division of the muscle and deeper strictures is necessary in cases that fail to respond or are missed in the neonatal period.

Thyroid swellings

(see Chapter 13)

PYLORIC STENOSIS

Though often called congenital, hypertrophic pyloric stenosis only very rarely has its onset of symptoms at birth and has never been described in a stillbirth. Vomiting normally commences around 2–3 weeks of age, becoming more frequent and projectile. The vomitus is of gastric content (milk) and is never bile stained. It may become brownish or visibly bloodstained due either to an accompanying gastritis or to rupture of capillaries in the gastric mucosa from frequent vomiting. The baby fails to thrive, becomes constipated and dehydrated, developing a hypochloremic alkalosis from the loss of gastric acid.

Examination reveals a hungry, worried looking baby and if recently fed, visible gastric peristalsis, with a wave traveling from the left hypochondrium towards the right, may be apparent (Fig. 36.24). The diagnosis is confirmed during a test feed. For this the surgeon and the nurse or mother sit facing in opposite directions, the surgeon to the left of the nurse (Fig. 36.25). The baby is fed with the bottle in the right hand or at the left breast of the nursing mother. The surgeon palpates the tumor with the left hand. It is felt as an olive-shaped mass which lies just to the right of the midline, in the right hypochondrium. Contraction of the tumor is noted with variation in palpability, thus confirming that one is not confusing it with a Riedel's lobe of liver, or similar anomaly. If difficulty is encountered in palpating the tumor, the passage of a nasogastric tube to wash out the stomach may facilitate the procedure (it may be that the filled gastric antrum has previously obscured the pylorus). This seemingly ritual routine not only enhances the chance of palpating the tumor but avoids the calamity of the baby vomiting over the examiner's trousers!

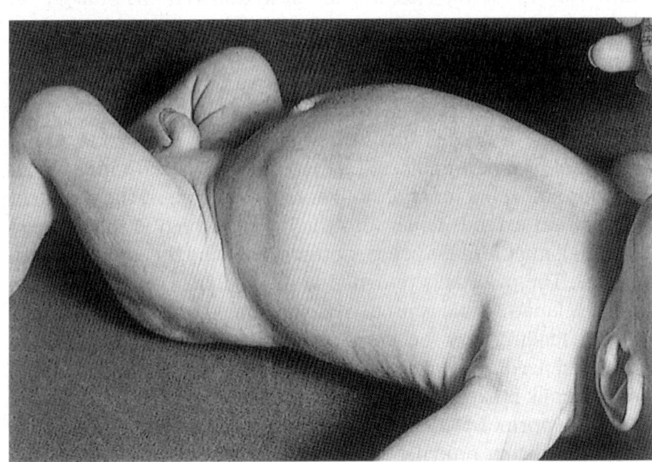

Fig. 36.24 Pyloric stenosis: visible peristalsis.

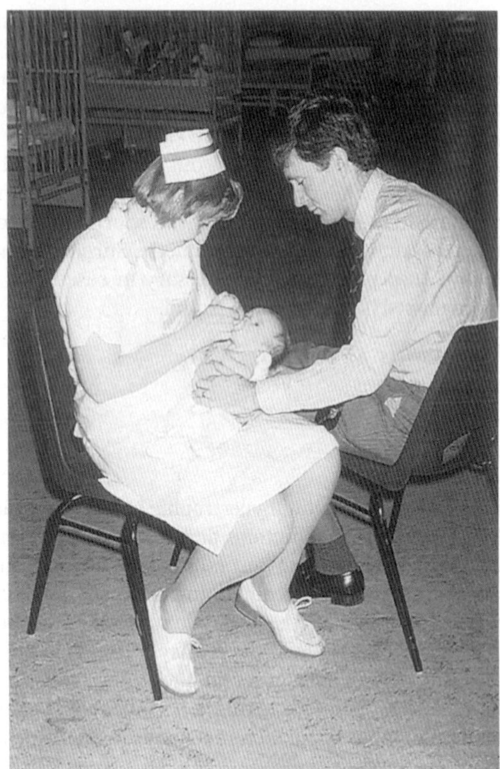

Fig. 36.25 Pyloric stenosis: test feed.

Most surgeons will only operate if they can palpate the tumor but if difficulty is encountered in palpation, ultrasound examination is now the diagnostic investigation of choice.

Treatment

First the hypochloremic alkalosis together with any associated hypokalemia is corrected by administering 5% dextrose in 0.45% saline with added potassium chloride if required. Although the use of 0.45% saline takes twice as long to correct the deficit as normal saline would, it is safer to administer. Preoperative gastric lavage is also performed and the nasogastric tube left in situ.

Once the electrolyte and acid–base deficit is corrected, surgery is performed under general anesthesia. The universally accepted operation of choice is the pyloromyotomy attributed to Ramstedt.[12] Actually the first recorded use of this procedure was by Sir Harold Stiles[13] in the Royal Hospital for Sick Children, Edinburgh on 3 February 1910, a year prior to Ramstedt's operation performed on 28 July 1911 and published in 1912. Unfortunately Stiles' patient died on the fourth postoperative day, either from gastroenteritis or delayed chloroform poisoning!

The pylorus is delivered through a right transverse upper abdominal or a periumbilical incision, and an incision made from the pyloroduodenal junction well onto the antrum of the stomach. The incision extends down into the muscle which is then spread bluntly, all muscle fibers being ruptured, allowing the intact mucosa to bulge. The pylorus is returned to the abdomen and the wound closed. A laparoscopic approach can be used in some centers.

Oral feeding can be commenced in 4 h. Some choose a graduated feeding regime of dextrose, half strength, then full strength milk introduced over 24–48 h. Others advise a more rapid return to normal feeds. Certainly breast-fed infants come to no harm from being returned to the breast initially for a short time, gradually increasing to normal feeding time.

Vomiting in the first 24 h postoperatively is not unusual and is presumably related to preoperative gastritis. If persistent it usually settles after gastric lavage. Most babies will be fit for discharge within 24–72 h after surgery.

GASTROESOPHAGEAL REFLUX

This is due to incompetence at the cardia and is another cause of vomiting that may commence as early as the neonatal period. The condition may or may not be associated with a hiatus hernia. The infant vomits effortlessly at any time, and usually appears unconcerned about the problem. The vomiting need not be related to feed times. The vomitus may be coffee ground or streaked with bright red blood if there is associated peptic esophagitis. The diagnosis is confirmed by barium studies and pH studies together with endoscopy if indicated. Most cases respond to conservative management of thickening the feeds, sitting the baby up at all times (although there is dispute about this) and the administration of an antacid such as Gaviscon. In more severe cases an H_2 antagonist or a proton pump inhibitor is used. If, however, the infant fails to thrive, has persistent peptic esophagitis, recurrent aspiration pneumonitis or a proven large 'sliding' hiatus hernia, then a surgical antireflux procedure is required. If an esophageal stricture has already developed it will usually resolve after surgery but in some cases bougienage or balloon dilation is required. Various antireflux operations have been devised, the most popular being the Nissen fundoplication. The esophagus and the gastric fundus is mobilized, the right crus of the diaphragm tightened and wrapped around the abdominal esophagus. This operation is now best performed laparoscopically,[14] reducing postoperative discomfort and length of hospital stay.

Children with severe neurological handicap are especially prone to gastroesophageal reflux and hiatus hernia. Usually their parents, or carers welcome the surgical treatment of these children, as their well-being is so obviously improved. Presumably they suffer a great deal of discomfort related to esophagitis and their frustration is increased by their inability to complain. The results of surgery in such cases is invariably rewarding.

INTUSSUSCEPTION

Intussusception is the invagination of part of the intestine into itself. An intussusception arising in the ileum may pass all the way round the large bowel to appear at the anus. The lead point is known as the intussusceptum, the sheath as the intussuscipiens and between these are the entering and returning layers of the bowel. Naturally, the mesentery with its vessels is drawn between the entering and returning layers, leading to engorgement of the vessels and diapedesis of red cells into the lumen of the bowel. Mucus is produced by the engorgement of the mucosal cells and, mixed with the red cells, creates the classical redcurrant jelly stool. Eventually a strangulating obstruction occurs and gangrene of the intussusceptum may result.

In infants the lead point is presumed to be an enlarged Peyer's patch, the lymphoid tissue presumably responding to a viral stimulant. This becomes the apex of the intussusception which then proceeds for a variable distance into the colon. The peak incidence is in infants 3–9 months of age. The timing has been attributed to a change in the bowel flora associated with weaning. In older children the lead point may be an invaginated Meckel's diverticulum, a polyp, an enteric cyst, or hemorrhage into the bowel wall in Henoch–Schönlein purpura or leukemia. It is more common in boys than in girls, some reporting a ratio as high as 5:1, but in Edinburgh the ratio is only 1.2:1. Some report seasonal variation, possibly related to infectious agents.

The presentation is with a painful cry, drawing up the knees and going pale, presumably in relation to colic (88% in our series). The colicky pain is intermittent and occurs with increasing frequency as the condition progresses, rather like labor pains. Vomiting is a common symptom (86%) and the passage of redcurrant jelly stools is frequent (56%).

On examination, between attacks of colic, an abdominal mass is usually palpable. This is typically sausage shaped and commonly palpable in the ascending or transverse colon. A small percentage of intussusceptions present at the anus.

Investigation

Plain abdominal X-ray will often show a filling defect corresponding to the intussusception and will demonstrate any obstruction by the presence of fluid levels within the bowel. Ultrasound can identify a 'target sign' corresponding to the layers of the intussusception. Occasionally a contrast enema may be used diagnostically in frankly obstructed cases.

Treatment

First an intravenous infusion is set up. Some collapsed infants require blood or plasma for primary resuscitation, others only require isotonic fluids. A nasogastric tube may be passed, especially if vomiting has been a marked symptom at presentation. Preparation is as for a surgical reduction; the operating room is arranged in case it is required but in most cases non-operative reduction is first attempted. The only contraindications to non-operative management are a seriously ill child with a prolonged history, marked intestinal obstruction or evidence of peritonitis (rare).

Hydrostatic reduction has been intermittently popular since first advocated by Hirschsprung in 1876. Nowadays a barium enema under X-ray screening is used as a therapeutic technique and is frequently successful. Recently air has been used for reduction rather than barium. (The method has for centuries found favor in China where fire bellows have traditionally been used.) Air is an excellent contrast medium and scientific control of the pressure is by attaching the rectal Foley catheter to a sphygmomanometer, increasing the pressure to 100 mmHg if necessary. This method appears to have a greater success rate than barium and in the rare occurrence of perforation, proves safer.

Surgical reduction is required for those in whom non-operative reduction fails. The intussusception is reduced manually by stripping it back from the point the apex has reached. Pulling on the entering layer of bowel can lead to serosal splitting or rupture of the bowel. Once the intussusception is reduced appendectomy is usually performed. This may help to prevent recurrence by adherence of the cecum in the right iliac fossa. If reduction proves impossible then a limited bowel resection may be required.

Recurrence rates of 2–4% have been recorded and seem unrelated to the method of reduction.

APPENDICITIS

This is the most common condition for which emergency abdominal surgery is required in childhood. Its symptomatology and management are similar to those in adults although in the very young child there may be difficulty in making the appropriate diagnosis. Appendicitis is still a condition with a significant morbidity and mortality. In a recent series, reporting on the last 5 years of the 1970s, there were four deaths related to appendicitis in children in Scotland. Delay in diagnosis can thus convert an eminently treatable condition into a lethal one.

Classically the condition presents with pain, vomiting and fever. The pain commences periumbilically, the distended appendix causing dull and poorly localized midgut pain via visceral nerve fibers to the tenth thoracic nerve root. The pathology of appendicitis is of spreading inflammation from the mucosa through the wall to the serosa. Serosal inflammation leads to peritoneal inflammation and the pain is accurately localized to the right iliac fossa – classically at McBurney's point (two-thirds along a line from the umbilicus to the anterior superior iliac spine). Atypical presentation leads to difficulty in diagnosis, especially in the very young. Neonatal appendicitis is exceedingly rare and the mortality rate is high. In the preschool child the diagnosis is also difficult and a high perforation rate is encountered. The preschool child may present with anorexia, listlessness, fever, vomiting and diarrhea.

Care must be taken in the examination of the child with suspected appendicitis. The tongue may be coated and there is a classical 'fetor oris', a sweet smell on the breath perhaps partly related to ketones. The child is reluctant to climb onto the examination couch. The chest is examined to exclude a right lower lobe pneumonia, which may easily lead to a mistaken diagnosis of appendicitis. Examination of the abdomen must be very gentle, starting in the left lower quadrant and gradually working round each quadrant to finish in the right iliac fossa. Clumsy technique can lose a child's confidence and lead to voluntary guarding. Tenderness at McBurney's point remains the cardinal sign of appendicitis.

Involuntary guarding and rigidity are reliable signs of peritonism or peritonitis. There is no excuse in endeavoring to elicit rebound tenderness as, if present, the child's confidence is immediately lost, the pain being so severe, thus precluding subsequent examination. Likewise, rectal examination should be reserved for cases with negative or equivocal abdominal findings, where it may be the only means of diagnosis of a pelvic appendicitis. It may otherwise confirm a diagnosis of constipation or, in females, gynecological disease. It must be remembered that the appendix can adopt a variety of intra-abdominal positions circumferentially around the attachment to the cecum. A retrocecal appendix may have few abdominal signs initially, although psoas spasm may be apparent.

There are no investigations that can prove the presence of appendicitis. The white cell count need not be raised and an X-ray, whilst occasionally showing a fecolith, is generally unhelpful. Ultrasound is now of value in recognizing a thickened appendix with surrounding edema.

The differential diagnosis includes intestinal diseases such as gastroenteritis, Crohn's disease and other causes of terminal ileitis such as *Yersinia* infection, Meckel's diverticulitis and leukemic typhlitis, mesenteric adenitis and deep iliac adenitis. In addition, gynecological problems such as salpingitis and ovarian cysts must be considered. Urinary tract infection may also be confused with appendicitis, the situation being further complicated by the possible occurrence of pyuria when an inflamed appendix is adjacent to the bladder. Finally, medical disorders such as right basal pneumonia, diabetes mellitus, Henoch–Schönlein purpura and sickle-cell disease have all been misdiagnosed as appendicitis. In fact almost all causes of acute abdominal pain in childhood must be considered but appendicitis is the commonest surgical emergency.

Treatment

If necessary, preliminary resuscitation of the patient by administration of intravenous fluids should be considered. Once the patient has been adequately hydrated then appendectomy is carried out through a skin crease incision an inch or more below McBurney's point to leave a neat scar well below the 'bikini line' or preferably a laparoscopic approach is used. At induction of anesthesia a single dose of broad spectrum antibiotics such as an aminoglycoside and metronidazole, to cover bowel flora including *Escherichia coli* and *Bacteroides fragilis*, is administered to endeavor to prevent postoperative complications such as wound infections and intra-abdominal abscesses, especially pelvic and subphrenic. If an appendix mass is palpated some prefer conservative management with bed rest, intravenous fluids and antibiotics with an interval appendectomy at 3 months. Others proceed to appendectomy appropriately covered by antibiotic therapy.

PRIMARY PERITONITIS

This has a similar presentation to appendicitis but without a history of central pain moving to the right iliac fossa. The abdominal signs are those of peritonitis especially in the lower abdomen. At operation diffuse peritonitis is found with peritoneal exudate, yet no obvious focus of infection. The commonest causative organisms are pneumococci and streptococci. The source of infection has been thought to be the genital tract, the condition being commoner in girls, but the occasional occurrence in boys leads one to suspect blood-borne spread. There may be a preceding or coexisting upper respiratory tract infection. The management is appropriate antibiotic therapy (usually penicillin).

MECKEL'S DIVERTICULUM

Meckel's diverticulum arises from the vitellointestinal duct, which leads from the primitive gut to the yolk sac. Persistence of the proximal end of the duct occurs in 2% of the population (the 2 foot from the ileocecal valve, 2 inch long story is erroneous: it may be a variable length and variable distance from the ileocecal valve).

The vitellointestinal duct can lead to a number of anomalies if it persists (Fig. 36.26). The duct itself may remain patent to the umbilicus and thus present as a fistula in neonates. Partial obliteration may give rise to cyst formation or a persistent fibrous cord from the umbilicus to the ileum may act as an axis for localized volvulus or lead to bowel obstruction.

A Meckel's diverticulum may become inflamed, lead to hemorrhage or invaginate into the ileum and cause intussusception. Meckel's diverticulitis has an identical presentation to acute appendicitis and must always be considered if a normal appendix is identified at surgery.

Bleeding in relation to a Meckel's diverticulum arises because the lining often contains heterotopic gastric mucosa (35–49%). This leads to peptic ulceration of the adjacent normal ileal mucosa (Fig. 36.27). Bleeding usually occurs in preschool children, especially toddlers. It may be intermittent passage of a small amount of altered blood in the stool, although massive hemorrhage with the passage of maroon or even bright red blood is more common. After adequate resuscitation, with blood replacement, a Meckel's scan should be performed. This is a ^{99m}Tc pertechnetate isotope scan which has an affinity for parietal cells. The stomach is visualized on the scan image, together with the bladder, as the isotope is excreted through the kidneys. A third 'blob' of isotope is likely to indicate ectopic gastric mucosa in a Meckel's diverticulum (or rarely in a duplicated segment of bowel). Priming the patient with cimetidine for a few days enhances the scan image. Laparoscopy can avoid the need for a scan and even in the absence of a Meckel's demonstrate the presence or absence of blood in the upper small bowel. An appropriate upper or lower gastrointestinal endoscopy can then be performed under the same anaesthetic.

The treatment is in all cases Meckel's diverticulectomy, the diverticulum being found on the antimesenteric aspect of the ileum 40–100 cm proximal to the ileocecal valve.

SUPERIOR MESENTERIC ARTERY SYNDROME

This syndrome, a cause of acute and chronic abdominal pain in childhood, is due to obstruction of the third part of the duodenum by the superior mesenteric artery. It has variously been called Cast syndrome, Wilkie's syndrome, chronic duodenal ileus and arteriomesenteric duodenal compression syndrome. It may be congenital or acquired, the latter being due to rapid growth without associated weight gain, rapid weight loss or from hyperextension of the vertebral column in a plaster cast. The presentation may be acute or chronic with acute obstructive symptoms or intermittent abdominal pain and vomiting. Contrast studies, if performed between attacks, may show little but if performed in an acute episode will demonstrate obstruction of the third part of the duodenum. The superior mesenteric artery normally subtends an angle of 45° with the aorta but under the conditions described above the angle may decrease to 15° thus occluding the underlying duodenum.

Management is conservative or surgical, the former being alteration of diet, nursing prone and removing or windowing a

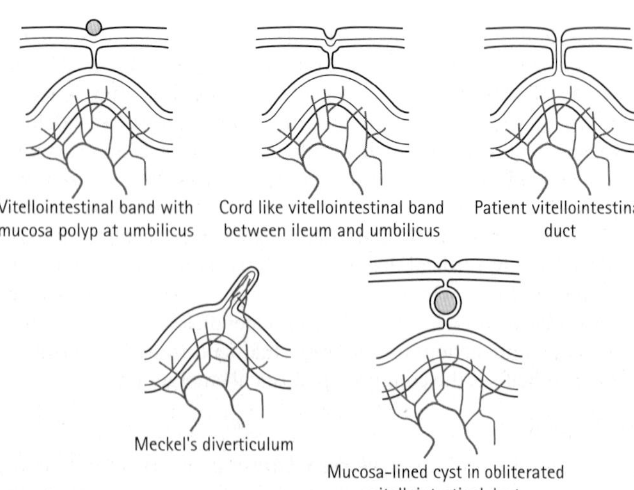

Fig. 36.26 Vitellointestinal remnants.

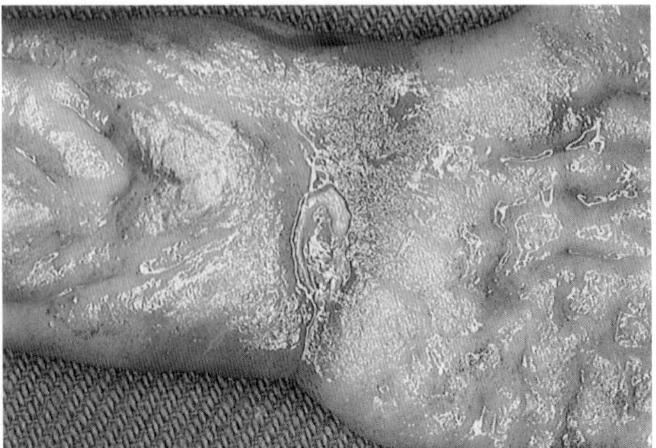

Fig. 36.27 Peptic ulcer at junction of gastric and ileal mucosa in Meckel's diverticulum.

plaster cast if present. Surgical management entails division of the ligament of Treitz and transposition of the small bowel to the right side in a position of nonrotation.[15]

CHOLEDOCHAL CYST

This is a cystic dilation of the choledochus (the common bile duct). The etiology is unknown but some believe it to be related to the reflux of pancreatic secretions into the common duct. The presentation may be in infancy with obstructive jaundice suggestive of biliary atresia, or in the older child with intermittent jaundice, abdominal pain and vomiting often associated with fever suggestive of ascending cholangitis. The diagnosis is by ultrasonography. Treatment consists of excision of the cyst and a Roux-en-Y choledochojejunostomy or hepaticojejunostomy. Failure to excise the entire cyst may result in carcinoma of the cyst wall in the long term.

CHOLELITHIASIS

Gallstones are uncommon in childhood but must be considered in children with hereditary spherocytosis. If metabolic stones develop then cholecystectomy is required, but in hemolytic disease the gallbladder is usually normal and simple cholecystotomy and removal of the stones is all that is required. This procedure should always be considered at the time of splenectomy in these children.

INGUINAL HERNIA AND HYDROCELE

These conditions have the same origin in childhood – the presence of a patent processus vaginalis. The only difference between them is the caliber of the processus (Fig. 36.28). If wide a hernia is produced, if narrow then peritoneal fluid may tract down to the tunica vaginalis. This explains the use of the term hydrocele from the Greek *hydro* = water, *kele* = hernia. (A similar derivation applies to encephalocele, omphalocele, ureterocele, etc.) Frequently hydrocele is spelt, erroneously, 'coele', even in textbooks: it is not derived from coelom (Greek *koiloma* = hollow).

The processus vaginalis is an outpouching of peritoneum drawn down by the descent of the testis. The distal portion persists as the tunica vaginalis but the intervening communication with the peritoneal cavity is normally obliterated. Persistence of a widely patent processus along its whole length results in a hernia of the 'complete' type – a scrotal hernia. Obliteration of the distal portion results in a 'funicular' hernial sac. Similarly, a hydrocele of the cord can arise, the distal portion being obliterated and the proximal communication narrowed.

These conditions are more common on the right side than the left, presumably related to the later descent of the right testis. They may also arise in girls, although hernias are less common. Occasionally an ovary may prolapse into a hernia – at surgery it must be inspected to confirm that it is indeed an ovary and not a testis in testicular feminization syndrome (Fig. 36.29). Chromosomal analysis may be of value in excluding this condition in girls with bilateral hernias but the incidence is extremely low. The hydrocele equivalent in a female is a hydrocele of the canal of Nuck – a small diverticulum of peritoneum accompanying the round ligament of the uterus through the inguinal canal.

In general, hydroceles are only treated surgically if they persist beyond the age of 1 year, the majority resolving spontaneously prior to that. In toddlers there is often a history of a hydrocele increasing in size towards the end of the day – the fluid slowly returns to the peritoneum through the narrow processus when the child is recumbent at night. Surgery consists of ligation and division of the patent processus vaginalis through a small inguinal incision.

Inguinal hernias are treated with a similar operation. If the hernia is not obvious on examination, despite a typical history, tickling may increase the intra-abdominal pressure to demonstrate the hernia, but its presence can be confirmed by rolling the spermatic cord over the pubic bone with the index finger, thickening being apparent in the presence of a hernia.

If a scrotal swelling is present, a hydrocele can usually be distinguished from a hernia by the fact that one can get above it. Rarely does a hydrocele extend up into the inguinal canal. Transillumination may be misleading, as the thin bowel wall, with intraluminal fluid in a young infant, will also transilluminate. The surgery is a semi-urgent herniotomy. There is no requirement for herniorrhaphy (repair).

Incarceration of an inguinal hernia implies irreducibility, which will lead to strangulation of the bowel if left untreated. Gentle reduction is attempted. Force must not be applied and unless reduction is easy the child should be sedated with i.m. morphine and tipped head down; occasionally gallows traction is of benefit. If reduction is unsuccessful, immediate surgical reduction and

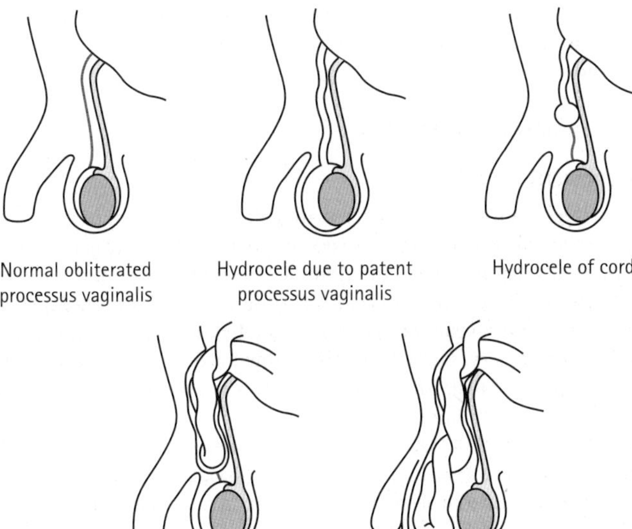

Fig. 36.28 Inguinal herniae and hydroceles.

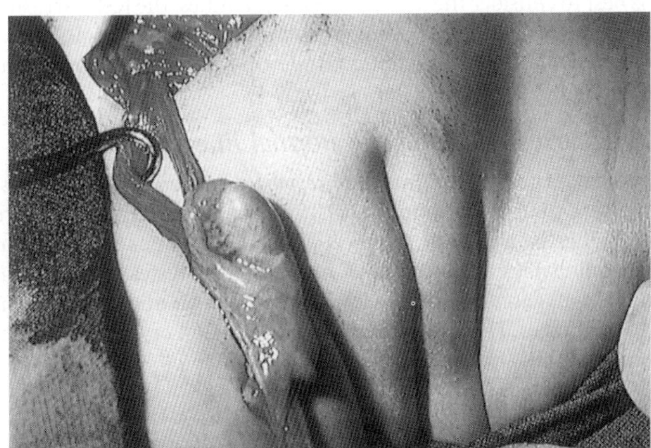

Fig. 36.29 External female genitalia and normal testis in testicular feminization syndrome.

herniotomy are necessary. If it is successfully reduced then herniotomy must be performed before the infant is discharged.

Confirmation of the previous incarceration may be made by observing an increase in testicular size on the affected side (a positive Robarts' sign). This results from venous obstruction of the pampiniform plexus which can result in testicular infarction in cases where the hernia is not urgently reduced.

FEMORAL HERNIA

This is uncommon in children but, as in adults, is recognized by the swelling lying below the inguinal ligament and lateral to the pubic tubercle. Femoral herniorrhaphy is required.

UMBILICAL HERNIA

By the time the umbilical cord has separated in the newborn the umbilical ring has usually closed but in a proportion of children a defect is left, resulting in an umbilical hernia. There is a higher incidence of this condition in blacks than in whites. Umbilical hernia occurs in Beckwith's syndrome, Hurler's syndrome, trisomy 18, and trisomy 13.

The vast majority of umbilical hernias will resolve spontaneously within the first 2 years of life. Incarceration and strangulation in umbilical hernias in childhood are so rare that they need not cause concern. Persistence of the hernia beyond the age of 2 years merits surgical repair, provided that care is taken to ensure that the incision lies within the umbilical folds.

A *paraumbilical hernia* usually lies in the linea alba immediately above the umbilical ring. This will not close spontaneously and surgical repair is required.

EPIGASTRIC HERNIA

An epigastric hernia occurs through the linea alba, usually midway between the xiphisternum and the umbilicus. It presents as a pea-sized swelling occasionally associated with pain and results from herniation of extraperitoneal fat through the defect. It is best treated surgically although it can safely be left alone.

SURGICAL ASPECTS OF THE GENITOURINARY TRACT

ANOMALIES OF TESTICULAR DESCENT

It is best to consider the following distinct entities: the testis arrested in the normal line of descent (true undescended); ectopic testes; and retractile testes. In addition, testes may be atrophic or absent (anorchia).

Testes arrested along the normal line of descent

The term cryptorchidism (Greek *cryptos* = hidden, *orchis* = testis) should be reserved for impalpable, usually abdominal, testes. There is a higher incidence of undescended testes in premature than in full-term babies. Two-thirds of undescended testes in newborn infants will descend, usually by 6 weeks in term and 3 months in preterm babies. There is an increased incidence of cryptorchidism in anencephalics and other cerebral anomalies.

Ectopic testes

These have descended as far as the external inguinal ring and then become deviated into the superficial inguinal, perineal (Fig. 36.30), suprapubic or femoral ectopic sites. The commonest by far is the superficial inguinal pouch, above and lateral to the external inguinal ring.

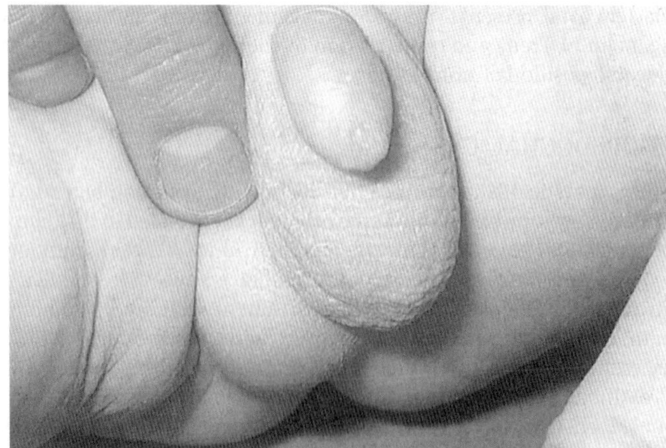

Fig. 36.30 Perineal ectopic testis.

Retractile testes

The cremasteric reflex in young children will draw the testes into the region of the superficial inguinal pouch very readily but they can be manipulated back down to the bottom of the scrotum. The testis would normally reside in the scrotum if such a child is in a warm bath or relaxed in bed.

Anorchia

Anorchia may be on one or both sides. If on one side alone there may be ipsilateral renal agenesis. If the baby is fully masculinized but both testes are absent it must be assumed that they have atrophied subsequent to torsion or infarction during development. Absence of testicular tissue and therefore lack of müllerian inhibitory hormone during early gestation can lead to müllerian development along female lines. The lack of androgenic stimulation (testosterone) from the testes leads to failure of wolffian duct development.

'Ascending testis'

Some boys with recorded testicular descent at routine clinic checks in infancy may be found later at preschool or school medicals to have an undescended testis. This phenomenon of the 'ascending testis' was noted first by Atwell.[16] It has been suggested that this is caused by failure of elongation of the spermatic cord during differential body growth, so that the testis is drawn up by absorption of the processus vaginalis.

Treatment

It has been shown that adverse morphological changes occur in undescended testes from the second year of life onwards with a statistically significant reduction of spermatogonia and tubular growth. Most surgeons therefore choose to perform orchidopexies between 2 and 3 years of age. An associated hernia is an indication for earlier surgery. There is no place now for delaying surgery until 9 or 10 years of age. Any testis, which has not descended in the first year of life, will not appear later.

The treatment of the true undescended testis and the ectopic testis is orchidopexy, the testis and cord being mobilized via an inguinal approach and usually fixed in the scrotum in a subdartos pouch.

Malignancy in the undescended testis

Testicular malignancy occurs in 0.0021% of adult males. Undescended testes occur in 0.28% of the population and 12% of cases of testicular malignancy are reported to occur in testes known to have been undescended. There is thus a 40 times greater incidence of malignancy in cryptorchid patients than in the general population. Orchidopexy probably does not eradicate the problem but at least the testis is placed in a position where early malignancy may be detected. In unilateral undescended testes there is also an increased risk of malignancy in the contralateral testis.

Fertility

Only one-third of those following bilateral orchidopexy and two-thirds of those after unilateral orchidopexy appear to have a sperm count sufficient to be potentially fertile. It is hoped, however, that these figures will be improved by the change in policy over the past few years to operate on the majority of cases in the second year of life.

THE ACUTE SCROTUM

This may result from torsion of the testis, torsion of a testicular appendage, epididymo-orchitis or idiopathic scrotal edema or, rarely, a testicular tumor.

Torsion of the testis

Torsion of the testis most commonly occurs in the neonatal period or at puberty, with a few cases presenting in the intervening years. In the neonate the torsion occurs outside the tunica vaginalis. In the neonatal period there is a plane of mobility between the tunica vaginalis and the outer layer of the scrotum. Presentation is with a reddened hemiscrotum with a hard, swollen, often indurated testis. This is not infrequently noted 24 h after birth although the torsion may have occurred at delivery. On exploration, through a groin incision, the testis is often black and infarcted but usually it is 'given the benefit of the doubt', untwisted and replaced in the scrotum, although the majority will atrophy.

After the newborn period, torsion occurs secondary to an abnormally high investment of the tunica, the testis often being described as having bell-clapper fixation. Presentation is with pain, which is usually testicular in position but theoretically, as testicular innervation is from T10, it should be felt centrally in the abdomen. Examination reveals a swollen hemiscrotum often with edema and erythema, depending on the length of history. There is exquisite tenderness on palpation. The treatment is emergency surgery as delay will affect the viability of the testis.

Preoperative isotope scanning or Doppler probing to confirm the diagnosis merely wastes time. The scrotum is explored, the testis derotated and, providing surgery is carried out within 6 h, the testis is likely to become pink under warm towels. It is then fixed in the scrotum. As the anomalous tunical attachment is likely to be bilateral, orchidopexy is also performed on the other side.

Torsion of testicular appendages

Embryological remnants are commonly attached to the testis. The hydatid of Morgagni is attached to the upper pole and is a müllerian duct remnant. It varies in size from a pinhead to a pea or may be absent. Other remnants include the appendix epididymis (a wolffian tubercle remnant), the paradidymis or organ of Giraldés (another mesonephric remnant) and the vas aberrans of Haller. The hydatid of Morgagni is the most common to undergo torsion which leads to less acute pain than testicular torsion, the pain being usually at the upper pole of the testis where occasionally a bluish nodule is seen through the scrotal skin. An infarcted hydatid can give rise to considerable swelling and inflammation and doubtful cases are best explored (Fig. 36.31) to exclude testicular torsion. In any case, the necrotic hydatid is best excised as an emergency, giving instant pain relief. If treated conservatively the pain lingers on for up to 2 weeks.

Epididymo-orchitis

This is rare in children unless there is an associated renal tract anomaly. If the latter has already been established then it is safe to treat with antibiotic therapy. If, however, the clinical picture cannot be distinguished from torsion of the testis, exploration is mandatory to establish the diagnosis.

Idiopathic scrotal edema

This is a fascinating entity presenting with erythema and edema of the scrotum suggestive of a possible underlying torsion. The erythema and edema spread beyond the scrotum however into the groin and perineum (Fig. 36.32). Usually the process is confined to one side of the scrotum and the adjacent groin and perineum.

The etiology is unknown. It may be an allergic phenomenon; it is occasionally associated with an eosinophilia and may respond to antihistamine therapy. Some suggest it may be caused by an insect bite. The testis is non-tender and the condition settles within a few days.

CIRCUMCISION

Routine circumcision of the newborn as commonly practiced in the USA is to be condemned, the incidence of complications, including death, far outweighing the supposed advantage of avoiding such problems as carcinoma of the penis. The latter is virtually unknown in those who practice adequate hygiene. The fact that it is 'more hygienic' is often used as an excuse for circumcision but one does not chop off the ears to save washing them, or the feet because they may smell! It has been suggested that lack of carcinoma of the cervix in Jewish women is related to male circumcision but Aitken-Swan & Baird[17] showed no difference in incidence in wives of circumcised and uncircumcised men. In 1975 a committee of the American Academy of Pediatrics stated: 'There is no absolute medical indication for the routine circumcision of the newborn. A program of good penile hygiene, simply retracting the foreskin to wash away accumulated smegma on a daily basis, would appear to offer all the advantages of circumcision without the attendant surgical risks or the increased risk of meatal stenosis'.[18]

Non-retractability of the prepuce, in childhood, should not be used as an excuse for 'lopping off an innocent and useful appendage'. Bokai[19] in 1869 was the first to draw attention to the physiological adherence of the foreskin, there being fusion of the glans and the prepuce developmentally. Diebert,[20] in 1933, showed that separation of the prepuce in the human penis is due to keratinization of the subpreputial epithelium, a process not complete at birth but accomplished during early childhood. Phimosis (a muzzling, from Greek *phimos* = muzzle) is thus physiological at birth.

Apart from religious or tribal reasons there are few indications for circumcision. The only valid one is a fibrous phimosis (Fig. 36.33). This may be due to inappropriate attempts at retraction at an early age, causing splitting and scarring of the preputial meatus, or perhaps is related to recurrent infections. In its most severe form it presents as balanitis xerotica obliterans with scarring of the underlying glans and urethral meatus. Meatal strictures also arise after neonatal circumcision secondary to meatitis which arises in the absence of the protective covering of the foreskin. Ballooning of the foreskin is often seen as an indication for circumcision but it will usually resolve in time. Recurrent balanitis or balanoposthitis is possibly related to partial separation of

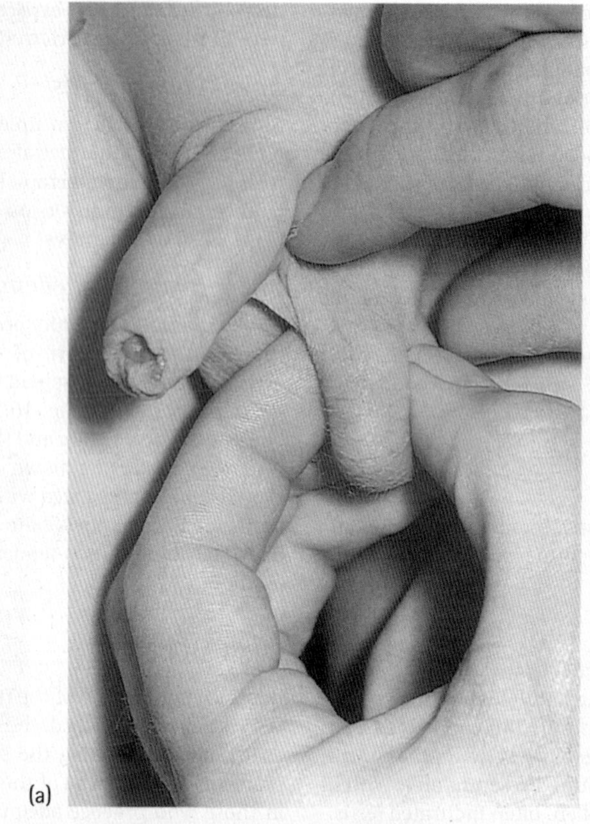

(a)

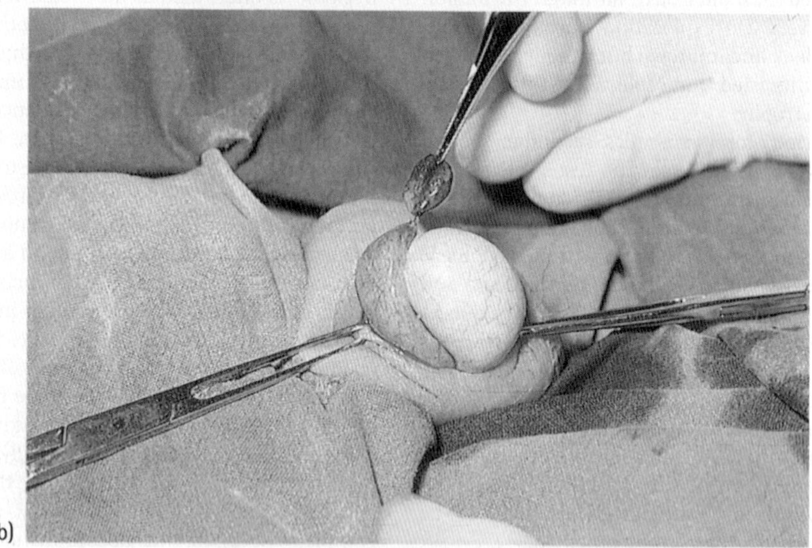

(b)

Fig. 36.31 Hydatid of Morgagni: (a) clinical appearance; (b) at operation.

preputial adhesion and infection of inadequately draining secretions. This can readily be resolved by separation of the adhesions. Previously this was normally carried out under general anesthesia but with the advent of EMLA cream (eutectic mixture of local anesthetics) the separation can readily be carried out painlessly and simply in the outpatient clinic or GP surgery.[21] Daily retraction with application of petroleum jelly for a few days to prevent readherence followed subsequently by normal preputial hygiene is all that is required.

In examination of the foreskin in small boys it often appears tight on attempted retraction. The simple technique advocated in 1950 by Sir James Spence[22] should be adopted: 'Retract the prepuce and you will see a pinpoint opening, but draw it forward and you will see a channel wide enough for all the purposes for which the infant needs the organ at that early age. What looks like a pinpoint opening at 7 months will become a wide channel of communication at 17 years.'

Operation

Circumcision is thus performed either for religious or tribal reasons, for fibrous phimosis or, perhaps most frequently, for remuneration! Hypospadias is a contraindication for neonatal circumcision, as is a buried penis. Neonatal circumcision is practiced, often without anesthesia using a plastibell or a Gomco clamp. In the former, a

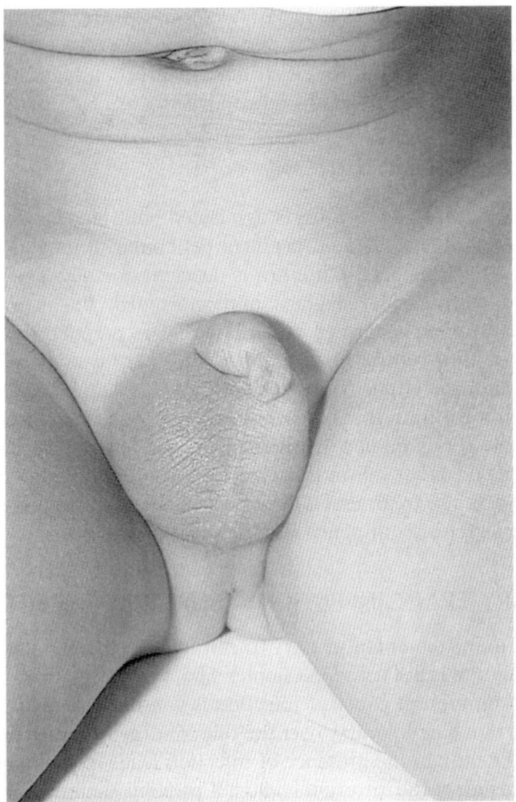

Fig. 36.32 Idiopathic scrotal edema.

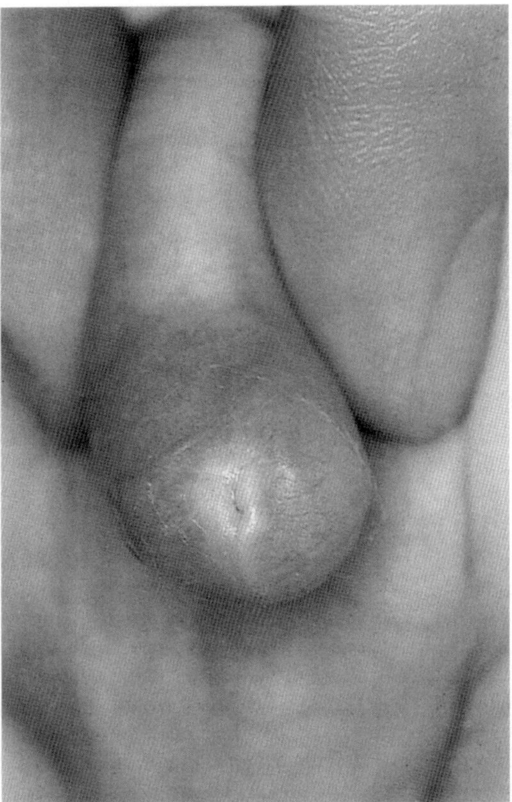

Fig. 36.33 Fibrous phimosis (balanitis xerotica obliterans).

plastic ring is placed under the foreskin and a string tied round the foreskin in a groove in the plastic device. Redundant skin together with the device separates off within a few days leaving a very neat cosmetic result. A Gomco clamp has a similar action but rather than the string, a cutting device removes the prepuce and compresses the skin edges causing them to fuse and prevent hemorrhage. In older children a surgical cutting technique with absorbable sutures is used. In many cases of phimosis a foreskin preserving preputioplasty is sufficient.

PARAPHIMOSIS

This occurs when a narrowed foreskin is retracted behind the corona glandis penis and cannot be returned. The constriction leads to engorgement of the glans and of a cuff of foreskin distal to the tight band but behind the corona (Fig. 36.34). Firm manual compression with gauze and EMLA cream will usually reduce the edema and facilitate return of the foreskin. If this fails, injection of hyaluronidase into the swollen ring of prepuce, under general anesthesia, followed by compression, allows reduction (Fig. 36.35). Occasionally the tight constricting band needs to be incised. Circumcision is frequently advocated following paraphimosis but, surprisingly, the foreskin is usually easily retractable a fortnight after the event and recurrence is exceptional.

HYPOSPADIAS (Greek *hypo* = below, *spadon* = rent)

This is one of the commonest congenital anomalies, occurring in one in 400 live male births. The meatus lies in an abnormal position on the ventral aspect of the penile shaft or even scrotally or perineally. The foreskin tends to be deficient in its ventral aspect and thus is described as 'hooded'. Thirdly, there is chordee, a ventral flexion of the penis, the incidence and degree of which increases as the meatus is more proximally placed. The meatus itself may be narrowed leading to potential problems of back pressure. In the majority of cases the meatus is coronal in position; rarely it is glandular. Of the remainder, most are on the penile shaft but a few lie more proximally still in the scrotum or perineum. It is often thought that hypospadias is frequently associated with upper renal tract anomalies but in fact the incidence of these is much the same as in the general population, except perhaps in the most severe types of the deformity. In those penoscrotal and perineal types there may be associated

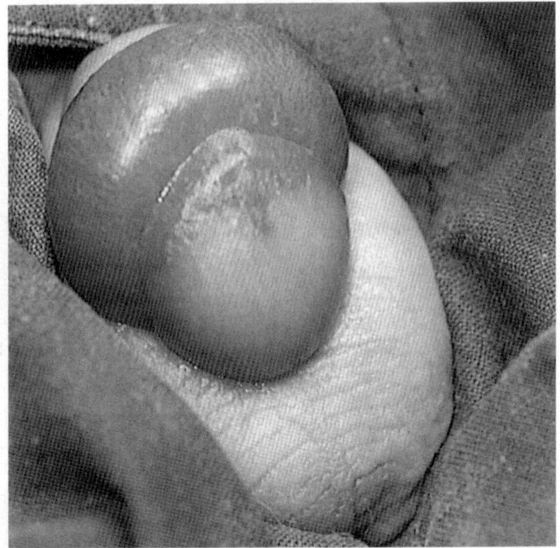

Fig. 36.34 Paraphimosis.

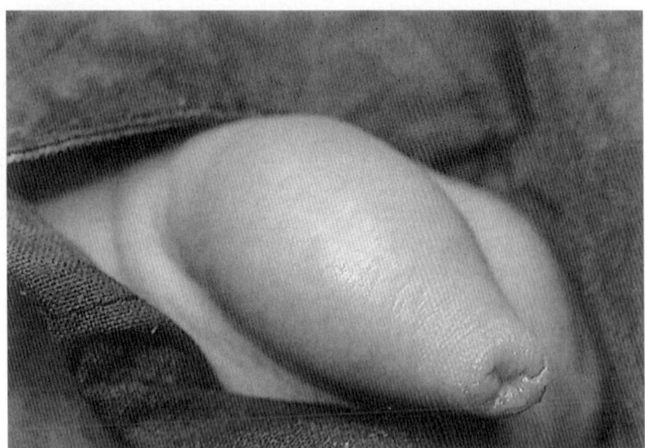

Fig. 36.35 Reduced paraphimosis.

undescended testes and the possibility of an intersex state must be investigated.

There are over 200 operations described in the literature for the correction of hypospadias. This gives some indication of the complication rate, each newly described repair aiming to be an improvement in this regard. The age for surgery is mainly the surgeon's preference. It has always been agreed that, where possible, correction should be complete by the time the boy starts school so that he may stand and pee like his peers! The more distally placed the meatus the easier it is to achieve a successful result. For a coronal hypospadias the MAGPI repair (meatal advancement and glanduloplasty incorporated) has become very popular and is generally carried out at a few months of age. The essential components to the repair of the more severe varieties are release of the chordee and urethral reconstruction. The chordee is related to tight fibrous bands distal to the meatus and thought possibly to relate to atrophy of that portion of the corpus spongiosium. It is, however, possible to have chordee without hypospadias so the etiology is uncertain. Fistula formation is unfortunately common following hypospadias repair and a few unfortunate cases require multiple interventions to achieve successful closure. The aim of all modern repairs is to create a terminal meatus on a well-formed glans and a penile shaft that is straight on erection together with a good cosmetic result (a good 'body image').

EPISPADIAS

In its most extreme form this is associated with bladder exstrophy. Otherwise it may be balanic, penile or penopubic. It may also occur in girls. In epispadias the urethra is deficient dorsally. The penis is flattened with a splayed glans and shortened, the crura being attached to often separated pubic bones. The prepuce is deficient dorsally with a ventral hood prepuce and there is dorsal chordee. Occasionally the problem is not obvious, the foreskin being complete and phimotic and the penis buried, but once the prepuce is retractable the condition is revealed. In the female the clitoris is duplicated on either side of the wide open urethra, defective dorsally (Fig. 36.36). The treatment is likewise dependent on sex and severity and the degree of continence and the success rate is variable.

URINARY TRACT INFECTION – SURGICAL ASPECTS

Medical management of urinary tract infections in neonates and in older children is discussed in Chapter 16.

The commonest cause of infection is *vesicoureteric reflux*. There remains much controversy over the role of surgery in vesicoureteric reflux.[23] Reflux in the presence of infection leads to pyelonephritis, the extension of the intrarenal reflux, if present, leading to scarring. If the child can be kept free of infection, the reflux may improve or resolve. Severe reflux should be treated surgically. This entails a transvesical operation to lengthen the submucosal tunnel of the ureter. It has a high rate of success but in a few cases leads to stenosis. More recently, a new technique involving the endoscopic injection of Teflon submucosally[24] beneath the ureteric orifice has been devised (STING – subureteric Teflon injection). This has proved very successful but long-term results have yet to be evaluated. Other substances such as bioplastique or collagen may be used as concern has been raised that Teflon may migrate to the brain or elsewhere, although the original authors refute this concept.

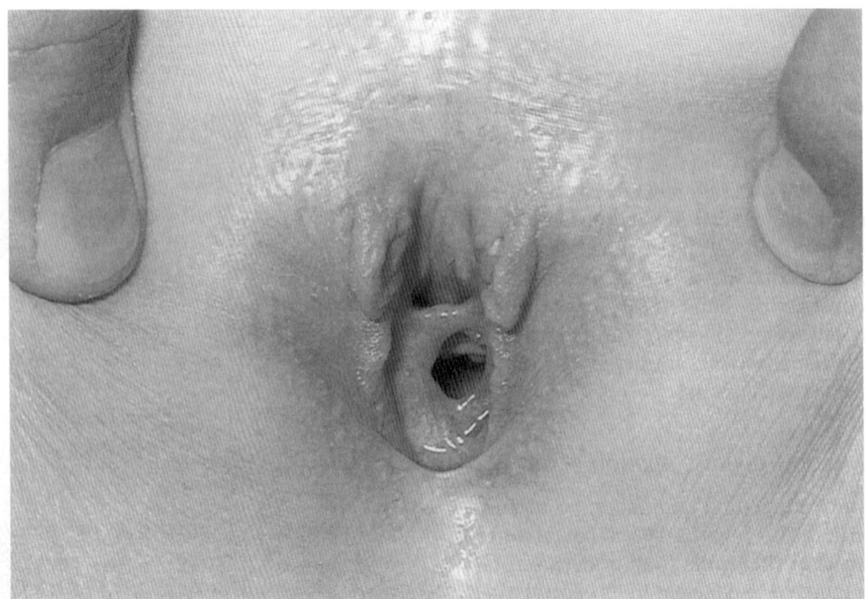

Fig. 36.36 Female epispadias.

Stenosis of the lower end of the ureter requires reimplantation, the stenotic segment being excised.

Duplex ureters may be an incidental finding without causing problems in the majority of cases. If detected in investigation of a urinary tract infection, there is usually an associated anomaly. The ureter from the upper pole tends to enter the bladder at a lower level. Thus the lower pole ureter has a shorter intramural course and a tendency to reflux. The upper pole ureter has a tendency to stenosis, an association with a ureterocele and a possible tendency to open below the bladder neck leading to incontinence. It may even open ectopically into the vagina.

If there is reflux of both ureters, reimplantation of both, in their common sheath, is usually the treatment of choice. Occasionally they join at a higher level leading to yo-yo reflux between the two and a predisposition to infection. This is treated either by heminephroureterectomy if one moiety is shown to have poor function on isotope studies, or else anastomosis at the level of the pelves may be advocated.

A *ureterocele* may arise in relation to the upper pole ureter. It represents herniation of the intramural portion of the ureter into the bladder. Its meatus may be stenosed, may open below the bladder neck or may even on occasion allow reflux. The ureterocele may obstruct the lower ureter or even lead to bladder outlet obstruction by prolapsing across the internal urethral meatus. The ureterocele may be incised endoscopically to relieve an acute problem, especially of value in the infant, or may be excised with ureteric reimplantation if appropriate. If an isotope scan shows minimal function in the affected moiety then partial nephroureterectomy may be the treatment of choice.

Hydronephrosis may be due to obstruction at the pelviureteric junction or, if the ureter is also dilated, to vesicoureteric obstruction or vesicoureteric reflux. Obstruction at the pelviureteric junction (PUJ) may be due to congenital narrowing, high insertion of the ureter, or aberrant renal vessels. The presentation is usually with investigation of a urinary tract infection. It may be diagnosed antenatally or in the older child may present with a Dietl's crisis, acute obstruction at the PUJ secondary to kinking after an abnormal fluid load. This may not present until the first beer-drinking spree in a young adult! In the neonate, antenatally diagnosed hydronephrosis may be a stable condition that can be monitored with serial ultrasound examinations and isotope studies as some infants will acquire normal drainage across the PUJ as they grow. At any age an isotope study will indicate whether the kidney has already suffered major damage. If its contribution to total renal function is less than 10% then nephrectomy is the treatment of choice. If there is doubt in an acute presentation, a percutaneous nephrostomy tube may be inserted under ultrasound guidance and further isotope studies, after draining for 1–2 weeks, may show improvement. If there is reasonable function but a definite PUJ obstruction then the treatment of choice is a pyeloplasty. This involves excision of the redundant extra renal pelvis and pelviureteric junction with reanastomosis of the proximal ureter to the dependent portion of the repaired pelvis.

CONGENITAL VASCULAR MALFORMATIONS

Haemangiomas

These are malformations of developing blood vessels. They commonly appear in the skin but may develop in any organ.

Strawberry naevus

These usually appear at about a week of age and may rapidly enlarge in the first few months of life. They then stop growing and usually resolve spontaneously by intravascular thrombosis. This process is normally complete by 5–7 years of age leaving only a minor blemish or none at all. Unless they are causing a problem such as occlusion of the eyelids, which can lead to permanent visual impairment, surgery is best avoided. The parents must be reassured that even the most unsightly facial lesions will resolve within a year or two of the child starting school. A few involute so rapidly that they become ulcerated. This is most common in lesions subject to trauma as on the perineum or back. Scarring will result from ulceration.

Stork mark

This is a superficial capillary hemangioma which may be seen on the forehead, bridge of the nose and upper eyelids. The lesion is often v-shaped pointing down to the nose and there is a corresponding mark on the nape of the neck. These marks presumably arise from the stork suspending the baby by the head in its beak! Again the parents can be reassured that the frontal lesion will resolve spontaneously although the nuchal one will commonly persist throughout life usually hidden by the hair.

Port wine stain (naevus flammeus)

Unlike a strawberry naevus this is present at birth and may be very disfiguring, as it becomes darker and increasingly nodular with age. In recent years laser treatment with a pulsed tuneable dye laser has considerably improved the appearance of these lesions in childhood.[25]

Sturge–Weber syndrome is a severe form of port wine stain on the scalp and face, in the distribution of one of the branches of the trigeminal nerve, associated with an underlying vascular anomaly of the arachnoid covering the cerebral hemisphere. This leads to epilepsy, hemiplegia and mental retardation.

Cavernous hemangioma

These may occur alone or in association with a capillary lesion in the overlying skin. They increase in size after birth but usually in proportion to the growth of the infant. Most resolve spontaneously but some persist requiring excision, if appropriate, or injection with sclerosants. Care must be taken in the latter option not to lead to ulceration of the skin. Very large lesions may lead to high output cardiac failure due to arteriovenous shunting. Embolization under radiological control may be required although some lesions regress on oral corticosteroid therapy.

Kasabach–Merritt syndrome

In the neonate, large or multiple hemangiomas are occasionally associated with a generalized bleeding disorder caused by the trapping of platelets within them which produces a profound thrombocytopenia. A course of prednisone, 2–4 mg/kg per 24 h can effect dramatic improvement, or, if this fails, embolization of the hemangioma can be considered.

Lymphangioma

These are similar to hemangiomas but involve lymphatics. They may also occur anywhere in the body but in particular they may present as a *cystic hygroma* most commonly arising in the cervical region (see above under 'head and neck').

Mixed *hamartomatous* lesions may contain hemangiomatous and lymphangiomatous elements.

CLEFT LIP AND PALATE

The main etiological factor in these anomalies is genetic. In about one-third of patients there is a family history. The incidence is about

1 in 700 births. The ratio of cleft lip (with or without cleft palate) to cleft palate alone is about 2:1.

The lip, alveolus and the portion of the hard palate anterior to the incisive foramen are derived from the maxillary and medial nasal processes. These fuse by the sixth week. The remainder of the palate forms from the palatine shelves. These grow from the maxillary swellings and fuse from anterior to posterior in the ninth to twelfth weeks. At the same time the nasal septum grows down to meet the palate.

Clefts result from failure of these lines of fusion. They vary in severity from a notch in the margin of the lip to a complete cleft in the maxilla. They may be unilateral or bilateral. Figure 36.37 illustrates the major types of cleft lip and palate.

Treatment is aimed at both a good cosmetic result with normal growth as well as a functional closure to facilitate swallowing and speech. The repair of the lip and alveolus is usually performed at around 3 months of age and the palatal defect between 6 and 15 months to give the best chance of normal speech. A multidisciplinary approach is required including a plastic surgeon, orthodontist, speech therapist, ENT surgeon, audiologist, etc.

BURNS

Thermal injury is a common childhood accident in all countries. Predisposing factors include primitive, poor or overcrowded housing, families under stress, flammable clothing, ignorance and lack of insight in parents.

The toddler, exploring his world on hands and knees or with unsteady gait, is a ready victim and boys are burned more often than girls. Scalding with hot liquids is by far the commonest cause of injury in this age group. Flame burns are less common than they were, but house fires still claim victims with the added risk of smoke inhalation injury. Other causes include contact with hot objects, chemicals, friction and electric current.

Severity of injury

This depends on three main factors:

1. ***Extent.*** Heat damages the underlying capillaries, causing them to leak protein-rich fluid. The resulting loss from the circulation reaches a critical level when the extent of the burn exceeds about 10% of the body surface area, and the child will require intravenous resuscitation. Extent is measured by using a chart (Fig. 36.38) or by taking the area of the hand as about 1%. Erythema should be discounted when making this measurement.
2. ***Depth.*** Healing depends on whether epithelial elements survive in the dermis. Partial thickness burns will heal by outgrowth of epithelial cells from hair follicles and sweat glands; they can be subdivided into superficial, which heal in less than 3 weeks and do not cause scars, and deep dermal which take longer to heal and cause hypertrophic scars. Deep or full thickness burns can heal only from the margins. The depth of tissue destruction is determined by the temperature of the agent, the duration of its contact, the skin thickness and the victim's age.
3. ***Site.*** Burns of the face and hands are particularly serious, and those of the perineum cause problems in management. While the skin is the site of injury in most instances, the epithelial linings of the respiratory and upper alimentary tracts may be damaged separately or together with a skin burn.

Pathophysiology

Local

The fluid loss from the circulation is at its maximum immediately after the burn and decreases over the following 48 h. A deep burn destroys significant numbers of red cells. The insulating and protective functions of skin are lost, and body heat, water and electrolytes pass from the body in much increased amounts. Nitrogen losses also rise.

General

There is a massive rise in the secretion of stress hormones.[26] Urinary water and sodium excretion fall and potassium and nitrogen losses increase. The larger the burn, the more profound the reaction tends to be. The catabolic phase lasts until the burn is healed.

Treatment

First aid

After separating the child from the source of the injury, clothing should be removed and the burn cooled by immersion in lukewarm

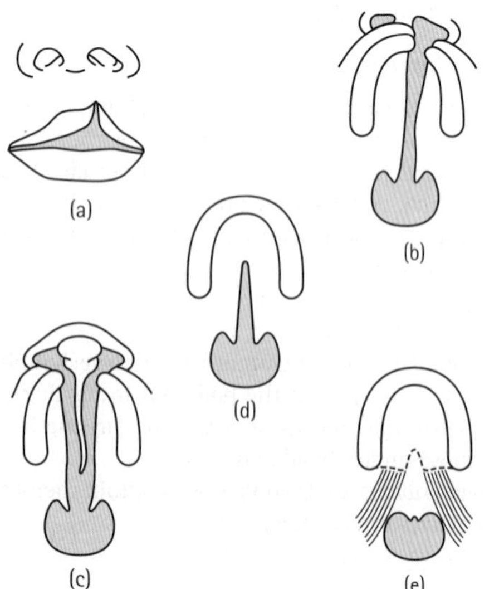

Fig. 36.37 (a) Incomplete unilateral cleft lip. (b) Complete unilateral cleft lip and palate. (c) Complete bilateral cleft lip and palate. (d) Isolated cleft of soft palate. (e) Submucous cleft palate.

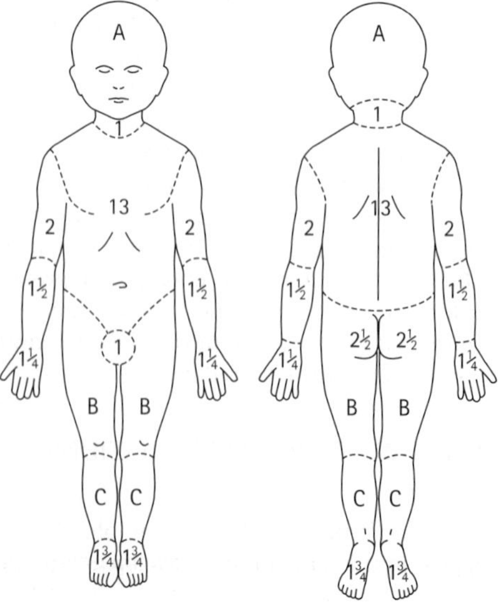

Fig. 36.38 Chart for calculating percentage area burned in childhood. A = 1/2 of head; B = 1/2 of one thigh; C = 1/2 of one leg. The percentages of these areas vary with age.

water or by use of a wet cloth (the risk of hypothermia must be remembered). The burn can then be covered with a clean cloth or clingfilm until definitive local treatment is possible.

Pain

A partial thickness burn is very painful, while deeply burned skin is anesthetic. Potent analgesia by the intramuscular or intravenous route is essential. Throughout treatment, attention must be focused on the avoidance of pain during practical procedures; analgesic or anesthetic drugs should be selected and used with precision.

Shock

Where the area burned exceeds 10% of the body surface, an intravenous infusion will be required. The restoration and maintenance of an effective circulation can be achieved with plasma, purified protein solution, dextran or balanced salt solutions. The quantities to be given vary with the weight of the child and the extent of the burn. The rate of administration is rapid initially and usually lasts for 36–48 h. Close patient observation, hourly urinary output measurement by an indwelling urethral catheter, and serial hemoglobin and hematocrit estimations provide adequate control data. A central venous pressure line can be helpful in the severe case, but it has been indicted as a major source of infection if maintained for days in the burned patient.

System management

Respiratory system

Where a child has been rescued from a burning building or where clothing has burned over the face, airway problems can be anticipated. Arterial blood gases should be monitored and intubation and assisted ventilation may be necessary. Bronchopneumonia is a frequent later complication of large burns.

Central nervous system

Toddlers with even minor scalds are liable to convulse in the first 2 days with serious or even fatal outcome. The cause is thought to lie with early fluid shifts and the lag that occurs within the brain and its meninges. Papilledema is not always present. Diazepam and mannitol (1 g/kg i.v. over 20 min) gain quick control of fits and brain swelling, and phenytoin sodium and dexamethasone prolong the effect. Focal neurological deficits may occur at any time, probably as a result of septic emboli.

Urinary system

In the first 2 days after injury increased levels of antidiuretic hormone limit urinary output. Infusion should be used circumspectly and a serum sodium level of not less than 130 mmol/L should be maintained.

In deep burns, thermal damage to red blood cells causes hemoglobinuria, which may lead to tubular necrosis and renal failure. If rapid restoration of circulating fluid volume does not clear the urine, a solute diuretic such as 20% mannitol should be given without delay. A catheter may be required to monitor urine output or avoid contamination of the burn. It should be removed as soon as possible.

Cardiovascular system

Electrical current injury may cause cardiac damage and an ECG examination is advisable after such an injury. General anesthesia is best avoided until the tracing has returned to normal.

Tachycardia persists throughout recovery from a large burn and is largely a product of a high metabolic rate to offset the high evaporative heat losses. Heat regulation is disturbed and the child must be kept warm to avoid hypothermia.

Hemopoietic system

Loss of red cells, destroyed by a deep burn, must be replaced by early transfusion. Further losses take place during surgery and erythropoiesis remains depressed until a large burn has healed. The red cell mass must be maintained by transfusion if the body is to achieve quick healing.

Alimentary system

Gastric stasis is common in the early hours after a large burn but oral intake should be started as soon as possible. Ranitidine has reduced the incidence of hemorrhagic gastritis and Curling's ulcer is now rarely seen.

Accurate naked weights, obtained twice weekly from admission, guide the clinician through the early weight gain of fluid retention, diuresis, the catabolic phase, and the anabolic phase that comes more quickly and strongly in the child.

Nutrition

Daily fluid intake must take account of increased losses through the burn wound. A high calorie intake is needed to balance heat loss and minimize lean tissue breakdown. A protein intake at the upper end of the normal range is adequate. Iron and vitamins C and B complex are supplemented to combat anemia and aid wound healing. The seriously burned child cannot take food in solid form and it is kinder and more effective to give most of this as a fortified liquid feed. A fine-bore nasogastric feeding tube for this purpose should be passed on all children with burns over 15%. The planned intake should be achieved stepwise over the first 1–2 weeks. Early forcing of high food intake may predispose to a post-stress diabetes which may be resistant to insulin. Neglect of food intake will result in a profound weight loss, hypoproteinemia, and failure of the burn to heal.

Musculoskeletal system

While immobilization may be unavoidable for practical reasons, its use will increase muscle wasting and delay the recovery of an effective musculature. Regular active exercises should be performed wherever possible. Joint positioning and joint movement require constant attention if severe, and possibly permanent, joint contracture is to be avoided.

Local care

Infection is the major complication of all but the smallest burn. It can destroy surviving epithelium and penetrate a deep burn, with a risk of invasive infection. The commonest organism is *Staphylococcus aureus* but the beta-hemolytic streptococcus is feared for its destructive capabilities and *Pseudomonas aeruginosa* can be dangerous on extensive burns. Constant monitoring, scrupulous hygiene and prevention of overcrowding are essential to control infection. Large burns should be isolated. Where appropriate, early excision and grafting can lead to healing before infection can occur. Local antibacterial agents are valuable but systemic antibiotics must be used with care as they can easily lead to superinfection with resistant organisms or fungi.

A superficial burn will, if protected from infection and trauma, heal in less than 3 weeks and is usually dressed with a well-padded gauze and cotton wool dressing with a Vaseline gauze inner layer. Deeper burns need skin grafting, unless very small.

Toxic shock syndrome

This can follow even very minor burns in the child[27] and can have a mortality of 11%.[28] It is therefore essential to recognize and treat it on suspicion. Signs are of an unwell, irritable child, 3 or more days after a burn, with pyrexia and three or more of the following: rash, hypotension, diarrhea or vomiting, inflamed mucous membranes, *Staphylococcus aureus* on wound swabs and occlusive dressings.

Treatment is with i.v. fluids, gammaglobulins (0.4 g/kg) or fresh blood or fresh frozen plasma (10 ml/kg over 4 h), exposure of the burn, topical antibacterial agent and i.v. antibiotics.

Scarring

A superficial burn should leave little physical trace; the healed skin will be dry and should be creamed several times a day. With deeper injuries, scarring is unavoidable. The hypertrophic scar reaction is most intense in childhood. On the face, it disfigures and distorts features. On the flexures, it limits joint movement. Unrelieved scar contracture impedes growth of that part and deforms the growing skeleton. Spontaneous resolution of the hypertrophic scar is slow, variable and incomplete. Its full development may be cut short and its regression accelerated by elastic compression, intralesional injection of steroid hormones, or application of silicone gel. Secondary surgical procedures are often required to replace the worst scars, their timing and scope being dictated by the physical, psychological and educational needs of the child.

Psychological support

A close rapport between child, nurse, parents and doctor is fundamental in such a taxing hospital stay, which can extend over months. The child deserves explanation, occupation, and freedom from recurring pain. The parents, whose guilt feelings should be appreciated, should be incorporated into the therapeutic effort. The help of an interested and experienced psychiatrist may be invaluable.

Prognosis

Intensive early therapy can resuscitate a child with the gravest of surface burns. However, long-term survival is rare where 70% or more of the skin is destroyed. A child who survives a burn with significant scarring faces the prospect of physical and psychological problems which will probably become worse during adolescence. Continued long-term support is needed for patient and family for many years.

REFERENCES (*Level 1 evidence)

1 Clements BS, Warner JO. Pulmonary sequestration and related bronchopulmonary vascular malformations: nomenclature and classification based on anatomical and embryological considerations. Thorax 1987; 42:401–408.

2 Bohn D, Tamura M, Perrin D, et al. Ventilatory predictors of pulmonary hypoplasia in congenital diaphragmatic hernia, confirmed by morphologic assessment. J Pediatr 1987; 111:423–431.

3 Sakai H, Tamura M, Hosokawa Y, et al. Effect of surgical repair on respiratory mechanics in congenital diaphragmatic hernia. J Pediatr 1987; 111:432–438.

4 MacKinlay GA, Burtles R. Oesophageal atresia: paralysis and ventilation in management of the wide gap. Pediatr Surg Int 1987; 2:10–12.

5 Hancock BJ, Wiseman NE. Congenital duodenal obstruction: the impact of an antenatal diagnosis. J Pediatr Surg 1989; 24:1027–1031.

6 Hirschsprung H. Stuhlragheit Neugeborener in Fotge von Dilation und Hypertrophie des Colons. Jahreb Kinderheilk 1887; 27:1–7.

7 Bodian M, Carter CO. A family study of Hirschsprung's disease. Ann Hum Genet 1963; 26:261–277.

8 Stephens FD. Wingspread Conference on Anorectal Malformations. Racine, Wisconsin; 1984.

9 de Vries PA, Pena A. Posterior sagittal anorectoplasty. J Pediatr Surg 1982; 17: 638–643.

10 Kasai M, Kimura S, Asakura Y. Surgical treatment of biliary atresia. J Pediatr Surg 1968; 3:665–675.

11 Ogita S, Tsuto T, Nakamura K, et al. OK-432 therapy for lymphangioma in children: why and how does it work? J Pediatr Surg 1996; 31:477–480.

12 Ramstedt C. Zur Operation der angeborenen Pylorusstenose. Medizinische Klinik (Berlin) 1912; 8:1702–1705.

13 Stiles HJ. (original operation note 3 February 1910 – personal possession) 1910.

14 Rothenburg SS. Experience with 220 consecutive laparoscopic Nissen fundoplications in infants and children. J Pediatr Surg 1998; 33:297–305.

15 Wilson-Storey D, MacKinlay GA. The superior mesenteric artery syndrome. J R Coll Surg Edin 1986; 31:175–178.

16 Atwell JD. Ascent of the testis: fact or fiction. Br J Urol 1985; 57:474–477.

17 Aitken-Swan J, Baird D. Circumcision and cancer of the cervix. Br J Cancer 1965; 19:217–227.

18 Report of the Ad Hoc Task Force on Circumcision. Pediatrics 1975; 56:610–611.

19 Bokai J. A fitma (preputium) sejtes adatapadasa a makkoz gyermakelnel. Orvosi Hetil 1869; 4: 583–587.

20 Diebert GA. The separation of the prepuce in the human penis. Anatomical Records 1933; 54:387–393.

21 MacKinlay GA. Save the prepuce. Painless separation of preputial adhesions in the outpatient clinic. BMJ 1988; 297:590–591.

22 Spence, Sir James (1950). Spence on circumcision. Lancet 1964; ii:902.

23 White RHR, O'Donnell B. Controversies in therapeutics. Management of urinary tract infection and vesico-ureteric reflux in children. 1. Operative treatment has no advantage over medical management (RHRW). 2. The case for surgery (BO'D). BMJ 1990; 300:1391–1394.

24 Puri P, Ninan GK, Sirana R. Subureteric Teflon injection (STING). Result of a European Survey. Eur Urol 1995; 27(1):71–73.

25 Tan OT, Sherwood K, Gilchrist BA. Treatment of children with port-wine stains using the flashlamp-pulsed tuneable dye laser. N Engl J Med 1989; 320:416–442.

26 Smith A, McIntosh N, Thomson M, et al. The stress effect of thermal injury on the hormones controlling fluid balance. Baillière's Clinical Paediatrics. London: Baillière; 1995.

27 Cole RP, Shakespeare PG. Toxic shock syndrome in scalded children. Burns 1990; 16:221–224.

28 de Saxe MJ, Hawtin P, Wieneke AA. Toxic shock syndrome in Britain – epidemiology and microbiology. Postgrad Med J 1985; 61:5–8.

37

Pain and palliative care

Ann Goldman, Richard Howard

PAIN

The overriding goals of medicine are the diagnosis and cure of disease but alongside these is the vital humanitarian aim of relieving distress and discomfort. In spite of this, until recently, there has been a remarkable lack of focus on pain management and research in children and also a persistence of myths and misinformation.

There have been widespread and firmly held beliefs in the past that children neither felt, responded to, nor remembered, painful experiences. However, extensive evidence now exists which indicates that, from the youngest preterm infant, children's nervous systems are able to perceive and respond to pain.[1] Fears about children being particularly vulnerable to strong analgesics have also been clarified and refuted by pharmacological and pharmacokinetic studies.[2] However, this increase in knowledge has not always led to the anticipated improvements in pain management and the undertreatment of pain remains commonplace. It is difficult to understand why this situation persists and perhaps it reflects the deep-seated nature of the myths and fears surrounding pain and analgesics. It may also relate to society's complex and ambivalent attitudes to pain; so that the need to provide pain relief is counteracted by feelings that pain is character building and that suffering now, may have benefits later in life or afterwards.

In this chapter we will consider pain assessment and the different pharmacological and non-pharmacological approaches to managing pain. We will look specifically at a number of situations where pain is a common problem and finally will consider the wider context of palliative care.

THE EXPERIENCE

Pain is a common part of all children's lives and a sensation they recognize easily. It has been defined by the International Association for the Study of Pain as 'an unpleasant sensory and emotional experience associated with actual or potential tissue damage or described in terms of such damage'.[3] This highlights that it is a subjective experience, not necessarily proportional to the underlying physiological damage and is powerfully influenced by psychological, social and cultural factors. Children's understanding of the multifactorial nature of pain develops early and evolves with their age, cognitive level and experience.[4]

Children may experience pain for many reasons and because of its complex nature a rigid system of classification is impossible. For practical purposes it can be helpful to consider painful experiences as acute, chronic and recurrent. Acute pain is often more clearly related to a physiological cause such as trauma or common illnesses, like ear and throat infections, appendicitis and sickle cell disease. Medical interventions are also an important cause of acute pain including immunization, procedures and postoperative pain. Chronic pain may also be associated with obvious underlying disease such as chronic rheumatological disorders, orthopedic problems in cerebral palsy and progressive malignant disease or may be less clearly associated with obvious tissue damage and behavioral factors may be more evident.

ASSESSMENT

A thorough assessment of pain forms the foundation for its management and has been extensively reviewed.[5] Children's age, developmental level and also the type of pain they are experiencing will influence the approach to assessment, and in all situations a broad picture acknowledging the complex nature of pain and the multiple factors which influence it needs to be constructed.

SELF-ASSESSMENT

Since pain is a subjective experience the ideal approach is one of self-report with as much information as possible about the pain coming from the child directly. A detailed history is especially important when the pain is chronic or difficult to understand and aims to discover the sites of the pain, its nature, frequency, severity, precipitating and relieving factors and other associated symptoms. Additional wider aspects to consider include the effect of the pain on the child and family's daily life, their coping skills and the meaning of the pain for them and within their culture. A variety of formal tools to measure pain have now been developed and validated.[5] The majority of these have been designed to help children quantify acute pain and pain severity. They can be valuable to include in the wider assessment and also to monitor the effectiveness of treatment. Regular use of practical and easy to administer tools in a clinical setting both helps the children to explain about their pain and also, if they are incorporated as routine in the clinical setting, encourages staff to focus on the child's pain regularly.[6,7]

Toddlers and young children

Toddlers and young children can provide simple information about their pain and its site but may not have the abstract concepts or verbal ability to describe its nature or intensity.[5] When using pain scales they have a tendency to choose the extreme ends of the scales. Scales which have proved successful for this age group include the use of a body outline, where the children can indicate the site of their pain on the body outline, and this can be combined with an indication of the severity of the pain by asking the child to choose different colored pencils to represent the level of severity of the pain. There are a variety of self-report scales using drawings or photographs of children's faces representing different degrees of pain and discomfort. Another example is the poker chip tool, which uses small plastic blocks to represent 'pieces of hurt' and the children can pick up between 1 and 4 to indicate pain severity.[8]

School age children

School age children can continue to use the same scales as the younger children but as they progress towards adolescence can also use visual analogue scales and more descriptive self-report scales such as the pediatric pain questionnaire, which was designed for children with chronic rheumatological disease.[9]

BEHAVIORAL SCALES

Infants, preverbal children and children with severe developmental delay are unable to report their own pain. Assessment depends on observation of the child and knowing them well. Health care workers consistently underestimate children's pain compared with children's own self-reports and although parents' ratings are closer to the children's own they still tend to underestimate the pain. The use of standardized observational scales can help staff produce pain assessments that are more closely matched to children's own ratings.[10]

In infants behavioral indicators for pain that have been studied include facial expression, cry, motor movements and changes in behavioral state and patterns.[5] Preterm infants' responses appear to be less vigorous than those of full-term infants and their expression of pain cues are more subtle. Evaluation of pain through facial expression is the most well established and typical characteristics expressing pain include eyes tightly closed, furrowed brows, broadened nasal root and deepened nasolabial furrow with a squared mouth and taut tongue. A variety of other multidimensional tools are also available.[11]

Assessment of pain in children with severe developmental delay has only recently been studied and interpreting these children's feelings poses a complex problem. Prior knowledge of the child is important as parents have been shown to identify pain through changes from their child's 'normal' range of facial expressions, muscle tone, movements, cry and mood.[12]

A number of behavioral scales have been developed for older children who are not cognitively impaired, for use primarily in acute pain and in research rather than clinical situations. These use observation of a variety of verbal expressions of pain, facial behavior, changes in tone and movement. Only one scale has attempted to consider the difference in assessing children with acute pain from chronic pain.[13] It tries to incorporate the observation that children with chronic severe pain often become withdrawn and spontaneous movements decrease and these children complain and express their pain less often than those in acute pain. It was specifically designed for children with malignant disease and is well validated in this situation.[13]

PHYSIOLOGICAL RESPONSES

Physiological responses to pain are activated by the autonomic nervous system and include tachycardia, sweating, increasing secretion of catecholamines and adrenocorticoid hormones. These have not proved clinically useful as they are part of a global response to stress and not specific to pain; also measurement of hormonal changes is invasive and slow.

CLINICAL MANAGEMENT OF PAIN

Both non-pharmacological and drug treatments of pain have a place in clinical pain management, the balance depending on the source and circumstances of pain.

NON-PHARMACOLOGICAL APPROACHES

Psychological

The unpleasant nature of pain and the many factors influencing it mean that in reality all pain and pain management is immersed in a psychological context. The choice for health care professionals is how to acknowledge and use this consciously, and how to incorporate psychological approaches constructively alongside other modalities of management.

Some approaches are very simple. Parents offer children the support they value most at times of stress, but they are still sometimes mistakenly excluded from the child's presence and care. Another obvious, but easily neglected, starting place is to ensure a high awareness, in clinical staff, of the distress and anxiety that pain causes children, particularly in the accident and emergency unit, postoperatively and on the wards. Simple and honest explanations of disease processes and thorough preparation for procedures and surgery can help reassure children and families, enhance feelings of control and so reduce anxiety.[14]

A variety of more formal techniques has also been used effectively and well validated in a wide range of clinical situations, including the use of relaxation, cognitive approaches including distraction, imagery and thought blocking and hypnosis.[15,16] Children are often very willing and cooperative subjects and enjoy the novelty of the techniques and sense of control they engender. Relaxation decreases muscle tension and has been used particularly successfully with headaches.[15] It is also often used alongside cognitive and hypnotherapy approaches, which have been demonstrated to be effective in a wide range of situations including both acute and chronic pain.[16] Distraction needs to be age appropriate and to actively involve the child. During procedures, blowing bubbles or pop-up books may engage younger children whilst competitive challenges with staff or computer games might help those who are older. Imagery involves the active use of the child's imagination and this can be intensified in older children to involve the induction of an altered state of consciousness that is hypnosis. These methods need a creative clinician with the skill to engage the imagination of the child and weave the child's individual interests into a relevant and absorbing experience in which the level of pain can be modulated.[15]

Family and individual psychotherapy may be used sometimes when it is felt that family conflict or an abnormally enmeshed or pathological family behavior is potentiating the child's pain. (see Ch. 33).

Physiotherapy

Physiotherapy has a range of useful techniques that can contribute to pain management and are particularly important for children with chronic pain. These aim to restore optimal physical function as well as to decrease pain. They include the use of active and passive exercise, often combined with goal setting and close monitoring. These may be used with heat and cooling, hydrotherapy, ultrasound and TENS (transcutaneous electrical nerve stimulation).[17] A TENS unit is a small (approximately 4 × 6 cm) portable box from which electrodes are applied to the skin to deliver imperceptible small electrical impulses which can help modulate the pain. TENS was developed to exploit the gate-control theory of pain, the constant low level of stimulation keeping the 'gate' in the spinal cord closed. Although the gate theory has to some extent been superseded, TENS can be very efficacious.[18]

PHARMACOLOGICAL APPROACHES

Selection of analgesics: multimodal analgesia

A relatively small range of analgesics is used in children. Selection of the most appropriate depends upon the cause and severity of the pain, the age and general condition of the patient, the setting and the facilities for supervision, monitoring and treatment of any side-effects.

The complex neurobiological mechanisms responsible for the clinical characteristics of both acute and chronic pain, and the influence of development on pain processing are becoming better understood. The increased pain sensitivity and tenderness (hyperalgesia and allodynia) at and near the site of injury are known to be the result of changes within the CNS involving many neural and chemical mediators. As these complexities are becoming better understood individual components of pain pathways can be targeted in a mechanistic and multimodal approach to analgesia.[19] A combination of analgesic drugs and techniques, with complementary modes of action, maximizes the therapeutic advantage of each whilst keeping the doses and side-effects to a minimum. This is the rationale underpinning the 'pain ladder' concept, new drugs being added as pain increases (Fig. 37.1).

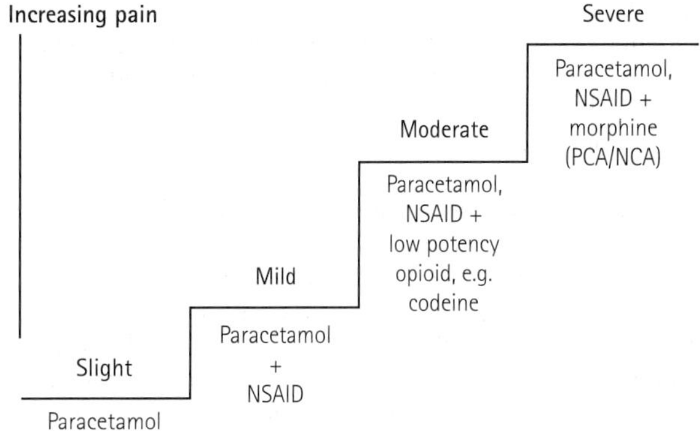

Fig. 37.1 Analgesic ladder. NCA, nurse controlled analgesia; PCA, patient controlled analgesia.

Mild analgesics

Paracetamol

Paracetamol is one of the most widely used drugs for children. It is regarded as a safe and effective mild analgesic, which can be used at every age including the neonate. Traditionally, paracetamol is thought to act centrally, analgesia is attributed to inhibition of cyclo-oxygenase and thereby prostaglandin production in the CNS. Other mechanisms have also been proposed including antagonism of serotonin (5HT) and at N-methyl D-aspartate (NMDA) receptors.

In the adult, several systematic reviews have demonstrated the analgesic efficacy of paracetamol for mild pain, but in fact there have been few studies specifically in children.[20,21] The efficacy of paracetamol is probably fairly low, the correct dosage is important for analgesia and for moderate or severe pain it is probably best combined with other agents, typically codeine and the non-steroidal anti-inflammatory drugs (NSAIDs).

Paracetamol is conjugated to glucuronide, sulfate or cysteine and excreted. In normal circumstances less than 10% is metabolized to a potentially hepatotoxic metabolite, N acetyl P amino benzoquinone imine (NAPQI). NAPQI is neutralized by combination with hepatic glutathione or with N acetyl cysteine and excreted harmlessly unless this pathway is saturated due to overdose or conjugates are in reduced supply. The P450 isoenzyme responsible for metabolism of paracetamol is developmentally regulated, with lower activity in the neonate, and this may confer some protection. However, reduced clearance in neonates may lead to accumulation of the drug and its metabolites and so a reduced daily dose is usually recommended in the newborn. Paracetamol hepatotoxicity is well recognized; typically it is a dose dependent complication associated with acute ingestion of more than 150 mg/kg. Chronic paracetamol treatment can also lead to toxicity at lower doses and it has been recommended that the drug should not routinely be given for more than 5 days at the maximum recommended dose.[22] Risk factors for toxicity include: chronic ingestion, especially in the malnourished due to reduced hepatic glutathione stores, pre-existing liver impairment (single doses are reasonably safe), hepatic enzyme induction and miscalculation or misinterpretation of commercial package labeling leading to accidental overdose.

The recommended total daily dose is 60 mg/kg in the newborn and 90 mg/kg in infants and older children.[23] This is usually given as 15 mg/kg or 20 mg/kg q.d.s. respectively. Absorption after oral paracetamol is excellent, rectal bioavailability is lower and more variable at 25–98%. In order to achieve therapeutic plasma levels a higher initial rectal dose is recommended (of the order of 30–40 mg/kg) followed by regular doses not exceeding maximum daily doses.

Propacetamol

Propacetamol is an intravenously injectable prodrug which is hydrolysed to paracetamol 2:1 (i.e. 1 g propacetamol yields 0.5 g paracetamol). It is useful when other routes of administration for paracetamol are not available. The pharmacokinetics of propacetamol have been studied in neonates and children, and it has been used for postoperative pain.[24,25] Transient but mild platelet dysfunction after propacetamol has been described. Contact dermatitis in health care workers may also occur.

Non-steroidal anti-inflammatory drugs (NSAIDS)

This group of drugs are thought to exert their effects both peripherally and centrally by cyclo-oxygenase inhibition (cf. paracetamol); they also inhibit the release of inflammatory mediators from neutrophils and macrophages. Cyclo-oxygenase helps to catalyse the conversion of arachidonic acid to prostaglandins, which modulate many autoregulatory physiological processes including sensitization of normally high threshold nociceptors at sites of inflammation. The NSAIDs ibuprofen, diclofenac and ketorolac were found to be safe and effective for postoperative analgesia in children in a recent systematically developed guideline.[26] They are also used widely for pain due to injury and many acute and chronic disease processes. These three drugs are used interchangeably in clinical practice, but their effect and side-effect profiles may differ slightly on an individual patient basis. Table 37.1 shows doses and routes. Ibuprofen is available 'over the counter' in the UK, diclofenac is presented in a convenient rectal formulation, and ketorolac is available parenterally.

Side-effects and toxicity

Asthma: caution is advised in the use of NSAIDs in the presence of wheezing as they are known to be cross-reactive with aspirin-induced asthma. The risks may have been overemphasized in children. Aspirin-induced asthma is very rare. A recent study found no deterioration in respiratory function after diclofenac in asthmatic children.[27]

Renal: kidney function is regulated by prostaglandins and two mechanisms of NSAID nephrotoxicity have been described. Functional renal failure can occur in a dose-dependent fashion, disappearing on withdrawal of the drug. Pre-existing poor function and dehydration may be contributing factors. Dose-independent interstitial nephritis with or without nephritic syndrome is rare; treatment is conservative or with corticosteroids.[28]

Coagulopathy: platelet function is altered by NSAIDs due to their reversible inhibition of thromboxane A2 and platelet endoperoxides. Gastrointestinal blood loss can occur, particularly associated with peptic ulceration. Increased intraoperative and postoperative blood loss, which is not usually clinically significant, may also occur.

Table 37.1 Non-steroidal analgesics

Drug	Routes of administration	Doses	Notes
Ibuprofen	Oral	20 mg/kg/day (5 mg/kg q.d.s.)	Max. 800 mg/day
Diclofenac	Oral or rectal	3 mg/kg/day (1 mg/kg t.d.s.)	Max.150 mg/day
Ketorolac	Oral Intravenous	0.5–1 mg/kg q.d.s. 0.5 mg/kg q.d.s.	Dosage restrictions apply in some countries. Max. 40 mg/day

Simultaneous prescription of H_2-receptor antagonists can help reduce the risk of gastrointestinal problems.[29]

Infants and neonates: NSAIDS are rarely given under the age of 6 months and are not usually used in neonates due to fears of possible interference with cerebral blood flow autoregulation and risk to immature renal function.[26]

Gastrointestinal: the normal protective function of the gastric mucosa is reduced by NSAIDS and this can lead to peptic ulceration. It is not usually a problem in short term use. Some newer drugs may be beneficial (see below).

NSAIDs and cyclo-oxygenase

Cyclo-oxygenase exists in two isoforms, COX-1 and COX-2. COX-1 is found in virtually all cell types. COX-2 is expressed in some organs notably the brain and lung but is specifically induced in inflammation in conjunction with a rapid rise in prostaglandin levels. The traditional NSAIDs are non-selective for these isoforms but individual drugs may differ slightly in their ability to depress activity. A new class of selective COX-2 inhibitors are now clinically available with reputedly fewer side-effects (particularly gastro-intestinal) in comparison with non-selective NSAIDs. Theoretically COX-2 type drugs may widen the indications for NSAIDs, but the exact consequences of their selectivity is not yet fully understood, for example, their use in the adult has been found to be associated with a possibly increased risk of adverse cardiovascular events and the incidence of renal complications may be similar to non-selective inhibitors. The use of COX-2 selective NSAIDs has not been studied in children.

Opioids and related drugs

Opioids exert their effects by acting at opioid receptors primarily in the spinal cord and brain. Despite the fact that morphine is one of the oldest and most widely used analgesics, opioid pharmacology is still not fully understood and many important questions remain unanswered. Opioids are the most powerful analgesics available with high efficacy for many types of acute and chronic pain, with the notable exception of neuropathic pain. Important considerations when prescribing opioids include their unpleasant and potentially dangerous side-effects and the development of tolerance which can be troublesome. Neonates, in particular, appear clinically to be more susceptible to the depressant effects of opioids; the causes of this are probably multifactorial but have not been fully explained (see below).

The doses and possible routes of administration of the commonly used opioids for children are shown in Table 37.2. Morphine has a fairly direct relationship between dose, efficacy and side-effects. The same is not true for all other opioids. Partial agonist drugs such as buprenorphine have a ceiling effect and others such as codeine and pethidine have unacceptable side-effect profiles at high doses which limit their use.

Morphine

Morphine is the prototype, high potency opioid and enormous experience in its use often makes it the drug of choice for severe pain. The pharmacokinetics and clinical use of morphine in children have been reviewed recently.[2] The pharmacokinetics and efficacy of morphine are developmentally regulated, although outside the neonatal period, which is characterized by high variability, efficacy is largely predictable and dose related.[30]

Morphine is well absorbed orally; formulations of morphine include a suspension and a slow-release compound (MST). Parenteral morphine is usually given intravenously either by intermittent dosing, continuous infusion or in a patient controlled analgesia (PCA) or nurse controlled analgesia (NCA) regimen (see Table 37.3). Subcutaneous

Table 37.2 Opioids

Drug	Routes of administration	Doses	Notes
Codeine	Oral	1 mg/kg q.d.s.	
	Rectal	1–1.5 mg/kg q.d.s.	
Oxycodone/hydrocodone	Oral	0.2 mg/kg q.d.s.	
Morphine	Oral	0.2–0.4 mg/kg q.d.s.	Long acting oral preparations available
	Intravenous	0.05 mg/kg	
	Subcutaneous	0.05 mg/kg	
	Epidural	0.02–0.05 mg/kg	
Fentanyl	OTFC (oral transmucosal)		See relevant product
	Transdermal	0.001–0.005 mg/kg	See relevant product
	Intravenous	0.001 mg/kg	Incremental dose
	Epidural	0.0001 mg/kg/h	Infusion
Pethidine	Oral	2 mg/kg q.d.s.	
	Intravenous	0.5–1 mg/kg	Incremental/loading dose
	Subcutaneous	0.5–1 mg/kg	Incremental/loading dose
Methadone	Oral	0.2 mg/kg t.d.s.	Useful long acting opioid
	Intravenous	0.1–0.2 mg/kg	

infusion of morphine is also used, particularly in palliative care. Preservative-free (as a precaution against chemical toxicity) morphine is also effective in the epidural space, usually combined with local anesthetic.[31]

Nausea and vomiting, sedation, and respiratory depression are the most frequently seen acute adverse effects of morphine. Itching also occurs especially after epidural morphine. Depression of gastrointestinal motility and constipation are a problem with prolonged use. In clinical practice, non-life-threatening side-effects can be treated by reducing the dosage of morphine, often in palliative care by waiting for tolerance to the side-effect to develop – drowsiness almost always wears off in a few days, or with appropriate therapy, e.g. antiemetics, antipruritics and laxatives. If necessary adverse effects of morphine can be reversed with the opioid antagonist, naloxone.

Fentanyl

Fentanyl is a synthetic, high potency (100× morphine), lipid soluble opioid. Its main use is during general anesthesia where its efficacy, rapid onset and short initial half-life are an advantage. Fentanyl is usually given intravenously. It is also a popular choice for ventilated neonates and infants on intensive care units (ICUs) (see below).

Table 37.3 Protocols for intravenous morphine administration

1. Morphine infusion		
Preparation:	Morphine sulfate 1 mg/kg in 50 ml solution	
Concentration:	20 mcg/kg/ml	
Initial dose:	2.5–5.0 ml (50–100 mcg/kg)	
Infusion:	0.5–1.5 ml/h (10–30 mcg/kg/h)	
2. PCA		
Preparation:	Morphine sulfate 1 mg/kg in 50 ml solution	
Concentration:	20 mcg/kg/ml	
Initial dose:	2.5–5.0 ml (50–100 mcg/kg)	
Programming	Background infusion:	0–0.2 ml/h (0–4 mcg/kg/h)
	PCA dose	0.5–1.0 ml (10–20 mcg/kg/h)
	Lockout interval:	5 min
3. NCA		
Preparation:	Morphine sulfate 1 mg/kg in 50 ml solution	
Concentration:	20 mcg/kg/ml	
Initial dose:	2.5–5.0 ml (50–100 mcg/kg)	
Programming	Background infusion:	0.5–1.0 ml/h (10–20 mcg/kg/h)
	NCA dose	0.5–1.0 ml (10–20 mcg/kg/h)
	Lockout interval:	20 min
4. Subcutanous morphine		
Preparation:	Morphine sulfate 1 mg/kg in 20 ml solution	
Concentration:	50 mcg/kg/ml	
	Initial dose:	1–2.0 ml (50–100 mcg/kg)
Programming	Infusion:	0.2–0.4 ml/h (10–20 mcg/kg/h)

Postoperatively fentanyl is commonly infused into the epidural space as its high lipid solubilty may limit rostral spread and reduce the incidence of some complications, notably respiratory depression, retention of urine and itching in comparison with morphine. Fentanyl is available as oral (transmucosal) and transdermal (fentanyl patch) preparations which can be used for procedural pain and pain in palliative care.

Fentanyl is very potent with a fast onset after intravenous administration. Opioid related side-effects of sedation, respiratory depression and itching are to be expected. High doses have also been associated with chest wall rigidity[32] and are usually only given when respiration is controlled.

Codeine

Codeine is a low potency opioid which can be used for mild to moderate pain including some postoperative pain and cancer pain. It is often combined with other analgesics for best effect, particularly paracetamol and the NSAIDs (see Fig. 37.1). Codeine is probably a morphine prodrug. The response to codeine is more variable than that to morphine and this may be due to genetic (and possibly developmental) differences in metabolizing capacity.[33] Ten per cent or more of individuals from some populations will not benefit from codeine analgesia. Despite this, they may experience some adverse effects as codeine can produce these without metabolism to morphine. Codeine should not be administered intravenously as it causes hypotension.

Oxycodone and hydrocodone

Oxycodone and hydrocodone are semisynthetic opioids suitable for mild to moderate pain especially in combination with paracetamol or NSAIDS. Sustained release formulations are also available but they have not been evaluated for use in children.

Tramadol

Tramadol is a synthetic moderate potency analgesic which has a novel dual mode of action by a combination of inhibition of serotonin and noradrenaline (norepinephrine) reuptake and mu-opioid receptor agonism by its active metabolite o-desmethyltramadol. Metabolism of tramadol is by the same cytochrome P450 enzyme subgroup responsible for codeine metabolism, and therefore may be subject to the same drawbacks (see above). Tramadol has been used for early postoperative analgesia in children with good effect. It has also been used in the caudal epidural space where it appears to have a slow onset (about 1 h) and moderate potency.

Pethidine

Pethidine is a synthetic opioid which has few advantages over morphine. Pethidine is metabolized to norpethidine which is neurotoxic, causing tremor, twitching, agitation and even convulsions. Norpethidine is probably also the cause of abnormal neurobehavioral tests in the neonate following maternal pethidine. High and repeated dosage and renal impairment are risk factors, but convulsions have been reported with low doses in the therapeutic range.[34] The use of pethidine in acute sickle cell pain has declined subsequent to reports of convulsions in children.

Pethidine was originally considered to induce less nausea and vomiting and to be less depressant to the respiratory center of the fetus and neonate than morphine. If it is administered in equi-analgesic dosage these differences are not apparent, although it remains popular in some centers.

Pethidine has also been recommended for use in pancreatitis as it was thought to be less likely to precipitate spasm of the sphincter of Oddi than morphine or other opioids. Evidence from adult literature does not support this hypothesis. The question has not been examined in children.

Novel systemic analgesics

Clonidine

Clonidine is an alpha2 adrenoceptor agonist with multiple effects including analgesia, sedation, antihypertension, antisialogogue, and others. Clonidine has a direct effect on spinal pre- and post-synaptic adrenoceptors in the dorsal horn. It also has many supraspinal effects which may also contribute to analgesia. The pharmacology, use and advantages of clonidine and other alpha2 adrenoceptor agonists in pediatrics has been recently recognized, particularly for postoperative pain. Sedation and hypotension are the principal side-effects of clonidine. Moderate dose independent reductions in blood pressure were found at doses within the therapeutic range 0.625–2.5 mcg/kg in children. The efficacy of clonidine in the neonate is not established. Severe respiratory depression after 2 mcg/kg caudal clonidine has been reported.

Ketamine

Ketamine is an antagonist at the glutamate NMDA receptor. The receptor is important in the generation of hyperalgesia in many pain states. High doses (1–2 mg/kg) have been used for many years as a general anesthetic. At 'low dose', < 1 mg/kg, ketamine has been found to be an effective analgesic or antihyperalgesic both systemically and epidurally. The use of low dose ketamine for postoperative pain in adults is fairly commonplace and has been reviewed. There are reports of its use in children, e.g. it has been used for analgesia–sedation in pediatric ICU with good effect,[35] and for postoperative pain. Ketamine in high doses induces neuro-behavioral and cognitive depression, sometimes accompanied by psychotomimetic effects characterized by bizzare dreams or hallucinations. This seems to be very rare at low doses.

Local anesthesia

Local anesthesia has a particularly important role in pediatric pain management as it is often extremely effective and avoids many of the complications of systemic analgesics. Local anesthetic creams and gels are widely used and are discussed in the section on procedural pain, below.

Bupivacaine

The amide-type local anesthetic bupivacaine is popular because of its long duration of action. Bupivacaine has been used widely for most types of local anesthetic procedure in children. It is almost universally the drug of choice for epidural analgesia where it can be infused for several days for postoperative pain, and sometimes longer for other indications. The pharmacokinetics of bupivacaine in children has been studied following wound infiltration – after trauma or surgery, peripheral nerve blocks and epidural analgesia. Neurotoxicity and cardiotoxicity have been reported but the incidence appears to be very low if dosage recommendations are not exceeded. Similar, newer and less toxic agents than bupivacaine, i.e. ropivacaine and l-bupivacaine are also available, and they may supersede bupivacaine for some indications.

MANAGEMENT OF ACUTE AND POSTOPERATIVE PAIN

Pain after surgery is largely a predictable event and therefore analgesia can be planned in advance according to the expected pain and postoperative setting. Pediatric anesthetists have special training in the use of systemic analgesics and local anesthetic techniques for surgery and they should also take some responsibility for postoperative pain management. Many of the principles and techniques used for postoperative pain may also be applied to other sources of acute or acute on chronic pain. Examples are post-traumatic injury, acute sickle cell crisis, mucositis and many others.

ANALGESIA FOR MINOR AND AMBULATORY OR DAY-CARE SURGERY

Most routine surgery in children is relatively minor and very often undertaken on a day case or day stay basis. Analgesia for day surgery should be effective and not delay discharge from hospital. The objective is to maximize comfort and mobility with little sedation or other side-effects. Postoperative nausea and vomiting (PONV) is a particular problem. In practice, this means limiting or avoiding the use of sedatives and opioids whilst encouraging the use of local anesthetic techniques. Health care workers need education and training to ensure that all runs smoothly and patients are pain free at discharge. Further analgesia will usually need to be continued at home for several days managed by parents who will need information and support in order to be able to do this effectively. Postoperative pain should be mostly treatable with 'over the counter' analgesics, which are safe and easily obtainable by parents at home. Otherwise the suitability of a procedure for day surgery must be questioned. Take home 'packs' containing analgesics and written information are often supplied to families at day surgery centers.

Local anesthetic techniques

Infiltration of the surgical wound can be used in many situations especially for very superficial surgery, its utility being limited mainly by the need for large volumes of local anesthetic and dosage restrictions. Infiltration is effective for a number of common pediatric procedures including herniotomy, eye surgery, dental surgery and tonsillectomy. A range of peripheral nerve blocks are frequently used. The ilioinguinal and iliohypogastric nerves, which supply the sensory innervation to the groin area, are easy to locate and block. Surgical exploration of the inguinal region includes hernia repair, ligation of patent processus vaginalis and orchidopexy. Recognized complications include quadriceps weakness due to spread of local anesthetic to the femoral nerve. The distal third of the penis is supplied by the dorsal nerves, which are easily blocked by an injection of local anesthetic at the base of the penis. Analgesia is suitable for circumcision, minor hypospadias repair and surgery on the urethral meatus. Dorsal nerve block has also been particularly advocated for neonatal circumcision, which is performed in some countries without general anesthesia.

Caudal block

There is an enormous literature extending back at least 30 years describing caudal epidural local anesthesia in children and has been reviewed recently.[36] Caudal block is effective for most operations below the level of the umbilicus – bupivacaine lasts 4–6 h. Recently other drugs, notably opioids, ketamine and clonidine have also been used either alone or in combination with local anesthetic, prolonging analgesia to 12 or more hours. The complications of caudal analgesia include temporary leg weakness, delayed micturition, vascular puncture, dural puncture, and inadvertent intravascular or intradural injection of local anesthetic. Epidural infection or neurological sequelae have not been reported after single caudal local anesthetic injections.

Systemic analgesia

Potent analgesia is likely to be necessary in the early postoperative period even after minor surgery. Institution of systemic analgesia after surgery should be planned to ensure a smooth and comfortable transition from the immediate postoperative and postanesthesia recovery phase. Drugs, timing and routes of administration selected are important. Reactive, PRN or 'as required' dosing schedules are not appropriate during the period of expected postoperative pain, and if used they are likely to lead to avoidable painful intervals while drugs are taking effect.

Nausea and vomiting

Nausea and vomiting is a common cause of morbidity after minor and day-care surgery. Its causes are multifactorial, associated with poor analgesia and not with preoperative anxiety. The etiology and management of postoperative nausea and vomiting (PONV) in children has been reviewed and a proactive approach to therapy is encouraged.[37] Risk factors for PONV include a previous history of PONV, general anesthesia, the use of opioids, early resumption of oral fluids and certain surgical procedures notably tonsillectomy and strabismus surgery.

ANALGESIA AFTER MAJOR SURGERY

Local anesthetic techniques, performed under general anesthesia before or after surgery can reduce analgesic requirements in the early postoperative period.[38] After major operations further analgesia can be accomplished by infusion of local anesthetic through a catheter located at the site of the block, e.g. continuous epidural analgesia. More commonly pain after major surgery is managed with morphine or other opioids. As the oral route is rarely available after major surgery for at least the first postoperative day, and often much longer after gastrointestinal operations, others must be used. Paracetamol, NSAIDs, codeine and morphine are all readily available in rectal formulations which have been popular. Rectal absorption for many drugs is known to be erratic and unpredictable, and a fatality following rectal morphine in a child has been reported. Nevertheless rectal administration of less potent drugs appears to be safe and is still widespread for paracetamol and NSAIDs.

Parenteral opioid infusion

Morphine infusion has been used safely for postoperative analgesia in children for more than 20 years. The dose range in non-ventilated children in general ward areas is around 10–30 mcg/kg/h. Either intravenous or subcutaneous routes can be used for morphine infusions, although the latter requires more concentrated solutions (Table 37.3). A wide range of morphine requirements after surgery in children has been observed and inadequate analgesia on the first postoperative day is more frequent at infusion rates < 20 mcg/kg/h.[39] Patient controlled analgesia (PCA) is popular for children 5 years or older. There is a substantial literature describing its use and efficacy.[40,41] Nurse controlled analgesia (NCA) is a modified continuous morphine infusion suitable for children who are unable to operate the PCA handset. Nursing staff can administer extra doses of morphine on the basis of pain assessments or before painful care or movement by operating the PCA handset. NCA increases flexibility, total morphine consumption and parent and nurse satisfaction with analgesia.[31] Protocols for morphine infusion, PCA and NCA are given in Table 37.3. Inadequate analgesia, nausea and vomiting, excessive sedation and respiratory depression can be troublesome problems in the postoperative period. Better pain assessment, appropriate dosing, multimodal analgesia and clear protocols should minimize poor efficacy and side-effects. Naloxone should always be available when opioids are being infused. Nausea and vomiting is increased with the use of opioids; 5HT antagonists (e.g. ondansetron) are popular treatment but may not be much more efficacious than cheaper, more traditional drugs such as cyclizine, the synthetic corticosteroid dexamethasone, which either alone or in combination has potent antiemetic effects. Combination antiemetic therapy is probably the most effective treatment (see Table 37.4).[37]

MANAGEMENT OF NEONATAL PAIN

Pain in the neonatal period requires special consideration because the immaturity of many body systems has a profound and often unpredictable influence on both the response to pain and analgesics. Advances in perinatal care have meant that many younger and smaller patients undergo diagnostic and therapeutic procedures and present for surgery in early life. The management of these painful situations is hindered by our inability to accurately measure pain in this group and a lack of information on the precise effects of many analgesics during early postnatal development. Research in the fields of pain assessment and the developmental neurobiology and pharmacology of pain may soon influence practice, but for the present pharmacological neonatal pain management is largely based on the empirical and judicious use of opioids (principally codeine, morphine, and fentanyl), paracetamol, and local anesthesia.[42]

OPIOIDS

Despite the fact that opioids are widely used in the neonatal period both for pain and sedation little is known of the thresholds for treatment or response in the term or preterm neonate. The pharmacokinetics of morphine and other opioids have been investigated and clear relationships between age and volume of distribution and plasma clearance have been established.[30] Underlying medical condition is probably also important as the maturation in morphine clearance observed in infants in the first few months of life is delayed in those undergoing cardiac surgery in comparison with age matched controls after other surgical procedures.[43] The lack of sensitive pain measurement tools and failure to correlate plasma morphine levels with analgesia has led some authors to use the emergence of side-effects such as respiratory depression to quantify the response to morphine.[43] Although there is no clear dose–response relationship between plasma morphine and respiratory depression, a common threshold in neonates and infants of around 20 ng/ml has been suggested and based on this, the dose of morphine to reach this target level has been investigated and found to be 5–15 mcg/kg/h in the neonate, some 25–50% lower than in older children.[44] Clearly, determination of the analgesic dose–response for opioids in the neonate is an important priority for further research. Suggested protocols are shown in Table 37.5.

PARACETAMOL

Paracetamol is considered to be safe and effective in the neonatal period although, as with adults and older children, the plasma level associated with analgesia is not known.

Table 37.4 Drug treatment of opioid side-effects

1. Respiratory depression		
Naloxone	4 mcg/kg	Intravenous
2. Nausea and vomiting		
Cyclizine	1 mg/kg	Oral/intravenous (max. 50 mg)
Ondansetron	0.1 mg/kg	Oral/intravenous (max. 8 mg)
Dexamethasone	0.1 mg/kg	Intravenous

Table 37.5 Suggested morphine infusion protocols in the neonate*

Neonatal morphine infusion		
Preparation:	Morphine sulfate 1.0 mg/kg in 50 ml solution	
Concentration:	20 mcg/kg/ml	
Initial dose:	0.5–5.0 ml (10–100 mcg/kg)	
Infusion:	0.1–0.7 ml/h (2–14 mcg/kg/h)	
Neonatal NCA		
Preparation:	Morphine sulfate 1 mg/kg in 50 ml solution	
	Concentration:	20 mcg/kg/ml
	Initial dose:	0.5–5.0 ml (10–100 mcg/kg)
Programming	Background infusion:	0.0–0.5 ml/h (0–10 mcg/kg/h)
	NCA dose	0.5–1.0 ml (10–20 mcg/kg/h)
	Lockout interval:	20 min

* With full cardiorespiratory monitoring in intensive care areas, higher doses may be appropriate when respiration is supported.

The majority of pharmacokinetic studies have assumed plasma levels associated with the antipyretic effect of paracetamol to be therapeutic, and therefore a guide to dosing schedules. The pharmacokinetics of paracetamol have been shown to be age dependent – neonates have a higher volume of distribution (174%) and lower clearance (62%) in comparison with older children.[45] Paracetamol is metabolized in the liver where it is conjugated to glucuronide, a small amount being oxidized by cytochrome P450 to a potentially hepatotoxic product (see above) which is conjugated to glutathione. Both these pathways are immature in the neonate and enhanced sulfation of paracetamol has been demonstrated which compensates for reduced glucuronidation. The current recommended dose of paracetamol in the neonate is 60 mg/kg/day, with some variation between different countries.[23] The route of administration is important as bioavailability is very variable. In term neonates 20 mg/kg rectal paracetamol 6 hourly (80 mg/kg/day) does not reliably achieve therapeutic plasma levels and an initial dose of 30 mg/kg is recommended.[46] In preterm neonates 20 mg/kg is effective but prolonged elimination results in accumulation if the dosing interval is less than 8 h.[46] Propacetamol, the injectable form of paracetamol, has also been used in the neonate; at less than 10 days old, 30 mg/kg/day of paracetamol (60 mg/kg/day of propacetamol) maintained plasma levels between 4 and 10 mg/L, whereas after 10 days double this dose was required.[24]

The analgesic efficacy of paracetamol in the neonate has not been well investigated. In a study of the response to heel lance, perhaps unsurprisingly, paracetamol was found to be ineffective.[47] Until further studies are available, paracetamol should be assumed to have similar potency in the neonate as in the older child and adult. Except in very mild pain it should probably be used in combination with other analgesics.

LOCAL ANESTHESIA

Local anesthesia is popular in the neonate as it avoids many of the problems associated with systemic drugs. Topical local anesthesia, infiltration and nerve blocks including epidural anesthesia can be used in the newborn. Neonates may be more susceptible to toxic effects of local anesthetics. Local anesthetics are extensively protein bound. The free (unbound) fraction is considered to be pharmacologically active and therefore also important for toxicity. The protein A- acid glycoprotein (AAG) and albumin are the most important plasma proteins involved and AAG levels are lower in neonates. Increased unbound bupivacaine has been demonstrated in the newborn and this may lead to increased susceptibility to toxicity and so lower doses are generally recommended. Prilocaine is a constituent of the topical formulation EMLA (see below – procedural pain) and its use in the neonate has been a cause for concern. A metabolite of prilocaine, orthotoluidine, is produced which leads to the development of methemglobin (oxidized hemoglobin), which has a reduced oxygen carrying capacity. Methemoglobin is reduced to hemoglobin by the enzyme methemoglobin reductase which is developmentally regulated. Neonates are also particularly susceptible because fetal hemoglobin is more easily oxidized than adult hemoglobin. Subsequent studies have shown that EMLA is safe for neonates provided the dose is limited proportionally.[48,49]

MANAGEMENT OF PROCEDURAL PAIN

Acutely painful procedures occur commonly in hospitalized patients particularly those receiving intensive care or with conditions requiring extended monitoring and treatment such as cancer, juvenile rheumatoid arthritis or epidermolysis bullosa.[50]

Invasive diagnostic and therapeutic procedures such as venepuncture, lumbar puncture, insertion of intravascular and other catheters, insertion and removal of drainage tubes, bone marrow aspiration and injections into joints are painful and potentially difficult to manage. Inadequate treatment of pain for a procedure will have implications for subsequent treatments, and management may become progressively more difficult. Psychological approaches, systemic or local analgesia with or without sedation and complementary therapies may all be useful.[18,51] For many children however, particularly the very young and uncooperative, there is little alternative to general anesthesia, which is quick, safe and effective but requires special facilities and personnel.

PSYCHOLOGICAL AND COMPLEMENTARY THERAPIES

Cognitive-behavioral and behavioral techniques have an important place in the management of procedural pain, often in combination with simple measures such as topical local anesthesia. There is a considerable literature describing the use and efficacy of such techniques. For a variety of procedures such as lumbar puncture and bone marrow aspiration cognitive-behavioral management in expert hands compares favorably with general anesthesia.[51] Transcutaneous electrical nerve stimulation (TENS), acupuncture, aromatherapy and massage therapy may also have a role although randomized, controlled comparisons with standard treatments in children are not available.

TOPICAL LOCAL ANESTHESIA

Topical local anesthetic, lidocaine- (lignocaine-) prilocaine cream (EMLA) or amethocaine gel (Ametop) have gained widespread acceptance for analgesia during venepuncture. Amethocaine gel has a more rapid onset and longer duration of action. It also causes vasodilatation which may be beneficial and is suitable for neonates. There is a small incidence of local reactions to amethocaine gel.

The use of EMLA has also been extended to other indications. EMLA was found to be effective for a variety of invasive procedures in neonates including arterial puncture, lumbar puncture and venous cannulation. It is also effective at reducing the postoperative pain of neonatal circumcision and at reducing pain from chest drain removal in infants and children.[52]

NITROUS OXIDE

Inhalation of a 50% mixture of nitrous oxide with oxygen (Entonox) can provide potent analgesia for short procedures in cooperative patients. A self-administration apparatus with a demand valve and safety features is available and is suitable for children of 5 years and above. Nitrous oxide–oxygen analgesia has been described for minor surgery, fracture reduction and many other procedures in accident and emergency departments.[53]

MANAGEMENT OF PAIN IN THE ICU

In the intensive care unit (ICU) sources of pain include the underlying condition, the presence of endotracheal and other tubes, drains and catheters and also the many procedures which such patients frequently undergo. (See sections on acute pain, neonatal pain and procedural pain for details of techniques.)

OPIOID INFUSIONS, TOLERANCE AND WITHDRAWAL

It is now normal practice for both neonates and older children to receive potent opioid analgesia as part of basic care in ICU areas. Opioid infusions are usually selected as they provide background analgesia, sedation, improve comfort and facilitate synchronization of respiration with artificial ventilation.[35] Morphine is the first choice analgesic for this use. Fentanyl is an alternative particularly if there is evidence or danger of pulmonary hypertension as it is thought to have less effect on the pulmonary vasculature.

A characteristic feature of opioid infusion after a few days of continuous use is progressive tolerance to both the analgesic and sedative effects. It is not uncommon for patients to receive doses far in excess of what is normally considered therapeutic. Intermittent administration is less likely to cause tolerance than continuous infusion but this can be impractical. A compromise of a background infusion with intermittent doses when necessary, e.g. for routine care, blood sampling, endotracheal suction and other procedures may be an advantage. Clearly this is very similar in concept to NCA (see above). Multimodal analgesia may also be helpful and the use of newer agents such as clonidine and low dose ketamine appear to retard the development of tolerance.

Abrupt withdrawal of opioids after 5 or more days of continuous use is very likely to result in the appearance of symptoms and signs of withdrawal. These are very unpleasant for the patient and family and may be dangerous as cerebral excitatory phenomena are prominent and convulsions may occur. Gradual reduction of infusion rates at 10–20% per day will normally avoid symptoms developing. This process should not delay extubation of the airway or discharge from ICU areas. If necessary oral preparations can be used and weaning from high doses continued in low dependency areas, even at home. Clonidine and benzodiazepines ameliorate the withdrawal syndrome associated with opioids. Some patients have also received high dose infusions of benzodiazepines, such as midazolam, and in such circumstances benzodiazepine withdrawal is also likely. Substitution of long acting benzodiazepines such as lorazepam and gradual withdrawal are therefore recommended.

PROCEDURES IN ICU AREAS

Children in ICU undergo numerous procedures. It is not safe to assume that background levels of analgesia will be sufficient for this incident acute pain and it should be actively managed with local anesthesia where possible or other suitable techniques (see section on procedural pain).

CHRONIC PAIN

There is no precise definition of when a pain becomes chronic and in many ways it relates more to the patient's perception of the situation and reaction to it than an objective measure. A number of the effects of pain on a person appear to differ depending on whether the pain is acute or chronic, and to form a continuum between. In acute pain the prevailing mood tends toward anxiety, whereas in chronic pain depression becomes predominant. Hope remains strong in acute pain whereas despair can dominate the chronic situation. In acute pain the person is able to focus on the pain itself but with chronic pain it pervades their whole life and their behavior and responses to the pain become incorporated into their everyday living.

Effective management in chronic pain therefore depends on recognizing the need to tackle both the underlying cause for the pain and also these wider manifestations, assessed on an individual basis. Sometimes the physical damage related to the pain is very clear and forms the focus for specific analgesic approaches. Pain may be constant, such as in progressive cancer or related to exacerbations in the illness, such as in rheumatological and connective tissue disorders. In other disorders a combination of background chronic pain occurs with acute episodes or pain from procedures superimposed. Examples include sickle cell disease, osteogenesis imperfecta and epidermolysis bullosa. Specific treatment aimed at reversing or relieving the underlying illness is ideally the most effective approach to relieving the pain but often this must be combined with appropriate short or long term analgesia. Analgesics are chosen according to the severity of the pain and whether it appears to be primarily related to tissue damage or to have inflammatory or neuropathic elements. Psychological assessment can indicate the role for appropriate introduction of cognitive and behavioral pain management skills.

SICKLE CELL DISEASE

The dual aspects of acute and chronic pain are particularly vividly represented by sickle cell disease, where the severe pain of each individual sickle cell crisis is typical of acute pain but the recurrent nature of the crises, their unpredictable nature and the life-long and incurable nature of the disease results in aspects characteristic of chronic intractable pain.[54] Management of pain for these children and young people has a poor record, with inappropriate fears of addiction and misunderstanding of cultural aspects of the illness, resulting in analgesics being underused and unnecessary suffering occurring. Current approaches have treated the acute pain more aggressively, recognizing the need to give the patients more credence and control, organizing systems to enable a more rapid response to pain at the start of a crisis and offering intravenous strong opioids by PCA. Alongside this, the increasing role of non-pharmacological approaches is contributing towards improving psychological support and daily living for these children.

CHRONIC PAIN SYNDROMES

A significant number of children present with symptoms of pain but where a physical cause for the pain is not evident, the pain seems disproportionate to the tissue damage or previous damage appears to have healed but the pain persists. In these children the typical aspects of chronic pain on the child and family are particularly overt.

One common picture, often occurring with limb pains, is that of increasing disability and associated sympathetically mediated features such as edema, decreased temperature and pallor or cyanotic coloring of the affected part, hyperesthesia of the skin, muscle wasting and eventually osteoporosis and atrophy. This has been called reflex sympathetic dystrophy (RSD) in the past but is now considered part of the spectrum of chronic regional pain syndrome (CRPS), in which sympathetic features may or may not be present and fatigue, widely disseminated pains and other symptoms are also common. Increasing malaise, disability, time off school and family disruption are common[55] and although children may be taking many analgesics they are rarely effective in relieving the pain.

Many of these children are labeled as malingering or disbelieved resulting in anger and frustration. A confident diagnosis of CRPS depends on careful exclusion of an observable underlying pathology, and then a recognition with the child and family of the complex and ill-understood nature of the problem, acknowledging the reality of the pain and symptoms. The causes are not clearly understood and appear to involve features of neuropathic pain, with a persistent and inappropriate up-regulation of pain perception, in the wider context of a biobehavioral response to the pain.[56] The most successful management is multidisciplinary.[57] As well as medical and nursing input it involves physiotherapy, psychology and pharmaceutical assessment followed by the development of a comprehensive treatment program, with the involvement of the child and family. Interventions usually aim to be outpatient based, but in severe situations intensive inpatient programs may be needed. Care includes the gradual withdrawal of inappropriate analgesics, and cautious use of medications effective in neuropathic pain such as the sodium channel blockers gabapentin and the tricyclic antidepressants.[58] Learning coping skills, cognitive and behavioral support, graded exercise, goal setting and regular support and monitoring. The course may be one of improvement and relapses. The use of sympathetic blocks is no longer routinely part of the care of CRPS patients.

PALLIATIVE CARE

Palliative care for children and young people is an active and total approach to care, embracing physical, emotional, social and spiritual elements. It focuses on enhancement of quality of life for the child and support for the family and includes the management of symptoms, provision of respite and care through death and bereavement.[59] Potentially all children with life-limiting illnesses and their families can benefit from palliative care. This includes a wide range of diagnoses, which can be thought of in four broad groups.

- Children with life-threatening conditions for which curative treatment may be possible but may fail; e.g. cancer.
- Children with illnesses where there are long periods of intensive treatment, aimed at prolonging quality life, but where premature death is anticipated; e.g. cystic fibrosis, muscular dystrophy.
- Children with progressive conditions where treatment is exclusively palliative and may extend over many years; e.g. Batten disease, mucopolysaccharidoses.
- Conditions with severe disability, often neurological, which cause extreme vulnerability to complications and where premature death is anticipated; e.g. severe cerebral palsy.

The exact number of children who fit into these groups has been underestimated in the past but recent data suggest a prevalence of between 1 and 2 per 1000 children.[59]

TRANSITION TO PALLIATIVE CARE

The transition to palliative care involves an acknowledgment that the prime focus of the child's care is increasingly, and eventually may be entirely, on the child's quality of life rather than treatments aimed at cure or significantly prolonging life. A model where palliative care is introduced as a late and last resort has predominated in the past[59] but a more flexible approach, where palliative care concepts are introduced earlier and incorporated alongside treatments to extend life is often much more appropriate (Fig. 37.2), especially in non-malignant diseases. This flexibility enables health care professionals to respond to the many complex, diverse and changing needs of children with life-threatening diseases, and can help both the family and professional staff in the difficult transition to palliative care (Fig. 37.2).

SYMPTOM MANAGEMENT

Symptom management is an essential part of palliative care. However, in spite of increasing awareness of the need for palliative care, many children still experience unresolved problems.[60] Symptom management should be approached systematically, through a careful and detailed history and assessment of the problems before making and instituting a management plan, which then needs to be reviewed and fine-tuned regularly. Formal assessment schemes are available and can help in evaluating pain[5] but these are only just beginning to be considered for other symptoms. Since quality of life for a child is so important at this time as well as considering the detailed nature of each symptom, clarifying its wider implications on the child and family's day to day living is particularly important in planning its management.

Although every child and family is unique the pattern of symptoms the child is likely to develop will be related to their underlying diagnosis. A child with inoperable congenital heart disease may be expected to suffer from fatigue, dyspnea and edema; a child with progressive malignant disease will probably have pain and a child with renal failure may be at risk of nausea, convulsions and itching. Awareness of potential problems enables carers to anticipate and plan ahead so medications which may be needed can be ordered ahead of time, preparations for different routes made readily available and discussion, even of a potentially difficult symptom, faced with the family. This can help avoid crisis management, feelings of panic and lack of control for both the family and health care workers and also unnecessary and unwanted hospital admissions.

In palliative care most medications, particularly analgesics need to be prescribed regularly and the oral route is the first choice. As the disease progresses initial oral therapy may no longer be possible, for example if the child is no longer able to absorb medication, they are too weak or their level of consciousness has declined and alternative routes must be used. Some children are prepared to have drugs rectally and prefer them to any 'needle'. More often they are given either subcutaneously, which is particularly convenient if the child is at home or intravenously if the child has a central intravenous line in situ. Most of the analgesics, antiemetics and sedatives commonly used in palliative care can be combined in solution for convenience. Whichever route is being used the least intrusive equipment should be chosen and unnecessary and inappropriate monitoring discouraged. Frequent review, negotiation with the family, flexibility and forward planning are vital for the child's well-being and to minimize the family's anxiety and distress.

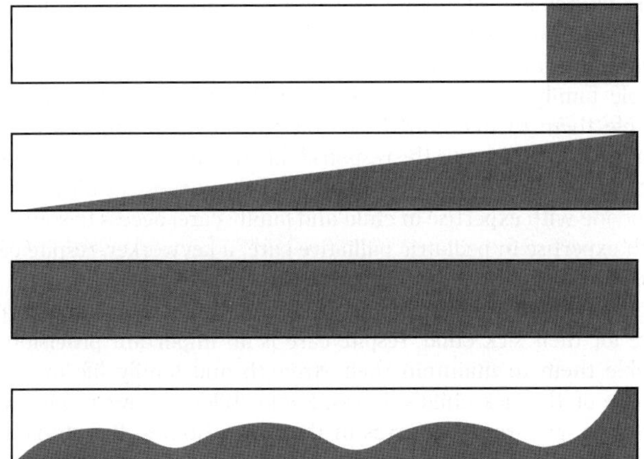

Fig. 37.2 Models of the relationship between palliative care and treatments aimed to cure or extensively prolong life. Palliative care represented as the filled area and curative treatments unfilled. During the course of illness different patterns relate to different needs and prognoses.

PAIN IN PALLIATIVE CARE

Pain is a prominent symptom for children with progressive cancer[60] and usually relates directly to the spread of the tumor. It can be anticipated that it will increase in severity as the illness progresses and it may include neuropathic elements or inflammatory pain from bony invasion, which have particular therapeutic implications. For children with other life-threatening illnesses pain, such as the spasms, musculoskeletal pains or gastroesophageal reflux in a child with severe cerebral palsy, may appear to be a less severe problem. However, parents have identified these pains as a major factor affecting their children's quality of life and can find it difficult to persuade professionals to recognize and treat them.

Plans for managing pain need to consider the widest aspects of pain and combine pharmacological and non-pharmacological approaches for maximum benefit. Sometimes treatment can be aimed to relieve the cause of pain, but more often the cause of the pain cannot be relieved and the approach is one of symptom relief, combining pharmacological and non-pharmacological approaches (Table 37.6). Inappropriate worries, for both families and staff, about the side-effects of strong opioids can inhibit good pain relief for the children, and need to be addressed by those with confidence and experience.

SYMPTOMS OTHER THAN PAIN

Many other symptoms occur commonly in children with life-threatening illnesses.[61] Understanding the cause of the problem can

Table 37.6 Pain management in palliative care

Treatments aimed to relieve the cause of pain
Intrathecal methotrexate for headaches of CNS leukemia
Antibiotics for non-life-threatening intercurrent infection
Surgery for severe hip pain in cerebral palsy
Pharmacological relief of pain
Analgesics according to the WHO ladder (Fig. 37.1); paracetamol, codeine, morphine, diamorphine, fentanyl
Non-steroidal anti-inflammatory drugs for musculoskeletal and bony pain
Gabapentin, amitriptyline, carbamazepine, phenytoin for neuropathic pain
Baclofen, diazepam for muscle spasm
Non-pharmacological approaches
Physiotherapy
TENS
Position, warmth, cold
Explanation and discussion
Distraction and hypnosis
Cognitive and behavioral management

help in making logical therapeutic choices but often symptoms need a flexible multidisciplinary team who can combine both medications and non-pharmacological approaches. Some problems are chronic, lasting many months or even years. Feeding can provide many problems with symptoms from gastroesophageal reflux, especially in children with neurodegenerative illnesses, including ethical issues about the role of gastrostomy or naso-gastric feeding and psychological stress for parents relating to their distress at being unable to nourish their child especially in the late stages of cancer. Consideration of the underlying goals of feeding, its contribution to the child's quality of life and negotiating plans with the family before a crisis occurs, can all help with potentially difficult decisions. Some symptoms such as convulsions, nausea and vomiting and increased secretions may be significantly helped by medications but others such as sensory impairment, intellectual deterioration and fatigue may not. In the latter situation care depends on multidisciplinary and practical support for the child and family, in order to help them cope with the situation as well as possible.

PSYCHOSOCIAL AND SPIRITUAL SUPPORT

The diagnosis of a life-threatening illness and the prospect of a child's impending death is one of the worst situations for any family to ever experience. This is heightened in developed economies by its relative rarity and by society's reluctance to acknowledge the transience of life and unwillingness to talk about death. A number of themes facing the sick child and family have been identified and these occur at diagnosis and then recur at different critical points throughout the course of the illness:

- families' needs for appropriate information;
- the importance of enabling children and families to identify and express their emotions and spiritual needs;
- recognition that emotional and spiritual needs and ways of coping vary between different members of the family and at different times during the illness;
- awareness of the difficulty for families of living with uncertainty;
- acknowledging the benefits of and enabling open and honest communication both within families and between families and professionals:
- the value of empowering families and enabling them to retain choices and a sense of control.

All children and young people facing death or with a reduced life expectancy deserve help in maintaining as much normal life as possible, ensuring good access to play, education and social experiences and assistance in focusing on and achieving appropriate goals in order to preserve their quality of life. For the parents and siblings of children with non-malignant diseases, especially those with severe physical and developmental delay, the prolonged time course and enormous nursing demands only increase the stress and practical difficulties. After a child's death follow-up for the parents and siblings through their bereavement with assessment of their path through grief and referral to appropriate support should be offered.

Awareness and attention to these difficulties and common themes can provide valuable support for families. Members of the multidisciplinary team need the ability and willingness to listen in depth, identify the issues and facilitate and contain the expression of emotion. Throughout the course of a child's illness and death family members are likely to experience a huge range of feelings, some of which they and their carers may have expected such as sadness, despair, depression, hopelessness, anger, bitterness and others which perhaps they may not, such as guilt, resentment of the sick child, isolation, and relief. Marital tension may be heightened and relations with grandparents and family strained. Siblings can also suffer and may feel a sense of exclusion and neglect though many also become very involved in care and also express positive experiences.[62] Families will also identify the fact that the illness has made them reassess their values and what is important in their lives and even that they may even have gained strength together.

Talking openly with families, and especially with the sick child themselves about the impending death is recognized as beneficial as this approach decreases the child's level of anxiety and improves the family's later adjustment.[63,64] However staff and families are extremely skilled at avoiding such difficult conversations and employ a variety of ways of distancing themselves.[65] Factors which need to be taken into account include the child's age and developmental level, their likely understanding of their illness and of death, the child and family's past experiences and the family's normal communication pattern and culture.

Most children are already aware, through their own interpretation of verbal and non-verbal cues, of much more about their illness and situation than most adults expect.[66] Listening to their cues, questioning their fears and worries, responding honestly but gradually and using a range of non-verbal approaches (play, stories, art) are all skills that can help and which members of the multidisciplinary palliative care team can bring to the family and child.

PROVISION OF CARE

Much thought has been given to developing services for children and young people with life-threatening illness in recent years.[59,67] The aim has been to provide flexible, coordinated, multidisciplinary care, tailored to the needs of the individual child and family, whatever the child's diagnosis and wherever they are being cared for.

Since most children have many needs and are often at the center of a complex network of health care providers, families have identified that a keyworker to coordinate care is very valuable. Some disease groups, such as cancer, cystic fibrosis and muscular dystrophy, have developed specialist nurses or therapists posts, to offer outreach from tertiary centers and take on this role. For children with other, rarer diseases pediatric community nurses often undertake this role.

For most children with a life-threatening illness their parents are the primary carers and the family prefer to spend as much of their time as possible at home. The professionals must work flexibly alongside the parents, negotiating a mutually acceptable care plan with them and offering information and expertise. However, the whole family will also need emotional and practical support to enable them to maintain their role. In order for families to feel confident to undertake the responsibility of care for the sick child at home they need to be sure that they have access at all times to someone with expertise in child and family care, access to someone with expertise in pediatric palliative care, a keyworker, respite care and the possibility of inpatient care if they need it.[68]

However willingly and lovingly families undertake the burden of care for their sick child, respite care is an important provision to enable them to maintain their strength and family life over the course of the sick child's illness. Some children have respite care provided by carers or nurses in their own homes. Respite is also offered by the charitably run children's hospices, of which there are now about 20 in the UK. These small, 8–10 bedded units offer nurse-led short-term breaks in an informal 'home from home' atmosphere. They also provide emotional support for parents and siblings, inpatient terminal care if it is the family's choice and bereavement follow-up.

As well as keyworkers for individual families it is recommended that each health district should have a specified pediatric health care professional, for example a senior nurse or a community pediatrician, to undertake responsibility for coordinating palliative care for all the children residing in that area, ensuring that keyworkers are appointed for families and that the multidisciplinary care team is established. This role is particularly important in ensuring both the practical and financial cooperation of health, social services and education in the families' needs.

CONCLUSION

Knowledge and skills in pain management and palliative care have been increasing in recent years. It will be essential to continue these developments and to increase the evidence-based information available, to challenge misinformation and to work towards enhancing pain management and reducing suffering for children throughout the world.

REFERENCES (* Level 1 Evidence)

1 Fitzgerald M, Anand KJS. Neuroanatomy and neurophysiology of pain. In: Schechter N, Berde C, Yaster M, eds. Pain in infants, children and adolescents. Baltimore: Williams and Wilkins; 1993:11–31.

2 Kart T, Christrup LL, Rasmussen M. Recommended use of morphine in neonates, infants and children based on a literature review: Part 1 – Pharmacokinetics. Paediatr Anaesth 1997; 7:93–101.

3 International Association for the Study of Pain, Subcommittee on Taxonomy. Pain terms: a list with definitions and notes on usage. Pain 1979; 6:249–252.

4 McGrath PJ. Annotation: aspects of pain in children and adolescents. J Child Psychol Psychiat 1995; 36(5):717–730.

5 Franck LS, Greenburg CS, Stevens B. Pain assessment in infants and children. Pediatr Clin North Am 2000; 47(3):487–512.

6 Ward SE, Gordon D. Application of American Pain Society quality assurance standards. Pain 1994; 56:299.

7 Miaskowski C, Jacox A, Hester N. Interdisciplinary guidelines for the management of acute pain: implications for quality improvement. J Nurse Care Qual 1992; 7:1.

8 Hester NO. The preoperational child's reaction to immunizations. Nurs Res 1979; 28:250.

9 Varni JW, Thompson KL, Hanson V. The Varni/Thompson pediatric pain questionairre. Chronic musculoskeletal pain in juvenile rheumatoid arthritis. Pain 1987; 28:27.

10 Colwell C, Clark L, Perkins R. Post operative use of pediatric pain scale: children's report vs nurse assessment of pain intensity and affect. J Pediatr Nurs 1996; 11:275.

11 Stevens B, Johnston CC, Petryshen P, et al. Premature infant profile: development and initial validation. Clin J Pain 1996; 12:13.

12 Breau LM, McGrath PJ, Camfield C, et al. Preliminary validation of an observational pain checklist for persons with cognitive impairments and inability to communicate verbally. Dev Med Child Neurol 2000; 42:609–616.

13 Gauvain-Piquard A, Rodary C, Francois P, et al. Validity assessment of the DEGR scale for observational rating of 2–6 year old child pain. J Pain Symptom Manag 1991; 6:171.

14 McGrath PA. Psychological aspects of pain perception. In: Schechter N, Berde C, Yaster M, eds. Pain in infants, children and adolescents. Baltimore: Williams and Wilkins; 1993:39–63.

15 Chen E, Jospeh MH, Zeltzer LK. Behavioral and cognitive interventions in the treatment of pain in children. Pediatr Clin North Am 2000; 47(3):513–525.

16 Kuttner L. Olomon R. Hynotherapy and imagery for managing children's pain. In: Schechter N, Berde C, Yaster M, eds, Pain in infants, children and adolescents. Baltimore: Lippincott, Williams and Wilkins; 2003.

17 McCarthy CF, Shea A, Sullivan P. Physical therapy management of pain in children. In: Schechter N, Berde C, Yaster M, eds, Pain in infants, children and adolescents. Baltimore: Lippincott, Williams and Wilkins; 2003:434–448.

18 Lander J, Fowler-Kerry S. TENS for children's procedural pain. Pain 1993; 52:209–216.

19 Fitzgerald M, Howard RF. The developmental neurobiology of pain. In: Schechter NL, Berde CB, Yaster M, eds. Pain in infants, children and adolescents. Baltimore: Lippincott, Williams and Wilkins; 2003:19–42.

*20 Moore A, Collins S, Carroll D, et al. Single dose paracetamol (acetaminophen), with and without codeine for postoperative pain. Cochrane Database Syst Rev 2000.

*21 de Craen AJ, Di Giulio G, Lampe-Schoenmaeckers JE, et al. Analgesic efficacy and safety of paracetamol–codeine combinations versus paracetamol alone: a systematic review. BMJ 1996; 313:321–325.

22 Hynson JL, South M. Childhood hepatotoxicity with paracetamol doses less than 150 mg/kg per day. Med J Aust 1999; 171:497.

23 Southall D. Prevention and control of pain in children – a manual for health care professionals. London: BMJ Publishing; 1997:56.

24 Autret E, Dutertre JP, Breteau M, et al. Pharmacokinetics of paracetamol in the neonate and infant after administration of propacetamol chlorhydrate. Dev Pharmacol Ther 1993; 20:129–134.

25 Granry JC, Rod B, Monrigal JP, et al. The analgesic efficacy of an injectable prodrug of acetaminophen in children after orthopaedic surgery. Paediatr Anaesth 1997; 7:445–449.

26 Rowbotham DJ. Guidelines for the use of nonsteroidal anti-inflammatory drugs in the perioperative period 1998.

27 Short JA, Barr CA, Palmer CD, et al. Use of diclofenac in children with asthma. Anaesthesia 2000; 55:334–337.

28 Robinson J, Malleson P, Lirenman D, Carter J. Nephrotic syndrome associated with nonsteroidal anti-inflammatory drug use in two children. Pediatrics 1990; 85:844–847.

*29 Rostom A, Wells G, Tugwell P, et al. The prevention of chronic NSAID induced upper gastrointestinal toxicity; a Cochrane collaboration metaanalysis of randomized controlled trial. J Rheumatol 2000; 27:2203–2214.

30 Hartley R, Levine MI. Opioid pharmacology in the newborn. In: Aynsley-Green AA, Ward Platt MP, Lloyd-Thomas AR, eds. Clinical pediatrics. London: Baillière Tindall; 1995: 467–494.

31 Lloyd-Thomas AR, Howard RF. A pain service for children. Paediatr Anaesth 1994; 4:3–15.

32 Fahnenstich H, Steffan J, Kau N, Bartmann P. Fentanyl-induced chest wall rigidity and laryngospasm in preterm and term infants. Crit Care Med 2000; 28:836–839.

33 Williams DG, Hatch DJ, Howard RF. Codeine phosphate in pediatric medicine. Br J Anesth 2001; 86:413–421.

34 Saneto RP, Fitch JA, Cohen BH. Acute neurotoxicity of meperidine in an infant. Pediatr Neurol 1996; 14:339–341.

35 Tobias JD, Rasmussen GE. Pain management and sedation in the pediatric intensive care unit. Pediatr Clin North Am 1994; 41:1269–1292.

36 Howard RF, Lloyd Thomas A. Pain management in children. In: Sumner E, Hatch DJ, eds. Paediatric Anaesthesia. London: Arnold; 2000a:317–338.

37 Rose JB, Watcha MF. Postoperative nausea and vomiting in pediatric patients. Br J Anaesth 1999; 83:105–117.

38 Markakis DA. Regional anesthesia in pediatrics. Anesthesiol Clin North Am 2000; 18:355–381, vii.

39 Esmail Z, Montgomery C, Courtrn C, et al. Efficacy and complications of morphine infusions in postoperative pediatric patients. Paediatr Anaesth 1999; 9:321–327.

40 Berde CB, Lehn BM, Yee JD, et al. Patient-controlled analgesia in children and adolescents: a randomized, prospective comparison with intramuscular administration of morphine for postoperative analgesia. J Pediatr 1991; 118:460–466.

41 Collins JJ, Geake J, Grier HE, et al. Patient-controlled analgesia for mucositis pain in children: a three-period crossover study comparing morphine and hydromorphone. J Pediatr 1996; 129:722–728.

42 Larsson BA. Pain management in neonates. Acta Paediatr 1999; 88:1301–1310.

43 Lynn A, Nespeca MK, Bratton SL, et al. Clearance of morphine in postoperative infants during intravenous infusion: the influence of age and surgery. Anesth Analg 1998; 86:958–963.

44 Lynn AM, Nespeca MK, Bratton SL, Shen DD. Intravenous morphine in postoperative infants: intermittent bolus dosing versus targeted continuous infusions. Pain 2000; 88:89–95.

45 Anderson BJ, Woollard GA, Holford NH. A model for size and age changes in the pharmacokinetics of paracetamol in neonates, infants and children. Br J Clin Pharmacol 2000; 50:125–134.

46 Van Lingen RA, Deinum HT, Quak CM, et al. Multiple-dose pharmacokinetics of rectally administered acetaminophen in term infants. Clin Pharmacol Ther 1999; 66:509–515.

***47** Shah V, Taddio A, Ohlsson A. Randomised controlled trial of paracetamol for heel prick pain in neonates. Arch Dis Child Fetal Neonatal Ed 1998; 79:F209–F211.

48 Brisman M, Ljung BM, Otterbom I. Methaemoglobin formation after the use of EMLA cream in term neonates. Acta Paediatr 1988; 87:1191–1194.

***49** Taddio A, Ohlsson A, Einarson TR, et al. A systematic review of lidocaine-prilocaine cream (EMLA) in the treatment of pain in neonates. Pediatr 1998; 101:E1.

50 Herod J, Denyer J, Goldman A, Howard RF. Epidermolysis bullosa in children: pathophysiology, anaesthesia and pain management. Paediatr Anaesth 2002; 12(5):388–397.

51 Ellis JA, Spanos NP. Cognitive-behavioral interventions for children's distress during bone marrow aspirations and lumbar punctures: a critical review. J Pain Symptom Manag 1994; 9:96–108.

52 Taddio A, Stevens B, Craig K, et al. Efficacy and safety of lidocaine-prilocaine cream for pain during circumcision. N Engl J Med 1997; 336:1197–1201.

53 Bruce E, Franck L. Self-administered nitrous oxide (Entonox) for the management of procedural pain. Pediatr Nurs 2000; 12:15–19.

54 Yaster M, Kost-Byerly S, Maxwell LG. The management of pain in sickle cell disease. Pediatr Clin North Am 2000; 47(3): 699–710.

55 Palermo T. Impact of recurrent and chronic pain on child and family daily functioning: a critical review of the literature. Dev Behav Pediatr 2000; 21(1):58–69.

56 Varni JW, Rapoff MA, Waldron S, et al. Chronic pain and emotional distress in children and adolescents. Dev Behav Pediatr 1996; 17(3):154–161.

57 Bennett SM, Chambers CT, Bellows D, et al. Evaluating treatment outcome in an interdisciplinary pediatric pain service. Pain Res Manag 2000; 5:169–172.

58 Kingery WS. A critical review of controlled clinical trials for peripheral neuropathic pain and CRPS. Pain 1999; 79:317–319.

59 A guide to the development of children's palliative care services. Report of a joint working party. Association for Children with life-threatening or terminal conditions and their families (ACT and the Royal College of Pediatrics and Child Health (RCPCH)). Published by and available from ACT, Orchard House, Orchard Lane Bristol BS1 5ST; 1997.

60 Wolfe J, Grier H, Klar N, et al. Symptoms and suffering at the end of life in children with cancer. N Engl J Med 2000; 342(5): 326–333.

61 Goldman A. Care of the dying child. Oxford: Oxford University Press; 1998.

62 Bluebond-Langner M. In the shadow of illness. Princeton, NJ: Princeton University Press; 1996.

63 Mulhern RK, Lauer ME, Hoffman RG. Death of a child at home or in hospital: subsequent adjustment of the family. Pediatrics 1983; 171:743–747.

64 Lauer ME, Mulhern RK,Wallskog JM, et al. A comparison study of parental adaptation following a child's death at home or in hospital. Pediatrics 1983; 171:107–112.

65 Goldman A, Christie D. Children with cancer talk about their own death with their families. Pediatr Haematol Oncol 1993; 10:223–231.

66 Bluebond-Langner M. The private worlds of dying children. Princeton, NJ: Princeton University Press; 1978.

67 Palliative care for young people aged 13–24 years. Report of the Association for Children with life-threatening or terminal conditions and their families (ACT) and the National Council for Hospice and Palliative Care Services and The Scottish Partnership for Palliative and Cancer Care. 2001. (Available from ACT, Orchard Lane, Bristol B5 5ST.)

68 Liben S, Goldman A. Home care for children with life-threatening illnesses. J Palliat Care 1998; 14(3):33–38.

Section 4

Investigation and therapy

38

Understanding and explaining practical procedures and their management

Steve Cunningham, Mary Rose, Ian A Laing

INTRODUCTION

The process of obtaining informed consent, specific for various tests and procedures, has become arguably more important with the public's wish and expectation that they can be involved in medical decisions. In requesting a test or procedure to a child, parents or other health professionals, it is important to know what is involved in that procedure. Understanding by the family will allow the child to be better prepared and will ensure the patient receives optimum benefit from each procedure. Even relatively simple medical words and phrases are difficult for most parents and children to understand, and innocent words can sound extremely frightening (murmur, tumor, anesthetic, etc). Children and parents may be reticent about asking for a 'translation' when the explanation is theoretically in their own language. Help them by considering the words you will use, in what context and how they might be misinterpreted. If you are explaining procedures to someone where your language is not their mother tongue, then use a translator (do not rely on relatives if this is an important procedure or one that carries significant risk).

Do not explain a procedure if you are not fully aware of what will be involved: find out about it. Why is the procedure necessary? When and where will it take place? What grade of staff will be performing it? What problems might be encountered and what risks are possible? Ensure that you are able to explain the balance of risk versus benefit of the procedure *in that child.*

In this chapter we will explain some common procedures, their benefits and the risks involved. There will be local variation in how procedures are performed, so find out how these differ in your locality. This will be important from the perspective of clinical governance. We will also discuss hazards to staff: if you are organizing the procedure then it may be your responsibility to warn members of staff of potential risks.

Know how to explain procedures to parents and children.

Do not explain procedures if you are not aware of exactly what will take place, and the possible problems/risks that might be encountered.

Local variation in procedures will be present. Try and find out how the procedures vary and give up to date information.

Be able to appreciate the hazards associated with procedures for both patients and staff, and therefore how to avoid them.

Do not perform procedures for which you are not adequately trained.

PREPARING PATIENTS FOR PROCEDURES

Issues of consent are dealt with in Chapter 4 of this book. Remember that issues of consent apply to both parents and children.

TALKING TO CHILDREN ABOUT PROCEDURES[1]

Misconceptions exist that delaying or not explaining procedures to children protects them from pain and fear. Similar fallacies construe that children will not understand or they are too young to be affected. Such mistaken beliefs often arise because staff and/or parents fail to appreciate the level of understanding of the child or because they have little ability to adapt their communication to language that the child will understand. If parents do not wish to have a procedure explained to their child, then those wishes must be respected, though parents should understand the procedure and not try to protect themselves by not telling the child. The parents should be made aware of the consequences of not discussing an important procedure with their child. Even if parents are present during a procedure, the child should be the focus of explanation. Do not ignore the child hoping they will pick up information given to the parents.

When talking to a child, introduce yourself and take account of the cognitive level of the child and their language. Don't patronize, and consider throughout the consultation whether you retain their interest and understanding. In your introduction, recognize (as the child will) your authority as an adult, but be respectful of the child's status. Give a clear introduction to the topic or plan to be discussed and be careful not to make promises you will not be able to keep (e.g. confidentiality etc.). Communicate on the same physical level, and begin the conversation with a non-threatening topic. Warn the child the main topic to be discussed is a serious one, and enquire as to what the child understands about that topic already. Always give adequate time for the child to respond or ask questions and listen carefully to their response, but do not pressurize the child into giving a response. Do not attempt to anticipate their answers. Go at the child's pace and check the child has understood. Any explanation should be a clear and simple, optimistic (but realistic) narrative of the events. There is a tendency to overestimate what information has been conveyed and how much has been understood, and a tendency to underestimate what the child has acquired from other sources. Be aware of cultural differences and how explanation and understanding may differ for that culture (ask the child about their culture!).

The child will often give clues as to when the conversation is over. If the procedure is complex, then it is often not possible to cover everything at one meeting and a further time can be arranged. End by summarizing what has been discussed, including the child's viewpoints; offer a plan. Explain that you are available to discuss the procedure and how the child (and parents) can contact you.

USE OF PLAY SPECIALISTS

Play specialist are a well trained and respected part of the pediatric team in any hospital. They have knowledge of infant and childcare, nursing and teaching. The play specialist is able to introduce different types of play and activities to individual children based on their age and development. Children use play as a medium to express feelings. Familiar play helps children to normalize a clinical environment, with reduction in their anxiety and stress.

Hospital play specialists have a significant role in preparing children for procedures during their stay in hospital. Preparation can be achieved by use of photobooks and role playing. Children can also be given the opportunity to touch and play with medical equipment in a safe and controlled environment, i.e. syringe painting, dolls fitted with cannulae, nasogastric tubes, etc. As a familiar face to the children, play specialists can have a significant effect in relaxing them during procedures using distraction methods.

THE MANAGEMENT OF PROCEDURAL PAIN

INTRODUCTION

Pain management is considered in detail in Chapter 37 but as procedural pain has been particularly common in the past we make no excuse for considering its management here. Good pain management will pay dividends in terms of later cooperation by the child and parents. Moral, humanitarian, ethical and physiological reasons dictate that every effort should be made to anticipate and safely and effectively control pain in all children, whatever their age, maturity or severity of illness.[2]

Pre-emptive pain control helps to minimize fear and anxiety associated with the procedure, reduces the stress response, prevents the 'wind up' phenomenon of central nervous system sensitization to noxious stimuli and tissue release of pain mediators.

Pain prevention should be tailored to the individual child's needs using a combination of non-drug techniques, local anesthetic, simple analgesics and opioids and sedation where appropriate. By using a multimodal approach one is able to reduce the doses required of stronger agents and thus reduce the incidence of adverse effects. Management of pain requires regular pain assessment and this must be linked to appropriate action.

PAIN ASSESSMENT

There are multiple tools for pain assessment. This reflects that none is ideal. Whichever pain assessment tool is chosen it must be appropriate for the child's stage of development and it must be part of a cycle of assessment–intervention–reassessment.

Listed below are examples of age specific pain assessment tools.

Neonates (up to 1 month; ex-preterm up to 60 weeks postconceptional age)

CRIES is one of the most widely used and tested pain assessment tools in neonates.[3] CRIES looks at five physiologic and behavioral indicators:

- Crying
- Requirement for oxygen
- Increased vital signs (heart rate and blood pressure)
- Expression
- Sleeplessness

Each indicator is rated on a 3 point score (0–2).

Infants (1 month–1 year) and toddlers (1–3 years)

The FLACC scale looks at five categories of pain behavior[4] (Table 38.1).

Children aged 3–7 years

Most 3 year olds can differentiate the presence or absence of pain and they can indicate pain intensity in broad categories such as mild, moderate, or severe.

The faces scale (Fig. 38.1) can work well.

Older children and adolescents

Older children are able to use a numerical scale as used in adults; for example 0–10 where 0 is no pain and 10 is the worst pain imaginable.

NON-PHARMACOLOGICAL TECHNIQUES

Non-drug approaches should supplement but not replace appropriate drug treatment. They may be categorized as:

- Supportive

Table 38.1 FLACC scale

Categories	Scoring		
	0	1	2
Face	No particular expression or smile	Occasional grimace or frown, withdrawn, disinterested	Frequent to constant quivering chin, clenched jaw
Legs	Normal position or relaxed	Uneasy, restless, tense	Kicking, or legs drawn up
Activity	Lying quietly, normal position, moves easily	Squirming, shifting back and forth, tense	Arched rigid or jerking
Cry	No cry	Moans or whimpers; occasional complaint	Crying steadily, screams or sobs
Consolability	Content, relaxed	Reassured by occasional touching, hugging or being talked to, distractible	Difficult to console

Fig. 38.1 FACES scale.

- Cognitive
- Behavioral
- Physical

Supportive therapies are aimed at empowering the child and the family by providing information and involving them in decision-making processes. Children should never be lied to about painful procedures or they will distrust and fear what will be done to them in the future.

Cognitive methods are intended to influence a child's thoughts and images using techniques such as distraction and imagery.

Behavioral methods include deep breathing and progressive relaxation, and are useful for controlling anticipatory anxiety for procedures such as venepuncture.

Physical methods include touch, heat and cold and sucrose analgesia. Sucrose analgesia has been shown to decrease crying in neonates undergoing painful procedures.[5]

REGIONAL ANESTHETIC TECHNIQUES

Local anesthetic techniques play a major part in the provision of procedural analgesia for children.

Topical local anesthesia of the skin should be used before all needle punctures in children.[6] EMLA cream is effective after 60–90 min application and is licensed for use in children over 1 year. An alternative preparation is amethocaine gel that is effective after 40 min application and has a longer duration of action once the cream has been removed. Amethocaine gel is not recommended for use in children below 1 month.[7] EMLA cream causes vasoconstriction whereas amethocaine causes vasodilatation. Both preparations are applied underneath an occlusive dressing. The application of these agents at lumbar puncture and bone marrow aspirate sites facilitates the subcutaneous injection of local anesthetic if these procedures are to be carried out awake and reduces the sedative or anesthetic requirement.

Other regional techniques include surgical wound infiltration, peripheral nerve blockade, plexus blockade and central neuraxial blockade (epidural and spinal analgesia). These techniques are generally combined with general anesthesia and have the benefit of reducing the requirement for anesthetic agents and opioids, thus allowing a more rapid recovery from anesthesia and a reduction in opioid induced side-effects.

Commonly used single nerve blocks are ilioinguinal for hernia repair, dorsal nerve of the penis for penile surgery and sciatic and femoral for lower limb procedures. Analgesia for procedures on the arm can be achieved by blocking the brachial plexus.

The most common central block is the caudal block. The epidural space is accessed via the sacral hiatus and local anesthetic is deposited around the nerve roots. Caudal analgesia is suitable for any surgery below the umbilicus. A caudal catheter may be inserted allowing prolongation of the block by infusion or top ups. In infants it is possible to thread the catheter to the thoracic region. The epidural space may also be accessed via the lumbar or thoracic route.

Spinal anesthesia is sometimes used as the sole anesthetic technique for hernia repair in premature neonates as this population are prone to general anesthesia induced postoperative apneas.[9] The use of a regional technique reduces but does not abolish apnea.

The above techniques all have potentially serious complications such as nerve damage, local anesthetic toxicity and inadvertent intravascular injection of local anesthetic and should therefore only be performed by personnel skilled in the techniques.

Additional problems associated with epidural analgesia include urinary retention, leg weakness, risk of pressure sores and epidural hematoma or infection.

The most commonly used local anesthetics are lidocaine (lignocaine) and bupivacaine. The doses of local anesthetic that may be administered are limited by toxicity. The maximum safe doses are increased by the addition of adrenaline (epinephrine). Maximum safe doses are:

- Lidocaine: 3 mg/kg (7 mg/kg with adrenaline)
- Bupivacaine: 2 mg/kg (3 mg/kg with adrenaline)

Bupivacaine has a longer duration of action than lidocaine (lignocaine) and is the drug most commonly used for blocks. However both central nervous system and cardiac toxicity can occur which has led to the search for safer local anesthetics. Two new local anesthetics have been introduced and registered for use in children down to the age of 12 years. Ropivacaine and levobupivacaine both appear to have a safer toxicity profile and to produce less motor block at equi-analgesic doses in adults.[4] The safety profile of these drugs in children is currently under investigation and it is likely that they may provide safer alternatives to bupivacaine.

PARACETAMOL

Paracetamol is safe and effective in children for mild to moderate pain and when given as a coanalgesic has a 20% opioid sparing effect.

Recommendations for oral dosing in children over one month are:

- 20 mg/kg loading dose, then 15 mg/kg 4–8 hourly to a maximum of 90 mg/kg/day.
- Absorption from the rectal route is slow and it is now realized that higher loading doses up to 40 mg/kg are required to achieve therapeutic plasma concentrations of 10–25 mcg/ml, and subsequent rectal doses of approximately 20 mg/kg 6 hourly are needed for maintenance.
- Total daily doses of 90 mg/kg/day may be safely used for up to 72 h in otherwise healthy children. In neonates and young infants the total daily dose should be reduced to 60 mg/kg/day.

The administration of paracetamol is limited by the occurrence of hepatotoxicity. Care should be taken in the febrile, hypovolemic, dehydrated child who will be more susceptible to the hepatotoxic effects.

NON-STEROIDAL ANTI-INFLAMMATORY DRUGS (NSAIDs)

NSAIDs have become increasingly important in the management of mild to moderate acute pain in children. Aspirin is the oldest NSAID, but the association of Reye's syndrome with the use of aspirin means it is no longer recommended for use in children under 16 years (19 years in the USA), except in the treatment of juvenile rheumatoid arthritis. There appears to be little difference between the analgesic efficacy of the different NSAIDs. Commonly used NSAIDs are:

- Diclofenac up to 1 mg/kg 8 hourly – available orally or rectally
- Ibuprofen 5 mg/kg 6 hourly – available orally and sublingual
- Ketorolac 1 mg/kg loading dose followed by 0.5 mg/kg 6 hourly for a maximum of 48 h – available intravenously.

When used in combination with paracetamol, NSAIDs have an additive analgesic effect and an opioid sparing effect. NSAIDs are contraindicated in:[13]

- Infants less than 1 year – because renal maturation is still occurring
- Renal impairment
- Dehydration or hypovolemia
- Impaired hepatic function
- Bleeding or coagulation disorders. NSAIDs affect platelet function and can prolong the bleeding time
- Peptic ulcer disease.

NSAIDs and asthma: NSAID-induced bronchospasm occurs in 5–10% of adult onset asthmatics, especially as part of the syndrome of asthma, hay fever and nasal polyps. Consequently NSAIDs should be used with caution in children with asthma.

NITROUS OXIDE

Inhaled nitrous oxide is a safe and effective method of providing rapid onset analgesia for short painful procedures such as dressing changes, lumbar puncture, suture insertion or removal, drain removal. Nitrous oxide is administered in 50% oxygen as Entonox. Nitrous oxide is insoluble in blood so is delivered quickly to the brain when inhaled. It achieves maximal analgesia after 2 minutes of use and produces an analgesic effect equivalent to that of intravenous morphine. Entonox works best in children over 5 years old. Contra-indications include: pneumothorax, bowel obstruction, recent head injury, chronic respiratory disease, uncorrected congenital heart disease and gastroesophageal reflux.

OPIOIDS

Opioids play a major role in the management of severe pain in children. This section deals with their use for procedural pain. Opioids have a narrow therapeutic index so their use is a balance between satisfactory analgesia and the degree of side-effects.

Morphine is the most commonly used opioid and is the yardstick against which all other opioids are assessed (Table 38.2).

Morphine can be given by the oral, intramuscular, intravenous, subcutaneous, rectal, epidural or spinal routes. In addition fentanyl may be given transdermally or transmucosally.

A slow release oral preparation of morphine is available for long term pain. When administered orally morphine is well absorbed from the gastrointestinal tract but is subject to first pass metabolism. Morphine is predominantly metabolized by the liver to morphine-3-glucuronide and morphine-6-glucuronide. The latter metabolite has twice the analgesic potency of morphine and a longer half-life. The glucuronide metabolites are excreted by the kidneys, so there is a risk of accumulation in renal impairment.

The use of opioids in neonates

Neonates are particularly sensitive to the adverse effects of opioids. In neonates aged 1–7 days the clearance of morphine is one-third that of older infants and the elimination half-life is 1.7 times longer. Enzyme systems mature rapidly and by the age of 1 month morphine clearance is equivalent to that of children aged 1–17 years.[14]

Administration of parenteral opioids

The administration of intramuscular injections is to be discouraged; the child's dislike of injections may lead them to under-report their pain.

The administration of an intravenous bolus will produce satisfactory analgesia within 5–10 min. The bolus dose of morphine for infants over 3 months is 100 mcg/kg. If pain is ongoing this should be followed by a continuous infusion of up to 40 mcg/kg/h. The administration of a bolus raises the plasma concentration of morphine to a therapeutic level and the infusion maintains levels in the therapeutic range. If an infusion is started without the administration of a bolus it can take up to 5 half-lives for the plasma concentration to reach therapeutic levels and the half-life of morphine is at least 3 h. Similarly if adverse effects occur the infusion should be discontinued until these effects have resolved and the infusion recommenced at a lower dose, usually 50% lower than the previous dose.[15]

Recommended dosing schedules for morphine infusions in non-ventilated neonates are:

0–1 month up to 4 mcg/kg/h

> 1–3 months up to 10 mcg/kg/h

It should be noted that the above dosage regimens are a guide and that the success of any opioid technique in children requires that it be titrated to the individual child's needs.

Monitoring: Children receiving opioids should be regularly checked for the efficacy of analgesia, and adverse effects. Any child receiving parenteral opioids should be nursed in a part of the ward

Table 38.2 Analgesic potency of opioids in relation to intravenous morphine

Opioid	IV/IM	Oral
Morphine	1	0.15–0.33
Diamorphine	2	–
Pethidine	0.1	0.025
Codeine	0.08	0.05
Fentanyl	100	–
Methadone	1	0.5

where they are easily visible and their monitors can be observed. Assessment should consist of:

- Pain assessment
- Oxygen saturation in air
- Respiratory rate
- Degree of sedation
- Nausea and vomiting

ANALGESIA IN THE INTENSIVE CARE AND NEONATAL UNIT

For a child (and their parents) the intensive care unit is a threatening environment, which generates anxiety and fear. The presence of drains and tubes and invasive procedures such as insertion of catheters, cannulae and tracheal tubes cause pain and discomfort. The most commonly used agents for sedation and analgesia are morphine and midazolam. Fentanyl, a shorter acting opioid is sometimes used in place of morphine. The respiratory depressant effect of opioids becomes beneficial by facilitating the use of intermittent positive pressure ventilation.

For neonates requiring invasive procedures such as blood sampling the simple technique of sucrose analgesia is beneficial.[5]

The long term use of opioid and benzodiazepine infusions leads to tolerance and abrupt cessation will result in withdrawal symptoms. Slow weaning of sedative agents by 10–20% of the dose per day will prevent this.

CONCLUSION

The management of pain in children should be by the simplest effective technique, multimodal, pre-emptive where possible and frequently reassessed and titrated to the child's needs.

Procedures

Clinical governance dictates that procedures should only be carried out by those who have had a fully supervised training. The descriptions provided here are insufficient to enable you to perform these tasks, but they should provide enough information for you to be familiar with what is involved so that you can describe them adequately to parents and patients.

NON-SPECIALIST PROCEDURES

Peripheral venous sampling

Procedure. The most common form of blood sampling takes blood from a peripheral vein. In children, the veins in the arm (brachial) and back of the hand are most frequently used. Neonates should be provided with, and children should be offered, local anesthetic cream to numb the pain.

Complications. Localized hematoma (bruise) may occur which will disappear in a few days. Tourniquets will produce false calcium estimation.

Hazards. In children, separate needle and syringe are still used more frequently than closed needle systems. These are more hazardous to users and patients in terms of needlestick injury. Needles with the hub broken off should not be used under any circumstances. Gloves should be worn during all blood taking procedures.

Peripheral capillary sampling

Procedure. This method of blood sampling is satisfactory for assessing arterialized carbon dioxide and pH in the peripheral blood. It can also be used for complete blood counts and glucose estimation. In the neonate the side of the heel is used and in older infants and children the finger tip. The procedure is quick and although some centers use an anesthetic cream for such intervention, this may cause blood vessel constriction that can reduce the amount of sample. A spring loaded lancet reduces damage to skin and is least painful. A capillary tube collects the sample from the skin (which is sometimes smeared with Vaseline to help localize the blood). The area is held with cotton wool following the procedure to stop bleeding.

Complications. Biochemical tests on capillary samples may have errors, especially of potassium and calcium measurements. In neonates, very deep stabs on the heel have been rarely associated with osteomyelitis.

Hazards. Automated spring loaded lancets need to be disposed of in a similar way to other 'sharps'. Blood sampling should be performed wearing gloves.

Peripheral arterial sampling

Procedure. This is required for measurement of arterial oxygen, and also carbon dioxide and pH. Transcutaneous oxygen and saturation monitoring has reduced the need for frequent arterial sampling to estimate arterial oxygen. The most common site for an arterial sample is the radial artery in the neonate and the older child, and the posterior tibial artery in the neonate. Other arteries can be used as long as an adequate alternative arterial supply can be demonstrated to that area of tissue. Fixed sampling syringes are now in common use which contain heparin to stop the sample clotting. Arterial sampling can be painful (use local anesthetic cream, or subcutaneous local anesthetic injection without adrenaline). The pulse is identified and the needle inserted at a 45° angle. Pressure will need to be applied to the site for up to 5 min after removal of the needle before bleeding stops.

Complications. Hematoma frequently forms during arterial sampling, either because of insufficient pressure applied to the overlying skin once the needle is withdrawn, or because the needle pierces the artery at an oblique angle, limiting blood drawn but damaging the vessel wall. Occasionally, arterial spasm can severely limit arterial supply to the limb peripheral to the sampling site: this should correct over a few minutes, though occasionally an arterial vasodilator may have to be infused.

Hazards. Sharps need to be disposed of appropriately. Gloves should be worn, and because of the possible spray of arterial blood users may wish to use protective eyewear.

Peripheral venous access

Procedure. A peripheral venous cannula is frequently placed in children (the drip). In neonates, veins may easily be seen but may be too small to cannulate, in toddlers veins may be too difficult to see because of subcutaneous fat. At all ages, knowledge of the distribution of large subcutaneous veins is valuable. Local anesthetic cream should be used where possible. A tourniquet may be applied to help fill veins, though it is often helpful to have a second person to apply a tourniquet with their hand (ensuring that little wriggles don't ruin your attempts to site the cannula). Parents should be warned that this technique is difficult and even in experienced hands several attempts may be required. In very young children with poor venous access, a scalp vein may be the most sensible option, though many parents may find it particularly distressing because hair in the region has to be shaved to enable fixation. Peripheral venous cannulation represents a standard technique to most doctors, yet is associated with significant stress to many parents. Children may need securing to ensure a quick and relatively painless procedure.

Complications. Hematoma formation is common. Occasionally, particularly when using scalp veins, an artery may be mistaken for a vein during cannulation. Any pulsatility of flow during cannulation is arterial and the cannula should be withdrawn (using 5 min of pressure) immediately.
Hazards. Sharps must to be disposed of appropriately. Gloves should be worn.

Peripheral venous cutdown access

Procedure. This procedure is used when no veins can be identified for percutaneous cannulation. Children needing this procedure are commonly in extremis, but every attempt should be made to ensure adequate explanation and pain relief. The sterile procedure usually cannulates the long saphenous vein just above the ankle, by making an incision in the skin and dissecting back the tissues until the vein is identified. A small slit in the vein then allows the cannula to be inserted. The catheter is sutured in place.
Complications. Bleeding at the site may occur when circulation is re-established if sutures are not secure enough.
Hazards. This is a sterile surgical procedure with full protection against blood biohazard.

Interosseous needle insertion

Procedure. This is an emergency procedure used when no veins can be identified for peripheral cannulation. In a shocked child with hypotension, this procedure should be performed after no more than two quick attempts at peripheral cannulation. The tibia is the most common site for insertion, though the femoral head and other sites are possible. The child is frequently in extremis and pain relief may not be possible without access in an unstable child. The position of insertion is just below the tibial tuberosity on the anteromedial aspect of the tibia. The needle is screwed steadily into bone until the outer cortex is felt to give way. The bone marrow that can be aspirated can be sent for blood glucose and electrolyte concentration, in addition to blood culture. All intravenous preparations can be given via intraosseous needle. Though the needle is fairly secure within the bone, it should be attached with tapes. When circulation is re-established, intravenous access should be obtained and the intraosseous needle withdrawn.
Complications. Leak of instilled fluid into the skin around the site of the needle may occur if the needle is not properly sited. The needle can occasionally exit the bone on the opposite side and this should be checked for before fluid is instilled.
Hazards. When dropped, intraosseus needles tend to fall on the handle exposing the needle upright: great care is needed to alert others in the vicinity if the needle is dropped. Sharps need to be disposed of appropriately. Gloves should be worn.

Peripheral arterial access

Procedure. This is only needed if a child requires intensive care. In older children the radial or femoral arteries are typically cannulated. In neonates the radial, posterior tibial and dorsalis pedis are most commonly used. As far as parents are concerned, the procedure is similar to peripheral venous cannulation. In practice, arterial cannulation is more difficult, particularly as the arterial pulse can sometimes be difficult to precisely localize, and the elastic wall of the artery and arterial spasm may impede cannulation. The small risk of peripheral ischemia following insertion of an arterial catheter should be balanced against the benefit of continuous arterial access (and the availability of continuous direct arterial blood pressure). Local anesthetic should be used for insertion. The cannula, once in place, needs careful and continued observation for signs of peripheral ischemia and localized hematoma or leak. Arterial spasm and peripheral ischemia are discussed in the section on arterial sampling (see above).
Complications. Peripheral ischemia. Blood loss from puncture site or misconnected blood pressure monitoring circuit.
Hazards. Sharps need to be disposed of appropriately. Gloves should be worn.

Central venous access: Seldinger catheterization technique

Procedure. This procedure is performed under general anesthetic in theater or intensive care, for administration of medicines and fluids into a central vein and/or measurement of central venous pressure. The most frequent sites are the deep veins of the neck and upper chest or the femoral veins. The Seldinger technique commonly used is a system of progressive dilation of a channel into which the catheter will be placed. Initially a long needle attached to a syringe locates the vessel. A guidewire is then fed through the needle to maintain a track to the vessel. The needle is then removed and a large dilator is pushed over the guidewire. Depending on the amount of dilatation required, a larger guidewire may be put through that dilator, and the initial dilator can then be replaced by a wider dilator to increase further the size of the tract. Finally, a catheter can be pushed over the guidewire, which is then removed and the deep venous catheter is fixed into position externally. The catheter can be single, double or even triple lumen. Each lumen can be attached to an 'octopus' (multiple access attachment): it must be remembered however that all fluids and medicines going into each lumen of the catheter must be compatible. The external part of the catheter is sometimes stitched into place, or in other centers simply adhered to the chest wall with transparent adhesive patches. A chest X-ray is taken following insertion to make sure that there is no pneumothorax and to identify the position of the tip of the catheter (it should optimally remain in a large vein and not the heart). Catheters may be removed by cutting stitches if present and pulling slowly and steadily on the catheter until it is removed: a patch of gauze should be applied over the area until bleeding ceases. No other special attention is needed and no X-ray is routinely required following removal. The technique for accessing central venous lines should be an aseptic technique, with handwashing, sterile gloves, etc.: each hospital should have a policy on this technique.
Complications. Catheters have an increased risk of infection after 2 weeks in situ and so should be considered for removal or replacement at that time. Care has to be taken during insertion that the catheter is not open to the atmosphere during inspiration, as this may result in significant air embolus.
Hazards. This is a sterile surgical procedure with full protection against blood biohazard.

Central venous access: tunneled line with external access

Procedure. This procedure is used when children require regular deep venous access for a prolonged period of time (i.e. oncology patients, parenteral nutrition patients). The most common site is the upper chest. The technique is surgical and involves the identification of a deep vein via a small incision on the upper chest wall. The catheter is then tunneled under the skin and into the central vein. A cuff of material is present around the central portion of the catheter that is placed in the subcutaneous tissues and helps to anchor the catheter in position. The catheters frequently have two or three lumens. Lines are fixed in place by transparent adhesive patches. A chest X-ray is routine after placing the line to identify its position. Catheters can usually be removed with pain relief but

without general anesthetic. Once removed, a patch of gauze is applied to the area to stop bleeding which is usually transient.
Complications. Line infections can be a cause of significant systemic illness in these children, and should be suspected in the event of pyrexia/unexplained illness. Great care should be taken in removing a central line that possibly has clot on or around it (identified by ultrasound): this is particularly true in infants with congenital heart disease where a shunt may lead to cerebral embolus. Clot formation around the catheter can result in significant obstruction to flow in neck veins.
Hazards. This is a sterile surgical procedure with full protection against blood biohazard.

Central venous access: tunneled line with subcutaneous access

Procedure. This technique is most often used in children who will require periodic, but regular deep venous access (e.g. cystic fibrosis patients). Most devices are single lumen. The most common site is the upper chest, so that the subcutaneous access plate is stable against the rib cage. The technique is a similar surgical technique to the tunneled line with external access, except that in this case the tunneled line from the deep vein is attached to an access plate that remains subcutaneous and the skin overlying this area is sutured. In order to use the catheter an external needle (with hub and line) must pierce the soft latex bubble on top of the subcutaneous access plate. The external portion can be fixed in place with a transparent adhesive patch. The external needle and hub can be put into position in theater and the line used soon after return from theater. The external needle and hub should be replaced every 2 weeks during long-term use. The system is not uncomfortable and is a very easy way of ensuring dependable deep vein access. A chest X-ray is routine after placing the line to identify its position. The line should be flushed every 4 weeks with a heparin solution if not in use. The external needle and hub can be removed by aseptic technique without pain relief. The internal portion of the system can only be removed surgically under anesthesia.
Complications. Teenage girls may find the bulge of access plate uncomfortable near breast tissue and may prefer it to be placed in the axilla. The line should flush easily, though it may not be possible to withdraw blood from the line depending on position. If the line will not flush, then it may be blocked with clot: there are a number of fibrinolytic options to unblock lumens and these should be tried as early as possible to save the line. If there is pain when flushing the line, the line may have become disconnected from the hub: obtain a contrast injection study in radiology. Clot formation and infection risks are the same as those discussed above.
Hazards. This is a sterile surgical procedure with full protection against blood biohazard.

Lumbar puncture

Procedure. A lumbar puncture enables access to the cerebrospinal fluid (CSF) surrounding the spinal cord. It is performed safely in the majority of children; however caution is needed if there is a question of raised intracranial pressure (i.e. meningism, headache, vomiting). Children with coagulopathy or respiratory instability are also at risk from the procedure. In children under 1 year of age with a soft patent anterior fontanelle the procedure is considered safe. In children without a patent anterior fontanelle, it is not possible to reliably identify raised intracranial pressure by fundoscopy alone and so a cranial CT may be required, or, if the index of suspicion of meningitis is high, then intravenous antibiotics can be started and a lumbar puncture performed at a later time. Children and infants usually lie on their side for the procedure, with oxygen saturation and heart rate monitoring. Local anesthetic cream should be used if possible. Complete aseptic technique should be used, including gown and sterile gloves. The key to success is having the back well flexed and perfectly perpendicular to the edge of the bed. An assistant who will maintain the position when the needle enters the back is very important. The needle is placed in the lower back (between L3 and L4) and fluid withdrawn (approximately 2 ml). Two or three attempts may be required to find the spinal fluid space, particularly if the child is active. Following removal of enough fluid, the central portion of the needle is replaced and the needle withdrawn: a sealant spray or liquid is quickly applied to close the puncture hole and a dressing or sticking plaster is placed over the site.
Complications. Occasionally a blood vessel close to the spine may be hit by the needle and the sample will be heavily bloodstained: these samples should still be sent for culture. If this occurs then a further attempt one intervertebral space higher may be attempted. Headache is a common side-effect following lumbar puncture, and should settle with simple pain relief over 48 h. In children with raised intracranial pressure a lumbar puncture may result in 'coning', where the base of the brain is pushed down into the base of the skull depressing the respiratory center and other autonomic control centers. This is a neurological emergency requiring urgent intensive care support.
Hazards. Sharps are used and should be disposed of appropriately. Cerebrospinal fluid should be considered an infected biohazard.

Clean catch urine sampling

Procedure. This is performed in children suspected of having a urinary tract infection (bag urine collection is frequently contaminated, and the result sets off a whole series of unnecessary investigations). The child should be well hydrated and be sat on a parent's knee with no diaper (nappy). The genitals should be cleaned with sterile water (not disinfectant) and left to dry. The hands of the person collecting the sample should be washed prior to collection. A small sterile container should be held ready, waiting for the child to pee and a sample (approximately mid stream) obtained as soon as the event occurs. Good observation is required, as the opportunity may not arise again for many more hours.
Complications. None.
Hazards. Hands should be thoroughly washed after sample collection as they may be contaminated with bodily fluids.

Suprapubic urine sampling

Procedure. This technique enables a rapid and clean sample of urine to be obtained. It is particularly useful if children are unwell with a suspected urinary tract infection and antibiotics need to be started. The bladder is an abdominal organ in the baby but becomes more and more pelvic as the infant grows. The child needs to be lying on their back with their legs kept still. The bladder should be palpated (or percussed), or alternatively can be identified on ultrasound: in an emergency the bladder can be sampled without these, but may contain no urine (a 'dry' tap). The suprapubic area should be cleaned with antiseptic fluid and then a small needle attached to a syringe is inserted perpendicular to the skin in the midline just above the symphis pubis in the infant but in the older child may need to be directed more into the pelvis. Urine is withdrawn into the syringe and the needle withdrawn. Pressure need only be applied to the area for a short time and then the area left without dressing if there is no bleeding.
Complications. 'Dry' tap: knowledge of when the infant/child last passed urine and good clinical practice should minimize the number of these. Hematuria may be noted for a short period after the procedure.

Occasionally adjacent bowel can be punctured; this typically does not cause a problem as the hole created is small and self-healing.
Hazards. Care should be taken as the child may move during the procedure if not correctly nursed, causing needlestick injury. Sharps should be disposed of carefully.

SPECIALIST PROCEDURES

NEONATAL

Umbilical catheterization

Umbilical arterial and venous catheters are commonly inserted in newborn infants who need intensive care. The arterial line is invaluable for obtaining blood samples, including those for arterial blood gas tensions, and also for intravascular continuous measurement of blood pressure. The venous catheter may also be used for blood sampling, but if appropriately positioned may also be used for administering drugs and parenteral nutrition. Umbilical catheters may also be used for exchange transfusions (see below).
Procedure. Ensure that the infant is kept warm, adequately restrained, and carefully monitored throughout. Before starting the procedure, estimate the length of catheter to be inserted: for venous cannulation measure the distance from umbilicus to mid-sternum, and for umbilical arterial catheterization measure the distance from umbilicus to shoulder tip and add 1 cm. Sterile technique is maintained throughout. A sterile gauze ribbon is tied around the stump of the umbilicus and is used to maintain hemostasis. A catheter (3.5 or 5.0 G) is filled with heparinized half-normal saline via a syringe and three-way tap. The umbilical cord is cut 0.5 cm from the skin. Small curved self-retaining artery forceps are applied to the umbilical surface and the vein and arteries are identified. The vein is frequently found cephalad to the arteries. The arteries are often side by side, thick-walled and smaller than the vein.

Cannulation of the vein is often very easy, and involves inserting the catheter and feeding it along the lumen of the vein. The tip of the cannula may be placed inferior to the liver if it is not intended to administer drugs by this route, but should be above the diaphragm if it is intended to use the catheter as a multipurpose central line. For a low position, during insertion of the catheter aspirate on the syringe and stop when venous blood is obtained easily. For a high position, ideally the venous line tip should be in the inferior vena cava above the ductus venosus. In practice the venous line will often cease to advance before the line is inserted to the premeasured distance. Pull the catheter gently back, 1 cm at a time until venous blood flows easily. Fix the catheter at that point. Tie the catheter firmly in place using a purse-string suture through the umbilical cord ideally avoiding the skin completely (the cord is painless, the skin very sensitive). The catheter may also be taped gently but firmly to the anterior abdominal wall to ensure that its position is secure even during handling.

Cannulation of an artery is more difficult. Identify the larger of the arteries, and use small, curved non-toothed forceps to open out the lumen so that it resembles a trumpet bell (this is much more difficult than it sounds). Once the lumen has been thus enlarged, the catheter is gently inserted and threaded along the artery. After the procedure, it is essential to confirm catheter tip site by ultrasonography or X-ray. The tip of the arterial catheter should be positioned at a level between the fifth and eighth thoracic vertebrae (T5–8), or between the third and fourth lumbar vertebrae (L3–4).
Complications. Infection is an important complication of insertion of all central lines. Such instrumentation is also associated with necrotizing enterocolitis. Umbilical arterial catheterization may cause ischemic changes over the buttocks, cyanosis of the toes and hematuria.
Hazards. If the tip of any venous catheter is placed in the heart, a pericardial effusion may occur and the resulting tamponade may cause collapse and death. Inadequate fixation of any umbilical line may cause the catheter to fall out with potentially life-threatening hemorrhage.

Chest drain

In the newborn period, a chest drain is most commonly used to treat a tension pneumothorax. It occasionally may be used to drain a pleural effusion, e.g. after rupture of the thoracic duct.
Procedure. Temporary alleviation of a tension pneumothorax may be achieved by inserting a butterfly needle, 23 G, into the appropriate side of the chest, choosing the second intercostal space in the midclavicular line. This needle is connected via a 3-way tap to a 20 ml syringe. Because this temporary measure brings clinical improvement, there is always time to provide sedation and analgesia for insertion of a formal chest drain which is a very painful procedure.

Every effort should be made to place the drain tip anteriorly in the chest. This may be most easily achieved by turning the infant so that the pneumothorax is uppermost. Full aseptic technique is used. Select the fifth intercostal space in the anterior axillary line. Infiltrate local anesthetic. Use a fine scalpel blade to make a transverse incision in the skin and to dissect through the intercostal muscles, just above the fifth rib. Clip a pair of forceps firmly on to the trocar and cannula 1 cm from the tip, thus ensuring that the trocar does not cause damage to lung, heart or mediastinum during drain insertion. The tip of the trocar and cannula is then inserted gently into the intrapleural space, the forceps are released, the trocar withdrawn and the cannula is slid anteriorly and connected immediately to an underwater-seal drainage system. Bubbling of the water indicates that gas is being successfully drained. Swinging of the water level indicates that the cannula is in the thoracic cavity but not draining air, because the lung has expanded. The cannula is secured to the skin of the chest wall by a purse-string suture and firm tape. If the drain neither bubbles nor swings, it is blocked.
Complications. Hemorrhage may occur from an intercostal artery. Pleurisy may follow particularly if the drain remains in situ for many days.
Hazards. Failure to secure the forceps on the trocar and cannula with uncontrolled insertion may result in the trocar damaging the visceral pleura which may cause a bronchopleural fistula or damage to the mediastinum, diaphragm, liver, spleen and heart.

Exchange transfusion

Exchange transfusions are carried out to treat hemolytic disease of the newborn, severe anemia, polycythemia and occasionally in an attempt to combat overwhelming sepsis. Hemolytic disease may require more than one exchange, and on each occasion the clinician may elect to exchange 160–200 ml/kg body weight of semi-packed red cells, in the hope of achieving a hematocrit of approximately 50%. If the etiology of the problem is rhesus disease, then the blood used in the exchange transfusion should be rhesus negative and cross-matched against the infant's blood grouping. If an exchange transfusion must be carried out at birth, the blood used should be group O rhesus negative red cells and with AB serum compatible with mother's serum. Anemia severe enough to cause cardiac failure may be treated with an exchange transfusion of packed cells, 20 ml/kg. Polycythemia which is symptomatic or results in a venous hematocrit greater than 70% may be treated with 20 ml/kg of colloid or crystalloid. There is limited experience in using exchange transfusion as a treatment for overwhelming sepsis and so the chosen amount of blood exchanged might be similar to that for hemolytic disease in the hope of eliminating most toxins from the bloodstream.

Procedure. Prior to carrying out an exchange transfusion it is essential to fully investigate the etiology of the problem as the transfusion itself may obscure the underlying cause of the hemolysis – all blood tests must be completed at the beginning of the first cycle.

Clinicians vary in their timing, route and method of choice. Exchanges of 20 ml/kg may be safely achieved in 30 min, while double-volume exchange transfusions may take 2 h or more. Some clinicians use an umbilical venous line for infusion and extraction, some use an umbilical artery, while some infuse through a venous line and extract via an artery. Continuous infusion and extraction of identical volumes may be used. It is also possible to divide the time allocated into 5 or 10 min cycles, during which individual cycles the clinician infuses and extracts a calculated small volume of blood, colloid or crystalloid.

If the exchange is done through an umbilical catheter then the procedure for insertion of the catheter is as described above. The cannula is connected to three linked 3-way taps. The first tap is directly connected to the infusate and a syringe, the second tap is connected to the effluent bag, and the third tap is connected to a syringe and the umbilical catheter.

Throughout the procedure the infant is fully monitored and cared for by a dedicated nurse and a doctor who have no other duties in the intensive care unit during the time allocated. The baby is nursed in its neutral thermal environment. Each volume infused or extracted is carefully measured and documented. The respiratory and heart rates are measured and documented every 10 min, and a near-patient testing measure of blood glucose concentrations should be recorded every 30 min. Clinical judgment dictates whether plasma electrolytes, calcium or blood gas tensions are measured and if so how often. Whatever infusate is used, it must be prewarmed to 37° Celsius prior to the procedure.

Complications. These include sepsis, necrotizing enterocolitis, electrolyte disturbances and loss of temperature control.

Hazards. Overheating or underheating of the infusate can be fatal. Infants in cardiac failure may tolerate the exchange poorly and may show cardiac rhythm disturbances including ventricular fibrillation and asystole.

GASTROINTESTINAL

Upper gastrointestinal endoscopy (gastroscopy)

Procedure. This is the visual examination of the lining of the esophagus, stomach and duodenum with a thin, flexible telescope with a camera and light source attached (endoscope). This procedure may be used for diagnostic and/or therapeutic purposes. Indications for upper endoscopy include unexplained vomiting, abdominal pain, intestinal malabsorption, upper gastrointestinal hemorrhage, removal of a foreign body and placement of enteral feeding tubes. Depending on the child's age, the procedure may be carried out under general anesthetic or intravenous sedation and in theater or in an endoscopy unit. Preparation involves a period of fasting. The endoscope is passed through the mouth, down the esophagus and into the stomach. The endoscope is then passed through the pylorus and into the duodenum. To allow inspection of all areas, the endoscopist will insufflate the area with some air. All areas are examined for abnormalities. The endoscope has a biopsy channel and biopsies can be obtained from any areas of concern. Random biopsies are obtained from various areas when no gross abnormalities are detected. The biopsies are then sent to pathology, biochemistry or bacteriology for closer inspection.

Other forceps may be used with the endoscope to allow retrieval of foreign bodies or for therapeutic procedures such as treating sites of bleeding. Upper endoscopy may also facilitate placement of tubes for feeding purposes, e.g. nasoduodenal or nasojejunal tubes, or for longer term feeding, a percutaneous endoscopic gastrostomy tube may be inserted.

Complications. Common complications include sore throat and feeling bloated. Major complications are rare but include perforation and bleeding. Most complications in children have occurred during therapeutic endoscopic procedures. These include infection and gastrocolic fistula post gastrostomy tube insertion. Perforation and esophageal stricture have been reported in children undergoing procedures for bleeding.

Hazards. Staff may come into contact with body fluid and blood biohazards and should be protected against them.

Lower gastrointestinal endoscopy (colonoscopy)

Procedure. This is the visual examination of the lining of the colon from the anus to the cecum and terminal ileum with a long thin flexible telescope with a camera and light source (colonoscope). This procedure may be used for diagnostic and therapeutic purposes. Indications include rectal bleeding, unexplained diarrhea and abdominal pain with abnormal growth or weight loss. It is also used to investigate abnormalities suspected on barium enema or small bowel follow through, e.g. inflammatory bowel disease. In children with suspected polyps, colonoscopy provides a method of diagnosis and therapy with endoscopic removal of the lesions.

Depending on the age of the child, the procedure may be carried out under general anesthetic or intravenous sedation. Preparation involves ensuring the colon is free of any fecal debris. Cooperation with bowel preparations in children can be difficult and can impede successful colonoscopy. A successful regimen includes a combination of stimulant laxatives and enemas or administration of colonic lavage solution via a nasogastric tube. The procedure is usually carried out in the theater area or an endoscopy unit. The child is placed in the left lateral position with the knees partially bent. The colonoscope is introduced through the anus into the rectum, and into the sigmoid, descending, transverse and ascending colon, cecum and then through the ileocecal valve and into the terminal ileum. All areas are examined for any abnormalities. Biopsies can be taken.

Polypectomy is the most common intervention performed during colonoscopy and is used for both diagnostic and therapeutic purposes. This is a minimally invasive procedure and prevents many patients undergoing major abdominal surgery.

Complications. Colonoscopy can result in complications such as perforation and bleeding. The risks are slightly higher when a polypectomy is carried out.

Hazards. Staff may come into contact with body fluid and blood biohazards and should be protected against them.

Percutaneous liver biopsy

Procedure. A small piece of liver tissue is obtained for pathological or bacteriological examination. Indications include differentiation of conjugated hyperbilirubinemia in infancy, chronic hepatitis, diagnosis of some hereditary conditions, e.g. Wilson's disease, diagnosis of metabolic or storage disorders and post transplant rejection.

The specimen is usually obtained via the abdominal wall using a Tru-cut or Menghini needle. In some cases, in small children (< 6 kg) or those with a bleeding disorder, the biopsy is obtained by routing through the internal jugular vein to the hepatic vein. Depending on the age of the child, the procedure may be carried out under general anesthetic or intravenous sedation with local anesthetic.

Preparation should include full blood count, clotting screen and blood group and blood saved for crossmatching for possible transfusion if required after the procedure. The child should also be fasted. An aspiration technique, using a Menghini needle, is the most commonly used in children as it is smaller. It is less likely to tear the liver capsule and reduces the risk of damage to the large intrahepatic blood vessels or bile ducts. The child is placed in a supine position with the right flank exposed and the right arm drawn up beside the head. The point of entry is marked (this may be done with aid of ultrasound) – this is the area of maximal dullness, usually between the seventh and ninth intercostal space. The area is cleaned and the needle tract infiltrated with local anesthetic. A small nick is then made in the skin with a small scalpel. A syringe is attached to the Menghini needle and the needle is introduced through the skin as far as the intercostal ligament. With the patient's breath in expiration and the syringe barrel in full suction, the needle is rapidly advanced into the liver and immediately withdrawn. At all times, the needle is directed at a right angle to the liver surface. Pressure is applied to the area and an occlusive dressing placed over the area and the child is placed on the right side for 4 h. Pulse, respiration, blood pressure and observation of the wound area are carried out on a regular basis, e.g. 1/4 hourly for 2 h, 1/2 hourly for 2 h, hourly for 4 h, then 4 h. The dressing remains in place for 24–48 h.

Complications. The most common complications are local pain and infection. More serious complications include bleeding, pneumothorax, and intraperitoneal bile leaks.

Hazards. Staff may be exposed to unprotected sharps and body fluids. Care should be taken when handling the automatically firing biopsy needles.

CARDIOLOGY

ECG

Procedure. This procedure records the small electrical impulses made by the heart. The different electrodes record this electrical activity from different parts of the heart. Children have to remove clothes from their chest for this procedure. Ten sticky electrodes are applied, one to each arm and leg, and then six across the chest. The electrodes are a little cold when applied, and a little uncomfortable being removed (like a small elastoplast being removed). They remain on for the duration of the record. Children have to lie still during the procedure to prevent artifact.

Complications and hazards. There are no complications or hazards associated with this procedure.

Blood pressure and four limb BP

Procedure. Blood pressure records the pressure of blood in the arteries as the blood is pumped from the heart, and then at its lowest point just before the heart is about to pump again. It can be measured at any point in the body, but is usually measured on the upper arm and can be done manually (a sphygmomanometer) or automatically (oscillometric: Dinamap). In both, a cuff is wrapped around the arm and inflated above the top pressure and then reduced until a pulse is just detected (the systolic pressure). It is then further reduced until the lowest pressure is detected, through a loss of sound at the stethoscope, or automatically through a loss of variation in the pulse dynamics. It may be necessary to repeat the test two or three times to obtain an accurate reading. If it is suspected that there is an obstruction to blood flow in the arterial system it may be useful to identify differences between blood pressure in all four limbs.

Complications. Blood pressure should not be measured in any limb that has recently had venepuncture as this may cause bleeding. Automatic blood pressure machines may be unable to identify patients with extreme hypertension as it is outside their range.

Hazards. Mercury in sphygmomanometers is considered a risk and care should be taken if the column is broken. Mercury is being replaced with alternatives in most modern sphygmomanometers.

24-h ECG

Procedure. This is a heart trace recording that helps to identify problems in heart rate rhythm. The skin in four small areas of the chest is roughened a little to give good attachment of the electrodes. Leads attached to these electrodes are connected to a recorder the size of a mobile cassette player ('Walkman') that is held in a pouch worn around the waist. For the next 24 h, the heart rate tracing is recorded onto a tape whilst children undergo all their usual activities, except for having a bath, shower or going swimming. After 24 h, the parents can remove the electrodes and bring the tape and recorder back to the hospital. The child does not need to come back to hospital with the recorder.

Complications and hazards. There are no significant complications or hazards associated with this procedure.

Echocardiography

Procedure. This is an ultrasound examination of the heart. Gel is put on the chest and a probe is used to look at the heart. Young children may require some short term sedation before the procedure to ensure that they remain still and good images are obtained. The scanning probe needs to be moved to different positions on the chest and upper abdomen. Sometimes pressing on the upper abdomen is a little uncomfortable, but this is not usually for more than a minute or two. Transesophageal echocardiography is a special technique that uses ultrasound to look at the heart from a different angle. Here a special ultrasound probe is passed down the esophagus so that the heart can be looked at from the back. Children require significant sedation or more usually a general anesthetic for this technique.

Complications and hazards. There are no significant complications or hazards associated with routine echocardiography. Esophageal perforation might result from the esophageal approach.

Cardiac catheterization

Procedure. This technique looks at the heart and major blood vessels in a number of ways. It can measure precise blood pressures in different parts of the heart, main blood vessels and lungs, and identify how these blood pressures change in response to changes in inspired oxygen or drug treatments. The technique can also take video pictures of the heart chambers pumping, when dye is injected into the heart chambers. Children can usually come into hospital the morning of the test. They should not eat for 6 h or drink for 4 h before the procedure. Children usually have a general anesthetic for this procedure, though it can be done under deep sedation. Depending on which part of the heart needs assessment, a catheter is put into a vein and/or an artery at the top of the leg. Through these catheters, smaller catheters can be placed that can move through the blood vessels up into the heart, and through the heart into the lungs. Blood pressure can be measured as the catheter moves to different areas. Following removal of the catheters, pressure has to be applied to the site at the top of the leg where they were placed. Children can generally go home later the same day.

Complications. Significant blood loss can rarely occur from the entry site. A hematoma will form if insufficient pressure is applied, or if the child has a bleeding tendency.

Hazards. The screening procedure involves radiation and pregnant women should not be present during video imaging. Blood exposure may be significant during this procedure and protective clothing, gloves and eye protection should be worn.

RESPIRATORY

Use of large volume spacer

Procedure. A large volume spacer is a holding device used most commonly for medicines that will help symptoms of wheeze, cough and chest tightness. Children who are young (< 4 years), or very breathless, will need to use a soft mask fitted to the spacer. The spacer has a valve near the mouthpiece which will click when the child breathes in and out. If children are too young to move this valve (their tidal volume is too small), then hold the spacer at a 45° angle down towards the child's mouth, so that the valve is always open. Take the metered dose inhaler and shake it before placing it at the end of the spacer, ask the child to take regular, deep breaths and press one dose of the inhaler into the spacer. The child should then take 5 (larger child) to 10 breaths (small child, low tidal volume). Remove the inhaler, shake again and repeat. Local policy will dictate how many times this should be repeated, but a multidose policy of 10 doses of salbutamol (100 mcg) over 10 min is commonly used. Small volume spacers are effective, particularly in younger children and are used in a similar fashion.

Complications. The dose provided from the spacer is dependent on the electrostatic charge inside the spacer. This can be reduced in a new spacer by pressing 10 doses of the inhaler into the spacer before its first use, to coat the inside of the spacer and reduce its charge. Spacers should be cleaned once per month by washing in soapy water and leaving to dry without rinsing off the soap (this reduces electrostatic charge).

Hazards. Large volume spacers need to be reviewed regularly as the valve can become blocked with time. A large volume spacer should be replaced every 6 months.

Replacing a tracheostomy tube (leaks/types/speaking valves)

Procedure. This is a skill which must be learnt from someone experienced in the technique. Once the tracheostomy track has epithelialized, however, it is relatively straightforward to replace a tube. Tracheostomies are placed for a number of reasons and it is possible that a child may be able to breathe adequately for some time without the tube until skilled hands arrive. A tube blocked by secretions will cause significant respiratory difficulties to a child so all carers should be taught how to replace the tube. Two people are usually required for replacement. Suction should be available and switched on. Add a little lubrication to the outside of the tube and move the introducer out and back into the tube to make sure it is not sticking. Explain what you are about to do to the child. Place the child flat with a pillow or similar object under the shoulders to extend the neck. Hold the chin in position keeping the neck steady. Place the neckband in position (to which the cotton tapes on the tracheostomy tube will be tied). Cut the cotton tapes securing the old tube. Remove the tube following the curve of the tube and insert the new tube immediately along the same curve. Then remove the introducer. Hold the tube in position using gentle pressure on the side wings. Tie the cotton tapes to the neckband onto each side of the tracheostomy tube using single hitch and bow (for quick release – no knots!). Check the tightness of the cotton tapes with the child sitting up. It should be possible to put one finger only between the neckband and the child's neck. Speaking valves are one-way valves attached to the tracheostomy tube allowing inspiration, but not expiration through the tube. They are placed if there is sufficient leak around the tracheostomy to enable expiration through the vocal chords. Children sometimes find the experience strange and difficult to cope with. Most children will learn to vocalize with a tracheostomy, often by blocking the tracheostomy off with their finger!

Complications. If when replacing a tracheostomy you have difficulty in replacing a tube of the same size, ensure that the child's neck is adequately extended, and replace with a tube that is one size smaller than the original and call for help. If the tracheostomy fistula is poorly formed (first week post op usually) then the tube should only be replaced by a skilled ENT surgeon, as a false passage may be created in the peritracheal tissues. Most children are able to eat and drink normally with a tracheostomy; however feeding issues often arise because children cannot taste food properly as they do not breathe through their noses.

Hazards. Secretions should be considered infective and gloves used at all times.

Drain of pleural effusion/empyema

Procedure. There are numerous methods of draining fluid from the chest and you should ask which method is being used locally: this description is for pigtail drainage. The area of maximal fluid should be identified using ultrasound or chest CT scan. The radiologist should be able to mark the optimal site on the chest wall for obtaining the fluid (you should tell the radiologist whether the child will be sitting or lying for the drainage procedure). In most children a general anesthetic will be required for these procedures and so they will be lying down, though teenagers can occasionally be cooperative with fluid sampling for diagnostic purposes, or the placement of a pigtail catheter (but not a large bore chest drain).

If a pigtail catheter is being placed, it is often done under radiological guidance with general anesthetic. The site marked is penetrated with a large bore needle attached to a syringe. Once through the chest wall, suction is applied to the syringe until fluid/pus is drained. With this position held, the syringe is removed keeping the needle in place, and a guidewire passed through the needle into the cavity. A dilator is then passed over the guidewire to stretch the hole made in the skin and chest wall: radiological screening can confirm the position of the guidewire in the cavity. A larger guidewire is then passed through the dilator and the pigtail catheter slipped over this guidewire. The pigtail catheter is straight when passed over the guidewire, but is curled in the pigtail position by tightening the fine suture that runs from its tip to the external hub. This suture can be fixed in position by tightening the hub, and the suture must be released by unscrewing the hub (or cutting the suture) before attempting to remove the pigtail from the chest. Pigtail catheters are fixed to the skin with tape and when removed do not need a purse-string suture as the dilation procedure ensures a small hole in the chest wall that will close without air leak.

Large bore catheters are usually placed by surgeons. Again the optimal site should have been identified radiologically. A small incision is made on the chest wall and then the hole is enlarged by blunt dissection until the pleural space is entered. The catheter is placed into the maximal area of fluid or pus and fixed with sutures, and a purse-string suture prepared around the base on the catheter to be tightened when the catheter is removed. Large bore catheters can be removed in a ward side room. Ensure adequate pain relief before the procedure. Begin by cutting the stay sutures and preparing the purse-string sutures to be tightened. If possible ask the patient to hold their breath, whilst rapidly removing the tube and tightening the purse-string suture. A dressing should be applied over the site.

Generally chest drains for fluid removal do not require suction. Significant pain relief is required and it is imperative to ensure early activity for recovery from the underlying chest disorder.

Complications. Introducers should not be used with any intrathoracic drain as inadvertent puncture of organs may occur. Pneumothorax may result from any drainage procedure. It can be identified on a chest X-ray following the procedure.
Hazards. Sharps are used in both procedures and should be identified and disposed of by the operator. Fluid from the chest should be considered infected and must be handled with gloves at all times.

Drainage of pneumothorax

Procedure. This procedure in children older than neonates is similar to that for large bore chest drain insertion (above). It is usually done under general anesthesia. Chest X-ray helps to locate the maximal area of air. Small pneumothoraces which are not under tension (i.e. not increasing in size) may resolve spontaneously over weeks as the gas is reabsorbed (so they may not require drainage). The insertion of the drain is as described above, except that the drain must always be connected to an underwater seal which remains below the level of the chest. The drainage set generally has 10–20 cm H_2O suction pressure applied to empty air from the thoracic cavity. The chest drain remains in situ until the drain has not bubbled for 24 h at least. Water swinging in the column demonstrates that the drain is communicating with the pleural space. If it is not swinging, then the drain is not communicating and is probably blocked. Pain relief is very important in children with chest drains and children should be encouraged to mobilize with their chest drain as soon as possible.
Complications. A persistent air leak may require further intervention, though this is unusual. Disconnection of the chest drain or the underwater seal may lead to air being sucked into the pleural space during inspiration. Raising the drain above the level of the chest may lead to water being sucked into the pleural space.
Hazards. Should a chest drain slip out of position, the whole chest drain should be replaced. Pushing the current drain back into the chest can lead to infection and septicemia.

Flexible bronchoscopy

Procedure. Bronchoscopy can be rigid (generally ENT surgeons) or flexible (generally respiratory pediatricians). Rigid bronchoscopy is able to give better manipulative access to the airways and is superior for foreign body removal and operative procedures. Flexible bronchoscopy gives better definition of lesions within the airway and can better identify dynamic and peripheral problems within the airway. Flexible bronchoscopy can be performed under sedation (common in the USA) or general anesthetic. No special preparation is required for the child, except for anesthetic considerations. Under general anesthetic the bronchoscope can be passed via a face-mask (giving good evaluation of the upper airways, and no distortion of the larynx and upper trachea), laryngeal mask, or endotracheal tube. If the procedure is for an anatomical diagnostic purpose then face-mask is the preferred method, with the child spontaneously breathing and local anesthetic applied to the vocal chords. If the procedure is to obtain accurate microbiological specimens, then laryngeal mask or endotracheal tube is preferred.

Bronchoalveolar lavage is often performed in children. If no specific area of interest is identified then samples are usually taken from the (right) middle lobe and the (left) lingula. The tip of the bronchoscope is lodged into the chosen peripheral airway and a volume (1–2 ml/kg) of warmed saline is instiled. Suction is then applied to recover liquid into a trap. Frequently, more than one sample is taken from each site in order to increase the chances of obtaining alveolar (as opposed to bronchial) lining fluid. Bronchial biopsy is unusual in children, but is used diagnostically in patients with lung transplant to identify rejection.
Complications. Flexible bronchoscopes can cause a significant obstruction to an airway, particularly in a small child. If such children develop significant hypoxia or hypercarbia then the procedure should be stopped. Following bronchoscopy, particularly with lavage, children may develop pyrexia (usually within 12 h; the children do not appear toxic and the temperature quickly resolves) or an oxygen requirement (rapidly resolving). Pulmonary hemorrhage is rare in children unless they are biopsied. It usually settles spontaneously or responds to topical adrenaline (epinephrine) applied via the suction channel of the bronchoscope.
Hazards. Secretions should be considered infected and gloves worn at all times. Sharps used by operators should be identified and removed.

Peak flow measurement

Procedure. Children need to stand (if possible) to perform peak flow measurement. The child should take as large a breath as possible, and then place lips tight around the mouthpiece and blow out, as fast and hard as possible. The best of three attempts should be recorded. The predicted value is based on height and sex. In children frequently using peak flow, the estimate of airway compromise should be taken from their personal best peak flow when well, rather than predicted values. Peak flow can be used to identify response to treatment in acute asthma (i.e. bronchodilator response) or can estimate long term control assessing morning and evening recordings: a peak flow and symptom diary should be provided.
Complications. The procedure may induce coughing and wheeze in children with unstable asthma. Obtaining a recording should not hold up emergency treatment of acute asthma.
Hazards. The mouthpieces are single patient use and should be considered infected by secretions when handled.

Spirometry (flow volume loop)

Procedure. Some machines require initial tidal breathing while others go straight into a full expiratory/inspiratory maneuver. Patients should stand and breathe in as much as possible. They then blow out as hard and long as possible until no more air is moving from their chest (can be seen on the spirometer) and then take an equally big breath in again without removing lips from the mouthpiece. The best of three attempts should be taken. The shape of the flow/volume loop may give valuable diagnostic information on the site of airway problems. The forced expiratory flow in 1 second (FEV_1) can be measured as can the vital capacity and tidal volume.
Complications. In small children in particular air leak from the nose may reduce the measurement; nose pegs, if tolerated, will help this. Poor cooperation may limit the value of this test in some children (the flow volume loop may help in identifying such children).
Hazards. Mouthpieces are single patient use and should be considered infected with secretions. Bacterial filters should be used to protect patients from cross infection, particularly children with cystic fibrosis.

Exercise induced bronchoconstriction

Procedure. Exercise induced bronchoconstriction is common in children with asthma and can be used as a confirmatory diagnostic test. The test uses a treadmill to increase ventilation whilst breathing dry air. Typically, children should perform at 60–70% of maximum ventilation for 4–8 min. Most tests use an incremental increase in speed and treadmill angle to induce gentle 'jogging' and mild breathlessness, usually for 6 min. Bronchoconstriction usually occurs at the end of the exercise period and in the 5–10 min following, so peak flow measurements are made before exercise,

every 2 min during exercise and then every 5 min following exercise for 30 min. A bronchodilator is sometimes given at the end of this period to assess whether peak flow returns fully back to baseline. FEV_1 may be used instead of peak flow as a measurement.
Complications. Children may cooperate poorly with a lengthy procedure and need much encouragement. Children with significant bronchoconstriction may need the procedure stopped to be provided with bronchodilator.
Hazards. Children may slip on the treadmill and observation is needed at all times.

Progressive exercise testing

Procedure. This procedure assesses cardiorespiratory reserve. Children are asked to exercise on a treadmill, where the angle of incline and speed are progressively increased. Heart rate and oxygen saturation are measured at each speed and angle. The angle is increased by 5° increments to a maximum 20°, and then the speed is increased from 1.9 miles per hour, to 2.5, 3.1 and finally 3.8 mph.
Complications. The exercise test will be stopped if children exceed 80% of maximal heart rate (220 beats per minute, minus age), or if significant desaturation occurs.
Hazards. Children may slip on the treadmill and careful observation is required at all times. Appropriate selection of children is essential for this test so that physical disabilities do not limit the test or endanger the child using a treadmill. Arrhythmias may occur in susceptible children.

Sweat test

Procedure. There are two main methods for obtaining sweat for chloride estimation in the diagnosis of cystic fibrosis: Gibson and Cooke, and the Macroduct Method.

Gibson and Cooke: Remove all clothes except for pants/diaper. A site is identified which is hair and wrinkle free and not broken or irritated. A magnesium sulfate lint pad is placed on the leg and the electrode (negative) strapped on. The pilocarpine lint pad and its electrode (positive) are placed on the child's back. The electrodes are attached to the iontophoresis box and the current increased to 4 milliamperes for 5 min. The current is then switched off and all pads and electrodes removed. The pilocarpine area is washed with sterile water and dried, taking great care not to contaminate the site. Sterile filter paper is then placed on the stimulated area using forceps and immediately covered with parafilm and tape. Replace all clothes and leave child to play for 30 min. Then remove the parafilm, and use sterile forceps to place the filter paper into a weighed sweat bottle. The sample is then immediately taken to Biochemistry for weighing and chloride assay.

Macroduct: This is the same as for Gibson and Cooke except that the sweat is collected in a 'Macroduct' sweat collector. This is a shallow concave disc with microbore tubing attached through a hole in the center of the disc, placed on the skin being stimulated. Sweat is forced through the central hole by hydrostatic pressure and is collected in the microbore tubing. After a 30 min collection period, the tubing is detached and the sweat is extracted into a collection cup.
Complications. Children < 2 weeks of age don't sweat well and it may not be possible to perform the test satisfactorily. Contamination of the site can cause significant error in results.
Hazards. This test should only be performed by adequately trained staff that maintain standards by performing the test regularly.

Skin prick allergy testing

Procedure. Any area of skin can be used, but it is typically the forearm or back. The area should be free of eczema. Steroid creams should not have been applied that day and oral antihistamines should not have been taken for 3 days. Standard skin test solutions are used. Boxes are drawn on the skin with a ballpoint. A single drop of test solution is placed in a box. Note which box contains which solution. A negative (saline) and positive (histamine) control solution is used. The skin is gently pierced (small scratch) through the solution with the tip of a small gauge needle or lancet. This allows the solution to enter the skin. A separate needle should be used for each solution. Leave for 15 min to identify any reaction, then blot the arm to remove any excess secretions. The size of the weal is then measured in millimeters. A reaction of 3 mm or more is generally considered important.
Complications. Localized irritation can persist and can be alleviated by antihistamine cream.
Hazards. Sharps should be identified and disposed of appropriately.

NEUROLOGY

EEG

Procedure. This is a method of monitoring electrical activity in the brain. The test takes about 90 min. After measuring the head, a number of scalp electrodes are placed at measured intervals on the scalp with a paste fixative. Once in place, children are encouraged to relax whilst the recording is made. They may be asked to take repeated deep breaths (hyperventilate) or be shown a strobe light flashing at different speeds, to stimulate electrical activity helpful in diagnosis. Children may also be observed during sleep (often with cardiorespiratory polysomnography) or over a prolonged period of time with video recording to associate electrical activity with movement (video telemetry). It is also possible to assess the effect of some medications on changing the electrical activity (this may require a cannula to be placed beforehand). The EEG is also used to help diagnose irreversible brain death.
Complications. Hair may need to be removed to fix electrodes and this can cause some discomfort and distress to children and parents.
Hazards. None of note.

Skin biopsy

Procedure. This is performed under local anesthesia in most children and may be taken from any area of skin. Local anesthetic cream and injection of local anesthetic can be used. A small ellipsoid portion of skin tissue is cut along skin lines, with the central tissue removed for assessment, and the two edges sutured together. A dressing is placed over the sutured wound.
Complications. A small amount of bleeding may occur, but should respond easily to gentle pressure.
Hazards. Sharps are used and should be disposed of appropriately. Full aseptic technique should be used.

Muscle biopsy

Procedure. This procedure can be done under local or general anesthetic. The most common sites are the buttocks, upper anterior thigh or shoulder. A small incision is made along skin lines and then the tissues dissected to reveal the muscle. A special muscle biopsy clamp is then used to hold a portion of muscle stretched at a constant tension. The muscle is then cut either side of this clamp and the clamp with the muscle in it goes for assessment. The cut muscle is then sutured to the fascia surrounding the muscle, and the wound edges sutured together.
Complications. Bleeding is relatively common and vessels can be cauterized or ligated.

Hazards. Sharps are used and should be disposed of appropriately. Full aseptic technique should be used.

Neonatal ventriculotomy

Enlargement of the cerebral ventricles may be due to shrinkage of surrounding cerebral matter. More frequently it is caused by failure of resorption of cerebrospinal fluid in the arachnoid space or blockage of the outflow of cerebrospinal fluid from the ventricles or in the aqueduct. Such enlargement may represent raised pressure within the ventricles and may be accompanied by a rapidly expanding occipitofrontal circumference. Most commonly this follows an intraventricular hemorrhage. While hydrocephalus usually is 'communicating' and therefore may be treated by lumbar puncture to release fluid, ventriculotomy may sometimes be needed to measure the intraventricular pressure and to drain ventricular fluid. Rarely ventriculotomy is carried out as a diagnostic test when encephalitis is suspected in the presence of hydrocephalus. Prior to the procedure careful ultrasonography of the brain should be carried out to assess the depth at which fluid is likely to be obtained.

Procedure. It is vital that sterile technique is maintained throughout. This procedure should not be carried out if the infant has a coagulopathy. If the enlargement of the ventricles is bilateral, then the right lateral corner of the anterior fontanelle is the chosen site for ventriculotomy. The hair of the baby's head should be shaved for a radius of 3 cm around the chosen site, and then a 'four minute clean' of the skin should be carried out. The ventriculotomy is carried out using a dedicated needle and cannula, and these are inserted into the skin and the needle tip is pointed medially and anteriorly towards the inner canthus of the ipsilateral eye. The needle and cannula are advanced 0.5 cm at a time and the needle withdrawn leaving the cannula in situ. If the hydrocephalus is significant and the cannula is inserted to the appropriate depth, there is rarely any difficulty in obtaining cerebrospinal fluid from the right ventricle. The pressure monitoring circuit is then attached to the cannula and a pressure reading obtained. If the pressure is elevated then cerebrospinal fluid is drained in order to bring the pressure towards the normal range (less than 5 mmHg in newborn infants), bearing in mind that this procedure may require to be carried out at regular intervals in the subsequent days. The pressure chosen at the end of the procedure and the volume removed are a matter of clinical judgment. The needle is then withdrawn and the ventriculotomy site is covered with sterile gauze.

Complications. The needle may traumatize a major artery or vein. There is evidence that recurrent tapping may be associated with formation of a porencephalic cyst.

Hazards. Poor technique may result in the introduction of infection, and bacterial encephalitis may follow.

Subdural tap

This procedure may be appropriate for the child less than 2 years of age whose coronal suture is still palpably patent, and where a subdural collection of fluid is to be diagnosed and drained. Older children will require a surgical burr hole to achieve these goals. The child with a bleeding diathesis should be carefully assessed.

Procedure. The child is wrapped firmly in a blanket, and the clinical condition is kept under close surveillance during the tap. A generous area over and around the anterior fontanelle is shaved and washed thoroughly with Betadine. Full aseptic precautions are taken. The needle used may be 20 G × 2.2 cm and must have a stylet and 'guard' which is fixed 5 mm from the tip, to prevent plunging inadvertently too deep into the tissues. A point is chosen on the coronal suture 3 cm from the mid-line and lateral to the anterior fontanelle. The firmness of the guard should be checked and the skin pierced. The skin is dragged laterally along the coronal suture by the needle tip which is then pushed firmly through the suture with a rotating action. The stylet is removed and any subdural collection will show itself as straw-colored or bloodstained fluid welling up the spinal needle. Samples from the effusion should be collected for bacteriological and biochemical investigation. A maximum of 30 ml of fluid should be allowed to flow and then the needle is removed. The previous lateral drag on the skin provides a natural seal, which is supplemented with firm pressure for 5 min using a sterile dry swab. The other side may then be explored in the same way. The practitioner should not allow the needle tip to penetrate deeper than 5 mm. Complications of the procedure include infection, subgalleal fluid collections, trauma to the cerebral cortex and laceration of the superior sagittal sinus.

Complications. Include infection, subgalleal fluid collections.

Hazards. Trauma to the cerebral cortex and laceration of the superior sagittal sinus. Blood exposure is a possible biohazard and so gloves should be worn at all times. This should be a surgically sterile procedure. Sharps are used and should be disposed of appropriately.

ENDOCRINOLOGY

Short Synacthen testing

Procedure. This is a test that assesses how well the body is able to produce natural steroids. Children will require an injection into a vein and will also require four venous blood samples. The simplest way to do this is to put a cannula into a vein at the start that can be used for both injecting and also taking samples. Children should be offered anesthetic cream before placing the cannula. No special preparation is required and the study can take place at any time, even after meals. Children are given an injection of Synacthen (0.5 mcg/m^2), a drug which stimulates the body to produce natural steroids. A blood sample will then be taken every 30 min for 2 h to look for the cortisol response to the injection. The level of response shows how well the body is able to produce natural steroids. Normal = a cortisol rise > 145 nmol above basal.

Complications. Certain medicines interfere with the test so a full drug history should be obtained.

Hazards. Blood exposure is a possible biohazard and so gloves should be worn at all times. Sharps are used and should be disposed of appropriately.

Glucose tolerance test

Procedure. This is a test to identify diabetes (diabetes mellitus). It is used when there is a question about the diagnosis, and not if children are known to have obvious diabetes. The test can be done as a day case. Children should have eaten well for the 5 days before the test (i.e. not been unwell and not hungry). Children should have nothing to eat overnight (4 h in babies), though they can drink plain water (no diluting juice). Five venous blood samples will be required so it is often easier to put a cannula into a vein so that samples can be easily taken. Local anesthetic cream can be used so that this is not painful. After a first blood sample has been taken, children are given a drink containing a known amount of sugar (1.75 g/kg). The body will absorb this sugar and should be able to control the amount that stays in the bloodstream. In diabetes, too much sugar stays in the bloodstream (a fasting level > 7.8 mmol/L or a 2 h level > 11.1 mmol/L). Blood samples are taken through the same cannula every 30 min for 2 h after the sugar drink. After the fifth sample is taken at 2 h the test is finished, the cannula can be removed and the child can go home.

Complications. This test should not be performed on patients known to be suffering from an infection, patients with uncontrolled thyroid dysfunction, or patients recovering from severe stress (e.g. surgery) as these alter insulin sensitivity.
Hazards. Blood exposure is a possible biohazard and so gloves should be worn at all times. Sharps are used and should be disposed of appropriately.

RADIOLOGY

Barium X-ray

Procedure. Barium is a contrast medium that can outline structures on X-ray. It is generally used in the gut.

Upper gastrointestinal studies: Children need to fast for 4 (barium swallow) to 6 (barium meal and follow through) hours. A gown covers their clothes in case barium spills. For a barium swallow children are given a barium drink and their pharynx and esophagus is observed on X-ray screening. A barium meal involves a similar drink though this time the radiologists are most interested in the stomach. Children may be given a white powder that fizzes (like sherbet) to create air bubbles in the stomach. These procedures take 15–30 min. A barium follow through is the same but takes longer, as the barium has to pass through the gut. To encourage barium to pass through the gut, children are encouraged to lie on their right side and X-rays are taken every 15–30 min. To get pictures of the whole small gut can take up to 4 h.

Lower gastrointestinal studies: A barium enema is a study of the large bowel when barium liquid is passed via a soft tube placed into the rectum.
Complications. Occasional aspiration of barium occurs during barium swallow. Typically this resolves spontaneously though occasionally such children may require suction.
Hazards. As with all X-ray studies anyone who is pregnant should not be present in the room.

Computed tomography (CT), with/without contrast

Procedure. Computed tomography is an X-ray technique for detailed imaging. Very young children can often be imaged whilst asleep, older children whilst awake and still some children may require general anesthetic, especially for chest CT views. The procedure is quick and painless and provided children have not required an anesthetic the procedure can be performed as an outpatient. The CT scanner usually has a bed with a giant hole (like a huge 'polo' mint) through which the bed slowly moves during the scan. The scanner can be quite noisy and children should be warned of this. If contrast medium is required to highlight blood vessels, then a cannula will need to be inserted (with anesthetic cream).
Complications. Some children feel excessively claustrophobic in such an environment: newer open scanners will be particularly useful for children.
Hazards. Significant doses of radiation are used in CT scanning: lead aprons must be provided to parents/carers staying in the room with children.

Magnetic resonance imaging (MRI)

Procedure. MRI does not involve radiation but generates a significant and strong magnetic field in its environment. It can be used to scan all body areas. The procedure is similar to CT scanning (see above). Contrast is not required in MRI scanning as blood/water differentiation can be made with technical manipulation of scanned signals. The procedure is quick and painless and provided children have not required an anesthetic they do not need admission.
Complications. There are no known risks to MRI.
Hazards. The intense magnetic field in an MRI suite can cause metal objects to fly through the air. Parents should be advised that all metal objects must be removed before entering such an area.

Ultrasound scans (USS)

Procedure. Ultrasound is considered to be completely safe, and is painless and straightforward. It can be used to investigate most tissues, though it is most adapted to neonatal cranial examination, abdominal examination and liver and gall bladder examination. Ultrasound of the chest for fluid/pus collection is also very useful. In all instances a small amount of warmed gel is applied to the skin overlying the area to be visualized. No discomfort is caused and the gel can be removed following the procedure. Infants < 6 months of age generally have a suitably large fontanelle to enable adequate views of the brain. Children requiring ultrasound of the abdomen should have a full bladder at the time of examination, but should not have been given fizzy (carbonated) drinks as these can disturb the pictures obtained. Those requiring liver and gall bladder ultrasound should have nothing to eat for 4 h before the appointment: drinks may be given, but not fizzy drinks or milk.
Complications. None.
Hazards. None.

White cell scan

Procedure. This is an isotope scan (low level radioactive 'dye') that is used to find a site of infection. Children are given the isotope by injection via a vein (anesthetic cream can be offered). Children are asked to arrive first thing in the morning, when a blood sample of 20 ml is taken. This blood is delivered to RadioPharmacy, where the white cells are separated out and isotope added to them. These radiolabelled white cells are reinjected into a vein at midday. A picture is taken 20 min after the injection and again at 3 h. Children do not have to undress for the procedure and only have to lie down on a special camera bed for a few minutes.
Complications. An injection of isotope into the tissues is not important (the radioactive dose is extremely small).
Hazards. Only trained staff should handle isotope mixtures. Sharps should be disposed of correctly.

Bone scan

Procedure. This is a radioactive isotope scan which is used to look at the skeleton. Children are given the isotope by injection into a vein (anesthetic cream can be offered). The child does not need to undress, but lies on a special gamma camera bed. Radiologists inject the isotope and take two pictures immediately; this part of the scan looks at blood flow through the heart and takes around 10 min. There is then a delay of approximately 3 h until the bones of the skeleton become visible. Children can usually leave the department and eat normally. They should be encouraged to drink plenty of fluids. When the bones are visible, a number of gamma camera pictures are taken (depending on how many areas need to be investigated), usually taking up to an hour.
Complications. An injection of isotope into the tissues is not important.
Hazards. Only trained staff should handle isotope mixtures. Sharps should be disposed of correctly.

DMSA scan

Procedure. This is a radioactive isotope scan that is used to look at kidney function. The isotope is given by intravenous injection (anesthetic cream can be offered). Once injected there is a delay until the kidneys are visible on the camera. This is at least 1.5 h, but not unusually 5 h and very occasionally children will be asked to come back 24 h after the injection so that the kidneys can be seen.

In the time period between injection of the isotope and the camera photos, families can usually leave the department and eat and drink as normal. When ready, three pictures are usually taken and this takes around 30 min. Children do not have to get undressed during this time, but they have to lie on a special gamma camera bed.
Complications. An injection of isotope into the tissues is not important. Children with intercurrent urinary tract infection should not have a DMSA scan.
Hazards. Only trained staff should handle isotope mixtures. Sharps should be disposed of correctly.

MAG3 scan

Procedure. This is a radioactive isotope scan that is used to look at the drainage of the kidneys and identify (but not grade) vesicoureteric reflux. Children are given the isotope by intravenous injection (anesthetic cream can be offered). The child does not have to undress, but has to lie on a special gamma camera bed. The radiologist will inject the isotope and start taking pictures immediately, continuing until all the isotope has drained through the kidneys. This usually takes 20–45 min. If the child is toilet trained, when the bladder is full they may be asked to pass urine into a container while sitting or standing in front of the camera. This identifies reflux of urine from the bladder to kidneys. This is an important component of the test and it may take some time to induce a child to empty their bladder.
Complications. An injection of isotope into the tissues is not important. Children with intercurrent urinary tract infection should not have a DMSA scan.
Hazards. Only trained staff should handle isotope mixtures. Sharps should be disposed of correctly.

Micturating cystourethrogram (MCU)

Procedure. This is an X-ray examination of the bladder. Children are asked to undress and lie on the X-ray table. A urinary catheter is passed through the urethra into the bladder. The tube is then connected to a bottle containing X-ray contrast medium. The contrast runs into the bladder until it is full and the child wants to pass urine. Babies may pee spontaneously, older children will use a potty or container. The bladder is X-rayed as urine is passed. The examination takes approximately 45 min.
Complications. Explanation beforehand may allay fears about catheterization. Catheterization may fail in some girls. Catheterization can rarely cause urethral trauma.
Hazards. Urine should be considered infected and gloves should be worn.

Direct cystogram

Procedure. This procedure is similar to the micturating cystourethrogram, but the bladder is directly accessed by suprapubic injection of contrast medium until the bladder is full. The needle can then be withdrawn whilst the child pees, and the study is completed in the same way as for MCU (above).
Complications. Anesthetic cream applied suprapubically can reduce discomfort with this test.
Hazards. Problems are rarely encountered. Sharps should be disposed of appropriately.

HEMATOLOGY/ONCOLOGY

Bone marrow aspiration

Procedure. Bone marrow examination may allow diagnosis of malignancy, aplasia or storage disorders. Although the procedure can be performed under local anesthetic with sedation, general anesthetic is used in most children. Children should have normal coagulation studies, or receive coagulation cover prior to the procedure. In children under 3 months of age, bone marrow is aspirated from the anterior tibia. Children older than this have marrow aspiration from the posterior iliac crest, just above the posterior superior iliac spine. A needle and trocar are inserted at the site by a twisting motion into the bone, and once the trocar is removed, strong suction is applied to a syringe attached to the needle. Generally only a small volume (0.2 ml) of marrow is required. The trochar is then reinserted, needle and trochar removed and pressure applied to the site for 5 min to stop bleeding.
Complications. If marrow cannot be aspirated, then the trocar is reinserted and the needle advanced a little further. Occasional pressure applied to the bone can cause a fracture (especially the tibia). Bleeding may cause a subperiosteal hematoma. Poor aseptic technique may result in osteomyelitis.
Hazards. Sharps and blood biohazard need dealing with during the procedure.

RENAL

Percutaneous renal biopsy

Procedure. Both kidneys are identified by ultrasound to make sure that a normal kidney is present on the other side (so if you get major complications you don't lose your only good kidney!). Under general anesthetic a spot is marked on the skin at a suitable place for needle entry to avoid bowel and pleura (with a fairly direct vertical route to the lower pole of the kidney). A second spot is marked where the ultrasound probe can be placed to observe needle entry into the lower pole. The distance from skin to kidney is measured. The skin is cleaned and sterile gloves put on and the ultrasound probe is cleaned. A small scalpel nick in the skin allows easy access for the needle. An automatic cutting needle is then inserted to the correct depth under direct observation with ultrasound. As soon as the needle is inside the kidney, the cutting needle is fired, preferably with the patient's breath held in inspiration (by the anesthetist). The aim is to get both cortex and medulla, aiming as far away as possible from the hilum: too low is below the kidney – no harm done; too high and the biopsy may enter a major vessel at the hilum – this will require emergency surgery. Three biopsy cores are required – for light microscopy, electron microscopy and immunohistochemistry. Following the procedure simple dressings are required and the patient will need careful cardiorespiratory observation.
Complications. Renal vascular bleed. Formation of an arterio-venous fistula (unlikely if the hilum is avoided). Infection is often quoted but rarely seen. The procedure will need to be repeated if there is an inadequate biopsy with no glomeruli present.
Hazards. Automatic firing biopsy needles should be handled with care. The procedure should be aseptic and protection will be required against bodily fluids.

RHEUMATOLOGY

Steroid joint injection

Procedure. This procedure is performed in children when joint inflammation is not settling with medication. Draining the fluid from the joint and injecting it with steroid is a very effective way of controlling the inflammation for anything up to 12 months from a single injection. The procedure is normally performed in theater, with the child asleep under a general anesthetic so that they do not feel any discomfort in the joint. It is often performed as a day case. Children are given a general anesthetic and the procedure usually takes about 10–20 min to complete. It is very important that children rest the injected joint for next 24 h following injection, in order to allow the steroid treatment to have the best chance of helping the joint. Moving around will not harm the child, but there is a reduced chance of the steroid staying in one place and helping the joint that has been treated. For younger children, and children where a few joints are treated at the same time it is sensible to keep them in hospital overnight simply to ensure that they do get the rest that they need. The treatment should help to reduce the joint inflammation whilst exercise and movement rehabilitation continues.

Complications. This form of steroid treatment is considered very safe, and does not cause any long term steroid side-effects such as failure to grow in height, weight gain, increase risk of infection, diabetes or osteoporosis (thinning) of the bones.

Hazards. Sharps used in this procedure should be identified and disposed of appropriately.

REFERENCES (* Level 1 evidence)

1 Alderson P, Montgomery J. Health care choices. Making decisions with children: Summary of conclusions. Bull Med Ethics 1996; 117:8–11.

2 Stevens B. Management of painful procedures in the newborn. Curr Opin Pediatr 1996; 8:102–107.

3 Freeman JA, Doyle E, Im NG, Morton NS. Topical anesthesia of the skin: a review. Paediatr Anaesth 1993; 3:495–510.

4 Lawson RA, Smart NG, Gudgeon AC, Morton NS. Evaluation of amethocaine gel preparation for percutaneous analgesia before venous cannulation in children. Br J Anaesth 1995; 7555:282–285.

5 Rowbotham DJ. Guidelines for the use of nonsteroidal anti-inflammatory drugs in the peri-operative period. London: Royal College of Anaesthetists; 1998.

6 Doyle E, Mottart KJ, Marshall C, Morton NS. Comparison of different bolus doses of morphine for patient controlled analgesia in children. Br J Anaesth 1994; 72:160–163.

7 Krechel SW, Bildner J. CRIES: a new neonatal postoperative pain measurement score. Initial testing of validity and reliability. Paediatr Anaesth 1995; 5:53–61.

8 Fitzgerald M. The developmental neurobiology of pain. In: Melzack R, Wall PD, eds. Textbook of pain. Edinburgh: Churchill Livingstone; 1999:233–252.

9 Compton P, Darakjian J, Miotto K. Screening for addiction in patients with chronic pain and substance abuse: evaluation of a pilot assessment tool. J Pain Symptom Manage 1998; 16:355–363.

10 Anand KJS, Hickey PR. Pain and its effects in the human neonate and fetus. N Engl J Med 1987; 317:1321–1329.

11 Anderson B. What we don't know about paracetamol in children. Paediatr Anaesth 1998; 8:451–460.

12 Merkel S, Voepel-Lewis T, Shayevitz J, Malviya S. The FLACC: a behavioral scale for scoring postoperative pain in young children. Pediatr Nurs 1997; 23:293–297.

13 Morton NS. Prevention and control of pain in children. Br J Anaesth 1999; 83:118–129.

14 Kehlet H, Werner M, Perkins F. Balanced analgesia: what is it and what are its advantages in postoperative pain? Drugs 1999; 58:793–797.

15 Morton NS. Development of a monitoring protocol for safe use of opioids in children. Paediatr Anaesth 1993; 3:179–184.

39

Practical aspects of diagnostic imaging

George M A Hendry, Alastair Graham Wilkinson

INTRODUCTION

Imaging of the pediatric patient will be influenced by the availability of equipment and expertise.

Imaging has been revolutionized with the introduction of ultrasound (US), computerized tomography (CT), radioisotope scanning (RIS), magnetic resonance imaging (MRI) and interventional techniques. However, the conventional techniques of plain X-rays and contrast studies are still of importance and, together with US, constitute the majority of investigations. The initial section of this chapter provides an insight into the various techniques available and the later sections discuss their applications to the various body systems.

GENERAL DISCUSSION

The child should be examined in a pleasant, friendly environment. The X-ray rooms and waiting areas can be decorated with posters, paintings and a supply of friendly 'animals' and toys should be available. In older children any procedure should be explained in understandable terms: this will often gain their cooperation. Parents are encouraged to be present in the room to comfort their child. Sedation is rarely necessary for conventional imaging techniques.

Trained personnel – radiologists, radiographers, nurses and anesthetists – are essential for a complete and successful pediatric imaging unit. In a general hospital at least two radiographers and one radiologist should be trained in, and have responsibility for, the investigation and interpretation of pediatric problems.

Strict radiation protection is critical in pediatric departments to avoid radiation damage to sensitive immature and developing structures and to avoid cumulative damage to the chromosomes of future generations. Ionizing radiation (medical exposures) regulations 2000 (IRMER) have been introduced requiring strict criteria for the justification of radiation procedures and the use of the lowest dose technique for the clinical situation. Radiation dose can be reduced by the correct choice of exposure factors, particularly low dose techniques in CT. High dose radiographic imaging of the spine and pelvis should be replaced by non-ionizing methods, particularly MRI, where appropriate. Accurate coning of the X-ray beam to the area of the body to be examined, lead shielding of the gonads and avoidance of film retakes are important. These factors obviously require the presence of an experienced pediatric radiographer.

Close liaison between the clinician and radiologist will lead to the correct examination for the clinical problem, thus avoiding unnecessary and repeat investigations. Investigations should also begin with the least invasive procedure and proceed along recognized flow channels.[1]

EQUIPMENT AND IMAGING MODALITIES

Any hospital concerned with the investigation of children must have conventional X-rays and real-time US available. It is also important to have easy access to CT, nuclear medicine and MRI. The latter modalities record images in digital format which has the advantage of easy data manipulation with changing of window levels and width. The information acquired can be fully utilized and transferred by digital link to other sites. The system allows the development of patient archiving and communication systems (PACS) which enables instant storage and retrieval of data. In the future all plain radiographs will be acquired in digital format.

Digitization also allows more flexible tissue analysis after a single exposure and eliminates retakes due to poor choice of exposure factors.

Careful positioning of the child for a radiological investigation is important. Immobilization may be necessary. The parent or helper in the department often will suffice by holding the child; bucky bands and foam pads may, however, be necessary. Pediatric screening units should have specialized cradles to secure the child. Radiographic views in different positions are thus possible without struggling, preventing excessive radiation exposure.

CONVENTIONAL X-RAYS

X-rays are high frequency electromagnetic waves. An image is produced by light exposure of the photographic film by fluorescent screens excited by the X-ray beam as it emerges from the patient. Plain films are almost universally used as the only or primary modality for investigation of suspected bony injury, pneumonia, mediastinal and lung masses and bowel obstruction or perforation. Healing of fractures is monitored by serial X-rays to confirm adequate union in a satisfactory position.

Fluoroscopy is a dynamic X-ray image produced when the emergent X-ray beam is directed onto a photomultiplier tube. The image can then be observed on a television monitor. The information from fluoroscopy can be digitized and the resultant data stored on hard disk with selected images transferred to hard copy film. Barium meals, enemas, cystograms and interventional procedures are performed under fluoroscopic control.

The image on the X-ray film depends on the contrast produced by differential absorption of X-rays in different body tissues. Air, fat, bone and soft tissues are the natural contrasts. The contrast differences can be enhanced by giving artificial media, such as barium or iodine as a water-soluble contrast. Non-ionic water-soluble contrasts are now routinely used for intravenous, intra-arterial and intrathecal examinations. Injection of this contrast enhances vascular structures and increases the contrast differentiation between body tissues. The benefits of non-ionic contrast are the low osmolality and diminished toxicity.[2]

Flavored non-ionic contrast media are used in the examination of swallowing mechanisms in suspected aspiration, tracheoesophageal fistula and in the diagnosis of bowel obstruction in the neonate. The contrast, being of low osmolality, is not diluted during passage through the gut. Traditionally sodium acetrizoate (Gastrografin), a hypertonic water-soluble contrast, has been used as a contrast medium in the diagnosis and treatment of meconium ileus, meconium plug syndrome and meconium ileus equivalent. As this contrast has 10 times the osmolality of plasma, it causes osmotic effects and dehydration, particularly in small children. Adequate fluid balance must therefore be maintained during the use of the contrast. This may necessitate intravenous fluids. Non-ionic water-soluble contrast is only 2–3 times the osmolality of plasma. It has been shown to be equally effective in treatment of these conditions.

Barium sulfate is an inert, dense, safe contrast medium. It is exclusively used for gastrointestinal studies. The contrast may be produced in liquid or powder form. Added flavoring is essential, as children may be reluctant to drink the contrast.

Double contrast barium studies combine the use of high-density barium and air. The latter may be swallowed in sufficient volume by an apprehensive child but can be supplemented by bicarbonate contained in the barium suspension or by giving additional bicarbonate powders or tablets. These procedures provide an excellent thin barium coating of the gut mucosa enabling superficial ulcerations or polyps to be detected. Low-density barium mixtures are suitable for examination of the small bowel. The small bowel enema is a procedure where the contrast is injected directly through a nasojejunal tube followed by saline or methylcellulose. This procedure may give more accurate assessment of mucosal detail.

ULTRASOUND

This non-invasive and inexpensive modality has revolutionized the imaging of pediatric diseases. A transducer produces high frequency sound waves of between 3.5 and 12 MHz which penetrate the tissues and are reflected from different tissue interfaces back to the transducer. Differing intensities of signal from varying interfaces in the tissue are then converted into a digital format, allowing a sectional image of the organ structure to be formed.

Several types of transducer are available. The sector scanner with a small head is useful when examining the brain through a small anterior fontanel or for an intercostal or subcostal approach to the chest and upper abdomen. Linear and curved linear array transducers have multiple crystals and are electronically controlled. In the former, the image produced is rectangular with excellent near-field detail which is useful for the examination of superficial structures. No known deleterious effects of ultrasound have been recorded in vivo. Recommended power levels are determined by advisory committees and a fail-safe governor is built into most US machines. Children rarely need sedation and feeding the baby before or while scanning leads to a quiet examination. Good transducer–skin contact using a coupling jelly is important. Reflection of ultrasound by gas can cause problems in the abdomen and chest and the lack of information behind bone makes it of limited value in intracranial investigation beyond infancy.

Real-time ultrasound is continuous sampling of the organs examined with a frame rate of 10–40 per second. Patient movement becomes therefore less significant. Ultrasound is a sectional technique and a mental image of the organ examined is formed during the procedure. Spot films can be made of any section.

Successful ultrasound is operator dependent and thus should only be performed by specialist trained sonographers.

Doppler ultrasound

Doppler ultrasound is a technique for assessing blood flow by measuring the frequency changes of sound reflected from flowing red blood cells. The information is presented as a spectrum of frequency versus time and, if the appropriate angle correction is made, velocity versus time. Duplex Doppler ultrasound refers to a simultaneous display of a two-dimensional ultrasound image together with the pulsed Doppler data. The Doppler signal can be sampled from any area of the cross-sectional image and this is facilitated if color Doppler is also available.

Color Doppler images both frequency shift and phase information. This allows red blood cell movement to be color encoded with hue dependent on the speed and direction of movement with respect to the transducer. Color imaging highlights blood flow against the gray background of the 2D image and has revolutionized the echocardiographic diagnosis of congenital heart disease, allowing small shunts to be detected accurately.

A further development in Doppler ultrasound is the so-called power Doppler. This technique measures the density rather than the velocity of the red blood cells in the sample area. The amplitude of the signal is governed by the amount of blood within the sample volume. Large amplitude signals are portrayed as a bright hue and weak signals as a dim color on the monitor.

The technique is independent of the angle of insonation and the flow velocity of the red blood cells. The technique is also called ultrasound angiography as it gives a detailed road map of blood flow in an organ. The technique is three times more sensitive than conventional Doppler and shows smaller blood vessels at deeper depths. It also provides better edge enhancement of blood vessels. The disadvantage is the inability to provide functional information such as direction of flow[3] and flow velocity measurements.

Contrast agents are now being developed for ultrasound. These require the injection of microbubbles of air into the circulation which cause echo enhancement in blood vessels. Vascular structures thus show enhancement during certain phases of circulation. Contrast microbubbles can also be injected into the bladder and vesicoureteric reflux demonstrated by increased echogenicity in the upper tracts.

The main indications for Doppler ultrasound are:

1. diagnosis of congenital heart disease (see Ch. 19);
2. demonstration of arterial and venous flow to confirm vessel patency;
3. investigation of hemodynamic disturbances in aneurysms and stenoses;
4. detection of physiological and pathological changes indicated by quantitative Doppler shifts;
5. measurement of absolute blood flow.[4]

The parameters commonly used in quantifying Doppler changes are the pulsatility or the resistive index, peak systolic velocity, diastolic velocity and mean flow velocity.

For example, in examination of the brain, decreased diastolic flow can be demonstrated in conditions such as hydrocephalus or cerebral edema where raised intracranial pressure is present. This is manifest by an increase in the resistance index or pulsatility index.[5]

Higher frequency shifts in systole indicating an increase in systolic velocity are noted at the site of arterial stenosis and this technique is useful in the investigation of renal and aortic vascular abnormalities in systemic hypertension and in demonstrating vascular thrombosis and stenosis following renal and hepatic transplantation.

It must always be remembered that associated physiological changes such as circulatory collapse and persistent ductus arteriosus can affect the Doppler spectrum and cause spurious abnormalities in the abovementioned parameters.[4]

COMPUTERIZED TOMOGRAPHY SCANNING (CT)

In this technique an X-ray fan beam rotates around the body placed in the central aperture of the scanner and detectors record the emergent beam from every angle. The information from multiple interactions of the X-rays with the tissues is computerized and presented as a 2D image of a slice through the body. Conventional scanners perform one slice at a time with each slice taking 1 second. Modern scanners can also operate in a spiral fashion and can complete a scan of the abdomen or chest within half a minute, allowing this to be completed within a single breath hold and enabling much more efficient use of a rapid bolus of i.v. contrast. The section thickness can be collimated between 1 and 10 mm and sections may be contiguous or spaced. Thin sections allow more detailed imaging with high resolution (at the expense of a poorer signal-to-noise ratio).[6] This fine section tomography is useful in the chest to assess bronchiectasis and interstitial lung disease or in the assessment of the petrous bone in suspected abnormalities of the middle and inner ears.[7]

Software packages can allow volume measurement (e.g. size of abdominal tumors) and 3D reconstructions are particularly useful for craniofacial abnormalities, airway and joint imaging. The data can be reformatted in any plane.

CT accounts for most medical radiation dose.[8] The dose should be reduced by tailoring the examination to the clinical problem.[9–11] Technical advances with improving sensitivity of the detectors and a specific policy to reduce the kV and mA in children also contribute to a reduction in dose.[11,12] Radiation doses are determined in relation to skin dose, bone marrow dose and gonadal dose.

CT scanners with fast scan times of under 1 sec/section are of value in children, to minimize artifact due to child movement and gut motility. Rapid reconstruction of the image also shortens the examination. Children are not ideal subjects for CT as fat (the natural contrast to define certain organs) is lacking. Preparation of the child for the procedure is important. An explanation to the child and parents often overcomes anxiety and the presence of trained pediatric staff in the unit is a necessity. In many centers general anesthesia is felt to be safer than sedation. During sedation or anesthesia the child must be adequately monitored with oxygen saturation, blood pressure and respiration continuously recorded. A person trained in pediatric resuscitation should be available. The child should be fasted for 5 hours before sedation or general anesthesia.

Contrast will allow differentiation of structures in the section. The gut is opacified with a 2–5% diluted solution of a non-ionic contrast (300 mg/ml) in a dose of 100–500 ml, depending on the age of the child. Three-quarters of the dose is given 1 h before the procedure, the remaining volume 15 min before. In pelvic examinations the rectum is opacified with a similar dilute contrast.

Intravenous non-ionic water-soluble contrast will enhance vascular structures and visualize the renal tract. Rapid injection and immediate CT examination is termed dynamic scanning.

CT is particularly useful in the investigation of head injuries, imaging of parenchymal and metastatic disease in the chest, and in acute abdominal trauma.[6,13] Orthopedic applications include the investigation of congenital abnormalities of the feet, bone tumors and spondylolysis. With specialized software, assessment of the mineral content of bone is possible.

MRI is now regarded as the primary imaging modality for the central nervous system and in skeletal abnormalities including tumors, osteomyelitis, osteochondritis and Perthes' disease.

NUCLEAR MEDICINE

Nuclear medicine studies involve the administration, usually intravenous, of a radionuclide bound to a carrier molecule which is organ specific. The radionuclide emits radiation usually in the form of gamma rays and the technique can be used for both diagnostic and therapeutic purposes.

The most commonly used radionuclide is technetium 99m, which has a physical half-life of 6 h and emits gamma energy of 140 keV. Iodine 123 (half-life 13 h), iodine 131 (half-life 8.04 days), xenon 133 (half-life 5.3 days) and krypton 81m (half-life 13 seconds) are occasionally used. The child receives a weight/surface area-related dose of the radionuclide and the radiation dose from this technique is frequently less than that received from equivalent X-rays.

Recently specific monoclonal antibodies, e.g. UJ13A, 3F8, or metaiodobenzylguanidine (MIBG) have been labeled with large doses of ^{131}I (beta particle emitter) and used in the treatment of neuroblastoma. The use of radionuclides for therapeutic purposes is a potential growth area. Unlike other imaging modalities which provide anatomical images, radionuclide studies provide functional information and are of value in the diagnosis of renal disease, gastrointestinal disorders, lung disease, skeletal abnormalities and in tumor staging.[14]

SINGLE PHOTON EMISSION TOMOGRAPHY (SPECT)

This is an allied technique which involves the use of the gamma camera rotating around the body during the examination, collecting data from multiple angles. Computer manipulation of these data produces a series of axial images allowing greater sensitivity in detecting smaller differences in activity and also more precise localization of abnormalities. This has multiple applications including more accurate detection of renal scars (^{99m}Tc DMSA), localizing a seizure focus in epileptic patients (^{99m}Tc HMPAO) and spinal abnormalities in patients with back ache (^{99m}Tc MDP) with particular reference to osteoid osteoma, osteomyelitis and spondylolysis.

MAGNETIC RESONANCE IMAGING (MRI)

This technique has imaging capabilities which are ideally suited to pediatrics and should become an essential feature of all pediatric centers. It depends on the ability of the nucleus of an atom to resonate under certain conditions in the presence of a magnetic field. The child is placed within a strong magnetic field and then exposed to a specific radiofrequency (RF) by means of a coil which fits the body part to be examined. This causes the nuclei in the subject to resonate about their equilibrium. When the RF pulse is terminated the nuclei continue to resonate with emission of RF detected as the MR signal, before returning to their original equilibrium position. The resonant or precession frequency becomes higher when the magnetic field strength increases. [Larmors equation.]

The signal originates from protons within the body (largely from free water in the tissues). Differing RF pulse sequences and repetition times can be used to produce resonance from which an image can be constructed. Maximum contrast between tissues can be achieved by the correct choice of these variables.

Several different types of magnet are available. The low field strength magnets operate at 0.18–0.23 Tesla and usually have an open configuration (Fig. 39.1) rather than a tunnel so are less claustrophobic for children and are also quiet. The low field strength, however, results in a lower signal-to-noise ratio and hence reduced resolution and longer acquisition time for the image. Sequences have been developed to counteract these problems.

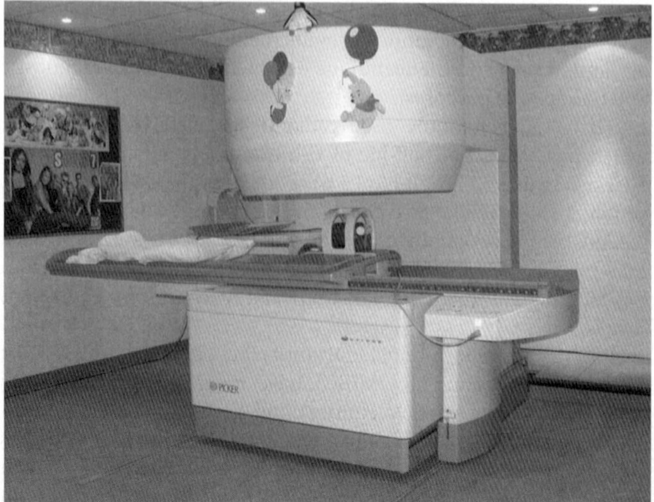

Fig. 39.1 Open magnetic resonance scanner.

Mid-range magnets and high field strength magnets have magnetic field strengths of 0.3–0.5 and 1–2 Tesla. These systems are supercooled with helium, are more expensive and are noisier during data acquisition and require more shielding for the magnetic field. The high field systems are nearly all of tunnel configuration with corresponding problems of claustrophobia and access, particularly during anesthesia. The advantages of the high field strength systems are the ability to acquire the image data in a shorter time with generally better resolution from an improved signal-to-noise ratio. Spectroscopy and functional brain studies are possible with magnetic field strengths of 1.5 Tesla and above.

The time for acquisition of the data during the examination also depends on the sequence chosen. This may vary from 1 to 9 minutes and usually three or more acquisitions are required to complete the examination. Fast scan techniques dramatically reduce the examination times making the modality more suitable for restless children and enabling dynamic studies to be carried out. Other sequences include turbo spin, fluid attenuation, fat suppression techniques and contrast-enhanced dynamic angiography.

MRI is the optimum modality for imaging of the central nervous system where detailed images cannot be achieved with other techniques. Newer sequences such as diffusion-weighted imaging allow earlier diagnosis of ischemic changes including periventricular leukomalacia.[15]

MRI also enables imaging of the heart and vascular system. In conventional spin echo images, flowing blood appears as a signal void which helps differentiate vessels from lymph nodes. Gradient echo images can be used to produce a high signal from flowing blood, allowing magnetic resonance angiography. With cardiac gating, cine loop images of the heart can be obtained to give detailed information on cardiac function and congenital abnormalities such as coarctation of the aorta and intracardiac defects. Volume acquisition techniques allow the blood vessels in a given volume to be examined in any plane. Postprocessing using the maximum intensity projection technique (MIP) allows 3D reconstruction of vessels which can be rotated to permit visualization from any angle. Standard spin echo T1 images in coronal, sagittal and axial planes will outline vascular rings, including the double aortic arch and aberrant innominate artery. The relationship of the vessel with the trachea is clearly identified.

In the lung, metastases are less well demonstrated than with CT. In cystic fibrosis, mucus plugs produce a bright signal, as do areas of inflammation. It is not possible, however, to obtain the same parenchymal detail as achieved with high resolution CT.

MRI is a useful technique for imaging abdominal masses, particularly those arising in the liver, kidney or retroperitoneal areas. Fluid-filled structures are easily identified using the appropriate sequences and the relation of major blood vessels to the tumor is beautifully demonstrated. Being a multiplanar imaging technique, MRI is valuable in the assessment of presacral masses, the demonstration of the uterus and ovaries in intersex and endocrine abnormalities[16] and the assessment of the pelvic floor muscles in anorectal atresia.

As yet it is not possible to examine the gastrointestinal tract as gut movement causes multiple artifacts. In future, this may be possible with the use of contrast media and antispasmodics. MRI is also a recognized technique in the diagnosis of diseases involving the musculoskeletal system. Although cortical bone produces a signal void, it is the changes in marrow signal which identify the pathology of osteomyelitis, trauma, bleeding or edema.

It is important to remember that the signal from the pediatric bone marrow changes with the aging of the child. As more fat accumulates with increasing age, there is a corresponding increase in the marrow signal.[17] MRI has been described as useful in the initial diagnosis of Perthes' disease where a low signal is seen in the epiphysis of the femur on T1 and T2 images. Growth plate injuries, osteomyelitis and involvement of the bone marrow in metastatic disease may all be diagnosed with this technique.[18,19]

INTERVENTIONAL PROCEDURES

These techniques have now been well integrated into pediatric practice.[20] Percutaneous nephrostomy with catheterization and drainage of a hydronephrosis initially involves the ultrasonic guidance of a fine 22G needle into the renal pelvis. Following aspiration of urine, water-soluble contrast may be injected for fluoroscopic identification of the pelvicalyceal system. A guidewire is then inserted through the needle. The tract is dilated and finally a 5–8 French catheter is coiled in the renal pelvis. The procedure is best performed under general anesthetic. Balloon dilatation of pelviureteric junction obstruction and postoperative strictures can be performed, though insertion of a temporary ureteric stent is necessary to prevent occlusion of the ureter by inflammatory changes.

Dilatation of esophageal strictures with a balloon catheter is now a well-described technique (Fig. 39.2). The procedure is performed under general anesthesia in conjunction with the surgical team. The stricture is initially outlined with contrast and the balloon catheter size selected.[21,22] A narrow feeding tube is then passed through the mouth and a guidewire fed through the feeding tube to cross the stricture. The preselected balloon catheter, varying in size from 6 mm to 20 mm, is passed over the guidewire and inflated with contrast under fluoroscopic control, until waisting at the stricture is abolished. Larger balloons of 30–35 mm have been used successfully in achalasia.[22] Continuous ECG monitoring is essential as esophageal dilatation can cause bradycardia or apnea.

A similar technique has been described for small bowel and colonic strictures. A record of screening time and number of procedures is essential to monitor radiation exposure.

The hydrostatic reduction of intussusception and treatment of meconium ileus with water-soluble contrast will be discussed in the relevant sections.

Foreign bodies in the esophagus may be removed with a balloon catheter. The catheter is inserted through the mouth and the balloon inflated distal to the foreign body. In the prone head-down position the catheter is pulled cranially and the foreign body is removed from the mouth with forceps.[23] Similarly magnetic material lying in the esophagus or stomach may be withdrawn using a magnet attached to a nasogastric tube. This is of particular value in withdrawing the small batteries now used in calculators and some coins which are now magnetic. Batteries if left in situ may disintegrate, causing corrosive strictures and perforations of the esophagus and stomach.[24]

Recently the transjugular intrahepatic portosystemic shunt (TIPS) procedure has been used in children with portal hypertension caused by liver disease. A stent is inserted in the liver substance to connect the portal vein to the hepatic vein, reducing portal venous pressure and preventing complications such as bleeding varices.

Arteriovenous malformations can be embolized following selective catheterization of feeding vessels at angiography. Steel coils, acrylic glue or various types of particulate matter can be used to reduce flow through the abnormality.

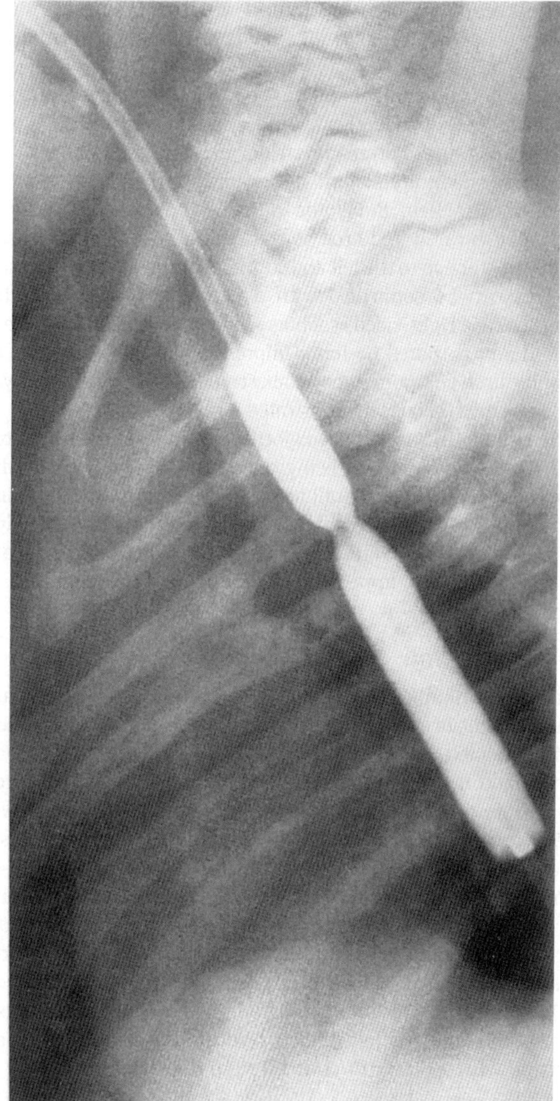

Fig. 39.2 Balloon dilatation of esophageal stricture. Note indentation on the contrast-filled balloon from the stricture.

BODY SYSTEMS

RESPIRATORY SYSTEM

Plain radiographs

Chest radiographs are the most frequently requested imaging procedure in children and there is opportunity for effective cost reduction and radiation protection by more careful vetting of requests. Radiographic technique is important and an acceptable chest radiograph must include the whole chest from the thoracic inlet to diaphragm and be sufficiently penetrated to show major spinal abnormalities through the mediastinal shadow. Younger children are usually examined supine and older cooperative children can be examined erect. The routine use of lateral chest radiographs is unnecessary. Lung segments which are collapsed or consolidated can be located by their interference with normal mediastinal or diaphragmatic contours. Overinflation is assessed by the effects on rib configuration and the diaphragm level and shape. Pleural effusions previously detected by means of decubitus films should be confirmed with ultrasound. In suspected foreign body aspiration, collapse or overinflation are the findings. A single anteroposterior (AP) film is all that is required. A normal chest X-ray may be found in 20% of cases of inhaled foreign bodies. The management is on clinical findings so if a foreign body is suspected then a bronchoscopy is indicated independent of the radiology.

When imaging children with stridor the standard radiographs are an AP chest radiograph, lateral neck radiograph and a high kV filter view of the trachea. Subglottic narrowing is seen in croup but radiography is rarely required. A right-sided aortic knuckle usually deviates the trachea to the left and suggests the presence of a vascular ring. This can be confirmed with a contrast swallow, the classic findings being a right-sided esophageal impression from a right aortic arch and an associated posterior impression on the esophagus from the double arch component or an aberrant left subclavian artery. The exact anatomy is clearly demonstrated with MRI.

The child with suspected epiglottitis should be admitted directly to the ward, the condition being diagnosed clinically or on direct laryngoscopy in theater. Fatalities have arisen secondary to airway obstruction during radiography of these children. Occasionally the diagnosis is confused clinically with croup, but the typical lateral neck radiographic appearance of a swollen epiglottis and aryepiglottic folds allows differentiation.

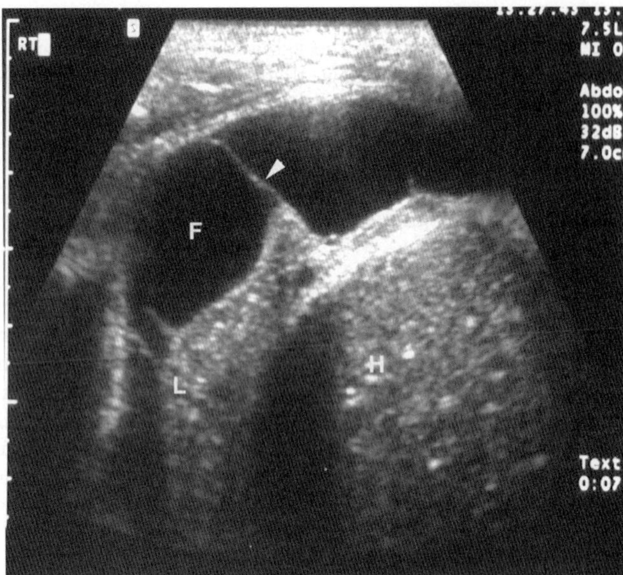

Fig. 39.3 Pleural effusion: transverse US showing fluid (F), collapsed lung (L), liver (H) and fibrin stranding (arrowhead).

Contrast swallow

The contrast mainly used is barium sulfate. The indications are in the assessment of mediastinal masses and stridor when a vascular ring is suspected.

In children with swallowing problems, such as in cerebral palsy, where aspiration is suspected, iso-osmolar non-ionic water-soluble contrast media should be used. This contrast does not provoke pulmonary edema if aspirated. Suspected 'H'-type tracheoesophageal fistulae are examined using video recording with the child in the prone or lateral position. A nasogastric tube is inserted into the esophagus. Contrast is injected to distend the esophagus during withdrawal of the tube from the carina to the pharynx. Contrast is seen to cross from the esophagus forwards and upwards into the trachea. Video recording is necessary to avoid confusion with spillover of contrast from the larynx.

Ultrasound

This non-invasive modality is the first-line investigation in congenital heart disease. The technique also provides a rapid method to determine the presence of a pericardial effusion. An opaque hemithorax, whether due to consolidation, pleural fluid (Fig. 39.3) or an underlying neoplasm, can be assessed. This avoids the need for further X-ray films. Ultrasound can differentiate between subpulmonary pleural fluid, subphrenic fluid and an elevated diaphragm and can assess diaphragmatic movement.

Pulmonary and mediastinal masses can be visualized with ultrasound if adjacent to the chest wall or heart. The consistency of the mass, whether cystic or solid, can be assessed. Sequestration of the lung is characterized by a solid or cystic mass in the lower zones and the supplying arterial vessel can often be visualized piercing the diaphragm. The characteristics of the blood flow in the vessel can be analyzed with a Doppler study. Contrast enhanced CT or MRI further identify the anatomy.

Computerized tomography scanning

This sectional technique is of value in the imaging of pulmonary and mediastinal masses.[25] The technique will display any calcification, fat or bone destruction associated with the abnormality. The differentiation of primary pulmonary consolidation, abscess formation and empyema can be made with this technique. Contrast enhancement will outline the vascular pleura leaving the contents of an empyema unopacified. Primary pulmonary diseases including bronchiectasis (Fig. 39.4), interstitial fibrosis and cystic adenomatoid malformation can also be assessed using thin section high-resolution technique.[7] In suspected air trapping sections on inspiration and expiration are evaluated. Artifacts from areas of atelectasis are produced in the lung fields if a general anesthetic is used. CT can also be used in the demonstration of tracheal and laryngeal anatomy.

MRI scanning of the chest

MRI can delineate the extent and the tissue nature of mediastinal masses, e.g. fluid in a cystic hygroma (Fig. 39.5) or fat in a teratoma. The technique can demonstrate intrathecal involvement of paravertebral masses such as neuroblastoma. The technique allows

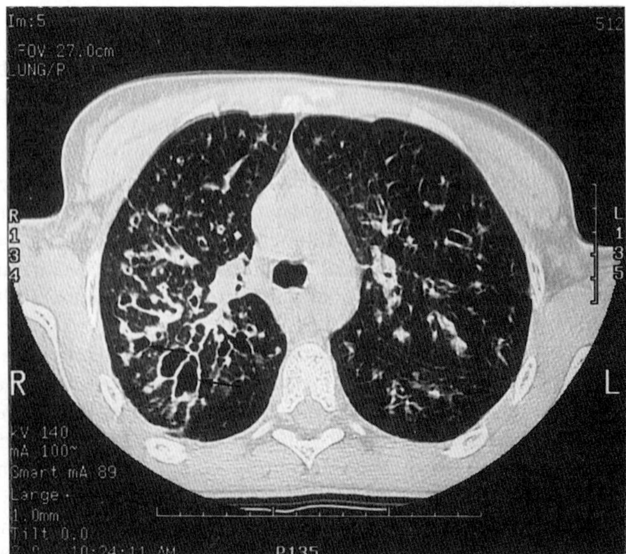

Fig. 39.4 High resolution computed tomography scan of the lungs demonstrating diffuse bronchiectasis.

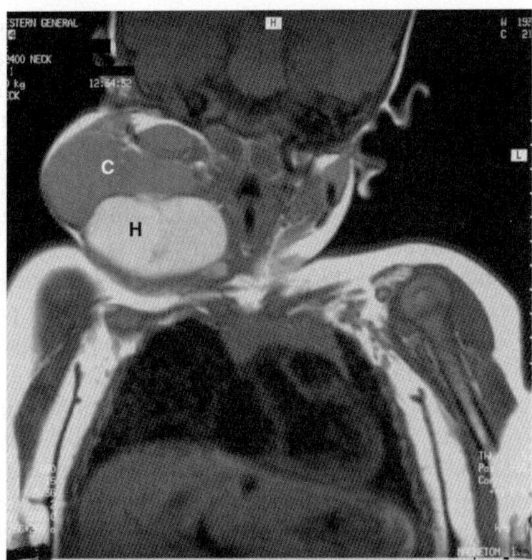

Fig. 39.5 Cystic hygroma: coronal T1-weighted image showing cysts (C) in soft tissues of the right side of the neck. Cyst with high signal indicates previous hemorrhage (H).

demonstration of arteries and veins without the need of contrast media and hence can be used to diagnose vascular rings causing stridor, and differentiate vessels from other masses causing compression, e.g. lymph nodes.[26]

The technique has the advantages of portraying the image in any plane (coronal, sagittal and axial) but does not as yet have the resolution of CT for the imaging of parenchymal lung disease. For the role of MRI in cardiac disease, see Chapter 19.

Radionuclide scanning

Radionuclide studies provide reliable information regarding lung perfusion and ventilation. Ventilation lung scans can be performed using xenon 133 or 127, with an aerosol ('Technegas') or krypton 81m. The use of xenon or an aerosol can be extremely difficult in a small, uncooperative child and, although difficult to obtain, krypton is particularly useful as it has a short half-life of 13 seconds, can be inhaled through a simple mask and provides better quality images. Perfusion scanning to assess the pulmonary blood flow to the lungs is usually carried out using technetium 99m macroaggregates of albumin (MAA). The pulmonary arterioles are temporarily occluded by the albumin particles. The number of arterioles and alveoli increase rapidly from about 4 months to 3 years before reaching the adult level at about 8 years. The number of particles injected should be reduced in proportion to the child's weight/surface area with a further 50% reduction if the child has a right to left shunt or pulmonary hypertension.

Lung scans are useful in the assessment of several congenital lung lesions, e.g. congenital lobar emphysema, or hypoplasia. They also have a role in the preoperative and postoperative assessment of some forms of congenital heart disease, e.g. right to left shunts and pulmonary artery hypoplasia. They are valuable in the follow-up of children with foreign body aspiration, previous collapse and/or consolidation, bronchiectasis and cystic fibrosis. They can be used in the diagnosis of the occasional child with suspected pulmonary emboli.

ALIMENTARY TRACT

The radiographic investigations with the lowest positive yield are those referred for vague abdominal pain, encopresis and constipation. Acute appendicitis is a clinical diagnosis which does not require the use of contrast studies although in young children more difficult diagnoses may be confirmed with ultrasound or CT although the latter has a high radiation dose.

Cradles are useful devices for immobilizing infants for alimentary tract examinations, reducing handling and inducing reassurance analogous to wrapping an infant in a shawl.

Conventional radiography

Plain films are useful in assessing mechanical obstructions from esophagus to rectum, whether congenital or acquired. Supine films sometimes require supplementation with horizontal beam films which can be taken with the child erect, decubitus with right side raised or with a lateral shoot-through view with the child supine or prone. These views may demonstrate air fluid levels and evaluate any free intraperitoneal air following perforation. In children over 1 year of age the nature of dilated bowel loops can be recognized by the same criteria used in adults – jejunum with complete transverse folds, ileum featureless and colon with haustrations which do not extend across the whole lumen. However, in infancy the site and number of dilated loops is a better guide and in anorectal atresia the rectum may not fill with swallowed air until 48 h after birth, best demonstrated with the baby lying prone over a pillow or wedge.

Intussusceptions can be identified on plain films as a soft tissue density mass anywhere along the line of the colon. A degree of small bowel obstruction is often present. Ultrasound clearly demonstrates the intussuscepting mass even when it is obscured on plain films due to dilated bowel loops and in many departments obviates the need for radiographs.

In necrotizing enterocolitis the plain film findings include thickened bowel mucosa, immotile bowel loops, intramural gas which has a linear or bubble-like pattern and, rarely, portal venous gas seen as a branching lucent appearance within the liver. Free intraperitoneal gas following perforation may be recognized on the supine film as a central lucency (Fig. 39.6), the so-called football sign, the central lace due to the outlined falciform ligament.

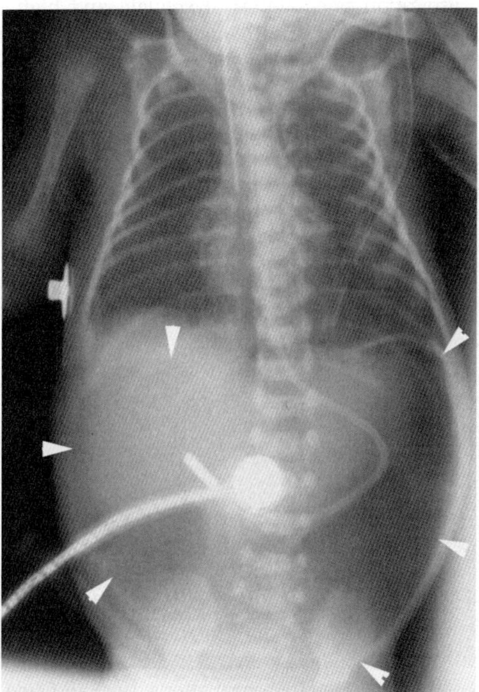

Fig. 39.6 Pneumoperitoneum: supine film showing large central lucency (arrowheads).

A gas-free abdomen is sinister in infancy – it may denote an infant so debilitated that the normal amount of air cannot be swallowed, a stomach filled with excess secretions in high obstruction or a high esophageal atresia without distal tracheoesophageal fistula. If there is clinical doubt a little air introduced through a nasogastric catheter will help to differentiate. A stiff opaque catheter held in the upper pouch during a plain film of the chest and upper abdomen is all that is required to confirm esophageal atresia (Fig. 39.7). The level of the atresia will be shown as well as any associated vertebral anomaly and the presence of a distal tracheoesophageal fistula will be confirmed by the presence of abdominal bowel gas. The position of the aortic knuckle is seen best on a penetrated chest film but US may be required for definitive visualization. This information is vital to the surgeon in planning the approach.

Peritoneal calcification in the newborn denotes prenatal perforation (calcification can become visible within 4 days of perforation at this age) and is commonly secondary to obstructive bowel disease including atresia and meconium ileus. Apart from swallowed foreign bodies fecoliths are the commonest intra-abdominal opacities in the UK and can be extremely helpful in the diagnosis of appendicitis.

Loss of definition or displacement of the normal preperitoneal fat and the psoas shadows in relation to inflammatory disease and neoplasm are useful in older children but are rarely seen in young infants.

Contrast studies

Barium sulfate is cheap and safe and is the most commonly used contrast in the alimentary tract. It is contraindicated in perforation as a leak may cause mediastinitis or peritonitis. It does not cause pulmonary edema if aspirated. When perforation is suspected low osmolality water-soluble contrast should be used. High osmolality water-soluble contrast should not be used in upper gastrointestinal (GI) studies in children due to the risk of pulmonary edema if aspirated.

Indications for barium studies in children include persistent vomiting, aspiration pneumonias, dysphagia and high intestinal obstructions particularly due to malrotation and volvulus. Milk isotope studies and pH monitoring have reduced the need for barium meals to detect gastroesophageal reflux and upper GI endoscopy is preferred to detect peptic ulceration. Fasting for 4 h is adequate preparation for barium meals and barium can be given from a bottle, feeder cup, beaker or straw. Barium is injected down a nasogastric tube when children cannot or will not swallow. High-density barium (e.g. 200% weight for volume) should be used for double contrast technique studies to detect fine mucosal abnormalities in the esophagus, stomach and duodenum. Low-density barium (50–100%) should be used for single contrast examinations to detect malrotation or for small bowel examinations. In a tiny premature neonate 5 ml of barium may suffice though an adolescent may require 500 ml to perform a small bowel examination.

The small bowel enema is a technique where contrast is injected directly into the jejunum through an appropriately placed nasojejunal tube. This is followed by methylcellulose, water, saline or air. Screening of the barium column as it passes through the gut improves visualization of individual bowel loops and is useful in the diagnosis of Crohn's disease and lymphoma.

Malabsorption is better investigated with biochemical techniques and biopsy studies. A symptomatic Meckel's diverticulum is rarely filled on barium follow-through investigation. In malrotation the position of the duodenojejunal flexure is low and to the right of the midline. If volvulus has occurred partial duodenal obstruction may be present or the spiral shape of the twisted midgut noted (Fig. 39.8). If the diagnosis is in doubt then a follow-through study with screening of the ileocecal region is necessary. A barium enema is no longer regarded as the best investigation for the diagnosis of malrotation.[27]

Endoscopy is now recognized as the first line investigation in inflammatory bowel disease particularly in situations where biopsy of the mucosa is required. However, barium contrasts are also commonly used to examine the colon and rectum. The double

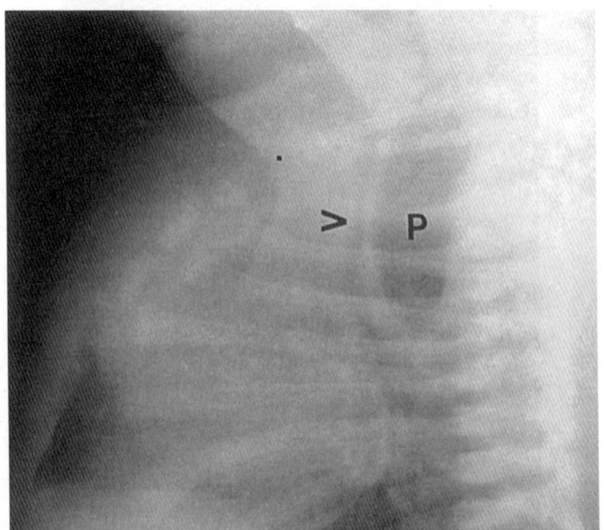

Fig. 39.7 Newborn with esophageal atresia. Note air filling the proximal esophageal pouch (P) indenting the trachea. Associated tracheal narrowing due to tracheomalacia (arrowhead).

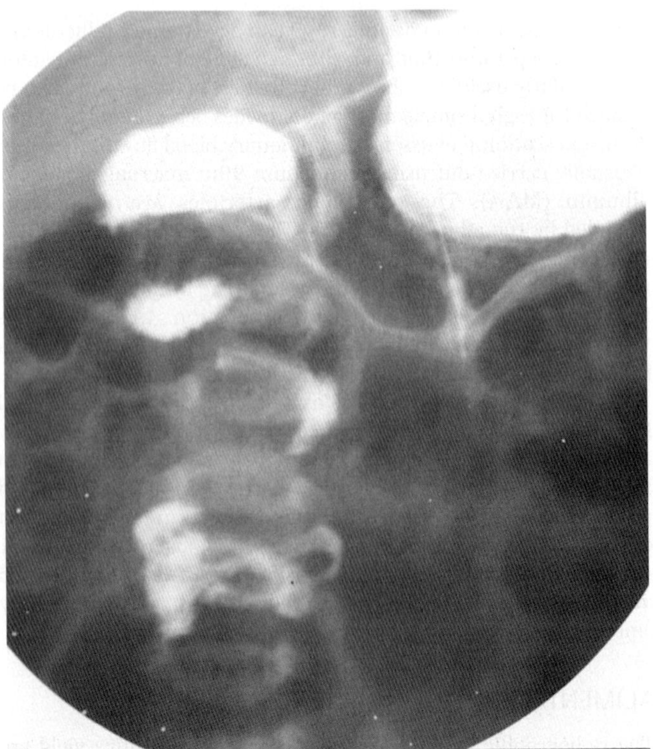

Fig. 39.8 Barium meal showing volvulus: 'corkscrew' appearance of proximal jejunum.

contrast technique requires excellent cleansing of the large bowel. Preparation involves a low-residue diet for 24 h, together with an orally effective laxative. High-density barium is used to fill the colon which is then drained to remove surplus contrast. Air is insufflated to distend the colon, leaving only a thin layer of barium coating the mucosa to demonstrate abnormalities such as ulceration or polyps (Fig. 39.9). Most information can be obtained with two decubitus views which should be inspected before other films are taken. The technique is best deferred for 7 days after full-thickness colonic biopsy. Unprepared single contrast enemas with low-density barium (50% w/v) may be performed in constipated children suspected of having Hirschsprung's disease to detect the zone of transition (Fig. 39.10) from the narrow aganglionic segment distally to the distended colon laden with feces proximally. Balloon catheters should not be used since this may obscure a transition zone in the rectum. A 24-h film may show delayed colonic clearance of barium which may be diagnostic of Hirschsprung's disease. Rectal biopsy provides histological confirmation.

Reduction of an intussusception with contrast is a well-recognized procedure in the correct clinical setting. Contraindications are complete bowel obstruction, the presence of perforation or peritonitis and an extremely sick child. Air is now preferred to barium[28] and insufflated into the rectum with a hand pump, using a small valve or a sphygmomanometer to limit the pressure to 120 mmHg. In some centers special pumps with flow rate and pressure controls have been devised. Air can be seen distending the distal colon and outlining the intussusception as a soft tissue mass that moves proximally. When the intussusception is reduced there is sudden loss of the soft tissue mass in the cecum and air distention of the terminal ileum (Fig. 39.11a & b). This endpoint of successful reduction can be more difficult to appreciate if there is gaseous distention of small bowel due to obstruction and a water-soluble contrast enema may then be helpful for confirmation. It is commonly observed that the child relaxes almost immediately following successful reduction.

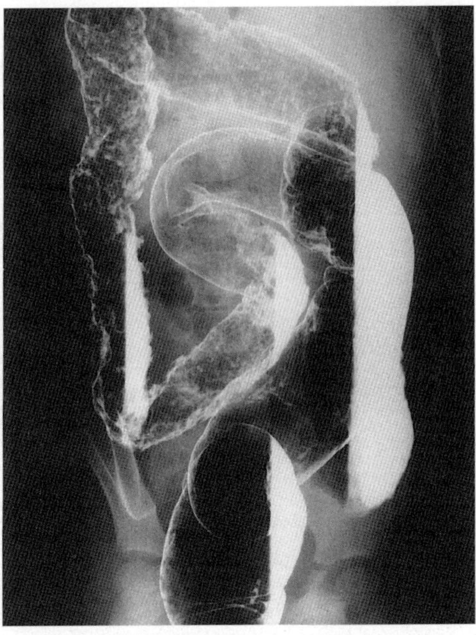

Fig. 39.9 Double contrast barium enema showing typical changes of ulcerative colitis with superficial and submucosal ulceration throughout the colon.

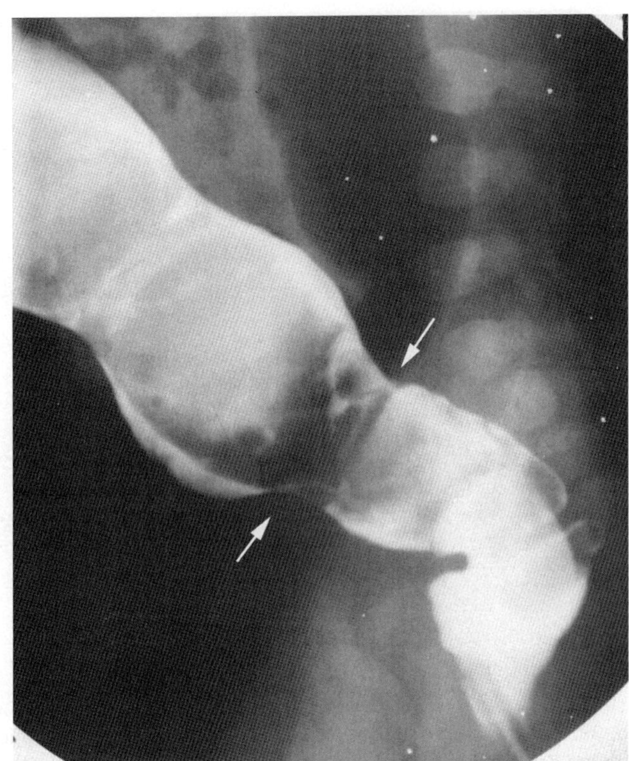

Fig. 39.10 Hirschsprung's disease: barium enema showing zone of transition (arrows).

The success rate of reduction is generally claimed to be higher for air than barium (over 90% for air). Perforation is rare and easily recognized by air outlining the liver. Perforation with air causes less peritoneal contamination and a smaller perforation defect as compared with barium.[29] Respiratory distress from abdominal distention following perforation has been reported, though if air insufflation is stopped immediately, this will not occur. If air reduction is not complete on the first attempt, a further attempt performed a few hours later may be successful. Reduction of intussusception using saline as the hydrostatic medium together with ultrasound monitoring has recently been reported with a 91% success rate.[30]

In the diagnosis and treatment of meconium ileus and meconium plug syndrome hypertonic water-soluble contrast is used.[31] This contrast lubricates the obstructing plugs and, being hypertonic, draws fluid into the gut lumen, softening the plug. Undiluted Gastrografin may cause mucosal ulceration and in our practice the contrast is diluted from an osmolality of 2150 to 700 mOsmol/L. The use of hypertonic contrast media requires simultaneous intravenous fluid replacement therapy to avoid dehydration in the small baby. Plain film evidence of perforation, either recent with free intraperitoneal air or old reflected by peritoneal calcification, is a contraindication to therapeutic enema. Perforation may indicate intestinal volvulus or small bowel atresia.[31] Liaison with the surgical team before therapeutic enema ensures that should perforation occur as a complication of the procedure, it can be dealt with promptly.

Ultrasound examination

The use of ultrasound examination in gastrointestinal problems is now well recognized. Ultrasound diagnosis of pyloric stenosis is 100% accurate in experienced hands and has replaced barium meal. The findings of the pyloric canal on ultrasound are of an

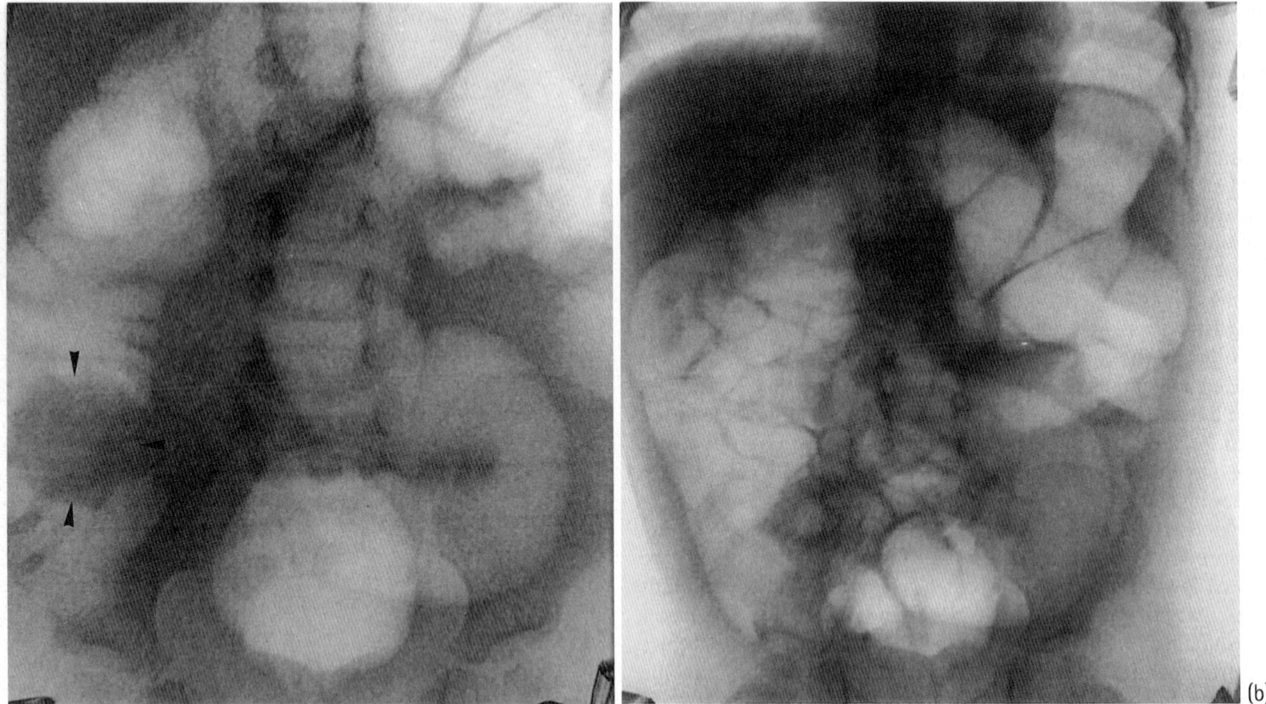

Fig. 39.11 Intussusception. (a) Air enema reduction of intussusception (arrowheads). (b) Final reduction showing free filling of the small bowel with gas and the disappearance of the soft tissue swelling of the intussusception.

elongated canal measuring over 14 mm in length, over 12 mm in diameter inclusive of muscle thickness of over 3.5 mm which fails to shorten and open in response to vigorous gastric peristalsis (Fig. 39.12). Ultrasound can also be used to diagnose intussusception and the typical appearances are of a target or 'donut' shaped intra-abdominal mass (Fig. 39.13). The examination is particularly useful in those children presenting with obstruction where the mass is not seen on the plain film.[32] Ultrasound can demonstrate free intraperitoneal fluid indicating transudate caused by venous engorgement; air reduction can still be successful but should be undertaken with care since free fluid can also indicate necrosis of the bowel wall. Risk factors for reduction also include intestinal obstruction, loss of Doppler flow in the intussusception,[33] and fluid trapped within the colon due to incarceration.[34]

The technique will also demonstrate duplication cysts of the bowel and dilated fluid-filled loops of gut in obstruction and ileus and evaluate mucosal thickening. Small amounts (more than 10 ml) of free intraperitoneal fluid can be clearly detected in the pelvis or subhepatic area.

Ultrasound is a sensitive and specific technique for the diagnosis of acute appendicitis. The criteria for diagnosis include non-compressibility of the appendix, a transverse diameter greater than 6 mm, mucosal edema and the presence of an appendicolith (Fig. 39.14).[35–37] In hemolytic uremic syndrome the clinical presentation of the child may be with abdominal pain and rectal bleeding. A target sign may be seen with ultrasound representing the hemorrhagic gut mucosa. This may be confused with an intussusception. Doppler ultrasound may reveal generalized avascularity of the gut[38] which is a manifestation of the ischemic vasculitis which occurs in this condition. It is worthy of note that the kidney parenchyma may be hyperechoic reflecting the glomerular vasculitis. It is to be noted that thickened mucosa can also be demonstrated on ultrasound in Crohn's disease (Fig. 39.15a & b) and ulcerative colitis.

The diagnosis of an intra-abdominal abscess is suggested by a thick-walled cystic lesion often sited in the pelvis. Ultrasound may also be used to assess upper gut obstruction and the injection of

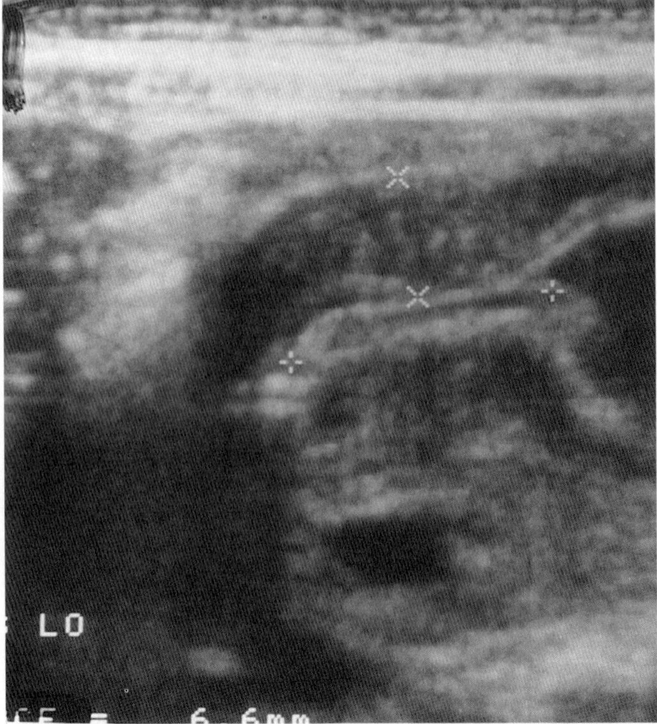

Fig. 39.12 Pyloric stenosis. Longitudinal ultrasound scan through the pylorus. The vertical crosses indicate the length of the canal, oblique crosses the thickness of the muscle layer.

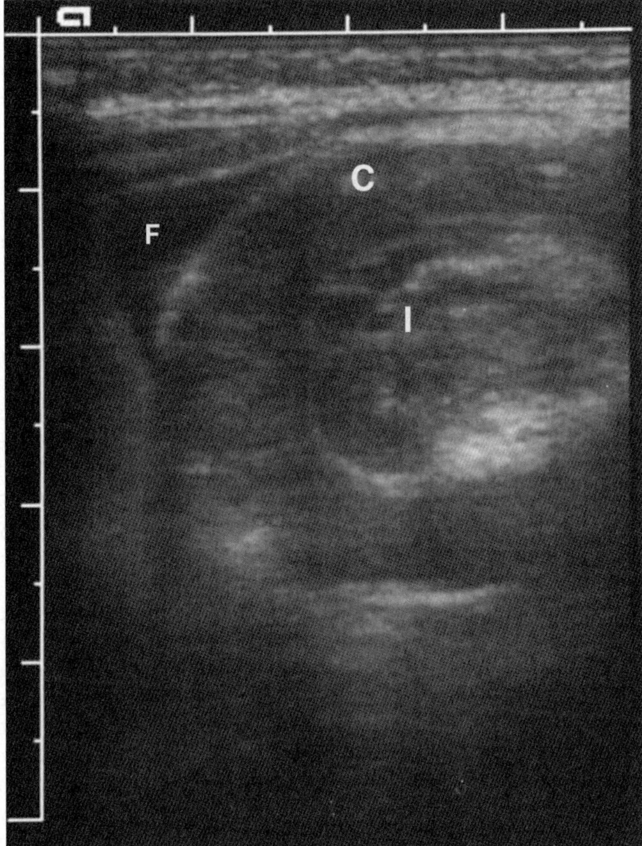

Fig. 39.13 Intussusception: transverse US showing 'donut' appearance with intussuscepted small bowel (I), colonic wall (C) and a little free intraperitoneal fluid (F).

fluid into the stomach through a nasogastric tube allows visualization of a dilated fluid-filled duodenum secondary to duodenal obstruction. In malrotation the anatomical relationships of the superior mesenteric artery and vein are usually altered. Thus the transverse US section at the level of the uncinate lobe of the pancreas reveals the vein situated to the left of the artery compared with its normal right anterolateral position. However US is not sufficiently reliable to replace the barium meal in the diagnosis of malrotation.[39] In anorectal atresia the fluid- or meconium-filled rectum can be identified as a transonic or mixed echoic structure. When scanning from the perineum the distance between the skin and the rectum can be measured directly. If this is less than 1 cm the atresia is unlikely to be complicated by the presence of a fistula and represents a so-called low lesion.

Nuclear medicine studies

Technetium 99m pertechnetate is taken up by the mucus secretory cells of gastric mucosa as well as by the thyroid gland and choroid plexus. Meckel's diverticulae or duplication cysts containing gastric mucosa will take up the radionuclide. The child should be fasted for 3–4 h prior to the examination. Some centers have found the use of cimetidine in a dose of 20 mg/kg in three divided doses on the day before the examination with a double dose on the morning of the examination to be helpful, as it blocks secretion of pertechnetate from the gastric mucosa and improves the lesion-to-background ratio. An area of abnormal uptake of the radionuclide should appear at the same time as stomach activity and may be found anywhere in the abdomen.

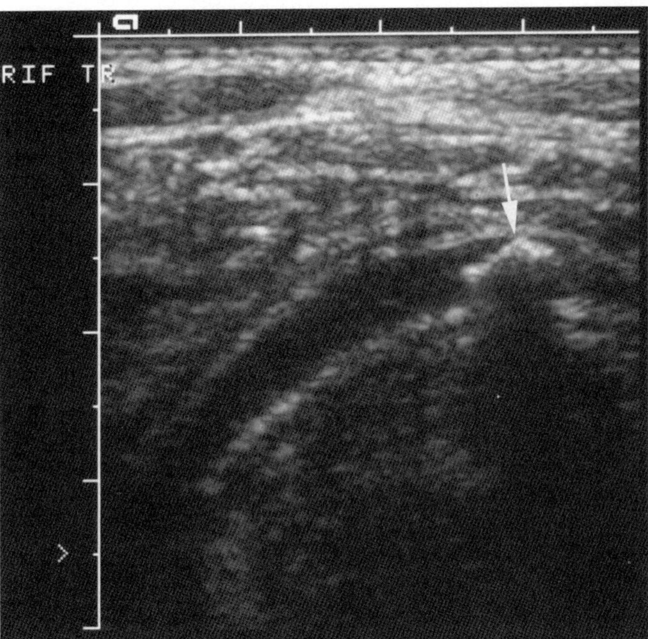

Fig. 39.14 Appendicitis: US in longitudinal plane of appendix showing appendicolith (arrow).

Technetium sulfur colloid can be added to milk and used in the assessment of gastroesophageal reflux or gastric emptying. Technetium HMPAO (hexamethylpropyleneamine oxime) labeled white cells have recently been used in the diagnosis of inflammatory bowel disease such as ulcerative colitis and Crohn's disease. Increased activity in the small and large bowel occurs in areas involved with the disease. The same radionuclide has replaced the use of indium 111 in the labeling of white blood cells for the investigation of suspected inflammatory lesions such as abdominal abscesses.

Computerized tomography

This has a limited place in gastrointestinal imaging, but is useful in the investigation of appendicitis, intraperitoneal abscess and trauma to the abdominal organs.[13] Contrast-enhanced CT has the ability to examine multiple organs as well as identifying free intraperitoneal air and coincidental damage to bony structures including the spine and pelvis.

LIVER AND BILIARY TRACT

The common clinical indications for radiological imaging of the liver are trauma, hepatomegaly, jaundice and portal hypertension. There are numerous causes of liver enlargement, including heart failure, hepatitis, septicemia, storage diseases, alpha1-antitrypsin deficiency and primary and secondary neoplasms. Plain X-rays are of little value.

Ultrasound is the initial imaging method and will define the liver size, shape and consistency. Decreased echoity generally or discrete hypoechoic masses are characteristic of leukemic and lymphomatous infiltration. Increased echoity is seen in fatty infiltration, cirrhosis and hemochromatosis. Cysts and abscesses have a mainly transonic appearance with a rim of variable thickness. Fungal infection occurs in immunocompromised children and can appear as multiple areas of increased or decreased echogenicity, target lesions (concentric high and low echogenicity) or diffuse abnormality of echotexture; these lesions can be biopsied

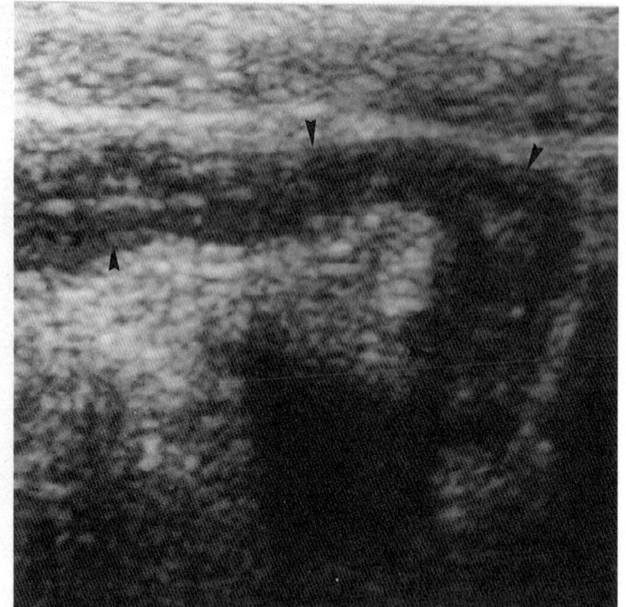
(a)

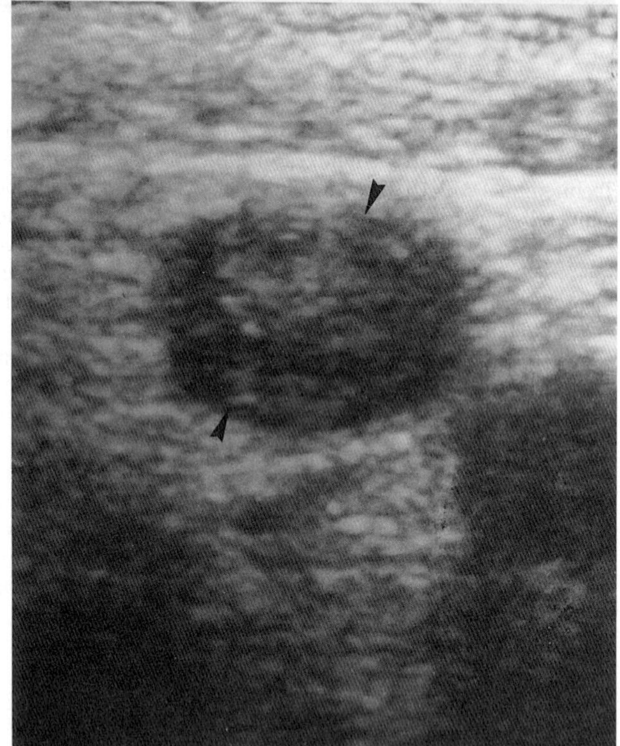
(b)

Fig. 39.15 Crohn's disease. Ultrasound scan through the terminal ileum showing hypoechoic edematous mucosa (arrowheads) representing the string sign: (a) longitudinal, (b) transverse sections.

under ultrasound guidance. Primary liver tumors are usually hyperechoic.[40] Areas of necrosis, however, impart a variable consistency with transonic and echoic features on ultrasound. Indeed, hemangioendotheliomas and mesenchymal hamartomas may have a large cystic component. Ultrasound can be used in the initial assessment of liver, splenic and renal trauma. Contusion or laceration may be seen and free intraperitoneal fluid identified.

Ultrasound is also the mainstay in imaging of the biliary tract. The patient should be fasted from fatty foods and maintain a clear fluid intake for 6 h before the examination. The bile-filled gall bladder is clearly demonstrated and the presence of gallstones and mucosal thickening assessed. An absent or small gall bladder is a feature of biliary atresia; the obliterated remains of the extrahepatic bile ducts may be seen on US as the triangular cord sign.[41] It is recognized that the presence of a choledochal cyst in the intrahepatic portal region is suggestive of an underlying biliary atresia. In less than 5% of cases, dilatation of the intrahepatic biliary ducts is seen. The diameter of the normal common bile duct should be less than 4 mm. Obstructive biliary disease is rare in children but is described secondary to gallstones (seen in hemolytic disease, inflammatory bowel disease, therapy with certain drugs, especially ciclosporin, or prolonged parenteral nutrition), enlarged portal lymph nodes, lymphoma, retroperitoneal sarcomas or primitive pancreatic tumors.

Choledochal cysts are characterized by a transonic cystic mass separate from the gall bladder and in the line of the common bile duct (Fig. 39.16). A dilated gall bladder has been described in Kawasaki's disease, secondary to parenteral nutrition and in acalculus cholecystitis and is a non-specific finding in many children who are sick from a variety of causes. Sludge and debris often layer along the gall bladder floor.

Analogs of iminodiacetic acid linked to technetium are excreted by hepatocytes and are used to assess biliary drainage. The third-generation derivative trimethyl bromoiminodiacetic acid (BROMIDA) is particularly useful in the jaundiced neonate suspected of having biliary atresia. The presence of radionuclide in the gut will exclude this diagnosis (Fig. 39.17), though its absence does not confirm the diagnosis as severe hepatitis can cause a similar picture. Uptake of the radionuclide is enhanced by giving the neonate a 5-day course of phenobarbital 5 mg/kg/day in divided doses. BROMIDA scanning is also valuable in the follow-up of children with portoenterostomies for biliary atresia.

Doppler ultrasound is useful in the assessment of liver disease, particularly in biliary cirrhosis, portal hypertension and after liver transplantation. The hepatic arterial blood flow, portal venous and hepatic venous flow is assessed. Color Doppler enables the direction of flow to be more easily determined. In thrombosis of the vessels no flow is recorded. In portal vein thrombosis the normal portal vein is absent and replaced by peripheral collaterals. In stenosis of the portal vein altered frequency shifts at the level of the narrowing are noted. In

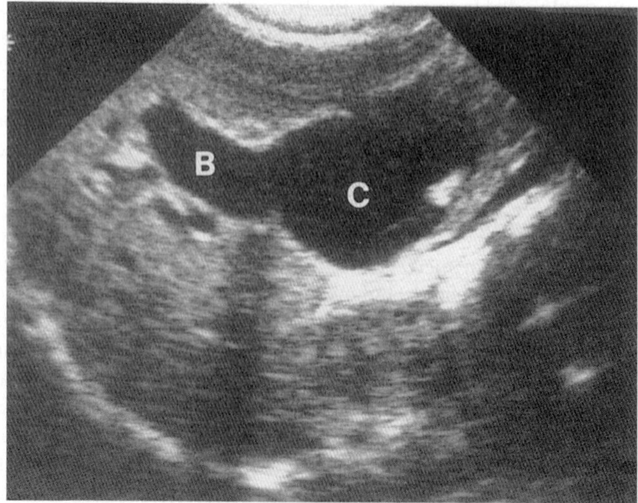

Fig. 39.16 Sagittal ultrasound section through the liver. Note transonic area representing the choledochal cyst (C) and associated dilatation of the common bile duct (B).

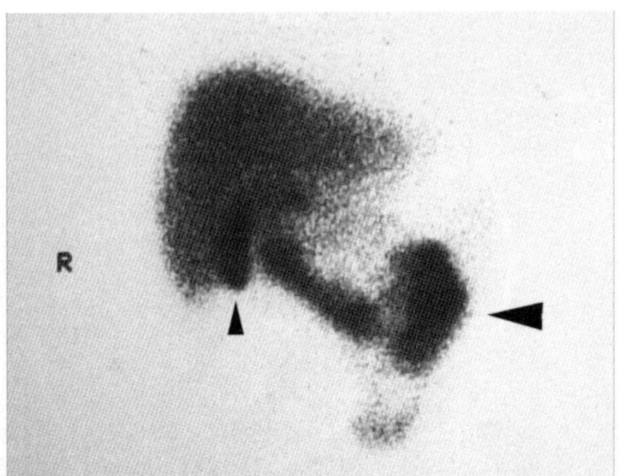

Fig. 39.17 HIDA scan: anterior 30-minute view showing normal drainage of activity into the gall bladder (small arrowhead) and small bowel (large arrowhead).

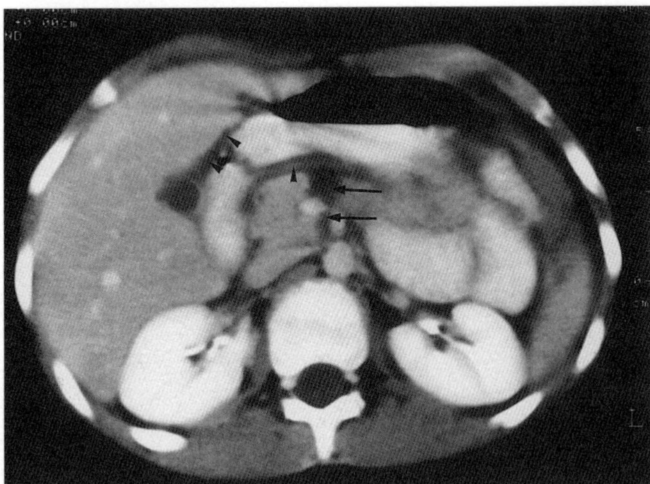

Fig. 39.18 Axial CT scans through the pancreas with contrast enhancement of the gut and kidney. Pancreatic laceration (long arrows), free fluid seen in the lesser sac and under the liver (arrowheads).

progressive biliary cirrhosis reduced diastolic flow in the hepatic artery may be found. Thickening of the lesser omentum and varices can be visualized. The technique cannot measure portal venous pressure.

CT scanning can further evaluate the extent of the liver masses but in children appears to be less sensitive in detecting disease than ultrasonic investigation.

MRI scanning is now the second line investigation after US in demonstrating hepatic abnormalities such as mass lesions and abnormal tissue characteristics such as fatty infiltration, iron overload and contrast enhancement. Superparamagnetic contrast agents based on manganese or iron are taken up by the reticular cells and can differentiate normal liver tissue from mass lesions.

Angiography may be indicated in the preoperative assessment of liver tumors and indirect portal venography is helpful if portosystemic shunting is being considered. Two-dimensional Doppler ultrasound is used, however, in the routine assessment of portal hypertension.

PANCREAS AND SPLEEN

These organs are best imaged with CT and ultrasound. The ultrasonic appearance of acute pancreatitis is characterized by a swollen pancreas of low echogenicity and ill-defined outline. Chronic pancreatitis as seen in cystic fibrosis is characterized by a small hyperechoic organ. Pancreatic pseudocysts following trauma or inflammation are clearly defined as transonic areas. Splenic enlargement may be an indication of reactive splenomegaly in systemic infection, portal hypertension, or splenic disease such as infiltration with leukemic tissue, or deposition diseases including mucopolysaccharidosis. Splenic involvement with lymphoma or leukemia is characterized by discrete or diffuse areas of low echogenicity. Splenic fungal abscesses may occur in immunocompromised children and can have increased or decreased echogenicity or target appearance. Both ultrasound and CT are of value in assessing abdominal trauma (Fig. 39.18). Scintigraphy with labeled denatured red cells will accurately delineate viable splenic tissue in suspected asplenia.

CENTRAL NERVOUS SYSTEM

Plain radiographs

Plain skull X-rays may be considered obsolete if CT services are available, but are still useful in the initial assessment of suspected craniostenosis, metastatic and metabolic bone disease and fractures of the skull vault. Conventional radiography is still requested after trauma to the skull and spine but its place after skull trauma is the subject of ongoing acrimonious debate. In children the relationship between skull fracture and intracranial injury is poor and CT when clinically indicated is becoming the first line imaging method in head trauma.[42]

Imaging of the spinal cord is now performed with MR. Plain films may be helpful in the immediate assessment of major spinal trauma, supplemented with CT if fractures and/or dislocation are suspected.

Ultrasound

A 7.5 MHz transducer is used in premature babies and neonates with access through the anterior fontanel, though a 5 MHz transducer is necessary to visualize the posterior fossa adequately in older babies. A high frequency (10–12 MHz) linear transducer should be used to assess the extra-axial spaces.

The indications for US are in the assessment of parenchymal changes following hypoxia in the neonate with detection and grading of intraventricular hemorrhage (Fig. 39.19). Acute severe hypoxic injury can occur without visible changes on ultrasound and CT or preferably MRI should be performed if there is clinical doubt. Periventricular leukomalacia is characterized by initial periventricular echogenicity followed by developing cystic changes and enlarging ventricles. The position of drainage catheters can also be assessed. Meningitis may be recognized by increased meningeal echogenicity, widened extra-axial spaces containing echogenic debris, secondary hydrocephalus and parenchymal echogenic areas representing complicating infarcts. Congenital brain abnormalities detectable on ultrasound include absence of the corpus callosum with a high midline 3rd ventricle and separation of the lateral ventricles, holoprosencephaly, midline brain cysts and the Arnold–Chiari malformations. Congenital brain tumors, papillomas and teratomas are rare.

Papillomas are of high echoity and usually present in the 3rd and lateral ventricles. Teratomas have a mixed echoity often with total disorganization of brain tissue. A widened subdural space is seen in children with macrocrania. This is often a benign appearance and in the absence of other clinical abnormalities, the appearance returns to normal with growth of the child. A wide space is also seen in the presence of pathological fluid collections following trauma or infection or associated with cerebral atrophy.

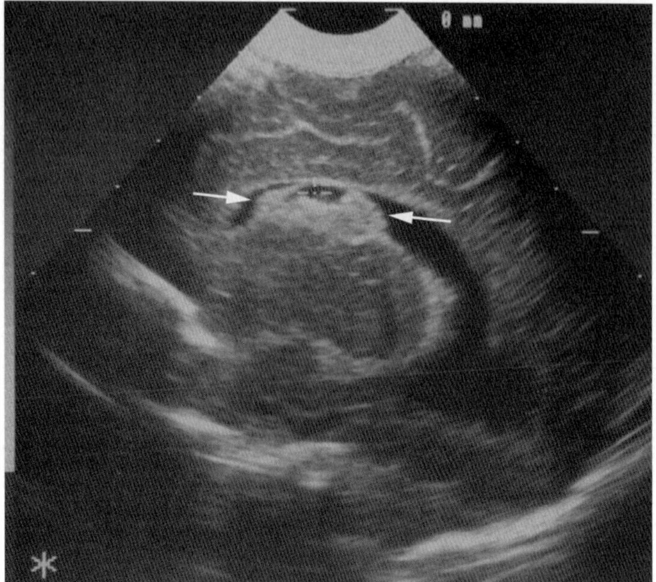

Fig. 39.19 Intraventricular hemorrhage: parasagittal US showing hemorrhage into the germinal matrix (between arrows) undergoing cystic (+) change.

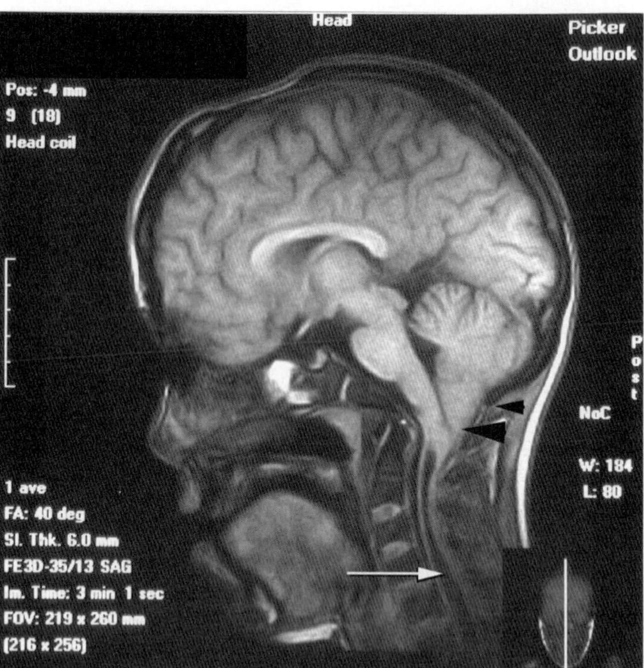

Fig. 39.20 Arnold–Chiari malformation: sagittal T1-weighted MR image showing tonsillar descent (large arrowhead) below the level of the foramen magnum (small arrowhead), and syringomyelia of the cervical cord (arrow).

It is possible to differentiate subdural from subarachnoid fluid collections; a network of vessels is seen within the arachnoid space and the arachnoid membrane itself can be visualized when using a modern high frequency linear probe.

Doppler ultrasound is helpful in the physiological assessment of cerebral abnormalities, including anoxia and cerebral hemorrhage, and diastolic flow may be reduced or absent in raised intracranial pressure. Doppler traces from the middle cerebral arteries can be obtained by scanning through the temporoparietal bones and the anterior cerebral arteries directly through the anterior fontanel. Assessment of arteriovenous malformations is possible demonstrating feeding arteries, draining veins and turbulent flow within the malformation.

The spinal cord and brainstem can be visualized with ultrasonic imaging in the neonate before the posterior vertebral elements ossify in the midline. The medullary pyramids and cerebellar vermis are assessed through either the anterior fontanel or foramen magnum. The position of the spinal cord, the conus and the cauda equina are assessed. In a child with obvious or occult spinal dysraphism, a tethered cord, the presence of a wide subarachnoid space or associated intraspinal lipoma may be recognized.

Computerized tomography

CT has largely been replaced with ultrasound and MRI but current indications for CT are acute trauma when complicated fractures (such as basal fractures and depressed fractures of the vault) and intracranial hemorrhage can be demonstrated. CT is occasionally useful in the further assessment of cerebral tumors, for example when the demonstration of fat or calcification is helpful. 3D reconstruction of CT scans may be helpful to the surgeon in complex craniofacial abnormalities. High resolution CT of the cochlea and vestibular structures is useful in the assessment of congenital deafness.

Magnetic resonance imaging

MR is now the cornerstone of brain imaging for suspected congenital abnormalities (Fig. 39.20), neoplasms (Fig. 39.21), epilepsy, developmental delay syndromes, infection, ischemia,[43] abscess formation, demyelination and the follow-up of trauma including non-accidental injury. MR can demonstrate the normal development of myelination[44] and abnormalities of white matter can be evaluated. Migration anomalies such as schizencephaly, cortical dysplasia and gray matter heteropia are demonstrated by MR.[45] T2-weighted MR images demonstrate brain edema with much greater sensitivity than CT and fluid attenuation inversion

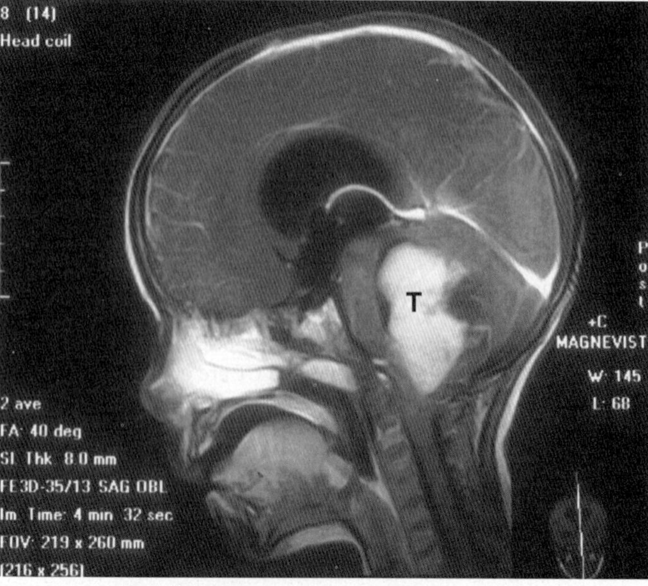

Fig. 39.21 Medulloblastoma: coronal T1-weighted MR image following injection of gadolinium showing tumor enhancement.

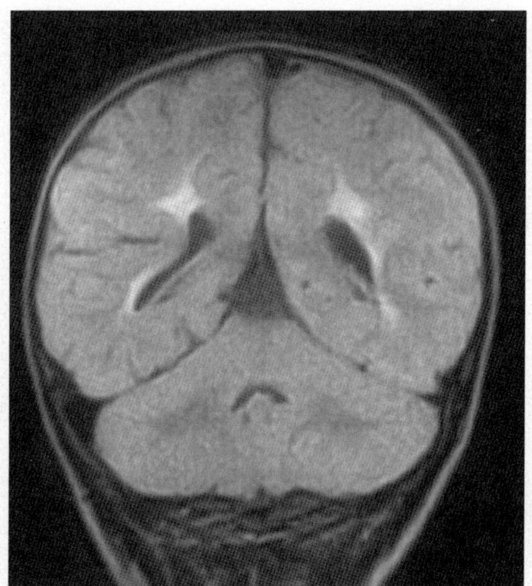

Fig. 39.22 Periventricular leukomalacia: coronal FLAIR MR image showing periventricular high signal.

recovery (FLAIR) sequences are particularly useful in demonstrating edema or gliosis in the periventricular white matter (Fig. 39.22). Early ischemic changes may best be appreciated with specialized MRI sequences such as diffusion weighted imaging which can detect changes as early as 6 h after injury. In diffusion weighted imaging there is signal hyperintensity in regions of restricted diffusion which is believed to reflect the shift of water from extracellular to intracellular compartments in compromised brain tissue.[46] Special sequences can be used for demonstration of CSF flow in the evaluation of hydrocephalus. MR angiography can demonstrate anomalies such as arteriovenous malformations, aneurysms and vessel occlusions.

Angiography

Cerebral angiography may still be indicated in the investigation of vascular malformations, intracranial aneurysms and occlusive disease of the intracranial vessels, particularly if intervention is anticipated. Selective catheterization through the femoral route is the safest and most usual method. Embolization of selected arteriovenous malformations and aneurysms may be possible.

Single photon emission computed tomography

SPECT scanning using 99m technetium HMPAO can be used in the assessment of regional cerebral blood flow. It is of particular value in localizing the focus of a seizure in children who fail to respond to medical therapy. There may be increased uptake of the radionuclide during an ictal scan with decreased uptake at the same site from an interictal study. It has been particularly useful in the assessment of children with temporal lobe epilepsy where surgery is contemplated.

URINARY TRACT

Ultrasound

US is the initial modality used in children presenting with urinary tract infection, hematuria, abdominal mass and enuresis. It is effective as a screen for congenital renal anomalies as part of chromosomal abnormalities and syndromes. The technique is also useful in assessing the natural history of fetal hydronephrosis and multicystic kidney.

The examination is of value in the diagnosis of congenital malformations, including horseshoe kidney, crossed renal ectopia or non-rotation. Duplex kidneys (Fig. 39.23) may be complicated by hydronephrosis, reflux and ureterocele. The dilated pelvicalyceal system, ureter and ureterocele can be directly visualized. Reflux nephropathy may produce a small kidney with an echogenic cortex. Localized renal scars are better demonstrated with ^{99m}Tc DMSA isotope scans.

Echogenic kidneys with or without loss of corticomedullary differentiation are seen in acute renal vein thrombosis, glomerular and interstitial disease and autosomal recessive polycystic kidney disease. The kidneys are also enlarged in the acute stages of these diseases.

Echogenic but small kidneys are seen in chronic glomerular disease, the later stages of renal vein thrombosis and renal dysplasia. Autosomal dominant polycystic kidney disease is characterized by discrete cysts in the renal cortex. However, it may be difficult to distinguish from autosomal recessive polycystic kidney disease in the earlier stages when the kidneys may be enlarged with small cysts in both conditions. Multicystic kidney disease is unusually unilateral and characterized by multiple non-communicating cysts.

Nephrocalcinosis (seen in renal tubular acidosis and hypercalcemia) is characterized by echogenic medullary pyramids. A similar appearance may be seen transiently as a normal appearance in the first few days of life.

US is extremely sensitive in detecting minor widening of the pelvicalyceal system. This can lead to difficulties in interpretation as it is a normal finding in well-hydrated children or secondary to ureteric distention from a full bladder. A false-positive diagnosis of early obstruction or vesicoureteric reflux may ensue. The AP diameter of the renal pelvis in the transverse scan should normally be less than 5–7 mm.

Renal calculi are easily seen in the parenchyma but small stones may be overlooked when sited in the non-dilated renal pelvis because of adjacent bright echoes from the renal sinus. Calculi lying in the focal plane of the transducer produce an acoustic shadow, allowing easier identification (Fig. 39.24). The bladder should be assessed and the presence of a ureterocele, trabeculation, residual urine or calculus identified. In posterior urethral valves, a dilated posterior urethra may be detected and examination of this area via

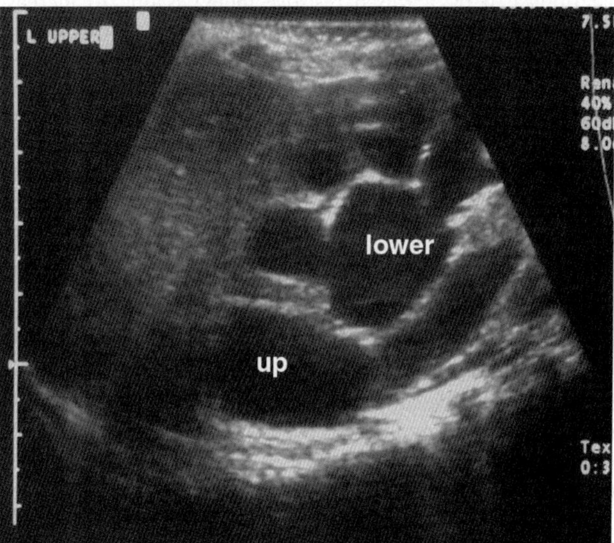

Fig. 39.23 Longitudinal US scan of duplex kidney showing upper (up) and lower (lower) moieties.

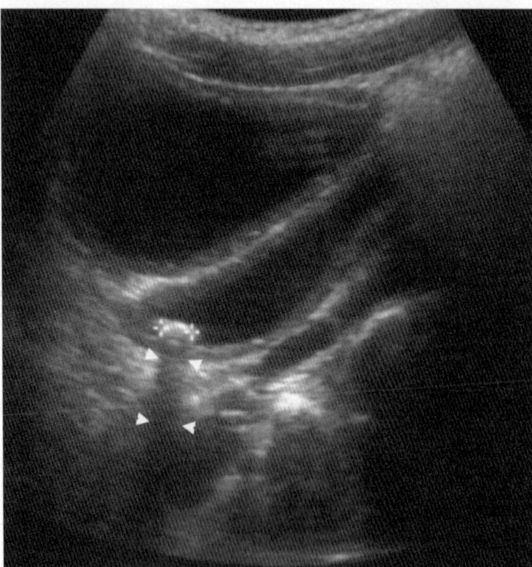

Fig. 39.24 Longitudinal US showing lower ureteric stone with acoustic shadowing (arrowheads).

a perineal approach is of value. Primary renal tumors, the most common being a nephroblastoma, are initially assessed with ultrasound where the size, shape and staging of the tumor is possible. Extension into the inferior vena cava (IVC) is well demonstrated especially with color Doppler ultrasound.

Sonographic detection of vesicoureteral reflux can be performed when US contrast agents containing microbubbles are injected into the bladder whilst US examination of the kidneys is performed. Increased echogenicity of urine in the renal pelvis indicates that reflux has occurred.[47]

Doppler ultrasound of the renal vessels is of value in the diagnosis of renal artery stenosis where changes in spectral profiles are seen at the site of stenosis and in the poststenotic area. The technique is also of value in the determination of renal vein patency in renal vein thrombosis. In hemolytic uremic syndrome, decreased flow in diastole is commonly seen in the active stages of the disease. Improvement in the RI usually precedes clinical recovery. Doppler ultrasound is used to monitor kidneys following renal transplantation; decreased diastolic flow (indicated by a raised resistive index) is due to increased resistance to perfusion which may be due to rejection, ciclosporin A toxicity, acute tubular necrosis, pyelonephritis, venous thrombosis or ureteric obstruction. Pelvicalyceal dilatation in a transplant kidney may be due to ureteric obstruction or reflux and differentiation may be impossible on US. Abnormalities of flow may be identified prior to the development of biochemical abnormalities and in the appropriate clinical context can indicate the need for biopsy which is best performed under US guidance.[48] Arterial occlusion is indicated by lack of flow within the transplanted organ.

Intravenous urography

The requirement for this examination has decreased with the advances in US and radioisotope and MR scanning. The indications are in the further evaluation of confusing results or for further imaging of an abnormality detected on ultrasound (Fig. 39.25). The technique may be required for further delineation of ureteric detail and assessment of congenital abnormalities.

In children under 2 years no preparation is required and in particular, dehydration is to be avoided. Non-ionic contrast media should be used in a concentration of 300 mg iodine/ml. The standard dose is 2–3 ml/kg up to a maximum of 50 ml. Following an initial plain film a 15-min full-length film of the renal tract often suffices for the examination. Delayed prone films may be indicated in the presence of obstruction. Lateral or oblique films or spot films under fluoroscopic control may occasionally be helpful.

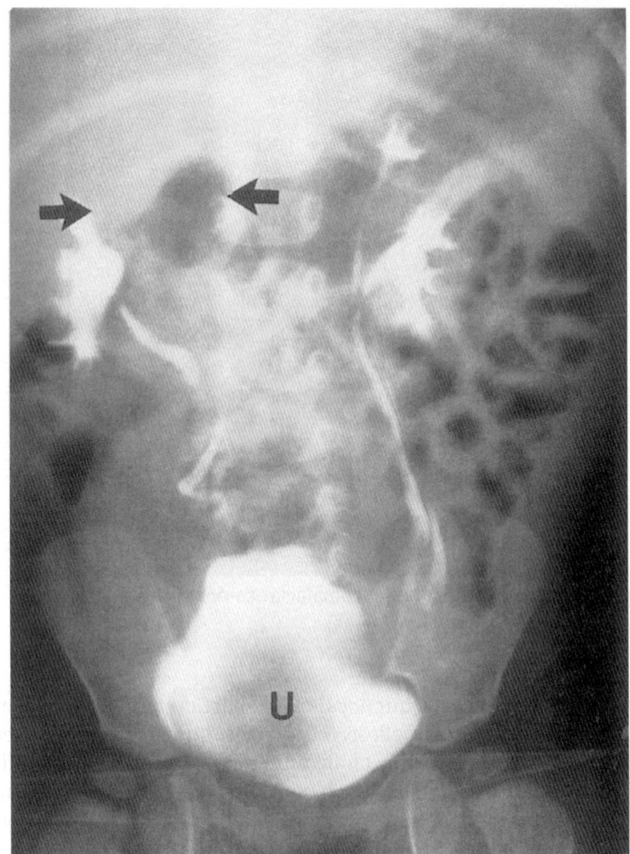

Fig. 39.25 Intravenous urogram in a child with bilateral duplex kidneys; note non-functioning upper moiety causing lateral deviation of lower moiety pelvis (arrows). Filling defect noted in the bladder representing ureterocele (U) associated with right upper moiety.

Micturating cystourethrography

The most common indication for MCU is in the investigation of urinary tract infection when reflux is suspected in a child less than 2 years of age. The examination is also indicated in those children found to have a dilated urinary tract on ultrasound. Vesicoureteric reflux is graded according to severity,[49] significant reflux being that reaching the kidney. Other indications for cystography include a child with a poor urinary stream and where abnormalities of the urethra are suspected.

Sedation is rarely required. Under sterile conditions a fine feeding tube is inserted into the bladder. If severe reflux is demonstrated during the procedure then the child should be started on antibiotics. The study is a dynamic process and a video recording of micturition with appropriate spot films is necessary. The configuration, shape and function of the bladder can be assessed and the presence of urethral abnormalities, valves, diverticula or strictures noted in addition to vesicoureteric reflux. Girls may be examined supine but to demonstrate the urethra boys must be rotated into an oblique or lateral position.

Nuclear medicine studies

Technetium 99m DMSA (dimercaptosuccinic acid) is taken up by the proximal renal tubular cells and demonstrates functional renal tissue. The radiation dose is very low. Differential renal function is routinely calculated and is normally within the range of 45–55%. It is particularly valuable in the workup of the child with a urinary tract infection as it is the most sensitive method of detecting renal scarring (Fig. 39.26).[14] Areas of reduced uptake of the radionuclide will be found in over 20% of children with acute pyelonephritis and animal studies have demonstrated that these areas progress to scarring in the absence of adequate treatment. DMSA scanning can thus be used to highlight the 'at risk' kidney. It can also be used to identify ectopic renal tissue and to assess horseshoe kidneys.

Technetium 99m MAG3 (mercaptoacetyltriglycine) is primarily excreted by the proximal convoluted tubules and is used to assess drainage though some functional information is also present on images obtained within the first 2 min after injection. Time–activity curves are plotted for the renal areas. These renogram curves will rise initially during extraction of the isotope from the blood, but should fall promptly and rapidly if the upper tract is neither dilated nor obstructed. The curve will be flat or continue to rise in the presence of obstruction. Prolongation of the rising phase will also be seen in kidneys with reduced function or dilatation of the upper tracts. If the system is known to be dilated, furosemide (frusemide) should be administrated simultaneously with the isotope. Due to the diuresis a dilated non-obstructed system should then clear isotope more quickly than an obstructed system.[50] If the result is still equivocal retrograde or antegrade pyelography may be necessary.

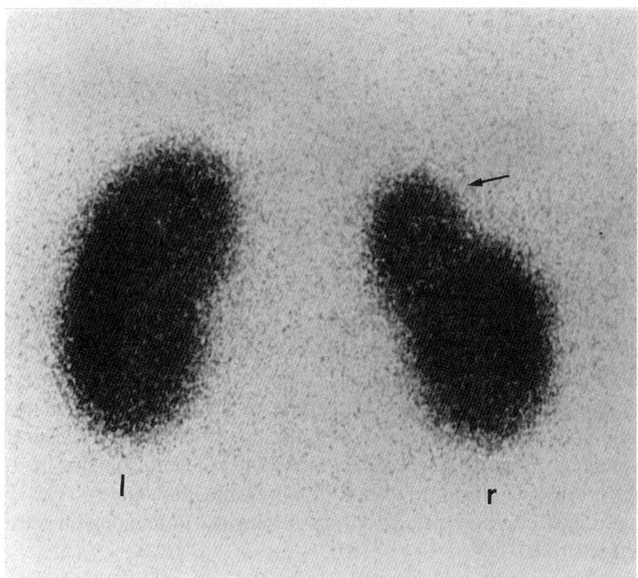

Fig. 39.26 Technetium 99m DMSA isotope scan of the kidney. This 2-h scan reveals decreased uptake in the upper pole of the right kidney compatible with scarring (arrow).

Isotope cystography either direct (by catheterization or suprapubic injection) (Fig. 39.27) or indirect (following MAG3 renography) can be used to assess vesicoureteric reflux. Reflux often occurs during micturition and is detected by an increase in the count rate in the renal area.

Computerized tomography

Contrast enhanced CT is of particular value in the investigation of renal trauma. Its role in the staging of primary renal masses, the most common being a Wilms' tumor (Fig. 39.28) is being superseded by MR. CT is of little value in the majority of urinary tract abnormalities.

Magnetic resonance

MR has an increasing role in investigation of the renal tract. Combined static-dynamic MR urography gives functional and morphological information in complex congenital renal anomalies and obstruction.[51] MR is now the primary modality for the staging of renal tumors. MR angiography and venography can demonstrate abnormalities of the renal vasculature. MR is likely to play an increasing part in the investigation of reflux nephropathy but currently this is curtailed by cost, limited access to machines and the need for sedation.[52]

Pyelography

This technique is useful in complex problems, particularly the anatomical demonstration of non-functioning duplex kidneys and the assessment of ureteric strictures. Retrograde (following placement of a ureteric catheter at cystoscopy) or antegrade (by direct puncture of the kidney under US guidance) pyelography can be used to exclude mechanical obstruction in dilated systems where the use of renography is inconclusive.

Angiography

This technique is occasionally needed in the investigation of hypertension following prior workup of the patient with ultrasound, isotope and MR investigations. The technique will reveal accurately the presence of renal arterial stenosis, segmental

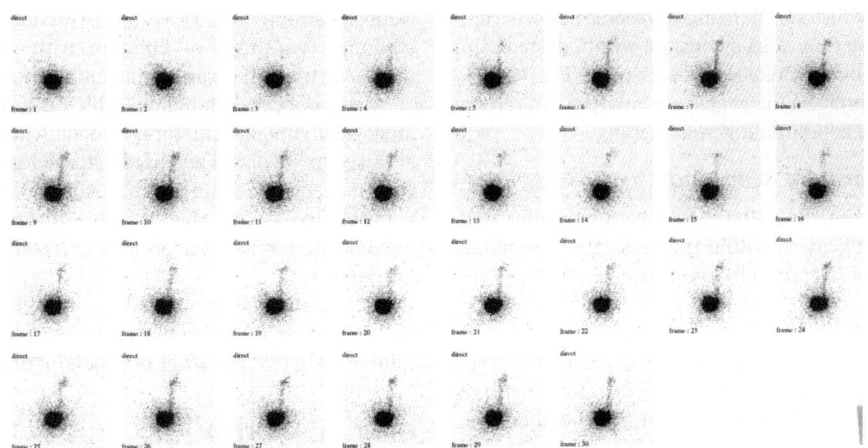

Fig. 39.27 Direct isotope cystogram: 30 10-second frames showing reflux into the right kidney during 5-minute period after injection of radionuclide suprapubically.

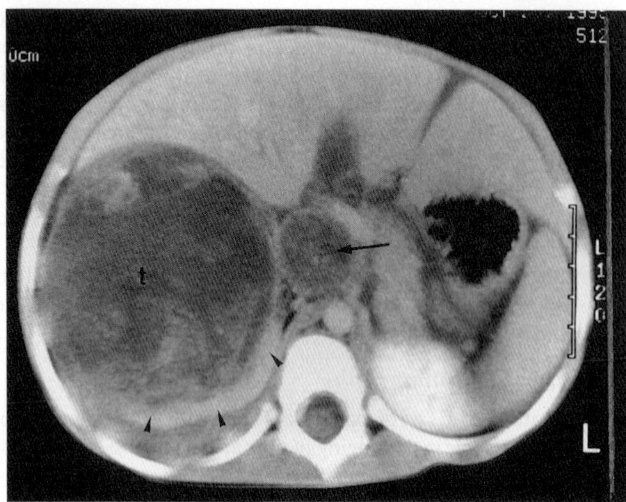

Fig. 39.28 Contrast enhanced CT of the abdomen. Large Wilms' tumor (t) arising from and destroying the right kidney (arrowheads). Extension of tumor into the IVC (long arrow).

or main branch, fibromuscular hyperplasia or aortic abnormalities such as narrowing in neurofibromatosis and Takayasu's disease.

RETROPERITONEUM

Investigation of the retroperitoneum will be required in primary adrenal gland masses, i.e. adenomas and carcinomas which commonly present with virilization. Other tumors include ganglioneuromas and neuroblastomas or cystic lesions, abscess or hemorrhage related to the gland. Primary retroperitoneal tumors include neurogenic masses, teratomas, lymphomas and rhabdomyosarcomas. Masses may also arise secondary to vertebral abnormalities such as osteomyelitis and primary vertebral neoplasms.

Plain radiographs

The basic imaging methods include plain abdominal films to visualize any calcification in the mass and identify secondary erosions in the vertebral bodies or fat or bone content in a teratoma.

Ultrasonic imaging

Ultrasonic imaging will clearly demonstrate a mass greater than 1.5 cm, but often fails to depict spread into the retroperitoneal structures, particularly if the lesion is calcified or hidden by bowel gas. In adrenal hemorrhage the history, changing ultrasonic pattern from sonolucent to echogenic or vice versa associated with a decrease in size obviates the need for further radiological assessment (Fig. 39.29). In congenital adrenal hyperplasia the glands are enlarged but return to normal size rapidly with appropriate steroid therapy.

Computerized tomography scanning

CT scanning is useful for the delineation of retroperitoneal masses if MRI is not available. Calcification within the mass and associated abnormalities of the vertebrae are well demonstrated.

Magnetic resonance imaging

MRI is now the modality of choice for the demonstration of retroperitoneal and paraspinal abnormalities. Encroachment of infection or tumor into the spinal canal is demonstrated without the need for myelographic contrast. Tissue contrast is superior to that achieved with CT, increasing sensitivity in the detection of abnormalities and allowing accurate diagnosis and staging of tumors

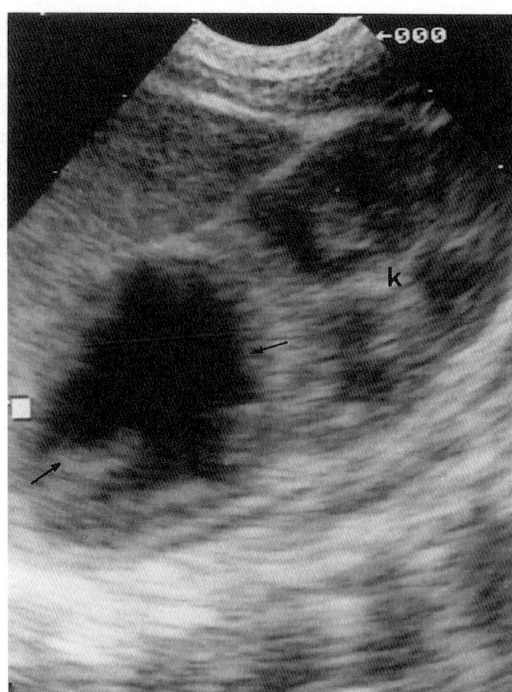

Fig. 39.29 Sagittal ultrasound scan through the right kidney (k) showing a hypoechoic area in the right suprarenal gland. This represents an adrenal hemorrhage (arrows).

(Fig. 39.30). Nephroblastoma distorts the kidney but does not generally cross the midline whereas neuroblastoma infiltrates the retroperitoneum on both sides of the midline displacing the aorta, the IVC and their branches anteriorly. Nephroblastoma can extend into the lumen of the IVC and metastasize to the liver. Focal or diffuse bone marrow metastases are common in neuroblastoma. Follow-up scans can assess response to therapy. Marrow abnormalities in the spine due to infection, tumor or abnormal hemopoiesis can be appreciated. Hemorrhage into the psoas muscle in hemophilia is well demonstrated.

Nuclear medicine studies

Bone scintigraphy using 99m technetium methylene diphosphonate is more sensitive than conventional radiography in the detection of bony metastatic disease, the deposits usually being identified as areas of increased uptake of the radionuclide. Neuroblastoma and rhabdomyosarcoma frequently metastasize to bone. Two-thirds of children with neuroblastoma will show uptake of the bone scanning agent in the primary tumor.

Metaiodobenzylguanidine (MIBG) is a synthetic neurotransmitter analog with uptake and storage similar to that of noradrenaline. It can be linked to ^{131}I or ^{123}I and used in the detection of neural crest tumors such as neuroblastoma and pheochromocytoma. More than 90% of neuroblastomas are able to concentrate MIBG. ^{123}I MIBG shows maximal tumor uptake at around 48 h and can be used for therapeutic purposes.

The somatostatin analog octreotide gives similar uptake to MIBG in patients with neuroblastoma or pheochromocytoma but its uptake is superior in other neuroendocrine tumors.

GENITAL SYSTEM

The uterus, ovaries and vagina can be clearly assessed using ultrasound (Fig. 39.31). This is dependent on visualization through

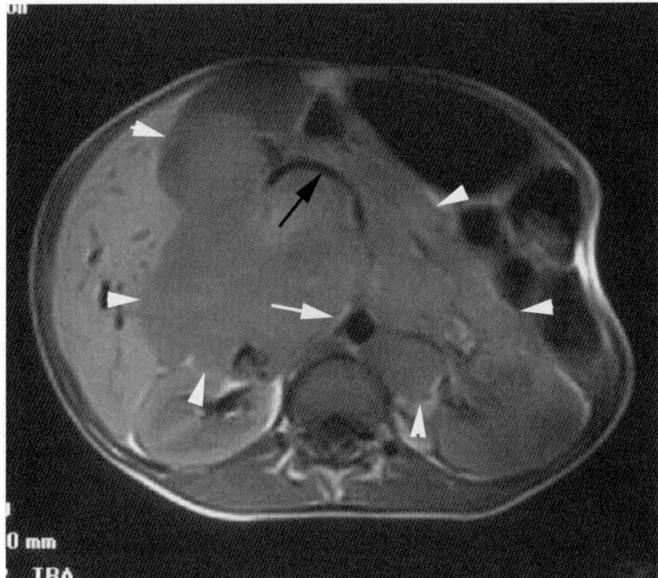

Fig. 39.30 Neuroblastoma: T1-weighted transverse MR image showing encasement of the aorta (white arrow) and hepatic artery (black arrow) by tumor (arrowheads).

a fluid-filled bladder. The developing ovary contains multiple follicles. Charts are available for normal ovarian and uterine sizes in relation to age.[53] The technique can thus be used to assess the internal organs in intersex states, precocious or delayed puberty and chromosomal abnormalities.

Uterine growth and vaginal mucosal thickness can be measured and related to hormone therapy. The presence of foreign bodies in the vagina as a cause of discharge can also be diagnosed. The imaging of ovarian and pelvic abnormalities may be improved by transvaginal ultrasound, but this is not normally performed in pediatric practice.

The imaging of cloacal and urogenital sinus abnormalities requires the technique of genitography where water-soluble contrast is injected into the perineal orifice followed by relevant radiographs (Fig. 39.32).

The scrotum and inguinal canal can be examined using a 7–12 MHz linear probe and abnormalities such as hydrocele, undescended testis, patent processus vaginalis, cyst of the spermatic cord and inguinal hernia demonstrated. When the clinical presentation is pain and swelling the differential diagnosis includes epididymitis, torted hydatid of Morgagni and testicular torsion. In acute torsion the testis is enlarged and hyperechoic with absent Doppler signal.[54] Both torted appendix of Morgagni and epididymitis cause swelling of the epididymis with increased Doppler flow signals although the former may sometimes be recognized as a cystic lesion adjacent to the epididymis.[55] Following trauma to the scrotum the testes can be examined for rupture. Varicoceles can be recognized as multiple vascular channels with increased blood flow.

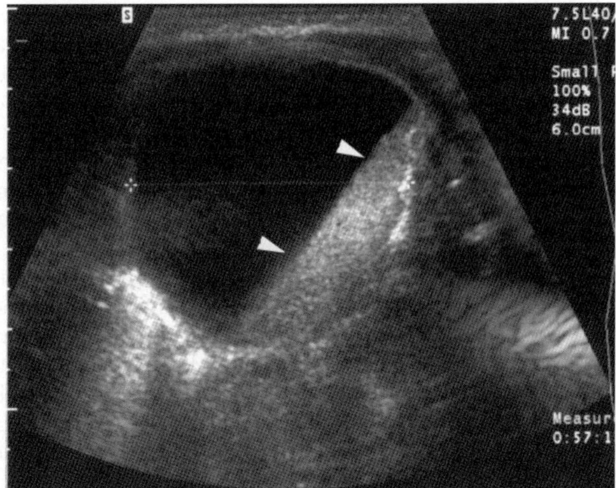

Fig. 39.31 Ovarian cyst: US showing fluid-fluid level of debris (arrowheads) within the cyst.

MRI is now being recognized as a multiplanar modality to image the uterus and ovaries. The technique can also be used to locate the position of undescended testes if US has been unsuccessful in demonstrating the testis in the inguinal canal.

SKELETAL SYSTEM

Plain radiographs

The commonest indication for radiography is in the assessment of trauma. It is important to include the joints at both ends of the bone being examined and to have two views at right angles to each other. Greenstick fractures are common in childhood and can be recognized by kinks in the cortex with or without significant deformity. Undisplaced spiral fractures of the tibia are common in toddlers. The diagnosis may only be made on a follow-up film at least 7 days following the trauma. Periosteal reaction is present and the fracture line may be visible. Requests for radiography in trauma should be vetted to prevent inappropriate examinations in trivial

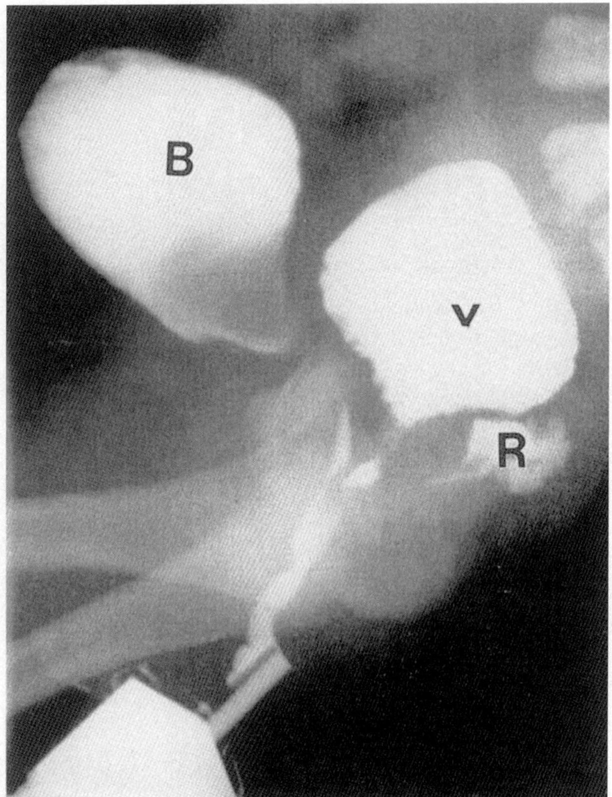

Fig. 39.32 Genitogram demonstrating persistent urogenital sinus with opening of the bladder (B), vagina (V) and rectum (R) into a common chamber.

trauma; this is particularly likely in minor skull, spine and chest injuries.

Views of the elbow with its six ossification centers are particularly difficult for inexperienced clinicians to interpret but a comparison view of the other elbow should rarely be necessary if the films are reviewed promptly by a pediatric radiologist. A range of normal films retained in the casualty department may be helpful. Plain films in osteomyelitis may be normal for several days after abnormalities are detectable by nuclear medicine, ultrasound or MRI.

Non-accidental injury to infants, often due to shaking, can be recognized by the characteristic metaphyseal fractures which can appear as 'corner' fractures (Fig. 39.33) or 'bucket handle' fractures depending upon the projection. Multiple fractures in various stages of healing[56] may be detected on skeletal survey. Rib fractures due to compression of the chest characteristically occur posteriorly where the rib is bent over the tip of the transverse process, in the midaxillary line or anteriorly. Skull fractures and subdural collections may be found. MRI is proving to be the most valuable technique in that dating of subdural and extradural hemorrhages is possible (Fig. 39.34). A skeletal survey should include AP and lateral skull, lateral spine, chest, pelvis and AP limb X-rays. Coned views of the knee, ankle, elbow and wrist joints may be required to confirm minor metaphyseal fractures.

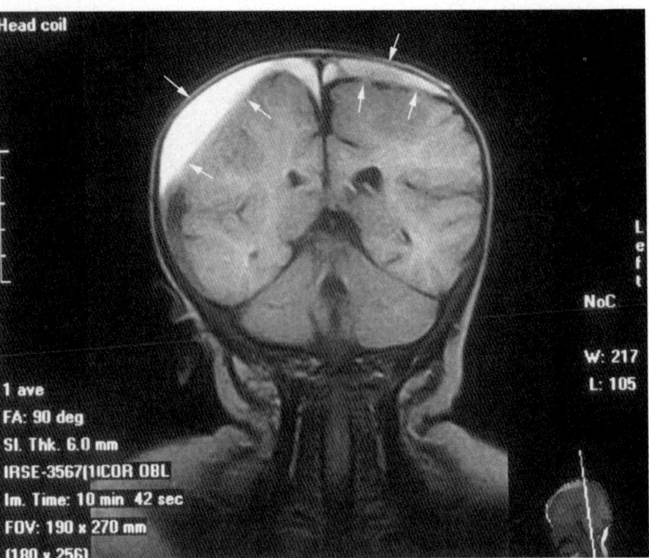

Fig. 39.34 Non-accidental injury of the brain: coronal FLAIR MR image showing bilateral subdural hematomata (arrows).

Skeletal survey is also performed in the assessment of bone dysplasias. The abnormality may be localized to the diaphyseal, metaphyseal or epiphyseal areas of the bones and may involve the spine. The survey for dysplasia need only include the limbs on one side of the body. Surveys for malignant disease are particularly useful in Langerhans' cell histiocytosis when the isotope scan may be unremarkable. In metabolic disease including rickets, hyperparathyroidism and lead poisoning a film of one wrist or knee is usually adequate for diagnosis and follow-up. Endocrine abnormalities may result in abnormal delay or advancement in bone age. This is usually assessed from a radiograph of the left hand and wrist by comparison with standards[57] or by computation of a score using specific criteria.[58]

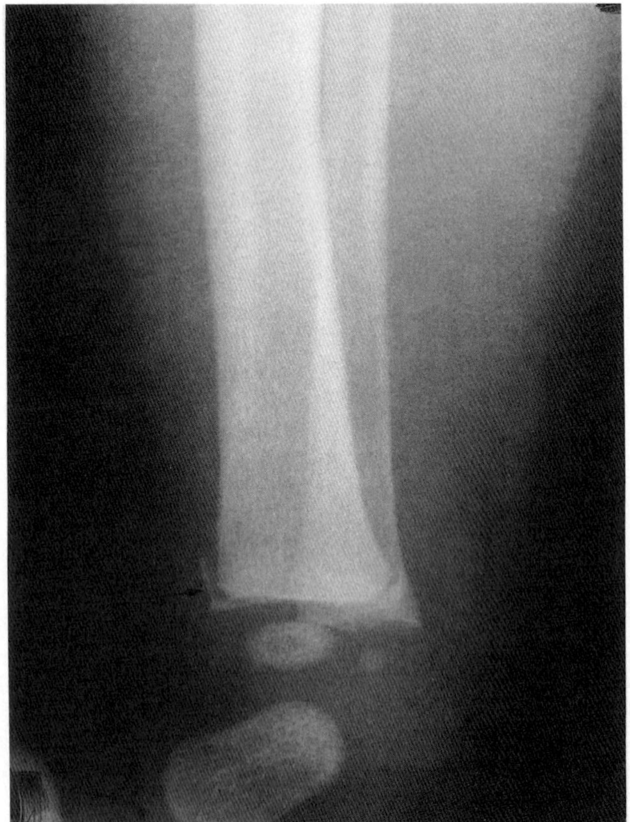
Fig. 39.33 Non-accidental injury. Lateral view of the tibia and fibula demonstrating the typical corner fractures at the lower end of the tibia (arrow) and soft tissue swelling anterior to the tibia.

Perthes' disease is common in children aged 5–8 years and plain films may show flattening of the epiphysis, but in the early stages subarticular lucency is usually only demonstrated on the 'frog' leg lateral film. Slipped upper femoral capital epiphysis occurs in children aged 10–16 years, and may occur with no history of trauma. The epiphysis may slip medially or posteriorly. Signs on the AP radiograph include reduced height of the epiphysis, loss of clarity of the growth plate, medial slip of the epiphysis with extrusion of the metaphysis from the acetabulum and reduced bone density. A 'frog' lateral is mandatory to detect cases in which the slip is predominantly posterior and should include both hips because the disease is not infrequently bilateral.

Back pain in children is a significant symptom and should be taken seriously. Plain spinal radiographs are useful in the detection of trauma, congenital abnormalities including hemivertebrae, fused vertebrae and scoliosis. Discitis is represented by a narrow disc space with eventual destruction of the vertebral body end plates. Radioisotope scanning using ^{99m}Tc phosphate compounds is more sensitive in detecting the abnormality early when plain films may be normal. MRI will clearly depict changes in the disc space and vertebral body marrow. The defects of spondylolysis and spondylolisthesis may be detected on plain X-ray or MR but CT is the most sensitive technique (Fig. 39.35). Secondary changes due to spinal canal masses or paraspinal masses, e.g. in neuroblastoma, may produce pedicle erosion. Many bone dysplasias, metabolic abnormalities and tumors have abnormalities revealed on plain radiographs. These include inferior beaking of the vertebral body in Hurler's syndrome, central and anterior beaking in spondyloepiphyseal dysplasia and vertebra plana in Langerhans' cell histiocytosis. Multiple vertebral body collapse and generalized osteoporosis are found in neuroblastoma and leukemia.

Imaging of the spinal cord is now performed with MRI. Plain films are helpful in the immediate assessment of major spinal trauma, supplemented with CT if fractures and/or dislocation are suspected.

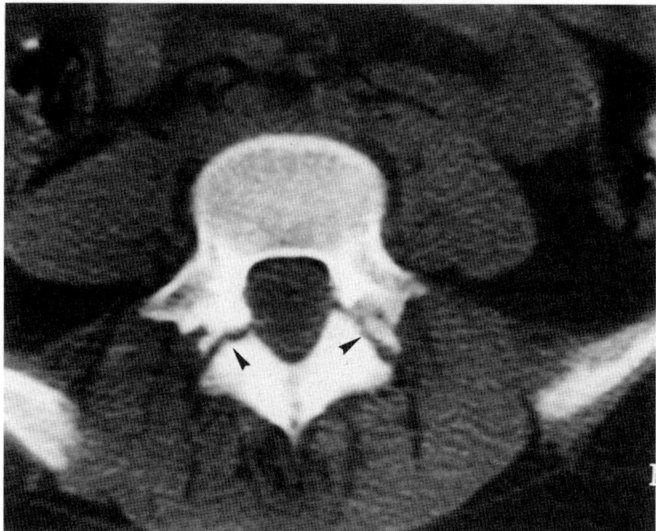

Fig. 39.35 Axial CT scan through the spine at the L5 level. Bilateral spondylolysis defects in the pars interarticularis (arrowheads).

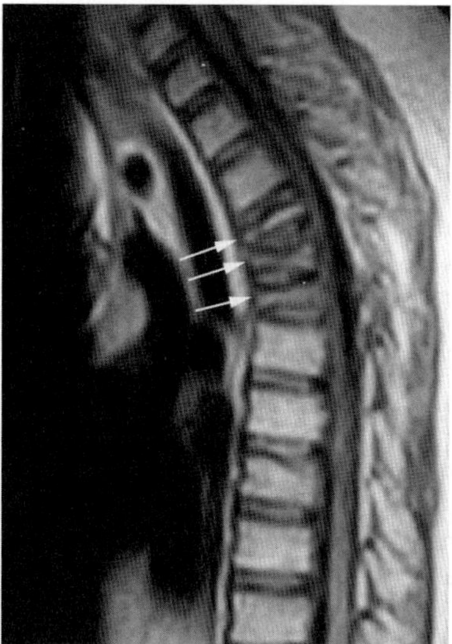

Fig. 39.36 Vertebra plana: longitudinal T1-weighted MR image showing complete collapse of three thoracic vertebrae due to Langerhans' cell histiocytosis (arrows) with preservation of the intervening discs.

Nuclear medicine studies

Technetium 99m diphosphonate compounds (usually methylene diphosphonate – MDP) are used in the investigation of bone disorders including infection, trauma, tumors and avascular necrosis. Uptake of the radionuclide is dependent on blood flow and osteoblastic activity. A triple bone scan is usually performed when osteomyelitis is suspected and consists of a blood flow study followed immediately by a blood pool study with static images some 3 h later. Within 12 h of the development of symptoms of osteomyelitis there will be increased blood flow, hyperemia and increased uptake of the radionuclide on the later images. False negative scans occur in the neonate or when there is a particularly destructive infection. Increased blood flow, hyperemia, with a more diffuse late uptake may occur with a septic arthritis. In Perthes' disease, where there is avascular necrosis of the femoral capital epiphysis, an area of reduced uptake of the radionuclide will be identified (cold area). A bone scan may detect unsuspected fractures in a child with non-accidental injury.

Bone scintigraphy can be of value in the diagnosis and localization of benign lesions such as osteoid osteoma. It plays an important role in the staging of neuroblastoma, rhabdomyosarcoma, osteogenic sarcoma, Ewing's sarcoma and histiocytosis and should be routinely performed in the workup of these children. Bony metastastic disease occurs less frequently with other tumors and a bone scan should only be performed in these children if they are experiencing bone pain, e.g. lymphoma or leukemia. Pulmonary metastatic deposits in a child with osteogenic sarcoma may show up as 'hot areas' in the lungs.

Magnetic resonance imaging

MR scanning with its excellent contrast definition is the best modality to demonstrate the extent of intraosseous and extraosseous spread of primary bone tumors, though CT gives excellent demonstration of bony architecture and is used to detect lung metastases. Knowledge of the normal variations in T1 and T2 signals of marrow related to age is essential. Detailed information on marrow abnormalities is crucial when contemplating reconstructive surgery with prostheses. MRI will also assess marrow abnormalities in other tumors such as neuroblastoma, leukemia and Langerhans' cell histiocytosis (Fig. 39.36). The extent of osteomyelitis can be accurately assessed, usually showing a decreased T1 signal and high T2 signal due to edema in the marrow and adjacent soft tissues in the acute stages (Fig. 39.37). MRI demonstrates ischemic change in Perthes' disease and sickle cell disease. MRI shows bone and soft tissue changes caused by hemorrhage in hemophilia and is used in the assessment of chronic arthropathy due to hemophilia and juvenile rheumatoid arthritis. Special sequences can demonstrate articular cartilage.

MRI has a developing role in the assessment of trauma, particularly in those injuries which are poorly demonstrated on plain films such as growth plate injuries, cartilage and ligament

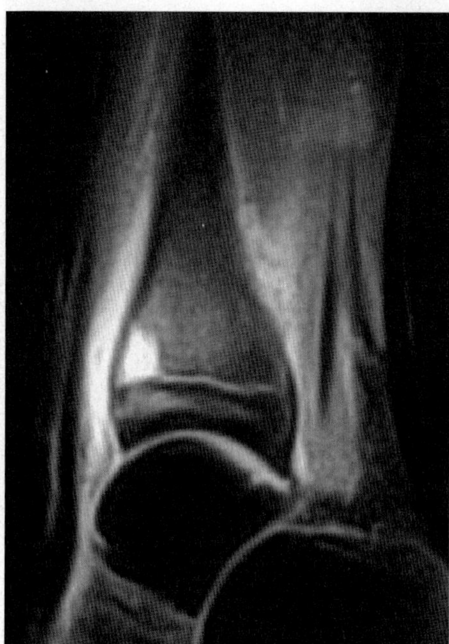

Fig. 39.37 Osteomyelitis: inversion recovery fat-suppression image showing high signal in localized abscess in the lower tibial metaphysis with inflammatory changes in the adjacent soft tissues.

injuries, the assessment of stability of fragments in osteochondritis dissecans, injury to the intra-articular structures of the knee and wrist and the assessment of spinal cord injury without radiological abnormality. In all these applications MRI elegantly demonstrates soft tissue injuries that may be of major clinical significance such as those causing spinal instability. MRI can also detect bone bruising or occult fractures which may be important in particular locations such as the scaphoid where fractures may be complicated by avascular necrosis.

Computerized tomography scanning

The role of CT in tumor staging has been superseded by MRI. CT can be useful in trauma of the spine or pelvis to demonstrate small displaced fragments of bone. Limited CT can be used to investigate suspected rotatory subluxation of the atlantoaxial joint. CT measurement of leg lengths and hip anteversion can be performed with low dose techniques (Fig. 39.38).

Ultrasound

Ultrasound examination of the infant hip is now well established as the method of choice in the investigation of congenital acetabular dysplasia. It can be performed up to the age of 6 months after which ossification of the femoral head obscures acetabular detail. It allows assessment of the acetabular morphology (Fig. 39.39) which can be graded according to Graf[59] or using the dynamic study of Harcke.[60] Stability can be assessed by stressing the hip during the ultrasound examination and observing the movement of the femoral head relative to the acetabulum. Increasingly treatment is influenced by the ultrasound examination rather than dictated by clinical features alone.

Ultrasound can assess the presence and size of effusion and guide aspiration if clinically indicated in the painful hip[61] (Fig. 39.40) and other joints. Traction injuries such as Osgood–Schlatter's disease can be identified by bony fragmentation, soft tissue swelling and increased color Doppler signals due to hyperemia. Soft tissue masses identified by ultrasound include lymph node enlargement, abscess formation, lipomata, hemangiomata, cystic hygromas and popliteal cysts. Other soft tissue masses may require biopsy for identification and this can be guided by ultrasound. Foreign bodies can be detected in the soft tissues (Fig. 39.41), including those which are radiolucent such as splinters of wood or plastic which are not detected on radiographs. Early osteomyelitis can be diagnosed with ultrasound, demonstrating the presence of soft tissue edema and subperiosteal fluid before abnormalities can be demonstrated on plain radiographs.

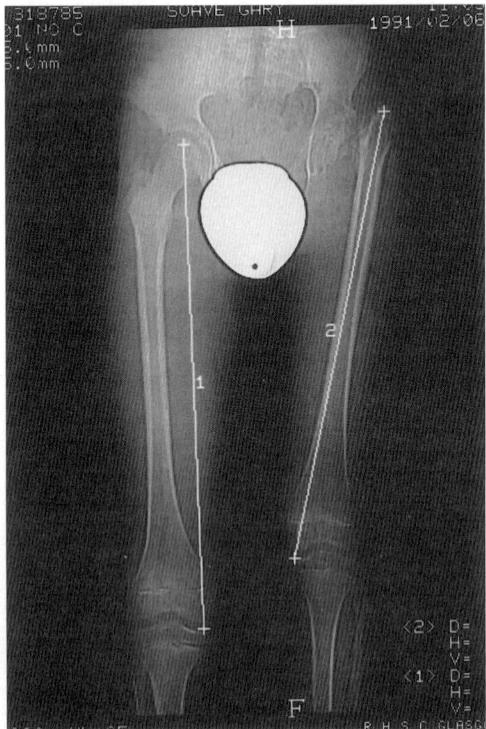

Fig. 39.38 The use of a CT scanogram in estimating leg length. Note destruction of the left femoral head. This was secondary to septic arthritis.

(a)
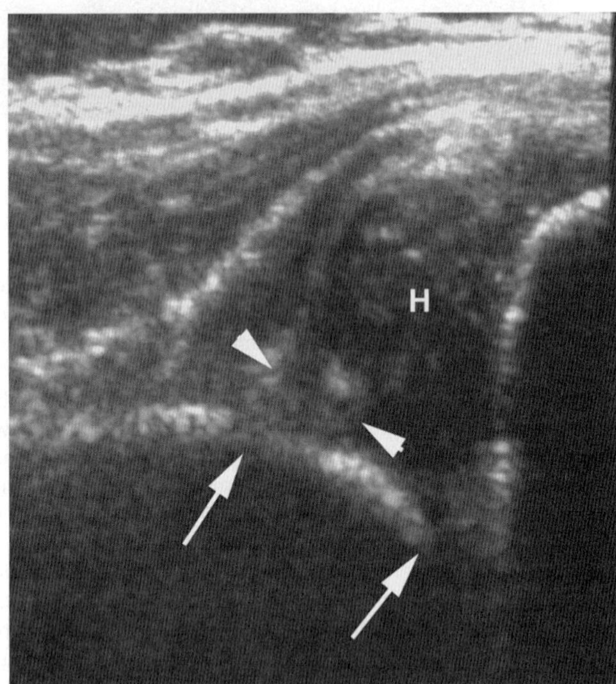

(b)
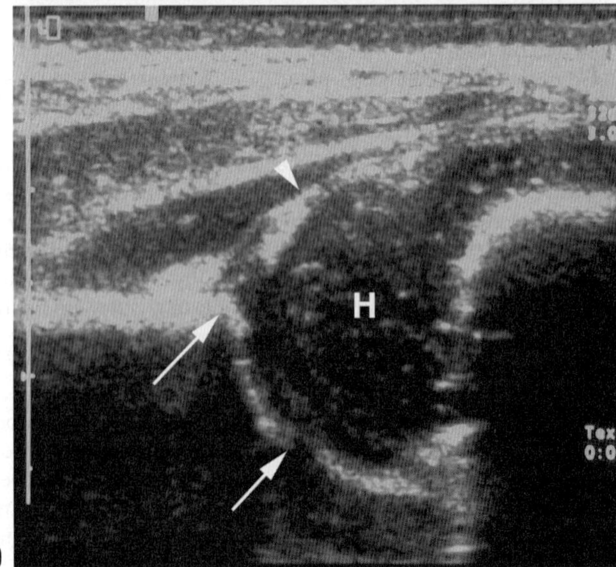

Fig. 39.39 (a) US of dysplastic hip (Graf type 4) showing shallow acetabulum (arrows), superior subluxation of femoral head (H) with interposition of the cartilaginous labrum (arrowhead). (b) Normal hip for comparison.

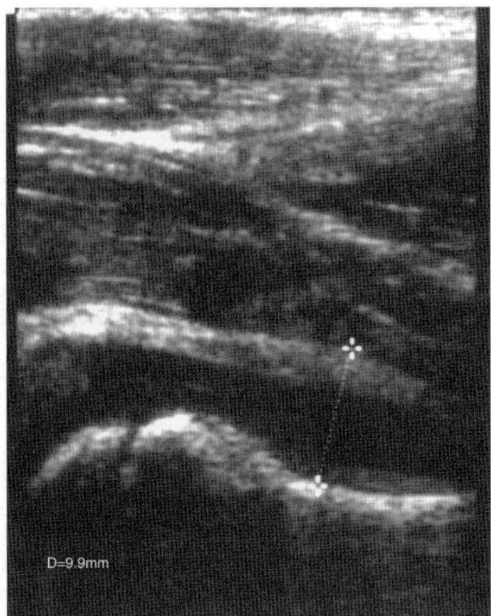

Fig. 39.40 Longitudinal US of hip showing effusion (callipers) anterior to the femoral neck.

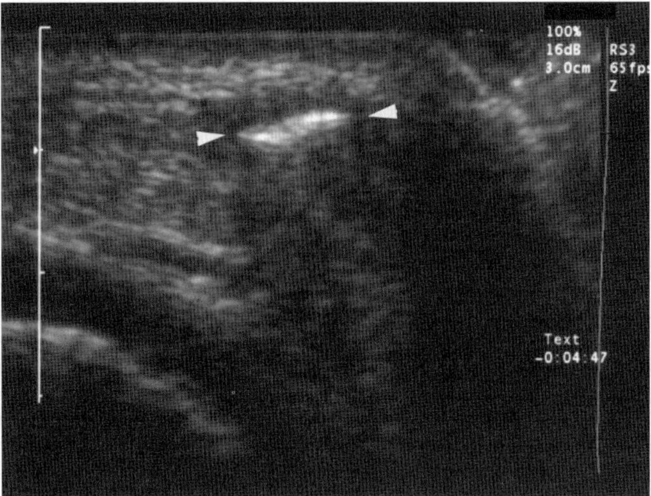

Fig. 39.41 US showing bright echo from foreign body (arrowheads) in soft tissues.

REFERENCES

1 Royal College of Radiologists. Making the best use of a department of clinical radiology. In: Guidelines for doctors, 4th edn. London: RCR; 1998.

2 Grainger RG. Low osmolar contrast media. BMJ 1984; 289: 144–145.

3 Babcock DS, Patriquin H, Lafortune M, Dauzat M. Power Doppler sonography: basic principles and clinical applications in children. Pediatr Radiol 1996; 26:109–115.

4 Winkler P, Helmke K. Major pitfalls in Doppler examination of the cerebral vascular system. Pediatr Radiol 1989; 19:267–268.

5 Goh D, Minns RA, Hendry GMA, et al. Cerebrovascular resistive index assessed by duplex Doppler sonography and its relationship to intracranial pressure in infantile hydrocephalus. Pediatr Radiol 1992; 22:246–250.

6 White KS. Helical/spiral CT scanning: a paediatric radiology perspective. Pediatr Radiol 1996; 26:5–14.

7 Kuhn JP. High resolution CT of paediatric pulmonary parenchymal disorders. Radiol Clin North Am 1993; 31:533–551.

8 Dixon AK, Dendy P. Spiral CT. How much does radiation dose matter? Lancet 1998; 352: 1082–1083.

9 Chan CY, Wong YC, Chau LF, et al. Radiation dose reduction in paediatric cranial CT. Pediatr Radiol 1999; 29:770–775.

10 Bremner DJ, Elliston CD, Hall EJ, Berdon WE. Response to the statement by the Society of Paediatric Radiology on radiation risks from pediatric CT scans. Pediatr Radiol 2001; 31:389–391.

11 Ambrosino MM, Genieser KJ, Roche A, et al. Feasibility of high resolution low dose chest CT in evaluating the pediatric chest. Pediatr Radiol 1994; 24:6–10.

12 Naidich DP. Helical CT of the thorax: clinical applications. Radiol Clin North Am 1994; 32:759–774.

13 Ruess L, Sivit CJ, Eichelberger MR, et al. Blunt hepatic and splenic trauma in children: correlation of a CT injury severity scale with clinical outcome. Pediatr Radiol 1995; 25: 321–325.

14 Gordon I. Effect of nuclear medicine on paediatric imaging. Br J Radiol 1993; 66:971–985.

15 Inder T, Huppi PS, Zientera GP, et al. Early detection of periventricular leukomalacia by diffusion weighted magnetic resonance imaging techniques. J Paediatr 1999; 134: 631–634.

16 Secaf E, Hricak H, Gooding CA, et al. Role of MRI in the evaluation of ambiguous genitalia. Pediatr Radiol 1994; 24:231–235.

17 Moore SG, Dawson KL. Red and yellow marrow in the femur: age related changes in appearance at MR imaging. Radiology 1990; 175:219–223.

18 Jaramillo D, Hoffer FA, Shapiro F, Rand F. MRI imaging of fractures of the growth plate. Am J Roentgenol 1990; 155: 1261–1265.

19 Darnman BC, Hoffer FA, Rand FF, O'Rourke EJ. Osteomyelitis in children. Gadolinium enhanced MR imaging. Radiology 1992; 182:743–748.

20 Towbin RB. Paediatric interventional procedures in the 1980s. A period of development, growth and acceptance. Radiology 1989; 170(3): 1081–1091.

21 Jayakrishnan VK, Wilkinson AG. Treatment of oesophageal strictures in children: a comparison of fluoroscopically guided balloon dilatation with surgical bouginage. Pediatr Radiol 2001; 31:98–101.

22 Wilkinson AG, Raine PAM. Pneumatic dilatation in childhood cardio-achalasia. Pediatr Radiol 1997; 27:60–62.

23 McDermott VGM, Taylor T, Wyatt JP, et al. Oro-gastric magnet removal of ingested disc batteries. J Paediatr Surg 1995; 31: 29–33.

24 Volle E, Beyer P, Kaufmann HJ. Therapeutic approach to ingested button type batteries. Magnetic removal of ingested button type batteries. Pediatr Radiol 1989; 19: 114–118.

25 Meza MP, Benson M, Slovis TL. Imaging of mediastinal masses in children. Radiol Clin North Am 1993; 31:583–604.

26 Hendry GMA. Magnetic resonance imaging of the paediatric chest. Pediatr Respir Rev 2000; 1:249–258.

27 Millar AJW, Rode H, Brown RA, Cywes S. The deadly vomit: malrotation and mid gut volvulus. Pediatr Surg Int 1987; 2:172–176.

28 Gu L, Alton DJ, Daneman A, et al. Intussusception reduction in children with rectal insufflation of air. Am J Roentgenol 1988; 150:1345–1348.

29 Shiels WE II, Kirks DR, Keller GL, et al. Colonic perforation by air and liquid enemas: comparison study in young pigs. Am J Roentgenol 1993; 160:931–935.

30 Rohrschneider WK, Troger T. Hydrostatic reduction of intussusception under ultrasound guidance. Pediatr Radiol 1995; 25: 530–534.

31 Leonidas JC, Berdon WE, Baker DH, Santulli TV. Meconium ileus and its complications. Am J Roentgenol 1970; 130:598–609.

32 Verschelden P, Filiatrault N, Garel L, et al. Intussusception in children: reliability of ultrasound in diagnosis. A prospective study. Radiology 1992; 184:741–744.

33 Lim HK, Bae SH, Lee KH, et al. Assessment of the reducibility of ileocolic intussusception in children: usefulness of colour Doppler sonography. Radiology 1994; 191:781–785.

34 Britton I, Wilkinson AG. Ultrasound features of intussusception predicting outcome of air enema. Pediatr Radiol 1999; 29: 705–710.

35 Puylaert JB. Acute appendicitis: ultrasound evaluation using graded compression. Radiology 1986; 158:355–360.
36 Vignault F, Filiatrault D, Brandt ML, et al. Acute appendicitis in children: evaluation with ultrasound. Radiology 1990; 176:501–504.
37 Siegel MJ. Appendicitis in children: ultrasound and diagnosis. Pediatr Surg Int 1995; 10:62–65.
38 Friedland JA, Herman T, Siegel MJ. Escherichia: O157–H7–associated haemolytic uraemic syndrome. Value of colonic colour doppler sonography. Pediatr Radiol 1995; 25:S65–S67.
39 Ashley LM, Allen S, Teele RL. A normal sonogram does not exclude malrotation. Pediatr Radiol 2001; 31:354–356.
40 Pobiel RS, Bisset JS III. Imaging of liver tumours in the infant and child (pictorial essay). Pediatr Radiol 1995; 25:495–506.
41 Kendrick APT, Phua KB, Subramaniam R. Making the diagnosis of biliary atresia using the triangular cord sign and gallbladder length. Pediatr Radiol 2000; 30:69–73.
42 Lloyd DA, Carty H, Patterson M, et al. Predictive value of skull radiography for intracranial injury in children with blunt head injury. Lancet 1997; 349:821–824.
43 Christophe C, Clercx A, Blum D, et al. Early MR detection of cortical and subcortical hypoxic ischaemic encephalopathy in full term infants. Pediatr Radiol 1994; 24: 581–584.
44 Staudt M, Schropp C, Staudt F, et al. MRI assessment of myelinization. An age standardisation. Pediatr Radiol 1994; 4: 122–127.
45 Leventer RJ, Phelan EM, Coleman LT. Clinical and imaging features of cortical malformations in childhood. Neurology 1999; 53(4):715–722.
46 Connelly A, Chong WK, Johnson CL, et al. Diffusion weighted magnetic resonance imaging of compromised tissue in stroke. Arch Dis Child 1997; 77(1):38–41.
47 Darge K, Troeger J, Duetting T, et al. Reflux in young patients: comparison of voiding US of the bladder and retrovesical space with echo enhancement versus voiding cystourethrography for diagnosis. Radiology 1999; 210(1):201–207.
48 Tublin ME, Dodd GD. Sonography of renal transplantation. Radiol Clin North Am 1995; 33:447–459.
49 Levitt SB. Medical versus surgical treatment of primary vesico-ureteric reflux. Report of the International Reflux Study Committee. Pediatrics 1981; 67:392–400.
50 Anderson PJ, Rangarajan V, Gordon I. Assessment of drainage in PUJ dilatation: pelvic excretion efficiency as an index of renal function. Nucl Med Commun 1997; 18(9): 823–826.
51 Rohrschneider WK, Becker K, Hoffend J, et al. Combined static-dynamic MR urography for the simultaneous evaluation of morphology and function in urinary tract obstruction. II. Findings in experimentally induced ureteric stenosis. Pediatr Radiol 2000; 30(8):523–532.
52 Chan Y-L, Chan K-W, Yeung C-K, et al. Potential utility of MRI in the evaluation of children at risk of renal scarring. Pediatr Radiol 1999; 29:856–862.
53 Salardi S, Orsini LF, Cacciari E, et al. Pelvic ultrasound in premenarchal girls. Relation to puberty and sex hormone concentrations. Arch Dis Child 1985; 60: 120–125.
54 Luker GD, Siegel MJ. Colour doppler sonography of the scrotum in children (pictorial essay). Am J Roentgenol 1994; 163:649–655.
55 Munden MM, Trautwein LM. Scrotal pathology in pediatrics with sonographic imaging. Curr Probl Diagn Radiol 2000; 29:185–205.
56 Nimkin K, Kleinman PK. Imaging of child abuse. Pediatr Clin North Am 1997; 44(3): 615–635.
57 Greulich WW, Pyle SI. Radiographic atlas of skeletal development of the hand and wrist, 2nd edn. California: Stanford University Press; 1984.
58 Tanner JM, Whitehouse RH, Cameron N. Assessment of skeletal maturity and prediction of adult height (TW2 method). London: Academic Press; 1983.
59 Graf R. Fundamentals of sonographic diagnosis of the infant hip. J Pediatr Orthop 1984; 4:735–741.
60 Harcke HT. Examination of the infant hip with real time ultrasonography. J Ultrasound Med 1984; 4:131–137.
61 Miralles M, Gonzalez G, Pulpeiro JR. Sonography of the painful hip in children. 500 consecutive cases. Am J Roentgenol 1989; 152:579–582.

40

Biochemical and physiological tables and reference ranges for laboratory tests

Neville R Belton

BIOCHEMICAL AND PHYSIOLOGICAL DATA

The *Système International d'Unités* or SI unit system has been widely adopted in basic sciences and medicine in many countries including the UK and, more recently, the USA.[1,2] In this chapter reference values are generally given in SI units followed by traditional units. In Tables 40.1, 40.2 and 40.3[3–5] a *multiplication factor* has been given for each substance. This is the number by which the values in *traditional units* need to be *multiplied* in order to convert to *SI units* (thus also if the values in *SI units* are divided by this factor, the result will be given in traditional units).

The SI unit of quantity is the mole.

$$\text{Concentration in moles} = \frac{\text{weight in grams}}{\text{molecular weight}}$$

The unit of volume commonly used in clinical biochemistry is the liter. Hence moles/Liter or mol/L is the standard unit used in these tables.

Similarly the smaller units are millimoles/L (mmol/L)
micromoles/L (μmol/L)
nanomoles/L (nmol/L)
and picomoles/L (pmol/L)

1 mole	=	10^3 millimoles
1 millimole	=	10^3 micromoles
1 micromole	=	10^3 nanomoles and
1 nanomole	=	10^3 picomoles

EXAMPLES OF CONVERSIONS

Urea has a molecular weight of 60

$$\therefore 180\ \text{mg/100 ml urea} = \frac{180 \times 10}{60} = 30\ \text{mmol/L}$$

(the factor 10 is used to convert from 100 ml to 1 liter).

Glucose has a molecular weight of 180

$$\therefore 90\ \text{mg/100 ml glucose} = \frac{90 \times 10}{180} = 5\ \text{mmol/L}$$

For *univalent* ions the units remain the same if the concentration was previously expressed in mEq/L

e.g. *sodium* 140 mEq/L = 140 mmol/L

For *divalent* ions, e.g. calcium, the old values are divided by two, the valency of calcium
10 mg/100 ml calcium

$$\text{i.e. } 5\ \text{mEq/L} = \frac{5}{2} = 2.5\ \text{mmol/L}$$

Thus

$$= \frac{10 \times 10\ \text{(i.e. to convert from 100 ml to l liter)}}{40\ \text{(molecular weight of calcium)}} = 25\ \text{mmol/L}$$

10 mg/100 ml calcium = 5 mEq/L calcium = 2.5 mmol/L

SI UNITS ENZYMES

In serum and other tissues enzymes are always measured by their enzymatic activity alone, and never by absolute quantities of the enzyme. The units in which enzyme activity is expressed vary widely, in many cases depending primarily on the units used by the investigators who first estimated the enzyme clinically.

The International Union of Biochemistry recommended in 1964 that enzyme activities be expressed in international units (IU) where 1 IU is that amount of enzyme which will catalyze the transformation of 1 micromole of substrate per minute. A further unit of enzyme activity is the *Katal* which is that amount of an enzyme which will catalyze the transformation of 1 mole of substrate per second under defined conditions. The Katal is not in common usage.

However, despite this system of units, and because of the range of methods available – which may use different substrates to measure the same enzyme – the clinician should always be aware of the normal range of values relevant to the method used in his hospital. Units/Liter or U/L is now in common use.

Table 40.1 Normal blood serum and plasma values

	Traditional units, normal ranges	Multiplication factor	SI units, normal ranges
Acetoacetate plus acetone (serum)	Up to 3.0 mg/100 ml	10	Up to 30 mg/L
Acid phosphatase (serum)	5.0–12.6 U/L 2.8–7.0 King-Armstrong units		
Adrenocorticotropic hormone (ACTH) (plasma)	10–80 g/L		<2–20 mU/L
Alanine aminotransferase (ALT) (glutamic-pyruvic transaminase) (serum)			
Infants	10–80 U/L		
Children	10–40 U/L 10–35 spectrophotometric (Wroblewski) units		
Aldolase (serum)	2.6–13.5 U/L 3.5–18.3 Bruns units		
Aldosterone (plasma)			
Infants	<108 ng/100 ml	27.7	<3000 pmol/L
Children	<36 ng/100 ml		<1000 pmol/L
Alkaline phosphatase (ALP) (serum)			
Newborns and infants	140–1100 U/L		
Children	250–800 U/L 8–27.5 King-Armstrong units		
Amino acids (serum) (all values are in non-fasting plasma, and may be up to two times higher in neonates; all other amino acid concentrations are normally less than 25 µmol/L)			
Alanine	1.6–4.3 mg/100 ml	112.4	180–480 µmol/L
α-Aminobutyrate	0.1–0.4 mg/100 ml	97.1	10–40 µmol/L
Arginine	0.5–2.3 mg/100 ml	57.5	30–130 µmol/L
Asparagine	0.4–1.2 mg/100 ml	75.8	30–90 µmol/L
Aspartate	<2.3 mg/100 ml	75.2	<170 µmol/L
Citrulline	0.4–1.2 mg/100 ml	57.1	20–70 µmol/L
Cystine	0.5–2.6 mg/100 ml	41.7	20–110 µmol/L
Glutamate	<1.9 mg/100 ml	68	<130 µmol/L
Glutamine	7.9–12.3 mg/100 ml	68.4	540–840 µmol/L
Glycine	0.8–2.9 mg/100 ml	133.3	100–390 µmol/L
Histidine	<3.6 mg/100 ml	64.5	<230 µmol/L
Isoleucine	0.3–1.3 mg/100 ml	76.3	20–100 µmol/L
Leucine	0.8–3.0 mg/100 ml	76.3	60–230 µmol/L
Lysine	1.6–4.1 mg/100 ml	68.5	110–280 µmol/L
Methionine	<1.2 mg/100 ml	67.1	<80 µmol/L
Ornithine	0.4–1.3 mg/100 ml	75.8	30–100 µmol/L
Phenylalanine	0.3–2.1 mg/100 ml	60.6	20–130 µmol/L
Proline	1.0–3.2 mg/100 ml	87	90–280 µmol/L
Serine	0.8–3.0 mg/100 ml	95.2	80–290 µmol/L
Taurine	0.1–1.8 mg/100 ml	80	10–140 µmol/L
Threonine	1.0–2.6 mg/100 ml	84	80–220 µmol/L
Tryptophan	0.2–2.0 mg/100 ml	49	10–100 µmol/L
Tyrosine	0.5–1.8 mg/100 ml	55.2	30–100 µmol/L
Valine	1.2–3.9 mg/100 ml	85.5	100–330 µmol/L
α-Amino nitrogen (plasma or serum)			
Newborns	3.7–11.7 mg/100 ml	0.714	2.6–8.4 mmol/L
6 weeks–11 years	3.0–7.5 mg/100 ml		2.1–5.4 mmol/L
(serum values are higher than those in plasma)			
Ammonia (blood)			
Newborns (higher in jaundiced and premature infants)	90–150 µg/100 ml	0.587	53–88 µmol/L
Infants and older children	35–80 µg/100 ml		21–47 µmol/L
Amylase (negligible at birth)			
Infants	<50 U/L		
Children	100–400 U/L 60–200 Somogyi units		

Table 40.1 *Cont'd*

	Traditional units, normal ranges	Multiplication factor	SI units, normal ranges
Androstenedione (serum)			
Infants	<86 ng/100 ml	0.035	<3 nmol/L
Post-puberty			
Male	58–230 ng/100 ml		2–8 nmol/L
Female	58–315 ng/100 ml		2–11 nmol/L
α_1-Antitrypsin (α_1-Antiprotease) (serum)	1.8–4.0 g/L	1	1.8–4.0 g/L
Arginine vasopressin (AVP)			
Newborns	<10 pg/ml	1.0	<10 pmol/L
Thereafter	<5 pg/ml		<5 pmol/L
Ascorbic acid (plasma)	0.5–1.5 mg/100 ml	56.8	28–85 μmol/L
Aspartate aminotransferase (AST) (glutamic-oxaloacetic transaminase)			
Newborns	10–75 U/L		
Children	10–45 U/L		
10–40 spectrophotometric (Karmen) units			
Atrial natriuretic peptide (ANP)			
Newborns	30–150 pg/ml	0.33	10–50 pmol/L
Thereafter	5–35 pg/ml		1.7–11.7 pmol/L
Base excess (blood) (usually below -2.5 mmol/L in newborn)	+2.5 to -2.5 mEq/L	1.0	+2.5 to -2.5 mmol/L
Bicarbonate or total CO_2 (plasma)			
Newborns	18–23 mEq/L	1.0	18–23 mmol/L
Thereafter	20–26 mEq/L		20–26 mmol/L
Bilirubin, total (serum)			
Cord blood	Up to 2.9 mg/100 ml	17.1	Up to 50 μmol/L
Cord blood (premature infants)	Up to 3.4 mg/100 ml		Up to 58 μmol/L
First 24 h (higher in premature infants)	Up to 6.0 mg/100 ml		Up to 103 μmol/L
2–5 days (in the newborn period virtually all the bilirubin is present as free (unconjugated) bilirubin)	Up to 12 mg/100 ml		Up to 205 μmol/L
After 1 month (mainly unconjugated)	0.1–1.5 mg/100 ml		1.7–26 μmol/L
Blood volume			
At birth	61–100 (mean 78) ml/kg	1.0	61–100 (mean 78) ml/kg
Values increase slightly during 1st week			
Higher values are found in premature infants and when there is delayed clamping of the umbilical cord			
Thereafter values gradually fall towards adult values	53–87 (mean 71) ml/kg		53–87 (mean 71) ml/kg
Body water (expressed as a % of body weight – mean values)			
Total			
At birth	79%		79%
6 months	68%		68%
1 year and thereafter	60%		60%
Extracellular			
At birth	44%		44%
6 months	28%		28%
1 year	26%		26%
Falling gradually thereafter to	20%		20%
Intracellular			
At birth	35%		35%
6 months	38%		38%
1 year	34%		34%
Rising again by 2 years to	40%		40%
Calcium (serum)			
Cord blood	9.3-12.2 mg/100 ml	0.25	2.33-3.05 mmol/L

Table 40.1 *Cont'd*

	Traditional units, normal ranges	Multiplication factor	SI units, normal ranges
1st week			
Breast-fed	8.2–12.2 mg/100 ml		2.05–3.05 mmol/L
Bottle-fed	7.4–11.0 mg/100 ml		1.85–2.75 mmol/L
Thereafter	8.8–11.0 mg/100 ml		2.20–2.75 mmol/L
(About 40% of the calcium is protein bound, the remainder being ionized or ultrafiltrable. A slightly lower amount, 30–35%, is protein bound in the newborn period)			
Calcium, ionized (plasma)	4.0–5.2 mg/100 ml	0.25	1.00–1.30 mmol/L
Carbon dioxide, total (serum)			
Newborns	14–23 mmol/L	1.0	14–23 mmol/L
Increasing during first few hours of life to	18–27 mmol/L		18–27 mmol/L
PCO_2 – carbon dioxide, partial pressure (arterial blood) (higher values are found in newborn infants and in venous blood)	35–45 mmHg	0.133	4.7–6.0 kPa
Carboxyhemoglobin			
Newborns (higher in infants with Rh or ABO incompatibilities)	Up to 1.5% of total hemoglobin		Up to 1.5% total of hemoglobin
Older children	Up to 5% of total hemoglobin		Up to 5% of total hemoglobin
Carotenes (serum)			
Up to 1 year	70–340 µg/100 ml	0.0186	1.3–6.3 µmol/L
1 year and older	100–150 µg/100 ml		1.9–2.8 µmol/L
Catecholamines (plasma)			
Noradrenaline (norepinephrine)			
Supine	100–400 pg/ml	5.911	591–2364 pmol/L
Standing	300–900 pg/ml		1773–5320 pmol/L
Adrenaline (epinephrine)			
Supine	<70 pg/ml	5.458	<382 pmol/L
Standing	<100 pg/ml		<546 pmol/L
Dopamine			
Supine and standing	<30 pg/ml	6.528	<196 pmol/L
Ceruloplasmin (serum, plasma)			
Newborns	0.05–0.2 g/L	6.67	0.3–1.3 µmol/L
Thereafter	0.2–0.4 g/L		1.3–2.7 µmol/L
Chloride (serum)	95–106 mEq/L	1.0	95–106 mmol/L
Cholesterol (serum)			
Cord blood	23–135 mg/100 ml	0.0259	0.6–3.5 mmol/L
1–6 weeks	93–217 mg/100 ml		2.4–5.6 mmol/L
Increasing gradually until 1 year and older	119–263 mg/100 ml		3.1–6.8 mmol/L
Copper (serum)			
Cord blood	48–142 µg/100 ml	0.157	7.6–22.4 µmol/L
Older children	77–185 µg/100 ml		12.1–29.1 µmol/L
Copper oxidase (serum)			
Values are as for ceruloplasmin			
Cortisol (plasma)			
At birth (normally 1/5 to 1/2 of maternal plasma) lower values are seen in infants born by cesarean section than by vaginal delivery)	3.4–22.1 µg/100 ml	27.6	94–610 nmol/L
12 h	16.0 (mean) µg/100 ml		440 (mean) nmol/L
24 h	7.0 (mean) µg/100 ml		193 (mean) nmol/L
Older children			
0800 h	8–26 µg/100 ml		200–720 nmol/L
2200 h (usually less than 50% of 0800 h value)	Below 7.4 µg/100 ml		Below 205 nmol/L
(There is considerable diurnal variation such that the highest values are at about 0800 h and lowest around 2200–2400 h. This diurnal variation is absent in newborn infants up to about 5–6 weeks)			
Creatine kinase (serum) (CK)			
Newborns	<300 units/L		
Children	<200 units/L		

Table 40.1 *Cont'd*

	Traditional units, normal ranges	Multiplication factor	SI units, normal ranges
Creatinine (plasma)			
Newborns (higher in preterm infants)	0.2–1.1 mg/100 ml	88.4	20–100 μmol/L
Thereafter	0.2–0.9 mg/100 ml		20–80 μmol/L
Dehydroepiandrosterone (DHA) (serum)			
Children 7–10 years	7–10 g		0.4–7 nmol/L
Children 11–14 years	11–14 g		1–20 nmol/L
Dehydroepiandrosterone sulfate (DHAS) (serum)			
Newborns			0.5–7 μmol/L
Thereafter			<1.4 μmol/L
1,25-Dihydroxyvitamin (plasma)	25–45 pg/ml	2.4	60–108 nmol/L
2,3-Diphosphoglycerate (blood)			
Newborn (1st day)	3.4–7.5 mmol/L red blood cells		3.4–7.5 mmol/L red blood cells
5th day	4.9–8.9 mmol/L red blood cells		4.9–8.9 mmol/L red blood cells
Decreasing thereafter until at 3 weeks and thereafter	3.9–6.8 mmol/L red blood cells		3.9–6.8 mmol/L red blood cells
Dopamine (plasma) } see Catecholamines			
Adrenaline (epinephrine) (plasma) } see Catecholamines			
Estradiol (serum)			
Newborns	27–52 ng/100 ml	36.7	1000–1900 pmol/L
Prepubertal	<1.9 ng/100 ml		<70 pmol/L
Adults			
Male	<4.1 ng/100 ml		<150 pmol/L
Female	>2.2 ng/100 ml		>80 pmol/L
Fats – see Lipids			
Fatty acids – see Lipids			
Ferritin			
Cord blood	70–200 ng/ml		
1 day–2 months	100–500 ng/ml		
Thereafter values fall to:			
4 months (mean)	100 ng/ml		
6 months (mean)	60 ng/ml		
1 year	16–100 ng/ml		
5–15 years	10–100 ng/ml		
α_1-Fetoprotein (serum)			
Newborns	<55 000 units/ml (may be higher if premature)		
Infants at 8 weeks	<3100 units/ml		
Infants at 20 weeks	<40 units/ml		
Children	<15 units/ml		
Fibrinogen (plasma)			
Newborns	150–350 mg/100 ml	0.0294	4.4–10.3 μmol/L
Older children	200–400 mg/100 ml		5.8–11.6 μmol/L
Fibrin/fibrinogen degradation products (serum)	2.3–19.5 μg/ml	1.0	2.3–19.5 mg/L
Folic acid (serum) (higher values, up to 40 nmol/L are found in newborns and up to 50 nmol/L in preterm infants)	5–15 ng/ml	2.27	11–34 nmol/L
Follicle-stimulating hormone (FSH) (plasma)			
Children	<3.0 U/L		
Galactose (blood)			
Newborns	0–20 mg/100 ml	0.0556	0–1.1 mmol/L
Thereafter	<4.3 mg/100 ml		<240 μmol/L
Galactose-1-phosphate (blood)			
Children	<0.6 μmol/g Hb		
Galactose-1-phosphate uridyltransferase (erythrocytes)	>20 units/g Hb		
In galactosemia	<6 units/g Hb		
(Carriers)	(10–15 units/g Hb)		

Table 40.1 *Cont'd*

	Traditional units, normal ranges	Multiplication factor	SI units, normal ranges
Glucose (blood)			
Fasting	60–100 mg/100 ml	0.0556	3.3–5.5 mmol/L
Newborns	40–80 mg/100 ml		2.2–4.4 mmol/L
(Transiently low values below 2.2 mmol/L are commonly seen on the first day of life. Persistently low values should be investigated)			
Glutamic-oxaloacetic transaminase (serum) – see under Aspartate aminotransferase			
Glutamic-pyruvic transaminase (serum) – see under Alanine aminotransferase			
γ-Glutamyltransferase (serum) (γGT)			
Newborns	<200 units/L		
Infants	<120 units/L		
Children	<35 units/L		
Glycogen (erythrocytes)			
Newborns	48–361 μg/g hemoglobin	1.0	48–361 μg/g hemoglobin
Older children	32–151 μg/g hemoglobin		32–151 μg/g hemoglobin
Growth hormone (serum)	<5 mU/L		
Peak value should be above 15 mU/L after appropriate stimulation			
Hemoglobin (blood) – see Table 40.9			
Hemoglobin, glycated (hemoglobin A_1)	4.7–7.9% of total Hb		
Haptoglobins (serum)	30–200 mg/100 ml	0.01	0.3–2.0 g/L
Hydrogen ion concentration (see also pH)	(pH 7.35–7.42)		38–45 nmol/L
17-α-Hydroxyprogesterone (serum)			
Cord blood	<5000 ng/100 ml	0.03	<150 nmol/L
Newborns	<1000 ng/100 ml		<30 nmol/L
Children	<200 ng/100 ml		<6 nmol/L
25-Hydroxyvitamin D (plasma) (there is a seasonal variation in values which are highest in summer and lowest in winter)	>10 ng/ml	2.5	>25 nmol/L
Immunoglobulins – see Proteins			
Insulin (serum)			
Fasting	5–40 μ units/ml	1.0	5–40 mU/L
Newborns (before first feed)	25–87 μ units/ml		25–87 mU/L
Iron (serum)			
Newborns	110–270 μg/100 ml	0.179	19.7–48.3 μmol/L
Falling in first 6 months, then rising by 3 years of age to	60–175 μg/100 ml		10.7–31.3 μmol/L
(Higher values are found if determinations are done by atomic absorption spectrophotometry)			
Iron-binding capacity (serum) (TIBC)			
Newborns	59–175 μg/100 ml	0.179	11–31 μmol/L
Rising gradually during first 6 months to	250–400 μg/100 ml		45–72 μmol/L
Ketones	Up to 3 mg/100 ml	10	Up to 30 mg/L
Lactate (blood)			
Newborns	Up to 3.0 mEq/L	1.0	Up to 3.0 mmol/L
Thereafter	1.0–1.8 mEq/L		1.0–1.8 mmol/L
Lactate dehydrogenase (serum) (LDH) (Values may be twice as high in newborns)	58–230 units/L or 120–480 spectrophotometric (Wroblewski) units		
Lactate dehydrogenase isoenzymes (serum)			
LDH_1 (heart)	24–34%		
LDH_2 (heart, red blood cells)	35–45%		
LDH_3 (muscle)	15–25%		
LDH_4 (liver, muscle)	4–10%		
LDH_5 (liver, muscle)	1–9%		

Table 40.1 *Cont'd*

	Traditional units, normal ranges	Multiplication factor	SI units, normal ranges
Lead (blood)	Up to 40 μg/100 ml	0.0483	Up to 1.9 μmol/L
Lipids (serum)			
Total			
Newborns	150–400 mg/100 ml	0.01	1.5–4.0 g/L
Thereafter	400–1000 mg/100 ml		4.0–10.0 g/L
Free (non-esterified) fatty acids			
Newborns	250–1000 μEq/L	1.0	250–1000 μmol/L
Older children	300–1450 μEq/L		300–1450 μmol/L
Phospholipids			
Cord blood	75–150 mg/100 ml	0.01	0.75–1.5 g/L
Newborns	170–250 mg/100 ml		1.7–2.5 g/L
Older children	150–300 mg/100 ml		1.5–3.0 g/L
Phospholipid phosphorus	5–10 mg/100 ml	0.323	1.6–3.2 mmol/L
Triglycerides (plasma) – fasting	100–1300 mg/100 ml	0.00133	0.6–1.7 mmol/L
Lipoproteins (serum)			
Newborns			
Alpha	71–176 mg/100 ml	0.01	0.71–1.76 g/L
Beta	51–158 mg/100 ml		0.51–1.58 g/L
Omega (chylomicrons)	48–106 mg/100 ml		0.48–1.06 g/L
Total	170–440 mg/100 ml		1.70–4.40 g/L
There is a fairly sharp rise in the first 10 days, then a further gradual rise until at 2 years and older			
Alpha	147–327 mg/100 ml	0.01	1.47–3.27 g/L
Beta	225–541 mg/100 ml		2.25–5.41 g/L
Omega (chylomicrons)	98–268 mg/100 ml		0.98–2.68 g/L
Total	490–1090 mg/100 ml		4.90–10.9 g/L
Luteinizing hormone (LH) (serum)			
Children	<1.9 U/L		
Magnesium (serum)			
Cord blood	1.50–2.50 mg/100 ml	0.41	0.62–1.03 mmol/L
Newborns	1.40–2.45 mg/100 ml		0.58–1.00 mmol/L
Older children	1.45–2.32 mg/100 ml		0.60–0.95 mmol/L
Methemoglobin (blood)	0–0.3 g/100 ml	10	0–3 g/L
In preterm infants	0–0.4 g/100 ml		0–4 g/L
Non-protein nitrogen (serum)			
Cord blood	24–38 mg/100 ml	0.714	17–27 mmol/L
Newborns	20–33 mg/100 ml		14–24 mmol/L
Children	25–40 mg/100 ml		18–29 mmol/L
Noradrenaline (norepinephrine) (plasma) – see Catecholamines			
Osmolality (serum)	275–295 mosmol/kg	1.0	275–295 mmol/kg
Oxygen capacity (blood)	1.335 ml oxygen/g hemoglobin	1.0	1.335 ml oxygen/g hemoglobin
Oxygen content (blood)			
Umbilical vein (umbilical artery values are usually 4–8 vol. % lower)	5.5–18.8 vol. %		
Children	13.7–17.5 vol. %		
Oxygen saturation (arterial blood)			
Umbilical artery	0–32%		
Umbilical vein	26–73% (mean 47%)		
Children	86–101%		
Oxygen saturation (venous blood)			
Newborns	30–80%		
Older children	60–85%		
Parathyroid hormone (plasma)	<0.2 U/L		
PCO_2 – see Carbon dioxide			
pH (arterial blood) (See also hydrogen ion) (Venous blood values are 0.03 lower)	7.35–7.42		
PO_2– oxygen tension (arterial blood)			
Umbilical vein	12.8–32.0 mmHg	0.133	1.7–4.3 kPa

Table 40.1 *Cont'd*

	Traditional units, normal ranges		Multiplication factor		SI units, normal ranges	
PO_2– oxygen tension (arterial blood) *Cont'd*						
Newborns after first 24 h	77–100 mmHg				9.3–13.3 kPa	
Older children	85–105 mmHg				11.3–14.0 kPa	
Phenylalanine (plasma)						
Umbilical vein	0.4–2.0 mg/100 ml		60.5		25–119 μmol/L	
Newborns (Transient values above 2.8 mg/100 ml may be found in the newborn period. Plasma concentrations are usually maintained at between 84 and 300 μmol/L in the treatment of phenylketonuria)	0.7–2.8 mg/100 ml				42–170 μmol/L	
Phospholipids (serum) – see Lipids						
Phosphorus, inorganic (serum)						
Cord blood	3.2–7.6 mg/100 ml		0.323		1.03–2.45 mmol/L	
Newborns, 1st week	5.8–9.0 mg/100 ml				1.87–2.91 mmol/L	
Newborns, 2nd week	4.9–8.9 mg/100 ml				1.58–2.87 mmol/L	
Up to 1 year	4.0–6.5 mg/100 ml				1.30–2.10 mmol/L	
Thereafter	3.6–5.9 mg/100 ml				1.16–1.91 mmol/L	
(Phosphorus values in the newborn period vary greatly depending very much on the type of milk feed; lower values are found in breast-fed infants)						
Plasma volume						
At birth	33.5–49.5 ml/kg		1.0		33.5–49.5 ml/kg	
Rising until at 3–6 months of age the mean value is about	54 ml/kg				54 ml/kg	
Thereafter it falls so that the range for older children is	31–54 ml/kg				31–54 ml/kg	
Potassium (serum)						
Umbilical vein	3.3–6.8 mEq/L		1.0		3.3–6.8 mmol/L	
Newborns	4.3–7.6 mEq/L				4.3–7.6 mmol/L	
Older children	3.5–5.6 mEq/L				3.5–5.6 mmol/L	
Progesterone (serum)						
Adults						
Male	<64 ng/100 ml		0.032		<2 nmol/L	
Female	<2800 ng/100 ml				<90 nmol/L	
Prolactin (serum)						
Newborns	<4000 mU/L					
Children	60–390 mU/L					
Proteins (serum)						
Values in g/100 ml	Total	Albumin	Globulins			
			α_1	α_2	β	γ
Newborns	4.6–7.7	2.5–5.0	0.1–0.3	0.4–0.6	0.3–0.6	0.8–1.2
1 year	5.6–7.3	3.5–5.0	0.2–0.4	0.4–1.0	0.5–1.0	0.5–1.3
4 years and over	6.0–8.0	3.7–5.0	0.2–0.4	0.4–1.0	0.6–1.1	0.5–1.8
Values in g/L (using multiplication factor of 10)						
Newborns	46–77	25–50	1–3	4–6	3–6	6–14
1 year	56–73	35–50	2–4	4–10	5–9	4–12
4 years and over	60–80	37–50	2–4	4–10	6–10	5–12
(Low total protein and albumin values are found in immature infants)						
Immunoglobulins (serum)	IgG		IgA		IgM	
	mg/100 ml	g/L	mg/100 ml	g/L	mg/100 ml	g/L
Newborns	650–1450	6.5–14.5	0–10	0–0.1	0–30	0–0.3
1–3 months	200–650	2.0–6.5	5–40	0.05–0.4	10–100	0.1–1.0
4–6 months	150–800	1.5–8.0	10–60	0.1–0.6	10–100	0.1–1.0
1 year	300–1200	3.0–12.0	20–80	0.2–0.8	40–200	0.4–2.0
3 years and older	500–1500	5.0–15.0	30–300	0.3–3.0	40–200	0.4–2.0
(Immunoglobulin values vary widely in children, particularly in the first 6 months of life. Care should be taken therefore in interpreting marginal differences from the normal)						
Pyruvate (blood)	0.05–0.09 mEq/L		1000		50–80 μmol/L	
Renin (plasma)	1.1–4.1 mg/ml/h					

Table 40.1 *Cont'd*

	Traditional units, normal ranges	Multiplication factor	SI units, normal ranges
Sodium (serum, plasma)			
Newborns	132–145 mEq/L	1.0	132–145 mmol/L
Thereafter	135–145 mEq/L		135–145 mmol/L
Standard bicarbonate (blood)			
Umbilical vein	12–21 mEq/L	1.0	12–21 mmol/L
Newborns	18–25		18–25 mmol/L
Thereafter	21–25		21–25 mmol/L
Sulfate (serum)	0.5–1.5 mg/100 ml	104.1	50–150 μmol/L
Testosterone (serum)			
Newborns (male)	Up to 200 mg/100 ml	0.0347	<7 nmol/L
Infants (male), 2–4 months	<375 mg/100 ml		<13 nmol/L
Boys			
Prepubertal	Up to 100 ng/100 ml	0.0347	Up to 3.5 nmol/L
Rising at puberty to	290–865 ng/100 ml		10–30 nmol/L
Girls	<100 ng/100 ml		<3.5 nmol/L
Thyrotropin or thyroid stimulating hormone – TSH (serum)			
Newborns	<25 mU/L		
Thereafter	0.3–5.0 mU/L		
Thyroxine – T_4 (serum)			
Cord blood and newborns	11–34 μg/100 ml	12.9	140–440 nmol/L
Infants	7–15 μg/100 ml		90–195 nmol/L
Children	5.4–14 μg/100 ml		70–180 nmol/L
Thyroxine, free (FT_4) (serum)	0.7–1.8 ng/100 ml	12.9	9–23 pmol/L
Triiodothyronine – T_3 (serum)			
Cord blood (values are well below maternal serum values)	10–45 ng/100 ml	0.0154	0.15–0.45 nmol/L
Newborns	50–400 ng/100 ml		0.8–6.2 nmol/L
Thereafter	100–250 ng/100 ml		1.5–3.8 nmol/L
Tyrosine (plasma)			
Cord blood	0.7–2.0 mg/100 ml	0.0552	39–110 μmol/L
Newborns (Transiently increased values may be found in the newborn, particularly in the immature infant. Markedly or persistently high values should be investigated)	0.7–5.6 mg/100 ml		39–309 μmol/L
Older children	0.7–1.1 mg/100 ml		39–61 μmol/L
Urea (blood) (Higher values are commonly seen during the first 6 months of life in infants fed on unmodified milks, i.e. those whose protein concentration is substantially above that of breast milk)	15–40 mg/100 ml	0.166	2.5–6.6 mmol/L
Urea nitrogen (blood) (See comment on protein intake under Urea as blood urea nitrogen also depends on protein intake as well as functional maturity of the kidneys)	7–19 mg/100 ml	0.357	2.5–6.8 mmol/L
Uric acid (serum)	2.0–7.0 mg/100 ml	0.0595	0.12–0.42 mmol/L
Vitamin A (serum)	20–100 μg/100 ml	0.0349	0.7–3.5 μmol/L
Vitamin C, ascorbic acid (plasma)	0.5–1.5 mg/100 ml	56.8	28–85 μmol/L
Vitamin E, α-tocopherol (plasma)			
Cord blood and newborn infants	0.2–0.6 mg/100 ml	23.2	5–14 μmol/L
Vitamin E concentrations increase slowly with age until at 2 years and older the normal range is	0.5–1.2 mg/100 ml		12–28 μmol/L
Newborn infants if artificially fed continue to have plasma concentrations similar to or slightly above the values quoted for cord blood. Breast-fed infants however have higher values similar to those of older children.Preterm infants have lower values than full-term infants			
Zinc (serum)			
Cord blood	72–212 μg/100 ml	0.153	11–32 μmol/L
Children	60–190 μg/100 ml		9–29 μmol/L

Table 40.2 Normal constituents of urine

	Traditional units, normal ranges	Multiplication factor	SI units, normal ranges
Acidity – see pH and Titratable acidity			
Adrenaline	0.02–0.7 μg/kg/24 h	5.46	0.11–0.38 nmol/kg/24 h
Aldosterone – see Steroids			
Amino acids (these values may be up to two times higher in neonates)			
Alanine	232–717 mg/g creatinine	0.099	23–71 μmol/mmol creatinine
α-Aminoadipate	18–145 mg/g creatinine	0.055	1–8 μmol/mmol creatinine
α-Aminobutyrate	23–93 mg/g creatinine	0.086	2–8 μmol/mmol creatinine
β-Aminoisobutyrate	23–581 mg/g creatinine	0.086	2–50 μmol/mmol creatinine
Arginine	59–216 mg/g creatinine	0.051	3–11 μmol/mmol creatinine
Asparagine	<90 mg/g creatinine	0.067	<6 μmol/mmol creatinine
Aspartate	106–455 mg/g creatinine	0.066	7–30 μmol/mmol creatinine
Citrulline	20–137 mg/g creatinine	0.051	1–7 μmol/mmol creatinine
Cystathionine			<20 μmol/mmol creatinine
Cystine	108–405 mg/g creatinine	0.037	4–15 μmol/mmol creatinine
Glutamate	<50 mg/g creatinine	0.060	<3 μmol/mmol creatinine
Glutamine	557–1459 mg/g creatinine	0.061	34–89 μmol/mmol creatinine
Glycine	958–4593 mg/g creatinine	0.118	113–542 μmol/mmol creatinine
Histidine	825–5754 mg/g creatinine	0.057	47–328 μmol/mmol creatinine
Isoleucine	15–90 mg/g creatinine	0.067	1–6 μmol/mmol creatinine
Leucine	30–164 mg/g creatinine	0.067	2–11 μmol/mmol creatinine
Lysine	115–475 mg/g creatinine	0.061	7–29 μmol/mmol creatinine
Methionine	34–153 mg/g creatinine	0.059	2–9 μmol/mmol creatinine
Ornithine	30–119 mg/g creatinine	0.067	2–8 μmol/mmol creatinine
Phenylalanine	74–315 mg/g creatinine	0.054	4–17 μmol/mmol creatinine
Phosphoethanolamine			2–25 μmol/mmol creatinine
Proline	<13 mg/g creatinine	0.077	<1 μmol/mmol creatinine
Serine	298–607 mg/g creatinine	0.084	25–51 μmol/mmol creatinine
Taurine	521–2281 mg/g creatinine	0.071	37–162 μmol/mmol creatinine
Threonine	149–338 mg/g creatinine	0.074	11–25 μmol/mmol creatinine
Tryptophan	23–186 mg/g creatinine	0.043	1–8 μmol/mmol creatinine
Tyrosine	102–306 mg/g creatinine	0.049	5–15 μmol/mmol creatinine
Valine	13–92 mg/g creatinine	0.076	1–7 μmol/mmol creatinine
α-Amino nitrogen			
Premature infants	10.0–26.8 mg/kg/24 h	71.4	714–1910 μmol/kg/24 h
Newborns	6.8–20.7 mg/kg/24 h		485–1480 μmol/kg/24 h
Infants	3.4–8.5 mg/kg/24 h		243–607 μmol/kg/24 h
Children (values are lower in breast-milk-fed babies than in those fed on cow's milk)	0.9–2.9 mg/kg/24 h		64–207 μmol/kg/24 h
Using creatinine as an index the normal values in children are	0.14–0.78 mg α-amino nitrogen/μmol creatinine nitrogen	631	88–492 μmol α-amino nitrogen/μmol creatinine nitrogen
δ-Aminolevulinic acid (high levels are found in lead poisoning and in some porphyrias)	Up to 0.5 mg/100 ml	7.63	Up to 38 μmol/L
Ammonia			
Newborns: 1st day	0.02–0.50 mEq/kg/24 h	1.0	0.02–0.50 mmol/kg/24 h
Newborns: 7th day	0.26–0.86 mEq/kg/24 h		0.26–0.86 mmol/kg/24 h
Children	0.52–1.08 mEq/kg/24 h or 7–34 μEq/min/1.73 m^2		0.52–1.08 mmol/kg/24 h 7–34 μmol/min/1.73 m^2
Ascorbic acid load test			
>5% of an oral dose of 20 mg/kg are excreted in 24 h			
Bicarbonate			
None when the pH is below 6.8			
Calcium			
Newborns (1st week of life)	0–0.7 mg/kg/24 h	25	0–17.5 μmol/kg/24 h
Infants	Up to 40 mg/24 h		Up to 1000 μmol/24 h
Older children	Up to 4 mg/kg/24 h or 30–150 mg/24 h		Up to 100 μmol/kg/24 h or 750–3750 μmol/24 h

Table 40.2 *Cont'd*

	Traditional units, normal ranges	Multiplication factor	SI units, normal ranges
Calcium : creatinine ratio (estimated on the second morning urine, i.e. the first specimen voided after the overnight urine has been passed)	Up to 0.25 mg/mg	2.82	Up to 0.7 mmol/mmol
Catecholamines			
Total	0.4–2.0 μg/kg/24 h	5.91	2.4–11.8 μmol/kg/24 h – calculated as noradrenaline
Adrenaline (epinephrine)	0.027–0.7 μg/kg/24 h	5.46	0.15–3.8 μmol/kg/24 h
Noradrenaline (norepinephrine)	0.4–1.6 μg/kg/24 h	5.91	2.4–9.5 μmol/kg/24 h
Cells			
Erythrocytes	0–2 mm^3	10^6	0–2 × 10^6/L
Leukocytes			
Males	0–4 mm^3		0–4 × 10^6/L
Females	0–20 mm^3		0–20 × 10^6/L
Chloride			
Newborn infant	Up to 3 g/L	28.2	Up to 85 mmol/L
Older children	Up to 4 mEq/kg/24 h or 170–250 mEq/L		Up to 4 mmol/kg/24 h or 170–250 mmol/L
Concentrating capacity – see Osmolality			
Copper	Up to 40 μg/24 h or <40 μg/100 ml	0.0157	Up to 0.6 μmol/24 h or <6.3 μmol/L
Coproporphyrin (increased excretion is found in lead poisoning, liver disease and some porphyrias)	Up to 0.1 μg/ml	1.53	Up to 0.15 μmol/L
Creatine			
Newborns	Up to 36 mg/kg/24 h	7.69	Up to 280 μmol/kg/24 h
Infants	Up to 15 mg/kg/24 h		Up to 115 μmol/kg/24 h
Values in girls are higher than those in boys			
There is a gradually decreasing creatine excretion with age to adult levels of	Up to 2 mg/kg/24 h		Up to 15 μmol/kg/24 h
Creatinine			
Newborns and infants	10–20 mg/kg/24 h	8.84	88–176 μmol/kg/24 h
Older children	5–40 mg/kg/24 h		44–354 μmol/kg/24 h
Creatinine clearance			
Newborns	40–65 ml/min/1.73 m^2		
Increasing gradually until at 1 year and older			
Males	98–150 ml/min/1.73 m^2		
Females	95–123 ml/min/1.73 m^2		
Galactose			
Infants on a milk diet may excrete up to	20–25 mg/100 ml	0.056	1.1–1.4 mmol/L
Much higher values are seen in galactosemia			
Glucose			
Newborns	Up to 20 mg/100 ml	0.056	Up to 1.1 mmol/L
Older children	Up to 5 mg/100 ml		Up to 0.28 mmol/L
Homovanillic acid (HVA) Increased in neuroblastoma	3–16 μg/mg creatinine		
5-Hydroxyindole acetic acid	1.4–13.2 mg/24 h	5.26	7–70 μmol/24 h
4-Hydroxy 3-methoxymandelate (HMMA) – see under Vanillylmandelic acid			
5-Hydroxytryptamine (serotonin)	43–123 μg/24 h		
Lead	1.5–22 μg/24 h	4.83	7–106 nmol/24 h
Magnesium			
Newborns (1st week of life)	Up to 10 mg/24 h	41.1	Up to 411 μmol/24 h
Older children	1.24–4.4 mg/kg/24 h		51–181 μmol/kg/24 h
Magnesium/creatinine ratio	Up to 0.41 mg/mg	0.215	Up to 0.09 mmol/mmol
Metanephrine (high values, above 0.2, are found in pheochromocytoma)	0.02–0.16 μg/mg creatinine		

Table 40.2 *Cont'd*

	Traditional units, normal ranges	Multiplication factor	SI units, normal ranges
Mucopolysaccharides (expressed as hexuronic acid)	Increasing from 0.5 mg/24 h at age 2 years to 2–12 mg/24 h at 14 years		
Normetanephrine (increased in pheochromocytoma)	0.05–0.6 μg/mg creatinine		
Osmolality			
Newborns			
Delivery urine	79–118 mosmol/kg	1.0	79–118 mmol/kg
Maximum in neonatal period	600 mosmol/kg		600 mmol/kg
After at least a 12-h thirst or in the 4 h after DDAVP the osmolality should be greater than 750 mosmol/kg (specific gravity 1.022)			>750 mmol/kg
Normal values of up to 1200 mosmol/kg may be observed but in newborns and young infants, until maturity of renal function is obtained, values of this order are not found			Up to 1200 mmol/kg
pH			
Newborns	5.0 or higher		
Older children	5.3–7.2		
Phosphorus			
Newborns (breast-fed) (values for cow's-milk-fed babies may be up to 10 times higher)	0–0.7 mg/24 h	0.0325	Up to 0.023 mg/kg/24 h
Infants	Up to 200 mg/24 h		Up to 6.5 mmol/24 h
Older children	15–20 mg/kg/24 h		0.49–0.65 mmol/kg/24 h
Porphobilinogen (no increase in lead poisoning)	Up to 0.2 mg/100 ml		
Potassium			
Newborns (breast-fed) (up to twice this value in infants fed on cow's milk formulae)	Up to 2.3 mEq/kg/24 h	1.0	Up to 2.3 mmol/kg/24 h
Older children (usually about half the sodium excretion)	Up to 2 mEq/kg/24 h		Up to 2 mmol/kg/24 h or 25–125 mmol/L
Protein			
Newborns	About 10 mg/24 h		
Older children	30–50 mg/24 h (about 25% albumin)		
Sodium			
Newborns (breast-fed)			
1st day	0.11–0.39 mEq/kg/24 h	1.0	0.11–0.39 mmol/kg/24 h
7th day	Up to 4.4 mEq/kg/24 h		Up to 4.4 mmol/kg/24 h or 1.5 mmol/h/1.73 m^2 (mean)
(Values are normally up to 50% above this level in infants fed on cow's milk formulae and in preterm infants)			
Older children	Up to 3.7 mEq/kg/24 h		Up to 3.7 mmol/kg/24 h or 40–225 mmol/24 h
Steroids			
Aldosterone	1–5 μg/24 h	2.774	2.7–14 nmol/24 h
17-Hydroxycorticosteroids (17-oxogenic steroids)			
Newborns	Up to 1 mg/24 h	3.47	Up to 3.5 μmol/24 h
Up to 6 years	2–6 mg/24 h		7–21 μmol/24 h
6–9 years	6–8 mg/24 h		21–28 μmol/24 h
10–14 years	8–10 mg/24 h		28–35 μmol/24 h
17-Ketosteroids (17-oxosteroids)			
Newborns (1st 2 weeks)	0.5–2.5 mg/24 h	3.47	1.7–8.7 μmol/24 h
2 weeks–2 years	0–0.5 mg/24 h		0–1.7 μmol/24 h
2–8 years	0–2.5 mg/24 h		0–8.7 μmol/24 h
8–10 years	0.7–4 mg/24 h		2.4–14 μmol/24 h
Thereafter there is a gradual increase during puberty to values of:			
Boys	2.5–13 mg/24 h		8.7–45 μmol/24 h
Girls	2.5–11 mg/24 h		8.7–38 μmol/24 h
Pregnanediol	0–1 mg/24 h	3.12	0.3–3 μmol/24 h

Table 40.2 *Cont'd*

	Traditional units, normal ranges	Multiplication factor	SI units, normal ranges
Pregnanetriol			
Newborns	0.2–0.3 mg/24 h	2.97	0.6–0.9 μmol/24 h
Older children	Up to 1.1 mg/24 h		Up to 3.3 μmol/24 h
Steroid ratio:			
11-Deoxysteroids / 11-Oxysteroids	>0.5 (first week of life >0.8)		
This steroid 11-oxygenation index is a reflection of the efficiency of the last stage of cortisol biosynthesis High values are found in congenital adrenal hyperplasia			
Testosterone (before puberty)	Up to 5 μg/24 h	3.47	Up to 17 nmol/24 h
Titratable acidity			
Newborns	45–110 μEq/min/1.73 m^2 or about 0.3 mEq/kg/24 h	1.0	45–110 μmol/min/1.73 m^2 or about 0.3 mmol/kg/24 h
Older children	35–70 μEq/min/1.73 m^2 or 1 mEq/kg/24 h		35–70 μmol/min/1.73 m^2 or 1 mmol/kg/24 h
Urea clearance (lower in newborns)	50–90 ml/min/1.73 m^2		
Urobilinogen	Up to 3 mg/24 h		
Vanillylmandelic acid (VMA) or 4-hydroxy-3-methoxymandelate (HMMA)			
Newborns–6 months	Up to 200 μg/kg/24 h	5.05	Up to 1010 nmol/kg/24 h
6 months–15 years	60–150 μg/kg/24 h or <6 mg/24 h		300–760 nmol/kg/24 h or <30 μmol/24 h
(Elevated levels are seen in children with neuroblastomas, gangliomas and pheochromocytomas)			
Volume			

1st and 2nd days:	15–60 ml	1–3 years:	500–600 ml
3–10 days:	50–300 ml	3–4 years:	600–700 ml
10 days–2 months:	250–450 ml	5–7 years:	650–1000 ml
2 months–1 year:	400–500 ml	8–14 years:	800–1400 ml

Many other substances which are either not normally present in the urine or which are present in small quantities may be estimated when appropriate. These include hemoglobin, homogentisic acid, phenylpyruvic acid, etc.

Table 40.3 Normal cerebrospinal fluid (CSF) values

	Traditional units, normal ranges	Multiplication factor	SI units, normal ranges
β-n-Acetylhexosaminidase	0–4 IU/L	1.0	0–4 IU/L
γ-Aminobutyric acid (GABA)			83–383 pmol/L
α-Amino nitrogen	1.0–1.5 mg/100 ml	0.714	0.7–1.1 mmol/L
Aspartate aminotransferase			
Newborns	1–10 Karmen spectrophotometric units (0.5–5.0 IU/L)		
Older children	2–20 Karmen units (1–10 IU/L)		
(In the normal child the CSF level of this enzyme is about half that of the serum level. Increased CSF levels of the enzyme occur in infants and children with various intracranial pathological conditions such as acute bacterial meningitis)			
Bicarbonate	21.3–25.9 mEq/L	1.0	21.3–25.9 mmol/L
Bilirubin			
Newborns (correlates with serum levels: most is unconjugated)	0.04–0.44 mg/100 ml	17.1	0.7–7.5μmol/L
Older children	None		None
(CSF concentrations vary with changes in serum concentration. Free bilirubin can be identified if present in significant quantity on a spectrophotometric scan due to its characteristic flattened			

Table 40.3 *Cont'd*

	Traditional units, normal ranges	Multiplication factor	SI units, normal ranges
Bilirubin *Cont'd*			
peak with a maximum at about 455 nm. Conjugated bilirubin (bilirubin glucuronides) has a maximum at 422 nm. Where bilirubin is present in increased amounts and there is spectrophotometric evidence of 'old' blood also, the most likely source of both is a CNS hemorrhage. Large amounts of bilirubin are seen in the CSF with no blood present in neonatal hyperbilirubinemia[3,4]			
Calcium			
Newborns	5.5–7.7 mg/100 ml	0.25	1.38–1.93 mmol/L
Older children	4.0–5.2 mg/100 ml		1.0–1.30 mmol/L
(Spinal fluid calcium concentration approximates to that of serum ionized calcium)			
Cell count			
Erythrocytes			
During the first 14 days of life	Up to 675/mm^3	10^6	Up to 675 × 10^6/L
Later	0–2/mm^3		0–2 × 10^6/L
Leukocytes: in newborns, particularly in premature infants	Up to 14/mm^3		Up to 14 × 10^6/L
In the first year of life	Up to 10/mm^3		Up to 10 × 10^6/L
After 1 year	Up to 5/mm^3		Up to 5 × 10^6/L
Chloride	116–128 mEq/L	1.0	116–128 mmol/L
The range is slightly lower in newborn and young infants	109–123 mEq/L		109–123 mmol/L
Carbon dioxide			
Combining power (see also PCO_2)	22–28 mEq/L	1.0	22–28 mmol/L
Cholesterol	219–571 μg/100 ml	0.0259	5.7–14.8 μmol/L
Newborns	Up to 220 μg/100 ml		Up to 5.7 μmol/L
(approximately 35% is free cholesterol and 65% esterified)			
Creatine kinase			
Newborns	0.7–2.0 IU/L	1.0	0.7–2.0 IU/L
Older children	0.2–1.6 IU/L		0.2–1.6 IU/L
Glucose (the CSF level is less than, but varies with, changes in blood glucose. It is often low in newborn infants and pathologically low when the CSF is infected)	50–80 mg/100 ml	0.0556	2.8–4.4 mmol/L
β-Glucuronidase	0–30 mIU/L	1.0	0–30 mIU/L
Glutamic-oxaloacetic transaminase – see Aspartate aminotransferase			
Homovanillic acid (HVA)	75–200 mg/ml		
5-Hydroxyindole acetic acid			
Birth–1 year	90–150 ng/ml	5.24	470–785 nmol/L
1 year onwards	30–90 ng/ml		160–470 nmol/L
Lactate	7.2–22.0 mg/100 ml	0.112	0.8–2.4 mmol/L
(lactate : pyruvate ratio 14.3–17.6. Higher values are found in newborns following intrauterine or neonatal asphyxia)			
Lactate dehydrogenase (LDH)			
Newborns	3–120 Wroblewski units (1.5–58 IU/L)	1.0	3–120 Wroblewski units (1.5–58 IU/L)
Older children	14–59 Wroblewski units (6.8–30 IU/L)		14–59 Wroblewski units (6.8–30 IU/L)
(Increased LDH activity in the CSF is observed in acute bacterial infections and in many cases of organic brain disease)			
Lipids			
Total	766–1740 μg/100 ml	0.01	7.7–17.4 mg/L
Free (non-esterified) fatty acids	42–98 μEq/L	1.0	42–98 μmol/L
Neutral fat (glycerides)	0–900 μg/100 ml	0.01	0–9 mg/L
Phospholipids	209–889 μg/100 ml	0.01	2.1–8.9 mg/100 ml
Magnesium			
Newborns	1.8–2.6 mEq/L	0.5	0.9–1.3 mmol/L
Older children	0.49–4.0 mEq/L		0.25–2.0 mmol/L

Table 40.3 *Cont'd*

	Traditional units, normal ranges	Multiplication factor	SI units, normal ranges
Non-protein nitrogen	11–20 mg/100 ml	10	110–200 mg/L
Osmolality	273–304 mosmol/kg (mean 285)	1.0	273–304 mmol/kg (mean 285)
(It has been suggested that if the CSF osmolality is considerably greater than that of the serum, severe neurological disturbance may occur. This is particularly true in hyperosmolar hypernatremic dehydration[5]			
PCO_2			
Newborns	38–63 mmHg (mean 49)	0.133	5.1–8.4 kPa (mean 6.5)
Thereafter	40–51 mmHg		5.3–6.8 kPa
pH	7.32–7.37		
Potassium	2.1–3.9 mEq/L	1.0	2.1–3.9 mmol/L
(Levels in spinal fluid are largely independent of serum values. Infants may have lower values than the range quoted)			
Phosphorus, inorganic			
Newborns	0.7–3.1 mg/100 ml	0.323	0.23–1.00 mmol/L
Older children	1.4–2.2 mg/100 ml		0.45–0.71 mmol/L
Pressure			
Newborns	50–80 mm water		
Infants	40–150 mm water		
Children	70–200 mm water		
Protein			
Lumbar fluid	20–40 mg/100 ml	10	200–400 mg/L
Lumbar fluid contains more protein than fluid from the cisterna magna which in turn contains more protein than ventricular fluid. Thus the upper limit of normal for cisternal fluid is	25 mg/100 ml		250 mg/L
And that for ventricular fluid	15 mg/100 ml		150 mg/L
Newborns (lumbar fluid)	25–90 mg/100 ml		250–900 mg/L
Reducing to upper limits of normal at 1 month	70 mg/100 ml		700 mg/L
And at 6 months	40 mg/100 ml		400 mg/L
Even higher values up to	250 or 300 mg/100 ml		2500–3000 mg/L
may be found in premature infants and in some term infants			
Protein electrophoresis			
Newborns:			
Albumin (+ prealbumin)	50%		
α_1-Globulins	7%		
α_2-Globulins	9%		
β-Globulins	14%		
γ-Globulins	20%		
Gradually changing until in			
Older children:			
Albumin (+ prealbumin)	52%		
α_1-Globulins	7%		
α_2-Globulins	9%		
β-Globulins	20%		
γ-Globulins	12%		
Pyruvate	0.4–0.7 mg/100 ml	113	40–80 μmol/L
Newborns	0.6–1.2 mg/100 ml		70–140 μmol/L
Sodium	130–157 mEq/L	1	130–157 mmol/L
Urea nitrogen	7–18 mg/100 ml	0.166	1.2–3.0 mmol/L
Uric acid	0.5–2.6 mg/100 ml	0.0595	0.03–0.15 mmol/L
Volume			
Infants	40–60 ml		
Young children	60–100 ml		
Older children	80–120 ml		
Adults	100–160 ml		
Water content	98.3–99.6 g/100 ml		

Table 40.4 Normal constituents of stools

Amount
Meconium: 70–90 g
Newborns: Breast-milk-fed: 15–25 g/24 h
Cow's-milk-fed: 30–40 g/24 h
2 months–6 years: 7–54 g/24 h
Older children: 30–200 g/24 h
(Amount is lower on a mainly meat diet, but may be higher than quoted values on a mainly vegetable diet)

Appearance
69% of healthy newborns have their first stools within 12 h and 94% within 24 h
Meconium: greenish-brown to black
Infants: golden yellow (due to bilirubin), on breast milk, turning green (biliverdin) on standing, brown (stercobilin) on cow's milk
Older children: brown (stercobilin, bilifuscin, mesobilifuscin) darkening on exposure to air; pitch black when hematin content is high due to stomach or upper intestinal tract hemorrhage; light gray when fat content is high, due to breakdown products of bile pigments

Bilirubin
Meconium: 430–1750 μmol/kg (252–1020 mg/kg)
The bilirubin content of stools falls as that of the plasma rises in the newborn period. This fall continues throughout the first year of life when adult values of 9–34 μg/kg (5–20 mg/24 h) are reached.
Disturbances of intestinal flora by antibiotics can cause an increase in bilirubin content

Blood
The Apt test for fetal hemoglobin may be performed on stool samples to show whether blood in the stool of a newborn infant is maternal in origin or from the infant[6]

Calcium
Meconium: 3.3–20 mmol/kg (130–800 mg/kg)
Infants: 6.5–8.25 mmol/24 h (200–300 mg/24 h) increasing in childhood towards adult values of 7.5–32.5 mmol/24 h (300–1000 mg/24 h)

Copper
Meconium: 157–393 μmol/kg (10–25 mg/kg) increasing to adult values of 0–79 μmol/24 h (0–5 mg/24 h)

Coproporphyrin
See Porphyrins

Fat and fatty acids
See Lipids

Iron
Meconium: 215–484 μmol/kg (12–27 mg/kg) increasing to adult values of 102–120 μmol/24 h (5.7–6.7 mg/24 h)

Lactic acid
Up to 0.44 mmol/24 h (40 mg/24 h)
Increased in carbohydrate malabsorption

Lipids
Total fats: in children greater than 90% of dietary fat should be absorbed where fat intake is normal. Although normal total fecal fat is usually less than 2 g/day, the upper limit of normal is usually set at about 4.5–5 g/day. In addition the proportion of fat is usually less than 50% of the fecal dry weight in young children up to 6 months and less than 25% in older children
Free fatty acids: up to 1.4 g per 24 h or about two-thirds of the total fat

Magnesium
Meconium: 9–30 mmol/kg (219–729 mg/kg) increasing to adult value of 5–15 mmol/24 h (122–365 mg/24 h)

Nitrogen
Meconium: 19 g/kg (mean value)
Newborn infants: breast-milk-fed: 160 mg/24 h
Cow's-milk-fed: 400 mg/24 h
Adult: 1–2 g/24 h

Organic acids
Up to 400 mmol/kg

pH
Meconium: 5.7–6.4
Newborns, breast-milk-fed: 4.6–5.2
In general while infants on breast milk have acid stools, those on cow's milk have neutral or alkaline stools
Older children: 5.0–8.8, but normally slightly alkaline (7.0–7.5)
Stools with a pH of less than 5 should be further examined for reducing substances, etc.

Phosphorus
Meconium: 2.4–7.9 mmol/kg (74–254 mg/kg)
Infants: 4.9–6.0 mmol/24 h (157–193 mg/24 h) increasing in childhood towards adult values of 10–24 mmol/24 h (310–775 mg/24 h)

Porphyrins
Coproporphyrin and protoporphyrin are found in stools in small quantities, usually less than 1–2 mg/24 h
Coproporphyrin is related to the amount of meat in the diet. See also Bilirubin and Urobilinogen

Potassium
Meconium: 12–51 mmol/kg

Protein
Small amounts, mainly undigested nutrient protein and bacterial proteins are found

Sodium
Meconium: 90–182 mmol/kg

Trypsin
Meconium: None
In a child of under 2 years of age, if a 1 in 50 dilution of fresh feces fails to digest gelatin, this finding is evidence of cystic fibrosis of the pancreas

Urobilinogen
Rarely found in stools in the first week of life and only in small quantities up to 1 year of age. Later up to 240 nmol (200 mg) of urobilinogen/24 h may be found normally

Water
Meconium: 68–82% of the total weight of stools
Newborn–3 months: 65–85% of the total weight of stools (slightly higher in breast-fed babies)
3 months–6 years: 82–86% of the total weight of stools

Table 40.5 Therapeutic ranges for commonly used drugs in children

Drug	Therapeutic range in blood (μmol/L unless stated otherwise)
Carbamazepine	12–50
Chloramphenicol	30–60
Diazepam	0.7–1.0
Digoxin	
Infants	Up to 5.1 nmol/L
Older children and adults	1.0–2.6 nmol/L
Ethosuximide	280–700
Gentamicin	7.5–9.0
Peak 15 min post i.v. or 60 min post i.m.	8.0–18.5
Trough-predose	<3.7
Paracetamol	
Toxic value at 4 h	>1300
Toxic value at 8 h	>650
Toxic value at 12 h	>300
Phenobarbital	60–130
For febrile convulsions	>60
Phenytoin	30–70
Primidone	23–55
Theophylline	55–110
For preterm apnea	30–70
Tobramycin	11–21
Sodium valproate	300–600

Table 40.6 Normal amniotic fluid values

Acetone bodies
0.20 mg/L

Calcium
1.6–2.1 mmol/L (6.4–8.2 mg/100 ml). Values above this range may be found near to term

Chloride
113 mmol/L (113 mEq/L) is the mean value up to 30 weeks' gestation decreasing to a mean value of 111 mmol/L (111 mEq/L) at term

Citrate
155–420 μmol/L (3.0–8.1 mg/100 ml)

Creatine kinase
4.5 ± 2.3 IU/L. No significant changes occur with increasing gestational age. Markedly elevated values (10–180 times normal) may be indicative of intrauterine death

Creatinine
Up to 28 weeks' gestation: <88 μmol/L (0.1 mg/100 ml) increasing gradually, 36 weeks–term, >141 μmol/L (1.6 mg/100 ml). Low values tend to be associated with stillborn infants or polyhydramnios. High values above 350 μmol/L (4.0 mg/100 ml) tend to be associated with toxemic and diabetic mothers. Creatinine concentration in amniotic fluid has been suggested as an index of fetal maturity as have several other substances such as uric acid, total protein, total hydroxyproline, and α-fetoprotein

Enzymes
Many enzymes have been detected and estimated in amniotic fluid At present the measurement of enzymes in cultured amniotic fluid cells is mainly used for the detection of inborn errors of metabolism

α-Fetoprotein
18 weeks: 2.4–23.8 mg/L (k units/ml)
25–42 weeks: 0–10.5 mg/L (k units/ml).
Values are high in spina bifida and anencephalus, but raised values have also been described in association with placental injury and fetal death, Turner's syndrome, congenital nephrosis, omphalocele and duodenal atresia

Glucose
See Sugar

5-Hydroxyindole acetic acid
8–42 nmol/g protein in the 1st and 2nd trimester, increasing to 79–315 nmol/g protein (15–60 ng/mg protein) in the last trimester. Normal values occur in polyhydramnios but low values occur in association with anencephalus and spina bifida

α-Ketoglutarate (2-oxoglutarate)
10–95 μmol/L (0.1–1.4 mg/100 ml)

Lactate
Generally higher levels are found in amniotic fluid than in peripheral venous blood. Two different ranges are available in the literature. They are 2.6–5.9 mmol/L (23–56 mg/100 ml) and 5.8-12 mmol/L (52–108 mg/100 ml). High levels appear to be associated with fetal distress or delay in onset of respiration. Lower values are found at cesarean sections

Lecithin : sphingomyelin ratio
This ratio has been shown to be a good index of pulmonary surfactant in the fetus. Normally this ratio is between 0.8 and 1.9 up to 32 weeks and then increases rapidly up to values of 5 or 6 at term. When this ratio is below 1.5 just before birth, the possibility of respiratory distress syndrome occurring is high (about 80%). If the ratio is above 2.0 respiratory distress is unlikely even in a preterm infant. When the ratio is between 1.5 and 2.0, about 20% of newborns develop respiratory distress

Magnesium
18 weeks' gestation: 0.7–0.95 mmol/L (1.4–1.9 mEq/L)
Term: 0.25–0.7 mmol/L (0.5–1.4 mEq/L)

Nitrogen
0.6 g/L – about half is non-protein nitrogen

Osmolality
About 280 mmol/kg (280 mosmol/kg) at 10 weeks' gestation gradually falling to 250–260 mmol/kg (250–260 mosmol/kg) at term

PCO_2
5.9–7.6 kPa (44–57 mmHg)

pH
7.04–7.20

Phosphorus, inorganic
0.42–0.81 (mean 0.65) mmol/L or 1.3–2.5 mg/100 ml (mean 2.0) at term

Potassium
3.3–5.2 mmol/L (3.3–5.2 mEq/L) – slight fall towards term

Protein, total
3–11 g/L (0.3–1.1 g/100 ml) mainly albumin (albumin : globulin ratio about 3.1)

Sodium
137 mmol/L (137 mEq/L) is the mean value up to 30 weeks' gestation decreasing to a mean value of 133 mmol/L (133 mEq/L) at term

Solids, total
0.9–1.7% at term. Probably similar throughout pregnancy

Standard bicarbonate
13.0–19.8 mmol/L (13.0–19.8 mEq/L)

Sugar, reducing
0–300 mg/L (0–30 mg/100 ml) with a mean value of 130 mg/L (13 mg/100 ml). Decreased in long pregnancy

Urea
2.1–6.2 mmol/L (12.7–37.1 mg/100 ml). Increases occur as pregnancy progresses but values are too widely scattered, particularly near term for this determination on its own to be a useful indicator of fetal maturity

Uric acid
2nd trimester: 0.12–0.33 mmol/L (2.1–5.5 mg/100 ml)
Term: 0.33–0.65 mmol/L (5.5–11.0 mg/100 ml)
This increasing uric acid output later in pregnancy reflects the increasing urinary output of the maturing fetus and its increasing muscle mass

Volume (mean values)
10 weeks' gestation: 30 ml
20 weeks' gestation: 250 ml
30 weeks' gestation: 600 ml
36 weeks' gestation: 1000 ml
Term: 800 ml
Polyhydramnios (>2000 ml) is commonly associated with intestinal obstruction and an increased incidence of congenital malformations. Oligohydramnios (<300 ml) is found in association with renal agenesis

Table 40.7 Function tests

Alanine load test
250 mg L-alanine/kg body weight orally, in cold water, is given to fasted patient. In patients with unimpaired gluconeogenesis there is normally a significant increase in the blood glucose concentration with little or no increase in lactic acid. Alanine levels reach a peak by about 1 h, then rapidly return to normal

Calcium loading test
Calcium, 1 g/1.73 m^2 body surface area, is given as calcium gluconate (Sandocal), and the patient is given, after fasting, a standard breakfast containing approximately 300 calories, 25 mmol sodium, 100 mg calcium, and 100 mg phosphorus. Normal children have urinary calcium: creatinine ratios below 0.8 before and in the 4 h after the calcium load

Creatinine clearance
Normal: 90–150 ml/min/1.73 m^2 (40–65 in newborns)

$$\text{Calculation: } \frac{\text{urine creatinine (mmol / L)} \times \text{vol / min}}{\text{Plasma creatinine (mmol / L)}} \times \frac{1.73}{\text{surface area}}$$

Dexamethasone suppression test (of adrenal corticosteroid secretion)
Low dose: 20 μg/kg/day in four equal doses at 6-hourly intervals for 2 days.
Plasma cortisol <1 nmol/L
Urine cortisol <50 nmol/24 h
Most patients with Cushing's syndrome give greater levels than stated, irrespective of etiology
High dose: 80 μg/kg/day in four equal doses at 6-hourly intervals for 2 days. Suppression by this higher dose but not the low dose is most frequently seen in pituitary-dependent bilateral adrenal hyperplasia (Cushing's disease)

Glucose tolerance test
Dose – 1.75 g/kg, not to exceed 75 g. Diabetes should be diagnosed only when the fasting plasma glucose is 7.8 mmol/L or higher, the 2 h concentration is 11.1 mmol/L or higher, and a value taken between these times is also 11.1 mmol/L or higher. Impaired glucose tolerance is present in children with a normal fasting plasma glucose and a 2 h concentration above 7.8 mmol/L, even if the 2 h level and another taken between 0 and 2 h both exceed 11.1 mmol/L

Growth hormone stimulation tests
Response to insulin hypoglycemia, arginine, clonidine or Bovril – peak >20 mU/L

Growth hormone (GH) releasing factor (GRF) test
Measurement of the plasma growth hormone response to biosynthetic GRF may be of value in assessing whether GH insufficiency, identified by the clonidine or insulin hypoglycemia tests is due to pituitary or hypothalamic dysfunction. After a baseline blood sample, 1 μg/kg body weight is given i.v. and blood samples collected at 15, 30, 45, 60, 75, 90 and 120 min. A normal response is a rise in GH greater than 30 mU/L, peaking at 15–30 min after GRF administration

Fat absorption
The normal daily fecal fat excretion in children is 14 mmol (4 g) or less when assessed in a 5-day collection

Renal functional capacity
GFR
Newborns: 40–65 ml/min/1.73 m^2 increasing steadily to 90–150ml/min/1.73m^2 in children aged 1 year or older
Maximum concentrating ability
Newborns: up to 600 mosm/kg
Infants after 6 months and children: 800–1200 mosm/kg
Minimum urinary pH: 5.3 (after acid load)

Synacthen screening test
Synacthen (Tetracosactrin BP) is given by intravenous injection (500 ng per 1.73 m^2) and blood samples collected at 30, 60, 90 and 120 min. Cortisol concentration at 30 min should reach at least 425 nmol/L, with an increase of at least 145 nmol/L above the basal concentration

Depot synacthen test
Dose 1 mg i.m. daily for 3 days. Plasma cortisol increases at least 3-fold over basal concentrations in normals. There is also a response in secondary adrenal insufficiency. An absent cortisol response is definitive evidence of primary adrenal insufficiency

Xylose absorption test
5 g dose xylose: normal urine excretion should be greater than 1 g/5-h period (>20% of dose). Normal plasma xylose >1.3 mmol/L, 1 h after 5 g xylose

(See Hindmarsh & Swift 1995[7] for a full assessment of growth hormone provocation tests and Walker & Hughes 1995[8] for endocrine tests and normal values)

Table 40.8 Conversion factors

Ionic concentration

$$\text{mmol / L} = \frac{\text{mg / 100ml} \times 10}{\text{molecular weight}}$$

$$\text{mEq / L} = \frac{\text{mg / 100ml} \times 10}{\text{equivalent weight}}$$

$$\left(\text{equivalent weight} = \frac{\text{atomic weight}}{\text{valency}}\right)$$

To convert mEq/L to mg/100 ml for the following ions:

Sodium	multiply by	2.30
Potassium	multiply by	3.91
Calcium	multiply by	2.00
Magnesium	multiply by	1.215
Phosphorus	multiply by	1.72 (at pH 7.4)
Chloride	multiply by	3.55
Bicarbonate	multiply by	6.1
Lactate	multiply by	9.0
Protein	multiply by	0.41

To convert mg/100 ml to mEq/L, divide by the conversion factors given in right-hand column

Temperature
To convert °Fahrenheit to °Centigrade subtract 32 and then multiply by 5/9
To convert °Centigrade to °Fahrenheit multiply by 9/5 and then add 32

Energy
To convert kilocalories (kcals) to kilojoules (kjoules) multiply by 4.18

Weight
To convert grams to pounds and ounces divide by 454 to obtain the complete number of pounds, divide the remainder by 28.4 to obtain number of ounces
To convert pounds and ounces to grams multiply pounds by 454, multiply ounces by 28.4 and add the two products together

Table 40.9a Normal blood count values from birth to 18 years

Age	Hb (g/dl)	RBC ($\times 10^{12}$/L)	Hct	MCV (fl)	WBC ($\times 10^9$/L)	Neutrophils ($\times 10^9$/L)	Lymphocytes ($\times 10^9$/L)	Monocytes ($\times 10^9$/L)	Eosinophils ($\times 10^9$/L)	Basophils ($\times 10^9$/L)	Platelets ($\times 10^9$/L)	Reticulocytes ($\times 10^9$/L)
Birth (term infants)	14.9–23.7	3.7–6.5	0.47–0.75	100–125	10–26	2.7–14.4	2.0–7.3	0–1.9	0–0.85	0–0.1	150–450	110–450
2 weeks	13.4–19.8	3.9–5.9	0.41–0.65	88–110	6–21	1.5–5.4	2.8–9.1	0.1–1.7	0–0.85	0–0.1	170–500	10–80
2 months	9.4–13.0	3.1–4.3	0.28–0.42	84–98	5–15	0.7–4.8	3.3–10.3	0.4–1.2	0.05–0.9	0.02–0.13	210–650	35–200
6 months	10.0–13.0	3.8–4.9	0.3–0.38	73–84	6–17	1–6	3.3–11.5	0.2–1.3	0.1–1.1	0.02–0.2	210–560	15–110
1 year	10.1–13.0	3.9–5.1	0.3–0.38	70–82	6–16	1–8	3.4–10.5	0.2–0.9	0.05–0.9	0.02–0.13	200–550	
2–6 years	11.0–13.8	3.9–5.0	0.32–0.4	72–87	6–17	1.5–8.5	1.8–8.4	0.15–1.3	0.05–1.1	0.02–0.12	210–490	
6–12 years	11.1–14.7	3.9–5.2	0.32–0.43	76–90	4.5–14.5	1.5–8.0	1.5–5.0	0.15–1.3	0.05–1.0	0.02–0.12	170–450	50–130
12–18 years												
Female	12.1–15.1	4.1–5.1	0.35–0.44	77–94	4.5–13	1.5–6	1.5–4.5	0.15–1.3	0.05–0.8	0.02–0.12	180–430	
Male	12.1–16.6	4.2–5.6	0.35–0.49	77–92								

Red cell values at birth derived from skin puncture blood; most other data from venous blood
Adapted from Hinchliffe 1999[9]

Table 40.9b Reference values for coagulation tests in healthy children aged 1–16 years compared with adults

	Age			
Coagulation tests	1–5 years Mean (boundary)	6–10 years Mean (boundary)	11–16 years Mean (boundary)	Adult Mean (boundary)
PT(s)	11 (10.6–11.4)	11.1 (10.1–12.1)	11.2 (10.2–12.0)	12 (11.0–14.0)
INR	1.0 (0.96–1.04)	1.01 (0.91–1.11)	1.02 (0.93–1.10)	1.10 (1.0–1.3)
APTT(s)	30 (24–36)	31 (26–36)	32 (26–37)	33 (27–40)
Fibrinogen (g/L)	2.76 (1.70–4.05)	2.79 (1.57–4.0)	3.0 (1.54–4.48)	2.78 (1.56–4.0)
Bleeding time (min)	6 (2.5–10)*	7 (2.5–13)*	5 (3–8)*	4 (1–7)
II (unit/ml)	0.94 (0.71–1.16)*	0.88 (0.67–1.07)*	0.83 (0.61–1.04)*	1.08 (0.70–1.46)
V (unit/ml)	1.03 (0.79–1.27)	0.90 (0.63–1.16)*	0.77 (0.55–0.99)*	1.06 (0.62–1.50)
VII (unit/ml)	0.82 (0.55–1.16)*	0.85 (0.52–1.20)*	0.83 (0.58–1.15)*	1.05 (0.67–1.43)
VIII (unit/ml)	0.90 (0.59–1.42)	0.95 (0.58–1.32)	0.92 (0.53–1.31)	0.99 (0.50–1.49)
VWF (unit/ml)	0.82 (0.60–1.20)	0.95 (0.44–1.44)	1.00 (0.46–1.53)	0.92 (0.50–1.58)
IX (unit/ml)	0.73 (0.47–1.04)*	0.75 (0.63–0.89)*	0.82 (0.59–1.22)*	1.09 (0.55–1.63)
X (unit/ml)	0.88 (0.58–1.16)*	0.75 (0.55–1.01)*	0.79 (0.50–1.17)*	1.06 (0.70–1.52)
XI (unit/ml)	0.97 (0.56–1.50)	0.86 (0.52–1.20)	0.74 (0.50–0.97)*	0.97 (0.67–1.27)
XII (unit/ml)	0.93 (0.64–1.29)	0.92 (0.60–1.40)	0.81 (0.34–1.37)*	1.08 (0.52–1.64)
PK (unit/ml)	0.95 (0.65–1.30)	0.99 (0.66–1.31)	0.99 (0.53–1.45)	1.12 (0.62–1.62)
HMWK (unit/ml)	0.98 (0.64–1.32)	0.93 (0.60–1.30)	0.91 (0.63–1.19)	0.92 (0.50–1.36)
XIIIa (unit/ml)	1.08 (0.72–1.43)*	1.09 (0.65–1.51)*	0.99 (0.57–1.40)	1.05 (0.55–1.55)
XIIIs (unit/ml)	1.13 (0.69–1.56)*	1.16 (0.77–1.54)*	1.02 (0.60–1.43)	0.97 (0.57–1.37)

All factors except fibrinogen are expressed as unit/ml, where pooled plasma contains 1.0 unit/ml. All data are expressed as the mean, followed by the upper and lower boundary encompassing 95% of the population. Between 20 and 50 samples were assayed for each value for each age group. Some measurements were skewed due to a disproportionate number of high values. The lower limit, which excludes the lower 2.5% of the population, is given.
APTT, activated partial thromboplastin time; HMWK, high molecular weight kininogen INR, international normalized ratio; PK, prekallikrein; PT, prothrombin time; VIII, Factor VIII procoagulant; VWF, von Willebrand factor.
*Values that are significantly different from adults
From Chalmers & Gibson 1999[10] with permission.

Table 40.10 Systolic blood pressure (mmHg) in awake children by age and cuff size

	4 cm cuff			8 cm cuff			12 cm cuff		
Age	No. of children	Mean (SD) blood pressure	95th centile	No. of children	Mean (SD) blood pressure	95th centile	No. of children	Mean (SD) blood pressure	95th centile
4 days*	171	76.2 (9.9)	95						
6 weeks*	1129	95.7 (10.7)	113						
6 months	129	104.8 (10.7)	124	738	88.5 (12.3)	109			
1 year				1323	93.4 (11.1)	112			
2 years				1322	95.5 (10.6)	115			
3 years				1218	96.8 (9.7)	115			
4 years				1149	97.4 (9.3)	113			
5 years				777	96.2 (9.4)	114	218	89.1 (9.3)	107
6 years				449	95.8 (9.1)	112	626	90.0 (8.2)	104
7 years				187	97.3 (9.2)	114	881	90.0 (8.6)	104
8 years				55	96.2 (8.6)	110	1042	91.9 (8.4)	105
9 years							963	92.3 (8.7)	106
10 years							449	94.3 (8.8)	111

*Some of the babies were asleep at time of measurement.
From de Swiet et al 1992[11]

Table 40.11 Diastolic blood pressure (mmHg) in awake children by age and cuff size*

	8 mm cuff			12 mm cuff		
Age (years)	No. of children	Mean (SD) blood pressure	95th centile	No. of children	Mean (SD) blood pressure	95th centile
5	777	62.3 (9.5)	78	218	57.8 (9.5)	73
6	442	63.6 (9.4)	70	621	59.6 (9.5)	74
7	179	66.2 (7.6)	81	839	60.6 (8.2)	75
8	55	65.2 (7.8)	78	1016	60.7 (7.6)	74
9				954	60.2 (7.6)	73
10				442	61.8 (7.2)	75

* The numbers of children studied are less than in Table 40.10 because the diastolic blood pressure (Korotkoff V) could not be determined for every child.
From de Swiet et al 1992[11]

Table 40.12 Blood pressure levels for the 90th and 95th percentiles of blood pressure for boys aged 1 to 17 years by percentiles of height

Age (years)	Blood pressure percentile*	Systolic blood pressure by percentile of height† (mmHg)							Diastolic blood pressure by percentile of height† (mmHg)						
		5%	10%	25%	50%	75%	90%	95%	5%	10%	25%	50%	75%	90%	95%
1	90th	94	95	97	98	100	102	102	50	51	52	53	54	54	55
	95th	98	99	101	102	104	106	106	55	55	56	57	58	59	59
2	90th	98	99	100	102	104	105	106	55	55	56	57	58	59	59
	95th	101	102	104	106	108	109	110	59	59	60	61	62	63	63
3	90th	100	101	103	105	107	108	109	59	59	60	61	62	63	63
	95th	104	105	107	109	111	112	113	63	63	64	65	66	67	67
4	90th	102	103	105	107	109	110	111	62	62	63	64	65	66	66
	95th	106	107	109	111	113	114	115	66	67	67	68	69	70	71
5	90th	104	105	106	108	110	112	112	65	65	66	67	68	69	69
	95th	108	109	110	112	114	115	116	69	70	70	71	72	73	74
6	90th	105	106	108	110	111	113	114	67	68	69	70	70	71	72
	95th	109	110	112	114	115	117	117	72	72	73	74	75	76	76
7	90th	106	107	109	111	113	114	115	69	70	71	72	72	73	74
	95th	110	111	113	115	116	118	119	74	74	75	76	77	78	78
8	90th	107	108	110	112	114	115	116	71	71	72	73	74	75	75
	95th	111	112	114	116	118	119	120	75	76	76	77	78	79	80
9	90th	109	110	112	113	115	117	117	72	73	73	74	75	76	77
	95th	113	114	116	117	119	121	121	76	77	78	79	80	80	81
10	90th	110	112	113	115	117	118	119	73	74	74	75	76	77	78
	95th	114	115	117	119	121	122	123	77	78	79	80	80	81	82
11	90th	112	113	115	117	119	120	121	74	74	75	76	77	78	78
	95th	116	117	119	121	123	124	125	78	79	79	80	81	82	83
12	90th	115	116	117	119	121	123	123	75	75	76	77	78	78	79
	95th	119	120	121	123	125	126	127	79	79	80	81	82	83	83
13	90th	117	118	120	122	124	125	126	75	76	76	77	78	79	80
	95th	121	122	124	126	128	129	130	79	80	81	82	83	83	84
14	90th	120	121	123	125	126	128	128	76	76	77	78	79	80	80
	95th	124	125	127	128	130	132	132	80	81	81	82	83	84	85
15	90th	123	124	125	127	129	131	131	77	77	78	79	80	81	81
	95th	127	128	129	131	133	134	135	81	82	83	83	84	85	86
16	90th	125	126	128	130	132	133	134	79	79	80	81	82	82	83
	95th	129	130	132	134	136	137	138	83	83	84	85	86	87	87
17	90th	128	129	131	133	134	136	136	81	81	82	83	84	85	85
	95th	132	133	135	136	138	140	140	85	85	86	87	88	89	89

* Blood pressure percentile was determined by a single measurement
† Height percentile was determined by standard growth curves
Reproduced by permission of Pediatrics 1996[12]

Table 40.13 Blood pressure levels for the 90th and 95th percentiles of blood pressure for girls aged 1 to 17 years by percentiles of height

Age (years)	Blood pressure percentile*	Systolic blood pressure by percentile of height† (mmHg)							Diastolic blood pressure by percentile of height† (mmHg)						
		5%	10%	25%	50%	75%	90%	95%	5%	10%	25%	50%	75%	90%	95%
1	90th	97	98	99	100	102	103	104	53	53	53	54	55	56	56
	95th	101	102	103	104	105	107	107	57	57	57	58	59	60	60
2	90th	99	99	100	102	103	104	105	57	57	58	58	59	60	61
	95th	102	103	104	105	107	108	109	61	61	62	62	63	64	65
3	90th	100	100	102	103	104	105	106	61	61	61	62	63	63	64
	95th	104	104	105	107	108	109	110	65	65	65	66	67	67	68
4	90th	101	102	103	104	106	107	108	63	63	64	65	65	66	67
	95th	105	106	107	108	109	111	111	67	67	68	69	69	70	71
5	90th	103	103	104	106	107	108	109	65	66	66	67	68	68	69
	95th	107	107	108	110	111	112	113	69	70	70	71	72	72	73
6	90th	104	105	106	107	109	110	111	67	67	68	69	69	70	71
	95th	108	109	110	111	112	114	114	71	71	72	73	73	74	75
7	90th	106	107	108	109	110	112	112	69	69	69	70	71	72	72
	95th	110	110	112	113	114	115	116	73	73	73	74	75	76	76
8	90th	108	109	110	111	112	113	114	70	70	71	71	72	73	74
	95th	112	112	113	115	116	117	118	74	74	75	75	76	77	78
9	90th	110	110	112	113	114	115	116	71	72	72	73	74	74	75
	95th	114	114	115	117	118	119	120	75	76	76	77	78	78	79
10	90th	112	112	114	115	116	117	118	73	73	73	74	75	76	76
	95th	116	116	117	119	120	121	122	77	77	77	78	79	80	80
11	90th	114	114	116	117	118	119	120	74	74	75	75	76	77	77
	95th	118	118	119	121	122	123	124	78	78	79	79	80	81	81
12	90th	116	116	118	119	120	121	122	75	75	76	76	77	78	78
	95th	120	120	121	123	124	125	126	79	79	80	80	81	82	82
13	90th	118	118	119	121	122	123	124	76	76	77	78	78	79	80
	95th	121	122	123	125	126	127	128	80	80	81	82	82	83	84
14	90th	119	120	121	122	124	125	126	77	77	78	79	79	80	81
	95th	123	124	125	126	128	129	130	81	81	82	83	83	84	85
15	90th	121	121	122	124	125	126	127	78	78	79	79	80	81	82
	95th	124	125	126	128	129	130	131	82	82	83	83	84	85	86
16	90th	122	122	123	125	126	127	128	79	79	79	80	81	82	82
	95th	125	126	127	128	130	131	132	83	83	83	84	85	86	86
17	90th	122	123	124	125	126	128	128	79	79	79	80	81	82	82
	95th	126	126	127	129	130	131	132	83	83	83	84	85	86	86

* Blood pressure percentile was determined by a single reading
† Height percentile was determined by standard growth curves
Reproduced by permission of Pediatrics 1996[12]

Table 40.14 Composition of infant milk and formula feeds (all values refer to the concentration per 100 ml of normally reconstituted feeds)

	Energy		Protein			Fat				Carbohydrate				Minerals					
Milk or formula (manufacturer)	KJ	kcal	Total (g)	Casein (%)	Whey (%)	Total (g)	Saturated (%)	Unsaturated (%)	Type	Total (g)	Lactose (g)	Malto dextrin (g)	Other (g)	Na (mg)	K (mg)	Ca (mg)	P (mg)	Mg (mg)	Fe (µg)
Human (breast) milk	293	70	1.1	32	68	4.2	51	49		7.0	7.0			15	60	35	15	2.8	76
Cow's milk	267	64	3.1	77	23	3.8	63	37		4.7	4.7			53	136	112	89	11	58
Modified milks – whey dominant																			
Aptamil First (Milupa)	280	67	1.5	40	60	3.6	49	51	Veg. oils, milk fat	7.2	7.2			26	82	60	38	5.2	700
Farley's First (Farley's)	284	68	1.45	40	60	3.82	35.9	64.1	Veg. oils, fish oils	7.0	7.0			17	57	39	27	5.2	650
Omneo Comfort 1 (Cow and Gate)	295	70	1.7	0	100	3.3	42	58	Veg. oils	8.4	2.9	4.0	1.5	23	66	53	29	5.7	500
Premium (Cow and Gate)	280	67	1.41	40	60	3.5	37	63	Veg. oils	7.5	7.4			19	64	52	26	5.0	500
SMA Gold (SMA Nutrition)	280	67	1.5	40	60	3.6	45	55	Veg. oils	7.2	7.2			16	70	46	33	6.4	800
Modified milks – casein dominant																			
Aptamil Extra (Milupa)	285	67	1.9	80	20	3.1	44	56	Veg. oils	8.1	8.1			20	88	84	56	8	700
Farley's Second (Farley's)	289	69	1.7	80	20	3.5	35.9	64.1	Veg. oils	7.7	7.7			18	78	56	45	5.5	730
Milumil (Milupa)	283	67	1.9	80	20	3.1	42	58	Veg. oils	8.1	6.1	1.9		25	97	76	46	8	700
Plus (Cow and Gate)	280	67	1.7	80	20	3.4	38	62	Veg. oils	7.3	7.2			21	82	80	45	5.4	500
SMA White (SMA Nutrition)	280	67	1.6	80	20	3.6	45	55	Veg. oils	7.0	7.0			22	80	56	44	5.3	800
Follow-on milks																			
Farley's Follow-on (Farley's)	285	68	2.1	64	36	3.4	36	63	Veg. oils, milk fat	7.4	7.4			30	88	72	58	7.2	1200
Forward (Milupa)	311	74	2.1	80	20	3.3	42	58	Veg. oils	9.0	7.0	2.0		30	127	87	62	7.0	1200
Hipp Organic (Hipp Nutrition)	287	69	2.1	55	45	3.5	3.7	63	Veg. oils	7.2	7.2			36	133	99	69	10.3	1200
Omneo Comfort 2 (Cow and Gate)	300	72	1.9	0	100	3.3	42	58	Veg. oils	8.7	3.0	4.0	1.7	29	83	92	54	6.8	1200
Progress (SMA Nutrition)	281	67	2.2	80	20	3.0	45	55	Veg. oils	7.8	7.8			33	107	90	62	8	1300
Step-Up (Cow and Gate)	290	70	1.8	80	20	3.4	38	62	Veg. oils	8.0	7.8			27	87	88	51	7	1300
Next Steps (Cow and Gate)	325	77	1.9	80	20	3.3	39	61	Veg. oils	9.9	6.6	2.1	1.2	30	84	92	54	6.8	1300
Preterm milks (for low birth weight babies)																			
Nutriprem 1 (Cow and Gate)	335	80	2.4	42	58	4.4	41	59	Veg. oils, marine oil	7.9	6.0	1.9		41	80	100	50	10	900
Nutriprem 2 (Cow and Gate)	310	75	2.0	40	60	4.1	39	61	Veg. oils marine oil	7.4	5.9	1.5		26	77	94	50	6.7	1200
OsterPrem (Farley's)	334	80	2.0	39	61	4.6	41.6	58.4	Veg. oils, milk fat	7.65	6.0	1.65		42	72	110	63	5	40
PreAptamil (Milupa)	335	80	2.4	40	60	4.4	43	57	Veg. oils	7.9	6.2	1.7		41	80	100	50	10	900
PremCare (Farley's)	301	72	1.85	39	61	3.96	42	58	Milk fat, veg. oils, fish oil	7.24	6.2	1.04		22	78	70	35	5.2	650

Minerals						Vitamins																
Cu (μg)	Zn (μg)	Mn (μg)	Cl (mg)	I (μg)	Se (μg)	A (μg)	B_1 (μg)	B_2 (μg)	Pantothenic acid (μg)	B_6 (μg)	B_{12} (μg)	Biotin (μg)	Folic acid (μg)	Niacin (μg)	C (mg)	D (μg)	E (mg)	K (μg)	Choline (mg)	Carnitine (mg)	Inositol (mg)	Taurine (mg)
39	295		43	7		60	16	31	260	5.9	0.01	0.76	5.2	230	3.8	0.01		0.35				
21	400	3	97	26		50	30	165	350	60	0.4	1.9	6	80	1.0	0.03		0.09				
40	500	10	51	10		60	40	120	400	40	0.2	1.0	10	1500	8	1.0	0.6	3.0				7.0
42	340	3.4	40	4.5	1.0	82	42	55	230	35	0.14	1.0	3.4	690	6.9	1.0	0.48	2.7	4.8			5.0
37	500	70	50	12	1.5	84	40	100	310	40	0.5	1.6	10	1200	8	1.4	0.8	4.9	7		3.5	5.1
40	500	10	43	10	1.5	65	40	100	300	40	0.2	1.7	11	750	8	1.4	1.1	5.1	7.4			6.3
33	600	5.0	43	10	1.4	75	100	150	300	60	0.2	2.0	8	900	9	1.1	0.74	6.7	10	1.3		4.7
30	500	4.0	63	9.1		63	40	80	400	40	0.2	1.0	11	1300	8	1.1	0.6	3.2				6.0
43	360	3.6	48	10	1.5	82	41	55	220	34	0.14	1.2	3.4	690	6.9	1.0	0.48	3.0	4.9			5.0
30	500	8	63	9.1		63	40	60	400	40	0.2	1.0	11	1300	8	1.1	0.6	3.2				6.0
40	500	10	53	10	1.5	65	40	110	300	40	0.2	1.5	11	750	8	1.4	1.1	5.0	8			5.4
33	600	5.0	55	10	1.4	75	100	150	300	60	0.2	2.0	8	900	9	1.1	0.74	6.7	6.7	0.6		4.7
41	400	3.6	5.8	10		80	40	150	360	40	0.2	3.0	7	650	10	1.1	0.48	2.9	4.8			5.0
70	600	10	71	12.4	1.5	62	50	160	400	50	0.2	1.0	11	1200	9.0	1.0	0.6	3.1				
21	700		69	14		73	60	270	560	30	0.3	2.5			8.6	1.2	0.4	1.1				
48	800	69	54	12	1.5	84	50	110	310	40	0.55	1.6	10	810	8.3	1.9	0.8	4.9	7.4		3.5	4.1
60	900	4.3	71	12	1.5	75	100	150	300	60	0.2	2.0	8	900	14	1.5	0.74	6.7	9	0.8		0.5
50	900	10	55	11	1.5	65	40	120	290	40	0.2	1.6	11	830	8.0	1.9	1.1	5	8.2			5.0
50	900	10	57	11	1.5	62	40	140	290	40	0.16	1.6	10	820	8	1.9	1.1	4.9	7.9			2.7
80	700	10	48	25	1.9	227	140	200	1000	120	0.2	3.0	48	3000	16	5	3.0	6.6	10	2	30	5.5
60	710	6.7	46	20	1.9	99	90	110	620	80	0.28	3.0	20	1700	16	1.6	1.9	5.9	32		29	4.9
96	880	3	60	20	1.4	100	95	180	500	100	0.2	2.0	50	1000	28	2.4	10.0	7	5.6	1.0	3.2	5.1
80	700	5.0	48	14		108	140	200	1000	120	0.2	3.0	48	3000	16	2.4	3	6.6	10	2	30	5.5
57	600	5.0	45	4.5	1.3	100	95	100	400	80	0.2	1.1	25	1000	15	1.3	1.5	6.0	1.1			5.1

Table 40.14 *Cont'd*

Milk or formula (manufacturer)	Energy KJ	Energy kcal	Protein Total (g)	Protein Casein (%)	Protein Whey (%)	Fat Total (g)	Fat Saturated (%)	Fat Unsaturated (%)	Fat Type	Carbohydrate Total (g)	Carbohydrate Lactose (g)	Carbohydrate Malto dextrin (g)	Carbohydrate Other (g)	Minerals Na (mg)	Minerals K (mg)	Minerals Ca (mg)	Minerals P (mg)	Minerals Mg (mg)	Minerals Fe (µg)
SMA Low Birth Weight (SMA Nutrition)	343	82	2.0	40	60	4.4	49	51	Veg. oils, MCT	8.6	4.3	4.3		35	85	80	42.5	8	800
Soya milks																			
Infasoy (Cow and Gate)	280	66	1.8			3.6	39	61	Veg. oils	6.7			6.7	18	65	54	27	5	800
Isomil (Abbott)	286	68	1.8			3.7	43	57	Corn oil, coconut oil	6.9		4.2	2.7	32	77	70	50	5	1000
Farley's Soya (Farley's)	293	70	1.95			3.8	37	63	Veg. oils	7.0			7.0	25	75	56	37	5.7	700
Prosobee (Mead Johnson)	283	68	2.0			3.6	43	57	Veg. oils	6.6			6.6	24	81	64	51	7.4	1200
Wysoy (SMA Nutrition)	280	67	1.8			3.6	45	55	Veg. oils				6.9	19	72	67	50	6.7	800

For powdered preparations, reconstitution is normally made by diluting one levelled scoop of powder in 30 ml of water. Only the scoop provided by the manufacturer for that powder should be used.

For further information on the composition of infant milks and foods see Department of Health and Social Security (1977, 1980, 1988),[13–15] Department of Health (1994),[16] ESPGAN (1977, 1981, 1982, 1987, 1990)[17–21] and Tsang et al (1993).[22]

Table 40.15 Composition of special formula infant feeds and supplements (all values refer to the concentration per 100 ml of normally reconstituted feeds except

Feed (manufacturer)	Type/clinical indications	Energy kJ (mg)	Energy kcal (µg)	Protein g (µg)	Protein Type	Fat g	Fat Type	Carbohydrate g	Carbohydrate Type
AL 110 (Nestlé)	Lactose free	280	67	1.9	Casein	3.3	Milk fat, corn oil	7.4	Maltodextrin from corn starch
Alfaré (Nestlé)	Hypoallergenic	301	72	2.5	Whey, amino acids	7.5	MCT, milk fat, corn oil	7.8	Maltodextrin, starch
Analog LCP (SHS*)	Phenylalanine free	300	72	1.95	Amino acids	3.5	LCPs	8.1	Glucose syrup
Caprilon (SHS)	For fat malabsorption	275	66	1.5	Whey, casein	3.6	MCT oil, Soy oil	7.0	Glucose syrup
Enfamil AR (Mead Johnson)	Prethickened, for posseting and reflux	287	69	1.7	Casein, whey	3.5	Veg. oils	7.55	Glucose polymer, lactose, rice starch
Galactomin 17 (SHS)	Low lactose, for galactosemia	280	67	1.9	Sodium + calcium caseinates	3.4	Palm, Canola, coconut and sunflower oils	7.4	Glucose syrup
Galactomin 19 (SHS)	Low lactose, for glucose-galactose intolerance	288	69	1.9	Casein	4.0		6.4	Fructose, trace of lactose
Generaid Plus (SHS)	For hepatic disorders	428	102	2.42	Whey, amino acids	4.2	MCT (35%)	13.6	Glucose syrup
HN 25 (Milupa)	Low lactose, for treatment of diarrhea	242	57	2.6	Milk protein	1.2	Vegetable fat	9.1	Maltodextrin starch
Infatrini (Nutricia)	High energy infant milk	420	100	2.6	Skimmed milk, whey	5.4	Vegetable oils	10.4	Maltodextrin, lactose
Locasol (SHS)	Low calcium for hypercalcemia	278	67	1.9	Casein, demineralized whey	3.4	Vegetable oils, milk fat	7.0	Lactose
MCT Pepdite 0–2 (SHS)	Free from lactose, gluten, fructose, sucrose	286	68	2.1	Hydrolyzed non-milk protein, amino acids	2.7	Coconut oil, sunflower oil	8.9	Glucose syrup
Monogen (SHS)	For lipid and lymphatic disorders	310	74	2.0	Whey, amino acids	2.0	MCT (93%), LCT (7%)	12	Glucose syrup
Neocate (SHS)	Free of protein, gluten, lactose and sucrose Hypoallergenic	298	71	1.95	Amino acids	3.5	Safflower, coconut and soya oils	8.1	Glucose syrup
Neocate Advance (SHS)	Hypoallergenic	420	100	2.5	Amino acids	3.5	Vegetable oils	14.6	Glucose syrup

Minerals						Vitamins																
Cu (μg)	Zn (μg)	Mn (μg)	Cl (mg)	I (μg)	Se (μg)	A (μg)	B_1 (μg)	B_2 (μg)	Pantothenic acid (μg)	B_6 (μg)	B_{12} (μg)	Biotin (μg)	Folic acid (μg)	Niacin (μg)	C (mg)	D (μg)	E (mg)	K (μg)	Choline (mg)	Carnitine (mg)	Inositol (mg)	Taurine (mg)
82.5	800	10	60	10		100	120	200	450	72	0.3	2.4	48	1320	11	1.5	1.2	8	15	2.6	4.5	4.7
40	620	40	45	13	1.0	80	40	100	300	40	0.2	1.5	10	900	8.0	1.4	0.9	5	7.9	1.5	3.5	5.3
50	800	40	59	10		99	70	60	500	40	0.3	3.0	13	700	7	1.14	1.7	5.5	8.0	1.2		4.5
42	540	34	50	8.4		100	42	56	240	36	0.15	1.1	3.5	700	9	1.1	0.50	2.8	4.9	0.85	4.0	5.1
51	810	17	54	10	1.5	61	54	61	340	41	0.2	2.0	11	680	8.1	1.0	1.4	5.4	8.1	1.4	11.5	4.1
33	600	20	43	12	1.4	75	100	150	300	60	0.2	3.5	8	900	9	1.1	0.74	10	8.5	1	10	4.7

where otherwise stated)

Minerals								Vitamins													
Na (mg)	K (mg)	Ca (mg)	P (mg)	Mg (mg)	Fe (μg)	Cu (μg)	Zn (μg)	A (μg)	B_1 (μg)	B_2 (μg)	Pantothenic acid (μg)	B_6 (μg)	B_{12} (μg)	Biotin (μg)	Folic (μg)	Niacin (μg)	C (mg)	D (μg)	E (μg)	K (μg)	Osmolality (mOsm/kg H_2O)
23	80	60	40	6.7	800	40	500	60	40	90	300	50	0.15	1.5	6	500	5.4	1.0	0.8	5.5	170 @ 13.3%
44	90	60	38	9	900	43	540	72	40	100	320	50	0.16	1.6	10	760	5.8	1.1	0.9	5.9	195 @ 15%
18	63	49	35	5.1	1050	70	750	79	60	90	400	80	0.19	3.9	5.7	680	6	1.3	0.7	3.1	353 @ 15%
18	65	54	27	5	500	40	400	80	40	100	300	40	0.2	1.5	10	760	7.6	2	0.8	5.1	233
24	85	55	44	5.4	800	44	700	61	54	61	340	41	0.2	2.0	11	670	8.1	1.0	1.4	5.4	230
27	97	83	55	6.6	500	80	400	79	40	100	300	40	0.2	1.6	10	900	8	1.1	0.9	5.2	210
20	66	55	27	8.0	500	79	400	81	40	100	300	40	0.2	1.5	10	900	8.1	1.3	1.0	5.3	487
15	103	69	52	9.5	900	60	590	60	40	60	220	40	0.11	2.8	3.9	450	5.2	0.7	0.4	2.2	215 @ 17%
39	109	66	48	8	1000	30	200	56	40	100	400	30	0.2	1	10	400	9	1.1	0.7	2	
23	100	80	40	8	800	60	600	100	60	150	450	60	0.3	2.3	15	1200	12	2	1.2	7.5	325
27	97	≤7	55	6.6	500	40	400	80	40	100	300	40	0.2	1.6	10.5	900	8	<0.004	0.8	5.2	310
35	58	45	35	5.1	830	60	600	80	60	90	250	50	0.15	3.9	5.8	680	6.2	1.1	0.7	6.8	277 @ 15%
35	58	45	35	5.1	800	60	600	80	60	90	250	50	0.15	3.9	5.8	680	6.1	1.1	0.7	6.7	280 @ 17.5%
18	63	49	34	5.1	1050	60	750	79	60	90	400	80	0.19	3.9	5.7	680	6.0	1.3	0.7	3.2	353
60	117	45	35	12.5	620	45	440	37	60	70	250	80	0.07	2	7	950	3.3	0.8	0.6	1.6	636 (1:4 dilution)

Table 40.15 *Cont'd*

Feed (manufacturer)	Type/clinical indications	Energy		Protein		Fat		Carbohydrate	
		kJ (mg)	kcal (µg)	g (µg)	Type	g	Type	g	Type
Nutramigen (Mead Johnson)	Free of protein, lactose and sucrose	284	68	1.9	Enzymatically hydrolyzed casein	3.4	Palm, soy, coconut and sunflower oils	7.4	Glucose polymers corn starch
Pepdite 0–2 (SHS)	Free from lactose, gluten, fructose, sucrose	297	71	2.1	Hydrolyzed non-milk protein, amino acids	3.5	Coconut oil, peanut oil, animal fat	7.8	Glucose syrup
Pepti-Junior (Cow and Gate)	Hypoallergenic	280	67		Whey hydrolysate		Corn oil, MCT oil		Glucose syrup, lactose
Pregestimil (Mead Johnson)	Free of protein, lactose and sucrose	284	68	1.9	Enzymatically hydrolyzed casein	3.8	Corn, soy, safflower and MCT oils		Glucose polymers, corn starch
Prejomin (Milupa)	Hypoallergenic	313	75	2.0	Hydrolysate	3.6	Vegetable fats	8.6	Maltodextrins, starch
SMA High Energy (SMA Nutrition)	High energy infant milk	382	91	2.0	Lactalbumin, casein	4.9	Vegetable oils	14.7	Lactose
SMA LF (SMA Nutrition)	Lactose free	281	67	1.5	Lactalbumin, casein	3.6	Vegetable oils	7.2	Glucose syrup
XP Analog (SHS)	Phenylalanine free, for PKU	300	72	1.95	Amino acids	3.5	Safflower, coconut and soya bean oils	8.1	Glucose syrup
Components used in special feeds									
Calogen (SHS)	High calorie fat emulsion	1850	450	–		50	Arachis oil, peanut oil	-	Gluclose polymer
Comminuted chicken meat (SHS)	Carbohydrate free	212–266	51–64	7.0–8.0	Chicken meat	2.5–3.5		-	None
Instant Carobel (Cow and Gate)	Instant feed thickener	†1065	†251	†2.4		†0.45		†59	Maltodextrin
Liquid Duocal (SHS)	Calorie supplement	661	158	–		7.1	Vegetable oils	23.4	Glucose syrup
Liquid Maxijul (SHS)	High energy supplement	1700	400	–		–		50	Glucose syrup
Liquigen (SHS)	Fat (MCT) supplement, for malabsorption	1850	450	–		50	MCT	–	
Maxijul LE (SHS)	Carbohydrate source	†1632	384					96	Glucose syrup
Maxipro (SHS)	Protein supplement, free from gluten, fructose, sucrose	332	79	16.0	Whey protein, amino acids	1.2		<1.0	Lactose
MCT Duocal (SHS)	Energy supplement, free of protein, lactose, gluten, sucrose	†2042	†486	–		†23.2	Vegetable oils, high in MCT	†74	Glucose syrup
MCT oil (SHS)	Medium chain triglycerides	3515	855			95	Medium chain triglycerides		
Nestargel (Nestlé)	Feed thickener	Does not add energy to feed							
Polycal (Nutricia)	Carbohydrate source	†1610	†380	–		–		†94.5	Maltodextrin, maltose, glucose
Scandishake (SHS)	High energy supplement	†2153	†514	†4.7		†24.7		†68.2	
Seravit, pediatric (SHS)	Vitamin, trace element and mineral mixture								
Solagen (SHS)	Soy oil emulsion	1776	432	–		48	Soy oil		
Super Soluble Duocal (SHS)	Free from gluten, protein, lactose	†2061	†492	–		†22.3	Vegetable oils	†72.7	Glucose syrup
Super Soluble Maxijul (SHS)	Carbohydrate source, lactose, sucrose free	†1615	†380	–		–	hydrolysate	†95	Corn starch hydrolysate
XP Maxamaid (SHS)	Phenylalanine free	†1311	†309	†25	Amino acids	<0.5		†51	Glucose syrup

* SHS = Scientific Hospital Supplies.
† Concentrations per 100 g.
‡ Concentrations per 17 g (recommended daily intake from 6 months)
All values refer to the normal dilution as recommended by the manufacturer.

Minerals								Vitamins													
Na (mg)	K (mg)	Ca (mg)	P (mg)	Mg (mg)	Fe (μg)	Cu (μg)	Zn (μg)	A (μg)	B_1 (μg)	B_2 (μg)	Pantothenic acid (μg)	B_6 (μg)	B_{12} (μg)	Biotin (μg)	Folic (μg)	Niacin (μg)	C (mg)	D (μg)	E (μg)	K (μg)	Osmolality (mOsm/kg H_2O)
32	74	64	43	7.4	1200	51	700	61	54	61	338	41	0.2	2	10.8	680	8.1	1.0	1.35	5.4	320
35	58	45	35	5.1	825	60	585	80	60	90	255	52	0.15	3.9	5.8	675	6.2	1.1	0.7	6.8	9.8
20	66	54	27	7.7	900	40	400	77	40	100	260	40	0.19	1.5	10	900	7.7	1.3	1.2	5.1	200
32	74	63	42	7.5	1200	66	470	78	66	60	320	40	0.37	2	11	850	7.5	1.1	1.6	11	320
42	92	57	29	11	1800	60	600	71	50	60	500	40	0.2	2.0	12	1100	7.5	1.2	0.8	4.7	225
22	88	57	42	9.1	1100	50	820	100	140	200	400	82	0.3	2.7	11	1200	12	1.4	1.0	9.1	415
16	70	55	37	6	800	33	600	75	100	150	300	60	0.2	2	8	900	9	1.1	0.7	6.7	198
18	63	49	34	5.1	1050	70	750	79	60	90	400	80	0.19	3.9	5.7	680	6	1.3	0.7	3.1	353
<10	50	9	45	8	400	50	200														131
8	240	130	20	50(contains carob bean gum flour)																	
20	30	30	15																1.7		
<23	<4		<5																		
28																					
23	4																				225 (1:5 dilution)
26	94	100	66																		
30	3.7																				
(MCT oil should always be diluted before use)																					
50	50	50	100																		
†140	570	130	400	94 (values for vanilla flavor; different values for other flavors)																	
‡<2	Trace	43.7	291	60.7	11700	780		7800	710	540	2890	580	1.46	36	52	5950	68		4.9	28.2	216 (1:10 dilution)
†69	470	312	235	43	4100	270	2700														310 (1:3 dilution)
<20	<5	<5	<5																		420 (1:3 dilution)
<20	<5		<5					525	1080	1200	3700	1400	3.9	120	240	12000	135	12	5.9	30	
580	840	810	810	200																	

Table 40.16 Examples of pediatric enteral feeds

		Composition per 100 ml						
		Protein	Energy		Fat	Carbohydrate		
Feed	Protein	g	kcal	kJ	g	g	Special features	Manufacturer
Nutrison Paediatric (Standard)	Caseinates	2.75	100	420	4.5	12.2		Cow & Gate
Nutrison Paediatric (Energy Plus)	Caseinates	3.4	150	630	6.8	18.8		Cow & Gate
Paediasure	Whey and caseinate	3.0	100	420	5.0	11.0		Abbott Laboratories
Elemental 028	Essential and non-essential amino acids	2.0	76	322	1.3	14.1	Severe GI tract impairment	Scientific Hospital Supplies
Elemental 028 Extra	Essential and non-essential amino acids	2.5	85	358	3.5	11.0	Severe GI tract impairment	Scientific Hospital Supplies
Generaid Plus	Whey and branched chain amino acids	2.42	102	428	4.2	13.6	Hepatic disorders. Fat: 35% MCT : 65% LCT	Scientific Hospital Supplies
Kindergen P.R.O.D.	Whey and essential amino acids	1.5	101	424	5.2	12.1	Chronic renal failure	Scientific Hospital Supplies
Peptide 2+	Soya and beef peptides	2.8	88	369	3.5	11.4	GI tract impairment	Scientific Hospital Supplies
MCT Peptide 2+	Soya and beef peptides	2.8	91	381	3.6	11.8	GI tract impairment + fat malabsorption. Fat: 83% MCT : 17% LCT	Scientific Hospital Supplies

Table 40.17 Estimated average requirements (EARs)[†] for energy

Age	EARs MJ/d (kcal/d)	
	Males	Females
0–3 months	2.28 (545)	2.16 (515)
4–6 months	2.89 (690)	2.69 (645)
7–9 months	3.44 (825)	3.20 (765)
10–12 months	3.85 (920)	3.61 (865)
1–3 years	5.15 (1230)	4.86 (1165)
4–6 years	7.16 (1715)	6.46 (1545)
7–10 years	8.24 (1970)	7.28 (1740)
11–14 years	9.27 (2220)	7.92 (1845)
15–18 years	11.51 (2755)	8.83 (2110)
19–50 years	10.60 (2550)	8.10 (1940)
51–59 years	10.60 (2550)	8.00 (1900)
60–64 years	9.93 (2380)	7.99 (1900)
65–74 years	9.71 (2330)	7.96 (1900)
75+ years	8.77 (2100)	7.61 (1810)
Pregnancy		+0.80*(200)
Lactation:		
1 month		+1.90 (450)
2 months		+2.20 (530)
3 months		+2.40 (570)
4–6 months (group 1)		+2.00 (480)
4–6 months (group 2)		+2.40 (570)
>6 months (group 1)		+1.00 (240)
>6 months (group 2)		+2.30 (550)

* Last trimester only.

Group 1 mothers: those breast-feeding for up to 6 months

Group 2 mothers: those breast-feeding for more than 6 months

[†] EAR, estimated average requirement of a group of people for energy or protein or a vitamin or mineral. About half will usually need more than the EAR, and half less.

From Department of Health 1991[23]

Table 40.18 Reference nutrient intakes* for protein

Age	Reference nutrient intake** (g/d)
0–3 months	12.5[†]
4–6 months	12.7
7–9 months	13.7
10–12 months	14.9
1–3 years	14.5
4–6 years	19.7
7–10 years	28.3
Males:	
11–14 years	42.1
15–18 years	55.2
19–50 years	55.5
50+ years	53.3
Females:	
11–14 years	41.2
15–18 years	45.0
19–50 years	45.0
50+ years	46.5
Pregnancy[‡]	+6
Lactation:[‡]	
0–4 months	+11
4+ months	+8

* These figures, based on egg and milk protein, assume complete digestibility.

[†] No values for infants 0–3 months are given by WHO. The RNI is calculated from the recommendations of COMA.

[‡] To be added to adult requirement through all stages of pregnancy and lactation.

** RNI, reference nutrient intake for protein or a vitamin or mineral. An amount of the nutrient that is enough, or more than enough, for about 97% of people in a group. If average intake of a group is at RNI, then the risk of deficiency in the group is very small. From Department of Health 1991[23]

Table 40.19 Reference nutrient intakes for vitamins and minerals

Age	Thiamin (mg/d)	Riboflavin (mg/d)	Niacin (nicotinic acid equivalent) (mg/d)	Vitamin B_6 (mg/d)§	Vitamin B_{12} (μg/d)	Folate (μg/d)	Vitamin C (mg/d)	Vitamin A (μg/d)	Vitamin D (μg/d)
0–3 months	0.2	0.4	3	0.2	0.3	50	25	350	8.5
4–6 months	0.2	0.4	3	0.2	0.3	50	25	350	8.5
7–9 months	0.2	0.4	4	0.3	0.4	50	25	350	7
10–12 months	0.3	0.4	5	0.4	0.4	50	25	350	7
1–3 years	0.5	0.6	8	0.7	0.5	70	30	400	7
4–6 years	0.7	0.8	11	0.9	0.8	100	30	500	–
7–10 years	0.7	1.0	12	1.0	1.0	150	30	500	–
Males									
11–14 years	0.9	1.2	15	1.2	1.2	200	35	600	–
15–18 years	1.1	1.3	18	1.5	1.5	200	40	700	–
19–50 years	1.0	1.3	17	1.4	1.5	200	40	700	–
50+ years	0.9	1.3	16	1.4	1.5	200	40	700	†
Females									
11–14 years	0.7	1.1	12	1.0	1.2	200	35	600	–
15–18 years	0.8	1.1	14	1.2	1.5	200	40	600	–
19–50 years	0.8	1.1	13	1.2	1.5	200	40	600	–
50+ years	0.8	1.1	12	1.2	1.5	200	40	600	†
Pregnancy	+0.1‡	+0.3	*	*	*	+100	+10	+100	10
Lactation:									
0–4 months	+0.2	+0.5	+2	*	+0.5	+ 60	+30	+350	10
4+ months	+0.2	+0.5	+2	*	+0.5	+ 60	+30	+350	10

* No increment.
† After age 65 the RNI is 10 μg/d for men and women.
‡ For last trimester only.
§ Based on protein providing 14.7% of EAR for energy.
** Phosphorus RNI is set equal to calcium in molar terms.
†† 1 mmol sodium = 23 mg.
‡‡ 1 mmol potassium = 39 mg.
§§ Corresponds to sodium 1 mmol = 35.5 mg.
*** Insufficient for women with high menstrual losses where the most practical way of meeting iron requirements is to take iron supplements.
From Department of Health 1991[23]

Calcium (mg/d)	Phosphorus** (mg/d)	Magnesium (mg/d)	Sodium (mg/d)††	Potassium (mg/d)‡‡	Chloride (mg/d)§§	Iron (mg/d)	Zinc (mg/d)	Copper (mg/d)	Selenium (μg/d)	Iodine (μg/d)
525	400	55	210	800	320	1.7	4.0	0.2	10	50
525	400	60	280	850	400	4.3	4.0	0.3	13	60
525	400	75	320	700	500	7.8	5.0	0.3	10	60
525	400	80	350	700	500	7.8	5.0	0.3	10	60
350	270	85	500	800	800	6.9	5.0	0.4	15	70
450	350	120	700	1100	1100	6.1	6.5	0.6	20	100
550	450	200	1200	2000	1800	8.7	7.0	0.7	30	110
1000	775	280	1600	3100	2500	11.3	9.0	0.8	45	130
1000	775	300	1600	3500	2500	11.3	9.5	1.0	70	140
700	550	300	1600	3500	2500	8.7	9.5	1.2	75	140
700	550	300	1600	3500	2500	8.7	9.5	1.2	75	140
800	625	280	1600	3100	2500	14.8***	9.0	0.8	45	130
800	625	300	1600	3500	2500	14.8***	7.0	1.0	60	140
700	550	270	1600	3500	2500	14.8***	7.0	1.2	60	140
700	550	270	1600	3500	2500	8.7	7.0	1.2	60	140
*	*	*	*	*	*	*	*	*	*	*
+550	+440	+50	*	*	*	*	+6.0	+0.3	+15	*
+550	+440	+50	*	*	*	*	+2.5	+0.3	+15	*

Table 40.20 Safe intakes

Nutrient	Safe intake*
Vitamins:	
Pantothenic acid	
Adults	3–7 mg/d
Infants	1.7 mg/d
Biotin	10–200 μg/d
Vitamin E	
Men	Above 4 mg/d
Women	Above 3 mg/d
Infants	0.4 mg/g polyunsaturated fatty acid
Vitamin K	
Adults	1 μg/kg/d
Infants	10 μg/d
Minerals:	
Manganese	
Adults	1.4 mg (26 μmol)/d
Infants and children	16 μg (0.3 μmol)/d
Molybdenum	
Adults	50–400 μg/d
Infants, children and adolescents	0.5–1.5 μg/kg/d
Chromium	
Adults	25 μg (0.5 μmol)/d
Children and adolescents	0.1–1.0 μg (2–20 μmol)/kg/d
Fluoride (for infants only)	0.05 mg (3 μmol)/kg/d

* Safe intakes have been set for some nutrients for which there are insufficient reliable data on human requirements to set any dietary reference values. However, these safe intakes were set particularly for infants and children. The safe intake was judged to be a level or range of intake at which there is no risk of deficiency, and below a level where there is a risk of undesirable effects
From Department of Health 1991[23]

Table 40.21 Food and Nutrition Board, National Academy of Sciences–National Research Council recommended dietary allowances* revised 1989. 'Designed for the maintenance of good nutrition of practically all healthy people in the United States'

		Weight†		Height†			Fat-soluble vitamins			
							Vitamin A	Vitamin	Vitamin E	Vitamin K
Category	Age (years) or condition	kg	lb	cm	in	Protein (g)	(μg RE)††	D (μg)**	(mg α-TE)§	(μg)
Infants	0.0–0.5	6	13	60	24	13	375	7.5	3	5
	0.5–1.0	9	20	71	28	14	375	10	4	10
Children	1–3	13	29	90	35	16	400	10	6	15
	4–6	20	44	112	44	24	500	10	7	20
	7–10	28	62	132	52	28	700	10	7	30
Males	11–14	45	99	157	62	45	1000	10	10	45
	15–18	66	145	176	69	59	1000	10	10	65
	19–24	72	160	177	70	58	1000	10	10	70
	25–50	79	174	176	70	63	1000	5	10	80
	51+	77	170	173	68	63	1000	5	10	80
Females	11–14	46	101	157	62	46	800	10	8	45
	15–18	55	120	163	64	44	800	10	8	55
	19–24	58	128	164	65	46	800	10	8	60
	25–50	63	138	163	64	50	800	5	8	65
	51+	65	143	160	63	50	800	5	8	65
Pregnant						65	800	10	10	65
Lactating	1st 6 months					65	1300	10	12	65
	2nd 6 months					62	1200	10	11	65

* The allowances, expressed as average daily intakes over time, are intended to provide for individual variations among most normal persons as they live in the USA under usual environmental stresses. Diets should be based on a variety of common foods in order to provide other nutrients for which human requirements have been less well defined.
† Weights and heights of reference adults are actual medians for the US population of the designated age, as reported by NHANES II (NHANES II = National Health and Nutrition Examination Survey (1976–1980)[25]). The median weights and heights of those under 19 years of age were taken from Hamill et al (1979).[26] The use of these figures does not imply that the height-to-weight ratios are ideal.
†† Retinol equivalent. 1 retinol equivalent = 1 μg retinol or 6 μg β-carotene. See text for calculation of vitamin A activity of diets as retinol equivalents.

Table 40.22 Estimated safe and adequate daily dietary intakes of selected vitamins and minerals*

Category	Age (years)	Vitamins		Trace elements†				
		Biotin (μg)	Pantothenic acid (mg)	Copper (mg)	Manganese (mg)	Fluoride (mg)	Chromium (μg)	Molybdenum (μg)
Infants	0–0.5	10	2	0.4–0.6	0.3–0.6	0.1–0.5	10–40	15–30
	0.5–1	15	3	0.6–0.7	0.6–1.0	0.2–1.0	20–60	20–40
Children and adolescents	1–3	20	3	0.7–1.0	1.0–1.5	0.5–1.5	20–80	25–50
	4–6	25	3–4	1.0–1.5	1.5–2.0	1.0–2.5	30–120	30–75
	7–10	30	4–5	1.0–2.0	2.0–3.0	1.5–2.5	50–200	50–150
	11+	30–100	4–7	1.5–2.5	2.0–5.0	1.5–2.5	50–200	75–250
Adults		30–100	4–7	1.5–3.0	2.0–5.0	1.5–4.0	50–200	75–250

* Because there is less information on which to base allowances, these figures are not given in Table 40.19 and are provided here in the form of ranges of recommended intakes.

† Since the toxic levels for many trace elements may be only several times usual intakes, the upper levels for the trace elements given in this table should not be habitually exceeded. From National Research Council 1989[24]

Water-soluble vitamins							Minerals						
Vitamin C (mg)	Thiamin (mg)	Riboflavin (mg)	Niacin (mg NE)ǂ	Vitamin B_6 (mg)	Folate (μg)	Vitamin B_{12} (μg)	Calcium (mg)	Phosphorus (mg)	Magnesium (mg)	Iron (mg)	Zinc (mg)	Iodine (μg)	Selenium (μg)
30	0.3	0.4	5	0.3	25	0.3	400	300	40	6	5	40	10
35	0.4	0.5	6	0.6	35	0.5	600	500	60	10	5	50	15
40	0.7	0.8	9	1.0	50	0.7	800	800	80	10	10	70	20
45	0.9	1.1	12	1.1	75	1.0	800	800	120	10	10	90	20
45	1.0	1.2	13	1.4	100	1.4	800	800	170	10	10	120	30
50	1.3	1.5	17	1.7	150	2.0	1200	1200	270	12	15	150	40
60	1.5	1.8	20	2.0	200	2.0	1200	1200	400	12	15	150	50
60	1.5	1.7	19	2.0	200	2.0	1200	1200	350	10	15	150	70
60	1.5	1.7	19	2.0	200	2.0	800	800	350	10	15	150	70
60	1.2	1.4	15	2.0	200	2.0	800	800	350	10	15	150	70
50	1.1	1.3	15	1.4	150	2.0	1200	1200	280	15	12	150	45
60	1.1	1.3	15	1.5	180	2.0	1200	1200	300	15	12	150	50
60	1.1	1.3	15	1.6	180	2.0	1200	1200	280	15	12	150	55
60	1.1	1.3	15	1.6	180	2.0	800	800	280	15	12	150	55
60	1.0	1.2	13	1.6	180	2.0	800	800	280	10	12	150	55
70	1.5	1.6	17	2.2	400	2.2	1200	1200	320	30	15	175	65
95	1.6	1.8	20	2.1	280	2.6	1200	1200	355	15	19	200	75
90	1.6	1.7	20	2.1	260	2.6	1200	1200	340	15	16	200	75

** As cholecalciferol. 10 μg cholecalciferol = 400 IU of vitamin D.

§ α-tocopherol equivalents. 1 mg *d*-α-tocopherol = 1 α-TE. See text for variation in allowances and calculation of vitamin E activity of the diet as α-tocopherol equivalents.

ǂ 1 NE (niacin equivalent) is equal to 1 mg of niacin or 60 mg of dietary tryptophan.

From National Research Council 1989[24]

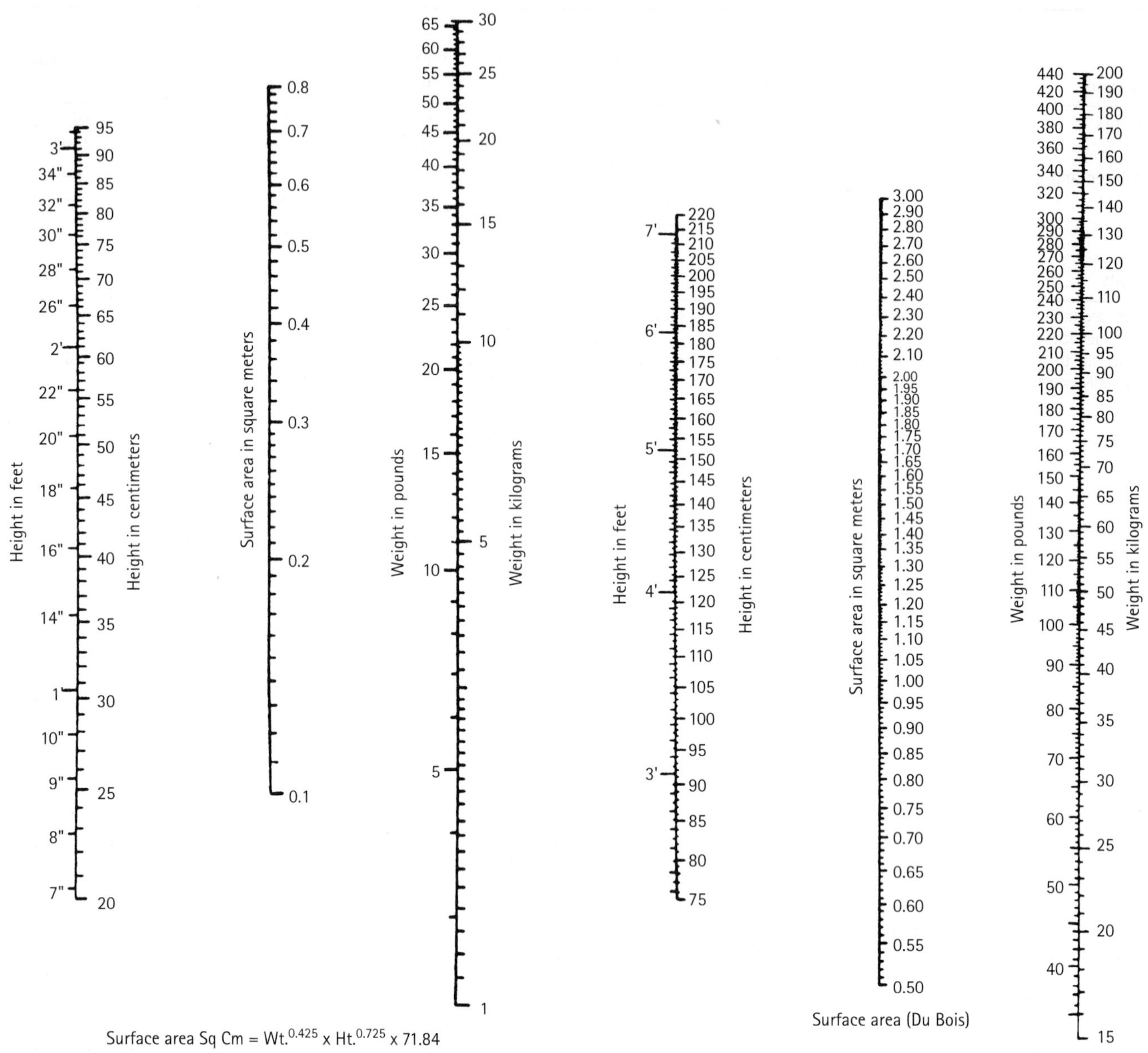

Fig. 40.1 Nomograms for body surface area [after du Bois & du Bois (1916)[27] and Crawford et al (1950)[28]]. A rapid rough method for estimating surface area from weight alone is: surface area $m^2 = (4W+7)/(W+90)$ (where W = weight in kilograms) (Costeff 1966).[29] (See also Fig. 40.2.)

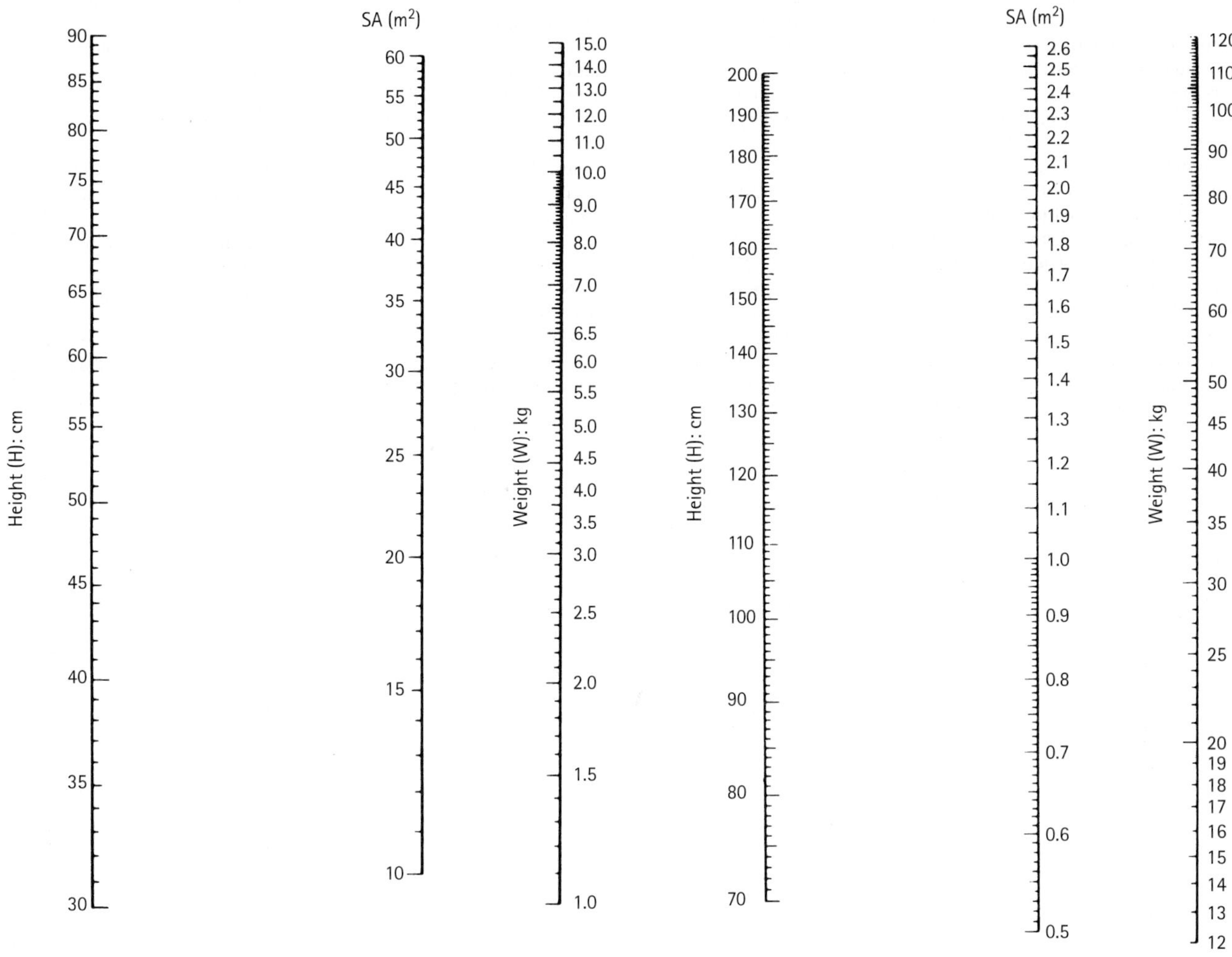

Fig. 40.2 Nomograms for body surface area (Haycock et al 1978).[30] Surface area was calculated geometrically from 34 body measurements and the following formula derived: surface area (m^2) = weight $(kg)^{0.5378} \times$ height $(cm)^{0.3964} \times 0.024265$.
Haycock et al state that as the du Bois formula (see Fig. 40.1) increasingly underestimates surface area as values fall below 0.7 m^2, their nomograms are more accurate in this lower range and particularly so for newborn infants.

REFERENCES

1 American Academy of Pediatrics. Committee on Hospital Care: metrication and SI units. Pediatrics 1980; 65:659–664.

2 American Academy of Pediatrics. Committee on Drugs: SI units. Pediatrics 1989; 83:129–131.

3 Kjellin KG. Bilirubin compounds in the CSF. J Neurol Sci 1970; 13:161–173.

4 Hellstrom B, Kjellin KG. The diagnostic value of spectrophotometry in the newborn period. Dev Med Child Neurol 1971; 13:789–797.

5 Habel AH, Simpson H. Osmolar relation between cerebrospinal fluid and serum in hypersomolar hypernatraemic dehydration. Arch Dis Child 1976; 51:660–666.

6 Apt L, Downey WS. Melena neonatorum. The swallowed blood syndrome. A simple test for the differentiation of adult and foetal haemoglobin in bloody stools. J Pediatr 1955; 47:6–12.

7 Hindmarsh PC, Swift PGF. An assessment of growth hormone provocation tests. Arch Dis Child 1995; 72:362–368.

8 Walker JM, Hughes IA. Tests and normal values in paediatric endocrinology. In: Brook CGD, ed. Clinical paediatric endocrinology. 3rd edn. Oxford: Blackwell Science; 1995:782–798.

9 Hinchliffe RF. Reference values. In: Lilleyman JS, Hann IM, Blanchette VS, eds. Paediatric haematology. 2nd edn. Edinburgh: Churchill Livingstone; 1999:1–20.

10 Chalmers EA, Gibson BES. Acquired disorders of hemostatis during childhood. In: Lilleyman JS, Hann IM, Blanchette VS, eds. Paediatric haematology. 2nd edn. Edinburgh: Churchill Livingstone; 1999.

11 de Swiet M, Fayers P, Shinebourne EA. Blood pressure in the first 10 years of life: the Brompton study. BMJ 1992; 304:23–26.

12 National High Blood Pressure Education Program Working Group on Hypertension Control in Children and Adolescents. Update on the 1987 Task Force Report on High Blood Pressure in Children and Adolescents: a working group report from the National High Blood Pressure Education Program. Pediatrics 1996; 98:649–658.

13 Department of Health and Social Security. The composition of human milk. Report on Health and Social Subjects No. 12. London: HMSO; 1977.

14 Department of Health and Social Security. Artifical feeds for the young infant. Report on Health and Social Subjects No. 18. London: HMSO; 1980.

15 Department of Health and Social Security. Present day practice in infant feeding: third report. Report on Health and Social Subjects No. 32. London: HMSO; 1988.

16 Department of Health. Weaning and the weaning diet. Report on Health and Social Subjects No. 45. London: HMSO; 1994.

17 ESPGAN Committee on Nutrition. Guidelines on infant nutrition I. Recommendations for the composition of an adapted formula. Acta Paediatr Scand Suppl 1977; 262:1–20.

18 ESPGAN Committee on Nutrition. Guidelines on infant nutrition II. Recommendations for the composition of follow-up formula and beikost. Acta Paediatr Scand Suppl 1981; 287:1–25.
19 ESPGAN European Society for Pediatric Gastroenterology and Nutrition. Recommendations for infant feeding. Acta Paediatr Scand Suppl 1982; 302:1–27.
20 ESPGAN Nutrition and feeding of preterm infants. Acta Paediatr Scand Suppl 1987; 336:1–14 and Oxford: Blackwell; 1987:1–248.
21 ESPGAN Committee on Nutrition. Comments on the composition of cow's milk based follow-up formulas. Acta Paediatr Scand 1990; 79:250–254.
22 Tsang RC, Lucas A, Uauy R, et al. Nutritional needs of the preterm infant. Baltimore: Williams & Wilkins; 1993.
23 Department of Health. Dietary values for food, energy and nutrients for the United Kingdom. Report on Health and Social Subjects No. 41. London: HMSO; 1991.
24 National Research Council. Recommended dietary allowances, 10th edn. Washington: National Academy Press; 1989.
25 National Health and Nutrition Examination Survey (1976–1980). Atlanta: National Center for Health Statistics, Centres for Disease Control and Prevention.
26 Hamill PVV, Drizd TA, Johnson CL, et al. Physical growth: National Center for Health Statistics percentiles. Am J Clin Nutr 1979; 32:607–629.
27 Du Bois D, Du Bois EF. Clinical calorimetry. Tenth paper. A formula to estimate the approximate surface area if height and weight be known. Arch Intern Med 1916; 17:863.
28 Crawford JD, Terry ME, Rourke GM. Simplification of drug dosage calculation by application of the surface area principle. Pediatrics 1950; 5:783–790.
29 Costeff H. A simple empirical formula for calculating approximate surface area in children. Arch Dis Child 1966; 41:681–683.
30 Haycock GB, Schwartz GJ, Wisotsky DH. Geometric method for measuring body surface area: A height–weight formula validated in infants, children and adults. J Pediatr 1978; 93:62–66.

41

Pediatric prescribing

George Rylance

Prescribing for children encompasses a number of knowledge-based skills and practical considerations. These include knowledge and understanding of inter- and intraindividual variation relating to age, body composition, differential maturation of body organs, and state of health.

Pharmacokinetics is the mathematical expression of the drug handling processes of absorption, distribution, metabolism and excretion which determine a medicine's disposition in the body. Pharmacodynamics describes what the medicine does to the body and therefore the processes linking the concentration of a drug in a body fluid with pharmacological effect. This is essentially the interaction of a drug with a receptor at the site of action.

DRUG HANDLING PROCESSES

Unless they are administered directly into the vascular system, all medicines need to be absorbed. Most will depend on absorption from the gastrointestinal tract.

GASTROINTESTINAL ABSORPTION

The rate and extent of gastrointestinal absorption is affected by gut pH and flora, gastric contents and emptying time, gut motility and absorptive surfaces. All vary somewhat according to age and with certain disease processes. After the neonatal period, there are a few differences with age and gastrointestinal absorption of medicines is usually predictable in rate and extent. The unpredictability of the newborn period relates to reduced gastric acid secretion, reduced gastric emptying time, and reduced intestinal motility and biliary function. The oral route is preferred for drug administration generally.

OTHER ROUTES OF DRUG ABSORPTION

Absorption from **muscle** is unpredictable. Drugs which are not water soluble tend to precipitate with resultant delayed or decreased absorption. The rate and extent is also compromised by poor perfusion in serious illness.

Absorption through **skin** is more important with regard to toxicity than benefit. Preterm skin represents much less of a barrier than that of a full term baby and hexachlorophene, aniline dye, and steroid toxicity have been reported. However, the same characteristics afford a potential for drug delivery via topical creams and patch formulations although these are limited in application.

DISTRIBUTION

The composition of body water compartments, protein binding, regional blood flow and membrane permeability are important determinants of drug distribution in the body. The relatively large total and extracellular body water compartments in the newborn and infancy period largely account for the greater drug distribution volumes in young children.

Drug distribution is also affected by the extent and characteristics of protein binding. The lower protein binding for drugs in particular in the newborn and infant probably relates to the amount of albumin available, different affinity, and competitive displacement by endogenous substances (e.g. bilirubin; free fatty acids). The greater free fraction at this age contributes to a larger distribution volume and increase in clearance. Although albumin is the major drug binding protein, lipoproteins and alpha-1 acid glycoprotein are important and their concentration is influenced by age, nutrition and disease processes.

METABOLISM

Removal of a drug from the body occurs as soon as it is absorbed. The process of removal for many drugs includes biotransformation into more water soluble compounds so facilitating elimination through the kidney or in bile. For most drugs, this process makes them less active or completely inactive although some 'parent' drugs are converted from active to other active compounds (theophylline to caffeine and morphine to morphine-6-glucuronide) and in some cases to more active compounds (carbamazepine to its 10′11 epoxide metabolite).

Most biotransformation processes occur in the liver although some occur in the intestine. There are two phases of metabolism, both occurring mainly within the hepatocyte. Phase I reactions are enzymatic and involve oxidation, reduction, hydroxylation or hydrolysis; Phase II reactions are mainly those of conjugation with glucuronide, sulfate or glycine.

The cytochrome P450 mixed function oxidase system is the most important biotransformation system incorporating many enzymes and isoenzymes. In general, these enzymes systems are immature at birth and particularly so in premature newborns. There is therefore relatively slow clearance of most metabolized drugs in the first 2 or 3 months of life. Between 2 and 6 months, clearance is more rapid than in adults and even more so for most drugs from 6 months to 2 years. From 2 to 12 years, somewhat faster clearance rates than in adults are maintained but after 12 years, adult values are the norm (Table 41.1).

EXCRETION

Glomerular filtration of drugs depends on renal blood flow, protein binding and the functionality of the glomeruli. The relatively low glomerular filtration rates in premature and full term newborns result in the half-lives of renal cleared drugs being approximately two to three times longer than those in adults, and this difference is maintained up to 1–2 weeks age. Thereafter, rates are similar in infants and adults up to 2 months. Half-lives are subsequently faster until about 2–3 years.

PHARMACOKINETICS

Pharmacokinetics refers to the mathematical expressions of drug changes in the body. **Bioavailability** describes the fraction (percentage) of drug reaching the systemic circulation of that presented to the body. For intravenously administered drugs, this is considered to be 1 (100%). For other routes of administration, values are usually somewhat less than 100% and this amount (and the rate of absorption) depends on a number of physicochemical properties of the drugs and other factors related to the patient. Reduced blood flow to the gut in intestinal and systemic illness tends to slow the rate and extent of absorption but food in the gut only tends to delay absorption.

Volume of distribution describes an apparent hypothetical volume within which a drug is distributed. It tends to be larger in babies, infants and young children than in adults. The relationship between dose (bioavailable dose = FD), volume of distribution (aV_d), and concentration (c) is given by the equation:

$$c = FD/aV_d \text{..........Equation 1}$$

In simplistic terms, it is like achieving a pink volume of liquid (c) when an amount of red dye (D) is put into a bucket of water (aV_d). In clinical terms, it determines what loading dose, either initially ($c \times aV_d$) or during maintenance therapy ((desired – measured concentration) $\times aV_d$) is required, e.g. to stop fitting using phenytoin.

The **(elimination) half-life ($t\frac{1}{2}$)** describes the time it takes for a drug concentration in any body fluid to reduce by half. It most frequently refers to blood. Mathematically its value is given by dividing 0.693 by the slope of the terminal portion of the log concentration-time 'curve' or elimination rate constant (k_e):

$$t\tfrac{1}{2} = 0.693/k_e.$$

Clearance is the volume from which drug is removed per unit time. The concept of renal clearance is well understood. Drug clearance usually refers to total body clearance (Cl) and is the product of apparent volume of distribution and the elimination rate constant:

$$Cl = K_e . aV_d \quad \text{or} \quad Cl = (0.693/t\tfrac{1}{2}) . aV_d.$$

PRESCRIBING PRINCIPLES

Choice of drugs depends on a number of factors. Of course, the benefit–risk assessment has to be positive, and the drug delivery needs to be practically feasible. This will depend on an assessment of handling, kinetics and formulation availability. For antibiotics the choice is further determined by the likely or known causal organism, the minimum inhibiting concentration (MIC), and the ability to reach the site of action.

In considering the **administration route** for most drugs, the oral route is preferred but is inappropriate if there is significant vomiting and when gut perfusion is compromised by systemic illness. Gut pathology and immaturity (first week or two of life) are significant and

Table 41.1 Approximate elimination half life ($t\frac{1}{2}$) and total clearance (Cl) for drugs in children relative to adult values for different elimination pathways (from published literature database)

		Preterm newborn	Full term newborn	1wk–2m	2m–6m	6m–2y	2y–12y	12y–18y
All drugs	t½	3.8	1.85	1.8	1.1	0.75	0.95	1.05
All drugs	Cl	0.5	0.7	0.75	1.2	1.7	1.35	1.0
Renally cleared drugs	t½	2.7	2.6	1.1	0.75	0.6	1.1	–
Metabolized drugs Cytochrome P450 Isoenzyme 1A2 (caffeine, theophylline)	t½	–	9.1	4.0	1.2	0.6	0.6	–
Metabolized drugs Cytochrome P450 Isoenzyme 3A	t½	5.1	1.9	1.75	0.35	0.5	0.75	0.75
Metabolized drugs Cytochrome P450 All isoenzymes	t½	4.4	1.75	3.5	1.25	0.6	0.75	0.95
Phase II glucuronidation drugs	t½	4.2	2.8	2.1	0.9	1.15	1.3	1.5

important considerations. The intramuscular route only serves the purpose of 'one-off' administration because of pain and unpredictable bioavailability. The skin route is more of a toxicity consideration but some benefit is afforded in the newborn and for a small but increasing number of drugs available as patches. Inhalation of antibiotics in cystic fibrosis, and steroid and/or beta-2 agonists in asthma are established examples for this route. The rectal route is more unpredictable than the oral route but affords possibilities in vomiting, 'nil by mouth', and upper gut pathologies. Rectal administration is well established in some acute situations (benzodiazepines in continuing fits) and in situations where skilled personnel are not available, e.g. home use of diazepam, paracetamol and antiemetics. More recent use of intranasal or buccal delivery has proved efficacious for midazolam as sedation and in stopping fits.

Some drugs are not stable when administrated orally but most drugs are and therefore should be given by this route. Liquids are most rapidly absorbed giving shorter times to peak concentrations. Tablets that require disintegration and dissolution are more slowly absorbed as a result. **Choice of formulation** is also important because of variation in palatability.

Dose determination is especially difficult given the wide inter- and intraindividual variability of pharmacokinetic parameters with age. Pharmacodynamic and receptor variability are less well worked out but are likely to be of similar or even greater importance. For drugs where there is only a small difference between appropriately effective and toxic concentrations (drugs with low or narrow **therapeutic indices**), individualization of dosage is even more important.

If there is a clear endpoint of efficacy (e.g. blood pressure lowering; stopping fits) and if there is a wide therapeutic index, titration with increasing doses is appropriate. For some problems and drugs, plasma concentration therapeutic ranges are established and doses are then determined by the target concentration. Pharmacokinetic knowledge determines dosage in these situations. For example, and using the rearranged Equation 1, the required single dose is the product of target concentration and apparent volume of distribution. For phenytoin use in a child who continues to convulse, the equation for an infant of 3 months could be:

$$\text{IV dose (mg/kg)} = aV_d\ (0.75\ \text{L/kg}) \times \text{desired concentration}\ (20\ \text{mg/L}) = 15\ \text{mg/kg}.$$

The repeated doses that are necessary are determined by a drug's clearance; the frequency of dosing by its half-life (for drugs for which there is a relationship between concentration in blood and clinical effect). The dose is given by:

$$\text{Dose} = \text{concentration (mg/L)} \times \text{clearance}\ (\text{L.kg.h}^{-1}) \times \text{dose interval (h)}.$$

The **frequency of dosing** will not result in wide fluctuation between doses if the dose interval approximates the half-life.

Many of these considerations relate to knowledge about the kinetics of the drug, and the recommended dose regimens in prescriber reference sources are based on these and other factors where such knowledge exists.

Therapeutic drug monitoring whereby drug concentrations are measured to determine dose regimens is not practically useful for drugs (the majority) which have clearly defined and easily measured clinical effects or endpoints. For the remainder, drug level monitoring is potentially useful but established therapeutic ranges are available for only a few. Phenytoin and gentamicin are the best known examples. Concentration monitoring is especially useful in potential drug–drug interaction scenarios, where the therapeutic index is narrow, and in situations of therapeutic failure or potential non-compliance.

Practical conditions for measurement include: 'steady state' concentrations (at least five elimination half-lives should have elapsed since starting therapy in chronic situations); time of likely peak concentration; whether measurement is primarily for efficacy or toxicity (peak or trough [pre dose] concentrations may be more related to one or the other).

Length of treatment is determined by published data related to the condition treated and individual patient response. **Compliance** with therapy in chronic situations may frequently be no more than 50% of that prescribed or intended. Its relevance in the assessment of therapeutic failure should not be underestimated.

DRUG INTERACTIONS

Drugs primarily interact with food and other drugs. However, for most drugs, food is not of major clinical significance.

Interactions with other drugs – the effects of one drug changed by another – are important if they lead to toxicity or reduced efficacy. Drug absorption interactions are relatively unimportant. However, other pharmacokinetic interactions based on protein binding or drug clearance are potentially of much greater clinical relevance. Drugs which are more than 90% protein bound and with relatively low volumes of distribution are those for which interactions should be considered although changes arising from displacement of one drug from protein binding sites by another and so increasing the amount of 'free drug' are rarely of clinical importance because of the transient nature of this effect.

Drugs which influence the metabolism of others by inhibiting or inducing the mixed function oxidase system are frequently of clinical concern. Rifampicin, carbamazepine, phenytoin and phenobarbital are examples of enzyme inducing drugs which lower the concentration of some other drugs. Cimetidine, erythromycin and sodium valproate are enzyme inhibiting drugs which increase the concentrations of those other drugs dependent on similar mechanisms for clearance.

DRUGS IN BREAST MILK

The context of consideration should always be 'which drugs should not be used or deserve special consideration in breast-feeding mothers?' rather than 'should mothers be allowed to breast-feed when taking these drugs?'. Few drugs require particular consideration. These are listed with effects and special considerations in Table 41.2. In general, the following considerations are relevant:

- Is a drug really necessary? If it is, a discussion between pediatrician and mother's doctor is necessary.
- If a drug is needed, choose one which is the safer of alternatives, e.g. warfarin rather than phenindione; paracetamol rather than aspirin.
- Consider the benefit of measuring the drug concentration in the baby.
- Drug exposure may be reduced by taking medication just before a baby's long sleep, or just after breast-feeding.

UNLICENSED MEDICINES AND THE USE OF LICENSED MEDICINES FOR UNLICENSED APPLICATIONS

More than 30% of medicines used in hospital practice are either unlicensed, or are used outwith the license indications.

Table 41.2 Drugs and breast milk

Problem area	Drug	Effect
Cytotoxics	Cyclophosphamide Ciclosporin Doxorubicin Methotrexate	Possible immunosuppression; unknown effect on growth or association with carcinogenesis
Abuse/social	Amfetamine	Irritability, poor sleeping
	Cocaine	Irritability; vomiting; seizures
	Heroin	Tremors; restlessness; poor feeding
	Phencyclidine	Potent hallucinogen
Radiopharmaceuticals (cessation of breastfeeding according to time of effect)	Copper 64 (^{64}Cu)	Radioactive 50 h (3 days)
	Gallium 67 (^{67}Ga)	Radioactive 2 wks (2 wks)
	Iodine 123 (^{123}I)	Radioactive 30 h (2 days)
	Iodine 125 (^{125}I)	Radioactive 12 days (2 wks)
	Iodine 131 (^{131}I)	Radioactive 2–14 days (2 wks)
	Technetium 99m (^{99m}Tc)	Radioactive 15 h–3 days (3 days)
Other drugs to be cautious about	Atenolol	Cyanosis; bradycardia
	Clemastine	Drowsiness; irritability; high pitched cry (1 case)
	Ergotamine	Vomiting; diarrhea; fits
	Lithium	Half therapeutic concentration
	Phenindione	Increased prothrombin time and partial prothrombin time

The Joint Standing Committee on Medicines of the Royal College of Paediatric and Child Health and the Neonatal and Paediatrics Pharmacists Group has recognized the need for those who prescribe for children to prescribe unlicensed medicines, or use medicines 'off label' and has provided the following information and guidance:

- Those who prescribe for a child should choose the medicine which offers the best prospect for the child, with due regard to cost.
- The informed use of licensed medicines for unlicensed applications, and unlicensed medicines is necessary in pediatric practice.
- Health professionals should have ready access to sound information on any medicine they prescribe, dispense or administer, and its availability.
- In general, it is not necessary to obtain explicit consent of parents, carers or child patients to prescribe or administer licensed medicines for unlicensed applications, or to prescribe unlicensed medicines.
- *Those with administrative responsibilities* should support therapeutic practices that are advocated by a respectable, responsible body of professional opinion.

WHAT PARENTS AND CHILDREN NEED TO KNOW ABOUT MEDICINES

The prescriber needs to recognize the need for information provision and the following is an appropriate and basic check list.

- Medicine generic/brand name.
- How the medicine is expected to help. What results are expected. How long it takes to start working.
- How much to take at one time and how often.
- For how long the medicine will need to be taken.
- When to take the medicine. Before or after meals? At bed time. At special times?
- How to take it. Can it be diluted. With juices? With food?
- Other medicine, foods, drinks which shouldn't be taken with the medicine.
- What restriction on activities are necessary.
- Possible side-effects. When might they occur? Can they be reduced? Will they go away by themselves?
- When to seek help if problems occur.
- What to do and how long to wait if things don't get better.
- How to keep the medicine safely and in what storage provision.
- Expiry date.
- How to renew the medicine by prescription.

FURTHER READING

American Academy of Pediatrics Committee on Drugs. Transfer of drugs and other chemicals into human milk. Pediatrics 2001; 108(3): 776–789.

Drug Information for the Health Care Professional 2002, 22nd edition. United States Pharmacopea Micromedex. Thomson Healthcare.

Ginsberg G, Hattis D, Sonawane B, et al. Evaluation of child/adult pharmacokinetic differences from a database derived from the therapeutic drug literature. Toxicol Sci 2002; 66:185–200.

Medicines for Children. Royal College of Paediatrics and Child Health and Neonatal and Paediatric Pharmacists Group. London: RCPCH; 1999.

Index

Notes to index: (1) Users are reminded of the *Biochemical and physiological tables* at the end of the text
Notes to index: (2) age-groups listed are: neonates; preterm infants; infants; preschool children; school children; adolescents